THE METABOLIC BASIS OF INHERITED DISEASE

Fifth Edition

John B. Stanbury, M.D.
Senior Physician, Massachusetts General Hospital
Division of Health Science and Technology and
Department of Nutrition and Food Science
Massachusetts Institute of Technology

James B. Wyngaarden, M.D.
Director, National Institutes of Health

Donald S. Fredrickson, M.D.
Scholar-in-Residence
National Academy of Sciences

Joseph L. Goldstein, M.D.
Paul J. Thomas Professor of Genetics and
Chairman, Department of Molecular Genetics
University of Texas Health Science Center at Dallas

Michael S. Brown, M.D.
Paul J. Thomas Professor of Genetics and
Director, Center for Genetic Disease
University of Texas Health Science Center at Dallas

McGraw-Hill Book Company

New York   St. Louis   San Francisco   Auckland   Bogotá   Guatemala   Hamburg   Johannesburg
Lisbon   London   Madrid   Mexico   Montreal   New Delhi   Panama   Paris
San Juan   São Paulo   Singapore   Sydney   Tokyo   Toronto

NOTICE

Medicine is an ever-changing science. As new research and clinical experience broaden our knowledge, changes in treatment and drug therapy are required. The editors and the publisher of this work have made every effort to ensure that the drug dosage schedules herein are accurate and in accord with the standards accepted at the time of publication. Readers are advised, however, to check the product information sheet included in the package of each drug they plan to administer to be certain that changes have not been made in the recommended dose or in the contraindications for administration. This recommendation is of particular importance in regard to new or infrequently used drugs.

THE METABOLIC BASIS OF INHERITED DISEASE

Copyright © 1983, 1978, 1972, 1966, 1960 by McGraw-Hill, Inc. All rights reserved. Printed in the United States of America. Except as permitted under the United States Copyright Act of 1976, no part of this publication may be reproduced or distributed in any form or by any means, or stored in a data base or retrieval system, without the prior written permission of the publisher.

234567890 DODO 898765432

ISBN 0-07-060726-5

This book was set in Sabon by Typographic Sales, Inc.; the editors were Richard S. Laufer, Ellen Warren, and Donna McIvor; the production supervisor was Jeanne Skahan; the designer was Murray Fleminger.
R. R. Donnelley & Sons Company was printer and binder.

Library of Congress Cataloging in Publication Data
Main entry under title:

The Metabolic basis of inherited disease.

   Bibliography: p.
   Includes index.
   1. Metabolism, Inborn errors of.   I. Stanbury,
John B. [DNLM: 1. Hereditary diseases.   2. Metabolic diseases.   3. Metabolism, Inborn errors.
WD 200 M587]
RC627.8.M47 1983   616.3'9042   82-8919
ISBN 0-07-060726-5   AACR2

CONTENTS

Part 4 Disorders of Lipoprotein and Lipid Metabolism

Part 5 Disorders of Lysosomal Enzymes

Part 13 Disorders of the Immune and Other Defense Systems

LIST OF CONTRIBUTORS

Björn A. Afzelius, Ph.D.

Professor, Wenner-Gren Institute, University of Stockholm, Stockholm, Sweden

D. Bernard Amos, M.D.

James B. Duke Professor, Division of Immunology, Duke University Medical Center, Durham, North Carolina

Constantine Anast, M.D.

Professor of Pediatrics, Harvard Medical School; Senior Associate in Medicine, Boston Children's Hospital, Boston, Massachusetts

Karl E. Anderson, M.D.

Associate Professor and Physician, The Rockefeller University Hospital, New York

W. French Anderson, M.D.

Chief, Hemoglobinopathy Branch, Hematology Division, National Heart, Lung and Blood Institute, National Institutes of Health, Bethesda, Maryland

Thomas E. Andreoli, M.D.

Professor and Chairman, Department of Internal Medicine; Professor of Physiology and Cell Biology, University of Texas Medical School at Houston; Chief of Medicine, Hermann Hospital, Houston, Texas

Stanley H. Appel, M.D.

Professor and Chairman, Department of Neurology, Baylor College of Medicine, Houston, Texas

Irwin M. Arias, M.D.

Professor of Medicine, Albert Einstein College of Medicine, New York

Gerd Assman, M.D.

Professor of Medicine and Director of the Central Laboratory, Westphalian-Wilhelms University, Munster, Germany

K. Frank Austen, M.D.

Theodore B. Bayles Professor of Medicine, Harvard Medical School; Chairman, Department of Rheumatology and Immunology, Brigham and Women's Hospital, Boston, Massachusetts

Bernard M. Babior, M.D.

Professor of Medicine, Tufts University School of Medicine; New England Medical Center Hospital, Division of Hematology-Oncology, Boston, Massachusetts

John A. Barranger, M.D.

Chief, Section on Clinical Investigations and Therapeutics, Developmental and Metabolic Neurology Branch, National Institute of Neurological and Communicative Disorders and Stroke, National Institutes of Health, Bethesda, Maryland

Arthur L. Beaudet, M.D.

Associate Professor of Pediatrics, Assistant Professor of Cell Biology, Baylor College of Medicine, Houston, Texas

Vladimir M. Berginer, M.D.

Soroka Medical Center, Ben Gurion University Hospital, Beer Sheba, Israel

Ronald W. Berninger, Ph.D.

Assistant Professor of Pediatrics, Boston Floating Hospital, Tufts University School of Medicine, Boston, Massachusetts

Ernest Beutler, M.D.

Chairman, Department of Clinical Research, Scripps Clinic and Research Foundation, La Jolla, California

John P. Blass, M.D., Ph.D.

Winifred Masterson Burke Professor of Neurology and Medicine and Chief, Division of Chronic and Degenerative Disease, Cornell University Medical College at The Burke Rehabilitation Center, White Plains, New York

Thomas H. Bothwell, M.D., D.Sc.

Professor and Head of Department of Medicine, University of the Witwatersrand Medical School; Director, Medical Research Council Iron and Red Cell Metabolism Unit, Johannesburg, South Africa

Roscoe O. Brady, M.D.

Chief, Section on Clinical Investigations and Therapeutics, Developmental and Metabolic Neurology Branch, National Institute of Neurological and Communicative Disorders and Stroke, National Institutes of Health, Bethesda, Maryland

Michael S. Brown, M.D.

Paul J. Thomas Professor of Genetics; Director, Center for Genetic Disease, University of Texas Health Science Center at Dallas, Dallas, Texas

Robert W. Charlton, B.Sc., M.D.

Professor of Experimental and Clinical Pharmacology, University of the Witwatersrand Medical School, Johannesburg, South Africa

Winston W. Chen, Ph.D.

Assistant Professor of Neurology, The Johns Hopkins University, Baltimore, Maryland

J. Roy Chowdhury, M.D.

Assistant Professor of Medicine, Albert Einstein College of Medicine, New York

James E. Cleaver, Ph.D.

Professor of Radiology (Radiobiology), Laboratory of Radiobiology and Environmental Health, University of California, San Francisco, San Francisco, California

Carol A. Crowley, M.D.

Assistant Professor of Pediatrics, Rhode Island Hospital, Providence, Rhode Island

Ronald G.`Crystal, M.D.

Chief, Pulmonary Branch, National Heart, Lung, and Blood Institute, National Institutes of Health, Bethesda, Maryland

R. Michael Culpepper, M.D.

Assistant Professor of Internal Medicine, University of Texas Medical School at Houston; Attending Physician, Hermann Hospital, Houston, Texas

David M. Danks, M.D.

Professor of Pediatrics, University of Melbourne, and Director, Birth Defects Research Institute, Royal Children's Hospital Research Foundation, Victoria, Australia

Robert J. Desnick, Ph.D., M.D.

Professor of Pediatrics and Genetics; Chief, Division of Medical Genetics, Mount Sinai School of Medicine, New York

Marc K. Drezner, M.D.

Associate Professor of Medicine, Department of Medicine, Duke University Medical Center, Durham, North Carolina

Jacques E. Dumont, M.D., Ph.D.

Scientific Office of European Community; Professor of Biochemistry, University of Brussels; Head, Institute of Interdisciplinary Research, Brussels, Belgium

Bo Dupont, M.D.

Member and Professor, Sloan-Kettering Institute for Cancer Research, New York

Douglas T. Fearon, M.D.

Associate Professor of Medicine, Harvard Medical School, Department of Rheumatology and Immunology, Brigham and Women's Hospital, Boston, Massachusetts

Thomas B. Fitzpatrick, M.D.

Department of Dermatology, Harvard Medical School, Massachusetts General Hospital, Boston, Massachusetts

Daniel W. Foster, M.D.

Professor of Internal Medicine, University of Texas Health Science Center at Dallas, Dallas, Texas

Donald S. Fredrickson, M.D.

Scholar-in-Residence, National Academy of Sciences, Washington, D.C.

James E. Gadek, M.D.

Senior Investigator, Pulmonary Branch, National Heart, Lung, and Blood Institute, National Institutes of Health, Bethesda, Maryland

Richard Gitzelmann, M.D.

Professor, Division of Metabolism, Department of Pediatrics, University of Zurich, Kinderspital Zurich, Zurich, Switzerland

Egil Gjone, M.D.

Professor of Medicine and Head, Medical Department A, Rikshospitalet National Hospital of Norway, Oslo, Norway

David N. Glass, M.D.

Associate Professor of Medicine, Harvard Medical School, Department of Rheumatology and Immunology, Brigham and Women's Hospital, Boston, Massachusetts

John A. Glomset, M.D.

Investigator, Howard Hughes Medical Institute; Professor of Medicine, Adjunct Professor of Biochemistry, and Core Staff Member Regional Primate Research Center, University of Washington, Seattle, Washington

Lowell A. Goldsmith, M.D.

James H. Sterner Professor of Dermatology and Chief, Dermatology Unit, The University of Rochester Medical Center, School of Medicine and Dentistry, Strong Memorial Hospital, Rochester, New York

Joseph L. Goldstein, M.D.

Paul J. Thomas Professor of Genetics and Chairman, Department of Molecular Genetics, University of Texas Health Science Center at Dallas, Dallas, Texas

Antonio M. Gotto, Jr., M.D.

Professor and Chairman, Department of Medicine, Baylor College of Medicine; The Methodist Hospital, Houston, Texas

Gary M. Gray, M.D.

Professor of Medicine and, Head, Division of Gastroenterology, Stanford University School of Medicine, Stanford, California

James E. Griffin, M.D.

Associate Professor of Internal Medicine, University of Texas Health Science Center at Dallas, Dallas, Texas

Kevin Grumbach, B.A.

Research Assistant, Cornell University Medical College, New York

Steven C. Hebert, M.D.

Assistant Professor of Internal Medicine, University of Texas Medical School at Houston; Attending Physician, Hermann Hospital, Houston, Texas

Peter N. Herbert, M.D.

Associate Professor, Brown University Program in Medicine; Director, Division of Nutrition and Metabolism, Miriam Hospital, Providence, Rhode Island

Michael S. Hershfield, M.D.

Associate Professor of Medicine and Assistant Professor of Biochemistry, Duke University Medical Center, Durham, North Carolina

R. Rodney Howell, M.D.

Professor and Chairman, Department of Pediatrics, The University of Texas Medical School at Houston, Houston, Texas

Edward W. Holmes, M.D.

Investigator, Howard Hughes Medical Institute; Professor of Medicine and Assistant Professor of Biochemistry, Duke University Medical Center, Durham, North Carolina

Ernst R. Jaffe, M.D.

Professor of Medicine, Albert Einstein College of Yeshiva University, New York

Yuet W. Kan, M.D.

Investigator, Howard Hughes Medical Institute; Professor of Medicine, University of California, San Francisco, San Francisco, California

Attallah Kappas, M.D.

Professor and Physician-in-Chief, The Rockefeller University Hospital, New York

William N. Kelley, M.D.

John G. Searle Professor and Chairman, Department of Internal Medicine; Professor, Department of Biological Chemistry, The University of Michigan Medical School, Ann Arbor, Michigan

Edwin H. Kolodny, M.D.

Associate Professor in Neurology at the Massachusetts General Hospital, Harvard Medical School; Associate Director, Eunice Kennedy Shriver Center for Mental Retardation, Inc., Walter E. Fernald State School, Waltham, Massachusetts

Donna D. Kostyu, Ph.D.

Medical Research Associate, Division of Immunology, Duke University Medical Center, Durham, North Carolina

Nicholas M. Kredich, M.D.

Investigator, Howard Hughes Medical Institute; Professor of Medicine and Assistant Professor of Biochemistry, Duke University Medical Center, Durham, North Carolina

Philip Leder, M.D.

Professor and Chairman, Department of Genetics, Harvard Medical School, Boston, Massachusetts

Mark Leshin, M.D.

Assistant Professor of Internal Medicine, The University of Texas Health Science Center at Dallas, Dallas, Texas

Lenore S. Levine, M.D.

Professor of Pediatrics, Cornell University Medical College, New York

Harvey L. Levy, M.D.

Assistant Neurologist and Associate Pediatrician, Massachusetts General Hospital; Associate Professor of Neurology, Harvard Medical School, Boston, Massachusetts

Samuel E. Lux, M.D.

Associate Professor of Pediatrics, Division of Hematology-Oncology, Children's Hospital Medical Center, Harvard Medical School, Boston, Massachusetts

Paul C. MacDonald, M.D.

Professor of Obstetrics and Gynecology and of Biochemistry; Director of the Cecil and Ida Green Center for Reproductive Biology Sciences; The University of Texas Health Science Center at Dallas, Dallas, Texas

Philip W. Majerus, M.D.

Professor of Medicine and Biological Chemistry, Washington University School of Medicine, St. Louis, Missouri

Rodger P. McEver, M.D.

Assistant Professor of Medicine, University of Texas Health Science Center, San Antonio, Texas

Patrick A. McKee, M.D.

Investigator, Howard Hughes Medical Institute; Professor of Medicine, Division of General Medicine, Duke University Medical Center, Durham, North Carolina

Victor A. McKusick, M.D.

William Osler Professor of Medicine and Director and Physician-in-Chief, Department of Medicine, The Johns Hopkins Hospital, Baltimore, Maryland

Alton Meister, M.D.

Professor of Biochemistry, Cornell University Medical College, New York

R. Curtis Morris, Jr., M.D.

Professor of Medicine and Pediatrics; Director, General Clinical Research Center, Department of Medicine, University of California Medical Center, San Francisco, California

Hugo W. Moser, M.D.

Professor of Neurology and Pediatrics, Johns Hopkins University; Director, John F. Kennedy Institute for Handicapped Children, Baltimore, Maryland

Björn Mossberg, M.D.

Associate Professor, Department of Medicine I, South Hospital, Stockholm, Sweden

Arno G. Motulsky, M.D.

Professor of Medicine and Genetics and Director, Center for Inherited Diseases, University of Washington, Seattle, Washington

S. Harvey Mudd, M.D.

Chief, Section on Alkaloid Biosynthesis, Laboratory of General and Comparative Biochemistry, National Institute of Mental Health, National Institutes of Health, Bethesda, Maryland

Saood Murad, Ph.D.

Medical Research Associate, Duke University Medical Center, Durham, North Carolina

Francis A. Neelon, M.D.

Associate Professor of Medicine, Department of Medicine, Duke University Medical Center, Durham, North Carolina

Elizabeth F. Neufeld, Ph.D.

Chief, Genetics and Biochemistry Branch, National Institute of Arthritis, Diabetes, and Digestive and Kidney Diseases, National Institutes of Health, Bethesda, Maryland

Maria I. New, M.D.

Professor and Chairman, Department of Pediatrics; Division Head, Pediatric Endocrinology, Harold and Percy Uris Professor of Pediatric Endocrinology and Metabolism, The New York Hospital-Cornell Medical Center, New York

Esko A. Nikkilä, M.D.

Third Department of Medicine, University of Helsinki, Helsinki, Finland

Kaare R. Norum, M.D.

Professor and Chairman, Institute of Nutrition Research, University of Oslo School of Medicine, Oslo, Norway

Walter Nutzenadel, M.D.

Associate Professor of Pediatrics, Universitats-Kinderklinik, Hofmeisterweg, Germany

William L. Nyhan, M.D., Ph.D.

Professor and Chairman, Department of Pediatrics, School of Medicine, University of California, San Diego, La Jolla, California

John S. O'Brien, M.D.

Professor of Neurosciences, Department of Neurosciences, School of Medicine, University of California, San Diego, La Jolla, California

Donald E. Paglia, M.D.

Professor, Division of Surgical Pathology, Department of Pathology, UCLA Center for the Health Sciences, UCLA School of Medicine, Los Angeles, California

Thomas L. Perry, M.D.

Professor of Pharmacology, Department of Pharmacology, University of British Columbia, Vancouver, British Columbia

James M. Phang, M.D.

Head, Endocrine Section, National Cancer Institute, National Institutes of Health, Bethesda, Maryland

Sheldon R. Pinnell, M.D.

Professor of Medicine and Dermatology, Duke University Medical Center, Durham, North Carolina

Walter C. Quevedo, Jr., Ph.D.

Professor of Biology, Division of Biology and Medicine, Brown University, Providence, Rhode Island

Howard Rasmussen, M.D., Ph.D.

Professor of Medicine, Physiology and Cell Biology, Yale University School of Medicine, New Haven, Connecticut

Allan L. Reiss, Ph.D.

Research Associate, Division of Hematology, Coney Island Hospital, New York

Fred S. Rosen, M.D.

James L. Gamble Professor of Pediatrics, Harvard Medical School, The Children's Hospital Medical Center, Boston, Massachusetts

Leon E. Rosenberg, M.D.

Professor of Pediatrics and Internal Medicine; C.N.H. Long Professor and Chairman, Department of Human Genetics, Yale University School of Medicine, New Haven, Connecticut

Beryl J. Rosenstein, M.D.

Associate Professor of Pediatrics, Johns Hopkins University School of Medicine, Baltimore, Maryland

Allen D. Roses, M.D.

Professor and Chief, Division of Neurology, Department of Medicine, Duke University Medical Center, Durham, North Carolina

Peter B. Rowe, M.D.

Lorimer Dods Professor and Director, The University of Sydney, Children's Medical Research Foundation, The Royal Alexandra Hospital for Children, Camperdown, Australia

Richard L. Sabina, Ph.D.

Research Associate, Department of Medicine, Duke University Medical Center, Durham, North Carolina

Gerald Salen, M.D.

Department of Medicine, College of Medicine and Dentistry, New

Jersey Medical School, Newark, New Jersey; Veterans Administration Hospital, East Orange, New Jersey

Shigeru Sassa, M.D., Ph.D.

Associate Professor and Physician, The Rockefeller University Hospital, New York

Jerry A. Schneider, M.D.

Professor of Pediatrics, Department of Pediatrics, School of Medicine, University of California, San Diego, La Jolla, California

Joseph D. Schulman, M.D.

Head, Section on Human Biochemical and Developmental Genetics, National Institute of Child Health and Human Development, National Institutes of Health, Bethesda, Maryland

Joel M. Schwartz, M.D.

Associate Professor of Medicine, State University of New York Downstate Medical Center; Chief, Division of Hematology, Coney Island Hospital, New York

Charles R. Scriver, M.D.

Professor of Biology, Genetics and Pediatrics, Le Belle Laboratory for Biochemical Genetics, McGill University-Montreal Children's Hospital Research Institute, Montreal, Quebec

Anthony A. Sebastian, M.D.

Associate Professor of Medicine, Associate Director, General Clinical Research Center, University of California, San Francisco, San Francisco, California

Stanton Segal, M.D.

Professor of Pediatrics and Medicine, University of Pennsylvania School of Medicine, Children's Hospital of Philadelphia, Philadelphia, Pennsylvania

Larry J. Shapiro, M.D.

Associate Professor of Pediatrics, UCLA School of Medicine, Division of Medical Genetics, Harbor-UCLA Medical Center, Torrance, California

Sarah Shefer, M.D.

Department of Medicine, College of Medicine and Dentistry of New Jersey, New Jersey Medical School, Newark, New Jersey

James B. Sidbury, M.D.

Scientific Director, National Institute of Child Health and Human Development, National Institutes of Health, Bethesda, Maryland

Olli Simell, M.D.

Lecturer, Department of Pediatrics, University of Helsinki, Helsinki, Finland

H. Anne Simmonds, Ph.D.

Purine Laboratory, Clinical Science Laboratories, Guy's Hospital Medical School, London, England

Lloyd H. Smith, Jr., M.D.

Professor of Medicine and Chairman, Department of Medicine, University of California Medical Center, San Francisco, California

Robert J. Smith, M.D.

Assistant Professor of Medicine, Harvard Medical School, Joslin Diabetes Foundation, Inc., Boston, Massachusetts

John B. Stanbury, M.D.

Senior Physician, Massachusetts General Hospital; Division of Health Science and Technology and Department of Nutrition and Food Science, Massachusetts Institute of Technology, Cambridge, Massachusetts

Daniel Steinberg, M.D., Ph.D.

Professor, Department of Medicine and Head, Division of Metabolic Disease, University of California, San Diego, La Jolla, California

Beat Steinmann, M.D.
Privatdozent, Division of Metabolism, Department of Pediatrics, University of Zurich, Kinderspital Zurich, Zurich, Switzerland

Kunihiko Suzuki, M.D.
Professor of Neurology and Neuroscience, The Saul R. Korey Department of Neurology, Department of Neuroscience, and the Rose F. Kennedy Center for Research in Mental Retardation and Human Development, Albert Einstein College of Medicine, New York

Yoshiyuki Suzuki, M.D.
Associate Professor of Pediatrics, Department of Pediatrics, Faculty of Medicine, The University of Tokyo, Tokyo, Japan

Judith L. Swain, M.D.
Assistant Professor of Medicine and Assistant Professor of Physiology, Duke University Medical Center, Durham, North Carolina

Charles C. Sweeley, Ph.D.
Professor and Chairman, Department of Biochemistry, Michigan State University, East Lansing, Michigan

Richard C. Talamo, M.D.
Professor and Chairman, Department of Pediatrics, Boston Floating Hospital, Tufts University School of Medicine, Boston, Massachusetts

Kay Tanaka, M.D.
Professor of Human Genetics, Department of Human Genetics, School of Medicine, Yale University, New Haven, Connecticut

Kouichi R. Tanaka, M.D.
Professor and Chief, Division of Hematology, Department of Medicine, Harbor-UCLA Medical Center, UCLA School of Medicine, Torrance, California

Samuel O. Thier, M.D.
Sterling Professor and Chairman, Department of Internal Medicine, Yale University School of Medicine, New Haven, Connecticut

Ara Tourian, M.D.
Associate Professor of Neurology, Department of Medicine, Neurogenetics and Cell Biology Laboratory, Duke University Medical Center, Durham, North Carolina

William N. Valentine, M.D.
Professor, Division of Hematology/Oncology, Department of Medicine, UCLA Center for the Health Sciences, UCLA School of Medicine, Los Angeles, California

David Valle, M.D.
Associate Professor of Pediatrics and Medicine and Director,

Pediatric Genetics Clinic, The Johns Hopkins University School of Medicine, The Johns Hopkins Hospital, Baltimore, Maryland

Karel J. Van Acker, M.D.
Professor, Department of Pediatrics, University of Antwerp, Wilrijk, Belgium

Georges Van Den Berghe, M.D.
Investigator, Laboratory of Physiological Chemistry, International Institute of Cellular and Molecular Pathology, Brussels; Consultant Physician, Department of Pediatrics, Catholic University of Leuven, Leuven, Belgium

Mackenzie Walser, M.D.
Professor of Pharmacology and Medicine, The Johns Hopkins University School of Medicine, Department of Pharmacology, Baltimore, Maryland

Robert A. Weisberg, M.D.
Head, Section on Microbial Genetics, Laboratory of Molecular Genetics, National Institute of Child Health and Human Development, National Institutes of Health, Bethesda, Maryland

Hibbard E. Williams, M.D.
Dean and Professor of Medicine, School of Medicine, University of California, Davis, California

Julian C. Williams, M.D., Ph.D.
Assistant Professor of Pediatrics, The University of Texas Medical School at Houston, Houston, Texas

Jean D. Wilson, M.D.
Professor of Internal Medicine, University of Texas Health Science Center at Dallas, Dallas, Texas

Robert M. Winslow, M.D.
Chief, Hemoglobinopathy Branch, Hematology Division, Center for Infectious Diseases, Department of Health and Human Services, Atlanta, Georgia

Carl J. Witkop, D.D.S.
Professor and Chairman, Division of Human Genetics and Department of Oral Pathology and Genetics, University of Minnesota, Health Sciences Unit A, Minneapolis, Minnesota

Allan W. Wolkoff, M.D.
Associate Professor of Medicine, Albert Einstein College of Medicine, New York

James B. Wyngaarden, M.D.
Director, National Institutes of Health, Bethesda, Maryland

PREFACE

The first edition of *The Metabolic Basis of Inherited Disease* was published in 1960, a time when the "inborn errors of metabolism" were being rediscovered and slowly converted to "molecular diseases." The book was designed to provide both clinicians and research scientists a base from which to track developments in a field that seemed likely to expand. A format was established which attempted to set a standard for completeness and clarity. The most important feature of planning was the recruiting of authors who were at the center of events and who could describe them with a perspective which extended from the past into the future. Space was allotted for detailed description of what was known and for speculation about what was yet to be learned. The authors were encouraged to be generous with bibliographies and illustrations.

None of those associated with the first volume, only a half-dozen of whom still remain among the one hundred and thirty-eight contributors to this fifth edition, could have foreseen the swiftness or the amount of change that the next four revisions of the text would record. The vantage point selected in the late 1950s was at the confluence of rising streams of information coming from molecular genetics and cell biology. The flood shows no sign of cresting and its impact upon understanding in human biology and medicine has been profound. Each succeeding edition has contained more chapters, and described more diseases, than the one before it. Expansion in the number of new disorders is now decreasing, but the depth of understanding steadily increases. The appreciation of allelism as a basis for heterogeneity arising from mutations at the same genetic locus continues to grow especially. Each increment of new detail in the structures of genes and their protein products

is accompanied by ever more precise awareness of how altered structure affects function. Virtually every human disease has received greater illumination by new technologies, most notably in the fields of molecular biology and immunology. Whole metabolic systems, such as the lysosomes, have been discovered and their points of dysfunction thoroughly mapped in the intervening years. Diagnosis continues to improve, and the detection of genetic abnormality in the fetal state and in normal-appearing carriers is constantly sharpening. More specific and effective therapies continue to be developed. It is now anticipated that the human genome will be largely mapped in a few years. Undoubtedly, means for replacement of some of the defective genes will soon be discovered.

This fifth edition reflects the intention of the editors and publishers to maintain the original goals of the book despite the revolutionary transformation of its contents. The foremost objective continues to be the critical synthesis of knowledge by the most expert, and presentation in a manner that provides the student, the clinician, or the scientist as much instruction as each seeks on how genes control metabolic processes, the abnormal states of which clarify the limits of the normal. There are changes in format to provide easier access to some important facts. A detailed summary now precedes each chapter. There is also a twenty-three-page tabular supplement summarizing useful data about the major metabolic diseases arising from mutation. Fourteen new chapters on diseases not covered in previous editions as well as two new introductory chapters, one on the fundamentals of molecular genetics and the other on the major histocompatibility complex, have been included in this edition. A few diseases (ten) whose knowledge base has not changed significantly since the last edition have been selected for presentation in summary form only, including citation of a few key references, so that valuable space may be shifted to more active areas of investigation. In all chapters, the authors have been encouraged to update bibliographies with a concentration on more recent publications. Clear reference is provided, however, to archives where older, more historical facts can be found. This necessary triage notwithstanding, the average bibliography in a chapter contains about as many entries as in previous editions. Readers are encouraged to guard their older editions of this book. They form a valuable series through which the evolution of knowledge of genetic structure and expression in humans can be traced in detail.

From one standpoint, the most important recent change made to cope with the contemporary challenge and to prepare for the future is the increase in number of the editors to five.

The three "senior" editors warmly welcome Joseph Goldstein and Michael Brown into harness and acknowledge their invaluable influence on this edition. To the seventy-eight new contributors and the fifty-five who have joined us again from the previous edition, we express our appreciation for their remarkable adherence to the deadlines and to the other standards set by previous publications. We also salute their predecessors upon whose contributions they have built. We must ultimately depend upon our readers, for whom this volume has been completely rewritten, to instruct us as to how we should best fashion its replacements.

John B. Stanbury M.D.
James B. Wyngaarden M.D.
Donald S. Fredrickson M.D.
Joseph L. Goldstein M.D.
Michael S. Brown M.D.

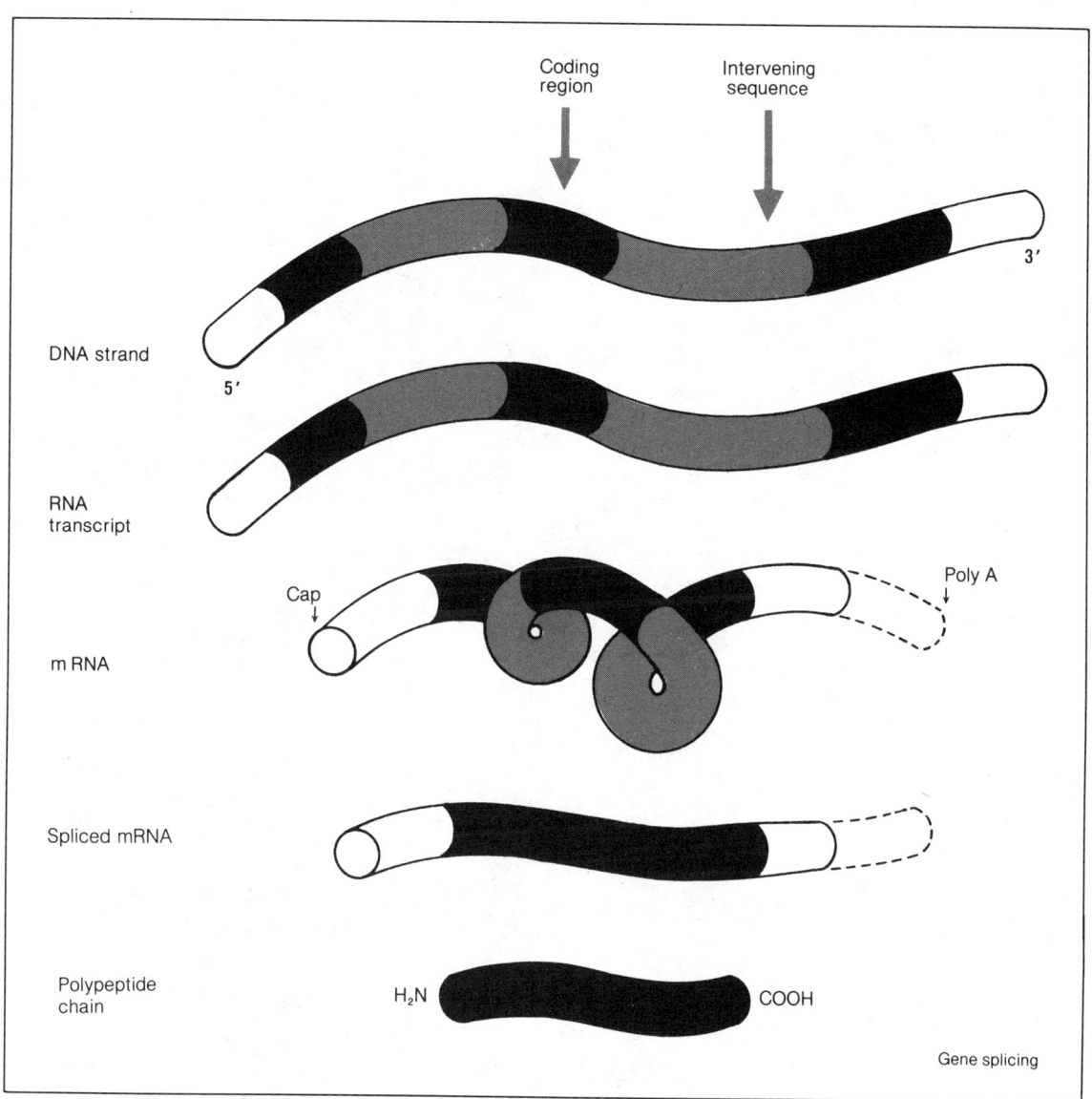

Coding region

Intervening sequence

DNA strand

5'

3'

RNA transcript

Cap

Poly A

mRNA

Spliced mRNA

Polypeptide chain

H₂N

COOH

Gene splicing

INTRODUCTION

1

INBORN ERRORS OF METABOLISM IN THE 1980s

THE EDITORS

The conceptual union of genetics and metabolism is perhaps the most fruitful development in biologic science of the past decades. Each of these disciplines has profound explanatory consequences for the other, and both have implications for the understanding of human disease. The intimate relation between genetics and metabolism is symbolized by the title of this volume: *The Metabolic Basis of Inherited Disease.* In the 1980s, it could just as easily be: *The Inherited Basis of Metabolic Disease.*

One outstanding product of the union of genetics and metabolism is the map of the human genome that is presented in Fig. 1-1 and in the accompanying key. As of early 1982, the chromosomal location of more than 350 genes had been identified [1, 2]. All of the 22 autosomes, as well as the X and Y chromosomes, contain at least one known gene. The localized genes include many that code for enzymes as well as many that code for nonenzymatic proteins such as hemoglobin and immunoglobulins. As McKusick has pointed out [1], the elucidation of the human gene map is a triumph of human anatomy analogous to the discovery that the kidney is the site of urine production and that the heart pumps blood.

The map of the human genome has direct relevance to the metabolic diseases that form the subject of this book. Through the use of this map, we can now locate the pathologic region of deoxyribonucleic acid (DNA) that is responsible for classic genetic diseases such as sickle-cell anemia and β thalassemia (short arm of chromosome 11), Tay-Sachs disease (long arm of chromosome 15), galactosemia (short arm of chromosome 9), and more than 30 others (see Table 1-1). When geneticists discuss one of these diseases, they are now talking about an anatomic derangement in the same concrete sense that urologists talk about a kidney stone or cardiologists talk about a stenotic mitral valve. This is quite an achievement for a field that started with a vague notion of heritable "factors" that somehow produced disease.

DEVELOPMENT OF THE CONCEPT OF INHERITED METABOLIC DISEASE

Inborn Error Concept (Garrod)

The history of human biochemical genetics begins at the turn of the twentieth century, when Sir Archibald Garrod initiated the brilliant studies of alkaptonuria that were to culminate in his Croonian Lectures in 1908 [3] and in his monograph, *Inborn Errors of Metabolism,* which appeared in 1909 and in modified form in 1923 [4].

Garrod had observed that patients with alkaptonuria excreted large, rather constant quantities of homogentisic acid throughout their lifetimes, whereas other persons excreted

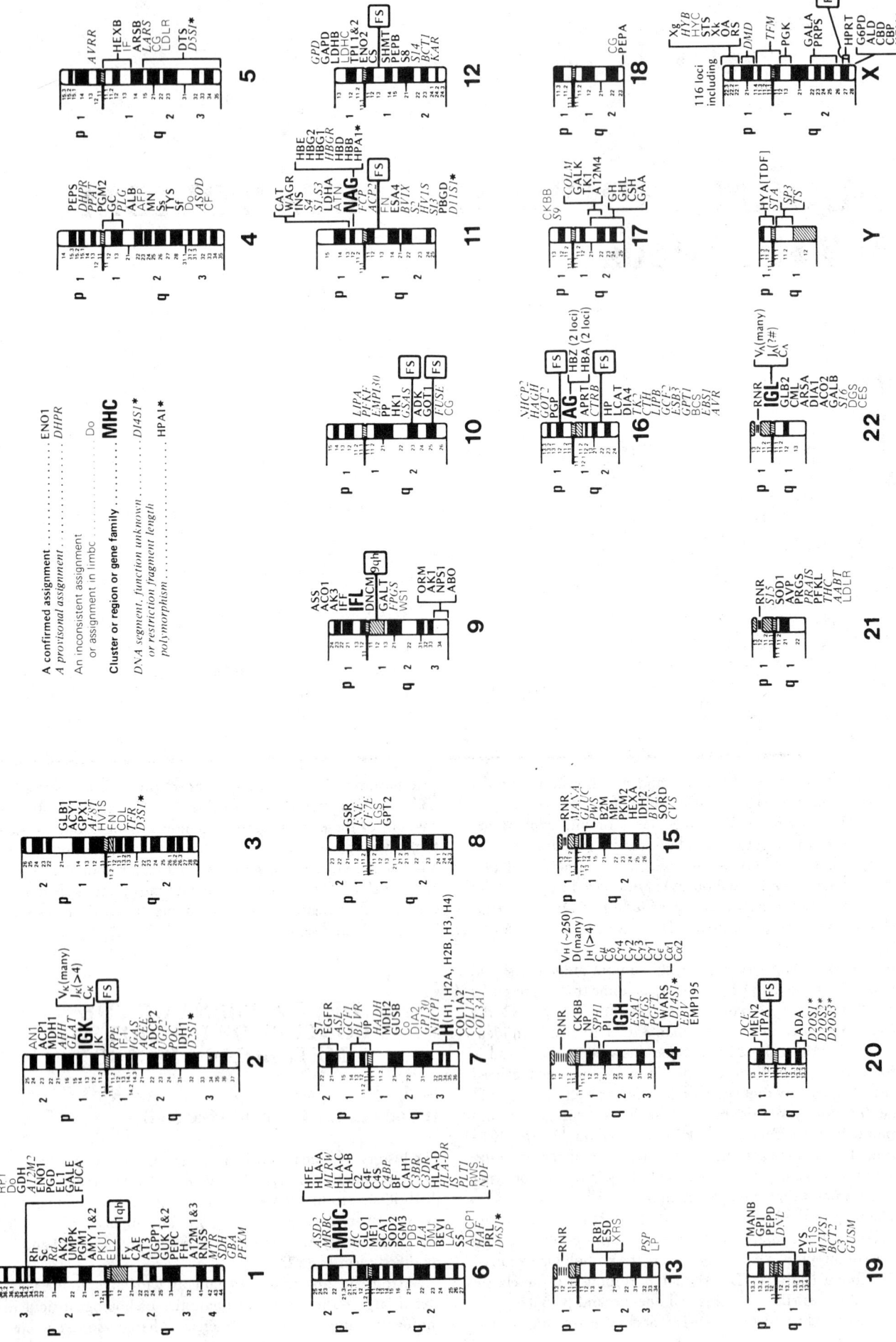

Figure 1-1 A diagrammatic synopsis of the gene map of the human chromosomes. The banding patterns and numbering of banded regions are those given in the International System for Human Cytogenetics Nomenclature, 1978. An assignment is considered confirmed if found in two laboratories or several families. It is considered provisional if based on evidence from only one laboratory. Inconsistent assignments based on conflicting evidence and assignments for which the evidence is weaker than that for provisional assignment are separately indicated (also termed "tentative" or "in limbo"). See Key below for gene locus symbols. (*Courtesy of Victor A. McKusick.*)

ABO = ABO blood group—9q34
ACEE = Acetylcholinesterase expression—chr. 2
ACON-M = Aconitase, mitochondrial—22q11-qter
ACON-S = Aconitase, soluble—9pter-p13
ACP1 = Acid phosphatase-1—2p23
#ACP2 = Acid phosphatase-2—11p12-cen
ACY1 = Aminoacylase-1—3pter-q13
#ADA = Adenosine deaminase—20q13-qter
ADCP1 = Adenosine deaminase complexing protein-1—chr. 6
ADCP2 = Adenosine deaminase complexing protein-2—chr. 2
ADK = Adenosine kinase—10q11-q24
#AH3 = Adrenal hyperplasia III (21-hydroxylase deficiency) (6p2105-6p23)
AHH = Aryl hydrocarbon hydroxylase—2p
AK1 = Adenylate kinase-1 (soluble)—9q34
AK2 = Adenylate kinase-2 (mitochondrial)—1p32-p34
AK3 = Adenylate kinase-3 (mitochondrial)—9pter-p13
AL = Lethal antigen: 3 loci—a1, a3 on 11p13-pter; a2 on 11q13-qter
#Alb = Albumin—4q11-q13
#ALD = Adrenoleukodystrophy—(Xq28; linked to G6PD)
AMY1 = Amylase, salivary—1p1
AMY2 = Amylase, pancreatic—1p1
#An1 = Aniridia, type 1 (chr. 2; linked to ACP1)
#APRT = Adenine phosphoribosyltransferase—16q
ARP-1* = Arbitrary (or anonymous) restriction polymorphism-1—chr. 14
#ARS-A = Arylsulfatase A—chr. 22
#ARS-B = Arylsulfatase B—chr. 5
#ASD2 = Atrial septal defect, secundum type (chr. 6; linked to HLA)
#ASH = Asymmetric septal hypertrophy (chr. 6; linked to HLA)
#ASL = Argininosuccinate lyase—7pter-q22
#ASOD = Anterior segment ocular dysgenesis (chr. 4; linked to MNSs)
#ASS = Argininosuccinate synthetase—chr. 9
#AT = Ataxia-telangiectasia—?chr. 14
AT3 = Antithrombin III (chr. 1)
AV12M1 = Adenovirus-12 chromosome modification site-1—1q42-43
AV12M2 = Adenovirus-12 chromosome modification site-2—1p36
AV12M3 = Adenovirus-12 chromosome modification site-3—1q21
AV12-17 = Adenovirus-12 chromosome modification site-17—17q21-q22
AVP = Antiviral protein—21q21-qter
AVr = Antiviral state regulator—chr. 5
β2M (B2M) = Beta-2-microglobulin—15q14-q21
BCT-1 = Branched chain amino acid transferase-1—chr. 12
BCT-2 = Branched chain amino acid transferase-2—chr. 19

BEVI = Baboon M7 virus infection—chr. 6
BF = Properdin factor B—chr. 6 (in MHC)
BVIN = BALB virus induction, N-tropic—chr. 15
BVIX = BALB virus induction, xenotropic—chr. 11
#C2 = Complement component-2—chr. 6 (in MHC)
#C4F = Complement component-4 fast—chr. 6 (in MHC)
#C4S = Complement component-4 slow—chr. 6 (in MHC)
#Cae = Cataract, zonular pulverulent (chr. 1; linked to Fy)
#CAT = Catalase—11p
CB = Colorblindness (deutan and protan) (Xq28)
CB3S = Coxsackie B3 virus susceptibility—chr. 19
CdL = Cornelia de Lange syndrome—?chr. 3
#CF7E = Clotting factor VII expression (chr. 8)
CG = Chorionic gonadotropin (chr. 10 and 18; chr. 5 or 6)
Ch = Chido blood group—same as C4S
#CHOL = Hereditary hypercholesterolemia—chr. 6
#CF = Cystic fibrosis—?chr. 2
CKBB = Creatine kinase, brain type—chr. 14
#CML = Chronic myeloid leukemia—22q12
Co = Colton blood group (chr. 7)
CO11 = Collagen I alpha-1 chain—chr. 7 and 17
CO12 = Collagen I alpha-2 chain—chr. 7 and 17
CO31 = Collagen III alpha-1 chain—chr. 7
CPNH = Chromosomal protein, nonhistone—chr. 16
CS = Citrate synthase, mitochondrial—chr. 12
CSMT (or CSH) = Chorionic somatomammotropin—chr. 17
DCE = Desmosterol-to-cholesterol enzyme—chr. 20
#DHPR = Quinoid dihydropteridine reductase—chr. 4
DIA-1 = NADH-diaphorase—chr. 22
#DMD = Duchenne muscular dystrophy—?Xp12-p21
#DMJ = Juvenile diabetes mellitus (chr. 6; ?linked to HLA)
DNC = Lysosomal DNA-ase—chr. 19
DNCM = Cytoplasmic membrane DNA—9qh
Do = Dombrock blood group (?chr. 1 or 4)
#DTS = Diphtheria toxin sensitivity—5q15-qter
E1 = Pseudocholinesterase-1—(?chr. 3; linked to Tf)
#E2 = Pseudocholinesterase-2—16cen-q22
E11S = Echo 11 sensitivity—19q
#EB51 = Epidermolysis bullosa, Ogna type (chr. 10)
#EBV = Epstein-Barr virus integration site—chr. 14
EGFR = Epidermal growth factor, receptor for—chr. 7
E11 = Elliptocytosis-1—(1p; linked to Rh)
E12 = Elliptocytosis-2—(? linkage to chr. 1 markers other than Rh)
EMP130 = External membrane protein-130—chr. 10
EMP195 = External membrane protein-195—chr. 14
ENO1 = Enolase-1—1p36-1pter
ENO2 = Enolase-2—chr. 12
Es-Act = Esterase activator—chr. 4 or 5

EsA4 = Esterase-A4—11cen-q22
EsD = Esterase D—13q14
FGRAT = Formylglycinamide riboride amidotransferase—chr. 4 or 5
FH = Fumarate hydratase—1q42-qter
FN = Fibronectin—chr. 3, 8, 11
FPGS = Folylpolyglutamate synthetase—chr. 9
FS = Fragile site, observed in cultured cells, with or without folate deficient medium, or BrdU—2q11; 9q33; 10q23; 10q25; 11q13; 16pl124; 16q22; 20p11; Xq27
#αFUC (FUCA) = Alpha-L-fucosidase—1p32-p34
FUSE = Polykaryocytosis inducer—chr. 10
#Fy = Duffy blood group—1q13
Gal+Act = Galactose + activator—chr. 2
#αGALA = Alpha-galactosidase A (Fabry disease)—Xq22-q24
αGALB = Alpha-galactosidase B—22q13-qter
#βGAL-1 = Beta-galactosidase-1—3pter-q13
βGAL-2 = Beta-galactosidase-2—22q13-qter
#GALE = Galactose-4-epimerase—1p21-pter
#GALK = Galactokinase—17q21-q22
#GALT = Galactose-1-phosphate uridyltransferase—9p13 or 9p22
GAPD = Glyceraldehyde-3-phosphate dehydrogenase—12p122-pter
GARS = Glycinamide ribonucleotide synthetase—chr. 21
#GBA = Acid beta-glucosidase—1p11-1qter
GC = Group-specific component—4q11-q13
GDH = Glucose dehydrogenase—1p21-pter (1p32-pter)
#GH = Growth hormone—chr. 17
#αGLU (GLUA) = Alpha-glucosidase—chr. 17
GLUC = Neutral alpha-glucosidase C—chr. 15
GLO1 = Glyoxylase I—6p21-6p22
GOT-M = Glutamate oxaloacetate transaminase, mitochondrial—chr. 16
GOT-S = Glutamate oxaloacetate transaminase, soluble—10q24-q26
#G6PD = Glucose-6-phosphate dehydrogenase—Xq28
GP130 = Granulocyte glycoprotein—7q22-qter
#GPI = Glucosephosphate isomerase—chr. 19
GPT1 = Glutamate pyruvate transaminase, soluble—chr. 10
#GPx1 = Glutathione peroxidase-1—3p13-q12
#GSR = Glutathione reductase—8p21
GSS = Glutamate-gamma-semialdehyde synthetase—chr. 10
GUK1 & 2 = Guanylate kinase-1 & 2—1q32-q42
#GUS = Beta-glucuronidase—chr. 7
H4 (+4 others) = Histone H4 and 4 other histone genes—chr. 7
HADH = Hydroxyacyl-CoA dehydrogenase—chr. 7
HaF = Hageman factor—7q35

(*Continued on p. 6*)

* An indication of chromosomal and in some instances regional locations of the gene is shown: e.g., 9q34 means band 34 of the long arm of chromosome 9; 2p23 means band 23 of the short arm of chromosome 2.

NOTE: The symbol (#) indicates that the locus so marked is the site of one or more mutations that cause disease.

Figure 1-1 (Continued)

#Hbα	=	Hemoglobin alpha chain—chr. 16
#Hbβ	=	Hemoglobin beta chain—11p1205-p1208
Hbδ	=	Hemoglobin delta chain—11p1205-p1208
HbγA,G	=	Hemoglobin gamma chains, ala or gly as AA 136—11p1205-p1208
Hbγr	=	Hemoglobin gamma regulator—11p1205-p1208
Hbε	=	Hemoglobin epsilon chain—11p1205-p1208
Hbζ	=	Hemoglobin zeta chain—chr. 16
#Hch	=	Hemochromatosis (chr. 6; linked to HLA)
#HEM-A	=	Classic hemophilia—(Xq28)
#HexA	=	Hexosaminidase A—15q22-15qter
#HexB	=	Hexosaminidase B—5cen-q13
#HGPRT	=	Hypoxanthine-guanine phosphoribosyltransferase—Xq26-qter
HHPFH	=	Heterocellular hereditary persistence of fetal hemoglobin—11p1205-p1208
#HK1	=	Hexokinase-1—10pter-q24
HLA (A-D)	=	Human leukocyte antigens—6p2105-p23
HLA-DR	=	Human leukocyte antigen, D-related—6p2105-p23
Hp	=	Haptoglobin—chr. 16
Hpa1*	=	Hpa I restriction endonuclease polymorphism—11p1205-p1208
#HVS	=	Herpes virus sensitivity (chr. 3 and 11)
H-Y	=	Y histocompatibility antigen (Y chr.)
IDH-M	=	Isocitrate dehydrogenase, mitochondrial—15q21-qter
IDH-S	=	Isocitrate dehydrogenase, soluble—2q11 or 2q32-qter
If	=	Interferon, chain unspecified—?chr. 13
If-1	=	Interferon-1—2p23-qter
If-2	=	Interferon-2 (chr. 5)
IF-F	=	Interferon, fibroblast (chr. 9)
IF-L	=	Interferon, leukocyte (chr. 9)
IgAS	=	Immunoglobulin heavy chains attachment site—chr. 2
IGH	=	Immunoglobulin heavy chain gene family—chr. 14
IGL	=	Immunoglobulin lambda light chain gene family—?chr. 21
Ins	=	Insulin—chr. 11
ITP	=	Inosine triphosphatase—20p
Jk	=	Kidd blood group—7q
Km	=	Kappa immunoglobulin light chains, Inv (chr. 7)
#LAP	=	Laryngeal adductor paralysis—(chr. 6; linked to HLA)
#LCAT	=	Lecithin-cholesterol acyltransferase—(16q22; linked to Hp alpha)
LDH-A	=	Lactate dehydrogenase A—11p1203-p1208
LDH-B	=	Lactate dehydrogenase B—12p121-p122
LDH-C	=	Lactate dehydrogenase C—(12p; linked to LDH-B in pigeon)
LGS	=	Langer-Giedion syndrome—?8q
LIPA	=	Lysosomal acid lipase-A—chr. 10
LIPB	=	Lysosomal acid lipase-B—chr. 16
Lp	=	Lipoprotein—Lp—chr. 13
LTRS	=	Leucyl-tRNA synthetase—chr. 5
β2M (B2M)	=	Beta-2-microglobulin—15q22-15qter (15q12-q21)
M7VS1	=	Baboon M7 virus sensitivity-1—chr. 19
αMAN-A	=	Cytoplasmic alpha-D-mannosidase—15q11-qter
#αMAN-B	=	Lysosomal alpha-D-mannosidase—19pter-q13
MDH-M	=	Malate dehydrogenase, mitochondrial—7p22-q22
MDH-S	=	Malate dehydrogenase, soluble—2p23
ME1	=	Malic enzyme, soluble—6p21-q16
MHC	=	Major histocompatibility complex—6p2105-p23
MLC-W	=	Mixed lymphocyte culture, weak (chr. 6)
MNSs	=	MNSs blood group—4q
MPI	=	Mannosephosphate isomerase—15q22-qter
MRBC	=	Monkey red blood cell receptor—chr. 6
#MTR	=	5-Methyltetrahydrofolate: L-homocysteine S-methyltransferase, or tetrahydropteroyl-glutamate methyltransferase—chr. 1
#NAG	=	Non-alpha globin region—11p1205-1208
#NDF	=	Neutrophil differentiation factor (chr. 6)
#NP	=	Nucleoside phosphorylase—14q13
#NPa	=	Nail-patella syndrome—(9q3; linked to AK-1)
#OA	=	Ocular albinism—(Xp22; linked to Xg)
#OPCAI	=	Olivopontocerebellar atrophy I—(chr. 6; linked to HLA)
P	=	P blood group (chr. 6)
PA	=	Plasminogen activator (chr. 6)
#PBGD	=	Phosphobilinogen deaminase—11q23-qter
#PDB	=	Paget disease of bone—(chr. 6; ?linked to HLA)
PepA	=	Peptidase A—18q23-qter
PepB	=	Peptidase B—12q21
PepC	=	Peptidase C—1q25, or 1q42
PepD	=	Peptidase D—chr. 19
PepS	=	Peptidase S—4pter-q12
PFK-F	=	Phosphofructokinase, fibroblast—chr. 10
PFK-L	=	Phosphofructokinase, liver—chr. 21
6PGD	=	6-Phosphogluconate dehydrogenase—1p34-pter
PGK	=	Phosphoglycerate kinase—Xq13
PGM1	=	Phosphoglucomutase-1—1p32; 1p221-p311; 1p33-p34
PGM2	=	Phosphoglucomutase-2—4p14-q12
PGM3	=	Phosphoglucomutase-3—6q
PGP	=	Phosphoglycolate phosphatase—16p
PK3	=	Pyruvate kinase-3—15q14-qter
#PKU	=	Phenylketonuria (1p; linked to AMY)
PL	=	Prolactin—chr. 6
POMC	=	Proopiomelanocortin—chr. 2
PP	=	Inorganic pyrophosphatase—10pter-q24
PRPPAT	=	Phosphoribosylpyrophosphate amidotransferase—4pter-q21
PRPPS	=	Phosphoribosylpyrophosphate synthetase—X chr.
PRAIS	=	Phosphoribosylaminoimidazole synthetase—chr. 21
#PVS	=	Polio virus sensitivity—19q
#PWS	=	Prader-Willi syndrome—15q11-q12
1qh	=	Paracentric heterochromatic segment, long arm, chr. 1
#RB1	=	Retinoblastoma-1—13q12-q14; 13q21-22
rC3b	=	Receptor for C3b—chr. 6 (in MHC)
rC3d	=	Receptor for C3d—chr. 6 (in MHC)
Rg	=	Rodgers blood group—same as C4F
#Rh	=	Rhesus blood group (1p32-pter)
RN5S	=	5S RNA gene(s)—1q42-q43
#RP1	=	Retinitis pigmentosa-1 (chr. 1)
rRNA	=	Ribosomal RNA—13p12, 14p12, 15p12, 21p12, 22p12
Rts	=	Retinoschisis—(?Xp22; linked to Xg)
#RwS	=	Ragweed sensitivity—(chr. 6; ?linked to HLA)
SA6	=	Surface antigen 6—chr. 6
SA7	=	Surface antigen 7—7p12-pter
SA11	=	Surface antigen 11—11p
SA12	=	Surface antigen 12—chr. 12
SA17	=	Surface antigen 17—chr. 17
SA21	=	Surface antigen 21—chr. 21
Sc	=	Scianna blood group—(1p32-p34)
SDH	=	Succinate dehydrogenase—chr. 1
Sf	=	Stoltzfus blood group—(4q; linked to MNSs)
SHMT	=	Serine hydroxymethyltransferase—chr. 12
SOD1	=	Superoxide dismutase, soluble—21q211
SOD2	=	Superoxide dismutase, mitochondrial—6q21
SORD	=	Sorbitol dehydrogenase—15pter-q21
#Sph 1	=	Spherocytosis, Denver type—(8p11 or chr. 12)
#SS	=	Steroid sulfatase—?Xp22-pter
#TC2	=	Transcobalamin II—(9q; ?linked to ABO)
TDF	=	Testis determining factor—prob. same as H-Y
Tfm	=	Testicular feminization syndrome—Xcen-p13
Tf	=	Transferrin—?chr. 3
TK-M	=	Thymidine kinase, mitochondrial—chr. 16
TK-S	=	Thymidine kinase, soluble—17q21-q22
#TPI-1 & 2	=	Triosephosphate isomerase-1 & 2—TPI-1 on 12p12.2-pter
tsAF8	=	Temperature-sensitive (AF8) complement—chr. 3
#Tyr	=	Tyrosinase—(?11p)
#Tys	=	Sclerotylosis—(4q; linked to MNSs)
UGPP1	=	Uridyl diphosphate glucose pyrophosphorylase-1—1q21-q23
UGPP2	=	Uridyl diphosphate glucose pyrophosphorylase-2—chr. 2
#UMPK	=	Uridine monophosphate kinase—1p32
UP	=	Uridine phosphorylase—chr. 7
#WAGR	=	Wilms tumor/aniridia/gonadoblastoma/retardation11p13
WTRS	=	Tryptophanyl-tRNA synthetase—chr. 14
#WS1	=	Waardenburg syndrome-1—(chr. 9; ?linked to ABO)
Xg	=	Xg blood group (X chr., ?Xp2)

Table 1-1 Metabolic diseases that have been mapped to specific autosomes

Disease	Chromosome*
Disorders of carbohydrate metabolism	
Glycogen storage disease, type II (Pompe's disease)	17q
Galactosemia	9q
Galactokinase deficiency	17q
Galactose-4-epimerase deficiency	1p
Disorders of amino acid metabolism	
Atypical phenylketonuria (dihydropteridine reductase deficiency)	4q
Argininosuccinic aciduria	7p
Citrullinemia	9p
Disorders of lipoprotein and lipid metabolism	
Familial lecithin: cholesterol acyltransferase deficiency	16q
Disorders of lysosomal enzymes	
Mucopolysaccharidosis, type VI (Maroteaux-Lamy syndrome)	5q
Mucopolysaccharidosis, type VII (β-glucuronidase deficiency)	7p
Fucosidosis	1p
Mannosidosis	19q
Wolman disease and cholesteryl ester storage disease	10q
Lysosomal acid phosphatase deficiency	11p
Metachromatic leukodystrophy	22q
Sandhoff disease	5q
Tay-Sachs disease	15q
Generalized gangliosidosis	3p
Disorders of steroid metabolism	
Adrenogenital syndrome (steroid 21-hydroxylase deficiency)	6p
Disorders of purine and pyrimidine metabolism	
Adenine phosphoribosyl transferase deficiency	16q
Adenosine deaminase deficiency	20q
Nucleoside phosphorylase deficiency	14q
Disorders of metal metabolism	
Hemochromatosis	6p
Acute intermittent porphyria	11q
Disorders of the blood and blood-forming tissues	
Glucosephosphate isomerase deficiency	19p
Hexokinase deficiency	10q
Triosephosphate isomerase deficiency	12p
Elliptocytosis	1p
Sickle-cell anemia and all other β-chain variants	11p
Hemoglobin constant spring and all other α-chain variants	16p
α Thalassemias	16p
β Thalassemias	11p
Disorders of immune and other defense systems	
C_2 deficiency	6p
C_4 deficiency	6p

* These numbers indicate the chromosome that carries the particular locus. The chromosome arm is indicated when known: p = short arm; q = long arm.
SOURCE: Data modified from McKusick [1].

none at all. [5]. He observed that this condition had a familial distribution and that while frequently one or more sibs were involved, parents and more distant relatives were normal. There was a high incidence of consanguine marriages in the parents of his patients, as well as in the parents of similar patients studied elsewhere. On conferring with Bateson, one of the earliest of the great school of British geneticists, Garrod learned that these observations could readily be explained if the defect were inherited as a recessive condition in terms of the recently rediscovered laws of Mendel [6, 7].

From his observations of patients with alkaptonuria, albi-

nism, cystinuria, and pentosuria, Garrod developed the concept that certain diseases of lifelong duration arise because an enzyme governing a single metabolic step is reduced in activity or missing altogether [8]. Garrod viewed the accumulation of homogentisic acid in alkaptonuria as evidence that this substance is a normal metabolite in the dissimulation of tyrosine, and he correctly attributed its accumulation to a failure of oxidation of homogentisic acid. A half-century later, Garrod's hypothesis was proved by the demonstration of unmeasurable activity of homogentisic acid oxidase in the liver of a patient with alkaptonuria [9].

Similarly, the failure of pigment formation in the skin in albinism, the excretion of large amounts of cystine in the urine in cystinuria, and the appearance of pentose in the urine in essential pentosuria were viewed by Garrod as the results of blocks in normal metabolic pathways. He attributed the first instance to failure of melanin formation and the other two to excretion of metabolites accumulating proximal to a metabolic block.

One Gene–One Enzyme Concept (Beadle and Tatum)

The term *gene* was first applied to the hereditary determinant of a unit characteristic by Johannsen in 1911 [10]. The relation between gene and enzyme attained clear definition in the one gene–one enzyme principle, first succinctly stated by Beadle in 1945 [11]. This formulation, now a biologic precept, emerged gradually from studies of eye color in the fruit fly, *Drosophila*, by Beadle and Tatum [12, 13] and Ephrussi [14]. It received extensive support from the classic studies of Beadle and Tatum on induced mutants of *Neurospora crassa*, in which acquisitions of requirements for specific metabolites in the culture medium were traced to losses of single chemical transformations, each dependent on a different enzyme [15, 16].

The one gene–one enzyme concept that developed from these experiments has been well expressed by Tatum [16] as follows:

1. All biochemical processes in all organisms are under genetic control.
2. These biochemical processes are resolvable into series of individual stepwise reactions.
3. Each biochemical reaction is under the ultimate control of a different single gene.
4. Mutation of a single gene results only in an alteration in the ability of the cell to carry out a single primary chemical reaction.

The one gene–one enzyme hypothesis has since been made more precise [17] and extended to cover proteins that are not enzymes, as well as complex proteins composed of nonidentical polypeptide chains linked in various ways. The functional unit of DNA which controls the structure of a single polypeptide chain is frequently called a *cistron* [18]. The one gene–one enzyme principle has been redefined as the one cistron–one polypeptide concept.

The one gene–one enzyme concept had immediate explanatory potential for the inborn errors of metabolism that Garrod had described. It appeared that inherited diseases such as alkaptonuria were produced by mutations in genes encoding enzymes in the same way that vitamin-dependent mutants of *Neurospora* lacked single enzymes required for vitamin synthesis. It was not until 1948 that the first enzyme defect in a human genetic disease was demonstrated by Gibson. This was the deficiency of the NADH-dependent enzyme required for the reduction of methemoglobin in recessive methemoglobinemia [19]. This was soon followed by the description in 1952 by Cori and Cori of glucose-6-phosphatase deficiency in von Gierke's disease (glycogen storage disease, type I) [20] and in 1953 by Jervis of phenylalanine hydroxylase deficiency in phenylketonuria [21].

Molecular Disease Concept (Pauling and Ingram)

Direct evidence that human mutations actually produce an alteration in the primary structure of proteins was first obtained in 1949 by Pauling and his associates [22]. Studying hemoglobin extracted from erythrocytes of patients with sickle-cell anemia, Pauling showed that sickle hemoglobin migrated differently in an electric field than did normal hemoglobin. Heterozygotes for the sickle-cell trait produced both normal and abnormal hemoglobin molecules. The subsequent studies of Ingram established that the electrophoretic abnormality arose because sickle-cell hemoglobin had a valine substituted for a glutamic acid residue at a particular point in the amino acid sequence [23]. This finding closed one era of discovery in human biochemical genetics: Inborn errors of metabolism were caused by mutant genes that produced abnormal proteins whose functional activities were altered.

MOLECULAR BASIS OF GENE EXPRESSION

The human genome is estimated to contain about 50,000 to 100,000 genes, each of which is composed of a linear polymer of DNA. The genes are assembled into lengthy linear arrays that together with certain proteins form rod-shaped bodies called *chromosomes*. All normal nucleated human cells other than sperm or ova contain 46 chromosomes, arrayed in 23 pairs, one of each pair derived from each of the individual's parents. The recent striking discovery that genes are not continuous sequences of DNA but consist of coding sequences (exons) interrupted by intervening sequences (introns) has led to a new view of gene expression that is discussed in detail in Chap. 2.

The genetic information carried on chromosomes is transmitted to daughter cells under two different sets of circumstances. One of these occurs whenever a somatic cell (i.e., a nongerm cell) divides. This process, called *mitosis*, functions to transmit two identical copies of each gene to each daughter cell, thus maintaining a uniform genetic makeup in all cells of a single organism. The other set of circumstances prevails when genetic information is to be transmitted from one individual to an offspring. This process, called *meiosis*, functions to produce germ cells (i.e., ova or spermatozoa) that possess only one copy of each parental chromosome, thus allowing for new combinations of chromosomes to occur when the ovum and sperm cell fuse during fertilization and restoring the *diploid* state.

During the process of meiosis, the 46 chromosomes of an immature germ cell arrange themselves in 23 pairs at the center of the nucleus, each pair being composed of one chromosome derived from the mother and its homologous chromosome derived from the father. At a specified point in the meiotic process, the two partner chromosomes separate, only one of each pair going into each daughter cell, or gamete. Thus, meiosis produces gametes with a reduction in the number of chromosomes from 46 to 23, each gamete having received one chromosome from each of the 23 pairs. The assortment of the chromosomes within each pair is random, so that each germ cell receives a different combination of maternal and paternal chromosomes. During the process of fertilization the fusion of ovum and sperm cell, each of which has 23 chromosomes, results ultimately in an individual with 46 chromosomes.

The independent assortment of chromosomes into gametes during meiosis produces an enormous diversity among the possible genotypes of the progeny. For each 23 pairs of chromosomes, there are 2^{23} different combinations of chromosomes that could occur in a gamete, and the likelihood that one set of parents will produce two offspring with the identical complement of chromosomes is one in 2^{23} or one in 8.4 million (assuming no monozygotic twins). Adding even further to the enormous genetic diversity in humans is the phenomenon of *genetic recombination* (discussed below; see page 11).

The Structure of DNA

DNA is composed of two long chains of nucleotides wrapped around each other to form a double helix. The nucleotides each consist of one of two purine bases (adenine and guanine) or two pyrimidine bases (cytosine and thymine) coupled to a molecule of deoxyribose phosphate. The nucleotides are joined to each other by phosphodiester linkages between the deoxyribose groups. These linkages are structured so that the bases are oriented toward the inside of the helix. To form the double helix, each base of one strand pairs with a base of the opposite strand through a series of hydrogen bonds. Each purine always pairs with a pyrimidine (adenine always with thymine, guanine always with cytosine). Thus, when the sequence of bases in one strand of DNA is known, the sequence of bases in the complementary strand can be predicted [24].

The double-helical model of DNA immediately suggested the manner in which genes could be replicated for transmission to offspring. The actual replication process is mechanically complex but conceptually simple. The two strands of DNA separate, and each is copied by a series of enzymes that inserts a complementary base opposite each base on the original strand of DNA. Thus, two identical double helices are generated from one [25].

In addition to its primary structure, the DNA is organized into a variety of secondary coils and loops under the influence of histone proteins that bind to the DNA. This organization may have great importance in the regulation of gene expression and is discussed in Chap. 2.

The Genetic Code

The sequence of bases in a specific gene ultimately dictates the sequence of amino acids in a specific protein. This collinearity between the DNA molecule and the protein sequence is achieved by means of the *genetic code* [25]. The four types of bases in DNA are arranged in groups of three, each triplet forming a code word or *codon* that signifies a single amino acid. Thus, the sequence adenine-adenine-adenine (or AAA) codes for phenylalanine, the sequence guanine-adenine-adenine codes for leucine, etc. In this manner, triplet codons exist for each of the 20 amino acids (Fig. 1-2). Inasmuch as 64 different triplets can be generated from the four bases and only 20 amino acids exist, the genetic code is said to be *degenerate*. That is, there are several codons for each amino acid. Each codon, however, is completely specific. Three codons, ATT, ATC, and ACT, do not code for amino acids. Rather, these codons are stop signals that indicate the termination of a polypeptide chain.

DNA-RNA-Protein

To translate its genetic information into a protein, a segment of DNA is first transcribed into messenger ribonucleic acid (messenger RNA). The messenger RNA contains a sequence of purine and pyrimidine bases that is complementary to the bases of the DNA. By this mechanism each adenine of DNA becomes a uridine of RNA, each cytosine of DNA becomes a guanine of RNA, each thymine of DNA becomes an adenine of RNA, and each guanine of DNA becomes a cytosine of RNA. Thus, each DNA triplet codon is translated into a corresponding RNA triplet codon.

The messenger RNA for each gene is processed extensively by modifying enzymes within the cell nucleus. It then crosses the nuclear membrane and enters the cytoplasm, where it serves as a template for the synthesis of a single protein [25]. To translate the messenger RNA code into a protein, the messenger RNA binds to a complex structure called a *ribosome*, which is composed of a different type of RNA (ribosomal

RNA) and a large number of proteins. In order to be inserted into its proper place in the protein sequence, each of the 20 amino acids is attached in the cytoplasm to an additional type of RNA (transfer RNA). Each amino acid is attached to a specific set of transfer RNAs. Each transfer RNA contains an "anticodon loop," which includes a sequence of three bases that is complementary to a specific codon in the corresponding messenger RNA. For example, phenylalanine is attached specifically to a transfer RNA whose anticodon loop contains the sequence AAA, which is complimentary to the messenger RNA codon UUU, which codes for phenylalanine.

Under the influence of a host of cytoplasmic factors (initiation factors, elongation factors, and termination factors), peptide bonds are formed between the various amino acids that are aligned along the messenger RNA chain. Eventually, a terminator codon is reached and the completed polypeptide is released from the ribosome. Inasmuch as the primary sequence of bases in the coding regions of the DNA determines the corresponding primary sequence of amino acids in the protein, the gene and its protein are said to be *collinear*. This means that any alteration of the sequence of bases in the gene will result in an alteration of the protein at a specific point in its sequence.

MUTATION AS THE ORIGIN OF GENETIC DISEASE

Broadly defined, a *mutation* is a stable, heritable alteration in DNA. From the viewpoint of evolution, mutations are essential for the generation of sufficient genetic diversity to permit species to adapt to their environment through the mechanism of natural selection.

Mutations can involve gross alterations in the structure of a chromosome, such as a duplication or deletion, or the translocation of a portion of one chromosome to another. On the other hand, mutations can be minute, involving a deletion, insertion, or replacement of a single base. Deletions or insertions of a single base give rise to *frame-shift mutations* because they alter the reading frame of the genetic code so that every

Figure 1-2 The genetic code. The DNA codons appear in boldface type; the complementary RNA codons are in italics. A = adenine, C = cytosine, G = guanine, T = thymine, U = uridine (replaces thymine in RNA). In RNA, adenine is complementary to thymine of DNA; uridine is complementary to adenine of DNA; cytosine is complementary to guanine, and vice versa. "Stop" = punctuation. The amino acids are abbreviated as follows: Ala = alanine, Arg = arginine, Asn = asparagine, Asp = aspartic acid, Cys = cysteine, Gln = glutamine, Glu = glutamic acid, Gly = glycine, His = histidine, Ile = isoleucine, Leu = leucine, Lys = lysine, Met = methionine, Phe = phenylalanine, Pro = proline, Ser = serine, Thr = threonine, Trp = tryptophan, Tyr = tyrosine, Val = valine.

First nucleotide		*Second nucleotide*										*Third nucleotide*
		A or *U*		G or *C*		T or *A*		C or *G*				
A or U	A	**AAA** *UUU*	Phe	**AGA** *UCU*		**ATA** *UAU*	Tyr	**ACA** *UGU*	Cys	A or *U*		
		AAG *UUC*		**AGG** *UCC*	Ser	**ATG** *UAC*		**ACG** *UGC*		G or *C*		
	U	**AAT** *UUA*	Leu	**AGT** *UCA*		**ATT** *UAA*	Stop	**ACT** *UGA* Stop		T or *A*		
		AAC *UUG*		**AGC** *UCG*		**ATC** *UAG*		**ACC** *UGG* Trp		C or *G*		
G or C	G	**GAA** *CUU*	Leu	**GGA** *CCU*		**GTA** *CAU*	His	**GCA** *CGU*	Arg	A or *U*		
		GAG *CUC*		**GGG** *CCC*	Pro	**GTG** *CAC*		**GCG** *CGC*		G or *C*		
	C	**GAT** *CUA*		**GGT** *CCA*		**GTT** *CAA*	Gln	**GCT** *CGA*		T or *A*		
		GAC *CUG*		**GGC** *CCG*		**GTC** *CAG*		**GCC** *CGG*		C or *G*		
T or A	T	**TAA** *AUU*	Ile	**TGA** *ACU*		**TTA** *AAU*	Asn	**TCA** *AGU*	Ser	A or *U*		
		TAG *AUC*		**TGG** *ACC*	Thr	**TTG** *AAC*		**TCG** *AGC*		G or *C*		
	A	**TAT** *AUA*		**TGT** *ACA*		**TTT** *AAA*	Lys	**TCT** *AGA*	Arg	T or *A*		
		TAC *AUG* Met		**TGC** *ACG*		**TTC** *AAG*		**TCC** *AGG*		C or *G*		
C or G	C	**CAA** *GUU*	Val	**CGA** *GCU*		**CTA** *GAU*	Asp	**CCA** *GGU*	Gly	A or *U*		
		CAG *GUC*		**CGG** *GCC*	Ala	**CTG** *GAC*		**CCG** *GGC*		G or *C*		
	G	**CAT** *GUA*		**CGT** *GCA*		**CTT** *GAA*	Glu	**CCT** *GGA*		T or *A*		
		CAC *GUG*		**CGC** *GCG*		**CTC** *GAG*		**CCC** *GGG*		C or *G*		

triplet distal to the mutation in the same gene is altered. When one base is replaced by another, the result is a *point mutation*. Point mutations may be of three types: (1) a *synonomous mutation* (comprising about 23 percent of random point mutations), in which the base replacement does not lead to a change in the amino acid, but only to the substitution of a different codon for the same amino acid [e.g., a replacement of the terminal adenine in the codon for phenylalanine (AAA) by a guanine, changing the codon to AAG, which still codes for phenylalanine]; (2) a *missense mutation* (73 percent of point mutations), in which the base replacement changes the codon from one amino acid to another [e.g., the replacement of the terminal adenine in the codon for phenylalanine (AAA) by a thymine, which would change the codon to leucine (AAT)]; and (3) a *nonsense mutation* (4 percent of point mutations), in which the base replacement changes the codon to one of the termination codons [e.g., the replacement of the terminal adenine in the codon for tyrosine [ATA] by a thymine, coverting the codon to a stop codon (ATT)] [26].

In addition to these point mutations, there are larger deletion mutations in which a portion of a gene is deleted. Such a deletion mutation can interrupt the coding region of a gene, causing the absence of its protein product. Alternatively, if the deletion bridges between the coding regions of two genes, it can produce a fusion of the two genes and result in the production of a hybrid protein containing the initial sequence of one protein followed by the terminal sequence of another protein.

When mutations occur in germ cells, the mutant gene does not affect the individual in whom the mutation occurs but becomes manifest only in subsequent generations. On the other hand, when mutations occur in somatic cells at an early developmental stage, they affect the individual harboring the mutation but are not passed to subsequent generations. The individual harboring such a somatic cell mutation is said to be a *mosaic* because he or she possesses two populations of cells: normal cells and cells harboring the mutant gene.

GENETIC DIVERSITY IN HUMANS: THE CONCEPT OF POLYMORPHISM

A striking discovery of the past 15 years is the realization that the gene for a given enzyme frequently exists in different forms in different normal individuals. The widespread nature of this genetic diversity first became apparent when it became possible to study enzymes by electrophoresis of crude cell extracts and thereby to detect structurally variant forms of enzymes without the necessity of purification. With the use of this technique, studies by Harris in humans [27] and by Lewontin and Hubby in *Drosophila* [28] demonstrated that many enzymes existed in two or more forms in the population. These multiple forms are due to the existence in the population of multiple genes (called *alleles*) at the same genetic locus coding for the same enzyme. At each genetic locus, each individual possesses two alleles, one derived from each parent. If the two alleles are identical, the individual is said to be *homozygous;* if they differ, he or she is *heterozygous*. The various alleles have been derived from a single precursor allele by mutations that have occurred during the evolution of the species; in general, they differ from each other only in the substitution of one base for another (missense mutations). In the vast majority of cases, the

enzymes produced by both alleles at a given locus are equally functional, i.e., the amino acid difference is "neutral" from the standpoint of natural selection.

Based on population studies of 71 enzymes and other proteins that lend themselves to analysis by electrophoresis or other techniques, Harris has found that 28 percent of genetic loci show multiple alleles in the population [26]. Moreover, the average individual is detectably heterozygous at 7 percent of his or her loci. Since most detection methods require a change in the charge of the protein, they can detect only about one-third of the actual base changes that are possible, since only one-third result in a substitution of an amino acid with a different charge. Thus, each individual may actually be heterozygous at as many as 20 percent of his or her loci.

Although the enzymes produced by these various alleles are all functional, they may differ in subtle ways, such as stability, affinity for substrates, level of activity, etc. It seems clear that this enormous degree of subtle genetic diversity among normal people accounts for the genetic component of the normal population distributions for quantitative and polygenic traits such as height, intelligence, and blood pressure.

At most genetic loci (such as that for the β chain of hemoglobin), there is one standard allele that accounts for the vast majority of the alleles in the population, whereas the alternate alleles are rare. At other genetic loci (such as that for the α chain of haptoglobin, a plasma protein), no single allele occurs with sufficient frequency to be designated as standard or normal. This latter situation represents an extreme example of genetic polymorphism. In strict terms, *polymorphism* is said to exist in a given population when the most common allele at a given locus accounts for fewer than 99 percent of the alleles in the population. By definition, when a polymorphism exists at a genetic locus, at least 2 percent of the population must be heterozygous at that locus [26]. Table 1-2 lists those plasma proteins and cellular enzymes for which electrophoretically determined polymorphisms have been demonstrated.

Harris's estimate that at least 28 percent of the genes in humans show polymorphism has recently been disputed on the basis of two-dimensional electrophoretic studies of homogenates of cultured human fibroblasts [29, 30]. This electrophoretic technique separates proteins on the basis of charge and size. The major proteins of fibroblast homogenates have been studied by this technique in several laboratories, and fewer than 2 percent are said to differ among different individuals [29, 30]. Inasmuch as individual proteins are identified by nonspecific techniques, the two-dimensional electrophoretic technique examines only those proteins that are relatively abundant in the cell. It is possible that polymorphisms are less frequent at the loci encoding these abundant structural proteins than they are at loci encoding enzymes.

GENETIC LINKAGE AND THE HUMAN GENE MAP

It is estimated that the DNA in the nucleus of each human cell codes for 50,000 to 100,000 structural genes. Only a small number of these genes have actually been identified. The most recent update of McKusick's catalog of *Mendelian Inheritance in Man* [31] indicates that more than 1350 single-gene-determined human diseases are known to exist, thus implying that at least 1350 of the 50,000 or so human genes have under-

Table 1-2 Plasma proteins and cellular enzymes that exhibit electrophoretically detectable polymorphisms

Protein	Locus name
Plasma proteins	
Haptoglobin (α chain)	Hp α
Transferrin	Tf
Vitamin D-binding protein	Gc (for group-specific component)
Ceruloplasmin	Cp
α-1-Antitrypsin	Pi (for protease inhibitor)
α-1-Acid glycoprotein	Oro (for orosomucoid)
β-2-Glycoprotein I	—
Properdin factor B	Bf
Complement	
Second component	C2
Third component	C3
Fourth component	C4
Sixth component	C6
Enzymes	
Pancreatic amylase	AMY_2
Cholinesterase	E_2
Red blood cell enzymes	
Acid phosphatase 1	ACP_1
Adenosine deaminase	ADA
Adenylate kinase	AK_1
Carbonic anhydrase 2	CA_2
Diaphorase (NADPH-dependent)	DIA_2
Esterase D	ESD
Galactose-1-uridyl transferase	GALT
Glucose-6-phosphate dehydrogenase	Gd
Glutamic-pyruvic transaminase	GPT
Glutathione peroxidase	GPX
Glutathione reductase	GSR
Glyoxalase I	GLO
Peptidase A	PEPA
Peptidase C	PEPC
Peptidase D	PEPD
Phosphoglucomutase 1	PG_{M1}
Phosphoglucomutase 2	PG_{M2}
Phosphogluconate dehydrogenase	PGD
Uridine monophosphate kinase	UMPK
White blood cell enzymes	
Aconitase (soluble)	$ACON_S$
Cytidine deaminase	CDA
α-L-Fucosidase	αFUC
α-Glucosidase	αGLUC
Glutamic-oxaloacetic transaminase mitochondrial	GOT_M
Hexokinase 3	HK_3
Malic enzyme (mitochondrial)	ME_M
Phosphoglucomutase 3	PG_{M3}

SOURCE: Data from Giblett [132].

gone mutation so as to cause human disease. The chromosomal location of more than 350 of these genes is now known (Fig. 1-1).

The ability to locate genes relative to each other on the human chromosomes grew out of the pioneering studies of Morgan and his school in the first two decades of this century

[32]. Using the fruit fly *D. melanogaster*, Morgan demonstrated that genes are aligned in a linear manner on the chromosomes and that if two genes are close together on the same chromosome, they do not assort independently at meiosis but are transmitted to the same gamete more than 50 percent of the time. Such genes are said to be *linked*. When two genes on a single chromosome are far apart, they are not genetically linked, even though they are physically linked by being on the same continuous chromosome. This lack of linkage is due to the phenomenon of *crossing-over*.

During the process of meiosis when homologous chromosomes are paired, bridges frequently form between corresponding regions of the chromosome pair. These bridges, or *chiasmas,* are regions in which the two chromosomes break at identical points along their length and subsequently rejoin, the distal segments having been switched from one homologous chromosome to the other. During this process of crossing-over, no net change in the amount of genetic material occurs. However, a *recombination* of genes does occur. For example, consider a chromosome with two loci, A and B, located at opposite ends of the same chromosome. On this particular chromosome, the A locus has a rare *x* allele and the B locus also has a rare *y* allele.

Without the phenomenon of recombination, every offspring that inherited the *x* allele at the A locus would also inherit the *y* allele at the B locus. However, if recombination occurs, the A locus with the *x* allele would then be on the opposite chromosome from the B locus with the *y* allele. In this case, any offspring that inherited the *x* allele at the A locus could not inherit the *y* allele at the B locus.

Crossing-over in humans occurs with great frequency in every meiosis, and the resultant recombination of genes may occur at any point on a chromosome. The farther apart two genes are on the same chromosome, the greater is the likelihood that a crossing-over will occur in the space between them. When two genes are on the opposite ends of a long chromosome, the probability of recombination is so great that their respective alleles are transmitted to offspring almost independently of one another, just as if the two gene loci were on different chromosomes. On the other hand, gene loci that are close together on the same chromosome are said to be *linked,* so that there is a great likelihood that offspring will inherit the same combination of alleles that is present on the parental chromosome.

Fig. 1-1 and its accompanying key give the chromosomal assignments of 240 autosomal loci, with indications of the confidence of the assignment. In addition, some 110 loci are known from pedigree studies to be located on the X chromosome. As illustrated in Fig. 1-1, the mapping of genes on chromosome 1 (the largest chromosome), on chromosome 6 (the chromosome containing the major histocompatibility or HLA locus), and on a small segment of the short arm of chromosome 11 (the chromosome containing the β chain of hemoglobin) is extensive.

Assignment of a locus to a specific chromosome is based on a variety of methods that have been reviewed in detail by McKusick and Ruddle [1, 2]. The nine most commonly used techniques are listed below, with an example of a linkage assignment that was made on the basis of the technique indicated in parentheses: (1) study of linkage of traits in large families with multiple alleles at two loci (e.g., linkage of the nail-patella syndrome and the ABO blood group); (2) cosegregation of specific proteins and single chromosomes in clones from somatic cell hybrids (e.g., thymidine kinase segregates with chromosome 17); (3) microcell-mediated gene transfer (e.g., type I procollagen is transferred by chromosome 17); (4) chromosome-mediated gene transfer (e.g., cotransfer of galactokinase and thymidine kinase); (5) DNA-RNA annealing or *in situ* hybridization (e.g., ribosomal RNA hybridizes to acrocentric chromosomes); (6) DNA/cDNA molecular hybridization in solution or "Cot analysis" of somatic cell hybrids containing a small number of human chromosomes (e.g., assignment of the β chain of hemoglobin to chromosome 11); (7) DNA restriction endonuclease techniques (e.g., fine structure of the β-globin region on chromosome 11); (8) deletion mapping (concurrence of chromosomal deletion and phenotypic evidence of hemizygosity); trisomy mapping (presence of three different alleles in the case of a highly polymorphic locus); or gene dosage effects (correlation of the triplicate state of part or all of a chromosome with 50 percent more gene product) (e.g., acid phosphatase-1 to chromosome 2 and glutathione reductase to chromosome 8); and (9) deductions from the amino acid sequence of proteins (e.g., linkage of δ- and β-hemoglobin loci inferred from the study of hemoglobin Lepore, a product of the fusion of the two loci).

About 60 percent of the assignments in Fig. 1-1 were obtained from somatic cell hybridization studies; about 25 percent emerged from study of the linkage of traits in families; and about 6 percent were made independently by both somatic cell hybridization and family studies. The remaining 11 percent of assignments were made on the basis of one of the other methods listed above [1, 2].

When the location of a gene is known, physicians can use the concept of gene linkage to predict which individual in a given family will be affected by a given trait. An example can be seen in the map of human chromosome 1 (Fig. 1-1). The locus for the gene specifying the Rh blood group factor and the locus for the gene producing one form of the dominant trait, hereditary elliptocytosis, occur in close proximity on this chromosome. Thus, if a subject with hereditary elliptocytosis transmits the disease to an offspring, the offspring will usually inherit the allele that is present at the Rh locus on this chromosome. If the Rh allele on this chromosome happens to be a rare one in the population (such as r'), one can assume that whichever offspring inherits the r' allele at the Rh locus will also inherit the abnormal allele at the elliptocytosis locus. On the other hand, if an offspring does not exhibit the r' allele, he or she will not usually have elliptocytosis. The concept of linkage does not imply an association between any particular set of Rh alleles and the disease state elliptocytosis, but rather a linkage between the two genetic loci. Thus, in different families the abnormal elliptocytosis allele may be associated with the R^1, R^0, r_2, or any other allele at the Rh locus, depending on the allele that happened to be at that locus when the elliptocytosis mutation occurred. Stated another way, the elliptocytosis locus is *linked* to the Rh locus in every family, but the particular Rh allele with which it is *associated* will differ from family to family.

The specific chromosomal localization of the genes responsible for at least 35 of the autosomally inherited inborn errors of metabolism discussed in this book is now known (Table 1-1). Included in this list are 12 lysosomal storage diseases (including Tay-Sachs disease), two disorders of the urea cycle, four disorders of carbohydrate metabolism (including galactosemia), and several immune deficiency disorders [1].

McKusick and Ruddle suggest that the entire human genome may be mapped in complete chemical detail by the end of the century [1, 2]. As discussed in Chap. 2, the sequencing of the nucleic acids of the genes has become technically easier than the sequencing of amino acids of the gene product. This fact, coupled with the use of DNA restriction enzyme analysis and hybridization for the identification of "restriction fragment length polymorphisms" (discussed below), makes McKusick and Ruddle's bold suggestion a realistic one.

CATEGORIES OF GENETIC DISORDERS

Genetic diseases generally fall into one of three categories. (1) *Chromosomal disorders* involve the lack, excess, or abnormal arrangement of one or more chromosomes, producing large amounts of excessive or deficient genetic material and affecting many genes. (2) *Mendelian or monogenic disorders* are determined primarily by a single mutant gene. Accordingly, these disorders display simple (Mendelian) inheritance patterns that can be classified into autosomal dominant, autosomal recessive, or X-linked types. (3) *Multifactorial disorders* are caused by an interaction of multiple genes and multiple exogenous or environmental factors. Although many of these multifactorial disorders, such as diabetes mellitus, gout, and cleft lip and palate, are said to run in families, the inheritance pattern is complex and the risk to relatives is much less than that seen in the single-gene (Mendelian) disorders. Each of the above three categories of genetic disease presents different problems with respect to causation, prevention, diagnosis, genetic counseling, and treatment [33].

Chromosomal Disorders

The *karyotype* of an individual (i.e., the number and structure of the chromosomes) can be ascertained from readily accessible body cells, such as peripheral blood lymphocytes or skin fibroblasts, by growing them in tissue culture until active proliferation occurs and then preparing single metaphase cells for examination of chromosomes by microscopy. Recent developments have made it possible to identify each individual chromosome by special staining of DNA sequences, by the affinity of fluorescent dyes (such as quinacrine hydrochloride) for certain chromosomal segments that can be visualized by fluorescence microscopy, and by treatment of the chromosomes with dyes (Giemsa) after treatment with proteolytic enzymes (trypsin). These techniques produce characteristic *banding patterns* for each chromosome (Fig. 1-3). The number of chromosomes in normal individuals is 46, of which 44 are the 22 pairs of *autosomes* and the other 2 are the *sex chromosomes*. Females have two X chromosomes (XX), and males have one X chromosome and one Y chromosome (XY). Each of the 22 pairs of autosomes and the 2 sex chromosomes can be distinguished on the basis of size, location of the centromere (which divides the chromosome into arms of equal or unequal length), and the unique banding pattern (Fig. 1-3). The relative length of the arms and the position of the centromere are used as criteria to divide the human chromosomes into seven groups (designated A to G) (Fig. 1-3).

Most chromosomal disorders found in humans can be classified into one of four groups: (1) excess or loss of one or more

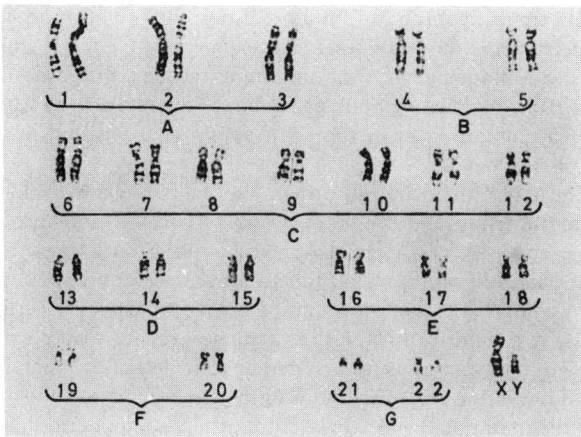

Figure 1-3 The karyotype of a normal male showing the chromosomes of a single somatic cell in the metaphase stage of cell division. The photographic images of the chromosomes have been cut out and arranged according to descending length and varying arm ratio. The chromosomes have been stained by the Giemsa technique, which allows each chromosome pair to be identified by its unique banding pattern. Chromosomes 1 to 22 are the autosomes. The sex chromosomes in this normal male are an X and a Y. The normal female has an identical karyotype except for the absence of the Y chromosome and the presence instead of a second X chromosome. *(Courtesy of K. Hirshhorn.)*

chromosomes *(aneuploidy);* (2) breakage and loss of a piece of a chromosome *(deletion);* (3) breakage of two chromosomes, with transfer and fusion of parts of the broken fragments onto each other *(translocation);* and (4) abnormal splitting of the centromere during mitosis so that one arm is lost and the other is duplicated to form one symmetrical chromosome with two genetically identical arms *(isochromosome formation).* In addition, chromosomal *mosaicism* may occur such that a single individual may possess two cell lines, or *clones,* each differing in its chromosomal constitution. For example, many patients with the Turner syndrome have been shown to possess some cells with a 45,XO constitution and other cells with a normal 46,XX. Their karyotype is symbolized 45,XO/46,XX.

The *autosomal* trisomies responsible for specific clinical syndromes include: (1) trisomy 21 (Down syndrome or mongolism), characterized by mental retardation, a characteristic facies, marked hypotonia, and many other abnormalities; (2) trisomy 13, characterized by ocular coloboma, cleft lip and palate, polydactyly, and an average life span of less than 1 year; and (3) trisomy 18, characterized by micrognathia, severe failure to thrive, multiple malformations, and a life span of less than 3 months.

The numerical aberrations of the sex chromosomes include three disorders with 47 chromosomes (47,XXY; 47,XYY; and 47,XXX) and one disorder with 45 chromosomes (45,XO). The XXY karyotype is found in patients with the Klinefelter syndrome, who are phenotypic males with testicular dysgenesis, infertility, gynecomastia, tall stature, and behavioral changes. Most individuals with a 47,XYY karyotype are normal fertile males; however, some may be unusually tall and show tendencies to criminality or other behavioral abnormalities. Most individuals with the 47,XXX karyotype are clinically normal females, but some may be mentally retarded and deficient in secondary sexual development. The 45,XO karyotype is found in about one-half of patients with the Turner syndrome, who are phenotypic females with ovarian dysgenesis, failure of secondary sexual development, short stature, renal anomalies, and pterygium colli. Patients with the Turner

syndrome who do not have a 45,XO karyotype may have either mosaicism (45,XO/46,XX or 45,XO/46,XY) or a structural abnormality of the X chromosome, such as an isochromosome X.

Little is known about the factors that cause chromosomal disorders in humans. The most important finding is the association between increasing maternal age and nondisjunction syndromes such as the Down syndrome (trisomy 21) and the Klinefelter syndrome (47,XXY). A possible etiologic role for other factors, such as genetic predisposition, autoimmune disorders (involving the thyroid gland, in particular), viruses, chemical mutagens, and radiation, has also been suggested [33].

The detected frequency of chromosomal aberrations in karyotypes of unselected newborn infants is 1 in 200 (0.5 percent), while among first-trimester spontaneous abortions the frequency of chromosomal defects is as high as 50 percent. Thus, the vast majority of fetuses with chromosomal abnormalities are lost in early fetal life. A high frequency of chromosomal aberrations has, however, been observed in patients with several clinical abnormalities, including (1) multiple congenital malformations (5 to 20 percent); (2) infertility and sterility (1 to 10 percent); (3) mental retardation (1 to 3 percent); and (4) certain forms of malignancy, such as chronic myelogenous leukemia, in which the long arm of chromosome 22 is translocated to one of the larger chromosomes, most often to the long arm of chromosome 9, producing the so-called *Philadelphia* chromosome.

In most instances, chromosomal disorders occur as new mutations. Both parents are usually normal, and the risk of recurrence in sibs is low. In those cases in which one parent is the carrier of a chromosomal rearrangement, such as in the translocation form of Down syndrome, the recurrence risk to subsequent children may be as high as 20 percent. Table 1-3 lists the most frequently encountered chromosomal abnormalities occurring among live-born infants.

A complete chromosome analysis is clinically indicated in the following situations: (1) in children with multiple congenital anomalies, with mental defects of unknown cause, or with failure to grow for unknown reasons; (2) in all children with suspected Down syndrome and in their parents if a balanced translocation is shown to exist; (3) in couples in whom the wife aborts repeatedly; (4) in families producing many congenitally abnormal children; (5) in women with primary amenorrhea; (6) in individuals with ambiguous external genitalia; and (7) in patients with hematologic malignancies, such as chronic myelogenous leukemia.

Table 1-3 Prevalence of chromosomal disorders among live-born infants

Disorder	Prevalence
Autosomal abnormalities	
Trisomy 21 (Down syndrome)	1 in 600
Trisomy 18	1 in 5000
Trisomy 13	1 in 15,000
Sex chromosome abnormalities	
Klinefelter syndrome (47,XXY)	1 in 450 males
XYY syndrome (47,XYY)	1 in 1000 males
Triple-X syndrome (47,XXX)	1 in 1000 females
Turner syndrome (45,XO, 46,XO/XX, 46,XO/XY, isochromosome X)	1 in 1500 females

SOURCE: Data modified from Vogel and Motulsky [33] and Galjaard [35].

For a more complete discussion of the etiology and clinical features of chromosomal abnormalities affecting humans, the reader is referred to Chap. 3 in the last edition of this book [34], as well as to Chap. 2 in *Human Genetics: Problems and Approaches* by Vogel and Motulsky [33].

Monogenic Disorders

Disorders caused by single mutant genes show one of three simple (or Mendelian) patterns of inheritance: (1) autosomal dominant, (2) autosomal recessive, or (3) X-linked. The distinction between "dominant" and "recessive" is one of convenience in pedigree analysis and does not imply a fundamental difference in genetic mechanism. The term *dominant* implies that a mutation will be clinically manifest when an individual has a single dose of this mutation (or is *heterozygous* for it), while *recessive* implies that a double dose (or *homozygosity*) is required for clinical detection. Genes are never dominant or recessive; their effects, however, produce clinical patterns that are classified as dominant or recessive. Despite their overall clinical "normality," individuals who are heterozygous for recessive genes often have biochemical abnormalities that are demonstrable in the laboratory. On the other hand, those who are homozygous for dominant genes are usually more severely affected than are the heterozygotes.

With few exceptions, each of the approximately 1400 Mendelian diseases is rare. As a group, these disorders constitute an important cause of morbidity and death, accounting directly for more than 5 percent of all pediatric hospital admissions [35]. The overall population frequency of monogenic disorders is about 10 per 1000 live births, comprising about 7 in 1000 dominants, about 2.5 in 1000 recessives, and about 0.4 in 1000 X-linked conditions [36]. Table 1-4 lists some of the most common Mendelian disorders.

If a particular disease shows one of the three Mendelian patterns of inheritance, its pathogenesis, no matter how complex, must be due to an abnormality in a single protein molecule. For example, in sickle-cell anemia, the entire clinical syndrome, including such seemingly unrelated disturbances as anemia,

Table 1-4 Prevalence of some common monogenic disorders among live-born infants

Disorder	Estimated prevalence
Autosomal dominant	
Familial hypercholesterolemia	1 in 500
Polycystic kidney disease	1 in 1250
Huntington's chorea	1 in 2500
Hereditary spherocytosis	1 in 5000
Marfan syndrome	1 in 20,000
Autosomal recessive	
Sickle-cell anemia	1 in 625 (U.S. blacks)
Cystic fibrosis	1 in 2000 (U.S. whites)
Tay-Sachs disease	1 in 3000 (U.S. Jews)
Phenylketonuria	1 in 12,000
Mucopolysaccharidoses (all types together)	1 in 25,000
Glycogen storage diseases (all types together)	1 in 50,000
X-linked	
Duchenne muscular dystrophy	1 in 7000
Hemophilia	1 in 10,000

SOURCE: Data modified from Galjaard [35], Carter [36], and Motulsky [133].

pain crises, nephropathy, and predisposition to pneumococcal infections, is the physiologic consequence of having thymine instead of adenine at a specific site in the gene that codes for the β chain of hemoglobin, producing a substitution of a valine for a glutamic acid in the sixth amino acid position in the protein sequence.

In many Mendelian disorders, especially those with dominant inheritance, it is not yet possible to demonstrate directly the protein that is altered by the mutation. In such cases (e.g., the Marfan syndrome and tuberous sclerosis), only the distal physiologic effects of the mutation are recognizable. Nevertheless, it is safe to assume that a single primary defect exists whenever a disease is transmitted by a single gene mechanism, and the various manifestations of the disease can all be related to the mutational event by a more or less complicated "pedigree of causes."

The basic biochemical lesions in monogenic disorders involve defects in a wide variety of proteins, including enzymes, receptors, transport proteins, peptide hormones, immunoglobulins, collagens, and coagulation factors. Of the approximately 250 human diseases whose biochemical basis has been defined, about 170 involve abnormalities in enzymes (Table 1-5).

Autosomal Dominant Disorders   Dominant diseases are manifest in the heterozygous state, i.e., when only one abnormal gene (*mutant allele*) is present and the corresponding partner allele on the homologous chromosome is normal. By definition, the gene responsible for an autosomal dominant disorder must be located on one of the 22 autosomes; hence, both males and females can be affected. Since alleles segregate independently at meiosis, there is a 1 in 2 chance that the offspring of an affected heterozygote will inherit the mutant allele.

Figure 1-4 shows a typical pedigree involving an autosomal dominant trait. The following features are characteristic: (1) each affected individual has an affected parent (unless the condition arose by a new mutation in the sperm or ovum that formed the individual or is mildly expressed in the affected parent); (2) an affected individual will bear, on the average, both normal and affected offspring in equal proportions; (3) normal children of an affected individual will have only normal offspring; (4) males and females are affected in equal proportions; (5) each sex is equally likely to transmit the condition to male and female offspring, with male-to-male transmission occurring; and (6) vertical transmission of the condition through successive generations occurs, especially when the trait does not impair the reproductive capacity.

NEW MUTATIONS   While half of the offspring of an individual with an autosomal dominant condition will inherit the disease, it is not necessarily true that each affected person must have an affected parent. In every autosomal dominant disease, a certain proportion of affected persons owe their disorder to a new mutation rather than to an inherited one. Since a rough estimate of the frequency of mutation is 5×10^{-6} mutations per gene per generation and since a dominant trait, by definition, requires a mutation in only one of a pair of alleles, one would expect that about 1 in 100,000 newborn persons would possess a new mutation at any given genetic locus. Many of these mutations either will not impair the function of the gene product or will involve a recessive function, so that the mutation will be clinically silent. Others, however, will cause a

Table 1-5 Disorders in which a deficient activity of a specific enzyme has been demonstrated in human beings

Condition	Enzyme with deficient activity	Condition	Enzyme with deficient activity
Acatalasia	Catalase	Glycogen storage disease IV	Amylo-(1, 4 to 1,6)-transglucosidase
Acetyl CoA carboxylase deficiency	Acetyl CoA carboxylase	Glycogen storage disease V	Muscle phosphorylase
Acid phosphatase deficiency	Acid phosphatase	Glycogen storage disease VI	Liver phosphorylase
Adrenal hyperplasia I	20,21-Desmolase	Glycogen storage disease VII	Muscle phosphofructokinase
Adrenal hyperplasia II	3-β-Hydroxysteroid dehydrogenase	Glycogen storage disease VIII	Liver phosphorylase kinase
Adrenal hyperplasia III	21-Hydroxylase	Gout, primary	Hypoxanthine-guanine phosphoribosyl transferase
Adrenal hyperplasia IV	11-β-Hydroxylase	Gout, primary	PP-ribose-P synthetase (increased)
Adrenal hyperplasia V	17-Hydroxylase		
Albinism	Tyrosinase	Granulomatous disease	NADPH oxidase
Aldosterone deficiency I	18-OH-Dehydrogenase	Hemolytic anemia	Adenosine triphosphatase
Alcaptonuria	Homogentisic acid oxidase	Hemolytic anemia	Adenylate kinase
Apnea, drug-induced	Pseudocholinesterase	Hemolytic anemia	Aldolase A
Argininemia	Arginase	Hemolytic anemia	Diphosphoglycerate mutase
Argininosuccinic aciduria	Argininosuccinase	Hemolytic anemia	γ-Glutamylcysteine synthetase
Aspartylglycosaminuria	Special hydrolase (AADG-ase)	Hemolytic anemia	Glucose-6-phosphate dehydrogenase
Ataxia, intermittent	Pyruvate decarboxylase		
Carnosinemia	Carnosinase	Hemolytic anemia	Glutathione peroxidase
Cholesteryl ester deficiency (Norum-Gjone disease)	Lecithin cholesterol acetyltransferase (LCAT)	Hemolytic anemia	Glutathione reductase
		Hemolytic anemia	Glutathione synthetase
Citrullinemia	Argininosuccinic acid synthetase	Hemolytic anemia	Hexokinase
Crigler-Najjar syndrome	Glucuronyl transferase	Hemolytic anemia	Hexosephosphate isomerase
Cystathioninuria	Cystathionase	Hemolytic anemia	6-Phosphogluconate dehydrogenase
2,8-Dihydroxyadenine nephrolithiasis	Adenine phosphoribosyl transferase		
		Hemolytic anemia	Phosphoglycerate kinase
Disaccharide intolerance I	Invertase	Hemolytic anemia	Pyrimidine 5′-nucleotidase
Disaccharide intolerance II	Invertase, maltase	Hemolytic anemia	Pyruvate kinase
Disaccharide intolerance III	Lactase	Hemolytic anemia	Triosephosphate isomerase
Ehlers-Danlos syndrome, type V	Lysyloxidase	Histidinemia	Histidase
Ehlers-Danlos syndrome, type VI	Collagen lysyl hydroxylase	Homocystinuria I	Cystathionine synthetase
		Homocystinuria II	N(5,10)-methylenetetra hydrofolate reductase
Ehlers-Danlos syndrome, type VII	Procollagen peptidase		
		2-Hydroxyglutaric aciduria	D-2-hydroxy-glutarate dehydrogenase
Fabry's disease	α-Galactosidase A		
Fanconi's panmyelopathy	Exonuclease	β-Hydroxyisovaleric aciduria and methylcrotonyl glycinuria	β-Methylcrotonyl CoA carboxylase
Farber's lipogranulomatosis	Ceramidase		
Formiminotransferase deficiency	Formiminotransferase	Hydroxyprolinemia	Hydroxyproline oxidase
Fructose intolerance	Fructose-1-phosphate aldolase	Hyper-β-alaninemia	β-Alanine-α-ketoglutarate aminotransferase
Fructosuria	Hepatic fructokinase		
Fucosidosis	α-L-Fucosidase	Hyperammonemia I	Carbamyl phosphate synthetase
Galactokinase deficiency	Galactokinase	Hyperammonemia II	Ornithine transcarbamylase
Galactose epimerase deficiency	Galactose epimerase	Hyperglycinemia, nonketotic form	Glycine formiminotransferase
Galactosemia	Galactose-1-phosphate uridyl transferase		
		Hyperlysinemia	Lysine-ketoglutarate reductase
Gangliosidosis, G_{M1}, type I or infantile	β-Galactosidase A, B	Hyperprolinemia I	Proline oxidase
		Hyperprolinemia II	δ-1-Pyrroline-5-carboxylate dehydrogenase
Gangliosidosis, G_{M1}, type II or juvenile	β-Galactosidase A, B		
		Hypoglycemia and acidosis	Fructose-1, 6-diphosphatase
Gangliosidosis, G_{M2}, (Tay-Sachs disease)	Hexosaminidase A	Hypophosphatasia	Alkaline phosphatase
		Ichthyosis, X-linked	Steroid sulfatase
Gangliosidosis, G_{M2}, juvenile	Hexosaminidase A	Immunodeficiency disease	Adenosine deaminase
Gangliosidosis, G_{M2}, adult	Hexosaminidase A	Immunodeficiency disease	Purine nucleoside phosphorylase
Gangliosidosis, G_{M2}, (Sandhoff's disease)	Hexosaminidase A, B	Intestinal lactase deficiency (adult)	Lactase
Gangliosidosis, G_{M3}	UDP-N-acetyl-galactosaminyl transferase	Isovaleric acidemia	Isovaleric acid CoA dehydrogenase
Gaucher's disease	Glucocerebrosidase	Ketoacidosis, infantile	Succinyl CoA:3-ketoacid CoA-transferase
G6PD deficiency (favism, primaquine sensitivity, etc.)	Glucose-6-phosphate dehydrogenase	β-Ketothiolase deficiency	α-Methylacetoacetyl CoA-β-ketothiolase
Glutathionemia	γ-Glutamyltransferase		
Glycogen storage disease I	Glucose-6-phosphatase	Krabbe's disease	Galactocerebroside β-galactosidase
Glycogen storage disease II	α-1,4-Glucosidase		
Glycogen storage disease III	Amylo-1, 6-glucosidase	Lactase deficiency	Lactase

Table 1-5 (Continued)

Condition	Enzyme with deficient activity	Condition	Enzyme with deficient activity
Lactosyl ceramidosis	Lactosyl ceramidase	Orotic aciduria II	Orotidylic decarboxylase
Leigh's necrotizing encephalomyelopathy	Pyruvate carboxylase	Oxalosis I (glycolic aciduria)	2-Oxo-glutarate-glyoxylate carboligase
Lesch-Nyhan syndrome	Hypoxanthine-guanine phosphoribosyl transferase	Oxalosis II (glyceric aciduria)	D-Glyceric dehydrogenase
		Pentosuria	L-Xylulose reductase
Lipase deficiency, congenital	Lipase (pancreatic)	Phenylketonuria	Phenylalanine hydroxylase
Lipoprotein lipase deficiency (type I hyperlipoproteinemia)	Lipoprotein lipase	Phenylketonuria	Dihydropteridine reductase
Lysine intolerance	L-Lysine:NAD-oxidoreductase	Porphyria, acute intermittent	Porphobilinogen deaminase
Male pseudohermaphroditism	Testicular 17,20-desmolase	Porphyria, congenital erythropoietic	Uroporphyrinogen III cosynthetase
Male pseudohermaphroditism	Testicular 17-ketosteroid dehydrogenese	Porphyria cutanea tarda	Uroporphyrinogen decarboxylase
Male pseudohermaphroditism	5α-Reductase	Porphyria, hereditary copro	Coproporphyrinogen oxidase
Mannosidosis	α-Mannosidase	Porphyria, proto-	Ferrochelatase
Maple sugar urine disease	Keto acid decarboxylase	Propionic acidemia	Propionyl CoA carboxylase
Maple syrup urine disease	Dihydrolipoyl dehydrogenese	Pulmonary emphysema, or cirrhosis	α-1-Antitrypsin
Metachromatic leukodystrophy I	Arylsulfatase A (sulfatide sulfatase)	Pyridoxine-dependent infantile convulsions	Glutamic acid decarboxylase
Metachromatic leukodystrophy II	Arylsulfatase A, B, C and steroid sulfatase	Pyridoxine-responsive anemia	δ-Aminolevulinic acid synthetase
Methemoglobinemia	NAD-methemoglobin reductase	Pyroglutamic aciduria	Glutathione synthetase
Methylmalonic aciduria I (vitamin B$_{12}$-unresponsive)	Methylmalonic CoA mutase	Pyruvate carboxylase deficiency	Pyruvate carboxylase
Methylmalonic aciduria II (vitamin B$_{12}$-responsive)	5' Deoxyadenosyl transferase	Pyruvate decarboxylase deficiency	Pyruvate decarboxylase
Methylmalonic aciduria III	Methylmalonyl-CoA racemase	Refsum's disease	Phytanic acid α-oxidase
Mucopolysaccharidosis IH (Hurler)	α-L-Iduronidase	Renal tubular acidosis with deafness	Carbonic anhydrase B
Mucopolysaccharidosis IS (Scheie)	α-L-Iduronidase	Richner-Hanhart syndrome	Tyrosine aminotransferase
Mucopolysaccharidosis II (Hunter)	Sulfo-iduronidase sulfatase	Rickets, vitamin D-dependent	25-Hydroxycholecalciferol 1-hydroxylase
Mucopolysaccharidosis IIIA (Sanfilippo)	Heparan sulfate sulfatase	Sarcosinemia	Sarcosine dehydrogenase
Mucopolysaccharidosis IIIB (Sanfilippo)	N-acetyl-α-D-glucosaminidase	Sucrase-isomaltase deficiency	Sucrase, isomaltase
		Sulfite oxidase deficiency	Sulfite oxidase
Mucopolysaccharidosis IV (Morquio)	6-Sulfatase	Thyroid hormonogenesis, defect in, II	Iodide peroxidase
Mucopolysaccharidosis VI (Maroteaux-Lamy)	Arylsulfatase B	Thyroid hormonogenesis, defect in, IV	Iodotyrosine dehalogenase (deiodinase)
Mucopolysaccharidosis VII	β-Glucuronidase	Trypsinogen deficiency	Trypsinogen
Myeloperoxidase deficiency with disseminated candidiasis	Myeloperoxidase	Tyrosinemia I	Para-hydroxyphenylpyruvate oxidase
Myopathy	Myoadenylate deaminase	Tyrosinemia II	Tyrosine transaminase
Niemann-Pick disease	Sphingomyelinase	Valinemia	Valine transaminase
Ornithinemia	Ornithine ketoacid aminotransferase	Wolman's disease	Acid lipase
		Xanthinuria	Xanthine oxidase
		Xanthurenic aciduria	Kynureninase
Orotic aciduria I	Orotidylic pyrophosphorylase and orotidylic decarboxylase	Xeroderma pigmentosum	DNA-specific endonuclease
		Xyloxidase deficiency	Xylosidase

defective gene product that gives rise to a dominant trait. The parent in whose germ cells the mutation arose will be clinically normal. Likewise, the sibs of the affected individual will be normal since the mutation will affect only a single germ cell. The affected individual will be able to transmit the disease, and half of his or her children will be affected.

The proportion of patients with dominant disorders that represent new mutations is inversely proportional to the effect of the disease on biologic fitness. The term *biologic fitness* refers to the ability of an affected individual to produce children who survive to adult life and reproduce. In the extreme case, if a dominant mutation produced absolute infertility,

then all observed cases would, of necessity, represent new mutations, and it would be impossible to prove the genetic transmission of the trait. In less severe disorders, as in tuberous sclerosis, the severe mental retardation reduces biologic fitness to about 20 percent of normal, and the proportion of cases due to new mutations is about 80 percent [37]. In dominant disorders such as familial hypercholesterolemia, in which there is no reduction in biologic fitness, virtually all affected persons have a family pedigree showing classic vertical transmission (Chap. 33).

Many new mutations appear to occur in the germ cells of fathers who are of relatively advanced age [38]. Such a "pater-

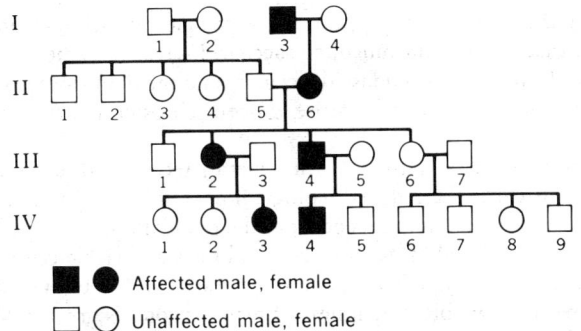

Affected male, female

Unaffected male, female

Figure 1-4 Pedigree pattern of an autosomal dominant trait. Note the *vertical* pattern of inheritance.

nal age effect" is seen, for example, in the Marfan syndrome, in which the average age of fathers of sporadic or "new mutation" cases (37 years) is in excess of the mean age of fathers generally (30 years) and also in excess of the age of fathers who transmit the Marfan disease due to an inherited mutation (30 years) [39].

Before one concludes that a dominant disorder in a given patient with unaffected parents is the result of a new mutation, it is important to consider two other possibilities: (1) the gene may be carried by one parent, in whom the disease is of low expressivity (discussed below), and (2) extramarital paternity may have occurred, since this is found in about 3 to 5 percent of randomly studied children in the United States.

CHARACTERISTICS OF DOMINANT TRAITS   Most autosomal dominant disorders show two characteristic features that are not usually seen in recessive syndromes: (1) *delayed age of onset* and (2) *variability in clinical expression*. Delayed age of onset is seen in disorders such as Huntington's chorea and adult polycystic kidney disease. These disorders do not become manifest clinically until adult life, even though the mutant gene is present from the time of conception. Variability in clinical expression is illustrated dramatically by the multiple endocrine adenoma-peptic ulcer syndrome [40]. Patients in the same family inheriting the same abnormal gene may have hyperplasia or neoplasia of one or all of a wide variety of endocrine tissues, such as the pancreas, parathyroid glands, pituitary gland, or adipose tissue. The resulting clinical manifestations are extremely diverse; different members of the same family may develop peptic ulcers, hypoglycemia, kidney stones, multiple lipomas of the skin, or bitemporal hemianopsia. Because of this variability, the recognition that each family member suffers from the same genetic abnormality can be difficult.

BIOCHEMICAL BASIS OF DOMINANT TRAITS   Since dominant mutations involve a type of gene product that in a 50 percent deficiency is capable of producing clinical symptoms in heterozygotes, the responsible mutations are likely to involve abnormalities in two classes of proteins (41): (1) those that regulate complex metabolic pathways, such as membrane receptors and rate-limiting enzymes in biosynthetic pathways under feedback control, and (2) key nonenzymic or structural proteins, such as hemoglobin or collagen. As discussed below, genetic defects in most enzymes do not cause symptoms in heterozygotes and hence do not produce dominant diseases.

Because they do not result from simple, easily measured enzyme deficiencies, the basic biochemical defects have been identified in only a handful of the approximately 600 autosomal dominant disorders. These include familial hypercholesterolemia (abnormal cell surface receptor that binds plasma low density lipoprotein and thereby regulates cholesterol metabolism); some types of hereditary methemoglobinemia and several hemolytic anemias due to unstable forms of hemoglobin (abnormal hemoglobin molecule); hereditary angioneurotic edema (abnormal protein inhibitor of an enzyme involved in the serum complement system); and acute intermittent porphyria (abnormal enzyme that catalyzes a rate-limiting step in the heme biosynthetic pathway).

Autosomal Recessive Disorders   Autosomal recessive conditions are those that are clinically apparent only in the homozygous state, i.e., when both alleles at a particular genetic locus are mutant alleles. By definition, the gene responsible for an autosomal recessive disorder must be located on one of the 22 autosomes; thus, both males and females can be affected.

Figure 1-5 shows a pedigree of a family with an autosomal recessive trait. The following features are characteristic: (1) the parents are clinically normal; (2) only sibs are affected, and vertical transmission does not occur; and (3) males and females are affected in equal proportions.

CHARACTERISTICS OF AUTOSOMAL RECESSIVE TRAITS   The relative infrequency of recessive genes in the population and the requirement for two abnormal genes for clinical expression combine to create special conditions for autosomal recessive inheritance: (1) the more infrequent the mutant gene in the population, the stronger the likelihood that affected individuals are the product of consanguine matings (see below); (2) if a husband and wife are both carriers for the same autosomal recessive gene, 25 percent of the children will be normal, 50 percent will be heterozygous carriers, and 25 percent will be homozygous and affected with the disease; (3) if an affected individual marries a heterozygote (as may occur with a common mutant gene or a consanguine marriage), half the children will be affected, and a pedigree simulating dominant inheritance will result; and (4) if two individuals with the same recessive disease marry, all their children will be affected.

The clinical picture in autosomal recessive disorders tends to be more uniform than that of dominant diseases, and onset often occurs early in life. As a general rule, recessive disorders are more commonly diagnosed in children, while dominant diseases are more frequently encountered in adults.

In recessive inheritance only one of four children in a sibship is expected to be affected; hence, multiple cases in a family may not occur. This is especially true in a society in which small families are common. Consider, for example, 16 families in which both parents are heterozygous for the same recessive disorder, such as cystic fibrosis. If each family has 2 children, 9

Figure 1-5 Pedigree pattern of an autosomal recessive trait. Note the *horizontal* pattern of inheritance.

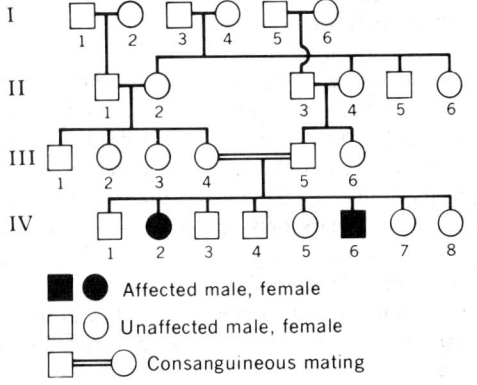

Affected male, female

Unaffected male, female

Consanguineous mating

of the 16 families will have no affected children, 6 will have 1 affected and 1 normal child, and only 1 of the 16 families will have 2 affected children. Because of the tendency toward small families in the United States, physicians usually see sporadic or isolated cases of a recessive disease without an affected sib to alert them to the possibility of a genetic disorder. Fortunately, because of the relatively uniform clinical picture of recessive disorders and because many can be diagnosed directly by biochemical tests, the diagnosis of a genetic disease can usually be made even when no other members of a family are clinically affected.

BIOCHEMICAL DEFECTS   Basic biochemical lesions underlying many autosomal recessive disorders have been identified. Mutations that give rise to recessive diseases usually involve enzymatic proteins, as opposed to nonenzymatic proteins. In these conditions, recessive inheritance occurs because a mutation that destroys the catalytic activity of an enzyme generally does not impair the health of a heterozygote (i.e., an individual who has one mutant allele specifying a functionless enzyme and one normal allele on the partner chromosome specifying a normal enzyme). In this situation, each cell in the body usually produces about 50 percent of the normal number of active enzyme molecules. However, normal regulatory mechanisms function to avert any clinical consequences of this 50 percent deficiency, and so heterozygotes for enzyme defects usually are clinically normal [41]. Frequently such compensation involves nothing more complicated than a simple two- to threefold increase in the substrate concentration for the enzyme. The concentration of a substrate is usually maintained at a point below saturation for the enzyme that metabolizes it. When the enzyme level is reduced 50 percent, as in a heterozygote for a functionless gene at that locus, the residual 50 percent of enzyme molecules can be made to function twice as fast as normal, simply by allowing the substrate concentration to increase twofold. If the twofold increase in substrate does not otherwise affect metabolism adversely, the heterozygote is clinically normal. On the other hand, when an individual inherits functionless alleles at both loci specifying an enzyme, the reduction in enzyme activity is too great for a compensatory mechanism to overcome the deficiency, and a disease results.

Phenylketonuria (PKU) is a well-documented example of heterozygote compensation. Heterozygotes for phenylalanine hydroxylase deficiency are clinically asymptomatic because the body compensates for the half-normal level of the enzyme by raising the phenylalanine concentration approximately twofold. Under these conditions, a normal amount of phenylalanine can be metabolized with no symptoms. On the other hand, the homozygote for PKU has such a severe reduction in phenylalanine hydroxylase activity that enormous levels of phenylalanine accumulate, with marked spillover into secondary metabolic pathways causing detrimental brain development.

The genetic enzyme deficiencies that produce recessive diseases tend to involve enzymes that participate in catabolic pathways. Frequently these enzymes degrade organic molecules that are ingested in the diet, such as galactose (galactosemia), phenylalanine (PKU), and phytanic acid (Refsum syndrome). A special class of such catabolic diseases is one in which the deficiency affects an acid hydrolase that occurs within lysosomes. In these *lysosomal storage disorders* [42, 43], the substrate, usually a complex lipid or polysaccharide, accumulates within swollen lysosomes in specific organs, giving the cells a foamy appearance. Examples of such lysosomal diseases include the mucopolysaccharidoses such as the Hurler syndrome (α-iduronidase deficiency) and the lipid storage diseases such as Gaucher disease (glucocerebrosidase deficiency).

POPULATION GENETICS   In general, recessive diseases are rare because the reduced biologic fitness of homozygotes acts to remove the mutant gene from the population. A few lethal recessive disorders, such as cystic fibrosis and sickle-cell anemia, are common. To explain this paradox, it has been postulated that the biologic fitness of heterozygotes is greater than that of noncarriers for these genes. In such a case, the frequency of the gene in the population depends on the balance between the increased fitness of the relatively numerous heterozygotes and the reduced fitness of the less common homozygotes. A small selective advantage of the heterozygote over the normal person results in a high gene frequency and hence a high birth frequency of homozygotes even when the disease is lethal [44]. Thus, about 1 in 22 Caucasians is a heterozygous carrier for the genetically lethal disease cystic fibrosis, and the disease occurs in about 1 in 2000 Caucasian births. In order to maintain such a high gene frequency, heterozygotes for cystic fibrosis must have a definite reproductive advantage over noncarriers, but the nature of this advantage is unknown. In sickle-cell anemia, another recessive disorder with high frequency among certain populations, heterozygotes are known to have increased resistance to malaria [44].

CONSANGUINITY   By definition, a recessive disease requires the inheritance of a mutation at the same genetic locus from each parent. When the genes are rare, the likelihood of any two parents being carriers for the same defect is small. If the parents have a common ancestor who carried a recessive gene, then the likelihood that two of the descendants would each have inherited the gene becomes relatively great. The less frequent the recessive gene, the stronger becomes the likelihood that an affected individual must have resulted from such a consanguine mating. On the other hand, certain recessive genes are so common in the population that the likelihood of two random parents being carriers is great enough to eliminate the need for consanguinity. For common traits such as sickle-cell anemia, PKU, cystic fibrosis, and Tay-Sachs disease, all of which have a high carrier frequency in certain populations, consanguinity is usually not present in the parents.

In general, consanguinity is an infrequent finding clinically in parents of patients with recessive diseases in the United States. This is because the prevalence of consanguinity in the population is very low. In most areas of the United States (as opposed to areas with relative geographic isolation, such as northern Norway and certain valleys in Switzerland), a disorder must indeed be rare before it is associated with an important frequency of consanguinity. For example, consanguinity is expected in a large proportion of families having children with very rare disorders, such as abetalipoproteinemia.

X-linked Disorders   The genes responsible for X-linked disorders are located on the X chromosome; therefore, the clinical risk and severity of the disease are different for the two sexes. Since a female has two X chromosomes, she may be either heterozygous or homozygous for a mutant gene, and the trait may demonstrate either recessive or dominant expression. Males, on the other hand, have only one X chromosome, so they can be expected to display the full syndrome

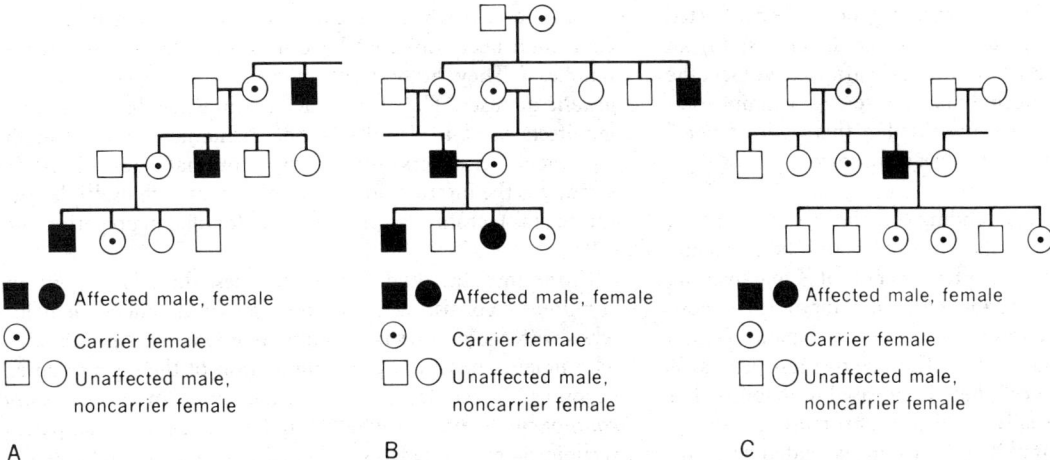

Figure 1-6 Pedigree patterns of an X-linked recessive trait. *A.* Note the oblique pattern of inheritance. *B.* An affected female can result from the mating of an affected male and a carrier female, as in the consanguine marriage shown here. *C.* An affected male mating with a normal noncarrier female has all normal sons and all carrier daughters.

whenever they inherit the gene regardless of whether the gene produces a recessive or dominant trait in the female. Thus, the terms *X-linked dominant* and *X-linked recessive* refer only to the expression of the gene in women.

An important feature of all X-linked inheritance is the absence of male-to-male (i.e., father-to-son) transmission of the trait. This follows because a male must always contribute his Y chromosome to his sons; hence, he can never contribute his X chromosome. On the other hand, a male contributes his sole X chromosome to all his daughters, and so all daughters of a male with an X-linked trait must inherit the mutant gene.

X-LINKED RECESSIVE TRAITS   The pedigree in Fig. 1-6 illustrates the characteristic features of X-linked recessive inheritance. (1) In contrast to the vertical distribution in dominant traits (parents and children affected) and the horizontal distribution in autosomal recessive traits (sibs affected), the pedigree pattern in X-linked recessive traits tends to be oblique; that is, the trait occurs in the maternal uncles of affected males and in male cousins who are descended from the mother's sisters who are carriers (Fig. 1-6A); (2) male offspring of carrier females have a 50 percent chance of being affected; (3) all female offspring of affected males are carriers, and affected males do not transmit the disease to their sons (Fig. 1-6C); (4) unaffected males do not transmit the trait to any offspring; and (5) affected homozygous females occur only when an affected male fathers the child of a carrier female (Fig. 1-6B).

Examples of X-linked recessive disorders in humans incude hemophilia A, nephrogenic diabetes insipidus, the Lesch-Nyhan syndrome, Duchenne muscular dystrophy, glucose-6-phosphate dehydrogenase deficiency, testicular feminization, and Fabry disease. Color blindness is also inherited as an X-linked recessive trait, but it is sufficiently frequent (occurring in about 8 percent of Caucasian males) that the occurrence of homozygous color-blind females is no rarity.

X-LINKED DOMINANT TRAITS   X-linked dominant inheritance is illustrated by the pedigree in Fig. 1-7. Its characteristic features are as follows: (1) females are affected about twice as often as males; (2) an affected female transmits the disorder to half of her sons and half of her daughters; (3) an affected male

transmits the disorder to all of his daughters and to none of his sons; and (4) the syndrome is more variable and less severe in heterozygous affected females than in hemizygous affected males. One common trait, the Xg(a+) blood group, is inherited as an X-linked dominant trait, as are a few diseases, such as vitamin D–resistant rickets (hypophosphatemic rickets).

Some rare conditions may be inherited as X-linked dominant traits in which there is lethality in the hemizygous male. The characteristics of this form of inheritance are illustrated by the pedigree in Fig. 1-8. (1) The disorder occurs only in females

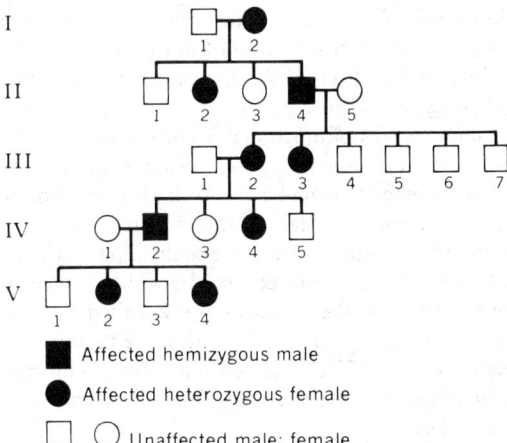

Figure 1-7 Pedigree pattern of an X-linked dominant trait.

Figure 1-8 Pedigree pattern of an X-linked dominant trait lethal in the hemizygous male.

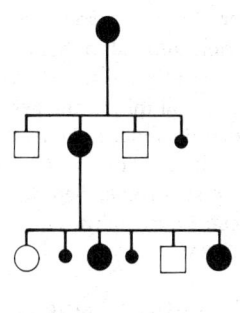

who are heterozygous for the mutant gene; (2) an affected mother transmits the trait to half of her daughters; (3) an increased frequency of abortions occurs in affected women, the abortions representing affected male fetuses. An example of a condition that appears to be transmitted by this mode of inheritance is ornithine transcarbamylase deficiency.

X INACTIVATION   Understanding of the mechanisms of expression of X-linked traits in females has been greatly advanced by knowledge of the phenomenon of X inactivation, or the so-called Lyon effect [45]. Early in embryonic development, one of the two X chromosomes in each somatic cell of a female is irreversibly inactivated. The inactivation process is random, so that for each cell there is an equal probability that the paternally or maternally derived X chromosome will be inactivated. The inactivated X chromosome is rendered permanently nonfunctional, so that all progeny of the initial cell inherit the same active and inactive X chromosomes. Thus, each female is a mosaic; on the average, half of her cells express the X chromosome of the father, and half express the X chromosome of the mother. If a mutation in a gene is carried on one of her X chromosomes, about one-half of the cells in each tissue will be normal and the other half will manifest the mutant phenotype. Chance or selection of one clone of cells may disturb these proportions in any given individual. Depending on the proportions of mutant and normal X chromosomes that are active in each tissue, a genetically heterozygous female may be clinically normal or she may have mild or severe manifestations of the disease. To illustrate, some mothers of boys with the X-linked recessive Duchenne form of muscular dystrophy may show mild manifestations of the disease, such as limb girdle weakness or hypertrophied calves.

In each female cell the nonfunctional X chromosome can be identified by several techniques. By ordinary staining, the inactivated X chromosome in metaphase appears heteropyknotic (condensed), and it replicates late in the mitotic cycle ("late labeling" with tritiated thymidine). In nondividing cells, the inactivated X chromosome can be observed as a clump of chromatin at the periphery of the nucleus—the so-called X chromatin or Barr body. In abnormal cells with more than two X chromosomes, such as 47,XXX, all but one of the X chromosomes are inactivated, so these cells may have multiple X-chromatin bodies.

FEMALE CARRIERS   In families in which only a single male is affected with an X-linked recessive disease, proper genetic counseling requires that the mother undergo tests, if available, to determine whether she is a carrier. If she is, half of her daughters will be carriers and half of her sons will be affected. On the other hand, if her affected son represents a new mutation, only his daughters will inherit the gene. At present, biochemical tests can identify female carriers for several severe X-linked diseases, including the Lesch-Nyhan syndrome, Fabry disease, Hunter syndrome, hemophilia, and the Duchenne form of muscular dystrophy.

Multifactorial Genetic Diseases

The common chronic diseases of adults (such as essential hypertension, gout, coronary heart disease, diabetes mellitus, peptic ulcer disease, and schizophrenia), as well as the common birth defects (such as cleft lip and palate, spina bifida, and congenital heart disease), have long been known to "run in families." They fit best into the category of *multifactorial genetic diseases*. The genetic element in these disorders rarely manifests itself in an all-or-none fashion, as it does in the monogenic disorders and in chromosomal aberrations. Instead, it is the interaction of multiple genes with multiple environmental factors that produces the familial aggregation [46, 47].

In the multifactorial genetic diseases, there is a *polygenic component* consisting of multiple genes at independent loci whose effects interact in a cumulative fashion. An individual who inherits just the right combination of these genes passes beyond a "threshold of risk," at which point an *environmental component* determines whether and to what extent that person is clinically affected [46, 47]. In order for another individual in the same family to express the same syndrome, a similar combination of genes must be inherited. Since sibs share half of their genes, the probability of a sib inheriting the same combination of genes is $(\frac{1}{2})^n$, where n is the number of genes required to express the trait (assuming that none of the genes is linked).

Inasmuch as the precise number of genes responsible for polygenic traits is unknown, the risk of inheritance for a relative of an affected individual is difficult to calculate, and the standard is based on empiric risk figures (i.e., a direct tally of the proportion of affected relatives in previously reported families). In contrast to the monogenic disorders, in which 25 or 50 percent of the first-degree relatives of an affected proband are at genetic risk, multifactorial genetic disorders are generally observed empirically to affect no more than 5 to 10 percent of first-degree relatives. Moreover, in contrast to Mendelian traits, the recurrence risk of multifactorial conditions varies from family to family, and its estimation is significantly influenced by two factors: (1) the number of affected persons already present in the family, and (2) the severity of the disorder in the index case. The greater number of affected relatives and the more severe their disease, the higher the risk to other relatives. For example, the risk of cleft lip in the sibs of a child with unilateral cleft lip is about 2.5 percent, but if the lesion in the index case is bilateral, the risk in the sibs rises to 6 percent [46, 47].

The hypothesis of a polygenic component in the inheritance of multifactorial diseases has been given a sound basis in recent years by the demonstration that at least 28 percent of all gene loci harbor polymorphic alleles that vary among individuals (discussed above). Such a large degree of variation in normal genes undoubtedly provides the substrate for variations in genetic predisposition with which environmental factors can interact. So far, the genetic loci most strikingly associated with predisposition to specific diseases are those that constitute the major histocompatibility locus or HLA (human leukocyte antigens) system [48]. The HLA gene complex is located on the short arm of chromosome 6. It consists of four closely linked but distinct loci (A, B, C, and D). The products of these genes are proteins that are found on the surface of body cells and that enable an individual's immune system to distinguish its own cells from those of someone else. Each HLA locus in the population consists of multiple alleles, each of which produces an immunologically distinct protein. For example, an individual may inherit any 2 of 21 alleles at the HLA-B locus. The inheritance of certain alleles predisposes to the development of certain diseases when the individual is exposed to an environmental challenge. For a more detailed discussion of the HLA locus and its role in disease susceptibility, the reader is referred to Chap. 3.

Multifactorial disorders are heterogeneous in the sense that the relative contribution of the polygenic factors ("risk genes") and environmental factors will vary greatly from patient to patient. Among common phenotypes which are largely multifactorial, a small proportion of cases may be created by major mutant genes. For example, although coronary heart disease is usually of multifactorial etiology, about 5 percent of subjects with premature myocardial infarctions are heterozygotes for familial hypercholesterolemia, a single-gene disorder that produces atherosclerosis in the absence of any extraordinary environmental factor [49].

INTERACTION BETWEEN SINGLE GENETIC AND ENVIRONMENTAL FACTORS

In addition to polygenic states, many single-gene mutations are known to create abnormal responses to environmental factors.

In particular, several inherited single-gene mutations have been shown to produce clinically significant and often life-threatening idiosyncratic responses to drugs.

Table 1-6 lists the most important of these *pharmacogenetic* disorders, which encompass all three of the Mendelian modes of inheritance [33, 50]. Perhaps the most common is glucose-6-phosphate dehydrogenase deficiency, an X-linked recessive trait in which a variety of drugs may precipitate a hemolytic anemia (Chap. 74). Plasma pseudocholinesterase deficiency and hepatic transacetylase deficiency are examples of autosomal recessive traits that alter drug catabolism so that when the muscle relaxant suxamethonium or the antituberculous drug isoniazid is administered, apnea or peripheral neuropathy may ensue. Malignant hyperthermia is an autosomal dominant trait in which acute hyperpyrexia, muscle rigidity, and hyperkalemic cardiac arrest may be induced by administration of any one of several anesthetic agents. Acute intermittent prophyria is another example of a single-gene disorder that is exacerbated by drugs such as barbiturates (Chap. 60).

Misinterpretation of adverse drug reactions may result in serious harm to patients. In general, all unusual idiosyncratic reactions should be considered to be genetically determined until proved otherwise. Fortunately, the pharmacogenetic disorders are a group of diseases for which therapy is straightfor-

Table 1-6 Examples of pharmacogenetic disorders

Disorder	Abnormal protein	Mode of inheritance	Prevalence	Drugs producing the abnormal response	Clinical effect
Slow inactivation of isoniazid	Isoniazid acetylase in liver	Autosomal recessive	Approximately 50% of U.S. population	Isoniazid, sulfamethazine sulfamaprine, phenelzine, dapsone, hydralazine, procainamide	Polyneuritis (isoniazid); lupuslike reaction (hydralazine)
Suxamethonium sensitivity or atypical pseudocholinesterase	Pseudocholinesterase in plasma	Autosomal recessive	Several mutant alleles; most common allele occurs 1 in 2500	Suxamethonium or succinylcholine	Apnea
Warfarin resistance	? Altered receptor or enzyme in liver with increased affinity for vitamin K	Autosomal dominant	Rare	Warfarin (coumadin)	Inability to achieve anticoagulation with usual doses of drug
Glucose-6-phosphate dehydrogenase deficiency	Glucose-6-phosphate dehydrogenase in erythrocytes	X-linked recessive	Approximately 100 million affected in world; occurs in high frequency where malaria is endemic; multiple alleles	Analgesics, sulfonamides, antimalarials, nitrofurantoin, other drugs	Hemolysis
Drug-sensitive hemoglobins Hemoglobin Zurich	Arginine substitution chain histidine at the 63d position of the β of hemoglobin	Autosomal dominant	Rare	Sulfonamides	Hemolysis
Hemoglobin H	Hemoglobin composed of four β chains; α chains missing	Autosomal dominant	Rare	Many different drugs	Hemolysis
Malignant hyperthermia	Unknown	Autosomal dominant	Approximately 1 in 20,000	Various anesthetics, especially halothane	Severe hyperpyrexia, muscle rigidity, death

SOURCE: Data modified from Vesell [50].

ward: avoidance of the noxious drug by the patient and relatives.

In addition to drugs, other factors in the environment may aggravate specific genetic traits. Cigarette smoke may have deleterious effects on persons homozygous and possibly heterozygous for α-1-antitrypsin deficiency, who are predisposed to the development of emphysema (Chap. 64). Patients with xeroderma pigmentosum are unusually sensitive to sunlight and high temperatures (Chap. 57). Avoidance of milk at an early age prevents many of the complications ordinarily seen in persons with galactosemia (Chap. 7).

Genetic-environmental interactions are particularly important in pregnancy. Women who are affected with PKU may develop high plasma phenylalanine levels during pregnancy, and thus their offspring may suffer from phenylalanine-induced birth defects even though the offspring may not themselves have PKU (Chap. 12). Other examples of diseases resulting from an adverse genetic relation between the mother and fetus include erythroblastosis caused by Rh incompatibility and diabetic embryopathy, a series of major birth defects occurring in about 5 percent of the offspring of women who are clinically diabetic during pregnancy.

GENETIC HETEROGENEITY

When two or more mutations produce a similar clinical syndrome, *genetic heterogeneity* is said to exist. Hemophilia is one example of such a genetically heterogeneous syndrome. A clinically similar bleeding disorder can be caused by mutations at either of two distinct loci on the X chromosome, one leading to a deficiency of factor VIII (classic hemophilia) and the other causing a deficiency of factor IX (Christmas disease). It is now generally believed that most, if not all, hereditary diseases, when carefully analyzed, will be shown to be genetically heterogeneous [51, 52].

Genetic heterogeneity may result from the existence of a series of different mutations at a single genetic locus *(allelic heterogeneity)* or from mutations at different genetic loci *(nonallelic heterogeneity)*. For example, drug-induced hemolysis of red blood cells can occur in patients with any one of several different allelic mutations at the glucose-6-phosphate dehydrogenase locus. On the other hand, hemophilia, as mentioned above, is an example of a syndrome in which nonallelic mutations can produce a similar clinical picture.

A striking example of genetic heterogeneity is provided by the syndrome of hereditary methemoglobinemia. This syndrome, which was once regarded as a homogeneous clinical entity, can be produced by at least 10 different mutations that occur at three distinct gene loci: two at the locus coding for the α chain of hemoglobin, three at the locus coding for the β chain of hemoglobin, and at least five at the NADH dehydrogenase locus (Chaps. 75 and 76).

In the past, it was generally assumed that if a given genetic disease segregated in families as a typical autosomal recessive trait, then the affected individuals were homozygous for a single mutant gene. In view of the multiple alleles that occur at virtually all genetic loci, it is clear that many so-called homozygotes may in fact be *genetic compounds*. In such individuals, the paternally derived and maternally derived alleles bear different alterations in the DNA of the same gene. The clinical

Table 1-7 Inherited metabolic diseases for which genetic compounds have been demonstrated

α-1-Antitrypsin deficiency
Cystinosis
Cystinuria
"Homozygous" familial hypercholesterolemia (LDL
  receptor-internalization defect)
Galactosemia (galactose-1-phosphate uridyl transferase deficiency)
Gaucher disease (glucocerebrosidase deficiency)
Glucosephosphate isomerase deficiency
Hemoglobin α-chain variants
Hemoglobin β-chain variants
Hurler-Scheie syndrome (α-L-iduronidase deficiency)
Iminoglycinuria
Metachomatic leukodystrophy (cerebroside sulfatase deficiency)
Hereditary methemoglobinemia (NADH dehydrogenase deficiency)
Phenylketonuria (phenylalanine hydroxylase deficiency)
Pseudocholinesterase deficiency
Pyruvate kinase deficiency

SOURCE: Data modified from McKusick [53].

syndrome in a genetic compound may resemble the syndrome that is produced by true homozygosity for one of the alleles. Frequently, however, the syndrome is intermediate between the syndromes produced by homozygosity for either allele. The classic examples of genetic compound states are provided by the hemoglobinopathies. For example, patients with SC disease, who have inherited the gene for hemoglobin S from one parent and the gene for hemoglobin C from the other parent, have a clinical syndrome that resembles in some ways the syndrome seen in true SS homozygotes but is usually distinct (Chap. 76). Among the mucopolysaccharide storage diseases, genetic compounds of the Hurler gene (severe allele) and Scheie gene (mild allele) produce a clinical syndrome whose severity is intermediate between those of the respective homozygous states (Chap. 36).

Table 1-7 lists those autosomal recessive inborn errors of metabolism for which genetic compounds have been identified on the basis of biochemical or somatic cell genetic evidence, or both. Many more are likely to emerge as analytical methods become more precise.

PATHOGENESIS OF GENETIC DISEASES

Every genetic disease results from a primary alteration in DNA structure. This alteration in DNA structure produces a disturbance in protein structure and function, and this in turn leads to a disruption in cell and organ function. Table 1-8 lists the different types of derangements that can occur at the sequential levels of DNA structure (level 1), protein function (level 2), and cell and organ function (level 3) and provides examples from the repertoire of human inherited diseases.

Level 1: Altered DNA Structure

Until recently, it was not possible to study directly the structure of mutant genes. The nature of several mutations has now been deduced from the amino acid sequences of mutant proteins and

Table 1-8 Pathogenesis of genetic diseases: Expression at three levels

Level of expression	Type of derangement	Example (chapter no.)*
I. *Altered DNA structure*	1. Deletion mutation	α Thalassemia (77)* Hemoglobin lepore (77)
	2. Missense mutation	Sickle-cell disease (76) G-6-PD deficiency (A-variant) (74)
	3. Nonsense mutation	β Thalassemia (rare variant) (77)
	4. Frame-shift mutation	Hemoglobin Wayne (76)
	5. Gene duplication	Hemoglobin Grady (76)

ENZYMES

II. *Disturbed protein function*	1. Absent activity a. Protein detectable immunologically	Galactosemia (7) Lesch-Nyhan syndrome (few variants) (51) Homocystinuria (half of variants) (25)
	b. No protein detectable immunologically	Lesch-Nyhan syndrome (most variants) (51) Homocystinuria (half of variants) (25)
	2. Reduced activity a. Decreased affinity for substrates	G-6-PD deficiency (Freiburg variant) (74) Citrullinemia (rare variant) (20)
	b. Decreased affinity for cofactors	G-6-PD deficiency (Cornell variant) (74) Homocystinuria (pyridoxine-responsive type) (25) Cystathionuria (rare variant) (25)
	c. Unstable structure	G-6-PD deficiency (most variants) (74) Steroid 5-α-reductase deficiency (Los Angeles variant) (48)
	3. Enhanced activity	G-6-PD Hektoen variant (74) Rare form of gout due to altered PRPP synthetase (50)

NONENZYMIC PROTEINS

	4. Defective posttranslational modification	α-1-Antitrypsin deficiency (ZZ variant) (64)
	5. Enhanced tendency to aggregation	Sickle-cell disease (76) CC disease (76)
	6. Defective ligand binding	Familial hypercholesterolemia (33) Testicular feminization (48)
III. *Disrupted cell and organ function*	1. Altered flux through metabolic pathways a. Accumulation of a toxic precursor (catabolic pathway)	Phenylketonuria (12) Alkaptonuria (14) Lysosomal storage diseases (36-46)
	b. Deficiency of product (anabolic pathway)	Familial goiter (11) Adrenogenital syndromes (47) Albinism (15)
	c. Overproduction of product (anabolic pathway)	Rare form of gout due to altered PRPP synthetase (50)
	2. Disordered feedback regulation of synthetic pathways a. Overproduction of end product due to decreased synthesis or availability of feedback regulator	Acute intermittent porphyria (60) Lesch-Nyhan syndrome (51) Familial hypercholesterolemia (33)
	3. Disordered membrane function a. Deficient transmembrane transport	Cystinuria (80) Hartnup disease (82)
	b. Deficient receptor-mediated endocytosis	Familial hypercholesterolemia (receptor-negative and receptor-defective variants) (33)
	c. Deficient generation of second messenger	Pseudohypoparathyroidism (69)
	4. Disordered intracellular compartmentation a. Accumulation of unprocessed protein	α-1-Antitrypsin deficiency (ZZ variant) (64)
	b. Mislocation of protein	I-cell disease (37) Familial hypercholesterolemia (internalization-defective variant) (33)
	5. Distorted cell or tissue architecture a. Alteration of cell shape	Sickle-cell disease (76) Hereditary spherocytosis (72)
	b. Alteration of organelle structure	Kartagener syndrome (91)
	c. Alteration of extracellular matrix	Ehlers-Danlos syndrome, type VI (lysylhydroxylase deficiency) (63)

* Abbreviations: G-6-PD, glucose-6-phosphate dehydrogenase; PRPP synthetase, phosphoribosylpyrophosphate synthetase.

the genetic code. Most of this amino acid sequence information has been obtained from studies of hemoglobin and glucose-6-phosphate dehydrogenase, two proteins that can be extracted from easily available red blood cells of affected individuals. At least four types of mutations have been delineated by this approach: deletions, duplications, missense mutations, and frame-shift mutations [26]. Examples of each are given in Table 1-8.

Another type of mutation, the nonsense mutation, has been demonstrated recently in humans using DNA restriction enzyme analysis and DNA sequencing techniques. Chang and Kan obtained the partial nucleotide sequence of β-globin messenger RNA isolated from a unique patient with one type of homozygous β° thalassemia [54]. At the position corresponding to amino acid 17, they found the replacement of an adenine by a uracil. This changed the RNA codon AAG, which codes for lysine in the normal β chain, to UAG, which is a termination codon. As a result, only a small portion (the first 16 amino acids) of the normal β chain was synthesized.

With the availability of DNA cloning techniques, it should soon be possible to study directly the altered DNA sequence in many human mutations, even those that involve genes that code for quantitatively minor proteins, such as most enzymes. It is also likely that these new techniques may also reveal mutations in the noncoding regions of DNA that affect the rates of synthesis, processing, or stability of messenger RNAs for specific proteins (see Chap. 2).

Level 2: Disturbed Protein Function

Localized mutations in DNA manifest themselves initially as abnormalities in the synthesis or structure of single enzymatic or nonenzymatic proteins. When the affected protein is an enzyme, the genetic defect results in an absent, reduced, or enhanced rate of a specific enzyme-catalyzed reaction (Table 1-8).

Theoretically, alterations in the amount of measurable enzymic activity might be due to a mutation in the *structural gene* for the enzyme (i.e., the gene that specifies the primary amino acid sequence of the enzyme protein) or to a mutation in a *control gene* (i.e., a region of DNA that controls the rate at which the structural gene is transcribed into messenger RNA or the rate at which the messenger RNA is processed and translated into protein). At present, almost nothing is known about the existence or function of control genes in eukaryotic organisms, including humans. It is clear that the synthetic rate for most important proteins is tightly regulated, often by specific metabolites or hormones, but the precise mechanisms for this regulation have remained obscure. [55].

In bacteria, protein synthesis is controlled at the level of the operon [56, 57]. This is a region of DNA that contains a linear sequence of genes that code for enzymes catalyzing sequential steps in an enzymatic pathway. A single polycistronic messenger RNA for all of the enzymes is synthesized under the control of a single closely linked operator locus. The rate of messenger RNA synthesis is controlled by a repressor, which is a protein produced by an unlinked regulatory gene. When the repressor binds to the operator, it blocks synthesis of the polycistronic messenger RNA. Binding of the repressor to DNA is controlled, in turn, by a low molecular weight inducer, which binds to the repressor and inactivates it. In the classic example

of such a system, that of the *lac operon*, the genes direct the synthesis of proteins necessary for the uptake and metabolism of lactose in *Escherichia coli*. The physiologic inducer in this system is lactose, which binds to the repressor, inactivates it, and thereby unblocks the synthesis of the enzymes necessary for lactose metabolism. Other metabolic pathways in bacteria are controlled by negative effectors which activate repressors rather than inactivating them, and hence function to suppress enzyme synthesis.

To date, a detailed search in eukaryotic cells has so far failed to find evidence for the existence of an operon analogous to those found in bacteria. Indeed, polycistronic messenger RNAs do not appear to exist in eukaryotic cells [82]. Moreover, enzymes that are functionally associated do not appear to be clustered together on the genome, or even to occur on the same chromosome [1, 2]. A striking example is the protein globin, in which the α and β subunits are on different chromosomes (numbers 16 and 11, respectively).

Considering the lack of knowledge about the existence of control genes in humans, it is not surprising that no diseases have been identified that are due to mutations in control genes. Whenever such a suggestion has been made, as in the case of hereditary persistence of fetal hemoglobin or in hereditary orotic aciduria, more detailed study revealed that these diseases are due to mutations in structural genes (Chaps. 76 and 56, respectively).

Positive evidence for the existence of structural gene mutations in humans emerges from the finding that affected individuals usually produce structurally abnormal proteins rather than small amounts of normal proteins [58]. Although no control gene mutations have yet been conclusively identified in humans, it seems likely that they exist. They may be found among the large number of poorly understood dominant disorders and may become apparent as the new techniques of molecular genetics are applied to human diseases (see Chap. 2).

In the case of genetic defects causing an absence of detectable enzyme activity, the defects at the protein level traditionally have been divided into two classes. In one class, the presence of a mutant protein is detectable immunologically, although not functionally. This class is designated *CRM-positive* (i.e., cross-reacting material positive). In the second class of mutants, no enzymic protein is detectable immunologically as well as functionally. This class is designated *CRM-negative*. In most cases in which mutant enzymes have been studied, cross-reacting material is detected [59], but a number of CRM-negative mutations have been reported, most notably in the Lesch-Nyhan syndrome and in about one-half of the cases of homocystinuria. The presence of CRM-positive material suggests that the genetic defect is due to a missense mutation with a consequent amino acid substitution that destroys the activity, but not the antigenicity, of the mutant enzyme.

In most genetic enzyme deficiency states, a reduced but detectable level of enzymatic activity can be measured by sensitive assays [59]. The residual enzyme activity can frequently be shown to be due to a catalytically abnormal enzyme. In many cases, the low enzyme activities are accompanied by a decreased affinity of the mutant enzyme for substrates or cofactors. In other cases, the catalytic activity of the mutant enzyme is normal but the enzyme is intrinsically unstable and is rapidly degraded in the cell. This relative instability can frequently be demonstrated by comparison of the rates of thermal inactivation of the mutant and normal enzymes when heated *in vitro*.

In the most extensively studied series of enzyme defects, i.e., those involving erythrocyte glucose-6-phosphate dehydrogenase, most of the mutations lead to decreased enzyme activity because they produce unstable enzymes whose activity decays as the red blood cell ages (Chap. 74). It is not clear whether enzyme instability is as frequent a cause of enzyme deficiency in other disorders that affect primarily nucleated cells. In contrast to the situation in the anucleate erythrocyte, an unstable enzyme in a nucleated cell can be replaced by new enzyme synthesis, and hence mutations that produce minor degrees of enzyme instability in nucleated cells may not cause disease. The various types of abnormalities that reduce enzymatic activity are not mutually exclusive, i.e., a mutant enzyme may have a reduced affinity for substrates as well as cofactors and also be unstable.

There are a few well-documented cases in which an apparent structural gene mutation can produce an enzyme with enhanced, rather than diminished, catalytic activity. In one such case involving phosphoribosylpyrophosphate synthetase, the enhanced enzyme activity leads to overproduction of uric acid and clinical gout (Chap. 50).

With the exception of the hemoglobinopathies, relatively few diseases have been shown to be due to mutations in genes coding for nonenzymatic proteins. This difference in frequency between defects involving enzymatic and nonenzymatic proteins probably reflects ascertainment bias in that genetic defects in enzymes are easier to demonstrate than are defects in nonenzymatic proteins. Nevertheless, several defects in nonenzymatic proteins have recently been identified. In one of these, the ZZ variant of α-1-antitrypsin deficiency, a missense mutation in the structural gene for α-1-antitrypsin leads to the production of an altered protein that is not susceptible to normal posttranslational processing [60]. As a result of the amino acid substitution, the carbohydrate is not added to the protein in the normal manner, and the defective glycoprotein accumulates in liver cells apparently because of a block in secretion [61].

Another class of defects in nonenzymatic proteins is that which leads to altered proteins with an enhanced tendency to aggregation. The classic example is the β-globin mutation in sickle-cell disease. A further type of defect involves receptor proteins whose normal function is to bind specific ligands and transmit signals. The two well-characterized examples are the abnormal plasma membrane receptor for low density lipoprotein (LDL) in familial hypercholesterolemia (Chap. 33) and the abnormal cytoplasmic androgen receptor in the complete form of testicular feminization (Chap. 48).

Level 3: Disrupted Cell and Organ Function

In general, genetic diseases first come to clinical attention because of disturbances at the third level of expression, i.e., the level of cell and organ function. Several types of derangements occur, and these are listed in Table 1-8.

Altered Flux through Metabolic Pathways Among the inborn errors of metabolism that have been characterized so far, the most frequently observed defect is an altered flux through a metabolic pathway that is directly attributable to the alteration in activity of a mutant enzyme. Most of the classic inborn errors of metabolism involve catabolic pathways, i.e., pathways that lead to the degradation of complex molecules. When such a pathway is blocked by virtue of a mutation, cell function is usually disrupted by the accumulation of a toxic precursor proximal to the metabolic block. A classic example is PKU, in which a reduced activity of phenylalanine hydroxylase causes the accumulation of a variety of derivatives of phenylalanine that cannot be metabolized normally. These substances, in turn, interfere with the normal production of myelin in the brain (Chap. 12). In one large class of such catabolic defects, individual lysosomal enzymes are genetically altered. These deficiencies lead to the accumulation of undigested substrates, usually complex polymers that cannot be hydrolyzed normally. The polymers accumulate within lysosomes. The tissues that are affected are those in which the substance in question is normally catabolized in the largest amounts (Chaps. 36 to 46).

When a mutation involves an anabolic pathway, symptoms are usually caused by a deficiency of the product. This is most notable in albinism, a disease in which melanin cannot be produced normally (Chap. 15), and in many of the familial goiter syndromes, in which thyroxine cannot be produced normally (Chap. 11). A much less frequent situation exists in which a product is actually overproduced as a direct result of an enzyme alteration. One example is a rare form of gout which is due to an altered phosphoribosylpyrophosphate synthetase enzyme that has enhanced catalytic activity, as a result of which uric acid is overproduced and gout ensues (Chap. 50).

Disordered Feedback Regulation of Synthetic Pathways In addition to a primary alteration of flux through a metabolic pathway, mutations may disrupt metabolism by disrupting the feedback regulation of synthetic pathways. Only a few such examples are known at present, but more are to be expected in the future. In the first type of defect, there is overproduction of an end product due to decreased synthesis of a feedback regulator. The classic example is acute intermittent porphyria, in which a deficiency of the enzyme porphobilinogen deaminase leads to a diminished production of heme. Inasmuch as heme is normally a feedback inhibitor of *de novo* porphyrin biosynthesis, the decreased production of heme leads to an overproduction of nonheme porphyrins, and this causes the syndrome of acute intermittent porphyria (Chap. 60). Overproduction of end products also results from the metabolic block in the Lesch-Nyhan syndrome and in familial hypercholesterolemia. In the former case, the deficiency of hypoxanthine guanine phosphoribosyl transferase leads to an accumulation of the substrate phosphoribosyl pyrophosphate, which is diverted into the *de novo* purine synthesis pathway, eventually causing overproduction of uric acid (Chap. 50). In familial hypercholesterolemia, cholesterol carried in plasma LDL cannot reach appropriate intracellular sites owing to a defect in the plasma membrane receptor for LDL. Since LDL-bound cholesterol is normally a feedback regulator of cholesterol biosynthesis, the receptor defect evokes cholesterol overproduction in cells that ordinarily would not be producing cholesterol, but rather would be using cholesterol derived from LDL (Chap. 33).

Disordered Membrane Function A third group of diseases exists in which the genetic defect leads to impairment of a specific function of a plasma membrane protein. In one type of defect the transmembrane transport of specific molecules is defective, apparently because the membrane carrier proteins are altered as a result of mutation. The affected substrates can be amino acids (as in cystinuria and Hartnup disease), carbohydrates (as in the Fanconi syndrome), or ions (as in renal tubular acidosis). When these diseases affect the transport systems of the kidney, they frequently lead to excessive loss of substrates in the urine since the kidney transport systems usually function to reabsorb solutes that are filtered at the glomeruli (Chaps. 80 to 84).

Whereas small molecules are transported directly across membranes by carrier-mediated processes, macromolecules, such as transport proteins and peptide hormones, enter cells by receptor-mediated endocytosis. The macromolecule binds to a cell surface receptor that fixes it at the plasma membrane, after which the membrane invaginates into the cell and pinches off to form an endocytic vesicle that carries the ligand into the cell [62]. One disease, familial hypercholesterolemia, is known to be due to a mutation in a gene that codes for a receptor that normally carries out receptor-mediated endocytosis. In this disease, a genetic defect in the LDL receptor prevents normal uptake and degradation of LDL by body cells and causes LDL, and its cholesterol, to accumulate in plasma. Eventually, the lipoprotein deposits in artery walls and atherosclerosis ensues (Chap. 33).

Still another type of primary membrane dysfunction has been observed recently in cells of patients with pseudohypoparathyroidism (Chap. 69). These cells have a genetic defect in a plasma membrane protein (the GTP-sensitive N protein) whose action is required in order for certain hormones to stimulate adenylate cyclase and thereby to regulate metabolism in target cells [63, 64]. Patients with pseudohypoparathyroidism who lack functional N protein have a complex syndrome in which their cells appear resistant to several peptide hormones. For some reason, the system that is most affected is the one by which parathyroid hormone interacts with bone and kidney cells to raise the serum calcium level. As a result, the most evident symptoms in these patients are hypocalcemia and tetany (Chap. 69).

It is of interest that the latter two syndromes, in contrast to nearly all of the others discussed in this chapter, are dominant as opposed to recessive traits. It may be that defects in signal generation by membrane receptors will often become clinically manifest in heterozygotes [41].

Disordered Intracellular Compartmentation   A fourth class of diseases are those in which the mutation results in disordered intracellular compartmentation. Studies over the past 30 years in cell biology have delineated a complex series of events by which cellular organelles are produced and by which proteins are directed to specific sites within each cell [65]. These pathways frequently involve chemical modifications of proteins that occur after the protein is synthesized. For example, most proteins that are destined for secretion are synthesized with an extra sequence of amino acids at the amino-terminal end, the *signal sequence* [66]. The signal sequence is the first part of the protein to be synthesized. As soon as the signal sequence is synthesized, it binds the messenger RNA-containing ribosome to the membranes of the endoplasmic reticulum. The signal sequence then crosses the membrane of the endoplasmic reticulum. As the remainder of the protein is synthesized, it is pulled linearly across the endoplasmic reticu-

lum membrane like a thread following a needle. After the main body of the protein has begun to traverse the endoplasmic reticulum membrane, the signal sequence is removed by proteolytic cleavage. The completed protein is sequestered on the cisternal side of the endoplasmic reticulum, where a series of carbohydrate molecules is added to form a glycoprotein. The glycoprotein is transported to the cell's Golgi complex, where the carbohydrate side chains are modified. The completed glycoprotein is then packaged into a secretory vesicle that fuses with the plasma membrane, discharging the glycoprotein into the extracellular fluid.

It is clear that mutations must occur in the genes that mediate all of these compartmentation events and that these mutations must be a cause of human disease. Such mutations are difficult to demonstrate because they do not manifest simply as enzyme deficiency states. Nevertheless, a few examples of primary defects in cell compartmentation are known. One of these, the ZZ type of α-1-antitrypsin deficiency, was discussed above. This disease was detected because α-1-antitrypsin, a normal plasma protein, is deficient in plasma. The disease is produced by a missense mutation in the structural gene for α-1-antitrypsin that produces an amino acid substitution in the protein [60]. The defective protein cannot be processed properly by the liver cell [61], and it accumulates within cell vesicles, apparently because it cannot be secreted normally.

In two other conditions, evidence for protein mislocation mutations exists. In one, I-cell disease, there is a primary deficiency of a processing enzyme that is normally responsible for the occurrence of mannose-6-phosphate residues in lysosomal enzymes ([67] and Chap. 37). Ordinarily, the mannose-6-phosphate residues are added after the lysosomal enzymes are synthesized. This carbohydrate moiety serves as a signal that allows the lysosomal enzymes to bind to a mannose-6-phosphate receptor that directs the lysosomal enzyme into the lysosome where it is activated. Owing to a defective processing enzyme, most of the lysosomal enzymes in the cells of I-cell patients do not have mannose-6-phosphate. Instead of binding to the receptor and entering lysosomes, these enzymes pass through the cell and are secreted into the plasma like a secretory protein. This defect is almost exactly the reverse of the one in α-1-antitrypsin deficiency. In I-cell disease, a processing defect results in the failure of retention of a protein rather than a failure of secretion.

An additional type of mislocation mutation occurs in a rare form of familial hypercholesterolemia. Two families have been observed to have an abnormal allele at the LDL receptor locus that produces a cell surface receptor that can bind LDL but cannot transport it into the cell ([68] and Chap. 33). In normal cells, uptake of LDL occurs because the LDL receptors move laterally within the plane of the membrane until they reach coated pits, which are regions of the cell surface that pinch off to form endocytic vesicles [62]. As the coated pits pinch off, they carry receptor-bound ligands into cells. The receptor produced by the *internalization-defective* allele cannot be incorporated into coated pits and hence cannot carry LDL into cells. In this type of mislocation mutation, the protein can reach the appropriate membrane (i.e., the plasma membrane) but cannot enter a segment of that membrane that is crucial for its function (i.e., the coated pit).

Distorted Cell or Tissue Architecture   A final category of cell and organ dysfunction is that which results from distorted cell or tissue architecture. In this category is sickle-cell disease, in which the abnormal hemoglobin aggregates, distorts cellular shape, and leads to hemolysis (Chap. 76). In another red cell disease, hereditary spherocytosis, abnormal red cell shape also contributes to hemolysis (Chap. 72).

A second type of defect in cellular architecture has been described recently in patients with the Kartagener syndrome ("immotile cilia syndrome") (Chap. 91). These patients have a defect in the gene encoding a structural protein called *dynein* [69]. This protein is found in cilia, where it forms arms that cross-link the microtubules. In the absence of dynein arms the microtubules cannot slide properly, the cilia cannot undulate, and the paralysis of cilia leads to a series of developmental and functional abnormalities. Homozygotes for this defect have immotile spermatozoa, situs inversus, bronchiectasis, chronic sinusitis, and anosmia. Interestingly, heterozygotes are asymptomatic.

Tissue architecture can also be distorted by genetic defects in the structure or processing of proteins that form the extracellular matrix. These abnormalities are particulary prominent in patients with a variety of connective tissue disorders that are grouped together as the Ehlers-Danlos syndromes (Chap. 63). One of these disorders (type VI) is due to a defect in the gene for proto-collagen lysylhydroxylase, an enzyme that is important for the cross-linking of collagen fibrils [70]. In homozygotes for this recessive syndrome, the collagen is deficient in hydroxylysine, normal cross-linking does not occur, and the patients suffer from severe scoliosis, recurrent joint dislocations, and serious ocular complications. Defects in the organization of collagen and other extracellular proteins such as elastin are suspected in other conditions in which connective tissue is weakened. The exact nature of these defects has been difficult to elucidate because there are few experimental systems in which to study the formation of complex structures by human tissues in vitro.

Pathogenesis of the Common Monogenic Diseases

A genetic disease can be considered to be fully understood when we comprehend the aberration at all three levels of expression, i.e., DNA, protein, and cell function. Such complete information is not available for any one genetic disease. The diseases that are closest to being understood at all levels are the hemoglobinopathies, thalassemias, and some types of glucose-6-phosphate dehydrogenase deficiency. For most diseases, information at one level is extensive, whereas information at the other levels is lacking. In general, for the diseases covered in this book, the missing or altered enzyme or nonenzymatic protein has been identified and the accumulated or deficient metabolites are known. Frequently, there is uncertainty as to how the metabolic alteration actually produces the disease. For example, in PKU we know that the accumulation of various phenylalanine derivatives somehow disrupts myelin formation in the brain, but how this occurs remains a mystery.

Table 1-9 lists the five most common monogenic diseases covered in this book and indicates the extent of knowledge at all three levels of expression. The diseases in Table 1-9 show the range from fairly detailed knowledge at all levels (sickle-cell anemia) to a woeful lack of insight at any level (cystic fibrosis).

TECHNIQUES FOR STUDYING METABOLIC DISEASES

Originally, inborn errors of metabolism attracted Garrod's attention because of the deficiency of a product (melanin in

Table 1-9 Pathogenesis of the five most prevalent monogenic diseases among certain populations in the United States

	Sickle-cell disease	Glucose-6-phosphate dehydrogenase deficiency (A⁻ variant)	Tay-Sachs disease	Familial hypercholesterolemia (receptor-negative variant)	Cystic fibrosis
Prevalence	1 in 625 U.S. blacks	1 in 20 U.S. blacks	1 in 3000 U.S. Jews	1 in 1000 All populations	1 in 2000 U.S. whites
Mode of inheritance	Autosomal recessive	X-linked recessive	Autosomal recessive	Autosomal dominant	Autosomal recessive
Mutant gene product	β chain of hemoglobin	Glucose-6-phosphate dehydrogenase	α chain of hexosaminidase A	Low density lipoprotein receptor	?
Chromosomal location	11p	Xq	15q	?	?
Expression					
Altered DNA structure	Missense mutation CTC⟶CAC (Glu)⟶(Val)	?	?	?	?
Disturbed protein function	Enhanced aggregation	Unstable enzyme	Absent enzyme activity	Absent receptor activity (homozygotes); ½-normal receptor activity (heterozygotes)	?
Disrupted cell and organ function	Alteration of cell shape leads to hemolysis	Deficiency of product (NADPH) leads to hemolysis	Accumulation of substrate (G_{M2} gaglioside) in lysosomes of neurons leads to brain dysfunction	Deficient receptor-mediated endocytosis causes LDL to accumulate in plasma and prevents body cells from using its cholesterol; hypercholesterolemia and atherosclerosis result	Primary abnormality unknown; secondary abnormalities involve exocrine cells

albinism) or the urinary excretion of an excess amount of a precursor (pentosuria, cystinuria, and alkaptonuria). Identification of the specific metabolite depended on the existence of qualitative chemical tests. This approach is still the basis for the detection of most biochemical genetic defects.

Identification of Accumulated or Missing Metabolites by Chemical Methods

A high index of suspicion on the part of the mother and the physician may provide clues that something is awry in an infant. Several inherited disorders are associated with specific urinary odors or with urinary crystals or unusual urinary colors [35, 71]. The majority of diagnostic procedures rely upon qualitative color tests of urine designed to identify an abnormal concentration of a potential metabolite, such as the ferric chloride test for phenylpyruvic acid. Other tests include the use of nitrosonaphthol for detection of tryosyl compounds; nitroprusside for detection of disulfides such as cystine, homocystine, or mercaptolactate; cetyltrimethylammonium bromide for detection of mucopolysaccharides; or reducing reagents for detection of mellituria. Most color tests are not specific, and a positive test result is only an indication for more detailed biochemical investigation of the patient. Other methods include amino acid paper or column chromatography and the separation of dinitrophenylhydrazines of keto acids by thin-layer chromatography.

Direct Enzyme Assay of Blood or Fresh Tissue

When a biochemical pathway is known, chemical identification of an accumulated metabolite frequently leads directly to recognition of the site of the metabolic derangement and to confirmation by direct assay for activity of the suspect enzyme. When the steps in a metabolic pathway are not well understood, full disclosure of the biochemical abnormality frequently has to await the elucidation of the normal pathways of synthesis and degradation of the compound. Indeed, metabolic errors have served as a stimulus and a source of insight for biochemists in defining pathways of normal metabolism, as in the case of the gangliosidoses. In many cases, the accumulation of a metabolite in a patient with an enzyme deficiency provides the first clue to the existence or importance of a pathway. An outstanding example is the deficiency of α-mannosidase in mannosidosis.

Diagnosis of an enzymatic defect may be made by direct assay of blood or tissue obtained by biopsy. Samples of intestinal mucosa may be readily obtained at a negligible risk, and biopsies of liver and thyroid have provided critical information in some instances in which such information would have been unobtainable in any other way. A particularly useful technique is enzyme assay in white blood cells. These cells are easily isolated from normal and affected individuals. They have been used to demonstrate the defect in a variety of disorders, such as maple syrup urine disease, methylmalonic aciduria, some of the glycogen storage diseases, orotic aciduria, and others. At least 35 disorders produce enzymatic or phenotypic abnormalities of the leukocyte [72]. An equally large number of inborn errors can be demonstrated in the red blood cells. Among these are deficiencies in many of the enzymes involving the glycolytic

and oxidative pathways of glucose metabolism, acatalasia, and of course the hemoglobinopathies.

Identification of Protein Variants

Polymorphisms of proteins have usually been detected on the basis of abnormal electrophoretic mobility, attributable to a change in the net charge of the molecule (see Table 1-2). It has been estimated that only one-third of amino acid substitutions result in a charge difference and altered mobility of protein on electrophoresis [26].

In enzyme deficiency states in which some residual activity is detected, certain observations may suggest an enzyme variant rather than a reduction in the number of normal enzyme molecules. Among these are changed electrophoretic behavior, abnormal kinetics disclosed by different Michaelis constants, altered response to substrates or cofactors, altered sensitivity to inhibitors, increased or decreased heat lability, or different pH optima. Immunologic procedures may disclose the presence of cross-reactive material (CRM), presumably representing a protein variant, in the absence of enzymatic activity. Combinations of these methods have revealed over 100 variants of erythrocyte glucose-6-phosphate dehydrogenase, most of which represent different amino acid substitutions in a single polypeptide chain.

Cell Culture Studies

The technology of cell culture has been standardized to the point where it is routine for many laboratories to grow somatic cells in vitro. The most readily cultured cells, skin fibroblasts, have been exploited widely in the study of genetics of human disorders [68, 73–75]. Single cells can be isolated and cloned. Cultures can be synchronized for study of events of the cell cycle. Biochemical studies of varying levels of complexity can be performed on the cells. A full potential of cell culture in the study of hereditary disease is just being realized. Over 150 strains of mutant human fibroblasts are available on request from the Institute for Medical Research, Camden, New Jersey [76].

Cultured fibroblasts perform a constellation of biosynthetic activities, including synthesis of purine and pyrimidine nucleotides; 7 of the 20 structural amino acids; DNA, RNA, and protein; and cholesterol and other membrane lipids. Many enzymes can be assayed and their kinetic properties, inhibition characteristics, and thermal stabilities studied. The enzymatic defect has been demonstrated in human skin fibroblasts for at least 100 inborn errors and in human long-term lymphoblastoid cells for at least 25 inborn errors [76].

The use of cell culture has proved essential in the elucidation of the biochemical defects for several metabolic disorders. The underlying defects in the mucopolysaccharidoses were first revealed in the now classic "cross-correction" studies of Neufeld and Fratantoni [74]. These workers found that the medium in which fibroblasts from a patient with the Hurler syndrome had grown was able to correct the defect in the cells from a patient with the Hunter syndrome. This was because the Hurler cells excreted induronate sulfatase, the lysosomal enzyme that was deficient in the Hunter cells. Conversely, the medium from the Hunter cells contained α-1-iduronidase, which corrected the defect of the Hurler cells. These observations were the first to indicate the nature of the biochemical defects in these two syndromes, viz., in each case a deficiency of a different enzyme involved in mucopolysaccharide catabolism (Chap. 36). Moreover, these experiments provided the first indication that lysosomal enzymes could exchange between cells, a finding that later led to the elucidation of the pathway for receptor-mediated endocytosis of lysosomal enzymes (Chap. 37).

In addition to the mucopolysaccharidoses, the use of cultured cells provided the first clue to the elucidation of the biochemical defects in several other genetic disorders, including familial hypercholesterolemia (Chap. 33), I-cell disease (Chap. 37), and xeroderma pigmentosum (Chap. 57).

The fibroblast culture technique, unfortunately, is not applicable to the study of all inborn errors, since the metabolic activity at fault may not be a property native to the fibroblast. For example, phenylalanine hydroxylase activity is confined to the hepatic parenchymal cell; accordingly, PKU cannot be diagnosed with fibroblast cultures.

With the newer techniques of molecular biology, it is possible to isolate radioactive probes for specific genes and to study by DNA hybridization the structure of these genes in cultured cells, even when the gene product is not synthesized (see Chap. 2). Thus, in the future, cultured fibroblasts may be useful for genetic analysis even when they do not produce a specific protein. A striking example is the work of Kan and Dozy [77], who made the prenatal diagnosis of sickle-cell anemia by studying the structure of the β-globin gene in amniotic fluid fibroblasts that do not produce globin (see below).

Cells in culture offer unique opportunities for testing genetic mechanisms. X-linked mutations have been used in cell cultures to test the X-inactivation hypothesis of Lyon. Studies of at least five X-linked loci, including the loci for glucose-6-phosphate dehydrogenase, hypoxanthine-guanine phosphoribosyl transferase (Lesch-Nyhan syndrome), phosphoglycerate kinase, ceramide trihexose α-galactosidase (Fabry disease), and phosphorylase-b-kinase (glycogen storage disease, type VIII), have shown random X inactivation of the paternal or maternal X chromosome in each cell of heterozygous females [78]. Similar inactivation does not occur in autosomal loci. Nor does it appear that inactivation of one X is necessarily complete at all loci. Present evidence suggests that in the case of at least two X-linked loci—the Xg(a) locus [79] and the steroid sulfatase locus [80]—both alleles are expressed in cells of heterozygous females.

Somatic cell hybrids whose nuclei contain genomes from different species, including serially propagated hybrids of mouse and human fibroblast cells, have been prepared in a number of laboratories [81–83]. Following hybridization, there is a gradual reduction in chromosome number in which human chromosomes are preferentially eliminated one by one. As mentioned earlier, this technology has been responsible for most of the genetic mapping of the human autosomes.

The cell hybridization technique has also been useful in defining heterogeneity of a number of inborn errors by complementation analysis [82, 83]. Cultured fibroblasts from two affected individuals with a similar phenotype are fused to form heterokaryons with the use of either Sendai virus or polyethylene glycol. By definition, if the abnormal phenotype of the two parental strains is corrected in the heterokaryon, the defects must involve different genes. On the other hand, a negative complementation test suggests that the defects in the two parental strains involve allelic mutations that are not mutually corrective. This approach has been skillfully used in the analysis of heterogeneity in several inborn errors, including xeroderma pigmentosum (Chap. 57), the methylmalonic acidemias (Chap. 23), the proprionic acidemias (Chap. 23), and the G_{M2} gangliosidoses (Chap. 46).

DNA Restriction Endonuclease Analysis

The most recent and potentially the most powerful technique for studying human inborn errors involves the use of DNA restriction enzymes [84]. These enzymes recognize specific sequences in DNA and catalyze endonucleolytic cleavages, yielding fragments of defined lengths. The restriction fragments can be separated by electrophoresis in agarose gels according to molecular size [85]. Restriction fragments encoding specific gene sequences can be detected on the agarose gels by the hybridization method developed by Southern [86]. In the Southern technique, the DNA fragments from an agarose gel are transferred to nitrocellulose paper and hybridized with radioactive complementary DNA or RNA sequences of known composition. Differences among individuals in the length of a particular restriction fragment can arise from either (1) a substitution of one or more bases in the DNA, resulting in the loss of a cleavage site or the formation of a new one or (2) insertion or deletion of blocks of DNA within a fragment.

This new technology, which is described in more detail in Chap. 2, has already made possible a number of advances in our understanding of the hemoglobinopathies and the thalassemias [87–90]. As discussed in Chaps. 2, 76, and 77, the restriction endonuclease technique has led not only to an explosion in the molecular genetics of the thalassemias but also to the discovery of a polymorphism in an *Hpa* I endonuclease recognition site adjacent to the β-globin structural gene [91], and this in turn has aided in the prenatal diagnosis of sickle-cell anemia [77].

DIAGNOSIS AND PREVENTION OF METABOLIC DISEASES

The present trend for couples to have smaller families has heightened the concern that children should be healthy and free of genetic diseases. Primary-care physicians are called upon to play a more active role in the prevention and treatment of hereditary diseases. In most clinical situations, genetic advice can be given by the primary physician once the relatively simple principles of medical genetics and genetic counseling have been mastered. For a more in-depth discussion of these principles, the reader is referred to Vogel and Motulsky's textbook entitled *Human Genetics: Problems and Approaches* [33].

Genetic Counseling

The prevention of genetic diseases requires the advance identification of matings that are capable of producing defective genotypes. These may involve matings in which one of the two individuals is carrying a dominant or X-linked gene mutation or a balanced translocation, or matings in which individuals carry a deleterious recessive gene at the same locus. Such individuals are usually identified through the birth of an affected child or near relative, in which case retrospective genetic counseling can be provided.

When advising family members about the risk of transmitting a disorder that has already affected someone in the family, the counselor's first step is to be certain of the *correct diagnosis*—in particular, to make certain that the problem in question is really of genetic origin. This is especially important in disorders that may have either a genetic or a nongenetic etiology, such as deafness or mental retardation. Second, if the disease has a hereditary element, the possiblity of genetic heterogeneity must be considered.

Estimation of the *recurrence risk* of a disease requires knowledge of the genetic mechanisms controlling the relevant disorder. When more than one genetic mechanism exists, or when environmental factors can cause clinically indistinguishable traits, the *relative probabilities* of the different mechanisms operating in the particular family are computed. For conditions determined by simple Mendelian inheritance, there is no difficulty in predicting the probability of an offspring's being affected, provided the genotypes of the parents can be recognized. Identification of the parental genotype is easiest for autosomal recessive and X-linked disorders since the basic lesions in the two forms of Mendelian inheritance ususally involve simple enzyme deficiencies for which biochemical tests are now available.

For autosomal dominant disorders, identification of the parental genotype is considerably more difficult since the basic defect is known for only a few of these disorders, and the diagnosis of the heterozygote for a dominant disorder depends almost exclusively on the clinical evaluation and a careful pedigree analysis. In counseling a family in which one relative is affected with a dominant disorder, it is important that appropriate clinical examination of all first-degree relatives and appropriately selected distant relatives be carried out. If relatives appear unaffected, there is the possiblity that the clinical symptoms may be masked by *delayed age of onset* and *variability in expression*. When no relatives are affected, the possiblity of a new dominant mutation must be entertained.

When advising families about multifactorial genetic diseases, such as diabetes mellitus, in which the inheritance pattern is not clear-cut, the physician must resort to empiric risk estimates that have been derived from retrospectively assembled data [33].

Once the parental genotypes are determined, the genetic prognosis is usually presented in terms of probability that a given couple will produce an affected offspring. The physician providing genetic counseling must make certain that the couple understands not only the meaning of such absolute risk figures but also the severity of the disease and the variability in clinical expression. In other words, in dealing with disorder such as α-1-antitrypsin deficiency, it is important for the parents to realize not only that they have a 25 percent risk of producing a child with this disorder but also that a certain proportion of children with the disorder have severe disease with both liver and pulmonary manifestations, a certain portion have mild disease with only pulmonary manifestations, etc. They should also have an understanding of the potential impact of the disease on their family. A disease that is lethal at birth might be classified by some as more "severe" than one that is lethal at

age 16, but the latter is likely to have a much more profound impact on the family.

In contrast to retrospective genetic counseling, in which advice is given after the birth of at least one affected family member, in prospective genetic counseling advice is provided to possible carriers of recessive genes before an affected individual is born. As a first step, the identification of heterozygous individuals by a population-screening procedure is required. Second, unmarried heterozygous persons are told about the risk of having affected children if they marry someone who is heterozygous for the same gene. Finally, if two heterozygous persons are already married, there is the possibility of preventing the birth of affected infants if the disease can be diagnosed in utero by amniocentesis.

Antenatal Diagnosis of Genetic Disease

The use of transabdominal amniocentesis permits diagnosis of certain genetic diseases at a stage early enough to terminate the pregnancy and to prevent the birth of a defective child. This procedure gives high-risk couples the opportunity to have unaffected children provided they are willing for the pregnancy to be terminated in the event that an abnormal fetus is detected.

Amniocentesis consists of the transabdominal apsiration of amniotic fluid from the uterus. The procedure involves minimal risk. Maternal mortality has not been observed, and morbidity has been minor. Fetal loss (due to death or spontaneous abortion) is no greater than in controls matched for maternal age, gravity, parity, race, religion, socioeconomic group, gestational age, and other features [33, 92, 93]. If a diagnostic amniocentesis is performed at the fifteenth week of gestation, the 4-week delay required for culture of an adequate number of cells for biochemical or cytogenetic study brings one only to the twentieth week, when pregnancy may still be terminated safely.

Direct examination of the amniotic fluid itself may be diagnostic. For example, an elevated level of α-fetoprotein is a relatively good indicator of the presence of spina bifida or some other related neural tube abnormality [94]. More frequently, prenatal diagnosis requires culture of the fetal cells in vitro, as mentioned above. By this means, the karyotype of the fetus can be determined, to ascertain fetal sex and to detect various chromosomal aberrations such as the Down syndrome.

Many inborn errors of metabolism can be detected by suitable assays of specific enzyme activities in the cultured fetal cells. Table 1-10 lists those enzyme deficiency states for which prenatal diagnosis is currently feasible. The development of appropriate standards for determining deficiencies in activity of various enzymes in cells derived prenatally is a paramount problem in the application of this important technique.

A most promising approach for increasing the number of metabolic diseases that can be diagnosed antenatally involves applying the detailed knowledge of the anatomy of the human genome. For example, the gene causing myotonic dystrophy is linked to the gene *secretor*, which determines the secretion of the ABO blood group substances into blood fluids, including saliva and amniotic fluid ([95] and Chap. 66). This linkage relationship makes it possible, in selected families, to perform amniocentesis for determination of the secretor status of the fetus and thereby to predict inheritance of the gene for myo-

Table 1-10 Inborn errors of metabolism for which prenatal diagnosis is feasible

Disorders of carbohydrate metabolism
  Glycogen storage diseases—types II, III, and IV
  Galactosemia
  Galactokinase deficiency
  Pyruvate decarboxylase deficiency
Disorders of amino acid metabolism
  Argininosuccinic aciduria
  Citrullinemia
  Homocystinuria
  Maple syrup urine disease
  Methylmalonic aciduria
  Isovaleric acidemia
  Ketotic hyperglycinemia
Disorders of lipoprotein and lipid metabolism
  Homozygous familial hypercholesterolemia (receptor-negative type)
  Refsum syndrome
Disorders of lysosomal enzymes
  Mucopolysaccharidosis, type I (Hurler syndrome)
  Mucopolysaccharidosis, type II (Hunter syndrome)
  Mucopolysaccharidosis, type III (Sanfilippo syndrome, types A and B)
  Mucopolysaccharidosis, type VI (Maroteaux-Lamy syndrome)
  Mucopolysaccharidosis, type VII (β-glucuronidase deficiency)
  I-cell disease
  Lysosomal acid phosphatase deficiency
  Wolman syndrome and cholesteryl ester storage disease
  Fabry disease
  Gaucher disease
  Krabbe disease (globoid cell leukodystrophy)
  Metachromatic leukodystrophy

  Niemann-Pick disease
  Tay-Sachs disease
  Sandhoff disease
  Generalized gangliosidosis
  Juvenile gangliosidosis
  Fucosidosis
  Mannosidosis
  Farber disease (lipogranulomatosis)
Disorders of steroid metabolism
  21-Hydroxylase deficiency—congenital adrenal hyperplasia
  Complete testicular feminization
  Steroid sulfatase deficiency (X-linked ichthyosis)
Disorders of purine and pyrimidine metabolism
  Lesch-Nyhan syndrome
  Hereditary orotic aciduria
  Xeroderma pigmentosum
  Adenosine deaminase deficiency (combined immunodeficiency)
Disorders of metal metabolism
  Menkes' syndrome
Disorders of porphyrin and heme metabolism
  Acute intermittent porphyria
Disorders involving connective tissue, molecules, and bone
  Hypophosphatasia (some types)
Disorders of the blood and blood-forming tissues
  Sickle-cell anemia
  α Thalassemias
  β Thalassemias
  Glucose-6-phosphate dehydrogenase deficiency
Disorders of transport
  Cystinosis

SOURCE: Date modified from Epstein and Golbus [93] and Galjaard [35].

tonic dystrophy [95]. There are three other disorders like myotonic dystrophy which cannot be diagnosed in cultured amniotic fluid cells by direct assay of the mutant gene product, but which can be diagnosed in the fetus by virtue of their linkage with a marker protein that itself can be detected in amniotic fluid or cells [1]. These include: classic hemophilia, which is linked to glucose-6-phosphate dehydrogenase (Chap. 70); the 21-hydroxylase deficiency type of congenital adrenal hyperplasia, which is linked to the HLA locus (Chap. 47); and sickle-cell anemia, which is linked to the *HpA* I restriction site mutation ([77] and Chap. 76).

Genetic Screening

Genetic screening represents the search in a population for persons possessing certain genotypes that are known to be associated with or to predispose to disease in the individuals or their descendants [96]. Screening is also employed for research purposes in order to ascertain distributions of traits, e.g., polymorphisms, not known to be associated with disease. In this section, we are concerned only with the identification of deleterious genes in individual members of populations.

Genetic disease accounts for a significant proportion of hospitalized children in referral centers. In studies in Montreal, Baltimore, and Newcastle, from 6 to 8 percent of diseases among hospitalized children were attributable to single gene defects and from 0.4 to 2.5 percent to chromosomal abnormalities; another 22 to 31 percent were considered gene-influenced [35, 97].

Identification of genetic disease in a newborn infant may allow the institution of a prophylactic program to supply that which is lacking or to remove that which is injurious to the child. Identification of couples at high risk of transmitting a serious genetic disease may permit a couple to forestall the birth of affected children, either through abortion after antenatal diagnosis or by being told about the probability of having an affected child, so that they may make an informed decision with regard to birth control.

Genetic Screening of Newborns This practice was initiated in order to identify PKU in infants in time to institute a low phenylalanine diet and thus prevent the devastating effects of the untreated disease [98]. Virtually all states have passed laws mandating screening for PKU, and some 90 percent of all infants born in the United States are now screened [99]. More than 13 million American newborns have been screened and more than 1100 affected individuals have been identified, giving an incidence of 1 per 11,500 live births [100]. Cost-effectiveness surveys in the United States [101] and England [102] have shown that screening programs for PKU can be justified in economic terms as well as on medical, ethical, and humanistic grounds. The costs of case identification are less than the costs of institutionalized care of affected individuals. Early problems that arose from the failure to recognize certain hyperphenylalaninemia variants (Chap. 12) have been solved, and PKU screening is now on a firm basis.

PKU screening can be performed by a urinary ferric chloride test, by the Guthrie microbiologic screen for elevated blood phenylalanine levels (which employs bacteria that require phe-

Table 1-11   Prevalence of some inborn errors of metabolism for which newborn screening tests are available

Disorder	Average prevalence per live-born infants
Congenital hypothyroidism	1 in 6000
Cystinuria	1 in 7000
α-1-Antitrypsin deficiency	1 in 8000
Phenylketonuria	1 in 12,000
Histidinemia	1 in 17,000
Iminoglycinuria	1 in 20,000
Hartnup disease	1 in 26,000
Hyperprolinemia	1 in 40,000
Galactosemia	1 in 57,000
Adenosine deaminase deficiency	< 1 in 100,000
Maple syrup urine disease	1 in 200,000
Homocystinuria	1 in 200,000

SOURCE: Data from Galjaard [35].

nylalanine for growth), or by column chromatography. When either of the first two tests is provisionally positive, a more definitive measurement of plasma phenylalanine concentration is warranted.

The Guthrie microbiologic assay for blood phenylalanine became available for mass screening in 1961 [98]. By 1972 Guthrie had further developed his procedures so that as many as 11 disorders could be detected from a single sample of dried blood collected on filter paper and submitted by mail [103]. These incude PKU, maple syrup urine disease, homocystinuria, tyrosinemia, histidinemia, valinemia, galactosemia, argininosuccinic aciduria, orotic aciduria, α-1-antitrypsin deficiency, angioneurotic edema (absence of inhibitor of C-1 esterase), and sickle-cell anemia. The population frequencies of some inborn errors of metabolism for which screening tests are available are shown in Table 1-11.

Screening Programs in High-Risk Populations

Tay-Sachs disease   The carrier frequency of this lethal disorder is 1 in 30 to 1 in 60 in the American Jewish population of northeastern European ancestry, approximately tenfold higher than in the population at large. Detection of Tay-Sachs heterozygotes is accomplished by assay of hexosaminidase A in white blood cells or by measurement of resistance of serum hexosaminidase A to heat inactivation [104]. Tay-Sachs disease is an ideal disorder for screening for reproductive counseling for the following reasons: (1) it is limited mainly to a defined population; (2) there is a simple, reliable, automated, and relatively inexpensive test for identifying the carrier state; (3) there are positive reproductive alternatives for couples, both of whom are carriers, because the disorder can be diagnosed antenatally following amniocentesis at a time when induced abortion can be safely performed. Thus, such couples can plan to have unaffected children while avoiding having children with the disease.

Up to 1979, more than 250,000 Jewish individuals, mainly in the United States, Canada, and Israel, and a smaller number in Great Britain and South Africa, had been tested [35]. Over 10,000 heterozygous carriers were identified; included in this group were 210 couples who had not yet given birth to affected children [35].

The advent of reliable screening procedures for heterozygote detection and antenatal diagnosis is particularly valuable in Tay-Sachs disease, in which 80 percent of cases are first cases. But amniocentesis also enables the prevention of the birth of a second affected child in a family in which one Tay-Sachs case has appeared and in which both parents are therefore known heterozygotes. In the San Diego area alone, 17 women in this situation became pregnant and were examined by amniocentesis. Nine affected fetuses were identified, and in eight cases therapeutic abortion was performed. In one instance, the procedure was carried out too late (in the third trimester), and the child later developed typical Tay-Sachs disease [104].

Lesch-Nyhan syndrome   There is no economically feasible method for identifying the female heterozygote carrier of this X-linked recessive disorder in population screening, but identification of the heterozygote state can be accomplished by tissue culture techniques in the case of sisters or daughters of known carriers [105]. In addition, antenatal diagnosis of a potentially involved fetus can be accomplished with cells obtained by amniocentesis [106]. The stimulus for such efforts is invariably the previous birth of one or more affected male infants in the family, so that the process does not avoid first cases.

Sickle-cell disease   Screening for sickle-cell anemia and sickle-cell trait is being conducted in many cities. The most reliable procedure is electrophoresis, which will also screen for other hemoglobinopathies. The three favorable features of screening for Tay-Sachs disease apply here also, except that the procedures for antenatal diagnosis of an affected fetus are less well developed and are available in only a few centers. There are two approaches to the antenatal diagnosis of sickle-cell disease. One approach is based on the expression of β chains in the fetus as early as the second month of gestation. Erythrocytes can be aspirated from the placental circulation by fetoscopy, but this is currently a specialized and somewhat hazardous research procedure. Both heterozygotes [107–109] and homozygotes [110, 111] for hemoglobin S have been identified with this technique. The second approach, discovered by Kan and Dozy [77], involves the direct analysis of genes in DNA extracted from fetal fibroblasts obtained by amniocentesis. In many cases, the sickle-cell globin mutation in the β-globin gene is linked to a restriction site polymorphism that can easily be identified by electrophoretic and hybridization techniques (Chap. 77). The ability to identify an SS fetus by these new techniques raises an ethical issue not present in Tay-Sachs disease because sickle-cell disease has such a variable expression. In some individuals mild disease may be compatible with a long and productive life.

Dominant diseases   In spite of the many advances that have been made in screening for genetic disease, there remain a number of important dominantly inherited disorders in which we are without a useful lead for antenatal diagnosis. An example is Huntington's chorea, which cannot be diagnosed in the potential victim until the disease strikes in adult life. There is one dominant disorder—familial hypercholesterolemia—in which the rare birth of severely affected homozygotes can be prevented by amniocentesis and prenatal diagnosis [112].

Heterozygote Detection

The necessities of family counseling highlight the need for methods of identifying the heterozygous carrier of X-linked or autosomal recessive traits. Considerable success has already been achieved. In some instances, measurements of a specific metabolite or an enzyme activity in the presumed heterozygote permit differentiation of "heterozygote values" from the distribution of normal values. In the presumed heterozygote for cystathioninuria, the excretion of cystathionine in the urine is elevated, but not as much as in the patient with the homozygous disease. In acatalasia type I, erythrocyte catalase activity values are approximately one-half normal in the heterozygous carrier. Ceramide trihexoside α-galactosidase activity in heterozygotes for Fabry disease is low in plasma, as is the activity of hexosaminidase A in leukocytes of carriers of Tay-Sachs disease.

Additional tests for the heterozygous state depend mainly on detection of a failure to handle an abnormal load of substrate. Thus, in presumed heterozygotes for PKU, there is reduced tolerance to an administered load of phenylalanine, which is a better discriminant than the slight elevation of phenylalanine levels in the blood. Such tolerance tests detect heterozygotes only in instances in which the intermediate activity value of the enzyme being tested can be limited. This is often not possible. For example, in alkaptonuria one cannot detect heterozygotes this way. Even if the activity of homogentisic acid oxidase is presumed to be half-normal in the liver of the heterozygote (this has not been studied), such a liver would be able to metabolize more than 500 g homogentisic acid per day. The homozygote excretes only 2 to 10 g per day.

Detection of the heterozygote for accessible proteins that can be studied by physical methods has been highly successful. Thus, the heterozygotes for abnormal hemoglobins and for the diseases characterized by abnormalities of circulating plasma proteins, such as α-1-antitrypsin, are now routinely identifiable.

Heterozygous female sibs or daughters of mothers who have given birth to male children with the Lesch-Nyhan syndrome may be identified by the study of fibroblasts in culture. The detection of cells lacking HGPRT (hypoxanthine-guanine phosphoribosyl transferase) activity may require preliminary incubation in a medium containing a toxic purine antimetabolite, such as thioguanine [124] or azaguanine, which will be destructive only to the normal cell capable of converting the analogue to its active ribonucleotide derivative.

It must be emphasized that the presence of a single gene for a recessive disease is not demonstrated conclusively by an abnormal result of a tolerance test or by a finding of depressed enzyme activity values alone. Such results must be correlated with pedigree data and, in addition, must be interpreted with care to exclude both nongenetic causes for the test abnormality and the homozygous state of a milder form of the disorder, as in the Duarte variant of galactosemia (i.e., galactokinase deficiency) [113].

TREATMENT OF METABOLIC DISEASES

Treatment of the patient with an inherited disorder depends upon accurate diagnosis and an understanding of the patho-

physiology of the disease. This understanding includes an appreciation of the interaction of genetic and environmental factors in many inherited diseases. Well-known examples include PKU, which predisposes to toxic reactions to dietary phenylalanine, and glucose-6-phosphate dehydrogenase deficiency, which predisposes to hemolysis following ingestion of fava beans and during the course of acute viral hepatitis and infectious mononucleosis or after administration of certain drugs, including aspirin and phenacetin. These are therapeutically challenging interactions, for in such instances, control of environmental factors may permit amelioration or even complete neutralization of the effect of the genetic change.

Table 1-12 lists examples of genetic diseases that can be successfully treated at the present time.

Dietary Restriction of the Substrate

Dietary restriction is often an effective way to reduce the excessive substrate that accumulates behind a metabolic block [114]. A general reduction in protein intake will improve the clinical manifestations and prevent brain damage in a number of rare disorders of the urea cycle associated with ammonia intoxication, including argininosuccinic aciduria and citrullinemia. A diet low in phenylalanine is effective in preventing growth and mental retardation in PKU, especially if started soon after birth. A fructose-free diet effectively controls the symptoms of hereditary fructose intolerance due to deficiency of fructose-1-phosphate aldolase. Similarly, a diet that is virtually galactose-free will avert brain damage and cataract formation in children with galactokinase or galactose-1-phosphate uridyl transferase deficiency. In Refsum's disease, the accumulation of phytanic acid can be prevented by control of the intake of this lipid, with significant improvement in neurologic and other deficits.

Replacement of the Deficient End Product

A metabolic block will not only result in accumulation of the substrate of the missing enzyme but will also lead to a decrease in the product of the reaction or later products of the sequence. When one of these products is biologically important, replacement may alleviate the deficiency state. Goiter resulting from a metabolic block in thyroxine production can be effectively treated and cretinism prevented by replacement of thyroid hormone. In the adrenogenital syndromes, corticosteroid administration not only supplies the missing hormone but also corrects the disordered steroidal secretory pattern and leads to remission of the clinical manifestations. In orotic aciduria, in which orotic acid cannot be transformed to uridine, administration of uridine supplies the pyrimidines needed for hematopoietic functions with correction of macrocytic anemia and also suppresses orotic acid synthesis, with a reduction in the tendency toward orotic acid urolithiasis. Administration of dietary copper will effectively combat the inherited copper deficiency of Menkes' syndrome.

Depletion of the Storage Substance

In some hereditary disorders the clinical consequences can be attributed to the accumulation of stored materials in the tissues

Table 1-12 Some examples of treatable inborn errors of metabolism

Method of treatment	Disorder
Dietary restriction of substrate	
Lactose	Lactase deficiency
Galactose	Galactosemia and galactokinase deficiency
Fructose	Fructose intolerance
Neutral fats	Familial lipoprotein lipase deficiency
Phytanic acid	Refsum syndrome
Phenylalanine	Phenylketonuria
Protein	Citrullinemia and other urea-cycle disorders
Replacement of deficient end product	
Copper	Menkes' syndrome
Vitamin D and phosphate	Hypophosphatemic rickets
Cortisol	Adrenogenital syndromes
Thyroxine	Familial goiters
Uridine	Orotic aciduria
Depletion of storage substance	
Sterol removal by bile-acid binding resins	Familial hypercholesterolemia
Cystine removal by D-penicillamine	Cystinuria
Copper removal by D-penicillamine	Wilson's disease
Iron removal by phlebotomy	Hemochromatosis
Uric acid removal by uricosuric agents	Gout
Amplification of enzyme activity	
Pyridoxine (vitamin B_6)	Homocystinuria
Vitamin B_{12}	Methylmalonic aciduria
Phenobarbital	Crigler-Najjar variant and other forms of unconjugated hyperbilirubinemia
Replacement of mutant protein	
Gamma globulin	Agammaglobulinemia
Factor VIII (AHG)	Hemophilia
Infusion of irradiated erythrocytes containing adenosine deaminase	Severe combined immunodeficiency disease
Organ transplantation	
Kidney	Fabry's disease, cystinosis, Alport syndrome, polycystic kidney disease (adult form)
Allogenic bone marrow	Lymphopenic hypogammaglobulinemia (Swiss type), Wiscott-Aldrich syndrome, severe combined immunodeficiency disease
Surgical removal	
Splenectomy	Hereditary spherocytosis
Portacaval shunt	Glycogen storage disease (type I) and homozygous familial hypercholesterolemia
Colectomy	Familial polyposis of colon
Thyroidectomy	Medullary thyroid carcinoma syndrome

of the body, and removal of the excess material may ameliorate the effects of the genetic lesion. Removal of stored copper in Wilson's disease by penicillamine and of excess iron in hemo-chromatosis by frequent phlebotomy illustrate this approach. Use of uricosuric agents to deplete the body of uric acid in tophaceous gout and of bile-acid binding resins to reduce plasma cholesterol levels in familial hypercholesterolemia are additional examples.

Use of Metabolic Inhibitors

In instances in which a toxic metabolite accumulates because of a metabolic error, it may be possible to control the production of the toxic substance by use of an appropriate metabolic inhibitor. Allopurinol is an effective inhibitor of xanthine oxidase and a successful agent for controlling uric acid production in gout and 2,8-dioxyadenine production in patients with homozygous adenine phosphoribosyltransferase deficiency and 2,8-dioxyadenine renal stones. Clofibrate, which inhibits the synthesis or release of triglycerides from the liver, reduces blood lipid levels to normal in type III hyperlipoproteinemia.

Amplification of Enzyme Activity

Many enzyme proteins require vitamin-derived or metal cofactors for biologic activity. In some inborn errors of metabolism, the mutation affects the ability of the apoenzyme to combine with its cofactor [115]. In other genetic disorders, there is a metabolic defect in the conversion of a precursor vitamin to its active cofactor form. In both situations, administration of the appropriate cofactor may alleviate the metabolic abnormality by increasing the catalytic activity of the apoenzyme. Pyridoxine (vitamin B_6) is a cofactor for the enzyme cystathionine synthetase. In more than one-half of patients with homocystinuria due to deficient activity of this enzyme, administration of large doses of pyridoxine partially overcomes the block in homocystine metabolism. Similarly, the metabolic ketoacidosis of some patients with methylmalonic aciduria is corrected by treatment with pharmacologic doses of vitamin B_{12}, and the clinical and hematologic abnormalities of patients with hereditary dihydrofolate reductase deficiency are corrected by administration of small doses of 5-formyltetrahydrofolate, which bypasses the metabolic block (replacement of the deficient end product).

Phenobarbital and certain other drugs increase production of smooth endoplasmic reticulum and of certain of its enzymes, including NADPH-cytochrome c reductase, cytochrome P-450, and several drug-hydroxylating enzymes [116]. Administration of phenobarbital to patients with unconjugated hyperbilirubinemia in a variant of the Crigler-Najjar syndrome or with Gilbert's syndrome may result in a fall in plasma bilirubin levels secondary to induction of hepatic glucuronyl transferase.

Replacement of the Mutant Protein

Direct replacement of the missing protein is an attractive approach to the treatment of recessively inherited diseases. Greater success has been achieved in deficiencies of nonenzymatic than of enzymatic proteins. Examples include replacement of gamma globulin in agammaglobulinemia, of albumin in analbuminemia, or of factor VIII in hemophilia. In each of these cases, the deficient gene product is a plasma protein. The metabolic and immunologic defects of patients with severe combined immunodeficiency due to adenosine deaminase deficiency are transiently corrected by infusion of irradiated erythrocytes containing normal levels of adenosine deaminase activity.

Much less success has attended efforts to replace missing enzymes that normally function within cells. Enzyme infusions have been attempted in the mucopolysaccharidoses, Gaucher's disease, Tay-Sachs disease, and Pompe's disease, but the therapeutic benefits are unproved. The lysosomal storage diseases are perhaps the best candidates for treatment by administration of exogenous enzymes, for body cells have highly specific mechanisms for taking up exogenous proteins and delivering them to lysosomes [62]. In order for this mechanism to be effective, the exogenous protein must be able to bind to a specific recognition site on the plasma membrane of the target cell so that it can be selectively internalized.

A number of attempts have been made to use naturally occurring receptors on the cell surface to achieve this binding. The most logical receptor is the one for the lysosomal enzymes themselves. The work of Sly's laboratory [67] and Neufeld's laboratory [117] has demonstrated that lysosomal enzymes contain covalently bound residues of mannose-6-phosphate. Many body cells such as hepatocytes, kidney cells, and fibroblasts have plasma membrane receptors that bind proteins that contain mannose-6-phosphate and facilitate their cellular uptake and delivery to lysosomes. This mannose-6-phosphate receptor system normally functions on intracellular membranes, where it plays a role in directing newly synthesized lysosomal enzymes to lysosomes. Since some of these receptors are on the cell surface, they should facilitate the delivery of intravenously administered lysosomal enzymes to cellular lysosomes. Such therapy in humans would require purification of large amounts of the appropriate mannose-6-phosphate-containing human lysosomal enzyme. Unfortunately, the most readily obtained source of human enzyme, the placenta, yields lysosomal enzymes that have already had their mannose-6-phosphate residues removed enzymatically [118]. Such removal normally occurs after the enzyme reaches the lysosome. Thus, it is unlikely that sufficient amounts of human mannose-6-phosphate-containing enzyme could be purified to permit successful therapy. An additional problem is tissue specificity. Even if large amounts of a mannose-6-phosphate-containing enzyme were available, some means would be necessary to direct it to specific cells. This delivery problem is particularly troublesome in the case of lysosomal storage disorders, such as Tay-Sachs disease, that affect the brain. Direct delivery of enzymes to the brain will require circumvention of the blood-brain barrier, a feat that may be accomplished through the intravascular administration of hypertonic mannitol solutions [119].

An alternative method for delivery of enzymes to lysosomes of specific tissues is to couple the enzymes covalently to another molecule for which the tissue contains receptors. If the receptors normally carry out receptor-mediated endocytosis, then the coupled lysosomal enzyme would be carried in "piggyback" fashion to cellular lysosomes along with the primary ligand [120]. One attractive aspect of this scheme is that one could use ligands for which receptors exist only in certain tissues. This would achieve specificity of cellular targeting as well as intracellular targeting.

A host of receptors are now known to engage in receptor-mediated endocytosis and would be useful for such delivery [62]. For example, one could use the mannose-6-phosphate receptor itself by coupling purified placental mannose-6-phosphate-deficient lysosomal enzymes with other proteins, such as yeast mannans, that contain such residues. Preferably the mannose-6-phosphate residues could be coupled directly with the lysosomal enzymes themselves, thus avoiding the necessity of a foreign protein.

Other receptor systems that could be used include the LDL receptor, the asialoglycoprotein receptor, and the α-2-macroglobulin receptor [62]. Particularly useful might be a recently described receptor that binds acetylated LDL [121]. This receptor is so far known to be expressed only on macrophagelike cells, including hepatic Kuppfer cells, peritoneal macrophages, and other tissue histiocytes. This receptor might be useful in foam-cell diseases such as Gaucher's disease, in which macrophages are a prominent focus of accumulation of the deposited material. Macrophage receptors for the Fc component of immunoglobulins could also be used for the same purpose.

Instead of coupling the lysosomal enzyme directly to the receptor-specific ligand, some investigators have incorporated the ligand into artificial phospholipid-cholesterol vesicles or liposomes [122, 123]. The surface of the liposome is then coated with a material that will direct the liposome to a target cell. Beutler and coworkers have modified this method by using vesicles made from hyptonically lysed and resealed red cells into which glucocerebrosidase has been incorporated [124]. These artificial cells remain in the circulation longer than do the liposomes, and eventually they are taken up by macrophages in the liver and spleen. Unfortunately, fairly extensive trials of this approach in patients with Gaucher's disease have not yet been successful.

In general, attempts at direct enzyme replacement in lysosomal enzyme deficiency diseases have so far not yielded positive therapeutic results. In many cases, the delivery methods used were not sophisticated. New knowledge of the normal mechanism of lysosomal enzyme delivery and of the process of receptor-mediated endocytosis may allow such therapy to succeed in the future.

Modification of the Mutant Protein

Many proteins can be modified by the addition of subgroups. For example, sickle-cell hemoglobin can be carbamylated by cyanate at the valine in position 1 of the β chain, which then blocks the hydrophobic bonding of the normal Val-1 to the mutant Val-6 of the β globin of hemoglobin S, thereby preventing sickling in vitro. Severe toxic reactions, such as peripheral neuropathy, sharply limit the clinical usefulness of cyanate therapy in patients with sickle-cell disease. Nevertheless, this approach holds promise for the future.

Organ Transplantation

Allotransplantation of the organ in which the deficient enzyme is normally synthesized has been attempted in a variety of inherited diseases. By far the greatest experience has involved renal transplantation, which has been performed in the Alport syndrome, the adult from of polycystic kidney disease, renal amyloidosis, cystinosis, Fabry's disease, Gaucher's disease, oxalosis, and some other conditions [125]. The results in most instances have paralleled those of renal transplantation for other forms of end-stage renal disease. There has been no evidence of reactivation of the renal lesion in patients with the Alport syndrome or of the development of cystinosis or Fabry's disease in the transplanted kidneys. Amyloidosis has recurred in the graft on rare occasions. By contrast, severe recurrent oxalosis has developed in a number of transplanted kidneys, and end-stage renal failure due to oxalosis is not now considered an indication for renal transplantation. Patients with Fabry's disease have developed measurable levels of the missing enzyme, ceramide trihexosidase, in plasma following renal transplantation, and there have been a few long-term survivals. Nevertheless, renal transplantation in patients with inborn errors of metabolism should be limited to replacement of failed kidneys. Results do not warrant the use of renal transplantation primarily for enzyme replacement.

Transplantation of allogenic marrow has successfully corrected a number of immunodeficiency states, including lymphopenic hypogammaglobulinemia (Swiss type), the Wiscott-Aldrich syndrome, and severe combined immunodeficiency disease [126–128].

Surgical Removal

Surgery also plays a role in certain hereditary disorders. Examples include splenectomy in hereditary spherocytosis and colectomy in preventing neoplastic transformation in familial polyposis of the colon. Also, surgery offers a quick and permanent cure for polydactyly as well as for certain other dominantly inherited structural defects.

Genetic Engineering

The conceptual and technological revolution in the realm of DNA has raised the real possibility of direct gene replacement in human genetic diseases [85, 129–131]. It is theoretically possible that a whole individual, or an isolated subset of his or her cells, could be infected with a virus carrying a normal copy of the mutated gene. The virus could be made to integrate into the host genome in such a way that the normal gene would be expressed. This therapeutic avenue, which would have been considered extremely visionary 5 years ago, is now a real possibility. A full discussion of this field is presented in Chap. 2.

REFERENCES

1. MCKUSICK VA: The anatomy of the human genome. *Am J Med* 69:267, 1980
2. MCKUSICK VA, RUDDLE FH: The status of the gene map of the human chromosomes. *Science* 196:390, 1977
3. GARROD AE: Inborn errors of metabolism (Croonian Lectures). *Lancet* 2:1, 73, 142, 214, 1908
4. GARROD AE: *Inborn Errors of Metabolism.* Oxford University Press, London, 1923
5. GARROD AE: A contribution to the study of alkaptonuria. *Proc R Med Chir Soc* 2, 130, 1899
6. GARROD AE: The incidence of alkaptonuria: A study in chemical individuality. *Lancet* 2:1616, 1902
7. MENDEL G: *Versuche über Pflanzenhybriden.* Leipzig, Engelmann, 1901
8. BEARN AG, MILLER ED: Archibald Garrod and the development of the concept of inborn errors of metabolism. *Bull Hist Med* 53:315, 1979
9. LADU BN, ZANNONI VA, LASTER L, SEEGMILLER JE: The nature of the defect in tyrosine metabolism in alcaptonuria. *J Biol Chem* 230:251, 1958
10. JOHANNSEN W: The genotype conception of heredity. *Am Nat* 45:129, 1911
11. BEADLE GW: Biochemical genetics. *Chem Rev* 37:15, 1945
12. BEADLE GW, TATUM EL: Experimental control of developmental reactions. *Am Nat* 75:107, 1941
13. BEADLE GW, TATUM EL: Genetic control of biochemical reactions in *Neurospora. Proc Natl Acad Sci USA* 27:499, 1941
14. EPHRUSSI B: Chemistry of "eye color hormones" of *Drosophila. Q Rev Biol* 17:327, 1942
15. BEADLE GW: Genes and chemical reactions in *Neurospora. Science* 129:1715, 1959
16. TATUM EL: A case history in biological research. *Science* 129:1711, 1959
17. HOROWITZ NH, LEUPOLD U: Some recent studies bearing on the one gene one enzyme hypothesis. *Symp Quant Biol* 16:65, 1951
18. BENZER S: The elementary units of heredity, in McElroy WD, Glass B (eds): *The Chemical Basis of Heredity.* Baltimore, Johns Hopkins University Press, 1957, p 70
19. GIBSON QH: The reduction of methaemoglobin in red blood cells and studies on the cause of idiopathic methaemoglobinaemia. *Biochem J* 42:13, 1948
20. CORI GT, CORI CF: Glucose-6-phosphatase of the liver in glycogen storage disease. *J Biol Chem* 199:661, 1952
21. JERVIS GA: Phenylpyruvic oligophrenia: Deficiency of phenylalanine oxidizing system. *Proc Soc Exp Biol Med* 82:514, 1953
22. PAULING L, ITANO HA, SINGER SJ, WELLS IC: Sickle cell anemia: A molecular disease. *Science* 110:543, 1949
23. INGRAM VM: A specific chemical difference between the globins of normal human and sickle cell anaemia haemoglobin. *Nature* 178:792, 1956
24. KORNBERG A: *DNA Replication.* San Francisco, WH Freeman & Co Publishers, 1980
25. WATSON JD: *Molecular Biology of the Gene,* ed 3. New York, WA Benjamin, Inc, 1976
26. HARRIS H: *The Principles of Human Biochemical Genetics,* ed 3. Amsterdam, North-Holland Publishing Co, 1980
27. HARRIS H: Enzyme polymorphisms in man. *Proc Roy Soc B* 174:1, 1966
28. LEWONTIN RC, HUBBY JL: A molecular approach to the study of genetic heterozygosity in natural populations. II. Amount of variation and degree of heterozygosity in natural population of *Drosophila pseudoobscura. Genetics* 54:595, 1966
29. WALTON KE, STYER D, GRUENSTEIN EI: Genetic polymorphism in normal human fibroblasts as analyzed by two-dimensional polyacrylamide gel electrophoresis. *J Biol Chem* 254:7951, 1979
30. MCCONKEY EH, TAYLOR BJ, PHAN D: Human heterozygosity: A new estimate. *Proc Natl Acad Sci USA* 76:6500, 1979
31. MCKUSICK VA: *Mendelian Inheritance in Man: Catalogs of Autosomal Dominant, Autosomal Research, and X-Linked Phenotypes,* ed 5. Baltimore, Johns Hopkins University Press, 1978
32. MORGAN TH: The relation of genetics to physiology and medicine, in Baltimore D (ed): *Nobel Lectures in Molecular Biology 1933–1975.* New York, Elsevier North-Holland Inc, 1977, p 3
33. VOGEL F, MOTULSKY AG: *Human Genetics: Problems and Approaches.* Berlin, Springer-Verlag, 1979
34. ENGEL E: The chromosomal basis of human heredity, in Stanbury JB, Wyngaarden JB, Fredrickson DS, (eds): *The Metabolic Basis of Inherited Disease.* New York: McGraw-Hill Book Co, 1978, p 51
35. GALJAARD H: *Genetic Metabolic Diseases: Early Diagnosis and Prenatal Analysis.* Amsterdam, Elsevier/North-Holland Biochemical Press, 1980
36. CARTER CO: Monogenic disorders. *J Med Genet* 14:316, 1977
37. BUNDEY S, EVANS K: Tuberous sclerosis—a genetic study. *J Neurol Neurosurg Psychiatr* 32:591, 1969
38. JONES KL, SMITH DW, HARVEY MAS, HALL BD, QUAN L: Older paternal age and fresh gene mutation: Data on additional disorders. *J Pediatr* 86:84, 1975
39. MURDOCH JL, WALKER BA, MCKUSICK VA: Parental age effects on the occurrence of new mutations for the Marfan syndrome. *Ann Hum Genet* 35:331, 1972
40. BALLARD HS, FRAME B, HARTSOCK RJ: Familial multiple endocrine adenoma-peptic ulcer complex. *Medicine* 43:481, 1964
41. BROWN MS, GOLDSTEIN JL: New directions in human biochemical genetics: Understanding the manifestations of receptor deficiency disorders. *Prog Med Genet* 1 (new series):103, 1976
42. HERS HG: Inborn lysosomal diseases. *Gastroenterology* 48:625, 1965
43. NEUFELD EF, TIMPLE WL, SHAPIRO LJ: Inherited disorders of lysosomal metabolism. *Ann Rev Biochem* 44:357, 1975

44. CAVALLI-STORZA LL, BODMER WF: *The Genetics of Human Populations.* San Francisco, WH Freeman & Co Publishers, 1971

45. LYON MF: X-Chromosome inactivation and developmental patterns in mammals. *Biol Rev* 47:1, 1972

46. CARTER CO: Genetics of common disorders. *Br Med Bull* 25:52, 1972

47. CARTER CO: Principles of polygenic inheritance. *Birth Defects: Original Article Series* 13:69, 1977

48. MCMICHAEL A, MCDEVITT H: The association between the HLA system and disease. *Prog Med Genet* 2 (new series):39, 1977

49. GOLDSTEIN JL, SCHROTT HG, HAZZARD WR, BIERMAN EL, MOTULSKY AG: Hyperlipidemia in coronary heart disease. II. Genetic analysis of lipid levels in 176 families and delineation of a new inherited disorder, combined hyperlipidemia. *J Clin Invest* 52:1544, 1973

50. VESELL ES: Pharmacogenetics: Multiple interactions between genes and environment as determinants of drug response. *Am J Med* 66:183, 1979

51. CHILDS B, DER KALOUSTIAN VM: Genetic heterogeneity. *N Engl J Med* 279:1205, 1267, 1968

52. HARRIS H: Genetic heterogeneity in inherited disease. *J Clin Pathol* 27, (suppl 8):32, 1974

53. MCKUSICK VA: Analytic review: Phenotypic diversity of human diseases resulting from allelic series. *Am J Hum Genet* 25:446, 1973

54. CHANG JC, KAN YW: β⁰ Thalassemia, a nonsense mutation in man. *Proc Natl Acad Sci USA* 76:2886, 1979

55. PAIGEN K: Acid hydrolases as models of genetic control. *Ann Rev Genet* 13:417, 1979

56. JACOB F, MONOD J: Genetic regulatory mechanisms in the synthesis of proteins. *J Mol Biol* 3:318, 1961

57. JACOB F, MONOD J: On the regulation of gene activity. *Symp Quant Biol* 38:193, 1963

58. DARNELL JE: Implications of RNA-RNA splicing in evolution of eukaryotic cells. *Science* 202:1257, 1978

59. SUTTON HE, WAGNER RP: Mutation and enzyme function in humans. *Ann Rev Genet* 9:187, 1975

60. YOSHIDA A, LIEBERMAN J, GAIDULIS L, EWING C: Molecular abnormality of human alpha₁-antitrypsin variant (Pi-ZZ) associated with plasma activity deficiency. *Proc Natl Acad Sci USA* 73:1324, 1976

61. HEREZ A, KATONA E, CUTZ E, WILSON JR, BARTON M: α₁-Antitrypsin: The presence of excess mannose in the Z variant isolated from liver. *Science* 201:1229, 1978

62. GOLDSTEIN JL, ANDERSON RGW, BROWN MS: Coated pits, coated vesicles, and receptor-mediated endocytosis. *Nature* 279:679, 1979

63. FARFEL Z, BRICKMAN AS, KASLOW HR, BROTHERS VM, BOURNE HR: Defect of receptor-cyclase coupling protein in pseudohypoparathyroidism. *N Engl J Med* 303:238, 1980

64. LEVINE MA, DOWNS RW, JR, SINGER M, MARX SJ, AURBACH GD, SPIEGEL AM: Deficient activity of guanine nucleotide regulatory protein in erythrocytes from patients with pseudohypoparathyroidism. *Biochem Biophys Res Comm* 94:1319, 1980

65. SILVERSTEIN SC (ed): *Transport of Macromolecules in Cellular Systems.* Berlin, Dahlem Konferenzen, 1978

66. BLOBEL G: Intracellular protein topogenesis. *Proc Natl Acad Sci USA* 77:1496, 1980

67. KAPLAN A, ACHORD DT, SLY WS: Phosphohexosyl components of a lysosomal enzyme are recognized by pinocytosis receptors on human fibroblasts. *Proc Natl Acad Sci USA* 74:2026, 1977

68. GOLDSTEIN JL, BROWN MS: The LDL receptor locus and the genetics of familial hypercholesterolemia. *Ann Rev Genet* 13:259, 1979

69. AFZELIUS BA: The immotile-cilia syndrome and other ciliary disorders. *Int Rev Exp Pathol* 19:1, 1979

70. KRONE SM, PINNELL SR, ERBE RW: Lysylprotocollagen hydroxylase deficiency in fibroblasts from siblings with hydroxylysine-deficient collagen. *Proc Natl Acad Sci USA* 69:2899, 1972

71. THOMAS GH, HOWELL RR: *Selected Screening Tests for Genetic Metabolic Diseases.* Chicago, Year Book Medical Publishers Inc, 1973

72. HSIA DY-Y: Study of hereditary metabolic diseases using in vitro techniques. *Metabolism* 19:309, 1970

73. KROOTH RS, DARLINGTON GA, VELAZQUEZ AA: The genetics of cultured mammalian cells. *Ann Rev Genet* 2:141, 1968

74. NEUFELD EF, FRATANTONI JC: Inborn errors of mucopolysaccharide metabolism. *Science* 169:141, 1970

75. CLEAVER JE, BOOTSMA D: Xeroderma pigmentosum: Biochemical and genetic characteristics. *Ann Rev Genet* 9:19, 1975

76. *The Human Genetic Mutant Cell Repository: List of Genetic Variants, Chromosomal Aberrations and Normal Cell Cultures Submitted to the Repository,* ed 7. Bethesda, Md, NIH Publication No 80-2011, 1980

77. KAN YW, DOZY AM: Antenatal diagnosis of sickle-cell anemia by DNA analysis of amniotic fluid cells. *Lancet* 2:910, 1978

78. BERG K: Inactivation of one of the X chromosomes in females is a biological phenomenon of clinical importance. *Acta Med Scand* 206:1, 1979

79. FIALKOW PJ, LISKER R, GIBLETT ER, ZAVALA C: Xg locus: Failure to detect inactivation in females with chronic myelocytic leukaemia. *Nature* 226:367, 1970

80. SHAPIRO LJ, MOHANDAS T, WEISS R: Non-inactivation of an X-chromosome locus in man. *Science* 204:1224, 1979

81. MIGEON BR, CHILDS B: Hybridization of mammalian somatic cells. *Prog Med Genet* 7 (old series):1, 1970

82. SAUNDERS M, SWEETMAN L, ROBINSON B, ROTH K, COHN R, GRAVEL RA: Biotin-response organicaciduria: Multiple carboxylase defects and complementation studies with propionicacidemia in cultured fibroblasts. *J Clin Invest* 64:1695, 1979

83. GRAVEL RA, LEUNG A, SAUNDERS M, HOSLI P: Analysis of genetic complementation by whole-cell microtechniques in fibroblast heterokaryons. *Proc Natl Acad Sci USA* 76:6520, 1979

84. SMITH HO: Nucleotide sequence specificity of restriction endonucleases. *Science* 205:455, 1979

85. NATHANS D: Restriction endonucleases, Simian virus 40, and the new genetics. *Science* 206:903, 1979

86. SOUTHERN EM: Detection of specific sequences among DNA fragments separated by gel electrophoresis. *J Mol Biol* 98:503, 1975

87. FLAVELL RA, BERNARDS R, KOOTER JM, DEBOER E, LITTLE PFR, ANNISON G, WILLIAMSON R: The structure of human β-globin gene in β-thalassaemia. *Nucleic Acids Res* 6:249, 1979

88. WEATHERALL DJ, CLEGG JB: Recent developments in the molecular genetics of human hemoglobin. *Cell* 16:467, 1979

89. FORGET BG: Molecular genetics of human hemoglobin synthesis. *Ann Intern Med* 91:605, 1979

90. BANK A, MEARS G, RAMIREZ F: Disorders of human hemoglobin. *Science* 207:493, 1980

91. KAN YW, DOZY AM: Evolution of the hemoglobin S and C genes in world populations. *Science* 209:388, 1980

92. MILUNSKY A: Prenatal diagnosis of genetic disorders. *N Engl J Med* 300:157, 1976

93. EPSTEIN CJ, GOLBUS MS: Prenatal diagnosis of genetic diseases. *Am Sci* 65:703, 1977

94. BROCK DJH: Biochemical and cytological methods in the diagnosis of neural tube defects. *Prog Med Genet* 2 (new series):1, 1977

95. GIBSON SLM, FERGUSON-SMITH MA: The use of genetic linkage in counselling families with dystrophia myotonica. *Clin Genet* 17:443, 1980

96. *Genetic Screening: Programs, Principles and Research.* Washington, DC, National Academy of Sciences, 1975

97. SCRIVER CR, NEAL JL, SAGINUR R, CLOW A: The frequency of genetic disease and congenital malformation among patients in a pediatric hospital. *Can Med Assoc J* 108:1111, 1973

98. MACCREADY RA, HUSSEY MG: Newborn phenylketonuria detection program in Massachusetts. *Am J Public Health* 54:2075, 1964

99. LEVY HL: Newborn metabolic screening: Past and prospect. *N Engl J Med* 293:824, 1975

100. LEVY HL: Genetic screening. *Adv Hum Genet* 4:1, 1973

101. Massachusetts Department of Public Health: Cost-benefit analysis of newborn screening for metabolic disorders. *N Engl J Med* 291:1414, 1974

102. RAINE DN: Inherited metabolic disease. *Lancet* 2:996, 1974

103. GUTHRIE R: Mass screening for genetic disease. *Hosp Pract* 7:93, 1972

104. KABACK MM, O'BRIEN JS: Tay-Sachs: Prototype for prevention of genetic disease, in McKusick VA, Claiborne R (eds): *Medical Genetics.* New York, HP Publishing Co, 1974, p 253

105. MIGEON BR: X-linked hypoxanthine-guanine phosphoribosyl transferase deficiency: Detection of heterozygotes by selective medium. *Biochem Genet* 4:377, 1970

106. BOYLE JA, RAIVIO KO, ASTRIN KH, SCHULMAN JD, GRAF ML, SEEGMILLER JE, JACOBSEN CB: Lesch-Nyhan syndrome: Preventive control by prenatal diagnosis. *Science* 169:688, 1970

107. KAN YW, DOZY AM, ALTER BP, FRIGOLETTO FD, NATHAN DG: Detection of the sickle gene in human fetus. Potential for intrauterine diagnosis of sickle-cell anemia. *N Engl J Med* 287:1, 1972

108. HOBBINS JC, MAHONEY MJ: In utero diagnosis of hemoglobinopathies. *N Engl J Med* 290:1065, 1974

109. CHANG H, HOBBINS JR, CIVIDALLI G, FRIGOLETTO FD, MAHONEY MJ, KAN YW, NATHAN DG: In utero diagnosis of hemoglobinopathies. Hemoglobin synthesis in fetal red cells. *N Engl J Med* 290:1067, 1974

110. KAN YW, GOLBUS MS, TRECARTIN R: Prenatal diagnosis of sickle-cell anemia. *N Engl J Med* 294:1039, 1976

111. ALTER BP, FRIEDMAN S, HOBBINS JC, MAHONEY MJ, SHERMAN AS, MCSWEENEY JF, SCHWARTZ E, NATHAN DG: Prenatal diagnosis of sickle-cell anemia and alpha G-Philadelphia. *N Engl J Med* 294:1040, 1976

112. BROWN MS, KOVANEN PT, GOLDSTEIN JL, ECKELS R, VANDENBERGHE K, VAN DEN BERGE H, TRYNS JP, CASSIMAN JJ: Prenatal diagnosis of homozygous familial hypercholesterolemia: Expression of a genetic receptor disease in utero. *Lancet* 1:526, 1978

113. BEUTLER E: The Duarte variant in galactosemia, in Hsia Dy-Y (ed): *Galactosemia.* Springfield, Ill, Charles C Thomas Publisher, 1969, p 163

114. HOLTZMAN NA: Dietary treatment of inborn errors of metabolism. *Ann Rev Med* 21:335, 1970

115. ROSENBERG LE: Vitamin-responsive inherited metabolic disorders. *Adv Hum Genet* 6:1, 1976

116. SCHIMKE RT, DOYLE D: Control of enzyme levels in animal tissues. *Ann Rev Biochem* 39:929, 1970

117. HASILIK A, NEUFELD EF: Biosynthesis of lysosomal enzymes in fibroblasts: Phosphorylation of mannose residues. *J Biol Chem* 255:4946, 1980

118. ACHORD DT, BROT FE, BELL CE, SLY WS: Human β-glucuronidase: In vivo clearance and in vitro uptake by a glycoprotein recognition system on reticuloendothelial cells. *Cell* 15:269, 1978

119. BARRANGER JA, RAPOPORT SI, FREDERICKS WR, PENTCHEV PG, MacDERMOT KD, STENSING JK, BRADY RO: Modification of the blood-brain barrier: Increased concentration and fate of enzymes entering the brain. *Proc Natl Acad Sci USA* 76:481, 1979

120. NEVILLE DM, JR, CHANG T-M: Receptor-mediated protein transport into cells. Entry mechanisms for toxins, hormones, antibodies, viruses, lysosomal hydrolases, asialoglycoproteins, and carrier proteins. *Curr Top Membr Transport* 10:65, 1978

121. BROWN MS, BASU SK, FALCK JR, HO YK, GOLDSTEIN JL: The scavenger cell pathway for lipoprotein degradation: Specificity of the binding site that mediates the uptake of negatively-charged LDL by macrophages. *J Supra Struct* 13:67, 1980

122. DESNICK RJ, THORPE SR, FIDDLER MB: Toward enzyme therapy for lysosomal storage diseases. *Physiol Rev* 56:57, 1976

123. DESNICK RJ: Prospects for enzyme therapy in the lysosomal storage diseases of Ashkenazi Jews, in Goodman RM, Motulsky AG (eds): *Genetic Diseases among Ashkenazi Jews*. New York, Raven Press, 1979, p 253

124. BEUTLER E: Gaucher disease, in Goodman RM, Motulsky AG (eds): *Genetic Diseases among Ashkenazi Jews*. New York, Raven Press, 1979, p 157

125. Renal transplantation in congenital and metabolic diseases: A report from the ASC/NIH renal transplant registry. *JAMA* 232:148, 1975

126. MEUWISSEN HJ, GATTI RA, TERASAKI PI, HONG R, GOOD RA: Treatment of lymphopenic hypogamma-globulinemia and bone-marrow aplasia by transplantation of allogeneic marrow. *N Engl J Med* 281:691, 1969

127. BACH FH, ALBERTINE RJ, JOO P, ANDERSON JL, BORTIN MM: Bone-marrow transplantation in a patient with the Wiskott-Aldrich syndrome. *Lancet* 2:1364, 1968

128. BUCKLEY RH, WHISNANT JK, SCHIFF RI, GILBERTSEN RB, HUANG AT, PLATT MS: Correction of severe combined immunodeficiency by fetal liver cells. *N Engl J Med* 294:1076, 1976

129. COHEN SN: Gene manipulation. *N Engl J Med* 294:883, 1976

130. PELLICER A, ROBINS D, WOLD B, SWEET R, JACKSON J, LOWRY I, ROBERTS JM, SIM GK, SILVERSTEIN S, AXEL R: Altering genotype and phenotype by DNA-mediated gene transfer. *Science* 209:1414, 1980

131. MULLIGAN RC, BERG P: Expression of a bacterial gene in mammalian cells. *Science* 209:1422, 1980

132. GIBLETT ER: Genetic polymorphisms in human blood. *Ann Rev Genet* 11:13, 1977

133. MOTULSKY AG: Frequency of sickling disorders in U.S. Blacks. *N Engl J Med* 288:31, 1973

SUMMARY TABLES FOR INBORN ERRORS OF METABOLISM

● DISORDERS OF CARBOHYDRATE METABOLISM ●

Name of disease	Chap. no.	Prevalence	Mode of inheritance	Mutant gene product	Chromosomal location	Altered DNA structure	Disturbed protein function	Disrupted cell and organ function
Diabetes mellitus, type 1 (insulin-dependent, ketosis-prone)	4	1 per 500	Unknown	Unknown	Susceptibility influenced by gene(s) linked to HLA locus on short arm of chromosome 6	Unknown	Unknown	Destruction of pancreatic β-cells by (?) virus or (?) autoimmune factors leads to insulin deficiency and relative glucagon excess. Hyperglycemia, ketoacidosis, angiopathy, and neuropathy result.
Diabetes mellitus, type 2 (insulin-dependent, ketosis-resistant)	4	1 per 130 Caucasians; uncertain in Blacks	Unknown	Unknown	Unknown	Unknown	Unknown	Impaired insulin secretion or resistance to insulin action leads to relative insulin deficiency and glucagon excess. Hyperglycemia, angiopathy, and neuropathy result.
Essential fructosuria	5	~ 1 per 130,000; more common in Jews	Autosomal recessive	Fructokinase	Unknown	Unknown	Deficient enzyme activity	Decreased conversion of fructose to fructose-1-phosphate leads to alimentary hyperfructosemia and fructosuria. No clinical dysfunction.
Hereditary fructose intolerance	5	1 per 20,000 in Switzerland	Autosomal recessive	Fructose-1-phosphate aldolase	Unknown	Unknown	Deficient enzyme activity	Ingestion of fructose leads to accumulation of fructose-1-phosphate, which inhibits glycogenolysis and gluconeogenesis, causing hypoglycemia.
Hereditary fructose-1,6-diphophatase deficiency	5	32 cases reported	Autosomal recessive	Fructose-1,6-diphosphatase	Unknown	Unknown	Absent or deficient enzyme activity	Gluconeogenesis is impaired, causing accumulation of gluconeogenic precursors such as amino acids, lactate, and ketones. This in turn leads to hypoglycemia, ketosis, and lactic acidosis.
Glycogen storage disease, type I (von Gierke's disease)	6	~ 1 per 100,000	Autosomal recessive	Glucose-6-phosphatase	Unknown	Unknown	Absent enzyme activity	Deficiency of product (glucose) leads to hypoglycemia. Accumulation of glycogen in liver and kidney causes organomegaly.
Glycogen storage disease, type II (Pompe's disease)	6	~ 1 per 100,000	Autosomal recessive	Lysosomal α-1,4-glucosidase	17 (long arm)	Unknown	Absent or deficient enzyme activity	Glycogen accumulates within lysosomes of muscle and heart. Muscle weakness and heart failure occur.
Glycogen storage disease, type III (Cori's disease, Forbes' disease)	6	~ 1 per 100,000	Autosomal recessive	Amylo-1,6-glucosidase (debrancher enzyme)	Unknown	Unknown	Deficient enzyme activity	Structurally abnormal glycogen accumulates in liver and muscle. Hepatomegaly and muscle weakness occur.
Glycogen storage disease, type IV (Andersen's disease)	6	1 per 500,000	Autosomal recessive	Amylo-(1,4:1,6)-transglucosidase (brancher enzyme)	Unknown	Unknown	Deficient enzyme activity	Accumulation of structurally abnormal glycogen in liver causes cirrhosis.
Glycogen storage disease, type V (McArdle's disease)	6	1 per 500,000	Autosomal recessive	Muscle phosphorylase	Unknown	Unknown	Absent or deficient enzyme activity	Accumulation of glycogen in muscle causes muscle cramps on exercise and myoglobinuria.
Glycogen storage disease, type VI (Hers' disease)	6	1 per 200,000	Autosomal recessive	Hepatic phosphorylase	Unknown	Unknown	Deficient enzyme activity	Accumulation of glycogen in liver causes hepatomegaly.

SUMMARY TABLES FOR INBORN ERRORS OF METABOLISM

Name of disease	Chap. no.	Prevalence	Mode of inheritance	Mutant gene product	Chromosomal location	Altered DNA structure	Disturbed protein function	Disrupted cell and organ function
							Expression	
Glycogen storage disease, type VII (Tauri's disease)	6	1 per 500,000	Autosomal recessive	Muscle phosphofructokinase	Unknown	Unknown	Deficient enzyme activity	Accumulation of glycogen in muscle. Exercise intolerance occurs.
Glycogen storage disease, type VIII (liver phosphorylase deficiency)	6	~ 1 per 100,000	X-Linked recessive	Phosphorylase-b-kinase	X	Unknown	Deficient enzyme activity	Accumulation of glycogen in liver causes hepatomegaly.
Galactosemia	7	1 per 62,000	Autosomal recessive	Galactose-1-phosphate uridyl transferase	9 (short arm)	Unknown	Absent enzyme activity	Accumulation of galactitol, galactose-1-phosphate, and galactonate causes cataracts, mental retardation, and liver and kidney dysfunction.
Galactokinase deficiency	7	~ 1 per 100,000	Autosomal recessive	Galactokinase	17 (long arm)	Unknown	Absent enzyme activity	Accumulation of galactitol causes cataracts.
Galactose epimerase deficiency	7	Unknown	Autosomal recessive	Uridine diphosphogalactose-4-epimerase	1 (short arm)	Unknown	Absent enzyme activity	Galactose-1-phosphate accumulates in red cells without clinical dysfunction.
Pentosuria	8	1 per 2500 Ashkenazi Jews	Autosomal recessive	L-Xylulose reductase	Unknown	Unknown	Deficient enzyme activity	Accumulation of substrate (L-xylulose) leads to its continuous excretion in the urine without apparent clinical dysfunction.
Pyruvate dehydrogenase complex deficiency	9	< 100 cases reported	Autosomal recessive	One of several proteins of pyruvate dehydrogenase complex	Unknown	Unknown	Deficient enzyme activity	Deficiency of product (acetyl CoA) leads to decreased synthesis of acetylcholine, thereby causing neurological abnormalities.
Pyruvate carboxylase deficiency	9	< 20 cases reported	Autosomal recessive	Pyruvate carboxylase	Unknown	Unknown	Absent or deficient enzyme activity	Deficiency of product (oxaloacetate) leads to decreased gluconeogenesis, causing: (1) fasting hypoglycemia and lactic acid acidosis and (2) decreased synthesis of amino acid neurotransmitters and neurological abnormalities.
Primary hyperoxaluria, type I	10	Uncommon, but not rare	Autosomal recessive	2-Oxoglutarate: glyoxylate carboligase (soluble)	Unknown	Unknown	Deficient enzyme activity	Block in metabolism of glyoxylate leads to precursor accumulation, causing hyperoxaluria with oxalosis and calcium oxalate nephrolithiasis.
Primary hyperoxaluria, type II	10	4 cases reported	Autosomal recessive	D-Glycerate dehydrogenase	Unknown	Unknown	Absent enzyme activity	Enzyme abnormality leads to excessive synthesis of oxalate, causing hyperoxaluria and calcium oxalate nephrolithiasis. Link between enzyme abnormality and oxalate overproduction is not established.

Disorder	Chromosome	Frequency	Inheritance	Defect	Location		Enzyme activity	Comments
Familial goiter (multiple disorders involving gene loci that produce defects in thyrotropin responsiveness, iodide transport, iodide organification, coupling of iodotyrosines, deiodination of iodotyrosines, synthesis of thyroglobulin, and thyroid hormone responsiveness)	11	Rare	Autosomal recessive	Unknown for most disorders Organification defects: thyroid peroxidase system Deiodination defects: iodotyrosine deiodinase system	Unknown	Unknown	Unknown for most disorders; absent or defective enzymes for organification and deiodination defects	Decreased secretion of thyroid hormone leads to enhanced secretion of thyrotropin, thus producing goiter with or without hypothyroidism.
Hyperphenylalanemia, type I (classic phenylketonuria)	12	1 per 11,000	Autosomal recessive	Phenylalanine hydroxylase	Unknown	Unknown	Absent enzyme activity	Accumulation of substrate (phenylalanine) or its metabolite(s) interferes with brain maturation (synaptogenesis) and myelination, causing brain dysfunction.
Hyperphenylalanemia, types II and III	12	1 per 43,000	Autosomal recessive	Phenylalanine hydroxylase	Unknown	Unknown	Deficient enzyme activity (1.5-35 percent of normal)	Same as type I except that patients are either mildly retarded (type II) or normal (type III).
Hyperphenylalanemia, type IV (dihydropteridine reductase deficiency)	12	~1 per 1 million	Autosomal recessive	Dihydropteridine reductase	4 (short arm)	Unknown	Absent enzyme activity	Same as in type I. In addition, deficiency of biogenic amine synthesis and impaired oxidation of long-chain alkyl ethers of glycerol contribute to brain dysfunction.
Hyperphenylalanemia, type V (dihydrobiopterin synthetase deficiency)	12	~1 per 30,000	Autosomal recessive	Dihydrobiopterin synthetase	Unknown	Unknown	Deficient enzyme activity	Same as in type IV.
Tyrosinemia, type I (hepatorenal tyrosinemia; tyrosinosis)	13	1 per 100,000 worldwide; 1 per 10,000 in French Canadian isolate	Autosomal recessive	(?) Hydrolase for fumarylacetoacetate and maleylacetoacetate	Unknown	Unknown	Absent enzyme activity	Enzyme abnormality leads to accumulation of succinylacetone and succinylacetoacetone and their precursors, which inhibit several hepatic enzymes. This, in turn, leads to Fanconi syndrome and cirrhosis.
Tyrosinemia, type II (Richner-Hanhart syndrome)	13	Rare	Autosomal recessive	Tyrosine aminotransferase	Unknown	Unknown	Absent enzyme activity	Accumulated substrate (tyrosine) crystallizes in epidermis and cornea, causing palmar and plantar keratosis and corneal ulcers.
Alcaptonuria	14	~1 per 250,000	Autosomal recessive	Homogentisic acid oxidase	Unknown	Unknown	Absent enzyme activity	Accumulation of substrate (homogentisic acid) leads to deposition of ochronotic pigment (polymeric homogentisic acid) in connetive tissue, causing calcified ear cartilage, pigmented sclerae, and arthritis.
Oculocutaneous albinism, tyrosinase-negative type	15	1 per 39,000 Caucasians; 1 per 28,000 Blacks	Autosomal recessive	Tyrosinase	Unknown	Unknown	Absent enzyme activity	Deficiency of product (melanin) leads to nystagmus, decreased visual acuity, and increased susceptibility of skin to ultraviolet radiation-induced damage and cancer.

SUMMARY TABLES FOR INBORN ERRORS OF METABOLISM

Name of disease	Chap. no.	Prevalence	Mode of inheritance	Mutant gene product	Chromosomal location	Altered DNA structure	Disturbed protein function	Expression
								Disrupted cell and organ function
Oculocutaneous albinism, tyrosinase-positive type	15	1 per 37,000 Caucasians; 1 per 15,000 Blacks; ~1 per 150 in certain American Indians	Autosomal recessive	Unknown (nonallelic with tyrosinase-negative oculocutaneous albinism)	Unknown	Unknown	Unknown	Deficiency and maldistribution of melanin leads to marked hypopigmentation of oculocutaneous structures. This leads to nystagmus, decreased visual acuity, and increased susceptibility of skin to ultraviolet radiation-induced damage and cancer.
X-linked ocular albinism	15	~1 per 50,000	X-Linked recessive	Unknown	X (short arm)	Unknown	Unknown	Deficient synthesis of melanin in optic fundus with some reduction in pigment in irides and skin, leading to nystagmus and decreased visual acuity.
Chediak-Higashi syndrome	15	Rare	Autosomal recessive	Unknown	Unknown	Unknown	Unknown	Abnormal fusion of lysosome-like organelles produces enlarged lysosomes and melanosomes. This is associated with hypopigmentation of oculocutaneous structures (causing nystagmus, and decreased visual acuity) and decreased chemotaxis of neutrophils (causing infections). Platelet abnormalities, progressive neuropathy, and lymphoreticular malignancy also occur.
Hermansky-Pudlak syndrome	15	~1 per 60,000 Caucasians; 1 per 5000 Puerto Ricans	Autosomal recessive	Unknown	Unknown	Unknown	Unknown	Hypopigmentation of oculocutaneous structures causes nystagmus, decreased visual acuity, and increased susceptibility of skin to ultraviolet radiation-induced damage and cancer. Abnormal platelet function leads to hemorrhagic diathesis.
Histidinemia	16	Rare	Autosomal recessive	Histidase	Unknown	Unknown	Absent enzyme activity	Decreased conversion of histidine to urocanic acid leads to speech and neurological abnormalities by an unknown mechanism.
5-Oxoprolinuria	17	Rare	Autosomal recessive	Glutathione synthetase	Unknown	Unknown	Deficient enzyme activity (most tissues)	Deficiency of product (glutathione) leads to increased formation of γ-glutamylcysteine and conversion of this intermediate to 5-oxoproline, which causes metabolic acidosis and 5-oxoprolinuria.
Glutathione synthetase deficiency without 5-oxoprolinuria	17	Rare	Autosomal recessive	Glutathione synthetase	Unknown	Unknown	Unstable enzyme (limited to erythrocytes)	Deficiency of product (glutathione) in erythrocytes causes compensated hemolytic anemia.
γ-Glutamylcysteine synthetase deficiency	17	Rare	Autosomal recessive	γ-Glutamylcysteine synthetase	Unknown	Unknown	Deficient enzyme activity	Deficiency of product (glutathione) leads to generalized glutathione deficiency and markedly reduced γ-glutamyl cycle, causing hemolytic anemia and neurological disease.

γ-Glutamyl transpeptidase deficiency	17	Rare	Autosomal recessive	γ-Glutamyl transpeptidase	Unknown	Unknown	Deficient enzyme activity	Accumulation and urinary excretion of glutathione, γ-glutamylcysteine, and cysteine.
Prolidase deficiency (hyperimidodipeptiduria)	18	<1 per 600,000	Autosomal recessive	Prolidase (imididodipeptidase)	Unknown	Unknown	Deficient enzyme activity	Excretion of imidodipeptide (X-proline) in urine associated with skin changes, dysmorphogenesis, and other consequences.
Hyperhydroxyprolinemia	18	<1 per 600,000	Autosomal recessive	4-Hydroxy-L-proline oxidase	Unknown	Unknown	Deficient enzyme activity	Accumulation of substrate (4-hydroxy-L-proline). No apparent clinical dysfunction.
Hyperprolinemia, types I and II	18	1 per 200,000	Autosomal recessive	Type I: proline oxidase; Type II: Δ'-pyrroline-5-carboxylate dehydrogenase	Unknown	Unknown	Deficient enzyme activity	Accumulation of substrate. No apparent clinical dysfunction.
Gyrate atrophy of the choroid and retina	19	91 cases reported; 1 per 50,000 in Finland	Autosomal recessive	Ornithine-δ-aminotransferase	Unknown	Unknown	Absent or deficient enzyme activity	Accumulation of substrate (ornithine) inhibits synthesis of Δ'-pyrroline-5-carboxylate, which leads to retinal abnormalities.
Hyperornithinemia-hyperammonemia-homocitrullinuria syndrome	19	10 cases reported	Autosomal recessive	Unknown	Unknown	Unknown	Impaired ornithine transport into mitochondria	Decreased availability of ornithine within mitochondria leads to decreased citrulline synthesis and impaired ammonia detoxification, causing hyperammonemia.
Carbamylphosphate synthetase deficiency	20	Rare	Autosomal recessive	Carbamylphosphate synthetase I	Unknown	Unknown	Absent or deficient enzyme activity	Impaired urea formation leads to hyperammonemia and coma.
Ornithine carbamyltransferase deficiency	20	Rare	X-Linked dominant	Ornithine carbamyltransferase	X	Unknown	Deficient enzyme activity	Impaired urea formation leads to hyperammonemia and coma.
Argininosuccinate synthetase deficiency	20	Rare	Autosomal recessive	Argininosuccinate synthetase	9 (short arm)	Unknown	Deficient enzyme activity	Accumulation of substrate (citrulline) in blood, urine, and cerebrospinal fluid leads to neurological dysfunction.
Argininosuccinate lyase deficiency	20	1 per 70,000	Autosomal recessive	Argininosuccinate lyase	7 (short arm)	Unknown	Deficient enzyme activity	Accumulation of substrate (argininosuccinate) in blood, urine, and cerebrospinal fluid leads to neurological dysfunction.
Argininemia	20	Unknown	Autosomal recessive	Arginase	Unknown	Unknown	Deficient enzyme activity	Accumulation of substrate (arginine) in blood and cerebrospinal fluid leads to neurological dysfunction.
Hyperlysinemia, periodic form	21	1 documented case	Unknown	(?) L-Lysine dehydrogenase	Unknown	Unknown	Deficient enzyme activity	Accumulation of substrate (lysine) leads to inhibition of arginase activity, thereby causing hyperammonemia and nervous system dysfunction.
Hyperlysinemia, persistent form	21	~12 cases reported	Autosomal recessive	L-Lysine: ketoglutarate reductase	Unknown	Unknown	Deficient enzyme activity	Link between enzyme deficiency and observed mental retardation is not established.
Hypervalinemia	22	1 case reported	(?) Autosomal recessive	(?) Valine transaminase	Unknown	Unknown	Deficient enzyme activity	Accumulation of valine leads to developmental retardation by an unknown mechanism.
Hyperleucine-isoleucinemia	22	2 cases reported (in sibs)	Autosomal recessive	(?) Leucine-isoleucine transaminase	Unknown	Unknown	Deficient enzyme activity	Accumulation of leucine, isoleucine, and proline leads to developmental retardation by an unknown mechanism.

SUMMARY TABLES FOR INBORN ERRORS OF METABOLISM

Name of disease	Chap. no.	Prevalence	Mode of inheritance	Mutant gene product	Chromosomal location	Altered DNA structure	Disturbed protein function	Disrupted cell and organ function
							Expression	
Maple syrup urine disease (branched-chain ketoaciduria)	22	1 per 216,000	Autosomal recessive	Branched-chain 2-ketoacid decarboxylase	Unknown	Unknown	Deficient enzyme activity	Accumulation of branched-chain ketoacids causes ketoacidosis and may lead to developmental retardation.
Isovaleric acidemia	22	37 cases reported	Autosomal recessive	Isovaleryl CoA dehydrogenase	Unknown	Unknown	Deficient enzyme activity	Accumulation of isovaleric acid leads to coma and maturation arrest of hematopoietic cells.
Glutaric aciduria, type II	22	6 cases reported	Autosomal recessive	Unknown	Unknown	Unknown	Deficiency of several acyl CoA dehydrogenases	Accumulation of precursors and secondary metabolites (dicarboxylic and short-chain fatty acids) produces severe acidosis and hypoglycemia.
3-Hydroxy-3-methylglutaryl CoA lyase deficiency	22	5 cases reported	Autosomal recessive	3-Hydroxy-3-methylglutaryl CoA lyase	Unknown	Unknown	Deficient enzyme activity	Accumulation of precursors and secondary metabolites leads to ketoacidosis and hypoglycemia.
3-Ketothiolase deficiency	22	7 cases reported	Autosomal recessive	Acetoacetyl CoA 3-ketothiolase	Unknown	Unknown	Deficient enzyme activity	Accumulation of precursors and their metabolites leads to ketoacidosis.
Propionic acidemia (2 nonallelic disorders designated *pcc A* and *pcc BC*)	23	Rare	Autosomal recessive	Propionyl CoA carboxylase (PCC)	Unknown	Unknown	Deficient enzyme activity (nonallelic variants probably reflect mutations in nonidentical subunits of PCC)	Accumulation of propionate and alternate pathway metabolites (methylcitrate, hydroxypropionate and propionylglycine) leads to ketoacidosis and developmental retardation.
Multiple carboxylase deficiency (two nonallelic forms)	23	Unknown	(?) Autosomal recessive	Unknown	Unknown	Unknown	Unknown	Defective biotin metabolism causes impairment of multiple biotin-dependent carboxylases, causing accumulation of propionate (and its by-products) and of β-methylcrotonylglycine. Ketoacidosis, alopecia, and eczematoid skin eruptions ensue.
Methylmalonic acidemia (two allelic variants designated *mut°* and *mut⁻*)	23	1 per 20,000	Autosomal recessive	Methylmalonyl CoA mutase (MUT) apoenzyme	Unknown	Unknown	Absent MUT activity in *mut°*; deficient MUT activity due to reduced affinity for cofactor (adenosylcobalamin) in *mut⁻*	Accumulation of methylmalonate, leading to metabolic ketoacidosis and developmental retardation.
Methylmalonic acidemia (two allelic variants designated *cbl A* and *cbl B*)	23	1 per 20,000	Autosomal recessive	*cbl A* form: unknown *cbl B* form: ATP:cobalamin¹ adenosyltransferase	Unknown	Unknown	Unknown in *cbl A*; absent or deficient enzyme activity in *cbl B*	Impaired adenosylcobalamin synthesis leads to deficient methylmalonyl CoA mutase (MUT) activity; clinical and chemical findings resemble those in apoprotein MUT deficiency.

Disorder		Incidence	Inheritance	Enzyme defect			Basic defect	Clinical and biochemical features
Methylmalonic acidemia and homocystinuria (two nonallelic forms designated *cbl* C and *cbl* D)	23	Rare	Autosomal recessive	Unknown	Unknown	Unknown	Unknown	Impaired synthesis of adenosylcobalamin and methylcobalamin leads to deficient activities of two cobalamin-dependent enzymes, $5N$-methyltetrahydrofolate: homocysteine methyltransferase and methylmalonyl CoA mutase. Hematologic and neurologic abnormalities prominent.
Congenital defect of folate absorption	24	Rare	Autosomal recessive	Unknown	Unknown	Unknown	Defective transport system for folate in intestinal mucosa	Deficiency of folate derivatives leads to neurological abnormalities.
Dihydrofolate reductase deficiency	24	Rare	Autosomal recessive	Dihydrofolate reductase	Unknown	Unknown	Absent or deficient enzyme activity	Decreased conversion of folate to its active form (tetrahydrofolate) leads to neurological abnormalities and megaloblastic anemia.
Methylene tetrahydrofolate reductase deficiency	24	Rare	Autosomal recessive	Methylene tetrahydrofolate reductase	Unknown	Unknown	Absent or deficient enzyme activity	Inability to transfer methyl groups causes reduced formation of methionine from homocysteine, which leads to homocystinuria and neurological disturbances.
Cystathioninuria	25	1 per 70,000 to 1 per 333,000	Autosomal recessive	γ-Cystathionase	Unknown	Unknown	Absent or deficient enzyme activity	Accumulation of cystathionine and its metabolites. No known clinical sequelae.
Homocystinuria	25	1 per 200,000	Autosomal recessive	Cystathionine β-synthase	Unknown	Unknown	Absent or deficient enzyme activity	Accumulation of precursors (homocyst(e)ine, methionine, and their metabolites) leads to dislocated optic lenses, thromboembolic diathesis, mental retardation, and osteoporosis.
Hypersarcosinemia	26	~ 12 cases reported	Autosomal recessive	Sarcosine dehydrogenase complex	Unknown	Unknown	Deficient enzyme activity	Accumulation of substrate (sarcosine). Link between enzyme defect and occasional neurological findings is not established.
Nonketotic hyperglycinemia	27	~ 1 per 250,000 in United States; 1 per 12,000 in northern Finland	Autosomal recessive	One of several proteins of glycine cleavage enzyme system	Unknown	Unknown	Deficient enzyme acitivity	Substrate (glycine) accumulates in body fluids, including cerebrospinal fluid. Severe retardation may be related to glycine's role as a neurotransmitter.
Hyper-β-alaninemia	28	Rare	Autosomal recessive	β-Alanine transaminase	Unknown	Unknown	Deficient enzyme activity	Central nervous system dysfunction of unknown mechanism.
Carnosinase deficiency	28	< 1 per 500,000	Autosomal recessive	Serum carnosinase	Unknown	Unknown	Deficient enzyme activity	Substrate (carnosine) accumulates. Relation between enzyme defect and neurological dysfunction is not known.
Homocarnosinosis	28	Rare	Autosomal recessive	Brain homocarnosinase	Unknown	Unknown	Absent enzyme activity	Substrate (homocarnosine) accumulates. Link between enzyme defect and neurological dysfunction is not established.

SUMMARY TABLES FOR INBORN ERRORS OF METABOLISM

● DISORDERS OF LIPOPROTEIN AND LIPID METABOLISM ●

Name of disease	Chap. no.	Prevalence	Mode of inheritance	Mutant gene product	Chromosomal location	Altered DNA structure	Disturbed protein function	Disrupted cell and organ function
							Expression	
Abetalipoproteinemia	29	~ 50 cases reported	Autosomal recessive	Unknown	Unknown	Unknown	Unknown	Lack of synthesis and/or secretion of apoprotein B prevents formation of chylomicrons, VLDL, and LDL. This leads to decreased vitamin E transport, which in turn causes neurologic and retinal abnormalities. Heterozygotes have normal plasma levels of apoprotein B.
Familial hypobetalipoproteinemia	29	7 cases reported	Autosomal recessive	Unknown	Unknown	Unknown	Unknown	Homozygotes have syndrome similar to abetalipoproteinemia. Heterozygotes have one-half of the normal levels of apoprotein B in plasma and are asymptomatic.
Tangier disease	29	26 cases reported	Autosomal recessive	Unknown	Unknown	Unknown	Unknown	Decreased synthesis and increased catabolism of the apoprotein components (apo A-I and apo A-II) of HDL. As a result, HDL is absent from plasma and other lipoproteins are abnormal. Cholesteryl esters accumulate in reticuloendothelial cells, causing tonsillar enlargement, splenomegaly, and neuropathy.
Familial lipoprotein lipase deficiency	30	~ 100 cases reported	Autosomal recessive	Lipoprotein lipase	Unknown	Unknown	Absent enzyme activity	Accumulation of substrate (chylomicrons) in plasma produces hypertriglyceridemia, pancreatitis, and eruptive xanthomas of skin.
Apolipoprotein C-II deficiency	30	~ 25 cases reported	Autosomal recessive	Apolipoprotein C-II (activator of lipoprotein lipase)	Unknown	Unknown	Decreased enzyme activity (lipoprotein lipase) due to absence of activator.	Accumulation of chylomicrons and VLDL in plasma produces hypertriglyceridemia, pancreatitis, and eruptive xanthomas of skin.
Familial type 5 hyperlipoproteinemia	30	Uncommon, but not rare	Autosomal dominant	Unknown	Unknown	Unknown	Unknown	Accumulation of chylomicrons and VLDL in plasma, producing hypertriglyceridemia, pancreatitis, and eruptive xanthomas of skin.
Familial lecithin:cholesterol acyltransferase (LCAT) deficiency	31	26 cases reported	Autosomal recessive	Plasma LCAT	16 (long arm)	Unknown	Absent enzyme activity	Accumulation of substrate (free cholesterol) in plasma and tissues leads to anemia, cataracts, proteinuria, and renal failure.
Familial type 3 hyperlipoproteinemia (dysbetalipoproteinemia)	32	~ 1 per 10,000	Susceptibility inherited as autosomal recessive trait; expression requires other genetic or environmental factors	Apoprotein E^D	Unknown	Missense mutation (arginine → cysteine)	Abnormal protein structure	Deficient binding of apoprotein E^D to hepatic lipoprotein receptors causes plasma accumulation of chylomicron and VLDL remnants. Hyperlipidemia and atherosclerosis result.

46

	Disorder	Frequency	Inheritance	Enzyme/Protein			Enzyme Activity	Comments
33	Familial hypercholesterolemia, three allelic types	Receptor-negative type: ~ 1 per 1,000 Receptor-defective type: ~ 1 per 1,000 Internalization type: rare	Autosomal dominant	LDL receptor	Unknown	Unknown	Absent or defective receptor activity (homozygotes); half-normal receptor activity (heterozygotes)	Deficient receptor-mediated endocytosis causes LDL to accumulate in plasma and prevents body cells from using its cholesterol. Hypercholesterolemia and atherosclerosis result.
34	Cerebrotendinous xanthomatosis	53 cases reported	Autosomal recessive	Hepatic sterol hydroxylase [(?)24-hydroxylase or 26-hydroxylase)]	Unknown	Unknown	Deficient enzyme activity	Reduced synthesis of cholic and chenodeoxycholic acids secondary to hydroxylase deficiency leads to compensatory increase in synthesis of cholesterol and cholestanol, which deposit in tissues.
34	Sitosterolemia with xanthomatosis	16 cases reported	Autosomal recessive	Unknown	Unknown	Unknown	Unknown	Increased intestinal absorption and decreased excretion of plant sterols (sitosterol and campesterol) and cholesterol lead to sterol deposition in tissues.
35	Phytanic acid storage disease (Refsum's disease)	~ 100 cases reported	Autosomal recessive	Phytanic acid α-hydroxylase	Unknown	Unknown	Absent enzyme activity	Accumulation of substrate (phytanic acid) causes retinitis pigmentosa, ataxia, and peripheral neuropathy.

● DISORDERS OF LYSOSOMAL ENZYMES ●

	Disorder	Frequency	Inheritance	Enzyme/Protein			Enzyme Activity	Comments
36	Mucopolysaccharidosis, type I (Hurler, Scheie, and Hurler-Scheie syndromes—three allelic disorders)	Hurler syndrome: ~ 1 per 100,000 Scheie syndrome: ~ 1 per 500,000 Hurler-Scheie syndrome: rare	Autosomal recessive	Lysosomal α-L-iduronidase	Unknown	Unknown	Absent enzyme activity (molecular difference accounting for allelic variants is unknown)	Defective lysosomal degradation of dermatan and heparan sulfates leads to storage of incompletely degraded mucopolysaccharides. This produces ocular cataracts in Scheie syndrome and widespread tissue abnormalities in Hurler and Hurler-Scheie syndromes.
36	Mucopolysaccharidosis, type II (Hunter syndrome)	~ 1 per 150,000	X-Linked recessive	Lysosomal iduronate sulfatase	X	Unknown	Absent enzyme activity	Defective lysosomal degradation of dermatan and heparan sulfates leads to storage of incompletely degraded mucopolysaccharides. Cellular function disrupted in many tissues.
36	Mucopolysaccharidosis, type III (Sanfilippo syndromes—four nonallelic disorders)	~ 1 per 24,000 (all four disorders combined)	Autosomal recessive	Type III A: lysosomal heparan N-sulfatase Type III B: lysosomal N-acetyl-α-D-glucosaminidase Type III C: lysosomal acetyl-CoA:α-glucosaminide N-acetyltransferase Type III D: lysosomal N-acetyl-α-D-glucosaminide 6-sulfatase	Unknown	Unknown	Absent or deficient enzyme activity	Defective intralysosomal degradation of heparan sulfate leads to storage of incompletely degraded mucopolysaccharides. Cellular function disrupted predominantly in central nervous system.

SUMMARY TABLES FOR INBORN ERRORS OF METABOLISM

Name of disease	Chap. no.	Prevalence	Mode of inheritance	Mutant gene product	Chromosomal location	Altered DNA structure	Disturbed protein function	Disrupted cell and organ function
						Expression		
Mucopolysaccharidosis, type IV (Morquio syndromes—two nonallelic disorders)	36	< 1 per 100,000 (both disorders combined)	Autosomal recessive	Type IV A: lysosomal galactosamine 6-sulfate sulfatase Type IV B: lysosomal β-galactosidase	Unknown	Unknown	Absent enzyme activity	Defective lysosomal degradation of keratan sulfate leads to storage of incompletely degraded mucopolysaccharides. Cellular function disrupted in skeletal and cardiovascular systems.
Mucopolysaccharidosis, type VI (Maroteaux-Lamy syndrome—several allelic types)	36	< 1 per 100,000	Autosomal recessive	Lysosomal arylsulfatase B	5 (long arm)	Unknown	Absent or deficient enzyme activity	Defective lysosomal degradation of dermatan sulfate leads to storage of incompletely degraded mucopolysaccharides. Cellular function disrupted in skeletal and cardiovascular systems.
Mucopolysaccharidosis, type VII (Sly syndrome)	36	~ 12 cases reported	Autosomal recessive	Lysosomal β-glucuronidase	7 (short arm)	Unknown	Absent or deficient enzyme activity	Defective lysosomal degradation of dermatan and heparan sulfates leads to storage of incompletely degraded mucopolysaccharides. Cellular function disrupted in many tissues.
I-Cell disease (mucolipidosis II) and pseudo-Hurler polydystrophy (mucolipidosis III)—two allelic disorders	37	Rare	Autosomal recessive	N-Acetylglucosaminyl phosphotransferase	Unknown	Unknown	Enzyme activity absent (I-cell disease) or deficient (pseudo-Hurler polydystrophy)	Deficiency of enzyme required for the synthesis of mannose-6-phosphate group attached to lysosomal enzymes. Lack of mannose-6-phosphate recognition marker prevents lysosomal enzymes from entering lysosomes. This leads to abnormal storage of mucopolysaccharides, glycoproteins, and glycolipids in cells, causing bone, joint, and psychomotor abnormalities.
Mannosidosis	38	50–100 cases reported	Autosomal recessive	Lysosomal α-D-mannosidase	19 (long arm)	Unknown	Deficient or unstable enzyme activity	Accumulation of oligosaccharides causes tissue damage.
Sialidosis	38	50–100 cases reported	Autosomal recessive	Lysosomal α-neuraminidase (glycoprotein substrate)	Unknown	Unknown	Deficient enzyme activity	Accumulation of oligosaccharides causes tissue damage.
Aspartylglycosaminuria	38	70–100 cases in Finland; extremely rare elsewhere	Autosomal recessive	Lysosomal aspartylglycosaminidase	Unknown	Unknown	Deficient enzyme activity	Accumulation of glycopeptides causes tissue damage.
Fucosidosis	38	30–60 cases reported	Autosomal recessive	Lysosomal α-L-fucosidase	1 (short arm)	Unknown	Deficient enzyme activity	Accumulation of glycolipid, glycopeptides, and oligosaccharides causes tissue damage.

No.	Disease	Frequency	Inheritance	Enzyme	Chromosome		Enzyme activity	Consequences
39	Acid lipase deficiency (Wolman's disease and cholesteryl ester storage disease—two allelic disorders)	Wolman's disease: 40 cases reported. Cholesteryl ester storage disease: 23 cases reported	Autosomal recessive	Lysosomal acid lipase	10 (long arm)	Unknown	Absent or deficient enzyme activity (molecular difference accounting for allelic variants is unknown)	Cholesteryl esters and triglycerides accumulate in lysosomes of body cells producing hepatic, intestinal, and adrenal dysfunction. Death in infancy in Wolman's disease. Hyperlipidemia and atherosclerosis with survival to early adulthood in cholesteryl ester storage disease.
40	Ceramidase deficiency (Farber's lipogranulomatosis)	27 cases reported	Autosomal recessive	Lysosomal acid ceramidase	Unknown	Unknown	Absent enzyme activity	Accumulation of substrate (ceramide) leads to granulomatous reaction in joints, subcutaneous tissues, larynx, and other tissues. Accumulation of ceramides and gangliosides in lysosomes of neurons leads to spinal cord and brain dysfunction.
41	Niemann-Pick disease	1 per 25,000 U.S. Jews	Autosomal recessive	Lysosomal sphingomyelinase	Unknown	Unknown	Deficient enzyme activity	Accumulation of substrate (sphingomyelin) in lysosomes leads to dysfunction of brain and parenchymal tissues (spleen, liver, lung, lymph nodes).
42	Gaucher's disease, type I	~1 per 2000 U.S. Jews	Autosomal recessive	Lysosomal glucocerebrosidase	Unknown	Unknown	Deficient enzyme activity	Accumulation of substrate (glucocerebroside) in lysosomes leads to splenomegaly, hepatomegaly and bone pain. Central nervous system damage occurs in occasional patients.
43	Galactosylceramide lipidosis (globoid cell leukodystrophy; Krabbe's disease)	1 per 50,000 in Sweden; much lower elsewhere	Autosomal recessive	Lysosomal galactosylceramidase	Unknown	Unknown	Absent enzyme activity	Accumulation of substrate (galactosylceramide) leads to disappearance of oligodendroglia and cessation of myelination, resulting in destruction of central nervous system white matter and peripheral neuropathy.
44	Metachromatic leukodystrophy (late-infantile, juvenile, and adult types—three allelic disorders)	~1 per 100,000 (all three types combined)	Autosomal recessive	Lysosomal arylsulfatase A	22 (long arm)	Unknown	Absent or deficient enzyme activity (molecular difference accounting for allelic variants is unknown)	Accumulation of substrate (cerebroside sulfate) in lysosomes of oligodendroglia and Schwann cells leads to demyelination, causing neurological symptoms.
44	Multiple sulfatase deficiency	Rare	Autosomal recessive	Unknown	Unknown	Unknown	Deficiency of multiple sulfatases, including arylsulfatase A, steroid sulfatase, and mucopolysaccharide sulfatases	Accumulation of substrates (cerebroside sulfate, steroid sulfates, and mucopolysaccharides) in lysosomes leads to clinical picture that combines features of metachromatic leukodystrophy, ichthyosis, and mucopolysaccharidoses. Central nervous system, skin, and bones affected.
45	Fabry's disease (α-galactosidase A deficiency)	~1 per 40,000	X-Linked recessive	α-Galactosidase A	X (long arm)	Unknown	Unstable or absent enzyme activity	Accumulation of substrates (globotriaosylceramide, galabiosylceramide, and blood group B glycosphingolipids), particularly in lysosomes of blood vessels, leads to renal failure, myocardial and cerebral vascular disease.

SUMMARY TABLES FOR INBORN ERRORS OF METABOLISM

Name of disease	Chap. no.	Prevalence	Mode of inheritance	Mutant gene product	Chromosomal location	Expression		
						Altered DNA structure	Disturbed protein function	Disrupted cell and organ function
G_{M1} Gangliosidosis	46	~ 130 cases reported	Autosomal recessive	Lysosomal acid β-galactosidase	3 (short arm)	Unknown	Absent enzyme activity	Accumulation of substrates (G_{M1} ganglioside and galactosyl glucoconjugates) leads to brain dysfunction and bony abnormalities.
Tay-Sachs disease	46	1 per 3000 U.S. Jews	Autosomal recessive	α-Chain of lysosomal hexosaminidase A	15 (long arm)	Unknown	Absent enzyme activity	Accumulation of substrate (G_{M2} ganglioside) in lysosomes of neurons leads to brain dysfunction.
● DISORDERS OF STEROID METABOLISM ●								
Congenital adrenal hyperplasia (21-hydroxylase deficiency)	47	~ 1 per 10,000	Autosomal recessive	21-Hydroxylase	6 (short arm)	Unknown	Deficient enzyme activity	Deficient cortisol secretion results in compensatory overproduction of cortisol precursors and adrenal androgens, leading to virilization; salt-wasting may occur secondary to aldosterone deficiency in some cases.
Congenital adrenal hyperplasia (11β-hydroxylase deficiency)	47	Rare	Autosomal recessive	11β-Hydroxylase	Unknown	Unknown	Deficient enzyme activity	Deficient cortisol secretion results in compensatory overproduction of cortisol precursors and adrenal androgens, leading to virilization and, in some cases, hypertension.
Disorders of the androgen receptor (complete testicular feminization, incomplete testicular feminization, Reifenstein syndrome—three allelic disorders)	48	1 in 64,000 male births (complete testicular feminization)	X-Linked recessive	Androgen receptor protein	X (long arm)	Unknown	Absent, unstable, or deficient protein	Failure of the androgen receptor complex to reach the nucleus of male target cells leads to androgen resistance and feminization in utero and in postembryonic life.
Steroid 5α-reductase deficiency	48	Rare	Autosomal recessive	Steroid 5α-reductase	Unknown	Unknown	Absent or unstable enzyme activity	Deficiency of product (dihydrotestosterone) leads to a form of male pseudohermaphroditism in which genetic males have male internal genitalia, but female external genitalia.
Steroid sulfatase deficiency (X-linked ichthyosis)	49	1 per 6000 males	X-Linked recessive	Steroid sulfatase	X (short arm)	Unknown	Absent enzyme activity	Deficient estrogen production from sulfated precursors during fetal life leads to delayed parturition. Postnatally, cholesterol sulfate accumulates in blood, skin, and other tissues. Ichthyosis may be related to cholesterol sulfate accumulation in skin.

● DISORDERS OF PURINE AND PYRIMIDINE METABOLISM ●

Page	Disorder	Incidence	Inheritance	Enzyme	Chromosome		Enzyme defect	Pathogenesis
50	Primary gout: Idiopathic	1 per 500 in Western populations; 1 per 50 in American males by age 60; 1 per 10 males and 1 per 25 females in some Polynesian groups	Multifactorial	Unknown	Unknown	Unknown	Unknown	Mixed pathogenesis: increased biosynthesis and reduced renal clearance of uric acid in most affected individuals.
50	Primary gout: Partial deficiency of hypoxanthine-guanine phosphoribosyltransferase (HPRT) (see Chap. 51)							
50	Primary gout: Superactive variant of phosphoribosylpyrophosphate (PP-ribose-P) synthetase	~10 families reported	X-linked recessive	PP-ribose-P synthetase	X (long arm)	Unknown	Enhanced enzyme activity	Increased production of PP-ribose-P leads to increased purine synthesis de novo, causing gout.
51	Hypoxanthine-guanine phosphoribosyltransferase (HPRT) deficiency (Lesch-Nyhan syndrome and partial HPRT deficiency—two allelic disorders)	Lesch-Nyhan syndrome: 1 per 10,000 males Partial HPRT deficiency: 1 per 100,000 males	X-Linked recessive	Hypoxanthine-guanine phospho-ribosyltransferase (HPRT)	X (long arm)	Unknown	Absent or deficient enzyme activity	Accumulation of substrate (phosphoribosylpyrophosphate) leads to enhanced purine biosynthesis de novo, causing gout. Cause of severe (Lesch-Nyhan syndrome) and mild (partial HPRT deficiency) central nervous system dysfunction is unknown.
52	Adenine phosphoribosyltransferase deficiency	11 cases reported	Autosomal recessive	Adenine phospho-ribosyltransferase	16 (long arm)	Unknown	Absent enzyme activity	Adenine is metabolized through an alternative pathway leading to accumulation of 2,8-dihydroxyadenine, a product that is insoluble in the kidney and urinary tract. Urolithiasis frequently results.
53	Adenosine deaminase deficiency with severe combined immunodeficiency disease	50 reported cases	Autosomal recessive	Catalytic subunit of adenosine deaminase	20 (long arm)	Unknown	Absent enzyme activity	Accumulation of substrates (adenosine and deoxyadenosine), which are toxic to lymphoid cells, leads to immunodeficiency.
53	Purine nucleoside phosphorylase deficiency with cellular immunodeficiency	9 cases reported	Autosomal recessive	Purine nucleoside phosphorylase	14 (long arm)	Unknown	Absent enzyme activity	Accumulation of substrates (primarily deoxyadenosine) is toxic to T lymphocytes, causing defective cellular immunity.
54	Myoadenylate deaminase deficiency	Rare	Autosomal recessive	AMP deaminase (isoenzyme A)	Unknown	Unknown	Absent enzyme activity in skeletal muscle	Disruption of purine nucleotide cycle leads to ATP depletion and postexercise fatigue, cramps, and myalgias.
55	Xanthinuria	1 per 45,000	Autosomal recessive	Xanthine dehydrogenase (xanthine oxidase)	Unknown	Unknown	Absent enzyme activity	Accumulated substrate (xanthine) crystallizes in urinary tract and muscle, causing nephrolithiasis and myopathy.

SUMMARY TABLES FOR INBORN ERRORS OF METABOLISM

Name of disease	Chap. no.	Prevalence	Mode of inheritance	Mutant gene product	Chromosomal location	Expression		
						Altered DNA structure	Disturbed protein function	Disrupted cell and organ function
Orotic aciduria	56	~ 10 cases reported	Autosomal recessive	Orotate phosphoribosyltransferase or orotidine 5'-phosphate decarboxylase	Unknown	Unknown	Deficient enzyme activity	Accumulation of orotic acid leads to stone formation. Deficiency of pyrimidine nucleotides associated with megaloblastic anemia, mental retardation, and growth retardation.
Xeroderma pigmentosum, multiple types involving multiple gene loci	57	1 per 250,000 (about 10 times more frequent in Egypt)	Autosomal recessive	At least eight enzymes that affect DNA repair and replication	Unknown	Unknown	Absent or deficient enzyme activity	Decreased capacity to repair or replicate DNA that is damaged by ultraviolet light or chemical carcinogens leads to multiple skin carcinomas.

● DISORDERS OF METAL METABOLISM ●

Name of disease	Chap. no.	Prevalence	Mode of inheritance	Mutant gene product	Chromosomal location	Altered DNA structure	Disturbed protein function	Disrupted cell and organ function
Wilson's disease	58	~1 per 50,000	Autosomal recessive	Unknown	Unknown	Unknown	Unknown	Defective biliary excretion of copper leads to accumulation of copper in liver (cirrhosis), cornea (Kayser-Fleischer ring), and basal ganglia (neurological disease).
Menkes' (steely-hair) disease	58	~ 1 per 100,000	X-Linked recessive	Unknown	Unknown	Unknown	Unknown	Defective transport of copper leads to deficiency of copper-containing enzymes and causes arterial and brain degeneration.
Idiopathic hemochromatosis	59	~1 per 400 is homozygous for idiopathic hemochromatosis gene (overt or unexpressed)	Autosomal recessive	Unknown	6 (short arm)	Unknown	Unknown	An abnormally high proportion of dietary iron is absorbed into the body. When the body iron content reaches massive proportions (> 15 g), many organs are damaged, including liver, heart, and pancreas. Most homozygotes do not accumulate such large amounts of iron and are asymptomatic.

● DISORDERS OF PORPHYRIN AND HEME METABOLISM ●

Name of disease	Chap. no.	Prevalence	Mode of inheritance	Mutant gene product	Chromosomal location	Altered DNA structure	Disturbed protein function	Disrupted cell and organ function
Congenital erythropoietic porphyria	60	Rare	Autosomal recessive	Uroporphyrinogen III cosynthase	Unknown	Unknown	Deficient enzyme activity	Accumulation of type I porphyrins in erythroid cells (causing hemolytic anemia) and in skin (causing marked cutaneous photosensitivity).
Erythropoietic protoporphyria	60	Rare	Autosomal dominant	Ferrochelatase	Unknown	Unknown	Deficient enzyme activity	Accumulation of substrate (protoporphyrin) in skin (causing mild photosensitivity) and in erythroid cells.
Acute intermittent porphyria	60	Uncommon, but not rare	Autosomal dominant	Porphobilinogen deaminase	11 (long arm)	Unknown	Deficient enzyme activity	Clinical expression is dependent on hormonal, drug, and nutritional factors that induce hepatic heme synthesis. When the disease is clinically expressed, substrate (porphobilinogen) and other intermediates accumulate in liver and are excreted in urine. Cause of neurological manifestations is poorly understood.

Disorder		Frequency	Inheritance	Enzyme	Chromosome		Defect	Comments
Hereditary coproporphyria	60	Rare	Autosomal dominant	Coproporphyrinogen oxidase	Unknown	Unknown	Deficient enzyme activity	Clinical expression is dependent on same factors as in acute intermittent porphyria. With clinical expression, substrate (coproporphyrinogen III) and other intermediates accumulate in liver. Neurological symptoms and skin photosensitivity may develop.
Variegate porphyria	60	Common in South Africa; rare in other parts of world	Autosomal dominant	Proporphyrinogen oxidase (or ferrochelatase)	Unknown	Unknown	Deficient enzyme activity	Clinical expression is dependent on same factors as in acute intermittent porphyria. With clinical expression, proporphyrin and other intermediates accumulate in liver. Neurological symptoms and skin photosensitivity may develop.
Porphyria cutanea tarda, familial form	60	Uncommon, but not rare	Autosomal dominant	Uroporphyrinogen decarboxylase	Unknown	Unknown	Deficient enzyme activity	Clinical expression dependent on a combination of the enzyme defect and an acquired factor, usually siderosis due to alcoholic liver disease. Porphyrinogen substrates of the decarboxylase accumulate in liver. These are transported to other tissues, including skin, where they cause skin photosensitivity.
Crigler-Najjar syndrome, type I	61	Rare	Autosomal recessive	Hepatic bilirubin UDP-glucuronyl transferase	Unknown	Unknown	Absent enzyme activity	Substrate (unconjugated bilirubin) accumulates in brain, resulting in kernicterus.
Crigler-Najjar syndrome, type II	61	Uncommon	(?) Autosomal recessive	Hepatic bilirubin UDP-glucuronyl transferase	Unknown	Unknown	Deficient enzyme activity	Partial ability to conjugate bilirubin leads to mild unconjugated hyperbilirubinemia with increased proportion of bilirubin monoglucuronide in bile. Usually benign disorder.
Gilbert's syndrome	61	~ 1 per 30	Autosomal dominant	Unknown	Unknown	Unknown	Unknown	Impaired hepatic uptake of bilirubin and reduced activity of hepatic bilirubin uridine diphosphoglucuronyl transferase lead to mild unconjugated hyperbilirubinemia and increased proportion of bilirubin monoglucuronide in bile. Benign disorder.
Dubin-Johnson syndrome	61	Rare worldwide; 1 per 1300 in Persian Jews	Autosomal recessive	Unknown	Unknown	Unknown	Unknown	Failure of biliary excretion of conjugated bilirubin produces mild conjugated hyperbilirubinemia.
Rotor's syndrome	61	Rare	Autosomal recessive	Unknown	Unknown	Unknown	Unknown	Partial failure of biliary excretion of conjugated bilirubin causes mild hyperbilirubinemia.
Acatalasemia	62	~ 1 per 1 million	Autosomal recessive	Catalase	11 (short arm)	Unknown	Absent, deficient, or unstable enzyme activity	Failure of degradation of H_2O_2 (which is produced by bacteria) causes hemoglobin to be oxidized, thereby depriving infected mucosal tissues of oxygen. Most affected individuals are asymptomatic but some have ulceration of the oral and nasal mucosa.

SUMMARY TABLES FOR INBORN ERRORS OF METABOLISM

● DISORDERS INVOLVING CONNECTIVE TISSUE, MUSCLE, AND BONE ●

Name of disease	Chap. no.	Prevalence	Mode of inheritance	Mutant gene product	Chromosomal location	Altered DNA structure	Expression	
							Disturbed protein function	Disrupted cell and organ function
Ehlers-Danlos syndromes, types I to IX	63	~1 per 50,000 (all types combined)	Types I, II, III, IVa, VIII: autosomal dominant; Types IVb, VI, VII, IX: autosomal recessive; Type V: X-linked recessive	Type VI: lysyl hydroxylase; Type VII: procollagen peptidase; Other types: unknown	Unknown	Unknown	Types VI and VII: deficient enzyme activity	Type VI: Hydroxylysine-deficient collagen is unable to form intermolecular crosslinks, causing marked joint hypermobility, kyphoscoliosis, and ocular fragility. Type VII: Incomplete conversion of procollagen to collagen leads to joint hypermobility and hip dislocation. Other Types: Abnormalities in structure or metabolism of collagen cause various combinations of skin fragility, joint hyperextensibility, easy bruisability, hernias, and rupture of arteries and bowel.
α_1-Antitrypsin deficiency (PiZZ variant)	64	~1 per 3500	Autosomal recessive	α_1-Antitrypsin	14 (long arm)	Missense mutation (glutamic acid→lysine)	Abnormal protein structure	Abnormal structure of α_1-antitrypsin prevents normal posttranslational glycosylation, thereby preventing its secretion from liver. Reduced levels of α_1-antitrypsin in plasma and lung cause lung tissue to be destroyed by neutrophil elastase.
Amyloid nephropathy associated with familial Mediterranean fever	65	1 per 3000 Sephardic Jews	Autosomal recessive	Unknown	Unknown	Unknown	Unknown	Deposition of amyloid fibrillar protein extracellularly in the kidney leads to nephrotic syndrome and renal failure.
Hereditary systemic amyloidoses—neuropathic and cardiac types	65	Rare	Autosomal dominant	Unknown	Unknown	Unknown	Unknown	Deposition of amyloid fibrillar proteins extracellularly leads to neural or cardiac dysfunction.
Duchenne's muscular dystrophy	66	~1 per 10,000 males	X-Linked recessive	Unknown	X (short arm)	Unknown	Unknown	Progressive dystrophy of skeletal muscles.
Myotonic dystrophy	66	~1 per 30,000	Autosomal dominant	Unknown	Unknown	Unknown	Unknown	Multiple membrane alterations, causing skeletal muscle dystrophy, myotonia, cataracts, cardiac conduction defects, mental retardation, etc.
Familial periodic paralyses—hypokalemic, normokalemic, and hyperkalemic types	67	~1 per 100,000 for hypokalemic type; other types less prevalent	Autosomal dominant	Unknown	Unknown	Unknown	Unknown	Alterations in resting membrane potential of muscle fibers lead to intermittent paralysis.
Hypophosphatasia	68	Uncommon, but not rare	Autosomal recessive	Alkaline phosphatase (bone enzyme)	Unknown	Unknown	Deficient enzyme activity	Decreased hydrolysis of pyrophosphates and other phosphate esters causes accumulation of inorganic phosphate and phosphoethanolamine in vesicles of developing bone, leading to defective bone formation.

No.	Disorder	Frequency	Inheritance	Gene product	Chromosome	Molecular defect	Protein/biochemical defect	Clinical consequences
69	Pseudohypoparathyroidism, several types	~ 1 per 50,000	Autosomal dominant, autosomal recessive, and X-linked recessive	Type 1A: guanosine nucleotide regulatory protein of adenyl cyclase complex Other types: unknown	Unknown	Unknown	Type 1A: defective regulatory protein leads to decreased adenyl cyclase activity	Insufficient intracellular generation of cyclic AMP (type 1) and failure to respond to cyclic AMP (type 2) leads to resistance to parathyroid hormone and other hormones. Hypocalcemia is outstanding symptom.
70	Classic hemophilia	1 per 10,000 males	X-Linked recessive	Factor VIII	X (long arm)	Unknown	Low or absent amount of factor VIII protein	Impaired function of coagulation system, leading to bleeding.
70	Von Willebrand's disease	Uncommon, but not rare	Autosomal dominant	Von Willebrand factor	Unknown	Unknown	Absence of von Willebrand protein in homozygotes and one-half normal level in heterozygotes.	Impaired function of coagulation system, causing severe bleeding in homozygotes and mild to no bleeding in heterozygotes.
71	Bernard-Soulier disease	~ 50 cases reported	Autosomal recessive	Platelet membrane glycoprotein Ib	Unknown	Unknown	Absent platelet membrane glycoprotein Ib (receptor for von Willebrand factor)	Failure of platelet membrane to bind plasma von Willebrand factor results in defective platelet adhesion to blood vessel subendothelium, causing mild bleeding.
71	Glanzmann's thrombasthenia	Uncommon, but not rare	Autosomal recessive	Platelet membrane glycoprotein IIb-IIIa	Unknown	Unknown	Absent or decreased platelet membrane glycoprotein IIb-IIIa (receptor for fibrinogen)	Failure of platelet membrane to interact with extracellular fibrinogen and intracellular contractile proteins results in defective platelet aggregation and clot retardation, causing mild bleeding.
72	Hereditary spherocytosis, several types	1 per 5000 Caucasians (less common in other ethnic groups)	Autosomal dominant	Spectrin—in some families; defect unknown in other families	Unknown	Unknown	Defective interaction of spectrin with protein 4.1 of red blood cell (in some families)	Weakened red cell membrane skeleton results in loss of membrane surface, formation of spherocytes, splenic sequestration, and hemolysis.
72	Hereditary elliptocytosis, several types	1 per 2500	Autosomal dominant	Unknown	1 (short arm) in one type; other types involve different gene loci	Unknown	Deficient or abnormal red blood cell membrane proteins	Weakened red cell membrane skeleton results in elliptocytosis, presumably due to abnormal plastic deformation. In severe cases, this leads to membrane fragmentation, poikilocytosis, splenic sequestration, and hemolysis.
73	Pyruvate kinase deficiency with hemolytic anemia	1 per 20,000 Caucasians	Autosomal recessive	Pyruvate kinase	Unknown	Unknown	Deficient enzyme activity	Deficiency of product (ATP) leads to hemolysis.
74	Glucose-6-phosphate dehydrogenase (G6PD) deficiency; multiple allelic disorders, including mild A – type and severe Mediterranean type	A – type: 1 per 11 U.S. Blacks Mediterranean type: common in Middle East and other Mediterranean countries	Susceptibility inherited as X-linked recessive trait; clinical expression requires precipitating factor.	G6PD	X (long arm)	Unknown	Unstable enzyme	Deficiency of product (NADHP) leads to mild hemolytic anemia after stress, such as ingestion of oxidant drugs, infections, or diabetic acidosis.

SUMMARY TABLES FOR INBORN ERRORS OF METABOLISM

Name of disease	Chap. no.	Prevalence	Mode of inheritance	Mutant gene product	Chromosomal location	Expression			
						Altered DNA structure	Disturbed protein function	Disrupted cell and organ function	
Hereditary methemoglobinemia (see Chap. 76 for related nonallelic disorders)	75	Uncommon, but not rare	Autosomal recessive	NADH cytochrome b₅ reductase	Unknown	Unknown	Deficient enzyme activity in erythrocyte cytosol (100 percent of cases) and in microsomes of many tissues (15 percent of cases)	Failure to reduce substrate (cytochrome b₅) leads to accumulation of methemoglobin in erythrocytes. Patients with generalized defect have secondary abnormalities in brain function.	
Sickle cell anemia	76	1 per 625 U.S. Blacks	Autosomal recessive	β-Globin	11 (short arm)	Missense mutation: CTC → CAC, Glutamic acid → valine	Aggregation of hemoglobin S	Aggregation of hemoglobin alters red cell shape, leading to sickling and hemolysis, which causes widespread tissue ischemia and infarction.	
Methemoglobinemias, several types involving two gene loci	76	Rare	Autosomal dominant	α-Globin and β-globin	16 (short arm) and 11 (short arm) for α-globin and β-globin genes, respectively	Point mutations	Disruption of hemoglobin bond	Oxidation of heme leads to cyanosis.	
Polycythemia, multiple types involving two gene loci	76	Rare	Autosomal dominant	α-Globin and β-globin	16 (short arm) and 11 (short arm) for α-globin and β-globin genes, respectively	Point mutations; missense mutations	Increase in affinity for oxygen	Decreased release of oxygen to tissues stimulates erythropoiesis, causing polycythemia.	
Unstable hemoglobins, multiple types involving two gene loci	76	Uncommon, but not rare	Autosomal dominant	α-Globin and β-globin	16 (short arm) and 11 (short arm) for α-globin and β-globin genes, respectively	Point mutations; insertions; deletions; missense mutations	Unstable protein (decreased solubility)	Hemoglobin precipitates, causing decreased cell flexibility and hemolytic anemia.	
α Thalassemia, multiple allelic disorders	77	High frequency in Mediterranean, African, and Asian populations	Autosomal recessive	α-Globin	16 (short arm)	Deletion of both α loci (α thalassemia 1); deletion of one α locus (α thalassemia 2); single nucleotide mutation of termination codon (Hb Constant Spring); nondeletion defects due to (1) mutation within intervening sequence and (2) unknown mutations	Deficiency of α-globin	Decreased α-globin synthesis leads to uncombined β-globin chains, which disrupts erythroid cell maturation and function, causing microcytosis, ineffective erythropoiesis, and hemolysis.	

No.	Disorder	Frequency / Population	Inheritance	Gene Product	Chromosome	Molecular Lesion	Defect	Pathophysiology / Clinical
77	β Thalassemia, multiple allelic disorders	High frequency in Mediterranean and Asian populations	Autosomal recessive	β-Globin	11 (short arm)	Gene deletion; nonsense mutation; frame shift mutation; mutation in intervening sequence causing abnormal processing	Decreased or absent β-globin	Decreased β-globin leads to uncombined α-globin chains, which disrupts erythroid cell maturation and function, causing microcytosis, ineffective erythrocytosis, and hemolysis.

● **DISORDERS OF TRANSPORT** ●

No.	Disorder	Frequency / Population	Inheritance	Gene Product	Chromosome	Molecular Lesion	Defect	Pathophysiology / Clinical
78	Intestinal lactase deficiency	1 per 10 Caucasians; majority of Asians, Africans, and American Blacks are affected	Autosomal recessive	Intestinal lactase	Unknown	Unknown	Deficient enzyme activity	Unabsorbed substrate (lactose) accumulates in intestinal lumen and exerts an osmotic effect. This in turn leads to abdominal fullness, cramping abdominal pain, and diarrhea.
78	Intestinal sucrase-α-dextrinase deficiency	Rare	Autosomal recessive	Sucrase-α-dextrinase	Unknown	Unknown	Absent enzyme activity	Unabsorbed substrates (sucrose and isomaltase) accumulate in intestinal lumen and exert an osmotic effect. This in turn leads to abdominal fullness, cramping abdominal pain, and diarrhea.
78	Glucose-galactose malabsorption	~ 20 cases reported	Autosomal recessive	Unknown	Unknown	Unknown	Defect in shared transport system for glucose and galactose in intestinal mucosa	Unabsorbed substrates (glucose and galactose) accumulate in intestinal lumen and exert an osmotic effect. This in turn leads to abdominal fullness, cramping abdominal pain, and diarrhea.
79	Vitamin D-dependent rickets	Rare	Autosomal recessive	25-Hydroxyvitamin D_3-1-hydroxylase	Unknown	Unknown	Deficient enzyme activity	Deficient formation of 1,25-dihydroxyvitamin D_3 in renal tubule leads to calciopenic rickets.
79	Familial hypophosphatemic (vitamin D-resistant) rickets	~ 1 per 25,000	X-Linked dominant	Unknown	X	Unknown	Defective phosphate transport system in renal tubule and intestinal mucosa.	Deficient renal tubular reabsorption of phosphate leads to calciopenic rickets.
80	Cystinuria, three allelic types	1 per 7000	Autosomal recessive	Unknown	Unknown	Unknown	Defect in shared transport system for cystine and diabasic amino acids (ornithine, arginine, lysine) in renal tubule and intestinal mucosa.	Elevated urinary excretion of cystine causes urinary tract calculi. Intestinal transport defect causes no clinical dysfunction.
81	Familial renal iminoglycinuria	1 per 15,000	Autosomal recessive	Unknown	Unknown	Unknown	Defect in shared transport system for imino amino acids and glycine in renal tubule	Aminoaciduria without clinical dysfunction.

57

SUMMARY TABLES FOR INBORN ERRORS OF METABOLISM

Name of disease	Chap. no.	Prevalence	Mode of inheritance	Mutant gene product	Chromosomal location	Expression		
						Altered DNA structure	Disturbed protein function	Disrupted cell and organ function
Hartnup disease	82	60 cases reported	Autosomal recessive	Unknown	Unknown	Unknown	Defect in shared transport system for neutral amino acids in renal tubule and intestinal mucosa	Renal transport defect causes characteristic pattern of aminoaciduria. Variable symptoms occur due to tryptophan loss, leading to nicotinamide deficiency and pellagra-like skin rash.
Renal glycosuria	83	Uncommon, but not rare	Autosomal recessive	Unknown	Unknown	Unknown	Kinetic abnormality in transport system for glucose in renal tubule	Renal transport defect leads to glycosuria without clinical dysfunction.
Renal tubular acidosis, type 1 (several different disorders)	84	Uncommon, but not rare	Autosomal dominant	Unknown	Unknown	Unknown	Defective acidification mechanism in distal tubule of nephron	Metabolic acidosis with or without hypercalciuria. Hypercalciuria leads to nephrocalcinosis.
Cystinosis	85	~ 1 per 100,000	Autosomal recessive	Unknown	Unknown	Unknown	Unknown	Cystine accumulates in lysosomes in multiple tissues. This is associated with renal tubular and glomerular dysfunction, retinopathy, hypothyroidism, and short stature.
Nephrogenic diabetes insipidus	86	Uncommon, but not rare	X-Linked recessive	Unknown	X	Unknown	Unknown	Renal tubular cells fail to accumulate cyclic AMP in response to vasopression. The resulting vasopression unresponsiveness leads to polyuria, hyposthenuria, and polydypsia.
Cystic fibrosis	87	1 per 2000 Caucasians; rare in other ethnic groups	Autosomal recessive	Unknown	Unknown	Unknown	Unknown	Dysfunction of exocrine cells leads to pulmonary infections, exocrine pancreatic insufficiency, meconium ileus, and atrophy of the vas deferens.

● DISORDERS OF THE IMMUNE AND OTHER DEFENSE SYSTEMS ●

Name of disease	Chap. no.	Prevalence	Mode of inheritance	Mutant gene product	Chromosomal location	Altered DNA structure	Disturbed protein function	Disrupted cell and organ function
X-Linked agammaglobulinemia	88	Uncommon, but not rare	X-Linked recessive	Unknown	X	Unknown	Unknown	Failure of synthesis of antibodies due to an absence of plasma cells in lymphoid tissue, bone marrow, spleen, and intestine. Recurrent pyogenic infections occur.
Hereditary angioedema ($\overline{C1}$ inhibitor deficiency)	89	Uncommon, but not rare	Autosomal dominant	Inhibitor protein of $\overline{C1}$, a component of complement	Unknown	Unknown	Low amount of $\overline{C1}$ inhibitor protein (85 percent of cases); normal amount of $\overline{C1}$ inhibitor protein with diminished function (15 percent of cases).	In absence of its inhibitor, active $\overline{C1}$ increases the permeability of blood vessels, leading to angioedema.

Disease	No.	Frequency	Inheritance	Defective protein	Chromosome		Laboratory finding	Consequences
C3b Inactivator deficiency	89	3 kindreds reported	Autosomal dominant	C3b Inactivator protein, a component of complement	Unknown	Unknown	Low serum levels of C3b inactivator	Decreased C3b inactivation leads to low levels of C3 and b. This in turn leads to diminished chemotaxis, opsonization, and bactericidal capacity of serum with resultant recurrent bacterial infections.
Chronic granulomatous disease (several types involving two gene loci)	90	Uncommon, but not rare	X-Linked recessive (most families) Autosomal recessive (few families)	One of several enzymes of NADPH oxidase complex	X (short arm) for X-linked recessive type; unknown for other type	Unknown	Absent or deficient enzyme activity in neutrophils	Deficiency of product (O_2^-) prevents neutrophils from expressing respiratory burst. This in turn leads to impaired bacterial killing and chronic infections.
Leukocyte G6PD deficiency	90	Rare	X-Linked recessive	G6PD	X (long arm)	Unknown	Absent enzyme activity in neutrophils	Deficiency of product (NADPH) prevents neutrophils from expressing respiratory burst. Impaired bacterial killing promotes infections.
Myeloperoxidase deficiency	90	~ 20 cases reported	Autosomal recessive	Myeloperoxidase	Unknown	Unknown	Absent enzyme activity	Deficiency of product (OCl^-, a potent antimicrobial oxidant) leads to impaired bacterial killing.
Immotile cilia syndrome (Kartagener's syndrome)	91	~ 1 per 20,000	Autosomal recessive	Unknown	Unknown	Unknown	Absence of structural and enzymatic proteins of cilia (dynein arms).	Ciliary immotility or dyskinesis causes abnormalities of the respiratory tract (bronchiectasis) and spermatozoa (male sterility).

2

FUNDAMENTALS OF MOLECULAR GENETICS

ROBERT A. WEISBERG

PHILIP LEDER

Classical genetics has established a connection between certain human diseases and heredity; indeed, that is the very substance of this volume. But until recently, the relationship between an inherited disease and the precise genetic alteration responsible for it has been virtually impossible to establish with certainty. Fortunately, classical genetics can now be complemented by a set of new and powerful techniques that have recently illuminated the structure and function of several human genes at the molecular level. Such knowledge will certainly bear on the diagnosis and eventually the treatment of genetic disease. The purpose of this chapter is, therefore, to present the salient principles and some of the techniques of molecular genetics, and to illustrate the powerful insights they can provide into the connections between genes and disease. In particular, we would like to advance a comprehensible picture of the chromosome in action by taking into account the major molecular events that are involved in the transmission and use of genetic information. Indeed, it is just these details that provide the excitement and beauty that are so much a part of the new genetics.

THE MOLECULAR FLOW OF INFORMATION

Because of the remarkable discoveries of the past 35 years, we now know a great deal about how living organisms store, transmit, and utilize their genetic information. The picture is most detailed for prokaryotic organisms such as the colon bacillus *Escherichia coli* and several of the viruses (called *bacteriophages*) that parasitize it. It is less detailed, and therefore more rapidly being filled in, for eukaryotic organisms such as

yeast, the fruit fly, and humans. In the brief account that follows, we shall first outline the principal steps of information processing and then describe each step in more detail. We shall draw most heavily on our knowledge of prokaryotes, but where eukaryotes are known to differ in important ways, we shall present the differences. We refer the reader to the textbooks by Watson [1] and Stent and Calendar [2] for a more systematic and comprehensive treatment than we can provide here.

Most organisms store their genetic information in *deoxyribonucleic acid (DNA)*. DNA is a linear polymer of four different monomeric units, collectively called *deoxyribonucleotides* or simply *nucleotides,* that are linked together in a chain by phosphodiester bonds (Fig. 2-1). A typical DNA molecule consists of two interwound polynucleotide chains, each containing several thousand to several million monomers (Fig. 2-2). Each nucleotide in one chain is specifically linked by hydrogen bonds to a nucleotide in the other chain. Only two nucleotide pairings are found in DNA: deoxyadenosine monophosphate with thymidine monophosphate (or A-T) and deoxyguanosine monophosphate with deoxycytidine monophosphate (or G-C). Thus, the sequence of nucleotides of one chain fixes the sequence of the other, and the two chains are therefore said to be *complementary* to each other.

The sequence of the four nucleotides along a polynucleotide chain varies among the DNAs of unrelated organisms and indeed is the molecular basis of their genetic diversity. Because most genetic characteristics are stably transmitted from parent to progeny, the sequence of nucleotides in DNA must be faithfully copied or replicated as the organism reproduces itself. This occurs by unwinding of the two chains and polymerization of two daughter chains along the separated parents. The nucleotide sequence and hence the genetic information is con-

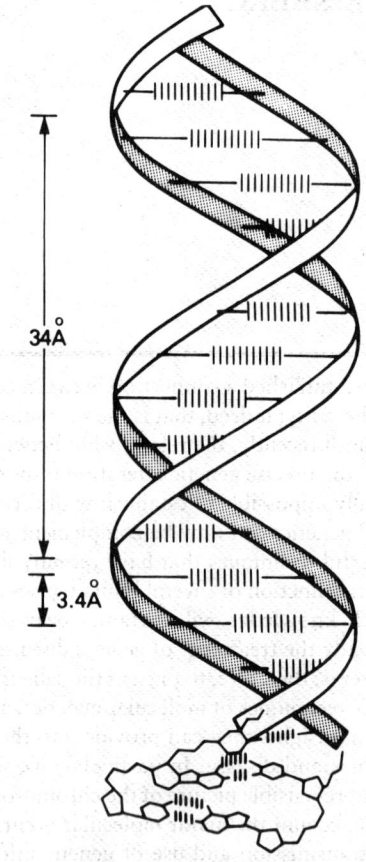

Figure 2-1 A polynucleotide chain. One of each of the four different monomeric units of DNA is present in this tetranucleotide. The monomers of DNA are, from top to bottom, deoxyguanosine monophosphate (or G), deoxycytidine monophosphate (or C), deoxyadenosine monophosphate (or A), and thymidine monophosphate (or T). Each nucleotide consists of a phosphate group, a deoxyribose moiety, and a heterocyclic base. G and A have purine bases, and C and T have pyrimidine bases. The phosphodiester bonds that link adjacent nucleotides extend from the 3′ position of one deoxyribose moiety to the 5′ position of the next; this gives the chain a chemical polarity. An abbreviated way of writing the same sequence is shown at the top right. In RNA (see text) ribose, which contains a 2′-hydroxyl group, replaces deoxyribose, and uridine monophosphate (or U) replaces T. U differs from T in the substitution of ribose for deoxyribose and in the loss of the 5-methyl group.

served during this process because each nucleotide in the daughter chains is paired specifically with its complement in the parental or template chains before polymerization occurs.

How does the sequence of nucleotides in DNA determine the observable hereditary characteristics (the phenotype) of an organism? First, the information stored in DNA is transcribed onto another polynucleotide chain of slightly different chemical composition called *ribonucleic acid* or *RNA*. Transcription is similar in many ways to replication. The monomers of the nascent RNA molecule are aligned in correct order during polymerization by complementary pairing to the appropriate chain of the DNA molecule. In some cases, the transcribed RNA is incorporated directly into cellular structures such as ribosomes, but most transcripts are used to specify the sequence of amino acids in polypeptide chains. These tran-

scripts are called *messenger RNAs* (or *mRNAs*). Nucleotide sequence determines amino acid sequence according to the triplet code given in Table 2-1. The translation of one sequence into the other requires a formidable array of macromolecules and will be described more fully below.

The amino acid sequence of a polypeptide chain determines the way it will fold into a three-dimensional structure and interact with other macromolecules. Such completed polypep-

Figure 2-2 The structure of DNA. In the top part of the figure, the two interwound hydrogen-bonded polynucleotide chains of DNA are shown. The hydrogen bonds are indicated by vertical hatches. The distance between adjacent nucleotide pairs is 3.4 Å. The distance between adjacent turns of the double helix is 34 Å or about 10 nucleotide pairs. The lower part of the figure shows an alternative representation in which the opposite chemical polarities of the two chains can be clearly seen. (*From Kornberg [3] by permission.*)

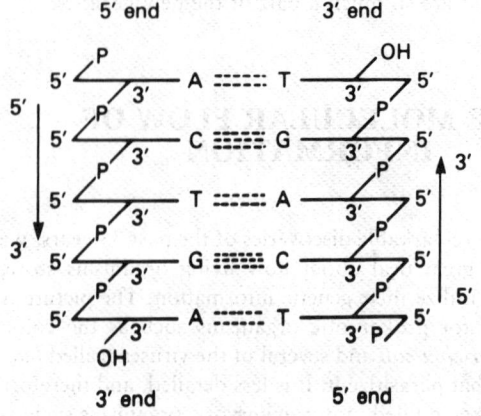

Table 2–1 The Genetic Code*

First base	Second base				Third base
	U	C	A	G	
U	Phe	Ser	Tyr	Cys	U
	Phe	Ser	Tyr	Cys	C
	Leu	Ser	Ter	Ter or Cys	A
	Leu	Ser	Ter	Trp	G
C	Leu	Pro	His	Arg	U
	Leu	Pro	His	Arg	C
	Leu	Pro	Gln	Arg	A
	Leu	Pro	Gln	Arg	G
A	Ile	Thr	Asn	Ser	U
	Ile	Thr	Asn	Ser	C
	Ile	Thr	Lys	Arg	A
	Met and FMET	Thr	Lys	Arg	G
G	Val	Ala	Asp	Gly	U
	Val	Ala	Asp	Gly	C
	Val	Ala	Glu	Gly	A
	Val or FMET	Ala	Glu	Gly	G

* Several code words, e.g. GUG, specify more than one amino acid. They are ambiguous. The basis for this ambiguity is not clearly understood. In the case of AUG, which specifies Met and FMET (FMET = formyl methionine; used as initial amino acid in prokaryotes), preference for one or another codon may be provided by a special sequence preceding the initial codon of a gene. If AUG is the initial codon, it specifies FMET in prokaryotes or a special MET-tRNA in eukaryotes.

tide chains, or *proteins,* form the enzymes and many of the structural components of cells. Thus, the array of proteins produced by an organism is of prime importance in determining its form and functions. A stretch of DNA that encodes a single polypeptide chain is called a *gene.* Each gene is expressed— that is, transcribed into mRNA and translated into protein— according to a program that is itself genetically determined. An organism is what it is only in part because of the proteins it can produce. The amount of each protein and the timing of its production during the life cycle are equally important. Some proteins are much more abundant than others, and many proteins are made only in response to specific internal or external stimuli. Therefore, in the sections that follow, we shall not only describe replication, transcription, and translation in more detail but also give examples of the regulation of each process.

THE STATE OF DNA IN EUKARYOTIC CHROMOSOMES: THE NUCLEOSOME [4, 5]

The DNA of higher organisms, separated from the great bulk of cellular components by a nuclear membrane, is wound into a tightly and regularly packed chromosomal structure consisting of nucleoprotein elements called *nucleosomes* (Fig. 2-3). Each of these nucleosomal elements is in turn composed of four (sometimes five) protein subunits, *histones,* that form a core structure about which are wound approximately 140 nucleotide pairs of genomic DNA. Histone structure is remarkably well conserved throughout the eukaryotic kingdom. Such

conservation argues strongly that strict functional requirements, presumably related to the detailed architecture of the nucleosome, impede divergent evolution. The nucleosomes, arranged as "beads on a string," become further organized into more highly ordered structures consisting of coils of many closely packed nucleosomes that in turn must form fundamental organizational units of the eukaryotic chromosome.

Nucleosomal structure may serve a variety of purposes, for example, in simply compacting the enormous amount of DNA (about 5×10^9 base pairs) comprising the human genome. Aside from such a packing function, this ubiquitous structure must also be reconciled with a train of enzymes that acts upon DNA to permit its orderly replication and transcription. Undoubtedly, these functions are subserved and modulated by other proteins that little resemble the monotonous structure of the histones and that recognize specific structural features of a DNA sequence. A fundamental question in eukaryotic molecular biology is how this nucleoprotein structure permits access to specific proteins and is differentially made available in the course of cellular growth and development.

Bacterial DNA, while by no means a naked nucleic acid polymer, is not organized into stable nucleosomes. Nevertheless, bacterial DNA-binding proteins exist that resemble histones in amino acid composition and may also play a role in compacting DNA.

THE REACTIONS

DNA Replication [3]

DNA synthesis typically begins at specific starting points called *origins.* Organisms with small genomes, such as viruses and bacteria, have one or a small number of origins, while organisms with larger genomes have many origins per chromosome. Studies with bacteria and bacteriophages have revealed that the set of enzymes that catalyzes the initiation of replication overlaps only partially with the set that catalyzes polynucleotide chain elongation, the second phase of replication. The initiating enzymes recognize the nucleotide sequence of the origin and promote the synthesis there of a short polynucleotide chain called a *primer.* In several cases, it has been shown that the primer consists of ribonucleotides, the building blocks of RNA, rather than deoxyribonucleotides. The substrates for polymerization are not the nucleotides themselves but activated derivatives: 5′-nucleoside triphosphates. The mechanism of polymerization is shown in Fig. 2-4. The addition of new monomers always occurs at the 3′ end of the primer, and chain growth is therefore said to proceed in a 5′ to 3′ direction. All known nucleotide polymerizing enzymes work in this way. The mechanism of termination of primer synthesis is not yet well understood, but at some point a new enzyme complex, whose principal component is DNA polymerase, extends the primer by adding deoxyribonucleotides to its 3′ end. The primer is subsequently degraded and replaced by deoxyribonucleotides.

A DNA molecule consists of two interwound polynucleotide chains of opposite chemical polarity. One chain is oriented 5′ to 3′, the other 3′ to 5′ (see Fig. 2-1). Therefore, a single initiation event leads to copying of only one of the chains. Copying of the second requires further initiations, and these occur as

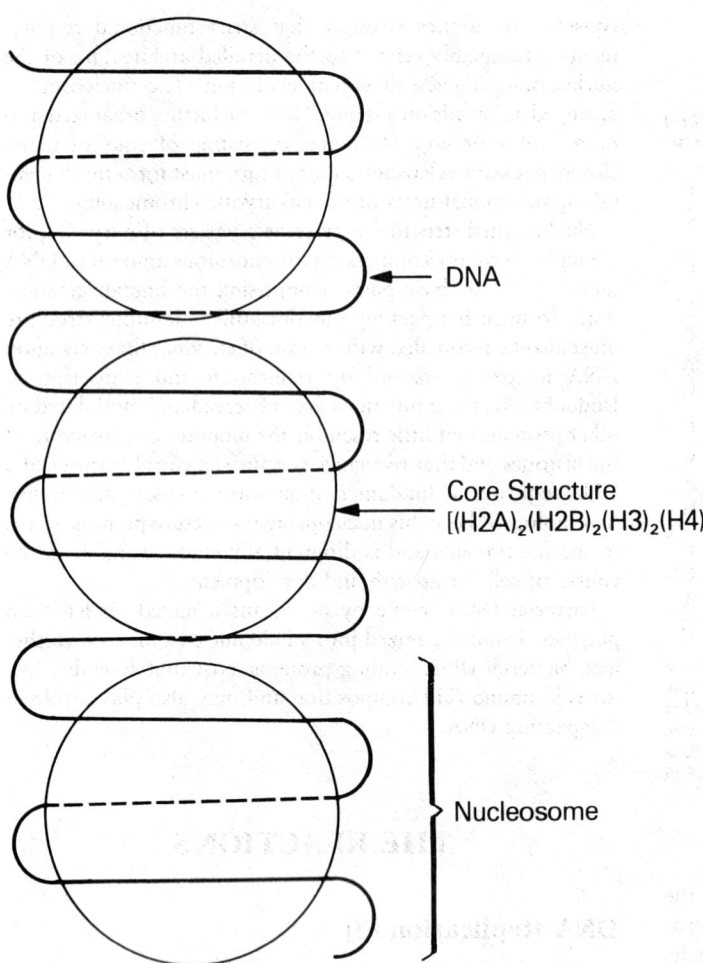

← DNA

← Core Structure [(H2A)₂(H2B)₂(H3)₂(H4)₂)]

Nucleosome

Figure 2-3 The fundamental unit of eukaryotic chromosomal structure: the nucleosome. The nucleosome is diagrammatically represented showing the core structure composed of two units of each of the basic histones: H2A, H2B, H3, and H4. A 140 base pair length of DNA is wrapped around each core structure. The structure has a width of approximately 100 Å and as shown is tightly packed in a "beads on a string" form. Higher organizational levels of nucleosomes are thought to consist of packs of nucleosomes arranged by being stacked into solenoidlike structures.

the two chains unwind, as shown in Fig. 2-5. Note that in any given region of a replicating molecule, copying of one of the chains occurs by continuous addition of nucleotides to a 3′ end, while copying of the other proceeds by a discontinuous series of initiations and elongations followed by enzymatic removal of the primers and linking up of the newly synthesized fragments.

DNA replication in bacteria appears to be controlled mainly at the level of initiation; the elongation rate is relatively constant over a wide range of growth rates. The mechanisms that link initiation rate with growth rate and that ensure proper

Figure 2-4 DNA polymerization. The addition of 5′-thymidine triphosphate to the 3′-hydroxyl group of the terminal A of a polynucleotide chain is shown. (*From Kornberg [3] by permission.*)

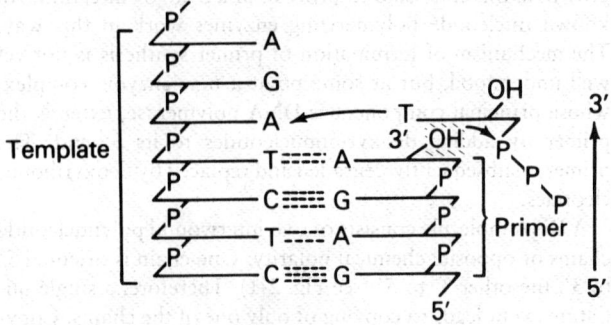

segregation of replicated chromosomes into daughter cells upon cell division are largely unknown.

The copying of genetic information is extremely accurate: The mutation rate is estimated to be about 10^{-9} per nucleotide pair per replication in bacteria, and in organisms with larger genomes it appears to be considerably less. The mutation rate is under genetic control. It can be increased or decreased by a mutation in a "mutator gene" [6]. Some mutator genes determine the synthesis of DNA polymerases, while the functions of others are as yet unknown. The extraordinarily low mutation rate and the properties of mutator genes and DNA polymerases suggest the existence of "proofreading systems" that increase the fidelity of DNA replication over what might be expected from the thermodynamics of nucleotide pairing. One step in proofreading probably occurs at the growing point of a replicating DNA molecule. As each new nucleotide is incorporated, its stereochemical relation to its partner in the parental chain is assayed. If the pairing is incorrect, the nucleotide is removed by enzymatic hydrolysis of the phosphodiester bond. In bacteria the nuclease that accomplishes this step is also the principal DNA polymerase of the cell. Another type of proofreading catches errors that are not at the ends of growing chains. In this case, incorrect pairing between nucleotides in otherwise complementary chains is recognized by an enzyme, one of the mismatched nucleotides excised, and the resulting gap filled in with the correct nucleotide. Recent work suggests that this proofreading system preferentially corrects the most

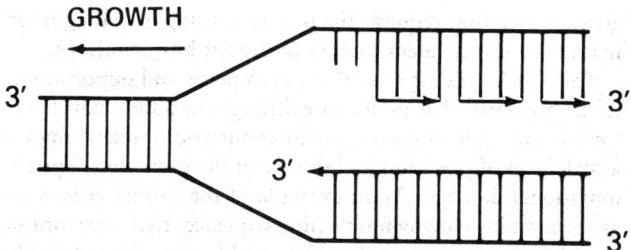

GROWTH

Figure 2-5 Continuous and discontinuous DNA synthesis. The diagram illustrates the region around the growing point of a DNA molecule. Unreplicated DNA lies to the left and replicated DNA to the right. The addition of deoxynucleotides to the 3' end of a growing chain can occur continuously, but synthesis of the complementary chain is discontinuous. It occurs by repeated initiations followed by growth of short chains (represented by a series of three short arrows) in a direction that is opposite to that of the overall direction of growth. The short chains are eventually linked up, with removal of any ribonucleotide primers.

recently synthesized chain, thus removing the newly incorporated mismatched nucleotide rather than the parental (and presumably nonmutant) nucleotide. The old and new chains of a DNA molecule can be distinguished by a chemical modification of DNA (methylation of adenine) that takes place only with some delay after synthesis and is therefore absent on a recently synthesized chain [7].

Transcription

Prokaryotes [8, 9]   Transcription of DNA into RNA is the first step in gene expression. The monomeric units of RNA, the ribonucleotides, differ from deoxyribonucleotides in that ribose replaces deoxyribose, and uridine monophosphate (or U) replaces thymidine monophosphate (see the legend to Fig. 2-1). In bacteria a single multisubunit enzyme, RNA polymerase, is responsible for almost all transcription. In the simplest case, RNA polymerase binds to DNA at a specific sequence called a *promoter* and initiates the polymerization of ribonucleotides in a 5' to 3' direction. The substrates for RNA synthesis, as in the case of DNA synthesis, are not the nucleotides themselves but activated derivatives: 5'-ribonucleoside triphosphates. The nascent RNA chain, unlike a nascent DNA chain, does not form a stably paired structure with the template chain of DNA; instead, pairing between RNA and DNA is transient and localized to a short region behind the growing point in which the two chains of DNA have unwound (Fig. 2-6). RNA synthesis proceeds until the enzyme encounters another specific sequence called a *terminator,* at which point chain elongation ceases, and the newly synthesized transcript is released.

RNA polymerase initiates transcription at some promoters only if an effector protein is present. The prototype of such effectors is the cyclic AMP receptor protein, which, in the presence of the nucleotide cyclic AMP, allows RNA polymerase to initiate transcription of genes that encode catabolic enzymes. Other well-studied effector proteins are synthesized after infection by certain viruses. Clearly, these proteins enable the cell or viruses infecting the cell to control gene expression by regulating the initiation of transcription.

How do effectors promote initiation of transcription? The best understood example to date involves the P_M promoter of bacteriophage λ. The effector, called λ *repressor* because of its

principal role in virus development (see below), binds to the DNA at sites immediately adjacent to the P_M. It appears likely that direct contact between bound repressor and RNA polymerase stimulates initiation of transcription [10].

Transcription termination is another point of control. Some viruses synthesize proteins that prevent termination at certain terminators, and in other cases termination is coupled to translation of the terminator region into protein [11]. Such translation-modulated terminators, called *attenuators,* are found before certain bacterial genes whose products are required for the biosynthesis of amino acids. Translation of the region immediately before the attenuator depends specifically on the supply of the amino acid whose corresponding biosynthetic genes lie immediately after the terminator. Therefore these genes are not transcribed when their products are not needed. We shall consider other examples of transcription control below.

The nucleotide sequences of many promoters, terminators, mutant promoters, and mutant terminators have been determined. Comparison of these sequences shows that nucleotides required for initiation and termination of RNA synthesis lie immediately before the first and last nucleotides, respectively, that are copied to give the transcript. In the case of promoters, we know that the required nucleotides are to a large extent the same as those that physically interact with RNA polymerase. Less is known about the mechanism of termination. The nucleotide sequence of terminators and the properties of attenuators suggest that the formation of intrachain paired regions—hairpinlike structures—at the ends of the transcripts is important for termination. The formation of such paired regions can be favored or blocked according to the movement of ribosomes along the RNA during translation. For some terminators a specific effector protein is required for efficient termination.

Figure 2-6   Initial steps in DNA transcription. The diagram illustrates the region around the growing point of an RNA transcript. The line terminated by an arrow represents a growing RNA chain. The 5'-nucleoside triphosphate at the other end is the start point of synthesis. RNA polymerase binds to a promoter site and initiates transcription in a 5' to 3' direction. The immediate product of transcription is a partially three-stranded structure containing a single polydeoxynucleotide chain opposite a region of DNA-RNA hybrid. The nascent RNA chain is subsequently released, with re-formation of double-stranded DNA.

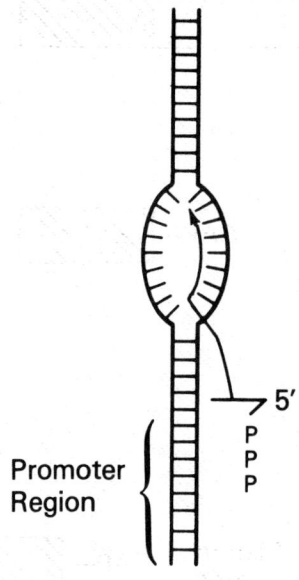

Promoter
Region

Eukaryotes [12, 13]   The biochemistry of transcription in higher organisms is not unlike that found in bacteria, but the enzymes involved and their arrangement within the cell differ in a most interesting way. First, the templates for transcription, the chromosomes, are separated by a nuclear membrane from the cytoplasm that contains the protein synthetic apparatus of the cell. This functional and morphologic segregation isolates the nuclear transcribing and processing enzymes that produce and finally export finished RNA from the cytoplasmic enzymes involved in their use.

In keeping with this morphologic separation, eukaryotic organisms appear to divide the tasks of transcription among three separate, highly specialized sets of RNA polymerases. Two of these, RNA polymerases I and III, are concerned with the transcription of RNA products vital to protein synthesis, the ribosomal and transfer RNAs, respectively (see below). These enzymes are not involved in the production of the protein-encoding mRNAs. This task falls to a third enzyme, RNA polymerase II, which seems to be responsible for the synthesis of precursors of the mRNAs.

In addition to the morphologic segregation of the transcriptional apparatus and the distribution of three specialized transcription functions among three sets of enzymes, there is another important difference between prokaryotic and eukaroytic RNA production. Eukaryotic mRNA requires a number of important processing steps or chemical modifications before it can emerge in functional form in the cytoplasm.

Perhaps the most intriguing of these processing steps follows from the fact that a large number of (but not all) genes in higher eukaryotes are interrupted [14]. That is, they are represented in discontinuous bits of coding sequence separated from one another by noncoding sequences called *intervening sequences* or *introns* (Fig. 2-7). It is now clear that transcription of these genes proceeds from a specific initiation site (analogous to a bacterial promoter) through the entire gene, coding and noncoding sequences, so as to produce a larger mRNA precursor from which the noncoding sequences must be removed to form a coherent mRNA. Thus an additional step is involved in the expression of genetic information from these

genes, a step that requires the precise splicing of coding information by the covalent joining of distant bits of mRNA.

This RNA splicing step offers both perils and opportunities to the organism. The perils arise through the additional chance for error provided by a reaction that must occur many times at a high level of precision and that is, at the same time, open to mutational damage. As an example of the former risk, some genes contain so many intervening sequences that an error rate of only a few percent per splice would markedly reduce the yield of coherent mRNA. As an example of the latter risk, a mutation might obliterate a splice signal or create a new splice signal in an inappropriate location. Opportunities arise because programmed flexibility in the splicing of coding regions would allow an array of coding sequences to be put together in a number of possibly useful combinations. It is now clear, for example, that the coding sequences of an immunoglobulin heavy chain can be brought together in two different ways, one to include, another to exclude, a coding sequence that specifies a part of the polypeptide chain that anchors an immunoglobulin molecule to the surface of a lymphocyte (Fig. 2-8) [15]. If mRNA splicing occurs so as to exclude the anchor peptide sequence, a circulating rather than a surface immunoglobulin is produced. So, while the splicing reactions place additional demands upon the system of information flow, they also provide a means of creating new genetic information by joining bits of linear genetic information in a variety of useful combinations

Creating additional genetic possibilities cannot be the only reason that some genes are split. Certain studies suggest that the splicing sequence is essential for an RNA transcript of certain mammalian genes to exit from the nucleus of the cell in a

Figure 2-7 Transcription of an interrupted gene and the maturation of its mRNA. A model globin gene is represented diagrammatically, indicating the initiation site for transcription (INI), the coding sequences (hatched) (sometimes called *exons*), the intervening sequences (IVS introns) and the poly(A) addition site (pA . . .). The gene is represented 5′ to 3′ (left to right). The primary transcript includes this entire gene. Maturation involves the addition of a 5′ cap structure (see text), a 3′ poly(A) tail, and the splicing out of its two intervening sequences with the covalent ligation of the coding sequences.

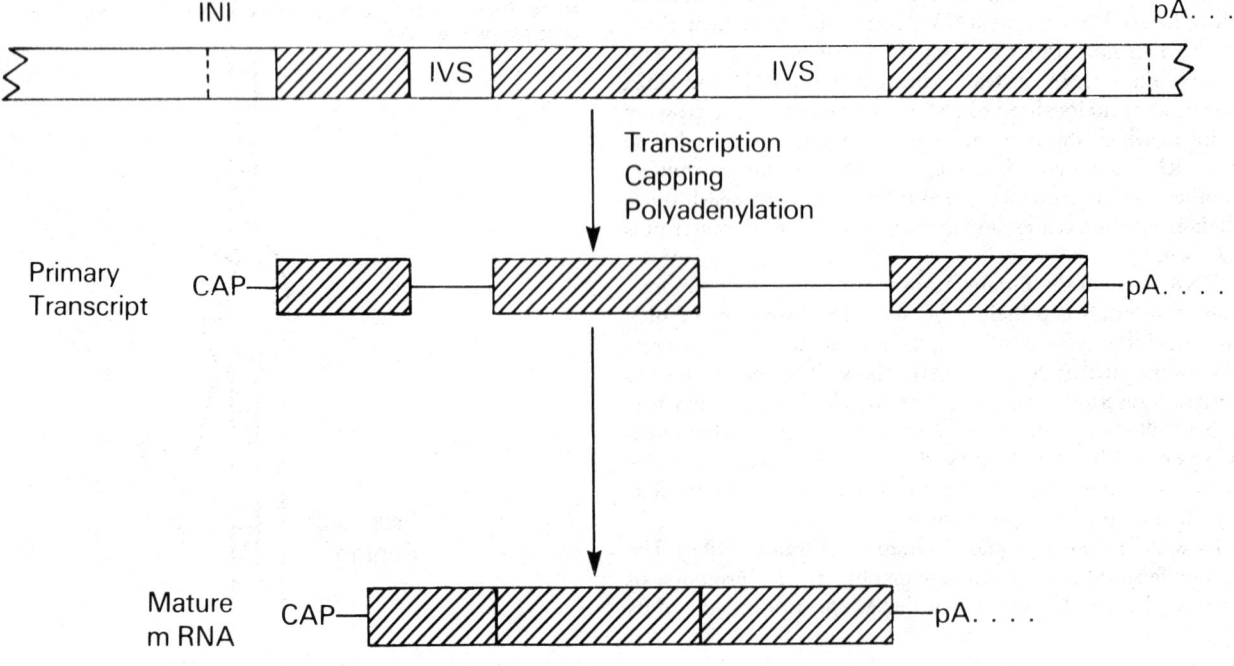

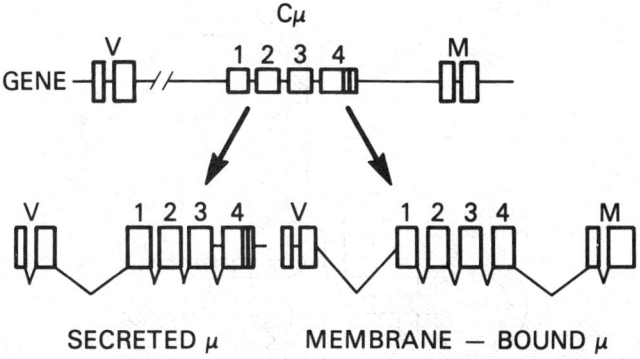

Figure 2-8 Alternative RNA splice modes in the immunoglobulin heavy chain gene. An immunoglobulin μ heavy chain gene is represented diagrammatically (*top*). The boxes represent coding sequences and the lines intervening or flanking sequences. V refers to the variable region sequences, while Cμ and the numbers refer to each μ constant region coding domain. The boxes under the letter M are coding regions corresponding to anchor peptides. The arrows point to alternative transcription and processing pathways. The anchor peptide coding segment is not spliced to the mRNA on the left but is spliced to the mRNA on the right. This option allows the same gene to direct the synthesis of a free or membrane-bound immunoglobulin. (*After Rogers et al. [15].*)

stable fashion (see Ref. 14). Still, a number of genes (e.g., those encoding histones, interferons, and Herpes virus thymidine kinase) are not split and are obviously expressed in a variety of cells, suggesting that there are at least two classes of genes and transcripts, whole and divided, and that these contain additional, as yet unrecognized features that employ different mechanisms to deliver RNA transcripts to the cytoplasm.

There are two additional modifications that occur during the maturation of a eukaryotic mRNA: the addition of a 7-methylguanosine by an unusual 5′-5′ pyrophosphate linkage to the 5′ terminal nucleotide of the mRNA (called a *cap*) and the addition of a variable-length tail of A residues to the 3′ end of the mRNA (Fig. 2-7) [16, 17]. Both of these modifications occur within the nucleus, apparently prior to the removal of the intervening sequences. Capping occurs in all eukaryote mRNAs thus far examined and seems to enhance the translation efficiency of the mRNA (at least in cell-free systems). Poly(A) addition is prevalent, but not universal (e.g., histone mRNAs are not polyadenylated), and has no as yet known role in posttranscriptional processes.

Perhaps it is unfair to note these modifications and processing steps as the hallmarks that distinguish higher and lower forms of life. Their precedents are clearly evident in the processing and modification steps that are involved in the production of ribosomal and tRNAs in both humans and bacteria. A further carryover from bacterial mechanisms is the promoter-

related sequences that are invariably associated with transcriptional initiation sites in mammalian genes. A ubiquitous hexanucleotide, TATAA^A_C, is found almost exactly three turns of a double helix (30 base pairs) from the capping signal of eukaryotic genes and appears to be an essential part of the eukaryotic promoter (Fig. 2-9). Another sequence (AATAA) has been identified close to the poly(A) addition site of many genes and may represent a critical signal for polyadenylation.

Translation and the Genetic Code [18–20]

Translation, the process whereby the genetic message directs the assembly of amino acids into specific arrays in the form of proteins, is by far the most complex of the reactions involved in the flow of information from gene to cytoplasm. The process requires over 100 different protein and RNA species, utilizing them as simple, soluble elements or in the form of particulate multienzyme complexes such as ribosomes. Ribosomes move along an mRNA molecule, translating each of its triplet code words or codons in a 5′ to 3′ direction to assemble a polypeptide from its NH$_3$ to its COOH ends. The instructional portion of the complex, the mRNA, is related to the protein product through the genetic code, an array of the 64 permutations of the four nucleotides taken three at a time (Table 2-1). Almost all of these 64 triplet code words specify an amino acid, but one (and rarely another, see below) designate a translational initiation point, while three others are stop signals, indicating that the polypeptide chain terminates at the point at which they occur. Moreover, this code is virtually universal, having the same meaning throughout the animal and plant kingdoms. An exception to the universality of this coding language occurs among certain mitochondrial genes in which codons that normally signify "stop" instead specify the insertion of a particular amino acid.

The Adaptor Molecules and Their Enzymes [21] The oligonucleotide code words do not interact with amino acids directly but rather through adaptor or tRNA molecules to which the amino acids are joined by a highly specific enzyme in an energy-rich bond. There is at least one, but often more than one, tRNA species corresponding to each of the 20 naturally occurring amino acids. Correspondingly, there are special and highly specific enzymes called *aminoacyl-tRNA synthetases* that covalently join amino acids to their cognate tRNAs. These enzymes perform a very special function, not only in activating amino acids but also in assuring that each amino acid is joined only to its cognate tRNA and to no other. The fidelity of the translation process depends upon the fidelity of these synthe-

Figure 2-9 Conserved signals thought to play a role in the transcription of mammalian genes. The globin genes of the mouse (called β-major, β-minor, and α-1) are diagrammatically represented together with their conserved signal sequences. The letters cAp. . . represent the initiation site for transcription and the first capped nucleotide of the mRNA. Each box represents a coding sequence and the numbers 1 and 2 over each line represent the two intervening sequences. The 5′ (*left*) TATAAA or TATAAG sequences are thought to be a part of the transcriptional initiation site. The conserved 3′ (*right*) AATAA pentanucleotide may be required as a poly(A) addition signal.

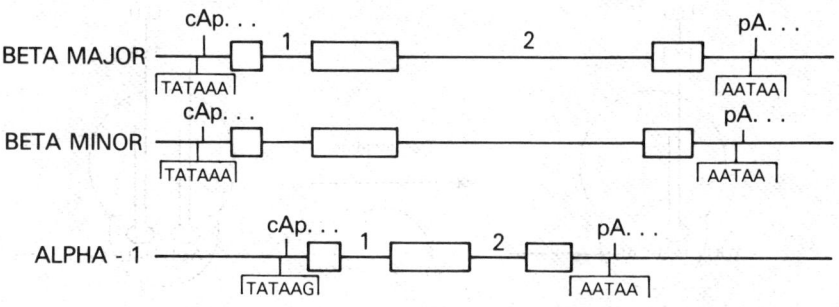

tases, and they constitute a family of enzymes, each of which specifies a single amino acid.

The primary as well as the three-dimensional structure of tRNA molecules is now known in considerable detail. Thus it is clear that a sequence of three nucleotides complementary to the codon, the *anticodon,* is exposed at one end of the folded tRNA molecule, while the amino acid acceptor site is exposed at the other (Fig. 2-10). The rules for complementary pairing between codons in mRNA and anticodons in tRNA differ somewhat from those for interchain pairing in DNA, especially in the third nucleotide position of the codon. Here U can pair with A or G, G can pair with C or U, and a derivative of G, inosine, can pair with U, C, or A. Such a relaxation of the steric requirements for nucleotide pairing is called *wobble.* Because of wobble, certain codons can be read in an ambiguous way (e.g., GUG can be read as either valine or methionine) and certain tRNAs can recognize more than one codon (e.g., phenylalanine tRNA; UUU or UUC). Amino acids are thus specified at two recognition steps; one in which a specific enzyme joins the amino acid to a specific tRNA, and another, in which the tRNA, serving as an adaptor molecule, is brought into the translation complex through a codon-anticodon interaction between the mRNA and the tRNA (Figs. 2-10 and 2-11).

Translational Initiation, Elongation, and Termination [*18, 19*]

The translation process itself involves a host of soluble enzymes or *factors,* a large particulate nucleoprotein element called a *ribosome,* as well as mRNAs and tRNAs. While the bacterial and eukaryotic protein synthetic elements differ somewhat, their common features can be considered together. The initiation point is usually encoded in mRNA by a single methionine codon, AUG, which, in bacteria, occurs about 10 nucleotides to the 3' side of a purine-rich sequence which is itself roughly complementary to a 7 to 9 base sequence in the

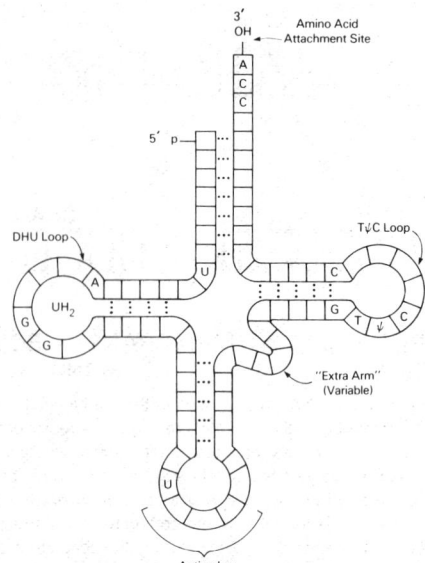

Figure 2-10 A diagrammatic representation of a tRNA molecule. Each base in the tRNA is represented by a box. The structure is shown with interacting complementary sequences indicated by a row of dots. Each conserved loop is shown (DHU, dehydrouridylic acid loop; TψC, thymidylic acid-pseudouridylic acid-cytidylic acid loop). The anticodon position is indicated. All tRNAs end with a CCA sequence at their 3' terminus that serves as the amino acid acceptor portion of the molecule. (*After Stryer* [22].)

RNA portion of the smaller of the two ribosomal subunits. This signal apparently distinguishes initiation from internal methionine codons, for there are also two different species of methionine-accepting tRNAs, one for initiation and one for internal use. In eukaryotic mRNAs the 5' cap modification appears to serve this function.

A number of soluble initiation factors, as well as the ribo-

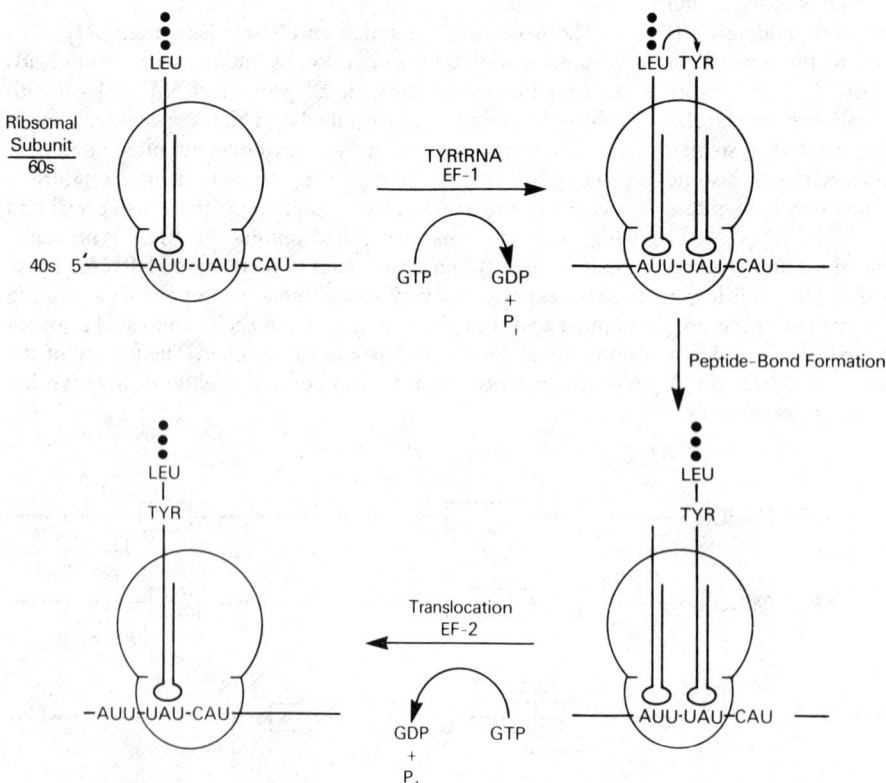

Figure 2-11 The elongation reactions in protein synthesis. The figure diagrammatically represents the ribosome (60 S and 40 S subunits), the tRNA moieties (hairpinlike structures), and the associated mRNAs. The first elongation intermediate (*upper left*) shows a peptidyl tRNA, the peptide portion of which is represented by leucine and three dots, at the donor site on the ribosome interacting with a leucine codon, AUU. In the presence of GTP and elongation factor 1 (EF-1), tyr-tRNA binds to the next available codon at the receptor site. The peptide is transferred to the oncoming tyr-tRNA by an enzymatic activity associated with the 60 S subunit of the ribosome. The next step involves release of the deacylated tRNA (leucine) and the translocation of the mRNA and the newly elongated peptidyl tRNA to the donor site, exposing the next available codon, CAU, for recognition. The later reaction requires elongation factor 2 (EF-2) and consumes GTP. The entire process is repeated until a termination codon is encountered, and the finished peptide is released in the presence of appropriate termination factors.

nucleotide guanosine triphosphate, are necessary to attach the initial met-tRNA to a ribosome and to begin the process of translation. Additional soluble protein factors, called *elongation factors,* are required for the elongation steps of protein synthesis, the process by which the ribosome moves across the mRNA one codon at a time, adding a single amino acid to the growing polypeptide chain at each translocation step (Fig. 2-11). The ribosome itself plays a role in catalyzing these reactions, supplying sites for peptide bond formation and translocation. Interestingly, diphtheria toxin specifically inactivates one of these factors, the translocase EF-2, by catalyzing the addition of adenosine diphosphoribose [23]. Treatment of polysomes (strings of ribosomes on a single mRNA molecule) by diphtheria toxin therefore "freezes" the ribosomes in place.

Termination, the final step of the translation reaction, occurs when one of the codons, UAA, UAG, or UGA, is reached. Since there are usually no tRNAs corresponding to these codons, the growing peptide chain is released (in the presence of appropriate termination factors) and, in most eukaryotic mRNAs, translation ends at this point. In contrast, prokaryotic organisms use mRNAs that encode several polypeptides. Here the ribosome releases each polypeptide as it encounters a termination codon, but it can remain associated with the (polycistronic) mRNA until the next initiator codon is reached.

Mutation and the Genetic Code   Most mutations, alterations in the structure of DNA (see below), manifest effects at the level of translation. Obviously, a single base change can alter the meaning of a codon, causing the substitution of one amino acid for another, e.g., the glutamic acid ($GA^A/_G$), valine ($GU^A/_G$) substitution seen in sickle-cell anemia. Other mutations, by introducing or deleting one or several bases, may cause a coding frameshift in which the frame of reading of the genetic code is thrown out of phase and its amino acid translation entirely changed; for example, the three codons AAU UUU CCC (Asn Phe Pro) can be converted to GAA AUU UCC C (Glu Ile Ser) by adding a single G to their 5' end. Usually these frameshift mutations also introduce a new in-phase termination (Ter) codon following a stretch of frameshifted missense reading, as in the conversion of CCC UUU AAA (Pro Phe Lys) to GCC CUU UAA A (Ala Leu Ter) by the addition of a single G. A number of amino acid codons are converted to termination codons by the alteration of a single base, e.g.,

$$[UUA(Leu) \rightarrow UAA(Ter)] \qquad (1)$$

Such a mutation would create a premature termination signal in mRNA, producing a foreshortened protein. Indeed, just such a mutation seems to be responsible for one of the β thalassemias in which β-globin chains are not synthesized [24]. Conversely, a mutation in a normal termination codon converting it to an amino acid codon

$$[UAA(Ter) \rightarrow CAA(Gln)] \qquad (2)$$

would produce an elongated protein by read-through, as in the case of hemoglobin Constant Spring, which is 31 amino acids longer than normal α-globin (see Chap. 76).

Suppression   One other type of mutation deserves consideration. Since codon recognition depends upon codon-anticodon (tRNA) interaction, a mutation changing a base in an anticodon should also alter the codon recognition properties of a tRNA. A normal tyrosine-tRNA will recognize the codon (5')UAC(3') because it possesses the complementary anticodon (3')AUG(5'). If the last nucleotide in the tyrosine-tRNA anticodon is converted to C, as in (3')AUC(5'), it should now recognize the termination codon (5')UAG(3') and insert a tyrosine at what would normally be a termination signal. Such mutant tRNA species have long been known to bacterial geneticists as a special class of suppressor (correcting) mutations. Suppressor tRNAs allow ribosomes to translate through termination codons that arise by mutation within other genes. Such termination suppressor tRNAs are also known to occur in yeast, and while as yet undiscovered in higher organisms, they are likely to occur throughout all living species.

The Control of Gene Expression

The proper rate and timing of the processes described above are essential for the adaptive responses of microorganisms to their environment, for the development of viruses after infection, for differentiation during embryogenesis, for the production of antibodies, and for many other adaptive and developmental phenomena. Disruption of proper control frequently leads to disease or death. Gene expression is regulated at several points: at the level of genetic structure, of initiation and termination of transcription, and of the stability and translatability of mRNA. We shall discuss each of these in turn, again using examples drawn from both lower and higher forms of life so as to anticipate as fully as possible mechanisms that may all eventually prove relevant to the genes of humans.

Control at the Level of DNA Structure

INVERSION AND INSERTION: SALMONELLA ANTIGENS AND PROPHAGE λ   We now know that the structure of genes changes more frequently than was once suspected. In some cases, the changes are predictable and play a role in gene expression. The variation of flagellar antigens (*flagella* are surface appendages required for cell motility) in the bacterium *Salmonella typhimurium* is a well-studied example [25, 26]. This organism can produce two alternative flagellar proteins. A clone of bacteria consists largely of individuals that express the flagellar antigen of their parent, but variants expressing the alternative antigen arise at frequencies that greatly exceed the mutation rate, and these variants can be recognized because they are not immobilized by antiserum raised against the parental antigen. The switch from production of one antigen to production of the other is correlated with the inversion of a short segment of DNA (Fig. 2-12). Inversion couples (or uncouples) the gene that encodes one of the flagellar antigens with (or from) its promoter. The same promoter also appears to be required for transcription of a regulatory gene whose product represses expression of the gene encoding the alternative flagellar antigen (which is located elsewhere on the bacterial chromosome). Thus the orientation of the DNA segment that contains the promoter governs which flagellar gene is expressed.

How does inversion occur? A plausible answer to this question is based on the analysis of the insertion of the bacteriophage λ chromosome into the chromosome of its host [27, 28]. After infection with λ, some cells survive and give rise to progeny that contain a quiescent form of the virus chromosome known as *prophage.* The prophage consists of a complete but

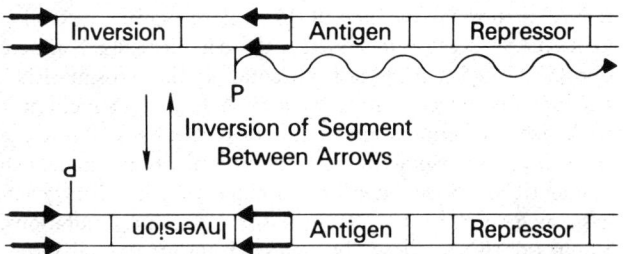

Figure 2-12 Gene control by inversion. The two pairs of horizontal lines represent a segment of the bacterial chromosome, and the wavy line terminated by an arrow represents an RNA transcript initiated from promoter P. The short arrows represent a 14-nucleotide pair sequence that is repeated in inverted order at each end of the invertible segment. The region marked "Inversion" encodes a product required for inversion, that marked "Antigen" encodes one of the alternative flagellar antigens, and that marked "Repressor" encodes a repressor of the gene for the other flagellar antigen. Inversion may occur by lining up the two 14-nucleotide pair regions in the same orientation followed by breakage, reciprocal exchange, and rejoining within this region (see text). Transcription of the antigen and repressor genes occurs only when the promoter is in the top orientation.

largely untranscribed virus chromosome (see below) that replicates in synchrony with the host because it is inserted at a specific site in the bacterial chromosome. Insertion is reversible and occurs by breakage, reciprocal exchange, and rejoining of polynucleotide chains, as shown in Fig. 2-13. The points of exchange lie within a 15-nucleotide pair sequence that is present in both the virus and the host chromosomes. After insertion, this sequence is found in two identically oriented copies at each end of the prophage. The reaction requires phage and host-encoded proteins that interact specifically with the DNA around the insertion sites and promote the exchange. The DNA inversion associated with flagellar antigen variation formally resembles λ insertion in having exchange points that lie within a 14-nucleotide pair sequence that is repeated in inverted order at each end of the segment. Inversion also requires a specific protein, which is encoded within the invertible segment. Although direct biochemical evidence is lacking, the two reactions could occur by a similar mechanism.

GENE SUBSTITUTION: YEAST MATING TYPE CONVERSION [26, 29]   A second type of regular change in genetic structure that plays a role in gene expression has been studied in yeast. Haploid yeast cells have one of two alternative mating types, *a* or *α*. In certain strains, *a* cells give rise to *a* progeny (and vice versa) with high frequency. Genetic and biochemical studies have shown that change in mating type is governed by a movement of genetic information from one location to another in yeast chromosome III. Phenotypic change occurs because the genetic information is expressed in the second (or *cassette*) locus, while it is silent in the first (or *library*) locus. There are two library loci on chromosome III; one normally contains *a* and the other *α* information. In contrast to *Salmonella* inversion and λ insertion, the change in yeast genetic structure is not reciprocal. When the switch occurs, the information at the library locus is conserved and the information at the cassette locus is discarded. Moreover, the choice of library locus is not random but depends on whether *a* or *α* information is being expressed in the cassette locus. Thus *a* switches to *α* and vice versa, with a probability that is greater than 0.5 per generation. Several important questions about this system remain to be answered. How is gene expression differentially controlled at the library and cassette loci? What is the mechanism of genetic change,

and what gives it its directionality? It already seems likely that the answers to the second question will differ substantially from those found for the *Salmonella* inversion and λ insertion systems.

RECOMBINATION WITH DELETION: THE ACTIVATION OF ANTIBODY GENES [30]   A third type of programmed change in gene structure is required for the activation of antibody genes in vertebrates. This alteration also compensates for the problem of creating an enormous repertoire of antibody molecules from what is, relatively speaking, a small and limited array of genes. The immunoglobulin light chain genes of humans present a striking example of this creative type of recombination. Formation of an active κ light chain gene requires a genetic rearrangement that joins one of several hundred gene segments that encode the NH_3^+ terminal 95 amino acids of the light chain (the variable or V region) to one of five short (about 13 codons) joining (J) segments of DNA. The J segments are located a few thousand bases away from the single segment

Figure 2-13 The mechanism of bacteriophage λ insertion. The concentric circles represent a circular form of the bacteriophage λ chromosome (which contains about 50,000 nucleotide pairs), the two horizontal lines, a segment of the *E. coli* chromosome, and the two pairs of arrows in the DNAs, a 15-nucleotide pair sequence that is present in both of them. Insertion occurs by breakage, reciprocal exchange, and rejoining of polynucleotide chains within the repeated sequence.

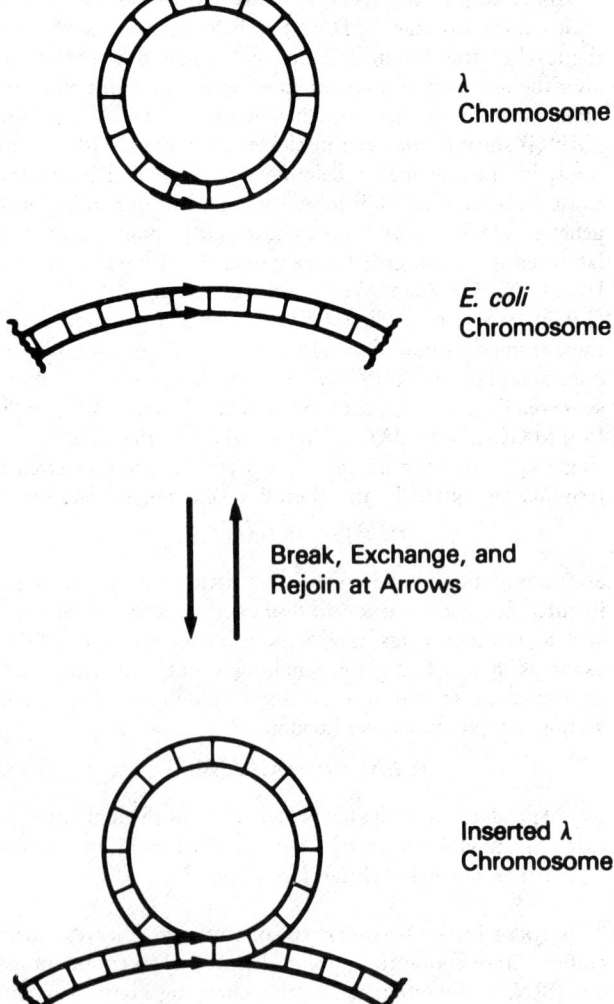

λ
Chromosome

E. coli
Chromosome

Break, Exchange, and
Rejoin at Arrows

Inserted λ
Chromosome

that encodes the last hundred or so amino acids of the κ light chain (the constant region) (Fig. 2-14). The fused variable J segment is subsequently joined to the constant region by RNA splicing before translation into protein.

By joining one of about 300 variable region segments to one of five J segments, one can generate $300 \times 5 = 1500$ different combinations or 1500 different light chain molecules. Thus this special recombination system not only activates genes but creates new genetic possibilities. In the case of immunoglobulin heavy chains, the possibility of generating additional diversity is further amplified because the complete variable region is assembled not from two but from three separately encoded bits of DNA. Also, as noted above, alternative RNA splicing pathways provide additional opportunities to use coding sequences in different combinations.

Control of DNA Transcription: The Phage λ Example

[*31*] Transcription is controlled both at its initiation and at its termination. In bacteria, transcripts initiating at particular promoters can be stimulated by effector proteins or depressed by repressor proteins, as discussed above. Several effectors, repressors, and promoters can be combined into a regulatory circuit that enables the organism to alter its development in response to internal or environmental signals. Such a regulatory circuit has been extensively studied in the bacteriophage λ.

Figure 2-14 The formation of an active immunoglobulin light chain gene. The immunoglobulin light chain gene is diagrammed such that boxes represent coding sequences and open, dotted, and hatched boxes represent variable, joining, and constant regions, respectively. Dashed lines indicate that the distances separating coding segments are not known. The upper figure indicates the immunoglobulin coding sequences in germline DNA. There are several hundred variable region genes, five joining region genes, and one constant region gene. A recombination event is necessary to form an active gene (shown below), and it involves the covalent joining of one of the variable region genes to one of the J-region genes (arrow). L, V, J, and C in the lower portion of the figure represent hydrophobic leader, variable, joining, and constant region genes, respectively.

Lambda propagates itself in two mutually exclusive ways: as a quiescent prophage, replicating in synchrony with the host (*lysogenic growth*), or as an autonomous genetic element, replicating much faster than the host, with consequent cell death and liberation of several hundred progeny virus particles (*lytic growth*). The prophage is quiescent in part because the λ repressor protein prevents the initiation of transcription at two λ promoters. It does this by binding to "operator" sites in the DNA adjacent to the promoters, thereby physically excluding RNA polymerase from the DNA. Among the repressed genes are some whose expression leads to rapid autonomous growth of the virus and death of the host cell. Bound repressor has a second function. It stimulates the initiation of transcription at a second promoter site that is responsible for transcription of its own gene. This ensures continued synthesis of repressor. When a λ particle infects a cell that contains no preexisting repressor, how is the choice between lytic and lysogenic growth made? In fact, a complicated regulatory circuit, consisting principally of three promoters and three virus regulatory proteins, ensures that the choice will be both decisive and responsive to environmental conditions, such as the nutritional state of the cell. Two of the promoters, together with their cognate effector proteins, allow the gene that encodes repressor to be transcribed either at the high rate needed to prevent killing of an infected cell or at the low rate suitable for the maintenance of an inserted prophage. The activity of the first effector is linked, in a still poorly understood way, to the health of the cell. The third regulatory protein depresses transcription of the repressor gene, thereby favoring lytic growth. We refer the reader to Ref. 31 for a more complete discussion of this complex transcriptional switch.

We noted above that transcription is also controlled at the level of termination. A particularly well-studied case is again found in phage λ. One of the genes that is expressed immediately after infection encodes an antiterminator protein. This

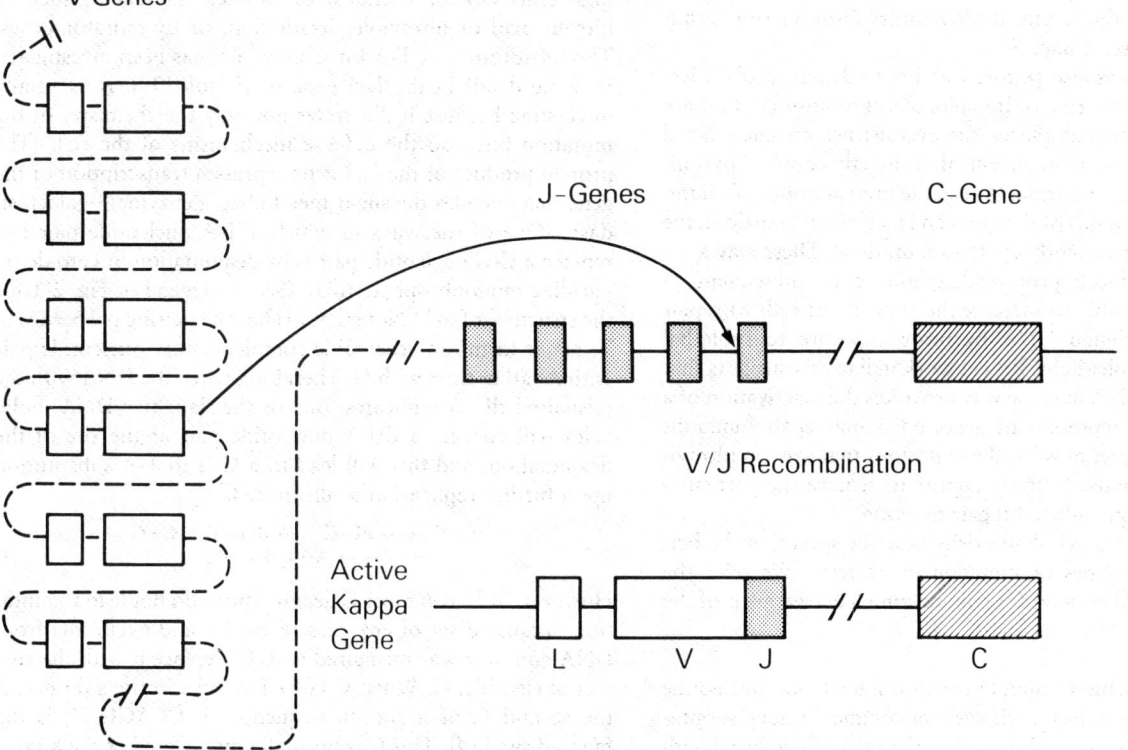

V Genes

J-Genes   C-Gene

V/J Recombination

Active
Kappa
Gene

L   V   J   C

protein allows RNA polymerase to ignore terminator sites in the DNA. Genes located distal to these sites are essential both for lytic virus growth and for the establishment of lysogeny.

MECHANISMS OF GENE CHANGE

Mutational Classes, Frequency, and Repair [3, 6, 32]

Mutations are of two classes: (1) point changes, such as substitution of one nucleotide for another and addition or deletion of a few nucleotides, and (2) larger changes (or chromosomal rearrangements) such as inversion, transposition, deletion, and addition of hundreds to millions of nucleotides. We now know a great deal about the basic mechanisms of both kinds of mutation in microorganisms, and it is not wildly optimistic to expect that in the near future the detailed enzymatic pathways that promote and prevent DNA change will also become known.

Mutations arise spontaneously in wild-type bacteria at an exceedingly low frequency—about 10^{-9} per nucleotide pair per replication—but can be induced with much higher efficiency by relaxing the proofreading standards of the DNA replication machinery, as discussed above, or by treatment with agents that damage DNA. Damage to DNA is not inevitably lethal. Repair mechanisms exist both in bacteria and in higher organisms that remove damaged nucleotides and replace them by copying the information present in the undamaged complementary polynucleotide chain. An example of such excision repair is shown in Fig. 2-15; in this case, irradiation with ultraviolet light of 260 nm has linked adjacent pyrimidine nucleotides in one chain via a cyclobutyl ring to form a pyrimidine dimer. Defects in an early step of the excision repair pathway are responsible for the extreme sensitivity to ultraviolet light shown by individuals with the hereditary disorder xeroderma pigmentosum (see Chap. 57).

Other processes also restore viability to damaged DNA: Recombination between two homologous chromosomes that are damaged at different places can reconstruct an undamaged chromosome, as can an enzyme that directly converts pyrimidine dimers to their normal state in the presence of visible light. Although some kinds of damage can be efficiently repaired, the restored DNA frequently contains mutations. These may arise because of reduced proofreading during or subsequent to repair. It is possible to increase the capacity of cells to repair ultraviolet-irradiated DNA by prior exposure to sublethal doses of ultraviolet light. Recent work in bacteria suggests that the damaged DNA in some way provokes the inactivation of a transcriptional repressor of genes encoding repair functions [33]. Interestingly, most of the mutations that arise in ultraviolet light-irradiated bacteria appear to require the participation of a damage-induced repair function.

In what follows, we shall briefly describe several of the better understood types of mutation in bacteria. We refer the reader to several reviews for a more complete treatment of the subject [6, 32–34].

Point Mutations   Simple substitution of one nucleotide pair for another appears relatively uncommon among spontaneously occurring mutations in *E. coli* but can be induced with

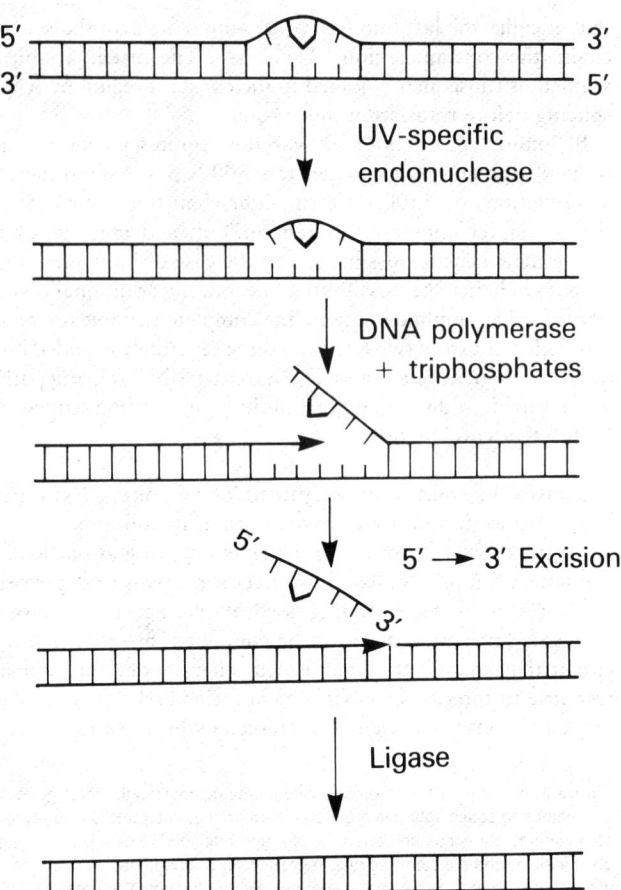

Figure 2-15   Excision repair of a pyrimidine dimer. The horizontal double line represents a DNA segment that is distorted at its center by an ultraviolet light-induced pyrimidine dimer. Repair of the damage is thought to occur by the steps shown. (*From Hanawalt et al. [32] by permission.*)

high efficiency by chemical or physical mutagens, such as nitrous acid or ultraviolet irradiation, or by mutator genes. The substitution of T-A for C-G, which has been investigated in some detail in the *lac*I gene of *E. coli* [34], is especially interesting because it illustrates not only the chemistry of the mutation but also the defense mechanisms of the cell. (The protein product of the *lac*I gene represses transcription of the gene that encodes the sugar metabolizing enzyme β-galactosidase.) One of the ways in which a T-A nucleotide pair can replace a C-G nucleotide pair is by deamination of C to deoxyuridine monophosphate (dU). (See the legend of Fig. 2-1 for the structure of dU.) Note that dU has the pairing properties of T, i.e., it forms an acceptable complementary nucleotide pair with A rather than with G. Therefore, when the DNA with the mispaired dU-G replicates, one of the daughter DNA molecules will contain a dU-A nucleotide pair at the site of the deamination, and this will lead to a C-G to T-A substitution upon further replication as illustrated:

$$C-G \longrightarrow dU-G \longrightarrow dU-T + C-G$$
$$\longrightarrow \longrightarrow A-T + C-G \qquad (3)$$

However, in *E. coli* most C deaminations do not lead to mutation because a set of enzymes recognize and excise dU from DNA and, if it was mispaired with G, replace it with the correct nucleotide, C. When C-G to T-A substitutions do occur, the second C of a specific sequence, 5'-CCAGG-3', is the favored site [34]. This C is normally methylated at the 5 position (see Fig. 2-1) by a DNA cytosine methylase that acts uniquely at this sequence. Deamination of 5-methyl C produces not dU but T, a normal constituent of DNA, and hence one that is more likely to persist until the region containing the mispaired T is replicated. After replication the newly introduced thymine would be correctly paired with A in one of the daughter molecules, and the mutation would therefore be fixed in the DNA. It seems possible that DNA contains T instead of dU in order to avoid the consequences of deamination of C, an event that may be relatively frequent inside cells. Although cytosine deamination is probably not the major cause of spontaneous point mutations in *E. coli,* several potent chemical mutagens, such as nitrous acid, bisulfite, and hydroxylamine, promote it.

A second kind of spontaenous point mutation, which is considerably more frequent than the first in the *lac*I gene, is the addition or deletion of a four-nucleotide pair unit that is part of a triple tandem repeat (Fig. 2-16A). It has been proposed that this type of mutation arises by "slipping" of one of the polynucleotide chains relative to the other at the growing point of a DNA molecule. The formation of a stable structure after slipping is favored by repeats in the DNA sequence (Fig. 2-16B).

As the above discussion suggests, the type and frequency of point mutations should depend on the sequence of nucleotides in the DNA. Indeed, the highly nonrandom distribution of mutations along the chromosome was noted many years before the molecular basis of some of the "hot spots" was revealed [37]. Each mutagen and mutator gene so far tested has its own specificity which, in many cases, is still poorly understood.

Chromosomal Rearrangements [35, 36] Chromosomal rearrangements in bacteria have recently been the subject of intense investigation, and we shall describe two cases in which some progress toward understanding the mechanism has been made. The first case is the generation of a class of DNA deletions. The nucleotide sequence of 12 spontaneously occurring

deletions within the *lac*I gene of *E. coli* has been determined, and the endpoints of seven fall within short sequences that were directly repeated in the undeleted gene (Fig. 2-17). Among the seven, the endpoints of one are unique and those of the other six are composed of three pairs of duplicates. Stimulation of DNA deletion by short repeated sequences could be explained either by slipped mispairing (Fig. 2-16) or by λ-type excision (Fig. 2-13).

The second case is the transposition of specific DNA segments from one location to another within or between chromosomes. Such transposed segments have a phenotype when they disrupt genes and are in fact responsible for an important fraction of all spontaneous mutations. These DNA segments, which are called *transposable elements* or *transposons,* fall into a small number of discrete classes as defined by nucleotide sequence. The lengths of the transposable elements analyzed to date range from 200 to about 6000 nucleotide pairs, and in most of them 20 to 40 nucleotide pairs at one end are repeated in inverted order at the other. Two transposable elements of the same class that are separated by a stretch of DNA form a unit called a *compound transposon* that, like the original element, can transpose in toto within or between chromosomes. Several transposable elements have been shown to encode proteins that are required for transposition. The proteins presumably act at the very ends of the elements since these also are required for transposition.

Two striking attributes of transposable elements should be mentioned. (1) Transposition appears to be nonreciprocal, i.e., the appearance of a transposable element in a new location does not entail its loss from its original location. Therefore, in all of the current molecular models of transposition, it is assumed that a replica, not the original transposable element, is inserted into the new location. (2) A stretch of 5 to 11 nucleotide pairs, the exact number depending on the element, is found in two copies adjacent to each end of the transposable element after transposition has occurred. These nucleotides were present only once at the target site (Fig. 2-18). Duplication of target sequences is characteristic of all bacterial trans-

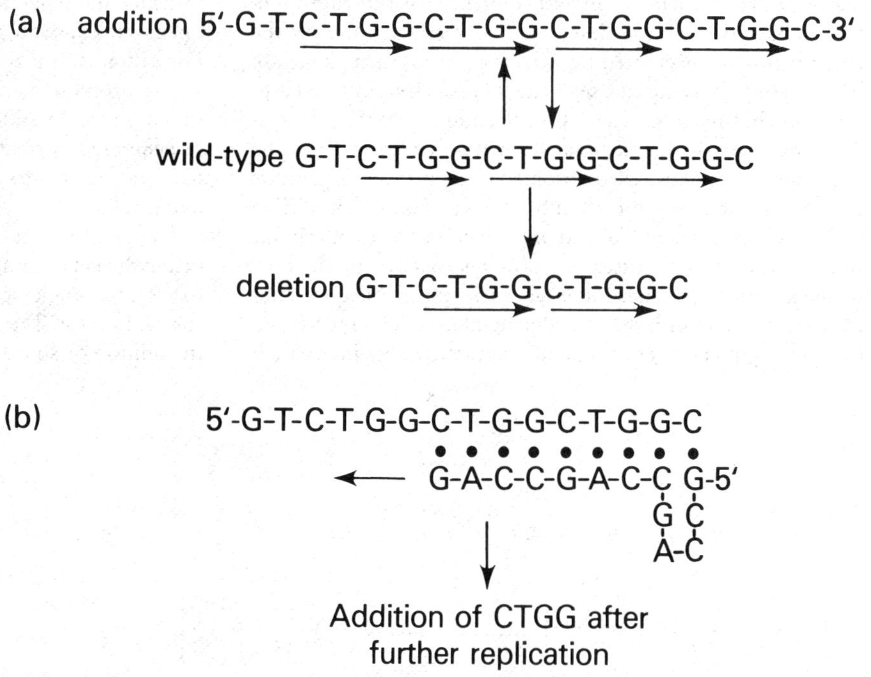

Figure 2-16 A "hot spot" for spontaneous mutation. (A) The wild-type sequence, shown in the middle line, is in the *lac*I gene of *E. coli.* The tetranucleotide CTGG (underlined arrow) is repeated three times. The indicated addition (above) or deletion (below) of a CTGG unit accounts for about two-thirds of all spontaneous mutations in this gene. (B) "Slipped mispairing," presumed to occur during DNA replication, may explain addition of a CTGG unit. The template chain is on the top and the growing chain on the bottom. The leftward arrow indicates the direction of chain growth. Filled circles indicate bonds between complementary nucleotide pairs. The tetranucleotide 3'-GACC in the bottom chain is not paired with the template chain because the growing chain has slipped back four nucleotides. After completion of the growing chain and a further round of replication, the sequence

5'-CTGG
GACC-5'

will be added to the genome at that point. A deletion would occur if the template rather than the daughter chain slipped and mispaired at the appropriate point during replication. ([A] *From Miller* [34] *by permission.*)

(a) addition 5'-G-T-C-T-G-G-C-T-G-G-C-T-G-G-C-T-G-G-C-3'

wild-type G-T-C-T-G-G-C-T-G-G-C-T-G-G-C

deletion G-T-C-T-G-G-C-T-G-G-C

(b) 5'-G-T-C-T-G-G-C-T-G-G-C-T-G-G-C

← G-A-C-C-G-A-C-C G-5'
                              G C
                              A-C

Addition of CTGG after
further replication

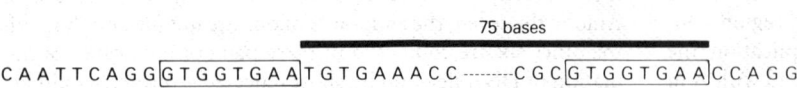

Figure 2-17 A sequence favoring deletions. Two independently isolated deletions among 12 analyzed in the *lac*I gene had endpoints within the eight-nucleotide pair, directly-repeated sequence (boxed). Thus, this sequence favors deletions (see text). The deletion mutant has lost one of the repeated sequences in addition to the 75 nucleotide pair interval between them. (*From Miller [34] by permission.*)

posable elements and transposons studied to date and has also been found adjacent to analogous sequences in animal tumor viruses and in yeast.

Although transposable elements are a significant source of spontaneous mutation in bacteria, they are important for other reasons as well. First, the activity responsible for transposition also promotes fusions and inversions between either end of the element and sequences elsewhere on the chromosome. Such rearrangements can create new transposons and new patterns of gene regulation. The mobility of transposons is important in the evolution of plasmids that carry clusters of genes determining resistance to many different antibiotics. (Plasmids are autonomously replicating circular DNA molecules found in many strains of bacteria.) It is believed that these plasmids were formed by multiple transpositions of antibiotic resistance genes onto plasmids that originally lacked them. The organization of these plasmids is one of the major causes of antibiotic resistance among strains of bacteria in hospitals. Finally, higher organisms such as yeast, *Drosophila,* maize, and mammals contain elements that appear similar to the transposable elements of bacteria. Indeed, the RNA tumor viruses, when incorporated into the chromosomes of certain vertebrates, have a structure precisely analogous to that of a compound transposon.

RECOMBINANT DNA METHODOLOGY AND THE NEW GENETICS

Much of the biochemical analysis of gene structure and function in bacteria we have described was made possible by the construction of specialized transducing phage. Such phage are hybrids; they carry specific segments of host DNA inserted into the virus chromosome. They allow the amplification and physical separation of the bacterial segments they carry from the remainder of the host chromosome. This purification permits the analysis of gene expression by the technique of annealing the transducing phage DNA to unpurified mixtures of cellular mRNAs [1]. In many cases, the proteins encoded by the host segments can be produced in large, easily purifiable quantities by infecting cells with the transducing phage. Such specialized transducing phage were originally constructed by in vivo ge-

netic recombination between virus and host, and this initially limited the technique to the analysis of bacterial gene expression and the production of bacterial gene products. It is through a decade-long application of this approach that so much has been learned about the regulated expression of bacterial genes and their viruses.

The Strategy and Usefulness of Gene Cloning [*38, 39*]

The analysis of gene structure and function in eukaryotes was originally limited by two factors: (1) the sheer complexity and size of the genome defied direct experimental analysis, and (2) the fact that naturally occurring viruses of higher organisms, unlike bacteriophages, could not be used to amplify and purify specific segments of the host genome. Recently, however, we have learned to recombine DNA fragments in vitro, and this has extended the possibility of analysis to any organism from which DNA or RNA can be obtained. The properties of two classes of enzyme are of critical importance for in vitro recombination: DNA ligases, which promote joining of DNA fragments at their ends, and restriction endonucleases, which cut DNA at sites that are specific for each enzyme. Thus, preselected fragments of "foreign" DNA, excised from larger molecules by the action of one or more restriction endonucleases, can be inserted into specific sites of "vector" chromosomes (Fig. 2-19). The vectors are typically plasmids or bacteriophage chromosomes. Once this has been done, the structure and function of the foreign DNA can be investigated using both the techniques that were originally applied with classic transducing phage and new techniques that have been developed to take advantage of the power of recombination in vitro. For example, it is now possible to insert fragments containing strong promoters adjacent to genes whose expression we wish to maximize. In addition, mutations in preselected regions can be generated by treating a DNA fragment with a mutagen prior to inserting it into a vector and assessing its functions in a living cell.

The great power of this constellation of techniques in analyzing the genes of humans comes from the ability to isolate or to clone a single specific DNA fragment carrying a gene of special interest. The gene can subsequently be amplified, free of the million or so other genes that occupy the human genome.

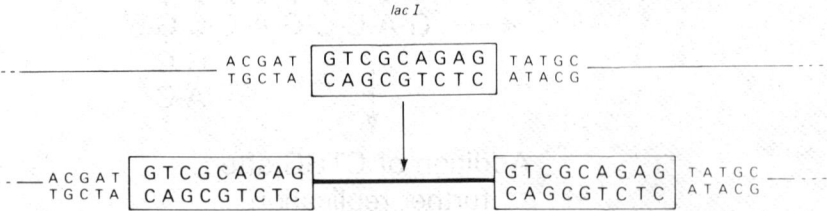

Figure 2-18 Repeated sequences, bracket-transposable elements. The top line shows the sequence of a segment of the wild-type *lac*I gene. The bottom line shows the sequence of a *lac*I insertion mutation. The insertion is represented by the heavy line; it is a 768-nucleotide pair long, transposable element called *IS1*. (*From Calos and Miller [35] by permission.*)

BACTERIAL VIRUS   **SOURCE OF MAMMALIAN DNA**

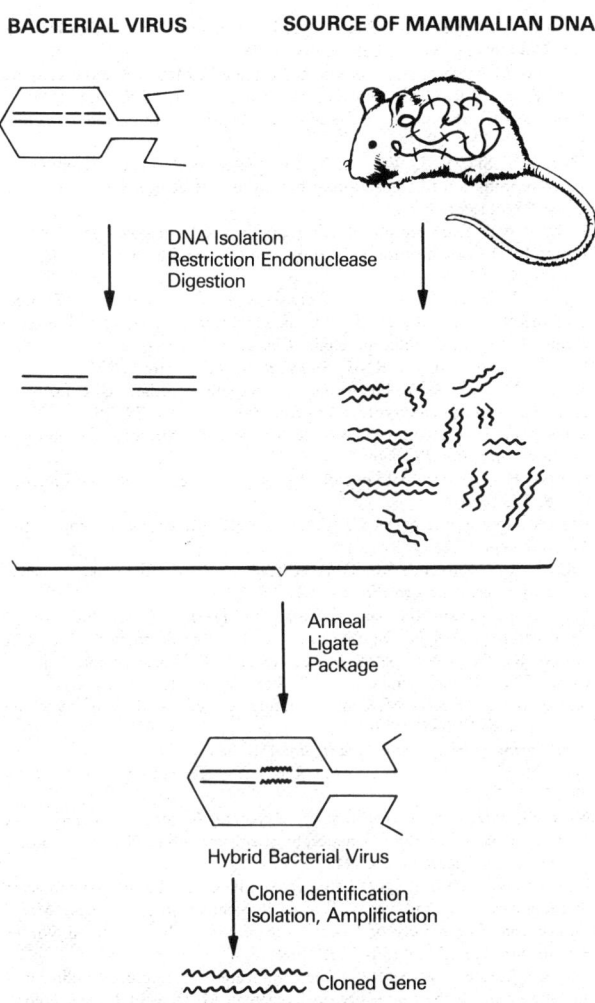

DNA Isolation
Restriction Endonuclease
Digestion

Anneal
Ligate
Package

Hybrid Bacterial Virus

Clone Identification
Isolation, Amplification

Cloned Gene

Figure 2-19 Strategy for DNA cloning. The process of gene cloning involves the creation of a vector (diagrammatically indicated here as a bacteriophage or bacterial virus, usually phage λ) with appropriate sites for cleavage with a restriction endonuclease. The indicated vector's DNA is cleaved twice in this case so as to produce three fragments of DNA. The middle fragment in the case of phage λ is dispensable and can be replaced by foreign DNA. The restriction enzymes recognize and cleave at specific sequences and cut double-stranded DNA in such a way as to leave a self-complementary, sticky end, e.g.:

```
. . .GAATTC. . .——→. . .G        + AATTC. . .
      | | | | | |              |              |
. . .CTTAAG              CTTAA          G. . .
```

These complementary ends, created in both the vector and foreign DNA, will anneal to one another and can be covalently linked using the enzyme DNA ligase. Once linked into a full phage-sized molecule, the DNA can be "packaged" into viral particles that can be assembled in vitro in the presence of ATP and appropriate head, tail, and packaging proteins. The assembled phage will each contain a fragment of the donor DNA and, if the donor is a human, approximately 250,000 such phages would carry the entire genome. A particular gene of interest can be selected from the mixture if an assay for its activity is available or if a complementary nucleotide sequence, such as an mRNA or cloned DNA copy of an mRNA (a cDNA), is available. Such screening techniques can easily detect one sought-after clone among a million. The cloned genes can be amplified directly using the bacteriophage.

Isolated, the nucleotide sequence of the gene and mutants derived from it can be determined using rapid chemical or enzymatic techniques. Those regions relevant to its ordered function—or dysfunction—can therefore be known in great detail. Moreover, genes that encode proteins of particular interest can be linked to transcriptional promoters and trans-

lational initiation sites of bacteria (or yeast) and forced to produce relatively large amounts of, e.g., insulin or interferon.

Gene Mapping and Diagnostic Applications

In addition to allowing the structure of genes to be determined, the recombinant DNA technology also permits us to determine the precise arrangement of genes at a complex locus. For example, the arrangement of immunoglobulin genes in humans has been determined by cloning overlapping segments of DNA carrying these genes and then aligning their structures by determining the specific positions of restriction endonuclease cleavage sites within each fragment [40]. Furthermore, this ability to identify a DNA fragment bearing a specific gene can be used to determine the chromosomal location of any cloned gene. One of the more effective ways of doing this involves forming hybrid cell lines between human and Chinese hamster cells that retain varying numbers of human chromosomes. Since a specific human gene can be identified in the hybrid cell line's DNA and since these hybrid cell lines tend to lose human chromosomes, the presence of the human gene can be correlated with the retention of the human chromosome that carries it. Both globin and immunoglobulin genes have been chromosomally mapped in this way (see Chap. 1).

These same techniques can be used to identify genetic polymorphisms that are not phenotypically recognizable. (A *polymorphism* is a difference in the structure of a given gene among individuals in a population.) One of the early lessons of gene cloning has been the recognition that DNA not directly involved in a coding or regulatory function undergoes rather rapid evolutionary change. Two individuals may have identical structural genes, e.g., for globin, but when the sequences that flank these genes are explored, differences are frequently discovered. Occasionally such individual differences—actually nucleotide sequence polymorphisms—will alter a restriction endonuclease cleavage site or change the size of a restriction fragment. The relevant fragment can be detected, as described in Fig. 2-20. Indeed, in certain individuals the β-globin S gene is associated with a nearby restriction site polymorphism and the genotype of the propositus of an affected family can be determined in utero from the DNA of a small sample of cells obtained from amniotic fluid [41] (see Chap. 76).

Gene Therapy

What about using these techniques to correct inborn errors of metabolism? Clearly, these techniques will allow us to determine the precise genetic basis of a variety of inherited disorders, pinpointing to the nucleotide pair the alteration responsible for the disease. With this knowledge and the normal gene in hand, one might expect gene therapy to be a simple matter. Several formidable barriers remain. While there are good techniques available for introducing genes into cells, there is still no predictable way to introduce them into a particular chromosomal location that assures their ordered and controlled expression. Further there is not yet a reliable way to reintroduce "corrected" cells into an organism so that they will survive, while analogous cells carrying the defective gene are safely eliminated. Nevertheless, the stage seems set for overcoming even these formidable barriers.

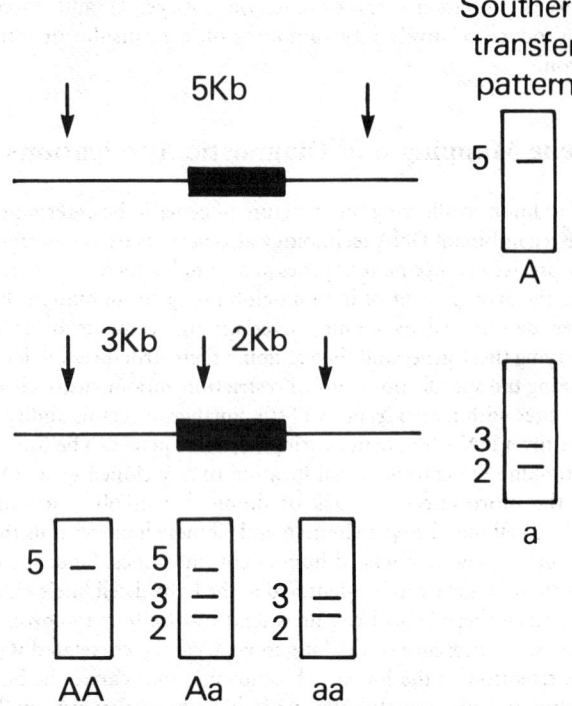

Figure 2-20 Identification of sequence polymorphism in genomic DNA. The figure diagrammatically represents a coding sequence (filled box) and its surrounding restriction sites (arrows) in genomic DNA. If DNA is derived from a homozygous individual and digested with a restriction endonuclease, it will yield a 5-kilobase (kb) fragment of DNA carrying the relevant sequence. This DNA can be separated from fragments of other sizes by gel electrophoresis and transferred to a nitrocellulose sheet by a technique developed by Southern [41]. The sheet is then incubated with a radioactive, cloned gene that will anneal only to the sequence represented by the filled box, thereby making it radioactive. The location of the radioactive DNA can, in turn, be detected by radioautography (see A). If there is a polymorphic form of the gene with an additional restriction site, as shown in a, digestion and analysis will reveal two bands, e.g., one 2 kb, the other 3 kb in length. The heterozygous offspring of two homozygous individuals will, of course, show all three fragments (Aa). The power of the technique derives from its ability to look directly at a nucleotide sequence to determine genotype, even if the region is phenotypically silent. As mentioned in the text, such an analysis can be used to detect the β^S mutation in certain sickle-cell patients [42].

REFERENCES

1. WATSON JD: *Molecular Biology of the Gene.* Menlo Park, Calif, WA Benjamin, Inc, 1976
2. STENT G, CALENDAR R: *Molecular Genetics,* ed 2. San Francisco, WH Freeman & Co, Publishers, 1978
3. KORNBERG A: *DNA Replication.* San Francisco, WH Freeman & Co, Publishers, 1980
4. McGHEE JD, FELSENFELD G: Nucleosome structure. *Ann Rev Biochem* 49:115, 1980
5. KORNBERG RD, KLUG A: The nucleosome. *Sci Am* 244:52, 1981
6. COX ES: Bacterial mutator genes and the control of spontaneous mutation. *Ann Rev Genet* 10:135, 1976
7. RADMAN M, WAGNER R, JR, GLICKMAN B, MESELSON M: DNA Methylation, mismatch correction and genetic stability, in Alacevic M (ed): *Progress in Environmental Mutagenesis.* New York, Elsevier North-Holland, Inc, 1980, pp 121–130
8. ROSENBERG M, COURT D: Regulatory sequences involved in the promotion and termination of RNA transcription. *Ann Rev Genet* 13:319, 1979
9. LOSICK R, CHAMBERLIN M (eds): *RNA Polymerase.* Cold Spring Harbor, NY, Cold Spring Harbor Laboratory, 1976
10. PTASHNE M, JEFFREY A, JOHNSON A, MAURER R, MEYER B, PABO C, ROBERTS T, SAUER R: How the λ repressor and cro work. *Cell* 19:1, 1980
11. YANOFSKY C: Attenuation in the control of expression of bacterial operons. *Nature* 289:751, 1981
12. MATSUI T, SEGALL J, WEIL A, ROEDER R: Multiple factors required for accurate initiation of transcription by purified RNA polymerase II. *J Biol Chem* 255:11992, 1980
13. FLAVELL RA: Transcription of eukaryotic genes. *Nature* 285:356, 1980
14. LEDER P: The organization and expression of cloned globin genes. *Harvey Lect* 74:81, 1980
15. ROGERS J, EARLY P, CARTER C, CALAME K, BOND M, HOOD L, WALL R: Two mRNAs with different 3' ends encode membrane-bound and secreted forms of immunoglobulin mu chain. *Cell* 20:303, 1980
16. PERRY RP: Processing of RNA. *Ann Rev Biochem* 45:605, 1976
17. REVELL M, GRONER Y: Post-transcriptional and translational controls of gene expression in eukaryotes. *Ann Rev Biochem* 47:1079, 1978
18. WEISSBACH H, OCHOA S: Soluble factors required for eukaryotic protein synthesis. *Ann Rev Biochem* 45:191, 1976
19. LODISH H: Translational control of protein synthesis. *Ann Rev Biochem* 45:39, 72, 1976
20. BRIMACOMBE R, STOFFLER G, WITTMANN HG: Ribosome structure. *Ann Rev Biochem* 47:217, 1978
21. RICH A, RAJ BHANDARY UL: Transfer RNA: Molecular structure, sequence and properties. *Ann Rev Biochem* 45:805, 1976
22. STRYER L: *Biochemistry.* San Francisco, WH Freeman & Co, Inc, 1981
23. PAPPENHEIMER AM JR: Diphtheria toxin. *Ann Rev Biochem* 46:69, 1977
24. CHANG JC, KAN YW, TRECARTIN RF, TEMPLE GF: Nonsense mutation as a cause of beta 0 thalassemia. *Ann NY Acad Sci* 344:113, 1980
25. SILVERMAN M, SIMON M: Phase variation: Genetic analysis of switching mutants. *Cell* 19:845, 1980
26. *Cold Spring Harbor Symp Quant Biol* 45, 1981
27. NASH HA: Integration and excision of bacteriophage λ. *Curr Top Micr Imm* 78:171, 1977
28. NASH H, MIZUUCHI K, ENQUIST L, WEISBERG R: Strand exchange in λ integrative recombination: Genetics, biochemistry and models. *Cold Spring Harbor Symp Quant Biol* 45:417, 1980
29. HERSKOWITZ I, RINE J, SPRAGUE G, JENSEN R: Control of cell type in yeast by genetic cassettes, in Scott W, Warner R, Schulz J, Joseph D (eds): *Mobilization and Reassembly of Genetic Information.* Miami, Miami Winter Symposium, vol 17, pp 133–153, 1980
30. LEDER P, MAX EE, SEIDMAN JG: The organization of immunoglobulin genes and the origin of their diversity, in Fougereau M, Dausset J (eds): *Fourth International Congress of Immunology, Immunology 80.* London, Academic Press, Ltd, 1980, p 34
31. HERSKOWITZ I, HAGEN D: The lysis-lysogeny decision of phage λ: Explicit programming and responsiveness. *Ann Rev Genet* 14:399, 1980
32. HANAWALT P, COOPER P, GANESAN A, SMITH C: DNA repair in bacteria and mammalian cells. *Ann Rev Biochem* 48:783, 1979
33. KENYON C, WALKER G: DNA damaging agents stimulate gene expression at specific loci in *Escherichia coli. Proc Natl Acad Sci USA* 77:2819, 1979
34. MILLER JH: The *lacI* gene: Its role in *lac* operon control and its use as a genetic system, in Miller JH, Reznikoff WS (eds): *The Operon.* Cold Spring Harbor, NY, Cold Spring Harbor Laboratory, 1978, p 31
35. CALOS MP, MILLER JH: Transposable elements. *Cell* 20:579, 1980
36. DRAKE JW: *The Molecular Basis of Mutation.* San Francisco, Holden-Day, Inc, 1970
37. BENZER S: On the topography of the genetic fine structure. *Proc Natl Acad Sci USA* 47:403, 1961
38. *Science* 209:No 4463, 1981
39. DENNISTON KJ, ENQUIST LW (eds): Recombinant DNA, in *Benchmark Papers in Microbiology,* Umbriet WW (series ed), New York, Academic Press, Inc, 1981, vol 15
40. HIETER PA, KORSMEYER SJ, HOLLIS GJ, MAX EE, MAIZEL JV JR, WALDMANN TA, LEDER P: Immunoglobulin light chain genes of mouse and man, in Janeway C, Sercarz EE, Wigzell H, Fox CF (eds): *Immunoglobulin Idiotypes and Their Expression,* ICN-UCLA Symposia on Molecular and Cellular Biology. New York, Academic Press, Inc, pp 33–48, 1981
41. SOUTHERN E: Detection of specific sequences among DNA fragments separated by gel electrophoresis. *J Molec Biol* 98:503, 1975
42. KAN YW, DOZY AM: Polymorphism of DNA sequence adjacent to human β-globin structural gene: Relationship to sickle mutation. *Proc Natl Acad Sci USA* 75:5631, 1978

3

THE HISTOCOMPATIBILITY COMPLEX: Genetic Polymorphism and Disease Susceptibility

DONNA D. KOSTYU

D. BERNARD AMOS

1. *HLA, the major histocompatibility complex (MHC) in humans, consists of a cluster of genes on chromosome 6. These genes have very different properties. The best known are those which determine serologically defined antigens. Others function in the generation and regulation of immune responsiveness, and genes throughout the cluster are associated with susceptibility or resistance to disease.*

2. *There are five internationally recognized, highly polymorphic components of the human MHC. HLA-A, -B, and -C are class 1 transmembrane glycoproteins found on most nucleated cells. They have a molecular weight of 44,000 and are associated with a nonpolymorphic polypeptide with a molecular weight of 11,000 called β_2-microglobulin. The class 2 HLA-DR antigens consist of two tightly bound transmembrane glycoproteins with molecular weights of 34,000 and 29,000. Expression is restricted primarily to B lymphocytes, monocytes, macrophages, and endothelial cells. The fifth component, HLA-D, is recognized through the complex proliferative responses to allogeneic cells in mixed lymphocyte cultures.*

3. *Newer attributes of the MHC include two new series of B-cell antigens designated MB and MT, and additional loci which cause restimulation in primed lymphocyte cultures or code for antigens which are recognized as target structures by cytolytic T cells.*

4. *Evidence for the involvement of the MHC in immune recognition and response came from studies with laboratory animals and is being confirmed, with some difficulty, in humans. The generation and control of an efficient immune response require specific collaboration (cooperation) between two or more subsets of lymphocytes which must be MHC identical, especially for the region coding for class 2 antigens. In addition, the recognition of virally infected or chemically modified cells appears to depend on the modification and subsequent recognition of altered self-MHC antigens. In this latter case, class 1 antigens are involved.*

5. *Evidence for the involvement of the MHC in disease processes has been striking. Different alleles of different loci are associated with a wide variety of diseases. Examples include the association of DR4 with type 1 insulin-dependent diabetes mellitus, HLA-B8 and DR3 with endocrine disorders, HLA-B27 with ankylosing spondylitis, and HLA-A3 with hemochromatosis. While these associations have been made most often at the population level, formal linkage has been demonstrated only for hemochromatosis and between HLA-B and 21-hydroxylase deficiency. Some diseases follow HLA inheritance within families but show no association with a particular antigen at the population level. Different ethnic groups are often characterized both by antigens largely restricted to that population and by diseases which may occur with those specificities.*

6. *There are probably numerous causes for such disease*

associations—the inclusion in the HLA region of genes regulating enzymes and complement components, the actual alteration of HLA antigens by infectious agents, or cross-reactivity between HLA components and viruses or bacterial products. Some genes in the MHC may determine predisposition to disease, while others may determine resistance. In particular, MHC genes determining the rates, levels, or balance of cellular and humoral immune responses may likewise affect the prognosis or complications of a disease.

HLA, the designation given to a cluster of genes located on the short arm of chromosome 6 (Fig. 3-1), is the major histocompatibility complex (MHC) of humans [1]. The MHC genes specify a set of antigenically active proteins that occupy the outer surfaces of cells. The genes at the MHC loci are highly polymorphic—that is, in the population at large there are many different alleles at each locus. Each individual in the population inherits two specific alleles at each locus and is thus genetically distinct. When exposed to cells from other individuals in the same species, individuals form antibodies (alloantibodies) against the antigens that are foreign.

All mammals and birds that have been adequately tested have an MHC which is surprisingly similar [2]. The evolution of a cluster of many genes into an MHC appears to have begun during the age of Amphibia and to have been well advanced by the development of Reptilia. That it has important functions is evidenced by its conservation during the divergence of birds from mammals and the early death from immunodeficiency of those few humans who lack MHC-specified antigens [3, 4]. *Histocompatibility* refers to the involvement of the MHC antigens in tissue or organ graft rejection. *Major* refers to the fact that rejection between two individuals of the same species who differ at the MHC is rapid and can be arrested only by extensive immune suppression of the recipient. This is in contrast to minor histocompatibility antigen involvement, in which incompatibility leads to a chronic rejection more easily controlled with immunosuppression. The system is *complex* because many genes of differing function are clustered together to form the MHC. Although the term *histocompatibility* is an old one, derived from allotransplants, it is entirely appropriate since MHC genes are intricately involved in the self-recognition processes, in lymphocyte interactions, and in the rejection of virally or chemically modified autologous cells, including transformed cells.

The term *HLA* refers to human leukocyte antigens, which were the first antigens of the human MHC to be studied. The earliest studies of human leukocyte antigens were greatly influenced by the discovery that hemolytic anemias could be caused by antibodies against the patient's own red cells. It therefore appeared logical to search for antibodies to white cells in leukopenia. It was not long before such antibodies were found, but, paradoxically, while leukocyte antibodies would react with cells from a panel of random donors, they seldom if ever reacted against the patient's own leukocytes. Eventually it was found that the antibody was formed in response to the leukocytes in the buffy coat of the blood transfused during therapy and that one group of the antibodies was directed against an antigen that was present on leukocytes from about 50 percent of subjects. The identification of this antigen as *MAC* [5], later

called *HLA-A2*, provided Jean Dausset with the first step that led eventually to his winning the Nobel Prize.

A separate impetus was provided by investigators working on tumor antigens responsible for skin and tissue rejection in experimental animals. A second Nobel laureate, George Snell, was responsible (with the late Peter Gorer) for the recognition of the most potent tissue antigens in the mouse, those of the H-2 system [6]. H-2 is the mouse homologue of HLA.

With the introduction of immunosuppressive drugs, human kidney transplantation became a practical therapeutic modality. Intrafamilial kidney grafts were often more successful than grafts from cadavers, and a genetic basis for rejection or acceptance was sought. Since compatibility for the red cell A and B antigens did not guarantee kidney graft compatibility, lessons learned from mouse transplantation genetics were applied to humans. Within less than 10 years, the importance and the complexity of HLA was realized.

Two new characteristics of the MHC have recently emerged which attest to the importance of HLA as a general regulator of the immune response. The first is the realization that a competent immune response is dependent upon the interaction of various types of cells within a single individual. These interactions are possible only when the MHC of these cells is identical. This *MHC restriction* pertains to interactions between T and B lymphocytes, between T cells and macrophages, and between cytotoxic T cells and virally or chemically modified target cells. The cytotoxic T cells of a host can kill cells bearing viral antigens and antigens introduced during transplantation only if the target cells share at least one HLA-A or -B allele with the host (see below). The second phenomenon concerns the finding that many diseases are associated with particular HLA antigens. This finding suggested that the HLA antigens themselves, or genes linked to HLA, play an important role in disease susceptibility. (For a general discussion of genetic linkage and association, see Chap. 1.)

This chapter will describe the components of the HLA system, their biochemistry when known, their polymorphic nature, and their involvement in and regulation of the immune response. We will then present some of the diseases known to be associated with these antigens and some of the problems in converting an association with HLA to genetic linkage to HLA.

OVERVIEW: HLA AS A SUPERGENE

The concept of a *supergene* originated in 1931 when Fischer [7] coined the term and defined it as a group of closely linked loci which have evolved together and function in concert. Selective interactions between the genes or their products maintain linkage. Cepellini introduced a helpful term, *haplotype*. This can be defined as the array of genes clustered together on a single chromosome that together constitute a functional unit, in this case the HLA. The HLA supergene is found on the sixth chromosome in humans. While the boundaries of HLA are commonly represented as HLA-DR on one side and HLA-A on the other (Fig. 3–1), new loci are being mapped on the centromeric side of HLA-D, and the existence of others on the telomeric side of HLA-A appears probable. Thus, the limits of HLA are not absolutely defined. The basic components of the HLA supergene include the following [8, 9].

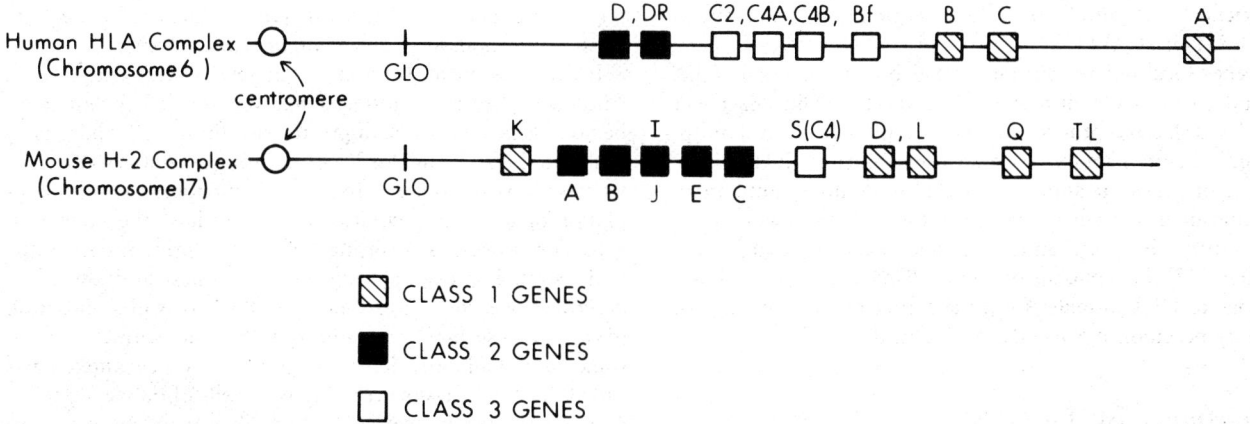

Figure 3-1 Schematic diagram of the homologous functional classes of MHC genes in humans and mouse. The exact sequence of the human complement genes, of HLA-D and DR, and of H-2D and L is not known. Distances are not exact.

HLA-A, -B, -C

These are the structural genes for three 44,000 molecular weight glycoproteins (gp44) found on most nucleated cells. Each is an integral component of the plasma membrane. Each gene contains one or more regions that exhibit polymorphism among individuals. The polymorphism leads to the production of proteins with differing antigenic sites, or *epitopes*, which are easily recognizable through antibody-dependent, complement-mediated lysis of peripheral blood lymphocytes or through other serologic tests. The HLA-A, -B, and -C antigens represent the most thoroughly understood and most easily detectable gene products of the HLA supergene. These products are often designated *class 1* antigens (Fig. 3–1) since there is presumptive evidence in humans and definitive evidence in the mouse for more genes close to or within the MHC region which code for similar cell membrane components.

HLA-D

The HLA-D alleles differ from the HLA-A, -B, and -C gene products in that they are definable only by a functional test called the *mixed lymphocyte culture* or *MLC* and not by serologic testing. An MLC consists of coculturing lymphocytes from two individuals for several days and measuring the resulting proliferation. The absence of proliferation implies identity at HLA-D. Only certain classes of cells will stimulate proliferation, notably B lymphocytes, macrophages, and endothelial cells. No HLA-D gene product has been isolated.

HLA-DR

First identified during attempted serologic definition of HLA-D, these alleles are usually recognized through antibody-dependent, complement-mediated cytotoxicity assays. The HLA-DR antigens are genetically and structurally dissimilar to the HLA-A, -B, and -C antigens and thus represent a second type *(class 2)* of MHC antigen. The HLA-DR antigens are found on a two-chain molecule, an α and a β chain with molecular weights of 34,000 and 29,000, respectively. Both subunits span the membrane, and both chains appear to be determined by genes closely linked in the MHC. Because these were originally thought to be the antigens stimulating the MLC response, and thus identical to HLA-D, they were called *DR* or *D-related* antigens. However, it is now recognized that the MLC response is a complex response independent of or only partially involving HLA-DR antigens.

Complement Components

Structural genes determining C2 [10] and C4 (both C4A and C4B loci) [11, 12] of the classic complement pathway, and Bf of the alternate complement pathway [13], are closely associated with HLA (see Chap. 89). These complement components have been designated *class 3* products of the MHC. Receptors for C3b and C3d, the breakdown fragments of C3, have also been linked to the MHC [14], as has a C8 deficiency in one study [15], although other studies have shown no linkage [16, 17]. Complement components which are not linked to HLA include Clr [18, 19], C1 inhibitor [20], C3 [21], C6 [18, 22], and C7 [23]. These linkages have been discussed in detail elsewhere [24, 25].

Glyoxalase

A locus determining alleles of the red cell enzyme glyoxalase is found approximately 5 centimorgans to the left of HLA-D [26]. A similar gene is linked to the mouse MHC [27]. This locus is designated GLO.

Possible New MHC Loci

One new identifiable MHC locus was first recognized and identified by Charmot et al. [28] and later independently described by Shaw et al. [29]. These antigens are identifiable by secondary stimulation in the mixed lymphocyte culture. This primed lymphocyte test (or PLT) seems to recognize, in addition to HLA-DR, new B-cell-specific antigens which have been designated *SB* by Shaw et al. and *PL* by Charmot et al. T-cell-specific antigens may also be determined by genes closely linked to the MHC.

Other genes showing linkage to the MHC include a locus determining congenital adrenal hyperplasia (21-hydroxylase deficiency) [30] and a locus for olivopontocerebellar ataxia (OPCA-1 or SCA) [31].

Genes localized to chromosome 6 but not close to HLA include superoxide dismutase 2 (SOD-2), malic enzyme 1 (ME1) [32], a receptor for monkey red blood cells [33], mitochondrial glutamate oxaloacetate transaminase (GOT_m) [34], a gene or genes for antigens detected with mouse antihuman chromosome 6 serums [35], genes for Ig heavy chains [36], α-1-antitrypsin [36], and adenosine-deaminase-complexing protein [37]. Phosphoglucomutase (PGM_3) shows very loose linkage to HLA in males [38]; the earlier reported linkage of urinary pepsinogen 5 to HLA is doubtful [39].

Inheritance of the MHC

Although there are many alleles at the HLA loci, the inheritance is simple since the entire cluster of genes, or haplotype, is inherited as a unit. For convenience the two paternal chromosomes or haplotypes are often designated *a* and *b* and the maternal haplotypes *c* and *d*. The children must therefore be *ac, ad, bc,* or *bd*. This segregation of haplotypes is illustrated in Fig. 3–2. Two sibs inheriting the same haplotypes (e.g., *ac* and *ac*) are designated *HLA identical*, sibs and parents sharing one haplotype (e.g., *bc* and *bd*) are *haploidentical*, and sibs sharing neither haplotype (e.g., *ac* and *bd*) are *haplodistinct*. These relationships have great relevance in kidney transplantation and in many immunologic reactions, including mixed lymphocyte stimulation.

HLA Terminology

As of 1980, 20 antigens had been designated at the HLA-A locus, 42 at HLA-B, 8 at HLA-C, 12 at HLA-D, and 10 at HLA-DR [40]. A current listing is given in Table 3-1. Serums thought to detect new antigens are distributed for testing during the periodic International Histocompatibility Testing Workshops. Such workshops have been held every 2 or 3 years since 1964 (1964, 1965, 1967, 1970, 1972, 1975, 1977, and 1980) [41–48]. Nomenclature reports updating some antigens and assigning new antigens are published by the World Health Organization as a bulletin following each workshop. These reports are also included in the later *Histocompatibility Test-*

ing volumes and in immunologic journals such as *Tissue Antigens, Transplantation,* and *Human Immunology.*

It can be seen in Table 3-1 that several new antigens are variants or "splits" of antigens that were previously thought to be homogeneous. For example, the two forms of A9 have been designated Aw23 and Aw24. By convention, antigens are split when serums are found to react with lymphocytes of a subpopulation of subjects previously thought to have the same antigen. The process of splitting has been continuous since the mid-1960s. For example, one of the earliest antigens to be described was the antigen 4a (now Bw4) of van Rood et al. [49]. Several serums were later found to react with the cells of some but not all individuals carrying 4a. This new antigen was called 4c. Next, serums reacting with cells of only a subset of 4c-positive subjects were identified. One of the antigens "included" in 4c was called HLA-B5, another HLA-B18. Still later, HLA-B5 was split into Bw51 and Bw52. Antibodies that react with several antigens, e.g., those reacting with 4a and 4c, are called *supertypic,* and antibodies reacting with one of the subsets, e.g., Bw51, are called *subtypic.* These antigens may also be called *public* and *private.*

Although the process of splitting may seem arbitrary, there are five reasons for supposing that the subtypic definition of specificities in HLA is meaningful. (1) The subtypic specificities segregate clearly and are inherited independently in families. (2) The presence of a subtypic specificity may be associated with susceptibility to disease, e.g., B27 and ankylosing spondylitis, while a highly cross-reactive but clearly different specificity, e.g., B7, shows no such association and may, in fact, have different disease associations. (3) Very specific antigenic differences, e.g., those between the two variants of B5, Bw51, and Bw52, can be clearly distinguished by the fundamentally different process of cell-mediated cytotoxicity. (4) Population studies often show that one subtypic antigen, e.g., Bw44, is very common in Caucasian populations, while the other B12 subtype, Bw45, is found predominantly in black populations. (5) The distinction between B-locus subtypic specificities is highly correlated with Bw4 or with Bw6.

This system of nomenclature ignores some broadly reactive serums that react with unusual groups of subtypic antigens. Although the serums that have been most intensely studied react only with alleles of one locus (e.g., HLA-B), many serums (especially those defining Bw4) also react with one or more A locus antigens (e.g., A9, Aw32) [50, 51]. In addition to these

Figure 3-2 Segregation of the HLA haplotype in a family.

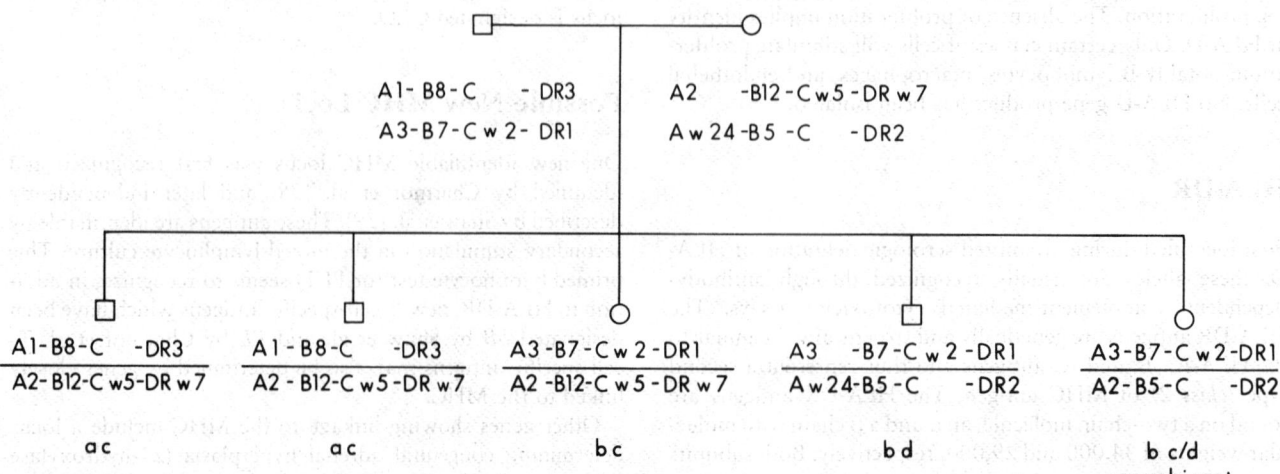

Table 3-1 Current HLA antigens

HLA-A locus	HLA-B locus	HLA-C locus	HLA-D locus	HLA-DR locus
A1	B5	Cw1 (T1, AJ)	Dw1 (LD101)	DRw1 (WIA1)
A2	Bw51 (5.1)	Cw2 (T2, SA532)	Dw2 (LD102, LD-7a)	DRw2 (WIA2)
A3	Bw52 (5.2)	Cw3 (T3, UPS)	Dw3 (LD103, LD-8a)	DRw3 (W IA3)
A9	B7	Cw4 (T4, Rh315)	Dw4 (LD104)	DRw4 (WIA4)
Aw23†	B8	Cw5 (T5)	Dw5 (LD105)	DRw5 (WIA5)
Aw24	Bw59 (HOK-1, 8.2)	Cw6 (T7)	Dw6 (LD106)	DRw6 (WIA6)
A10	B12	Cw7 (CVE, TOK)	Dw7 (LD107)	DRw7 (WIA7)
A25	Bw44 (12 not TT*)	Cw8 (T8, T9)	Dw8 (LD108)	DRw8 (8W DRw8)
A26	Bw45 (TT*)		Dw9 (TB9, OH)	DRw9 (WIA 4 × 7)
A11	B13		Dw10 (LD16)	DRw10 (ST-1, LTM)
A28	B14 (Maki)		Dw11 (LD17)	
Aw19 (Li)‡	B15 (LND)		Dw12 (DB4, DHO)	
A29 (w19.1)	Bw62 (15.1, 15B)			
Aw30 (w19.3)	Bw63 (15.2, 15A)			
Aw31 (w19.4)	Bw16			
Aw32 (w19.5)	Bw38 (16.1)			
Aw33 (w19.6)	Bw39 (16.2)			
Aw34 (Malay 2)	B17 (Mapi)			
Aw36 (Mo*, LT)	Bw57 (17.1, 17A, 17 long)			
Aw43 (BK)	Bw58 (17.2, 17B, 17 short)			
	B18 (CM)			
	Bw21			
	Bw49 (w21. 1, SL-ET)			
	Bw50 (w21. 2, ET*)			
	Bw22 (AA)			
	Bw55 (22.1)			
	Bw56 (22.2)			
	B27 (FJH)			
	Bw35 (W5, R*)			
	B37 (TY)			
	B40 (w10, BB)			
	Bw60 (40.1)			
	Bw61 (40.2)			
	Bw41 (Sabell, LK, Da34)			
	Bw42 (MWA)			
	Bw46 (HS, SIN 2)			
	Bw47 (407*, Mo66, Cas, Bw40c)			
	Bw48 (KSO, JA, Bw40.3)			
	Bw53 (HR)			
	Bw54 (Sapi, Bw22J)			
	Bw4 (4a)			
	Bw6 (4b)			

† Splits or variants of an antigen are listed as indentations below the original antigen. The small "w" (for workshop) indicates an antigen that has been accepted provisionally at an international workshop as a specific HLA antigen. When the specificity of such an HLA antigen has been established, the w is deleted.

‡ Previous designations are listed in parentheses.

NOTE: The asterisks that appear are part of the locus name and do not refer to a footnote.

alloantigenic sites, there are also antigenic determinants or *epitopes* which are common to all A-locus or all B-locus molecules. These "core" or framework specificities are identified by cross-species antibodies (xenoantibodies) produced in rabbits or monoclonal antibodies produced in mice [52].

THE HLA-A, -B, AND -C ANTIGENS

The HLA-A, -B, and -C antigens are antigenic sites or epitopes on integral membrane glycoprotein molecules present on most nucleated cells. These molecules are believed to have arisen from gene duplication since they exhibit similar biochemical structures and have extensive homologies. Consequently, the

HLA-A, -B, and -C molecules are considered together here. However, their function is unknown, and during evolution the functions of -A, -B, and -C may have diverged.

Tissue Distribution and Expression

The HLA-A, -B, and -C antigens are codominantly expressed on nearly all lymphocytes, macrophages, fibroblasts, platelets, endothelial cells, cells of the spleen, heart, liver, lung, intestine, and kidney, and most other nucleated human cells [53]. These antigens are also present in the placenta but are not on the trophoblast [54]. The red cell Bennett-Goodspeed antigens correlate with several known HLA antigens: Bg^a with HLA-B7, Bg^b with HLA-B17, and Bg^c with HLA-A28 [55], but chemical identity has not been established. The Rogers and

Chido antigens represent C4A and C4B on the red cell surface [11, 12]. Other HLA antigens on the red cell have been detected only through the use of the Auto Technicon and appear to be present in trace quantitites, possibly on reticulocytes.

Peripheral blood T lymphocytes have approximately 10^3 to 10^4 HLA molecules per antigen per cell, while cultured B lymphoblastoid cells may have 5 to 13 times as many [56, 57]. Interferon-treated cells are also reported to have enhanced expression of HLA [58]. HLA-A and -B antigens have been found in soluble form in saliva, serum, and plasma [53, 59], urine [60], seminal plasma [61], and in low concentration in colostrum and milk [62].

Two families with HLA deficiency have been reported. Van Rood and his colleagues have described a Turkish family in which two children had severe hypogammaglobulinemia [3]. Both children lacked detectable HLA-A, -B, and -C antigens on lymphocytes, platelets, and fibroblasts. An immunodeficient child from a Middle Eastern family was also described by Betuel and coworkers [4]. Circulating lymphocytes lacked all HLA-A, -B, and -C antigens. HLA types were determinable from serum. Ceppellini has described a chimeric individual who carried both HLA haplotypes of both parents and thus had twice as many antigens as normal [63]. Mayr et al [64] have presented another example of abnormal heredity in a mother with apparent gonadal mosaicism. The HLA-A, -B, and -C haplotypes passed on to her children were not expressed on her circulating lymphocytes but were present in the maternal grandmother.

A more common and apparently normal absence of particular HLA-B and -C antigens is characteristic of platelets [65] and fibroblasts of some individuals [66]. This deficiency is not known to be related to any immunologic abnormality. Recent studies of membrane markers on early lymphoid stem cells have shown that the HLA-A, -B, and -C antigens are not present at detectable levels [67].

A secondary deficiency of HLA-A, -B, and -C expression in vitro is due to the absence of β_2-microglobulin, since β_2-microglobulin is necessary for membrane transport of the HLA antigens and insertion into the membrane. The most notable example is that of the Daudi cell line [68].

Biochemistry

The HLA-A, -B, and -C molecules are each composed of two noncovalently bound polypeptides, the larger of which is an integral membrane component (Fig. 3-3) [69]. This larger "heavy" chain, determined by the HLA region, is a glycoprotein with a molecular weight of 44,000 (gp44). The smaller "light" chain is β_2-microglobulin, with a molecular weight of 11,600 that is determined by a gene on chromosome 15. β_2-Microglobulin polymorphism has not been reported. The antigenicity of the HLA molecules is due to multiple, noncontinuous amino acid substitutions on the gp44 chain. The probability of multiple antigenic sites (epitopes) per molecule is of interest and will be discussed later.

Biochemical analysis of the HLA molecules required the introduction of several innovative techniques, e.g., the use of enzymes such as ficin or papain, which selectively cleave the antigen-bearing portion of the molecules, the use of detergents to solubilize cell membranes, and lectin affinity purification [69]. One molecule, HLA-B7, has been completely sequenced. Several others have been extensively sequenced, and the cumulative description of these molecules is as follows [69].

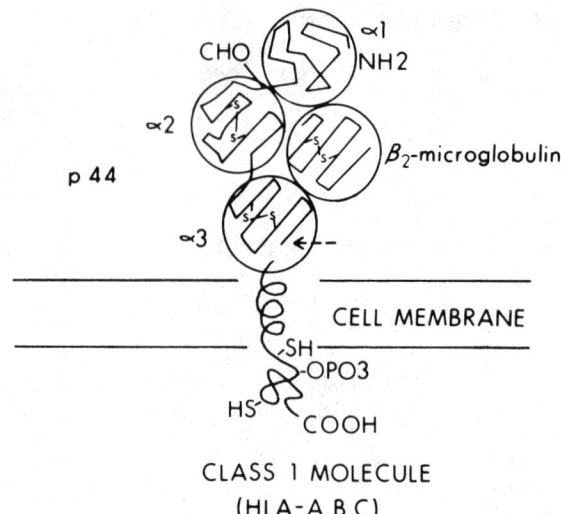

Figure 3-3 Schematic drawing of an HLA-A, -B, or -C molecule. The arrow designates a papain-sensitive cleavage site. (*Modified from Owen MJ, Crumpton MJ: Biochemistry of major human histocompatibility antigens. Immunol Today 1:117, 1980.*)

HLA-A and HLA-B (presumably also the less well studied HLA-C) have an α1 domain (an amino terminal portion of approximately 110 amino acids), two disulfide-bonded loops or "domains" (α2 and α3) of 63 and 36 amino acids, a short sequence of amino acids responsible for membrane insertion, and a cytoplasmic carboxy terminal end of approximately 30 amino acids (Fig. 3-3).

Information on HLA-C is sketchy due to the difficulties encountered in isolation and purification. While HLA-C has the same approximate molecular weight as HLA-A and HLA-B, the carbohydrate is reported to be more heterogeneous and the molecule to be less stable and more easily degraded [70]. As noted earlier, fewer HLA-C antigens have been defined. This has prompted Ferrara et al., who extensively immunized against HLA-C and failed to produce antibodies, to conclude that null genes or null antigens for HLA-C exist [71]. Inherent instability and low immunogenicity are other possibilities.

In addition to the homologous structures in the mouse (H-2D, K, and L), other antigens are determined by genes near H-2. These antigens also have a class 1 structure (β_2-microglobulinlike chain and gp44). Two of those proteins, the Qa and Tl antigens, are differentiation antigens found on T cells and on some leukemia cells [72, 73].

Typing Procedures

Typing for HLA-A, -B, and -C is most frequently based on the reaction of lymphocytes with specific HLA antiserums in a complement-dependent lytic assay [74]. The current assay requires incubating 0.001 ml lymphocytes with 0.001 ml human antiserum in the wells of a microtiter tray. After 30 min and an optional wash, 0.005 ml rabbit serum is added as a source of complement. Then, 60 min later, cell viability is measured. The degree of cell death can be measured in several ways, such as by uptake of a vital dye (e.g., trypan blue or eosin), release of a fluorescent material (e.g., fluoroscein diacetate), or release of a radioactive label (e.g., ^{51}Cr). The sensitivity of the complement-mediated test can be increased by washing the sensitized cells before adding complement, with the addition of antiglobulin [75], or by extending the incubation time. These two procedures tend to favor cross-reactivity.

Other types of assays are used sporadically. These include direct or indirect immunofluorescence [76] or incubation with ^{125}I-labeled protein A from *Staphylococcus aureus* [77], which binds to human IgG. Other older, less reproducible methods have included leukoagglutination and mixed hemagglutination. HLA typing in the future will probably be based on the reaction of monoclonal antibodies and new techniques, such as enzyme-linked immunoassay (ELISA) or radioimmunoassay. At the time of writing, only a few monoclonal antibodies are giving reactions comparable to those of the alloantibodies, and these are being used in lytic tests.

Lymphocytes are obtained from peripheral blood by ficoll-hypaque density gradient sedimentation [78]. They can be used immediately and can be depleted of macrophages or further divided into T and B lymphocytes. Other types of cells that may be tested in a complement-mediated assay include fibroblasts and B and T lymphoblastoid cell lines, macrophages, and possibly platelets. One very sensitive, albeit indirect, way to ascertain HLA antigens is by absorption of a single antiserum by the cell in question. The absorbed serum is then retested on a known positive lymphocyte to see if antibody activity has been removed [79].

HLA typing serums come from several sources, most commonly from multiparous women who have been sensitized to paternal antigens on the fetus during pregnancy [80]. Unfortunately, sensitization is often to more than one HLA antigen. Since the HLA antibodies tend to be cross-reactive, the majority of maternal antiserums are not sufficiently specific to give reactions which conform to the generally accepted concept of HLA. Other serum donors include individuals on dialysis, those who have received multiple blood transfusions, and those who have been experimentally immunized with human lymphocytes [81]. The active immunoglobulin in most HLA alloantiserums is generally IgG. Titers are usually low, in the range of 1:1 or 1:16, depending on the method of testing. HLA antibodies are very rarely encountered in the absence of immunization with allogenic cells but are occasionally found [82, 83].

A new method that is actively being explored in many centers is the isolation of monoclonal antibodies from the fusion of antibody-producing cells with myeloma cells [84]. These antiserums will be invaluable, since they bypass the usual problems of mixtures of antibodies, and they can be constructed to react with rare antigens. They do present their own problems, however. Relatively few monoclonal antibodies are cytotoxic, so that direct binding assays must often be used. Because immunization is dependent upon the injection of human cells or cell products into the mouse, antibodies are likely to be formed to structural parts of the HLA proteins that are shared by many of the proteins. Such antibodies are therefore irrelevant to HLA typing. Despite the interest being devoted to hybridoma antibody production it will apparently be some years before monoclonal antiserums become widely useful in HLA typing.

Cross-reactivity

Numerous cross-reactive families or groups of HLA antigens (CREGs) are widely recognized. Perhaps best known are the HLA-B7, B27; HLA-B5, Bw35, Bw51, Bw52, Bw53, B18; the A3, A11, A10; and the A2, A28 CREGs. Serums recognizing CREGs are often designated *multispecific*. Some of the serums may contain antibodies of differing specificity, but most

appear to be oligospecific. In part, cross-reactivity depends upon reactivity with antigens that are similar but not identical.

Unusual HLA-ABC Antigens

As mentioned previously, it has been assumed by most investigators that only one antigen exists per HLA molecule. The possibility of several epitopes per molecule has now been established beyond a reasonable doubt, and "antigens" which may represent separate epitopes on a single molecule will be briefly listed here.

Bw4, Bw6 All HLA-B molecules apparently carry two HLA antigens, a public antigen (which is either Bw4 or Bw6) and a private or subtypic antigen. Bw4 and Bw6 (formerly 4a and 4b) represent a diallelic system, one of which is expressed on every HLA-B molecule [49, 85, 86]. Although these antigens were recognized as long ago as 1962, their significance was largely overlooked, since they appeared to represent examples of multispecificity. However, as van Rood et al. pointed out [49], Bw4 and Bw6 split many known HLA-B antigens. For example, B16 exists as two variants, Bw38 (16.1) and Bw39 (16.2). All individuals who are Bw38+ are Bw4+, and all Bw39+ individuals are Bw6+. Similar divisions have been documented for the variants of B12, B15, and Bw21.

Public Antigens The term *public antigens* arose from mouse studies in which an antigen restricted to one mouse strain was designated a *private antigen*, while one found in two or more dissimilar strains (and sometimes present at both H-2 D and K) was designated a *public antigen*. In the human, the terms *public* (or *supertypic*) and *private* (or *subtypic*) similarly refer to the antigens that are found on several of the HLA gene products, in contrast to those found on a more restricted set of proteins. For instance, the B5 antigen might now be referred to as a supertypic antigen, since there are at least two types of B5: Bw51 and Bw52 [87]. Some of the public HLA antigens that have been described include:

1. Antigen LHe, present on Bw4, A9 (both Aw23 and Aw24 variants), and Aw32 [50, 51].
2. Antigen ST, present on HLA-B8, -B15, -B17, and the 4c antigens [88].
3. An antigen common to Bw6 and A11 [89].
4. An unnamed specificity on HLA-A2 and HLA-B17 molecules that is recognized by a murine monoclonal antibody [90]. Similar reactivity by alloantiserums has not been observed.
5. The antigenic site recognized by a monoclonal antibody (MB40.1) that reacts with both HLA-A and HLA-B antigens, e.g., A28, B7, B8, and B40 [91].

THE HLA-D COMPLEX

The HLA-D antigens are definable by mixed lymphocytic culture (MLC) (reviewed in Refs. 92, 93), a technically simple assay in which lymphocytes from the individual to be typed (responder cells) are mixed with lymphocytes from a series of donors known to be homozygous for HLA-D (stimulator cells). The responder fails to give a proliferative reaction if the cells possess the HLA-D allele present on the stimulator cells.

HLA-D Typing

A mixed lymphocyte culture consists of culturing 10^5 responding cells and 10^5 stimulating lymphocytes together for 5 to 7 days [92, 93]. The stimulating cells are inactivated by γ irradiation or mitomycin C to prevent proliferation. During this time, HLA-D disparity results in proliferation, which is measurable by incorporation of radiolabeled nucleotides such as [³H]thymidine.

HLA-D typing has become possible only through the use of lymphocytes from individuals who carry two identical HLA-D specificities. These lymphocytes are HTCs, or homozygous typing cells [94, 95]. HLA-D homozygous individuals occur very rarely in populations. They are more common in first-cousin marriages, in which the children have an appreciable chance of inheriting two copies of the same chromosome from the great-grandparent, or in incestuous matings. For HLA-D typing, a person is set up as a responder, with the stimulators being Dw1 HTCs, Dw2 HTCs, etc. The responding cells will react with all stimulators except those carrying D alleles identical to the responder's. Thus a person who fails to respond to the Dw2 and Dw3 HTCs but responds to all others would be considered Dw2, Dw3 positive.

The degree of proliferation is usually assessed by measurement of the incorporation of [³H]thymidine into DNA. The data can be presented in several ways, e.g., the stimulation index, a ratio of counts per minute (cpm) in the experimental combination of cells versus cpm in the autologous combination. Because some lymphocytes have high intrinsic levels of thymidine incorporation and because of other factors, such as the side effects of therapy for disease, the degree of proliferation may vary. Also, some HTCs provide very clear separation into positive and negative responses, while many others do not. Several modifications have been introduced. Instead of comparing the experimental cpm with background, the experimental cpm are compared with the maximum possible stimulation, determined by using a pool of stimulating cells or by the response to cells from three or more unrelated individuals. Thus, the relative response (RR) has a maximum value of 100 percent and values less than some arbitrary value (e.g., 25 percent) are by convention considered "negative." For certain purposes, such as the definition of new specificities, an extended matrix of stimulatory and responder cells is included in a massive experiment, and inherent differences in responsive and stimulatory capacity are compensated for by double normalization of the data [46, 96]. The HTCs giving the best typing responses include those from first-cousin marriages, in which the two haplotypes have recent common ancestry. Since it is now realized that at least two additional loci can, on occasion, induce stimulation, it appears probable that the overlapping values given by the poorer HTCs may be due to heterozygosity at these new loci.

Tissue Distribution

Only certain types of cells will stimulate in MLC. HLA-D-positive cells include B lymphocytes and B lymphoblastoid cell lines [97], Langerhans cells of the skin [98], monocytes and macrophages [99], and endothelial cells [100].

THE HLA-DR COMPLEX

The HLA-DR antigens (Fig. 3-4) are commonly referred to as *B-cell antigens* or *Ia antigens* (equivalent to the immune associated antigens of the mouse). These antigens, present on B lymphocytes, were originally detected by their reaction with fluorescent antibodies. They were considered to be equivalent to the functionally defined HLA-D antigens. Nomenclature was designed to be consistent between the two sets: a Dw1 HTC carries the DR1 antigens, etc. Unfortunately, a simple correspondence is not always found, and the terminologies are now diverging. Correlations between D and DR are not consistent in American Indians, Orientals, and blacks [101–105]. There is also evidence for at least two other allelic systems, MB [106] and MT [107] antigens on the molecular complex that carries the DR epitope [40]. The genetics of the B-cell antigens will be important, since the DR antigens probably play a role in immune responses and since many diseases are associated with HLA D-DR specificities.

HLA-DR Typing Procedures

Typing for HLA-DR in many ways is similar to HLA-A, -B, and -C typing. Both rely on human antiserums and rabbit serum as a source of complement. In HLA-DR typing, however, the target is the B lymphocyte, incubation times are sometimes lengthened, and the rabbit serum must be carefully selected to avoid the high background often seen when B cells or B cell lines are tested. Only the B-cell subfraction of peripheral blood lymphocytes is used by most laboratories, and contaminating HLA-A, -B, and -C antibodies must be removed from the alloantiserums [108].

Figure 3-4 Schematic drawing of the HLA-DR (class 2) molecule. The arrows designate papain-sensitive cleavage sites. (*Modified from Strominger et al.* [69].)

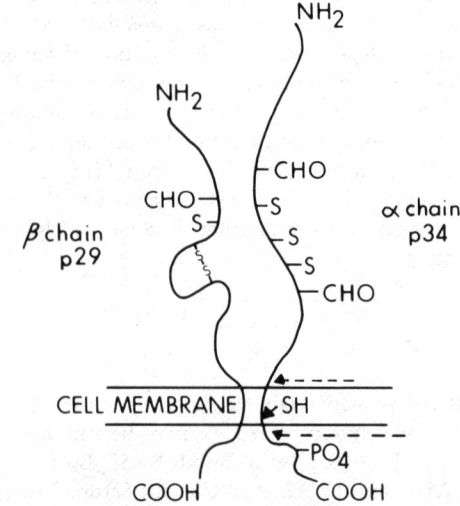

Both positive and negative selective measures can be used to isolate a pure B-cell population [40]. B cells constitute less than 15 percent of the usual peripheral blood lymphocytes. Selective depletion of T cells can be performed by rosetting with sheep red blood cells [109]. Positive selection of B cells can be accomplished by taking advantage of their membrane receptor for the Fc portion of immunoglobulins [110], their surface immunoglobulin [111], their adherence to nylon fibers [112], or their ability to form rosettes in the presence of a monoclonal anti-Ia antibody [113].

Modification of the dye exclusion cytotoxicity assay is continually being attempted. Two-color fluorescence is one alternative [114] which is time-consuming but does not require separation of B cells from T cells. In this procedure, B cells are labeled with a fluorescein-coupled Ig (green) before the cytotoxicity assay is performed. After cytotoxicity occurs, the dead cells are stained with ethidium bromide (red). The dead B cells can be identified by their content of both green and red fluorescence, as ascertained by the alternative use of UV and visible light.

The addition of an anti-β_2-microglobulin serum to B cells clears the surface of HLA-A, -B, and -C antigens and thereby eliminates reactivity with HLA-A, -B, and -C antiserums. Complement-mediated cytotoxicity to DR antigens proceeds unimpeded [115]. DR typing has also been performed on mitogen-activated peripheral blood lymphocytes [116].

Antiserums

Human serums having anti HLA-A, -B, or -C reactivity often include antibodies to HLA-DR antigens. Since peripheral blood lymphocytes are usually mostly T cells which do not express DR antigens, the inclusion of anti-DR antibodies in a serum gives little trouble in ABC typing. In contrast, since B cells carry the A, B, and C antigens in addition to DR, the A, B, and C activity must be removed before DR typing. This is accomplished by platelet absorption (platelets carry HLA-A and generally HLA-B antigens, but not DR) or by T-cell lines [108]. Absorption is a time-consuming and expensive procedure, since each absorbed serum must be retested to ensure that absorption was complete. Monoclonal antibodies do not require absorption. Xenoantiserums, which recognize a nonpolymorphic "framework" antigen, are useful in the classification of cells as DR$^+$ or DR$^-$, e.g., in subtyping leukemias.

Tissue Distribution

The HLA-DR-positive cells include B lymphocytes, B lymphoblastoid cell lines, monocytes and macrophages, Langerhans cells, and endothelial cells [117–119]. Ia-like antigens have also been found on activated T cells [116], on early but not late myeloid cells [120], and on some cultured or fresh malignant melanoma cells [121]. Thus, the DR antigens most often, but possibly not always, are characteristic of cells with an immune function. Due to their position on endothelial and Langerhans cells, they can be potent transplantation antigens. In addition, Ia-like antigens (identified by indirect immunofluorescence using monoclonal antibodies that detect framework determinants) have been reported to be located on normal tissues of differing embryonic origin, including the epithelium of both

the gastrointestinal tract and the mammary gland, urinary bladder, bronchial glands, thymic reticuloepithelial cells of entodermic origin, acinar cells of the parotid, astrocytes, Kupffer cells, and endometrium [122]. Natali et al. have suggested that since these Ia-like antigens are found in mammary cells and endometrium [122], their expression may be under hormonal control. It remains to be established that these antigens are identical to the DR antigens of blood lymphocytes. It is conceivable that some of them may be tissue-specific differentiation antigens.

Serology

HLA-DR seems complex for many reasons—including the probability of multiple, closely linked loci and the possibility of cross-reactivity. There are 11 known DR antigens [40], with suggestions that at least DR6 can be split. Two loci more recently described are MB and MT [40, 106, 107]. Both are less polymorphic than DR, and because they show association with or include specific DR antigens (Fig. 3-5), their presence has often been ascribed to cross-reactivity. For example, serums detecting MB1 react with most DR-1, -2, and -6-positive cells from Caucasians. MT1 serums react similarly. The most convincing evidence that MB and MT do represent the products of separate loci is based on biochemical data from two-dimensional gel analysis, isoelectric focusing, and immunoprecipitation [123, 124]. In the homologous system in the mouse, four loci exist on the same chromosome, two determining α chains and the other two determining β chains [6, 125]. It is likely that a similar arrangement occurs on the human chromosome 6.

Biochemistry

The HLA-DR, -MB, and -MT antigens are epitopes on a molecule that is formed from the association of two glycoproteins [69, 125, 126] (Fig. 3-4). The larger α chain and smaller β chain have molecular weights of approximately 34,000 and 29,000, respectively. Both are glycosylated, integral membrane components, and both chains appear to be determined by genes within the MHC. DR antigenicity has been attributed to the α chain by some investigators and to the β chain by others. While some think that antigenicity is due to variable amino acid sequences, others, using different antiserums and different methods have found evidence that some of the murine Ia anti-

Figure 3-5 Associations of the MB, MT, and DR antigens.

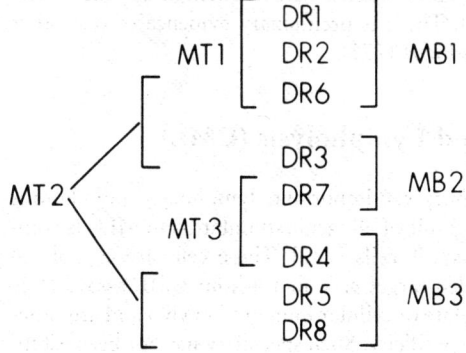

gens are carbohydrates, possibly glycolipids [127]. It is also reported that the DR found on activated T cells may not be identical to that found on the autologous B cells [128], and the possibility that there exist two sets of DR molecules, one carrying the DR and MB antigens and the other DR and MT, remains strong. Analysis of the genetics and biochemistry of DR is complicated by the strong (but not covalent) binding of the two chains; the antigen association or overlap is high.

NEW MHC LOCI

Primed Lymphocyte Typing (PLT)

Lymphocytes that have responded in a primary mixed lymphocyte response (MLR) can be restimulated in a secondary MLR using the same or different stimulating cells [129]. These "primed" lymphocytes will proliferate more rapidly upon secondary challenge (e.g., 1 to 2 days rather than 5 to 7 days) with cells presenting the same antigen. Priming can be used to produce highly specific PLT responding cells capable of recognizing HLA-D/-DR antigens, as well as new antigens. For example, if a father (Dw1, Dw2) responds in MLR with his daughter (Dw1/Dx) or his son (Dw1/Dw3), his primed PLT cells will recognize a Dx in one case or a Dw3 in another. The PLT cells, once generated, can then be used to test a whole cell panel.

MLR combination		Specificity of PLT response
Responding cell	Stimulating cell	
Father Dw1, Dw2	Daughter Dw1, Dx	Dx
Father Dw1, Dw2	Son Dw1, Dw3	Dw3

The response in PLT, as in MLR, is complex, and at least two other loci (in addition to D/DR) are responsible for PLT reactivity. One allelic series has been examined by Charmot et al. [28] and by Shaw et al. [29]. The latter group has studied cells from individuals who are HLA-A, -B, -C, -D, -DR, and -MB identical but who nevertheless generate a strongly positive PLT. If the responses are grouped, a single locus with at least five alleles is postulated. Shaw et al. called this locus the *SB* or *secondary B* cell locus (Charmot et al. have termed theirs *PL*). The SB antigens are (1) expressed on B cells, not on T cells; (2) coded for by a gene between HLA-B and GLO (Fig. 3-1); (3) stimulate little primary cellular response; but (4) stimulate strong PLT and strong secondary cytotoxic T-cell responses. Disease associations appear probable, as certain combinations of HLA-B and SB are frequent in dermatitis herpetiformis [130]. There is preliminary evidence of one other PLT-stimulating locus [131].

Cell-mediated Lympholysis (CML)

One of the minor, yet important, lymphocyte populations responding as a result of allogenic stimulation in MLC is composed of cytotoxic T cells [132]. These cells are capable of lysing radiolabeled target cells in a 4-hour CML assay. They are a likely correlate of cellular immunity in vivo and are capable of exquisite specificity. Such specificity has not been established in graft rejection.

The generation of cytotoxic T cells requires I region identity in the mouse (so presumably D/DR identity in humans) between the T helper cells and T precursor cytotoxic cells [133]. The target antigens include the Class 1 (HLA-A, -B, and -C) antigens. Cytotoxic lymphocytes can be exquisitely specific. They can discriminate between the antigenic variants of B5 (Bw51, Bw52, and a new variant called *B5.y*) [134]. Other specific cytotoxic lymphocytes have been raised against HLA-A2 [135]. Cytotoxic lymphocytes raised against a whole haplotype difference have much broader specificity, from which it can be inferred that additional HLA loci, functioning as target antigens in CML, are determined by genes in the chromosomal segment between D/DR and GLO, e.g., HDr, which was suggested to be a CML target several years ago [136].

T-cell-specific Antigens

In the mouse, there are loci close to H-2 that also code for differentiation antigens which have a class 1-like structure. These antigens, the TL^a and Qa series, are expressed on T-cell subsets and on some leukemic cells. These genes map to the right of H-2 D/L and are markers for what is known as the TL^a-Qa-2 region [137].

Several searches for homologous molecules on human T cells have provided suggestive evidence that T-cell-specific antigens are determined by genes near or within HLA [138, 139]. Molt 4, an "early" T-cell line, seems to express an antigen distinct from HLA-A, -B, and -C but associated with β_2-microglobulin [140]. Some quantitative binding assays have found the concentration of β_2-microglobulin to be higher on these cells than can be accounted for by HLA-A, -B, and -C [141], although others have not [56]. Even peripheral blood T lymphocytes, after mitogen stimulation, are reported to show activity distinct from HLA-A, -B, -C, and -DR [142].

POPULATION GENETICS AND LINKAGE DISEQUILIBRIUM

As early as 1967, it was realized that the HLA antigens characteristic of one population could be completely absent in another [143]. Consequently, the 1972 Histocompatibility Workshop was designed to "HLA type the populations of the world" [45]. Included were Eskimos, American Indians, African pygmies, Nepalese Sherpas, Australian aborigines, Easter Islanders, and many more. Because of the intricacies of the Oriental HLA haplotypes and because of extreme differences in disease associations, an Asian Pan Oceanian Histocompatibility Testing Workshop was held in 1979 and a second one in 1981 [144, 145]. Some antigens, such as A2 and Bw35, are found in nearly all populations. The A1, A3, B8, and B27 antigens are found in Caucasians and blacks, but seldom if ever in Orientals. Where present, their introduction from the outside cannot be excluded. Certain antigens are found almost exclusively in blacks, e.g., Aw43 or Bw45 [146], or in Chinese e.g., Bw46 [47]. A summary of HLA gene frequencies in several ethnic groups is given in Table 3-2.

Bodmer and Thomson have calculated the number of possible arrangements of HLA alleles forming the Caucasion haplotype [147]. In 1975, based on 19 HLA-A antigens, 26 HLA-B

Table 3-2 HLA-A, -B, -C, -D, and -DR gene frequencies*

	European Caucasians	N. American Caucasians	American blacks	African blacks	Japanese	American Indians
HLA-A	(228)†	(290)	(128)	(102)	(195)	(89)
A1	15.8%	16.1%	8.1%	3.9%	1.2%	2.5%
A2	27.0	28.0	16.3	9.4	25.3	45.3
A3	12.6	14.1	7.0	6.4	0.7	0.6
Aw23 ⎱ A9	2.4	1.9	10.6	10.8		
A9					37.2	23.2
Aw24 ⎰	8.8	7.3	5.1	2.4		
A25 ⎱ A10	2.0	2.6	0.4	3.5		
A10					12.7	0.6
A26 ⎰	3.9	3.4	2.3	4.5		
A11	5.1	5.1	2.8	‡	6.7	‡
A28	4.4	4.2	5.8	8.9	‡	2.8
A29	5.8	3.6	2.3	6.4	0.2	0.6
Aw30	3.9	2.9	13.0	22.1	0.5	1.1
Aw31	2.3	4.5	2.8	4.2	8.7	19.9
Aw32	2.9	3.7	1.9	1.5	0.5	1.1
Aw33	0.7	1.2	5.1	1.0	2.0	0.6
Aw43	‡	‡	‡	‡	‡	‡
Blank	2.2	1.3	16.5	11.0	4.2	1.8
HLA-B	(228)†	(290)	(128)	(102)	(195)	(89)
B5	5.9%	5.9%	4.9%	3.0%	20.9%	14.0%
B7	10.4	10.5	12.6	7.3	7.1	0.6
B8	9.2	10.4	5.5	7.1	0.2	1.7
B12	16.6	13.8	14.0	12.7	6.5	1.7
B13	3.2	2.6	0.4	1.5	0.8	‡
B14	2.4	5.1	4.6	3.6	0.5	‡
B18	6.2	3.1	3.6	2.0	‡	0.6
B27	4.6	5.6	0.8	‡	0.3	6.2
B15	4.8	5.9	4.7	3.0	9.3	13.7
Bw38 ⎱ Bw16	2.0	2.5	0.4		1.8	
Bw16				1.5		14.5
Bw39 ⎰	3.5	1.4	0.4		4.7	
B17	5.7	4.9	11.2	16.1	0.6	‡
Bw21	2.2	3.8	4.4	1.5	1.5	‡
Bw22	3.6	2.3	3.9	‡	6.5	0.6
Bw35	9.9	8.6	12.5	7.2	9.4	22.1
B37	1.1	1.7	1.2	‡	0.8	‡
B40	8.1	9.2	3.9	2.0	21.8	16.6
Bw41	‡	‡	‡	1.5	‡	‡
Bw42	‡	‡	‡	12.3	‡	‡
Blank	3.6	2.8	11.0	17.9	7.6	7.8
HLA-C	(321)†	(271)	(107)	(101)	(203)	(89)
Cw1	4.8%	3.7%	1.9%	‡	11.1%	10.1%
Cw2	5.4	6.0	9.2	11.4	1.4	4.6
Cw3	9.4	11.4	8.8	5.5	16.3	16.6
Cw4	12.6	10.2	12.9	14.2	4.3	23.4
Cw5	8.4	5.2	1.4	1.0	1.2	1.1
Cw6	12.6	11.3	‡	17.7	2.1	‡
Blank	46.7	52.1	65.8	50.2	53.5	44.2
HLA-D	(99)†	(125)				
Dw1	7.9%	6.8%				
Dw2	9.5	11.7				
Dw3	9.5	9.0				
Dw4	5.1	5.2				
Dw5	9.0	6.1				
Dw6	11.5	8.9				
Dw7	5.8	9.8				
Dw8	2.5	1.6				
Blank	39.1	40.9				
HLA-DR	(334)‡	(273)	(110)	(77)	(164)	(69)
DR1	6.2%	5.2%	7.3%	‡	4.5%	‡
DR2	11.2	13.9	13.8	8.7	16.5	8.4
DR3	8.9	11.8	12.4	11.7	‡	9.1
DR4	7.8	16.5	7.2	3.5	14.4	21.5
DR5	15.1	11.9	15.4	7.4	5.4	6.0

Table 3-2 HLA-A, -B, -C, -D, and -DR gene frequencies* *(Continued)*

	European Caucasians	N. American Caucasians	American blacks	African blacks	Japanese	American Indians
DRw6	8.6	11.5	19.1	9.9	6.7	5.9
DR7	15.6	12.4	12.0	6.6	‡	3.7
DRw8	5.6	4.2	7.5	7.2	7.2	12.9
Blank	21.2	12.6	5.3	45.0	45.3	32.5

* From Bodmer et al. [47]. The percentage of individuals with each allele is given.
† Number of individuals typed.
‡ Alleles not present.

antigens, 6 HLA-C antigens, and 8 HLA-D alleles, 26,676 haplotypes, 33,194,624 phenotypes, and 355,817,826 genotypes would be possible. Some of these haplotypes may never be found. In contrast, certain haplotypes, such as A1-B8-DR3 and A3-B7-DR2, are extremely frequent. The association of antigens more frequently than would be expected by chance is called *linkage disequilibrium*. It is given a numerical value referred to as *delta*. The reasons for linkage disequilibrium are disputed [147–150]. It has been attributed to selective forces (e.g., infectious disease) acting either on the HLA antigens themselves or on closely linked loci. Linkage disequilibrium has also been thought to be an artifact of population expansion, migration, and an admixture of heterogeneous populations (lack of time for equilibration). Observations on the mouse suggest two further possibilities: (1) A series of semi-lethal genes (the T/t complex regulating embryonic differentiation) effectively suppresses recombination along the chromosome carrying H-2 [151]. (2) Recombination in some hybrids is 200 times as frequent as recombination in other crosses [152]. Similar phenomena may occur in humans. A locus regulating spinal development has been mapped to the sixth chromosome [153], and several nuclear families include more than one recombinant. One 10-sib family includes no fewer than five recombinants in the HLA region, with a sixth recombination in the next generation.

THE MHC AND IMMUNE RESPONSIVENESS

Some of the ways in which the MHC is tied to immune responsiveness have been mentioned. For example, the HLA-A, -B, -C, and -DR molecules are potent histocompatibility antigens and can function as targets for both alloantibody and alloreactive cytotoxic T cells. The haplotype provides a powerful target for allograft rejection. HLA-D/DR, MB, and MT alleles are differentiation antigens commonly found on immunoreactive cells and are structurally homologous to the Ia antigens of H-2.

In the mouse, a unique set of genes controls the magnitude of the immune response to thymus-dependent antigens (e.g., those requiring helper T-cell recognition). There is presumptive evidence for the existence of similar genes in humans. These immune response or Ir genes are capable of determining the level (e.g., responder versus nonresponder status) of antibody production and of effector T-cell activation [154, 155]. Mouse Ir genes map to the H-2 I region which determines B-cell antigens. Human Ir genes appear to be associated with

HLA but have not been localized to any particular region. For example, Greenberg et al. [156] reported that individuals with the antigen HLA-B5 are high responders to streptococcal antigens. HLA-B5 individuals are also reported to have higher levels of immune complexes in acute rheumatic fever [157]. Certain HLA antigens have also been associated with acute post-streptococcal glomerulonephritis [158] and with high and low responses to schistosomal antigens [159]. Sensitivity to ragweed [160], cellular responses in vitro to influenza [161] and responses in vitro to insulin [162] as a complication of insulin therapy in diabetics have also been reported to exhibit HLA associations.

Unsuccessful attempts at defining Ir gene functions, including those using synthetic polypeptides, vaccinia, influenza A, measles, and tetanus toxoid, can be attributed to many causes—failure to use a discriminating antigen dose, antigenic complexity, failure to use family members for the studies, or inability to control for sensitization from previous exposure. Multigenic effects may be especially difficult to deal with. The Ir1 gene of the H-2 complex is only one of five or more different Ir genes of the mouse.

One further function of the MHC involves the generation and regulation of the immune response. An effective immune response requires specific cooperation between two or more subsets of lymphocytes. These lymphocyte populations must be MHC compatible for effective interaction (*MHC restriction*). In some cases, identity of Class 1 antigens (H-2 D or K in the mouse; HLA-A or -B in the human) is required. At other times, class 2 antigens (H-2I, HLA-DR) must be identical. An abbreviated list is given in Table 3–3.

The efficient interaction between T helper cells (T_H), which help "present" antigen to cytotoxic T cells, and B cells leads to the differentiation and proliferation of specific cytotoxic T cells and antibody-secreting plasma cells [163]. This interaction requires class 2 MHC compatibility. Similarly, the inflammatory response characteristic of delayed type hypersensitivity requires H-2 I region identity [163]. Soluble "helper" and "suppressor" factors produced by T cells carry I-A or I-J determinants, respectively [164]. Of importance is the observation that T cells recognize an antigen only when it is associated with MHC determinants.

The dual recognition of both "self-MHC" and antigen has been explained by two different models [165]. The first, the *dual receptor* model, postulates two separate receptors on T cells, one for the MHC product and one for the antigen. A second model postulates an alteration of the MHC product upon binding of antigen. This *altered-self* hypothesis requires a single T-cell receptor which binds an antigen-MHC complex (Fig. 3-6). In either case, the reaction requires that the T cell be "instructed" by the thymus [166].

It is of great interest to see if, as a result of Ir genes, susceptibility to certain infections will show DR associations. The increased reactivity of B5$^+$ individuals to streptococcal antigens has been mentioned [158]. Rheumatic fever also appears to be associated with certain HLA alleles, e.g., the increase of immune complexes in B5$^+$ rheumatic fever patients [157], and an increased reactivity of a particular B-cell serum in Bogota, Columbia, and New York City [157]. Japanese workers have found an increase of the HLA-D En allele in individuals with acute poststreptococcal glomerulonephritis [158]. This antigen has not been identified outside Japan. A functional Fc-receptor defect, leading to an impaired ability to clear IgG-containing immune complexes from the circulation, has been associated with the B8-DR3 antigens in patients with dermatitis herpetiformis [185].

Diseases Associated with the Haplotype

In cases of loose linkage or polygenic diseases with one gene linked to HLA, any association with a particular HLA antigen would be slight and likely to be missed in a population study. Only families will be informative in these cases. An example is leprosy, in which the lepromatous and tuberculoid forms segregate with the HLA haplotype in families. No association with a specific HLA antigen has been found [186]. There are many diseases in which only a slight HLA association has been documented, e.g., in malignancies, as mentioned earlier. Further studies with other HLA markers (e.g., SB antigens) in families could be extremely informative.

It is also worth noting that some diseases are found almost exclusively with a particular haplotype. A striking example is that of C2 deficiency, which is found with an A25-B18-Dw2 haplotype (see Chap. 89) [187]. Many of the individuals with total C2 deficiency are A25-B18-Dw2 homozygous. The C2 gene has been placed between HLA-B and DR.

Speculations about the HLA-disease Associations

HLA-disease associations can be grouped into the following categories: (1) malignant diseases, for which there is little definitive evidence; (2) inflammatory diseases, such as ankylosing spondylitis and Reiter's disease, which are associated with B27; (3) inborn errors of metabolism, such as hemochromatosis and steroid 21-hydroxylase deficiency; (4) complement-deficiency syndromes; (5) diseases of abnormal differentiation, e.g., congenital neutropenia [188], (6) autoaggressive and endocrine diseases associated with D/DR; and (7) other diseases, such as leprosy, which may be related only to the HLA haplotype and not to any specific allele. It is most unlikely that any unifying cause exists because of the variety of types of disease—from hemochromatosis to psoriasis to Graves' disease—and because different regions of the haplotype appear to be central to certain types of disease (see Table 3-4). Worth mentioning is the possibility that HLA-linked genes may affect the development of a disease or might even determine resistance. For example, retrospective studies of a lethal disease may include a high frequency of long-term survivors. Hence an HLA association would be for increased survival and not for disease susceptibility.

Some of the suggested mechanisms which would account for the observed HLA-disease associations or linkage are given in Table 3-5. For further information, the reader is referred to specific reviews [173, 189–191].

Table 3-4 Examples of HLA-disease associations

Antigen associated	Disease	Relative risk	Comments
A3	Hemochromatosis	4	Recessive inheritance with >95% penetrance; linked to HLA; most common haplotype is A3-C -B14 -BfF -DRw6
B27	Ankylosing spondylitis	90	Associated in all populations
Bw47	Steroid 21-hydroxylase deficiency	15	Late-onset 21-hydroxylase deficiency linked to B14-DR1
DR7	Psoriasis	43	Association with DR7 in Caucasians and in Japanese, especially in early-onset disease; no clear linkage with HLA in 13 multiplex families; Cw6 also associated
DR4 only		6	DR3 associated with type II disease and
DR3 only	Diabetes mellitus	3	DR4 with type I disease; inheritance
Both DR3 and DR4		33	not simple dominant or recessive; seen in Caucasians, blacks, and Japanese
DR3, B8	Chronic active hepatitis	2	Especially in young females with auto-antibodies
DR3, B8	Myasthenia gravis	3	HLA association varies with race; association with thymic disease and complications rather than susceptibility
DR3	Celiac disease	17	Recessive inheritance; DR7 also associated
DR2	Multiple sclerosis	4	At least one more HLA gene important in susceptibility

SOURCE: Modified from Terasaki [40].

Table 3-5 Possible mechanisms for HLA disease associations

Molecular mimicry—cross-reactivity between viruses, bacteria, or environmental agents and HLA antigens

Immune-response genes linked to HLA

Complement genes linked to HLA

Enzyme genes linked to HLA

HLA antigens functioning as virus pathogen receptors

Linked genes determining or controlling differentiation processes

Alteration or modification of HLA antigen as a result of an infectious agent, drug, or environmental agent

---

FUTURE DEVELOPMENTS

For a disease such as hemochromatosis, in which the disease phenotype is expressed in over 90 percent of homozygotes, it should be possible to determine the nature of the genetic defect through studies of abnormalities in iron absorption and transport. For those diseases such as congenital adrenal hyperplasia (steroid 21-hydroxylase deficiency), in which an enzymatic defect can be demonstrated, it should soon be possible to clone the abnormal gene. Where abnormal regulation is implicated, cloning may be more difficult, and we may have to await cloning of the haplotype or regions of the haplotype. We believe that abnormal immune regulation and enzymatic defects will be frequent causes of diseases attributed to genes in the D-DR segment. It is also likely that many new associations will emerge when new markers are identified in the GLO-DR segment (Fig. 3-1). At the present time, this region can be studied only imperfectly because of the limited polymorphism of Glo and because the only identification of other genes is by functional studies with lymphocytes. This approach is not cost-effective for screening populations.

Information will be gained not only on HLA association but also on the definition and classification of disease, the etiology and pathogenic mechanisms of disease, and genetic, racial, and familial predispositions. It is not unlikely that knowledge of HLA associations will be useful in treatment, prognosis, diagnosis, or identification of those individuals at risk.

REFERENCES

1. AMOS D B, KOSTYU DD: HLA—A central immunological agency of man. *Adv Hum Genet* 10:137, 1980
2. GOTZE D (ed): *The Major Histocompatibility System in Man and Animals.* New York, Springer-Verlag, New York, 1977
3. SCHURMANN RKB, VAN ROOD JJ, VOSSEN JM, SCHELLEKENS P TH A, FELTKAMP-VROOM TH M, DOYER E, GMELLING-MAYLING F, VISSNER HKA: Failure of lymphocyte-membrane HLA-A and B expression in two siblings with combined immunodeficiency. *Clin Immunol Immunopath* 14:418, 1979
4. BETUEL H, TOURAINE JL, SOUILLET G, JEUNE M: Absence of cell-membrane HLA antigens in an immunodeficient child. *Tissue Antigens* 11:68, 1978
5. DAUSSET J: Iso-leucoanticorps. *Acta Haemat (Basel)* 20:156, 1958
6. KLEIN J: The major histocompatibility complex of the mouse. *Science* 203:516, 1979
7. FISHER RA: *Genetical Theory of Natural Selection*, ed 2. New York, Dover Publications, Inc, 1958
8. FRANCKE U, WEITKAMP LR: Report of the committee on the genetic constitution of chromosome 6. *Cytogenet Cell Genet* 25:32, 1979
9. BAKKER E, PEARSON PL, MEERA KHAN P, SCHREUDER GM TH, MADAN K: Orientation of major histocompatibility (MHC) genes relative to the centromere of human chromosome 6. *Clin Genet* 15:198, 1979
10. WARD FE, LEVY SB, PINNELL SR: Mixed lymphocyte responses in a four generation C2 deficiency family. *Transplant Proc* 9:1733, 1977
11. O'NEILL GJ, YANG SY, DUPONT B: Two HLA-linked loci controlling the fourth component of human complement. *Proc Natl Acad Sci USA* 75:5165, 1978
12. O'NEILL GJ, MINITER P, POLLACK MS, DUPONT B: Different HLA antigen associations for the functionally active and inactive products of the complement C4F$_1$ allele. *Hum Immunol* 1:23, 1980
13. ALBERT ED, RITTNER C, SCHOLZ S, KUNTZ B, MICKEY MR: Three point association of HLA-A, B Bf haplotypes deduced in 200 parents of 100 families. *Scand J Immunol* 6:459, 1977
14. CURRY RA, DIERICH MP, PELLEGRINO MA, HOCH JA: Evidence for linkage between HLA antigens and receptors for complement components C3b and C3d in human-mouse hybrids. *Immunogenetics* 3:465, 1976
15. MERRITT AD, PETERSEN BH, BIEGEL AA, MEYERS DA, BROOKES GF, HODES ME: Chromosome 6: Linkage of the eighth component of complement (C8) to the histocompatibility region (HLA), in Baltimore Conference (1975), Third International Workshop on Human Gene Mapping. *Birth Defects: Original Article Series* 12, p 364. New York, The National Foundation, 1976
16. GIRALDO G, DEGOS L, BETH E, SASPORTES M, MARCELLI A, GHARBI R, DAY NK: C8 deficiency in a family with xeroderma pigmentosum. Lack of linkage to the HLA region. *Clin Immunol Immunopathol* 8:377, 1977
17. JERSILD C, RUBENSTEIN P, DAY NK: The HLA system and inherited deficiencies of the complement system. *Transplant Rev* 32:43, 1976
18. MITTAL KK, WOLSKI DP, LIM D, GEWURZ A, GEWURZ H, SCHMID FR: Genetic independence between the HLA system and deficiency of the first and sixth components of complement. *Tissue Antigens* 7:97, 1976
19. DAY NK, RUBENSTEIN P, DEBRACCO M, MONEADA B, HANSEN JA, DUPONT B, THOMSEN M, SVEJGAARD A, JERSILD C: Hereditary Clr deficiency: Lack of linkage to HLA in two families, in Kissmeyer-Nielsen F (ed): *Histocompatibility Testing 1975,* Copenhagen: Munksgaard, 1976, p 960
20. RITTNER C: Genetic loci of components of the classical and alternated pathway of complement activation: A new dimension of the immunogenetic linkage group (HLA) on chromosome 6 in man. *Hum Genet* 35:1, 1976
21. OSOFSKY SG, THOMPSON BH, GEWURZ H, SCHMID FR, MITTAL KK: Evidence for lack of linkage between HLA and C3 deficiency in man. *Immunogenetics* 4:195, 1977
22. HOBART MJ, COOK PJL, LACHMANN PJ: Linkage studies with C6. *J Immunogenet* 4:423, 1977
23. DELAGE JM, BERGERON P, SIMARD J, LEHNER-NETSCH G, PROCHAZKA E: Hereditary C7 deficiency. Diagnosis and HL-A studies in a French-Canadian family. *J Clin Invest* 60:1061, 1977
24. DUPONT B, GOOD RA, HAUPTMANN G, SCHREUDER I, SELIGMANN M: Immunopathology, immunodeficiencies, and complement deficiencies, in Dausset J, Svejgaard A (eds): *HLA and Disease.* Copenhagen: Munksgaard, 1977, p 233
25. LACHMANN PJ, HOBART MJ: Complement genetics in relation to HLA. *Br Med Bull* 34:247, 1978
26. OLAISEN B, GEDDE-DAHL JR T, THORSBY E: Localization of the human GLO gene locus. *Humangenetik* 32:301, 1976
27. MEO T, DOUGLAS T, RIJNBECK AM: Glyoxalase I polymorphism in the mouse: A new genetic marker linked to H-2. *Science* 198:311, 1977
28. CHARMOT D, MAWAS C, KRISTENSEN T, MERCIER P: The HLA-D system: At least two loci and four distinct phenotypic traits per haplotype. Introduction to component typing in families and population by primed lymphocyte typing. *Immunogenetics,* 13:57, 1981
29. SHAW S, POLLACK MS, PAYNE SM, JOHNSON AH: HLA-linked B cell alloantigens of a new segregant series: Population and family studies of the SB antigens. *Hum Immunol* 1:177, 1980
30. LARON Z, POLLACK MS, ZAMIR R, ROITMAN A, DICKERMAN Z, LEVINE LS, LORENZEN F, O'NEILL GJ, PANG S, NEW MI, DUPONT B: Late onset 21-hydroxylase deficiency and HLA in the Ashkenazi population: A new allele at the 21-hydroxylase locus. *Hum Immunol* 1:55, 1980
31. JACKSON JF, CURRIER RD, TERASAKI PI, MORTON NE: Spinocerebellar ataxia and HLA linkage. *New Engl J Med* 296:1138, 1977
32. VAN SOMEREN H, WESTERVELD A, HAGEMEIJER A, MEES JR, MEERA KHAN P, ZAALBERG OB: Human antigen and enzyme markers in man-Chinese hamster somatic cell hybrids: Evidence for synteny between the HL-A, PGM$_3$, ME$_1$, and IPO-B loci. *Proc Natl Acad Sci USA* 71:962, 1974
33. PELLEGRINO MA, CURRY RA, PELLEGRINO AG, HOCK JA: Linkage between the B-cell specific receptor for monkey red blood cells and HL-A. *Immunogenetics* 2:543, 1975
34. CRAIG IW, TOLLEY E, BOBROW M: Assignment of a gene necessary for the expression of mitochondrial glutamate oxaloacetate transaminase in human-mouse hybrid cells. Fourth International Workshop in Human Gene Mapping, Winnipeg, Canada, 1977

35. KNOWLES BB, MAUSNER R, ADEN DP: Preliminary characterization of human cell surface molecules controlled by human chromosomes 7 and 6. Fourth International Workshop on Human Gene Mapping, Winnipeg, Canada, 1977

36. SMITH M, HIRSCHHORN K: Location of genes for human heavy chain immunoglobulin to chromosome 6. *Proc Natl Acad Sci USA* 75:3367, 1978

37. KOCH G, SHOWS TB: A gene on human chromosome 6 functions in assembly of tissue-specific adenosine deaminase isozymes. *Proc Natl Acad Sci USA* 75:3876, 1978

38. LAMM LU, KISSMEYER-NIELSEN F, HENNINGSEN K: Linkage and association studies of two phosphoglucomutase loci (PGM₁ and PGM₃) to eighteen other markers. *Hum Hered* 20:305, 1970

39. WEITKAMP LR: Further data concerning the linkage relationships of loci for urinary pepsinogen and HLA. Fourth International Workshop on Human Gene Mapping, Winnipeg, Canada, 1977

40. TERASAKI PI (ed): *Histocompatibility Testing 1980.* Los Angeles, UCLA Tissue Typing Laboratory, 1980

41. RUSSELL PS, WINN HJ (eds): *Histocompatibility Testing 1965.* Washington, D.C., National Academy of Sciences of the USA publ 1229, 1965

42. BALNER H, CLETON FJ, EERNISSE JG (eds): *Histocompatibility Testing.* Baltimore, Williams & Wilkins, 1966

43. CURTONI ES, MATTIUZ PL, TOSI RM (eds): *Histocompatibility Testing 1967.* Copenhagen, Munksgaard, 1967

44. TERASAKI PI (ed): *Histocompatibility Testing 1970.* Copenhagen, Munksgaard, 1970

45. DAUSSET J, COLOMBANI J (eds): *Histocompatibility Testing 1972.* Copenhagen, Munksgaard, 1973

46. KISSMEYER-NIELSEN F (ed): *Histocompatibility Testing 1975.* Copenhagen, Munksgaard, 1976

47. BODMER WF, BATCHELOR JR, BODMER JG, FESTENSTEIN H, MORRIS PJ (eds): *Histocompatibility Testing 1977.* Copenhagen, Munksgaard, 1977

48. *Tissue Antigens,* vol 5, pp 291–466, 1975

49. VAN ROOD JJ, VAN LEEUWEN A, ZWEERUS R: The 4a and 4b antigens, do they or don't they? in TERASAKI PI (ed): *Histocompatibility Testing 1970,* Copenhagen, Munksgaard, 1970

50. LEGRAND L, DAUSSET J: The complexity of the HL-A gene product. II. Possible evidence for a "public" determinant common to the first and second HL-A series. *Transplantation* 19:177, 1975

51. KOSTYU DD, CRESSWELL P, AMOS DB: A public HLA antigen associated with HLA-A9, Aw32 and Bw4. *Immunogenetics* 10:433, 1980

52. PARHAM P, BARNSTABLE CJ, BODMER WF: Properties of an anti-HLA-A, -B, -C monoclonal antibody. Use of a monoclonal antibody (W6/32) in structural studies of HLA-A, -B, -C antigens. *J Immunol* 123:242, 1979

53. ALBERT ED, GOTZE D: The major histocompatiblity system in man, in Gotze D (ed): *The Major Histocompatibility system in Man and Animals.* New York, Springer-Verlag New York, 1977, p 7

54. FAULK WP, SANDERSON AR, TEMPLE A: Distribution of MHC antigens in human placental chorionic villi. *Transplant Proc* 9:1379, 1977

55. MORTON JA, PICKLES MM, SUTTON L, SKOV F: Identification of further antigens on red cells and lymphocytes: Association of Bgᵇ with w17 (Te 57) and Bgᶜ with w28 (Da15, Ba⁺). *Vox Sang* 21:141, 1971

56. BRODSKY FM, PARHAM P, BARNSTABLE CJ, CRUMPTON MJ, BODMER WF: Monoclonal antibodies for analysis of the HLA system. *Immunol Rev* 47:3, 1979

57. TRUCCO M, DEPETRIS S, GAROTTA G, CEPPELLINI R: Quantitative analysis of cell surface HLA structures by means of monoclonal antibodies. *Hum Immunol* 1:233, 1980

58. HERON I, HOKLAND M, BERG K: Enhanced expression of β₂-microglobulin and HLA antigens on human lymphoid cells by interferon. *Proc Natl Acad Sci USA* 75:6215, 1978

59. BILLING RJ, SAFANI M, PETERSON P: Soluble HLA antigens present in normal human serum. *Tissue Antigens* 10:75, 1977

60. REISFELD RA, PELLEGRINO MA, FERRONE S: The immunologic and molecular profiles of HLA antigens isolated from urine. *J Immunol* 118:264, 1977

61. MITTAL KK: Human histocompatibility (HL-A) antigens in semen and their role in reproduction. *Fertil Steril* 26:704, 1975

62. DAWSON JR, SHASBY SS, AMOS DB: The serological detection of HL-A antigens in human milk. *Tissue Antigens* 4:76, 1974

63. CEPPELLINI R: Old and new facts and speculations about transplantation antigens of man. *Prog Immunol* 1:973, 1971

64. MAYR MR, PAUSCH V, SCHNEDL W: Human chimaera detectable only by investigation of her progeny. *Nature (Lond)* 277:210, 1979

65. ASTER RH, SZATKOWSKI N, LIEBERT M, DUQUESNOY RJ: Expression of HLA-B12, HLA-B8, w4 and w6 on platelets. *Transplant Proc* 9:1695, 1977

66. POLLACK MS, MAURER D, LEVINE LS, NEW MI, PANG S, DUCHON MA, OWENS RP, MERKATZ IR, NITOWSKY HM, SACHS G, DUPONT B: HLA typing of amniotic cells: The prenatal diagnosis of congenital adrenal hyperplasia (21-OH-deficiency type). *Transplant Proc* 11:1726, 1979

67. BROWN G, BIBERFELD P, CHRISTENSSON B, MASON DY: The distribution of HLA on human lymphoid, bone marrow and peripheral blood cells. *Eur J Immunol* 9:272, 1979

68. ARCE-GOMEZ B, JONES EA, BARNSTABLE CJ, SOLOMON E, BODMER WF: The genetic control of HLA-A and B antigens in somatic cell hybrids: Requirement for β₂-microglobulin. *Tissue Antigens* 11:96, 1978

69. STROMINGER JL, ENGELHARD VH, FUKS A, GUILD BC, HYAFIL F, KAUFMAN JF, KORMAN AJ, KOSTYK TG, KRANGEL MS, LANCET D, LOPEZ DE CASTRO JA, MANN DL, ORR HT, PARHAM PR, PARKER KC, PLOEGH HL, POBER JS, ROBB RJ, SHACKELFORD DA: The biochemical analysis of products of the major histocompatibility complex, in Benacerraf B, Dorf M (eds): *The Role of the Major Histocompatibility Complex in Immunobiology,* New York: Garland Publishing Co, 1981, p 115

70. SNARY D, BARNSTABLE CJ, BODMER WF, CRUMPTON MJ: Molecular structure of human histocompatibility antigens: The HLA-C series. *Eur J Immunol* 8:580, 1977

71. FERRARA G, TOSI R, LONGO A, CASTELLANI A, VIVIANI C, CARMINATI G: Silent alleles at the HLA-C locus. *J Immunol* 121:731, 1978

72. VITETTA ES, UHR JW, BOYSE EA: Association of a β₂-microglobulin-like subunit with H-2 and TL alloantigens on murine thymocytes. *J Immunol* 114:252, 1975

73. MICHAELSON J, FLAHERTY L, VITETTA E, POULIK MD: Molecular similarities between the Qa-2 alloantigen and other gene products of the 17th chromosome of the mouse. *J Exp Med* 145:1066, 1977

74. AMOS DB, POOL P, GRIER J: HLA-A, HLA-B, HLA-C, and HLA-DR, in Rose NR, Friedman H (eds): *Manual of Clinical Immunology,* Washington, DC, American Society for Microbiology, 1980, p 978

75. JOHNSON AH, ROSSEN RD, BUTLER WT: Detection of allo-antibodies using a sensitive antiglobulin microcytotoxicity test: Identification of low levels of preformed antibodies in accelerated allograft rejection. *Tissue Antigens* 2:215, 1972

76. DECARY F, VERMEULEN A, ENGELFRIET CP: A look at HL-A antisera in the indirect immunofluorescence technique (IIFT), in Kissmeyer-Nielsen F (ed): *Histocompatibility Testing 1975,* Copenhagen, Munksgaard, 1975, p 380

77. DORVAL G, WELSH KI, NILSSON K, WIGZELL H: Quantitation of β₂-microglobulin and HLA on the surface of human cells. I. T and B lymphocytes and lymphoblasts. *Scand J Immunol* 6:255, 1977

78. BOYUM A: Separation of leukocytes from blood and bone marrow. *Scand J Clin Lab Invest* (suppl) 97:21, 1968

79. YUNIS EJ, AMOS DB, EGURO SY, DORF ME: Cross-reactions of HL-A antibodies. I. Characterization by absorption and elution. *Transplantation* 14:474, 1972

80. DOUGHTY DW, GELSTHORPE K: Some parameters of lymphocyte antibody activity through pregnancy and further eluates of placental material. *Tissue Antigens* 8:43, 1976

81. AMOS DB, CORLEY RB, KOSTYU DD: The production of antibody against HL-A antigen. *Symp Ser Immunobiol, Standardization Intern Symp HL-A Reagents* 18:1, 1972

82. COLLINS ZV, ARNOLD PF, PEETOOM F, SMITH GS, WALFORD RL: A naturally occurring monospecific anti-HL-A 8 isoantibody. *Tissue Antigens* 3:358, 1973

83. LEPAGE V, DEGOS L, DAUSSET J: A natural anti-HLA-A2 antibody reacting with homozygous cells. *Tissue Antigens* 8:139, 1976

84. RH KENNETT, TJ MCKEARN, KB BECHTOL (eds): *Monoclonal Antibodies, Hybridomas: A New Dimension in Biological Analyses,* New York, Plenum Press, 1980

85. AYRES J, CRESSWELL P: HLA-B specificities and w4,w6 specificities are on the same polypeptide. *Eur J Immunol* 6:794, 1976

86. BRIGHT S: Second locus HL-A antigens and 4a or 4b. *Tissue Antigens* 7:23, 1976

87. PAYNE R, AMOS B, KOSTYU D, ENGELFRIET CP, VAN DEN BERG-LOONEN PM, CURTONI ES, RICHIARDI P: Subdivisions of the HLA-B5 and Bw35 complex. *Tissue Antigens* 11:302, 1978

88. VERGHESE MW, WARD FE: Absorption, elution and blocking studies with the complex antiserum ST. *Tissue Antigens* 12:239, 1978

89. BELVEDERE M, MATTIUZ P, CURTONI ES: An antibody cross-reacting with LA and FOUR antigens of the HL-A system. *Immunogenetics* 1:538, 1975

90. MCMICHAEL AJ, PARHAM P, RUST N, BRODSKY F: A monoclonal antibody that recognizes an antigenic determinant shared by HLA-A2 and B17. *Hum Immunol* 1:121, 1980

91. PARHAM P, MCLEAN J: Characterization, evolution and molecular basis of a polymorphic antigenic determinant shared by HLA-A and B products. *Hum Immunol* 1:131, 1980

92. DUPONT B, HANSEN JA, YUNIS EJ: Human mixed lymphocyte culture reaction: Genetics, specificity and biological implications. *Adv Immunol* 23:108, 1976

93. BRADLEY BA, FESTENSTEIN H: Cellular typing. *Br Med Bull* 34:223, 1978

94. VAN DEN TWEEL JG, VAN OUD ALBLAS AB, KEUNING JJ, GOULMY E, TER-MIJTELEN A, BACH ML, VAN ROOD JJ: Typing for MLC (LD). I. Lympho-cytes from cousin marriage offspring as typing cells. *Transplant Proc* 5:1535, 1973

95. JORGENSEN F, LAMM LU, KISSMEYER-NIELSEN F: Mixed lymphocyte cul-tures with inbred individuals: An approach to MLC typing. *Tissue Anti-gens* 3:323, 1973

96. JENSEN EB, KRISTENSEN T, JORGENSEN F, LAMM LU: HLA-D typing homo-zygous typing cells. A statistical analysis of experimental and biological variation. *Tissue Antigens* 10:83, 1977

97. LOHRMANN HP, NOVIKOVS L, GRAW RL JR: Stimulatory capacity of human T and B lymphocytes in the mixed leukocyte culture. *Nature (Lond)* 250:144, 1974

98. THORSBY E, ALBRECHTSEN D, HIRSCHBERG H, KAAKINEN A, SOLHEIM BG: MLC-activating HLA-D determinants: Identification, tissue distribu-tion, and significance. *Transplant Proc* 9:393, 1977

99. KAAKINEN A, HIRSCHBERG H: Stimulation of human lymphocytes by allo-geneic macrophages *in vitro*. *Tissue Antigens* 10:306, 1977

100. HIRSHBERG H, EVENSON SA, HENRIKSEN T, THORSBY E: Stimulation of human lymphocytes by allogenic endothelial cells *in vitro*. *Tissue Antigens* 4:257, 1974

101. RICHIARDI P, BELVEDERE M, BORELLI T: Split of HLA-DRW2 into sub-typic specificities closely correlated to two HLA-D products. *Immunoge-netics* 7:57, 1978

102. TROUP GM, JAMESON J, THOMSEN M, SVEJGAARD A, WALFORD RL: Stud-ies of HLA alloantigens of the Navajo Indians of North America. *Tissue Antigens* 12:44, 1978

103. LAYRISSE Z, SIMONEY N, PARK MS, TERASAKI PI: HLA-D and DRw deter-minants in an American indigenous isolate. *Transplant Proc* 11:1788, 1979

104. SEKIGUCHI S, KOBAYASHI K, KONOEDA Y, TAKATA H: Two components of the Ia4 × 7 B lyphocyte antigen found in Japanese, in Terasaki PI (ed): *Histocompatibility Testing 1980*, Copenhagen: Munksgaard, 1980, p 836

105. SUCIU-FOCA N, WERNER J, ROHOWSKY C, MCKIERNAN P, SUSINNO E, RUBENSTEIN P: Indications that Dw and DRw determinants are controlled by distinct (but closely linked) genes. *Transplant Proc* 10:799, 1978

106. DUQUESNOY RJ, MARRARI M, ANNEN K: Identification of an HLA-DR associated system of B-cell antigens. *Transplant Proc* 11:1757, 1979

107. PARK MS, TERASAKI PI, NAKATA S, AOKI D: Supertypic DR groups MT1, MT2, and MT3. *Eighth International Workshop Newsletter* 16:20, 1979

108. VAN ROOD JJ, VAN LEEUWEN A, KEUNING JJ, VAN OUD ALBLAS AB: The serological recognition of the human MLC determinants using a modified cytotoxicity technique. *Tissue Antigens* 5:73, 1975

109. MENDES NF, TOINAI MEA, SILVEIRA NPA, GILBERTSEN RB, METZGAR RS: Technical aspects of the rosette tests used to detect human complement receptor (B) and sheep erythrocyte-binding (T) lymphocytes. *J Immunol* 111:860, 1973

110. MANN DL, ABELSON L, HARRIS S, AMOS DB: Detection of antigens specific for B-lymphoid cultured cell lines with human alloantisera. *J Exp Med* 142:84, 1975

111. GRIER JO, ABELSON LA, MANN DL, AMOS DB, JOHNSON AH: Enrichment of B lymphocytes using goat anti-human F(ab')₂. *Tissue Antigens* 10:236, 1977

112. LOWRY R, GOGUEN J, CARPENTER CB, STROM TB, GAROVOY MR: Improved B cell typing for HLA-DR Using nylon wool column enriched B lymphocyte preparations. *Tissue Antigens* 14:325, 1979

113. STOCKER JW, GAROTTA G, HAUSMAN B, TRUCCO M, CEPPELLINI R: Sep-aration of human cells bearing HLA-DR antigens using a monoclonal anti-body rosetting method. *Tissue Antigens* 13:212, 1979

114. VAN ROOD JJ, VAN LEEUWEN A, PLOEM JS: A method to detect simulta-neously two cell populations by 2 colour fluorescence. *Nature (Lond)* 262:795, 1976

115. HUNTER SV, BENSON JW, BULL RW, POULIK MD: Use of turkey anti-human β₂-microglobulin antisera for identification of DR antibodies. *Transplant Proc* 10:853, 1978

116. DEWOLF WC, SCHLOSSMAN SF, YUNIS EJ: DRw antisera react with acti-vated T cells. *J Immunol* 122:1780, 1979

117. WINCHESTER RJ, KUNKEL HG: The human Ia system. *Adv Immunol* 28:221, 1979

118. BODMER JG, PICKBOURNE P, RICHARDS S: Ia serology, in Bodmer WF, Batchelor R, Bodmer JG, Festenstein H, Morris PJ (eds): *Histocompati-bility Testing 1977*. Copenhagen, Munksgaard, 1978, p 35

119. WALFORD RL: Human B-cell alloantigenic systems: Their medical and bio-logical significance, in Ferrara GB (ed): *HLA System—New Aspects*, New York, Elsevier North-Holland, Inc, 1977, p 105

120. WINCHESTER RJ, ROSS GD, JAROWSKI CI, WONG CY, HALPER J, BROX-MEYER HE: Expression of Ia-like antigen molecules on human granulo-cytes during early phases of differentiation. *Proc Natl Acad Sci USA* 74:4012, 1977

121. WINCHESTER RJ, WANG C-Y, GIBOFSKY A, KUNKEL HG, LLOYD KO, OLD LJ: Expression of Ia-like antigens on cultured human malignant melanoma cell lines. *Proc Natl Acad Sci USA* 75:6235–6239, 1978

122. NATALI PG, DE MARTINO C, QUARANTA V, NIRCOTRA MR, FREZZA F, PELLEGRINO MA, FERRONE S: Expression of Ia-like antigens in normal human nonlymphoid tissues. *Transplantation* 31:75, 1981

123. MARKET ML, CRESSWELL P: Polymorphism of human B-cell alloantigens: Evidence for three loci within the HLA system. *Proc Natl Acad Sci USA* 77:6101, 1980

124. TOSI R, TANIGAKI N, CENTIS D, FERRARA GB, PRESSMAN D: Immunolog-ical dissection of human Ia molecules. *J Exp Med* 148:1592, 1978

125. The antigens of the major histocompatibility complex and their biological functions, in *New Initiatives in Immunology*. Washington, DC, National Institutes of Health pub no 81–2215, 1981, p 121

126. KAUFMAN JF, ANDERSEN RL, STROMINGER JL: HLA-DR antigens have polymorphic light chains and invariant heavy chains as assessed by lysine-containing tryptic peptide analysis. *J Exp Med* 152:54s, 1980

127. PARISH CR, HIGGINS TJ, MCKENZIE IFC: Comparison of antigens recog-nized by xenogeneic and allogeneic anti-Ia antibodies: Evidence for two classes of Ia antigens. *Immunogenetics* 6:343, 1978

128. YU DTY, MCCUNE JM, FU SM, WINCHESTER RJ, KUNKEL HG: Two types of Ia-positive cells. *J Exp Med* 152:89s, 1980

129. SHEEHY MJ, BACH FH: Primed LD typing (PLT)—Technical considera-tions. *Tissue Antigens* 8:157, 1976

130. SHAW S, HALL RP, DUQUESNOY RJ, KATZ SI: Interaction between HLA-SB and HLA-DR phenotypes in determining the risk of dermititis herpetifor-mis. *Hum Immunol* in press, 1981

131. ECKELS DD, HARTZMAN RJ: Evidence for a primed lymphocyte (PLT) re-stimulating determinant encoded by a new gene linked to HLA. Submit-ted

132. KRISTENSEN T: Studies on the specificity of CML. Report from a CML workshop. *Tissue Antigens* 11:330, 1978

133. SPRENT T, KORNGOLD R, MOLNAR-KIMBER K: T cell recognition of anti-gen *in vivo*. Role of the H-2 complex. *Springer Semin Immunopathol* 3:213, 1980

134. ROBINSON MA, NOREEN HJ, AMOS DB, YUNIS EJ: Target antigens of cell-mediated lympholysis. Discrimination of HLA subtypes by cytotoxic lymphocytes. *J Immunol* 121:1486, 1978

135. ANDREOTTI PE, APGAR JR, CRESSWELL P: HLA-A2 as a target for cell-mediated lympholysis: Evidence from immuno selected HLA-A2 negative mutant cell lines. *Hum Immmunol* 1:77, 1980

136. YUNIS EJ, AMOS DB: Three closely linked genetic systems relevant to trans-plantation. *Proc Natl Acad Sci USA* 68:3031, 1971

137. KLEIN J, FLAHERTY L, VANDE BERG JL, SHREFFLER DC: H-2 haplotypes, genes, regions and antigens: First listing. *Immunogenetics* 6:489, 1978

138. GAZIT E, TERHORST C, MAHONEY RJ, YUNIS EJ: Alloantigens of the human T(HT) genetic region of the HLA linkage group. *Hum Immunol* 1:97, 1980

139. BILLING RJ, CLARK B, TERASAKI PI: Characterization of three different human T cell membrane antigens, two being present on T lymphocyte subpopulations. *Hum Immunol* 1:141, 1980

140. TADA N, TANIGAKI N, PRESSMAN D: Human cell membrane components bound to β₂-microglobulin in T cell type cell lines. *J Immunol* 120:513, 1978

141. TRUCCO M, DEPETRIS S, GAROTTA G, CEPPELLINI R: Quantitative analysis of cell surface HLA structures by means of monoclonal antibodies. *Hum Immunol* 1:233, 1980

142. KIM SJ, CHRISTIANSEN FT, GOSAR I, SILVER DM, POLLACK M, DUPONT B: Frequency of alloantibodies reacting with PHA-activated T lymphocytes, unexplainable by known HLA activities. *Hum Immunol* 1:347, 1980

143. RUBINSTEIN PR, COSTA A, VAN LEEUWEN A, VAN ROOD JJ: The leukocyte antigens of the Mapuche Indians, in Curtoni ES, Mattiuz PL, Tosi RM (eds): *Histocompatibility Testing 1967*, Copenhagen, Munksgaard, 1967, p 251

144. Proceeding of the Second Asia and Oceania Histocompatiblity Workshop and Conference. Japan HLA Association, Tsuju K, Komori K (eds) Hakone, Japan, October 1979

145. Proceeding of the Second Asia and Oceania Histocompatibility Workshop and Conference. 1981, in press

146. WARD FE, AMOS DB, DEJONGH D, JOHNSON AH: B cell antigens of Black Americans. *Tissue Antigens* 13:290, 1979

147. BODMER W, THOMSON G: Population genetics and evolution of the HLA system, in Dausset J, Svejgaard A (eds): *HLA and Disease*, Copenhagen, Munksgaard, 1977, p 280

148. BODMER WF: Evolutionary significance of the HL-A system. *Nature* 237:139, 1972

149. BODMER WF, BODMER JG: Evolution and function of the HLA system. *Br Med Bull* 34:309, 1978

150. DEGOS L, DAUSSET J: Human migrations and HL-A linkage disequilibri-um. *Immunogenetics* 1:195, 1974

151. BENNET D: The T-locus of the mouse. *Cell* 6:441, 1975

152. SHREFFLER DC, DAVID CS: Studies on recombination within the mouse H-2 complex. *Tissue Antigens* 2:232, 1972

153. AMOS DB, RUDERMAN R, MENDELL NR, JOHNSON AH: Linkage between HL-A and spinal development. *Transplant Proc* 7:93, 1975

154. MUNRO A, WALDMANN H: The major histocompatibility system and the immune response. *Br Med Bull* 34:253, 1978

155. UHR JW, CAPRA D, VITETTA E, COOK RG: Organization of the immune response genes. *Science* 206:292, 1979

156. GREENBERG LJ, GRAY ED, YUNIS EJ: Association of HL-A 5 and immune responsiveness *in vitro* to streptococcal antigens. *J Exp Med* 141:935, 1975

157. PATARROYO ME, WINCHESTER RJ, VEJERANO A, GIBOFSKY A, CHALEM F, ZABRISKIE JB, KUNKEL HG: Association of a B-cell alloantigen with susceptibility to rheumatic fever. *Nature* 278:173, 1979

158. SASAZUKI T, HAYASE R, IWAMOTO I, TSUCHIDA H: HLA and acute post-streptococcal glomerulonephritis. *New Engl J Med* 301:1184, 1979

159. TULIKAINEN A: On the way to understanding the pathogenesis of HLA-associated diseases. *Focus on Medical Biology* 58:53, 1980

160. MENDELL NR, AMOS DB, BLUMENTHAL MN, GLEICH GJ, YUNIS EJ: The association of Ra3 skin test response with HLA-A2. Evidence of an interaction with antigen E skin test response rather than IgE. *Hum Immunol*, in press, 1981

161. SHAW S, BIDDISON WE: HLA-linked genetic control of the specificity of human cytotoxic T cell responses to influenza virus. *J Exp Med* 149:565, 1979

162. ROSENTHAL AS: Regulation of the immune response—Role of the macrophage. *New Engl J Med* 303:1153, 1980

163. EICHMANN K (ed): Cell communication between subsets of lymphocytes. *Springer Semin Immunopathol*, vol. 3. New York, Springer-Verlag, 1980

164. GERMAIN RN, BENACERRAF B: Helper and suppressor T cell factors. *Springer Semin Immunopathol* 3:93, 1980

165. BURAKOFF, SJ: Specificity of cytolytic T-cells responses, in Dorf ME (ed): *The Role of the Major Histocompatibility Complex in Immunobiology*, New York, Garland Press, 1981, p 343

166. ZINKERNAGEL RM, DOHERTY PC: MHC-restricted cytotoxic T cells. Studies on the biologic role of polymorphic major transplantation antigens determining T-cell restriction-specificity, function and responsiveness. *Adv Immunol* 27:52, 1979

167. AMIEL JL: Study of the leucocyte phenotypes in Hodgkin's disease, in Curtoni ES, Mattiuz PL, Tosi RM (eds): *Histocompatibility Testing 1967*, Copenhagen, Munksgaard, 1967, p 79

168. KOURILSKY FM, DAUSSET J, FEINGOLD N, DUPUY JM, BERNARD J: Etude de la repartition des antigenes leucocytaires chez des malades atteints de leucemie aigue en remission, in Dausset J, Hamburger J, Mathe G (eds): *Advance in Transplantation*, Copenhagen, Munksgaard, 1967, p 515

169. SIMONS MJ, AMIEL JL: HLA and malignant diseases, in Dausset J, Svejgaard A (eds): *HLA and Disease*. Copenhagen, Munksgaard, 1977, p 212

170. deWOLF WC, LANGE PH, SHEPHERD R, MARTIN-ALOSCO S, YUNIS EJ: Association of HLA and renal cell carcinoma. *Hum Immunol* 2:41, 1981

171. deWOLF WC, LANGE PH, EINARSON ME, YUNIS E: HLA and testicular cancer. *Nature* 277:216, 1979

172. SVEJGAARD A, RYDER LP: Associations between HLA and Disease, in Dausset J, Svejgaard A (eds): *HLA and Disease*. Copenhagen, Munksgaard, 1977, p 46

173. DAUSSET J, SVEJGAARD A (eds): *HLA and Disease*. Copenhagen, Munksgaard, 1977

174. EDWARDS CQ, CARTWRIGHT GE, SKOLNICK MH, AMOS DB: Genetic mapping of the hemochromatosis locus on chromosome six. *Hum Immunol* 1:19, 1980

175. LIPINSKI M, HORS J, SALEUN JP, SADDI R, PASSA P, LAFAURIE S, FEINGOLD N, DAUSSET J: Idiopathic hemochromatosis: Linkage to HLA. *Tissue Antigens* 11:471, 1978

176. ELSTON RC, SOBEL E: Sampling considerations in the gathering and analysis of pedigree data. *Am J Hum Genet* 31:62, 1979

177. KRAVITZ K, SKOLNICK M, CANNINGS C, CARMELLI D, BATY B, AMOS B, JOHNSON JA, MENDELL N, EDWARDS C, CARTWRIGHT G: Genetic linkage between hereditary hemochromatosis and HLA. *Am J Hum Genet* 31:601, 1979

178. MARSH DG, BIAS WB: Basal serum IgE levels and HLA antigen frequencies in allergic subjects. II. Studies in people sensitive to rye grass group I and ragweed antigen E and of postulated immune response (Ir) loci in the HLA region. *Immunogenetics* 5:235, 1977

179. SCHLOSSTEIN L, TERASAKI PI, BLUESTONE R, PEARSON CM: High association of an HL-A antigen, w27, with ankylosing spondylitis. *New Engl J Med* 288:704, 1973

180. BREWERTON DA, CAFFREY M, HART FD, JAMES DCO, NICHOLLS A, STURROCK RD: Ankylosing spondylitis and HL-A 27. *Lancet* 1:904, 1973

181. SACHS JA, STERIOFF S, RABINETTE M, WOLF E, CURRY HLF, FESTENSTEIN H: Ankylosing spondylitis and the major histocompatibility system. *Tissue Antigens* 5:129, 1975

182. BREWERTON DA, ALBERT E: Rheumatology, in Dausset J, Svejgaard A (eds): *HLA and Disease*. Copenhagen, Munksgaard, 1977, p 94

183. DRUERY C, BASHIR H, GECZY AF, ALEXANDER K, EDMONDS J: Search for *Klebsiella* cell wall components cross-reactive with lymphocytes of B27+AS+individuals. *Hum Immunol* 1:151, 1980

184. AWDEK Z, RAUM D, FLEISCHNICK E, CRIGLER JF, GERALD PS, ALPER CA: MHC-linked complement haplotypes (complotypes) in congenital adrenal hyperplasia (CAH), *Clin Res* 29:287a, 1981

185. LAWLEY TJ, HALL RP, FAUCI AS, KATZ SI, HAMBURGER MI, FRANK MM: Defective Fc receptor functions associated with the HLA-B8/DRw 3 haplotype. *New Engl J Med* 304:185, 1981

186. deVRIES RRP, NIJENHUIS LE, Lai A Fat RFM, van ROOD JJ: HLA-linked genetic control of host response to *Mycobacterium leprae. Lancet* 2:1328, 1976

187. AGNELLO V: Complement deficiency states. *Medicine* 1:57, 1978

188. HANSEN JA, DUPONT B, L'ESPERANCE P, GOOD RA: Congenital neutropenia: Abnormal neutrophil differentiation associated with HLA. *Immunogenetics* 4:327, 1977

189. DAUSSET J, DEGOS L, HORS J: The association of the HL-A antigens with diseases. *Clin Immunol Immunopathol* 3:127, 1974

190. AMOS DB, WARD FE: Theoretical considerations in the association between HLA and Disease, in Dausset J, Svejgaard A (eds): *HLA and Disease*. Copenhagen, Munksgaard, 1977, p 269

191. MURPHY GP (ed): *HLA and Malignancy*, New York, Alan R. Liss, Inc. 1977

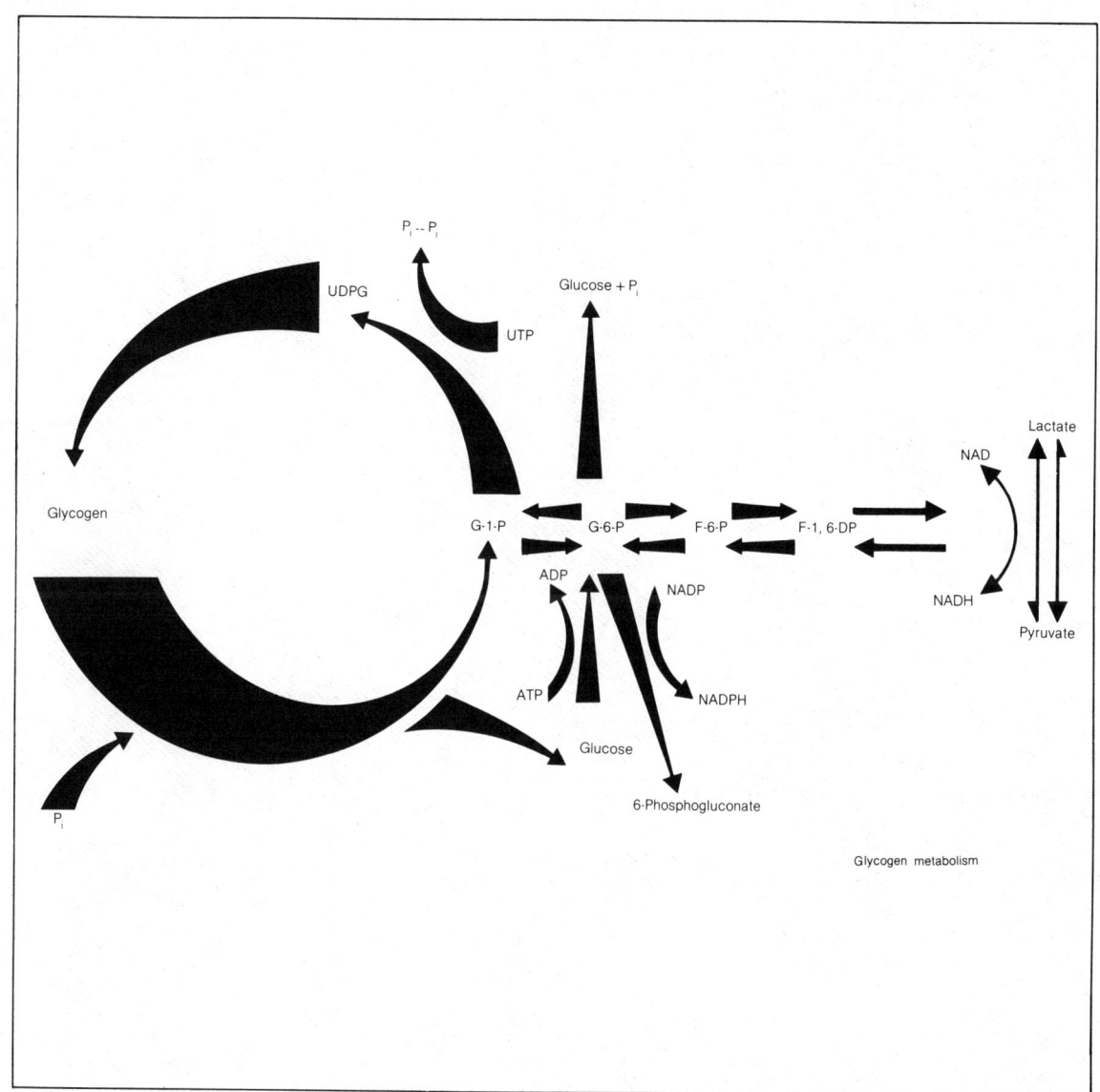

PART 2

Glycogen metabolism

DISORDERS OF CARBOHYDRATE METABOLISM

4

DIABETES MELLITUS

DANIEL W. FOSTER

1. Primary diabetes mellitus is a disease characterized by relative or absolute insulin deficiency and relative or absolute glucagon excess. These hormonal derangements produce a set of metabolic abnormalities and a complement of long-term complications involving the eyes, kidneys, nerves, and blood vessels.

2. There are two major forms of the primary illness: insulin-dependent diabetes mellitus (type 1) and non-insulin-dependent diabetes mellitus (type 2). The former is characterized by susceptibility to ketoacidosis in the absence of administered insulin, while the latter is not. Heterogeneity probably exists within both forms. Hyperglycemia occurring in the context of some other disease or genetic abnormality is termed secondary diabetes. The prevalence of diabetes is about 10 per 1000 in the general population, with one-fourth being insulin-dependent and the remainder non-insulin-dependent.

3. Type 1 diabetes (insulin-dependent) appears to require a permissive genetic background coupled with an external factor which may be viral. Islet cell antibodies are common in the first few months after diagnosis. In most cases, they probably arise in response to β-cell injury with leakage of cellular antigens, but in some patients they may represent primary autoimmune disease.

4. Type 2 diabetes (non-insulin-dependent) seems to be almost completely determined by genetic factors. No relationship to viruses has been postulated, and islet cell antibodies are not present. Insulin resistance appears to play a major role, although impaired insulin release from the β cell is also present. Insulin resistance is due to both a decrease in insulin receptor number on target cells and a poorly defined postreceptor defect.

5. Type 1 and type 2 appear to be genetically distinct. Neither major form follows simple patterns of Mendelian inheritance, but a series of HLA associations demonstrated in type 1 disease suggests that a susceptibility gene(s) for diabetes resides on the sixth human chromosome. Studies of inheritance of HLA haplotypes in sibs concordant for diabetes imply that at least two genes may be involved. No HLA associations have been found in type 2 diabetes.

6. The preeminent metabolic abnormality of diabetes is hyperglycemia caused by consistent overproduction of glucose in the liver (inappropriate gluconeogenesis) coupled with inefficient disposal of glucose in peripheral tissues. Ketogenesis in insulin-dependent subjects is due to accelerated mobilization of free fatty acids from the adipose mass and concomitant activation of the fatty acid oxidizing system in the liver. Both hyperglycemia and ketogenesis result from a combination of insulin deficiency and glucagon excess. Insulin defi-

ciency is primarily responsible for the defect in disposal of glucose and increased rates of lipolysis in adipocytes, while glucagon excess manifests itself by altering the hepatic capacity for gluconeogenesis and ketogenesis. The reason that ketogenesis is not activated in non-insulin-dependent diabetes is not known.

7. *The cause of late degenerative complications in diabetes remains obscure. Recognition of widespread non-enzymatic glycosylation of body proteins such as hemoglobin and albumin, together with the observation that rates of glycosylation increase in direct proportion to plasma glucose concentrations, has led to the hypothesis that elevated glucose itself is the mediator of these complications. Therapeutic trials utilizing more physiologic insulin delivery systems and improved monitoring techniques may provide the necessary evidence to answer this important question.*

The term *diabetes mellitus* is not precisely defined. In practice, any condition in which there is an elevation of the plasma glucose under fasting conditions tends to be called *diabetes*. Several diseases are associated with persistent hyperglycemia and thus qualify for the diagnosis. While many physicians consider *abnormal glucose tolerance* to be equivalent to diabetes, since stress of any type (physical or emotional) can cause abnormal metabolism of glucose sufficient to suggest a diabetic state, diagnoses and classifications based on response to a glucose load must be considered imprecise. The operative mechanism for glucose intolerance in normal persons is probably stress-induced epinephrine release [1].

This chapter will focus on what might best be called *primary diabetes mellitus*, a human illness characterized by relative or absolute insulin deficiency, relative or absolute glucagon excess, a set of metabolic abnormalities caused by these hormonal derangements, and a complement of long-term complications involving the eyes, kidneys, nerves, and blood vessels. All other hyperglycemic states will be considered *secondary*, meaning that they are associated with, and presumably caused by, some other primary disease or genetic abnormality.

DIAGNOSIS

The diagnosis of symptomatic diabetes is quite simple since hyperglycemia-induced osmotic diuresis and its associated thirst are easily recognizable. There is also little controversy about diagnoses based on elevated concentrations of glucose in plasma after an overnight fast even if the patient is asymptomatic. The difficulty comes in those subjects considered to be candidates for diabetes in whom the diagnosis is based on the oral glucose tolerance test. It is now widely recognized that the standard test overdiagnoses diabetes, particularly if the original criteria of Fajans and Conn [2] are utilized [3]. This has resulted in two sets of problems. First, many patients have been given a false diagnosis of serious disease, with resultant high costs in both emotional and economic terms. Second, and more important for the concerns of this chapter, a number of research studies have been rendered suspect because patients

were labeled diabetic who probably never had the disease. A case in point is the University Group Diabetes Program report on the effectiveness and dangers of oral antidiabetic drugs [4]. For the same reason, the spectrum of diseases labeled secondary diabetes may be far too broad, i.e., the glucose intolerance reported in many conditions may not be an intrinsic feature of the illness but simply the consequence of stress-induced hormonal changes which impair the response to a glucose challenge nonspecifically. In an attempt to deal with these problems, the National Diabetes Data Group has published a new set of standards for the diagnosis of diabetes [3]. These standards have also been accepted by the World Health Organization. They are as follows:

1. Fasting plasma glucose concentration (venous) ≥ 140 mg/dl on at least two separate occasions.

2. Plasma glucose concentrations (venous) ≥ 200 mg/dl at 2 h and one other intervening point after oral ingestion of 75 g glucose.

In evaluating older studies, the new standards must be applied in retrospect. Glucose values obtained on venous whole blood must be increased 15 percent to be equivalent to plasma concentrations; a similar correction is applied to capillary whole blood in the fasting state, but not after glucose ingestion [3]. While the newly suggested criteria for diagnosis in the asymptomatic patient render the chance of developing symptomatic disease much higher, they are not absolute and some normal persons will still be included.

A second diagnostic category, designated *impaired glucose tolerance* (2-h venous plasma glucose between 140 and 200 mg/dl plus one other value ≥ 200 mg/dl), is of uncertain significance since, as mentioned, such values can be produced by stress-induced changes in the hormones regulating glucose metabolism in nondiabetic subjects.

CLASSIFICATION

An overall classification of diabetes is given in Table 4-1. The scheme basically follows the recommendations of the National Diabetes Data Group [3] except that the terms *primary* and *secondary* are retained to indicate the absence or presence of an associated disease. *Insulin-dependent* means that in the absence of insulin, ketoacidosis will supervene. Insulin is frequently required to control hyperglycemia in *non-insulin-*

Table 4-1 Classification of diabetes

A. Primary
  1. Insulin-dependent diabetes mellitus (IDDM, type 1)
  2. Non-insulin-dependent diabetes mellitus (NIDDM, type 2)
    a. Nonobese NIDDM
    b. Obese NIDDM
B. Secondary
  1. Pancreatic disease
  2. Hormonal abnormalities
  3. Drug- or chemical-induced
  4. Insulin receptor abnormalities
  5. Genetic syndromes
  6. Other

SOURCE: Based on National Diabetes Data Group [3].

dependent diabetic subjects, but such patients do not develop ketoacidosis on insulin withdrawal. Other characteristics of the two primary types of diabetes will be considered below. There are numerous conditions that fit into the category of secondary diabetes. Some produce only mild glucose intolerance, while others cause a full-blown diabetic syndrome even to the point of ketoacidosis. *Pancreatic diseases,* the most common of which is chronic pancreatitis in alcoholics, induce hyperglycemia because the β-cell mass is decreased in the generalized destructive process, resulting in hypoinsulinemia. *Hormonal diabetes* may result from primary endocrine disease (acromegaly, Cushing's syndrome, pheochromocytoma) or as a consequence of the administration of hormones for therapeutic purposes. Mechanisms include both inhibition of insulin release and induction of insulin resistance. Numerous *drugs* act in similar fashion (a list is available in Ref. 3). An interesting secondary syndrome is glucose intolerance due to *dysfunction of insulin receptors* in the plasma membranes of cells; one type, due to antibodies against the receptor, will be discussed subsequently. A variety of *genetic syndromes* are associated with clinical diabetes or abnormal glucose tolerance. The best known are the lipodystrophic states, ataxia telangiectasia, and myotonic dystrophy. The category designated *other* is undefined, the only condition listed by the National Diabetes Data Group being severe malnutrition.

PREVALENCE

The prevalence of diabetes mellitus is difficult to determine accurately because of the problems of diagnosis outlined above. Further, rates differ according to the race, age, and sex of the sample under study. For example, Pima Indians of the United States have an overall prevalence for diabetes of 19 percent, but the peak prevalence is 47 percent in men between the ages of 65 and 74 and increases to 69 percent in women between ages 55 and 64 [5]. By contrast, hyperglycemia and glucose intolerance are extremely rare in Alaskan Indians and Eskimos at any age [6]. If one considers prevalence without regard to the type of diabetes, rough estimates can be obtained from screening procedures in normal populations. In a massive diabetes detection program in Cleveland, 307,208 subjects (essentially all > 20 years of age) had glucose concentrations determined in whole blood obtained by a capillary stick 2 h after ingesting 75 g glucose [7]. A value of greater than 140 mg/dl (7.8 mM) was obtained in 12,600 (4.1 percent). Of these, 40 percent were 180 mg/dl (10 mM) or higher. Since 180 mg/dl is close to the 200 mg/dl (11.1 mM) 2-h postprandial value considered the diagnostic level for diabetes after glucose tolerance testing by the National Diabetes Data Group, the prevalence in this population would appear to be about 1.6 percent of the adult population. The percentage of abnormal test results increased with age, a reproducible finding in all studies of glucose tolerance in large populations. Support for the Cleveland estimate comes from a random sample of 295 normal persons drawn from the general population of Bedford, England, who were given a glucose tolerance test with 50 g glucose [8]. Five of the group had 2-h capillary values of greater than 180 mg/dl, suggesting a prevalence of 1.7 percent for diabetes in an adult English population. A quoted estimate for prevalence of diabetes in Sweden made by the Swedish

Board of Social Health and Welfare is 1.5 percent, although the data upon which the estimate was based were not cited [9]. Thus there is a remarkable similarity in estimates of prevalence for unclassified diabetes in three Western societies. These figures, while lower than the 2 to 4 percent prevalence cited in major textbooks of medicine (e.g., [10]), are probably still too high, since a 5-year follow-up of subjects with 2-h postglucose values of ≥ 180 mg/dl showed a progression to overt diabetes in only 31 percent in the Cleveland study [11]. It seems possible that the true prevalence is somewhere around 1 percent, with symptomatic diabetes being even less. Solid estimates for overall rates of appearance of diabetes are virtually nonexistent, although a figure of 140 per 100,000 annually has been claimed in Sweden [9].

Data on prevalence in children are much more reliable since ascertainment is usually based on the development of symptomatic disease or elevated fasting plasma glucose values rather than on glucose tolerance testing. A registry of newly diagnosed diabetics under the age of 16 in Great Britain indicated a yearly appearance rate of 8 per 100,000 [12]. A similar study in New Zealand found the annual prevalence to be 10.4 per 100,000 in subjects under 20 years of age [13]. Rates between ages 11 and 19 were double those of ages 1 to 9, the peak occurring in the 10 to 15-year range. The most thorough study in the United States was carried out in Allegheny County, Pennsylvania, between 1965 and 1976 [14]. All cases under the age of 20 were identified from hospital records and surveys of pediatric practices in the county. The number of persons at risk under the age of 20 was a little over a half million. Annual rates were (per 100,000): white males, 16; white females, 15; nonwhite males, 10; and nonwhite females, 11. The highest prevalence in all groups was between 10 and 14 years of age. The authors cited 10 population-based surveys of the prevalence of type 1 diabetes. The lowest rate was 3.7 per 100,000 per year in France, while the highest was 19.6 per 100,000 per year in Sweden. Utilizing 13 per 100,000 as an average annual rate of appearance (based on the Pittsburgh study), the prevalence of type 1 diabetes in the United States at age 20 should be approximately 0.26 percent (20 × 0.013 percent). Walker and Cudworth estimated the prevalence in England at age 16 to be 0.22 percent [15]. Comparison of these figures with the total estimate of the prevalence of diabetes in adults (about 1 percent) suggests that about one-fourth of the total cases will represent type 1 disease while three-fourths will be other forms, the bulk of which represent primary type 2 illness. Ratios of type 1 to type 2 diabetes are higher in young populations and much lower in the older age range.

GENETICS

The genetics of primary diabetes is extremely complicated and must be considered unsolved despite extensive study and speculation [16]. That the disease has a genetic background in most cases is not arguable, but the nature and mechanisms of that genetic contribution remain clouded and controversial. There are three major reasons. First, there is the previously cited difficulty regarding diagnosis of diabetes. Many studies are based on unacceptable diagnostic criteria, which confound evaluation of inheritance patterns and estimates of gene frequency. Second, there is considerable evidence that neither type 1 nor type 2 categories of primary diabetes mellitus represent single disease entities [17]. Thus, the phenotypic expressions "insulin-dependent diabetes mellitus" and "non-insulin-dependent diabetes mellitus" probably represent several distinct genotypes which may or may not exhibit similar inheritance patterns. Third, the product(s) of the diabetes susceptibility gene(s) are unknown. It is thus not possible to trace transmission of the gene(s) through families or populations. Some clues are available for type 1 disease because of HLA associations that seem firm (see below), but no such relationships exist with type 2 diabetes.

The only form of diabetes in which the inheritance is generally accepted as established is *maturity onset diabetes of the young* (MODY), in which simple Mendelian dominance of the autosomal type appears to operate [18, 19]. This disease is characterized by a very mild hyperglycemia, onset early in life, resistance to ketosis, relative insulinopenia, and normal absolute values for glucagon and growth hormone (although concentrations of both tend to be high for the concentration of plasma glucose present). Friedman and Fialkow [20] have summarized the evidence that the pattern of inheritance is autosomal dominant in type:

1. Over 20 families have been studied with three-generation direct transmission of the hyperglycemic trait; in six of these families, four or five generations were affected.
2. A 1:1 ratio of diabetic and nondiabetic offspring has been found when one parent was diabetic.
3. Among 37 obligate carriers in the pedigree studied by Tattersall [21], only 5 did not have overt diabetes.
4. Direct male-to-male transmission was observed, precluding X-linked inheritance.

Genetics of Insulin-dependent Diabetes Mellitus

Twin Studies and Pedigree Analysis   Studies of diabetes in monozygotic twins have proven of interest. When onset is under age 40, the concordance rate is 50 percent or less [22, 23], i.e., if one twin has overt diabetes, the chance of the second twin developing the disease is less than half. It is extremely unfortunate that evaluation in these studies has focused on age of onset. It is assumed that most subjects whose disease began prior to age 40 had type 1 diabetes. However, as noted above, peak incidence of insulin-dependent diabetes is between 10 and 15 years of age and falls off subsequently. It is therefore entirely possible that the cohort of twins with onset under age 40 actually consisted of a mixture of type 1 and type 2 patients. Since the concordance rate in the latter approaches 100 percent (see below), true concordance in insulin-dependent twins may be far less than 50 percent. Regardless of the absolute figure, the studies strongly suggest that diabetes of the insulin-dependent type is not the simple consequence of genetic makeup alone but that in most cases some extragenetic (environmental) insult is also required. Such a formulation does not preclude the existence of more nearly pure genetic forms or those in which disease results almost exclusively from environmental damage to the pancreas, since it has already been argued that type 1 diabetes is heterogeneous. That the genetic effect in most insulin-dependent patients is largely permissive (rather than causal) is suggested by the observation that diabetes is uncommon in first-degree relatives of concordant twins

under the age of 40, in contrast to their older counterparts [23].

It has been possible to examine the children of two parents with diabetes in a fairly large number of cases [24, 25]. The problem, from the standpoint of type 1 disease, is that most of the conjugal couples with diabetes had the non-insulin-dependent variety of the illness. There is no series reporting the prevalence of diabetes in the children of two parents who have type 1 disease. The prevalence of diabetes in children of two parents with diabetes does not appear to be increased if one of the parents has type 1 disease (compared to both parents with non-insulin-dependent diabetes), although the percentage of insulin-dependent disease increases [25, 26]. Interestingly, 1 to 2 percent of children from marriages in which both parents have type 2 disease develop insulin-requiring diabetes [25, 26]. This would appear to be somewhat higher than the estimated prevalence of insulin-dependent disease in the general population of 0.25 percent. The discrepancy may be accounted for by a bias of ascertainment in families in which the disease is known, since it has been established that diabetic children are much more likely to know of other cases of diabetes in the family than are nondiabetic children [26, 27].

When family histories of classic insulin-dependent diabetic patients are examined, evidence of vertical transmission is relatively rare and the incidence of diabetes in sibs is low. For example, in 35 such families reported by Tattersall and Fajans [18], only 41 (11 percent) of the index cases had a parent who was known to have diabetes and only 21 had diabetic grandparents (6 percent). Of 99 sibs of the diabetic children, only 6 had overt diabetes. These and similar studies argue against simple Mendelian inheritance patterns of either the dominant or recessive type in insulin-dependent diabetes mellitus unless extremely low penetrance rates are postulated [15].

HLA Relationships   Since the early 1970s, it has been recognized that insulin-dependent diabetes mellitus is associated with certain human leukocyte antigens (HLA). The genes for these antigens are located on the short arm of the sixth human chromosome and represent the major histocompatibility determinants in humans. Four loci are currently recognized, A, B, C, and D, with a number of alleles identified at each site [20]. Antigens are identified by notation of locus and number, e.g., HLA-B8. If the antigen is considered unequivocally defined by members of the International Histocompatibility Workshop, no other notation is given. A small w after the locus (e.g., HLA-Dw3) indicates provisional acceptance of the antigen; the w is removed once identification is considered definite. Antigens at the D locus were originally identified using mixed lymphocyte cultures for typing and are designated HLA-D. Subsequently a serologic test was developed [28], and typing via this procedure is designated HLA-DR. It is not yet known whether D and DR antigens are identical. At the time of this writing there are 10 defined and 10 provisional antigens at the A locus, 12 defined and 30 provisional antigens at the B locus, and 8 antigens, all provisional, at the C site. At the D locus, 12 D and 10 DR antigens have been recognized. All of the former and four of the latter remain provisional.

On the basis of many studies, it is now clear that some HLA alleles are associated with an increased risk for type 1 diabetes, while others are present in diabetic subjects with much lesser prevalence than in the general population [20, 29, 30]. A summary of the known associations in Caucasians, averaged from multiple studies, is given in Table 4-2. Major alleles conferring

Table 4-2 Associations between HLA antigens and type 1 diabetes in Caucasians*

HLA antigens	Relative risk
A2	1.33
A11	0.46
Aw30	2.48
B5	0.57
B7	0.48
B8	2.67
B12	0.70
B15	1.95
B18	1.76
Bw35	0.56
Cw3	1.44
Dw2	0.04
Dw3	2.69
Dw4	4.80
DR2	0.36
DR3	4.77
DR4	2.63

* Data represent a summary of multiple studies of HLA associations and relative risks. *Relative risk* refers to the chance of developing diabetes with a given HLA phenotype relative to the chance in a random control sample of a population with the same ethnic makeup. All of the associations shown are statistically significant, but risks close to 1.0 are probably biologically trivial.
SOURCE: Adapted from Friedman and Fialkow [20].

enhanced risk include HLA-B8, HLA-B15, HLA-B18, HLA-Dw3, HLA-Dw4, HLA-DR3, and HLA-DR4. Current opinion is that the D-DR locus is of primary importance and that other associations are due to linkage disequilibrium between B and A sites and the D-DR region [29–34]. The term *linkage disequilibrium* refers to a nonrandom association between alleles at two linked loci. Thus, if allele X (an alternative gene) at locus A has a gene frequency of 0.2 and allele Y at locus B has a gene frequency of 0.3, then the combination of XY should occur with a frequency of 0.06. If the frequency of XY is not equal to the product of the frequencies of the respective alleles, then the two genes are said to be in linkage disequilibrium. The association may be positive or negative depending on whether the XY product is greater or less than expected. The HLA antigens found much less frequently in association with type 1 diabetes than in the nondiabetic population are B7, Dw2, and DR2 [20, 34, 35]. While these genes have been considered "protective" [35], it is probable that they are really "low-risk" genes because they bear an inverse relationship with the presence of Dw3 and/or Dw4, i.e., the presence of Dw2 (DR2) or B7 makes it unlikely that Dw3 or Dw4 will be present [34].

Most authors report that homozygosity for an HLA antigen having a positive association with type 1 diabetes does not further increase the risk, while the presence of two separate alleles with a positive association has a more than additive effect [20, 29, 35]. Thus, in the study shown in Table 4-3, the presence of homozygous Dw3 is associated with a relative risk of 3.7, while the relative risk of homozygous Dw4 is 4.9; by contrast, the Dw3/Dw4 phenotype increases relative risk to 9.4. If relative risk is calculated not against a general nondia-

betic population but against a subset of that population not having the predisposing antigen, much higher risk values are obtained [36]. Representative figures for the D locus from the 1980 International Histocompatibility Workshop using this type of calculation were: DR3, 3.3; DR4, 6.3; DR3/DR3, 10.5; DR4/DR4, 15.6; DR3/DR4, 33.1. The results suggest some increased risk for DR3 and DR4 homozygosity, with an unequivocal increase conferred by the combined presence of DR3 and DR4 [36].

The HLA genes themselves are not thought to confer susceptibility to diabetes. Rather, the putative diabetic gene(s) is considered to be located in close proximity to the D region within the major histocompatibility complex. This conclusion is drawn from the fact that a number of different HLA antigens are associated with the disease and that HLA associations vary from family to family and in different populations [20, 37, 38]. Moreover, it is possible to have insulin-dependent diabetes in the absence of high-risk HLA antigens. The same conclusion can be drawn from studies of diabetic multiplex families (families with at least two sibs having the disease) in which occasionally concordant sibs have entirely different HLA haplotypes [20].

Inheritance The pattern of inheritance of insulin-dependent diabetes is not yet known for reasons previously discussed. It is entirely possible that different mechanisms exist in different families (or populations) because the disease is heterogeneous [17].

Relatively few investigators hypothesize that type 1 diabetes is inherited in *autosomal dominant* fashion. An ingenious argument for such inheritance has been put forth by MacDonald [39] on the basis of an evaluation of the frequency of insulin-dependent diabetes in black Americans. Since diabetes is rare in west African blacks (whence the black American population is largely derived), he argues that its appearance in Americans of that ethnic derivation must be due to the infusion of Caucasian genes. MacDonald points out that such a flux of genes has occurred, that it is unidirectional (white → black), and that about 20 percent of the total gene pool in blacks is

Table 4-3 Relative risks of developing type 1 diabetes with combinations of HLA antigens

HLA phenotype	Relative risk
B15/B15*	2.1
B15/X†	2.5
B8/B8	3.1
B8/X	2.5
B8/B15	9.8
Dw3/Dw3‡	3.7
Dw4/Dw4	4.9
Dw3/Dw4	9.4

* Homozygosity as shown in the table actually means that only a single antigen was found at the B or D locus. It is theoretically possible that some unknown antigen not detectable by current techniques was present, but this seems unlikely.
† X refers to a B locus antigen other than 8 or 15.
‡ DR antigens were not assessed in this study.
SOURCE: Adapted from Nerup [29].

Caucasian-derived. If susceptibility to diabetes was inherited as a recessive trait, then the frequency of the disease should be about $\frac{1}{25}$ that of whites ($\frac{1}{5} \times \frac{1}{5}$) since presumably 80 percent of the gene pool would not contain the diabetic trait. Actually, American blacks develop diabetes at a rate at least as great as the percent of the Caucasian gene pool. This fact, together with the observation that predisposing HLA genes are identical in the two populations, suggested a dominant mode of inheritance (i.e., the ratio of diabetes to genetic inheritance is much higher than would be expected with a recessive disease). In actuality, the prevalence of type 1 diabetes in blacks is probably considerably higher than estimated by MacDonald (60 to 70 percent of the rate in whites if the results of the Pittsburgh diabetes registry apply generally in the United States) [14]. Since the relative prevalence of the disease in blacks is higher than the estimated transfer of Caucasian genes, it is possible that environmental rather than genetic factors account for its appearance; i.e., the genetic background might have been present in Africa while the necessary environmental insult was missing. The strongest argument against the dominant hypothesis is the fact that only 5 to 11 percent of insulin-dependent diabetics have a parent with the disease [18, 32].

Most recent attempts at genetic clarification have involved the use of HLA phenotypes (and genotypes) as the closest available markers for the putative diabetes susceptibility gene(s). The argument for *autosomal recessive* inheritance is based primarily on the fact that essentially all studies of multiplex families show a high frequency of HLA identity (two shared haplotypes) in concordant sibs with type 1 diabetes. Thus, two copies of the putative susceptibility gene appear to enhance the chance of having diabetes [15, 20]. Rubinstein, Suciu-Foca, and Nicholson, in an analysis of 31 families using D locus typing as the discriminator, concluded that inheritance was recessive with 50 percent penetrance (appearance of overt disease) [40]. Their argument for recessivity focused on HLA identity in concordant sibs and deviation in the pattern of distribution of maternal and paternal haplotypes in nondiabetic, non-HLA-D identical sibs from that expected with a single dominant gene. Penetrance of 50 percent was deduced from the fact that only half the HLA-D identical sibs were concordant. The presumption was that penetrance required an environmental factor similar to that postulated in cited studies of young identical twins. A strong argument against simple recessive inheritance is the observation that in most studies, homozygosity for a positively associated allele (e.g., B8/B8, B15/B15) confers little or no increased risk for diabetes, while the presence of two distinct positively associated alleles (e.g., B8/B15, Dw3/Dw4) does so [29, 36]. Increased risk (greater than additive) conferred by two different genes at the same locus is called *overdominance* (the same phenomenon caused by genes located at different sites is termed *epistasis*). It has been pointed out that in family studies overdominance may mimic recessive inheritance, but that when demonstrated directly, as in the examination of the inheritance of HLA haplotypes, its presence is strong evidence against autosomal recessive inheritance due to a single gene defect [29]. Rubinstein et al. [40] found that homozygosity for both DW3 and B8 alleles caused increased risk for the appearance of diabetes in backcross and intercross families, a result supportive of the recessive pattern. They thus downplay the possibility of overdominance. The reason their findings differ from those of most workers is not known.

An alternative to the autosomal recessive hypothesis suggests that at least two different genes confer susceptibility to diabetes [15, 29]. The two genes could be alleles at the same site or nonallelic. Studies of HLA haplotypes are entirely compatible with such an interpretation and could also acount for the clinical picture of overdominance or epistasis [15]. An interesting variant of the two-gene model has been constructed [41, 42]. The model assumes a single diabetes susceptibility locus tightly linked to the HLA region, with two predisposing alleles for diabetes, S_1 and S_2, and one or more nondiabetogenic alleles designated s. It is assumed that S_1 and S_2 confer risks for different clinical forms of insulin-dependent diabetes and that they segregate in linkage disequilibrium with different HLA alleles. Thus S_1 predisposes to autoimmune diabetes and is linked to the HLA-B8, Dw3 locus, while S_2 confers risk for nonautoimmune diabetes and segregates with HLA-B15, DW4 (see Table 4-4). In principle this model is genetically *intermediate* (neither dominant nor recessive). While published mathematical solutions [41, 42] are suspect because certain of the input observations (e.g., prevalence of diabetes) are questionable, the model can account for family and population studies suggesting dominant [32, 39] or recessive [40, 43] inheritance, the phenomenon of overdominance, and clinical evidence of diabetic heterogeneity. Some form of the two-gene intermediate model would appear to have the greatest explanatory potential for the genetics of insulin-dependent diabetes, given present knowledge regarding this disease. One gene would be sufficient to confer risk for diabetes, but two genes would significantly enhance that risk. Discovery of specific markers for the susceptibility gene(s) of diabetes will be required for final clarification.

No specific comments will be made regarding *multifactorial* inheritance, although it is obviously a possibility.

Genetics of Non-insulin-dependent Diabetes Mellitus

Twin Studies and Pedigree Analysis   In contrast to the situation with younger monozygotic twins, concordance rates for diabetes are greater than 90 percent when the index twin develops the disease after the age of 40 [20, 22, 23]. This finding strongly suggests that the genetic influence is powerful in non-insulin-dependent diabetes. Indeed, in nonobese subjects it may be essentially exclusive (no environmental insult required) [3]. Family studies of non-insulin-dependent diabetics have been reported to show the disease in 26 percent of sibs and 33 percent of children [44]. Children of two parents with

Table 4-4   Heterogeneity in type 1 diabetes—postulated syndromes

Syndrome	1A	1B
HLA association	B15, DR4*	B8, DR3†
Islet cell antibodies	Transient	Persistent
Immune endocrinopathy	Normal frequency	Increased frequency
Insulin antibodies	Low responders	High responders
Age of onset	Early years	Any age
Microangiopathy	Not increased	? Increased
Etiology	Virus, chemical	Autoimmune

* Haplotype may commonly be DR4-Dw4-B15(Bw62)-Cw3-A2 (see text).
† Haplotype may commonly be DR3-Dw3-B8-Cw7-A1 (see text).
SOURCE: Adapted from Rotter and Rimoin [17]. Type 1A and 1B nomenclature from Bottazzo, Cudworth, Moul, Doniach, and Festenstein [66].

type 2 diabetes have been reported to inherit the disease with frequencies varying from 3 to 30 percent [24–26]. The accuracy of these figures is not known since modern diagnostic standards were not applied. Almost certainly the inheritance rates are inflated, particularly when ascertainment was based on glucose tolerance tests.

HLA Relationships   There are no HLA relationships in non-insulin-dependent diabetes (including MODY), with the possible exception of the Xhosa tribe of South Africa [45].

Inheritance   Only two patterns of inheritance have been seriously entertained: autosomal recessive and multifactorial. The single-gene autosomal recessive pattern would require the appearance of diabetes in 100 percent of the offspring of two parents manifesting the disease. Since the children of parents who both have diabetes probably have true diabetes only 3 to 10 percent of the time, the recessive hypothesis appears unlikely unless penetrance is extremely low (which would not appear to be the case from twin studies). At present, multifactorial inheritance appears most likely [20] but, as in the case of insulin-dependent diabetes, the issue can be settled only when a specific marker for the diabetic susceptibility gene(s) is identified.

EPIDEMIOLOGY

Insulin-dependent Diabetes Mellitus

The mechanisms by which genetic susceptibility to insulin-dependent diabetes is translated into overt disease are not known, but interest has focused on viruses and immune phenomena.

Viruses and Diabetes   The fact that most young patients with insulin-dependent diabetes have no family history and that concordance rates for monozygotic twins are 50 percent or less has spotlighted the role of the environment in this disease. The possibility that viruses might be involved was initially raised because there seemed to be more than a chance occurrence between the onset of diabetes and recent infections with mumps, hepatitis, infectious mononucleosis, congenital rubella, and Coxsackie virus B [25, 46, 47]. Moreover, a seasonal variation in onset has been widely reported [46]. Epidemiologic studies are suggestive but inconclusive. For example, antibody to Coxsackie B4 was found much more frequently in serums of 162 patients with insulin-dependent diabetes of recent onset than in 319 control subjects [48]. On the other hand, when serums were collected from 49 pairs of identical twins (27 discordant, 22 concordant), no differences were found in antibody titers to mumps, cytomegalovirus, rubella, Coxsackie virus types B1 to B5, or *Mycoplasma pneumoniae* between affected and nonaffected twins; i.e., the twins with overt diabetes did not have higher titers to the viruses tested than the unaffected sibs [49]. An obvious problem with all serologic studies is that viral infection might initiate a process (such as an immune response) which could induce disease at a much later time when antibody titers had returned to normal.

Direct support for virus-induced diabetes in humans was provided by isolation of Coxsackie B virus from the pancreas of a 10-year-old boy, previously healthy, who died from complications of ketoacidosis following a flulike illness [50]. Rising titers of neutralizing antibody to the virus indicated recent infection. Inoculation of the agent into normal mice produced hyperglycemia, and viral antigens were demonstrated in the β cells. The infecting agent appeared to be related to Coxsackie B4 and could be reisolated from infected cells of several species. This report strongly suggests that viruses alone can cause diabetes in humans if the proper genetic background is present (there was a strong family history of diabetes in the patient). The conclusion is not unequivocal since presumably a severe viral illness might precipitate ketoacidosis in a type 1 diabetic subject whose insulin deficiency had not yet reached the symptomatic phase.

Additional support for the possibility that viruses play a role in the induction of diabetes has come from studies in animals [47]. A variety of viral agents (e.g., encephalomyocarditis M variant, Coxsackie B, reovirus) have the capacity to induce hyperglycemia in rodents. It has been shown that there is a marked difference in susceptibility to development of diabetes for the same inoculum of virus in different strains of mice and rats. This differential susceptibility is not limited to one viral strain, i.e., mice or rats susceptible to Coxsackie B virus are also susceptible to induction by encephalomyocarditis virus and vice versa [51]. A predisposition to develop diabetes following infection with encephalomyocarditis virus is inherited as an autosomal recessive trait [52], but susceptibility appears to be uninfluenced by the major histocompatibility complex (H-2) in mice [53]. All viruses inducing diabetes in experimental animals infect the β cell but not the α cell [54, 55]. Recovery of viral antigens from pancreatic monolayers prepared from different strains of mice after infection with encephalomyocarditis virus parallels the patterns of resistance-susceptibility in vivo [56]. The susceptibility gene for diabetes was originally thought to act primarily by controlling the number of viral receptors on the surface of the β cell [56], but it now appears that additional factors play a role. This is illustrated by an intriguing experiment in which a susceptible strain of mice (DBA/2) was crossed with a resistant strain (C57BL/6) [57]. The hybrids were treated with streptozotocin to destroy their own pancreatic islets, after which they developed diabetes. Transplants of neonatal pancreas from either the susceptible or resistant parental strains were then carried out (the genetic design of the experiment prevented rejection of either type of pancreas). Hyperglycemia was reversed by the pancreatic transplants. Four weeks later, the transplanted animals and nontransplanted controls were inoculated with encephalomyocarditis virus. Surprisingly, diabetes was reinduced in hybrids containing either resistant or susceptible pancreas. In other words, placement of pancreas from a resistant animal in a susceptible species made it vulnerable to destruction by the diabetogenic virus. This experiment strongly suggests that host factors distinct from the number of viral receptors on the pancreas play a role in determining susceptibility to viral diabetes. Similar conclusions derive from an experiment in which resistant C57BL/6 mice were rendered sensitive to viral-induced diabetes by introducing the obesity gene from ob/ob mice [58]. Another factor of potential importance is the observation that diabetogenic viruses passed repeatedly through pancreatic β-cell cultures show a markedly increased capacity to cause diabetes in the same recipient strain, i.e., they become more virulent [51].

On the basis of these studies, it can be seen that susceptibility to diabetes as a consequence of viral infection can be influenced at several levels. First, there may be genetically controlled differences in whole-organism susceptibility to viral infection (e.g., ability to produce interferon). Second, the same strain of virus may vary widely in virulence, possibly because of passage through the pancreas of several human hosts. Third, target organs in the infected host may vary in susceptibility to attack or destruction by virus (given equivalent inocula) through genetic control of the number of viral receptors on the β cell or other host factors. One of the latter might be the capacity to develop autoantibodies against the pancreas (see the next section). While it cannot yet be accepted as proven that viruses represent the major inducing factor for the appearance of insulin-dependent diabetes mellitus in humans, the evidence is strong enough to warrant continuing aggressive investigation of the problem.

Autoimmunity in Diabetes   It has long been known that there is a relationship between diabetes mellitus and the immune endocrinopathy syndrome. The prevalence of plasma antibodies to thyroid gland and gastric mucosa is three times higher in insulin-dependent diabetic subjects than in age- and sex-matched control subjects. Similarly, antibodies to adrenal cortex occur 30 times more frequently in insulin-requiring diabetics than in normal subjects. The prevalence of diabetes mellitus in idiopathic Addison's disease is 10 times that of the general population. Aware of this fact, in 1974 Bottazzo, Florin-Christensen and Doniach [59] tested the plasma for circulating antibodies to pancreatic islet cells in 171 subjects at risk for autoimmune disease. Of these, 124 had organ-specific antibodies in the plasma and a number had endocrine deficiency syndromes. Of the 171 serums, 13 gave uniform cytoplasmic immunofluorescence when tested on unfixed human pancreas obtained at autopsy. The antibody proved to be IgG in type and reaction was seen with α, β, and δ cells. Ten of the patients with positive antibodies had overt diabetes, and most had at least one other autoimmune disorder. Only 1 month later, five additional patients with insulin-dependent diabetes mellitus and coexistent autoimmunity characterized by IgG antibodies to pancreatic islet cells were reported [60]. In both series, far more patients with diabetes were negative for antibodies than had them. It was then shown that when serum was obtained from children with diabetes of recent onset, the percentage positive for antibodies dramatically increased [61]. On the basis of studies in much larger numbers of patients, a modified concept of the role of islet cell antibodies has now emerged. All investigators concur that the prevalence of islet antibodies is extremely high in newly diagnosed diabetes, in the range of 60 to 90 percent [62, 63]. If one correlates the presence of antibodies with the duration of disease, the prevalence falls to about 20 percent by 5 years, and after 10 to 20 years it is only 5 to 10 percent. Those patients with persistent islet cell antibodies have a high incidence of concurrent polyendocrine disease.

Subsequently a different type of islet antibody was described which binds to the plasma membrane of islet cells rather than to membrane components of the cytoplasm, as is the case with the original antibody [64]. The surface antibody appears to be present with approximately the same frequency as the original islet cell cytoplasmic antibody but has the additional capacity to induce lysis of β cells in the presence of complement, i.e., it is cytotoxic [65].

It has been pointed out that those patients with persistent islet cell antibodies and a tendency to develop immune endocrinopathy also have a high frequency of the HLA-DR3-Dw3-

B8-Cw7-A1 haplotype, while those who rapidly clear plasma antibodies are more likely to be associated with HLA-DR4-Dw4-B15(Bw62)-Cw3-A2 [15, 66]. On the basis of these differences, there has been a tendency to divide insulin-dependent diabetes into two types (Table 4-4). Conceptually, the group of patients carrying the D4-B15 alleles are considered to develop antibodies in response to some external injury (e.g., viral, chemical) which causes leakage of tissue antigens. By contrast, those subjects associated with the HLA-D3-B8 alleles are considered to have a purely autoimmune form of diabetes [17, 66]. These syndromes should be accepted only tentatively. Certainly the clinical phenotypes are not solely determined by the HLA-associated diabetes susceptibility genes since the capacity to respond to insulin injections with anti-insulin antibody formation reputed to be characteristic of the B8-DR3 phenotype, is at least partially determined by the IgG heavy-chain gene complex [67]. Moreover, evidence has now been adduced that antibodies to the gastric mucosa and thyroid gland (frequent accompaniments of the immune endocrinopathy syndrome) may not be controlled by the locus postulated to regulate susceptibility to an autoimmune form of diabetes [68].

In spite of the suggestion that at least one form of type 1 diabetes is an autoimmune disease, with insulin deficiency produced as a consequence of the autoantibodies, the role of the latter in pathogenesis is not yet certain. Evidence bearing on the problem is as follows. "Insulitis," an infiltrate of lymphocytes and large mononuclear cells in and around the islets, is common in pancreases of young persons dying within 6 months of the clinical onset of diabetes. Insulitis can also be induced in experimental animals infected with diabetogenic viruses or treated with β-cell toxins. Since similar infiltrates had been recognized in endocrine glands affected by autoimmune endocrinopathies, the presence of insulitis has been considered consistent with an autoimmune mechanism [64, 69].

An experimental model compatible with an autoimmune component can be produced by administration of subdiabetogenic doses of streptozotocin. When given in large amounts, this β-cell toxin rapidly induces diabetes with complete destruction of the pancreas. Animals die (in a large percentage of the cases) in acute diabetic ketoacidosis. On the other hand, if streptozotocin is administered in subdiabetogenic doses for five injections, the appearance of hyperglycemia is delayed for approximately 2 weeks and develops in association with insulitis. Acute toxic effects of streptozotocin can be prevented by prior administration of 3-0-methyl-d-glucose (3-OMG). When 3-OMG was given simultaneously with small doses of streptozotocin, late insulitis and hyperglycemia still appeared. By contrast, when 3-OMG was combined with antilymphocyte serum (ALS), diabetes was completely prevented provided ALS administration was sufficiently prolonged [69]. This experiment strongly suggests that low-dose streptozotocin induces diabetes by direct action (prevented by 3-OMG) and lymphocyte-mediated inflammatory islet cell lesions (prevented by ALS). The streptozotocin model is a complicated one, however, since males are much more sensitive to the toxin than females [70], a situation which does not pertain in human diabetes, in which male/female ratios are near unity [14]. It may not, therefore, be a model of the human illness. Moreover, the quantitative contribution of the presumed autoimmune (insulitis) element of this model is clouded by the observation that islet cell number and volume decrease (together with an 84 percent fall in insulin secretory capacity) prior to the onset of insulitis [71]. A somewhat similar toxin-induced diabetes is seen in humans in whom the ingestion of a rodenticide (Vacor) is followed by insulin-dependent diabetes. These patients demonstrate islet cell surface antibodies, but a causal role in pathogenesis cannot be proven [72].

Cell-mediated cytotoxicity may also participate in the induction of insulinopenic diabetes since lymphocytes from type 1 diabetic subjects are capable of attacking insulinoma cells in culture [73]. The fact that athymic (nude) mice develop hyperglycemia equivalent to that of controls following streptozotocin injection [74] would seem to indicate that thymus-derived lymphocytes are not required. However, it is now known that T-cell function is not completely absent from such animals, presumably because some populations of pre-T cells can subsume, at least qualitatively, normal T-cell function. For this reason, experiments in the athymic mouse cannot be used as definitive evidence against a role for cell-mediated immunity in the induction of diabetes. On the other hand, the absence of insulitis in these animals does suggest that lymphocytic infiltration of the pancreas is unnecessary for impairment of β-cell function [74].

It has been reported that diabetes could be passively transferred by injection of spleen cells from streptozotocin-treated animals into nondiabetic recipients [75] and that T lymphocytes were the inducing agents [76]. The same authors indicated that similar transfer could be accomplished using human diabetic lymphocytes in athymic mice [77]. Unfortunately, other workers have failed to reproduce the findings [74, 78].

Summary An attractive scenario for the epidemiology of insulin-dependent diabetes can be constructed [25]. According to this formulation, susceptibility to diabetes is genetically determined and inherited as a permissive factor. Given the proper genetic background, injury to the β cell can be produced by an environmental agent which might be either chemical or viral. Size of the inoculum, duration of exposure, virulence of the infective agent, and host responses to infectious or noxious stimuli would all play modulating roles in determining the appearance of overt disease. Subsequent to β-cell injury, antigens would be released into the bloodstream. The autoantibodies produced would then attack the β cell, completing the damage sequence. A single exposure to an inciting agent might not be sufficient to cause disease. For example, an infection with mumps virus might produce clinically inapparent damage to the pancreas, while a subsequent infection with Coxsackie B4 virus could produce enough additional damage to initiate hyperglycemia. In some cases, it would be possible to develop insulin-dependent diabetes without the necessity of external factors. This form of the disease might be truly autoimmune in the sense that antibodies arise spontaneously. Its hallmark would be the presence of antibodies against other endocrine tissues, the presence of endocrine disease of the immune type, or both.

Appealing as this formulation may be, it should be accepted with caution. Serious questions remain regarding every aspect of the scheme. Genetic mechanisms are mysterious, the role of viruses has not been proved, and it is conceivable that the antibodies are only markers of some underlying disease process.

Non-insulin-dependent Diabetes Mellitus

There is no suggestion that viruses or autoimmunity are involved in the induction of non-insulin-dependent diabetes mellitus. The high concordance rate in identical twins strongly suggests that a genetic factor(s) primarily determines its appearance. Obesity is common [3] and together with increased caloric intake doubtless is a major external precipitating factor. Certainly decreased caloric intake and weight loss can reverse elevated plasma glucose concentrations and return β-cell function toward normal in obese diabetic subjects [79]. Obesity is not the total explanation since non-insulin-dependent diabetes may occur in individuals with normal weight.

A characteristic feature of type 2 diabetes is insulin resistance [80]. The effectiveness of the hormone in disposing of a glucose load is impaired whether fasting insulin levels are low, normal, or high [81]. In patients with overt disease (fasting hyperglycemia), insulin release in response to glucose loads is almost always blunted. Thus, there is a β-cell defect in addition to insulin resistance [80]. Insulin resistance is often due to concomitant obesity but is also present in individuals of normal weight. In either case, there is a decreased number of insulin receptors on target cells. Subjects with severe insulin resistance also appear to have a postreceptor defect. The nature of the postreceptor defect is unknown, but it may be secondary to effective insulin deficiency at the tissue level since the defect can be reversed by insulin therapy in some patients without change in weight [80, 81a]. A remarkable report has appeared from Scandinavia indicating that in men with impaired glucose tolerance, progression to overt diabetes can be prevented for up to 10 years by treatment with 1.5 g tolbutamide daily prior to the development of hyperglycemia [9]. This study has not been confirmed and, because of its prolonged nature, it may never be. Nevertheless, the possibility that β-cell function might be preserved pharmacologically in persons at risk for type 2 diabetes deserves further study, particularly if future developments allow reliable identification of the prediabetic state. For reasons discussed earlier, glucose tolerance testing is not adequate in this regard.

Summary The chain of events leading to symptomatic non-insulin-dependent diabetes is not known. Insulin resistance is an important component, especially when obesity is present. The nature of the intrinsic resistance (unrelated to obesity) remains obscure but could be related to prolonged functional inadequacy of insulin in target tissues, with consequent loss or inactivation of glucose-metabolizing enzymes or a deficit in microsome-bound glucose transport units which normally are recruited into the plasma membrane when insulin is present [81b] (see below). Genetically determined β-cell damage almost certainly is important in overt disease, since severe obesity with marked insulin resistance does not cause hyperglycemia in nondiabetic subjects. This suggests that the normal pancreas has sufficient reserves to overcome the resistant state, while the diabetic pancreas does not. The nature of the pancreatic defect and its relation to hormone resistance await clarification.

METABOLIC ASPECTS

Of the multiple metabolic abnormalities that characterize uncontrolled diabetes, two are of preeminent importance from the standpoint of producing acute symptoms: *disturbed glucose metabolism*, which results in hyperglycemia, obligatory osmotic diuresis, thirst, and weight loss, and *accelerated ketone body production* (in type 1 disease), which results in ketoacidosis. Other abnormalities (e.g., hypertriglyceridemia, disturbances in the renin-angiotensin axis with hyperkalemia, altered leukocyte function) are of lesser immediate importance, although they contribute to the composite clinical picture of primary diabetes in both insulin-dependent and independent subjects. The metabolic changes of diabetes are hormonally induced. In this section, these hormonal alterations and their effects on glucose metabolism and ketogenesis will be briefly reviewed.

Hormonal Changes

Six hormones are important in regulating fuel metabolism in humans: insulin, glucagon, epinephrine, norepinephrine, cortisol, and growth hormone. In broad terms, insulin can be considered the primary anabolic hormone (linked with synthesis and storage of body fuels), while the other five subserve catabolic functions (the breakdown and oxidation of stored fuels for the provision of energy in the absence of food intake). Since their biologic effects are, in general, opposite to those of insulin, they have been called *counterregulatory*. Basal plasma concentrations of cortisol, epinephrine, and growth hormone tend to be normal in diabetic subjects [82–84]; when plasma is sampled repeatedly throughout a 24-h period, integrated values for epinephrine, norepinephrine, and growth hormone (but not cortisol) are slightly elevated in young insulin-dependent patients [85, 86]. During physical or emotional stress, or in response to hypoglycemia, concentrations of the counterregulatory hormones in plasma rise, sometimes to very high levels [87, 88]. Under these circumstances, they contribute to the development of both hyperglycemia and ketosis.

The primary hormones involved in diabetes are insulin and glucagon. In untreated diabetic subjects (regardless of type) there is relative or absolute hypoinsulinemia and relative or absolute hyperglucagonemia so that the ratio of glucagon to insulin is increased even under basal conditions [89, 90]. The deficiency and excess, respectively, of the β- and α-cell hormones become exaggerated during stress. While the role of glucagon has been controversial [91], it now seems overwhelmingly likely that the metabolic changes of uncontrolled diabetes are not due solely to insulin deficiency but that glucagon plays a critical role in initiating and controlling the hyperglycemic and ketogenic processes [89–91]. Hyperglucagonemia is probably a secondary consequence of insulin deficiency since glucagon concentrations can be restored to normal by aggressive insulin therapy [92, 93]. Insulin is considered to act primarily in nonhepatic target cells to accelerate transport of glucose, amino acids, and other ions through the plasma membrane [94], to inhibit the hormone-sensitive lipase of adipose tissues such that free fatty acid mobilization is impaired [95], and to stimulate the synthesis of protein, fat, and glycogen [95–97]. The role of insulin in the liver is complicated; while there is no doubt that it can reverse the increased hepatic production of glucose and ketones that occur in fasting and uncontrolled diabetes, increasing evidence suggests that its major effect is to antagonize glucagon-induced activation of these processes [97, 98]. In other words, the effects of insulin on hepatocytes not activated by glucagon (or catecholamines) are small. The mechanisms by which insulin acts at the molecular level after binding to its receptor remain unknown despite extensive work. Current thought focuses on changes in the glu-

cose transport unit of the plasma membrane and on release of activators and inhibitors of phosphorylation-dephosphorylation reactions inside the cell [94, 99–101].

While the primary actions of insulin are on nonhepatic (peripheral) tissues, the major effects of glucagon are exerted in the liver [89]. Hepatic responses include activation of the enzymes of glycogen breakdown and gluconeogenesis [102, 103] and derepression of the fatty acid oxidizing-ketogenic machinery [104]. These actions are probably exerted primarily through phosphorylation of key enzymes (e.g., [105]). How the protein kinases that carry out these reactions are activated is currently unclear. For some time, it was assumed that glucagon and catecholamines operated through the generation of cyclic AMP in the cell through β-adrenergic mechanisms. Studies in rodents now indicate that the catecholamines can alter glycogenolysis and gluconeogenesis through α-adrenergic receptors without the necessity for a rise in cyclic AMP, probably by inducing changes in concentration or distribution of intracellular calcium [97, 102, 103, 106]. It is not known whether similar phenomena operate in human liver or whether glucagon can act via the alternate pathway.

Altered Glucose Metabolism

The hyperglycemia of diabetes is the consequence of both increased hepatic production and diminished peripheral utilization of glucose. In the first few hours of a fast in humans, the bulk of hepatic glucose production comes from glycogen breakdown [107]. As glycogen stores are depleted, endogenous glucose production occurs by gluconeogenesis in both the liver and the kidney, but quantitatively the former is significantly more important [108]. The same sequence operates following the withdrawal of insulin in diabetic subjects [109]. Although hepatic overproduction of glucose accounts for fasting hyperglycemia and initiates the osmotic diuresis of uncontrolled diabetes, diminished utilization of hexose plays an increasingly important role as the period of insulin withdrawal becomes more prolonged [109, 110]. This progressive decrease in glucose utilization causes plasma concentrations to remain high in spite of the fact that hepatic production rates are maximal several hours after insulin withdrawal and subsequently decline (although remaining elevated) [109]. The reason for the diminished rate of glucose production with time is not known, but glycogen depletion may be involved; that is, after glycogen stores have been dissipated, the residual rate of glucose production reflects gluconeogenesis, presumably a slower process. How insulin deficiency causes impaired glucose utilization in peripheral target tissues is unknown. There is disagreement over whether the hormone normally increases movement of glucose into the cell by causing transfer (recruitment) of cryptic glucose transport units from microsomes into the plasma membrane [111a] or simply activates the transport molecules already present [112]. Whatever the mechanism, absence of insulin presumably deactivates the transport system and subsequent oxidative events such that the rate of removal of glucose from the plasma and interstitial fluid is slowed.

While terms such as *insulin deficiency* or *insulin withdrawal* are frequently used to indicate the cause of decompensation in diabetes, glucagon is crucial for initiating hepatic overproduction of glucose and ketones. This was shown most explicitly by a classic experiment in which somatostatin was infused in type 1 diabetic subjects taken off insulin. Under these circumstances, hyperglycemia and ketoacidosis were markedly delayed in appearance compared to control experiments in which saline was infused [113]. Somatostatin has the capacity to block both insulin and glucagon release from the pancreas, but in insulinopenic patients its only significant effect is to lower plasma glucagon levels. Along the same lines, only glucagon, of all the counterregulatory hormones, increases in parallel with a rise in glucose and ketones during the developmental stage of diabetic ketoacidosis [109]. Many other experiments are in accord with the conclusion that glucagon has powerful hyperglycemic and ketogenic effects [89, 109, 110].

The interrelationships between glucagon and insulin are shown schematically in Fig. 4-1. The two hormones form an integrated metabolic unit for the control of plasma glucose concentration and ketone body production [114, 115]. In the liver (and possibly other tissues), the two hormones exert opposing effects. Large changes in concentrations are not required to produce major metabolic responses. Thus, a decrease in insulin occurring against the background of a normal glucagon concentration may result in the same change in liver metabolism that would be seen with a major absolute increase of glucagon coupled with a normal or elevated insulin concentration. This has led to the concept that the molar ratio of glucagon to insulin is more important than the absolute level of either [104, 114, 115]. Also, α- and β-cell hormones are believed to interact in paracrine fashion within the islets of Langerhans; insulin inhibits the release of glucagon while glucagon stimulates secretion of insulin [89, 115]. Similar relationships exist with somatostatin-secreting δ cells. While δ cells appear to be increased in islets from insulin-dependent diabetic subjects [116], techniques for assay of somatostatin in plasma are not yet reliable enough to allow us to draw firm conclusions regarding its role in the metabolic changes of human diabetes [117]. The complex interrelationships between glucagon and insulin existing both within the islets and in target tissues have rendered interpretation of in vivo studies extremely difficult. This is because perturbation of either hormones or substrates induces multiple changes in other hormones and substrates such that primary and secondary changes are difficult to dissect [110]. Nevertheless, it appears safe to state that the hyperglycemia of insulin-dependent diabetes mellitus (and probably all forms of endogenous hyperglycemia) is due to relative or absolute deficiency of insulin coupled with relative or absolute excess of glucagon [115].

Ketogenesis

The same hormonal changes that cause glycogen breakdown and increased gluconeogenesis in uncontrolled diabetes also induce hepatic ketogenesis in insulin-dependent subjects [104, 118]. The substrate for acetoacetate and β-hydroxybutyrate production in the liver is long-chain fatty acids mobilized in response to hypoinsulinemia with or without a concomitant rise in lipolytic counterregulatory hormones. Fatty acids taken up by the liver in the normal fed state or in the well-controlled diabetic subject are reesterified to form triglycerides and are largely transported back into the plasma as very low density lipoproteins [118]. This is because the system of enzymes that oxidize fatty acids is inactive when the [glucagon]: [insulin] ratio is low. Following a fast of several hours or in uncontrolled diabetes, a shift in this ratio favoring glucagon activates the oxidative sequence for fatty acids in the liver and preferentially shunts incoming free fatty acids into ketone body production.

The mechanism whereby glucagon exerts its action is now well understood [119]. The rate-limiting step for fatty acid oxidation is transport of substrate across the inner mitochondrial membrane (Fig. 4-2). Long-chain fatty acyl CoA molecules cannot traverse the barrier membrane, but fatty acids bound to carnitine are freely permeable. Transesterification of the acyl CoA to its carrier molecule is accomplished through the action of carnitine acyltransferase I (carnitine palmitoyltransferase I), with reversal of the process inside the mitochondrion under the influence of carnitine acyltransferase II (carnitine palmitoyltransferase II). Since the β-oxidative sequence for fatty acids is a high-capacity system, and presumably is fully active at all times, entry of fatty acids into the mitochondrion is followed by the obligatory production of ketone bodies because only a minor fraction of the acetyl CoA formed from fatty acids enters the tricarboxylic acid cycle [120].

Carnitine acyltransferase I is a regulated enzyme which is powerfully inhibited in the presence of a low [glucagon]: [insulin] ratio (see Fig. 4-3). This inhibition is exerted by malonyl CoA, the primary substrate for fatty acid synthesis [121]. When glucagon concentrations rise, malonyl CoA levels drop precipitously because the α-cell hormone inhibits key enzymes on the pathway of fatty acid synthesis from glucose (e.g., phosphofructokinase, pyruvate kinase, and acetyl CoA carboxylase) [119a]. Under these circumstances, carnitine acyltransferase I is activated and long-chain fatty acyl CoA molecules are rapidly and efficiently taken into the mitochondrion for oxidation to acetoacetic and β-hydroxybutyric acids. The process is further facilitated by a rise in the hepatic concentration of carnitine, which tends to drive the reaction by mass action [122]. Once the hepatic ketone-synthesizing machinery is activated, the rate of ketogenesis is determined by the concentration of fatty acids present in the liver according to first-order kinetics. Hepatic uptake of fatty acids is the passive consequence of plasma concentrations. Since free fatty acid levels in plasma are high in uncontrolled diabetes (the consequence of activated lipolysis in adipocytes), major ketone production is assured. Hepatic overproduction of ketones appears to be the primary cause of ketoacidosis, although the capacity to oxidize aceto-

Figure 4-1 Insulin-glucagon relationships in normal persons and diabetics. As indicated in panel a, within the islets insulin inhibits glucagon release, while glucagon stimulates insulin secretion. In target tissues such as the liver, the two hormones are biologic antagonists. In diabetes (panel b), destruction or dysfunction of the β cell removes the inhibitory influence of insulin on glucagon release in the islets and allows unrestrained activity of the α-cell hormone in target tissues. (*From Unger and Orci* [115]. *Reprinted by permission of the New England Journal of Medicine.*)

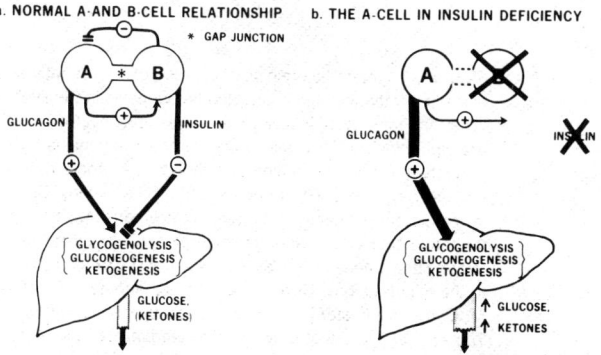

a. NORMAL A- AND B-CELL RELATIONSHIP   b. THE A-CELL IN INSULIN DEFICIENCY

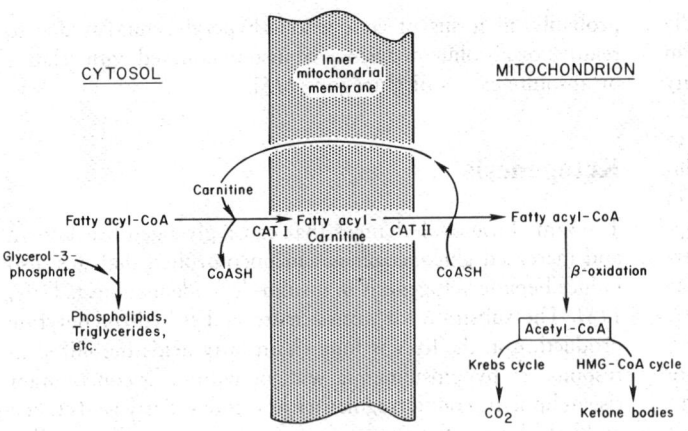

Figure 4-2 The oxidation of fatty acids in liver. Fatty acyl CoA must be esterified to carnitine in order to cross the inner mitochondrial membrane. This reaction is catalyzed by carnitine acyltransferase I (CAT I). Inside the mitochondrion the reaction is reversed by carnitine acyltransferase II. (CAT II). See text for details. (*From McGarry JD: New perspectives in the regulation of ketogenesis. Diabetes 28:517, 1979. Reproduced by permission of the American Diabetes Association.*)

acetate and β-hydroxybutyrate in peripheral tissues appears to become saturated at high plasma concentrations [109]. Following administration of insulin, all metabolic abnormalities are reversed.

Metabolic Crises

The diabetic patient is vulnerable to three major types of crises: ketoacidosis; hyperosmolar, nonketotic coma; and hypoglycemia. All three of these may lead to serious consequences. *Diabetic ketoacidosis* is the end result of decompensated control in insulin-dependent diabetic subjects. Its characteristics are extracellular volume depletion, dehydration, and severe metabolic acidosis [123–125]. The fluid abnormalities are due to the development of hyperglycemia for the reasons outlined above. Glucose enters the renal tubule by glomerular filtration and is reabsorbed proximally. The tubular maximum for reabsorption is about 225 mg/min, which means that with a glomerular filtration rate of 120 ml/min, glycosuria will appear at a plasma glucose concentration of 180 to 190 mg/dl. If glomerular filtration rates fall because of intrinsic renal disease or volume depletion, higher plasma concentrations are required to induce glycosuria. Unreabsorbed glucose causes an osmotic diuresis which progresses in severity as hyperglycemia increases. During osmotic diuresis, obligate loss of free water together with electrolytes accounts for both volume depletion and dehydration [126]. The fluid deficit in diabetic ketoacido-

sis is usually limited (3 to 5 liters) because nausea and vomiting or Kussmaul breathing signal the onset of illness and bring the patient to the hospital; only occasionally are fluid losses equivalent to those characteristic of hyperosmolar coma. The metabolic acidosis is accounted for almost exclusively by the ketone bodies, although modest elevations of lactate contribute to the anion gap [125].

Hyperosmolar coma occurs in type 2 diabetic subjects who are resistant to ketosis. The clinical picture of extreme hyperglycemia, profound volume depletion (on average 10 to 12 liters), altered central nervous system function (stupor, coma, convulsions), hyperviscosity with diffuse intravascular coagulation and hemorrhage, and ultimate vascular collapse is due to prolonged and unrestrained osmotic diuresis [125, 127]. A frequent complication is septicemia or pneumonia due to gram-negative organisms [128]. The reason for the absence of ketoacidosis in non-insulin-dependent diabetics, even when stress is extreme, is unknown. Limited mobilization of free fatty acids and an antiketogenic effect of dehydration have been evoked, but both appear untenable as sole explanations since some patients with the syndrome have extremely high levels of fatty acids in plasma and since full-blown ketoacidosis can occur in type 1 patients in the face of severe hyperosmolarity [127]. It is possible that portal vein insulin levels in these patients are sufficiently high to prevent activation of fatty acid oxidation in the liver. Such an explanation is not very convincing, however, since with severe stress residual insulin release should be blocked by catecholamines, with a concomitant rise in gluca-

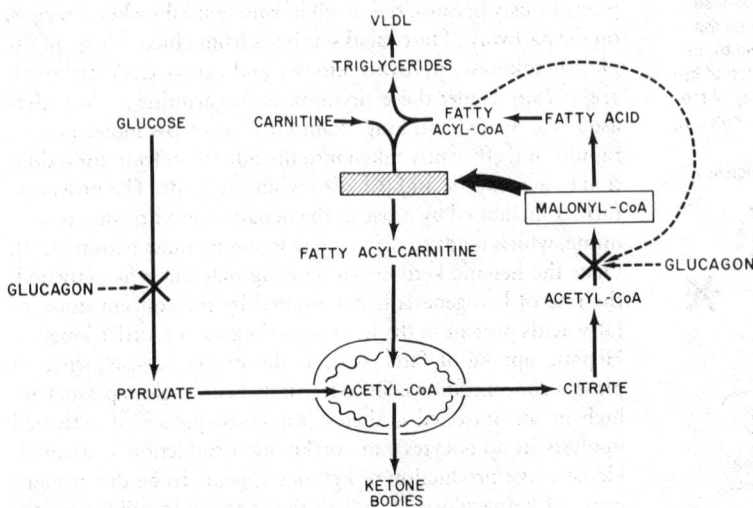

Figure 4-3 Interrelationships of glucose oxidation, fatty acid oxidation, fatty acid synthesis, and ketogenesis in the liver. When the [glucagon]:[insulin] ratio is low, malonyl CoA levels are high, blocking fatty acid oxidation and ketogenesis through inhibition of carnitine acyltransferase I and driving fatty acid synthesis. Glucagon excess blocks malonyl CoA formation, thereby activating carnitine acyltransferase I and the fatty acid oxidative-ketogenic sequence with cessation of fatty acid synthesis. High levels of fatty acyl CoA contribute to the fall of malonyl CoA in uncontrolled diabetes. (*From McGarry and Foster [119] Reproduced by permission of The Annual Review of Biochemistry, Annual Reviews, Inc.*)

gon providing the necessary change in the [glucagon]: [insulin] ratio required for activation of ketogenesis. A more reasonable explanation might be a genetically determined resistance of the fatty acid oxidation-ketogenic sequence to activation by glucagon. The site could be carnitine acyltransferase I or beyond. While such an abnormality has not been demonstrated in humans, partial hepatic resistance to glucagon has been observed in the ob/ob mouse, a genetically obese animal with certain biochemical characteristics reminiscent of human type 2 diabetes [129]. *Hypoglycemia* in the diabetic is almost always the consequence of imbalance between administration of insulin and food intake. It is particularly common when "tight" control is attempted by traditional forms of therapy or insulin infusion pumps. It may even occur during use of the artificial external pancreas unless protective dextrose or glucagon infusion mechanisms are provided [130]. Hypoglycemia may cause distressing symptoms when severe or simply worsen diabetic control in the absence of symptoms if less severe (Somogyi effect). The latter occurs because counterregulatory mechanisms in diabetics are not impaired [131]. Plasma glucagon has been reported not to increase in response to a fall in plasma glucose concentration in some studies, but levels were already elevated [132, 133]. In some diabetics epinephrine, cortisol, and growth hormone release appears to be induced by a fall in glucose concentration even if absolute hypoglycemia does not occur [133]. Insulin-dependent diabetics also appear to be hypersensitive to the counterregulatory hormones, responding to their infusion with higher rates of hepatic glucose production than occurs in normal controls [134]. Hyperresponsiveness to release signals and enhanced sensitivity of glucose mobilization doubtless contribute to metabolic instability in some insulin-dependent patients. On the basis of these observations, it can be concluded that diabetics are not vulnerable to hypoglycemia because of an intrinsic abnormality in hormonal defense mechanisms. Rather, the problem is a manifestation of nonideal therapy wherein the administration of sufficient insulin to control postprandial hyperglycemia provides too much hormone between meals. Hypoglycemia due to sulfonylurea therapy in non-insulin-dependent subjects is rare but usually severe when it occurs [125]. The reasons for this severity are not understood.

LATE COMPLICATIONS

The major problem in long-term diabetes is the development of degenerative complications which cause devastating morbidity and death. Emphasis is usually placed on retinopathy, nephropathy, neuropathy, and atherosclerosis. The first three are ordinarily categorized as *microangiopathy* (although it is by no means certain that the complications are solely due to small-vessel disease), while the latter is termed *macroangiopathy* [135]. The exact prevalence of these complications is unknown, although it seems clear that they increase with the duration of disease. In patients who had diabetes for more than 40 years, retinopathy was found in up to 75 percent, while estimates of nephropathy and neuropathy ranged from 8 to 48 percent [136, 137]. These patients may not reflect the general diabetic population, most of whom do not live so long with their disease. In one cohort of 372 insulin-dependent subjects followed prospectively by the same team of physicians

from the time of diagnosis, nephropathy (clinically diagnosed by the presence of proteinuria) was present in 4 percent after 16 years and 14 percent after 26 years [138]. Equivalent figures for retinopathy were 27 and 85 percent, respectively. The former percentage may be low since retinal angiography was not available in the early phases of the study. Whatever the exact incidence, it is clear that the problem of late complications is huge. Diabetes is a major cause of new blindness in the United States [139] and represents a significant portion of all persons with renal failure. Unpublished estimates indicate that up to 50 percent of patients on chronic hemodialysis may eventually become diabetics.

While not generally considered long-term complications, many other abnormalities may be present throughout the course of the disease and contribute directly or indirectly to the development of degenerative lesions. These include hyperlipoproteinemia, altered immune responses, abnormal platelet function, imbalance in the prostacyclin-thromboxane system, defective leukocyte defense mechanisms, increased blood viscosity, and abnormalities of fibrinolysis. Interested readers are referred to an excellent review of some of these problems [140]. One caveat seems warranted. Many experiments reporting abnormalities in blood and its formed elements have been carried out in vitro and may not apply in vivo. For example, increased platelet adhesiveness and aggregation demonstrated in vitro does not appear to be accompanied by altered platelet half-life in vivo [141]. Along the same lines, certain assays such as those used to measure prostacyclin and thromboxane generation are questionable because of lack of linearity with time and other problems. Caution is indicated, therefore, in accepting all claimed abnormalities in diabetes as established facts [140].

The critical issue is whether the four major complications develop as a consequence of the metabolic manifestations of the disease (in particular, hyperglycemia) or whether they arise independently. The question has been extensively discussed but at present is unanswerable. In favor of a positive relationship are a variety of clinical studies suggesting a correlation between the degree of control and the appearance of complications [135, 140], reports of improved motor nerve conduction times [142], and thinning of capillary basement membranes [143] after normalization or near-normalization of plasma glucose for only a few months, and evidence that transplantation of presumably normal kidneys into diabetic recipients results in the early appearance of arteriolar hyalinosis of both afferent and efferent vessels compatible with the changes seen in spontaneously occurring diabetic nephropathy [144]. Evidence suggesting that complications may not be causally linked to poor diabetic control is derived from other clinical studies [145], from the observation that as many as 25 percent of patients with long-term diabetes never develop retinopathy regardless of the degree of control [146, 147], from reports that typical diabetic retinopathy may be present at diagnosis [148] or prior to the development of hyperglycemia [149], and from suggestions that the aforementioned capillary basement membrane thickening may appear in normoglycemic subjects presumed to have a high chance of carrying a diabetic gene [149–151]. The meaning of the last observation is clouded because of controversy regarding the assessment and interpretation of capillary basement membrane thickening [135, 140].

The view that elevated plasma glucose values themselves might be harmful has been strengthened by the observation that nonenzymatic glycosylation of proteins is common in the body and that the rate of glycosylation increases as a direct function of the degree of hyperglycemia. The most widely studied of the glycosylated proteins is hemoglobin A_{Ic} (Hb A_{Ic}), a fast-moving minor hemoglobin present in normal persons which increases several fold in uncontrolled diabetes. Elevated levels are reversed by aggressive insulin therapy [152]. The amino acids primarily glucosylated are valine and lysine. In addition to Hb A_{Ic}, glucose-lysine adducts have been found in human serum albumin [153], erythrocytic membranes [154], lens protein [155], and basic myelin protein [156]. The presumption has been made that such glycosylation could produce abnormal structure and function of proteins and contribute to or cause degenerative complications [152, 157]. While conceptually attractive, such speculations should not be facilely accepted in the absence of much stronger experimental support than is now available.

Previous attempts to answer the question of whether good control would prevent the appearance of late complications were not definitive for two reasons: It was not possible to assess accurately the degree of control, and in most patients it was not possible to normalize the plasma glucose throughout the day [135]. Both difficulties can now be overcome. It seems clear that reasonable estimates of mean levels of glucose in plasma can be obtained by measurement of Hb A_{Ic} [152] or glycosylated albumin [153, 158]. The former, with a longer half-life, would reflect changes over a period of 6 to 10 weeks, while the latter molecule, which turns over much more rapidly, would indicate the degree of control over the previous 10 to 21 days. Some confusion has developed regarding use of the Hb A_{Ic} concentrations because of reports that its concentration changes rapidly with short-term alterations in the level of plasma glucose. This finding is explained by the mechanism of formation of Hb A_{Ic} shown in Fig. 4-4 (from Ref. 152).

When glucose binds to the terminal valine of the β chain of hemoglobin A, it first forms an aldimine (Schiff base) before undergoing Amadori rearrangement to the ketoamine form of the molecule. As indicated by the k values, the aldimine, which has been called *pre-Hb A_{Ic}*, forms and dissociates rapidly and can thus be considered labile. The ketoamine forms much more slowly but once produced is stable. It is the aldimine fraction that changes rapidly (hours) with a rise or fall in plasma glucose. Removal of pre-Hb A_{Ic} by overnight dialysis of red cell

hemolysates or incubation of whole red cells in saline obviates the problem, leaving only stable Hb A_{Ic} which is not affected by immediate changes in glucose concentration [152, 159]. *Pre-Hb A_{IC}* can be removed even more rapidly by preincubation with semicarbazide and aniline [159a].

A second way of assessing control is by home glucose monitoring using capillary blood obtained by finger sticks and a reflectance meter [160, 161]. By measuring glucose concentrations several times a day, a reasonably accurate estimate of mean diurnal concentrations can be obtained. An alternate advance that may allow meaningful clinical trials to be undertaken is the newly developed capability of delivering insulin in a physiologic pattern with normalization or near normalization of the plasma glucose. This can be done with portable insulin infusion pumps which deliver insulin at a constant basal rate coupled with preprandial bursts [162] or a schedule of multiple injections of regular insulin given in combination with a small amount of a long-acting preparation [163]. It should be possible in the immediate future to carry out a prospective study in which two groups of newly diagnosed insulin-dependent diabetic patients are compared—one treated traditionally and the other tightly controlled using these techniques. Accurate assessment of the degree of control would come from regular measurement of Hb A_{Ic} or glycosylated albumin, possibly initially supplemented by home monitoring of the plasma glucose. While it is unlikely that established major complications can ever be reversed by such treatment, it is conceivable that their appearance may be prevented or severely restricted if plasma glucose (or some as yet unidentified factor that changes in parallel with the plasma glucose during periods of inadequate treatment) is maintained in the normal range. This possibility clearly should be tested. On the other hand, it is also possible that the appearance of nephropathy, retinopathy, and neuropathy is genetically regulated and only marginally influenced by the metabolic abnormalities. A third possibility is that both genetic and metabolic factors are important, in which case prophylactic measures focusing on control of the plasma glucose might be helpful in some patients but not universally effective in preventing degenerative changes.

Finally, it should be noted that aggressive insulin therapy may be harmful in some patients. There are two preliminary reports of rapid worsening of retinopathy during therapy with insulin infusion pumps [164, 165].

Figure 4-4 Mechanism of the formation of Hb A_{Ic}.

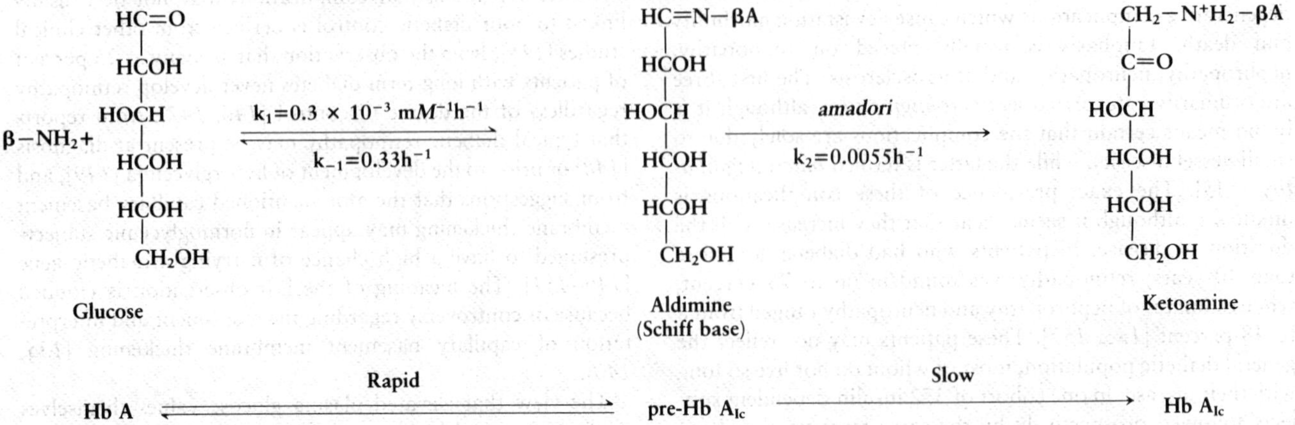

RARE FORMS OF DIABETES

Diabetic syndromes other than the two common primary types discussed in the bulk of this chapter are rare. Two are of considerable importance because they provide insights into the genetics, biochemistry, and physiology of insulin synthesis and action. The first is diabetes due to an *abnormal insulin* [166, 167]. The patient had modest fasting hyperglycemia and hyperinsulinemia, suggesting insulin resistance, but responded normally to exogenous insulin. No inhibitor of insulin action was found in plasma. When the patient's insulin was purified, it was found to have a diminished capacity to bind to insulin receptors on IM-9 lymphocytes and isolated adipocytes, and its biologic activity was 15 percent of normal. Subsequent studies showed that the defect was due to substitution of a leucine for phenylalanine at position 24 of the β chain (see Fig. 4-5 for the normal structure of insulin) [168, 169]. A mutation at the arginine sites binding the β chain to the connecting peptide results in familial hyperproinsulinemia [170], but this abnormality does not cause clinical diabetes.

It is now known that the insulin gene is located on the short arm of the eleventh chromosome in humans [171, 172]. By exploiting mutations in human insulin and recombinant DNA techniques, it should soon be possible to dissect transcription-translation-posttranslation mechanisms in insulin synthesis and to answer such fundamental questions as whether the connecting peptide contributes to the immunologic and biologic properties of the hormone [173]. Details of insulin synthesis are available in the review by Chan, Kwok, and Steiner [174].

A second condition which is much more important than its clinical prevalence would indicate is insulin resistance (and diabetes) due to *insulin receptor antibodies*. Occurring in patients with an underlying immunologic disease (lupuslike)

and acanthosis nigricans, the defect may be mild or severe [175]. From a physiologic standpoint, the importance of these antibodies is that they exhibit both agonist and antagonist activity with the receptor and thus may serve as a powerful tool to dissect receptor structure and function [176, 177]. They can be used to precipitate solubilized membranes and to identify the intra-receptor insulin binding sites. On the basis of studies to date, it appears that the insulin receptor is oligomeric, consisting of subunits with molecular weights of 95 and 130 k [177]. It is hoped that an understanding of its structure and function will allow solution of the critical unsolved problem in insulin action, namely, how receptor binding is linked to changes in intracellular metabolism.

REFERENCES

1. HAMBURG S, HENDLER R, SHERWIN RS: Influence of small increments of epinephrine on glucose tolerance in normal humans. *Ann Intern Med* 93:566, 1980
2. FAJANS SS, CONN JW: The early recognition of diabetes mellitus. *Ann NY Acad Sci* 82:208, 1959
3. NATIONAL DIABETES DATA GROUP: Classification and diagnosis of diabetes mellitus and other categories of glucose intolerance. *Diabetes* 28:1039, 1979
4. UNIVERSITY GROUP DIABETES PROGRAM: A study of the effect of hypoglycemic agents on vascular complications in patients with adult-onset diabetes: I. Design, methods, and baseline characteristics. *Diabetes* 19 (suppl 2):747, 1970
5. BENNETT PH, RUSHFORTH NB, MILLER M, LECOMPTE PM: Epidemiologic studies of diabetes in the Pima Indians. *Recent Prog Horm Res* 32:333, 1976
6. MOURATOFF GJ, CARROLL NV, SCOTT EM: Diabetes mellitus in Athabaskan Indians in Alaska. *Diabetes* 18:29, 1969
7. GENUTH SM, HOUSER HB, CARTER JR, JR, MERKATZ I, PRICE JW, SCHUMACHER OP, WIELAND RG: Community screening for diabetes by blood glucose measurement. Results of a five year experience. *Diabetes* 25:1110, 1976
8. Diabetes survey in Bedford 1962. *Proc R Soc Med* 57:193, 1964
9. SARTOR G, SCHERSTEN B, CARLSTRÖM S, MELANDER A, NORDEN Å, PERSSON G: Ten-year follow-up of subjects with impaired glucose tolerance. Prevention of diabetes by tolbutamide and diet regulation. *Diabetes* 29:4l, 1980
10. CAHILL GF, JR: Diabetes mellitus, in Beeson PB, McDermott W, Wyn-

Figure 4-5 Human proinsulin. (*Modified from Gabbay KH: The insulinopathies. N Engl J Med 302:165, 1980.*)

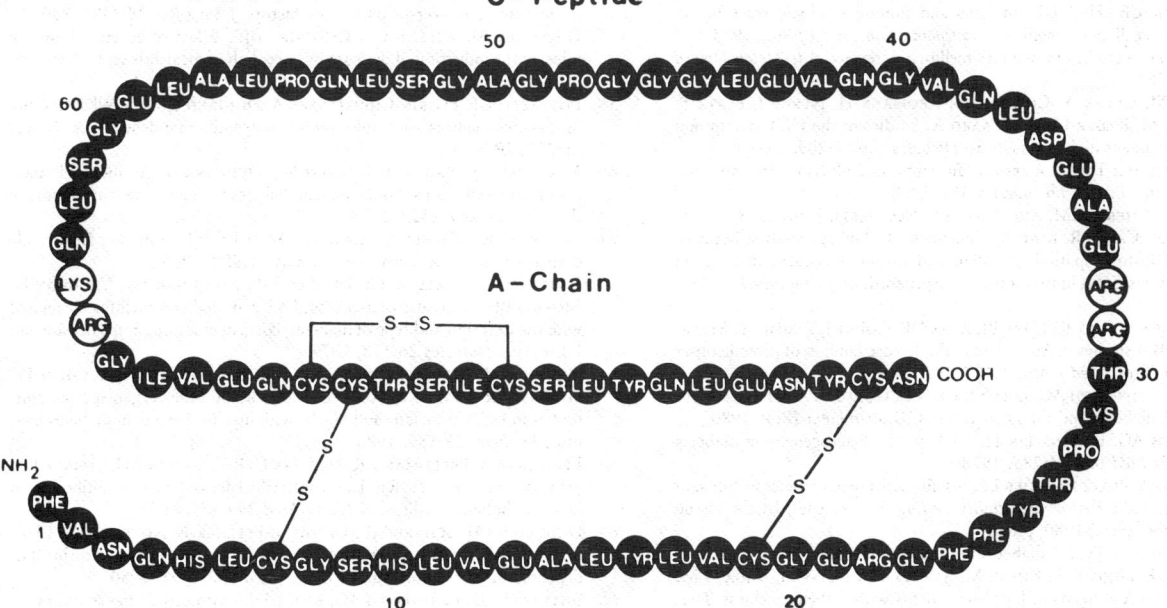

gaarden JB (eds): *Cecil Textbook of Medicine,* Philadelphia, WB Saunders Co, 1979, p 1969

11. GENUTH SM, HOUSER HB, CARTER JR, JR, MERKATZ IR, PRICE JW, SCHUMACHER OP, WIELAND RG: Observations on the value of mass indiscriminate screening for diabetes mellitus based on a five-year follow-up. *Diabetes* 27:377, 1978

12. BLOOM A, HAYES TM, GAMBLE DR: Registry of newly diagnosed diabetic children. *Br Med J* 3:580, 1975

13. CROSSLEY JR, UPSDELL M: The incidence of juvenile diabetes mellitus in New Zealand. *Diabetologia* 18:29, 1980

14. LAPORTE RE, FISHBEIN HA, DRASH AL, KULLER LH, SCHNEIDER BB, ORCHARD TJ, WAGENER DK: The Pittsburgh insulin dependent diabetes mellitus (IDDM) registry. The incidence of insulin dependent diabetes mellitus in Allegheny County, Pennsylvania (1965–1976). *Diabetes* 30:279, 1981

15. WALKER A, CUDWORTH AG: Type 1 (insulin-dependent) diabetic multiplex families. Mode of genetic transmission. *Diabetes* 29:1036, 1980

16. NEEL JV: Diabetes mellitus—a geneticist's nightmare, in Creutzfeldt W, Köbberling J, Neel JV (eds): *The Genetics of Diabetes Mellitus.* New York, Springer-Verlag New York, Inc, 1976 p1

17. ROTTER JI, RIMOIN DL: Heterogeneity in diabetes mellitus—update, 1978. *Diabetes* 27:599, 1978

18. TATTERSALL RB, FAJANS SS: A difference between the inheritance of classical juvenile-onset and maturity-onset type diabetes of young people. *Diabetes* 24:44, 1975

19. BARBOSA J, RAMSAY R, GOETZ FC: Plasma glucose, insulin, glucagon, and growth hormone in kindreds with maturity-onset type of hyperglycemia in young people. *Ann Intern Med* 88:595, 1978

20. FRIEDMAN JM, FIALKOW PJ: The genetics of diabetes, in Steinberg AG, Bearn AG, Motulsky AG, Childs B (eds): *Progress in Medical Genetics IV.* Philadelphia, WB Saunders Co, 1980, p 199

21. TATTERSALL R: The inheritance of maturity-onset type diabetes in young people, in Creutzfeldt W, Köbberling J, Neel JV (eds): *The Genetics of Diabetes Mellitus.* New York, Springer-Verlag New York, Inc, 1976, p 88

22. TATTERSALL RB, PYKE DA: Diabetes in identical twins. *Lancet* 2:1120, 1972

23. PYKE DA, NELSON PG: Diabetes mellitus in identical twins, in Creutzfeldt W, Köbberling J, Neel JV (eds): *The Genetics of Diabetes Mellitus* New York, Springer-Verlag New York, Inc, 1976, p 194

24. TATTERSALL R: Diabetes in the offspring of conjugal diabetic parents, in Creutzfeldt W, Köbberling J, Neel JV (eds): *The Genetics of Diabetes Mellitus.* New York, Springer-Verlag New York, Inc, 1976, p 188

25. GANDA OP, SOELDNER JS: Genetic, acquired and related factors in the etiology of diabetes mellitus. *Arch Intern Med* 137:461, 1977

26. BALLY C, SOELDNER JS, GLEASON RE: Frequency of diabetes in offspring (OFF) of diabetic couples (DC). *Diabetes* 25 (suppl 1):335, 1976

27. TATTERSALL RB, FAJANS SS: Prevalence of diabetes and glucose intolerance in 199 offspring of thirty-seven conjugal diabetic parents. *Diabetes* 24:452, 1975

28. GAROVOY MR, BARBOSA J, REDDISH M, MARTIN S, NOREEN H, YUNIS EJ, CARPENTER CB: HLA-DR antigens and unique serologic reactions in juvenile-onset diabetes mellitus. *Transplantation Proc* 10:967, 1978

29. NERUP J: HLA studies in diabetes mellitus: A review. *Adv Metab Disord* 9:263, 1978

30. CHRISTY M, GREEN A, CHRISTAU B, KROMANN H, NERUP J, PLATZ P, THOMSEN M, RYDER LP, SVEJGAARD A: Studies of the HLA system and insulin-dependent diabetes mellitus. *Diabetes Care* 2:209, 1979

31. CUDWORTH AG: The HLA system, autoimmune endocrinopathy and diabetes mellitus. *Eur J Clin Invest* 8:355, 1978

32. BARBOSA J, CHERN MM, ANDERSON VE, NOREEN H, JOHNSON S, REINSMOEN N, MCCARTY R, KING R, GREENBERG L: Linkage analysis between the major histocompatibility system and insulin-dependent diabetes in families with patients in two consecutive generations. *J Clin Invest* 65:592, 1980

33. SERJEANTSON S, KIRK RL, DRY PJ, RYAN DP, COURT J, ZIMMET P, STEPANAS AV: HLA studies in Australian multiple-case families of juvenile onset diabetes millitus. *Med J Aust* 1:107, 1980

34. SACHS JA, CUDWORTH AG, JARAQUEMADA D, GORSUCH AN, FESTENSTEIN H: Type 1 diabetes and the HLA-D locus. *Diabetologia* 18:4l, 1980

35. CUDWORTH AG, FESTENSTEIN H: HLA genetic heterogeneity in diabetes mellitus. *Br Med Bull* 34:285, 1978

36. SVEJGAARD A, PLATZ P, RYDER LP: Insulin-dependent diabetes mellitus, in Terasaki PJ (ed): *Histocompatibility Testing.* Los Angeles, UCLA Tissue Typing Laboratory, 1980, p 638

37. CUDWORTH AG: Type 1 diabetes mellitus. *Diabetologia* 14:281, 1978

38. NAKAO Y, FUKUNISHI T, KOIDE M, AKASAWA K, IKEDA M, YAHATA M, IMURA H: HLA antigens in Japanese patients with diabetes mellitus. *Diabetes* 26:736, 1977

39. MACDONALD MJ: Hypothesis: The frequencies of juvenile diabetes in American blacks and caucasians are consistent with dominant inheritance. *Diabetes* 29:110, 1980

40. RUBINSTEIN P, SUCIU-FOCA N, NICHOLSON JF: Genetics of juvenile diabetes mellitus. A recessive gene closely linked to HLA D and with 50 percent penetrance. *N England J Med* 297:1036, 1977

41. HODGE SE, ROTTER JI, LANGE KL: A three allele model for heterogeneity of juvenile onset insulin dependent diabetes. *Ann Hum Genet* 43:399, 1980

42. ROTTER JI, HODGE SE: Response: Racial differences in juvenile-type diabetes are consistent with more than one mode of inheritance. *Diabetes* 29:115, 1980

43. BARBOSA J, KING R, NOREEN H, YUNIS EJ: The histocompatibility system in juvenile, insulin-dependent diabetic multiplex kindreds. *J Clin Invest* 60:989, 1977

44. KÖBBERLING J: Genetic heterogeneities within idiopathic diabetes, in Creutzfeldt W, Köbberling J, Neel JV (eds): *The Genetics of Diabetes Mellitus.* New York, Springer-Verlag New York, Inc, 1976, p 79

45. BRIGGS BR, JACKSON WPU, DUTOIT ED, BOTHA MC: The histocompatibility (HLA) antigen distribution in diabetes in Southern African blacks (Xhosa). *Diabetes* 29:68, 1980

46. GAMBLE DR: A possible virus etiology for juvenile diabetes, in Creutzfeldt W, Köbberling J, Neel JV (eds): *The Genetics of Diabetes Mellitus.* New York, Springer-Verlag New York, Inc, 1976, p 95

47. RAYFIELD EJ, SETO Y: Viruses and the pathogenesis of diabetes mellitus. *Diabetes* 27:1126, 1978

48. GAMBLE DR, TAYLOR KW, CUMMING H: Coxsackie viruses and diabetes mellitus. *Br Med J* 4:260, 1973

49. NELSON PG, PYKE DA, GAMBLE DR: Viruses and the aetiology of diabetes: A study in identical twins. *Br Med J* 4:249, 1975

50. YOON J-W, AUSTIN M, ONODERA T, NOTKINS AL: Virus-induced diabetes mellitus. Isolation of a virus from the pancreas of a child with diabetic ketoacidosis. *N Engl J Med* 300:1173, 1979

51. YOON J-W, ONODERA T, NOTKINS AL: Virus-induced diabetes mellitus. XV. Beta cell damage and insulin-dependent hyperglycemia in mice infected with Coxsackie virus B4. *J Exp Med* 148:1068, 1978

52. ONODERA T, YOON J-W, BROWN KS, NOTKINS AL: Evidence for a single locus controlling susceptibility to virus-induced diabetes mellitus. *Nature (London)* 274:693, 1978

53. KROMANN H, LERNMARK Å, VESTERGAARD BF, EGEBERG J, NERUP J: The influence of the major histocompatibility complex (H-2) on experimental diabetes in mice. *Diabetologia* 16:107, 1979

54. ONODERA T, JENSON AB, YOON J-W, NOTKINS AL: Virus-induced diabetes mellitus: Reovirus infection of pancreatic β cells in mice. *Science* 201:529, 1978

55. STEFAN Y, MALAISSE-LAGAE F, YOON J-W, NOTKINS AL, ORCI L: Virus-induced diabetes in mice: A quantitative evaluation of islet cell population by immunofluorescence technique. *Diabetologia* 15:395, 1978

56. CHAIREZ R, YOON J-W, NOTKINS AL: Virus-induced diabetes milletus. X. Attachment of encephalomyocarditis virus and permissiveness of cultured pancreatic β-cells to infection. *Virology* 85:606, 1978

57. DAFOE DC, NAJI A, PLOTKIN SA, BARKER CF: Susceptibility to diabetogenic virus: Host versus pancreatic factors. *J Surg Res* 28:338, 1980

58. D'ANDREA BJ, WILSON GL, CRAIGHEAD JE: Effect of genetic obesity in mice on the induction of diabetes by encephalomyocarditis virus. *Diabetes,* 30:451, 1981

59. BOTTAZZO GF, FLORIN-CHRISTENSEN A, DONIACH D: Islet-cell antibodies in diabetes mellitus with autoimmune polyendocrine deficiencies. *Lancet* 2:1279, 1974

60. MACCUISH AC, BARNES EW, IRVINE WJ, DUNCAN LJP: Antibodies to pancreatic islet cells in insulin-dependent diabetes with coexistent autoimmune disease. *Lancet* 2:1529, 1974

61. LENDRUM R, WALKER G, GAMBLE DR: Islet-cell antibodies in juvenile diabetes mellitus of recent onset. *Lancet* 1:880, 1975

62. IRVINE WJ, MCCALLUM CJ, DUNCAN LJP, FARQUHAR JW, VAUGHAN H, MORRIS PJ: Pancreatic islet-cell antibodies in diabetes mellitus correlated with the duration and type of diabetes, coexistent autoimmune disease and HLA type. *Diabetes* 26:138, 1977

63. NEUFELD M, MACLAREN NK, RILEY WJ, LEZOTTE D, MCLAUGHLIN JV, SILVERSTEIN J, ROSENBLOOM AL: Islet cell and other organ-specific antibodies in U.S. caucasians and blacks with insulin-dependent diabetes mellitus. *Diabetes* 29:589, 1980

64. LERNMARK Å, FREEDMAN ZR, HOFMAN C, RUBENSTEIN AH, STEINER DF, JACKSON RL, WINTER RJ, TRAISMAN HS: Islet-cell-surface antibodies in juvenile diabetes mellitus. *N Engl J Med* 299:375, 1978

65. DOBERSEN MJ, SCHARFF JE, GINSBERG-FELLNER F, NOTKINS AL: Cytotoxic autoantibodies to beta cells in the serum of patients with insulin-dependent diabetes mellitus. *N Engl J Med* 303:1493, 1980

66. BOTTAZZO GF, CUDWORTH AG, MOUL DJ, DONIACH D, FESTENSTEIN H: Evidence for a primary autoimmune type of diabetes mellitus. *Br Med J* 2:1253, 1978

67. NAKAO Y, MATSUMOTO H, MIYAZAKI T, MIZUNO N, ARIMA N, WAKISAKA A, OKIMOTO K, AKAZAWA Y, TSUJI K, FUJITA T: IgG heavy-chain (Gm) allotypes and immune response to insulin in insulin-requiring diabetes mellitus. *N Engl J Med* 304:407, 1981

68. GORSUCH AN, DEAN BM, BOTTAZZO GF, LISTER J, CUDWORTH AG: Evidence that type I diabetes and thyrogastric autoimmunity have different genetic determinants. *Br Med J* 280:145, 1980

69. ROSSINI AA, WILLIAMS RM, APPEL MC, LIKE AA: Complete protection from low-dose streptozotocin-induced diabetes in mice. *Nature* 276:182, 1978

70. MACLAREN NK, NEUFELD M, MCLAUGHLIN JV, TAYLOR G: Androgen sensitization of streptozotocin-induced diabetes in mice. *Diabetes* 29:710, 1980

71. BONNEVIE-NIELSEN V, STEFFES MW, LERNMARK Å: A major loss in islet mass and B-cell function preceeds hyperglycemia in mice given multiple low doses of streptozotocin. *Diabetes*, 30:424, 1981

72. KARAM JH, LEWITT PA, YOUNG CW, NOWLAIN RE, FRANKEL BJ, FUJIYA H, FREEDMAN ZR, GRODSKY GM: Insulinopenic diabetes after rodenticide (Vacor) ingestion. A unique model of acquired diabetes in man. *Diabetes* 29:971, 1980

73. HUANG S-W, MACLAREN NK: Insulin-dependent diabetes: A disease of autoaggression. *Science* 192:64, 1976

74. BEATTIE G, LANNOM R, LIPSICK J, KAPLAN NO, OSLER AG: Streptozotocin-induced diabetes in athymic and conventional BALB/c mice. *Diabetes* 29:146, 1980

75. BUSCHARD K, RYGAARD J: Passive transfer of streptozotocin induced diabetes mellitus with spleen cells. *Acta Pathol Microbiol Scand [C]* 85:469, 1977

76. BUSCHARD K, RYGAARD J: T-lymphocytes transfer streptozotocin induced diabetes mellitus in mice. *Acta Pathol Microbiol Scand [C]* 86:277, 1978

77. BUSCHARD K, MADSBAD S, RYGAARD J: Passive transfer of diabetes mellitus from man to mouse. *Lancet* 1:908, 1978.

78. NEUFELD M, MCLAUGHLIN J, MACLAREN NK, ROSENBLOOM E, DONNELLY W: Failure to transfer diabetes mellitus from man to mouse. *N Engl J Med* 301:665, 1979

79. GENUTH SM: Insulin secretion in obesity and diabetes: An illustrative case. *Ann Intern Med* 87:714, 1977

80. OLEFSKY JM: Insulin resistance and insulin action. An *in vitro* and *in vivo* perspective. *Diabetes* 30:148, 1981

81. REAVEN GM, BERNSTEIN R, DAVIS B, OLEFSKY JM: Nonketotic diabetes mellitus: Insulin deficiency or insulin resistance? *Am J Med* 60:80, 1976

81a. GINSBERG H, RAYFIELD EJ: Effect of insulin therapy on insulin resistance in Type II diabetic subjects. Evidence for heterogeneity. *Diabetes* 30:739, 1981

81b. KARNIELI E, HISSIN PJ, SIMPSON IA, SALANS LB, CUSHMAN SW: A possible mechanism of insulin resistance in the rat adipose cell in streptozotocin-induced diabetes mellitus. Depletion of intracellular glucose transport systems. *J Clin Invest* 68:811, 1981

82. SPERLING MA, BACON G, KENNY FM, DRASH AL: Cortisol secretion in acidotic and nonacidotic diabetes mellitus. *Am J Dis Child* 124:690, 1972

83. CRYER PE, SILVERBERG AB, SANTIAGO JV, SHAH SD: Plasma catecholamines in diabetes. The syndromes of hypoadrenergic and hyperadrenergic postural hypotension. *Am J Med* 64:407, 1978

84. SANTIAGO JV, CLARKE WL, SHAH SD, CRYER PE: Epinephrine, norepinephrine, glucagon and growth hormone release in association with physiological decrements in the plasma glucose concentration in normal and diabetic man. *J Clin Endocrinol Metab* 51:877, 1980

85. HAYFORD JT, DANNEY MM, HENDRIX JA, THOMPSON RG: Integrated concentration of growth hormone in juvenile-onset diabetes. *Diabetes* 29:391, 1980

86. ZADIK Z, KAYNE R, KAPPY M, PLOTNICK LP, KOWARSKI AA: Increased integrated concentration of norepinephrine, epinephrine, aldosterone and growth hormone in patients with uncontrolled juvenile diabetes mellitus. *Diabetes* 29:655, 1980

87. SCHADE DS, EATON RP: The controversy concerning counterregulatory hormone secretion. A hypothesis for the prevention of diabetic ketoacidosis? *Diabetes* 26:596, 1977

88. CRYER PE: Glucose counter-regulation in man. *Diabetes* 30:261, 1981

89. UNGER RH: The milieu interieur and the islets of Langerhans. *Diabetologia* 20:1, 1981

90. UNGER RH, ORCI L: Hypothesis. The essential role of glucagon in the pathogenesis of diabetes mellitus. *Lancet* 1:14, 1975

91. UNGER RH: Role of glucagon in the pathogenesis of diabetes: The status of the controversy. *Metabolism* 27:1691, 1978

92. RASKIN P, PIETRI A, UNGER RH: Changes in glucagon levels after four to five weeks of glucoregulation by portable insulin infusion pumps. *Diabetes* 28:1033, 1979

93. KAWAMORI R, SHICHIRI M, KIKUCHI M, YAMASAKI Y, ABE H: Perfect normalization of excessive glucagon responses to intravenous arginine in human diabetes mellitus with the artificial beta-cell. *Diabetes* 29:762, 1980

94. CZECH MP: Insulin action and the regulation of hexose transport. *Diabetes* 29:399, 1980

95. KHOO JC, STEINBERG D, THOMPSON B, MAYER SE: Hormonal regulation of adipocyte enzymes. The effects of epinephrine and insulin on the control of lipase, phosphorylase kinase, phosphorylase and glycogen synthase. *J Biol Chem* 248:3823, 1973

96. JEFFERSON LS: Role of insulin in the regulation of protein synthesis. *Diabetes* 29:487, 1980

97. STRICKLAND WG, BLACKMORE PF, EXTON JH: The role of calcium in alpha-adrenergic inactivation of glycogen synthase in rat hepatocytes and its inhibition by insulin. *Diabetes* 29:617, 1980

98. BOYD ME, ALBRIGHT EB, FOSTER DW, MCGARRY JD: *In vitro* reversal of the fasting state of liver metabolism in the rat. Reevaluation of the roles of insulin and glucose. *J Clin Invest*, 68:142, 1981

99. LARNER J, GALASKO G, CHENG K, DEPAOLI-ROACH AA, HUANG L, DAGGY P, KELLOGG J: Generation by insulin of a chemical mediator that controls protein phosphorylation and dephosphorylation. *Science* 206:1408, 1979

100. JARETT L, SEALS JR: Pyruvate dehydrogenase activation in adipocyte mitochondria by an insulin-generated mediator from muscle. *Science* 206:1407, 1979

101. CHENG K, GALASKO G, HUANG L, KELLOGG J, LARNER J: Studies on the insulin mediator. II. Separation of two antagonistic biologically active materials from fraction II. *Diabetes* 29:659, 1980

102. HUTSON NJ, BRUMLEY FT, ASSIMACOPOULOS FD, HARPER SC, EXTON JH: Studies on the α-adrenergic activation of hepatic glucose output. Studies on the α-adrenergic activation of phosphorylase and gluconeogenesis and inactivation of glycogen synthase in isolated rat liver parenchymal cells. *J Biol Chem* 251:5200, 1976

103. BLACKMORE PF, ASSIMACOPOULOS-JEANNET F, CHAN TM, EXTON JH: Studies on α-adrenergic activation of hepatic glucose output. Insulin inhibition of α-adrenergic and glucagon actions in normal and calcium depleted hepatocytes. *J Biol Chem* 254:2828, 1979

104. MCGARRY JD, WRIGHT PH, FOSTER DW: Hormonal control of ketogenesis. Rapid activation of hepatic ketogenic capacity in fed rats by anti-insulin serum and glucagon. *J Clin Invest* 55:1202, 1975

105. WITTERS LA, KOWALOFF EM, AVRUCH J: Glucagon regulation of protein phosphorylation. Identification of acetyl coenzyme A carboxylase as a substrate. *J Biol Chem* 254:245, 1979

106. BIRNBAUM MJ, FAIN JN: Activation of protein kinase and glycogen phosphorylase in isolated rat liver cells by glucagon and catecholamines. *J Biol Chem* 252:528, 1977

107. RUDERMAN NB, AOKI TT, CAHILL GF, JR: Gluconeogenesis and its disorders in man, in Hanson RW, Mehlman MA (eds): *Gluconeogenesis: Its Regulation in Mammalian Species*. New York, John Wiley & Sons, Inc, 1976, p 515

108. OWEN OE, PATEL MS, BLOCK BSB, KREULEN TH, REICHLE FA, MAZZOLI MA: Gluconeogenesis in normal, cirrhotic, and diabetic humans, in Hanson RW, Mehlman MA (eds): *Gluconeogenesis: Its Regulation in Mammalian Species*. New York, John Wiley & Sons, Inc, 1976, p 533

109. MILES JM, RIZZA RA, HAYMOND MW, GERICH JE: Effects of acute insulin deficiency on glucose and ketone body turnover in man. Evidence for the primacy of overproduction of glucose and ketone bodies in the genesis of diabetic ketoacidosis. *Diabetes* 29:926, 1980

110. CHERRINGTON AD, WILLIAMS PE, LILJENQUIST JE, LACY WW: The control of glycogenolysis and gluconeogenesis *in vivo* by insulin and glucagon, in Pierluissi J (ed): *Endocrine Pancreas and Diabetes*. Amsterdam, Excerpta Medica, 1979, p 172

111. CUSHMAN SW, WARDZALA LJ: Potential mechanism of insulin action on glucose transport in the isolated rat adipose cell. Apparent translocation of intracellular transport systems to the plasma membrane. *J Biol Chem* 255:4758, 1980

111a. KARNIELI E, ZARNOWSKI MJ, HISSIN PJ, SIMPSON HJ, SALANS LB, CUSHMAN SW: Insulin-stimulated translocation of glucose transport systems in the isolated rat adipose cell. Time course, reversal, insulin concentration dependency, and relationship to glucose transport activity. *J Biol Chem* 256:4772, 1981

112. CARTER-SU C, CZECH MP: Reconstitution of D-glucose transport activity from cytoplasmic membranes. Evidence against recruitment of cytoplasmic membrane transporters into the plasma membrane as the sole action of insulin. *J Biol Chem* 255:10382, 1980

113. GERICH JE, LORENZI M, BIER DM, SCHNEIDER V, TSALIKIAN E, KARAM JH, FORSHAM PH: Prevention of human diabetic ketoacidosis by somatostatin. Evidence for an essential role of glucagon. *N Engl J Med* 292:985, 1975

114. UNGER RH: Diabetes and the alpha cell. *Diabetes* 25:136, 1976

115. UNGER RH, ORCI L: Glucagon and the A-cell: Physiology and pathophys-

iology. *N Engl J Med,* 304:1518 and 1575, 1981

116. ORCI L, BAETENS D, RUFENER C, AMHERDT M, RAVAZZOLA M, STUDER P, MALAISSE-LAGAE F, UNGER RH: Hypertrophy and hyperplasia of somatostatin-containing D-cells in diabetes. *Proc Natl Acad Sci USA* 73:1338, 1976

117. MACKES K, ITOH M, GREEN K, GERICH J: Radioimmunoassay of human plasma somatostatin. *Diabetes,* 30:728, 1981

118. MCGARRY JD, FOSTER DW: Hormonal control of ketogenesis. Biochemical considerations. *Arch Intern Med* 137:495, 1977

119. MCGARRY JD, FOSTER DW: Regulation of hepatic fatty acid oxidation and ketone body production. *Ann Rev Biochem* 49:395, 1980

119a. UYEDA K, FURUYA E, LUBY LJ: The effect of natural and synthetic D-fructose 2,6-bisphosphate on the regulatory kinetic properties of liver and muscle phosphofructokinases. *J Biol Chem* 256:8394, 1981

120. MCGARRY JD, FOSTER DW: The regulation of ketogenesis from octanoic acid. The role of the tricarboxylic acid cycle and fatty acid synthesis. *J Biol Chem* 246:1149, 1971

121. MCGARRY JD, LEATHERMAN GF, FOSTER DW: Carnitine palmitoyltransferase I. The site of inhibition of hepatic fatty acid oxidation by malonyl-CoA. *J Biol Chem* 253:4128, 1978

122. MCGARRY JD, ROBLES-VALDES C, FOSTER DW: Role of carnitine in hepatic ketogenesis. *Proc Natl Acad Sci USA* 72:4385, 1975

123. MCGARRY JD, FOSTER DW: Regulation of ketogenesis and clinical aspects of the ketotic state. *Metabolism* 21:471, 1972

124. KREISBERG RA: Diabetic ketoacidosis: New concepts and trends in pathogenesis and treatment. *Ann Intern Med* 88:681, 1978

125. FOSTER DW: Diabetes mellitus, in Isselbacher KJ, Adams RD, Braunwald E, Petersdorf RG, Wilson JD (eds): *Harrison's Principles of Internal Medicine,* ed. 9. New York, McGraw-Hill Book Co, 1980, p 1741

126. FEIG PU, MCCURDY DK: The hypertonic state. *N Engl J Med* 297:1444, 1977

127. FOSTER DW: Insulin deficiency and hyperosmolar coma. *Adv Intern Med* 19:159, 1974

128. ARIEFF AI, CARROLL HJ: Nonketotic hyperosmolar coma with hyperglycemia: Clinical features, pathophysiology, renal function, acid-base balance, plasma-cerebrospinal fluid equilibria and the effects of therapy in 37 cases. *Medicine* 51:73, 1972

129. MA GY, GOVE CD, HEMS DA: Effects of glucagon and insulin on fatty acid synthesis and glycogen degradation in the perfused liver of normal and genetically obese (ob/ob) mice. *Biochem J* 174:761, 1978

130. MARLISS EB, MURRAY FT, STOKES EF, ZINMAN B, NAKHOODA AF, DENOGA A, LEIBEL BS, ALBISSER AM: Normalization of glycemia in diabetics during meals with insulin and glucagon delivery by the artificial pancreas. *Diabetes* 26:663, 1977

131. SANTIAGO JV, CLARKE WL, SHAH SD, CRYER PE: Epinephrine, norepinephrine, glucagon and growth hormone release in association with physiological decrements in plasma glucose concentration in normal and diabetic man. *J Clin Endocrinol Metab* 51:877, 1980

132. SACCA L, SHERWIN R, HENDLER R, FELIG P: Influence of continuous physiologic hyperinsulinemia on glucose kinetics and counterregulatory hormones in normal and diabetic humans. *J Clin Invest* 63:849, 1979

133. DEFRONZO RA, HENDLER R, CHRISTENSEN N: Stimulation of counterregulatory hormonal responses in diabetic man by a fall in glucose concentration. *Diabetes* 29:125, 1980

134. SHAMOON H, HENDLER R, SHERWIN RS: Altered responsiveness to cortisol, epinephrine, and glucagon in insulin-infused juvenile-onset diabetics. A mechanism for diabetic instability. *Diabetes* 29:284, 1980

135. RASKIN P: Diabetic regulation and its relationship to microangiopathy. *Metabolism* 27:235, 1978

136. PAZ-GUEVARA AT, HSU T-H, WHITE P: Juvenile diabetes mellitus after forty years. *Diabetes* 24:559, 1975

137. OAKLEY WG, PYKE DA, TATTERSALL RB, WATKINS PJ: Long-term diabetes. A clinical study of 92 patients after 40 years. *Quart J Med* 169:145, 1974

138. LESTRADET H, PAPOZ L, HELLOUIN DE MENIBUS C, LEVAVASSEUR F, BESSE J, BILLAUD L, BATTISTELLI F, TRIC P, LESTRADET F: Long-term study of mortality and vascular complications in juvenile-onset (Type 1) diabetes. *Diabetes* 30:175, 1981

139. LIANG JC, GOLDBERG MF: Treatment of diabetic retinopathy. *Diabetes* 29:841, 1980

140. BROWNLEE M, CAHILL GF, JR: Diabetic control and vascular complications, in Paoletti R, Gotto AM, Jr (eds): *Atherosclerosis Reviews.* New York, Raven Press, 1979, vol 4, p 29

141. JONES RL, PARADISE C, PETERSON CM: Platelet survival in patients with diabetes mellitus. *Diabetes,* 30:486, 1981

142. PIETRI A, EHLE AL, RASKIN P: Changes in nerve conduction velocity after six weeks of glucoregulation with portable insulin infusion pumps. *Diabetes* 29:668, 1980

143. PETERSON CM, JONES RL, ESTERLY JA, WANTZ GE, JACKSON RL: Changes in basement membrane thickening and pulse volume with improved glucose control and exercise in patients with insulin-dependent diabetes mellitus. *Diabetes Care* 3:586, 1980

144. MAUER SM, BARBOSA J, VERNIER RL, KJELLSTRAND CM, BUSELMEIER TJ, SIMMONS RL, NAJARIAN JS, GOETZ FC: Development of diabetic vascular lesions in normal kidneys transplanted into patients with diabetes mellitus. *N Engl J Med* 295:916, 1976

145. KNOWLES HC: The problem of the relationship of the control of diabetes to the development of vascular disease. *Trans Am Clin Climatol Assoc* 76:142, 1964

146. BURDITT AF, CAIRD FI, DRAPER GJ: The history of diabetic retinopathy. *Quart J Med* 37:303, 1968

147. MALONE JI, VAN CADER TC, EDWARDS WC: Diabetic vascular changes in children. *Diabetes* 26:673, 1977

148. SOLER NG, FITZGERALD MG, MALINS JM, SUMMERS ROC: Retinopathy at diagnosis of diabetes, with special reference to patients under 40 years of age. *Br Med J* 3:567, 1969

149. HUTTON WL, SNYDER WB, VAISER A, SIPERSTEIN MD: Retinal microangiopathy without associated glucose intolerance. *Trans Am Acad Ophth Otol* 76:968, 1972

150. SIPERSTEIN MD, UNGER RH, MADISON LL: Studies of muscle capillary basement membranes in normal subjects, diabetic, and pre-diabetic patients. *J Clin Invest* 47:1973, 1968

151. MARKS JF, RASKIN P, STASTNY P: Increase in capillary basement membrane width in parents of children with type I diabetes mellitus. Association with HLA-DR4. *Diabetes,* 30:475, 1981

152. BUNN HF: Evaluation of glycosylated hemoglobin in diabetic patients. *Diabetes,* 30:613, 1981

153. DAY JF, THORPE SR, BAYNES JW: Nonenzymatically glucosylated albumin. *In vitro* preparation and isolation from normal human serum. *J Biol Chem* 254:595, 1979

154. MILLER JA, GRAVALLESE EG, BUNN HF: Nonenzymatic glycosylation of erythrocyte membrane proteins. Relevance to diabetes. *J Clin Invest* 65:896, 1980

155. STEVENS VJ, ROUZER CA, MONNIER VM, CERAMI A: Diabetic cataract formation: Potential role of glycosylation in lens crystalline. *Proc Natl Acad Sci USA* 75:2918, 1978

156. FLÜCKIGER R, WINTERHALTER KH: Glycosylated hemoglobins, in Caughey WS (ed): *Biochemical and Clinical Aspects of Hemoglobin Abnormalities.* New York, Academic Press, Inc, 1978, p 205

157. PETERSON CM, JONES RL: Minor hemoglobins, diabetic "control," and diseases of postsynthetic protein modification. *Ann Intern Med* 87:489, 1977

158. DOLHOFFER R, WIELAND OH: Increased glycosylation of serum albumin in diabetes mellitus. *Diabetes* 29:417, 1980

159. COMPAGNUCCI P, CARTECHINI MG, BOLLI G, DE FEO P, SANTEUSANIO F, BRUNETTI P: The importance of determining irreversibly-glycosylated hemoglobin in diabetics. *Diabetes,* 30:607, 1981

159a. NATHAN DN, AVEZZANO ES, PALMER JL: A rapid chemical means for removing labile glycohemoglobin. *Diabetes* 30:700, 1981

160. TATTERSALL RB: Home blood glucose monitoring. *Diabetologia* 16:71, 1979

161. PETERSON CM, JOVANOVIC LB, BROWNLEE M, JONES RL, CERAMI A: Closing the loop: Practical and theoretical. *Diabetes Care* 3:318, 1980

162. CHAMPION MC, SHEPHERD GAA, RODGER NW, DUPRE J: Continuous subcutaneous infusion of insulin in the management of diabetes mellitus. *Diabetes* 29:206, 1980

163. PETERSON CM, JONES RL, DUPUIS A, LEVINE BS, BERNSTEIN R, O'SHEA M: Feasibility of improved blood glucose control in patients with insulin-dependent diabetes mellitus. *Diabetes Care* 2:329, 1979

164. DRASH AL, DANEMAN D, TRAVIS L: Progressive retinopathy with improved metabolic control in diabetic dwarfism (Mauriac's syndrome). *Diabetes* 29 (suppl 2):1A, 1980

165. TAMBORLANE W, SHERWIN R, BERGMAN M, EBERSOLE J, PUKLIN J, FELIG P: Can treatment of diabetes with a portable insulin pump reverse diabetic complications? *Diabetes* (suppl 2):18A, 1980

166. TAGER H, GIVEN B, BALDWIN D, MAKO M, MARKESE J, RUBENSTEIN A, OLEFSKY J, KOBAYASHI M, KOLTERMAN O, POUCHER R: A structurally abnormal insulin causing human diabetes. *Nature (London)* 281:122, 1979

167. GIVEN BD, MAKO ME, TAGER HS, BALDWIN D, MARKESE J, RUBENSTEIN AH, OLEFSKY J, KOBAYASHI M, KOLTERMAN O, POUCHER R: Diabetes due to secretion of an abnormal insulin. *N Engl J Med* 302:129, 1980

168. OLEFSKY JM, SAEKOW M, TAGER H, RUBENSTEIN AH: Characterization of a mutant human insulin species *J Biol Chem* 255:6098, 1980

169. KWOK SC, CHAN SJ, RUBENSTEIN AH, POUCHER R, STEINER DF: Loss of a restriction endonuclease cleavage site in the gene of a structurally abnormal human insulin. *Biochem Biophys Res Com* 98:844, 1981

170. GABBAY KH, BERGENSTAL RM, WOLFF J, MAKO ME, RUBENSTEIN AH: Familial hyperproinsulinemia: Partial characterization of circulating proinsulin-like material. *Proc Natl Acad Sci USA* 76:2881: 1979

171. OWERBACH D, BELL GI, RUTTER WJ, SHOWS TB: The insulin gene is located on chromosome 11 in humans. *Nature (London)* 286:82, 1980
172. OWERBACH D, BELL GI, RUTTER WJ, BROWN JA, SHOWS TB: The insulin gene is located on the short arm of chromosome 11 in humans. *Diabetes* 30:267, 1981
173. BAUMAN WA, YALOW RS: Immunologic potency of recombined A- and B-chains of synthetic human and pancreatic pork insulins. *Diabetes* 30:265, 1981
174. CHAN SJ, KWOK SCM, STEINER DF: The biosynthesis of insulin: Some genetic and evolutionary aspects. *Diabetes Care* 4:4, 1981

175. FLIER JS, KAHN CR, ROTH J: Receptors, antireceptor antibodies and mechanisms of insulin resistance. *N Engl J Med* 300:413, 1979
176. GRUNFELD C, VAN OBBERGHEN E, KARLSSON FA, KAHN CR: Antibody-induced desensitization of the insulin receptor. Studies of the mechanism of desensitization in 3T3-L1 fatty fibroblasts. *J Clin Invest* 66:1124, 1980
177. KASUGA M, VAN OBBERGHEN E, YAMADA KM, HARRISON LC: Autoantibodies against the insulin receptor recognize the insulin binding subunits of an oligomeric receptor. *Diabetes* 30:354, 1981

5

ESSENTIAL FRUCTOSURIA, HEREDITARY FRUCTOSE INTOLERANCE, AND FRUCTOSE-1,6-DIPHOSPHATASE DEFICIENCY

RICHARD GITZELMANN

BEAT STEINMANN

GEORGES VAN DEN BERGHE

1. *Fructose is an important source of dietary carbohydrates. In Western societies, the average daily intake is presently about 50 to 100 g. The liver, kidney, and small intestine are the main sites of fructose metabolism, but adipose tissue participates. Fructose, given intravenously in high doses, is clearly toxic and causes hyperuricemia, hyperlactatemia, and ultrastructural alterations in liver and intestinal cells.*

2. *Essential fructosuria is a benign, asymptomatic metabolic anomaly caused by the absence of fructokinase. Alimentary hyperfructosemia and fructosuria are the principal signs. In spite of the interruption of the specific fructose pathway, up to nine-tenths of the administered fructose is retained by fructokinase-deficient subjects.*

3. *Hereditary fructose intolerance is characterized by severe hypoglycemia and vomiting shortly after the intake of fructose. Prolonged fructose ingestion in infants leads to poor feeding, vomiting, hepatomegaly, jaundice, hemorrhage, a proximal renal tubular syndrome, and finally, hepatic failure and death. Patients develop a strong distaste for sweet food. A chronic course is, therefore, observed only in the preschool-age child. Fructose-1-phosphate aldolase of liver, kidney cortex, and small intestine is deficient. Hypoglycemia after fructose ingestion is caused by fructose-1-phosphate inhibiting glycogenolysis at the phosphorylase*

level and gluconeogenesis at the mutant aldolase level. Patients remain healthy on a fructose- and sucrose-free diet.

4. *Hereditary fructose-1,6-diphosphatase deficiency is characterized by episodic spells of hyperventilation, apnea, hypoglycemia, ketosis, and lactic acidosis, with a precipitous and often lethal course in the newborn infant. Later episodes are often triggered by fasting and febrile infections. Due to the enzyme defect, gluconeogenesis is severely impaired. Gluconeogenic precursors such as amino acids, lactate, and ketones accumulate as soon as liver glycogen stores are depleted. Patients do not vomit after fructose intake and do not develop aversion to sweets. Their tolerance to fasting grows with age. Patients past early childhood seem to develop normally.*

5. *All three defects are inherited as autosomal recessive traits.*

Three inherited abnormalities of fructose metabolism are known. Two of these are caused by a defect of one of the enzymes of the specialized fructose pathway: *essential fructosuria* and *hereditary fructose intolerance*, the former a harmless and the latter a potentially lethal condition. Although not a defect of the specialized fructose pathway, the more recently described hepatic *fructose-1,6-diphosphatase deficiency* is usually classified as an error of fructose metabolism. The defect of this enzyme of the gluconeogenic pathway becomes clinically manifest through hypoglycemia and lactic acidosis on fasting and may also be life-threatening. The description of the clinical symptoms and biochemical anomalies in the three inborn errors of metabolism will be preceded by an outline of the metabolism of fructose. The potential toxic effects of fructose loads on normal organisms will also be discussed since their comprehension is essential for the understanding of the pathophysiology of hereditary fructose intolerance and of fructose-1,6-diphosphatase deficiency.

METABOLISM OF FRUCTOSE

Sources and Uses of Fructose

The ketohexose fructose is a natural component of many plants and honey. As the free monosaccharide, it is widely distributed among vegetables and fruits, where it can account for up to 40 percent of the dry weight. As the disaccharide sucrose, which consists of one molecule each of glucose and fructose, it is found in even more numerous nutrients and thus constitutes an important source of dietary carbohydrate. Lists of the fructose content of various foodstuffs are available [1, 2].

Fructose, as sucrose or the free monosaccharide, is widely used for nutrition or as a sweetening additive in foods and medications and even in infant formulas. In Western societies, its average daily intake is presently about 50 to 100 g. Recent statistics reveal a trend toward further increases of the consumption of free fructose [3]. This may be explained by its sweetening power, which, for the same caloric intake, is approximately 1.7-fold that of sucrose, and by the development of new technologies for its industrial production. In view of animal and human observations indicating that the ketohexose may elevate plasma triglycerides, the increase in the consumption of fructose has provoked concern and has been discussed at several symposiums [4–6].

Medical uses for fructose have also been advocated. The observation by Minkowski in 1893 [7] that the utilization of fructose does not require insulin resulted in the still widespread belief that fructose is an adequate sweetening agent in the diet of patients with diabetes mellitus, an issue outside the scope of this chapter. The development of intravenous nutrition in the early fifties has led to the utilization of fructose as a source of energy. Solutions of equimolar amounts of fructose and glucose, prepared by the hydrolysis of sucrose and known as *invert sugar,* as well as solutions of pure fructose, sometimes named *levulose,* are available. The infusion of both solutions carries important risks to normal individuals and becomes life-threatening in hereditary fructose intolerance and fructose-1, 6-diphosphatase deficiency. Their use as glucose substitutes for parenteral nutrition should be discouraged.

The polyol sorbitol constitutes another source of fructose. It is converted to fructose in the liver by sorbitol dehydrogenase, and its further metabolism is thus identical to that of the ketose. Although less abundant than fructose, sorbitol is also widely distributed in fruits and vegetables. Its chemical stability has led to its use as a substitute for glucose in infusion solutions. It is also widely used as a sweetener for diabetic

patients. For the same reasons as noted for fructose and invert sugar, it should not be used for parenteral nutrition. Insulin, a polymer of fructose, is present in vegetables such as chicory and sweet potatoes. It may be hydrolyzed to fructose in acid at high temperature, but only insignificant quantities are split and absorbed as fructose in the intestine. Fructose is also present in the tri- and tetrasaccharides raffinose and stachyose, but these play no role in human nutrition.

Detection, Identification, and Measurement of Fructose

The reducing capacity of fructose is approximately 98 percent that of glucose. Fructose is detected by all reactions based on the reducing properties of sugars. The older term, *levulose,* indicates its optical levorotatory power. Fructose is fermented by yeast but is not attacked by glucose oxidase. The Seliwanoff reaction, based on the conversion of fructose to hydroxymethylfurfural and condensation with resorcinol in hot acid, was adapted by Roe et al. [8] and by Higashi and Peters [9] for the quantitative determination of fructose in blood and urine. It is not entirely specific for fructose. Pentoses, and to a lesser extent glucose, may interfere. The prior removal of glucose by incubation with glucose oxidase has proved valuable. The osazones of fructose and glucose are identical.

In order to prove that a reducing substance which gives a positive Seliwanoff reaction is fructose, one must resort to identification by chromatography. The best quantitative and entirely specific assay for fructose uses the enzymes hexokinase, phosphoglucose isomerase, and glucose-6-phosphate dehydrogenase. After the conversion of glucose to 6-phosphogluconate, phosphoglucose isomerase is added to the incubation mixture, allowing fructose-6-phosphate to be converted to 6-phosphogluconate and to be measured by the stoichiometric reduction of nicotinamide adenine dinucleotide phosphate (NADP).

Fructose Transport

The study of the membrane transport of fructose is complicated by the possibility of the ketohexose being rapidly utilized after its cellular penetration, especially in tissues which possess the specialized enzymes of fructose metabolism. In the small intestine, investigations of fructose absorption are further confounded by species differences. In humans [10] and the rat [11], a large proportion of the ingested fructose appears to be absorbed unchanged, but in the guinea pig [11, 12], hamster [13], and dog [14], the ketohexose is metabolized further in the intestinal wall. Most investigations support the existence of a specific intestinal transport system for D-fructose, which is distinct from that of glucose and operates more slowly. Fructose influx is a saturable function of concentration that conforms to Michaelis-Menten kinetics. In the rat intestine, the concentration of the ketohexose required for half-maximal influx is approximately 100 mM [15, 16], but lower values have been determined in other species. There is considerable controversy concerning the dependence of intestinal fructose transport on energy. A carrier-mediated diffusion process [15, 17, 18] as well as an active transport mechanism [16, 19–21] has been proposed.

Fructose does not enter the hepatocyte freely, as evidenced

by the steep gradient between its extra- and intracellular concentrations [22, 23]. Computations from the kinetics of fructose uptake and metabolism in the perfused rat liver [23] are in accordance with a carrier-mediated transport with a K_m of 67 mM and a V_{max} equal to 30 μmol/min per gram of tissue. Even higher K_m values have been obtained by direct measurement of transport rates in isolated hepatocytes [24].

Investigations of fructose uptake in adipose tissue indicate that the ketohexose can be transported by two different carriers [25–27]. A specific carrier for fructose, with a half-saturation concentration of 25 mM, is insensitive to glucose inhibition and independent of insulin. Fructose can also be transported, although only in the absence of glucose, by the glucose carrier which has a fivefold lower K_m and also a lower V_{max}, which is increased by insulin.

Investigations of the utilization of fructose in humans have shown that there is virtually no renal threshold for this ketose, since it is lost even at low blood levels [28–31]. These urinary losses account, nevertheless, for only a few percent of the administered dose.

The extracellular concentrations of fructose after its oral or intravenous administration are lower than the affinity constants of the different fructose carriers. After fructose ingestion, the concentration of fructose in hepatic portal blood reaches about 1.5 mmol/liter (27 mg/dl) in humans [32] and animals [33, 34]. When the ketohexose is administered by continuous infusion, its concentration in peripheral blood increases linearly with the infusion rate. In men, at rates of 0.5, 1.0, and 1.5 g fructose per kilogram per hour, fructosemia reaches 42, 87, and 140 mg/dl, and renal loss amounts to 2.0, 5.0, and 5.7 percent of the administered dose [29, 31]. The plasma concentration of fructose will thus control the rate of entry of fructose into the cell. It will also determine the rate of phosphorylation of fructose in the tissues that possess fructokinase, since this enzyme has a similar V_{max} but an approximately hundred-fold higher affinity for fructose (see below) than the carrier-mediated transport of the ketohexose.

Sites of Fructose Metabolism

In humans and laboratory animals the liver, and to a smaller extent the kidney and small intestine, are the main sites of fructose metabolism [34–38]. These tissues possess a specialized pathway composed of three enzymes: fructokinase, aldolase type B, and triokinase, that convert fructose to intermediates of the glycolytic-gluconeogenic pathway (Fig. 5-1). The ketohexose is thus metabolized mainly to glucose and lactate. Fructokinase phosphorylates fructose into fructose-1-phosphate. The high affinity for its substrates and the high activity of the enzyme explain the preferential utilization of fructose by the organs mentioned above, a process long known to be independent of insulin [7, 28, 39].

In other tissues fructose can in theory be utilized after phosphorylation to fructose-6-phosphate by hexokinase. Conversion is limited in vivo by the physiologic level of glucose, since the affinity of hexokinase for glucose exceeds that for fructose by several orders of magnitude [40, 41]. The capacity of various tissues to metabolize fructose has been investigated by Froesch and Ginsberg [25, 26]. Normal human erythrocytes and leukocytes metabolize fructose nearly as fast as glucose, but solely in the absence of glucose. In rat diaphragm, the utilization of fructose is only 50 percent inhibited by the addition

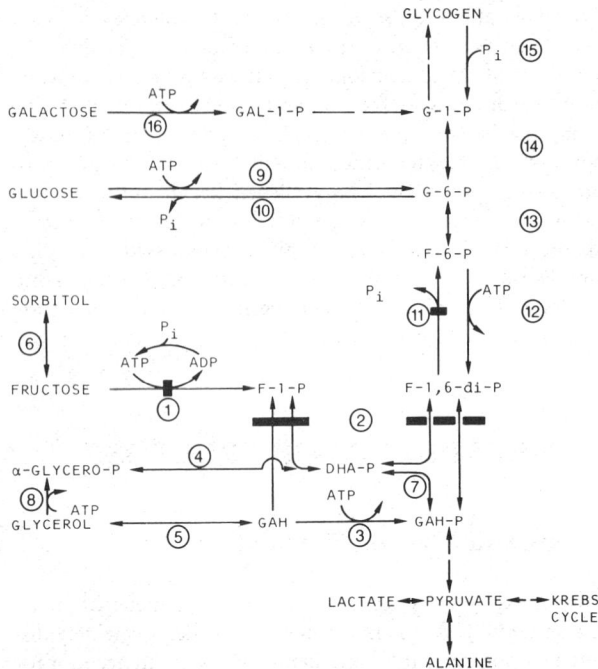

Figure 5-1 The pathway of fructose metabolism in the liver and its defects. DHA, dihydroxyacetone; GAH, glyceraldehyde; (1) fructokinase, (2) aldolase, (3) triokinase, (4) α-glycerophosphate dehydrogenase, (5) alcohol dehydrogenase, (6) sorbitol dehydrogenase, (7) triose phosphate isomerase, (8) glycerol kinase, (9) hexokinase, (10) glucose-6-phosphatase, (11) fructose-1,6-diphosphatase, (12) phosphofructokinase, (13) phosphohexose isomerase, (14) phosphoglucomutase, (15) glycogen phosphorylase, (16) galactokinase.

of glucose at physiologic concentrations. This is explained by the low intracellular concentration of free glucose. The participation of muscle in the metabolism of fructose is of little significance since it utilizes fructose at no more than one-fifth of the rate for glucose. Adipose tissue, in contrast, may participate in fructose uptake. Indeed, fructose metabolism proceeds almost as fast as glucose metabolism in this tissue, with little or no inhibition by glucose. This can be explained by the virtual absence of free glucose in the adipocyte because of the binding of the hexose to its carrier.

Studies of the metabolism of fructose in the body as a whole demonstrate that the ketohexose is also utilized by peripheral tissues after its conversion to glucose in the liver [42–44]. This peripheral utilization evidently requires insulin.

Enzymes of Fructose Metabolism

The properties of the specialized enzymes of fructose metabolism will only be summarized here. A detailed account of the experiments that led to the elucidation of the fructose pathway can be found in a monograph by Hers [45]. Most studies have been performed with liver enzymes, although these reactions have also been located in the kidney and small intestine.

Fructokinase (EC 2.7.1.3) Fructokinase catalyzes the phosphorylation of fructose to fructose-1-phosphate [46–48]. The phosphoryl donor is ATP as the Mg^{2+} complex [49]. The enzyme requires high concentrations of KCl and has a high affinity for fructose, with a K_m of about 0.5 mM [48, 50–52]. Affinity constants for Mg^{2+}-ATP, obtained by different authors, vary between 0.2 and 1 to 2 mM [50–53]. Measurements of V_{max} in crude extracts from rat liver provided values of 2.2 to 3.1 μmol/min per gram of tissue at 22 to 25 °C [22, 51, 54, 55]. Fructokinase is not specific for fructose [48, 51, 52, 56, 57] since it also catalyses the phosphorylation of L-sorbose, D-tagatose, D-xylulose, and L-galactoheptulose. It can therefore be regarded as a ketohexokinase.

Aldolase (EC 2.1.2.13)   Liver aldolase splits fructose-1-phosphate to D-glyceraldehyde and dihydroxyacetone phosphate [58, 59]. The same enzyme catalyzes the splitting of fructose-1,6-diphosphate to D-glyceraldehyde-3-phosphate and dihydroxyacetone phosphate and the condensation of the trioses. Liver aldolase has the same maximal activity with fructose-1, 6-diphosphate as with fructose-1-phosphate [58]. Vertebrates possess three homologous fructaldolases termed *A, B,* and *C* which are distinct proteins, structurally closely related but immunochemically distinguishable without cross reactions [60, 61]. The proteins are composed of four subunits of the three known monomer types A, B, and C to form the prevalent homopolymers with molecular weights of 160,000 [62]. Hybrids are also formed [63], but at least in skeletal muscle, subunit exchange does not occur in vivo [64]. An interesting developmental transition from the predominance of aldolase A toward that of aldolase B is observed in the human liver, kidney, and small intestine [65, 66]. As the catalytic properties of aldolases A, B, and C are different [62, 67] (see Table 5-4), the transition suggests adaptation to the specific metabolic needs during ontogeny. It is of special interest that in small intestinal epithelium, aldolase A predominates in the rapidly dividing crypt cells and aldolase B in the absorptive villus cells [68]. In the kidney, aldolase B appears primarily in the proximal tubules, whereas aldolase A is predominant in the distal tubules and glomeruli [69, 70].

The kinetic parameters of liver aldolase are similar to those of fructokinase: The V_{max} reaches 1.6 [54] to 3.4 μmol/min per gram of tissue [22] at 25 °C. Michaelis constants appear to vary between humans and animals. The K_m of human aldolase B was given as 7.5 mM for fructose-1-phosphate and as 0.01 mM for fructose-1,6-diphosphate [62]. Liver aldolase is inhibited by a series of metabolites, inosine monophosphate (IMP) being the most potent one [22].

Triokinase (2.7.1.28)   This enzyme catalyzes the phosphorylation of D-glyceraldehyde into D-glyceraldehyde-3-phosphate [58]. The preferential phosphoryl donor is adenosine triphosphate (ATP), but studies by Frandsen and Grunnet [71] have shown that inosine triphosphate (ITP) can be utilized at 14 percent and guanosine triphosphate (GTP) at 10 percent of the rate of utilization of the adenine nucleotide. The maximal activity of the rat liver enzyme is approximately 1.5 μmol/min/g at 37 °C [72], while the K_m values are 0.01 mM for D-glyceraldehyde [73] and 0.77 mM for Mg^{2+}-ATP [71].

Alternate Pathways   Two alternate pathways have been proposed for the conversion of D-glyceraldehyde to a triose phosphate: (1) reduction to glycerol by NADH and alcohol dehydrogenase or by NADPH and aldose reductase, followed by phosphorylation to α-glycerophosphate and subsequent oxidation to dihydroxyacetone phosphate; and (2) oxidation to glyceric acid and conversion to phosphoglycerate. As was discussed by Hers [45], studies of the randomization of the fructose carbons indicate that D-glyceraldehyde is utilized by

triokinase in vivo. This conclusion was confirmed by a kinetic study of the glyceraldehyde-metabolizing enzymes [73] and by experiments with [4-^{3}H, 6-^{14}C] fructose [74].

Fructose-1,6-diphosphatase (Fructose-1,6-bisphosphatase, Hexose Diphosphatase, EC 3.1.3.11)   Hexose diphosphatase catalyzes the splitting of fructose-1,6-diphosphate to fructose-6-phosphate and P_i. The reaction is irreversible and allows the Embden-Meyerhof pathway to proceed in the direction of gluconeogenesis. Hexose diphosphatase is subjected to complex regulation (for a review, see Ref. 75). It is inhibited allosterically by physiologic concentrations of adenosine monophosphate (AMP). The reaction products fructose-6-phosphate and P_i are competitive inhibitors. The divalent cation Mg^{2+} is required for activity and modulates the inhibition by AMP. Purification of the human liver enzyme has been reported recently [76]. Hexose diphosphatase antagonizes the reaction catalyzed by phosphofructokinase, i.e., the formation from fructose-6-phosphate and ATP of fructose-1,6-diphosphate and adenine diphosphate (ADP). This reaction is also irreversible and is the main regulatory step of glycolysis. Both enzymes thus play an essential role in directing the metabolic flux through the Embden-Meyerhof pathway toward glycolysis or gluconeogenesis. Much attention has been devoted in recent years to the possiblity that phosphofructokinase and hexose diphosphatase could operate simultaneously in the liver. This should give rise to a so-called futile cycle without net flux of metabolites, but resulting in a wasteful hydrolysis of ATP. There is now good experimental evidence (see Ref. 77 for a review) that recycling between fructose-6-phosphate and fructose-1,6 diphosphate occurs in the liver of fed rats but little or none in starved ones. In isolated hepatocytes, the degree of recycling can be decreased by the addition of glucagon. This hormone effect appears to be mediated by a newly discovered low molecular weight regulator, fructose-2,6-bisphosphate [78], which stimulates phosphofructokinase [79] and inhibits hexose diphosphatase [80]. Incubation of hepatocytes with glucose induces the accumulation of fructose-2,6-bisphosphate, whereas the addition of glucagon provokes its disappearance. Glucagon and glucose, respectively, stimulate and inhibit gluconeogenesis in the liver and have the reverse effect on glycolysis. These effects can thus be explained by the opposite actions of fructose-2,6-bisphosphate on phosphofructokinase and fructose-1,6-diphosphatase.

End Products of Fructose Metabolism

Studies with the perfused rat liver [81] have shown that after 1 h of perfusion with 20 mM fructose, 52 percent of the keto-hexose was recovered as glucose. This conversion results in a usually modest increment in glycemia in normal human subjects [43, 82]. Lactate and pyruvate accounted for 18 percent and glycogen for 8 percent. The remaining 22 percent were assumed to be metabolized to triglycerides, CO_2, ketone bodies, and small amounts of glycerol and sorbitol. Additional details concerning the further metabolism of fructose in liver can be found elsewhere [83].

Biosynthesis of Fructose

Mention should be made of the metabolic pathway by which

the accessory glands of the male reproductive tract and the placenta synthesize fructose from glucose by way of sorbitol. Hers has detected two enzymes catalyzing these reactions, i.e., sorbitol dehydrogenase and aldose reductase [84]. These two enzymes have since also been detected in nervous tissue and blood vessels. During prolonged hyperglycemia, sorbitol accumulates intracellularly to a considerable extent.

TOXICITY OF FRUCTOSE

After the discovery of hereditary fructose intolerance [85], fructose toxicity was first thought to be limited to individuals with the enzyme defect. In the late 1960s, deleterious effects of high doses of intravenous fructose were also clinically recognized in healthy persons. Hyperuricemia [86] and lactic acidosis [87] were the prominent findings. These observations have led to the recommendation of great caution in the use of fructose in parenteral nutrition [88–91]. Numerous experimental studies designed to elucidate the pathogenesis of the deleterious effects have been done. Effects can be traced to the very rapid rates of fructose metabolism reached after its parenteral administration. When fructose is given intravenously in humans, it disappears from the circulation twice as fast as glucose, its half-life being about 18 min [29] as compared to 43 min for glucose [92]. This is due to (1) the rapid rate of fructose transport at high extracellular concentrations of the ketose and to (2) the higher activity of fructokinase in comparison with the glucose-phosphorylating capacity of hexokinase plus glucokinase. The first consequence of the rapid metabolism of fructose is the accumulation of fructose-1-phosphate, which was first recognized in the liver. Within minutes after a parenteral fructose load, the concentration of the fructose ester, normally not detectable, may reach 10 μmol/g [22, 93–99]. Fructose-1-phosphate accumulates because fructokinase acts much more rapidly than the metabolic pathways converting triose phosphates to glucose and lactate. This accumulation provokes important changes in the concentration of several other metabolites that explain the toxic effects of fructose.

The Hyperuricemic Effect of Fructose

In 1967, Perheentupa and Raivio [86] reported that the intravenous administration of 0.5 g fructose per kilogram of body weight provoked hyperuricemia and hyperuricosuria not only in patients with hereditary fructose intolerance but also in normal children. This observation has been repeatedly confirmed [100, 101] in patients as well as in healthy adult volunteers, especially with infusion rates above 1.0 to 1.5 g/kg·h [102]. Although other authors have not observed the effect with lower infusion rates [103, 104], a rise in the serum uric acid level has been found after the infusion of as little as 0.16 g fructose per kilogram per hour in critically ill subjects [105]. Other studies [106, 107] show that the urinary excretion of uric acid, expressed as the creatinine ratio, is a more sensitive indicator of the effect of fructose than is hyperuricemia.

Investigations in animals by Mäenpää et al. [108] and later in humans [97, 109] demonstrated that the hyperuricemic effect of fructose results from degradation of the adenine nucleotide pool. Indeed, within 2 min after a parenteral fructose load to rats, the concentration of ATP falls to 40 percent of its normal value without an equivalent increase of ADP and AMP [108]. There is also a marked decrease in the concentration of P_i preceding that of ATP. The decrease of ATP is explained by its utilization in the fructokinase reaction. The P_i depletion results from its participation in the rephosphorylation of ADP in mitochondria (Fig. 5-2). The concentrations of several other nucleotides: uridine-5′-diphosphate (UTP), UDP-glucose [110, 111], and guanosine triphosphate (GTP) [99] are also diminished. The decrease of GTP may be due to its utilization in the triokinase reaction [71]. The accumulation of IMP, observed by Woods et al. [22], denotes an increase in the reaction rate of AMP deaminase and can contribute to the buildup of fructose-1-phosphate by its inhibitory effect on aldolase. It cannot explain the initial accumulation of the fructose ester, since the accumulation of fructose-1-phosphate precedes that of IMP [99].

Detailed investigations of the degradation of the adenine nucleotide pool leading to hyperuricemia have shown that it is explained exclusively by the deinhibition of hepatic AMP deaminase (for reviews, see Refs. 83 and 112). Although the catabolism of the hepatic adenine nucleotides could theoretically also begin by dephosphorylation of AMP followed by deamination of adenosine by adenosine deaminase [22, 113a, 114], kinetic studies of the cytoplasmic 5′-nucleotidase in rat liver [115] and experiments with isolated rat hepatocytes [116] demonstrate that this pathway does not operate. Moreover, the membranous and lysosomal 5′-nucleotidases do not qualify for a role in the catabolism of the cytoplasmic purine nucleotides.

Studies of the kinetics of rat liver AMP deaminase [99], confirmed by experiments with isolated rat hepatocytes [116], have led to the conclusion that AMP deaminase is the limiting step in hepatic adenine nucleotide breakdown (Fig. 5-3). The enzyme has complex allosteric properties and is strongly influenced by various metabolites: ATP is a potent activator, whereas P_i and GTP are inhibitory. At physiologic concentrations of its substrate and effectors, the enzyme is 95 percent inhibited. The fructose-induced degradation of the hepatic adenine nucleotide pool can thus be explained by a release of the physiologic inhibition of AMP deaminase, caused by a decrease in the concentrations of P_i and GTP during fructose metabolism (Fig. 5-3). Depletion of high energy phosphates has also been observed in other fructose-metabolizing tissues, namely the small intestine [117] and kidney [111, 118], after the administration of the ketose. Recent studies with single rat nephrons have shown that in accordance with the localization of the fructokinase and fructose-1-phosphate aldolase activi-

Figure 5-2 The mechanism of fructose-induced hyperuricemia.

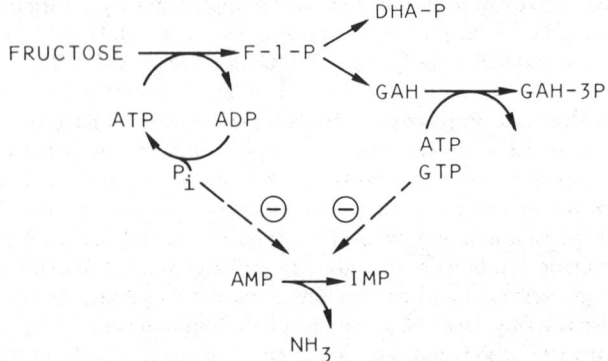

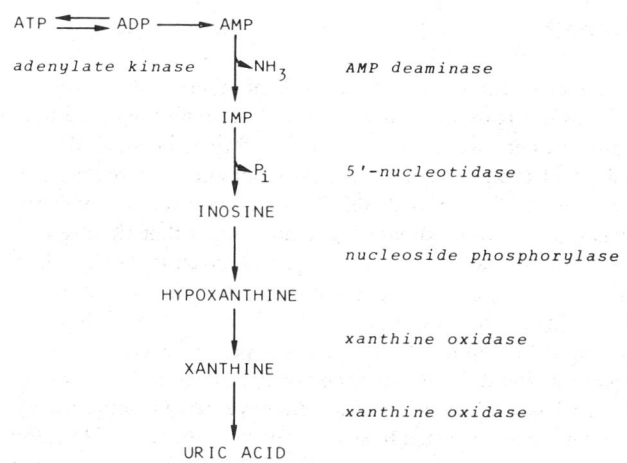

Figure 5-3 The pathway of the degradation of adenine nucleotides in the liver.

ties, the effects of fructose are confined to the proximal tubule [70]. The contribution of the kidney and small intestine to the hyperuricemic effect of fructose is difficult to assess since in humans, xanthine oxidase is found only in the liver and in small intestinal mucosa [119].

The catabolism of the adenine nucleotides ATP, ADP, and AMP which are freely interconvertible by the adenylate kinase reaction should be kept to a minimum for two reasons: (1) adenine nucleotides play a major role in the energy metabolism of the cell, and (2) the low solubility of uric acid, coupled to its limited renal excretion, entails the danger of crystal precipitation with the damaging consequences seen in gout. The fructose-induced hyperuricemia should thus not be considered a harmless phenomenon but a reflection of the loss of high energy phosphate.

The depletion of ATP, the main "energy currency" of the cell, is mirrored by a selective loss of Mg^{2+} from the liver and, to some extent, from the kidney [120] and results in a series of disturbances in fructose-metabolizing tissues, most of which were demonstrated in the liver of experimental animals. They include inhibition of protein [97, 108, 121] and RNA [97] synthesis, disaggregation of ribosomes [120], interference with the formation of cyclic AMP [98] and the detoxication of ammonia [122]. The marked ultrastructural lesions such as loss of ribosomes and intracellular membrane redistribution in rat hepatocytes [123] and the smooth endoplasmic reticulum proliferation seen in mouse jejunal absorptive cells [124] are most likely related phenomena.

The degradation of adenine nucleotides may theoretically be prevented by the administration of phosphate. Data obtained in animals indicate that, although the infusion of phosphate largely prevents the fructose-induced degradation of adenine nucleotides in the kidney cortex, it is much less effective in the liver, probably because of its limited entry into this tissue [118].

The Increase of Blood Lactate Provoked by Fructose

Whereas the infusion of glucose usually does not elevate the concentration of blood lactate more than twofold, increases of two- to fivefold have been reported after the infusion of fructose in healthy volunteers and in patients [104, 107, 125, 126].

This may also be explained by the more rapid utilization of fructose as compared with glucose in the liver. Besides the high activity of fructokinase, two other factors may play a role in the accumulation of lactic acid: (1) the metabolism of fructose bypasses the enzyme phosphofructokinase, the regulatory step of glycolysis, and (2) the stimulation of pyruvate kinase by fructose-1-phosphate [127]. The individual variation in the increase of the lactatemia after fructose infusions and the observation of a bimodal distribution have led to the suggestion of genetic differences in the metabolism of fructose [128].

The fructose-induced increase in lactic acid may provoke metabolic acidosis in adults [87, 129] as well as in children [130, 131]. Metabolic acidosis has also been reported in the fetus of mothers receiving intravenous fructose during labor [132]. It may become life-threatening in liver failure, as exemplified by the case reports provided by Craig and Crane [129] and by Woods et al. [89]. Fructose is therefore an unsatisfactory substitute for glucose in parenteral nutrition. Anoxia, liver disease, diabetes mellitus, inborn errors of fructose, lactate and ammonia metabolism, and glycogenosis type I are absolute contraindications.

ESSENTIAL FRUCTOSURIA—HEPATIC FRUCTOKINASE DEFICIENCY

Historical Note and Definition [133]

This rare and benign error of metabolism was first described in 1876 independently by Czapek [134] and by Zimmer [135] in a man also suffering from diabetes mellitus. In 1961, Laron [136] counted 50 published cases and Steinitz in 1969 fewer than 80 [137]. Since the disorder is asymptomatic and harmless, many cases may remain undetected and the detected ones unpublished. The original name of the disorder, *essential fructosuria*, became obsolete in 1961–1962 when the fructokinase defect was discovered, but it is still in use. A nonalimentary fructosuria of obscure etiology has been observed in one child [138].

Laboratory Findings, Biochemical Defect, Functional Studies

Affected persons are usually discovered on routine urinalysis by the presence of a reducing substance. They are healthy and have otherwise normal liver function and alimentary fructosuria. Fructosuria depends on the time and amount of fructose and sucrose intake, and thus it is inconstant. After an overnight fast, fructose is measurable only in small quantities, if at all, in the blood of the affected persons, just as in normal persons. The misdiagnosis of diabetes mellitus [139, 140] or renal diabetes [140] is avoided only when the nonglucose nature of the sugar is recognized. This can be done by means of thin-layer or paper chromatography.

The disorder is caused by the inherited deficiency of fructokinase (EC 2.7.1.3) normally present in the liver, intestine, and kidney cortex [54, 70, 141, 142]. The deficiency was demonstrated in the liver of an adult by Schapira et al. [143] using the assay designed by Hers and Joassin [144]. Assays of intestinal or kidney cortex fructokinase have to our knowledge not been done in persons with essential fructosuria. Thus the block appears to be as follows:

$$\text{Fructose} \xrightarrow[\text{fructokinase}]{\quad//\quad} \text{fructose-1-phosphate} \quad (1)$$

After an oral or intravenous load, e.g., with 1 g per kilogram of body weight, blood fructose rises rapidly far beyond the level of 10 to 30 mg/100 ml seen in controls, falls slowly, and does not disappear for 6 h or longer [136, 145]. Between 10 and 20 percent of the administered dose is excreted in urine [136, 146] compared to 1 to 2 percent [136] or less [145] in normal subjects. Blood glucose, lactate, pyruvate, and urate change little, in contrast to the rise of these metabolites in normal persons; phosphorus, magnesium, standard bicarbonate, free fatty acids, and insulin remain constant [145–148] (Fig. 5-4). The rise of the respiratory quotient (RQ) after fructose ingestion in fasted patients with essential fructosuria is less than in normal subjects [139, 147]. These findings indicate a slower than normal utilization of fructose. An 8-year-old girl weighing 40 kg, on a 1-h-long continuous fructose infusion retained from 40 to 60 mg of the sugar per minute [136]. The nine-tenths of a dose of fructose which is retained by fructosuria subjects after a bolus is most probably metabolized via fructose-6-phosphate in adipose tissue and skeletal muscle. As in normal subjects, oral D-sorbitol is converted to fructose, which becomes measurable in blood (Fig. 5-4) [145, 149]; urinary loss as fructose is only about one-half that seen after a fructose load [145, 149]. Almost 80 percent of a 5-g sorbose load was lost in urine by a fructosuric woman [139].

Figure 5-4 Oral fructose and sorbitol tolerance tests in two sibs with essential fructosuria. Fructose: ■ R.K. ♂, 16 years; ● A.K. ♀, 19 years; --- Controls (N = 5). Sorbitol: □ R.K. In the probands, phosphorus, magnesium, standard bicarbonate, free fatty acids, and insulin remained unchanged. (*From Steinmann et al. [145].*)

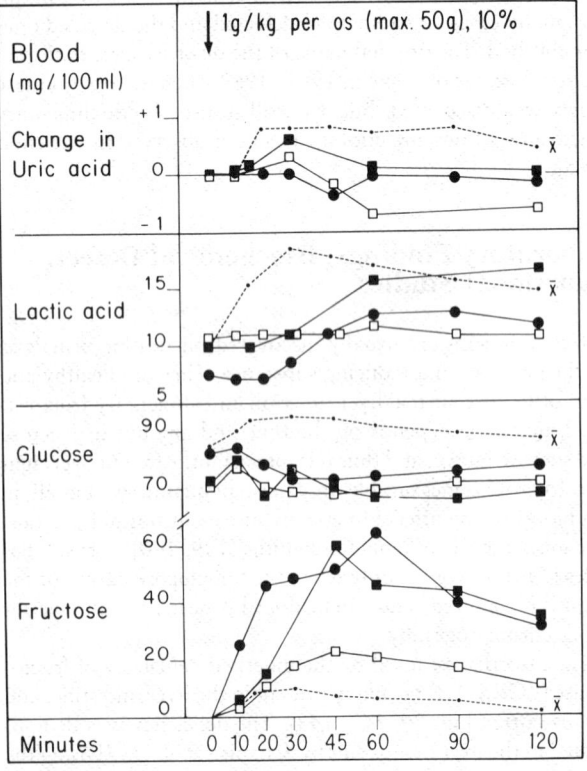

Genetics

The most careful study of the mode of inheritance of essential fructosuria is that of Lasker [150]. After reviewing the literature and her own cases, she concluded that the anomaly was inherited as an autosomal recessive trait and occurred perhaps once in 130,000 individuals. She gave good reasons why this was only an approximate figure and stated that the disorder may be even rarer. On the other hand, given its benign character, it may escape discovery during a lifetime. Marble [151] reported only four cases among 29,000 cases of mellituria seen at the Joslin Clinic. Heterozygotes appear to excrete no more fructose after an oral load than normal subjects [152]. Fructokinase has not been assayed in heterozygotes. Essential fructosuria has been reported from many parts of the world [150]. By 1961, the proportion of Jews in the known and proven cases of this disorder was 18 out of 50 cases [136].

HEREDITARY FRUCTOSE INTOLERANCE

Historical Note and Definition

In 1956 Chambers and Pratt [153] described a case of "idiosyncrasy to fructose" in a 24-year-old woman whose only complaints were feelings of anxiety and attacks of nausea and vomiting after eating food containing fruit or cane sugar. Froesch et al. [85] reported the typical syndrome of hereditary fructose intolerance in 1957 in two sibs and two relatives. Both groups recognized that this disorder of fructose metabolism was distinct from essential fructosuria. Froesch et al. suspected a deficiency of aldolase as the cause. The defect was shown by Hers and Joassin in 1961 on two liver biopsy specimens to consist in a loss of the ability of the enzyme to split fructose-1-phosphate [144]. By 1971, 100 cases were reported in the literature [154] from Europe and the United States, and since then, reports have been numerous. The disorder, once considered a rare inborn error of metabolism, is sufficiently common for certain centers to have collected the records of dozens of patients [155–157].

Only in 1970 was hereditary fructose-1,6-diphosphatase deficiency recognized as a separate disorder [158] also causing intolerance to fructose. After a reinvestigation in 1972, "familial galactose and fructose intolerance," originally described in 1961, must now be questioned as a disease entity [159].

Clinical and Laboratory Findings

Infants and adult patients with hereditary fructose intolerance are perfectly healthy and asymptomatic as long as they do not ingest any food containing fructose or sucrose. Thus during breast feeding, no metabolic derangement occurs. At weaning, with the intake of fruits and vegetables, the first symptoms appear. The younger the child [160] and the higher the dietary fructose load, the more severe the reaction. The newborn infant who is not breast-fed but receives a cow's milk formula with fructose or sucrose substituting for lactose is in danger of death.

In the infant and small child [155, 156], leading symptoms are poor feeding, vomiting, and failure to thrive (Table 5-1). All other symptoms occur less frequently but are more specific and indicative of gastrointestinal discomfort, hypoglycemia, shock, and liver disease. As the clinical presentation is multifaceted in the small infant, the diagnosis is easily missed. If the intake of the noxious sugar persists, hypoglycemic episodes recur and liver and kidney failure progress, eventually leading to death. In one series [155], clinical findings in the order of decreasing frequency were hepatomegaly, pallor, hemorrhages such as melena, hematemesis, suffusions, trembling and jerks, shock, jaundice, edema, tachypnea, ascites, oliguria or anuria as signs of severe shock, splenomegaly, fever, and rickets. Laboratory findings are those of liver failure, of proximal renal tubular dysfunction, and of certain derangements of intermediary metabolism (Table 5-2).

The child survives and symptoms regress when the formula is changed to a nonnoxious one or replaced by intravenous infusions with glucose as the carbohydrate. If the patient escapes diagnosis at this point, the disease takes a protracted, uphill-downhill course. By experience, certain mothers learn quickly how to select harmless formulas and foods for their affected child. The protracted course is also typical for the patient whose first exposure to fructose occurs at regular weaning. Here the prominent features are abdominal distention, hepatomegaly, and poor growth. Acute episodes become rarer as the child develops a distinct aversion to discomfort-causing sweetened foods and drinks. Aversion to sweet food is neither general nor indiscriminate [153] but selective and directed at particular sweetened foods or drinks. Thus it is not innate but acquired by learning. For instance, a fructose-intolerant medical student not knowing her diagnosis disliked all desserts with the exception of glucose candies. A 4-year-old boy refused sweets but loved one brand of peppermints; surprisingly, they were made of sucrose [174]. Children usually adopt peculiar feeding habits which protect them but are not always understood by surrounding persons, who sometimes resort to forcing sweet foods [161–163]. Diagnosis at this period is usually made during examination for suspected storage disorder or sometimes for anomalous behavior [161] (Fig. 5-5) and only after carefully taking the nutritional history. Other patients, following a self-imposed low fructose diet, go on undiagnosed into adulthood and may be discovered by chance.

Table 5-1 Symptoms and signs in hereditary fructose intolerance

Acute exposure	Chronic exposure
Sweating	Poor feeding, vomiting
Trembling	Failure to thrive
Dizziness	Incessant crying, irritability
Nausea	Drowsiness, apathy
Vomiting	Jaundice
Apathy, lethargy, coma	Abdominal distention
Convulsions	Hepatomegaly
	Hemorrhages
	Diarrhea
	Tremor, jerking
	Edema, ascites
	Poor growth

Sequelae: Protracted fibrosis, cirrhosis, steatosis of the liver; aversion to sweets and peculiar feeding habits; lack of dental caries.

Table 5-2 Laboratory findings in chronically exposed patients with hereditary fructose intolerance

Liver	Decreased serum levels of coagulation factors
	Increased serum levels of hepatic enzymes
	Hypoproteinemia
	Increased plasma methionine, tyrosine, etc.
	Hyperbilirubinemia
	Fructosemia and fructosuria
Kidney	Glucosuria
	Proteinuria
	Hyperphosphaturia and hypophosphatemia
	Loss of bicarbonates, high urinary pH, and acidosis
	Hyperaminoaciduria
	Hyperkaliuria and hypokalemia
Intermediary metabolism	Hypoglycemia
	Hypophosphatemia
	Hypokalemia
	Lactic acidosis and organic aciduria
	Hyperuricemia
	Hypermagnesemia
Others	Anemia
	Thrombocytopenia
	Acanthocytes, fragmentocytes

Approximately half of all adults with hereditary fructose intolerance are completely free of caries [160, 162, 164–166], a fact indicating that dietary sucrose is the chief caries-promoting agent. It also leads dentists to suspect hereditary fructose intolerance [163]. Some adult patients are diagnosed during a family investigation after the discovery of an affected young relative [163, 164, 167], sometimes their own child [168, 169]. Yet other undiagnosed fructose-intolerant children and adults are less fortunate and receive infusions of fructose, sorbitol, or invert sugar, sometimes for unrelated health reasons [170, 171], e.g., after routine surgery. Some die from acute poisoning [172, 173].

It must be stressed that in the two casuistic reviews [155, 156] comprising 75 children, hypoglycemia was documented only in a minority. It correlated poorly with jerking and trembling in the infant. Hypoglycemia, while considered a major and dangerous metabolic manifestation of hereditary fructose intolerance, is short-lived, lasting only a limited time after each ingestion of fructose. It thus easily escapes detection.

Histologic examination of the liver performed by diagnostic biopsy shows diffuse steatosis of liver cells, necrosis of a few scattered hepatocytes, periportal and intralobular fibrosis and, in more advanced stages of the disease, cirrhosis [156, 175, 176]. At autopsy, findings include hepatic dystrophy and necrosis [176–178]. In the kidney, histologic changes are remarkably discrete. They include some granulation and perhaps vacuolization of epithelial cells lining the proximal tubules, which may be slightly dilated [177, 178]. In the small intestine, gross inspection and microscopic examination may reveal submucosal or serosal hemorrhages. Intracranial [156, 160] and intraocular hemorrhages [155] have been reported.

Ultrastructural studies on liver biopsy specimens of fructose-intolerant children have been done. Spycher [179] found in all three specimens studied that hepatocytes and sometimes Kupffer cells contained polymorphous cytoplasmic inclusions of different size, in part membrane-bound and probably lysosomal. Inclusions contained amorphous, electron-dense masses and numerous concentric membranous arrays varying

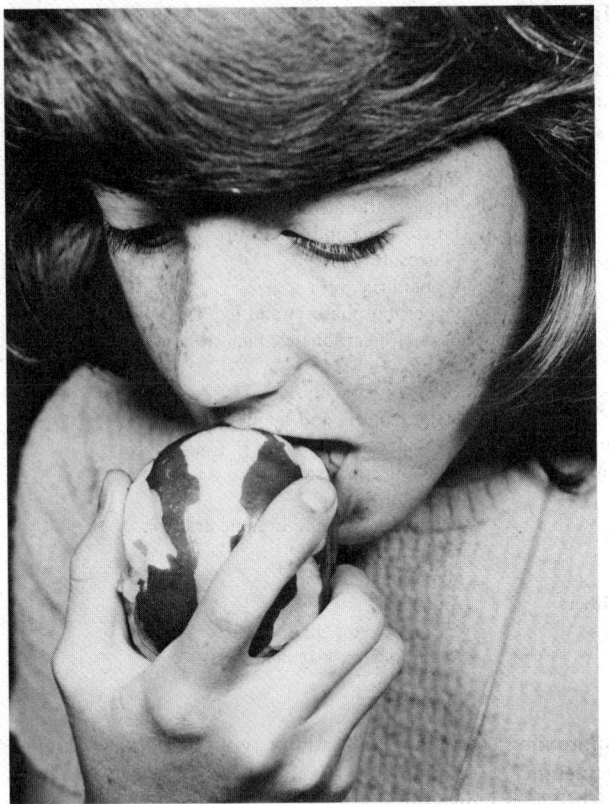

Figure 5-5 A 12-year-old girl with hereditary fructose intolerance "eating" an apple. She had been referred for anomalous behavior at age 8 years.

greatly in size and often surrounded by an electron-lucent halo. Similar findings had been reported earlier [180].

Biochemical Defect

The enzyme defect (Fig. 5-1) is that of fructose-1-phosphate aldolase B (fructose-bisphosphate aldolase, EC 2.1.2.13) of the liver, kidney cortex, and small intestine. Aldolase A and C [60, 61, 181], prevalent in other organs such as skeletal muscle and brain, are not affected. The activity of the liver enzyme is reduced to 15 percent of normal or less with fructose-1-

phosphate and to a distinctly lesser degree with fructose-1,6-diphosphate. A representative sample of measurements on biopsy specimens is shown in Table 5-3. It confirms the findings of an earlier series [182] and shows that in the patients, the activity ratio of fructose-1,6-diphosphate to fructose-1-phosphate aldolase is increased, a fact of diagnostic value originally pointed out by Hers and Joassin [144] and Schapira et al. [143]. Fructose-1-phosphate aldolase activity was undetectable in 5 of 35 biopsy specimens in one series [157] but was never absent in the 34 biopsy specimens of another series [182]. The activities of liver fructokinase [143, 144, 183] and fructose-1,6-diphosphatase (Table 5-3) are normal. A similar reduction of fructaldolase activities is found in biopsied jejunal mucosa and in kidney cortex at operation and at autopsy (Table 5-4).

The significance of residual fructaldolase activities in liver, kidney and intestine of patients with hereditary fructose intolerance is still controversial. Mature human liver contains all three forms of fructaldolase, but B predominates with 98 percent of the protein [181]. Aldolase A, with less than 2 to 3 percent of protein [181, 182], contributes 15 percent of the total activity [182] due to its higher specific activity. Residual liver fructose-1,6-diphosphate aldolase has been attributed variably to a persisting fetal enzyme, shortly to be recognized as aldolase A [144, 183, 184], and to aldolase C [182]. Both are unaffected by the mutation and have a higher fructose-1,6-diphosphate aldolase/fructose-1-phosphate aldolase activity ratio (13 and 7) than normal aldolase B (0.9) [62]. Conceivably, the partially inactive mutant aldolase B itself has an increased activity ratio. In the majority of biopsy specimens studied, a cross-reacting material was present [157, 182], and an abnormally high K_m for fructose-1,6-diphosphate [185] and fructose-1-phosphate [182], and decreased heat stability [157] of mutant human aldolase have been reported. Furthermore, a certain restoration of fructose-1-phosphate aldolase in extracts of biopsied liver was achieved in vitro by reducing agents [182], and in a minority of tissue specimens, antibodies to aldolase B activated the residual enzyme [157, 186]. At any rate, the residual aldolase activity never appears to become rate-limiting in glycolysis or gluconeogenesis except after fructose loading. Normal functioning of gluconeogenesis is amply documented by the prompt rise of blood glucose after oral dihydroxyacetone [145, 187–189] and by the patients' normal tolerance to fasting.

Table 5-3 Fructaldolase and fructose-1,6-diphosphatase measured in liver biopsy specimens of children with hereditary fructose intolerance (HFI) and controls (IU per gram wet weight)

		Fructaldolase			
		FDP (a)	F-1-P (b)	a/b	FDPase
HFI	x̄ (median)	0.46	0.11	(3.9)	3.82
	SD	0.16	0.09		1.66
	Range	0.13–0.82	0.00–0.36	1.7–∞	1.71–7.20
	N	35	35	35	24
Controls*	x̄	2.61	2.40	1.1	3.78
	SD	0.46	0.49	0.1	0.74
	Range	2.07–3.79	1.82–3.40	1.0–1.2	2.73–4.98
	N	10	10	10	7

* Nine adult organ donors and one child with a histologically normal liver.
SOURCE: From Steinmann and Gitzelmann [157].

Table 5-4 Activity ratio, fructose-1,6-diphosphate to fructose-1-phosphate aldolase, measured in tissues of patients with hereditary fructose intolerance and controls, at biopsy or autopsy, and in isolated human aldolases A, B, and C

	Controls			Hereditary fructose intolerance			
	Mean	Range	(N)	Mean (median)	Range	(N)	Ref.
Liver	1.0	0.9–1.1	(5)	6.2; 6.2		(2)	144
	1.1	1.0–1.2	(10)	(3.9)	1.8–∞	(33)	157
				1.7; 11*		(2)	157
		1.0–1.2		6.6	2.9–11.0	(34)	182
	~1.7		(11)				54
Intestine	1.9	1.0–2.5	(28)	(26.7)	3.1–∞	(8)	274
				1.8		(1)	160
		3.5–4.0	(4)				142
	1.7	1.1–2.3	(7)	32.6; 3.5		(2)	275
				9.1		(1)	276
Kidney cortex	2.8		(5)				141
	1.3		(1)				277
	3.2	2.6–4	(6)	∞		(1)	278
	1.7; 2.5		(2)	18		(1)	157
	2.7						69
Kidney medulla	6		(4)				141
	23		(1)				277
	5.8; 9.6		(2)				157
	3.4						69
Aldolase A	13						62
Aldolase B	0.9						62
Aldolase C	7						62

*Values in italics refer to measures at autopsy.

Functional Studies

In individuals with hereditary fructose intolerance, both the ingestion and the injection of fructose cause chemical changes, symptoms, and signs, some of which are also seen in normal persons, albeit to a far lesser degree. After an intravenous load, patients and healthy persons [190] experience dull epigastric pain which is unexplained; it usually starts 2 to 3 min after a bolus and tapers off after 10 min. Only the patients report a nagging hunger feeling toward and during the second hour [157]. An oral fructose load causes occasional diarrhea in control persons but no other ill effects. In contrast, patients become limp, and nauseated and vomit, sometimes with blood, are covered with cold sweat, and develop signs of shock and hypoglycemia. The ill effects are dose dependent [85, 153] and may last for several hours. Proteinuria, generalized aminoaciduria, a rise of serum transaminases, and jaundice may appear and last for several days [175, 191, 193].

The chemical signs provoked by fructose in the patient consist of a rapid fall first of serum phosphate and then of blood glucose and a rise of urate and magnesium. Blood alanine, lactate, glycerol, and nonesterified fatty acids rise [163, 164, 194]. Insulin remains constant or falls [160, 164, 165, 195, 196], while growth hormone rises [164, 196], probably in response to hypoglycemia. Effects are clearly dose dependent [189]. The degree of fructose intolerance may diminish with age [85], but considerable differences in the individual patient have also been recorded [161]. Because of the ill effects of oral loads and the unreliability of results, tests should not be done orally. Figs. 5-6 and 5-7 illustrate the course of intravenous tolerance tests in normal and fructose-intolerant children and

adults [157]. The small dose of 200 mg/kg is recommended. Fructose-intolerant children and adults extract fructose from the blood normally [157] except when the administered dose is excessive [192]. In intolerant children, chemical responses are generally more prompt and pronounced than in adult patients. After an equal per weight fructose dose (i.e., a higher per unit surface area dose), hypoglycemia in the adults is milder and somewhat delayed, and thus is not an independent diagnostic criterion. One girl, repeatedly tested, was found to convert to the adult type of blood response between ages 12 and 18½ years [157]. Adults experience a short-lived hyperkalemia [157] followed by a potassium decline [157, 165], and this was also seen in one child [157]. Urinary excretion of lactate, alanine, urate, and magnesium increases after the load [145, 157], changes also seen after an oral load [193]. That intravenous fructose tests are not at all harmless even when fructose is given in a small dose must be concluded from the observation of a test-induced proximal renal tubular syndrome in adult patients [157, 197]. Acute fructose hepatotoxicity for the fructose-intolerant subject is evident from the investigations by Odièvre [198]. Four-hour infusions of fructose in children caused clotting factors II, V, VII, and X to drop after 2 to 4 h; they reverted to normal levels only after 24 to 48 h. Interesting morphologic observations in the liver and small intestine of an adult patient 2 h after an oral load with 50 g fructose were made by Phillips et al. [199]. By light microscopy, there were no changes, but electron microscopy revealed striking fine structural alterations reminiscent of those seen in fructose-loaded laboratory animals [200] (see "Toxicity of Fructose," above). They included concentric and irregularly disposed membranous arrays in and marked rarefaction of the hyalo-

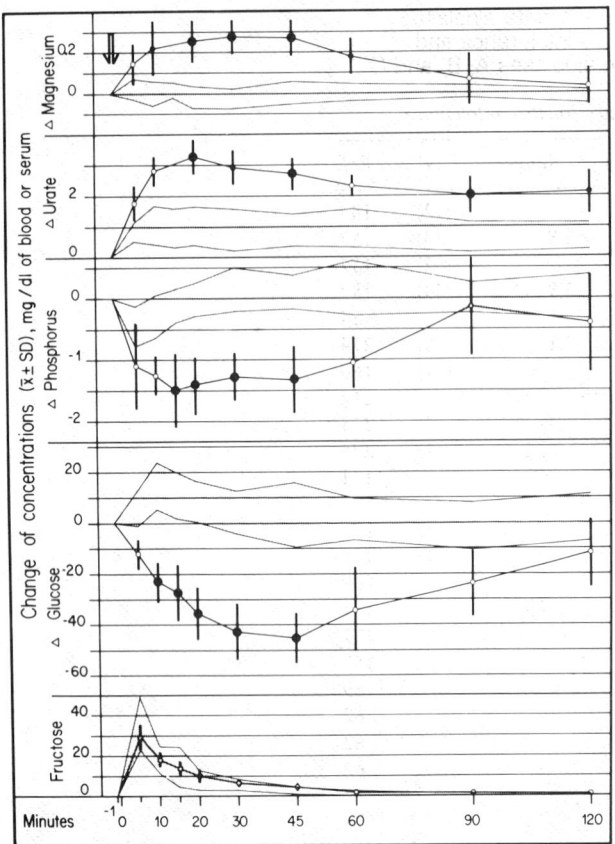

Figure 5-6 Intravenous fructose tolerance tests (200 mg/kg; 20 percent solution) in 10 children with hereditary fructose intolerance and 16 contrast children. The shaded areas comprise means ± 1 SD of the contrasts; bars represent the means ± 1 SD in the patients. Symbols: ● mean; no overlap between the two groups; ◐ mean; the extreme values of both groups coincided; ○ mean; overlap occurred between the two groups. (*From Steinmann and Gitzelmann [157].*)

plasm of hepatocytes. Concentric arrays of smooth endoplasmic reticulum were visible in the supranuclear region of enterocytes.

The intravenous loading with sorbitol causes the same chemical changes in the patient, but only insignificant fructosemia [157] or none at all [165]. This documents the fact that intravenous sorbitol is rapidly converted to fructose in the liver and that fructosemia is not a prerequisite for hypoglycemia and the other observed changes (Fig. 5-8). It is noteworthy that the test does not appear to cause epigastric discomfort [165].

The disappearance of L-sorbose from the blood of normal subjects is somewhat slower than that of fructose. This would be expected from the fact that liver fructokinase phosphorylates fructose faster than sorbose and in preference to this ketose [57]. The half-life of sorbose, calculated from data of Froesch et al. [165], lies between 24 and 29 min. In two normal subjects about 30 percent of the administered L-sorbose was excreted in urine, compared to 1 to 2 percent with fructose [165]. In patients with hereditary fructose intolerance, the sorbose level rose higher and fell more slowly, with a half-life of approximately 64 min, and accordingly these patients excreted over 80 percent of the administered sorbose in the urine within 24 h. The ability to assimilate sorbose obviously was greatly impaired, but patients had no symptoms and neither blood glucose nor inorganic phosphorus changed [165, 168, 195].

Furthermore, prior administration of sorbose did not alter or delay the response of patients with hereditary fructose intolerance to subsequent administration of fructose [165]. One might speculate that because of the small affinity of fructokinase for sorbose, only a small amount of sorbose-1-phosphate accumulates in the liver cells, too little to cause the metabolic effects attributed to fructose-1-phosphate accumulation (see below).

Sucrose tolerance tests are not routinely done when hereditary fructose intolerance is suspected. One 10-month-old boy suspected of having intestinal sucrose-isomaltase deficiency was given an oral sucrose load (50 g/m²). He developed hypoglycemia, whereupon the correct diagnosis was made (unpublished). A fructose-intolerant women volunteered for an oral raffinose loading test (42 g) when it was not clear whether this fructose-containing trisaccharide of vegetable origin could be hydrolyzed in the human small intestine [201]. She experienced no hypoglycemia, although with equivalent dose of oral fructose (12 g) she did (unpublished). In contrast to sucrose, raffinose is not hydrolyzed in the intestine and thus is safe for consumption by fructose-intolerant persons.

The fructose-induced hypoglycemia seen in these patients is not due to hyperinsulinism [160, 164, 165, 192, 195] and is not corrected by exogenous glucagon [98, 164, 165, 189, 194, 202] or dibutyryl cyclic AMP [98]. On the other hand, when administration of oral or intravenous fructose is accompanied [188] or followed [164, 189] by oral or intravenous galactose, the fructose-induced hypoglycemia is prevented or corrected. Neither dihydroxyacetone [188, 189] nor inorganic phosphate [154, 189, 195, 202] has a corrective effect. These facts dem-

Figure 5-7 Intravenous fructose tolerance tests (200 mg/kg; 20 percent solution) in six adults with hereditary fructose intolerance and six controls. For symbols, see Fig. 5-6. (*From Steinmann and Gitzelmann [157].*)

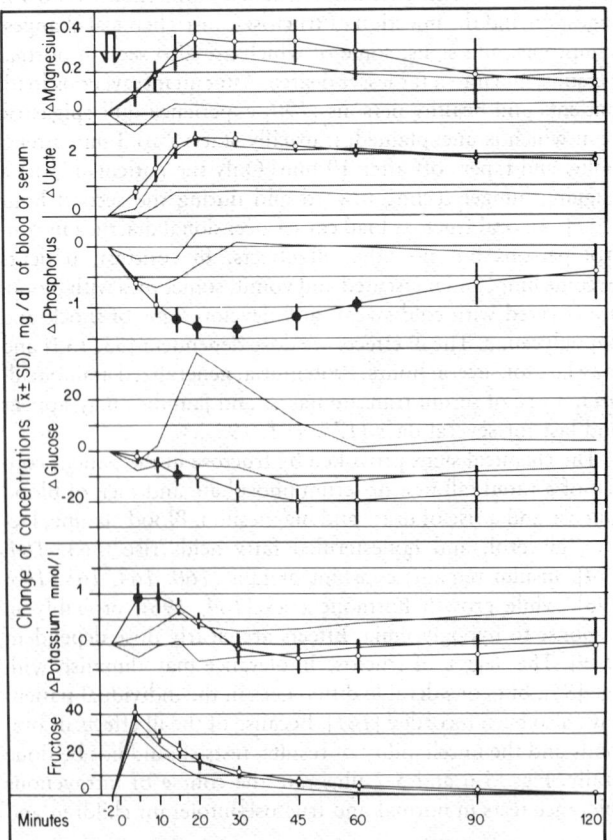

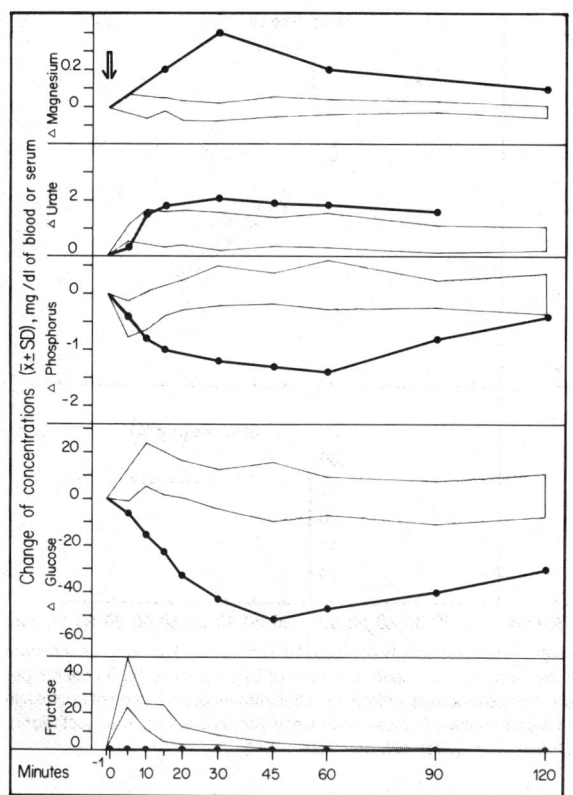

Figure 5-8 Intravenous sorbitol tolerance test (200 mg/kg; 40 percent solution) in a 12-year-old fructose-intolerant girl. Shaded areas represent means ± 1 SD of 16 contrast children after intravenous fructose, as in Fig. 5-6. (*Unpublished*.)

onstrate that during a limited period of time after the fructose load, hepatic glucose formation by way of glycogenolysis or gluconeogenesis is impaired.

Pathophysiology

The enzyme defect results in the accumulation of fructose-1-phosphate in the liver, kidney, and small intestine and in an inability to convert fructose to blood glucose. Fructose-1-phosphate accumulates even after the ingestion of small physiologic amounts of fructose. The pathophysiologic findings constitute marked exaggerations of the deleterious effects of fructose observed in normal individuals. Direct proof that the changes in intracellular metabolites observed after fructose loads in animals also occur in patients with hereditary fructose intolerance is, of course, scarce for ethical reasons. The accumulation of fructose-1-phosphate has been verified [203, 204]. A depletion of intracellular P_i can be inferred from the long-lasting fall of serum inorganic phosphate in the patients after fructose. For instance, it was calculated that the conversion of 6.6 mmol (= 1.2 g) fructose to fructose-1-phosphate by an infant patient weighing 8.8 kg requires more P_i than the amount present in the entire extracellular fluid [165]. The increase of serum magnesium after fructose in the patients [160, 205] probably reflects the loss of ATP from the fructose-metabolizing tissues. Indeed, ATP is a strong Mg^{2+} chelator, and a decrease in its concentration is likely to result in a release of cellular Mg^{2+}. Undoubtedly, several of the toxic effects of fructose in the patients are caused by the depletion of ATP. The

loss of hepatic ATP, by its inhibitory effect on protein synthesis, may explain the hyperaminoacidemia, the decrease in blood clotting factors, and the other signs of liver failure. The complex renal tubular dysfunction resembling the Fanconi syndrome [206] may be caused by the degradation of ATP in the kidney. A modulation of the renal dysfunction by the level of parathyroid hormone has been reported [197]. The metabolic acidosis is due to both lactic acidosis and proximal renal tubular acidosis, the former being far more important [193].

The profound fructose-induced hypoglycemia is seen only in patients with hereditary fructose intolerance or fructose-1,6-diphosphatase deficiency (see below), although the rapid intravenous infusion of fructose may exceptionally induce a slight lowering of blood glucose in normal newborn infants [207] and in healthy adults [208]. Its mechanism is not immediately apparent and has been the subject of extensive investigations. It is not due to increased glucose utilization by the peripheral tissues but is caused by a block of glucose release from the liver. This was demonstrated by Dubois et al. [192] (Fig. 5-9). After the injection of tracer amounts of [1-^{14}C]glucose into a normal child, specific radioactivity of the blood glucose decreased exponentially, indicating dilution of the label by nonradioactive glucose released from the liver. This decrease was not influenced by the administration of fructose (right panel). In a patient studied by the same protocol, the administration of fructose resulted in the temporary arrest of the decrease in specific radioactivity which paralleled the hypoglycemia (left panel). Impairment of glucose release by the liver could be due to an inhibition of glycogenolysis, gluconeogenesis, or both.

Decreased gluconeogenesis is apparent from the fact that the fructose-induced hypoglycemia cannot be corrected by dihydroxyacetone, which enters the glycolytic-gluconeogenic pathway at the triokinase step. The hindrance of dihydroxyacetone conversion to glucose may be due to several mechanisms. Inhibition by fructose-1-phosphate of two gluconeogenic enzymes, glucose-6-phosphate isomerase [209] and liver aldolase [209a] has been reported. When residual aldolase was assayed in the direction of condensation of the triose phosphates to fructose-1,6-diphosphate, inhibition was observed in patient liver homogenate but not in control liver. The inhibition of glucose-6-phosphate isomerase by fructose-1-phosphate may account for the occasional occurrence of a transient decrease in blood glucose upon rapid infusion of the ketose in normal subjects [207, 208]. Depletion of ATP may also explain decreased gluconeogenesis. Indeed, studies of perfused rat liver have shown that this rate depends upon the concentration of ATP up to the physiologic level, a half-maximal effect being observed at 0.6 mM ATP [210]. Even complete inhibition of gluconeogenesis cannot, by itself explain the rapid, fructose-induced fall in blood glucose characteristic of hereditary fructose intolerance. Several hours of fasting are required for patients with fructose-1,6-diphosphatase deficiency to become hypoglycemic (see below). Furthermore, a higher dose of fructose is required to provoke a lowering of blood glucose in these patients.

A block of glycogenolysis during fructose-induced hypoglycemia is evidenced by the inability of glucagon to correct the blood glucose. The increase of liver glycogen in a biopsy done by Cain and Ryman [211] is in keeping with this observation. Inhibition of phosphoglucomutase by fructose-1-phosphate in vitro was suggested by Sidbury [212]; since fructose-induced hypoglycemia can be corrected by galactose, conversion of glucose-1-phosphate to glucose-6-phosphate and free glucose

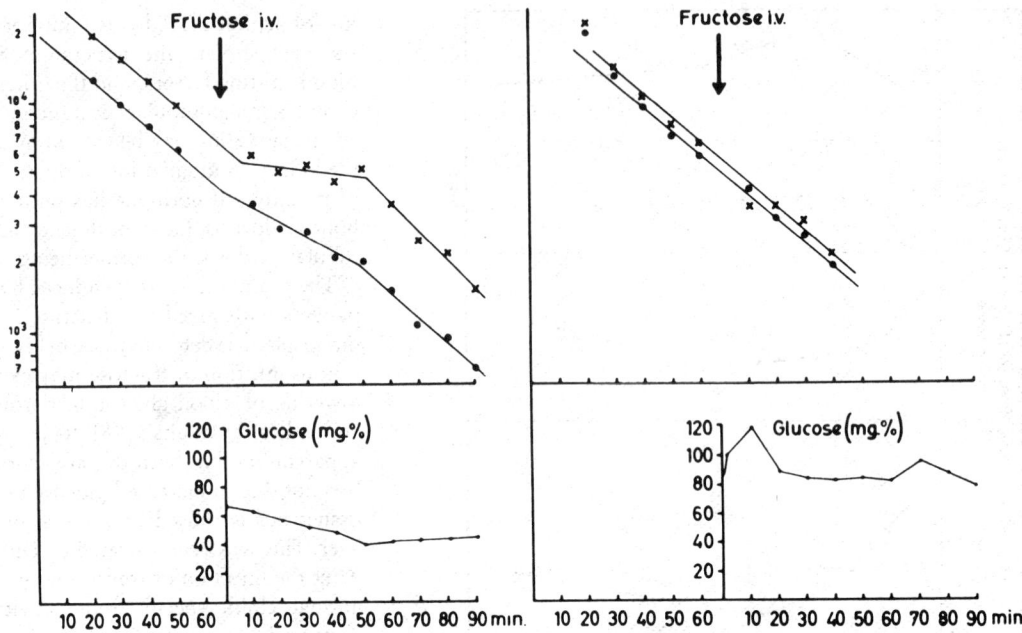

Figure 5-9   Total radioactivity of blood [1-^{14}C]glucose (·) (in counts per minute per milliliter of blood) and specific activity of blood glucose (x) (in counts per milligram of blood glucose), before and after intravenous injection of fructose in a patient with hereditary fructose intolerance (*left*) and a normal subject (*right*). (*From Dubois et al. [192] with permission.*)

is not impaired in vivo [164]. Therefore, breakdown of liver glycogen must be blocked at the level of phosphorylase.

The action of glucagon on the complex phosphorylase regulatory system involves the following sequence: (1) The hormone stimulates liver adenylate cyclase, causing a large increase of hepatic cyclic AMP reflected in plasma and urine [213]; (2) cyclic AMP induces the conversion of inactive phosphorylase b to the active form a through successive stimulation of protein kinase and phosphorylase kinase; and (3) phosphorylase a reacts with glycogen and P_i, producing glucose-1-phosphate. The effects of fructose on the different steps have been investigated in detail [98, 214] (for reviews, see Refs. 83 and 214a). The glucagon-induced accumulation of cyclic AMP is markedly reduced by prior administration of fructose. This effect was observed in the urine of patients after a diagnostic dose of iv fructose and in the livers of rats receiving fructose loads, where it correlated with the decrease of ATP, the substrate of adenylate cyclase. Slowed formation of cyclic AMP did not explain the suppression of the hormonal effect, since fructose-induced hypoglycemia was not corrected by the injection of dibutyryl cyclic AMP. Furthermore, the amount of cyclic AMP formed in the livers of experimental animals was still sufficient to bring about the conversion of phosphorylase b to the active form a. Competitive inhibition of phosphorylase a from animal liver by fructose-1-phosphate was demonstrated [98, 215–218]. It is enhanced by lowering the concentration of P_i. The inhibition seemed insufficiently pronounced at the concentration of fructose-1-phosphate and P_i prevailing in the livers of experimental animals after fructose administration to account for complete abolition of the phosphorolytic degradation of glycogen. Total inhibition of phosphorylase a could nevertheless be evidenced in animals in vivo [214a, 218]. Van den Berghe [83] used rats loaded with tagatose, since in the liver this fructose isomer produces similar changes which last longer because of slower metabolism of tagatose-1-phosphate. In control rats, glucagon increased hepatic glucose-6-phosphate three fold within 10 min, reflecting the breakdown of glycogen. The increase was completely abolished in rats which had received tagatose prior to the hormone, despite normal activation of phosphorylase. It can thus be concluded that part

of the total P_i measured may be bound and consequently unavailable for phosphorylase a, resulting in the enhancement of the inhibitory effect of fructose-1-phosphate. From these animal experiments, it may be inferred that hypoglycemia in patients is an exaggeration of physiologic events brought about by the inability to convert fructose to glucose. The absence of a corrective effect of phosphate infusions may be related to the limited entry of P_i into the liver.

In spite of the loss of the ability of the liver, kidney, and small intestine to metabolize fructose beyond fructose-1-phosphate, only 10 to 20 percent of the administered ketohexose is excreted in the patients' urine. This led to an investigation of their metabolism of fructose. As expected, red and white blood cells metabolize fructose normally by way of hexokinase. In liver tissue, oxidation of [U-^{14}C]fructose to $^{14}CO_2$ and incorporation of the label into glycogen is only 1 to 6 percent normal [165] (Table 5-5). Studies in vivo by Landau et al. [219] indicate that this limited metabolism occurs by phosphorylation of fructose to fructose-6-phosphate. The amount of fructose utilized by the liver of these patients is too small to explain why as much as 90 percent of the administered

Table 5-5   Metabolism of [U-^{14}C]fructose by liver biopsy tissue of two patients with hereditary fructose intolerance and five normal subjects*

Subject	Oxidation to $^{14}CO_2$	Incorporation into glycogen
Normal subjects	1.75 (0.60–2.56)	14.66 (8.6–23.1)
Patient 1	0.109	0.151
Patient 2	0.078	0.812

* [U-^{14}C]fructose and unlabeled glucose were present in the incubation medium in a concentration of 100 mg/100 ml. The figures represent micromoles of fructose carbon incorporated into glycogen or oxidized to $^{14}CO_2$ per gram of tissue per total incubation period. In the normal subjects, the mean and range are indicated.

SOURCE: Froesch et al. [165].

fructose is assimilated. It has therefore been suggested that adipose tissue is the main site of fructose utilization in patients with hereditary fructose intolerance as well as in those with essential fructosuria [25, 26].

Diagnosis, Treatment, Course

The diagnosis of hereditary fructose intolerance can be suspected from a detailed nutritional history and the clinical picture [155, 175]. A high degree of clinical awareness is often needed for prompt diagnosis, as the spectrum of symptoms and signs is wide and nonspecific [155, 156, 170, 198, 220]. Small infants are referred for vomiting of unknown etiology, possible pyloric stenosis or gastroesophageal reflux, or toxic disorders, while older infants and small children are referred for hepatomegaly [155, 156, 221]. Usually, hepatitis, intrauterine infection, septicemia, hemolytic-uremic syndrome, tumor of the liver or storage disorder, galactosemia, tyrosinosis, and Wilson's disease are considered. Suspicion is fostered by the presence of reducing substances in the urine (glucose or fructose, or both) or by hyperaminoaciduria and high blood methionine and tyrosine, discovered by selective screening. It is important to know that fructosuria may have disappeared at the time of urinalysis.

As soon as fructose intolerance is suspected, all sucrose, fructose and sorbitol must be eliminated at once from the diet and from medications. The beneficial effect of withdrawal, usually seen within days, is the first positive element of diagnosis. It must be confirmed, preferably after several weeks of fructose abstinence, by an intravenous fructose tolerance test (200 mg/kg) (Figs. 5-6 and 5-7) and, in case of doubt, by the assay [222] of fructaldolase in a biopsy of liver or perhaps small intestine (Tables 5-3 and 5-4). Fructaldolase activities in the serum of patients are only slightly diminished and hence of no diagnostic value [223]. Enzymatic diagnosis from blood cells is not possible, and the same must be said of cultivated skin fibroblasts, since they express predominantly aldolase A [224].

Treatment consists of the elimination from the diet of all sources of sucrose and fructose [1, 2, 225, 226]. Supportive measures such as infusion of fresh frozen plasma or exchange transfusion may alleviate the clotting disorder and restore complement deficiency [227]. Recovery of renal and hepatic functions takes days. Small infants recover more slowly than older ones and may yet die of hepatic failure several days after the withdrawal of fructose. Once recovery is made, the further course is uneventful, intellectual development is unimpaired, and catch-up growth proceeds [175, 228]. Starting during the second half of their first year of life, patients protect themselves by a self-imposed exclusion diet.

Small children usually have hepatomegaly for months or years in spite of adequate treatment [156]. The reason for this is unclear, but it may be connected with a particularly high degree of intolerance during childhood [85] and also with hidden sources [166] of dietary fructose and sucrose. It is interesting that a group of adult patients on the average consumed 2.5 g sucrose daily, i.e., 5 percent of what was consumed by controls [166]. A rapid disappearance of intralobular hepatic fibrosis and a decrease of periportal fibrosis were observed in serial liver biopsy specimens, but fatty vacuolization of liver cells persisted or increased, and its distribution changed from diffuse to periportal [156, 225].

The oldest known patient was born in 1886 and was properly recognized toward the end of the last century as intolerant to sugar, although never reported. She had lived sugar-free and died at age 83 of an unrelated cause. The diagnosis was verified biochemically on postmortem liver examination [229].

Patients (or their parents) should state their intolerance to fructose on any hospital admission. Infusion solutions containing fructose, sorbitol, or invert sugar, still widely used in hospitals, e.g., after routine surgery, constitute an immediate threat to the life of patients. Such accidents, fatal and nonfatal, have been published [155, 170–173, 230], and a number of unpublished [231–234] iatrogenic deaths are known.

Genetics

The majority of cases have been reported from Europe and North America. One child was Indian [235]. The true incidence is not known but has been estimated at approximately 1:20,000 for Switzerland [226]. In recent years, evidence has grown that considerable numbers of children and adult patients must live undiagnosed in the general population. This can be concluded from the following facts: reports of iatrogenic accidents and deaths following infusions of fructose, invert sugar, and sorbitol in hospitals, published and unpublished; the surfacing of undiagnosed patients among older sibs and other relatives of young probands during extended family investigations [163, 164, 175, 191]; the self-diagnosis of medical students during a lecture on hereditary fructose intolerance (unpublished); and the frequent occurrence of parent-child [163, 167–169, 231, 236–239] or grandparent-grandchild [240] cases. Hereditary fructose intolerance occurs in all parts of the world except perhaps for Israel [137]. Sex distribution among the affected is even. Affected monozygotic twins have been observed [167, 197]. The overwhelming majority of parents are unaffected. Consanguinity of parents is not uncommon. One couple of affected parents produced four children, all affected [172]. The mode of inheritance is thus autosomal recessive. An apparently dominant case may be the child of an affected homozygous parent and a healthy heterozygote (pseudodominance). All parents examined so far have had normal liver fructaldolase activity [241], a fact incompatible with dominant inheritance.

Heterozygotes for hereditary fructose intolerance cannot be identified. Oral or intravenous fructose tolerance tests have been done in six sets of parents [160, 164, 241], in another parent and his healthy grandchild, who was the daughter of a patient [163]. The results were normal, without exception. In one set of parents given a continuous fructose infusion, fructose blood clearance was diminished when compared to that of controls [242]. This could not be confirmed in 11 parents [145, 154, 192]. In seven, significant differences were not found even though blood glucose, standard bicarbonate, phosphorus, lactate, urate and urinary urate/creatinine, and magnesium/creatinine ratios were determined [145].

Given the variation of liver enzyme activities between patients, Levin et al. [160] speculated that there may be more than one genotype involved. Koster et al. suspected the same from different K_m values for fructose-1-phosphate between patients [185]. Stronger evidence for genetic heterogeneity stems from studies by Gitzelmann et al. [186], who found that antibodies to normal aldolase B stimulated fructose-1-phosphate cleavage in liver homogenates of some patients but not others. These studies have been augmented recently [157]. Wide variations of heat stability of the residual FDP-aldolase were discovered. Antibody activation of mutant fructaldolase has since been reported [243].

FRUCTOSE-1,6-DIPHOSPHATASE DEFICIENCY

Historical Note

Fructose-1,6-diphosphate deficiency was first described in 1970 by Baker and Wingrad [158]. Two further reports appeared within a year [187, 244] and were followed by a continuing string of observations [245–261]. We are now aware of 21 published reports of patients and 11 affected sibs, all children, in 19 families. A variant form of fructose-1,6-diphosphatase deficiency in a woman and her daughter [262] and combined fructose-1,6-diphosphatase and glucose-6-phosphatase deficiency in another female [263] have been observed.

Clinical and Laboratory Findings

Fructose-1,6-diphosphatase deficiency is a severe disorder of gluconeogenesis causing life-threatening episodes in newborn infants and small children. Approximately one-half of the afflicted children had their first symptoms between their first and fourth day of life and the remainder in equal numbers before and after their sixth month. The latest manifestation, with one exception, was at age 4 years [258]. In the newborn, hyperventilation is the commonest symptom, usually caused by profound acidosis. Irritability, somnolence or coma, apneic spells, dyspnea and tachycardia, muscular hypotonia, and a moderate hepatomegaly may be observed. Hypoglycemia may be an isolated chemical sign [255] but is usually detected when sought, together with ketonuria. The first attacks in the newborn period are promptly overcome by the administration of glucose and sodium bicarbonate. Weeks or many months of apparent well-being can pass between the first and further attacks.

Later episodes are usually triggered by febrile infections. Refusal to feed and vomiting, which often accompany febrile infections in children, precipitate the onset. The evolution is usually dramatic: Hyperventilation, trembling, lethargy, coma, and convulsions follow in short succession within a few hours and reflect profound acidosis, ketosis, and hypoglycemia. Apnea and cardiac arrest have been observed [187]. Flushing [187] and hematemesis [248, 249] have occurred exceptionally. Lactate, ketones, alanine, and uric acid [256, 257] are elevated in the blood and appear in the urine [187, 249]. Blood glucose is low, but attacks of ketoacidosis without hypoglycemia have been observed [256, 257]. Hepatomegaly and muscle weakness are often present. Failure to thrive is the exception [257]. In one child, the clinical and biochemical presentation and course were suggestive of tyrosinosis [244, 245], with liver dysfunction, hyperaminoaciduria, wasting, sepsis, and death. In contrast to hereditary fructose intolerance, disturbances of liver function are the exception [252], and renal tubular function and blood coagulation are undisturbed. EEG

tracings may be abnormal during attacks but later return to normal. A slow wave pattern has been described [261]. Two sibs had a peculiar low amplitude pattern with slowed background activity and intermittent, spindle-shaped, fast-activity bursts [187]. The third sib had multifocal spikes and sharp waves on low background activity.

Most affected children experience a number of acute attacks before the diagnosis is made. Once the diagnosis is established and treatment begins, the course is favorable. The patients do not develop an aversion to sweet foods; in fact, they may even enjoy eating fruits and sweets [158]. Hepatomegaly regresses slowly or more rapidly, but lapses occur [248, 256, 260] and may be related to the intake of fructose and sucrose. Somatic, psychomotor, and intellectual development seems unimpaired.

The clinical features of the unusual mother-child cases of Taunton et al. [262] differed from the common ones. The mother presented at age 20 years with emotional lability, dizziness, fatigability, and symptomatic hypoglycemia and the child at age 13 months with unresponsiveness and confusion.

Biochemical Defect, Functional Studies, Pathogenesis

Deficiency of fructose-1,6-diphosphatase (hexose diphosphatase, fructose-1,6-bisphosphatase, EC 3.1.3.11) can be demonstrated in the liver and also in the jejunum [247], kidney [244, 249], and probably the leukocytes [249]. In two-thirds of the children, liver fructose-1,6-diphosphatase activity was either absent or reduced to a trace and in the others was reduced to one-fifth or less. Inactivity of fructose-1,6-diphosphatase in the liver and the active enzyme in skeletal muscle was demonstrated in one patient [246]; in another, the enzyme activity was absent in the liver, kidney, and leukocytes but was present in skeletal muscle extract [249]. These findings, together with further biochemical evidence, demonstrate that muscle contains a distinct enzyme not involved in this disorder.

Liver glycogen was normal in four liver biopsy specimens but was increased in two others [187, 249]. Liver glucose-6-phosphatase was measured and was normally active in 10 children. The combined deficiency of fructose-1,6-diphosphatase and glucose-6-phosphatase observed in an adult [263] is thus exceptional. Other enzymes examined in the liver included aldolase, pyruvate kinase, phosphoenolpyruvate carboxykinase, phosphorylase, phosphoglucomutase, phosphofructokinase, amylo-1,6-glucosidase, and acid maltase. They were normal.

Fructose-1,6-diphosphatase is a key enzyme of gluconeogenesis. Its inactivity prevents the endogenous formation of glucose from the precursors lactate, glycerol, and gluconeogenic amino acids such as alanine. It is not surprising that more than half of the afflicted infants become symptomatic within the first week of life when they are dependent on gluconeogenesis [264]. On subsequent days, higher milk volume and more frequent feedings seem to postpone further manifestations until insufficient food intake together with higher energy expenditure during infectious fever induces further episodes.

Dependence of fructose-1,6-diphosphatase-deficient children on exogenous glucose can easily be demonstrated. During fasting, maintenance of blood glucose depends initially on glycogenolysis, and the duration of normoglycemia therefore on the amount of available liver glycogen. Blood glucose may drop within a few hours [249] or only after 14 h or more [158, 187]. Simultaneously, lactate and pyruvate rise [158, 187, 249] and their ratio increases. Blood ketones and alanine also rise. When hypoglycemia is reached, the blood glucose level is irresponsive to injected glucagon. This indicates that liver glycogen stores have been depleted (Fig. 5-10). In the fed state, patients have a normal hyperglycemic response to glucagon. Feeding a diet excessively high in protein or fat equally provokes hypoglycemia, acidosis, and ketonemia [246]. High lactate/pyruvate and α-glycerophosphate/dihydroxyacetone phosphate ratios, demonstrated in biopsied liver, indicate the accumulation of glyceraldehyde-3-phosphate and insufficient reoxidation of NADH [246].

Fructose-1,6-diphosphatase-deficient patients have reduced tolerance to fructose and sorbitol, but generally it is higher than in patients with hereditary fructose intolerance. For instance, one infant tolerated 5 g sucrose per kilogram per day in his formula [145]. Fructose-1,6-diphosphatase-deficient patients do not develop gastrointestinal symptoms after an oral load [158, 187]. As in hereditary fructose intolerance, blood glucose and phosphorus drop after the load, while lactate, urate, magnesium, and alanine rise (Figs. 5-11 and 5-12). Fructose-induced hypoglycemia is not related to insulin release [158, 187, 246, 248, 253] and cannot be corrected by injecting glucagon [158, 248, 255, 261] or epinephrine [249]. The response to fructose is similar when given intravenously or orally and is clearly dose dependent [187, 255, 256]. Although, in fructose-1,6-diphosphatase-deficient children, fructose-induced changes of blood metabolites seem somewhat less drastic than they are in children with hereditary fructose intolerance, fructose tolerance tests are not without risk. The 20-month-old patient studied by Corbeel et al. [261] became comatous after the injection of 500 mg/kg fructose. Repeated sorbitol infusions in a 2-year-old patient were deleterious [265, 266] (Fig. 5-13).

Oral administration of glycerol [158, 187, 246, 247, 250, 253, 255, 257, 259, 260] provokes a response quite similar to that seen after fructose administration. Hypoglycemia is paral-

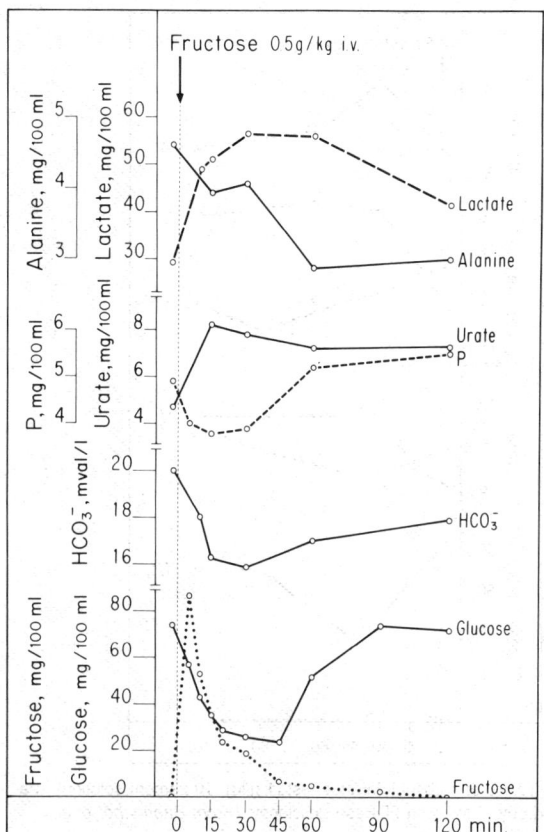

Figure 5-11 Intravenous fructose tolerance test in a 21-month-old boy (T.M.) with FDPase deficiency [187] with the high dose of 500 mg/kg. The lower dose of 200 mg/kg is preferable [157]. (*From Steinmann and Gitzelmann [273]*.)

leled by a drop in phosphorus and bicarbonate; lactate rises. In contrast, children with intact gluconeogenesis respond with an increase of blood glucose but not of lactic acid [246]. Hypoglycemia is again unrelated to insulin release [158, 246] and is refractory to glucagon [158]. Alanine, given intravenously or orally, can cause a similar though milder hypoglycemic response [246, 253, 255, 256] or none at all [247, 248, 253, 260]. The responses to alanine infusion after 6 and after 12 h of fasting were divergent in Pagliara's patient [246]. After a 6-h fast, alanine caused a rise of glucose and after a 12-h fast a late fall. The handling of a dihydroxyacetone load (1 g/kg orally) was tested in only one patient on two occasions [145, 187]. During the first half hour blood glucose fell in the patient but rose in adult controls and in a child with hereditary fructose intolerance [145]. In all, blood lactate rose and phosphorus and bicarbonate fell. The adult controls had a delayed hypoglycemic response due to hyperinsulinism [145].

Fructose-1,6-diphosphatase-deficient children have normal galactose tolerance. Injection or ingestion is followed by normoglycemia or mild hyperglycemia, indicating normal assimilation of this sugar. Since lactose provides approximately 40 percent of the energy in human milk, breast-fed infant patients remain asymptomatic from the end of their first week.

Hypoglycemia occurs after prolonged fasting when glycogen stores are depleted and the liver switches from glycogen breakdown to glucose production from gluconeogenic precursors. Precursors cannot be converted to glucose, and lactate accumulates and causes metabolic acidosis. Blood levels of precursors such as pyruvate, ketones, and alanine also rise. The

Figure 5-10 Prolonged fasting in a 17-month-old boy (T.M.) with FDPase deficiency. (*From Baerlocher et al. [187]*.)

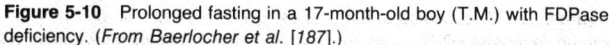

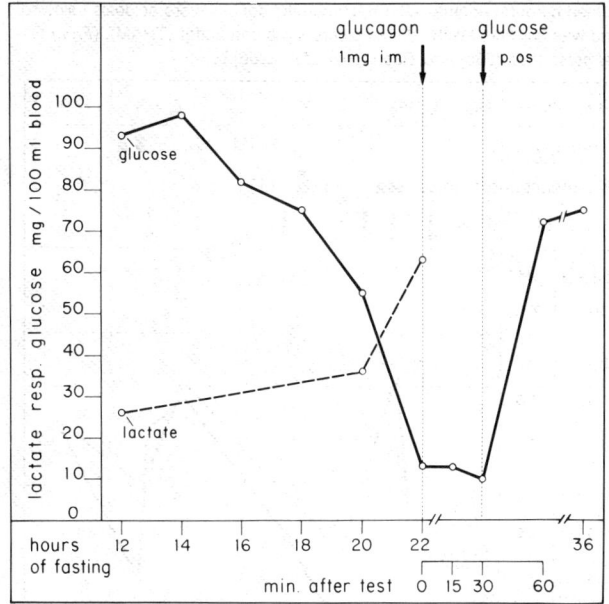

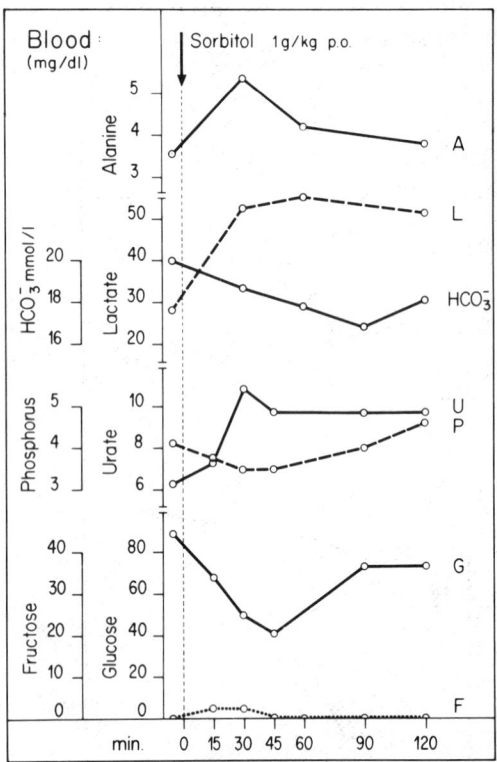

Figure 5-12 Oral sorbitol tolerance test (1 g/kg; 10 percent solution) in a 4-year-old boy (T.M.) with FDPase deficiency. (*From Baerlocher et al.* [*187*].)

newborn patient is particularly prone to hypoglycemia and acidosis during the first few days, when food intake is limited and only a little glycogen is available in the liver. The patient's tolerance to fasting depends on the size of the glycogen stores and is shortened in situations of increased catabolism and energy expenditure, e.g., in febrile infections. Tolerance to fasting, although limited, is not nil (Fig. 5-14). It seems to improve somewhat with age. A correlation with residual fructose-1,6-diphosphatase activity in the liver should exist but has not been documented.

Reactive hypoglycemia after fructose, sorbitol, glycerol, dihydroxyacetone, and alanine is somewhat more complex (Fig. 5-1). As in hereditary fructose intolerance, glycolytic phosphate esters may accumulate intracellularly and inhibit glycogen phosphorylase. This presumption is supported by the glucagon refractiveness of hypoglycemia.

Liver phosphorylase is inhibited in various ways by fructose-1-phosphate, fructose-1,6-diphosphate, and α-glycerophosphate [98, 215, 216, 218]. Inhibition is more pronounced as intracellular inorganic phosphate drops. Hyperuricemia and hypermagnesemia reflect adenine nucleotide breakdown (see section on the pathophysiology of hereditary fructose intolerance, above).

The cause of hepatomegaly and of fatty infiltration of the liver is uncertain. Fat deposition is likely to result from a constant flooding with amino acids and glycerol that can either be released as lactate or converted to fat and stored.

Diagnosis, Treatment, Prognosis

Fructose-1,6-diphosphatase deficiency must be suspected in full-term newborns of normal birth weight suffering from

hyperventilation, convulsions, and coma accompanied by hypoglycemia, ketosis, and acidosis, especially when signs of neonatal infection, cerebral hemorrhage, and left heart failure are absent. The disorder must also be suspected in small children suffering from episodic hypoglycemia triggered by febrile infection or starvation. Other defects of glyconeogenesis, such as the deficiencies of glucose-6-phosphatase, pyruvate carboxylase, pyruvate dehydrogenase, and phosphoenolpyruvate carboxykinase [267] may be difficult to exclude. Fasting tests (Fig. 5-10) and tolerance tests with fructose (Fig. 5-11), sorbitol (Fig. 5-12), glycerol, alanine, or dihydroxyacetone [145, 266] must be postponed until remission and should be carried out with adequate monitoring. A fructose load should not be given by mouth unless hereditary fructose intolerance is definitely excluded. The use of a moderate dose, e.g., 200 mg/kg intravenously is recommended [157], since higher doses may be dangerous [261]. Aversion to sweets and signs of a proximal renal tubular syndrome after fructose (or sorbitol) exposure, as seen in hereditary fructose intolerance, are absent in fructose-1,6-diphosphatase deficiency.

The diagnosis is established by demonstrating an enzyme deficiency in a liver biopsy specimen [222]. Although the defect has also been demonstrated in leukocytes by some investigators [249, 250, 256, 260, 268], others [269], including ourselves, have attempted this in vain in peripheral leukocytes and in Epstein-Barr virus-transformed lymphoblasts (unpublished data). After criticism [269], the originally reported activities of leukocytes [249, 270] were corrected [271]. Difficulties seem to have been due to the extremely low activity in white blood cells. Culturing peripheral lymphocytes increased the specific fructose-1,6-diphosphatase activity considerably [272]; this may become of diagnostic use. Fructose-1,6-diphosphatase deficiency has also been documented in jejunal biopsy material [247] and in the kidney at autopsy [244, 249]. Results of enzyme assays on tissues obtained at autopsy must be interpreted with caution, since the enzyme inactivates rapidly due to autolysis [Ref. 157 and unpublished data]. Fructose-1,6-diphosphatase is unmeasurable in cultured skin fibroblasts and in amniotic fluid cells [270]. Prenatal diagnosis is thus impossible.

Figure 5-13 Final course of a 2-year-old girl, M.M., older sib of T.M. [187], with undiagnosed FDPase deficiency after repeated sorbitol infusions for assumed cerebral edema. After each sorbitol dose, severe acidosis followed and was corrected with sodium bicarbonate and buffer (THAM). (*From Gitzelmann et al.* [*265*] *and Baerlocher et al.* [*266*].)

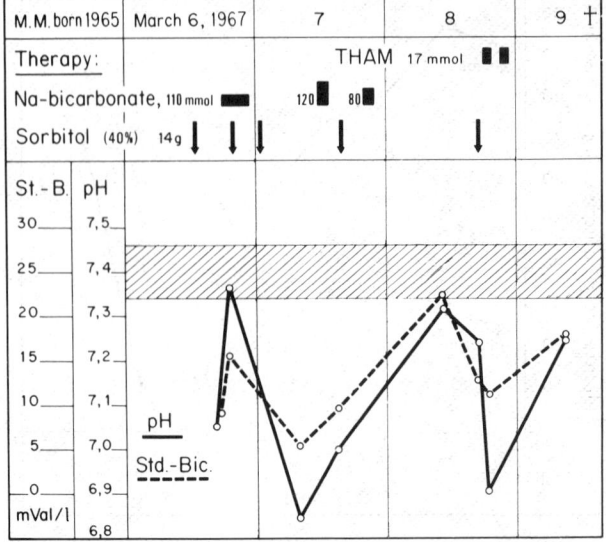

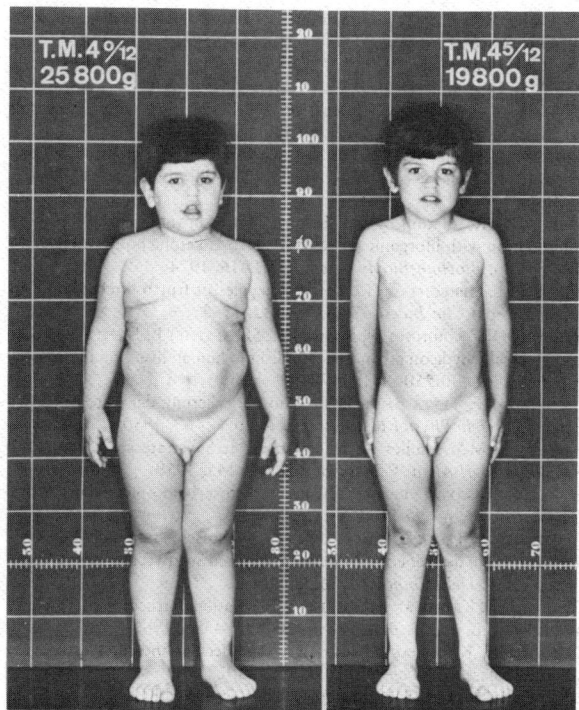

Figure 5-14 Patient T.M. [187], FDPase deficient, aged 4 years and obese because of overnutrition. Five months later, he had lost 6 kg by dieting (800–900 kcal/m²·day; carbohydrates 66 percent, proteins 22 percent, fat 12 percent).

Light microscopy of biopsied and autopsied liver usually reveals fatty infiltration, but neither fibrosis nor disturbed architecture, as is common in hereditary fructose intolerance. Electron-microscopic findings [187, 248, 258] have not been revealing.

Treatment of acute attacks consists of correction of hypoglycemia and acidosis by intravenous infusion and is usually rapidly successful. Later, avoidance of fasting prevents further episodes. Fructose and sucrose should be eliminated from the diet. The degree of intolerance to fructose may vary considerably between patients and even in the individual [248]. Acute episodes may be precipitated by fructose or sucrose ingestion. For instance, one newborn gained weight on a sucrose-containing formula during his first and further weeks of life [187], and another infant had her second and repeated attacks at age 7 months when weaned to baby food [246]. An 8-year-old boy, in remission for 2 years, suffered a relapse which led to diagnosis upon being prescribed a fructose-containing syrup for asthenia [258]. The liver size usually diminishes, but lapses occur [248, 252, 256, 258, 260]. Substitution of part of the dietary fat with carbohydrates and reduction of protein to the basic requirement have been recommended [246]. Treatment with folic acid was advocated [247] and repeatedly tried in typical cases [250, 258] as well as in the "new mild variant" [262], but its benefit remains to be proved.

As a rule, the firstborn child with the disease dies or suffers more than the following children, who profit from the experience gained by parents and physicians with the first. Once the diagnosis is established, the course seems benign, and growth and development are normal. Lapses during febrile infections are controlled easily by glucose, either alone or in combination with sodium bicarbonate. Baker and Wingrad [158] have the clinical impression that tolerance to fasting increases with age, and our experience supports this impression. It may be assumed that undiagnosed fructose-1,6-diphosphatase-

deficient adults exist in the general population. These persons, like those with undiagnosed hereditary fructose intolerance, may be endangered by the indiscriminate use of fructose, invert sugar, or sorbitol in infusion solutions.

Genetics

The incidence of fructose-1,6-diphosphatase deficiency is still unknown. In the 11 years since its first description, a total of 21 probands in 19 families have been reported, all but one diagnosed by enzyme assay in biopsied liver. (The unusual cases of Taunton et al. [262] and Service et al. [263] are not counted here.) A syndrome strongly suggestive of the disorder had existed in 11 sibs. Nine were older than the probands and had died under circumstances similar to those which led to the hospital admission of the probands. A total of 38 patients are now known to us [279]. Of these, 12 are boys and 26 are girls, involving 24 families in the United States and Europe and 1 in Japan. One patient was a black North American [247] and one an Indian child living in England [251, 252].

Parental consanguinity was mentioned three times [244, 245, 254]. The parents are healthy. One couple had normal responses to intravenous fructose and glycerol [246]. All three parents tested had intermediate fructose-1,6-diphosphatase activity in the liver [248, 265], but results of activity measurements in leukocytes were less than conclusive [249, 260, 270]. The mode of inheritance appears to be autosomal recessive. The excess of female patients is unexplained but may be chance. At any rate, increased fetal loss (e.g., of affected males) has not been reported.

REFERENCES

1. HARDINGE MG, SWARNER JB, JULIA B, CROOKS H: Carbohydrates in foods. *J Am Diet Assoc* 46:197, 1965
2. SOMOGYI JC, TRAUTNER K: Der Glukose-, Fruktose- und Saccharosegehalt verschiedener Gemüsearten. *Schweiz Med Wschr* 104:177–182, 1974
3. BOHANNON NV, KARAM JH, FORSHAM PH: Endocrine responses to sugar ingestion in man. *J Am Diet Assoc* 76:555–560, 1980
4. NIKKILÄ EA, HUTTUNEN JK (eds): Clinical and metabolic aspects of fructose. *Acta Medica Scand* (suppl) 542, 1972
5. SIPPLE HL, McNUTT KW (eds): *Sugars in Nutrition.* New York, Academic Press, Inc 1974
6. GUGGENHEIM B (ed): *Health and Sugar Substitutes.* Basel, S. Karger, 1979
7. MINKOWSKI O: Untersuchungen uUber den Diabetes mellitus nach Exstrirpation des Pankreas. *Arch Exp Pathol Pharmakol* 31:85–189, 1893
8. ROE JH, EPSTEIN JH, GOLDSTEIN NP: A photometric method for the determination of inulin in plasma and urine. *J Biol Chem* 178:839, 1949
9. HIGASHI A, PETER L: A rapid colorimetric method for the determination of inulin in plasma and urine. *J Lab Clin Med* 35:475, 1950
10. COOK GC: Absorption and Metabolism of D (−) fructose in man. *Am J Clin Nutr* 24:1302–1307, 1971
11. GINSBURG V, HERS HG: On the conversion of fructose to glucose by guinea pig intestine. *Biochem Biophys Acta* 38:427–434, 1960
12. DARLINGTON WA, QUASTEL JH: Absorption of sugars from isolated surviving intestine. *Arch Biochem Biophys* 43:194–207, 1953
13. WILSON TH, VINCENT TN: Absorption of sugars in vitro by the intestine of the golden hamster. *J Biol Chem* 216:851–866, 1955
14. SHOEMAKER WC, YANOF HM, TURK LN, WILSON TH: Glucose and fructose absorption in the unanesthesized dog. *Gastroenterology* 44:654–663, 1963
15. SIGRIST-NELSON K, HOPFER U: A distinct D-fructose transport system in isolated brush border membrane. *Biochim Biophys Acta* 367:247–259, 1974
16. CROUZOULON G: Les propriétés cinétiques du flux d'entrée du fructose à travers la bordure en brosse du jéjunum du rat. Effect d'un régime riche en fructose. *Arch Int Physiol Biochim* 86:725–740, 1978
17. SCHULTZ SG, STRECKER CK: Fructose influx across the brush border of rabbit ileum. *Biochim Biophys Acta* 211:586–588, 1970

18. HONEGGER P, SEMENZA G: Multiplicity of carriers for free glucalogues in hamster small intestine. *Biochim Biophys Acta* 318:390–410, 1973

19. GRACEY M, BURKE V, OSHIN A: Active intestinal transport of D-fructose. *Biochim Biophys Acta* 266:397–406, 1972

20. MACRAE AR, NEUDOERFFER TS: Support for the existence of an active transport mechanism of fructose in the rat. *Biochim Biophys Acta* 288:137–144, 1972

21. MAVRIAS DA, MAYER RJ: Metabolism of fructose in the small intestine. 2. The effect of fructose feeding on fructose transport and metabolism in guinea pig small intestine. *Biochim Biophys Acta* 291:538–544, 1973

22. WOODS HF, EGGLESTON LV, KREBS HA: The cause of hepatic accumulation of fructose-1-phosphate on fructose loading. *Biochem J* 119:501–510, 1970

23. SESTOFT L, FLERON P: Determination of the kinetic constants of fructose transport and phosphorylation in the perfused rat liver. *Biochim Biophys Acta* 345:27–38, 1974

24. CRAIK JD, ELLIOTT KRF: Transport of D-fructose and D-galactose into isolated rat hepatocytes. *Biochem J* 192:373–375, 1980

25. FROESCH ER, GINSBERG JL: Fructose metabolism of adipose tissue. 1. Comparison of fructose and glucose metabolism in epididymal adipose tissue of normal rats. *J Biol Chem* 237:3317–3324, 1962

26. FROESCH ER: Fructose metabolism of adipose tissue of normal and diabetic rats, in *Handbook of Physiology. vol 52*, Adipose Tissue, by Renold AE, Cahill GF Jr (eds) Washington, DC, American Physiology Society, 1965, pp 281–293

27. SCHOENLE E, ZAPF J, FROESCH ER: Transport and metabolism of fructose in fat cells of normal and hypophysectomized rats. *Am J Physiol* 237:E325–E330, 1979

28. MILLER M, DRUCKER WR, OWENS JE, CRAIG JW, WOODWARD H JR: Metabolism of intravenous fructose and glucose in normal and diabetic subjects. *J Clin Invest* 31:115–125, 1952

29. SMITH LH, ETTINGER RH, SELIGSON D: A comparison of the metabolism of fructose and glucose in hepatic disease and diabetes mellitus. *J Clin Invest* 32:273–282, 1953

30. LANE HC, DODD K: Use of glucose, invert sugar and fructose for parenteral feeding of children. *Pediatrics* 20:668–675, 1957

31. ZÖLLNER N, HEUCKENKAMP P-U, NECHWATAL W: Ueber die Verwertung und renale Ausscheidung von Fructose während ihrer langdauernden intravenösen Zufuhr. *Klin Wschr* 46:1300–1308, 1968

32. HOLDSWORTH CD, DAWSON AM: Absorption of fructose in man. *Proc Soc Exp Biol Med* 118:142–145, 1965

33. CROSSLEY JN, MacDONALD I: The influence in male baboons of a high sucrose diet on the portal and arterial levels of glucose and fructose following a sucrose meal. *Nutr Metab* 12:171–178, 1970

34. TOPPING DL, MAYES PA: The concentration of fructose, glucose and lactate in the splanchnic blood vessels of rats absorbing fructose. *Nutr Metab* 13:331–338, 1971

35. BOLLMAN JL, MANN FC: The physiology of the liver. 14. The utilisation of fructose following complete removal of the liver. *Am J Physiol* 96:683–695, 1931

36. REINECKE RM: The kidney as a locus of fructose metabolism. *Am J Physiol* 141:669–676, 1944

37. MENDELOFF AI, WEICHSELBAUM TE: Role of the human liver in the assimilation of intravenously administered fructose. *Metabolism* 2:450–458, 1953

38. WOLFE BM, AHUJA SP, MARLISS EB: Effects of intravenously administered fructose and glucose on splanchnic aminoacid and carbohydrate metabolism in hypertriglyceridemic man. *J Clin Invest* 56:970–977, 1975

39. LEVINE R, HUDDLESTUN B: The comparative action of insulin on the disposal of intravenous fructose and glucose. *Fed Proc* 6:151–152, 1947

40. SOLS A, CRANE RK: Substrate specificity of brain hexokinase. *J Biol Chem* 210:581–595, 1954

41. KATZEN HM, SCHIMKE RT: Multiple forms of hexokinase in the rat: Tissue distribution, age dependency and properties. *Proc Natl Acad Sci USA* 54:1218–1225, 1965

42. FROESCH ER, ZAPF J, KELLER U, OELZ O: Comparative study of the metabolism of U-14C-fructose, U-14C-sorbitol and U-14C-xylitol in the normal and streptozotocin-diabetic rat. *Eur J Clin Invest* 2:8–14, 1971

43. KELLER U, FROESCH ER: Metabolism and oxidation of U-14C-glucose, xylitol, fructose and sorbitol in the fasted and in the streptozotocin-diabetic rat. *Diabetologia* 7:349–356, 1971

44. KELLER U, FROESCH ER: Vergleichende Untersuchungen über den Stoffwechsel von Xylit, Sorbit und Fruktose beim Menschen. *Schweiz Med Wschr* 102:1017–1022, 1972

45. HERS HG: *Le Métabolisme du Fructose*. Brussels, Editions Arscia, 1957

46. LEUTHARDT F, TESTA E: Die Phosphorylierung der Fructose in der Leber. II. Mitteilung. *Helv Chim Acta* 34:931–938, 1951

47. CORI GT, OCHOA S, SLEIN MW, CORI CF: The metabolism of fructose in liver. Isolation of fructose-1-phosphate and inorganic phyrophosphate. *Biochim Biophys Acta* 7:304–317, 1951

48. HERS HG: La fructokinase du foie. *Biochim Biophys Acta* 8:316–423, 1952

49. HERS HG: Rôle du magnésium et du potassium dans la réaction fructokinasique. *Biochim Biophys Acta* 8:424–430, 1952

50. PARKS, RE, BEN-GERSHOM E, LARDY HA: Liver fructokinase. *J Biol Chem* 227:231–242, 1957

51. ADELMAN RC, BALLARD FJ, WEINHOUSE S: Purification and properties of rat liver fructokinase. *J Biol Chem* 242:3360–3365, 1967

52. SANCHEZ JJ, GONZALEZ NS, PONTIS HG: Fructoskinase from rat liver. 2. The role of K+ on the enzyme activity. *Biochim Biophys Acta* 227:79–85, 1971

53. SESTOFT L: Regulation of fructose metabolism in the perfused rat liver. Interrelation with inorganic phosphate, glucose, ketone body and ethanol metabolism. *Biochim Biophys Acta* 343:1–16, 1974

54. HEINZ F, LAMPRECHT W, KIRSCH J: Enzymes of fructose metabolism in human liver. *J Clin Invest* 47:1826–1832, 1968

55. THIEDEN HID, GRUNNET N, DAMGAARD SE, SESTOFT L: Effect of fructose and glyceraldehyde on ethanol metabolism in human liver and in rat liver. *Eur J Biochem* 30:250–261, 1972

56. LEUTHARDT F, TESTA E: Ueber die Phosphorylierung der Ketosen in der Leber (1.). *Helv Physiol Pharmacol Acta* 8:C67–69, 1950

57. KUYPER ChMA: Studies on fructokinase. 1. Substrate specificity. *Proc Koninkl Nederl Akad Wetenschap* 62:137–145, 1959

58. HERS HG, KUSAKA T: Le métabolisme du fructose-1-phosphate dans le foie. *Biochim Biophys Acta* 11:427, 1953

59. LEUTHARDT F, TESTA E, WOLF HP: Der enzymatische Abbau des Fructose-1-phosphats in der Leber. 3. Mitteilung über den Stoffwechsel der Fructose in der Leber. *Helv Chim Acta* 36:227, 1953

60. PENHOET EE, KOCHMAN M, RUTTER WJ: Isolation of fructose diphosphate aldolases A, B, and C. *Biochemistry* 8:4391–4395, 1969

61. PENHOET EE, KOCHMAN M, RUTTER WJ: Molecular and catalytic properties of aldolase C. *Biochemistry* 8:4396–4402, 1969

62. DIKOW AL, JECKEL D, PFLEIDERER G: Isolierung und Charakterisierung von Aldolase A, B und C aus menschlichen Organen. *Hoppe Seyler's Z Physiol Chem* 352:1151–1156, 1971

63. PENHOET E, RAJKUMAR T, RUTTER WJ: Multiple forms of fructose diphosphate aldolase in mammalian tissues. *Proc Natl Acad Sci USA* 56:1275–1282, 1966

64. LEBHERZ HG: Evidence for the lack of subunit exchange between aldolase tetramers in vivo. *J Biol Chem* 250:7388–7391, 1975

65. LEBHERZ HG, RUTTER WJ: Distribution of fructose diphosphate aldolase variants in biological systems. *Biochemistry* 8:109–121, 1969

66. REHBEIN-THÖNER M, PFLEIDERER G: The changes in aldolase isoenzyme pattern during development of the human kidney and small intestine—demonstrated in organ extracts and tissue sections. *Hoppe Seyler's Z Physiol Chem* 358:169–180, 1977

67. PENHOET EE, RUTTER WJ: Catalytic and immunochemical properties of homomeric and heteromeric combinations of aldolase subunits. *J Biol Chem* 246:318–323, 1971

68. WACHSMUTH ED: Differentiation of epithelial cells in human jejunum: Localization and quantification of aminopeptidase, alkaline phosphatase and aldolase isozymes in tissue sections. *Histochemistry* 48:101–109, 1976

69. PFLEIDERER G, THÖNER M, WACHSMUTH ED: Histological examination of the aldolase monomer composition of cells from human kidney and hypernephroid carcinoma. *Beitr Pathol* 156:266–279, 1975

70. BURCH HB, CHOI S, DENCE CN, ALVEY TR, COLE BR, LOWRY OH: Metabolic effects of large fructose loads in different parts of the rat nephron. *J Biol Chem* 255:8239–8244, 1980

71. FRANDSEN EK, GRUNNET N: Kinetic properties of triokinase from rat liver. *Eur J Biochem* 23:588–592, 1971

72. HERS HG: "Triokinase" in Colowick SP, Kaplan NO (eds): *Methods in Enzymology*. New York, Academic Press, Inc, 1962, vol 5, pp 362–364

73. SILLERO MAG, SILLERO A, SOLS A: Enzymes involved in fructose metabolism in liver and the glyceraldehyde metabolic crossroads. *Eur J Biochem* 10:345–350, 1969

74. HUE L, HERS HG: The conversion of [4-3H]fructose and of [4-3H]glucose to liver glycogen in the mouse. An investigation of the glyceraldehyde crossroads. *Eur J Biochem* 29:268–275, 1972

75. HORECKER BL, MELLONI E, PONTREMOLI S: Fructose 1, 6-bisphosphatase: Properties of the neutral enzyme and its modification by proteolytic enzymes. *Adv Enzymol* 42:193–226, 1975

76. DZUGAJ A, KOCHMAN L: Purification of human liver fructose-1, 6-bisphosphatase. *Biochem Biophys Acta* 614:407–412, 1980

77. HUE L: The role of futile cycles in the regulation of carbohydrate metabolism. *Adv Enzymol* 52:247–331, 1981

78. VAN SCHAFTINGEN E, HUE L, HERS HG: Fructose 2,6-bisphosphate, the probable structure of the glucose- and glucagon-sensitive stimulator of phosphofructokinase. *Biochem J* 192:897–901, 1980

79. VAN SCHAFTINGEN E, HUE L, HERS HG: Control of the fructose 6-phosphate/fructose 1, 6-bisphosphate cycle in isolated hepatocytes by glucose and glucagon. Role of low-molecular-weight stimulator of phosphofructokinase. *Biochem J* 192:887–895, 1980

80. VAN SCHAFTINGEN E, HERS HG: Inhibition of fructose 1, 6-bisphosphatase by fructose 2, 6-bisphosphate. *Proc Natl Acad Sci USA* 78:2861–2863, 1981

81. EXTON JH, PARK CR: Control of gluconeogenesis in liver. 1. General features of gluconeogenesis in the perfused livers of rats. *J Biol Chem* 242:2622–2636, 1967

82. ATWELL ME, WATERHOUSE C: Glucose production from fructose. *Diabetes* 20:193–199, 1971

83. VAN DEN BERGHE G: Metabolic effects of fructose in the liver. *Curr Top Cell Regul* 13:97, 1978

84. HERS HG: L'Aldose-réductase. Le méchanisme de la formation du fructose séminal et du fructose foetal. *Biochim Biophys Acta* 37:120–126, 127–138, 1960

85. FROESCH ER, PRADER A, LABHART A, STUBER HW, WOLF HP: Die hereditäre Fructoseintoleranz, eine bisher nicht bekannte kongenitale Stoffwechselstörung. *Schweiz Med Wschr* 87:1168–1171, 1957

86. PERHEENTUPA J, RAIVIO K: Fructose-induced hyperuricaemia. *Lancet* 2:528–531, 1967

87. BERGSTRÖM J, HULTMAN E, ROCH-NORLUND AE: Lactic acid accumulation in connection with fructose infusion. *Acta Med Scand* 184:359–364, 1968

88. HERS HG: Misuses for fructose. *Nature* 227:241, 1979

89. WOODS HF, EGGLESTON LV, KREBS, HA: The cause of hepatic accumulation of fructose 1-phosphate on fructose loading. *Biochem J* 119:501–510, 1970

90. SESTOFT L: Fructose—en advarsal. *Ugeskr Laeger* 134:571, 1972

91. VAN DEN BERGHE G, HERS HG: Dangers of intravenous fructose and sorbitol. *Acta Paediatr Belg* 31:115–123, 1978

92. CONARD V: Mesure de l'assimilation du glucose: Bases théoriques et applications cliniques. *Acta Gastroenterol Belg* 18:655–705, 1955

93. KJERULF-JENSEN K: The phosphate esters formed in the liver tissue of rats and rabbits during assimilation of hexoses and glycerol. *Acta Physiol Scand* 4:249–258, 1942

94. GÜNTHER MA, SILLERO A, SOLS A: Fructokinase assay with a specific spectrophotometric method using 1-phosphofructokinase. *Enzymol Biol Clin* 8:341–352, 1967

95. HEINZ F, JUNGHÄNEL J: Metabolitenmuster in Rattenleber nach Fructose aplikation. *Hoppe Seylers' Z Physiol Chem* 350:859–866, 1969

96. SESTOFT L, TONNESEN K, HANSEN FV, DAMGAARD SE: Fructose and D-glyceraldehyde metabolism in the isolated perfused pig liver. *Eur J Biochem* 30:542–552, 1972

97. BODE JC, ZELDER O, RUMPELT HJ, WITTKAMP U: Depletion of liver adenosine phosphates and metabolic effects of intravenous infusion of fructose or sorbitol in man and in the rat. *Eur J clin Invest* 3:436–441, 1973

98. VAN DEN BERGHE G, HUE L, HERS HG: Effect of the administration of fructose on the glycogenolytic action of glucagon. An investigation of the pathogeny of hereditary fructose intolerance. *Biochem J* 134:637–645, 1973

99. VAN DEN BERGHE G, BRONFMAN M, VANNESTE R, HERS HG: The mechanism of adenosine triphosphate depletion in the liver after a load of fructose. A kinetic study of liver adenylate deaminase. *Biochem J* 162:601–609, 1977

100. FOX IH, KELLEY WN: Studies on the mechanism of fructose-induced hyperuricaemia in man. *Metabolism* 21:713–721, 1972

101. NARINS RG, WEISBERG JS, MYERS AR: Effects of carbohydrates on uric acid metabolism. *Metabolism* 23:455–465, 1974

102. HEUCKENKAMP PV, ZÖLLNER N: Fructose-induced hyperuricaemia. *Lancet* 1:808–809, 1971

103. CURRERI PW, PRUITT BA JR: Absence of fructose-induced hyperuricaemia in men. *Lancet* 1:839, 1970

104. HESSOV I: Effects of fructose and glucose infusions on blood acid-base equilibrium in the postoperative period. *Acta Chir Scand* 140:347–351, 1974

105. PEASTON MJT: Dangers of intravenous fructose. *Lancet* 1:266, 1973

106. KOGUT MD, ROE TF, WON NG, DONNELL GN: Fructose-induced hyperuricaemia: Observations in normal children and in patients with hereditary fructose intolerance and galactosemia. *Pediatr Res* 9:774–778, 1975

107. SAHEBJAMI D, SCALETTAR R: Effects of fructose infusion on lactate and uric acid metabolism. *Lancet* 1:366–369, 1971

108. MÄENPÄÄ PH, RAIVIO KO, KEKOMÄKI MP: Liver adenine nucleotides: Fructose-induced depletion and its effect on protein synthesis. *Science* 161:1253–1254, 1968

109. HULTMAN E, NILSSON LH, SAHLIN K: Adenine nucleotide content of human liver. Normal values and fructose-induced depletion. *Scand J Clin Lab Invest* 35:245–251, 1975

110. BURCH HB, MAX P JR, CHYU K, LOWRY OH: Metabolic intermediates in liver of rats given large amounts of fructose or dihydroxyacetone. *Biochem Biophys Res Commun* 34:619–626, 1969

111. BURCH HB, LOWRY OH, MEINHARDT L, MAX P JR, CHYU K: Effects of fructose, dihydroxyacetone, glycerol, and glucose on metabolites and related compounds in liver and kidney. *J Biol Chem* 245:2092–2102, 1970

112. VAN DEN BERGHE G: Metabolic effects of fructose in the liver. *Curr Top Cell Regul* 13:97–135, 1978

113. VAN DEN BERGHE G: Regulation of purine catabolism, in Hue L, Van de Werve (eds): *Short Term Regulation of Liver Metabolism.* Amsterdam, Elsevier North-Holland, 1981, pp 361–376

113a. FOX IH: Purine ribonucleotide catabolism: Clinical and biochemical significance. *Rev Nutr Metab* 16:65–78, 1974

114. FOX IH, KELLEY, WN: The role of adenosine and 2-deoxyadenosine in mammalian cells. *Ann Rev Biochem* 47:655, 1978

115. VAN DEN BERGHE G, VON POTTELSBERGHE C, HERS HG: A kinetic study of the soluble 5'-nucleotidase of rat liver. *Biochem J* 162:611–616, 1977

116. VAN DEN BERGHE G, BONTEMPS F, HERS HG: Purine catabolism in isolated rat hepatocytes. Influence of coformycin. *Biochem J* 188:913–920, 1980

117. LAMERS JMJ, HÜLSMANN WC: The effect of fructose on the stores of energy-rich phosphate in rat jejunum in vivo. *Biochim Biophys Acta* 313:1–8, 1973

118. MORRIS RC JR, NIGON K, REED EB: Evidence that the severity of depletion of inorganic phosphate determines the severity of the disturbance of adenine nucleotide metabolism in the liver and renal cortex of the fructose-loaded rat. *J Clin Invest* 61:209–220, 1978

119. WATTS RWE, WATTS JEM, SEEGMILLER JE: Xanthine oxidase activity in human tissues and its inhibition by allopurinol (4-hydroxypyrazolo (3, 4-d) pyrimidine). *J Lab Clin Med* 66:688–697, 1965

120. MÄENPÄÄ PH: Fructose-induced alterations in liver polysome profiles and Mg^{2+} levels. *FEBS Lett* 24:37–40, 1972

121. MÄENPÄÄ PH: Fructose and liver protein synthesis. *Acta Med Scand* 542 (suppl):115–118, 1972

122. VAN DEN BERGHE G, VINCENT MF: Effect of fructose on the metabolization of ammonia. Presented at the Annual Meeting of the European Society for Paediatric Research, Turku (Finland), June 25–29, 1978

123. YU DT, BURCH HB, PHILLIPS MJ: Pathogenesis of fructose hepatotoxicity. *Lab Invest* 30:85–92, 1974

124. HUGON JS, MAESTRACCI D, MÉNARD D: Smooth endoplasmic reticulum proliferation in mouse enterocytes induced by fructose feeding. *Histochemie* 29:189–197, 1972

125. ASHARE R, MOORE R, ELLISON EH: Utilization of glucose, fructose and invert sugar. Comparison in diseases of the liver and pancreas. *Arch Surg* 70:428–435, 1955

126. KAYE R, WILLIAMS ML, BARBERO G: Comparative study of glucose and fructose metabolism in infants with reference to utilization and to the accumulation of glycolytic intermediates. *J Clin Invest* 37:752–762, 1958

127. EGGLESTON LV, WOODS HF: Activation of liver pyruvate kinase by fructose-1-phosphate. *FEBS Lett* 6:43–45, 1970

128. COOK GC, JACOBSON J: Individual variation in fructose metabolism in man. *Br J Nutr* 26:187–195, 1971

129. CRAIG GM, CRANE CW: Lactic acidosis complicating liver failure after intravenous fructose. *Br Med J* 4:211–212, 1971

130. ANDERSSON G, BROHULT J, STERNER G: Increasing metabolic acidosis following fructose infusion in two children. *Acta Paediatr Scand* 58:301–304, 1969

131. ODIÉVRE M, POIRIER C, LEVILLAIN P, MODIGLIANI E, STRAUCH G: Etude des réponses glucosémiques, lactacidémiques et insulinémiques après administration intraveineuse rapide de doses variables de fructose chez l'enfant normal. *Arch Fr Pediatr* 27:1057–1068, 1970

132. PEARSON JF, SHUTTLEWORTH R: The metabolic effects of a hypertonic fructose infusion on the mother and fetus during labor. *Am J Obstet Gynecol* 111:259–265, 1971

133. KRANE SM: Fructosuria, in: Stanbury JB, Wyngaarden JB, Fredrickson DS (eds): *The Metabolic Basis of Inherited Disease, ed. 1.* New York, McGraw-Hill Book Co, 1960, pp 144–155

134. CZAPEK F: Eine seltene Form von Diabetes mellitus. *Prager Med Wschr* 1:245–249, 265–270, 1876

135. ZIMMER K: I. Levulose im Harn eines Diabetikers. *Dtsch Med Wschr* 1:329–332, 1876

136. LARON Z: Essential benign fructosuria. *Arch Dis Child* 36:273–277, 1961

137. STEINITZ H, MIZRAHY O: Essential fructosuria and hereditary fructose intolerance. *N Engl J Med* 280:222, 1969

138. KHACHADURIAN AK: Nonalimentary fructosuria. *Pediatrics* 32:455–457, 1963

139. HEERES PA, VOS H: Fructosuria. *Arch Intern Med* 44:47–64, 1929

140. LENZNER AR: Fructosuria: Report of a case. *Ann Int Med* 45:702–706, 1956

141. HEINZ F, SCHLEGEL F, KRAUSE PH: Enzymes of fructose metabolism in human kidney. *Enzyme* 19:85–92, 1975

142. HEINZ F, SCHLEGEL F, KRAUSE PH: Enzymes of fructose metabolism in human small intestine mucosa. *Enzyme* 19:93–101, 1975

143. SCHAPIRA F, SCHAPIRA G, DREYFUS J-C: La lésion enzymatique de la fructosurie bénigne. *Enzymol Biol Clin* 1:170–175, 1961–1962

144. Hers HG, Joassin G: Anomalie de l'aldolase hépatique dans l'intolérance au fructose. *Enzymol Biol Clin* 1:4–14, 1961

145. Steinmann B, Baerlocher K, Gitzelmann R: Hereditäre Störungen des Fruktosestoffwechsels: Belastungsproben mit Fruktose, Sorbitol und Dihydroxyaceton. *Nutr Metab* 18 (suppl 1):115–132, 1975

146. Sachs B, Sternfeld L, Kraus G: Essential fructosuria. Its pathophysiology. *Am J Dis Child* 63:252–269, 1942

147. Regenberger HJ, Chambers WH, Blatherwick NR: Respiratory metabolism in fructosuria. *J Nutr* 21:553–564, 1941

148. Baylon H, Schapira F, Wegmann R, Dreyfus J-C, Moulias R, Poyart C, Coumel Ph: Note préliminaire sur l'étude clinique, biologique, histochimique et enzymatique de la fructosurie familiale essentielle. *Rev Fr Etud Clin Biol* 7:531–534, 1962

149. Silver S, Reiner M: Essential fructosuria. Report of three cases with metabolic studies. *Arch Int Med* 54:412–426, 1934

150. Lasker M: Essential fructosuria. *Hum Biol* 13:51–63, 1941

151. Marble A: The diagnosis of the less common melliturias. *Med Clin North Am* 31:313–325, 1947

152. Leonidas JC: Essential fructosuria. *NY State J Med* 65:2257–2259, 1965

153. Chambers RA, Pratt RTC: Idiosyncrasy to fructose. *Lancet* 2:340, 1956

154. Perheentupa J, Raivio KO, Nikkilä EA: Hereditary fructose intolerance. *Acta Med Scand* 542 (suppl):65–75, 1972

155. Baerlocher K, Gitzelmann R, Steinmann B, Gitzelmann-Cumarasamy N: Hereditary fructose intolerance in early childhood: A major diagnostic challenge. *Helv Paediatr Acta* 33:465–487, 1978

156. Odièvre M, Gentil C, Gautier M, Alagille D: Hereditary fructose intolerance in childhood. *Am J Dis Child* 132:605–608, 1978

157. Steinmann B, Gitzelmann R: The diagnosis of hereditary fructose intolerance. *Helv Paediatr Acta* 36:297, 1981

158. Baker L, Wingrad AI: Fasting hypoglycaemia and metabolic acidosis associated with deficiency of hepatic fructose-1, 6-diphosphatase activity. *Lancet* 2:13–16, 1970

159. Turner RC, Spathis GS, Nabarro JDN, Dormandy TL: Familial fructose and galactose intolerance. *Lancet* 2:872, 1972

160. Levin B, Snodgrass GJAI, Oberholzer VG, Burgess EA, Dobbs RH: Fructosaemia. Observations on seven cases. *Am J Med* 45:826–838, 1968

161. Swales JD, Smith ADM: Adult fructose intolerance. *Q J Med* 35:455–473, 1966

162. Marthaler TM, Froesch ER: Hereditary fructose intolerance. Dental status of eight patients. *Br Dent J* 123:597–599, 1967

163. Köhlin P, Melin K: Hereditary fructose intolerance in four swedish families. *Acta Paediatr Scand* 57:24–32, 1968

164. Cornblath M, Rosenthal IM, Reisner SH, Wybregt SH, Crane RK: Hereditary fructose intolerance. *N Engl J Med* 269:1271–1278, 1963

165. Froesch ER, Wolf HP, Baitsch H, Prader A, Labhart A: Hereditary fructose intolerance. An inborn defect of hepatic fructose-1-phosphate splitting aldolase. *Am J Med* 34:151–167, 1963

166. Newbrun E, Hoover C, Mettraux G, Graf H: Comparison of dietary habits and dental health of subjects with hereditary fructose intolerance and control subjects. *J Am Dent Assoc* 101:619–626, 1980

167. Rampa M, Froesch ER: Eleven cases of hereditary fructose intolerance in one Swiss family with a pair of monozygotic and dizygotic twins. *Helv Paediatr Acta* 36:317, 1981

168. Wolf H, Zschocke D, Wedemeyer FW, Hübner W: Angeborene hereditäre Fructose-Intoleranz. *Klin Wschr* 37:693–696, 1959

169. Barry RGG, St Colum S, Magner JW: Hereditary fructose intolerance in parent and child. *J Irish Med Assoc* 61:308–310, 1968

170. Lameire N, Mussche M, Baele G, Kint J, Ringoir S: Hereditary fructose intolerance: A difficult diagnosis in the adult. *Am J Med* 65:416–423, 1978

171. De Vroede M, Mozin M-J, Cadranel S, Loeb H, Heimann R: Découverte d'une fructosémie á l'occasion d'une insuffisance hépatique aigue chez un enfant de 16 mois. *Pédiatrie* 35:353–358, 1980

172. Schulte M-J, Lenz W: Fatal sorbitol infusion in patient with fructose-sorbitol intolerance. *Lancet* 2:188, 1977

173. Hackl JM, Balogh D, Kunz F, Dworzak E, Puschendorf B, Decristoforo A, Maier F: Postoperative Fruktoseintoleranz. *Wiener Klin Wschrift* 90:237–240, 1978

174. Leonard JV: Personal communication

175. Black JA, Simpson K: Fructose intolerance. *Br Med J* 4:138–141, 1967

176. Roschlau G: *Leberbiopsie im Kindesalter*. G Fischer Verlag Jena, 1978, pp 80–83

177. Dubois R, Loeb H, Malaisse-Lagae F, Toppet M: Etude clinique et anatomo-pathologique de deux cas d'intolérance congénitale au fructose. *Pédiatrie* 20:5–14, 1965

178. Briner H, Schneider J: Personal communication

179. Spycher MA: Unpublished data

180. Rossner JA, Feist D: Hereditäre Fruktoseintoleranz. *Verh Dtsch Ges Pathol* 55:376–385, 1971

181. Pfleiderer G, Dikow AL, Falkenberg F: Quantitative Bestimmung genetisch determinierter Isoenzyme mittels Immunititration. Verteilungsmuster der Aldolase A, B und C in menschlichen Organ- und Gewebsextrakten sowie in normalen und pathologischen Seren. *Hoppe Seyler's Z Physiol Chem* 355:233–238, 1974

182. Schapira F, Hatzfeld A, Gregori C: Studies on liver aldolases in hereditary fructose intolerance. *Enzyme* 18:73–83, 1974

183. Schapira F, Dreyfus J-C: L'aldolase hépatique dans l'intolérance au fructose. *Rev Fr Etudes Clin Biol* 12:486–489, 1967

184. Schapira F, Nordmann Y, Gregori C: Hereditary alterations of fructose metabolizing enzymes. *Acta Med Scand* 542 (suppl):77–83, 1972

185. Koster JF, Slee RG, Fernandes J: On the biochemical basis of hereditary fructose intolerance. *Biochem Biophys Res Commun* 64:289–294, 1975

186. Gitzelmann R, Steinmann B, Bally C, Lebherz HG: Antibody activation of mutant human fructosediphosphate aldolase B in liver extracts of patients with hereditary fructose intolerance. *Biochem Biophys Res Commun* 59:1270–1277, 1974

187. Baerlocher K, Gitzelmann R, Nüssli R, Dumermuth G: Infantile lactic acidosis due to hereditary fructose 1, 6-diphosphatase deficiency. *Helv Paediatr Acta* 26:489–506, 1971

188. Gentil C, Colin J, Valette AM, Alagille D, Lelong M: Mémoires. Etude du métabolisme glucidique au cours de l'intolérance héréditaire au fructose. Essai d'interprétation de l'hypoglycosémie. *Rev Fr Etudes Clin Biol* 9:596–607, 1964

189. Rossier A, Milhaud G, Colin J, Job J-C, Brault A, Beauvais P, Lemerle J: Intolérance congénitale au fructose. Deuz cas familiaux avec étude biochimique in vitro. *Arch Fr Pediatr* 23:533–552, 1966

190. Saxon L, Papper S: Abdominal pain occurring during the rapid administration of fructose solutions. *N Engl J Med* 256:132–133, 1957

191. Froesch ER, Prader A, Wolf HP, Labhart A: Die hereditäre Fructoseintoleranz. *Helv Paediatr Acta* 14:99–112, 1959

192. Dubois R, Loeb H, Ooms, HA, Gillet P, Bartman J, Champenois A: Etude d'un cas d'hypoglycémie fonctionelle par intolérance au fructose. *Helv Paediatr Acta* 16:90–96, 1961

193. Richardson RMA, Little JA, Patten RL, Goldstein MB, Halperin ML: Pathogenesis of acidosis in hereditary fructose intolerance. *Metabolism* 28:1133–1138, 1979

194. Perheentupa J, Pitkänen E, Nikkilä EA, Somersalo O, Hakosalo J: Hereditary fructose intolerance. A clinical study of four cases. *Ann Paediatr Fenn* 8:221–235, 1962

195. Nivelon J-L, Mathieu M, Kissin C, Collombel C, Cotte J, Béthenod M: Intolérance au fructose. Observation et méchanisme physiopathologique de l'hypoglucosémie. *Ann Pédiatr Paris* 43:817–824, 1967

196. Modigliani E, Strauch G, Odièvre M: Hormonal response to intravenous fructose in normal and fructosaemic children: A study of insulin and growth hormone secretion. *Rev Eur Etudes Clin Biol* 15:882–887, 1970

197. Morris RC, McSherry E, Sebastian A: Modulation of experimental renal dysfunction of hereditary fructose intolerance by circulating parathyroid hormone. *Proc Natl Acad Sci USA* 68:132–135, 1971

198. Odièvre M: Les difficultés du diagnostic de l'intolérance héréditaire au fructose chez le nourrisson. *Arch Fr Pediatr* 26:5–19, 1969

199. Phillips MJ, Path MC, Little JA, Ptak TW: Subcellular pathology of hereditary fructose intolerance. *Am J Med* 44:910–921, 1968

200. Phillips MJ, Yu DT, Burch HB: Animal model of human disease: Hereditary fructose intolerance. *Am J Pathol* 75:591–594, 1974

201. Gitzelmann R, Auricchio O: The handling of soya α-galactosides by a normal and a galactosemic child. *Pediatrics* 36:231–235, 1965

202. Desbuquois B, Lardinois R, Gentil C, Odièvre M: Effets d'une surcharge en phosphate de sodium sur l'hypoglucosémie dans onze observations d'intolérance héréditaire au fructose. *Arch Fr Pediatr* 26:21–35, 1969

203. Pitkänen E, Perheentupa J: Eine biochemische Untersuchung über zwei Fälle von Fructoseintoleranz. *Ann Paediatr Fenn* 8:236–244, 1962

204. Hue L: Unpublished data

205. Levin B, Oberholzer VG, Snodgrass GJAI, Stimmler L, Wilmers MJ: Fructosaemia. An inborn error of fructose metabolism. *Arch Dis Child* 38:220–230, 1963

206. Morris RC Jr: An experimental renal acidification defect in patients with hereditary fructose intolerance. 2. Its distinction from classic renal tubular acidosis; its resemblance to the renal acidification defect associated with the Fanconi syndrome of children with cystinosis. *J Clin Invest* 47:1648–1663, 1968

207. Schwartz R, Gamsu H, Mulligan PB, Reisner SH, Wybregt SH, Cornblath M: Transient intolerance to exogenous fructose in the newborn. *J Clin Invest* 43:333–340, 1964

208. Renold AE, Winegrad AI, Froesch ER, Thorn GW: Studies on the site of action of the aryl sulfonyl ureas in man. *Metabolism* 5:757–767, 1956

209. ZALITIS J, OLIVER IT: Inhibition of glucose phosphate isomerase by metabolic intermediates of fructose. *Biochem J* 102:753–759, 1967

209a. BALLY C, LEUTHARDT F: Unpublished data

210. WILKENING J, NOWACK J, DECKER K: The dependence of glucose formation from lactate on the adenosine triphosphate content in the isolated perfused rat liver. *Biochim Biophys Acta* 392:299–309, 1975

211. CAIN ARR, RYMAN BE: High liver glycogen in hereditary fructose intolerance. *Gut* 12:929–932, 1971

212. SIDBURY JB: Zur Biochemie der hereditären Fructoseintoleranz. *Helv Paediatr Acta* 14:317–318, 1959

213. BROADUS AE, KAMINSKY NI, NORTHCUTT RC, HARDMAN JG, SUTHERLAND EW, LIDDLE GW: Effects of glucagon on adenosine 3′, 5′-monophosphate and guanosine 3′, 5′-monophosphate in human plasma and urine. *J Clin Invest* 49:2237–2245, 1970

214. RAMBAUD P, JOANNARD A, BOST M, MARCHAL A, RACHAIL M, ROGET J: Trouble de la glycogénolyse dans l'intolérance héréditaire au fructose. Etude de deux observations chez l'enfant. *Arch Fr Pediatr* 30:1051–1062, 1973

214a. VAN DEN BERGHE G: Biochemical aspects of hereditary fructose intolerance in Hommes FA, van den Berg CJ (eds): *Normal and Pathological Development of Energy Metabolism.* London, Academic Press, Ltd. pp 211–226, 1975

215. MADDAIAH VT, MADSEN NB: Kinetics of purified liver phosphorylase. *J Biol Chem* 241:3873–3881, 1966

216. KAUFMANN U, FROESCH ER: Inhibition of phosphorylase-a by fructose-1-phosphate, α-glycerophosphate and fructose-1, 6-diphosphate. Explanation for fructose-induced hypoglycaemia in hereditary fructose intolerance and fructose-1, 6-diphosphatase deficiency. *Eur J Clin Invest* 3:407–413, 1973

217. THURSTON JH, JONES EM: Decrease and inhibition of liver phosphorylase (LP) after fructose: An experimental model for the study of hereditary fructose intolerance (HFI), abstracted. *Pediatr Res* 5:392, 1971

218. THURSTON JH, JONES EM, HAUHART RE: Decrease and inhibition of liver glycogen phosphorylase after fructose. An experimental model for the study of hereditary fructose intolerance. *Diabetes* 23:597–604, 1974

219. LANDAU BR, MARSHALL JS, CRAIG JW, HOSTETLER KY, GENUTH SM: Quantitation of the pathways of fructose metabolism in normal and fructose-intolerant subjects. *J Lab Clin Med* 78:608–618, 1971

220. MERCIER J-C, BOURRILLON A, BEAUFILS F, ODIÈVRE M: Intolérance héréditaire au fructose à révélation précoce. *Arch Fr Pediatr* 33:945–953, 1976

221. PERHEENTUPA J, PITKÄNEN E: Symptomless hereditary fructose intolerance. *Lancet* 1:1358–1359, 1962

222. GITZELMANN R: D. Enzymes of fructose and galactose metabolism; galactose-1-phosphate in Curtius H Ch, Roth M (eds): *Clinical Biochemistry: Principles and Methods.* Berlin, New York, de Gruyter 1974, pp 1236–1251

223. HUE L, VAN HOOF F, HERS H-G: Serum aldolase in Tay-Sachs disease and in fructose intolerance. *Am J Med* 51:785–787, 1971

224. BURTON BK, CHACKO CM, NADLER HL: Aldolase in cultivated human fibroblasts. *Proc Soc Exp Biol Med* 146:605–607, 1974

225. ODIÈVRE M, GAUTIER M, RIEU D: Intolérance héréditaire au fructose du nourrisson. Evolution des lésions histologiques hépatiques sous traitement diététique prolongé. (Etude de huit observations) *Arch Fr Pediatr* 26:433–443, 1969

226. CORNBLATH M, SCHWARTZ R: *Disorders of Carbohydrate Medtabolism in Infancy,* ed 2. Vol 3 in the series *Major Problems in Clinical Pediatrics.* Philadelphia, WB Saunders Co, 1976

227. WYKE RJ, RAJKOVIC IA, EDDLESTON ALWF, WILLIAMS R: Defective opsonization and complement deficiency in serum from patients with fulminant hepatic failure. *Gut* 21:643–649, 1980

228. NÜSSLI R: Das Wachstum von Patienten mit hereditärer Fruktoseintoleranz oder hereditärer Saccharose-Isomaltose-Malabsorption. *Helv Paediatr Acta* 26:637–648, 1971

229. BRAUMAN J, KENTOS P, FRISQUE P, GEPTS W, VERBANCK M: Intolérance héréditaire au fructose chez une femme de 83 ans. *Acta Clin Belg* 26:65–77, 1971

230. HEINE W, SCHILL H, TESSMANN D, KUPATZ H: Letale Leberdystropyhie bei drei Geschwistern mit hereditärer Fruktoseintoleranz nach Dauertropffinfusionen mit sorbitolhaltigen Infusionslösungen. *Dtsch Gesundheitsw* 24:2325–2329, 1969

231. BLOM W, FERNANDES J: Unpublished data

232. MÜLLER-WIEFEL DE, SCHÄRER K: Unpublished data

233. GIRGENSOHN H: Unpublished data

234. TROST C: Personal communication

235. SITADEVI C, RAMAIAH Y, ASKARI Z: Fructose intolerance associated with congenital cataract. *Ind J Pediatr* 35:496–498, 1968

236. GITZELMANN R, BAERLOCHER K: Vorteile und Nachteile der Fructose in der Nahrung. *Pädiatr Fortbildk Praxis* 37:40–55, 1973

237. LINDÉN AL, NISELL J: Hereditär fructosintolerans. *Svensk Läk-Tidn* 61:3185–3195, 1964

238. KURZ R, HÄCHL G, HOHENWALLNER W, BERGER H: Hereditäre Fruktoseintoleranz mit vermutlich dominantem Erbgang. *Arch Kinderheilk* 183:233–239, 1971

239. VON RUECKER A, ENDRES W, SHIN YS, BUTENANDT I, STEINMANN B, GITZELMANN R: A case of fatal hereditary fructose intolerance. Misleading information on formula composition. *Helv Paediatr Acta* 36:(Nr 6), 1981

240. LEUPOLD D: Unpublished data

241. RAIVIO K, PERHEENTUPA J, NIKKILÄ EA: Aldolase activities in the liver in parents of patients with hereditary fructose intolerance. *Clin Chim Acta* 17:275–279, 1967

242. BEYREISS K, WILLGERODT H, THEILE H: Untersuchungen bei heterozygoten Merkmalsträgern für Fruktoseintoleranz. *Klin Wschr* 46:465–468, 1968

243. SCHAPIRA F: Kinetic and immunological abnormalities of aldolase B in hereditary fructose intolerance. *Biochem Soc Trans* 3:232–234, 1975

244. HÜLSMANN WC, FERNANDEZ J: A child with lactacidemia and fructose diphosphatase deficiency in the liver. *Pediatr Res* 5:633–637, 1971

245. BAKKER HD, DE BREE PK, KETTING D, VAN SPRANG FJ, WADMAN SK: Fructose-1,6-diphosphatase deficiency: Another enzyme defect which can present itself with the clinical features of "tyrosinosis." *Clin Chim Acta* 55:41–47, 1974

246. PAGLIARA AS, KARL IE, KEATING JP, BROWN BI, KIPNIS DM: Hepatic fructose-1,6-diphosphatase deficiency. A cause of lactic acidosis and hypoglycemia in infancy. *J Clin Invest* 51:2115–2123, 1972

247. GREENE HL, STIFEL FB, HERMAN RH: "Ketotic hypoglycemia" due to hepatic fructose-1,6-diphosphatase deficiency. *Am J Dis Child* 124:415–418, 1972

248. SAUDUBRAY J-M, DREYFUS J-C, CEPANEC C, LE LO 'CH H, TRUNG PH, MOZZICONACCI P: Acidose lactique, hypoglycémie et hépatomégalie par déficit héréditaire en fructose-1,6-diphosphatase hépatique. *Arch Fr Pediatr* 30:609–632, 1973

249. MELANÇON SB, KHACHADURIAN AK, NADLER HL, BROWN BI: Metabolic and biochemical studies in fructose 1, 6-diphosphatase deficiency. *J Pediatr* 82:650–667, 1973

250. DE ROSAS FJ, WAPNIR RA, LIFSHITZ F, SILVERBERG M, OLSON M: Folic acid enhanced gluconeogenesis in glycerol induced hypoglycemia and fructose-1, 6-diphosphatase deficiency. Presented at the 56th Annual Meeting of the Endocrine Society, Atlanta, 1974

251. EAGLE RB, MACNAB AJ, RYMAN BE, STRANG LB: Liver biopsy data on a child with fructose 1, 6-diphosphatase deficiency that closely resembled many aspects of glucose 6-phosphatase deficiency (von Gierke's type I glycogen-storage disease). *Biochem Soc Trans* 2:1118–1121, 1974

252. STACEY TE, STRANG LB, FLEISCHMAN A, EAGLE R, RYMAN BE: Treatment of fructose-1, 6-diphosphatase deficiency, abstracted. International Symposium on Inborn Errors of Metabolism in the Human. *J Inherited Metab Dis* in press

253. ODIÈVRE M, BRIVET M, MOATTI N, DREYFUS J-C, BEAUFILS F, LEJEUNE C, FEFFER J: Déficit en fructose-1, 6-diphosphatase chez deux soeurs. *Arch Fr Pediatr* 32:113–122, 1975

254. RETBI J-M, GABILAN J-C, MARSAC C: Acidose lactique et hypoglycémie à début néonatal par déficit congénital en fructose-1, 6-diphosphatase hépatique. *Arch Fr Pediatr* 32:367–380, 1975

255. RETBI J-M: Acidose lactique et hypoglycémie par déficit congénital en fructose 1, 6 diphosphatase hépatique. *These Med,* Paris, Université René-Descartes, 1972

256. CORBEEL L, EGGERMONT E, EECKELS R, JAEKEN J, CASTEELS-VAN DAELE M, DEVLIEGER H, DELMOTTE B: Recurrent attacks of ketotic acidosis associated with fructose-1, 6-diphosphatase deficiency. *Acta Paediatr Belg* 29:29–34, 1976

257. HOPWOOD NJ, HOLZMAN I, DRASH AL: Fructose-1, 6-diphosphatase deficiency. *Am J Dis Child* 131:418–421, 1977

258. DE PRÀ M, LAUDANNA E: La malattia di Baker-Winegrad. *Minerva Pediatr* 30:1973–1986, 1978

259. RALLISON ML, MEIKLE AW, ZIGRANG WD: Hypoglycemia and lactic acidosis associated with fructose-1,6-diphosphatase deficiency. *J Pediatr* 94:933–936, 1979

260. KINUGASA A, KUSUNOKI T, IWASHIMA A: Deficiency of glucose-6-phosphate dehydrogenase found in a case of hepatic fructose-1,6-diphosphatase deficiency. *Pediatr Res* 13:1361–1364, 1979

261. CORBEEL LM, EGGERMONT E, BETTENS W, CASTEELS-VAN DAELE M, TIMMERMANS J: Fructose intolerance with normal liver aldolase. *Helv Paediatr Acta* 25:626–633, 1970. NOTE: The FDPase activity, reported to be low in the Note-added-in-Proof, was later reinvestigated by more refined techniques and found deficient.

262. TAUNTON OD, GREENE HL, STIEFEL FB, HOFELDT FD, LUFKIN EG, HAGLER L, HERMAN Y, HERMAN RH: Fructose-1,6-diphosphatase deficiency, hypoglycemia, and response to folate therapy in a mother and her daughter. *Biochem Med* 19:260–276, 1978

263. SERVICE FJ, VENEZIALE CM, NELSON RA, ELLEFSON RD, GO VLW: Combined deficiency of glucose-6-phosphatase and fructose-1,6-diphospha-

tase. Studies of glucagon secretion and fuel utilization. *Am J Med* 64:696–706, 1978

264. PAGLIARA AS, KARL IE, HAMMOND M, KIPNIS DM: Hypoglycemia in infancy and childhood, Parts I and II. *J Pediatr* 82:365–379, 558–577, 1973

265. GITZELMANN R, BAERLOCHER K, PRADER A: Hereditäre Störungen im Fructose- und Galactosestoffwechsel. *Mschr Kinderheilk* 121:174–180, 1973

266. BAERLOCHER K, GITZELMANN R, STEINMANN B: Clinical and genetic studies of disorders in fructose metabolism, in Burman D, Holton JB, Pennock CA (eds): *Inherited Disorders of Carbohydrate Metabolism.* Lancaster, MTP Press, LTD 1980 pp 163–190

267. ROBINSON BH, TAYLOR J, SHERWOOD WG: The genetic heterogeneity of lactic acidosis: Occurrence of recognizable inborn errors of metabolism in a pediatric population with lactic acidosis. *Pediatr Res* 14:956–962, 1980

268. SCHRIJVER J, HOMMES FA: Activity of fructose-1,6-diphosphatase in human leukocytes. *N Engl J Med* 292:1298–1299, 1975

269. CAHILL J, KIRTLEY ME: FDPase activity in human leukocytes. *N Engl J Med* 292:212, 1975

270. MELANCON SB, NADLER HL: Detection of fructose-1,6-diphosphatase deficiency with use of white blood cells. *N Engl J Med* 286:731–732, 1972

271. MELANCON SB, NADLER HL: FDPase activity in human leukocytes. *N Engl J Med* 292:212–213, 1975

272. FONG W-F, HYNIE I, LEE H, MCKENDRY JBR: Increase of fructose-1,6-diphosphatase activity in cultured human peripheral lymphocytes and its suppression by phytohemagglutinin. *Biochem Biophys Res Commun* 88:222–228, 1979

273. STEINMANN B, GITZELMANN R: Fruktose und Sorbitol in Infusionsflüssigkeiten sind nicht immer harmlos, in Ritzel G, Brubacher G (eds): *Monosaccharides and Polyalcohols in Nutrition, Therapy and Dietetics. Int J Vitam Nutr Res* (suppl 15):289–294, 1976

274. STREB H, POSSLET HG, WOLTER K, BENDER SW: Aldolase activities of the small intestinal mucosa in malabsorption states and hereditary fructose intolerance. *Eur J Pediatr* 37:5, 1981

275. NISELL J, LINDÉN L: Fructose-1-phosphate aldolase and fructose-1-6-diphosphate aldolase activity in the mucosa of the intestine in hereditary fructose intolerance. *Scand J Gastroenterol* 3:80–82, 1968

276. MÉTAIS P, JUIF J, SACREZ R: Etude biochimique d'un cas d'intolérance héréditaire au fructose. *Ann Biol Clin* 20:801–811, 1962

277. KRANHOLD JF, LOH D, MORRIS RC: Renal fructose-metabolizing enzymes: Significance in hereditary fructose intolerance. *Science* 165:402–403, 1969

278. MORRIS RC, UEKI I, LOH D, EANES RZ, MCLIN P: Absence of renal fructose-1-phosphate aldolase activity in hereditary fructose intolerance. *Nature* 214:920–921, 1967

279. DE BARSY T, HUG G. Unpublished observations

6

THE GLYCOGEN STORAGE DISEASES

R. RODNEY HOWELL

JULIAN C. WILLIAMS

Inherited defects may affect many enzymes involved in the synthesis and degradation of glycogen. A broad clinical spectrum is presented by the recognized clinical types of glycogen storage disease.

1. Von Gierke's disease is caused by a deficiency of glucose-6-phosphatase. Patients with the disorder are characterized by massive hepatomegaly, failure to thrive, and severe hypoglycemia, particularly during infancy. They have increased plasma concentrations of lactic acid and hyperlipidemia. Administration of epinephrine or glucagon causes a subnormal rise in blood glucose and further increases in blood lactate. Hyperuricemia occurs regularly, and many patients have clinical gout in young adulthood. Renal enlargement is seen roentgenographically. Inheritance is autosomal recessive. The diagnosis is established by demonstrating an increased content of glycogen with normal structure in a liver biopsy and absent glucose-6-phosphatase activity. Although treatment is symptomatic, continuous infusion of glucose by nasogastric tube has been helpful.

2. Infants with generalized glycogen storage disease have massive cardiomegaly and hypotonia but no muscle wasting. The disease is inherited as an autosomal recessive trait. The diagnosis is made by finding an increased concentration of glycogen of normal structure in virtually all tissues and by demonstrating an absence of lysosomal α-1,4-glucosidase (acid maltase) activity. Cardiorespiratory failure causes death by 2 years of age. In less common forms of the disease, there is no significant cardiac involvement and the patients survive well into adulthood. This disease can be diagnosed in utero by amniocentesis and enzyme studies on the cultured amniotic fluid cells.

3. Deficiency of the debrancher enzyme has a clinical course similar to that in glucose-6-phosphatase deficiency but is usually milder. Massive hepatomegaly is present in young children and diminishes with age, and some older patients lack hepatic enlargement. Hypoglycemia is variable, as are responses to epinephrine and glucagon. A variety of biochemical subtypes based on tissue variability are described in this condition. Muscle, liver, and erythrocyte glycogen are elevated, and the glycogen has short outer branches. Deficiency of the debrancher enzyme is inherited in an autosomal recessive fashion. Muscle wasting and weakness are features in some patients.

4. A deficiency of branching enzyme in Andersen's disease produces an accumulation of abnormal glycogen with long outer branches. Clinically, there is progressive cirrhosis with hepatosplenomegaly and ascites. Death from liver failure occurs usually before 2 years of

141

age in this rare form of glycogen storage disease. It is inherited as an autosomal recessive. Muscle hypotonia may dominate the clinical features.

5. *Limitation of strenuous exercise by painful cramps is the presenting feature in patients with McArdle's disease. The symptoms do not usually appear until 20 years of age. Myoglobinuria occurs in half the patients after strenuous exercise. Renal failure may follow. Findings on physical examination are normal. There is no hypoglycemia. Muscular exercise fails to cause an increase in venous lactate. Muscle biopsy shows absent phosphorylase activity and increased glycogen content. Inheritance is autosomal recessive.*

6. *Hepatic glycogen storage disease was established as a category for patients considered to have liver phosphorylase deficiency. Patients have a mild clinical course; phosphorylase deficiency is striking, but the activating system is normal.*

7. *Patients with Tarui's disease (muscle phosphofructokinase deficiency) are clinically identical to those with McArdle's disease. After exercise these patients have painful cramps and sometimes myoglobinuria. Muscle biopsies show deficiency in phosphofructokinase activity and increased glycogen concentration. Inheritance appears to be autosomal recessive.*

8. *A deficiency of liver phosphorylase kinase characterizes one form of hepatic glycogen storage disease. Symptoms and findings include mild hepatomegaly, increased liver glycogen, and mild hypoglycemia. Diagnosis is made by the demonstration of deficient leukocyte or hepatic phosphorylase b kinase. The disease is X-linked in most cases and is fully manifested only in males.*

The dramatic physical findings which often accompany the glycogen storage diseases led to the clinical and pathologic recognition of these disorders as long ago as 1929 [1]. It was evident early that among diagnosed patients there were some with prominent liver involvement ("hepatic" glycogen storage disease or von Gierke's disease) and others with a more generalized storage of glycogen, including a striking cardiac involvement [2].

In 1952 the Coris [3] demonstrated a specific deficiency of glucose-6-phosphatase in a patient with the hepatic form of glycogen storage disease. This was the first proof of a hepatic enzyme deficiency in humans. In 1963 Hers formulated the concept of a lysosomal storage disease based upon the finding of α-glucosidase deficiency in the generalized glycogenosis with cardiac involvement. As further enzyme studies have been performed on tissues from patients with the glycogen storage diseases, it has become clear that deficiencies of a variety of enzymes involved in glycogen synthesis and degradation can produce diseases that are not readily distinguishable clinically. On the other hand, it is also remarkable that genetic abnormalities in glycogen metabolism can produce such a vast spectrum of clinical disorders. The glycogen storage diseases may present themselves as disorders primarily of the liver, heart, or musculoskeletal system. We are now aware of at least eight groups of inherited abnormalities in glycogen metabolism in

humans that can be defined clinically or biochemically; additional abnormalities will undoubtedly be defined in the future.

GLYCOGEN AND GLYCOGEN METABOLISM

Structure and Function

Glycogen is the principle storage form of carbohydrate in animals and is found in varying concentrations in virtually all cells. Starches, the storage carbohydrates of plants, contain both amylose (which has exclusively 1,4 linkages between its constituent glucose molecules) and amylopectin (which has, in addition, 4 percent 1,6 branch point linkages). Glycogen has 7 to 8 percent 1,6 linkages, which permits a highly branched polymeric structure. This highly branched structure imparts considerably greater solubility to mammalian glycogen than is possessed by the starches, decreases the osmotic pressure exerted by the carbohydrate constituents, and may, via water of hydration, aid in water storage by organisms.

Glycogens are simpler molecules than proteins or nucleic acids, since glucose is their only building block [4]. Glycogen differs from most other important macromolecules in humans in that it is quite polydisperse and lacks a fixed molecular weight [5]. There is controversy about its exact macromolecular structure. French has pointed out that it is particularly difficult to construct a physical model of glycogen based on a more or less regularly branching pattern when the molecular size becomes large [6]. If one begins at the reducing end and increases the molecular size by elongating the straight chain and branching it, there is room to spare. But as the molecule increases in size, there comes a point at which the periphery is so densely packed that it is sterically impossible to continue regular branching. Since virtually all models with extensive branching would allow adequate space in the interior of the molecule, it is assumed that glycogen does indeed have many chains that terminate in the interior. These buried chains might well be resistant to enzymes because of steric protection. French has also pointed out that formation of the 1,6 branch points at the expense of 1,4 links is highly favored thermodynamically [6]. Since glycogen has less than 10 percent of its glucose residues in 1,6 linkage, the branching enzyme must be severely hindered sterically (Fig. 6-1). Enzymatic digestion has shown that 10 percent of the glucose residues in the glycogen polymer occupy nonreducing end positions and that 60 percent are in the outer chains [7]. Brammer et al. have demonstrated that there are clusters of very dense branching and short inner chains (i.e., an average inner chain length of 4 residues), while the average outer chain length is 10 to 14 residues [8]. This absence of very long chains agrees with the model of glycogen structure proposed by Gunja-Smith et al. [9].

Glycogen extracted under gentle conditions in cold water has molecular weights ranging from a few million to well over several hundred million [10]. Physical evidence (such as viscosity measurements) suggests that glycogen is nearly spherical and is extensively hydrated. If the molecule is at all hydrated and regularly branched, a molecular weight of 5 to 6 million would be about the largest possible. This consideration has led

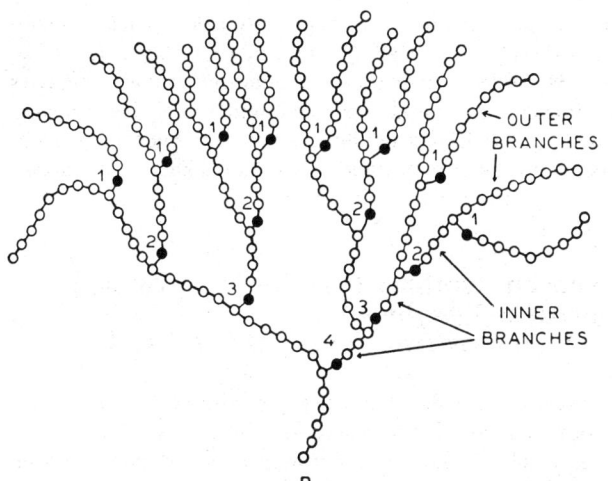

Figure 6-1 Schematic representation of part of a glycogen molecule. Each circle represents a glucose molecule; the open circles represent the linear portions of glycogen with the glucoses in a 1,4 linkage. Branch points in the glycogen (α-1,6 linkage) are represented by closed circles. R = reducing end group. The terminal glucose in the outer branches is nonreducing. *(From G.T. Cori [247], with permission.)*

to the suggestion that the extraordinarily large molecular weight species are in reality aggregates of molecules of smaller size [6]. The exact nature of the forces holding the large molecules together is not known, but Leloir has suggested that native glycogen may contain a non-1,4/non-1,6 linkage that is very labile [11]. When visualized under the electron microscope, these large particles appear to consist of single units that range in size from 1 to 5 million. It would appear, therefore, that glycogen as it exists in vivo is composed of small, nearly spherical, highly branched units that have molecular weights of several million. These units, in turn, are aggregated by forces that are currently not clearly understood.

Glycogen Content of Human Tissues

There is limited information on the glycogen content of normal, fresh human liver and muscle. Preparation for biopsy often includes prolonged fasts and infusions of glucose; infusion of fructose, particularly, will elevate the hepatic glycogen concentration. In addition, a wide variety of physiologic stimuli affect the tissue glycogen concentration. Muscle biopsy specimens from highly trained athletes contain greatly increased glycogen levels when compared with controls [12]. Certain of the glycogen storage diseases may on occasion have normal or near normal tissue glycogen content. The usual concentration of glycogen in liver is less than 5 to 7 g per 100 g wet weight; muscle glycogen is usually under 2 g per 100 g wet weight.

Human fetal liver begins to accumulate glycogen during the final trimester of pregnancy [13]. The usual amount of branching is found in the earliest samples. Liver glycogen levels fall rapidly in the newborn period, in association with an increase in phosphorylase activity [13]. Adult levels are reached by 2 to 3 weeks of age.

In view of these findings, measurement of tissue glycogen content may fail to establish or rule out a diagnosis of a glycogen storage disease except when high concentrations of gly-

cogen or abnormal glycogen structure are encountered. As Öckerman has wisely emphasized, if tissue staining is used for glycogen quantitation, even greater caution must be exercised, since this is at best a semiquantitative method.

Although liver glycogen content reflects to a considerable degree the nutritional status of the subject, there is no firm evidence that hyperalimentation alone can lead to excessive deposition of liver glycogen [14].

Glucokinase (EC 2.7.1.2) and the Hexokinases (EC 2.7.1.1)

The phosphorylation of glucose,

$$\text{Glucose} + \text{ATP} \xrightarrow{\text{Mg}^{2+}} \text{glucose-6-phosphate} + \text{ADP}$$

is catalyzed in mammalian tissues by several kinases with different distributions and properties. In liver there is a highly specific glucokinase in addition to other hexokinases. The glucokinase activity of liver falls dramatically during fasting and in alloxan diabetes. Refeeding (after fasting) or treatment with insulin (in diabetes) causes a prompt increase in glucokinase [15]. Adrenalectomy, cortisone, and thyroid hormone have no effect on glucokinase activity [16]. Muscle contains only less specific hexokinases and has no detectable specific glucokinase activity [17]. Certain of the properties of glucokinase and the hexokinases are summarized in Table 6-1 [14]. The rate of phosphorylation of glucose by the liver is well correlated with glucokinase activity. As its activity is affected by a series of physiologic stimuli, its role in the regulation of glycogen synthesis is apparent. It is estimated that in the normal, well-fed animal, glucokinase accounts for 80 percent of hepatic phosphorylation of glucose [19].

Phosphoglucomutase (EC 2.7.5.l)

Phosphoglucomutase catalyzes the reversible transfer of a phosphate group between the 1 and 6 positions of glucose (see Fig. 6-2). There is no known complete deficiency of this enzyme in human beings. This is the only reversible step in glycogen synthesis and breakdown; its central position suggests that total deficiency of the enzyme might be lethal.

At 30°C, the equilibrium lies far toward glucose-6-phos-

Table 6-1 Comparative properties of glucokinase and hexokinases in rat liver

Property	Glucokinase	Hexokinases
Michaelis constant for glucose	10 mM	0.01–0.1 mM
Allosteric inhibition by glucose-6-phosphatase	No	Yes
Ability to phosphorylate fructose	Poor	Good
Ability to phosphorylate glucosamine	None	Good
Molecular weight	50,000	96,000
Typical activity in normal fed animals, μmoles per g liver per minute at 30°C	3	1
Activity in starved animals	Decreased	Normal

SOURCE: Data from Sols [18].

phate (94 to 95 percent of the total glucose phosphate). The enzyme mechanism has been established as [20, 21]

$$\alpha\text{-Glucose-1-phosphate} + \text{phosphoenzyme} \rightleftharpoons$$
$$\alpha\text{-Glucose-1,6-diphosphate} + \text{dephosphoenzyme} \rightleftharpoons$$
$$\alpha\text{-Glucose-6-phosphate} + \text{phosphoenzyme}$$

The requirement for glucose-1,6-diphosphate is well established. It functions as a "primer," or as a true coenzyme, and is required only in catalytic amounts [20]. Glucose-1,6-diphosphate can also be synthesized by phosphoglucokinase (ATP-D-glucose-1-phosphate 6-phosphotransferase), and this intermediate has been implicated in the postulated pathway of glycogen synthesis from glucose without the involvement of glucose-6-phosphate [22]. Phosphoglucomutase is not thought to be a site of physiologic regulation of glycogen synthesis or degradation.

Uridine Diphosphate (UDP)-Glucose Pyrophosphorylase (EC 2.7.7.9)

Enzyme activity is especially high in the liver. As much as 0.3 percent of the extractable protein (from calf liver) has pyrophosphorylase activity [23]. The reaction catalyzed by the enzyme is (Fig. 6-2)

$$\text{Glucose-1-phosphate} + \text{UTP} \longrightarrow \text{UDP-glucose} + \text{PP}_i \qquad (3)$$

The reaction provides UDP-glucose for glycogen synthase and is involved in galactose metabolism and glucuronide synthesis [22]. The pyrophosphorylase can use other nucleoside sugars as substrates but at much lower rates.

This large enzyme (molecular weight 400,000) is competitively inhibited by uridine diphosphate. The large quantity of

this enzyme in the liver, in addition to its low Michaelis constant for UTP (2.2×10^{-4} M) and glucose-1-phosphate (5.5×10^{-5} M) and the high turnover number (83,000), indicates that this enzyme would rarely be limiting in glycogen formation [23]. Since UDP is inhibitory, it must be removed (by conversion to UTP or by further degradation). There is no known deficiency of this enzyme in humans.

Glycogen Synthase (Uridine Diphosphate Glucose:α-1,4-Glucan α-1,4-Glucosyltransferase) (EC 2.4.1.11)

It was once contended that the enzyme phosphorylase is active in both the synthesis and degradation of glycogen. It is primarily responsible for the phosphorolysis of glycogen by breaking terminal 1,4 linkages to release glucose-1-phosphate (see the section "Phosphorylases"). The difficulty in this concept was in understanding what might control the direction of this reaction so that it would go toward either synthesis or degradation. The reaction is in equilibrium when the ratio of inorganic phosphate to glucose-1-phosphate is 3.5 at pH 7. At higher ratios, glycogen degradation occurs (in rat diaphragm the ratio is about 300). Also, agents which are known to activate phosphorylase (e.g., epinephrine and glucagon) always induce glycogenolysis.

In 1957, Leloir and Cardini [24] first demonstrated that synthesis of glycogen occurs in liver extracts incubated with uridine diphosphate-glucose (UDPG). Synthesis of glycogen in human muscle *not involving phosphorylase* was first clearly shown in studies of patients lacking muscle phosphorylase (McArdle's disease). This synthesis reaction, catalyzed by glycogen synthase, is (Fig. 6-2)

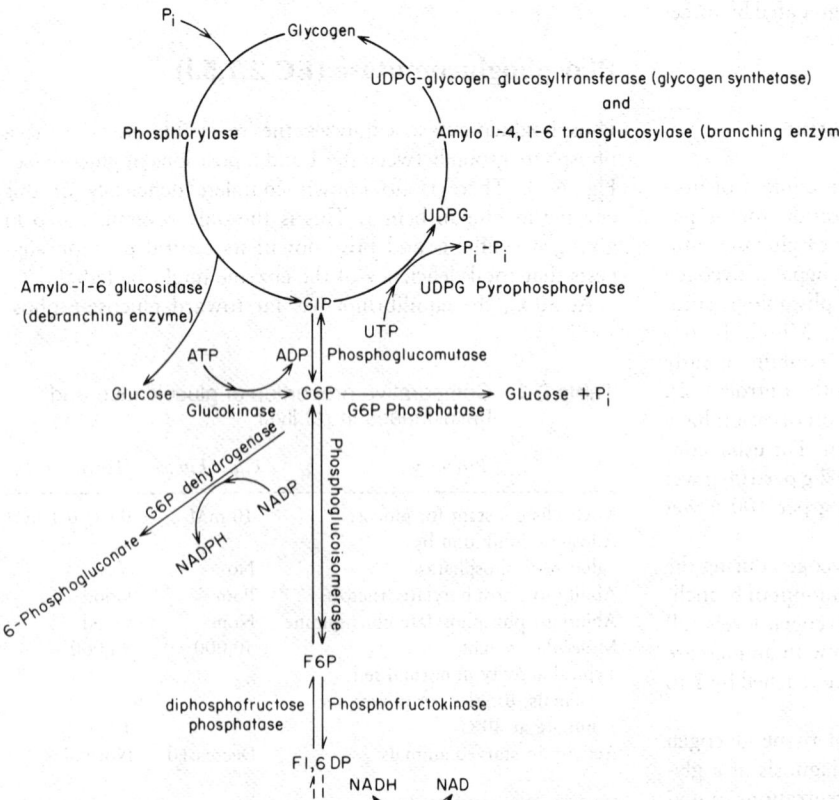

Figure 6-2 Major pathways in the synthesis and degradation of glycogen. The broken line indicates several steps which have been omitted between fructose-1,6-diphosphate and pyruvate. (*Modified from Bueding and Colocci* [248].)

$$UDPG + G_n(\text{glycogen primer}) \longrightarrow G_{(n+1)} + UDP \qquad (4)$$

The equilibrium of this reaction strongly favors glycogen synthesis.

Activity of the most highly purified glycogen synthase is wholly dependent on the addition of glycogen as primer [25, 26]. The nature of the primer in vivo is unknown. Although the enzyme does not require a metal ion, it is stimulated two-fold by $MgCl_2$.

Pioneering studies in Larner's laboratories have clearly shown that glycogen synthase exists in two distinct forms, initially termed D (dependent) and I (independent) [27]. This nomenclature referred to the fact that the I form is little stimulated in vitro by glucose-6-phosphate, whereas the D form is dependent on it for activity. It has now been realized that this terminology is a misnomer and an artifact due to the in vitro assay conditions employed. Mersmann and Segal [28] have suggested that a be used for the form (synthase I) active in vivo and b for the physiologically inactive form (synthase D). De Wulf et al. [29] and Gold [30] have demonstrated that in liver the primary metabolites controlling synthases a and b are P_i and ATP. Adenine nucleotides strongly inhibit synthase a, while P_i activates, and only at nonphysiologic concentrations does glucose-6-phosphate partially reverse this inhibition. Synthase b is activated by glucose-6-phosphate at nonphysiologic concentrations, but in muscle, physiologic levels of glucose-6-phosphate partially reverse the ATP inhibition of synthase a [31]. Glucose-6-phosphate also appears to increase the affinity of both synthases for UDPG.

In the presence of higher concentrations of glucose-6-phosphate and P_i, the enzyme is relatively insensitive to changes in the concentration of either of these ligands. The a form functions at about one-half to full capacity under all conditions which are likely to exist in vivo. If one compares the activity of synthase a and b at physiologic concentrations of ATP, UDPG, glucose-6-phosphate, and P_i, one finds a ratio of about 15:1 in specific activities. As extracted from normal fed animals, the enzyme appears to be entirely in the b (inactive) form. Insulin converts a substantial portion to the a form; this effect is reversed by glucagon [32].

DeWulf and Hers [33, 34] have found that intravenous administration of glucose stimulates fifteen- to twentyfold the conversion of glucose to glycogen by the liver. This is associated with a sharp increase in glycogen synthase activity. The rate of glycogen synthesis is not correlated with liver glucose content but is highly correlated with glycogen synthase activity

The interconversion of synthases a and b have been shown to be enzymatically mediated.

$$\text{Glycogen synthase } a + {}_n\text{ATP} \xrightarrow[\text{Mg}^{2+}]{\text{kinase}} \text{glycogen synthase } b + {}_n\text{ADP}$$
$$(\text{active})$$

$$\text{Glycogen synthase } b \xrightarrow{\text{phosphatase}} \text{glycogen synthase } a + {}_n P_i$$
$$(\text{inactive})$$
$$(5)$$

During glycogen breakdown adenosine-3',5'-monophosphate (cyclic AMP) exerts control by initiating the activation of phosphorylase b kinase, which in turn activates the degradation enzyme (see the section "Muscle Phosphorylase"). This cyclic nucleotide also stimulates the kinase which converts the a (active) form of glycogen synthase to the b (inactive) form [35]. Huijing and Larner [35] suggest that Mg^{2+} causes an allosteric activation of glycogen synthase a kinase and that cyclic AMP increases the degree of affinity of the allosteric site of the

enzyme for Mg^{2+}. Recent data suggest that the glycogen synthase a kinase is identical to phosphorylase b kinase-kinase [22]. Thus, cyclic AMP levels, mediated by hormonal control of adenyl cyclase, coordinately regulate the pathways of glycogen synthesis and degradation.

Glycogen synthase exists bound to particulate glycogen (as does phosphorylase and branching enzyme) and is primarily associated with the smooth endoplasmic reticulum [36]. On fasting, there is a progressive decrease in glycogen synthase activity associated with the smooth endoplasmic reticulum. The kinase responsible for converting the a form of glycogen synthase to the b form is also contained in the smooth endoplasmic reticulum fraction of liver.

Branching Enzyme (α-1,4-Glucan:α-1,4-Glucan 6α-Glycosyltransferase) (EC 2.4.1.18)

A deficiency of the enzyme catalyzing the branching of glycogen was postulated by Cori in a patient reported in 1952 by Andersen and demonstrated in 1966 by Brown and Brown [37].

Branching of glycogen is effected by the transfer of a segment of at least six α-1,4-linked glucosyl units from the outer chains of glycogen or amylopectin into a 1,6 position [38]. It is not known whether transfer occurs to the same or to neighboring chains [38]. The purified enzyme (90 percent pure) has a broad pH optimum and a molecular weight of 100,000. Structural studies are consistent with the enzyme's having placed each new branch point at an average position four glucose units away from the nearest preexisting outer branch point of the parent polysaccharide [38].

Phosphorylases (α-1,4 Glucan: Orthophosphate α-Glucosyltransferase) (EC 2.4.1.1)

Glycogen phosphorylases catalyze the stepwise cleavage of glucosyl units from the nonreducing end of the α-1,4-glucosyl chain of glycogen, liberating glucose-1-phosphate. It is by activation of this enzyme that epinephrine and glucagon play their important roles in controlling glycogenolysis. Although the catalyzed reaction is reversible in vitro, conditions in vivo probably result only in glycogen degradation.

Phosphorylase attacks the glycogen molecules from the nonreducing terminus of each chain, releasing successive glucose residues as glucose-1-phosphate until about four residues remain on each branch. Phosphorylase can proceed no further until the α-1,4 trisaccharide is transferred from the 1,6-linked glucose moiety to a terminal 1,4 glucose unit by an oligo-(1,4→1,4)-glucan transferase. Removal of the glucose attached in a 1,6 linkage by an amylo-1,6-glucosidase permits phosphorylase to continue until the next branch point is reached [39] (Fig. 6-3). Since liver and muscle phosphorylases are distinct proteins [40], they will be considered separately.

Muscle Phosphorylase Muscle phosphorylase, first crystallized from the rabbit, exists in an active (phosphorylase a) and an inactive (phosphorylase b) form. Phosphorylase in resting muscle is predominantly in the b (inactive) form [41]. The conversion of the b to a form of phosphorylase occurs as

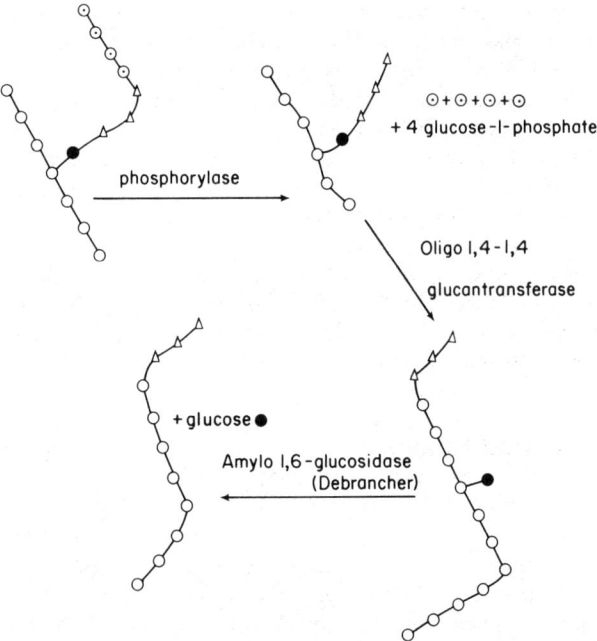

Figure 6-3 Schematic representation of the enzymatic debranching of glycogen. Only a small segment of a glycogen molecule is represented. In order for debrancher to work, the three glucose residues attached to the branched glucose (α-1,6-linked) after phosphorylase action must be transferred by an oligo-(1,4→1,4)-glucan transferase. Note that the debrancher yields free glucose, while phosphorylase produces glucose-1-phosphate.

$$\text{Phosphorylase } b + 4\text{ATP} \xrightarrow[\text{Mg}^{2+}]{\text{active phosphorylase kinase}}$$

$$\text{Phosphorylase } a + \text{ADP} \tag{6}$$

This phosphorylation of the inactive enzyme in the presence of ATP is catalyzed by a specific kinase, phosphorylase b kinase. This kinase itself exists in both an active and an inactive form and is activated by 3′,5′-cyclic AMP-dependent phosphorylase b kinase-kinase (identical to glycogen synthase kinase). The activation of phosphorylase by epinephrine (and glucagon in the liver) is mediated through changes in tissue levels of cyclic AMP [42].

Phosphorylase a formation is stimulated without changes in cyclic AMP or phosphorylase b kinase at low levels (4×10^{-15} M) of isoproterenol. Tetanic electrical stimulation also rapidly enhances phosphorylase a formation without change in cyclic AMP or phosphorylase b kinase [42].

The reverse reaction (phosphorylase dephosphorylation and inactivation) is catalyzed by a highly specific phosphatase [43] which is inhibited by cyclic AMP in concentrations as low as $10^{-5}M$.

Tryptic peptide analyses of phosphorylase have shown that seryl residues undergo phosphorylation during phosphorylase activation [44]. The seryl phosphate residue is in different amino acid sequences in liver and muscle.

Cyclic AMP is required for any activity in vitro of phosphorylase b, and it increases phosphorylase a activity by about 30 to 40 percent [44]. No change in the molecular weight of phosphorylase b in the presence of cyclic AMP is perceived by light-scattering techniques. Since the sedimentation constant of the nonphosphorylated enzyme is changed in the presence of cyclic AMP, this nucleotide probably produces conformational changes in the b protein.

At one time, it was thought that the active muscle phosphor-

ylase a existed solely as a tetramer with a molecular weight of 500,000, and that phosphorylase b is a dimer with a molecular weight of 250,000. Treatment of the enzymes with SH-binding reagents forms subunits with a molecular weight of 125,000. The tetrameric form of phosphorylase a contains four phosphate groups, four groups of pyridoxal-5′-phosphate, and binds four cyclic AMP units. Later studies have shown that at high protein concentrations, phosphorylase a exists in equilibrium between a high activity and a low activity form and that the active form is a dimer with a molecular weight of about 250,000. The tetrameric form of phosphorylase a (molecular weight 500,000) cannot bind to glycogen, and therefore the only active form of phosphorylase in vivo is the dimer [45].

Although aggregation of phosphorylase into a tetramer appears to follow phosphorylation closely, the exact relationship is unclear. Tryptic digests of phosphorylase a show that at the sight of phosphorylation the peptide chain has a high positive charge. It is suggested that aggregation follows phosphorylation by neutralizing the charges at this site. This would allow interaction between interpeptide chains previously statically repulsed [46]. Aggregation would also be favored by high protein concentrations.

At high ionic strength and low protein concentrations, the tetrameric form of phosphorylase a dissociates into a dimeric species of higher catalytic activity [47]. It has also been shown that the conversion of the dimeric species of phosphorylase a into the tetrameric form (inactive) is effectively blocked by glycogen [48].

There is considerable difficulty in the determination of molecular weights of associating systems such as that of phosphorylase. The molecular weights of phosphorylase a and b have been reinvestigated by Seery et al. [49] using a variety of conditions favoring association and dissociation. They found a molecular weight of 185,000 to 188,000 for phosphorylase b and 370,000 for phosphorylase a. Their data fit more closely than previous data with regard to stoichiometry of pyridoxal-5′-phosphate.

Liver Phosphorylase   Liver phosphorylase also exists in an active and an inactive form. In a similar fashion, the activation of this phosphorylase is accomplished by phosphorylation (via a protein-phosphate covalent bond) of the enzyme by phosphorylase b kinase which requires ATP and Mg^{2+}. Unlike muscle phosphorylase, liver phosphorylase does not appear to undergo molecular weight change during activation. It has a molecular weight of about 237,000 in either the active or inactive condition [50].

Liver phosphorylase is inactivated by a highly specific phosphatase. Numerous studies have suggested that this phosphatase is identical to the enzyme removing the phosphate group from phosphorylase b kinase and glycogen synthase [51]. The dephosphorylated liver phosphorylase is not greatly activated by the addition of AMP [52]. Phosphorylated liver phosphorylase activity is increased by up to 40 percent by AMP in vitro. Although cysteine and reduced glutathione do not stimulate phosphorylase activity, they do protect against inhibition by glucagon and epinephrine through their stimulatory effect on phosphorylase b kinase, while the muscle phosphorylase is activated only by epinephrine.

The phosphorylase b kinase activation by glucagon is affected by increasing the tissue concentrations of cyclic AMP. The plasma membrane of hepatic parenchymal cells contains an adenyl cyclase system which is stimulated by glucagon [53].

Epinephrine and ACTH do not stimulate this adenyl cyclase. This suggests that glucagon exerts its regulatory action in the liver by stimulating adenyl cyclase activity in the plasma membrane [53]. This, in turn, would increase tissue levels of cyclic AMP, which would activate phosphorylase *b* kinase and thereby produce the active form of the phosphorylase.

Amylo-1,6-glucosidase (Debrancher) (EC 3.2.1.33)

After extensive phosphorylase action on glycogen, the molecule contains four glucose residues in α-1,4 glucosidic bonds attached by a 1,6 link to the glycogen molecule (see Fig. 6-3). This molecule is called the *phosphorylase limit dextrin* [54]. In order for amylo-1,6-glucosidase (debrancher) to act on this molecule, three of these glucose residues must be removed to expose the 1,6-linked glucose at the branch point. This is accomplished by an oligo-(1,4 → 1,4)-glucan transferase, which transfers these three glucose residues (probably as a unit) to another glycogen chain, with resynthesis of the α-1,4 bond [55] (Fig. 6-3). The most highly purified preparations of amylo-1,6-glucosidase contain significant oligo-(1,4 → 1,4)-glucan transferase activity, and this enzyme has appropriately been called a *glucosidase transferase*. During purification and heat inactivation these enzyme activities remain in a constant ratio [56]. Yet, rabbit muscle amylo-1,6-glucosidase is not a single enzyme species but is thought of as two enzymes with different pH optima [57]. Possibly debrancher is a single protein with two catalytic activities, but until this is clarified, it is assumed to be a multienzyme complex.

The action of debrancher on the limit dextrin yields free glucose. Since glycogen contains about 8 percent branch points (1,6 links), extensive glycogen degradation by phosphorylase and debrancher yields about 8 percent free glucose. The debrancher reaction is reversible, and [^{14}C]glucose can be incorporated into glycogen by this enzyme. The reverse reaction has a different pH optimum (broad, about pH 8.0) from the forward reaction, i.e., the liberation of glucose from a phosphorylase limit dextrin (pH optimum near 6.0) [51].

The several assays used for measuring the debrancher enzyme clearly do not measure the same activities; this is established by the variability in data obtained using different assays for debranching enzyme in human tissues. Nothing is known about the physiologic variables that affect the tissue levels of this enzyme.

Glucose-6-phosphatase (EC 3.1.3.9)

Glucose-6-phosphatase is a microsomal enzyme that catalyzes the irreversible reaction (Fig. 6-2)

$$\text{Glucose-6-phosphate} + H_2O \longrightarrow \text{glucose} + P_i \qquad (7)$$

As with most microsomal enzymes, it has not been highly purified, and its molecular properties are not known [58].

Glucose-6-phosphatase shows quite broad specificity and multiplicity of function. None of the alternative hexose phosphates is hydrolyzed at a rate of more than one-fifth that of glucose-6-phosphate [59]. Incubation for several minutes at pH 5.0, 37°C, destroys the ability of this enzyme to hydrolyze glucose-6-phosphate without loss of the nonspecific hydrolase activity [60, 61]. This finding has been of practical value in correcting for nonspecific phosphatase activity when assaying liver tissues from patients. The enzyme is normally present in human liver, kidney, and intestinal mucosa. By histochemical techniques it has also been demonstrated in the pancreatic β cells, localized in the cisternae of the endoplasmic reticulum and the nuclear membrane [62].

Glucose-6-phosphatase possesses several other enzymatic properties, two of which are [59, 63]:

1. The ability to cleave inorganic pyrophosphate hydrolytically

2. The ability to transfer phosphate from inorganic pyrophosphate to glucose, thereby forming glucose-6-phosphate.

There are both purification data [59] and considerable genetic data which indicate that these activities reside in a single protein [63].

In animals a 300 percent increase in glucose-6-phosphatase activity is seen after 48 h of fasting [64]. With continued fasting, activity returns to near-basal levels by 124 h. Alloxan diabetic rats have increased liver glucose-6-phosphatase activity, which returns to normal during insulin treatment [65]. The increase in liver glucose-6-phosphatase that occurs on a diet rich in fructose and protein can be blocked by including 1 percent ethionine in the diet [61].

Hydrocortisone administration increases the activity of this enzyme in rat liver [66]. Ethanol administration in rats produces a considerable increase in glucose-6-phosphatase activity [67]. There is also a large increase in liver glucose-6-phosphatase activity in hereditary fructose intolerance, in which there is a deficiency of aldolase activity.

Phosphofructokinase (EC 2.7.1.11)

This enzyme catalyzes the irreversible conversion of fructose-6-phosphate to fructose-1,6-diphosphate. At normal tissue substrate concentrations, phosphorylation of fructose-6-phosphate is a controlling step in glycolysis [68].

Citrate and ATP are inhibitors of liver and brain phosphofructokinase. Inhibition by ATP and citrate can be overcome by fructose diphosphate (FDP), P_i, fructose-6-phosphate, AMP, 3',5' AMP, or ADP. A fall in ATP or a rise in P_i or AMP within the cell activates phosphofructokinase and therefore enhances glycolysis [68]. At the usual levels of ATP in the cell, phosphofructokinase is in an inactive state (as long as P_i, AMP, and FDP are at low levels) [68]. This enzyme, which has a molecular weight of about 360,000, exhibits kinetics typical for allosteric inhibition in the presence of high concentrations of ATP [69].

α-1,4-Glucosidase (Acid Maltase) (EC 3.2.1.20)

The potential importance of the activity of this enzyme was realized only after it was found by Hers [70] to be deficient in generalized glycogenosis. Alpha-1,4-glucosidase is compartmentalized within the lysosomes and sediments during cell fractionation in the lysosome-rich, light mitochondrial fraction. In human liver the α-glucosidase activity at neutral pH is only one-tenth to one-third that at pH 4.0 [71]. It hydrolyzes maltose and other linear oligosaccharides, as well as glycogen, to yield free glucose [61].

Many hydrolytic enzymes have the same distribution during ultracentrifugation and the same structure-linked latency pattern (e.g., acid ribonuclease, acid deoxyribonuclease, cathepsin, aryl sulfatases, β-galactosidase, and β-N-acetyl-glucosaminidase). The lysosomal localization of acid maltase has been confirmed by equilibration centrifugation in density gradients, by its structure-linked latency, and by its release under controlled damage [72].

Widespread distribution of this activity in human tissues, including fibroblasts growing in vitro as well as in leukocytes, has made it relatively easy to diagnose genetic deficiencies of this enzyme.

Control of Glycogen Metabolism

As described in the previous section, there are multiple positive and negative effectors of the individual enzymes responsible for glycogen. This control is mediated by metabolite levels, hormonal balance, ionic effects, and neural discharge. Thus, the control of glycogen concentration and metabolism is regulated by the summation of these factors, as reviewed in detail by Newsholme and Start [73] and by Hers [74]. The primary regulators are cyclic AMP, glucose, and glycogen. As illustrated in Fig. 6-4, a complex cascade for coordinate control of glycogen synthesis and glycogenolysis has been elucidated. Hormonally initiated changes in cyclic AMP trigger the cascade amplification system. Perhaps neglected is the role of glycogen itself. High glycogen concentrations favor glycogenolysis by inhibiting the glycogen synthase phosphatase and phosphorylase a phosphatase while stimulating phosphorylase b kinase. But the intracellular level of phosphorylase, the rate-limiting enzyme of glycogen breakdown, remains as the

primary indicator of the state of glycogen metabolism. Phosphorylase a also regulates the activity of glycogen synthase phosphatase and consequently the level of glycogen synthase a and the rate of glycogen synthesis.

INHERITED ABNORMALITIES IN GLYCOGEN METABOLISM

In 1952, the Coris [3] demonstrated directly a deficiency of liver glucose-6-phosphatase in patients with von Gierke's disease. This, the first demonstrated inherited deficiency of a liver enzyme in humans, marked the beginning of such studies on a variety of hereditary diseases. There is now known a series of inherited defects involving glycogen metabolism in liver, muscle, and other tissues. The Coris began a system of numbering these diseases sequentially. Since their original classification, other forms of glycogen storage disease have been described, and numerous conflicting numbering systems have evolved. In order to avoid this confusion and because the enzymatic deficiencies are known, we prefer to abandon all numbering classifications and to refer to the diseases by the nature of the enzyme deficiency. The eponyms will also be given for historical completeness.

Glucose-6-phosphatase Deficiency

Clinical Features Children with this disorder, which is also called *hepatorenal glycogen storage disease* and *von*

Figure 6-4 Cascade for coordinate activation-inactivation of the enzymes of glycogen synthesis and degradation. The respective phosphorylation-dephosphorylation mechanisms are indicated.

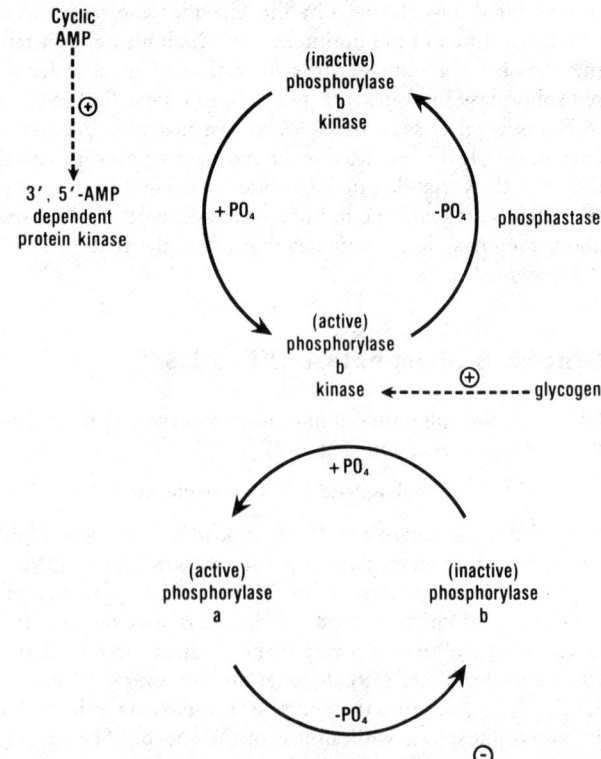

Gierke's disease, have short stature without disproportion of head, limbs, or trunk length [75]. The abdomen is huge and round because of massive enlargement of the liver. Liver enlargement is found in the newborn and persists throughout life (Fig. 6-5). As the patient grows older, the abdomen becomes less prominent. There is a tendency to adiposity, with generous accumulations of fat in the cheeks, buttocks, and subcutaneous tissues. The musculature is flabby and poorly developed [76]. Although the kidneys are enlarged, they cannot be palpated because of the massive hepatic enlargement. Radiographically, the kidney enlargement is readily appreciated (Fig. 6-6). The spleen is only rarely enlarged. Fine et al. [77] have reported multiple, bilateral, symmetric, yellowish, discrete paramacular lesions in the fundi of three of five patients. We find these fundal changes quite specific for this disorder. Osteoporosis is usually present and possibly is secondary to a negative calcium balance related to the chronic acidosis.

Xanthomas appear commonly over the extensor surfaces of the extremities. These lesions are similar to those seen in patients with disorders of lipoprotein metabolism resulting in high circulating levels of very low density lipoprotein. Since these patients always have hyperuricemia, xanthomas must be distinguished from gouty tophi, which may have a similar distribution.

Bleeding may be a major clinical problem. Frequent, severe nosebleeds and persistent oozing of blood after surgery are troublesome. Although a variety of problems of hemostatsis have been reported, impaired platelet function seems to underlie the bleeding problem. This is manifested by prolonged bleeding time, reduced platelet adhesion, and defective collagen and epinephrine-induced aggregation [78]. Hutton et al. have found low adenine nucleotide levels in patients with glucose-6-phosphatase and fructose-1,6-diphosphatase deficiency [79]. These abnormalities, as well as platelet dysfunctions, were corrected when normoglycemia was maintained by glucose infusion. They suggested that abnormal platelet function is due to depleted nucleotide pools secondary to hypoglycemia. Often an abundance of small superficial vessels is visible in the skin of these patients.

Fine et al. [80] and Howell et al. [76] have reported an increased frequency of intermittent episodes of diarrhea in patients with glucose-6-phosphatase deficiency. Milla et al. have suggested that this is due to glucose malabsorption [81]. We found no abnormality in fat absorption in one of our patients suspected of malabsorption [76]. But loss of haustration and smooth walls have been demonstrated in the colon of von Gierke's patients [82]. Liver function test results (transaminases, Bromsulphalein conjugation) are normal.

The degree of hypoglycemia is extremely variable. In addition to fasting hypoglycemia and unresponsiveness to epinephrine and glucagon, there is a striking elevation in levels of blood lactate, pyruvate, triglycerides, phospholipids, cholesterol, and uric acid [76]. The disease is compatible with reasonably long life, and many adult patients are known [83, 84]. Ketosis has long been considered a hallmark of this disease, but only rarely have elevated blood ketone values been published [76]. Fernandez and Pikaar [85] and Binkiewicz and Senior [86] have studied extensively the problem of ketosis in children with von Gierke's disease. They have shown quite conclusively that these children are resistant to ketosis, which they have attributed to high pyruvate providing adequate oxaloacetate and thereby preventing acetyl CoA accumulation.

Recent data by McGarry and Foster demonstrating the reg-

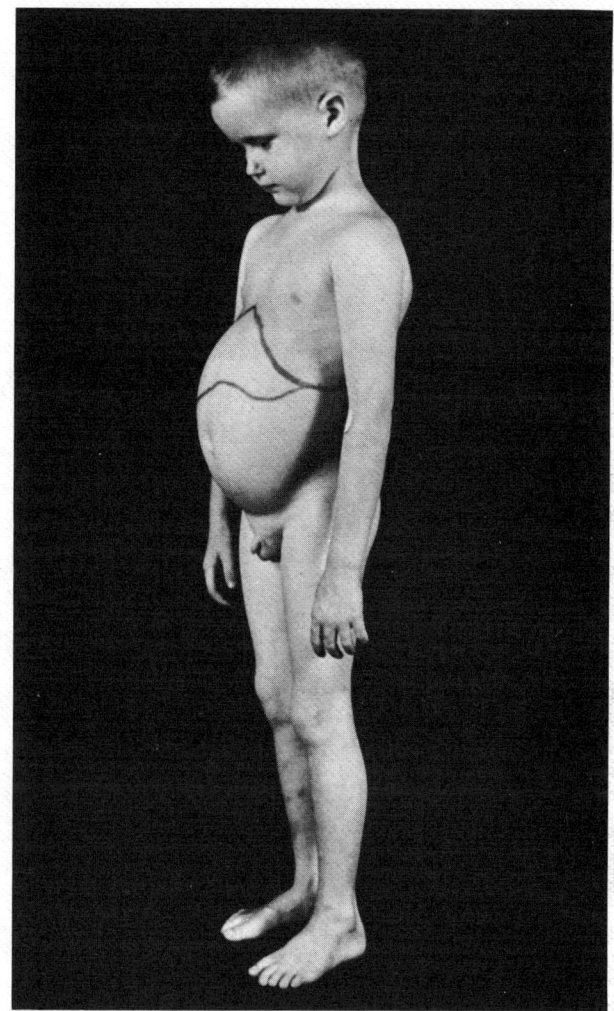

Figure 6-5 Seven-year-old boy (D.M.) with glucose-6-phosphatase deficiency glycogen storage disease. The massive liver is outlined on the protuberant abdomen. In addition to short stature, there are generous fat deposits in the cheeks. We have previously published biochemical data on this boy [76].

ulatory role of malonyl CoA in the suppression of ketogenesis [87] suggest that in glucose-6-phosphatase deficiency, ongoing hepatic glycolysis would inhibit ketogenesis via carnitine palmityltransferase and fatty acid synthesis. Suppression of β oxidation in the presence of an increased fatty acid flux results in increased ω oxidation of fatty acids, producing elevated levels of dicarboxylic acids [88].

Convulsions accompanying severe hypoglycemia may occur during the first years of life. In some patients, profound hypoglycemia is seen without clinical symptoms; patients may be asymptomatic with blood glucose concentrations under 10 mg/100 ml. It has been suggested that these patients, like starved obese patients [89], have replaced glucose with β-hydroxybutyrate and acetoacetate as the primary fuel of the brain. The absence of ketosis makes this explanation unlikely, but alternate substrates could play a role.

A Fanconi-like syndrome (aminoaciduria, glycosuria, and phosphaturia) with abnormal galactose metabolism occurs in patients with glucose-6-phosphatase deficiency [90]. In normal mammals glucose-6-phosphatase is found in the proximal and distal convoluted tubules. In these patients glucose-6-phosphatase is deficient in the kidney, and glycogen accumulates there.

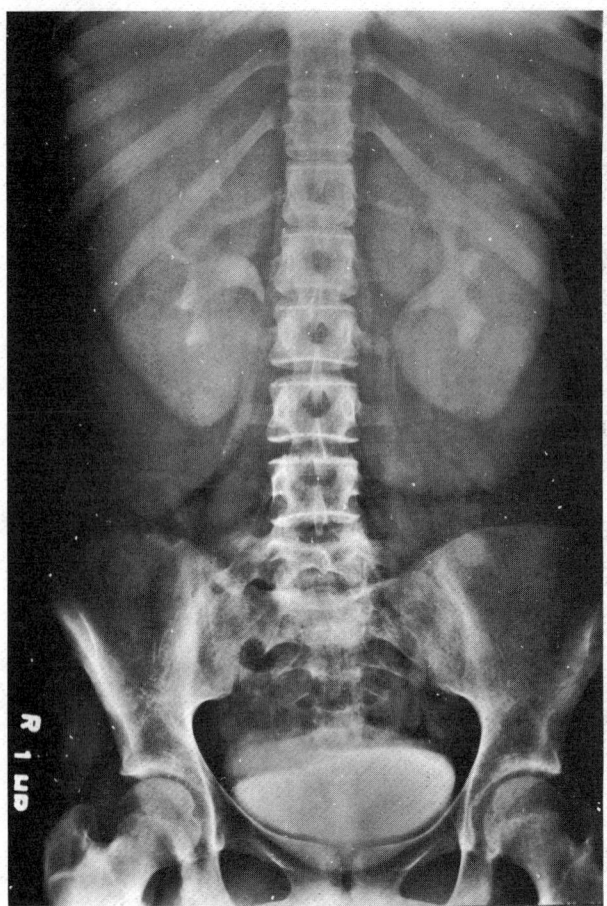

Figure 6-6 Abdominal roentgenogram taken during an intravenous pyelo-gram of a young woman with glucose-6-phosphatase deficiency glycogen storage disease. The nephrogram shows the large kidneys. The outline of the enormous liver can be seen bilaterally just above the pelvis. It is clear from this film why the enlarged kidneys are rarely palpable.

If this enzyme were essential for energy-requiring renal processes, problems in renal transport would be expected. Fanconi's syndrome, which occurs rarely in von Gierke's disease (never in our experience), is seen regularly in hereditary fructose intolerance, in which there is increased liver glycogen; care must be exercised to distinguish between these two diseases.

The Mechanisms of the Lipid Abnormalities Hyperlipidemia may be a dominant feature in these patients [76, 91]. The operation of the glycolytic pathway and Krebs cycle results in production of NADH, while that of the oxidative pathway results in production of NADPH. Reduction of pyruvate to lactate requires either NADH or NADPH; fatty acid synthesis requires both these nucleotide cofactors. NADPH is required in cholesterol synthesis, in which it may indeed be the rate-limiting factor. Fatty acid and cholesterol synthesis require acetyl CoA, which is produced in abundance from the pyruvate generated by glycolysis. The existing conditions of increased flux of fatty acid from adipose tissue to the liver, inhibition of ketogenesis, and increased hepatic levels of glycerol-1-phosphate result in increased triglyceride and lipoprotein synthesis. Thus, the substrates and the reduced coenzymes necessary for synthesis of lactate, fatty acids, and cholesterol are made available in quantity by high-level operation of the glycolytic and oxidative pathways, and these synthetic

processes, in turn, regenerate the oxidized coenzymes necessary for sustaining active operation of these carbohydrate pathways. Thus, elevated levels of serum triglycerides, phospholipids, and cholesterol are possible consequences of glycogenolytic and gluconeogenic responses to hypoglycemia in liver containing abundant glycogen, a block in glucose-6-phosphatase function, and active glycolytic and phosphogluconic oxidative pathways [76].

The elevation of free fatty acid levels in serum is probably a direct consequence of hypoglycemia. Hypoglycemia is a potent stimulus to the release of free fatty acids by adipose tissue, and the high free fatty acid levels observed probably reflect mobilization from the periphery [76]. Öckerman [92, 93] has also observed that serum concentrations of glycerol are elevated in these patients.

Patients with glucose-6-phosphatase deficiency have diminished triglyceride elimination rates and 5-min postheparin lipoprotein lipase activity [94].

Lactic Acidosis and Substrate Cycling In glucose-6-phosphatase deficiency, there exists the paradox of a liver in the fed state and a fasted peripheral tissue bed. Gluconeogenic precursors produced in the periphery are transported to the liver and incorporated into glycogen. Hypoglycemia in a milieu of decreased insulin levels and hyperglucagonemia promotes glycogenolysis [95]. Small amounts of free glucose are released by the action of debrancher enzyme, but the absence of glucose-6-phosphatase commits the glucose-1-phosphate produced by phosphorylase to glycolytic catabolism. This results in increased lactate production and turnover [96, 97]. Urinary lactate in patients with von Gierke's disease is elevated 10- to 300-fold [98]. Thus, substrate cycling of glucose-6-phosphate $\rightarrow$ lactate $\rightarrow$ glucose-1-phosphate $\rightarrow$ glycogen $\rightarrow$ glucose-1-phosphate $\rightarrow$ glucose-6-phosphate occurs at a phenomenal rate. Although this process appears futile, it is the only way that free glucose can be produced (via debrancher enzyme). If so, the faster the rate of cycling, the greater the rate of glucose production.

Glucose Tolerance and Insulin Output Results of glucose tolerance tests in these patients are characteristically diabetic in type [76]. Earlier, it was thought that this was due to the competitive inhibition of hexokinase by glucose-6-phosphate, which was thought to accumulate in the liver. Although liver glucose-6-phosphate concentration is moderately elevated [99], this would probably not inhibit hexokinase. More important, glucokinase, which is probably responsible for most hepatic glucose phosphorylation, is not inhibited by glucose-6-phosphate. Basal plasma insulin levels were found to be approximately 50 to 60 percent of normal in five older patients with von Gierke's disease [100]. Three well-known stimuli for secretion of insulin in normal humans (glucose, glucose plus a protein meal, and arginine infusion) resulted in outputs of insulin significantly less than normal in these patients (Fig. 6-7). Okada et al. found similar results in 10 patients with hepatic glycogenosis along with normal glucagon secretion [101]. These authors suggested that persistent hypoinsulinism may contribute to the growth failure of these patients.

The Mechanisms of Hyperuricemia Hyperuricemia in association with von Gierke's disease has been reported in a

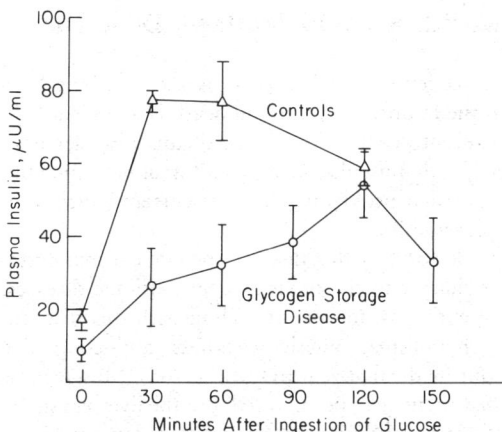

Figure 6-7 Plasma insulin levels after the ingestion of glucose in 15 normal subjects and 5 adolescent or adult patients with glucose-6-phosphatase deficiency. Values are the means ± standard errors of the means. The reduced insulin output in this group of patients disease is clear. (*From Lockwood et al.* [*100*].)

large number of patients since the association was first described by Kolb et al. in two patients in 1955 [102]. In such patients, hyperuricemia appears in early infancy but rarely becomes symptomatic before the end of the first decade of life. This was originally attributed to a decreased excretion of uric acid because of competitive inhibition of renal tubular urate secretion by lactate, which frequently is elevated in the serum. This suggestion was supported by the demonstration of reduced urate clearance in these patients [76], though renal function was normal as measured by other parameters. Fine et al. [103] and Alepa et al. [84] studied urate clearances in five patients with glucose-6-phosphatase deficiency and found that glucose infusions increased the clearance of uric acid. However, both groups observed that the increase in urate clearance occurred at a time when serum lactic acid concentration had not yet changed appreciably. Fine et al. suggested that since renal glucose-6-phosphatase was deficient in these patients, glucose was unavailable to the renal tubules as an energy source.

The finding by Jeune et al. [104] that several patients with hyperuricemia and glycogen storage disease actually had normal or increased uric acid clearance indicated that extrarenal factors might also be important. Uric acid production was studied [84, 105, 106] in five patients and found to be increased. There was an increase in specific activity of urinary uric acid after [1-14C]glycine administration in several patients studied this way. The cumulative incorporation of isotopic glycine into urinary uric acid observed in three patients was greater than that observed in most patients with primary gout due to the excessive production of uric acid. The precise mechanism by which a deficiency of glucose-6-phosphatase causes the excessive production of uric acid remains unknown. It has been suggested that an increased synthesis of phosphoribosylpyrophosphate (PRPP) results from a deficiency of glucose-6-phosphatase [107, 108]. Alternatively, recent studies have documented decreased concentrations of purine nucleotides in von Gierke's disease [109]. Glucose-6-phosphatase deficiency results in increased levels of phosphorylated glycolytic intermediates and diminished hepatic levels of ATP and P_i. Continuous glycogenolysis depletes ATP stores and results in enhanced adenine nucleotide degradation (see Chap. 50).

Functional Tests Characteristically, these patients have a much diminished rise in blood glucose after administration of glucagon or epinephrine, as would be anticipated with a deficiency of glucose-6-phosphatase activity. The major product of glycogenolysis in these patients is lactic acid rather than glucose. Glucagon and epinephrine tolerance tests are rarely completely "flat"; this is probably related to the fact that in glycogenolysis, the 1,6-linked glucosyl residues are released as free glucose by debrancher activity. Because of the variability of individual responses to tolerance tests, we do not feel that diagnosis of a specific glycogen storage disease can be made by these criteria and that specific enzymatic assay is necessary.

Biochemical Diagnosis In all instances in which a glycogen storage disease is suspected, final diagnosis should be made by direct assay of appropriate tissue. In von Gierke's disease, a liver biopsy is desirable. Although a diagnosis can be made on needle biopsy material, an open biopsy is preferred except under unusual circumstances. Correction of metabolic derangements prior to and during general anesthesia is essential in order to avoid intractable acidosis and its complications [110]. The open biopsy affords adequate tissue for glycogen determination, glycogen structure analyses, and replicate assays of the various enzymes, as well as for light and electron microscopy. More important, direct vision permits control of bleeding, should any occur. Enzyme analysis should be done on fresh, unfrozen, unfixed tissue in a laboratory in which these assays are well established. The glycogen content is usually elevated and has a normal structure. Glucose-6-phosphatase activity is characteristically totally absent. Also absent are the other enzymatic activities associated with glucose-6-phosphatase, i.e., pyrophosphate-glucose phosphotransferase, carbamyl phosphate-glucose phosphotransferase, and inorganic pyrophosphatase [63].

Van Hoof et al. [111] have presented an ingenious method for glucose-6-phosphatase assay in vivo. Following the intravenous infusion of a mixture of [U-14C] and [2-3H] glucose into a normal subject, the half-life of [U-14C] glucose was 1.6 times as great as that of [2-3H] glucose, so the ratio of 3H to 14C progressively declined. This reduction in ratio requires glucose-6-phosphatase; therefore, in patients deficient in glucose-6-phosphatase, the ratio remains 1. This technique has been applied by Sann et al. to a study of what has been termed *glycogenosis type IB* [112]. These patients are clinically identical to glucose-6-phosphatase-deficient patients but have normal enzyme activity in frozen tissue in vitro. Sann et al. demonstrated a defect in glucose-6-phosphatase activity in vivo by this isotope technique. The puzzle of glycogenosis type IB has recently been solved by Narisawa et al. [113], who found that unfrozen liver in one of these patients had greatly reduced glucose-6-phosphatase activity and that detergents restored the activity to normal. This suggested a defect in glucose-6-phosphate transport across the hepatic microsomal membrane.

Genetics There are many examples of this disorder among sibs, both male and female, whose parents are clinically normal. In addition, several patients affected with glucose-6-phosphatase deficiency (both male and female) have had phenotypically normal children [83, 84]. Studies on intestinal glucose-6-phosphatase activity in patients with von Gierke's disease and their families support an autosomal recessive inheritance scheme [114]. Field and Drash [114], who studied the parents of five children with hepatorenal glycogenosis, found that all had reduced intestinal glucose-6-phosphatase, while another brother and the maternal grandmother had normal values.

Adenomas A morphologic abnormality of the liver, only infrequently appreciated in the past, is the development of adenomatous nodules within the liver parenchyma. In a study of eight patients aged 3 to 23 years, we demonstrated (using radioisotopic scans) depressed isotope uptake in all but a single preteen patient [115]. These areas of depressed isotope uptake, initially diffuse, evolved into discrete nodular areas which increased in number and size with age. The biopsy specimens of three patients were studied. In each case, only an adenomatous change was observed, but one patient later developed hepatocellular carcinoma in one of these nodules and died from this disease. Miller et al. have confirmed these findings in their studies of 15 patients with glucose-6-phosphatase deficiency [116].

The presence of hepatomegaly with discrete or diffuse nodules on liver scans should suggest von Gierke's disease. The development of hepatocellular carcinoma in one of these nodules suggests that they should be considered premalignant [115].

Treatment Glucagon and thyroxine have been suggested for treatment of this disease but they appear at best to be of questionable benefit [104]. Frequent feedings are helpful if there is hypoglycemia. Since these patients have a limited capacity for converting amino acids to free glucose, a high-protein diet is not of special value.

Portal diversions have been employed in at least 20 patients [117]. A 20-year follow-up is available for Starzl's first patient. A high mortality diminished interest after the first few patients had surgery. The discovery of Folkman et al. [118] that long term intravenous alimentation prior to surgery reduced the liver size dramatically and returned bleeding factors and other metabolic conditions toward normal has greatly expedited the surgery.

After surgery, most (but not all) of the patients have had a substantial growth spurt, reduction in liver size (due to delipidation), reduction in serum urate and lipids, and improvement in bleeding parameters. Fasting hypoglycemia remains a troublesome feature. The technical difficulty of the surgery, as well as postoperative management, call for careful consideration of the benefits for each patient and limitation of this procedure to a few specialized centers.

Portacaval shunting is less effective than continous intragastric feeding [119]. This technique has come into widespread use in recent years. Nocturnal continuous nasogastric feeding plus frequent daytime high-carbohydrate meals corrects the metabolic and hormonal abnormalities of glucose-6-phosphatase deficiency [120]. The remarkable clinical improvement and growth spurt that occur after initiation of this therapy appear to be due to correction of hypoglycemia and suppression of glycogenolytic-glycolytic cycling.

The benefits of these treatments can be dramatic, particularly on growth. They should be performed only under conditions which permit complex metabolic monitoring. Recent studies have demonstrated regression of the hepatomas during such treatment. This is perhaps the most important benefit [121].

α-1,4-Glucosidase (Acid Maltase) Deficiency

Generalized glycogenosis, or Pompe's disease, has long been recognized in the infant; early cardiac death is a clinical hallmark [2]. In recent years, other forms of this disorder have been described, with muscular wasting and weakness and minimal or absent cardiac problems. There are currently three general clinical presentations.

In the infantile form of this disease, the clinical manifestations contrast sharply to the other glycogen storage diseases. The usual presenting symptoms of a child with this disorder are profound hypotonia, muscle weakness, and congestive heart failure during the first year of life (Fig. 6-8). Muscle mass is normal. The tongue may be enlarged, but the liver is usually of normal size prior to the onset of cardiac decompensation. The heart is strikingly enlarged (Fig. 6-9). The electrocardiogram (ECG) shows the specific change of gigantic QRS complexes in all leads and a shortened PR interval [122] (Fig. 6-10). Cardiac failure without cyanosis is common in the first year of life. There are no significant murmurs [119], and cardiac catheterization frequently shows biventricular hypertrophy with left outflow tract obstruction [123]. There are no abnormalities of glucose homeostasis, and blood lactate, uric acid, and lipid levels are normal.

Symptoms appear between birth and 6 months of age, and most patients are dead by 1 year of age. The cause of death is cardiorespiratory failure, pneumonia, or aspiration. At autopsy, a massive increase in glycogen is found in most tissues as well as a basophilic material digestible by amylase and containing phosphate (Fig. 6-11) [124]. Besides glycogen accumulation in the liver, muscle, and heart, there is extensive deposition in the motor nuclei of the brainstem and anterior horn cells of the spinal cord [125]. Only slight deposition occurs in cortical neurons; such storage is present by the eighteenth week of gestation [126]. Although there is increased glycogen in Schwann cells of peripheral nerves, no apparent clinical dysfunction occurs. Electromyography reveals pseudomyotonic discharges, fibrillations, and high-frequency discharges in all three clinical forms of the disease [127].

In a second group of patients, the disease appears in infancy

Figure 6-8 Seven-month-old female infant (D.B.) with generalized glycogenosis (α-glucosidase deficiency). The profound hypotonia is evident. Studies of muscle biopsy specimens in our laboratory showed increased glycogen (10 g per 100 g wet weight of tissue) of normal structure, normal phosphorylase and debrancher activity, and absent α-1,4-glucosidase activity. (*Photograph courtesy of Dr. M. Museles.*)

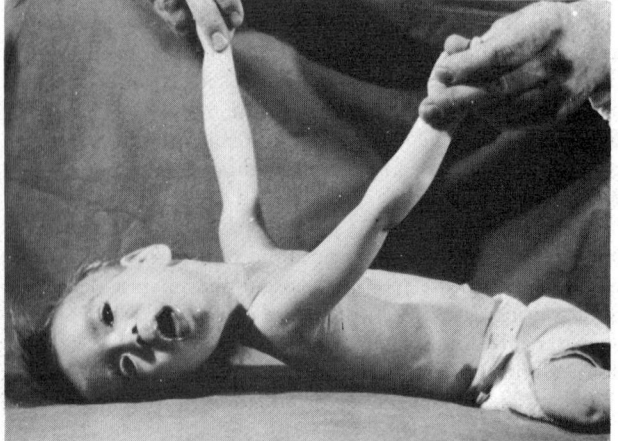

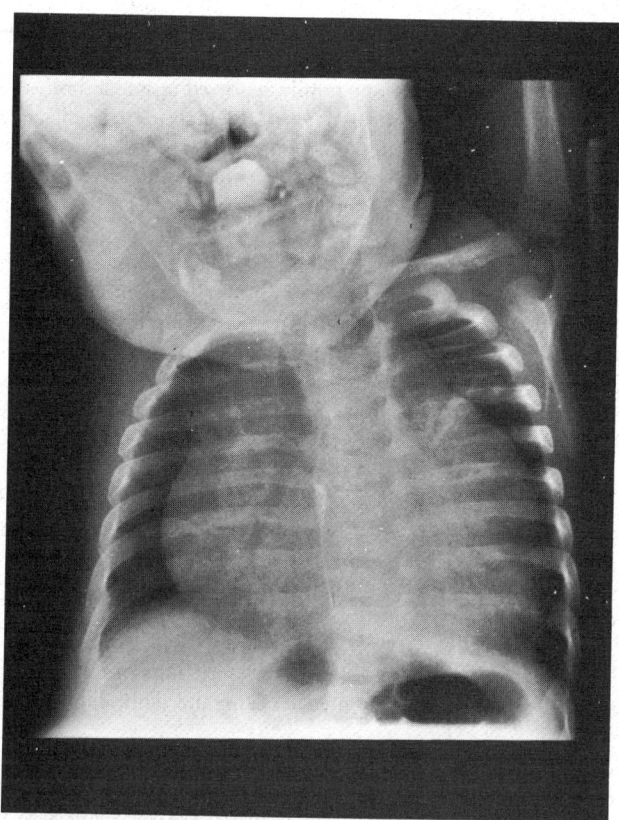

Figure 6-9 Chest roentgenogram of a 4-month-old female infant (A.M.) with generalized glycogen storage disease. The massive heart dominates the film with a cardiothoracic index of 0.80 to 0.85.

or early childhood and progresses much more slowly than the infantile form. The symptoms are primarily muscle weakness and hypotonia without clinical cardiac disease [128, 129]. No patient has survived beyond 19 years. Death usually results from pneumonia and respiratory failure [125].

The third group of patients do not present until the second to fourth decades of life, although in retrospect they may have had decreased muscle strength. The primary complaint is muscle weakness, but some patients have acute respiratory failure [130]. The disease is slowly progressive and mimics other chronic myopathies [128, 131–133]. Cardiac abnormalities are absent or minimal. Electromyographic findings are similar to those seen in the infantile form.

The reasons for the differences in clinical findings cannot be readily resolved, since lysosomal α-1,4-glucosidase activity is deficient in all tissues from patients in all three groups [128, 132, 133]. Puzzling is the absence of glycogen accumulation in the heart, liver, and brain of adult patients even though enzyme activity is severely deficient. Such glycogen accumulation is variable among different muscles in the same patient and correlates with the degree of clinical weakness [132]. It has been suggested that the small residual acid maltase activity found in adult tissues, in contrast to those of infantile patients, may explain the differences in age of onset, severity, or selective involvement of skeletal muscle in the adult [133]. It is difficult to believe that glycogen would be stored in muscle but not in the liver with similar degrees of enzyme deficiency.

Pompe's disease was the basis for the formulation of the concept of lysosomal storage disease by Hers [134]. The usual enzymes of glycogen synthesis and degradation were found to be normal. Hers [70] demonstrated that tissues from normal

persons contain an acid α-1,4-glucosidase (acid maltase) and that this enzyme activity is absent in patients with generalized glycogen storage disease. In normal tissues the enzyme has a pH optimum of 4.5, sediments with lysosomes during tissue fractionation, and is considered to be a lysosomal enzyme. Baudhuin et al. [135], in an elegant electron-microscopic study of the liver of a child affected with Pompe's disease, demonstrated that there is a dual localization of glycogen in the parenchymal cells. As in normal liver, part of the glycogen was freely dispersed within the cell, but in this liver specimen a large fraction was segregated in vacuoles surrounded by a single membrane (Fig. 6-12). The diameter of the vacuoles was as large as 8 μm. They have various shapes and are not seen in the hepatic parenchymal cells in other types of glycogenosis [135].

The simultaneous absence of a lysosomal α-glucosidase and the finding of an intravacuolar accumulation of glycogen indicate that there is a causal relationship between these two findings and strongly suggests that the vacuoles are lysosomes engorged with glycogen [134].

Presumably, during lysosomal development, cell components which accumulate within lysosomes are degraded by the enzymes which are localized therein. In generalized glycogen storage disease, glycogen may accumulate because of a deficiency of the lysosomal acid maltase, while other cell components (e.g., RNA, protein) are degraded. The lysosomal glycogen, enclosed by a membrane, would not be accessible to the other glycogenolytic enzymes, which are present at normal levels within the cytoplasm.

Garancis [136] found lysosomal glycogen most abundant in liver and kidneys and only a few engorged lysosomes in muscle and myocardium. This suggested a defect other than that of the α-1,4-glucosidase, but no direct evidence supports this concept. Hug [126] has stressed that the cytoplasmic glycogen in acid maltase deficiency is abnormally increased but can be mobilized with epinephrine or glucagon. He and other authors have suggested that the α-1,4-glucosidase deficiency may be

Figure 6-10 Electrocardiogram of the patient A.M. There are gigantic complexes, here reduced to one-fifth, in leads V_5, V_6, and V_8. This suggests massive biventricular hypertrophy. The PR interval (0.04 s) is short.

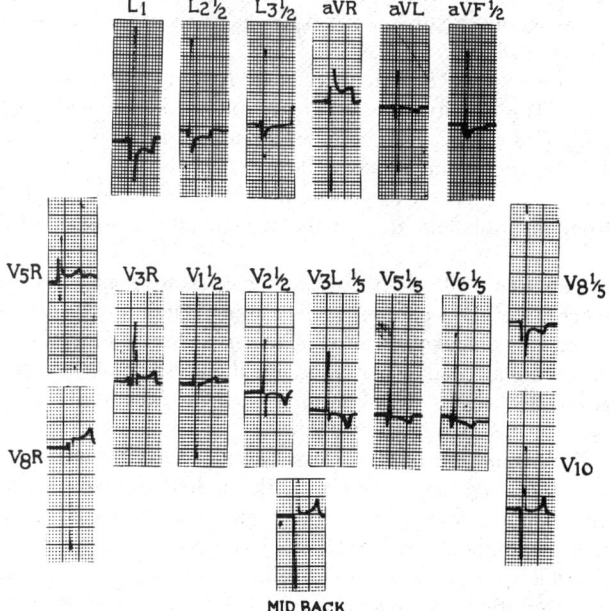

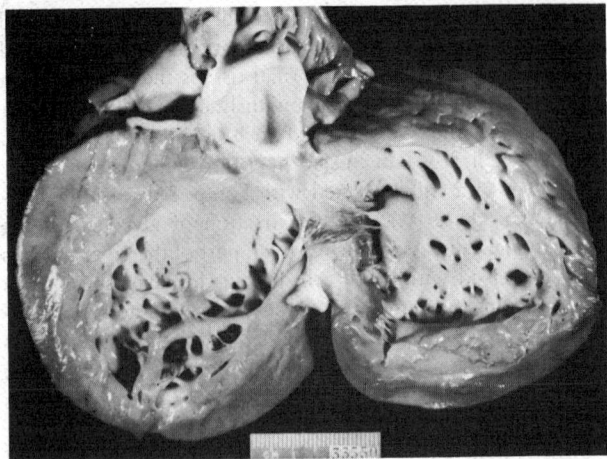

Figure 6-11   The heart of the patient A.M. (see Figs. 6-9 and 6-10) at autopsy (age at death, 5 months). The heart is greatly enlarged, with thickened ventricles, due to extensive glycogen infiltration. There is some endocardial thickening.

secondary to another as yet unidentified lesion. Martin et al. contend that the increase in cytoplasmic glycogen is more apparent than real [124]. The glycogen that accumulates in generalized glycogenosis has been reported to be of normal structure [70], but the internal part of the molecule may have an increased branching [137]. Possibly the increased urinary excretion of oligosaccharides with α-1,6 linkages by patients with generalized glycogenosis and with debrancher deficiency reflects this proposed structure [138].

Diagnosis   In a patient with appropriate clinical findings, the diagnosis is established by the demonstration of an increased tissue concentration of glycogen and an acid α-1,4-glucosidase deficiency. Muscle biopsy specimens are usually studied. Leukocyte acid maltase has usually been (but not always) deficient [139]. These variable findings have been resolved by the demonstration of a renal α-1,4-glucosidase with a broad pH optimum which overlaps that of the lysosomal enzyme. Dreyfus and Poënaru have shown that this renal isoenzyme is present in leukocytes in amounts that vary from person to person [140]. This interfering activity can be removed by isoelectric precipitation at pH 5.0, allowing the unambiguous use of leukocytes for diagnosis of the lysosomal enzyme deficiency [141].

Normal urine is rich in renal α-1,4-glucosidase activity [132]. This activity probably arises from shed, disrupted renal cells. This observation precludes the use of direct assay of α-1,4-glucosidase in amniotic fluid (which arises from fetal urine) as a prenatal diagnostic method. Fibroblasts cultured from amniotic fluid are reliable for prenatal diagnosis [142].

Genetics   All family studies suggest autosomal recessive inheritance. Some parents (both fathers and mothers) have had reductions in leukocyte enzyme activity, whereas others have been normal. Studies that allow for the presence of the renal enzymatic activity will likely improve the usefulness of leukocytes for heterozygote detection.

Enzyme activity in fibroblasts developed from skin biopsy specimens of patients' families with children affected with α-glucosidase deficiency were compatible with autosomal recessive inheritance. Presumed heterozygotes have reduced but detectable fibroblast α-1,4-glucosidase activity [143]. There is an interesting and unexplained preponderance of affected males. In heterozygote studies, care must be exercised not to confuse the residual lysosomal enzyme activity with the microsomal neutral maltase present in all tissues [144].

There has been only one family reported in which both the infantile and adult forms of α-1,4-glucosidase deficiency occurred [145]. It seems likely that some of the less severe infantile forms and the juvenile forms of the disease represent genetic compounds of different abnormal alleles.

Treatment   Purified acid maltase isolated from *Aspergillus niger* has been administered without clinical success [135]. There were no apparent immunologic complications associated with infusion of α-1,4-glucosidase purified to homogeneity from human placenta [146]. The enzyme activity was recovered only in liver biopsies, not muscle. There was no clinical or morphologic improvement. The technical and theoretical problems of enzyme replacement therapy are great [147]. The primary difficulty is targeting the enzyme to the desired site of action. New experimental techniques may ultimately prove successful [148]. At present, prenatal diagnosis by enzyme assay offers the only form of management of this condition.

Ethanolaminosis   A recently described storage disease which presents with cardiomegaly, generalized muscular hypo-

Figure 6-12   Electron micrograph of a portion of a hepatic parenchymal cell from a liver biopsy of a patient with α-glucosidase deficiency. Two vacuoles filled with glycogen are seen at magnification ×69,000. A membrane can be followed around most of the periphery of the vacuoles. (*From P. Baudhuin, H.G. Hers, and H. Loeb [135], with permission.*)

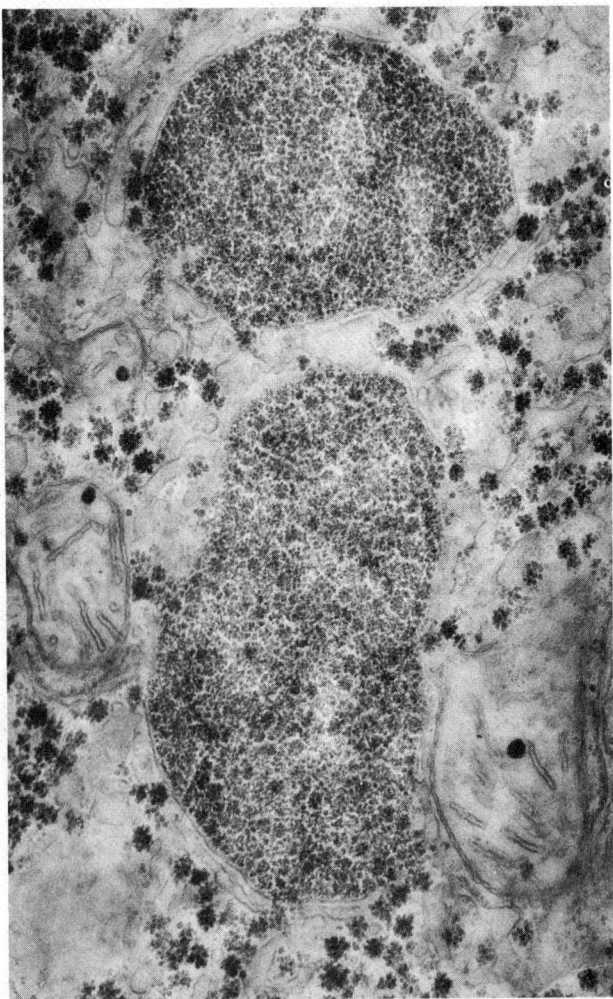

tonia, cerebral dysfunction, failure to thrive, and early death resembles generalized glycogen storage disease. Widespread tissue deposition of ethanolamine (PAS-positive) due to a deficiency of ethanolamine kinase has been seen. There is no abnormality of glycogen [149].

Amylo-1,6-glucosidase (Debrancher) Deficiency

In this form of glycogen storage disease, also named *limit dextrinosis* and *Cori's disease,* a polysaccharide accumulates with a structure resembling that of the limit dextrin produced by degradation of glycogen by phosphorylase which is free of debrancher (amylo-1,6-glucosidase) activity [60]. By physical examination alone, these patients cannot be reliably distinguished from patients with glucose-6-phosphatase deficiency. Early in life, hepatomegaly and growth retardation may be striking. In contrast to patients with von Gierke's disease, moderate enlargement of the spleen sometimes occurs [150].

Glycogen of abnormal structure accumulates in muscle as well as in the liver and may cause a myopathy [150, 151].

Muscle wasting and weakness is a feature in some patients [151]; rapid walking and climbing results in weakness without cramps. A group of patients with debrancher deficiency who do not present until adult life have recently been well characterized [151, 152]. Their primary symptoms are progressive muscle weakness. In these patients, as well as the infantile form, glycogen may accumulate in the heart. The ECG shows hypertrophy; sudden death may occur [153].

Generally the clinical course of this disease is milder than that of glucose-6-phosphatase deficiency. Severe hypoglycemia and convulsions may appear. Although remarkable and difficult to explain, it is well documented that the liver size returns to normal at puberty [60] in at least some of these patients (Fig. 6-13). There is no renal enlargement in this disease; this fact distinguishes the disorder from glucose-6-phosphatase deficiency. Children with debrancher deficiency and renal tubular acidosis resulting in severe failure to thrive have been described [154].

Serum lipid levels are variably elevated [155]. Serum uric acid concentration is usually normal, and adult patients have not had symptoms of gout.

Serum transaminase levels are consistently elevated in young children and normal in adults. Mild inflammatory disease of the liver is common, and cirrhosis, usually mild, occurs in this disease [150]. Frank cirrhosis is not unknown [117].

Function Studies   Galactose and fructose are readily con-

Figure 6-13 Growth and development in a young man (R.G.) with debrancher deficiency. Left, the patient at age 7, with the enlarged liver outlined on the abdomen. The abdomen at this age was not as protuberant as when the patient was younger. Right, the same patient at age 17. Growth has been completely normal, the liver is now not enlarged, and the patient is asymptomatic. (*Photographs courtesy of Dr. Harriet G. Guild.*)

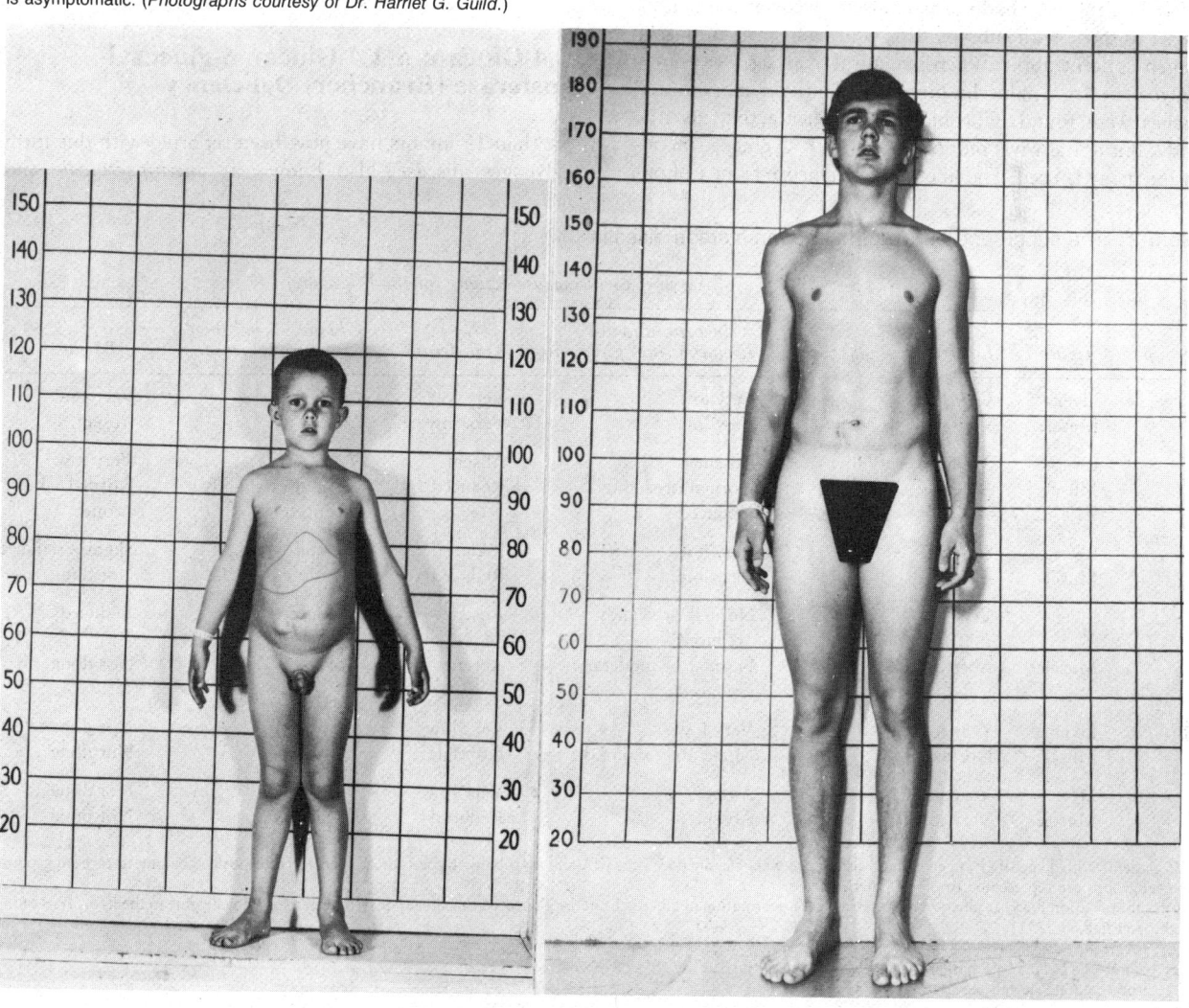

verted to glucose by these patients; similarly, protein and amino acid mixtures given orally induce a small and prolonged rise in blood glucose level. The rise in blood sugar level after epinephrine and glucagon is variable. Hug et al. [156] found a normal glucagon response 2 h after feeding and no response after a 14-h fast. This was interpreted as indicating availability after feeding of glucose from the elongated outer branches of glycogen, which could be degraded by phosphorylase in the absence of debranching activity. It is not a consistent finding.

Biochemical Investigations Liver glycogen concentration is often much increased (up to 17.4 g/per 100 g tissue) in this disorder [60]. We routinely find modest reductions in hepatic glucose-6-phosphatase activity. The glycogen is found to have short outer branches and resembles a phosphorylase limit dextrin.

A series of techniques is available for measuring debrancher activity. These assays clearly do not measure the same enzyme activity. Methods currently used are (1) liberation of glucose from a phosphorylase limit dextrin, (2) incorporation of [^{14}C]glucose into glycogen, (3) 1,4 → 1,4 transfer of an oligoglucan (glucan transferase activity), and (4) hydrolysis of singly branched oligosaccharides.

Using these various methods, Hers and associates [157] have described a series of biochemical subtypes of debrancher deficiency. These are summarized in Table 6-2. Some of the patients studied by van Hoff and Hers (e.g., subtypes IIIB, IIIE, and IIIF in Table 6-2) had normal muscle glycogen content, in contrast to those with subtype IIIA, who had elevated muscle glycogen concentration. When structural analyses were done on glycogen from muscle biopsy specimens, short outer branches were found. Fibroblast debrancher activity is frequently, but not always, reduced when the ^{14}C-glucose incorporation assay is used. The liberation of glucose from a phos-

phorylase limit dextrin correlates with the pressure of absence of debrancher enzyme activity in fibroblasts [158].

Genetics All the available data suggest an autosomal recessive inheritance of this disease. Some investigators have shown intermediate levels of leukocyte debrancher in presumed heterozygotes [159, 160], while others have not been able to identify heterozygotes [161]. There is widespread variability in tissue enzyme activity even within single affected families [140, 151]. Some discrepancies undoubtedly arise from the use of different assay techniques.

In Israel this disease accounts for 73 percent of the glycogen storage disorders. It was found to have a minimal prevalence of 1:5420 in a non-Ashkenazi Jewish community which originated in North Africa. No debrancher deficiency has been seen in the Ashkenazi Jews [162].

Treatment Frequent feedings and a high protein diet are indicated for a child with symptoms of debrancher deficiency. Patients who have had a portacaval transposition apparently benefited from this procedure [117]. Nocturnal nasogastric feedings have had a very beneficial effect similar to the results obtained in glucose-6-phosphatase deficiency. The young man shown in Fig. 6-13 is now asymptomatic, has no hypoglycemia, and has normal responses to epinephrine. The outlook for a long life is good, judging from the group of relatively asymptomatic adults who are known. The development of myopathy and cardiac hypertrophy remains a concern.

α-1,4-Glucan: α-1,4-Glucan 6-glucosyltransferase (Brancher) Deficiency

More than 15 infants have now been reported with this form of glycogen disease, also known as *amylopectinosis* and

Table 6-2 The subgroups of Type III glycogen storage disease*

		Amylo-1,6-glucosidase activity (method of assay)				
Subgroup	Tissue	Limit dextrin glucose	Incorporation of ^{14}C glucose into glycogen	Transferase	Glucosyl-Schardinger dextrin glucose	B$_5$ glucose†
IIIA	Liver	Very low	Very low	Very low	Absent	Very low
	Muscle	Very low	Very low	Very low	Absent	Absent
IIIB	Liver	Absent or very low	Absent	Absent	Very low	Very low
	Muscle	Absent	Normal or slightly reduced	Reduced	Normal or slightly reduced	Normal when done
IIIC	Liver	Absent	Very low	Reduced	Normal	Slightly reduced
	Muscle	Absent	Very low	Reduced	Very low	Not done
IIID	Liver	Very low	Normal or slightly reduced	Absent	Reduced	Reduced
	Muscle	Absent	Normal or moderately reduced	Absent	Normal	Not done
IIIE‡	Liver	Very low	Very low	Very low	Very low	Not done
	Muscle	Normal	Moderately reduced	Normal	Normal	Not done
IIIF§	Liver	Very low	Absent	Very low	Absent	Not done
	Muscle	Very low	Absent	Reduced	Reduced	Not done

* Of 45 patients with Type III glycogen storage disease, 34 were classified as Type IIIA and 6 probably fit best into Type IIIB [151]. Others belong to rare subgroups; some subgroups are represented by a single patient.
† B$_5$ is the abbreviation for 6^3-α-glucosyl maltotetraose. The formation of glucose from the glucosyl-Schardinger dextrin or B$_5$ is specifically due to the hydrolysis of the 1,6-glucosyl linkage [151].
‡ Case 6 [151].
§ Cases 10 and 11 [151]. These patients are dizygotic male twins.
SOURCE: From the data of van Hoof and Hers [151].

Andersen's disease [66, 163–165]. The clinical histories of these children are similar; they appear normal at birth but soon fail to thrive. Hepatomegaly is seen in the first few months of life. There is poor weight gain and increasing size of the liver and spleen (Fig. 6-14). The child follows a course of progressive cirrhosis of the liver, with death in the second year of life. Only one child has survived until age 4 years. Polysaccharide accumulates in the heart, but only nonspecific ECG abnormalities have been reported. Heart dilatation has been reported in several cases, and death from cardiac tamponade and failure occurred in one instance [164–166]. McMaster et al. have emphasized the clinical neurologic dysfunction manifested as poor development, hypotonia, muscular atrophy, and decreased or absent deep tendon reflexes, and correlated the findings with autopsy data on nervous system accumulation of amylopectin [167].

There are increases in serum transaminase activities, as would be expected in such severe liver disease. Glucose tolerance test results are normal; epinephrine and glucagon test results have been variable. It might be expected that these functional tests would be abnormal in severe liver disease even without a basic defect in glycogen metabolism.

The glycogen concentration is usually not increased in any tissues. The glycogen is abnormal in structure. The long outer chains, similar to those of amylopectin, give the name *amylopectinosis*. Reduced branching makes the glycogen much less soluble. The cirrhosis may be due to a foreign-body reaction to the abnormal glycogen.

Clinically, this form of glycogen disease is distinctive because of the early cirrhosis with liver failure and the splenomegaly. A young boy with brancher deficiency whom we have studied is shown in Fig. 6-14.

Biochemical Studies Illingworth and Cori, after studying the glycogen in Andersen's original patient [165], suggested that there was a deficiency of the branching enzyme. Brown and Brown [37] have shown brancher deficiency in the liver and leukocytes of a 15-month-old Indian girl with amylopectinosis.

Glycogen from these patients has an abnormal iodine spectrum (with λ max around 525 nm, like amylopectin), as well as an increased degradation by phosphorylase. These findings indicate long outer branches. Mercier and Whelan have studied in detail the abnormal polysaccharide that accumulates in brancher deficiency [168]. They have emphasized that this material differs from amylopectin in having shorter inner chains and larger outer chains. Brown and Brown [37] found that muscle glycogen was normal in content and structure in their patient. If the branching enzyme is absent, how does the branching that is present arise? It has been suggested that there might be two branching activities with different substrate requirements [37, 164]. Also, branching enzyme activity which is no longer active could have been present during fetal development. More likely, the few branches found in this abnormal glycogen are due to a reversal of debrancher enzyme [168].

Genetics The preponderance of male patients probably reflects simply the small number of patients recognized. Two pairs of sibs are reported, and consanguinity is known in at least two families. The parents of Levin's patient [169] and of our patient (Fig. 6-14) had normal leukocyte brancher activity.

Howell et al. found brancher activity in normal skin fibroblasts but found it deficient in skin fibroblasts derived from the

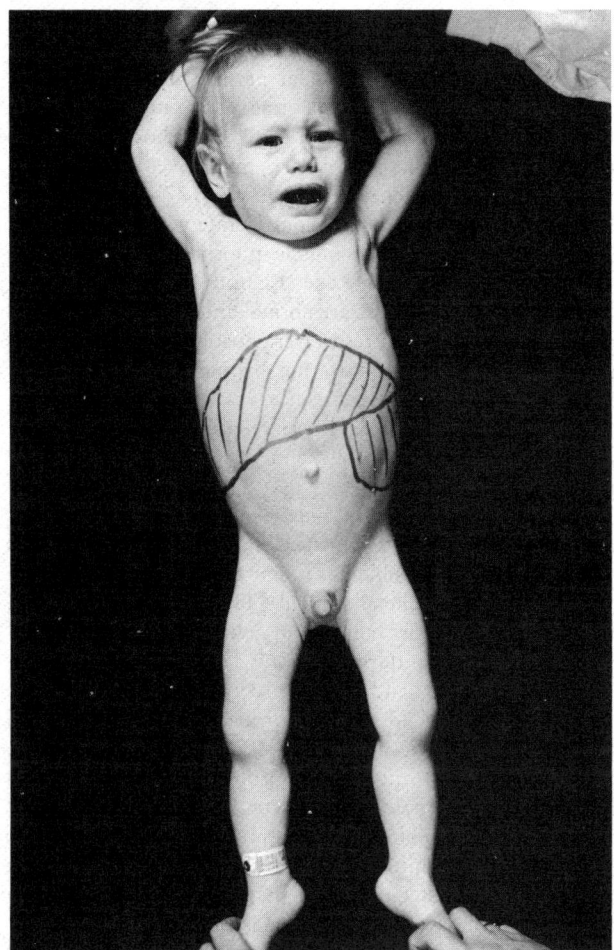

Figure 6-14 Fifteen-month-old boy with debrancher deficiency glycogen storage disease. The patient has marked hepatomegaly (with cirrhosis histologically) and considerable splenic enlargement. The liver and spleen are outlined. Venous distention was prominent over the abdomen but is not visible here. Brancher activity in the leukocytes of this patient was less than 10 percent of normal values.

patient shown in Fig. 6-14 [170]. Brancher activity in skin fibroblasts from parents was less that that of controls. This strongly suggests autosomal recessive inheritance.

Treatment The treatment is that for liver failure and ascites. Parenteral administration of α-1,4-glucosidase from *A. niger* [171] has been tried without benefit, although the liver glycogen content decreased. One patient died 24 h after portacaval transposition [169]. The identification of the defect in fibroblasts has enabled successful prenatal diagnosis of this disorder (B.I. Brown, personal communication).

Muscle Phosphorylase Deficiency

The patients who have been reported with deficiency of muscle phosphorylase have shown a striking history of limited ability to perform strenuous exercise because of painful muscle cramps [172]. Myoglobinuria has appeared in over half these patients following episodes of exercise and muscle cramps. This disorder was delineated clinically by McArdle in 1951 [173]. He studied a patient who during ischemic exercise had no increase in venous lactate from the exercised extremity.

McArdle suggested a defect in the degradation of glycogen to lactate. Mommaerts et al. [174] and Schmid et al. [175, 176] demonstrated in clinically similar patients a lack of muscle phosphorylase (0.5 percent of normal), high muscle glycogen concentrations, and normal muscle phosphorylase kinase activities. Other studies in these patients showed normal activity of other glycogen enzymes in muscle [177]. Pearson et al. [178] also found no rise in venous lactate with exercise (Fig. 6-15) and an absence of muscle phosphorylase. All these patients tolerated moderate exercise normally.

Clinically, these patients are normal and well developed and have no abnormalities at rest. Liver phosphorylase presumably is normal. These patients are not hypoglycemic and have a normal response to glucagon. Since, as discussed earlier, muscle and liver phosphorylase differ in many properties, it is not surprising that these two phosphorylases are under separate genetic control.

During muscular exercise, the use of ATP increases perhaps several-hundred-fold [178]. Aerobic metabolism generates ATP as rapidly as possible but is limited by the diffusion rates of fuel and oxygen. The additional ATP required for sustained vigorous exercise must come from glycogenolysis (by way of phosphorylase); only during stressful exercise is muscle phosphorylase essential and its lack clinically evident. These patients have not had clinical cardiac problems, but ECG abnormalities have been recorded [178–179]. Rowland et al. [172] have pointed out that the profusion of muscle action potentials characteristic of muscle cramps in other situations is absent during the painful contractures experienced by these patients. ATP is required for muscle relaxation in two different reactions. Rowland et al. studied tissue ATP concentrations in order to see whether a deficiency in tissue ATP levels might be responsible for the painful contractures characteristic of this disorder [180]. Normal ATP concentrations were found.

If an exercising subject with McArdle's syndrome can sustain the exercise after symptoms appear, the symptoms will lessen or disappear; this has been called the *second wind* phenomenon [175, 181]. Pernow et al. [181] found that this phenomenon is closely related to the prevailing levels of fatty acids and increased blood flow to muscle and postulated that these changes improved energy sources for the muscle.

Within hours after strenuous exercise, lactate dehydrogenase, aldolase, and creatine phosphokinase activities in patients' serum increase dramatically [182]. This need not imply tissue death but may be due only to reversible metabolic conditions within the muscle which compromise the ability of the cell to maintain membrane competence [183]. The muscle damage due to strenuous exercise is readily demonstrable by radionuclide scan [184]. The need to avoid exceeding the exercise tolerance is demonstrated by the reports of acute renal failure following the myoglobinuria associated with excessive exercise by these patients [185].

While normal exercising muscles put out alanine [186], the muscles of patients affected with McArdle's disease take up alanine during exercise. This might well serve as an auxilliary fuel. The increase in muscle phosphoenolpyruvate carboxykinase [187] would support this theory.

It is remarkable that this defect, although undoubtedly present from birth, produces either mild or no symptoms whatever during childhood. Indeed, it has been diagnosed in only one patient before 10 years of age (at 4 years), and that was due to his being part of a family study [172]. Some affected children have tolerated extraordinary exercise (basketball, lacrosse) without symptoms.

The clinical history of patients with this disease has been arbitrarily but usefully divided into three phases [175]. The first phase occurs in childhood and adolescence, when one finds increased fatigability and few other symptoms. During the second period (20 to 40 years of age), severe cramps and myoglobinuria develop. In the third period (beginning at about age 40), cramps and myoglobinuria are less conspicuous, and wasting and weakness appear with increasing severity. Older patients have very significant weakness and wasting.

DiMauro and Hartlage have described a new variant of muscle phosphorylase deficiency [188]. Their 4-week-old female patient had generalized, rapidly progressive muscle weakness which resulted in death at 13 weeks of age from respiratory insufficiency. Biochemical investigation showed a muscle glycogen content of 3.1 g per 100 g tissue, no detectable phosphorylase activity, and normal debrancher and acid maltase enzyme levels. The female sib of this patient died at 4 months of age with a similar picture [189]. Electrophoretic separation of phosphorylase isoenzymes showed only one band in the heart which corresponded to one of the three normal cardiac isoenzymes. Addition of normal muscle homogenate to the patient's heart homogenate resulted in the appearance of the three bands normally seen in the heart. This indicates that in normal heart the three bands correspond to a muscle isoenzyme, a cardiac isoenzyme, and a heart muscle hybrid. We have recently seen a male infant who presented at birth with a similar clinical picture and died in the newborn period of respiratory failure [190].

The single functional test of value is the demonstration that venous lactate from a limb performing ischemic exercise fails to increase (Fig. 6-16).

Histologic studies of the muscle with PAS (periodic acid-Schiff) and Best's carmine stains show numerous well-defined round or oval collections of staining material under the sarcolemmal membrane [191]. Electron micrographs display disor-

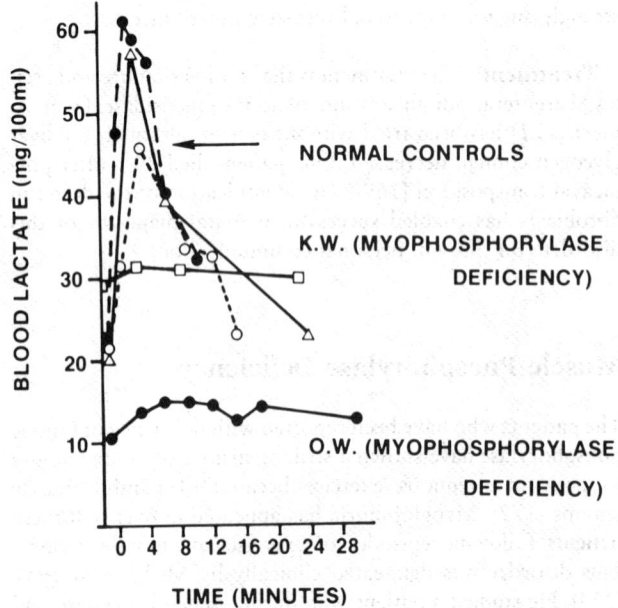

Figure 6-15 Blood lactate concentrations obtained from the antecubital vein after ischemic forearm muscle work. Patients O.W. and K.W. both have McArdle's disease (muscle phosphorylase deficiency) and have no rise in venous blood lactate levels, as do control subjects.

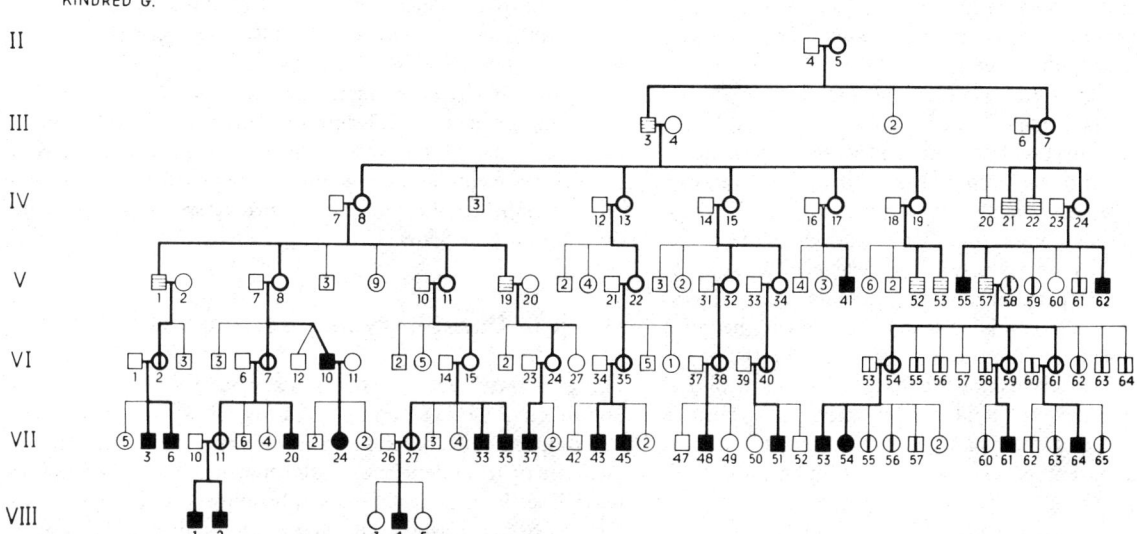

■, ● GSD SYMPTOMS, ENZYME ASSAYS POSITIVE

☐ GSD REPORTED OR BY INFERENCE

○ CARRIER OF DEFECTIVE TRAIT (BY INFERENCE, NO RECORDED HISTORY OF GSD)

◫, ◑ NO SYMPTOMS, ENZYME ASSAYS PERFORMED

☐, ○ NO RECORDED GSD SYMPTOMS, NO ENZYME ASSAYS

④, ④ NUMBER OF (OTHER) DESCENDANTS WITHOUT RECORDED HISTORY OF GSD AND ENZYME ASSAYS

INFERRED TRANSFER OF DEFECTIVE TRAIT INDICATED BY BOLD LINES

KINDRED G.

Figure 6-16 Pedigree of cases of liver glycogenosis due to hepatic phosphorylase *b* kinase deficiency. These data suggest an X chromosomal inheritance; the two females with mild symptoms and moderate reduction in enzyme activity are thought to be heterozygotes. (*From F. Huijing and J. Fernandes [215], with permission.*)

ganization of myofibrils at the level of the I band. This is because of compression of myofibrils by excess glycogen in the intermyofibrillar space [191]. After exercise, some mitochondria contain vacuoles or collections of particles that resemble glycogen [191].

Biochemical Studies It is important to demonstrate directly a deficiency of phosphorylase, since any defect in the glycolytic pathway could generate superficially similar clinical findings. Glycogen of normal structure accumulates in moderate amounts (up to 4 g/100 g) in muscle. Modest depressions of other muscle enzyme activities occur [176] but are usually secondary defects. Some patients with McArdle's disease have no immunologic cross-reactive material (CRM) to normal phosphorylase, while others have CRM and, in one instance, low, unstable phosphorylase activity [192]. Other investigators have demonstrated inactive myophosphorylase subunits in the muscle of some McArdle's patients by sodium dodecyl sulfate polyacrylamide gel electrophoresis [193, 194].

A puzzling aspect of myophosphorylase deficiency is that activity can be demonstrated histochemically in regenerating muscle fibers both in vivo and in vitro in tissue from affected patients [195, 196]. Further immunologic and electrophoretic studies of muscle in culture have shown that this activity is due to a fetal isoenzyme which must be under different genetic control than the adult muscle enzyme [197, 198].

Genetics A large pedigree with well-studied patients was collected by Dawson et al. [199]. It strongly supported an autosomal recessive inheritance. Certain family members, who could have been heterozygotes, had cramps after exercise. There has been a marked preponderance of males in the liter-

ature. This could be merely a reflection of small numbers and sampling effects. Women are known to have myophosphorylase deficiency; one has been followed through a normal pregnancy which proceeded without complication. Many of the patients were not studied well enough to permit ruling out deficient phosphorylase *b* kinase.

Treatment Avoidance of extreme exercise is the best treatment and is essential because of the risk of myoglobinuria and secondary renal failure [185]. Administration of oral glucose and fructose (to increase muscle energy supplies) has given variable results. Pernow et al. [181] reported some success with isoproterenol. This drug increased the serum concentration of free fatty acids and blood flow to the muscle.

Hepatic Phosphorylase Deficiency

In a study of a large group of patients with hepatic forms of the glycogen storage diseases, Hers [200] segregated certain patients with increased hepatic glycogen and a reduction to about 25 percent of normal hepatic phosphorylase activity. This form of the disease is also known as *Hers' disease*. These patients clinically were like those with mild forms of glucose-6-phosphatase deficiency. Some, but not all, were deficient in leukocyte phosphorylase [201]. Leukocyte phosphorylase activities in family members were variable and somewhat confusing with regard to genetic transmission. Koster et al. have described two brothers with a deficiency of hepatic phosphorylase and normal phosphorylase *b* kinase activity. In white blood cells, phosphorylase activity was reduced to 20 percent of normal, and one isoenzyme was missing upon electrophoresis. Fibroblasts from these patients did not reflect the hepatic enzyme deficiency [202].

The difficulty in assessing the reported cases of hepatic phosphorylase deficiency lies in their inadequate enzymologic evaluation. In most cases, the phosphorylase-activating system has not been assayed or the assays have been incomplete, which makes it impossible to differentiate phosphorylase deficiency from that of phosphorylase *b* kinase. Also, there is a major problem in assaying total liver phosphorylase activity in that the amount of active phosphorylase is variable and the activation of phosphorylase *b* by AMP in vitro is incomplete. Measurement of phosphorylase activity before and after heat inactivation would clarify this aspect.

Baussan et al. have evaluated 24 patients with reduced hepatic phosphorylase activity [203]. The authors could not discriminate phosphorylase from phosphorylase *b* kinase deficiency (contrary to previous reports) [204] by an intravenous glucagon tolerance test. Using erythrocyte hemolysates, they could subclassify their patients into two categories: (1) 16 boys and 1 girl with phosphorylase *b* kinase deficiency and (2) 2 girls and 5 boys with primary phosphorylase deficiency. Hers and van Hoof [71], after studying many patients with hepatic glycogenoses, is of the opinion that classification on the basis of low phosphorylase level is not adequate and that low phosphorylase is not a constant finding even among sibs. Future investigations should evaluate patients with increased liver glycogen and an apparent deficiency of hepatic phosphorylase more carefully.

Muscle Phosphofructokinase Deficiency

Tarui et al. [205] reported a muscle glycogen storage disease in Japan. They studied three sibs with clinical histories identical to McArdle's (muscle phosphorylase deficiency) disease. One had experienced myoglobinuria. Ischemic exercise caused no rise in venous lactate level. These patients showed marked increases in the concentrations of glucose-6-phosphate and fructose-6-phosphate in their muscles but had low muscle fructose-1,6-diphosphate. Muscle phosphofructokinase activity was 1 to 3 percent of normal. Increased activity of both glycogen synthase and uridine diphosphoglucose (UDPG) pyrophosphorylase contributed to glycogen storage in the muscle [206]. In a fourth patient from the United States with similar clinical and biochemical findings, and phosphofructokinase deficiency, Layzer et al. [207] found no component in the biopsy of their patient that reacted with an antibody against purified human muscle phosphofructokinase.

These four patients showed similar reductions of erythrocyte phosphofructokinase activity [205, 207]. Immunologic studies by Tarui et al. [208] showed at least two components of erythrocyte phosphofructokinase. About 50 percent of the total activity is attributable to a form of the enzyme immunologically identical to muscle phosphofructokinase. They attribute the reduced erythrocyte life span (13 to 16 days by ^{51}Cr labeling) to erythroid hyperplasia and the reticulocytosis (3.8 to 6.5 percent) seen in their patients to the deficiency of the muscle form of phosphofructokinase in the erythrocyte, which results in 50 percent reduction of total erythrocyte phosphofructokinase activity [208]. The occurrence in sibs of both sexes, with consanguinity in one set of parents, suggests autosomal recessive inheritance. The reduction of erythrocyte phosphofructokinase activity in the parents also supports this view.

Several additional cases have been reported [209], including two with "severe congenital muscular dystrophy" and "painful joint stiffness" resulting in death for one patient at 6 months of age from respiratory complications [210]. Hyper-

uricemia and gout were found in one patient with phosphofructokinase deficiency [211]. It was suggested that accumulation of glucose-6-phosphate and fructose-6-phosphate results in the shunting of these intermediates into the pentose phosphate pathway and increased phosphoribosylpyrophosphate synthesis yielding an overproduction of purines and pyrimidines. This patient also accumulated an abnormal polysaccharide in muscle which histochemically resembled that seen in amylopectinosis and in Lafora disease.

Erythrocytes from patients with phosphofructokinase deficiency are deficient in 2,3-diphosphoglycerate. The reason for glycogen accumulation in this disorder is unclear. Glucose-6-phosphate accumulates and may activate glycogen synthase while inhibiting phosphorylase. Further studies of this phenomenon are indicated [212].

Hepatic Phosphorylase *b* Kinase Deficiency

Phosphorylase requires specific enzymes for both activation and inactivation. The finding of a low phosphorylase activity in a biopsy might therefore arise from phosphorylase deficiency per se or from deficiency of the enzymes that activate phosphorylase. Patients deficient in phosphorylase *b* kinase have recently been described. They have reduced liver and leukocyte phosphorylase and clearly can now be removed from the heterogeneous group of hepatic glycogen disease. Hug et al. [213] have reported five children with no symptoms except hepatomegaly and increased liver glycogen concentrations. Slow activation of phosphorylase was found in vitro, and it was inferred that there was about a 90 percent deficiency of phosphorylase *b* kinase. There was a normal response to glucagon and shrinkage of the liver in response to glucagon.

By direct assay, Huijing [214] found low activity of phosphorylase *b* kinase in the leukocytes of a group of patients with "phosphorylase" deficiency. Huijing and Fernandes [215] have collected histories of 32 patients with phosphorylase *b* kinase deficiency. Enzyme data and the extensive pedigree of the patients support the theory of an X-linked inheritance (Fig. 6-16). These patients have had only mild symptoms. Three females with large livers and moderately reduced leukocyte enzyme concentrations were considered to be heterozygotes; they showed minimal manifestations of the disease [215]. Low leukocyte phosphorylase *b* kinase activity seems to reflect low activity of this enzyme in the liver [216].

The studies of Migeon and Huijing [217] suggest that there are two populations of cells in cultured fibroblasts of mothers of patients with phosphorylase *b* kinase deficiency. Their biochemical data were not conclusive but suggested an X-linked inheritance. Lederer et al. have completely evaluated nine patients, all males, with phosphorylase *b* kinase deficiency using erythrocyte and leukocyte lysates in conjunction with liver and muscle biopsies [218]. These authors have also identified two pairs of sibs, in both cases brother and sister, who displayed partial deficiency of phosphorylase *b* kinase in red blood cells and leukocytes but total deficiency in the liver. They considered these patients to be examples of autosomal recessive inheritance.

The mechanism of phosphorylase activation has been of considerable interest. Mice deficient in phosphorylase *b* kinase have a small amount (0.3 percent) of residual activity [219]. Other mechanisms of phosphorylase activation have been defined which could explain the normal glucagon test. At least one patient had a normal muscle phosphorylase-activating system, although deficient in liver [220].

Other Possible Inherited Defects in Glycogen Metabolism

Spencer-Peet, Lewis, and Stewart [221] described identical twins with profound hypoglycemia, low (but not absent) liver glycogen, and absence of liver glycogen synthase. These children had diabetic-type glucose tolerance test results. The hypoglycemia appeared only after long fasting. When the children were in a fed state, their response to glucagon was normal. When the children were hypoglycemic after fasting, glucagon produced no rise in their blood sugar level. These patients clearly were able to synthesize glycogen, as proved by the presence of glycogen in their livers and a normal response to the glucagon when fed. They have improved with age [222]. Two of three sibs also had frequent episodes of hypoglycemia, glucose intolerance, and diminished response to glucagon in the fasted state. Others have recently reported a brother and sister with fasting hypoglycemia and hyperketonemia [223, 224]. While they were being fed, their blood glucose and lactate levels were elevated and their alanine level corresponded to their blood glucose level. In the girl, glycogen synthase was deficient in the liver but normal in muscle.

Clinically, the findings in these children fit well with the syndrome of ketotic hypoglycemia, a poorly understood but relatively common form of hypoglycemia in children. It appears that ketotic hypoglycemia patients (and the Spencer-Peet et al. patients) have a defect involving gluconeogenesis or the ability of muscle to release sufficient alanine rather than a primary disorder of glycogen metabolism. Some patients with ketotic hypoglycemia have extremely low concentrations of liver glycogen and low serum insulin values [225, 226]. Since glycogen synthase activity is regulated by insulin, low liver glycogen synthase activity would be expected to accompany low serum insulin concentrations. In addition, Hers has emphasized the lability of glycogen synthase when isolated in the presence of low tissue concentrations of glycogen [227]. One would not expect that glycogen synthase activity would be deficient in all children with ketotic hypoglycemia. It may occur with some frequency in that group with very low serum insulin concentrations. Although inherited deficiencies of glycogen synthase may be documented in the future, existing data do not establish such an entity. It would be of interest to measure glycogen synthase activity (rich in normal fibroblasts) in fibroblasts derived from these patients.

Individual patients with a partial deficiency of phosphoglucomutase in liver and muscle [228] and in muscle alone have been reported. No direct assay was made in the patient with the muscular form of the disease. Some of these reports are brief but substantial [228]. The defect, either in muscle or in liver, may well require individual classification in the future.

A patient with diffuse nodular cirrhosis causing death at 14 months of age, glycogen storage in all organs as visualized histochemically, and normal glycogen-metabolizing enzymes has been described [229]. The glycogen has been extensively characterized as having a low molecular weight (8000 to 15,000) and an average chain length of 17 to 18 glucose units [230]. This glycogen was also a poor primer for glycogen synthase

[231]. The molecular defect in this patient has not been elucidated.

Hug et al. have reported one female child with asymptomatic hepatomegaly, normoglycemia, and no response to glucagon [232]. Glycogen was accumulated in the liver and muscle. The authors postulated a deficiency of cyclic AMP-dependent kinase.

Multiple Enzymatic Defects

Many examples of multiple enzymatic defects have been reported in the glycogen storage diseases. They have been summarized by Auerbach and DiGeorge [233]. Many may be artifactual because of improper handling of tissues and inadequate assays.

There are several examples of the simultaneous occurrence of debrancher deficiency and marked reduction of glucose-6-phosphatase activity in the same family or the same individual. Modest reductions of glucose-6-phosphatase are seen regularly with debrancher deficiency. One of these is clearly the primary genetic event, the other being secondary or adaptive. In order to prove a double genetic defect in an individual, it must be demonstrated that both parents are heterozygous for both defects. This would occur with great rarity, even in highly inbred kindreds.

It is surprising that putative multiple defects are not found more frequently since the tissues are so frequently disorganized by glycogen and lipid deposition. The genetic implications of multiple enzyme deficiencies are so important that reports should be examined critically.

Animal Models of Glycogen Storage Diseases

Ethical and technical difficulties prohibit many studies of glycogen storage diseases in humans. Certainly, ascertainment of the mechanisms of secondary metabolic compensations and of the efficacy of new therapeutic protocols would be more practical if animal models were readily available. Erickson et al. [234] have studied albino mice with four radiation-induced alleles for glucose-6-phosphatase, which are fatal in the newborn period if present in the homozygous state. These mice lack glucose-6-phosphatase activity in the liver and kidney. Liver glycogen was lower in the affected animals (1.9 g/100 g) than in controls (5.9 g/100 g). The short life of these mice makes further study difficult. Perhaps supportive parenteral nutrition or continuous nasogastric feeding will allow the development of a viable model for von Gierke's disease.

There have been reports of a generalized glycogen storage disease, presumably due to α-glucosidase deficiency in the dog [235], cat [236], and sheep [237]. In all cases, the tissues were fixed and no enzyme studies were possible. Also, no parents of these animals could be identified and thus the mutation was lost. Fortunately, α-glucosidase deficiency has recently been well documented in an Australian line of Shorthorn cattle [238]. The pathologic changes appear similar to the human infantile form of α-glucosidase deficiency, but the age of onset and infrequency of clinical cardiac manifestations suggest a closer resemblance to the human juvenile variant [239]. A deficiency of lysosomal α-glucosidase has been demonstrated, as well as glycogen accumulation in all tissues. Heterozygotes were readily detected and a screening program was undertaken [240]. Under the direction of Professor John Howell, a breeding herd of heterozygotes has been established at Murdoch University, Western Australia, and detailed clinical, pathologic, and biochemical studies are underway on the natural history of the disease and the effects of enzyme replacement therapy [241].

Storage of glycogen with the characteristic short outer chains of debrancher enzyme deficiency has been described in German Shepherd dogs [242, 243]. Debrancher activity is 0 to 7 percent of normal. A deficiency of phosphorylase *b* kinase in mice has been well documented [219, 244] and is inherited as an X-linked mutation. An autosomal recessive deficiency of phosphorylase *b* kinase has recently been described in a strain of rats [245, 246].

Certain of the authors' studies were funded by grants from the National Institutes of Health and the Muscular Dystrophy Association of America.

REFERENCES

1. VON GIERKE E: Hepato-nephro-megalia glykogenia (Glykogenspeicherkrankheit der Leber und Nieren). *Beitr Pathol Anat* 82:497–513, 1929
2. POMPE JC: Over idiopatische hypertrofie van het hart. *Ned Tijdschr Geneeskd* 76:304–311, 1932
3. CORI GT, CORI CF: Glucose-6-phosphatase of the liver in glycogen storage disease. *J Biol Chem* 199:661–667, 1952
4. CORI GT: Glycogen structure and enzyme deficiencies in glycogen storage disease. *Harvey Lect* 48:145–171, 1954
5. STETTEN DEW, JR, STETTEN MR: Glycogen metabolism. *Physiol Rev* 40:505–537, 1960
6. FRENCH D: Structure of glycogen and its amylolytic degradation, in Whelan WJ (ed): *Control of Glycogen Metabolism*. Boston, Little, Brown & Co, 1964, p 7
7. STEINITZ K: Laboratory diagnosis of glycogen diseases. *Adv Clin Chem* 9:227–354, 1967
8. BRAMMER GL, ROUGVIE MA, FRENCH D: Distribution of α-amylase resistant regions in the glycogen molecule. *Carbohydr Res* 24:343–354, 1972
9. GUNJA-SMITH Z, MARSHALL JJ, MERCIER L, SMITH EE, WHELAN WJ: A revision of the Meyer-Bernfeld model of glycogen and amylopectin. *FEBS Lett* 12:101–104, 1970
10. ORRELL SA, JR, BUEDING E, REISSIG M: Physical characteristics of undegraded glycogen, in Whelan WJ (ed): *Control of Glycogen Metabolism*. Boston, Little, Brown & Co, 1964, p 29
11. PARODI AJ, MORDOH J, KRISMAN CR, LELOIR LF: In vitro synthesis of particulate glycogen from uridine diphosphate glucose. *Arch Biochem Biophys* 132:111–117, 1969
12. MORGAN TE, SHORT FA, COBB LS: Muscle adaptation to exercise in man: Effects in glycogen and lipid. *J Clin Invest* 47:A71, 1968
13. DAWES GS, SHELLEY HJ: Physiologic aspects of carbohydrate metabolism in the fetus and newborn, in Dickens F, Randle PJ, Whelan WJ (eds): *Carbohydrate metabolism and Its Disorders*. New York, Academic Press, Inc, 1968, vol 2, p 87
14. FIELD RA: Glycogen deposition diseases, in Stanbury JB, Wyngaarden JB, Fredrickson DS (eds): *The Metabolic Basis of Inherited Disease*, 2d ed. New York, McGraw-Hill Book Co, 1966, p 141
15. SOLS A, SALAS M, VIÑUELA E: Induced biosynthesis of liver glucokinase. *Adv Enzyme Regul* 2:177–188, 1964
16. SHARMA C, MANJESHWAR R, WEINHOUSE S: Hormonal and dietary regulation of hepatic glucokinase. *Adv Enzyme Regul* 2:188–200, 1964
17. SOLS A: Hexokinase and glucokinase, in Whelan WJ (ed): *Control of Glycogen Metabolism*. Boston, Little, Brown & Co, 1964, p 301
18. SOLS A: Phosphorylation and glycolysis, in Dickens F, Randle PR, Whelan WJ (eds): *Carbohydrate Metabolism and Its Disorders*. New York, Academic Press, Inc, 1968, vol 1, p 53
19. LONDON WP: A theoretical study of hepatic glycogen metabolism. *J Biol Chem* 241:3008–3022, 1966
20. SMITH EE, TAYLOR PM, WHELAN WJ: Enzymic process in glycogen metabolism, in Dickens F, Randle PJ, Whelan WJ (eds): *Carbohydrate Metabolism and Its Disorders*. New York, Academic Press, Inc, 1968, vol 1, p 89
21. RAY WJ, JR, ROSCELLI GA: The phosphoglucomutase pathway. An investigation of phospho-enzyme isomerization. *J Biol Chem* 239:3935–3941, 1964
22. RYMAN BE, WHELAN WJ: New aspects of glycogen metabolism. *Adv Enzymol* 34:285–443, 1971
23. ALBRECHT GJ, BASS ST, SEIFERT LL, HANSEN RG: Crystallization and properties of uridine diphosphate glucose pyrophosphorylase from liver. *J Biol Chem* 241:2968–2975, 1966
24. LELOIR LF, CARDINI CE: Biosynthesis of glycogen from uridine diphosphate glucose. *J Am Chem Soc* 79:6340–6341, 1957
25. HAUK R, BROWN DH: Preparation and properties of uridine diphosphoglucose-glycogen transferase from rabbit muscle. *Biochim Biophys Acta* 33:556–559, 1959
26. MCVERRY PH, KIM KH: Purification and kinetic mechanism of rat liver glycogen synthase. *Biochemistry* 13:3505–3511, 1974
27. FRIEDMAN DL, LARNER J: Studies on UDPG-α-glucan transglucosylase III. Interconversion of two forms of muscle UDPG-α-glucan tranglucosylase by a phosphorylation-dephosphorylation reaction sequence. *Biochemistry* 2:669–675, 1963
28. MERSMANN JJ, SEGAL HL: An on-off mechanism for liver glycogen synthetase activity. *Proc Natl Acad Sci USA* 58:1688–1695, 1967
29. DE WULF H, STALMANS W, HERS HG: The influence of inorganic phosphate, adenosine triphosphate and glucose-6-phosphate on the activity of liver glycogen synthetase. *Eur J Biochem* 6:545–551, 1968
30. GOLD AH: On the possibility of metabolite control of liver glycogen synthetase activity. *Biochemistry* 9:946–952, 1970
31. PIRAS R, ROTHMAN LB, CABIB E: Regulation of muscle glycogen synthetase by metabolites. Differential effects in the I and D forms. *Biochemistry* 7:56–66, 1968
32. BISHOP JS, LARNER J: Rapid activation-inactivation of liver uridine diphosphate glucose-glycogen transferase and phosphorylase by insulin and glucagon in vivo. *J Biol Chem* 242:1354–1356, 1967
33. DE WULF H, HERS HG: The stimulation of glycogen synthesis and of glycogen synthetase in the liver by the administration of glucose. *Eur J Biochem* 2:50–56, 1967
34. HERS HG, DE WULF H: The regulation of glycogen synthesis in the liver, in Whelan WJ (ed): *Control of Glycogen Metabolism*. New York, Academic Press, Inc, 1968, p 65
35. HUIJING F, LARNER J: On the mechanism of action of adenosine 3',5'-cyclophosphate. *Proc Natl Acad Sci USA* 56:647–653, 1967
36. VARDANIS A: Glycogen-bound enzymes: A new method of isolation. *Arch Biochem Biophys* 130:408–412, 1969
37. BROWN BI, BROWN DH: Lack of an α-1,4-glucan:α-1,4-Glucan 6-glycosyl transferase in a case of type IV glycogenosis. *Proc Natl Acad Sci USA* 56:725–729, 1966
38. VERHUE W, HERS HG: A study of the reaction catalysed by the liver branching enzyme. *Biochem J* 99:222–227, 1966
39. WHITE A, HANDLER P, SMITH EW: *Principles of Biochemistry*, 4th ed. New York, McGraw-Hill Book Co, 1968, p 436
40. HENION WF, SUTHERLAND EW: Immunological differences of phosphorylases. *J Biol Chem* 224:477–488, 1957
41. FISCHER EH, KREBS EG: The isolation and crystallization of rabbit skeletal muscle phosphorylase b. *J Biol Chem* 231:65–71, 1958.
42. STULL JT, MAYER SE: Regulation of phosphorylase activation in skeletal muscle in vivo. *J Biol Chem* 246:5716–5723, 1971
43. KELLER PJ, CORI GT: Purification and properties of the phosphorylase-rupturing enzyme. *J Biol Chem* 214:127–134, 1955
44. FISHER EH, APPLEMAN MM, KREBS EG: The structure of phosphorylases, in Whelan WJ (ed): *Control of Glycogen Metabolism*. Boston, Little, Brown & Co, 1964, p 94
45. METZGER B, HELMREICH E, GLASER L: The mechanism of activation of skeletal muscle phosphorylase a by glycogen. *Proc Natl Acad Sci USA* 57:994–1001, 1967
46. FISCHER EH, GRAVES DJ, CRITTENDEN ERS, KREBS EG: Structure of the site phosphorylated in the phosphorylase b to a reaction. *J Biol Chem* 234:1698–1704, 1959
47. WANG JH, GRAVES DJ: The relationship of the dissociation to the catalytic activity of glycogen phosphorylase a. *Biochemistry* 3:1437–1445, 1964
48. HELMREICH E, MICHAELIDES MC, CORI CF: Effects of substrates and a substrate analog on the binding of 5'-adenylic acid to muscle phosphorylase a. *Biochemistry* 6:3695–3710, 1967
49. SEERY VL, FISCHER EH, TELLER DC: A reinvestigation of the molecular weight of glycogen phosphorylase. *Biochemistry* 6:3315–3327, 1967
50. SUTHERLAND EW, WOSILAIT WD: The relationship of epinephrine and glucagon to liver phosphorylase; liver phosphorylase, preparation and properties. *J Biol Chem* 218:459–468, 1956
51. KATO K, SATO S: Glycogen synthetase-D phosphatase. 1. Some new properties of the partially purified enzyme from the rabbit skeletal muscle. *J Biol Chem* 247:7420–7429, 1972
52. WOSILAIT WD, SUTHERLAND EW: The relationship of epinephrine and glucagon to liver phosphorylase; enzymatic inactivation of liver phosphorylase. *J Biol Chem* 218:469–481, 1956

53. POHL SL, BIRNBAUMER L, RODBELL M: Glucagon-sensitive adenyl cyclase in plasma membrane of hepatic parenchymal cells. *Science* 164:566–567, 1969

54. HERS HG, VERHUE W, MATHIEU M: The mechanism of action of amylo-1,6-glucosidase, in Whelan WJ (ed): *Control of Glycogen Metabolism*. Boston, Little, Brown & Co, 1964, p 151

55. ABDULLAH M, TAYLOR PM, WHELAN WJ: The enzymic debranching of glycogen and the role of transferase, in Whelan WJ (ed): *Control of Glycogen Metabolism*. Boston, Little, Brown & Co, 1964, p 123

56. BROWN DH, ILLINGWORTH B: The role of oligo-1,4 → 1,4-glucan transferase and amylo-1,6-glucosidase in the debranching of glycogen, in Whelan WJ (ed): *Control of Glycogen Metabolism*. Boston, Little, Brown & Co, 1964, p 139

57. TAYLOR PM, WHELAN WJ: Rabbit muscle amylo-1,6-glucosidase: Properties and evidence of heterogeneity, in Whelan WJ (ed): *Control of Glycogen Metabolism*. New York, Academic Press, Inc, 1968, p 101

58. CORI CF, GARLAND RC, CHANG HW: Purification of particulate glucose-6-phosphatase. *Biochemistry* 12:3126–3130, 1973

59. NORDLIE RC: Metabolic regulation by multifunctional glucose-6-phosphatase. *Curr Top Cell Regul* 8:33–117, 1974

60. BROWN BI, BROWN DH: The glycogen storage diseases: Types I, III, IV, V, VII and unclassified glycogenoses, in Whelan WJ (ed): *Carbohydrate Metabolism and Its Disorders*. New York, Academic Press, Inc, 1968, vol 2, p 123

61. HERS HG: Glycogen storage disease. *Adv Metabolic Disorders* 1:1–44, 1964

62. LAZARUS SS, BARDEN H: Specificity and ultrastructural localization of pancreatic β cell glucose-6-phosphatase. *Diabetes* 14:146–156, 1965

63. HEFFERAN PM, HOWELL RR: Genetic evidence for the common identity of glucose-6-phosphatase, pyrophosphate-glucose phosphotransferase, carbamyl phosphate-glucose phosphotransferase and inorganic pyrophosphatase. *Biochim Biophys Acta* 496:431–435, 1977

64. ARION WJ, NORDLIE RC: Liver glucose-6-phosphatase and pyrophosphate-glucose phosphotransferase: Effects of fasting. *Biochem Biophys Res Commun* 20:606–610, 1965

65. NORDLIE RC, ARION WJ: Liver microsomal glucose-6-phosphatase, inorganic pyrophosphatase, and pyrophosphate-glucose phosphotransferase. 3. Associated nucleoside triphosphate- and nucleoside diphosphate-glucose phosphotransferase activities. *J Biol Chem* 240:2155–2164, 1965

66. SIDBURY JB, JR, MASON J, BURNS WB, JR, RUEBNER BH: Type IV glycogenosis: Report of a case proven by characterization of glycogen and studied at necropsy. *Bull Hopkins Hosp* 111:157–181, 1962

67. ISHII H, JOLY JG, LIEBER CS: Increase of microsomal glucose-6-phosphatase activity after chronic ethanol administration. *Metabolism* 22:799–806, 1973

68. PASSONNEAU JV, LOWRY OH: The role of phosphofructokinase in metabolic regulation. *Adv Enzyme Regul* 2:265–274, 1964

69. WHITE A, HANDLER P, SMITH EM: *Principles of Biochemistry*, 4th ed. New York, McGraw-Hill Book Co, 1968, p 395

70. HERS HG: α-Glucosidase deficiency in generalized glycogen storage disease (Pompe's disease). *Biochem J* 86:11–16, 1963

71. HERS HG, VAN HOOF F: Glycogen storage diseases: Type II and type VI glycogenosis, in Dickens F, Randle PJ, Whelan WJ (eds): *Carbohydrate Metabolism and Its Disorders*. New York, Academic Press, Inc, 1968, p 151

72. LEJEUNE N, THINÉS-SEMPOUX D, HERS HG: Tissue fractionation studies. 16. Intracellular distribution and properties of α-glucosidases in rat liver. *Biochem J* 86:16–21, 1963

73. NEWSHOLME EA, START C: Regulation of glycogen metabolism, in *Regulation in Metabolism*. London, John Wiley & Sons, Ltd, 1973, p 146

74. HERS HG: The control of glycogen metabolism in the liver. *Ann Rev Biochem* 45:167–189, 1976

75. DONNELL GN: Growth in glycogen storage disease type I. Evaluation of endocrine function. *Am J Dis Child* 117:169–177, 1969

76. HOWELL RR, ASHTON DM, WYNGAARDEN JB: Glucose-6-phosphatase deficiency glycogen storage disease. Studies on the interrelationships of carbohydrate, lipid and purine abnormalities. *Pediatrics* 29:553–565, 1962

77. FINE RN, WILSON WA, DONNELL GN: Retinal changes in glycogen storage disease type I. *Am J Dis Child* 115:328–331, 1968

78. CORBY DG, PUTMAN CW, GREENE HL: Impaired platelet function in glucose-6-phosphatase deficiency. *J Pediatr* 85:71–76, 1974

79. HUTTON RA, MACNAB AJ, RIVERS PA: Defect of platelet function associated with chronic hypoglycemia. *Arch Dis Child* 51:49–55, 1976

80. FINE RR, KOGUT MB, DONNELL GN: Intestinal absorption in type I glycogen storage disease. *J Pediatr* 75:632–635, 1969

81. MILLA PJ, ATHERTON DA, LEONARD JV, WOLFF OH, LAKE BD: Disordered intestinal function in glycogen storage disease. *J Inherited Metab Dis* 1:155–157, 1978

82. FELLOWS RP, BERDON WE, BAKER DH, HARRIS R: Barium enema findings in type I hepatorenal glycogen storage disease. *Pediatr Radiol* 3:75–77, 1975

83. VAN CREVELD S: Clinical course of glycogen storage disease. *Chemi Weekblad* 57:445, 1961

84. ALEPA FP, HOWELL RR, KLINENBERG JR, SEEGMILLER JE: Relationships between glycogen storage disease and tophaceous gout. *Am J Med* 42:58–66, 1967

85. FERNANDES J, PIKAAR NA: Ketosis in hepatic glycogenosis. *Arch Dis Child* 47:41–46, 1972.

86. BINKIEWICZ A, SENIOR B: Decreased ketogenesis in von Gierke's disease (type I glycogenosis). *J Pediatr* 83:973–978, 1973

87. MCGARRY JD, FOSTER DW: Regulation of hepatic fatty acid oxidation and ketone body production. *Ann Rev Biochem* 49:395–420, 1980

88. DOSMAN J, CRAWHALL JC, KLASSEN GA, MAMER OA, NEUMANN P: Urinary excretion of C6-C10 dicarboxylic acids in glycogen storage disease types I and III. *Clin Chim Acta* 51:93–101, 1974

89. OWEN OE, MORGAN AP, KEMP HG, SULLIVAN JM, HERRERA MG, CAHILL GF, JR: Brain metabolism during fasting. *J Clin Invest* 46:1589–1595, 1967

90. GARTY R, COOPER M, TABACHNIK E: The Fanconi syndrome associated with hepatic glycogenosis and abnormal metabolism of galactose. *J Pediatr* 85:821–823, 1974

91. FERNANDES J, PIKAAR NA: Hyperlipemia in children with liver glycogen disease. *Am J Clin Nutr* 22:617–627, 1969

92. ÖCKERMAN PA: Glucose, glycerol and free fatty acids in glycogen storage disease type I: Blood levels in the fasting and non-fasting state. Effect of glucose and adrenalin administation. *Clin Chem Acta* 12:370–382, 1965

93. ÖCKERMAN PA: In vitro studies of adipose tissue metabolism of glucose, glycerol and free fatty acids in glycogen storage disease type I. *Clin Chim Acta* 12:383–388, 1965

94. FORGET PP, FERNANDES J, BEGEMANN PH: Triglyceride clearing in glycogen storage disease. *Pediatr Res* 8:114–119, 1974

95. SARCIONE EJ, SOKAL JE, LOWE CU: Hepatic glycogenolysis induced by glucagon in a patient with type I liver glycogen disease. *Biochem Med* 3:337–343, 1970

96. SADEGHI-NEJAD A, PRESENTE E, BINKIEWICZ A, SENIOR B: Studies in type I glycogenosis of the liver. The genesis and disposition of lactate. *J Pediatr* 85:49–54, 1974

97. ZUPPINGER K, ROSSI E: Metabolic studies in liver glycogen disease with special reference to lactate metabolism. *Helv Med Acta* 35:406–422, 1970

98. FERNANDES J, BLOM W: Urinary lactate excretion in normal children and in children with enzyme defects of carbohydrate metabolism. *Clin Chim Acta* 66:345–352, 1976

99. ÖCKERMAN PA: Assay by a spectrofluorimetric method of glucose-6-phosphate in the liver in glycogen storage disease type I. *Clin Chem Acta* 12:455–452, 1965

100. LOCKWOOD DH, MERIMEE TJ, EDGAR PJ, GREENE ML, FUJIMOTO WY, SEEGMILLER JE, HOWELL RR: Insulin secretion in type I glycogen storage disease. *Diabetes* 18:755–758, 1969

101. OKADA S, SEINO Y, KODAMA H, YUTAKA T, INUI K, ISHIDA M, YABUUCHI H, SEINO Y: Insulin and glucagon secretion in hepatic glycogenoses. *Acta Pediatr Scand* 68:735–738, 1979

102. KOLB FO, DE LALLA OF, GOFMAN JW: The hyperlipidemias in disorders of carbohydrate metabolism: Serial lipoprotein studies in diabetic acidosis with xanthomatosis and in glycogen storage disease. *Metabolism* 4:310–317, 1955

103. FINE RN, STRAUSS J, DONNELL GN: Hyperuricemia in glycogen storage disease type I. *Am J Dis Child* 112:572–576, 1966

104. JEUNE M, FRANCOIS R, JARLOT B: Contribution a l'étude des polycories glycogéniques du foie. *Rev. Internat Hepatol* 9:1–33, 1959

105. JAKOVCIC S, SORENSEN LB: Studies of uric acid metabolism in glycogen storage disease associated with gouty arthritis. *Arthritis Rheum* 10:129–134, 1967

106. KELLEY WN, ROSENBLOOM FM, SEEGMILLER JE, HOWELL RR: Excessive production of uric acid in type I glycogen storage disease. *J Pediatr* 72:488–496, 1968

107. HOWELL RR: The interrelationship of glycogen storage disease and gout. *Arthritis Rheum* 8:780–785, 1965

108. HOWELL RR: Hyperuricemia in childhood. *Fed Proc* 27:1078–1082, 1968

109. GREENE HL, WILSON FA, HEFFERAN P, TERRY AB, MORAN JR, SLONIM AE, CLAUS TH, BURR IM: ATP depletion, a possible role in the pathogenesis of hyperuricemia in glycogen storage disease type I. *J Clin Invest* 62:321–328, 1978

110. EDELSTEIN G, HIRSHMAN CA: Hyperthermia and ketoacidosis during anesthesia in a child with glycogen storage disease. *Anesthesiology* 52:90–92, 1980

111. VAN HOOF F, HUE L, DE BARSY T, JACQUEMIN P, DEVOS P, HERS HG: Glycogen storage diseases. *Biochimie* 54:745–752, 1972

112. SANN L, MATHIEU M, BOURGEOIS J, BIENVENU J, BETHENOD M: In vivo

evidence for defective activity of glucose-6-phosphatase in type IB glycogenosis. *J Pediatr* 96:691–694, 1980

113. NARISAWA K, IGARASHI Y, OTOMO H, TADA K: A new variant of glycogen storage disease type I probably due to a defect in the glucose-6-phosphatase transport system. *Biochem Biophys Res Commun* 83:1360–1364, 1978

114. FIELD JB, DRASH AL: Studies in glycogen storage disease. II. Heterogeneity in the inheritance of glycogen storage diseases. *Trans Assoc Am Physicians* 80:284–296, 1967

115. HOWELL RR, STEVENSON RE, BEN-MENACHEM Y, PHILIKY RL, BERRY DH: Hepatic adenomata in patients with type I glycogen storage disease (von Gierke's). *JAMA* 236:1481–1484, 1976

116. MILLER JH, GATES GF, LANDING BH, KOGUT MD, ROE TF: Scintigraphic abnormalities in glycogen storage diseases. *J Nucl Med* 19:354–358, 1978

117. STARZL TE, PUTNAM CW, PORTERN KA, HALGRIMSON CG, CORMAN J, BROWN BI, GOTLIN RW, RODGERSON DO, GREENE HL: Portal diversion for the treatment of glycogen storage disease in humans. *Ann Surg* 178:525–539, 1973

118. FOLKMAN J, PHILIPPART A, TZE WJ, CRIGLER J: Portacaval shunt for glycogen storage disease. Value of prolonged intravenous hyperalimentation before surgery. *Surgery* 72:306–314, 1972

119. BURR IM, O'NEILL JA, KARZON DT, HOWARD LJ, GREENE HL: Comparison of the effects of total parenteral nutrition, continuous intragastric feeding and portacaval shunt on a patient with type I glycogen storage disease. *J Pediatr* 85:792–795, 1974

120. GREENE HL, SLONIM AE, BURR IM: Type I glycogen storage disease: A metabolic basis for advances in treatment. *Adv Pediatr* 26:63–92, 1979

121. GREENE HL: Personal communication

122. GILLETTE PC, NIHILL MR, SINGER DB: Electrophysiological mechanism for the short PR interval in Pompe disease. *Am J Dis Child* 128:622–626, 1974

123. EHLERS KH, HAGSTROM JWC, LUKAS DS, REDO SF, ENGLE MA: Glycogen storage disease of the myocardium with obstruction to left ventricular outflow. *Circulation* 25:96–109. 1962

124. MARTIN JJ, DE BARSY T, VAN HOOF F, PALLADINI G: Pompe's disease: An inborn lysosomal disorder with storage of glycogen. A study of brain and striated muscle. *Acta Neuropathol (Berl)* 23:229–244, 1973.

125. GAMBETTI P, DIMAURO S, BAKER L: Nervous system in Pompe's disease: Ultrastructure and biochemistry. *J Neuropathol Exp Neurol* 30:412–430, 1971

126. HUG G: Pre- and postnatal pathology, enzyme treatment and unresolved issues in five lysosomal disorders. *Pharmacol Rev* 30:565–591, 1979

127. LENARD HG, SCHAUB J, KEUTEL J, OSANG M: Electromyography in type II glycogenosis. *Neuropaediatrie* 5:410–424, 1974

128. ENGEL AG, GOMEZ MR, SEYBOLD ME, LAMBERT EH: The spectrum and diagnosis of acid maltase deficiency. *Neurology* 23:95–106, 1973

129. TANAKA K, SHIMAZU S, OYA N, TOMISAWA M, KUSUNOKI T, SOYAMA K, ONO E: Muscular form of glycogenosis type II (Pompe's disease). *Pediatrics* 63:124–129, 1979

130. ROSENOW EC, ENGEL AE: Acid maltase deficiency in adults presenting as respiratory failure. *Am J Med* 64:485–491, 1978

131. ENGEL AG: Acid maltase deficiency in adults: Studies in four cases of a syndrome which may mimic muscular dystrophy or other myopathies. *Brain* 93:599–616, 1970

132. MARTIN JJ, DE BARSY T, DEN TANDT WR: Acid maltase deficiency in non-identical adult twins: A morphological and biochemical study. *J Neurol* 213:105–118, 1976

133. DIMAURO S, STERN LZ, MEHLER M, NAGLE RB, PAYNE C: Adult onset acid maltase deficiency: A postmortem study. *Muscle Nerve* 1:27–36, 1978

134. HERS HG: Inborn lysosomal diseases. *Gastroenterology* 48:625–633, 1965

135. BAUDHUIN P, HERS HG, LOEB H: An electron microscopic and biochemical study of type II glycogenosis. *Lab Invest* 13:1139–1152, 1964

136. GARANCIS JC: Type II glycogenosis. Biochemical and electron microscope study. *Am J Med* 44:289–300, 1968

137. ILLINGWORTH B, LARNER J, CORI GT: Structure of glycogens and amylopectins. 1. Enzymatic determination of chain length. *J Biol Chem* 199:631–640, 1952

138. LENNARTSON G, LUNDBLAD A, LUNDSTEN J, SVENSSON S, HAGER A: Glucose-containing oligosaccharides in the urine of patients with glycogen storage disease type II and type III. *Eur J. Biochem* 83:325–334, 1978

139. KOSTER JF, SLEE RG, HULSMANN WC: The use of leukocytes as an aid in the diagnosis of a variant of glycogen storage disease type II (Pompe's disease). *Eur J. Clin Invest* 2:467–471, 1972

140. DREYFUS JC, POËNARU L: Alpha glucosidases in white blood cells with reference to the detection of acid α-1,4-glucosidase deficiency. *Biochem Biophys Res Commun* 85:615–622, 1978

141. BROADHEAD DM, BUTTERWORTH J: α-Glucosidase in Pompe's disease. *J Inherited Metab Dis* 1:153–154, 1978

142. BUTTERWORTH J, BROADHEAD DM: Diagnosis of Pompe's disease in cultured skin fibroblasts and primary amniotic fluid cells using 4-methylumbelliferyl-α-D-glucopyranoside as substrate. *Clin Chim Acta* 78:335–342, 1977

143. NITOWSKY HM, GRUNFIELD A: Lysosomal α-glucosidase in type II glycogenosis: Activity in leukocytes and cell cultures in relation to genotype. *J Lab Clin Med* 69:472–484, 1967

144. MEHLER M, DIMAURO S: Residual acid maltase activity in late onset acid maltase deficiency. *Neurology* 27:178–184, 1977

145. BUSCH HFM, KOSTER JF, VAN WEERDEN TW: Infantile and adult onset acid maltase deficiency occurring in the same family. *Neurology* 29:415–416, 1979

146. DE BARSY T, VAN HOOF F: Enzyme replacement therapy with purified human acid α-glucosidase in type II glycogenosis, in Tager JM, Hooghwinkel GJM, Daems WT (eds): *Enzyme Therapy in Lysosomal Storage Diseases.* Amsterdam, North Holland, 1974, p 277

147. DESNICK RJ, THORPE SR, FIDDLER MB: Toward enzyme therapy for lysosomal storage diseases. *Physiol Rev* 56:57–99, 1976

148. WILLIAMS JC, MURRAY AK: Enzyme replacement in Pompe's disease with an α-glucosidase: Low density lipoprotein complex, in Desnick RJ, Paul NW, Dickman F (eds): *Enzyme Therapy in Genetic Disease. 2. Birth Defects.* Original Series XVI. New York, Alan R Liss, Inc, 1980, p 415

149. VIETOR KW, HAVSTEEN B, HARMS D, BUSSE H, HEYNE K: Ethanolaminosis: A newly recognized, generalized storage disease with cardiomegaly, cerebral dysfunction and early death. *Eur J Pediatr* 126:61–75, 1977

150. BRANDT IK, DELUCA VA, JR: Type III glycogenosis: A family with an unusual tissue distribution of the enzyme lesion. *Am J Med* 40:779–784, 1966

151. BRUNBERG JA, MCCORMICK WF, SCHOCHET SS: Type III glycogenosis: An adult with diffuse weakness and muscle wasting. *Arch Neurol* 25:171–178, 1971

152. DIMAURO S, HARTWIG GB, HAYS A, EASTWOOD AB, FRANCO R, OLARTE M, CHANG M, ROSES AD, FETELL M, SCHOENFELDT RS, STERN LZ: Debrancher deficiency: Neuromuscular disorder in five adults. *Ann Neurol* 5:422–436, 1978

153. MILLER CG, ALLEYNE GA, BROOKS SEH: Gross cardiac involvement in glycogen storage disease type III. *Br Heart J* 34:862–864, 1972

154. CHEN J, FRIEDMAN M: Renal tubular acidosis associated with type III glycogenosis. *Acta Pediatr Scand* 68:779–782, 1979

155. VÍTEK B, ŠRÁČKOVÁ D, TOMAN M, KRATKY J, VOGNAREK J: Hyperlipidemia in type III glycogenosis. *Acta Pediatr Scand* 59:701–705, 1970

156. HUG G, KRILL CE, JR, PERRIN EV, GUEST GM: Cori's disease (amylo-1, 6-glucosidase deficiency). Report of a case in a Negro child. *N Engl J Med* 268:113–120, 1963

157. VAN HOOF F, HERS HG: The subgroups of type III glycogenosis. *Eur J Biochem* 2:265–270, 1967

158. BROWN DH, WAINDLE LM, BROWN BI: The apparent activity in vivo of the lysosomal pathway of glycogen catabolism in cultured human skin fibroblasts from patients with type III glycogen storage disease. *J Biol Chem* 253:5005–5011, 1978

159. WILLIAMS C, FIELD JB: Studies in glycogen storage disease. III. Limit dextrinosis: A genetic study. *J Pediatr* 72:214–221, 1968

160. WILLIAMS HE, KENDIG EM, FIELD JB: Leukocyte debranching enzyme in glycogen storage disease. *J Clin Invest* 42:656–660

161. HUIJING F, KLEIN OBBINK HJ, VAN CREVELD S: The activity of the debranching enzyme system in leukocytes. A study of glycogen storage disease type III. *Acta Genet (Basel)* 18:128–136, 1968

162. LEVIN S, MOSES SW, CHAYOTH R, JAGODA N, STEINITZ K: Glycogen storage disease in Israel. A clinical, biochemical and genetic study. *Isr J Med Sci* 3:397–410, 1967

163. ANDERSEN DH: Familial cirrhosis of the liver with storage of abnormal glycogen. *Lab Invest* 5:11–20, 1956

164. LANDING BH, REED GB, DIXON JFP, NEUSTEIN HB, DONNELL GN: Type IV glycogenosis: Patient with absence of a branching enzyme α-1,4-glucan: α-1,4-glucan 6-glycosyl transferase. *Lab. Invest.* 19:546–547, 1968

165. ILLINGWORTH B, CORI GT: Structure of glycogens and amylopectins. III. Normal and abnormal human glycogen. *J Biol Chem* 199:653–660, 1952

166. CRAIG SM, UZMAN LL: A familial metabolic disorder with storage of an unusual polysaccharide complex. *Pediatrics* 22:20–32, 1958

167. MCMASTER KR, POWERS JM, HENNIGAR GR, WOHLTMANN HJ, FARR GH: Nervous system involvement in type IV glycogenosis. *Arch Pathol Lab Med* 103:105–111, 1979

168. MERCIER C, WHELAN WJ: Further characterization of glycogen from type IV glycogen storage disease. *Eur J Biochem* 40:221–223, 1973

169. LEVIN B, BURGESS EA, MORTIMER PE: Glycogen storage disease type IV: Amylopectinosis. *Arch Dis Child* 43:548–555, 1968

170. HOWELL RR, KABACK MM, BROWN BI: Type IV glycogen storage disease: Branching enzyme deficiency in skin fibroblasts and possible heterozygote detection. *J Pediatr* 78:638–642, 1971

171. FERNANDES J, HUIJING F: Branching enzyme deficiency glycogenosis:

Studies in therapy. *Arch Dis Child* 43:347–352, 1968

172. ROWLAND LP, LOVELACE RE, SCHOTLAND DL, ARAKI S, CARMEL P: The clinical diagnosis of McArdle's disease: Identification of another family with deficiency of muscle phosphorylase. *Neurology* 16:93–100, 1966

173. McARDLE B: Myopathy due to a defect in muscle glycogen breakdown. *Clin Sci* 10:13–35, 1951

174. MOMMAERTS WFHM, ILLINGWORTH B, PEARSON CM, GUILLORY RJ, SERAYDARIAN K: A functional disorder of muscle associated with the absence of phosphorylase. *Proc Natl Acad Sci USA* 45:791–797, 1959

175. SCHMID R, MAHLER R: Chronic progressive myopathy with myoglobinuria: Demonstration of a glycogenolytic defect in the muscle. *J Clin Invest* 38:2044–2058, 1959

176. SCHMID R, ROBBINS PW, TRAUT RR: Glycogen synthesis in muscle lacking phosphorylase. *Proc Natl Acad Sci USA* 45:1236–1240, 1959

177. LARNER J, VILLAR-PALASI C: Enzymes in a glycogen storage myopathy. *Proc Natl Acad Sci USA* 45:1234–1235, 1959

178. PEARSON CM, RIMER DG, MOMMAERTS WFHM: A metabolic myopathy due to absence of muscle phosphorylase. *Am J Med* 30:502–517, 1961

179. SALTER RH: The muscle glycogenoses. *Lancet* 1:1301–1304, 1968

180. ROWLAND LP, ARAKI S, CARMEL P: Contracture in McArdle's disease. *Arch Neurol* 13:541–544, 1965

181. PERNOW BB, HAVEL RJ, JENNINGS DB: The second wind phenomenon in McArdle's syndrome. *Acta Med Scand* (suppl) 472:294–307, 1967

182. HAMMETT JF, BALE P, BASSER LS, NEALE FC: McArdle's disease: Three cases in an Australian family. *Proc Aust Assoc Neurol* 4:21–25, 1966

183. HOWELL RR: The diagnostic value of serum enzyme measurements. *J Pediatr* 68:122–134, 1966

184. SWIFT TR, BROWN M: Tc-99m pyrophosphate muscle labeling in McArdle's syndrome. *J Nucl Med* 19:295–297, 1978

185. BANK WJ, DiMAURO S, ROWLAND LP: Renal failure in McArdle's disease. *N Engl J Med* 287:1102, 1972

186. WAHREN J, FELIG P, HAVEL RJ, JORFELDT L, PERNOW B, SALTIN B: Amino acid metabolism in McArdle's syndrome. *N Engl J Med* 288:774–777, 1973

187. NOLTE J, SCHOLLMEYER P: Metabolic adaptation in muscle of phosphorylase deficiency (McArdle's disease). *Klin Wochenschr* 51:250–251, 1973

188. DiMAURO S, HARTLAGE PL: Fatal infantile form of muscle phosphorylase deficiency. *Neurology* 28:1124–1129, 1978

189. MIRANDA AF, NETTE EG, HARTLAGE PL, DiMAURO S: Phosphorylase isoenzymes in normal and myophosphorylase-deficient human heart. *Neurology* 29:1538–1541, 1979

190. DE LA MARZA M, PATTEN BM, WILLIAMS JC, CHAMBERS JP: Myophosphorylase deficiency: A new cause of infantile hypotonia simulating infantile muscular atrophy. *Neurology* 30:402, 1980

191. SCHOTLAND DL, SPIRO D, ROWLAND LP, CARMEL P: Ultrastructural studies of muscle in McArdle's disease. *J Neuropathol Exp Neurol* 24:629–644, 1965

192. DREYFUS JC, PROUX D, ALEXANDRE Y: Molecular studies on glycogen storage diseases. *Enzyme* 18:60–72, 1974

193. FEIT H, BROOKE MH: Myophosphorylase deficiency: Two different molecular etiologies. *Neurology* 26:963–967, 1976

194. KOSTER JF, SLEE RG, JENNEKENS FGI, WINTZER AR, van BERKEL TJC: McArdle's disease: A study on the molecular basis of two different etiologies of myophosphorylase deficiency. *Clin Chim Acta* 94:229–235, 1979

195. ROELOFS RI, ENGEL WK, CHAUVIN PB: Histochemical phosphorylase activity in regenerating muscle fibers from myophosphorylase-deficient patients. *Science* 177:795–797, 1972

196. MITSUMOTO H: McArdle disease: Phosphorylase activity in regenerating muscle fibers. *Neurology* 29:258–262, 1979

197. SATO K, IMAI F, HATAYAMA I, ROELOFS RI: Characterization of glycogen phosphorylase isoenzymes present in cultured skeletal muscle from patients with McArdle's disease. *Biochem Biophys Res Commun* 78:663–668, 1977

198. DiMAURO S, ARNOLD S, MIRANDA A, ROWLAND LP: McArdle's disease: The mystery of reappearing phosphorylase activity in muscle culture—a fetal isoenzyme. *Ann Neurol* 3:60–66, 1978

199. DAWSON DM, SPONG FL, HARRINGTON JF: McArdle's disease: Lack of muscle phosphorylase. *Ann Intern Med* 69:229–235, 1968

200. HERS HG: Etudes enzymatiques sur fragments hepatiques. Application a la classification des glycogenoses. *Rev Int Hepatol* 9:35–55, 1959

201. ÖCKERMAN PA, JELKE H, KAIJSER K: Glycogenosis type 6 (liver phosphorylase deficiency). A case followed for ten years with normal phosphorylase activity in white blood cells and jejunal mucosa. *Acta Pediatr Scand* 55:10–16, 1966

202. KOSTER JF, SLEE RG, DAEGELEN D, MEIENHOFER MC, DREYFUS JC, NIERMEYER MF, FERNANDES J: Isoenzyme patterns of phosphorylase in white blood cells and fibroblasts from patients with liver phosphorylase deficiency. *Clin Chim Acta* 69:121–125, 1976

203. BAUSSAN C, MOATTI N, ODIEVRU M, LEMONNIER A: Liver glycogenosis caused by a defective phosphorylase system: Hemolysate analysis. *Pediatrics* 67:107–112, 1981

204. FERNANDES J, KOSTER JF, GROSE WFA, SORDEDRAGER N: Hepatic phosphorylase deficiency. *Arch Dis Child* 49:186–191, 1974

205. TARUI S, OKUNO G, IKURA Y, TANAKA T, SUDA M, NISHIKAWA M: Phosphofructokinase deficiency in skeletal muscle: A new type of glycogenosis. *Biochem Biophsy Res Commun* 19:517–523, 1965

206. OKUNO G, HIZUKURI S, NISHIKAWA M: Activities of glycogen synthetase and UDPG pyrophosphorylase in muscle of a patient with a new type of muscle glycogenosis caused by phosphofructokinase deficiency. *Nature* 212:1490–1491, 1966

207. LAYZER RB, ROWLAND LP, RANNEY HM: Muscle phosphofructokinase deficiency. *Arch Neurol* 17:512–523, 1967

208. TARUI S, KONO N, NASU T, NISHIKAWA M: Enzymatic basis for the coexistence of myopathy and hemolytic disease in inherited muscle phosphofructokinase deficiency. *Biochem Biophys Res Commun* 34:77–83, 1969

209. DUPOND JL, ROBERT M, CARBILLET JP, LECONTE DES FLORIS R: Glycogenose musculaire et anemie hemolytique par deficit enzymatique chez deus germains. *Neur Presse Med* 6:2665–2668, 1977

210. GUIBAUD P, CARRIER H, MATHIEU M, DORCHE O, PARCHOUX B, BETHENOD M, LARBRE F: Observation familiale de dystrophie musculaire congenitale par deficit en phosphofructokinase. *Arch Fr Pediatr* 35:1110–1115, 1978

211. AGAMANOLIS DP, ASKARI AD, DiMAURO S, HAYS A, KUMOR K, LIPTON M, and RAYNOR A: Muscle phosphofructokinase deficiency: Two cases with unusual polysaccharide accumulation and immunologically active enzyme protein. *Muscle Nerve* 3:456–467, 1980

212. TARUI S, KONO N, KUWAJIMA M, IKURA Y: Type VII glycogenosis (muscle and erythrocyte phosphofructokinase deficiency). *Monogr Hum Genet* 9:42–47, 1978

213. HUG G, SCHUBERT WK, CHUCK G: Deficient activity of dephosphophosphorylase kinase and accumulation of glycogen in the liver. *J Clin Invest* 48:704–715, 1969

214. HUIJING F: Phosphorylase kinase in leukocytes of normal subjects and of patients with glycogen storage disease. *Biochim Biophys Acta* 148:601–603, 1967

215. HUIJING F, FERNANDES J: X chromosomal inheritance of liver glycogenosis with phosphorylase kinase deficiency. *Am J Hum Genet* 21:275–284, 1969

216. HUIJING F, SANDBERG DH: Phosphorylase kinase defect: A generalized disorder. *South Med J* 63:1482, 1970

217. MIGEON BR, HUIJING F: Glycogen storage disease associated with phosphorylase kinase deficiency: Evidence for X inactivation. *Am J Hum Genet* 26:360–368, 1974

218. LEDERER B, van HOOF F, van den BERGHE G, HERS H: Glycogen phosphorylase and its converter enzymes in hemolysates of normal human subjects and of patients with type VI glycogen storage disease: A study of phosphorylase kinase deficiency. *Biochem J* 147:23–35, 1975

219. GROSS SR, MAYER SE: Characterization of the phosphorylase b to a converting activity in skeletal muscle extracts of mice with the phosphorylase b kinase deficiency mutation. *J Biol Chem* 249:6710–6718, 1974

220. MORISHITA Y, NISHYAMA K, YAMAMURA H, KODAMA S, NEGISHI H, MATSUO M, MATSUO T, NISHIZUKA Y: Glycogen phosphorylase kinase deficiency: A survey of enzymes in phosphorylase activating system. *Biochem Biophys Res Commun* 54:833–841, 1973

221. SPENCER-PEET J, LEWIS GM, STEWART KM: Glycogen synthetase deficiency, in Whelan WJ (ed): *Control of Glycogen Metabolism*. Boston, Little, Brown & Co, 1964 p 377

222. DYKES JRW, SPENCER-PEET J: Hepatic glycogen synthetase deficiency. Further studies in a family. *Arch Dis Child* 47:558–563, 1972

223. AYNSLEY-GREEN A, WILLIAMSON DH, GITZELMANN R: Hepatic glycogen synthase deficiency. Definition of syndrome from metabolic and enzyme studies in a nine year old girl. *Arch Dis Child* 52:573–579, 1977

224. AYNSLEY-GREEN A, WILLIAMSON DH, GITZELMANN R: Asymptomatic hepatic glycogen synthase deficiency. *Lancet* 2:147–148, 1978

225. KOGUT MD, BLASKOVICS M, DONNELL GN: Idiopathic hypoglycemia: A study of twenty-six children. *J Pediatr* 74:853–871, 1969

226. SAULS HS: Ketotic hypoglycemia: Quantitation of ketosis and liver glycogen during the ketogenic test diet. Program, Society for Pediatric Research, Atlantic City, NJ 1966, p 190

227. HERS HG: Comments, in Whelan WJ (ed): *Control of Glycogen Metabolism*. Boston, Little, Brown & Co, 1964, p 386

228. ILLINGWORTH B, BROWN DH: Glycogen storage diseases, types III, IV and VI, in Whelan WJ (ed): *Control of Glycogen Metabolism*. Boston, Little, Brown & Co, 1964, p 336

229. KRIVIT W, SHARP HL, LEE JC, LARNER J, EDSTROM R: Low molecular weight glycogen as a cause of generalized glycogen storage disease. *Am J Med* 54:88–97, 1973

230. EDSTROM RD: Stucture of a low molecular weight form of glycogen iso-

lated from the liver in a case of glycogen storage disease. *J Biol Chem* 247:1360–1367, 1972

231. SHEN LC, EDSTROM RD, LARNER J: Primer activity of a low molecular weight glycogen from a patient with an unusual glycogen storage disease. *Physiol Chem Phys* 4:56–60, 1972

232. HUG G, SCHUBERT WK, CHUCK G: Loss of cyclic 3′,5′-AMP dependent kinase and reduction of phosphorylase kinase in skeletal muscle of a girl with deactivated phosphorylase and glycogenosis of liver and muscle. *Biochem Biophys Res Commun* 40:982–988, 1970

233. AUERBACH VH, DiGEORGE AM: Genetic mechanisms producing multiple enzyme defects. A review of unexplained cases and a new hypothesis. *Am J Med Sci* 249:718–747, 1965

234. ERICKSON RP, GLUECKSOHN-WAELSCH S, CORI CF: Glucose-6-phosphatase deficiency caused by radiation-included alleles at the albino locus on the mouse. *Proc Natl Acad Sci USA* 59:437–444, 1968

235. MOSTAFA IE: A case of glycogenic cardiomegaly in a dog. *Acta Vet Scand* 22:197–208, 1970

236. SANDSTROM B, WESTMAN J, ÖCKERMAN PA: Glycogenosis of the central nervous system in the cat. *Acta Neuropathol (Berl)* 14:194–200, 1969

237. MANKTELOW BW, HARTLEY WJ: Generalized glycogen storage disease in sheep. *J Comp Pathol* 85:139–145, 1975

238. RICHARDS RB, EDWARDS JR, COOK RD, WHITE RR: Bovine generalized glycogenosis. *Neuropathol Appl Neurobiol* 3:45–56, 1977

239. EDWARDS JR, RICHARDS RB: Bovine generalized glycogenosis type II: A clinico-pathological study. *Br Vet J* 135:338–348, 1979

240. JOLLY RD, VAN DE WATER NS, RICHARDS RB, DORLING PR: Generalized glycogenosis in beef shorthorn cattle—heterozygote detection. *Aust J Exp Biol Med Sci* 55:141–150, 1977

241. HOWELL JM, DORLING PR, COOK RD, ROBINSON WF, BRADLEY S, GAWTHORNE JM: Infantile and late onset form of generalized glycogenosis type II in cattle (in press), 1981

242. RAFIQUZZAMAN M, SVENKERUD R, STRANDE A, HAUGE JG: Glycogenosis in the dog. *Acta Vet Scand* 17:210–222, 1976

243. CEH L, HAUGE JG, SVENKERUD R, STRANDE A: Glycogenosis type III in the dog. *Acta Vet Scand* 17:196–209, 1976

244. GROSS SR: Animal models of glycogen storage conditions—their relations to human disease. *West J Med* 123:194–201, 1975

245. MALTHUS R, CLARK DG, WATTS C, SNEYD JGT: Glycogen storage disease in rats, a genetically determined deficiency of liver phosphorylase kinase. *Biochem J* 188:99–106, 1980

246. CLARK DG, TOPPING DL, ILLMAN RJ, TRIMBLE RT, MALTHUS RS: A glycogen storage disease (gsd/gsd) rat: Studies in lipid metabolism, lipogenesis, plasma, metabolites and bile acid secretion. *Metabolism* 29:415–420, 1980

247. CORI GT: Biochemical aspects of glycogen deposition diseases. *Bibl Paediatr* 3:344–358, 1958

248. BUEDING E, COLACCI AV: Enzymes of glycogen metabolism in mammalian fetal liver, in Barnes AC (ed): *Intrauterine Development*. Philadelphia, Lea & Febiger, 1968, p 233

7

DISORDERS OF GALACTOSE METABOLISM

STANTON SEGAL

1. Two inherited disorders of galactose metabolism resulting in galactosemia have been delineated. They are transmitted by autosomal recessive inheritance.

2. The genetic disturbance is expressed as a cellular deficiency of either galactokinase or galactose-1-phosphate uridyl transferase, the enzymes catalyzing the first and second reactions in the unique pathway by which galactose is converted to glucose.

3. The clinical manifestations are toxicity syndromes resulting from exposure of the patients to galactose. Toxicity in galactokinase deficiency is milder and is mainly manifested by cataracts. In transferase deficiency, galactose ingestion is characterized by inanition, failure to thrive, vomiting, liver disease, cataracts, and mental retardation.

4. The diagnosis is suggested by the detection of galactose in the blood or urine and is established by demonstration of the enzyme deficiency in the peripheral blood cells. Adequate procedures are available for screening large populations for transferase deficiency.

5. In these disorders, there is an alternative metabolic route of galactose metabolism through reduction to galactitol and oxidation to galactonate. Galactitol is not further metabolized but is excreted by the kidney. Transferase deficiency is associated with the accumulation of galactose-1-phosphate in the tissues in addition to galactitol and galactonate accumulation.

6. Most patients with galactose-1-phosphate uridyl transferase deficiency can oxidize only a small fraction of galactose to carbon dioxide. This ability does not increase with age, and it seems unlikely that alternative metabolic pathways involving sugar nucleotides develop to circumvent the block in galactose conversion to glucose. There is, however, a group of galactosemic patients, all of whom are black, who in spite of the absence of transferase in the red cells can oxidize limited amounts of galactose. These patients have about 10 percent of normal transferase activity in the liver and intestine. Several other clinical variants of transferase deficiency with altered electrophoretic mobility of the enzyme have been described.

7. In transferase-deficient red cells a protein immunologically identical to the active enzyme has been found. Chemical characterization of the protein reveals no gross differences from the normal enzyme. This suggests a structural mutation involving an amino acid near the active site.

8. The cause of the entire toxicity syndrome in transferase deficiency is uncertain. On present evidence, it is reasonable to conclude that the cataract formation in both disorders of galactose metabolism is secondary to galactitol formation in the lens.

9. A condition has been found in which there is a deficiency of red cell uridine diphosphate galactose-4-epimerase without involvement of other tissues. The

absence of galactosemia and other symptoms indicates that this is a benign disorder which may be detected by screening procedures for blood galactose which also react with red cell galactose-1-phosphate.

The name *galactosemia* has been given to a toxicity syndrome associated with the administration of galactose to patients with an inherited disorder of galactose utilization [1–5]. The constellation of nutritional failure, liver disease, cataracts, and mental retardation results from a deficiency of galactose-1-phosphate uridyl transferase [6], one of several enzymes in the galactose metabolic pathway. Another inherited syndrome of elevated plasma galactose concentration associated with galactosuria and juvenile cataracts has been described as resulting from galactokinase deficiency [7]. The possibility exists that disorders of other enzymes in the galactose metabolic sequence could also result in "galactosemia." The term *galactosemia*, therefore, has become inadequate. Also the name *galactose diabetes* for galactokinase deficiency [8] seems inappropriate. It appears reasonable to qualify the descriptive term *galactosemia* with the appropriate enzyme fault. The two known syndromes of disordered galactose metabolism will be designated *transferase deficiency galactosemia* and *galactokinase deficiency galactosemia* and will be discussed as such in this chapter.

THE BIOCHEMISTRY AND PHYSIOLOGY OF GALACTOSE UTILIZATION

The Uridine Nucleotide Pathway

The main dietary source of galactose is the disaccharide lactose, the principal carbohydrate of mammalian milk. Hydrolysis of lactose by the galactosidase, lactase, of the intestinal microvillae results in release of the monosaccharides, glucose and galactose. These two sugars differ only by the configuration of the hydroxyl group about the fourth carbon (Fig. 7-1). The main pathway of galactose metabolism in humans is the

conversion of galactose to glucose, without disruption of the carbon skeleton, by the epimerization of the hydroxyl group of carbon 4. This requires several enzymatic steps, as elucidated by Leloir and associates [9–11] and Kalckar and coworkers [12], and is shown in Fig. 7-2.

Galactokinase   This enzyme has been described in yeast [9, 13, 14], bacteria [15, 16], and mammalian tissues [10]. Galactose reacts with ATP to form galactose-1-phosphate and ADP; Mg^{2+} is required. The equilibrium is far in the direction of sugar phosphorylation, but the reaction is reversible [17]. The *Escherichia coli* enzyme has been purified, the amino acid composition found, and the molecular weight determined to be 40,000 [16]. The reaction of the bacterial enzyme is of the random bimolecular type [18]. Protection by thiols is a property common to the bacterial and liver enzyme. The yeast enzyme has also been purified and has properties similar to those of the *E. coli* enzyme, with a monomeric structure and a molecular weight of 58,000 [19]. A DNA fragment containing the galactokinase gene has been maintained and shown to be expressed in a mutant of *E. coli* with deletion of its own gene [20].

The mammalian enzyme has been studied in detail in tissue homogenates or purified preparations in rat [21, 22] and pig liver [23], human red cells [24, 25], human leukocytes, and cultured human fibroblasts [26, 27], human placenta [28], and various human fetal tissues in which it is detected after the seventh week of gestation [29]. Liver enzyme reacts with galactosamine and 2-deoxygalactose, but the yeast enzyme is more specific for galactose. In the rat, activity of the liver enzyme is inhibited by high levels of both substrate and product, regulatory phenomena which would tend to decrease formation of galactose-1-phosphate, a possible toxic metabolite. The specific activity of rat liver enzyme increases after birth to a maximum at about 5 days of age, followed by a progressive fall (Fig. 7-3) [21, 22]. This decrease in specific activity is compensated for by increased organ size, so that the total activity in liver increases to a maximum at about 20 days of age [30]. In the human fetus, the liver-specific enzyme activity increases progressively from the seventh week until term without change in the enzyme K_m [29]

The developmental changes in liver activity do not appear to be regulated by dietary galactose. Normal human fibroblasts

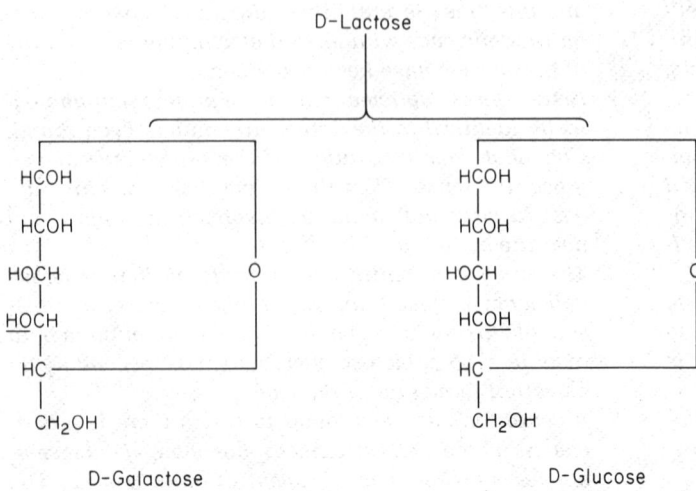

Figure 7-1   Structure of galactose and glucose, the monosaccharides in lactose. Note the difference in the spatial relation of the hydroxyl group on the fourth carbon.

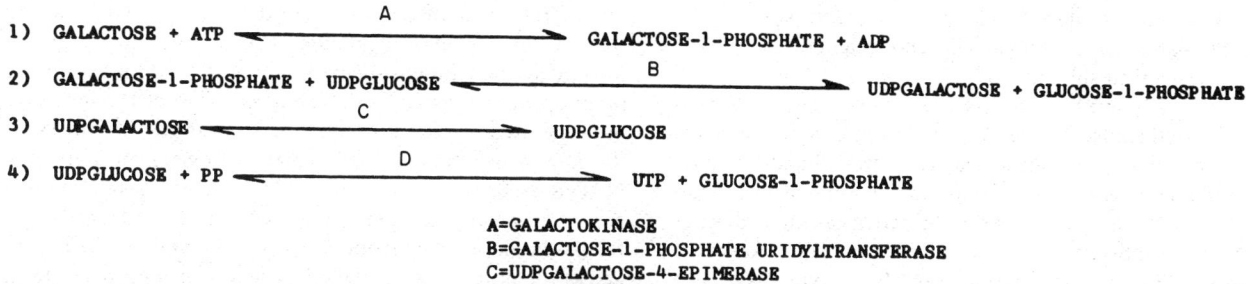

Figure 7-2 Reactions of the pathway of galactose metabolism responsible for the galactose-glucose interconversion.

in tissue culture show enhanced galactokinase when grown in the presence of galactose [31]. Galactokinase activity is higher in red blood cells from newborn human in infants than in cells from adults [24]. The red cell enzyme has been purified over 3000-fold and found to have a dimeric structure, the monomers having a molecular weight of 25,000 to 27,000 [32]. The red cell enzyme resembles that of other mammalian tissue galactokinase in its substrate affinities but differs from that of *E. coli*. The red cell enzyme, like that of liver, undergoes substrate and product inhibition [25]. This type of regulation would tend to decrease the formation of galactose-1-phosphate. Higher galactokinase activity in newborn erythrocytes than in adults may be related to differences in substrate affinity [25]. Tedesco et al. [33] have presented evidence for racial polymorphism within the black population, noting three levels of red cell galactokinase activity. The assignment of the gene for galactokinase has been made to human chromosome 17, and its regional localization on the chromosome has been assigned to band q21-22 [34]. The red cell enzymes of various mammals have been compared [35] and a gene locus controlling galactokinase activity in mouse blood has been described [36]. In the mouse the interstrain difference in blood galactokinase was not reflected, however, by parallel differences in activity of the liver enzymes [37].

Galactokinase synthesis has been carried out in vitro,

employing bacteriophage DNA coding for the enzyme and a cell-free extract prepared from a Gal deletion strain of *E. coli* [38]. Cyclic adenosine monophosphate is required for the process in vitro [39]. 3′,5′ Cyclic adenosine monophosphate stimulates *E. coli* galactokinase activity [40] as well as that of the animallike protozoan, Tetrahymena [41]. Although there has been doubt that cyclic nucleotide plays a role in the expression in vivo of the galactose operon in *E. coli* [42], recent work has shown the importance of cyclic AMP and its receptor protein in regulation of the galactose operon [43].

Galactose-1-phosphate Uridyl Transferase This enzyme catalyzes the second step in the galactose-glucose interconversion in which the product of the galactokinase reaction, galactose-1-phosphate, reacts with uridine diphosphate glucose (UDP-glucose) to give UDP-galactose and glucose-1-phosphate [12]. The enzyme is present in bacteria [44] and most mammalian tissues [45]. Bacterial transferase has been purified to homogeneity and consists of two structural subunits of 40,000 mol. wt. [46]. The enzymatic mechanism of the bacterial enzyme is of the ping-pong type [47]. The stereochemical course [48] and N-terminal and C-terminal amino acid sequences of the *E. coli* enzyme have been determined [49]. The nucleophile to which the uridylyl group is bonded in the bacterial enzyme intermediate has been found to be imidazole

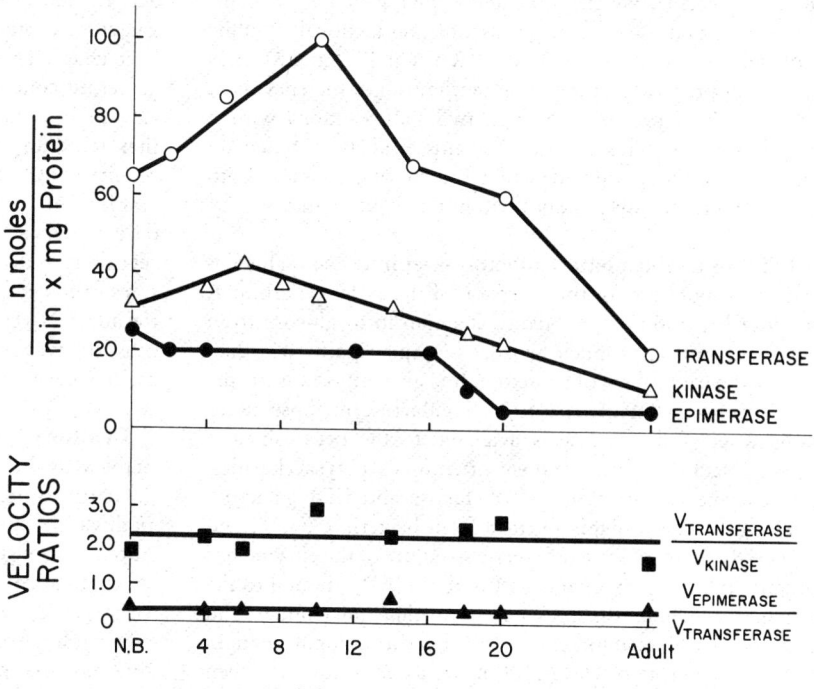

Figure 7-3 The specific activity of galactokinase, galactose-1-phosphate uridyl transferase, and epimerase in rat liver as a function of age. *(From P. Cuatrecasas and S. Segal [21], D. Bertoli and S. Segal [45], and R. Cohn and S. Segal [96].)*

N^3 of a histidine residue [50]. Highly purified yeast enzyme is similar to that of *E. coli* with a molecular weight of 86,100 and with two identical subunits [51].

Calf [52, 53] and human liver [54, 55] enzymes have been partially purified. Isoelectric focusing indicates a microheterogeneity of human liver transferase, with several bands of activity on acrylamide gel [56]. Transferase is present in human fetal tissues, the liver enzyme-specific activity being highest at 28 weeks gestation with unchanging K_m values throughout gestation [29]. The properties of rat liver enzyme have also been examined [45]. Liver transferase has a K_m for UDP-glucose of 0.1 to 0.2 mM, a value within the physiologic range of liver UDP-glucose concentration [57]. Thus, the rate of the reaction may be regulated by substrate concentration and limited by UDP-glucose substrate inhibition of the transferase observed at higher levels. Glucose-1-phosphate is a potent inhibitor of the enzyme [45]. Uridine nucleotides such as uridine di- and triphosphate are extremely powerful competitive inhibitors of substrate UDP-glucose [58]. Substantial data indicate that the enzyme is influenced by the general state of carbohydrate metabolic processes. During perfusion with galactose of suckling but not adult liver, transferase-specific activity is initially increased but falls to low levels after 90 min [59]. This phenomenon is also observed when glucose is perfused.

Dietary and hormonal influences on the liver enzyme have not been reported. Transferase has been examined extensively in both human [60] and rat intestine [61], including developmental characteristics in the rat [61]. Feeding a high-galactose diet increases transferase activity in rat intestinal mucosa [62]. Properties of the enzyme in human diploid fibroblasts in culture and amniotic fluid cells have been delineated [63–66]. Hammersen, Mandell, and Levy have shown that the fibroblast enzyme consists of four activity bands on starch-gel electrophoresis [67].

The most extensive studies have been made of purified human red cell enzyme [55, 68–70]. The kinetic characteristics of the pure enzyme are similar to those in crude preparations. Although Tedesco [55] postulated a trimeric structure with a 90,000 molecular weight, Dale and Popjak [69] and Williams [70] found that the enzyme consists of two identical subunits with a molecular weight of 88,000. Wu et al. [71] and Markus et al. [72] proposed a ping-pong mechanism in the enzymatic activity which proceeds through two half-reactions with a uridylyl-enzyme intermediate. Williams et al. [73], based on inhibition studies, concluded that the enzyme contains both cysteinyl and histidyl residues within its active center.

Uridine Diphosphate Galactose-4-epimerase   This enzyme is responsible for the inversion of the hydroxyl group at the fourth carbon of the hexose chain to form glucose from galactose and has a much broader biologic significance than merely the catabolism of galactose. It is also important for the conversion of UDP-glucose to UDP-galactose in those situations where only glucose is available to the organism and where galactose is a constituent of complex polysaccharides. The enzyme is specific for UDP-glucose and UDP-galactose [74] and has been highly purified from bacteria [75–77] and yeast [78, 79] in which a polymeric structure of the enzyme has been found. In these organisms 1 mol of NAD is bound to the enzyme, which in the presence of uridine nucleotides and galactose exhibits fluorescence and conformational changes [80, 81]. The role of UMP and sugars as activators has been studied by Kang et al. [82] and by Ketley and Schellenberg

[83]. Circular dichroism spectra of the *E. coli* enzyme indicate that the conversion of the bound NAD to NADH is accompanied by an increase in α-helix structure [84] and alteration in binding characteristics [85]. The mechanism of the inversion has generated considerable interest. Kalckar [86] has reviewed the data, which indicate that neither hydrogen from water nor NAD is exchanged with hydroxyl hydrogen at carbon 4. Oxygen 18 from isotopic water is not involved. A novel mechanism for oxidation and reduction at carbon 4 involving the hydrogen of the uracil ring of UDP-glucose has been proposed [87]. Maitra and Ankel [88] and Adair and Gabriel [89] have evidence that a 4-ulose is involved in an oxidoreductase mechanism.

For liver enzyme activity, exogenous NAD is required, and NADH is a potent inhibitor of the enzyme [90]. At equilibrium the ratio of UDP-galactose to UDP-glucose is 1:3. Epimerase from calf liver has been purified 3000-fold and found to be a dimer of 70,000 mol wt [91]. NAD binds to the enzyme and induces a conformation resulting in enzyme activity. It has been calculated that in a normal catalytic cycle NAD dissociates once in every 9000 catalytic events. Metabolic control of galactose metabolism by regulation of liver epimerase activity is likely. Any process disturbing the NAD/NADH ratio, such as ethanol metabolism which generates NADH, will impair galactose utilization [92]. Since greater NADH inhibition occurs at physiologic pH than at the alkaline pH optimum of the enzyme, intracellular pH may be an important factor in the rate of the reaction. In this regard, intact cells with a high glycolytic rate show little epimerase activity, whereas broken cell preparations have considerable enzyme function [93]. Cellular levels of UDP-glucose, as well as other uridine nucleotides, may also exert rate-regulating effects [94, 95]. Animal age appears important, since the liver of newborn rats has a higher activity, which remains elevated during the period of milk ingestion [96] (Fig. 7-3). The data of Fig. 7-3 suggest that epimerase may be the rate-limiting enzyme in rat liver. Epimerase activity of intestinal mucosa is low during the suckling period and increases with age [96]. The intestinal enzyme activity can be enhanced by feeding diets high in glucose or galactose content [62]. The enzyme in human fibroblasts has been characterized, and activity was found not to be related to galactose concentration of the incubation medium [97]. The enzyme in human red cells has a higher activity in newborns than in adults, and hemolysate activity of newborns does not require exogenous NAD, as does that of adults [98]. Considerable NAD remains in hemolysates because NAD nucleosidase is deficient in the newborn. Starch-gel electrophoresis reveals two distinct activity bands for epimerase in hemolysates from newborn, but only one band of different mobility in the adult. NAD added to the gel caused the enzyme of the adult cells to have a two-banded pattern [98]. The gene for epimerase has been assigned to human chromosome 1 [99, 100].

Uridine Diphosphate Glucose Pyrophosphorylase   The activity of this enzyme not only enables the carbon chain of galactose originally phosphorylated (Fig. 7-2) to enter the pathway of glucose metabolism as glucose-1-phosphate but also is responsible for the important function of the synthesis of UDP-glucose from UTP and glucose. Originally found in yeast [101, 102], it is abundant in mammalian liver, from which it has been crystallized [103]. A polymeric subunit structure has been determined [104]. The crystalline enzyme from human liver reacts to some extent with other sugar nucleotides besides UDP-glucose, including UDP-galactose. Bovine mammary gland enzyme is inhibited by galactose-1-phosphate [105]. Certain E. coli strains with defective galactose metabolism have been shown to have an absence of this enzyme [106, 107]. The molecular weight of the mammalian enzyme is approximately 400,000, with eight identical subunits [108].

Alternative Pathways of Galactose Metabolism

Reduction to Galactitol The presence of galactitol in the tissues of animals fed galactose [109–111] and in the tissues [112, 113] and urine of patients with both transferase [114] and galactokinase deficiency galactosemia [115] demonstrates the importance of the reduction of galactose in mammalian metabolism (Fig. 7-4). Reduction of sugars to the polyol, first described by Hers in the seminal vesicle and placenta of sheep [116], may be catalyzed by two enzymes found in most animal tissues [117]. One is aldose reductase or polyol: NADP-oxidoreductase, which reacts with a variety of aldehydes, glyceraldehyde being the principal substrate [118, 119]. The K_m values for galactose of highly purified enzymes from lens [118] and brain [120] are 12 and 20 mM, respectively. The other enzyme, L-hexonate dehydrogenase [121] or L-gulonate: NADP-oxidoreductase, is an enzyme whose preferred substrates are uronic acids and their lactones, but which acts on galactose with much less affinity than aldose reductase. The K_m of purified brain enzyme for galactose is 159 mM [120]. The very high K_m values indicate that only when tissue levels of galactose are much elevated would reduction be important, being catalyzed primarily by aldose reductase. Under normal circumstances galactose would be phosphorylated by way of galactokinase.

The tissue distribution of both reductive enzymes has been demonstrated by starch-gel electrophoresis [117]. Lens is the only tissue with aldose reductase activity exclusively. In peripheral nerve, aldose reductase has been localized to the Schwann cells [122] and in kidney primarily in the renal papillae [123]. Aldose reductase activity of lens and other tissues is stimulated by sulfate ions [118] and ATP [124]. It is inhibited by various keto and fatty acids [94] and ADP [124]. Increased enzyme activity has been observed in rat brain after birth [125].

Oxidation of Galactose to Galactonate Patients with transferase-deficient galactosemia excrete galactonate in urine after galactose is administered [126], and rats fed a high galactose diet not only excrete galactonate in urine but accumulate galactonic acid in several tissues, including liver, intestine, heart, and kidney [127]. Galactonate accumulates in suckling rat liver perfused with high concentrations of galactose [128].

The difference in the rate of radioactive CO_2 formation from oxidation of [1-^{14}C]galactose and [2-^{14}C]galactose by transferase-deficient patients led Segal and Cuatrecasas to postulate that a direct oxidative pathway may play a role in galactose disposition when the normal pathway is blocked [129].

A pathway of galactose metabolism in rat liver has been described in which galactose reacts with NAD to form galactonic acid [130]. The latter compound is then oxidized to form β-ketogalactonic acid, which undergoes decarboxylation to D-xylulose, a sugar capable of further metabolism [130]. The initial enzyme was characterized in the soluble cell fraction as a galactose dehydrogenase with a K_m of 26 mM [131, 132]. Srivastava and Beutler [133] failed to demonstrate the oxidation of galactose to galactonate but showed the formation of galactose-6-phosphate and its subsequent oxidation to 6-phosphogalactonic acid. Rancour et al. [127] recently demonstrated that rat liver microsomes produce galactonic acid when incubated with 30 mM galactose. Oxygen was not required, and formation of hydrogen peroxide was observed. A liver sample obtained at autopsy from a transferase-deficient galactosemic patient contained galactonate, suggesting that a similar system might be responsible for galactonate production when galactose metabolism is blocked by the Leloir pathway [127].

Uridine Diphosphate Galactose Pyrophosphorylase This enzyme, first detected in yeast [12] and subsequently identified in mammalian liver [134, 135], catalyzes the reaction of galactose-1-phosphate with uridine triphosphate to form UDP-galactose and pyrophosphate. Function of this enzyme could circumvent the block in galactose metabolism due to transferase deficiency, and indeed, preliminary data indicated that this could be the case [134]. However, the activity of this enzyme in human liver is low and does not increase with age [136]. There is now considerable doubt that catalysis is due to an enzyme with a unique affinity for galactose-1-phosphate. It is probable that the enzyme performing this function is UDP-glucose pyrophosphorylase [103]. The enzyme has been found to be present in human fibroblasts in tissue culture [137].

Physiologic Aspects of Galactose Metabolism

Human beings are capable of metabolizing large quantities of galactose given orally or intravenously, as demonstrated by the rapid elimination of galactose from blood [138] and the oxidation of radioactive galactose to $^{14}CO_2$ [139]. A rise in the level of plasma glucose is found after galactose loading, because of the conversion of galactose to glucose through the sugar nucleotide pathway. When tracer amounts of radioactive galactose are given intravenously to normal subjects, 50 percent of the radioactivity may be found in the body glucose

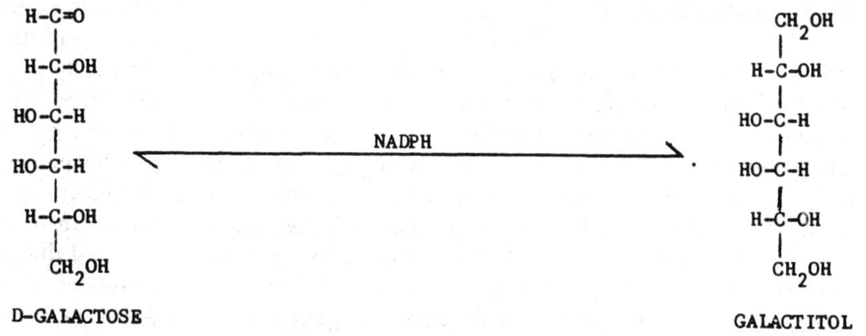

Figure 7-4 The conversion of galactose to galactitol by aldose reductase.

pools within 30 min. Curves of $^{14}CO_2$ excretion in expired air closely resemble those seen after the administration of radioactive glucose itself [139]. Plasma galactose is so rapidly removed by the liver that the rate of galactose clearance is a measure of hepatic blood flow [140]. The mechanism appears to be saturated at plasma levels of 50 mg/dl. Tygstrup [141] and Keiding [142] estimate that the capacity of hepatic elimination corresponds to the limits of the ability of galactokinase to phosphorylate the sugar. Urinary elimination is not a significant factor in the disposition of galactose loads [143]. Studies of the resorption of galactose by the human kidney reveal a low and incomplete threshold at plasma levels of 10 to 20 mg/dl.

Galactose tolerance tests have been used to estimate impaired liver function [144] and have shown that clearance of intravenously administered galactose is slow and the oxidation of isotopic galactose impaired in the presence of liver damage [145, 146]. Ethanol administration slows galactose elimination from blood in both humans [138, 139, 147] and rats [148], the effect presumably being due to tissue elevation of NADH and inhibition of UDP-galactose-4-epimerase [92].

Age may have some influence on galactose metabolism. Maximal utilization of galactose by rat liver in vitro occurs in tissue from the newborn and young [149]. This corresponds to the elevated enzyme levels shown in Fig. 7-3. Haworth and Ford [150] and Mulligan and Schwartz [151] have demonstrated that human neonates have a higher elevation of blood glucose after galactose administration than adults. The elimination of intravenous galactose in the neonate has been reported by some to be slower than in the adult [151, 152], while others report no difference [153]. Vink and Kroes reported the elimination rate to be faster in young children than in adults [154].

The importance of galactose in metabolism of the young animal has been emphasized in recent studies involving perfusion of the immature liver. Sparks et al. [155] have reported that galactose infused into the isolated near-term monkey fetal liver regulates glycogen metabolism by enhancing the activity of glycogen synthetase and inhibiting phosphorylase, a phenomenon also seen in the adult [156]. In a series of studies of galactose infusion into liver of suckling 15-day-old rats, greater glucose output in the young compared to the adult was observed [157]. Almost quantitative conversion of galactose to glucose and a suppression of glucose formation from endogenous precursors occur in perfused suckling rat liver [158]. In addition, there is a lability of galactose metabolizing enzymes, especially galactokinase and galactose-1-phosphate uridyl transferase, which is not observed during perfusion of adult rat liver [59].

Galactose Enzymes and Mutations in Microorganisms

Studies of metabolism and genetic regulation in microorganisms have contributed greatly to modern concepts of gene function and enzyme synthesis. The work done with galactose mutants in bacteria, especially E. coli, deserves some mention in a consideration of disorders of galactose metabolism in human beings. Although the direct application of E. coli genetics cannot be made to humans, the knowledge gives a greater conceptual framework for viewing the human mutations.

Normally the ability of E. coli to metabolize galactose is inducible, i.e., incubation in solutions containing galactose is followed by the appearance of high levels of the enzymes of the sugar nucleotide pathway, galactokinase, galactose-1-phosphate uridyl transferase, and UDP-Gal-4-epimerase [159–161]. Numerous mutants have been described that are unable to metabolize galactose, the so-called Gal$^-$ mutants [162]. Analysis of these mutants has shown an absence of one or more of the enzymes of the pathway. In addition, Gal$^-$ mutants have been described with defective UDP-glucose pyrophosphorylase [106, 107]. Constitutive mutants have been described in which galactose no longer needs to be added to the media in order that the enzymes be present [163]. Genetic mapping of the galactose genes on the E. coli chromosome has been done. The sequence of the genes is kinase, transferase, epimerase, and operator (K-T-E-O) [164–166]. The UDP-glucose pyrophosphorylase maps in a different position on the E. coli chromosome. The K-T-E-O genes function as an operon, with a regulator gene that is not linked to the Gal region being present elsewhere on the chromosome [163]. Some constitutive mutations are located at the regulator gene site, but one has been described that is a mutation in the terminal region of the epimerase gene. This is a so-called operator constitutive mutation which no longer recognizes the ability of the product of the regulator gene to repress initiation of enzyme synthesis [163]. Recent studies indicate that two overlapping promotors control the expression of the gal operon in E. coli and that cyclic AMP and its receptor protein regulate promotor activity. In addition, DNA mapping and sequencing of the operator of the E. coli operon have been reported [43]. The works of Wilson and Hogness characterizing the protein structure of E. coli galactokinase [16] and UDP-galactose-4-epimerase [76] suggest that the genes are made up of 1100 base pairs. The molecular expression and regulation of galactose pathway enzymes in yeast have also been reported [167–170].

The effects of galactose on mutants with various enzyme deficiencies have been studied [171, 172]. The presence of galactose does not impair the growth of galactokinase-deficient organisms but does impede the growth of transferase-deficient organisms. Galactose-1-phosphate accumulates in the latter bacteria, and this inhibits glycerolkinase formation [173]. Epimerase-deficient [174, 175] and UDP-glucose pyrophosphorylase-deficient [106, 107] organisms have marked alterations in the composition of polysaccharides in their cell walls.

Perhaps the most fascinating aspect of E. coli galactose operon genetics is that a lysogenic bacteriophage called λ may incorporate the whole or a part of the galactose region of the E. coli chromosome into its own gene complement [176]. These phage particles have been termed λ dg. The λ dg phage is able to transduce the genes of the galactose operon into E. coli Gal$^-$ mutants [177]. That is, the λ dg may bring into a cell genetic material that will function to produce the galactose enzymes which the mutant was not able to do because of the genetic makeup in its own galactose operon. Such phenomena may ultimately have application to human genetic engineering for the correction of inherited metabolic defects. In theory at least, it seems possible that nonpathogenic viruses may be found which when grown on normal human fibroblasts will incorporate specific genetic material and on injection will infect body cells with reparative genes. Indeed, Merril et al. [178] have reported that bacterial virus infection with λ phage of transferase-deficient human fibroblasts can express the viral gene by detection of transferase activity.

TRANSFERASE DEFICIENCY GALACTOSEMIA

Clinical Aspects

The first detailed description of this syndrome by Mason and Turner in 1935 [1] was followed over the ensuing 25 years by numerous case descriptions that clearly established the clinical entity. The first reports of large groups of patients followed over a period of time appeared in 1961, when Hsia and Walker [179] discussed the variable clinical manifestations in 45 patients and Donnell et al. [180] described the growth of 24 affected children. The findings in 55 patients have been reported by Nadler and associates [181], and in 39 patients by Donnell et al. [182]. In 1970 Komrower and Lee reported a long-term follow-up of the 60 known cases of the disease in Great Britain [183]. Fishler et al. [184] updated the 27-year experience of the Los Angeles group in 1980.

The most common initial clinical symptom is failure to thrive. This occurs in almost all cases (Fig. 7-5). Vomiting or diarrhea was found in 52 out of 55 patients, usually starting

Figure 7-5 Patients with galactose-1-phosphate uridyl transferase deficiency. The left picture shows a child age 3½ months with inanition and hepatomegaly. In the middle is the same child after galactose restriction for 3 months. On the right is a 30-year-old man diagnosed in infancy by Mason and Turner [1].

within a few days of milk ingestion [181]. Signs of deranged liver function, either jaundice or hepatomegaly, are present almost as frequently after the first week of life. The jaundice of intrinsic liver disease may be accentuated by the severe hemolysis which may occur in some patients. Indeed, the peripheral blood picture may resemble that of erythroblastosis. Ascites may develop and is usually found in those infants who succumb. Cataracts have been observed within a few days of birth. These may be found only on slit-lamp examination by the ophthalmologist and are missed with an ophthalmoscope, since they consist of punctate lesions in the fetal lens nucleus. Retarded mental development may be apparent after the first several months of life. There appears to be a high frequency of neonatal death due to *E. coli* sepsis, with a fulminant course [185]. This may be due to inhibition of leukocyte bactericidal activity [186].

Occasionally, patients found to be homozygous for the disorder in the course of genetic studies have been asymptomatic while ingesting milk. These patients, in many instances, are black, and may be capable of metabolizing galactose [187]. There may be other patients who do not present a failure-to-thrive syndrome and are seen months after birth with motor retardation, hepatomegaly, and cataracts. The physician may be confronted with a child several years old with mental retardation and cataracts who proves to have this disorder. These children frequently have a history of partial treatment with

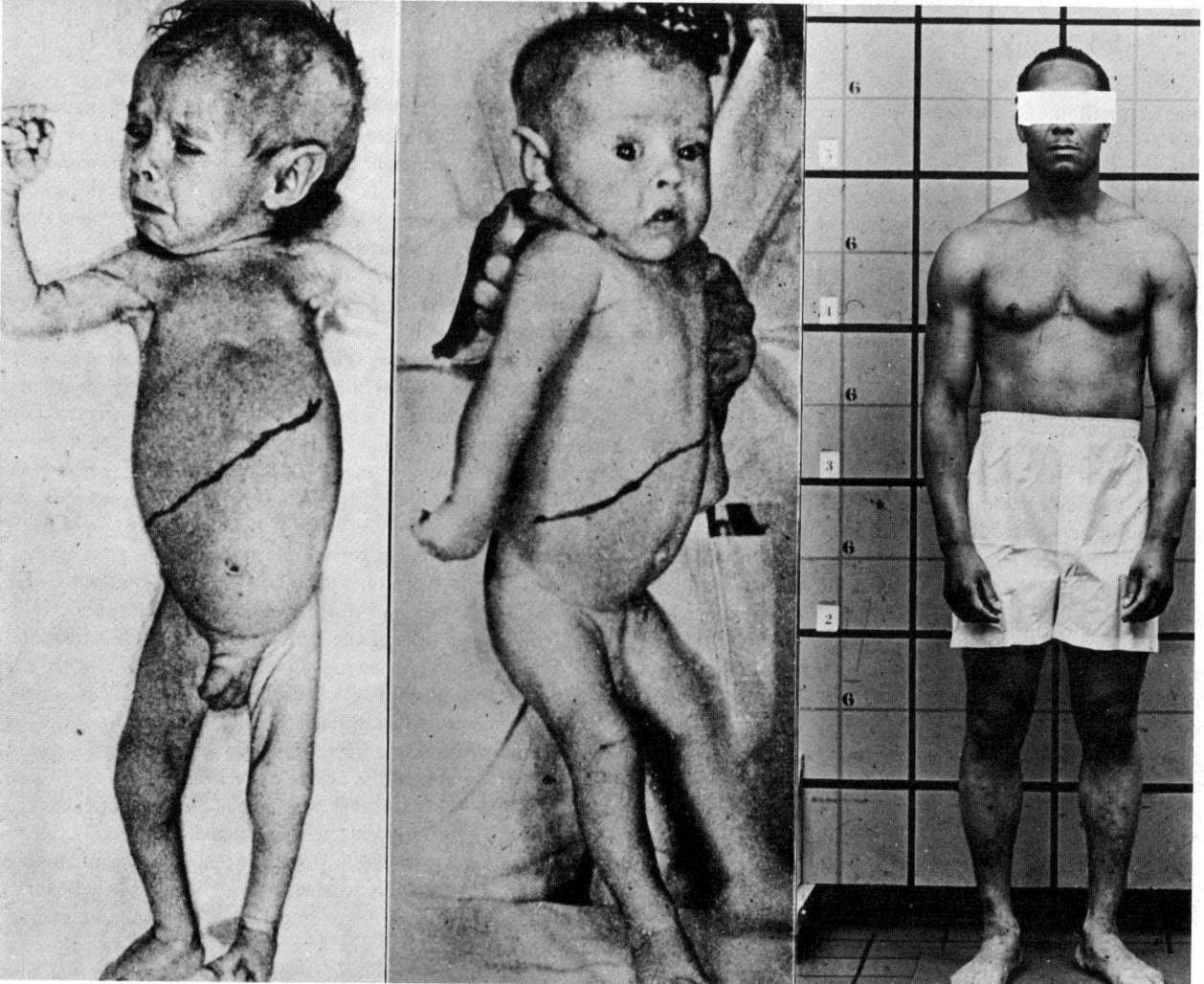

milk substitutes and reduced milk intake instituted because of vomiting on milk formulas.

The chemical findings, besides those of deranged liver function, include elevated blood galactose level, galactosuria, hyperchloremic acidosis, albuminuria, and aminoaciduria [2, 3]. On rare occasions, there may be a depression of blood glucose concentration. Hyperchloremic acidosis may be secondary to the gastrointestinal disturbance and poor food intake but can be a result of renal tubular dysfunction and a defect in urine acidification mechanisms [2]. The albuminuria [3] and the generalized renal aminoaciduria [188, 189] are manifestations of a renal toxicity syndrome. The galactosuria may be intermittent because of poor food intake or may disappear within 3 or 4 days with the use of intravenous glucose feeding. The finding of a urinary reducing substance which does not react in a glucose oxidase test is the alerting sign for considering a diagnosis of galactosemia. Yet these latter findings do not establish the diagnosis, since lactosuria also occurs in intestinal lactate deficiency, and severely impaired liver function due to viral or other causes may be accompanied by diminished galactose metabolism and galactosuria and be confused with galactosemia. The liver of affected patients has a characteristic acinar formation, so that liver biopsy on occasion has been helpful in establishing the diagnosis [190].

Management of Patients and Subsequent Course

At present the management of patients with galactosemia rests on the elimination of galactose from the diet. Failure to eliminate this sugar will usually result in progressive liver failure and death. Complete elimination of the sugar is the desired goal, but this may be difficult to accomplish. The preparations employed in infancy are Nutramigen, a casein hydrolysate, and soybean milks. Nutramigen may contain small amounts of lactose since it is prepared from milk, but this appears not to affect the therapeutic efficacy of the preparation. The use of soybean milk has been questioned because of the presence of sugars containing galactose such as raffinose and stachyose. However, Gitzelmann and Auricchio have shown that these galactose oligosaccharides are not hydrolyzed to their component sugars by human intestinal mucosa [191]. Furthermore, Donnell et al. have employed a soybean preparation in the treatment of several patients and have concluded there was no absorption of galactose [182].

As the children grow it is important to be aware of sources of galactose in foods other than milk. A list of permitted foods has been published [192]. The success of the procedure depends on parent education. There is no good evidence that at a prescribed age the diet can be relaxed. In childhood the ingestion of milk will result in gastrointestinal symptoms. It has frequently been observed that after puberty milk ingestion is tolerated without symptoms. Such findings have been interpreted as indication of the development of a metabolic capability. On the contrary, there are data to suggest that the patient with transferase-deficient galactosemia does not develop the ability to metabolize galactose as he increases in age [187]. In older patients, there may be psychologic problems associated with the adherence to stringent galactose restriction, and permission to include cakes, bread, and similar food should be considered. Milk restriction should be maintained. Schwarz [193] and Donnell and associates [182, 194] have

advocated assays of erythrocyte galactose-1-phosphate for monitoring adherence to the diet.

There is no evidence that dietary galactose restriction is harmful. Since the UDP-galactose-4-epimerase reaction is reversible and UDP-glucose can be converted to UDP-galactose, the body is able to provide adequately for the galactose component for brain cerebrosides and complex polysaccharides. Human intestinal lactase, does not appear to be diminished in patients with galactosemia who have not ingested lactose for many years [195].

Recently attention has focused on the restriction of dietary galactose during the pregnancies of women who have had children with galactosemia. This has stemmed from observations that the galactosemic syndrome is present at birth [179], from experimental evidence that the pups of pregnant rats fed high galactose diets are born with cataracts, and from other findings of galactose toxicity [196, 197]. Donnell et al. have carried out this restriction in 11 pregnancies resulting in transferase-deficient infants [182]. One had cataracts at birth but the other 10 were normal.

In those children with the manifestations of the toxicity syndrome, the galactose-free diet will cause a striking regression of all the symptoms and signs. Nausea and vomiting cease and weight gain ensues. Liver abnormalities clear; galactosuria, proteinuria, and aminoaciduria disappear. Cataracts will regress, and those visible with the ophthalmoscope may revert to small lesions seen only on slit-lamp examination. If the initial cataracts are not extensive, galactosemic patients who are well treated do not have impairment of sight because of cataracts. Subsequent growth and physical development appear to be within the normal range according to the findings in the large American groups [181, 182, 184]. The British experience [183] seems to be different, with most patients being below the 50th percentile in height and many below the 10th percentile. The explanation for this may be that the British collection of patients included many who were on poorly controlled diets and who were not cared for by the capable physicians who performed the survey. The experience of observers in this country has been that poor dietary control is associated with poor growth.

Mental retardation is the most significant outcome of clinical toxicity. The extent of retardation in transferase deficiency galactosemia differs from that of phenylketonuria in that extremely low IQ values are not generally seen even in those patients whose dietary therapy is started late in the first year. Of 41 patients followed by Donnell and associates [182], 29 had an IQ greater than 85 and 7 had an IQ within the 70 to 84 range. Only 3 were severely retarded. In this group, those whose mothers were on a galactose-free diet and who were treated from birth had normal IQ values. One patient first treated at 14 months of age also had a normal IQ. Nadler and coworkers [181], reviewing 44 patients, found 8 with IQs below 70 and 10 with IQs between 71 and 89. Those in the normal range as a group had lower IQs than their sibs. The correlation with time of institution of therapy and IQ was not clear in this series. In the British experience the average IQ of 32 patients on a good diet was 84, and of 22 patients on a moderately or poorly galactose-restricted diet was 77. Komrower and Lee [183] seem pessimistic about the outcome of dietary therapy. The eventual level of intelligence may be influenced by varying degrees of intrauterine damage due to fetal exposure to galactose. The best results are those of Donnell's group in whom intrauterine exposure to galactose was prevented by restricting lactose intake during pregnancy [182].

The assessment of long-term development published in 1972 [198] has recently been updated by Donnell's group. Table 7-1 summarizes the intelligence, visual-perceptual ability, and electroencephalogram findings in 60 patients. Children identified at birth to 1 month of age maintained the highest level of intellectual progress. Of 30 patients tested in the group, 15 had abnormal visual-perceptual status and 8 of 29 tested had abnormal electroencephalograms [184].

The actual measurement of IQ does not reveal the entire mental picture of these patients. Many with normal IQs are one or more grades behind in school and have specific learning disability involving spatial relationships and mathematics. Behaviorial problems are frequent because of short attention span. Psychologic problems seem to be prevalent, with inadequate drive, shyness, and withdrawal [181, 183]. These children may perform much better with close teacher supervision.

A recent new finding in the follow-up of transferase-deficient galactosemic patients is the high incidence of hypergonadotropic hypogonadism in females [199]. Ultrasonography of the pelvis showed that ovarian tissue was diminished or absent. There was no correlation of clinical course with ovarian function, but the frequency of hypogonadism was higher in females in whom diet therapy was delayed. All eight males examined had normal gonadal function. It appears that ovarian atrophy is an important manifestation of transferase deficiency galactosemia.

Detection of the Enzymatic Deficiency

The observation of Schwarz and associates [200] that galactose-1-phosphate levels were elevated in the red cells of patients with galactosemia was an important clue to the nature of the enzymatic defect. These observations suggested that the enzyme defect was in the subsequent metabolism of galactose-1-phosphate. Analysis of the enzymes catalyzing galactose conversion to glucose by Isselbacher et al. [6] subsequently demonstrated that these red blood cells specifically lacked the enzyme galactose-1-phosphate uridyl transferase. The deficiency of this enzyme has been demonstrated also in the white blood cells [201], skin fibroblasts [202], intestinal mucosa [60], and liver [54, 203] of these patients. Preliminary data suggested that the red cells of these patients contain a protein capable of neutralizing antibody to liver transferase [204].

Although an abnormally high amount of red cell galactose-1-phosphate has been used as a diagnostic criterion, the direct assay of red cell transferase activity provides the definitive diagnosis. The development of the red cell uridine diphosphate glucose consumption test by Anderson et al. [205] provided the

means of making the diagnosis and has been used extensively over the last decade. This procedure is based on the assay of UDP-glucose before and after incubation with galactose-1-phosphate and red cell hemolysate by measurement of the NAD formed in the conversion of UDP-glucose to UDP-glucuronic acid by UDP-glucose dehydrogenase. The kinetics of the reaction have subsequently been improved by increasing the substrate levels [206] and stabilizing the enzyme with sulfhydryl compounds [207]. With this procedure a complete absence of red cell transferase in homozygous patients is found and intermediate levels appear to characterize heterozygous carriers [208]. Several studies utilizing the UDP-glucose consumption test have been summarized by Hsia [209]. Normal red cell values are 6 μmol UDP-glucose consumed per hour per milliliter of RBC, or 25 μmol UDP-glucose consumed per hour per gram of hemoglobin.

Other approaches to the assay of Gal-1-P-uridyl transferase have involved the use of radioactive galactose [210] and galactose-1-phosphate as substrates, with an assay of the UDP-[^{14}C]galactose formed [201, 203, 211, 212]. This procedure has proved valuable for the study of reaction kinetics [45]. The oxidation of [^{14}C] galactose to $^{14}CO_2$ has also been used to assess a defect of galactose metabolism in various tissues [213, 214]. Employing this procedure, Ng and associates have shown that the red cells of three patients with absent transferase by the UDP-glucose consumption test had detectable $^{14}CO_2$ liberation and formation of small amounts of labeled UDP-galactose [215]. This type of test does not specifically determine a deficiency of transferase and may give abnormal results in galactokinase deficiency or any other deficient step in the series of reactions by which galactose is converted to CO_2.

Numerous methods for detection of the reaction product of the transferase reaction, glucose-1-phosphate, have been devised. These depend on conversion to glucose-6-phosphate and an assay of the NADPH formed when glucose-6-P dehydrogenase is added. This reaction has been coupled to the reduction of methylene blue [216], but NADPH may also be determined fluorometrically [217]. In galactosemic cells there is no dye decolorization, whereas in normal red cells the dye decolorizes in a fixed time interval (Fig. 7-6). This has been shown to be an effective screening method [216, 218], as has the spot test devised by Beutler and Baluda in which the NADPH formed a bright fluorescence under UV light in normal samples but was absent in cells from transferase-deficient galactosemic patients [219, 220].

The presumptive diagnosis of galactosemia may be made by the identification of galactose in the urine and blood of affected individuals. The finding of a reducing substance in urine which does not react with glucose oxidase reagents, such as Clinistix, is consistent with the presence of galactose, but lac-

Table 7-1 Distribution of intelligence, visual-perceptual ability, and EEG findings in galactosemic patients[*]

Group number	Group cases	Age range, years	DQ/IQ range	Mean DQ/IQ	Standard deviation	Visual-perceptual status		EEG status	
						Normal	Abnormal	Normal	Abnormal
I	13	0–5	70–125	102	12.8	4	—	4	1
II	25	6–16	50–117	91	17.5	7	18	12	12
III	22	17–29	72–119	94	18.2	14	8	17	5
Total sample				95	16				

[*]N = 60.
SOURCE: From Fishler, Koch, Donnell, and Wenz [184].

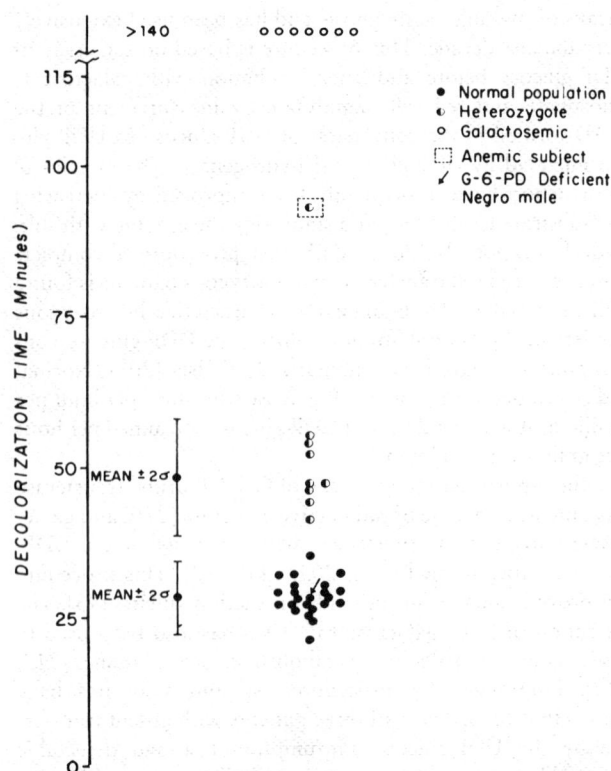

Figure 7-6 Reduction of methylene blue by venous blood samples as a detection method for transferase deficiency. Methylene blue is converted to its leuko form by the formation of NADPH resulting from the transferase assay procedure. The color change is detected visually. (*From E. Beutler, M. Baluda, and G. N. Donnell [216].*)

performed by glucose oxidase methods. Relatively specific methods for determining galactose in blood and urine with the use of galactose oxidase [145, 224–226] and galactose dehydrogenase [227] have been introduced. Dahlqvist has devised a paper impregnated with galactose oxidase which is very sensitive and when dipped in urine will permit detection of abnormal amounts of galactose [227, 228]. This appears to be useful in routine screening for galactosuria. It should be pointed out that many normal infants [227, 229], especially premature infants [227, 230] in the postnatal period have a physiologic melituria. Normal newborns have up to 60 mg galactose per deciliter urine in the first 5 days of life, while this level may be detected well into the second week of life in premature infants [227]. Some children with a high consumption of milk may have galactosuria [231]. The demonstration of galactosemia and galactosuria by the performance of a galactose tolerance test is not desirable as a diagnostic procedure.

Galactose Metabolism in Patients with Transferase Deficiency

Early attempts to measure the ability of galactosemic patients to metabolize galactose depended upon determination of the fraction of ingested galactose excreted in the urine. This ranged from 15 to 60 percent in 24 h; the remainder presumably was stored in the body or metabolized [3, 232]. A more accurate quantitative assessment has been devised in which the conversion of intravenously administered [14C]galactose to $^{14}CO_2$ is measured for a period of 5 h [129, 187, 233]. Of a group of 14 patients so studied, 9 converted the sugar slowly to $^{14}CO_2$, excreting 0 to 8 percent of the administered ^{14}C; and 5 oxidized the sugar at near-normal rates (Fig. 7-7). The ability to metabolize galactose to CO_2 was not related to sex, age, or puberty (Table 7-2). Those patients in the first group were reevaluated at intervals over a period of several years and did not develop greater ability to carry out the conversion. All these patients were Caucasian. The five subjects who oxidized significant amounts of galactose in spite of an absence of red cell transferase were all black. One of these was the patient reported by Mason and Turner in 1935. [1] in the first careful delineation of the galactosemic syndrome associated with transferase deficiency (Fig. 7-5). One of these black subjects

tose, fructose, and pentose may give similar results. The identification of the sugar may be made by paper chromatography [221] or gas-liquid chromatography [222, 223]. The intermittent nature of the galactosuria may make its detection difficult, and the sugar may not be detected in extremely dilute urine. Perhaps a greater hazard is the fact that many hospital laboratories routinely test urine only for glucose, with commercial glucose oxidase preparations which will not detect galactose. The unwary physician may believe the urine to be sugar-free. The same possibility holds for missing high blood galactose levels in hospital laboratories where a blood glucose test is

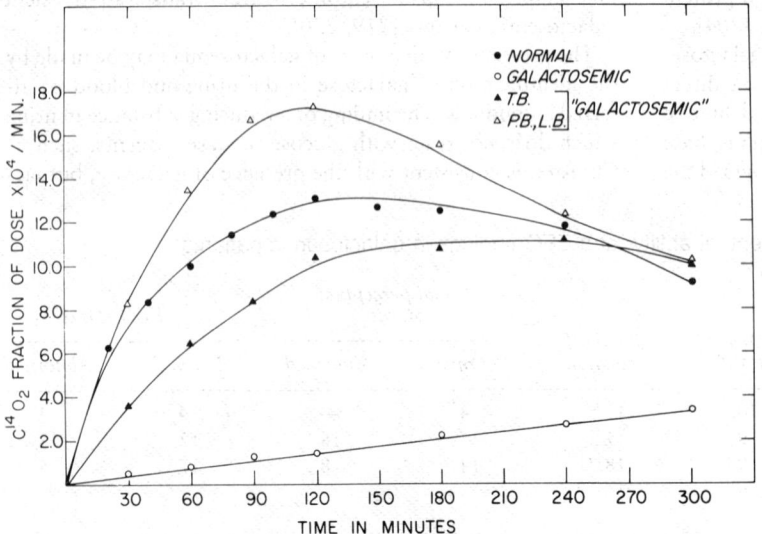

Figure 7-7 The excretion of $^{14}CO_2$ in expired air by normal subjects and patients with transferase deficiency after intravenous administration of 1-g quantitites of sugar containing [1-^{14}C]galactose. (*From S. Segal, A. Blair, and H. Roth [187].*)

Table 7-2 The oxidation of intravenous [1-^{14}C]galactose by normal subjects and patients with transferase deficiency galactosemia

Subject	Age, yr	Sex	Race*	Amount,* g	Administered ^{14}C in expired ^{14}CO$_2$ in 5 h, % injected[†]
Patients					
W.Wa	3	M	N	TR	21
	8			1.0	27
J.O.	6	M	C	TR	1
M.Wa	7	M	N	1.0	28
B.A.	7	M	C	1.0	8
L.F.	7	F	C	TR	8
E.W.	9	M	C	TR	0
P.R.	9	F	C	TR	3
	11			1.0	7
	15			1.0	7
P.Br.	10	F	N	TR	45
				1.0	42
L.J.	11	M	C	TR	1
	15			TR	5
	19			1.0	11
L.Br.	11	M	N	TR	36
				1.0	35
H.T.	14	M	C	TR	5
	17			1.0	5
J.S.	16	M	C	1.0	2
J.D.	16	M	C	TR	3
				1.0	5
T.B.	30	M	N	TR	19
				1.0	26
				2.0	28
				10.0	19
Normals[‡]					
3	18–21	M	C	TR	30–35
2	25–35	M	C	1.0	31–33
1	18	M	C	10.0	29
3	18–21	M	C	20.0	25–27

* TR = tracer, 1 to 5 mg; N = Negro; C = Caucasian.
† Patients received 1 to 3 μCi of ^{14}C sugar; normals, 5 μCi.
‡ Total number of normal subjects studied.
SOURCE: From Segal, Blair, and Roth [187]; Segal and Cuatrecasas [129]; Baker et al. [233]; and some unpublished data of the author.

was asymptomatic while ingesting galactose; his condition was detected only by family screening [233]. A similar black patient has been described by Hsia [209]. The ability of one subject to metabolize 10 g given intravenously was limited, but he could ingest 40 g galactose per day for 5 days without developing elevated blood galactose levels [234]. This patient converted galactose to blood glucose [187], demonstrated ethanol inhibition of galactose metabolism [187], and oxidized [1-^{14}C]galactose and [2-^{14}C]galactose in a normal pattern [129]. These observations are consistent with the function of the sugar nucleotide pathway. Liver biopsy specimens from two black patients oxidized [1-^{14}C]galactose to ^{14}CO$_2$ [233, 235]. Assay for the transferase activity of intestinal mucosa [60] and liver tissue [54] from black subjects has disclosed levels of about 10 percent of normal (Table 7-3). Caucasian patients have no enzyme detectable in these tissues. The findings strongly indicate that the capacity of black patients with galactosemia to metabolize limited amounts of galactose is based on residual transferase activity in visceral tissue. While the ability to metabolize galactose is correlated with race, a genetic basis is not truly established. The fact that sibs are involved favors a genetic origin. Why the black may have a galactose toxicity syndrome in the neonatal period is not known; perhaps this

phenomenon is due to the large amount of galactose ingested relative to the limited enzyme capacity.

Why any galactose oxidation is seen in Caucasian patients when no transferase is detectable in tissues is also unanswered. Measurements of ^{14}CO$_2$ for up to 9 h after the administration of labeled sugar have shown a progressive increase in the amount oxidized [129]. In these patients, one finds a different pattern and yield of ^{14}CO$_2$ when C-1 and C-2 labeled sugar is given. This is consistent with the direct oxidation of galactose to galactonate and the subsequent decarboxylation of C-1 [130]. Indeed, these patients excrete galactonate in urine after galactose is administered [108]. There is no indication that UDP-galactose pyrophosphorylase, which could circumvent the block at the transferase step, is active in these patients. Abraham and Howell [136] have demonstrated that this enzyme activity, which is very low, does not increase with age as postulated by Isselbacher [134], and Segal et al. [54] have shown insignificant activity in biopsy specimens of the liver of patients with galactosemia.

Several attempts have been made to stimulate galactose oxidation in Caucasian patients. Progesterone [236] and menthol [237] administration have enhanced the oxidation of tracer amounts of ^{14}C-labeled galactose, but the effect was not

Table 7-3 Activity of human liver and intestinal galactose-1-phosphate uridyl transferase

Subject	Age, yr	Race	Sex	Transferase activity, nmol/protein (min·mg)	
				Liver	Intestine
Controls					
B	41	C	F	11.8	
S	37	C	F	17.2	
C	2	C	F	16.1	
K	9	C	M	14.7	
U	4 (mo)	C	F	15.0	
S	23	C	M		15.2
D	21	C	M		12.2
H	22	C	F		8.9
M	22	C	F		12.3
L	22	C	M		15.8
Galactosemia*					
L.W.	7 (mo)	N	F		1.0
W.Wa	9	N	M	1.3	0.5
M.Wa	8	N	M	1.8	1.6
C.Wi	5	C	F	Nondetectable	Nondetectable
F.R.	2	C	M	Nondetectable	Nondetectable

* Nondetectable red blood cell transferase.
SOURCE: From Segal, Rogers, and Holtzapple [54]; Rogers, Holtzapple, Mellman, and Segal [60].

observed when larger amounts of the sugar were given [238]. Corticosteroids in high dosage cause no acceleration of impaired galactose metabolism [238]. Administration of orotic acid has been reported to be therapeutic when given to children showing galactose toxicity [239]; but under experimental conditions the oral administration of orotic acid seemed to have no influence on [14C]galactose oxidation [240].

The alternate route which is clearly functioning is that in which galactose is reduced by the enzyme aldose reductase to form the sugar alcohol, galactitol [118, 119]. Galactitol has been isolated from the tissues and urine of patients [112–114], and radioactive galactose given to a patient was converted to galactitol [241]. The sugar alcohol is not further metabolized or converted to carbon dioxide. After the administration of [14C]galactitol to normal subjects, all of the label is excreted in the urine, with none appearing as $^{14}CO_2$ [242]. Galactitol excretion in the urine continues for several days after galactosuria disappears. This seems to be the main route of elimination. Tissue accumulation of galactitol may be important in galactose toxicity.

In 1962 Inouye et al. demonstrated the presence of galactose-6-phosphate in galactosemic erythrocytes [243]. Presumably this ester could be formed from galactose-1-phosphate by the action of phosphoglucomutase. The galactose-6-phosphate can be oxidized further to 6-phosphogalactonate by an enzyme, hexose-6-phosphate dehydrogenase, found in red cells [243] and liver [244–245]. The significance of this pathway is unknown.

Galactose-1-phosphate can be generated in erythrocytes of transferase-deficient patients by pyrophosphorolysis of UDP-galactose, which is formed by the epimerization of UDP-glucose [246, 247]. Thus, galactose-1-phosphate accumulation in red cells is not necessarily due to phosphorylation of galactose by galactokinase.

Galactose utilization has been examined in cultured human fibroblasts from transferase-deficient [248–250] and galacto-

kinase-deficient patients [250]. When incubated with radioactive galactose, transferase-deficient cells produce $^{14}CO_2$ but at a very slow rate. Since little labeled carbon dioxide is obtained from galactokinase-deficient cells, it appears that the metabolic pathway involved utilizes galactose-1-phosphate. The clinical significance of these observations is open to question, since the substrate concentrations used are so minute as to have no physiologic significance. Transferase-deficient cells accumulate galactose-1-phosphate whether they are grown with galactose or glucose [249]. Pulse-chase studies with radioactive galactose indicate that galactose is taken up and phosphorylated, with the resulting galactose-1-phosphate then dephosphorylated to free galactose. Galactose then leaves the cell in a futile cycle of phosphorylation and dephosphorylation. Radioactive galactose incorporation in cell-surface glycoproteins of lymphocytes from transferase-deficient patients is only 7 percent of normal [251]. Despite this fact, there is no evidence for a deficiency of cell-surface galactose groups with good response to galactose-binding mitogens and sensitivity to galactose-binding toxic lectin.

Variants of Transferase Deficiency Galactosemia

In addition to the black variant described above, other variants have been found (Table 7-4). In 1965 Beutler and associates [252, 253], employing more sensitive methods, described another mutation at the transferase locus, termed the *Duarte* variant, which results in diminished red cell transferase activity but no clinical disorder. While screening a large number of blood samples for transferase activity, these workers found a number of specimens in which the enzyme level was 50 percent of normal. This was suggestive of heterozygosity for galactosemia, but pedigree studies revealed that the red cells of parents of these propositi had about 75 percent of normal enzyme levels. This was inconsistent with the genetics of the standard form of transferase deficiency galactosemia [254] (Fig. 7-8). Subsequent investigation of the enzyme of this variant showed that it is indistinguishable from normal with regard to the pH optimum, thermal stability, and Michaelis constant [68], but that it migrates faster on starch-gel electrophoresis [255]. Ng et al. [256] have demonstrated two distinct enzyme bands for the Duarte red cell enzyme, which migrate faster on gel electrophoresis than the single normal enzyme band. The enzyme activity of a sample from a parent of a subject homozygous for the Duarte variant reveals three bands, the normal and two bands for the variant enzyme.

All the data are consistent with the Duarte gene's being allelic with the normal and galactosemic gene. Indeed, Beutler et al. [254], Mellman and associates [257], and Gitzelmann and coworkers [258] have described individuals with lower levels of red cell transferase than the 50 percent of normal of either the galactosemic heterozygote or the Duarte homozygote. These subjects with 25 percent of normal enzyme activity are mixed heterozygotes, with one Duarte gene and one galactosemia gene (Fig. 7-8). Levy et al. [259] reported that the compound heterozygote for the Duarte variant and classic galactosemic gene is the most common abnormality detected by screening newborn infants for uridyl transferase deficiency. In none of the 10 subjects studied by Levy et al [259] were clinical abnormalities observed, although small amounts of galactose were present in 2 subjects after milk ingestion. On the other

Table 7-4   Characteristics of galactose-1-phosphate uridyl transferase variants

Variant	Erythrocyte transferase activity (% of normal)	Starch-gel electrophoretic mobility (compared to normal)	Other characteristics
Homozygotes			
"Classic"	0	Nondetected	
Duarte	50	Faster	
"Negro"	0	Nondetected	10% activity in liver & intestine
Münster	30	Nondetected	Inhibition by glucose-1-P
Heterozygotes			
Indiana	0–45	Slower	Unstable enzyme
Rennes	7	Slower	
Los Angeles	140	Faster	
Chicago	27	Faster	

hand, Kelly [260], who also observed 10 such genetic compound individuals, believes that this condition is not entirely benign early in life. One subject exhibited clear-cut signs of galactose toxicity for a brief period after birth, and three others had high blood galactose levels after several days of milk feeding. Adults with both allelic genes appear healthy. In those infants with high blood galactose levels, treatment with a low galactose diet seems prudent for the first few months of life.

Schapira and Kaplan [261] have reported two Congolese sibs living in France, ages 2 and 16 months, with the usual features of transferase deficiency galactosemia in the first few weeks of life. Red cell transferase was about 7 percent of normal, and starch-gel electrophoresis of the red cell enzyme revealed a fluorescence band which moved more slowly (i.e., had less anodic mobility) than the normal enzyme. The name *Rennes* was given to this variant. Hammersen, Houghton, and Levy [262], during the course of screening newborns for transferase deficiency, detected a Caucasian baby with about 10 percent of normal transferase activity in both erythrocytes and skin fibroblasts. The enzyme mobility during starch-gel electrophoresis was slower than normal and corresponded to that of the Rennes variant. The child was apparently healthy during

the first 3 weeks of life while on milk in spite of moderate galactosemia. Blood galactose levels after an oral galactose tolerance test rose to levels above 50 mg/dl, but the sugar was cleared from the blood by 3 h, contrary to what happens in subjects with classic uridyl transferase deficiency. The child's parents had enzyme activity in red cells and fibroblasts between 35 and 60 percent of normal, but no abnormal transferase was found on electrophoresis of hemolysates of either parent. Fibroblast enzyme from the mother, however, showed an elecrophoretic pattern suggesting that she is a carrier for the slowly moving Rennes variant. The best explanation is that the child was a double heterozygote (genetic compound) for "classic" transferase deficiency galactosemic gene and the Rennes variant.

A variant designated *Indiana* has been described [263] in an 18-month-old Caucasian girl who, when challenged with milk, had galactosemia, galactosuria, and galactose-1-phosphate elevation in her red cells. She had been on a galactose-free diet from birth because a sib had died at age 6 weeks with symptoms consistent with those of transferase deficiency galactosemia. Her erythrocyte transferase activity, which was approximately 35 percent of normal, was highly unstable, with rapid

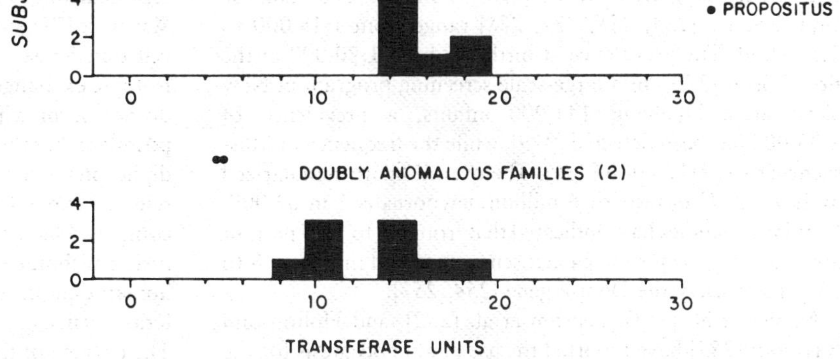

Figure 7-8 Distribution of transferase enzyme activity in patients and children of families with the galactosemia gene, who are designated type G, and those with the Duarte gene, who are labeled type D. In type G the propositi are heterozygous carriers for galactosemia (Gt+/gt). In the doubly anomalous families the propositi are thought to be heterozygous for both abnormal genes (GtD/gt). (*From E. Beutler* [253].)

loss of activity in heparin or in isotonic phosphate buffer. No activity of transferase was detected on electrophoresis of a hemolysate from this child's blood, probably because of instability. Erythrocyte transferase activities in the mother and maternal grandmother were 75 percent of normal, and showed instability on storage and a decreased mobility on electrophoresis. Pedigree analysis suggested that the father was a carrier for the classic uridyl deficiency galactosemia gene, while the mother carried the Indiana variant gene, which would make the patient a double heterozygote.

Ng, Bergren, and Donnell [264] have detected six families with a variant enzyme termed *Los Angeles*, and Ibarra et al. [265] have reported an additional family. Homozygotes and heterozygotes have erythrocyte transferase activity higher than normal but with an electrophoretic pattern similar to that observed with the Duarte variant enzyme. There is no associated abnormality of galactose metabolism. In the pedigree analyses subjects were found who appeared to be double heterozygotes for Los Angeles and Duarte variants, as well as for Los Angeles and classical uridyl transferase deficiency galactosemia. Of 418 presumed-normal Caucasian adults, 4.5 percent were found to be Los Angeles variant carriers. Several new variants have been described. One has been termed *Chicago*, an apparent genetic compound in which there is about 27 percent normal red cell activity and a faster electrophoretic pattern [266]. Of particular interest is what appears to be a homozygous entity described from Munster, West Germany [267]. Within the first 2 weeks of life, the patient developed vomiting, jaundice, failure to thrive, and hepatosplenomegaly which were reversed on a galactose-free diet. Analysis of red cell transferase indicated 30 percent of normal activity in a standard assay [268]. The enzyme became inactivated within 30 min of incubation. This was attributed to inhibition by the product, glucose-1-phosphate, an inhibition also produced by addition of other sugar phosphates. The enzyme exhibited a lowered affinity for galactose-1-phosphate, non-Michaelis-Menten kinetics with UDP-glucose. and was not detected on Collogel electrophoretograms.

Genetics and the Genetic Defect

Numerous investigations of red and white cell transferase of family members have indicated that the disorder is transmitted as an autosomal recessive trait [269–273]. Obligate heterozygotes have about 50 percent of normal activity [208, 210, 211, 216, 269–273]. The detection of the genotype in cultured fibroblasts and leukocytes is more accurate if the transferase/galactokinase ratio is determined [274]. Estimates of the prevalence of transferase-deficient galactosemia based on the detection of heterozygotes in Wales [275], Denmark [276], and the United States [254, 258, 277, 278] range from 1:18,000 to 1:180,000. The prevalence at birth has been 1:70,000 in the British Isles [270]. In a large-scale screening program in New York State involving 141,000 infants, a prevalence of 1:35,000 has been detected [279], while the frequency in Massachusetts is 1:190,000 [280]. The overall figure summarized by Levy [281] in tests of 6 million newborns is 1 in 62,000. Population studies have indicated that from 0.9 to 1.25 percent are heterozygous for the galactosemia gene and that from 8 to 13 percent carry the Duarte gene [254, 257].

Nadler et al. [181], Fensom et al. [282], and Holton and Raymont [283] have reported the use of amniocentesis for the

intrauterine diagnosis of the homozygote. This procedure has less significance here than for the potentially lethal and untreatable metabolic diseases, since the placement of pregnant heterozygous women on galactose-free diets and the dietary treatment of the infant may result in normal children. Normal pregnancy and childbirth have been described in galactosemic woman [284, 285].

The location of the gene for transferase activity was postulated by Brandt et al. [286] to be on human chromosome 21, since patients with Down's syndrome and trisomy 21 had transferase activity in whole blood specimens which was about 40 percent higher than that of normal subjects. Hsia et al. [287] found raised transferase activity in the white but not the red blood cells of patients with Down's syndrome. Rosner et al. [288], on the contrary, found elevation of the enzyme activity in red cells. A deletion of the long arm of chromosome 21, the so-called Philadelphia chromosome, is not associated with a decrease in transferase activity [289]. The finding that other leukocyte enzymes, such as galactokinase [290], acid phosphatase [291], and X-linked glucose-6-phosphate dehydrogenase [291], are elevated in patients with Down's syndrome has prompted the interpretation that the enzyme changes are secondary to a generalized derangement of white cells in this disease. Dahlqvist et al. [292] have found transferase elevations not only in trisomy 21 but also in patients with the Cornelia de Lange syndrome without chromosomal aberration. The assignment for the transferase gene locus has been made to human chromosome 9 [293–295]. Galactokinase was asyntenic with transferase and has been shown independently to segregate with chromosome 17 [34].

Significant studies have been made concerning the genetic defect at the molecular level. Tedesco and collaborators [296, 297], by double immunodiffusion techniques, have shown that rabbit antibody to purified human red cell galactose-1-phosphate uridyl transferase reacts with protein from patients with no red cell enzyme activity, thus establishing that there is an immunologic cross-reacting material identical to the normal enzyme but devoid of catalytic activity. Red cell extracts from Duarte-variant individuals give precipitin bands of complete identity against rabbit antibody to the human enzyme [55]. Duarte-variant erythrocyte transferase required twice as much antibody for complete precipitation of enzyme activity as the normal enzyme. These data suggest that the Duarte molecule is a protein identical to normal transferase but with less efficient catalytic activity. Dale and Popjak [69] isolated the inactive protein from transferase-deficient red cells in a pure state by affinity chromatography and have shown that peptide maps made after tryptic hydrolysis are identical to similarly prepared normal enzyme. All the data indicate that the inactive transferase results from a structural gene mutation resulting in the replacement of an amino acid, possibly near the catalytic site. Wu et al. [71] and Markes et al. [72] present evidence that red cell transferase may utilize a ping-pong mechanism and that isotopic exchange reactions carried out by the normal enzyme do not occur with enzyme of transferase-deficient cells; they postulate that the mutant enzyme either has a defective uridine diphosphate hexose binding site or is unable to cleave or release hexose-1-phosphate from an enzyme-nucleotide sugar complex. Nadler, Chacko, and Rachmeler [65], employing cell fusion technique, have found that hybrid cells formed from human diploid fibroblasts from different patients with transferase deficiency galactosemia demonstrate enzyme activity. The enzyme of these hybrid cells was similar to the normal in regard to K_m, pH, and electrophoretic mobility, but differed in V_{max}, specific activity, and thermal lability. They postulated interallelic complementation in the hybrid cells. Other interpretations are possible, especially with the demonstration that the enzyme consists of a dimeric structure [69, 70].

Pathogenesis of Galactose Toxicity

Since the patient with transferase deficiency exhibits a toxicity syndrome on ingestion of galactose, it has been assumed that the patient never exposed to the sugar should have no abnormalities. Long-term follow-up seems to indicate that this is not the case [184]. Galactose-1-phosphate can be elevated in red cells of patients not exposed to the sugar [246, 247] and can be formed from uridine diphosphogalactose by pyrophosphorylytic cleavage. This led Gitzelmann and Hansen [298] to postulate that galactosemics may have a continuous self-intoxication and that there may be uncontrolled biosynthesis of galactose from glucose even in well-treated infants. The fact that galactose-1-phosphate is the metabolite which accumulates behind the metabolic block has suggested that high levels of this substance cause derangements of cellular metabolism [299]. With the discovery that galactitol, the product of an alternate route, also accumulates in tissues, the emphasis has shifted to the toxic effects of this polyol. The biochemical cause for the toxicity in any organ may differ and be dependent on the peculiar metabolic patterns and structure of the organ. Investigation of the underlying disruption of cellular processes has depended mainly on changes induced in animals, especially young rats [196, 197, 300, 301] and chicks [302–305], which are fed diets abnormally high in galactose. In making use of these animal models, one must not lose sight of the fact that the enzymes of the sugar nucleotide pathway are present but in limiting quantity. Since the kinetics of the multienzyme galactose pathway and the rate-limiting step have not been clearly delineated, the situation is not entirely analogous to a complete metabolic block at the transferase step. For example, UDP-glucose appears to be depleted and UDP-galactose increased in tissues of these galactose-fed animals, a situation which may not obtain in the human disease [306, 307].

The Lens Investigations to elucidate the cause of the cataract provide a panoramic view of research in this field. The feeding of a 40 to 50 percent galactose diet to weanling rats uniformly induces cataracts within 2 to 3 weeks [236, 300, 308]. The amount of galactose in the diet and the age of the rat are critical, cataracts being induced most readily in the fetal rats whose mother is fed a high galactose diet [196] and with greater difficulty in older rats. Diets containing less than 30 percent galactose may induce cataracts only in some weanling rats and only after prolonged feeding [236]. A high fat diet [309], progesterone administration [236], and hypophysectomy [310] decrease the incidence of cataract induced by galactose. Galactose-1-phosphate is increased in the lens of the rat fed galactose [311], as well as in the lens of patients with galactosemia [312]. Early observations by Lerman [313] attempted to explain the cataract as a result of the inhibition by galactose-1-phosphate of glucose-6-phosphate dehydrogenase with a consequent decrease in glucose metabolism, but this has not been confirmed. Cataracts induced by feeding galactose to rats are reversible when galactose is removed from the diet. The reverse process has been well studied [314, 315, 316].

The demonstration by van Heyningen [109] that galactitol accumulates in the lens of rats fed galactose was followed by the work of Kinoshita and his associates, who demonstrated the presence of aldose reductase in the lens [118] and also demonstrated that the cataracts were closely associated with the imbibition of water by the lens as galactitol accumulated [317, 318]. Galactitol is formed within the lens and becomes osmotically active because it diffuses from the lens with difficulty. Experiments with the lens in vitro have shown that balancing the osmolality of the incubation media to the osmotic properties of galactitol prevents cataract formation. In experiments with an inhibitor of aldose reductase, 3,3-tetramethyleneglutaric acid, Kinoshita et al. found that prevention of polyol accumulation blocked the water accumulation and resulted in a transparent lens after 3 day's incubation in galactose [319] (Fig. 7-9). Many biochemical alterations occur concurrently in the lens undergoing galactose-induced cataract formation. These include alteration in protein synthesis [320, 321], amino acid transport [322–324], ion fluxes [325, 326], inositol content [324, 327, 328], carbohydrate enzymes [329], glutathione reductase [330], and abnormal phase separation of lens fiber cytoplasm. [331]. The change that appears first after the increased fluid uptake is a marked decrease in lens glutathione [318]. ATP changes occur late in the process and do not appear to be involved with the fundamental changes [332]. Glycolysis and respiration of the lens are reduced about 30 percent after 2 days of galactose feeding and remain at this level until cataracts occur [329]. It seems conclusive that the initiator of the cataractous process in rats is galactitol, not galactose-1-phosphate, the latter accumulating only late in the process. Substantiating evidence is found in patients with galactokinase deficiency who have cataracts in the absence of galactose-1-phosphate formation [7]. The formation of cataracts in galactose-fed rats can be prevented by nutrient supplements [333]. This suggests the nutrient imbalance may be a prime etiologic factor in the toxicity of galactose, especially in the lens.

Liver If the cause of cataracts seems clear, the reason for toxicity in the liver remains obscure. The severe liver damage seen in transferase deficiency is not observed in rats fed a high-galactose diet. Although the liver of children with galactosemia has elevated levels of galactose-1-phosphate [193] and galactitol [113], the livers of rats fed galactose accumulate galactose-1-phosphate but not galactitol [110]. Chicks fed galactose accumulate large amounts of galactitol without severe liver damage [111]. Patients with galactokinase deficiency who ingest large quantities of galactose and who form galactitol have no liver damage [7]. It may be that an as yet unknown metabolite is responsible for the liver damage. Of importance may be the recent demonstration of galactonate in the liver of galactose-fed rats and a galactosemic patient [127]. Galactosamine is known to induce liver damage in animals [334, 335], and 2-deoxy-D-galactose injection in rats is associated with inorganic phosphate and ATP depletion, which is associated with liver abnormalities [336, 337]. This may serve as a model for the study of liver cell injury in galactosemia.

Though microscopic liver damage is not seen in animals given galactose, biochemical abnormalities have been observed. In rats there is a decrease in liver glycogen [338] and diminished hexose phosphorylation [338], and in chicks an abnormal glycogen-containing galactose [339]. No decrease in ATP levels occurs. The hypoglycemia sometimes seen clinically and induced by feeding galactose to patients may be related to

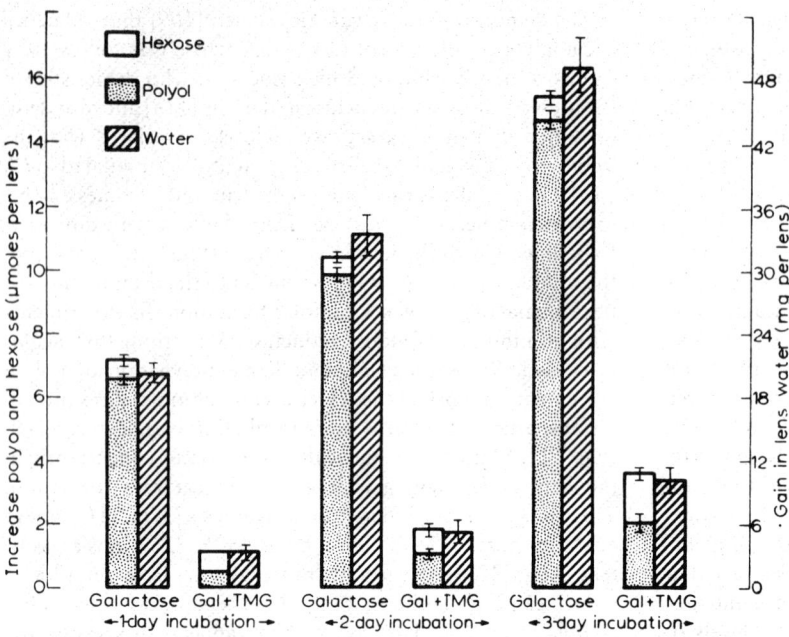

Figure 7-9 Prevention of galactitol formation and water accumulation by rabbit lens incubated with galactose. In 30 m*M* galactose solution, the lens which has been incubated for 3 days with 10 m*M* 3.3-tetramethylene glutaric acid (TMG), an aldose reductase inhibitor, remains clear. (*From J. H. Kinoshita, D. Dvornik, M. Kraml, and K. H. Gabbay [319].*)

deranged hepatic metabolism, since galactose does not stimulate the release of insulin from the pancreas [340, 341]. Sidbury postulated galactose-1-phosphate inhibition of phosphoglucomutase as an explanation [299], but this can only be shown in vitro in the absence of cofactor glucose-1-6-diphosphate. Patients given galactose have impaired hepatic glucose output [342] and do not respond normally to glucagon administration [343]. In a biopsy specimen from a single patient, the formation of glycogen from glucose was impaired [344].

Kidney Galactose-1-phosphate [193] and galactitol [113] have been detected in the kidney of patients with galactosemia. Galactitol accumulates in the kidney of rats fed galactose, large quantities being found in the renal papillae [123]. The aminoaciduria of transferase deficiency has not been seen in patients with galactokinase deficiency, by whom large amounts of galactitol are excreted in the urine [7]. Aminoaciduria has been induced in rats fed a high galactose diet [345], and in normal human subjects to whom galactose was given intravenously [346]. The incubation of slices of kidney cortex with galactose produces impairment of amino acid accumulation by tubule cells [347]. The inhibition, which is noncompetitive in nature, has been observed also in the intestinal mucosa of rats [348], a tissue which accumulates galactose-1-phosphate during galactose feeding [349].

Brain The one manifestation of galactose toxicity which may not be reversible is mental retardation. In patients with transferase deficiency, galactitol is found in the brain [112], and in rats fed galactose, galactitol accumulates to a greater extent in the brain than in any other tissue except the lens [110]. Enzymes of galactitol formation are active in nerve tissue [120]. The weanling or adult rat develops no apparent brain abnormality when fed galactose, but the fetuses of pregnant rats fed galactose have decreased brain development [350] and decreased amounts of brain DNA, especially in the cerebrum [351]. Wells and Wells have shown an impaired conversion of glucose to inositol in brain slices from newborn rats exposed to galactose in utero [352]. No impairment of glucose

conversion to inositol or alteration in inositol concentration was observed in isolated synaptosomes from similarly exposed animals [353], which may suggest that nonneuronal cellular elements may be responsible for the findings in brain slices. Some of the effects on brain development may reflect the smaller body weight and placentas which occur in this model [196]. Decreased nerve conduction has been reported in toxic rats [354, 355].

The chick given galactose in water develops ataxia and convulsions, followed by death [79, 111, 302–303, 356–358]. The findings are more severe in females and in certain strains and are associated with both galactose-1-phosphate [357], galactose-6-phosphate [359], and galactitol accumulation in brain [111]. They are reversible if the galactose is removed. This suggests that the changes seen pathologically in these brains [360] may be secondary.

Wells and his colleagues [358, 361–367] have performed an elegant series of biochemical studies of the effect of galactose feeding on chick brain metabolism. The changes resulting from galactose administration were a diminution of ATP and energy charge, diminution of brain glucose and glycolytic intermediates, redistribution of hexokinase, enhanced fragility of neural lysosomes, and a decrease in fast axoplasmic transport. Slight decrease in brain amino acid pools occurred, but polyribosomal profiles and protein synthesis were unaltered. The administration of glucose to the neurotoxic chick resulted in temporary cessation of symptoms [363], with brain ATP and glucose concentration returning to normal. Malone, Wells, and Segal [368] reported that the chick neurotoxicity syndrome correlated with hyperosmolar dehydration resulting from galactose feeding, and also showed decreased entry of glucose into brain [369]. They did not find a significant depletion of ATP. The decrease in ATP and energy charge observed by Granett et al. [362], although less than 10 percent, was statistically significant. The chick galactose toxicity syndrome may result from several factors, such as plasma hyperosmolarity and change in energy metabolism resulting from galactose phosphorylation or interference with transport of glucose into brain. Whether the chick neurotoxicity syndrome is related to the mental retardation observed in humans is open to question. Its acuteness and reversibility lead one to think it may not be. The rat does not respond to galactose administration with acute brain toxicity, although a decrease in brain glucose [125] and amino acids has been observed [370]. The finding of pseudotumor cerebri as a toxicity manifestation of both human transferase [371] and galactokinase [372] deficiency indicates changes relative to osmolality of brain tissue and biologic fluids. Detailed studies of inositol and phosphatidylinositol metabolism in synaptosomes from galactose-fed rats have indicated that there is an impaired response to acetylcholine in increasing the incorporation of inositol into phosphatidylinositol [353]. Incorporation of inorganic phosphate as a response to acetylcholine was not impaired. This suggests that the effect of galactose feeding is at a biochemical site distal to the acetylcholine receptor [373]. Woolley has suggested that serotonin depletion in the brain is a basic cause of mental retardation in various toxic states [374]. Woolley and Gommi explain the retardation of galactosemia on the basis of decreased serotonin receptors [375]. No abnormality has been observed on direct measurement of serotonin uptake by synaptosomes from galactose intoxicated rats [376], which raises some doubt about the Woolley and Gommi hypothesis.

Cell Toxicity   Galactose toxicity has been demonstrated in tissue culture [377]. The growth of fibroblast cultures from patients with transferase deficiency is inhibited by galactose. Electron microscopy of transferase-deficient cells incubated with galactose reveals striking dilatation of the endoplasmic reticulum, and cytoplasmic degeneration and cell death within 72 h. Fibroblasts from transferase-deficient cells have impaired incorporation of radioactive sulfate when exposed to galactose [378]. Red cells with the defect have impaired oxygen uptake when incubated with galactose [200]. A decrease in ATP described under these conditions [379] has not been confirmed [380]. The fact that mutants of *E. coli* deficient in transferase have an impaired growth in galactose media, while galactokinase mutants do not, implies that galactose-1-phosphate is related to the toxicity in bacteria [171, 172].

GALACTOKINASE DEFICIENCY GALACTOSEMIA

Clinical Aspects

This disorder was first described in 1965 [7, 8]. Since the first reports, there have been several others [381–390]. The wealth of knowledge garnered about the transferase deficiency disorder over the past 3 decades has not yet been duplicated in galactokinase deficiency.

The first patient recognized to have galactokinase deficiency was a male 44 years old at the time of biochemical diagnosis by Gitzelmann [7, 8]. Galactosuria after milk ingestion was detected when he was treated for cataracts in 1932 at the age of 9. Investigations at that time led Fanconi to call the patient's condition *galactose diabetes* [391]. His sisters had been seen in 1909 at ages $5\frac{1}{2}$ and $7\frac{1}{2}$ by ophthalmologists because of cataracts, but melituria had not been recognized. The impression by physicians was that both girls were mentally retarded. Dietary restrictions were never imposed, and the patients

developed recurrent cataracts, poor vision, and blindness. Both females married and had several children. When studied, the 44-year-old male was ingesting 3 qt of milk a day without obvious effects. He was blind and complained of weakness and pain in his extremities which was attributed to neurofibromatosis. No IQ tests were performed on any of these patients, but the impression was that though they were illiterate, their intelligence as adults was normal. There was never any evidence of jaundice or liver disease, and no aminoaciduria or proteinuria was detected [7].

The newborn with this disorder reported by Thalhammer et al. [383] was an apparently normal female who on a routine screen of capillary heel blood at 7 days of life was found to have 100 mg galactose per deciliter of blood. Routine examination at the time revealed no hepatosplenomegaly or gastrointestinal disturbance. When the infant was 17 days old and still on milk feedings, the liver and spleen were felt just below the costal margin. Ophthalmologic examination revealed circumscript opacities along the posterior lens suture, but they were not thought to be abnormal. Jaundice was not present. Total serum bilirubin was 2.0 mg/dl (direct, 1.2 mg/dl). Serum enzyme tests of liver function were normal. The infant was placed on a galactose-free diet on day 20 and at age $4\frac{1}{2}$ months was found to be thriving and without other abnormalities.

The 9-year-old child reported by Monteleone et al. [381] had cataracts and red cells deficient in galactokinase, but no evidence of liver or renal disease or mental retardation. The two 4-month-old twins of McVie et al. [382] were admitted to a hospital for hernia repair and were discovered incidentally to have high blood galactose levels and high urinary galactitol, but no liver disease or aminoaciduria. Ophthalmologic examination revealed bilateral perinuclear zonular cataracts in both infants. Pickering and Howell [389] have described a patient in whom development was normal (except for cataracts) until age 17, when there was the onset of uncontrollable generalized seizures and severe debilitation. The relationship, however, of the neurologic involvement to the enzyme deficiency is unclear, especially since the patient had been on an essentially galactose-free diet from an early age. Two sibs have been described with galactokinase deficiency who are quite retarded mentally [392].

Diagnosis

The absence of inanition, gastrointestinal dysfunction, and jaundice in the newborn period and the appearance of cataracts in the older patients on unrestricted diets differentiate this disorder from transferase deficiency galactosemia. In the absence of severe manifestations, it is apparent that the diagnosis in early infancy will depend upon the routine screening of blood and urine for galactose. Since cataracts may be the first and only abnormality, this disorder should be suspected in any child with cataracts. Galactokinase deficiency should also be considered in patients with pseudotumor cerebri [372].

The presence of a reducing substance in the urine may be identified as galactose by the methods described above for transferase deficiency. Thalhammer and coworkers [319] indicate that high blood galactose levels are best detected after milk feedings and that the level may be low in morning fasting specimens. The diagnosis can be made by the finding of normal amounts of galactose-1-phosphate uridyl transferase and an absence of galactokinase in the red blood cells [7]. Like transferase-deficient red cells, those with no galactokinase will be unable to oxidize galactose ^{14}C to ^{14}CO$_2$ [7]. The urine of all young patients with cataracts should be examined for sugar with methods other than those using glucose oxidase; there should also be an assay of the red cells for the defect. In the kindred reported by Monteleone et al. [381], cataracts developed later in life in heterozygous relatives. This led Beutler et al. [393] to suggest that heterozygotes may be at risk for cataracts. In a subsequent survey of galactokinase activity of blood of 210 patients who developed cataracts before the age of 40, Beutler et al. [394] found two patients with absence of galactokinase. These patients developed cataracts in the first year of life. There was a statistically significant lowering of enzyme activity among 92 other patients whose cataracts developed during the first year of life. Skalka and Prchal [395] have also found a significant reduction of red cell galactokinase in 47 percent of patients age 50 or under who had bilateral cataracts. Therapy for the disorder should be aimed at galactose restriction, as in transferase deficiency.

Galactose Metabolism in Galactokinase Deficiency

Gitzelmann studied the 44-year-old male with this disorder by milk loading and found that large quantities of ingested galactose were excreted as galactitol [7]. After ingesting 360 g galactose over a period of 5 days without ill effects, he excreted 192 g as galactose and 48 g as galactitol. On most test procedures the urinary galactitol to galactose ratio was about 1:4.

The author, in collaboration with Dr. Gitzelmann and Dr. H. J. Wells, has studied the metabolism of galactose in the same male patient by injection of radioactive galactose and determination of ^{14}CO$_2$ expired over a 5-h period [396]. After injection of [1-^{14}C]galactose, only 5 percent of the label appeared in expired air, an amount similar to that seen in Caucasian transferase-deficient patients (Table 7-2). Essentially no label was excreted as CO$_2$ after the injection of [^{14}C]galactitol or galactonate. The low yield of ^{14}CO$_2$ from galactose indicated that galactokinase deficiency exists in tissues other than the peripheral blood cells, the only type of cells directly assayed. This finding indicates that lack of severe galactose-induced toxicity is not due to a situation similar to that seen in black subjects with transferase deficiency, where the subjects lack the enzyme in the blood cells but have residual enzyme activity in the liver (Table 7-3) and can metabolize the sugar (Table 7-2 and Fig. 7-7). The lack of galactitol oxidation and almost total excretion of the labeled galactitol in urine are consistent with galactitol being an end product in galactose metabolism.

Genetics and Screening

Gitzelmann's erythrocyte assay for galactokinase among the kindred of the three adult patients revealed several members with values intermediate between those of the patients and a group of 100 normal subjects [7]. Mayes and Guthrie [397] have screened the red blood cells of 642 persons for galactokinase and have found the cells in 6 of them to have half the normal activity. Their data are consistent with an autosomal recessive inheritance. The estimate of heterozygotes is 1:107

and for homozygous births is about 1:40,000. The newborn described by Thalhammer and colleagues [383] with complete deficiency was the first detected with galactosemia after the analysis of 35,770 blood samples for galactose. It is interesting that the first four patients described were members of unrelated gypsy families. Tedesco et al. [33, 278] have observed a racial polymorphism for erythrocyte galactokinase, with activity being about 30 percent lower in pregnant black females than in white females. Their genetic analysis [278] suggests that there is a variant gene in the black population. Mellman et al. [398] have reported that some individuals heterozygous for galactokinase deficiency may have an abnormal galactose tolerance test. The results of screening 6 million infants worldwide reported by Levy [281] indicate the detection of only 6 infants with galactokinase deficiency, in contrast to 97 with transferase deficiency. Pickering and Howell [389] have assessed galactokinase activity in human fibroblasts [from a homozygous patient and obligate heterozygotes. Fibroblasts from the patient had no detectable activity, while heterozygote cells had about half the normal activity.

Toxicity Factors

The basis of the galactose toxicity syndromes has been discussed above under "Transferase Deficiency Galactosemia." The topic is considered again here because of the contribution to the understanding of galactose-induced toxicity by the discovery of galactokinase deficiency. It seems clear that cataracts are the chief result of failure to phosphorylate galactose, with the reduction of galactose to galactitol through an alternative metabolic route. The absence of liver and kidney damage in galactokinase deficiency and the presence of damage to these organs in transferase deficiency make it likely that toxicity is in some way associated with galactose-1-phosphate formation. Not enough information is at hand to dissociate conclusively the mental retardation from galactokinase deficiency, although the evidence suggests that retardation is not a feature. If this is true, then brain damage in transferase deficiency would be the result of galactose phosphorylation and of the failure of galactose-1-phosphate to be further metabolized.

Animal Models   Galactose toxicity has been studied in the galactose-fed rat and chick, as indicated earlier. In both these instances, the enzymes of galactose metabolism are normal but their capacity is exceeded by the large amounts of ingested sugar. These models, therefore, are not entirely comparable to patients with single enzyme deficiencies. Stephens et al. [399, 400] have detected what may be a suitable animal model. They reported the occurrence of cataract formation and diarrhea in orphan kangaroos fed cow's milk during rearing. The red cells of the gray kangaroo were found to contain only about 10 percent of the galactokinase and uridyl transferase activity of human red cells. Red kangaroo erythrocytes contain 10 percent of human cell galactokinase activity and 50 percent of the human cell transferase activity. A subsequent study was made of galactose handling by the kangaroo [401]. Galactose tolerance of young kangaroos was greatly impaired but improved markedly at the stage at which definitive structure of the ruminant type of stomach in adults is formed. Cataract formation was seen only in pouch-young animals. Erythrocyte enzymes have been analyzed in a variety of marsupial species. Many show both galactokinase and transferase deficiency. The koala and wombat have primarily a transferase deficiency and may be suitable models for transferase deficiency galactosemia. Kangaroo milk contains little lactose, so that the enzymatic deficiencies are of no physiologic concerns except when the animals are given lactose-containing milk.

URIDINE DIPHOSPHATE GALACTOSE-4-EPIMERASE DEFICIENCY

Gitzelmann [402] has reported a newborn child who was found by a bacterial screening procedure for blood galactose to have elevated galactose levels but who had normal uridyl transferase and galactokinase levels. Red cell epimerase was absent. Subsequent investigation revealed that the level of galactose was not elevated in the blood but that the level of red cell galactose-1-phosphate was elevated. (The bacterial assay was capable of detecting the phosphorylated compound.) A 2-year follow-up report of the patient by Gitzelmann and Steinmann [403] revealed normal growth and development, with normal ability to metabolize ingested galactose. The only metabolic consequence of galactose ingestion was the elevation of galactose-1-phosphate in red cells, without any resulting red cell abnormality.

Epimerase activity was absent in both erythrocytes and leukocytes but was normal in cultured skin fibroblasts and in a liver biopsy specimen from the patient. Thirty-nine members of the family were examined for red cell enzyme activity. The related parents both have levels of epimerase activity below the range of normal, and the pedigree analysis was consistent with a recessive inheritance of the trait. Gitzelmann et al. [404] have now reported eight cases of epimerase deficiency in three families. All persons were healthy and had normal galactose tolerance, the only abnormality being a rise in red cell galactose-1-phosphate. The deficiency was restricted to circulating blood cells.

Mitchell et al. [405] have reported that phytohemagglutinin stimulation of leukocytes from these patients results in the appearance of epimerase activity. The enzyme activity is also present in lymphocytes maintained in long-term culture. Properties of the enzyme in such cultures are similar to those of the normal enzyme except for heat stability at 40°C. The mutant enzyme appears to be unstable and to require higher NAD concentration for maximum activity [404].

Supported by Grant AM 10894 from the National Institutes of Health.

REFERENCES

1. MASON HH, TURNER ME: Chronic galactosemia. Am J Dis Child 50:359, 1935
2. KOMROWER GM, SCHWARZ V, HOLZEL A, GOLDBERG L: A clinical and biochemical study of galactosemia. Arch Dis Child 31:254, 1956
3. HOLZEL A, KOMROWER GM, SCHWARZ V: Galactosemia. Am J Med 22:703, 1957
4. ISSELBACHER, KJ: Galactose metabolism and galactosemia. Am J Med 26:715, 1959
5. HOLZEL A: Galactosemia. Br Med Bull 17:213, 1961
6. ISSELBACHER KJ, ANDERSON EP, KURAHASHI K, KALCKAR HM: Congeni-

tal galactosemia, a single enzymatic block in galactose metabolism. Science 123:635, 1956
7. GITZELMANN R: Hereditary galactokinase deficiency, a newly recognized cause of juvenile cataracts. Pediatr Res 1:14, 1967
8. GITZELMANN R: Deficiency of erythrocyte galactokinase in a patient with galactose diabetes. Lancet 2:670, 1965
9. CAPUTIO R, LELOIR LF, TRUCCO RE: Lactase and lactose fermentation in S. fragilis. Enzymologia 12:350, 1948
10. CARDINI CE, LELOIR LF: Enzymatic phosphorylation of galactosamine and galactose. Arch Biochem Biophys 45:55, 1953
11. LELOIR LF: Enzymatic transformation of uridine diphosphate glucose into galactose derivative. Arch Biochem Biophys 33:186, 1951
12. KALCKAR HM, BRAGANCA B, MUNCH-PETERSEN A: Uridyl transferases and the formation of uridine diphosphate galactose. Nature (Lond.), 172:1038, 1953
13. WILKINSON JF: The pathway of the adaptive fermentation of galactose by yeast. Biochem J 44:460, 1949
14. HEINRICH MR: The purification and properties of yeast galactokinase. J Biol Chem 239:50, 1964
15. SHERMAN JR, ADLER J: Galactokinase from E. coli. J Biol Chem 238:874, 1963
16. WILSON D, HOGNESS D: The enzymes of the galactose operon in E. coli. III. The size and composition of galactokinase. J Biol Chem 244:2137, 1969
17. ATKINSON M, BARTON R, MORTON R: Equilibrium constant of phosphoryl transfer from adenosine triphosphate to galactose in the presence of galactokinase. Biochem J 78:813, 1961
18. GULBINSKY J, CLELAND W: Kinetic studies of Escherichia coli galactokinase. Biochemistry 7:566, 1968
19. SCHELL MA, WILSON DB: Purification and properties of galactokinase from Saccharomyces cerevisiae. J Biol Chem 252:1162, 1977
20. CITRON BA, FEISS M, DONELSON JE: Expression of the yeast galactokinase gene in Escherichia coli. Gene 6:251, 1979
21. CUATRECASAS P, SEGAL S: Mammalian galactokinase. J Biol Chem 240:2382, 1965
22. WALKER DG, KHAN HH: Some properties of galactokinase in developing rat liver. Biochem J 108:169, 1968
23. BALLARD FJ: Purification and properties of galactokinase from pig liver. Biochem J 98:347, 1966
24. NG WG, DONNELL GN, BERGREN WR: Galactokinase activity in human erythrocytes of individuals at different ages. J Lab Clin Med 66:115, 1965
25. MATHAI C, BEUTLER E: Biochemical characteristics of galactokinase from adult and fetal human red cells. Enzymologia 33:14, 1967
26. TEDESCO TA, MELLMAN WJ: Galactose-1-phosphate uridyltransferase and galactokinase activity in cultured human diploid fibroblasts and peripheral blood leukocytes. I. Analysis of transferase genotypes by the ratio of the activities of the two enzymes. J Clin Invest 48:2390, 1969
27. CHACKO CM, MCCRONE L, NADLER HL: A study of galactokinase and glucose 4-epimerase from normal and galactosemic skin fibroblasts. Biochim Biophys Acta 284:552, 1972
28. SRIVASTAVA SK, BLUME KG, VAN LOON C, BEUTLER E: Purification and kinetic properties of galactokinase from human placenta. Arch Biochem Biophys 150:191, 1972
29. SHIN-BUEHRING YS, BEIER T, TAN A, OSANG M, SCHAUB J: The activity of galactose-1-phosphate uridyltransferase and galactokinase in human fetal organs. Pediat Res 11:1003, 1977
30. COHN R, SEGAL S: Galactose metabolism and its regulation. Metabolism 22:627, 1973
31. ZACCHELLO F, BENSON PF, BROWN S, CROLL P, GIANNELLI F: Induction of galactokinase in fibroblasts from heterozygous and homozygous subjects. Nature [New Biol] 239:95, 1972
32. BLUME KG, BEUTLER E: Purification and properties of galactokinase from human red blood cells. J Biol Chem 246:6507, 1971
33. TEDESCO TA, BONOW R, MILLER K, MELLMAN WJ: Galactokinase: Evidence for a new racial polymorphism. Science 178:176, 1972
34. ELSEVIER SM, KUCHERLAPATI RS, NICHOLS EA, CREAGAN RP, GILES RE, RUDDLE FH, WILLECKE K, MCDOUGALL JK: Assignment of the gene for galactokinase to human chromosome 17 and its regional localisation to band q21-22. Nature (Lond) 251:633, 1974
35. MAGNANI M, CUCCHIARINI L, STOCCHI V, BOSSU M, DACHA M, FORNAINI G: Comparative studies of galactokinase activity on mammal's red blood cells. Comp Biochem Physiol 64B:267, 1979
36. MISHKIN JD, TAYLOR BA, MELLMAN WJ: Glk: A locus controlling galactokinase activity in the mouse. Biochem Gene 14:635, 1976
37. ROGERS S, KIRSCH S, SEGAL S: Enzymes of galactose metabolism in erythrocytes and liver of inbred strains of mice. Life Sci 24:2159, 1979
38. PARKS JS, GOTTESMAN M, PERLMAN RL, PASTAN I: Regulation of galactokinase synthesis by cyclic adenosine 3',5'-monophosphate in cell-free extracts. J Biol Chem 246:2419, 1971

39. NISSLEY SP, ANDERSON WB, GOTTESMAN ME, PERLMAN RL, PASTAN I: *In vitro* transcription of the gal operon requires cyclic adenosine monophosphate and cyclic adenosine monophosphate receptor protein. *J Biol Chem* 246:4671, 1971

40. TAO M, SCHWEIGER M: Stimulation of galactokinase synthesis in *Escherichia coli* by adenosine 3',5' cyclic monophosphate. *J Bacteriol* 102:38, 1970

41. ROBERTS CT, JR, MORSE DE: Genetic regulation of galactokinase in *Tetrahymena* by cyclic AMP, glucose, and epinephrine. *Proc Natl Acad Sci USA* 75:1810, 1978

42. ROTHMAN-DENES LB, HESSE JE, EPSTEIN W: Role of cyclic adenosine 3',5'-monophosphate in the *in vitro* expression of the galactose operon of *Escherichia coli*. *J Bacteriol* 114:1040, 1973

43. DILAURO R, TANIGUCHI T, MUSSO R, DE CROMBRUGGHE B: Unusual location and function of the operator in the *Escherichia coli* galactose operon. *Nature* 279:494, 1979

44. KURAHASHI K, SUGIMURA A: Purification and properties of galactose-1-phosphate uridyl transferase from *E. coli*. *J Biol Chem* 235:940, 1960

45. BERTOLI D, SEGAL S: Developmental aspects and some characteristics of mammalian galactose-1-phosphate uridyl transferase. *J Biol Chem* 241:4023, 1966

46. SAITO S, OZUTSUMI M, KURASHASHI K: Galactose-1-phosphate uridyl transferase of *E. coli*. *J Biochem* 242:2362, 1967

47. WONG LJ, FREY PA: Galactose-1-phosphate uridyl transferase: Rate studies confirming a uridyl-enzyme intermediate on the catalytic pathway. *Biochemistry* 13:3889, 1974

48. REX SHEU KF, RICHARD JP, FREY PA: Stereochemical courses of nucleotidyltransferase and phosphotransferase action. Uridine diphosphate glucose pyrophosphorylase, galactose-1-phosphate uridylyltransferase, adenylate kinase, and nucleoside diphosphate kinase. *Biochemistry* 18:5548, 1979

49. RAYCHOWDHURY R, SCHLESINGER DH, WILSON DB: *E. coli* galactose-1-phosphate uridyl transferase: N-terminal and C-terminal sequences. *Molec Cellular Biochem* 23:167, 1979

50. YANG S-LL, FREY PA: Nucleophile in the active site of *Escherichia coli* galactose-1-phosphate uridylyltransferase: Degradation of the uridyl-enzyme intermediate to N³-phosphohistidine. *Biochemistry* 18:2980, 1979

51. SEGAWA T, FUKASAWA T: The enzymes of the galactose cluster in *Saccharomyces cerevisiae*. *J Biol Chem* 254:10707, 1979

52. KURAHASHI K, ANDERSON E: Galactose-1-phosphate uridyl transferase, its purification and application. *Biochim Biophys Acta* 29:498, 1958

53. MAYER JS, HANSON RG: Galactose-1-phosphate uridyl transferase, in Wood WA (ed): *Methods of Enzymology*. New York, Academic Press, Inc, 1966, vol 9, p 708

54. SEGAL S, ROGERS S, HOLTZAPPLE PG: Liver galactose-1-phosphate uridyl transferase: Activity in normal and galactosemic subjects. *J Clin Invest* 50:500, 1971

55. TEDESCO TA: Human galactose-1-phosphate uridyl transferase. *J Biol Chem* 247:6631, 1972

56. SCHAPIRA F, GREGORI C, BANROQUEST J: Microheterogeneity of human galactose-1-phosphate uridyl transferase. Isoelectrofocusing results. *Biochem Biophys Res Commun* 80:291, 1978

57. KEPPLER D, FROHLICH J, REUTER W, WIELAND O, DECKER K: Changes in uridine nucleotides during liver perfusion with D-galactosamine. *FEBS Lett* 4:278, 1969

58. SEGAL S, ROGERS S: Nucleotide inhibition of mammalian liver galactose-1-phosphate uridyl transferase. *Biochim Biophys Acta* 250:351, 1971

59. ROGERS S, SEGAL S: Changing activities of galactose metabolizing enzymes during perfusion of suckling rat liver. *Am J Physiol* 240:E333, 1981

60. ROGERS S, HOLTZAPPLE PG, MELLMAN WJ, SEGAL S: Characteristics of galactose-1-phosphate uridyl transferase in intestinal mucosa of normal and galactosemic humans. *Metabolism* 19:701, 1970

61. KOO C, ROGERS S, SEGAL S: Developmental aspects of galactose-1-phosphate uridyltransferase in rat intestine. *Biol Neonate* 27:153, 1975

62. STIFEL FB, HERMAN RH, ROSENWEIG NS: Dietary regulation of galactose metabolizing enzymes: Adaptive changes in rat jejunum. *Science* 162:692, 1968

63. TEDESCO TA, MELLMAN WJ: The UDP glucose consumption assay for gal-1-P uridyl transferase, in Hsia DYY (ed): *Galactosemia*. Springfield, Ill, Charles C Thomas, Publisher, 1969, p 66

64. TEDESCO TA, MELLMAN WJ: Galactose-1-phosphate uridyl transferase and galactokinase activity in cultured human diploid fibroblasts and peripheral blood leukocytes. *J Clin Invest* 48:2390, 1969

65. NADLER HL, CHACKO CM, RACHMELER M: Interallelic complementation in hybrid cells derived from human diploid strains deficient in galactose-1-phosphate uridyl transferase activity. *Proc Natl Acad Sci USA* 67:976, 1970

66. SHIN-BUEHRING Y, LEITNER H, HENSELEIT H, WIRTZ A, HAAS B, SCHAUB J: Characteristics of galactokinase and galactose-1-phosphate uridyltransferase in cultivated fibroblasts and amniotic fluid cells. *Hum Genet* 48:31, 1979

67. HAMMERSEN G, MANDELL R, LEVY HL: Galactose-1-phosphate uridyl

transferase in fibroblasts: Isozymes in normal and variant states. *Ann Hum Genet* 39:147, 1975

68. BEUTLER E, BALUDA M: Biochemical properties of human red cell galactose-1-phosphate uridyl transferase (UDP glucose: α-D Galactose-1-phosphate uridyl transferase) from normal and mutant subjects. *J Lab Clin Med* 67:947, 1966

69. DALE GL, POPJAK G: Purification of normal and inactive galactosemic galactose-1-phosphate uridylyl transferase from human red cells. *J Biol Chem* 251:1057, 1976

70. WILLIAMS VP: Purification and some properties of galactose 1-phosphate uridylyltransferase from human red cells. *Arch Biochem Biophys* 191:182, 1978

71. WU JW, TEDESCO TA, KALLEN RG, MELLMAN WJ: Human galactose-1-phosphate uridylyltransferase. *J Biol Chem* 249:7038, 1974

72. MARKUS HB, WU JW, BOCHES FS, TEDESCO TA, MELLMAN WJ, KALLEN RG: Human erythrocyte galactose-1-phosphate uridylyltransferase. *J Biol Chem* 252:5363, 1977

73. WILLIAMS VP, FRIED C, POPJAK G: Human red cell galactose 1-phosphate uridylyltransferase: Effects of site-specific reagents on catalytic activity. *Arch Biochem Biophys* 206:353, 1981

74. SALO W, NORDIN J, Peterson D, BEVILL R, KIRKWOOD S: The specificity of UDP-glucose 4-epimerase from the yeast *Saccharomyces fragilis*. *Biochim Biophys Acta* 151:484, 1968

75. WILSON D, HOGNESS D: The enzymes of the galactose operon in *E. coli*. I. Purification and characterization of uridine diphosphogalactose-4-epimerase. *J Biol Chem* 239:2469, 1964

76. WILSON D, HOGNESS D: The enzymes of the galactose operon in *E. coli*. II. The subunits of uridine diphosphoglucose-4-epimerase. *J Biol Chem* 244:2132, 1969

77. DEELEY R, BLACKBURN P, FERDINAND W: The first enzyme of the *gal* operon in inducible and operator-constitutive strains of *Escherichia coli*. A comparison of the properties and amino-terminal sequences of UDP galactose 4-epimerase. *Eur J Biochem* 60:371, 1975

78. DARROW R, RODSTROM R: Subunit association and catalytic activity of uridine diphosphate galactose-4-epimerase from yeast. *Proc Natl Acad Sci USA* 55:205, 1966

79. DARROW R, RODSTROM R: Uridine diphosphate galactose 4-epimerase from yeast. *J Biol Chem* 245:2036, 1970

80. BERTLAND A, BUGGE B, KALCKAR H: Fluorescence enhancement of uridine diphosphogalactose 4-epimerase induced by specific sugars. *Arch Biochem Biophys* 116:280, 1966

81. BERTLAND A, KALCKAR H: Reversible changes of ordered polypeptide structures in oxidized and reduced epimerase. *Proc Natl Acad Sci USA* 61:629, 1968

82. KANG UG, NOLAN D, FREY PA: Uridine diphosphate galactose 4-epimerase. *J Biol Chem* 250:7099, 1975

83. KETLEY JN, SCHELLENBERG KA: Substrate stereochemical requirements in the reductive inactivation of uridine diphosphate galactose 4-epimerase by sugar and 5'-uridine monophosphate. *Biochemistry* 12:315, 1973

84. WONG SS, CASSIM JY, FREY PA: *Escherichia coli* uridine diphosphate galactose 4-epimerase: Circular dichroism of the protein and protein bound dihydronicotinamide adenine dinucleotide. *Biochemistry* 17:516, 1978

85. WONG SS, FREY PA: Uridine diphosphate galactose 4-epimerase: Nucleotide and 8-anilinolnaphthalenesulfonate binding properties of the substrate binding site. *Biochemistry* 17:3551, 1978

86. KALCKAR HM: Uridine diphosphogalactose metabolism, enzymology and biology. *Adv Enzymol* 20:111, 1958

87. DE ROBICHON-SZULMAJSTER H: Sur un nouveau mécanisme d'oxydoréduction, appliqué à la réaction d'epimérisation: uridinediphosphogalactose uridine diphosphoglucose. *J Molec Biol* 3:253, 1961

88. MAITRA US, ANKEL H: Uridine diphosphate-4-keto-glucose, an intermediate in the uridine diphosphate-galactose-4-epimerase reaction. *Proc Natl Acad Sci USA* 68:2660, 1971

89. ADAIR WL, JR, GABRIEL O: 4-Uloses as intermediates in enzyme-nicotinamide adenine dinucleotide-mediated oxidoreductase mechanisms. I. Uridine diphosphate-galactose-4-epimerase. *J Biol Chem* 248:4653, 1973

90. MAXWELL E: The enzymatic interconversion of uridine diphosphogalactose and uridine diphosphoglucose. *J Biol Chem* 229:139, 1957

91. LANGER R, GLASER, L: Interaction of nucleotides with liver uridine diphosphate-glucose-4'-epimerase. *J Biol Chem* 249:1126, 1974

92. ISSELBACHER KJ, KRANE SM: Studies on the mechanism of the inhibition of galactose oxidation by ethanol. *J Biol Chem* 236:2394, 1961

93. ROBINSON E, KALCKAR H, TROEDSON H: Metabolic inhibitions of mammalian uridine diphosphate galactose-4-epimerase in cell cultures and tumor cells. *J Biol Chem* 241:2737, 1966

94. COHN R, SEGAL S: Regulation of mammalian liver uridine diphosphogalactose-4-epimerase by pyrimidine nucleotides. *Biochim Biophys Acta* 222:533, 1970

95. GEREN CR, GEREN LM, EBNER KE: Inhibition and inactivation of bovine mammary and liver UDP-galactose-4-epimerases. *J Biol Chem* 252:2089, 1977

96. COHN R, SEGAL S: Some characteristics and developmental aspects of rat

uridine diphosphogalactose-4-epimerase. *Biochim Biophys Acta* 171:333, 1969

97. CHACKO CM, MCCRONE L, NADLER HL: A study of galactokinase and glucose epimerase from normal and galactosemic skin fibroblasts. *Biochim Biophys Acta* 284:552, 1972

98. BERGEN WR, NG WG, DONNELL GN: Uridine diphosphate galactose-4-epimerase in human and other mammalian hemolysates. *Biochim Biophys Acta* 315:464, 1973

99. LIN MS, OIZUMI J, NG WG, ALFI OS, DONNELL GN: Assignment of the gene for uridine diphosphate galactose-4-epimerase to human chromosome 1 by human-mouse somatic cell hybridization. *Somatic Cell Genet* 5:363, 1979

100. BENN PA, SHOWS TB, D'NCONA GG, CROCE CM, ORKWISZEWSKI KG, MELLMAN WJ: Assignment of a gene for uridine diphosphate galactose-4-epimerase to human chromosome 1 by somatic cell hybridization, with evidence for a regional assignment to 1pter→ 1p21. *Cytogenet Cell Genet* 24:138, 1979

101. MUNCH-PETERSEN A, KALCKAR H, CUTOLO E, SMITH E: Uridyl transferases and the formation of uridine triphosphate. *Nature (Lond)* 172:1036, 1953

102. MUNCH-PETERSEN A: Investigations of the properties and mechanism of the uridine diphosphate glucose pyrophosphorylase reaction. *Acta Chem Scand* 9:1523, 1955

103. KNOP J, HANSEN R: Uridine diphosphate glucose pyrophosphorylase. IV. Crystallization and properties of the enzyme from human liver. *J Biol Chem* 245:2499, 1970

104. LEVINE S, GILLETT TA, HOGEMAN E, HANSEN RG: Uridine diphosphate glucose pyrophosphorylase. II. Polymeric and subunit structure. *J Biol Chem* 244:5729, 1969

105. STEELMAN VS, EBNER KE: The enzymes of lactose biosynthesis. I. Purification and properties of UDPG pyrophosphorylase from bovine mammary tissue. *Biochim Biophys Acta* 128:92, 1966

106. SUNDARARAJAN TA, RAPIN AM, KALCKAR HM: Biochemical observations on E. coli mutants defective in uridine diphosphoglucose. *Proc Natl Acad Sci USA* 48:2187, 1962

107. FUKASAWA T, JOKURA K, KURAHASHI H: Mutations in E. coli that affect uridine diphosphate glucose pyrophosphorylase activity and galactose fermentation. *Biochim Biophys Acta* 74:608, 1963

108. TURNQUIST RL, GILLETT TD, HANSEN RG: Uridine diphosphate glucose pyrophosphorylase. *J Biol Chem* 249:7695, 1974

109. VAN HEYNINGEN R: Formation of polyols by the lens of the rat with "sugar" cataracts. *Nature (Lond.)* 184:194, 1959

110. QUAN-MA R, WELLS W: The distribution of galactitol in tissues of rats fed galactose. *Biochem Biophys Res Commun* 20:486, 1965

111. WELLS H, SEGAL S: Galactose toxicity in the chick: Tissue accumulation of galactose and galactitol. *FEBS Lett* 5:121, 1969

112. WELLS W, PITTMAN T, WELLS H, EGAN T: The isolation and identification of galactitol from the brains of galactosemia patients. *J Biol Chem* 240:1002, 1965

113. QUAN-MA R, WELLS H, WELLS W, SHERMAN F, EGAN T: Galactitol in the tissues of a galactosemic child. *Am J Dis Child* 112:477, 1966

114. WELLS W, PITTMAN T, EGAN T: The isolation and identification of galactitol from the urine of patients with galactosemia. *J Biol Chem* 239:3192, 1964

115. GITZELMANN R, CURTIUS HC, MULLER M: Galactitol excretion in the urine of a galactokinase deficient man. *Biochem Biophys Res Commun* 22:437, 1966

116. HERS HG: L'Aldose-reductase. *Biochim Biophys Acta* 37:120, 1960

117. CLEMENTS R, WEAVER J, WINEGRAD A: The distribution of polyol: NADP oxidoreductase in mammalian tissues. *Biochem Biophys Res Commun* 37:347, 1969

118. HAYMAN S, KINOSHITA JH: Isolation and properties of lens aldose reductase. *J Biol Chem* 240:877, 1965

119. HAYMAN S, LOU M, MEROLA L, KINOSHITA JH: Aldose reductase activity in the lens and other tissues. *Biochim Biophys Acta* 128:474, 1966

120. MOONSAMMY G, STEWART M: Purification and properties of brain aldose reductase and L-hexonate dehydrogenase. *J Neurochem* 14:1187, 1967

121. MANO Y, SUZUKI K, YAMADA K, SCHIMAZONO N: Enzymic studies on TPN L-hexonate dehydrogenase from rat liver. *J Biochem (Tokyo)* 49:618, 1961

122. GABBAY K, O'SULLIVAN J: The sorbitol pathway: Enzyme localization and content in normal and diabetic nerve and cord. *Diabetes* 17:239, 1968

123. GABBAY K, O'SULLIVAN J: The sorbitol pathway in diabetes and galactosemia: Enzyme and substrate localization and changes in kidney. *Diabetes* 17:300, 1968

124. CLEMENTS R, WINEGRAD A: Modulation of mammalian polyol: NADP oxidoreductase activity by ADP and ATP. *Biochim Biophys Res Commun* 36:1006, 1969

125. WELLS WW: Galactitol metabolism, in Hsia DYY (ed): *Galactosemia*. Springfield, Ill, Charles C Thomas, Publisher, 1969, p 227

126. BERGREN W, NG W, DONNELL G: Galactonic acid in galactosemia. *Science* 176:683, 1972

127. RANCOUR NJ, HAWKINS ED, WELLS WW: Galactose oxidation in liver. *Arch Biochem Biophys* 193:232, 1979

128. LICHTENSTEIN G, ROGERS S, SEGAL S: Unpublished results

129. SEGAL S, CUATRECASAS P: The oxidation of C14 galactose by patients with congenital galactosemia. *Am J Med* 44:340, 1968

130. CUATRECASAS P, SEGAL S: Galactose conversion to D-xylulose: An alternate route of galactose metabolism. *Science* 153:549, 1966

131. CUATRECASAS P, SEGAL S: Mammalian galactose dehydrogenase. I. Identification and purification in rat liver. *J Biol Chem* 241:5904, 1966

132. CUATRECASAS P, SEGAL S: Mammalian galactose dehydrogenase. II Properties, substrate specificity and developmental changes. *J Biol Chem* 241:5910, 1966

133. SRIVASTAVA SK, BEUTLER E: Auxiliary pathways of galactose metabolism. *J Biol Chem* 244:6377, 1969

134. ISSELBACHER KJ: Evidence for an accessory pathway of galactose metabolism in mammalian liver. *Science* 126:652, 1957

135. ISSELBACHER K: A mammalian uridinediphosphate galactose pyrophosphorylase. *J Biol Chem* 232:429, 1958

136. ABRAHAM H, HOWELL R: Human hepatic uridine diphosphate galactose pyrophosphorylase. *J Biol Chem* 244:545, 1969

137. CHACKO CM, MCCRONE ML, NADLER HL: Uridine diphosphoglucose pyrophosphorylase and uridine diphosphogalactose phosphorylase in human skin fibroblasts from normal and galactosemic individuals. *Biochim Biophys Acta* 268:113, 1972

138. STENSTAM T: Peroral and intravenous galactose tests: Comparative study of their significance in different conditions. *Acta Med Scand.* (suppl.):177, 1946

139. SEGAL S, BLAIR A: Some observations on the metabolism of D-galactose in normal man. *J Clin Invest* 40:2016, 1961

140. TYGSTRUP N, WINKLER K: Galactose blood clearance as a measure of hepatic blood flow. *Clin Sci* 17:1, 1958

141. TYGSTRUP N: Determination of the hepatic elimination capacity (Lm) of galactose by single injection. *Scand J Clin Lab Invest* (Suppl) 18:92, 118, 1966

142. KEIDING S: Galactose elimination capacity in the rat. *Scand J Clin Lab Invest* 31:319, 1973

143. TYGSTRUP N: The urinary excretion of galactose and its significance in clinical intravenous galactose tolerance tests. *Acta Physiol Scand* 51:263, 1961

144. COLCHER H, PATEK AJ, KENDALL FE: Galactose disappearance from the blood stream: Calculation of a galactose removal constant and its application as a test of liver function. *J Clin Invest* 25:768, 1946

145. TENGSTRÖM B: An intravenous galactose tolerance test with an enzymatic determination of galactose: A comparison with other diagnostic aids in hepatobiliary diseases. *Scand J Clin Invest* 18:132, 1966

146. SHREEVE WW, SHOOP JD, OTT DG, MCINTEER BB: Test for alcoholic cirrhosis by conversion of [14C]- or [13C]galactose to expired CO2. *Gastroenterology* 71:98, 1976

147. TYGSTRUP N, LUNDQUIST F: The effect of ethanol on galactose elimination in man. *J Lab Clin Med* 59:102, 1962

148. SALASPURO MP, SALASPURO AE: The effect of ethanol on galactose elimination in rats with normal and choline-deficient fatty livers. *Scand J Clin Lab Invest* 22:49, 1968

149. SEGAL S, ROTH H, BERTOLI D: Galactose metabolism by rat liver tissue: Influence of age. *Science* 142:1311, 1963

150. HAWORTH JC, FORD JD: Variation of the oral galactose tolerance test with age. *J Pediatr* 63:276, 1963

151. MULLIGAN PB, SCHWARTZ R: Hepatic carbohydrate metabolism in the genesis of neonatal hypoglycemia. *Pediatrics* 30:125, 1962

152. HJELM M, SJÖLIN S: Changes in the elimination rate from blood of intravenously injected galactose during the neonatal period. *Scand J Clin Invest* (Suppl) 18:92, 126, 1966

153. THEODORE GM, FORD JD, HAWORTH JC: The intravenous galactose tolerance test in infancy. *Arch Dis Child* 39:505, 1964

154. VINK CDL, KROES AA: Liver function and age. *Clin Chim Acta* 4:674, 1959

155. SPARKS JW, LYNCH A, CHEZ RA, GLINSMANN W: Glycogen regulation in isoalted perfused near term monkey liver. *Pediatr Res* 10:51, 156.

156. SPARKS JW, LYNCH A, GLINSMANN WH: Regulation of rat liver glycogen synthesis and activities of glycogen cycle enzymes by glucose and galactose. *Metabolism* 25:47, 1976

157. BERMAN W, ROGERS S, BAUTISTA J, SEGAL S: Galactose and glucose metabolism in the isolated perfused 15-day old and adult rat liver. *Metabolism* 27:1721, 1978

158. BERMAN W, ROGERS S, BAUTISTA J, SEGAL S: Galactose metabolism in isolated perfused suckling rat liver. *Am J Physiol* 236(6):E633-637, 1979

159. JORDAN E, YARMOLINSKY MB, KALCKAR HM: Control of inducibility of enzymes of the galactose sequence in *Escherichia coli*. *Proc Natl Acad Sci USA* 48:32, 1962

160. BUTTIN G: MÉCANISMES regulateurs dans la biosynthèse des enzymes du metabolisme du galactose chez E. coli K-12: I. La biosynthèse induite de la

galactokinase et l'induction simultanée de la séquence enzymatique. *J Molec Biol* 7:183, 1963

161. WU HCP, KALCKAR HM: Endogenous induction of the gal operon in *E coli* K-12. *Proc Natl Acad Sci USA*, 55:622, 1966

162. KALCKAR HM, KURAHASHI K, JORDAN E: Hereditary defects in galactose metabolism in *E coli* mutants 1. Determination of enzyme activities. *Proc Natl Acad Sci USA* 45:1776, 1959

163. BUTTIN G: Mecanismes regulateurs dans la biosynthèse des enzymes du metabolisme du galactose chez. *E coli* K-12. II. Le déterminisme génétique de la régulation. *J Molec Biol* 7:183, 1963

164. MORSE ML: Preliminary genetic map of seventeen galactose mutations in *E. coli* K-12. *Proc Natl Acad Sci USA*. 48:1314, 1962

165. BUTTIN G: Sur la structure de l'opéron galactose chez *E coli* K-12. *CR Acad Sci (Paris)* 255:1233, 1962

166. ADLER J, KAISER AD: Mapping of the galactose genes of *Escherichia coli* by transduction with phage PI. *Virology* 19:117, 1963

167. HOPPER JE, BROACH JR, ROWE LB: Regulation of the galactose pathway in *Saccharomyces cerevisiae*: Induction of uridyl transferase mRNA and dependency on *GAL4* gene function. *Proc Natl Acad Sci USA* 75:2878, 1978

168. BROACH JR: Galactose regulation in *Saccharomyces cerevisiae*. The enzymes encoded by the *GAL7, 10, 1* cluster are co-ordinately controlled and separately translated. *J Molec Biol* 131:41, 1979

169. MATSUMOTO K, TOH-E A, OSHIMA Y: Genetic control of galactokinase synthesis in *Saccharomyces cerevisiae*: Evidence for constitutive expression of the positive regulatory gene *gal4*. *J Bacteriol* 134:446, 1978

170. HOPPER JE, ROWE LB: Molecular expression and regulation of the galactose pathway genes in *Saccharomyces cerevisiae*. *J Biol Chem* 253:7566, 1978

171. KURAHASHI K, WAHBA AJ: Interference with growth of certain *E. coli* mutants by galactose. *Biochim Biophys Acta* 30:298, 1958

172. YARMOLINSKY MB, WIESMEYER H, KALCKAR HM, JORDAN E: Hereditary defects in *E. coli* mutants. II. Galactose induced sensitivity. *Proc Natl Acad Sci USA* 45:1786, 1959

173. SUNDARARAJAN TA: Interference with glycerokinase induction in mutants of *E. coli* accumulating Gal-1-P. *Proc Natl Acad Sci USA* 50:463, 1963

174. FUKASAWA T, NIKAIDO H: Galactose sensitive mutants of *Salmonella*. I. Metabolism of galactose. *Biochim Biophys Acta* 48:460, 1961

175. FUKASAWA T, NIKAIDO H: Galactose sensitive mutants of *Salmonella*. II. Bacteriolysis induced by galactose. *Biochim Biophys Acta* 48:470, 1961

176. MORSE ML, LEDERBERG EM, LEDERBERG J: Transduction in *E. coli* K-12. *Genetics* 41:142, 1956

177. ADLER J, TEMPLETON B: The amount of galactose genetic material in Δ dg bacteriophage with different densities. *J Molec Biol* 7:710, 1963

178. MERRIL CR, GEIER MR, PETRICCIANI JC: Bacterial virus gene expression in human cells. *Nature (Lond.)* 233:398, 1971

179. HSIA DYY, WALKER FA: Variability in the clinical manifestations of galactosemia. *J Pediatr* 59:872, 1961

180. DONNELL GN, COLLADO M, KOCH R: Growth and development of children with galactosemia. *J Pediatr* 58:836, 1961

181. NADLER HL, INOUYE T, HSIA DYY: Clinical galactosemia: A study of fifty-five cases, in Hsia DYY (ed): *Galactosemia*. Springfield, Ill, Charles C Thomas, Publisher, 1969, p 127

182. DONNELL GN, KOCH R, BERGREN WR: Observations on results of management of galactosemic patients, in Hsia DYY (ed): *Galactosemia*. Springfield, Ill, Charles C Thomas, Publisher, 1969, p 247

183. KOMROWER GM, LEE DH: Long term follow-up of galactosemia. *Arch Dis Child* 45:367, 1970

184. FISHLER K, KOCH R, DONNELL GN, WENZ E: Developmental aspects of galactosemia from infancy to childhood. *Clin Pediatr* 19:38, 1980

185. LEVY HL, SEPE SJ, SHIH VE, VAWTER GF, KLEIN JO: Sepsis due to *Escherichia coli* in neonates with galactosemia. *N Engl J Med* 297:823, 1977

186. LITCHFIELD WJ, WELLS WW: Effect of galactose on free radical reactions of polymorphonuclear leukocytes. *Arch Biochem Biophys* 188:26, 1978

187. SEGAL S, BLAIR A, ROTH H: The metabolism of galactose by patients with congenital galactosemia. *Am J Med* 38:62, 1965

188. HOLZEL A, KOMROWER GM, WILSON VK: Aminoaciduria in galactosemia. *Br Med J* 1:194, 1952

189. CUSWORTH DC, DENT CE, FLYNN FV: The aminoaciduria in galactosemia. *Arch Dis Child* 30:150, 1955

190. SMETANA HF, OLEN F: Hereditary galactose disease. *Am J Clin Pathol* 38:3, 1962

191. GITZELMANN R, AURICCHIO S: The handling of soya alpha galactosides by a normal and a galactosemic child. *Pediatrics* 36:231, 1965

192. KOCH R, ACOSTA P, DONNELL GN, LIEBERMAN E: Nutritional therapy of galactosemia. *Clin Pediatr (Phila)* 4:571, 1965

193. SCHWARZ V: The value of galactose phosphate determinations in the treatment of galactosemia. *Arch Dis Child* 35:428, 1960

194. DONNELL GN, BERGREN WR, PERRY G, KOCH R: Galactose-1-phosphate in galactosemia. *Pediatrics* 31:802, 1963

195. KOGUT MD, DONNELL GN, SHARO KNF: Studies of lactose absorption in patients with galactosemia. *J Pediatr* 71:75, 1967

196. SEGAL S, BERNSTEIN H: Observations on cataract formation in the new-born offspring of rats fed a high-galactose diet. *J Pediatr* 62:363, 1963

197. SPATZ M, SEGAL S: Transplacental galactose toxicity in rats. *J Pediatr* 67:438, 1965

198. FISHLER K, DONNELL GN, BERGREN WR, KOCH R: Intellectual and personality development in children with galactosemia. *Pediatrics* 50:412, 1972

199. KAUFMAN FR, KOGUT MD, DONNELL GN, GOEBELSMANN U, MARCH C, KOCH R: Hypergonadotropic hypogonadism in female patients with galactosemia. *N Engl J Med* 304:994, 1981

200. SCHWARZ V, GOLDBERG L, KOMROWER GM, HOLZEL A: Some disturbances of erythrocyte metabolism in galactosemia. *Biochem J* 62:34, 1956

201. INOUYE T, NADLER HL, HSIA DYY: Galactose-1-phosphate uridyl transferase in red and white blood cells. *Clin Chim Acta* 19:169, 1968

202. KROOTH R, WINBERG AN: Studies on cell lines developed from the tissues of patients with galactosemia. *J Exp Med* 113:1155, 1961

203. ANDERSON EP, KALCKAR HM, ISSELBACHER KJ: Defect in the uptake of galactose-1-phosphate into liver nucleotides in congenital galactosemia. *Science* 125:113, 1957

204. MAYES JS: Thesis for the Ph.D. degree, Michigan State Univ., 1965. Quoted by Hansen RG: Some chemical aspects of galactosemia, in Hsia DYY (ed): *Galactosemia*. Springfield, Ill, Charles C Thomas, Publisher, 1969, p 55

205. ANDERSON EP, KALCKAR HM, KURAHASHI K, ISSELBACHER KJ: A specific enzymatic assay for the diagnosis of congenital galactosemia, *J Lab Clin Med* 50:569, 1957

206. BEUTLER E, BALUDA MC: Improved method for measuring galactose-1-phosphate uridyl transferase activity of erythrocytes. *Clin Chim Acta* 13:369, 1966

207. MELLMAN WJ, TEDESCO TA: An improved assay of erythrocyte and leukocyte galactose-1-phosphate uridyl transferase: Stabilization of the enzyme by a thiol protective reagent. *J Lab Clin Med* 66:980, 1965

208. DONNELL GN, BERGREN WR, BRETTHAUER MS, HANSEN RG: The enzymatic expression of heterozygosity in families of children with galactosemia. *Pediatrics* 25:572, 1960

209. HSIA DYY: Clinical variants of galactosemia. *Metabolism* 16:419, 1967

210. ROBINSON A: The assay of galactokinase and galactose-1-phosphate uridyl transferase activity in human erythrocytes. *J Exp Med* 118:359, 1963

211. NG WG, BERGREN WR, DONNELL GN: Galactose-1-phosphate uridyl transferase assay by use of radioactive galactose-1-phosphate. *Clin Chim Acta* 10:337, 1964

212. NG WG, BERGREN WR, DONNELL GN: An improved procedure for the assay of hemolysate galactose-1-phosphate uridyl transferase activity by the use of ^{14}C labeled galactose-1-phosphate. *Clin Chim Acta* 15:489, 1967

213. WEINBERG AN: Detection of congenital galactosemia and the carrier state using galactose C^{14} and blood cells. *Metabolism* 10:728, 1961

214. EGGERMONT E, HERS HG: Une nouvelle méthode de détection de la galactosémie congénitale. *Clin Chim Acta* 7:437, 1962

215. NG WG, BERGREN WR, DONNELL GN: Galactose-1-phosphate uridyl-transferase activity in galactosaemia. *Nature (Lond)* 203:845, 1964

216. BEUTLER E, BALUDA M, DONNELL GN: A new method for the detection of galactosemia and its carrier state. *J Lab Clin Med* 64:694, 1964

217. COPENHAVER JH, BAUSCH LC, FITZGIBBONS JF: A fluorometric procedure for estimation of galactose-1-phosphate uridyl transferase activity in red blood cells. *Anal Biochem* 30:327, 1969

218. GATTI R, MANFIELD P, HSIA DYY: Screening for galactosemia in the newborn. *J Pediatr* 69:1126, 1936

219. BEUTLER E, BALUDA MC: A simple spot screening test for galactosemia. *J Lab Clin Med* 68:137, 1966

220. NELSON K, HSIA DYY: Screening for galactosemia and glucose-6-phosphate dehydrogenase deficiency in newborn infants. *J Pediatr* 71:582, 1967

221. HAWORTH JC, BARCHUK NH: A simple chromatographic screening test for the detection of galactosemia in newborn infants. *Pediatrics* 39:608, 1967

222. WELLS WW, CHIN T, WEBER B: Quantitative analysis of serum and urine sugars by gas chromatography. *Clin Chim Acta* 10:352, 1964

223. COPENHAVER JH: Quantitative analysis of plasma galactose and glucose by gas-liquid chromatography. *Anal Biochem* 17:76, 1966

224. DE VERDIER CH, HJELM M: A galactose oxidase method for the determination of galactose in blood plasma. *Clin Chim Acta* 7:742, 1962

225. ROTH H, SEGAL S, BERTOLI D: The quantitative determination of galactose—an enzymatic method using galactose oxidase with application to blood and other biological fluids. *Anal Biochem* 10:32, 1965

226. TENGSTROM B: Enzymatic determination of glucose and galactose in urine. *Scand J Lab Invest* 18 (suppl):92, 104, 1966

227. DAHLQVIST A, SVENNINGSEN NW: Galactose in the urine of newborn infants. *J Pediatr* 75:454, 1969

228. DAHLQVIST A: Test paper for galactose in urine. *Scand J Clin Lab Invest* 22:87, 1968

229. BICKEL H: Mellituria, a paper chromatographic study. *J Pediatr* 59:641, 1961

230. HAWORTH JC, MACDONALD MS: Reducing sugars in urine and blood of premature babies. *Arch Dis Child* 32:417, 1952

231. HALL WK, CRAVEY CE, CHEN PT, OOSTENDORFF ME, HOLLOWELL JG, JR, THEVAOS TG: An evaluation of galactosuria. *J Pediatr* 77:625, 1970

232. BRUCK E, RAPOPORT S: Galactosemia in an infant with cataracts: Clinical observations and carbohydrate studies. *Am J Dis Child* 70:267, 1945

233. BAKER L, MELLMAN WJ, TEDESCOTA, SEGAL S: Galactosemia: Symptomatic and asymptomatic homozygotes in one Negro sibship. *J Pediatr* 68:551,1966

234. SEGAL S: The Negro variant of congenital galactosemia, in Hsia DYY (ed): *Galactosemia*. Springfield, Ill, Charles C Thomas, Publisher, 1969, p 176

235. TOPPER YJ, LASTER L, SEGAL S: Galactose metabolism: Phenotype differences among tissues of a patient with congenital galactosemia. *Nature (Lond)* 196:1106, 1962

236. PESCH LA, SEGAL S, TOPPER Y: Progesterone effects on galactose metabolism in prepubertal patients with congenital galactosemia and in rats maintained on high galactose diets. *J Clin Invest* 39:178, 1960

237. ELDER TD, SEGAL S, MAXWELL ES, TOPPER Y: Some steroid hormone like effects of menthol. *Science* 132:255, 1960

238. SEGAL S: Isotopic studies of galactose oxidation in galactosemia, in Hsia DYY (ed): *Galactosemia*. Springfield, Ill, Charles C Thomas, Publisher, 1969 p. 42.

239. TADA K, KUDO Z, OHNO T, AKABONE J, CHICA R: Congenital galactosemia and orotic acid therapy with promising results. Preliminary report. *Tohoku J Exp Med* 77:340, 1962

240. SEGAL S, ROTH H, BLAIR A: Observations of orotic acid on galactose metabolism in congenital galactosemia. *J Pediatr* 68:135, 1966

241. EGAN TJ, WELLS WW: Alternate metabolic pathway in galactosemia. *Am J Dis Child* 111:400, 1966

242. WEINSTEIN AN, SEGAL S: The metabolic fate of 1.^{14}C galactitol in mammalian tissue. *Biochim Biophys Acta* 156:9, 1965

243. INOUYE T, TANNENBAUM M, HSIA DYY: Identification of galactose-6-phosphate in galactosemic erythrocytes. *Nature (Lond)* 193:67, 1962.

244. INOUYE T, SCHNEIDER JA, HSIA DYY: Enzymatic oxidation of galactose-6-phosphate. *Nature (Lond)* 204:1304, 1964

245. OHNO S, PAYNE HW, MORRISON M, BEUTLER E: Hexose-6-phosphate dehydrogenase found in human liver. *Science* 153:1015, 1966

246. GITZELMANN R: Formation of galactose-1-phosphate from uridine diphosphate galactose in erythrocytes from patients with galactosemia. *Pediatr Res* 3:279, 1969

247. GITZELMANN R, HANSEN RG: Galactose biogenesis and disposal in galactosemics. *Biochim Biophys Acta* 372:374, 1974

248. PETRICCIANI JC, BINDER MK, MERRIL CR, GEIER MR: Galactose utilization in galactosemia. *Science* 175:1368, 1972

249. MAYES JS, MILLER LR: The metabolism of galactose by galactosemic fibroblasts *in vitro*. *Biochim Biophys Acta* 313:9, 1973

250. FRIEDMAN TB, YARKIN RJ, MERRIL CR: Galactose and glucose metabolism in galactokinase deficient, galactose-1-*p*-uridyl transferase deficient and normal human fibroblasts. *J Cell Physiol* 85:569, 1974

251. BROWN E, HUGHES RC, WATTS RWE: Biochemical expression of the galactosemic defect in lymphocytes and the effects on glycoprotein synthesis. *Metabolism* 26:1047, 1977

252. BEUTLER E, BALUDA MC, STURGEON P, DAY RW: A new genetic abnormality resulting in galactose-1-phosphate uridyl transferase deficiency. *Lancet* 1:353, 1965

253. BEUTLER E: The Duarte variant in galactosemia, in Hsia DYY (ed): *Galactosemia*. Springfield, Ill, Charles C Thomas, Publisher, 1969, p 163

254. BEUTLER E, BALUDA MC, STURGEON P, DAY RW: The genetics of galactose-1-phosphate uridyl transferase deficiency. *J Lab Clin Med* 68:646, 1966

255. MATHAI CK, BEUTLER E: Electrophoretic variation of galactose-1-phosphate uridyl transferase. *Science* 154:1179, 1966

256. NG WG, BERGREN WR, FIELD M, DONNELL GN: An improved electrophoretic procedure for galactose-1-phosphate uridyl transferase: Demonstration of multiple activity bands with the Duarte variant. *Biochem Biophys Res Commun* 37:354, 1969

257. MELLMAN WJ, TEDESCO TA, FEIGL P: Estimation of the gene frequency of the Duarte variant of galactose-1-phosphate uridyl transferase. *Ann Hum Genet* 32:1, 1968

258. GITZELMANN R, POLEY JR, PRADER A: Partial galactose-1-phosphate uridyltransferase deficiency due to a variant enzyme. *Helv Paediatr Acta* 22:252, 1967

259. LEVY HL, SEPE SJ, WALTON DS, SHIH VE, HAMMERSEN G, HOUGHTON S,

260. BEUTLER E: Galactose-1-phosphate uridyl transferase deficiency due to Duarte/galactosemia combined variation: Clinical and biochemical studies. *J Pediatr* 92:390, 1978

261. KELLY S: Significance of the Duarte/classical galactosemia genetic compound. *J Pediatr* 94:937, 1979

262. SCHAPIRA F, KAPLAN JC: Electrophoretic abnormality of galactose-1-phosphate uridyl transferase in galactosemia. *Biochem Biophys Res Commun* 35:451, 1969

263. HAMMERSEN G, HOUGHTON S, LEVY HL: Rennes-like variant of galactosemia: Clinical and biochemical studies. *J Pediatr* 87:50, 1975

264. CHACKO CM, CHRISTIAN JC, NADLER HL: Unstable galactose-1-phosphate uridyl transferase: A new variant galactosemia. *J Pediatr* 78:454, 1971

265. NG WG, BERGREN WR, DONNELL GN: A new variant of galactose-1-phosphate uridyltransferase in man: The Los Angeles variant. *Ann Hum Genet* 37:1, 1973

266. IBARRA B, VACA G, SANCHEZ-CORONA J, HERNANDEZ A, RAIMEREZ ML, CNTU JM: Los Angeles variant of galactose-1-phosphate uridyltransferase (EC 2.7.7.12) in a Mexican family. *Hum Genet* 48:121, 1979

267. CHACKO CM, WAPPNER RS, BRANDT IK, NADLER HL: The Chicago variant of clinical galactosemia. *Humangenetick* 37:261, 1977

268. MATZ D, ENZENAUER J, MENNE F: Uber einen Fall von Atypischer Galaktosamie. *Humangenetik* 27:309, 1975

269. LANG A, GROEBE H, HELLKUHL B, VON FIGURA K: A new variant of galactosemia: Galactose-1-phosphate uridyltransferase sensitive to product inhibition by glucose 1-phosphate. *Pediatr Res* 14:729, 1980

270. KIRKMAN HN, BYNUM E: Enzymatic evidence of a galactosemic trait in parents and galactosemic children. *Ann Hum Genet* 23:117, 1959

271. SCHWARZ V, WELLS AR, HOLZEL A, KOMROWER GM: A study of the genetics of galactosemia. *Ann Hum Genet* 25:179, 1961

272. HUGH-JONES K, NEWCOMB AL, HSIA DYY: The genetic mechanism of galactosemia. *Arch Dis Child* 35:521, 1960

273. WALKER FA, HSIA DYY, SLATIS HM, STEINBERG AG: Galactosemia: A study of 27 kindreds in North America. *Ann Hum Genet* 25:287, 1962

274. GITZELMANN R, HODORN R: Zur biochemischen Genetik der Galaltosämie. *Helv Paediatr Acta* 16:1, 1961

275. MELLMAN WJ, TEDESCO TA: Galactose-1-phosphate uridyl transferase and galactokinase activity in cultured human diploid fibroblasts and peripherial blood leukocytes. *J Clin Invest* 48:2391, 1969

276. MCGUINESS R, SAUNDERS RA: Erythrocyte galactose-1-phosphate uridyl transferase and glucose-6-phosphate dehydrogenase activity in the population of Rhonda Foch. *Clin Chim Acta* 16:221, 1967

277. BRANDT NJ: Frenquency of heterozygotes for heriditary galactosemia in a normal population. *Acta Genet (Basel)* 17:289, 1967

278. HANSEN RG, BRETTHAUER RK, MAYES J, NORDIN JH: Estimation of frequency of occurrence of galactosemia in the population. *Proc Soc Exp Biol Med* 115:560, 1964

279. TEDESCO TA, MILLER KL, RAWNSLEY BE, MENNUTI MT, SPIELMAN RS, MELLMAN WJ: Human erythrocyte galactokinase and galactose-1-phosphate uridyltransferase: A population survey. *Am J Hum Genet* 27:737, 1975

280. KELLY S, KATZ S, BURNS J, BOYLAN J: Screening for galactosemia in New York State. *Public Health Rep* 85:575, 1970

281. SHIH VE, LEVY HL, KAROLKEWICZ V, HOUGHTON S, EFRON ML, ISSELBACHER KJ, BEUTLER F, MACCREADY RA: Galactosemia screening of newborns in Massachusetts. *N Engl J Med* 284:753, 1971

282. LEVY HL: Screening for galactosaemia, in Burman D, Holton JB, Pennock CA (eds): *Inherited Disorders of Carbohydrate Metabolism*. Lancaster, England, MTP Press Ltd, Falcon House, 1980, p 133

283. FENSOM AH, BENSON PF, BLUNT S: Prenatal diagnosis of galactosemia. *Br Med J* 4:386, 1974

284. HOLTON JB, RAYMONT CM: Prenatal diagnosis of classical galactosaemia, in Burman D, Holton JB, Pennock CA (eds): *Inherited Disorders of Carbohydrate Metabolism*. Lancaster, England, MTP Press Ltd, Falcon House, 1980, p 141

285. TEDESCO TA, MORROW G, MELLMAN WJ: Normal pregnancy and childbirth in galactosemic woman. *J Pediatr* 81:1159, 1972

286. SARDHARWALL KB, KOMROWER GM, SCHWARZ V: Pregnancy in classical galactosaemia, in Burman D, Holton JB, Pennock CA (eds): *Inherited Disorders of Carbohydrate Metabolism*. Lancaster, England, MTP Press Ltd, Falcon House, 1980, p 125

287. BRANDT NJ, FORLAND A, MIKKELSEN M, NIELSEN M, NIELSEN A, TOLSTRUP N: Galactosaemia locus and the Down's syndrome chromosome. *Lancet* 2:700, 1963

288. HSIA DYY, INOUYE T, WONG P, SOUTH A: Studies on galactose oxidation in Down's syndrome. *N Engl J Med* 270:1085, 1964

289. ROSNER F, ONG BH, PAINEY RS, MAHANAND D: Biochemical differentiation of trisomic Down's syndrome (mongolism) from that due to translocation. *N Engl J Med* 273:1356, 1965

289. WANG MYFW, DESFORGES JF: The Philadelphia chromosome and galactose-1-phosphate uridyl transferase. *Blood* 29:790, 1967

290. KRONE W, WOLF U, GOEDDE HW, BAITSCH H: Untersuchungen über der aktivität der galaktokinase im blut von normal personen und von patienten mit G$_{DO}$-trisomie. *Hum Genet* 1:279, 1965

291. MELLMAN WJ, OSKI FA, TEDESCOTA, HARRIS H: Leucocyte enzymes in Down's syndrome. *Lancet* 2:674, 1964

292. DAHLQVIST A, HALL B, KÄLLÉN B: Blood galactose-1-phosphate uridyl transferase activity in dysplastic patients with and without chromosomal aberrations. *Hum Hered* 19:628, 1969

293. MOHANDAS T, SPARKES RS, SPARKES MC, SHULKIN JD: Assignment of the human gene for galactose-1-phosphate uridyltransferase to chromosome 9: Studies with Chinese hamster-human somatic cell hybrids. *Proc Natl Acad Sci USA* 74:5628, 1977

294. MOHANDAS T, SPARKES RS, SPARKES MC, SHULKIN JD, TOOMEY KE, FUNDERBURK SJ: Regional localization of human gene loci on chromosome 9: Studies of somatic cell hybrids containing human translocations. *Am J Hum Genet* 31:586–600, 1979

295. SPARKES RS, SPARKES MC, FUNDERBURK SJ, MOEDJONO S: Expression of GALT in 9p chromosome alterations: Assignment of GALT locus to 9cen → 9p22. *Ann Hum Genet* 43:343, 1980

296. TEDESCO TA, MELLMAN WJ: Galactosemia: Evidence of a structural gene mutation. *Science* 172:727, 1971

297. TEDESCO TA, WU JW, BOCHES FS, MELLMAN WJ: The genetic defect in galactosemia. *N Engl J Med* 292:737, 1975

298. GITZELMANN R, HANSEN RG: Galactose metabolism, hereditary defects and their clinical significance, in Burman D, Holton JB, Pennock CA (eds): *Inherited Disorders of Carbohydrate Metabolism*. Lancaster, England, MTP Press Ltd, Falcon House, 1980

299. SIDBURY JB, JR: The role of galactose-1-phosphate in the pathogenesis of galactosemia, in Gardner LE (ed): *Molecular Genetics and Human Disease*. Springfield, Ill, Charles C Thomas, Publisher, 1960, p 61

300. MITCHELL HS: Cataract in rats fed on galactose. *Proc Soc Exp Biol Med* 32:971, 1935

301. CRAIG J, MADDOCK C: Observations on nature of galactose toxicity in rats. *AMA Arch Pathol* 55:118, 1953

302. DAM H: Galactose-poisoning in chicks. *Proc Soc Exp Biol Med* 55:57, 1944

303. RUTTER WJ, KRICHEVSKY P, SCOTT HM, HANSEN RG: The metabolism of lactose and galactose in the chick. *Poult Sci* 32:706, 1953

304. PERRY J, MOORE A, THOMAS D, HIRD F: Galactose intolerance: Observations on an experimental animal. *Acta Paediatr* 45:228, 1956

305. NORDIN JH, WILKIN DR, BRETTHAUER RK, HANSEN RG, SCOTT HM: A consideration of galactose toxicity in male and female chicks. *Poult Sci* 39:802, 1960

306. HANSEN RG, FREELAND RA, SCOTT HM: Lactose metabolism. V. The uridine nucleotides in galactose toxicity. *J Biol Chem* 219:391, 1956

307. KLETHI J, MANDEL P: Uridine diphosphate hexoses of lens from rats on a galactose rich diet. *Biochim Biophys Acta* 57:379, 1962

308. PATTERSON JW: Cataractogenic sugars. *Arch Biochem* 58:24, 1955

309. PATTERSON JW, PATTERSON ME, KENSEY VE, REDDY DVN: Lens assay on diabetic and galactosemic rats receiving diets that modify cataract development. *Invest Ophthalmol* 4:98, 1965

310. COTLIER E: Hypophysectomy effect on lens epithelium mitosis and galactose cataract development in rats. *Arch Ophthalmol* 67:476, 1962

311. SCHWARZ V, GOLDBERG L: Galactose-1-phosphate in galactose cataract. *Biochim Biophys Acta* 18:310, 1955

312. GITZELMANN R, CURTIUS HC, SCHNELLER I: Galactitol and galactose-1-phosphate in the lens of a galactosemic infant. *Exp Eye Res* 6:1, 1967

313. LERMAN S: Pathogenic factors in experimental cataract. Part I. *Arch Ophthalmol* 63:128, 1960

314. UNAKAR NJ, GENYEA C, REDDAN JR, REDDY VN: Ultrastructural changes during the developmental and reversal of galactose cataracts. *Exp Eye Res* 26:123, 1978

315. UNAKAR NJ, SMART T, REDDAN JR, DEVLIN I: Regression of cataracts in the offspring of galactose fed rats. *Ophthal Res* 11:52, 1979

316. BEYER-MEARS A, FARNSWORTH PN: Regional analyses of the opaque galactose cataract and the reversal process. *Metab Pediatr Ophthalmol* 4:9, 1980

317. KINOSHITA JH, MEROLA LO: Hydration of the lens during the development of galactose cataract. *Invest Ophthalmol* 3:577, 1964

318. SIPPEL TO: Changes in the water, protein and glutathione contents of the lens in the course of galactose cataract development in rats. *Invest Ophthalmol* 5:568, 1966

319. KINOSHITA JH, DVORNIK D, KRAML M, GABBAY KH: The effect of aldose reductase inhibition on the galactose exposed rabbit lens. *Biochim Biophys Acta* 158:472, 1968

320. DISCHE Z, ZELMENIS G, YOULOUS J: Studies on protein and protein synthesis—during the development of galactose cataract. *Am J Ophthalmol* 44:332, 1957

321. KADOR PF, ZIGLER JS, KINOSHITA JH: Alterations of lens protein synthesis in galactosemic rats. *Invest Ophthalmol Vis Sci* 18:696, 1979

322. KINOSHITA JH, MEROLA LO, HAYMAN S: Osmotic effects on the amino acid concentration mechanisms in the rabbit lens. *J Biol Chem* 240:310, 1965

323. REDDY D: Amino acid transport in the lens in relation to sugar cataracts. *Invest Ophthalmol* 4:700, 1965

324. KINOSHITA JH, BARBER GW, MEROLA LO, TUNG B: Changes in levels of free amino acids and myo-inositol in the galactose-exposed lens. *Invest Ophthalmol* 8:625, 1969

325. COTLIER E, BECKER B: Rubidium 86 accumulation and dulcitol distributions in lens of galactose-fed rats. *Exp Eye Res* 4:340, 1965

326. KINOSHITA JH, MEROLA LO, TUNG B: Changes in cation permeability in the galactose-exposed rabbit lens. *Exp Eye Res* 7:80, 1968

327. BROCKHUYSE R: Changes in myo-inositol permeability in the lens due to cataractous condition. *Biochim Biophys Acta* 163:269, 1968

328. STEWART M, KURIEN M, SHERMAN W, COTLIER E: Inositol changes in nerve and lens of galactose fed rats. *J Neurochem* 15:941, 1968

329. SIPPEL TO: Enzyme of carbohydrate metabolism in developing galactose cataracts of rats. *Invest Ophthalmol* 6:59, 1967

330. KORC I: Biochemical studies on cataracts in galactose fed rats. *Arch Biochem* 94:196, 1961

331. ISHIMOTO C, GOALWIN PW, SUN S-T, NISHIO I, TANAKA T: Cytoplasmic phase separation in formation of galactosemic cataract in lenses of young rats. *Proc Natl Acad Sci USA* 76:4414, 1979

332. SIPPEL T.O: Energy metabolism in the lens during development of galactose cataract in rats. *Invest Ophthalmol* 5:576, 1966

333. BEFFLEY JD, WILLIAMS RJ: The nutritional teamwork approach Prevention and regression of cataracts in rats. *Proc Natl Acad Sci USA* 71:4164, 1974

334. KEPPLER D, RUDIQIER J, REUTTER W, LESCH R, DECKER K: Orotate prevents galactosamine hepatitis. *Hoppe Seylers Z Physiol Chem* 35:102, 1970

335. KEPPLER D, DECKER K: Studies on the mechanism of galactosamine hepatitis. *Eur J Biochem* 10:219, 1969

336. STARLING JJ, KEPPLER DOR: Metabolism of 2-deoxy-d-galactose in liver induces phosphate and uridylate trapping. *Eur J Biochem* 80:373, 1977

337. LATTKE H, KOCH HK, LESCH R, KEPPLER DOR: Consequences of recurrent phosphate trapping induced by repeated injections of 2-deoxy-DO galactose. *Virchows Arch B Cell Path* 30:297, 1979

338. LANDAU B, HASTINGS A, ZOTTA S: Studies on carbohydrate metabolism in rat liver slices. *J Biol Chem* 233:1257, 1958

339. NORDIN J, HANSEN RG: Isolation and characterization of galactose from hydrolysates of glycogen. *J Biol Chem* 238:489, 1963

340. GRODSKY CM, BATIS AA, BENNETT II, VOELLA C, MCWILLIAMS NB, SMITH DF: Effects of carbohydrates on secretion of insulin from isolated rat pancreas. *Am J Physiol* 205:638, 1963

341. GITZELMANN R, ILLIC R: Inability of galactose to metabolize insulin in galactokinase deficient individuals. *Diabetologia* 5:143, 1969

342. DUBOIS R, LOEB H, OOMS HA: Etude de métabolisme glucidique dans la galactosémie et la fructosémie. *Rev Fr Etud Clin Biol* 7:509, 1962

343. GENTH C, VALLETTE AM, LEMONNIER A, COLIN J, ODIENRE M, LELUC R, THUONG TRILU C, ALAGILLE D: Etude de métabolisme glucidique an ecours de la galactosémie congénitale. *Arch Fr Pediatr* 23:509, 1966

344. TADA K: Glycogenesis and glycolysis in the liver from congenital galactosemia. *Tohoku J Exp Med* 82:168, 1964

345. ROSENBERG I, WEINBERG A, SEGAL S: The effect of high galactose diets on urinary excretion of amino acids in the rat. *Biochim Biophys Acta* 48:500, 1961

346. FOX M, THIER S, ROSENBERG L, SEGAL S: Impaired renal tubular function induced by sugar infusion in man. *J Clin Endocrinol* 24:1318, 1964

347. THIER S, FOX M, ROSENBERG L, SEGAL S: Hexose inhibition of amino acid uptake in the rat-kidney-cortex slice. *Biochim Biophys Acta* 93:106, 1964

348. SAUNDERS S, ISSELBACHER KJ: Inhibition of intestinal amino acid transport by hexoses. *Biochim Biophys Acta* 102:397, 1965

349. DIEDRICH D, ANDERSON L: Galactose 1-phosphate in the intestinal tissue of the rat during galactose absorption. *Biochim Biophys Acta* 43:490, 1960

350. HAWORTH JC, FORD JD, YOUNOSZAL MK: Effect of galactose toxicity on growth of the rat fetus and brain. *Pediatr Res* 3:441, 1969

351. HAWORTH JC, FORD JD, HO, HK: The effect of galactose toxicity on growth of the developing rat brain. *Brain Res* 21:385, 1970

352. WELLS HJ, WELLS WW: Galactose toxicity and myomositol metabolism in developing rat brain. *Biochemistry* 6:1168, 1967

353. WARFIELD A, SEGAL S: Myoinositol and phosphatidylinositol metabolism in synaptosomes from galactose-fed rats. *Proc Natl Acad Sci USA* 75:4568, 1978

354. GABBAY KH, SNIDER JJ: Galactosemic neuropathy: A model for diabetic neuropathy. *Diabetes* 19:357, 1970

355. MYERS RR, COSTELLO ML, POWELL HC: Increased endoneurial fluid pressure in galactose neuropathy. *Muscle Nerve* 299, 1979

356. KOZAK LP, WELLS WW: Effect of galactose on energy and phospholipid metabolism in the chick brain. *Arch Biochem Biophys* 135:371, 1969

357. MAYES JS, MILLER IR, MYERS FK: The relationship of galactose-1-phosphate accomulation and uridyltransferase activity to the differential galactose toxicity in male and female chicks. *Biochem Biophys Res Commun* 39:661, 1970

358. WELLS HJ, GORDON M, SEGAL S: Galactose toxicity in the chick: Oxidation of radioactive galactose. *Biochim Biophys Acta* 222:327, 1970

359. MUSICK WDL, WELLS WW: Studies on galactose metabolism on heart and brain: The identification of D-galactose 6-phosphate in brains of galactose-intoxicated chicks and rat hearts perfused with galactose. *Arch Biochem Biophys* 165:217, 1974

360. RIGDON RH, COUCH JR, CREGES CR, FERGUSON TM: Galactose intoxication pathologic study in the chick. *Experientia* 19:349, 1963

361. KOZAK LP, WELLS WW: Studies on the metabolic determinants of D-galactose-induced neurotoxicity in the chick. *J Neurochem* 18:2217, 1971

362. GRANEIT SE, KOZAK LP, McINTYRE JP, WELLS WW: Studies on cerebral energy metabolism during the course of galactose neurotoxicity in chicks. *J Neurochem* 19:1659, 1972

363. KNULL HR, WELLS WW: Recovery from galactose-induced neurotoxicity in the chick by the administration of glucose. *J Neurochem* 20:415, 1973

364. BLOSSER JC, WELLS WW: Enhanced fragility of neural lysosomes from chicks suffering from galactose toxicity. *J Neurochem* 19:1539, 1972

365. BLOSSER JC, WELLS WW: Studies on amino acid levels and protein metabolism in the brains of galactose-intoxicated chicks. *J Neurochem* 19:69, 1972

366. KNULL HR, TAYLOR WF, WELLS WW: Effects of energy metabolism on in vivo distribution of hexokinase in brain. *J Biol Chem* 248:5414, 1973

367. KNULL HR, LOBERI PF, WELLS WW: Galactose neurotoxicity in chicks. Effects on fast axoplasmic transport. *Brain Res* 79:524, 1974

368. MALONE J, WELLS H, SEGAL S: Decreased uptake of glucose by brain of the galactose toxic chick. *Brain Res* 43:700, 1972

369. MALONE J, WELLS HJ, SEGAL S: Galactose toxicity in the chick: Hyperosmolality. *Science* 174:952, 1971

370. CARVER NJ: Disturbances by galactose of the free amino acids of fetal rat brain. *Biochim Biophys Acta* 130:514, 1966

371. HETIENLOCHER PR, HILLMAN RE, HSIA YE: Pseudotumor cerebri in galactosemia. *J Pediatr* 76:902, 1970

372. LITMAN N, KANTER A, FINBERG L: Galactokinase deficiency presenting as pseudotumor cerebri. *J Pediatr* 86:410, 1975

373. BERRY G, YANDRASITZ J, SEGAL S: Experimental galactose toxicity: Effects on synaptosomal phosphatidyl-inositol metabolism. *J Neurochem* 37:888, 1981

374. WOODLEY DW: *Biochemical Basis of Psychosis or the Serotonin Hypothesis about Mental Diseases.* New York, John Wiley & Sons, Inc, 1962

375. WOOLLEY DW, GOMMI BW: Serotonin receptors. IV. Specific deficiency of receptors in galactose toxicity and its possible relationship to the idiocy of galactosemia. *Proc Natl Acad Sci USA* 52:14, 1964

376. YANDRASITZ JR, HWANG SM, COHN R, SEGAL S: On the involvement of serotonin in galactose brain toxicity. *J Neurochem* 33:1321,

377. MILLER LR, GORDON GB, BENCH KG: Cytologic alterations in hereditary metabolic disorders. I. The effects of galactose on galactosemia fibroblasts *in vitro. Lab Invest* 19:428, 1968

378. TEDESCO TA, MILLER KL: Galactosemia: Alterations in sulfate metabolism secondary to galactose-1-phoshate uridyltransferase deficiency. *Science* 205:1395, 1979

379. PENNINGTON JS, PRANNERD TAJ: Studies of erythrocyte phosphate enter metabolism in galactosemia. *Clin Sci* 17:385, 1958

380. ZIPURSKY A, ROWLAND M, FORD, JD, HAWORTH JC, ISRAELS LG: Erythrocyte metabolism in galactosemia. *Pediatrics* 35:126, 1965

381. MONTIFLEONE JA, BRUTLER F, MONTELEONE PL, URZ CI, CASEY FC: Cataracts galactosemia in hypergalactosemia due to galactokinase deficiency. *Am J Med* 50:403, 1971

382. OLAMBIWONNI NO, McVIE R Nc, WC, FRASIER SD, DONNELL GN: Galactokinase deficiency in twine clinical and biochemical studies. *Pediatrics* 53:314, 1974

383. THALHAMMER O, GIFZELMANN R, PANTILFESCRO M: Hypergalactosemia and galactosuria due to galactokinase deficiency in a newborn. *Pediatrics* 42:441, 1968

384. DAHLQVIST A, GAMSTORP I, MADSEN H: A patient with hereditary galactokinase deficiency. *Acta Paediatr Scand* 59:669, 1970

385. LINNEWEH F, SCRAUMLOFFEI F, VETRELLA M: Galaktokinase-defelt bei einem Neugeborenen. *Klim Wochenschbr* 48:31, 1970

386. VIGNFRON C, MARCHAL C, DEIFTS C: Deficit partiel et transitoire en galactokinase erythrocytaire chez un nouveau ne: étude biochimique. *Arch Fr Pediatr* 27:523, 1970

387. COOK JGH, DON NA, MANN, TP: Hereditary galactokinase deficiency. *Arch Dis Child* 46:465, 1971

388. LEVY NS, KRILLE AF, BEUTLER F: Galactokinase deficiency and cataracts. *Am J Ophthalmol* 74:41, 1972

389. PICKERING WR, HOWELL RR: Galactokinase deficiency: Clinical and biochemical findings in a new kindred. *J Pediatr* 81:50, 1972

390. KALOUD H, SITZMANN FC, AYER, R, PALINUF F: Klinische and biochemische Befunde bei emen Kleinkind mit hereditarem Galakto-kimasdefekt. *Klin Padiatr* 185:18, 1973

391. FANCONI G: Hochgradiage galaktose-Intoleranz galacktose-Diabetes bei einem Kinde Unit Neurofibromatosim Recklinghansen. *Jahrb Kinderheilkd* 138:1, 1933

392. SEGAL S, RUTMAN JY, FRIMPTER GW: Galactokinase deficiency and mental retardation. *J Pediatr* 95:750, 1979

393. REULIER F, KRILL A, COMINGS D, TRINIDAD F: Galactokinase deficiency: An important cause of familial cataracts in children and young adults. *J Lab Clin Med* 76: 1006, 1970

394. BEUTLER F, MAISUMOTO F, KUM W, KRILL A, LEVY N, SPARKES R. DEGNIS M: Galactokinase deficiency as a cause of cataracts. *N Engl J Med* 288:1203, 1973

395. SKALKA HW, PRCHAL JT: Presenile cataract formation and decreased activity of galactosemic enzymes. *Arch Ophthalmol* 98:269, 1980

396. GITZELMANN R, WELLS HJ, SEGAL S: Galactose metabolism in a patient with hereditary galactokinase deficiency. *Eur J Clin Invest* 4:79, 1974

397. MAYES JS, GUTHRIE R: Detection of heterozygotes for galactokinase deficiency a human population. *Biochem Genet* 2:219, 1968

398. MELIMAN WJ, RAWNSLEY BE, NICHOLS CW, NEEDLEMAN B, MENNUTI MT, MALONE J, TEDESCO TA: Galactose tolerance studies of individuals with reduced galactose pathway activity. *Am J Hum Genet* 27:748, 1975

399. STEPHENS T, IRVINE S, MUTTON P, GUPTA JD, HARLEY JD: Deficiency of two enzymes of galactose metabolism in kangaroos. *Nature (Lond.)* 248:524, 1974

400. STEPHENS T, IRVINE S, MUTTON P, GUPTA JD, HARLEY JD: The case of the cataractous kangaroo. *Med J Aust* 2:910, 1974

401. STEPHENS T, CROLLINE C, MUTTON P, GUPTA JD, HARTLEY JD: Galactose metabolism in relation to cataract formation in marsipials. *Aust J Exp Biol Med Sci* 53:233, 1973

402. GITZELMANN R: Deficiency of uridine diphosphate galactose 4-epimerase in blood cells of an apparently healthy infant. *Helv Paediat Acta* 27:125, 1972

403. GITZELMANN R, STEINMANN B: Uridine diphosphate galactose 4-epimerase deficiency. H. Clinical follow-up. *Helv Paedtr Acta* 28:49, 1973

404. GITZELMANN R, STEINMANN B, MITCHELL B, HAIGIS E: Uridine diphosphate galactose 4'-epimerase deficiency. *Helv Paediat Acta* 31:441, 1976

405. MITCHELL B, HAIGIS F, STEINMAN B, GITZELMANN R: Reversal of UDP galactose 4-epimerase deficiency of human leukocytes in culture. *Proc Natl Acad Sci USA* 72:5026, 1975

8

PENTOSURIA

This summary is adapted from the summary written by
Howard H. Hiatt for the fourth edition of this book. [1].

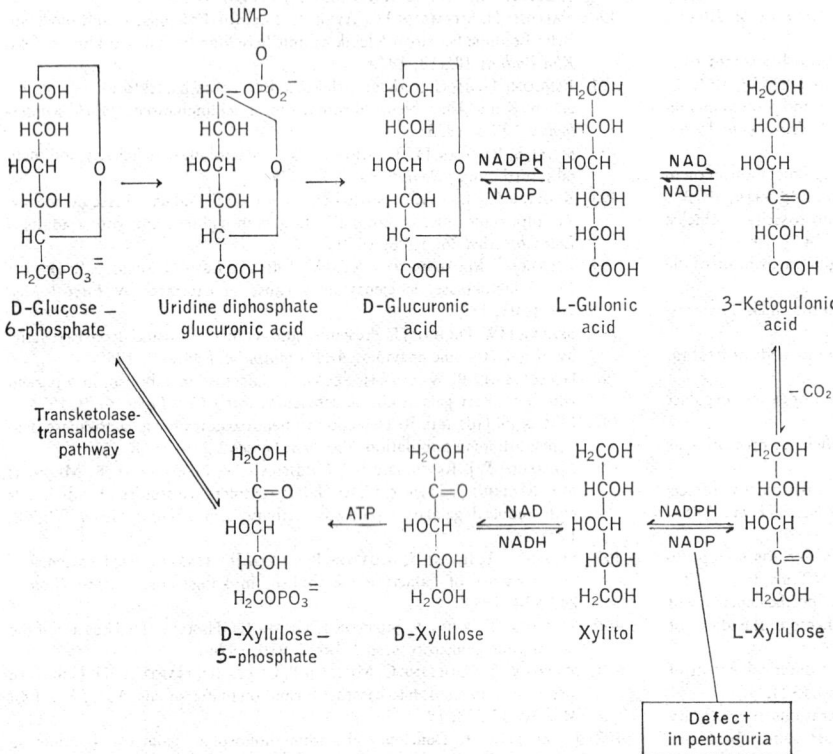

The glucuronic acid oxidation pathway, illustrating
the enzymatic site of the metabolic block in pentosuria.

---

1. Essential pentosuria *is an inborn error of metabolism in which large amounts (1 to 4 g) of the pentose L-xylulose is excreted in the urine each day. It is a benign disturbance which occurs principally in Jews and which behaves genetically as an autosomal recessive trait.*
2. *This disorder bears no relationship to diabetes mellitus and is easily distinguished from several other varieties of pentosuria in which milligram quantities of a number of pentoses other than L-xylulose appear in the urine.*
3. *Essential pentosuria is the result of a defect in the glucuronic acid oxidation pathway. In this route of carbohydrate metabolism the carboxyl carbon atom of D-glucuronic acid is removed in a series of reactions, giving rise to the pentose L-xylulose. This latter compound may then be converted to its stereoisomer, D-xylulose, which in turn may be phosphorylated. D-Xylulose-5-phosphate may participate in reactions of the pentose phosphate pathway which lead to its conver-*

sion to hexose phosphate (glucuronic acid → L-xylulose → xylitol → D-xylulose → pentose phosphate pathway → hexose phosphate). The glucuronic acid oxidation pathway serves no essential function in humans.
4. *The metabolic block in pentosuria results from reduced activity of L-xylulose reductase, the enzyme that catalyzes the conversion of L-xylulose to xylitol.*
5. *Heterozygotes can be recognized by demonstrating either an intermediate level of erythrocyte activity of L-xylulose reductase or increased urinary or serum L-xylulose, or both, in a glucuronolactone loading test.*

REFERENCE

1. HIATT HH: Pentosuria, in Stanbury JB, Wyngaarden JB, Frederickson DS (eds): *The Metabolic Basis of Inherited Disease*, ed 4. New York, McGraw-Hill Book Co, 1978, p 110

9

INBORN ERRORS OF PYRUVATE METABOLISM

JOHN P. BLASS

1. *Two inborn errors of pyruvate metabolism are recognized. One is a deficiency of pyruvate dehydrogenase, the enzyme system that catalyzes the oxidation of pyruvate to CO_2 and acetyl CoA. The other is a deficiency of pyruvate carboxylase, the enzyme system that catalyzes the fixation of CO_2 to pyruvate to form oxaloacetate. Both disorders appear to be inherited by an autosomal recessive mechanism.*

2. *Deficiencies of pyruvate dehydrogenase have been reported in over 50 patients. The most striking clinical abnormality involves the nervous system, causing ataxia and psychomotor retardation. Lactic acidosis is prominent in the most severe (infantile) cases. Pyruvate dehydrogenase is a complicated enzyme system involving three proteins, three substrates, and a complex regulation of inactivation and reactivation by a phosphorylation-dephosphorylation cycle. The site of the mutation in individual cases has not been clarified, but it is likely that extensive genetic heterogeneity is operative.*

3. *Pyruvate carboxylase deficiency occurs in infants with severe psychomotor retardation and lactic acidosis. A partial deficiency is also found in fibroblasts cultured from some children with subacute necrotizing encephalomyelopathy or with inborn errors of biotin metabolism, but the relation between the enzyme abnormality and the underlying disease is not known.*

4. *Diagnosis of a hereditary disorder of pyruvate metabolism is difficult. In a wide variety of clinical states the blood pyruvate level rises, apparently as a result of acquired decreases in the activities of pyruvate dehydrogenase and pyruvate decarboxylase. Such disorders include thiamine deficiency, shock, and Reye's syndrome. Distinguishing between primary and secondary syndromes requires enzyme assays of cultured fibroblasts, which are not yet standardized for clinical use.*

5. *The nervous system abnormalities in the disorders of pyruvate metabolism appear to be caused by deficiencies in the synthesis of neurotransmitters, rather than by inadequate production of ATP and related high energy compounds. For example, in pyruvate dehydrogenase deficiency, the impaired oxidation of pyruvate leads to decreased generation of acetyl CoA, which in turn causes a decreased synthesis of acetylcholine. In the pyruvate carboxylase deficiencies, the enzyme defect impairs the production of oxaloacetate, which in turn impairs gluconeogenesis, leading to decreased synthesis of amino acid neurotransmitters, such as aspartate, glutamate, and γ-aminobutyric acid.*

6. *Beneficial effects of various dietary and drug regimens have been described in individual case reports. None is well established.*

Pyruvic acid sits in the center of most charts of cellular metabolism (Fig. 9-1). It is a key intermediate in glycolysis and gluconeogenesis and in the main pathway by which glucose is oxidized to CO_2 and H_2O. Many metabolic disorders alter pyruvate metabolism indirectly. It is now clear that there are also two genetic disorders which directly affect the enzyme systems for which pyruvate is a major physiologic substrate, namely, the pyruvate dehydrogenase complex and pyruvate carboxylase. The inborn errors resulting from deficiencies of these two enzyme systems are discussed in this chapter.

DEFICIENCY OF THE PYRUVATE DEHYDROGENASE COMPLEX (PDHC)

Deficiency of the pyruvate dehydrogenase complex (PDHC) has been reported in over 50 patients [1] and confirmed independently in 2 [2–4]. The complexity of the chemistry and the inadequacy of available clinical assays make some of the reports hard to interpret. This syndrome appears to be inherited as an autosomal recessive trait, although this has not been clearly established.

Biochemistry of PDHC

No enzyme system more complicated than PDHC has yet been characterized [5, 6]. This enzyme complex catalyzes the oxidation of pyruvate to CO_2 and acetyl CoA with concomitant production of NADH (Figs. 9-1 and 9-2). To do so, it utilizes five cofactors: thiamine pyrophosphate (TPP), lipoic acid (dithiooctanoic acid), coenzyme A, flavine adenine dinucleotide (FAD), and NAD^+. It requires Mg^{2+}. The overall reaction is carried out by an ordered sequence of reactions catalyzed by three proteins: pyruvate dehydrogenase (PDH; EC 1.2.4.1),

Figure 9-1 Main pathways of carbohydrate metabolism: (1) pyruvate dehydrogenase complex (PDHC); (2) pyruvate carboxylase (PC).

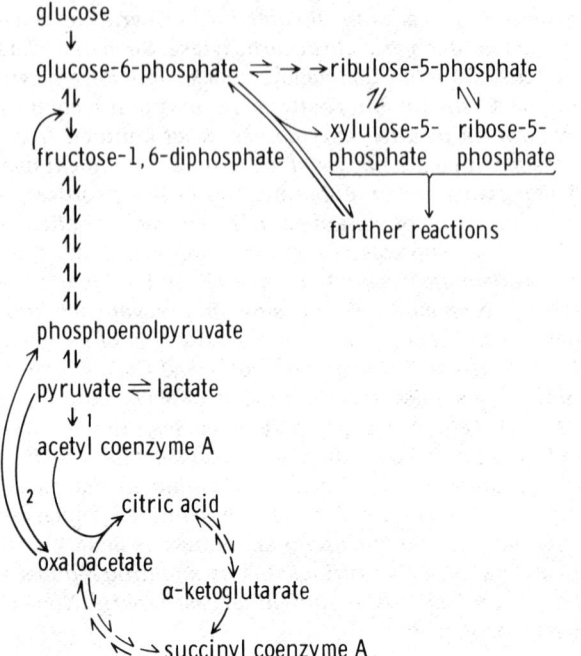

dihydrolipoyltransacetylase (DLT; EC 2.3.1.12), and dihydrolipoyl dehydrogenase (LAD; EC 1.6.4.3). They are arranged in an ordered array, as a pentagonal dodecahadron with icosahedral symmetry. The core consists of 60 DLT chains, to which 20 to 30 PDH molecules and 5 to 6 LAD molecules are attached noncovalently. These statements are based on the bovine enzymes. The human enzyme has not yet been purified to homogeneity despite intensive efforts [7]. The published nomenclature for this enzyme is confusing. The abbreviations PDH and PDC have been used to refer to either the whole complex or its pyruvate dehydrogenase component, which has also been erroneously called *pyruvate decarboxylase* [2]. LAD has commonly been referred to as *lipoamide dehydrogenase*.

The PDH component oxidatively decarboxylates pyruvate to form CO_2 while attaching the remaining 2-carbon fragment to TPP to form hydroxyethylthiamine (Fig. 9-2). PDH is a tetramer of $\alpha_2\beta_2$ structure. The α subunit binds TPP tightly but not covalently; the apparent K_m for the animal enzyme is 1 μm or less, while that for the human enzyme appears to be up to twentyfold greater [7a]. While artificial electron acceptors such as $Fe(CN)_6^{3-}$ can oxidize the hydroxyethylthiamine and regenerate the original active enzyme, they do so much less efficiently than the DLT enzyme of the complex. The α subunit of PDH is a major site of regulation of PDHC, as discussed below.

The DLT core enzyme catalyzes the transfer and simultaneous oxidation of the 2-carbon fragment of hydroxyethylthiamine to CoA, forming acetyl CoA (Fig. 9-2). In the process, the disulfide ring of covalently bound lipoic acid is reduced to the dihydro form and simultaneously oxidizes the acetaldehyde equivalent to an acetic acid equivalent [5, 6].

LAD reoxidizes the dihydrolipoic acid to the oxidized form by transferring hydrogens from dihydrolipoic acid to enzyme-bound FAD and from $FADH_2$ to soluble NAD^+ [8, 9]. The transfer of reducing equivalents from FAD to NAD^+ is the reverse of the usual direction of redox enzymes. LAD is a dimer of two apparently identical subunits. It is a transhydrogenase, catalyzing the transfer of reducing equivalents among a number of electron acceptors, including natural compounds such as NAD^+ and $NADP^+$ and artificial acceptors such as dichlorophenolindophenol and methylene blue. Indeed, Straub originally described it as a diaphorase [10]. Subsequent studies showed that it has LAD activity [11] and is a constituent of the pyruvate, ketoglutarate, and branched chain keto acid dehydrogenase complexes [5, 9, 12]. The amount of LAD in mitochondria is far in excess of that in the dehydrogenase complexes, suggesting that it might have other functions as well [9, 13]. Trace concentrations of Cu^{2+} oxidize a critical sulfhydryl group, transforming the enzyme from a two-electron transhydrogenase to a one-electron catalase [14, 15]. Thus, minimal impurities in laboratory water supply can alter the properties of the enzyme as usually assayed. There are important species variations [9]. The human enzyme has not been isolated.

Regulation of PDHC is intricate [5, 6]. Fine, moment-to-moment regulation appears to depend primarily on end product inhibition by NADH (competitively with NAD^+) and acetyl CoA (competitively with CoA). Covalent modification may be a more important regulatory mechanism [5, 6]. The α subunit of PDH is phosphorylated by a specific kinase (PDH$_a$ kinase, EC 2.7.1.99) and dephosphorylated by a specific phosphatase (PDH$_b$ phosphatase, EC 3.1.3.43), (Fig. 9-2). Phosphorylation inactivates PDH; dephosphorylation reactivates it. Numerous effectors alter the pitch of this regulatory system

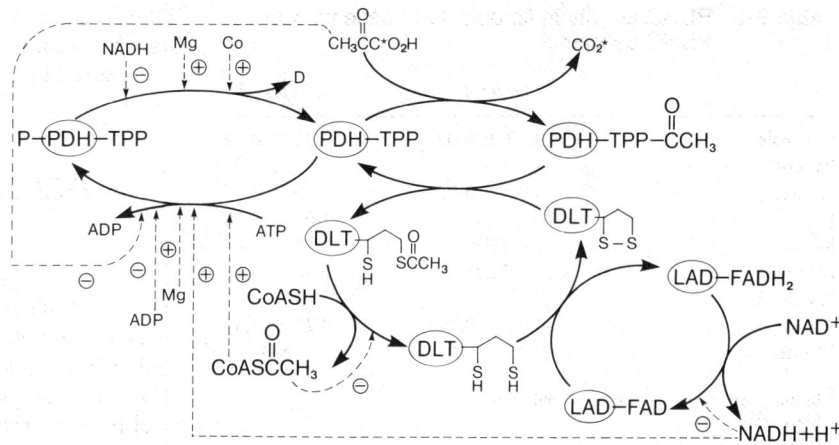

Figure 9-2 Pyruvate dehydrogenase complex—scheme: PDH, pyruvate dehydrogenase (EC 1.2.4.1); DLT, dihydrolipoyltransacetylase (EC 2.3.1.12); LAD, dihydrolipoyldehydrogenase (EC 1.6.4.3); Dotted lines indicate effectors; ⊕ enhances activity, ⊖ reduces activity.

(Fig. 9-2), but the most important single factor appears to be the ATP/ADP ratio inside the mitochondrion [4, 5, 16, 17]. The kinase incorporates the γ-phosphate of ATP into three specific serines in the α subunit of PDH. Phosphorylation at any of these sites inactivates PDHC [18–20]. Site 1 may be phosphorylated more readily than sites 2 and 3 [18], and phosphorylation of sites 2 and 3 have been reported to slow dephosphorylation of site 1 in some studies [6, 20] but not with highly purified enzyme [5, 18, 19]. Whether the inner mitochondrial membrane which surrounds PDHC in vivo affects the availability of the three sites for phosphorylation is not known. Recently, Morgan and Routtenberg [21] have reported that training leads to dephosphorylation of brain PDH, and Browning and coworkers [22] have reported that habituation can have the same effect. Also, insulin activates PDHC by favoring dephosphorylation [5, 6], perhaps via the action of an intermediate peptide [23].

Clinical Assays of PDHC

Given the complexity of PDHC, it is no surprise that measuring its activity in clinical samples has not been straightforward. Most clinical assays have been radiochemical, depending on the cofactor-dependent conversion of [1-^{14}C]pyruvate to $^{14}CO_2$ by cell-free extracts [1–4, 24]. They are technically demanding. The radioactive substrate is unstable [24, 25], and even the techniques for disrupting cells can dramatically alter activity [26].

In cultured skin fibroblasts, reported activities in controls have varied widely—from about 0.02 nmol/minute per milligram of protein [27] to about 1.0 [28]. Recently, Utter and Sheu [4, 29] have succeeded in activating (dephosphorylating) PDHC in cultured fibroblasts and obtained activities of about 2 nmol/minute per milligram of protein in cells from adults to about 5 in cells from newborn infants. Previous studies apparently examined largely the residual activity of inactivated enzyme. Sorbi and Blass [30] have combined the activation techniques of Utter et al. [4, 29] with a spectrophotometric-coupled enzyme assay for PDHC, using pigeon liver arylamine acetyltransferase to follow the production of acetyl CoA. Published studies of PDHC activity in leukocytes suffer from analogous drawbacks to published studies of cultured fibroblasts.

PDHC activity has been measured in biopsied human muscle [31] and in human liver obtained at biopsy or autopsy [28, 32,

33]. The relatively large amounts of tissue available have allowed the use of techniques well standardized on animal tissues, including activation. Compared to cultured cells, these tissues have the drawback that changes in PDHC may occur secondary to the disease process in both patients and controls. Neuromuscular diseases can change both the ratio of type 1 to type 2 muscle fibers and the number and properties of muscle mitochondria [34]. Liver contains protease(s) which acts on PDHC [35] and secondary changes in hepatic PDHC have been reported in Reye's syndrome [36].

PDHC is relatively stable post mortem in animal [37] and human [38] brain. However, reported activities of PDHC in autopsy human brain were very low [38].

LAD activity has been assayed in human autopsy tissues [39] and in serum [40], platelets [40–42], and cultured fibroblasts [41, 43]. Some assays appear chemically straightforward [39, 41]. Others appear nonspecific in that the measured activity is insensitive to known inhibitors of LAD [44].

This dreary catalog of technical problems provides the framework in which reports of PDHC deficiencies should be considered.

Clinical Characteristics

The two original patients with independently confirmed PDHC deficiencies typify the spectrum of clinical presentations in other reported cases.

Lactate Acidosis Consanguine parents, one of whose children had died in infancy, had a baby girl. She had decreased movement in her third trimester in utero and then fed poorly. Slow development was noted by age 7 months and lactate acidosis at age 18 months. When examined at age 3 years, she had severe psychomotor retardation with microcephaly, optic atrophy, muscular hypotonia despite hyperactive reflexes and scissoring, and poor coordination. She died before age 6. There was no autopsy. Activity of PDHC was 15 percent of the control mean in the original study and 7 percent in the studies of Sheu et al. (Table 9-1).

Ataxic Encephalopathy A boy born to unrelated parents began at age 16 months to have episodes of ataxia lasting up to a week and precipitated by nonspecific stresses such as intercurrent upper respiratory infections. [2, 45]. Initially he seemed normal between attacks except perhaps for mild clum-

Table 9-1 PDHC activity in fibroblasts*of patients with PDHC deficiency

	Series 1[†]	Series 2[‡]
Controls	0.39 ± 0.03	3.98 ± 0.24
Patient 1		
(ataxia)	0.04 ± 0.02	0.10 ± 0.05
Father	ND	1.05 ± 0.08
Mother	ND	0.74 ± 0.04
Brother	ND	2.30 ± 0.18
Patient 2		
(acidosis)	0.06 ± 0.01	0.28 ± 0.51
Mother	0.23 ± 0.06	ND

* In nmol/min per milligram of fibroblast protein.
† Blass et al. [2, 3, 131].
‡ Sheu et al. [4].
NOTE: Activity in series 1 was measured without activation [2, 3, 131]. In series 2, it was measured in the same cell lines after activation with dichloroacetate [4]. Values are nmol/min per milligram of fibroblast protein ± SEM. ND = not determined. See original references for details.

siness, but he has subsequently developed optic atrophy and a high arch. He has done well in school and is attending a demanding college. Activity of PDHC in his cultured fibroblasts was 11 percent of the control mean in the original studies and 2.5 percent by the methods of Sheu et al. (Table 9-1). Cells from his parents have activities intermediate between his and those of controls. This suggests that they each have a single deficient gene for PDHC, while he has two mutant genes.

Many reports of PDHC deficiency have not yet been confirmed by newer methods (Table 9-2). In one patient, activity of LAD was deficient by direct assay of liver, brain, and kidney obtained at autopsy, but fibroblasts from this child failed to grow and family studies were not done [39]. There is a possibility that the defect in the tissues was secondary to the disease process.

In patients with more severe PDHC deficiencies, the general clinical pattern is one of psychomotor retardation of early onset, with increasingly severe signs of dysfunction of much of the nervous system and death within the first decade. Levels of lactate are variable and in part reflect the diet. One patient nearly died on a high carbohydrate diet but has been relatively stable on a high fat diet and outlived his affected sibs [46]. Few of these patients have come to autopsy. Small brains with lack of white as well as gray matter were reported in two patients [46]. Two and possibly three [39] had the neuropathology of subacute necrotizing encephalomyelopathy or Leigh disease [28, 47]. Another had agenesis of the corpus callosum [101].

Milder PDHC deficiencies have tended to be associated with prominent ataxia, as well as other signs of widespread dysfunction of the nervous system [45, 48], i.e., with "ataxic encephalopathies" [49]. Whether mutations of PDHC occur in classic spinocerebellar syndromes such as Friedreich's ataxia is controversial [26, 27, 31, 40–43, 50] and depends in part on the definitions used for *patients* and *controls* [26, 31, 41, 48, 50].

DeVivo et al. [28] described a patient with autopsy-proven Leigh disease in whose liver, obtained post mortem, PDHC was unusually difficult to activate. PDHC activity in fibroblasts appeared normal, even after attempted activation. Butterworth and Melancon [47] made similar observations on the liver of another child with autopsy-proven Leigh disease.

Fibroblasts from two other children with Leigh disease may have had a subtle abnormality of PDHC [51, 52]. Leigh disease is discussed in greater detail below.

DEFICIENCY OF PYRUVATE CARBOXYLASE

Deficiency of pyruvate carboxylase (PC) has been unequivocally demonstrated in two severely retarded infants with congenital lactate acidosis [53–56] and reported in several others [57–65]. The syndrome appears to be inherited as an autosomal recessive trait.

Biochemistry of Pyruvate Carboxylase

This enzyme catalyzes the fixation of CO_2 to pyruvate to form oxaloacetate (Fig. 9-1). This is the first reaction of gluconeogenesis. It also provides 4-carbon compounds to "prime" the Kreb's tricarboxylic acid cycle, thereby providing the carbon skeleton for the putative neurotransmitter amino acids glutamate, aspartate, and γ-aminobutyric acid and also contributing to lipogenesis and ketogenesis.

The mammalian enzyme is tetrameric, with a molecular weight of about 70,000 [66]. The reaction mechanism is complex, probably involving two catalytic sites [66] and enzyme-bound biotin.

Acetyl CoA is a critical positive effector [66–69]. With saturating concentrations of substrates, addition of 50 μM acetyl CoA increases activity of the human enzyme over thirtyfold. The requirement for acetyl CoA is probably absolute under physiologic conditions. A divalent cation is needed in excess of that complexed by ATP or ADP. Monovalent cations also activate PC; K^+ is the most effective for the human enzyme (K_A 2.27 μM), while Na^+ is ineffective or possibly a mild inhibitor [68]. Millimolar concentrations of phenylpyruvate and *p*-hydroxyphenylpyruvate inhibit the human enzyme. Incubation in dilute solution at less than 20°C inactivates the human enzyme, but more slowly than it does the avian enzyme [68]. There do not appear to be tissue-specific isoenzymes; hereditary deficiencies affect all tissues examined in humans [53–56], and antibodies to the purified enzyme cross-react with all rat tissues studied [70]. Human PC is located inside mitochondria [71].

Standardized conditions [53–55] to assay human PC appear adequate to detect carriers (Table 9-3).

Clinical Characteristics of PC Deficiency

The two patients, one male and one female, with definite PC deficiency [53–56] were born to unrelated, clinically normal white parents with no family history of neurologic disease. They seemed normal at birth but developed seizures at age 3 months. Despite appropriate and intensive therapy, they deteriorated progressively, showing psychomotor retardation, poor head control, hypotonia, and bizarre posturing. Their courses were stormy. Both had lactic acidosis (up to 17 μM versus normal <2), elevated blood pyruvate levels (0.2 to 0.8

Table 9-2 Reports of PDHC deficiency

Patient	Presentation	PDHC[a] (percent)	Tissue[b]	Reference
1	Ataxia	3–10	Fibroblasts	2, 4, 45
2	Ataxia	8	Fibroblasts	132, 133
3	Ataxia	33	Fibroblasts	132, 133
4[c]	Acidosis, retardation	3–15	Fibroblasts	3, 4
5[d]	Leigh disease	"Partial"	Fibroblasts	51
6	Acidosis, retardation	10	Liver	134
7	Acidosis, retardation	Activation defect	Liver	135
8	Acidosis	0	Liver, brain	136
9[e]	Acidosis, retardation	15	Fibroblasts	46
10	Ataxia, retardation	36	Fibroblasts, platelets	120
11	Ataxia, retardation	32	Fibroblasts, platelets	120
12[f]	Acidosis, retardation	13	Fibroblasts	137
13[g]	Acidosis	11	Fibroblasts	138
14	Ataxia	22–28	Fibroblasts, white cells	129
15[d]	Leigh disease	15–50	Fibroblasts	52
16[h]	Leigh disease	26	Fibroblasts	52
17	Ataxia	49	Fibroblasts	139
18	Ataxia	27	Fibroblasts	139
19	Ataxia	44	Fibroblasts	139
20	Ataxia	46	Fibroblasts	139
21	Ataxia[i]	43	Fibroblasts	139
22	Acidosis, hypoglycemia	3–16	Liver, muscle, brain, kidney, heart	39
23	Acidosis, Ataxia	2	Fibroblasts	101
24	Ataxia, hypotonia	44	Fibroblasts	101
25	Acidosis, retardation	5	Fibroblasts, liver	141
26	Acidosis, retardation	37	Fibroblasts	33
27	Leigh disease[d]	Activation defect	Liver	56
28–37[j]	Acidosis, retardation, ataxia	5–50	Fibroblasts	142
38–46[k]	Neuropathy/ataxia	42–60	Fibroblasts	143
47–58[l]	Ataxia	27–45	Platelets	144
59–62[m]	Ataxia	22–38	Platelets	145
63–67[j]	Acidosis	8–39	Fibroblasts	146

[a] Activity as percent of control in each study.
[b] Tissues in which low activities were demonstrated.
[c] One sib died with a similar syndrome.
[d] Autopsy confirmed.
[e] Two sibs died with a similar syndrome.
[f] Two sibs died with a similar syndrome. The defect was replicated in two studies of these cells but not in two others.
[g] Loss of gray and white matter at autopsy after being on a respirator.
[h] Sib died with a similar syndrome and Leigh disease at autopsy. The defect was demonstrated in ferricyanide-linked but not in NAD-linked assays.
[i] Not confirmed in independent studies of platelets [140].
[j] Published clinical information on these patients is limited.
[k] Cells from patient with fatigue and no neurologic deficit, 42 percent of control mean activity; replicate biopsies from three "deficient" patients had normal activity.
[l] Activities calculated as ratios LAD to cytochrome-c-oxidase. Deficiencies of PDHC were not replicated in independent studies of two of these patients (140).
[m] Three other deficient patients also reported in [144]; in two of them, the defect was not independently replicated [140].

μM versus norm of 0.03 to 0.08), excessive blood and urine alanine levels, and intermittent hypoglycemia and ketosis. An alanine load failed to induce the normal gluconeogenetic response (in the boy).

Activity of PC was <1 percent of the control mean in fibroblasts from these patients, <17 percent in liver, and <0.1 percent in the brain and renal cortex of the one patient in whom it was measured. Activity in parental fibroblasts and lymphocytes was intermediate between patients and controls, indicating that the clinically normal parents each had a single abnormal gene for PC and the patients two abnormal genes.

Autopsy on the boy [53] demonstrated marked reductions in cerebral white matter, depletion of cerebral cortical neurons, numerous ectopic neurons, gliosis, and other degenerative changes. There was minimal hepatic portal fibrosis; earlier electron microscopy of a liver biopsy demonstrated abnormalities of the endoplasmic reticulum and paracrystalline inclusions in mitochondria. The renal tubular cells at autopsy contained vacuoles and fine granules. A muscle biopsy at 28 months showed rounded cross sections of muscle cells instead of the normal polygons and excessive lipid droplets in type I fibers.

Other reports of PC deficiency (Table 9-4) are not definitive, since they depend on measurements of PC activity in biopsy or

Table 9-3 Pyruvate carboxylase activities in fibroblasts in patients with PC deficiency and parents

	Patient 1[†] (0.02)	Patient 2[‡] (0)
Father	0.41	0.32
Mother	0.33	0.37
Controls	0.95–1.85	0.50

† PC[Portland] [55].
‡ PC[St. Louis] [56].
NOTE: Activities were measured in cultured fibroblasts from two families, by Atkin et al. and DeVivo et al. [55, 56]. Values are nmol/minute per milligram of protein; controls were studied in parallel with patients. For details, see original references.

autopsy liver. Hepatic PC activity can be low or absent in one sample of liver and normal in another sample from the same patient [59; 59a].

Two patients listed in Table 9-4 require further comment. Patient 5 reportedly responded to thiamine clinically, but PC in her liver was reported to lack a low-K_m component. Scrutton and White [68] have argued that this child had a deficiency of PDHC, with secondary abnormalities of PC due to a deficiency of the acetyl CoA activator. The Japanese patient (6) of Tada et al. [62] had a syndrome which can be classified as a severe ataxic encephalopathy. Finally, there are several patients in whom PC deficiency was reported to be associated with Leigh disease.

Leigh disease is a complicated entity. In 1951, Dennis Leigh described a child who died at 7 months after an illness which included somnolence and spasticity [72]. At autopsy, the brain showed changes very similar to those of Wernicke-Korsakoff syndrome, even though the child had apparently been well nourished. Subsequently, others recognized similar patients [73]. The definition has broadened to include not only the original infantile form but also adult forms which can resemble progressive ataxic encephalopathies or other degenerative dis-

eases of the nervous sytem [74–77]. Some clinicians now believe that they can detect patients with Leigh disease on the basis of certain unusual signs, such as rotary nystagmus and a peculiar waxing and waning of symptoms. Others require autopsy confirmation to accept the diagnosis. Even pathologic criteria are not straightforward [74, 77]. The neuropathologic changes of Wernicke-Korsakoff syndrome (and therefore of adult Leigh disease) occurred 5 to 10 times more often than did the clinical diagnosis in unselected patients coming to autopsy [78, 79].

A number of biochemical changes have been associated with this confusing clinical entity. Many workers have described elevated levels of lactate and pyruvate in the blood of patients with Leigh disease [28, 56, 57, 73]. DeVivo [73a] has suggested that normal cerebrospinal fluid lactate excludes the diagnosis.

A small portion of the thiamine in brain and other tissues exists as the triphosphate derivative. Pincus et al. [80] found none of this compound in the brain of a child with autopsy-proven Leigh disease. They reported that urine and tissues of such patients inhibited the kinase enzyme which forms thiamine triphosphate by phosphorylating thiamine pyrophosphate [81]. Murphy [82] reported that the "inhibitor" also occurs in cultured cells from these patients. Pincus and coworkers [83] have proposed a diagnostic test for Leigh disease based on assay of the inhibitor. Unfortunately, the proportion of false positives and false negatives has increased as experience has grown. Also, it is not clear what is being inhibited. Radioactivity from γ-phosphate-labeled radioactive ATP does not accumulate in thiamine triphosphate under conventional conditions of assay. There appears to be net phosphorylation of membrane-bound thiamine diphosphate [84], but as yet, there are no reports of whether or not the "inhibitor" inhibits phosphorylation of the natural substrate. As noted above, abnormalities of PDHC have been described in several cases of Leigh disease [28, 47, 51, 52], as well as of other enzymes in single case reports [85, 86].

Table 9-4 Reports of pyruvate carboxylase deficiency

Patient	Presentation[a]	Activity[b]	Tissue[c]	Reference
1	Leigh disease	<1	Liver	57
2	Retardation, acidosis	21	Liver	58
3	Leigh disease	<2	Liver	61
4[d]	Leigh disease	2–5	Liver, brain	59
5[e]	Retardation, acidosis	Kinetic	Liver	60
6	Retardation, ataxia	31	Liver	62
7	Leigh disease	2	Kidney	63
8[f]	Retardation (?) Leigh disease	21	Liver	147
9[g]	Acidosis, retardation	<1	Liver	64
10[h]	Acidosis, retardation	2	Kidney	64
11[i]	Retardation	Kinetic	Liver	65
12	Acidosis, retardation	0–7	Liver, fibroblasts, WBC	56
13	Acidosis, retardation	0–17	Liver, brain, kidney, fibroblasts, WBC	53

[a] Original authors' description. See original references for details.
[b] As percent of controls in same series.
[c] Tissues in which defects were demonstrated.
[d] Activity in a liver biopsy was normal; deficiency was demonstrated in autopsy tissues.
[e] Low K_m activity absent, high K_m normal.
[f] Sister with similar syndrome.
[g] Sister of patient 10.
[h] Brother of patient 9.
[i] Alper's syndrome.

One postulate consistent with the published reports on Leigh disease is that an inhibitor accumulates which can impair a number of enzymes.

SECONDARY ABNORMALITIES AFFECTING PYRUVATE METABOLISM

A number of secondary disorders affecting pyruvate metabolism are recognized. As discussed below, these secondary disorders must be distinguished clinically from the two rare inborn errors of pyruvate metabolism. One category of secondary disorders involves hereditary abnormalities of enzymes which catalyze steps in oxidative pathways subsequent to PDHC or in gluconeogenesis subsequent to PC (Fig. 9-1).

The list of hereditary abnormalities of mitochondrial oxidative metabolism is lengthening rapidly [87, 88]. The clinical syndromes vary but typically involve progressive disease of skeletal muscle, often mixed with damage to the nervous system—"neuromyopathies," sometimes resembling ataxic encephalopathies [87–91]. Biochemically, these disorders are generally not defined at the level of the aberrant protein—not even as well as PDHC or PC deficiencies.

Hereditary deficiencies have also been described for each of the distinctive enzymes of gluconeogenesis, i.e., those which do not also catalyze reactions of glycolysis (Fig. 9-1). The numbers of patients are small. Limited studies demonstrating deficiency of phosphoenolpyruvate carboxykinase in samples of autopsy liver [92, 93] do not rule out the possibility that the phosphoenolpyruvate carboxykinase deficiency is secondary, analogous to that in some cases of hepatic PC deficiency. Deficiencies of other gluconeogenic enzymes [94, 95] are discussed in Chaps. 5 and 6.

Another category of secondary disorders altering pyruvate metabolism consists of acquired abnormalities not due to primary mutations of enzymes of carbohydrate metabolism [1, 96, 97]. Such conditions are common. Any disorder which impairs transport of oxygen to tissues—including shock—can impair pyruvate oxidation. Dietary thiamine deficiency is a classic cause of elevated blood pyruvate. Lactic acidosis can complicate diabetes. In Reye's disease, infection can lead to reduced activities of PDHC and PC [36]. Inborn errors of biotin metabolism can lead to PC deficiency [98–100].

Patients may have mixtures of primary, inherited predispositions and acquired, environmental disorders. Wick et al. [101] have suggested that some patients require abnormally large amounts of dietary thiamine due to a hereditary abnormality of PDHC.

Since so many disorders can alter pyruvate metabolism, one cannot diagnose a hereditary disorder of pyruvate metabolism simply by the presence in blood or urine of excessive amounts of pyruvate or of its derivatives, lactate and alanine.

DIAGNOSIS

The diagnosis of one of the inborn errors of pyruvate metabolism is difficult. [1, 102–104]. In any patient suspected of having a primary or secondary syndrome, the first task is to be sure that the supply of oxygen to the tissues is adequate and that there is no external reason for impaired oxygen utilization (e.g., unrecognized toxins or occult sepsis).

Pyruvate and its derivatives, lactate and alanine, tend to occur in excessive amounts in the physiologic fluids of patients with hereditary disorders of pyruvate metabolism (i.e., primary or secondary pyruvate dysmetabolism syndromes). In general, but certainly not invariably, the ratios of pyruvate to lactate tend to remain in the normal range [1, 105]. Variability can be marked between patients and for the same patient at different times. One retarded boy with only minimal elevations of blood lactate at rest developed life-threatening lactic acidosis after $1\frac{1}{2}$ days on a diet containing 60 percent of its calories as carbohydrates [46]. Hypoglycemia has not been noted so much more often in patients with PC deficiency or other gluconeogenetic defects than in patients with PDHC deficiency and other oxidative defects as to be reliable for differential diagnosis.

Patients with PDHC deficiency usually develop excessive increases in blood pyruvate after a glucose load [1, 46, 48, 104]. Patients with PC deficiency or other gluconeogenetic defects typically do not increase their blood glucose levels appropriately after an alanine load [53, 56].

Muscle biopsy may be a useful procedure, particularly with histochemistry and search for "ragged-red" fibers[1] [34, 87, 88, 90]. Liver biopsy has often been done. Both can provide clinically useful information.

Definitive diagnosis requires enzymology. Clinical tests of white cells and fibroblasts for PC deficiency appear reliable [54, 55]. The newer procedures for assaying PDHC in fibroblasts may prove reliable and sensitive [4, 30]. However, since both these enzymes have complicated regulatory mechanisms and kinetics, it is unlikely that any single set of artificial assay conditions will suffice to detect all clinically significant mutations for either enzyme. Similar considerations apply to secondary pyruvate dysmetabolism syndromes, notably abnormalities of the electron transport chain [87, 88].

PATHOPHYSIOLOGY

Disease of the nervous system is usually the most striking clinical abnormality in these patients, presumably because the central nervous system depends more on continuous oxidation of pyruvate than do other organs [1, 96, 97]. Ketone bodies cannot completely replace pyruvate even in infants, and do so less efficiently as individuals grow into adults [106]. Close examination of these patients does reveal impaired development and poor function of organs other than the nervous system.

Surprisingly, mild to moderate impairment of cerebral carbohydrate metabolism appears to reduce biosynthetic activities more than it does the supply of energy, even though carbohydrates are the main fuels burned by the brain. Experimentally, hypoxia and other conditions which interfere with cerebral carbohydrate oxidation can severely impair neurologic function without altering ATP levels [107]. This observation was

---

[1] The defining characteristic of ragged-red fibers is excessive staining by histochemical procedures of mitochondrial enzymes (such as menadione succinate dehydrogenase). They are typically due to an excessive number or size of mitochondria.

made in 1953 and has been extensively confirmed. Of course, severe enough impairment of pyruvate oxidation does reduce cerebral ATP levels, but in that situation cells die, and so, often, do the animals.

Neurotransmitters derived from glucose play a critical role in neurologic function and turn over relatively rapidly. The synthesis of cerebral acetylcholine is exquisitely sensitive to impairment of carbohydrate oxidation [96, 97]. Impairing pyruvate oxidation proportionally reduces acetylcholine synthesis, even though less than 1 percent of the pyruvate oxidized to CO_2 is incorporated into the acetyl group of acetylcholine. The close linkage appears to reflect compartmentation of carbohydrate metabolism with respect to acetylcholine synthesis [108]. Gibson et al. [109] have recently reported that the synthesis of putative neurotransmitter amino acids is as sensitive to hypoxia as that of acetylcholine. The biosynthesis of 5-hydroxytryptamine (serotonin) and of catecholamines can also be reduced by hypoxia [110] and other conditions which impair carbohydrate catabolism [111].

Severe impairment of carbohydrate catabolism also impairs the biosynthesis of macromolecules [107, 112–114]. It is not known whether or not mild to moderate impairment does so directly, rather than by reducing neurotransmission and therefore brain activity.

PC deficiency can impair cerebral carbohydrate oxidation in at least two ways. Like other gluconeogenetic defects, it can cause fasting hypoglycemia, thereby reducing the supply of substrate. PC deficiency can also impair the supply of 4-carbon compounds to "prime" the tricarboxylic acid cycle. This mechanism would be expected to lead directly to deficiency of the putative neurotransmitter amino acids, aspartate, glutamate, and γ-aminobutyric acid (GABA). Net biosynthesis of these compounds in the brain requires the PC reaction [115].

Fragmentary data in the literature suggest that excessive lactic acid can damage tissue apart from its effect on pH [116–119].

The brain appears to adjust to impairments of carbohydrate catabolism in part by reducing function in order to maintain permanent structure [1, 96, 97]. This assumption implies some hope for therapy of at least the milder pyruvate dysmetabolism syndromes.

TREATMENT

The hereditary disorders of pyruvate metabolism typically result from partial deficiencies of highly regulated reactions. One may hope that dietary or other rational biochemical manipulations may benefit some of these patients. Several approaches have been tried in single patients in a few cases.

Provision of Product

A direct approach is to try to provide in the diet the product of the deficient reaction. The acetyl CoA which is the product of the PDHC reaction can also be made in the brain by burning ketone bodies, particularly in the young [106]. Several patients appear to have benefited from ketogenic diets, which were rich enough in fat to make the patient ketonemic and ketonuric but not acidotic or hypoglycemic, i.e., about 50 percent fat, 20 percent carbohydrate [46, 120]. Blood levels of ketones and glucose should be monitored while the diet appropriate for each patient is being established. Such diets may slow but do not stop the progression of the neurologic disease. They appear to make the course less stormy, perhaps by providing fat or by reducing the load of sugar to be burned. They can harm patients with gluconeogenetic defects [56].

The 4-carbon chain which is the product of the PC reaction can be provided in the diet as the amino acids, aspartate and glutamate, which are then transaminated to form tricarboxylic acid cycle intermediates [59]. Both of these amino acids can cross the blood-brain barrier after amidation in nonneural tissues (to asparagine and glutamine). Striking and sustained improvements have been reported in patients treated with these amino acids in whom PC deficiency was assumed but documented only in liver biopsies [59, 61]. In at least one such patient, PC activity was normal on rebiopsy after treatment [59a].

Activation

Two agents which favor activation (dephosphorylation) of PDHC have been tried. Large doses of thiamine may benefit some patients; some may have mutations of PDHC which decrease its affinity for thiamine pyrophosphate [101, 121]. McKahn [121a] has used dichloroacetate (DCA) in a patient with presumed PDHC deficiency [122]. It allowed this boy to go off a ketogenic diet without developing lactic acidemia but did not stop the progression of the neurologic disease.

Other Approaches

Acetazolamide prevented recurrent attacks of ataxia in patients from at least three kindreds, one of whom had a documented abnormality of pyruvate metabolism [123–125]. Lecithin [126, 127] and other cholinergic agents [128] have been reported to be of mild benefit to some patients with hereditary ataxia, including some with elevated blood pyruvate. The clinical changes have not been striking. Rather low amounts of citrate were reported to benefit a Japanese patient who was reported to have PDHC deficiency [129]. Menkes used short courses of steroids to reduce dramatically the severity and length of attacks in the first patient with a well-documented PDHC deficiency [2, 45]. Steroids may also have benefited a girl who died with a "ragged-red" neuromyopathy and lactic acidosis [130]. Mechanisms by which steroids might help such patients are not known.

Indeed, all therapeutic approaches tried in these patients are still at best experimental.

IMPLICATIONS

Study of the inborn errors of pyruvate metabolism is at an early stage. Most statements about them must still be tentative and conjectural. In 1932, Quastel [131] proposed that abnormalities of carbohydrate metabolism might contribute to disease of the nervous system, which is particularly dependent on carbohydrate oxidation. It is now clear that hereditary abnormalities of major pathways of carbohydrate metabolism can exist, at least in rare patients. Detailed studies are needed to specify their nature, frequency, and significance.

REFERENCES

1. BLASS JP: Pyruvate dehydrogenase deficiencies, in Burman D, Holton JB, Pennock CA (eds): *Inherited Disorders of Carbohydrate Metabolism.* Lancaster, UK, MTP Press, Ltd, 1980, p 239

2. BLASS JP, AVIGAN J, UHLENDORF BW: A defect in pyruvate decarboxylase in a child with an intermittent movement disorder. *J Clin Invest* 49: 423, 1970

3. BLASS JP, SCHULMAN JD, YOUNG DS, Hom E: An inherited defect affecting the tricarboxylic acid cycle in a patient with congenital lactic acidosis. *J Clin Invest* 51: 1545, 1972

4. SHEU KF, Hu CC, UTTER MF: Pyruvate dehydrogenase complex activity in normal and deficient fibroblasts. *J Clin Invest* 67: 1463, 1981

5. REED LJ, PETTIT FH, YEAMAN SJ, TEAGUE WM, BLEILE DM: Structure, function and regulation of the mammalian pyruvate dehydrogenase complex. *Proc Eur Biochem Soc* 60: 47, 1980

6. RANDLE PJ, SUGDEN PH, KERBEY AL, RADCLIFFE PM, HUTSON NJ: Regulation of pyruvate oxidation and the conservation of glucose. *Biochem Soc Symp* 43: 67, 1979

7. STANSBIE D: Regulation of the human pyruvate dehydrogenase complex. *Clin Sci Mol Med* 51: 445, 1976

7a. GIBSON: Unpublished results

8. MATTHEWS RG, BALLOU DP, WILLIAMS CH: Reactions of pig heart lipoamide dehydrogenase with pyridine nucleotides. *J Biol Chem* 254: 4974, 1979

9. WILLIAMS CH: Lipoamide dehydrogenase, in Boyer PD (ed): *The Enzymes.* New York, Academic Press, Inc, vol 13, p 106

10. STRAUB FB: Isolation and properties of a flavoprotein from heart muscle tissue. *Biochem J* 33: 787, 1939

11. MASSEY V: The identity of diaphorase and lipoyl dehydrogenase. *Biochim Biophys Acta* 37: 314, 1960

12. PETTIT FH, YEAMAN SJ, REED LJ: Purification and characterization of branched-chain α-keto acid dehydrogenase complex of bovine kidney. *Proc Natl Acad Sci USA* 75: 4881, 1978

13. STEIN AM, KAUFMAN BT, KAPLAN NO: On the mechanism of the transhydrogenase reaction catalyzed by a beef heart flavoprotein. *Biochem Biophys Res Commun* 2: 354, 1960

14. THORPE C, WILLIAMS CH: Modification of a pig heart lipoamide dehydrogenase by cupric ions. *Biochemistry* 14: 2419, 1975

15. NAKAMURA M, YAMAZAKI I: Salts-induced oxidase activity of lipoamide dehydrogenase from pig heart. *Eur J Biochem* 96: 417, 1979

16. OLSON MS, DENNIS SC, DEBUYSERE MS, PADMA A: The regulation of pyruvate dehydrogenase in the isolated perfused rat heart. *J Biol Chem* 253: 7369, 1978

17. JOPE R, BLASS JP: A comparison of the regulation of pyruvate dehydrogenase in mitochondria from rat brain and liver. *Biochem J* 150: 397, 1975

18. YEAMAN SJ, HUTCHESON ET, ROCHE TE, PETTIT FH, BROWN JR, REED LJ, WATSON DC, DIXON GH: Sites of phosphorylation on pyruvate dehydrogenase from bovine kidney and heart. *Biochemistry* 17: 2364, 1978

19. TEAGUE WM, PETTIT FH, YEAMAN SJ, REED LJ: Function of phosphorylation sites on pyruvate dehydrogenase. *Biochem Biophys Res Commun* 87: 244, 1979

20. SUGDEN PH, RANDLE PJ: Regulation of pig heart pyruvate dehydrogenase by phosphorylation. Studies on the subunit and phosphorylation stoichiometries. *Biochem J* 173: 659, 1978

21. MORGAN DG, ROUTTENBERG A: Evidence that a 41,000 dalton brain phosphoprotein is pyruvate dehydrogenase. *Biochem Biophys Res Commun* 95: 569, 1980

22. BROWNING M, BAUDRY M, BENNETT W, KELLY P, LYNCH G: Evidence that high frequency stimulation influences the phosphorylation of pyruvate dehydrogenase, and that the activity of this enzyme is linked to mitochondrial calcium sequestration. *Neurosci Abstr* 6: 197, 1980

23. SEALS JR, CZECH MP: Evidence that insulin activates an intrinsic plasma membrane protease in generating a secondary chemical mediator. *J Biol Chem* 255: 6529, 1980

24. BLASS JP, CEDERBAUM SD, KARK RAP: Rapid diagnosis of pyruvate and ketoglutarate deficiencies in platelet-enriched preparations from blood. *Clin Chim Acta* 75: 21, 1976

25. SILVERSTEIN E, BOYER PD: Instability of pyruvate-C^{14} in aqueous solutions as detected by enzymic assay. *Anal Biochem* 8: 470, 1964

26. BERTAGNOLIO B, UZIEL G, BOTTACHI E, CRENNA G, D'ANGELO A, DiDONATO S: Friedreich's ataxia in northern Italy. II. Biochemical studies in cultured cells. *Can J Neurol Sci* 7: 413, 1980

27. MELANCON SB, POTIER M, DALLAIRE L, ROLLIN R, FONTAINE G, GRENIER B: Pyruvate dehydrogenase, lipoamide dehydrogenase, and citrate synthase activity in fibroblasts from patients with Friedreich's and Charlevoix Saguenay ataxias. *Can J Neurol Sci* 6: 241, 1979

28. DeVIVO DC, HAYMOND MW, OBERT KA, NELSON JS, PAGLIARA AS: Defective activation of the pyruvate dehydrogenase complex in subacute necrotizing encephalomyelopathy (Leigh disease). *Ann Neurol* 6: 483, 1979

29. UTTER MF, SHEU KFR: Biochemical mechanism of biotin and thiamin action and relationships to genetic disease, in Desnick RJ (ed): *Enzyme Therapy in Genetic Diseases.* New York, Alan R Liss, Inc, p 289

30. SORBI S, BLASS JP: Abnormal activation of the pyruvate dehydrogenase complex in Leigh disease fibroblasts. *Neurology,* in press

31. EVANS OB: Muscle pyruvate oxidation in spinocerebellar degenerations. *Ann Neurol* 8: 129, 1980

32. STRÖMME JH, BORUD O, MOE PJ: Fatal lactic acidosis in a newborn attributable to a congenital defect of pyruvate dehydrogenase. *Pediatr Res* 10: 60, 1976

33. WENDEL U, PRZYREMBEL H, BECKER K, WALTHER B, BERGER R, BREMER HJ: Pyruvatdehydrogenase-Mangel-letaler Verlauf im Sälings-alter. *Mschr Kinderheilk* 126: 140, 1978

34. DUBOWITZ V, BROOKE H, NEVILLE HE: *Muscle Biopsy: A Modern Approach.* London: WB Saunders Co, Ltd, 1973

35. LYNEN A, SEDLACZEK E, WIELAND OH: Partial purification and characterization of a pyruvate dehydrogenase-complex-inactivating enzyme from rat liver. *Biochem J* 169: 321, 1978

36. ROBINSON BH, GALL DG, CUTZ E: Deficient activity of hepatic pyruvate dehydrogenase and pyruvate carboxylase in Reye's syndrome. *Pediatr Res* 11: 279, 1977

37. REYNOLDS SF: *Distribution of Pyruvate Dehydrogenase in the Cat Central Nervous System in Relation to Normal and Abnormal Neural Functions,* PhD thesis. UCLA, 1974 (Univ Microfilms 74-18, 808)

38. PERRY EK, PERRY RH, TOMLINSON BE, BLESSED G, GIBSON PH: Coenzyme A-acetylating enzymes in Alzheimer's disease: Possible cholinergic compartment of pyruvate dehydrogenase. *Neurosci Lett* 18: 105, 1980

39. ROBINSON BH, TAYLOR J, SHERWOOD WG: Deficiency of dihydro-lipoyl dehydrogenase (a component of the pyruvate and α-keto-glutarate dehydrogenase complexes): A cause of congenital chronic lactic acidosis in infancy. *Pediatr Res* 11: 1198, 1977

40. FILLA A. BUTTERWORTH RF, GEOFFREY G, LEMIEUX B, BARBEAU A: Serum and platelet lipoamide dehydrogenase in Friedreich's ataxia. *Can J Neurol Sci* 5: 111, 1978

41. STUMPF DA, PARKS J: Friedreich ataxia. II. Normal kinetics of lipoamide dehydrogenase. *Neurology* 29: 820, 1979

42. KARK RAP, RODRIGUEZ-BUDELLI M, PERLMAN S, GULLEY WF, TOROK K: Preclinical diagnosis and carrier detection in ataxia associated with abnormalities of lipoamide dehydrogenase. *Neurology* 30: 502, 1980

43. MELANCON SB, POTIER M, DALLAIRE L, FONTAINE G, GRENIER B, LEMIEUX B, GEOFFROY G, BARBEAU A: Lipoamide dehydrogenase in Friedreich's ataxia fibroblasts. *Can J Neurol Sci* 5: 115, 1978

44. BLASS JP, HINMAN L, SORICELLI A: Clinical assays of lipoamide dehydrogenase. *Neurology* 31: 763, 1981

45. BLASS JP, KARK RAP, ENGEL WK: Clinical studies of a patient with pyruvate decarboxylase deficiency. *Arch Neurol* 25: 449, 1971

46. CEDERBAUM SD, BLASS JP, MINKOFF N, BROWN WJ, COTTON ME, HARRIS SH: Sensitivity to carbohydrate in a patient with familial intermittent lactic acidosis and pyruvate dehydrogenase deficiency. *Pediatr Res* 10: 713, 1976

47. BUTTERWORTH R, MELANCON S: Personal communication

48. BLASS JP: Spinocerebellar disorders, in Appel S (ed): *Current Neurology.* Boston, Houghton Mifflin Co, 1981, vol 3, p 66

49. DiDONATO S, RIMOLDI M, MOISE A, BERTAGNOLIO B, UZIEL G: Fatal ataxia encephalopathy and carnitine acetyltransferase deficiency: A functional defect of pyruvate oxidation. *Neurology* 29: 1578, 1979

50. WILLIAMS LL: Pyruvate oxidation in Charcot-Marie-Tooth disease. *Neurology* 29: 1492, 1979

51. FARMER TW, VEATH L, MILLER AL, O'BRIEN JS, ROSENBERG RM: Pyruvate decarboxylase deficiency in a patient with subacute necrotizing encephalomyelopathy. *Neurology* 23: 429, 1973

52. BLASS JP, CEDERBAUM SD, DUNN HG: Biochemical defect in Leigh's disease. *Lancet* 1: 1237, 1976

53. ATKIN BM, BUIST NRM, UTTER MF, LEITER AB, BANKER BQ: Pyruvate carboxylase deficiency and lactic acidosis in a retarded child without Leigh's disease. *Pediatr Res* 13: 109, 1979

54. ATKIN BM, UTTER MF, WEINBERG, MB: Pyruvate carboxylase and phos-

phoenolpyruvate carboxykinase activity in leukocytes and fibroblasts from a patient with pyruvate carboxylase deficiency. *Pediatr Res* 13: 38, 1979

55. ATKIN BM: Carrier detection of pyruvate carboxylase deficiency in fibroblasts and lymphocytes. *Pediatr Res* 13: 1101, 1979

56. DEVIVO DC, HAYMOND MW, LECKIE MP, BUSSMAN YL, McDOUGAL DB, PAGLIARA AS: The clinical and biochemical implications of pyruvate carboxylase deficiency. *J Clin Endocrinol Metab* 45: 1281, 1977

57. HOMMES FA, POLMAN HA, REERINK JD: Leigh's encephalopathy: An inborn error of gluconeogenesis. *Arch Dis Child* 43: 423, 1968

58. YOSHIDA T, TADA K, KONNO T, ARAKAWA T: Hyperalaninemia with pyruvicemia due to pyruvate carboxylase deficiency of the liver. *Tohoku J Exp Med* 99: 121, 1969

59. GROVER WD, AUERBACH VH, PATEL MS: Biochemical studies and therapy in subacute necrotizing encephalomyelopathy (Leigh's syndrome). *J Pediatr* 81: 39, 1972

59a. HOMMES F: Personal communication

60. BRUNETTE MG, DELVIN E, HAZEL B, SCRIVER CR: Thiamin-responsive lactic acidosis in a patient with deficient low-Km pyruvate carboxylase activity in liver. *Pediatrics* 50: 702, 1972

61. TANG TT, GOOD TA, DYKEN PR, JOHNSEN SD, McCREADIE SR, LARDY HA, RUDOLPH FB: Pathogenesis of Leigh's encephalopathy. *J Pediatr* 81: 189, 1972

62. TADA K, SUGITA K, FUJITANI K, UESAKAI T, TAKADA G, OMURA K: Hyperalaninemia with pyruvicemia in a patient suggestive of Leigh's encephalomyelopathy. *Tohoku J Exp Med* 109: 13, 1973

63. GRUSKIN AB, PATEL MS, LINSHAW M, ETTENGER R, HUFF D, GROVER W: Renal function studies and kidney pyruvate carboxylase in subacute necrotizing encephalomyelopathy (Leigh's syndrome). *Pediatr Res* 7: 832, 1973

64. SAUDUBRAY JM, MARSAC C, CHARPENTIER C, CATHELINEAU L, BESSON LEAUD M, LEROUX JP: Neonatal congenital lactic acidosis with pyruvate carboxylase deficiency in two siblings. *Acta Paediatr Scand* 65: 717, 1976

65. TOMMASI M, JOUVET-TELINGE A, KOPP N, PIALAT J, GILLY J: Poliodystrophie cerebrale infantile d'Alpers-Un cas avec anomalie de la pyruvat-carboxylase hepatique. *Ann Anat Pathol* 22: 337, 1976

66. SCRUTTON MF, YOUNG MR: Pyruvate carboxylase, in Boyer PD (ed): *The Enzymes*, ed 3. New York, Academic Press, Inc, 1972, vol 6, p 1

67. MAHAN DE MUSHAHWAR IK, KOEPPE RE: Purification and properties of rat brain pyruvate carboxylase. *Biochem J* 145: 25, 1975

68. SCRUTTON MD, WHITE MD: Purification and properties of human liver pyruvate carboxylase. *Biochem Med* 9: 271, 1974

69. McCLURE WR, LARDY HA: Rat liver pyruvate carboxylase, IV. Factors affecting the regulation in vivo. *J Biol Chem* 246: 3591, 1971

70. BALLARD FJ, HANSON RW, RESHEF L: Immunochemical studies with soluble and mitochondrial pyruvate carboxylase activities from rat tissues. *Biochem J* 119: 735, 1970

71. WIELAND O, EVERTZ-PRÜSSE E, STUKOWSKI B: Distribution of pyruvate carboxylase and phosphoenol-pyruvate carboxykinase in human liver. *FEBS Lett* 2: 26, 1968

72. LEIGH D: Subacute necrotizing encephalomyelopathy in an infant. *J Neurol Neurosurg Psychiatr* 14: 216, 1951

73. MONTPETIT VJA, ANDERMAN F, CARPENTER S, FAWCETT JS, ZBOROWSKA-SLUIS D, GIBERSON HR: Subactue necrotizing encephalomyelopathy. *Brain* 94: 1, 1971

73a. DEVIVO DC: Personal communication

74. SIPE JC: Leigh's syndrome: The adult form of subacute necrotizing encephalomyelopathy with predilection for the brain stem. *Neurology* 23: 1030, 1973

75. DUNN HG, DOLMAN CL: Necrotizing encephalomyelopathy; report of a case with relapsing polyneuropathy and hyperalaninemia and with manifestations resembling Friedreich's ataxia. *Neurology* 19: 536, 1969

76. EXSS R, GULOTTA F, KALLFELZ HC, VÖLPEL M: Wernicke's encephalopathy and Friedreich's ataxia. *Neuropaediatrie* 5: 162, 1974

77. KALIMO H, LUNDBERG PO, OLSSON Y: Familial subacute necrotizing encephalomyelopathy of the adult form (adult Leigh syndrome). *Ann Neurol* 6: 200, 1978

78. HARPER CJ: Wernicke's encephalopathy: A more common disease than realized. *J Neurol Neurosurg Psychiatry* 42: 226, 1979

79. ANONYMOUS: Wernicke's preventable encephalopathy. *Lancet* 1: 1122, 1979

80. PINCUS JH, SOLITARE GB, COOPER JR: Thiamine triphosphate levels and histopathology. Correlation in Leigh's disease. *Arch Neurol* 33: 759, 1976

81. PINCUS JH, COOPER JR, PIROS K, TURNER V: Specificity of the urine inhibitor test for Leigh's disease. *Neurology* 24: 885, 1974

82. MURPHY JV: Subacute necrotizing encephalomyelopathy (Leigh's disease): Detection of the heterozygous carrier state. *Pediatrics* 51: 710, 1973

83. PINCUS JH, COOPER JR, PIROS K, TURNER V: Specificity of the urine inhibitor test for Leigh's disease. *Neurology* 24: 885, 1974

84. RUENWONGSA P. COOPER JR: The role of bound thiamine pyrophosphate in the synthesis of thiamin triphosphate in rat liver. *Biochim Biophys Acta* 482: 64, 1977

85. CLAYTON BE, DOBBS RH, PATRICK AD: Leigh's subacute necrotizing encephalopathy: Clinical and biochemical study, with special reference to therapy with lipoate. *Arch Dis Child* 42: 467, 1967

86. WILLEMS JL, MONNENS LAM, TRIJBELS JMF: Leigh's encephalomyelopathy in a patient with cytochrome-c-oxidase deficiency in muscle tissue. *Pediatrics* 60: 850, 1977

87. DIMAURO S: Metabolic myopathies, in Vinken PJ, Bruyn GW (eds): *Handbook of Clinical Neurology*. Amsterdam, North Holland Publishing Co, 1979, vol 41, p 175

88. DIMAURO S, SCHOTLAND DL, BONILLA E, LEE CP, DIMAURO PMM, SCARPA A: Mitochondrial myopathies: Which and how many? in Milhorat AT (ed): *Exploratory Concepts in Muscular Dystrophy*. Amsterdam, Exerpta Medica-Elsevier, 1974, vol 2, p 506

89. KARPATI G, CARPENTER S, LABRISSEAU A, LAFONTAINE R: The Kearns-Shy syndrome. A multisystem disease with mitochondrial abnormality demonstrated in skeletal muscle and skin. *J Neurol Sci* 19: 133, 1973

90. OLSON W, ENGEL WK, WALSH GO, EINAUGLER R: Oculocraniosomatic neuromuscular disease with "ragged-red" fibers. *Arch Neurol* 26: 193, 1972

91. ENGEL WK: Histochemical abnormalities of skeletal muscle in patients with acute psychoses. *Science* 168: 273, 1970

92. HOMMES FA, BENDIEN K, ELEMA JD, BREMER HJ, LOMBECK I: Two cases of phosphoenolpyruvate carboxykinase deficiency. *Acta Paediatr Scand* 65: 233, 1976

93. FISER RH, MELSHER HL, FISHER DA: Hepatic phosphoenol pyruvate carboxykinase (PEPCK) deficiency—a new cause of hypoglycemia in childhood. *Pediatr Res* 10: 60, 1974

94. PAGLIARA AS, KARL IE, KEATING JP, BROWN BI, KIPNIS DM: Hepatic fructose-1, 6-diphosphatase deficiency. *J Clin Invest* 51: 2145, 1972

95. MELANCON SB, KHACHADURIAN AK, NADLER HL, BROWN BI: Metabolic and biochemical studies in fructose-1,6-diphosphatase deficiency. *J Pediatr* 82: 650, 1973

96. BLASS JP, GIBSON GE: Carbohydrates and acetylcholine synthesis: Implications for cognitive disorders, in Davis KL, Berger PA (eds): *Brain Acetylcholine and Neuropsychiatric Disease*. New York, Plenum Publishing Corp, 1979, p 215

97. BLASS JP, GIBSON GE: Consequences of mild, graded hypoxia. *Adv Neurol* 26: 229, 1979

98. GOMPERTZ D, DRAFFAN GH, WATTS JL, HULL D: Biotin-responsive beta-methylcroton-glycinuria. *Lancet* 2: 22, 1971

99. SANDER JE, MALAMUD N, COWAN MJ, PACKMAN S, AMMAN AJ, WARA DW: Intermittent ataxia and immunodeficiency with multiple carboxylase deficiencies: A biotin-responsive disorder. *Ann Neurol* 8: 544, 1980

100. COWAN MJ, WARA DM, PACKMAN S: Multiple biotin-dependent carboxylase deficiencies associated with defects in T cell and B cell immunity. *Lancet* 2: 115, 1979

101. WICK H, SCHWEIZER K, BAUMGARTNER R: Thiamine dependency in a patient with congenital lacticacidemia due to pyruvate dehydrogenase deficiency. *Agents Actions* 7: 405, 1978

102. LEROUX JP, MARSAC C, SAUDUBRAY JM: Hyperlactacidemies congenitales enzymopathiques. *Ann Biol Clin* 34: 151, 1976

103. CAVANAGH NP: Cerebellar ataxia in infancy and childhood related to a disturbance of pyruvate and lactate metabolism. *Dev Med Child Neurol* 20: 672, 1978

104. STANSBIE D, SHERRIFF RJ, DENTON RM: Fructose load test—an in vivo screening test designed to assess pyruvate dehydrogenase activity and interconversion. *J Inherited Metab Dis* 1: 163, 1978

105. CHALMERS RA, LAWSON AM, BORUD O: Urinary organic acids in a case of congenital lactic acidosis due to pyruvate decarboxylase deficiency. *J Int Metab Dis* 1: 15, 1978

106. ITOH T, QUASTEL JH: Acetoacetate metabolism in infant and adult rat brain in vitro. *Biochem J* 116: 641, 1970

107. SIESJÖ BK: *Brain Metabolism*. New York: John Wiley & Sons, Inc, 1978

108. GIBSON GE, BLASS JP, JENDEN DJ: Measurement of acetylcholine turnover using glucose as precursor. Evidence for compartmentation of glucose metabolism in brain. *J Neurochem* 30: 71, 1978

109. GIBSON GE, PETERSON C, SANSONE J: Decreases in amino acid and acetylcholine metabolism during hypoxia. *J Neurochem* 37: 192, 1981

110. DAVIS JN, GIRON LT, STANTON E, MAURY W: The effect of hypoxia on brain neurotransmitter systems. *Adv Neurol* 26: 219, 1979

111. PLAITAKIS A, NICKLAS WJ, BERL S: Thiamine deficiency: Selective impairment of the cerebellar serotonergic system. *Neurology* 28: 691, 1978

112. GIBSON GE, BLASS JP: A relation between [NAD$^+$]/[NADH] potentials

and glucose utilization in rat brain slices. *J Biol Chem* 251: 4127, 1976

113. YANAGAHIRA T: Cerebral anoxia: Effect on transcription and translation. *J Neurochem* 22: 113, 1974

114. VOLPE JJ, MARASA JC: A role for thiamine in the regulation of fatty acid and cholesterol biosynthesis in cultured cells of neural origin. *J Neurochem* 30: 975, 1978

115. HOMMES FA, BERGER R, LUIT-DE-HAAN G: The effect of thiamine treatment on the activity of pyruvate dehydrogenase: Relation to the treatment of Leigh's encephalomyelopathy. *Pediatr Res* 7: 616, 1973

116. KOWALOFF EM, PHANG JM, GRANGER AS, DOWNING SJ: Regulation of proline oxidase activity by lactate. *Proc Natl Acad Sci USA* 74: 5368, 1977

117. PITTS FN, McCLURE JN: Lactate metabolism in anxiety neurosis. *New Engl J Med* 277: 1329, 1967

118. HALSAM MT: The relationship between the effect of lactate infusion and anxiety states, and their amelioration by carbon dioxide inhalation. *Br J Psychiatr* 125: 88, 1974

119. ARMIGER LC, GAVIN JB, HERDSON PB: Mitochondrial changes in dog myocardium induced by neutral lactate *in vitro. Lab Invest* 31: 29, 1974

120. FALK RE, CEDERBAUM SD, BLASS JP, PRUSS RJ, CARRELL RE: Ketonic diet in the management of pyruvate dehydrogenase deficiency. *Pediatrics* 58: 713, 1976

121. BUTLER JH, PETTIT FH, DAVIS PF, REED LJ: Binding of thiamin thiazolone pyrophosphate to mammalian pyruvate dehydrogenase and its effect on kinase and phosphatase activities. *Biochem Biophys Res Commun* 74: 1667, 1977

121a. McKAHN G: Personal communication

122. STACPOOLE PW, MOORE GW, KORNHAUSER CM: Metabolic effects of dichloroacetate in patients with diabetes mellitus and hyperproteinemia. *N Engl J Med* 298: 526, 1978

123. EVANS OB, KILROY AW, FENICHEL GM: Acetazolamide in the treatment of pyruvate dysmetabolism syndromes. *Arch Neurol* 35: 302, 1978

124. GRIGGS RC, MOXLEY RT, LAFRANCE RA, McQUILLEN J: Hereditary paroxysmal ataxia: Response to acetazolamide. *Neurology* 28: 1259, 1978

125. DONAT JR, AUGER R: Familial periodic ataxia. *Arch Neurol* 36: 568, 1979

126. BARBEAU A: Emerging treatments: Replacement therapy with choline or lecithin in neurologic diseases. *Can J Neurol Sci* 5: 157, 1978

127. REDING MJ, BLASS JP, DI PONTE P, STERN HD: Lecithin in hereditary ataxias. *Neurology,* 31: 363, 1981

128. KARK RAP, BLASS JP, SPENCE A: Physostigmine in patients with familial ataxias. *Neurology* 27: 70, 1975

129. OKA Y, MATSUDA I, ARASHIMA S, ANAKURA M, MITSUYAMA T, NAGAMATSU I; Citrate treatment in a patient with pyruvate decarboxylase deficiency. *Tohoku J Exp Med* 118: 131, 1976

130. SHAPIRA Y, CEDERBAUM SD, CANCILLA PA, NIELSEN D, LIPPE BM: Familial poliodystrophy, mitochondrial myopathy and lactate acidemia. *Neurology* 25: 614, 1975

131. QUASTEL JH: Biochemistry and mental disorder. *Lancet* 2: 1417, 1932

132. BLASS JP, GIBSON GE, KARK RAP: Pyruvate decarboxylase deficiency, in Gubler, CJ, Fujiwara, M, Dryfus PM (eds): *Thiamine.* New York, John Wiley & Sons, Inc, 1976, p 321

133. BLASS JP, LONSDALE D, UHCENDORF BW, HOM E: Intermittent ataxia with pyruvate-decarboxylase deficiency. *Lancet* 1: 1302, 1971

134. WILLEMS JL, MONNENS LAH, TRIJBELS JMF, SENGERS RAC, VEERKAMP JH: Pyruvate decarboxylase deficiency in liver. *New Engl J Med* 290: 406, 1974

135. ROBINSON BH, SHERWOOD WG: Pyruvate dehydrogenase phosphatase deficiency. Cause of congenital chronic lactic acidosis in infancy. *Pediatr Res* 9: 935, 1973

136. FARRELL DF, CLARK AF, SCOTT RC, WENNBERG RP: Absence of pyruvate decarboxylase activity in man: A cause of congenital lactic acidosis. *Science* 187: 1082, 1975

137. HAWORTH JC, PERRY TL, BLASS JP, HANSEN S, URQUHART ND: Lactic acidosis in three sibs due to defects in both pyruvate dehydrogenase and α-ketoglutarate dehydrogenase complexes. *Pediatrics* 58: 564, 1976

138. STRÖMME JH, BORUD O, MOE P: Fatal lactic acidosis in a newborn attributable to a congenital defect of pyruvate dehydrogenase. *Pediatr Res* 10: 60, 1976

139. BLASS JP, KARK RAP, MENON NK: Low activities of the pyruvate and oxoglutarate dehydrogenase complexes in 5 patients with Friedreich's ataxia. *New Engl J Med* 295: 62, 1976

140. CONSTANTOPOULOS G, CHANG CSC, BARRANGER JA: Normal pyruvate dehydrogenase complex activity in patients with Friedreich's ataxia. *Ann Neurol* 8: 636, 1980

141. KURODA Y, KLINE J, SWEETMAN L, NYHAN WL, GROSHONG TD: Abnormal pyruvate and α-ketoglutarate dehydrogenase complexes in a patient with lactic acidemia. *Pediatr Res* 13: 928, 1979

142. BLASS JP, CEDERBAUM SD, KARK RAP: Pyruvate dehydrogenase deficiency: Summary of results with 25 patients. *Trans Am Soc Neurochem* 7: 167, 1976

143. WILLIAMS LL: Pyruvate oxidation in Charcot-Marie-Tooth disease. *Neurology* 29: 1492, 1979

144. KARK RAP, RODRIGUEZ-BUDELLI MM: Clinical correlations of partial deficiency of lipoamide dehydrogenase. *Neurology* 29: 1006, 1979

145. KARK RAP, RODRIGUEZ-BUDELLI M: Pyruvate dehydrogenase deficiency in spinocerebellar degenerations. *Neurology* 29: 126, 1979

146. ROBINSON BH, TAYLOR J, SHERWOOD GW: The genetic heterogeneity of lactic acidosis: Occurrence of recognizable inborn errors of metabolism in a pediatric population with lactic acidosis. *Pediatr Res* 14: 956, 1980

147. MAESAKA H, KAZUHIKO K, MISUGI K, TADA K: Hyperalaninemia, hyperpyruvicemia and lactic acidosis due to pyruvate carboxylase deficiency of the liver; treatment with thaimine and lipoic acid. *Eur J Pediatr* 122: 159, 1976

10

PRIMARY HYPEROXALURIA

HIBBARD E. WILLIAMS

LLOYD H. SMITH, JR.

1. Primary hyperoxaluria *is a general term for two rare genetic disorders characterized clinically by recurrent calcium oxalate nephrolithiasis and nephrocalcinosis, frequently leading to progressive renal insufficiency and death before the age of 20. Symptoms of renal stone disease begin usually before the age of 5, although there are variations in age of onset and in severity of clinical symptoms. Calcium oxalate deposits may be found in extrarenal tissues, a pathologic condition termed* oxalosis.

2. *The disease is characterized biochemically by the continuous excessive synthesis and excretion of oxalic acid. The demonstration of different patterns of urinary organic acid excretion has allowed classification of this disease into two specific types. In type I (glycolic aciduria), excessive amounts of glyoxylic and glycolic acids are also found in the urine. In type II (L-glyceric aciduria), large amounts of L-glyceric acid but normal amounts of glyoxylic and glycolic acids are excreted.*

3. *In type I primary hyperoxaluria, the excessive synthesis of oxalate and glycolate results from a block in the metabolism of their immediate precursor, glyoxylate. In five patients with this disorder, a deficiency of a soluble α-ketoglutarate:glyoxylate carboligase has been demonstrated in preparations from liver, spleen, and kidney.*

4. *In type II primary hyperoxaluria, a defect in hydroxypyruvate metabolism results in its excessive reduction to L-glyceric acid, catalyzed by lactic dehydrogenase. A deficiency of leukocyte D-glyceric dehydrogenase has been demonstrated in four patients with this disorder.*

5. *The cause of excessive oxalate synthesis in primary hyperoxaluria type II has not been completely clarified. Studies suggest that hydroxypyruvate accumulation, secondary to D-glyceric dehydrogenase deficiency, may indirectly increase oxalate synthesis from glyoxylate. The reduction of hydroxypyruvate to L-glycerate enhances the oxidation of glyoxylate to oxalate in a coupled reaction catalyzed by lactic dehydrogenase.*

6. *The inheritance of both types of primary hyperoxaluria is presumed to be autosomal recessive. This conclusion is based on genetic analyses in type I and on limited leukocyte enzyme studies in type II heterozygotes. No consistent test for heterozygosity is available for the type I disease.*

7. *Treatment of primary hyperoxaluria is directed toward decreasing oxalate excretion by inhibition of oxalate synthesis and toward increasing calcium oxalate solubility at a given urinary concentration of oxalate. Pyridoxine in large doses has been successful in reducing oxalate synthesis in some patients with primary hyper-*

oxaluria. Inhibitors of oxalate synthesis from glyoxylate have been effective in vitro, but their efficacy has not been established in vivo. The use of phosphate or magnesium or both, agents which increase calcium oxalate solubility in vivo, may reduce the rate of new stone formation. Renal homotransplantation has not proved successful in the management of chronic renal insufficiency complicating primary hyperoxaluria in most cases.

Primary hyperoxaluria is a general term for two rare genetic disorders of glyoxylate metabolism which are characterized by recurrent calcium oxalate nephrolithiasis, chronic renal failure, and early death from uremia [1–4]. Nephrocalcinosis and extrarenal deposits of calcium oxalate, termed *oxalosis,* characterize the pathologic findings in this disorder. Patients with the major form of this disease (type I, also called *glycolic aciduria*) excrete in the urine excessive amounts of oxalic, glycolic, and glyoxylic acids. The biochemical basis of the disease is a defect in glyoxylate metabolism, which leads to increased synthesis and excretion of oxalic acid. The disorders of oxalate metabolism are illustrated in Fig. 10-1. The pattern of inheritance of primary hyperoxaluria type I suggests its transmission as an autosomal recessive trait.

A second type of primary hyperoxaluria has been described. Although the clinical findings do not distinguish this variant, there are differences in the pattern of urinary organic acids and in the basic metabolic defect [5]. In this disorder, termed L-*glyceric aciduria* (or *primary hyperoxaluria type II*), oxalic and glyceric acids are excreted in excess in the urine, but glycolic acid excretion is normal. A defect in hydroxypyruvate metabolism has been demonstrated. The disorder is presumably transmitted by an autosomal recessive mode of inheritance.

In this report emphasis will be placed on the biochemical pathogenesis and classification of these genetic disorders. Oxalate metabolism will be reviewed as it pertains to the biochemical basis for continued hyperoxaluria.

HISTORY

Oxalate was recognized in certain plants as early as the eighteenth century, but is was not until 1839 that calcium oxalate crystals were identified in urine [6]. Somewhat earlier, certain renal stones were found to contain calcium oxalate [7]. Methods for the measurement of oxalate content of urine were introduced early in this century and led to an interest in the "oxalate diathesis," which was thought to be related to many cases of rheumatism, neurasthenia, and dyspepsia. Unfortunately, the plethora of such disorders described exceeded the reliability of the oxalate measurements.

Primary hyperoxaluria, first described by Lepoutre in 1925 [8], was rarely reported until the 1950s, when the clinical and pathologic entity was accurately characterized. Despite these early studies, there was disagreement about the relationship between oxalosis and hyperoxaluria until 1960 [9]. It is now agreed that oxalosis is simply the tissue-storage complication of excessive oxalate synthesis (and presumed increased concentration), comparable to sodium urate deposits in tophaceous gout.

The first detailed report of a case of oxalosis appeared in 1950 [10]. In this case, a child had had renal stones and nephrocalcinosis beginning at the age of 2 years and died of renal failure at age 12. At postmortem examination, numerous calcium oxalate crystals were found in the bones and kidneys. Primary hyperoxaluria was first diagnosed during life in 1953, when a child with recurrent nephrolithiasis was found to have increased urinary excretion of oxalate [11]. In 1954 the report of hyperoxaluria and oxalosis in identical twins dying of chronic renal failure emphasized the familial nature of the disease [12]. Since these early cases, primary hyperoxaluria has been reported with increasing frequency, and in 1964 an extensive review summarized data on 63 typical and 42 atypical cases [3]. Subsequent reports have emphasized the clinical and biochemical heterogeneity of this disorder [3, 4, 13, 14, 15, 16].

CLINICAL FEATURES

Patients with primary hyperoxaluria type 1 typically develop the initial symptoms of the disease at an early age. The onset of symptoms may occur before the age of 5 (approximately 65 percent of patients) or even before the age of 1 (12 percent). There appears to be no significant difference in the sex incidence of reported cases, the male/female ratio being 1.3:1.

Initial symptoms generally relate to the presence of calcium oxalate nephrolithiasis, with typical renal colic or asymptom-

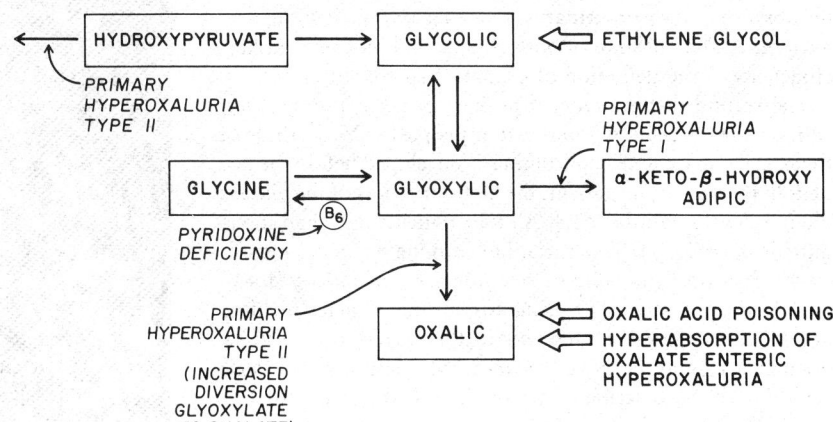

Figure 10-1 Disorders of oxalate metabolism in humans. The open arrows indicate exogenous causes of hyperoxaluria. The boldface arrows indicate the known acquired and hereditary enzyme defects or mechanisms leading to hyperoxaluria. *(From Williams and Smith [4], with permission of the publisher.)*

atic gross hematuria being the most common. Less frequently, patients may pass large numbers of small renal calculi with little discomfort. In a few male infants, urethral meatotomy has been necessary for relief of blockage by small concretions.

In a minority of patients, symptoms secondary to uremia may be the initial clinical manifestations of the disease. In such patients growth retardation is a frequent finding, and some patients with short stature have had features suggestive of secondary renal tubular acidosis. Symptoms are present for less than 10 years in over 90 percent of patients who die of the disease. Over 80 percent of patients die of renal failure before they reach the age of 20. This high mortality may reflect the method of ascertainment.

Other rarer clinical manifestations of primary hyperoxaluria include acute arthritis and symptoms referable to cardiac involvement. Attacks of joint pain have been diagnosed as gout [17, 18], supported in part by hyperuricemia, which is found frequently in this disease. Although this feature has been observed most commonly after the onset of the uremic phase of the disease, some patients have had both hyperuricemia and joint symptoms before renal insufficiency has appeared [12]. Sodium urate microcrystals have not yet been demonstrated in joint fluid from patients with primary hyperoxaluria. Since calcium oxalate crystals have been found in synovial membranes, it has been suggested that joint symptoms in these patients may be secondary to calcium oxalate crystallization in joint fluid. In some patients with primary hyperoxaluria [19, 20] the development of complete atrioventricular block has been related to the deposition of calcium oxalate crystals near the myocardial conduction system, a pathologic feature which has been substantiated in several reports [19, 21–23]. These patients may also exhibit severe peripheral vascular insufficiency [24].

A number of patients with hyperoxaluria do not show the typical pattern of onset or progression of the disease [3, 13, 15]. In these patients the disease may become manifest initially in adult life, even after the age of 40, the renal damage progressing less rapidly. Urinary oxalate excretion has been measured reliably in some but not all of these patients, so that the diagnosis of primary hyperoxaluria has not always been established conclusively. A few of these cases may be examples of pyridoxine deficiency (see "Classification of Hyperoxaluric States"). Another group of suspected hyperoxaluric subjects have died before the age of 1 year with renal insufficiency, nephrocalcinosis, and, in some, extrarenal oxalate deposition. As in the former group, the diagnosis of primary hyperoxaluria has been presumptive but unproved in these infants because of the absence of data on urinary oxalate excretion. Such reports have raised the question of both clinical and biochemical heterogeneity in the definition of primary hyperoxaluria.

The second distinct type of primary hyperoxaluria, L-*glyceric aciduria,* has been found in four people [5, 25]. In three of them, calcium oxalate nephrolithiasis developed before the age of 2. In the remaining patient, the first symptoms of the disease did not develop until age 24. All four patients have had intermittent microscopic hematuria, but in none has renal insufficiency developed, in spite of symptoms for over 15 years in two. In the oldest patient, insulin-requiring diabetes mellitus developed at age 34. Differences in the excretion of urinary organic acids and the site of the metabolic defect in L-glyceric aciduria will be described later in "The Pathogenesis of Primary Hyperoxaluria Type II."

There are no specific physical findings in patients with primary hyperoxaluria. Growth retardation reflects renal failure,

and acute arthritis and atrioventricular block are extremely rare. In the early stages of the disease, the development of hydronephrosis may lead to palpable renal enlargement. Calcium oxalate crystals in the eye have been reported in some patients, although many patients have been examined carefully for such crystals with negative results [26–29].

Roentgenographic features are confined largely to the genitourinary tract and the skeletal system. Urolithiasis and nephrocalcinosis are the abnormalities most frequently encountered. Radiopaque calcium oxalate densities may be observed both in the collecting system of the kidneys and within the renal parenchyma. In the uremic phase of the disease, secondary hyperparathyroidism may develop and lead to the roentgenographic bone changes of that disorder and to other forms of renal osteodystrophy.

PATHOLOGIC FEATURES

Nephrectomy specimens [9] from patients with hyperoxaluria have revealed nephrolithiasis, hydronephrosis, acute and chronic pyelonephritis, and tubular deposits of calcium oxalate. Nephrocalcinosis may not be present, and decreased renal function may be secondary to chronic obstruction and infection.

At postmortem examination [30], the kidneys of such patients are usually found to be small and to have thickened capsules that strip with difficulty. The surfaces are granular and contain focal depressed scars. They usually cut with noticeably increased resistance, and in most cases there is a gritty sensation, as though one were cutting through sand. On the cut surface the cortex is thin, and the pelves frequently contain calculi. Small crystals may sometimes be seen in the parenchyma with the naked eye.

On microscopic examination, interstitial fibrosis and interstitial nephritis may be found. Refractile crystals of various sizes are seen, primarily in the proximal convoluted tubules (Fig. 10-2). The tubular epithelium may be compressed or destroyed (Fig. 10-3), and the crystals may extend into the interstitial spaces [20, 30]. At times, large crystalline masses

Figure 10-2 Calcium oxalate crystals in the proximal convoluted tubules of a 34-year-old man dying of oxalosis and renal insufficiency. (Polarization microscopy ×175.) *(The authors are indebted to Dr. David Porter for permission to publish this photomicrograph.)*

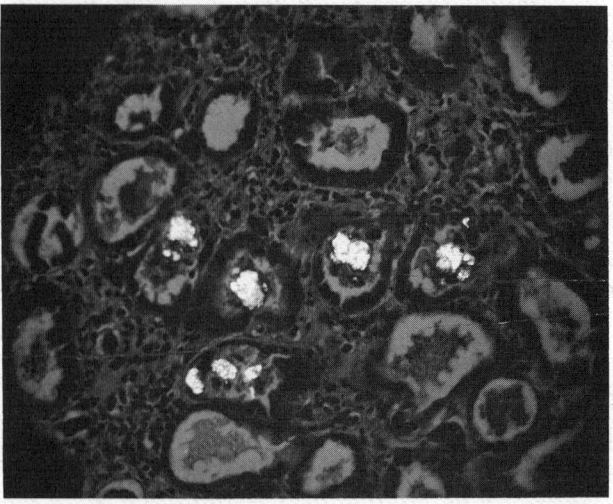

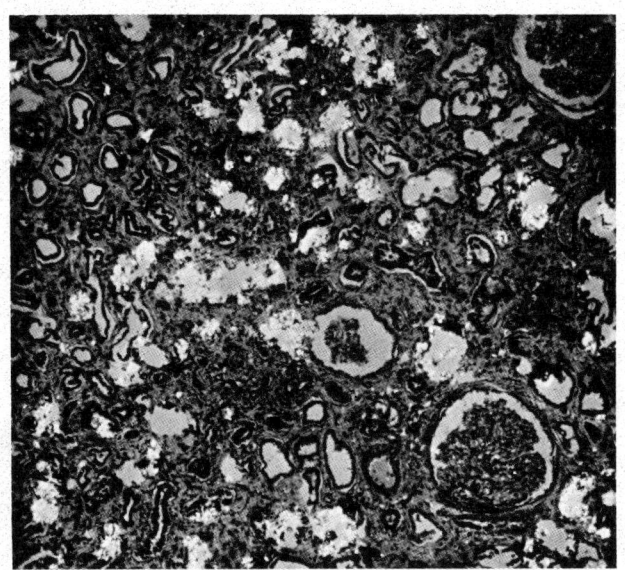

Figure 10-3 Oxalate nephrocalcinosis from a patient with primary hyperoxaluria and oxalosis. Most of the calcium oxalate crystals are related to the remains of renal tubules. (Half-crossed Nicol prisms ×70.) *(From Scowen et al. [30], with permission of the authors and publishers.)*

accompanied by heavy scarring are found in the tunica media and adventitia of small renal arteries and arterioles. The glomeruli are usually normal except for moderate pericapsular fibrosis and a rare hyalinized glomerulus.

Extrarenal deposits of calcium oxalate are variable in location and extent. The major sites of predilection are bone, heart, and the male urogenital system. In bone, crystal deposits occur in both the Haversian system and the marrow (Fig. 10-4) [10, 12, 30-34]. They may also occur in cartilage (Fig. 10-5) [35]. The myocardium may contain scattered deposits of calcium oxalate crystals and rarely may be heavily involved [21–23, 35]. The testis is a common site of extrarenal deposits. Crystals are frequently found in the walls of veins, arteries, and arterioles in this location and elsewhere. This finding has been noted particularly in hyperoxaluric patients undergoing long-term hemodialysis for chronic renal failure [36]. There appears to be a predilection for sites of tissue injury, such as foci of fibrosis or of chronic granulomatous inflammation in lungs or lymph nodes, but calcium oxalate crystals may also occur in these sites in subjects without hyperoxaluria. In addition, deposits have been described in the thyroid, spleen, liver, thymus, pituitary, adrenal, pancreas, and parathyroids [1, 3, 9–12, 20, 32, 35, 37–39]. Often these deposits are limited to the arterial and arteriolar walls within these organs. In some cases of primary hyperoxaluria, deposits have been found within the central nervous system [30, 31]. At death, the concentration of oxalate in the spinal fluid may be elevated [40]. In some patients with hyperoxaluria, peripheral neuropathy has been associated with intraaxonal deposits of oxalate in peripheral nerves [41–44].

On microscopic examination, the crystals appear round and globular or rhomboidal in shape and have a radial rosettelike pattern. They have a slight yellowish tinge and are doubly refractile under polarized light (Fig. 10-6). They do not stain with hematoxylin and eosin or, generally, with special techniques such as that of von Kossa unless calcium carbonate or phosphate has coprecipitated with oxalate [1, 32, 38, 39, 45].

The crystals may be identified in histologic sections by various chemical techniques. They are soluble when unstained deparaffinized sections are tested with concentrated hydro-

chloric or sulfuric acid, and are insoluble with lithium carbonate, glacial acetic acid, concentrated ammonium hydroxide, or concentrated potassium hydroxide. When the crystals are dissolved in concentrated sulfuric acid, small needlelike crystals of calcium sulfate may occasionally form [45]. If paraffin sections of tissue are first incinerated at 450°C for 30 min, calcium oxalate is oxidized to the carbonate, and small bubbles of carbon dioxide may be seen microscopically when concentrated sulfuric acid is allowed to run under the cover slip [46].

The crystals may be identified as calcium oxalate monohydrate by optical examination. The average width of single-needle crystals is 0.005 mm, and the average length is 0.05 mm. They have a birefringence of about 0.15 and an extinction angle of approximately 30° with respect to the length of the crystal. Calcium oxalate crystals have also been identified by x-ray diffraction in several cases of oxalosis [32, 35, 37, 45, 47].

DIAGNOSIS

The diagnosis of primary hyperoxaluria is based largely on the measurement of urinary oxalate excretion. Routine urinalysis is rarely of help in suggesting the diagnosis. Although calcium oxalate crystalluria is common in patients with hyperoxaluria, identical crystals occur in the urine of normal subjects, patients with calcium oxalate stones due to other causes, and patients with a variety of other renal abnormalities. Other nonspecific findings include microscopic hematuria, evidence of urinary tract infection, and (when renal failure supervenes) proteinuria and hyposthenuria.

The single most consistent laboratory finding in primary hyperoxaluria is an increased amount of urinary oxalate in the absence of pyridoxine deficiency, the excessive ingestion of oxalate or one of its immediate precursors (Fig. 10-7), or bowel disease with excessive absorption. Urinary oxalate excretion in normal humans varies between 10 and 50 mg/24 h using the isotope dilution method [48]. When corrected for body surface area, the excretion of oxalate in children is comparable to that in adults [48, 49]. In patients with primary hyperoxaluria, urinary oxalate excretion has averaged 240 mg/24 h and has exceeded 400 mg/24 h in some patients [48]. In our experience it has been distinctly unusual to find urinary oxalate levels of less than 100 mg/24 h in patients with this disorder in the

Figure 10-4 Calcium oxalate crystals in vertebral bone marrow from a patient with oxalosis (×150). *(From Dunn [32], with permission of the author and publisher.)*

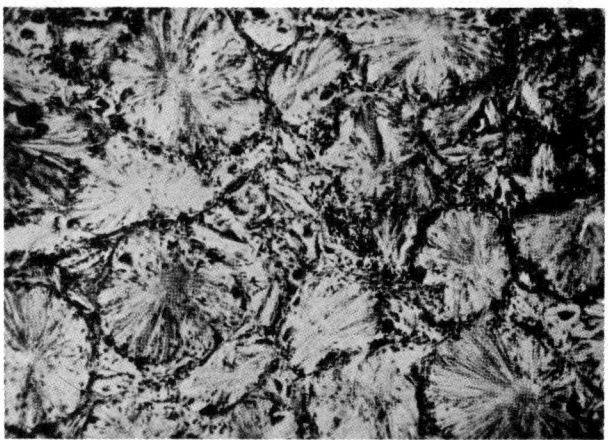

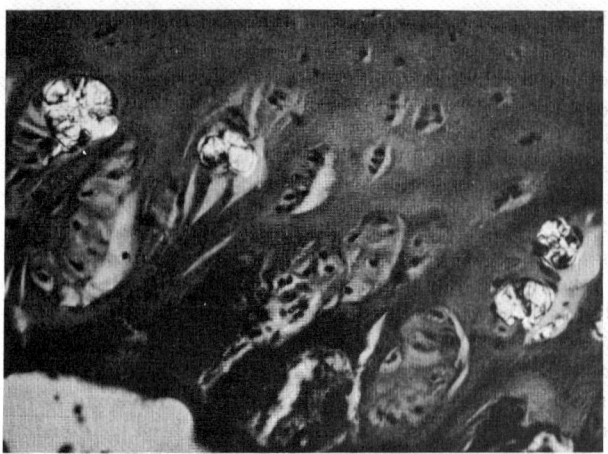

Figure 10-5 Calcium oxalate crystals in costochondral cartilage of a patient with primary hyperoxaluria and oxalosis, visualized under partial polarization (×175). *(From Godwin et al. [35], with permission of the authors and publisher.)*

absence of renal failure. After renal failure develops, urinary oxalate excretion decreases, and in the late stages of the disease it may fall within the normal range. Consequently, the diagnosis of primary hyperoxaluria in the terminal uremic stage of the disease may be difficult to document by current methods.

Numerous reports of the oxalate content of human plasma have appeared in the past 35 years, with wide variations in the absolute values found. An early permanganate-titration method gave levels of 2 to 4 mg/100 ml [50]. Using more demanding extraction methods, Barber and Gallimore [51] found plasma oxalate levels of 0.4 to 0.6 mg/100 ml. In 1961 Crawhall and Watts [52], utilizing a preparation of *Collybia velutipes* oxalic acid decarboxylase, found normal plasma oxalate concentrations to be less than 0.8 mg/100 ml, the lower limit of sensitivity of the method. These investigators were able to measure elevated levels of plasma oxalate in patients with primary hyperoxaluria only during the terminal oliguric phase of the disease. Zarembski and Hodgkinson [53], using a fluorometric method, found that serum oxalate levels in 17 normal adults ranged from 344 to 687 μg/100 ml. In only one of six subjects with primary hyperoxaluria was serum oxalate increased above this normal range. More recent reports by these investigators record the concentration of serum oxalate in normal adults as 100 to 235 μg/100 ml [54, 55]. Assuming no protein binding of oxalic acid at physiologic pH, the concentration of serum oxalate in normal subjects, studied with continuous intravenous infusion of isotopic oxalate, has been calculated as being approximately 15 μg/100 ml [56–59]. These latter values approach more closely those calculated on the basis of the total miscible pool of oxalate (assuming homogeneous distribution of oxalate throughout body water) of 7 to 15 μg/100 ml [59a]. In one study in which a gas chromatographic method was used to determine plasma oxalate, the concentration in normal subjects was 14.5 ± 8.9 μg/ml, a value 10 times higher than that reported in most other recent studies using other methods [60].

Recently Constable et al. [58a] studied plasma oxalate using both a radioisotopic infusion method and an enzymatic method. These results confirm the above calculated normal values of approximately 7 to 15 μg/100 ml and also documented elevated plasma oxalate levels both in patients with primary hyperoxaluria and in patients with chronic renal failure. Of note in this study was the finding that plasma oxalate was always higher at any level of plasma creatinine in patients with primary hyperoxaluria than in patients without hyperoxaluria who had chronic renal failure. This suggests the usefulness of plasma oxalate determinations in the diagnosis of primary hyperoxaluria. Akcay and Rose [59] have recently demonstrated that normal blood spontaneously generates oxalate on standing. In their careful enzymatic method the mean value for plasma oxalate was reported at 2126 umvl/L, or approximately 20 ug/100 ml.

The determination of the quantity of other urinary organic acids may be helpful in establishing the diagnosis of primary hyperoxaluria. Urinary glycolic acid excretion has been uniformly increased in all nonuremic patients with primary hyperoxaluria type I, i.e., the patients who did not exhibit L-glyceric aciduria. Excretion of glycolic acid in normal subjects varies between 15 and 60 mg/24 h [48], with some variation in the normal values based on methodology [61]. In primary hyperoxaluria type I, it usually exceeds 100 mg/24 h. There is no constant relationship between the amounts of oxalic and glycolic acids excreted. In the variant of primary hyperoxaluria, L-glyceric aciduria (type II), glycolic acid excretion is within the normal range. In these latter patients, large amounts (200 to 600 mg/24 h) of L-glyceric acid are found in the urine [62]. This organic acid cannot be measured in normal urine by methods now available. In some but not all patients with primary hyperoxaluria, glyoxylic acid excretion in the urine may be increased [48]. The lability of this compound and its nonenzymatic reaction with other urinary constituents have impaired the accuracy and usefulness of its determination. In six patients with primary hyperoxaluria, Zarembski et al. have reported elevations in urinary lactic acid excretion [14]. Using a specific isotope dilution method for urinary lactate, Williams et al. have not been able to confirm this finding in five patients with type I primary hyperoxaluria [63].

Extrarenal deposition of calcium oxalate crystals is a frequent accompaniment of primary hyperoxaluria, but such crystals cannot be considered pathognomonic of these diseases. Calcium oxalate crystals have been found in the kidney in a number of disorders, including chronic glomerulonephritis, chronic pyelonephritis, renal tubular acidosis, and acute tubular necrosis. In two reports, the incidence of calcium oxalate crystals in postmortem kidney specimens was 6.4 and 6.2 percent, respectively [64, 65]. In one study no statistical correlation was observed between the presence of crystalline deposits of oxalate in the kidney and the existence of renal disease

Figure 10-6 Calcium oxalate crystals from the lung of the patient of Fig. 10-2. (Polarization microscopy ×1500.) *(Courtesy of Dr. David Porter.)*

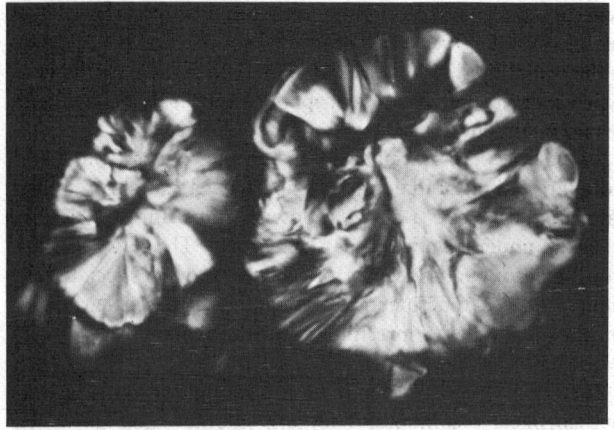

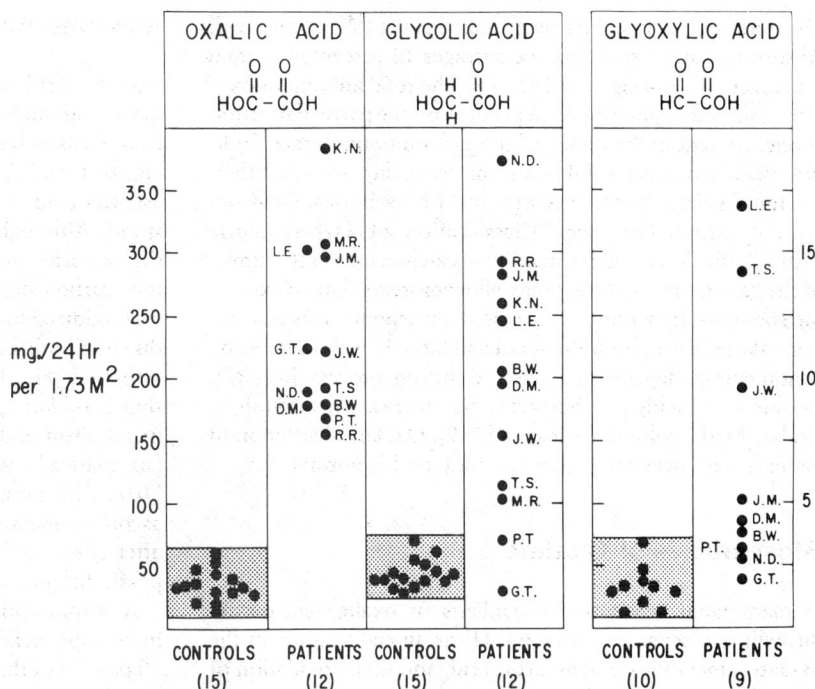

Figure 10-7 Urinary metabolites in primary hyperoxaluria. Patients P.T. and G.T. are sibs with L-glyceric aciduria (primary hyperoxaluria, type II). *(From Hockaday et al. [3], with permission of the publisher.)*

[64]. Crystals have been found in the myocardium of 5 of 50 patients who died from uremia [66]. Deposition of calcium oxalate may occur in other extrarenal sites, particularly in damaged tissues, in the absence of any disorder of oxalate metabolism [67–70]. Although oxalosis may be much more extensive in patients with primary hyperoxaluria, in the individual patient it is difficult to utilize this pathologic feature as a diagnostic criterion of the disease. One recent report suggests the usefulness of percutaneous bone biopsy in establishing the diagnosis of primary hyperoxaluria in view of the characteristic histologic picture [33]. However, it is not yet clear that this technique is specific for the genetic hyperoxaluric disorders.

The elucidation of the specific enzyme defects in patients with the two genetic variants of primary hyperoxaluria may allow the diagnosis to be made with greater specificity and accuracy in the future [4]. At the present time, these techniques for enzymatic assay are not readily available. The pattern of urinary excretion of organic acids remains the major basis for diagnosis.

OXALIC ACID

Oxalic acid is a relatively strong dicarboxylic acid with K_{a_1} of 6.5×10^{-2} and K_{a_2} of 6.1×10^{-5}. It may be crystallized as a dihydrate which loses water at 100°C. It forms acid and neutral salts, mono- and diesters, a monoamide known as *oxamic acid,* and a diamide called *oxamide.* Oxamate inhibits the enzymatic conversion of glyoxylate to oxalate catalyzed by lactic dehydrogenase [71]. Oxamide has been used in the experimental production of kidney stones [72].

The free acid is soluble in water to the extent of 8.7 g per 100 g water at 20°C. At neutral or alkaline pH, the calcium salt of oxalate exhibits very low solubility in water (0.67 mg per 100 g water at pH 7, 13°C). The precipitation of calcium oxalate is inhibited by a number of compounds, including urea, various ions [73] such as magnesium, iron, copper, zinc, citrate, sul-

fate, and lactate, certain colloids [74], and certain low-molecular-weight polypeptides [75]. Inorganic pyrophosphate also inhibits the precipitation of calcium oxalate from aqueous solutions. Although urine is frequently supersaturated with calcium oxalate under physiologic conditions, precipitation is presumably prevented by the large number of inhibitors present in normal urine.

The oxidation of oxalic acid by potassium permanganate has been used for its quantitative determination. In the presence of zinc and sulfuric acid, oxalic acid is successively and quantitatively reduced to glyoxylic and glycolic acids. A specific enzyme, oxalic acid decarboxylase, catalyzes the conversion of oxalate to carbon dioxide and formate [76]. Calcium oxalate is a common constituent of renal stones, being found in approximately 67 percent of all calculi [77]. In calculi it occurs as both the mono- and dihydrate, and rarely as the trihydrate. Calcium oxalate monohydrate, or whewellite, is the most common form found in stones [77]. The typical ditetragonal pyramid crystals, or "envelope" crystals, found commonly in urine samples represent the dihydrate form (weddellite) [77].

Absorption of Oxalate

Although oxalic acid is found in high concentration is certain plants, its biochemical function has not been established. Oxalate is present in highest concentration in spinach, rhubarb, parsley, cocoa, and tea. Smaller amounts are found in beans, carrots, and celery [78]. The content of oxalate in a typical diet has been reported as ranging from 97 to 930 mg [78–80]. This wide discrepancy calls for further study.

The recent finding of hyperoxaluria in patients with small-bowel disease has shed a great deal of light on the absorption of oxalate [81]. Early studies showed that ingested oxalate is poorly absorbed from the gastrointestinal tract; only 2.3 to 4.5 percent of ingested sodium oxalate (800 to 3200 mg) was absorbed by normal subjects in the fasting state as judged by the resulting increases in urinary oxalate [79]. More recently, absorption of oxalate has been studied using [^{14}C]oxalic acid. Absorption of the radioisotope averages 12 percent in normal humans in the fasting state [81, 82]. The total amount of oxalate absorbed appears to be dependent on the particular cation species present in the lumen of the gastrointestinal tract. Sodium oxalate is more soluble and more readily absorbed than calcium oxalate. In patients with small-bowel disease and significant steatorrhea (see "Classification of Hyperoxaluric States"), the decreased availability of calcium ions in the lumen of the gastrointestinal tract may allow more oxalate to exist as the sodium salt, leading to increased absorption. This absorption takes place in both the small and large bowels [83, 84] by a non-energy-dependent passive diffusion process [85–87]. Certain fatty acids and bile acids may increase absorption of oxalate by the colonic mucosa [85–89]. Oxalate absorption in patients with primary hyperoxaluria type I is normal [90].

Biosynthesis of Oxalate

In mammalian systems the synthesis of oxalic acid occurs through two separate pathways: (1) as an end product in the oxidative metabolism of ascorbic acid, and (2) by oxidation of glyoxylic acid. Although oxalate may be formed from a number of other precursors in microorganisms, particularly oxaloacetate, oxalosuccinate, and β-ketoadipate [91], in humans the major precursor of oxalate is glyoxylate. Evidence suggests that glyoxylate is formed primarily from glycine, glycolic acid, and α-keto-γ-hydroxyglutamic acid in humans, although other precursors have not been excluded. In microorganisms isocitric acid is the major source of glyoxylic acid, its cleavage being catalyzed by isocitrate ligase [92]. This enzyme has not yet been identified in mammalian systems. Although tryptophan has been described as a source of oxalate in humans [93], it is likely that such a conversion occurs through interconversion with serine and eventually glyoxylate. However, studies in perfused rat liver suggest that tryptophan conversion to oxalate may not involve serine as an obligatory intermediate [94]. There is no evidence that tryptophan is quantitatively important as an oxalate precursor in humans. In the rat, glycolate appears to be a more effective precursor of oxalate than glyoxylate [94]. Also, in the rat, phenylalanine and tyrosine give rise to oxalate, presumably by autooxidation of their respective α-keto analogues [95]. Recently, hydroxypyruvate has been shown to be a precursor of oxalate in the rat, presumably by conversion to glycoaldehyde and glycolate [96].

Ascorbic Acid Pathway

Ascorbic acid is a precursor of urinary oxalate in several laboratory animals and in humans [97–100]. Studies in vivo with isotopic ascorbate indicate that oxalate is derived from carbon atoms 1 and 2 of the parent compound. The pathways of ascorbic acid metabolism in humans are not thoroughly understood. Although some controversy exists, it seems probable that ascorbic acid is not metabolized significantly to respiratory carbon dioxide in humans [101]. Ascorbate is probably first oxidized to dehydroascorbate and then hydrolyzed to 2,3-diketogulonic acid, with subsequent conversion to oxalate and L-threose (Fig. 10-8) [101]. There is some evidence, however, that 2,3-diketogulonic acid is not an intermediate in ascorbate metabolism and that cleavage of the C2-C3 bond may occur enzymatically while the ascorbate lactone ring is still intact [101]. The question of whether glyoxylate is an intermediate in ascorbate metabolism is unresolved, but the absence of ^{14}CO$_2$ after administration of [^{14}C]ascorbate to humans makes this possibility unlikely.

Ascorbic acid has been established as an oxalate precursor by isotope techniques as noted, accounting for perhaps 35 to 50 percent of that normally excreted. Synthesis of oxalate from ascorbate must be maximally operative under normal conditions, since ingestion of relatively large amounts of ascorbic acid (less than 4 g) does not increase urinary oxalate [102, 103]. Ingestion of more than 4 g ascorbic acid per day has been reported to produce a variable increase in urinary oxalate excretion [104]. The mechanisms of control of oxalate synthesis from ascorbic acid have not been studied.

Glyoxylic Acid Pathway

The conversion of glyoxylate to oxalate may be catalyzed by three enzymes—glycolic acid oxidase, xanthine oxidase, and lactic dehydrogenase. The first enzyme, a flavoprotein, catalyzes both the conversion of glycolate to glyoxylate [105, 106] and that of glyoxylate to oxalate [107]. This latter step is functionally irreversible. Xanthine oxidase, also a flavoprotein which has been studied extensively in humans [108], similarly catalyzes the oxidation of glyoxylate to oxalate in mammalian tissues [109]. Studies of this reaction in human liver tissue indicate that xanthine oxidase plays only a minor role, if any, in the overall production of oxalate from glyoxylate in the intact human subject [110]. Administration of the xanthine oxidase

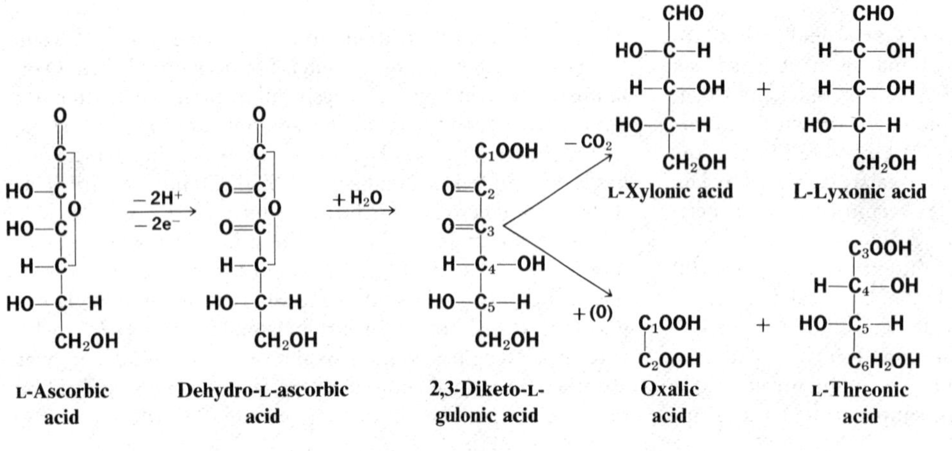

Figure 10-8 Pathways of ascorbic acid metabolism.

inhibitor allopurinol to gouty subjects did not alter the daily excretion of oxalate [110], and two patients with hereditary xanthinuria, with a genetic deficiency of xanthine oxidase, have had normal oxalate excretion [110].

Glyoxylate is a substrate for lactic dehydrogenase [111–114], and this enzyme is probably the most important one in controlling oxalate synthesis in humans [115]. This enzyme can bring about the reversible conversion of glyoxylate and glycolate, although the equilibrium of this reaction is far in the direction of the reduced substrate. In the presence of NAD (nicotinamide adenine dinucleotide), glyoxylate may also be oxidized to oxalate by lactic dehydrogenase [112]. In lactic dehydrogenase preparations from rat and humans, K_m values for both lactate and glyoxylate are similar, $1.5 \times 10^{-3}M$ [112].[1] Oxalate is an inhibitor of both glycolic acid oxidase and lactic dehydrogenase. Reports of dismutation reactions of glyoxylate to glycolate and oxalate may be accounted for by lactic dehydrogenase [118]. No specific mutase for glyoxylate has been demonstrated. Some dismutation of glyoxylic acid to oxalic and glycolic acids occurs nonenzymatically in vitro at neutral pH. Glyoxylate may be trapped and nonenzymatically decarboxylated by certain sulfhydryl compounds [119].

PRECURSORS OF GLYOXYLATE

Three immediate precursors of glyoxylate in man are known: glycine, glycolic acid, and α-keto-γ-hydroxyglutarate (Fig. 10-9). Although other pathways may exist, they have not as yet been described. Glycine is a major precursor of oxalate and therefore presumably of glyoxylate in humans. In an important study, Crawhall et al. administered [1-¹³C]glycine every 6 h to a control subject over a period of 4 days and in this manner obtained constant isotopic enrichment of the free glycine pool, as judged by the content of urinary glycine [120]. At equilibrium urinary oxalate was approximately 40 percent as highly labeled as urinary free glycine (Fig. 10-10). If urinary free glycine is a valid sample of the first glycine pool, these data indicate that a similar percentage of oxalate normally derives from glycine. [¹⁴C]Glycine has also been demonstrated as an oxalate precursor in five normal subjects, with approximately 0.05 percent of that administered appearing in urinary oxalate [49]. In a study by Dean and coworkers [121], the conversion of both [1-¹³C]glycine and [2-¹³C]glycine into urinary oxalate was studied in a single patient with primary hyperoxaluria. Estimations based on the degree of isotope dilution between free urinary glycine and urinary oxalate indicated that about 10 percent of oxalate derived from glycine. The rate of disappearance of ¹³C from urinary oxalate could be resolved into a single exponential component following [1-¹³C]glycine administration, and into two exponential components following [2-¹³C]glycine administration. These studies were thought to be consistent with the operation of two metabolic pathways in the conversion of glycine to oxalate, one by direct conversion of glycine to glyoxylate and oxalate, and a second involving the interconversion of glycine with serine, followed by the formation of ethanolamine, glycolaldehyde, glycolate, glyoxylate, and oxalate (Fig. 10-9).

Although glycine is an important source of urinary oxalate, it is unlikely that a large proportion of glycine is metabolized by way of the glyoxylate pathway. In a 72-kg normal subject, a first glycine pool of 5.8 g was found, with a turnover rate of 0.5 to 1.0 g glycine/(kg·day) [122]. It can be calculated, with certain assumptions discussed elsewhere [3], that not more than 0.5 to 1.0 percent of the turnover of glycine is accountable by glyoxylate formation. This is consistent with the minimal changes in oxalate excretion that occur in normal subjects or in patients with primary hyperoxaluria when glycine is administered [90]. In three patients with hyperoxaluria and small-bowel disease (see "Classification of Hyperoxaluric States"), oral glycine loading did increase urinary oxalate excretion nearly twofold [123], perhaps by intraluminal conversion of glycine to glyoxylate and oxalate with increased absorption of these organic acids.

Glycine can be converted directly to glyoxylate by oxidative deamination catalyzed by glycine oxidase or by transamination of glycine with a number of keto acids. It may be converted indirectly to glyoxylate by the serine-glycolate pathway (Fig. 10-9). Glycine oxidase, originally described in 1944 in mammalian liver and kidney preparations [124], oxidizes glycine to glyoxylate in the presence of flavin adenine dinucleotide. Evidence based on parallel activities during purification procedures suggests that this is the same enzyme as D-amino acid oxidase [125]. It belongs to the class of aerobic oxidases and yields H_2O_2 as a by-product.

$$\underset{\text{Glycine}}{\overset{\text{COOH}}{\underset{|}{\overset{|}{CH_2NH_2}}}} + O_2 + H_2O \rightarrow \underset{\text{Glyoxylic acid}}{\overset{\text{COOH}}{\underset{|}{\overset{|}{CHO}}}} + NH_3 + H_2O_2$$

Although in theory glycine may also be converted to glyoxylate by reversible transamination reactions, all cases so far described have equilibria far in the direction of glycine synthesis. This is consistent with the finding that deficiency of pyridoxine, a cofactor in these reactions as pyridoxal phosphate, leads to increased rather than decreased oxalate synthesis [126, 127]. The transamination reactions of glyoxylate to form glycine will be described further in this chapter in the section "Pathways of Glyoxylate Metabolism."

Glycolic acid is both a precursor and a product of glyoxylate. It is formed early in photosynthesis and so is present in plants, where it is the probable precursor of oxalate, glycine, and serine [128]. Administration of glycolic acid to the rat may lead to oxalosis and death from uremia [129]. The normal occurrence of glycolate in urine has been noted above (Fig. 10-7). Following the intravenous administration of a trace amount of [¹⁴C]glycolate, two normal control subjects excreted 1.03 percent as oxalate and 2.4 percent as unchanged glycolate over the subsequent 24 h [3]. The only metabolic fate established for glycolate in humans is its oxidation to glyoxylate and subsequent participation in the reactions summarized in Fig. 10-9. This oxidation is catalyzed by glycolic acid oxidase, a flavoprotein present in animals, plants, and microorganisms [104, 105]. In mammals the only known precursor of glycolate, other than glyoxylate, is glycolaldehyde. Glycolaldehyde may be formed from serine by way of ethanolamine [105] or from hydroxypyruvate catalyzed by pyruvate oxidase [130]. Glycolaldehyde also exists as a cofactor-bound intermediate in the transketolase reaction of the pentose-phosphate shunt pathway [131]. Oxidation of ethylene glycol, demonstrated as a component of a complex mammalian lipid [132], probably proceeds by way of glycolaldehyde. The oxidation of glycolal-

---

[1] See also Williams and Smith [116], and Smith et al. [117].

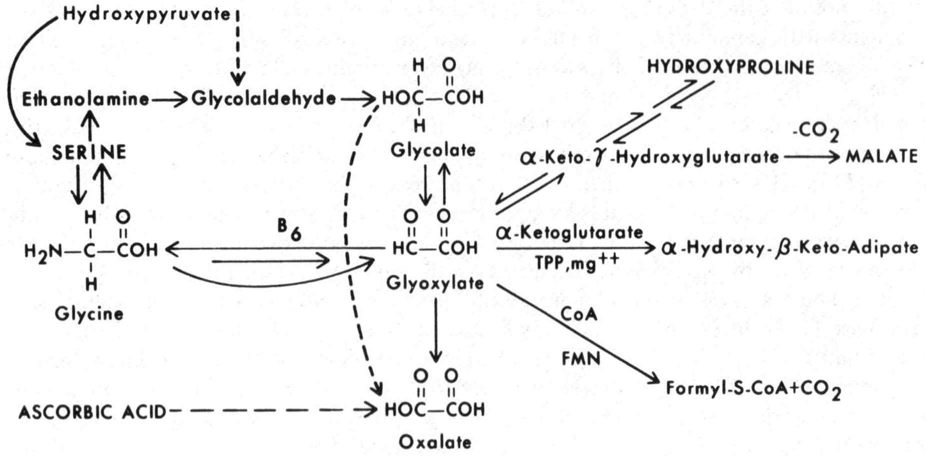

Figure 10-9 Pathways of oxalate metabolism in humans. The dotted pathways have not been proved in humans.

dehyde to glycolic acid is catalyzed by both aldehyde oxidase and dehydrogenases. The quantitative importance of the glycolaldehyde→glycolate→glyoxylate→oxalate pathway in humans has not been determined.

Studies in the isolated, perfused rat liver has shown glycolate to be a more effective precursor of oxalate than glyoxylate at low concentrations of glycolate in the perfusate [94]. As glycolate concentration increases, glyoxylate assumes a more important role in oxalate synthesis. This finding has suggested the possibility of either a separate metabolic pathway from glycolate to oxalate not involving glyoxylate as an intermediate or differences in the affinity of glycolate and glyoxylate for glycolic acid oxidase.

The concept of a separate pathway from glycolate to oxalate not involving glyoxylate has received further support in rat liver perfusion studies [96], and studies in isolated rat hepatocytes [279]. In these studies hydroxypyruvate and glycolate inhibited the oxidation of uniformly labeled [14C]glyoxylate to [14C]oxalate but stimulated total oxalate synthesis. [3-14C]hydroxypyruvate but not [1-14C]hydroxypyruvate was found to be a precursor of 14C oxalate in these rat liver perfusion studies. This observation has raised questions about the mechanisms of the hyperoxaluria in type II primary hyperoxaluria (see "The Pathogenesis of Primary Hyperoxaluria, Type II).

In addition to glycine and glycolic acid α-keto-γ-hydroxyglutarate is an immediate precursor of glyoxylate in mammalian systems (Fig. 10-9). This compound, formed during hydroxyproline catabolism, is reversibly converted to glyoxylate and pyruvate catalyzed by a specific aldolase [133]. It may also undergo oxidative decarboxylation to form malate [134]. Hydroxyketoglutarate aldolase activity is present but is low in human tissues [135]. In conditions associated with increased protein turnover and hydroxyprolinuria, no increase in urinary oxalate excretion has been observed, and administration of large doses of hydroxyproline to hyperoxaluric subjects failed to increase oxalate excretion [136]. In summary, current evidence does not suggest that hydroxyproline is an important precursor of glyoxylate and therefore of oxalate.

PATHWAYS OF GLYOXYLATE METABOLISM

The alternate pathways of glyoxylate metabolism are important, as they relate to possible mechanisms for in vivo accumulation of this oxalate precursor. Glyoxylate is an extremely versatile metabolic intermediate (Table 10-1), although not all its reactions can be demonstrated in mammalian systems. The oxidation of glyoxylate to oxalate has already been discussed. Glyoxylate may undergo transamination to glycine, with pyridoxal phosphate as a cofactor, a reaction or group of reactions extensively studied in preparations of animals, plants, and microorganisms [137,138]. It has been reported that the most active amino donor in rat liver is glutamate, and partial purification of glutamate:glycine transaminase from human liver has been obtained (139). In studies on transamination reactions of glyoxylate in human liver and kidney preparations from the laboratory of Williams and Smith, alanine was found to be the most active amino donor in both supernatant and particulate fractions [140]. Glyoxylate:ornithine transaminase was found only in the particulate fraction. Other amino acids, such as glutamine, arginine, and methionine, may be amino donors. In all these reactions the equilibrium lies far in the direction of glycine synthesis.

Glyoxylate may be reversibly reduced to glycolate (Fig. 10-9) in reactions catalyzed by three separate enzymes: lactic dehydrogenase [113], an NADH-linked glyoxylate reductase [141], and a separate NADPH-linked glyoxylate reductase [142]. The presence of specific glyoxylate reductases in humans has not been established. Lactic dehydrogenase catalyzes a dismutation of glyoxylate [143] with partial reduction to glycolate and conversion in vivo of [14C]glyoxylate to

Figure 10-10 13C content of urinary oxalate (height of stippled columns) and of urinary glycine (combined heights of hatched and stippled columns) of a patient with primary hyperoxaluria. *(From Crawhall et al. [120], with permission of the authors and publisher.)*

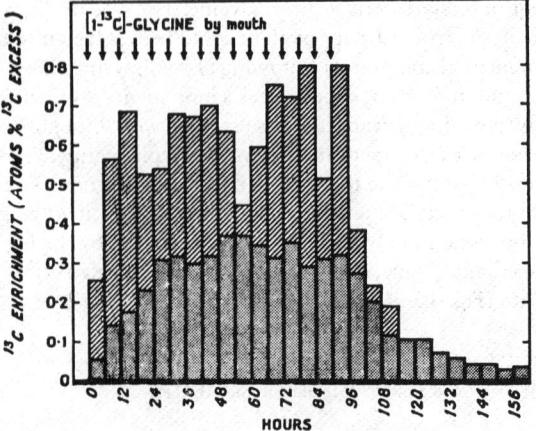

Table 10-1 Enzymatic reactions in glyoxylate metabolism*

1. Glyoxylate + [0] → oxalate

2. Glyoxylate + L-glutamate $\underset{}{\overset{B_6}{\rightleftharpoons}}$ glycine + α-ketoglutarate

3. Glyoxylate + L-ornithine $\underset{}{\overset{B_6}{\rightleftharpoons}}$ glycine + glutamic-γ-semialdehyde

4. Glyoxylate + other amino acids $\underset{}{\overset{B_6}{\rightleftharpoons}}$ glycine + keto acid

5. Glyoxylate $\underset{-H}{\overset{+H}{\rightleftharpoons}}$ glycolate

6. Glyoxylate + α-ketoglutarate $\xrightarrow{TPP}$ α-hydroxy-β-ketoadipate

7. Glyoxylate + pyruvate ⇄ 2-keto-4-hydroxyglutarate

8. Glyoxylate + CoA $\xrightarrow{FMN}$ formyl-S-CoA + CO_2

9. Glyoxylate + acetyle CoA → malate + CoA

10. Glyoxylate + glyoxylate $\xrightarrow{TPP}$ tartronic semialdehyde + CO_2

11. Glyoxylate + urea → glyoxylurea

12. Glyoxylate + glycine → β-hydroxyaspartate

13. Glyoxylate + propionyl CoA → α-hydroxyglutarate + CoA

14. Glyoxylate + butyryl CoA → β-ethylmalate + CoA

15. Glyoxylate + valeryl CoA → β-η-propylmalate + CoA

16. Glyoxylate + succinte ⇄ isocitrate

17. Glyoxylate + pyruvate → lactaldehyde

* The first eight reactions have been found in mammalian systems. The remaining reactions have been described so far only in microorganisms or plants.
SOURCE: From Williams and Smith [4], with permission of the publisher.

[14C]glycolate in human subjects. An average of 3.7 percent of administered [14C]glyoxylate was excreted as urinary [14C]glycolate within 24 h in three control subjects [3]. This does not establish the percentage of glyoxylate normally reduced to glycolate, since control subjects excrete only 2.4 percent of injected [14C]glycolate as unaltered glycolate [3]. The reversible aldolase-catalyzed condensation of pyruvate and glyoxylate to form α-keto-γ-hydroxyglutarate has been described above.

In an important pathway glyoxylate and α-ketoglutarate undergo synergistic decarboxylation. The first observations indicated a complex enzymatic reaction, or reactions, for glyoxylate, requiring NAD, thiamine pyrophosphate, L-glutamate, and manganese (Mn^{2+}) for optimal activity, yielding carbon dioxide and N-formyl glutamate [144]. Further studies by Crawhall and Watts demonstrated that α-ketoglutarate was more effective than glutamate in this reaction [145]. No formylglutamate was found as a reaction product. More recently, α-keto-β-hydroxyadipate was proposed as the primary product of this carboligase reaction, with decarboxylation of α-ketoglutarate [146]. A partially purified enzyme from pig liver mitochondria catalyzed the synergistic decarboxylation of glyoxylate and α-ketoglutarate, but the products of the reaction were not identified [147]. Koch and coworkers have developed an assay for the activity of α-ketoglutarate: glyoxylate carboligase and have characterized the product as α-hydroxy-β-ketoadipate [148]). Activity was present in rat liver mito-

chondria and in cytoplasmic and mitochondrial fractions of human liver, kidney, and spleen. Both the cytoplasmic and mitochondrial enzymes had a similar pH optimum (6.5), and both required thiamine pyrophosphate and Mg^{2+} for full activity. Lower levels of enzyme activity could also be detected in soluble and particulate fractions of skeletal muscle and in the particulate fraction of disrupted human leukocytes.

In studies of rat and rabbit tissues, the cellular distribution of the carboligase was examined using marker enzymes of known localization in order to monitor the composition of subcellular fractions obtained by differential centrifugation [149]. Using this technique, it was not possible to demonstrate a separate soluble carboligase in the cytoplasm of these tissues. The distribution pattern of the α-ketoglutarate: glyoxylate carboligase was similar to that of α-ketoglutarate dehydrogenase complex. The subsequent reactions and the purpose of the α-hydroxy-β-ketoadipate pathway have not been established.

Glyoxylate may react with CoA in the presence of flavin mononucleotide (FMN) to form formyl-S-CoA and carbon dioxide. This reaction, much less active in rat liver mitochondria than the carboligase reaction described in the previous paragraph [150], has not as yet been demonstrated in human tissue preparations.

CONTROL OF OXALATE SYNTHESIS

Oxalate is a metabolic end product in humans. All of the oxalate that is synthesized is excreted in the urine. It has no known function even in leafy plants, where its concentration may reach levels of 14 g per 100 g dry weight [80]. Its synthesis in mammalian systems appears to be the infortuitous result of the substrate versatility of glyoxylate for oxidation by enzymes with other primary catalytic functions: lactic dehydrogenase [111–114], glycolic acid oxidase [106], and xanthine oxidase [109]. As previously noted, the quantitative significance of these enzymes (or even the presence or absence of others) in glyoxylate oxidation has not been established. Recent studies of oxalate synthesis from glyoxylate in a dialyzed erythrocyte hemolysate preparation and in human liver and heart supernatant fractions indicate that lactic dehydrogenase is the major enzyme responsible for this conversion in these preparations in vitro [151, 152]. Studies of rat liver suggest that glycolic acid oxidase may be the most important enzyme controlling oxalate synthesis in that species [94]. Xanthine oxidase seems of least importance, since oxalate excretion is normal in hereditary xanthinuria [100] and allopurinol administration does not reduce oxalate excretion [110]. In three normal subjects only a small fraction, 11.7 percent, of intravenously administered [14C]glyoxylate was converted to oxalate, as judged by the urinary excretion of [14C]oxalate over the subsequent 24 h. An increased percentage of glyoxylate is oxidized to oxalate when the glyoxylate pool is expanded in vitro, as demonstrated in the early studies of Nakada and Weinhouse [138], or in vivo as seen in primary hyperoxaluria (see "In Vivo Studies of Glyoxylate Metabolism in Primary Hyperoxaluria").

Oxalate exhibits product inhibition of its synthesis from glyoxylate catalyzed by partially purified glycolic acid oxidase [89] or by lactic dehydrogenase [71, 153]. The inhibition of oxalate synthesis in human erythrocytes may reflect oxalate inhibition of lactic dehydrogenase [154]. Oxalate inhibition of glyoxylate oxidation by glycolic acid oxidase is competitive in nature, with a K_i of 3.1×10^{-3} at pH 7.3 [106]. Inhibition of lactic dehydrogenase by oxalate demonstrates more complex kinetics, suggesting competition and also the formation of an inactive complex [71]. Pharmacologic agents which inhibit oxalate synthesis will be described later in this chapter under "Treatment."

The oxidation of glyoxylate to oxalate by lactic dehydrogenase may be enhanced by pyruvate [143] or by hydroxypyruvate [117]. It is likely that this occurs through the reoxidation of the LDH (lactate dehydrogenase)-NADH complex. Enhancement of oxalate synthesis from glyoxylate by intact human erythrocytes, erythrocyte hemolysates, and rat liver supernatant can be demonstrated by the addition of hydroxypyruvate to the medium [117]. In partially purified lactic dehydrogenase preparations in the presence of NADH, both hydroxypyruvate and pyruvate increase the synthesis of oxalate from glyoxylate [117]. This may be one mechanism to explain the increased oxalate synthesis in L-glyceric aciduria (see "The Pathogenesis of Primary Hyperoxaluria Type II").

CATABOLISM OF OXALATE

Oxalate may be further metabolized in microorganisms by direct decarboxylation [155] or by the intermediate formation of oxalyl-coenzyme A [156]. In humans it is a nonessential end product of metabolism. Radioactive oxalate administered to rats is excreted unchanged in urine and feces, and respiratory CO_2 and urinary hippurate are not labeled [98, 157, 158]. Small amounts of oxalate may be stored in bone following large doses. [^{14}C]Oxalate given intravenously to normal humans does not label respiratory CO_2, and 89 to 99 percent is recovered unchanged in the urine [59]. It is possible that a small amount of oxalate may be excreted in succus entericus and bile, with subsequent bacterial degradation in the intestinal lumen, a mechanism analogous to that of urate degradation. If so, the amounts destroyed must be small. The normal synthetic rate of oxalate can be calculated from its pool size (3.5 to 6.1 mg) and turnover rate (biologic half-time of 2.2 to 2.8 h) as being 24 to 46 mg per day [59]. This figure agrees closely with the normal urinary excretory rate.

EXCRETION OF OXALATE

In humans, oxalate is excreted almost exclusively in the urine. Studies of the renal clearance of oxalate in humans and laboratory animals have led to different conclusions. In the dog, using isotopic oxalate, Cattell and coworkers [159] have demonstrated three mechanisms in the renal excretion of oxalate: glomerular filtration, secretion in the proximal part of the nephron, and reabsorption by passive back-diffusion. Net tubular secretion of oxalate was demonstrated with an oxalate:inulin clearance ratio averaging 1.28. Clearance of oxalate was reduced by carinamide, probenecid, and para-aminohippurate but was unaffected by urine pH. In contrast to these findings, Zarembski and Hodgkinson [53] reported the renal clearance of oxalate in normal adults to be 3.4 to 5.0 ml/min and found an oxalate clearance of 12.4 to 51.3 ml/min

in seven hyperoxaluric subjects, with oxalate:creatinine clearance ratios varying between 0.23 and 0.94. These studies have suggested a renal tubular defect in the reabsorption of oxalate in primary hyperoxaluria, but such a defect alone could not account for accumulation of calcium oxalate in the body in the face of excessive excretion. The renal clearance of oxalate in normal adults and patients with primary hyperoxaluria (types I and II) has been restudied by Williams et al. [56], using an isotopic oxalate method similar to that used by Cattell and coworkers in the dog [159]. With this technique the calculated clearance of oxalate in humans averaged 169 ml/min, with an oxalate:inulin clearance ratio of 1.6. In patients with both types of primary hyperoxaluria, the renal clearance of oxalate and the ratio of oxalate clearance to inulin clearance were not significantly different from those in normal subjects [56]. Similar findings using an isotopic oxalate method have been reported by others [57, 58, 160, 161]. Recently, Weinman et al. have demonstrated in micropuncture studies the secretion of oxalate in the early proximal tubule, with bidirectional flow in the mid-proximal tubule of the rat nephron [162]. These differences in the reported oxalate clearance in humans appear to be related to differences in methods of study. The results with isotopic oxalate in humans, consistent with previous studies in the dog, support the accuracy of current methods for determining plasma oxalate [58].

THE PATHOGENESIS OF PRIMARY HYPEROXALURIA TYPE I (GLYCOLIC ACIDURIA)

Excessive accumulation of oxalate, or for that matter of any metabolite in the body, could result from one or a combination of the four variables listed in Table 10-2: increased absorption, decreased excretion, decreased catabolism, or increased biosynthesis.

Two patients with primary hyperoxaluria absorbed 1.2 to 5.4 percent of administered sodium oxalate, amounts comparable to those in a control series [90]. If figures of dietary content of oxalate are correct, even complete absorption could not account for the excessive amounts excreted in primary hyperoxaluria [3]. Reduction in excretion cannot account primarily for the accumulation of oxalate, since continued excessive excretion is the diagnostic hallmark of these genetic disorders. Reduced excretion may exacerbate oxalosis after renal failure occurs. Although increased clearance of oxalate has been reported in patients with primary hyperoxaluria [53], more recent results have demonstrated normal renal clearances in this disorder [56, 57]. Furthermore, increased clearance of

Table 10-2 Metabolic derangements which might result in oxalate accumulation, contrasted with condition in primary hyperoxaluria

Derangement	Primary hyperoxaluria
1. Increased gastrointestinal absorption of oxalate	Normal gastrointestinal absorption
2. Decreased excretion of oxalate	Persistent hyperoxaluria
3. Decreased catabolism of oxalate	Not metabolized in humans
4. Increased biosynthesis of oxalate	Increased biosynthesis

oxalate could not account for its pathologic accumulation as oxalosis. Since oxalate is not normally catabolized in humans, the continued excessive excretion of oxalate characteristic of primary hyperoxaluria must result from its increased rate of biosynthesis.

As reviewed in the section "Biosynthesis of Oxalate," the only known immediate precursors of oxalate in humans are ascorbate and glyoxylate. In an important study using [1-^{13}C]ascorbic acid, Atkins and coworkers demonstrated that the pool size, turnover rate, and metabolic conversion of ascorbate to urinary oxalate were similar in a control subject and in two patients with primary hyperoxaluria [163]. Less than 10 percent of the urinary oxalate in the patients derived from the oxidation of ascorbate, the absolute amount of ascorbate converted to oxalate being normal. Administration of large amounts of ascorbate to patients with primary hyperoxaluria failed to increase urinary oxalate [102, 103]. An abnormality of ascorbic acid metabolism cannot, therefore, be implicated as contributing to the excessive oxalate synthesis in these genetic disorders. By elimination, increased oxidation of glyoxylate offers the most likely explanation for enhanced oxalate synthesis in primary hyperoxaluria. Such increased synthesis might result from (1) an increased activity of the enzymes that oxidize glyoxylate to oxalate or (2) an increased concentration of glyoxylate, most probably secondary to a block in an alternate pathway of metabolism.

Quantitative in vitro studies of the activities of enzymes that oxidize glyoxylate to oxalate in humans are complicated by lack of information concerning their relative importance [151]. Within these limitations, it has been demonstrated that glyoxylate conversion to oxalate is not enhanced in preparations of liver mitochondria [145], whole homogenates of liver and kidney [2], or erythrocytes [154] from patients with primary hyperoxaluria type I (glycolic aciduria). In addition, no abnormality in oxalate inhibition of oxalate synthesis from glyoxylate was found in erythrocytes from hyperoxaluric patients. Secondary enhancement of enzyme activity may be the proximate cause of increased oxalate synthesis in L-glyceric aciduria but does not appear to contribute to that of glycolic aciduria. The evidence for accumulation of glyoxylate secondary to its impaired metabolism in vivo and the studies in vitro of the site of the enzymatic defect will now be reviewed briefly.

In Vivo Studies of Glyoxylate Metabolism in Primary Hyperoxaluria

Early studies of the pathogenesis of primary hyperoxaluria were directed toward establishing the presence of glyoxylate accumulation in the disease and compiling evidence for its impaired metabolism. The measurement of glyoxylate in biologic fluids was found to be unreliable because of its nonenzymatic reactivity with a number of other normal metabolites [48]. Within these limitations the excretion of glyoxylate was found to be elevated above the normal range [0.5 to 4.4 mg/(24 h · 1.73 m^2)] in six of seven patients with primary hyperoxaluria type I (Fig. 10-7). Reports to the contrary notwithstanding [164], in our opinion no reliable method is now available for measuring glyoxylate in blood or plasma. It was reasoned that if the glyoxylate pool were expanded, increased reduction to glycolate might occur, in line with its increased oxidation to oxalate. As described in the section "Diagnosis," hyperglycolic aciduria was found to be as characteristic of the

disorder as hyperoxaluria (Fig. 10-7) [37]. In fact its demonstration is the most direct method for the diagnosis of the type I variant of the disease.

The metabolism of [1-^{14}C]glyoxylate (1μmol/kg of body weight intravenously) is altered in primary hyperoxaluria, with a diminished rate of conversion to respiratory CO_2 (Fig. 10-11) and increased excretion as urinary oxalate and glycolate Table 10-3 [165]. In these same studies three of four parents of patients with primary hyperoxaluria demonstrated rates of CO_2 production from [^{14}C]glyoxylate less than those of the control subjects. This suggested a partial defect in these presumed heterozygotes [165]. One of the parents metabolized glyoxylate at a normal rate. A similar impairment of [^{14}C]glyoxylate metabolism to CO_2, together with increased urinary excretion as glycolate and oxalate, was found during constant intravenous infusion of the isotope over a 6-h period in order to obtain equilibrium rates [3].

Because of the close precursor-product relationship of glycolate with glyoxylate, similar in vivo studies of glycolate metabolism were performed in patients with primary hyperoxaluria [3]. In confirmation of the results with glyoxylate, the metabolism of intravenously administered [1-^{14}C]glycolate to respiratory CO_2 was reduced, while its conversion to urinary oxalate and its excretion as unaltered [^{14}C]glycolate were increased when compared with control subjects (Table 10-4).

The contribution of glycine to urinary oxalate has been studied by two different methods in patients with primary hyperoxaluria [57, 120]. [1-^{13}C]Glycine was administered over 4 days in order to obtain constant isotope enrichment of the free glycine pool, as reflected in the isotopic content of urinary glycine [120]. At equilibrium the fractions of urinary oxalate derived from glycine were 50 and 32 percent, respectively, in two patients with primary hyperoxaluria, values comparable to that found in a control subject (40 percent). In another patient with primary hyperoxaluria the cumulative incorporation of [^{14}C]glycine (given as a single oral tracer dose) into urinary oxalate was 0.22 percent, a value about four times higher than that found in five control subjects (0.05 percent) [59]. Because the degree of the increased incorporation of isotope approximated the degree of hyperoxaluria, the interpretation was made that the fractional contribution of glycine to

Figure 10-11 Metabolism of carboxyl-labeled [^{14}C]glyoxylic acid. (From Frederick et al. [165], with permission of the publisher.)

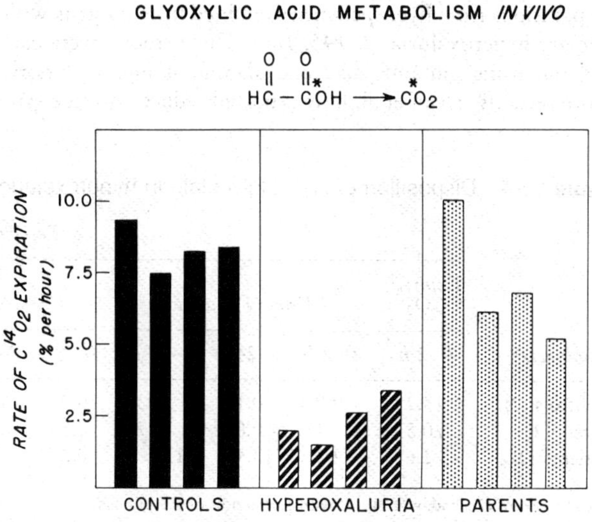

GLYOXYLIC ACID METABOLISM *IN VIVO*

Table 10-3 Incorporation of [1-^{14}C]glyoxylate into urinary oxalate and glycolate

| | Percentage of isotope administered | | | | | |
| | Urinary oxalate | | | Urinary glycolate | | |
Subjects	0–2 h	2–24 h	0–24 h	0–2 h	2–24 h	0–24 h
Controls (3)	5.3	6.4	11.7	3.0	0.7	3.7
Parents (4)	14.1	6.1	20.2	2.7	0.5	3.2
Patients (4)	9.7	15.6	25.3	5.4	9.4	14.8

SOURCE: From Frederick et al. [144].

oxalate synthesis was unchanged in the patient with primary hyperoxaluria. This observation, confirmatory of the [^{13}C]glycine studies cited above, would be more consistent with a defect in the further metabolism of glyoxylate than with a selective overproduction of glyoxylate from one of its precursors.

In the studies with [^{14}C]glyoxylate and [^{14}C]glycolate the incorporation of isotope into urinary glycine was found to be diminished (Table 10-4) [3]. It has been established that pyridoxine deficiency results in hyperoxaluria in experimental animals [126] and in humans [127]. This presumably represents a block in one or more of the transamination reactions that convert glyoxylate to glycine in which pyridoxal phosphate serves as a cofactor. On the basis of these in vivo studies it seemed most likely that the enzymatic defect would be found in one of the transamination reactions, representing biochemically the apoenzyme equivalent of pyridoxine deficiency. As noted in the next section, this has not been confirmed.

In Vitro Studies of the Enzymatic Defect in Glyoxylate Metabolism

Studies of glyoxylate metabolism in vitro have been carried out using tissue preparations of liver, kidney, spleen, erythrocytes, and leukocytes from patients with primary hyperoxaluria type I. Because of the studies in vivo outlined in the previous section, particular attention has been directed to the transamination reactions (with various amino donors) for the conversion of glyoxylate to glycine. Studies from two laboratories have failed to demonstrate any impairment of glycine synthesis from glyoxylate in whole homogenates or soluble or particulate preparations from liver specimens obtained from patients with primary hyperoxaluria [2, 145, 166]. These studies were carried out using glutamic acid and alanine as amino donors. More recently, Dean et al. have reported reduced glycine synthesis from glyoxylate in kidney homogenates from two patients with primary hyperoxaluria [167, 168], one of whom had normal hepatic glyoxylate transaminase activity [168]. Low levels of renal transaminase activity were similarly found in kidney preparations from three patients by Williams et al., but control specimens from uremic patients demonstrated equally reduced activities [140]. It is clear that the enzymatic defect of primary hyperoxaluria cannot be confined to the kidneys, since excessive oxalate synthesis continues following bilateral nephrectomy in association with renal transplantation [169]. We conclude that no defect in glyoxylate transamination has been firmly established in vitro. It is possible that the wrong amino donors have been used or that a defect in the kinetics of the reaction(s) has been overlooked. The partial reversal of hyperoxaluria by excess pyridoxine (see "Treatment") may represent cofactor enzyme induction or stabilization, or possibly may indicate another pyridoxine dependency syndrome [170]. The requirement for added pyridoxal phosphate could not be demonstrated in vitro. In view of the demonstrated defect in the soluble carboligase reaction to be described, it seems most probable that the studies in vivo indicating reduced conversion of [^{14}C]glyoxylate to urinary [^{14}C]glycine reflect the expanded glyoxylate pool together with the small amount of the daily glycine pool that is excreted (<1 percent).

The reaction of glyoxylate with α-ketoglutarate to form α-hydroxy-β-ketoadipate has been described earlier in "Pathways of Glyoxalate Metabolism" (Fig. 10-9). This reaction sequence leads to the synergistic decarboxylation of glyoxylate and α-ketoglutarate. No abnormality in the activity of this pathway was found in liver mitochondria from three patients with primary hyperoxaluria by Crawhall and Watts [166]. Subsequently, Koch et al. studied the activity of α-ketoglutarate:glyoxylate carboligase in cytoplasmic and mitochondrial preparations from the liver, kidney, and spleen from five patients with primary hyperoxaluria compared with control

Table 10-4 Disposition of [1-^{14}C]glycolate in hyperoxaluric and control subjects

| | Percentage of isotope administered | | | | | | | | | | | | |
| | Expired CO$_2$ | Urinary oxalate | | | Urinary glyoxylate | | | Urinary hippurate | | | Urinary glycolate | | |
Subjects	0–2 h	0–2 h	2–24 h	0–24 h	0–2 h	2–24 h	0–24 h	0–2 h	2–24 h	0–24 h	0–2 h	2–24 h	0–24 h
Controls (2)	18.2	0.9	0.13	1.03	0.09	0.03	0.12	2.50	0.48	2.98	2.3	0.1	2.4
Parent (1)	20.5	1.1	0.07	1.17	0.16	0	0.16	5.8	0.42	6.22	2.8	0.1	2.9
Patients (2)	2.6	4.1	13.4	17.5	0.27	0.12	0.39	0.29	0.22	0.51	12.2	26.0	38.2

SOURCE: From Hockaday et al. [3] with permission of the publisher.

subjects undergoing renal homotransplantation because of uremia secondary to chronic glomerulonephritis [148]. In confirmation of the work of Crawhall and Watts, enzyme activity in mitochondria was found to be within the control range. In contrast, the activity of soluble δ-ketoglutarate:glyoxylate carboligase was reduced markedly in all three organs (Fig. 10-12). No inhibition of activity was found on mixing hyperoxaluric and control enzyme preparations, nor was carboligase activity inhibited by oxalate or glycolate, which are overproduced in primary hyperoxaluria [3]. These data indicate a specific defect in the cytoplasmic carboligase, presumably an isoenzyme of the mitochondrial enzyme, as the cause of glyoxylate accumulation in primary hyperoxaluria. This concept of the disease is illustrated in Fig. 10-1. The consequences of this defect suggest that the cytoplasmic carboligase is of major importance in the further metabolism of glyoxylate. At the present time, no studies have been carried out on the activity of soluble α-ketoglutarate:glyoxylate carboligase in preparations from presumed heterozygotes of primary hyperoxaluria. The finding by O'Fallon and Brosemer [149] that α-ketoglutarate:glyoxylate carboligase activity is located exclusively within the mitochondria in rat and rabbit tissues may represent species differences in the subcellular localization of this enzyme between *Homo sapiens* and other mammalian species.

Bourke et al. [171] found normal activity of α-ketoglutarate:glyoxylate carboligase in both mitochondrial and soluble cytoplasmic fractions of skeletal muscle from a 10-year-old patient with type I primary hyperoxaluria. Although other tissues were not examined in this patient, Bourke et al. suggested that this finding indicated further biochemical heterogeneity in primary hyperoxaluria.

THE PATHOGENESIS OF PRIMARY HYPEROXALURIA TYPE II (L-GLYCERIC ACIDURIA)

Four patients (three of them sibs) have been found to have excessive excretion of oxalate but normal excretion of glycolate. By chromatographic techniques a new organic acid was found in their urine that was identified as L-glyceric acid by color reaction with chromotropic acid, quantitative conversion to glyoxylate by periodate oxidation, purification to constant specific activity after the addition of [^{14}C]glycerate, substrate specificity with D-glyceric dehydrogenase and lactic dehydrogenase, and optical rotatory dispersion curves [5]. By an isotope dilution method, L-glycerate excretion was found to be between 225 and 638 mg/(24 h · 1.73 m^2) in the urine of patients with this disorder [49]. No L-glycerate was found in normal urine using this isotope dilution technique. Urinary glyoxylate level was not elevated in the two patients studied [3]. A consideration of the pathogenesis of L-glyceric aciduria requires a brief review of glyceric acid and hydroxypyruvic acid metabolism.

Glyceric Acid and Hydroxypyruvic Acid Metabolism

Glyceric acid is a relatively weak acid, with many properties similar to those of lactic and glycolic acids. The L form of

2-OXO-GLUTARATE: GLYOXYLATE CARBOLIGASE

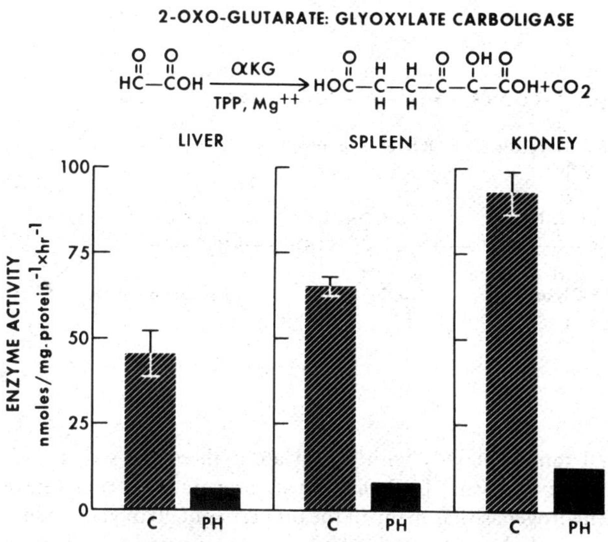

Figure 10-12 α-Ketoglutarate:glyoxylate carboligase activity in tissues from patients with primary hyperoxaluria, type I (P. H.), and control subjects (C). (*From Williams and Smith [4], with permission of the publisher.*)

glyceric acid forms calcium salts that are soluble in water to the extent of 1 g in 10 ml water. The D form also forms calcium salts that are somewhat less soluble. The free acid is soluble in water, alcohol, and acetone. It can be prepared either by oxidation of glyceraldehyde or by the action of nitrous acid on serine.

The major source of glyceric acid in both plants and mammals is hydroxypyruvic acid (Fig. 10-13). D-Glyceric acid is produced from hydroxypyruvate by the enzyme D-glycerate dehydrogenase (hydroxypyruvate reductase). This enzyme has been studied extensively in plant, animal, and microbial systems [172–174]. The enzyme purified from calf liver utilizes NADH and NADPH equally well as hydrogen donors [174]. L-Glycerate, L-lactate, and glycolate will not serve as substrates for the enzyme. Glyoxylate is reduced to glycolate by this enzyme but more slowly than is hydroxypyruvate. The relative K_m values are hydroxypyruvate—4.5×10^{-5} M (with NADH) and 2.0×10^{-5} M (with NADPH), and glyoxylate—1.4×10^{-4} M (with NADH) and 2.5×10^{-4} M (with NADPH). The equilibrium of the reaction between hydroxypyruvate and glycerate strongly favors the reduced product, although the oxidative reaction is shifted to favor hydroxypyruvate synthesis at pH 9 in the presence of carbonyl-trapping reagents. D-Glycerate dehydrogenase purified from spinach leaves differs from the mammalian enzyme in its specificity for NADH [175]. Similar to the calf liver enzyme, the spinach preparation utilizes both hydroxypyruvate and glyoxylate as substrates, but the maximal rate of reduction of hydroxypyruvate is four to five times that observed with glyoxylate. Crystalline D-glycerate dehydrogenase prepared from *Pseudomonas acidovorans* utilizes only hydroxypyruvate as substrate; no activity is observed with either pyruvate or glyoxylate [176]. A flavoprotein enzyme, D-α-hydroxy acid dehydrogenase, has been reported in yeast and mammalian liver and kidney mitochondria [177]. This enzyme has a wide specificity for many hydroxy acids, including D-glycerate, D-lactate, D-α-hydroxybutyrate, and D-malate.

Evidence in plants and bacteria has suggested the similarity of D-glycerate dehydrogenase and the NADH-linked glyoxylate reductase [175]. This latter enzyme has activity with both glyoxylate and hydroxypyruvate as substrates, but the maxi-

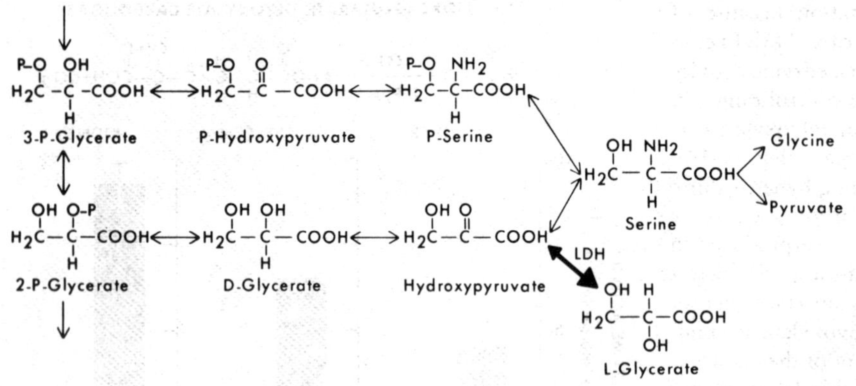

Figure 10-13 Pathways of serine and glycerate metabolism in mammalian systems. LDH, lactic dehydrogenase. *(From Williams and Smith [62], with permission of the publisher.)*

mal rate of activity with glyoxylate is three times that with hydroxypyruvate. In *Pseudomonas* preparations, D-glycerate dehydrogenase has many of the properties of glyoxylate reductase, including stimulation at high ionic strength, similar pH optimum, and inhibition with dihydroxyfumarate [176]. At present, the question of whether glyoxylate reductase and D-glycerate dehydrogenase represent different enzymes in mammalian systems has not been resolved.

In mammalian systems L-glyceric acid is the product of the reduction of hydroxypyruvate by lactic dehydrogenase in the presence of NADH [172]. L-Glycerate is as effective a substrate as L-lactate for the lactate dehydrogenases of skeletal and heart muscle [178]. The equilibrium of the oxidation-reduction of L-glycerate and hydroxypyruvate catalyzed by lactic dehydrogenase favors the reduced product.

As discussed, hydroxypyruvate is a substrate for both D-glyceric acid and lactic dehydrogenase. It is the only known immediate precursor of L-glycerate. The major source of hydroxypyruvate is serine, an interconversion catalyzed by an alanine:hydroxypyruvate transaminase described in mammalian liver preparations, including adult and fetal human liver [179]. Glutamine has also been described as an effective amino donor for this enzyme.

Hydroxypyruvate is an important intermediate in both the synthesis and metabolism of serine (Fig. 10-13). In animals both phosphorylated and nonphosphorylated pathways exist for serine biosynthesis, the relative activity of the enzymes involved in these pathways varying widely in the species studied [180]. The regulation of these pathways, which has been studied extensively in animals, involves dietary factors, pyruvate, and product inhibition [173, 180]. In rats fed high protein diets, depression of 3-phosphoglycerate dehydrogenase and phosphoserine dehydratase activities have been observed [173]. On low protein diets, an inverse relationship of these enzymes exists. With dietary manipulations, no change in D-glycerate dehydrogenase was observed. In contrast, cortisone treatment of rats produced a 60 percent decrease in D-glycerate dehydrogenase activity and an 80 percent decrease in 3-phosphoglycerate dehydrogenase activity [181]. These studies have suggested that in the rat, the phosphorylated pathway is more important for serine biosynthesis and the nonphosphorylated pathway for gluconeogenesis and serine catabolism. Similar findings have been reported in beef and chicken liver, although considerable serine biosynthesis occurs by both pathways in pig liver and dog kidney [180]. The relative importance of these two pathways for the biosynthesis of serine in humans has not been fully resolved.

Studies in Vivo

The excretion of excessive amounts of L-glyceric acid in primary hyperoxaluria type II suggested an abnormality in hydroxypyruvate metabolism, with its secondary reduction catalyzed by lactic dehydrogenase. This would be analogous to the excessive reduction of glyoxylate to glycolate in primary hyperoxaluria type I. In order to determine precursor-product relationships, [l-^{14}C]hydroxypyruvate was given intravenously to a patient with L-glyceric aciduria [5]. Approximately 15 percent of the injected isotope was recovered in urinary L-glycerate, establishing hydroxypyruvate as a glycerate precursor in vivo. In this study none of the isotope was found in urinary oxalate. Recently, Richardson recovered radioactively labeled oxalate in urine after administration of [3-^{14}C]hydroxypyruvate to rats. This suggests that hydroxypyruvate can function as a significant precursor of oxalate in laboratory animals [182]. Such a possibility in humans must await further studies of [3-^{14}C]hydroxypyruvate metabolism.

In order to determine if a precursor-product relationship exists between glyoxylate and hydroxypyruvate, [1-^{14}C]glyoxylate was given intravenously to a patient with L-glyceric aciduria [5]. Comparative studies were conducted in normal subjects and patients with hyperoxaluria type I. The patient with L-glyceric aciduria incorporated excessive amounts of [1-^{14}C]glyoxylate into urinary oxalate, a finding similar to that in patients with primary hyperoxaluria with glycolic aciduria (Table 10-3). In contrast, decreased amounts of isotope were recovered in urinary glycolate when compared with normal subjects and patients with primary hyperoxaluria and glycolic aciduria. This finding implies a partial defect in the conversion of glyoxylate to glycolate in L-glyceric aciduria. No isotope incorporation from [l-^{14}C]glyoxylate into urinary L-glycerate was found in the patient with L-glyceric aciduria. This latter finding, together with the absence of any incorporation from [l-^{14}C]hydroxypyruvate into urinary oxalate, suggested the lack of a close precursor-product relationship between glyoxylate and hydroxypyruvate in L-glyceric aciduria. However, the recent finding by Liao and Richardson [96] that [3-^{14}]hydroxypyruvate but not [l-^{14}C]hydroxypyruvate is a precursor of oxalate in the rat has raised a question about the precursor-product relationship of hydroxypyruvate and oxalate in humans and indicates the importance of further [3-^{14}C]hydroxypyruvate studies in human subjects.

The studies carried out in vivo are consistent with a defect in hydroxypyruvate metabolism, although they fail to explain the mechanism of the accompanying increased oxalate synthesis.

No method for measuring hydroxypyruvate in urine or blood has been developed. The lability of hydroxypyruvate interferes with such studies. Attention was therefore directed toward the demonstration in vitro of a defect in hydroxypyruvate metabolism.

Studies in Vitro

Hydroxypyruvate might accumulate because of a block in its transamination to serine (alanine:hydroxypyruvate transaminase) or in its reduction to D-glycerate (D-glyceric dehydrogenase) (Fig. 10-13). The activity of D-glyceric dehydrogenase with NADP as a cofactor was measured in leukocyte preparations from 4 patients with L-glyceric aciduria, the 2 parents of three sibs with the disorder, and 14 normal control subjects [5]. No enzyme activity was detectable in leukocytes from the four patients with glyceric aciduria (Fig. 10-14). Enzyme activity was low in leukocytes from the mother but was within the normal range in leukocytes from the father of the three sibs with L-glyceric aciduria. In one patient with primary hyperoxaluria and glycolic aciduria, leukocyte D-glyceric dehydrogenase activity was within the normal range. The presence of an enzyme inhibitor in patients with L-glyceric aciduria was ruled out by the failure of inhibition of normal enzyme activity in leukocyte preparations from patients mixed with preparations from normal subjects.

This enzyme defect in L-glyceric aciduria allows an explanation for the excessive synthesis and excretion of L-glyceric acid, presumably arising from hydroxypyruvate (Fig. 10-13). The cause of the hyperoxaluria in these patients is not directly clarified by this enzyme defect. As noted earlier in "Glyceric Acid

Figure 10-14 D-Glyceric dehydrogenase activity in leukocytes from four patients with L-glyceric aciduria (primary hyperoxaluria, type II), parents of three sibs with this syndrome, and control subjects. *(From Williams and Smith [5], with permission of the publisher.)*

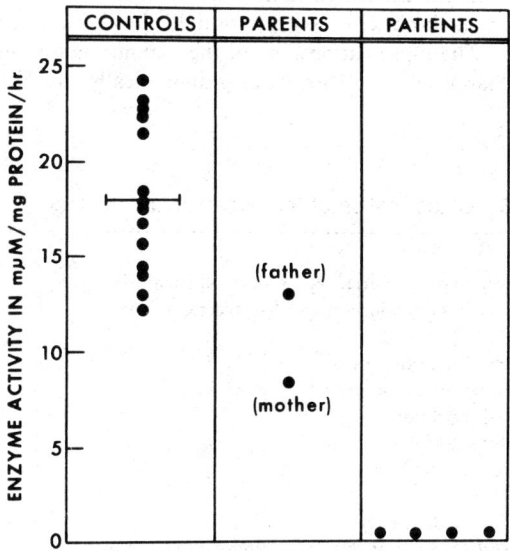

and Hydroxypyruvate Metabolism," there is some evidence in plants and bacteria to suggest the similarity of D-glyceric dehydrogenase and glyoxylate reductase [175]. It was postulated that the enzyme defect in L-glyceric aciduria may account for a block in the reduction of glyoxylate to glycolate as well as for a block in the reduction of hydroxypyruvate to D-glycerate. Such a parallel defect in these two metabolic pathways might explain the observed combination of L-glyceric aciduria and hyperoxaluria in the absence of hyperglycolic aciduria. A primary defect in glyoxylate metabolism leading to excessive hydroxypyruvate synthesis by some interconnecting pathway seems unlikely in view of the studies in vivo and in vitro. The possibility that hydroxypyruvate or L-glycerate accumulation might inhibit glyoxylate metabolism has not been fully investigated, but no inhibition of α-ketoglutarate:glyoxylate carboligase by hydroxypyruvate or glycerate was demonstrated [5]. The speculations above are based on the assumption that a deficiency of D-glyceric dehydrogenase with accumulation of hydroxypyruvate (reflected one step removed by L-glyceric aciduria) is somehow linked with a block in glyoxylate metabolism. A second mechanism to explain the relationship of hydroxypyruvate accumulation to increased oxalate synthesis should also be considered. As noted earlier, an increased activity of the enzyme or enzymes that oxidize glyoxylate to oxalate might also result in increased synthesis of oxalate in the absence of glyoxylate accumulation. The urinary glyoxylate level was not elevated in either patient with L-glyceric aciduria in whom it was determined. Metabolism of [l-^{14}C]glyoxylate to respiratory CO_2 was not as much impaired in a patient with L-glyceric aciduria as in four patients with primary hyperoxaluria type I, in spite of an even greater shunting of isotope into oxalate [5]. In studies on human erythrocytes and leukocytes and in partially purified lactic dehydrogenase preparations, it has been demonstrated that hydroxypyruvate enhances oxalate synthesis and diminishes glycolate synthesis from glyoxylate, presumably through reduction of lactic dehydrogenase-NADH (Fig. 10-15) [116]. It seems most likely, therefore, that the increased oxalate synthesis of D-glyceric dehydrogenase deficiency is the indirect consequence of coupled oxidation-reduction of glyoxylate and hydroxypyruvate through their common nonspecific reactivity with certain enzymes, especially lactic dehydrogenase.

Animal studies with [3-^{14}C]hydroxypyruvate have suggested a precursor-product relationship between hydroxypyruvate and oxalate [96, 182]. This raises questions about the etiology of the hyperoxaluria in the type II syndrome. If such an interconversion exists in humans, then accumulation of hydroxypyruvate may lead more directly to increased oxalate excretion. Two findings speak against this hypothesis in humans: the low glycolate excretion in the type II syndrome and the [^{14}C]glyoxylate infusion studies that have demonstrated increased conversion of glyoxylate to oxalate and decreased conversion of glyoxylate to glycolate [5]. Further studies on human beings will be needed to evaluate this hypothesis.

The study of D-glyceric dehydrogenase deficiency in patients with L-glyceric aciduria has implications relating to the pathway of serine biosynthesis in humans. Both phosphorylated and nonphosphorylated pathways for serine biosynthesis have been found in mammalian preparations [180]. In one patient with L-glyceric aciduria, serine was found in normal concentrations in plasma and urine [5]. The accumulation of hydroxypyruvate rather than D-glycerate in this disorder and

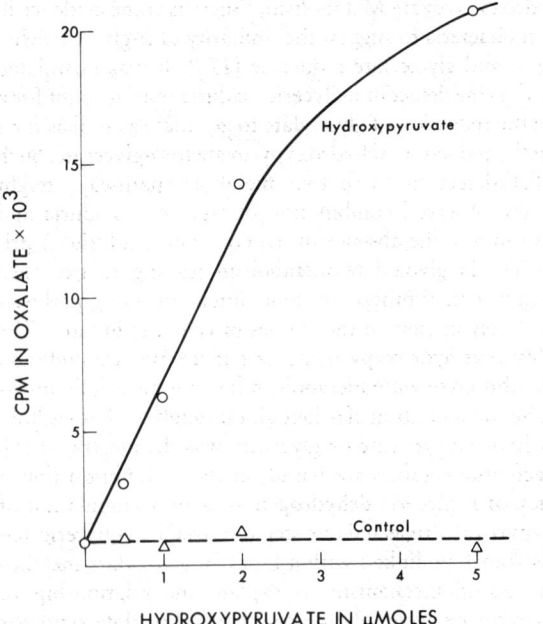

Figure 10-15 The effect of hydroxypyruvate on [^{14}C]oxalate synthesis from [^{14}C]glyoxalate catalyzed by lactic dehydrogenase.

the normal concentration of serine support the concept that the nonphosphorylated pathway of serine metabolism normally operates in the direction of gluconeogenesis in humans (Fig. 10-13), serine biosynthesis occurring by way of the phosphorylated pathway.

CLASSIFICATION OF HYPEROXALURIC STATES

Hyperoxaluria in humans may be divided into primary (or genetic) and secondary types, the latter related to an abnormal nutritional state. The increased production of oxalate in type I results indirectly from a block in glyoxylate metabolism. It is analogous to the accumulation of phenylpyruvate, phenyllactate, and phenylacetate in phenylketonuria. In the type II disease, hyperoxaluria seems most likely to result from enhanced shunting from glyoxylate to oxalate through coupled oxidation-reduction with hydroxypyruvate. Table 10-5 compares these two genetic disorders as studied by Williams and Smith. Other forms of genetic hyperoxaluria may exist.

In addition to these genetically determined conditions, several secondary or acquired disorders result in hyperoxaluria (Fig. 10-1). Oxalosis may be produced experimentally by the feeding or parenteral administration of oxalate to laboratory animals, and rare cases of oxalate poisoning have been described in human beings.

Glycolic acid is a source of glyoxylate and therefore of oxalate in humans. The dietary content of glycolate and its absorption have not been studied in human beings, but it has been demonstrated that excessive ingestion of glycolic acid by the rat may lead to oxalosis and death from uremia [129]. The ingestion of ethylene glycol, a precursor of glycolate, increases urinary oxalate in experimental animals and in humans [183–185]. Excessive ingestion of ethylene glycol leads to extensive

crystallization of calcium oxalate in renal tubules and within the renal parenchyma [184]. Fatal cases of ethylene glycol poisoning in humans exhibit similar pathologic lesions in the kidney, and this probably accounts for the acute renal insufficiency of this syndrome [188].

Thiamine pyrophosphate is a cofactor in the synergistic decarboxylation of glyoxylate and α-ketoglutarate by α-ketoglutarate:glyoxylate carboligase. Since a deficiency of the cytoplasmic enzyme results in the clinical syndrome of primary hyperoxaluria type I, a deficiency of the cofactor for this reaction should result in a similar metabolic derangement. The glyoxylate level has been reported elevated in the blood of two patients with presumed vitamin deficiencies, but no studies of oxalate excretion were mentioned [164]. Thiamine deficiency in the rat increases glyoxylate concentration in various organs and its excretion in the urine [187, 188]. Thiamine deficiency in rats may also result in decreased oxaluria [189]. Neither hyperoxaluria nor oxalosis has been found in thiamine-deficient human subjects [190]. Normal urinary oxalate was found in several patients with the Wernicke-Korsakov syndrome [4]. More systematic studies of glyoxylate and oxalate metabolism in thiamine deficiency are required.

In close analogy to the genetic disorders, pyridoxine deficiency in experimental animals leads to hyperoxaluria and oxalosis, presumably because of the reduced transamination of glyoxylate to glycine [126]. The induction of pyridoxine deficiency in humans also results in a progressive increase in urinary oxalate [127]. In studies in vivo, pyridoxine-deficient rats converted labeled ethanolamine and ethylene glycol to oxalate to a greater extent than normal controls [191]. Surprisingly, these studies and more recent ones [94] did not show greater conversion of [^{14}C]glyoxylate into labeled urinary oxalate in pyridoxine-deficient animals. In liver and kidney homogenates, oxalate synthesis from glycolate was similar in control and pyridoxine-deficient animals. Carbon dioxide production from [^{14}C]glyoxylate was impaired in kidney but not in liver homogenates from pyridoxine-deficient animals [191]. The possibility has been emphasized that some previously described cases of hyperoxaluria represent pyridoxine deficiency. It is interesting that patients with pyridoxine-responsive seizures have no abnormality of oxalate metabolism.

Reduction in oxalate excretion during treatment of patients with primary oxaluria with excess pyridoxine has been noted (Fig. 10-16). The interrelationships of these abnormalities in oxalate metabolism are shown diagrammatically in Fig. 10-1.

Table 10-5 Classification of the hyperoxaluric states

I. Genetic
   A. Primary hyperoxaluria, type I—glycolic aciduria
   B. Primary hyperoxaluria, type II—glyceric aciduria
II. Acquired
   A. Increased ingestion of oxalate
   B. Increased intake of an oxalate precursor
      1 Methoxyflurane
      2 Ethylene glycol
      3 Ascorbic acid
      4 Xylitol
   C. Pyridoxine deficiency
   D. Hyperabsorption of oxalate—enteric hyperoxaluria

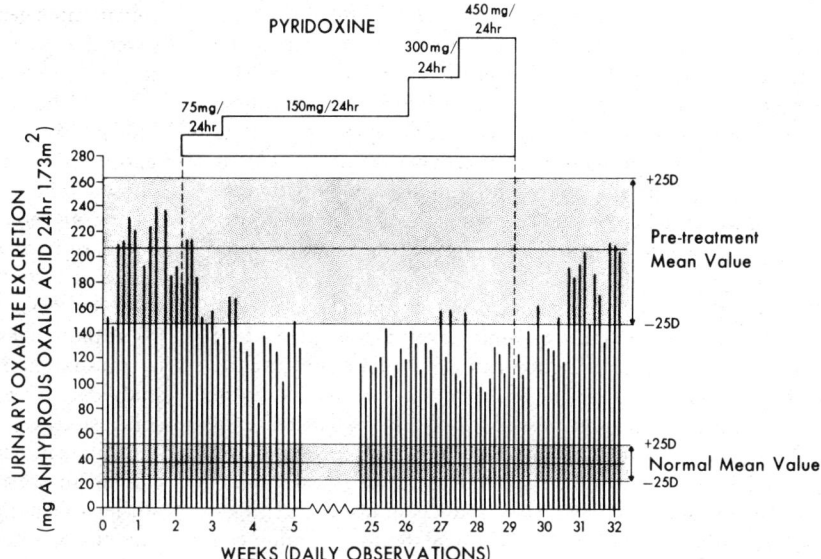

Figure 10-16 The effect of pyridoxine hydrochloride therapy on daily urinary oxalate excretion in a patient with primary hyperoxaluria, type I. *(From Gibbs and Watts [192], with permission of the authors and publisher.)*

Hyperoxaluria and deposits of oxalate in the kidney have recently been found to occur after administration of the anesthetic agent methoxyflurane [193–198]. This 2-carbon fluorinated compound is presumably converted in vivo to oxalate, which is then both excreted in excess in the urine and deposited in the renal parenchyma, leading to transient renal failure. We observed a patient with extensive burns who received small doses of methoxyflurane periodically during wound debridement [199]. Renal failure gradually developed, oxalate crystals appeared in the urine, and hyperoxaluria in excess of 250 mg/24 h occurred. Urinary oxalate eventually returned to normal levels over a 2-week period after discontinuation of the drug.

An interesting hyperoxaluric syndrome has been defined in a group of patients with a variety of malabsorptive states [200–203]. The syndrome was originally recognized in patients with ileal resection of greater than 50 cm. The recurrent calcium oxalate nephrolithiasis that developed in these patients soon after surgery was related to marked hyperoxaluria in the absence of glycolic or glyceric aciduria. The syndrome has been recognized in patients with significant fat malabsorption secondary to a variety of chronic gastrointestinal disorders, i.e., chronic inflammatory bowel disease, chronic pancreatic and biliary tract diseases, bacterial overgrowth syndrome, and after jejunoileal bypass procedures. Hyperoxaluria in these patients usually ranges from 100 to 300 mg/24 h.

Patients with this syndrome hyperabsorb dietary oxalate [204, 205]. Most patients absorbed more than 40 percent of an orally administered dose of isotopic oxalate, compared with a mean of 12 percent in normal subjects (Fig. 10-17) [81]. This degree of hyperabsorption and the amount of oxalate excreted in the urine appear to be proportional to the degree of fat malabsorption [81, 206–209]. Control of the fat malabsorption by dietary administration of medium-chain triglycerides, reduction of dietary oxalate, and administration of oral calcium supplements reduce oxalate excretion to normal levels in these patients [210–213]. These findings have suggested the following hypothesis to explain the oxalate hyperabsorption and hyperoxaluria in these patients: Oxalate and fatty acids in the lumen of the small intestine compete for intraluminal cal-

cium ions. In the presence of normal fat absorption and adequate intraluminal calcium, most oxalate in the intestine exists as the insoluble and relatively nonabsorbable calcium salt. This accounts for the very small amount of oral oxalate absorbed in normal subjects. In the presence of significant fat malabsorption, the intraluminal fatty acid concentration increases dramatically, binding calcium to form calcium-fatty acid soaps and lowering the concentration of intraluminal free calcium ions. This leaves more oxalate in solution as the sodium salt, which has been shown to be freely diffusible across the gastrointestinal wall [85], enabling hyperabsorption of oxalate. This hypothesis is supported by studies in vitro of oxalate solubility in the presence of fatty acids [214] and by the previously cited studies in vivo, in which luminal concentrations of fatty acids, oxalate, and calcium were altered in patients with the syndrome.

A number of studies have emphasized the role of the colon in the hyperabsorption of oxalate in the enteric hyperoxaluria

Figure 10-17 Absorption of [^{14}C]oxalate from the gastrointestinal tract in normal subjects with enteric hyperoxaluria after ileal resection (minimal ≤ 50 cm, extensive ≥ 100 cm). *(From Earnest et al. [81], with permission of the publisher.)*

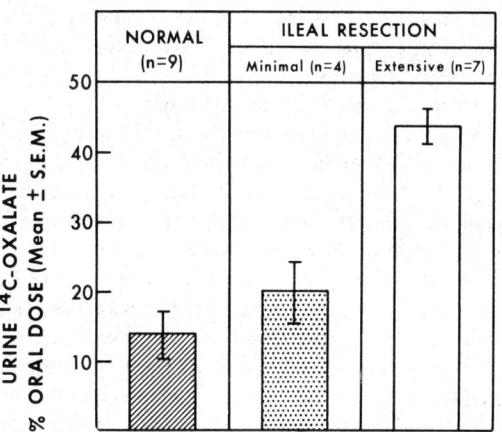

syndrome [84, 215]. The finding that certain bile acids and fatty acids may stimulate the transport of oxalate across the colonic mucosa [85–89, 216], and the finding that cholestyramine administration may decrease the hyperoxaluria in these patients, have emphasized increased colonic uptake of oxalate as an important mechanism in the hyperoxaluria [216]. It seems likely that both increased intraluminal solubility of oxalate and increased colonic absorption of oxalate play varying roles in the hyperoxaluria of patients with the enteric hyperoxaluria syndrome [217].

Most patients with recurrent calcium oxalate stone disease do not have hyperoxaluria. Some investigators [218–220] have reported higher excretion rates of oxalate (but usually within the normal range) in recurrent stone formers than in normal subjects. It is quite possible that such small increases in oxalate excretion could be important in the pathogenesis of the stone disease in view of the major effect of oxalate concentration on calcium oxalate activity products in urine [221]. Perhaps relatively minimal increases in oxalate concentration can lead to periods of oxalate crystalluria and eventual crystal growth and stone formation. If such a mechanism is operative, then reduction of oxalate excretion could play a major role in the treatment of idiopathic stone disease.

Oxalosis in the absence of hyperoxaluria has been observed in a number of patients given large doses of xylitol by intravenous infusion [222]. In some of these patients, massive deposits of calcium oxalate have been found in the kidneys and central nervous system. It has been hypothesized that the xylitol is metabolized to active glycoaldehyde and then to glycolic acid, leading to hyperglycolic aciduria [223]. The mechanism for the massive tissue oxalate deposition remains unknown. The studies of Hauschildt and Watts do not support the concept that xylitol is a precursor of urinary oxalate [224, 225].

INHERITANCE

On the basis of a number of family studies, type I primary hyperoxaluria appears to be inherited as an autosomal recessive character. In at least 16 families, hyperoxaluria has been documented in two or more sibs without evidence of the disease in their parents [3]. The incidence of consanguine marriages is ten- to twentyfold that found in the general population. In 13 families in which the disease was present, 30 sibs had hyperoxaluria and 29 had no evidence of the disease [3]. This deviation in the expected ratio of 1:3 in recessive transmission is probably related to bias in case selection.

The heterozygous state cannot be determined in type I primary hyperoxaluria. In nearly all instances in which it has been studied, urinary oxalate excretion has been normal in parents of patients with the disease [3]. Studies of α-ketoglutarate:glyoxylate carboligase activity have not been reported in presumed heterozygotes for type I primary hyperoxaluria.

Although an autosomal recessive mode of inheritance seems most likely in this disorder, dominant inheritance has been suggested by some studies. This suggestion is based on the noted 1:1 ratio of sib involvement and by the occasionally modestly increased oxalate excretion in parents of patients with the disorder [226–228]. In at least four instances hyperoxaluria has been detected in successive generations, and in one family, possibly in three generations [226–229]. These findings have suggested possible genetic heterogeneity in primary hyperoxaluria.

The inheritance pattern of type II primary hyperoxaluria is difficult to determine because of the small number of cases reported. The disease has been found in three sibs (both sexes) whose parents did not show increased excretion of either oxalic or glyceric acids. Leukocyte D-glyceric dehydrogenase studies of two parents have demonstrated a definite reduction in enzyme activity in the mother's leukocytes; enzyme activity in the leukocytes of the father was at the lower range of normal [5]. Although it seems likely that type II primary hyperoxaluria is transmitted as an autosomal recessive character, further study of a large series of patients is necessary before definite conclusions can be reached.

Oxalate is a component of nearly two-thirds of all renal calculi but the vast majority of patients with recurrent stones do not have hyperoxaluria [230]. A diurnal variation in oxalate excretion has been reported to be more evident in patients with renal calculi than in normal subjects [231]. Since normal urine is often supersaturated with calcium oxalate, it is not surprising that oxalate stone disease is so common. In an extensive study of familial calcium oxalate stone disease, Resnick et al. found higher frequencies of renal calculi among 625 parents and sibs of 106 subjects with recurrent calcium oxalate stones when compared with corresponding relatives of spouses of the propositi [232]. Analysis of the data ruled out monogenic inheritance, but the findings were compatible with inheritance by a polygenic system, with a lesser risk for females. One implication of these data suggested by Resnick et al. is that no single biochemical variable will be found that will account for a calcium oxalate stone diathesis.

TREATMENT

Because of the progressive renal failure that eventually develops in most patients with primary hyperoxaluria, early diagnosis is essential if therapeutic measures are to prevent early demise. The major approaches to therapy have been directed either toward reduction in oxalate synthesis and excretion or toward prevention of calcium oxalate stone formation at a given level of urinary oxalate. Both methods have apparently met with some success, but long-term studies are necessary to evaluate fully the effects of any therapeutic program.

A number of attempts to reduce oxalate synthesis and excretion have been undertaken, with variable degrees of success. Reduction of the availability of glycine, a major precursor of oxalate, by dietary protein restriction or by trapping glycine as hippurate with benzoate has been attempted [9, 90]. Because of the extremely high turnover rate and low fractional conversion of glycine to oxalate, protein restriction has not met with success. Trapping of glycine with benzoate may reduce oxalate excretion modestly, but this effect has been temporary and, therefore, not useful for long-term treatment [233]. Although D-amino acids might competitively inhibit the oxidation of glycine to glyoxylate, large oral doses of D,L-glutamate and D,L-histidine have failed to reduce urinary oxalate levels in patients with primary hyperoxaluria [234].

Because hyperoxaluria has been observed to accompany

pyridoxine deficiency, several attempts have been made to utilize this vitamin in the treatment of primary hyperoxaluria. In experimental animals pyridoxine administration may increase the transamination of glyoxylate to glycine, presumably by inducing synthesis of the transaminase apoenzyme or inhibiting its catabolism [235]. The administration of pyridoxine to normal subjects and mentally deficient patients without hyperoxaluria has been reported to reduce urinary oxalate excretion [234, 189]. Thiamine administration did not affect oxalate excretion in three patients with primary hyperoxaluria [236].

Studies by Smith and Williams [234] and by Gibbs and Watts [192, 236] have demonstrated a definite decrease in the excretion of urinary oxalate in patients with primary hyperoxaluria given large doses of pyridoxine (Fig. 10-15). A similar finding has been reported by Giertz in a single hyperoxaluric subject given 400 mg/day of pyridoxine [237]. This promising approach should receive more extensive evaluation with larger numbers of patients.

The use of aldehyde dehydrogenase inhibitors to reduce oxalate synthesis and excretion was introduced by Solomons and coworkers in 1967 [169]. These investigators reported a significant reduction in urinary oxalate with calcium carbimide in a 12-year-old patient with primary hyperoxaluria undergoing renal transplantation. These authors subsequently commented on the successful use of this drug in two other patients and postulated that the effect on oxalate synthesis was due to inhibition of glycol aldehyde conversion to glycolate [238]. Zarembski and coworkers [239] were unable to demonstrate a consistent reduction in urinary oxalate in three hyperoxaluric subjects treated with calcium carbimide. Other workers have also failed to confirm the effectiveness of aldehyde dehydrogenase inhibitors in reducing oxalate excretion in primary hyperoxaluria [240]. Gibbs and Watts [241] found no effect of disulfiram on oxalate excretion in a single patient when the drug was given alone or in combination with allopurinol. Similarly, in studies in vitro disulfiram did not inhibit the oxidation of glyoxylate to oxalate in human erythrocytes [154], the supernatant fraction of human liver [241], or the supernatant and particulate fractions of liver obtained from a patient with primary hyperoxaluria [241]. In our opinion, the usefulness of aldehyde dehydrogenase inhibitors in the treatment of primary hyperoxaluria has not been established. The report of a 40 percent reduction in oxalate excretion in a single hyperoxaluric subject with the monamine oxidase inhibitor isocarboxazide [171] has not been confirmed in other studies [236], and isocarboxazide did not inhibit oxalate synthesis in vivo in rats [118].

A similar approach to the treatment of primary hyperoxaluria has been the inhibition of glyoxylate oxidation to oxalate, analogous to the inhibition of uric acid synthesis from xanthine and hypoxanthine with allopurinol. As mentioned previously, the oxidation of glyoxylate to oxalate is catalyzed by three enzymes: glycolic acid oxidase, xanthine oxidase, and lactic dehydrogenase. Oxalate excretion is not affected by allopurinol, nor is oxalate excretion increased in patients with hereditary xanthinuria [110, 242].

Several compounds inhibit the oxidation in vitro of glyoxylate to oxalate by glycolic acid oxidase. The most active are hydroxymethanesulfonic acid and hydroxymethanesulfinic acid [243, 244]. Inhibition of oxalate synthesis from glyoxylate in human liver particulate and supernatant fractions with the former compound has been reported by Gibbs and Watts [241]. In erythrocyte hemolysates the synthesis of oxalate from glyoxylate can be inhibited by oxamate [117]. Since this compound is a potent inhibitor of lactic dehydrogenase, the inhibition of oxalate synthesis in this system is probably related to the effect of oxamate on lactic dehydrogenase rather than glycolic acid oxidase. In addition, a number of other analogues of oxalate are potent inhibitors of lactic dehydrogenase–catalyzed oxalate synthesis [117]. Oxalatehydrazide and oxamatehydrazide have been shown to inhibit oxalate synthesis in vivo in the rat. Diminished oxidation of glyoxylate to oxalate by a partially purified glycolic acid oxidase preparation from rat liver and human erythrocytes has been observed with hydroxymethanesulfonic acid [117]. Attempts to demonstrate reduction of urinary oxalate in laboratory animals with the use of this compound in vivo have not been successful [244]. Sodiumhydroxybutanesulfonate did not reduce urinary oxalate excretion in monkeys [236]. Oral administration of tris-hydroxymethylaminomethane (THAM) to two normal subjects and one patient with primary hyperoxaluria failed to alter significantly urinary oxalate excretion [245], in spite of the effectiveness of this compound as an inhibitor of glycolic acid oxidase in vitro [246]. Recently, n-heptanoate and phenyllactate, inhibitors of glycolic acid oxidase in vitro, have been shown to reduce oxalate synthesis in the perfused rat liver, and the latter compound reduced oxalate synthesis from ethylene glycol in the rat in vivo [247]. No evident reduction of urinary oxalate excretion could be demonstrated in two patients with phenylketonuria and excessive phenyllactate excretion [248], although more recently oxalate excretion has been reported to be low in patients with phenylketonuria [96]. The use of agents that inhibit oxalate synthesis would be a logical method for the treatment of patients with primary hyperoxaluria as well as of other patients with recurrent idiopathic calcium oxalate nephrolithiasis. Further studies of their effectiveness in vivo and their possible toxicity are necessary in order to establish the usefulness of this pharmacologic approach.

A second approach to the treatment of hyperoxaluria has been directed toward reducing the tendency to calcium oxalate stone formation at any given level of urinary oxalate concentration. As with other causes of recurrent nephrolithiasis, maintenance of large urine volumes is important. Because urinary calcium is little affected by wide variations in dietary calcium and because urinary oxalate may increase somewhat with calcium restriction, alterations in dietary calcium should not be carried out in these patients [249–251]. Several studies have emphasized the inhibitory effect of various metal ions, particularly magnesium, on kidney stone formation. Lyon and coworkers [252, 253] found inhibition of calcium oxalate stone formation in rats made hyperoxaluric by pyridoxine deficiency with the use of magnesium supplements, although occasional magnesium acid phosphate stones were found in the bladder of animals on the high magnesium intake. Gershoff and Prien [254] have reported the successful use of daily magnesium oxide and pyridoxine in patients with recurrent calcium oxalate nephrolithiasis. No recurrence of stones was found in 30 to 36 patients for periods of up to 5 years, and urine obtained from treated subjects had an increased capacity to maintain calcium oxalate in solution. Magnesium oxide therapy has also been reported to be beneficial in a small number of patients with both types of primary hyperoxaluria [255, 256].

Several studies have emphasized the usefulness of a high phosphate intake in the treatment of recurrent calcium oxalate stone disease [257–259]. This therapeutic program has been supported by the demonstration that oral administration of orthophosphate to patients with recurrent kidney stone disease inhibits the ability of their urine to mineralize rachitic rat cartilage. Although the mechanism of this inhibition has not been clearly established, factors such as reduction of urinary calcium, increase in urinary pyrophosphate, and increase in certain protective polypeptides may play a role. The supplementary phosphate program has seemed to reduce new stone formation in the series of patients with this serious disorder who have been followed up by us for the past several years, and Smith et al. [260] have reported similar success in seven patients with primary hyperoxaluria. Reports of the effectiveness of tyrosine [261] in lowering urinary oxalate require further study and confirmation in patients with primary hyperoxaluria before it can be recommended.

Succinimide has recently been reported to reduce oxaluria in the rat treated with ethylene glycol [262] and in patients with hyperoxaluria [263, 264]. Watts and coworkers were not, however, able to demonstrate a significant decrease in oxalate or glycolate excretion in three patients with primary hyperoxaluria type I [236]. The presumed mechanism for an effect of succinimide on oxalate excretion and the confirmation of a definite effect in hyperoxaluric subjects require further study.

Finally, renal transplantation has been used in the treatment of several uremic patients with primary hyperoxaluria. Several reports have recorded lack of success with this procedure, apparently related to the rapid reaccumulation of oxalate crystals in the transplanted kidney [265–274]. Three other patients with primary hyperoxaluria known to us died shortly after renal transplantation. Although most reported patients with hyperoxaluria who have undergone renal transplantation have not survived more than 18 months, a few cases of primary hyperoxaluria have been reported in whom good renal function was maintained 24 months or more after transplantation [271–273]. Until successful methods for inhibition of oxalate synthesis become available, renal homotransplantation from a surviving donor does not seem indicated in primary hyperoxaluria. Chronic hemodialysis has now been attempted in several patients with primary hyperoxaluria [36, 275–278]. Although good control of uremia has been achieved, oxalosis has continued unabated with continued deposits of calcium oxalate crystals in peripheral nerves, bones, myocardium, and the walls of small superficial skin vessels, often leading to ischemic infarcts of subcutaneous tissue in the extremities. Although oxalate is easily dialyzable, neither hemodialysis nor peritoneal dialysis [276] removes sufficient oxalate to keep up with production rates in vivo.

Many of the studies referred to in this chapter were supported by Research Grant GM-19527 from the Public Health Service.

REFERENCES

1. ARCHER HE, DORMER AE, SCOWEN EF, WATTS RWE: Primary hyperoxaluria. Lancet 2:320, 1957
2. WYNGAARDEN JB, ELDER TD: Primary hyperoxaluria and oxalosis, in Stanbury JR, Wyngaarden JB, Fredrickson DS (eds): The Metabolic Basis of Inherited Disease, ed 2. New York, McGraw-Hill Book Co, 1966
3. HOCKADAY, TDR, CLAYTON, JE, FREDERICK EW, SMITH IH, JR: Primary hyperoxaluria. Medicine, 43:315, 1964
4. WILLIAMS HE, SMITH, LH, JR: Disorders of oxalate metabolism. Am J Med 45:715, 1968
5. WILLIAMS HE, SMITH LH, JR: L-Glyceric aciduria: A new genetic variant of primary oxaluria. N Engl J Med 278:233, 1968
6. DONNÉ MA: Tableau de differents dépôts de matières salines et de substance organiées qui se font dans les urines, presentant les caractères propre à les distinguer entre eux et à reconnaitre leure nature. CR Acad Sci [D] (Paris) 6:419, 1838
7. WOLLASTON WH: On cystic oxide, a new species of urinary calculus. Phil Trans (Lond) 100:223, 1810
8. LEPOUTRE C: Calculs multiples chez un enfant. Infiltration due parenchyme rénal par des cristaux. J Urol 20:424, 1925
9. DANIELS RA, MICHELS R, AISEN P, GOLDSTEIN G: Familial hyperoxaluria. Am J Med 29:820, 1960
10. DAVIS JS, KLINGBERG WG, STOWELL RE: Nephrolithiasis and nephrocalcinosis with calcium oxalate crystals in kidneys and bones. J Pediatr 36:323, 1950
11. NEWNS GH, BLACK JA: A case of calcium oxalate nephrocalcinosis. Great Ormond St J 5:40, 1953
12. APONTE GE, FETTER TR: Familial idiopathic oxalate nephrocalcinosis. Am J Clin Pathol 24:1363, 1954
13. COCHRAN M, HODGKINSON A, ZAREMBSKI PM, ANDERSON CK: Hyperoxaluria in adults. Br J Surg 55:121, 1968
14. ZAREMBSKI PM, HODGKINSON A, COCHRAN M: Urinary excretion of lactic acid and other organic acids in patients with primary hyperoxaluria, in Hodgkinson A, Nordin BEC (eds): Renal Stone Research Symposium. London, Churchill, Livingstone, Ltd, 1969, p 319
15. HELIN I: Primary hyperoxaluria An analysis of 17 scandanavian patients. Scand J Urol Nephrol 14:61, 1980
16. HOLMGREN G, HORNSTROM T, JOHANSSON S, SAMUELSON G: Primary hyperoxaluria (glycolic acid variant): A clinical and genetical investigation of eight cases. UPS J Med Sci 83:65, 1978
17. McLAURIN AW, BEISEL WR, McCORMICK GJ, SCALETTAR R, HERMAN RH: Primary hyperoxaluria. Ann Intern Med 55:70, 1961
18. SMITH LH, JR: Unpublished cases.
19. ANTOINE B, SLAMA R, JOSSO F, DE MONTERA H, HABIB R, RICHET G: La déstruction du parenchyme rénal par envahissement de cristau d'oxalates de calcium: Deux nouvelles observations d'oxalose rénale. Presse Méd 68:803, 1960
20. STAUFFER M: Oxalosis: Report of a case, with a review of the literature and discussion of the pathogenesis. N Engl J Med 263:386, 1960
21. WEST RR, SALYER WR, HUTCHINS GM: Adult-onset primary oxalosis with complete heart block. Johns Hopkins Med J 133:195, 1973
22. COLTART DJ, HUDSON REB: Primary oxalosis of the heart: A cause of heart block. Br Heart J 33:315, 1971
23. PIKULA B, PLAMENAC P, ĆURČIĆ B, NIKULIN A: Myocarditis caused by primary oxalosis in a 4-year-old child. Virchows Arch [Pathol Anat] 358:99, 1973
24. ARBUS GS, SNIDERMAN S: Oxalosis with peripheral gangrene. Arch Pathol 97:107, 1974
25. WILLIAMS HE, SMITH LH, JR: L-Glyceric aciduria, in Hodgkinson A, Nordin BEC (eds): Renal Stone Research Symposium. London, Churchill Livingstone, Ltd, 1969, p 309
26. BURI, J-F: l'Oxalose, Helvet Paediatr Acta 17, (suppl) 11:1, 1962
27. BULLOCK JD, ALBERT DM, SKINNER HCW, MILLER WH, GALLA JE: Calcium oxalate retinopathy associated with generalized oxalosis: X-ray diffraction and electron microscopic studies of crystal deposits. Invest Ophthalmol 13:256, 1974
28. CAINE R, ALBERT DM, LAHAV M, BULLOCK J: Oxalate retinopathy: An experimental model of a flecked retina. Invest Ophthalmol 14:359, 1975
29. TOUSSAINT D, VEREERSTRAETEN P, GOFFIN P, VANLANDUYT P, JEDWAB J, LEGRAND JM: Primary hyperoxaluria. Clinical, histological and crystallographic study of the ocular lesions. Arch Ophtalmol (Paris) 36:97, 1976
30. SCOWEN EF, STANSFIELD AG, WATTS RWE: Oxalosis and primary hyperoxaluria. J Pathol Bact 77:195, 1959
31. HAQQANI MT: Crystals in brain and meninges in primary hyperoxaluria and oxalosis. J Clin Pathol 30:16, 1977
32. DUNN HG: Oxalosis: Report of a case with review of the literature. Am J Dis Child 90:58, 1955
33. MATHEWS M, STAUFFER M, CAMERON EC, MALONEY N, SHERRARD DJ: Bone biopsy to diagnose hyperoxaluria in patients with renal failure. Ann Intern Med 90:777, 1979
34. GHERARDI G, POGGI A, SISCA S, CALDERARO V, BONUCCI E: Bone oxalosis and renal osteodystrophy. Arch Pathol Lab Med 104:105, 1980
35. GODWIN JT, FOWLER MF, DEMPSEY EF, HENNEMAN PH: Primary hyperoxaluria and oxalosis: Report of a case and review of the literature. N Engl J Med 259:1099, 1958
36. BOQUIST L, LINDQVIST B, OSTBERG Y, STEEN L: Primary oxalosis. Am J Med 54:673, 1973
37. CHISHOLM GD, HEARD BE: Oxalosis. Br J Surg 50:78, 1962

38. BURKE EC BAGGENSTOSS AH, OWEN CA, JR, POWER MH, LOHR OW: Oxalosis. *Pediatrics* 15:383, 1955

39. NEUSTEIN HR, STEVENSON SS, KRAINER L: Oxalosis with renal calcinosis due to calcium oxalate. *J Pediatr* 47:624, 1955

40. HALL EG, SCOWEN EF, WATTS RWE: Clinical manifestations of primary hyperoxaluria. *Arch Dis Child* 35:108, 1960

41. MOORHEAD PJ, COOPER DJ, TIMPERLEY WR: Progressive peripheral neuropathy in patient with primary hyperoxaluria. *Br Med J* 2:312, 1975

42. BILBAO JM, BERRY H, MAROTTA J, ROSS RC: Peripheral neuropathy in oxalosis. A case report with electron microscopic observations. *Can J Neurol Sci* 3:63, 1976

43. MOORHEAD PM, COOPER DM, TIMPERLEY WR: Progressive peripheral neuropathy in patient with primary hyperoxaluria. *Br Med J* 2:312, 1975

44. HALL BM, WALSH JC, HORVATH JS, LYTTON DG: Peripheral neuropathy complicating primary hyperoxaluria. *J Neurol Sci* 29:343, 1976

45. EDWARDS DL.: Idiopathic familial oxalosis. *Arch Pathol* 64:546, 1957

46. JOHNSON F.: A method for demonstrating calcium oxalate in tissue sections. *J Histochem Cytochem* 4:404, 1956

47. MARSHALL VF, HORWITH M.: Oxalosis. *J Urol* 82:278, 1959

48. HOCKADAY TDR, FREDERICK EW, CLAYTON JE, SMITH LH, JR: Studies on primary hyperoxaluria. II. Urinary oxalate, glycolate, and glyoxylate measurement by isotope dilution method. *J Lab Clin Med* 65:677, 1965

49. GIBBS DA, WATTS RWE.: The variation of urinary oxalate excretion with age. *J Lab Clin Med* 73:901, 1969

50. MERZ W, MAUGERI S: Uber das Vorkommen und die Bestimmung der Oxalsäure im Blut. *Hoppe-Seyler Z Physiol Chem* 201:31, 1931

51. BARBER HH, GALLIMORE EJ: The metabolism of oxalic acid in the animal body. *Biochem J* 34:144, 1940

52. CRAWHALL JC, WATTS RWE: The oxalate content of human plasma. *Clin Sci* 20:357, 1961

53. ZAREMBSKI PM, HODGKINSON A: The renal clearance of oxalic acid in normal subjects and in patients with primary hyperoxaluria. *Invest Urol* 1:87, 1963

54. ZAREMBSKI PM, HODGKINSON A: Fluorimetric determination of oxalic acid in blood and other biological material *Biochem J* 96:717, 1965

55. HODGKINSON A: Determination of oxalic acid in biological material. *Clin Chem* 16:547, 1970

56. WILLIAMS HE, JOHNSON GA, SMITH LH, JR: The renal clearance of oxalate in normal subjects and patients with primary hyperoxaluria. *Clin Sci* 41:219, 1971

57. HODGKINSON A, WILKINSON R, NORDIN BEC: The concentration of oxalic acid in human blood, in Cifuentes Delatte L, Rapaldo A, Hodgkinson A (eds): *Urinary Calculi: Recent Advances in Aetiology, Stone Structure and Treatment.* Basel, S Karger, 1973, pp 18-23

58. CONSTABLE AR, JOEKES AM, KASIDAS GP, O'REGAN P, ROSE GA: Plasma level and renal clearance of oxalate in normal subjects and in patients with primary hyperoxaluria or chronic renal failure or both. *Clin Sci Mol Med* 56:299, 1979

59. AKCAY T, ROSE G, ALAN: The real and apparent plasma oxalate. *Clin Chim Acta* 101:305, 1980

59a. ELDER TD, WYNGAARDEN JB: The biosynthesis and turnover of oxalate in normal and hyperoxaluric subjects. *J Clin Invest* 39:1337, 1960

60. RUSSELL JC, CHAMBERS M: A specific assay for plasma oxalate. *Clin Biochem* 6:22, 1973

61. NIEDERWIESER A, MATASOVIC A, LEUMANN EP: Glycolic acid in urine. A colorimetric method with values in normal adult controls and in patients with primary hyperoxaluria. *Clin Chim Acta* 89:13, 1978

62. WILLIAMS HE, SMITH LH, JR: Identification and determination of glyceric acid in human urine. *J Lab Clin Med* 71:495, 1968

63. WILLIAMS HE, JOHNSON G, MORRIS RC: To be published.

64. BENNINGTON JL, HABER SL, SMITH JV, WARNER NE: Crystals of calcium oxalate in the human kidney: Studies by means of electronmicroprobe and X-ray diffraction. *Am J Clin Pathol* 41:8, 1964

65. FANGER H, ESPARZA A: Crystals of calcium oxalate in the kidney in uremia. *Am J Clin Pathol* 41:597, 1964

66. BENNETT B, ROSENBLUM C: Calcium oxalate crystals in the myocardium in uremic patients. *Lab Invest* 10:947, 1961

67. GROSS S: Granulomatous thyroiditis with anisotropic crystalline material. *Arch Pathol* 59:412, 1955

68. COGAN DG, KUWABARA T, SILBERT J, KERN H, MCMURRARY V, HURLBERT C: Calcium oxalate and calcium phosphate crystals in detached retinas. *Arch Opthalmol* 60:366, 1958

69. GLYNN LE: Crystalline bodies in tunica media of middle cerebral artery. *J Pathol Bact* 51:445, 1940

70. SALYER WR, KEREN D: Oxalosis as a complication of chronic renal failure. *Kidney Int* 4:61, 1973

71. NOVOA WB, WINER AD, GLAID AJ, SCHWERT GW: Lactic dehydrogenase. V. Inhibition by oxamate and by oxalate. *J Biol Chem* 234:1143, 1959

72. VERMEULEN CW, LYON ES: Mechanisms of genesis and growth of calculi. *Am J Med* 45:684, 1968

73. ELLIOT JS, EUSEBIO E: Calcium oxalate solubility: The effect of trace metals. *Invest Urol* 4:428, 1967

74. MACLAGAN NF, ANDERSON AJ: Some observations on urinary colloids in relation to urinary calculi. *Br J Urol* 30:269, 1958

75. HOWARD JE, THOMAS WC, JR: Control of crystallization in urine. *Am J Med* 45:693, 1968

76. JAKOBY WB: Oxalate decarboxylation: Oxalate → formate + CO_2, in Colowick SP, Kaplan NO (eds): *Methods in Enzymology*, vol 5, *Preparation and Assay of Enzymes*. New York, Academic Press, Inc, 1962, p 637

77. PRIEN EL, PRIEN EL JR: Composition and structure of urinary stone. *Am J Med* 45:654, 1968

78. ZAREMBSKI PM, HODGKINSON A: The oxalic acid content of English diets. *Br J Nutr* 16:627, 1962

79. ARCHER HE, DORMER AE, SCOWEN EF, WATTS RWE: Studies on the urinary excretion of oxalate by normal subjects. *Clin Sci* 16:405, 1957

80. ZAREMBKSI PM, HODGKINSON A: The determination of oxalic acid in food. *Analyst* 87:698, 1962

81. EARNEST DL, JOHNSON G, WILLIAMS HE, ADMIRAND WH: Hyperoxaluria in patients with ileal resection: An abnormality in dietary oxalate absorption. *Gastroenterology* 66:1114, 1974

82. CHADWICK VS, MODHA K, DOWLING RH: Mechanism for hyperoxaluria in patients with ileal dysfunction. *N Engl J Med* 289:172, 1973

83. EARNEST D, WILLIAMS HE: Unpublished observations

84. DOBBINS JW, BINDER HJ: Importance of the colon in enteric hyperoxaluria. *N Engl J Med* 296:298, 1977

85. BINDER, HJ: Intestinal oxalate absorption. *Gastroenterology* 67:441, 1974

86. SCHWARTZ SE, STAUFFER JO, BURGESS LW, CHENEY M: Oxalate uptake by everted sacs of rat colon. Regional differences and the effects of Ph and ricinoleic acid. *Biochim Biophys Acta* 593:404, 1980

87. CASPARY WF: Intestinal oxalate absorption. I. Absorption in vitro. *Res Exp Med (Berlin)* 171:13, 1977

88. DOBBINS JW, BINDER HJ: Effect of bile salts and fatty acids on the colon absorption of oxalate. *Gastroenterology* 70:1096, 1976

89. FAIRCLOUGH PD, FEEST TG, CHADWICK VS, CLARK ML: Effect of sodium chenodeoxycholate on oxalate absorption from the excluded human colon—a mechanism for 'enteric' hyperoxaluria. *Gut* 18:240, 1977

90. ARCHER, HE, DORMER AE, SCOWEN EF, WATTS RWE: The aetiology of primary hyperoxaluria. *Br Med J* 1:175, 1958

91. KORNBERG HL, ELSDEN SR: The metabolism of 2-carbon compounds by microorganisms, in Nord FF (ed): *Advances in Enzymology*. New York, Interscience, 1961, p 401

92. LIAO LL, RICHARDSON KE: The metabolism of oxalate precursors in isolated perfused rat livers. *Arch Biochem Biophys* 153:438, 1972

93. MADSEN NB: Test for isocitritase and malate synthetase in animal tissues. *Biochim Biophys Acta* 27:199, 1958

94. FARAGALLA FF, GERSHOFF SN: Occurrence of C^{14}-oxalate in rat urine after administration of C^{14}-tryptophane. *Proc Soc Exp Biol Med* 114:602, 1963

95. COOK DA, HENDERSON LM: The formation of oxalic acid from the side chain of aromatic amino acids in the rat. *Biochim Biophys Acta* 184:404, 1969

96. LIAO LL, RICHARDSON KE: The synthesis of oxylate from hydroxypyruvate by isolated perfused rat liver. The mechanism of hyperoxaluria in L-glyceric aciduria. *Biochim Biophys Acta* 538:76, 1978

97. CURTIN CO, KING CG: The metabolism of ascorbic acid-I-^{14}C and oxalic acid-^{14}C in the rat. *J Biol Chem* 216:539, 1955

98. BANAY M, DIMANT E: On the metabolism of L-ascorbic acid in the scorbutic guinea-pig. *Biochim Biophys Acta* 59:313, 1962

99. ART AF, VON SCHUCHING S, ENNS T: L-Ascorbic-l-C^{14} acid catabolism in the rhesus monkey. *Nature (Lond)* 193:1178, 1962

100. HELLMAN L, BURNS JJ: Metabolism of L-ascorbic acid l-^{14}C in man. *J Biol Chem* 230:923, 1958

101. BAKER EM, SAARI JC, TOLBERT BM: Ascorbic acid metabolism in man. *Am J Clin Nutr* 19:371, 1966

102. LAMBDEN MP, CHRYSTOWSKI GA: Urinary oxalate excretion by man following ascorbic acid ingestion. *Proc Soc Exp Biol Med* 85:190, 1954

103. TAKENOUGHI K, ASO K, KAWASE K, ICHIKAWA H, SHIOMI T: On the metabolites of ascorbic acid, especially oxalic acid, eliminated in urine, following the administration of large amounts of ascorbic acid. *J Vitamin (Kyoto)* 12:49, 1966

104. BRIGGS MH, GARCIA-WEBB P, DAVIES P: Urinary oxalate and vitamin-C supplements. *Lancet* 2:201, 1973

105. CLAGETT CO, TOLBERT NE, BURRIS RH: Oxidation of α-hydroxy acids by enzymes from plants. *J Biol Chem* 178:977, 1949

106. KUN E, DECHARY JM, PITOT HC: The oxidation of glycolic acid by a liver enzyme. *J Biol Chem* 210:269, 1954

107. RICHARDSON KE, TOLBERT NE: Oxidation of glyoxylic acid to oxalic acid by glycolic acid oxidase. *J Biol Chem* 236:1280, 1961

108. ENGELMAN K, WATTS RWE, KLINENBERG JR, SJOERDSMA A, SEEGMILLER JE: Clinical, physiological, and biochemical studies of a patient with xanthinuria and pheochromocytoma. *Am J Med* 37:839, 1964

109. BOOTH, VH: The specificity of xanthine oxidase. *Biochem J* 32:494, 1938

110. GIBBS DA, WATTS RWE: An investigation of the possible role of xanthine oxidase in the oxidation of glyoxylate to oxalate. *Clin Sci* 31:285, 1966

111. KRAKOW G, VENNESLAND B: The stereospecificity of glyoxylate reduction in leaves. *Biochem Z* 338:31, 1963

112. SAWAKI S, HATTORI N, YAMADA K: Reduction of nicotinamide adenine dinucleotide by glyoxylate in animal organs. *J Vitamin (Kyoto)* 12:303, 1966

113. BANNER MR, ROSALKI SB. Glyoxylate as a substrate for lactate dehydrogenase. *Nature (Lond)* 213:726, 1967

114. SAWAKI S, HATTORI N, MORIKAWA N, YAMADA K: Oxidation and reduction of glyoxylate by lactate dehydrogenase. *J Vitamin (Kyoto)* 13:93, 1967

115. GIBBS DA: The separation and characterization of the enzymes which oxidize glyoxylate to oxalate in the liver. *Clin Sci* 41:3P, 1971

116. WILLIAMS HE, SMITH LH, JR.: Possible pathogenic mechanism for hyperoxaluria in L-glyceric aciduria. *Science* 171:390, 1971

117. SMITH LH, JR, BAUER RL, CRAIG JC, WILLIAMS HE: Inhibition of oxalate synthesis: In vitro studies using analogues of oxalate and glycolate. *Biochem Med* 6:317, 1972

118. KLEINZELLER A: Oxidation of acetic acid in animal tissues. *Biochem J* 37:674, 1943

119. O'KEEFFE CM, CIES L, SMITH LH, JR: Inhibition of oxalate biosynthesis: In vivo studies in the rat. *Biochem Med* 7:299, 1973

120. CRAWHALL JC, SCOWEN EF, WATTS RWE: Conversion of glycine to oxalate in primary hyperoxaluria. *Lancet* 2:806, 1959

121. DEAN BM, WATTS RWE, WESTWICK WJ: The conversion of [1-^{13}C] glycine and [2-^{13}C] glycine to [^{13}C] oxalate in primary hyperoxaluria: Evidence for the existence of more than one metabolic pathway from glycine to oxalate in man. *Clin Sci* 35:325, 1968

122. WATTS RWE, CRAWHALL JC: The first glycine metabolic pool in man. *Biochem J* 73:277, 1959

123. WILLIAMS HE, EARNEST D, ADMIRAND W: Mechanism of hyperoxaluria in bowel disease, in Cifuentes Delatte L, Rapado A, Hodgkinson A (eds): *Urinary Calculi: Recent Advances in Aetiology, Stone Structure and Treatment.* Basel, S Karger, 1973, pp 41-45

124. RATNER S, NOCITO V, GREEN DE: Glycine oxidase. *J Biol Chem* 152:119, 1944

125. NEIMS AH, HELLERMAN L: Specificity of the D-amino acid oxidase in relation to glycine oxidase activity. *J Biol Chem* 237:976, 1962

126. GERSHOFF SN, FARAGALLA FF, NELSON DA, ANDRUS SB: Vitamin B₆ deficiency and oxalate nephrocalcinosis in the cat. *Am J Med* 27:72, 1959

127. FABER SR, FEITLER WW, BLEILER RE, OHLSON MA, HODGES RE: The effects of an induced pyridoxine and pantothenic acid deficiency on excretions of oxalic and xanthurenic acids in the urine. *Am J Clin Nutr* 12:406, 1963

128. WHITTINGHAM CP, PRITCHARD GG: The production of glycolate during photosynthesis in *Chlorella. Proc R Soc [Biol]* 157:366, 1963

129. SILBERGELD S, CARTER HE: The toxicity of glycolic acid in male and female rats. *Arch Biochem* 84:183, 1959

130. DAFONSECA-WOLLHEIM F, BOCK KW, HOLZER H: Preparation of "active-glycolic aldehyde" [2-1,2-dihydroxyethyl] thiamine pyrophosphate] from hydroxypyruvate and thiamine pyrophosphate with a preparation of pyruvic oxidase from pig-heart muscle. *Biochem Biophys Res Commun* 9:466, 1962

131. HOLZER H, KATTERMAN R, BUSCH D: A thiamine pyrophosphate-glycolaldehyde compound ("active glycolaldehyde") as intermediate in the transketolase reaction. *Biochem Biophys Res Commun* 7:167, 1962

132. CARTER HE, JOHNSON P, TEETS DW, YU RK: Isolation of ethylene glycol from the lipids of beef lung. *Biochem Biophys Res Commun* 13:156, 1963

133. DEKKER EE, MAITRA U: Conversion of γ-hydroxglutamate to glyoxylate and alanine; purification and properties of the enzyme system. *J Biol Chem* 237:2218, 1962

134. HOCKADAY TDR, CLAYTON JE, SMITH LH, JR: The metabolic error in primary hyperoxaluria. *Arch Dis Child* 40:485, 1965

135. PAYES B, LATIES CG: The enzymatic conversion of γ-hydroxy-α-ketoglutarate to malate: A postulated step in the cyclic oxidation of glyoxylate. *Biochem Biophys Res Commun* 13:179, 1963

136. SMITH LH, JR: Unpublished observations

137. CAMMARATA PS, COHEN PP: The scope of the transamination reaction in animal tissues. *J Biol Chem* 187:439, 1950

138. NAKADA HI, WEINHOUSE S: Non-enzymatic transamination with glyoxylic acid and various amino-acids. *J Biol Chem* 204:831, 1953

139. THOMPSON JS, RICHARDSON KE: Isolation and characterization of a glutamate-glycine transaminase from human liver. *Arch Biochem* 117:599, 1966

140. WILLIAMS HE, WILSON KM, SMITH LH, JR: Studies on primary hyperoxaluria. III. Transamination reactions of glyoxylate in human tissue preparations. *J Lab Clin Med* 70:494, 1967

141. ZELITCH I: Oxidation and reduction of glycolic and glyoxylic acids in plants. II. Glyoxylic acid reductase. *J Biol Chem* 201:719, 1953

142. ZELITCH I, GOTTO AM: Properties of a new glyoxylate reductase from leaves. *Biochem J* 84:541, 1962

143. ROMANO M, CERRA M: The action of crystalline lactate dehydrogenase from rabbit muscle on glyoxylate. *Biochim Biophys Acta* 177:421, 1969

144. NAKADA HI, SUND LP: Glyoxylic acid oxidation by rat liver. *J Biol Chem* 233:8, 1958

145. CRAWHALL JC, WATTS RWE: The metabolism of glyoxylate by human and rat liver mitochondria. *Biochem J* 85:163, 1962

146. KAWASAKI H, OKUYAMA M, KIKUCHI G: α-Ketoglutarate-dependent oxidation of glyoxylic acid in rat mitochondria. *J Biochem* 59:419, 1966

147. STEWART PR, QUAYLE JR: The synergistic decarboxylation of glyoxylate and 2-oxoglutarate by an enzyme from mammalian liver. *Biochem J* 98:43p, 1966

148. KOCH J, STOKSTAD ELR, WILLIAMS HE, SMITH LH, JR: Deficiency of 2-oxoglutarate:glyoxylate carboligase activity in primary hyperoxaluria. *Proc Natl Acad Sci USA* 57:1123, 1967

149. O'FALLON JV, BROSEMER RW: Cellular localization of alpha-ketoglutarate:Glyoxylate carboligase in rat tissues. *Biochim Biophys Acta* 499:321, 1977

150. KOCH J, STOKSTAD ELR: Personal communication

151. SMITH LH, JR, BAUER RL, WILLIAMS HE: Oxalate and glycolate synthesis by hemic cell. *J Lab Clin Med* 78:245, 1971

152. WATTS RWE: Oxalate biosynthesis in primary hyperoxaluria, in Cifuentes Delatte L, Rapado A, Hodgkinson A (eds): *Urinary Calculi; Recent Advances in Aetiology, Stone Structure and Treatment.* Basel, S Karger, 1973, pp 13-17

153. ZEWE V, FROMM HJ: Kinetic studies of rabbit muscle lactate dehydrogenase. II. Mechanism of the reaction. *Biochemistry* 4:782, 1965

154. FISHER V, WATTS RWE: The metabolism of glyoxylate in blood from normal subjects and patients with primary hyperoxaluria. *Clin Sci* 34:97, 1968

155. SHIMAZONO H, HAYAISHI O: Enzymatic decarboxylation of oxalic acid. *J Biol Chem* 227:151, 1957

156. QUAYLE JR, KEECH DB, TAYLOR GA: Carbon assimilation by *Pseudomonas oxalaticus* (OX1). 4. Metabolism of oxalate in cell-free extracts of the organism grown on oxalate. *Biochem J* 78:225, 1961

157. WEINHOUSE S, FRIEDMANN B: Metabolism of labeled 2-carbon acids in the intact rat. *J Biol Chem* 191:707, 1951

158. BRUBACHER G, JUST M, BODUR H, BERNHARD K: Zur Biochemie der Oxalsaure. *Z Physiol Chem* 304:173, 1956

159. CATTELL WR, SPENCER G, TAYLOR GW, WATTS RWE: The mechanism of the renal excretion of oxalate in the dog. *Clin Sci* 22:43, 1962

160. OSSWALD H, HAUTMANN R: Renal elimination kinetics and plasma half-life of oxalate in man. *Urol Int* 34:440, 1979

161. PRENEN JA, MEES EJ, BOER P, ENDEMAN HJ, EPHRAIM, KH: Oxalic acid concentration in serum measured by isotopic clearance technique. Experience in hyper- and normooxaluric subjects. *Proc Eur Dial Transplant Assoc* 16:566, 1979

162. WEINMAN EJ, FRANKFURT SJ, INCE A, SANSOM S: Renal tubular transport of organic acids. *J Clin Invest* 61:801, 1978

163. ATKINS GL, DEAN BM, GRIFFIN WJ, SCOWEN EF, WATTS RWE: Quantitative aspects of ascorbic acid metabolism in patients with primary hyperoxaluria. *Clin Sci* 29:305, 1965

164. BUCKLE RM: The glyoxylic acid content of human blood and its relationship to thiamine deficiency. *Clin Sci* 25:207, 1963

165. FREDERICK EW, RABKIN, MT, RICHIE RH, JR, SMITH LH, JR: Studies on primary hyperoxaluria. I. *In vivo* demonstration of a defect in glyoxylate metabolism. *N. Engl J Med* 269:821, 1963

166. CRAWHALL JC, WATTS RWE: The metabolism of [1-^{14}C]-glyoxylate by the liver mitochondria of patients with primary hyperoxaluria and non-hyperoxaluric subjects. *Clin Sci* 23:163, 1962

167. DEAN BM, GRIFFIN WJ, WATTS RWE: Primary hyperoxaluria. *Lancet* 1:406, 1966

168. DEAN BM, WATTS RWE, WESTWICK WJ: Metabolism of [1-^{14}C] glyoxylate, [1-^{14}C] glycollate, [1-^{14}C] glycine, and [2-^{14}C] glycine by homogenates of kidney and liver tissue from hyperoxaluric and control subjects. *Biochem J* 105:701, 1967

169. SOLOMONS CC, GOODMAN SI, RILEY CM: Calcium carbimide in the treatment of primary hyperoxaluria. *N Engl J Med* 276:207, 1967

170. SCRIVER CR, HUTCHINSON JH: The vitamin B₆ deficiency syndrome in human infancy: Biochemical and clinical observations. *Pediatrics* 31:240, 1963

171. BOURKE E, FRINDT G, FLYNN P, SCHREINER GE: Primary hyperoxaluria with normal α-ketoglutarate:glyoxylate carboligase activity. *Ann Int Med* 76:279, 1972

172. DAWKINS PD, DICKENS F: Oxidation of D- and L-glycerate by rat liver. *Biochem J* 94:353, 1965

173. FALLON HJ, HACKNEY EJ, BYRNE WL: Serine biosynthesis in rat liver: Regulation of enzyme concentration by dietary factors. *J Biol Chem* 241:4157, 1966

174. WILLIS JE, SALLACH HJ: Evidence for mammalian D-glyceric dehydrogenase. *J Biol Chem* 237:910, 1962

175. SALLACH HJ: D-Glycerate dehydrogenase of liver and spinach, in Wood WA (ed): *Methods in Enzymology*, vol 9, *Carbohydrate Metabolism*. New York, Academic Press, Inc, 1966, p 221

176. KOHN LD, JAKOBY WB: Hydroxypyruvate reductase (D-gllycerate dehydrogenase; crystalline) *Pseudomonas*, in Wood WA (ed): *Methods in Enzymology*, vol 9, *Carbohydrate Metabolism*. New York, Academic Press, Inc, 1966, p 229

177. CREMONA T, SINGER TP: D-α-Hydroxy acid dehydrogenase, in Wood WA (ed): *Methods in Enzymology*, vol 9, *Carbohydrate Metabolism*. New York, Academic Press, Inc, 1966, p 327

178. ANDERSON SR, FLORINI, JR, VESTLING CS: Rat liver lactate dehydrogenase. III. Kinetics and specificity. *J Biol Chem* 239:2991, 1964

179. CHEUNG GP, COTROPIA JP, SALLACH HJ: Comparative studies of enzymes related to serine metabolism in fetal and adult liver. *Biochim Biophys Acta* 170:334, 1968

180. WALSH DA, SALLACH HJ: Comparative studies on pathways for serine biosynthesis in animal tissues. *J Biol Chem* 24:4068, 1966

181. FALLON HJ, BYRNE WL: Depression of enzyme activity by cortisone: An effect on serine metabolism. *Endocrinology* 80:847, 1967

182. RICHARDSON KE, LIAO, LI: Formation of oxalate from hydroxypyruvate by isolated perfused rat liver. *Fed Proc* 32:565, 1973

183. POHL J: Ueber den oxydativen Abbau der Fettkörper im thierischen Organismus. *Arch Exp Path Pharmkol* 37:413, 1896

184. LYON ES, BORDEN TA, VERMEULEN CW: Experimental oxalate lithiasis produced with ethylene glycol. *Invest Urol* 4:143, 1966

185. PARRY MF, WALLACH R: Ethylene glycol poisoning. *Am J Med* 57:143, 1974

186. FRIEDMAN EA, GREENBERG JB, MERRILL JP, DAMMIN GJ: Consequences of ethylene glycol poisoning. *Am J Med* 32:891, 1962

187. LIANG C: Studies on experimental thiamine deficiency: Trends of keto-acid formation and detection of glyoxylic acid. *Biochem J* 82:429, 1962

188. TAKASAKI E: The urinary excretion of oxalic acid in vitamin B_1 deficient rats. *Invest Urol* 7:150, 1969

189. GERSHOFF SN: Vitamin B_6 and oxalate metabolism. *Vitam Horm (NY)* 22:581, 1964

190. SALYER WR, SALYER DC: Thiamine deficiency and oxalosis. *J Clin Pathol* 27:558, 1974

191. RUNYAN TJ, GERSHOFF SN: The effect of vitamin B_6 deficiency in rats on the metabolism of oxalic acid precursors. *J Biol Chem* 240:1889, 1965

192. GIBBS D, WATTS RWE: The action of pyridoxine in primary hyperoxaluria. *Clin Sci* 38:277, 1970

193. FRASCINO JA, VANAMEE P, ROSEN PP: Renal oxalosis and azotemia after methoxyflurane anesthesia. *N Engl J Med* 283:676, 1970

194. MAZZE RI, COUSINS MJ: Methoxyflurane anesthesia. *Arch Pathol* 92:484, 1971

195. AUFDERHEIDE AC: Renal tubular calcium oxalate crystal deposition: Its possible relation to methoxyflurane anesthesia. *Arch Pathol* 92:162, 1971

196. SILVERBERG DS, McINTYRE WR, ULAN RA, GAIN EA: Oxalic acid excretion after methoxyflurane and halothane anesthesia. *Can Anaesth Soc J* 18:496, 1971

197. BERGSTRAND A, COLLSTE LG, FRANKSSON C, GLAS JE, LÖFSTRÖM B, MAGNUSSON G, NORDENSTAM H, WERNER B: Oxalosis in renal transplants following methoxyflurane anaesthesia. *Br J Anaesth* 44:569, 1972

198. McINTYRE JWR, RUSSELL JC, CHAMBERS M: Oxalemia following methoxyflurane anesthesia in man. *Anesth Analg* 52:946, 1973

199. JENSEN P, WILLIAMS HE: Unpublished observations

200. ADMIRAND W, EARNEST D, WILLIAMS HE: Hyperoxaluria and bowel disease. *Trans Assoc Am Phys* 84:307, 1972

200a. ADMIRAND WH: Hyperoxaluria and bowel disease. *N Engl J Med* 286:1412, 1972

201. SMITH LH, FROMM H, HOFMANN AF: Acquired hyperoxaluria, nephrolithiasis, and intestinal disease: Description of a syndrome. *N Engl J Med* 286:1371, 1972

202. DOWLING, RH, ROSE GA, SUTOR DJ: Hyperoxaluria and renal calculi in ileal disease. *Lancet* 1:1103, 1971

203. EARNEST DL: Enteric hyperoxaluria. *Adv Intern Med* 24:407, 1979

204. CHADWICK VS, MODHA K, DOWLING, RH: Pathogenesis of secondary hyperoxaluria in ileal resection. *Gut* 13:840, 1972

205. STAUFFER JO, HUMPHREYS MH, WEIR GJ: Acquired hyperoxaluria with regional enteritis after ileal resection: Role of dietary oxalate. *Ann Intern Med* 79:383, 1973

206. ANDERSSON H: Letter to the editor: Hyperoxaluria with ileal dysfunction. *N Engl J Med* 290:107. 1974

207. RAMPTON DS, KASIDAS GP, ROSE GA, SARNER M: Oxalate loading test: A screening test for steatorrhoea. *Gut* 20:1089, 1979

208. CASPARY WE, TONISSEN J: Enteric hyperoxaluria. I. Intestinal oxalate absorption in gastrointestinal diseases (Author's translation). *Klin Wochensch* 56:607, 1978

209. ANDERSSON H, FILIPSSON S, HULTEN L: Urinary oxalate excretion related to ileocolic surgery in patients with Crohn's disease. *Scand J Gastroenterol* 12:465, 1978

210. EARNEST D, WILLIAMS HE: Personal communication

211. HOLST, PEDERSEN J, SITTEN J: The effect of calcium on hyperoxaluria following jejunoileal bypass in morbid obesity. *Scand J Gastroenterol* 14:97, 1979

212. CASPARY WE, TONISSEN J, LANKISCH PG: 'Enteral' hyperoxaluria. Effect of cholestyramine, calcium, neomycin, and bile acids on intestinal oxalate absorption in man. *Acta Hepatogastroenterol (Stuttg)* 24:193, 1977

213. STAUFFER JQ: Hyperoxaluria and intestinal disease. The role of steatorrhoea and dietary calcium in regulating intestinal oxalate absorption. *Am J Dig Dis* 22:921, 1977

214. EARNEST D: In preparation

215. MODIGLIANI R, LABAYLE D, AYMES C, DENVIL R: Evidence for excessive absorption of oxalate by the colon in enteric hyperoxaluria. *Scand J Gastroenterol* 13:187, 1978

216. STAUFFER JQ: Hyperoxaluria and calcium oxalate nephrolithiasis after jejunoileal bypass. *Am J Clin Nutr* 30:64, 1977

217. BARILLA DE, NOTZ C, KENNEDY D, PAK CY: Renal oxalate excretion following oral oxalate loads in patients with ileal disease and with renal and absorptive hypercalciurias. Effect of calcium and magnesium. *Am J Med* 64:579, 1978

218. MARSHALL RW, COCHRAN M, HODGKINSON A: Relationships between calcium and oxalic acid intake in the diet and their excretion in the urine of normal and renal-stone-forming subjects. *Clin Sci* 43:91, 1972

219. HODGKINSON A: Relations between oxalic acid, calcium, magnesium, and creatinine excretion in normal men and male patients with calcium oxalate kidney stones. *Clin Sci Mol Med* 46:357, 1974

220. MARSHALL RW, BARRY H: Urine saturation and the formation of calcium-containing renal calculi: The effects of various forms of therapy, in Cifuentes Delatte L, Rapado A, Hodgkinson A (eds): *Urinary Calculi: Recent Advances in Aetiology, Stone Structure and Treatment*. Basel, S Karger, 1973, pp 164–169

221. ROBERTSON WG, PEACOCK M, NORDIN BEC: Measurement of activity products in urine from stone-formers and normal subjects, in Finlayson B, Hench LL, Smith LH (eds): *Urolithiasis: Physical Aspects*. Washington, DC, National Academy of Science, 1972

222. SCHRÖDER R, DELACROIX WF, FRANZEN U, KLEIN PJ, MÜLLER, W: Therapiebedingte Form einer reno-cerebralen Oxalose? *Acta Neuropathol (Berl)* 27:181, 1974

223. CHALMERS RA, LAWSON AH, HAUSCHILDT S, WATTS RWE: The urinary excretion of glycolic acid and threonic acid by xylitol-infused patients and their relationship to the possible role of active glycolaldehyde in the transketolase reaction in vivo. *Biochem Soc Trans* 3:518-521, 1975

224. HAUSCHILDT S, WATTS RWE: Studies on the effect of xylitol on oxalate formation. *Biochem Pharmacol* 25:27-29, 1976

225. WATTS RW, HAUSCHILDT S, CHALMERS RA, LAWSON AM: Metabolic investigations during xylitol infusion. *Int J Vit Nutr Res* 15:216, 1975

226. DE TONI G, DURAND P: Observations on two opposite clinical situations: Renal acidosis and alkalosis. *Ann Paediat* 193:257, 1959

227. LAGRUE G, LAUDAT MH, MEYER P, SAPIR M, MILLIEZ P: Oxalose familiale avec acidose hyperchlorémique secondaire. *Sem Hôp Paris* 35:2023, 1959

228. ÕIGAARD H, SÓDERHJELM L, HÓGLUND NJ, WERNER I: Familial oxalosis. II. *Acta Soc Med Upsal* 68:55, 1963

229. SHEPARD TH, II, LEE LW, KREBS EG: Primary hyperoxaluria. II. Genetic studies in a family. *Pediatrics* 25:869, 1960

230. HODGKINSON A, ZAREMBSKI PM: Oxalic acid metabolism in man: A review. *Calcif Tissue Res* 2:115, 1968

231. ZAREMBSKI PM, HODGKINSON A: Some factors influencing the urinary excretion of oxalic acid in man. *Clin Chim Acta* 25:1, 1969

232. RESNICK M, PRIDGEN DB, GOODMAN HO: Genetic predisposition to formation of calcium oxalate renal calculi. *N Engl J Med* 278:1313, 1968

233. SWARTZ D, ISRAELS S: Primary hyperoxaluria. *J Urol* 90:94, 1963

234. SMITH LH, JR, WILLIAMS HE: Treatment of primary hyperoxaluria. *Mod Treat* 4:522, 1967

235. GREENGARD O, GORDON M: The cofactor-mediated regulation of apoenzyme levels in animal tissues. I. The pyridoxine-induced rise of rat liver tyrosine transaminase level *in vivo*. *J Biol Chem* 238:3708, 1963

236. WATTS RW, CHALMERS RA, GIBBS DA, LAWSON AM, PURKISS P, SPELLACY E: Studies on some possible biochemical treatments of primary hyperoxaluria. *QJ Med* 48:259, 1979

237. GIERTZ G: [Hyperoxaluria.] Urologists' Correspondence Club Karolinska Sjukhuset, Stockholm 60, Sweden), Jan. 2, 1970

238. SOLOMONS CC, GOODMAN SI, RILEY CM: Treatment of hyperoxaluria. *N Engl J Med* 277:1425, 1967

239. ZAREMBSKI PM, HODGKINSON A, COCHRAN M: Treatment of primary hyperoxaluria with calcium carbimide. *N Engl J Med* 277:1000, 1967

240. SMITH LH, JONES JD, KEATING FR, JR: Primary hyperoxaluria, in Hodgkinson A, Nordin BEC (eds): *Renal Stone Research Symposium.* London, Churchill Livingstone, Ltd, 1969, p 297

241. GIBBS DA, WATTS RWE: Oxalate formation from glyoxylate in primary hyperoxaluria: Studies on liver tissue. *Clin Sci* 32:351, 1967

242. KING JS, JR, WAINER A: Glyoxylate metabolism in normal and stone-forming humans and the effect of allopurinol therapy. *Proc Soc Exp Biol Med* 128:1162, 1968

243. FREDERICK EW, RABKIN MT, SMITH LH, JR: Primary hyperoxaluria: A defect in glyoxylate metabolism. *J Clin Invest* 41:1358, 1962

244. BAUER R, WILLIAMS HE, SMITH LH, JR: Unpublished observations

245. WILLIAMS HE, SMITH LH, JR: Unpublished observations

246. BAKER AL, TOLBERT NE: Glycolate oxidase (ferredoxin-containing form), in Wood WA (ed): *Methods in Enzymology,* vol 9, *Carbohydrate Metabolism.* New York, Academic Press, Inc, 1966, p 338

247. LIAO LL, RICHARDSON KE: The inhibition of oxalate biosynthesis in isolated perfused rat liver by DL-phenyllactate and N-heptanoate. *Arch Biochem Biophys* 154:68, 1973

248. WILLIAMS HE, SMITH LH, JR: Unpublished observations

249. HODGKINSON A, PYRAH LN: The urinary excretion of calcium and inorganic phosphate in 344 patients with calcium stone of renal origin. *Br J Surg* 46:10 1958

250. NORDIN BEC, BARRY H, BULUSU L, SPEED R: Dietary treatment of recurrent calcium stone disease, in Cifuentes Delatte L, Rapado A, Hodgkinson A (eds): *Urinary Calculi: Recent Advances in Aetiology, Stone Structure and Treatment.* Basel, S Karger, 1973, pp 170–176

251. PEACOCK M, KNOWLES F, NORDIN BEC: Effect of calcium administration and deprivation on serum and urine calcium in stone-forming and control subjects. *Br Med J* 2:729, 1968

252. LYON ES, BORDEN TA, ELLIS JE, VERMEULEN CW: Calcium oxalate lithiasis produced by pyridoxine deficiency and inhibition with high magnesium diets. *Invest Urol* 4:133, 1966

253. BORDEN TA, LYON ES: The effects of magnesium and pH on experimental calcium oxalate stone disease. *Invest Urol* 6:412, 1969

254. GERSHOFF SN, PRIEN EL: Effect of daily MgO and vitamin B_6 administration to patients with recurrent oxalate kidney stones. *Am J Clin Nutr* 20:393, 1967

255. DENT CE, STAMP TCB: Treatment of primary hyperoxaluria. *Arch Dis Child* 45:735, 1970

256. SILVER L, BREUDLER H: Use of magnesium oxide in management of familial hyperoxaluria. *J Urol* 106:274, 1971

257. HOWARD JE, THOMAS WC, JR, MUKAI T, JOHNSTON RA, JR, PASCOE BJ: Calcification of cartilage by urine, and a suggestion for therapy in patients with certain kinds of calculi. *Trans Assoc Am Physicians* 75:301, 1962

258. HOWARD JE, THOMAS WC, JR: Control of crystallization in urine. *Am J Med* 45:693, 1968

259. THOMAS WC, JR, MILLER GH, JR: Inorganic phosphates in the treatment of renal calculi. *Mod Treat* 4:494, 1967

260. SMITH LH, THOMAS WC, JR, ARNAUD CD: Orthophosphate therapy in calcium renal lithiasis, in Cifuentes Delatte L, Rapado A, Hodgkinson A (eds): *Urinary Calculi: Recent Advances in Aetiology, Stone Structure and Treatment.* Basel, S Karger, 1973, pp 188–197

261. ZINSSER HH, KARP F: How to diminish endogenous oxalate excretion. I. tyrosine administration. *Invest Urol* 10:249, 1973

262. THOMAS J, DUBURQUE MT, CHAMPAGNAC A, JEAN S: Effect of succinimide on hyperoxaluria in the rat estimated value of the different dosing methods of oxaluria. *Urol Int* 32:1, 1977

263. THOMAS J, MELON JM, THOMAS E, STEG A, ABOULKER P: The role of oxalic acid in oxalate nephrolithiasis, in Cifuentes Lelatte, Rapado A, Hodgkinson A (eds): *Urinary Calculi: Recent Advances in Aetiology, Stone Structure and Treatment.* Basel, S Karger, 1973, pp 57–66

264. HAUTMANN R, HERING FJ, LUTZEYER W: Calcium oxalate stone disease: Effects and side effects of cellulose phosphate and succinate in long-term treatment of absorptive hypercalciuria or hyperoxaluria. *J Urol* 120:712, 1978

265. DEODHAR SD, TUNG KSK, ZÜHLKE V, NAKAMOTO S: Renal homotransplantation in a patient with primary familial oxalosis. *Arch Pathol* 87:118, 1969

266. KLAUWERS J, WOLF PL, COHN R: Failure of renal transplantation in primary oxalosis. *JAMA* 209:551, 1969

267. SAXON A, BUSCH GJ, MERRILL JP, FRANCO V, WILSON RE: Renal transplantation in primary hyperoxaluria. *Arch Intern Med* 133:464, 1974

268. MAHONY JF, STOREY BG, MCCARTHY SW, STEWART JH: Letter to the editor: Treatment of oxaluric renal failure. *N Engl J Med* 287:1252, 1972

269. KOCH B, IRVINE AH, BARR JR, POZNANSKI WJ: Three kidney transplantations in a patient with primary hereditary hyperoxaluria. *Can Med Ass J* 106:1323, 1972

270. JACOBSEN E, MOSBAEK N: Primary hyperoxaluria, treated with haemodialysis and kidney transplantation. *Dan Med Bull* 21:72, 1974

271. MORGAN JM, HARTLEY MW, MILLER AC, DIETHELM AG: Successful renal transplantation in hyperoxaluria. *Arch Surg* 109:430, 1974

272. FREI, D, BINSWANGER U, KEUSCH G, BRINER J, LARGIADER E: Intact function of a transplanted kidney 3 years after organ transplantation with primary oxalosis. *Schweiz Med Wochenschr* 109:979, 1979

273. LEUMANN EP, WEGMANN W, LARGIADER F: Prolonged survival after renal transplantation in primary hyperoxaluria of childhood. *Clin Nephrol* 9:29, 1978

274. HALVERSTADT, DB, WENZL JE: Primary hyperoxaluria and renal transplantation. *J Urol* 111:398, 1974

275. WALLS J, MORLEY AR, KERR DNS: Primary hyperoxaluria in adult siblings: With some observations on the role of regular haemodialysis therapy. *Br J Urol* 41:546, 1969

276. ZAREMBSKI PM, ROSEN SM, HODGKINSON A: Dialysis in the treatment of primary hyperoxaluria. *Br J Urol* 41:530, 1969

277. SAXON A: Hemodialysis for oxaluric renal failure. *N Engl Med* 288:526, 1973

278. BLACKBURN WE, MCROBERTS JW, BHATHENA D, VAZQUEZ M, LUKE RG: Severe vascular complications in oxalosis after bilateral nephrectomy. *Ann Intern Med* 82:44, 1975

279. ROFE AM, EDWARD JB: Oxalate synthesis in isolated rat hepatocytes: The effects of hydroxypyruvate and amino oxyacetate. *Biochem Med* 20:323, 1978

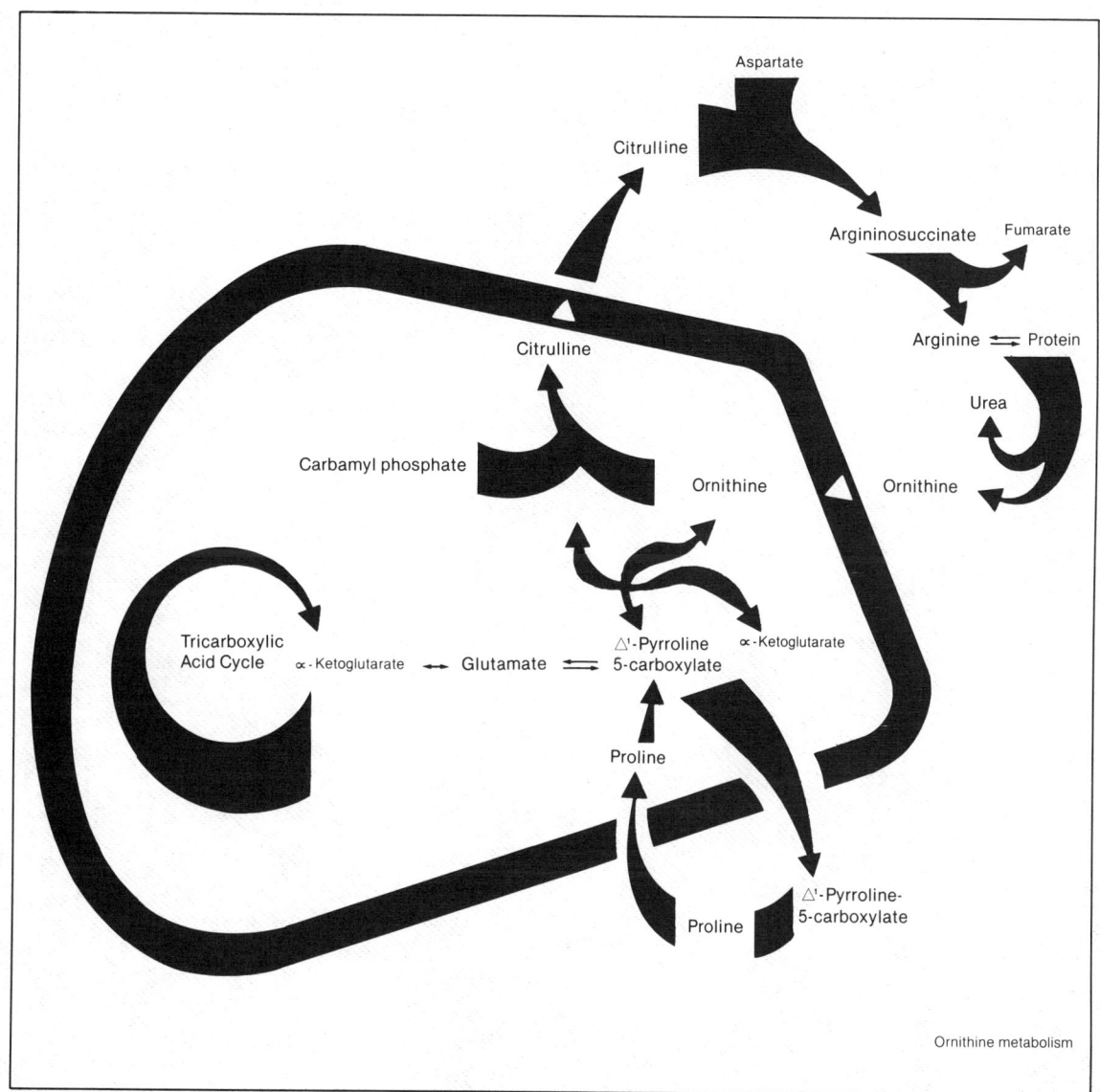

PART 3

Ornithine metabolism

DISORDERS OF AMINO ACID METABOLISM

11

FAMILIAL GOITER AND RELATED DISORDERS

J. B. STANBURY

J. E. DUMONT

1. *Synthesis, storage, secretion, delivery, and utilization of the thyroid hormones involve a complex sequence of metabolic events, many of which are dependent upon specific enzymatic activity. Thyroid disease may result from blockage at many steps in this metabolic process. The thyroid operates under hypothalamic-pituitary control; inherited disorders in control may also cause thyroid disease.*

2. *Studies of a cretinous patient from a consanguine marriage have indicated a limited response to thyrotropin (TSH), both in synthesis of the specific thyroid protein thyroglobulin and in cell growth and division. Other similar patients have been described with no response of adenyl cyclase activity to TSH. An analogous familial disorder has been observed in a strain of mice.*

3. *Familial goiter and hypothyroidism may occur when there is failure of the thyroid cell to transport iodide and maintain a favorable concentration gradient inside the follicle (iodide transport defect). The salivary and gastric glands of these patients are also unable to concentrate iodide.*

4. *Familial goiter may also result from failure to convert inorganic iodide into iodine in the thyroid gland (organification defect). This may happen in different patients because of the absence of thyroid peroxidase, abnormal peroxidase, or perhaps because of a diminished supply of peroxide. Accumulated iodide is pre-*

cipitously discharged from the gland upon administration of $ClO_4{}^-$. A group of patients with goiter and congenital nerve deafness (Pendred's syndrome) have iodine in the gland which is partially discharged following administration of $ClO_4{}^-$.

5. *Several families of patients have been studied who have a defect in the coupling of iodotyrosines into iodothyronines (coupling defect). The disease can be suspected when it is shown that iodothyronines fail to appear in biopsy specimens of thyroid tissue which has a normal or nearly normal concentration of iodine.*

6. *Family groups are known to be unable to deiodinate iodotyrosines (iodotyrosine deiodinase defect). Loss of hormone precursors from the gland into the urine accounts for hypothyroidism and compensatory goiter. Goitrous but otherwise normal relatives of such patients may deiodinate diiodotyrosine (DIT) less well than normal individuals. The condition is most convincingly diagnosed by the demonstration that intravenously administered, labeled DIT is excreted intact in the urine.*

7. *Familial goiter may occur in humans and sheep because of impaired synthesis of thyroglobulin. Some such patients may iodinate other proteins within the thyroid cell. In others, the thyroid may synthesize abnormal forms of thyroglobulin.*

8. *A syndrome of familial goiter, nerve deafness, and*

stippled epiphyses has been described. The results of investigations are consistent with an impaired ability of body cells to respond adequately to thyroid hormone. Other patients also have had impaired response of the peripheral cells to thyroid hormone but have differed somewhat both clinically and physiologically. In one, the diminished sensitivity appeared to be confined to the thyrotroph cells of the anterior pituitary.

9. *Familial hypothyroidism may arise from several different disorders of hypothalamic or pituitary control of the thyroid. Abnormalities of thyroid hormone transport are recognized but usually are not accompanied by any clinical disorder.*

10. *In most of the above conditions, errors are inherited as autosomal recessive traits. Because of the rarity of the genes responsible for each disorder, a high proportion of cases occur as a consequence of consanguine matings.*

Laboratory investigations of many subjects with familial thyroid disease have made it possible to classify some according to specific and identifiable biochemical lesions. In each of the categories reviewed here, the lesion is specific and distinct, but the net effect is the same: Synthesis, delivery, or effectiveness of thyroid hormones is inadequate (Fig. 11-1). Before considering these groups individually, it is appropriate to survey certain aspects of the metabolism of iodine that seem relevant to each. A schema of the metabolic circuit of iodine appears in Fig. 11-2. Competent general reviews are available elsewhere [1–3]. For a relevant older bibliography, the earlier edition of this chapter may be consulted [4].

THYROID PHYSIOLOGY AND METABOLISM: AN OVERVIEW

Iodide[1] ion is absorbed through the gastrointestinal tract and is rapidly distributed throughout the extracellular fluid of the

body. The volume of distribution is approximately 30 percent of body weight. Iodinated thyronines and tyrosines may be absorbed intact but are partially (T_3: 5 percent; T_4: 50 percent) or almost totally (iodotyrosines: 95 percent) deiodinated prior to absorption. Upon absorption, thyroxine (T_4) and 3,5,3'-triiodothyronine (T_3) are confined to the vascular compartment because of binding to carrier proteins in the plasma.

Except in the postprandial state, the iodide concentration of the plasma is less than 0.2 µg/dl. The inorganic iodide of the plasma is removed almost entirely by the kidney and the thyroid. Renal clearance of iodide is normally about 35 ml/min and is independent of the iodine supply in humans. Thyroidal clearance varies widely, depending on the functional state of the gland but normally lies between 10 and 35 ml/min. The iodide cleared from the plasma by the salivary and gastric glands is returned after absorption in the small intestine. Small amounts of iodide are removed by the mammary glands during lactation, and some organic iodine is lost in the feces and urine.

The function of the thyroid follicle cell is to trap iodide from the blood and to use it for the synthesis of the thyroid hormones T_4 and T_3. The thyroid cell synthesizes principally one exportable glycoprotein, thyroglobulin, which is secreted by exocytosis into the follicular lumen. Iodide is trapped at the basal membrane of the cell and concentrated in the lumen; it is oxidized and bound to the tyrosyl residue of thyroglobulin by a peroxidase presumably at the apical membrane of the cell (Fig. 11-3). The H_2O_2 required by the peroxidase is supplied by a still poorly defined H_2O_2-generating system. Thyroperoxidase also catalyzes the oxidative coupling of iodotyrosines into iodothyronines, T_4 and T_3, within the matrix of thyroglobulin. Thyroglobulin slowly diffuses within the follicular lumen to ensure the relative homogeneity of the luminal content, the colloid. Thyroid colloid thus constitutes a store of sequestered iodine, the iodotyrosyls, and thyroid hormones. In the secretory process, thyroglobulin is endocytosed by the follicular cell by micropinocytosis or macropinocytosis and digested into its constituent amino acids in secondary lysosomes. While the iodothyronines are released, presumably by diffusion, the

---

[1] In this chapter, *iodine* is used in a generic sense to encompass all forms and oxidation states unless otherwise indicated.

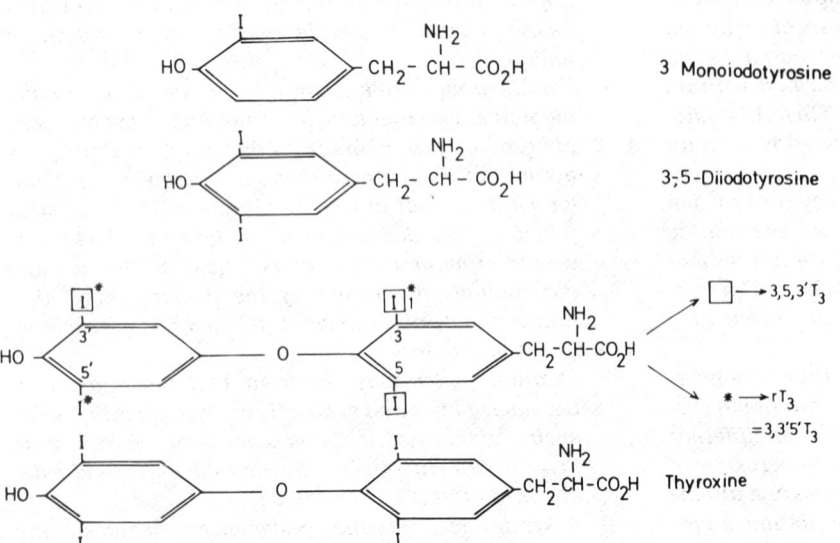

3 Monoiodotyrosine

3,5-Diiodotyrosine

Thyroxine

Figure 11-1 Iodinated amino acids of the thyroid. rT_3 = reverse triiodothyronine.

DATA EXPRESSED AS μG OF IODINE

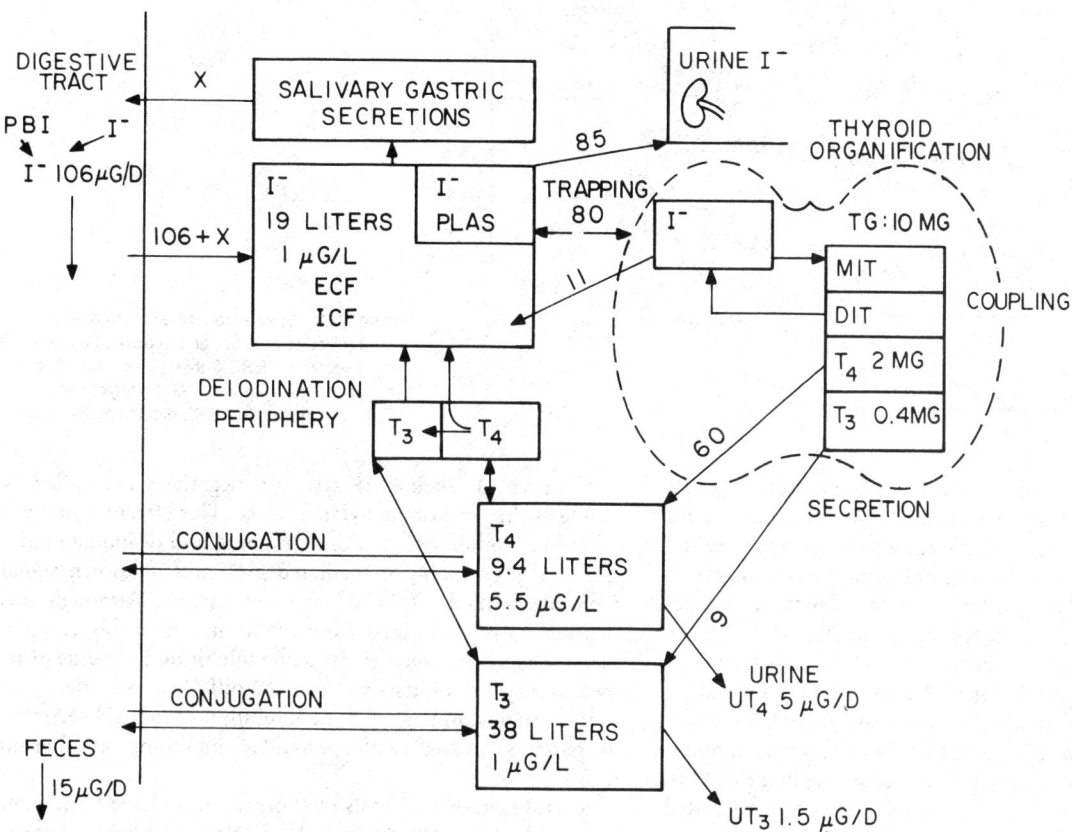

Figure 11-2 Iodine metabolism in humans. Fluxes of iodine expressed in micrograms of iodine per day. For each compartment, the distribution space and concentration are given. PBI, protein-bound iodine; TG, thyroglobulin; X, flux of iodine through the digestive tract cycle; UT$_3$, UT$_4$, urinary excretions; ECF, extracellular fluid; ICF, intracellular fluid.

iodotyrosines are deiodinated in the cell, thus allowing the re-utilization of their iodine.

All the metabolic steps of the follicular cell, as well as its growth, are controlled by TSH (thyrotropin), which acts mainly by enhancing the generation of cyclic AMP. The levels of TSH in the plasma are the result of positive hypothalamic control exerted through TRH (thyrotropin-releasing hormone), and negative control by circulating iodothyronines on TSH synthesis and secretion by the pituitary thyrotrophs.

The thyroid hormones are transported mostly bound to thyroxine-binding proteins (TBG: thyroxine-binding globulin. TBPA: thyroxine-binding prealbumin, and albumin). T$_4$, which must be considered a prohormone, is deiodinated to the active hormone T$_3$ or to an inactive species rT$_3$ at the periphery. The action of thyroid hormone on the peripheral cells, exerted mostly at the level of protein synthesis, is to enhance certain components of cellular intermediary metabolism and to sustain growth and development.

Most of the metabolic steps outlined here involve several different proteins. Regulatory defects may be expected for any of the proteins involved in any one metabolic step, but the phenotypic expression of such defects will be virtually identical. In this chapter, defects will be classified on the basis of the function involved, i.e., of the phenotypic expression. It will be understood that each of these classes may encompass several different genetic defects.

THYROTROPIN AND THYROID FUNCTION

Thyroid function and growth are controlled by TSH. Several accessory circuits (involving neurotransmitters, acetylcholine, norepinephrine, prostaglandins, and iodine) are superimposed on the main control. Thus control is exerted by a complex regulatory network (Fig. 11-4). TSH acutely stimulates the binding of iodide to proteins, iodotyrosine oxidative coupling, thyroid hormone release, and many pathways of intermediary metabolism, such as the oxidation of glucose by the pentose phosphate pathway. With a delay of several hours, TSH enhances the trapping of iodide and the synthesis of proteins, RNA, and so on. Chronically administered, it induces cell growth and multiplication, i.e., thyroid hyperplasia and cell hypertrophy [5].

TSH interacts with the cell at the level of the plasma membrane by binding to specific receptors coupled to effectors or catalytic units (Fig. 11-5). One such system, thyroid adenylate cyclase, is now well known. It represents for the thyroid and TSH the application of the Sutherland model of hormone action. TSH binds to a receptor and activates it; the activated receptor, in turn, activates a nucleotide-binding protein (N) (also called G/F) which binds GTP; the GTP-activated N protein binds to and activates the catalytic unit, i.e., the cyclase which catalyzes the generation of cyclic AMP from ATP (turn on). The action of the hormone is terminated by the hydrolysis

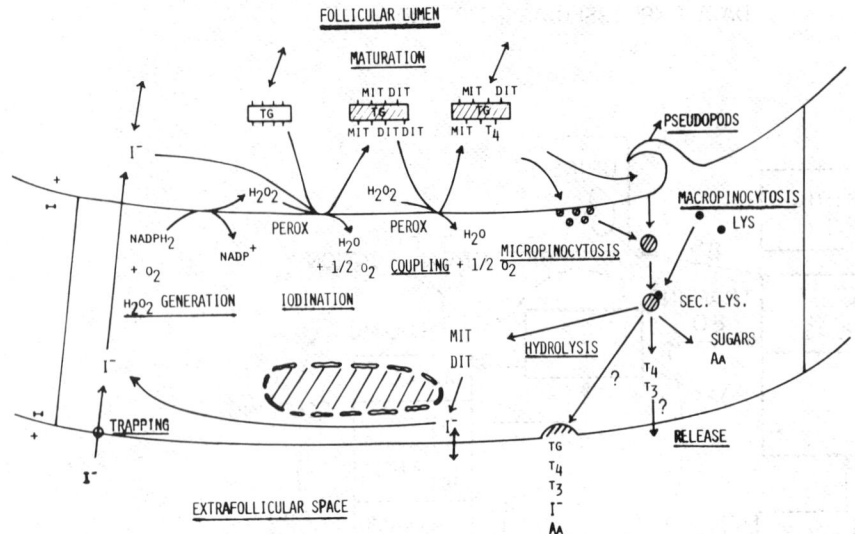

Figure 11-3 Specialized metabolism of the thyroid follicular cell. Aa, amino acids; Lys, primary lysosome; PEROX, thyroperoxidase; Sec Lys, secondary lysosome; TG, thyroglobulin; MIT, monoiodotyrosine; DIT, diiodotyrosine.

of bound GTP by GTPase activity of the N protein (turn off) [6, 7]. It is presumed that the receptor, N protein, and cyclase are independent proteins freely floating and interacting in the two-dimensional plane of the membrane. In the cytosol, cyclic AMP binds to cyclic AMP-dependent protein kinases by a reaction $R_2C_2 + 4$ cyclic AMP $\rightleftharpoons R_2$(cyclic AMP)$_4$ + 2C. R is the regulatory subunit and C the catalytic subunit. At least two such kinases have been identified: I and II. R, the regulatory subunit of the kinases, blocks enzyme activity, while the binding of cyclic AMP to R releases the active catalytic subunit, which phosphorylates specific protein substrates in the cell [8]. While in the dog thyroid 12 such proteins are phosphorylated in this way in response to TSH, only one of these, the histone H_1, has been identified, and the relations of these phosphorylations to the physiologic effects of the hormone are still unknown [9]. It has been demonstrated that this scheme accounts for most of the effects of TSH on the dog thyroid, including, at least in part, promotion of growth. In the human thyroid, TSH stimulates iodination and glycogenolysis by activating cyclase, but which other effects of the hormone are mediated by cyclic AMP is not known.

Some effects of TSH are not mediated by cyclic AMP, among them activation of phosphatidylinositol turnover. The role of this effect, as in other systems, is still unknown. Thus TSH has both cyclic AMP-dependent and -independent effects. By analogy with the adrenergic system, we call them *B* and *A effects*. This could be explained by the existence of two different receptors for TSH (A and B versus α and β receptors of norepinephrine) or two effector systems coupled to one receptor [10].

Chronic stimulation of the thyroid by TSH leads to a decrease in the response (e.g., secretion) to the hormone (desensitization). Several mechanisms could account for this: acute (after 30 min) decrease in the stimulation of adenylate cyclase, exhaustion of the apical membranes available for phagocytosis, and a later (after days) down regulation of the number of TSH receptors [11, 12].

Several other physiologic agents activate thyroid adenylate cyclase, among these norepinephrine acting on β receptors and E prostaglandins. Compared to those of TSH, their effects are in general of lower amplitude, shorter duration, and unknown role. The thyroid-stimulating immunoglobulins, TSI, which reproduce all the effects of TSH and bind to the same receptors, are believed to be the cause of hyperthyroidism in Graves' disease [12].

The thyroid cyclic AMP system is negatively controlled by iodide at the level of adenylate cyclase. This effect of iodide is relieved by inhibitors of iodide trapping and of iodide oxidation and presumably is mediated by a still unknown signal molecule termed *XI*, which contains iodine. Although this mechanism is undoubtedly important, it is probably complemented by others, such as the acute inhibition by iodide of its own transport, of its oxidation (Wolff-Chaikoff effect), of iodotyrosine coupling, and the inhibition of thyroid secretion in patients treated with peroxidase-inhibiting antithyroid drugs.

Several negative controls of short duration have been demonstrated in the dog thyroid gland. Norepinephrine exerts a direct action through the α receptors on the cyclase. Also, acetylcholine and PGF$_{2\alpha}$, by increasing Ca^{2+} influx in the thyroid, inhibit secretion directly, activate guanylate cyclase—whose product, cyclic GMP, activates cyclic nucleotide phosphodiesterase—and activate arachidonate release and prostaglandin synthesis [13]. These mechanisms have not yet been studied in the human thyroid [14]. Other extracellular signal molecules, vasointestinal peptide (VIP), TRH, and thyroid growth-inducing immunoglobulins, have some effects on the thyroids of some species, but their role, if any, in the human thyroid remains undefined.

TSH action on the human thyroid can be studied at different levels. The best indexes may be the normal functional effects of the hormone in vivo, i.e., the acute stimulation of hormone release and the delayed enhancement of iodide trapping. Such tests give no clue concerning the mechanisms involved. An absent secretory response may reflect stimulation that is already maximal, deficient hormone synthesis, iodine overexposure, etc. Moreover, they provide only one result (positive or negative). With one piece of tissue in vitro, several results can be obtained, but it cannot be overemphasized that, whatever the parameter measured, information must be obtained on the kinetics of the response and concentration effects. Also, in order to validate a negative result, it is essential that a positively responding tissue be tested at the same time with the same reagents. Studies on intact cells, such as slices or cultured cells, will give fewer artifacts but more complex responses than studies on acellular systems. The parameters investigated can be cyclic AMP accumulation, protein iodination, and glucose [^{14}C] oxidation. The two latter measurements explore the whole sequence of events between hormone binding and terminal effects. The effect of TSH on protein iodination in human thyroid slices is not constantly reproducible, and with regard to glucose oxidation it should be remembered that the effect of TSH on normal tissue is biphasic. Thus, glucose [^{14}C] oxidation is decreased by TSH at low hormone concentrations (reflecting glucose phosphate pool dilution by glycogenolysis) and increased only at high concentrations. This latter effect is not reproduced by dibutyryl cyclic AMP and may be an A effect of TSH [15]. It would be useful if more precise functional responses to TSH could be developed, and if they were mimicked by analogues of cyclic AMP, one might be able to pinpoint defects prior to cyclic AMP or subsequent to this step in the regulatory sequence.

Studies with acellular systems bear on the binding of TSH to thyroid membranes and on TSH activation of adenylate cyclase in membranes. For binding studies, it is essential that relevant binding be measured. Many binding studies have been carried out under conditions which failed to demonstrate the receptor [16]. The specificity of binding should be assured by chase experiments. For studies of adenylate cyclase activation, it should be noted that all artifacts (such as disruption by heavy homogenization) will tend to decrease or to erase the TSH response. Damaged preparations of thyroid adenylate cyclase with normal basal activity, NaF activation, and TSH binding are easily obtained, but they may show no effect of TSH on the enzyme. It is therefore advisable in similar studies to investigate the TSH response by several different methods; otherwise, a defect in TSH response is not fully demonstrated.

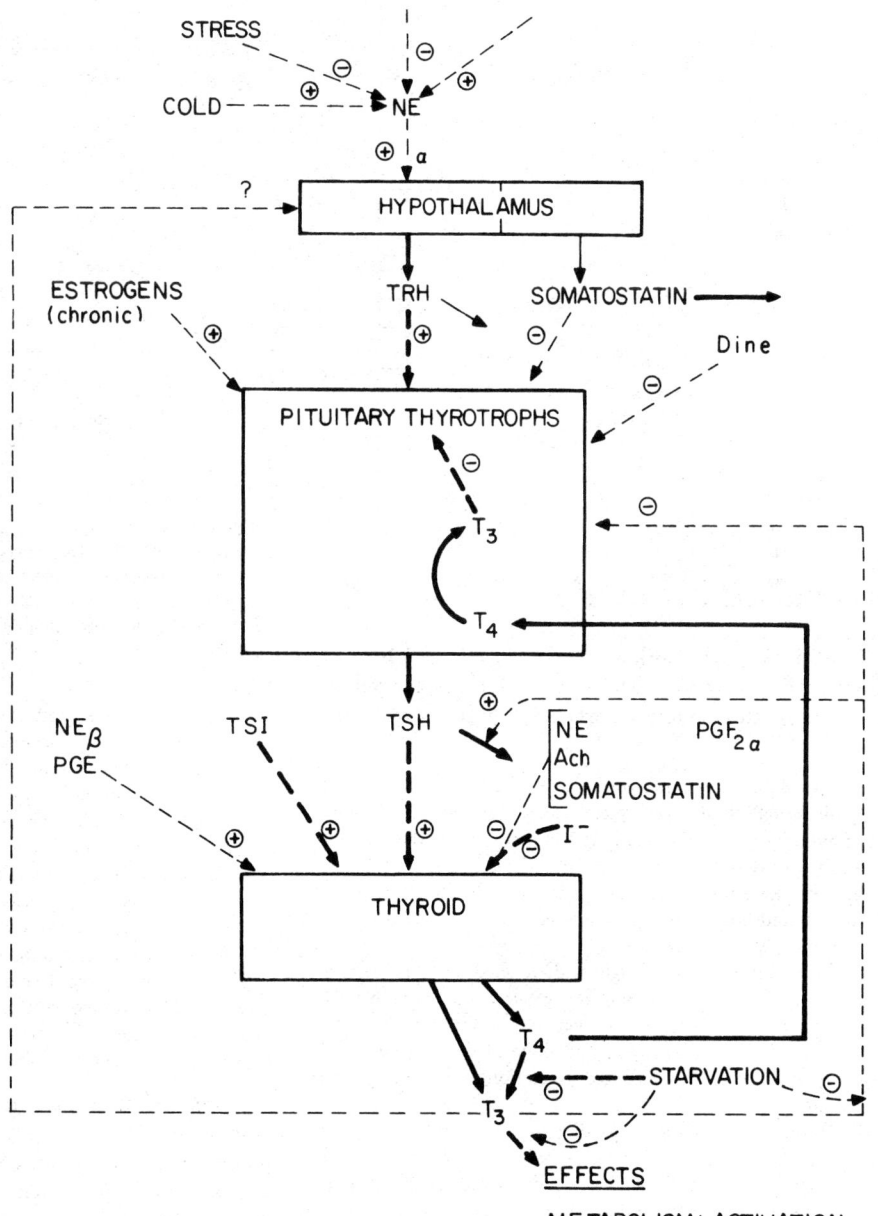

Figure 11-4 Control of thyroid hormone action. Uninterrupted arrows indicate chemical transformations or transports. Interrupted arrows indicate controls: ⊕ stimulations, ⊖ inhibitions. The dominating elements of the system are indicated by heavy arrows. NE, norepinephrine acting through receptors; Dine, dopamine; Ach, acetylcholine; TSI, thyroid-stimulating immunoglobulins.

NE = NOREPINEPHRINE

ACH = ACETYLCHOLINE

α β: α and β receptors of NE

EFFECTS

METABOLISM: ACTIVATION

GROWTH: REQUIRED

MENTAL DEVELOPMENT: REQUIRED

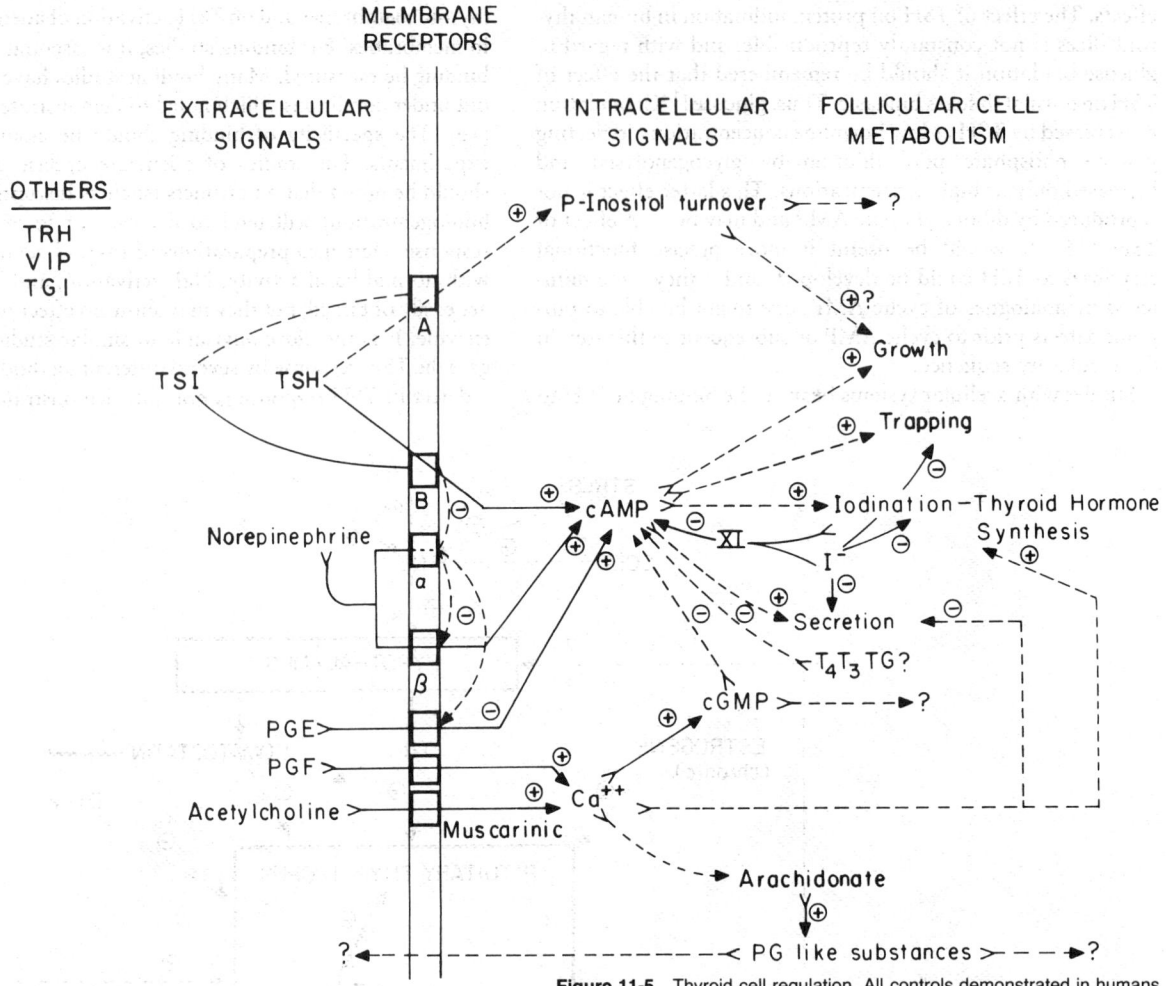

Figure 11-5 Thyroid cell regulation. All controls demonstrated in humans are represented by uninterrupted lines. Controls demonstrated only in the dog are represented by interrupted lines; + and − stand for positive and negative controls. TG, thyroglobulin; TSI, thyroid-stimulating immunoglobulins; TGI, thyroid growth-promoting immunoglobulins; VIP, vasointestinal peptide; XI, unknown mediator of the iodide inhibitory effect.

Related Clinical Disorders

Congenital Hypothyroidism with Impaired Thyroid Response to Thyrotropin   This is a rare form of congenital hypothyroidism. Reasonable criteria have been satisfied for three patients.

An 8-year-old boy appeared normal at birth, but by 6 months of age retarded intellectual development was recognized [17]. A diagnosis of hypothyroidism was made at 2 years of age, and treatment was begun with desiccated thyroid.

The parents were first cousins once removed. They had three normal children and one other who was said to be retarded but who had a normal PBI.

The patient was 110 cm in height and weighed 19.3 kg. He was able to feed and dress himself and to say a few intelligible words. The bone age was $3\frac{1}{2}$ years. The face was typically cretinoid. Hearing was normal. The isthmus and right lobe of the thyroid gland were easily palpable but not enlarged. Excretion of [127]I in the urine was normal.

The PBI concentration was 1.0 μg/dl in one study and 2.4 μg/dl in another. Uptake of ^{131}I was 37 percent during a first study and 27 percent during a second. A perchlorate discharge test result was normal. TSH failed to increase the ^{131}I uptake. Diiodotyrosine was metabolized normally. No labeled iodine corresponding to any component other than iodide was found in the urine after administration of radiodine.

The TBG capacity was slightly low, but the TBPA capacity was normal. Radioimmunoassay and bioassay for TSH gave very high values.

The thyroid weighed about 5 g. It was normally vascularized. Slices from a biopsy specimen incubated with L-[14C]glucose did not respond to TSH (1 unit). No thyroglobulin could be detected by physical or immunologic means.

The microscopic picture was unusual. There was a diffuse increase in the stroma. Between the thickened fibrous septums, the follicles were generally small to medium in size but displayed a wide variation in the lining cells. Some follicles filled with colloid had cells that were very flat and involuted or even atrophic. Other follicles, often adjacent to the inactive ones, were lined with hypertrophied, large, cuboidal cells typical of reactive hyperplasia. There was a heterogeneous mixture of these two follicular patterns. Another feature of interest was the frequency of atypical nuclear forms, often bizarre in shape and hyperchromatic.

A remarkably similar patient has been studied by Codaccioni et al. [18]. This 17-year-old male, a product of consanguine parents, was retarded at 18 months of age but progressed with thyroid replacement therapy. Plasma thyroid hormone levels were very low, and the TSH concentrations were much elevated. Uptake of ^{131}I by the thyroid was not stimulated by TSH but was increased by an intravenous injection of dibutyryl cyclic AMP. Thyroid membranes prepared from a biopsy specimen bound TSH normally, and labeled TSH was normally displaced by stable TSH. Cyclase activity was normally stimulated by NaF, but stimulation by TSH was much decreased compared to normal membranes. There was a much reduced concentration of thyroglobulin in the gland. The thyroid parenchymal cells were devoid of colloid droplets. The basal plasma membrane and basal membranes were scalloped, thickened, and infolded. The gland was not enlarged.

The dissociation between the lack of response to TSH on the one hand and the response to NaF and dibutyryl cyclic AMP on the other led Codaccioni et al. to suggest an error in coupling between the TSH receptor and adenyl cyclase stimulation. They pointed out the possibility of the similar dissociation in some patients with pseudohypoparathyroidism [19, 20].

Farfel et al. [21] have found a reduced amount of the N protein component of the adenyl cyclase system in some patients with pseudohypoparathyroidism [22]. This abnormality is reflected by multiple endocrine insufficiencies, including hypothyroidism. The N protein mediates cyclase stimulation by NaF, and since the response to NaF was normal in the membranes from the patient of Codaccioni et al. and receptor binding of TSH was normal, the disorder must be between the TSH receptor binding site and the receptor-cyclase coupling protein.

The patient of Medeiros-Neto et al. [23] was a 19-year-old severely retarded, hypothyroid male. Plasma thyroid hormone concentrations were low, and plasma TSH was high and gave an exaggerated response to TRH. There was no in vitro response to TSH administration. Tissue slices from a biopsy specimen did not respond as well to TSH as did controls by increasing the thyroid to medium ^{131}I ratio, nor was there a response in adenyl cyclase activity. No thyroglobulin could be detected.

A 4-year-old retarded, hypothyroid male has been described by Job et al. [24]. The thyroid of this patient was not enlarged. Uptake of ^{131}I was low and failed to respond to TSH administration. While it seems possible that this patient was an example of TSH unresponsiveness, the lack of in vitro studies leaves the diagnosis in doubt.

A strain of mice has been found with an autosomal recessive mutation characterized by retarded growth, low thyroid hormone concentration, and elevated TSH [25]. These mice fail to respond to TSH but respond to thyroid hormone. This gene has been mapped.

A rat thyroid tumor developed by Wolman of the National Cancer Institute (line 1-8) has been studied [26, 27]. Basal and fluoride-sensitive adenyl cyclase activities were normal, but plasma membranes from the tumor failed to respond to TSH and bound TSH poorly, although the small amount of TSH which was bound was more tightly bound than in controls [28]. It appeared that its failure to respond to TSH was due to a change in the TSH receptor. The rat tumor membranes lacked a transferase required for synthesis of more complex gangliosides. As gangliosides were thought by these authors to be important components of the receptor, they hypothesized that the lack of transferase explained the defect [28]. However, the scarce evidence that complex gangliosides are part of the receptor has not been substantiated. TSH binding and response to NaF may be retained by differentiated thyroid tumors [29, 30] or may be reduced [31].

INTERPRETATION The patients who appear to have had thyroids unresponsive to TSH have had certain unusual features. In spite of severe clinical hypothyroidism and low serum hormone concentrations, the avidity of the thyroid for iodine was normal. Although the TSH levels in the blood were high and there was much cellular hypertrophy in the biopsy specimens, there was no goiter. No evidence for a protein resembling thyroglobulin could be found.

The abnormalities suggest a failure of the thyroid glands to respond adequately to TSH. Crucial for the diagnosis is the combination of high TSH levels and low thyroid response in vivo, as shown by low or normal iodide uptake and absence of goiter. An almost normal thyroid size in the absence of a TSH effect is conceivable because TSH does not appear to be necessary for differentiation and early growth in utero. Of course, such a picture could result from inflammation followed by fibrosis at an early age. In this case, the thyroid would be fully activated but would not grow. One would expect a very fast turnover of a small pool of thyroid iodine and follicular cell hypertrophy, as, for example, in Congolese myxedematous endemic cretinism or in the lingual thyroid. Lack of response of intact cells to TSH after a preincubation to wash out bound TSH would support the diagnosis of a defect in TSH responsivity.

Thyroid membranes from a biopsy specimen of the patient of Codaccioni et al. [18] responded to NaF and bound TSH but did not respond to TSH. These findings suggest that the error was not in binding by the TSH receptor but in another component of the specific membrane adenyl cyclase system. The error in the 1-8 rat thyroid tumor would seem to be in the receptor. There is no evidence regarding the specific defect in other patients with the syndrome of TSH unresponsiveness.

A suggested set of diagnostic criteria for this syndrome appears in Table 11-1. In addition, as opportunities arise, a detailed study of the thyroid membrane preparations will provide useful information and refine the molecular diagnosis. Given the complexity of the receptor and the adenyl cyclase system, one may anticipate that there are several subsets of this syndrome. Also, since goiter is not a feature of the syndrome, it is possible that some patients carrying a diagnosis of sporadic cretinism in fact belong to this group.

Table 11-1 Diagnostic criteria for thyrotropin insensitivity

In vivo
  1. Hypothyroid; no goiter, thyroid in normal position
  2. Normal or low normal ^{131}I uptake
  3. Slow iodine turnover and small iodine pool in the thyroid
  4. No in vivo response to TSH (hormone release, iodine uptake)
  5. Plasma TSH high by bioassay
In vitro
  Thyroid biopsy
  1. Little colloid; no thyroglobulin
  2. Epithelial cells abnormal; no cell division
  3. No response of slices to TSH
     a. No cyclic AMP accumulation
     b. No functional effect; no appearance of colloid droplets, no decrease, and no increase in glucose (1^{14}C) oxidation, etc.

If the defect involved adenylate cyclase, analogues of cyclic AMP should elicit the functional effect of TSH. In this event, studies of TSH binding by thyroid membranes should permit investigation of the receptor. Measurement of cyclase activity with Mn ATP as substrate would assess the integrity of the catalytic unit of the enzyme, and measurement of cyclase activity in the presence of NaF or GPP NHP would assess the activity of the N GTPase. The whole operation of the receptor cyclase complex could be assessed by measurement of cycylase activity in the presence of TSH and GTP.

The observation that two of the three patients were products of consanguine matings suggests the possibility of autosomal recessive inheritance for this rare disorder.

IODIDE TRANSPORT

The first step of iodine metabolism in the thyroid is the trapping of iodide by the follicles. The uptake, which takes place even in the absence of any further metabolism of iodine, results from an active transport mechanism. At normal plasma iodine ion concentrations, the trapping of iodide is the limiting step of iodine metabolism in the thyroid.

Iodide uptake, as measured by its clearance, depends upon thyroid blood flow and the iodide extraction ratio [(A−V)/A], where A and V are the arterial and venous concentrations, respectively, of iodide. Since the blood transit time in the thyroid is smaller than the half-life of iodide in red cells [32], this extraction ratio cannot be greater than 0.55 to 0.60, even if 99 percent of the plasma iodide is eventually taken up. Such ratios are obtained in iodine-deficient dogs, and in these preparations iodide trapping is limited by the thyroid blood flow [33, 34]. In normal humans, the extraction ratio is estimated at around 0.20 [33].

The iodide extraction ratio in the thyroid reflects the activity of an iodide transport mechanism commonly called the *iodide pump*. Pump efficiency is generally evaluated, in tissues in which iodide oxidation has been blocked, by the ratios T/M, T/S, or C/M, where T, C, M, and S are the radioactivities per unit volume of labeled iodide in the thyroid, in isolated cells, in the incubation medium, or in the serum, respectively. At equilibrium, and if the thyroid is considered as one compartment, these ratios are equal to C/M ÷ KTB where C/M is the unidirectional iodide clearance per unit weight of tissue and KTB is the rate constant for unidirectional iodide efflux [35].

Autoradiography, as well as compartmental analysis of uptake kinetics, shows that the thyroid follicle concentrates radioiodide in its lumen. This requires follicle integrity and implies a flux through both the basal and apical membranes of the cell. The electrical polarity of the cell is such that iodide has to overcome an electrical gradient to enter the cell, but it may flow downhill with the gradient to accumulate in the lumen. This, and the fact that isolated cells also concentrate iodide, indicates the existence of an active transport mechanism in the basal membrane. Kinetic and radioautographic experiments showing that under certain conditions perchlorate and radioiodide first accumulate in the cell suggest that transport may also take place at the apical membrane [34, 36, 37] (Fig. 11-3).

The characteristics of the iodide transport system have been established in the thyroids of several species [35]:

1. It concentrates iodide as such against a chemical and electrical gradient.
2. It is saturable and obeys Michaelis-Menten kinetics with an apparent K_m of $3 \times 10^{-5} M$.
3. It depends on the availability of ATP derived from oxidative phosphorylation or glycolysis.
4. It concentrates other anions (ClO_4^-, BF_4^-, etc.) which compete with iodide, having a similar charge and ionic volume.
5. It is inhibited by thiocyanate and inhibitors of the Na^+/K^+-activated ATPase such as ouabain.

Mechanisms with similar characteristics have been demonstrated in digestive glands, such as the salivary glands and gastric mucosa, and in other tissues, such as the mammary gland and choroid plexus. The fact that concentration of iodide by these glands disappears in congenital cretins with a defect of iodide trapping supports the hypothesis that the same protein is involved in these transports. Iodide is not oxidized or bound to proteins in these glands [38].

The biochemical mechanism of iodide transport is unknown. The fact that Na^+ in the extracellular medium is required and that there is a delay in the inhibitory action of metabolic inhibitors and ouabain suggests that an ion gradient generated by the Na^+/K^+-activated ATPase rather than the enzyme itself may be the motive force for the transport [39–42]. There is good evidence in favor of a model in which Na^+ influx would be coupled to I^- influx [34, 40, 43] by a mobile carrier. A role for an iodide-binding phospholipid has been postulated but not yet supported [44]. Such a model explains why thiocyanate and perchlorate not only block iodide uptake but also release iodide already trapped in the gland.

Iodide trapping is decreased and then increases following stimulation by TSH. The former effect reflects an increased efflux presumably caused by increased cell permeability; the latter effect reflects an increased influx by enhancement of the V_{max}. The TSH action is inhibited by inhibitors of RNA and protein synthesis. This suggests induction at the level of transcription. Both effects of TSH are reproduced by cyclic AMP analogues [45]. Chronic treatment with TSH considerably increases iodide trapping, while excess iodine depresses it, even in hypophysectomized animals.

Iodide trapping can be evaluated in vivo by iodide clearance under methimazole treatment or, more conveniently but qualitatively, by the uptake of pertechnetate, a nonmetabolizable analogue. The transport mechanism can also be studied in digestive glands, such as the salivary gland, by the salivary/plasma (S/P) radioiodide or SCN^- ratios.

Transport of iodide in vitro must be studied with intact cells. It can be measured in the presence of peroxidase inhibitors (methimazole, propylthiouracil) at equilibrium by the T/M ratio in thyroid slices or by the C/M ratio of isolated cells. It should be remembered that these ratios can be modified by factors other than changes in the transport mechanism itself. For instance, iodide uptake in slices will be much decreased if follicles are opened by the slicing procedure itself, which releases proteolytic enzymes. The probability of opening will increase with the size of the follicles (e.g., in colloid goiter) and the thinness of the slices [46].

Related Clinical Disorders

Hypothyroidism from Failure to Transport Iodide (Iodide Transport Defect) Iodide transport depends on the integrity of Na^+/K^+-activated ATPase, of the ATP supply, and of the transport system itself. Defects in the first two processes would have consequences for many other cell types which would overshadow their thyroid aspects. The transport system itself probably involves two steps at most and perhaps only one. Thus inherited defects in transport may involve only a single protein.

A male patient with an iodide transport defect was 15 years old at the time of the study [47]. Birth was at full term after a normal pregnancy. Birth weight was 4.3 kg. A small umbilical hernia noticed at birth was surgically repaired at 3 years of age. Early milestones of development were normal, but progress in school was slow. At age 8, the basal metabolic rate was −29 percent, and the serum cholesterol level was 560 mg/dl. Roentgenograms of the bones disclosed a delay in maturation of 3 years. The patient responded well to 65 mg thyroid daily, and growth and school performance became normal. Puberty was normal. A small goiter was observed 2 months before admission, and thyroid was discontinued. He quickly became lethargic, gained 9 kg, and became constipated.

His only sib was normal. The family was closely intermarried, and several members of both the paternal and maternal forebears had had goiter (Fig. 11-6).

The skin was dry and moderately pigmented. The thyroid was about three times the normal size and contained numerous small nodules. The BMR was −39 percent. Total serum iodine concentration was 1.5 μg/dl and PBI 0.5 μg/dl. The sella turcica was at the upper limit of normal or slightly larger than normal size. Bone age was consistent with the chronological age. Biopsy of the thyroid disclosed numerous small nodules. Some were cystic, but most were cellular. There was intense hyperplasia of the parenchymal elements. Scarcely any colloid could be seen.

The uptake of ^{131}I was 11.4 percent at 24 h. At 48 h, 7.8 percent was in the gland. Of the administered ^{131}I, 67 percent appeared in the urine within the first 24 h and 86.3 percent in the first 48 h. The concentration of iodide in saliva was not significantly different from that in the serum (S/P ratio). Both parents, a sister, and a maternal aunt of the patient had S/P ratios higher than 20 and were comparable to those of control subjects.

The S/P ratios for SCN⁻ indicated little, if any, active concentration by the salivary glands. The ratio of ^{131}I in gastric fluid collected 5 h after administration of the ^{131}I and 30 min after introduction of a gastric tube to that of plasma was 0.8. The pH of the gastric fluid was 2. Tissue slices from the biopsy fragments failed to accumulate ^{131}I from a medium in which they were incubated. On the other hand, a small amount of protein-bound ^{131}I initially present in the slices was formed from the two tracer doses of ^{131}I administered several days before biopsy. Over 90 percent of the ^{131}I precipitated under the conditions of thyroglobulin precipitation.

The patient was discharged on a dose of 1 mg potassium iodide three times daily. Within 4 weeks his BMR had risen steadily to +8, and his thyroid enlargement had virtually disappeared. He has remained well and euthyroid on this program for the intervening 20 years. He is a practicing attorney.

INTERPRETATION   The abnormality of this patient may be a missing component of the iodide transport system, a component common to the transport systems of the thyroid, the salivary gland, and the gastric mucosa. It is possible that some undetected inhibitor of the transport process was present. If so, it could not have been SCN⁻, because the amount of SCN⁻ in the saliva was less than normal.

The defect must have been one which is fairly specific for transport of iodide and related anions, and at the same time one which is not essential to more general transport processes in the cell and their energy sources because apart from iodide transport, those cells were evidently functioning quite normally. One may surmise that the iodide gradient is dependent on a specific binding substance whose structure or orientation is maintained by an expenditure of cell energy. No such substance has been described, except possibly the iodinated lipid of Vilkki [44].

Figure 11-6 Family history of a 15-year-old male with failure of iodide transport. Note the several consanguine marriages.

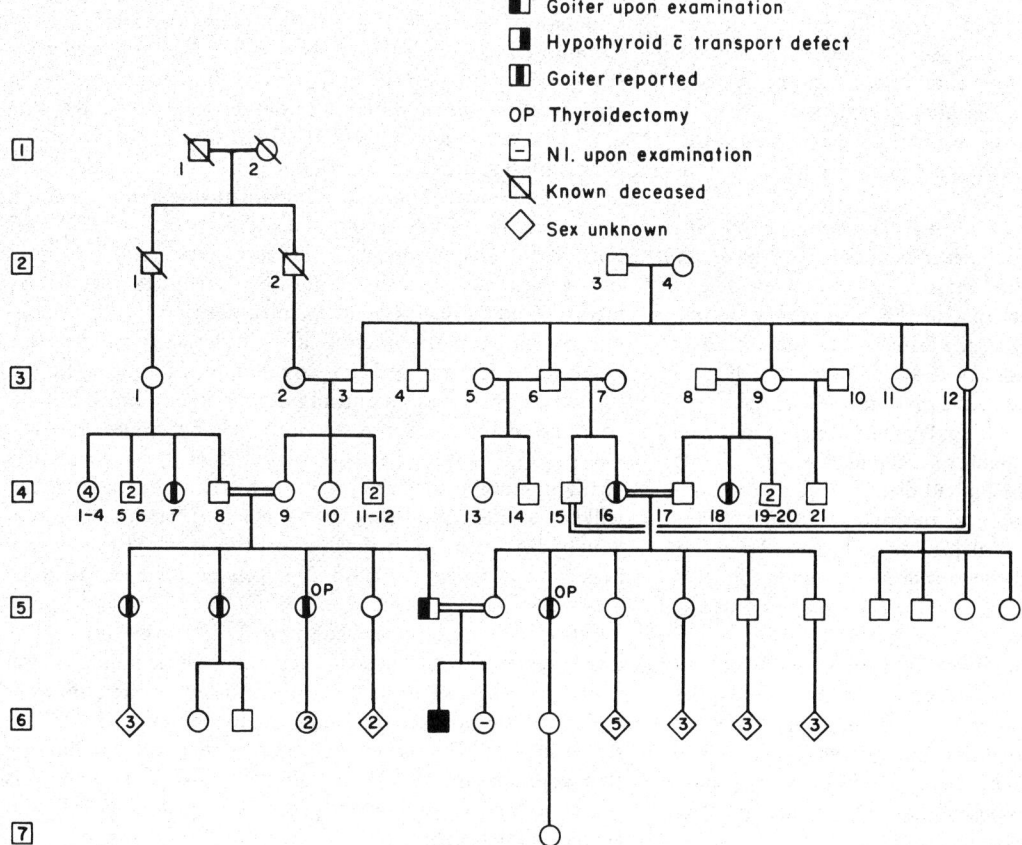

- ■ Goiter upon examination
- ◧ Hypothyroid c̄ transport defect
- ◫ Goiter reported
- OP Thyroidectomy
- ⊟ N l. upon examination
- ⊠ Known deceased
- ◇ Sex unknown

OTHER SIMILAR CASES   This form of familial goiter seems to be quite rare. Federman et al. [48] in 1958 reported a 19-month-old infant with cretinism and a goiter who had failed to accumulate iodine in the gland. They surmised that the thyroid of their patient might be unable to take iodine from the blood. Later studies on this same patient confirmed this conclusion [49].

Two brothers whose parents were not consanguine have been reported by Gilboa et al. [50]. One was age 14. Myxedema had been diagnosed at age 1 month, and in the intervening years thyroid had been given and development had been normal. A goiter had appeared. The patient had the signs and symptoms of myxedema 5 weeks after withdrawal of medication. The ^{131}I uptake was 11.5 percent at 24 h. Tissue slices from a thyroid biopsy specimen failed to concentrate iodide from the suspending medium. Administration of Lugol's solution was followed by a prompt disappearance of the findings of hypothyroidism, but continued medication resulted in thyrotoxicosis. With reduction in dosage, the patient became normal. The 24-year-old brother had a large goiter. He had always taken thyroid and became hypothyroid when this was withdrawn. His ^{131}I uptake at 4 h was only 3 percent after medication was discontinued.

Five Japanese patients, three from a sibship, have been studied by Toyoshima et al. [51]. Three of the five were retarded, but only one of these was from the sibship. The ^{131}I saliva/serum ratios were approximately 1.0. All were euthyroid when treated with potassium iodide. A 50-year-old retarded woman with recurrent goiter and myxedema has been reported from South Africa. The ^{131}I S/P ratio was 0.83 [52]. Two such patients have been reported from Norway [53] and another from Japan [53a].

The block in transport of iodide may not necessarily be complete. Papadopoulos et al. [54] reported a 9-year-old male with goiter and retardation who had a partially defective iodide transport system. The ratio of iodide in the saliva to that in the plasma had a mean value of 17.2, far lower than the mean of 84.3 in our normal subjects. Serum T_4 iodine was 0.5 μg/dl, and tissue slices from a biopsy specimen achieved a concentration ratio of only 1.7 against the suspending medium, as compared to a normal value of 7.1.

It is interesting that the patient of Papadopoulos et al. [54] was retarded and had a partial defect, whereas others have not been permanently retarded and yet have had a complete defect. The reason for this may be that in this instance the iodine intake was low, as shown by a daily urinary excretion of 16 μg. The thyroid clearance of iodide was 4.5 ml/min (normal, 8 to 40), and the absolute uptake by the thyroid was 0.7 μg/h (normal, 0.5 to 6.0). Thus, even with only a partial defect in iodide transport, this patient was unable to accumulate enough iodine in the thyroid because of the limited dietary availability. Similar considerations may apply to the two retarded patients reported by Medeiros-Neto et al. [55]. In both, the S/P ratio for ^{131}I was less than 8.0, and they resided in a region which is deficient in iodine.

Genetics   The consanguinity of the parents of our patient and the appearance of the disorder in sibs in the families reported by Gilboa and Struwe suggest autosomal recessive inheritance. Eight of the reported patients were males, and there were seven females. These were from nine different families, three of which were consanguine. Autosomal recessive inheritance seems most probable.

Table 11-2   Diagnostic criteria for the complete iodide transport defect

Required	*Helpful and confirmatory*
1. Goiter; hypothyroid or compensated hypothyroid	1. No concentration of iodide by the gastric mucosa
2. Little if any uptake of radioiodine	2. No concentration of thiocyanate by the salivary glands

3. No concentration of iodide by the salivary glands	3. Thyroid biopsy
	  a. Hyperplasia
	  b. Low iodine content and concentration

	4. Metabolic response to iodide medication

Diagnosis   Identification of this defect depends on demonstration of low iodide clearance by the thyroid, hypothyroidism, hyperplastic goiter, and reduced transport of iodide by the salivary glands. Diagnostic criteria for the complete defect appear in Table 11-2. Diagnosis of a partial defect would depend upon establishing the fact that transport by the thyroid and other transporting systems is less than normal.

IODIDE OXIDATION AND BINDING TO PROTEINS; IODOTYROSINE COUPLING

Most of the iodine stored in the thyroid is covalently bound to 19 S thyroglobulin as components of amino acids: the thyroid hormones (T_3, T_4) and their precursors, the iodotyrosines (monoiodotyrosine, MIT, and diiodotyrosine, DIT). Thyroglobulin also contains minor amounts of 3,3',5'-iodothyronine (rT_3), 3,3'-diiodothyronine (T'_2), and monoiodohistidine. A few percent of the thyroglobulin is in the form of a dimer with a 27 S sedimentation coefficient. Other organic forms are found: particulate insoluble iodoproteins (a few percent of the iodine) and traces of iodinated lipids. The role of these forms is unknown. The concentrations of iodide (less than 0.25 percent) and of free hormones or iodotyrosines are very low.

The synthesis of thyroid hormones requires several elements: iodide, thyroglobulin as substrates, an H_2O_2-generating system, and thyroperoxidase. At least three steps are involved: generation of H_2O_2, oxidation of iodide and binding to the tyrosyl residues of thyroglobulin, and the oxidative coupling of these iodotyrosyls into iodothyronines. The last two steps take place in a sequential manner within the matrix of thyroglobulin; they are catalyzed by the same enzymes and will be considered together in this section. Iodination and oxidative coupling are posttranslational processes. They are independent of protein synthesis. (For general reviews, see Refs. 56–58.)

When iodination is allowed to proceed, the thyroid, despite a very active iodide transport, accumulates little iodide. Moreover, it is necessary to overload the transport system in order to demonstrate any activation of protein iodination [59, 60]. In the normal thyroid, iodide transport is therefore the limiting step in iodide uptake; the machinery of protein iodination is geared to lock any iodide trapped by the gland efficiently into covalent linkage [61].

The iodinating systems which can be demonstrated in thyroid homogenates are found in the sedimenting particulate fractions. This suggests that iodination takes place at the level of cell structures. On the other hand, autoradiography of glands exposed in vivo or in vitro to radioiodide always shows the protein-labeled material in the colloid lumen. The obvious explanation of this apparent paradox is that iodination occurs at the interface between the follicular cells and the colloid lumen, i.e., at the level of the apical membrane and its microvilli [61]. This hypothesis is supported by the autoradiographic demonstration by both light and electron microscopy of rings of radioiodine-labeled proteins at the periphery of the colloid and on the apical cell membrane early after in vivo administration of radioiodide, as well as by the reported relative enrichment of iodinating activity in preparation of apical cell membranes [56, 57, 62, 63]. Histochemic staining demonstrates peroxidase activity on the apical cell surface [64]. This localization fits the location of the substrates of protein iodination, iodide, and thyroglobulin, which are concentrated in the lumen, and of the cytosol coenzymes NADPH and NADH of the H_2O_2-generating system. It also explains the nice correlation between iodinating capacity and follicular structure during ontogenesis and findings in cell cultures. This arrangement also sequestrates H_2O_2 and possibly oxygen radicals and an iodinating system that might otherwise iodinate cell lipids and proteins themselves in the absence of the proper substrate thyroglobulin [65]. Under some circumstances, iodination can take place inside the follicular cells, e.g., in isolated cells and in some tumors [66]. Peroxidase staining may also be observed in several cell locations. Although such a mechanism may operate in some pathologic conditions, its physiologic significance is doubtful. On the other hand, whether iodination at the apex of the cell can also take place during exocytosis in these vesicles remains an open question [67].

All the peroxidases need H_2O_2 in order to oxidize I^- and to bind it to proteins. Protein iodination in acellular thyroid particulate systems is inhibited by catalase. The source of H_2O_2 in the follicular cell is termed the H_2O_2-generating system, but its nature is poorly known. As in leukocytes, NADH and NADPH, mostly the latter, stimulate iodination in acellular systems. Accordingly, it has been postulated that the system might be a NADPH (NADH) oxidase. NADPH cytochrome c reductase could be a part of the system, since antibodies against this enzyme inhibit iodination in vitro [61]. Since the enzyme is not thought to interact directly with O_2, other autooxidizable factor(s) must be involved. Vitamin K_3, cytochrome b, and flavin have been suggested. H_2O_2 could be formed from O_2^- as a precursor by superoxide dismutase, and thyroid cells, like all cells, contain such enzymes. Thyroid NADPH cytochrome c reductase has not been found to produce O_2^-, and superoxide dismutase does not inhibit iodination in acellular systems [58]. Monoamine oxidase and xanthine oxidase have also been proposed as thyroid H_2O_2-generating systems.

In intact cell, as in acellular systems, H_2O_2 always greatly enhances iodination; catalase inhibits iodination; and stimulation by TSH of iodination in dog thyroid slices is accompanied by a stimulation of H_2O_2 formation. These facts suggest that H_2O_2 generation may be the limiting step, i.e., the regulated step in iodination [65].

Inorganic iodide must lose an electron before it can displace hydrogen from tyrosyl residues. This is accomplished in the presence of H_2O_2 by thyroid peroxidase. The substances, such as most antithyroid drugs and goitrogens, which inhibit protein iodination in vivo or in intact cells, inhibit the peroxide-peroxidase system. Thyroid peroxidase is a membrane-bound enzyme which has been purified from iodinating particulates. It is similar in many aspects to other peroxidases, such as lactoperoxidase and horseradish peroxidase. It is a hemoprotein of 100,000 daltons with rather broad specificity. It is active only in the presence of H_2O_2, but excess H_2O_2 inhibits it. The enzyme catalyzes the iodination of free or bound tyrosines, and it also catalyzes the oxidation of I^- to I_2 and that of tyrosine to bityrosine. Nunez and Pommier have shown that these reactions involve two closely related binding sites which bind either tyrosine or iodide, oxidize them to free radicals, and then bind these covalently [58].

$$E + H_2O_2 + \left\langle \begin{array}{c} 1 \\ 2 \end{array} \right. + I^- + Tyr \longrightarrow E \left\langle \begin{array}{c} I^0 \\ Tyr^0 \end{array} \right. \longrightarrow E + MIT \quad (1)$$

This explains why each time I_2 is formed in the reaction, iodination is inhibited, and thus why high levels of iodide inhibit iodination. Inhibition of iodination by thiourea and similar drugs is attributed to two reactions. In the absence of iodide, the drug inactivates the peroxidase irreversibly, and in the presence of iodide the enzyme catalyzes the oxidation of the drug, thus partially preventing enzyme inactivation. In the latter case, antithyroid drugs behave as competitors of iodination [56, 57].

Thyroid peroxidase, like other peroxidases, is also able to catalyze the intramolecular coupling of thyroglobulin iodotyrosyl groups in vitro. The same antithyroid agents which inhibit iodination in intact cells and in acellular systems also inhibit oxidative coupling in these systems. Iodothyronine synthesis by intermolecular coupling of free 3,5-diiodo-4-hydroxyphenylpyruvic acid (DIHPPA) to iodotyrosines bound in thyroglobulin is possible, but there is little evidence that this mechanism operates in vivo, and all the available data on coupling can be explained without postulating this supplementary hypothesis [56].

Thyroid peroxidase may couple two iodotyrosines by the same mechanism as that of iodination. Two iodotyrosyl groups bound to the two enzyme-binding sites would be coupled after oxidation to iodotyrosyl radicals. The coupling would thus result in the replacement in the peptidic chains of thyroglobulin of one iodotyrosine by an iodothyronine and the other by a dehydroalanine. Thyroid peroxidase is the only enzyme of this class which catalyzes iodination and coupling at physiologic pH. Other peroxidases catalyze the two reactions at different pHs. Coupling requires iodotyrosines and H_2O_2 and also iodide [58].

The formation of iodotyrosines and iodothyronines in thyroglobulin does not follow a simple MIT, DIT, T_3, and T_4 precursor-product relationship. In fact, the kinetics suggest that iodination and coupling proceed in a rigid sequential manner, so that only four to eight tyrosyl groups, which are among the first to be iodinated, can be coupled into iodothyronines. T_3 is preferentially formed at low levels of iodination but never exceeds 0.4 mole T_3 per mole of thyroglobulin. A large part of the 110 tyrosyl groups in thyroglobulin are not iodinated, while only part of the MIT can be transformed into DIT. There is a maximal number of iodothyronines synthesized in thyroglobulin (three to four). All these facts indicate that there are rigid structural and spatial requirements for tyrosyl iodination and coupling; they are imposed by the thyroglobulin structure itself [56, 68, 69].

Iodination of thyroglobulin is accompanied by important structural changes in the protein. There is an increase in the sedimentation coefficient (17 to 19 S), differences in shape (from ovoid to cylindrical), lower dissociability, etc. These changes reflect the effects of the addition of iodine, but also those of cystine formation and structural changes in the protein.

In species in which the limiting step in iodination is the generation of H_2O_2 the main or first-line regulation of the system should bear on this mechanism. Indeed, TSH and cyclic AMP analogues enhance iodination and H_2O_2 generation in dog thyroid slices [5]. The inhibitory effect of iodide on adenylate cyclase after its oxidation to an unknown intermediate certainly affects this system, but other effects of iodide are not excluded [79]. Thyroid peroxidase itself is also inhibited by excess iodide, which competes with tyrosine for the second substrate site of the enzyme. The latter effect, alone or in combination with the former, could explain the well-known Wolff-Chaikoff effect, in which excess iodide inhibits protein iodination in intact cells. No evidence has been found of an action of TSH or cyclic AMP on thyroid peroxidase. Two biochemical controls of the isolated peroxidase have been demonstrated: a requirement for iodide in the coupling reaction and an activation of the enzyme by very low levels (10^{-7} M) of DIT. The physiologic relevance of these controls remains to be elucidated [56].

In normal humans, radioiodide is organified immediately after trapping. The thyroid radioactivity curve rises while the plasma curve decreases, and no radioiodide can be chased from the thyroid by thiocyanate or perchlorate. In the case of a complete block of protein iodination, thyroid radioactivity declines in parallel with plasma radioiodide, and this radioactivity is completely released within minutes after administration of anions such as SCN^- and ClO_4^-. It is thus easy to detect qualitatively in vivo a complete block of protein iodination. With partial defects, the perchlorate discharge test is not very sensitive, and quantitative measurements in vivo of protein iodination capacity are needed. This requires a protocol in which this parameter could be measured (as radioiodide uptake or clearance) under conditions in which this step becomes rate limiting, i.e., at relatively high ($\sim 10^5$ M) iodide concentrations.

Iodinating activity can be studied in intact cells at high concentrations of iodide (10^{-5} to $10^{-4}M$). The activation of this step in metabolism by an exogenous H_2O_2-generating system would indicate that the H_2O_2 supply is limiting in the tissue and would be an argument for the normality of thyroid peroxidase [70]. The effect of H_2O_2 can also be investigated in acellular preparations. The function of thyroid peroxidase can be studied in particulate or solubilized preparations, employing guaiacol oxidation, oxidation of I^- to I_2, binding of I^- to thyroglobulin, and coupling of iodotyrosines into thyroglobulin which contains iodotyrosines but little iodothyronines either in the presence or absence of hematin [58].

Related Clinical Disorders

Familial Goiter from Failure to Form Organic Iodine Organification Defect; Peroxidase Defect A number of patients have been studied who have an impairment in the organification of iodine. They belong to a category of inherited thyroid metabolic error which is illustrated by the following case reports.

A female patient was 16 years old in 1949 at the time of the initial studies. She was dwarfed and grossly retarded mentally [71]. The thyroid was enlarged five or six times the normal size, nodular, and firm. A bruit and thrill were present, and the skin over the thyroid felt warm to the touch. The PBI concentration of the blood was 1.0 μg/dl. The patient had three normal sibs and three who were similarly affected. The parents were consanguine (Fig. 11-7).

When the patient had been without thyroid medication for 3 weeks, ^{131}I was given orally. The labeled iodine in the gland reached a high plateau in less than 2 h. A 1-g dose of KSCN was given by mouth 27 h later. This caused an immediate and striking fall in the concentration of labeled iodine in the gland (Fig. 11-8). At the end of 2 h, the count had fallen to 25 percent of the previous level.

At thyroidectomy, the gland weighed 97 g. There was intense hyperplasia, coupled with cystic degeneration and fibrosis. An analysis of the tissue disclosed a PBI concentration of 1.4 μg/100 g. The normal thyroid gland, weighing about 20 g, contains from 4 to 15 mg iodine, of which 1 to 2 percent at most is inorganic.

The mother, one of the normal sibs, and three of the affected sibs of this patient were similarly studied. Thyroid function in the mother and the normal sibs was normal, but two of the three sibs with hypothyroidism and goiter had thyroid abnormalities entirely similar to those of this patient. The third sib was not available for physiologic studies; his huge goiter had been removed several years earlier.

Identical twin girls (grandnieces of patient VI 5 of Fig. 11-7) were brought for study at age 10½ years [72]. Both had thyroids which had been observed to be enlarged at age 1 month. Growth and development seemed normal, but bone age was retarded. The thyroids were four to five times the normal size. There were no clinical signs of hypothyroidism. Serum T_4 concentrations were 7.4 μg/dl and 7.5 μg/dl in the sibs.

Each patient was given 5 μCi radioactive iodine orally while fasting. The labeled iodine accumulated rapidly reaching a plateau of 91 percent uptake at 4 h. At 5½ h, 500 mg $KClO_4$ was given orally. As may be seen in Fig. 11-8, there was a rapid loss of labeled iodine which continued for 2 h, when 22 percent of the administered dose remained in the gland. Administration of propylthiouracil occasioned no noteworthy acceleration of the rate of loss of labeled iodine from the gland or appearance of labeled iodine in the urine.

Since these two children were the product of a nonconsanguine marriage, the findings were interpreted as indicating a partial peroxidase defect resulting from compound heterozygosity for two different abnormal alleles.

The patients described in the preceding paragraphs illustrate the usual clinical and laboratory findings for placing them in the organification defect category. Further experience and laboratory studies have demonstrated biochemical and presumably genetic heterogeneity, as might have been anticipated in view of the complex nature of the process of thyroid iodine organification. A number of additional reports have appeared [73–78].

This disorder can now be subdivided into five subgroups according to distinctly different biochemical characteristics; these subgroups are not clearly homogeneous within themselves.

ABSENT, INACTIVE, OR ABNORMAL THYROID PEROXIDASE

A 17-year-old mentally deficient male patient studied by Pommier et al. was found to be hypothyroid at age 6 months [79]. A goiter had been present for at least 5 years. The plasma thyroxine concentration was 1.2 μg/dl, the T_3 was 85 μg/dl, and the ^{131}I uptake was 26 percent at 2 h, with rapid turnover. Administration of 400 mg $KClO_4$ resulted in the disappearance of 90 percent of the ^{131}I from the gland in 45 min. Serum TSH concentrations were high and reached high levels after administration of TRH.

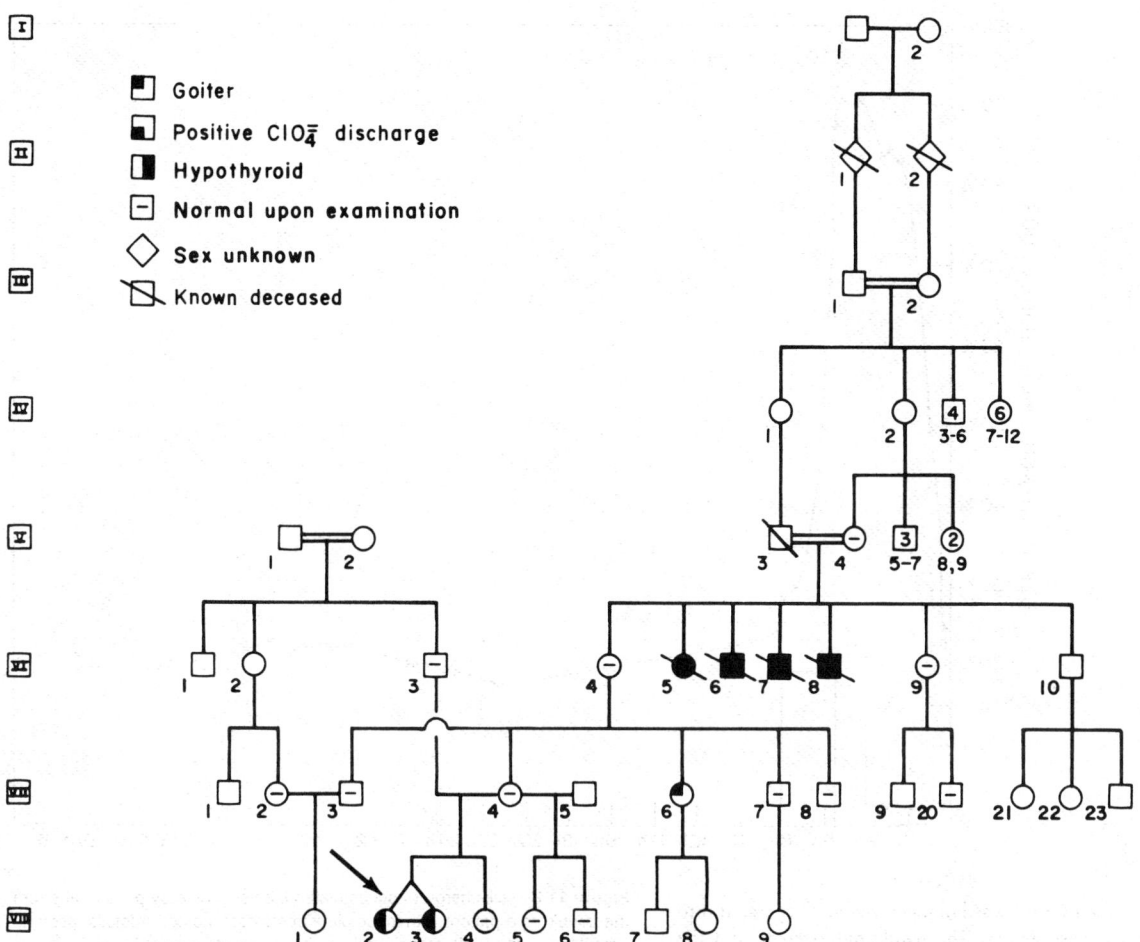

Figure 11-7 Family tree of a kindred with the peroxidase defect. The arrow points to the twins described in the test who have a partial defect; their maternal aunt and three uncles as shown had complete peroxidase defects.

Microscopic examination of a large excised thyroid lobe disclosed "colloid goiter" without nodules or fibrosis. It was not possible to demonstrate peroxidase activity either before or after solubilization with trypsin and digitonin when tested by guaiacol peroxidation, by iodination using poorly iodinated thyroglobulin as substrate, or by the $I^- \rightarrow I_2$ reaction. Activity could not be enhanced by preincubation with hematin. A normal amount of thyroglobulin was present which was almost lacking in iodine. The findings were interpreted as resulting from an absence of peroxidase.

Several other mentally deficient, hypothyroid patients with goiter have been described who also appeared to lack thyroid peroxidase [80–83]. The mother of one of these patients was euthyroid but had a goiter which had reduced peroxidase activity [82]. In some instances [80, 83] it is not clear whether the peroxidase was in fact absent, or whether it was masked and might have been available if the enzyme had been solubilized by treatment with trypsin and a detergent, as in the patient described by Pommier et al. [79].

An abnormal peroxidase was evidently responsible for a large goiter in a euthyroid patient studied by Nunez et al. [84]. The solubilized preparation peroxidized I^- to I_2, but the K_m was low. It did not peroxidize guaiacol nor did it iodinate an iodine-poor thyroglobulin, and it was abnormal in some of its physical properties. The thyroglobulin from the gland was virtually free of iodine. The total lack of iodinating activity and the euthyroid state of the patient was an unresolved discrepancy. Another euthyroid patient with goiter and diminished peroxidase activity has been described [85]. The thyroid of a

retarded female was studied by Niepomniszcze et al. [86] and found to have almost no peroxidase activity, even after solubilization and reincubation with hematin. The thyroglobulin from this gland could not be iodinated enzymatically by human or bovine peroxidase but could be iodinated chemically to normal iodination levels. It contained little iodine initially. Thus there appeared to be two defects: almost absent peroxidase and a thyroglobulin which was not iodinated by normal peroxidase. The latter defect was attributed to a possible failure of oxidation of some part of the thyroglobulin molecule, but other thyroglobulin obtained from glands without peroxidase activity is readily iodinated enzymatically [79]. A possible explanation for the resistance of this thyroglobulin is the presence of a firmly attached inhibitor such as that described by Pommier et al. [87].

From the foregoing, it may be concluded that the organification defect may be attributed to absent, reduced, or abnormal peroxidase and that the defect may be complete or incomplete.

PEROXIDASE APOENZYME-PROSTHETIC GROUP DEFECT
Two patients have been described with reduced peroxidase activity which was restored by incubation of the enzyme complex with its prosthetic group, hematin.

A 16-year-old girl was found at age 6 years to have a goiter [88, 106]. A thyroidectomy was done at age 12, but the goiter returned. She was entirely euthyroid. Serum concentrations of T_4 and TSH were normal. Administration of perchlorate resulted in a loss of half the ^{131}I in the gland.

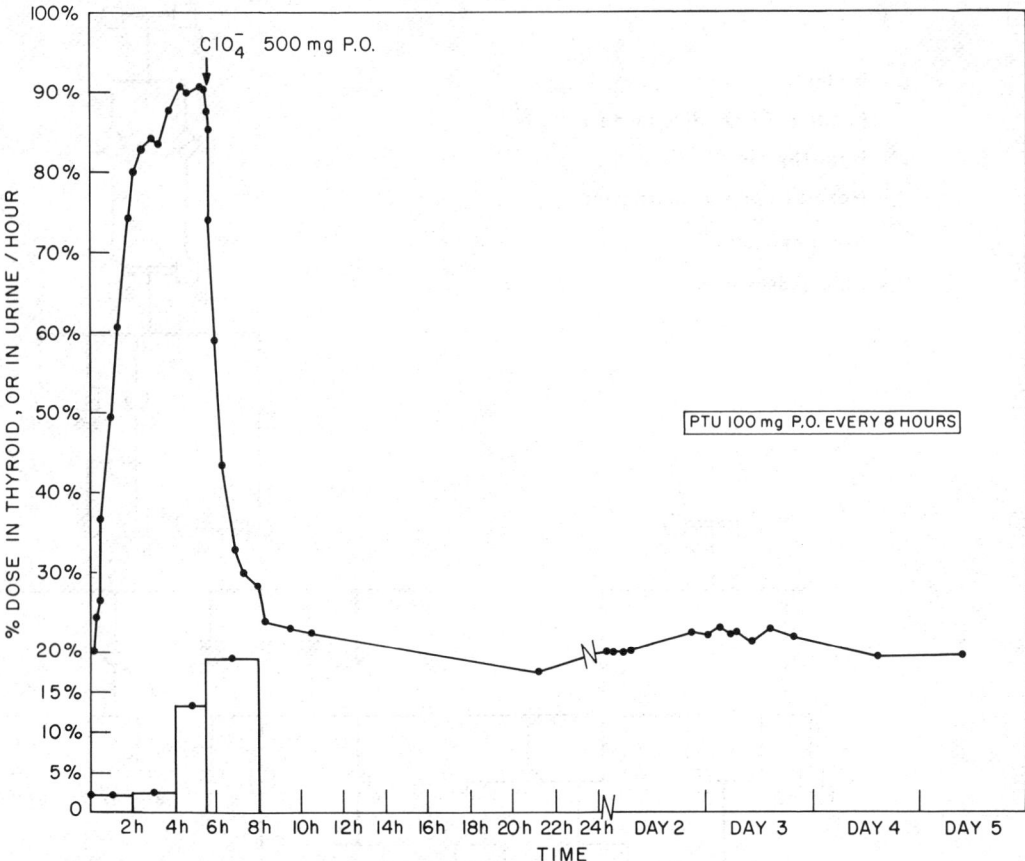

Figure 11-8 Discharge of accumulated labeled iodide by perchlorate from the thyroid of a patient with incomplete peroxidase defect. Administration of propylthiouracil (PTU) occasioned no change in retention of iodine by the thyroid or increased renal excretion (bars).

A specimen of the thyroid was homogenized and separated into fractions for peroxidase assays. The whole homogenate and the fractions had no peroxidase activity by the triiodide assay and did not iodinate tyrosine. A digitonin-solubilized preparation behaved similarly and also failed to peroxidize guaiacol. Some evidence of doubtful significance was found for an inhibitor with the triiodide and guaiacol assays but not in the tyrosine iodinase and hydroxyphenyl pyruvic acid assays. Preincubation of the solubilized enzyme preparation restored peroxidase activity to normal levels in the tyrosine iodinase assay but caused only a negligible change in the triiodide assay. Presumably, in vivo there was enough peroxidase activity in the large goiter to produce an adequate amount of hormone; the binding of peroxidase to its prosthetic group seemed to be faulty.

A second patient has been reported who evidently had a similar defect. The patient was hypothyroid [89]. Peroxidase activity both in crude particulate and in a trypsin/deoxycholate-solubilized preparation was restored toward, but not to, normal by incubation with hematin. Improvement in activity was evident in the iodide peroxidase, tyrosine, tyrosine iodinase, and guaiacol assays. The enzyme seemed abnormally sensitive to H_2O_2 in the iodide peroxidase assay system.

PEROXIDASE INHIBITED OR IN AN ABNORMAL INTRACELLULAR LOCATION

An enlarged thyroid had been observed in a 25-year-old mother of two normal children [84, 90]. She appeared to be euthyroid, but the total serum thyroxine concentration while on no medication was 1.2 μg/dl. The radioiodine uptake was elevated, and a third of that accumulation was promptly discharged by administration of $KClO_4$. A subtotal thyroidectomy yielded 500 g thyroid tissue.

Thyroid particles prepared from the homogenized thyroid were "pseudosolubilized" by treatment with digitonin or solubilized by treatment also with trypsin. The peroxidase was similar in its physical properties to hog thyroid peroxidase. The K_m for oxidation of I^- to I_2 with the solubilized enzyme was the same as that for hog enzyme. The K_m values for peroxidation of guaiacol were similar. Iodination of iodine-poor thyroglobulin was substantially lower than that of hog peroxidase if the two preparations were normalized with respect to iodide peroxidation, and relatively less iodothyronine was formed. The pseudosolubilized enzyme was much less active in all systems than in the preparation which was treated with both trypsin and digitonin. Thyroglobulin was present and normal, but with a low iodine concentration. At least a partial explanation for the findings in this patient is that the thyroid peroxidase was abnormally bound in the thyroid particles, from where it was released by initial treatment with trypsin. This does not explain the reduced capacity of the solubilized enzyme to iodinate thyroglobulin or to catalyze the iodotyrosine coupling reaction.

Another patient with a much reduced thyroid peroxidase activity has been described [89]. The peroxidase had a normal K_m H_2O_2, but the peroxidase was found largely in pellets sedimenting between 39,000 and 105,000 g, whereas usually it is found in the highest specific activity in the 39,000-g pellet. A cytostructural abnormality has also been proposed as an explanation for the thyroid abnormality in a large sibship from Brazil [91]. Three members had goiter and were euthyroid, while five had goiter and were hypothyroid. The thyroids of three with positive perchlorate tests were available for study. Peroxidase activity was normal or elevated by three assay methods in all three, but in one, approximately half the activity was found in the 105,000-*g* supernatant, whereas normally it resides primarily in the pellet.

These accounts, in which an abnormality in the availability of peroxidase was described, do not lead to a clear concept of the basic disorder. The peroxidase in the first patient was abnormal even after solubilization and purification, and in the other two, the only abnormality was altered distribution in centrifugal cuts.

DEFICIENCY IN H_2O_2 PRODUCTION While a deficiency in the production of H_2O_2 has been suggested several times as a cause of impaired iodide organification, in only one instance has strong evidence been offered [92]. A 37-year-old euthyroid woman developed a goiter in the course of a pregnancy. The plasma T_4 concentration was normal and the TSH was elevated. Thyroid uptake of ^{131}I was rapid and high, and most of it was quickly discharged by administration of thiocyanate. The gland was composed of well-differentiated follicles lined with cuboidal cells.

Incorporation of iodide into protein occurred only slightly in homogenate of the thyroid but was increased to near-normal levels by the addition of H_2O_2, an H_2O_2-generating system, FAD, or the reduced form of cytochrome b_5. Microsomal NADPH cytochrome b_5 reductase activity was low. The major protein of the thyroid was thyroglobulin, which had a moderately reduced iodine content. It was normally iodinated by horseradish peroxidase and an H_2O_2-generating system.

Administration of large doses of FAD (250 mg per day) seemed to reduce the goiter size and restore normal thyroid function. Riboflavin was without effect. This is puzzling, since FAD administered orally is resolved in the intestine to riboflavin before absorption. The author suggested that enough of the FAD might have been absorbed intact to reach the thyroid, where as cofactor it could support the cytochrome b_5 reductase. Thus, the evidence might suggest a defect of the synthesis of FAD, with resulting reduced production of H_2O_2, and deficient thyroglobulin iodination or impaired binding of FAD by its apoprotein cytochrome b_5 reductase.

RECEPTOR ABNORMALITY There are several reports of apparent peroxidase deficiency, as suggested by positive perchlorate tests, when in fact peroxidase seemed to be normal when tested. However, the fault appeared to be attributable to abnormality or inaccessibility of the receptor, thyroglobulin.

Kusakabe [92a] described his studies on a 51-year-old woman whose development had been normal. The goiter was of recent onset. Radioiodine uptake was 33 percent at 2 h and fell precipitously to 4 percent with administration of thiocyanate. The removed thyroid showed no evidence of lymphocytic infiltration. Particulates prepared from the thyroid homogenate showed normal peroxidase activity in the pyrogallol and triiodine assays and iodinated thyroglobulin normally, and these activities were not significantly enhanced by addition of a peroxide-generating system. The receptor protein, on the other hand, seemed distinctly abnormal. It was much less well iodinated by the particulates or by horseradish peroxidase than was normal thyroglobulin. The thyroglobulin was unusually readily dissociated into subunits, even during the initial ultracentrifugation. More than half the thyroglobulin had an $s_{20,w}$ of 3.0 and the rest an $s_{20,w}$ of 18.1. Curiously and inexplicably, the dissociated thyroglobulin appeared to precipitate with antihuman albumin antiserum, whereas prior to dissociation it was completely precipitable with antithyroglobulin antiserum. When the thyroglobulin was iodinated with I_2 and analyzed spectrophotometrically, a

normal amount of MIT was found, but the number of DIT and tyrosine residues found was much smaller than in normal thyroglobulin. The native thyroglobulin had a low normal iodine content.

A different type of abnormality has been observed in two enlarged thyroids from patients who had organification defects [87]. Thyroglobulin prepared from these glands had a low content of iodine. They were not iodinated by hog thyroid peroxidase and an H_2O_2-generating system in the presence of iodide. They were normal by analytical ultracentrifugation and by Sephadex G 200 and agarose chromatography. After extensive dialysis, the thyroglobulin was normally iodinated by the hog peroxidase system. The dialyzable inhibitor was thermostable, but its identity was not established.

Absence of the normal receptor protein has been suggested as a cause of the deficiency of peroxidase activity [93]. Two sisters with congenital goiter and positive perchlorate tests appeared to have normal or elevated thyroid peroxidase activity by the usual assay methods. No thyroglobulin could be detected. Nevertheless, a number of other patients have been described who had no thyroglobulin but who had negative perchlorate discharge tests.

INTERPRETATION Patients similar or identical to those described in the preceding paragraphs have been reported [94–99], and thyroid tumors have been described which concentrated iodine without organification [70, 100]. Neel et al. [101] surveyed 50 sibships containing at least one patient with congenital hypothyroidism and found only one family with an organification defect as demonstrated by a positive SCN^- test. In another study from the same laboratory, positive SCN^- tests were found in 7 of 56 Michigan cretins [102]. The potential malignancy of congenital goiters with organification defect has been noted by Salabe et al. [103].

The common denominator of the patients in this group is the release of labeled iodine from the thyroid gland upon administration of KSCN or $KClO_4$. The clinical findings have not been uniform. Some patients have been severely cretinous, with profound retardation of structural and intellectual development. Those reported by Clayton et al. [104] and by others were clinically euthyroid, as confirmed by laboratory examination.

The release of labeled iodine from the thyroid by SCN^- or ClO_4^- indicates a store of inorganic iodide in the gland which can be readily displaced. Normally, virtually none of the accumulated iodine can be displaced in this way. Those patients who show a release of labeled iodine appear to have a metabolic defect which impairs the conversion of accumulated iodide to organically bound iodine. Since this limits or prevents hormone synthesis, compensatory hypertrophy and hyperplasia of the thyroid occur, as well as the consequences of an insufficient hormonal supply.

There is biochemical as well as clinical diversity within this class of inherited disorders of the thyroid. In some, it has not been possible to identify peroxidase activity [83, 86, 100, 105, 106]. In others, peroxidase activity is demonstrable only after addition of hematin [88, 106] or after solubilization of the enzyme by treatment of tissue homogenate with trypsin and digitonin [84, 90]. No information is available regarding possible allelism of the various subtypes of the disorder. Minimal diagnostic criteria for clinical and laboratory ascertainment appear in Table 11-3.

The occurrence of goiter without hypothyroidism in family

Table 11-3 Diagnostic criteria for the peroxidase defect

Required	Helpful and confirmatory
1. Goiter; hypothyroid or compensated hypothyroid	1. Thyroid biopsy a. Hyperplasia
2. Developmental retardation usually	b. Low iodine content and concentration
3. Rapid accumulation and turnover of radioiodine	c. Little if any organic iodine
4. Rapid discharge of radioiodine from the thyroid after administration of SCN^- or ClO_4^-	d. Little iodinating activity in intact cells e. Absence of the effect of exogenous H_2O_2 (peroxidase defect)
5. Low T_4 is usual; elevated TSH or enhanced TSH response to TRH	f. Absent or abnormal peroxidase activity (with or without hematin) 2. In vivo kinetics consistent with an expanded inorganic iodide pool

members of index patients [72] has suggested that thyroid disease may be a manifestation of the heterozygous state of a condition which, when homozygous, results in hypothyroidism, goiter, and retardation. Perchlorate discharge tests have failed to disclose significant iodide discharge in these patients as an indication of limited peroxidase activity. Perhaps a more stringent test of peroxidase activity in the thyroids of obligate heterozygotes would disclose a partial defect. On the other hand, Baschieri et al. [109] tested a large number of patients with thyroid disease and their relatives with ClO_4^- after administration of ^{131}I. A significant number of normal relatives of patients who had positive discharge test results also had positive test results, whereas no relatives of patients with negative results had positive results. The authors suggested that by this method of ascertainment, the character has dominant transmission.

Familial Goiter and Deaf Mutism (Pendred's Syndrome)

A 67-year-old retired craftsman, a deaf mute, had always been well [110]. A goiter was found incidentally. Five of eight sibs were deaf. The parents were not consanguine. The patient was intelligent. His thyroid was diffusely enlarged to about three times the normal size. There was no clinical suggestion of hypothyroidism. Findings from routine clinical laboratory studies were within normal limits, except for mild glucose intolerance. Hearing loss was in the range of 95 to 100 decibels in both ears and was sensorineural in type.

Histologic examination of a thyroid biopsy specimen disclosed a variable pattern of small nodules. Follicles varied in size and contained colloid. The epithelium was infolded slightly in focal areas, and the cell height indicated moderate hyperplasia.

A 62-year-old brother also had findings typical of Pendred's syndrome. His health had always been good. Physical examination disclosed normal findings, except for deafness and a diffuse goiter enlarged two to three times. Routine clinical laboratory findings, chest roentgenogram, and electrocardiogram were within normal limits. Hearing loss was complete and was sensorineural in type.

Measurements of PBI, BEI, and total and free T_4 were low normal. The ^{131}I uptake was 22.7 percent at 4 h and 41.6 percent at 24 h. The serum PB ^{131}I conversion ratio and the half-life of labeled T_4 and plasma TSH were normal. Antithyroid antibodies were absent. TBG and TBPA capacities proved to be slightly lower than normal.

Sodium perchlorate given 2 h after ^{131}I resulted in a 25 percent fall

in the counting rate over the thyroid by 30 min and a 31 percent fall by 60 min.

Studies on the patient's brother (who also had Pendred's syndrome) were normal, except that the result of the perchlorate discharge test was not positive.

Analysis of the thyroid biopsy disclosed that more than 90 percent of ^{131}I was in the soluble fraction. The MIT/DIT ratio for the soluble fraction was 5.4 for ^{131}I, given 19 days before surgery, and 4.9 for ^{125}I, given 2 days before the biopsy. Not more than 3 percent of the labeled iodine was present as iodothyronines. T_3 probably represented about one-third of the thyronine fraction.

Since Brain reported five families with congenital goiter and deafness in 1927 [111], many other families have been reported with this association of diseases [112–113]. With few exceptions, the clinical pattern has been uniform. Goiter has been apparent either at birth or within the first decade or two of life, and nerve deafness has been present from birth or has developed during childhood. Intelligence and growth have usually, but not always, been normal. Vestibular function has been normal or somewhat impaired, and the tympanic membranes have been intact.

These patients have usually not had huge goiters. Thyroid function, as assessed by the usual clinical and laboratory data, has been normal in most of them. The serum concentrations of PBI in most of the affected persons of Johnsen's kindreds were distinctly low [116], and the mean value of the 15 patients of Thould and Scowen was 3.36 μg/dl [115]. Two of the four affected members of the sibship of Elman [116] developed invasive adenocarcinoma, and Roberts' patient [117] had a localized histologic change suggestive of malignant alteration. Two of the four patients in Thieme's sibship also had a local malignant change without evidence of distant extension [118].

Morgans and Trotter [119] first showed that ClO_4^- causes an appreciable discharge of iodide from the thyroids of patients with Pendred's syndrome, and this abnormality has become a hallmark of the disease. The fraction of the radioiodine which accumulates in the thyroid within the first hour or two and which is discharged with ClO_4^- is usually 25 to 50 percent. Discharge is not so complete as in the patients with complete organification defect described in the preceding sections.

Medeiros-Neto et al. studied the thyroids from two patients with congenital goiter and deafness from Brazil [120]. Both showed a large fraction of the iodine present as a dense particulate iodoprotein. Less than 15 percent of the iodine was present as 19 S protein. A euthyroid female with deafness and a huge goiter, studied by Shane et al. [121], demonstrated the expected radioiodine discharge with thiocyanate. No T_3 or T_4 was found in the thyroid protein, and a defect both in organification of iodine and in iodotyrosine coupling was considered. Ljungren et al. [122], on the other hand, found normal peroxidase in two thyroids from patients with Pendred's syndrome, as have others [123, 124], and suggested a defect in the production of H_2O_2.

The deafness remains puzzling. Changes have been induced in the middle ear of developing chicks by injections of propylthiouracil into the yolk sac, and these changes are prevented by simultaneously administering T_4 [125]. Similarly, changes in the hair cells and tectorial membranes of the cochlea appear in the pups of mice whose mothers are given PTU, and these changes also fail to appear if T_4 is given [126, 127].

There have been few opportunities to study thyroid specimens from patients with this disease. The usual histologic pattern has been that of nodular goiter. The principal iodoprotein of our patient was a 19 S soluble component, while that of Medeiros-Neto et al. was an insoluble complex, and that of Desai et al. [128] was a more slowly sedimenting (15.2 to 16.8 S) protein with immunologic and solubility properties of thyroglobulin. Cave and Dunn [124] have described heterogeneity in amino acid composition in three specimens of thyroglobulin prepared from the gland of a patient with Pendred's syndrome, but the thyroglobulin was similar to normal thyroglobulin in physical properties. Both our patients [110] and that of Shane et al. [121] had a high ratio of MIT to DIT. Our patient had T_4 in the gland, whereas the patient of Shane et al. had none. Our patient and his brother with Pendred's syndrome seemed unusually sensitive to perchlorate in that inhibition of radioiodine uptake was abnormally prolonged after administration of perchlorate; this observation has been confirmed in a large kindred in rural Brazil [129], but its significance is unclear. The same phenomenon has been observed in a patient with peroxidase defects without deafness [129a]. Suggested diagnostic criteria appear in Table 11-4.

INTERPRETATION The patients of the Pendred group appear to differ from those with the full organification defect in several particulars. (1) They are not myxedematous, and most but not all [130] are clinically euthyroid, whereas the patients with the full organification defect (who are not deaf) are usually cretinous. Nevertheless, an exaggerated response to TRH suggests a compensated or borderline hypothyroid state [131], and instances of retardation are reported [132]. (2) The patients with Pendred's syndrome usually do not have large goiters. (3) The discharge of labeled iodine from the gland is neither so precipitous nor so complete. (4) The pathogenetic relationship between the aural changes and those in the thyroid is entirely obscure. There is no evidence for fetal hypothyroidism in the Pendred syndrome, and yet only by inducing fetal hypothyroidism in the experimental animal can changes be induced in the ear. (5) The curious hypersensitivity to perchlorate also remains unexplained.

GENETICS Fraser et al. [133] summarized their studies up to 1960. They found 113 affected patients among 72 families. Johnsen's two families included 24 members, 21 of whom were personally examined [114]. Of these, 12 exhibited goiter and deafness. Of Johnsen's patients, four were the result of intermarriage of two affected members of two families, and in this kindred, the disease appeared in successive generations. Fraser et al. [133] reported the appearance of the disease among the children of a marriage between two persons with Pendred's

syndrome. The disease had appeared only within a single generation in all other recorded instances. While in most instances the pattern is that of an autosomal recessive inheritance with tight concordance between goiter and deafness, there are reports of dissociation within kindreds of deafness and goiter [134]. Approximately one-half the sibs in the reported families have been afflicted, but if a correction is applied for inadequate ascertainment, then the ratio of affected to nonaffected sibs is almost 1:3 and accordingly fits the pattern of autosomal recessive inheritance [135]. A discordant note is patient 18 of Johnsen's family, and we do not know whether or not her husband had Pendred's syndrome. It is well known that the social intimacy among the deaf and blind often leads to marriage.

Congenital Hypothyroidism with Failure of Coupling of Iodotyrosines

Defective coupling of MIT and DIT into T_3 and T_4 appeared to be the cause of hypothyroidism and goiter in a 25-year-old retarded female [136]. A diagnosis of hypothyroidism was made at age 4, and desiccated thyroid was prescribed but taken only intermittently. A goiter was first observed at age 17. At 22, her PBI was 3.5 μg/dl. Earlier studies had disclosed an unusually rapid uptake of ^{131}I to values in excess of 95 percent. The labeled iodine in the thyroid was not dislodged by administration of KSCN. The daily excretion of ^{127}I was normal at a time when the patient had ingested no desiccated thyroid for the previous 8 weeks. A total thyroidectomy was performed. The specimen displayed extreme hyperplasia. There were two first-cousin marriages in the patient's immediate antecedents. A sister, 4 years older, suffered from an identical disorder.

Studies included measurements of the kinetics of iodine metabolism and chemical examination of the histologic specimen at the time of surgery. Radioiodine uptake reached a maximum of 99.3 percent within the first 2 h and was released at a rate approaching 3 percent per day. When methimazole was given, there was a sharp increase to 7.3 percent per day. Iodine clearance by the kidney was normal. The renal excretion rate of labeled iodine rose sharply upon administration of methimazole.

Chromatographic analysis of serial serum samples taken between 7 and 79 h after administration of ^{131}I disclosed T_4 and T_3 in all samples. Yet in spite of heavy labeling of the gland and a rapid turnover of iodine by the gland, it was impossible to demonstrate more than a trace of T_4 in the surgical thyroid specimen taken 79 h after administration of ^{131}I, although iodide and abundant MIT and DIT were demonstrated with ease.

Two lines of investigation indicated that the primary fault in this thyroid was an impaired ability to couple MIT and DIT into T_3 and T_4. Serial chromatographic analyses of the serum for many hours after the administration of ^{131}I demonstrated the early appearance of T_4 and T_3, whereas analysis of the glandular tissue failed to disclose labeled T_4 or T_3. Only when the whole gland was subjected to chemical analysis was it possible to identify a trace of T_4. Yet at the same time, abundant quantities of MIT and DIT were found. Thus it appeared that while this gland was making ample MIT and DIT and was storing them in large amounts, the T_4 and T_3 which were produced were not stored but were immediately released into the blood.

Supporting information was obtained from kinetic studies of iodine metabolism. For the details of these observations and their interpretation, the reader may consult the original publication [136]. It was possible to view the release of iodine from the gland in two ways. During administration of methimazole, the specific activity of the labeled iodine which appeared in the urine was extremely high: 17 percent per milligram at a time

Table 11-4 Diagnostic criteria for Pendred's syndrome

Required	Helpful and confirmatory
1. Goiter and nerve deafness; no iodide deficiency	1. Thyroid biopsy
2. Mild hypothyroid or compensated hypothyroid condition usually	a. Normal to slight hyperplasia
	b. Low concentration of iodine
3. Partial discharge of radioiodine from thyroid by SCN^- or ClO_4^-	c. MIT/DIT ratio high; iodotyrosine/iodothyronine ratio high
4. Hypersensitivity to ClO_4^- (?) (see text)	d. Thyroglobulin present and normal

when the specific activity of the gland was only 2.9 percent per milligram. This finding indicated that methimazole was blocking the reutilization of labeled iodine derived from a pool of high specific activity, whereas most of the labeled iodine in the thyroid was in a pool of low specific activity.

The amount of unlabeled iodine leaving the gland daily was calculated to be at least 1 mg (normal, 50 to 150 μg). Only a small fraction of the iodine leaving the gland could have been in the form of thyroid hormone, because otherwise the patient would have been thyrotoxic. Accordingly, the thyroid must have been releasing iodide or a readily metabolized iodinated substance which was quickly broken down, either by the gland itself or in the periphery, to yield iodine.

The simplest formulation to account for the facts was that the coupling of DIT to yield T_4 took place only to a limited degree. The T_4 which was formed was rapidly secreted. The highly stimulated gland maintained an exceedingly rapid flux of some of its own iodine. Some went on to form hormone, some was retained for storage as MIT and DIT, and a large fraction—perhaps in the form of MIT—was formed and released for deiododination, either in the gland or the periphery, or both.

Other patients with similar clinical and biochemical findings have been reported [133–139]. A woman with goiter since childhood but no hypothyroidism described by Pommier et al. had a thyroid with normal peroxidase K_m and V_{max} for the reaction $I^- \rightarrow I_2$ [84, 90]. It catalyzed the iodination of poorly iodinated thyroglobulin slightly less well than with controls but was markedly inefficient in catalyzing the peroxidase-directed coupling reaction. These observations indicated that peroxidation of iodide, thyroglobulin iodination, and coupling are separate functions of the peroxidase, and that in this patient there was a true coupling failure based on enzyme functional deficiency. Cooper et al. [139a] have reported studies on two subjects from a sibship of 14 who were goitrous, possibly mildly hypothyroid but with normal stature and intelligence, and had developed metastatic thyroid carcinoma. Kinetic studies disclosed a leak of nonhormonal iodine from the glands. It seems possible that the iodide leak was a result of impaired iodotyrosyl coupling, rapid turnover of glandular iodotyrosyl residues, and escape of the iodine from this pool into the plasma.

Coupling defect is a term which has been employed when goiter has been accompanied by a reduced rate of thyroid hormone synthesis but no impairment in the formation of MIT or DIT. It has been inferred that these findings arise from defective coupling of hormone precursors into finished hormone.

INTERPRETATION Coupling is a complex biochemical event which is doubtless vulnerable and is impaired by anything that dilutes the iodine in the thyroglobulin molecule. A paradigm of this is severe iodine deficiency [140].

The complexity of the coupling reaction suggests several hypothetical causes for the coupling defect. Apart from the causes of defective iodination which necessarily entail a coupling defect, the following mechanisms might be considered: a defect in the activation of the enzyme by iodide or DIT; defects in thyroglobulin structure which would prevent access of the involved tyrosyl groups to the peroxidase or would not satisfy the rigid spatial requirements of coupling; absence of thyroglobulin, etc. Such mechanisms could be classified into two categories: defects at the peroxidase level and at the thyroglobulin level. A distinction between these categories could be established by the joint crossed study of oxidative coupling in patient and normal thyroglobulin as catalyzed by patient and normal thyroid peroxidase, using the methods proposed by Nunez et al. [98]. The distinction between the coupling defect and the defect in some patients with impaired thyroglobulin synthesis may be blurred. It is possible to set up certain criteria which should be met if one is to localize a defect at this level (Table 11-5).

Little can be said regarding the genetics of this poorly defined group, which is almost surely heterogeneous. Consanguinity and family clustering are found in those consigned to this category. Both sexes are represented. The most probable pattern is autosomal recessive.

THYROGLOBULIN SYNTHESIS

Thyroglobulin is a large globular glycoprotein with a molecular weight of 660,000 and a sedimentation coefficient of approximately 19 S. It usually comprises about 75 percent of the total proteins of the mammalian thyroid, but this amount is subjected to wide variations depending on the activity of the gland. Thyroglobulin is secreted by thyroid cells into the lumen of the thyroid follicles, where, after iodination and coupling of a fraction of its tyrosyl residues, it becomes a storage form of T_3 and T_4. The carbohydrate moieties of thyroglobulin make up about 10 percent of the molecule, and they are organized into four types of carbohydrate units [10, 141]. The 27 and 37 S thyroglobulins are dimers and trimers of 19 S thyroglobulins formed during oxidation and iodination of the protein. They therefore result from the same pathway of genetic expression [142, 143] and will not be considered independently here.

The amino acid composition of thyroglobulin is not at all exceptional. It does not contain unusual amounts of tyrosines (2 percent; 122 residues per mole), but it has a large component of cysteine [230] mostly in the disulfide form. The coupling of iodotyrosines into iodothyronines is more efficient in iodinated thyroglobulin than in other artificially iodinated proteins. This suggests that there is a specific tertiary structure of the molecule. Biochemical models of the coupling mechanisms have been proposed, but the actual structural characteristics of the system are awaiting precise information about thyroglobulin structure [10, 58, 69].

Table 11-5 Diagnostic criteria for the coupling defect

1. Goiter; hypothyroid or compensated hypothyroid
2. Exclusion of other recognized defects
3. Thyroid biopsy 4 or more days after radioiodine
   a. High MIT/DIT ratio; little iodothyronine
   b. Hyperplasia
   c. Normal or altered thyroglobulin
   d. Normal or low, but not very low, iodine concentration and content
   e. Normal iodide peroxidase activity, but reduced catalysis of coupling in normal, low iodine thyroglobulin or reduced catalysis of coupling by normal peroxidase in the patient's thyroglobulin
4. For several days, higher urine iodine specific activity than total plasma specific activity
5. Possible demonstration by iodine kinetics of a substantial iodide "leak" and a rapid intrathyroidal recycling of iodine

The quaternary structure of thyroglobulin itself has been a controversial subject for many years. Studies dealing with the translation of thyroglobulin mRNA have indicated that thyroglobulin is a dimer composed of 300,000-dalton polypeptide subunits [10]. Some questions remain unanswered. Do thyroglobulin subunits contain identical polypeptide chains? Is there a single species of thyroglobulin molecule? Experiments dealing with the analytical characterization of the protein have yielded conflicting results. Recent data involving the restriction mapping of a synthetic thyroglobulin gene suggest the existence of a major class of thyroglobulin molecules containing identical polypeptide subunits [144].

Information regarding the thyroglobulin primary structure is scarce. Dunn et al. have obtained evidence that the hormonogenic portion of the molecule is located on a relatively short fragment of the polypeptide chains [145]. Analyses of peptides generated by proteolysis of thyroglobulin have provided evidence that the subunits contain repetetive structures [146], but cross-hybridization was not observed between three independent thyroglobulin cDNA fragments together representing 70 percent of the structural gene. This suggests that internal repetition, if present, must be far from precise. [147].

There are only a few copies of the thyroglobulin gene in the mammalian genome (probably a single copy per haploid genome) [144]. It is interspersed with numerous intervening sequences [144a] (Fig. 11-9).

Little is known about the transcription of thyroglobulin gene(s). Since the mRNA for thyroglobulin is quite stable ($t_{1/2}$: 220 h), its rate of synthesis need not be too rapid. Now that cloned cDNA fragments are available, this process will become accessible to a direct experimental approach.

Since synthesis of thyroglobulin accounts for at least 50 percent of the total protein synthesis in the thyroid, one would expect to find a major population or populations of polyribosomes of homogeneous size engaged in the synthesis of thyroglobulin subunits in the thyroid. Thyroglobulin is an "export" protein synthesized only by polyribosomes bound to the endoplasmic reticulum. When care is taken to isolate intact membrane-bound polyribosomes, a relatively large population of very large polysomes is observed in the thyroid of various mammals, and these nascent peptides are immunologically related to thyroglobulin [10, 141].

mRNA that contains a polyadenylated sequence has been purified from thyroglobulin-synthesizing polyribosomes isolated from the cow and has been characterized. With a sedimentation coefficient of 33 S and a molecular weight of about 2.8×10^6 (8600 bases), this mRNA is about 10 times larger than the average eukaryotic mRNA. It could code for a polypeptide with a maximal molecular weight of 330,000. The actual informational content of the 33 S mRNA was tested by microinjection into oocytes of *Xenopus laevis*. The batrachian oocyte translated the bovine 33 S mRNA into a 300,000-dalton polypeptide (or polypeptides) that was (or were) immunologically and chemically related to bovine thyroglobulin. The primary translation product or products corresponded to 12 S half-thyroglobulin molecules that spontaneously formed 19 S dimers of thyroglobulin. From these results, it may be concluded that the synthesis of 19 S thyroglobulin involves only transitory 12 S precursor(s) that correspond to the protomeric chain(s) [10].

After synthesis, thyroglobulin subunits are discharged into the cistern of the endoplasmic reticulum. It is not known whether this phenomenon involves the synthesis of a signal

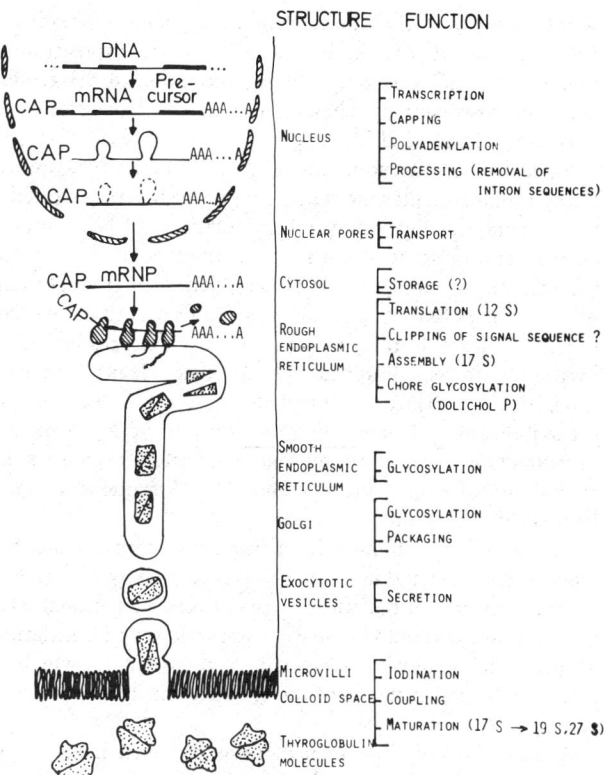

STRUCTURE   FUNCTION

Figure 11-9 Steps in the expression of the thyroglobulin gene. Dolichol P, dolichol phosphate.

peptide transiently attached to thyroglobulin polypeptide chains.

Glycosylation of thyroglobulin occurs in the rough endoplasmic reticulum during its transfer to the Golgi apparatus. Once believed to involve the stepwise attachment of carbohydrate units to the polypeptide, glycosylation has been shown to involve the synthesis of a core carbohydrate chain (containing two N-acetylglucosamine, five mannose, and two glucose residues) attached to the membrane as a dolichol derivative. The core carbohydrate is then transferred to the thyroglobulin chain (asparagine or serine). Subsequently, it undergoes a multistage process to yield the four types of carbohydrate units found in complete thyroglobulin molecules. This involves a sequential enzymatic removal of glucose and some mannoses, followed by the addition of N-acetylglucosamine, galactose, and N-acetylneuraminic acid (sialic) to form the asparagine-linked saccharide units [148–150]. Sialic acid is added as the final residue to some of the chains, so that normal human thyroglobulin contains 23 sialic acid residues per 19 S molecule. It has been suggested that the release of thyroglobulin into the follicular space depends on the presence of sialic acid in the molecule, since certain rat thyroid tumors lacking sialyl transferase are defective in thyroglobulin secretion and iodination [15]. Nevertheless, this observation could reflect other abnormalities in these profoundly altered tumor cells, since secretion of many polypeptides, such as albumin, prolactin, and growth hormone, does not seem to involve any glycosylated intermediates.

Thyroglobulin is secreted into the colloid space by the fusion of exocytotic vesicles with the apical membrane of the cell. These vesicles contain not only noniodinated thyroglobulin molecules but also peroxidase, so that both the enzyme and one of the substrates of the iodination reaction are delivered simultaneously to the apical membrane, where iodination is believed to occur [11, 67]. Iodination is the major posttranslational event and is accompanied by oxidation of SH groups, decreased dissociability, changes in structure (from cylindrical to ovoid), etc. [142, 152].

A parallel between stimulation by TSH and the development of the rough endoplasmic reticulum has been demonstrated in the frog and the dog. An overall stimulation of RNA synthesis occurs concomitantly with an actinomycin D–sensitive increase in protein synthesis. Accumulation of thyroglobulin mRNA occurs following stimulation by TSH both in vivo and in tissue culture. In the absence of TSH, the expression of the thyroglobulin gene disappears [10]. It is not clear whether the TSH effect involves a true stimulation of mRNA synthesis or the stabilization of preexisting messages, or both. By permitting direct measurement of thyroglobulin mRNA synthesis, the availability of cloned thyroglobulin cDNA sequences should help clarify this point.

TSH stimulates amino acid incorporation into thyroid proteins both in vivo and in vitro. This is mediated by cyclic AMP, and at least part of the effect occurs at the translational level. The mechanisms could involve phosphorylation of translational factors by a ribosome-associated protein kinase, which, in turn, would lead to the recruitment of previously inactive ribosomes.

Analyses of polyribosomal patterns obtained from bovine thyroid tissue incubated in the presence of TSH have shown a specific increase in the amount of the large thyroglobulin-synthesizing polyribosomes accompanied by a decrease in the amount of free monoribosomes. The effect was rapid (30 min) and could be mimicked by dibutyryl cyclic AMP. No change in the average size of the thyroglobulin-synthesizing polyribosomes was observed. These results suggest that TSH specifically stimulates thyroglobulin synthesis at the translational level by promoting the translation of a pool of inactive thyroglobulin mRNA [10].

The intracellular movements of thyroglobulin from the rough endoplasmic reticulum to its storage place in the colloid space are controlled by TSH. Thyroid tissue from T_4-suppressed mice accumulates exocytotic vesicles near the apical membrane of the cell. Administration of TSH to these animals stimulates the secretion of thyroglobulin by promoting fusion of the exocytotic vesicles with the apical membrane. Stimulation by TSH of thyroglobulin transfer along the membrane system of the cell has also been demonstrated morphologically and biochemically [10, 11, 67].

Defects in thyroglobulin synthesis could take place at any of the levels of gene expression: regulation of transcription, initiation of transcription, processing of the nuclear RNA, transport, translation, or posttranslational processing. Such disorders, if generalized for all proteins, would be lethal. Their specificity for thyroglobulin would imply the existence of specific steps for the expression of this gene. Mutations in the leader, intervening, or coding sequences of the gene could certainly lead to such specific defects. For example, the integrity of the postulated signal peptide sequence is probably required for thyroglobulin release into the cisternae of the rough endoplasmic reticulum. Such defects would all cause a decrease or an absence of thyroglobulin synthesis. The consequences of such a decrease would be inadequate iodination, diminished iodine storage, and reduced iodotyrosine coupling. This could be partially obviated in stimulated thyroids by the use of substitute protein substrates, such as albumin synthesized or introduced (by leakage into the lumen?) into the thyroid.

Point mutations in thyroglobulin sequence, on the other hand, could be important if they altered the structure of the protein so as to impair oxidative coupling of iodotyrosines. Such defects would also fall into the class of oxidative coupling defects.

The molecular diagnosis of defects in thyroglobulin synthesis obviously requires the in vitro study of thyroid cells. The absence of thyroglobulin in a thyroid biopsy specimen has little meaning as such, since chronic stimulation of the thyroid per se leads to fast turnover of a very small pool of this protein. Only gross alterations of the protein can be demonstrated by immunologic or classic biochemical investigations of protein sedimentation coefficients, dissociability, precipitability by $(NH_4)_2SO_4$, amino acid composition, etc. Study of oxidative coupling in defective thyroglobulin as catalyzed by normal thyroid peroxidase should reveal a structural impairment of iodothyronine synthesis. Absence of a thyroglobulin gene, or a defect at any level of its expression, should be revealed by the study of labeled amino acid incorporation into immunoprecipitable thyroglobulin in intact cells or of labeled nucleosides or nucleotide incorporation into mRNA hybridizable to thyroglobulin cDNA probes in intact cells or nuclei. Such probes can also be used to measure thyroglobulin coding sequences at the various levels (DNA, RNA in nuclei, polysomes, etc.). Finally, thyroglobulin cDNA probes will permit separation and analysis by restriction mapping, electron-microscopic analysis, and even direct sequencing of the thyroglobulin gene itself with its noncoding sequences.

Related Clinical Disorders

Familial Goiter with Diminished or Altered Thyroglobulin Synthesis   Thyroglobulin is a large, complex protein which is synthesized exclusively in the thyroid. It is entirely probable that there are errors in thyroglobulin structure which are at the root of human disease. An extreme form of error would be one in which no identifiable protein is produced. A presumed defect in thyroglobulin synthesis is illustrated in the following account [153].

Three members of a sibship of four had goiter. The gland of the mother was two times the normal size, and that of the father was $1\frac{1}{2}$ times normal. They were not consanguine. ^{131}I uptake by the thyroid glands of both parents was normal. The oldest sib was a 20-year-old male. An enlarged thyroid was noted shortly after birth. Growth and development were normal. The thyroid was estimated to weigh 100 g. A 12-year-old female sib developed normally. There was no significant enlargement of the thyroid, and uptake of ^{131}I was normal. A 7-year-old male sib was hypothyroid. The thyroid was estimated to weigh 40 g. Bone age at age 6 was $2\frac{1}{2}$ years. Free T_4 was low, and ^{131}I uptake was high. The serum concentration of TSH was high. Rapid improvement followed T_4 therapy.

The principal subject of investigation was a 16-year-old female who had an enlarged thyroid at birth. It had slowly increased in size over the years. Growth was within normal limits, but walking and talking seemed slightly delayed. There were no clinical signs of hyper- or hypothyroidism. The thyroid was estimated to weigh 150 g. A bruit was heard over the gland. When treated with L-thyroxine, the patient became tense and nervous and lost 2.3 kg. Serum PBI and serum free thyroxine were normal; radioiodine uptake by the thyroid was elevated. Serum TSH concentration was normal. Of the plasma-labeled iodine, 25 percent was not extracted into acid butanol. On a second occasion during thyroxine therapy, over 40 percent of the serum iodine was not butanol-extractable. The serum T_4-binding globulin level and T_3 resin uptake were within normal limits.

A large, multinodular goiter was removed. Histologic examination disclosed large follicles with cuboidal to columnar epithelium.

Most of the iodine was in the soluble fraction of the homogenized specimen. The MIT/DIT ratio was approximately 0.3. Significant labeling above background was associated with T_4 in the chromatograms of the trypsin digests of the soluble fraction.

Sucrose density gradient centrifugation of the soluble fraction showed only one absorbance peak in the 4 S position. There were no peaks at the 12 or 19 S positions. Most of the labeled iodine coincided with the absorbance peak at 4 S, but there was a small rise in the amount of labeled iodine between the 12 and 19 S positions. Thus, there appeared to be a virtual absence of stable thyroglobulin from the gland and little if any labeled thyroglobulin.

Salting-out curves showed no sharp zone of precipitation as is seen with thyroglobulin between 1.6 and 1.9 M. Starch-gel electrophoresis of the soluble supernatant showed no detectable staining in the band customarily occupied by thyroglobulin. The soluble fraction gave a strong reaction with rabbit antihuman albumin antiserum on Ouchterlony plates, but none of the labeled iodine was precipitated by antihuman thyroglobulin.

Thyroglobulin might be undetectable in the thyroid because of failure of synthesis, rapid turnover, escape, or degradation of subunits before aggregation into the dimeric structure. Several findings suggested that fast turnover was not the cause of the absence of thyroglobulin from this gland. The follicular spaces at the time of surgery were amply large, and the gland did not resemble others in which metabolic blocks caused hyperplasia of the cells to such a degree as to fill the space normally occupied by the colloid. If turnover were unusually rapid, then one would not expect to find an ample follicular space. The low MIT/DIT ratio (0.3) was also not compatible with rapid synthesis and turnover of the iodoamino acids. Iodine deficiency and other causes of thyroid hyperplasia are generally associated with an MIT/DIT ratio higher than 1.0. Furthermore, serial in vivo measurements over the thyroid, extending over several days, gave no evidence of unusually rapid turnover of iodine.

Other Reports A number of reports have suggested that thyroglobulin was either absent from the thyroid or had altered characteristics; in others, the predominant iodinated component was some other iodinated protein, such as iodoalbumin [154–157]. Iodoalbumin may comprise a substantial fraction of the total soluble iodoprotein of sporadic goiter. McGirr et al. [158] found an abnormal iodinated protein in a patient with familial goiter which was resistant to trypsin and chymotrypsin. In three thyroids from hypothyroid patients, Michel et al. [159] found abnormal soluble iodoproteins. One of these was less soluble in ammonium sulfate than is thyroglobulin. A 15-year-old euthyroid female with a congenital goiter had no detectable thyroglobulin but did have a small amount of ^{131}I-labeled 4 S protein [160]. The gland was intensely hyperplastic. A large amount of labeled iodine sedimented with the cell nuclei. Thyroglobulin was not detected. Pittman and Pittman reported two goitrous and cretinous sibs with low plasma thyroxine concentrations and evidence of thyroid hyperplasia [161]. Less than 8 percent of the labeled protein in the thyroid was thyroglobulin. The principal component was iodoalbumin. Other reports have appeared with similar observations [162–167].

Some of these thyroids have had reduced amounts of thyroglobulin, or none at all, or immunoreactive molecules which presumably were subunits of 19 S thyroglobulin. Some of the patients were hypothyroid, while others made sufficient hormone for metabolic compensation. Dinsart et al. [168] used DNA complementary to bovine thyroglobulin mRNA as a probe for mRNA from one of the congenital goiters studied by Wagar et al. [165] which contained no thyroglobulin. Molecular hybridization disclosed that thyroglobulin-related sequences were present but at only about one-thirtieth that in RNA from normal thyroids. Perhaps the simplest hypothesis is that the related sequences in the DNA were not being transcribed as rapidly as normal, or that because of a sequence error they were less stable than normal.

A 17-year-old hypothyroid female studied by Monaco et al. [169] had a large goiter which had a relatively larger than normal amount of iodoprotein which was membrane-bound and a less than normal amount which was soluble. The sialic acid component, the terminal carbohydrate moiety, was much decreased. These findings led to the speculation that there was defective secretion into the follicular lumen of the thyroglobulin which was being incompletely glycosylated.

The thyroid of the patient of Bernal and Obregon [170] had 37 percent of the thyroglobulin-like antigens in the particulate fraction, and this was largely 12 S protein. Kusakabe [171] has reported a patient with a thyroglobulin which was normal in many physical properties but appeared to be abnormal in that it could be iodinated less readily than normal thyroglobulin in its normally folded state. Lissitzky et al. [172] have proposed that goiter in two brothers was a result of a defect in transport of thyroglobulin from the endoplasmic reticulum cisternae into the follicular lumen. Two types of thyroglobulin were identified. One, found in small amounts, was completely immunoreactive. The other, 30 times more abundant, was only partially immunoreactive, had a normal iodoamino acid composition, and was present in overdistended cisternae of the rough endoplasmic reticulum. Both forms had abnormal amino acid compositions, but the component in lesser amounts had reduced carbohydrate content. Sialyl and galactosyl transferase activities were normal. Abnormally structured thyroglobulin, for example, in the postulated signal peptide sequences may have been the central abnormality in these subjects. A similar patient and a similar interpretation have been reported by Monaco et al. [172a], and the sib pair with congenital goiter reported by Pittman and Pittman may have had a similar defect [172b].

There are three well-studied animal models of inherited thyroglobulin deficiency. Falconer et al. [173], studying tissue slices from a strain of congenitally goitrous merino sheep from South Australia, found impaired incorporation of labeled amino acids into the protein component which had the salt solubility characteristics of thyroglobulin. Merino sheep with what appeared to be the same disorder have been studied in New Zealand [174]. Dolling and Good found a thyroglobulin immunoreactive iodoprotein in goiters from these sheep, but it had a sedimentation coefficient of 8 S and a molecular weight estimated at 170,000. Other iodoproteins were present which had the immunologic properties of albumin and immunoglobulin G [175].

A strain of Afrikander cattle also displays congenital goiter

[176, 177]. These thyroids contain an abnormal thyroglobulin which reacts with antithyroglobulin antibody but differs in its physical properties from thyroglobulin. The 12 S component reacts with antithyroglobulin antibody, but it does not associate to form a 19 S structure, and 4 and 18 S components contain no iodine. The amino acid composition of the 12 S component resembled that of thyroglobulin [178, 179]. On polyacrylamide gels, it resolved into 14 polypeptide components. Glycosylation of iodoproteins was normal [180, 181].

The most thoroughly studied animal model is that of a strain of hypothyroid goats from the Netherlands [182, 183]. While it was possible to detect a trace of thyroglobulin (about $\frac{1}{10,000}$ of the normal) in the glands from these animals by immunological methods, it was not possible to demonstrate thyroglobulin by ultracentrifugation or other means. Employing DNA complementary to beef thyroglobulin as a probe [184], it was possible to identify the mRNA sequence for thyroglobulin, but at a concentration of only about one-tenth to one-fortieth that of normal thyroids. In addition, this mRNA was in a much higher concentration in the nuclei than elsewhere relative to the distribution in normal glands. No thyroglobulin-synthesizing polysomes were observed. Interestingly, addition of iodide to the diet restored the euthyroid state, but the amount of thyroglobulin was not increased [185–187]. A number of explanations for these findings come readily to mind, but the error is in the rate of synthesis of thyroglobulin mRNA or somewhere in its metabolism. It is interesting that the euthyroid state can be restored in animals with this disorder by administration of iodide, presumably by enabling synthesis of T_4 and T_3 in the abnormal iodoproteins [181].

The thyroglobulin rat tumor lines 1CZ of Wollman show very little formation of soluble thyroglobulin. That which is formed remains bound to cell membranes [188]. Although there was some incorporation of acetylglucosamine into membrane-bound thyroglobulin, there was no sialic acid in the soluble thyroglobulin. Sialotransferase activity was virtually absent [188]. The findings were consistent with defective thyroglobulin release because of the absence of incorporation of sialic acid into thyroglobulin in this tumor. The analogy with the patient of Monaco et al. [169, 189] is striking.

It is apparent that this category of thyroid disease is heterogeneous. Diagnosis rests principally on laboratory examination of a thyroid tissue specimen. Suggested diagnostic criteria appear in Table 11-6.

Cretinism with Abnormal Iodinated Polypeptides in the Serum   This is probably not a tenable nosologic entity. Patients were put into this grouping because of the appearance in the blood of iodinated amino acids in peptide linkage which were not extractable with acid butanol. Most if not all patients previously so grouped [190] would probably be given another diagnosis at the present time. Analyses of the circulating peptide have usually if not invariably indicated its similarity or perhaps identity with iodinated serum albumin. A similar and perhaps identical albuminlike protein has been identified in the plasma of certain patients with endemic goiter [191], Hashimoto's disease [192], cancer of the thyroid [193], Graves' disease [194], and nodular goiter [195]. Strong evidence identifying it as iodoalbumin has been obtained in Graves' disease.

It seems probable that the synthesis of this protein, or family of proteins, is a normal event in the thyroid and that under special circumstances, perhaps as a result of hyperplasia, it spills into the blood perfusing the gland. This might occur pari

Table 11-6   Diagnostic criteria for impaired thyroglobulin synthesis

1. Goiter; hypothyroid or compensated hypothyroid
2. Radioiodine uptake normal or high
3. Rigorous exclusion of other defects
4. Thyroid biopsy
   a. Colloid spaces present; cell hyperplasia
   b. No thyroglobulin
   c. Abnormal light iodoproteins present
   d. Thyroglobulin 3 to 8 S subunits demonstrated immunologically (type of Robbins and Van Zyl)
   e. Abnormal total content, subcellular localization, or structure of the thyroglobulin-coding nuclear or mRNA (by hybridization with thyroglobulin cDNA).

passu with increased metabolic activity of the gland from any cause, or as a result of any block in normal synthesis through the thyroglobulin pathway. The possibility is by no means excluded that the plasma component is plasma albumin iodinated as it passes through the thyroid, or perhaps albumin that diffuses into the thyroid cell, becomes iodinated, and then diffuses out again [196].

Finding an iodinated peptide in the blood of a patient with familial goiter is only an indication to search for some cause for the glandular hyperplasia. The finding itself at present does not specify any particular category of metabolic disease.

SECRETION OF THYROID HORMONE AND IODINE RECYCLING

The synthesized thyroid hormones, T_4 and T_3, are stored in the thyroglobulin of the follicular lumen. Their secretion involves endocytosis and hydrolysis of thyroglobulin rather than exocytosis, as in other secretory glands. Whereas thyroglobulin contains iodotyrosines (about 80 percent of its iodine) and iodothyronines, the products of secretion are mostly T_4 and T_3, some iodide, and thyroglobulin itself. This implies that the major part of thyroglobulin is completely hydrolyzed and that a large part of the iodotyrosines are deiodinated and their iodine recycled in the follicular cells. Iodothyronines and iodide appear in the venous overflow and thyroglobulin mostly in the thyroid lymphatics. The turnover of the colloid in humans is normally about 1 percent per day, but this may be increased or decreased, depending on the level of activity of the gland. In the chronically strongly stimulated gland, the colloid lumen virtually disappears, and the thyroglobulin pool is almost nonexistent. This suggests that the whole storage process is short-circuited and that thyroglobulin is iodinated and hydrolyzed within a very short time [10, 197].

The secretion of intact thyroglobulin represents a sizable proportion of the total amount of this protein which is synthesized in the thyroid ($\pm$ 7 percent) [198]. The mechanism of this secretion is unknown, but it appears to be an active process following a different pathway from iodothyronine secretion [10, 199].

The endocytosis of the colloid in the follicular cells takes place by macro- and micropinocytosis. Macropinocytosis accounts for thyroid secretion after an acute stimulation by TSH. Within minutes pseudopods develop, mostly at the margin of follicular cells. Their size depends on the level of TSH.

The lateral and apical borders of the pseudopods progressively fuse, engulfing the colloid indiscriminately. This is a process similar to phagocytosis, and indeed, isolated thyroid cells carry on active ingestion of latex particles. It is inhibited by inhibitors of microtubules and microfilaments. This indicates involvement of tubulin and actomyosin in the process. The resulting colloid droplets are interiorized and later fuse with primary lysosomes to form secondary lysosomes in which hydrolysis can take place. In fully stimulated dog follicular cells, the lifetime of the colloid droplet may extend to 40 min. Although endocytosis is obviously the limiting step in secretion, under acute stimulation of cells filled with colloid droplets, thyroglobulinolysis may become limiting [5, 197, 200–202]. Thyroid secretion is not fully accounted for by macropinocytosis. For example, the very active secretion of chronically hyperstimulated follicular cells is not inhibited by inhibitors of macropinocytosis; moreover, it is not accompanied by morphologic evidence of this process (pseudopods, colloid droplets, etc., as shown by transmission or scanning electron microscopy). On the other hand, micropinocytosis of proteins demonstratable by electron microscopy (ferritin, for example) has been demonstrated in follicular cells [203, 204]. There is, therefore, little doubt that this process plays an important (probably the major) role in basal thyroid secretion [67, 201]. Experiments in vitro suggest some selectivity in this process, the mature and more iodinated molecules being taken up more rapidly. Thyroglobulin receptors and binding of desialated thyroglobulin could be involved. The fate of the vesicles depends upon their protein content. Thus, cationized ferritin reaches the Golgi cisternae, and this indicates that membrane patches involved in micropinocytosis could be recycled through the Golgi and secretory vesicles to the plasma membrane [204]. This suggests an orderly traffic of vesicles and a sophisticated signal system.

During endocytosis of colloid, a large surface of the apical membrane is interiorized. This is possible only because exocytosis of newly formed thyroglobulin by fusion of secretory microvesicles with the membrane supplies the necessary membranes. In fact, the two processes of exocytosis and endocytosis are coupled, exocytosis preceding endocytosis after TSH stimulation. Under several circumstances, such as after chronic T_4 treatment, the supply of secretory vesicles becomes limiting for endocytosis. Thus the secretory cycle is similar in the follicular cell to that in other protein-secreting cells if one considers that protein secretion is directed toward the follicular lumen [11, 67, 81]. Endocytosis and iodination take place at the periphery of the colloid lumen. It is clear that more recently iodinated thyroglobulin molecules have more chance to be taken up and hydrolyzed than the others. Slow diffusion of the colloid enhances this phenomenon, which is referred to as the *last come, first served hypothesis* [67, 197].

The fact that excretory vesicles, as well as apical membranes at the bases of microvilli but not pseudopod or colloid droplet membranes, contain peroxidase shows that in both exocytosis and endocytosis extensive membrane reshuffling takes place [197, 204].

The hydrolysis of thyroglobulin droplets resulting from micro- and macropinocytosis takes place in the lysosomes (called *secondary lysosomes* when they result from the fusion of a large ingested droplet and a primary lysosome). These cell organelles contain all the enzymes necessary to hydrolyze completely glycoproteins at acid pH: proteases, glycoside hydrolases, peptidyl amino acid hydrolases, dipeptide hydrolases,

and so on. Thyroglobulinolysis in intact lysosomes is activated by glutathione. This suggests that reduction of the single-stranded bonds in the protein could be a limiting step [206]. The amino acids released by thyroglobulin hydrolysis in lysosomes are probably mixed with the cellular pools, causing a dilution of exogenous amino acids taken up by the cells. After intense stimulation a spillover of amino acids into venous blood is observed. The carbohydrate moieties of thyroglobulin are digested, as evidenced by the loss of PAS staining. The released carbohydrates are presumably recycled in the cells, although some sialic acid is released into the blood [197].

Free iodotyrosines, but not iodothyronines, are rapidly deiodinated by a deiodinase constituted of a ferredoxin, NADPH ferredoxin reductase and a flavin mononucleotide-containing deiodinase [207, 208]. The same system operates in thyroid and in peripheral tissues (e.g., kidney, liver). It is inhibited competitively by dinitrotyrosine and blocked by any agent which oxidizes NADPH, such as menadione. The exact localization of this "microsomal" system has not been elucidated. The iodide released from iodotyrosines is largely reutilized in the thyroid, mixing with the trapped exogenous iodide. Part of this iodide leaks out of the gland. The importance of this leakage is related to the iodine content of the thyroid. In cases of intense or acute TSH stimulation, some iodotyrosines escape the deiodinase and spill over into the venous effluent of the gland. The iodothyronines (T_4, T_3 and small amounts of rT_3) are excreted by an unknown mechanism. Since there is no evidence of lysosomal exocytosis at the basal membrane, it is believed that the iodothyronines are secreted by passive diffusion or, since they are charged amino acids, by passive mediated transport [67, 197]. The T_4/T_3 ratio in the thyroid secretion is lower than in thyroglobulin, especially early after TSH stimulation. This reflects two mechanisms: an earlier release of T_3 during thyroglobulinolysis and a partial deiodination of T_4 by an enzymatic system inhibited by propylthiouracil, similar to the peripheral system [209, 210].

Thyroid secretion is controlled by TSH. In the dog, basal secretion, mostly involving micropinocytosis of thyroglobulin, may not require cyclic AMP, while secretion after acute TSH administration, involving macropinocytosis, is mediated by cyclic AMP [10, 201]. Secretion is inhibited by iodide even in patients treated with antiperoxidase drugs [9].

Thyroid secretion can be best studied in vivo by the serum T_4, T_3, and thyroglobulin response to TSH administration [211]. No reliable in vitro method exists. The presence of an active dehalogenating system can also be studied in vivo. In patients presenting a defect in dehalogenase activity, labeled iodotyrosines will be found in the plasma and urine after radioiodine administration. Moreover, a large proportion of injected radioiodine-labeled DIT or MIT will be recovered after 1 and 2 h in the urine as iodotyrosines and not iodide. Deiodination of iodotyrosines can also be studied in vitro using slices or homogenates of thyroid tissue. Normal tissue incubated in the presence of dinitrotyrosine should also fail to deiodinate the labeled DIT.

In spite of the large number of steps and proteins involved in thyroid secretion, no true congenital defect has been observed for this process. This is perhaps due to the relative nonspecificity of the secretion machinery: Defects in actomyosin, tubulin, membrane or lysosomal proteins would have very general consequences in all cells. It is therefore not surprising that the only well-defined defect involves the deiodinase system, which is important only for the metabolism of iodotyrosines. It may be hypothesized that specific defects involving thyroid secretion could exist. If such a defect involved endocytosis, it would lead to distension of the colloid lumen and colloid goiter; if localized beyond endocytosis, a defect would lead to a thyroid lysosomal disease with accumulation of precursors such as thyroglobulin upstream of the metabolic block. Under such circumstances, it would be of great interest to know whether increased thyroglobulin secretion could compensate for the defects.

Related Clinical Disorders

Congenital Hypothyroidism from Failure of Iodotyrosine Deiodinase Activity

A 27-year-old male had a goiter at birth [212]. Thyroid medication was given for many years but was discontinued 4 years prior to entering the hospital because of tuberculosis. From that time on, the goiter increased in size. The serum concentration of PBI was 0.5 μg/dl. The patient's parents were not consanguine and were normal, as was an older brother, but a younger brother had a goiter at birth and was retarded, both physically and mentally.

The initial study concerned the fate of an administered dose of ^{131}I [212, 213]. Labeled iodine accumulated unusually rapidly in the thyroid (Fig. 11-10). Within 70 min, 74 percent had appeared in the neck region, and during this time there was a rapid fall in the serum concentration of labeled iodine. After 70 min the labeled iodine began to leave the thyroid and to appear in the blood as a component which was partially precipitable with trichloroacetic acid. By 48 h, only 25 percent of the administered dose remained in the gland. The serum concentration of labeled iodine had risen to 0.5 percent per liter, and from that point it slowly fell during succeeding days. Nearly identical in vivo retention and release curves were obtained from the patient's brother.

Serial specimens of serum were chromatographed. In successive specimens there were increasing amounts of labeled iodine, which had the chromatographic mobility of MIT and DIT.

The gland was removed because of pressure symptoms. The histologic pattern was that of intense hyperplasia, but some areas showed a tendency to form colloid, and there were also areas of cystic degeneration and fibrosis. The gland weighed 198 g at operation; 3.4 percent of the labeled iodine was recovered as T_4, and the remainder in small amounts as iodine and in large amounts as MIT and DIT.

The fate of injected labeled MIT and DIT was ascertained [214]. Only a small fraction of the labeled iodine was removed and excreted in the urine as free iodide, whereas normal subjects excreted the label almost entirely as free iodide. There was no evidence that any of the DIT was deiodinated, and there was little evidence of conjugation or deamination. In the first 24 h after administration,

78.6 percent of the injected labeled DIT was recovered unchanged in the urine.

The thyroid gland of the patient's brother was removed because of pressure symptoms. Tissue slices were incubated in the presence of ^{131}I-labeled DIT, and the rate of deiodination was compared with that of calf thyroid slices and with human control tissue from a patient with nodular goiter measured simultaneously. A normal amount of deiodination was demonstrated in the nodular goiter and in the calf slices, but the thyroid tissue slices from the patient failed to deiodinate the substrate DIT [215].

OTHER REPORTS   Other patients with the dehalogenase defect have been described [216–225]. Administration of desiccated thyroid [226] and iodide [227, 228] has induced remissions that have persisted long after withdrawal of medication.

Kusakabe and Miyake [229] studied six patients with simple goiter in Japan who appeared to have partial defects in deiodination in the thyroid and in other organs. Four others had defective deiodination in other organs, but deiodination of three of these, as ascertained by thyroid biopsy, was normal. They have also reported three sisters from a first-cousin marriage who were goitrous but otherwise normal [230]. DIT was deiodinated by the thyroid glands but not by other organs. Dissociation of the deiodinating capacity between the thyroid and other tissues has not been reported elsewhere.

Three sibs from a consanguine family from Iran [231] had a partial defect in deiodinating activity but were euthyroid. They deiodinated MIT but not DIT. Presumed heterozygotes had deiodinating activity which was intermediate between the presumed homozygotes and controls.

INTERPRETATION   Patients in this category share a defect in their capacity to deiodinate MIT and DIT. The deiodinating enzyme occurs normally not only in the thyroid but also in the liver, kidney, and other organs. The metabolic defect is usually both intra- and extrathyroidal, for not only are the afflicted patients unable to deiodinate MIT and DIT in their thyroid glands, but when these substances are administered either before or after thyroidectomy or to the patient receiving full doses of desiccated thyroid, the labeled iodotyrosine appears almost quantitatively in an unchanged form in the urine or (in the case of MIT) as conjugates. Continued leakage of hormone precursors from both the gland and the body depletes iodine stores and sets up a vicious cycle of iodine loss, thyroid hyperplasia, and increasing synthesis and secretion of hormone precursors. Diagnostic criteria appear in Table 11-7.

GENETICS   An unusual opportunity to study the genetics of this kind of goitrous cretinism has been beautifully exploited by Hutchison and McGirr [221, 232, 233]. They have traced the complex family history of their Scottish patients through 160 years. The original male member came from Ireland and married his first cousin. There had been little marriage subsequently outside the tinker group; close intermarriage within the group has been extremely frequent. Ten goitrous cretins are known to have appeared among 31 persons in four sets of sibs.

A study of the family tree shows that this form of cretinism with goiter behaves as a simple autosomal recessive trait. There is no sex predilection. The marriages which resulted in afflicted persons were all consanguine, but in no case was a parent afflicted. The inheritance ratio was somewhat in excess of the expected 1:3 in that there were 10 afflicted sibs and 21 normal children in four sibships, but Hutchison and McGirr point out

Figure 11-10 Metabolism of iodine in patient with the dehalogenase defect. ^{131}I was given orally at zero time, and serial counts were made over the thyroid and in the serum.

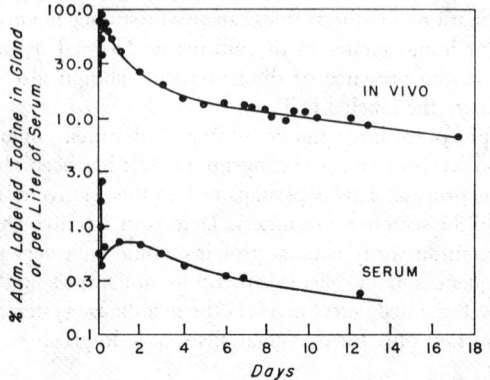

Table 11-7 Diagnostic criteria for the dehalogenase defect

Required	Helpful and confirmatory
1. Goiter; hypothyroid or compensated hypothyroid	1. Thyroid biopsy
2. Mental retardation usually	a. No deiodination of MIT or DIT
3. Rapid and high uptake of radioiodine; rapid turnover (unless compensated for by therapy)	b. Hyperplasia; normal thyroglobulin
4. MIT, DIT and conjugates, and derivatives in plasma and urine	c. Abundant MIT and DIT; little or no iodothyronine
5. No deiodination of injected MIT or DIT	2. Temporary restoration of normal thyroid hormone production by thyroid or iodide medication

that undoubtedly a number of unafflicted sibs were lost to genetic study [221]. There have been no marriages of the afflicted members of this kindred, so that there has been no opportunity to test inheritance from phenotypes. On the other hand, relatives of some of these patients [214] demonstrated defective DIT deiodinase activity and had evidence of thyroid disease but without mental or skeletal retardation. These relatives presumably were heterozygotes. Rochiccioli and Dutau [225] have been able to identify carriers of the trait by giving stable DIT along with the labeled DIT. Carriers are less efficient in deiodinating the DIT. Similarly, Codaccioni et al. [234] have studied relatives of patients with dehalogenase deficiency. They gave 20 to 25 mg stable DIT along with labeled DIT and found that the best discrimination was achieved when the first 2-h excretion of undeiodinated labeled DIT was measured. The relatives of patients excreted 20.4 percent during this time, whereas normal subjects excreted 11.4 percent, and the patients with dehalogenase deficiency excreted 52 to 79 percent.

Diminished Thyroid Protease Activity   Diminished thyroid protease activity has been suggested as a cause of familial goiter [235]. Uncertainty regarding the exact nature of the thyroid proteases concerned with hormone mobilization has limited exploration of this promising possibility for definition of additional metabolic errors of the thyroid.

TRANSPORT AND METABOLISM OF THYROID HORMONES

Transport

Thyroid hormones are transported in the plasma mainly bound by noncovalent interactions to three proteins: thyroxine-binding globulin (TBG), prealbumin (TBPA), and albumin. The presence of these proteins has three main physiologic consequences:

1. The concentration of free hormone is very low compared to total hormone (0.04 percent for T_4, 0.4 percent for T_3). Since it is the free hormone which is acting on cells or transported across epithelia, the transported hormones may be considered a circulating storage form.

2. Since dissociation rates are much faster than blood disappearance rates, the system behaves as an important buffer against fluctuations in hormone level due to variations in secretion or metabolism.

3. The metabolism of thyroid hormones is much slower for thyroid hormones than for unbound amino acids (9 percent per day for T_4, 75 percent for T_3).

From mass law equations for each type of binding site and for the iodothyronines, the level of bound and free hormone can be calculated for any set of hormone and protein concentrations. In general, free hormone levels are proportional to total concentrations. As total iodothyronines increase, the proportion bound to TBG decreases, while TBPA and albumin increase their share of bound hormones. When total T_4 increases, both free T_4 and T_3 increase, whereas when total T_3 increases, only free T_3 levels rise.

TBG is an acidic protein, an inter α-globulin with a molecular weight of about 60,000 which is composed of a single polypeptide chain and four carbohydrate side chains. It is a compact, symmetric molecule with approximately half of the peptide groups equally distributed in α-helical and β-pleated sheet structures. It contains a single high affinity specific binding site for T_4, with an affinity of $6 \times 10^9 \ M^{-1}$ for T_4 and $0.33 \times 10^9 \ M^{-1}$ for T_3. TBG is synthesized in hepatocytes. Synthesis is enhanced by estrogens and at physiologic levels by thyroid hormones. It is decreased by high concentrations of T_4 or T_3. TBG is probably also catabolized after desialytation by the hepatocytes.

TBPA is a protein with a molecular weight of 55,000 which is composed of four identical polypeptide subunits containing no carbohydrate. It is the fastest-migrating serum protein on electrophoresis. The subunits form a double trumpet-shaped molecule with an inside continuous open channel. The two thyroid hormone binding sites are located at each side of this channel, bearing the alanine side chain of the hormone oriented toward the outside. They are highly specific, present a lower affinity than those of TBG ($3.2 \times 10^8 \ M^{-1}$ for T_4, $0.25 \times 10^8 \ M^{-1}$ for T_3), and show negative cooperativity for the second binding. Prealbumin synthesis, probably in the liver, is decreased by stress and protein deficiency.

Albumin has one relatively high affinity site for T_4 ($1.3 \times 10^6 \ M^{-1}$ for T_4, $0.2 \times 10^6 \ M^{-1}$ for T_3) which is not very specific and other lower affinity sites.

As shown by the fact that deficiency of these transport proteins has no known detrimental health effect, their role is certainly not crucial. Whatever their concentration, the pituitary thyroid feedback system maintains constant or restores the free hormone levels. Until now, therefore, the main clinical interest of these proteins has been their effect on the measurement of plasma hormone levels.

Transport proteins are easily measured by counting paper electrophoretograms of serum incubated with labeled T_4 and various concentrations of T_4 [236] or TBG by radioimmunoassay.

Metabolism of Thyroid Hormones

All the available evidence suggests that at least for the delayed nuclear-mediated effects, T_3 is the active thyroid hormone; T_4 should be considered a prohormone; and rT_3 is inactive [237]. Indeed, three effects—the suppression of TRH-induced TSH secretion, the synthesis of growth hormone, and the increased activity of liver α-glycerophosphate dehydrogenase—are correlated with T_3 and not T_4 levels in experiments in which conversion of T_4 to T_3 has been increased (exposure to cold) or decreased (treatment with propylthiouracil or iopanoic acid), with opposite effects on the tissue hormone levels. This conclusion is in conceptual agreement with the fact that nuclear receptors have a higher affinity for T_3 than for T_4. The fact that parameters of biologic activity often correlate better with serum levels of T_4 than T_3 does not argue against this conclusion. Indeed, the circulating levels of T_3 do not reflect faithfully the amounts of T_3 which reach the nuclear receptors, since T_3 nuclear levels are largely influenced by T_4 to T_3 intracellular conversion [237].

The main pathways of deiodination in peripheral tissues involve the deiodination of T_4 (3,5,3',5' T_4) to T_3 (3,5,3' T_3) or rT_3 (3,3'5' T_3) and subsequent deiodination of rT_3 and T_3 to 3,3' T_2, and then to 3' T_1. It is probable that the same enzyme, an iodothyronine-5'-deiodinase, catalyzes the conversion of T_4 to T_3 and rT_3 to T_2; another enzyme, an iodothyronine-5-deiodinase, catalyzes the conversion of T_4 to rT_3 and T_3 to T_2. Both enzymes require thiol compounds, probably reduced glutathione. Inhibition of the first enzyme would channel T_4 metabolism to rT_3, with an accumulation of rT_3 [238, 239]. In adults the production rates of T_3 and rT_3 are similar, while before birth almost all T_4 is converted to rT_3.

Conversion of T_4 to T_3 is very low in the fetus up to 30 weeks of gestation. The T_3 level is therefore unmeasurable, while the rT_3 level is high (250 mg/dl). Thereafter T_3 slowly rises while rT_3 slowly decreases. This suggests the progressive functioning of 5'-iodothyronine deiodinase activity. This evolution continues after birth. It is probable that the maturational increase in hepatic conversion of T_4 to T_3 is induced by cortisol and involves both induction of the enzyme and increased availability of cofactor (e.g., glutathione) [265].

Reciprocal changes in serum rT_3 and T_3 levels have been well demonstrated. Dietary restriction, systemic illness, propranolol, amidarone, propylthiouracil, and high levels of cortisol induce a reduction of T_3 and an elevation of rT_3 levels, T_4 remaining constant [238]. This is sometimes called the *low T_3 syndrome*. The controlled peripheral conversion of T_4 to T_3 thus allows individual cells to regulate their content of active hormone according to their needs. Channeling of T_4 molecules to inactive rT_3 would, therefore, be the ultimate safeguard of the cell against possible toxic effects of thyroid hormone.

Glucuronidation, mostly of T_4, and sulfoconjugation, mostly of T_3, with enterohepatic circulation of the former, account for only a moderate fraction (less than 25 percent) of iodothyronine metabolism. Side chain reactions, i.e., deamination and decarboxylation of the alanine side chain of the iodothyronines, also play a role in this metabolism [236]. Their physiologic relevance is unknown.

Undoubtedly, the complex enzymatic pathway of T_4 metabolism could be the object of genetic deficiency, but none has been discovered so far.

Related Clinical Disorders

Familial Disorders of Thyroid Hormone Transport
The abnormalities of thyroid hormone transport by the carrier proteins have usually been quantitative in nature, but qualitative changes have also been described. Lee et al. [240] described a patient with low serum TBG but a binding protein with low T_4 affinity and high capacity which cochromatographed with TBG on DEAF Sephadex but had the electropho-

retic mobility of albumin. The trait appeared to be inherited as an autosomal dominant. Genetic polymorphism of TBPA occurs in monkeys [241, 242].

Generally alterations in the transport proteins are not related to a change in clinical state or the appearance of thyroid disease, and measurements of free hormones in the plasma have been within normal limits or slightly altered [243–248]. Horwitz and Refetoff found that 5 out of 12 patients with TBG deficiency had Graves' disease [249]. The 12 were identified from among approximately 20,000 subjects screened in a busy thyroid clinic. Others have also reported thyrotoxicosis in association with altered TBG [250, 251]. Alterations in TBG have been reported in a number of nonthyroidal disorders [252]. Shane et al. [253] studied members of four generations with TBG excess and goiter but concluded from their genetic analysis that the traits were distinct. Reported association between familial hyperlipidemia and TBG deficiency may have been an example of loose linkage or coincidence [254].

FAMILIAL DEFICIENCY OF TBG   Among the affected families with TBG deficiency, TBG has been undetectable in males and approximately half normal in females. In one of these families, an XO subject was found who proved to have no TBG. These findings, the absence of male-to-male transmission, and transmission to females by an affected male all indicate X-linked transmission. There is one instance of a female with absent TBG which remains unexplained [255, 256].

Bigazzi et al. [257] have identified a female with X-linked T_4-binding globulin deficiency. She was indistinguishable from males with the deficiency in the family. Pedigree analysis and laboratory studies indicated that this patient's father had TBG deficiency and that her mother was heterozygous for the trait.

FAMILIAL REDUCED TBG   In this variant, TBG is reduced but not absent in males [258, 259]. Since the quantitative changes in TBG are less striking in this variant than in the complete deficiency syndrome, it is more difficult to assign genotypes. Bode, using the product of T_4 and TBG, was able to indicate genetic concordance in 15 of 16 females in a large kindred, and the last had not reproduced. The available information on the families described is consistent with inheritance on the X chromosome.

FAMILIAL EXCESS OF TBG OR TBPA   Approximately 10 families have been reported with TBG sharply elevated in males, often to four or more times normal [260]. Affected females have an intermediate value of about two to two and a half times normal. Present information is consistent with X-linked inheritance. Moses et al. have described a family with excess TBPA [261].

ACTIONS OF THYROID HORMONES

Physiologic and Growth Effects

In mammals the main roles of thyroid hormones are to sustain normal body growth and maturation, including cerebral development, and to enhance metabolic activity. In utero, the hormones are not necessary for the growth of a normal embryo, but their absence leads to partially reversible growth retardation and delay in bone maturation at the end of pregnancy and after birth. Hypothyroidism during fetal and early neonatal life induces an irreversible failure in brain maturation. Thus, even when corrected in adult life, congenital hypothyroidism is characterized by growth failure, i.e., dwarfism and idiocy. Such patients are called *cretins*. The thyroid hormones accelerate but do not increase overall growth. Excess does not lead to gigantism, as growth hormone does in acromegaly [262–264].

Thyroid hormones enhance the activity of many metabolic pathways in many tissues. In general, their effect on anabolic pathways predominates at low doses, whereas the action on catabolic pathways is preponderant at high doses (e.g., on glycogen, lipid, and protein metabolism). This often confers a biphasic character on the hormone action on many metabolic variables. Thus low doses increase while high doses decrease liver glycogen. Also, the nature of T_4 effects varies according to the tissue. For instance, it enhances oxygen consumption of liver and muscle but not brain tissue. A general characteristic of these effects is their delay, which reflects the fact that these effects are the final consequence of a long chain of biochemical events [237, 262, 265].

The peripheral action of thyromimetic substances is intimately related to structure. An ether or thio ether bridge between the two rings is necessary. The *p*-hydroxyl substituent can be replaced by a methoxy group, and the alanine side chain can be radically altered, with reduction but not deletion of action. Various substitutions of nitro, amino, alkyl, halogen, and hydroxyl groups can be made for the iodines, but almost always with diminution of activity. The crucial point about these facts is that iodine as such is not necessary for the action of the iodothyronines, thus, 3,5,3′,5′-tetramethylthyronine is fully thyromimetic. These molecules therefore act by themselves and not as carriers of iodine [266]. Removal of one iodine from the 5 position reduces activity, and in general removal of the 5′ substituent from substances with thyromimetic activity enhances the activity. Structural alteration may have differing metabolic effects depending on which of several assays is employed. This is not surprising when one considers that a structural change may alter absorption, protein binding, cell penetrance, or degradation of the compound and that different assays may measure different effects of the substances in question [263, 266].

Thyroid hormone is required for growth. The fact that thyroid hormone induces the synthesis of growth hormone in the pituitary and that plasma of hypothyroid patients is almost devoid of this hormone may partially explain the growth effect of T_4. Nevertheless, growth hormone administration alone does not restore growth in cretins [262]. Thyroid hormone may also directly enhance somatomedin secretion. Moreover, the hormone directly enhances growth and multiplication in various cell culture systems [262, 263].

Thyroid hormone is necessary for the development of the nervous system [267]. One possible mechanism of the retardation in hypothyroid animals is the delay in the morphogenesis of neurons and in the growth of axons due to a delay in the normal appearance of some microtubule-associated proteins in this tissue [268]. Retardation of myelination is also involved. Failure of maturation at the critical period leads to irreversible damage, which at the level of the brain is expressed as mental deficiency. Thyroid hormone deprivation in the embryo may also lead to other defects of the nervous system. For instance,

propylthiouracil causes specific lesions of the sensory brain cells of acoustic papillae and of the tectorial membrane of the organ of Corti in chicks and rats.

Biochemical Effects

The complexity of the metabolic effects of thyroid hormones is perhaps best exemplified by the description of the actions on adipose tissue:

1. Increased activity of adenylate cyclase.
2. Decreased activity of particulate low K_m cyclic AMP-specific cyclic nucleotide phosphodiesterase, which enhances the cyclic AMP response to agents that activate adenylate cyclase, such as norepinephrine.
3. Decreased activity of the enzymes of the hexose monophosphate pathway (hexokinase, glucose-6-phosphate dehydrogenase, 6-phosphogluconate dehydrogenase), i.e., of the $NADPH_2$ supply.
4. Decreased activity of the enzymes of fatty acid synthesis (ATP citrate lyase, acetyl CoA carboxylase, fatty acid synthetase). All these effects bear on the V_{max}, i.e., on the level of the enzymes and thus presumably on their synthesis. This coordinated action will lead to increased lipolysis and decreased lipogenesis: By increasing cyclic AMP, levels 1 and 2 will activate the lipolytic enzymes (lipase) and inactivate the three main lipogenetic enzymes; and by decreasing the supply of the main coenzymes $NADPH_2$ and the enzymes, levels 3 and 4 will decrease lipogenesis [269–271]. Thus, in this tissue, the hormone acts by enhancing coordinately the synthesis and thus the levels of multiple, specific key enzymes which all contribute complementarily to the general action required, which in this case is lipolysis.

Besides such multiple coordinated effects on the composition of the enzymatic machinery of the target cell, thyroid hormones also act by modifying the synthesis, catabolism, and receptors for other hormones. Thus, for example, insulin catabolism and the number of insulin receptors are both increased in the hyperthyroid animal. The well-known increase in the biologic response to catecholamines induced by T_3 is a general phenomenon caused, depending on the organ and the species, by an increased number of receptors, increased coupling of the receptor with adenylate cyclase, decreased cyclic nucleotide phosphodiesterase activity, and so on [269, 272].

The most thoroughly studied general action of thyroid hormones is their stimulation of the basal metabolic rate, i.e., of tissue respiration. Several known biochemical effects can account for this, but there is still controversy regarding their relative importance. Among these are:

1. Induction of a cytosolic glycerophosphate dehydrogenase which catalyzes the shuttle of reducing equivalents from cytosol $NADH_2$ to the mitochondrial electron transport chain
2. Increased density of mitochondria secondary to enhanced mitochondriogenesis in muscle, liver, etc. [273]
3. Increase in the activity of Na^+/K^+-activated ATPase in the liver, skeletal muscle, and kidney by activation of its biosynthesis [274]
4. Increased response to catecholamines
5. Increased protein synthesis
6. Increased work of the heart [275]

Many direct biochemical effects of thyroid hormones in acellular preparations have been reported: uncoupling of oxidative phosphorylation, activation of coupled mitochondrial respiration, inhibition of Zn-containing enzymes by chelation of the metal, activation of diphosphoglycerate mutase in the erythrocyte, dissociation of glutamate dehydrogenase, activation of adenylsuccinate synthetase, and so on. However, for none of these effects has the physiologic or even pharmacologic relevance been established.

Mechanisms of Biochemical Action

The initial point of interaction of a hormone with a cell is, by definition, the receptor of the hormone. Such a molecule should bind the hormone in significant amounts at the physiologic concentrations of the hormone, and this interaction should cause the primary effect, i.e., the biochemical action which by a more or less complex sequence of causal relationships will lead to the complete pattern of hormone actions. The concept of a receptor involves both binding and action. In the case of thyroid hormones, specific high affinity, saturable binding sites have been demonstrated in the nucleus, but no direct biochemical consequence of this binding has yet been shown. Nevertheless, there are many arguments in favor of the hypothesis that these acceptor molecules are receptors.

1. Acceptors are found in high concentrations in target but not in unresponsive cells. These nuclear acceptors constitute the only site where T_3 is retained after injection.
2. Binding and activity of different analogues are correlated.
3. Occupancy in vivo of the acceptors parallels the level and general action of the hormones.
4. Little or no acceptor is found in cells of congenital cretins with resistance to thyroid hormones.

The receptor has a binding affinity constant for T_3 of about $0.2 \times 10^{10} M^{-1}$ and a capacity of about 2 ng/g of liver. Affinity for T_3 is four- to tenfold that for T_4, but DT_3 binds with the same affinity as LT_3 [275]. In the physiological range of hormone concentration, about 30 percent [263, 276] of the receptors are occupied, predominantly by T_3. Thyroid receptors appear at different times in different organs during ontogenesis: in the fetal brain and after birth in the liver [265]. It seems probable that prior to binding to the nuclear receptor, thyroid hormones have to pass the plasma membrane by a mediated transport mechanism, and that in the cytosol they may bind to lower affinity receptors [277, 278].

Little is known about the mechanism of action of the thyroid hormone "receptor." Its nuclear location and the fact that the first observed biochemical effects of the hormone in vivo take place in the nucleus (e.g., activation of RNA polymerases, RNA synthesis, etc.) suggest a primary effect on the transcription machinery. This hypothesis is supported by our more precise knowledge of the sequence of events in one well-studied system: the induction by T_3 of growth hormone (GH) synthesis in rat pituitary. In this case, it has been shown quite clearly that T_3 in physiologic doses enhances the concentration GH mRNA and the synthesis of GH itself. Similar effects have been obtained in vitro [279, 280]. This clearly suggests but does not prove that the effect of the hormone is on transcription. It is evident that such a mechanism will apply to other mRNAs and proteins, but the pattern of synthesized mRNAs and proteins synthesized in different tissues will be different. Hybridization experiments suggest that the expression of many genes is enhanced by T_3 [266].

Apart from effects at the level of transcription, it is probable, although much debated, that thyroid hormones may also affect directly the plasma membrane and mitochondria. The action at the level of the membrane would explain the very early effects of the hormones on substrate transport [278].

The biochemical actions of T_3 in any tissue will be regulated by many other factors. For instance, starvation inhibits many but not all T_3 effects [266].

Defects in thyroid hormone action could take place at any of the steps of its biochemical sequence: mediated transport, nuclear and possibly cytoplasmic receptors, interaction with chromatin, affected genes, and so on. The action of these hormones in humans can be best studied in vivo as the response to T_3 and T_4 administration. Various endpoints may be used—plasma TSH decrease, BMR, etc.—but it is evident that we lack specific tests of the various actions of thyroid hormones. In vitro, what is needed is a measurement in intact cells of a definite effect of the hormones (such as the induction of one enzyme). Such a test, which would explore the whole causal sequence of at least one effect of the hormone, is still to be developed. On the other hand, the application to nuclear preparations of lymphocytes or cultured fibroblasts of labeled T_3-binding measurements permits one to study reliably that step of hormone action.

Related Clinical Disorders

Familial Disorders of Thyroid Hormone Effects   At least eight sets of studies have indicated resistance of target organs to the thyroid hormones, and others have been studied but not yet published [281]. In six there appeared to be resistance on the part of all peripheral cells, whereas in one the pituitary appeared insensitive to the normal inhibitory effect of T_3.

The most extensive study is that of Refetoff et al. [281–285]. In 1967 they first described two of six children of a consanguine marriage who had deaf mutism, delayed bone age, stippled epiphyses, and elevated plasma levels of T_4 with normal plasma TBG concentrations. A third child, 8 weeks old at the time, has followed a similar clinical course until the present [284]. This family has been thoroughly studied since the original observations were reported.

There was no other history of goiter, deafness, or other congenital abnormalities in the family. The father and mother were first cousins once removed. Three half-sibs from a previous marriage of the mother are normal. Both parents are third-generation Americans of Mexican extraction.

The oldest child was a 14-year-old male at the time of the initial study. Early development was somewhat delayed, and deafness was noted during early infancy. At school he was above average in general performance. He had normal body proportions and normally erupted teeth. The thyroid gland was estimated to be about four times the normal size. Findings on otoscopic examination were normal. There were no stigmata suggestive of thyroid dysfunction. His sister, 4 years younger, and an affected brother, 13 years younger, have been entirely similar.

The striking finding was the discrepancy between the euthyroid clinical state and the clinical laboratory evidence consistent with hyperthyroidism. The initial mean PBI levels were 14.0, 20.8, and 19.38 µg/dl for the three sibs. These results were confirmed on repeated determinations, and similar values were obtained from different laboratories. The PBI of the mother during the last trimester of gestation was 8.1 μg/dl. Measurements of BEI and T_4 confirmed the PBI values. Free T_4 values were 6.2 and 7.6 μg/dl for the older sibs (normal 2.5 ± 0.4). TBG and TBPA capacities were within normal limits. The 24-h uptake of ^{131}I fell within the hyperthyroid range in one of the patients (70 percent) and was borderline for the other two (49 and 51 percent, respectively). Scans of the neck showed a somewhat irregular distribution of radioiodine throughout symmetric thyroid glands. The basal metabolic rates were normal, as were serum enzyme assays and plasma lipids. Dentition was normal and growth steady.

Electrocardiograms and chest and skull roentgenograms were all within normal limits, except for epiphyseal dysgenesis. The dysgenesis in the oldest sib improved strikingly as he matured, and his laboratory values tended toward normal. All three affected sibs had delayed bone age [281, 282]. Serum protein electrophoretic patterns were normal. Antithyroglobulin titers were negative at 1:16 dilution. A summary of the principal laboratory findings appears in Table 11-8.

The distribution space of iodide was increased, thyroid iodide clearance from plasma was elevated, and renal clearance was normal. The disappearance rate of labeled iodine from the serum was increased, as was the thyroid uptake fraction. The rate of release of iodine from the thyroid was increased. Serum PB ^{131}I at 48 h was normal, but the conversion ratio was high. The peripheral degradation rate of thyroid hormone was several times normal. The thyroid of one of the sibs was only partially suppressed by daily administration of 1 mg T_4 daily or 375 μg T_3. Studies with labeled hormone indicated that these entered the tissues, including the liver. Lymphocyte nuclei from the youngest affected sib had a single binding site with a binding affinity constant of $0.43 \times 10^9 \, M^{-1}$ compared with a value of $8.9 \pm 7.1 \times 10^9 \, M^{-1}$ for control nuclei. The binding capacity was comparable to control values. Thus, the defect appeared to be due to a defect at the nuclear receptor level [285]. Mean TSH values have been normal, but at times individual values have been slightly elevated in spite of elevated levels of T_3 and T_4. LATS has not been detected, nor have anticytoplasmic or anticolloid antibodies appeared. Uptake of ^{131}I has been elevated at times and not dischargeable with perchlorate.

Baseline responses of TSH and prolactin to TRH were normal in spite of the sharply elevated plasma T_4 and T_3 concentrations. Although the response was at times blunted by administration of T_3, it was still present, and in some observations it was increased. The T_4 concentration was not suppressed by administration of T_3. Prednisone rapidly suppressed T_4 and T_3 concentrations and obliterated the response to TRH. Thus the pituitary was resistant to the specific suppressing effect of thyroid hormone but not to nonspecific suppression by glucocorticoid. Cultured fibroblasts from one of these

patients showed normal conversion of T_4 to T_3. Thus it appears that the defect in the affected members resides in a defective high affinity nuclear T_3 binding protein. Unexplained are the deafness, the curious stippled epiphyses, and the tendency toward recovery from some of the features of the syndrome with the passage of time.

A similar but not identical patient has been described by Bode et al. [286]. This 8-year-old euthyroid male child of a consanguine marriage had a small goiter, an initial T_4 level of 19.5 μg/dl, free T_4 of 4 μg/dl, and T_3 of 505 ng/dl. TSH and T_4 binding protein concentrations were normal. There was a brisk response to injected TRH, both in plasma TSH and in T_3 concentration. There was a fall in ^{131}I uptake and in TRH sensitivity with administration of 50 μg T_3 three times daily. Measurements of BMR were normal. The patient was not deaf, and the epiphyses and bone age were normal. Thus this patient and those described above were resistant but not completely resistant to thyroid hormone, but there were interesting clinical differences.

The patient of Lamberg [287] was a 25-year-old woman with goiter dating from birth. Concentrations of total and free T_4 and T_3 were approximately twice normal, and T_4 turnover was rapid. The response of TSH to TRH and of TRH to T_3 administration were normal. Daily 100-μg doses of T_3 suppressed ^{131}I uptake and serum TSH levels. The affinity constant for T_3 of lymphocyte nuclei was low normal and was considered presumptive evidence for an abnormally low affinity of the receptor for the hormone [288]. The patient was not deaf and had no bone changes. Thus, while she was seemingly resistant to thyroid hormone, the degree of resistance seems to have been considerably less than in the patients of Refetoff et al. A similar patient has been described by Schneider et al. [289]. Three members of a family with peripheral resistance to thyroid hormone were also described by Lamberg et al. [290]. Each was normal, except for goiter in two of them. Plasma concentrations of T_4 and T_3 were elevated, but the response to TRH was normal. Two had been operated on under a presumably erroneous diagnosis of thyrotoxicosis. As in Lamberg et al.'s earlier patient, the lymphocyte nuclear affinity for T_3 was within normal limits, but low, and suggestive of a mild deficiency of nuclear receptor protein [291]. Another family with mild manifestations in which inheritance appeared to have a dominant pattern has been described by Liewendahl et al. [292].

An 18-year-old woman with recurrent thyrotoxicosis and goiter has been reported who had TSH concentrations which were inappropriately high for the plasma levels of T_3 [243]. Peripheral responses to thyroid hormones were normal, and the pituitary responded to TRH in spite of the thyrotoxic state. It was concluded that the thyrotropic cells of the pituitary were less than normally sensitive to the negative feedback control exerted by T_3. Other sim-

Table 11-8 Syndrome of familial resistance to the action of thyroid hormone

Tests related to thyroid function	Sib 1, M.G.		Sib 2, V.G.		Sib 3, Ma.G.		Mother J.G., normal
	Age, years		Age, years		Age, years		
Serum	14	16½	10	12½	1	9.5	
Total iodine, μg/dl	13.6	11.6	17.0	16.0	16.8	—	7.0
Protein-bound iodine, μg/dl	12.8	10.2	12.6	15.8	—	—	6.8
Butanol-extractable iodine, μg/dl	10.4	—	—	14.0	14.0	—	5.8
Total T_4, μg/dl	17.5	14.8	20.2	16.8	—	24.	—
Total T_3, ng/dl	—	280	450	—	—	370	—
Free T_4, ng/dl	—	6.7	7.6	—	—	—	2.2
T_4-binding globulin capacity, μg/dl	18.1	18.0	18.1	18.0	—	—	24.7
T_4-binding prealbumin capacity, μg/dl	193	—	176	—	—	—	212
Immunoreactive serum TSH, microunits/ml	—	4.0	—	5.0	5	1.2	—
Cholesterol	—	208	—	168	166	—	174

ilar patients have been described by Agerbaek [294] by Elewarut et al. [295], and by Kaplowitz et al. [295a].

The patients who appear to be resistant to the peripheral effects of the thyroid hormones do not conform to a single pattern either clinically or from the laboratory point of view. Some, but not all, are hypothyroid clinically and are retarded in growth. Some are deaf, and some have goiter. The impaired responsiveness in some is confined to the pituitary, whereas in most it is manifest in all tissues, but to a varying degree. The common feature is a plasma concentration of TSH which is inappropriate to the concentration of T_4 and T_3 in the plasma, or a response to TRH which is inappropriate, or both. The defect or defects may be at the level of the nuclear receptor, or it may lie anterior to it, or in the chain of events which follows the receptor interaction with the hormone.

A set of diagnostic criteria for a diagnosis of general tissue reduced responsiveness to thyroid hormones appears in Table 11-9. Different criteria would be required for a diagnosis of resistance confined to the thyrotropic cells of the pituitary.

THYROID CONTROL

The thyroid system is controlled at five levels: the brain, hypothalamus, hypophysis, thyroid, and periphery by the conversion of prohormone T_4 to T_3 [296]. Various controls are exerted on the TRH-secreting neurons largely through positive α-adrenergic and perhaps serotonin receptors. The pituitary thyrotrophs are stimulated by TRH and inhibited by somatostatin and dopamine. T_4 after transformation to T_3 also exerts a delayed and long-term inhibition. Chronic administration of estrogens activates the thyrotrophs. TSH stimulates the thyroid, as described earlier in detail. The catabolism of TSH depends on thyroid hormone action.

Effects at the level of the hypothalamus are of the neural type, i.e., immediate and of short duration. At the lower levels, effects are more delayed and of longer duration. For example, the first effects of T_3 take place hours after hormone administration and persist for days. Desensitization to TRH and TSH actions contributes to termination of their action. Control of the hypothalamo-hypophyseal thyroid system matures only at the end of fetal life and the beginning of neonatal life [265].

Impulses from the brain influence the hypophysiotropic TRH secretory neurons through an ill-defined neural network. Adrenergic neurons probably constitute the final common pathway for diverse positive (e.g., cold), negative (e.g., stress, morphine), or alternative (e.g., nyctohemeral rhythms) stimuli. Norepinephrine acts on the TRH-secreting neurons through α-adrenergic receptors [296]. A positive neural control through serotonin has been suggested [297]. Positive as well as negative feedback of thyroid hormones on these neurons has been proposed.

TRH is a tripeptide (pyroglutamyl-histidyl-prolinamide). Little is known about its biosynthesis. TRH neurons are located in the thyrotropic area of the hypothalamus, i.e., in the area where electrical excitation causes TSH release. They extend from the paraventricular and supraoptic nuclei to the anterior border of the median eminence. TRH granules are transported down the axon by axoplasmic flow and are secreted at the level of the median eminence, where TRH penetrates fenestrated capillaries into the hypophyseal portal neuron system, to be carried to the anterior lobe of the hypophysis [296].

Apart from its role in the hypothalamo-hypophyseal system, TRH is a general neurotransmitter found in various areas of the brain and in the periphery (e.g., in the pancreas) [298]. It is inactivated in the serum within minutes. Thus it is a local hormone.

The action of TRH on the thyrotrophs is very rapid. Binding to its receptor triggers a depolarization and an influx of calcium into the cytosol, which by the classic stimulus-secretion coupling mechanism causes TSH secretion. TRH also activates adenylate cyclase, which may complement the first mechanism or account for other effects [299, 300]. TRH also activates TSH synthesis and glycosylation, and probably the growth and multiplication of thyrotrophs. TRH also activates prolactin secretion, but whether this effect has a physiologic meaning remains controversial [296].

There is good evidence that hypothalamic somatostatin is a physiologic inhibitor of TSH secretion. Little is known about its origin, its control, and its locus and mechanism of action (hypothalamus or pituitary) [296].

TSH is a glycoprotein of molecular weight 28,000. It is composed of two subunits, α (MW: 14,700, two oligosaccharide moieties) and β (MW: 15,600, one oligosaccharide moiety). The α subunit is common to TSH, FSH, and LH, while the β subunit is specific for each of these hormones. The subunit thus confers on the hormone its biologic specificity and is the major determinant of immunologic specificity. Separate α and β subunits have no thyroid effect [301]. The α and β subunits are synthesized on different polysomes; there is no common precursor protein [302]. Their biosynthesis is comparable to that of other glycoproteins, such as thyroglobulin. Thus, there is synthesis of a preprotein with a signal sequence on the rough ergastoplasm, release in the lumen of the ergastoplasm with hydrolysis (clippase) of this sequence, core glycosylation by dolichol phosphate intermediates, removal of some glucoses, and further glycosylation in the reticulum. The α subunits are synthesized in large excess compared to β, but the β subunits have to be glycosylated in order to combine [303]. In normal humans TSH and its β subunit are secreted, but when the thyrotrophs are stimulated, as in hypothyroidism, α subunits are also secreted [301].

The thyrotrophs are mainly controlled by the antagonistic control of TRH and thyroid hormones. Hypothalamic control accounts for the TSH nyctohemeral rhythm, with its nocturnal maximum, and for the cold-induced TSH, T_4, and T_3 secretion immediately after birth [265].

TSH secretion is tightly controlled by the level of free thyroid hormone. Small relative changes result in altered TSH secretion over the entire physiologic range. The inhibiting effect of thyroid hormone has a delay period of several hours, requires new protein synthesis, and is exerted both acutely and

Table 11-9 Diagnostic criteria for syndrome of generalized thyroid hormone unresponsiveness

1. Hypothyroid or compensated hypothyroid; small goiter
2. High plasma T_4 and T_3 levels; normal plasma
3. Subnormal response to large doses of T_3 or T_4; diminished response to normal thyroid suppression test
4. Response to TRH inappropriate to plasma T_3 and T_4 levels
5. Rigorous exclusion of endemic goiter and iodine deficiency

chronically on the number of TRH receptors, TSH secretion, TSH synthesis, and even the growth and multiplication of thyrotrophs [296, 304]. The inhibition of secretion is faster and will induce TSH accumulation in a first phase [305].

T_3 inhibits the thyrotrophs directly, but at the physiologic level the main external agent of control is T_4, which, through deiodination in the thyrotrophs themselves, provides the inhibiting cellular T_3 [306]. Chronic primary hypothyroidism leads to increased TSH levels but also to hypertrophy and multiplication of the thyrotrophs (which normally represent about 2 percent of the cell population of the anterior lobe) and to enlargement of the sella turcica.

Estrogens enhance the responsiveness of the thyrotrophs to TRH in animals and possibly in humans [307]. Dopamine exerts negative control on TSH secretion in humans, probably at the level of the thyrotrophs [308, 309]. The metabolism of TSH is rapid (half-life about 1 h). It is accelerated by hyperthyroidism and decreased in hypothyroidism. It is principally metabolized in the kidney [307].

Investigation of the thyroid system can be carried out in vivo. Plasma levels of TRH, TSH, and thyroid hormones can be measured. TRH levels reflect largely the secretion of TRH from organs other than the hypothalamus [298]. On the other hand, the effects of TRH and TSH can be measured, as well as the feedback of thyroid hormones. Pharmacologic testing of the hypothalamus itself is not yet developed.

Related Clinical Disorders

Hypothalamic Hypothyroidism   While it seems probable that there are inherited defects in the synthesis or secretion of TRH, these have not yet been described. Hypothyroidism arising from TRH deficiency has often been described in isolated cases [310] and is presumed if the pituitary of a hypothyroid subject with low TSH responds to TRH with a rise in TSH.

Familial Pituitary Hypothyroidism   Hypothetically, familial TSH deficiency would be caused by failure of the TSH-secreting cells to bind or respond to TRF, impaired synthesis or secretion of TSH, or abnormal sensitivity to inhibition by circulating thyroid hormone. TSH deficiency could arise from a failure of the cells specifically concerned with TSH supply or because the pituitary as a whole is functioning poorly.

Six syndromes of familial pituitary hypothyroidism are recognized (Table 11-10). These are only briefly described here because so little is known about the intimate biochemical disturbance which is responsible for each.

ISOLATED TSH DEFICIENCY   Only one family has been reported [311]. Two of three sibs from a consanguine mating were hypothyroid and had no detectable TSH. The third sib had died at age 3 years of pneumonia. The thyroids of both children responded to TSH, but the pituitary did not respond to TRF. Other indicators of pituitary function were normal. The precise cause of the TSH deficiency in these two patients is unknown.

FAMILIAL PANHYPOPITUITARISM   These patients have evidence, usually obvious, of deficiencies of other anterior pituitary hormones, and the clinical impression of hypothyroidism may not be striking. There is almost invariably deficiency of

human growth hormone (HGH), and gonadotropic hormones are often lacking [312, 313]. Stress may elicit evidence of ACTH deficiency. It is possible that some of these patients have congenital lack of multiple releasing factors. The failure of the patients of Adler-Bier et al. [313] to respond to TRH or to LH-RH tends to place the defect in the pituitary.

There are two forms of familial panhypopituitarism. The more common form has been reported in approximately 20 families from Canada, Switzerland, Morocco, and Yugoslavia [312, 313]. It is inherited as an autosomal recessive trait. Another variant affects only males [314–316]. Available information is consistent with X-linked inheritance, but sex-limited autosomal inheritance has not been ruled out.

FAMILIAL ABSENCE OF THE PITUITARY   A number of patients in several families have been reported with a syndrome of pituitary agenesis [317–319]. Although weight and length at birth were usually normal, they developed a uniform clinical presentation, with early lethargy, cyanosis, hypoglycemia, convulsions, and collapse. Prolonged jaundice is present in those who survive beyond the first days of life. Administration of TRH causes no increase in the low TSH levels. Most have died within the first days or weeks of life. Two sibs who survived into their teens showed extreme physical and mental retardation [318]. Two affected sibs, younger children of an affected sibship, were developing normally on replacement therapy [319]. Earlier reports have been reviewed [317].

Radiologically, the sella turcica is small but normally shaped. Autopsy findings include absent anterior pituitary tissue, absent posterior pituitary, atrophic gonads in 50 to 60 percent, and atrophic thyroids in about 90 percent of the patients. The occurrence of the syndrome in consanguine parents suggests autosomal recessive inheritance [318].

FAMILIAL ABSENCE OF THE SELLA TURCICA   Two pairs of sisters have been described with a virtual absence of the sella turcica, growth failure, hypoglycemia, and hypothyroidism [320, 321]. One pair died in infancy [321]. Three others were mentally retarded. Response tests indicated that some pituitary tissue was present.

FAMILIAL ENLARGEMENT OF THE SELLA TURCICA   Three sibs, one male and two females, with short stature and hypothyroidism have been described who had enlarged sella turcicas [322]. The TSH response to TRH was impaired, and there was evidence of GH deficiency. The parents were not consanguine.

UNCLASSIFIED TYPES OF FAMILIAL THYROID DISEASE WITH HYPOTHYROIDISM

A number of case reports have appeared from time to time concerning individuals or families with thyroid disease and hypothyroidism which do not fall conveniently into any of the groups delineated earlier in this chapter. In each instance, the disease is presumably the result of an inborn error in one of the metabolic pathways of the thyroid system, and in each case the error has defied precise definition.

An unusual family has been described by Murray et al. [323]

Table 11-10 The inherited syndromes of pituitary insufficiency which are accompanied by hypothyroidism

	Inheritancy	Congenital hypothyroidism	Measurable TSH	Response to TRH	Associated pituitary deficiencies
Isolated TSH deficiency [285]	Autosomal recessive	Yes	No	No	No
Panhypopituitarism:					
Autosomal recessive [312, 313]	—	Yes [313]	Yes Low or no [313]	Yes‡ No [313]	FSH, HGH, LH ACTH
X-linked recessive [314–316]	—	Yes	ns* Yes†	ns	HGH, FSH, LH, ACTH
Pituitary agenesis [317–319]	Autosomal recessive	Yes	No	ns	ns
Panhypopituitarism with absent sella turcica [320, 321]	Autosomal recessive	Yes	Yes	ns	HGH, FSH, LH, ACTH
Panhypopituitarism with enlarged sella turcica [322]	Autosomal recessive	Yes	No	No	GH

*ns: not studied.
† This patient appeared to be hypothyroid (T_4 = 2.1 μg/dl) and had evidence of other pituitary deficiencies. The plasma TSH was 9 μU/ml.
‡ An unreported 35-year-old prepubertal, myxedematous, hypoadrenal female with two affected male sibs showed a small delayed peak in TSH after TRH stimulation. After treatment with physiologic doses of T_4 and cortisone acetate she failed to respond. (Courtesy of G. Segre, Massachusetts General Hospital.)
SOURCE: Dr. M. Harbison, revised and with additions.

in which nontoxic goiter occurred in five generations and in four of five members of the sibship of the propositus. The thyroid glands were characterized by nodularity and by calcification which was strikingly evident on roentgenographic examination. None of the recognized abnormalities of thyroid function was present. There was evidence of increased uptake and turnover of iodine, and the distribution of iodoamino acids in these thyroid glands was normal. A possibly similar infant with neonatal hypothyroidism and a calcified goiter has been described by Courpotin et al. [324].

Greig et al. [325] have reported two pairs of monozygotic twins, one pair of which was athyreotic and the other had ectopic thyroid tissue. They also reported a mother-daughter pair who were athyreotic. Familial nonendemic, athyreotic cretinism has been occasionally reported elsewhere. There is the possibility that some of these patients may have had thyroids unresponsive to TSH or one of the syndromes of TSH deficiency. Cross et al. [326] studied a hypothyroid sib pair, one of whom had thyroid tissue in a normal position by technetium scanning. A feature was muscular hypotrophy, which qualified the pair for inclusion in the Debré-Semelaigne syndrome. There was no response to TSH administration.

Savoie et al. have identified mono- and diiodohistidine in the thyroids and urine of four unrelated patients with congenital goitrous hypothyroidism [327]. The T_4 content of the goiters was very low; the iodohistidine appeared to be in the albumin of the gland. The authors suggested that some form of thyroglobulin defect resulted in inappropriate iodination of histidyl residues of albumin.

DIAGNOSIS OF FAMILIAL THYROID DISEASE

These patients usually attract attention because of hypothyroidism, goiter, or both. They may be detected in the course of screening programs, or early in the postnatal period because of failure to thrive and some of the other manifestations of hypothyroidism, or they may be undetected until much later.

If hypothyroidism is established in the postnatal period or during the first important developmental months, then in general it is probably unwise to undertake extensive investigation. Rather, the child should be vigorously treated. Some years later, medication can be withdrawn and an effort made to ascertain the precise type of hypothyroidism.

At the time of critical evaluation, a TSH measurement is invaluable in indicating whether the origin of the hypothyroidism is in the pituitary or elsewhere. If elsewhere, a radioiodide or technetium scan will indicate the size and position of the functional thyroid, if present. For this purpose, especially in the young, technetium is preferred.

The most useful observation thereafter is the uptake and retention of labeled iodine by the thyroid. Characteristically these patients, except those with the transport defect and TSH unresponsiveness, have an unusually rapid uptake curve, which reaches high levels within the first hour or two following administration. Measurements of turnover and of the effects of ClO_4^- and methimazole may give further clues to diagnosis. Analysis of the pattern of metabolism of the iodoamino acids in the peripheral blood also may be helpful. Most important is histological and biochemical analysis of the thyroid itself. Study of one of these patients may rapidly become a major research project.

The discussion thus far has centered largely on the diagnosis in patients who have a complete defect, i.e., homozygous expression. An important problem, and a more difficult one from many points of view, is the diagnosis of a specific genetic defect in a patient who may be heterozygous for that defect. Thus in the deiodinase-defect group the heterozygous state may cause disease. There is also evidence that heterozygotes for the transport and organification defects may also have goiter. Clearly, much further research is needed so that heterozygotes may be detected and the contribution of the heterozygous state of these defects to mild thyroid disease determined.

TREATMENT

Satisfactory treatment depends on the stage of development of the local disease and the degree to which irreversible changes have occurred in the skeleton and central nervous system. Remarkable shrinkage of the goiter (if present) may be expected from treatment with thyroid hormone in usual maintenance doses, provided irreversible changes of degeneration, cyst formation, and fibrous replacement have not taken place. The goiter will inevitably recur if medication is discontinued.

Care should be exercised in managing a patient with a familial goiter in view of the tendency of some goiters to undergo malignant change. In general, it would be wise to remove any nodule which fails to shrink after several weeks of replacement therapy. Unfortunately, this is often the case with well-established goiters, so that more often than not these patients eventually require surgery. Thyroid hormone is required after thyroidectomy, unless it is desirable to maintain the patient in a hypothyroid state.

Unless treatment is begun early within the first few weeks of life, there is risk of permanent retardation of intellectual development or skeletal growth. There is reason to suspect that damage may occur in utero, so that no amount of replacement therapy may prevent developmental arrest and permanent retardation.

Medication should be sufficient. Perhaps a safe rule is to give increasing doses of hormone until the first signs of overdosage appear (tachycardia, hyperactivity) and then to reduce the dosage slightly. Particular attention should be paid to newborn sibs of patients who have familial goiter.

Management of the patients with fully developed goiter, hypothyroidism, and permanent retardation is unsatisfactory. Little is accomplished in the adult by replacement therapy, and as often as not unacceptable aggressiveness or other undesirable behavior may be the result of full thyroid medication. In these patients the dosage is best adjusted to that which keeps the patients active and comfortable without arousing unwanted side effects.

A few patients with familial goiter, such as some of those who have associated VIIIth nerve deafness, appear to manufacture adequate amounts of hormone and to develop normally. They require thyroid substance only to prevent growth of the small goiters to which they are predisposed.

Special problems arise if the hypothyroid state is a result of deficient TSH. Immediate and vigorous replacement medication with thyroid hormone may precipitate an adrenal cortical crisis, if the adrenal cortical system has reduced function. Adequacy of this system must be established before hypothyroidism is treated in patients with hypothyroidism accompanied by low TSH.

REFERENCES

1. DEGROOT LJ (ed): *Endocrinology.* New York, Grune & Stratton, Inc, 1979, vol 1
2. DE VISSCHER M (ed): *The Thyroid Gland.* New York, Raven Press, 1980
3. GREER MA, SOLOMON DH: *Handbook of Physiology,* Sec 7, *Endocrinology.* Washington, DC, American Physiological Society, 1974, vol 3
4. STANBURY JB: Familial goiter, in Stanbury JB, Wyngaarden JB, Fredrickson DS (eds): *The Metabolic Basis of Inherited Disease,* ed 4. New York, McGraw-Hill Book Co, 1978, p 206
5. DUMONT JE: The action of thyrotropin on thyroid metabolism, *Vit Horm* 29:287-412, 1971
6. ROSS EM, HAGA T, HOWLETT AC, SCHWARZMEIER J, SCHLEIFER LS, GILMAN AG: Hormone-sensitive adenylate cyclase: Resolution and reconstitution of components necessary for regulation of the enzyme, *Adv Cycl Nucl Res* 9:53-68, 1978
7. SWILLENS S, DUMONT JE: A unifying model of current concepts and data on adenylate cyclase activation by β-adrenergic agonists, *Life Sci* 27:1013-1028, 1980
8. CORBIN JD, LINCOLN TM: Comparison of cAMP- and cGMP-dependent protein kinases, *Adv Cycl Nucl Res* 9:159-170, 1978
9. DUMONT JE, BOEYNAEMS JM, DECOSTER C, ERNEUX C, LAMY F, LECOCQ R, MOCKEL J, UNGER J, VAN SANDE J: Biochemical mechanisms in the control of thyroid function and growth, *Adv Cycl Nucl Res* 9:723-734, 1978
10. VAN HERLE AJ, VASSART G, DUMONT JE: Control of thyroglobulin synthesis and secretion, *N Engl J Med* 301:239-249, 307-314, 1979
11. EKHOLM R: Thyroid hormone secretion, *Hormones Cell Regul* 1:51-110, 1977
12. FIELD JB, MUTO H, CHOU MCY: The adenylate cyclase-cyclic AMP system in Graves' disease, *Adv Cycl Nucl Res* 12:359-372, 1980
13. DUMONT JE, BOEYNAEMS JM, VAN SANDE J, ERNEUX C, DECOSTER C, VAN CAUTER E, MOCKEL J: Cyclic AMP, calcium and cyclic GMP in the regulation of thyroid function, *Horm Cell Regul* 1:171-194, 1977
14. VAN SANDE J, MOCKEL J, BOEYNAEMS JM, DOR P, ANDRY G, DUMONT JE: Regulation of cyclic nucleotide and prostaglandin formation in normal human thyroid tissues and in autonomous nodules, *J Clin Endoc Metab* 50:776-785, 1980
15. OTTEN J, DUMONT JE: Glucose metabolism in normal human thyroid tissue in vitro, *Eur J Clin Invest* 2:213-219, 1972
16. PEKONEN F, WEINTRAUB BD: Thyrotropin receptors on bovine thyroid membranes: Two types with different affinities and specificities, *Endocrinology* 105:352-359, 1979
17. STANBURY JB, ROCMANS P, BUHLER UK, OCHI Y: Congenital hypothyroidism with impaired thyroid response to thyrotropin, *N Engl J Med* 279:1132, 1968
18. CODACCIONI JL, CARAYON P, MICHEL-BECHET M, FOUCAULT F, LEFORT G, PIERRON H: Congenital hypothyroidism associated with thyrotropin unresponsiveness and thyroid cell membrane alterations, *J Clin Endocrinol Metab* 50:932, 1980
19. MARX SJ, HERSHMAN JM, AURBACH GD: Thyroid dysfunction in pseudohypoparathyroidism, *J Clin Endocrin Metab* 33:822, 1971
20. WOLFSDORF JI, ROSENFIELD RL, FANG VS, KOBAYASHI R, RAZDAN AK, KIM MH: Partial gonadotrophin-resistance in pseudohypoparathyroidism, *Acta Endocrinol (Kbh)* 88:321, 1978
21. FARFEL Z, BRICKMAN AS, KASLOW HR, BROTHERS VM, BOURNE HR: Defect of receptor-cyclase coupling protein in pseudohypoparathyroidism. *Mass Med Soc* 303:237, 1980
22. KASLOW HR, JOHNSON GL, BROTHERS VM, BOURNE HR: A regulatory component of adenylate cyclase from human erythrocyte membranes. *J Bio Chem* 255:3736, 1980
23. MEDEIROS-NETO GA, KNOBEL M, BRONSTEIN MD, SIMONETTI J, FILHO FF, MATTAR E: Impaired cyclic-AMP response to thyrotrophin in congenital hypothyroidism with thyroglobulin deficiency. *Acta Endocrinol* 92:62, 1972
24. JOB JC, CANLORBE P, THOMASSIN N, VASSAL J: L'hypothyroidie infantile à début précoce avec glande en place, fixation fiable de radio-iode et défaut de réponse à la thyrostimuline. *Ann Endocrinol* 30:696, 1979
25. BEAMER WG, EICHER EM, MALTAIS LJ, SOUTHARD JL: Inherited primary hypothyroidism in mice, *Science* 212:61 1981
26. MACCHIA V, MELDOLESHI MF, CHIARIELLO M: Adenyl-cyclase in a transplantable thyroid tumor: Loss of ability to respond to TSH. *Endocrinology* 90:1483, 1972
27. MANDATO E, MELDOLESI MF, MACCHIA V: Diminished binding of thyroid stimulating hormone in a transplantable rat thyroid tumor as a possible cause of hormone unresponsiveness. *Cancer Res* 35:3089, 1975
28. MELDOLESI MF, FISHMAN PH, SALVATORE MA, KOHN LD, BRADY RO: Relationship of gangliosides to the structure and function of thyrotropin receptors: Their absence on plasma membranes of a thyroid tumor defective in thyrotropin receptor activity. *Proc Natl Acad Sci USA* 73:4060, 1976
29. ABE Y, ICHIKAWA Y, HOMMA M, ITO K, MIMURA T: TSH receptor and adenylate cyclase in undifferentiated thyroid carcinoma. *Lancet* 2:506, 1977
30. CARAYON P, THOMAS-MORVAN C, CASTANAS E, TUBIANA M: Human thyroid cancer: Membrane thyrotropin binding and adenylate cyclase activity. *J Clin Endocrinol Metab* 51:915, 1980
31. TAKAHASI H, JIANG N, GORMAN CA, LEE CY: Thyrotropin receptors in normal and pathological human thyroid tissues. *J Clin Endocrinol Metab* 47:870, 1978
32. MERIN RM, WOLLMAN SH: Transparent-chamber studies of vessels circu-

lation, and follicles in thyroid grafts in unanesthetized mice, *J Natl Cancer Inst* 34:415, 1965

33. SODERBERG U: Temporal characteristics of thyroid activity, *Physiol Rev* 39:777, 1959

34. ROCMANS PA, PENEL JC, CANTRAINE FR, DUMONT JE: Kinetic analysis of iodide transport in dog thyroid slices: Perchlorate-induced discharge, *Am J Physiol* 232:E343, 1977

35. WOLFF J: Transport of iodide and other anions in the thyroid gland, *Physiol Rev* 44:45, 1964

36. ANDROS G, WOLLMAN SH: Autoradiographic localization of radioiodide in the thyroid gland of the mouse, *Am J Physiol* 213:198, 1967

37. CHOW SY, WOODBURY DM: Kinetics of distribution of radioactive perchlorate in rat and guinea-pig thyroid glands, *J Endocrinol* 47:207, 1970

38. BROWN-GRANT K: Extrathyroidal iodide concentrating mechanisms, *Physiol Rev* 41:189, 1961

39. WOLFF J: Iodide concentrating mechanism, in Rall JE, Kopin IJ (eds): *The Thyroid and Biogenic Amines.* Amsterdam, Elsevier North-Holland Biomedical Press, 1972, vol 8, p 115

40. BAGCHI N, FAWCETT DM: Role of sodium ion in active transport of iodide by cultured thyroid cells. *Biochim Biophys Acta* 318:235, 1973

41. TYLER DD, GONZE J, LAMY F, DUMONT JE: Influence of mitochondrial inhibitors on the respiration and energy-dependent uptake of iodide by thyroid slices, *Biochem J* 106:123, 1968

42. SHISHIBA Y, SOLOMON DH: Effect of amphotericin B on thyroidal iodide concentration, *Endocrinology* 81:467, 1967

43. IFF HW, WILBRANDT W: Die Abhangigkeit der Jodakkumulation in Schilddrusenschnitten von der ionalen Zusammensetzung des Inkubationsmediums und ihre Beeinflussung durch Herzglykoside, *Biochim Biophys Acta* 70:711, 1963

44. VILKKI P, JAAKONMAKI I: Role of fatty acids in iodide-complexing lecithin, *Endocrinology* 78:453, 1966

45. KNOPP J, STOLC V, TONG W: Evidence for the induction of iodide transport in bovine thyroid cells treated with thyroid stimulating hormone and dibutyryl cyclic adenosine 3′5′—monophosphate, *J Biol chem* 245: 4403, 1970

46. JORTAY AM, CANTRAINE FRL, DUMONT JE: Iodide trapping by thyroid slices in vitro, *Horm Metab Res* 6:309, 1974

47. STANBURY JB, CHAPMAN EM: Congenital hypothyroidism with goitre: Absence of an iodide-concentrating mechanism. *Lancet* 1:1162, 1960

48. FEDERMAN D, ROBBINS J, RALL JE: Some observations on cretinism and its treatment. *N Engl J Med* 259:610, 1958

49. WOLFF J, THOMPSON RH, ROBBINS J: Congenital goitrous cretinism due to absence of iodide-concentrating ability. *J Clin Endocrinol Metab* 24:699, 1964

50. GILBOA V, BER A, LEWITIS Z, HASENFRATZ J: Goitrous myxedema due to iodide trapping defect. *Arch Intern Med* 112:212, 1963

51. TOYOSHIMA K, MATSUMOTO Y, NISHIDA M, YABUUCHI H: Five cases of absence of iodide concentrating mechanism. *Acta Endocrinol* 84:527, 1977

52. PANNALL PR, STEYN AF, VAN REENEN O: Iodide-trapping defect of the thyroid. *S Afr Med J* 53:414, 1978

53. STRUWE FR E, SESEKE G, KEMPE H, HOFFMAN G: Seltene form der hypothyreose bei geschwietern (jodakkumulationsstorung), *Mschr Kinderheilk* 117:189, 1969

53a. SAITO K, YAMAMOTO K, YOSHIDA S, MANABE S, SUZUKI M, TAKAI T, SAITO T, KUZUYA T, MORIYAMA S: Goitrous hypothyroidism due to iodide-trapping defect. *J Clin Endocrinol Metab* 53:1267, 1981

54. PAPADOPOULOS SN, VAGENAKIS AG, MOSCHOS A, KOUTRAS DA, MATSANIOTIS N. MALAMOS B: A case of a partial defect of the iodide trapping mechanism. *J Clin Endocrinol Metab* 30:302, 1970

55. MEDEIROS-NETO GA, BLOISE W, ULHOA-CINTRA AB: Partial defect of iodide traping mechanism in two siblings with congenital goiter and hypothyroidism. *J Clin Endocrinol Metab* 35:370, 1972

56. NUNEZ J: Iodination and thyroid hormone synthesis, in De Visscher M (ed): *The Thyroid Gland.* New York, Raven Press, 1980, pp 39–59

57. TAUROG A: Hormone synthesis, in DeGroot L (ed): *Endocrinology.* New York, Grune & Stratton, Inc, 1979, pp 331–342

58. NUNEZ J, POMMIER J: Formation of thyroid hormones, *Vit Horm* 1981 (in press)

59. ROSENBERG IN, ATMANS JC, ISAACS GH: Studies on thyroid iodine metabolism. *Rec Progr Horm Res* 21:33, 1965

60. RODESCH F, NEVE P, WILLEMS C, DUMONT JE: Stimulation of thyroid metabolism by thyrotropin, cyclic 3′5′-AMP, dibutyryl cyclic 3′5′-AMP and prostaglandin E. *Eur J Biochem* 8:26, 1969

61. DEGROOT LJ, NIEPOMNISZCZE H: Biosynthesis of thyroid hormone: Basic and clinical aspects, *Metabolism* 26:665, 1977

62. STEIN O, GROSS J: Metabolism of ^{125}I in thyroid gland studied with electron microscopic autoradiography. *Endocrinology* 75:787, 1964

63. HILDERSON HJ, VAN DESSEL G, LAGROU A, DIERICK W: The subcellular biochemistry of thyroid. *Subcell Biochem* 7:213, 1980

64. TICE LW, WOLLMAN SH: Ultrastructural localization of peroxidase activity on membranes of the typical thyroid epithelial cells, *Lab Invest* 26:63, 1972

65. RODESCH FR, DUMONT JE: Metabolic properties of isolated sheep thyroid cells. *Exp Cell Res* 47:386, 1967

66. ROUSSET B, PONCET CH, DUMONT JE, MORNEX R: Intracellular and extracellular sites of iodination in dispersed hog thyroid cells, *Biochem J* 192:801, 1980

67. ERICSON LE: Exocytosis and endocytosis in the thyroid follicle cell, *Mol Cell Endocrinal* 22:1, 1981

68. POMMIER J: Structure-function relationship in thyroglobulin, *Horm Cell Regul* 2:180, 1978

69. CANTRAINE FRL, DUMONT JE: Models of in vitro thyroglobulin iodination, *Mol Cell Endocrinol* 2:233, 1975

70. DEMEESTER-MIRKINE N, VAN SANDE J, CORVILAIN J, DUMONT JE: Benign thyroid nodule with normal iodide trap and defective organification. *J Clin Endocrinol Metab* 41:1169, 1975

71. STANBURY JB, HEDGE AN: A study of a family of goitrous cretins. *J Clin Endocrinol Metab* 10:1471, 1950

72. PEREZ-CUVIT E, CRIGLER JF Jr, STANBURY JB: Partial and total iodide organification defect in different sibships in a kindred. *Am J Hum Genet* 29:142, 1977

73. HADDAD HM, SIDBURY JB Jr: Defect of the iodinating system in congenital goitrous cretinism: Report of a case with biochemical studies. *J Clin Endocrinol Metab* 19:1446, 1959

74. SCHULTZ A, FLINK EB, KENNEDY BJ, ZIEVE L: Exchangeable character of accumulated I^{131} in the thyroid gland of a goitrous cretin. *J Clin Endocrinol Metab* 17:441, 1957

75. CLAYTON GW, SMITH JD, LEISER AL: Familial goiter with defect in intrinsic metabolism of thyroxine without hypothyroidism. *J Pediatr* 52:129, 1958

76. FURTH ED, CARVALHO M, VIANNA B: Familial goiter due to an organification defect in euthyroid siblings. *J Clin Endocrinol* 27:1137, 1967

77. LELONG M, JOSEPH R, CANLORBE P, JOB JC, PLAINFOSSE B.: L'hypothyroidic par anomalie congenitale de l'hormonogenese (cinq observations). *Arch Fr Pediatr* 13:1, 1956

78. MOURIZ J, RIESCO G, USOBIAGA P: Thyroid proteins in a goitrous cretin with iodide organification defect. *J Clin Endocrinol Metab* 29:942, 1969

79. POMMIER J, TOURNIAIRE J, RAHMOUN B, DEME D, PALLO D, BORNET H, NUNEZ J: Thyroid iodine organification defects: A case with lack of thyroglobulin iodination and a case without any peroxidase activity. *J Clin Endocrinol Metab* 42:319, 1976

80. VALENTA LJ, BODE H, VICKERY AL, CAULFIELD JB, MALOOF F: Lack of thyroid peroxidase activity as the cause of congenital goitrous hypothyroidism. *J Clin Endocrinol Metab* 36:830, 1973

81. EGGO MC, BURROW GN, ALEXANDER NM, GORDON JH: Iodination and the structure of human thyroglobulin., *J Clin Endocrinol Metab* 51:7, 1980

82. MEDEIROS-NETO GA, KALLAS WG, TAUROG A, KNOBEL M, BISI H, CALALIERE H, MATTAR E: Familial thyroid peroxidase deficiency associated with retinitis pigmentosa. Submitted to *Clin Endocrinol (London)*, 1981, in press

83. MEDEIROS-NETO GA, KNOBEL M, YAMAMOTO K, CAVALIERE H, KALLAS W: Deficient thyroid peroxidase causing organification defect and goitrous hypothyroidism. *J Endocrinol Invest* 2:353, 1979

84. NUNEZ J, POMMIER J, DOMINICI R, RAHMOUN B, DEME D, TOURNIAIRE J: Peroxidase and thyroglobulins from different goiters. Thyroid Research, 7th International Thyroid Conference, 1976, p 467

85. NIEPOMNISZCZE H, DEGROSSI OJ, SCAVINI LM, CURUTCHET HP: Familial goiter with partial iodine incorporation block and euthyroidism due to the deficient peroxidase defect. Thyroid Research, 7th International Thyroid Conference, 1976, p 470

86. NIEPOMNISZCZE H, CASTELLS S, DEGROOT LJ, REFETOFF S, KIM OS, RAPOPORT B, HATI R: Peroxidase defect in congenital goiter with complete organification block. *J Clin Endocrinol Metab* 36:347, 1973

87. POMMIER J, DOMINICI R, BOUGNERES P, RAHMOUN B, NUNEZ J: A dialysable inhibitor bound to thyroglobulin and from two goiters with iodine organification defect. *J Mol Med* 2:169, 1977

88. NIEPOMNISZCZE H, ROSENBLOOM AL, DEGROOT LJ, SHIMAOKA K, REFETOFF S, YAMAMOTO K: Differentiation of two abnormalities in thyroid peroxidase causing organification defect and goitrous hypothyroidism. *Metabolism* 24:57, 1975

89. NIEPOMNISZCZE H, DEGROOT LJ, HAGEN GA: Abnormal thyroid peroxidase causing iodide organification. *J Clin Endocrinol Metab* 34:607, 1972

90. POMMIER J, TOURNIAIRE J, DEME D, CHALENDAR D, BORNET H, NUNEZ J: A defective thyroid peroxidase solubilized from a familial goiter with iodine organification defect. *J Clin Endocrinol Metab* 39:69, 1974

91. MEDEIROS-NETO GA, NAKASHIMA T, TAUROG A, KNOBEL M, SIMONETTI JP, MATTAR E: Congenital goitre and hypothyroidism with impaired

iodide organification and high thyroid peroxidase concentration. *Clin Endocrinol* 11:123, 1979

92. KUSAKABE T: Deficient cytochrome b₅ reductase activity in nontoxic goiter with iodide organification defect. *Metabolism* 24:1103, 1975

92a. KUSAKABE T: Goitrous subject with defective synthesis of diiodotyrosine due to thyroglobulin abnormalities. *J Clin Endocrinol Metab* 37:317, 1973

93. NIEPOMNISZCZE H, MEDEIROS-NETO GA, REFETOFF S, DEGROOT LJ, FANG VS: Familial goitre with partial iodine organification defect, lack of thyroglobulin and high levels of thyroid peroxidase. *Clin Endocrinol* 6:27, 1977

94. LELONG M, JOSEPH R, CANLORBE P, JOB JC, PLAINFOSSE B: L'hypothyroidie par anomalie congenitale de l'hormonogenese (cinq observations). *Arch Fr Pediatr* 13:1, 1956

95. GARDNER JV, HAYLES AB, WOOLNER LB, OWEN CA: Iodine metabolism in goitrous cretins. *J Clin Endocrinol Metab* 19:638, 1959

96. KONIG MP, BAUMANN TH, SCHARER K, HERREN CH: Familiare kongenitale Storung der Schilddrusnwnhormonsynthese: Fehlerhafte Oxydation von anorganischen Jod. *Schweiz Med Wochenschr* 94:319, 1964

97. JACKSON ADM: Non-endemic goitrous cretinism. *Arch Dis Child* 29:571, 1954

98. PENA J, BELMONTE AV, TOJO R: Hipotiroidismo bocioso por defecto en el proceso de organificatión del iodo: Una observación en gemelos. *Rev Esp Pediatr* 21:103, 1965

99. MOURIZ J, RIESCO G, USOBIAGA P: Thyroid proteins in a goitrous cretin with iodide organification defect. *J Clin Endocrinol Metab* 29:942, 1969

100. VALENTA L: Metastatic thyroid carcinoma in man concentrating iodine without organification. *J Clin Endocrinol Metab* 26:1317, 1966

101. NEEL JV, CARR EA, BEIERWALTES WH, DAVIDSON RT: Genetic studies on the congenitally hypothyroid. *Pediatrics* 27:269, 1971

102. CARR EA, BEIERWALTES WH, NEEL JV, DAVIDSON R, LOWRY GG, DODSON VN, TANTON JH: The various types of thyroid malfunction in cretinism and their relative frequency. *Pediatrics* 28:1, 1961

103. SALABE BG, PINCHERA A, BACHIERI L, MONACO F: The potential malignancy of thyroid nodules with organification defect. Report of a case. *Folia Endocrinol* 22:23, 1969

104. CLAYTON GW, SMITH JD, LEISER A: Familial goiter with defect in intrinsic metabolism of thyroxine without hypothyroidism. *J Pediatr* 52:129, 1958

105. VALENTA LJ, BODE H, VICKERY AL, CAULFIELD JB, MALOOF F: Lack of thyroid peroxidase activity as the cause of congenital goitrous hypothyroidism. *J Clin Endocrinol* 36:830, 1973

106. HAGEN GA, NIEPOMNISZCZE H, HAIBACH H, BIGAZZI M, HATI R, RAPOPORT B, JIMENIZ C, DEGROOT LJ, FRAWLEY TE: Peroxidase deficiency in familial goiter with iodide organification defect. *N Engl J Med* 285:1394, 1971

109. BASCHIERI L, BENEDETTI G, DELUCA F, NEGRI M: Evaluation and limitations of the perchlorate test in the study of thyroid function. *J Clin Endocrinol Metab* 23:786, 1963

110. MILUTINOVIC PS, STANBURY JB, WICKEN JV, JONES EW: Thyroid function in a family with the Pendred syndrome. *J Clin Endocrinol Metab* 29:962, 1969

111. BRAIN WR: Heredity in simple goiter. *Q J Med* 20:303, 1927

112. NILSSON LR, BORGFORS N, GAMSTROP I, HOLST HE, LIDEN G: Nonendemic goitre and deafness. *Acta Paediatr* 53:117, 1964

113. BAX GM: Het Krop-Doofheid Syndroom van Pendred. Amsterdam, Drukkerij Wed, G van Soest N V, 1965

114. JOHNSEN S: Familial deafness and goitre in persons with a low level of protein-bound iodine. *Acta Otolaryngol (Stock)* (suppl) 140:168, 1958

115. THOULD AK, SCOWEN EF: The syndrome of congenital deafness and simple goitre, in Pitt-Rivers R (ed): *Advances in Thyroid Research.* Elmsford, NY, Pergamon Press, Inc, 1961

116. ELMAN DS: Familial association of nerve deafness with nodular goiter and thyroid carcinoma. *N Engl J Med* 259:219, 1958

117. ROBERTS KD: Thyroid carcinoma in childhood in Great Britain. *Arch Dis Child* 32:58, 1957

118. THIEME ET: A report of the occurrence of deaf-mutism and goiter in four of six siblings of a North American family. *Ann Surg* 146:941, 1957

119. MORGANS ME, TROTTER WR: Association of congenital deafness with goitre. *Lancet* 1:607, 1958

120. MEDEIROS-NETO GA, NICOLAU W, KIEFFER J, CINTRA ABU: Thyroidal iodoproteins in Pendred's syndrome. *J Clin Endocrinol Metab* 28:1205, 1968

121. SHANE SR, JONES JE, FLINK EB: Familial goiter and congenital nerve deafness. *J Clin Endocrinol Metab* 25:1085, 1965

122. LJUNGREN J-G, LINDSTROM H, HJERN B: The concentration of peroxidase in normal and adenomatous human thyroid tissue with special reference to patients with Pendred's syndrome. *Acta Endocrinol* 72:272, 1973

123. BURROW GN, SPAULDING SW, ALEXANDER NM, BOWER BF: Normal peroxidase activity in Pendred's syndrome. *J Clin Endocrinol Metab* 36:522, 1973

124. CAVE WT JR, DUNN JT: Studies on the thyroidal defect in an atypical form of Pendred's syndrome. *J Clin Endocrinol Metab* 41:590, 1975

125. BARGMAN GJ, GARDNER LI: Otic lesions and congenital hypothyroidism in the developing chick. *J Clin Invest* 46:1828, 1967

126. DEOL MS: An experimental approach to the understanding and treatment of hereditary syndromes with congenital deafness and hypothyroidism. *J Med Genet* 10:235, 1973

127. DEOL MS: Congenital deafness and hypothyrodism. *Lancet* 2:105, 1973

128. DESAI KB, MEHTA MN, PATEL MC, RAMANNA L, GANATRA RD: Thyroidal iodoproteins in Pendred's syndrome. *J Endocrinol Metab* 63:409, 1974

129. ALMEIDA F, TEMPORAL A, CAVALCANTI N, NETO SL, ALBUQUERQUE R, SA TC: Pendred's syndrome in an area of endemic goiter in Brazil: Genetic and metabolic studies, in Dunn JT, Medeiros-Neto GA (eds): *Endemic Goiter and Cretinism: Continuing Threats to World Health.* Washington, DC, World Health Organization, 1974, p 167

129a. NIEPOMNISZCZE H: Personal communication

130. SAFAR A, CHAUSSAIN J-L, VASSAL J, CANLORBE P, DAILLY R, DE MENIBUS CH, SAVIOE J-C, JOB JC: Hypothyroidie précoce majeure, partiellement regressive, dans deux cas de syndrome de Pendred. *Arch Fr Pediatr* 30:843, 1973

131. GOMEZ-PAN A, EVERED DC, HALL R: Pituitary-thyroid function in Pendred's syndrome. *Br Med J* 2:152, 1974

132. THOMPSON J, MAGUIRE NC, HURWITZ LJ: A family with deafness, goitre, epilepsy, and low intelligence segregating independently. *Ir J Med Sci* 3:427, 1970

133. FRASER GR, MORGANS ME, TROTTER WR: The syndrome of sporadic goitre and congenital deafness. *Q J Med* 29:279, 1960

134. PAPASOV VG: Untersuchungen uber das wesen des Pendred-syndroms. *Z Gesamte Inn Med* 24:766, 1969

135. TROTTER WR: The association of deafness with thyroid dysfunction. *Br Med Bull* 16:92, 1960

136. STANBURY JB, OHELA K, PITT-RIVERS R: The metabolism of iodine in two goitrous cretins compared with that in two patients receiving methimazole. *J Clin Endocrinol Metab* 15:54, 1955

137. STANBURY JB: Familial goiter, in Stanbury JB, Wyngaarden JB, Fredrickson DS (eds): *The Metabolic Basis of Inherited Disease,* ed 3. New York, McGraw-Hill Book Co, 1972, p 233

138. JACOBSEN BB: Normal serum T3 value in one of two siblings with goitrous hypothyroidism and dyshormonogenesis. *Dan Med Bull* 20:192, 1973

139. MORRIS JH: Defective coupling of iodotyrosine in familial goiters. *Arch Int Med* 114:417, 1964

139a. COOPER DS, AXELROD L, DEGROOT LJ, VICKERY AL, MALOOF F: Congenital goiter and the development of metastatic follicular carcinoma with evidence for a leak of nonhormonal iodide: Clinical, pathological, kinetic, and biochemical studies and a review of the literature. *J Clin Endocrinol Metab* 52:294, 1981

140. ERMANS AM, KINTHAERT J, CAMUS M: Defective intrathyroidal iodine metabolism in nontoxic goiter: Inadequate iodination of thyroglobulin. *J Clin Endocrinol Metab* 28:1307, 1968

141. DENAYER P, VASSART G: Structure and biosynthesis of thyroglobulin, in De Visscher M (ed): *The Thyroid Gland.* New York, Raven Press, 1980, p 21

142. SALVATORE G, STANBURY JB, RALL JE: Inherited defects of thyroid hormone biosynthesis, in De Visscher M (ed): *The Thyroid Gland.* New York, Raven Press, 1980, p 443

143. MARRIQ C, ROLLAND M, LISSITZKY S: Polypeptide chains of 19-S thyroglobulin from several mammalian species and of porcine 27-S iodoprotein. *Eur J Biochem* 79:143, 1977

144. VASSART G, BROCAS H: Restriction mapping of synthetic thyroglobulin structural gene as a means of investigating thyroglobulin structure. *Biochim Biophys Acta* 610:189, 1980

145. DUNN JT, DUNN AD, HEPPNER DG JR, KIM PS: A discrete thyroxine-rich iodopeptide of 20,000 daltons from rabbit thyroglobulin. *J Biol Chem* 256:942, 1981

146. MARRIQ C, STEIN A, ROLLAND M, LISSITZKY S: Probable internal homology in thyroglobulin peptide chain. *Eur J Biochem* 87:275, 1978

147. CHRISTOPHE D, BROCAS H, GANNON F, DE MARTYNOFF G, PAYS E, VASSART G: Molecular cloning of bovine thyroglobulin complementary DNA; Characterization of 2500-base-pair and 1900-base-pair fragments. *Eur J Biochem* 111:419, 1980

148. SPIRO MJ: Preferential response of thyroid glycosyltransferases to changes in thyrotropin stimulation. *Arch Biochem Biophys* 202:35, 1980

149. SPIRO RG, SPIRO MJ, BHOYROO VD: Processing of carbohydrate units of glycoproteins. Characterization of thyroid glucosidase. *J Biol Chem* 254:7659, 1979

150. RONIN D, BOUCHILLOUX S: Cell-free labeling in thyroid rough microsomes of lipid-linked and protein-linked oligosaccharides: I. Mannosylated units. *Biochim Biophys Acta* 539:470, 1978

151. MONACO F, D'ARMIENTO M, ROBBINS J: Incorporation of carbohydrates into abnormal thyroglobulin in an experimental rat thyroid tumor. *Endocrinology* 94:1445, 1974

152. BERG G, BJORKMAN U, EKHOLM R: Conformational change of the thyroglobulin molecule induced by oxidation in vitro. *Mol Cell Endocrinol* 17:139, 1980

153. RIDDICK FA JR, DESAI KB, STANBURY JB, MURISON PJ: Familial goiter with diminished synthesis of thyroglobulin. *Z Exp Med* 150:203, 1969

154. MOURIZ J, RIESCO G, USOBIAGA P: Thyroid proteins in a goitrous cretin with iodide organification defect. *J Clin Endocrinol Metab* 29:942, 1969

155. STANBURY JB: The iodoproteins of the normal and abnormal thyroid gland. *Adv Clin Biochem Res* 4:5, 1968

156. LIZARRALDE G, JONES B, SEAL US, JONES JE: Goitrous cretinism with chromosomal aberration and defect in thyroglobulin synthesis. *J Clin Endocrinol Metab* 26:1227, 1966

157. ALEXANDER NM, BURROW GN: Thyroxine biosynthesis in human goitrous cretinism. *J Clin Endocrinol Metab* 30:308, 1970

158. McGIRR EM, HUTCHISON JH, CLEMENT WE, KENNEDY JS, CURRIE AR: Goitre and cretinism due to the production of an abnormal iodinated thyroid compound. *Scott Med J* 5:189, 1960

159. MICHEL R, RALL JE, ROCHE J, TUBIANA M: Thyroidal iodoproteins in patients with goitrous hypothyroidism. *J Clin Endocrinol Metab* 24:352, 1964

160. DEGROOT LJ, STANBURY JB: The syndrome of congenital goiter with butanol-insoluble serum iodide. *Am J Med* 27:586, 1959

161. PITTMAN CS, PITTMAN JA JR: A study of the thyroglobulin, thyroidal protease, and iodoproteins in two congenital goitrous cretins. *Am J Med* 40:49, 1966

162. ALEXANDER NM, BURROW GN: Thyroxine biosynthesis in human goitrous cretinism. *J Clin Endocrinol Metab* 30:308, 1970

163. SULTAN CH, BISMUTH J, CASTAY M, DUMAS R, MICHEL-BECHET M, LISSITZKY S, JEAN B: Hypothyroidie par anomalie congenitale de synthèse de la thyroglobuline. *Arch Fr Pediatr* 31:11, 1974

164. LELONG M, CANLORBE P, MICHEL R, TUBIANA M, JOB JC: Un cas d'hypothyroidie par anomalie de l'hormonogenèse. *Arch Fr Pediatr* 17:105, 1960

165. WAGAR G, LAMBERG BA, SAARINEN P: Congenital goitre with thyroglobulin deficiency, in Robbins J, Braverman LE (eds): *Thyroid Research.* Amsterdam, Excerpta Medica, 1966, p 463

166. RIESCO G, BERNAL J, SANCHEZ-FRANCO F: Thyroglobulin defect in a human congenital goiter. *J Clin Endocrinol Metab* 38:33, 1974

167. FOREST JC, BENARD B, BELLABARBA D, PARE G: Iodoproteins in congenital goitre with elevated levels of serum TSH and T3. *Acta Endocrinol* 76:89, 1974

168. DINSART C, WAGAR G, VOORTHUIZEN VAN F, VASSART G: Thyroglobulin complementary DNA as a means to investigate congenital goiters with impaired thyroglobulin synthesis. *Ann Endocrinol* 39:133, 1979

169. MONACO F, ANDREOLI M, BERETTA-ANGUISSOLA A: Isolation and characterization of soluble and particulate thyroid iodoproteins in human congenital goiter. *Horm Res* 5:141, 1974

170. BERNAL J, OBREGON MJ: Thyroglobulin-like antigens in a goiter with impaired thyroglobulin biosynthesis. *J Clin Endocrinol Metab* 39:592, 1974

171. KUSAKABE T: A goitrous subject with structural abnormality of thyroglobulin. *J Clin Endocrinol Metab* 35:785, 1972

172. LISSITZKY S, TORRESANI J, BURROW GN, BOUCHILLOUX S, CHABAUD O: Defective thyroglobulin export as a cause of congenital goiter. *Clin Endocrinol* 4:363, 1975

172a. MONACO F, ANDREOLI M, BERETTA-ANGUISSOLA A: Isolation and characterization of soluble and particulate thyroid iodoproteins in human congenital goiter. *Horm Res* 5:141, 1974

172b. PITTMAN CS, PITTMAN JA: A study of the thyroglobulin, thyroidal protease and iodoproteins in two congenital goitrous cretins. *Am J Med* 40:49, 1966

173. FALCONER IR, ROITT IM, SEAMARK RF, TORRIGIANI G: Studies of the congenitally goitrous sheep: Iodoproteins of the goitre. *Biochem J* 117:417, 1970

174. RAC R, HILL GN, PAIN RW, MULHEARN CJ: Congenital goitre in merino sheep due to an inherited defect in the biosynthesis of thyroid hormone. *Vet Sci* 9:209, 1968

175. DOLLING CE, GOOD BF: Congenital goitre in sheep: Isolation of the iodoproteins which replace thyroglobulins. *J Endocrinol* 71:179, 1976

176. ROBBINS J, VAN ZYL A, VAN DER WALT K: Abnormal thyroglobulin in congenital goiter of cattle. *Endocrinology* 78:1213, 1966

177. VAN ZYLE A, SCHULZ K, WILSON B, PANSEGROUW D: Thyroidal iodine and enzymatic defects in cattle with congenital goiter. *Endocrinology* 76:353, 1965

178. THERON CN, VAN JAARSVELD PP: Immunochemical properties of a thyroglobulin-like 12S iodoprotein in a congenital bovine goiter. *S Afri Med J* 46:756, 1972

179. THERON CN, VAN JAARSEVELD PP: The thyroidal serum iodoproteins in a congenital bovine goitre. *S Afr Med J* 42:756, 1975

180. VAN JAARSVELD P, VAN DER WALT B, THERON CN: Afrikander cattle congenital goiter: Purification and partial identification of the complex iodoprotein pattern. *Endocrinology* 91:470, 1972

181. PAMMENTER M, ALBRECHT C, LIEBENBERG NVDW, VAN JAARSVELD P: Afrikander cattle congenital goiter: Characteristics of its morphology and iodoprotein pattern. *Endocrinology* 102:954, 1978

182. VAN VOORTHUIZEN WF, DINSART C, FLAVELL RA, DEVIJLDER JJ, VASSART G: Abnormal cellular localization of thyroglobulin mRNA associated with hereditary congenital goiter and thyroglobulin deficiency. *Proc Natl Acad Sci USA* 75:74, 1978

183. DE VIJLDER JJ, VAN VOORTHUIZEN WF, VAN DIJK JE, RIJNBERK A, TEGELAERS WHH: Hereditary congenital goiter with thyroglobulin deficiency in a breed of goats. *Endocrinology* 102:1214, 1978

184. DINSART C, VAN VOORTHUIZEN F, VASSART G: Reverse transcription of thyroglobulin 33-S mRNA, *Eur J Biochem* 78:175, 1977

185. RIJNBERK A, DEVIJLDER JJ, VAN DIJK JE, JORNA TJ, TEGELAERS WHH: Congenital defect in iodothyronine synthesis: Clinical aspects of iodine metabolism in goats with congenital goitre and hypothyroidism. *Br Vet J* 133:495, 1977

186. VIJLDER JJ, VAN VOORTHUIZEN WF, VAN DIJK JE, VASSART G, TEGELAERS WHH: Hereditary congenital goiter in an inbred strain of goats, in Hommes FA (ed): *Models for the Study of Inborn Errors of Metabolism.* New York, Elsevier North-Holland Biomedical Press, 1979

187. VAN VOORTHUIZEN WF, DEVIJLDER JJ, VAN DIJK JE, TEGELAERS WHH: Euthyroidism via iodide supplementation in hereditary congenital goiter with thyroglobulin deficiency. *Endocrinology* 103:2105, 1978

188. MONACO F, ROBBINS J: Membrane-bound thyroglobulin in an experimental thyroid tumor of rats. *Biochim Biophys Acta* 279:118, 1972

189. MONACO F, ROBBINS J: Defective thyroglobulin synthesis in an experimental rat thyroid tumor. *J Bio Chem* 218:2328, 1973

190. SNARSKI A, SLISZ J, GOCKOWSKI K: Przpadk wrodzonej niedoczynnosci tarczycy z defektem tyreoglobuliny i zastepczym jodowaniem albuminy. *Endokrynologia Polska* 29:316, 1978

191. LAMBERG B-A, HINTZE G, KARLSSON R: Non-butanol extractable iodine in the serum of eumetabolic adult goitre patients. *Acta Endocrinol(Kbh)* 44:291, 1963

192. OWEN CA JR, McCONAHEY WM: An unusual iodinated protein of the serum in Hashimoto's thyroiditis. *J Clin Endocrinol Metab* 16:1570, 1956

193. ROBBINS J, RALL JE, RAWSON RW: A new serum iodine component in patients with functional carcinoma of the thyroid. *J Clin Endocrinol Metab* 15:1315, 1955

194. STANBURY JB, JANSSEN M-A: Labeled iodoalbumin in the plasma in thyrotoxicosis after I^{125} and I^{131}. *J Clin Endocrinol Metab* 23:1056, 1963

195. CREENSPAN FS, LOWENSTEIN JM, SPIKER P, CRAIG S: Abnormal iodoprotein in nontoxic goiter. *N Engl J Med* 269:830, 1963

196. LISSITZKY S, BISMUTH J, CODACCIONI JL, CARTOUZOU G: Congenital goiter with iodoalbumin replacing thyroglobulin and defect of deiodination of iodotyrosines: Serum origin of the thyroid iodoalbumin. *J Clin Endocrinol Metab* 28:1797, 1968

197. VANDENHOVE E, VANDENBROUCKE MF: Secretion of thyroid hormones, in De Visscher M (ed): *The Thyroid Gland.* New York, Raven Press, 1980, p 61

198. IZUMI M, LARSEN PR: Metabolic clearance of endogenous and radioiodinated thyroglobulin in rats. *Endocrinology* 103:96, 1978

199. UNGER J, VAN HEUVERSWYN B, DECOSTER C, CANTRAINE F, MOCKEL J, VAN HERLE A: Thyroglobulin and thyroid hormone release after intravenous administration of bovine thyrotropin in man. *J Clin Metab* 51:590, 1980

200. WOLLMAN SH: Secretion of thyroid hormones, in Dingle ZT, Fell MS (eds): *Lysosomes in Biology and Pathology.* Amsterdam, Elsevier North-Holland Biomedical Press, 1969, vol 2, p 483

201. UNGER J, BOEYNAEMS JM, KETELBANT-BALASSE P, DUMONT JE, MOCKEL J: Kinetics of dog thyroid secretion in vitro. *Endocrinology* 103:1597, 1978

202. DUMONT JE, WILLEMS C, VAN SANDE J, NEVE P: Regulation of the release of thyroid hormones: Role of cyclic AMP. *Ann NY Acad Sci* 185:291, 1971

203. SELJELID R, REITH A, NAKKEN KF: The early phase of endocytosis in rat thyroid follicle cells. *Lab Invest* 23:595, 1970

204. HERZOG V, MILLER F: Membrane retrieval in epithelial cells of isolated thyroid follicles. *Eur J Cell Biol* 19:203, 1979

205. CONSIGLIO E, SALVATORE G, RALL JE, KOHN LD: Thyroglobulin interactions with thyroid plasma membranes. The existence of specific receptors and their potential role. *J Biol Chem* 254:5065, 1979

206. PISAREV MA, DUMONT JE: The role of reduced glutathion in thyroglobulin proteolysis in vitro. *Acta Endocrinol* 79:76, 1975

207. GOSWAMI A, ROSENBERG IN: Characterization of a flavoprotein iodityrosine deiodinase from bovine thyroid. Flavin nucleotide binding and oxidation-reduction properties. *J Biol Chem* 254:12326, 1979

208. GOSWAMI A, ROSENBERG IN: Ferredoxin and ferredoxin reductase activities in bovine thyroid. Possible relationship to iodotyrosine deiodinase. *J Biol Chem* 256:893, 1981

209. GREEN WL: Metabolism of thyroid hormones by rat thyroid tissue in vitro. *Endocrinology* 103:826, 1978

210. LAURBERG, P: The effect of propylthiouracil on thyroid-stimulating hormone-induced alterations in iodothyronine secretion from perfused dog thyroids. *Biochim Biophys Acta* 588:351, 1979

211. UNGER J, VAN HEUVERSWYN B, DECOSTER C, CANTRAINE F, MOCKEL J, VAN HERLE A: Thyroglobulin and thyroid hormone release after intravenous administration of bovine thyrotropin in man. *J Clin Endocrinol Metab* 51:590, 1980

212. STANBURY JB, KASSENAAR, AAH, MEIJER JWA, TERPSTRA J: The occurrence of mono- and diiodotyrosine in the blood of a patient with congenital goiter. *J Clin Endocrinol Metab* 15:1216, 1955

213. STANBURY JB, MEIJER JWA, KASSENAAR AAH: The metabolism of iodotyrosines. II. The metabolism of mono- and di-iodotyrosine in certain patients with familial goiter. *J Clin Endocrinol Metab* 16:848, 1956

214. STANBURY JB, KASSENAAR AAH, MEIJER JWA: The metabolism of iodotyrosines. I. The fate of mono- and di-iodotyrosine in normal subjects and in patients with various diseases. *J Clin Endocrinol Metab* 16:735, 1956

215. QUERIDO A, STANBURY JB, KASSENAAR, AAH, MEIJER JWA: The metabolism of iodotyrosines. III. Di-iodotyrosine dehalogenating activity of human thyroid tissue. *J Clin Endocrinol Metab* 16:1096, 1956

216. STANBURY JB: Familial goiter, in Stanbury JB, Wyngaarden JB, Fredrickson DS (eds): *The Metabolic Basis of Inherited Disease,* ed 3. New York, McGraw-Hill Book Co, 1972, p 233

217. MCGIRR EM, HUTCHISON JH: Radioactive iodine studies in non-endemic goitrous cretins. *Lancet* 1:1117, 1953

218. HUTCHISON JH, MCGIRR EM: Hypothyroidism as an inborn error of metabolism *J Clin Endocrinol Metab* 14:869, 1954

219. STANBURY JB, MEIJER JWA, KASSENAAR AAH: The metabolism of iodotyrosines. II. The metabolism of mono- and di-iodotyrosine in certain patients with familial goiter. *J Clin Endocrinol Metab* 16:848, 1956

220. CHOUFOER JC, KASSENAAR AAH, QUERIDO A: The syndrome of congenital hypothyroidism with defective dehalogenation of iodotyrosines: Further observations and discussion of the pathophysiology. *J Clin Endocrinol Metab* 20:983, 1960

221. HUTCHISON JH, MCGIRR EM: Sporadic nonendemic goitrous cretinism. *Lancet* 1:1035, 1956

222. MCGIRR EM, CLEMENT WE, CURRIE AR, KENNEDY JS: Impaired dehalogenase activity as a cause of goitre with malignant changes. *Scott Med J* 4:232, 1959

223. HORST W: Radiojoddiagnostik van Struma und Schilddrüsenkrebs und Untersuchungen zur Frage einer Jodfehlverwertung in deren Pathogenese. Verh. d. 4 Jahrestagung des Deutschen Zentralaus-Schusses für Krebsbekämfung und Krebsforschung, edited by A. Dietrich. *Sonderbd. zur Strahlentherapie* 34:150, 1956

224. CODACCIONI JL, PIERRON H, ROUAULT F, BISMUTH J, AQUARON R: Hypothyroïdie infantile par defaut d'iodotyrosine-déshalogenase. I. Quatre nouveaux cas. *Ann Endocrinol.* (Paris), 31, 1161, 1970

225 ROCHICCIOLI P, DUTAU G: Trouble de l'hormonosynthèse thyroïdienne par déficit en iodotyrosine-déshalogenase. *Arch Fr Pediatr.* 31:25, 1974

226. CHOUFOER JC: Further observations on congenital hypothyroidism with defective dehalogenation of iodotyrosines, in Pitt-Rivers R (ed): *Advances in Thyroid Research.* Elmsford, NY, Pergamon Press, Inc, 1961, p 36

227. CODACCIONI JL, PIERRON H, ROUAULT F, AQUARON R, JAQUET P: Hypothyroïdie infantile par défaut d'iodotyrosine-déshalogenase. II. Résultats du traitement par l'iode de 5 cas. *Ann Endocrinol (Paris)* 31:1174, 1970

228. VAGUE J, CODACCIONI JL: Bilan de 7 ans de traitement par l'iode d'un premier cas d'hypothroidie infantile par défaut de désiodation des iodotyrosines. *Ann Endocrinol (Paris)* 31:1156, 1970

229. KUSAKABE T, MIYAKE T: Defective deiodination of I^{131}-labeled L-diiodotyrosine in patients with simple goiter. *J Clin Endocrinol Metab* 23:132, 1963

230. KUSAKABE T, MIYAKE T: Thyroidal deiodination defect in three sisters with simple goiter. *J Clin Endocrinol Metab* 24:456, 1964

231. ISMAIL-BEIGI F, RAHIMIFAR M: A variant of iodotyrosine-dehalogenase deficiency. *J Clin Endocrinol Metab* 44:499, 1977

232. MCGIRR EM, HUTCHISON JH, CLEMENT WE: Sporadic goitrous cretinism: Dehalogenase deficiency in the thyroid gland of a goitrous cretin and in heterozygous carriers. *Lancet* 2:823, 1959

233. MURRAY P, THOMSON JA, MCGIRR EM, WALLACE TJ, MACDONALD EM, MACCABE HJ: Absent and defective iodotyrosine deiodination in a family some of whose members are goitrous cretins. *Lancet* 1:183, 1965

234. CODACCIONI JL, RINALDI JP, BISMUTH J: The test of overloading of 1-diiodotyrosine (DIT) in the screening of iodotyrosine dehalogenase deficiency. *Acta Endocrinol* 87:95, 1978

235. REINWEIN D: Hormonsynthese und Enzymspectrum bei Erkrankungen der menschlichen Schilddrusse. *Acta Endocrinol (Kbh)* (suppl) 47:94, 1964

236. GERSHENGORN MC, GLINOER D, ROBBINS J: Transport and metabolism of thyroid hormones, in De Visscher M (ed): *The Thyroid.* New York, Raven Press, 1980, p 81

237. BERNAL J, OBREGON MJ, RODRIGUEZ-PERA A, MALLOL J, HERNANDEZ P, ESCOBAR DEL RAY F, MORREALE DE ESCOBAR G: Metabolism and action of thyroid hormone. *Horm Cell Regul* 5:107, 1981

238. VISSER TJ: A tentative review of recent in vitro observations of the enzymatic deiodination of iodothyronines and its possible physiological implications. *Mol Cell Endocrinol* 10:241, 1978

239. CHOPRA IJ: Sulfhydryl groups and the monodeiodination of thyroxine to triiodothyronine. *Science* 199:904, 1978

240. LEE, PWN, GOLDEN MP, VAN HERLE AJ, LIPPE GM, KAPLAN SA: Inherited abnormal thyroid hormone-bindings protein causing selective increase of total serum thyroxine. *J Clin Endocrinol Metab* 49:292, 1979

241. BERNSTEIN RS, ROBBINS J, RALL JE: Polymorphism of monkey thyroxine-binding prealbumin (TBOA): Mode of inheritance and hybridization. *Endocrinology* 86:383, 1970

242. ALPER CA, ROBIN NI, REFETOFF S: Genetic polymorphism of rhesus thyroxine-binding prealbumin: Evidence for tetrameric structure in primates. *PNAS* 63:775, 1969

243. BEIERWALTES WH, ROBBINS J: Familial increase in the thyroxine binding sites in serum alpha globulin. *J Clin Invest* 38:1683, 1959

244. NIKOLAI TF, SEAL US: X-chromosome linked inheritance of thyroxine binding globulin deficiency. *J Clin Endocrinol Metab* 27:1515, 1967

245. JONES JE, SEAL US: X-chromosome linked inheritance of elevated thyroxine-binding globulin. *J Clin Endocrinol Metab* 27:1521, 1967

246 NICOLOFF JT, DOWLING JT, PATTON DD: Inheritance of decreased thyroxine-binding by the thyroxine-binding globulin. *J Clin Endocrinol Metab* 24:294, 1964

247. DUSSAULT JM, FISHER DA, NICOLOFF JT, ROW VV, VOLPE, R: The effect of alterations of thyroxine binding capacity of the dialysable fractions of triiodothyronine in circulation. *Acta Endocrinol* 72:265, 1973

248. DAUGBJERG PS, ASFELD VH: Familial low thyroxine-binding globulin capacity. *Dan Med Bull* 25:257, 1978

249. HORWITZ DL, REFETOFF S: Thyrotoxicosis associated with inherited thyroxine binding globulin deficiency in five patients. *Proceedings, 57th Annual Meeting of the Endocrine Society,* New York, no 159, p 130, 1975

250. WAHNER HW, EMSLANDER RF, GORMAN CA: Thyroid overactivity and TBG deficiency simulating "T3 hyperthyroidism." *J Clin Endocrinol* 33:93, 1971

251. GERSTNER JB, CAPLAN RH: Hyperthyroidism with normal concentrations of total serum thyroxine and thyrodothyronine. *J Clin Endocrinol Metab* 42:64, 1976

252. REFETOFF S: Thyroid hormone transport, in DeGroot LJ (ed): *Endocrinology.* New York, Grune & Stratton, Inc, p 347

253. SHANE SR, SEAL US, JONES JE: X-chromosome linked inheritance of elevated thyroxine-binding globulin in association with goiter. *J Clin Endocrinol Metab* 32:587, 1971

254. LAMBERTS, SWJ, CASPARIE AF, MIEDEMA K, HENNEMANN G, HULSMANS HAM: Thyroxine binding globulin deficiency in a family with Type I hyperlipoproteinaemia *Clin Endocrinol* 6:197, 1977

255. REFETOFF S, SELENKOW HA: Familial thyroxine binding globulin deficiency in a patient with Turner's syndrome (XO): Genetic study of a kindred. *N Engl J Med* 278:1081, 1968

256. NUSYNOWITZ ML, CLARK RE, STRADER WJ, ESTRIN HM, SEAL VS: Thyroxine binding globulin deficiency in three families and total deficiency in a normal woman. *Am J Med* 50:458, 1971

257. BIGAZZI M, RONGA R, OLIVOTTI AL, SCARSELLI G, REFETOFF S: Inherited X chromosome linked thyroxine-binding globulin (TBG) deficiency in a homozygous female. *J Endocrinol Invest* 4:349, 1980

258. MOLOSHOK RE, HSU LYF, SEAL US, HIRSCHHORN K: Partial thyroxine binding globulin deficiency in a family. *Pediatrics* 44:518, 1969

259. BODE HH, ROTHMAN KJ, DANON M: Linkage of thyroxine binding globulin deficiency to other X-chromosome loci. *J Clin Endocrinol Metab* 37:25, 1973

260. HODGSON SF, WAHNER HW: Hereditary increased thyroxine binding globulin capacity. *Proc Mayo Clin* 47:720, 1972

261. MOSES AC, LAWLOR JF, HADDOW JE, JACKSON IMD: A new syndrome of familial euthyroid hyperthyroxenemia: Elevated thyroxine caused by increased immunoreactive thyroid-binding prealbumin (TBPA). Abstract, 56th meeting, American Thyroid Association, November 5–8, 1980, San Diego

262. GREENBERG AH, NAJJAR S, BLIZZARD RM: Effects of thyroid hormone on growth, differentiation and development, in Greer MA, Solomon DH (eds): *Handbook of Physiology.* Washington, DC, American Physiological Society, 1974, section 7, vol 3, p 377

263. BERNAL J, DEGROOT LJ: Mode of action of thyroid hormones, in De Visscher M (ed): *The Thyroid.* New York, Raven Press, 1980, p 123

264. DEGROOT L: Thyroid hormone action, in DeGroot L (ed): *Endocrinology.* New York, Grune & Stratton, Inc, 1979, p 357

265. FISCHER, DA, KLEIN AH: Thyroid development and disorders of thyroid function in the newborn. *N Engl J Med* 304:702, 1981

266. OPPENHEIMER JH: Thyroid hormone action at the cellular level. *Science* 203:971, 1979

267. LENNON AM, OSTY J, NUNEZ J: Cytosolic thyroxine-binding protein and brain development. *Mol Cell Endocrinol* 18:201, 1980

268. MARECK A, FELLOUS A, FRANCON J, NUNEZ J: Changes in composition and activity of microtubule-associated proteins during brain development. *Nature* 284:353, 1980

269. NUNEZ J, CORREZE C: Interdependent effects of thyroid hormones and cyclic AMP on lipolysis and lipogenesis in the fat cell. *Adv Cycl Nucl Res* 14:539, 1981

270. VERHAEGEN M, CORREZE C, KRUG E, NUNEZ J: Cyclic AMP and lipogenesis in fat cells from thyroidectomized rat. *Mol Cell Endocrinol* 14:167, 1979

271. NUNEZ J, PLAS C, CORREZE C: Cell competence and cell sensitivity to hormonal stimulation: Two concepts discussed with two systems, the fetal hepatocyte and the adult adipocyte. *Horm Cell Regul* 1:119, 1977

272. MALBON CC: The effects of thyroid status on the modulation of fat cell β-adrenergic receptor agonist affinity by guanine nucleotides. *Mol Pharmacol* 18:193, 1980

273. BOUHNIK J, CLOT JP, BAUDRY M, MICHEL R: Early effects of thyroidectomy and triiodothyronine administration on rat-liver mitochondria. *Mol Cell Endocrinol* 15:1, 1979

274. ISMAIL-BEIGI F, BISSEL DM, EDELMAN I S: Thyroid thermogenesis in adult rat hepatocytes in primary monolayer culture. Direct action of thyroid hormone in vitro. *J Gen Physiol* 73:369, 1979

275. SESTOFT L: Metabolic aspects of the calorigenic effect of thyroid hormone in mammals. *Clin Endocrinol* 13:489, 1980

276. SCHWARTZ HL, OPPENHEIMER JH: Nuclear triiodothyronine receptor sites in brain: Probable identity with hepatic receptors and regional distribution. *Endocrinology* 103:267, 1978

277. RAO GS: Mode of entry of steroid and thyroid hormones into cells. *Mol Cell Endocrinol* 21:97, 1981

278. STERLING K: Thyroid hormone action at the cell level. *Med Prog* 300:117, 1979

279. SEO H, BROCAS H, VASSART G, REFETOFF S: Early in vitro induction of rat pituitary GH mRNA by T$_3$[1]. *Endocrinology* 103:1506, 1978

280. SEO H, WUNDERLICH C, VASSART G, REFETOFF S: Growth hormone responses to thyroid hormone in the neonatal rat. Resistance and anamnestic response. *J Clin Invest* 67:569, 1981

281. REFETOFF S: Resistance to thyroid hormone, in Oppenheimer JH (ed): *Thyroid Today.* 1980, vol 3, p 1

282. REFETOFF S, DEGROOT L J, BENARD B, DEWIND LT: Studies of a sibship with apparent hereditary resistance to the intracellular action of thyroid hormone. *Metabolism* 21:732, 1972

283. REFETOFF S, DEWIND L T, DEGROOT LJ: Familial syndrome combining deaf-mutism, stippled epiphyses, goiter and abnormally high PBI: Possible target organ refractoriness to thyroid hormone. *J Clin Endocrinol* 27:279, 1967

284. REFETOFF S, DEGROOT L J, BARSANO CP: Defective thyroid hormone feedback regulation in the syndrome of peripheral resistance to thyroid hormone. *J Clin Endocrinol Metab* 51:41, 1980

285. BERNAL J, REFETOFF S, DEGROOT LJ: Abnormalities of triiodothyronine binding to lymphocyte and fibroblast nuclei from a patient with peripheral tissue resistance to thyroid hormone action. *J Clin Endocrinol Metab* 47:1266, 1978

286. BODE HH, DANON M, WEINTRAUB BD, MALOOF E, CRAWFORD JD: Partial target organ resistance to thyroid hormone. *J Clin Invest* 52:776, 1973

287. LAMBERG BA: Congenital euthyroid goitre and partial peripheral resistance to thyroid hormones. *Lancet* 1:854, 1973

288. LIEWENDAHL K: Triiodothyronine binding to lymphocytes from euthyroid subjects and a patient with peripheral resistance to thyroid hormone. *Acta Endocrinol* 83:64, 1976

289. SCHNEIDER G, KEISER HR, BARDIN CW: Peripheral resistance to thyroxine: A cause of short stature in a boy without goitre. *Clin Endocrinol* 4:111, 1975

290. LAMBERG BA, SANDSTROM R, ROSENGARD S, SAARINEN P, EVERED DC: Sporadic and familial partial peripheral resistance to thyroid hormone, in Harland WA, Orr JS (eds): *Thyroid Hormone Metabolism.* London, Academic Press, Ltd, 1975, p 139

291. LAMBERG BA, ROSENGARD S, LIEWENDAHL K, SAARINEN P, EVERED DC: Familial partial peripheral resistance to thyroid hormones. *Acta Endocrinol* 87:303, 1978

292. LIEWENDAHL K, ROSENGARD S, LAMBERG BA: Nuclear binding of triiodothyronine and thyroxine in lymphocytes from subjects with hyperthyroidism, hypothyroidism and resistance to thyroid hormones. *Clin Chim Acta* 83:41, 1978

293. GERSHENGORN MC, WEINTRAUB BD: Thyrotropin-induced hyperthyroidism caused by selective pituitary resistance to thyroid hormone. *J Clin Invest* 56:633, 1975

294. AGERBAEK H: Congenital goiter presumably resulting from tissue resistance to thyroid hormones. *Israel J Med Sci* 8:1859, 1972

295. ELEWARUT A, MUSSCHE M, VERMEULEN A: Familial partial target organ resistance to thyroid hormone. *J Clin Endocrinol Metab* 43:575, 1976

295a. KAPLOWITZ PB, D'ERCOLE AJ, UTIGER RD: Peripheral resistance to thyroid hormone in an infant. *J Clin Endocrinol Metab* 53:958, 1981

296. DEMEESTER-MIRKINE N, DUMONT JE: The hypothalamo-pituitary thyroid axis, in De Visscher M (ed): *The Thyroid.* New York, Raven Press, 1980, p 145

297. JORDAN D, PONCET C, MORNEX R, PONSIN G: Participation of serotonin in thyrotropin release. I. Evidence for the action of serotonin on thyrotropin releasing hormone release. *Endocrinology* 103:414, 1978

298. ENGLER D, SCANLON MF, JACKSON IMD: Thyrotropin releasing hormone in the systemic circulation of the neonatal rat is derived from the pancreas and other extraneural tissues. *J Clin Invest* 67:800, 1981

299. TARASKEVICH PS, DOUGLAS WW: Action potentials occur in cells of the normal anterior pituitary gland and are stimulated by the hypophysiotropic peptide thyrotropin-releasing hormone. *Proc Natl Acad Sci USA* 74:4064, 1977

300. SCHREY MP, BROWN BL, EKINS RP: Studies on the role of calcium and cyclic nucleotides in the control of TSH secretion. *Mol Cell Endocrinol* 11:249, 1978

301. WILBER JF: Human pituitary thyrotropin, in DeGroot LJ (ed): *Endocrinology.* New York, Grune & Stratton, Inc, 1979, vol 1, p 141

302. KOURIDES IA, WEINTRAUB BD: mRNA-directed biosynthesis of α subunit of thyrotropin: Translation in cell-free and whole cell systems. *Proc Natl Acad Sci USA* 76:298, 1978

303. WEINTRAUB BD, STANNARD BS, LINNEKIN D, MARSHALL M: Relationship of glycosylation to de novo thyroid-stimulating hormone biosynthesis and secretion by mouse pituitary tumor cells. *J Biol Chem* 255:5715, 1980

304. GERSHENGORN MC, GERAS E, MARCUS-SAMUELS BE, REBECCHI MJ: Receptor affinity and biological potency of thyroid hormones in thyrotropic cells. *Am Physiol Soc* 237:E142, 1979

305. SPIRA O, BIRKENFELD A, AVNI A, GROSS J, GORDON A: TSH synthesis and release in the thyroidectomized rat. *Acta Endocrinol* 92:502, 1979

306. LARSEN PR, BAVLI SZ, CASTONGUAY M, JOVE R: Direct radioimmunoassay of nuclear 3,5,3' triiodothyronine in rat anterior pituitary. *J Clin Invest* 65:675, 1980

307. MORNEX R, JORDAN D: Contrôle hypothalamique de la sécrétion de TSH. Méthodes actuelles d'exploration et perspectives d'avenir. *C R Soc Biol* 173:496, 1979

308. SCANLON MF, RODRIGUEZ-ARNAO MD, POURMAND M, SHALE D J, WEIGHTMAN DR, LEWIS M, HALL R: Catecholaminergic interactions in the regulation of thyrotropin (TSH) secretion in man. *J Endocrinol Invest* 3:125, 1980

309. FOORD SM, PETERS J, SCANLON MF, REES SMITH B, HALL R: Dopaminergic control of TSH secretion in isolated rat pituitary cells. *FEBS Lett* 121:257, 1980

310. PITTMAN JA, HAIGLER ED, HERSHMAN JM, PITTMAN CS: Hypothalamic hypothyroidism. *N Engl J Med* 285:844, 1971

311. MIYAI K, AZUKIZAWA M, KUMUHARA Y: Familial isolated thyrotropin deficiency with cretinism. *N Engl J Med* 285:1043, 1971

312. RIMOIN DL, SCHIMKE RN: *Genetic Disorders of the Endocrine Glands.* St Louis, CV Mosby Co, 1971, p 29

313. ADLER-BIER M, PERTZELAND A, LARON Z, LIEBERMAN E, MOSES S: Multiple Pituitary Hormone Deficiencies in Eight Siblings of One Jewish Moroccan Family. *Acta Pediatr Scand* 68:401, 1979

314. SCHIMKE RN, SPAULDING JJ, HOLLOWELL JG: X-linked congenital panhypopituitarism, in *Birth Defects.* Baltimore, Williams and Wilkins Co, 1971, vol 7, no 6, p 21

315. PHELAN PD, CONELLY J, MARTIN FIR, WETTENHALL HNB: X-linked recessive hypopituitarism, in *Birth Defects.* Baltimore, Williams and Wilkins Co, 1971, vol 7, no 6, p 24

316. ZIPF WB, KELCH RP, BACON GE: Variable X-linked recessive hypopituitarism with evidence of gonadotropin deficiency in two pre-pubertal males. *Clin Genet* 11:249, 1977

317. SADEGHI-NEJAD A, SENIOR B: A familial syndrome of isolated "aplasia" of the anterior pituitary. *J Pediatr* 84:79, 1974

318. STEINER MM, BOGGS JD: Absence of pituitary gland, hypothyroidism, hypoadrenalism and hypogonadism in a 17-year-old dwarf. *J Clin Endocrinol* 25:1591, 1965

319. STEINER MM: Rare dwarfism with chronic hypoglycemia and convulsions. *J Clin Endocrinol* 13:283, 1953

320. FIERRIER PE, STONE EF, Jr: Familial pituitary dwarfism associated with an abnormal sella turcica. *Pediatrics* 43:858, 1969

321. SIPPONEN P, SIMILA S, COLLAN Y, AUTERE T, HERVA R: Familial syndrome with panhypopituitarism, hypoplasia of the hypophysis, and poorly developed sella turcica. *S Arch Dis Child* 53:664, 1978

322. PARKS JS, TENORE A, BONGIOVANNI AM, KIRKLAND RT: Familial hypopituitarism with large sella turcica. *N Engl J Med* 298:698, 1978

323. MURRAY IPC, THOMSON JA, McGIRR EM, MacDONALD EM, KENNEDY

JS, McLennan I: Unusual familial goiter associated with intrathyroidal calcification. *J Clin Endocrinol Metab* 26:1039, 1966

324. Courpotin C, Iniguez M, Labrune B: *Nozv. Press Med* 6:3984, 1977

325. Greig WR, Henderson AS, Boyle JA, McGirr EM, Hutchison JH: Thyroid dysgenesis in two pairs of monozygotic twins and in a mother and child. *J Clin Endocrinal Metab* 26:1309, 1966

326. Cross HE, Hollander CS, Rimoin DL, McKusick VA: Familial agoitrous cretinism accompanied by muscular hypertrophy. *Pediatrics* 41:413,1968

327. Savoie JC, Massin JP, Savoie F: Studies on mono- and diiodohistidine, II. Congenital goitrous hypothyroidism with thyroglobulin defect and iodohistidine-rich iodoalbumin production. *J Clin Invest* 52:116, 1973

12

PHENYLKETONURIA AND HYPERPHENYLALANINEMIA

ARA TOURIAN

JAMES B. SIDBURY

1. Impaired oxidation of phenylalanine can be the result of absent or deficient phenylalanine hydroxylase, dihydropteridine reductase, or dihydrobiopterin synthesis. The respective clinical phenotypes are classic phenylketonuria (PKU), hyperphenylalaninemia types II and III, and hyperphenylalaninemia types IV and V.

2. In classic PKU the most important and consistent feature is mental retardation. This becomes evident in midinfancy, and in later childhood 98 percent of untreated patients have an IQ below 70. Other manifestations include seizures, psychotic behavior, eczema, dermatographia, "mousy" odor, and pigment dilution. None of these signs is seen in patients diagnosed early and treated properly. In classic PKU there is no detectable activity of phenylalanine hydroxylase. In hyperphenylalaninemia types II and III, phenylalanine hydroxylase activity is present but much reduced; affected patients are clinically normal or may be retarded. In type IV (dihydropteridine reductase deficiency) and type V (dihydrobiopterin synthetase deficiency) the clinical manifestations start in the first year of life, with major neurologic deficits. Hyperphenylalaninemia, neurotransmitter synthesis deficit, and impaired oxidation of long-chain alkyl ethers of glycerol contribute to brain dysfunction. Other variants of hyperphenylalaninemia (types VI to VIII) produce dif-

ferent manifestations and are based on other defects of phenylalanine metabolism.

3. Phenylalanine hydroxylase is a dimer with a molecular weight of 110,000 in rat liver and 100,000 in human liver. Two nonidentical subunits of approximately 50,000 comprise the dimer. Tetrahydrobiopterin is the natural cofactor. The initial reduction of dihydrobiopterin to tetrahydrobiopterin requires dihydrofolate reductase. Once the biopterin is reduced to the tetrahydro form, it shuttles back and forth between the quinonoid and tetrahydro forms through the mediation of dihydropteridine reductase. Dihydrobiopterin synthetase is required for the synthesis of biopterin.

4. Three isoenzymes of liver phenylalanine hydroxylase in the rat have been identified by immunologic and isoelectric focusing methods. The kidney isoenzyme cross-reacts with antibody to one of the liver isoenzymes, but it is not identical. Phosphorylation of rodent phenylalanine hydroxylase generates two isoenzymes. Thus, a nonphosphorylated dimer with a molecular weight of 100,000, a fully phosphorylated dimer, and an intermediate half-phosphorylated dimer can be generated. These observations on rodent phenylalanine hydroxylase have not been reported on human enzyme.

5. No cross-reacting material to phenylalanine hydroxy-

lase antibody can be detected in classic PKU or type II hyperphenylalaninemia. No cross-reacting material to dihydropteridine reductase can be detected in type IV hyperphenylalaninemia.

6. *All of the hyperphenylalaninemic states are transmitted as autosomal recessive conditions except type VI, which appears to be X-linked.*

7. *Heterozygotes of types I and II can be ascertained with a high degree of accuracy using postprandial plasma phenylalanine/tyrosine ratios. Determination of liver phenylalanine hydroxylase levels in types I and II hyperphenylalaninemic subjects and their parents has provided results showing a lack of gene dosage effect. This suggests the possibility that the affected individuals may be allelic compounds.*

8. *Dietary restriction of phenylalanine intake is the only practical therapy of classic PKU at present. Reduction of hyperphenylalaninemia to about 4 to 10 mg/dl, when begun as soon as possible after birth, allows normal physical and mental development in types I and II. In types IV and V, 5-hydroxytryptophan and L-dihydroxyphenylalanine supplements are also required, as this condition is otherwise usually lethal by the fifth year, even with good dietary control of hyperphenylalaninemia. In type V, relacement therapy with tetrahydrobiopterin is required in addition to dietary restrictions of phenylalanine intakes. Long-term results of treatment of these variants (types IV and V) are not yet available.*

Phenylketonuria (PKU) and *hyperphenylalaninemia* designate a group of inborn errors of metabolism of phenylalanine that share the common feature of impaired phenylalanine oxidation, which results in elevated tissue and serum phenylalanine. The primary enzymatic defect may be localized to phenylalanine hydroxylase or dihydropteridine reductase, or to one of the sequential enzymatic steps in the synthesis of the cofactor biopterin.

Excess phenylpyruvic acid in the urine was identified by Fölling [1] in 1934 in the urine of patients with a condition that was named *phenylketonuria* by Penrose and Quastel [2] 3 years later. Jervis in 1947 [3] identified the metabolic error by showing that feeding phenylalanine to such patients did not result in tyrosine production. Subsequently in 1953 [4] he showed that a liver extract from such a patient was deficient in the ability to convert phenylalanine to tyrosine (Fig. 12-1). A diet therapy comprising phenylalanine restriction was reported by Bickel et al. in 1953 [5]. The development of a simple method for determining blood phenylalanine concentration has facilitated the mass screening of neonates for hyperphenylalaninemia [6–8]. A spectrum of phenylalanine hydroxylase deficiency [9–11] has been defined, as well as defects in dihydropteridine reductase [12], the cofactor reducing enzyme, and defects in the synthesis of the cofactor biopterin [13–15] (Fig. 12-1).

PKU has been the model for the study of mental retardation consequent to an inborn error of metabolism, partly because of the degree of success with animal models [16] and partly because dietary modification can prevent the mental retardation that is almost inevitable in the untreated individual [5, 9, 10].

The success of nutritional intervention in preventing brain damage in this inherited metabolic disease underscores the interplay of genetic constitution with the environment. It also suggests that the brain of a fetus with classic PKU develops normally in intrauterine life in spite of the total lack of fetal hepatic phenylalanine hydroxylase activity. The critical period of human brain growth and development extends over the first 6 months of the neonatal period [17]. Little cell division takes place in the human brain after 5 months of age, and further growth occurs by increases in the protein, DNA, and lipid content of cells. Myelination may not be completed until 5 or 6 years of age. Elevated tissue levels of phenylalanine or its metabolites could be the mediators of an altered biochemical environment causing the arrest of differentiation of the central nervous system of the neonate and resulting in retardation. Once the process of maturation of the brain is completed, discontinuation of the low phenylalanine diet should not have a devastating effect on future intellectual ability or emotional behavior [18], but recent clinical observation suggests that early discontinuation may result in some deterioration of intellectual ability and emotional behavior and that continuation of the diet may be necessary to a later age than previously suggested [18–21]. This approximates the experience with well-controlled, treated cases of PKU, but exceptions have been recorded (Table 12-1, types IV, V, VI). The biologic basis of these exceptions is under active investigation, which has already opened a new chapter in the understanding of hyperphenylalaninemia [12–15].

METABOLISM OF PHENYLALANINE IN MAMMALIAN TISSUES

Phenylalanine is an essential amino acid for protein synthesis in mammalian tissues [22]. The proportion of dietary phenylalanine that is utilized for protein synthesis varies with age. It is about 50 percent of the daily intake during early growth and decreases as the growth rate declines [9]. Physiologically, the most significant pathway of phenylalanine degradation is through hydroxylation to tyrosine [23–25] (Fig. 12-2). Feeding experiments with [^{14}C] phenylalanine have demonstrated unequivocally that L-phenylalanine is hydroxylated in the 4 position of the phenyl ring [24]. The reverse reaction, tyrosine to phenylalanine, does not take place even when a phenylalanine-deficient diet is fed to mice [25]. This hydroxylation is limited to the liver, kidney, and pancreas in mammalian tissues [26]; surgical biopsy specimens from human kidney also have this activity [27]. Tyrosine, the product of the hydroxylation, is also essential for protein synthesis in mammalian tissues. In the central nervous system, tyrosine is an essential amino acid and a precursor of such biogenic amines as dopamine and norepinephrine. Tyrosine also serves as a substrate for thyroxine and melanin synthesis (Fig. 12-2).

The Hydroxylase Reaction

The presence of phenylalanine hydroxylase activity in the soluble fraction of mammalian liver extracts, the requirement for atmospheric oxygen and NADH, and the specificity of this reaction for L-phenylalanine were first demonstrated by Uden-

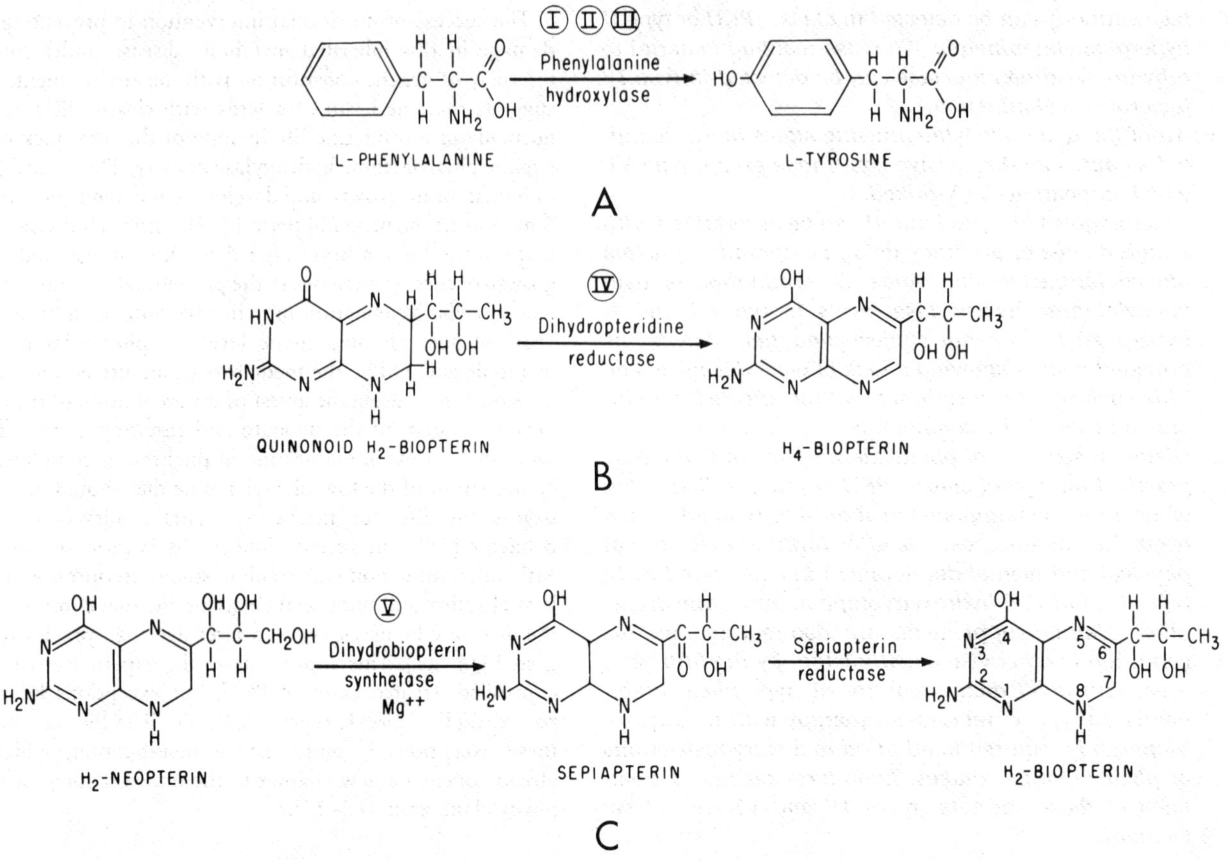

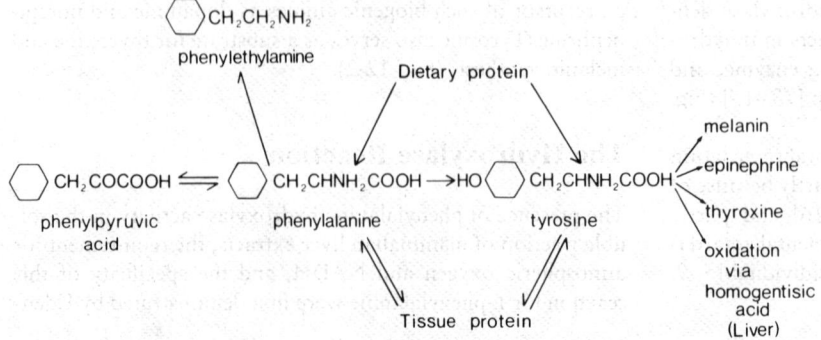

L-PHENYLALANINE   L-TYROSINE

A

QUINONOID H₂-BIOPTERIN   H₄-BIOPTERIN

B

H₂-NEOPTERIN   SEPIAPTERIN   H₂-BIOPTERIN

C

Figure 12–1 *A.* The blocked reaction of phenylalanine to tyrosine in classic phenylketonuria, type I, and hyperphenylalaninemia, types II and III. *B.* The blocked reaction of quinonoid H_2-biopterin to H_4-biopterin due to deficiency of dihydropteridine reductase, hyperphenylalaninemia type IV. *C.* The blocked reaction of H_2-neopterin to sepiaterin due to dihydrobiopterin synthetase, hyperphenylalaninemia type V.

friend and Cooper [28]. The hydroxylating system was resolved into two protein components by Mitoma [29].

The next major breakthrough came when Kaufman identified the structure of tetrahydrobiopterin, an obligatory cofactor, and traced its transformations during the hydroxylation reaction [30–33] (Fig. 12-3).

Bublitz [34] developed a simple assay for phenylalanine hydroxylase using dithiothreitol, which was based on Kaufman's [33] observation that certain reductants can rapidly reduce the oxidized *synthetic cofactor* pterin. Dithiothreitol not only regenerates the tetrahydropteridine from dihydropteridine but also effectively protects the system from peroxide formed during the aerobic oxidation of tetrahydropteridine. This system has greatly helped in developing some of the newer concepts of the biology of phenylalanine hydroxylase by other investigators that are noted in this chapter.

Studies with aromatic substrates labeled in specific positions with deuterium or tritium have uncovered a fundamental property of aromatic hydroxylation reactions [35]: A frequent consequence of hydroxylation is an intramolecular shift of the

group displaced by hydroxyl to an adjacent position on the aromatic ring. This is in contrast to the classic concept of aromatic substitution, in which the group at the site of substitution would be lost by direct displacement [36].

Biopterin Structure, Activity, and Synthesis The cofactor isolated from the liver is dihydrobiopterin, 7,8-dihydro-2-amino-4-hydroxy-6-[1,2-dihydroxypropyl (L-erythro)]-pteridine [31–33]. The reduction of dihydrobiopterin to tetrahydrobiopterin requires an NADPH-dependent dihydrofolate reductase [31–33]. Once the biopterin is reduced to the tetrahydro form, it shuttles back and forth between the quinonoid and tetrahydro forms and requires an NADH-dependent dihydropteridine reductase [37] for this reduction. In crude liver extracts, and presumably in the liver cell, the cofactor exists

phenylethylamine

Dietary protein

melanin

epinephrine

phenylpyruvic acid   phenylalanine   tyrosine

thyroxine

oxidation via homogentisic acid (Liver)

Tissue protein

Figure 12–2 The metabolic flow of phenylalanine and tyrosine.

predominantly in a form that is active in the hydroxylating system without dihydrofolate reductase (either the tetrahydro or the quinonoid dihydro form) [32]. In the purification procedure tetrahydrobiopterin oxidizes and tautomerizes to the 7,8-dihydro compound [32]. Dihydrofolate reductase may function in the biosynthesis of biopterin [32].

Biopterin is synthetized from guanosine triphosphate (GTP) in sequential enzymatic steps [38–40] (Fig. 12-3). Biopterin is the obligatory cofactor for hydroxylation of the aromatic amino acids phenylalanine, tyrosine, and tryptophan [32,41,42]. The cofactor is an electron donor in the system, and, although a number of synthetic reduced pteridines can serve the same function, tetrahydrobiopterin has the highest K_m, 0.0045 mM, and is thought to be the natural cofactor [32]. PKU patients have higher plasma levels of biopterin than do normal persons.

An oral load of phenylalanine given to normal subjects leads to four- to five-fold increase in biopterin-related compounds. Biopterin-deficient patients (hyperphenylalaninemia type V) do not respond with a rise of serum biopterin to a similar phenylalanine load [15].

Physical Properties of Phenylalanine Hydroxylase

Phenylalanine hydroxylase has been purified from rat [43–46], human [44, 47–50], and monkey [51] liver. The native enzyme at first was thought to be an equilibrium mixture of components with molecular weights of 110,000 and 210,000 [43], but native rat liver phenylalanine hydroxylase was found to consist of a single species of molecular weight 110,000 and not a mixture in a study [52] done with a fraction from rat liver partially purified by the procedure of Kaufman. Fisher et al.

Table 12–1 Classification of hyperphenylalaninemia

Type	Condition	Clinical aspects	Defect	Blood Phe	Blood Tyr	Urine	Treatment
I	Phenylketonuria	Mental retardation and associated symptoms if untreated	Phe hydroxylase absent	>20 mg/100 dl on regular diet	Normal–low	Elevation of Phe metabolites	Low Phe diet
II	Persistent hyperphenylalaninemia	Normal; may show retardation without treatment in more severe cases	Decreased Phe hydroxylase	May be same as PKU early; later 4–20 mg/100 dl on regular diet	Normal–low	Normal or transiently increased Phe metabolites	None—or temporary dietary therapy
III	Transient mild hyperphenylalaninemia	Normal	Maturational delay of hydroxylase	May be same as PKU early; progressively declines toward normal	Normal–low	Same as type II	Same as type II
IV	Dihydropteridine reductase deficiency	Initially normal; seizures, abnormal development evident within first year of life	Deficient or absent dihydropteridine reductase	Variable—may be as in type I	Normal	Variable, dependent on age and Phe concentration in blood	Dopa, 5-OH-tryptophan, carbidopa
V	Abnormal dihydrobiopterin function	Myoclonus, uncontrolled movements, tetraplegia, greasy skin, recurrent hyperthermia	Dihydrobiopterin synthesis defect	May be >20 mg/100 dl	Normal	Abnormal biopterin metabolites	Dopa, 5-OH-tryptophan, carbidopa
VI	Persistent hyperphenylaninemia and tyrosinemia	Progressive ataxia and seizures appearing between 12 and 18 months of age	? Catabolism tyrosine	10 mg/100 dl	Elevated	Phenylethylamine, mandelic acid, p-OH mandelic acid	Reduced Phe intake
VII	Transient neonatal tyrosinemia	Associated with low birth weight, high protein intake	p-Hydroxyphenyl pyruvic oxidase inhibition	Transiently 4–12 mg/100 dl	Transiently elevated: 5–50 mg/100 dl	Gross aminoaciduria, Tyr metabolites	Vitamin C
VIII	Hereditary tyrosinemia	Chronic liver disease	Deficiency: 1. p-OH phenylpyruvate deoxygenase 2. Cytoplasmic tyrosine aminotransferase 3. Fumarylacetoacetate	2–8 mg/100 dl	4 mg/100 dl	1, 2. Gross aminoaciduria Tyr metabolites. 3. 5-Amino-levulinate	1, 2. Low Tyr diet. 3. Low Tyr diet plus glutathione injections

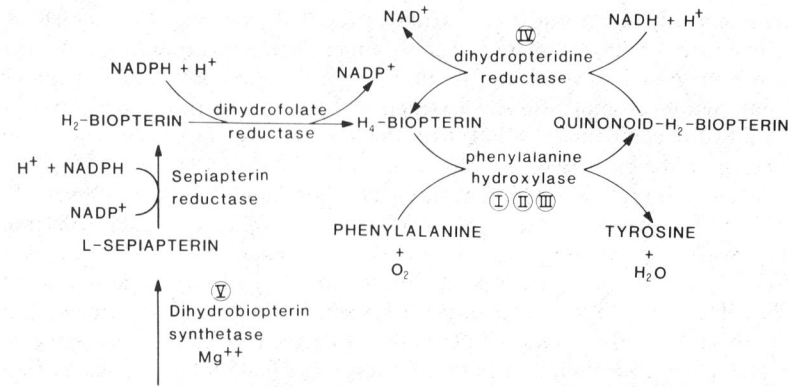

q-D-ERYTHRO-7, 8-DIHYDRONEOPTERIN TRIPHOSPHATE

Figure 12–3 Scheme of phenylalanine hydroxylation and cofactor transformations. The coenzyme H_2-biopterin as isolated from the liver is reduced by an NADPH-dependent dihydrofolate reductase. The reduced H_4-biopterin participates with L-phenylalanine and O_2 in the phenylalanine hydroxylase reaction. The oxidized cofactor (quinonoid-H_2-biopterin) is then regenerated by an NADH-dependent dihydropteridine reductase, without any further need for the action of dihydrofolate reductase [37]. H_2-Biopterin is synthesized from guanosine triphosphate in sequential enzymatic steps which include q-D-erythro-7, 8-dihydroneopterin triphosphate to L-sepiapterin through the action of dihydrobiopterin synthetase and NADPH-dependent sepiapterin reductase [38–40]. The Roman numerals indicate the sites of enzymatic block in the designated hyperphenylalaninemia. *(Figure adapted in part from Kaufman S, The phenylalanine hydroxylating system from mammalian liver.* Adv Enz Related Areas Molec Biol 35:245, 1971, by permission of the publishers, John Wiley and Sons, Inc., New York.)

[53] confirmed this result using purified rat liver enzyme. Since then, a number of investigators using sucrose density sedimentation, acrylamide gel electrophoresis, and Sephadex G-200 gel filtration have shown that both rat and human liver phenylalanine hydroxylase have a native molecular weight of 100,000 to 110,000 [45, 48, 49, 53]. However, Shiman et al. [46] and Choo et al. [50] have reported a native molecular weight of 265,000. Glass wool filtration of the liver extract removes fatty materials, which induces the native enzyme to aggregate to 250,000 molecular weight [48.] Possibly other agents can also aggregate phenylalanine hydroxylase nonspecifically in vitro but have no biologic role in liver cells.

Each molecule of rat liver phenylalanine hydroxylase contains two atoms of iron [53]. Removal of the iron results in loss of enzymatic activity, and activity can be restored by the addition of ferrous chloride. The ferric iron may participate in transfer of electrons from tetrahydrobiopterin to oxygen [53]. An analysis of purified phenylalanine hydroxylase disclosed only 0.2 g atom copper per mole [53]. Others have reported that the rat liver enzyme contains one atom of copper and one molecule of FAD [45]; this remains to be verified. Human phenylalanine hydroxylase seems to be similar to the rat enzyme [44, 48–50]. The molecular weight of human fetal liver phenylalanine hydroxylase is 100,000 [48]. The K_m for phenylalanine is 0.04 mM, for biopterin 0.003 mM, and for O_2 0.95 percent when the reaction velocity is measured in the presence of lysolecithin [47]. When the synthetic cofactor is used, the K_m, for phenylalanine is 1.6 mM, for phenylalanine is 1.6 mM, for tetrahydropteridine (synthetic cofactor) 0.05 mM, and for oxygen 3.40 percent [47].

Regulation of Phenylalanine Hydroxylase Activity
Phenylalanine is an essential amino acid for protein synthesis in mammalian cells [22]. The intermittent dietary intake of protein results in major shifts in the level of this amino acid in tissues [54, 55]. Membrane transport of amino acids and synthesis of protein require critical minimum and maximum phenylalanine and tyrosine concentrations in tissues and in brain [56]. Liver phenylalanine hydroxylase regulates the levels of phenylalanine and tyrosine. The breakdown of concentration boundaries and the consequent devastating effect on brain development are well documented in classic PKU (type I), in which liver phenylalanine hydroxylase is nonfunctional because of mutation [4, 50, 57]. The reverse situation, hypophenylalaninemia, can also result in devastating brain damage, seen when a diet severely restricted in phenylalanine is administered to PKU babies [5, 10].

Liver cells possess a variety of means for maintaining tissue phenylalanine level homeostasis by modification of phenylalanine hydroxylase enzyme activity to cope with major changes in the environment. The immediate and short-term regulation of the activity of the enzyme is achieved by modulation via the substrate phenylalanine and the cofactor biopterin [33, 52, 58, 59] and by phosphorylation of the enzyme [60, 61, 78] (Table 12-2). The long-term activity regulation, in the range of days, is effected by changes in the steady-state level of phenylalanine hydroxylase by synthesis *de novo* or by altered rates of degradation [54, 55, 62] (Table 12-3). Enzyme synthesis *de novo* is induced by insulin, dexamethasone, and a protein factor in serum [63–65]. Their additive effects can alter the constitutive level of the enzyme by at least ten- to twentyfold in hepatoma cells in culture, but whether they are also operative in the liver of the intact organism is unknown. In neonatal rat liver, but not kidney, phenylalanine hydroxylase can also be induced by hydrocortisone [66].

Substrate and Cofactor Modification of the Catalytic Activity of Phenylalanine Hydroxylase The concept of substrate inhibition of phenylalanine hydroxylase at high levels of phenylalanine has been around ever since the first kinetic study by Udenfriend and Cooper in 1952 [28]. More recent kinetic data in vitro do show inhibition of hydroxylation in the presence of the natural cofactor biopterin when the phenylalanine concentration is greater than 0.5 mM [33, 43]. The view of an inhibitory role of phenylalanine on phenylalanine hydroxylase has now been replaced by the newer concept that phenylalanine activates and regulates the activity of phenylalanine hydroxylase [52, 58, 59].

Phenylalanine hydroxylase is an allosteric enzyme, and its activity is modified by phenylalanine, which binds to a site distinct from its catalytic site [52, 58, 59]. A distinct activation site of the enzyme was first suggested when an initial lag in the

Table 12–2 Regulation of the catalytic activity of phenylalanine hydroxylase

Modifier/species	Mechanism	Effect
1. Phenylalanine/rodent		
Tourian [52]	Monomer → dimer	Activation of
Ayling and Helfand [58]	Independent Phe activation site on enzyme	phenylalanine hydroxylase
Shiman and Gray [59]	Induces enzyme to absorb to hydrophobic surface	Activation of phenyl-alanine hydroxylase
2. Glucagon/rodent		
Donlon and Kaufman [60, 61, 78]	Phosphorylation of PH	↑ V_{max} 4×
	Conversion of multiple forms to a single form	↑ V_{max} 2–3×
Abita et al. [87] isolated hepatocytes	Phosphorylation by a cyclic AMP-dependent protein kinase promotes phosphorylation of PH	
3. Pterine, biopterin/rodent		
Tourian [52] (pterin)	Reversal of Phe, activation of PH	Reversal of activation by Phe (↓ V_{max})
Ayling and Hefland [58] (biopterin)	Negative modifier of activation of PH by Phe	Reversal of activation by Phe
4. Lysolecithin, chymotrypsin/rodent		
Fisher and Kaufman [72]	Sigmoid Phe saturation curve of Phe → hyperbolic	↑ V_{max} K_m 0.2→ 0.1 mM
Ayling and Hefland [58]	Desensitization of Phe activation site of PH	K_m 0.2→ 0.1 mM
Lysolecithin Shiman and Gray [59]	Induce PH to adsorb to hydrophobic surface (action similar to Phe)	Activation of phenylalanine hydroxylase
5. Phenylalanine hydroxylating-stimulating protein (PHS/rodent) Huang et al. [74]	Reverses the phenomenon of decrease in specific activity of PH with increasing Phe concentration	Stimulates phenylalanine hydroxylase

Abbreviations: Phe = phenylalanine; PH = phenylalanine hydroxylase; PHS = phenylalanine hydroxylase-stimulating protein.

velocity of the reaction was noted which could be corrected by phenylalanine but not by tetrahydropterin, the lag time being inversely correlated with phenylalanine concentration [52]. Tetrahydropterin did not activate the enzyme. An initial lag in the velocity of the reaction had also been noted by Kaufman [68], Christensen [69], and Nielsen [70], but its significance was not appreciated. The activation rate constant is dependent on time, phenylalanine (or fluorophenylalanine) concentration, and temperature [52] and is described by the exponential equation

$$V_a = V_f + (V_o - V_f)e^{-\alpha t} \qquad (1)$$

where V_o is the fully activated rate, V_a is the activation rate at time t, V_f is the final equilibrium rate achieved, and α is a complex rate constant that depends on substrate concentration [52]. Kinetic analysis of the effect of phenylalanine concentration on the initial reaction rate (V) resulted in a parabolic curve which could be fitted as a straight line when plotted as $1/S^2$, suggesting that two independent sites, a catalytic site and an activation site, existed on the enzyme molecule [52]. Ayling and Helfand [58] showed that activation of phenylalanine hydroxylase by phenylalanine is even more dramatic in the presence of the natural cofactor *biopterin* and confirmed the $1/S^2$ phenylalanine to $1/V$ relationship. They also showed that under selected conditions p-chlorophenylalanine can serve as an activator but a poor substrate for phenylalanine hydroxylase. This observation supports the concept of two distinct sites, one activating and the other catalytic.

The kinetic measurements were done at phenylalanine and biopterin concentrations that were, respectively, one and two orders of magnitude above the recorded tissue values. Estimates of biopterin and phenylalanine concentrations in the liver are 10^{-6} M and 2×10^{-4} M, respectively [71]. Thus, the biologic role of the activation phenomenon may be more important in vivo than is apparent from the studies in vitro. Phenylalanine shifted the sedimentation velocity of phenylalanine hydroxylase from that of a slower-sedimenting species (S value, 6.1) to that of a faster one (S value, 9.14), with molecular weights of 110,000 and 177,000, respectively [52,58]. Ayling and Helfand have confirmed the shift in sedimentation velocity of phenylalanine hydroxylase from human liver and kidney when exposed to phenylalanine [58]. Self-association of the monomer could possibly also result in activated polymer species of phenylalanine hydroxylase, but if that were the case, then increasing the concentration of monomer should result in a parabolic activity curve, which was not observed. Hence, it was proposed that the probable mechanism of phenylalanine activation of phenylalanine hydroxylase involves a shift of dimer to tetramer. This is at variance with the original postulate of tetramer-to-dimer shift for more active form of the enzyme [43].

More recently, it has been shown that phenylalanine-activated phenylalanine hydroxylase binds tightly and reversibly to hydrophobic chromatography support [59]. This remarkable property has resulted in a simplified single-step purification procedure. Since the continuous presence of phenylalanine is

Table 12–3 Regulation of the steady-state activity of phenylalanine hydroxylase in the liver and hepatoma cells in culture

Animal studies

Modifier/species	Mechanism	Effect
1. Phenylalanine/rodent		
Freedland et al. [54]	Reduced degradation of PH?	Activity increased
Greengard and DelValle [66]	Synthesis *de novo* not inhibited by actinomycin	Activity increased
2. Casein/cockerels		
Ohno and Tasaki [55]	Unknown Reduced degradation or synthesis *de novo*?	Activity increased
3. Hydrocortisone/neonatal rats		
Greengard and DelValle [66]	Synthesis *de novo*, actinomycin inhibited	Activity increased
4. Biopterin/human		
Leeming et al. [15]	Biopterin elevated in PKU and hyperphenyl alaninemia	Activity increased

Tissue culture (hepatoma cells)

1. Insulin		
Phase I	Cycloheximide inhibited	Activity increased
Phase II	Actinomycin and	Activity increased
Tourian [65]	cycloheximide inhibited	
2. Serum		
Phase I	Cycloheximide inhibited	Activity increased
Phase II	Actinomycin and	
Tourian [65]	cycloheximide inhibited	
Haggerty et al. [63]		
3. Dexamethasone,		
hydrocortisone	Cycloheximide	Activity increased
N^6,O^2-dibutyryl-3′:5′-cyclic	inhibited	threefold
adenosine monophosphate	Synthesis *de novo*	
Haggerty et al. [63]		

required to maintain the enzyme in an adsorbed state, it was argued that the phenylalanine activation site and the hydrophobic site must be physically distinct.

A more detailed look at the substrate activation phenomenon in the presence of *6-methylpterin* (a synthetic cofactor) has added some new models to the kinetics of the reaction [59]. Ayling and Helfand [58] had already shown that the structure of the cofactor modifies the kinetics of the reaction with respect to phenylalanine. Lysolecithin and phenylalanine appear to effect the same functional changes in phenylalanine hydroxylase: Both compounds activate the enzyme for hydroxylation of phenylalanine, both induce an ability in the enzyme to adsorb to hydrophobic surfaces, and both stimulate hydroxylation of tryptophan by phenylalanine hydroxylase [59].

Tetrahydrobiopterin may act as a negative modifier of phenylalanine hydroxylase. This phenomenon was reported with the synthetic cofactor tetrahydropterin [52], but it is more dramatically illustrated by the time course of nonactivated phenylalanine hydroxylase in the presence of biopterin [58].

The catalytic activity of phenylalanine hydroxylase can also be modified by lysolecithin and α-chymotrypsin [67]. In the presence of the natural cofactor (tetrahydrobiopterin), rat liver phenylalanine hydroxylase has a sigmoidal saturation curve (Hill coefficient 2.0). Lysolecithin or chymotrypsin increases the maximum velocity and decreases twofold the K_m of the hydroxylase for phenylalanine. Without lysolecithin the K_m is about 0.2 mM. In the presence of lysolecithin, the phenylalanine saturation curve becomes hyperbolic and the K_m is 0.09

mM. Plasma concentration of phenylalanine is in the range of 0.03 to 0.12 mM. Lysolecithin exposes the sulfhydryl group of the hydroxylase and appears to alter the conformation of the enzyme. Chymotrypsin partially hydrolyzes the hydroxylase, reducing its size from molecular weight 100,000 to 67,000 [67].

It has been suggested that the role of lysolecithin and chymotrypsin in vivo is to regulate hydroxylase activity homeostatically during liver damage, when lysosomal digestive enzymes are released. The disruption of lysosomes might also reversibly activate phenylalanine hydroxylase through the release of phospholipase A [73], an enzyme that converts the hydroxylase inhibitor lecithin [72] to the hydroxylase activator lysolecithin.

A protein factor named *phenylalanine hydroxylase stimulator (PHS)* has been purified from rat liver extracts. It is heat-stable and has a molecular weight of 51,000 [74]. At pH values above neutrality, or in the presence of phospholipids such as lysolecithin and the natural cofactor tetrahydrobiopterin, the specific activity of phenylalanine hydroxylase decreases with increasing enzyme concentration. The reason for the stimulating effect of PHS is that, when it is present, this decrease in specific activity does not occur.

Mild detergents or aging of phenylalanine hydroxylase desensitize the phenylalanine-activating site, so that the enzyme can no longer be activated by preincubation with phenylalanine [58]. There is a threefold reduction of the K_m value with no effect on the V_{max}. It is likely that this same mechanism is operative in the modification of the catalytic activity of phenylalanine hydroxylase by lysolecithin and α-chymotrypsin [72]. The shift of phenylalanine saturation kinetics from sigmoidal to hyperbolic signifies inactivation of the "activating" site of the enzyme by a variety of mechanisms such as desensitization or inactivation by aging, detergents, lysolecithin, and α-chymotrypsin.

Regulation of the Steady-state Activity of Phenylalanine Hydroxylase

Control of Phenylalanine Hydroxylase Activity   The long-term regulation, in the range of days, of phenylalanine metabolism in mammalian liver is effected by changes in the steady-state level of phenylalanine hydroxylase. Tissue culture and animal studies have uncovered some of the metabolites, hormones, and components in the diet that can modulate phenylalanine hydroxylase activity (Table 12-3).

Control of Phenylalanine Hydroxylase Activity in Tissue Culture   Control of the steady state of phenylalanine hydroxylase by hormones and serum factors has been demonstrated directly in tissue cultures of hepatic explants and in hepatoma cell cultures. In 22-day-gestation fetal hepatic explants the phenylalanine hydroxylase activity decays with a half-time of 6 h, while a high baseline of tyrosine aminotransferase activity and hydrocortisone inducibility of this activity is maintained for 72 h. This observation suggests that phenylalanine hydroxylase activity requires extrahepatic factors for induction and maintenance of a high tissue steady state [62].

The second line of evidence is derived from minimal deviation H4-II-E-C3 hepatoma cell culture studies [63–65]. Phenylalanine hydroxylase activity is present in two clonal cell lines (H4-II-E-C3 and MH$_1$C$_1$) derived from rat hepatomas in culture [63]. The levels of phenylalanine hydroxylase in these cell lines were stimulated threefold by hydrocortisone, dexamethasone, or N^6-O$^{2'}$-dibutyryl-3',5'-cyclic adenosine monophosphate [63]. The induction of the enzyme activity by hydrocortisone in the H4-II-E-C3 line was shown to depend on protein synthesis de novo, since it was inhibited by cycloheximide. Elegant immunologic methods have shown half-times of phenylalanine hydroxylase of hepatoma cells in culture of 7.4 to 8.2 h. These do not change with hydrocortisone induction, indicating that the rate of synthesis of phenylalanine hydroxylase is increased during induction [75].

Stationary phase, minimal deviation hepatoma H4-II-E-C3 cell cultures that are deprived of serum respond to dialyzed fetal calf serum or insulin with a biphasic time course of phenylalanine hydroxylase induction [65]. These two agents induce phenylalanine hydroxylase additively during both the initial 3-h and the delayed 24-h phases. The initial phase of induction by insulin is inhibited by cycloheximide but not by actinomycin D. The delayed induction by both dialyzed fetal calf serum and insulin, which represents 80 percent of the induced enzyme activity, is inhibited by 10^{-6} M cycloheximide and 0.20 μg per milliliter of actinomycin D. This observation suggests that gene transcription and protein synthesis mediate the serum and insulin effects.

Fractionation of fetal calf serum localizes most of the phenylalanine hydroxylase-inducing activity in the fraction that precipitates between 33 and 50 percent of saturation with ammonium sulfate. Heating for 20 min destroys 90 percent of the activity at 75°C and all of it at 100°C.

H4-II-E-C3 cells in culture do not synthesize the factor(s) in serum that induces phenylalanine hydroxylase. The studies of fetal explants and minimal deviation hepatoma cultures can best be interpreted in the following manner: Mammalian hepatic phenylalanine hydroxylase is maintained at a low constitutive level. An extrahepatic inductive factor, probably a protein, induces phenylalanine hydroxylase. Induction cannot take place in a resting G_0 phase liver cell, as shown by (1) the time lag of induction, (2) the correlation of enzyme induction with DNA synthesis in H4-II-E-C3 cell cultures, and (3) the absence of induction in fetal explant cultures [62], which do not divide and hence cannot go through an S phase (DNA synthesis) of the cell cycle [65].

Mouse erythroleukemia cells, which have no detectable phenylalanine hydroxylase, express this activity when fused to hepatoma cytoplast. The resulting cybrid is capable of growing in tyrosine-free medium [76]. Preliminary results suggest that the cytoplasmic regulatory factor is RNA in nature [77].

Animal Studies   The level of liver phenylalanine hydroxylase in rodents can be modulated by changes in dietary phenylalanine [54]. Injection of phenylalanine increased by 2.5-fold in 9 h the hepatic activity of 6-day-old and adult rats that had been pretreated 24 h earlier with p-chlorophenylalanine [66]. Administration of a single dose of p-chlorophenylalanine (360 mg/kg) to rats leads to the irreversible loss of 90 percent of hepatic phenylalanine hydroxylase activity [66, 79]. Without such pretreatment, phenylalanine did not raise the enzyme concentration. Puromycin inhibited the substrate-induced increase in phenylalanine hydroxylase. p-Chlorophenylalanine does not alter the rate of synthesis or the rate of degradation of phenylalanine hydroxylase, and there is no detectable p-chlorophenylalanine in the enzyme molecule [79]. The half-life of rat liver phenylalanine hydroxylase measured by specific antiserum titration with prelabeled enzyme is 2 days [79].

Activities of liver amino acid-catabolizing enzymes and liver and plasma-free amino acid concentrations in adult cockerels fed diets containing 3 to 12 percent casein were determined 2 h after a meal. Phenylalanine hydroxylase activity increases with increase in dietary casein from 3 to 12 percent and thereafter remains unchanged. Reflecting the change in phenylalanine hydroxylase activity, phenylalanine increases in the liver and decreases in the plasma. Liver tyrosine is not influenced by the dietary casein level, whereas plasma tyrosine increases sharply, from 3 to 12 percent of dietary casein [55]. Thus, the difference between liver and plasma-free phenylalanine and tyrosine in response to a protein load clearly illustrates the very tight control that seems to operate in catabolizing phenylalanine.

The injection of cortisol was without effect on the liver in adult rats but caused a threefold rise in phenylalanine hydroxylase activity in immature rats. The effects of cortisol and phenylalanine were additive. Actinomycin inhibited the cortisol-induced increase but not the substrate-induced increase in phenylalanine hydroxylase. Cortisol and phenylalanine do not induce renal phenylalanine hydroxylase. Thus either the genetic or the cellular control of the renal enzyme is different from that of the liver enzyme [66].

The Effect of Glucagon on Phenylalanine Metabolism and Phenylalanine-degrading Enzymes   Phenylalanine oxidation is stimulated and urinary phenylalanine excretion is depressed when rats are treated with glucagon subcutaneously for 10 days and an oral load of phenylalanine is administered [80]. Glucagon induces liver dihydropteridine reductase more than twofold [80]. Rats pretreated with glucagon show a time-dependent increase in phenylalanine hydroxylase activity only when this activity is measured in the presence of tetrahydrobiopterin [78]. A maximum fourfold stimulation of hydroxylase activity occurs. The rise in activity can be correlated with phosphorylation and conversion of multiple forms of the enzyme to a single form [78].

Alternative Mechanism of Regulating Tissue Phenylalanine   When tissue levels of phenylalanine, tyrosine, or tryptophan are elevated, decarboxylation becomes a major route of metabolism [81]. When inhibitors of L-amino acid decarboxylase are administered together with large oral doses of the appropriate amino acids, blood levels of amino acids are further elevated approximately twofold. The inhibitors by themselves do not alter plasma levels of the aromatic amino acids and do not inhibit other major routes of metabolism, such as transamination in the case of tyrosine [81].

Isoenzymes and Immunology of Rat Liver, Kidney, and Hepatoma Phenylalanine Hydroxylase   The first evidence for rat liver phenylalanine hydroxylase isoenzymes was presented by Kaufman and Fisher [43]. They found two isoenzymes with identical molecular weights (110,000) but different charges, each having full enzymatic activity.

We have reported three immunologically distinct and non-cross-reacting isoenzymes of rat liver [83]. The isoenzymes were distinguished by (1) isoelectric focusing [84], (2) immunotitration, (3) double immunodiffusion, and (4) immunoabsorption [83]. Only a single isoenzyme could be distinguished for rat kidney and minimal deviation hepatoma phenylalanine hydroxylase, even when hepatoma cells were induced by hydrocortisone prior to tissue extract preparation.

Isoelectric focusing of partially purified fractions of rat liver phenylalanine hydroxylase prepared either by the method of Kaufman and Fisher [43] or of Gillam et al. [45] gave three identical isoenzyme peaks with pIs of 5.20, 5.30, and 5.60. Isoelectric focusing of kidney and H4-II-E-C3 hepatoma phenylalanine hydroxylase gave single peaks for each, with pIs of 5.35 and 5.20, respectively [84]. Thus the claim by Gillam et al. [45] that the two isoenzymes of rat liver PH demonstrated by Kaufman and Fisher [43] using acrylamide gel electrophoresis are artifacts of the purification procedure has not been substantiated.

We have proposed an epigenetic modification of phenylalanine hydroxylase structure, e.g., by phosphorylation of serine residues, addition of carbohydrate groups, or removal of components of the polypeptide chains by proteolytic enzymes, as a possible explanation of immunologically distinct isoenzymes because of difficulty in reconciling our observations in the rodent with the concept of a single gene lesion in PKU [83].

Barranger et al. [82] and DelValle and Greengard [85] have identified three isoenzymes of rat liver phenylalanine hydroxylase by using calcium phosphate gel and hydroxyapatite chromatography. These isoenzymes had identical molecular weights and kinetic constants but different charges [82]. Donlon and Kaufman [60] have shown that phosphorylation of phenylalanine hydroxylase could explain the multiple forms of rodent enzyme isolated by Barranger et al. [82]. The two major forms of rat liver phenylalanine hydroxylase resolved by calcium phosphate gel chromatography contain dissimilar amounts of protein-bound phosphate. The hydroxylase activity of these forms, assayed in the presence of tetrahydrobiopterin, can be differentially stimulated by treatment with Mg^{2+}, ATP, cyclic

AMP, and protein kinase [86]. This results in the production of chromatographically distinct species of the two forms, leading to a new form which contains 1 mole of phosphate per subunit (molecular weight 50,000). In addition, phosphorylation in vitro eliminates the heterogeneity displayed by the isolated forms [61]. Glucagon (10^{-9} M) added to isolated rat hepatocytes increases the level of cyclic AMP inside the cells and the activity of phenylalanine hydroxylase [87]. Thus, a nonphosphorylated dimer with a molecular weight of 100,000, a fully phosphorylated dimer, and an intermediate half-phosphorylated dimer species of phenylalanine hydroxylase can be generated by this model: 00 $\rightleftharpoons$ 00-P $\rightleftharpoons$ P-00-P [61].

No immunologically distinct isoenzymes were identified by Freidman et al. [88] or Ayling et al. [44]. The resuspended antigen-antibody complex lost 60 percent of its initial activity, which suggested that the enzyme was unstable, or alternatively, that immune serum had an inhibitor under the conditions of titration [88]. The antigen-antibody complex required more than 48 h to precipitate and achieve 50 percent inhibition, during which the enzyme was unstable [44]. Because of this instability, a differential precipitation of antigen-antibody complex with 35 percent ammonium sulfate was used. In our hands this procedure precipitates significant amounts of phenylalanine hydroxylase with nonimmune control globulin and therefore is not a reliable method of titration.

Three hypothetical models of rodent phenylalanine hydroxylase isoenzymes can be formulated from the immunologic, gel electrophoresis, and isoelectric focusing data, plus phosphorylation data.

1. If the isoenzymes have identical molecular weights but differ in charge [43], with two nonidentical subunits of molecular weight 54,000 [72], then the isoenzymes would have the following structure:

$$\alpha\alpha, \ \alpha\beta, \ \beta_\iota\beta_\iota \ \text{(liver)}, \ \beta_\kappa\beta_\kappa \ \text{(kidney)} \qquad (2)$$

2. If the subunits are identical [43], then the isoenzymes would have the following structure:

$$\alpha\alpha, \ \beta\beta, \ \text{and} \ \gamma_\iota\gamma_\iota \ \text{(liver), and} \ \gamma_\kappa\gamma_\kappa \ \text{(kidney)} \qquad (3)$$

3. If the isoenzymes are generated through epigenetic modification of the enzyme structure by phosphorylation and have identical subunits (a single allelic locus), then the polypeptide chains will have the $\alpha\alpha$ structure. If they have nonidentical subunits (two nonallelic loci), then the isozymes will have the $\alpha\beta$ structure.

The autosomal recessive nature of PKU would argue in favor of the epigenetic modification of protein structure as the basis of isoenzymes of liver phenylalanine hydroxylase in humans. This argument cannot resolve the issue of the rodent liver and kidney isoenzymes [83, 84]. The measurement of phenylalanine hydroxylase in the presence of synthetic cofactor does not distinguish the species of phosphorylated from nonphosphorylated enzyme [89], and the phosphorylation phenomenon cannot explain the existence of rodent isoenzymes characterized by immunologic and isoelectric focusing methods observed by Tourian et al. [83, 84]. Additionally, it has not been reported in the literature that the human isoenzymes observed by Barranger et al. [82] can be similarly explained by phosphorylation and dephosphorylation.

Immunology of Human Phenylalanine Hydroxylase in Phenylketonuria and Hyperphenylalaninemia   Antibody to rat liver phenylalanine hydroxylase cross-reacts with human phenylalanine hydroxylase on double immunodiffusion with complete fusion of the immunoprecipitin lines [90], but no immunoprecipitin line forms in a cross reaction with liver extract of the ammonium sulfate fraction from PKU or hyperphenylalaninemic human liver [90]. No protein corresponding to either intact phenylalanine hydroxylase or its subunits could be purified from extracts from two PKU patients prepared by affinity chromatography [50]. Choo et al. [50], using an affinity column procedure for purification of human phenylalanine hydroxylase, have identified two nonidentical subunits with molecular weights of 50,000, in addition to four (degradation product) protein spots of molecular weight 49,000 on two-dimensional gels under dissociating conditions. They found no cross-reacting material from extracts of liver tissue of two PKU patients to any of these subunits. Bartholome and Ertel [91] have detected a cross-reacting immunoprecipitin line on double diffusion with monkey liver phenylalanine hydroxylase antibody. It is difficult to reconcile this observation with previous results [90, 50].

Fetal Developmental Biology of Human Phenylalanine Hydroxylase   Human fetal liver phenylalanine hydroxylase activity was first demonstrated by perfusion techniques measuring the conversion of [3-^{14}C]phenylalanine to [^{14}C]tyrosine [92]. Direct measurements on liver extracts from 11- to 20-week-gestation human abortuses have demonstrated both phenylalanine hydroxylase and dihydropteridine reductase activity, as well as the presence of a natural cofactor [93]. The K_m values for phenylalanine and the synthetic cofactor were identical to those of adult liver [93, 94]. Phenylalanine hydroxylase activity in hepatic tissue approaches adult levels at a fetal age of 7 weeks [95].

The kidneys of 8- to 20-week-gestation fetuses have no detectable phenylalanine hydroxylase activity. Thus, the ontogeny of kidney phenylalanine hydroxylase is different from that of the liver enzyme in humans [48].

Experimental Models of PKU   The reader is referred to the previous edition of this chapter [96].

THE HYPERPHENYLALANINEMIA SYNDROMES

When screening for PKU was established, the simple goal was to detect and treat infants having PKU. It soon became evident that a significant number of infants with hyperphenylalaninemia did not have PKU [7, 11]. The phenylalanine hydoxylase deficiency was less severe. These infants needed to be distinguished from the PKU patients because their management is different. Subsequently, a third subset became evident—less frequent, but having a more somber course, necessitating prompt discrimination from the earlier recognized entities. These patients were shown to have a defect in the metabolism of tetrahydrobiopterin. Table 12-1 presents a classification of hyperphenylalaninemias which may be encountered in the course of neonatal screening.

Hyperphenylalaninemia, Type I: Classic PKU

One of the compelling reasons for screening for PKU in the neonatal period is that infants with this condition only rarely

have symptoms that would lead the clinician to suspect metabolic disease [97–99] (Table 12-4). Eczema is observed in approximately 25 percent of untreated patients during the first year of life, but this finding is nonspecific and, indeed, is a rare cause of eczema in infants. The musty odor due to phenylacetic acid may occur relatively early in the first year of life, but it may not be a complaint of the parent. The dilution of pigment due to inhibition of tyrosinase is similarly not often helpful because this is primarily a disease of Caucasians. The lack of symptoms in the first year of life is relevant in that without proper dietary control the PKU patient will lose 50 IQ points in that year [10].

After the first year, the pigment dilution, eczema, delayed psychomotor development, failure to walk or talk, seizures, hyperactivity, agitated and aggressive behavior, muscular hypertoxicity, tremor, microcephaly, prominent maxilla with widened interdermal spaces, enamel hypoplasia, decalcification of the long bones, and decreased rate of growth form a constellation of symptoms that indicate PKU [100]. Ultimately, 96 to 98 percent of untreated PKU patients will have an IQ of less than 50.

The phenylalanine hydroxylase in the liver of PKU patients is approximately 0.27 percent of normal activity. In contrast to the hydroxylase from the liver of normal individuals, it is not inhibited by 0.1 mM phenylalanine or stimulated as well by lysolecithin [57].

Hyperphenylalaninemia: Types II and III

Patients with non-PKU persistent hyperphenylalaninemia form phenotypically a continuum ranging from those difficult to distinguish from classic PKU to the more mildly affected, with a blood phenylalanine concentration of 4 to 10 mg/dl. In general, but not invariably, the hydroxylase activity in the liver correlates with the blood phenylalanine level [102]. The activity found in these patients has varied from 1.5 to 34.5 percent of normal [102, 103]. Distinguishing the varying levels of functional activity is important since dietary management is adjusted accordingly. Guttler [104] classifies the hyperphenylalaninemias according to dietary tolerance for phenylalanine and the response to a phenylalanine load. Classic PKU has a phenylalanine tolerance of less than 0.13 mmol/kg per day; mild PKU a tolerance of 0.14 to 0.30 mmol/kg per day; and persistent hyperphenylalaninemia a normal phenylalanine tolerance, i.e., 0.7 mmol/kg per day. This method separates those with transient hyperphenylalaninemia with normal tolerance from the persistent hyperphenylalaninemias. Phenylalanine toler-

Table 12–4   Prevalence of phenylketonuria in different countries

Australia	1:9000	Ireland	1:4500
Austria	1:11,000	Israel	1:19,000
Belgium	1:6000	Japan	1:60,000
Canada	1:15,000	New Zealand	1:16,000
Czechoslovakia	1:7000	Norway	1:13,700
Denmark	1:9000	Poland	1:8000
France	1:13,000	Sweden	1:38,000
West Germany	1:6000	Switzerland	1:16,600
Finland	1:100,000	U.S.	1:11,000
Great Britain		Yugoslavia	1:13,000
England	1:12,000		
N. Ireland	1:10,000		
Scotland	1:6000		

ance can be used as a functional basis for classification. Guttler [104] found, as did a collaborative study [105], that proper classification frequently is not possible on the basis of the blood phenylalanine levels and evaluation of urinary metabolites. It was necessary to test phenylalanine loading at 4 to 6 months and again at 12 and 18 months in order to determine which children required continuation of the diet. The important point is that dietary management should be instituted until the classification can be established.

Transaminase Deficiency

Patients reported as having possible transaminase deficiency were able to maintain a normal blood phenylalanine level except when exposed to a high protein intake [106]. Kaufman [107] has reasoned that these patients may, indeed, have had a transient mild deficiency of the dihydropteridine reductase enzyme. He also argues convincingly that a transaminase deficiency alone would not lead to hyperphenylalaninemia.

Hyperphenylalaninemia Due to Coenzyme Defects: Types IV, V

The most important advances in understanding the hyperphenylalaninemias have been made in defining the defects associated with deficiency of the phenylalanine hydroxylase coenzyme, tetrahydrobiopterin. A deficiency of dihydropteridine reductase was first demonstrated enzymatically [12] in a patient with feeding difficulties beginning shortly after birth, choking attacks progressive from the neonatal period, developmental delay apparent by 5 months of age, seizures beginning in the first year of life, and failure of control of the symptoms with a low phenylalanine diet [108].

Subsequently, Leeming et al. [109] reported a different defect in an infant with a blood phenylalanine level of 30 mg/dl at 7 days of age and 49 mg/dl at 13 days. During the first 2 months of life, she responded poorly to stimuli. At 3 months of age, the deep tendon reflexes were hyperactive and the torso and extremities were hypertonic. By 6 months, athetoid movements of the arms, myoclonia, frequent yawning, difficulty in swallowing, and increased salivation had appeared. The abnormal movements disappeared around 1 year of age and she became completely inactive, with loss of reflexes. The EEG was diffusely abnormal. The patient was shown to have reduced biopterins in the urine and blood and a distribution different from normal. Additional reports confirmed that this was a new entity which appeared to be due to a defect in dihydrobiopterin synthetase [14, 110]. It is not clear that each of the biopterin synthesis defects is at the same enzymatic site. Theoretically, each of the sequential steps could be the site of a mutation resulting in clinical hyperphenylalaninemia (Fig. 12-3). One report [111] was sobering in indicating that the affected infant did not have an elevated blood phenylalanine level at 6 days of age, whereas it was 20 mg/dl at age 6 months after neurologic symptoms were apparent.

Distinguishing patients with these forms, estimated to comprise 1 to 3 percent of those with hyperphenylalaninemia, is particularly important because the outcome without treatment is poor [12, 109], and the mode of treatment is different from that of the usual forms of hyperphenylalaninemia [112, 113]. The coenzyme for phenylalanine hydroxylase, tyrosine hydroxylase, and tryptophan hydroxylase catalyzes the synthesis of tyrosine and the important neurotransmitters dopa, adrenaline, noradrenaline, and serotonin. The tetrahydro form of an unconjugated pteridine is the obligatory cofactor for an enzyme system in the liver which catalyzes the oxidation of long-chain alkyl ethers of glycerol to fatty acids and free glycerol [114]. Whereas the deficiency of putative neurotransmitters has been proposed to be responsible for the brain symptoms, it is likely that abnormal fatty acid and glycerol metabolism, which has not been evaluated in this condition, also contributes to the neurologic picture.

Increased Phenylalanine and Tyrosine

Rennert et al. [115] have described two brothers with increased phenylalanine and tyrosine in the plasma who had progressive clinical deterioration, with ataxia and seizures appearing between 12 and 18 months of age. They had increased urinary concentrations of phenylethylamine, mandelic acid, and p-hydroxymandelic acid. Two additional families have been studied since the original report. These children survive without further deterioration on a diet of moderate phenylalanine intake (60 mg/kg) [116].

Transient neonatal tyrosinemia is benign. It is most frequently encountered in the premature infant. It was found by Kretchmer [117] to reflect a partial impairment of p-hydroxyphenylpyruvic acid oxidase (see L.A. Goldsmith, Chap. 13). The disorder responds to ascorbic acid administration [118]. The prevalence of this type of tyrosinemia is approximately 1 in 400 [104].

Hyperphenylalaninemia may be secondary to one of the hereditary tyrosinemias. Three enzymatic defects of tyrosine have been identified: (1) p-hydroxyphenylpyruvate deoxygenase deficiency [119, 120], (2) cytoplasmic tyrosine aminotransferase deficiency [121], and (3) fumarylacetoacetate deficiency [122]. (See Chap. 13.)

These conditions emphasize the need to measure tyrosine when the blood phenylalanine is found to be elevated.

Diagnosis

There are no pathognomonic symptoms in a newborn infant with hyperphenylalaninemia. If it is accepted that early dietary management is important, the only way to accomplish this is by neonatal screening. Two methods have been widely used for screening for elevated blood phenylalanine levels: (1) The method of Guthrie [7] is a bacterial inhibition assay which uses a phenylalanine competitive inhibitor, β-2-thienylalanine, in the agar. The rate of growth of the organisms is a function of the level of phenylalanine in the sample. (2) The second method is fluorometric determination of phenylalanine [8]. In order not to confuse the phenylalaninemias with the disorders of tyrosine metabolism in the screening process, it is important that tyrosine also be measured when the confirmatory tests for elevated phenylalanine are processed.

There are two major issues in screening. First, the overall success will depend on the completeness of testing of all infants after birth. Second, testing should be done after the infant has had a significant protein intake, since the PKU infant has normal blood levels at birth and until exposed to 24 h of protein intake [N.A. Holtzman, cited in Ref. 123]. The claim that the infant must be exposed to at least 24 h of protein feeding in order to obtain an elevated blood phenylalanine has been challenged in a limited, controlled study [124].

If a second blood test reveals elevated blood phenylalanine, the infant is admitted to the hospital for a challenge of 3 days with a 1:2 dilution of evaporated milk formula. If the blood phenylalanine rises to 20 mg/dl or greater during the 3-day period, the infant is placed on a phenylalanine-deficient diet, with the phenylalanine adjusted to tolerance. The infant is given a challenge at 4 to 6 months with a diet containing 180 mg phenylalanine per kilogram of body weight. If the blood phenylalanine rises above 20 mg/dl again, the restrictive diet is resumed. At 12 to 18 months the challenge is repeated with phenylalanine or a diet with an equivalent amount at 180 mg per kilogram of body weight. If the phenylalanine level does not return to normal within 72 h, the diet is resumed. The challenge is repeated every 6 to 8 months. Occasionally, patients may not show a return of tolerance for several years.

For clinical purposes, the questions to be answered are these: Is the hyperphenylalaninemia persistent or transient? What is the tolerance for dietary phenylalanine?

The coenzyme defects require a more specific approach. Dihydropteridine reductase can be assayed in liver, fibroblasts [12], and blood cells [125]. The measurement of defects in biopterin synthesis is more difficult. The simplest approach, were it readily available, would be the administration of 2.0 to 2.5 mg/kg tetrahydrobiopterin by mouth, with the measurement of blood phenylalanine before and 6 h after administration. Hyperphenylalaninemia consequent to a defect of phenylalanine hydroxylase will show no effect, whereas coenzyme defects will show a dramatic fall in blood phenylalanine [113, 125, 126]. If 2 mg/kg dihydrobiopterin is given by mouth, patients with PKU or dihydropteridine reductase deficiency show no fall in phenylalanine level, whereas patients with defective biopterin synthesis will do so [111, 127]. In the biopterin synthesis defect, there is low urine biopterin, large amounts of neopterin, and small amounts of dihydroneopterins. Normal patients have no neopterin, whereas patients with dihydropteridine reductase deficiency excrete increased amounts of dihydrobiopterin as well as traces of biopterin and neopterin [128]. Tetrahydrobiopterin is the major pteridine of the biopterin series in the urine of normal individuals and those with PKU [128]. The introduction of high performance liquid chromatography will facilitate the identification of these compounds in the urine [129, 130].

Treatment

The symptoms important in PKU relate to cerebral dysfunction. Control of the blood phenylalanine concentration prevents the progressive, irreversible loss of cerebral development [131]. The earlier treatment is instituted, the better the ultimate outcome [131]. The irreversible effects of exposure to high phenylalanine levels in utero emphasize the great susceptibility of the developing brain and the irreversibility of the effects on the immature brain (see below) [132].

The patient with PKU has a virtually total block in catabolism through the hydroxylase pathway. The phenylalanine required is that which is necessary for protein synthesis. The requirement for phenylalanine varies with age, from 47 to 90 mg/kg per day in the infant 2 to 4 months of age to approxi-

mately 27 mg/kg per day after 1 year of age [133]. The diet prescribed in infancy is based on approximately 90 percent of the protein coming from a low phenylalanine milk preparation such as Lofenelac. Patients with phenylalanine hydroxylase variants will handle larger amounts of phenylalanine. The amount varies from individual to individual depending on the amount of enzyme activity. The diet is adjusted according to the tolerance of the individual as judged from the blood phenylalanine level. The blood level can safely be maintained in the range for normal individuals [133], and studies comparing the IQ of those maintained below 5.5 mg/dl with those monitored between 5.5 and 10 mg/dl showed a higher IQ at 42 to 48 months in the former group [131]. Maintaining the blood phenylalanine level below normal has been associated with poor growth, retarded bone age, hepatomegaly, repeated infections, hypoglycemia, and neurologic symptoms [134].

Blood phenylalanine is monitored weekly for the first year and every 2 to 4 weeks thereafter as needed. Other foods, specifically fruits and vegetables, are introduced at the usual times. After the first year of life, the question arises as to when the diet can be discontinued. Since the last edition of this volume [96], the answer is still not definitive. It is clear that there is a wide variation in response to diet withdrawal in different children [20]. Some children taken off the diet at $4\frac{1}{2}$ years of age showed no loss in IQ scoring, but others lost as many as 19 IQ points. The current inclination is slowly to decrease strict control at 8 to 10 years of age, reinstituting it if there is retrogression [19, 21].

The oral administration of phenylalanine ammonia lyase has been suggested and shown to effect a fall of blood phenylalanine in a few subjects under controlled circumstances [135]. It is difficult to see how this approach would be useful generally since the effect would be variable with a fixed dose and varying phenylalanine intake. If the phenylalanine intake can be controlled, the enzyme would be superfluous. It may have a beneficial role in those children who are erratically maintained on a diet or may make more palatable the low phenylalanine diets for pregnant PKU patients.

The basic approach to therapy, which is the maintenance of a near normal blood level of phenylalanine, is designed to prevent a rise in a metabolite(s) which leads to permanent damage to the central nervous system. The metabolite(s) which might be considered as the "toxic" culprit has been thoroughly reviewed [56, 136]. In addition to theoretical considerations [137–140], the fact that there is an effect on the IQ at $4\frac{1}{2}$ years, when the level of blood phenylalanine is kept below 12 mg/dl, below the concentration which would give rise to significant levels of alternate phenylalanine metabolites, suggests that phenylalanine itself is the likely offending agent. The paradox is that newborn patients having hyperphenylalaninemia with levels below 20 mg/dl do not appear to require dietary management. Either there is something unique to the PKU patient during the first 3 to 4 years of life with a level of 15 mg/dl phenylalanine or, more probably, there is a lack of precise data to determine whether the hyperphenylalaninemic patient who has a blood concentration of 15 mg/dl would, in fact, have a higher IQ were the phenylalanine concentration kept below 5 mg/dl in the first several years of life. The mechanism which seems most reasonable at this point is that the elevated phenylalanine competes with other amino acids for the transport system into the neurons and creates an amino acid imbalance within the cell which inhibits protein synthesis and synaptogenesis. Myelin reduction would be secondary to reduced myelin protein synthesis. If this hypothesis is reasonable, there follows an imperative for close control and monitoring of these patients.

Therapy for patients with coenzyme defects has two phases. The elevated phenylalanine needs to be carefully controlled for the same reasons given for PKU patients. Also, since the coenzymes are essential to the endogenous production of neurotransmitters by tryptophan hydroxylase and tyrosine hydroxylase, and to the oxidation of glyceryl ethers, treatment should be directed toward the deficiency of the monoamine neurotransmitters and toward the faulty oxidation of glyceryl ethers. Treatment is said to be effective with L-dopa, 5-hydroxytryptophan, and carbidopa, an inhibitor of dopa decarboxylase [110, 141]. The long-term results cannot be assessed at this time.

Maternal Phenylketonuria

The success of the screening for elevated blood phenylalanine in neonates and the successful management of those identified as having hyperphenylalaninemia have created another problem. Some of the women who were treated early have now reached reproductive age. Most of the infants born to untreated PKU mothers have shown mental retardation and other anomalies, even though the infant did not have PKU. Lenke and Levy [132], using their own data and the responses to a questionnaire sent to international investigators, have analyzed the data from sufficient numbers of pregnancies to be able to discern definite trends. Table 12-5 presents the findings. Fetal brain damage is a function of maternal blood phenylalanine levels. There appears to be a threshold effect for congenital heart disease and low birth weight.

The diets of 34 women were managed at some point before or during pregnancy. Only three were under management before conception. One of the progeny had an IQ of 80. The children of 7 of 11 mothers whose dietary management was initiated in the first trimester had IQ evaluations. The average was 103, with a range of 74 to 127. When management was initiated in the second and third trimesters, the IQs of those tested were 84 and 79, respectively. The results from untreated pregnancies appear in Table 12-5.

Clearly, there is benefit from management of the blood level of phenylalanine in pregnancy. The best results appear to follow early initiation of dietary management.

The most surprising finding in the survey of Lenke and Levy [132] was the high frequency of hyperphenylalaninemic offspring of these mothers. Affected children were born to 27 out of 155 mothers, and 40 of 423 children had hyperphenylalaninemia. With a gene frequency of 1:50 for PKU or hyperphenylalaninemia, one would expect that 1 in every 100 births of three mothers to have PKU. In seven families there was a substantial difference between the blood phenylalanine levels of the mother and infant. One PKU mother had two infants with mild hyperphenylalaninemia; three mothers with mild hyperphenylalaninemia had infants with PKU. Three hyperphenylalaninemic mothers had one infant with PKU and one with hyperphenylalaninemia. A number of hypotheses can be offered to explain these important and surprising observations. By definition, all of the children born to PKU mothers are obligate heterozygotes. From Table 12-6, it can be seen that the phenylalanine hydroxylase activity of parents with hyperphenylalaninemic children ranges from 4.4 to 23 (moles of tyrosine formed per gram of protein per hour), and yet these parents do not suffer from hyperphenylalaninemia. Is it possible that maternal PKU prevents the normal expression of liver phenylalanine hydroxylase during fetal development, resulting in a condition of phenotypic hyperphenylalaninemia even in the absence of the double dose of the PKU gene? Alternately, is it possible that if obligate heterozygote parents of hyperphenylalaninemic children were tested during the neonatal period, they would in fact show hyperphenylalaninemia? This seems unlikely since the heterozygote sibs of PKU children do not suffer from neonatal hyperphenylalaninemia. The true reason for this observation remains to be discovered.

Electroencephalogram (EEG)

The incidence of seizures in untreated or late-treated PKU patients is between 37 and 50 percent [142, 143]. An abnormal EEG was reported in 89 and 96 percent [142, 144]. In a study

Table 12–5   Frequency of spontaneous abortion and abnormalities in the offspring of women with phenylketonuria or hyperphenylalaninemia untreated during pregnancy

Complication (%)	Groupings of maternal phenylalanine levels				
	>20 mg/dl	16–19 mg/dl	11–15 mg/dl	3–10 mg/dl	Frequency (%) in normal population
	Percentage affected in each group				
Spontaneous abortions	24	30	0	8	15–20
Mental retardation	92	73	22	21	5.0
Microcephaly	73	68	35	24	4.8
Congenital heart disease	12	15	6	0	
Birth weight <2500 g	40	52	56	13	9.6

SOURCE: After Lenke and Levy [132].

Table 12-6 Results of phenylalanine hydroxylase assays on the liver from normal subjects and patients with phenylketonuria and hyperphenylalaninemia

Subject	Number of subjects	Age, yr	Enzyme activity mol tyr formed (g protein, h)
Control	3	10–86	58.8–96
	6	20–60	48.0–96
	13	2–70	63.6–134
PKU	12	1/12–9	0
Hyperphenylalanemia	1	3/12	6.3
	3		2.7, 3.8, 4.7
	2		6.0, 24.7
	16	1/12–19	
	12	1/12–19	1.5–6.2
	4	1–4	14.9, 31.8, 34.5, 8.7
Parents of hyperphenylalanine-mic children	6		23, 7.2, 4.4, 7.7, 5.8, 11.4

of the EEG in 90 early-treated, late-treated, and variant children, it was found that 73 percent of early-treated and 62 percent of the variant children had a normal EEG, whereas 69 percent of the late-treated group had an abnormal EEG. Of the children, 40 had more than one EEG, and in 10 of these one EEG was normal and the other abnormal [145].

When seizures occur in untreated patients with PKU, dietary regulation of the blood phenylalanine level will usually control them. The effect requires several months of therapy [100].

Pathology

Few abnormalities were found in the brains of five patients ranging in age from 16 months to 67 years [146]. There was some astrocytosis in the older patients but no abnormality of myelination. The younger patients showed reduced myelin staining. Structural alteration in the white matter myelin of eight patients of varying age has been reported [147]. The younger patients had spongy lesions with reduced myelination. Older patients had frankly demyelinating lesions.

There is less lipid in the brains of these patients even when no abnormality of myelin staining can be demonstrated. Lipids associated with myelin, particularly galactolipids, are notably decreased [148]. Recovery of myelin from the white matter was significantly less than that from subjects mentally retarded from other causes [149]. Proteolipids are also depressed in the brains of individuals with PKU [150, 151]. The ratio of mono-enoic unsaturated fatty acids to saturated acids is decreased and there is a deficiency of hydroxy fatty acid in glycolipids, especially sulfatides [152].

Genetics

Mass screening had identified an unexpectedly large number of patients with hyperphenylalaninemia who do not have PKU. Non-PKU phenylalaninemia is estimated to have approximately half the frequency of PKU and segregates among population groups [104]. Coenzyme defects account for 3 percent of hyperphenylalaninemias [112].

All of the hyperphenylalaninemias appear to be autosomal

recessive, except for type VI, which has been seen only in males in the three families studied [116]. The coenzyme defects also appear to be autosomal recessive, with the expected gene dosage effect in heterozygotes of dihydropteridine reductase deficiency [153]. The gene for dihydropteridine reductase has been assigned to the short arm of chromosome 4 in banding region q1 [McKusick, cited in Ref. 99]. No attempts have been made to demonstrate heterozygosity in the biopterin synthesis defect.

Although the phenylalanine hydroxylase defects appear to be autosomal recessive, there is no proportional gene expression in the heterozygote (see Table 12-6). Heterozygotes show 10 percent of normal activity rather than the 50 percent expected. The unexpectedly high incidence of children with PKU and hyperphenylalaninemia born of mothers with PKU raises questions which have not been resolved (see "Maternal Phenylketonuria" above).

Kaufman [107] has explained the anomalous phenylalanine hydroxylase gene dosage effect by negative intraallelic or interallelic interaction between subunits of a homopolymeric or heteropolymeric phenylalanine hydroxylase enzyme. Another suggestion offered is that there may be a third allele at the phenylalanine hydroxylase locus [154]. Liver biopsy hydroxylase activity in hyperphenylalaninemic patients and parents has allowed some insight into the complexity of gene dosage, but little progress has been made beyond that. Culturing hepatic cells and cloning the gene from different variants would be the most direct method of elucidating the genetics of the hyperphenylalaninemias.

REFERENCES

1. FÖLLING A: Uber ausscheidung von Phenylbrenztraubensaure in den Harn als Stoffwechselanomalie in Verbindung mit Imbezillitat. *Hoppe-Seyler's Z Physiol Chem* 227:169, 1934

2. PENROSE L, QUASTEL JH: Metabolic studies in phenylketonuria. *Biochem J* 31:266, 1937

3. JERVIS GA: Studies on phenylpyruvic oligophrenia: The position of the metabolic error. *J Biol Chem* 169:651, 1947

4. JERVIS GA: Phenylpyruvic oligophrenia deficiency of phenylalanine-oxidizing system. *Proc Soc Exp Biol Med* 82:514, 1953

5. BICKEL H, GERRARD J, HICKMANS EM: Influence of phenylalanine intake on phenylketonuria. *Lancet* 2:812, 1953

6. GUTHRIE R: Blood screening for phenylketonuria. *JAMA* 178:863, 1961

7. GUTHRIE R, SUSI A: A simple phenylalanine method for detecting phenylketonuria in large populations of newborn infants. *Pediatrics* 32:338, 1963

8. McCAMAN MW, ROBINS E: Fluorimetric method for the determination of phenylalanine in serum. *J Lab Clin Med* 59:885, 1962

9. SCRIVER CR, ROSENBERG LE: *Amino Acid Metabolism and Its Disorders.* Philadelphia, WB Saunders Co, 1973, pp 290–337

10. KOCH R, BLASKOVICS M, WENZ E, FISHLER K, SCHAEFFLER G: Phenylalaninemia and phenylketonuria, in Nyhan, WL (ed): *Heritable Disorders of Amino Acid Metabolism.* New York, John Wiley & Sons, Inc, 1974, pp 109–140

11. COMMITTEE FOR THE STUDY OF INBORN ERRORS OF METABOLISM, NATIONAL RESEARCH COUNCIL: *Genetic Screening: Programs, Principles and Research.* Washington, DC, National Academy of Sciences, 1975, pp 21–93

12. KAUFMAN S, HOLTZMAN NA, MILSTIEN S, BUTLER IJ, KRUMHOLZ A: Phenylketonuria due to a deficiency of dihydropteridine reductase. *New Engl J Med* 293:785, 1975

13. REY F, HARPEY JP, LEEMING RJ, BLAIR JA, AICARDI J, REY J: Les hyperphenylalaninemics avec activite normale de la phenylalanine hydroxylase. *Arch Fr Pediatr* 34 (suppl): 109, 1977

14. KAUFMAN S, BERLOW S, SUMMER GK, MILSTIEN S, SCHULMAN JD, ORLOFF S, SPIELBERG S, PUESCHEL S: Hyperphenylalaninemia due to a deficiency of biopterin. *New Engl J Med* 299:673, 1978

15. LEEMING RJ, BLAIR JA, GREEN A, RAINE DN: Biopterin derivatives in normal and phenylketonuric patients after oral loads of L-phenylalanine, L-tyroxine, and L-tryptophan. *Arch Dis Child* 51:771, 1976

16. LIPTON MA, GORDON R, GUROFF G, UDENFRIEND S: p-Chlorophenylalanine-induced chemical manifestations of phenylketonuria in rats. *Science* 156:248, 1967

17. WINICK M: Malnutrition and brain development. *J Pediatr* 74:667, 1969

18. HOLTZMAN NA, WELCHER DW, MELLITS ED: Termination of restricted diet in children with phenylketonuria: A randomized controlled study. *New Engl J Med* 293:1121, 1975

19. WILLIAMSON M, KOCH R, BERLOW S: Diet discontinuation in phenylketonuria (letter to the editor). *Pediatrics* 63:823, 1979

20. CABALSKA B, DUCZYŃSKA N, BORZYMOWSKA J, ZORSKA K, KOŚLACZ-FOLGA A, BOŻKOWA K: Termination of dietary treatment in phenylketonuria. *Eur J Pediatr* 126:253, 1977

21. SMITH I, LOBASCHER ME, STEVENSON JE, WOLFF OH, SCHMIDT H, GRUBEL-KAISER S, BICKEL H: Effect of stopping low-phenylalanine diet on intellectual progress of children with phenylketonuria. *Br Med J* 2:723, 1978

22. WOMACK M, ROSE WC: Feeding experiments with mixtures of highly purified amino acids. VI. The relation of phenylalanine and tyrosine to growth. *J Biol Chem* 107:449, 1934

23. EMBDEN G, BALDES K: Uber den Abbau des Phenylalanins im tierischen Organismus. *Biochem Z* 55:301, 1913

24. MOSS AR, SCHOENHEIMER R: The conversion of phenylalanine to tyrosine in normal rats. *J Biol Chem* 135:415, 1940

25. GRAU CR, STEELE R: Phenylalanine and tyrosine utilization in normal and phenylalanine-deficient young mice. *J Nutr* 53:59, 1954

26. TOURIAN A, GODDARD J, PUCK TT: Phenylalanine hydroxylase activity in mammalian cells. *J Cell Physiol* 73:159, 1969

27. AYLING JE, HELFAND GD, PIRSON WD: Phenylalanine hydroxylase from human kidney. *Enzyme* 20:6, 1975

28. UDENFRIEND S, COOPER JR: The enzymatic conversion of phenylalanine to tyrosine. *J Biol Chem* 194:503, 1952

29. MITOMA C: Studies on partially purified phenylalanine hydroxylase. *Arch Biochem Biophys* 60:476, 1956

30. KAUFMAN S: A new cofactor required for the enzymatic conversion of phenylalanine to tyrosine. *J Biol Chem* 230:931, 1958

31. KAUFMAN S: The structure of the phenylalanine-hydroxylation cofactor. *Proc Natl Acad Sci USA* 50:1085, 1963

32. KAUFMAN S: Metabolism of phenylalanine hydroxylation cofactor. *J Biol Chem* 242:3934, 1967

33. KAUFMAN S: The phenylalanine hydroxylating system from mammalian liver. *Adv Enzymol* 35:245, 1971

34. BUBLITZ C: A direct assay for liver phenylalanine hydroxylase. *Biochim Biophys Acta* 191:249, 1969

35. GUROFF G, REIFSNYDER CA, DALY J: Retention of deuterium in p-tyrosine formed enzymatically from p-deuterophenylalanine. *Biochem Biophys Res Commun* 24:720, 1966

36. GUROFF G, DALY JW, JERINA DM, RENSON J, WITKOP B, UDENFRIEND S: Hydroxylation-induced migration: The NIH shift. *Science* 157:1524, 1967

37. CRAINE JE, HALL ES, KAUFMAN S: The isolation and characterization of dihydropteridine reductase from sheep liver. *J Biol Chem* 247:6082, 1972

38. BROWN GM: The biosynthesis of pteridines. *Adv Enzymol* 35:35, 1971

39. ETO I, FUKUSHIMA K, SHIOTA T: Enzymatic synthesis of biopterin from D-erythrodihydroneopterin triphosphate by extracts of kidneys from Syrian golden hamsters. *J Biol Chem* 251:6505, 1976

40. GAL EM, NELSON JM, SHERMAN AD: Biopterin: III. Purification and characterization of enzymes involved in the cerebral synthesis of 7, 8-dihydrobiopterin. *Neurochem Res* 3:69, 1978

41. SHIMAN R, AKINO M, KAUFMAN S: Solubilization and partial purification of tyrosine hydroxylase from bovine adrenal medulla. *J Biol Chem* 246:1330, 1971

42. FRIEDMAN PA, KAPPELMAN AH, KAUFMAN S: Partial purification and characterization of tryptophane hydroxylase from rabbit hindbrain. *J Biol Chem* 247:4165, 1972

43. KAUFMAN S, FISHER DB: Purification and some physical properties of phenylalanine hydroxylase from rat liver. *J Biol Chem* 245:4745, 1970

44. AYLING JE, PIRSON WD, AL-JANABI JM, HELFAND GD: Kidney phenylalanine hydroxylase from man and rat: Comparison with the liver enzyme. *Biochemistry* 13:78, 1974

45. GILLAM SS, WOO SLC, WOOLFE LI: The isolation and properties of phenylalanine hydroxylase from rat liver. *Biochem J* 139:731, 1974

46. SHIMAN R, GRAY DW, PATER A: A simple purification of phenylalanine hydroxylase by substrate-induced hydrophobic chromatography. *J Biol Chem* 254:11300, 1979

47. FRIEDMAN PA, KAUFMAN S: Some characteristics of partially purified human liver phenylalanine hydroxylase. *Biochim Biophys Acta* 293:56, 1973

48. WOO SLC, GILLAM SS, WOOLF LI: The isolation and properties of phenylalanine hydroxylase from human liver. *Biochem J* 139:741, 1974

49. WOOLF LI: The isolation, properties, and assay of phenylalanine hydroxylase from human and rat liver. *Biochem Med* 16:284, 1976

50. CHOO KH, COTTON RGH, DANKS DM, JENNINGS IG: Genetics of mammalian phenylalanine hydroxylase system. *Biochem J* 181:285, 1979

51. COTTON RGH: Phenylalanine hydroxylase of *Macaca irus:* Purification of two components of the enzyme. *Biochem Biophys Acta* 235:61, 1971

52. TOURIAN A: Activation of phenylalanine hydroxylase by phenylalanine. *Biochim Biophys Acta* 242:345, 1971

53. FISHER DB, KIRKWOOD R, KAUFMAN S: Rat liver phenylalanine hydroxylase, an iron enzyme. *J Biol Chem* 247:5161, 1972

54. FREEDLAND RA, KRAKOWSKI MC, WAISMAN HA: Effect of age, sex and nutrition on liver phenylalanine hydroxylase activity in rats. *Am J Physiol* 202:145, 1962

55. OHNO T, TASAKI I: Relation between liver amino acid-catabolizing enzymes and free amino acids of liver and plasma in adult cockerels fed diets containing graded levels of protein. *J Nutr* 107:829, 1977

56. GAULL GE, TALLAN HH, LAJTHA A, RASIN D: Pathogenisis of brain dysfunction in inborn errors of amino-acid metabolism, in Gaull GE (ed): *Biology of Brain Dysfunction.* New York, Plenum Publishing Corp, 1975, vol 3, p 47

57. FREIDMAN PA, FISHER DB, KANG ES, KAUFMAN S: Detection of hepatic phenylalanine 4-hydroxylase in classical phenylketonuria. *Proc Natl Acad Sci USA* 70:552, 1973

58. AYLING JE, HELFAND GD: Effect of pteridine cofactor structure on regulation of phenylalanine hydroxylase activity, in Pfleiderer W (ed): *Chemistry and Biology of Pteridines.* New York, Walter de Gruyter, 1975, p 304

59. SHIMAN R, GRAY DW: Substrate activation of phenylalanine hydroxylase. *J Biol Chem* 255:4793, 1980

60. DONLON J, KAUFMAN S: Modification of the multiple forms of rat hepatic phenylalanine hydroxylase by *in vitro* phosphorylation. *Biochem Biophys Res Commun* 78:1011, 1977

61. DONLON J, KAUFMAN S: Relationship between the multiple forms of rat hepatic phenylalanine hydroxylase and degree of phosphorylation. *J Biol Chem* 255:2146, 1980

62. TOURIAN A: Phenylalanine hydroxylase activity in foetal hepatic organ culture. *Biochim Biophys Acta* 309:44, 1973

63. HAGGERTY D, YOUNG PL, POPJAK G, CARNES WH: Phenylalanine hydroxylase in cultured hepatocytes. I. Hormonal control of enzyme levels. *J Biol Chem* 248:223, 1973

64. TOURIAN A: The effect of serum factors and hormones on phenylalanine hydroxylase synthesis, in *Transactions of the Fifth Meeting of the American Society for Neurochemistry,* New Orleans, 1974, p 127

65. TOURIAN A: Control of phenylalanine hydroxylase synthesis in tissue culture by serum and insulin. *J Cell Physiol* 87:15, 1976

66. GREENGARD O, DELVALLE JA: The regulation of phenylalanine hydroxylase in rat tissues *in vivo.* Substrate- and cortisol-induced elevations in phenylalanine hydroxylase activity. *Biochem J* 154:619, 1976

67. FISHER DB, KAUFMAN S: The stimulation of rat liver phenylalanine hydroxylase by phospholipids. *J Biol Chem* 247:2250, 1972

68. KAUFMAN S: The enzymatic conversion of phenylalanine to tyrosine. *J Biol Chem* 226:571,1957

69. CHRISTENSEN PJ: On the determination of phenylalanine hydroxylase activity in crude liver extracts. *Scand J Clin Lab Invest* 14:623, 1962

70. NIELSEN KH: Rat liver phenylalanine hydroxylase: A method for the measurement of activity, with particular reference to the distinctive features of the enzyme and the pteridine cofactor. *Eur J Biochem* 7:360, 1969

71. KAUFMAN S: Biopterin and metabolic disease, in Kisliuk RL, Brown GM (eds): *Chemistry and Biology of Pteridines, Developments in Biochemistry.* Amsterdam, Elsevier North Holland Publishing Co, 1979, vol 4, p 117

72. FISHER DB, KAUFMAN S: The stimulation of rat liver phenylalanine hydroxylase by lysolecithin and alpha-chymotrypsin. *J Biol Chem* 248:4345, 1973

73. DE DUVE C: The lysosome concept, in De Reuck AVS, Cameron MP (eds): *Ciba Foundation Symposium on Lysosomes.* Boston, Little, Brown & Co, 1963, p 1

74. HUANG CY, MAX EE, KAUFMAN S: Purification and characterization of phenylalanine hydroxylase-stimulating protein from rat liver. *J Biol Chem* 248:4235, 1973

75. BAKER RE, SHIMAN R: Measurement of phenylalanine hydroxylase turnover in cultured hepatoma cells. *J Biol Chem* 254:9633, 1979

76. GOPALAKRISHNAN TV, ANDERSON WF: Epigenetic activation of phenylalanine hydroxylase in mouse erythroleukemia cells by the cytoplast of rat hepatoma cells. *Proc Nat Acad Sci USA* 76:3932, 1979

77. GOPALAKRISHNAN TV: The identification of the chemical nature of the cytoplasmic regulatory factor for phenylalanine hydroxylase gene. *J Cell Biol* 87:Abstract 2219, 1980

78. DONLON J, KAUFMAN S: Glucagon stimulation of rat hepatic phenylalanine hydroxylase through phosphorylation in vivo. *J Biol Chem* 253:6657, 1978

79. CHANG N, KAUFMAN S, MILSTIEN S: The mechanism of the irreversible inhibition of rat liver phenylalanine hydroxylase due to treatment with p-chlorophenylalanine. *J Biol Chem* 254:2665, 1979

80. BRAND LM, HARPER AE: Effect of glucagon on phenylalanine metabolism and phenylalanine-degrading enzymes in the rat. *Biochem J* 142:231, 1974

81. DAVID J-C, DAIRMAN W, UDENFRIEND S: On the importance of decarboxylation in the metabolism of phenylalanine, tyrosine and tryptophan. *Arch Biochem Biophys* 160:561, 1974

82. BARRANGER JA, GEIGER PJ, HUZINO A, BESSMAN SP: Isozymes of phenylalanine hydroxylase. *Science* 175:903, 1972

83. TOURIAN A, TREIMAN L, ABE K: Three immunologically distinct isozymes of phenylalinine hydroxylase. *Biochemistry* 14:4055, 1975

84. TOURIAN A: The unique identity of rat hepatoma phenylalanine hydroxylase. *Biochem Biophys Res Commun* 68:51, 1976

85. DELVALLE JA, GREENGARD O: Isoenzyme composition of hepatic phenylalanine hydroxylase in developing rats after treatment with cortisol, alpha-methylphenylalanine and p-chlorophenylalanine in vivo. *Biochem Med* 20:247, 1978

86. ABITA J-P, MILSTIEN S, CHANG N, KAUFMAN S: In vitro activation of rat liver phenylalanine hydroxylase by phosphorylation. *J Biol Chem* 251:5310, 1976

87. ABITA J-P, CHAMRAS H, ROSSELIN G, REY F: Hormonal control of phenylalanine hydroxylase activity in isolated rat hepatocytes. *Biochem Biophys Res Commun* 92:912, 1980

88. FRIEDMAN PA, LLOYD T, KAUFMAN S: Production of antibodies to rat liver phenylalaine hydroxylase crossreactivity with other pterin-dependent hydroxylases. *Mol Pharmacol* 8:501, 1972

89. KAUFMAN S: Oral communication. Heidelberg Workshop on Molecular Basis of PKU, Sept 1979

90. FREIDMAN PA, KAUFMAN S, KANG ES: Nature of the molecular defect in phenylketonuria and hyperphenylalaninemia. *Nature (London)* 240:157, 1972

91. BARTHOLOME K, ERTEL E: Immunological detection of phenylalanine hydroxylase in phenylketonuria. *Lancet* 2:862, 1976

92. RYAN WL, ORR W: Phenylalanine conversion to tyrosine by the human fetal liver. *Arch Biochem Biophys* 113:684, 1966

93. JAKUBOVIC A: Phenylalanine-hydroxylating system in the human fetus at different developmental ages. *Biochim Biophys Acta* 237:469, 1971

94. KAUFMAN S: Phenylalanine hydroxylase of human liver: Assay and some properties. *Arch Biochem Biophys* 134:249, 1969

95. RÄIHÄ NCR: Phenylalanine hydroxylase in human liver during development. *Pediatr Res* 7:1, 1973

96. TOURIAN A, SIDBURY JB: Phenylketonuria, in Stanbury JB, Wyngaarden JB, Frederickson DS (eds): *The Metabolic Basis of Inherited Disease,* ed 4. New York, McGraw-Hill Book Co, 1978, p 240

97. PUESCHEL SM, ROTHMAN KJ: Birth weight analysis of children with phenylketonuria. *Pediatr Res* 10:419, 1976

98. SAUGSTAD LF: Birthweights in children with phenylketonuria and in their siblings. *Lancet* 1:809, 1972

99. KANG ES, KENNEDY JL, JR, GATES L, BURWASH I, MCKINNON A: Clinical observations in phenylketonuria. *Pediatrics* 35:932, 1965

100. KNOX WE: Phenylketonuria, in Stanbury JB, Wyngaarden JB, Fredrickson DS (eds): *The Metabolic Basis of Inherited Disease,* ed 3. New York, McGraw-Hill Book Co, 1972, p 266

101. CHOO KH, COTTON RGH, JENNINGS IG, DANKS DM: Observations indicating the nature of the mutation in phenylketonuria. *J Inherited Metab Dis* 2:79, 1979

102. BARTHOLOME K, LUTZ P, BICKEL H: Determination of phenylalanine hydroxylase activity in patients with phenylketonuria and hyperphenylalaninemia. *Pediatr Res* 9:899,1975

103. KANG ES, KAUFMAN S, GERALD PS: Clinical and biochemical observations of patients with atypical phenylketonuria. *Pediatrics* 45:83: 1970

104. GUTTLER F: Hyperphenylalaninemia. Diagnosis and classification of various types of phenylalanine hydroxylase deficiency in childhood. *Acta Paediatr Scan (Suppl)* 280:3–80, 1980

105. WILLIAMSON M, DOBSON JC, KOCH R: Collaborative study of children treated for phenylketonuria: Study design. *Pediatrics* 60:815, 1980

106. AUERBACH VH, DIGEORGE AM, CARPENTER GG: Phenylalaninemia: A study of the diversity of disorders which produce elevation of blood concentrations of phenylalanine, in Nyhan WC (ed): *Amino Acid Metabolism and Genetic Variation.* New York, McGraw-Hill Book Co, 1967, p 11

107. KAUFMAN S: Phenylketonuria: Biochemical mechanisms. *Adv Neurochem* 2:1, 1976

108. SMITH I: Atypical phenylketonuria accompanied by a severe progressive neurological illness unresponsive to dietary treatment. *Arch Dis Child* 49:245, 1974

109. LEEMING RJ, BLAIR JA, REY F: Biopterin derivatives in atypical phenylketonuria. *Lancet* 1:99, 1976

110. BARTHOLOME K, BYRD DJ, KAUFMAN S: Atypical phenylketonuria with normal phenylalanine hydroxylase and dihydropteridine reductase activity in vitro. *Pediatrics* 59:757, 1977

111. SCHAUB J, DAUMLING S, CURTIUS H-CH, NIEDERWIESER A, BARTHOLOME K, VISCONTINI M, SCHIRCKS B, BIERI JH: Tetrahydrobiopterin therapy of atypical phenylketonuria due to defective dihydrobiopterin biosynthesis. *Arch Dis Child* 53:674, 1978

112. DANKS DM, BARTHOLOME K, CLAYTON BE, CURTIUS H, GROBE H, KAUFMAN S, LEEMING R, PFLEIDERER W, REMBOLD H, REY F: Malignant hyperphenylalaninaemia—current status (June 1977). *J Inherited Metab Dis* 1:49, 1978

113. CURTIUS H-CH, NIEDERWIESER A, VISCONTINI M, OTTEN A, SCHAUB J, SCHEIBENREITER S, SCHMIDT H: Atypical phenylketonuria due to tetrahydrobiopterin deficiency. Diagnosis and treatment with tetrahydrobiopterin, dihydrobiopterin and sepiapterin. *Clin Chim Acta* 93:251, 1979

114. TIETZ A, LINDBERG M, KENNEDY EP: A new pteridine-requiring enzyme system for the oxidation of glyceryl ethers. *J Biol Chem* 239:4081, 1964

115. RENNERT O, JULIUS R, AYLSWORTH A, WILLIAMS C, GREER M: A new disorder of phenylalanine metabolism associated with ataxia, convulsions and retardation. Combined abstracts, *Am Pediatr, Soc, Soc Pediatr Res,* Atlantic City, NJ, 1971

116. RENNERT O: Personal communication

117. KRETCHMER N: Enzymatic patterns during development. *Pediatrics* 23:606, 1959

118. LEVINE SZ, MARPLES E, GORDON HH: A defect in the metabolism of aromatic amino acids in premature infants: The role of vitamin C. *Science* 90:620, 1939

119. MEDES G: A new error of tyrosine metabolism: Tyrosinosis. The intermediary metabolism of tyrosine and phenylalanine. *Biochem J* 26:917, 1932

120. LINDBLAD B, LINDSTEDT G, LINDSTEDT S, RUNDGREN M: Metabolism of p-hydroxyphenylpyruvate in hereditary tyrosinemia, in Stern J, Trothill C (eds): *Organic Acidurias.* Edinburgh and London, Churchill Livingstone, Ltd, 1972, p 63

121. KENNAWAY NG, BUIST NRM: Metabolic studies in a patient with hepatic cytosol tyrosine aminotransferase deficiency. *Pediatr Res* 5:287, 1971

122. LINDBLAD B, LINDSTEDT S, STEEN G: On the enzymic defects in hereditary tyrosinemia. *Proc Natl Acad Sci, USA* 74:4641, 1977

123. SCRIVER CR, CLOW CL: Phenylketonuria: Epitome of human biochemical genetics. *New Engl J Med* 303:1336–1342, 1394–1400, 1980

124. MERYASH DL, LEVY HL, GUTHRIE R, WARNER R, BLOOM S, CARR JR: Prospective study of early neonatal screening for phenylketonuria. *New Engl J Med* 304:294, 1981

125. FIRGAIRA FA, COTTON RGH, DANKS DM: Dihydropteridine reductase deficiency diagnosis by assays on peripheral blood-cells. *Lancet* 2:1260, 1979

126. DANKS DM, SCHLESINGER P, FIRGAIRA F, COTTON RGH, WATSON BM, REMBOLD H, HENNINGS G: Malignant hyperphenylalaninemia—clinical features, biochemical findings, and experience with administration of biopterins. *Pediatr Res* 13:1150, 1979

127. NIEDERWIESER A, CURTIUS H-CH, BETTONI O, BIERI J, SCHIRCKS B, VISCONTINI M, SCHAUB J: Atypical phenylketonuria caused by 7, 8-dihydro-biopterin synthetase deficiency. *Lancet* 1:131, 1979

128. KAUFMAN S: Differential diagnosis of variant forms of hyperphenylalaninemia. *Pediatrics* 65:840, 1980

129. KUKUSHIMA T, NIXON JC: Reverse phase high-performance liquid chromatographic separation of unconjugated pterins and pteridines, in Kisliuk

RL, Brown GM, (eds): *Chemistry and Biology of Pteridines*. Amsterdam, Elsevier North Holland, 1979, vol 4, p 35

130. MILSTIEN S, KAUFMAN S, SUMMER GK: Hyperphenylalaninemia due to dihydropteridine reductase deficiency: Diagnosis is by measurement of oxidized and reduced pterins in urine. *Pediatrics* 65:806, 1980

131. DOBSON JC, WILLIAMSON ML, AZEN C, KOCH R: Intellectual assessment of 111 four-year-old children with phenylketonuria. *Pediatrics* 60:822, 1977

132. LENKE RR, LEVY HL: Maternal phenylketonuria and hyperphenylalaninemia: An international survey of the outcome of untreated and treated pregnancies. *New Engl J Med* 303:1202, 1980

133. SYNDERMAN SE: The amino acid requirements of the infant, in Nyhan WL (ed): *Heritable Disorders of Amino Acid Metabolism*, ed 4. New York, John Wiley & Sons, Inc. 1974, p 64

134. DODGE PR, PRENSKY AL, FEIGIN RD, HOLMES SJ: Phenylketonuria, in *Nutrition and the Developing Nervous System*. St. Louis, CV Mosby Co, 1975, p 481

135. HOSKINS JA, JACK G, WADE HE, PEIRIS RJD, WRIGHT EC, STARR DJT, STERN J: Enzymatic control of phenylalanine intake in phenylketonuria. *Lancet* 1:392, 1980

136. BLAU K: Phenylalanine hydroxylase deficiency: Biochemical, physiological and clinical aspects of phenylketonuria and related phenylalaninemias, in Youdim MBH (ed): *Aromatic Amino Acid Hydroxylases and Mental Disease*. New York, Wiley, 1980, p 77

137. HARPER KE, LEUNG P, YOSHIDA A, ROGERS QR: Some new thoughts on amino acid imbalance. *Fed Proc* 23:1087, 1964

138. APPEL SH: *In vitro* inhibition of brain protein synthesis: An approach to the molecular pathology of maple syrup urine disease and phenylketonuria. *J Clin Invest* 44:1026, 1965

139. HUGHES JV, JOHNSON TC: The effects of hyperphenylalaninaemia on the concentrations of aminoacyl-transfer ribonucleic acid *in vivo*: A mechanism for the inhibition of neural protein synthesis by phenylalanine. *Biochem J* 162:527, 1977

140. ADRIAENSSENS K, ALLEN RJ, LOWENTHAL Y, MARDENS Y, TOURTELLOTTE WW: Brain and cerebrospinal fluid free amino acids in phenylketonuria. *J Genet Hum* 17:223, 1969

141. BREWSTER TG, MOSKOWITZ MA, KAUFMAN S, BRESLOW JL, MILSTIEN S, ABROMS IF: Dihydropteridine reductase deficiency associated with severe neurologic disease and mild hyperphenylalaninemia. *Pediatrics* 63:94, 1979

142. FOIS A, ROSENBERG C, GIBBS FA: The electroencephalogram in phenylpyruvic oligophrenia. *Electroencephalogr Clin Neurophysiol* 7:569, 1955

143. DEGEN R, LAESKER G, THEILE H: EEG-Befunds bei phenylketonurie. *Kinderaerztl Prax* 40:97, 1972

144. POLEY JR, DUMERMUTH G: EEG findings in patients with PKU, in Holt KS, Coffey VP (eds): *Some Recent Advances in Inborn Errors of Metabolism*. Edinburgh, Churchill Livingstone, Ltd, 1968, p 61

145. ROLLE-DAYA H, PUESCHEL SM, LOMBROSO CT: Electroencephalographic findings in children with phenylketonuria. *Am J Dis Child* 129:896, 1975

146. ALVORD EC JR, STEVENSON LD, VOGEL FS, ENGLE RL JR: Neuropathological findings in phenyl-pyruvic oligophrenia (phenylketonuria). *J Neuropathol Exp Neurol* 9:298, 1950

147. MALAMUD N: Neuropathology of phenylketonuria. *J Neuropathol Exp Neurol* 25:254, 1966

148. AGRAWAL HC, DAVISON AN: Myelination and amino acid imbalance in the developing brain, in Himwich WA (ed): *Biochemistry of Developing Brain*. New York, Marcel Dekker Inc, 1973, p 143

149. SHAH SN, PETERSON NA, McKEAN CM: Lipid composition of human cerebral white matter and myelin in phenylketonuria. *J Neurochem* 19:2369, 1972

150. MENKES JH: Cerebral proteolipids in phenylketonuria. *Neurology* 18:1003, 1968

151. PRENSKY AL, CARR S, MOSER HW: Development of myelin in inherited disorders of amino acid metabolism. *Arch Neurol* 19:552, 1968

152. MENKES JH: Cerebral lipids in phenylketonuria. *Pediatrics* 37:967, 1966

153. MILSTIEN S, HOLTZMAN NA, O'FLYNN ME, THOMAS GH, BUTLER IJ, KAUFMAN S: Hyperphenylalaninemia due to dihydropteridine reductase deficiency. *J Pediatr* 89:763, 1976

154. WOOLF LI, GOODWIN BL, CRANSTON WI, WADE DN, WOOLF, F, HUDSON FP, McBEAN MS: A third allele at the phenylalanine-hydroxylase locus in mild phenylketonuria (hyperphenylalaninemia). *Lancet* 1:114, 1968

155. PAUL TD, BRANDT IK, ELSAS LJ, JACKSON CE, MAMUNES P, NANCE CS, NANCE WE: Phenylketonuria heterozygote detection in families with affected children. *Am J Hum Genet* 30:293, 1978

13

TYROSINEMIA AND RELATED DISORDERS

LOWELL A. GOLDSMITH

A. Tyrosinemia II *(Richner-Hanhart Syndrome)*

1. *Tyrosinemia II is an inherited disease associated with a deficiency of hepatic tyrosine aminotransferase (TAT), the rate-limiting enzyme of tyrosine catabolism.*

2. *Tyrosinemia, tyrosinuria, and increases in urinary phenolic acids, N-acetyltyrosine, and tyramine persist for life. The metabolism of other amino acids and renal and hepatic functions are otherwise normal.*

3. *Corneal erosions and plaques, palm and sole erosions, and hyperkeratoses usually occur during the first months of life and do not respond to conventional therapy. Mental retardation sometimes occurs.*

4. *Intracellular crystallization of tyrosine initiates inflammation.*

5. *The disease has autosomal recessive inheritance; the carrier state has not been detected biochemically.*

6. *Therapy with a low tyrosine, low phenylalanine diet is curative.*

7. *The syndrome occurs as an autosomal recessive trait in ranch mink and is reproduced by feeding rats a low protein, high tyrosine diet.*

B. Neonatal Tyrosinemia

1. *Asymptomatic tyrosinemia associated with increased excretion of tyrosine and its metabolites is found (usually by amino acid screening programs) in 0.2 to 10 percent of neonates. It is more common in premature*

and less common in breast-fed infants. The tyrosine level decreases to normal within weeks to months.

2. *The long-term sequelae of this tyrosinemia are moot and may include mild mental retardation.*

3. *Dietary restriction of protein rapidly decreases plasma tyrosine to normal. The efficacy of ascorbic acid supplementation is questionable.*

4. *The enzymatic nature of the defect is unknown since there are no direct measurements of the hepatic enzymes from these relatively healthy infants.*

C. Tyrosinosis

1. *Tyrosinosis is probably an inherited defect of fumarylacetoacetate (FAA) hydrolyase and maleylacetoacetate (MAA) hydrolyase. Succinylacetoacetone and succinylacetone accumulate and inhibit renal tubular function, some hepatic enzymes of tyrosine catabolism, and porphobilinogen synthetase; and decrease glutathione levels.*

2. *The acute form of the disease, due to severe enzyme deficiency, is associated with liver failure, a cabbage-like odor, and often death by age 1 year. In the chronic form of the disease, renal tubular dysfunction, vitamin D–resistant rickets, and acute intermittent porphyria-like symptoms may be present. Hepatoma is a late complication.*

3. *Anemia, abnormal liver function, increased plasma α-fetoprotein, moderate increases in plasma tyrosine and*

its metabolites, and increased plasma methionine are present. The urine contains succinylacetone and succinylacetoacetone. Generalized aminoaciduria, phosphaturia, glycosuria, and uricosuria occur.

4. *FAA hydrolase and MAA hydrolase activities are decreased and may be the primary defects in this disease. Fructose-1-phosphate aldolase deficiency and galactose-1-phosphate uridyl transferase deficiency produce similar renal and hepatic abnormalities.*

5. *The disease has autosomal recessive inheritance. It has a worldwide distribution and a high prevalence in Quebec, especially in the Chicoutini-Lac St. Jean region.*

6. *Therapy with a low tyrosine, low phenylalanine diet, often combined with a low methionine diet, has been helpful. Recently, treatment with cysteine supplementation has been used.*

Tyrosinemia, tyrosinuria, and phenolaciduria accompany several inborn errors of metabolism. A major effort in the past 50 years has been to separate and establish the enzymatic basis of the individual diseases having this chemical phenotype. This chapter presents the current state of knowledge of these disorders and of normal tyrosine metabolism.

Tyrosinemia II (Richner-Hanhart syndrome), a disease probably caused by a genetic deficiency in hepatic tyrosine aminotransferase (TAT), in which there is accumulation of tyrosine and its metabolites following classic Garrodian principles, is discussed first, since its metabolic basis is best established. The second major disease discussed, *tyrosinosis (tyrosinemia I)*, has a more complicated pathophysiology since metabolic products accumulate which inhibit many transport functions and enzymatic activities, including those related to tyrosine metabolism. The consequences of decreased activity of tyrosine catabolism in the neonatal period are discussed as well.

Several patients with abnormal tyrosine metabolism, of an as yet undiscovered cause, including a patient studied by Medes over 50 years ago, complete the coverage of the chapter.

TYROSINEMIA II (RICHNER-HANHART SYNDROME)

Clinical Aspects

Richner and Hanhart recognized a distinctive oculocutaneous syndrome associated with tyrosinemia II 35 years before its metabolic basis was determined (see Ref. 10). Restudy of some of their original patients confirmed the association. The patients were biochemically proven to have the syndrome, and some of their clinical and biochemical features are listed in Table 13-1. Cases of the syndrome before its biochemical basis was recognized have been reviewed [26].

Biochemically diagnosed cases have been described from several countries. Both parents of several of the probands have been Italian or have had Italian ancestry. The probands of Italian background have been reported from Italy [12, 18, 19],

Australia [16], Canada [5], Lausanne, Switzerland [20], and the United States [10]. Probands of non-Italian ancestry have been reported from Switzerland [25], Spain [25], southwestern France [22], Norway [13], the United States [1, 9, 15, 24], and a Turkish family living in Germany [21].

Eye Lesions These usually begin during the first few months of life. Symptoms may be limited to lacrimation, photophobia, and redness (Fig. 13-1). Signs may include mild corneal herpetiform erosions, dendritic ulcers, and, rarely, corneal and conjunctival plaques [11]. Neovascularization may be prominent. The ulcers stain poorly, if at all, with fluorescein, and bacterial and viral studies are negative. Lesions have occurred in a corneal transplant [19]. Long-term effects include corneal scarring [1], nystagmus [5, 26], exodeviation, and glaucoma [20].

Skin Lesions These begin with or after the eye lesions (Fig. 13-2). In some cases, no skin lesions are reported. The lesions are painful, nonpruritic, and sometimes associated with hyperhidrosis; they are limited to the palms and soles, especially the tips of the digits and the thenar and hypothenar eminences. They may be linear or subungual. They begin as blisters or erosions which crust and become hyperkeratotic. One patient was symptom-free in the morning, worse during the day, and developed erythema and pain during a tyrosine tolerance test [16]. Hyperkeratosis of the tongue is reported [22]. Hyperpigmentation is not present.

Neurologic Features These include mental retardation. Among the classic cases of Richner-Hanhart syndrome, retardation is an inconstant feature [12]. In those with biochemically proved tyrosinemia II, retardation to a mild to moderate degree has been reported (Table 13-1), but this may reflect an ascertainment bias. Self-mutilating behavior has occurred [1], as have disturbances of fine coordination [20]. Language defects have been more prominent than mathematical defects (unpublished observations in families 7 and 14, Table 13-1).

Other organ involvement has been limited to one child with multiple congenital anomalies, including cleft lip and palate, microcephaly, inguinal hernias, talipes equinovarus, and the presence of one kidney [1]. One patient had femoral streakiness [5, 27].

Histopathology

Skin biopsy is not diagnostic. It may show hyperkeratosis, acanthosis, and parakeratosis. An electron micrograph showed 2- to 3-μm lipidlike granules with 10-nm filaments and myelinlike figures intermixed with the granules [10]. A conjunctival plaque showed increased bundles of keratofibrils and alcian blue-positive inclusions [11]. Endothelial cells contained similar inclusions and whorled membranous structures. Fine, needlelike crystals were seen in the fibroblasts.

Biochemical Features

Tyrosinemia and Tyrosinuria Tyrosinemia is a diagnostic feature of the syndrome. The tyrosine level has been higher in younger patients (Table 13-1). The plasma tyrosine levels (mg/dl) (mean ± SD) for patients aged up to 7 years were 43.4

Table 13-1 Tyrosinemia with eye and epidermal disease

| Family | Sex | Age at onset of symptoms | | Age at diagnosis of tyrosinemia* | Mental state | Tyrosine level† | | Reference |
		Eye	Skin			Plasma mg/dl	Urine mg/mg creatinine‡	
1	M	2 wk	Present (onset?)	2	Retarded	up to 62	0.32 (65 mg/24 h)	1–4
2	F	Infancy	8 mo	13	Retarded	25	0.35	5–8
3	M	Early infancy	—	10.5	Retarded	16–27	0.29	9
4	M	8 yr	6 yr	11.5	Retarded	25–30	0.56	10, 11
5	F	<4 mo	—	4 mo		48	140 mg/24 h	12
6	F	10 days	None	4 mo	Normal at 4½ yr	51		13, 14
7	F	5 wk	4 mo	14 mo	Mildly retarded at age 7	36–52	3.2	15
8	F	3 mo	15 mo	14	Low normal	24.6	0.19	16, 17
9	F	5 mo	15 mo	3.5	IQ = 73	35	—	18
	F	No	Yes	28	? Minimally retarded	30	—	18
10	M	1 mo	1 mo	29	Normal	14–15	—	19
	F	1 mo	1 mo	26	Normal	14–16.5	—	19
11	M	40 days	<7 mo	3.2	IQ = 57 at age 7	32	0.29	20
12	M	—	—	6	—	31.1	—	21
13	F	15 days	5 mo	1	Severe retardation	52	66 mg/24 h	22, 23
14	M	7 yr	7 yr	55	Mild retardation	21.7	0.8	24
		?	10 yr	51	Normal	20.3		24
15	M	1 yr	1–2 yr	36	IQ = 75	33.5	345 mg per liter	25
16	F	—	14 yr	33	IQ = 85	21	709 mg per liter	25
	M	—	15 yr	36	No retardation	20.5	331 mg per liter	25

— Not reported; ? unknown.
* Years unless specified.
† Recalculated from original data in μmol when necessary; normal plasma tyrosine = <2.5 mg/dl; normal urine tyrosine = <0.05 mg/mg creatinine.
‡ mg/mg creatinine unless indicated.

± 10.97 ($n = 8$) and for ages 8 to 55 were 23.0 ± 5.3 ($n = 12$). The means differ at the $p < 0.001$ level of significance. Many of the older patients have had skin and eye lesions at blood tyrosine levels at which younger patients have been completely asymptomatic. These findings suggest that in this disease tyrosine levels decrease with age, with the opening of alternative metabolic pathways for tyrosine, and that local tissue factors which influence disease may have age-associated changes. Skin abnormalities have been most apparent in older patients [24, 25]. The tyrosinemia rapidly responds to a low tyrosine diet [28] (Fig. 13-3).

Tyrosine is the only amino acid increased in the urine in these patients. Tyrosine clearance is essentially normal, with renal tubular absorption of over 99 percent of filtered tyrosine [10, 29]. Routine liver and renal studies are normal. In three patients, cerebral spinal fluid tyrosine levels ranged from 3.5 to 8 mg/dl, with blood tyrosine values of 25 to 52 mg/dl [5, 20, 23].

Figure 13-1 Corneal changes in tyrosinemia II. Cornea of patient in family 7 of Table 13-1. *A.* Corneal opacity and neovascularization in eye before therapy. *B.* Eye after 6 weeks of therapy with a low tyrosine, low phenylalanine diet. *(From Goldsmith LA, in Fitzpatrick TB et al (eds): Dermatology in General Medicine. New York, McGraw-Hill Book Co, 1979, p 1042, with permission.)*

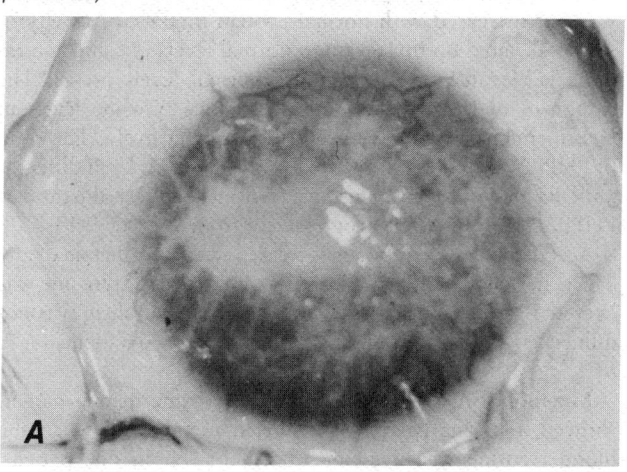
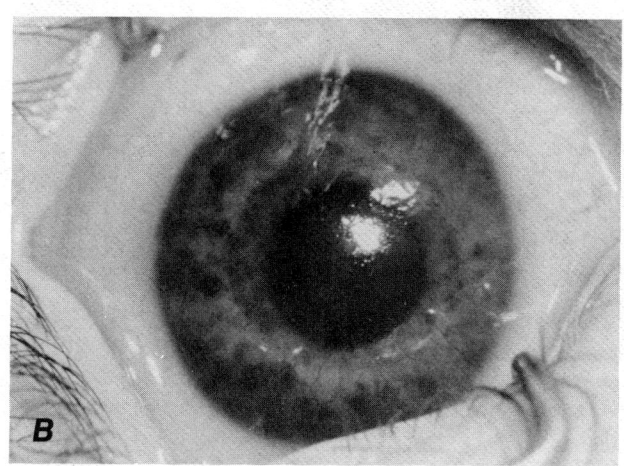

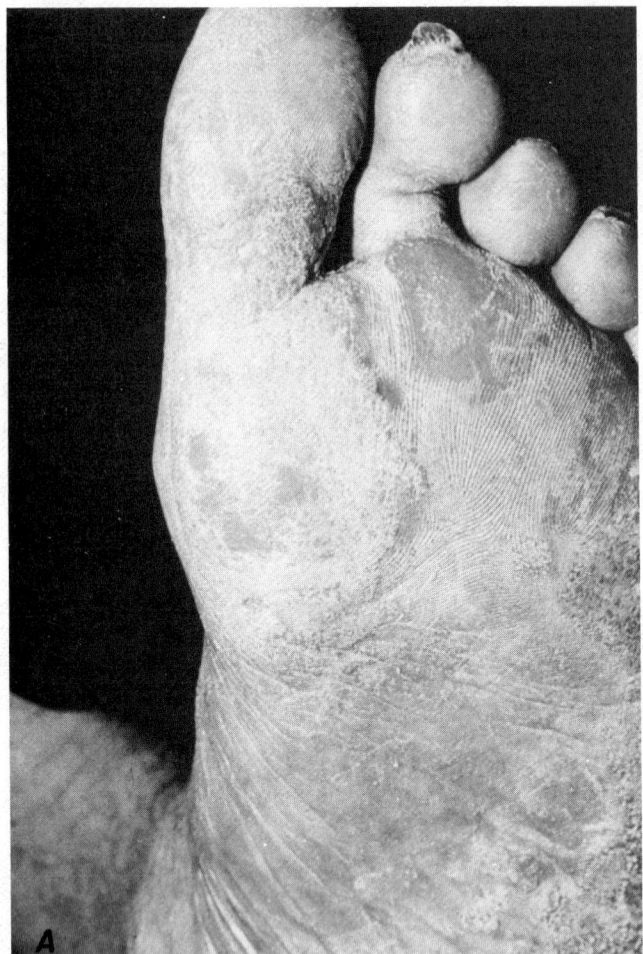

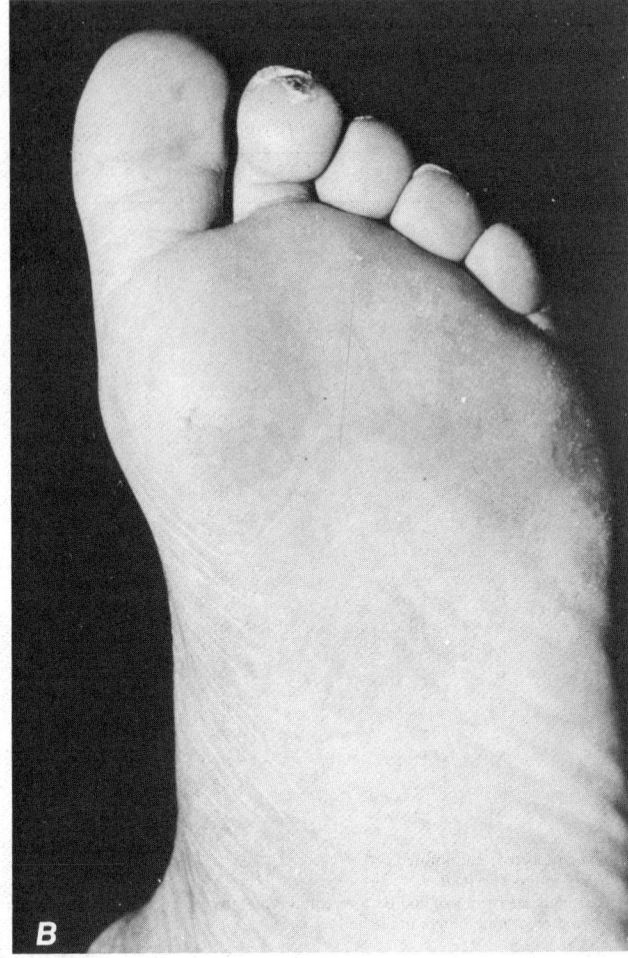

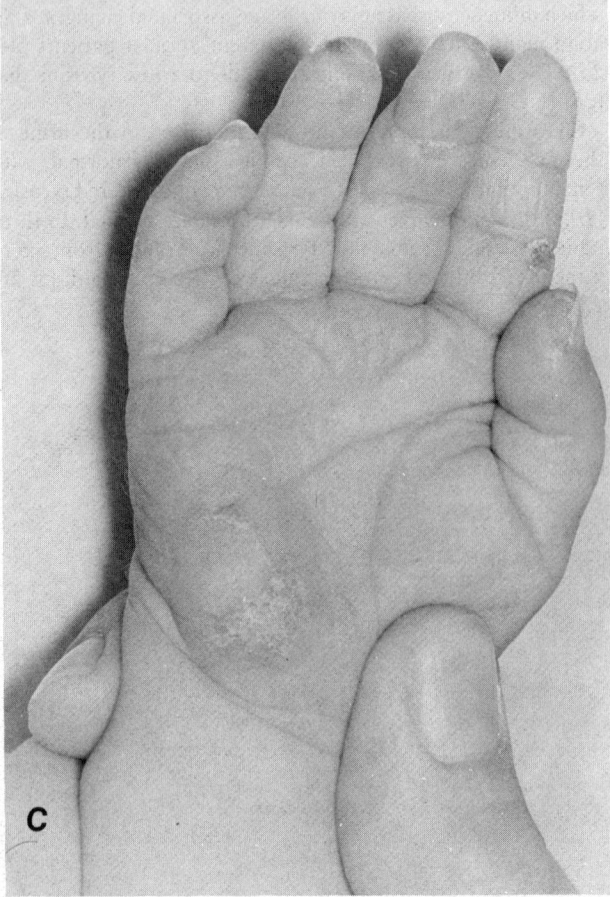

Figure 13-2   Skin abnormalities in tyrosinemia II. *A.* Soles of 55-year-old male with tyrosinemia II (family 14 in Table 13-1) before therapy. *B.* Soles after 2 months of a low tyrosine, low phenylalanine diet. *(A and B from Goldsmith LA, Thorpe JM, and Roe CR [24], by permission of the J Invest Dermatol.) C.* Hyperkeratotic and erosive lesions in 13-month-old girl with tyrosinemia II (family 7, Table 13-1) *(From Goldsmith LA in Fitzpatrick TB et al (eds): Dermatology in General Medicine. New York, McGraw-Hill Book Co, 1979, p 1042, with permission.)*

The urinary tyrosine metabolites, *p*-hydroxyphenylpyruvic acid (PHPPA), *p*-hydroxyphenyllactic acid (PHPLA), *p*-hydroxyphenylacetic acid (PHPAA), N-acetyltyrosine, and *p*-tyramine (Fig. 13-5) are increased from 88 to 170 times normal levels [4, 5, 7, 9, 10, 17, 20, 22, 23]. In one patient [5], PHPPA was not increased with normal protein intake. N-Acetyltyrosine is elevated up to 160 times normal levels [4], and *p*-tyramine is elevated up to 88 times normal levels [4, 7]. The responses of these metabolites to various tyrosine levels in tyrosinemic patients have been studied extensively. The ratio of PHPPA to PHPLA has varied from 0.16 to 1.14 in different patients [4, 17, 20, 23]. During a tyrosine load test, the ratio of PHPPA to PHPLA fell progressively from 1.14 to 0.13 [20]. N-Acetyltyrosine excretion is increased with tyrosinemia of any cause. In one patient [4] 75 percent of unoxidized tyrosine was excreted as N-acetyltyrosine. *p*-Tyramine metabolism was not influenced by sterilization of the intestine in two patients [4, 7, 8].

Metabolic studies with deuterated tyrosine in one patient showed a normal pattern of labeled metabolites when the blood tyrosine was five times normal [17]. In one patient, plasma phenylalanine which was elevated fivefold became normal with treatment [23].

The plasma PHPAA concentration is normally not measurable but was 0.36 mg/dl in one patient [4].

Pattern of Urinary Metabolites in Tyrosinemia Multiple metabolic pathways [29, 30] are available for tyrosine (Figs. 13-4, 13-5). This obfuscates attempts to predict enzyme deficiencies on the basis of urinary metabolites. PHPPA can be formed by deamination of tyrosine in the kidney and directly excreted [30]. Even in the absence of TAT, tyrosine can be oxidized to PHPPA in tissues (e.g., liver, kidney, heart, muscle, and brain) which contain significant amounts of mitochondrial TAT (aspartate aminotransferase) (Fig. 13-6) [3, 31, 32]. Since three of these tissues (heart, muscle, and brain) lack *p*-hydroxyphenylpyruvate oxidase (hydroxylase), PHPPA cannot be metabolized further and may appear in the circulation and be filtered directly by the kidney. PHPPA can be reduced in the liver to PHPLA by lactic dehydrogenase or aromatic keto acid reductase [30] and then excreted. Since the renal clearance of PHPPA is two to three times higher than the creatinine clearance, tubular secretion accounts for some of the urinary metabolites [29].

Hepatic Enzymes in Tyrosinemia II Tyrosine aminotransferase (E.C.2.6.1.5) activity has been assayed in the supernatant of liver homogenates in four patients with tyrosinemia

II [2, 17, 23, 24]. Activity was absent in two patients [2, 23] and reduced but present in two others [17, 24]. Other transaminases may have been responsible for the activity in the oldest patient studied [24], and technical criticisms of one of the studies have been made [33, 34].

Mitochondrial aspartate aminotransferase was normal in one patient [2] and slightly increased in two patients [23, 24]; the increase in its activity may represent a compensatory response to high plasma tyrosine levels.

Liver *p*-hydroxyphenylpyruvate hydroxylase was normal in one patient [2].

Genetics of Tyrosinemia II

Consanguinity occurred in five families of Table 13-1 [7, 10, 15, 18, 24]. Involved sibs with normal parents appeared in families 10, 14, and 16. The sexes are equally affected. All data are consistent with autosomal recessive inheritance as is information from the classic cases of the syndrome [26]. The pedigree from a large North Carolina kindred containing families 7 and 15 of Table 13-1 shows consanguinity (Fig. 13-7).

Treatment

A low tyrosine, low phenylalanine diet [28] (e.g., Mead Johnson 3200 AB) has been used successfully in several patients [1, 5, 10, 13, 15, 25], with rapid resolution of the clinical symptoms and signs (Fig. 13-3). Pyridoxine [1, 10, 15], vitamin C

Figure 13-3 Response of elevated plasma tyrosine to low tyrosine, low phenylalanine diet in patient of family 7 in Table 13-1. *(From Goldsmith LA in Fitzpatrick TB et al (eds): Dermatology in General Medicine. New York, McGraw-Hill Book Co, 1979, p 1042, with permission.)*

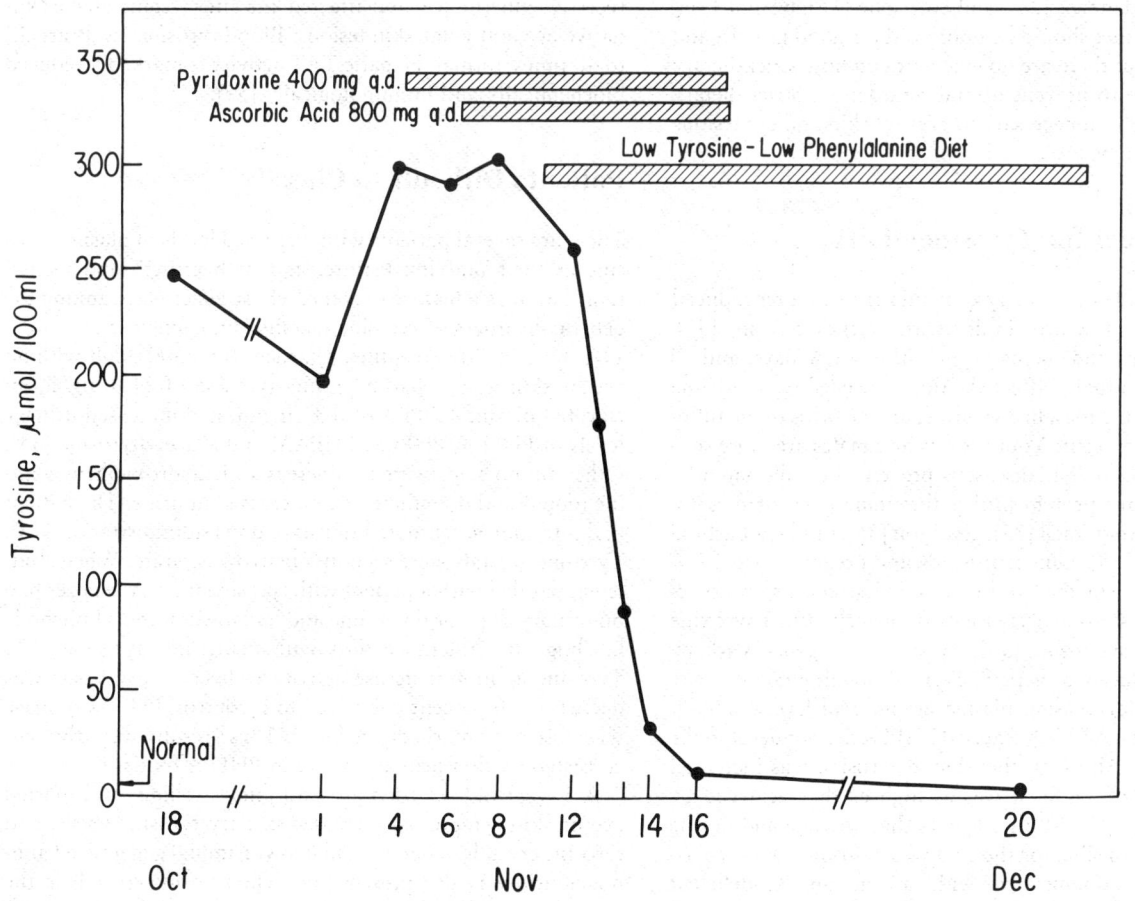

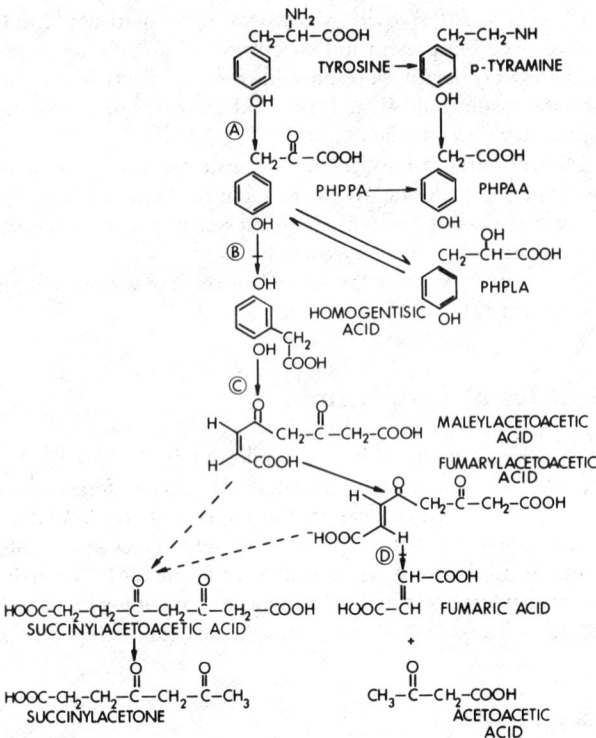

Figure 13-4 Major pathway for tyrosine catabolism. Major tyrosine metabolites include p-tyramine, PHPPA (p-hydroxyphenylpyruvic acid), PHPAA (p-hydroxyphenylacetic acid), PHPLA (p-hydroxyphenyllactic acid), and homogentisic acid. Enzymes include (A) tyrosine aminotransferase, (B) p-hydroxyphenylpyruvate oxidase (hydrolyase), (C) homogentisic acid oxidase, (D) fumarylacetoacetate (FAA) hydrolyase.

[4, 9, 10, 15], danazol [24], and cortisone [1] have not been successful. The diet should be optimized for good growth and development, but there are no guidelines on how strict dietary control must be to prevent mental retardation. Strict dietary control has not been necessary to prevent skin and eye lesions [15, 21, 24] (see below).

Animal Model for Tyrosinemia II

The phenotypic features of tyrosinemia II can be reproduced by feeding rats a low protein diet with excess L-tyrosine [35]. Corneal erosions and edema begin within a few days, and all animals are eventually affected. Alopecia, cheilitis, erythema and swelling of the toes, brown urine, and arthritis of the tibiotarsal joints also occur. Younger rats and males are more seriously affected [35]. The disease is prevented or alleviated by increasing dietary protein [36], L-threonine [37], or methionine [38] or by thiouracil [35], glucagon [36], or phenobarbital administration [39]. Glucocorticoids and pregnenolone-16-α-carbonitrile prevent the syndrome; ethylestrenol, spironolactone, and progesterone decrease its frequency [39]. Thyroxine aggravates the syndrome [35]. Most of the agents work by increasing the levels of hepatic TAT, although glucagon may act by directly decreasing plasma amino acid levels, since it does not induce TAT [36]. Rats fed PHPPA did not develop the syndrome [40]. Although their blood tyrosine was increased (back reaction of TAT), it was as high as that achieved by tyrosine feeding. This study suggests that tyrosine and not its products is responsible for the clinical syndrome. Desoxypyridoxine, when administered with a vitamin B_6–deficient

diet, produced tyrosinemia (up to 52 mg/dl in lactating females) [41].

Mechanism for Tissue Damage The evolution of the eye lesions in tyrosinemic rats has been investigated [42–44]. Long, slender (0.5- to 1.1-μm) birefringent crystals with prismatic shapes are limited to damaged areas in the corneal epithelium. Similar shapes are seen in electron micrographs. The crystals pass through the cell and nuclear membranes. Levels of tyrosine in the aqueous humor parallel and are slightly less than serum tyrosine levels [42]. Edema occurs within 24 h, and polymorphonuclear leukocytes infiltrate the stroma and cause opacities. By 7 days, new blood vessels invade the corneal epithelium [43].

Skin lesions follow a similar course, are limited to volar surfaces, and are associated with dense polymorphonuclear infiltrates [45].

Intracellular crystallization is proposed as the mechanism for tissue damage [44–46]. Tyrosine levels in plasma exceed saturation, and the levels of amino acids in the epidermis may exceed those in plasma [47]. Since tyrosine crystals destabilize lysosomes [48] and break erythrocyte membranes [48], release of cellular proteolytic enzymes may be the initial step in the inflammatory cascade. This pathogenic mechanism is consistent with the clearing of skin and eye lesions while tyrosine levels are still many times normal, since it implies that a critical threshold for tyrosine must be exceeded for the appearance of clinical disease.

Tyrosinemia II in the Mink Ranch mink (*Mustela vison*) have an inherited disease with many of the features of human tyrosinemia II [50, 52]. The disease has autosomal recessive inheritance, and affected kits after weaning have exudative eye and volar skin lesions. Blood tyrosine levels are 35 to 40 times normal. Hepatic TAT activity is markedly reduced biochemically and immunologically [52].

Patients Difficult to Classify

There are several patients with increased levels of plasma tyrosine as their unifying feature, and with growth and mental retardation as a feature of some, whose exact place among the genetic disorders of tyrosine metabolism is unclear.

A short (< 3d percentile), retarded (IQ = 46) adult with no eye or skin lesions had a plasma tyrosine of 21.6 mg/dl, an elevated plasma PHPPA of 0.37 mg/dl, and increased urinary levels of PHPPA, PHPLA, PHPAA, and N-acetyltyrosine [53]. Other amino acids were not increased. Dihydroxyphenylalanine (dopa) and dopamine were increased in urine. The patient had a tremor accentuated during L-dopa administration [17]. Tyrosine crystals were seen in a marrow aspirate. When studied in parallel with a patient with tyrosinemia II, the latter had no urinary dopa or dopamine and had lower levels of phenolic labeling after tolerance tests with deuterated tyrosine [17]. Tyrosine aminotransferase activity in liver biopsy tissue was decreased 30 percent compared to a control. PHPPA oxidase was absent or markedly reduced. These results were thought consistent with a primary defect in PHPPA oxidase.

A 3½-year-old retarded girl had joint swelling, no reported eye or skin symptoms, increased urinary tyrosine levels, and tyrosine crystals in her bone marrow. Familial generalized aminoaciduria was also present [54]. The tyrosine crystals in the

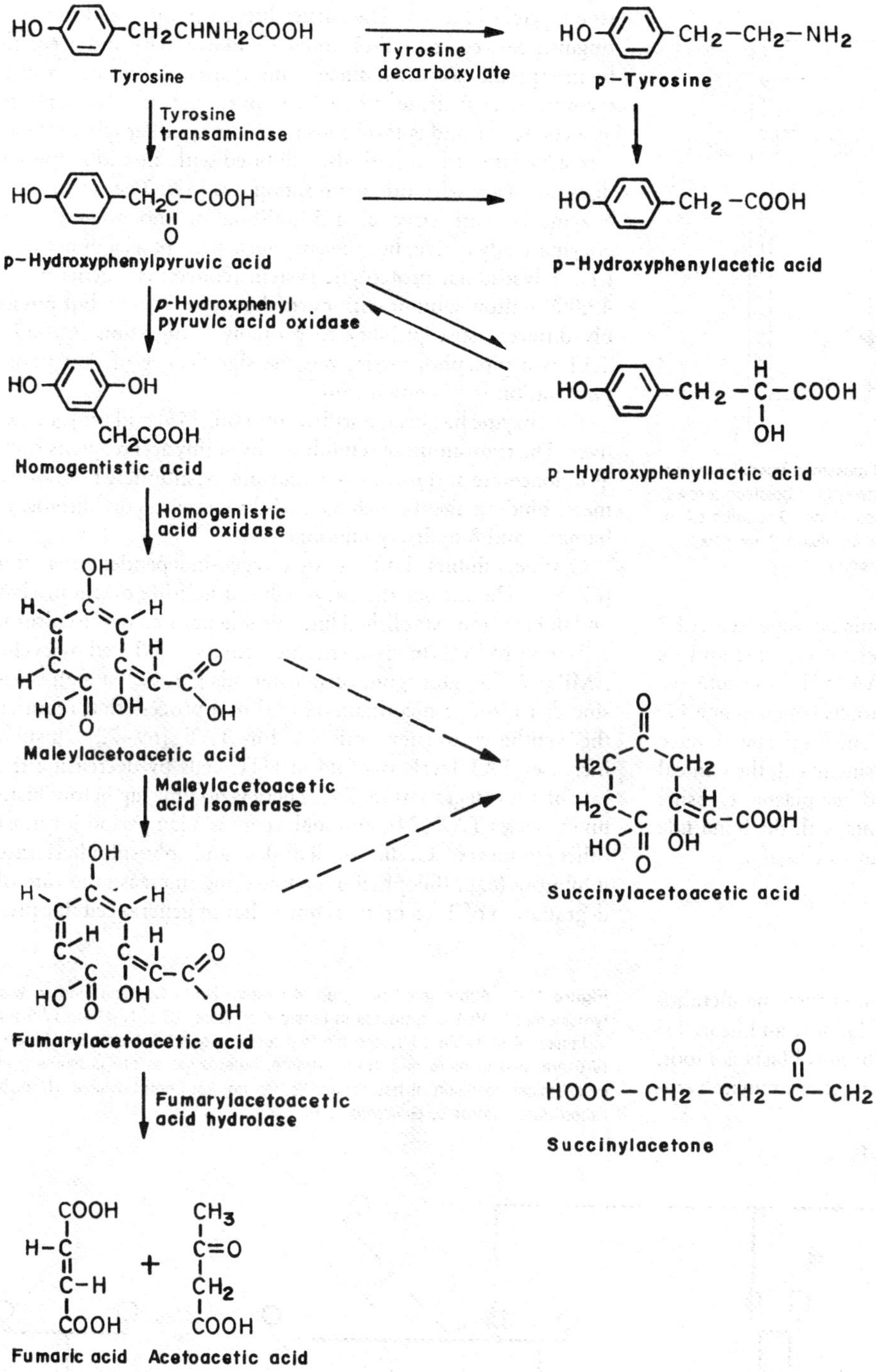

Tyrosine

Tyrosine decarboxylate

p-Tyrosine

Tyrosine transaminase

p-Hydroxyphenylpyruvic acid

p-Hydroxyphenylacetic acid

p-Hydroxphenyl pyruvic acid oxidase

p-Hydroxyphenyllactic acid

Homogentistic acid

Homogenistic acid oxidase

Maleylacetoacetic acid

Succinylacetoacetic acid

Maleylacetoacetic acid isomerase

Fumarylacetoacetic acid

$HOOC-CH_2-CH_2-C-CH_2-C-CH_3$

Succinylacetone

Fumarylacetoacetic acid hydrolase

Fumaric acid   Acetoacetic acid

Figure 13-5 Metabolic pathways for tyrosine.

marrow may have reflected only the high blood levels. Marrow aspiration on patients with documented tyrosinemia II has not been reported.

A 3½-year-old native Canadian Indian girl without known consanguinity developed seizures at 8 months and had motor, language, and social delay by age 6 months. No skin or eye lesions were present. At 11 months, her plasma tyrosine concentration was 16.3 mg/dl; other plasma amino acids were normal [55]. Urinary tyrosine was 3½ to 7 times normal, and plasma PHPLA was 0.09 mg/dl (normally undetectable). Urinary PHPPA, PHPLA, and PHPAA were increased. Soluble TAT was decreased in fibroblasts. The TAT in fibroblasts had a K_m for pyridoxal phosphate a hundredfold higher than nor-

mal and a normal K_m for tyrosine. Patients with tyrosinemia II usually have higher plasma tyrosine levels in childhood. This child may have had a deficiency of another aminotransferase (not TAT) important for tyrosine metabolism.

Over 50 years ago, Medes studied a 49-year-old male with myasthenia gravis who had high levels of urinary PHPPA which increased with a high protein or a high tyrosine diet. With the high tyrosine diet, dopa was excreted in the urine. Despite extensive study at the time and extensive speculation [56] since then, this patient cannot be identified with any of the currently described disorders of tyrosine metabolism. No similar patient has been described.

An 18-year-old severely retarded girl with microcephaly and

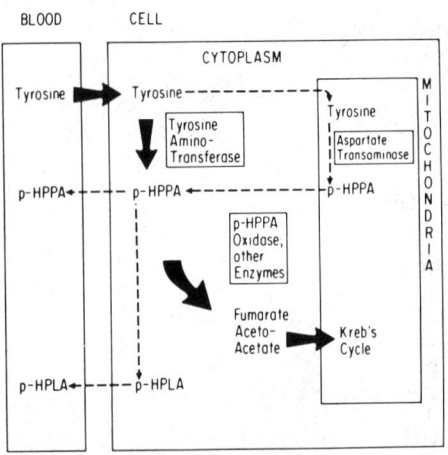

Figure 13-6 Proposed pathways of tyrosine metabolism in normal individuals and those with tyrosinemia II. The normal pathway is in boldface arrows and the metabolism in tyrosinemia II in broken lines. *(From Goldsmith LA in Fitzpatrick TB et al (eds): Dermatology in General Medicine. New York, McGraw-Hill Book Co, 1979, p 1042, with permission.)*

retardation had growth retardation, plasma tyrosine levels of 7 to 11 mg/dl, and increased urinary levels of tyrosine and its metabolites PHPPA, PHPLA, and PHPAA [57]. No acute eye or skin symptoms were present, but cataracts began at age 17. Although several authors, including this one (in the past), have considered this patient to have had tyrosinemia II, the clinical picture is atypical for that disorder, and her plasma tyrosine would be the lowest of any of the patients with the bona fide syndrome. She remains a patient difficult to classify.

Tyrosine Metabolism

Hepatic TAT is the rate-limiting enzyme in tyrosine metabolism. It is found predominantly in liver, kidney, and heart [3] and is absent in skin [58]; its presence in fibroblasts is moot. The normal physiologic role of TAT is to transaminate tyro-

sine to yield PHPAA. The earlier literature often did not distinguish between true TAT and TAT-like activity and needs to be interpreted critically, since many transaminases can utilize tyrosine as a substrate [59]. TAT requires pyridoxal phosphate as a coenzyme and is fastidious in requiring α-ketoglutarate as a cosubstrate; it is specifically inhibited with an antibody that does not react with other transaminases [59]. The rat hepatic enzyme is synthesized as a 53,000-dalton monomer that is enzymatically active, but the enzyme is present as a dimer [60, 61]. A lysosomal proteolytic system (convertase) generates a 49,000-dalton subunit with normal enzyme activity but possibly different susceptibility to proteolytic digestion [60–65]. TAT is a phosphoprotein, but the significance of that phosphorylation is unknown [66].

The enzyme has been purified from dog [56] and rat [60, 61] liver. The transaminase is inhibited by sulfhydryl reagents such as iodoacetate and p-chloromercuriphenylsulfonate but not by metal binding agents such as α,α'-dipyridyl, diethyldithiocarbamate, and δ-hydroxyquinoline [56].

Cystine inhibits TAT as an oxygen-independent reaction [67, 68]. The rat hepatic enzyme has a half-life of 2 h in vivo and in HTC (an established line of rat hepatoma tissue culture) cells in vitro [61]. In vivo, enzyme activity is induced by cyclic AMP [69, 70], glucagon, corticosteroids [71, 72], a high tyrosine diet [36], or nicotinamide [73] in a process that requires the synthesis of new mRNA for TAT [69–72]. Insulin increases TAT levels twofold in HTC cells by decreasing the rate of TAT degradation [74]. There is no time lag before insulin increases TAT [74], although there is a lag period for most other inducers. Cyclic nucleotides and phosphodiesterase inhibitors (e.g., theophylline, papaverine) increase the rate of degradation of TAT up to 2½ times that of general cellular pro-

Figure 13-7 Abbreviated pedigree of eastern North Carolina kindred with tyrosinemia II. VI-1 is a patient in family 7 of Table 13-1; IV-4 and IV-5 are in family 14 in Table 13-1, and his feet are in Fig. 13-3 *A* and *B*. IV-2 and IV-6 are said to have had the syndrome; heterozygotes are presumed, as biochemical definition of heterozygotes has not yet been possible. *(Unpublished data, Thorpe J, Goldsmith LA.)*

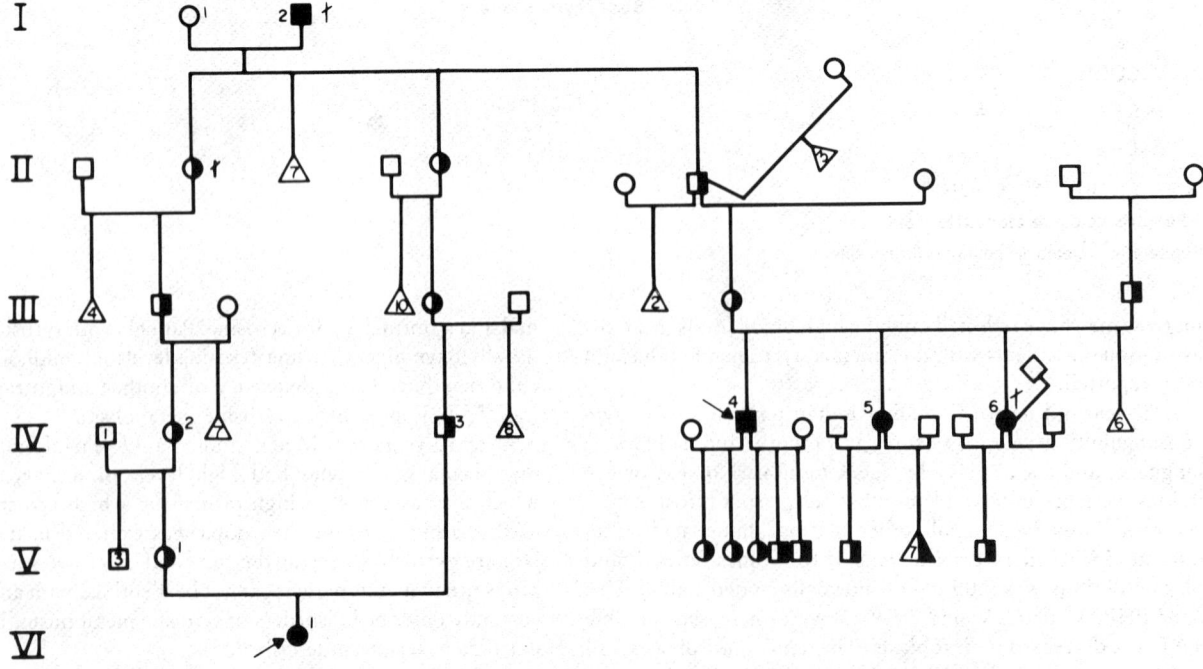

tein [75]. Genetic variants of HTC lacking TAT activity but responding to corticosteroids have been described [76].

Messenger RNA for TAT has been prepared and translated in vitro using both the wheat germ and reticulocyte cell-free systems. The increased TAT activity seen after hydrocortisone or dibutyryl cyclic AMP administration is due to a specific increase in the level of functional mRNA for the enzyme [69–72]. Dibutyryl cyclic AMP also appears to increase the rate of TAT-specific peptide chain elongation [77]. Messenger RNA for TAT has an estimated half-line of 1.2 h [72]. Inhibitors of protein synthesis (cycloheximide, puromycin, emetine) increase TAT-mRNA levels [78–80]. Actinomycin D causes superinduction by decreasing the activity of a TAT-degrading enzyme [81]. The increase in mRNA for TAT in the presence of inhibitors of protein synthesis suggests that the synthesis of other new proteins is not a necessary step in the inductive process. Thus TAT enzyme synthesis is regulated in a complex fashion involving transcriptional, posttranscriptional, and translational controls. TAT activity is very low in fetal life but is inducible by tyrosine, dexamethasone, and cyclic AMP [82, 83].

In the next enzyme in the metabolism pathway, PHPAA oxidase (hydroxylating) (E.C.1.14.2.2) catalyzes the oxidation of PHPAA to homogentisic acid. This enzyme is present in the liver and kidney of various mammalian species, including hogs, rabbits, rats, dogs, and humans [56]. It is not present in muscle, heart, or brain [32]. Purified PHPAA oxidase has been prepared from beef, pig, dog, chicken, rat, and human liver [56]. Properties of the enzyme have been summarized [56]. Since the conversions of phenylpyruvate to o-hydroxyphenylpyruvate, and of PHPPA to homogentisic acid, remain constant during purification, it is assumed that the same enzyme performs both oxidations [56].

The conversion of PHPAA to homogentisic acid requires two atoms of oxygen and the liberation of one molecule of CO_2. The reaction mechanism is complex and involves hydroxylation of the aromatic ring, migration of the side chain, and oxidation and decarboxylation of the side chain from pyruvate to acetate [56].

p-Hydroxyphenylpyruvate oxidase in vitro requires nonstoichiometric amounts of ascorbic acid or one of the group of compounds that can replace the vitamin, such as the reduced form of 2,6-dichlorophenolindophenol. These agents appear to prevent a gradual inhibition of the enzyme by its substrate [56]. In vitro, the substrate p-hydroxyphenylpyruvate generates peroxide in the presence of oxygen and the H_2O_2 inhibits the enzyme. Catalase and horseradish peroxidase protect the enzyme. It is undecided whether inhibition of the enzyme occurs in vivo [32].

The enzyme can be inhibited by relatively low concentrations of diethyldithiocarbamate and 1,10-phenanthroline and by sulfhydryl-binding agents, such as p-chloromercuribenzoic acid [56].

The amount of tyrosine which follows other metabolic pathways has been debated. Most investigators agree that only 0.3 to 1.0 percent of dietary tyrosine is decarboxylated to tyramine [84].

New tyrosine metabolites, Hawkinsin [(2-cystein-S-y1-1,4-dihydroxy-cyclohex-5-en-lyl) acetic acid], and cis and trans 4-hydroxycyclohexylacetic acid have been described in a family with transient tyrosinemia in which the infant had prolonged acidosis [85, 87] (Fig. 13–8). It has been postulated [87] that

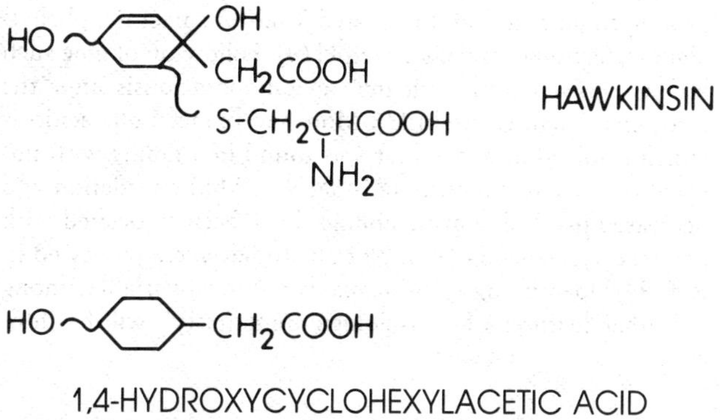

HAWKINSIN

1,4-HYDROXYCYCLOHEXYLACETIC ACID

Figure 13-8   Two recently discovered tyrosine metabolites. Hawkinsin and its desulfurated product, 1,4-dihydroxycyclohexylacetic acid, have been found in a family with a presumptive abnormality in p-hydroxyphenylpyruvate oxidase.

these metabolites are derived from an intermediate in the 4-hydroxyphenylpyruvate hydroxylase.

Tyrosine Tolerance Tests

Tyrosine tolerance tests are complicated by the insolubility of tyrosine and must be critically evaluated. Phenylalanine tolerance tests have been proposed, overcoming the problems with solubility. Tolerance tests with deuterated L[^{2}H$_2$]tyrosine and L[^{2}H$_5$]phenylalanine indicated that plasma and liver tyrosine are not in equilibrium [88]. Analysis of the labeling pattern further suggested that synthesis of labeled tyrosine from labeled phenylalanine in liver is unlikely [88] and that labeling occurred in several distinct anatomic compartments, consistent with the hypotheses used to explain the pattern of urinary metabolites in tyrosinemia II.

NEONATAL TYROSINEMIA

Clinical Features

Neonatal asymptomatic tyrosinemia and increased excretion of tyrosine and its metabolites are not uncommon. Males and premature infants are more frequently affected [14, 89]. The prevalence of this diagnosis varies in different populations from 0.2 to 10 percent according to feeding practices [24]. In Belgium, with over 30,000 newborns screened annually, there was a decrease in neonatal tyrosinemia from 0.7 to 0.2 percent in infants over 2500 g and from 3.6 to 0.4 percent in infants under 2500 between 1972 and 1977 [14]. Similar decreases occurred in Scandinavia. This was correlated with more breast feeding and more feeding of low protein ("humanized") cow's milk [14]. In the Inuit, living in Canada, who breast-feed their children, the incidence of tyrosine levels over 7.5 mg/dl was 14.8 and 6.2 percent in two separate studies performed in 1970–1972, and 1973–1974, respectively [90]. Although initially associated with low ascorbate levels, other genetic factors probably are involved since ascorbate supplementation did not significantly affect the incidence [91].

Children with neonatal tyrosinemia may be somewhat lethargic and have difficulty drinking, impaired motor activity, prolonged jaundice, and increased levels of galactose, phenylalanine, histidine, and cholesterol [14]. Follow-up of nine such infants showed four with mild metabolic acidosis after the tyrosinemia had cleared [92]. More severe metabolic acidosis which resolved at age 1 year was found in a family with unusual tyrosine metabolites [85–88, 93]. Mild retardation and decreased psycholinguistic abilities have been associated with neonatal tyrosinemia [94]. Not all studies agree [reviewed in Ref. 94]. Identifying tyrosinemia as a critical variable among the other features of "physiologic immaturity" will be difficult.

Biochemistry

Blood tyrosine, blood phenylalanine, urine tyrosine, PHPAA, PHPLA, PHPPA, N-acetyltyrosine, and p-tyramine are all increased [95].

Etiology

It is usually assumed that this disorder is due to a relative deficiency of p-hydroxyphenylpyruvate oxidase [30]. High protein diets with resulting high tyrosine and phenylalanine levels stress this enzyme. It is assumed that ascorbate protects the enzyme from substrate inhibition, although there is no evidence that this occurs in vivo [32]. The response of some patients to ascorbate and the increase of tyrosine metabolites in scorbutic animals and people is consistent with this hypothesis, as are studies in vitro with p-hydroxyphenylpyruvate oxidase [32]. With no real study of this enzyme and tyrosine aminotransferase in patients with neonatal tyrosinemia, this is a hypothesis at best. Since tyrosine aminotransferase is the rate-limiting enzyme of tyrosine metabolism and since the mechanism proposed by Fellman et al. [31] can explain the increased levels of tyrosine metabolites, the basic defect in neonatal tyrosinemia is still to be determined.

Therapy

Most cases are controlled by reducing protein to 2 to 3 g/kg per day or by breast feeding. The value of ascorbic acid supplementation at 100 mg four times a day has been questioned [95] and supported. Since some patients respond dramatically to vitamin C therapy, there may be two kinds of neonatal tyrosinemia. Establishing whether there is more than one form would be important, since patients with neurologic sequelae may represent a distinct subset.

TYROSINOSIS

Tyrosinosis, although not a primary disorder of tyrosine metabolism, is accompanied by elevated levels of tyrosine and its metabolites. Over 100 instances of the syndrome are reported [56]. Synonyms for the syndrome are: *tyrosyluria* and *hypermethioninemia* in an infant with hepatic cirrhosis and *nodular hyperplasia, hypermethioninemia, tyrosinosis, tyrosinose congenitale, tyrosinemia, hereditary tyrosinemia, inborn*

hepatorenal dysfunction, and *tyrosinemia I* [56]. Renaming it when a definite etiology is established will be useful. The term *tyrosinosis* is proposed until its exact metabolic basis is defined.

Clinical Features

Acute and chronic forms of the disease occur within the same family. In the acute form, during the first few weeks to months of life there is failure to thrive, vomiting, diarrhea, and a cabbagelike odor. Hepatomegaly, fever, edema, melena, and epistaxis are frequent. If untreated, death from liver failure ensues in 6 to 8 months [39, 56].

Similar but milder features characterize the chronic form. Chronic liver disease, renal tubular dysfunction (deToni-Fanconi syndrome; see Chap. 84), and vitamin D–resistant rickets dominate the clinical features by 1 year of age. Death occurs usually during the first decade. Hypertension may appear. Abdominal crises and polyneuropathy are related to acute, intermittent, porphyrialike chemical abnormalities [96]. Hepatoma is a late complication in 37 percent of patients [97]. Hypoglycemia which is unresponsive to glucagon may be present.

Laboratory Findings

Normocytic anemia and leukocytosis are always present, and the platelet count may be increased [30, 56]. Serum bilirubin and hepatic enzymes are increased, cholesterol is decreased, and prothrombin time is prolonged. α-Fetoprotein [60] and plasma renin are increased [96].

Plasma tyrosine is increased up to 6 to 12 mg/dl, methionine is increased, especially in the acute form, up to 1 to 5 mg/dl, and other amino acids may be increased as well [30, 56]. Urinary excretion of tyrosine and its metabolites, including PHPPA and PHPLA, are increased [30, 56]. Hematuria may be present. Glycosuria, phosphaturia, and a generalized aminoaciduria [30, 56], as well as an increase in glyceraldehyde, are also present [98]. The urine, as well as serum, contains succinylacetoacetate and succinylacetone [99, 100]. Urinary δ-amino levulinic acid [96] and catecholamines [96] are increased.

The amino acids excreted in excessive amounts, in decreasing order, are tyrosine (64 to 150 times normal), proline (10 to 125), threonine (10 to 37), alanine (9 to 30), glycine (8 to 20), phenylalanine (8 to 16), α-aminobutyric acid (7 to 30), isoleucine (5 to 24), serine (5 to 8), leucine and aspartic acid (3 to 10), and methionine (2 to 14) [56].

The red blood cell reduced glutathione level is decreased, as is the plasma cystine level [101].

The liver shows chronic active hepatitis [56], with fatty infiltration and tubular or pseudoacinar structures, lobular regeneration, and frequently hepatoma [102]. These is cellular swelling in the kidneys and astrogliosis in the white matter of the brain [102]. The pancreatic islets commonly are hyperplastic.

Diagnosis

Tyrosinosis should be considered in the differential diagnosis of liver failure in childhood. If a high tyrosine level is detected in infancy and childhood, tyrosinosis, neonatal tyrosinemia, and tyrosinemia II must be considered, along with fructose-1, 6-diphosphatase deficiency, fructose-1-phosphate aldolase deficiency, galactose-1-phosphate uridyl transferase deficiency, giant cell hepatitis, and neonatal infections. Urinary tests for succinylacetone and hepatic biopsies and assay for fumarylacetoacetate hydrolase establish the diagnosis [100].

Treatment

A low tyrosine, low phenylalanine (and often low methionine) diet has been the mainstay of therapy on the assumption that tyrosine, methionine, and their metabolites play significant roles in the toxicity [103]. Tyrosine and its metabolites seem unlikely candidates for such roles considering the experience with tyrosinemia II. Cysteine supplementation has helped at least one patient [101].

A phenylalanine-tyrosine deficiency syndrome associated with growth failure, anorexia, lethargy, hypotonia, and an increase in plasma nonaromatic amino acids should be avoided if the low tyrosine, low phenylalanine diet is used [104].

Liver homotransplantation has been accomplished in an effort to prevent hepatoma. It was also effective treatment for the metabolic abnormalities [105].

Pathogenesis

A deficiency of fumarylacetoacetate (FAA) hydrolase is proposed as the basis of the disease [99, 100]. Activity of this enzyme was 6 percent of control levels in six patients with the acute form of the disease and 20 percent of control levels in two patients with the chronic form [100]. Maleylacetoacetate (MAA) hydrolase is decreased as well [100]. The genetic basis for a decrease in both enzyme activities is speculative [99]. These enzyme activities are not decreased in other forms of liver failure. It is proposed that the degree of residual enzyme activity determines whether the disease will be acute or chronic in any affected homozygote. TAT and p-hydroxyphenylpyruvate oxidase are decreased in this disease and in other forms of liver disease. It is hypothesized that with deficiencies of the primary enzymes and disposal of FFA and MAA, these substrates would be increased and, in tissues with 4-hydroxyphenylpyruvate dioxygenase activity, that enzyme forms succinylacetone and succinylacetoacetate from FAA and MAA. Succinylacetone is structurally similar to maleic acid, a known inhibitor of renal tubular function, and may cause the renal tubular defects.

Succinylacetone, a structural analogue of δ-amino levulinic acid, markedly inhibits porphobilinogen synthetase (δ-amino acid dehydratase) [99, 106] and leads to increased levels of δ-amino levulinic acid and symptoms of acute intermittent porphyria. Succinylacetone inhibits cell growth [106]. Reduced glutathione may react with MAA and FAA, leading to decreased glutathione levels, which may interfere with glutathione-dependent detoxification mechanisms [100].

The high K_m form of S-adenosylmethionine may be inhibited by a "toxic metabolite" from MAA or FAA [107] and may be responsible for the abnormal methionine metabolism and hepatic dysfunction.

Identification of succinylacetone and related products, as well as the low plasma cystine and low erythrocyte glutathione

levels in patients, have led to treatment with cysteine supplementation or penicillamine [101, 108]. It was thought [99] that SH-containing compounds would form adducts with MAA and FAA and inhibit these potentially toxic compounds. The long-term effect of therapy remains to be determined.

Loading tests with homogentisic acid stress FAA hydrolase, leading to accumulation of succinylacetone, which was detected by a decrease in red cell δ-dehydrogenase levels [108a]. Heterozygotes had more pronounced disease than controls, a finding which strengthened the presumption that FAA hydrolase was the prime defect in the disease.

In fructose-1-phosphate aldolase deficiency (Chap. 53) and galactose-1-phosphate uridyl transferase deficiency (Chap. 7), similar but less extreme liver and renal damage occurs and is presumably also due to toxic metabolites. A tyrosinosislike syndrome has been produced by administration of chloral hydrate [109].

Genetics

This disorder has autosomal recessive inheritance. Consanguine matings have been frequent [110]. Both sexes are equally affected. There is a high prevalence of the trait in the French-Canadian population of Quebec, with an overall prevalence in Quebec of 0.8 per 10,000 births. In the Chicoutini Lac-St. Jean region of Quebec the heterozygote prevalence is 1:14, with one in 685 having the disease. A founder effect is documented for the high gene frequency in this region [110]. Screening studies have established a prevalence of the disease of 1:120,000 in Sweden and 1:100,000 in Norway [14].

Personal investigations were supported by the National Institutes of Health, Grant AM-17253 and General Clinical Research Center RR-30. Publication No. 99 of the Dermatological Research Laboratories at Duke University Medical Center.

REFERENCES

1. BURNS RP: The tyrosine aminotransferase deficiency: An unusual cause of corneal ulcers. *Am J Ophthal* 73:400, 1972
2. BURNS RP, GIPSON IK, MURRAY MJ: Keratopathy in tyrosinemia. *Birth Defects: Original Article Series* XII:169, 1976
3. FELLMAN JH, VANBELLINGHEN PJ, JONES RT, KOLER RD: Soluble and mitochondrial forms of tyrosine aminotransferase. Relationship to human tyrosinemia. *Biochemistry* 8:615, 1969
4. KENNAWAY NG, BUIST NRM: Metabolic studies in a patient with hepatic cytosol tyrosine aminotransferase deficiency. *Pediatr Res* 5:287, 1971
5. HILL A, ZALESKI WA: Tyrosinosis: Biochemical studies of an unusual case. *Clin Biochem* 4:263, 1971
6. ZALESKI WA, HILL A, KUSHNIRUK W: Skin lesions in tyrosinosis: Response to dietary treatment. *Br J Dermatol* 88:335, 1973
7. HOAG GN, HILL A, ZALESKI W: Urinary p-tyramine in hereditary tyrosinemia: I. Levels as compared to normal individuals, effect of diet, and relationship to urinary tyrosine. *Clin Biochem* 10:24, 1977
8. HOAG GN, HILL A, ZALESKI W: Urinary p-tyramine in hereditary tyrosinemia: II. Origin of urinary p-tyramine. *Clin Biochem* 10:26, 1977
9. HOLSTON JL Jr, LEVY HL, TOMLIN GA, ATKINS RJ PATTON TH, HOSTY TS: Tyrosinosis: A patient without liver or renal disease. *Pediatrics* 48:393, 1971
10. GOLDSMITH LA, KANG E, BIENFANG DC, JIMBOW K, GERALD P, BADEN HP: Tyrosinemia with plantar and palmar keratosis and keratitis. *J Pediatr* 83: 798, 1973
11. BIENFANG DC, KUWABARA T, PUESCHEL SM: The Richner-Hanhart syndrome. Report of a case with associated tyrosinemia. *Arch Ophthal* 94:1133, 1976
12. ZAMMARCHI E, LA CAUZA C, CALZOLARI C: Un caso di ipertirosinemia con tirosiluria. *Minerva Pediatr* 26:203, 1974
13. SANDBERG HO: Bilateral keratopathy and tyrosinosis. *Acta Ophthal* 53:760, 1975

14. HALVORSEN S: Screening for disorders of tyrosine metabolism, in Bickel H, Guthrie R, Hammersen G (eds): *Neonatal Screening for Inborn Errors of Metabolism*, New York, Springer-Verlag, New York, Inc, 1980, p 45

15. GOLDSMITH LA, REED J: Tyrosine-induced eye and skin lesions. *JAMA* 236:382, 1976

16. BILLSON FA, DANKS DM: Corneal and skin changes in tyrosinaemia. *Aust J Ophthal* 3:112, 1975

17. FAULL KF, GAN I, HALPERN B, HAMMOND J, IM S, COTTON RGH, DANKS DM: Metabolic studies on two patients with nonhepatic tyrosinemia using deuterated tyrosine loads. *Pediatr Res* 11:631, 1977

18. GARIBALDI LR, SILIATO F, DE MARTINI I, SCARSI MR, ROMANO C: Oculocutaneous tyrosinosis. Report of two cases in the same family. *Helv Paediatr Acta* 32:173, 1977

19. BARDELLI AM, BORGOGNI P, FARNETANI MA, FOIS A, FREZZOTTI R, MATTEI R, MOLINELLI M, SARGENTINI I: Familial tyrosinaemia with eye and skin lesions. *Opthalmologica* 175:5, 1977

20. PELET B, ANTENER I, FAGGIONI R, SPAHR A, GAUTIER E: Tyrosinemia without liver or renal damage with plantar and palmar keratosis and keratitis (Hypertyrosinemia type II). *Helv Paediatr Acta* 34:177, 1979

21. JAEGER W, GALLASCH G, SCHNYDER UW, LUTZ P, SCHMIDT H: Tyrosinemia and bilateral pseudokeratitis dendritica (Richner-Hanhart-syndrome). *Metab Pediatr Ophthal* 3:111, 1979

22. LARREGUE M, DE GIACOMONI PH, BRESSIEUX J-M, ODIÈVRE M: Syndrome de Richner-Hanhart ou tyrosinose oculo-cutanée. *Ann Dermatol Venereol* 106:53, 1979

23. LEMONNIER F, CHARPENTIER C, ODIÈVRE M, LARRÈGUE M, LEMONNIER A: Tyrosine aminotransferase isoenzyme deficiency. *J Peds* 94:931, 1979

24. GOLDSMITH LA, THORPE JM, ROE CR: Hepatic enzymes of tyrosine metabolism in tyrosinemia II. *J Invest Dermatol* 73:530, 1979

25. HUNZIKER N: Richner-Hanhart syndrome and tyrosinemia type II. *Dermatologica* 160:180, 1980

26. FRANCESCHETTI AT, SCHNYDER UW, FELGENHAUER WR: Die cornea beim Richner-Hanhart syndrom. *Bericht uber die 71, Zusammenkunft der Deutschen Ophthalm Gesellschaft in Heidelberg*, 1971 p 109

27. ZALESKI WA, HOUSTON CS, HILL A: Unusual radiological changes in tyrosinosis. *Lancet* 2:46, 1972

28. HILL A, NORDIN PM, ZALESKI WA: Dietary treatment of tyrosinosis. *J Am Diet Assoc* 56:308, 1970

29. BUIST NRM, KENNAWAY NG, FELLMAN JH: Disorders of tyrosine metabolism, in Nyhan WR (ed): *Heritable Disorders of Amino Acid Metabolism: Patterns of Clinical and Genetic Variation*. New York, John Wiley & Sons, Inc, 1974, p 160

30. SCRIVER CR, ROSENBERG LE: Tyrosine, in Scriver Cr, Rosenberg LE (eds): *Amino Acid Metabolism and Its Disorders*, Philadelphia, WB Saunders Co, 1973, p 338

31. FELLMAN JH, BUIST NRM, KENNAWAY NG, SWANSON RE: The source of aromatic ketoacids in tyrosinaemia and phenylketonuria. *Clin Chim Acta* 39:243, 1972

32. FELLMAN JH, FUJITA TS, ROTH ES: Assay, properties an tissue distribution of *p*-hydroxyphenylpyruvate hydroxylase. *Biochim Biophys Acta* 284:90, 1972

33. BUIST NRM, FELLMAN JH, KENNAWAY N: Letter to the editor: Metabolic studies in tyrosinemia. *Pediatr Res* 12:56, 1978

34. DANKS DM: Letter to the editor: Reply to Dr. Buist. *Pediatr Res* 12:57, 1978

35. SCHWEIZER W: Studies on the effect of l-tyrosine on the white rat. *J Physiol* 106:167, 1947

36. IP CCY, HARPER AE: Effects of dietary protein content and glucagon administration on tyrosine metabolism and tyrosine toxicity in the rat. *J Nutr* 103:1594, 1973

37. ALAM SQ, BECKER RV, STUCKI WP, ROGERS QR: Effect of threonine on the toxicity of excess tyrosine and cataract formation in the rat. *J Nutr* 89:91, 1968

38. YAMAMOTO Y, TOYOSHIMA R, MURAMATSU K: Effect of additional protein or methionine and threonine on tyrosine catabolism in rats fed diets high in tyrosine. *Agric Biol Chem* 43:2585, 1979

39. SELYE H: Steroids influencing the toxicity of L-tyrosine. *J Nutr* 101:515, 1971

40. BOCTOR AM, HARPER AE: Tyrosine toxicity in the rat: Effect of high intake of *p*-hydroxyphenylpyruvic acid and of force-feeding high tyrosine diet. *J Nutr* 95:535, 19

41. EASTON EJ SIMPSON I, MARTIN, JK, CAMPBELL DJ: Tyrosinemia induced by a pyridoxine antagonist, desoxypyridoxine. *Clin Chem* 18:161, 1972

42. RICH LF, BEARD ME, BURNS RP: Excess dietary tyrosine and corneal lesions. *Exp Eye Res* 17:87, 1973

43. BEARD ME, BURNS RP, RICH LF, SQUIRES E: Histopathology of keratopathy in the tyrosine-fed rat. *Invest Ophthal* 13: 1037, 1974

44. GIPSON IK, BURNS RP, WOLFE-LANDE JD: Crystals in corneal epithelial lesions of tyrosine fed rats. *Invest Ophthal* 14:937, 1975

45. GOLDSMITH LA: Molecular biology and molecular pathology of a newly described molecular disease—tyrosinemia II (The Richner-Hanhart syndrome). *Exp Cell Biol* 46:96, 1978

46. GOLDSMITH LA: Tyrosine-induced skin disease. *Br J Dermatol* 98:119, 1978

47. TABACHNICK J: Labadie JH: Studies on the biochemistry of epidermis. IV. The free amino acids, ammonia, urea, and pyrrolidone carboxylic acid content of conventional and germ-free albino guinea-pig epidermis. *J Invest Dermatol* 54:24, 1970

48. GOLDSMITH LA: Hemolysis and lysosomal activation by solid state tyrosine. *Biochem Biophys Res Commun* 64:558, 1975

49. GOLDSMITH LA: Haemolysis induced by tyrosine crystals. Modifiers and inhibitors. *Biochem J* 158:17, 1976.

50. SCHWARTZ TM, SCHACKELFORD RM: Pseudodistemper is apparently new ailment of mink. *US Fur Rancher* 52:6, 1973

51. CHRISTENSEN K, FISCHER P, KNUDSEN KEB, LARSEN S, SØRENSEN H, VENGE O: A syndrome of hereditary tyrosinemia in mink (*Mustela vison Schreb*). *Can J Comp Med* 43:333, 1979

52. GOLDSMITH LA, THORPE JM, MARSH RF: Tyrosine aminotransferase deficiency in mink (*Mustela vison*): A model for human tyrosinemia II. *Biochem Genet* (in press), 1981

53. LOUIS WJ, PITT DD, DAVIES H: Biochemical studies in a patient with "Tyrosinosis." *Aust NZ J Med* 4:281, 1974

54. JAISWAL RB, BHAI I, NATH N, NATH MC: Tyrosinosis—Part 1: Clinical, radiological and biochemical aspects. *Indian Pediatr* 6:1, 1969

55. DEGROOT GW, DAKSHINAMURTI K, ALLAN L, HAWORTH JC: Defect in soluble tyrosine aminotransferase in skin fibroblasts of a patient with tyrosinemia. *Pediatr Res* 14:896, 1980

56. LA DU BN, GJESSING LR: Tyrosinosis and tyrosinemia, in Stanbury JB, Wyngaarden JB, Fredrickson DS (eds): *Metabolic Basis of Inherited Disease*, ed 4. New York, McGraw-Hill Book Co, 1978, p 256

57. WADMAN SK, VAN SPRANG FJ, MAAS JW, KETTING D: An exceptional case of tyrosinosis. *J Ment Defic Res* 12:269, 1968

58. THORPE JM, GOLDSMITH LA: Tyrosine aminotransferase activity in skin. *J Invest Dermatol* 75:371, 1980

59. SPENCER CJ, GELEHRTER TD: Pseudoisozymes of hepatic tyrosine aminotransferase. *J Biol Chem* 249:577, 1974

60. LEE K-L, ROBERSON LE, KENNEY FT: Properties of tyrosine aminotransferase from rat liver. *Anal Biochem* 95:188, 1979

61. HARGROVE JL, DIESTERHAFT M, NOGUCHI T, GRANNER DK: Identification of native tyrosine aminotransferase and an explanation for the multiple forms. *J Biol Chem* 255:71, 1980

62. RUBENSTEIN PA, IVARIE RD: Isolation of two different molecular weight polypeptides copurifying with rat liver tyrosine aminotransferase. *Arch Biochem Biophys* 194:299, 1979

63. SMITH GJ, PEARCE PH, OLIVER IT: A lysosomal factor that interconverts multiple forms of rat liver tyrosine aminotransferase. *Life Sci* 19: 1763, 1976

64. BOCTOR A, GROSSMAN A: Tyrosine aminotransferase converting factor. Kinetic properties, cellular localization, and tissue distribution. *Biochem Biophys Acta* 543:137, 1978

65. GOHDA E, PITOT HC: Purification and characterization of a factor catalyzing the conversion of the multiple forms of tyrosine aminotransferase from rat liver. *J Biol Chem* 255:7371, 1980

66. LEE K-L, NICKOL JM: Phosphorylation of tyrosine aminotransferase in vivo. *J Biol Chem* 249:6024, 1974

67. FEDERICI G, DI COLA D, SACCHETTA P, DI ILIO C, DEL BOCCIO G, POLIDORO G: Reversible inactivation of tyrosine aminotransferase from guinea pig liver by thiol and disulfide compounds. *Biochem Biophys Res Commun* 81:650, 1978

68. BUCKLEY WT, MILLIGAN LP: Participation of cysteine and cystine in inactivation of tyrosine aminotransferase in rat liver homogenates. *Biochem J* 176:449, 1978

69. ERNEST MJ, FEIGELSON P: Increase in hepatic tyrosine aminotransferase mRNA during enzyme induction by $N^6,O^{2'}$-dibutyryl cyclic AMP. *J Biol Chem* 253:319, 1978

70. NOGUCHI T, DIESTERHAFT M, GRANNER D: Dibutyryl cyclic AMP increases the amount of functional messenger RNA coding for tyrosine aminotransferase in rat liver. *J Biol Chem* 253:1332, 1978

71. OLSON PS, THOMPSON EB, GRANNER DK: Regulation of hepatoma tissue culture cell tyrosine aminotransferase messenger ribonucleic acid by dexamethasone. *Biochemistry* 19:1705, 1980

72. NICKOL JM, LEE K-L, KENNEY FT: Changes in hepatic levels of tyrosine aminotransferase messenger RNA during induction by hydrocortisone. *J Biol Chem* 253:4009, 1978

73. KROGER, VH, GRATZ R: Induktion der tyrosin-aminotransferase (EC 2.5.1.5) in der rattenleber durch nicotinsäureamid. *J Clin Chem Clin Biochem* 16:525, 1978

74. SPENCER CJ, HEATON JH, GELEHRTER TD, RICHARDSON KI, GARWIN JL: Insulin selectively slows the degradation rat of tyrosine aminotransferase. *J Biol Chem* 253:7677, 1978

75. STELLWAGEN RH, SAILOR RD, KOHLI KK: Acceleration of the degradation of tyrosine aminotransferase in rat hepatoma (HTC) cells by inhibitors of cyclic nucleotide phosphodiesterase. *Biochem Biophys Res Commun* 78:1162, 1977

76. THOMPSON EB, GRANNER KD, GELEHRTER TD, HAGER GL: Unlinked control of multiple glucocorticoid-sensitive processes in spontaneous HTC cell variants, in Sato GH, Ross R (eds): *Hormones and Cell Culture.* Cold Spring Harbor, NY, Cold Spring Harbor Laboratory, 1979, p 339

77. ROPER MD, WICKS WD: Evidence for acceleration of the rate of elongation of tyrosine aminotransferase nascent chains by dibutyryl cyclic AMP. *Proc Natl Acad Sci USA* 75:140, 1978

78. ERNEST MJ, DELAP L, FEIGELSON P: Induction of hepatic tyrosine aminotransferase mRNA by protein synthesis inhibitors. *J Biol Chem* 253:2895, 1978

79. HOFER E, SEKERIS CE: Cycloheximide causes increase accumulation of translatable mRNA for tyrosine aminotransferase and tryptophan oxygenase in livers of cortisol-treated rats. *Eur J Biochem* 86:547, 1978

80. LIU AY-C: Role of cyclic AMP-dependent protein kinase in the induction of tyrosine aminotransferase. *J Biol Chem* 255:4421, 1980

81. KRÖGER H, DONNER I, VOSS H, PLOTZE G: Superinduction of tyrosine aminotransferase in RLC-cells. *Biomedicine* 31:89, 1979

82. COUFALIK AH, MONDER C: Regulation of the tyrosine oxidizing system in fetal rat liver. *Arch Biochem Biophys* 199:67, 1980

83. ANDERSSON SM, RAIHA CR, OHISALO JJ: Regulation of tyrosine aminotransferase in foetal rat liver. *Biochem J* 186:609, 1980

84. FELLMAN JH, ROTH ES, FUJITA TS: Decarboxylation to tyramine is not a major route of tyrosine metabolism in mammals. *Arch Biochem Biophys* 174:562, 1976

85. NIEDERWIESER A, MATASOVÍC A, TIPPETT P, DANKS DM: A new sulfur amino acid, named Hawkinsin, identified in a baby with transient tyrosinemia and her mother. *Clin Chim Acta* 76:345, 1977

86. NIEDERWIESER A, MATASOVÍC A, NEUHEISER F, WETZEL E: New tyrosine metabolites in humans: Hawkinsin and *cis-* and *trans*-4-hydroxycyclohexylacetic acids. Unusual adsorption of deuterated and non-deuterated Hawkinsin during gas chromatography. *J Chromat* 146:207, 1978

87. NIEDERWIESER A, WADMAN SK, DANKS DM: Excreton of *cis-* and *trans*-4-hydroxycyclohexylacetic acid in addition to Hawkinsin in a family with a postulated defect of 4-hydroxyphenylpyruvate dioxygenase. *Clin Chim Acta* 90:195, 1978

88. FELL V, HOSKINS JA, POLLITT RJ: The labelling of urinary acids after oral doses of deuterated L-phenylalanine and L-tyrosine in normal subjects. Quantitative studies with implications for the deuterated phenylalanine load test in phenylketonuria. *Clin Chim Acta* 83:259, 1978

89. WONG, PWK, LAMBERT AM, KOMROWER GM: Tyrosinaemia and tyrosyluria in infancy. *Dev Med Child Neurol* 9:551, 1967

90. CLOW CL, LABERGE C, SCRIVER CR: Neonatal hypertyrosinemia and evidence for deficiency of ascorbic acid in Arctic and subarctic peoples. *CMA J* 113:624, 1975

91. SCRIVER CR, PERRY JRT, LASLEY L, CLOW CL, COULTER D, LABERGE C: Neonatal tyrosinemia (NT) in the Eskimo. Result of protein polymorphism. *Pediatr Res* 11:411, 1977

92. FERNBACH SA, SUMMONS RF, PEREIRA WE, DUFFIELD AM: Metabolic studies of transient tyrosinemia in premature infants. *Pediatr Res* 9:172, 1975

93. DANKS DM, TIPPETT P, ROGERS J: A new form of prolonged transient tyrosinemia presenting with severe metabolic acidosis. *Acta Paediatr Scand* 64:209, 1975

94. MAMUNES P, PRINCE PE, THORNTON NH, HUNT PA, HITCHCOCK ES: Intellectual deficits after transient tyrosinemia in the term neonate. *Pediatrics* 57:675, 1976

95. BAKKER HD, WADMAN SK, VAN SPRANG FJ, VAN DER HEIDEN C, KETTING D, DE BREE PK: Tyrosinemia and tyrosyluria in healthy prematures: Time courses not vitamin C-dependent. *Clin Chim Acta* 61:73, 1975

96. STRIFE CF, ZUROWESTE EL, EMMETT EA, FINELLI VN, PETERING HG, BERRY HK: Tyrosinemia with acute intermittent porphyria: aminolevulinic acid dehydratase deficiency related to elevated urinary aminolevulinic acid levels. *J Ped* 90:400, 1977

97. WEINBERG AG, MIZE CE, WORTHEN HG: The occurrence of hepatoma in the chronic form of hereditary tyrosinemia. *J Ped* 88:434, 1976

98. TOMER KB, ROTHMAN R, YUDKOFF M, SEGAL S: Unusual pattern of metabolites in the urine of a child with tyrosinemia: Glyceraldehyde. *Clin Chim Acta* 81:109, 1977

99. LINDBLAD B, LINDSTEDT S, STEEN G: On the enzymic defects in hereditary tyrosinemia. *Proc Natl Acad Sci USA* 74:4641, 1977

100. LESCAULT A, LABERGE C, GRENIER A, GAGNÉ R, MAMER OA: Deficiency of liver fumarylacetoacetate hydrolase in acute and chronic hereditary tyrosinemia. In press.

101. SØIRDAHL S, LIE SO, JELLUM E, STOKKE O: Increased need for L-cysteine in hereditary tyrosinemia. *Pediatr Res* 13:74, 1979

102. CARSON NAJ, BIGGART JD, BITTLES AH, DONOVAN D: Hereditary tyrosinaemia. Clinical, enzymatic, and pathological study of an infant with the acute form of the disease. *Arch Dis Child* 51:106, 1976

103. MICHALS K, MATALON R, WONG PWK: Importance of methionine restriction. Dietary treatment of tyrosinemia type I. *J Am Diet Assoc* 73:508, 1978

104. COHN RM, YUDKOFF M, YOST B, SEGAL S: Phenylalanine-tyrosine deficiency syndrome as a complication of the management of hereditary tyrosinemia. *Am J Clin Nutr* 30:209, 1977

105. FISCH RO, McCABE ERB, DOEDEN D, KOEP LJ, KOHLHOFF JG, SILVERMAN A, STARZL TE: Homotransplantation of the liver in a patient with hepatoma and hereditary tyrosinemia. *J Ped* 93:592, 1978

106. EBERT PS, HESS RA, FRYKHOLM BC, TSCHUDY DP: Succinylacetone, a potent inhibitor of heme biosynthesis: Effect on cell growth, heme content and δ-aminolevulinic acid dehydrase activity of malignant murine erythroleukemia cells. *Biochem Biophys Res Commun* 88:1382, 1979

107. LIAU MC, CHANG CF, BELANGER L, GRENIER A: Correlation of isozyme patterns of S-adenosylmethionine synthetase with fetal stages and pathological states of the liver. *Can Res* 39:162, 1979

108. FÄLLSTRÖM S-P, LINDBALD B, LINDSTEDT S, STEEN G: Hereditary tyrosinemia—fumarylacetoacetase deficiency. *Pediatr Res* 13:78a, 1979

108a. LABERGE: Personal communication

109. WATTS RWE, CHALMERS RA, LIBERMAN MM, LAWSON AM: Some biochemical effects of chloral hydrate in an infant with a tyrosinemia-like syndrome. *Pediatr Res* 9:875, 1975

110. BERGERON P, LABERGE C, GRENIER A: Hereditary tyrosinemia in the province of Quebec: Prevalence at birth and geographic distribution. *Clin Genet* 5:157, 1974

14

ALKAPTONURIA

This summary is adapted from the summary written by Bert N. La Du for the fourth edition of this book [1].

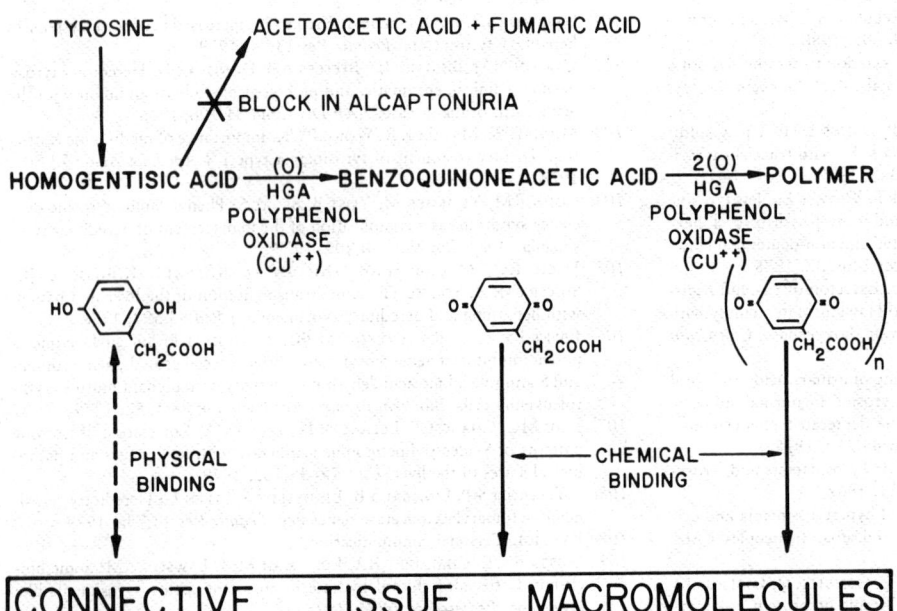

Postulated scheme for the formation of ochronotic pigment in alcaptonuria. The metabolic block in alcaptonuria results from a deficiency of homogentisic acid oxidase.

1. Alkaptonuria *is a rare hereditary metabolic disease in which homogentisic acid, an intermediary product in the metabolism of phenylalanine and tyrosine, cannot be further metabolized. The accumulation of homogentisic acid causes a characteristic triad of homogentisic aciduria, ochronosis (pigmentation of connective tissue), and arthritis.*
2. *The cause of the disease is a lack of the enzyme homogentisic acid oxidase. This enzyme normally functions primarily in the liver and kidney. It requires oxygen, ferrous ion, and sulfhydryl groups in order to open the ring of homogentisic acid.*
3. *The condition is inherited as an autosomal recessive trait. No method for the detection of heterozygotes has been devised.*
4. *The relationship between the metabolic defect and the clinical complications of ochronosis and arthritis*

remain a challenging research problem. Even though the lack of homogentisic acid oxidase and the resultant accumulation of homogentisic acid are no doubt the ultimate causes of these complications, the cellular mechanisms that bring them about are unknown.
5. Alkaptonuria *enjoys the historic distinction of being the human disease that led to elucidation of the concept of "inborn errors of metabolism" by A. E. Garrod in 1902.*

REFERENCES

1. LA DU BN: Alkaptonuria, in Stanbury JB, Wyngaarden JB, Fredrickson DS (eds): *The Metabolic Basis of Inherited Disease*, ed 4. New York, McGraw-Hill Book Co, 1978, p 286
2. SŘSEŇ S: Alkaptonuria. *Johns Hopkins Med J* 145:217, 1979

15

ALBINISM AND OTHER DISORDERS OF PIGMENT METABOLISM

CARL J. WITKOP, JR.

WALTER C. QUEVEDO, JR.

THOMAS B. FITZPATRICK

1. *Albinism is a generic designation covering a variety of clinical syndromes exhibiting hypomelanosis based on heritable metabolic defects in the pigment cell (melanocyte) system of the eye and skin. In human albinos (with the exception of the BADS syndrome), melanocytes appear to be normally distributed throughout the eye and skin but fail to synthesize adequate amounts of melanin.*

2. *Oculocutaneous albinism (OCA) in humans exists in 10 distinct forms which have in common decreased pigmentation of the skin, hair, and eyes; decreased visual acuity; and hypoplasia of the fovea, with varying degrees of nystagmus and photophobia. These forms have been designated tyrosinase-positive albinism; tyrosinase-negative albinism; yellow mutant albinism; Chédiak-Higashi syndrome; Hermansky-Pudlak syndrome; Cross syndrome; brown albinism; autosomal dominant albinism; rufous albinism; and black locks-albinism-deafness of sensorineural type (BADS syndrome). All but the dominant form are inherited as autosomal recessive traits.*

3. *Ocular albinism (OA) occurs as an autosomal recessive trait at least as frequently as it occurs as an X-linked trait. X-linked ocular albinos and heterozygotes have macromelanosomes in the melanocytes of skin, but they have not been observed in the autosomal recessive form. In females heterozygous for X-*

linked OA (Nettleship variety), the retinas show a mosaic pattern of pigment distribution due to random X-chromosome inactivation early in development. The metabolic defects leading to hypomelanosis of the retinal and uveal tracts in the various forms of OA are unknown. Skin pigmentation appears to be slightly altered.

4. *Oculocutaneous albinoidism is inherited as an autosomal dominant trait. With rare exceptions, patients do not have associated nystagmus or photophobia or markedly decreased visual acuity.*

5. *All 10 forms of OCA can be distinguished from one another on the basis of their incidence as well as their clinical, biochemical, ultrastructural, and genetic characteristics.*

6. *Tyrosinase-negative (ty-neg) albinos have a constant phenotype that does not vary with ethnic background. The phenotype is characterized by a complete absence of visible pigment. Hair bulbs incubated in L-tyrosine do not form pigment, and melanocytes contain only stage I and stage II unpigmented melanosomes.*

7. *Tyrosinase-positive (ty-pos) albinos have some visible pigment, although in infancy this may not be clinically apparent in Caucasoids. Hair color is usually white-yellow to yellow-tan, and lightly pigmented nevi may be present. Hair bulb melanocytes may con-*

301

tain up to early stage III, lightly pigmented melanosomes, which when incubated in L-tyrosine deposit black eumelanin and are converted to stage IV melanosomes.

8. *Yellow mutant albinos phenotypically have yellow to yellow-red hair, but hair bulbs do not form black eumelanin upon incubation with L-tyrosine. When hair bulbs are incubated with L-tyrosine plus L-cysteine, there is an intensification of the yellow-red (pheomelanin) color of their unevenly pigmented stage III melanosomes. The melanogenic defect in yellow mutant albinism may be tied in some way to pheomelanogenesis rather than to eumelanogenesis. It appears to be allelic with ty-neg albinism.*

9. *The Hermansky-Pudlak syndrome (HPS) is a ty-pos type of albinism. In addition, it has a mild bleeding diathesis due to storage pool-deficient platelets which lack normal levels of nonmetabolic adenine nucleotides and serotonin, but whose aggregation defect can be corrected by epinephrine stimulation of the membrane-modulated aggregation pathway. There is also a storage defect in which ceroidlike material and lipids accumulate in reticuloendothelial tissue, in urine, in the oral and gastrointestinal mucosa, and in the lung, where they lead to restrictive lung disease. Patients may develop ulcerative colitis. Hair bulb melanocytes in HPS may contain pheomelanosomes as well as eumelanosomes, and they differ in this feature from hair bulb melanocytes in ty-pos albinism.*

10. *The Cross syndrome is characterized by features of OCA, small eyes, and severely retarded mental and physical development. Hair bulb melanocytes contain reduced numbers of melanosomes of all stages. The melanosomes frequently form small clusters. After incubation in L-tyrosine, most melanosomes are converted to fully pigmented stage IV melanosomes.*

11. *The Chédiak-Higashi syndrome (CHS), usually fatal in childhood, is characterized by pigment dilution, the presence of giant peroxidase-positive secondary lysosomal granules in leukocytes which do not degranulate and which impede chemotaxis, and a marked susceptibility to infection. Children surviving early infections frequently develop a terminal lymphoreticular malignancy. The reduced hair, skin, and eye color is associated with giant melanosomes in melanocytes and keratinocytes. The number of melanosomes within keratinocytes is reduced. The giant melanosomes appear to be degraded by lysosomal hydrolases within melanocytes. Melanosomes of more normal size are transferred to keratinocytes, where they form unusually large phagolysosomes. The cutaneous hypopigmentation of CHS appears to result from the reduced number of melanosomes within keratinocytes and possibly from the grouping of melanosomes into aggregates of abnormal size. A defect in killer cell function is found in CHS lymphocytes.*

12. *The brown and rufous OCA phenotypes have been distinguished with certainty only among deeply pigmented populations of Africa and New Guinea. Both types have mild nystagmus and visual defects.*

13. *Autosomal dominant albinism is distinguished from autosomal dominant albinoidism by the presence of nystagmus.*

14. *The BADS syndrome, in contrast to all other forms of albinism, lacks melanocytes in the white skin and hair. The defect appears to be a disorder of migration of neural crest cells to their peripheral sites.*

15. *All human albinos tested have normal visual fields but do not have binocular vision. The absence of binocular vision in human albinos appears to result from abnormal optic pathways, with most fibers from the temporal retina crossing to the side of the brain opposite the eye of origin, and rearrangements in the geniculocortical projections. This contrasts to the situation in normally pigmented individuals, in whom the temporal retina fibers pass instead to the same side of the brain as the eye of origin. Neurophysiologic as well as direct morphologic studies in humans support this interpretation.*

16. *Animal models provide perspective in the elucidation of human albinism. The pink-eyed dilution (p/p) mutant variety of coat color in the mouse closely approximates ty-pos albinism in humans. Human ty-neg albinism is strikingly paralleled in expression by the albinism in mice regulated by a recessive c-locus allele. The comparative approach permits speculations on the possible mechanisms operative at the molecular level in human albinism. The c locus in mice appears to be a regulatory rather than a structural locus.*

17. *Albino and hypopigmented animals may be inappropriate models for certain types of research involving vision, hearing, behavior, otic and optic neuroanatomic and physiologic functions, and drug testing.*

18. *Similarities in the expression of albinism in humans and mice may reflect the existence of gene loci maintained in common by both species throughout broad periods of the evolutionary diversification of mammals.*

HISTORICAL INTRODUCTION

Albinism comprises a heterogeneous group of heritable disorders of the melanin pigmentary system, found throughout the animal kingdom. In humans, all forms of albinism are characterized by hypoplasia of the fovea, photophobia, nystagmus, and decreased visual acuity, in addition to absent or decreased melanotic pigment in skin, hair, and eyes (oculocutaneous albinism, OCA) or eye (ocular albinism, OA). The term *albinoidism* refers to hypomelanotic conditions without nystagmus, photophobia, and decreased visual acuity [1, 2]. Ten disorders with the clinical features of OCA (Table 15-1) and four disorders with features of OA (Table 15-2) have been described. These disorders can be identified by their clinical, genetic, and ultrastructural features [2–4] and by the response of anagen hair bulbs incubated in L-tyrosine for their ability to produce pigment [5].

Historical reviews of albinism can be found in the comprehensive monographs by Pearson et al. [6] and in more recent summaries by Froggatt [7, 8] and Witkop [4]. The term *albino* is derived from the Latin adjective *albus*, "white," and was first applied by Balthazar Tellez to certain "white" Negroes whom he observed on the west coast of Africa near present-day Lagos, Nigeria [6]. Recognizable accounts of albinism dating from the first century A.D. are to be found in Pliny [9] and Aulus Gellius [10]. According to Sorsby [11], the Pseudoepigraphic description of the birth of Noah in the Book of Enoch the Prophet indicates that he was possibly an albino, and Revelation 1:14 describes an albino phenotype. The essential clinical features of albinism are well summarized in the following description, published in 1699 by Lionel Wafer [12]:

> There is one complexion so singular . . . that I never saw nor heard of any like them in any part of the world. . . . They are white . . . 'tis rather a milk-white, lighter than the colour of any [Europeans], and much like that of a white horse. . . . From their seeing so clear as they do in a moon-shiny night, we us'd to call them moon-ey'd. For they see not very well in the sun, poring in the clearest Day; their eyes being but weak, and running with water if the sun shine towards them; so that in the day-time they care not to go abroad. . . . When moon-shiny night's come, they are all life and activity, running abroad, and into the woods, skipping about like wild-bucks, and running as fast by moon-light, even in the gloom and shade of the woods, as the other [Indians] by Day, being as nimble as they, tho' not so strong and lusty. . . . Neither is the child of a man and woman of these white [Indians], white like the parents, but copper-colour'd as their parents were. . . . They were but short-lived.

The outstanding characteristics are the "milk-white" color and photophobia, with "eyes being but weak, and running with water if the sun shine towards them." The recessive inheritance is suggested by the fact that "neither is the child of a man and woman of these white [Indians], white like the parents, but copper-colour'd." The striking contrast of albino skin with the normal darkly pigmented skin of Indians and Negroes sets them apart, and many myths were conjured up about these strange "moon-ey'd" people. Several albino heroes are prominent in the mythology of the Cuna tribe of Indians residing on the San Blas Islands off the coast of Panama.

By 1913, the general outlines of what we now know about albinism and melanin production had been established or predicted. Albinism was one of the first inherited anomalies in humans to be investigated statistically on the basis of a population ascertainment by Raseri in 1879 [13]. Ehrmann [14] demonstrated that melanin was formed intracellularly by "melanoblasts" (now called *melanocytes*) and transferred to epithelial cells by "protoplasmic threads" which connected melanoblasts to epithelial cells (keratinocytes). He indicated that light was necessary to stimulate pigment production. Florence Durham [15], in 1904, demonstrated that tyrosinase activity could be found in the skin of pigmented animals but was absent in albino animals. Considerable experimental evidence on the nature of the defect in albinism led Sir Archibald Garrod [16] to speculate that albinism, among other disorders, was an inborn error of metabolism. In 1908, when enzyme chemistry was in its infancy, Garrod wrote:

> Three possible explanations of the phenomenon of albinism suggest themselves. We might suppose that the cells which usually contain pigment fail to take up melanins formed elsewhere; or that the albino has an unusual power of destroying these pigments; or again that he fails to form them. . . . It is very unlikely that the melanin is conveyed to the pigmented cells and there deposited, for all the evidence available indicates that the pigment is formed *in situ*, probably by the action of intracellular enzymes. . . . Only certain specialised cells appear to have the power of forming melanin. . . . Taking all the known facts into consideration, the theory that what the albino lacks is the power of forming melanin which is normally

possessed by certain specialised cells is that which has most in its favour and is probably the true one. If so, an intracellular enzyme is probably wanting in the subjects of this anomaly, an explanation which . . . brings albinism into line with some other inborn metabolic errors, of which a similar explanation is at least a possible one.

Pearson et al. [6] and Stannus [17] reported in 1913 their results of a worldwide survey of albinism and hypomelanotic disorders and proposed that albinism was ascribable to either the absence of "melanoblasts" or to the absence of tyrosinase activity, but they favored the theory that albinism was due to a structural defect. As will be seen, the various forms of albinism in which patients have decreased or absent melanotic pigment in skin, hair, or eyes with nystagmus, photophobia, and decreased visual acuity result in most albinotic disorders from an intracellular block in melanogenesis and in one type from an absence of pigment-forming cells (melanocytes) in peripheral tissues. This chapter, devoted to albinism in humans, reexamines Garrod's [16] proposal in the light of recent research in pigment-cell biology.

Albinism is found in fishes, amphibians, reptiles, and birds, as well as in humans and other mammals [18–23].

DEFINITION AND CLASSIFICATION

Melanocytes are distinctive, specialized dendritic cells in which the biosynthesis of melanin takes place. During embryonic development in mammals, precursor melanocytes, except in the retinal pigment epithelium, arise in the neural crest and actively migrate to peripheral sites (Fig. 15-1). The melanocytes of the retinal pigment epithelium are derived from the outer layer of the optic cup and differ morphologically from the melanocytes in other sites. In humans, mature melanocytes are normally present in certain characteristic regions: *skin* (hair bulbs, dermis, and the dermoepidermal junction), *mucous membranes, nervous system* (pia-arachnoid), *eye* (uveal tract and retinal pigment epithelium), *inner ear, cochlea* (wall of the modiolus, spiral lamina, Reissner's membrane and stria vascularis), and *vestibular system* (saccule, utricle, and ampullae) [24]. Melanin pigment is synthesized in specialized cytoplasmic organelles called *melanosomes*. The enzymatic conversion of the amino acid tyrosine to melanin is catalyzed by the aerobic oxidase *tyrosinase* (EC 1.14.18.1). Melanogenesis will be summarized later in this chapter. All melanocytes with the exception of those in the hair bulbs, retinal pigment epithelium, and inner ear appear to have the ability to form malignant melanomas.

The metabolic defects that are manifested as albinism may involve the entire melanocyte system (OCA) or melanocytes at a specific site (OA). The terminology used in the classification of the different types of albinism should clearly reflect the extent and, when possible, the nature of pigmentary involvement. One goal of human genetics is to relate specific variations in expressed characteristics (phenotype) to the hereditary information coded within the genome. Genetic terminology should reflect the precision of this knowledge. Use of the term *albinism* should be restricted to congenital heritable hypomelanosis that is limited to the eye (OA) or involves the eye and integument (OCA) and in which nystagmus, photophobia, and decreased visual acuity are present. In albinoidism there is

Table 15-1 Comparison of the characteristics of hypomelanotic diseases with features of oculocutaneous albinism

Characteristic	Ty-neg	Ty-pos	Ym	HPS	CHS
Hair color	White throughout life	White, yellow-tan; darkens with age	White at birth; yellow-red by 6 months	White, red, brown	Blond to dark brown; steel gray tint
Skin color	Pink to red	Pink-white to cream	White at birth; cream, slight tan on exposed skin	Cream-gray to light normal	Pink to pink-white
Pigmented nevi and freckles	Absent	May be present and numerous	Present	Present	Present
Susceptibility to skin neoplasia	++++	+++	Unknown	+++	++
Eye color	Gray to blue	Blue, yellow-brown; age- and race-dependent	Blue in infancy; darkens with age	Blue-gray to brown; age- and race-dependent	Blue to dark brown
Transillumination of iris	No visible pigment	Pigment cartwheel effect at pupil and limbus	Cartwheel effect in adults	None to cartwheel effect	Cartwheel effect to normal
Red reflex	Present	May be absent in dark-race adults	Present	Present in light Caucasians; not in dark races	Present, less after 5 years
Fundal pigment	0	0 to + in adults	0 to + in adults	0 to + in adults	+ to +++
Nystagmus	++++	++ to +++	+ to +++	+ to +++	0 to ++
Photophobia	++++	++ to +++	+ to ++	+ to ++++	0 to ++
Visual acuity	Most, legally blind; constant or worse with age; 20/200 to 20/400+	Children, severe defect; adults, same or better; 20/60 to 20/400+	Same as ty-neg; may improve with age; 20/90 to 20/400	20/70 to 20/400	Normal to moderate decrease
Serum tyrosine levels	Normal	Low normal to normal	Normal	Normal	Normal
β-Melanocyte-stimulating hormone levels	Normal	Normal	Unknown	Unknown	Unknown
Melanosome in hair bulbs	Stages I and II only	To early stage III, polyphagosomes	To stage III polyphagosomes	To stage III, polyphagosomes, pheomelanosomes	Giant to normal stage IV
Incubation of hair bulbs in tyrosine	No pigmentation	Pigmentation	None to questionable increase	Pigmentation	Pigmentation
Other	Heterozygotes have less than half normal tyrosinase activity	³HOH test suggests heterogeneity in ty-pos albinos	Hair bulb test shows increased red or yellow with tyrosine-cysteine incubation	Platelet defect; ceroid storage; cytoplasmic bodies in monocytes	Susceptibility to infection; giant lysosomal-like granules; lymphoreticular like malignancy

hypomelanism in skin and eye, but there is no nystagmus or decreased visual acuity. As will be shown subsequently, this clinical division is more than an arbitrary classification, since those forms with nystagmus and decreased visual acuity all have anomalous optic neuronal tracts, while those without nystagmus or reduced visual acuity do not show these defects. Most forms of OCA and OA have a defect in intracellular melanogenesis manifested by a partial or total reduction of melanin deposition on melanosomes and, in some forms, morphologically abnormal melanosomes. This definition would, for example, exclude circumscribed (spotty) hypomelanosis of the skin [25], which has erroneously been called *cutaneous albinism* but should more correctly be called *piebaldism*. The justification for this restriction of terminology is to be found in a number of recent studies with the electron microscope and with enzyme histochemistry.

The currently recognized types of OCA and OA in humans are listed in Tables 15-1 and 15-2, along with a summary of

their major clinical and histologic features. Although there is evidence that melanosomes in skin may be involved in some forms of OA [26, 27], the proposed classification provides some advantages over any used previously. Later, each of the various types of human albinism will be considered in detail. Basic to this survey is an understanding of the major features of melanin metabolism within the normal oculocutaneous melanocyte system of humans.

MELANIN AND NORMAL MELANIN PIGMENTATION

Epidermal Melanin Unit and Skin Color

Color variation in human skin derives chiefly from the presence within the epidermis of specialized melanin-bearing

Cross syndrome	Brown OCA	Rufous OCA	Autosomal dominant OCA	Black locks-albinism-deafness syndrome
White to light blond	Beige to light brown in Africans	Mahogany red to deep red	White to cream with reddish tint	Snow white with pigmented locks
Pink to pink-white	Cream to light tan on exposed skin	Reddish brown	White to cream	White with melanized macules
Present	May be present	May be present	May be present	May be present in macular areas
Unknown	Similar to Caucasians in Africa +	Low	Unknown	Unobserved, but probably ++++
Gray-blue	Hazel to light brown	Reddish brown to brown	Gray to blue	Gray-blue
Unknown; cataracts	Cartwheel effect	Slight	Translucent to cartwheel effect	No visible pigment
Unknown; cataracts	Present in children; may be absent in adults	Unknown	Present in children	Present in children and adults
Unknown; cataracts	+ to ++ in adults	+ to +++	0 to +	0
+++ to ++++	+ to ++	0 to ++	++ to +++	++++
Unknown	+ to ++	0 to ++	++ to +++	++++
Blind	20/30 to 20/100	Normal to 20/100	20/70 to 20/200	20/300 to 20/400+
Normal	Unknown	Unknown	Unknown	Unknown
Unknown	Unknown	Unknown	Unknown	Unknown
Scanty; stage III; some stage IV	Stage I to stage III, some lightly pigmented stage IV, polyphagosomes	Unknown	Stage I to early stage III; no structural abnormality	No melanocytes in white hair and skin; normal melanocytes and melanosomes in pigmented hair and skin;
Pigmentation	Pigmentation	Pigmentation	Pigmentation. Increased tyrosine activity in Golgi	White hair—0; pigmented hair—pigment increases
Oligophrenia; microphthalmia; gingival fibromatosis; athetosis	This defect recognized to date only in Africans and New Guineans	Seen in New Guineans and Africans	Melanocytes present in normal numbers	Profound sensorineural deafness; probably due to failure of embryonic neural elements to migrate from crest to ear

organelles, the melanosomes. Tanning of human skin on exposure to ultraviolet radiation (UVR) results from the presence of increased amounts of melanin within the epidermis. Melanosomes synthesized by melanocytes are passed to keratinocytes and transported within them to the epidermal surface. *Melanin must be present in keratinocytes* to impart a brown color, as viewed in the living skin. In some cases, the melanosomes are catabolized en route. New information indicates that the multicellular *epidermal melanin unit* (melanocyte and associated pool of keratinocytes), rather than the melanocyte alone, is the focal point for the control of melanin metabolism within mammalian epidermis (Fig. 15-2). Gross human skin color derives from the visual impact of the summed melanin pigmentation of the many epidermal melanin units [28].

Melanin pigmentation of human skin is divisible into two components: (1) *constitutive skin color* designates the cutaneous melanin pigmentation generated in accordance with cellular genetic programs in the absence of direct influences by ultraviolet radiation and is generally taken to be the level of pigmentation in those parts of the body habitually shielded from light; (2) *facultative (inducible) skin color* or "tan" characterizes the immediate and delayed tanning reactions elicited by direct exposure of the skin to UVR. Facultative color change is reversible in that the hyperpigmentation of the skin tends to decline toward the constitutive level when exposure to UVR is discontinued. Skin hyperpigmentation induced by endocrine changes, as in pregnancy and Addison's disease, also represents a type of facultative color change. Alterations in endocrine balance may significantly influence the response of human skin to UVR. Accordingly, facultative color changes in humans arise from the complex interplay of light, hormones, and the "tanning potential" set by the individual's genetic constitution.

The full extent of genetic involvement in *facultative color change* is not known. The capacity for facultative color change is broadly related to levels of constitutive skin color. In addi-

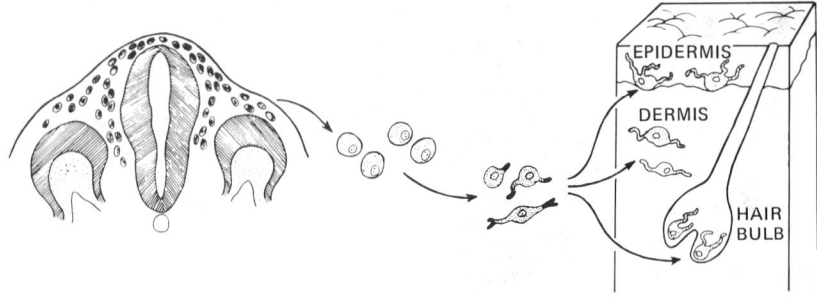

NEURAL CREST   MELANOBLASTS "MELANOGONIA"   MELANOCYTES

Figure 15-1 Schematic representation of embryonic derivation of melanocytes from the neural crest.

tion, the marked variation in the ability of very light-skinned individuals to tan on exposure to UVR suggests that gene action beyond that presently detectable in constitutive skin color is involved. The concepts of constitutive and facultative skin color as defined above are used throughout this chapter.

Constitutive Melanin Pigmentation

It has been estimated that the additive interaction of genes at three or four loci (i.e., three to four gene pairs) is sufficient to account for the variation in skin color between black and white Americans [29]. The range of color encompassed by this scheme is so broad that the same number of loci interacting might account for the difference in constitutive skin color throughout the human race. Reasons for believing that the actual situation may be considerably more complicated have been advanced by Harrison [30]. In addition to the polygenetic series that, through additive interactions determines levels of cutaneous pigmentation, other genes are known, as in albinism, to act "individually in partly or completely deleting melanin pigmentation." In mice, more than 147 genes at approximately 62 loci affect skin and hair color [23]. Genetic influences on human melanin pigmentation may be equally complex.

Melanin Biosynthesis

Melanin is synthesized by melanocytes in membrane-bound

Table 15-2 Comparison of the characteristics of the various forms of ocular albinism

Characteristic	X-linked (Nettleship)	Autosomal recessive ocular albinism	X-linked (Forsius-Eriksson)	OA-lentigines-deafness
Hair color	Normal to slight lightening	Normal	Normal	Normal
Skin color	Normal to mottled	Normal	Normal	Normal
Pigmented nevi and freckles	Present	Present	Present	Lentigines
Susceptibility to skin neoplasia	No	No	No	Unknown
Eye color	Normal range	Normal range	Normal range	Normal range
Transillumination of iris	Cartwheel, males; diaphanous, females	Cartwheel to diaphanous	Diaphanous males; normal females	Cartwheel to diaphanous
Red reflex	Present, males	Present, males	Present, males	Present
Fundal pigment	Males, 0; females, mosaic fundus	Males and females, 0 to +	Males, 0	0
Nystagmus	++ to ++++	++ to +++	++ to ++++	+++
Photophobia	++ to +++	++ to +++	++ to ++++	+++
Visual acuity	Moderate to severe decrease; 20/50 to 20/400	Moderate to severe decrease; 20/100 to 20/400	Moderate	20/200
Serum tyrosine levels	Unknown	Unknown	Unknown	Unknown
β-Melanocyte-stimulating hormone levels	Unknown	Unknown	Unknown	Unknown
Melanosomes	Abnormal giant and normal	Normal	Unknown; probably normal	Macromelanosomes in lentigines
Incubation of hair bulbs in tyrosine	Pigmentation	Pigmentation	Unknown; probably normal	Unknown
Other	X-linked; severely affected males; in carrier females, mosaic retina	Autosomal recessive; males and females equally affected	X-linked; males: protanopia; females: no mosaic retina; high axial myopia	Sensorineural deafness; autosomal dominant

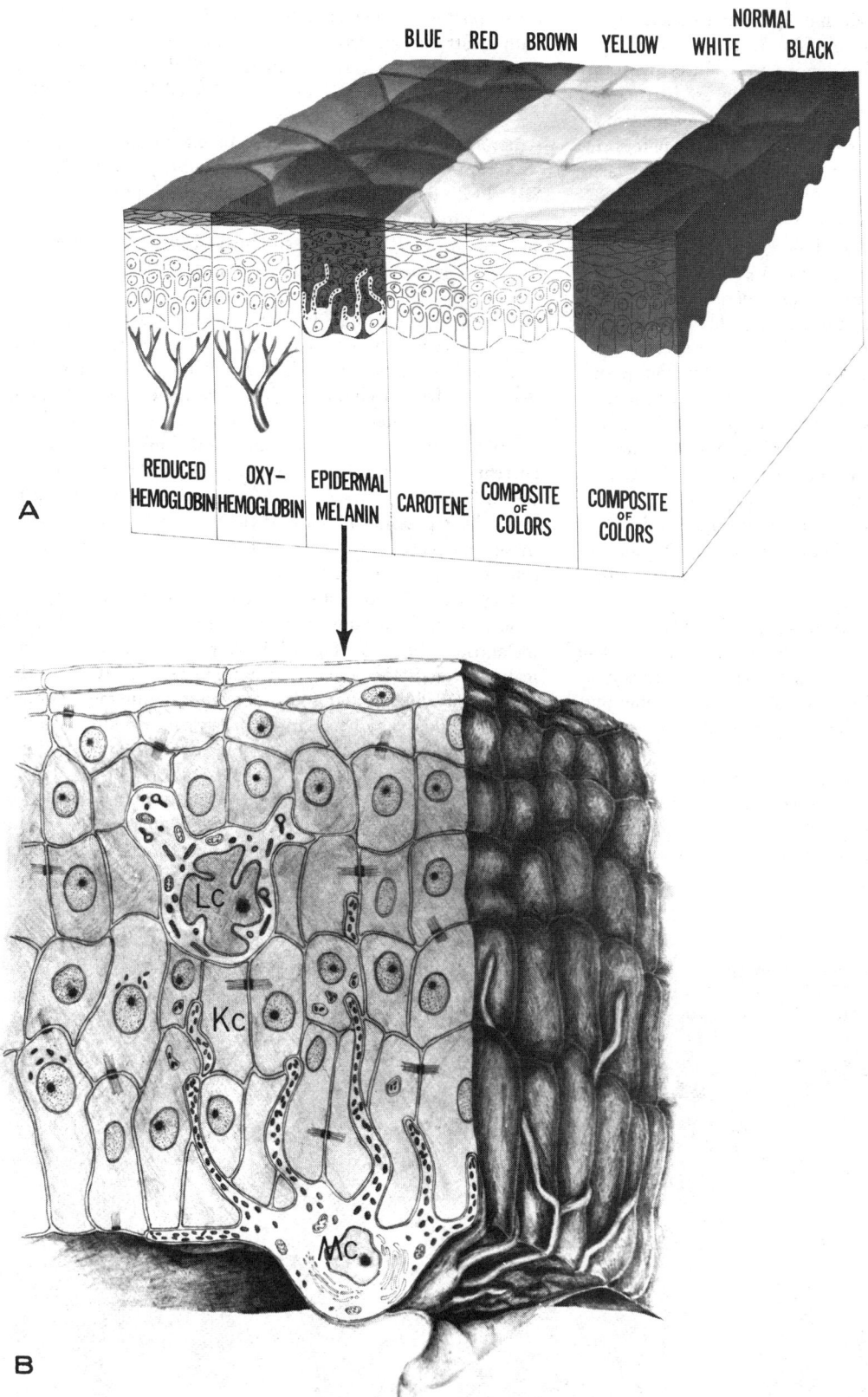

Figure 15-2 *A.* Schematic representation of the components of normal skin color. *B.* Epidermal melanin unit consisting of a melanocyte and associated pool of keratinocytes. Langerhans cell is located among the suprabasal keratinocytes. MC, melanocyte; KC, keratinocyte; LC, Langerhans cell.

particles, the melanosomes, which in epidermal structures are then transferred to keratinocytes [31] (Fig. 15-3). Electron microscopically fully formed melanosomes from brown- and black-pigmented hair appear as round to ellipsoid structures on which pigment is evenly distributed and are recognized as eumelanosomes. Melanosomes from red or yellow hair show an uneven distribution of pigment in a spotty or granular fashion and are recognized as pheomelanosomes.

Pheomelanosomes and eumelanosomes of follicular melanocytes at their earliest stage of development (stage I) are identical, i.e., multivesicular bodylike structures, round in shape, with a limiting membrane surrounding microvesicles (globulovesicular bodies) and filaments [32]. The filaments have a periodicity of approximately 100 Å. In eumelanogenesis, the stage II melanosome is oval in shape, and its numerous filaments become aligned parallel to the long axis of the melanosome. Melanin is subsequently deposited within the melanosome (stage III), ultimately producing a more or less homogeneous darkening of its interior (stage IV). Round, membrane-limited microvesicles (vesiculoglobular bodies) may be found within eumelanosomes at all stages of development. Electron-lucent spherical bodies are frequently found in the stage IV melanosome [32, 33]. One interpretation is that the electron-lucent bodies of stage IV melanosomes are microvesicles that are embedded in eumelanin that has been deposited on their surfaces but not within their interiors. The exact relationship between microvesicles within melanosomes and the electron-lucent bodies is unknown. It is possible that microvesicles are related to the incorporation of tyrosinase into the developing melanosomes [34].

The pheomelanosomes of human red hair apparently parallel eumelanosomes in their development but have pheomelanin deposited in irregular patches on the filamentous matrix [35, 36]. In some redheads the pheomelanosomes may have a granular rather than a filamentous interior [37].

The morphology of eumelanosomes and pheomelanosomes

forms part of the evidence that they have a two-step origin, with contributions from the rough endoplasmic reticulum/smooth endoplasmic reticulum (RER/SER) and Golgi endoplasmic reticulumlike/GOLGI (GERL/GOLGI) complex [34, 38–40]. A variety of evidence suggests that the filamentous structural matrix proteins of the eumelanosomes are synthesized on the RER and packaged in membranes in the RER or SER [33]. In turn, tyrosinase synthesized on the RER is enclosed in membrane-limited microvesicles at one or more sites in the GERL/GOLGI complex. The tyrosinase-bearing microvesicles are thought to fuse with the structural premelanosomes of RER/SER origin, yielding a melanosome fully equipped with tyrosinase [33, 34]. Biochemical and cytochemical studies indicate that tyrosinase may be located in the limiting membrane as well as in the matrix of the melanosome [41, 42]. The mechanisms that determine the abilities of melanosome-related vesicles to recognize each other and fuse to form complete melanosomes are totally unknown. Based on current knowledge of epidermal and follicular melanocytes, the RER, SER, and GERL/GOLGI complex, as in other secretory cells, represents a highly efficient system for the rapid synthesis and packaging of melanosomes for export to receptor cells, in this case, keratinocytes.

The chemical conversion of the substrate amino acid, tyrosine, to both eumelanin and pheomelanin occurs within the melanosome [43–45] (Fig. 15-4). At the heart of the biochemical pathway is the copper-containing enzyme tyrosinase (EC 1.14.18.1), which initiates melanogenesis within melanosomes by catalyzing the hydroxylation of L-tyrosine to L-β-3, 4-dihydroxyphenylalanine (dopa) and the oxidation of dopa to dopaquinone [32, 33, 44].

A branch point occurs at the dopaquinone step, leading to either eumelanogenesis (slow reaction) or pheomelanogenesis (fast reaction). The intermediate dopaquinone may alternatively react with cysteine [45, 46], leading to the formation of cysteinyldopa intermediates and eventually pheomelanin, or

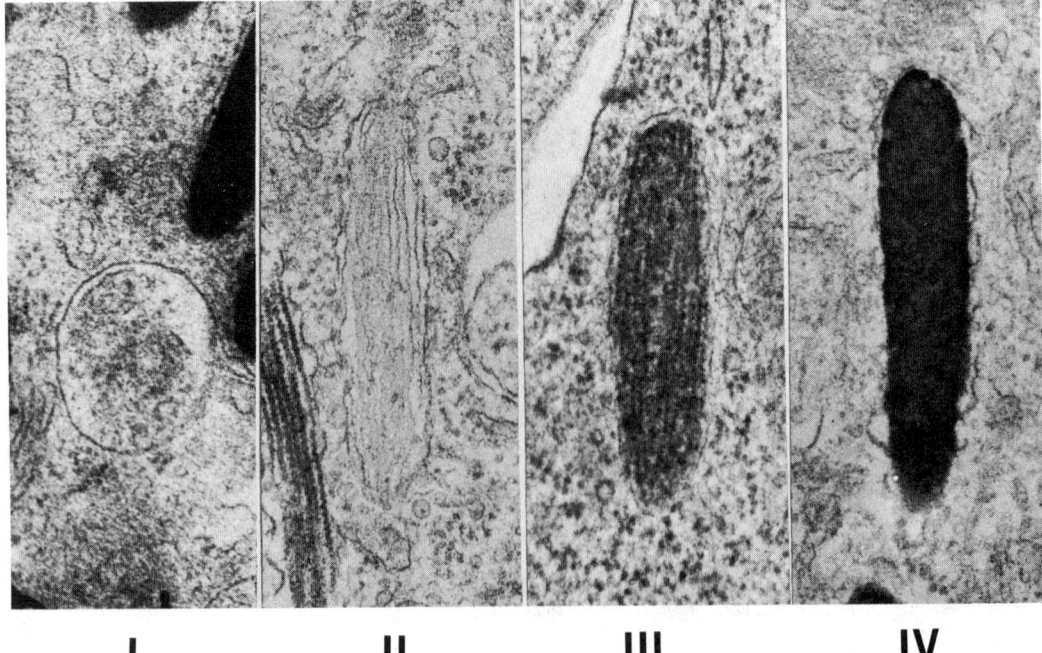

I   II   III   IV

Figure 15-3 Stages in the development of the eumelanosome (see text for detailed description).

Figure 15-4 Postulated metabolic pathways of eumelanin and pheomelanin biosynthesis. Both begin with the enzymatic (tyrosinase) conversion of tyrosine to dopa to dopaquinone. Numbers indicate points in the pathways that present evidence suggests may be under regulatory control. (1) The tyrosinase step is present in epidermal melanocytes and under genetic control (c locus in mice) and is the step defective in ty-neg OCA. (2) The tyrosine hydroxylase step initiates the catechol pathway, is present in the CNS-adrenal system, and appears intact in albinos; all have had normal pigmentation in the CNS. (3) Pheomelanogenesis is initiated by the addition of cysteine (or glutathione-minor) to dopaquinone and appears to be under genetic control, possibly through regulation of the melanocyte environment control of cysteine levels [475–477]. Points 4, 5, and 6 are possible sites of posttyrosinase control within the melanocyte. (4) Dopachrome conversion factor is thought to accelerate the conversion of dopachrome to 5,6-dihydroxyindole. (5) 5,6-Dihydroxyindole conversion factor postulated to accelerate melanin formation under melanotropin influence. (6) A blocking factor which restricts melanogenesis at this step [50–52]. Most melanin polymers in vivo contain elements of both pheo- and eumelanogenesis in varying proportions. The dotted arrows indicate possible incorporation of intermediates in eumelanin polymers. The eumelanin pathway was adapted from Mason [478]; the pheomelanin pathway was adapted from Prota [45, 46].

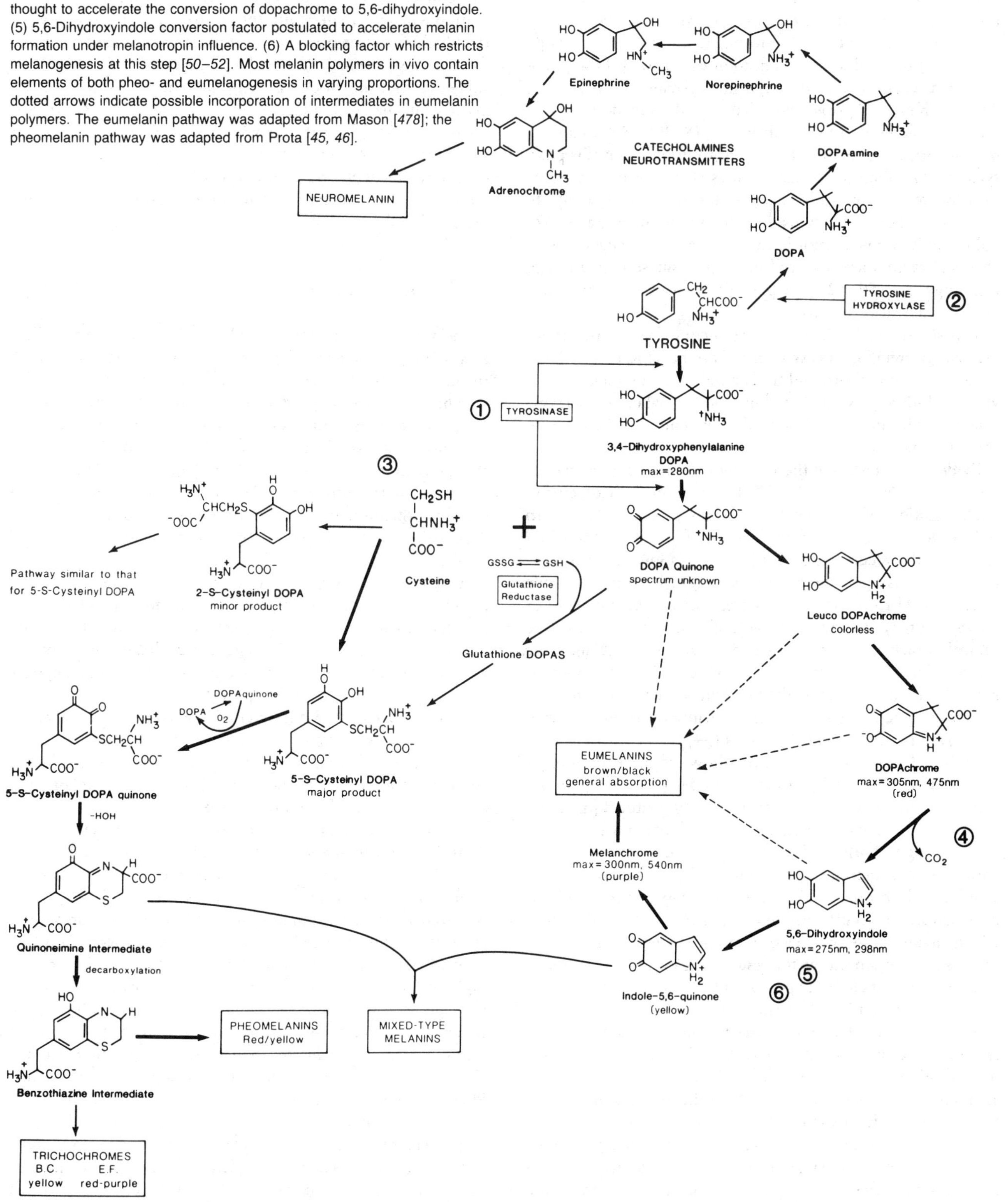

proceed to form the colorless intermediate leukodopachrome and eventually eumelanin (Fig. 15-4). All reactions subsequent to the synthesis of dopaquinone generally have been considered to occur spontaneously in vivo through auto-oxidation, but a number of observations in humans and animals have suggested that posttyrosinase regulation of melanogenesis exists in vivo and that some regulatory steps are under genetic control. Genetic control at the dopaquinone step is adduced from the poorly understood inheritance of red hair in humans and from various mouse mutants which produce mostly pheomelanins. Yellow mutant human albinism probably involves a mutation of a gene regulating this switch point, since yellow mutant hair bulbs fail to pigment in tyrosine or dopa solutions but produce intensification of red or yellow pheomelanins when incubated in tyrosine-cysteine mixtures [47]. Siberian hamsters grow white hairs in the fall despite high tyrosinase activity in their hair bulbs [48, 49]. Melatonin has been identified as the probable agent to bring about this posttyrosinase inhibition of melanogenesis [49]. The initial interaction of melatonin with melanocytes involves binding to receptors either in the cytosol or the plasma membrane [49]. Subsequent events are not known. Recent work suggests that chemical factors are involved in posttyrosinase regulation of melanogenesis [50–52]. The possible role of these factors will be discussed subsequently.

Tyrosinase (EC 1.14.18.1) is a bifunctional, copper-containing glycoprotein [53, 54] synthesized on the RER, glycosolated in the Golgi apparatus, and transferred to the premelanosome via GERL-derived vesiculoglobular bodies, where the enzyme functions physiologically to produce melanin on the melanosome matrix [55–58].

Evidence suggests that there are two atoms of copper in each human tyrosinase molecule [53]. Dopa serves as a cofactor in the utilization of tyrosine by tyrosinase, possibly acting to reduce divalent copper to the cuprous form [44]. The exact role played by cuprous ions in the oxidation of tyrosine is unknown. Based on the reactivity of cuprous ions in simple systems in vitro, it has been suggested that cuprous ions of tyrosinase may interact with molecular oxygen to form free radicals which oxidize tyrosine to dopa and other melanogenic intermediates [59]. Carbohydrates, which constitute about 20 per unit of purified mammalian tyrosinase, may serve in binding the enzyme to the melanosomal membrane or matrix or in stabilizing the enzyme at these sites [54].

Mammalian tyrosinase has been shown to occur in three or four different forms by polyacrylamide gel electrophoresis [60–63]. The isoenzymes are currently designated T_1 through T_4, with T_1 having the greatest anodal mobility and T_4 remaining close to the origin [54, 64]. Amino acid analyses of the various isoenzymes are virtually identical, and the molecular weights of the protein chains based on amino acid content indicate identical molecular weights of approximately 65,000 [64]. Kinetic identity [54] and electrophoretic evidence indicate that these isoenzymes occur as the result of posttranslational modifications of a single basic polypeptide chain or as an electrophoretic artifact [54]. The isoenzymes are immunologically identical [65, 66]. These data suggest that the isoenzymes are encoded by a single genetic locus [64]. T_4 is a relatively insoluble membrane-bound tyrosinase associated with the melanosomal matrix. Dissociation of T_4 from the melanosomal membrane converts it to soluble T_1. T_2 appears to be an artifact caused by deamination of T_3 under electrophoretic conditions [52]. Current evidence suggests that the de novo form of tyrosinase is synthesized as T_3 (soluble). Neutral sugars and sialic acid are added, forming T_1 (soluble), which is then bound to the melanosomal matrix, forming T_4 (insoluble) [52, 54].

Several factors are involved in posttyrosinase regulation of melanogenesis [50–52] (Fig. 15-4). These factors are currently designated: (1) dopachrome conversion factor, which promotes the reduction: decarboxylation of dopachrome to 5,6-dihydroxyindole; (2) 5,6-dihydroxyindole conversion factor, which promotes the oxidation of 5,6-dihydroxyindole to indole-5,6-quinone; and (3) blocking factor, which inhibits oxidation of 5,6-dihydroxyindole to indole-5,6-quinone. The two conversion factors increase the rate of visible pigment formation when incubated with the appropriate substrates, while the blocking factor prevents melanin formation and results in the colorless compound 5,6-dihydroxyindole [50, 51]. It is suggested that the blocking factor is bound to T_1 and may be involved in enzyme inhibition during transfer of the enzyme to the melanosome [52]. If posttyrosinase factors are involved in regulatory control in melanocytes, they provide additional sites in the biosynthetic pathway at which the process may be interrupted and may be of significance in certain forms of albinism to be discussed shortly.

Melanin Structure

Eumelanins are intractably insoluble, black-brown in color, and of high molecular weight. Pheomelanins are yellow through reddish brown in color and also of high molecular weight but are readily soluble in dilute alkali. Closely related to the pheomelanins, and frequently grouped with them, are the low molecular weight trichochromes. Both are derived from the interaction of cysteine with dopaquinone [45, 46]. Eumelanin is now thought to be a heteropolymer derived from the copolymerization of 5,6-dihydroxyindole and several of its precursors, such as dopaquinone and dopachrome [32] (Fig. 15-4).

As eumelanin polymerization progresses, the developing polymer is thought to entrap free radicals and to undergo partial degradation by hydrogen peroxide generated during the auto-oxidative process [67]. These complicated interactions alter the structure of eumelanin, making molecular analysis extremely difficult [45, 46, 67]. Blosis [67] maintains that the free radicals generated during eumelanin synthesis are the key to explaining why it contains several types of monomers and covalent bonds, has an irregular structure, contains entrapped, stabilized free radicals, and has a complex pattern of light absorption resulting in a black appearance.

Pheomelanins and trichochromes which are present primarily in hair and feathers are derived from the addition of cysteine to dopaquinone to form cysteinyldopa in two isomeric forms, 5-S-cysteinyldopa and 2-S-cysteinyldopa, which are oxidized to cysteinylquinone [45, 46]. The latter undergoes cyclization and reduction by cysteinyldopa to form dihydrobenzothiazine, which is then converted into trichochromes or high molecular weight pheomelanins by covalent bonding through poorly understood oxidative processes. Although the structure of some trichochromes has been established, little is known about the high molecular weight of pheomelanins. Trichochromes are modified dimers of dihydrobenzothiazine. Pheomelanins and eumelanins are generally thought to be complexed in vivo with proteins of the melanosomal matrix to form melanoprotein, a property which adds further complications to their chemical analysis [32]. Whittaker has concluded that melanin is not covalently linked to protein in chick embryo melanosomes [68]. The distinction between pheomelanins and eumelanins may not be as clear-cut as the foregoing statements would seem to indicate. Cysteinyldopa is synthesized by eumelanocytes as well as pheomelanocytes and may have a role in the melanization of melanosomes in both [32].

Transfer and Fate of Melanosomes within Keratinocytes

Melanosomes synthesized by melanocytes are transferred to keratinocytes of the skin and hair by means of dendritic processes [32]. The melanocytes of the epidermal-dermal interface and of the matrix of the hair bulb project their dendrites between each keratinocyte. In the epidermis, each melanocyte supplies melanosomes to a group of approximately 36 keratinocytes. This partnership of a single melanocyte and its constellation of keratinocytes is expressed in the term *epidermal melanin unit* (Fig. 15-2). It denotes the functional as well as structural integration of a melanocyte and associated keratinocytes at levels of biologic organization that transcend those of the individual component cells [69].

Melanosomes within keratinocytes occur as discrete particles (nonaggregated) or as aggregates of two or more melanosomes within membrane-limited organelles (Fig. 15-3). These melanosome-containing organelles, previously termed *melanosome complexes*, resemble the membrane-limited, melanosome-containing organelles identified as phagolysosomes within macrophages. Aggregated melanosomes in keratinocytes appear to undergo gradual degradation into small electron-dense particles. This phenomenon of aggregation of melanosomes into complexes or alternatively occurring as single melanosomes in keratinocytes is variable, and the factors that determine it are not completely understood [70]. Aggregation appears to be a size-dependent phenomenon [71], inasmuch as small ellipsoidal melanosomes aggregate in the form of a secondary lysosome and undergo degradation. Larger ellipsoidal melanosomes do not appear to aggregate within keratinocytes. Each phagocytized large melanosome forms part of a secondary lysosome and is possibly less prone to degradation than are melanosomes forming complexes. While there is a general tendency for large melanosomes to exist as single nonaggregated melanosomes in keratinocytes and for small melanosomes to aggregate into phagolysosomes [70, 71], there is no agreement as to the critical size above which melanosomes are arranged singly within keratinocytes. Estimates range from 0.4 to 1 μm [72]. Further, while melanosomes in keratinocytes of unexposed skin from Australian aborigines and African blacks tend to occur as single large melanosomes, whereas those from Caucasians, Orientals, and Amerindians are smaller and predominantly aggregated in phagolysosomes [70–75], this difference is not absolute and the pattern can be altered by trauma, UVR, and other factors [76, 77].

The biosynthesis of melanosomes within melanocytes depends on cues arising in the dermis and throughout the complex levels of biologic organization which characterize the epidermal melanin unit [78]. The reported changes in lysosomes alone suggest that the metabolic activity of keratinocytes is significantly altered by the arrival of melanosomes from melanocytes. These metabolic changes possibly extend beyond those associated with lysosomes and, by feedback control, affect the melanocytes in which the melanosomes originated. Products derived from melanosome degradation or from other sources within keratinocytes can conceivably pass downward by way of the dendrites or the intercellular spaces [78, 79] to regulate melanocyte function.

Facultative Melanin Pigmentation: Action of Light

Physiologic Responses   Solar radiation profoundly influences facultative skin color. The increase in melanin pigmentation after exposure of human skin to sunlight or to UVR from artificial sources is familiarly known as "tanning." Tanning involves two distinct biologic phenomena: (1) immediate tanning and (2) delayed tanning. Immediate tanning is optimally produced by both long UVR (320 to 380 nm) and visible (400 to 700 nm) light, and delayed tanning is optimally stimulated by exposure to the so-called sunburn spectrum (290 to 320 nm) and to a lesser extent by exposure to long-wave UVR and visible radiation.

Immediate tanning can best be seen in moderately to heavily pigmented individuals or in the previously exposed (tanned) areas of fair-skinned individuals. The skin begins to become hyperpigmented within 5 to 10 min on exposure to the midday summer sun and is maximally pigmented after 1 h of irradiation. The hyperpigmented areas, when withdrawn from exposure to light, fade rapidly within the first 30 min, and thereafter the color usually fades gradually, so that after 3 to 4 h, the irradiated areas are barely hyperpigmented. Sometimes, after prolonged sun exposure (90 to 120 min), residual hyperpigmentation may be visible for as long as 24 to 36 h, after which time newly synthesized melanin (delayed tanning) begins to pigment the skin.

Delayed tanning involves new production of melanosomes and therefore appears slowly over a period of days after exposure to UVR. An increased tyrosinase reaction is demonstrable histochemically at 48 to 72 h following exposure. No increased tyrosinase reaction is evident in immediate tanning because new melanosomes are not synthesized.

Light Exposure and the Epidermal Melanin Unit   The immediate tanning reaction involves (1) a rapid transfer of melanosomes from melanocytes to keratinocytes elicited by the active, motive force of microfilaments and microtubules; (2) rapid redistribution of melanosomes in melanocytes; and (3) an increase in the degree of melanization of melanosomes due either to photo-oxidation of melanin in melanosomes or to the enzyme-mediated oxidation of melanin.

Hyperpigmentation of the skin in delayed tanning is due to the following seven changes in the normal process of melanin pigmentation: (1) an increase in the number of functional melanocytes as the result of proliferation of melanocytes and also possibly the activation of dormant or resting melanocytes; (2) hypertrophy of melanocytes and increased arborization of their dendrites; (3) augmentation of melanosomal synthesis manifested by an increase in the number of stages I to IV melanosomes; (4) an increase in the rate of melanization in melanosomes; (5) an increase in the transfer of melanosomes from melanocytes to keratinocytes as the result of increased turnover of keratinocytes; (6) most notably in Caucasoids and Mongoloids, an increase in the size of melanosome complexes and possibly altered melanosome degradation within keratinocytes; and (7) activation of tyrosinase as a result of the direct effect of radiation on the tyrosinase-inhibiting sulfhydryl compounds of the epidermis [80].

TYPES OF ALBINISM IN HUMANS

Oculocutaneous forms of albinism (OCA) are hereditary disorders in which there is a congenital absence or reduction of melanin pigment in the skin, hair, and eyes, accompanied by hypoplasia of the fovea, nystagmus, photophobia, and decreased visual acuity [1, 2, 4, 81]. Ten disorders have been identified in humans which show these clinical features, but with some variation in the severity of each [2, 82]. These include tyrosinase-negative (ty-neg) OCA [15, 16, 83, 84]; tyrosinase-positive (ty-pos) OCA [4, 5, 83, 84]; Hermansky-Pudlak syndrome (HPS) [82–85]; Chédiak-Higashi syndrome (CHS) [86–89]; Cross syndrome [90–93]; brown OCA [94]; rufous OCA [3, 6, 95, 96]; autosomal dominant (AD-OCA) [2, 97]; black locks, albinism, and deafness of sensorineural type (BADS) [2]; and yellow mutant (ym) OCA [47, 98]. With the exception of AD-OCA, all are inherited as autosomal recessive traits [2, 99]. They can be distinguished from one another on the basis of clinical and biochemical criteria [2, 3, 47, 100], as well as by their genetic characteristics as determined by matings of albinos of different genotypes [4, 84, 101–104] and distribution in various populations [2, 4, 7, 8, 82, 105–111]. Thus, the classic description of albinism as an autosomal recessive trait due to a defect in a single enzyme, tyrosinase [112], must be modified to include a number of distinct genetic diseases, most of which show tyrosinase activity [4, 82].

Patients with ocular forms of albinism have hypopigmented irides and fundi, and hypoplasia of the fovea accompanied by nystagmus, photophobia, and decreased visual acuity. The skin is normal to slightly hypopigmented. Giant abnormal melanosomes [26, 113], occur in dermal and fundal melanocytes in the X-linked Nettleship-Falls (XOAN) form of the trait [114–117] while in autosomal recessive ocular albinism (AROA) [26, 81] dermal melanosomes are normal. Traditionally, two X-linked types of OA have been recognized. In the more common form, XOAN [114, 115], the heterozygous females usually show mosaic patterns of retinal pigment compatible with a Lyonization effect of genes on the X chromosome [115, 118, 119]. In the Forsius-Eriksson type [120],

which may not represent a true type of OA [121], retinal mosaicism has not been observed [120, 122].

Albinoidism [2], which lacks nystagmus, photophobia, and decreased visual acuity, may occur in oculocutaneous forms [123, 124], associated with deafness [125], secondary to a metabolic error, as in Menkes' syndrome [126], as an inconsistent feature in Apert syndrome [127], and in a Waardenburglike condition [128].

Piebaldism [129] (leukism) [22], heterochromia irides, and white hair locks [8, 130] are conditions in which portions of the skin, hair, and eyes are congenitally hypopigmented. Many of these "spotty" forms of depigmentation are associated with deafness. Vitiligo, in which the skin is normally pigmented at birth but becomes depigmented later in life, often shows a distinct inheritance pattern compatible with an autosomal dominant trait [131, 132]. All these conditions and those metabolic conditions in which the patient is normally pigmented at birth but may later become depigmented (e.g., Menkes' syndrome [126], phenylketonuria [133–135], and kwashiorkor [4]) are not considered forms of albinism and will not be included here. (See Ref. 136 for a review of hypomelanotic disorders.)

The general clinical, biochemical, and genetic features of the various forms of OCA and OA are summarized in Tables 15-1 and 15-2.

Oculocutaneous Albinism

Tyrosinase-negative (Ty-neg) Oculocutaneous Albinism [5, 83, 84] This form of albinism (approximate synonyms: *complete perfect albinism* [6, 137–139], *albinism* [15, 140], and *albinism I* [141, 142]) may be considered the classic Garrod [16] type of albinism in that there is no clinically detectable pigment in skin, hair, or eyes, nor is there evidence of tyrosinase activity in tissues incubated in L-tyrosine or L-dopa [4, 83, 84, 100]. Hair bulbs from patients with this type of albinism do not have pigment discernible by light (Fig. 15-5A) or electron microscopy (Fig. 15-6A). Melanocytes are present in skin, hair, and eyes, but they contain only stage I and stage II melanosomes, with no evidence of pigment accumula-

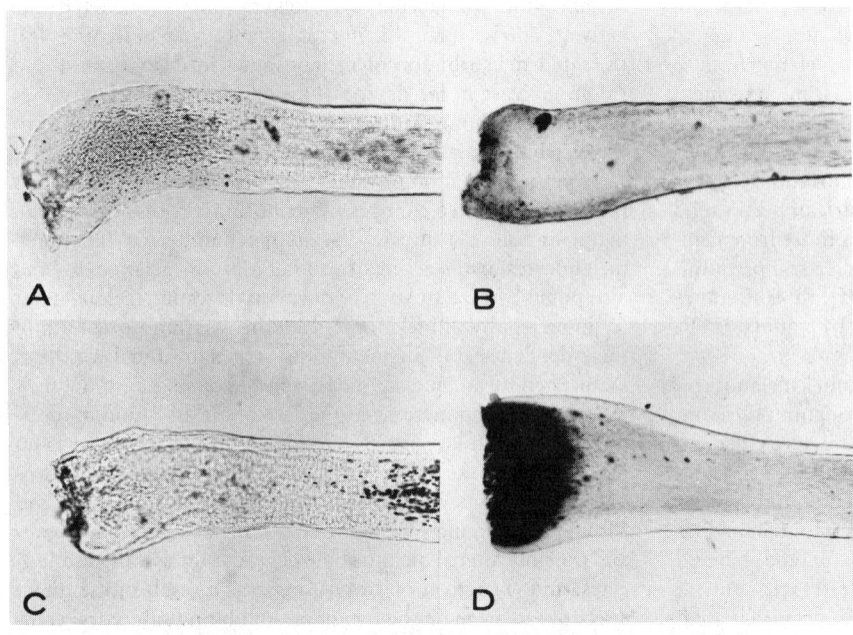

Figure 15-5 Comparison of hair bulbs from a ty-neg and a ty-pos albino. Hair bulbs from a ty-neg albino: *A*, freshly epilated; *B*, after incubation in 80 mg L-tyrosine per 100 dl of 0.1 *N* phosphate buffer, pH 6.8, for 12 h. Similarly treated hair bulbs from a ty-pos albino: *C*, freshly epilated; *D*, after incubation in L-tyrosine as above. No pigmentation is formed in the ty-neg hair bulb, while the ty-pos hair bulb forms adequate pigment. *(From Witkop et al. [84].)*

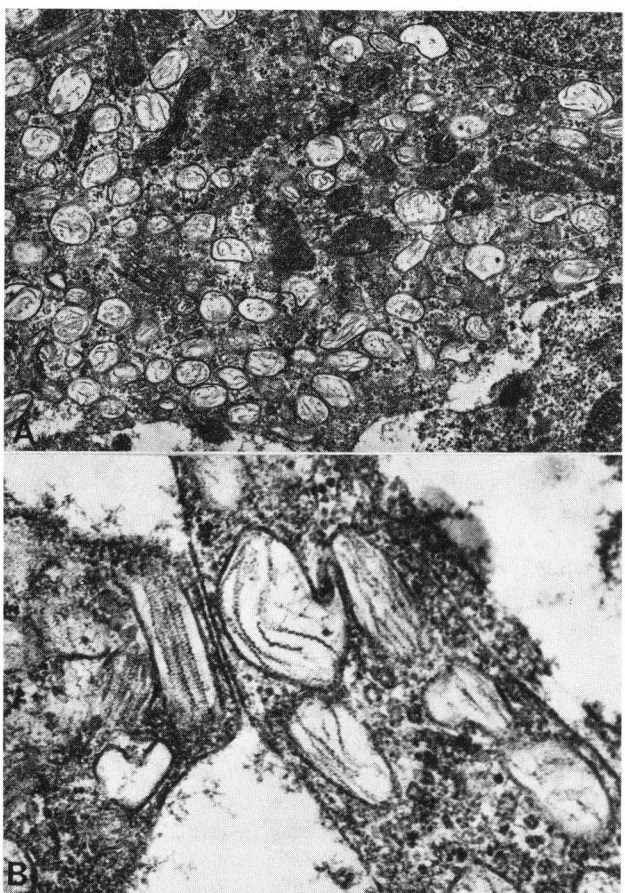

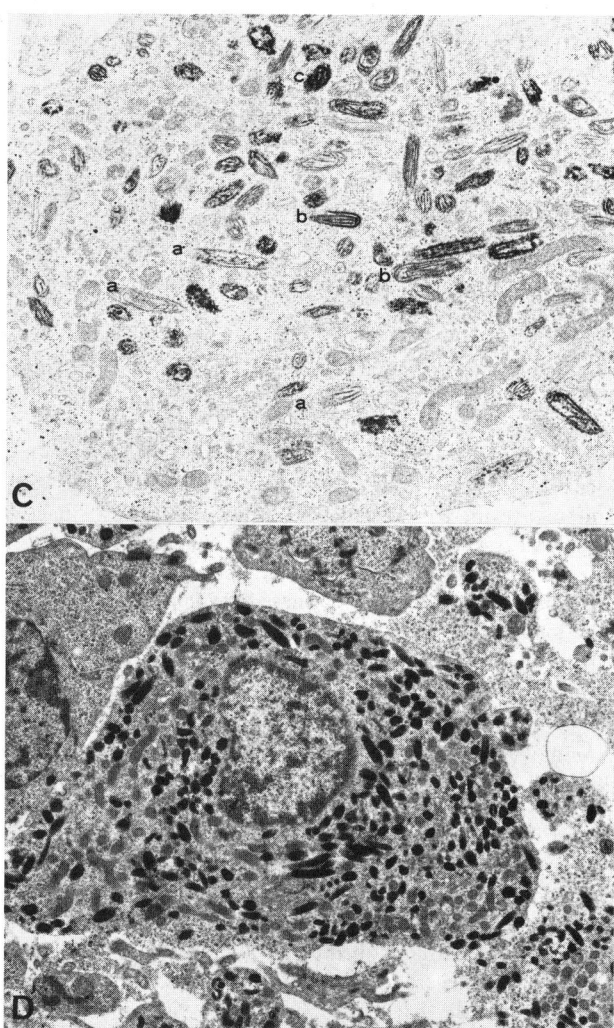

Figure 15-6 Thin-section electron photomicrographs of ty-neg (*A* and *B*) and ty-pos (*C* and *D*) hair bulbs. *A.* Freshly epilated hair bulb from a ty-neg albino, and *(B)* after incubation in L-tyrosine as above, showing stage II melanosomes containing no pigment on the matrix. *A.* ×48,000; *B,* ×66,000. *C.* Freshly epilated hair bulb from a ty-pos albino showing (a) stage II unpigmented melanosomes, (b) lightly pigmented early stage III melanosomes, and, rarely, (c) pigmented stage IV melanosomes. ×27,500. *D.* After incubation in L-tyrosine, nearly all melanosomes have been converted to stage IV melanosomes. ×10,250. *(From Witkop et al. [84].)*

tion on the melanosomal matrix (Fig. 15-6*A*). Hair bulbs incubated in L-tyrosine or L-dopa by the method of Kugelman and van Scott [5] do not form pigment discernible visually (Fig. 15-5*B*) or by electron-microscopic means (Fig. 15-6*B*). (See "Differential Diagnosis and Hair Bulb Incubation Test" below.)

Ty-neg albinos from various pigmentary (racial) backgrounds have similar phenotypic characteristics. All have snow-white hair; pink-white skin; gray to blue-gray irides in tangential illumination; a prominent red reflex from a completely unmelanized fundus (giving a "pink-eye" appearance); very diaphanous irides with no cartwheel effect on transillumination and through which the lens is visible [4, 143]; severe nystagmus and photophobia [3, 4]; and a markedly decreased visual acuity [3, 144]. Hypoplasia of the macula is always present. The foveal pit is absent. There is absence of pigment in the macula lutea, and the normal hyperpigmentation surrounding the fovea is lacking [145] (Table 15-3). After prolonged exposure to sunlight, the hair tips may turn a light yellow, which has been interpreted as a change in the keratin configuration. Brown-pigmented nevi are not found on the skin, but accumulations of nevus cells are detectable as small reddish or purplish-red spots on the skin. The two most impor-

tant clinical signs of ty-neg OCA are lack of pigment in the irides and absence of pigment in skin and hair.

Approximately 90 percent of ty-neg albinos have a moderate to severe strabismus. Most frequent is esotropia (80 percent); the remainder are exotropic. Exposure of the patient to bright sunlight will accentuate both the nystagmus and the strabismus. The visual acuity of most ty-neg albinos has been 20/200 or greater, with most patients remaining the same or becoming worse with age [3].

Electron photomicrographs of ty-neg albino hair bulbs show that they contain numerous melanocytes filled with stage I intermediate vesicles, and stage II early melanosomes, in which the unmelanized matrix is plainly visible [84, 146, 147]. In this unmelanized stage, a prominent melanosomal matrix may be distinguished. The cross-linked fibers of the melanosomal matrix closely resemble the matrix found in stage II melanosomes from normal hair types. Following incubation in L-tyrosine or L-dopa, there is no evidence of any increased pigmentation in the stage II melanosomes, nor is there any evidence of enzyme activity in the GERL apparatus, endoplasmic reticulum, or vesicular bodies [4, 84, 147]. In this disease, melanosomes do not develop past stage II. Premelanosomes are found lying in the cytoplasm of the melanocyte or packed into its dendrites and are passed into keratinocytes [82].

Serum levels of L-tyrosine, copper, and β-melanocyte-stimulating hormone (β-MSH) in ty-neg albinos are within normal

Table 15-3   Ophthalmologic findings in Ty-neg albinos

	No. tested	Mean acuity	Range of acuity	Mean trans-illumination	Mean nystagmus	Fundus pigment
Homozygotes						
Caucasian	31	20/300	200–400	3.0	3.0	0
Negro	8	20/300	200–400	3.0	3.0	0
Heterozygotes						
Caucasian	44			0.6 (26 individuals were +)		
Negro	10			0.3 (3 individuals were +)		

limits. There is no evidence of a pigment inhibitor in the serum of ty-neg albinos [4, 47]. Hair bulbs from normal red-haired individuals and from ty-pos albinos incubated in serum of ty-neg albinos readily form pigment [47].

All available evidence indicates a mutation of the tyrosinase locus such that no active tyrosinase is synthesized [4, 47, 84], and further, there is no evidence of the synthesis of an inactive tyrosinase protein. In this respect, ty-neg human albinism resembles c-locus albinism in mice. Recent evidence strongly suggests that the c locus (tyrosinase locus) in mice is a regulatory locus rather than a locus affecting the structure of the tyrosinase protein [148]. Tyrosinase isolated from various c-locus mutants in mice appears to be identical in structure and function but varies in amount [148].

Caucasian ty-neg heterozygotes may have detectable clinical differences in iris translucency from normal [116, 117]. While abnormal iris translucency is found in some ty-neg Caucasian heterozygotes, it is rarely encountered in Negro heterozygotes (Table 15-3). Even among Caucasians, this sign is not sufficiently precise to make it a reliable indicator of the carrier state [3, 143]. Chemical detection of the heterozygote state of ty-neg albinism has been developed by King and Witkop [100, 149], utilizing a micromethod adapted from Pomerantz [150], which depends upon the detection of [³H]OH production from a tritiated tyrosine substrate. The test utilizes anagen hair bulbs as the tissue source of enzyme activity. Ty-neg albino hair bulbs produce no increase in [³H]OH when incubated in [³H]tyrosine (Fig. 15-7). The obligate heterozygotes of ty-neg albinism produce less than half the amount of tritiated water produced by normally pigmented subjects [149]. This test determines the free unbound tyrosinase (T_1, T_3). Because the heterozygotes are normally pigmented, it is postulated that T_1 tyrosinase is immediately bound to the melanosome as T_4 in the heterozygote, leaving no excess unbound, soluble enzyme. Hence the test indicates little or no enzymatic activity in the heterozygote rather than the 50 percent activity expected theoretically in carriers of the gene.

While ty-neg albinism in humans appears to be the homologue of the c-locus albinism in animals, certain reservations must be entertained. Tissues from c/c mice show essentially the same ultrastructural features of melanocytes and melanosomes found in humans and react to L-tyrosine and L-dopa incubation and enzyme activity in a manner similar to that of human ty-neg tissue. Linkage studies in mice and rats show that the albinism (c-locus) and β-hemoglobin loci are linked [151, 152]. What may have been ty-neg albinism and sickle-cell hemoglobin have been observed to segregate in the same human kindred [153]. Ty-pos albinism and sickle-cell hemoglobin show no evidence for linkage [4].

Tyrosinase-positive (Ty-pos) Oculocutaneous Albinism [4, 5, 82–84]   Adults with this form of albinism (approximate synonyms: *complete imperfect albinism* [137, 138] *albinoidism* [83], and *albinism II* [141, 142]) usually have some clinically detectable pigment. Patients have evidence of tyrosinase activity when tissues such as hair bulbs are incubated in L-tyrosine or L-dopa [3–5, 83, 100, 149]. Hair bulbs from patients with ty-pos albinism frequently have a few pigment granules discernible with the light microscope (Fig. 15-5C), and lightly pigmented stage III melanosomes can be observed in thin-section electron photomicrographs (Fig. 15-6C). Hair bulbs incubated by the method of Kugelman and van Scott [5] form increased amounts of pigment discernible with a light microscope (Fig. 15-5D), and increased pigmentation of melanosomes can be seen with the electron microscope (Fig. 15-6D). (See "Differential Diagnosis and Hair Bulb Incubation Test" below.)

The major clinical feature distinguishing ty-pos albinism from ty-neg albinism is that some melanin pigment is formed in skin, hair, and eyes. The onset of visible pigment formation is delayed, so that infants with this form of albinism, regardless of their ethnic (pigmentary) background, may phenotypically resemble the ty-neg albino infant. The ty-pos albino accumulates small amounts of pigment with age. The intensity of the pigment accumulated depends upon the pigmentary (racial) background of the patient. Phenotypically, the clinical characteristics of the ty-pos albino overlap those of both the ty-neg albino and normal lightly pigmented individuals. Many ty-pos Caucasian albino infants and some adults may phenotypically resemble ty-neg Caucasian albinos. Some ty-pos adult Negro albinos have been observed to have skin color darker than that of some normal blond Caucasians. Although most ty-pos albi-

Figure 15-7   Mean tyrosine oxidized in pmoles per 120 min for hair bulbs from normal persons with different hair colors and from various types of oculocutaneous albinos (OCAs). Bar = mean for each hair color; square = ty-neg OCA; triangle = ty-pos OCA; diamond = ym OCA; star = HPS. *(From King et al. [195].)*

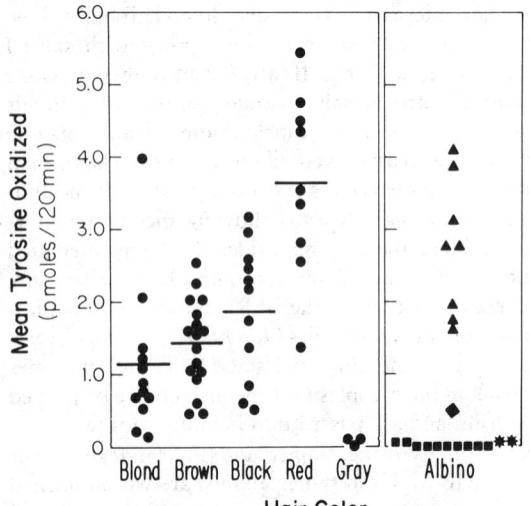

nos of all racial backgrounds have white hair in infancy, they frequently gradually accumulate pigment, so that the hair color turns to yellow or light tan with age.

A history is frequently obtained of a change in eye color from light gray to blue or yellow, hazel, or even light brown and a change in hair color from white to cream, tan, or light yellow-brown. A red eye reflex is usually easily elicited in all infants, but in children and adults among American Indian and African ty-pos albinos it may be absent or diminished. It is usually retained in adult Caucasian ty-pos albinos. Adult Caucasian albinos usually have a lighter retina than do adult Negro and Indian albinos of this type, but even in these individuals some darkening can be noted with age. The foveal reflex is usually absent or markedly diminished. Among 52 ty-pos albinos from the Brandywine isolate, approximately 10 percent had questionable macular reflexes [4]. Mesodermal remnants on the anterior surface of the iris and the posterior surface of the cornea were seen on slit-lamp examination in 25 percent of this group. Strabismus, usually esotropic, was found in 60 percent. The irides are diaphanous on transillumination, with a prominent cartwheel effect showing pigment accumulation, particularly at the pupillary border and the limbus of the iris [4]. The irides are less diaphanous in the ty-pos type than in the ty-neg type of albino [3, 143]. Horizontal or rotary nystagmus and photophobia have been observed in all subjects but appear to be less severe than in the ty-neg type of albino (Tables 15-3 and 15-4). Some subjects have maintained that photophobia and nystagmus have decreased with age [139].

Visual acuity shows a greater range among ty-pos albinos, but in general the mean acuity value is less than among ty-neg albinos [3] and nystagmus is less severe [3] (Tables 15-3 and 15-4). Ty-pos albino adults may have better visual acuity and less severe nystagmus than they had as children [3, 154], while ty-neg albinos tend to have the same defects as adults that they had as children, or more severe ones. The prognosis for vision is somewhat better for a ty-pos than for a ty-neg albino.

The central nervous system of ty-pos albinos is normally pigmented [155]. Brain tissue shows normal pigmentation of the locus ceruleus and substantia nigra. Thus neuromelanin is present in these structures, as noted previously in albinos of unknown type [156, 157].

Thin-section electron photomicrographs of freshly epilated ty-pos hair bulb and skin melanocytes show numerous stage I intermediate vesicles, stage II melanosomes, and partially pigmented stage III melanosomes. Fully pigmented stage IV melanosomes are rarely seen [84] (Fig. 15-6C).

Melanocytes from ty-pos albinos frequently contain one or more polyphagosome complexes (Table 15-5) in which aggregates of melanosomes, at various stages of development, and strands of endoplasmic reticulum are observed undergoing destruction in the cytoplasm of the melanocyte. Partially pig-

mented, early stage III melanosomes are found in dendrites of the ty-pos melanocyte, and melanosomes in various stages of development are passed to keratinocytes, where they occupy a normal position over the nucleus [107].

Hair bulbs from ty-pos albinos prefixed in 1 percent glutaraldehyde and incubated in 80 mg L-tyrosine per deciliter of phosphate buffer (pH 6.8) for 10 h and then stained in 1 percent osmic acid and 1 percent glutaraldehyde show that nearly all melanosomes have been converted to the fully pigmented stage IV condition (Fig. 15-6D). This incubation procedure often results in staining of the terminal layers of the Golgi cisternae (GERL) and indicates that tyrosinase uncomplexed in melanosomes is present in this structure, just as it is in the GERL from normally pigmented subjects and animals [82, 158, 159]. Pigmented stage II to stage IV melanosomes are passed to keratinocytes, where they lie individually or in phagolysosomes over the nucleus of the keratinocyte.

Serum copper levels and serum β-MSH levels have been found normal in ty-pos albinos; the tyrosine levels have varied from low normal to normal [47, 84]. A study by Zipkin et al. [160] on the transport of tyrosine from plasma into saliva suggested that there is possibly a transport defect of tyrosine in this type of albinism. Tyrosine is actively transported across salivary membrane barriers. Normal subjects have approximately twice the concentration of tyrosine in parotid saliva as in their serums. Ty-pos albinos have approximately half the normal concentration of salivary tyrosine (normal, 7.3 ± 0.4 mg/dl; obligate ty-pos heterozygotes, 8.2 ± 2.4 mg/dl; ty-pos albinos, 3.7 ± 0.5 mg/dl). Hair bulb incubation studies using a dilution gradient of substrate concentration suggest that there is no substrate transport defect in ty-pos albinism [47].

King and Witkop [149] assayed the activity of tyrosinase in hair bulbs from a number of albinos whose hair bulbs formed increased pigment when tested by the method of Kugelman and von Scott [5]. The results suggest that there are two types of ty-pos albino. Although the hair bulb test [5] shows increased pigmentation formed after incubation in L-tyrosine in CHS, HPS, and CS, King and Witkop [149] found that two types of ty-pos albinos could be distinguished among hair test-positive albinos without features of these syndromes. Type I ty-pos albinos showed a two- to fourfold increase in tyrosinase activity when compared with hair bulb assays of normal blond, brown, and black hair, while in Type II ty-pos albinos the activity fell within the range of values of normally pigmented subjects (Fig. 15-7). This study suggests that biochemical and genetic heterogeneity may exist within the present classification of ty-pos albinism. Further, the kinetic property of the enzyme isolated from ty-pos albinos was identical to that of normally pigmented patients [161].

Pigmentation can be induced in vivo in the skin of ty-pos albinos by stripping the skin with cellulose tape to minute

Table 15-4 Ophthalmologic findings in Ty-pos albinos

	No. tested	Mean acuity	Range of acuity	Mean trans-illumination	Mean nystagmus	Fundus pigment
Homozygotes						
Caucasian	40	20/225	70–400	1.9	2.0	0
Negro	82	20/200	70–400	1.4	1.8	+
Amerindian	20	20/200	60–400	1.5	2.0	+
Heterozygotes						
Caucasian	62			0.3 (5 individuals were +)		
Negro	75			0		
Amerindian	13			0		

Table 15-5 Laboratory findings in various types of albinos: Number tested/number with abnormalities

Type	Chromosome breaks	Polyphagosomes in melanocytes	Absent platelet dense bodies	Abnormal platelet aggregometry	High urinary GI-1†	Abnormal urinary chromatogram
Ty-neg	5/0	17/0	7/0	18/0	3/0	1/0
Ty-pos	28/1*	25/8	15/0	23/2	5/2	4/0
Ym	3/1*	6/0	5/0	5/1	0/0	5/0
HPS	4/0	14/0	25/25	15/15	3/0	3/0

* Patient with infectious mononucleosis; on retesting, no breaks were found.
† Glycolipid fraction one.

bleeding points and packing the area with wet gauze strips containing a solution of L-tyrosine and L-dopa for 1 week, followed by UVR [154]. The metabolic block has not been overcome by oral L-dopa. One ty-pos albino subject was given L-dopa, 5.5 g daily for 100 days, but no increased pigmentation of skin, hair, or eyes was noted. The addition of 500 mg pyridoxine for 2 weeks to this treatment also had no effect on pigmentation [82].

The basic defect in ty-pos albinism is unknown. The serum levels of the substrate amino acids tyrosine and phenylalanine are within the normal range [47, 82]. Inhibitors of pigmentation are not present in ty-pos serum since hair bulbs from ty-pos albinos will pigment in vitro in their own serum without added substrate, as will normal blond hair bulbs [47]. Hair bulb incubation studies show that the minimum substrate concentration needed to induce visible or microscopic pigment formation in 12 h is no different from that for normally colored hair [4, 47]. The tyrosinase activities of hair bulbs assayed in vitro range from normal to a fourfold increase compared with hair bulbs from patients with normally colored hair [100, 149], and enzyme kinetic studies indicate that tyrosinase from ty-pos hair bulbs is identical to normal enzymes [161]. Prolonged oral administration of L-dopa and UVR does not increase pigment in vivo. These facts suggest several possible sites of the block, which may include, among others, a defect in an intracellular inhibitor or a defective feedback control mechanism.

Heterozygotes for ty-pos albinism have not been identifiable by clinical or biochemical tests which have an acceptable reliability. Estimates of iris translucency in ty-pos obligate heterozygotes fall within the range of values of normally pigmented subjects [3, 143] (Table 15-4). Tyrosinase activity as measured by the conversion of [³H]tyrosine to L-dopa and [³H]OH in hair bulbs of ty-pos obligate heterozygotes is indistinguishable from normal [100, 149, 161]. The basic biochemical defect is unknown.

The Hermansky-Pudlak Syndrome (HPS) [85] The approximate synonym is *albinism with hemorrhagic diathesis* [85]. This syndrome consists of the triad of ty-pos OCA, hemorrhagic diathesis due to storage pool-deficient platelets, and an accumulation of a ceroidlike material in the reticuloendothelial system, lung, oral and intestinal mucosa, and urine [81, 82, 85, 162–177]. Restrictive lung disease and ulcerative colitis develop in the third and fourth decades of life [85, 178]. Approximately 200 patients with the disorder have been reported or are known to the authors. HPS has been reported in diverse ethnic populations (see table 15-7 in Ref. 81). Reports have included Japanese [179, 180], Argentinians [181], Czechs [182], Belgians [183], Italians [184], and Swiss [185]. The authors have examined previously unreported HPS

patients who were Finnish, Hasidic and Ashkenazic Jewish, English, Scottish, German, and American whites and blacks. The condition is unusually prevalent among Puerto Ricans. Of 92 albino Puerto Rican patients who have come to our attention, 90 have had HPS. In addition to the Dutch patients from Apeldorn [186, 187], several American kindreds have traced their ancestry to progenitors from this area of Holland.

Hermansky and Pudlak [85] first described the essential features of the syndrome in two 33-year-old albino patients who throughout life had suffered episodes of epistaxis, bruising, or prolonged bleeding following tooth extraction. The reports of Firth [162] of red-headed albinos with bleeding diathesis and of Horler and Witts [188] and Larsen et al. [189] may represent examples of the disorder, but details on these patients are insufficient to warrant their inclusion as definite examples.

What basic genetically determined defect can account for the diverse alterations in pigment formation, the defect in platelet storage pool, and storage of an abnormal ceroidlike material? The segregation of all three defects as a unit trait within kindreds indicates that these defects are ascribable to a pleiotropic effect of a single autosomal gene mutation [82] and are not the result of two or more closely linked mutations [171]. Since recessively inherited traits usually involve defects in enzymatic proteins, whereas dominant traits most often represent mutations affecting structural proteins [190], one may suppose that the basic defect in HPS involves an enzyme alteration.

CLINICAL FEATURES OF HPS The pigment disorder in HPS has a variable phenotypic expression depending upon age and racial ancestry. Patients of Northern European ancestry may closely resemble the ty-neg phenotype, while those from India and Puerto Rico resemble normal Northern Europeans in their pigmentary features. It is only when patients from deeply pigmented stocks are compared with their parents and when nystagmus and photophobia are also noted that the essential depigmented condition of the HPS patient is recognized.

The Irish patient reported by White and colleagues [170], the Dutch patients of Verloop and associates [191], and the American-Ukranian patients of Witkop et al. [82] were extremely blond and resembled closely the ty-neg type of albino. These patients had light gray-blue eyes with little evidence of a cartwheel effect on transillumination and no visually detectable pigment in their hair or skin. All of these patients had marked nystagmus, a prominent red reflex, and a completely depigmented iris and were thought on initial examination to be ty-neg albinos. The patients of Hermansky and Pudlak [85] were intermediate in their phenotypic expression and had some obvious pigment in their irides. The Dutch patients examined by Gerritsen and colleagues [186, 187] were from relatively darkly pigmented parents and had reddish-brown hair. The pigmentary features alone, without the findings of nystagmus, photophobia, and bleeding defect in these families, were insufficient to raise a high degree of clinical suspicion that these patients were unusual.

Puerto Rican patients frequently show considerable deposits of pigment in skin, eyes, and hair, the hair often being red or red-brown. The patient of Muñiz and associates [169] and the man reported by Garay and associates [178] had reddish-brown hair, mottled brown irides, pigmented nevi, freckles, and deposits of pigment in the skin exposed to sunlight. Muñiz's patient [169] had been a sugar cane cutter exposed to intense sunlight and showed dermatization of "granular" melanin similar to that seen in patients with xeroderma pigmentosum. His irides had deposits of brown pigment, especially at the limbus and the pupillary borders. A red reflex could be elicited but was not a prominent feature [82]. Patients of East Indian (Madras) extraction [82] and Hasidic Jewish patients have resembled normal United States Caucasians, with cream-colored skin with some tanning effect, light brown hair, green to hazel eyes, frank or latent nystagmus, photophobia, depigmented fundi, and the biochemical features of HPS (Table 15-6).

Mild hemorrhagic episodes are a cardinal feature of the syndrome. Most patients have a history of mild bleeding events, but in a few, massive fatal bleeding has occurred [82, 192]. Most frequently reported is ease of bruisability, epistaxis, gingival bleeding (Fig. 15-8), prolonged bleeding following tooth extraction, and hemoptysis. Women with the disorder have had massive bleeding following delivery [82, 187, 190, 191]. The kindred of the patient of Muñiz and associates [169] was reinvestigated by Witkop et al. [82]. An affected sister of the propositus married an unaffected cousin and had an affected daughter. The sister died of massive hemorrhage following the birth of her affected daughter. The daughter developed gastric symptoms at age 26 and died after taking a proprietary antacid which contained large amounts of aspirin. Other examples have been observed in which administration of aspirin may have resulted in intensifying the hemorrhagic defect, resulting in fatal bleeding [192]. Among the first 39 patients reported with HPS, 31 had prolonged bleeding following tooth extraction.

Ceroidlike material appears in the reticuloendothelial system, lung, and oral and gastrointestinal mucosa. A few patients have been observed with papillary lesions of the palate with white centers resembling gouty tophi (Fig. 15-8). These lesions contain cellular inclusions of ceroidlike material [177].

Commencing in the third decade, many patients, particularly those of Puerto Rican extraction, develop deposits of the material in the lung [82, 164, 178] associated with the radiographic changes of interstitial fibrosis and the development of restrictive lung disease [81, 82, 85, 178, 183, 193]. The origi-

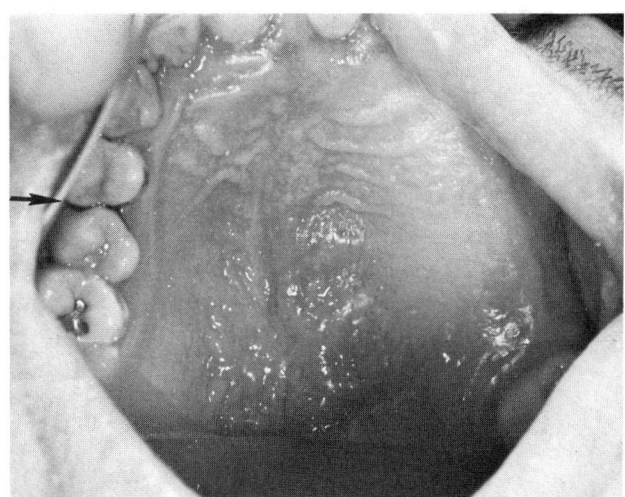

Figure 15-8 Palate of a patient with HPS shows spontaneous gingival hemorrhage (arrow) and palatal lesions which may have a white center resembling gouty tophi. These lesions contain ceroidlike material and are found in some patients with HPS. *(From Witkop et al. [177].)*

nal patients described by Hermansky and Pudlak [85] had lung changes diagnosed on chest radiographs as interstitial pulmonary fibrosis, and at autopsy they had extensive pulmonary deposits of ceroidlike material in the lung [163, 164]. Patients with similar radiographic changes in the lungs (Fig. 15-9) and deposition of golden ceroidlike material in the alveolar macrophages have been observed by Witkop and associates [81, 82], Garay et al. [178], and Davies and Tuddenham [193].

Davies and Tuddenham [193] described cryptogenic fibrosing alveolitis in four sibs aged 35 to 44, the offspring of first-cousin parents, who showed progressive breathlessness and markedly reduced transfer factor for carbon monoxide but marginally reduced or normal vital capacities, total lung capacity, and forced expiratory volume. In contrast, the Puerto Rican patients described by Garay and colleagues [178], who ranged from 20 to 43 years of age, showed a dramatic reduction on pulmonary function tests, a reduction in lung volumes, decreased diffusing capacity (DL_{CO}), resting hypoxemia which worsened with exercise, and maximum expiratory flow-volume curves with contours typical of restrictive interstitial lung disease. Restrictive interstitial lung disease as an integral progressive symptom of HPS in the third to fourth decades is probably more common than has been realized in the past and may account for cases diagnosed as the Hamman-Rich syndrome [183].

Granulomatous colitis occupies a similar status as a previously unrecognized component of HPS [178, 194]. While ceroidlike material was found within macrophages in the

Table 15-6 Ophthalmologic findings in ym and HPS albinos

	No. tested	Mean acuity	Range of acuity	Mean transillumination	Mean nystagmus	Fundus pigment
Homozygotes						
ym						
Caucasian	11	20/200	90–400	1.5	1.0	+
Negro	3	20/200		1.0	1.0	++
Hermansky-Pudlak						
Caucasian	15	20/200	70–400	2.5	3.0	+
Heterozygotes						
Caucasian HPS	8	20/20		2.0	0	+++
Indian HPS	2	20/50	20–100	1.5	0	++++

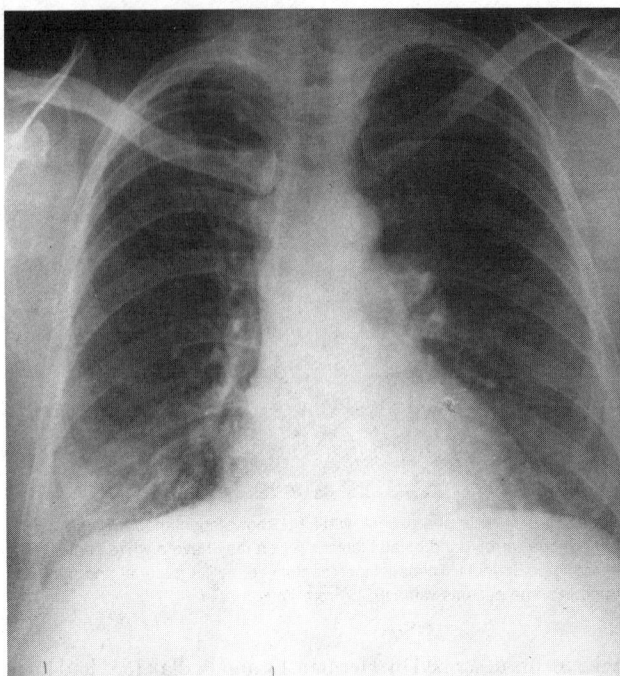

Figure 15-9 Radiograph of a Dutch woman with HPS shows diffuse streaking and nodular radiopaque areas interpreted as compatible with lipid storage disease. Patients with similar chest findings have had massive infiltrations of ceroidlike pigment in lung tissues at autopsy. (From Witkop et al. [82].)

colonic wall in Hermansky and Pudlak's original patients [85], no associated symptoms were reported. Schinella and coworkers [194] found that five of nine Puerto Rican HPS patients had colitis. These patients were also those reported to have restrictive lung disease by Garay et al. [178]. Since this initial report, an additional sibship from Puerto Rico has been observed by the authors in which two males, aged 33 years, have had both restrictive lung disease and ulcerative colitis. Schinella and coworkers [194] documented the onset of colitis in these patients as beginning at 12 years of age and requiring surgical resection as early as age 17. The onset of episodes of fever, abdominal pain, and bloody diarrhea has occurred from 12 to

30 years of age in Puerto Rican patients. With one exception, colitis has not been reported or observed among the North American, Dutch, or English patients examined by the authors. The colitis is refractive to medical treatment and involves primarily the ileum and sigmoid and rectosigmoid colons, requiring surgical resection [194]. The gross appearance of the colon showed multiple bleeding points with longitudinal superficial and deep ulcerations and induration of the bowel wall.

Kidney disease may constitute another unrecognized complication of HPS. A 62-year-old patient of Finnish extraction, seen by the authors, until the age of 58 had minimal radiographic evidence of fibrosis in his lung. At this time, he developed signs of kidney failure, which by age 62 required dialysis. The kidneys were small and diffusely radiopaque. Chest radiographs at 62 years of age showed massive fibrotic changes of the lungs. Bednar et al. [163, 164] described a massive accumulation of ceroidlike material in the kidneys in the original patients. Thus the possibility exists that accumulation of storage material in lungs is secondary to kidney failure and failure of the kidney to clear the material.

THE PIGMENT DEFECT IN HPS   The hair bulb incubation test of Kugelman and van Scott [5] shows a minimal increased pigmentation after incubation in L-tyrosine or L-dopa among Caucasians [3, 82]. Electron photomicrographs of thin sections of freshly epilated hair bulbs from HPS patients show numerous atypical, irregularly pigmented pheomelanosomes resembling those seen in normal red-haired patients (Fig. 15-10). Melanosomes up to stage III are abundant, but fully formed stage IV melanosomes are rare [3, 82, 177, 185, 193]. Atypical large melanosomes with matrix fibers running at various angles are also encountered. The melanosomes in keratinocytes occur as individual organelles and in membrane-bound aggregates, within which they are found in varying stages of formation [3, 82, 185].

After hair bulbs are incubated in L-tyrosine, nearly all the early melanosomes are converted to fully pigmented melanosomes. Microassay of tyrosinase activity usually ranges from zero to low normal values [195]. Thus these cells have the ability to form mature melanosomes, and the tyrosinase step is intact but reduced in activity. Pigmentation of the terminal

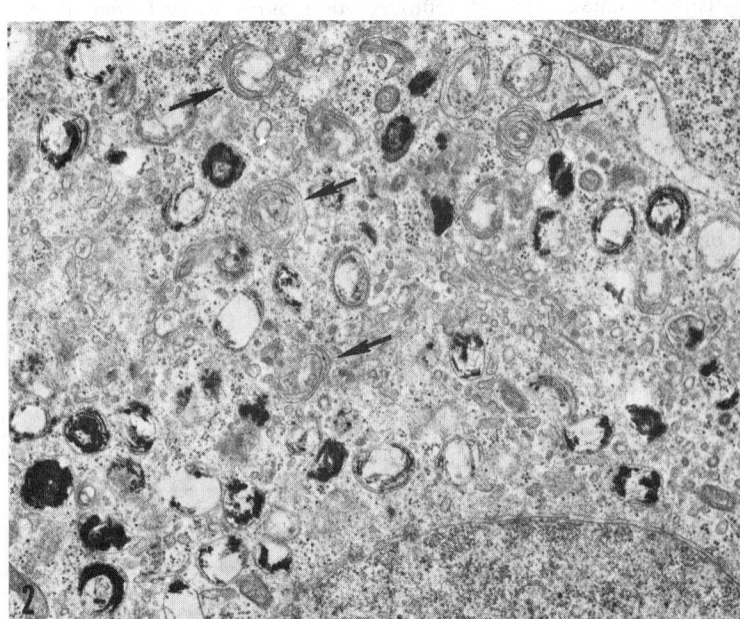

Figure 15-10 Electron photomicrograph of a hair bulb melanocyte from a Dutch woman with HPS, demonstrating numerous pheomelanosomes similar to those in normal subjects with red hair. Unpigmented round melanosomes (arrow) and unevenly pigmented pheomelanosomes are common. ×20,000. (From Witkop et al. [177].)

cisterna layer of the Golgi apparatus after incubation in L-tyrosine [82] (Fig. 15-11A) indicates the presence of tyrosinase uncomplexed with melanosomal matrix in this structure [158].

An occasional melanocyte may contain vacuoles resembling the lipid inclusion vacuoles seen in macrophages and epithelial cells in this disease (Fig. 15-11B). Normal melanosomes from the skin of HPS patients are greatly reduced or absent. The melanocytes are weakly dopa positive but increase in pigment after tyrosine-cysteine and dopa-cysteine incubation [3, 185]. Macromelanosomes similar to those observed in X-linked OA (Nettleship) (XOAN) and neurofibromatosis have been observed by Frenk and Lattion [185] in the skin from HPS patients (Fig. 15-27).

THE PLATELET DEFECT IN HPS   Platelets from patients with HPS have morphologic, chemical, and functional defects [82, 165–167, 170–174, 196, 197]. Normal platelets in thin sections have an average of 1.1 to 1.4 dense bodies per platelet [198–200] (Table 15-7). These are the storage organelles for serotonin (5-hydroxytryptamine, or 5-HT), adenine nucleotides (ADP and ATP), and calcium. Platelets from HPS patients have a marked decrease in the number of dense bodies [166, 170, 174, 196, 197, 200] (Fig. 15-12; Table 15-7). Platelets from rabbits can be depleted of dense bodies by reserpine but can recruit dense bodies when exposed to serotonin-rich plasma [201]. When HPS platelets are exposed to 5-HT-rich plasma, the initial uptake of 5-HT is normal [172, 173, 202], but it rapidly diverges from the uptake curve of normal platelets [172–174, 180, 182, 184], and significant numbers of dense bodies do not form. Platelets from patients with HPS contain 10 percent or less of normal levels of 5-HT [166, 167, 172–174, 182, 186, 189, 196, 200, 202–204] (Table 15-7). Analysis of nucleotides by high-pressure liquid chromatography shows a marked reduction of ADP in the HPS platelet, while AMP is unchanged and ATP falls within the range of low normal to deficient values [179, 184, 186, 203, 204] (Table 15-7). Accordingly, the HPS platelet shows a striking elevation of the ATP/ADP ratio [172, 173, 179, 180, 182, 184, 186, 193, 203–205] (Table 15-7). HPS platelets thus meet the requirements of storage pool-deficient platelets. Other types of storage pool-deficient disorders are known [202, 206, 207], but these are not associated with albinism.

Platelets from HPS patients also show a decrease in calcium content [208]. The morphologic abnormality of absent dense bodies (storage organelles) in HPS platelets thus correlates with the observed chemical deficiencies of 5-HT, ADP, and calcium. Several studies have addressed the problem of uptake and metabolism of 5-HT by HPS platelets. Maurer and coworkers [174] found that orally administered L-tryptophan,

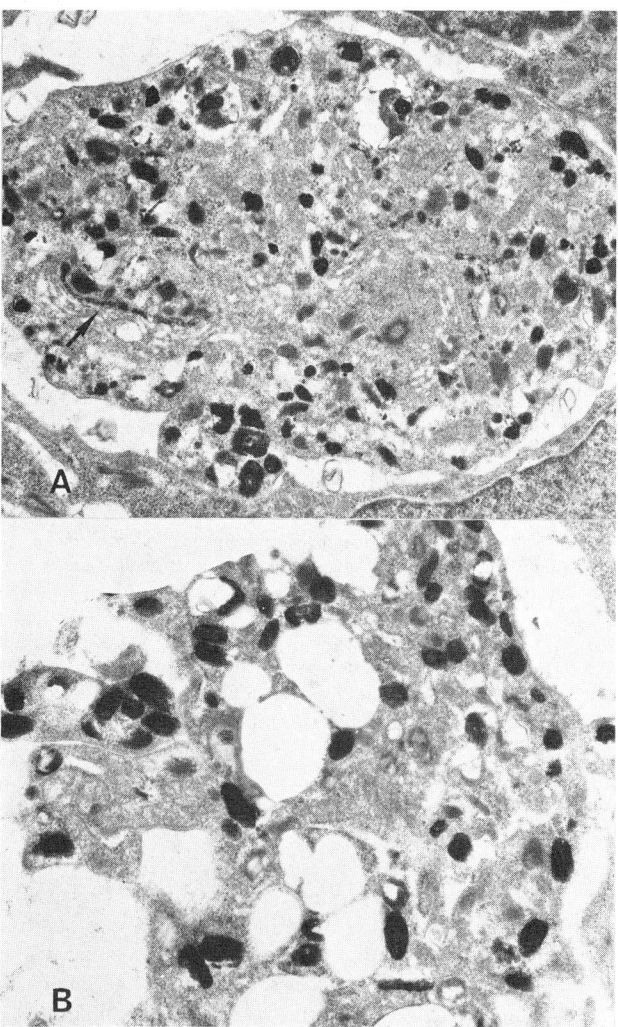

Figure 15-11 *A.* Melanocyte from a patient with HPS after incubation in L-tyrosine shows that nearly all the melanosomes have been converted to stage IV. Note also the pigmentation in the terminal layer of the Golgi, indicating that tyrosinase uncomplexed with melanosomes is present in this structure. ×17,000. *B.* Melanocyte from an HPS patient shows numerous vacuoles resembling the lipid vacuoles seen in bone marrow macrophages. ×22,000. *(From Witkop et al. [177].)*

the precursor of 5-HT, results in a rapid increase and retention over a 4-h period of 5-HT in normal platelets, but in only a slight rise followed by a rapid loss in HPS platelets. The urinary excretion of the chief metabolite of serotonin synthesis, 5-hydroxyindoleacetic acid (5-HIAA) is normal in HPS. This suggests that the synthetic pathway in the gastrointestinal tract is intact.

The uptake of ^{14}C-labeled serotonin by HPS platelets in

Table 15-7 Comparative values for adenine nucleotides, 5-hydroxytryptamine, and dense bodies seen in thin sections of platelets from patients with HPS and in normal subjects

Sample	ATP	ADP	AMP	Total	ATP/ADP	5HT	No. of dense bodies
Normal*	7.4	4.0	3.0	14.5	1.8	464 ± 79	1.1/platelet
Patient 1	10.2	2.0	1.7	13.9	5.1	23	1/100 platelets
Patient 2	7.0	1.2	0.8	9.1	5.7	36	1/75 platelets
Patient 3	4.0	0.9	1.9	6.8	4.3		

* Normal values represent the means of three replicate determinations from eight donors each; from Rao et al. [203] and Gerrard et al. [205].

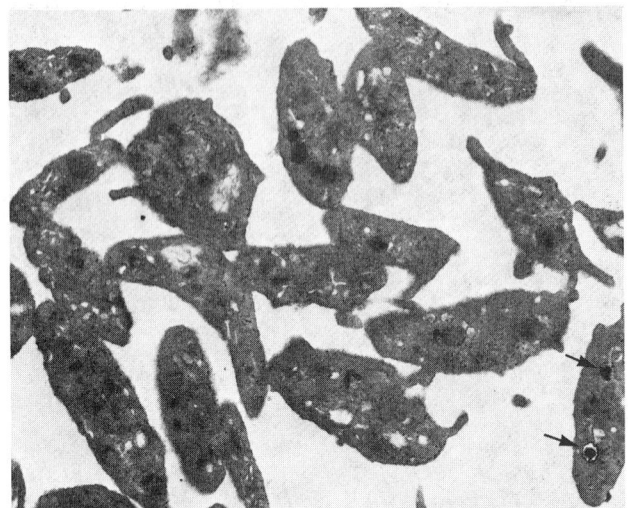

Figure 15-12 Thin-section electron photomicrograph of platelets from a patient with HPS illustrates the virtual absence of dense bodies (arrow). ×15,000. *(From White et al. [170].)*

vitro is at first rapid but quickly reaches saturation at a level much below that of normal platelets [172, 202]. Further, the metabolism of the $[^{14}C]$5-HT is rapid. When HPS platelet-rich plasma is incubated with $[^{3}H]$5-HT, the metabolites 5-HIAA and others are formed rapidly and in large amounts, and the ratio of $[^{3}H]$ metabolites to $[^{3}H]$5-HT is elevated far above normal [182, 202].

Smith [209], with Hardisty and Mills [172], found that both the uptake and release of $[^{3}H]$epinephrine in HPS platelets was similar to the uptake and release of 5-HT. This suggests that epinephrine, like serotonin, is deficient in the HPS platelet. The metabolism of epinephrine was also abnormal, since approximately half the activity in normal platelets was found in the epinephrine fraction, whereas in the HPS platelets it was almost all covered in the metabolite fraction (Fig. 15-13). The content of dopamine, noradrenaline, and adrenaline in HPS platelets is also subnormal [184].

For many years, "irreversible" aggregation of normal platelets was believed to depend upon the release of storage pool constituents (5-HT, ADP, ATP, calcium) residing in platelet organelles, the dense bodies. The release of ADP was considered to be the final mediator in all forms of platelet aggregation. The discovery that arachidonic acid (AA), the prostaglandin (PG) precursor, induced aggregation of platelets because it was transformed into labile aggregating substances, PGG_2, PGH_2, and thromboxane A_2 (TXA_2) (Fig. 15-14), led to the hypothesis that TXA_2 is either a second final mediator or the agent of granule release and, hence, the release of ADP [210–213]. Aspirin (ASA) acetylates cyclo-oxygenase, blocks synthesis of endoperoxides and thromboxanes [214, 215], and inhibits the second "irreversible" wave of response to aggregating agents which in relatively low concentrations cause biphasic, irreversible clumping of non-ASA-treated normal platelets [216, 217]. ASA-treated platelets are refractory to aggregation by AA but can undergo the release reaction and irreversible aggregation at high concentrations of thrombin and collagen [218]. Thrombin-induced degranulated normal platelets [219, 220], as well as HPS platelets, which lack storage organelles [205], aggregate in response to AA and TXA_2. Thus, ADP is not required for aggregation. Thrombin-degranulated platelets do not aggregate with thrombin itself but aggregate with ADP [218, 221].

These observations, among others, led Vargaftig and co-workers [222] to postulate that platelet aggregation is a complex event involving at least three mechanisms for aggregation: release of ADP, formation of TXA_2, and a mechanism involving platelet aggregating factor (PAF), which may be the basic mediator of the ASA-resistant third pathway of platelet aggregation. PAF appears to be a 1-alkyl, 2-acetyl glycerophosphocholine released from macrophages and basophils. Aggregation and release reactions by PAF are inhibited by drugs which increase intracellular cAMP, such as prostacyclin (PGI_2) but may not be a major pathway in human platelets.

Recently it has been shown that ADP irreversibly aggregated platelets can dissociate when exposed to agents such as PGI_2 and a calmodulin-binding agent, trifluoperazine; are refractory to further aggregation by ADP, thrombin, AA, and calcium iontophore, A23187; and have elevated cAMP levels [223, 224]. Exposure of these dissociated platelets to low levels of epinephrine did not cause reaggregation but reduced the high levels of cAMP and restored their sensitivity to aggregation by AA, thrombin, ADP, and A23187 [223, 224]. Further, concentrations of ADP, thrombin, and AA that do not produce aggregation of ASA-treated normal platelets produce irreversible aggregation when the ASA-treated normal platelets are pretreated with epinephrine [225]. These findings prompted Rao and associates [226, 227] to postulate another major pathway of platelet aggregation, that of membrane modulation mediated by α-adrenergic receptors cooperatively linked to the endoperoxide and thromboxane receptor(s) which can secure

Figure 15-13 Uptake and release of $[^{3}H]$epinephrine by platelets. The three columns at the left show the platelet content of epinephrine (A) and epinephrine metabolite (M) before incubation and after 60- and 120-min incubation with $[^{3}H]$epinephrine. The two right-hand columns show the activity released into the supernatant (S) and remaining in the platelets (P) after incubation of labeled platelets with saline solution or thrombin. *(From Smith [209].)*

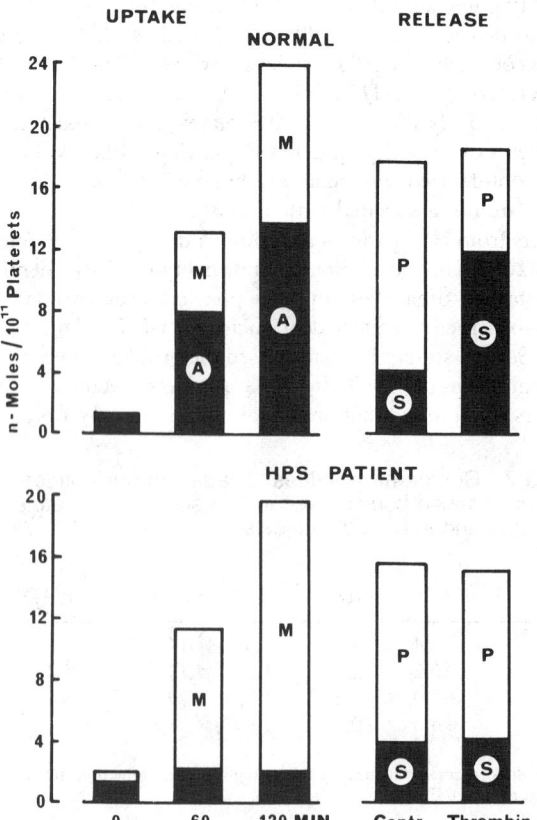

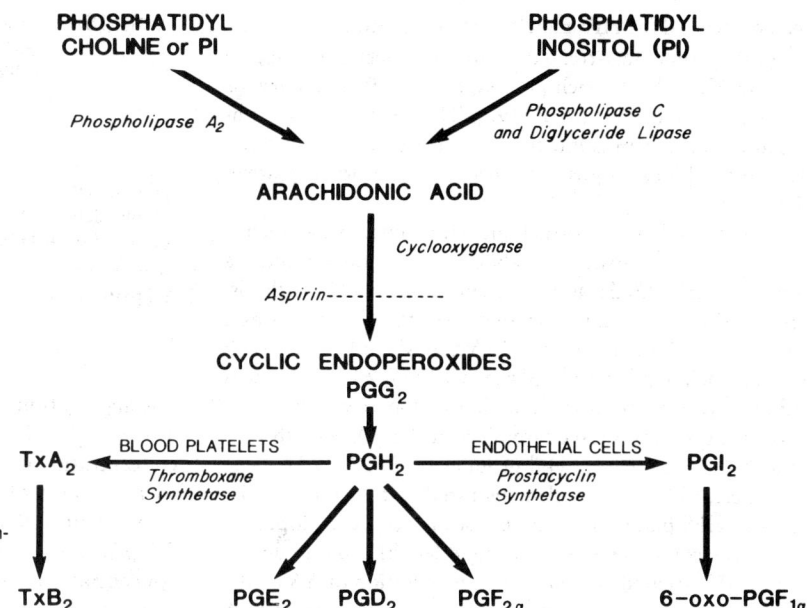

Figure 15-14 Schematic representation of prostaglandin (PG) synthesis in activated platelets and endothelial cells indicates steps that may be influenced in disorders of platelet aggregation. *(From Cohen [479].)*

irreversible aggregation of normal and HPS platelets, despite the absence of secretion and PG synthesis.

We will now examine the platelet defect in HPS in the light of these recent advances in knowledge of normal platelet functions and the contributions these unique platelets have made to our understanding of normal platelet function and thrombosis.

Aggregation studies of HPS platelets show that they have abnormal responses to potent aggregating agents such as ADP, epinephrine, thrombin, collagen, or bacteria. Aggregating agents added to platelet-rich plasma of normal subjects show an initial narrowing and upward deflection of the nephelometer pen (Fig. 15-15), which indicates an initial change in shape of the platelets. If the stimulus is sufficiently strong, the platelets then go through a massive irreversible aggregation, indicated by the second wave tracing (Fig. 15-15). The normal secondary wave depends upon the release by platelets of the nucleotides, serotonin, and calcium stored in the platelet organelles. Platelets from HPS patients show the initial shape change but do not go through the massive second irreversible wave when challenged by concentrations of agents sufficient to elicit this response in normal platelets (Fig. 15-15). With some variation, the platelets from the typical ASA-free HPS patient will not have a secondary wave of irreversible aggregation when stimulated by dilute solutions of collagen, epinephrine, and ADP but will aggregate with AA and variably with thrombin. The storage pool of the HPS platelets is insufficient to cause the secondary wave of aggregation [165, 169–171, 197]. The addition of only 10 percent of normal platelets to platelet-rich HPS plasma is sufficient to restore the collagen-induced aggregation curve to normal [82, 197] (Fig. 15-16). This suggests that when sufficient storage pool constituents are present, HPS platelets will aggregate.

Nephelometric tracings similar to those of HPS platelet-rich plasma are obtained from ASA-treated normal platelets [216, 228–231] (Fig. 15-16). The ASA-treated normal platelet differs from the HPS platelet in that it has normal dense bodies and contains a normal storage pool, but the effect of ASA is to block the platelet granule release mechanism [209]. The release mechanism is intact in the HPS platelet, but the HPS platelet has a deficient storage pool [197]. The ASA-treated normal

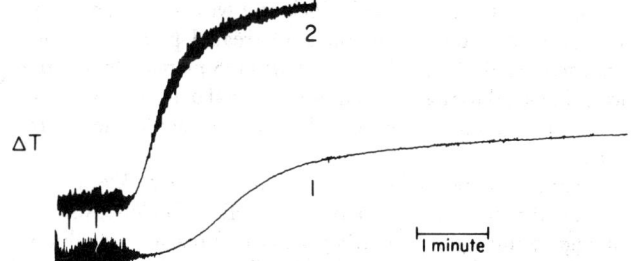

Figure 15-15 The aggregometer response of a patient's citrated platelet-rich plasma (C-PRP) to the addition of collagen in tracing 1 is compared with the response of a normal sample of C-PRP to the same agent shown in tracing 2. Narrowing of the baseline in both samples indicates that the HPS platelet, like the normal platelet, undergoes an initial shape change. However, the HPS tracing did not reach a maximal decrease in optical density, suggesting inadequate availability of secretory products essential for rapid development of irreversible aggregation. ΔT, change in light transmission. *(From White et al. [170].)*

Figure 15-16 Correction of collagen-induced aggregation response of ASA-treated normal platelets by storage pool-deficient HPS platelets. The tracings of HP platelets (1) and aspirin (ASA)-treated normal platelets (2) are similar, both lacking the irreversible component. However, mixing HPS and ASA C-PRP in the proportion of 6:4 results in an essentially normal tracing, indicating that the HPS platelets supply a component that overcomes the inhibitory effect of ASA, releasing the storage pool constituents from the ASA-treated normal platelets. ΔT, change in light transmission. *(From White and Witkop [197].)*

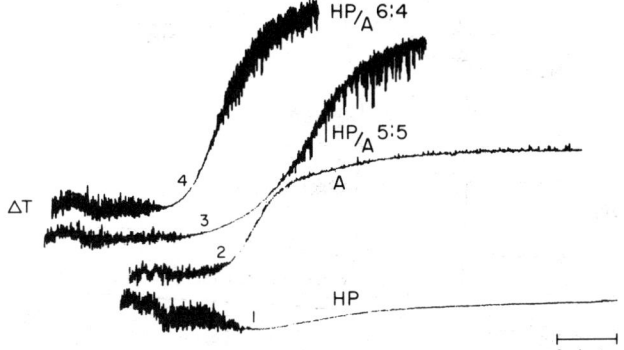

platelet defect and the HPS platelet defect are mutually correctable. If 30 percent ASA-treated normal platelets are added to 70 percent HPS platelet-rich plasma, the aggregation curve is indistinguishable from normal [197]. These experiments indicate that a mechanism is intact in the HPS platelet which can overcome the block imposed by ASA in the normal platelet [232].

A series of studies on normal and HPS platelets has identified the releasing substance (labile aggregation-stimulating substance, LASS) [205] as an intermediate in PG synthesis. Willis and Kuhn [233, 234] demonstrated that LASS acts as a chemical trigger for aggregation. ASA and ASA-like drugs such as indomethacin inhibit cyclo-oxygenase [235, 236]. LASS was found to consist of structurally similar endoperoxide intermediates of PG synthesis derived from precursor AA, with thromboxane A_2 as the effective end product [213, 233, 237] (Fig. 15-14). Gerrard et al. [205] demonstrated that the microsomal fraction of HPS platelets is a potent source of PG endoperoxides that overcome the ASA-blocking effect in collagen aggregation of ASA-treated normal cells. The addition of AA or the enzyme prostaglandin synthetase (cyclo-oxygenase) from HPS platelets alone did not correct the defect (Fig. 15-17). Further, the HPS LASS added to ASA-treated normal platelets was sufficient to overcome the ASA block and was accompanied by a release of serotonin from the ASA-treated platelets without collagen (Table 15-8). The action of HPS platelet endoperoxide is identical to that derived from normal platelets and causes a direct stimulation of the platelet contractile mechanism [200].

A series of experiments by Rao and associates [226] defined the membrane modulation system in HPS platelets. Addition of aggregating agents to HPS platelet-rich plasma in high concentrations, arachidonate (1.2 μM), thrombin (0.5 U/ml), and collagen (100 ng/ml), causes irreversible aggregation [226]. Addition of arachidonate at low concentration (0.45 μM), which effects aggregation in normal platelets, causes irrevers-

Table 15-8 The release of [^{14}C]5HT from aspirin-treated normal platelets using HP LASS without collagen*

	Pellet (× 10³ cpm)	Supernatant (× 10³ cpm)	Release %
AT platelets	23.4	0.3	1.3
AT platelets + HP LASS	16.3	9.3	36.3
AT platelets + HPS synthetase	25.4	0.5	1.9
AT platelets + arachidonate	23.8	1.0	4.0

* After Gerrard and others [205, 232].

ible aggregation in HPS platelets but no secretion of ADP (Fig. 15-18). HPS platelets do not respond with aggregation to any concentration of epinephrine and develop only primary waves to the action of threshold concentrations of thrombin (0.2 μg/ml) and ADP (2.0 μM). Pretreatment of HPS platelets with 2.5 μM of epinephrine and subsequent exposure to threshold concentrations of thrombin and ADP produce irreversible aggregation. ASA-treated storage pool-deficient HPS platelets, which cannot form TXA_2 or undergo release reaction on stimulation by AA, can still undergo irreversible aggregation in response to thrombin and ADP if treated first with epinephrine [226] (Fig. 15-19). On the other hand, ASA-treated HPS platelets do not aggregate with AA following treatment with epinephrine, while ASA-treated normal platelets do.

These findings indicate that HPS platelets, as well as normal platelets, possess the mechanism of intrinsic membrane modulation which is capable of restoring sensitivity to refractory cells and securing irreversible aggregation, even when PG synthesis is blocked and secretion cannot and does not take place. They further suggest that the receptor site for AA bypasses the membrane modulation system, and that some portion of the system may be altered in HPS. The findings are in accord with the concept of Huang and Detwiler [238], who have suggested that secretion is the result of irreversible aggregation, not its cause. These findings also explain why some HPS patients have had no indications of unusual bleeding episodes or only mild consequences of their platelet problem.

STORAGE DEFECT IN HPS   Two types of storage material accumulate in reticuloendothelial, oral mucosal, and other

Figure 15-17 Correction by HPS-LASS of the aspirin (ASA) defect in collagen (COLL)-induced aggregation. Normal (NL) platelets undergo irreversible aggregation when exposed to collagen. Incubation of normal platelets with 100 μM ASA for 15 min completely inhibits platelet aggregation. Addition of LASS generated from an HPS platelet microsomal fraction corrects the ASA-produced defect in collagen-induced aggregation, whereas addition of HPS-synthetase or arachidonate alone has no effect. ΔT, change in light transmission. (From Gerrard et al. [205].)

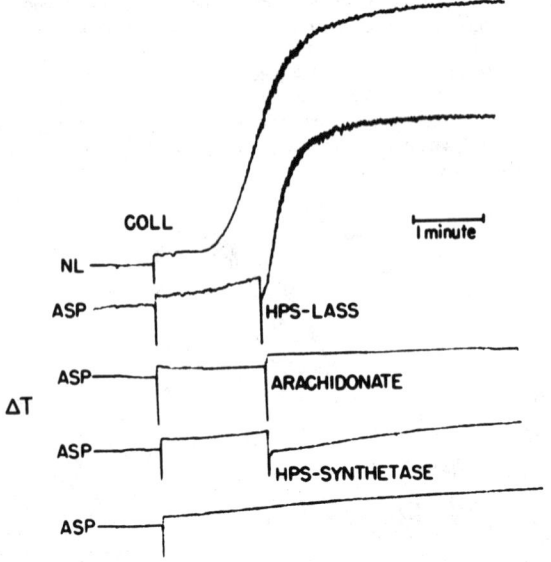

Figure 15-18 Response of normal (N) and Hermansky-Pudlak syndrome (HP) platelets to arachidonate (0.45 mM). Normal control platelets stirred with arachidonate respond with aggregation and release of ADP. HP platelets respond to arachidonate with irreversible aggregation, but without any detectable release of ADP. ΔT, change in light transmission. (From Rao et al. [226].)

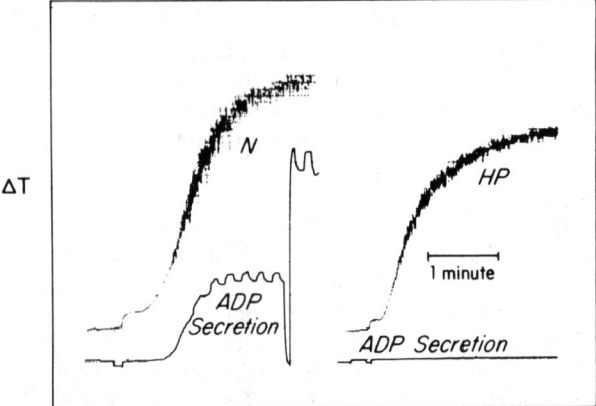

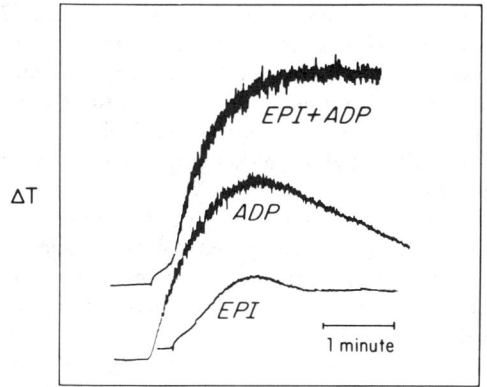

Figure 15-19 Influence of epinephrine (5 μM) on ADP (2 μM)-induced aggregation of aspirin-treated Hermansky-Pudlak syndrome platelets. ASA-treated HP platelets stirred with epinephrine or ADP respond with primary waves only. However, when these platelets are stirred with a combination of epinephrine and ADP, irreversible aggregation is obtained. Similar aggregation curves were obtained when epinephrine and thrombin were the stimulants. ΔT, change in light transmission. *(From Rao et al. [226].)*

cells and can be found in urine sediment [3, 82, 85, 163, 164, 166, 168, 169, 172, 174, 177, 191, 193, 196, 239] (Table 15-9). One fraction is soluble in chloroform:methanol and consists primarily of neutral fats, fatty acids, cholesterol, and cholesterol esters [177]. The other fraction, insoluble in chloroform:methanol, consists of clumps of golden-yellow pigmented granular material that resembles ceroid and lipofuscin [177] but probably respresents a unique storage substance differing from either.

Unsaturated fatty acids are believed to be precursors of both ceroid and the lipofuscins [240–243]. Bednar and coworkers [163] and Bednar and Jirasek [164] noted the ceroidlike accumulations in pigmented macrophages in the spleen, liver, and lungs of HPS patients. White et al. [176] described the ultrastructural and histochemic properties of the inclusions in bone marrow macrophages, circulating leukocytes, and urinary sed-

iment (Figs. 15-20 to 15-22). Witkop et al. [177] found the material in oral epithelial cells (Fig. 15-23). All studies suggest that the source of the abnormal pigment is phagocytized erythrocytes and that it is a complex lipid or a catechol.

Fresh untreated specimens of bone marrow, buccal mucosa, and, to a lesser extent, urinary sediment give histochemic reactions characteristic of neutral lipids, take lipofuscin stains, and have a bright yellow fluorescence in UVR [177] (Fig. 15-22; Table 15-9). After removal of soluble lipids by chloroform:methanol extraction, the material no longer stains with simple fat stains but retains its fluorescent characteristics and lipofuscin-staining qualities [168, 177] (Table 15-9). The staining qualities of the ceroidlike-lipid complex vary somewhat depending upon the source of the material. In bone marrow macrophages there is a close association of the golden-yellow granular ceroidlike material and lipid-filled vacuoles. Tissues in which this association occurs (liver, spleen, lung, oral epithelium) show histochemic reactions for fatty acids, neutral lipids, and ceroid-lipofuscin. Where the ceroidlike material is separated from the lipid, the fat stains are less intense or absent. The amount of ceroidlike material recovered from tissue or urinary sources varies from patient to patient. Bednar et al. [163] found that renal epithelium gives the strongest reaction for ceroid. The patient of Halon and Mitus [168] had abundant golden-yellow Schmorl-positive material in urine, as did the Dutch patients [82, 177, 187, 191]. Puerto Rican patients showed massive amounts in marrow and in the urinary sediment [82, 177], while English patients had relatively small amounts in urinary sediment at comparable ages.

Bone marrow contains pigment-laden macrophages which stain a sea-blue color with azure dyes [3, 82, 85, 163, 164, 168, 172, 191]. As a result, the disorder has been classified under the syndrome of the sea-blue histiocyte [244], but the inclusions in the HPS macrophages are unlike all other examples of sea-blue histiocytes examined in the electron microscope [82, 243, 245]. Abnormal lipids and unusual levels of normal lipids

Table 15-9 Histochemic reactions for material stored in tissue or urine and buccal epithelial cells in HPS patients*

Test	Tissue (bone marrow)	Urine or buccal cells	
		Before C:M ext.†	After C:M ext.†
Schmorl reaction	+ (varies by pH)	+ (varies by pH)	+ (varies by pH)
Ziehl-Neelsen	+	+	+
Periodic acid-Schiff (PAS)	+	+	+
PAS-diastase digestion	+	+	+
Acetylation-PAS	−		
Luxol fast blue	+	+	+
Nile blue (Lillie)	+ (blue-green)	+ (blue-green)	±
Ferrous iron (Lillie)	−	−	−
Prussian blue	−	−	
Toluidine blue	+ (varies by pH)	+ (dark blue)	
Oil red 0	+	±	−
Sudan black B	+	±	−
Fluorescence UV	+ (yellow)	+ (intense yellow)	+ (intense yellow)
Ammoniacal silver (Masson)	Weak		
Acid phosphatase	+		
Beta-glucuronidase	+		
Alkaline phosphatase	−		
Peroxidase	−		
Solubility in 2% EDTA		−	−

*See also Bednar et al. [163].
†Chloroform:methanol extraction.

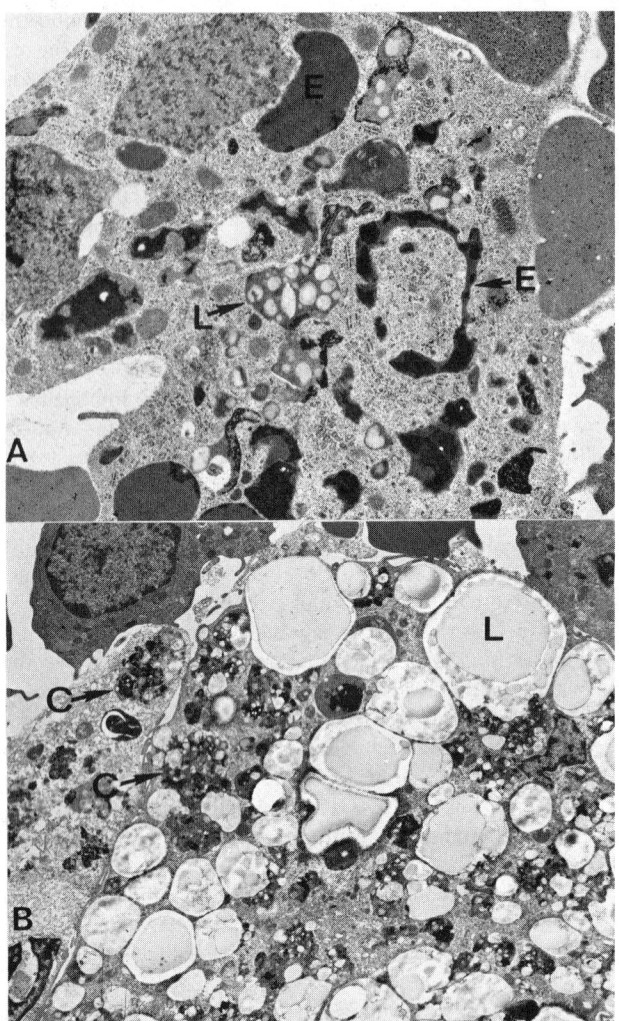

Figure 15-20 Bone marrow macrophages from a patient with HPS. *A.* Early stages of erythrocyte (E) digestion and globular electron-dense, lipidlike material with included vacuoles (L). ×11,500. *B.* Late stage showing the macrophage cytoplasm filled with many clear vacuoles (L), resembling those seen in lipid storage diseases, and numerous electron-dense inclusions (C) resembling ceroid. ×14,500. *(From White et al. [175].)*

have not been found in the plasma (serum) of HPS patients [82, 177, 246] (Table 15-10).

INCLUSIONS IN CIRCULATING LEUKOCYTES Two types of inclusions have been noted in the cytoplasm of peripheral leukocytes. One type resembles the ceroidlike-lipid complex observed in bone marrow macrophages (Fig. 15-20), and the other is a membrane-bound particle with an electron-dense core and peripheral fibrillar material (Fig. 15-24).

Halon and Mitus [168] found small vesicles and vacuoles in the peripheral lymphocytes of their patient. White et al. [175, 175] described ceroidlike-lipid complexes in circulating monocytes (Fig. 15-21) which were not observed in bone marrow monocytes. A second type of inclusion was also noted in circulating monocytes (Fig. 15-24) but not in bone marrow cells [176]. No cells were observed to contain both types of inclusions. These membrane-bound particles have an electron-dense core with peripherally arranged, electron-dense fibrils which resemble apatite crystals. A similar mass of fibrils was identified in the keratinocytes of a patient with ym albinism (Fig.

15-25) but not in the hair cells of the HPS patients [82, 176]. These inclusion bodies closely resemble structures found in melanocytes of leaf frogs. In frogs, these structures were believed to represent a new type of melanosome producing a red pigment which was neither pheomelanin nor eumelanin [247] but represented a pteridine-containing rhodomelanochrome [248].

HPS heterozygotes have a statistically significant lowered 5-HT content in platelets compared to normal subjects, but the range of values for the HPS heterozygotes overlaps the lower range of normal values sufficiently to make this an unreliable test for the carrier [186].

THE BASIC DEFECT IN HPS The basic defect in HPS is unknown. A large number of enzymes and metabolic products are normal in HPS patients (Tables 15-10 to 15-13). Witkop et al. [177] postulated that a defect in glutathione peroxidase could account for all the features of the disorder, but subsequent investigation by Gerritsen and coworkers [246] failed to find any abnormality in this or other platelet enzymes.

Although Rao et al. [226] demonstrated that ASA-treated HPS platelets will aggregate after exposure to low levels of epinephrine, and hence probably are not seriously compromised in vivo, it is still considered advisable to have the HPS patient avoid ASA and PG-inhibiting drugs. Cryoprecipitate infusion has been reported to be effective in lowering bleeding times for up to 24 h in some patients [249, 250].

Chédiak-Higashi Syndrome (CHS) [86–89, 251] Approximate synonyms are *Béguez Cesar-Steinbrinck-Chédiak-Higashi syndrome, congenital gigantism of peroxidase granules, granulation anomaly of leukocytes,* and *hereditary gigantism of cytoplasmic organelles.* This is often a fatal disease of childhood characterized by an imperfect OCA (pigment dilution) with giant melanosomes [252–254], giant peroxidase-positive lysosomal granules in leukocytes [86, 255–257] and giant granules in Schwann cells [253, 258] and other tissues, and a marked susceptibility to infections [86, 251, 259–262]. During the course of the disease, children may

Figure 15-21 Thin-section electron photomicrograph of a peripheral monocyte from a patient with HPS contains abnormal particulate deposits of ceroidlike material. Lamellar structures characteristic of phospholipids are not seen. ×12,300. *(From White et al. [176].)*

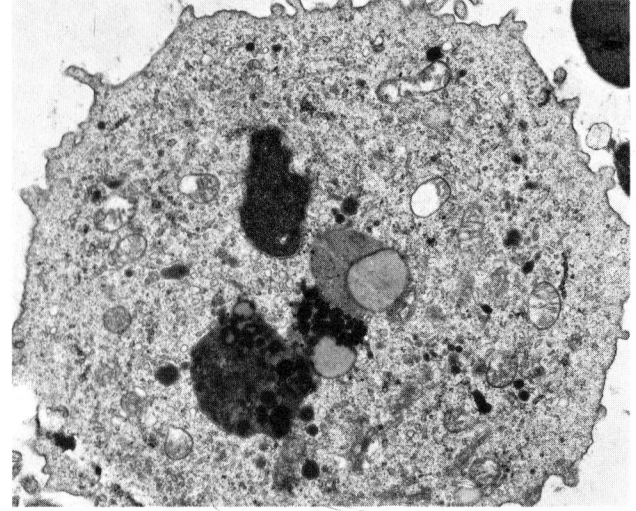

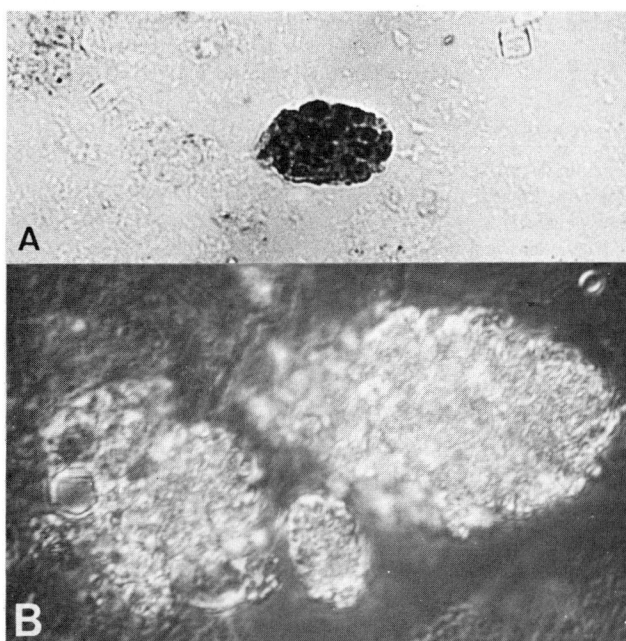

Figure 15-22 *A.* Unstained granule of golden-yellow ceroidlike material from the urine sediment of a patient with HPS. ×312. *B.* Ceroidlike material from the urine sediment shows intense yellow fluorescence when viewed by ultraviolet illumination. ×1,200. *(From Witkop et al. [177].)*

develop a peripheral neuropathy [253, 261, 263]. Children surviving the early infectious episodes, i.e., children of ages 8 to 18 years, most frequently develop a terminal lymphoreticular malignancy [86, 253, 258, 261, 264, 265]. A few patients have survived to age 20 years [265–267].

The color of the hair may vary from light blond to brunette, but it has an unusually striking, metallic, frosted gray sheen. The skin color varies from light cream to slate gray. The skin usually burns easily, even after moderate exposure to sunlight. Pigmented and papillary lesions of the skin occur in high frequency. The eyes are usually pigmented and vary from a pale blue-violet to brown, the latter especially if the parents are also dark-eyed. In contrast to what is seen in the ty-neg type of albinism, transillumination of the ocular bulb shows definite accumulations of pigment in the iris. Most patients show a moderate photophobia, squint, and nystagmus, but in dark-eyed patients these may be absent [252]. Funduscopic examination may show a moderate to markedly decreased pigmentation of the retina [252, 268, 269], the optic nerve head may be elevated by edema [267, 268], the electroretinogram (ERG) negative and positive responses are abnormal, and visually evoked potential (VEP) latency is increased [270].

Young children have repeated infections, usually with gram-positive organisms of the staphylococcal and streptococcal type [267]. At about 5 years of age a progressive neuropathy frequently develops, manifested by cranial and peripheral neuropathy, and a wide-based, stamping gait [261, 263] accompanied by muscle weakness, foot drop, decreased muscle stretch reflexes, sensory loss, diffusely abnormal electroencephalogram, abnormal electromyogram, decreased motor nerve conduction velocity, and occasionally convulsions [271].

The accelerated phase of the disease is a lymphohistiocytic proliferation of unknown origin that has occurred in a majority of cases [271]. As the disease progresses, anemia, thrombo-

cytopenia, and absolute neutropenia develop. Poor prognostic signs of the lymphoreticular malignancy are mediastinal and hilar lymphadenopathy, jaundice, marked splenomegaly, moderate hepatomegaly, a leukemic type of gingivitis, and pseudomembranous sloughing of the buccal mucosa [263, 271, 272]. Previously normal tests of liver function, coagulation immunoglobulins, and cellular immunity may become abnormal. At autopsy, infiltration of mature lymphocytes and histiocytes but without significant numbers of plasma cells, eosinophils, or neutrophils may involve the perivascular architecture of nearly all tissues. A majority of patients have had bruising, epistaxis, gastrointestinal bleeding, and prolonged bleeding times not always accompanied by the thrombocytopenia of the accelerated phase. Platelets from some patients with or without bleeding may have a storage pool deficiency of nucleotides, serotonin, and releasable divalent cations [273–276]. ADP is decreased, the ATP/ADP ratio is increased, and the uptake and retention of 5-HT are impaired [274–276]. Giant granulation of platelets may be absent or vary to as high as 5 percent of platelets [273].

Melanocytes from CHS patients appear normal in number

Table 15-10   Laboratory values in HPS patients

	Patient A.M.P.	Patient J.R.V.
Age	53	32
Sex	F	M
Hemoglobin	14.9 g/dl	15.2 g/dl
White cell count	5900	7100
Polymorphonuclear leukocytes	64%	77%
Lymphocytes	27%	15%
Monocytes	7%	3%
Eosinophils	1%	5%
Basophils	1%	0%
Reticulocyte count	1.9%	
Bleeding time	—	6.5 min
Platelet count	270,000	290,000
Prothrombin time	11 s	10.9 s
Partial thromboplastin time	34 s	36.6 s
Thrombin time	15.6 s	14.4 s
Blood urea nitrogen	18 mg/dl	16 mg/dl
Creatinine	0.8 mg/dl	1 mg/dl
Fasting blood glucose	81 mg/dl	81 mg/dl
Serum calcium	9.1 mg/dl	9.5 mg/dl
Serum phosphorus	2.6 mg/dl	3.3 mg/dl
Serum cholesterol	249 mg/dl	155 mg/dl
Repeat	209 mg/dl	175 mg/dl
Triglycerides	124 mg/dl	62 mg/dl
Repeat	174 mg/dl	84 mg/dl
Phospholipids	267 mg/dl	195 mg/dl
Total lipids	744 mg/dl	444 mg/dl
Protein electrophoresis		
Albumin	4.03 g/dl	4.34 g/dl
Alpha$_1$ globulins	0.4 g/dl	0.29 g/dl
Alpha$_2$ globulins	0.59 g/dl	0.75 g/dl
Beta globulins	0.69 g/dl	0.87 g/dl
Gamma globulins	1.43 g/dl	1.04 g/dl
Serum vitamin A	145 μg	41 μg
Serum vitamin E	12 μg/ml	5 μg/ml
Serum vitamin C	0.68 mg/dl	1.1 mg/dl
^{14}C glycolytic screening	No deficiency in red cell glycolysis	No deficiency in red cell glycolysis

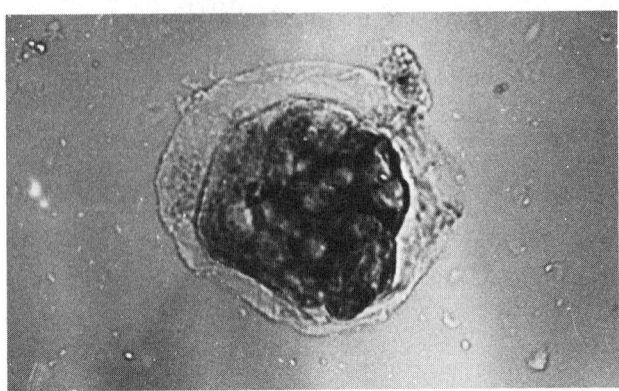

Figure 15-23 Oral epithelial cell from a patient with HPS shows a large inclusion of ceroidlike material resembling that seen in bone marrow, circulating monocytes, and urinary sediment. ×500. *(From Witkop et al. [177].)*

Table 15-11 Range of enzyme determinations in platelets of three patients with HPS and three normal subjects in μmol/(min·10^{11} platelets)*

Enzyme	Normal	HPS
Lactate dehydrogenase	99.0–148.7	108.8–132.3
Pyruvate kinase	219.0–140.3	202.7–226.7
Hexokinase	14.9–18.3	15.2–16.6
Glyceraldehyde-3-phosphate dehydrogenase	191.2–235.2	190.4–221.2
Phosphofructokinase	6.8–10.5	7.5–13.1
Aldolase	14.2–21.8	13.1–16.4
Glucose-6-phosphate dehydrogenase	16.2–25.6	14.3–19.1
6-Phosphate gluconate dehydrogenase	4.7–6.0	4.4–5.5
Glutathione reductase	10.8–12.6	10.1–11.7
3-Phosphate glycerate kinase	159.0–209.4	167.7–189.6

* Enzyme determinations by Jan-Willem N. Akkerman, Ph.D., Division of Hemostasis and Thrombosis, Department of Hematology, State University Hospital, Utrecht, The Netherlands.

and distribution, and they have tyrosinase activity. The hair bulb test of Kugelman and van Scott [5, 277] gives a positive result and produces fully pigmented stage IV melanosomes [47, 252, 257, 263]. The microassay for tyrosinase of King and Witkop [100] shows high activity of the enzyme in hair bulbs. The majority of the melanosomes are abnormally large structures that can be passed only with difficulty to the keratinocyte [252, 253, 257] (Fig. 15-26A), but some normal-sized melanosomes are formed [278]. The giant granules found in this disease were first studied in leukocytes, which stain for acid phosphatase and peroxidase [256–258], known to be localized in lysosomes. Abnormal membrane-bound lysosomal-like organelles may appear in infancy and have been found in cells of the buccal mucosa, Schwann cells, pancreas, liver, gastric and duodenal mucosa, adrenal, pituitary, spleen, kidney, bone marrow, hair, skin, iris, and conjunctiva [253, 258, 270, 271, 279]. Many of these organelles show fragility of their limiting membranes and undergo fragmentation and degeneration within leukocytes, Schwann cells, melanocytes, and keratinocytes [253, 265, 279].

Neutrophils from CHS patients contain a few giant (up to 4 μm) (Fig. 15-26B) azurophilic-staining granules. Neutrophils show reduced migration into inflammatory sites in vivo and defective chemotaxis in vitro [267, 280–282]. The leukotaxis defect has been attributed to an imbalance of cyclic nucleotides [282, 283] and a consequent inability to assemble microtubules, correctable in vitro and in vivo by ascorbic acid [284, 285]. The effect of filter pore size on migration in the standard Boyden chamber using zymosan-activated serum or an AA gradient showed that CHS neutrophils had a significant reduction in migratory response when 5-μm filters were used, but the dif-

ference from normal neutrophil migration was eliminated when 8-μm filters were employed [286]. This study indicated that the chemotactic defect was largely due to a mechanical impediment provided by the giant cytoplasmic granules and that the surface receptor and motility systems of the CHS neutrophil are intact [286].

Following bacterial ingestion there is delayed degranulation of leukocytes, accompanied by an absence of peroxidase activity and reduced bactericidal activity [268, 280, 281, 287–289]. Lysosomal enzymes (alkaline phosphatase, β-glucuronidase, and myeloperoxidase) [268] are reduced, and the cell is unable to deliver them to normal phagocytic vacuoles. The giant granules resemble the normal granules of the specific cell type in both fine structure and cytochemic reactions [290–300] and may show morphologic variability from one cell type to another, such as a ring-shaped lysosome in monocytes [301]. The variability in the intensity of cytochemic stains of the giant inclusions, even within the same cell, suggests that most giant granules undergo transformation to secondary lysosomes, which are unable to participate in the degranulation process [300]. The giant granules result from fusion of small primary granules which begins in the neutrophil precursors within the bone marrow and continues during cell maturation [302]. Present evidence indicates that the underlying

Figure 15-24 A. Low magnification (×10,250) of a circulating monocyte from a patient with HPS showing an electron-dense inclusion surrounded by a distinct membrane in the cytoplasm. B. At high magnification (×41,500), this inclusion consists of an electron-dense core surrounded by fibrillar material. Each fiber is 70 to 240 Å in diameter, straight or slightly curved. *(From White et al. [176].)*

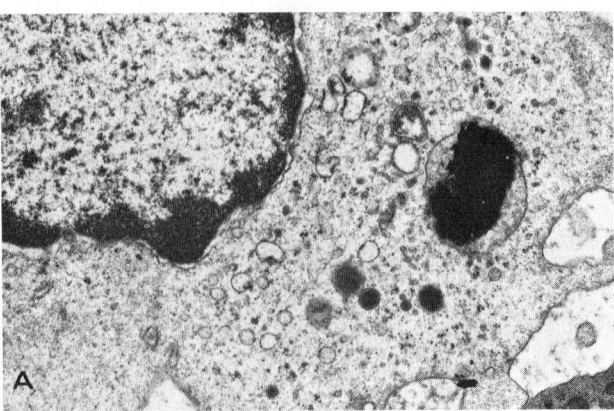

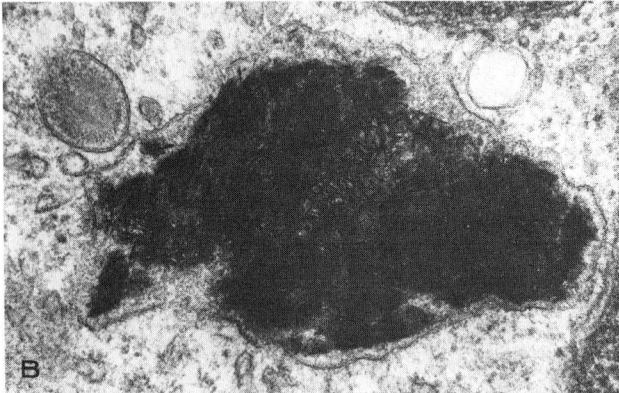

Table 15-12 Lysosomal enzymes in leukocytes of HPS patients and controls in nmol
p-nitrophenol liberated per milligram of protein per hour

Enzymes	Patient 1	Patient 2	Patient 5	Controls (mean $\pm$ SD)		
Arylsulfatase A	127.6	86.7	44.6	104	$\pm$	34
β-D-galactosidase pH 4.4	195.6	397	190	245	$\pm$	78
α-D-galactosidase	91.0	83.5	43.6	68	$\pm$	20
N-acetyl-β-D-glucosaminidase A	3330	3021	1225	1684	$\pm$	622
N-acetyl-β-D-glucosaminidase B	1152	not done	378	845	$\pm$	405
β-D-glucuronidase	402	197	326	316	$\pm$	92
α-D-glucosidase	59.2	72.8	22.1	38	$\pm$	12
α-L-fucosidase	135.7	258	100.8	91	$\pm$	24
α-D-mannosidase	447.6	880	315.5	381	$\pm$	154
Acid phosphatase	2580	2080	2078	3878	$\pm$	2190

SOURCE: From Gerritsen et al. [246].

defect in the CHS neutrophil involves an organelle membrane abnormality which fosters the giant granule formation [273, 302]. This membrane defect may be linked in some way to microtubule assembly, which has been found defective by some authors [282, 285], particularly in the beige mouse, thought to be homologous with the human disease. Abnormalities of cyclic nucleotide metabolism and microtubule assembly were postulated when it was observed that concanavalin A–induced capping took place spontaneously in the beige mouse leukocytes, a phenomenon which occurs in normal mouse cells only after treatment with microtubule poisons, such as colchicine [303]. The capping defect in the beige mouse cells could be corrected by treating cells in vitro with agents such as ascorbic acid and carbamylcholine, which elevated cellular levels of cGMP [282–285]. Human leukocytes were found to have normal levels of cGMP, however, and elevated levels of cAMP, which fell to normal values with ascorbic acid treatment [284]. Treatment with ascorbic acid in vitro and in vivo increased the number of centriole-associated microtubules and improved leukocyte function [282–284, 304, 305]. Additional support for a microtubule defect came from studies on beige mouse embryonic fibroblasts, human CHS monocytes in tissue culture [282], human CHS fibroblasts in culture [306], and human platelets [307]. The concept that microtubule formation underlies the defect present in all cell systems known to be abnormal in this disorder has been challenged. While platelets from CHS patients are functionally defective, share the cyclic nucleotide abnormality reported in CHS leukocytes, and possess giant granules [275, 276, 307, 308], the number of microtubules in platelets and their reassembly after depolymerization were identical to those of normal human platelets [307]. Microtubules associated with the centriole in CHS lymphocytes and monocytes were found to be numerically identical to those in normal cells [309]. Frankel et al. [310] were unable to detect differences from normal in the beige mouse in microtubule number and distribution, using indirect immunofluorescence in peritoneal macrophages and fibroblasts. Ostlund et al. [311] found the cytoplasmic microtubular network of cultured CHS fibroblasts quantitatively and qualitatively similar to normal human cultured fibroblasts. Further, there is no known defect in cell division in any organ system in CHS patients [312], a process which requires assembly of microtubules into mitotic spindles. At present, the role of a microtubule defect in CHS is unclear.

Patients with CHS may have a defect in cellular immunity. Roder [313] described a marked impairment in splenic natural killing (NK) function and antibody-dependent, cell-mediated cytolysis (ADCC) of tumor cells in beige mice. Other forms of cell-mediated lysis were normal [314]. Extension of this work to humans with CHS showed that the NK activity was profoundly impaired and did not result from an alteration of an antitarget selectivity pattern, or of the kinetics of lysis, of suppressor cells, of a lack of ability to respond to interferon, or a lack of target-cell recognition [315]. Lymphocyte-mediated ADCC against tumor-cell targets was also defective in the human cells, whereas ADCC mediated by mononuclear and polymorphonuclear leukocytes against erythrocyte targets was normal [316]. Thus CHS also shares a defect of the immune system with another pigment anomaly, the Griscelli syndrome [317, 318].

The classic pathognomonic feature of this syndrome is the presence of giant peroxidase-positive lysosomal granules in granulocytes of the peripheral blood. Giant granules which resemble those of CHS by light microscopy occur occasionally in chronic myelogenous leukemia and acute myeloid leukemias [319–321]. Electron microscopically, these giant granules are formed by fusion of azurophilic granules, as in CHS, but contain numerous microcrystalline structures resembling Auer bodies but with a different periodicity [321].

Treatment with high doses of ascorbic acid (200 mg in infants to 6 g in adults per day) has been advocated as a long-term regimen for patients with CHS [284]. Boxer et al. [284] reported clinical improvement as well as improved functions of

Figure 15-25 Section through a hair bulb keratinocyte of a patient with ym type albinism shows electron-opaque fibrils resembling those seen in circulating monocytes in HPS patients (Fig. 15-18). ×41,500. *(From White et al. [176].)*

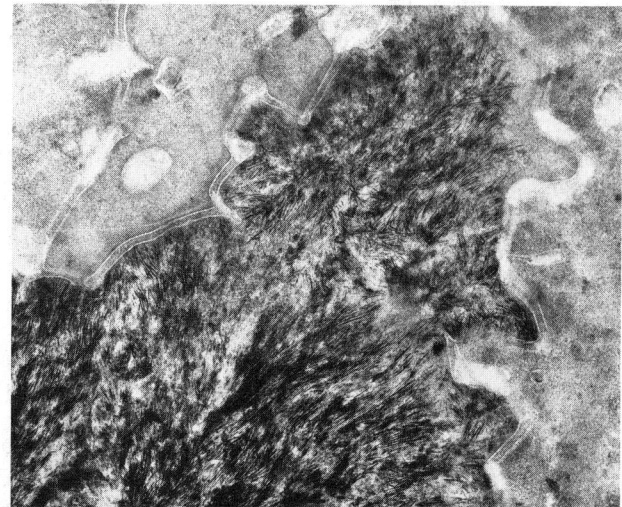

Table 15-13   Phospholipids of HPS-platelet membranes

Individuals	PS	PI	LyPC	Sph	PC	PE
Patient 1	14.3	1.3	1.5	19.6	37.5	25.8
Patient 2	12.7	1.5	2.3	18.0	39.0	26.5
Control	14.0	0.4	2.8	19.9	37.0	26.9
Control	14.2	1.0	1.8	18.8	40.0	24.2

The values are expressed as percentage of total lipid phosphorus.
PS = phosphatidylserine; PI = phosphatidylinositol; LyPC = lysophosphatidylcholine; Sph = sphingomyelin; PC = phosphatidylcholine and PE = phosphatidylethanolamine.
SOURCE: From Gerritsen et al. [246].

cells in vitro in an infant on ascorbic acid, but Gallin et al. [322] found no clinical improvement in two adult patients placed on ascorbic acid for 8 months. There was no improvement in phagocytic cell chemotaxis, bactericidal activity, or lymphocyte function after ascorbic acid in vivo, nor were the investigators able to demonstrate an effect in vitro on leukocyte chemotaxis or bactericidal activity. Their studies on the beige mouse, however, showed that ascorbic acid significantly protected both normal and CHS mice from a challenge lethal infection with *Candida albicans*, but the survival rate of beige mice was significantly less than that of controls. The ascorbic acid-treated beige mice had improved chemotaxis and bactericidal activity but no morphologic changes in giant lysosomal granules in polymorphonuclear leukocytes. No abnormality in cAMP or cGMP was found in the beige mouse leukocytes [322].

Heterozygotes for CHS occasionally show giant lysosomal granules in peripheral leukocytes, but not with sufficient frequency to make this a reliable test for the carrier.

A defect similar to that seen in CHS human patients has been observed in Aleutian mink [279, 281, 323], Hereford cattle [323, 324], a killer whale [325], cats [326], and beige mice [279].

The primary gene product defect in CHS is unknown.

Cross Syndrome [90]   This extremely rare syndrome (approximate synonyms: *oculocerebral-hypopigmentation syndrome* [90]; *hypopigmentation and microphthalmia* [4]; *gingival fibromatosis, hypopigmentation, microphthalmia, oligophrenia,* and *athetosis,* [91–93]) has been described in a girl and two boys from a multiply consanguine Amish family in Ohio [90]. An additional affected child from Uruguay has come to our attention. The affected children have extremely blond hair with a slight yellow-gray metallic sheen. The skin is dead white and turns pink on even a few minutes' exposure to sunlight. Lightly pigmented nevi may be present. Hypopigmentation is present at birth. The children have small eyes, cloudy corneas, and a coarse, jerky nystagmus. By 3 months of age, patients develop writhing motions of the extremities; they have constant sucking movements and high-pitched, weak cries. Affected children are unable to sit unaided, are below the third percentile for height and weight, and are severely retarded mentally. By late infancy, all children develop opacified and vascular corneas. Gingival fibromatosis develops concomitantly with eruption of the primary teeth [91, 92].

No chemical abnormalities have been found in urine, serum, or cerebrospinal fluid. The serum tyrosine concentration was within high normal limits by the method used (2.6 mg/dl), as was that of phenylalanine (0.1 mg/dl) [90]. One child died at 12 years of age from inanition and respiratory failure. Routinely prepared, formalin-fixed tissue specimens showed no abnormal inclusions in the brain, liver, spleen, or bone marrow [81].

No pigment is observed in fresh hair bulbs by means of visual microscopy [4]. The hair bulb test of Kugelman and van Scott gives a weakly positive result, showing a distribution of a few L-tyrosine- or L-dopa-positive melanocytes in the hair bulb. Electron photomicrographs show that melanocytes are scanty and contain small clusters of melanosomes of all stages. After incubation in L-tyrosine, most melanosomes are converted to fully pigmented stage IV melanosomes [4, 82].

The basic defect in Cross syndrome is unknown. The condition shares the hypopigmentation and microphthalmic features seen in mice homozygous for genes (*mi*) of the microphthalmia locus, which have been called *mock albinos* because of a deficiency of melanocytes [21].

Brown Oculocutaneous Albinism [94]   This phenotype has been identified in Africans [94] and New Guineans [327]. Brown oculocutaneous albinos are darker than ty-pos albinos, with medium brown hair, light brown to olive-colored skin, hazel eyes, moderate nystagmus which is elicited in some only after dark adaptation, and slight photophobia. Of the 23

Figure 15-26   *A.* Melanocyte from a hair bulb of a patient with CHS contains numerous giant melanosomes, as well as a few of normal size. ×20,000. *B.* Leukocyte from the same patient contains giant lysosomal granules, as well as a few granules of normal size. ×13,000. *(From Witkop et al. [82].)*

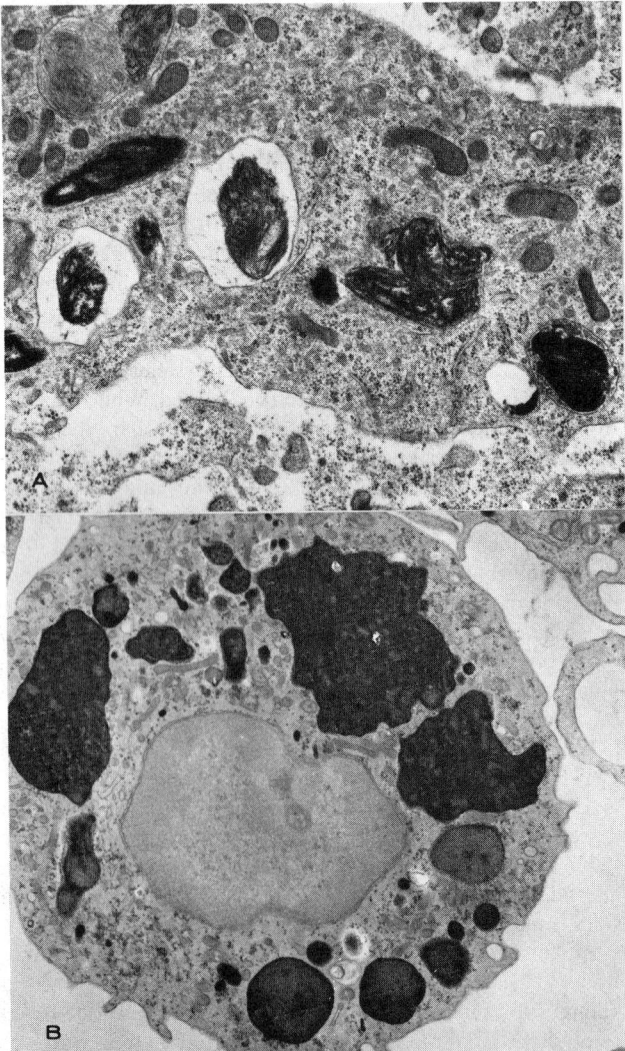

brown albinos studied by King et al. [94], 96 percent had nystagmus, 52 percent had strabismus, and 87 percent showed diaphanous irides. Approximately 35 percent of the brown Nigerian albinos had blue irides, 22 percent hazel, and 43 percent light brown. Light retinal pigment was present in 86 percent of the patients examined but was undetectable in 14 percent. In contrast to the ty-pos albino, there was little accumulation or change in pigment in the eyes or skin with age, and only one brown albino showed goose-foot lentigines on sun-exposed skin, as was found in approximately half of the African ty-pos albinos. Visual acuity was mildly reduced and ranged from 20/30 to 20/100. A few brown albinos had mild pachydermia and premalignant keratoses, but none was found with squamous cell carcinoma. Epilated hair bulbs contain eumelanosomes in all stages of formation but have only a slight increase in pigment formation following incubation in L-tyrosine. While earlier reports in the literature mention xanthous albinos [6], which include the brown albino and the red or rufous albino, the genotype has only recently been well delineated among Nigerians [94] and natives of New Guinea [327]. Brown albinos constitute approximately 6 percent of all types of OCA among the Ibo population. Brown albinism has a gene frequency of approximately 0.021 ± .004 in the Malalaua District of New Guinea [327]. The condition is clinically and ultrastructurally distinct from the "red skin" or rufous albino. The condition is inherited as an autosomal recessive trait.

Rufous Albinism [95]   Rufous albinism was mentioned by Pearson et al. [6] and was described in detail in natives of New Guinea by Walsh [95] and Harvey [96], and in Africans and American blacks [3]. The skin color is a mahogany reddish-brown, and the hair color varies from a deep mahogany red to a sandy red. The irides are reddish brown to brown with slight translucency on transillumination. About 80 percent of the patients have very mild nystagmus which is elicited primarily on lateral gaze or after dark adaptation. Only a mild photophobia is present. The fundus shows a definite light reddish-brown pigment. Visual acuity ranges from 20/20 to 20/100. The hair bulb test is positive. The condition is inherited as an autosomal recessive trait.

Autosomal Dominant Oculocutaneous Albinism [97] Frenk and Calme [97] reported a Swiss kindred of three generations in which patients had the clinical criteria of OCA and which was similar to a four-generation kindred observed by King and the author [2]. In these families hair color varied from white to white with slight red tints. Skin color ranged from white to light cream with pigmented nevi. The irides were gray to gray-blue in color, with marked translucency on transillumination. Nystagmus and photophobia were present in all cases and were about equal in severity to those in the ty-pos albino. Visual acuity ranged from 20/70 to 20/200. Ultrastructurally, the skin and hair contained normal numbers of melanocytes, and no structural abnormality of the melanosomes was observed. Frenk and Calme [97] believed that the activity of tyrosinase was increased in the regions of the Golgi and in premelanosomes in stage I.

Black Locks, Oculocutaneous Albinism, and Deafness of the Sensorineural Type (BADS Syndrome) [2]   This combination of defects was first recognized as unique by Efron, Beasley, and Witkop [2] in a kindred with an affected girl and boy. An additional kindred with an affected boy and girl has been observed by Kimberling [328]. Patients with this disorder have hypoplasia of the fovea, marked nystagmus, photophobia, transparent gray irides, a prominent red reflex, and visual acuity which ranges from 20/250 to 20/400. While the skin and hair are dead white, the patients show clusters of black hair occurring in locks and coin-shaped brown macules on the skin. Because of their profound congenital sensorineural deafness and marked decrease in visual acuity, patients may be socially retarded. One patient in one family had a complete sensorineural deafness in one ear and a 50-dB loss in the other. Above the ear, which retained some hearing, was a large black hair lock. In contrast to all other forms of albinism, melanocytes are absent in the white hair and white portions of the skin but are present and form normal eumelanosomes in the black locks and pigmented areas of the skin [2, 329]. There is either a failure of melanoblasts to migrate or of melanocytes to survive in the peripheral sites of skin, hair, eyes, and inner ear. Hair bulb incubation tests and hair bulb tyrosinase assay [100] were negative for white hairs, but pigmented hairs formed increased melanin following incubation and had normal ranges of tyrosinase activity for black hair. One obligate heterozygote showed a white blaze in the midscalp (not a forelock) and an unusual lesion of the fundus. Large, geometric patterns of hyperpigmentation of the fundus covered the entire posterior pole out to the equator. There were circles and lines separating zones of hyper- and hypopigmentation. The diameter of many of the zones approximated one-half the diameter of the optic disk. While in the homozygote the parietal vasculature was easily detected, in the obligate heterozygote the retinal vasculature was not visible. In the heterozygote the extent of the pigmentary changes but not the pattern was similar to that seen in Sjogren's reticular dystrophy of the retinal pigment epithelium. The condition is probably inherited as an autosomal recessive trait.

Yellow Mutant Oculocutaneous Albinism (ym) [4, 98] Approximate synonyms for this type of albinism are *Amish albinism* [98] and *xanthous albinism* [17, 139]. The yellow type of albino has yellow to yellow-red or yellow-brown hair and a slight tanning effect in skin exposed to sunlight. The result of the hair bulb test of Kugelman and van Scott [5] is either negative or equivocal. Melanocytes are present in skin, hair, and eyes, but melanosomes develop only to stage III and show an uneven pigmentation of the melanosomal matrix.

The phenotypic expression of the ym gene varies with the ethnic origin of the patient. Caucasian ym albinos at birth appear to have no visible pigment and resemble ty-neg albino infants. The hair is dead white but gradually turns a bright yellow between the ages of 6 weeks and 6 years. In addition, at approximately the same time, the skin turns a very light cream color and shows a minimal but distinct tanning effect when exposed to sunlight. In Negro patients with the ym mutation, the skin has a definite dark-cream color, frequently with numerous pigmented nevi, and the hair may vary from dark yellow to yellow-brown. By midinfancy, the irides usually have some detectable pigment, and by 3 years of age there is a distinct, easily detectable cartwheel effect on transillumination of the ocular bulb. Photophobia and nystagmus, although always present and distinctive features of the condition, are in general less severe than those seen in the ty-pos type of albino (Table 15-6). A slight amount of retinal pigment may be detected on funduscopic examination of Negro ym albinos but may be absent in Caucasian ym albinos. The macular reflex is absent or markedly diminished.

The main feature distinguishing ty-pos from ym albinos is in the response of the latter to hair bulb incubation tests. In the ym albinos, the result of the hair bulb incubation test is equivocal or negative, but there are nearly always microscopically distinguishable pigment granules in the hair bulb and often in the hair shaft. In the freshly epilated hair bulbs from Caucasian ym albinos, the pigment has a definite golden tint, and the color of the hair shaft varies from light to bright yellow. In Negro ym albinos the hair bulbs range from bright yellow to yellow-brown, frequently with reddish tints. On incubation in L-tyrosine or L-dopa, the hair bulbs from the ym albino do not form black eumelanin. Occasional hair bulbs will show some slight darkening. Frequently these hair bulbs are from ym albinos from more deeply pigmented families, but they lack the definite dark pigmentation seen in the ty-pos type of albino. Hair bulbs from ym subjects show intensification of the yellow-red pheomelanin when incubated in a solution of 40 mg L-tyrosine and 40 mg L-cysteine per deciliter of a 0.1 M phosphate buffer at pH 6.8. Hair bulbs of ty-pos and normal blond subjects incubated in the serum of ym albinos form increased pigment.

Thus the ym albino serum does not contain inhibitors for pigment formation [47]. The melanocytes appear to be packed with abnormal numbers of melanosomes in various stages of development. Many small, round, unevenly pigmented forms and elongated forms showing partial pigmentation of the matrix resembling the pheomelanosomes of red hair are present in melanocytes and in phagolysosomes in keratinocytes. Specimens incubated in tyrosine and viewed with the electron microscope do not show an increased density of melanosomes, as in the ty-pos type [4], but melanosomes become darker in an unevenly distributed pattern following tyrosine-cysteine incubation. Keratinocytes contain a fibrillar material resembling that found in melanophores of leaf frogs (Fig. 15-25).

The ym OCA gene is most likely allelic with the gene for ty-neg OCA [330]. Hu et al. [330] reported a kindred in which the unaffected mother was a first cousin of a biochemically proven ty-neg albino. She had three daughters with clinical, chemical, and ultrastructural features of ym albinism. It was postulated that the father was genotypically ym/+ and the mother ty-neg/+. The children, who appear to have the genotype ym/ty-neg, show typical ty-neg stage II melanosomes in freshly epilated hair bulbs. Following incubation in tyrosine-cysteine solutions, the small, round melanosomes showed a pheomelanin spotty type of pigment accumulation. Subsequent study of this family by the author showed that the tyrosinase activity in the hair bulbs of the mother was essentially zero, as has been found in obligate heterozygotes for ty-neg OCA [149]. The father, who was presumed to be an obligate heterozygote for ym albinism, also had low tyrosinase activity, which has been observed in this laboratory in obligate heterozygotes for ym OCA.

Ocular Albinism (OA)   Patients with OA usually fall within the range of normal pigmentation of hair and skin, but relatively mild cutaneous manifestations of pigmentary dilution are frequently found in all types of OA when the affected individuals are compared with their sibs, and in some forms, such as the X-linked OA described by Nettleship (XOAN) [114], there is histologic evidence of abnormalities in melanogenesis in skin [26, 113] as well as eyes [26, 145]. Classically, OA has been recognized as an X-linked trait [114], wherein the obligate heterozygotes show a mosaic pigment pattern of their

fundi [115] compatible with a Lyonization effect of genes on the X chromosome. A review of our clinic admissions and a study of a population of albinos at Moorfield's Eye Hospital indicate that the autosomal recessive form of ocular albinism (AROA) is at least as frequent as XOAN.

X-linked Ocular Albinism (Nettleship) (XOAN) [114, 115]   X-linked OA of the Nettleship-Falls type [114, 115] has also been described as hereditary sex-linked nystagmus [331, 332]. Pigmentation other than in the eyes is normal or slightly reduced [145, 333]. Hemizygous males are severely affected, while heterozygous females generally show minor pigmentary changes in the irides and retina. Giant round abnormal melanosomes are found in fundal and epidermal melanocytes [26, 113, 145].

Affected males have reduced pigmentation in the irides, which may vary from pale blue to light green, with an occasional patient showing brown pigment most prominent at the pupillary border. Eye color frequently becomes darker with age. The irides are diaphanous. Pigment is usually detectable at the pupillary borders and limbus. Nystagmus is nearly always present in the primary position and is most frequently either a combined rotary and horizontal or a horizontal type. Nystagmus has been reported to diminish with age, this improvement being accompanied by increased darkening of the iris color [334]. Head nodding and heat tilt are prominent in about half the affected males [334]. Photophobia is usually severe, and nystagmus becomes more prominent on exposure to light after dark adaptation. Visual acuity is usually 20/50 or less, seldom being worse than 20/300 in whites, but may be as good as 20/25 in blacks and does not improve with age [145]. Near vision is relatively better; most patients can read N5 or N6 type at 4 to 5 in. Refraction anomalies are common. Strabismus is found in about 60 percent of patients, with exotropia being about four times more frequent than esotropia [334]. In ty-pos albinism esotropia is about four times more frequent than exotropia [4].

The background color of the fundus is pale yellow to pale yellow-orange, not dead white, as in choroideremia [141, 334]. The choroidal vessels are easily visualized and the perifoveal vessels have a normal distribution [145], as seen in ty-pos OCA [335]. The ERG is usually normal [336, 337] but occasionally a supernormal scotopic ERG [336] and an electrooculogram ratio [338] may be recorded, the frequencies of these findings being greater in the ty-neg OCA than in the XOAN patients. The most constant clinical diagnostic feature is ophthalmoscopic evidence of foveal hypoplasia [145, 339]. This is especially helpful in diagnosing XOAN in blacks, in whom the irides often do not transilluminate and the fundus is moderately pigmented [145, 339]. Hemizygous blacks may show hypopigmented macules of the skin, most prominently on the torso [145, 339]. These features are important to recognize in black patients, since they are often misdiagnosed as having motor-defect congenital nystagmus [339].

Macromelanosomes are found in fetal retinal pigment epithelium and in the skin in both the hemizygous male and the heterozygous female [26, 145, 339] (Fig. 15-27).

Females heterozygous for X-chromosomal OA usually show a mosaic pattern of pigment distribution in the fundus and translucent irides [26, 115–119, 145, 334, 339–341]. The mosaic appearance of the fundus has been described as tigeroid, pigment dusting, or "splashes of mud" [115, 118, 119] and is attributed to Lyonization [342]. Occasionally a

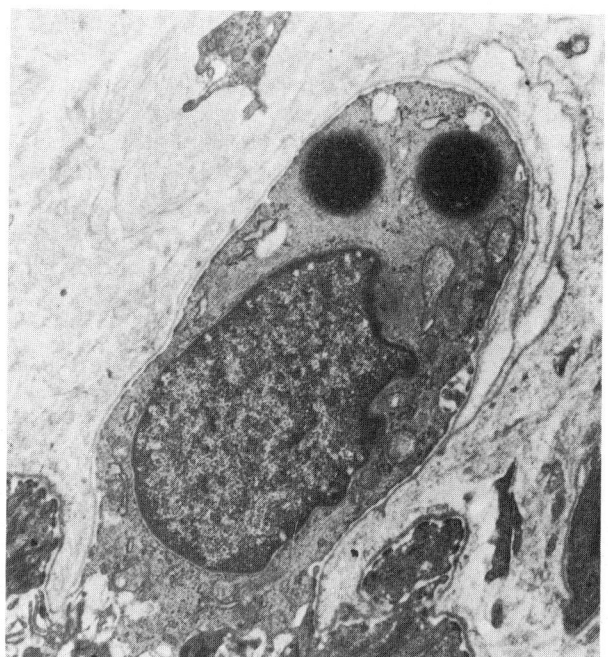

Figure 15-27 Macromelanosomes from the skin of a patient heterozygous for X-linked ocular albinism (OA). Similar macromelanosomes have been reported in skin biopsy specimens of patients with HPS and ocular albinism-lentigines-deafness syndrome. They differ from those in CHS (Fig. 15-26A). *(Courtesy of Dr. Francis E. O'Donnell, Jr.)*

female within a kindred may be affected as severely as a male, with nystagmus and photophobia in addition to severe iris and fundal hypopigmentation [117, 343]. These examples probably represent the chance selection by nearly all progenitor optic pigment cells of the X chromosome which bears the mutant gene on the active X chromosome.

Linkage between OA and the Xg blood group from combined kindreds has led to estimates of a recombination fraction of 0.15 [344–346]. A mating between a father with XOAN and a mother with autosomal recessive OA (AROA) showed complementation in the children. The female children had the heterozygous features of XOAN [104]. Similarly, matings observed by the author, of XOAN men with ty-pos women and with ty-neg women, have shown a similar complementation, with no detectable differences between the doubly heterozygous females and XOAN heterozygotes.

Autosomal Recessive Ocular Albinism (AROA) [81, 347]   AROA was initially described by Witkop et al. [81] in four families in which females were as severely affected as males, and the kindreds were not compatible with X-linked inheritance. Subsequent detailed studies on these families and others by O'Donnell et al. [347] showed that the patients had all the features of OA, including decreased visual acuity, prominent red reflex, hypoplasia of the fovea, photophobia, nystagmus, strabismus, diaphanous irides, and light yellow fundi. Three patients had a mildly subnormal scotopic ERG but were myopic. Visual acuity has ranged from 20/100 to 20/400 [347].

Seventeen families with this disorder have been studied by the authors, and others have come to our attention. The mothers have not had affected male relatives, and they have no mosaic pigment patterns in their fundi. Parents have shown diaphanous irides in some cases, but this has not been detectable in deeply pigmented families. Two of the families were

Amish, and the parents were multiply consanguine. The authors have also observed ym albinism [98], Cross syndrome [90, 91], and ty-neg OCA among Amish families, but the OA did not resemble these disorders. There was no evidence of Turner syndrome in the affected women. Buccal Barr body counts were normal, and chromosomal analysis of lymphocytes in one patient showed a normal female karyotype. A similarly affected female with no familial or chromosomal evidence of X linkage was described by Scialfa [348].

Pigmentation of the skin and hair is within normal limits, but affected patients generally have slightly lighter skin and hair color than their unaffected sibs [347]. Reticulated macular hypopigmentation of the skin seen in XOAN males has not been observed. The hair bulb tyrosine incubation test is positive. Electron-microscopic features of hair bulbs and skin are not unusual, and macromelanosomes which occur in the skin of XOAN patients have not been found [347]. It should be noted that macromelanosomes found on light microscopy of skin biopsy specimen and verified by electron microscopy is the preferred method of differentiating XOAN from AROA. Macromelanosomes occur in a number of disorders: HPS [185], ocular albinism-lentigines-deafness syndrome [349], both of which have nystagmus, nevus spilus [350], generalized lentigines [351], xeroderma pigmentosum [352], and neurofibromatosis [353]. The giant melanosomes of CHS have a different ultrastructural appearance (cf. Figs. 15-26A and 15-27) from all of the above.

Ocular Albinism-Lentigines-Deafness Syndrome [349] Seven affected males and five affected females were found in three consecutive generations of a Caucasian kindred in a pattern compatible with autosomal dominant inheritance [349]. Affected patients had reduced visual acuity, photophobia, congenital nystagmus, translucent irides, strabismus, hypermetropic refractive errors, and albinotic fundi with hypoplasia of the fovea. In addition, the patients had multiple cutaneous lentigines which histologically contained macromelanosomes which were absent in normal skin. The patients had congenital sensorineural deafness and vestibular abnormalities.

Forsius-Eriksson Syndrome [120] The approximate synonyms are *Åland eye disease and ocular albinism, Forsius Eriksson type.* Forsius and Eriksson [120] described an extensive kindred with an X-linked "fundusalbinismus" among families from the Åland Islands in the Gulf of Bothnia. The major features which distinguish the Åland disorder from the Nettleship type of X-linked OA are that in males the hypopigmentation is less severe in the former, males show a high frequency of protanomalous color blindness and high degrees of axial myopia, and female carriers do not have mosaic pigment patterns in the fundus [122, 354, 355]. Females may show slight color discrimination defects and latent nystagmus. The dyschromatopsia was found to be variable within kindreds and may be due to association with X-linked color blindness [356].

Reinvestigation of this kindred by O'Donnell et al. [121] showed that the patients lacked macromelanosomes, that the melanosomes of the skin were normal, and that the constant features of the syndrome are its X-linked inheritance, hypoplasia of the fovea, and nystagmus. They were unable to differentiate between a defective induction of retinal pigment and stretching of retinal pigment epithelium due to high-grade axial myopia, as alternatives for the observed hypopigmentation of the fundus. The condition must be differentiated from XOAN, X-linked nyctalopia and myopia [357], and isolated hypoplasia of the fovea [358].

Linkage studies with the Xg blood group show a recombination fraction of about 0.12 [359] and suggest that this type may be allelic or pseudoallelic (adjacent locus) to XOAN [355].

Albinoidism

Oculocutaneous and ocular forms of albinoidism are distinguished clinically from various types of albinism by the absence of hypoplasia of the fovea, nystagmus, photophobia and, with rare exceptions, by a lack of decreased visual acuity [2, 136]. Only two of these conditions will be dealt with in this text since they have been confused with several types of albinism. For detailed discussions of various forms of albinoidism and other pigment disorders, readers are referred to general texts [136, 360].

Oculocutaneous Albinoidism [81, 124, 361]   This rare form of ocular and oculocutaneous hypopigmentation has been described in only a few families [81, 124, 361]. Early reports may have described the same disorder [22, 139]. The condition differs from all forms of true OA in that it is inherited as an autosomal dominant trait and, with one exception, that patients do not have associated nystagmus, photophobia, or markedly decreased visual acuity. The hair is white to slightly yellow or reddish tinged. The skin is pink-white and becomes erythematous on short exposure to sunlight. A very slight tanning effect has been noted [361]. Hair bulbs from these patients incubated in L-tyrosine form increased pigment [81, 361]. The irides are blue in tangential light and are translucent. A foveal reflex is present.

No members of the affected families have been deaf. A dominantly inherited hypopigmentation with deafness was described by Tietz [125] and others [362] in which the phenotypic appearance of the patients resembled that of patients with autosomal dominant albinoidism. There are other reports of OA albinos with albino parents who probably represent pseudodominance of a recessive oculocutaneous albinism arising from inbreeding [4, 6, 363, 364].

Punctate Oculocutaneous Albinoidism [123]   A single kindred was described by Bergsma and Kaiser-Kupfer [123] in which patients were blond, had a very mild visual acuity defect of 20/30, dilated pupils, and anisocoria. Cone thresholds were slightly elevated. The irides showed a punctate type of transillumination, and a similar punctate pattern of windows in the retinal pigment epithelium was found on fluorescein angiography. Hair bulb tests were positive. The condition may be inherited as a dominant trait.

Hypopigmentation-Immunodeficiency Disease (Griscelli Syndrome) [317]   Griscelli and coworkers [317] and Siccardi et al. [365] described the association of pigmentary dilution with frequent pyogenic infections, hepatosplenomegaly, neutropenia, thrombocytopenia, and evidence of immunodeficiency. These patients from two kindreds were initially thought to have CHS because of the history of repeated infections and silvery gray hair [317].

Patients have pale skin, sometimes with a gray hue, silvery

gray hair, and no photophobia, nystagmus, or OA, although one patient showed depigmented spots in the retina. Skin biopsy specimens show melanin-congested melanocytes surrounded by hypopigmented keratinocytes at the dermal-epidermal junction. Melanocytes contain numerous granules but lack normal dendrites, few extending beyond the second layer of keratinocytes. In the hair shaft there are numerous large clumps of pigment which give the hair a leopard-skin appearance. Electron microscopically, the cytoplasm of the melanocytes is packed with normal-appearing melanosomes, but only a few isolated melanosomes can be identified in the adjacent keratinocytes, which lack phagolysosomes. This type of pigment defect is similar to that seen in the homozygous dilute mouse (d^l/d^l) [21].

Patients have an adequate number of T and B lymphocytes, but they have hypogammaglobulinemia and deficient antibody production and are incapable of manifesting delayed skin hypersensitivity or of rejecting skin grafts. The leukocytes do not stimulate normal lymphocytes and cannot generate cytotoxic cells during the mixed leukocyte reaction. T lymphocytes are unable to exert a helper effect on the maturation of B lymphocytes into immunoglobulin-containing cells following stimulation with pokeweed mitogen in vitro. Immune interferon titers from supernatants of mixed-leukocyte cultures and the NK activity are markedly reduced [318]. There is no morphologic abnormality of granulocytes, of which the bactericidal activity is only moderately reduced [365]. There is an elevation of polymorphonuclear leukocytes with capping of concanavalin A receptors. Brambilla et al. [366] reported an increased hemophagocytosis of bone marrow macrophages and increased erythrophagocytosis of an affected infant's red blood cells when suspended in the infant's serum and tested against normal monocytes from healthy donors.

This condition bears some resemblance to familial hemophagocytic reticulosis, from which it must be differentiated. There is no specific treatment for this disorder. The condition is inherited as an autosomal recessive trait.

The Central Nervous System in Albinos

Optic Neurologic Defects in Albinos   In vertebrates with laterally placed eyes and panoramic vision, such as in most fish, amphibians, reptiles, and birds [367], there is a complete decussation of optic fibers at the chiasma. As the eyes shift to a frontal position and develop stereoscopic vision, the proportion of optic fibers that originates in the temporal retina and does not decussate increases (rat, 10 percent; dog and horse, 20 percent; cat, 30 to 40 percent) [367–369]. Primates and humans have from 45 to 50 percent uncrossed fibers [370].

Albino animals and humans with all types of OCA (ty-neg, ty-pos, ym, HPS, brown) and OA (XOAN, AROA) [94, 155, 371–375] have abnormal optic neuronal pathways in that most fibers from the temporal retina, which in normally pigmented animals course to the same side of the brain as the eye of origin, cross to the opposite side [376–386]. Approximately 10 to 15 percent of albino animals and humans do not show VEP evidence of a decussation defect, and the proportion of rearranged fibers is somewhat variable. These anatomic abnormalities in the albino optic neuronal pathway result in behavioral [387] and electrophysiologic abnormalities [368, 388, 389]. The defect is independent of species and has been demonstrated in various animals with mutations at the c locus (tyrosinase locus), including the albino (c/c) guinea pig [368, 382], rat [376, 381, 387–390], rabbit [377, 385, 391], mink [385, 386], ferret [380], Siamese (c^s/c^s) cat [378, 379, 392–394], and chinchilla (c^{ch}/c^{ch}) white tiger [383].

Initially, it was postulated that the neuronal defect resulted from a nonpigmentary function of tyrosinase, which is defective or deficient in these animals, but the defect is not confined to animals with mutations at the c locus. This was demonstrated by Creel and collaborators [371, 375] in various types of human albinos. Monocularly stimulated, visually evoked potentials recorded from occipital leads over the right and left visual cortices give approximately symmetric responses in normal humans, reflecting the underlying approximately symmetric division of the optic tract. Creel et al. [371, 375] demonstrated asymmetric monocularly stimulated responses with reduction in the ipsilateral recordings in ty-pos, ym, brown, and HPS albinos, as well as in ty-neg human albinos, the last possibly the human homologue of c-locus albino animals [4]. Since ty-neg and ty-pos albinism and HPS and ty-pos albinism are not allelic, and since ty-pos, brown, and HPS melanocytes have tyrosinase activity varying from low normal to three times normal levels, Witkop et al. [82] and Creel et al. [371, 375] postulated that the optic defect is associated with any defect which results in the absence of pigment in the developing optic cup regardless of the underlying genetic mechanism. Sanderson and coworkers [386] tested mink with a variety of genes controlling pigment at different loci and demonstrated that any gene resulting in hypopigmentation of the fundi was associated with the optic defect.

Subsequent studies, including those determining localization of cerebral glucose utilization in the brain visual system of albino rats [395], VEP studies of human albinos with XOAN and AROA [372], and anatomic studies of albino human [155] and primate brains [396] showed evidence of disorganization of the retinogeniculate tracts.

The normal human lateral geniculate nuclei are organized into six layers, two magnocellular and four parvocellular (Fig. 15-28). Anatomic investigations to date of three brains from human albinos (ty-pos and ty-neg) showed defects in the size, orientation, and layered segments of the lateral geniculate nuclei [155]. Grossly, the geniculate ganglions appeared absent. The characteristic swelling did not show because the nucleus was rotated rostrolaterally about 30° to the frontal plane within the brain tissue, and the lateral tip was elevated. Abnormal fusions were found in the parvocellular layers, and only a single magnocellular layer was found in most sections (Fig. 15-28). The defects in human albino brains were similar to those found in an albino monkey [396].

Initially, it was believed that the fawn hooded rat was an exception to the emerging generalization that the decussation defect was associated with a lack of fundal pigment, since this animal has reduced ipsilateral tracts and the adult animal has pigmented fundi [376]. However, fundal pigment is lacking at birth and does not develop until after the major portion of the postnatal specification time for the final optic neuronal arrangement is past. While the details of how pigment is involved in the development of the optic system are unknown, the present evidence indicates that pigment in the optic cup is necessary for directing optic neurons to normal brain targets and for the development of a normal fovea, a relationship anticipated by Ida Mann as early as 1937 [397].

The proportion of neurons rearranged in albinos varies. Approximately 10 to 15 percent of animals and humans do not

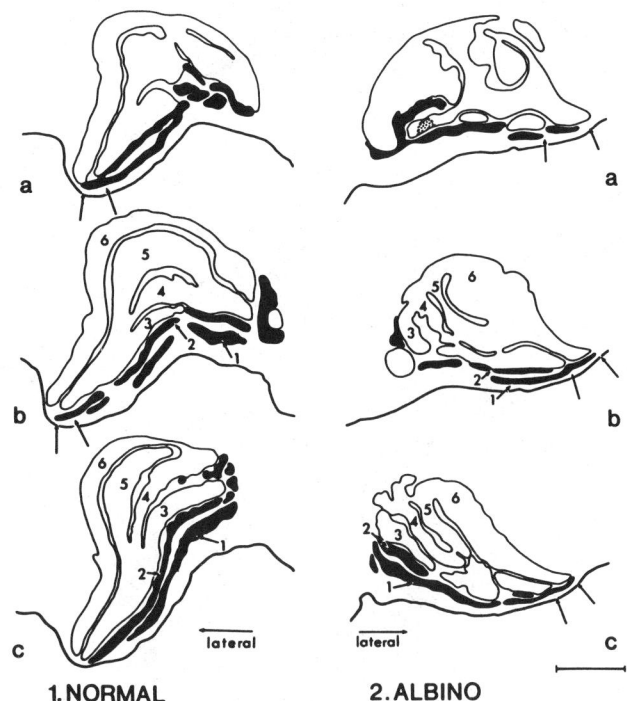

Figure 15-28 Drawings of frontal sections taken at comparable levels through the lateral geniculate nuclei of a normal (1) and a ty-pos albino (2) brain. The most rostral sections (level a) pass through the zone in which the six-layered and the four-layered segments are fusing. The magnocellular layers are shown in black, and the conventional numbering is indicated where six layers are evident. The bilaminar part of the nucleus is indicated by unlabeled arrows. Notice the small size of the albino nucleus, absence of the swelling adjacent to the tip, and disruption and fusion of layers compared with the normal. Scale = 2 mm. *(From Guillery et al. [155].)*

show evidence of a major rearrangement [371, 372]. Evidence from Siamese cats suggests that the midportions of the temporal retina are most susceptible to the anomaly [393, 394]. As a result of the decussation defect, most human albinos lack the internal mechanism for binocular vision.

Evidence that the pathways from the lateral geniculate ganglion to the visual cortex, the geniculocortical tracts, are also anomalous in albinos was demonstrated electroencephalographically by Guillery [378] and Hubel and Wiesel [398], and anatomically in Siamese (a c-locus mutation) cats by Guillery [393] and Kaas and Guillery [394]. Guillery and coworkers [399, 400] reasoned that given the initial decussation defect of the retinogeniculate pathway and normal connections from the lateral geniculate nucleus to the cortex, there would be a disruption of the order of the visual field segments, an inversion of a portion of the visual field as a reversal of normal such that there would be an ascending sequence in one layer of the cortex and a descending sequence in the same layer, and a noncorrespondence or mismatching of two adjacent layers (Fig. 15-29). It was found that partial compensation for these abnormalities was achieved in two ways in cats. In "Midwestern" cats the input to the cortex from the A_1 layer of the lateral geniculate nucleus (normally, temporal retinal nondecussated input) was suppressed. In "Boston" cats a rerouting of axons occurred, reversing the order of the misdirected mid-half-field segments [399, 400] (Fig. 15-30). While both patterns partially correct the order of the field projection in the cortex, they are incompatible with a binocular visual mechanism. Carroll and associates [401, 402], utilizing visually evoked potentials simultaneously recorded from multiple electrodes over the

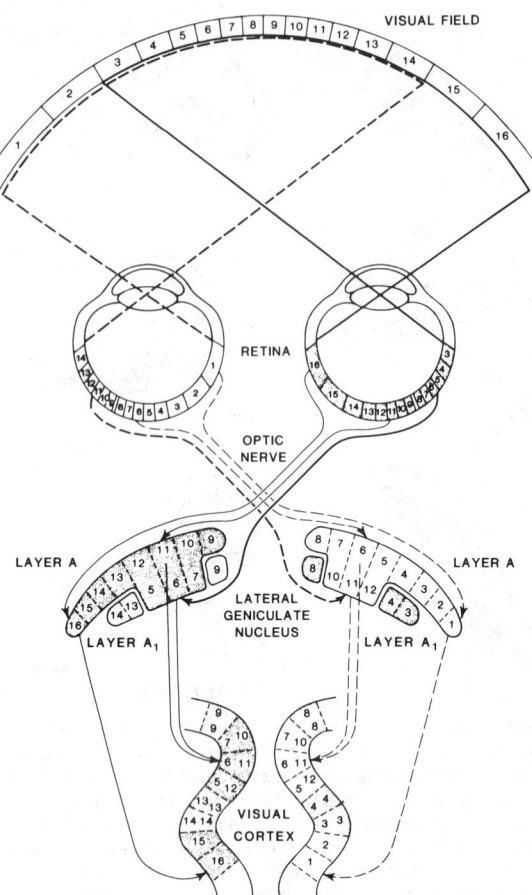

VISUAL FIELD

RETINA

OPTIC NERVE

LAYER A   LAYER A

LATERAL GENICULATE NUCLEUS

LAYER A₁   LAYER A₁

VISUAL CORTEX

Figure 15-29 Schematic representation of abnormal pathways (heavy arrows) to the lateral geniculate nuclei in the Siamese cat. If the connections from the lateral geniculate nuclei were normal, then the effects shown in the visual cortex would be expected. Projections from the two layers of the lateral geniculate would conflict, so that neural activity at a single point in the cortex would be interpreted as stimuli in two parts of the visual field, such as in segments 5 and 12. *(From Guillery [400].)*

visual cortex area of human albinos, found two patterns of response which were suggestive of a Boston or a Midwestern model. The particular type of pattern was not associated with a particular type of ty-pos or ty-neg albinism, but both patterns were found in various mutants. Cooper and Blasdel [403] examined the visual field map in the region of the 17/18 border and suggest that the two patterns, Boston and Midwestern, may represent ends of a continuum. They suggest that geniculocortical axons carrying aberrant ipsilateral field information in a given Siamese cat contain fibers directed by both mechanisms. Thus, although individual aberrant fibers within a single cat may fall into two distinct patterns on the basis of cortical termination, there could be a continuous variation between cats in the degree to which one or the other mechanism predominates within the total population of aberrant geniculocortical abberant fibers.

Collewijn et al. [404] found that in albino rabbits, restricting visual contrast to the anterior sector of the visual field—this sector being binocular in pigmented rabbits and somewhat homologous to the temporal retina in humans—resulted in a dramatically increased nystagmus. When a target was moved, horizontal optokinetic eye movements were inverted and the direction of pursuit by the eye was opposite to that of the stimulus. The researchers postulated that the optokinetic inversion could be causally associated with nystagmus in mam-

mals, particularly cats and humans, in which large proportions of temporal neurons remain ipsilateral in normal pigmented subjects but are rerouted to the contralateral side in the albino.

Otic Neurologic Defects in Albinism

The auditory system in mammals, while more complex, is somewhat analogous to the optic system in that pigment is normally found in the inner ear [405] and there are both decussated and nondecussated neuronal paths in the brain. The amount of pigment in the inner ear is correlated directly with the amount of pigment in the iris [406] and is lacking in albinos [405]. Evidence that an analogous decussation defect may exist in the auditory system of human ty-neg, ty-pos, and HPS albinos was presented by Creel et al. [407]. Brainstem auditorily evoked potentials in human albinos indicated a significant hemispheric asymmetry symptomatic of differences between decussated and nondecussated auditory pathways approximately at the level of the superior olivary nuclei, and most likely the medial superior olive (Fig. 15-31). There is a strong correlation in many species between the size of the medial superior olive and the size of the abducens nucleus that innervates the lateral rectus muscle of the eye [408]. The ratio of the size of the olive to the abducens nucleus varies markedly between animals with predominantly rod or predominantly cone foveae [408] but also reflects differences between animals with panoramic vision and less developed temporal retinas and those with binocular vision and well developed temporal retinas. The medial superior olive has been regarded as "a visual auditory system, having evolved as an adjunct to vision" [409]. On the basis of these considerations, Creel et al. [407] proposed that the development of the abducens nucleus may be

Figure 15-30 Schematic representation of two types of patterns in the geniculocortical projections in Siamese cats which compensate for the disrupted projections in the lateral geniculate nucleus, illustrated here for the left side of the brain. In a "Midwestern" cat the input to the cortex from layer A is largely suppressed, eliminating the misdirected segments 5 to 7. Thus, the misdirected part of the visual field, although projected to the wrong cortex, "reads" correctly as a more or less continuous picture of the outside world. *(From Guillery [400].)*

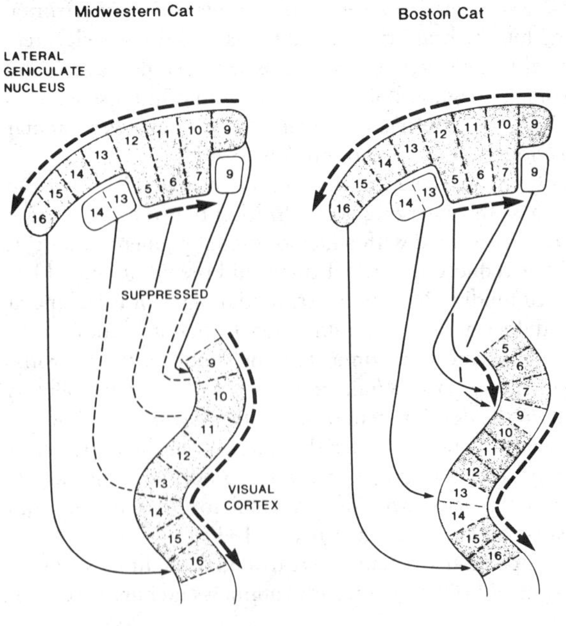

Midwestern Cat   Boston Cat

LATERAL GENICULATE NUCLEUS

SUPPRESSED

VISUAL CORTEX

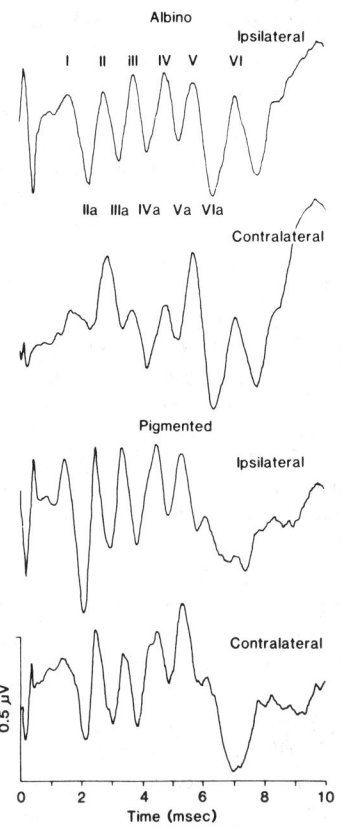

Figure 15-31 Brainstem auditorily evoked potentials recorded from hemispheres ipsilateral and contralateral to the stimulated ear in a human ty-neg albino and a pigmented subject showing over 50 percent attenuation of component III in the contralateral potential in the albino. The medial superior olive is most likely the primary generator of component III. *(From Creel et al. [407].)*

anomalous in albino mammals, as has been found in the Duane retraction syndrome with strabismus [410, 411]. If these considerations are correct, then when combined with the findings by Collewijn [404] on optokinetic inversion in albino rabbits, they suggest that a brainstem component may be involved in the nystagmus and strabismus seen in albinos, rather than simple hypoplasia of the fovea. It should be noted that animals with poorly defined foveae alone, such as the pigmented ground squirrel, do not have nystagmus, but the albino does.

Hood et al. [412], on the basis of temporary threshold shift (TTS) following intense noise challenge, postulated that melanin in the inner ear acts as a protective mechanism for noise trauma. Possibly melanin acts through its role as a semiconductor with high redox potential [413], attenuating sound energy peaks by converting them to thermal energy [414]. Garber et al. [415] showed that ty-pos, ty-neg, and HPS albinos had significantly greater TTS following 100- and 110-dB challenges than did blue- or brown-eyed normal subjects. Further, albinos had significant differences from pigmented subjects in dichotic hearing tasks which were compatible with a possible decussation defect in the auditory tract.

Other Central Nervous System Considerations

The central nervous system in albinos is normally pigmented.

The locus ceruleus and substantia nigra contain neuromelanin [155, 157] which is synthesized by tyrosine hydroxylase rather than tyrosinase.

Although an occasional albino will show both oligophrenia and some type of albinism, these situations probably arise as chance associations, particularly in kindreds in which parents are consanguine, or secondary to severe visual and auditory defects, as in BADS. Albinos in general have the same range of IQ scores as normally pigmented persons [416, 417].

DIFFERENTIAL DIAGNOSIS AND THE HAIR BULB INCUBATION TEST

The ocular findings are the most important signs and symptoms in making a diagnosis of any form of albinism. In order of constancy, they are: hypoplasia of the fovea; nystagmus; transillumination of the irides; photophobia; depigmentation of the fundi; and decreased visual acuity. In addition, hypopigmentation of the hair, skin, and eyes, particularly when the patient is compared with sibs or persons of similar ethnic background, should be present in order to make a diagnosis of OCA. The clinical, histologic, and chemical features of the various forms of albinism appear in Tables 15-1 and 15-2.

The hair bulb tyrosine incubation test is of value in distinguishing ty-neg OCA from ty-pos types. The original test solution used by Kugelman and van Scott [5] contained 80 mg L-tyrosine in 100 ml 0.1 M phosphate buffer at pH 6.8. The problem with this solution is the difficulty in solubilizing this amount of tyrosine at pH 6.8. The buffer is prepared from two stock solutions. A contains 28.392 g per liter of Na_2HPO_4 and B contains 27.598 g per liter of NaH_2PO_4. The working solution is made by combining 24.5 ml of A and 25.5 ml of B and bringing the volume to 1 dl with distilled water. Eighty milligrams L-tyrosine is added to 85 ml of the working buffer. The solution is heated and mixed with a few drops of concentrated HCl until all the tyrosine is in solution. The pH is adjusted to 6.8 with dilute NaOH, and sufficient working buffer is added to bring the volume up to 1 dl. The solution has a working life of 2 weeks. Hairs are plucked from the scalp to obtain those with well-developed anagen bulbs (Fig. 15-5). From 8 to 10 hair bulbs are incubated at 37°C for 12 to 24 h and compared under a dissecting microscope in *reflected light* for pigment formation with fresh or formalin-fixed controls from the patient. Light scattering from keratin bundles and spaces in the hair when viewed by transmitted light give a false impression of pigment. Methods of ty-neg heterozygote detection using tritiated tyrosine are available [89]. The pigment system in Caucasian infants and young children may not mature until 2 to 6 years of age. We recommend that the test be delayed until the child is 1.5 to 2 years of age, and, if negative, repeated at older ages or combined with electron microscopy. Ty-neg melanocytes contain only up to stage II melanosomes, while other types have stage III and stage IV melanosomes.

Ty-neg albinos have no visible pigment in skin, hair, and eyes, and hair bulbs incubated in L-tyrosine do not form pigment. Ty-pos albinos may have visible pigment, pigmented nevi, and freckles, and the hair bulb test is positive. Usually, HPS patients have a history of mild bleeding, abnormal platelet aggregation, and ceroidlike material in bone marrow and urine sediment. ASA and ASA-like drugs interfere with normal platelet aggregation, so that one must wait at least 1 week following the administration of any ASA-like drug before doing aggregation studies. Ym albinos have pigment in hair, skin, and eyes, exhibit a slight tanning effect, and have a faintly positive or negative reaction to the tyrosine hair bulb test but show an intensification of yellow, yellow-brown, or red pigment when incubated in 40 mg L-tyrosine:40 mg L-cysteine solution. Electron microscopically, ym melanocytes contain many small, round melanosomes with uneven distribution of pigment on the matrix. CHS patients have repeated infections, giant peroxidase-positive granules in leukocytes, steel-gray sheen to the hair, and, in some older children, neurologic findings. The Cross syndrome comprises severe oligophrenia, athetosis, gingival fibromatosis, and microphthalmia. Patients with BADS have profound sensorineural deafness and black locks.

Other depigmenting conditions may occasionally be encountered. Severe protein-calorie malnutrition may be accompanied by depigmentation. The eye color is dark, and the children do not have nystagmus or other ocular findings of albinism. Children with Menkes' syndrome or phenylketonuria may become depigmented but are normally pigmented at birth. Depigmentation, due to the copper absorption defect, usually occurs at 6 weeks to 6 months of age, and the children develop neurologic signs, most frequently opisthotonos. The mothers of X-linked OA males usually have mosaic pigment patterns in their ocular fundi, and macromelanosomes are present in skin biopsy specimens of both hemizygous males and heterozygous females. Autosomal recessive OA affects males and females with equal severity. Consanguinity may be present in the parents, mosaic fundi are absent in female heterozygotes, and macromelanosomes are not found in skin melanocytes.

CARCINOMA IN ALBINOS

OCAs, especially from tropical climates, are susceptible to neoplastic skin lesions [94, 108, 418–420]. The primary lesions are found almost exclusively on sun-exposed sites, such as the head, neck, and arms, with a predilection for the malar ridges, cheek, scalp, ear, and neck [94]. Ty-pos and HPS albinos develop goose foot-shaped lentigines, solar keratoses, and squamous cell carcinoma [94, 108, 420]. While albinos have been reported with melanomas [418, 421, 426], and we have seen a patient with HPS with melanomas, these tumors are rare and are probably not more frequent in albinos than in normally pigmented persons. Skin carcinomas in albinos are primarily squamous cell tumors arising from solar keratoses [94, 108, 420]. Among 512 albinos studied in Nigeria, 50 percent had developed solar keratoses by 14 years of age and 50 percent had developed squamous cell carcinoma by 26 years of age. No patient beyond 40 years of age was found in this albino population, nearly all having died of their malignancies prior to that age. None had melanomas, and basal cell carcinoma was rare [94, 420]. The carcinomas tend to be well differentiated histologically and to metastasize late. Ty-pos albinos did not show an increased frequency of chromosomal abnormalities in their lymphocytes or fibroblasts [3, 427]. CHS patients have a predilection for pigmentary and papillary lesions of the skin [89, 255, 259, 428, 429], but lymphoreticular malignancy is their major neoplastic problem.

PREVALENCE OF ALBINISM

Prevalence estimates of ty-neg and ty-pos albinism based upon detailed surveys of nonisolated general populations of North Carolina, Michigan, Maryland, Tennessee, and Minnesota show that the most commonly encountered form of OCA in the United States is the ty-pos type, but that it varies with race (Table 15-14). Froggatt [8] gave a somewhat higher prevalence for albinism of all types (1:10,000) among the Irish. Pearson and coworkers [6] gave 1:20,000 as an estimate for all types combined for the general world population. Ty-pos OCA occurs in the highest prevalence in a nonisolate general population in Africa [4, 17, 108, 110, 430].

Isolated populations may have unusually high prevalences of a particular type of albinism, although occasionally, as with the Amish and Mennonite populations, more than one type has been encountered (Table 15-15). All Amerindians, including the Tele Cuna of San Blas, Panama, and Chinese albinos tested in our laboratories have been ty-pos.

Ym albinism occurs in high prevalence among the Amish and has been observed in Polish, German, and English Caucasians and in U.S. blacks and Africans.

HPS occurs in diverse populations [81, 82]. Thus far, all but 2 of 92 Puerto Rican albino patients examined in our laboratory have had HPS, most originating from the Arecibo-Aguadilla area. HPS is at least five times as common as CHS. The condition also occurs in high prevalence in Dutch patients in southern Holland and in Madras State in India.

Cross syndrome has been described only in one Amish family and in a Uruguayan.

CHS has been described most frequently among patients of European ancestry [87, 254, 260, 264, 278, 284, 322, 431–434], particularly of Spanish descent [86, 259, 261, 428, 429, 435], and among Orientals [89, 251, 433].

Brown OCA has been identified with certainty only among Ibos of Nigeria [94], where it occurs with a prevalence of approximately 1:20,000, and in New Guinean indigenes [327].

Rufous albinism occurs in Africans and in high prevalence among New Guinean natives [95].

The prevalence of the various forms of albinism is especially high among patients in schools for the partially sighted. Fraser [436] estimated that some form of albinism accounted for 4 percent of the severely visually handicapped children in Australia. Witkop surveyed institutions for the partially sighted in five states in the United States and found that 10 percent of the

Table 15-14 Estimates of prevalence of ty-pos and ty-neg albinos in the general population of the United States by race*

Population	Albinism prevalence		
	Ty-neg	Ty-pos	Combined
Caucasian	1:39,000	1:37,000	1:19,000
Afro-American	1:28,000	1:15,000	1:10,000
Total United States	1:37,000	1:31,000	1:16,800

* Corrected for 88 percent Caucasian and 12 percent Negro, disregarding other racial components.
SOURCE: Revised from Witkop [4].

Table 15-15 Estimates of prevalence of albinism by type in population isolates

Isolate	Type of albinism	Estimated prevalence
Brandywine, Md 106	Ty-pos	1:85
Tele Cuna, San Blas, Panama 109	Ty-pos	1:143
Quiche-Maya, Guatemala 4	Ty-pos	1:6500
Zuni Amerindians 105, 107	Ty-pos	1:240
Hopi Amerindians 105	Ty-pos	1:227
Jemez 105	Ty-pos	1:140
Puerto Rico (West) 82	HPS	1:2000
Lencóis, Maranhão, Brazil 474	Probably HPS	1:300
Transkei 110	Mixed types	1:3000
Nigerians 108	Ty-pos	1:15,000
Ibo, Nigerians 2420	Ty-pos	1:1100
Ibo, Nigerians 94	Brown	1:10,000

patients had some form of albinism. OA accounted for about 1 percent of all children with visual handicaps, and about 9 percent had some type of OCA [3, 4, 84].

CLINICAL MANAGEMENT OF ALBINISM

The three major problems encountered by patients with albinism are their sensitivity to sunlight, with susceptibility to skin cancers, their visual acuity defect [373], and their psychosocial difficulties [373, 437, 438].

Albinos should avoid direct sunlight whenever possible, especially during the 2 h before and after solar noon during summer months. Sunscreen lotions, particularly those containing 5 percent p-aminobenzoic acid, applied to areas of skin exposed to the sun are helpful in avoiding major skin damage. The skin of older albinos should be inspected at yearly intervals for premalignant and malignant lesions. Protective clothing, such as denim, should be worn. It is important to realize that not all materials are as effective as others in blocking damaging radiation. The structure of the material is more important than the weight [438]. Carcinoma of the skin occurs in albinos who also have carotenemia and high serum levels of β-carotene. It does not appear that oral administration of β-carotene offers significant protection against the genesis of squamous cell carcinoma [420].

Tinted glasses may be helpful in reducing photophobia. Photochromatic lenses have met with variable acceptance by our patients and those of Taylor [373]. Haptic contact lenses with opaque scleral portions and painted irides have been tried with questionable success [373, 439]. Near vision is functionally better than far vision in most albinos, who have little difficulty reading N10 or N8 print or better. Print contact magnifiers have been used by a number of our patients whose work required fine, detailed reading. Operations for strabismus can be done for cosmetic purposes, but because of the decussation anomaly in the optic tract, binocular vision will not improve. Since near vision is functionally better than far vision, most albinos do quite well in a public school setting with the judicious use of special assistance. In general, albinos educated in public school settings do better than those in special institutions for the partially sighted [3, 373].

The use of high doses of ascorbic acid may be of benefit to patients with CHS.

HPS patients should avoid ASA or ASA-like drugs, which block the release of their reduced platelet storage pool constituents. Platelet transfusion may be necessary in the event of major surgery or massive bleeding.

COMPARATIVE DEVELOPMENTAL GENETICS OF ALBINISM

The nature of the genetic control of pigmentation in mammals has been clarified by study of the laboratory mouse. Numerous sites of gene action in the origin, distribution, and differentiation of melanoblasts during embryonic development have been identified in this species. In addition, it is now possible to outline in a preliminary fashion the biochemical pathways that translate hereditary information coded within the genome into the specialized pigmented organelles (melanosomes) elaborated by melanocytes [28, 38, 440, 441]. In view of the structural similarity of the melanocytes and melanosomes of mice and human beings, it is highly probable that the basic features of the genetic mechanisms that regulate melanocyte performance in the two species are comparable.

Many of the numerous gene mutations associated with altered hair and skin color in mice have been preserved by selective breeding and thereby provide a valuable source of material for experimental analysis. Four factors are of paramount importance in determining melanocyte form and function: (1) the genotype of the melanoblast; (2) the genotype of the environmental cells; (3) the environmental history of the melanocyte; and (4) the characteristics of the differentiated environmental cells [38, 442–444]. These factors, acting singly or in combination, influence such diverse events as the origin and differentiation of melanoblasts; melanocyte structure and number; size, shape, and color of melanosomes; specific stages in the biosynthesis of tyrosinase and melanosome assembly; and the patterns of transport of melanosomes within receptor cells. Detailed morphologic and biochemical analyses of numerous coat-color mutants of the house mouse have provided a clear insight into the step-by-step action of genes in the morphogenesis of pigment patterns [23]. Attention will be focused here on selected alleles at two gene loci that not only affect the pigmentation of mice but have relevance to the problem of albinism in humans. Recent papers summarize current knowledge on the nature and action of various genes on pigmentation in the mouse [38, 442–444].

The c locus in the mouse is of particular importance because the manifestations of its activities have parallels in human ty-neg OCA. It had been thought that alleles at this locus regulate the structure of tyrosinase and, consequently, the overall intensity of pigmentation. The dominant allele at the c locus permits formation of the full color appropriate to the remaining genotype. The lowest allelic member, when present in the homozygous state (c/c), produces albinism with absence of melanin pigment in the hair, skin, and eyes. The intermediate alleles bring about gradations of coat pigmentation between albinism and full color. Albino mice produce melanosomes within which no melanin is deposited. These pseudostage II melanosomes appear normal with respect to their structural proteins, but active tyrosinase is lacking. Albino melanocytes transfer these melanosomes to the keratinocytes of the hair follicle [445]. It was thought that alleles at the c locus, through their influence on the structure of tyrosinase, ultimately regulated the number and size of melanosomes and the amount of melanin deposited on each [440]. Studies with radioactive tyrosine in vivo and in vitro have demonstrated that tyrosinase activity increases within the melanosome when allelic substitutions are made progressively from c/c to C/C [446].

Studies by Pomerantz and Li [447] and Hearing [448] questioned elements of the foregoing conclusions. These investigators found evidence of tyrosinase activity in the skin and eyes of albino mice. Hearing has accordingly suggested that the c locus might more correctly be designated a regulatory than a structural locus for tyrosinase. Evidence that the c locus in mice is a regulatory locus for tyrosinase comes from the work of Townsend et al. [148]. The c-locus mutations influenced both the total tyrosinase activity and the subcellular distribution of the enzyme, while the kinetic parameters of the enzyme extracted from various mutants were essentially identical.

A recessive allele at the p locus in mice brings about a reduction in the amount of melanin within the eyes and hair coat, the absolute amount of pigment being determined by other gene loci. In overall features, the pink-eyed dilution mutation shows considerable resemblance to ty-pos OCA in humans. According to Sidman and Pearlstein [449] and Moyer [450], the p/p melanosomes in retinal melanocytes are abnormal in structure as a result of a defective alignment and cross-linkage of many compound fibers. Sidman and Pearlstein [449], on the basis of studies in vitro, concluded that the restricted melanin deposition within p/p melanosomes is caused primarily by limitations in the amount of tyrosine available for melanin synthesis, not by an impaired tyrosinase (enzyme) system. In contrast to p/p retinal melanocytes [449], the p/p follicular melanocytes appear to contain melanosomes with essentially normal matrixes [451]. Hearing et al. [452] reported that the structure of the melanosomal matrix in pigmented tissues of the eyes and hair follicles of p/p mice is essentially normal. In contrast to other investigators, they conclude that cross-linking of fibers normally does not occur in mouse melanosomes. Accordingly, the precise action of the pink-eyed dilution allele on the melanosome structure is not clear. The melanosomal matrix of ty-pos human albino does not appear unusual by electron microscopy.

The Inappropriate Use of Albino Animals as Models in Research

Albino and hypopigmented animals are the most frequently used models in animal research. Considerable evidence suggests that for many research problems, these types of animals have anatomic, biochemical-metabolic, and behavioral differences that make them unsuitable for the questions posed [453–455]. Most strains of albino rats and mice are also recessive for nonagouti. Nonagouti is associated with docility [456], and albinos from agouti strains are vicious, like wild rats [457]. Megacolon, with anomalies of Auerbach's plexus, occurs in white-spotted animals [458] and in humans with Waardenburg syndrome [459]. Deafness and inner ear anomalies occur in white cats and various spotted mouse mutants [460]. Comparisons of albino (c/c) mutation with congenic wild-type mice showed an association of albinism and susceptibility to audio-

genic seizures [461, 462]. If the recent evidence from ty-neg and ym human albinos, which may be homologues of the animal c locus, concerning evidence for a decussation defect in the auditory tract [407] is substantiated, a serious question would be raised concerning the use of the chinchilla as a model in acoustic and auditory research.

All types of human OAs and OCAs as well as a wide variety of animals with mutations at the c locus, have demonstrated anomalous visual systems with reduced numbers of uncrossed optic neurons to the lateral geniculate nuclei, pretectal nuclei and superior colliculus, and anomalous projections from the dorsal lateral geniculate nucleus to the visual cortex [454]. The visual system is abnormal in all types of albinism. Tyrosine has been reported to have a higher turnover in the liver of albinos than in pigmented animals [463], and differences in liver cytochrome P-450 levels were found in lethal albino deletions [464]. C57BL/6J albino mice have longer sleep times than congenic pigmented mice treated with ethanol or pentobarbital [453, 465–467]. The ML-50 dose of pentobarbital administered to a variety of pigmented rats was significantly less than the ML-100 dose for a variety of albino rat strains [468]. Behavioral differences in albino mice are significantly different in many respects from those in pigmented mice. Thiessen et al. [469] documented 20 out of 41 behaviors that were different in the albino from those in the pigmented animal. Psychologists concerned with learning ability in the rat using visual discrimination came to divergent conclusions, which retrospectively were probably due to anatomic differences in the optic tracts of albino versus pigmented animals. [371]. Perhaps the most relevant area in which albino animals are inappropriate models is in testing of drugs, particularly those which bind to melanin. Lindquist [470] studied the uptake and retention of a variety of drugs by melanized tissues of the rat. Kanamycin, hydroxychloroquine, chloroquine, chlorpromazine, quinine, dihydrostreptomycin, streptomycin, and viomycin were among the drugs which showed significant differences in the uptake and retention in the pigmented versus the albino animal (see Refs. 454, 455, and 471 for reviews). Melanin acts as a free radical receptor, and its absence may profoundly affect reactions where free radicals are generated.

Albinism in the Perspective of Evolutionary Biology

The diverse groups of mammals extant today have arisen from closely related ancestral stocks in the distant past and thus share genes in common. Although it is impossible to identify homologous genes in members of different species by standard breeding tests, it is possible to demonstrate gene homology at the molecular (DNA) level [472, 473]. The evidence indicates that considerable genic homology exists among the various classes of vertebrates [472, 473].

OA is broadly distributed among mammals [99]. It is possible that the similarities of expression of ty-neg OCA in humans and in the mouse may reflect the existence of gene loci maintained in common by both species throughout broad periods of evolutionary diversification. The recent identification of possible allelism between the genes for ty-neg albinism and ym albinism in humans [330] offers somewhat ambiguous evidence for homology between the ty-neg locus in humans and the c locus in mice. The two loci correspond in that they control levels of tyrosinase activity. The pheomelaninlike pigment of ym human albinos has no *c*-locus equivalent in mice; this finding might be taken as evidence against gene homology.

As with other functions of the body, evolution may have acted conservatively to preserve in unaltered form many "core" genes central to the occurrence and control of melanin pigmentation. It may have been somewhat more permissive of variation in the case of other pigmentary genes ("luxury" genes) which influenced the melanogenetic mechanisms in more subtle ways. This interpretation explains the striking similarities in the features of melanogenesis in many mammalian species. The variations may reflect the mutation and selection of luxury genes in adaptation to specialized modes of life.

Various phases of the author's work reported herein were supported by U.S. Public Health Service Grants GM 22167, GM 24558, and N1-AM 7-2200.

REFERENCES

1. FITZPATRICK TB, QUEVEDO WC JR: Albinism, in Stanbury JB, Wyngaarden JB, Fredrickson DS (eds): *The Metabolic Basis of Inherited Disease*, ed 3. New York, McGraw-Hill Book Co, 1972, p 326

2. WITKOP CJ, JR: Depigmentations of the general and oral tissues and their genetic foundations. *Ala J Med Sci* 16:331, 1979

3. WITKOP CJ JR, HILL CW, DESNICK SJ, THIES JK, THORN HL, JENKINS M, WHITE JG: Ophthalmologic, biochemical, platelet, and ultrastructural defects in the various types of oculocutaneous albinism. *J Invest Dermatol* 60:443, 1973

4. WITKOP CJ JR: Albinism, in Harris H, Hirschhorn K (eds): *Advances in Human Genetics*. New York, Plenum Publishing Corp, 1971, vol 2, pp 61–142

5. KUGELMAN TP, VAN SCOTT EJ: Tyrosinase activity in melanocytes of human albinos. *J Invest Dermatol* 37:73, 1961

6. PEARSON K, NETTLESHIP E, USHER CH: *A Monograph on Albinism in Man*. Drapers' Company Research Memoirs, Biometric Series 6, 8, 9: parts 1, 2, 4. London, Dulau, 1911–1913

7. FROGGATT P: *Albinism: A Statistical, Genetical and Clinical Appraisal Based upon a Complete Ascertainment of the Condition in Northern Ireland*, thesis. Trinity College, Dublin, 1957

8. FROGGATT P: Albinism in northern Ireland. *Ann Hum Genet* 24:213, 1960

9. PLINIUS SECUNDUS THE ELDER: *The Natural History of Pliny*, Rackman H (trans). London, William Heineman, Ltd, book 7, 1942

10. GELLIUS A: *The Attic Nights*, Rolfe JC (trans). London, William Heineman, Ltd, book 9, 1952

11. SORSBY A: Noah-an albino. *Br. Med J* 2:1587, 1958

12. WAFER L: *New Voyage and Description of the Isthmus of America, Giving an Account of the Author's Abode There*. London, 1699, p 134. (Cited by Pearson et al [6], part I, pp 17–18)

13. RASERI E: Materiali per l'etinologica Italiana. *Arch l'antropol Florence* 9:259, 1879

14. EHRMANN S: *Das melanotische Pigment und die pigmentbildenden Zellen des Menschen und der Wirbeltiere in ihrer Entwickelung nebst Bemerkungen über Blutbildung und Haarwechsel*. Cassel, T. G. Fisher, 1896

15. DURHAM FM: On the presence of tyrosinases in the skin of some pigmented vertebrates. *Proc Roy Soc* 74:310, 1904

16. GARROD AE: Inborn errors of metabolism, Croonian Lectures, Lecture I. *Lancet* 2:1–7, 1908

17. STANNUS HS: Anomalies of pigmentation among natives of Nyasaland: A contribution to the study of albinism. *Biometrika* 9:333, 1913

18. SHUFELDT RW: Albinism in American animals. *Proc Zool Soc Lond* 540, 1916

19. LITTLE CC: Coat color genes in rodents and carnivores. *Q Rev Biolol* 33:103, 1958

20. NOBLE GK: *The Biology of the Amphibia*. New York, Dover Publications, Inc, (1931) 1954, p 577

21. SEARLE AG: *Comparative Genetics of Coat Colour in Mammals*. London, Logos; New York, Academic Press, Inc, 1968

22. WAARDENBURG PJ: *Remarkable Facts in Human Albinism and Leukism*. The Netherlands, Assen, Van Gorcum, 1970

23. SILVERS WK: *The Coat Colors of Mice. A Model for Mammalian Gene Action and Interaction*. New York, Springer-Verlag, 1979

24. LAFERRIERE KA, ARENBERG IK, HAWKINS JE, JR, JOHNSSON LG: Melanocytes of the vestibular labyrinth and their relationship to the microvasculature. *Ann Otol* 83:685, 1974

25. JIMBOW K, FITZPATRICK TB, SZABO G, HORI Y: Congenital circumscribed hypomelanosis: A characterization based on electron microscopic study of tuberous sclerosis, nevus depigmentosis and piebaldism. *J Invest Dermatol* 64:50, 1975

26. O'DONNELL FE, JR, HAMBRICK GW, GREEN WR, ILIFF WJ, STONE DL: X-linked ocular albinism. An oculocutaneous macromelanosomal disorder. *Arch Ophthalmol* 94:1883, 1976

27. GARNER A, JAY BS: Macromelanosomes in X-linked ocular albinism. *Histopathology* 4:243, 1980

28. QUEVEDO WC JR, FITZPATRICK TB, PATHAK MA, JIMBOW K: Role of light in human skin color variation. *Am J Phys Anthropol* 43:393, 1975

29. STERN C: Model estimates of the number of gene pairs involved in pigmentation variability of the Negro-American. *Hum Hered* 20:165, 1970

30. HARRISON GA: Differences in human pigmentation: Measurement, geographic variation, and causes. *J Invest Dermatol* 60:418, 1973

31. SEIJI M, FITZPATRICK TB, SIMPSON RT, BIRBECK MSC: Chemical composition and terminology of specialized organelles (melanosomes and melanin granules) in mammalian melanocytes. *Nature* 197:1082, 1963

32. FITZPATRICK TB, SZABO G, SEIJI M, QUEVEDO WC JR: Biology of the melanin pigmentary system, in Fitzpatrick TB, Eisen AZ, Wolff K, Freedberg IM, Austen KF (eds): *Dermatology in General Medicine*, ed 2. New York, McGraw-Hill Book Co, 1979, pp 131–163

33. JIMBOW K, QUEVEDO WC JR, FITZPATRICK TB, SZABO G: Some aspects of melanin biology: 1950–1975. *J Invest Dermatol* 67:72, 1976

34. VARGA JM, MOELLMANN G, FRITSCH P, GODAWSKA E, LERNER AB: Association of cell surface receptors for melanotropin with the Golgi region in mouse melanoma cells. *Proc Natl Acad Sci USA* 73:559, 1976

35. MOTTAZ JH, ZELICKSON AS: Ultrastructure of hair pigment, in Montagna W, Dobson RL (eds): *Advances in Biology of Skin*, vol 9, *Hair Growth*. Oxford, Pergamon Press, Ltd, 1969, pp 471–489

36. STANKA P: Ultrastructural study of pigment cells of human red hair. *Cell Tissue Res* 150:167, 1974

37. BIRBECK MSC, BARNICOT NA: Electron microscope studies on pigment formation in human hair follicles, in Gordon M (ed): *Pigment Cell Biology*. New York, Academic Press, Inc, 1959

38. QUEVEDO WC JR: Genetic control of melanin metabolism within the melanin unit of mammalian epidermis. *J Invest Dermatol* 60:407, 1973

39. SUKURAI T, OCHIAI H, TAKEUCHI T: Ultrastructural change of melanosomes associated with agouti pattern formation in mouse hair. *Dev Biol* 47:466, 1975

40. QUEVEDO WC JR: Normal pigmentation: Histology, cellular biology, and chemistry. *Ala J Med Sci* 16:305, 1980

41. TODA K, FITZPATRICK TB: Ultrastructural and biochemical studies of the formation of melanosomes in the embryonic chick retinal pigment epithelium, in Riley V (ed): *Pigmentation: Its Genesis and Biologic Control*. New York, Appleton-Century-Crofts, 1972, pp 125–141

42. HEARING VJ, NICHOLSON JM, MONTAGUE PM, EKEL TM, TOMECKI KJ: Mammalian tyrosinase. Structural and functional interrelationships of isozymes. *Biochim Biophys Acta* 522:327, 1978

43. CLEFFMAN G: Function specific changes in the metabolism of agouti pigment cells. *Exp Cell Res* 35:590, 1964

44. LERNER AB: Metabolism of phenylalanine and tyrosine. *Adv Enzymol* 14:73, 1953

45. PROTA G: Recent advances in the chemistry of melanogenesis in mammals. *J Invest Dermatol* 75:122, 1980

46. PROTA G, THOMSON RH: Melanin pigmentation in mammals. *Endeavour* 35:32, 1976

47. WITKOP CJ JR, WHITE JC, NANCE WE, UMBER RE: Mutations in the melanin pigment system in man resulting in features of oculocutaneous albinism, in Riley V (ed): *Pigmentation: Its Genesis and Biologic Control*. New York, Appleton-Century-Crofts, 1972, pp 359–377

48. LOGAN A, WEATHERHEAD B: Pelage color changes and hairfollicle tyrosinase activity in the Siberian hamster. *J Invest Dermatol* 71:295, 1978

49. LOGAN A, WEATHERHEAD B: Post-tyrosinase inhibition of melanogenesis by melatonin in hairfollicles *in vitro*. *J Invest Dermatol* 74:47, 1980

50. KÖRNER AM, PAWELEK J: Dopachrome conversion: A possible control point in melanin biosynthesis. *J Invest Dermatol* 75:192, 1980

51. PAWELEK J, KÖRNER A, BERGSTROM A, BOLOGNA J: New regulators of melanin biosynthesis and the autodestruction of melanoma cells. *Nature* 286:617, 1980

52. HEARING VJ, KÖRNER AM, PAWELEK J: Mammalian tyrosinase: Association with post-tyrosinase controls, personal communication

53. NISHIOKA K: Particulate tyrosinase of human malignant melanoma. Solubilization, purification following trypsin treatment, and characterization. *Eur J Biochem* 85:137, 1978

54. HEARING VJ, NICHOLSON JM, MONTAGUE PM, EKEL TM, TOMECKI KJ: Mammalian tyrosinase. Structural and functional interrelationships and isozymes. *Biochim Biophys Acta* 522:327, 1978

55. JIMBOW K, FITZPATRICK TB: Characterization of a new melanosomal structural component—the vesicular body. *J Ultrastruct Res* 48:269, 1974

56. MAUL GG, BRUMBAUGH JA: On the possible function of coated vesicles in melanogenesis of the regenerating fowl feather. *J Cell Biol* 48:41, 1971

57. JIMBOW K, OIKAWA O, SUGIYAMA S, TAKEVICHI T: Comparison of eumelanogenesis and pheomelanogenesis in retinal and follicular melanocytes: Role of vesiculoglobular bodies in melanosome differentiation. *J Invest Dermatol* 73:278, 1979

58. MISHIMA Y, IMOKAWA G, OGURA H: Functional and three-dimensional differentiation of smooth membrane structures in melanogenesis, in Klaus SN (ed): *Pigment Cell Biologic Basis of Pigmentation*. Basel, S. Karger, 1979, vol 4, pp 277–290

59. OSTER G, OSTER F: Dopa stimulation of melanin formation. *Tenth International Pigment Cell Conference Abstracts. Yale J Biol Med* 50:574, 1977

60. BURNETT JB, SEILER H, BROWN IV: Separation and characterization of multiple forms of tyrosinase from mouse melanoma. *Cancer Res* 27:880, 1967

61. HOLSTEIN TJ, BURNETT JB, QUEVEDO WC JR: Genetic regulation of multiple forms of tyrosinase in mice. Action of *a* and *b* loci. *Proc Soc Exp Biol Med* 126:415, 1967

62. BURNETT JB, HOLSTEIN TJ, QUEVEDO WC JR: Electrophoretic variations of tyrosinase in follicular melanocytes during the hair growth cycle. *J Exp Zool* 171:369, 1969

63. POMERANTZ SH, LI JPC: Purification and properties of tyrosinase isoenzymes from hamster melanoma. *Yale J Biol Med* 46:541, 1973

64. HEARING VJ, EKEL TM, MONTAGUE PM: Mammalian tyrosinase: Isozymic forms of the enzyme. *Int J Biochem* 13:99, 1981

65. OHTAKI N, MIYAZAKI K: Immunologic homogeneity and electrophoretic heterogeneity of mouse melanoma tyrosinase. *J Invest Dermatol* 61:339, 1973

66. MIYAZAKI K, OHTAKI N: Tyrosinase as glycoprotein. *Arch Dermatol Forsch* 252:211, 1975

67. BLOSIS MS: The melanins: Their synthesis and structure, in Smith KC (ed): *Photochemical and Photobiological Reviews*. New York, Plenum Publishing Corp, 1978, vol 3, pp 115–134

68. WHITTAKER JR: Absence of a direct melanin-protein relationship in chick embryo melanocytes. *Biochim Biophys Acta* 583:378, 1979

69. FITZPATRICK TB, BREATHNACH AS: Das epidermale Melanin-Einheit-System. *Dermatol Wochenschr* 147:481, 1963

70. SZABO G, GERALD AB, PATHAK MA, FITZPATRICK TB: Racial differences in the fate of melanosomes in human epidermis. *Nature (Lond)* 222:1081, 1969

71. TODA K, PATHAK MA, PARRISH JA, FITZPATRICK TB, QUEVEDO WC JR: Alteration of racial differences in melanosome distribution in human epidermis after exposure to ultraviolet light. *Nature (New Biol)* 236:143, 1972

72. OLSON RL, GAYLOR J, EVERETT MA: Skin color, melanin, and erythema. *Arch Dermatol* 108:541, 1973

73. MITCHELL RE: The skin of the Australian aborigine: A light and electron-microscopical study. *Aust J Dermatol* 9:314, 1968

74. SZABO G, GERALD AB, PATHAK MA, FITZPATRICK TB: The ultrastructure of racial color differences in man, in Riley V (ed): *Pigmentation: Its Genesis and Biologic Control*. New York, Appleton-Century-Crofts, 1972, pp 23–41

75. KONRAD K, WOLFF K: Hyperpigmentation, melanosome size, and distribution patterns of melanosomes. *Arch Dermatol* 107:853, 1973

76. OLSON RL, EVERETT MA: Alterations in epidermal lysosomes following ultraviolet light exposure, in Urbach F (ed): *The Biologic Effects of Ultraviolet Radiation*. Oxford, Pergamon Press, Ltd, 1969, pp 473–476

77. MOTTAZ JH, THORNE EG, ZELICKSON AS: Response of the epidermal melanocyte to minor trauma. *Arch Dermatol* 104:611, 1971

78. QUEVEDO WC JR: Genetic regulation of pigmentation in mammals, in Kawamura T, Fitzpatrick TB, Seiji M (eds): *Biology of Normal and Abnormal Melanocytes*. Tokyo, University of Tokyo Press, 1971, pp 99–115

79. WOLFF K, HÖNIGSMANN H: Permeability of the epidermis and the phagocytic activity of keratinocytes: Ultrastructural studies with thorotrast as a marker. *J Ultrastruct Res* 36:176, 1971

80. PATHAK MA, HORI Y, SZABO G, FITZPATRICK TB: The photobiology of melanin pigmentation in human skin, in Kawamura T, Fitzpatrick TB, Seiji M (eds): *Biology of Normal and Abnormal Melanocytes*. Tokyo, University of Tokyo Press, Tokyo, 1971, pp 149–167

81. WITKOP CJ JR, QUEVEDO WC, JR, FITZPATRICK TB: Albinism, in Stanbury JB, Wyngaarden JB, Fredrickson DS (eds): *The Metabolic Basis of Inherited Disease*, ed 4. New York, McGraw-Hill Book Co, 1978, pp 283–316

82. WITKOP CJ JR, WHITE, JG, KING RA: Oculocutaneous albinism, in Nyhan WL (ed): *Heritable Disorders of Amino Acid Metabolism*. New York, John Wiley & Sons, Inc, 1974, pp 177–261

83. WITKOP CJ JR, VAN SCOTT EJ, JACOBY GA: Evidence for two forms of autosomal recessive albinism in man, in *Proceedings of the Second International Congress of Human Genetics*. Rome, Institute Gregor Mendel, 1961, pp 1064–1065

84. WITKOP CJ JR, NANCE WE, RAWLS RF, WHITE JG: Autosomal recessive oculocutaneous albinism in man: Evidence for genetic heterogeneity. *Am J Hum Genet* 22:55, 1970

85. HERMANSKY F, PUDLAK P: Albinism associated with hemorrhagic diathesis and unusual pigmented reticular cells in the bone marrow: Report of two cases with histochemical studies. *Blood* 14:162, 1959

86. BÉGUEZ-CESAR A: Neutropénia crónica maligna familiare con granulaciones atípicas de los leucocitos. *Bol Soc Cubana Pediatr* 15:900, 1943

87. STEINBRINCK W: Uber eine neue Granulationsanomalie der Leukocyten. *Dtsch Arch Klin Med* 193:577, 1948

88. CHÉDIAK M: Nouvelle anomalie leucocytaire de caractère constitutionnel et familial. *Rev Hematol* 7:362, 1952

89. HIGASHI O: Congenital gigantism of peroxidase granules. *Tohoku J Exp Med* 59:315, 1954

90. CROSS HE, MCKUSICK VA, BREEN W: A new oculocerebral syndrome with hypopigmentation. *J Pediatr* 70:398, 1967

91. WITKOP CJ, JR: Heterogeneity in gingival fibromatosis, in Bergsma D (ed): *Orofacial Structures*, Part 11, *Birth Defects Original Article Series*. Baltimore, Williams & Wilkins Co, 1971, vol 7, no 7, p 210

92. WITKOP CJ JR: Heterogeneity in inherited dental traits: Gingival fibromatosis and amelogenesis imperfecta. *South Med J* (suppl)1:64, 16, 1971

93. WITKOP CJ JR, CROSS HE: Gingival fibromatosis, hypopigmentation, microphthalmaia, oligophrenia and athetosis, in Bergsma D (ed): *Birth Defects Atlas and Compendium*. Baltimore, Williams & Wilkins Co, 1973, pp 434–435

94. KING RA, CREEL D, CERVENKA J, OKORO AN, WITKOP CJ: Albinism in Nigeria with delineation of new recessive oculocutaneous type. *Clin Genet* 17:259, 1980

95. WALSH JR: A distinctive pigment of the skin in New Guinea indigenes. *Ann Hum Genet (Lond)* 34:379, 1971

96. HARVEY RG: The "redskins" of Lufa sub-district. Further observations on the distinctive skin pigmentation of some New Guinea indigenes. *Hum Biol Oceania* 1:103, 1971

97. FRENK E, CALME A: Hypopigmentation oculo-cutanée familiar à transmission dominante due à un trouble de la formation des mélanosomes. *Schweiz Med Wochenschr* 107:1964, 1977

98. NANCE WE, JACKSON CE, WITKOP CJ JR: Amish albinism: A distinctive autosomal recessive phenotype. *Am J Hum Genet* 22:579, 1970

99. WITKOP CJ JR: Albinism. *Nat Hist* 84:48, 1975

100. KING RA, WITKOP CJ JR: Hairbulb tyrosinase activity in oculocutaneous albinism. *Nature* 263:69, 1976

101. TREVOR-ROPER PD: Marriage of two complete albinos with normally pigmented offspring. *Br J Ophthalmol* 36:107, 1952

102. TREVOR-ROPER PD: Albinism. *Proc R Soc Med Sec Ophthalmol* 56:21, 1963

103. GRAGG GW: Albinoidism and albinism, Part 8, Eye, in Bergsma D (ed): *Birth Defects Original Article Series*. Baltimore, Williams & Wilkins Co, 1971, vol 7, no 3, pp 203–204

104. JAEGER C, JAY B: X-linked ocular albinism. A family containing a manifesting heterozygote, and an affected male married to a female with autosomal recessive ocular albinism. *Hum Genet* 56:299, 1981

105. WOOLF CM: Albinism among Indians in Arizona and New Mexico. *Am J Hum Genet* 17:23, 1965

106. WITKOP CJ JR, MACLEAN CJ, SCHMIDT PJ, HENRY JL: Medical and dental findings in the Brandywine isolate. *Ala J Med Sci* 3:382, 1966.

107. WITKOP CJ JR, NISWANDER JP, BERGSMA DR, WORKMAN PL, WHITE JG: Tyrosinase-positive oculocutaneous albinism among the Zuni and the Brandywine triracial isolate: Biochemical and clinical characteristics and fertility. *Am J Phys Anthropol* 76:397, 1972

108. OKORO AN: Albinism in Nigeria. *Br J Dermatol* 92:485, 1975

109. KEELER CE: The Caribe Cuna moon-child and its heredity. *J Hered* 44:163, 1953

110. ROSE EF: Pigment anomalies encountered in the Transkei. *S Afr Med J* 48:2345, 1974

111. FREIRE-MAIA N, CAVALLI IJ: Genetic investigations in a Northern Brazilian island. I. Population structure. *Hum Hered* 28:386, 1978

112. KNOX WE: Sir Archibald Garrod's "inborn errors of metabolism." III. Albinism. *Am J Hum Genet* 10;249, 1958

113. GARNER A, JAY BS: Macromelanosomes in X-linked ocular albinism. *Histopathology* 4:243, 1980

114. NETTLESHIP E: On some hereditary diseases of the eye. *Trans Ophthalmol Soc UK* 29:59, 1909

115. FALLS HF: Sex-linked ocular albinism displaying typical fundus changes in female heterozygote. *Am J Ophthalmol* 34:41, 1951

116. WAARDENBURG PJ: Herkenbaarheid van latente overdragers van albinismus universalis en albinismus oculi. *Ned Tijdschr Geneeskd* 91:1863, 1947

117. WAARDENBURG PJ, VAN DEN BOSCH J: X-chromosomal ocular albinism in a Dutch family. *Ann Hum Genet* 21:101, 1956

118. GILLESPIE FD, COVELLI B: Carriers of ocular albinism with and without ocular changes. *Arch Ophthalmol* 70:121, 1963

119. KRILL AE: X-chromosomal–linked disease affecting the eye. Status of the heterozygous female. *Ophthalmol Soc* 67:535, 1969

120. FORSIUS H, ERIKSSON AW: Ein neues Augensyndrom mit X-chromosomaler Transmission. Eine Sippe mit Fundusalbinismus. Foveahypoplasie, Nystagmus, Myopie, Astigmatismus und Dyschromatopsie. *Klin Monatsbl Augenheilkd* 144:447, 1964

121. O'DONNELL FE, GREEN WR, MCKUSICK VA, FORSIUS H, ERIKSSON AW: Forsius-Eriksson syndrome: Its relation to the Nettleship-Falls X-linked ocular albinism. *Clin Genet* 17:403, 1980

122. WAARDENBURG PJ: Some notes on publications of Professor Arnold Sorsby and on Åland eye disease (Forsius-Eriksson syndrome). *J Med Genet* 7:194, 1970

123. BERGSMA DR, KAISER-KUPFER M: A new form of albinism. *Am J Ophthalmol* 77:837, 1974

124. DONALDSON DD: Transillumination of the iris. *Tr Am Ophthalmol Soc* 72:89, 1974

125. TIETZ W: A syndrome of deaf-mutism associated with albinism showing dominant autosomal inheritance. *Am J Hum Genet* 15:259, 1963

126. MENKES JH, ALTER M, STEIGLEDER GK, WEAKLEY DR, SUNG JS: A sex-linked recessive disorder with retardation of growth, peculiar hair and focal cerebral and cerebellar degeneration. *Pediatrics* 29:764, 1962

127. MARGOLIS S, SIEGEL IM, CHOY A, BREINING M: Depigmentation of hair, skin, and eyes associated with the Apert syndrome, in Summitt RL, Bergsma D (eds): *Recent Advances and New Syndromes, 1977. Birth Defects Original Article Series*, New York, Alan R Liss, Inc, 1978, vol 14, no 6C, p 341

128. BARD LA: Heterogeneity in Waardenburg's syndrome. *Arch Ophthalmol* 96:1193, 1978

129. COMINGS DE, ODLAND GF: Partial albinism. *JAMA* 195:510, 1966

130. FRANCOIS J, VERRIEST G: Anomalies of pigmentation, in Francois J (ed): *Heredity in Ophthalmology*. St. Louis, CV Mosby Co, 1961, p 519

131. MERENLENDER J, RYWLIN JA: A propos de l'hérédité du vitiligo acquis (vitiligo dans 3 générations). *Acta Dermatovener (Stockholm)*, 21:583, 1940

132. LERNER AB: Vitiligo. *J Invest Dermatol* 32:285, 1959

133. COWIE V, PENROSE LS: Dilution of hair colour in phenylketonuria. *Ann Eugen (Lond)* 15:297, 1951

134. SNYDERMAN SE, NORTON P, HOLT EL: "Effect" of tyrosine administration in phenylketonuria. *Fed Proc* 14:450, 1955

135. MIYAMOTO M, FITZPATRICK TB: Competitive inhibition of mammalian tyrosinase by phenylalanine and its relationship to hair pigmentation in phenylketonuria. *Nature (Lond)* 179:199, 1957

136. WITKOP CJ JR: Abnormalities of pigmentation, in Emery AEH, Rimoin DL (eds): *The Principles and Practice of Medical Genetics*. Edinburgh, Churchill Livingstone, Ltd, 1982

137. SAINT HILAIRE IG: *Histoire générale et particulière des anomalies de l'organisation chez l'homme et les animaux*. Paris, JB Ballière, 1832–1836

138. SAINT HILAIRE IG: Sur l'albinisme et le mélanisme. *La Lancette Française Gazette des Hôpitaux Civils et Militaires* 9:128, 509, 1839

139. NIEDELMAN ML: Abnormalities of pigmentation in the Negro. *Arch Dermatol Syphilol* 51:1, 1945

140. KLEIN D: Les diverse formes héréditaires de l'albinisme. *Bull Schweiz Akad Med Wiss* 17:351, 1961

141. WAARDENBURG PJ: in Waardenburg PJ, Fransehetti A, Klein D (eds): *Genetics and Ophthalmology*. Springfield, Ill, Charles C Thomas, Publisher, 1961, vol 1, pp 704–740

142. MCKUSICK VA: *Mendelian Inheritance in Man Catalogs of Autosomal Dominant, Autosomal Recessive, and X-linked Phenotypes*. ed 5. Baltimore, Johns Hopkins University Press, 1978, p 408

143. WIRTSCHAFTER JD, DENSLOW GT, SHINE IB: Quantification of iris translucency in albinism. *Arch Ophthalmol* 90:274, 1973

144. JAY B, CARRUTHERS J, TREPLIN MCW, WINDER AF: Human albinism, in Bergsma D, Bron AJ, Cotlier E (eds): *The Eye and Inborn Errors of Metabolism. Birth Defects Original Article Series*, New York, Alan R Liss Inc, 1976, vol 12, no 3, pp 415–426

145. O'DONNELL FE JR, GREEN WR: The eye in albinism, in Duane TD (ed): *Clinical Ophthalmology*. Hagerstown, Md, Harper & Row, Publishers, Inc, 1979

146. BIRBECK MSC, BARNICOT, NA: Electron microscope studies on pigment formation in human hair follicles, in Gordon M (ed): *Pigment Cell Biology*. New York, Academic Press, Inc, 1959, pp 549–562

147. JUNG EG, ANTON-LAMPRECHT I: Investigation of a case of oculocutaneous albinism, in Bergsma D (ed): *Birth Defects Original Article Series*, Part 12, *Skin, Hair and Nails*. Baltimore, Williams & Wilkins Co, 1971, vol 7, no 8, pp 26–30

148. TOWNSEND D, WITKOP CJ JR, MATTSON J: Tyrosinase subcellular distribution and kinetic parameters in wild type and *c*-locus mutant C57BL/6J mice. *J Exp Zool* 216:113, 1981

149. KING RA, WITKOP CJ: Detection of heterozygotes for tyrosinase-negative oculocutaneous albinism by hairbulb tyrosinase assay. *Am J Hum Genet* 29:164, 1977

150. POMERANTZ SH: L-Tyrosine-3,5-^{3}H assay for tyrosinase development in skin of newborn hamsters. *Science* 164:838, 1969

151. POPP RA: Studies of the mouse hemoglobin locus. II. Position of the hemoglobin locus with respect to albinism and shaker-1 loci. *J Hered* 53:73, 1962

152. BRDICKA R: Evidence for linkage between hemoglobin and chromagen loci. *Folia Biol (Praha)* 12:305, 1966

153. MASSIE RW, HARTMAN RC: Albinism and sicklemia in a Negro family. *Am J Hum Genet* 9:127, 1957

154. WITKOP CJ JR, WHITE, JG, NANCE, WE, JACKSON, CE, DESNICK S: Classification of albinism in man, in Bergsma D (ed): *Skin, Hair and Nails. Birth Defects Original Article Series*. Baltimore, The National Foundation, Williams & Wilkins Co, 1971, vol 7, no 8, pp 13–25

155. GUILLERY RW, OKORO AN, WITKOP CJ JR: Abnormal visual pathways in the brain of a human albino. *Brain Res* 96:373, 1975

156. FOLEY JH, BAXTER D: On the nature of pigment granules in the cells of the locus caeruleus and substantia nigra. *J Neuropathol* 17:586, 1958

157. KENNEDY BJ, ZELICKSON AS: Melanoma in an albino. *JAMA* 186:839, 1963

158. BRUMBAUGH JA, ZIEG RH: The ultrastructural effects of the dopa reaction upon developing retinal and epidermal melanocytes in the fowl, in Riley V (ed): *Pigmentation: Its Genesis and Biologic Control*. New York, Appleton-Century-Crofts, 1972, pp 107–123

159. MISHIMA Y, TAKAHASHI M, COOPER M: Intracytoplasmic activities in malignant melanoma: Viral, melanogenic and anti-melanogenic, in Kawamura T, Fitzpatrick TB, Seiji M (eds): *Biology of Normal and Abnormal Melanocytes*. Baltimore, University Park Press, 1971, pp 279–301

160. ZIPKIN I, HAWKINS GR, MAZZARELLA M: The tyrosine, tryptophan, and protein content of human parotid saliva in oral and systemic disease: Use of ultraviolet absorption technics, in Screebny LM, Meyer J (eds): *Salivary Glands and Their Secretions*. Oxford, Pergamon Press, 1964

161. KING RA, OLDS DP, WITKOP CJ JR: Characterization of human hairbulb tyrosinase: Properties of normal and albino enzyme. *J Invest Dermatol* 71:136, 1978

162. FIRTH D: Red-headed albinos. *Proc R Soc Med* 17:25, 1924

163. BEDNAR B, HERMANSKY F, LOJDA Z: Vascular pseudohemophilia associated with ceroid pigmentophagia in albinos. *Am J Pathol* 45:283, 1964

164. BEDNAR B, JIRASEK A: Cerebral ceroidosis in albinos. *Pathol Eur* 3:341, 1968

165. HARDISTY RM, HUTTON RA: Bleeding tendency associated with "new" abnormality of platelet behavior. *Lancet* 1:983, 1967

166. MAURER HM, WOLFF JA, BUCKINGHAM S, HOROWITZ HI, SPIELVOGEL A, SITARZ A: Heterogeneous hemostatic defect in albinism. *Abstr Soc Pediatr Res* 102, 1967

167. MILLS DCB, HARDISTY RM: The nature of the platelet defect in albinos with a bleeding tendency, abstracted. *Proceedings of the 13th Congress, International Society of Hematology*, Munich, 1970, p 31

168. HALON PJ, MITUS WJ: Ceroid storage in albinism. *Proceedings of the 13th Congress, International Society of Hematology*, Munich, 1970, p 322

169. MUÑIZ FJ, FRADERA J, MALDONADO N, PEREZ-SANTIAGO E: Albinism, bleeding tendency and abnormal pigmented cells in the bone marrow: A case report. *Texas Rep Biol Med* 28:167, 1970

170. WHITE JG, EDSON JR, DESNICK SJ, WITKOP CJ JR: Studies of platelets in a variant of the Hermansky-Pudlak syndrome. *Am J Pathol* 63:319, 1971

171. LOGAN LJ, RAPAPORT SI, MAHER I: Albinism and abnormal platelet function. *N Engl J Med* 284:1340, 1971

172. HARDISTY RM, MILLS DCB: The platelet defect associated with albinism. *Ann NY Acad Sci* 201:429, 1972

173. HARDISTY RM, MILLS DCB, KETSA-ARD K: The platelet defect associated with albinism. *Br J Haematol* 23:679, 1972

174. MAURER HM, WOLFF JA, BUCKINGHAM S, SPIELVOGEL AR: "Impotent" platelets with prolonged bleeding times. *Blood* 39:490, 1972

175. WHITE JG, WITKOP CJ JR, GERRITSEN SM: The Hermansky-Pudlak syndrome: Ultrastructure of bone marrow macrophages. *Am J Pathol* 70:329, 1973

176. WHITE JG, WITKOP CJ JR, GERRITSEN SM: The Hermansky-Pudlak syndrome: Inclusions in circulating leucocytes. *Br J Haematol* 24:761, 1973

177. WITKOP CJ JR, WHITE JG, GERRITSEN SM, TOWNSEND D, KING RA: Hermansky-Pudlak syndrome (HPS): A proposed block in glutathione peroxidase. *Oral Surg* 35:790, 1973

178. GARAY SM, GARDELLA JE, FAZZINI EP, GOLDRING RM: Hermansky-Pudlak syndrome. Pulmonary manifestations of a ceroid storage disease. *Am J Med* 66:737, 1979

179. MORI K, YODA B, SAKAI H, GOTO Y: A case of "storage-pool disease" associated with albinism (Hermansky-Pudlak syndrome). *Acta Haematol Jap* 41:992, 1978

180. TANOUE K: Defective platelet functions in a patient with albinism and storage pool disease. *Acta Haematol Jap* 41:1000, 1978

181. KLEIMANS M, SASSETTI B, KORDICH L: Disfunción plaquetaria y albinismo. Presentación de dos casos. *Sangre* 21:181, 1976

182. HERMANSKY F, CIESLAR P: Thrombopathies héréditaires par trouble de libération. *Rev Franc d'Hematol* 16:413, 1976

183. HOSTE P, WILLEMS J, DEVRIENDT J, LAMONT H, VAN DER STRAETEN M: Familial diffuse interstitial pulmonary fibrosis associated with oculocutaneous albinism. Report of two cases with a family study. *Scand J Respir Dis* 60:128, 1979

184. LOREZ HP, RICHARDS JG, DAPRADA M, PICOTTI GB, PARETI FI, CAPITANIO A, MANNUCCI PM: Storage pool disease: Comparative fluorescence microscopical, cytochemical and biochemical studies on amine-storing organelles of human blood platelets. *Br J Haematol* 43:297, 1979

185. FRENK E, LATTION F: The melanin pigmentary disorder in a family with Hermansky-Pudlak syndrome. *J Invest Dermatol* (in press)

186. GERRITSEN SM, AKKERMAN JWN, Nijmeijer B, Sixma JJ, Witkop CJ, White J: The Hermansky-Pudlak syndrome. Evidence for a lowered 5-hydroxytryptamine content in platelets of heterozygotes. *Scand J Haematol* 18:249, 1977

187. GERRITSEN SM: *The Hermansky-Pudlak Syndrome,* Proefschrift, Rijksuniversiteit Te Utrecht, Drukkerij Biblo B. V.—s'Hertogenbosch, Utrecht, June 6, 1978

188. HORLER AR, WITTS LJ: Hereditary capillary purpura (Von Willebrand's disease). *Q J Med* 27:173, 1958

189. LARSEN MC, LEY AB, ZUCKER MB, LOSEKE LE: The association of albinism with pseudohemophilia. *Ann Intern Med* 56:504, 1962

190. WITKOP CJ JR: Genetics. *Schweiz Monatsschr Zahnheilkd* 82:917, 1972

191. VERLOOP MCV, WIERINGEN A, VUYLSTEKE J, HART HC, HUIZINGA J: Albinismus, haemorrhagische Diathese und anomale Pigmentzellen im Knochenmark. *Med Klin* 59:408, 1964

192. THEURING F, FIEDLER J: Fatal bleeding following tooth extraction. Hermansky-Pudlak syndrome. *Dtsch Stomatol* 23:52, 1973

193. DAVIES BH, TUDDENHAM GD: Familial pulmonary fibrosis associated with oculocutaneous albinism and platelet function defect. A new syndrome. *Q J Med* (new series)45:219, 1976

194. SCHINELLA RA, GRECO MA, COLBERT BL, DENMARK LW, COX RP: Hermansky-Pudlak syndrome with granulomatous colitis. *Ann Intern Med* 92:20, 1980

195. KING RA, OLDS DP, WITKOP CJ JR: Enzyme studies in human oculocutaneous albinism, in Klaus SN (ed): *Pigment Cell Pathophysiology of Melanocytes.* Basel, S. Karger, 1979, vol 5, pp 16—20

196. MAURER HM, BUCKINGHAM S, MCGILVRAY E, SPIELVOGEL A, WOLFF JA: Prolonged bleeding time, abnormal binding of platelet serotonin (5-HT), absent platelet "dark body," defective platelet factor-3 activation, bone marrow inclusions and chromosome breaks in albinism. *Twelfth Congress, International Society of Hematology,* New York, 1968, p 198

197. WHITE JG, WITKOP CJ JR: Effects of normal and aspirin platelets on defective secondary aggregation in the Hermansky-Pudlak syndrome: A test for storage pool deficient platelets. *Am J Pathol* 68:57, 1972

198. WHITE JG: Fine structure alterations induced in platelets by adenosine diphosphate. *Blood* 31:604, 1968

199. WHITE JG: Dense bodies in human platelets: Inherent electron opacity of serotonin storage organelles. *Blood* 33:598, 1969

200. GERRARD JM, WHITE JG: The influence of prostaglandin endoperoxides on platelet ultrastructure. *Am J Pathol* 80:189, 1975

201. TRANZER JP, DAPRADA M, PLETSCHER A: Ultrastructural localization of 5-hydroxytryptamine in blood platelets. *Nature (Lond)* 212:1574, 1966

202. WEISS HJ, TSCHOPP TB, ROGERS J, BRAND H: Studies of platelet 5-hydroxytryptamine (serotonin) in storage pool disease and albinism. *Clin Invest* 54:421, 1974

203. RAO GHR, WHITE JG, JACHIMOWICZ AA, WITKOP CJ JR: Nucleotide profiles of normal and abnormal platelets by high-pressure liquid chromatography. *J Lab Clin Med* 84:839, 1974

204. RAO GHR, WHITE JG, JACHIMOWICZ AA, WITKOP CJ JR: An improved method for the extraction of endogenous platelet serotonin. *J Lab Clin Med* 87:129, 1976

205. GERRARD JM, WHITE JG, RAO GHR, KRIVIT W, WITKOP CJ JR: Labile aggregation stimulating substance (LASS): The factor from storage pool deficient platelets correcting defective aggregation and release of aspirin treated normal platelets. *Br J Haematol* 29:657, 1975

206. HOLMSEN H, WEISS HJ: Hereditary defect in the platelet release reaction caused by a deficiency in the storage pool of platelet adenine nucleotides. *Br J Haematol* 19:643, 1970

207. HOLMSEN H, WEISS HJ: Further evidence for a deficient storage pool of adenine nucleotides on platelets from some patients with thrombocytopathia—"storage pool disease." *Blood* 39:197, 1972

208. DAY HJ, HOLMSEN H, SCRUTTON MC, WEISS HJ: Metal content of platelets obtained from patients with storage pool deficiency. *Fourth International Congress of Thrombosis and Hemostasis.* Vienna, G. Gistel, 1973, p 297

209. SMITH B: Studies reported in R. M. Hardisty and D. C. B. Mills. The platelet defect associated with albinism. *Ann NY Acad Sci* 201:429, 1972

210. WILLIS AL, KUHN DC: A new potential mediator of arterial thrombosis whose biosynthesis is inhibited by aspirin. *Prostaglandins* 4:127, 1973

211. VARGAFTIG BB, ZIRINIS P: Platelet aggregation induced by arachidonic acid is accompanied by release of potential inflammatory mediators distinct from PGE$_2$ and PGF$_2$. *Nature (New Biol)* 244:114, 1973

212. SMITH JB, INGERMAN C, KOCSIS JJ, SILVER MJ: Formation of an intermediate in prostaglandin biosynthesis and its association with the platelet release reaction. *J Clin Invest* 53:1468, 1974

213. HAMBERG M, SVENSSON J, SAMUELSSON B: Thromboxanes: A new group of biologically active compounds derived from prostaglandin endoperoxides. *Proc Nat Acad Sci USA* 72:2994, 1975

214. SMITH JB, WILLIS AL: Aspirin selectively inhibits prostaglandin production in human platelets. *Nature* 231:235, 1971

215. ROTH GJ, STANFORD N, MAJERUS PW: Acetylation of prostaglandin synthase by aspirin. *Proc Natl Acad Sci USA* 72:3073, 1975

216. O'BRIEN JR: Effects of salicylates on human platelets. *Lancet* 1:779, 1968

217. ZUCKER MB, PETERSON J: Effect of acetylsalicylic acid, and other nonsteroidal anti-inflammatory agents, and dipyridamole on human blood platelets. *J Lab Clin Med* 76:66, 1970

218. VARGAFTIG BB: Carrageenan and thrombin trigger prostaglandin synthetase-independent aggregation of rabbit platelets: Inhibition by phospholipase A$_2$ inhibitors. *J Pharm Pharmacol* 29:222, 1977

219. KINLOUGH-RATHBONE RL, REIMERS HJ, MUSTARD JF, PACKHAM MA: Sodium arachidonate can induce platelet shape changes and aggregation which are independent of the release reaction. *Science* 192:1011, 1976

220. CHARO IF, FEINMAN RD, DETWILLER TC, SMITH JB, INGERMAN CM, SILVER MJ: Prostaglandin endoperoxides and thromboxane A$_2$ can induce platelet aggregation in the absence of secretion. *Nature (Lond)* 269:66, 1977

221. REIMERS HJ, KINLOUGH-RATHBONE RL, CAZENARE JP, SENYI AF, HIRSCH J, PACKHAM MA, MUSTARD JF: In vitro and in vivo functions of thrombin-treated platelets. *Thrombos Haemostas (Stutt)* 35:151, 1976

222. VARGAFTIG BB, CHIGNARD M, LECOUEDIC JP, BENVENISTE J: One, two, three or more pathways for platelet aggregation. *Acta Med Scand* (suppl) 642:23, 1980

223. RAO GHR, REDDY KR, WHITE JG: The influence of epinephrine on prostacyclin (PGI$_2$) induced dissociation of ADP aggregated platelets. *Prostaglandins Med* 4:385, 1980

224. RAO GHR, REDDY KR, WHITE JG: Influence of trifluoperazine on platelet aggregation and disaggregation. *Prostagland Med* 5:221, 1980

225. RAO GHR, JOHNSON GJ, WHITE JG: Influence of epinephrine on the aggregation response of aspirin-treated platelets. *Prostaglandins Med* 5:45, 1980

226. RAO GHR, GERRARD JM, WITKOP CJ, WHITE JG: Platelet aggregation independent of ADP release or prostaglandin synthesis in patients with Hermansky-Pudlak syndrome. *Prostaglandins Med* 6:459, 1981

227. RAO GHR, REDDY KR, WHITE JG: Modification of human platelet response to sodium arachidonate by membrane modulation. *Prostaglandins Med* 6:75, 1981

228. WEISS HJ, ALEDORT LM: Impaired platelet connective tissue reaction in man after aspirin ingestion. *Lancet* 2:495, 1967

229. WEISS HJ, ALEDORT LM, KOCHWA S: The effect of salicylates on the hemostatic properties of platelets in man. *J Clin Invest* 47:2169, 1968

230. ZUCKER MB, PETERSON J: Inhibition of adenosine diphosphate—induced secondary aggregation and other platelet functions by acetylsalicylic acid ingestion. *Proc Soc Exp Biol Med* 127:547, 1967

231. EVANS G, NISHIZAWA EE, PACKHAM MA, MUSTARD JF: The effect of acetylsalicylic acid (aspirin) on platelet function. *Blood* 30:550, 1967

232. GERRARD JM, WHITE, JG: The influence of aspirin and indomethacin on the platelet contractile wave. *Am J Pathol* 82:513, 1976

233. WILLIS AL, KUHN DC: A new potential mediator of arterial thrombosis whose biosynthesis is inhibited by aspirin. *Prostaglandins* 4:12, 1973

234. WILLIS AL: Isolation of a chemical trigger for thrombosis. *Prostaglandins* 5:1, 1974

235. SMITH JB, WILLIS AL: Formation and release of prostaglandins in response to thrombin. *Br J Pharmacol* 40:545, 1970

236. SILVER MJ, HERNANDOVICH J, INGERMAN C, KOCSIS JJ, SMITH JB: Persistent inhibition by aspirin of collagen-induced platelet prostaglandin formation, in Scriabine A, Sherry S (eds): *Platelets and Thrombosis.* Baltimore, University Park Press, 1974, pp 91—98

237. HAMBERG M, SVENSSON J, WAKABAYASHI T, SAMUELSSON B: Isolation and structure of two prostaglandin endoperoxides that cause platelet aggregation. *Proc Natl Acad Sci USA* 71:345, 1974

238. HUANG EM, DETWILER TC: Reassessment of the evidence for the role of secreted ADP in biphasic platelet aggregation. *J Lab Clin Med* 95:59, 1980

239. CIESLAR P, HEŘMANSKÝ F, SMETANA K, PROKEŠ J: Platelet functions and ultrastructure in the Heřmanský-Pudlák syndrome. *Folia Haematol (Leipz),* 101:553, 1974

240. SIAKOTOS AN, GOEBEL HH, PATEL V, WATANABE I, ZEMAN W: The morphogenesis and biochemical characteristics of ceroid isolated from cases of neuronal ceroid-lipofuscins, in Volk BW, Aronson SM (eds): *Advances in Experimental Medicine and Biology.* New York, Plenum Publishing Corp, 1972, pp 53—61

241. ENDICOTT KM: Similarity of the acid-fast pigment ceroid and oxidized unsaturated fat. *AMA Arch Pathol* 37:49, 1944

242. HARTROFT WS, PORTA EA: Ceroid. *Am J Med Sci* 250:324, 1965

243. PORTA EA, HARTROFT WS: Lipid pigments in relation to aging and dietary factors (lipofuscins), in Wolman M (ed): *Pigments in Pathology*. New York, Academic Press, Inc, 1969, pp 192–235

244. SAWITSKY A, ROSNER F, CHADSKY S: The sea-blue histiocyte syndrome, a review: Genetic and biochemical studies. *Semin Hematol* 9:285, 1972

245. JACOBSEN CD, GJONE E, HOVIG T: Sea-blue histiocytes in familial lecithin: cholesterol acyltransferase deficiency. *Scand J Haematol* 9:106, 1972

246. GERRITSEN SM, AKKERMAN JWN, STAAL G, ROELOFSEN B, KOSTER JF, SIXMA JJ: Biochemical studies in Hermansky-Pudlak syndrome. *Scand J Haematol* 23:161, 1979

247. BAGNARA JT, TAYLOR JD, PROTA G: Color changes, unusual melanosomes, and a new pigment from leaf frogs. *Science* 182:1034, 1973

248. MISURACA G, PROTA G, BAGNARA JT, FROST SK: Identification of the leaf-frog melanophore pigment, rhodomelanochrome, as pterorhodin. *Comp Biochem Physiol* 57B:41, 1977

249. GERRITSEN SW, AKKERMAN J-WN, SIXMA JJ: Correction of the bleeding time in patients with storage pool deficiency by infusion of cryoprecipitate. *Br J Haematol* 40:153, 1978

250. MACKIE I, BULL H, BROZOVÍC M, HUSSEIN M: Hermansky-Pudlak syndrome and factor VIII ristocetin cofactor. *Br J Haematol* 41:449, 1979

251. SATO A: Chediak and Higashi's disease: Probable identity of "a new leucocytal anomaly (Chediak)" and "congenital gigantism of peroxidase granules (Higashi)." *Tohoku J Exp Med* 61:201, 1955

252. WINDHORST DB, ZELICKSON AS, GOOD RA: A human pigmentary dilution based on a heritable subcellular structural defect—the Chédiak-Higashi syndrome. *J Invest Dermatol* 50:9, 1968

253. LOCKMAN LA, KENNEDY WR, WHITE JG: The Chediak-Higashi syndrome: Electrophysiologic and electron microscopic observations on the peripheral neuropathy. *J Pediatr* 70:942, 1967

254. DONOHUE WL, BAIN HW: Chediak-Higashi syndrome—a lethal familial disease with anomalous inclusions in the leucocytes and constitutional stigmata—report of a case with necropsy. *Pediatrics* 20:416, 1957

255. BERNARD J, BESSIS M, SELIGMANN M, CHASSIGNEUX J, CHOME J: Un cas de maladie de Chediak-Steinbrinck-Higashi: Étude Clinique et cytologique. *Presse Med* 68:563, 1960

256. BESSIS M, BERNARD J, SELIGMANN M: Étude cytologique d'un cas de maladie de Chediak. *Nouv Rev Fr Hematol* 1:422, 1961

257. WHITE JG: The Chediak-Higashi syndrome: A possible lysosomal disease. *Blood* 28:143, 1966

258. MYERS JP, SUNG JH, COWAN D, WOLFF A: Pathological findings in the central and peripheral nervous systems in Chediak-Higashi's disease and the finding of cytoplasmic neuronal inclusions. *J Neuropathol Exp Neurol* 22:357, 1963

259. MAGGI R, GUTIERRIZ E, PENALBER J, DI MENNA A, ROCCATAGLIAT M, MATERA F, ETCHEGARAY E, MILLAN J: Sindrome de Beguez Cesar-Chediak-Higashi. Presentación de dos casos. *Arch Argent Pediatr* 48:323, 1957

260. SCHNEIDER LA: Chediak-Higashi syndrome, in *Proceedings of the Seventh Congress, Society of International Hematology*. Rome, 1958, p 430

261. KRITZLER RA, TERNER JY, LINDENBAUM J, MAGIDSON J, WILLIAMS R, PREISIG R, PHILIPS GB: Chediak-Higashi syndrome—cytologic and serum lipid observations in a case and family. *Am J Med* 36:583, 1964

262. PADGETT GA, REIQUAM CW, HENSON JB, GORHAM JR: Comparative studies of susceptibility to infection in Chediak-Higashi syndrome. *J Pathol Bacteriol* 95:509, 1968

263. WITKOP CJ Jr: The face and oral structures, in Rubin A (ed): *Handbook of Congenital Malformations*. Philadelphia, WB Saunders Co, 1967, pp 103–156

264. EFRATI P, JONAS W: Chediak's anomaly of leucocytes in malignant lymphoma associated with leukemic manifestations: Case report with necropsy. *Blood* 13:1063, 1958

265. DENT PB, FISH, LA, WHITE JG, GOOD RA: Chediak-Higashi syndrome: Observations on the nature of the associated malignancy. *Lab Invest* 15:1634, 1966

266. LASCANO FD, FERREYRA ME, SEOANE MR: Enfermedad de Chediak-Higashi. *Rev Clin Esp* 110:329, 1968

267. WOLFF SM, DALE DC, CLARK RA, ROOT RK, KIMBALL HR: The Chediak-Higashi syndrome: Studies of host defenses. *Ann Intern Med* 76:293, 1972

268. BREGEAT P, DHERMY P, HAMARD H: Manifestations oculaires du syndrome de Chediak-Higashi. *Arch Ophthalmol (Paris)* 23:661, 1966

269. JOHNSON DL, JACOBSON LW, TOYAMA R, MONAHAN RH: Histopathy of eyes in Chediak-Higashi syndrome. *Arch Ophthalmol* 75:84, 1966

270. BENEZRA D, MENGISTU F, CIVIDALLI G, WEIZMAN Z, MERIN S, AUERBACH E: Chediak-Higashi syndrome: Ocular findings. *J Pediatr Ophthalmol Strabismus* 17:68, 1980

271. BLUME RS, WOLFF SM: The Chediak-Higashi syndrome: Studies in four patients and a review of the literature. *Medicine* 51:247, 1972

272. McLELLAND R, ESTEVEZ JM: The Chediak-Higashi syndrome: *J Assoc Can Radiol* 19:78, 1968

273. CLAWSON CC, WHITE JG: Chediak-Higashi syndrome, in Buyse M (ed): *Birth Defects Compendium*, ed 3. New York, Alan R Liss, Inc, 1982

274. BUCHANAN GR, HANDIN RI: Platelet function in the Chediak-Higashi syndrome. *Blood* 47:941, 1976

275. BELL TG, MEYERS KM, PRIEUR DJ, FAUCI AS, WOLFF SM, PADGETT GA: Decreased nucleotide and serotonin storage associated with defective function in Chediak-Higashi syndrome cattle and human platelets. *Blood* 48:175, 1976

276. BOXER GJ, HOLMSEN H, ROBKIN L, BANG NU, BOXER LA, BAEHNER RL: Abnormal platelet function in Chediak-Higashi syndrome. *Br J Haematol* 35:521, 1977

277. STEGMAIER OC, SCHNEIDER LA: Chediak-Higashi syndrome: Dermatologic manifestations. *Arch Dermatol* 91:1, 1965

278. WINDHORST DB, ZELICKSON AS, CLAWSON CC, DENT PB, POLLARA B, GOOD RA: The Chediak-Higashi anomaly and the Aleutian trait in mink: Homologous defects of lysosomal structure. *Ann NY Acad Sci* 155:818, 1968

279. LUTZNER MA, TIERNEY JH, BENDITT EP: Giant granules and widespread cytoplasmic inclusions in a genetic syndrome of Aleutian mink. *Lab Invest* 14:2063, 1965

280. CLARK RA, KIMBALL HR: Defective granulocyte chemotaxis in the Chediak-Higashi syndrome. *J Clin Invest* 50:2645, 1971

281. CLARK RA, KIMBALL HR, PADGETT GA: Granulocyte chemotaxis in the Chediak-Higashi syndrome of mink. *Blood* 39:644, 1972

282. OLIVER JM: Impaired microtubule function correctable by cyclic GMP and cholinergic agonist in the Chediak-Higashi syndrome. *Am J Pathol* 85:395, 1976

283. ZURIER RB: Cyclic nucleotides and the Chediak-Higashi syndrome, in Hamet P, Sands H (eds): *Advances in Cyclic Nucleotide Research*. New York, Raven Press, 1980, vol 12, pp 173–179

284. BOXER LA, WATANABE AM, RISTER M, BESCH HR, ALLEN J, BAEHNER RL: Correction of leukocyte function in Chediak-Higashi syndrome by ascorbate. *N Engl J Med* 295:1041, 1976

285. OLIVER JM, ZURIER RB: Correction of characteristic abnormalities of microtubule function and granule morphology in Chediak-Higashi syndrome with cholinergic agents. *J Clin Invest* 57:1239, 1976

286. CLAWSON CC, WHITE JG, REPINE JE: The Chédiak-Higashi syndrome. Evidence that defective leukotaxis is primarily due to an impediment by giant granules. *Am J Pathol* 92:745, 1978

287. CLAWSON CC, REPINE JE, WHITE JG: Chediak-Higashi syndrome: Quantitation defect in bactericidal capacity. *Blood* 38:814, 1971

288. CLAWSON CC, REPINE JE, WHITE JG: Quantitation of bactericidal capacity in normal and abnormal human neutrophils. *Pediatr Res* 6:367, 1972

289. CLAWSON CC, REPINE JE, WHITE JG: The Chediak-Higashi syndrome. Quantitation of a deficiency in maximal bactericidal capacity. *Am J Pathol* 94:539, 1979

290. BLUME RS, BENNETT JM, YANKEE RA, WOLFF SM: Defective granulocyte regulation in the Chediak-Higashi syndrome. *N Engl J Med* 279:1009, 1968

291. MAURI C, SILINGARDI V: A cytological and cytochemical study of Chediak's leukocytic anomaly. *Acta Haematol* 32:114, 1964

292. PAGE AR, BERENDES H, WARNER J, GOOD RA: The Chediak-Higashi syndrome. *Blood* 20:330, 1962

293. SADAN N, YAFFEE D, ROZENSZAN L, ADAR H, SOROKER B, EFRATI R: Cytochemical and genetic studies in four cases of Chediak-Higashi-Steinbrinck syndrome. *Acta Haematol* 34:20, 1965

294. WHITE JG: Virus-like particles in the peripheral blood cells of two patients with Chediak-Higashi syndrome. *Cancer* 19:877, 1966

295. WINDHORST DB, ZELICKSON AS, GOOD RA: Chediak-Higashi syndrome, hereditary gigantism of cytoplasmic organelles. *Science* 151:81, 1966

296. ASH P, LOUTIT JF, TOWNSEND KMS: Giant lysomes, a cytoplasmic marker in osteoclasts of beige mice. *Am J Pathol* 130:237, 1980

297. RAUSCH PG, PRYZWANSKY KB, SPITZNAGEL JK: Immunocytochemical identification of azurophilic and specific granule markers in the giant granules of Chediak-Higashi neutrophils. *New Engl J Med* 298:693, 1978

298. PARMLEY RT, POON M-C, CRIST WM, MALLUH A: Giant platelet granules in a child with the Chediak-Higashi syndrome. *Am J Hematol* 6:51, 1979

299. WHITE JG, CLAWSON CC: The Chediak-Higashi syndrome: Spectrum of giant organelles in peripheral blood cells. *Henry Ford Hosp Med J* 27:286, 1979

300. WHITE JG, CLAWSON CC: Chediak-Higashi syndrome: Variable cytochemical reactivity of giant inclusions in polymorphonuclear leukocytes. *Ultrastruct Pathol* 1:223, 1980

301. WHITE JG, CLAWSON CC: The Chediak-Higashi syndrome. Ring-shaped lysosomes in circulating monocytes. *Am J Pathol* 96:781, 1979

302. WHITE JG, CLAWSON CC: The Chediak-Higashi syndrome: The nature of the giant neutrophile granules and their interactions with cytoplasm and foreign particulates. *Am J Pathol* 98:151, 1980

303. OLIVER JM, ZURIER RB, BERLIN RD: Concanavalin A cap formation on polymorphonuclear leukocytes of normal and beige (Chediak-Higashi) mice. *Nature* 253:471, 1975

304. BOXER LA, RISTER M, ALLEN JM, BAEHNER RL: Improvement of Chediak-Higashi leukocyte function by cyclic guanosine monophosphate. *Blood* 49:9, 1977

305. BOXER LA, ALBERTINI DF, BAEHNER RL, OLIVER JM: Impaired microtubule assembly and polymorphonuclear leucocyte function in Chediak-Higashi syndrome correctable by ascorbic acid. *Br J Haematol* 43:207, 1979

306. HINDS K, DANES BS: Microtubular defects in Chediak-Higashi syndrome. *Lancet* 2:146, 1976

307. BUCHANAN GR, HANDIN RI: Platelet function in the Chediak-Higashi syndrome. *Blood* 47:941, 1976

308. WHITE JG: Platelet microtubules and giant granules in the Chediak-Higashi syndrome. *Am J Med Tech* 44:273, 1978

309. WHITE JG, CLAWSON CC: The Chediak-Higashi syndrome: Microtubules in monocytes and lymphocytes. *Am J Hematol* 7:349, 1979

310. FRANKEL FR, TUCKER RW, BRUCE J, STENBERG R: Fibroblasts and macrophages of mice with the Chediak-Higashi-like syndrome have microtubules and actin cables. *J Cell Biol* 79:401, 1978

311. OSTLUND RE, LEUNG JT, TUCKER RW: Abnormal lysosome-microtubule interaction in Chediak-Higashi syndrome. *Clin Res* 27:303A, 1979

312. KLEBANOFF SJ, CLARK RA: *The Neutrophil: Function and Clinical Disorders.* New York, Elsevier North-Holland, Inc, 1978, pp 735–792

313. RODER JC: The beige mutation in the mouse I. Stem cell predetermined impairment in natural killer cells. *J Immunol* 123:2168, 1979

314. RODER JC, LOHMANN-MATTHES M-L, DOMIZIG W, WIGZELL H: The beige mutation in the mouse II. Selectivity of the natural killer (NK) cell defect. *J Immunol* 123:2174, 1979

315. HALIOTIS T, RODER J, KLEIN M, ORTALDO J, FAUCI AS, HERBERMAN RB: Chédiak-Higashi gene in humans I. Impairment of natural-killer function. *J Exp Med* 151:1039, 1980

316. KLEIN M, RODER J, HALIOTIS T, KOREC S, JETT JR, HERBERMAN RB, KATZ P, FAUCI AS: Chédiak-Higashi gene in humans II. The selectivity of the defect in natural-killer and antibody-dependent cell-mediated cytotoxicity function. *J Exp Med* 151:1049, 1980

317. GRISCELLI C, DURANDY A, GUY-GRAND D, DAGUILLARD F, HERTZOG C, PRUNIERAS MA: A syndrome associating partial albinism and immunodeficiency. *Am J Med* 65:691, 1978

318. VIRELIZIER J-L, LIPINSKI M, TURSZ T, GRISCELLI C: Defects of immune interferon secretion and natural killer activity in patients with immunological disorders. *Lancet* 2:696, 1979

319. VAN SLYCK EJ, REBUCK JW: Pseudo-Chediak-Higashi anomaly in acute leukemia. *Am J Clin Pathol* 62:673, 1974

320. GORMAN AM, O'CONNELL LG: Letter to the editor. Pseudo-Chediak-Higashi anomaly in acute leukemia. *Am J Clin Pathol* 65:1030, 1976

321. TULLIEZ M, VERNANT JP, BRENTON-GORIUS J, IMBERT M, SULTAN C: Pseudo-Chediak-Higashi anomaly in a case of acute myeloid leukemia: Electron microscopic studies. *Blood* 54:863, 1979

322. GALLIN JI, ELIN RJ, HUBERT RT, FAUCI AS, KALINER MA, WOLFF SM: Efficacy of ascorbic acid in Chediak-Higashi syndrome (CHS): Studies in humans and mice. *Blood* 53:226, 1979

323. PADGETT GA, LEADER RW, GORHAM JR, O'MARY CC: The familial occurrence of the Chediak-Higashi syndrome in mink and cattle. *Genetics* 49:505, 1965

324. PADGETT GA: The Chediak-Higashi syndrome. *Adv Vet Sci Comp Med* 12:239, 1968

325. TAYLOR RE, FARRELL RK: Light and electron microscopy of peripheral blood neutrophiles in a killer whale affected with Chediak-Higashi syndrome. *Fed Proc* 32:822, 1973

326. KRAMER JW, DAVIS WC, PRIEUR DJ: Chediak-Higashi syndrome of cats. *Lab Invest* 36:554, 1977

327. HALL AJ, SESEBE T, CARDOZO RL, NURSE GT: A high-frequency albinism variant on the gulf coast of Papua. *Ann Hum Genet* (in press)

328. KIMBERLING WJ: Personal communication, 1979

329. WITKOP CJ JR, EFRON M, BEASLEY P, WHITE JG, KING RA: A syndrome of black locks, albinism and deafness of the sensory neural type (BADS): A defect apparently in migration of neuroectodermal cells, submitted

330. HU F, HANIFIN JM, PRESCOTT GH, TONGUE AC: Yellow mutant albinism: Cytochemical, ultrastructural, and genetic characterization suggesting multiple allelism. *Am J Hum Genet* 32:387, 1980

331. ENGELHARD CF: Eine Familie mit hereditarem Nystagmus. *Zentralbl Gesamte Neurol Psychiatr* 28:319, 1915

332. LEIN JN, SITWART CT, MALL FC: Sex-linked hereditary nystagmus. *Pediatrics* 18:214, 1956

333. WALKER BA, MARTYN LJ, COFFMAN T: X-linked ocular albinism, in Bergsma D (ed): *Eye*, Part 8, *Birth Defects Original Article Series.* Baltimore, Williams & Wilkins Co, 1971, vol 7, no 3, p 200

334. JOHNSON GJ, GILLAN JG, PEARCE WG: Ocular albinism in Newfoundland. *Can J Ophthalmol* 6:237, 1971

335. GREGOR Z: The perifoveal vasculature in albinism. *Br J Ophthalmol* 62:554, 1978

336. KRILL AE, LEE GB: The electroretinogram in albinos and carriers of the ocular albino trait. *Arch Ophthalmol* 69:32, 1963

337. TOMEI F, WIRTH A: Letter to Editors. The electroretinogram of albinos. *Vision Res* 18:1465, 1978

338. REESER F, WEINSTEIN GW, FEIOCK KB: Electrooculography as a test of retinal function. *Am J Ophthalmol* 70:505, 1970

339. O'DONNELL FE JR, GREEN WR, FLEISCHMAN JA, HAMBRICK GW: X-linked ocular albinism in blacks: Ocular albinism cum pigmento. *Arch Ophthalmol* 96:1189, 1978

340. FRANÇOIS J, DEWEER JP: Albinisme oculaire lié au sexe et altérations caractéristiques du fond d'oeil chz les femmes hétérozygotes. *Ophthalmologia* 126:209, 1953

341. GILLESPIE FD: Ocular albinisim with report of a family with female carriers. *Arch Ophthalmol* 66:774, 1961

342. LYON MF: Sex chromatin and gene action in the mammalian X-chromosome. *Am J Hum Genet* 14:135, 1962

343. PEARCE WG, JOHNSON GJ, SANGER R: Ocular albinism and Xg (Letter). *Lancet* 1:1072, 1971

344. FIALKOW PJ, GIBLETT ER, MOTULSKY AG: Measurable linkage between ocular albinism and Xg. *Am J Hum Genet* 19:63, 1967

345. PEARCE WG, SANGER R, RACE RR: Ocular albinism and Xg. *Lancet* 1:1282, 1968

346. PEARCE WG, JOHNSON GJ, GILLAN JG: Nystagmus in a female carrier of ocular albinism. *J Med Genet* 9:126, 1972

347. O'DONNELL FE, KING RA, GREEN WR, WITKOP CJ JR: Autosomal recessively inherited ocular albinism. *Arch Ophthalmol* 96:1621, 1978

348. SCIALFA AC: Ocular albinism in a female. *Am J Ophthalmol* 73:943, 1972

349. Lewis RA: Ocular albinism and deafness. *Twenty-ninth Annual Meeting, American Society of Human Genetics.* Vancouver, 1978, p 57A

350. KONRAD K, WOLFF K, HONIGSMANN H: The giant melanosome: A model of deranged melanosome-morphogenesis. *J Ultractruct Res* 48:102, 1974

351. ZEISLER EP, BECKER SW: Generalized lentigo: Its relation to systemic nonelevated nevi. *Arch Dermatol Syphilol* 33:109, 1936

352. GUERRIER CJ, LUTZNER MA, DEVICO V, PRUNIERAS M: An electron microscopical study of the skin in 18 cases of xeroderma pigmentosum. *Dermatologica* 146:211, 1973

353. BENEDICT PH, SZABO G, FITZPATRICK TB, SINESI SJ: Melanotic macules in Albright's syndrome and in neurofibromatosis. *JAMA* 205:618, 1968

354. SCIALFA A: Albinisme oculaire et dyschromatopsie. *Arch Ophthalmol* 27:483, 1967

355. WAARDENBURG PJ, ERIKSSON AW, FORSIUS H: Åland eye disease (syndroma Forsius-Eriksson). *Prog Neuro-Ophthalmol* 2:336, 1969

356. WARBURG M: Ocular albinism and protanopia in the same family. *Acta Ophthalmol* 42:444, 1964

357. MERIN S, ROWE H, AUERBACH E, LANDAU J: Syndrome of congenital high myopia with nyctalopia. Report of findings in 25 families. *Am J Ophthalmol* 70:541, 1970

358. CURRAN RE, ROBB RN: Isolated foveal hypoplasia. *Arch Ophthalmol* 94:48, 1976

359. RACE RR, SANGER R: *Blood Groups in Man*, ed. 5. Philadelphia, FA Davis Co, 1968, p 549

360. FITZPATRICK TB, EISEN AZ, WOLFF K, FREEDBERG IM, AUSTEN KF (eds): *Dermatology in General Medicine*, ed 2. New York, McGraw-Hill Book Co, 1979

361. FITZPATRICK TB: Pigmentary diseases. Method of T. B. Fitzpatrick, in Conn HF (ed): *Current Therapy*. Philadelphia, WB Saunders Co, 1958, pp 514–516

362. REED WB, STONE VM, BODER E, ZIPRKOWSKI L: Pigmentary disorders in association with congenital deafness. *Arch Dermatol* 95:176, 1967

363. PIPKIN AC, PIPKIN SB: Albinism in Negroes. *J Hered* 33:419, 1942

364. PIPKIN AC, PIPKIN SB: Ear pits and albinism in a Negro family. *J Hered* 34:240, 1943

365. SICCARDI AG, BIANCHI E, CALLIGARI A, CLIVIO A, FORTUNATO A, MAGRINI U, SACCHI F: A new familial defect in neutrophil bactericidal activity. *Helvet Paediatr Acta* 33:401, 1978

366. BRAMBILLA E, DECHELETTE E, STOEBER P: Partial albinism and immunodeficiency: Ultrastructural study of haemophagocytosis and bone marrow erythroblasts in one case. *Pathol Res Pract* 167:151, 1980

367. POLYAK S: in Klüver H (ed): *The Vertebrate Visual System.* Chicago, University of Chicago Press, 1957

368. CREEL DJ, GIOLLI RA: Retinogeniculostriate projections in guinea pigs: Albino and pigmented strains compared. *Exp Neurol* 36:411, 1972

369. HAYHOW WR, WEBB C, JERVIE A: The accessory optic fiber system of the rat. *J Comp Neurol* 115:187, 1960

370. KUPFER C, CHUMBLEY L, DOWNER JC: Quantitative histology of optic nerve, optic tract, and lateral geniculate nucleus of man. *J Anat* 101:393, 1967

371. CREEL D, WITKOP CJ JR, KING RA: Asymmetric visually evoked potentials in human albinos. Evidence for visual system anomalies. *Invest Ophthalmol* 13:430, 1974

372. CREEL D, O'DONNELL FE JR, WITKOP CJ JR: Visual system anomalies in human ocular albinos. *Science* 201:931, 1978

373. TAYLOR WOG: Eldridge-Green Lecture, 1978. Visual disabilities of oculocutaneous albinism and their alleviation. *Trans Ophthalmol Soc UK* 98:423, 1978

374. COLEMAN J, SYDNOR CF, WOLBARSHT ML, BESSLER M: Abnormal visual pathways in human albinos studied with visually evoked potentials. *Exp Neurol* 65:667, 1979

375. CREEL D, KING RA, WITKOP CJ JR, OKORO AN: Visual system anomalies in human albinos, in Klaus SN (ed): *Pigment Cell. Pathophysiology of Melanocytes.* New Haven, Conn, S. Karger, 1979, pp 21–27

376. LUND RD: Uncrossed visual pathways of hooded and albino rats. *Science* 149:1506, 1965

377. GIOLLI RA, GUTHRIE MD: The primary optic projections in the rabbit: An experimental degeneration study. *J Comp Neurol* 136:99, 1969

378. GUILLERY RW: An abnormal retinogeniculate projection in Siamese cats. *Brain Res* 14:739, 1969

379. CREEL DJ: Visual system anomaly associated with albinism in the cat. *Nature (Lond)* 231:465, 1971

380. GUILLERY RW: An abnormal retinogeniculate projection in the albino ferret *(Mustela furo). Brain Res* 33:482, 1971

381. GUILLERY RW, SITTHI AMORN C, EIGHMY BB: Mutants with abnormal visual pathways: An explanation of anomalous geniculate laminae. *Science* 174:831, 1971

382. GIOLLI RA, CREEL DJ: The primary optic projections in pigmented and albino guinea pigs: An experimental degeneration study. *Brain Res* 55:25, 1973

383. GUILLERY RW, KAAS JH: Genetic abnormality of the visual pathways in a "white" tiger. *Science* 180:1287, 1973

384. GUILLERY RW, SCOTT GL, CATTANACH BM, DEOL MS: Genetic mechanisms determining the central visual pathways of mice. *Science* 179:1014, 1973

385. SANDERSON KJ: Normal and abnormal retinogeniculate pathways in rabbits and mink. *Anta Rec* 172:398, 1972

386. SANDERSON KJ, GUILLERY RW, SHACKLEFORD RM: Congenitally abnormal visual pathways in mink *(Mustela vison)* with reduced retinal pigment. *J Comp Neurol* 154:225, 1974

387. CREEL DJ, SHERIDAN CL: Monocular acquisition and interocular transfer in albino rats with unilateral striate ablations. *Psychonomic Sci* 6:89, 1966

388. MONTERO VM, BRUGGE JF, BEITEL RE: Relation of the visual field to the lateral geniculate body of the albino rat. *J Neurophysiol* 31:221,1968

389. CREEL DJ, DUSTMAN RE, BECK EC: Differences in visually evoked responses in albino versus hooded rats. *Exp Neurol* 29:298, 1970

390. CUNNINGHAM TJ, LUND RD: Laminar patterns in the dorsal division of the lateral geniculate nucleus of the rat. *Brain Res* 34:394, 1971

391. GIOLLI RA, GUTHRIE MD: Organization of subcortical projections of visual areas I and II in the rabbit: An experimental degeneration study. *J Comp Neurol* 142:351, 1971

392. CREEL DJ: Differences of ipsilateral and contralateral visually evoked responses in the cat: Strains compared. *J Comp Physiol Psychol* 77:161, 1971

393. GUILLERY RW, KAAS JH: A study of normal and congenitally abnormal retinogeniculate projections in cats. *J Comp Neurol* 143:73, 1971

394. KAAS JH, GUILLERY RW: The transfer of abnormal visual field representation from the dorsal-lateral geniculate nucleus to the visual cortex in Siamese cats. *Brain Res* 59:61, 1973

395. BATIPPS M, MIYAOKA M, SHINOHARA M, SOKOLOFF L, KENNEDY C: Comparative rates of local cerebral glucose utilization in the visual system of conscious albino and pigmented rats. *Neurology (New York)* 31:58, 1981

396. GROSS KJ, HICKEY TL: Abnormal laminar patterns in the lateral geniculate nucleus of an albino monkey. *Brain Res* 190:231, 1980

397. MANN I: *Developmental Abnormalities of the Eye.* Cambridge, Cambridge University Press, 1937, p 155

398. HUBEL DH, WIESEL TN: Aberrant visual projections in the Siamese cat. *J Physiol* 218:33, 1971

399. GUILLERY RW, CASAGRANDE VA, OBERDORFER MD: Congenitally abnormal vision in Siamese cats. *Nature* 252:195, 1974

400. GUILLERY RW: Visual pathways in albinos. *Sci Am* 230:44 1974

401. CARROLL WM, JAY BS, McDONALD WI, HALLIDAY AM: Two distinct patterns of visual evoked response asymmetry in human albinism. *Nature* 286:604, 1980

402. CARROLL WM, JAY BS, McDONALD WI, HALLIDAY AM: Pattern evoked potentials in human albinism. *J Neurol Sci* 48:265, 1980

403. COOPER ML, BLASDEL GG: Regional variation in the representation of the visual field in the visual cortex of the Siamese cat. *J Comp Neurol* 193:237, 1980

404. COLLEWIJN H, WINTERSON BJ, DUBOIS MFW: Optokinetic eye movement in albino rabbits: Inversion in anterior visual field. *Science* 199:1351, 1977

405. WOLFF D: Melanin in the inner ear. *Arch Otolaryngol* 14:195, 1931

406. BONACCORSI P: Il colore dell'iride come "test" di valutazione qualitativa, nell'uomo, della concentrazione de melanina nella stria vascolare. *Annali Laringol Otol Rinol Faringol* 64:725, 1965

407. CREEL D, GARBER SR, KING RA, WITKOP CJ JR: Auditory brainstem anomalies in human albinos. *Science* 209:1253, 1980

408. HARRISON JM, HOWE ME: Auditory system. Anatomy, physiology (ear), in Keidel W, Neff W (eds): *Handbook of Sensory Physiology.* New York, Springer-Verlag, 1974, vol 5, pp 284–336

409. IRVING R, HARRISON JM: The superior olivary complex and audition: A comparative study. *J Comp Neurol* 130:77, 1967

410. JAY WM, HOYT CS: Abnormal brain stem auditory-evoked potentials in Stilling-Türk-Duane syndrome. *Am J Ophthalmol* 89:814, 1980

411. HOTCHKISS MG, MILLER NR, CLARK AW, GREEN WR: Bilateral Duane's retraction syndrome. A clinical-pathologic case report. *Arch Ophthalmol* 98:870, 1980

412. HOOD J, POOLE J, GREEDMAN L: Eye color and susceptibility to TTS. *J Acoust Soc Am* 59:706,1976

413. McGINNESS J, CORRY P, PROCTOR P: Amorphous semiconductor switching in melanins. *Science* 183:853, 1974

414. LYTTKENS L, LARSSON B, GÖLLER H, ENGLESSON S, STAHLE J: Melanin capacity to accumulate drugs in the inner ear. A study on lidocaine, bupivacaine and chloropromazine. *Acta Otolaryngol (Stockholm)* 80:61, 1979

415. GARBER SR, TURNER CW, CREEL D, WITKOP CJ JR: Auditory system abnormalities in human albinos. *Ear Hearing,* in press

416. BECKHAM AS: Albinism in Negro children. *J Genet Psychol* 69:199, 1946

417. STEWART HF JR, KEELER CE: A comparison of the intelligence and personality of moon-child albino and control Cuna Indians. *J Genet Psychol* 106:319, 1965

418. OETTLÈ AG: Skin cancer in Africa. *National Cancer Institute (USA) Monograph No. 10,* 1963, p 197

419. KEELER CE: Albinism, xeroderma pigmentosum, and skin cancer. *National Cancer Institute (USA) Monograph No. 10,* 1963, p 349

420. WITKOP CJ JR: Epidemiology of skin cancer in man. Genetic factors, in Laerum D, Iverson OH (eds): *Biology of Skin Cancer.* Geneva, International Union Against Cancer, Tech Report Series, 60, 1981

421. BHENDE YM: Malignant amelanotic melanoma of skin in albino. *Indian J Med Sci* 6:755, 1952

422. YOUNG TE: Malignant melanoma in an albino. *Arch Pathol* 64:186, 1957

423. LEONARDI R, GRASSO S: Melanoblastoma in albino: Histological findings. *Minerva Dermatol* 33:24, 1958

424. DURON RA: Malignant melanoma in albinos. *Rev Med Hondur* 33:149, 1965

425. GARRINGTON GE, SCOFIELD HH, CORNYN J, LACY GR: Intraoral malignant melanoma in a human albino. *Oral Surg* 24:224, 1967

426. ALPERT LI, DAMJANOV I: Malignant melanoma in an albino: Diagnosis supported by ultrastructure. *Mt Sinai J Med* 45:447, 1978

427. CERVENKA J, WITKOP CJ, JR OKORO AN, KING RA: Chromosome breaks and sister chromatid exchanges in albinos in Nigeria. *Clin Genet* 15:17, 1979

428. DOS SANTOS SOBINHO BJ, MOURAO OG: Chediak-Higashi syndrome—presentation of two cases. *J Pediatr (Rio de Janeiro)* 24:341, 1959

429. PIERINI DO, ABULAFIA J: Manifestaciones cutáneas del sindrome de Chediak-Higashi. *Arch Argent Dermatol* 8:23, 1958

430. BARNICOT NA: Albinism in southwestern Nigeria. *Ann Hum Genet* 17:38, 1952

431. GILLOON JR, PEASE GL, MILLS SD: Chediak-Higashi anomaly of the leucocytes: Report of a case. *Mayo Clin Proc* 35:635, 1960

432. SPENCER WH, HOGAN MJ: Ocular manifestations of Chediak-Higashi syndrome: Report of a case with histopathologic examination of ocular tissues. *Am J Ophthalmol* 50:1197, 1960

433. TAY CH, LOPEZ CG, LAZARUS AR: The Chediak-Higashi syndrome. *Med J Aust* 2:1024, 1970

434. SHERAMATA W, KOTT HS, CYR DP: The Chediak-Higashi-Steinbrinck syndrome. *Arch Neurol* 25:289,1971

435. SARAIVA LG, AZEVEDO M, CORREA JM, CARVALHO G, PROSPERO JD: Anomalous panleucocytic granulation. *Blood* 14:1112, 1959

436. FRASER GR: The causes of severe visual handicap among school children in South Australia. *Med J Aust* 1:615, 1968

437. CAMERON D: On being an albino: A personal account. *Br Med J* 1:28, 1979

438. BERNE B, FISCHER T: Protective effects of various types of clothes against UV radiation. *Acta Dermatovener (Stockholm)* 60:459, 1980

439. FONDA G: Characteristics and low-vision corrections in albinism. *Arch Ophthalmol* 68:754, 1962

440. WOLFE HG, COLEMAN DL: Pigmentation, in Green EL (ed): *Biology of the Laboratory Mouse,* ed 2. New York, McGraw-Hill Book Co, 1966, p 405

441. FITZPATRICK TB, QUEVEDO WC JR: The melanocyte system, in Fitzpatrick TB, Arndt KA, Clark WH Jr, Eisen AZ, Van Scott EJ, Vaughan JH (eds): *Dermatology in General Medicine.* New York, McGraw-Hill Book Co, 1971, p 146

442. MARKERT CL, SILVERS WK: The effects of gentoype and cell environment on melanoblast differentiation in the house mouse. *Genetics* 41:429, 1956

443. SILVERS WK: Genes and the pigment cells of mammals. *Science* 134:368, 1961

444. MINTZ B: Gene control of mammalian differentiation. *Ann Rev Genet* 8:411, 1974

445. PARAKKAL PE: Transfer of premelanosomes into the keratinizing cells of albino hair follicle. *J Cell Biol* 35:473, 1967

446. COLEMAN D : Effect of gene substitution on the incorporation of tyrosine into the melanin of mouse skin. *Arch Biochem Biophys* 96:562, 1962

447. POMERANTZ SH, LI JP-C: Tyrosinase in the skin of albino hamsters and mice. *Nature (Lond)* 252:241, 1974

448. HEARING VJ: Tyrosinase activity in subcellular fractions of black and albino mice. *Nature (New Biol)* 245:81, 1973

449. SIDMAN RL, PEARLSTEIN R: Pink-eyed dilution (*p*) gene in rodents: Increased pigmentation in tissue culture. *Dev Biol* 12:93, 1965

450. MOYER PH: Electron microscope observations on the origin, development and genetic control of melanin granules of the mouse eye, in Smelser GK (ed): *The Structure of the Eye. Proceedings of a Symposium, April 11–13, 1960, during the Seventh International Congress of Anatomists, New York.* New York, Academic Press, Inc, 1961, pp 469–486

451. RITTENHOUSE E: Genetic effects on fine structure and development of pigment granules in mouse hair bulb melanocytes. II. The *c* and *p* loci, and *ddpp* interaction. *Dev Biol* 17:366, 1968

452. HEARING VJ, PHILLIPS P, LUTZNER MA: The fine structure of melanogenesis in coat color mutants of the mouse. *J Ultrastruct Res* 43:88, 1973

453. WITKOP CJ JR, KING RA, CREEL DJ: The abnormal albino animal, in Riley V (ed): *Pigment Cell.* Basel, S. Karger, 1976, vol 3, pp 201–210

454. CREEL D: Review. Inappropriate use of albino animals as models in research. *Pharmacol Biochem Behav* 12:969, 1980

455. LOCKARD RB: The albino rat: A defensable choice or a bad habit? *Am Psychol* 23:734, 1968

456. KEELER CE: The association of the black (nonagouti) gene with behavior. *J Hered* 33:371, 1942

457. KEELER CE, KING HD: Multiple effects of coat color genes in the Norway rat, with special reference to the "marks of domestication." *Anat Rec* 81:48, 1941

458. WEBSTER W: Embryogenesis of the enteric ganglia in normal mice and in mice that develop congenital aganglionic megacolon. *J Embryol Exp Morph,* 30:573, 1973

459. OMENN GS, MCKUSICK VA: The association of Waardenburg syndrome and Hirschsprung megacolon. *Am J Med Genet* 3:217,1979

460. DEOL MS: The relationship between abnormalities of pigmentation and of the inner ear. *Proc R Soc* 175:201, 1970

461. HENRY KR, HAYTHORN MM: Albinism and auditory function in the lab-oratory mouse. I. Effects of single-gene substitutions on auditory physiology, audiogenic seizures, and developmental processes. *Behav Genet* 5:137, 1975

462. MAXSON SC: Strain differences in lateralization of acoustic primary for susceptibility to audiogenic seizures. *Exp Neurol* 63:436, 1979

463. MOJAMDAR MV, SHARMA KS, SHAH VC: A comparative study on tyrosine metabolism in livers of albino and black mice. *Indian J Biochem Biophys* 13:237, 1976

464. GLUECKSOHN-WAELSCH S: Genetic control of morphogenic and biochemical differentiation: Lethal albino deletions in the mouse. *Cell* 16:225, 1979

465. KING RA, RUSH WA: Alcohol sensitivity in the albino animal, in Riley V (ed): *Pigment Cell.* Basal, S. Karger, 1976, vol 3, pp 211–219

466. RANDALL CL, LESTER D: Differential effects of ethanol and pentobarbital on sleep time in C57BL and BALB mice. *J Pharmacol Exp Therap* 188:27, 1974

467. WESTENBERG IS, PAKALNIS R: Response to pentobarbital of pigmented vs. albino C57BL/6J-c^{2J} mice: A within strain comparison of sleeptimes and lethal doses. *Behav Neural Biol* 27:552, 1979

468. SHEARER D, CREEL D, WILSON CE: Strain differences in the response of rats to repeated injections of pentobarbital sodium. *Lab Anim Sci* 23:662, 1973

469. THIESSEN DD, OWEN K, WHITSETT M: Chromosome mapping of behavioral activities, in Lindsey G, Thiessen DD (eds): *Contributions to Behavior. Genetic Analyses: The Mouse as a Prototype.* New York, Appleton-Century-Crofts, 1970, pp 161–204

470. LINDQUIST NG: Accumulation of drugs on melanin. *Acta Radiol* 325 (suppl): 5, 1973

471. BARZA M, KANE A, BAUM J: Marked differences between pigmented and albino rabbits in the concentration of Clindamycin in iris and choroid-retina. *J Infect Dis* 139:203, 1979

472. KINEBUCHI S, HORI Y, TODA K, FITZPATRICK TB, KOBORI T: Unpublished data

473. DOBZHANSKY T: *Genetics of the Evolutionary Process.* New York and London, Columbia University Press, 1970

474. FREIERE-MAIA N, et al: Medical and genetic studies of the population of Lençois Island, Maranhão. *Twenty-fourth Annual Meeting, Brazilian Society of Advances in Science and Culture* 180 (suppl): 24, 1972

475. BRUMBAUGH JA: Differentiation of black-red melanin in the fowl: Interaction of pattern genes and feather follicle milieu. *J Exp Zool* 166:11, 1967

476. BRUMBAUGH JA: The ultrastructural effects of the *I* and *S* loci upon black-red melanin differentiation in the fowl. *Dev Biol* 24:392, 1971

477. PROTA G, SEARLE AG: Biochemical sites of gene action for melanogenesis in mammals. *Ann Genet Selection Anamale* 10:1, 1978

478. MASON HS: Comparative biochemistry of the phenolase complex. *Adv Enzymol* 16:105, 1955

479. COHEN I: Platelet structure and function. Role of prostaglandins. *Ann Clin Lab Sci* 19:187, 1980

16

HISTIDINEMIA

This summary is adapted from the summary written by Bert N. La Du for the fourth edition of this book [1].

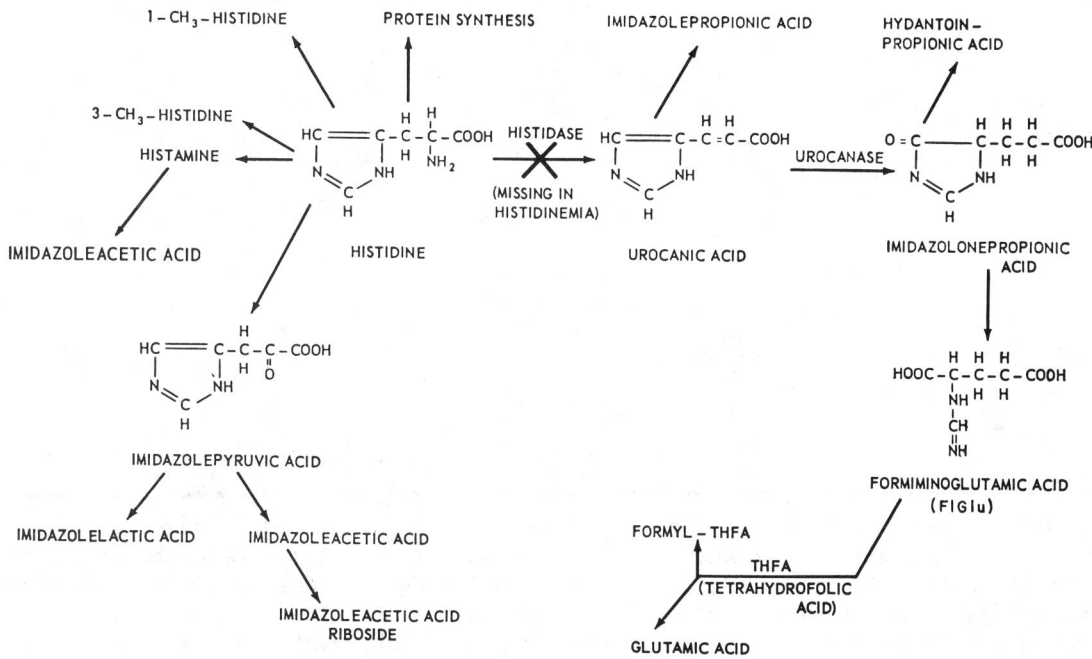

Pathways of histidine metabolism, illustrating the site of the enzymatic defect in histidinemia.

1. Histidinemia *is a rare disorder of histidine metabolism characterized by an elevation of the histidine concentration of the blood and an excessive excretion of histidine, imidazole pyruvic acid, and other imidazole metabolites in the urine.*

2. *Over half of the histidinemic subjects who have been described are mentally retarded, and more than half have a characteristic speech defect.*

3. *The biochemical disturbance in histidinemia results from the lack of the enzyme histidase (also called* histidine α-deaminase*), which converts histidine to urocanic acid. Direct demonstration of this enzymatic deficiency has been made in skin and liver biopsies from affected children.*

4. *In most cases, histidinemia is inherited as an autosomal recessive trait. One kindred may be an example of histidinemia inherited as an autosomal dominant trait.*

REFERENCES

1. La Du BN: Histidinemia, in Stanbury JB, Wyngaarden JB, Fredrickson DS (eds): *The Metabolic Basis of Inherited Disease,* ed 4. New York, McGraw-Hill Book Co, 1978, p 317
2. Kuroda Y, Osawa T, Ito M, Watanabe T, Takeda E, Toshima K, Miyao M: Relationship between skin histidase activity and blood histidine response to histidine intake in patients with histidinemia. *J Pediatr* 97:269, 1980

17

5-OXOPROLINURIA (PYROGLUTAMIC ACIDURIA) AND OTHER DISORDERS OF THE γ-GLUTAMYL CYCLE

1. 5-Oxoprolinuria, an inborn error of glutathione metabolism, is characterized by massive urinary excretion of 5-oxoproline, elevated levels of 5-oxoproline in the blood and cerebrospinal fluid, severe metabolic acidosis, tendency toward hemolysis, and defective central nervous system function. The enzymatic defect is at the glutathione synthetase step of the γ-glutamyl cycle; the generalized deficiency of glutathione synthetase leads to glutathione deficiency. Glutathione normally regulates its own biosynthesis by inhibiting γ-glutamylcysteine synthetase, the enzyme that catalyzes the first step in the synthesis of glutathione. Therefore, when there is marked reduction of glutathione levels, there is increased formation of γ-glutamylcysteine, which is converted to 5-oxoproline by the action of γ-glutamyl cyclotransferase (Figure 17-1). The overproduction of 5-oxoproline exceeds the capacity of 5-oxoprolinase to convert this substrate to glutamate, and some of the 5-oxoproline is therefore excreted in the urine. The metabolic defect leads to a modified γ-glutamyl cycle in which there is a futile synthesis of γ-glutamylcysteine followed by its conversion to 5-oxoproline and cysteine.

2. Glutathione synthetase deficiency, apparently restricted to the erythrocyte, is associated with reduced erythrocyte glutathione levels and well-compensated-for hemolytic disease. 5-Oxoprolinuria does not occur. This inborn error is associated with synthesis of an unstable glutathione synthetase molecule. The turnover of such a defective but active enzyme is apparently sufficiently rapid in most tissues to compensate for the defect, but this is not the case in the erythrocyte, in which protein synthesis does not take place.

3. In the inborn error associated with γ-glutamylcysteine synthetase deficiency, the patients exhibit hemolytic anemia, spinocerebellar degeneration, peripheral neuropathy, myopathy, and aminoaciduria. The patients have generalized glutathione deficiency and marked deficiency in the synthesis of γ-glutamyl compounds.

4. Patients with inborn deficiency of γ-glutamyl transpeptidase exhibit central nervous system involvement, glutathionemia, and urinary excretion of substantial amounts of glutathione, γ-glutamylcysteine, and cysteine moieties.

5. Individuals with an inborn deficiency of 5-oxoprolinase excrete moderate amounts of 5-oxoproline in their urine and have higher than normal blood plasma levels of 5-oxoproline. The patients thus far studied do not have acidosis or other symptoms clearly related to the biochemical defect.

Glutathione is a tripeptide (L-γ-glutamyl-L-cysteinylglycine) which is present in many mammalian tissues in relatively high concentrations. It is found intracellularly in millimolar concentrations; blood plasma and urine contain much lower levels.

348

The intracellular concentration of glutathione is far greater than that of cysteine and cystine; glutathione therefore seems to serve as a storage form of these sulfur-containing amino acids.

The glutathione molecule has two characteristic structural features: a γ-glutamyl linkage and a sulfhydryl group. These moieties of the tripeptide facilitate its participation in an impressive number and variety of functions. Glutathione is a participant in transhydrogenation reactions that function in the formation and maintenance of the sulfhydryl groups of other molecules (e.g., coenzyme A, various enzymes, and other proteins). It also provides a reducing capacity for other reactions, e.g., the formation of deoxyribonucleotides by ribonucleotide reductase. In addition, glutathione functions in the detoxication of hydrogen peroxide, other peroxides, and free radicals. Glutathione also functions in the detoxication of a variety of foreign compounds which interact with glutathione, and which are ultimately excreted in the urine or feces in the form of mercapturic acids. Similar derivatives of glutathione are formed in endogenous metabolism, e.g., in the metabolism of steroids, prostaglandins, leukotrienes, and melanins. There is also evidence that the γ-glutamyl moiety of glutathione plays a role in the transport of amino acids and possibly also of peptides and amines.

The synthesis and degradation of glutathione to its constituent amino acids take place by the reactions of the γ-glutamyl cycle (Fig. 17-2). Since this cycle leads to the synthesis of glutathione, its operation is closely connected with the several metabolic and physiologic functions that are performed by this ubiquitous tripeptide. Glutathione undoubtedly has important functions in the central nervous system, and it is notable that many of the patients with defects of the γ-glutamyl cycle are mentally retarded and exhibit other brain defects. The functions and metabolism of glutathione have been reviewed [1–5].

The intracellular synthesis of glutathione from its constituent amino acids, which occurs in virtually all mammalian tissues, takes place by reactions 1 and 2 [6].

$$\begin{array}{c}\text{L-Glutamate + L-cysteine + ATP} \\ \xrightarrow[\text{synthetase}]{\text{γ-glutamylcysteine}} \text{L-γ-glutamyl-L-cysteine + ADP + P}_i \end{array} \quad (1)$$

$$\begin{array}{c}\text{L-γ-Glutamyl-L-cysteine + glycine + ATP} \\ \xrightarrow[\text{synthetase}]{\text{glutathione}} \text{glutathione + ADP + P}_i \end{array} \quad (2)$$

Patients who exhibit a deficiency of the synthesis of glutathione are of three general types [7]:

1. Those with glutathione synthetase deficiency in whom the defect seems to be restricted to the erythrocytes.

2. Those in whom glutathione synthetase deficiency is generalized. Because patients of this type have greatly increased urinary excretion of 5-oxo-L-proline (synonyms: L-pyroglutamate, L-2-pyrrolidone-5-carboxylate), this condition has been called *5-oxoprolinuria* (or *pyroglutamic aciduria*). This disease is interesting because the enzymatic block greatly reduces synthesis of glutathione, which normally inhibits γ-glutamylcysteine synthetase by feedback control. The block thus increases the activity of the latter enzyme, and it is this effect which leads to the massive excretion of 5-oxoproline (Fig. 17-1).

3. Those with γ-glutamylcysteine synthetase deficiency, apparently generalized; two such patients have been described.

Although the three groups of patients listed above are defi-

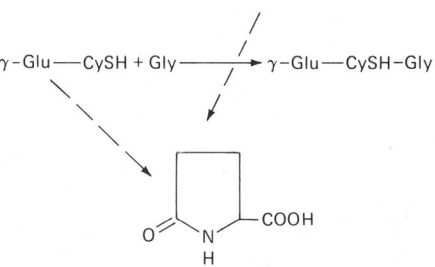

Figure 17-1 In 5-oxoprolinuria, glutathione synthetase is blocked. The consequent deficiency of glutathione (a feedback inhibitor of γ-glutamylcysteine synthetase) leads to excessive production of γ-glu-cySH, the γ-glu moiety of which is converted to 5-oxoproline.

cient in either of the enzymes required for glutathione synthesis and exhibit markedly reduced levels of erythrocyte glutathione, they differ substantially with respect to other biochemical findings and in their clinical manifestations. These patients must be distinguished from those who have enzymatic defects such as glucose-6-phosphate dehydrogenase deficiency, in whom glutathione can be synthesized from its constituent amino acids normally, but in whom there is a deficiency in maintaining glutathione in a reduced form (see Chap. 74) [8].

The initial step in the degradation of glutathione is catalyzed by γ-glutamyl transpeptidase, which catalyzes transfer of the γ-glutamyl moiety of glutathione to an amino acid or a peptide acceptor (which may be glutathione itself); cystine is among the best acceptors of the γ-glutamyl moiety (reaction 3).

$$\begin{array}{c}\text{Glutathione + L-cystine}\rightleftarrows\text{L-γ-glutamyl-L-cystine +} \\ \text{L-cysteinylglycine}\end{array} \quad (3)$$

Another reaction involved in the metabolism of glutathione by the γ-glutamyl cycle is catalyzed by 5-oxo-L-prolinase (reaction 4).

$$\text{5-oxo-L-proline + ATP + 2 H}_2\text{0} \rightarrow\text{L-glutamate + ADP + P}_i \quad (4)$$

Individuals with deficiencies of the enzyme activities that catalyze reactions 3 and 4 have been reported (see below).

THE γ-GLUTAMYL CYCLE

The synthesis of glutathione and its utilization are linked by a series of six enzyme-catalyzed reactions which have been termed the *γ-glutamyl cycle* (Fig. 17-2) [4, 5, 9]. The action of the membrane-bound enzyme γ-glutamyl transpeptidase, which catalyzes reaction 3, leads to formation of cysteinylglycine, which is cleaved to cysteine and glycine by dipeptidase. γ-Glutamyl amino acids are converted to the corresponding free amino acids and 5-oxoproline by the action of γ-glutamyl cyclotransferase. 5-Oxoproline is decyclized to yield glutamate (reaction 4). The equilibrium between 5-oxoproline and glutamate at pH values near neutrality markedly favors cyclization [10–12], and thus energy is required for decyclization. The mechanism of the coupling between ATP cleavage and that of the internal peptide bond of 5-oxoproline, which may involve an enzyme-bound phosphorylated derivative of 5-oxoproline [2, 13], requires further study.

γ-Glutamyl transpeptidase, the only membrane-bound enzyme of the cycle, is concentrated in the epithelia of tissues that are extensively involved in transport, e.g., the nephron,

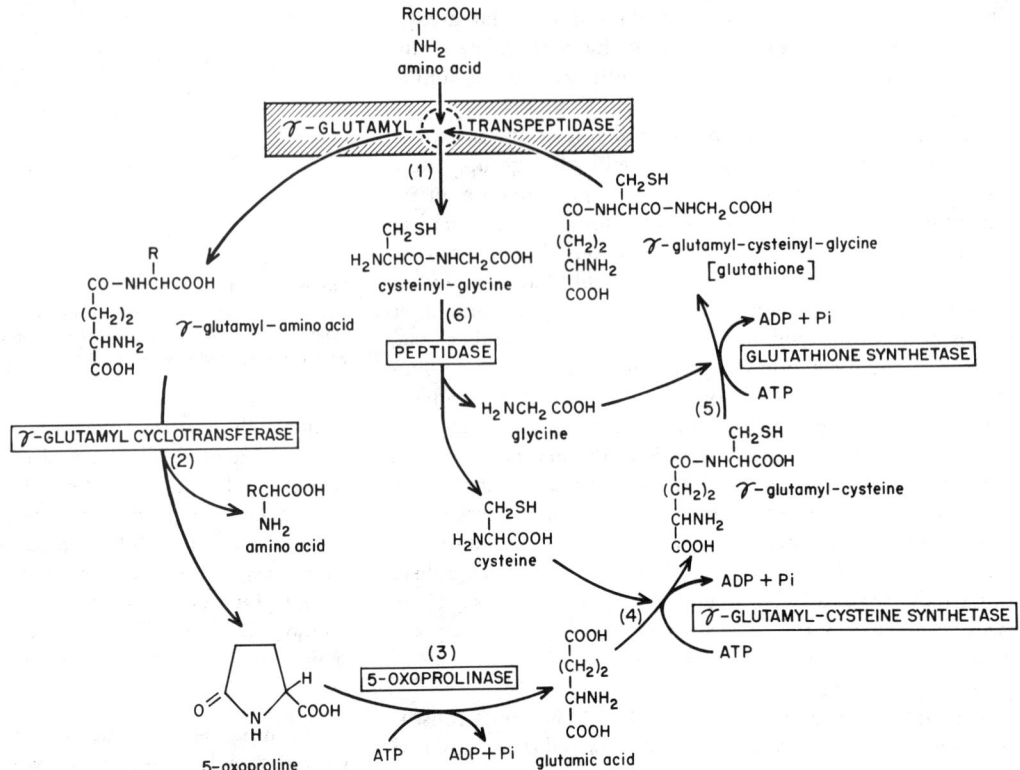

Figure 17-2. The γ-glutamyl cycle.

choroid plexus, jejunum, and ciliary body [14]. Although γ-glutamyl transpeptidase can catalyze hydrolysis of glutathione and other γ-glutamyl compounds in vitro, there is substantial evidence that transpeptidation is a major function of the enzyme in vivo [15]. The most active amino acid acceptors include cystine [16], glutamine, methionine, and other neutral amino acids [17]. Transpeptidase is localized on the cell membrane surface, and glutathione is found predominantly intracellularly. The finding of an enzyme on one side of a membrane and of its substrate on the other led to the postulate that there must be a mechanism for transporting intracellular glutathione to the membrane-bound enzyme [18]. When transpeptidase is inhibited in vivo by injecting animals with inhibitors of this enzyme, there is extensive glutathionuria [19]. These and other studies [4, 5] show that transported renal glutathione is a substrate of the transpeptidase. Such transport of glutathione undoubtedly occurs at the other anatomic sites at which transpeptidase is localized. Thus, transport of glutathione is a discrete step in the γ-glutamyl cycle. Transport of glutathione out of cells has been observed in liver perfusion studies [20] and in cells grown in tissue culture [21, 22], and it now appears that such transport of glutathione is a general phenomenon. In the kidney and at other sites at which transpeptidase is concentrated, intracellular glutathione is transported to the membrane-bound enzyme and the products of enzyme action are taken up by the cell. Tissues that have low transpeptidase activity, such as liver and muscle, transport glutathione to the blood plasma. Administration of an inhibitor of glutathione synthesis such as buthionine sulfoximine [23] leads to a prompt decrease in the tissue levels of glutathione and thus to decreased plasma glutathione levels. On the other hand, when an inhibitor of transpeptidase is given, plasma glutathione levels increase. Plasma glutathione levels are in the micromolar range (rat: approx. 25 μM; human: 1 to 3 μM) [24].

Glutathione is removed from plasma by the action of trans-peptidase, much of which is located in the kidney. Kidney uses glutathione that is transported from renal cells (intraorgan-cycle) as well as glutathione present in the plasma. Experiments on anephric animals treated with transpeptidase inhibitors show that about two-thirds of the plasma glutathione is used by the kidney and the remainder by extrarenal transpeptidase [25]. Further evidence for interorgan translocation of glutathione is that hepatic vein plasma has a much higher glutathione level than does arterial plasma [26]. Since about 80 percent of arterial plasma glutathione is removed during passage through the kidney, there is a mechanism apart from glomerular filtration for removing glutathione [26, 27]. The nonfiltration mechanism seems to involve the activity of transpeptidase not located in the renal tubule [26]. Extracellular oxidation of glutathione to glutathione disulfide is mainly a nonenzymatic process [28].

Direct evidence for transport of γ-glutamyl amino acids has been obtained [29]. Kidney and probably other cells have a transport mechanism for γ-glutamyl amino acids which is separate from those that transport free amino acids. The membrane transport of γ-glutamyl amino acids may be analogous to the transport of certain other dipeptides [30].

Modifications of the general scheme given in Fig. 17-2 have been considered [4, 5, 9]. Thus, it is possible that some of the γ-glutamyl amino acids formed are hydrolyzed to glutamate and amino acids. Successive transpeptidation reactions may also take place; γ-glutamyl amino acids can serve as acceptors of the γ-glutamyl group, leading to formation of di-γ-glutamyl amino acids. It is notable that γ-glutamyl cyclotransferase is most active toward the L-γ-glutamyl derivatives of the L isomers of several amino acids, e.g., glutamine, methionine, alanine, cysteine, cystine, and serine. This enzyme is also highly active toward a wide variety of di-γ-glutamyl amino acids, which may be formed by the action of transpeptidase [31].

Studies on the 5-oxoprolinase activities of tissue extracts

indicate that this enzyme has a lower activity than the activities found in vitro for the other enzymes of the cycle [32]. The activities observed in vitro for glutathione synthetase, γ-glutamylcysteine synthetase, and γ-glutamyl transpeptidase seem to be greater than those which probably occur in vivo. Caution must be exercised in basing conclusions about phenomena in vivo on the values of enzymatic activities determined under optimal conditions in vitro. Nevertheless, the reaction catalyzed by 5-oxoprolinase appears to be the slowest step in the γ-glutamyl cycle and may therefore be rate-limiting, but there seems to be sufficient 5-oxoprolinase to maintain the 5-oxoproline concentration of various mammalian tissues at their relatively low steady-state levels (20 to 50 μM) [32, 33, 34]. Even a complete block of 5-oxoprolinase activity would not stop the function of the cycle since glutamate can be produced by other pathways, such as hydrolysis of glutamine and transamination or reductive amination of α-ketoglutarate.

γ-Glutamylcysteine synthetase is nonallosterically inhibited by glutathione [35]. Studies on rat kidney γ-glutamylcysteine synthetase show that glutathione is a competitive inhibitor with respect to glutamate; the apparent K_i value for glutathione (2.3 mM) is about equivalent to the concentration of glutathione in rat kidney. γ-Glutamyl-α-aminobutyrate and γ-glutamyl-α-aminobutyrylglycine inhibit the enzyme much less than do the corresponding sulfhydryl compounds. This suggests that glutathione also binds to another site on the enzyme and that its sulfhydryl group is involved in such binding; glutathione may bind to both the glutamate and cysteine binding sites of the enzyme. The data on kidney γ-glutamylcysteine synthetase activity thus show that this enzyme is inhibited by glutathione under conditions similar to those that prevail in vivo; a physiologically significant feedback control mechanism is therefore indicated. It is likely that this is a general mechanism, since inhibition by glutathione of γ-glutamylcysteine synthetase from erythrocytes [36, 37] and liver [38] has been noted. The biosynthesis of glutathione is undoubtedly affected by other metabolic phenomena, especially by variations of the intracellular concentration of cysteine. The apparent K_m value for L-cysteine for γ-glutamylcysteine synthetase (0.35 mM) is not far from the range of the usual intracellular concentrations of cysteine.

Blocks of the γ-glutamyl cycle have been achieved in experimental animals by the use of specific enzyme inhibitors [4, 5, 9]. For example, administration of a competitive inhibitor of 5-oxoprolinase to mice leads to an appreciable increase in the tissue concentrations of 5-oxoproline and to urinary excretion of this compound. When an L-amino acid was given together with the inhibitor, there was a substantial increase of 5-oxoproline accumulation and excretion [33]. Administration of amino acids increases transpeptidation and thus the amount of 5-oxoproline formed by γ-glutamyl cyclotransferase. Similar results obtained in studies in which animals were also given inhibitors of γ-glutamyl cysteine synthetase, indicating that the formation of 5-oxoproline by the combined activities of γ-glutamylcysteine synthetase and γ-glutamyl cyclotransferase is not normally a major pathway for 5-oxoproline formation, but such a pathway occurs in 5-oxoprolinuria, as discussed below.

Although administration of small amounts of amino acids does not depress glutathione levels [39] because of rapid resynthesis of glutathione, administration of larger amounts of amino acids leads to a decrease of renal glutathione levels [40]. This decrease does not occur after administration of inhibitors of γ-glutamyl transpeptidase. When a competitive inhibitor of

γ-glutamyl cyclotransferase is given to animals, there is a marked decrease in the 5-oxoproline level of the kidney, and studies with a model substrate showed that this is due to in vivo inhibition of cyclotransferase [41]. γ-Glutamylcysteine synthetase may be inhibited in vivo by giving the specific inhibitor buthionine sulfoximine [23]. Methionine sulfoximine also inhibits this enzyme [39] as well as glutamine synthetase [42]. However, buthionine sulfoximine inhibits only the synthesis of glutathione. α-Ethylmethionine sulfoximine specifically inhibits glutamine synthetase and has no effect on γ-glutamylcysteine synthetase [43]. Experimental animals treated with inhibitors of γ-glutamyl transpeptidase exhibit biochemical phenomena which have also been observed in a patient with γ-glutamyl transpeptidase deficiency. The effects of inhibition of γ-glutamyl transpeptidase in vivo and of deficiency of this enzyme are considered below.

Inhibition of the cycle in vivo has been observed after administration of inhibitors of γ-glutamyl transpeptidase, γ-glutamylcysteine synthetase, 5-oxoprolinase, and γ-glutamyl cyclotransferase. Specific deficiencies of γ-glutamyl transpeptidase, γ-glutamylcysteine synthetase, glutathione synthetase, and 5-oxoprolinase have been observed in the diseases discussed below. Defects in amino acid transport have been thus far observed in γ-glutamylcysteine synthetase deficiency and in γ-glutamyl transpeptidase deficiency. That dramatic amino acid transport defects have not always been observed in such enzyme deficiencies or after inhibition of the enzymes is not surprising since the blocks thus far observed or achieved are far from complete. In addition, it is well established that there are multiple amino acid transport systems that overlap in specificity.

5-OXOPROLINURIA (PYROGLUTAMIC ACIDURIA)

Patient 1: The first patient with *5-oxoprolinuria* was reported in 1970 by Jellum et al. [44], who described a 19-year-old boy of normal height and weight who had been mentally retarded since childhood. Physical examination revealed signs of organic cerebral damage with spastic quadraparesis and cerebellar disturbances. Findings included increased resistance to passive movement, predominantly of the pyramidal type, retarded voluntary movements, pronounced tremor, and impaired coordination. Speech was simple, childlike, and dysarthric. The IQ (Wechsler) was estimated to be about 60. At age 17, the patient was treated surgically for a diaphragmatic hernia [45]. Postoperatively, he developed life-threatening acidosis, which was successfully treated with daily infusions containing potassium and bicarbonate ions. Later he was maintained on oral sodium bicarbonate. The patient excreted between 24 and 34.5 g (0.19 to 0.27 mol) of 5-oxoproline per day in his urine. The excretion of urea was 11.8 g/day, a value considered to be 35 to 45 percent of that expected normally. Urinary 5-oxoproline was identified by thin-layer chromatography, gas-liquid chromatography, and mass spectrometry. The serum contained 5-oxoproline and another glutamic acid derivative which was not identified.

Jellum et al. [44] tentatively concluded that the patient had a defect in one of the steps in the urea cycle. Administration of ammonium bicarbonate, sodium glutamate, or glutamine did not influence urinary excretion of 5-oxoproline [46]. An apparent correlation existed between the excretion of urinary ammonia and 5-oxoproline; the molar excretion of ammonium was about half that of 5-oxoproline even when the urinary pH was brought to the alkaline range by oral administration of sodium bicarbonate. Evidence was obtained that the patient converted ammonia to urea in a normal manner; thus he responded normally to a high calorie, low protein diet, with a sharp decrease in urea excretion, and when given a large dose of glutamine orally, he excreted extra nitrogen in the form of urea. When the patient was given an intravenous infusion containing a mixture of 19 amino acids, the blood concentrations of the amino acids increased substantially, about as expected, and the excretion of 5-oxoproline in the urine increased about twofold. Both the patient and a normal control subject were given an intravenous injection of a tracer dose of uniformly labeled 5-oxo-L-[^{14}C]proline, and the excretion of radioactive respiratory carbon dioxide was determined. The control subject excreted 17 percent of the injected radioactivity in 2.5 h; a total of only 1.7 percent of the administered radioactivity was excreted in 3 h by the patient. These and other observations made by Eldjarn et al. [46] led them to conclude that the patient had a block at the 5-oxoprolinase step of the γ-glutamyl cycle. This interpretation, which rested heavily on the studies with radioactive 5-oxoproline, had to be abandoned later when it was discovered that the blood plasma level of 5-oxoproline in the patient was 50 mg/dl (3.9 mM) [47], rather than one-tenth this value, as initially reported [44, 46, 48]. Thus, the markedly reduced excretion of ^{14}CO$_2$ by the patient after administration of a tracer dose of labeled 5-oxoproline could be explained by the very great dilution of the injected material.

The concentration of 5-oxoproline in the cerebrospinal fluid was reported to be 30 mg/dl (2.3 mM). The patient did not have aminoaciduria. The blood serum concentration of proline was reported to be 6.4 mg/dl a value considered to be about three times higher than normal. The serum concentrations of the other amino acids were normal. In a study in which the patient was given [^{14}C]pyruvate or [^{14}C]glutamate, a compound was found on thin-layer chromatography of the urine which became labeled prior to labeling of urinary 5-oxoproline; this compound yielded labeled glutamate on acid hydrolysis. The possible structure of this compound is discussed below.

Patient 2: Hagenfeldt et al. [49] described a female infant with 5-oxoprolinuria who developed severe metabolic acidosis on the third day of life. This acidosis was corrected by intravenous administration of sodium bicarbonate; discontinuation of treatment led to return of acidosis. Subsequently, the patient has been treated continuously with sodium bicarbonate. Examination at 11 and 14 months of age revealed no neurologic or other abnormalities; psychomotor development was normal. The patient was found to excrete between 48 and 54 mmol of 5-oxoproline per day, and this was shown to be of the L configuration by assays done with L-glutamate dehydrogenase after conversion of 5-oxoproline to glutamate by acid hydrolysis. The blood plasma concentration of 5-oxoproline was 58 mg/dl (4.5 mM). Aminoaciduria was not found, nor were any unusual peptides detected in the urine. The blood amino acid levels were normal. The formation of urinary urea increased as the protein content of the diet was increased, whereas the excretion of pyroglutamate seemed to decrease somewhat. The excretion of ammonia varied between 40 and 50 percent of the 5-oxoproline excretion (on a molar basis).

The turnover of 5-oxoproline was examined in studies in which an intravenous injection of radioactive 5-oxoproline was given. This revealed a daily synthesis of about 210 mmol of 5-oxoproline, of which about 50 mmol was excreted in the urine, indicating an endogenous utilization of 5-oxoproline of about 75 percent. The 5-oxoprolinase activity of the peripheral leukocytes was within the normal range. The patient became anemic during the neonatal period. Thus, on the third day of life, the hemoglobin concentration was 15 g/dl blood; the hemoglobin level decreased continuously to 7 to 8 g/dl at 3 weeks of age. The anemia disappeared spontaneously after 2 months, although some reticulocytosis was observed. At age 2 years and 10 months, there was a mild macrocytic anemia with a hemoglobin concentration of 8.5 to 11.5 g/dl. At this age development was normal, there were no neurologic symptoms, and the electroencephalogram and motor nerve conduction velocity were normal.

The Enzymatic Defect in 5-Oxoprolinuria

The enzyme defect in this inborn error of metabolism was identified by determinations of the enzyme activity carried out on the cultured skin fibroblasts of patient 2, erythrocytes from patient 2 and from the younger sister of this patient (patient 3), and the placenta obtained at the delivery of patient 3 [50]. This third patient [51] with 5-oxoprolinuria exhibited clinical and laboratory findings that were similar to those found with patient 2. The acid-base balance of the third patient was normal for 4 h after birth, but she then developed metabolic acidosis, and by 20 h of age, the blood pH had decreased to 7.3. She has been maintained on regular oral doses of sodium bicarbonate. A urine sample collected during the first hours of life prior to feeding contained 26 mM 5-oxo-L-proline. Jaundice, which developed at 50 h of age, disappeared in the course of the first week of life. Both this patient and her older sister had an increased rate of hemolysis.

Studies on several enzyme activities of the placenta and cultured skin fibroblasts of patients with 5-oxoprolinuria and controls are summarized in Table 17-1. The placenta of patient 3 showed activity of both γ-glutamylcysteine synthetase and γ-glutamyl cyclotransferase similar to control levels. However, the glutathione synthetase activity of the placenta was only about 2 percent of normal. Extracts of the cultured fibroblasts from patient 2 contained activities of γ-glutamylcysteine synthetase, γ-glutamyl cyclotransferase, and 5-oxoprolinase that

Table 17-1 Enzyme activities of placenta and cultured fibroblasts of patients with 5-oxoprolinuria*

Enzyme activity	Placenta		Fibroblasts	
	Patient	Control	Patient	Controls
γ-Glutamylcysteine synthetase	79	63	83	47
Glutathione synthetase	1.7	77	<2.0	46,72
γ-Glutamyl cyclotransferase	198	163	83	40
5-Oxoprolinase	. . .	. . .	6.1	3.5

* The activities are expressed as nanomoles per hour per milligram of protein.
SOURCE: Wellner et al. [50].

were somewhat greater than the corresponding activities found in fibroblasts obtained from a 1.5-year-old control subject. By contrast, the glutathione synthetase activity of the patient's fibroblasts was less than 5 percent of the control's. Studies on the erythrocytes of patients 2 and 3, their parents, and controls are summarized in Table 17-2. Erythrocytes from the patients and their parents had γ-glutamylcysteine synthetase and γ-glutamyl cyclotransferase activities similar to those in control samples. However, a marked deficiency of glutathione synthetase was found in erythrocytes from the patients: The values were about 5 to 10 percent of those in control samples. The erythrocyte glutathione synthetase of the father was appreciably less, and the value for the mother's erythrocytes was somewhat lower than that of controls. Determinations of glutathione synthetase activity of mixtures of extracts obtained from patients and the control subjects gave strictly additive results. The erythrocytes from patients 2 and 3 were found to have very low concentrations of glutathione. Similarly, the placenta (patient 3) contained 0.16 mM glutathione (control: 0.56 mM).

The enzyme studies indicate a marked deficiency of glutathione synthetase activity in several types of tissue obtained from two patients with 5-oxoprolinuria. The deficiency was found in erythrocytes, placenta, and cultured skin fibroblasts and suggested a generalized glutathione synthetase deficiency and thus a generalized deficiency of glutathione. It is notable that the erythrocytes of the father and possibly also of the mother of the patients exhibited glutathione synthetase activity intermediate between that of the patients and of the control subjects. This finding indicates that the condition, which is apparently autosomal recessive, may be detected in heterozygotes (see also Ref. 52).

Patients 2 and 3 were anemic and had an increased tendency toward hemolysis early in life. This finding is consistent with the low erythrocyte glutathione concentrations observed. Patient 1 was jaundiced during the early neonatal period and was very ill for 2 weeks after birth [45]. When the data obtained from the studies in which this patient was given labeled 5-oxoproline are recalculated using the corrected value for the serum concentration of 5-oxoproline, the endogenous production of 5-oxoproline is approximately 60 to 80 g/day, or more than twice the amount excreted in the urine [53]. These considerations indicate that this patient, like patient 2, produced a substantial amount of 5-oxoproline which was metabolized. In addition, intact fibroblasts cultured from skin biopsy specimens obtained from this patient metabolized 5-oxoproline to carbon dioxide at a normal rate, and the 5-oxoprolinase activity levels of the fibroblasts were also within the normal range [54].

An understanding of the way in which a block of glutathione synthetase can produce 5-oxoprolinuria involves consideration of the γ-glutamyl cycle and certain properties of the enzymes involved. Glutathione is not a substrate of γ-glutamyl cyclotransferase, and therefore this tripeptide may accumulate in cells in substantial concentrations, as it does under normal conditions. In contrast, γ-glutamylcysteine is an excellent substrate of γ-glutamyl cyclotransferase as well as of γ-glutamyl transpeptidase and glutathione synthetase (Fig. 17-3). The normal tissue concentration of γ-glutamylcysteine is very low, perhaps less than 1 percent that of glutathione. It is possible that normally γ-glutamylcysteine is protected from the action of γ-glutamyl cyclotransferase, perhaps by close linkage between the two synthetases or by compartmentalization within the cell

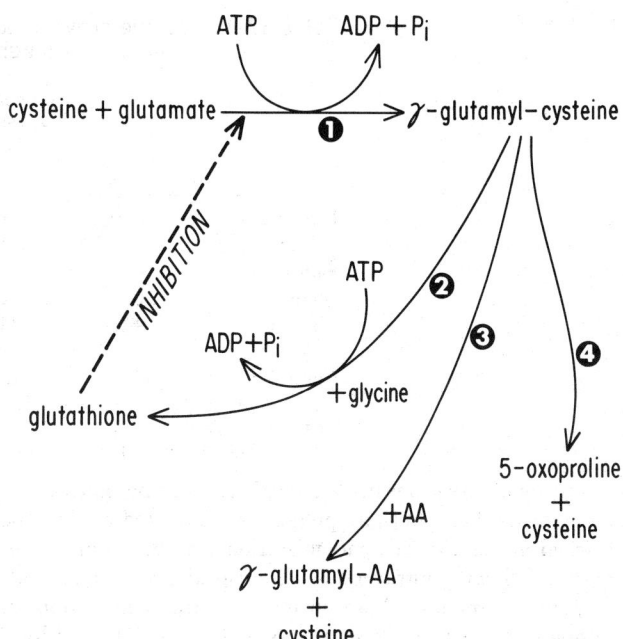

Figure 17-3 Metabolic interrelationships in glutathione biosynthesis. (1) γ-glutamylcysteine synthetase; (2) glutathione synthetase; (3) γ-glutamyl transpeptidase; (4) γ-glutamyl cyclotransferase. (*From Richman and Meister* [35], *with permission.*)

[9]. The affinity of glutathione synthetase for γ-glutamylcysteine may be greater than the affinities of the other enzymes that can act on this substrate. Since γ-glutamylcysteine is a good substrate for γ-glutamyl transpeptidase [17], this dipeptide might serve in place of glutathione as a γ-glutamyl donor in transpeptidation reactions with amino acids (reaction 3, Fig. 17-3). However, γ-glutamylcysteine which is not used for glutathione synthesis or for transpeptidation reactions would be converted to 5-oxoproline and cysteine (reaction 4, Fig. 17-3). A block in glutathione synthesis would lead to 5-oxoprolinuria if more than normal amounts of γ-glutamylcysteine were formed and converted to 5-oxoproline by the action of γ-glutamyl cyclotransferase, and if the overproduction of 5-oxoproline exceeded the capacity of 5-oxoprolinase to convert this substrate to glutamate [9]. This indeed seems to be the mechanism of 5-oxoprolinuria. It appears that γ-glutamylcysteine synthetase normally functions at substantially less than its maximal capacity because of feedback inhibition by glutathione. In the absence or marked reduction in the concentration of glutathione there is increased formation of γ-glutamylcysteine, which is efficiently converted to 5-oxoproline. This is an interesting example of a metabolic block that prevents the synthesis of a compound which functions normally as a feedback inhibitor. The compound that accumulates as a result of the block is derived from the immediate precursor of the feedback inhibitor. The metabolic defect in 5-oxoprolinuria therefore leads to a modified γ-glutamyl cycle (Fig. 17-4) in which γ-glutamylcysteine synthesis is followed by its conversion to 5-oxoproline and cysteine. In the modified cycle, γ-glutamylcysteine replaces glutathione as a γ-glutamyl donor for transpeptidation reactions, and cysteine is recycled. The modified γ-glutamyl cycle proposed for 5-oxoprolinuria is mediated by the actions of only four enzymes; neither cysteinylglycinase nor glutathione synthetase activity is required. It would be interesting to learn whether patients with 5-oxoprolinuria have secondary abnormalities involving glycine metabolism.

Table 17-2 Enzyme activities and glutathione content of erythrocytes from 5-oxoprolinuria patients, their parents, and controls

	Age, yr	Glutathione synthetase	γ-Glutamylcysteine synthetase	γ-Glutamyl cyclotransferase	Glutathione, mM*
			nmols/(h · mg hemoglobin)		
Patient 2	0.25	1.5	58	44	<0.01
Patient 3	3	1.3	59	44	<0.01
Father	30	8.6	50	40	
Mother	30	12	52	41	
Control ♀	4	24	61	39	
Control ♂	36	15	61	41	

* Normal range, 1 to 2 mM.
SOURCE: Wellner et al. [50].

Certain observations made on patient 1 may be explained in terms of the data and interpretations considered above. The marked increase in this patient's urinary excretion of 5-oxoproline following intravenous administration of amino acids may have represented an increase in transpeptidation in response to the increase in amino acid levels, followed by a corresponding increase in conversion of γ-glutamyl amino acids into 5-oxoproline, with "overflow" of the latter compound into the urine. This patient had low levels of glutathione; γ-glutamylcysteine could function as the γ-glutamyl donor for transpeptidation in this disorder. The glutamate-containing compound found in the blood and urine of patient 1 could have been γ-glutamylcysteine, but definite identification was not made.

The acidosis characteristic of 5-oxoprolinuria is readily explained by the marked accumulation of 5-oxoproline, which reaches levels as high as 3 to 6 mM in the plasma and cerebrospinal fluid. Presumably, high concentrations are also present in the tissues, including those of the central nervous system. It is possible, based on the findings on patient 1, that untreated 5-oxoprolinuria is associated with mental retardation and other central nervous system disturbances. This patient presumably had untreated chronic acidosis for about 17 years. Although it is possible that the brain defects were related largely to acidosis, the effects of acidosis as opposed to those of 5-oxoprolinemia and glutathione deficiency per se cannot be distinguished at this time. Further observations on patients 2 and 3, who have been treated with sodium bicarbonate since birth, will be interesting. These patients also show evidence of generalized glutathione deficiency, and it is notable that patients with generalized glutathione deficiency due to a block at the γ-glutamylcysteine synthetase step of the γ-glutamyl cycle (see below) have severe central nervous system disease.

The hemolytic anemia of 5-oxoprolinuric patients appears to be adequately explained by the markedly decreased concentrations of erythrocyte glutathione. Even so, hemolytic disease is not one of their major clinical problems.

Other Aspects and Possible Therapies for 5-Oxoprolinuria

Some additional and interesting observations were made on patient 1 when he was 24 years old [55]. His condition had gradually deteriorated neurologically, and he began to have frequent seizures. He continued to be treated with sodium bicarbonate and was also given potassium salts, chlorpromazine, and clonazepam. The glutathione synthetase activity of his erythrocytes was found to be less than 2 percent of that of controls. Most remarkably, it was found [55] that his erythrocytes were loaded with free amino acids in concentrations that were 5 to 100 times the normal levels. Thus, marked elevations in the concentrations of threonine, serine, asparagine, glutamate, proline, glycine, alanine, valine, methionine, isoleucine, leucine, tyrosine, phenylalanine, tryptophan, ornithine, lysine, histidine, and arginine were found in three different specimens of the patient's blood. The erythrocytes contained no detectable glutathione at the time of analysis. On at least two occasions, a substantial amount of methionine sulfoxide was found in the erythrocytes. Deproteinized extracts of the patient's erythrocytes were hydrolyzed in 6M hydrochloric acid *in vacuo* for 16 h at 105° C. Analyses of the hydrolysates revealed increases in a number of amino acids that could not be accounted for by hydrolysis of glutathione, 5-oxoproline, glutamine, and asparagine. No such amino acid accumulation occurred in the patient's skeletal muscle, in which the glutathione level was found to be about 3 percent of normal. A repetition of this study carried out about 1 year after the initial observations showed erythrocyte glutathione levels 5 to 10 percent of normal. At this time much lower levels of amino acids were found, although several continued to be present in elevated concentrations [56]. Similar studies were later carried out on patients 2 and 3 [57] and on another patient with 5-oxoprolinuria [58]. The erythrocytes of these patients contained glutathione levels that were 2 to 17 percent of normal. There were only minor changes in the amino acid levels.

Figure 17-4 Modified γ-glutamyl cycle in 5-oxoprolinuria. (*From Wellner et al.* [50] *with permission.*)

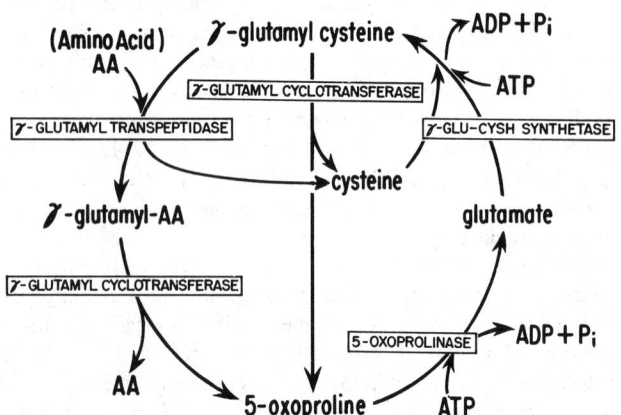

There is as yet no satisfactory explanation for the marked concentration of amino acids in the erythrocytes found at one time during the life of patient 1. A number of possible explanations have been put forth [55–57, 59], but none of these seems consistent with all of the currently available facts about glutathione metabolism and function. Although it has been suggested that there is a relationship between the level of erythrocyte glutathione and the remarkable incorporation of free amino acids (and apparently also of peptides) into erythrocytes, this has not been conclusively demonstrated, and other explanations for the findings are conceivable. It would clearly be important to examine the levels of amino acids in the erythrocytes of 5-oxoprolinuric patients as a routine in order to acquire more information about this phenomenon. A number of experimental approaches to this problem seem feasible and should be explored.

Patient 1 died at the age of 28. Pathologic examination showed selective atrophy of the granule cell layer of the cerebellum and focal lesions in the frontoparietal cortex and bilaterally in the visual cortex and the thalamus. The type and distribution of the lesions resembled those seen after mercury intoxication, and it was therefore suggested that treatment with an antioxidant might be of value in 5-oxoprolinuria [60].

Additional patients with 5-oxoprolinuria were reported in the literature between 1977 and 1980 [58, 61–63]. All have markedly decreased erythrocyte glutathione synthetase activity and decreased erythrocyte glutathione levels. Most exhibit an increased rate of hemolysis and many, but not all, have central nervous system involvement. It is notable that two patients had mild 5-oxoprolinuria without clinical acidosis or neurologic disease [62]. Even in the small group of patients thus far studied, there is considerable variability in the chemical and clinical findings, reflecting substantial biochemical heterogeneity, as has been noted in a number of other inborn errors of metabolism.

5-Oxoprolinuria is more common than initially believed, and its prevalence may be greater than currently appreciated. The diagnosis should be considered in patients with unexplained metabolic acidosis. Detection of heterozygotes is possible by determining erythrocyte glutathione synthetase activity or by measuring erythrocyte glutathione levels [50].

There is currently no convenient screening method available for the detection of 5-oxoproline in urine. 5-oxoproline does not give a color reaction with ninhydrin. Normal human urine contains variable amounts of 5-oxo-D-proline [formed by enzymatic cyclization of D-glutamate, which probably arises from dietary or bacterial sources (11,12)], and this may complicate the interpretation of analyses of urine for 5-oxoproline. Increased excretion of 5-oxoproline has been reported in patients with burns and allergic conditions [64]. Normal human skin contains large amounts of 5-oxoproline [65, 66]. Somewhat elevated levels of 5-oxo-L-proline and 5-oxo-D-proline have been found in the plasma of patients with renal insufficiency [67].

The activity of thioredoxin and of its reductase were normal in extracts of skin fibroblasts obtained from patients with 5-oxoprolinuria. This suggests that the levels of glutathione and thioredoxin are regulated independently [68]. Similar results were obtained with fibroblasts obtained from a cystinotic patient. Treatment of fibroblasts from a patient with 5-oxoprolinuria with L-serine and borate [a combination known to inhibit γ-glutamyl transpeptidase (69, 70)] caused more than a twofold increase in the content of cellular glutathione [71]. [A similar result was observed in the kidneys of mice treated with serine and borate (40).] Such treatment decreased the formation of 5-oxoproline from glutamate in 5-oxoprolinuric fibroblasts [71]. These findings led to the suggestion that inhibition of γ-glutamyl transpeptidase may be a useful approach to alleviating the effects of glutathione synthetase deficiency. Other inhibitors such as L-(αS, 5S)-α-amino-3-chloro-4,5-dihydro-5-isoxazoleacetic acid (AT-125) might also be considered. Another potentially useful therapeutic approach for 5-oxoprolinuria and perhaps other diseases associated with deficiency of glutathione consists of the administration of high doses of vitamin E [72, 73]. Therapeutic doses of vitamin E were reported to increase erythrocyte survival, an effect presumably associated with the antioxidant effect of this vitamin (see also Ref. 60). Another therapy that might be considered is a drug that would partially inhibit γ-glutamylcysteine synthetase. Moderate doses of buthionine sulfoximine [23] might decrease overproduction of γ-glutamylcysteine (without stopping synthesis completely), and thus decrease 5-oxoproline formation and ameliorate acidosis [75].

GLUTATHIONE SYNTHETASE DEFICIENCY WITHOUT 5-OXOPROLINURIA

A large family with a number of members with reduced erythrocyte glutathione concentrations and well-compensated-for hemolytic disease was described [76, 77], and later, two unrelated patients with hemolytic anemia and decreased erythrocyte glutathione levels were reported [78]. A similar patient was found to have a marked deficiency of erythrocyte glutathione synthetase activity. The erythrocytes from the parents and children of these patients had glutathione synthetase activity levels that were about half of those of controls [79]. This latter patient, as well as his heterozygous relatives, had normal levels of erythrocyte γ-glutamylcysteine synthetase activity. There are no indications in these or later reports on such patients that any of these individuals appeared to be ill during the neonatal period. Later studies on several patients showed that they do not have 5-oxoprolinuria [80]. It therefore appears that glutathione synthetase deficiency in these patients [76–79] is restricted to the erythrocyte. This would account for the relatively mild nature of this form of glutathione synthetase deficiency as compared to 5-oxoprolinuria.

Evidently in the mild form of glutathione deficiency the genetic lesion leads to synthesis of an unstable glutathione synthetase molecule. The rate of replacement of such a defective, but active, enzyme would appear to be sufficiently rapid in most tissues to compensate for the defect. However, such a compensatory mechanism would not be possible in the erythrocyte, in which protein synthesis does not take place. This interpretation is supported by recent studies on erythrocytes, leukocytes, and skin fibroblasts obtained from patients with glutathione synthetase deficiency with and without 5-oxoprolinuria [81]. In the cells from a patient with 5-oxoprolinuria, glutathione synthetase activity was grossly deficient in erythrocytes and in nucleated cells. In the milder disease, the mutant enzyme was active but unstable in both erythrocytes and nucleated cells.

γ-GLUTAMYLCYSTEINE SYNTHETASE DEFICIENCY

A syndrome of hemolytic anemia, spinocerebellar degeneration, peripheral neuropathy, myopathy, and aminoaciduria associated with glutathione deficiency was described in two sibs [82, 83]. One patient, examined initially at age 27, had mild hemolytic anemia associated with erythrocyte glutathione deficiency. The only physical abnormalities were absent reflexes in the lower extremities. Two years later, she developed psychotic behavior and a decrease in blood hemoglobin after receiving a sulfonamide for a urinary tract infection. By age 35, she had developed mild ataxia with impaired coordination and dysmetria in the upper and lower extremities. Her brother, at age 29, had hemolytic anemia and erythrocyte glutathione deficiency. By age 36, he developed muscular weakness, ataxia, and decreased vibratory and position sensation in both the upper and lower extremities, with dysmetria and dysdiadochokinesis. Deep-tendon reflexes were absent or sluggish, and by age 37 he had developed irregular staccato speech and painful myoclonic spasms of his right calf and foot.

Both patients had erythrocyte glutathione levels that were less than 3 percent of normal. The glutathione content of the peripheral leukocytes was less than one-half normal, and the glutathione content in the muscle was about 25 percent of normal. There was a marked reduction of γ-glutamylcysteine synthetase activity of the erythrocytes [9, 83], and both patients had generalized aminoaciduria [9, 83].

These patients have generalized deficiency of glutathione due to decreased γ-glutamylcysteine synthetase activity. In contrast to the patients with 5-oxoprolinuria, the patients with γ-*glutamylcysteine synthetase deficiency* have a severely impaired ability to synthesize γ-glutamyl compounds. Thus, whereas a block of glutathione synthetase leads to a modified γ-glutamyl cycle in which transpeptidation is possible with γ-glutamylcysteine, a block of γ-glutamylcysteine synthetase would be expected to reduce markedly the activity of the γ-glutamyl cycle. The finding of aminoaciduria in these patients is therefore of interest.

γ-GLUTAMYL TRANSPEPTIDASE DEFICIENCY

Two patients with apparently generalized γ-*glutamyl transpeptidase deficiency* have been described [84, 85]. The first of these is a moderately retarded man first studied at the age of 33, who was found to excrete glutathione in his urine and to have glutathionemia [84]. Subsequent studies of this patient's cultured skin fibroblasts showed an extreme reduction in the activity of γ-glutamyl transpeptidase [86]. He excreted about 850 mg glutathione in his urine per day. The serum amino acid concentrations were reported to be normal except for a reduction in the sum of asparagine and glutamine and a roughly comparable increase in glutamic acid, which was thought to reflect hydrolysis of glutamine to glutamate during sample storage and preparation. (This conclusion may not be valid, since nonenzymatic destruction of glutamine at pH values near neutrality leads to formation of 5-oxoproline rather than glutamate.) Renal reabsorption was calculated to be normal for 14 amino acids but fell slightly below the normal range for serine, tyrosine, phenylalanine, and the sum of asparagine and glutamine [86]. The data are consistent with a deficiency of glutamine transport [4]. The percentage of excretion of glutamine (plus asparagine) was about fivefold higher than the corresponding values for four amino acids (serine, alanine, tyrosine, and methionine), which were slightly above normal. The uptake kinetics for cystine, glutamine, methionine, and alanine were determined in studies on the cultured fibroblasts from this patient. No significant differences were found in the kinetics of uptake for each of these as compared with the results obtained with fibroblasts from a normal individual. The levels of phenylalanine, cystine, and cysteine in the mutant cells were significantly increased [87].

The second patient with γ-glutamyl transpeptidase deficiency is a mentally retarded young woman with severe behavioral problems [85]. No γ-glutamyl transpeptidase activity was detected in the urine, plasma, or cultured skin fibroblasts, but a slight activity was reported for the leukocytes. There was substantial glutathionuria and an elevated plasma glutathione level.

The initial reports on the two patients with γ-glutamyl transpeptidase deficiency indicated that both had glutathionuria and glutathionemia. Amino acid analysis of their urine was stated not to show unusual features other than the presence of glutathione. However, the reported data on the second patient indicate some degree of cystinuria [85]. Additional studies [88] of the urine of the second patient disclosed a substantial amount of γ-glutamylcysteine as well as an unusually large amount of cysteine. Both compounds were in disulfide form. Amino acid analysis of the urine was carried out after treatment with dithiothreitol and 2-vinylpyridine. A similar approach had previously been used in animals treated with inhibitors of γ-glutamyl transpeptidase [19]. The urine of animals whose transpeptidase activity was markedly inhibited by administration of L-γ-glutamyl-(o-carboxy)phenylhydrazide or AT-125 contained high concentrations of glutathione (3 to 28 mM) and about half as much γ-glutamylcyst(e)ine and cyst(e)ine. The finding of markedly increased urinary excretion of glutathione, cysteine, and γ-glutamylcysteine moieties in γ-glutamyl transpeptidase deficiency in humans and animals suggests that the physiologic function of γ-glutamyl transpeptidase is associated with the metabolism or transport (or both) of these sulfur-containing compounds. At least three pathways could account for the appearance of urinary γ-glutamylcysteine. (1) γ-Glutamylcysteine formed intracellularly by γ-glutamylcysteine synthetase might be translocated from cells to the blood plasma and the glomerular filtrate; (2) the small amount of active transpeptidase present in both the patient and the experimental animal may catalyze the extracellular formation of γ-glutamylcyst(e)ine from glutathione and cyst(e)ine; and (3) γ-glutamylcyst(e)ine may be formed by cleavage of the CYS-GLY bond of glutathione (or glutathione disulfide).

Pathway (1) is unlikely since there are two highly active intracellular enzymes (glutathione synthetase and γ-glutamyl cyclotransferase) that can utilize this dipeptide. Furthermore, in 5-oxoprolinuria the excess γ-glutamylcysteine formed intracellularly is effectively converted into 5-oxoproline by the cyclotransferase, and little if any γ-glutamylcysteine is found extracellularly. In addition, the absence of 5-oxoprolinuria in γ-glutamyl transpeptidase deficiency indicates that there is little or no increase in the intracellular level of γ-glutamylcysteine. Pathway (3) appears to be excluded by recent studies

[89], which also support pathway (2). The evidence strongly suggests that transpeptidation between glutathione and cystine occurs in vivo, and also that this reaction constitutes a significant physiologic function of the enzyme. The finding of the 2-vinylpyridine derivatives of cysteine and γ-glutamylcysteine after treatment of the urine of the second patient with dithiothreitol and 2-vinylpyridine is consistent with the presence of γ-glutamylcystine in the urine. Accumulation of γ-glutamylcystine and excretion of this compound would be expected if the rate of γ-glutamylcystine formation exceeds that of its transport into cells. The transport of γ-glutamyl amino acids has been found to be inhibited by high concentrations of glutathione. The appearance of large amounts of γ-glutamylcystine in the urine may therefore reflect an inhibitory effect of glutathione on the transport of γ-glutamylcystine. Intracellular reduction of γ-glutamylcystine would lead to formation of γ-glutamylcysteine and cysteine [16], both of which are substrates for glutathione biosynthesis. The findings [89] also indicate that γ-glutamyl transpeptidase activity is not completely absent in a patient [85] found to have a deficiency of this enzyme, and they show that the activity of the enzyme is not abolished in experimental animals treated with potent γ-glutamyl transpeptidase inhibitors. It will be important to carry out studies on the blood plasma concentrations of γ-glutamylcysteine and cysteine, (and the disulfide forms of these compounds) in such patients. It has been reported that normal human blood contains low but significant levels of γ-glutamyl-cyst(e)ine [90] and cystinylglycine [91].

5-OXOPROLINASE DEFICIENCY

Three individuals with *5-oxoprolinase deficiency* have recently been reported [92, 93]. Two of these [92], brothers aged 16 and 11, had enterocolitis and urolithiasis (a stone from one patient contained calcium oxalate and carbonate) and exhibited excessive excretion of 5-oxo-L-proline (39 to 71 mmole per day). One patient had a plasma 5-oxoproline level of about 0.18 mM. These patients, who did not have acidosis, neurologic symptoms, or hemolysis, had normal erythrocyte glutathione levels. The glutathione synthetase activities of their erythrocytes, leukocytes, and cultured skin fibroblasts were normal. The γ-glutamyl cyclotransferase activity and the activity of γ-glutamylcysteine synthetase of the erythrocytes were also within normal limits. The cultured skin fibroblasts of both patients and the leukocytes of one exhibited very low levels of 5-oxoprolinase. In the cultured fibroblasts the activity was about 2 percent of that of controls, whereas the activity found in the cells of the parents of the patients had a level of activity that was intermediate between that of the patients and the controls. Addition of extracts prepared from the cells to those of controls gave additive results. The affinity of glutathione synthetase from the patient for γ-glutamyl-α-aminobutyrate was normal and feedback inhibition of the patient's γ-glutamylcysteine synthetase by glutathione was also normal.

The third individual found to have 5-oxoprolinase deficiency was discovered in the course of study of her child, who had prolinemia and birth defects [93]. The mother was found to excrete large quantities of 5-oxoproline (28.6 ± 1.55 mmole per day). The father and the child had daily urinary 5-oxoproline excretion that was less than 1 mmole per day. The moth-

er's plasma 5-oxoproline level was nine times greater than that of controls. The erythrocyte glutathione synthetase activities of the mother and child were normal, and kinetic analysis showed no decrease in apparent affinity for ATP and glycine. The mother's blood glutathione level was normal. A skin biopsy specimen from the deltoid region of her arm and her cultured skin fibroblasts had about 2 percent of the 5-oxoprolinase activity of controls. Oral proline loading tests were performed on the mother, father, and child. Although the plasma proline values after the load were no different in the mother, father, and child than in controls, the family members all excreted pipecolic acid after the proline load. Lysine loading in the mother and child produced no pipecolic acid excretion. It is notable that the patient with 5-oxoprolinase deficiency (the mother) was apparently healthy, but her IQ was 67.

The clinical findings in the first two patients (enterocolitis, urolithiasis [92]) were quite different from those found in the third [93]. The urinary excretion of 5-oxoproline was about the same in all of these patients, as was the level of 5-oxoprolinase in their cultured skin fibroblasts. The evidence supports the conclusion that 5-oxoprolinase is an inherited recessive trait, but the associated phenomena, both clinical and biochemical, need to be studied further before definite conclusions can be drawn.

These patients do not seem to have abnormalities of amino acid transport associated with the γ-glutamyl cycle, nor do they have acidosis, apparently because accumulation of 5-oxoproline is not great. Although 5-oxoprolinase deficiency would decrease conversion of 5-oxoproline to glutamate, there is no deficiency of glutamate, which is available from the diet, and by reductive amination and transamination of α-ketoglutarate. A deficiency of glutathione would not be expected, therefore, nor has it been found. The values for total daily excretion of 5-oxoproline in these patients (29 to 71 mmoles) could be taken as *minimal* estimates of the amounts of glutathione that is metabolized per day via 5-oxoproline. The total formation of 5-oxoproline is undoubtedly much greater than such calculated minimal values because these patients do not have a complete lack of 5-oxoprolinase. The levels of 5-oxoprolinase activity in the various tissues of the patients are not yet known. The situation may be analogous to that seen in patients who have a deficiency in one of the urea cycle enzymes, but who nevertheless can synthesize urea at a substantial rate (see Chap. 20).

REFERENCES

1. SIES H, WENDEL A (eds): Glutathione, functions in liver and kidney, Berlin, Heidelberg, New York, Springer-Verlag, 1978
2. JAKOBY WB, ARIAS I (eds): Workshop on glutathione, Krok Symposium, Santa Barbara, Calif, June 2–3, 1975. New York, Raven Press, 1976
3. MEISTER A: Biochemistry of glutathione, in Greenberg DM (ed): *Metabolism of Sulfur Compounds.* New York, Academic Press, Inc, 1975, pp 101–288
4. MEISTER A, TATE SS: Glutathione and related γ-glutamyl compounds: Biosynthesis and utilization. *Ann Rev Biochem* 45:559–604, 1976
5. MEISTER A: On the cycles of glutathione metabolism and transport, in Horecker B, Stadtman E (eds): *Symposium on Biological Cycles (Honoring Sir Hans A. Krebs). Current Topics in Cellular Regulation.* vol 18, 1981, pp 21–57
6. MEISTER A: Glutathione synthesis, in *The Enzymes,* ed 3. vol 10, 1974, pp 671–697
7. MEISTER A: The γ-glutamyl cycle: Diseases associated with specific enzymatic deficiencies. *Ann Intern Med* 81:247–253, 1974
8. See Chap. 74, "Glucose 6-phosphate Dehydrogenase Deficiency," by Ernest Beutler, in this volume

9. MEISTER A: On the enzymology of amino acid transport. *Science* 180:33–39, 1973

10. WILSON H, CANNAN RK: The glutamic acid-pyrrolidonecarboxylic acid system. *J Biol Chem* 119:309–331, 1937

11. MEISTER A, BUKENBERGER MW: Enzymic conversion of D-glutamic acid to D-pyrrolidone carboxylic acid by mammalian tissues. *Nature (Lond)* 194:557–559, 1962

12. MEISTER A, BUKENBERGER MW, STRASSBURGER M: The optically specific enzymatic cyclization of D-glutamate. *Biochem Z (Otto Warburg Festband)* 338:217–229, 1963

13. VAN DER WERF P, GRIFFITH OW, MEISTER A: 5-Oxo-L-prolinase (L-pyroglutamate hydrolase); Purification and catalytic properties. *J Biol Chem* 250:6686, 1975

14. MEISTER A, TATE SS, ROSS LL: Membrane bound γ-glutamyl transpeptidase, in Martinosi A (ed): *The Enzymes of Biological Membranes.* New York, Plenum Publishing Corp, 1976, vol 3, pp 315–347

15. ALLISON D, MEISTER A: Evidence that transpeptidation is a significant function of γ-glutamyl transpeptidase. *J Biol Chem* 256:2988–2992, 1981

16. THOMPSON GA, MEISTER A: Utilization of L-cystine by the γ-glutamyl transpeptidase γ-glutamyl cyclotransferase pathway. *Proc Natl Acad Sci USA* 72:1985–1988, 1975

17. TATE SS, MEISTER A: Interaction of γ-glutamyl transpeptidase with amino acids, dipeptides, and derivatives and analogs of glutathione. *J Biol Chem* 249:7593–7602, 1974

18. MEISTER A: Current status of the γ-glutamyl cycle, in *Functions of Glutathione in Liver and Kidney.* Berlin, Heidelberg, New York, Springer-Verlag, 1978, pp 43–59

19. GRIFFITH OW, MEISTER A: Translocation of intracellular glutathione to membrane-bound γ-glutamyl transpeptidase as a discrete step in the γ-glutamyl cycle: Glutathionuria after inhibition of transpeptidase. *Proc Natl Acad Sci USA* 76:268–272, 1979

20. BARTOLI GM, SIES H: Reduced and oxidized glutathione efflux from liver. *FEBS Letts* 86:89–91, 1978

21. BANNAI S, TSUKEDA H: The export of glutathione from human diploid cells in culture. *J Biol Chem* 254:3444–3450, 1979

22. GRIFFITH OW, NOVOGRODSKY A, MEISTER A: Translocation of glutathione from lymphoid cells that have markedly different γ-glutamyl transpeptidase activities. *Proc Natl Acad Sci USA* 76:2249–2252, 1979

23. GRIFFITH OW, MEISTER A: Potent and specific inhibition of glutathione synthesis by buthionine sulfoximine (S-n-butyl homocysteine sulfoximine). *J Biol Chem* 254:7558–7560, 1979

24. ANDERSON ME, MEISTER A: Dynamic state of glutathione in blood plasma. *J Biol Chem* 255:9530–9533, 1980

25. GRIFFITH OW, MEISTER A: Glutathione: Interorgan translocation, turnover and metabolism. *Proc Natl Acad Sci USA* 76:5606–5610, 1979

26. ANDERSON ME, BRIDGES RJ, MEISTER A: Direct evidence for inter-organ transport of glutathione and that the non-filtration renal mechanism for glutathione utilization involves γ-glutamyl transpeptidase. *Biochem Biophys Res Commun* 96:848–853, 1980

27. HABERLE D, WAHLLANDER A, SIES H: Assessment of the kidney function in maintenance of plasma glutathione concentration and redox state in anesthetized rats. *FEBS Letts* 108:335–340, 1979

28. GRIFFITH OW, TATE SS: The apparent glutathione oxidase activity of γ-glutamyl transpeptidase. *J Biol Chem* 255:5011–5014, 1980

29. GRIFFITH OW, BRIDGES RJ, MEISTER A: Transport of γ-glutamyl amino acids: Role of glutathione and γ-glutamyl transpeptidase. *Proc Natl Acad Sci USA* 76:6319–6322, 1979

30. Peptide transport and hydrolysis. *CIBA Foundation Symposium, New Series.* New York, Elsevier North-Holland, Excerpta Medica, 1977, vol 50

31. TANIGUCHI N, MEISTER A: γ-Glutamyl cyclotransferase from rat kidney: Sulfhydryl groups and isolation of a stable form of the enzyme. *J Biol Chem* 253:1799–1806, 1978

32. VAN DER WERF P, MEISTER A: The metabolic formation and utilization of 5-oxo-L-proline (L-pyroglutamate, L-pyrrolidone carboxylate). *Adv Enzymol* 43:519–556, 1975

33. VAN DER WERF P, STEPHANI RA, MEISTER A: Accumulation of 5-oxoproline in mouse tissues after inhibition of 5-oxoprolinase and administration of amino acids: Evidence for function of the γ-glutamyl cycle. *Proc Natl Acad Sci USA* 71:1026–1029, 1974

34. SEKURA R, MEISTER A: Glutathione turnover in the kidney. Considerations relating to the γ-glutamyl cycle and the transport of amino acids. *Proc Natl Acad Sci USA* 71:2969–2972, 1974

35. RICHMAN P, MEISTER A: Regulation of γ-glutamylcysteine synthetase by nonallosteric feedback inhibition by glutathione. *J Biol Chem* 250:1422–1426, 1975

36. JACKSON RC: Studies in the enzymology of glutathione metabolism in human erythrocytes. *Biochem J* 111:309–315, 1969

37. WENDEL A: Biosynthesis of glutathione, in Flohe L, Benohr H Ch, Sies H, Waller HD, Wendel A (eds): *Symposium on Glutathione, Tubingen, March 1973.* Stuttgart, Thieme, 1973, pp 69–71

38. DAVIS JS, BALINSKY JB, HARRINGTON JS, SHEPHERD JB: Assay, purification, properties and mechanism of action of γ-glutamylcysteine synthetase from the liver of the rat and *Xenopus laevis. Biochem J* 133:667–678, 1973

39. PALEKAR AG, TATE SS, MEISTER A: Decrease in glutathione levels of kidney and liver after injection of methionine sulfoximine into rats. *Biochem Biophys Res Commun* 62:651–657, 1975

40. GRIFFITH OW, BRIDGES RJ, MEISTER A: Evidence that the γ-glutamyl cycle functions *in vivo* using intracellular glutathione: Effects of amino acids and selective inhibition of enzymes. *Proc Natl Acad Sci USA* 75:5405–5408, 1978

41. BRIDGES RJ, GRIFFITH OW, MEISTER A: L-γ-(Threo-β-methyl) glutamyl-L-α-aminobutyrate, a selective substrate of γ-glutamyl cyclotransferase: Inhibition of enzyme activity by β-aminoglutaryl-L-α-aminobutyrate. *J Biol Chem* 255:10,787–10,792, 1980

42. RONZIO R, MEISTER A: Phosphorylation of methionine sulfoximine by glutamine synthetase. *Proc Natl Acad Sci USA* 59:164–170, 1968

43. GRIFFITH OW, MEISTER A: Differential inhibition of glutamine and γ-glutamylcysteine synthetases by α-alkyl analogs of methionine sulfoximine that induce convulsions. *J Biol Chem* 253:2333–2338, 1978

44. JELLUM E, KLUGE T, BORRESEN HC, STOKKE O, ELDJARN L: Pyroglutamic aciduria—a new inborn error of metabolism. *Scand J Clin Lab Invest* 26:327–335, 1970

45. KLUGE T, BORRESEN HC, JELLUM E, STOKKE O, ELDJARN L, FRETHEIM B: Esophageal hiatus hernia and mental retardation: Life-threatening postoperative metabolic acidosis and potassium deficiency linked with a new inborn error of nitrogen metabolism. *Surgery* 71:104–109, 1972

46. ELDJARN L, JELLUM E, STOKKE O: Pyroglutamic aciduria: Studies on the enzymic block and on the metabolic origin of pyroglutamic acid. *Clin Chim Acta* 40:461–476, 1972

47. ELDJARN L, JELLUM E, STOKKE O: Hammes FA, Van Den Bern CJ (eds): Pyroglutamic aciduria, in *Inborn Errors of Metabolism.* New York, Academic Press, Inc, 1973, pp 255–260

48. ELDJARN L, STOKKE O, JELLUM E: Pyroglutamic aciduria. A new inborn error of metabolism possibly in the "γ-glutamyl cycle" proposed for amino acid transport, in Stern J, Toothill C (eds): *Organic Acidurias.* Baltimore, Williams & Wilkins Co, 1972, pp 113–120

49. HAGENFELDT L, LARSSON A, ZETTERSTROM R: Pyroglutamic aciduria. *Acta Paediatr Scand* 63:1–8, 1974

50. WELLNER VP, SEKURA R, MEISTER A, LARSSON A: Glutathione synthetase deficiency, an inborn error of metabolism involving the γ-glutamyl cycle in patients with 5-oxoprolinuria (pyroglutamic aciduria). *Proc Natl Acad Sci USA* 71:2505–2509, 1974

51. LARSSON A, ZETTERSTROM R, HAGENFELDT L, ANDERSSON R, DREBORG S, HORNELL H: Pyroglutamic aciduria (5-oxoprolinuria), an inborn error in glutathione metabolism. *Pediatr Res* 8:852–856, 1974

52. LARSSON A, ZETTERSTROM R, HORNELL H, PORATH U: Erythrocyte glutathione synthetase in 5-oxoprolinuria: Kinetic studies of the mutant enzyme and detection of heterozygotes. *Clin Chim Acta* 73:19–23, 1976

53. ELDJARN L, JELLUM E, STOKKE O: Pyroglutamic aciduria: Rate of formation and degradation of pyroglutamate. *Clin Chim Acta* 49:311–323, 1973

54. STROMME JH, ELDJARN L: The metabolism of L-pyroglutamic acid in fibroblasts from a patient with pyroglutamic aciduria: The demonstration of an L-pyroglutamate hydrolase system. *Scand J Clin Lab Invest* 29:335–342, 1972

55. MARSTEIN S, JELLUM E, HALPERN B, ELDJARN L, PERRY TL: Biochemical studies of erythrocytes in a patient with pyroglutamic acidemia (5-oxoprolinemia). *N Engl J Med* 295:406–412, 1976

56. MARSTEIN S, PERRY TL: Studies of amino acid content and transport in glutathione-deficient erythrocytes from a patient with pyroglutamic acidemia (5-oxoprolinemia). *Clin Chim Acta* 109:13–20, 1981

57. HAGENFELDT L, LARSSON A, ANDERSSON R: The γ-glutamyl cycle and amino acid transport. *N Engl J Med* 299:587–591, 1978

58. MENDELSON IS, ZALESKI WA, CASEY RE, CHRISTIE EJ, WELLNER VP, MEISTER A: Ataxia in 5-oxoprolinuria: Is there a connection between the γ-glutamyl cycle and GABA function?, abstracted. *Eleventh International Congress of Biochemistry,* Toronto, 1979

59. BEUTLER E: Editorial: Glutathione deficiency, pyroglutamic acidemia and amino acid transport. *N Engl J Med* 295:441–443, 1976

60. SKULLERUND K, MARSTEIN S, SCHRADER H, BRUNDELET PJ, JELLUM E: The cerebral lesions in a patient with generalized glutathione deficiency and pyroglutamic aciduria (5-oxoprolinuria). *Acta Neuropathol (Berl)* 52:235–238, 1980

61. SPIELBERG SP, KRAMER LI, GOODMAN SI, BUTLER J, TIETZE F, QUINN P, SCHULMAN JD: 5-Oxoprolinuria: Biochemical observations and case report. *J Pediatr* 91:237–241, 1977

62. BOIVIN P, GALAND C, SCHAISON G: Deficit en glutathion-synthetase avec 5-oxoprolinruie. Deux nouveaux cas et revue de la litterature. *Nouv Presse Med* 7:1531–1535, 1978

63. PORATH U, SCHREIER KL: Eine familie mit pyroglutaminacidurie. *Dtsch Med Wschr* 103:939–942, 1978

64. THAM R, NYSTROM I, HOLMSTEDT B: Identification by mass spectrometry

of pyroglutamic acid as a peak in the gas chromatography of human urine. *Biochem Pharmacol* 17:1735–1738, 1968

65. PASCHER G: Die wasserloslichen bestandteile der peripheren hornschicht (Hautoberflache). Quantitative analysen. III. α-Pyrrolidoncarbonsaure. *Arch Klin Exp Dermatol* 203:234–238, 1956

66. LADEN L, SPITZER R: Identification of a natural moisturizing agent in skin. *J Soc Cosmet Chem* 18:351–360, 1967

67. PALEKAR AG, TATE SS, SULLIVAN J, MEISTER A: Accumulation of 5-oxo-L-proline and 5-oxo-D-proline in the blood plasma in end stage renal disease. *Biochem Med* 14:339–345, 1975

68. LARSSON A, HOLMGREN A, BRATT I: Thioredoxin and glutathione in cultured fibroblasts from human cases with 5-oxoprolinuria and cystinosis. *FEBS Letts* 87:61–64, 1978

69. REVEL JP, BALL EG: The reaction of glutathione with amino acids and related compounds as catalyzed by γ-glutamyl transpeptidase. *J Biol Chem* 234:577–582, 1959

70. TATE SS, MEISTER A: Serine-borate complex as a transition-state inhibitor of γ-glutamyl transpeptidase. *Proc Natl Acad Sci USA* 75:4806–4809, 1978

71. SPIELBERG SP, BUTLER J DeB, MacDERMOTT K, SCHULMAN JD: Treatment of glutathione synthetase deficient fibroblasts by inhibiting γ-glutamyl transpeptidase activity with serine and borate. *Biochem Biophys Res Commun* 89:504–511, 1979

72. SPIELBERG SP, BOXER LA, CORASH LM, SCHULMAN JD: Improved erythrocyte survival with high-dose vitamin E in chronic hemolyzing G6PD and glutathione synthetase deficiencies. *Ann Intern Med* 90:53–54, 1979

73. CORASH L, SPIELBERG S, BARTSOCAS C, BOXER L, STEINHERZ R, SHEETZ M, EGAN M, SCHLESSELMAN J, SCHULMAN JD: Reduced chronic hemolysis during high-dose vitamin E administration in mediterranean-type glucose-6-phosphate dehydrogenase deficiency. *N Engl J Med* 303:416–420, 1980

74. OSKI FA: Editorial: Vitamin E—a radical defense. *N Engl J Med* 303:454–455, 1980

75. GRIFFITH OW, LARSSON A, MEISTER A: Inhibition of γ-glutamyl-cysteine synthetase by cystamine: An approach to a therapy of 5-oxoprolinuria (Pyroglutamic aciduria). *Biochem Biophys Res Commun* 79:919–925, 1977

76. OORT M, LOOS JA, PRINS HR: Hereditary absence of reduced glutathione in the erythrocytes—a new clinical and biochemical entity?. *Vox Sang* 6:370–373, 1961

77. PRINS HK, OORT M, LOOS JA, ZURCHER C, BECKERS T: Congenital nonspherocytic hemolytic anemia associated with glutathione deficiency of the erythrocytes. *Blood J Hematol* 27:145–166, 1966

78. BOIVIN P, GALAND C: La synthese du glutathion au cours de l'anemie hemolytique congenitale avec deficit en glutathion reduit. *Nouv Rev Fr Hematol* 5:707–720, 1965

79. MOHLER DN, MAJERUS PW, MINNICH V, HESS CE, GARRICK MD: Glutathione synthetase deficiency as a cause of hereditary hemolytic disease. *N Engl J Med* 283:1253–1257, 1970

80. BOIVIN P: Personal communication

81. SPIELBERG SP, GARRICK MD, CORASH LM, BUTLER J DeB, TIETZE F, ROGERS LV, SCHULMAN JD: Biochemical heterogeneity in glutathione synthetase deficiency. *J Clin Invest* 61:1417–1420, 1978

82. KONRAD PN, RICHARDS F II, VALENTINE WN, PAGLIA D: γ-Glutamyl-cysteine synthetase deficiency. *N Engl J Med* 286:557–561, 1972

83. RICHARDS F II, COOPER MR, PEARCE LA, COWAN RJ, SPURR CL: Familial spinocerebellar degeneration, hemolytic anemia, and glutathione deficiency. *Arch Intern Med* 124:534–537, 1974

84. GOODMAN SI, MACE JW, POLLACK S: Serum γ-glutamyl transpeptidase deficiency. *Lancet* 234–235, 1971

85. WRIGHT EC, STERN J, ERSSER R, PATRICK AD: Glutathionuria: γ-Glutamyl transpeptidase deficiency. *J Inher Metab Dis* 2:3–7, 1979

86. SCHULMAN JD, GOODMAN SI, MACE JW, PATRICK AD, TIETZE F, BUTLER EJ: Glutathionuria: Inborn error of metabolism due to tissue deficiency of γ-glutamyl transpeptidase. *Biochem Biophys Res Commun* 65:68–74, 1975

87. PELLEFIGURE F, BUTLER J DeB, SPIELBERG SP, HOLLENBERG MD, GOODMAN SI, SCHULMAN JD: Normal amino acid uptake by cultured human fibroblasts does not require γ-glutamyl transpeptidase. *Biochem Biophys Res Commun* 73:997–1002, 1976

88. GRIFFITH OW, MEISTER A: Excretion of cysteine and γ-glutamyl-cysteine moieties in human and experimental animal γ-glutamyl transpeptidase deficiency. *Proc Natl Acad Sci USA* 77:3384–3387, 1980

89. GRIFFITH OW, BRIDGES RJ, MEISTER A: Formation of γ-glutamylcyst(e)ine *in vivo* is catalyzed by γ-glutamyl transpeptidase. *Proc Natl Acad Sci USA* 1981, in press

90. HAGENFELDT L, ARVIDSSON A, LARSSON A: Glutathone and γ-glutamylcysteine in whole blood, plasma and erythrocytes. *Clin Chim Acta* 85:167–173, 1978

91. ARMSTRONG, MD: The occurrence of cystinylglycine in blood plasma. *Biochim Biophys Acta* 584:542–544, 1979

92. LARSSON A, MATTSSON B, WAUTERS EAK, VAN GOOL JD, DURAN M, WADMAN SK: 5-Oxoprolinuria due to hereditary 5-oxoprolinase deficiency in two brothers—A new inborn error of the γ-glutamyl cycle. *Acta Paediatr Scand*, 1980

93. ROSEL RA, HOMMES FA, SAMPER L: Pyroglutamic aciduria (5-oxoprolinuria) without glutathione synthetase deficiency and with decreased pyroglutamate hydrolase activity, abstracted. *International Symposium of Inborn Errors of Metabolism in Humans*. Interlaken, Switzerland, Sept. 2–5, 1980

18

DISORDERS OF PROLINE AND HYDROXYPROLINE METABOLISM

CHARLES R. SCRIVER

ROBERT J. SMITH

JAMES M. PHANG

1. *Hyperprolinemia comprises two distinct conditions, both apparently autosomal recessive, each due to mutations at separate genetic loci. Both traits are believed to be harmless. Proline oxidase activity is deficient in type I hyperprolinemia; Δ^1-pyrroline-5-carboxylate (P5C) dehydrogenase is deficient in type II hyperprolinemia. Only proline degradation is impaired in the type I trait; proline and free 4-hydroxyproline oxidation are affected in the type II condition. The plasma proline concentration is generally higher in the type II proband than in type I hyperprolinemia for several reasons, possibly including the relative severity of the enzyme defect (apparently greater in the type II defect), the position of the block, and the normal steady-state equilibriums regulating biosynthesis and degradation of proline. For reasons not yet understood, type I heterozygotes may exhibit mild hyperprolinemia; under endogenous conditions, type II heterozygotes do not.*

2. *Hyperhydroxyprolinemia is an autosomal recessive trait resulting from hydroxyproline oxidase deficiency. Proline metabolism is normal in probands. The condition does not affect collagen metabolism itself and is considered harmless. Hydroxyproline does not accumulate with a deficiency of P5C dehydrogenase (in type II hyperprolinemia), although the enzyme is common*
to the second step of proline and hydroxyproline catabolism.

3. *L-Proline biosynthesis and degradation are catalyzed by Δ^1-pyrroline-5-carboxylate reductase (EC 1.5.1.2) and proline oxidase (no EC number assigned), respectively. Δ^1-Pyrroline-5-carboxylate (P5C), which is the only intermediate shared by the biosynthetic and degradative limbs of proline metabolism, links the urea cycle (through ornithine) with the tricarboxylic acid cycle (through glutamate); ornithine-δ-transaminase (EC 2.6.1.13) and P5C dehydrogenase (EC 1.5.1.12) catalyze the respective steps for P5C "outflow." The transaminase and P5C "synthase" sustain proline biosynthesis via the shared P5C intermediate.*

4. *4-Hydroxy-L-proline is an intermediate of collagen metabolism. Its principal route of biosynthesis is by hydroxylation of the third-position proline in the prevalent tripeptide Gly-Pro-Pro in the nascent procollagen polypeptide chain. Free hydroxyproline is derived largely from cleavage of oligopeptides released during collagen turnover. Degradation of hydroxyproline resembles that of proline. Degradation to Δ^1-pyrroline-3-hydroxy-5-carboxylate is catalyzed by an independent catalytic activity:hydroxyproline oxidase (no EC number assigned). The subsequent pyrroline dehydrogenation step may be irreversible and is catalyzed by*

the same enzyme that serves P5C dehydrogenation. The principal route for subsequent disposal of hydroxyproline intermediates is cleavage by an aldolase reaction to yield glyoxylate and pyruvate. 3-Hydroxy-L-proline results from posttranslational hydroxylation of the Pro residue in the collagen sequence Gly-Pro-Hypro. The imino acid is a useful marker of basement membrane collagen. At least the first two steps of 3-hydroxyproline degradation are independent of those used by 4-hydroxyproline since abnormalities of 3-hydroxyproline metabolism are not seen in type II hyperprolinemia or in hyperhydroxyprolinemia.

5. *Prolidase deficiency is an autosomal recessive trait with a characteristic clinical syndrome which includes chronic dermatitis, mental retardation, and recurrent infections. Deficient cleavage of imino acid-containing peptides causes excessive urinary excretion of X-Pro dipeptides; hydroxyproline-containing peptides are also increased in urine. The proline peptide/hydroxyproline peptide excretion ratio is increased above normal at all ages. Activity of prolidase (EC 3.4.13.9) in leukocytes and erythrocytes is severely deficient (<6 percent normal) in probands and half normal in symptomless obligate heterozygotes.*

Proline and hydroxyproline are nonessential amino acids. They have only one hydrogen on the nitrogen atom inserted in a pyrrolidine ring (Fig. 18-2) and are usually designated by the trivial name *imino acid*. The principal form of hydroxyproline in humans is 4-hydroxy-L-proline, and its major source is collagen; 3-hydroxy-L-proline is present in much smaller amounts in body fluids. Proline is prominent in its free form, while hydroxyproline is relatively more abundant as an oligopeptide. Important pathways provide for the biosynthesis and degradation of free proline; analogous pathways of less quantitative significance also exist, in part, for free hydroxyproline metabolism. Proline and 4-hydroxyproline share the second step of their degradation. Hydroxyproline originating in peptide linkage is derived exclusively from the proline already present in peptide linkage.

Several inborn errors of imino acid metabolism are known (Fig. 18-1), and each has served to elucidate more clearly the metabolic interrelationships in humans. The *hyperprolinemias* comprise two separate disorders of proline oxidation. Type I involves proline dehydrogenase (oxidase); type II involves Δ¹-pyrroline-5-carboxylic acid dehydrogenase. *Hyperhydroxyprolinemia* is a disorder of free hydroxyproline catabolism, involv-

ing the step catalyzed by "hydroxyproline oxidase." Hydroxyproline metabolism is compromised in type II hyperprolinemia, but only its pyrroline metabolites accumulate in this phenotype. *Prolidase deficiency* is a disorder of oligopeptide cleavage associated with a complex clinical syndrome and massive urinary excretion of proline-containing dipeptides.

METABOLISM OF THE IMINO ACIDS

L-Proline is exceeded in concentration only by glutamine and alanine as an itinerant free amino acid in body fluids of the adult subject. D-Proline does not occur naturally in human metabolism. The principal isomer of hydroxyproline is 4-hydroxy-L-proline; the configurations at carbon 2, relative to the C—N bond, and at carbon 4, relative to the C—O bond, are both L (Fig. 18-2).

Collagen is a major reservoir for the two imino acids, but proline is ubiquitous in many other species of protein. Collagen is the only significant store of hydroxyproline and about half the pool of body proline in vertebrates. Proline accounts for 110 to 130 residues per 1000 residues in mammalian collagen, while 4-hydroxyproline occurs at about 80 to 100 residues per 1000 residues [1]. Collagen also contains small amounts of 3-hydroxy-L-proline [2] (Fig. 18-2).

The secondary amino group of the imino acids confers upon them distinctive roles as residues in protein [3–5] and as free metabolites [6]. The absence of a primary amino group excludes the imino acids from those pyridoxal-5′-phosphate coenzyme-catalyzed reactions which are otherwise of general importance for amino acid metabolism [7, 8]. As a result, decarboxylation and transamination reactions play no role in the metabolism of proline and hydroxyproline, as they do in the metabolism of the related 5-carbon amino acids, L-glutamate and L-ornithine. Although racemization could be catalyzed by microorganisms in the human intestinal tract at carbon 2 of both proline [9] and hydroxyproline [10], organisms utilize a nonpyridoxal mechanism instead of the customary pyridoxal-phosphate-dependent racemase. On the other hand, the general amino acid oxidase reactions are evident in mammalian tissues. D-Proline [11] and 4-hydroxy-D-proline [12] are substrates for mammalian D-amino acid oxidase activity. They yield Δ¹-pyrroline-2-carboxylate and Δ¹-pyrroline-4-hydroxy-2-carboxylate, respectively. Corrigan and colleagues [13] have noted that hydroxy-D-proline (threo or erythro isomer) is a sensitive substrate to test for D-amino acid oxidase activity by virtue of the high color yield of the Ehrlich-positive pyrrole-2-carboxylic acid which can be formed readily from the pyrroline product of the imino acid oxidation. The well-known L-amino acid oxidase activity in mammalian kidney, which is present in mitochondria [14], also oxidizes L-proline [15] to yield Δ¹-pyrroline-2-carboxylic acid; its action on hydroxyproline has not been reported. L-Proline ranks third among 16 amino acids with respect to relative affinity as substrate for L-amino acid oxidase in kidney [16].

Figure 18-1 Schematic diagram of principal outflow pathways in metabolism of L-proline, 4-hydroxy-L-proline, and L-ornithine. The sites of deficient enzyme activity are shown for: (A) type I hyperprolinemia (proline oxidase deficiency); (B) hyperhydroxyprolinemia (hydroxyproline oxidase deficiency); (C) type II hyperprolinemia (Δ¹-pyrroline-5-carboxylate dehydrogenase deficiency) (note sharing with hydroxyproline pathway); (D) hyperornithinemia with gyrate atrophy (ornithine-keto acid transaminase deficiency). See Chap. 17 for details.

Proline Metabolism

The pathways of proline metabolism in mammalian cells are summarized in Fig. 18-3. Proline can be synthesized from orni-

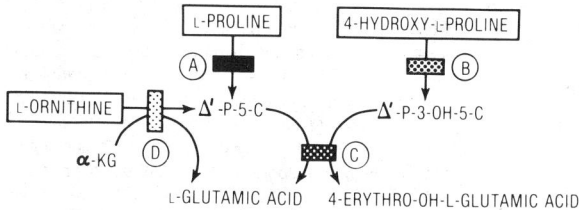

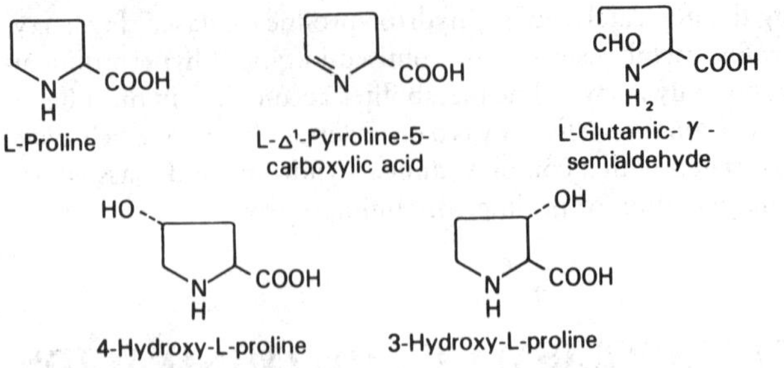

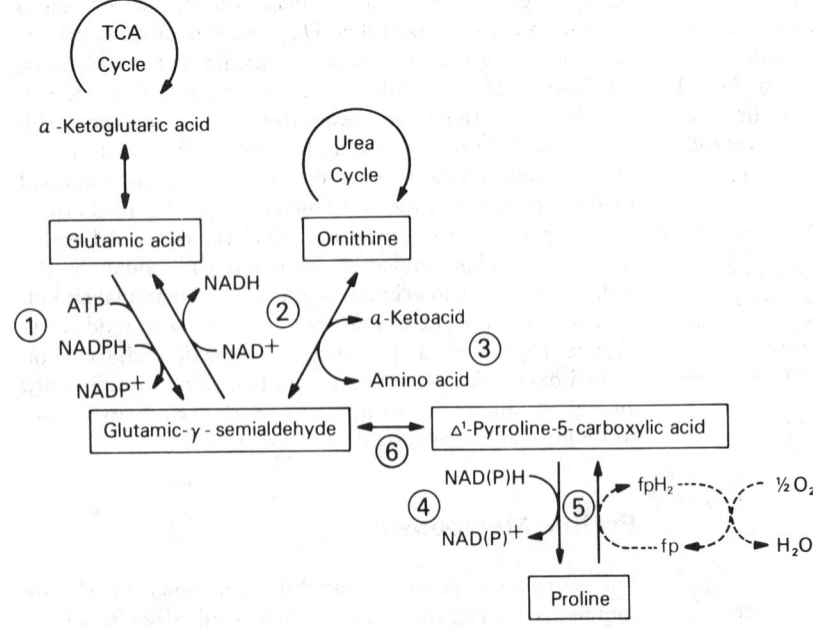

Figure 18-2   Schematic structures for proline, intermediates in the proline metabolic pathways, and the two forms of hydroxyproline present in mammalian tissues.

thine or glutamic acid via the common intermediates glutamic-γ-semialdehyde and pyrroline-5-carboxylic acid (P5C). The latter two compounds are in spontaneous equilibrium. Proline can also be degraded to P5C, glutamic acid, and probably ornithine. The reaction catalyzed by ornithine aminotransferase is potentially reversible, but there is considerable uncertainty about the direction of flow through the pathway in vivo. All of the other reactions depicted in Fig. 18-3 are irreversible, with separate enzymes catalyzing the synthetic and degradative steps. It should be noted that P5C is not only an intermediate in proline metabolism but also provides a link between the urea and tricarboxylic acid cycles. Stetten [17], Adams [6], and recently Adams and Frank [18] have published extensive reviews of prokaryotic and eukaryotic proline metabolism.

Biosynthesis   A study published 30 years ago first established the fact that radioisotopically labeled glutamate is converted to labeled proline in intact mammals [19]. Using *Escherichia coli* mutants, Vogel and Davis [20] then demonstrated that P5C is an intermediate between glutamate and proline and suggested the reaction sequence that is presently accepted for mammalian tissues (Fig. 18-3). Only recently has the formation of P5C from glutamate by cell-free preparations been verified. Using homogenates of rat small intestinal mucosa, Ross et al. described the formation of radioactive ornithine from radioactive glutamate in the presence of ATP, Mg^{2+}, and

NADPH [21]. Although neither P5C nor proline formation was measured, presumably ornithine was formed through ornithine aminotransferase via intermediate P5C. Subsequently, Smith et al. developed a method for measuring P5C formation from glutamate catalyzed by homogenates of cultured fibroblasts and designated this activity *P5C synthase* [22]. The requirement for ATP and NADPH is consistent with the two-step reaction sequence originally proposed by Strecker [23].

$$\text{Glutamate} \longrightarrow \begin{array}{c}\gamma\text{-Glutamyl}\\\text{Phosphate}\end{array} \longrightarrow \begin{array}{c}\text{Glutamic-}\gamma\text{-}\\\text{semialdehyde}\end{array} \longrightarrow \begin{array}{c}\text{Pyrroline-5-}\\\text{carboxylate}\end{array} \quad (1)$$

Further evidence for the two sequential reactions of P5C synthase derives from indirect assays of each step in bacteria [24–28]. Absolute identification of the γ-glutamyl phosphate intermediate apparently has been prevented by its instability [23].

The final step in proline synthesis, conversion of P5C to proline by P5C reductase (EC 1.5.1.2), is well defined. This is a soluble, largely cytosolic enzyme of wide tissue distribution [29] that utilizes reduced pyridine nucleotides [30]. Early work suggested that NADH is the preferred cofactor, since the rate of proline formation is highest with saturating concentrations of NADH and is inhibited if NADH and NADPH are added simultaneously [30, 31]. NADPH may be the preferred cofactor *in situ* since its K_m is fivefold lower than the K_m for NADH [30]. In addition, the affinity for P5C is much higher when NADPH is the cofactor [30]. Determination of P5C reductase activity in tissue homogenates has been complicated by its apparent cold lability [29], which may be attributable to a heat-labile inhibitor [31].

In addition to glutamate, ornithine is a precursor of proline via intermediate P5C [32, 33]. This occurs through reversible transfer of the δ-amino group of ornithine to α-ketoglutarate, catalyzed by a pyridoxal phosphate-dependent ornithine aminotransferase (EC 2.6.1.13). Studies of Chinese hamster ovary cells in culture indicate that ornithine can serve as an important source of proline. Mutant Chinese hamster ovary cells that lack P5C synthase activity, but have ornithine aminotransferase activity comparable to that of other fibroblasts, convert

Figure 18-3   Summary of the pathways of proline synthesis and degradation in mammalian tissues. The enzymes are: (1) P5C synthase; (2) P5C dehydrogenase; (3) ornithine aminotransferase; (4) P5C reductase; and (5) proline oxidase. Step 6 is spontaneous. The mechanism of coupling of proline oxidase to flavin nucleotides and electron transport has not been fully characterized.

enough ornithine to proline to grow at normal rates in proline-free medium [34]. Furthermore, in a number of different connective tissues where the demand for proline incorporation into collagen is high, there is a good correlation between ornithine aminotransferase and P5C reductase activities [35, 36].

Other quantitatively important pathways of proline biosynthesis are not believed to exist in mammalian cells. D-Proline can potentially be isomerized to L-proline in kidney via conversion to pyrroline-2-carboxylic acid by D-amino acid oxidase [37] and then reduction to L-proline by pyrroline-2-carboxylate reductase [38]. Species distribution of the latter enzyme is not entirely known, but it appears to be absent from mammalian tissues. Ornithine α-transaminase, a source of pyrroline-2-carboxylate that may exist in plants, has not been demonstrated in mammalian tissues (see Ref. 18 for review).

Degradation Proline is converted to P5C and then to either glutamic acid or ornithine. The enzymes catalyzing these respective interconversions are proline oxidase (EC number not assigned), P5C dehydrogenase (EC 1.5.1.12), and ornithine aminotransferase (EC 2.6.1.13). Although these enzymes are catabolic relative to proline, their metabolic function may not be limited to the utilization of proline carbons (see below).

Proline oxidase, which catalyzes the conversion of proline to P5C [39–41], has a number of unusual features. The enzyme is tightly bound to mitochondrial inner membranes and interacts with the electron transport chain presumably through a flavoprotein [40, 42]. Although the enzyme has been solubilized with detergents, it has not been purified to homogeneity [43]. Thus, the molecular mechanisms mediating the oxidation of proline and the transfer of electrons to the putative flavoprotein and then into the electron transport chain remain undefined.

Unlike the other enzymes of the pathway, proline oxidase is not ubiquitous but is restricted in location to the liver, kidney, heart, and brain [41, 44]. It may be that a low level of activity is masked by inhibitors in certain other tissues, such as pancreas [45]. In most cultured cells, proline oxidase is undetectable even when cells are derived from tissues with enzyme activity. Only LLC-RK1 cells, a line derived from rabbit kidney, have measurable activity [46].

P5C dehydrogenase, which catalyzes the conversion of P5C to glutamate [47, 48], may be present in both cytosol and mitochondria [49]. Catalytic activity requires oxidized pyridine nucleotide as cofactor. The hepatic P5C dehydrogenase exhibits kinetic properties which favor the utilization of NAD^+ rather than $NADP^+$. Most tissues as well as cultured cells have P5C dehydrogenase activity [50]. The level of activity differs widely among tissues [44]. In general, central tissues, such as liver and kidney, have higher levels than peripheral tissues, such as muscle, bone, and cartilage [44, 50, 51]. The red cell, with its high level of P5C reductase, has undetectable P5C dehydrogenase activity [52, 53].

The reversible formation of ornithine from P5C by ornithine aminotransferase readily occurs in vitro [54, 55]. Studies using purified ornithine aminotransferase show that the equilibrium constant (K_{eq}) of the enzyme markedly favors the formation of P5C from ornithine [56]. Furthermore, the finding of hyperornithinemia in patients with gyrate atrophy of the choroid and retina, in which a deficiency of ornithine aminotransferase is the primary defect [57, 58] (see Chap. 19), suggests that the flux from ornithine to P5C predominates. Nevertheless, when the mitochondrial redox state has been made reduced with rotenone, proline can be a source of ornithine.

Regulation of Proline Metabolism

Biosynthesis (Regulation) Regulation of proline biosynthesis is likely to be complex, since the P5C intermediate is common to both the synthetic and degradative pathways. In addition, recent studies suggest that these pathways may influence cell energetics and the redox state [59, 60]. Therefore, interpretation of regulatory events may require consideration of both cellular proline requirements and indirect effects of the intermediates on more distant pathways. P5C reductase is competitively inhibited by low concentrations of proline in cultured fibroblasts ($K_i = 2 \times 10^{-4}$ M) [61], and thus proline could regulate its own formation. In homogenates of mammalian liver, kidney, and brain, however, P5C reductase is not significantly inhibited by physiologic proline concentrations ($K_i = 10^{-2}$ M) [30, 31]. In these tissues, the reduction of P5C to proline may not be rate-limiting, and the rate of P5C formation may regulate proline synthesis. In addition, proline biosynthesis may also be influenced by the tissue content of P5C reductase, which is relatively high in collagen-forming tissues [35] and higher in young, rapidly growing animals than in older animals [62].

The regulation of the pathway from ornithine to P5C has been difficult to characterize because of the reversibility of the reaction. Although the equilibrium constant determined with purified enzyme activity favors P5C formation ($K_{eq} = 71$) [56], the reaction in situ may be more readily reversible because intracellular concentrations of the amino accepting α-ketoacids are approximately thirtyfold lower than the corresponding amino acids [63]. Therefore, in some tissues, ornithine aminotransferase may catalyze the net formation of ornithine from P5C. Although the enzyme activity has been shown to vary in response to dietary and hormonal stimuli [64–67], a hypothesis linking the regulation of ornithine aminotransferase to varying cellular requirements for proline has not emerged.

Until recently, it has not been possible to study the regulation of P5C synthase directly. Using intact cultured fibroblasts, Eagle and coworkers obtained indirect evidence for P5C synthase sensitivity to proline inhibition [68]. They followed the appearance of ^{14}C-labeled proline derived from [14C]ornithine or [14C]glutamate. Addition of proline to the culture medium inhibited proline formation from glutamine (100 percent inhibition with 10 mM proline) but did not decrease proline formation from ornithine. Since the final step in proline biosynthesis, P5C conversion to proline, is shared by the two precursors, the P5C synthase reaction presumably was inhibited. In a recent study on P5C synthase in homogenates of Chinese hamster ovary cells, the enzyme was 100 percent inhibited by 0.2 M proline [22]. The effect of lower concentrations of proline has not been reported. Data published in preliminary form [69] indicate that P5C synthase in cultured cells is also reversibly inhibited by low concentrations of ornithine ($K_i = 0.37$ mM).

With this knowledge, a hypothetical model for the overall regulation of proline biosynthesis can be constructed (Fig. 18-4). When intracellular proline levels are adequate, proline could regulate its own rate of formation by inhibiting P5C reductase. When ornithine levels are high, P5C synthase activity would be inhibited and P5C would be derived primarily

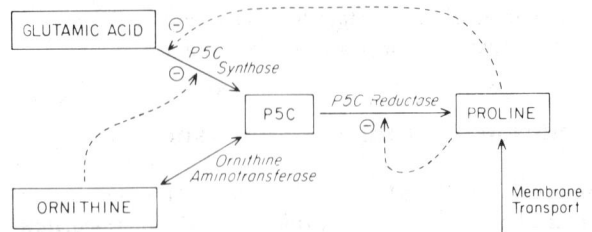

Figure 18-4 Hypothetical scheme for the regulation of proline biosynthesis in cultured cells. Dashed arrows and negative signs (−) indicate inhibitory effects.

from ornithine and then converted to proline by P5C reductase. When ornithine levels are low, P5C synthase would be active. A cell requiring proline could then preferentially convert glutamic acid to P5C, which is further reduced to proline. Overproduction of P5C from glutamic acid would be prevented through the inhibition of P5C synthase by proline. While these concepts may explain the regulation of proline biosynthesis, it is to be emphasized that the observations are largely limited to cultured cell systems. The specific pattern of regulation may be expected to vary in differentiated mammalian tissues.

Degradation (Regulation) Extensive regulation of proline oxidase in tissues has been described. Enzyme activity increases with growth and development in both liver and kidney [62]. Corticosteroids are necessary for full expression of proline oxidase activity. Decreased enzyme activity in animals either hypophysectomized or adrenalectomized can be restored with physiologic doses of corticosteroids; pharmacologic doses further increase enzyme levels [70]. The effect of steroids on proline oxidase activity in cultured LLC-RK1 cells suggests that the hormone directly induces synthesis of enzyme [71]. Lactate at physiologic concentrations and pyruvate to a lesser degree directly inhibit proline oxidase activity [43]. The inhibition by lactate is reversible, competitive relative to proline, and demonstrable in both mitochondrial particles and solubilized preparations. Long-chain fatty-acyl-coenzyme A moieties [72] and free fatty acids [45] inhibit enzyme activity. The masking of low levels of activity in certain tissues may be due to these inhibitors [45].

In spite of the paucity of studies on the regulation of P5C dehydrogenase, an interesting mechanism has been elucidated. In preparations of the enzyme from bovine kidney, a variety of amino acids inhibit enzyme activity [73]; different groups of amino acids inhibit additively. For example, in the presence of saturating concentrations of a branched chain amino acid, additional inhibition is produced by alanine. These studies suggest that there are saturable binding sites specific to each group of amino acids.

Metabolic Interlocks Although proline is readily converted to glucose and CO_2 by hepatocytes in vitro, the physiologic contribution of proline carbons to intermediates of the TCA and urea cycles and glucose remains uncertain. Measurements of arteriovenous differences across the splanchnic bed show relatively little difference in proline concentration [74]. Furthermore, a number of mechanisms regulating proline degradation cannot be related simply to the demand for proline as a source of carbons.

Recent studies suggest the possibility that interconversions of glutamate, ornithine, and proline not only mediate the transfer of carbons but also may regulate redox-dependent

pathways [52, 59, 60, 75]. It is proposed that proline and P5C function metabolically as a redox couple. In cultured cells [59] and erythrocytes [52] the addition of P5C to the incubation medium markedly stimulates glucose metabolism through the hexose-monophosphate-pentose (HMP) pathway. The effect is due to the P5C-dependent turnover of $NADP^+$ catalyzed by P5C reductase [15]. The preferential linkage to the NADPH/NADP redox system may reflect the markedly higher affinity of P5C reductase for NADPH [53]. Depending on the complement of enzymes in a given tissue, P5C can be produced from proline, ornithine, or glutamate. The synthesis of P5C from glutamate by P5C synthase also generates oxidizing potential in the form of $NADP^+$ [76].

In tissues with proline oxidase, the interconversions of P5C and proline catalyzed by P5C reductase and proline oxidase may constitute a cycle which allows for the generation of cytosolic oxidizing potential [60, 75]. Furthermore, the transfer of oxidizing potential occurs not only in cell-free systems [60] but also between intact cells with differing capacities for proline metabolism [75]. Isolated hepatocytes convert proline to P5C and release P5C into the incubation medium. Erythrocytes cannot produce P5C, but they readily accumulate it and can use it as a source of oxidizing potential. Thus, the hepatocyte can generate oxidizing potential which is transferred into red cells via the proline cycle and can utilize it for oxidation of glucose through the HMP pathway. It is likely that the physiologic role of P5C in stimulating HMP activity may have the synthesis of purine nucleotides as its endpoint. Since the formation of phosphoribosylpyrophosphate is dependent on ribose-5-P produced by the HMP pathway [77–79], P5C produced from ornithine, glutamate, or proline could act as a metabolic signal coordinating the availability of amino acids and the formation of nucleotides.

Some of these considerations may serve as a basis for interpreting regulatory mechanisms which may not have only the exchange of carbons as the regulatory endpoint. For example, the inhibition of proline oxidase by lactate [43] and fatty acids [45] and the inhibition of P5C reductase by ATP [30, 31] and NADP [30, 31, 53] may be more closely related to the contribution of proline to redox turnover and energetics than to the carbon pool. Similarly, the induction of ornithine aminotransferase by estrogens in kidney [66, 67] and the regulation of P5C dehydrogenase by amino acids [73] may relate more to the function of P5C as oxidizing potential for coordinating amino acid with nucleotide metabolism than to the conservation of P5C for proline biosynthesis. Again, the effect of hormones (insulin, glucagon) on proline transport [80, 81] may be related more to the regulatory functions of P5C than to the contribution of proline to the available carbon pool.

4-Hydroxyproline Metabolism

Biosynthesis The principal route of 4-hydroxy-L-proline biosynthesis in mammals is posttranslational hydroxylation of proline on nascent chains of procollagen [82]. The proline residue in the third position of the prevalent Gly-Pro-Pro triplet sequence is the preferred site for hydroxylation by prolyl hydroxylase in a reaction requiring ferrous iron, α-ketoglutarate, and O_2 [83]. Collagen biosynthesis and proline hydroxylation are discussed in detail in Chap. 16.

Although collagen is the major source of 4-hydroxyproline, it occurs in other proteins: elastin [84], the Clq component of complement [85], acetylcholinesterase [86], and several other partially characterized proteins [18]. Hydroxylation is also presumed to occur posttranslationally in these proteins since mammalian transfer RNA for hydroxyproline has not been identified. Whether enzymes distinct from collagen prolyl hydroxylase are involved is not known.

Free hydroxyproline is believed to arise exclusively from collagen and other hydroxyproline-containing proteins. It could theoretically be formed by condensation of glyoxylate and pyruvate (Fig. 18-5), but the essential step converting 4-erythrohydroxy-L-glutamate to Δ^1-3-hydroxy-5-carboxylic acid has not been demonstrated.

Degradation   The major pathway for the degradation of free hydroxy-L-proline parallels that for proline (Figs. 18-1, 18-5). Hydroxyproline is oxidized to Δ^1-pyrroline-3-hydroxy-5-carboxylic acid by an enzymatic mechanism similar to that mediating proline oxidation [17, 18, 87]. The pyrroline product is then converted to 4-erythro-hydroxy-L-glutamate by an NAD-dependent dehydrogenase [87], and hydroxyglutamate is subsequently transaminated with oxalacetate, forming 3-hydroxy-2-oxoglutarate [88]. Here, the parallelism with proline ends; hydroxy-oxoglutarate is cleaved to form 2-carbon and 3-carbon fragments. Thus, the final intermediates of hydroxyproline catabolism are glyoxylate and pyruvate [89], whereas that for proline is oxoglutarate. Despite the similarities in reaction mechanisms for the degradation of the two imino acids, the analogous reactions are catalyzed by distinct enzymes, with one notable exception [90]: A single enzyme catalyzes the dehydrogenation of both pyrroline-5-carboxylate and pyrroline-3-hydroxy-5-carboxylate [91]. The common dehydrogenase may explain the presence of both proline and hydroxyproline metabolites in the urine of patients with deficiency of this enzyme in type II hyperprolinemia [92].

A relatively minor degradative pathway for hydroxyproline occurs through the formation of pyrroline-4-hydroxy-2-carboxylic acid by L-amino acid oxidase. This pyrroline compound is spontaneously converted to pyrrole-2-carboxylic acid, which can be found in the urine of patients with enzyme deficiencies in the major degradative pathway.

3-Hydroxyproline Metabolism

Knowledge of 3-hydroxyproline metabolism is still limited because of its infrequent occurrence in collagen and difficulties in detection and quantification [18]. 3-Hydroxyproline occurs at relatively high levels in basement membrane collagens (20 to 25 residues of 3-hydroxyproline per 1000 residues) [93]. In interstitial collagens, it occurs at extremely low frequencies (e.g., one residue of 3-hydroxyproline in type Iα1 chains of calf collagen) [94]. Formation of 3-hydroxyproline results from posttranslational hydroxylation of proline, analogous to he formation of 4-hydroxyproline [95, 96]. The 3-hydroxyproline reaction appears to occur only on the second residue of the Gly-Pro-Hyp sequence in all collagen types [93], and presumably it can occur only after the third residue has been 4-hydroxylated [97]. The possible structural functions of 3-hydroxyproline in collagen are unknown, although its limitation to specific Gly-Pro-Hyp triplets in collagens [18] suggests that 3-hydroxylation is much more specific than 4-hydroxylation. Cofactor requirements are similar for the 3- and 4-prolyl hydroxylases [98], but they appear to be separate enzymes. The ratio of the two activities differs in a number of animal tissues [99], the sensitivity to inhibitors and 4-prolyl hydroxylase antibodies varies [98], and prolyl-3-hydroxylase activity has been selectively increased by purification from rat kidney [100].

The release of 3-hydroxyproline residues from collagen and subsequent degradation of free 3-hydroxyproline have not been fully characterized. Following injection of [14C]3-hydroxyproline into rats, 65 percent of the label appeared as CO_2 and only 5 percent appeared in the urine after 48 h, consistent with an active degradation system [101]. In rat kidney slice experiments, [14C]proline was identified as a product, but intermediates and other products have not been identified [101].

3-Hydroxyproline is, for the most part, limited to basement membrane collagen. Accordingly, the 3-hydroxyproline/4-hydroxyproline ratio in tissues has been used to estimate the ratio of basement membrane collagen to total collagen [102–

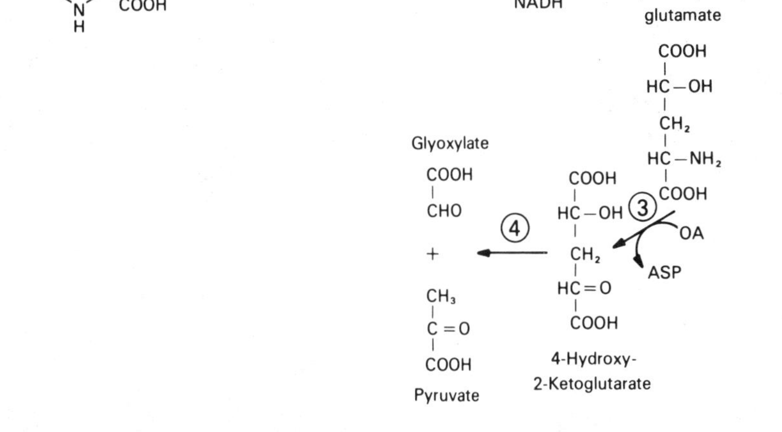

Figure 18-5   The pathways for the degradation of 4-hydroxy-L-proline in mammalian tissues. Major pathway: Although reaction 1 is analogous to that for proline oxidation, it is catalyzed by an enzyme distinct from that for proline [18]. Reaction 2, however, is catalyzed by a dehydrogenase common to the hydroxyproline and proline pathways [91]. The enzymes and their enzyme classification are: (1) hydroxy-L-proline oxidase (EC number not assigned); (2) Δ^1-pyrroline-3-hydroxy-5-carboxylate dehydrogenase (EC 2.6.1.12); (3) glutamic-aspartic acid aminotransferase probably (EC 2.6.1.1); and (4) 4-hydroxy-2-oxoglutaric acid lyase (EC 4.1.3.16). Minor pathway: Reaction 5 is catalyzed by L-amino acid oxidase, and reaction 6 is spontaneous. Pyrrole-2-carboxylic acid is found in the urine of patients with a defective major pathway (type II hyperprolinemia).

104]. The measurement of 3-hydroxyproline excretion in urine may be useful as a selective index of basement membrane collagen turnover. Two studies [105, 106] provide similar data for 24-h urinary 3-hydroxyproline excretion in normal adults (1.6 to 1.8 mg/24 h) but markedly different values in children. Another study describes elevated urinary excretion of peptides which probably contain 3- and 4-hydroxyproline in three children with oligopeptiduria [107]. As more information is accumulated about the distribution of 3-hydroxyproline in different collagens, and about the factors influencing its degradation and excretion in both peptide-bound and free forms, urinary excretion data may prove to be a valuable probe of the turnover of specific collagen species.

Distribution of Imino Acids in Body Fluids

Free Proline The normal concentration of proline in human plasma is between 0.1 and 0.45 mM [108]; values are lower in the rodent [109]. The average concentration is at the lower end of the range during the period of growth in children and is higher in the mature subject. Beyond early infancy there is virtually no proline in normal urine. Neonatal iminoglycinuria is a normal phenomenon; postnatal prolinuria is due to immaturity of the tubular transport systems for proline reclamation (see Chap. 81). The concentration of proline in cerebrospinal fluid is negligible (0 to 4.2 μmol/liter) [108]; the normal plasma: cerebrospinal fluid proline ratio exceeds 300. Proline is present in human amniotic fluid at an unchanging low concentration throughout pregnancy.

Free Hydroxyproline Only about one-fifth to one-quarter of plasma hydroxyproline is in the free form [110]. The age-dependent pattern of hydroxyproline excretion in urine parallels that of proline (see Chap. 81). Hydroxyproline is a negligible constituent of other body fluids.

Urinary Imino Acids in the Bound Form There is a large literature on the urinary excretion of peptide-bound hydroxyproline and proline [6, 112]. The ratio of urinary total proline: total hydroxyproline ("total" meaning free plus bound imino acid fractions) rises from an average of about 1.2 in childhood to about 2.4 in adults [113].

During periods of rapid growth (infancy and adolescence), peptide-bound hydroxyproline excretion is increased (Table 18-1) and reflects the enhanced rate of endogenous collagen turnover [112]. Free hydroxyproline excretion does not change concordantly at such times.

A wide variety of proline-containing oligopeptides is present in normal urine [113]. The predominant hydroxyproline-containing peptides are prolylhydroxyproline and glycylprolylhydroxyproline, which account for about 60 to 75 percent of the bound hydroxyproline excretion [112]. The latter accounts for 96 percent of the total hydroxyproline excretion in urine in the period beyond early infancy [114].

Membrane Transport of the Imino Acids

A brief résumé is given here for interpretation of the findings in hyperprolinemia, hydroxyprolinemia, and disorders of iminopeptide metabolism. Membrane transport of the free imino acids is described in detail in Chap. 81.

Free Imino Acids L-Proline and hydroxy-L-proline are taken up by tissues on stereo-specific, energy-coupled, substrate-specific membrane transport systems. These systems have been documented in detail for kidney (Chap. 81) and fetal bone [118, 119]. The former tissue highlights the nature of epithelial transport of the imino acids; the latter delineates how imino acids permeate tissues committed to collagen synthesis. Proline interacts competitively with hydroxyproline and glycine on a common membrane carrier, which serves their uptake preferentially at concentrations in excess of 0.1 mM. In kidney, and probably in bone as well, there is a second system, preferentially used by imino acids at concentrations of solute below 0.1 mM, that excludes glycine. The latter exhibits age-specific variation in activity in human kidney, being inactive at birth and maturing to full activity only during the first 100 days of life [108].

Proline [120] and hydroxyproline [121] both exhibit maximum rates of renal tubular absorption (Tm) in humans. The Tm_{Pro} is between 180 and 300 μmol/(min·1.73 m^2) and the Tm_{Hypro} is between 60 and 135 μmol/(min·1.73 m^2). The venous plasma threshold (concentration) at which prolinuria occurs is about 0.8 mM proline, and for hydroxyprolinuria it is

Table 18-1 Urinary excretion of imino acid-containing peptides on gelatin-free diets (per 24 h)

Hydroxyproline excretion*		Imino acid peptide excretion ratio†	
Age, yr	Hydroxyproline,‡ mg/(24 h·m^2) (±2 SD from mean)	Age, yr	Total Pro/total Hypro ratio (mean)
0–12 mo	40–191	1–4	1.28
1–2	40–121	4–9	1.21
2–10	34–93	8–12	1.31
11–14	40–113	12–16	1.39
18–21	13–28	16–20	1.58
22–65	9–23	20–40	2.13
>65	7–20	40–60	2.55

* Data of Kivirikko and Laitinen [115], Laitinen et al. [116], and Uitto et al. [117].
† Data of Nusgens and Lapiere [113].
‡ Data are for total (bound + free) hydroxyproline, which after the first 3 months of life is >95 percent peptide-bound for age-dependent excretion; data uncorrected for surface area (see Kivirikko [112]).

about 0.4 mM hydroxyproline. At the normal plasma concentration of the two imino acids, which is well below these levels, the urine is free of imino acids in healthy adults. A "combined" hyperaminoaciduria occurs at concentrations of the specific imino acid above the threshold level. As either imino acid proceeds to saturate its renal transport system, competitive inhibition of the transport of the other imino acid and of glycine occurs. Analogous observations have been made by Finerman et al. [118, 119] for bone. These workers also observed that collagen synthesis in fetal bone could be inhibited significantly when the extracellular concentration of hydroxyproline was sufficiently elevated (to 0.2 mM or more) to inhibit the transport of L-proline [at a quasiphysiologic concentration (0.14 mM) in the medium] and thus to deplete the intracellular concentration of the latter.

Peptide-linked Imino Acids Imino acids in oligopeptides are transported by systems independent of those used by the free imino acids. Rubino et al. [122] and Ganapathy et al. [123] described a typical dipeptide-serving mechanism used by glycylproline in the intestine. There is no interaction between this dipeptide and the respective free imino acid transport systems. Whereas dipeptide membrane systems operate efficiently under the conditions of intestinal absorption, their ability to reclaim imino acid-containing peptides from urine is poor in kidney. This may reflect the character of their activity in kidney as compared with intestine as well as a relative dearth of peptide hydrolysis activity in kidney epithelium. Proline-containing dipeptides are cleared into urine at high rates in humans [124], and the same is true of the hydroxyproline-containing oligopeptides [125]. The discrepancy between the efficiency of free imino acid reclamation and the inefficiency of peptide reabsorption largely accounts for the proportionately large peptide fraction in human urine (>95 percent of the total imino acid excretion).

THE HYPERPROLINEMIAS

Clinical Phenotypes

Nineteen families containing one or more members with hyperprolinemia are known to the authors (Table 18-2). On the basis of the findings in these families and pedigrees, the hyperprolinemia trait can be divided into two forms: type I hyperprolinemia, caused by deficient proline dehydrogenase (oxidase) activity, and type II hyperprolinemia, caused by deficient Δ^1-pyrroline-5-carboxylic acid dehydrogenase activity.

Type I Hyperprolinemia This trait has come to attention in several probands during investigation of renal disease. This was the case for the original proband in pedigree A and also in pedigrees B, C, E, H, and K. Coincidental association of renal disease with hyperprolinemia has persuaded casual observers that hyperprolinemia may offer an explanation for some forms of nephropathy. That this association is unlikely on clinical grounds alone should be apparent from the diversity of associated renal problems in the various probands and their relatives: an Alport-like syndrome and congenital hypoplasia in pedigree A; the nephrotic syndrome in proband B; congen-

ital ureteral obstruction and uremia in proband C; Wilm's tumor in proband E; Alport's syndrome in the H pedigree; obstructive uropathy in proband H; and pyelonephritis in proband K. A variety of other clinical diagnoses are reported in probands: ocular dystrophia in proband S, seizures in probands A, I, and K; and mental retardation in probands A, C, E, I, P, and Q.

Bias in ascertainment of associated hyperprolinemia probably accounts for the unwarranted assumption that hyperprolinemia and renal disease have a cause-and-effect relationship. Although it is not generally the case in uremia [154, 155], some types of renal disease might perturb proline metabolism. Renal parenchyma plays a significant role in proline uptake and metabolism in the mammal [109, 156, 157]. But to propose that hyperprolinemia is secondary to loss of renal parenchyma is to state the common clinical misconception in reverse. Moreover, the Pro/Re mouse with proline-oxidase deficiency (see below) has no abnormality of renal structure or function [158].

Genetic evidence is even more compelling than the clinical data against any association between hyperprolinemia and renal disease in type I hyperprolinemia. The original case report [127] was careful to delineate and stress the independent segregation of the dominantly inherited gene causing an Alport-like syndrome with nephropathy and the apparently recessive allele responsible for the hyperprolinemia (Fig. 18-6). Nonetheless, that report launched the popular misconception. So much for perspicacity among readers of the article. Claims of a correlation between "hyperprolinemia" and renal disease are still found in the literature [159, 160]. Care was not taken to prove that hyperprolinemia was actually present in the "probands" of these reports. Only "iminoglycinuria" was described, and iminoglycinuria may occur for many reasons other than hyperprolinemia.

Two lines of evidence firmly impugn any consistent relationship between an abnormality of proline oxidation and clinical disease. The first (pedigrees B, E, K, J, K, P, and Q) notes that sibs and relatives of probands are found who have hyperprolinemia without clinical abnormalities (Table 18-2). Conversely, there are relatives in these and other pedigrees who have clinical findings but do not have hyperprolinemia. The second line of evidence is found in pedigrees J and N, where routine metabolic screening led coincidentally to the diagnosis of hyperprolinemia in the probands. Subsequent investigation revealed that they and numerous hyperprolinemic relatives were healthy. The latter evidence has now been reiterated many times in newborn screening programs [161].

Type II Hyperprolinemia The probands in pedigrees D, F, G, and L came to medical attention because of neurologic symptoms that included retarded mental development and seizures. Probands M, O, and R had no significant clinical illness. Hyperprolinemia has been observed in otherwise healthy sibs in pedigrees F and R. Proline is a constituent of brain metabolism [162], but an interdependence between normal metabolism of proline and normal brain function remains to be proven. Cerebrospinal fluid proline is elevated in type II hyperprolinemia [147], as it is in type I hyperprolinemia [129], where CNS manifestations are less prevalent. Since the plasma: cerebrospinal fluid proline ratio is probably not diminished in hyperprolinemia, the change in cerebrospinal fluid proline may reflect primarily the change in plasma proline [108]. In sum-

Table 18-2 The hyperprolinemia pedigrees (types I and II)

Pedigree	Reference	Presumed type*	Age at diagnosis, yr	Sex	Plasma Proline, mM†
A	Scriver et al. [126] Schafer et al. [127]	I	5	M	0.67
B	Kopelman et al. [128]	I(?)	13	M	0.51[a]
C	Efron [129]	I	33	M	1.15–1.8
E	Perry et al. [130]	I	3	M	0.79–1.26
H	Goyer et al. [131]	I(?)	14	F	0.81
I	Piesowicz [132] Harries et al. [133]	I	6/12	M	2.2–2.6
J	Fontaine [134] Fontaine et al. [135]	I	9/12	F	0.72–1.0
K	Woody et al. [136]	I	3/12	M	1.3–1.85[b]
N	Mollica et al. [137]	I	20/12	F	1.07
P	Dodinval et al. [138] Haimaut et al. [139]	I	23/12	M	0.7–1.05
Q	Potter & Waickman [140]	I	1	M	1.75
S	Fusco et al. [152]	I	13	M	1.05
D‡	Berlow & Efron [141] Efron [142, 143] Selkoe [144]	II	19/22	M	3.7
F	Similä & Visakorpi [145] Similä [146]	II	6/12	M	3.5
G	Emery et al. [147]	II	18	F	1.75–2.6
L	Jeune et al. [148]§	II	4/12	M	0.47–1.2
M	Goodman [149]; Goodman et al. [92]; Valle et al. [50]	II	9	F	1.65
O	Applegarth et al. [150, 151]	II	5	M	2.75
R	Pavone et al. [153]	II	10	F	2.68

* Type I = block at proline oxidase; type II = block at Δ^1 pyrroline-5-carboxylic acid (PC) dehydrogenase: ? = PC excretion not mentioned; presumed that defect is type I.
† Normal values (range) for all ages, infant to adult; 0.1–0.45 mM [108]. Results obtained by quantitative analysis by elution chromatography on ion-exchange resin columns, except in pedigrees B and K (a, b), where direct chemical methods were used for proline analysis.

mary, we and others [93, 135, 137, 140, 151, 152] believe that the hyperprolinemias are benign conditions.[1]

Biochemical and Enzymatic Phenotypes

Type I Hyperprolinemia The level of hyperprolinemia rarely exceeds 2 mM in type I probands (Table 18-2, Fig. 18-7). This fact is important for comparison with the biochemical phenotype of type II hyperprolinemia.

Type I hyperprolinemia reflects a block in the degradation of proline. Since P5C does not accumulate in the blood or urine of these patients, hyperprolinemia should be the result of deficient proline dehydrogenase (oxidase) activity. A single report [129] on the assay of proline oxidation in a type I hyperprolinemia proband supports this hypothesis.

[1] An instance of asymptomatic hyperprolinemia was discovered incidentally in a proband and her sister during investigation of hypophosphatasia in the proband. The serum proline level in the two sibs was about 0.9 mM. Type I hyperprolinemia was presumed to be the diagnosis. The heterozygous type I phenotype was not excluded. (DeVries HR, Duran M, DeBree PK, Wadman SK: A patient with hypophosphatasia and hyperprolinemia. *Neth J Med* 21:28, 1978.)

Liver from propositus C (Table 18-2) was obtained at autopsy approximately 1 h post mortem [129]. The tissue was homogenized according to the method of Adams and Goldstone [87], incubated with L-proline and 4-hydroxy-L-proline, and assayed for production of Δ^1-pyrroline-5-carboxylic acid and Δ^1-pyrroline-3-hydroxy-5-carboxylic acid measured by the o-aminobenzaldehyde reaction [23]. Other aliquots were incubated with L-[14C]proline and labeled DL-hydroxyproline, and the recovery of [14C] in isolated glutamic acid and γ-hydroxyglutamic acid was measured. The results, when compared with 23 control human liver samples, indicated reduced proline oxidation [0.016 to 0.036 absorbance units at 440 cm (mean value, 0.025) compared to 0.093 to 1.6 absorbance units at 440 nm (mean value, 0.665) in control liver]. Conversion of proline to glutamate was estimated to be no more than 10 percent of normal in the patient. The combined results clearly indicated that degradation of proline to glutamic acid through the pyrroline intermediate was deficient in the patient with type I hyperprolinemia. The block was placed at the first step of proline degradation, that is, in the production of Δ^1-pyrroline-5-carboxylate from proline [129].

Since there was considerable variation in the proline oxidase

Table 18-2 The hyperprolinemia pedigrees (types I and II) *(Continued)*

Associated biochemical and clinical features

In probands			In relatives			
Renal disease	Mental retard.	Seizures or Abn. EEG	Cosanguine parents	Proline defect (alone)	Clinical disease (alone)	Proline defect and clinical disease
+	+	+	0	0	19	3
+	0	0	?	2	(1)?	1
+	+	0	0	0	5	3
+	+	0	+	5	3	5
+	0	0	+	0	10	2
0	+	+	0	2	0	0
0	0	0	0	6	0	0
+	—	+	+	4	Many	3
0	0	0	0	6	0	0
0	+	+	0	1	0	2
0	+	0	?	5	0	0
0	+	0	0?	1	5	3
					(= Ocular dystrophia)	
0	+	+	0	0	0	0
0	+	+	+	0	?	1**
0	+	+	+	0	0	(1)?
0	+	+	0	0	0	1
0	0	0	0	0	0	0
0	0	0¶	0	0	0	0
0	0	0	+	2	0	0

‡ An additional patient with type II hyperprolinemia and convulsions is mentioned by Efron [143]; the details on this appear to be equivalent to those presented by Selkoe [144].

§ A coexistent leucine transaminase defect in propositus caused hyperleucine-isoleucinemia. Thus the patient has a double aminoacidopathy.

¶ One seizure with fever at 2 years of age; EEG mildly abnormal at 13 years, suggesting epileptic disorder without localizing features.

** Mildly abnormal EEG only; otherwise normal.

activity of the control patients in this study [129], in both the biopsy and autopsy specimens, it was not possible to document the presumed heterozygous phenotype in liver biopsy material obtained from the father of proband C.

The oxidation of hydroxyproline was normal or near normal in the liver of proband C with type I hyperprolinemia [129]. This important observation indicates that "proline oxidase" and "hydroxyproline oxidase" enzymes are not identical in humans. The fact that human brain has proline oxidase but no hydroxyproline oxidase activity further suggests that the respective catalytic activities are different [129, 181].

Of additional interest in the studies of Efron [129] was evidence that [^{14}C]-labeled proline yields [^{14}C]-labeled glutamate in human liver (and kidney) in accordance with the degradative pathways proposed for mammalian systems (Fig. 18-3).

Future studies in human subjects will depend on parenchymal tissues as a source of enzyme since proline oxidase is not present in skin fibroblasts or blood leukocytes. Performance of the assay should recognize recent advances that delineate two components in the oxidase system [18, 163].

Type II Hyperprolinemia   Hyperprolinemia is greater in the type II trait than in type I. With few exceptions, patients with the former condition have plasma proline concentrations in excess of 1.5 mM (Fig. 18-7). Plasma hydroxyproline is not increased in type II hyperprolinemia.

Type II hyperprolinemia reflects a block at the second step of proline catabolism catalyzed by Δ^1-pyrroline-5-carboxylic acid dehydrogenase. Probands with this type of hyperprolinemia excrete Δ^1-pyrroline-5-carboxylic acid at all times [92, 142, 144, 146, 151, 152] in addition to very large amounts of proline. The amount of pyrroline substance excreted is approximately 40 times normal, while that of proline is several hundred times normal.

An o-aminobenzaldehyde-reacting pyrroline derivative of hydroxyproline is present in the urine of type II probands. This material has been identified as Δ^1-pyrroline-3-hydroxy-5-carboxylic acid [92, 164, 165]. The observation is interesting. It suggests that the deficient enzyme in type II hyperprolinemia is common to proline and hydroxyproline degradation. Goodman et al. [92] and Similä [165] examined hydroxyproline clearance from blood after giving an oral load of 4-hydroxy-L-proline (100 mg/kg) to control subjects and type II probands. The subsequent clearance of hydroxyproline from blood was

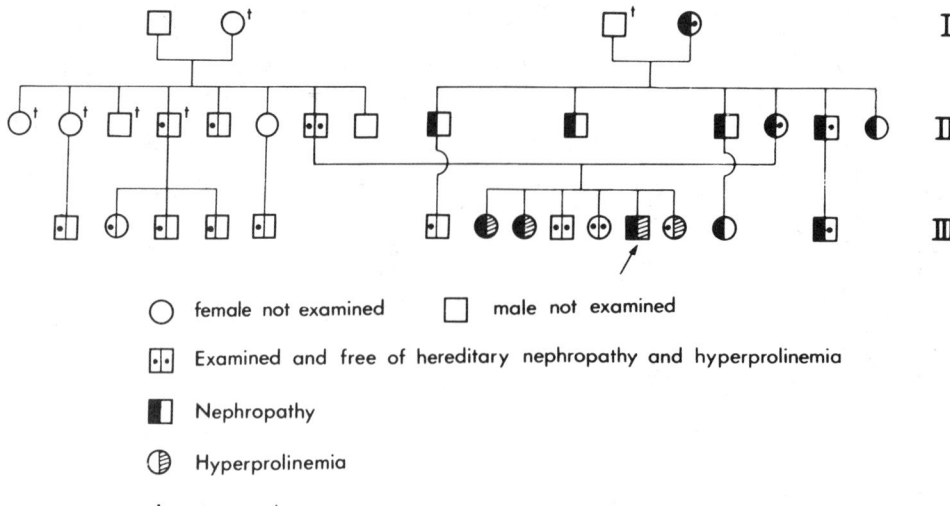

○ female not examined   □ male not examined

⊡ Examined and free of hereditary nephropathy and hyperprolinemia

◧ Nephropathy

◔ Hyperprolinemia

† deceased

Figure 18-6 Abbreviated pedigree of proband A with type I hyperprolinemia, showing dominant inheritance of familial nephropathy and apparent autosomal recessive inheritance of the hyperprolinemia. Clinical and genetic evidence suggests that there is no cause-and-effect relationship between the hyperprolinemia and the nephropathy. (*Redrawn from [127], with permission.*)

markedly attenuated, resembling that observed in hydroxyprolinemia itself (see below). The excretion of Δ^1-pyrroline-3-hydroxy-5-carboxylate increased after the loading test. The amount in urine under these conditions rose to 300 times the excretion rate observed in normal subjects following a comparable load of hydroxyproline [92, 165].

The enzyme defect in type II hyperprolinemia has been demonstrated in vitro [50, 90, 91]. Valle and colleagues [50, 90] measured the activity of the dehydrogenase in cultured skin fibroblasts from three probands (D, M and O, Table 18-2). Type II hyperprolinemia skin fibroblasts and leukocytes completely lack Δ^1-pyrroline-5-carboxylate dehydrogenase activity. Ornithine-δ-transaminase and Δ^1-pyrroline-5-carboxylate reductase activities are normal. Valle and colleagues [91] later showed that Δ^1-pyrroline-3-hydroxy-5-carboxylate dehydrogenase activities are equally deficient in type II probands. Heterozygotes have partial deficiency of both dehydrogenase activities in leukocytes and fibroblasts [50, 90]. These findings delineate the enzyme defect in type II hyperprolinemia and confirm that the second step in their degradative pathways is shared by proline and 4-hydroxyproline. The fact that plasma hydroxyproline is not increased in type II hyperprolinemia indicates that the shared dehydrogenase does not play the same role in regulating the free proline and hydroxyproline pools.

Mechanism of Hyperprolinemia

An interesting distinction between the two forms of hyperprolinemia remains to be clarified, i.e., that proline accumulation in plasma is greater in type II hyperprolinemia. Applegarth et al. [151] and Similä [166] observed that the major metabolite accumulation behind the block in type II hyperprolinemia is proline and not Δ^1-pyrroline-5-carboxylate. Ornithine is diverted to the pyrroline metabolite and then to proline in type II hyperprolinemia [165, 167]. Moreover, the ornithine pool may actually be increased in type II hyperprolinemia [92]. Nevertheless, the finding does not explain the disproportionate accumulation of proline. It follows that the pyrroline compound must be preferentially converted to proline in type II hyperprolinemia. Peisach and Strecker [30] and Valle et al. [50] have observed that the total activity of Δ^1-pyrroline-5-carboxylate reductase in liver is greater than that of proline

oxidase. Moreover, the K_m value of the former is lower than that of the latter (2×10^{-4} and 2×10^{-3} M, respectively). Therefore, in the presence of sufficient NADH, the steady-state equilibrium will favor proline formation from the pyrroline intermediate, rather than the reverse.

Mechanism of the Hyperaminoaciduria in Hyperprolinemia

Hyperaminociduria in the hyperprolinemia trait is specific and comprises an "iminoglycinuria" (proline, hydroxyproline, and glycine) (Fig. 18-8). When the plasma proline concentration exceeds 0.8 mM, which is the venous plasma threshold value for generating hyperprolinuria [126], the intensity of the iminoglycinuria is directly proportional to the degree of hyperprolinemia.

Hyperprolinuria results from progressive saturation of the proline reabsorption sites in the renal tubule. Prolinuria thus occurs by an "overflow" mechanism [120, 168]. At the same time, glycine and hydroxyproline are displaced from a site shared by the three substrates through competitive inhibition of the system by proline [120, 168]. The coexistence of overflow and competitive mechanisms in the generation of the characteristic iminoglycinuria of hyperprolinemia suggested the term *combined hyperaminoaciduria* to classify its origin [120, 168]. Hyperprolinemia was the first hereditary aminoacidopathy for which this mechanism of hyperaminoaciduria was demonstrated in humans.

The Pro/Re Mouse: An Animal Model of Type I Hyperprolinemia

There are few nonhuman vertebrate models of human inborn errors of amino acid metabolism [169, 170]. The Pro/Re mouse [157, 158, 163, 171, 172] with hyperprolinemia and hyperprolinuria is one of these. Residual hepatic proline dehydrogenase (oxidase) activity is < 10 percent of control strains [163, 172]. Loss of proline oxidase activity represents expression of an autosomal allele at the locus designated *pro-1* for control of component-1 activity in the proline dehydrogenase complex of the inner mitochondrial membrane [163]. Residual activity in Pro/Re tissue represents intact component 2 of proline dehydrogenase [163]. The component-2 activity might derive from hydroxyproline oxidase with activity for proline [18]. F_1 hybrid mice have intermediate hepatic enzyme activity and a normal or elevated endogenous proline concentration in blood [158, 163, 171]. Since proline oxidase activity in the kidney and brain of Pro/Re mice is also deficient, the disturbance of tissue proline metabolism is probably generalized.

The residual hepatic activity in Pro/Re mice is comparable to that in human liver in type I hyperprolinemia [129]. The defect in proline oxidation in Pro/Re is located at the step corresponding to type I hyperprolinemia in humans; urinary excretion of Δ^1-pyrroline-5-carboxylic acid is normal in both mutant counterparts. Thus Pro/Re mouse and human traits appear to be homologous in their effects on proline metabolism. No abnormalities of renal morphology are apparent in the mouse [158].

Three interesting features of proline metabolism have been delineated in the Pro/Re mutant. First, steady-state proline oxidation in kidney cortex slices is still substantial [157] and probably is due to component-2 proline dehydrogenase activ-

ity. Less than 4 percent of residual enzyme activity sustains about 20 percent of the normal rate of proline oxidation of physiologic concentrations of substrate (about 0.1 mM proline in extracellular fluid). The principal site of proline oxidation in kidney coincides with its major site of reabsorption. Second, proline oxidation rates increase toward normal at higher proline concentrations [173]. Since renal uptake of proline is normal [157], the finding indicates some compensation for the effect of the mutant allele by normal expression of the second locus controlling component-2 activity. Third, urinary excretion of proline in vivo is far in excess of that expected from the level of proline in plasma. Intracellular proline in Pro/Re kidney cortex is elevated about fourfold [157]. Whereas uptake of proline in vitro is not altered by the mutation in kidney cortex slices [157], reclamation of proline from urine in vivo is impaired. In this instance, the block in proline metabolism influences net proline reabsorption through its effect on the intracellular pool of proline which, in its expanded state, enhances the unidirectional backflux at the luminal membrane. The proline that leaks into the moving column of urine cannot be reclaimed and appears in bladder urine. The Pro/Re mutation thus reveals that intracellular metabolic "runout" of an amino acid, under normal conditions, assists its tubular reclamation and will influence the rate of net reabsorption [157, 173]. (This concept is discussed in further detail in Chap. 81.)

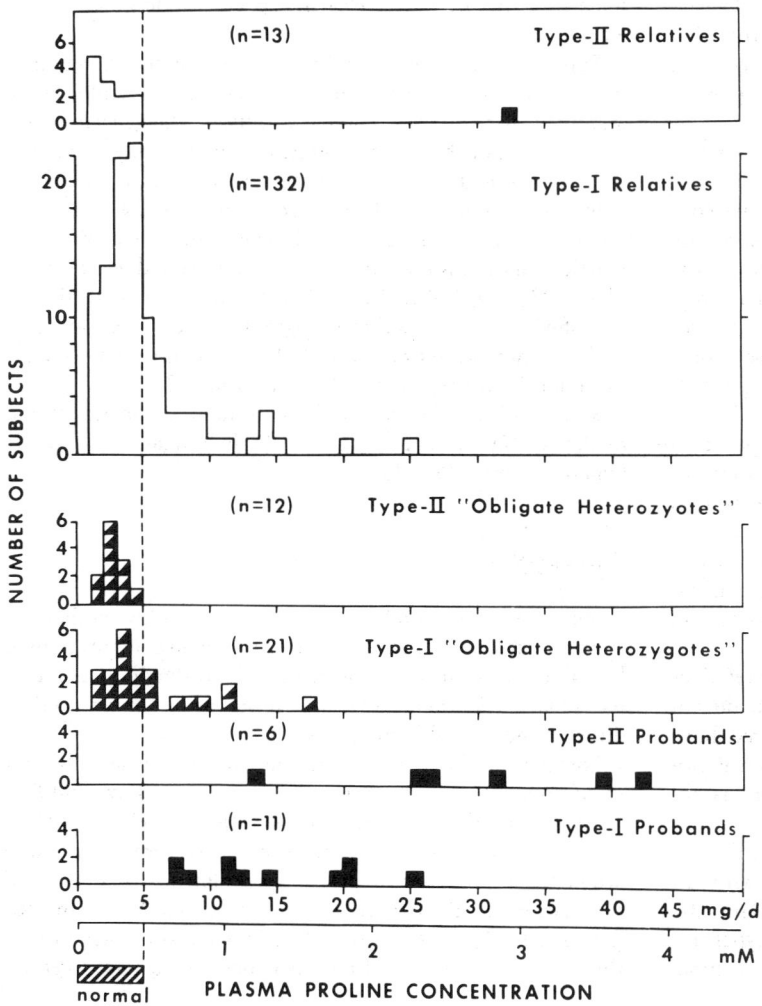

Figure 18-7 Distribution diagram of plasma proline concentration in type I and type II hyperprolinemia probands, their parents ("obligate heterozygotes," assuming autosomal recessive inheritance), and relatives of probands. (Data compiled from all reports cited in Table 18-2. Thirty-seven additional subjects in the type I pedigree K [136], whose plasma proline concentrations all fell in the normal range, are not included on the graph.)

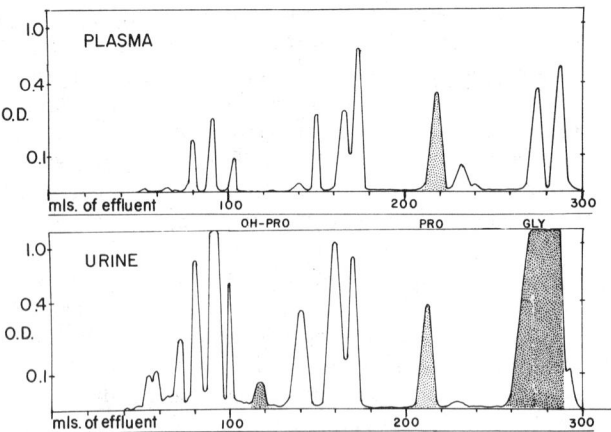

Figure 18-8 Profile of amino acids in plasma and urine of proband A (with type I hyperprolinemia) [126, 127] following elution chromatography on an ion-exchange resin column. The specific hyperaminoaciduria (hydroxyproline, proline, and glycine) is initiated by the elevated plasma proline concentration and reflects a "combined" mechanism comprising partial saturation of proline reabsorption leading to "overflow" prolinuria and competitive inhibition of hydroxyproline and glycine reabsorption on a common carrier in the presence of excess proline [120].

Genetics of the Hyperprolinemias

Type I and type II hyperprolinemia are the result of alleles at different genetic loci, because different enzymes are involved in the two traits. Both traits are inherited in autosomal recessive fashion. Consanguine matings have been identified in parents of type I and type II probands (Table 18-2).

Classification of the presumed phenotype (and genotype) is relatively easy in type II hyperprolinemia. Probands and sibs with hyperprolinemia (usually in excess of 1.5 mM) are considered to be homozygotes. The parents of the subjects are "obligate heterozygotes" but do not have endogenous hyperprolinemia (Fig. 18-7). These individuals experience mild hyperprolinemia only under conditions of an exogenous proline load [146]. Nonhyperprolinemic relatives of type II probands are considered to be either normal homozygotes or heterozygotes.

The situation is far less clear among relatives of type I probands because parents of these subjects can have hyperprolinemia (Fig. 18-8). The median plasma proline concentration of obligate heterozygotes is elevated above the normal mean value, and 9 of 21 type I parents have hyperprolinemia. There are six fathers (pedigrees E, H, I, J, K, and N) and three mothers (pedigrees I, K, and N) with hyperprolinemia. Among 132 relatives of type I probands, 35 have hyperprolinemia (Fig. 18-7). Since the data exclude 37 nonhyperprolinemic relatives described in pedigree K, and because all close and distant relatives in whom the plasma proline was measured have been combined in the graph, the segregation fraction is not meaningful, other than to indicate that the frequency is abnormal.

Is type I hyperprolinemia a dominantly inherited trait with incomplete penetrance? Type I probands K and I, with the highest recorded plasma proline concentrations (1.85 and 2.06 mM, respectively), are the offspring of parents with hyperprolinemia. On the other hand, probands C and O, with compa-

rable hyperprolinemia (1.8 and 1.75 mM, respectively), are the children of nonhyperprolinemic parents. Since numerous matings between individuals carrying a rare dominant allele are unlikely, it is reasonable to propose that type I hyperprolinemia is an autosomal recessive trait (Fig. 18-6) in which some heterozygotes exhibit hyperprolinemia for reasons that are not yet understood.

Is it possible that the hyperprolinemic and nonhyperprolinemic heterozygotes with the type I hyperprolinemia gene have different alleles? This hypothesis is not supported by data from consanguine matings (pedigrees F, H, and K). Only in pedigree K do the parents have the same phenotype (hyperprolinemia), while in pedigrees E and H, the consanguine parents have different phenotypes.

Diagnosis

Type I hyperprolinemia (> 0.45 mM; Ref. 108) is identified by the presence of persistent hyperprolinemia. The attendant finding of iminoglycinuria is dependent on the degree of hyperprolinemia and is not an obligatory feature of the phenotype. Δ^1-Pyrroline-5-carboxylate is not excreted in urine of type I subjects. Standard chemical methods and partition and ion-exchange elution chromatographic methods for the identification of proline are available (see previous editions). The preferred method is quantitative ion-exchange chromatography. Diagnosis is dependent on the demonstration of hyperprolinemia: hyperprolinuria is a nonspecific finding (see Chap. 81).

Type II hyperprolinemia is distinguished by the excretion of Δ^1-pyrroline-5-carboxylate in urine. This compound may be identified by the yellow color it produces when reacted with o-aminobenzaldehyde (0.5 percent weight/volume) and trichloroacetic acid (5 percent volume/volume) in alcohol. A 2-ml volume of o-aminobenzaldehyde reagent is mixed with a 1-min volume of urine diluted to 2 ml. The optical density of this reaction mixture is read at 440 nm and corrected for the urine blank [23, 129, 174]. Δ^1-Pyrroline-5-carboxylate may also be identified by partition chromatography followed by location with acid ninhydrin or isatin [23]. Discrimination between Δ^1-pyrroline-5-carboxylate and Δ^1-pyrroline-3-hydroxy-5-carboxylic acid can be achieved by column chromatographic methods [92] and is advisable in the investigation of type II hyperprolinemia [92, 151].

Therapy

Proline is a nonessential amino acid that is readily synthesized from precursors (Fig. 18-2). Nearly all protein contains proline [lactalbumin is an exception (175)]. Accordingly, one anticipates that dietary management by protein restriction would be difficult and probably ineffective.

Fortunately, the hyperprolinemias can be considered benign conditions that do not warrant treatment (see above and Ref. 176). In a particularly cogent observation, Whelan and Connors [177] have studied the outcome of two pregnancies in a woman with untreated type I hyperprolinemia; neither child was harmed by the maternal hyperprolinemia. Where investigators [132, 133, 143, 166, 178, 179] have attempted dietary therapy of the type I and type II hyperprolinemias, a certain degree of biochemical control was achieved and no apparent harm attended the "treatment," but no control of associated disease was apparent either.

It is interesting that dietary therapy can reduce proline accumulation at all. This finding suggests that endogenous proline synthesis is not sufficient to support its total requirement, particularly in young infants [133, 166]. The question may be raised of whether proline is a limiting amino acid during rapid growth.

(HYPER)HYDROXYPROLINEMIA

Clinical Phenotype

Hydroxyprolinemia is a metabolic disorder characterized by the accumulation of free 4-hydroxyproline to high levels in plasma. *Hyperhydroxyprolinemia* is a more accurate term, since hydroxyproline is a normal constituent of blood plasma, usually present at low levels (< 0.01 mM). Clinical evidence from probands and sibs suggests that the condition is harmless [180–188].

The disorder was first reported [180–182] in a retarded white American female, age 12 years, whose mother was also retarded. The father of the proband was believed to be an uncle. There were no other significant clinical findings. Unusual events associated with collagen metabolism affecting, for example, skin turgor, wound healing, and hernias, were not apparent in the patient's medical history.

The second proband [183, 184] was a Finnish woman, age 31 years, who came to medical attention because of a large nodular goiter. Studies of urinary hydroxyproline excretion in thyroid disease [112] led to the discovery of an excessive amount of free hydroxyproline in the patient's urine. During investigation of the pedigree, her healthy brother was discovered to have excessive hydroxyproline excretion. He was assumed to be hyperhydroxyprolinemic, but his plasma hydroxyproline concentration has not been reported [184].

The third proband [185, 186] was an English girl who had been investigated for mental retardation, hyperactivity, and abnormal behavior. Hyperhydroxyprolinemia was discovered in the course of biochemical investigations in the sixth year of life.

A fourth proband has been reported from India [187]. The patient was a male child, age 8 years, whose hydroxyprolinemia was identified in the course of routine investigation of mental retardation and behavioral disturbance. The patient's severe retardation (DQ about 20) may have resulted from a difficult perinatal course. The parental relationship was consanguine.

The fifth proband [188] was diagnosed at 51 years of age. She had had meningitis at 15 months, retarded development thereafter, and was admitted for custodial care at age 30 years. Incidental investigations revealed hyperhydroxyprolinemia (0.23 mM). Investigation of the family revealed elevated plasma hydroxyproline (0.25 mM) in an older sister whose only medical problem was recurrent eczema.

This limited clinical experience suggests that the association between hydroxyprolinemia and mental retardation that attracted attention in the first instance [180] occurred by chance. When a search for hydroxyprolinemia is made among retarded patients and yields probands with hydroxyprolinemia, it will, of course, confirm the association of hydroxyprolinemia with mental retardation. On the other hand, the discovery of coincidental hydroxyprolinemia in healthy persons [183, 184] disputes such an association. We also have the evidence that hydroxyprolinemia coincidentally discovered by newborn screening [161] behaves as a benign condition on long-term follow-up. On present evidence, it seems reasonable to accept the opinion that hydroxyprolinemia is probably a benign biochemical trait [184, 189].

Biochemical Phenotype

In Plasma The 4-hydroxyproline concentration in plasma is elevated more than fifteenfold above the normal range. Values in probands have been recorded over the range of 0.14 to 0.5 mM (normal < 0.01 mM). The concentration of other amino acids in plasma is normal in the trait. The erythrocyte hydroxyproline pool is also increased above normal [188].

In Cerebrospinal Fluid Cerebrospinal fluid hydroxyproline is not elevated in hydroxyprolinemia.

In Urine Urinary free hydroxyproline is greatly elevated. Excretion rates from 285 to 550 mg/24 h have been reported in three subjects ranging in age from 12 to 31 years [181, 184]. These values are greatly elevated, only trace amounts being found in the urine of normal subjects in the same age range. Renal reabsorption of free hydroxyproline exhibits normal saturability in hyperhydroxyprolinemic subjects [188]. Excretion of peptide-bound hydroxyproline (about 25 to 40 mg/24 h) by subjects with hydroxyprolinemia is normal [181, 182, 184], and the peptide excretion pattern is also normal [182]. However, the bound hydroxyproline fraction expressed in relation to total hydroxyproline in urine is diminished; the fraction is > 0.95 in normal subjects, whereas it is < 0.15 in the hydroxyprolinemia trait [181, 184].

Assuming that the block in free hydroxyproline oxidation is complete in hydroxyprolinemia, the urinary excretion data imply that about 90 percent of hydroxyproline released during collagen turnover is degraded by the free hydroxyproline pathway in the normal state. This flux represents the metabolism of at least 2 g or more of collagen daily under normal circumstances [112, 182, 184]. Estimates that fall in this range, and up to 5 g per day, have been derived from the study of proline peptide excretion in prolidase deficiency.

Metabolic Studies

4-Hydroxyl-L-proline loading (100 to 200 mg/kg by mouth) causes plasma hydroxyproline to rise higher in subjects with hydroxyprolinemia than in control subjects and to remain at elevated levels long after the loading procedure [181, 184, 188]. Up to 50 percent of the hydroxyproline is excreted directly into urine in the 24-h period after the load [184, 188]. Examination of urine for o-aminobenzaldehyde-reacting material prior to and after the load reveals no increase in the excretion of material corresponding to Δ^1-pyrroline-3-hydroxy-5-carboxylic acid in hydroxyprolinemia [181, 184, 188]. Excretion of such material after a hydroxyproline load characterizes the normal subject (Fig. 18-9). The rise in plasma proline after a load of L-proline (100 mg/kg by mouth) is normal in hydroxyprolinemia [181]. Pyrrole-2-carboxylic acid is excreted following the ingestion of allohydroxy-D-proline (3mg/kg) in hydroxyprolinemia [181]. These studies indicate that proline metabolism and D-amino acid oxidase activity (allohydroxyproline preferring) are both normal in hydroxyprolinemia. Pyrrole-2-carboxylate is excreted in increased amounts in hyperhydroxyprolinemia [190]. The source of this metabolite is the labile intermediate Δ^1-pyrroline-4-hydroxy-2-carboxylate [37] (viz. Fig. 18-5). This pathway may dispose of any hydroxyproline accumulating in type II hyperprolinemia [165].

3-Hydroxyproline metabolism is not perturbed in the hyperhydroxyprolinemia phenotype [105].

Hyperhydroxyprolinemia provides an opportunity to examine biosynthesis of this imino acid in humans. Labeling of urinary free hydroxyproline has been measured [182] following intravenous infusion of [1-^{14}C]glyoxylate. Small amounts of labeled hydroxyproline, 4-hydroxyglutamate, and 4-hydroxy-2-oxoglutarate (accounting in all for <0.2 percent of the administered radioactivity) were excreted in the 24-h period after the infusion. According to these results, a slight biosynthesis from glyoxylate may occur in humans. In view of the difficulties encountered in the attempt to demonstrate significant hydroxyproline synthesis with rat liver in vitro [191], it is difficult to know whether the human data provide any real insight into its synthesis in humans. The minimal transfer of label to hydroxyproline following an intravenous pulse of [^{14}C]glyoxylate could have occurred by an indirect route, such as the cycling of label through proline and collagen pools, with subsequent release of hydroxyproline. Labeling of the peptide hydroxyproline pool in urine was not studied in order to examine this possibility. Adams [6] has interpreted the studies of

Efron and colleagues [182] as evidence against significant biosynthesis of free hydroxyproline through reversal of the degradative pathway in humans.

Probable Nature of the Enzyme Defect in Hydroxyprolinemia

Tissue enzyme studies have not been reported in hydroxyprolinemia. The absence of Δ^1-pyrroline-3-hydroxy-5-carboxylate from urine of subjects with the trait [181, 184] and the failure to sustain the normal formation of this substance, and other metabolites in the main degradative pathway after loading with 4-hydroxy-L-proline [181, 188], places the presumed enzyme defect at the oxidation step converting 4-hydroxy-L-proline to Δ^1-pyrroline-3-hydroxy-5-carboxylic acid. Since proline metabolism is clearly normal [143] in the hydroxyprolinemia trait, it is likely that "proline oxidase" and "hydroxyproline oxidase" are independent catalytic activities. Additional evidence for this conclusion is found in the absence of hydroxyproline oxidase activity in mammalian brain cortex and cerebellum, both of which contain proline oxidase activity [129, 181].

Iminoaciduria in Hyperhydroxyprolinemia

Free hydroxyproline excretion is increased and its endogenous renal clearance is also elevated in the trait [181, 184, 188]. These findings are expected when the filtered load of hydroxyproline is elevated sufficiently to initiate saturation of its tubular transport systems [121, 168].

Renal clearance of proline and glycine is not abnormal in patients with hydroxyprolinemia [181, 184]. Although hydroxyproline, proline, and glycine share a common reabsorp-

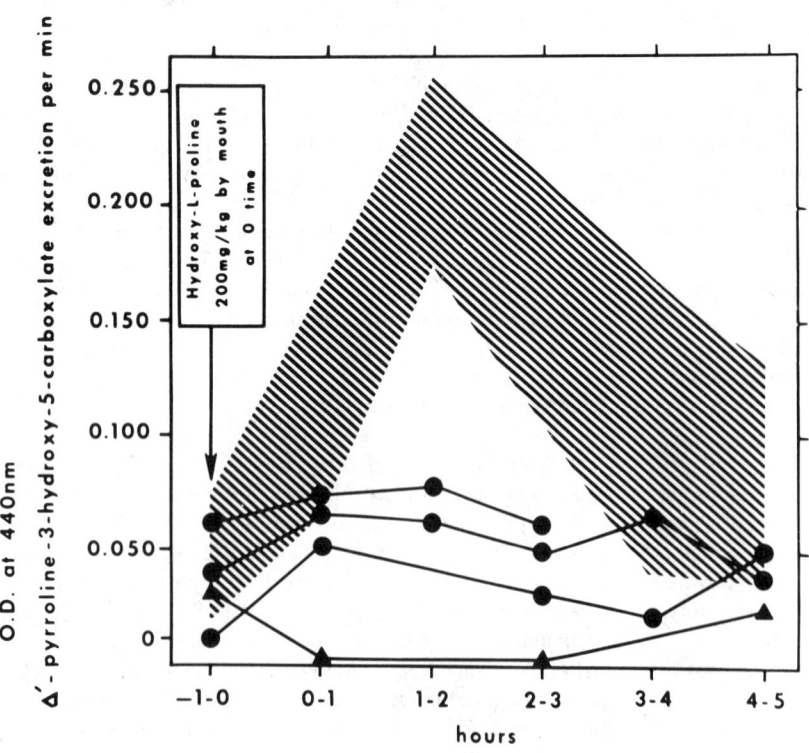

Figure 18-9 Excretion of Δ^1-pyrroline-3-hydroxy-5-carboxylate in urine by normal subjects (shaded area, $n = 13$) and by proband A (o—o) [181], studied three times, and proband B (Δ—Δ) [184] before and after receiving a hydroxyproline load (200 mg per kilogram of body weight orally). The results are presented as optical density readings for 1-min aliquots of urine from timed (1 to 2 h) collections. The urine sample was adjusted to a final volume of 2.0 ml (by dilution or evaporation); 2.0 ml of o-aminobenzaldehyde reagent was added [181], and the OD at 440 nm was measured to estimate the pyrroline content of the sample.

tion system and the clearance rates of hydroxyproline and glycine are usually increased in hyperprolinemia, the lack of evidence for competitive inhibition of proline and glycine reabsorption in hydroxyprolinemia is to be expected. The steady-state plasma concentration of hydroxyproline should exceed 0.4 mM before such inhibition occurs [121]. The endogenous hydroxyproline concentration has rarely exceeded this threshold value in the hydroxyprolinemia trait. Actually, it is rather surprising that hydroxyproline was ever found in urine in such excess, when the customary plasma concentrations ranged from 0.18 to 0.4 mM in the first three reported subjects [181–186]. The explanation for hydroxyprolinuria in hydroxyproline oxidase deficiency may depend in part on a defect in the renal metabolism of hydroxyproline. Oxidation of free hydroxyproline is prominent in normal mammalian kidney [39, 87], and the free hydroxyproline content of normal mammalian kidney cortex is negligible [181a]. Therefore a block in renal oxidation of hydroxyproline, leading to an elevated concentration of intracellular free hydroxyproline in tubular epithelium, could come to inhibit the net reabsorptive capacity by enhancing undirectional backflux into urine across the luminal membrane (see "The Pro/Re Mouse: An Animal Model of Type I Hyperprolinemia" above and Chap. 81).

Genetics

Apparent consanguinity in parents and appearance of the trait in both sexes and among sibs of probands suggest that the condition is autosomal recessive. There is no reason to suspect that the condition is not inherited.

Parents of probands do not have an elevated endogenous hydroxyproline concentration in plasma [181, 184, 188]. Clearance of hydroxyproline from plasma after a loading test is delayed in the heterozygote [188]. A presumably heterozygous 2-year-old child of the affected brother of the second proband [184] excreted more hydroxyproline in the free form (16.5 to 18 percent of the total) than is normal (< 5.2 percent; Ref. 116). Although the possibility of renal iminoglycinuria (see Chap. 81) was not ruled out in this subject, the original interpretation of the finding is of interest [184]. The investigators drew attention to the known attenuation of hydroxyproline oxidation in the postnatal period [192] and speculated that a heterozygote with only one normal allele for hydroxyproline oxidase activity might be compromised during infancy and thus might show a change in the composition of total urinary hydroxyproline. Six older and presumably obligate heterozygotes of the same pedigree had normal hydroxyproline excretion patterns [184].

Diagnosis

Diagnosis of hyperhydroxyprolinemia should be obtained on the blood sample. When the plasma hydroxyproline concentration is not greatly elevated, urine hydroxyproline may not be prominent because of the high venous plasma threshold that determines its escape in urine. Measurement of hydroxyproline in body fluids is possible with a variety of chemical and chromatographic methods (see previous editions). Quantitative analysis is reliably obtained by elution chromatography on an ion-exchange column.

The presence of hydroxyprolinuria does not constitute a diagnosis of hydroxyprolinemia. The former is a normal finding in the infant for at least 3 months after birth [108]. It is also a component of the urinary phenotype in hyperprolinemia (see above) and in renal iminoglycinuria (see Chap. 81). Hydroxyprolinemia of a modest degree (up to 0.1 mM) and exaggerated hydroxyprolinuria are normal findings in the postnatal period [192, 193]. Studies on the excretion of intermediates in the oxidation pathway of free hydroxyproline (Fig. 18-5) have yet to be done in the immature subject in seeking to identify the effect of impaired oxidation. Examination of the peptide pattern and of the peptide-bound/free hydroxyproline excretion ratio by appropriate methods will also clarify the nature of the disordered hydroxyproline metabolism in the hydroxyprolinemia phenotype.

Therapy

A correlation between hydroxyprolinemia and clinical disease has not been demonstrated. The prospect for therapy for this trait is not encouraging [143, 181, 182, 185], nor is it indicated. A diet free of hydroxyproline does not lower the concentration of hydroxyproline in body fluids. Since collagen breakdown is the principal endogenous source of free hydroxyproline, extracellular hydroxyproline will not be lowered by dietary limitations or manipulation of its renal excretion [185, 186] in hydroxyprolinemia.

PROLIDASE DEFICIENCY WITH HYPERIMIDODIPEPTIDURIA

Imino acid-containing dipeptides are released during collagen degradation. Two enzymes, prolidase and prolinase, cleave the soluble dipeptides. Prolidase (imidodipeptidase, EC 3.4.13.9) splits imidodipeptides with C-terminal proline or hydroxyproline residues. About one-quarter of the peptide bonds of collagen are imido bonds. Prolinase (iminodipeptidase, EC 3.4.13.8) splits N-terminal imino acids from dipeptides.

Prolidase acts only on imido bonds, which lack a hydrogen atom on the nitrogen forming the peptide linkage. The enzyme requires that the amino and carboxyl groups be free [194]. Prolidase is widely distributed in tissues and can be assayed readily in leukocytes, erythrocytes, and intestinal mucosa. The enzyme is believed to play an important role in the intestinal absorption of the imino acid-containing portion of dipeptides. Oligopeptides comprise a major fraction of the nitrogen absorbed from dietary protein [195].

Following the initial reports of a patient with probable prolidase deficiency (proband A) [196, 197], two other patients with proven prolidase deficiency were described [probands B (198, 199) and C (200)], and at least eight additional subjects with proven or suspected prolidase deficiency have been reported [113, 200–205] (Table 18-3). Proband F is described in the original reports [113, 202] as a "probable case or protocollagen proline hydroxylase deficiency." That patient is included here because the diagnosis of prolidase deficiency seems more reasonable.

Clinical Phenotype

A clinical syndrome is apparent in prolidase deficiency (Table 18-3). Chronic dermatitis, recurring leg ulcers, splenomegaly, characteristic facial features (viz. fig. 1, Ref. 196), and mental retardation are the most common findings. The dermatitis includes crusting erythematous lesions on the face, soles, and palms, an ecchymotic or fine purpuric rash, and chronic leg ulcers. The craniofacial features include prominent skull sutures, ptosis of the eyelids, and ocular proptosis. Mental retardation (IQ/DQ values, 45 to 90) was present in probands A, B, and D. Additional features include recurrent infections of the upper and lower respiratory tracts, joint laxity, waddling gait, protuberant abdomen, odd posture, and mild osteoporosis of the long bones. On histologic examination of the spleen [196], there is a widening of the cords of Billroth, swelling of sinusoidal lining cells, and thickening of arteriolar walls. Goodman and colleagues [196] used the term *lathyritic* to characterize the syndrome. The clinical signs are not obligatory manifestations of prolidase deficiency because at least two subjects (in pedigrees H and I, Table 18-3) are symptomless.

Biochemical Phenotype

Peptiduria   There is a characteristic massive increase in the excretion of imino acid-containing peptides. The proline/hydroxyproline peptide excretion ratio is significantly elevated relative to age-specific control data (Table 18-3). Characterization of the urinary dipeptides [197, 198, 201, 205] reveals an X-Pro pattern, i.e., an imidodipeptiduria. The X residue may be any one of many different amino acids, including aspartic acid, threonine, serine, proline, glutamate, glycine, alanine, valine, isoleucine, leucine, tyrosine, and phenylalanine among the major constituents. Glycylproline comprises one-fifth of the total proline-containing dipeptides excreted.

The excretion of peptide-bound hydroxyproline is also increased, but less strikingly than the excretion of proline peptides. The hydroxyprolinuria persists even when patients are examined on gelatin-free diets. Following the ingestion of a gelatin load, hydroxyproline peptide excretion is abnormally augmented [199] and comprises between 39 and 47 percent of the hydroxyproline in the load. By comparison, normal subjects excrete only about 6 percent of such a load as hydroxyproline-containing peptides. Imidopeptiduria is also prolonged for many hours after the gelatin load in patients with prolidase deficiency when compared with the normal response.

These findings with respect to imidodipeptide metabolism are compatible with a deficiency of prolidase activity in all tissues, including the intestinal epithelium. The observations deriving from gelatin feeding indicate that imidodipeptide uptake from the intestinal lumen proceeds even in the absence of intracellular imidodipeptidase activity. This is in keeping with the belief that the transport phase and the cleavage activity, both of which determine absorption of imino acid-containing peptides, are independent events [122–124].

Table 18-3   The prolidase deficiency syndrome with hyperimidodipeptiduria

Proband (reference)	Age (yr)	Sex	Fa	D	Sk	Sp	In	MR	Proline μmol/24 h (mg 24h)	Hypro μmol/24 h (mg 24h)	Pro/Hypro ratio (mg/mg)	Prolidase activity, % of control
A 196, 197	48	M	+	+	+	+	0	+/−	27,500 (3150)	2,130 (278)	11.4	Not assayed
B 198, 199	7	M	+	+	?	+	+	+/−	15,342 (1760)	5624;4660 (733;608)	2.4	0–7 (WBC) 0–2 (RBC)
C 199	? (Child)	F	+	+	?	+	+	?		1,620 (211)		"Deficient" (serum; WBC)
D 200	3¼	F	+	+	+	+	+	+	5170 (595)	840 (N) (110) (N)	5.4	<2 (RBC)
E 201	22	M	?	+	?	?	?	?			25.2	Not assayed
F 113, 202	? Adult	M	?	+	?	?	?	?	23,900 (2725)	1,205 (205)	13.3	Not assayed
G 203		M	?	+	?	?	?	+				
H	(Older sister)			+					↑	↑		0 (RBC) 0 (WBC)
204	6	F	0	0	0	0	0	0	↑	↑	↑	0 (RBC) 4 (WBC)
I	23	F		+					1.92	0.21	9.1	3 (RBC)
205	26	M	0	0	0	0	0	0	~1.3	~0.1	↑	6 (RBC)

* Key: Fa, typical facial features (see fig. 1, Ref. 196); D, dermatitis; Sk, skeletal and tendenous abnormalities; Sp, splenomegaly; In, frequent infections; MR, retarded mental development (see text for description).
† Imino acids in bound fraction, determined by hydrolysis. All values are abnormally high except the Pro/Hypro peptide excretion ratio in proband D. (N = normal for age). Normal values for hydroxyproline excretion are given in Table 18-1. The urinary peptide proline/peptide hydroxyproline ratio does not exceed 3.0 at any age and is below 2.0 up to late puberty [113].

Renal handling of N-terminal proline dipeptides is inefficient [124, 196], and the clearance rate of these substrates is high. Goodman et al. [196] found the renal clearance rates for glycylproline to be far in excess of the glomerular filtration rate in their patient with prolidase deficiency. On the other hand, the dipeptide clearance rate did not exceed the glomerular filtration rate in another patient with glycylprolinuria caused by metabolic bone disease [124], in whom prolidase activity was probably normal. Since dipeptides can be taken up from the blood at the antiluminal surface of tubular epithelium [206], it is possible that glycylproline appears in urine in prolidase deficiency, not only from the glomerular filtrate from which it is poorly reclaimed but also by leakage across the brush border from tubular epithelium, where it has escaped hydrolysis after uptake and has thus gained an elevated intracellular concentration.

The Enzyme Defect

Prolidase activity can be measured in erythrocytes or leukocytes. In prolidase deficiency the residual activity is less than 6 percent of normal (Table 18-3). Prolinase activity is normal. Symptomless patients do not necessarily have greater residual prolidase activity. The addition of purified prolidase enzyme to the urine of proband A permitted cleavage of the imidopeptides that were present in excess in the sample [197].

Genetics

Normal sex distribution, occurrence of the disorder in sibs (pedigrees H and I, Table 18-3), and consanguinity (pedigree I) are compatible with autosomal recessive inheritance.

The presumed heterozygotes do not have abnormal imidopeptide excretion [199], but prolidase activity in erythrocytes and leukocytes of presumed heterozygotes is about half normal [198, 204, 205].

Comment

A calculation of the collagen turnover required to sustain the degree of peptiduria observed in probands [197, 199, 200] yields estimates ranging from about 1 g/day for proband D ($3\frac{1}{4}$ years old) to 6 g/day in proband B (7 years), with an intermediate value of about 4.5 g/day in proband A (48 years). These values exceed the estimates (2 g/day) based on hydroxyproline excretion referred to above [6, 112, 182].

The prevalence of respiratory tract infection in prolidase-deficient subjects may be related to a change in the Clq complement factor which contains collagenlike amino acid sequences [85]. This component of complement has not been studied in prolidase deficiency. Jackson and colleagues [200] have interpreted the prolidase deficiency syndrome as a reflection of impaired recycling of collagen amino acids. Ubiquitous intracellular prolidase would be an essential end-stage component in the cellular recycling of collagen that can reclaim 90 to 95 percent of collagen proline [207]. Prolidase deficiency would block the normal reclamation of imido-linked imino acids and could thus alter the equilibrium of collagen metabolism.

OTHER IMINOACIDOPATHIES

A report [208] in Polish described type I hyperprolinemia in a $3\frac{1}{2}$ year-old female proband who presented with pneumonia and renal disease. Four of her nine sibs and her father had pyuria and hematuria, and two of them and the proband also had slight hyperprolinuria. The authors state that the proband had hyperprolinemia (32.5 μg/ml or 0.28 mM), as did one sib and the father. The proline value for the proband, while just outside the age-specific normal range recorded by the authors, is normal by other standards [108]. The Polish report is not included in the bibliography on hyperprolinemia until further information is available.

Another report [209] described a proband with hyperdicarboxylicaminoaciduria and mild fasting hyperprolinemia (0.4 to 0.9 mM).

The parents and four sibs had normal proline values. The hyperprolinemia was considered to be coincidental, with no apparent relationship to the renal transport abnormality affecting glutamate and aspartate.

REFERENCES

1. EASTOE JE: Composition of collagen and allied proteins, in Ramachandran GN (ed): *Treatise on Collagen I. Chemistry of Collagen.* New York, Academic Press, Inc, 1967, p 1
2. OGLE JD: ARLINGHAUS RB, LOGAN MA: 3-Hydroxy-proline, a new amino acid of collagen. *J Biol Chem* 237:3667, 1962
3. PERUTZ MF, KENDREW JC, WATSON HC: Structure and function of haemoglobin II. Some relations between polypeptide chain configuration and amino acid sequence. *J Mol Biol* 13:669, 1965
4. HARRINGTON WF, VON HIPPEL PH: The structure of collagen and gelatin. *Adv Protein Chem* 16:1, 1961
5. SZENT-GYORGYI AG, COHEN C: Role of proline in polypeptide chain configuration of proteins. *Science* 126:697, 1951
6. ADAMS E: Metabolism of proline and hydroxyproline. *Int Rev Connect Tissue Res* 5:1, 1970
7. SNELL EE: Chemical structure in relation to biological activity of vitamin B_6. *Vitam Horm* 16:77, 1958
8. WILLIAMS MA: Vitamin B_6 and amino acids—Recent research in animals. *Vitam Horm* 22:561, 1964
9. CARDINALE GJ, ABELES RH: Purification and mechanism of action of proline racemase. *Biochemistry* 7:3970, 1968
10. ADAMS E, NORTON IL: Purification and properties of inducible hydroxyproline 2-epimerase from Pseudomonas. *J Biol Chem* 239:1525, 1964
11. KREBS, HA: The oxidation of d (+) proline by d-amino acid oxidase. *Enzymologia* 7:53, 1939
12. RADHAKRISHNAN AN, MEISTER A: Conversion of hydroxyproline to pyrrole-2-carboxylic acid. *Biol Chem* 226:559, 1957
13. CORRIGAN JJ, WELLNER D, MEISTER A: Determination of D-amino acid oxidase activity in insect tissues using D-allohydroxyproline as substrate. *Biochim Biophys Acta* 73:50, 1963
14. NAKAMO M, DANOWSKI TS: Crystalline mammalian L-amino acid oxidase from rat kidney mitochondria. *J Biol Chem* 241:2075, 1966
15. BLANCHARD M, GREEN DE, NOCITO V, RATNER S: L-Amino acid oxidase in animal tissue. *J Biol Chem* 155:421, 1944
16. KREBS HA: The metabolic fate of amino acids, in Munro HN, Allison JB (eds): *Mammalian Protein Metabolism.* New York, Academic Press, Inc, 1964, vol 1, p 125
17. STETTEN MR: Metabolic relationship between glutamic acid, proline, hydroxyproline and ornithine, in McElroy WD, Glass B (eds): *Amino Acid Metabolism.* Baltimore, Johns Hopkins University Press, 1955, p 277
18. ADAMS E, FRANK L: Metabolism of proline and the hydroxyprolines. *Ann Rev Biochem* 49:1005, 1980
19. SALLACH HJ, KOEPPE RE, ROSE WC: The in vivo conversion of glutamic acid into proline and arginine. *J Am Chem Soc* 73:4500, 1951
20. VOGEL HJ, DAVIS BD: Glutamic acid γ-semialdehyde and Δ¹-pyrroline-5-carboxylic acid, intermediates in the biosynthesis of proline. *J Am Chem Soc* 74:109, 1952
21. ROSS G, DUNN D, JONES ME: Ornithine synthesis from glutamate in rat

intestinal mucosa homogenates: Evidence for the reduction of glutamate to γ-glutamyl semialdehyde. *Biochem Biophys Res Commun* 85:140, 1978

22. SMITH RJ, DOWNING SJ, PHANG JM, LODATO RF, AOKI TT: Pyrroline-5-carboxylate synthase activity in mammalian cells. *Proc Natl Acad Sci USA* 77:5221, 1980

23. STRECKER HJ: The interconversion of glutamic acid and proline I. The formation of Δ¹-pyrroline-5-carboxylic acid from glutamic acid in *Escherichia coli*. *J Biol Chem* 225:825, 1957

24. BAICH A: Proline synthesis in *Escherichia coli*. A proline-inhibitable glutamic acid kinase. *Biochim Biophys Acta* 192:462, 1969

25. BAICH A: The biosynthesis of proline in *Escherichia coli*. Phosphate-dependent glutamate γ-semialdehyde dehydrogenase (NADP), the second enzyme in the pathway. *Biochim Biophys Acta* 244:129, 1971

26. HAYZER DJ, MOSES V: The enzymes of proline biosynthesis in *Escherichia coli*. Their molecular weights and the problem of enzyme aggregation. *Biochem J* 173:219, 1978

27. KRISHNA RV, LEISINGER T: Biosynthesis of proline in *Pseudomonas aeruginosa*. *Biochem J* 181:215, 1979

28. KRISHNA RV, BEILSTEIN P, LEISINGER T: Biosynthesis of proline in *Pseudomonas aeruginosa*. Properties of γ-glutamyl phosphate reductase and 1-pyrroline-5-carboxylate reductase. *Biochem J* 181:223, 1979

29. HERZFELD A, MEZL VA, KNOX WE; Enzymes metabolizing Δ¹-pyrroline-5-carboxylate in rat tissues. *Biochem J* 166:95, 1977

30. PEISACH J, STRECKER HJ: The interconversion of glutamic acid and proline: V. The reduction of Δ¹-pyrroline-5-carboxylic acid to proline. *J Biol Chem* 237:2255, 1962

31. SMITH ME, GREENBERG DM: Preparation and properties of partially purified glutamic semialdehyde reductase. *J Biol Chem* 226:317, 1957

32. PERAINO C, PITOT HC: Ornithine-δ-transaminase in the rat. I. Assay and some general properties. *Biochim Biophys Acta* 73:222, 1963

33. PERAINO C: Functional properties of ornithine-ketoacid aminotransferase from rat liver. *Biochim Biophys Acta* 289:117, 1972

34. SMITH RJ, PHANG JM: The importance of ornithine as a precursor for proline in mammalian cells. *J Cell Physiol* 98:475, 1979

35. SMITH RJ, PHANG JM: Proline metabolism in cartilage: The importance of proline biosynthesis. *Metabolism* 27:685, 1978

36. SMITH RJ, REDDI AH, PHANG JM: Changes in proline synthetic and degradative enzymes during matrix-induced cartilage and bone formation. *Conn Tissue Res* 27:275, 1979

37. HEACOCK AM, ADAMS E: Formation and excretion of pyrrole-2-carboxylic acid. Whole animal and enzyme studies in the rat. *J Biol Chem* 250:2599, 1975

38. GREENBERG DM: Pyrroline-5-carboxylate reductase. *Methods Enzymol* 5:959, 1962

39. TAGGART JV, KRAKAUR RB: Studies on the cyclophorase system: V. The oxidation of proline and hydroxyproline. *J Biol Chem* 177:641, 1949

40. JOHNSON AB, STRECKER HJ: The interconversion of glutamic acid and proline: IV. The oxidation of proline by rat liver mitochondria. *J Biol Chem* 237:1876, 1962

41. KRAMAR R, FITSCHA P: Studies on the dehydrogenation of proline and hydroxyproline in animal tissues. *Enzymologia* 39:101, 1970

42. MEYER J: Proline transport in rat liver mitochondria. *Arch Biochem Biophys* 178:387, 1977

43. KOWALOFF EM, PHANG JM, GRANGER AS, DOWNING SJ: Regulation of proline oxidase activity by lactate. *Proc Natl Acad Sci USA* 74:5368, 1977

44. STETTEN MR, SCHOENHEIMER R: The metabolism of L-proline studied with the aid of deuterium and isotopic nitrogen. *J Biol Chem* 153:113, 1944

45. KADOWAKI H, PATTON GM, KNOX WE: Proline oxidase inhibition by free fatty acids of rat pancreas. *Biochim Biophys Acta* 614:294, 1980

46. DOWNING SJ, PHANG JM, KOWALOFF EM, VALLE D, SMITH RJ: Proline oxidase in cultured mammalian cells. *J Cell Phys* 91:369, 1977

47. STRECKER HJ: The interconversion of glutamic acid and proline: III. Δ¹-pyrroline-5-carboxylic acid dehydrogenase. *J Biol Chem* 235:3218, 1960

48. ADAMS E, GOLDSTONE A: Hydroxyproline metabolism. IV. Enzymatic synthesis of γ-hydroxyglutamate from Δ¹-pyrroline-3-hydroxy-5-carboxylate. *J Biol Chem* 235:3504, 1960

49. BRUNNER G, NEUPERT W: Localisation of proline oxidase and Δ¹-pyrroline-5-carboxylic acid dehydrogenase in rat liver. *FEBS Lett* 3:283, 1969

50. VALLE DL, PHANG JM, GOODMAN SI: Type II hyperprolinemia: Absence of Δ¹-pyrroline-5-carboxylic acid dehydrogenase activity. *Science* 185:1053, 1974

SMITH RJ, PHANG JM: Proline metabolism in cartilage: The importance of proline biosynthesis. *Metabolism* 27:685, 1978

PHANG JM: The function of pyrroline-5-carboxylate reductase in —ocytes. *Biochem Biophys Res Commun* 94:450, 1980

RRIS SC, PHANG JM: Pyrroline-5-carboxylate reductase in ocytes: A comparison of differential regulation. *J Clin Invest* 81

54. SMITH AD, BENZIMAN M, STRECKER HJ: The formation of ornithine from proline in animal tissues. *Biochem J* 104:557, 1967

55. McGIVAN JD, BRADFORD NM, BEAVIS AD: Factors influencing the activity of ornithine amino-transferase in isolated rat liver mitochondria. *Biochem J* 162:147, 1977

56. STRECKER HJ: Purification and properties of rat liver ornithine-δ-transaminase. *J Biol Chem* 240:1225, 1965

57. VALLE D, KAISER-KUPFER MI, DEL VALLE LA: Gyrate atrophy of the choroid and retina: Deficiency of ornithine aminotransferase in transformed lymphocytes. *Proc Natl Acad Sci USA* 74:5159, 1977

58. TRIJBELS JMF, SENGERS RCA, BAKKEREN JAJM, DE FORT AFM, DEUTMAN AF: L-Ornithine-ketoacid-transaminase deficiency in cultured fibroblasts of a patient with hyperornithinemia and gyrate atrophy of the choroid and retina. *Clin Chim Acta* 79:371, 1977

59. PHANG JM, DOWNING SJ, YEH GC, SMITH RJ, WILLIAMS JA: Stimulation of the hexose-monophosphate pentose pathway by Δ¹-pyrroline-5-carboxylic acid in human fibroblasts. *Biochem Biophys Res Commun* 87:363, 1980

60. PHANG JM, DOWNING SJ, YEH GC: Linkage of the HMP pathway to ATP generation by the proline cycle. *Biochem Biophys Res Commun* 93:462, 1980

61. VALLE D, DOWNING SJ, PHANG JM: Proline inhibition of pyrroline-5-carboxylate reductase: Differences in enzymes obtained from animal and tissue culture sources. *Biochem Biophys Res Commun* 54:1418, 1973

62. KOWALOFF EM, GRANGER AS, PHANG JM: Alterations in proline metabolic enzymes with mammalian development. *Metabolism* 25:1087, 1976

63. KREBS HA: The role of chemical equilibria in organ function, in Weber G (ed): *Advances in Enzyme Regulation*. New York, Pergamon Press, Inc, 1974, vol 13, p 449

64. WALDORF MA, HARPER AE: Metabolic adaptations in higher animals. VIII. Effect of diet on ornithine-α-ketoglutarate transaminase. *Proc Soc Exp Biol Med* 112:955, 1963

65. VOLPE P, STRECKER HJ: Amphi-directional control of a reversible reaction common to two enzyme sequences. *Biochem Biophys Res Commun* 32:240, 1968

66. LYONS RT, PITOT HC: Hormonal regulation of ornithine amino-transferase biosynthesis in rat liver and kidney. *Arch Biochem Biophys* 180:472, 1977

67. HERZFELD A, KNOX WE: The properties, developmental formation, and estrogen induction of ornithine aminotransferase in rat tissues. *J Biol Chem* 243:3327, 1968

68. EAGLE H, WASHINGTON CL, LEVY M: End product control of amino acid synthesis by cultured human cells. *J Biol Chem* 240:3944, 1965

69. SMITH RJ, DOWNING SJ, PHANG JM: Sources of proline in mammalian cells. Regulation of pyrroline-5-carboxylate synthase by ornithine. *Fed Proc* 38:353, 1979

70. KOWALOFF EM, GRANGER AS, PHANG JM: Glucocorticoid control of hepatic proline oxidase. *Metabolism* 26:893, 1977

71. KOWALOFF EM, PHANG JM, GRANGER AS, DOWNING SJ: Glucocorticoid induction of proline oxidase in LLC-RK₁ cells. *J Cell Phys* 97:153, 1978

72. PHANG JM, DOWNING SJ, SMITH RJ, YEH GC: The inhibition of proline oxidase by long-chain fatty acyl-Coenzyme As. *Fed Proc* 37:1480, 1978

73. LUNDGREN DW, OGUR M: Amino acid inhibition of a Δ¹-pyrroline-5-carboxylate dehydrogenase preparation from beef kidney mitochondria. *Biochem Biophys Res Commun* 49:147, 1972

74. FELIG P, OWEN OE, WAHREN J, CAHILL GF JR: Amino acid metabolism during prolonged starvation. *J Clin Invest* 48:584, 1969

75. PHANG JM, YEH GC, HAGEDORN CH: The intercellular proline cycle. *Life Sci* 28:53, 1981

76. SMITH RJ, DOWNING SJ, PHANG JM, LODATO RF, AOKI TT: Pyrroline-5-carboxylate synthase activity in mammalian cells. *Proc Natl Acad Sci USA* 77:5221, 1980

77. REITZER LJ, WICE BM, KENNEL D: The pentose cycle: Control and essential function in HeLa cell nucleic acid synthesis. *J Biol Chem* 255:5616, 1980

78. SMITH ML, BUCHANAN JM: Nucleotide and pentose synthesis after serum stimulation of resting 3T6 fibroblasts. *J Cell Phys* 101:293, 1979

79. HERSHKO A, RAZIN A, MAGER J: Regulation of the synthesis of 5-phosphoribosyl-1-pyrophosphate in intact red blood cells and in cell-free preparations. *Biochim Biophys Acta* 184:64, 1969

80. LE CAM A, FREYCHET P: Effect of catecholamines on amino acid transport in isolated rat hepatocytes. *Endocrinology* 101:379, 1978

81. FEHLMANN M, LE CAM A, FREYCHET P: Insulin and glucagon stimulation of amino acid transport in isolated rat hepatocytes. *J Biol Chem* 254:10431, 1979

82. PROCKOP DJ, BERG RA, KIVIRRIKO KI, UITTO J: Intracellular steps in the biosynthesis of collagen, in Ramachandran GN, Reddi AH (eds): *Biochemistry of Collagen*. New York, Plenum Publishing Corp, 1976

83. CARDINALE GJ, UDENFRIEND S: Prolyl hydroxylase. *Adv Enzymol* 41:245, 1974

84. BENTLEY JP, HANSON AN: The hydroxyproline of elastin. *Biochim Biophys Acta* 175:339, 1969

85. PORTER RR, REID KBM: The biochemistry of complement. *Nature* 275:699, 1978

86. ANGLISTER L, ROGOZINSKI S, SILMAN L: Detection of hydroxyproline in preparations of acetylcholinesterase from the electric organ of the electric eel. *FEBS Lett* 69:129, 1976

87. ADAMS E, GOLDSTONE A: Hydroxyproline metabolism: Enzymatic preparation and properties of Δ^1-pyrroline-3-hydroxy-5-carboxylate. *J Biol Chem* 235:3492, 1960

88. GOLDSTONE A, ADAMS E: Metabolism of gamma-hydroxyglutamic acid. *J Biol Chem* 237:3476, 1962

89. ROSSO RG, ADAMS E: 4-Hydroxy-2-ketoglutarate aldolase at rat liver purification, binding of substrates, and kinetic properties. *J Biol Chem* 242:5524, 1967

90. VALLE D, GOODMAN SI, APPLEGARTH DA, SHIH VE, PHANG JM: Type II hyperprolinemia. Δ^1-Pyrroline-5-carboxylic acid dehydrogenase deficiency in cultured skin fibroblasts and circulating lymphocytes. *J Clin Invest* 58:598, 1976

91. VALLE D, GOODMAN SI, HARRIS SC, PHANG JM: Genetic evidence for a common enzyme catalyzing the second step in the degradation of proline and hydroxyproline. *J Clin Invest* 64:1365, 1979

92. GOODMAN SI, MACE JW, MILES BS, TENG CC, BROWN SB: Defective hydroxyproline metabolism in Type II hyperprolinemia. *Biochem Med* 10:329, 1974

93. GRYDER RM, LAMON M, ADAMS E: Sequence position of 3-hydroxyproline in basement membrane collagen. Isolation of glycyl-3-hydroxyprolyl-4-hydroxyproline from swine kidney. *J Biol Chem* 250:2470, 1975

94. PIEZ KA: Primary structure, in Ramachandran GN, Reddi AH (eds): *Biochemistry of Collagen.* New York, Plenum Publishing Corp, 1976 p 1

95. KAPLAN A, WITKOP B, UDENFRIEND S: Conversion of proline-^{14}C to collagen trans-3-hydroxyproline-^{14}C in the chick embryo. *J Biol Chem* 239:2259, 1964

96. FUJIMOTO D, ADAMS E: Proline incorporation into the proline and hydroxyproline of earthworm-cuticle collagen. *Biochim Biophys Acta* 107:232, 1965

97. RISTELI J, TRYGGVASON K, KIVIRRIKO KI: A rapid assay for prolyl-3-hydroxylase activity. *Anal Biochem* 84:423, 1978

98. RISTELI J, TRYGGVASON K, KIVIRRIKO KI: Prolyl-3-hydroxylase: Partial characterization of the enzyme from rat kidney cortex. *Eur J Biochem* 73:485, 1977

99. TRYGGVASON K, MAJAMAA K, KIVIRRIKO KI: Prolyl-3-hydroxylase and 4-hydroxylase activities in certain rat and chick embryo tissues and age-related changes in their activities in the rat. *Biochem J* 178:127, 1979

100. TRYGGVASON K, RISTELI J, KIVIRRIKO KI: Separation of prolyl-3-hydroxylase and 4-hydroxylase activities and the 4-hydroxyproline requirement for synthesis of 3-hydroxyproline. *Biochem Biophys Res Commun* 76:275, 1977

101. RAMASWAMY SG, CHUNG AC, ADAMS E: Metabolism of 3-hydroxyproline in the rat. *Fed Proc* 39:1790, 1980

102. MAN M, ADAMS E: Basement membrane and interstitial collagen content of whole animals and tissues. *Biochim Biophys Res Commun* 66:9, 1975

103. MAN M, NAGLE RB, ADAMS E: Chemical estimation of interstitial and basement membrane collagen in obstructive nephropathy. *Exp Mol Pathol* 29:144, 1978

104. DEYL Z, MACEK K, ADAM M: Changes in the proportion of collagen Type IV with age—possible role in transport processes. *Exp Gerontol* 13:263, 1978

105. ADAMS E, RAMASWAMY S, LAMON M: 3-Hydroxy-proline content of normal urine. *J Clin Invest* 61:1482, 1978

106. SZYMANOVICZ A, POULIN G, RANDOUX A, BOREL JP: A method for the evaluation of 3-hydroxyproline in the urine. *Clin Chim Acta* 91:141, 1979

107. STEINER W, NIEDERWIESER A: Peptide analysis as amino alcohols by gas chromatography-mass spectrometry. Application to hyperoligopeptiduria. Detection of Gly-3Hyp-4Hyp and Gly-Pro-4Hyp-Gly. *Clin Chim Acta* 92:431, 1979

108. SCRIVER CR, ROSENBERG LE: *Amino Acid Metabolism and Its Disorders.* Philadelphia, WB Saunders Co, 1973

109. MOHYUDDIN F, SCRIVER CR: Amino acid transport in mammalian kidney: multiple systems for imino acids and glycine in rat kidney. *Am J Physiol* 219:1, 1970

110. KIBRICK AC, KITAGAWA G, MASKALERIS ML, GAINES R JR, MILHORAT AT: Hydroxyproline in human blood: forms in which it is present. *Proc Soc Exp Biol Med* 119:622, 1965.

111. ØYE I: The amount of free hydroxyproline in human blood serum. *Scand J Clin Lab Inves* 14:259, 1962

112. KIVIRIKKO KI: Urinary excretion of hydroxyproline in health and disease. *Int Rev Connect Tissue Res* 5:93, 1970

113. NUSGENS B, LAPIERE CH M: The relationship between proline and hydroxyproline urinary excretion in human as an index of collagen metabolism. *Clin Chim Acta* 48:203, 1973

114. MEILMAN E, URIVETZKY MM, RAPOPORT CM: Urinary hydroxyproline peptides. *J Clin Invest* 42:40, 1963

115. KIVIRIKKO KI, LAITINEN O: Clinical significance of urinary hydroxyproline determinations in children. *Ann Paediatr Fenn* 11:148, 1965

116. LAITINEN O, NIKKILÄ EA, KIVIRIKKO KI: Hydroxyproline in the serum and urine. Normal values and clinical significance. *Acta Med Scand* 179:275, 1966

117. UITTO J, LAITINEN O, LAMBERG BA, KIVIRIKKO KI: Further evaluation of the significance of urinary hydroxyproline determinations in the diagnosis of thyroid disorders. *Clin Chim Acta* 22:583, 1968

118. FINERMAN GAM, ROSENBERG LE: Amino acid transport in bone: Evidence for separate transport systems for neutral amino and imino acids. *J Biol Chem* 241:1487, 1966

119. FINERMAN GAM, DOWNING S, ROSENBERG LE: Amino acid transport in bone. II. Regulation of collagen synthesis by perturbation of proline transport. *Biochim Biophys Acta* 135:1008, 1967

120. SCRIVER CR, EFRON ML, SCHAFER IA: Renal tubular transport of proline, hydroxyproline and glycine in health and in familial hyperprolinemia. *J Clin Invest* 43:374, 1964

121. SCRIVER CR, GOLDMAN H: Renal tubular transport of proline, hydroxyproline and glycine. II. Hydroxy-L-proline as substrate and as inhibitor in vivo. *J Clin Invest* 45:1357, 1966

122. RUBINO A, FIELD M, SCHWACHMAN H: Intestinal transport of amino acid residues of dipeptides. I. Influx of the glycine residue of glycyl-L-proline across mucosal border. *J Biol Chem* 246:3542, 1971

123. GANAPATHY V, MENDICINO JF, LEIBACH FH: Transport of glycyl-L-proline into intestinal and renal brush border vesicles from rabbit. *J Biol Chem* 256:118, 1981

124. SCRIVER CR: Glycyl-proline in urine of humans with bone disease. *Can J Physiol Pharmacol* 42:357, 1964

125. BENOIT FL, WATTEN RH: Renal tubular transport of hydroxyproline peptides: Evidence for reabsorption and secretion. *Metabolism* 17:20, 1968

126. SCRIVER CR, SCHAFER IA, EFRON ML: New renal tubular amino acid transport system and a new hereditary disorder of amino acid metabolism. *Nature* 192:672, 1961

127. SCHAFER IA, SCRIVER CR, EFRON ML: Familial hyperprolinemia, cerebral dysfunction and renal anomalies occurring in a family with hereditary nephritis and deafness. *N Engl J Med* 267:51, 1962

128. KOPELMAN H, ASATOOR AM, MILNE MD: Hyperprolinaemia and hereditary nephritis. *Lancet* 2:1075, 1964

129. EFRON ML: Familial hyperprolinemia. Report of a second case, associated with congenital renal malformations, hereditary hematuria and mild mental retardation, with demonstration of an enzyme defect. *N Engl J Med* 272:1243, 1965

130. PERRY TL, HARDWICK DF, LOWRY RB, HANSEN S: Hyperprolinemia in two successive generations of a North American Indian family. *Ann Hum Genet* 31:401, 1968

131. GOYER RA, REYNOLDS J, BURKE J, BURKHOLDER P: Hereditary renal disease with neurosensory hearing loss, prolinuria and icthyosis. *Am J Med Sci* 256:166, 1968

132. PIESOWICZ AT: Hyperprolinaemia. *Arch Dis Child* 43:748, 1968

133. HARRIES JT, PIESOWICZ AT, SEAKINS JWT, FRANCIS DEM, WOLFF OH: Low proline diet in Type-I hyperprolinaemia *Arch Dis Child* 46:72, 1971

134. FONTAINE G: Personal communication, May 1969

135. FONTAINE G, FARNIAUX JP, DAUTREVAUX M: L'hyperprolinémie de Type I. Etude d'une observation familiale. *Helv Paediatr Acta* 25:165, 1970

136. WOODY NC, SNYDER CH, HARRIS JA: Hyperprolinemia: Clinical and biochemical family study. *Pediatrics* 44:554, 1969

137. MOLLICA F, PAVONE L, ANTENER I: Pure familial hyperprolinemia: Isolated inborn error of amino acid metabolism without other anomalies in a Sicilian family. *Pediatrics* 48:225, 1971

138. DODINVAL P, WILLEMS A, HEUSDEN A, HAINAUT H, GOTTSCHALK CH: Clearance rénale des acides aminés chez un enfant hyperprolinémique. *J Génét Hum* 17:297, 1969

139. HAINAUT H, HARIGA J, WILLEMS C, HEUSDEN A, CHAPELLE P: Hyperprolinémie essentielle familale. *Presse Méd.* 79:945, 1971

140. POTTER JL, WAICKMAN FJ: Hyperprolinemia. I. A study of a large family. *J Peds* 83:635, 1973

141. BERLOW S, EFRON ME: A new cause of hyperprolinemia associated with the excretion of Δ^1-pyrroline-5-carboxylic acid. *Proc Soc Pediatr Res, 34th Annual Meeting.* Seattle, 1964, p. 43

142. EFRON ML: Disorders of proline and hydroxyproline metabolism, in Stanbury JB, Wyngaarden JB, Fredrickson DS (eds): *The Metabolic Basis of Inherited Disease,* ed 2. New York, McGraw-Hill Book Co, 1966, p 376

143. EFRON ML: Treatment of hydroxyprolinemia and hyperprolinemia. *Am J Dis Child* 113:166, 1967

144. SELKOE DJ: Familial hyperprolinemia and mental retardation. A second metabolic type. *Neurology* 19:494, 1969

145. SIMILÄ S, VISAKORPI JK: Hyperprolinemia without renal disease. *Acta Paediatr Scand* (suppl.)177:122, 1967

146. SIMILÄ S: Hyperprolinemia Type II. *Ann Clin Res* 2:143, 1970

147. EMERY FA, GOLDIE L, STERN J: Hyperprolinaemia Type II. *J Ment Defic Res* 12:187, 1968

148. JEUNE M, COLLOMBEL C, MICHEL M, DAVID M, GUIBAULT P, GUERRIER G, ALBERT J: Hyperleucinisoleucinémie par défaut partiel de transamination associe à une hyperprolinémie de Type II. Observation familiale d'une double aminoacidopathie. *Semaine Hôp (Ann Pédiatr)* 17:85, 1970

149. GOODMAN SI: Personal communication, November 1970

150. APPLEGARTH DA, INGRAM P, HINGSTON J, STURROCK S, HARDWICK DF: Hyperprolinemia Type II. *Proceedings of the Thirteenth International Congress of Pediatrics,* 1971, vol 5, p 249, 1971

151. APPLEGARTH DA, INGRAM P, HINGSTON J, HARDWICK DF: Hyperprolinemia Type II. *Clin Biochem* 7:14, 1974

152. FUSCO G, CARLOMAGNO S, ROMANO A, RINALDI E, CEDROLA G, CIANCIARUSO L, CURTO A, ROSOLIA S, AURICCHIO G: Type-I hyperprolinemia in a family suffering from aniridia and severe dystrophia of ocular tissues. *Ophthalmologica* 173:1, 1976

153. PAVONE L, MOLLICA F, LEVY HL: Asymptomatic type-II hyperprolinemia associated with hyperglycinaemia in three sibs. *Arch Dis Child* 50:637, 1975

154. CONDON JR, ASATOOR AM: Amino acid metabolism in uraemic patients. *Clin Chim Acta* 32:333, 1971

155. MCGALE THF, PICKFORD JC, ABER GM: Quantitative changes in plasma amino acid uptake with renal disease. *Clin Chim Acta* 38:395, 1972

156. HOLTZAPPLE P, GERD M, REA C, SEGAL S: Metabolism and uptake of L-proline by human kidney cortex. *Pediatr Res* 7:818, 1973

157. SCRIVER CR, MCINNES RR, MOHYUDDIN F: Role of epithelial architecture and intracellular metabolism in proline uptake and transtubular reclamation in PRO/Re mouse kidney. *Proc Natl Acad Sci USA* 72:1431, 1975

158. KANWAR YS, KRAKOWER CA, MANALIGOD JR, JUSTICE P, WONG PW: Biochemical, morphological and hybrid studies in hyperprolinemic mice. *Biomedicine* 22:209, 1975

159. FUHRMANN W: Das syndrome der erblichen Nephrophathie mit Innenohrschwerhörigkeit (Alport-Syndrom). *Dtsch Med Wochenschr* 88:525, 1963

160. ROKKONES T, LØKEN AC: Congenital renal dysplasia, retinal dysplasia and mental retardation associated with hyperprolinuria and hyper-OH-prolinuria. *Acta Paediatr Scand* 57:225, 1968

161. LEVY HL: Genetic screening, in Harris H, Hirschhorn K (eds): *Advances in Human Genetics.* New York, Plenum Publishing Corp, 1973, vol 4, p 1

162. SPORN MB, DINGMAN W, DEFALCO A, DAVIES RK: The synthesis of urea in the living rat brain. *J Neurochem* 5, 62, 1959

163. BLAKE RL, HALL JG, RUSSELL ES: Mitochondrial proline dehydrogenase deficiency in hyperprolinemic PRO/Re mice: Genetic and enzymatic analyses. *Biochem Genet* 14:739, 1976

164. DOOLEY KC, APPLEGARTH DA: Hyperprolinemia Type II: Evidence of the excretion of 3-hydroxy delta 1-pyrroline 5-carboxylic acid. *Clin Biochem* 12:62, 1979

165. SIMILÄ S: Hydroxyproline metabolism in Type-II hyperprolinaemia. *Ann Clin Biochem* 16:177, 1979

166. SIMILÄ S: Dietary treatment in hyperprolinemia type II. *Acta Paediatr Scand* 63:249, 1974

167. SIMILÄ S: The catabolism of ornithine after intravenous loading in normal subjects and two patients with hyperprolinemia type II. *Clin Chim Acta* 28:457, 1970

168. SCRIVER CR, BERGERON M: Amino acid transport in kidney. The use of mutation to dissect membrane and transepithelial transport, in Nyhan WL (ed): *Heritable Disorders of Amino Acid Metabolism.* New York, John Wiley & Sons, Inc, 1974, p 515

169. LUSH IE: The biochemical genetics of vertebrates except man, in Neuberger A, Tatum EL (eds): *Frontiers of Biology.* Amsterdam, North-Holland, 1967, vol 3

170. BULFIELD G: Inherited metabolic disease in laboratory animals: A review. *J Inher Metab Dis* 3:133, 1980

171. BLAKE RL, RUSSELL ES: Hyperprolinemia and prolinuria in a new inbred strain of mice, PRO/Re. *Science* 176:809, 1972

172. BLAKE RL: Animal model for hyperprolinemia: Deficiency of mouse proline oxidase activity. *Biochem J* 129:987, 1972

173. SIMELL O, SCRIVER CR, MOHYUDDIN F: Structural relationships between metabolism and transport of proline in the nephron, abstracted. *Pediatr Res* 10:444, 1976

174. STRECKER HJ: The interconversion of glutamic acid and proline. II. The preparation and properties of Δ^1-pyrroline-5-carboxylic acid. *J Biol Chem* 235:2045, 1960

175. BLOCKS RJ, BOLLING D: *The Amino Acid Composition of Proteins and Foods.* Springfield, Ill, Charles C Thomas, Publisher, 1951

176. MOLLICA F, PAVONE L: Hyperprolinemia: A disease which does not need treatment? *Acta Paediatr Scand* 65:206, 1976

177. WHELAN DT, CONNORS WC: Maternal hyperprolinemia. *Lancet* 1:981, 1980

178. GOYER RA, MITCHELL BJ, LEONARD DL: Dietary reduction of hyperprolinemia. *J Lab Clin Med* 73:819, 1969

179. BERLOW S, LEPP P, SELKOE D, EFRON M: Hyperprolinemia, Type II: Δ^1-pyrroline-5-carboxylic acid dehydrogenase deficiency. Personal communication, September 1969

180. EFRON ML, BIXBY EM, PALATTAO LG, PRYLES CV: Hydroxyprolinemia associated with mental deficiency. *N Engl J Med* 267:1193, 1962

181. EFRON ML, BIXBY EM, PRYLES CV: Hydroxyprolinemia. II. A rare metabolic disease due to a deficiency of the enzyme "hydroxyproline oxidase." *N Engl J Med* 272:1299, 1965

181a. SCRIVER CR, unpublished data

182. EFRON ML, BIXBY EM, HOCKADAY TDR, SMITH LH JR, MESHORER, E: Hydroxyprolinemia. III. The origin of free hydroxyproline in hydroxyprolinemia. Collagen turnover. Evidence for a biosynthetic pathway in man. *Biochim Biophys Acta* 165:238, 1968

183. PELKONEN R, LÄHDEVIRTA J, VISAKORPI JK, KIVIRIKKO KI: Hydroxyprolinemia: A case without mental deficiency. *Scand J Clin Lab Invest* 23(suppl 108):21, 1969

184. PELKONEN R, KIVIRIKKO KI: Hydroxyprolinemia. *N Engl J Med* 283:451, 1970

185. RAINE DN: Personal communication, July 1969

186. RAINE DN: Defects in renal tubular reabsorption, in Benson PF (ed): *Defects in Cellular Organelles and Membranes in Relation to Mental Retardation.* London, Churchill, Livingston, Ltd, Institute for Research into Mental Retardation Study Group No. 2, 1971, p 43

187. RAMA RAO BS, SUBHASH MN, MARAYANAN HS: Hydroxyprolinemia: A case report. *Indian Pediatr* 11:829, 1974

188. ROESEL RA, BLANKENSHIP PR, LYNCH WR, CORYELL ME, THEVAOS TS, HALL WK: Hydroxyproline metabolism in two sisters with hydroxyprolinemia. *Hum Hered* 29:364, 1979

189. PROCKOP DJ: Hydroxyprolinemia as an illustration of nonessential enzymes in man. *N Engl J Med* 283:487, 1970

190. HEACOCK AM, ADAMS E: Formation and excretion of pyrrole-2-carboxylate in man. *J Clin Invest* 54:810, 1974

191. GOLDSTONE A, ADAMS E: Further metabolic reactions of γ-hydroxyglutamate: Amidation of γ-hydroxyglutamine possible reduction to hydroxyproline. *Biochem Biophys Res Commun* 16:71, 1964

192. MORROW G III, KIVIRIKKO KI, PROCKOP DJ: Catabolism and excretion of free hydroxyproline in infancy. *J Clin Endocrinol* 27:1365, 1967

193. MORROW G III, KIVIRIKKO KI, PROCKOP DJ: Hydroxyprolinemia and increased excretion of free hydroxyproline in early infancy. *J Clin Endocrinol* 26:1012, 1966

194. ADAMS E, SMITH EL: Peptidases of erythrocytes. II. Isolation and properties of prolidase. *J Biol Chem* 198:671, 1952

195. ADIBI SA, MERCER DW: Protein digestion in human intestine as reflected in luminal, mucosal and plasma amino acid concentration after meals. *J Clin Invest* 52:1586, 1973

196. GOODMAN SI, SOLOMONS CC, MUSCHENHEIM F, MCINTYRE CA, MILES B, O'BRIEN D: A syndrome resembling lathyrism associated with iminodipeptiduria. *Am J Med* 45:152, 1968

197. BUIST NRM, STRANDHOLM JJ, BELLINGER JF, KENNAWAY NG: Further studies on a patient with iminopeptiduria: A probable case of prolidase deficiency. *Metabolism* 21:1113, 1972

198. POWELL GF, RASCO MA, MANISCALCO RM: A prolidase deficiency in man with iminopeptiduria. *Metabolism* 23:505, 1974

199. POWELL GF, MANISCALCO RM: Bound hydroxyproline excretion following gelatin loading in prolidase deficiency. *Metabolism* 25:503, 1976

200. JACKSON SH, DENNIS AW, GREENBERG M: Iminopeptiduria: A genetic defect in recycling collagen. A method for determining prolidase in red blood cells. *Can Med Assoc J* 113:759, 1975

201. JOHNSTONE RAW, POVALL TJ, BATY JD, ROUSSET JL, CHARPENTIER C, LEMONNIER A: Determination of dipeptides in urine. *Clin Chim Acta* 52:137, 1974

202. LAPIERE CH M, NUSGENS B: Plaies cutanées torpides et trouble du metabolisme du collagene. *Arch Belg Dermatol Syph* 25:353, 1969

203. FAULL KF, SCHIER GM, SCHLESINGER P, HALPERN B: The mass spectrometric identification of dipeptides in the urine of a patient suffering from chronic skin ulceration and edema. *Clin Chim Acta* 70:313, 1976

204. UMEMURA S: Studies on a patient with iminodipeptiduria. II. Lack of prolidase activity in blood cells. *Physiol Chem Phys* 10:279, 1978

205. ISEMURA M, HANYO T, GEJYO F, NAKAZAWA R, IGARASHI R, MATSUO S, IKEDA K, SATO Y: Prolidase deficiency with imidopeptiduria. A familial case with and without clinical symptoms. *Clin Chim Acta* 93:401, 1979

206. NUTZENADEL W, SCRIVER CR: Transport and metabolism of β-alanyl-L-histidine (L-carnosine) by rat intestinal enterocytes, kidney cortex and striated muscle in vitro. Role in nutrition. *Am J Physiol* 230:643, 1976

207. JACKSON SH, HEININGER JA: Proline recycling during collagen metabolism as determined by concurrent $^{18}O_2$ and ^3H. *Biochim Biophys Acta* (In press)

208. Okninska A, Grygalewicz J, Kowalewska-Kantecka B, Iwanska J: Hyperprolinaemia familiaris-obserwaja rodziny (Familial hyperprolinaemia—observations of a family). *Pol Arch Med Wewn* 51:189, 1974

209. Teijema HI, van Gelderen HH, Giesberts MAH, Lawent de Angulo MSL: Dicarboxylic aminoaciduria: An inborn error of glutamate and aspartate transport with metabolic implications in combination with hyperprolinemia. *Metabolism* 23:115, 1974

19

THE HYPERORNITHINEMIAS

DAVID VALLE

OLLI SIMELL

1. Ornithine is a nonprotein amino acid that is the substrate or product of five enzymatic reactions and is transported by a transmitochondrial transport protein. Two of these enzymes, ornithine-δ-aminotransferase and ornithine decarboxylase, catalyze reactions which consume ornithine. The former catalyzes the major catabolic reaction for ornithine. The source of ornithine is arginine in dietary protein, although under certain circumstances de novo synthesis of ornithine apparently occurs by a reversal of the normal flux in the ornithine-δ-aminotransferase reaction.

2. There are two distinct genetic disorders which result in hyperornithinemia: gyrate atrophy of the choroid and retina and the hyperornithinemia-hyperammonemia-homocitrullinuria syndrome.

3. Gyrate atrophy of the choroid and retina is an autosomal recessively inherited form of progressive chorioretinal degeneration caused by a deficiency of ornithine-δ-aminotransferase. We know of 91 biochemically documented cases, half of which are Finnish. There is myopia, night blindness, and loss of peripheral vision starting late in the first decade, proceeding to tunnel vision and eventual blindness by the third and fourth decades. Posterior subcapsular cataracts are present ⁿⁿrly all patients by the end of the second decade. ⁿlar fundus exhibits sharply demarcated circu-
s of complete chorioretinal degeneration which

start in the midperiphery and gradually extend to the posterior pole. Tubular aggregates are present in the type II fibers of skeletal muscle. Plasma ornithine values range from 400 to 1400 μM and 0.5 to 10 mmols of ornithine are excreted daily. Plasma glutamate, glutamine, lysine, creatine, and creatinine concentrations are modestly reduced. Ornithine-δ-aminotransferase activity in the cells and tissues of patients is from 0 to 6 percent that in controls, and obligate heterozygotes have intermediate values. Four patients have had both in vitro and in vivo responses to pharmacologic doses of pyridoxal-phosphate or pyridoxine. Additional therapeutic approaches have included an arginine-restricted diet which in some patients has lowered plasma ornithine to normal values. Ophthalmologic abnormalities have not progressed in patients on pyridoxine or with significantly reduced ornithine values on the diet, and two patients on the diet have had some evidence of improved visual function. Pharmacologic doses of L-lysine or α-aminoisobutyric have increased renal losses of ornithine but have not been as effective as the diet in lowering plasma ornithine. Creatine administration has resulted in improvement of the histologic abnormalities in muscle.

4. The hyperornithinemia-hyperammonemia-homocitrullinuria syndrome is an autosomal recessively inherited disorder which has been described in 10 patients. The

clinical symptoms are related to the hyperammonemia and resemble those of the urea cycle disorders. No visual problems or fundus changes are present. Plasma ornithine concentrations range from 380 to 630 μM on a self-restricted protein diet and in general are slightly lower than in gyrate atrophy. The pathophysiology of the disease may involve diminished ornithine transport into the mitochondria, resulting in ornithine accumulation in the cytoplasm and reduced ability to clear carbamoyl phosphate and ammonia. The moderate reductions in leukocyte and liver carbamoyl phosphate synthetase I and in fibroblast ornithine decarboxylase, which have been reported in some of these patients, are probably not the primary defects. Ornithine-δ-aminotransferase is normal. Homocitrulline is thought to originate from transcarbamoylation of lysine. Its excretion is increased by lysine supplementation. The patients tolerate 1.2 to 1.5 g/kg protein daily without hyperammonemia. Further elevation of plasma ornithine by ornithine supplementation reduced the blood ammonia in one patient, but oral and intravenous ornithine did not reduce hyperammonemia caused by alanine infusions in another. The long-term efficacy of ornithine supplementation is unknown.

Ornithine is a nonprotein amino acid which plays an important role in the metabolism of urea, creatine, and polyamines. The pathways of ornithine metabolism are closely linked with those of proline (see Chap. 18). Together they allow the exchange of molecules between the urea (see Chap. 20) and tricarboxylic acid cycles. The major source of ornithine is arginine in dietary protein. The fates of the ornithine carbon atoms include incorporation into protein as arginine, proline, glutamate, or any of the α-ketoglutarate-derived nonessential amino acids; conversion to the polyamines and γ-aminobutyric acid; and oxidation in the tricarboxylic acid cycle.

There are two inherited disorders which result in hyperornithinemia: gyrate atrophy of the choroid and retina, with symptoms limited mainly to the eye; and the hyperornithinemia-hyperammonemia-homocitrullinuria syndrome, with symptoms resulting from ammonia accumulation and protein aversion. The former condition is due to a deficiency of the mitochondrial matrix enzyme ornithine-δ-aminotransferase (Fig. 19-1), while the basic defect in the latter has not been defined but may be an impairment in the carrier-mediated entry of ornithine into mitochondria.

ORNITHINE METABOLISM

Ornithine is either a substrate or a product of five enzymes and a mitochondrial transport protein (Fig. 19-2). The chemical characteristics of these proteins are listed in Table 19-1. Ornithine metabolism can be considered in four sections: the urea cycle; polyamine biosynthesis; creatine synthesis; and the ornithine-δ-aminotransferase reaction. Depending on the circumstances, the last reaction functions as a component in arginine degradation, proline biosynthesis, or *de novo* ornithine synthesis.

The Urea Cycle

In most instances, ornithine acts as a catalyst in the urea cycle, providing the molecular foundation upon which urea is assembled from the nitrogens provided by ammonium and aspartate and the carbon of bicarbonate. Each molecule of ornithine converted to citrulline in the mitochondrial matrix is eventually re-formed from arginine in the cytoplasm. Stoichiometric or noncatalytic utilization of ornithine in the urea cycle occurs in two special circumstances: (1) when the urea cycle is interrupted by inherited enzyme deficiencies which lead to the accumulation of citrulline, argininosuccinate, or arginine and result in the urinary loss of ornithine carbon skeletons in the form of the accumulated intermediate; and (2) when dietary arginine is less than that required for protein accretion. In this instance, ornithine and the reactions of the urea cycle are utilized for arginine synthesis.

Citrulline Synthesis Citrulline is formed in the mitochondrial matrix by the transfer of the carbamoyl moiety of carbamoyl phosphate to the δ-amino nitrogen of ornithine. The reaction is catalyzed by ornithine transcarbamoylase and is markedly influenced by the pH, with maximal rates between pH 8 and 9. This pH dependence suggests that zwitterionic ornithine, with an un-ionized δ-amino group (~10 percent of the total isoelectric form at physiologic pH), is the actual substrate for ornithine transcarbamoylase [1, 2]. Although substrate specificity is high at pH 8, some homocitrulline is formed by transcarbamoylation of L-lysine at pH 9 [3].

The ornithine transcarbamoylase reaction is regulated at both the substrate and gene levels. Within the matrix, ornithine concentrations are set by ornithine entry and the action of ornithine transcarbamoylase and ornithine-δ-aminotransferase [4]. The actual concentrations of ornithine and carbamyl

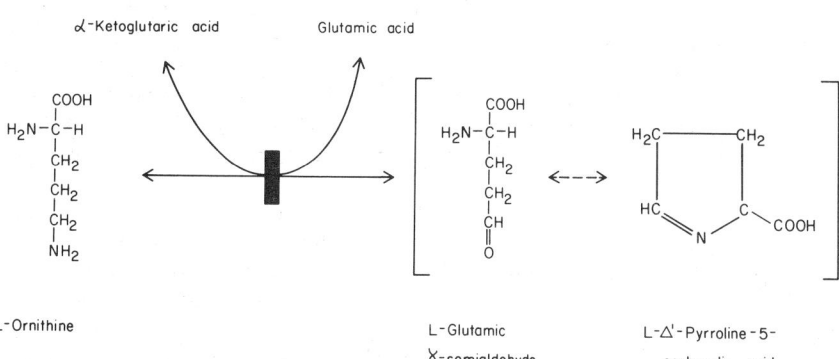

Figure 19-1   Deficiency of ornithine-δ-aminotransferase: the primary enzymatic defect in gyrate atrophy of the choroid and retina.

L-Ornithine   L-Glutamic γ-semialdehyde   L-Δ¹-Pyrroline-5-carboxylic acid

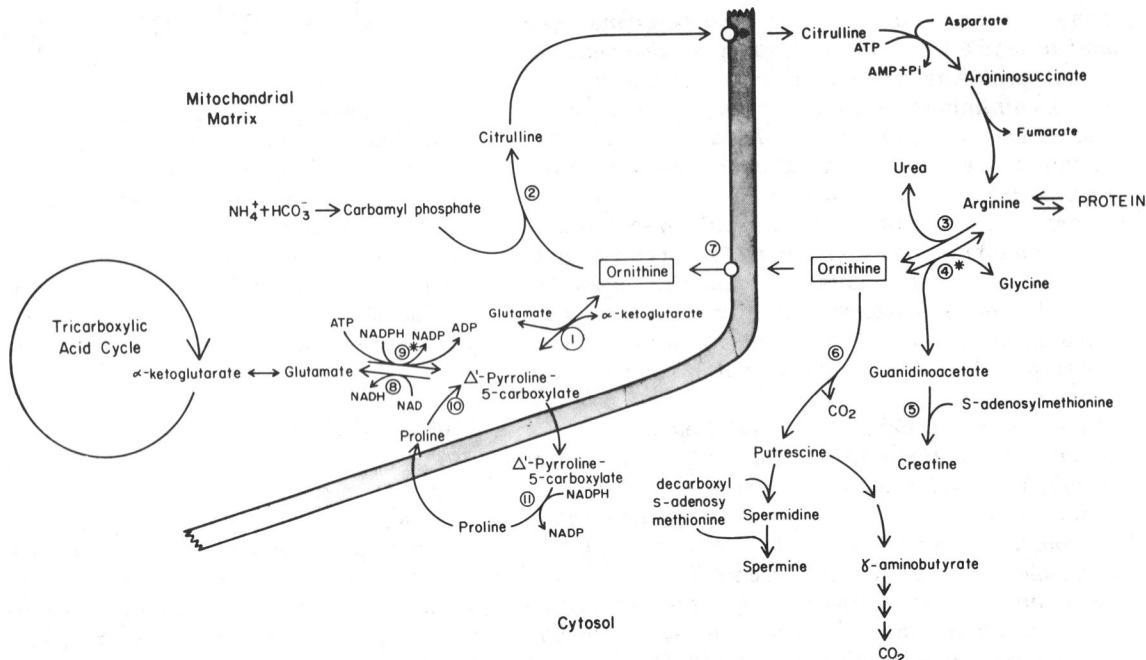

Figure 19-2 Ornithine metabolism and subcellular compartmentation. The shaded zone denotes the inner and outer mitochondrial membranes and the intermembranous space. The numbers refer to the following enzymes or proteins: ① , ornithine-δ-aminotransferase; ② , ornithine transcarbamoylase; ③ , arginase; ④ , glycine transamidinase; ⑤ , S-adenosylmethionine:guanidinoacetate N-methyltransferase; ⑥ , ornithine decarboxylase; ⑦ , ornithine transport protein in the inner mitochondrial membrane; ⑧ , Δ¹-pyrroline-5-carboxylate dehydrogenase; ⑨ , Δ¹-pyrroline-5-carboxylate synthase, ⑩ , proline oxidase; ⑪ , Δ¹-pyrroline-5-carboxilate reductase. *subcellular localization not established; in rat kidney, glycine transamidinase may be located on the outer (cytoplasmic) aspect of the inner mitochondrial membrane [223].

phosphate in this subcellular compartment, although of great interest, have not been directly measured. Raijman has suggested that ornithine is low in relation to the availability of carbamoyl phosphate [5], while others suggest that the latter usually limits the transcarbamoylase reaction and that ornithine by an uncertain mechanism may stimulate carbamoyl phosphate production [6, 7]. These conflicting views may indicate that either substrate can regulate citrulline synthesis depending on the circumstance. As in other urea cycle enzymes, the long-term regulation of ornithine transcarbamoylase activity is directly related to the quantity of dietary protein [8, 9].

An X-linked deficiency of ornithine transcarbamoylase has been described in humans (Chap. 20) and in the sparse fur mouse [10]. In both species, affected males exhibit protein intolerance, with lethargy, vomiting, hyperammonemia, coma, and orotic aciduria. Because ornithine catabolism by ornithine-δ-aminotransferase is intact, neither humans nor mice with this inborn error have significant increases in the plasma ornithine concentration.

Arginase   Biochemical, electrophoretic, immunologic, and genetic evidence suggests that there are at least two forms of arginase [11-14]. The activity in the cytosol of hepatic cells in ureotelic animals functions in the urea cycle and is remarkable for its high activity (highest of all urea cycle enzymes) [15] and low substrate affinity (Table 19-1). Ornithine and lysine are weak inhibitors [11, 16]. A second form of arginase, also weakly inhibitable by ornithine, has been found in the kidney, small intestine, pancreas, and mammary gland [11, 13, 17]. In most tissues, this form of arginase probably functions as the initial enzyme in a sequence of reactions which converts arginine to proline [17, 18].

Arginase deficiency has been described in several children with mental retardation, neuromuscular abnormalities, and hyperargininemia [20-22]. Arginase activity is deficient in the erythrocytes and presumably in the liver of these patients. Normal activity was found in the kidney of one [14]. Plasma ornithine concentrations are normal or only minimally reduced, in

part because renal arginase and glycine transamidinase provide alternatives for the conversion of arginine to ornithine.

Subcellular Compartmentation and Transport of Ornithine.   Three of the urea cycle enzymes, argininosuccinic acid synthetase, argininosuccinic acid lyase, and arginase, are cytosolic, while ornithine transcarbamoylase and carbamoyl phosphate synthetase are found in the mitochondrial matrix. Thus, a complete turn of the urea cycle requires the transport of ornithine into citrulline out of the mitochondrion. The mitochondrial boundary is composed of an inner and outer membrane with an intervening intermembrane space. The outer membrane is readily permeable to amino acids, while the inner is the true permeability barrier [23]. Ornithine transport into liver mitochondria is mediated by a specific carrier, which does not recognize L-arginine or L-lysine [4, 24, 25]. There is a disagreement on the energy requirements for this process. Gamble and Lehninger found that mitochondria accumulated cationic L-ornithine if respiratory energy (e.g., provided by succinate or glutamate) and a permeant proton yielding anion (HPO$_4^=$, H$_2$PO$_4^-$, acetate, or bicarbonate) were available [24]. Nonrespiring mitochondria were impermeable to either cationic ornithine (the dominant form of ornithine at physiologic pH), or the electroneural analogue, N-acetylornithine. In contrast, McGivan and coworkers found that the distribution of ornithine across the mitochondrial membrane was correlated with the transmitochondrial pH gradient, and that the intramitochondrial concentration of ornithine barely exceeded that in the medium when the catabolism of matrix ornithine by ornithine-δ-aminotransferase was blocked by amino-oxyacetate [4]. These results suggest that cationic ornithine is transported electroneutrally in exchange for H$^+$, without dependency on respiratory energy. Bradford and McGivan have also suggested that an ornithine/citrulline antiporter is present in liver mitochondria, which ensures tight coupling of the transmitochondrial fluxes of these substrates [25]. Extrapolation of the maximal mitochondrial ornithine transport to the in vivo situation suggests that this process may limit ornithine availability for transamination or citrulline synthesis, or both [4, 5, 26, 27].

Putrescine Synthesis

The physiologic roles of putrescine and other polyamines are poorly understood, but as polycations they readily associate with nucleic acids and phospholipids and seem to be important in cell replication and membrane stability [28, 29]. Putrescine (diaminobutane) is formed from ornithine in an irreversible reaction catalyzed by the pyridoxal phosphate-dependent enzyme, ornithine decarboxylase. Condensation of putrescine with propylamino moieties provided by decarboxy-S-adenosylmethionine forms the polyamines spermidine [H$_2$N-(CH$_2$)$_4$NH(CH$_2$)$_3$NH$_2$] and spermine [H$_2$N(CH$_2$)$_3$NH-(CH$_2$)$_4$NH(CH$_2$)$_3$NH$_2$] [30]. Approximately 0.5 mmole of spermidine is synthesized daily in normal adult humans [31, 32]. The activity of ornithine decarboxylase and the S-adenosylmethionine decarboxylating enzyme are thought to be major regulatory factors in polyamine synthesis rather than availability of substrate [28, 33, 34]. Ornithine decarboxylase activity is low in nondividing and high in rapidly proliferating cells

(e.g., embroylogic tissues, malignant tumors, and the stem cells of bone marrow and intestinal mucosa). A rapid and substantial (>10X) increase in ornithine decarboxylase activity is one of the earliest events following stimulation of resting cells to proliferate and leads to increases in the cellular levels of putrescine [29, 35]. Degradation of the enzyme is rapid and nearly constant, with a half-life of 10 to 20 min [28, 30]. The increment in ornithine decarboxylase is due to increased synthesis, which in some tissues results from an increased concentration of cyclic AMP [36].

Ornithine decarboxylase is specifically inhibited by a putrescine-induced protein (antizyme) [37, 38] and by pharmacologic agents including the enzyme-activated, irreversible inhibitor DL-α-difluromethylornithine and related compounds [39–41]. Pharmacologic inhibition of ornithine decarboxylase results in lower tissue polyamine levels and interferes with cell proliferation [40, 42] and growth [43].

Putrescine is also a precursor for the synthesis of γ-aminobutyric acid. More commonly, this neurotransmitter is synthesized directly from glutamic acid by glutamic acid decarboxylase [44]. Two reaction sequences which convert putrescine to γ-aminobutyrate have been described. One involves direct deamination by diamine oxidase (histaminase), while the other utilizes n-acetylated intermediates [44, 45]. De Mello and coworkers [46] found that a significant fraction of chick retina γ-aminobutyrate was derived from ornithine in early embryonic chicks, while glutamate became the major precursor by the time of hatching. In the adult rat brain, ornithine is efficiently converted to γ-aminobutyrate in nerve terminals [47]. The degradation of γ-aminobutyrate involves transamination by γ-aminobutyrate transaminase to form succinate semialde-

Table 19-1 Enzymes of ornithine metabolism

Enzymes	Subcellular compartment	Molecular weight	Cofactors	Kinetic parameters§	Equilibrium constant	Organ distribution
Ornithine aminotransferase* (EC2.6.1.13)	Mitochondrial matrix	180,000 tetramer	Pyridoxal phosphate	$K_{m_{orn}}$ = 2.8 × 10^{-3} M $K_{m_{\alpha kg}}$ = 0.28 × 10^{-3} M $K_{m_{P5C}}$ = 0.7 × 10^{-3} M $K_{m_{glu}}$ = 25.0 × 10^{-3} M	$\dfrac{\text{P5C + glu}}{\text{orn + }\alpha\text{KG}} = 70$	General
Ornithine carbamoyltransferase† (EC2.1.3.3)	Mitochondrial matrix	108,000 trimer	—	$K_{m_{orn}}$ = 4.7 × 10^{-4} M†† $K_{m_{cap}}$ = 7.0 × 10^{-4} M	$\dfrac{\text{cit}}{\text{orn + CAP}}$ = 6 × 10^5	Primarily liver; low activity in gut, brain, kidney
Ornithine decarboxylase* (EC4.1.1.17)	Cytoplasmic	70,000	Pyridoxal phosphate	$K_{m_{orn}}$ = 1 × 10^{-4} M	$\dfrac{\text{put}}{\text{orn}} = 1 \times 10^5$	General; high in rapidly dividing tissues
Arginase† (EC3.5.3.1)	Cytoplasmic	120,000 tetramer	Mn^{2+}	$K_{m_{arg}}$ = 1 × 10^{-2} M	—	Liver; gut and kidney 5 percent of hepatic; erythrocytes
Glycine transaminidase‡ (EC2.1.4.1)	**	100,000	—	$K_{m_{arg}}$ = 1.3 × 10^{-3} M $K_{m_{glu}}$ = 2.4 × 10^{-3} M $K_{m_{orn}}$ = 1.0 × 10^{-4} M $K_{m_{GAA}}$ = 3.9 × 10^{-3} M	$\dfrac{\text{orn + GAA}}{\text{arg + gly}} = 1.1$	Pancreas, liver, kidney‡‡

* Rat liver.
† Human liver.
‡ Hog kidney.
§ Values are representative for the enzyme source.
†† Marked pH dependency.
** Subcellular location in human tissues not known; in rat kidney, reported to be on the cytoplasmic side of the inner mitochondrial membrane [223].
‡‡ Low activity in human brain, no activity in rat brain [188].
Abbreviations: αkg, α-ketoglutarate; arg, arginine; cap, carbamoyl phosphate; cit, citrulline; GAA, guanidino acetate; glu, glutamate; gly, glycine; orn, ornithine; P5C, Δ^1-pyrroline-5-carboxylate; put, putrescine.
SOURCES: Ornithine-δ-aminotransferase data from Strecker [56], Matsuzawa [57], and Sanada et al. [65]; ornithine carbamoyl transferase data from Snodgrass [1] and Conboy et al. [97]; ornithine decarboxylase data from Williams-Ashman et al. [30]; arginase data from Soberon and Palacios [12] and Glass and Knox [18]; glycine transamidinase data from Ratner and Rochovansky [51] and Walker [48].

hyde, which is further oxidized to succinate and eventually to CO_2. Thus, the conversion of putrescine to γ-aminobutyrate provides a pathway for the oxidation of ornithine to CO_2 independently of the ornithine-δ-aminotransferase.

Creatine Synthesis

The first reaction in creatine synthesis, transfer of the amidino group of arginine to glycine to form guanidinoacetate and ornithine, is catalyzed by glycine transamidinase (Fig. 19-2) [48]. Guanidinoacetate is N-methylated by S-adenosylmethionine:guanidinoacetate N-methyltransferase to form creatine. The transamidinase reaction is readily reversible in vitro, but low tissue levels of guanidinoacetate probably prevent a significant reverse reaction in vivo. Creatine has no effect on the transamidinase in vitro but functions as an end product repressor in vivo [48–50]. Ornithine is a potent competitive inhibitor of the transamidinase [51–53].

In humans, both glycine transamidinase and the methyltransferase are present in high activity in the liver and pancreas, while in other mammals the kidney is the major site of the transamidinase [48]. Available information suggests that creatine is synthesized in these central organs, transported to muscle and nerve, and there phosphorylated to form the high-energy phosphagen creatine phosphate. The interesting possibility that other tissues, including brain, may be capable of creatine synthesis has been suggested and requires further study [54, 55].

The majority of total body creatine-creatine phosphate pool is located in muscle and amounts to approximately 120 g (915 mmol) in a 70-kg person. Both creatine and creatine phosphate undergo a first-order, nonenzymatic cyclization to creatinine at fractional rates of 0.011/day and 0.026/day, respectively [48]. Thus, in order to maintain the creatine-creatine phosphate pool, an amount of creatine equal to the amount of creatinine formed daily (approximately 2 g in an adult male) must be provided from either dietary sources or by endogenous synthesis. The relative contributions from these two sources are difficult to estimate, but studies of individuals on creatine-free diets indicate that endogenous synthesis can meet the entire requirement [48]. The relative magnitude of the synthetic pathway is indicated by the fact that creatine synthesis is quantitatively the major consumer of S-adenosylmethionine donated methyl groups in the body [31].

Ornithine-δ-aminotransferase Pathway

Ornithine-δ-aminotransferase is a pyridoxal phosphate-requiring Ω-transaminase, which catalyzes the reversible conversion of ornithine and α-ketoglutarate to Δ^1-pyrroline-5-carboxylate and glutamate (Fig. 19-1). Glutamate semialdehyde is the initial product formed by removal of the δ-amino group of ornithine; however, it cyclizes spontaneously to form Δ^1-pyrroline-5-carboxylate. Kinetic studies suggest that the cyclization is rapid and reversible [56–58]. Thus, in the subsequent discussions we consider Δ^1-pyrroline-5-carboxylate the reaction product, with the tacit assumption that it is in equilibrium with glutamate semialdehyde.

Chemistry Ornithine-δ-aminotransferase activity was first described in animal tissues by Quastel and Witty [59] and Meister [60]. Subsequently, ornithine-δ-aminotransferase has

been purified from rat liver [56, 61–65] and kidney [66–68]. Rat liver holo-ornithine-δ-aminotransferase is a tetramer with a molecular weight of 180,000, a sedimentation coefficient of 9.2 $S_{20,w}$ [65], and one molecule of pyridoxal phosphate per subunit [67, 69]. The protomers are identical in size (molecular weight 45,000) [65] and amino acid composition [64, 65]. The amino acid sequence is not known.

Although the reaction is reversible, the equilibrium constant favors the formation of Δ^1-pyrroline-5-carboxylate (Table 19-1) [56]. The complete reaction involves two half-reactions [69].

Ornithine + pyridoxal-ornithine-δ-aminotransferase $\longrightarrow$
Δ^1-pyrroline-5-carboxylate +
pyridoxamine-ornithine-δ-aminotransferase   (1)

Pyridoxamine - ornithine-δ-aminotransferase + α-ketoglutarate $\longrightarrow$
glutamate + pyridoxal - ornithine-δ-aminotransferase   (2)

The pH optimum of the overall reaction measured in the forward direction (pH 8.15) is a compromise between the more alkaline optimum of reaction 1 (~ pH 9) and the more acidic optimum of reaction 2 (~ pH 7). The optimum for the reverse reaction is pH 6.5 [57]. The pyridoxamine enzyme is unstable and can spontaneously release its amino group, allowing the formation of Δ^1-pyrroline-5-carboxylate to exceed that of glutamate under certain conditions [69]. High concentrations of pyridoxal phosphate inhibit the catalytic activity and increase the amount of bound cofactor to approximately four molecules per protomer [69]. The enzyme has high specificity for ornithine. Lysine, the one-carbon-longer homologue, has no effect on the reaction. Pyruvate and glyoxylate are poor substitutes for α-ketoglutarate. High concentrations of ornithine (> 25 mM), and particularly α-ketoglutarate (> 3 mM), are inhibitory [56]. Other low molecular weight compounds which at a concentration of 25 mM inhibit activity by at least 40 percent in the presence of saturating ornithine concentrations include L-valine, α-ketoisovalerate, α-ketoisocaproate, γ-aminobutyrate, and norvaline [56, 57]. Additional inhibiting compounds include nonspecific inhibitors of all vitamin B_6– dependent enzymes, e.g., canaline, cycloserine, hydroxylamine, and thiosemicarbazide [62, 70].

Jung and Seiler [71] and others [72] pointed out the similarity of ornithine-δ-aminotransferase and γ-aminobutyrate transaminase-catalyzed reactions. Both involve Ω-transamination of structurally related substrates. Thus, two supposedly specific, enzyme-activated, irreversible inhibitors ("suicide substrates") of γ-aminobutyrate transaminase, 4-aminohex-5-ynoic acid and 5-amino-1,3-cyclohexadienyl-carboxylic acid (gabaculine), also irreversibly inhibit ornithine-δ-aminotransferase both in vitro and in vivo in mice. A third, 4-aminohex-5-enoic acid, has no effect on ornithine-δ-aminotransferase. In the development and use of inhibitors of either enzyme, careful consideration should be given, therefore, to possible interactions with the other.

Ornithine-δ-aminotransferase Assays Two general methods of assaying ornithine-δ-aminotransferase activity have been utilized [56, 73]. The most widely used method depends on the quantitative formation of a dihydroquinozolinium derivative when Δ^1-pyrroline-5-carboxylate is reacted with o-aminobenzaldehyde. This derivative is measured spectrophotometrically with an extinction coefficient variously reported as 2.71 [56] and 2.59 [58] at 441 nM. One caution in interpreting results obtained with this assay is that o-aminobenzaldehyde reacts with several Δ^1-pyrroline compounds, including Δ^1-pyrroline-2-carboxylate, the cyclized form of the α-keto acid of ornithine [60, 74, 75]. Thus, under certain conditions, some of the apparent product measured by this assay may be other than Δ^1-pyrroline-5-carboxylate. A modification of this method utilizing high performance liquid chromatography has increased sensitivity and possibly also specificity [76].

A second method of measuring ornithine-δ-aminotransferase activity involves the use of radiolabeled ornithine and separation of this precursor from the product Δ^1-pyrroline-5-carboxylate by ion-exchange chromatography [73]. This method can be adapted to either low or high substrate concentrations and has the additional advantages of greater sensitivity and specificity than the standard spectrophotometric assay. The sensitivity of the assay is increased by purifying commercially available, radiolabeled ornithine by ion-exchange chromatography. This removes contaminants (e.g., γ-aminobutyrate) which may be inhibitory to ornithine-δ-aminotransferase activity.

Tissue Distribution Rat kidney, liver, and small intestine have high ornithine-δ-aminotransferase activity [61, 77–79]. The kidneys of animals exposed to estrogen (either normal females or gonadectomized males treated with estrogen) have the highest activity [77]. Lower levels of ornithine-δ-aminotransferase are present in the pancreas, submaxillary gland, heart, brain, spleen, adrenal, lung, mammary gland, cartilage, and skeletal muscle [19, 77–80]. Chick retina has high ornithine-δ-aminotransferase activity [81], and in cows the activity in the retina is the same as in the kidney [82]. Similar results have been observed in rabbit tissues [83]. Human cadaver neural retina and pigment epithelium have measurable levels of ornithine-δ-transferase [83], but human skeletal muscle obtained by biopsy of three normal adults had no detectable ornithine-δ-transferase activity [84].

Regulation of Ornithine-δ-aminotransferase Activity
In addition to the regulation by small molecules described above, ornithine-δ-aminotransferase activity varies greatly with changes in developmental, nutritional, and hormonal status. In rat liver and kidney, ornithine-δ-aminotransferase activity is barely detectable prenatally or during the first 2 postnatal weeks, but by 30 days of age it increases approximately fifteen-fold to adult levels [77, 85]. In the small intestine, ornithine-δ-aminotransferase activity is two to five times higher in the first 3 weeks of life than in adult intestine or liver [78].

After the first few weeks of life, liver ornithine-δ-aminotransferase activity in rats is markedly influenced by dietary protein intake. An increase in dietary protein from 20 to 70 percent by weight results in increased ornithine-δ-aminotransferase-specific activity within 1 day and by 4 days a peak activity sixfold higher than baseline levels. Concomitant high glucose feedings prevents this induction [66, 86]. Decreasing protein intake to 5 percent causes a twofold reduction in activity. Renal and small intestinal ornithine-δ-aminotransferase are not affected by variations in dietary protein [66]. Ornithine-δ-aminotransferase activity in the liver increases in response to glucagon, while activity in the kidney of gonadectomized rats increases four-fold in response to estrogen [87]. Thyroid hormone augments the estrogen response [87].

The perturbations of ornithine-δ-aminotransferase activity by nutritional and hormonal factors are due to quantitative changes in the amount of enzyme resulting from increased synthesis rather than decreased degradation [66, 87, 88]. The degradation in liver is faster than in kidney, with a half-life of 0.9 to 1.9 days in liver as compared to 4.0 days in kidney [89–92].

Cell Biology The well-documented autosomal recessive inheritance of ornithine-δ-aminotransferase deficiency (see below) indicates that the gene(s) for this enzyme, like those for nearly all mitochondrial matrix proteins, are encoded in the nucleus [93, 94]. This is in contrast to the genes for a small number of mitochondrial structural proteins and some elements of the electron transfer chain, which are encoded in mitochondrial DNA [93–95]. The protomers of ornithine-δ-aminotransferase, like those of other matrix proteins, must be synthesized on cytoplasmic ribosomes and then must enter the mitochondrion, assemble, and combine with pyridoxal phosphate. Studies of matrix proteins in *Neurospora* [93, 94, 96] and of human ornithine transcarbamylase [97] indicate that most but not all [98] mitochondrial proteins are synthesized as larger molecular weight precursors apparently with a signal peptide which directs them to the mitochondrial matrix [99]. The signal peptide is removed as the precursor enters the mitochondrion. Degradation of ornithine-δ-aminotransferase has been proposed to involve a specific neutral protease located within the matrix [100], but recent reports cast doubt on this hypothesis [101]. In any event, it should be obvious that the final phenotype of ornithine-δ-aminotransferase activity represents the summation of several steps and that a defect in any one of these steps could markedly alter the enzyme activity.

Metabolic Roles of the Ornithine-δ-aminotransferase Pathway The bridging position of the ornithine-δ-aminotransferase reaction as a link between the urea cycle on the one hand and proline metabolism and the tricarboxylic acid cycle on the other results in its involvement in several different metabolic processes.

ORNITHINE AND ARGININE CATABOLISM The relationships which predict ariginine and ornithine catabolism are shown in the following scheme:

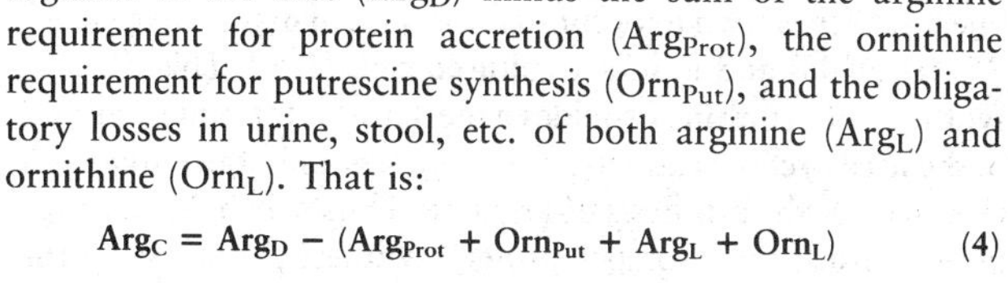

$$\text{Dietary protein} \rightarrow \text{arginine} \rightarrow \text{ornithine} \rightarrow \Delta^1\text{pyrroline-5-carboxylate}$$

urine, stool, and skin losses

protein accretion   putrescine   (3)

Thus in molar units, the amount of arginine catabolized daily to Δ^1-pyrroline-5-carboxylate (Arg_C) equals the amount of arginine in the diet (Arg_D) minus the sum of the arginine requirement for protein accretion (Arg_{Prot}), the ornithine requirement for putrescine synthesis (Orn_{Put}), and the obligatory losses in urine, stool, etc. of both arginine (Arg_L) and ornithine (Orn_L). That is:

$$Arg_C = Arg_D - (Arg_{Prot} + Orn_{Put} + Arg_L + Orn_L) \quad (4)$$

In healthy adults in nitrogen balance, there is no net increase in body protein, and the amount of arginine required for protein accretion approaches zero. In contrast, growing children or adults recovering from an episode of negative nitrogen balance may utilize significant arginine for Arg_{Prot}. Orn_{Put} has not been measured directly but is estimated to be small (less than 0.5

mmol/day in an adult) [31]. Normally, Orn_L and Arg_L are negligible but are significant in patients with overflow ornithinuria. These considerations indicate that in a healthy adult, Arg_C by way of the ornithine-δ-aminotransferase pathway is nearly equal to Arg_D. If dietary protein equals 1.5 g protein per kilogram of body weight per day, and if the arginine content of protein approximately equals 5 percent, then the daily ornithine-δ-aminotransferase flux equals ~0.4 mmol/kg or 28 mmol in a 70-kg man.

PROLINE SYNTHESIS Δ^1-Pyrroline-5-carboxylate, the immediate precursor of proline, can be synthesized either from glutamate in a reaction catalyzed by Δ^1-pyrroline-5-carboxylate synthase or from ornithine in a reaction catalyzed by ornithine-δ-aminotransferase (Fig. 19-2). The regulation of the relative contributions is of interest. Lodato and coworkers [102] have shown that physiologic concentrations of ornithine inhibit Δ'-pyrroline-5-carboxylate synthase. Therefore, high ornithine concentrations should favor the ornithine-δ-aminotransferase-mediated pathway of proline synthesis. In certain cells and tissues this pathway seems to be the preferred or only pathway of proline synthesis. In hormonally stimulated rat mammary gland, arginase, ornithine-δ-aminotransferase, and Δ'-pyrroline-5-carboxylate reductase activities increase coordinately in response to hormonal stimulation, and arginine (via ornithine) is a major biosynthetic precursor for the proline utilized in milk protein synthesis [18, 19]. The proline auxotrophy of Chinese hamster ovary cells is due to a deficiency of both pyrroline-5-carboxylate synthase and ornithine-δ-aminotransferase [103]. Prototrophic revertants with either ornithine-δ-aminotransferase or Δ'-pyrroline-5-carboxylate synthase activity grow normally. Finally, the work of Ertel and Isseroff suggests that the ornithine-δ-aminotransferase pathway is the major contributor to the tremendous proline biosynthetic capacity of the liver fluke, *Fasciola hepatica* [105]. To summarize, in some cells and tissues the ornithine-δ-aminotransferase-mediated pathway can be shown to play the major role in proline synthesis, although the relative contribution in most tissues with both proline biosynthetic pathways intact and normal substrate concentrations is still not known.

ORNITHINE AND ARGININE SYNTHESIS   As indicated above, the flow of substrates in the ornithine-δ-aminotransferase pathway is usually toward Δ^1-pyrroline-5-carboxylate. Reversal of this reaction, despite the unfavorable equilibrium constant, provides the only known pathway of *de novo* ornithine synthesis in mammalian cells. An alternative pathway of ornithine synthesis involving *N*-acetylated intermediates is present in microorganisms but has not been found in mammalian tissues [106, 75]. Synthesis of ornithine from glutamate or proline has been shown to occur in the tissues of mammals [57, 60, 75, 107, 108] and in intact cultured cells [109]. This *de novo* synthesis of ornithine provides a mechanism for replenishment of the urea cycle of catalytic intermediates and, if the urea cycle is intact, for the synthesis of arginine. Thus, when dietary arginine is insufficient for net protein synthesis, "reverse" ornithine-δ-aminotransferase assumes major importance. This capability probably explains the nonessentiality of arginine in human infants [110] and the fact that some patients with argininosuccinic acid lyase deficiency excrete more argininosuccinate than can be accounted for by arginine intake [111, 112].

The factors which favor reverse ornithine-δ-aminotransferase flux are unknown. Matsuzawa showed that the reverse reaction has a much lower pH optimum than the forward reaction and that it may be limited by a very low affinity for glutamate (see Table 19-2) [57]. In some animals (e.g., rat, cat) arginine is essential and failure to provide it results in growth failure, orotic aciduria, and hyperammonemia [113, 114]. These animals have ornithine-δ-aminotransferase activity [115]. Thus, the presence of ornithine-δ-aminotransferase is a necessary but not sufficient requisite for arginine synthesis.

DIFFERENTIAL DIAGNOSIS OF HYPERORNITHINEMIA

In normal individuals, fasting morning plasma ornithine concentrations range from 40 to 120 μM with a mean value of 60 to 80 μM. Two distinct entities are associated with significant increases in the plasma ornithine concentration: gyrate atrophy of the choroid and retina, and the hyperornithinemia-hyperammonemia-homocitrullinuria syndrome. In patients with gyrate atrophy, visual symptoms are apparent by late childhood and ornithine concentrations in plasma range from 400 to 1400 μM. Plasma ammonia is not elevated. In the hyperornithinemia-hyperammonemia-homocitrullinuria syndrome the plasma ornithine is often slightly lower than in gyrate atrophy (380 to 630 μM), but values overlap. Plasma ammonia concentrations are increased particularly after ingestion of a protein load. Urinary excretion of ornithine and its δ-lactam is increased in both types of hyperornithinemia, while homocitrulline, an amino acid usually not present in urine, is found only in the hyperammonemic type. The age of onset of hyperornithinemia in both these disorders is not known. One patient with hyperornithinemia-hyperammonemia-homocitrullinuria had a normal ornithine value in a neonatal screening sample [116]. Thus a normal ornithine in the neonatal period may not exclude the hyperornithinemias.

Moderate hyperornithinemia (~3x normal) was also present in two sibs reported by Bickel et al. [117]. At ages 7 and 3 years these patients had mental retardation, renal tubular dysfunction, abnormal liver function tests, and a 60 to 80 percent reduction in hepatic ornithine-δ-aminotransferase activity possibly because of an unexplained liver disease. Currently the boy is 9 and the girl is 15 years old. They are severely retarded; the girl is deaf and has petit mal epilepsy. Both have normal ocular examinations, normal plasma ornithine, normal liver function tests, generalized aminoaciduria, polyuria, isosthenuria, elevation of serum creatinine, and hypertension. The etiology of this syndrome remains unknown [118].

Nongenetic causes of modestly increased plasma ornithine concentrations include isoniazid therapy [119] and spurious elevations due to prolonged standing of the blood sample at room temperature due to conversion of arginine to ornithine by erythrocyte arginase.

In most urinary amino acid screening systems a similar pattern is observed in hyperornithinemias, cystinurias, lysinuric protein intolerance, other hyperdibasicaminacidurias, hyperlysinemias, and possibly in argininemia. The δ-lactam of ornithine, causing a faint brownish spot with ninhydrin, helps differentiate hyperornithinemias from the others, although plasma amino acids have to be measured quantitatively to confirm that diagnosis.

Table 19-2 Concentrations of selected amino acids in body fluids of patients with gyrate atrophy of the choroid and retina

Amino acid	Plasma (μM)		Cerebrospinal fluid (μM)		Aqueous humor (μM)	
	Patients* (n)	Controls† (n)	Patients* (n)	Controls* (n)	Patients* (n)	Controls* (n)
Ornithine	916 (51) 400– 1339	75 ± 5 (22)	274 (5) 217–314	8 (5) 6–11	898 (7) 763–987	63 (4) 38–84
Lysine	84 (51) 40–160	207 ± 9 (22)	17 (5) 12–20	26 16–44 (3)	82 (7) 73–92	145 (4) 128–158
Glutamate	20 (11) 5–43	35 ± 7 (22)	—	—	—	—
Glutamine	475 (11) 322–731	669 ± 21 (22)	—	—	—	—

* Mean over range.
† Mean ± SE.
SOURCES: Data from Takki [129], McCulloch et al. [134], Yatziv et al. [145], Stoppolini et al. [147], Kennaway et al. [155], Valle et al. [158]; Valle et al. [159], Berson et al. [222].

GYRATE ATROPHY OF THE CHOROID AND RETINA

Historical Note

The first description of a patient with gyrate atrophy of the choroid and retina, as defined by the characteristic appearance of the ocular fundus and a typical history of visual deterioration, was probably that of Jacobsohn in 1888 [120]. His report of a case of "atypical retinitis pigmentosa" includes a striking, hand-drawn view of the fundus showing the characteristic lesions of gyrate atrophy. Cutler in 1895 [121] and Fuchs in 1896 [122] were the first ophthalmologists to recognize this condition as a distinct entity. Fuchs bestowed on the disorder its euphonious appellation. Usher reviewed 26 cases in 1935, emphasizing the genetic aspects [123]. Several additional clinical reviews have been published [124, 125], and in 1974 Takki was able to collect nearly 100 patients from the literature [126]. Hyperornithinemia and ornithinuria were not recognized as the biochemical counterparts of this disorder until the report by Simell and Takki in 1973, 85 years after the initial ophthalmologic description [127]. Ironically, an earlier spark of insight into the nature of this disorder, the observation in 1960 of an abnormally large lysine-ornithine spot in the urine of a patient with gyrate atrophy, did not succeed in lighting the fires of scientific investigation [124, 128].

Clinical Picture

There are 91 biochemically confirmed cases of gyrate atrophy reported or known to us [129–152]. The major clinical problem in these patients is a slowly progressive loss of vision leading to blindness, usually by the fourth decade of life [129–132]. Myopia and decreased night vision are the earliest symptoms, usually noted before the end of the first decade. Reduced peripheral vision with constriction of the visual fields is obvious in the second decade. Nearly all patients develop posterior subcapsular cataracts late in the second decade or early in the third. The combination of the cataracts and constricted visual fields may result in severe visual impairment during the third decade. By the fourth to fifth decade, most patients are blind.

In a rare patient the visual deterioration proceeds more rapidly, with nearly complete loss of vision by age 20.

The changes in the ocular fundus parallel the development of the visual symptoms (Fig. 19-3). Myopia or decreased night vision often bring the patient to the attention of an ophthalmologist in late childhood or around the time of puberty. At this age sharply demarcated, circular areas of chorioretinal degeneration are present in the midperiphery of the ocular fundus. There may be increased pigmentation around the margins of these lesions. When observed over time, the lesions can be seen to start as punctate yellowish "dots" which gradually enlarge to the more typically circular areas of one- to two-disk diameters in size [132]. In the second decade, the retinal degeneration seems to proceed at a more rapid pace [131, 132]. The lesions enlarge, coalesce, and extend toward the posterior pole of the fundus. The margins of the lesions remain discrete and are often densely pigmented. The few choroidal vessels traversing the atrophic areas are markedly narrowed. In some patients additional foci of atrophy develop in the peripapillary area. By the third decade much of the fundus is involved. Increased pigmentation is common in the macular area, while the optic disk remains pink and does not become atrophic. There are filamentous vitreous opacities. The cornea and iris remain normal in appearance. In older patients there is complete chorioretinal degeneration, with a few thin strands of pigmented material traversing the fundus. Early in the clinical course, the appearance of the fundus is pathognomonic for gyrate atrophy. In the final stages the appearance is less specific and may easily be confused with the end stage of several other forms of chorioretinal degeneration, especially the X-linked disorder known as choroideremia [153].

The standard tests of visual function become abnormal at an irregular rate, with periods of rapid progression interspersed with periods of relatively stable function [129–132]. Visual acuity decreases gradually over several decades in some patients and abruptly over a few years in others [131]. Visual fields are progressively and concentrically reduced. Those patients with peripapillary atrophy have ring scotoma in addition to peripheral constriction. The electroretinogram, which may be normal at a time when there are a few atrophic patches in the periphery, eventually diminishes in amplitude and usually is totally extinguished well before the atrophy becomes complete. The electro-oculogram, a test of rod function, is also

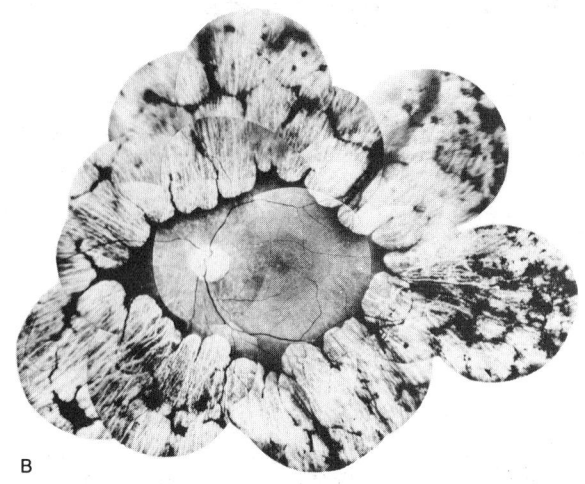

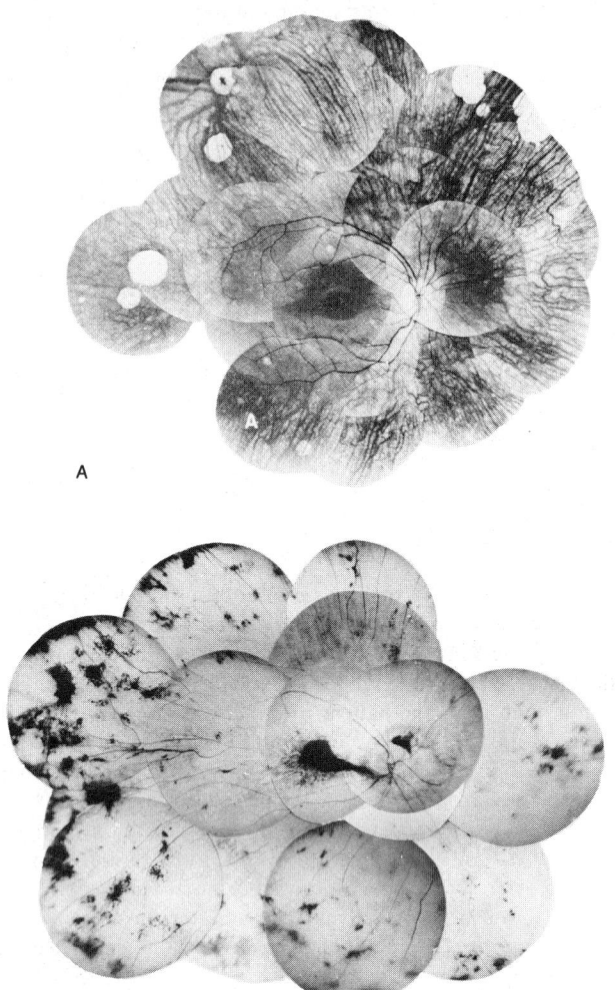

Figure 19-3 Progression of chorioretinal degeneration in the ocular fundi of patients with gyrate atrophy. *A.* Separate, circular areas of chorioretinal atrophy in the midperiphery of the fundus of an 8-year-old boy. *B.* Fused and enlarged atrophic areas in a 22-year-old woman. *C.* Complete atrophy of the choroid and retina in a 51-year-old man. An abundance of fine, velvetlike pigmentation is present in the macula and periphery. The retinal vessels are extremely narrow, and the disc is pink but not atrophic, as in retinitis pigmentosa. (*From Takki, K, Simmell O: Gyrate atrophy of the choroid and retina with hyperornithinemia (HOGA). In Bergsma D, Bron AJ, Cotlier E (eds): The Eye and Inborn Errors of Metabolism. New York, Alan R Liss, Inc, for the National Foundation-March of Dimes, BD: OAS 12(3):373–384, 1976.*)

severely diminished. Dark adaptometry is abnormal, with both an increase in the final threshold and prolongation of the time required to reach the threshold. In some patients fluorescein angiography has demonstrated a narrow concentric ring around the completely atrophic areas in which an abnormally granular retinal pigment epithelium overlays a normal-appearing choroid [129]. This suggests that the initial insult may involve the pigment epithelium of the retina.

Aside from visual impairment, patients with gyrate atrophy are for the most part asymptomatic. Despite this, histologic and ultrastructural abnormalities in mitochondria and skeletal muscle fibers have been described in many patients. Mitochondria in liver have shown nonspecific morphologic abnormalities, with elongation, branching, and segmentation [134]. The functional significance of these abnormalities is not known. Nearly all patients studied have had histologic abnormalities of the type 2 (fast twitch) fibers in skeletal muscle [133, 134, 138, 154, 155] (Fig. 19-4). These fibers are reduced in diameter and contain accumulations of abnormally staining material demonstrable by hematoxylin-eosin, Gomori ATPase, or NAD^+-tetrazolium reductase techniques. These accumulations vary in size from small subsarcolemmal deposits to large collections occupying nearly the entire cross-sectional area of the fiber. By electron microscopy, this abnormal material is formed by aggregates of parallel oriented tubules formed by one or, more typically, two concentric membranes with diam-

eters of 50 to 70 nm for the outer and 25 nm for the inner ("tubular aggregates"; see Ref. 156). The type 1 fibers are normal on examination by both light and electron microscopy. Their number relative to the type 2 fibers increases with age in patients with gyrate atrophy, while in normal subjects the ratio remains constant with age.

Tubular aggregates are not specific for gyrate atrophy. Identical histologic abnormalities have been observed in patients with the various forms of periodic paralysis, hyperthyroidism, porphyria cutanea tarda, myasthenia gravis, myotonic dystrophy, postviral infections, and alcoholism. They have also been observed in low numbers in the muscle of apparently normal male children and adults with nonspecific muscle complaints [156, 157]. Aside from patients with gyrate atrophy, they have not been observed in females.

In addition to these histologic abnormalities, many patients with gyrate atrophy have abnormal electromyograms with short-duration, low amplitude action potentials of the myopathic type [154]. Despite this, muscle strength and serum creatine phosphokinase activity are normal [133, 138, 154].

Additional abnormalities include mild to moderate diffuse slowing on electroencephalography in one-third or less of the patients [129, 133, 138]. Seizures do not occur with increased frequency, and the majority of patients are of normal intelligence [133, 138]. Abnormalities of scalp and body hair have been reported [138].

Biochemical Abnormalities

The discovery by Simell and Takki of ten- to twentyfold elevations of ornithine in plasma, cerebrospinal fluid, and aqueous humor and overflow ornithinuria was the first clue to the nature of the primary defect in gyrate atrophy [127, 130] (Table 19-2). Modest decreases in the plasma concentrations of other amino acids, including lysine, glutamic acid, and glutamine, have been described [130, 134, 145, 155, 158, 159]. Plasma lysine levels in patients ingesting a normal diet average about 40 percent of the normal mean and are often below normal range. Cerebrospinal fluid levels of lysine are in low normal range [130, 158].

Urinary excretion of ornithine in adult patients on a regular diet ranges from 0.5 to 10 mmol/day [145, 147, 158, 159] (Table 19-3). The excretion of arginine and lysine is also slightly increased [147, 158]. An unusual compound first identified as ornithine-methyl ester [160] and subsequently shown to be 3-aminopiperid-2-one, the cyclic δ-lactam of ornithine which forms spontaneously from ornithine methyl ester [152, 161] (Fig. 19-5), is found in gyrate atrophy and other conditions associated with hyperornithinemia. The fact that the plasma concentration of this component has been variously reported as low [162] to unmeasurable [158] suggests that it may originate in the kidney.

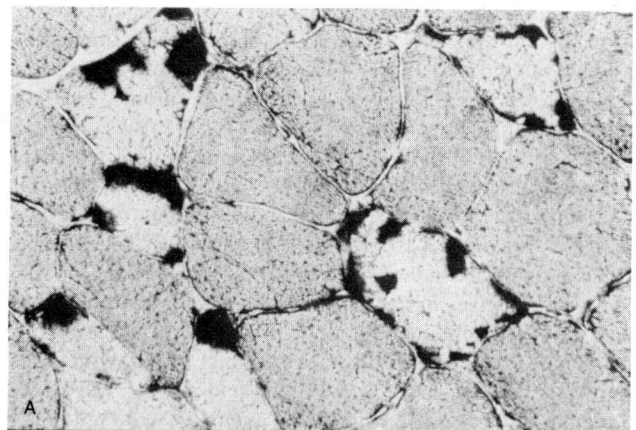

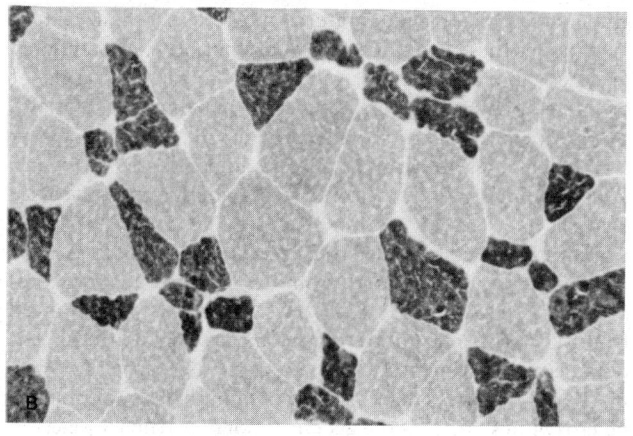

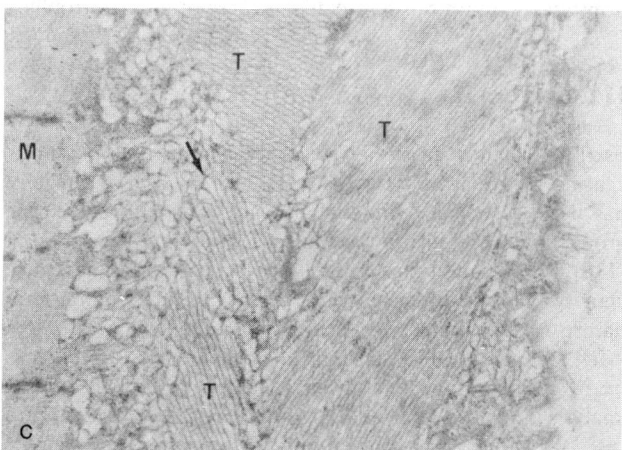

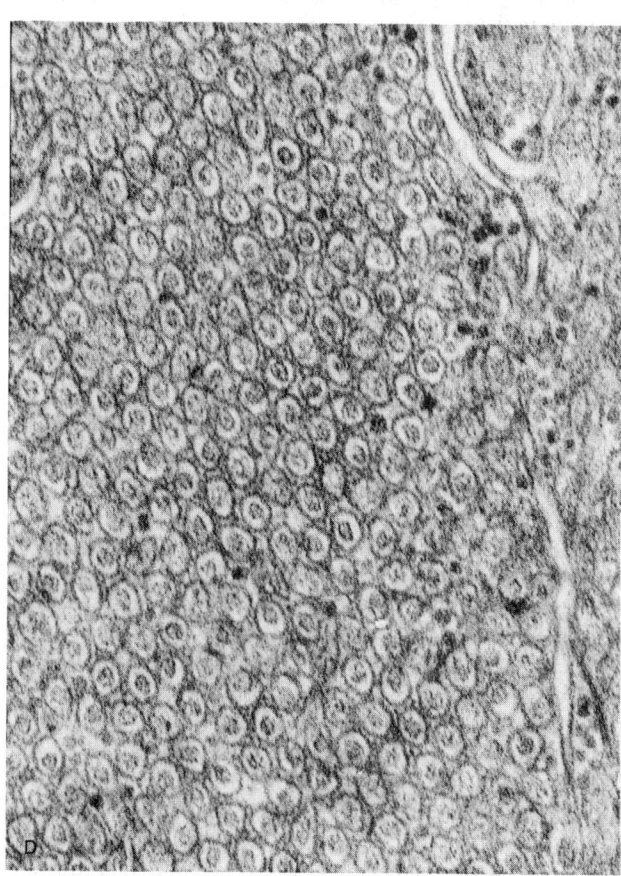

Figure 19-4 Histologic and ultrastructural abnormalitites in the skeletal muscle of gyrate atrophy patients. *A.* NADH-tetrazolium reductase stain demonstrates abnormal, irregular dark areas in the type 2 fibers, which at higher power can be shown to be tubular aggregates. X340. *B.* ATPase stain with preincubation at pH 9.1 stains the type 2 fibers dark and demonstrates several that are atrophic with ragged borders due to lack of enzyme activity in the tubular aggregates. X136. *C.* Ultrastructure of the tubular aggregates in the type 2 fibers showing bundles of parallel tubules (tubular aggregates). The zone between the myofibrils (M) and the regularly aligned tubules (T) consists of haphazardly oriented tubulovesicular structures. The ends of some tubules appear dilated in drumstick fashion. X20,000. *D.* Cross section of the tubules, most of which contain an inner tubule. X58,000. (*From Sipila et al. [154]; reprinted with permission of the authors and Neurology.*)

Table 19-3 Urinary excretion of basic amino acids in gyrate atrophy patients

	n	Excretion (μmol/day)			
		Ornithine	Arginine	Lysine	δ-Lactam of ornithine
Patients*	9	3130 (490–7500)	180 (50–3800)	1300 (400–2300)	1090 (520–3100)
Controls†	14	18 ± 23	10 ± 6	155 ± 114	—

* Mean (range).
† Mean ± SD.
SOURCE: Data for patients from Valle et al. [225]; data for controls from Holmgren [224].

The Enzyme Deficiency

The discovery of hyperornithinemia in gyrate atrophy directed attention to the enzymes of ornithine metabolism, particularly those catalyzing reactions which consume ornithine (Fig. 19-2). Deficiency of ornithine-δ-aminotransferase has been documented in cultured skin fibroblasts [150, 151, 155, 163, 164, 165], in phytohemagglutinin-stimulated lymphocytes [166], in primary skeletal muscle cultures [84], in liver biopsy material [167], and in hair roots [226]. We are aware of ornithine-δ-aminotransferase activity measurements in the fibroblasts of 13 patients in the literature (spectrophotometric assay) plus 19 from our own experience (Table 19-4). The ornithine-δ-aminotransferase activity in these 32 cell lines ranged from undetectable to 5.7 percent that of the mean of controls. Low level ornithine-δ-aminotransferase activity was also detected in liver obtained by percutaneous biopsy from two Finnish patients [167]. The residual activity had a greatly reduced affinity for ornithine (K_m, 200 mM). No studies have been performed in affected sibs to see if the presence or absence of residual activity is familial. Such a finding would suggest that differences in residual activity reflect different mutant alleles. No evidence has been found for ornithine-δ-aminotransferase inhibitors when gyrate atrophy and control cell or tissue extracts have been mixed [165–167]. Ornithine decarboxylase, the other enzyme which catalyzes an ornithine-consuming reaction, was normal in one patient [166].

The ornithine-δ-aminotransferase activity in 5 (including two sibs) of the 32 assayed cell lines has appeared to increase in the presence of very high concentrations of pyridoxal phosphate in the assay mixture [155, 165]. At usual assay concentrations of pyridoxal phosphate (16 to 40 μM), the ornithine-δ-aminotransferase activity in these five cell lines ranged from 1.2 to 5.7 percent of normal by spectrophotometric assay. The measured activity increased to as much as one-third that of controls, with assay pyridoxal phosphate concentrations of between 1 and 4 mM. Unfortunately, there has been no confirmation that the o-aminobenzaldehyde reactive material produced under these conditions was Δ^1-pyrroline-5-carboxylate

Figure 19-5 3-Aminopiperid-2-one, the δ-lactam of L-ornithine. The mechanism of its formation from ornithine is not known.

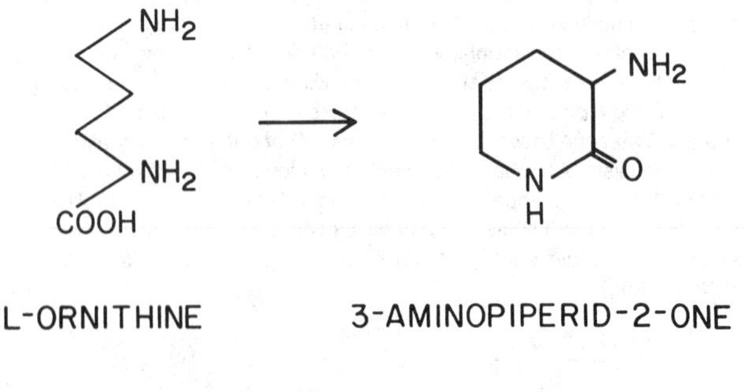

L-ORNITHINE   3-AMINOPIPERID-2-ONE

or that there was a requirement for α-ketoglutarate (see "Chemistry" p. 386). Four of the five patients with an in vitro response had partial reductions in plasma ornithine (average 47 percent) when given pharmacologic doses of pyridoxine (500 to 1000 mg/day) [155, 165]. Three also responded to relatively low doses (15 to 18 mg/day) [142, 155]. One patient described by Kennaway et al. [155] had an in vitro response without an in vivo response, while Valle et al. [159] described a patient with an in vivo response without an in vitro response. Despite the above reservations, the fact that only some cell lines show the in vitro response and that four of these five patients also had a partial in vivo reponse does suggest that some patients are indeed responsive to pyridoxal phosphate.

An alternative measure of ornithine-δ-aminotransferase activity can be obtained by incubating intact fibroblasts in a medium containing radiolabeled ornithine. Cells with ornithine-δ-aminotransferase activity synthesize radiolabeled proline and glutamate from precursor ornithine (see Fig. 19-2), while gyrate atrophy fibroblasts make little or no proline or glutamate. A report that gyrate atrophy cells synthesize glutamate under these conditions [151] has not been substantiated in other laboratories [168, 169]. This "intact cell" assay of ornithine-δ-aminotransferase function not only substantiates the direct enzyme assay but also provides the methodology for a complementation assay of genetic differences in the mutations leading to reduced ornithine-δ-aminotransferase (see below).

Ornithine-δ-aminotransferase activity has also been assayed in cultured skin fibroblasts from 13 obligate heterozygotes (Table 19-4) [151, 155, 165, 168]. The activity has ranged from 32 to 61 percent of the normal mean. A similar result was obtained in transformed lymphocytes [166]. This approximately 50 percent reduction in activity in the cells of obligate heterozygotes provides the genetic proof of a primary defect in ornithine-δ-aminotransferase as the cause of gyrate atrophy.

Heterogeneity

Factors which suggest heterogeneity among the mutations causing gyrate atrophy include: the fact that gyrate atrophy has been observed in individuals of several different ethnic groups; the variability in the clinical severity of gyrate atrophy [136]; the variability in residual ornithine-δ-aminotransferase activity and pyridoxine responsiveness; and the complicated nature of the biology of ornithine-δ-aminotransferase (see "Cell Biology," p. 387). Direct genetic evidence of heterogeneity in gyrate atrophy has been sought by complementation analysis [168, 169]. Fibroblasts from two different patients are fused, and the resulting heterokaryons are tested for recovery of ornithine-δ-aminotransferase by being incubated in radiolabeled ornithine and the amount of radioactivity incorporated into protein quantified. No complementation has been found in pairwise fusions of 10 gyrate atrophy patients (including one pyridoxine-responsive patient) [168, 169]. This result suggests either that the mutations in all 10 patients are identical or, more likely, that different mutations are occurring in the same structural gene and that interallelic complementation does not take place [170].

Pathophysiology

Biochemical Abnormalities Deficiency of ornithine-δ-aminotransferase explains most of the biochemical abnormalities observed in patients with gyrate atrophy. Hyperornithinemia is a direct result of the block in the ornithine-δ-aminotransferase reaction. An adult with gyrate atrophy ingesting 1.5 g/kg per day has an arginine intake of approximately 28 mmol/day. Little if any of this arginine is utilized for protein accretion. Arginine is converted to ornithine by arginase and to a lesser extent by glycine transamidinase (Fig. 19-2). A fraction of the ornithine is utilized for the synthesis of putrescine and polyamines (an estimated 0.5 mmol/day), and the remainder accumulates. Ornithine excretion increases concomitantly, particularly at plasma concentrations of more than 600 μM [159]. The high renal filtered load of ornithine also results in increased renal clearances of lysine, arginine, and cystine [158].

The total urinary excretion of arginine-derived carbon skeletons (arginine, ornithine, the δ-lactam of ornithine, citrulline, and argininosuccinic acid) by patients with gyrate atrophy is much less than the estimated arginine intake (Table 19-3). Therefore, as much as 75 percent of the ingested arginine cannot be accounted for in these patients [158]. Possible explanations for this include residual ornithine-δ-aminotransferase activity [167], gastrointestinal losses, greater flux to putrescine than estimated, or some unanticipated pathway for the catabolism of arginine, ornithine, or any of the urea cycle intermediates. Alpha transamination of arginine or ornithine would provide such an alternative degradation pathway, but there is no evidence that this occurs in humans [60, 171]. The extent of the conversion of ornithine to putrescine by ornithine decarboxylase may have been underestimated by data from studies measuring polyamine excretion [31, 32] since putrescine may also be converted to CO_2 via γ-aminobutyrate and succinate (Fig. 19-2). The enzymes necessary for this reaction sequence are present in mammalian tissues [45–47]. Ornithine decarboxylase is so highly regulated by factors related to the growth of cells [30] that it probably limits significant catabolism by this pathyway.

The extent of ornithine accumulation in patients with this disorder has not been determined since the compartments in which ornithine has been measured (plasma, cerebrospinal fluid, and aqueous humor) represent only a small fraction (~10 percent) of the total body ornithine pool [172]. The major portion of the free pool of most amino acids is located in the intracellular fluid of skeletal muscle and liver. In normal humans the intracellular ornithine concentration in muscle is fivefold that in plasma [173]. Lower values have been reported for rat muscle [174, 175]. If the former ratio is maintained in gyrate atrophy, the total body pool of ornithine in an adult could be as high as 100 to 150 mmol. A comparison of the intracellular versus plasma fractions of the total body orni-thine pool emphasizes the fact that a minor change in ornithine distribution can lead to a major change in plasma concentration without a change in total body ornithine. A temporary shift of ornithine from plasma to intracellular fluid may explain the transient, acute reduction of plasma ornithine in gyrate atrophy patients following a glucose load [133, 155, 158].

Hyperornithinemia and ornithine accumulation may also account for some of the abnormal concentrations of other plasma metabolites. The hypolysinemia may result from the increased renal clearance of lysine or an effect of ornithine on the catabolism or distribution of lysine [158]. The explanation for the reduced levels of glutamate and glutamine is not known, although it has been suggested that this is due to an alteration in the balance between urea precursors (glutamate, glutamine, ammonia) and urea production due to the increased concentration of ornithine [158]. Thus, instead of ornithine availability limiting urea production, the availability of urea precursors is limiting.

Mechanism of the Chorioretinal Degeneration How a deficiency of ornithine-δ-aminotransferase and subsequent ornithine accumulation lead to the chorioretinal degeneration and cataract formation is not known. Any hypothesis must explain the slowly progressive nature of this disorder, the minimal involvement of other organ systems, and the lack of ocular involvement in patients with the hyperornithinemia-hyperammonenia-homocitrullinuria syndrome. Possibilities include a toxic effect of the accumulated precursor (ornithine) or of one of its metabolites, or a deficiency of the reaction product (Δ^1-pyrroline-5-carboxylate) or one of its metabolites. The fact that ornithine-δ-aminotransferase activity is present in both neural retinal tissue and retinal pigment epithelium [81, 82] suggests that the enzyme function may be important in these tissues but does not discriminate between these two general mechanisms.

An additional problem in determining the mechanism of the chorioretinal degeneration is that there are no descriptions of the ocular pathology in humans with gyrate atrophy. Indeed, it is not known for certain which of the many specialized types of cells found in the choroid and retina are the first to be affected. Most attention has centered on the retinal pigment epithelial cells which form the outermost cell layer of the retina [176, 177]. The inner aspect of these cells surrounds the outer segments of the photoreceptor cells and performs a number of functions necessary for the well-being of the receptor cells. The choroidal aspect of the pigment epithelial cells rests on Bruch's membrane, a complex structure which is composed of basement membrane components of both the pigment epithelium and the choriocapillaris. The nutrient supply to the outermost third of the retina, including the pigment epithelium, is provided by specialized, dilated capillaries, the choriocapillaris, located just beneath Bruch's membrane. Metabolites such as glucose and amino acids move through Bruch's membrane and then must be transported across the retinal pigment epithelium to the photoreceptor cells. Because of these close relationships, damage to any of these components may destroy the others secondarily. Pathologic studies in a cat with gyrate atrophy and advanced retinal degeneration showed extensive involvement of the pigment epithelium, neuroretina, and choriocapillaris [178]. The observation in humans by Takki of areas of pigment epithelial cell damage with intact choriocapillaris suggests that the pigment layer is the site of the initial insult in gyrate atrophy [129]. Furthermore, Kuwabara and colleagues have shown that intravitreal injection of ornithine results in degeneration of the pigment epithelial cells in both rats and monkeys [179].

Two hypotheses on the pathophysiology of gyrate atrophy have recently been presented (Fig. 19-6). Sipila and coworkers [53, 154] have proposed that deficiency of creatine and creatine phosphate may account for both the histologic abnormalities in muscle and the chorioretinal degeneration. They suggest that the high ornithine concentrations inhibit glycine transamidinase, thereby reducing creatine synthesis and causing a reduction in total body creatine and creatine phosphate. Evidence supporting this hypothesis includes the well-documented sensitivity of glycine transamidinase to ornithine in vitro [51–53] and the observations that fasting serum creatine and creatinine, daily creatinine excretion, and the excretion of guanidinoacetate and creatine following an arginine load are all reduced in gyrate atrophy patients as compared to normal subjects [180] (Fig. 19-7). These observations suggest that glycine transamidinase is inhibited in vivo as well as in vitro and that there is a reduction of the total body creatine-creatine phosphate pool in gyrate atrophy. The extent of this reduction is not known. Creatinine excretion, although statistically reduced, overlaps with the normal range [180], and direct measurements of tissue creatine-creatine phosphate concentrations have not been performed. This hypothesis would explain the lack of ophthalmologic abnormalities in the hyperornithinemia-hyperammonemia-homocitrullinuria syndrome if the subcellular location of the transamidinase is within the mitochondria and if the defect in this syndrome is an abnormality of ornithine transport into mitochondria (Fig. 19-2). The recent observations of histologic improvement in the muscles of gyrate atrophy patients given exogenous creatine [181] and of improved visual function in patients whose plasma ornithine has been reduced by means of an arginine-restricted diet [137, 158, 182, 183] are compatible with this hypothesis.

Unfortunately, little is known about the role of creatine and creatine phosphate in retinal function. These compounds, as well as guanidinoacetate, are present in mammalian brain [48, 54, 184, 185] and appear to cross the blood-brain barrier

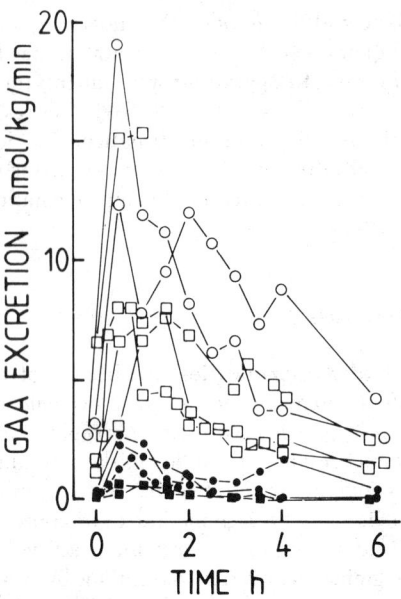

Figure 19-7 Guanidinoacetate (GAA) excretion after intravenous infusion of 1.1 mmol per kilogram body weight of arginine in (■) male and (●) female gyrate atrophy patients and (□) male and (○) female controls. (*From Sipila et al. [180] with permission of the authors and The Journal of Clinical Investigation.*)

slowly [186, 187]. Thus, local synthesis of creatine may be important in the brain and retina. Low glycine transamidinase activity has been found in the human brain [188] but has not been measured in the retina. The recent work with pharmacologic agents which deplete tissues of creatine phosphate [186, 187] and the possible reduction of creatine synthesis in other human and animal disorders [189] provide possibilities for additional study of the role of creatine depletion in the pathophysiology of gyrate atrophy. Finally, creatine phosphate has been implicated as an important energy source for phagocytosis by peritoneal macrophages [190]. This is intriguing in view of the highly phagocytic nature of the retinal pigment epithelium, although there is no direct evidence of phagocytic abnormalities in gyrate atrophy.

A second hypothesis on the pathophysiology of gyrate atrophy involves the deficient synthesis of Δ^1-pyrroline-5-carboxylate resulting from the genetic deficiency of ornithine-δ-aminotransferase and the inhibitory effects of ornithine on Δ^1-pyrroline-5-carboxylate synthase, the enzyme while catalyzes the formation of Δ'-pyrroline-5-carboxylate from glutamate (Fig. 19-6). The observations which support this model include the recent findings that Δ^1-pyrroline-5-carboxylate synthase is inhibited in vitro by near-physiologic concentrations of L-ornithine [102] and that ornithine is toxic to gyrate atrophy fibroblasts at concentrations which are tolerated by control cells [191, 192]. This toxic effect of ornithine is prevented by amino acids which inhibit Δ^1-pyrroline-5-carboxylate dehydrogenase, a Δ^1-pyrroline-5-carboxylate-consuming enzyme, and is partially prevented by the addition of exogenous Δ^1-pyrroline-5-carboxylate [193]. This hypothesis, therefore, suggests that the genetic defect in gyrate atrophy prevents the synthesis of Δ^1-pyrroline-5-carboxylate from ornithine and causes the accumulation of an inhibitor (ornithine) of the alternative pathway of Δ^1-pyrroline-5-carboxylate synthesis. The reduced availability of Δ^1-pyrroline-5-carboxylate may be detrimental either by resulting in decreased proline synthesis or because of disruption of the regulatory roles that Δ^1-pyrroline-

Figure 19-6 Schematic diagram of two different, nonexclusive hypotheses for the pathophysiology of gyrate atrophy of the choroid and retina. In one, high ornithine concentrations inhibit glycine transamidinase, causing a deficiency of guanidinoacetate and creatine. In the other, the combination of the inherited deficiency of ornithine-δ-aminotransferase and the inhibitory effect of ornithine on Δ^1-pyrroline-5-carboxylate synthase results in decreased formation of Δ^1-pyrroline-5-carboxylate and proline.

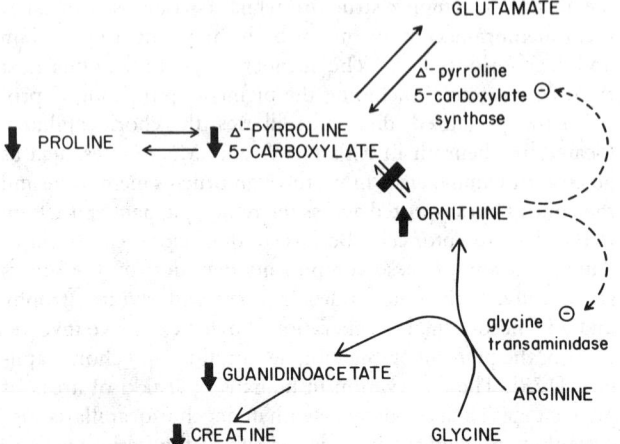

5-carboxylate and its metabolic interconversions have been shown to exert on the intracellular redox level and hexose monophosphate shunt activity [194, 195]. Depending on the mechanism, cells with access to extracellular fluid proline or with the ability to synthesize Δ^1-pyrroline-5-carboxylate from proline by the proline oxidase reaction would be predicted to be unscathed in gyrate atrophy. Thus most cells and tissues would be spared. Retinal pigment epithelium and neural retinal tissue lack proline oxidase [196], and although the availability of proline in the extracellular fluid of the retina is not known, it may be low judging from the fact that proline crosses the blood-brain barrier poorly [197] and is virtually absent from the cerebrospinal fluid [172].

This hypothesis would explain lack of ocular abnormalities in the hyperornithinemia-hyperammonemia-homocitrullinuria syndrome on the basis of normal Δ^1-pyrroline-5-carboxylate production from ornithine by intact ornithine-δ-aminotransferase. The beneficial effects of the reduction of ornithine accumulation [137, 182, 183] would be due to relieving the ornithine inhibition of Δ^1-pyrroline-5-carboxylate synthase. As with the first hypothesis, more information on retinal amino acid and energy metabolism in normal subjects and in gyrate atrophy patients is necessary for further evaluation.

Additional abnormalities of possible pathologic significance in gyrate atrophy include the modest reductions in the plasma concentrations of glutamate, glutamine, and lysine [129, 158]. Of these, only lysine is reduced below the normal range. The hypolysinemia seems unlikely to be related to the chorioretinal degeneration since it probably does not indicate a true lysine deficiency [158] and because other conditions with hypolysinemia (e.g., lysinuric protein intolerance) are not associated with ocular problems [198]. Abnormalities of polyamines or their metabolites could also play a pathologic role in gyrate atrophy. The fragmentary data available suggest that serum spermine, spermidine, and putrescine concentrations are in the normal range [155].

Treatment

The slow progression of the degenerative changes in gyrate atrophy and the difficulty in measuring small changes in ocular function objectively make evaluation of any therapy difficult [140]. Biochemical parameters (e.g., plasma amino acid concentrations) can be accurately measured, but until the pathophysiology is understood there is no assurance that correction of biochemical abnormalities in plasma will actually be beneficial. Three general approaches to the therapy of gyrate atrophy have been attempted: stimulation of residual ornithine-δ-aminotransferase activity with pharmacologic doses of pyridoxine; correction of ornithine accumulation by reducing the intake of its precursor arginine or increasing renal ornithine losses; and administration of creatine.

A response to pyridoxine, particularly if complete, should be an effective therapy regardless of the pathophysiologic mechanisms since the end result is a reduction in the accumulated precursor (ornithine) and an increased production of the reaction product (Δ^1-pyrroline-5-carboxylate). Administration of pharmacologic doses of pyridoxine hydrochloride (500 to 1000 mg/day) has been associated with a significant reduction in plasma ornithine in four patients from three sibships [139–142]. The actual reduction has averaged about 50 percent, although interpretation of this result is somewhat obscured by

the apparent lack of close regulation of arginine intake during these trials. In all instances plasma lysine returned to normal coincident with the decrease in plasma ornithine. Weleber and associates found that 15 to 20 mg/day of pyridoxine hydrochloride was just as effective as the higher dosage in their patients [142]. Fibroblast ornithine-δ-aminotransferase activity in these four patients responded in vitro to the addition of high concentrations of pyridoxal phosphate to the assay mixture [155, 165]. There has been no deterioration of vision in patients receiving pyridoxine, and one of Weleber's patients had improved electroretinograms while on pyridoxine [142].

A second approach to the therapy of gyrate atrophy has involved correction of the ornithine accumulation either by restricting the dietary intake of arginine or by augmenting renal losses of ornithine. The former has been accomplished by reducing protein intake to approximately 0.2 g/kg per day and supplying necessary amounts of essential amino acids, calories, minerals, and vitamins [140, 158, 159, 183]. On this regimen, plasma ornithine values have decreased two- to sixfold as ornithine is lost in the urine and consumed for putrescine synthesis, and at least three patients have maintained normal to near-normal ornithine values for extended periods of time (Fig. 19-8) [159]. The secondary abnormalities in plasma lysine, glutamate, glutamine, and ammonia have improved coincident with a reduction in plasma ornithine. Care must be taken to avoid excessive restriction of arginine, which can lead to hypoargininemia, hypoornithinemia, and acute hyperammonemia, particularly if nitrogen intake is high [159, 183]. Two patients, one of whom has been on the diet for over 3 years, have had modest improvement in subjective and objective tests of visual function [137, 182, 183] (including patient ZF in Fig. 19-8). None of the patients with a significant reduction in ornithine has had a progression of chorioretinal degeneration while on the diet. Although these results with diet therapy are encouraging, more experience with this therapy is necessary before final conclusions can be reached. The diet is very restrictive, and only highly motivated patients with good nutritional and medical management can maintain it.

Increasing the renal losses of ornithine by administration of compounds known to interfere with dibasic amino acid transport has been attempted, alone or in combination with diet therapy. Lysine [145, 158, 189] and the nonmetabolizable amino acid, α-aminoisobutyric acid, [158, 159] have been utilized for this purpose (Fig. 19-8). Both have been shown to increase ornithine excretion especially when plasma ornithine concentrations are high. As plasma ornithine concentrations decrease (particularly below 300 μM), these compounds become much less effective [158, 159]. No studies of the long-term efficacy of this approach have been reported.

A final form of therapy for gyrate atrophy derives from the hypothesis that creatine deficiency plays a pathophysiologic role in this disorder. Sipila and coworkers have administered 1.5 g creatine daily to seven gyrate atrophy patients for 1 year [181]. In all, there was improvement in the histologic abnormalities in muscle, but four of the seven had some progression in their ophthalmologic abnormalities documented by fundus photography. Whether this progression would have been even more extensive if the patients had not been taking creatine is impossible to say. These results indicate that creatine depletion does play a role in the muscle abnormalities. The progression of the ocular abnormalities despite administration of creatine suggests either that the pathophysiology of the chorioretinal degeneration is on a different basis or that at the dose used an

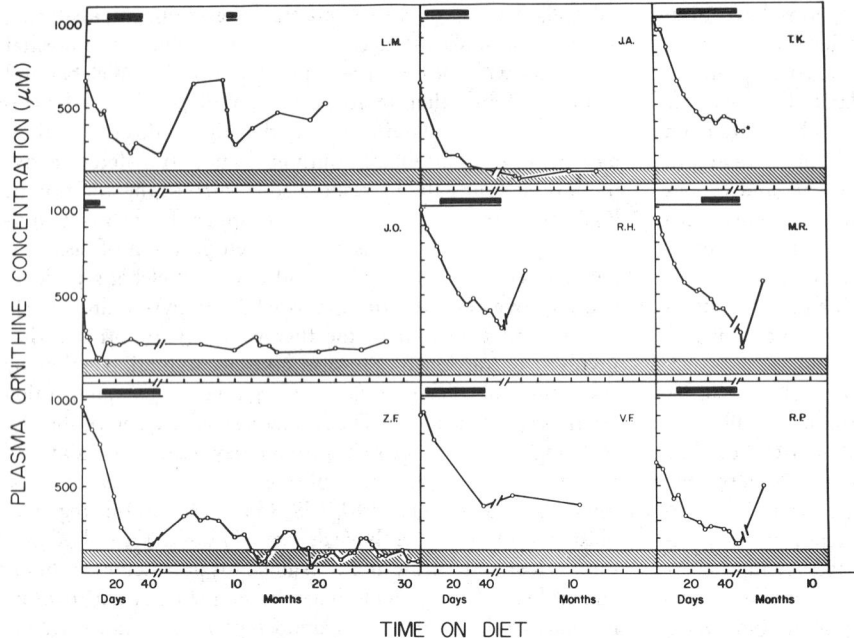

Figure 19-8 The response of plasma ornithine to an arginine-restricted diet and increase of renal ornithine losses by α-aminoisobutyric acid in nine gyrate atrophy patients. The thin horizontal bars along the top of each plot indicate time in the hospital longer than 5 days. The thick bars indicate times when the patients were taking α-aminoisobutyric acid. The cross-hatched areas indicate the normal range of plasma ornithine concentration. The value for plasma ornithine on day 0 of the diet represents the mean of at least three determinations on a regular diet. *, diet terminated. (*From Valle et al.* [159] *with modifications by permission of Ophthalmology.*)

inadequate amount of creatine reached the sensitive cells in the eye. Additional long-term studies of this innovative therapeutic approach are necessary.

Genetics

The inheritance of gyrate atrophy is clearly autosomal recessive. Males and females are equally affected, consanguinity is not uncommon [123, 200], and obligate heterozygotes have partially reduced ornithine-δ-aminotransferase activity (Table 19-4).

Gyrate atrophy is rare, with a total of 91 biochemically confirmed cases known to us. The nationality of the patients has included Finnish, Spanish, Italian, Dutch, English, Welsh, Portuguese, and Japanese. No cases have been reported in blacks. The incidence is apparently highest in Finland, with approximately 50 documented cases in a population of 4.8 million. Assuming 50 percent ascertainment, an estimated frequency of the disorder in Finland would be 1 in 50,000 individuals and the estimated heterozygote frequency would be 1 in 110 individuals. In the United States, the disorder is much rarer.

HYPERORNITHINEMIA-
HYPERAMMONEMIA-
HOMOCITRULLINURIA SYNDROME

Including the original patient of Shih et al. in 1969 [116], five male and three female subjects have been described with a syndrome chemically characterized by increased plasma ornithine concentration, postprandial hyperammonemia, and homocitrullinuria [201–203]. We are aware of two additional patients with typical findings of this syndrome [204, 205]. Six of the patients are from the same consanguine kindred, a fact which strongly suggests autosomal recessive inheritance [203]. All have a history typical of intermittent hyperammonemia. Pregnancy is uncomplicated, birth size normal, and the neona-

tal course uneventful if the children are breast-fed. Many refuse to eat and have episodes of vomiting, lethargy, and coma when fed a high protein formula. Growth is inadequate and developmental milestones are delayed. After infancy, most spontaneously select a low protein diet, avoiding milk and meat. The final mental outcome has varied from low normal to severe retardation. Seizures have occurred in four, beginning between the ages of 10 months and 18 years. The ocular fundi have been normal in all patients except one, who had papilledema, ataxia, hemiplegia, and choreoathetotic movements during an acute episode of hyperammonemia [203]. In another, the liver was slightly enlarged and firm. On biopsy, the hepatic architecture was normal microscopically, but ultrastructurally the mitochondria were elongated, had bizarre shapes and peculiar periodicity below the level of the inner limiting membrane. The longest mitochondria contained "crystalloid" structures, probably representing elongated systems of cristae or tubules [203].

One patient, maintained on 1 g/kg per day protein restriction during the whole pregnancy has given birth to a normal child [203].

Table 19-4 Ornithine-δ-aminotransferase activity in cultured skin fibroblasts of gyrate atrophy patients and heterozygotes*

Group	(n)	Enzyme activity† (nmol/hr/mg)	Percent of control
Controls	(22)	108.6 ± 19	100
Patients			
No activity	(13)	None detectable	0
Residual activity	(6)	1.8 (0.4–3.9)	2
Obligate heterozygotes	(7)	54.3 (37.8–79.4)	50

* Ornithine-δ-aminotransferase activity was assayed radioisotopically with both substrates present at 0.7 mM and 16 μM pyridoxal phosphate [73]. The division of patient cell lines into groups with no detectable activity and residual activity was unaffected by increasing the substrate concentrations to 15 mM ornithine and 2.5 mM α-ketoglutarate ± 0.6 mM pyridoxal phosphate. The ethnic origin of the patients included Finnish, English, Welsh, Scottish, Portuguese, Spanish, Japanese, and Indian.
† Expressed as mean ± SD or mean (range).

Biochemical Findings

Plasma ornithine concentrations as high as 915 μM have been reported in these patients [116]. In general, on a self-restricted protein diet, plasma ornithine values have ranged from 380 to 630 μM [116, 201–205]. Thus, although there is overlap, the hyperornithinemia in these patients tends to be less than in those with gyrate atrophy. Plasma arginine is normal, lysine moderately decreased, and glutamine and alanine often increased, as in other hyperammonemic states (see Chap. 20). Blood ammonia may be normal during fasting but is abnormally high following protein ingestion. High protein diets result in chronic hyperammonemia. Oral loading tests with 0.1 or 0.2 g/kg ornithine cause normal or slightly greater than normal increases in plasma ornithine and a slow return to initial concentrations. The responses of plasma citrulline and ornithine to citrulline loads, plasma lysine to lysine loads, and plasma and urinary homocitrulline to homocitrulline loads are indistinguishable from normal [116, 203].

There is mild to severe ornithinuria ranging from 73 to 8160 μmol/g creatinine. The highest excretions have been measured during acute exacerbations of hyperammonemia. Urinary homocitrulline greatly exceeds normal (patients range from 148 to 1190; mean ± SD in controls, 51 ± 38 μmol/g creatinine). Homocitrulline excretion seems to correlate with the amount of lysine ingested and is not influenced by citrulline loading. Renal homocitrulline reabsorption is normal [203]. The δ-lactam of ornithine, 3-amino-piperid-2-one, first believed to be ornithine methyl ester, has been detected in the urine of these patients in amounts ranging from 130 to 1050 μmol/g creatinine, whereas only traces are found in normal urine [152, 160, 161]. The origin and physiologic significance of this substance are unknown. Orotic acid excretion, believed to reflect carbamoyl phosphate accumulation, was elevated in half of the patients studied (mean and range, 31.6 and 8.2 to 109 mg/g creatinine; mean ± SD in controls, 8.3 ± 5.7 mg/g creatinine), suggesting that carbamoyl phosphate synthesis is intact in these patients [203].

The possibility of an enzymatic deficiency as the cause of this syndrome has been investigated, but no consistent or convincing defects have been demonstrated. The mean leukocyte carbamoyl phosphate synthetase I (mitochondrial; N-acetylglutamate dependent) in four patients was 13 percent of the mean of the controls, whereas leukocyte carbamoyl phosphate synthetase II (cytoplasmic; N-acetylglutamate independent) and the other urea cycle enzymes were normal. Carbamoyl phosphate synthetase I was 20 percent of the normal mean in a liver biopsy (just below the −2 SD value of the controls), while the cytoplasmic carbamoyl phosphate synthetase II was markedly and the other urea cycle enzymes slightly elevated as compared with control values [203]. Ornithine decarboxylase, measured in cultured fibroblasts of another patient, was also low at 20 to 30 percent of the normal mean [206]. Ornithine-δ-aminotransferase activity is normal in the cultured fibroblasts of patients [203, 207]. No enzyme activity measurements in the heterozygotes have been reported.

Pathophysiology

Ammonia accumulation can be reduced or prevented in vitro in isolated hepatocytes and in vivo in animals and patients with other types of urea cycle disorders by increasing the availability of the urea cycle intermediates arginine, ornithine, or citrulline [209–214]. Thus, the paradoxical combination of hyperornithinemia and hyperammonemia in this disease is fascinating.

Several possibilities have been proposed for the primary defect. Some patients have had moderate reduction in carbamoyl phosphate synthetase I activity [203], but deficiency of this enzyme is an unlikely explanation for this disease. Patients with well-documented carbamoyl phosphate synthetase I deficiency do not accumulate ornithine, nor do they excrete orotic acid or homocitrulline (see Chap. 20). The importance of the reported decreased activity remains obscure. Alternatively, deficient formation of N-acetylglutamate, an activator of carbamoyl phosphate synthetase I, might be the primary problem in this disorder. Neither the concentration nor the synthesis of N-acetylglutamate has been measured in these patients, and deficiency of N-acetylglutamate synthetase has been described in a hyperammonemic patient who lacked hyperornithinemia and homocitrullinuria [215].

In 1974 Fell and coworkers suggested that a defect in the transport of ornithine into mitochondria might explain the findings in this syndrome [202]. The entry of ornithine into liver mitochondria is mediated by one or possibly two specific carriers, one of which may be dependent on respiratory energy [4, 24, 25] (see "Subcellular Compartmentation and Transport of Ornithine," p. 384). Diminished entry of ornithine into mitochondria would decrease citrulline synthesis and impair ammonia detoxification. Furthermore, since ornithine-δ-aminotransferase, the major ornithine-catabolizing enzyme, is also within the mitochondria, diminished entry of ornithine would lead to ornithine accumulation in the cytosolic and extracellular fluids. This hypothesis predicts that increasing the cytosolic ornithine might drive transmitochondrial ornithine transport and improve the patient's urea cycle function. With this rationale in mind, Fell and coworkers supplemented their patient with 6 g ornithine daily. This doubled the plasma ornithine concentration and clearly reduced the plasma ammonia concentration [202]. However, in another patient the hyperammonemia induced by alanine infusion remained unaltered even when the test was preceded by daily supplementation of 6 g ornithine for 1 week and intravenous infusion of ornithine for 2 h prior to and during the alanine load [204]. This difference in response to ornithine supplementation may indicate heterogeneity of this syndrome. No direct measurements of mitochondrial ornithine fluxes are available in these patients, but suggestive evidence in favor of such a mitochondrial transport defect has been obtained in cultured fibroblasts [216, 217].

The origin of homocitrulline in these patients is uncertain. Infants ingesting heat-treated milk products excrete homocitrulline, which apparently is formed spontaneously from lysine when milk is heated [218]. Excessive amounts of homocitrulline are also excreted by some patients with hyperlysinemia and saccharopinuria [219–221]. The hypothesis of Fell et al. for the pathophysiology of this syndrome predicts that lysine uptake into mitochondria is normal and that the increased lysine/ornithine ratio in the mitochondrial matrix leads to ornithine transcarbamoylase-catalyzed conversion of lysine to homocitrulline. Indeed, lysine supplementation in one patient was followed by a significant rise in homocitrulline excretion [202]. The blood ammonia concentration increased simultaneously and suggested that this pathway cannot be used for removal of excessive carbamoyl phosphate and ammonia in these patients.

Treatment

Protein restriction to less than 1.2 g/kg per day results in decreased concentrations of ornithine in plasma and prevents postprandial hyperammonemia [116, 201–203]. If decreased ornithine transport into the mitochondria is the primary abnormality in this syndrome, the patients may also benefit from ornithine supplementation. In one patient, the addition of 6 g ornithine or 7.5 g arginine daily to the diet decreased blood ammonia to normal or near-normal values, while fasting plasma ornithine rose to as high as 1.5 mM [202]. The long-term effects of ornithine supplementation in these patients have not been documented and should be carefully evaluated in view of the association of hyperornithinemia with the chorioretinal degeneration in gyrate atrophy.

Genetics

The large Canadian pedigree of Gatfield et al. [203] with six affected subjects from both sexes strongly suggests autosomal recessive inheritance of the hyperornithinemia-hyperammonemia-homocitrullinuria syndrome. Since the primary biochemical derangement in the homozygotes is unknown, no biochemical tests are available to confirm the heterozygous status. The parents of one patient had normal plasma and urine amino acid concentrations and normal plasma ornithine responses to oral ornithine loads.

Supported in part by Grant EYO2948 from the National Institutes of Health, the Howard Hughes Medical Institute (DV), and the Retinitis Pigmentosa Foundation (OS).

REFERENCES

1. SNODGRASS PJ: The effects of pH on the kenetics of human liver ornithine-carbamyl phosphate transferase. *Biochemistry* 7:3047, 1968
2. MARSHALL M, COHEN PP: Ornithine transcarbamylase from *Streptococcus faecalis* and bovine liver. *J Biol Chem* 247:1654, 1972
3. MARSHALL M: Ornithine transcarbamylase from bovine liver, in Grisolia S, Baguena R, Mayor F (eds): *The Urea Cycle*. New York, John Wiley & Sons, Inc, 1976, p 169
4. MCGIVAN JD, BRADFORD NM, BEAVIS AD: Factors influencing the activity of ornithine aminotransferase in isolated rat liver mitochondria. *Biochem J* 162:147, 1977
5. RAIJMAN L: Enzyme and reactant concentrations and the regulation of urea synthesis in Grisolia S, Baguena R, Mayor F (eds): *The Urea Cycle*. New York, John Wiley & Sons, Inc, 1976, p 243
6. STEWART PM, WALSER M: Short term regulation of ureagenesis. *J Biol Chem* 255:5270, 1980
7. MEIJER AJ: Regulation of carbamoyl-phosphate synthase (ammonia) in liver in relation to urea cycle activity. *Trends Biochem Sci* 4:83, 1979
8. SCHIMKE RT: Adaptive characteristics of urea cycle enzymes in the rat. *J Biol Chem* 237:459, 1962
9. NUZUM CT, SNODGRASS PJ: Urea cycle enzyme adaptation to dietary protein in primates. *Science* 172:1042, 1971
10. DE MARS R, LE VAN SL, TREND BL, RUSSELL LB: Abnormal ornithine carbamoyl transferase in mice having the sparse-fur mutation. *Proc Natl Acad Sci USA* 73:1693,1976
11. REDDI PK, KNOX WE, HERZFELD A: Types of arginase in rat tissues. *Enzyme* 20:305, 1975
12. SOBERON G, PALACIOS R: Arginase in Grisolia S, Baguena R, Mayor F (eds): *The Urea Cycle*. New York, John Wiley & Sons, Inc, 1976, p 221
13. HERZFELD A, RAPER SM: The heterogeneity of arginases in rat tissues. *Biochem J* 153:469, 1976
14. SPECTOR EB, RICE SCH, CEDARBAUM SD: Evidence for two genes encoding human arginase. *Pediatr Res* 15:569, 1981
15. AEBI H:Coordinated changes in enzymes of the ornithine cycle and response to dietary conditions, in Grisolia S, Baguena R, Mayor F (eds):

The Urea Cycle. New York, John Wiley & Sons, Inc, 1976, p 275
16. BEDINO ST: Allosteric regulation of beef liver arginase activity by L-ornithine. *Ital J Biochem* 26:264, 1977
17. KAYSEN GA, STRECKER HJ: Purification and properties of arginase of rat kidney. *Biochem J* 133:779, 1973
18. GLASS RD, KNOX WE: Arginase isoenzymes of rat mammary gland, liver and other tissues. *J Biol Chem* 248:5785, 1973
19. MEZL VA, KNOX WE: Metabolism of arginine in lactating rat mammary gland. *Biochem J* 166:105, 1977
20. TERHEGGEN HG, LAVINHA F, COLUMBO JP, VAN SANDE M, LOWENTHAL A: Familial hyperargininemia. *J Genet Hum* 20:69, 1972
21. CEDARBAUM SD, SHAW KN, VALENTE M: Hyperargininemia. *J Pediatr* 90:569, 1977
22. SNYDERMAN SE, SANSARICO C, CHEN WJ, NORTON PM, PHANSALKAR SV: Argininemia. *J Pediatr* 90:563, 1977
23. KLINGENBERG M: Metabolic transport in mitochondria: An example for intracellular membrane function. *Essays Biochem* 6:119, 1970
24. GAMBLE JG, LEHNINGER AL: Transport of ornithine and citrulline across the mitochondrial membrane. *J Biol Chem* 248:610, 1973
25. BRADFORD NM, MCGIVAN JD: Evidence for the existence of an ornithine/citrulline antiporter in rat liver mitochondria. *FEBS Letters* 113:294, 1980
26. RAIJMAN L: Citrulline synthesis in rat tissues and liver content of carbamoyl phosphate and ornithine. *Biochem J* 138:225, 1974
27. BRYLA J, HARRIS EJ: Accumulation of ornithine and citrulline in rat liver mitochondria in relation to citrulline formation. *FEBS Lett* 72:331, 1976
28. RAINA A, JANNE J: Physiology of the natural polyamines putrescine, spermidine and spermine. *Medic Biol* 53:121, 1975
29. CAMPBELL RA, MORRIS DR, BARTOS D, DAVES GD, BARTOS F: Advances in Polyamine Research, vol 2, New York, Raven Press, 1978
30. WILLIAMS-ASHMAN HG, COPPOC GL, SCHEONONE A, WEBER G: Aspects of polyamine biosynthesis in normal and malignant eukaryotic cells, in Russell DH (ed): *Polyamines in Normal and Neoplastic Growth*. New York, Raven Press, 1973 p 181
31. MUDD SH, POOLE JR: Labile methyl balances for normal humans on various dietary regimens. *Metabolism* 24:721, 1975
32. MUDD SH, EBERT MH, SCRIVER CR: Labile methyl group balances in the human: The role of sarcosine. *Metabolism* 29:707, 1980
33. PEGG AE, WILLIAMS-ASHMAN HG: Biosynthesis of putrescine in the prostate gland of the rat. *Biochem J* 108:533, 1968
34. PEGG AE, LOCKWOOD DH, WILLIAMS-ASHMAN HG: Concentrations of putrescine and polyamines and their enzymic synthesis during androgen-induced prostatic growth. *Biochem J* 117:17, 1970
35. NISSLEY SP, PASSAMANI J, SHORT P: Stimulation of DNA synthesis, cell multiplication and ornithine decarboxylase in 3T3 cells by multiplication stimulating activity (MSA). *J Cell Physiol* 89:393, 1976
36. BYUS CV, RUSSELL DH: Ornithine decarboxylase activity: Control by cyclic nucleotides. *Science* 187:650, 1975
37. FONG WF, HELLER JS, CANELLAKIS ES: The appearance of an ornithine decarboxylase inhibitory protein upon the addition of putrescine to cell cultures. *Biochim Biophys Acta* 428:456, 1976
38. HELLER JS, FONG WF, CANELLAKIS FS: Induction of a protein inhibitor to ornithine decarboxylase by the end products of its reaction. *Proc Natl Acad Sci USA* 73:1858, 1976
39. METCALF BW, BEY P, DANZIN C, JUNG MJ, CASARA P, VERERT JP: Catalytic irreversible inhibition of mammalian ornithine decarboxylase (EC4.1.1.17) by substrate and product analogues. *J Am Chem Soc* 100:2551, 1978
40. MAMONT PS, DUCHESNE MC, JODER-OHLENBUSCH AM, GROVE J: Effects of ornithine decarboxylase inhibitors on cultured cells, in Seiler N, Jung MJ, Koch-Weser J (eds): *Enzyme-Activated Irreversible Inhibitors*. New York, Elsevier North-Holland Biomedical Press, 1978, p 43
41. O'LEARY MH, HERREID RM: Mechanism of inactivation of ornithine decarboxylase by α-methylornithine. *Biochemistry* 17:1010, 1978
42. FOZARD JR, PART ML, PRAKASH NJ, GROVE J, SCHECHTER PJ, SJOERDSMA A, KOCH-WESER J: L-Ornithine decarboxylase: An essential role in early mammalian embryogenesis. *Science* 208:505, 1980
43. BARTOLOME J, HUGUENARD J, SLOTKIN TA: Role of ornithine decarboxylase in cardiac growth and hypertrophy. *Science* 210:793, 1980
44. BAXTER CF: Some recent advances in studies of GABA metabolism and compartmentation in GABA, in Roberts E, Chase TN, Tower DB (eds): *Nervous System Function*. New York, Raven Press, 1976, p 61
45. SEILER N, AL-THERIB MJ: Putrescine catabolism in mammalian brain. *Biochem J* 144:29, 1974
46. DE MELLO FG, BACHRACH U, NIRENBERG M: Ornithine and glutamic acid decarboxylase activities in the developing chick retina. *J Neurochem* 27:847, 1978
47. MURRIN LC: Ornithine as a precursor for γ-aminobutyric acid in mammalian brain. *J Neurochem* 34:1779, 1980
48. WALKER JB: Creatine: Biosynthesis, regulation and function. *Adv Enzymol* 50:177, 1979

49. WALKER MS, WALKER JB: Repression of transamidinase activity during embryonic development. *J Biol Chem* 237:473, 1962

50. VAN PILSUM JF, CANFIELD TM: Transamidinase activities, in vitro, of kidneys from rats fed diets supplemented with nitrogen-containing compounds. *J Biol Chem* 237:2574, 1962

51. RATNER S, ROCHOVANSKY O: Biosynthesis of guanidinoacetic acid. I. Purification and properties of transamidinase. *Arch Biochem Biophys* 63:277, 1956

52. RATNER S, ROCHOVANSKY O: Biosynthesis of guanidinoacetic acid. II. Mechanism of amidine group transfer. *Arch Biochem Biophys* 63:296, 1956

53. SIPILA I: Inhibition of arginine-glycine aminodiotransferase by ornithine. *Biochim Biophys Acta* 613:79, 1980

54. DEFALCO AJ, DAVIES RK: The synthesis of creatine by the brain of the intact rat. *J Neurochem* 7:308, 1961

55. PARDRIDGE WM, DUDUCGIAN-VARTAVARIAN L, CASANELLO-ERTL D, JONES MR, KOPPLE JD: Amino acid and creatine metabolism in adult rat skeletal muscle cells in tissue culture. *Fed Proc* 39:1179, 1980

56. STRECKER HJ: Purification and properties of rat liver ornithine-δ-transaminase. *J Biol Chem* 240:1225, 1965

57. MATSUZAWA T: Characteristics of the inhibition of ornithine-δ-aminotransferase by branched-chain amino acids. *J Biochem* 75:601, 1974

58. MEZL VA, KNOX WE: Properties and analysis of a stable derivative of pyrroline-5-carboxylic acid for use in metabolic studies. *Anal Biochem* 74:430, 1976

59. QUASTEL JH, WITTY R: Ornithine transaminase. *Nature* 167:556, 1951

60. MEISTER A: Enzymatic transamination reactions involving arginine and ornithine. *J Biol Chem* 206:587, 1954

61. PERAINO C, PITOT HC: Ornithine-δ-transaminase in the rat. I. Assay and some general properties. *Biochim Biophys Acta* 73:222, 1963

62. KATUNUMA N, MATSUDA Y, TOMINO I: Studies on ornithine-ketoacid transaminase. I. Purification and properties. *J Biochem* 56:499, 1964

63. MATSUZAWA T, KATSUNUMA T, KATUNUMA N: Crystallization of ornithine transaminase and its properties. *Biochem Biophys Res Commun* 32:161, 1968

64. PERAINO C, BUNVILLE LG, TAHMISIAN TN: Chemical, physical and morphological properties of ornithine aminotransferase from rat liver. *J Biol Chem* 244:2241, 1969

65. SANADA Y, SHIOTANI T, OKUNO E, KATUNUMA N: Coenzyme-dependent conformational properties of rat liver ornithine aminotransferase. *Eur J Biochem* 69:507, 1976

66. SANADA Y, SUEMORI I, KATUNUMA N: Properties of ornithine aminotransferase from rat liver, kidney and small intestine. *Biochim Biophys Acta* 220:42, 1970

67. KALITA CC, KERMAN JD, STRECKER HJ: Preparation and properties of ornithine-oxo-acid aminotransferase of rat kidney. *Biochim Biophys Acta* 429:780, 1976

68. YIP MCM, COLLINS RK: Purification and properties of rat kidney and liver ornithine aminotransferase. *Enzyme* 12:187, 1971

69. PERAINO C: Functional properties of ornithine-ketoacid aminotransferase from rat liver. *Biochim Biophys Acta* 289:117, 1972

70. KITO K, SANADA Y, KATUNUMA N: Mode of inhibition of ornithine aminotransferase by L-canaline. *J Biochem* 83:201, 1978

71. JUNG MJ, SEILER N: Enzyme activated irreversible inhibitors of L-ornithine:2-oxoacid aminotransferase. *J Biol Chem* 253:7431, 1978

72. JOHN RA, JONES ED, FOWLER LJ: Enzyme-induced inactivation of transaminases by acetylenic and vinyl analogues of 4-aminobutyrate. *Biochem J* 177:721, 1979

73. PHANG JM, DOWNING SJ, VALLE D: A radioisotopic assay for ornithine-δ-transaminase. *Anal Biochem* 55:272, 1973

74. VALLE D, GOODMAN SI, HARRIS SC, PHANG JM: Genetic evidence for a common enzyme catalyzing the second step in the degradation of proline and hydroxyproline. *J Clin Invest* 64:1365, 1970

75. ADAMS E, FRANK L: Metabolism of proline and the hydroxyprolines. *Ann Rev Biochem* 49:1005, 1980

76. O'DONNELL JJ, SANDMAN RP, MARTIN SR: Assay of ornithine aminotransferase by high-performance liquid chromatography. *Anal Biochem* 90:41, 1978

77. HERZFELD A, KNOX WE: The properties, developmental formation and estrogen induction of ornithine aminotransferase in rat tissues. *J Biol Chem* 243:3227, 1968

78. HERZFELD A, RAPER S: Enzymes of ornithine metabolism in adult and developing rat intestine. *Biochim Biophys Acta* 428:600, 1976

79. HERZFELD A, RAPER S: Amino acid metabolizing enzymes in rat submaxillary gland, normal or neoplastic, and in pancrease. *Enzyme* 21:471, 1976

80. SMITH RJ, PHANG JM: Proline metabolism in cartilage: The importance of proline biosynthesis. *Metabolism* 27:685, 1978

81. BAICH A, RATZLAFF K: Ornithine aminotransferase in chick embryo tissues. *Invest Ophthalmol Vis Sci* 19:411, 1980

82. HAYASAKA S, SHIONO T, TAKAKU Y, MIZUNO K: Ornithine ketoacid aminotransferase in the bovine eye. *Invest Ophthalmol* 19:1457, 1980

83. VALLE D, STEEL G, TANAKA Y: Unpublished observations

84. ASKANAS V, VALLE D, KAISER-KUPFER MI, TAKKI K, ENGEL WK, BLUMENKOPF B: Cultured muscle fibers of gyrate atrophy patients: Tubules, ornithine toxicity and 1-ornithine-2-oxoacid aminotransferase deficiency. *Neurology* 30:368, 1980

85. RAIHA NCR, KEKOMAKI MP: Studies on the development of ornithine-ketoacid aminotransferase activity in rat liver. *Biochem J* 108:521, 1968

86. PERAINO C, PITOT HC: Studies on the induction and repression of enzymes in rat liver. *J Biol Chem* 239:4308, 1964

87. LYONS RT, PITOT HC: Hormonal regulation of ornithine aminotransferase biosynthesis in rat liver and kidney. *Arch Biochem Biophys* 180:472, 1977

88. WU C: Estrogen induction of ornithine aminotransferase in rat kidney slices. *Biochem Biophys Res Commun* 82:782, 1978

89. IP MM, CHEE PY, SWICK RW: Turnover of hepatic mitochondrial ornithine aminotransferase and cytochrome oxidase using ^{14}C-carbonate as tracer. *Biochim Biophys Acta* 354:29, 1974

90. CHEE PY, SWICK RW: Effect of dietary protein and tryptophan on the turnover of rat liver ornithine aminotransferase. *J Biol Chem* 251:1029, 1976

91. KOBAYASHI K, KITO K, KATUNUMA N: Effects of estrogen on the turnover rates of ornithine aminotransferase in rat liver and kidney. *J Biochem* 79:787, 1976

92. AUGUSTINE SL, SWICK RW: Turnover of total proteins and ornithine aminotransferase during liver regeneration in rats. *Am J Physiol* 238:46, 1980

93. SCHATZ G: How mitochondria import proteins from the cytoplasm. *FEBS Lett* 103:203, 1979

94. CHUA N, SCHMIDT GW: Transport of proteins into mitochondria and chloroplasts. *J Cell Biol* 81:461, 1979

95. LOCKER J, RABINOWITZ M: An overview of mitochondrial nucleic acids and biogenesis, in Fleischer S, Packer L (eds): *Methods in Enzymology.* New York, Academic Press, Inc, 1979, vol 56, p 3

96. MACCECCHINI M, RUDIN Y, SCHATZ G: Transport of proteins across the mitochondrial outer membrane. *J Biol Chem* 254:7468, 1979

97. CONBOY JG, KALOUSEK F, ROSENBERG LE: In vitro synthesis of a putative precursor of mitochondrial ornithine transcarbamoylase. *Proc Natl Acad Sci USA* 76:5724, 1979

98. MORI M, MORRIS SM, COHEN PP: Cell-free translation and thyroxine induction of carbamoylphosphate synthetase I messenger RNA in tadpole liver. *Proc Natl Acad Sci USA* 76:3179, 1979

99. MARX JL: Newly made proteins zip through the cell. *Science* 207:164, 1980

100. KOMINAMI E, KATUNUMA N: Studies on new intracellular proteases in various organs of rats: Participation of proteases in degradation of ornithine aminotransferase *in vitro* and *in vivo*. *Eur J Biochem* 62:425, 1976

101. GRISOLIA S, KNECHT E, HERNANDEZ-YAGO J, WALLACE R: Turnover and degradation of mitochondria and their proteins, in *Protein Degradation in Health and Disease.* New York, Ciba Foundation Symposium 75, Excerpta Medica, 1980, p 167

102. LODATO RF, SMITH RJ, VALLE D, PHANG MJ, AOKI TT: Regulation of proline biosynthesis: The inhibition of pyrroline-5-carboxylate synthase activity by ornithine. *Metabolism* 21:908, 1981

103. VALLE D, DOWNING SJ, HARRIS SC, PHANG JM: Proline biosynthesis: Multiple defects in Chinese hamster ovary cells. *Biochem Biophys Res Commun* 53:1130, 1973

104. SMITH RJ, PHANG JM: The importance of ornithine as a precursor for proline in mammalian cells. *J Cell Physiol* 98:475, 1979

105. ERTEL J, ISSEROFF H: Proline in Fascioliasis. I. Comparative activities of ornithine-δ-transaminase and proline oxidase in *Fasciola* and in mammalian livers. *J Parasitol* 60:574, 1974

106. SMITH AD, BENZIMAN M, STRECKER HJ: The formation of ornithine from proline in animal tissues. *Biochem J* 104:557, 1967

107. ROSS G, DUNN D, JONES ME: Ornithine synthesis from glutamate in rat intestinal mucosa homogenates: Evidence for the reduction of glutamate to γ-glutamyl semialdehyde. *Biochem Biophys Res Commun* 85:140, 1978

108. WINDMUELLER HG, SPAETH AE: Intestinal metabolism of glutamine and glutamate from the lumen as compared to glutamine from blood. *Arch Biochem Biophys* 171: 662, 1975

109. VALLE D, PHANG JM, DOWNING SJ: Unpublished observations

110. SNYDERMAN SE, BOYER A, HOLT LE: The arginine requirement of the infant. *Am J Dis Child* 97:78, 1959

111. MOSER HW, EFRON ML, BROWN H, DIAMOND R, NEUMAN CG: Argininosuccinic aciduria. Report of two new cases and demonstration of intermittent elevation of blood ammonia. *Am J Med* 42:9, 1967

112. BRUSILOW SW, BATSHAW ML: Personal communication

113. MORRIS JG, ROGERS QR: Ammonia intoxication in the near-adult cat as a result of a dietary deficiency of arginine. *Science* 199:431, 1978

114. MORRIS JG, ROGERS QR: Arginine: An essential amino acid for the cat. *J Nutr* 108:1944, 1978

115. STEWART PM, WALSER M, BATSHAW M, VALLE D: Effects of arginine-free meals on ureagenesis in cats. *Am J Physiol* 241:310, 1981

116. SHIH V, EFRON ML, MOSER HW: Hyperornithinemia, hyperammonemia, and homocitrullinuria. A new disorder of amino acid metabolism associated with myoclonic seizures and mental retardation. *Am J Dis Child* 117:83, 1969

117. BICKEL H, FEIST D, MULLER H, QUADBECK G: Ornithinamie, eine weiter aminosaurenstoff-Wechselsturung mit hirnschadijgung. *Dtsch Med Wochenschr* 47:2247, 1968

118. GRUBNER R: Personal communications

119. PERRY TL, HANSEN S: Biochemical effects in man and rat of three drugs which can increase brain GABA content. *J Neurochem* 30:679, 1978

120. JACOBSOHN E: Ein fall von Retinitis pigmentosa atypica. *Klin Monatsbl Augenheilkd* 26:202, 1888

121. CUTLER CW: Drei ungewohnliche Falle von Retinochorioideal degeneration. *Arch Augenheilkd* 30:117, 1895

122. FUCHS E: Ueber zwei der retinitis pigmentosa verwandte Krankheiten (retinitis punctata albescens und atrophia gyrata choriodeae et retinae). *Arch Augenheilkd* 32:111, 1896

123. USHER CH: The Bowman Lecture—On a few hereditary eye affections. *Trans Ophthalmol Sco UK* 55:164, 1935

124. KURSTJENS JH: Choroideremia and gyrate atrophy of the choroid and retina. Brief historical review. *Documenta Ophthalmol* 19:1, 1965

125. FRANCOIS J: Heredity of the choroidal dystrophies. *Adv Ophthalmol* 35:1, 1978

126. TAKKI K: *Gyrate atrophy of the choroid and retina associated with hyperornithinemia.* Thesis, University of Helsinki, Helsinki, 1975.

127. SIMELL O, TAKKI K: Raised plasma ornithine and gyrate atrophy of the choroid and retina. *Lancet* 1:1031, 1973

128. FRANCOIS J, BARBIER F, DE ROUCK A: Les conducteurs de gene de l'atrophia gyrata chorioideae et retinae de Fuchs (anomalie d'Alder). *Acta Med Genet Med Gemell* 9:74, 1960

129. TAKKI K: Gyrate atrophy of the choroid and retina associated with hyperornithinemia. *Br J Ophthalmol* 58:3, 1974

130. TAKKI K, SIMELL O: Gyrate atrophy of the choroid and retina with hyperornithinemia. *Birth Defects* 12:373, 1976

131. TAKKI K, MILTON RC: The natural history of gyrate atrophy of the choroid and retina. *Ophthalmology* 88:292, 1981

132. FRANCOIS J: Gyrate atrophy of the choroid and retina. *Ophthalmologica, (Basel)* 178:311, 1979

133. MCCULLOCH C, MARLISS EB: Gyrate atrophy of the choroid and retina with hyperornithinemia. *Am J Ophthalmol* 80:1047, 1975

134. MCCULLOCH JC, ARSHINOFF SA, MARLISS EB, PARKER JA: Hyperornithinemia and gyrate atrophy of the choroid and retina. *Ophthalmology* 85:918, 1978

135. KAISER-KUPFER MI, VALLE D, DEL VALLE LA: A specific enzyme defect in gyrate atrophy. *Am J Ophthalmol* 85:200, 1978

136. KAISER-KUPFER MI, VALLE D, BRON AJ: Clinical and biochemical heterogeneity in gyrate atrophy. *Am J Ophthalmol* 89:219, 1980

137. KAISER-KUPFER MI, DE MONASTERIO F, VALLE D, WALSER M, BRUSILOW SW: Visual results of a long-term trial of a low-arginine diet in gyrate atrophy of the choroid and retina. *Ophthalmology* 88:307, 1981

138. KAISER-KUPFER MI, KUWABARA T, ASKANAS V, BRODY L, TAKKI K, DVORETZKY I, ENGEL WK: Systemic manifestations of gyrate atrophy of the choroid and retina. *Ophthalmology* 88:302, 1981

139. BERSON EL, SCHMIDT SY, SHIH VE: Ocular and biochemical abnormalities in gyrate atrophy of the choroid and retina. *Ophthalmology* 85:1018, 1978

140. BERSON EL, SHIH VE, SULLIVAN PL: Ocular findings in patients with gyrate atrophy on pyridoxine and low-protein, low-arginine diets. *Ophthalmology* 88:311,1981

141. WELEBER RG, KENNAWAY NG, BUIST NR: Vitamin B₆ in management of gyrate atrophy of choroid and retina. *Lancet* 2:1213, 1978

142. WELEBER RG, KENNAWAY NG: Clinical trial of vitamin B₆ for gyrate atrophy of the choroid and retina. *Ophthalmology* 88:316, 1981

143. JAEGER W, KETTLER JV, LUTZ P, HILSDORF C: Differential diagnosis of gyrate atrophy of the choroid and retina (gyrate atrophy of the choroid and retina with and without hyperornithinemia) *Metab Pediatr Ophthalmol* 3:189, 1979

144. HODES DT, MUSHIN AS, LAURANCE BM, OBERHOLZER VG, BRIDDON A: Hyperornithinemia with gyrate atrophy of the choroid and retina in two siblings. *J R Soc Med* 73:588, 1980

145. YATZIV S, STATTER M, MERIN S: Metabolic studies in two families with hyperornithinemia and gyrate atrophy of choroid and retina. *J Lab Clin Med* 93:749, 1979

146. IANNETTI F: Hyperornithinemia in the gyrate atrophy of the retina and choroid. *Ann Ottal Clin Ocul* 12:555, 1976

147. STOPPOLONI G, PRISCO F, SANTINELLI R, TOLONE C: Hyperornithinemia and gyrate atrophy of choroid and retina. *Helv Paediatr Acta* 33:429, 1978

148. RINALDI E, STOPPOLONI GP, SAVASTANO S, RUSSO S, COTTICELLI L:

149. AKIYA S, OHSAWA M, OGATA T: Gyrate atrophy of the choroid and retina. Long-term observation of two brothers of gyrate atrophy of the choroid and retina with hyperornithinaemia. *Acta Soc Ophthalmol Jap* 81:310, 1978

150. TRIJBELS JMF, SENGERS RCA, BAKKEREN JAJM, DE KORT AFM, DUTMAN AF: L-Ornithine-ketoacid-transaminase deficiency in cultured fibroblasts of a patient with hyperornithinemia and gyrate atrophy of the choroid and retina. *Clin Chim Acta* 79:371, 1977

151. O'DONNELL JJ, SANDMAN RP, MARTIN SR: Gyrate atrophy of the retina: Inborn error of L-ornithine:2-oxoacid aminotransferase. *Science* 200:200, 1978

152. OBERHOLZER VG, BRIDDON A: 3-Amino-2-piperidone in the urine of patients with hyperornithinemia. *Clin Chim Acta* 87:411, 1978

153. KRILL AE: Clinical characteristics, in *Krill's Hereditary Retinal and Choroidal Diseases*, ed 7. New York, Harper & Row, Publishers, Inc, 1977, p 1012

154. SIPILA I, SIMELL O, RAPOLA J, SAINIO K, TUUTERI L: Gyrate atrophy of the choroid and retina with hyperornithinemia: Tubular aggregatates and type 2 fiber atrophy in muscle. *Neurology* 29:996, 1979

155. KENNAWAY NG, WELEBER RG, BUIST NRM: Gyrate atrophy of the choroid and retina with hyperornithinemia: Biochemical and histologic studies and response to vitamin B₆. *Am J Hum Genet* 32:529, 1980

156. ENGEL WK, BISHOP DW, CUNNINGHAM GG: Tubular aggregates in type II muscle fibers: Ultrastructural and histochemical correlation. *J Ultrastruct Res* 31:507, 1970

157. MARON BJ, FERRANS VJ: Aggregates of tubules in human cardiac muscle cells. *J Mol Cell Cardiol* 6:249, 1974

158. VALLE DL, WALSER M, BRUSILOW SW, KAISER-KUPFER MI: Gyrate atrophy of the choroid and retina: Amino acid metabolism and correction of hyperornithinemia with an arginine deficient diet. *J Clin Invest* 65:371, 1980

159. VALLE D, WALSER M, BRUSILOW S, KAISER-KUPFER M, TAKKI K: Gyrate atrophy of the choroid and retina: Biochemical considerations and experience with an arginine-restricted diet. *Ophthalmology* 88:325, 1981

160. GORDON BA, GATFIELD PD, TALLER E: Ornithine methyl ester. An unusual metabolite encountered in the urine of patients with a urea cycle disorder characterized by hyperammonemia, hyperornithinemia, and homocitrullinuria. *Clin Biochem* 10:78, 1977

161. FELL V, POLLITT RJ: 3-Aminopiperid-2-one, an unusual metabolite in the urine of a patient with hyperammonaemia, hyperornithinaemia and homocitrullinuria. *Clin Chim Acta* 87:405, 1978

162. OBERHOLZER VG: Personal communication

163. KENNAWAY NG, WELEBER RG, BUIST NRM: Gyrate atrophy of the choroid and retina: Deficient activity of ornithine ketoacid aminotransferase in cultured skin fibroblasts. *N Engl J Med* 297:1180, 1977

164. O'DONNELL JJ, SANDMAN RP, MARTIN SR: Deficient L-ornithine: 2-Oxoacid aminotransferase activity in cultured fibroblasts from a patient with gyrate atrophy of the retina. *Biochem Biophys Res Commun* 79:396, 1977

165. SHIH VE, BERSON EL, MANDELL R, SCHMIDT SY: Ornithine ketoacid transaminase deficiency in gyrate atrophy of the choroid and retina. *Am J Hum Genet* 30:174, 1978

166. VALLE D, KAISER-KUPFER MI, DEL VALLE LA: Gyrate atrophy of the choroid and retina: Deficiency of ornithine aminotransferase in transformed lymphocytes. *Proc Natl Acad Sci USA* 74:5159, 1977

167. SIPILA I, O'DONNELL JJ, SIMELL O: Gyrate atrophy of the choroid and retina with hyperornithinemia: Characterization of mutant liver-L-ornithine: 2-Oxoacid aminotransferase kinetics. *J Clin Invest*, in press

168. VALLE D, BOISON AP, KAISER-KUPFER MI: Complementation analysis of gyrate atrophy of the choroid and retina. *Pediatr Res* 13:427, 1979

169. SHIH VE, MANDELL R, JACOBY LB, BERSON EL: Genetic complementation analysis in fibroblasts from gyrate and atrophy and the syndrome of hyperornithinemia, hyperammonemia and homocitrullinuria. *Pediatr Res* 15:569, 1981

170. ROSENBERG LE: Progress in understanding autosomal recessive diseases, in Goodman RM, Motulsky AG (eds): *Genetic Diseases among Askenazi Jews.* New York, Raven Press, 1979, p 105

171. STETTEN MR: Mechanism of the conversion of ornithine into proline and glutamic acid in vivo. *J Biol Chem* 189:499, 1951

172. SCRIVER CR, ROSENBERG LE: *Amino Acid Metabolism and Its Disorders.* Philadelphia, WB Saunders Co, 1973, p 39

173. BERGSTROM J, FURST P, NOREE LO, VINNARS E: Intracellular free amino acid concentration in human muscle tissue. *J Appl Physiol* 36:693, 1974

174. GOPALAKRISHNA R, NAGARAJAN B: A modified method for estimation of ornithine in biological samples. *Anal Biochem* 101:472, 1980

175. MATSUZAWA T, ITO M, ISHIGURO I: Enzymatic assays of L-ornithine and L-Δ'-pyrroline-5-carboxylate in tissues and ornithine-load test in human subjects. *Anal Biochem* 106:1, 1980

Gyrate atrophy of choroid associated with hyperornithaenemia: Report of the first case in Italy. *J Pediatr Ophthalmol Strabismus* 16:133, 1979

176. COHEN AI: The retina and optic nerve, in Moses RA (ed): *Adler's Physiology of the Eye.* St. Louis, CV Mosby Co, 1975, p 367

177. ZINN KM, MARMOR MF: *The Retinal Pigment Epithelium.* Cambridge, Mass, Harvard University Press, 1979

178. VALLE DL, BOISON AP, JEZYK P, AGUIRRE G: Gyrate atrophy of the choroid and retina in a cat. *Invest Ophthalmol Vis Sci* 20:251, 1981.

179. KUWABARA T, ISHIKAWA Y, KAISER-KUPFER MI: Experimental model of gyrate atrophy in animals. *Ophthalmology* 88:331, 1981

180. SIPILA I, SIMELL O, ARJOMAA P: Gyrate atrophy of the choroid and retina with hyperornithinemia. Deficient formation of guanidinoacetic acid from arginine. *J Clin Invest* 66:684, 1980

181. SIPILA I, RAPOLA J, SIMELL O, VANNAS A: Supplementary creatine as a treatment for gyrate atrophy of the choroid and retina. *N Engl J Med* 304:867, 1981

182. KAISER-KUPFER MI, DE MONASTERIO FM, VALLE D, WALSER M, BRUSILOW S: Gyrate atrophy of the choroid and retina: Improved visual function following reduction of plasma ornithine by diet. *Science* 210:1128, 1980

183. MCINNES RR, ARSHINOFF SA, BELL L, MARLISS EB, MCCULLOCH JC: Hyperornithinaemia and gyrate atrophy of the retina: Improvement of vision during treatment with a low-arginine diet. *Lancet* 1:513, 1981

184. MORI A, KATAYAMA Y, HIGASHIDATE S, KIMURA S: Fluorometrical analysis of guanidino compounds in mouse brain. *J Neurochem* 32:643, 1979

185. MATSUMOTO M, KOBAYASHI K, MORI A: Distribution of guanidino compounds in bovine brain. *J Neurochem* 32:645, 1979

186. WOZNICKI DT, WALKER JB: Formation of a supplemental long time-constant reservoir of high energy phosphate by brain in vivo and in vitro and its reversible depletion by potassium depolarization. *J Neurochem* 33:75, 1979

187. WOZNICKI DT, WALKER JB: Utilization of cyclocreatine phosphate and analogue of creatine phosphate by mouse brain during ischemia and its sparing action on brain energy reserves. *J Neurochem* 34:1247, 1980

188. METHFESSEL J: Zur organ-und subzellularverteilung der transamidinase bei mensch und ratte. *Acta Biol Med Ger* 35:309, 1976

189. HARVEY JC: Reduced renal arginine-glycine transamidinase activity in myotonic goats and in patients with myotonic muscular dystrophy. *Johns Hopkins Med J* 125:270, 1969

190. LOIKE JD, KOZLER VF, SILVERSTEIN SC: Increased ATP and creatine phosphate turnover in phagocytosing mouse peritoneal macrophages. *J Biol Chem* 254:9558, 1979

191. VALLE D, BOISON AP, KAISER-KUPFER MI: Increased sensitivity of gyrate atrophy fibroblasts to ornithine toxicity. *Pediatr Res* 13:426, 1979

192. VALLE D, ASKANAS V, KAISER-KUPFER MI, TAKKI K, ENGEL K: Increased sensitivity of gyrate atrophy fibroblasts and cultured muscle cells to ornithine toxicity. *Pediatr Res* 14:528, 1980

193. VALLE D, BOISON AP, PHANG JM, SMITH RJ, KAISER-KUPFER MI: Unpublished observations

194. PHANG JM, DOWNING SJ, YEH GC, SMITH RJ, WILLIAMS JA: Stimulation of the hexose-monophosphate pentose pathway by Δ^1-pyrroline-5-carboxylic acid in human fibroblasts. *Biochem Biophys Res Commun* 87:363, 1979

195. YEH GC, HARRIS SC, PHANG JM: Pyrroline-5-carboxylate reductase in human erythrocytes. *J Clin Invest* 67:1042, 1981

196. MATSUZAWA T, ISHIGURO I: Hyperornithinemia with gyrate atrophy and enzymes involved in ornithine metabolism of the eye. *Biochem Int* 1:179, 1980

197. OLDENDORF WH: Brain uptake of radiolabeled amino acids, amines and hexoses after arterial injection. *Am J Physiol* 221:1629, 1971

198. RAJANTIE J, SIMELL O, PERHEENTUPA J: Lysinuric intolerance. Basolateral transport defect in renal tubuli. *J Clin Invest* 67:1078, 1981

199. GIORDANO C, DE SANTO NG, PLUVIO M, SANTINELLI R, STOPPOLONI G: Lysine in treatment of hyperornithinemia. *Nephron* 22:97, 1978

200. TAKKI K, SIMELL O: Genetic aspects in gyrate atrophy of the choroid and retina with hyperornithinemia. *Br J Ophthalmol* 58:907, 1974

201. WRIGHT T, POLLITT R: Psychomotor retardation, epileptic and stuporous attacks, irritability and ataxia associated with ammonia intoxication, high blood ornithine levels and increased homocitrulline in the urine. *Proc Roy Soc Med* 66:221, 1973

202. FELL V, POLLITT R, SAMPSON GA, WRIGHT T: Ornithinemia, hyperammonemia and homocitrullinuria. A disease associated with mental retardation and possiblily caused by defective mitochondrial transport. *Am J Dis Child* 127:752, 1974

203. GATFIELD PD, TALLER E, WOLFE DM, HAUST M: Hyperornithinemia, hyperammonemia and homocitrullinuria associated with decreased carbamyl phosphate synthetase I activity. *Pediatr Res* 9:488, 1975

204. SIMELL O, SCRIVER CR: Personal observations

205. HOMMES F: Personal observations

206. SHIH VE, MANDELL R: Metabolic defect in hyperornithinaemia. *Lancet* 2:1522, 1974

207. SHIH VE, SCHULMAN JO: Ornithine-ketoacid transaminase activity in human skin and amniotic fluid cell culture. *Clin Chim Acta* 27:73, 1970

208. SIMELL O, VALLE D: Personal observations

209. BRIGGS S, FREEDLAND RA: Effect of ornithine and lactate on urea synthesis in isolated hepatocytes. *Biochem J* 160:205, 1976

210. GREENSTEIN JP, WINITZ M, GULLINO P, BIRNBAUM SM, OTEY MC: Studies on the metabolism of amino acids and related compounds in vivo. III. Prevention of ammonia toxicity by arginine and related compounds. *Arch Biochem Biophys* 64:342, 1956

211. NATHANS D, FAHEY JL, SHIP AG: Sites of origin and removal of blood ammonia formed during glycine infusion: Effect of L-arginine. *J Lab Clin Med* 51:124, 1958

212. BRUSILOW SW, BATSHAW ML: Arginine therapy of argininosuccinase deficiency. *Lancet* 1:124, 1979

213. SIMELL O, PERHEENTUPA J, RAPOLA J, VISAKORPI JK, ESKELIN LE: Lysinuric protein intolerance. *Am J Med* 59:229, 1975

214. RAJANTIE J, SIMELL O, RAPOLA J, PERHEENTUPA J: Lysinuric protein intolerance: A two-year trial of dietary supplementation therapy with citrulline and lysine. *J Pediatr* 97:927, 1980

215. BACHMANN C, KRAHENBUHL S, COLOMBO JP, SCHUBIGER G, JAGGI KH, TONZ O: N-acetylglutamate synthetase deficiency: A disorder of ammonia detoxication. *N Engl Med* 304:543, 1981

216. SHIH VE, MANDELL R, HERZFELD A: Defective ornithine metabolism in the syndrome of hyperornithinemia, hyperammonemia and homocitrullinuria. International Symposium of Inborn Errors of Metabolism in Human. Interlaken, 1980

217. HOMMES FA, HO CK, GORDON BA, ROESEL RA, CORYELL ME: Decreased transport of ornithine across the inner mitochondrial membrane as a cause of hyperornithinemia. *J Inher Met Dis*, in press

218. GERRITSEN T, VAUGHN JG, WAISMAN HA: Origin of homocitrulline in the urine of infants. *Arch Biochem Biophys* 100:298, 1963

219. CARSON NA, SCALLY BG, NEILL DW, CARRE IJ: Saccharopinuria: A new inborn error of lysine metabolism. *Nature (Lond)* 218:679, 1968

220. SIMELL O, VASAKORPI JK, DONNER M: Saccharopinuria. *Arch Dis Child* 47:52, 1972

221. SIMELL O, SIPILA I, RAJANTIE J: Hyperlysinemia with hyperammonemia and homocitrullinuria. *Pediatr Res* 14:174, 1980

222. BERSON EL, SCHMIDT SY, RABIN AR: Plasma amino acids in hereditary retinal disease: Ornithine, lysine, and taurine. *Br J Ophthalmol* 60:142, 1976

223. MAGRI E, BALDONI G, GRAZI E: On the biosynthesis of creatine, intramitochondrial localization of transamidinase from rat kidney. *FEBS Lett* 55:91, 1975

224. HOLMGREN G: Effect of low, normal and high dietary protein intake on urinary amino acid excretion and plasma aminogram in children. *Nutr Metab* 16:223, 1974

225. VALLE D, WALSER M, BRUSILOW S, KAISER-KUPFER MI: Unpublished observations

226. JANSSEN AJM, PLAKKE T, TRIJBELS FJM, SENGERS RCA, MONNENS LAH: L-Ornithine ketoacid-transaminase assay in hair roots of homozygotes and heterozygotes for gyrate atrophy. *Clin Chim Acta* 113:213, 1981

20

UREA CYCLE DISORDERS AND OTHER HEREDITARY HYPERAMMONEMIC SYNDROMES

MACKENZIE WALSER

1. The biosynthesis of urea, a process which occurs almost exclusively in the liver, involves six enzymatic reactions. The first three occur in mitochondria: (1) the synthesis of N-acetylglutamate from acetyl CoA and glutamate; (2) the synthesis of carbamoyl phosphate from bicarbonate and ammonium ions, a reaction requiring the presence of N-acetylglutamate; and (3) the condensation of carbamoyl phosphate with ornithine to yield citrulline. The next three reactions occur in the cytosol: (1) the condensation of citrulline with aspartate to yield argininosuccinate; (2) hydrolysis of argininosuccinate to arginine and fumarate; and (3) hydrolysis of arginine to ornithine and urea.

2. Regulation of urea biosynthesis involves (1) substrate effects, (2) rapid activation of carbamoyl phosphate synthesis secondary to substrate-induced increments in N-acetylglutamate, (3) enzyme induction and repression; and (4) hormonal effects. In urea cycle enzymopathies, urea production continues mainly because of (1) accumulation of the substrate proximal to the metabolic block (in partial defects) and (2) urea production from arginine (except in arginase deficiency).

3. Hyperammonemia, the characteristic biochemical manifestation of these disorders, is toxic to the brain by virtue of its effects on carbohydrate metabolism and on neurotransmitters.

4. Therapy of complete as well as partial deficiencies of urea cycle enzymes is now feasible using essential amino acids or their keto-analogues in combination with severe protein restriction, arginine supplementation, sodium benzoate (to induce hippurate excretion), and N-carbamoylglutamate (to activate carbamoyl phosphate synthetase). Early diagnosis and treatment of hyperammonemic crises remain problems.

5. One case of N-acetylglutamate synthetase deficiency has recently been reported in brief.

6. At least 26 cases of carbamoyl phosphate synthetase deficiency including 18 neonatal cases have been reported. Pronounced hyperammonemia in the absence of orotic aciduria is characteristic. The disorder is inherited as an autosomal recessive trait.

7. Ornithine carbamoyl phosphate deficiency, an X-linked dominant trait, has been reported in at least 110 cases, including 40 to 45 males with virtually complete deficiency and neonatal onset (five of whom nevertheless survived for some months or years with treatment), 18 males with later onset of symptoms, and many females with varying degrees of partial deficiency. Hyperammonemia with pronounced orotic aciduria is characteristic.

8. Argininosuccinate synthetase deficiency, an autosomal recessive trait, has been reported in at least 53 symptomatic cases, including 22 neonatal cases and

23 cases of a late onset variant seen almost exclusively in Japan. Citrullinemia, with or without hyperammonemia and orotic aciduria, is the characteristic finding. Prenatal diagnosis is possible.

9. *Argininosuccinic aciduria, an autosomal recessive trait, is relatively common in the United States but uncommon elsewhere. A total of about 60 symptomatic cases has been described. Asymptomatic cases are also reported. Hyperammonemia is less frequent but may occur, especially when arginine deficiency develops due to defective arginine synthesis and loss of arginine in the urine as argininosuccinate. Prenatal diagnosis is possible. Optimal therapy has yet to be defined.*

10. *Arginase deficiency, another autosomal recessive trait, has been reported in 13 patients, 7 of whom are of Spanish-American origin. Argininemia and argininuria are pronounced; hyperammonemia occurs only occasionally, but orotic aciduria is common, although unexplained. A unique and consistent clinical syndrome is seen in untreated cases. Dietary therapy abolishes all signs of the disease.*

11. *Lysinuric protein intolerance is an autosomal recessive trait seen most often in Finland. The basic defect is impaired transport of basic amino acids in the intestine and kidney. Unexplained hyperammonemia and a variety of other clinical manifestations are seen. Basic amino acids are subnormal in plasma and increased in urine, but cystinuria is mild or absent. Citrulline supplementation, with or without lysine, is useful but does not eliminate all manifestations of the disease.*

12. *Transient hyperammonemia may occur in infancy and lead to the erroneous diagnosis of a urea cycle enzyme defect. Possible causes include developmental delay in argininosuccinate synthetase, asphyxia, and parenteral infusions.*

THE UREA CYCLE

General Properties of the Urea Cycle Enzymes

The urea-synthesizing enzyme system consists of four enzymes that operate in a cyclic manner, using ornithine as the substrate that is regenerated with each turn of the cycle and two enzymes whose combined action produces carbamoyl phosphate (CP), the substrate that first enters the cycle to combine with ornithine (Fig. 20-1) through the action of ornithine carbamoyl transferase (OCT). The other nitrogen atom of urea is derived from aspartate, which is condensed with citrulline (the condensation product of ornithine and carbamoyl phosphate) to yield argininosuccinate (ASA) by argininosuccinate synthetase (ASAS). The latter compound is hydrolyzed to arginine and fumarate by argininosuccinate lyase (ASAL), and arginine is hydrolyzed to urea and ornithine by arginase.

Two distinct carbamoyl phosphate synthetases exist: a cytosolic form (CPS II) that uses glutamine (or ammonia) as a substrate and produces CP as a precursor for pyrimidine synthesis;

and a mitochondrial form (CPS I) that uses ammonia, not glutamine, and requires N-acetylglutamate (AGA) for activation. The CP produced by CPS I is used entirely or (almost entirely) for ureagenesis except when mitochondrial CP levels become abnormally high. Under these circumstances, substantial quantities of CP escape into the cytosol and are channeled into pyrimidine synthesis.

AGA synthetase (AGAS), the enzyme that produces AGA, is as much a part of the metabolic path to urea as the other enzymes, because CPS I is completely inactive in the absence of AGA. AGAS is also mitochondrial in location. Its substrates are acetyl CoA and glutamate. Its product, AGA, escapes into the cytosol, where it is hydrolyzed by acylases.

Other enzymes and enzyme systems are intimately linked to the biosynthesis of urea:

1. Glutamate dehydrogenase, which maintains the ratio $[NH_4]$ $[\alpha\text{-ketoglutarate}]/[\text{glutamate}]$ close to its equilibrium value within the mitochondrion, a value which is in turn dependent on the ratios $NADH/NAD^+$ and $NADPH/NADP^+$

2. Aspartate:α-ketoglutarate aminotransferase and alanine:α-ketoglutarate aminotransferase, which maintain the ratios [glutamate] [oxaloacetate]/[α-ketoglutarate] [aspartate] and [glutamate] [pyruvate]/[α-ketoglutarate] [alanine], respectively, near their equilibrium values

3. The tricarboxylic acid cycle, which is the source of oxaloacetate that is transaminated to aspartate and then condenses with citrulline, the sink for fumarate and the source as well as the sink for α-ketoglutarate, depending on the conditions

4. Ornithine aminotransferase (OAT), an anapleurotic enzyme that can either remove excess ornithine by reaction with α-ketoglutarate or can synthesize ornithine from pyrroline-5-carboxylate and glutamate

5. Arginine-glycine transamidinase, which operates almost exclusively in the direction of production of guanidinoacetate and ornithine

6. The enzymes of pyrimidine biosynthesis, which channel off excess CP, as noted above

7. Pyruvate carboxylase, as a source of oxaloacetate, which can become rate-limiting for aspartate formation

In addition to these enzymes and enzyme systems, transport processes are obviously important in ureagenesis. For example, for every molecule of urea produced, a molecule of citrulline must leave the mitochondrion and a molecule of ornithine (produced by arginase action on arginine in the cytosol) must enter the mitochondrion. Bradford and McGivan [1] have characterized a citrulline-ornithine antiporter in the mitochondrial membrane and have presented evidence that ornithine may also enter via electroneutral exchange for H^+ whenever transamination of ornithine via OAT occurs. Although citrulline enters the mitochondrion rapidly at high concentrations in the absence of other permeant ions [1a], it does so only slowly at low concentrations [1].

Tissue Distribution of Urea Cycle Enzymes

It is generally held that no organ other than the liver is capable of synthesizing urea from ammonia and aspartate to any significant extent [2], although the possibility that other organs may do so has not been rigorously excluded. Portions of the

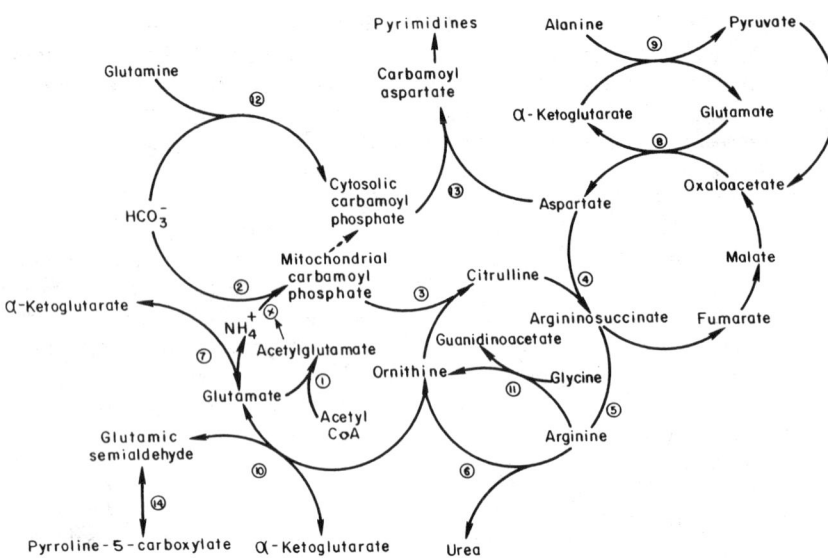

Figure 20-1 Principal reactions of the urea cycle and related reactions. The enzymes are (1) acetylglutamate synthetase, (2) carbamoyl phosphate synthetase I, (3) ornithine carbamoyl transferase, (4) argininosuccinate synthetase, (5) argininosuccinate lyase, (6) arginase, (7) glutamate dehydrogenase, (8) glutamate-oxaloacetate transaminase, (9) glutamate-pyruvate transaminase, (10) ornithine aminotransferase, (11) arginine-glycine transamidinase, (12) carbamoyl phosphate synthetase II, (13) aspartate carbamoyltransferase. Reaction 14 occurs spontaneously.

urea cycle are found in many tissues, and the complete cycle is demonstrable in several cell lines in culture [3]. The most physiologically important extrahepatic sites of the urea cycle enzymes are as follows:

The Intestine Here, the mitochondrial enzymes AGAS, CPS, and OCT are present at low levels [4–6], and citrulline is produced at a rate approximately one-twentieth the hepatic rate of ureagenesis [7–9]. The nitrogen for citrullinogenesis in the intestine is derived from glutamine. Ornithine also can be synthesized at this site by the operation of OAT in the reverse direction from which it commonly operates in the liver [10–12]. The cytosolic enzymes of the urea cycle are not present in significant quantities in the intestine, and consequently urea production apparently does not occur in this organ.

The Kidney Here, ASAS, ASAL, and arginase are all present [3]. OCT and CPS are present in only minute amounts [5]. ASAS and ASAL are responsible for a substantial uptake of citrulline by the kidney (about 8 mmol/day per 70 kg) in normal humans [13] and the release of a nearly equal quantity of arginine [13–15]. Evidence has been presented that the kidneys synthesize a larger proportion of the endogenous arginine used for body protein synthesis than does the liver [16]. Arginine also reacts with glycine, chiefly in the kidney, via arginine-glycine transamidinase, to yield guanidinoacetic acid and ornithine. It is possible that renal arginase may, under some conditions, catalyze the synthesis of small quantities of urea, since it is believed to be a source of ornithine derived from arginine [17]. Direct evidence for urea production by the kidney is lacking. Renal arginase is distinguishable from hepatic arginase by physical means as well as substrate specificity [17, 18].

The Brain Here, ASAS and ASAL are present in substantial amounts [3]. Arginase is also demonstrable [19, 20] in two distinct forms: one with kinetic properties distinct from liver arginase and another with physical properties distinct from liver arginase but the same kinetic properties [21]. The physiologic significance of the presence of these enzymes in the brain is uncertain, since neither citrulline uptake nor arginine release by the human brain is demonstrable [22, 23]. Indirect evidence for a functional role of brain arginase in producing urea has been obtained by study of the genetically spastic mouse, in which brain arginase activity is elevated. Brain arginine is

reduced and brain urea is increased in comparison with normal mice [24]. Arginase activity is highest in the cerebellum, while ASAS and ASAL are highest in the cerebral cortex [19]. A very low level of CPS is present in brain, but OCT is undetectable [5, 25]; hence *de novo* urea synthesis should not occur. Despite the low level of CPS, carbamoyl phosphate is reported to increase rapidly in the brain of animals injected with ammonium salts, and it has been suggested as a possible factor in the neurotoxicity of ammonia [26, 27].

Erythrocytes These contain a low level of ASAL activity [28] but significant arginase activity [29]. Presumably continuous conversion of arginine to ornithine and urea at a low rate takes place in the circulation, catalyzed by this enzyme, although probably at a rate no greater than 1 percent of hepatic ureagenesis. Indirect evidence for this conclusion comes from the study of macaque monkeys with erythrocytic arginase deficiency, in whom red cell arginine concentration approaches 1 mM [30]. Arginase activity is also demonstrable in normal muscle, lung, heart, salivary gland, and breast [2].

The Heart According to one report, urea synthesis from ammonium can occur in this organ [31].

Normal Levels of Urea Cycle Enzymes and Their Properties

Tables 20-1 and 20-2 list the maximal activities of the urea cycle enzymes in normal human liver and the most important kinetic properties of these enzymes as observed in human liver. A summary of these values as observed in liver of other animals is given by Meijer and Hensgens [58].

The Enzymes

N-ACETYLGLUTAMATE SYNTHETASE (EC 2.3.1.1)   This exclusively mitochondrial enzyme catalyzes the reaction

$$\text{Acetyl CoA} + \text{glutamate} \rightarrow \textit{N}\text{-acetylglutamate} + \text{CoA} \quad (1)$$

Arginine is a positive effector with an activation constant (K_A) of 30 μM in the rat [59]. Since this is in the range of hepatic arginine concentration, the possibility that arginine might exert a positive feedback effect on ureagenesis needs to be considered [60]. Substrate effects on AGA synthesis secondary to variations in mitochondrial acetyl CoA and glutamate are also possible sites of regulation. The inhibition of ureagenesis caused by a variety of organic acids may be the result of competitive inhibition of AGA synthetase by thioesters such as propionyl CoA [61], a substrate effect on AGA synthetase caused by acetyl CoA depletion [62, 63], or a direct inhibitory effect on CPS I of these thioesters [64]. This phenomenon is discussed in detail in Chap. 23. The enzyme also exhibits product inhibition by AGA ($K_i = 0.3$ mM) [64a].

CARBAMOYL PHOSPHATE SYNTHETASE (EC 6.3.4.16) CPS I catalyzes the reaction

$$NH_4^+ + HCO_3^- + 2MgATP \rightarrow CP + 2MgADP + P_i \text{ (Fig. 20-2) (2)}$$

The properties of the two binding sites for ATP have been studied in detail [64b]. The reaction requires AGA, Mg^{2+}, and K^+. Here K^+ decreases the K_m values for NH_4^+, AGA, and ATP in frog liver [65]. Glutamate and α-ketoglutarate are competitive inhibitors of AGA binding to CPS I with K_i values of 1 mM and 3 mM, respectively [66]. N-carbamoyl-L-glutamate and α-acetoxyglutarate are also activators; glutamate, α-ketoglutarate, glutarate, and α-hydroxyglutarate are inhibitors [65]. It is subject to product inhibition by MgADP ($K_i = 0.6$ to 1.3 mM) and by CP ($K_i = 10$ to 19 mM) [77] and is inhibited by acyl CoA esters [64]. Calcium at low concentration inhibits its activation by magnesium [78, 79]. Activation by AGA is associated with rapid changes in the conformation and subunit structure of the enzyme [67, 68] and an increased proportion of monomer [69]. Glutamine is inactive as a substrate. The

Table 20-1 Maximal activities of urea cycle enzymes in human liver

Age range, no. of observations, reference	AGAS	CPS I	OCT	ASAS	ASAL	Arginase
30–70 yr, $n = 8$ [32, 33]		279 ± 66 (1.91 ± 0.27)	6,600 ± 1,600 (44.2 ± 7.8)	90 ± 12 (0.62 ± 0.14)	220 ± 26 (1.49 ± 0.27)	85,600 ± 9,280 (579 ± 106)
9 hr–10 mo, $n = 6$ [34]		192 ± 68 (1.30 ± 0.40)	2,700 ± 680 (18.1 ± 4.9)	67 ± 11 (0.49 ± 0.09)	94 ± 28 (0.64 ± 0.15)	21,200 ± 8,600 (152 ± 56)
Adults, $n = 3–5$ [35]		108 ± 42	4310 ± 120	52 ± 7	102 ± 29	4993 ± 52
Neonates, $n = 3$ [36]		112 − 230 (0.81 − 1.41)	3950 − 4480 (25 − 32)	28 − 39 (0.21 − 0.30)	64 − 91 (0.39 − 0.66)	33,000 − 53,700 (233 − 410)
Adults, $n = 6$ [36]		242 ± 60 (1.49 ± 0.39)	5500 ± 810 (33.1 ± 4.0)	55 ± 44 (0.34 ± 0.27)	158 ± 20 (0.95 ± 0.15)	40,800 ± 10,100 (243 ± 29)
Adults, $n = ?$ [37]		(0.84 − 2.88)	(6.2 − 40.5)			
Adults, $n = 5–16$ [38]		232 ± 72	3120 ± 660		162 ± 43	49,400 ± 16700
Adults, $n = 10$ [39]				31 ± 4 (0.21 ± 0.04)		
Adults, $n = 4–12$ [40]		84 ± 115 (0.79 − 1.31)	1350 − 3200 (15.2 − 21.5)		100 − 202	11,400 − 42,000 (118 − 520)
Adults, $n = 19$ [41]		45 ± 13	6,670 ± 450	73 ± 6	142 ± 11	75,600 ± 7,300
Adults, $n = 12$ [42, 234]	0.33 − 1.98 (0.002 − 0.012)	110 − 356 (0.60 − 2.1)	2500 − 5700 (95 − 33.3)	38 −78 (0.09 − 0.41)	128 − 294 (0.7 − 2.1)	5300 − 14,600 (35 − 99)
Infants, $n = 8$ [42a]	(0.007 ± 0.001)					
Adults, $n = 10$ [43]		(0.90 ± 0.30)	(36 ± 10)		(1.0 ± 0.3)	(435 ± 120)
Adults, $n = ?$ [44]		234 ± 121	3100 ± 1030	40 ± 17	102 ± 30	18,400 ± 2800
3–50 yr, $n = 7$ [45]		(2.9 ± 0.6)	(42 ± 6)			(369 ± 112)
Adults(?), $n = 8$ [46]		(1.9 ± 0.3)	(44 ± 8)	(0.62 ± 0.14)	(1.5 ± 0.3)	(579 ± 106)
Adults, $n = 4$ [47]		110 ± 44	4350 ± 350	14 ± 2	84 ± 17	8720 ± 880
Neonates–adults ($n = 4–9$) [48]		200 ± 75	5430 ± 720			
Adults(?), $n = 5$ [49]		(2.2 ± 0.8)	(17.6 ± 4.4)		(1.5 ± 0.7)	(53 ± 16)
Adults, $n = 8$ [50]		246 ± 114	3360 ± 1260	29 ± 5	108 ± 42	22,300 ± 10,800
Adults(?), $n = 3$ [51]					(1.0 ± 0.3)	(1.5 ± 0.5)

NOTES: Values given are means ± standard deviation or range.
Units are μmoles per hour per gram wet weight or in parentheses, μmoles per hour per milligram protein.
Where age range of subjects is not specified, they are indicated as Adults (?).
Abbreviations: AGAS, acetylglutamate; CPS I, carbamoyl phosphate synthetase, mitochondrial form; OCT, ornithine carbamoyl transferase; ASAS, argininosuccinate synthetase; ASAL, argininosuccinate lyase.

Figure 20-2 The carbamoyl phosphate synthetase (CPS) reaction.

$$NH_4^+ + HCO_3^- + 2\,ATP^{\cdots\cdots} \rightleftharpoons NH_2CO_2PO_3^{--} + 2\,ADP^{\cdots} + P_i^{--} + 2\,H^+$$

kinetic constants *in situ* for CPS I may be substantially different from those observed in vitro [70]. Traces of heavy metals may be responsible for this discrepancy.

The monomeric unit of the human enzyme consists of a single polypeptide with a molecular weight of about 165,000 [52] and is apparently the predominant form of the enzyme [69, 71]. A protein some 5500 daltons larger is synthesized in the cytosol [72] and moves through the cytosol to the mitochondrion in an exclusively posttranslational manner [73]. The human liver enzyme has an apparant molecular weight of 178,000 to 190,000, reflecting an equilibrium between monomeric and dimeric forms [52, 53]. The mature enzyme comprises 15 to 26 percent of the total matrix protein of liver mitochondria, and its concentration is estimated to be 0.4 to 1.5 mM [71, 74–76].

ORNITHINE CARBAMOYLTRANSERASE (ORNITHINE TRANSCARBAMYLASE) (EC 2.1.3.3)   This catalyzes the reaction

Carbamoyl phosphate + ornithine ⇌ citrulline + P_i (Fig. 20-3)   (3)

The reaction is reversible, but the equilibrium greatly favors citrulline formation. It is inhibited by several amino acids [54, 80, 81] and by phosphate [81a]. The enzyme is a trimer of identical polypeptide subunits with a molecular weight of about 38,000 [54, 55, 81–83]. A precursor protein about 4000 daltons larger is synthesized in the cytosol and then transported to the mitochondrial matrix [84], where it is immediately processed to the mature enzyme [84a]. Although the maximal activity of OCT, as assayed in vivo, is 30 to 40 times greater than that of CPS I, its concentration in the mitochondrial matrix is about one-tenth as great [82, 85].

ARGININOSUCCINATE SYNTHETASE (EC 6.3.4.5)   This catalyzes the reaction

Citrulline + aspartate + ATP ⇌
argininosuccinate + AMP + PP_i (Fig. 20-4)   (4)

Figure 20-3 The ornithine carbamoyl transferase (OCT) reaction.

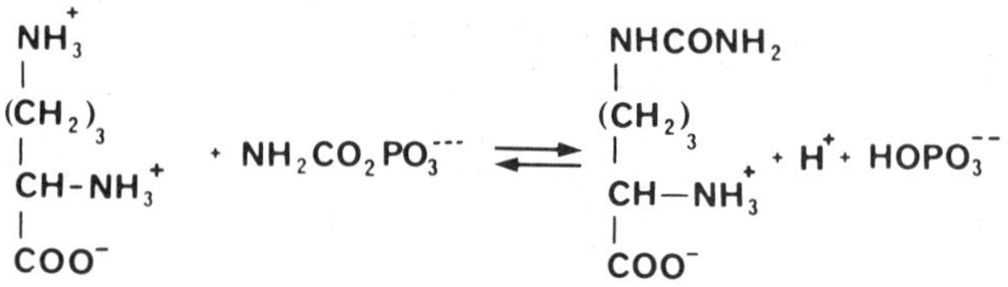

$$
\begin{array}{ccc}
\overset{+}{N}H_3 & & NHCONH_2 \\
| & & | \\
(CH_2)_3 & + NH_2CO_2PO_3^{---} \rightleftharpoons & (CH_2)_3 \\
| & & | \\
CH\text{-}\overset{+}{N}H_3 & & CH\text{-}\overset{+}{N}H_3 \\
| & & | \\
COO^- & & COO^-
\end{array} + H^+ + HOPO_3^{--}
$$

The enzyme is located in the cytosol. The reaction is effectively driven in a forward direction by the destruction of PP_i through the action of cytosolic inorganic pyrophosphatase [86]. Kinetic analysis has shown that each of the three substrates exhibits negative cooperativity with the enzyme, thus ensuring a response to each over a wide range of concentrations [87–90]. The enzyme is inhibited by several amino acids [90] including alanine [91] and saccharopine but not lysine [92]. It consists of four apparently identical subunits with a molecular weight of about 45,000 [88, 93]. Takada et al. [89] concluded from a study of rat liver ASAS that there are two kinds of subunits, which they designate *A* and *B*. Subunit A can bind two moles of ASA, but subunit B cannot bind ASA. They were able to identify three forms of ASAS: one containing two subunits each of A and B (designated *ASAS I*), one consisting of four subunits of A (*ASAS II*), and a third consisting of four subunits of B (*ASAS III*).

ARGININOSUCCINATE LYASE (ARGININOSUCCINASE) (EC 4.3.2.1)   This catalyzes the reaction

Argininosuccinate ⇌ arginine + fumarate (Fig. 20-5)   (5)

The reaction is readily reversible [3]. The enzyme is cytosolic in location. GTP has no effect on the human enzyme [56] but is an allosteric effector of the beef liver enzyme. The enzyme consists of four identical subunits of molecular weight 49,000 [2, 56]. Immunologically, the human liver enzyme is indistinguishable from the enzyme in skin fibroblasts [56].

ARGINASE (EC 3.5.3.1)   This catalyzes the reaction

Arginine → ornithine + urea (Fig. 20-6)   (6)

It is effectively irreversible because of the large free energy change. It is located in the cytosol but may be closely associated with mitochondria [17, 94]. The enzyme consists of four identical subunits of molecular weight 50,000 [2, 95]. It is inhibited by norvaline [96], ornithine, lysine, and branched chain amino acids, but not by their keto-analogues [97].

Metabolism of Urea Cycle Intermediates   Normal levels of urea cycle intermediates as found in rat liver are summarized by Meijer and Hensgens [58]. Some controversy exists as to the concentration of CP, which is in the range of 0.1 to 2 mM. Cohen et al. [98] report a steady-state CP concentration is saturating. Except for CP and AGA, which are presumably almost exclusively mitochondrial, and ASA, which is exclusively cytosolic, the distribution of the other intermediates between cytosolic and mitochondrial compartments is uncertain. This fact makes difficult attempts to delineate mathematical models of the urea cycle or to interpret experiments in

Table 20-2 Michaelis constants and activation constants of urea cycle enzymes in human liver

Enzyme*	Reagent or activator	K_m or K_a, mM, and reference
AGAS	Acetyl CoA	4.3 [64a], 0.7 [42a]
	Glutamate	7.7 [64a], 1.0 [42a]
	Arginine	0.03 [64a], 0.25 [42a]
CPS I	NH$_4^+$	0.8 [52], 1.3 [53]
	HCO$_3^-$	6.7 [52], 2.2 [53]
	MgATP^{2-}	1.1 [52]
	ATP	0.26 [53]
	AGA	0.1 [52], 0.15 [53]
OCT	Ornithine	0.2 [54], 0.4 [55]
	CP	0.09 [54], 0.16 [55]
ASAS	Citrulline	0.03 [35]
	Aspartate	0.03 [35]
	MgATP^{2-}	0.2 [35]
ASAL	ASA	0.2 [56]
	Fumarate	5.3 [56]
	Arginine	3.0 [56]
Arginase	Arginine	10(pH 9.5) [57]

*Abbreviations: See Table 20-1.

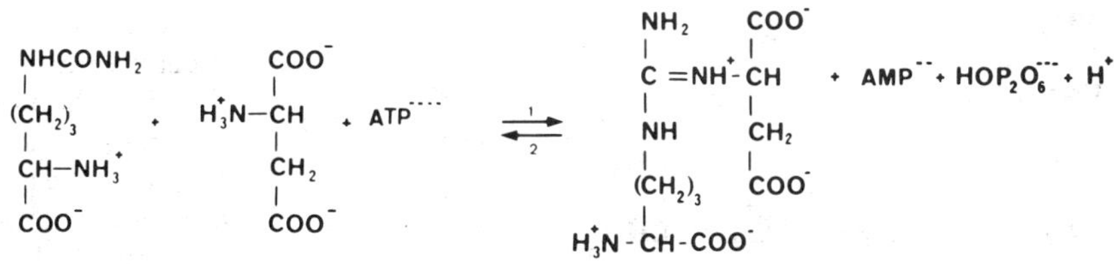

$$\begin{array}{ccc}
\text{NHCONH}_2 & \text{COO}^- & \\
| & | & \\
(\text{CH}_2)_3 & \text{H}_3\overset{+}{\text{N}}-\text{CH} & + \text{ATP} \\
| & | & \\
\text{CH}-\overset{+}{\text{NH}_3} & \text{CH}_2 & \\
| & | & \\
\text{COO}^- & \text{COO}^- &
\end{array}
\;\rightleftharpoons\;
\begin{array}{cc}
\text{NH}_2 & \text{COO}^- \\
| & | \\
\text{C}=\overset{+}{\text{NH}}-\text{CH} & + \text{AMP} + \text{HOP}_2\text{O}_6 + \text{H}^+ \\
| & | \\
\text{NH} & \text{CH}_2 \\
| & | \\
(\text{CH}_2)_3 & \text{COO}^- \\
| & \\
\text{H}_3\overset{+}{\text{N}}-\text{CH-COO}^- &
\end{array}$$

Figure 20-4 The argininosuccinate synthetase (ASAS) reaction.

which whole liver concentrations of these substances are measured. Techniques for estimating mitochondrial and cytosolic concentrations directly are now becoming available [99, 100].

AMMONIA   This is reported to be 0.7 to 0.9 μmol per gram wet weight of liver [101] but largely bound [102, 103]. Thus, when ammonia is added to suspensions of hepatocytes or isolated mitochondria [102] or is injected into intact rats [26], the increment in hepatocyte concentration, intramitochondrial concentration, or hepatic concentration is about the same as in medium, despite an initial concentration ratio of about 8 to 40:1. Liver ammonia returns to initial values sooner than does blood ammonia in intact rats [26]. CPS I may be responsible for at least some of the bound ammonia in liver mitochondria [103].

The major extrahepatic source of ammonia is the intestine, where ammonia is produced from arterial glutamine by intestinal metabolism and from urea and dietary protein by bacteria [8, 104–106]. During exercise, another major source is skeletal muscle [105], where ammonia is probably produced by the purine nucleotide cycle [107]. The rate of release of ammonia into the bloodstream by the kidney is usually small, but it may amount to as much as 7 mmol/h or 168 mmol/day [108]. Alkalinization of the urine increases the rate of release of ammonia into the renal vein [108].

While the liver is responsible for removing most of the ammonia produced in these organs from the blood, skeletal muscle may also remove substantial amounts during rest [109].

N-ACETYLGLUTAMATE   This is synthesized intramitochondrially. It is degraded to glutamate and acetate in the cytosol [110–112]. Efflux from mitochondria is slow, but whether it is limited by mitochondrial permeability or by its rate of destruction in the cytosol is uncertain [112–114]. AGA transport across the mitochondrial membrane is essentially unidirectional and energy-coupled [115]. AGA concentration in rat liver mitochondrial matrix is estimated to be about 0.02 to 0.3 mM [59, 63].

CARBAMOYL PHOSPHATE   This substance, synthesized by CPS I, accumulates intramitochondrially when the urea precursor concentration is high [26, 116], especially if the ornithine concentration is low [98, 117] or urea cycle enzymes

beyond CPS I are operating at a maximal rate or are inhibited [26, 118]. Although the permeability of the mitochondrial membrane to CP is low [98, 119], it may escape into the cytosol under these circumstances [60, 118–121], leading to substantial increments in pyrimidine biosynthesis and increased urinary excretion of orotic acid, uridine, and uracil. The increment in circulating glutamine that usually accompanies hyperammonemia may also contribute to increased flux through the pyrimidine pathway via CPS II under these circumstances. Some CP may escape from the mitochondrion even at physiologic concentrations of ornithine [119], but evidence against this view has been presented [26].

ORNITHINE   This is used catalytically in the urea cycle, and only a small quantity should be adequate for continued operation of the cycle provided no loss of compounds containing the ornithine skeleton from the liver occurs, and no degradation of ornithine itself occurs within the liver. Indeed, it is not at all clear from mathematical modeling of the urea cycle [122] whether any increase in the rate of ureagenesis should be expected from increments in hepatic ornithine above physiologic levels. Such increments lower the steady-state concentration of CP in rat liver [26] but should have little or no effect on the steady-state rate of citrulline production and therefore on urea biosynthesis. Pretreatment of rats with ornithine prevents the increase in liver CP that results from injection of ammonium salts [26]. On the other hand, when the ornithine concentration in liver slices, hepatocytes, or isolated perfused liver is reduced far below the normal level, as it is in such preparations unless precautions are taken to avoid it, the resulting accumulation of CP may be sufficiently great to cause product inhibition of the CPS I reaction (see above), or a significant rate of hydrolysis of CP by carbamoyl phosphate phosphatases or both [123], thus reducing the steady-state rate of ureagenesis. A minor direct stimulatory effect of ornithine on the CPS I reaction [75] is probably too small (about 15 percent) to be of physiologic significance. Ornithine is not incorporated into protein in mammalian tissues.

Whether loss of citrulline from the liver, which would deplete ornithine, occurs to any appreciable extent is uncertain. Clearly, most of the citrulline coming to the liver from the intestine [7–9, 124] passes through the liver. No uptake or release of ASA by the liver has been reported. Some arginine uptake by the liver occurs [124], providing a source of ornithine.

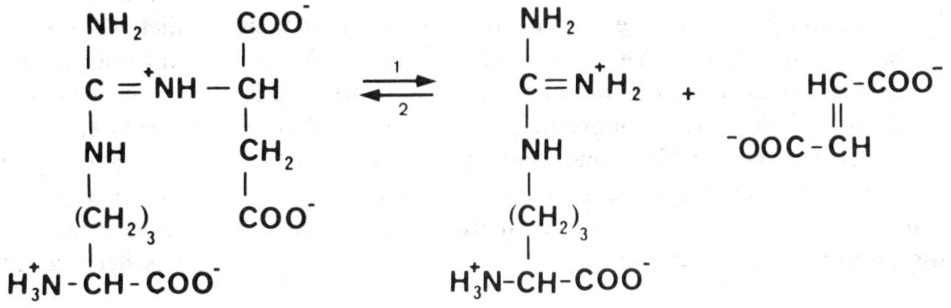

$$\begin{array}{cc}
\text{NH}_2 & \text{COO}^- \\
| & | \\
\text{C}=\overset{+}{\text{NH}}-\text{CH} & \\
| & | \\
\text{NH} & \text{CH}_2 \\
| & | \\
(\text{CH}_2)_3 & \text{COO}^- \\
| & \\
\text{H}_3\overset{+}{\text{N}}-\text{CH-COO}^- &
\end{array}
\;\rightleftharpoons\;
\begin{array}{c}
\text{NH}_2 \\
| \\
\text{C}=\overset{+}{\text{N}}\text{H}_2 \\
| \\
\text{NH} \\
| \\
(\text{CH}_2)_3 \\
| \\
\text{H}_3\overset{+}{\text{N}}-\text{CH-COO}^-
\end{array}
\; + \;
\begin{array}{c}
\text{HC-COO}^- \\
\| \\
^-\text{OOC-CH}
\end{array}$$

Figure 20-5 The argininosuccinate lyase (ASAL) reaction.

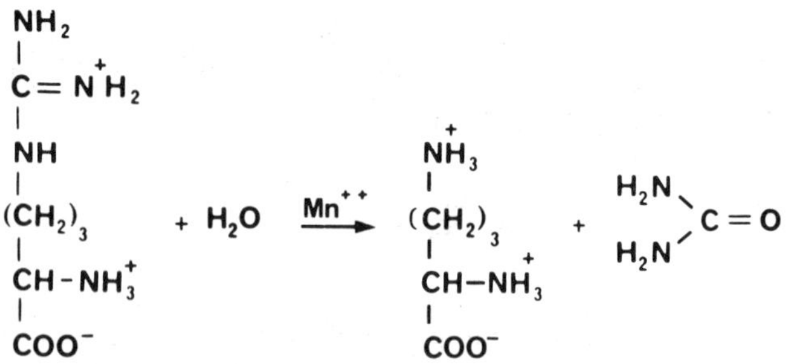

Figure 20-6 The arginase reaction.

Ornithine is produced in the liver (and to a greater extent in the kidney and heart) by arginine-glycine transamidinase. Nevertheless, no net release of ornithine from the normal human kidney *in situ* is demonstrable [13]. No uptake or release from the leg occurs [125].

Ornithine is transaminated in the liver to glutamate semialdehyde (which is in equilibrium with its cyclic form, pyrroline-5-carboxylate) by the OAT reaction [126]:

$$\text{Ornithine} + \alpha\text{-ketoglutarate} \rightleftharpoons$$
$$\text{glutamic semialdehyde} + \text{glutamate} \quad (7)$$

It is metabolized at a substantially lower rate by ornithine decarboxylase, which catalyzes the reaction

$$\text{Ornithine} \longrightarrow \text{putrescine} + CO_2 \quad (8)$$

Factors controlling these reactions are discussed in detail in Chap. 19. As noted above, the OAT reaction probably operates in the forward direction in liver and in the reverse direction in intestine and possibly in kidney [126]. In other tissues, its activity is low. Because of the effects on urea synthesis exerted in particular by changes in hepatic ornithine, it is clear that these enzymes (particularly OAT) have a potentially important role in the regulation of ureagenesis. For example, ornithine may be utilized to sustain ATP levels during energy deficiency states, with a resulting decrease in ureagenesis and hyperammonemia [127].

CITRULLINE   This is produced not only in the liver as an intermediate in urea biosynthesis but also in the intestine. Little uptake by the liver of portal venous citrulline occurs. It is taken up at a more or less comparable rate by the kidney, where it is largely converted to arginine, which is released into the renal vein. The same process also occurs to a minor extent in peripheral tissues [125]. It is not incorporated into protein in mammals.

ARGININOSUCCINATE   This is produced in the liver, where it apparently is converted quantitatively to arginine and thence to urea (neither uptake nor release having been reported). In the rat, ASA is normally present in the liver at a concentration of about 0.034 μmol per gram wet weight and in the serum at 0.01 μmol/ml [128]. Small amounts are excreted in the urine by normal human subjects [129]. It is probably produced in the brain, although this has never been proven, nor is its fate known in this organ. ASA in aqueous solution undergoes reversible ring closure to form two different anhydrides (Fig. 20-7). Anhydride II is the more stable of the two. All three forms are found in the blood and urine of patients with ASAL deficiency. Neither anhydride is attacked by ASAL. The chemical properties and interconversion of these three forms are discussed in detail by Ratner [3].

ARGININE   This is produced in the liver from ammonia and aspartate through the reactions of the urea cycle. It is also produced in the kidney from citrulline. A small portion of the arginine produced reacts with arginine-glycine transamidinase, but by far the greater portion reacts with arginase. The former enzyme may catalyze the production of arginine from guanidinoacetate under certain circumstances [131]. Both reactions produce stoichiometrically equivalent quantities of ornithine. In healthy adults, there is no necessary exogenous or endogenous arginine requirement for protein synthesis, since protein degradation and synthesis are equal. Nevertheless, there is a requirement for arginine intake or synthesis, to produce guanidinoacetate and thence creatine.

Using formulas for creatinine clearance in adult normal subjects proposed by Cockroft and Gault [132], who studied 249 hospitalized subjects, it is possible to derive expressions for creatinine production, P, (and therefore creatine production), in mmoles per kilogram per day (where A is age in years):

$$P = 0.25 - 0.0018A \text{ in males}$$
$$P = 0.21 - 0.0015A \text{ in females} \quad (9)$$

Since arginine intake in a 70-kg adult eating 50 g per day of protein is about 0.2 mmol/kg/day, it appears that the arginine requirement for creatine synthesis is barely met by dietary arginine in adults unless protein intake is substantial. A small but unknown fraction of creatinine output is derived from dietary creatine (and also dietary creatinine in cooked meat). In children under 4 years of age, creatinine output (E) in mmoles per day is a linear function of intracellular water (ICW) [133], in liters:

$$E = -0.35 + 0.35 \text{ ICW} \quad (10)$$

If ICW increases during growth at 15 ml/day, an additional 0.45 mmol/kg per day of arginine can be calculated to be required for the increasing creatine pool in muscle. Thus a 3-kg neonate requires approximately 0.25 mmol/kg per day of arginine (plus creatine), or the amount of arginine present in 0.8 g/kg per day of protein. The same inference is reached: Minimal dietary protein requirements barely meet the arginine requirement for creatine synthesis. Similar inferences can be drawn from normal rates of creatinine excretion in older children [133].

It follows that, in children with complete or nearly complete defects in AGAS, CPS, OCT, ASAS, or ASAL, provision of a very low protein intake supplemented by essential amino acids or keto acids but lacking arginine will induce creatine deficiency as well as arginine deficiency.

Even on an arginine-free diet, adequate arginine can be synthesized in normal infants (via OAT, ASAS, and ASAL) to prevent significant arginine deficiency [134]. Nevertheless, there is suggestive evidence for transient liver damage in adults fed diets free of arginine and histidine [135].

In contrast, most animal species studied to date require exogenous arginine for adequate growth and develop orotic aciduria and sometimes hyperammonemia on an arginine-free diet [136]. Ornithine or citrulline prevents the orotic aciduria, but only citrulline restores normal growth [136].

The domestic cat, in particular, is sensitive to arginine lack and often develops severe or even fatal hyperammonemia after a single arginine-free meal [137]. Although this and other observations suggest that failure of OAT to operate in the reverse direction in this species might be responsible, evidence has been reported that OAT is functional in the cat [138].

Apparently the unusually low hepatic ornithine level that occurs in some cats is the explanation, although why it is so low is unexplained.

Regulation of Ureagenesis

Substrate Regulation In the absence of any inherent regulatory mechanisms, ureagenesis will vary with the concentrations of ammonia and amino acids brought to the liver by the hepatic artery and portal vein. In the case of ammonia, the inference that all of the measured mitochondrial ammonia is freely available for enzymatic reactions [139] might suggest that the CPS I reaction is operating near its maximal rate. As pointed out by Sainsbury [102] and Wanders et al. [103], the appropriate value to use for mitochondrial ammonia in such calculations is one calculated from the extramitochondrial ammonia concentration and the pH difference between this compartment and the mitochondrial space, or about 0.03 mM (instead of 0.8 mM). Normal intramitochondrial ammonia, calculated in this way is far from saturating for the CPS I reaction. Mitochondrial aspartate may be saturating for the ASAS reaction, since normal liver aspartate [58] is many times higher than the K_m of this enzyme for aspartate, 0.03 mM (Table 20-2).

Alanine is the most important amino acid precursor of urea. Portal ammonia, derived in part from the action of bacterial urease within the intestine on urea diffusing inward from body fluids [140], partly from bacterial action on ingested protein [104, 105] and also from intestinal metabolism [8, 9], probably accounts for about 25 percent of the nitrogen incorporated into urea [141]. A number of other amino acids also contribute [124]. These mechanisms alone would suffice to rid the body of waste nitrogen derived from single loads of protein or amino acids that are not so great that hyperammonemia immediately supervenes. There is evidence that changes in urea production in response to varying dietary protein quality are mediated by changes in amino acid levels rather than by the activity of urea cycle enzymes [142]. There are two difficulties with regulation exclusively of this form: (1) the time needed to rid the body of excess nitrogen derived from large loads would be excessive; and (2) in the absence of protein loads, ureagenesis would continue, progressively depleting the circulating amino acid pool as well as inducing hypoammonemia.

The possibility that adenine nucleotide levels may play a role in regulating synthesis of CP has been discussed by several workers [58, 143, 144].

Substrate-induced Activation It has been pointed out [60, 78, 110, 113, 114] that changes in the concentration of

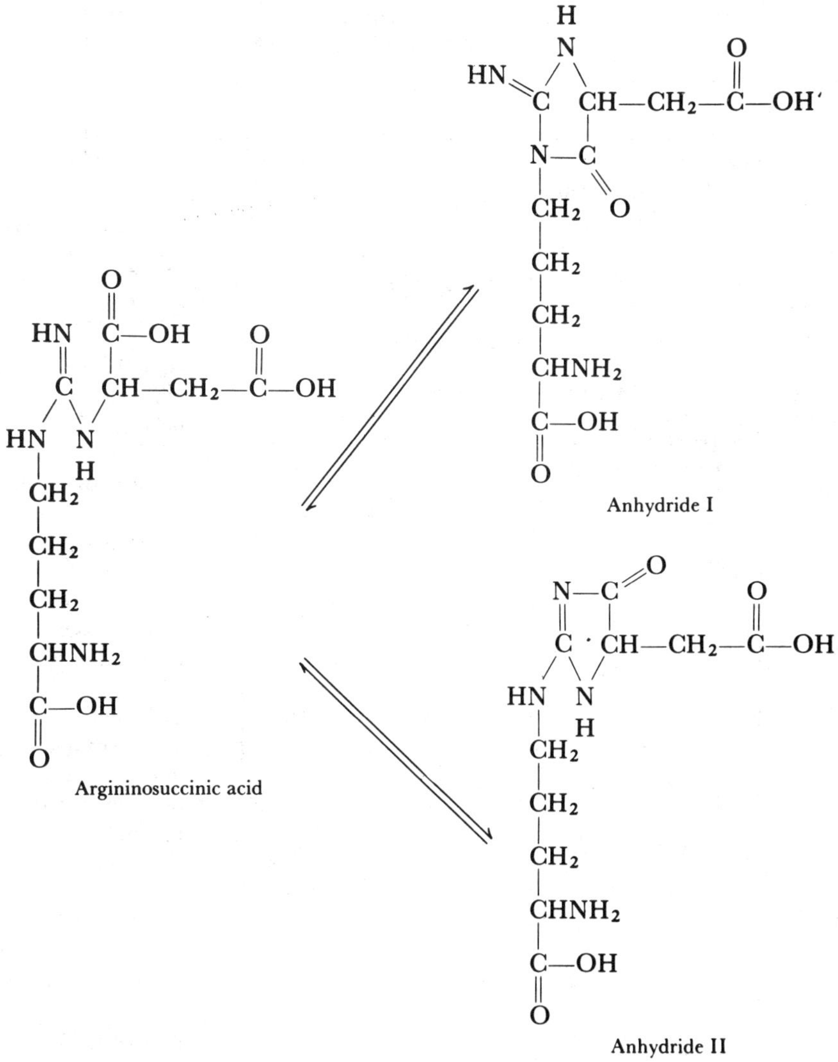

Figure 20-7 The interconversion of argininosuccinate to its two anhydrides, I and II. (*From Kennedy [130], with permission.*)

AGA represent a likely mechanism for rapid activation of the urea cycle following nitrogenous loads. The normal mitochondrial AGA concentration is suboptimal for CPS I activation [58, 59], and CPS I is completely inactive when AGA is absent. Direct evidence for short-term regulation of ureagenesis via rapid changes in AGA concentration has recently been presented by several workers [59, 145, 146]. Within a few minutes after intraperitoneal loads of 20 amino acids in rats, liver AGA content increases several-fold, concomitant with a sharp increase of CPS I activity as assayed in intact mitochondria (with their endogenous AGA content) (Figs. 20-8, 20-9). Since liver glutamate concentration rises equally rapidly, a substrate effect exerted by glutamate on AGA synthesis seems the most likely explanation [59, 145]. No changes in liver ATP were observed during these conditions. A similarly rapid increase in liver AGA is seen following loads of ammonium salts in rats [147].

Thus it appears that single protein loads activate the urea cycle by increasing CPS I activity toward the maximum as assayed in vivo. Similarly, carbohydrate feeding evidently reduces AGA levels and thus CPS I activity [148]. In this way, the rate of ureagenesis as a function of circulating amino acid concentration becomes a curve similar to that of positive cooperativity: Within a certain range of total amino acid concentration, apparently including the usual physiologic levels, small changes in amino acid concentration induce proportionally much greater changes in CPS I activity and therefore presumably in the rate of urea synthesis. At low circulating amino acid concentrations, ureagenesis nearly ceases, thus protecting the body pool of amino acids from depletion.

The applicability of this relationship to normal human subjects is suggested by the studies of Rafoth and Onstad [149], who measured the rate of urea production as a function of total plasma amino acid concentration in normal subjects. An approximately linear relationship with an intercept on the horizontal axis was observed, suggesting again that an increment in the nitrogen load leads to a proportionally greater increase in the rate of ureagenesis. No maximal rate of urea synthesis

Figure 20-8 Liver *N*-acetylglutamate (AGA) concentration at intervals following intraperitoneal injection into rats of 1.5 g/kg of a complete mixture of 20 amino acids (squares) or a mixture lacking arginine (circles). A rapid increase is seen whether or not arginine is present. (*From Steward and Walser* [59], *with permission.*)

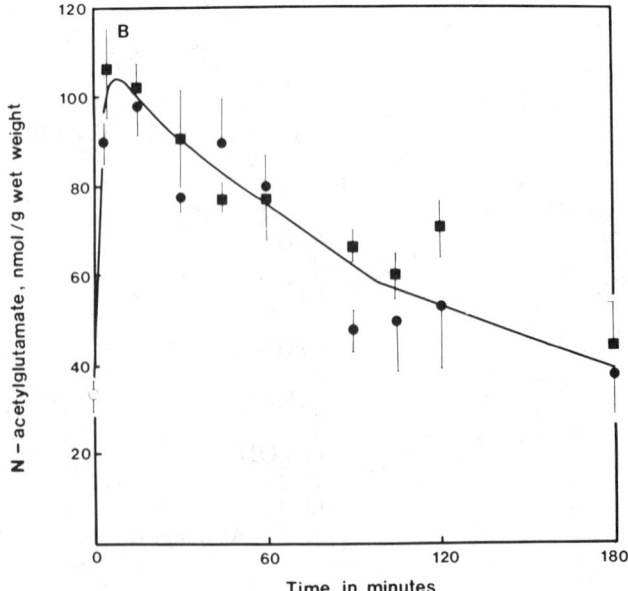

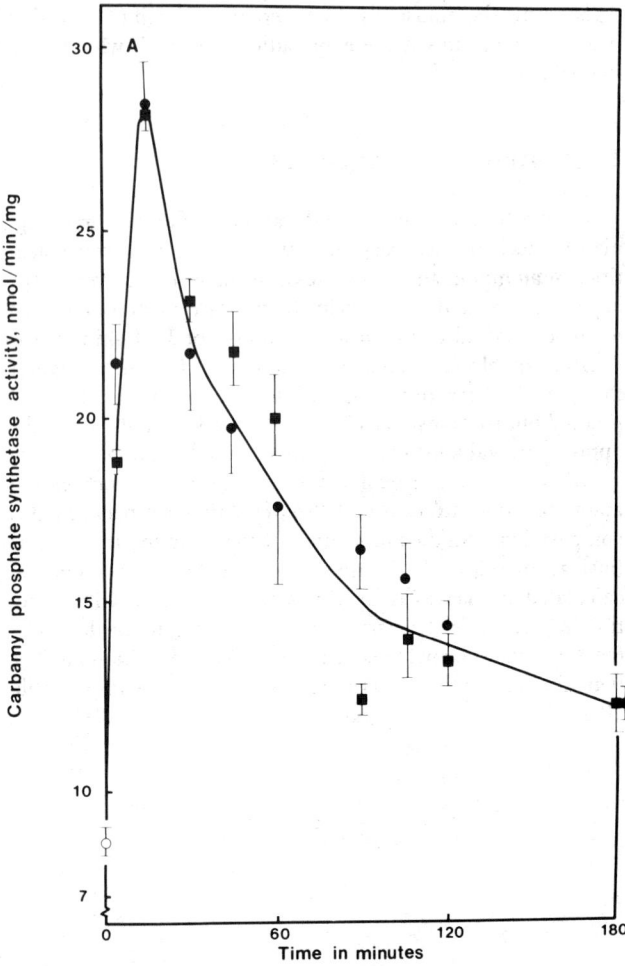

Figure 20-9 Carbamoyl phosphate (CP) synthetase activity of intact mitochondria isolated from livers of rats at varying intervals after injecting 1.5 g/kg of amino acids. Symbols as in Fig. 20-8. The rapid increase in activity is attributable to the increase in *N*-acetylglutamate concentration shown in Fig. 20-8. (*From Stewart and Walser* [59], *with permission.*)

could be demonstrated in these experiments. Earlier studies in which a maximal rate apparently had been demonstrated in normal humans [150] subsequently have been seen to be technically in error by the same workers [151].

Much debate has taken place as to which enzyme of the urea cycle is rate-limiting for urea synthesis. When all of the enzymes are operating at a rate less than maximal, it is clear that the rate of reaction is the same for all five enzymes (excepting AGAS). Under these conditions, determination of which enzyme is rate-determining (not rate-limiting) requires complete information about the concentration of intermediates (including AGA) at the active site of each enzyme, as well as knowledge of the relevant kinetic parameters. Clearly, no single enzyme exclusively determines the rate of ureagenesis under these conditions, but the kinetic parameters may well be such that one enzyme plays a more important role than the others. Most probably, CPS I is predominantly rate-determining, since it is the first committed step in ureagenesis [152].

When one of the enzymes is operating at maximal capacity but enzymes earlier in the cycle are operating at a higher rate, an unstable state exists and the substrate(s) of this enzyme must accumulate rapidly until the rate of generation of urea precursors falls below the maximal rate of this particular enzyme, thus permitting the accumulated intermediates to be metabolized.

In isolated liver or hepatocytes, ASAS often is found to become rate-limiting for the ASAS reaction, such as when lactate is not present or when ammonium and ornithine are present in excess [153].

Enzyme Induction and Repression   The classic work of Schimke [154–156] established that coordinate changes in the activities of CPS I, OCT, ASAS, ASAL, and arginase occur in rats in response to alterations in dietary protein intake. Similar adaptive changes have been reported in primates, including humans [32]. Das and Waterlow [157] showed that adaptive changes in ASAS, ASAL, and arginine occurred within 30 h. The half-life of CPS I in the rat has been estimated as 3 to 7 days [158]. The level of AGAS activity and the hepatic content of AGA also vary with protein intake [60, 114, 159]. The biochemical mechanisms of these changes in enzyme activity have been reviewed recently by Cohen [160].

Hormonal Effects on Urea Cycle Enzymes   Many hormones, including corticosteroids [156, 161–166], glucagon [146, 165, 167–172], growth hormone [161], thyroid hormone [166, 173, 174], and cyclic AMP [162, 163, 165, 170], affect the levels or activities of the urea cycle enzymes. A review of these effects is beyond the scope of this chapter.

The Lysine-Urea Cycle   Evidence from several sources has established that lysine can be converted to homocitrulline under as yet ill-defined circumstances. For example, lysine loads lead to the appearance of urinary homocitrulline in normal subjects [175]. Isolated rat liver exposed to lysine produces homocitrulline after 4 h [176]. Rat liver homogenate converts lysine to a compound tentatively identified as homocitrulline with a K_m of 2.2 mM [177] in a reaction dependent on the presence of CP. Homocitrulline may be excreted as a cyclic derivative of its α-keto analogue, α-keto-ϵ-ureidocaproate [178]. Homocitrullinuria is common in citrullinemia (see below). Strandholm et al. [179] have demonstrated homoargininosuccinate synthesis from homoarginine and fumarate. Paik et al. [180] found that the K_m for lysine of OCT was 10 times greater than that for ornithine, and the K_m of arginase for homoarginine was 200 times greater than that for arginine (in rat liver). Neither kidney nor liver homogenates converted labeled homocitrulline to labeled lysine. Thus, there is no evidence for a complete lysine-urea cycle in mammals, although some of the reactions can occur.

Urea Production in Urea Cycle Defects

It is commonly observed that the plasma urea concentration and the rate of urea excretion are normal or nearly normal in patients with these disorders. Subnormal plasma urea concentrations are seen only in neonates with complete or virtually complete defects, or in children receiving treatment specifically aimed at reducing the requirement for ureagenesis.

Several factors contribute to the continued urea production in these patients. Obviously, a partial deficiency of the liver enzyme or the presence of significant activity of the enzyme in other organs, such as the kidney, is one possible explanation. The most important factor is probably the increased substrate concentration proximal to the metabolic block. Unless enzyme deficiency is complete, the rate of ureagenesis easily can be normal when the substrate concentration becomes sufficiently high.

Kuchel et al. [122] have attempted to analyze this problem quantitatively by means of a mathematical model of the urea cycle. They used the relevant kinetic parameters available at the time but did not take AGA into account. They assumed that CP production was a constant. Despite these limitations, the results are of considerable interest. Tenfold reductions in OCT, ASAS, ASAL, or arginase activities had no significant effect on ureagenesis in this model but caused marked alterations in the steady-state concentration of the other intermediates. When they assumed that CP production fell by 80 percent, ureagenesis fell the same amount but ornithine rose and the steady-state citrulline concentration fell markedly. Further studies along these lines will be useful in attempting to understand the pathophysiology of these disorders.

Another source of urea in patients with urea cycle defects other than argininemia is dietary arginine. Urea production from arginine does not rid the body of waste nitrogen; on the contrary, it leaves an equivalent amount of nitrogen (as ornithine) for disposal. The contribution of this source to urea production is difficult to estimate.

Finally, it has been postulated that urea may be produced in some patients by an "alternate urea cycle" in which lysine replaces ornithine as the regenerated substrate. The cyclically produced intermediates would then become homocitrulline, homoargininosuccinate, and homoarginine. While there is evidence for the production of homocitrulline from lysine, as noted above, it is not clear why this cycle would operate when the ornithine cycle is impaired, unless it uses a different group of enzymes. So far, no such enzymes have been identified.

EFFECTS OF HYPERAMMONEMIA

Hyperammonemia is the predominant cause of symptoms in urea cycle enzymopathies. The causes, manifestations, and treatment of hyperammonemia in children have been reviewed recently by Cathelineau [181].

The mechanisms of the neurotoxicity of ammonia have been partially clarified by recent studies. The brain "detoxifies" ammonia chiefly by glutamine formation [182]:

$$\alpha\text{-Ketoglutarate} + \text{NH}_4^+ + \text{NADH} \rightleftharpoons \text{glutamate} + \text{NAD}^+ \quad (11)$$

$$\text{Glutamate} + \text{NH}_4^+ + \text{ATP} \longrightarrow \text{glutamine} + \text{ADP} + \text{P}_i \quad (12)$$

The first step is a reductive amination of α-ketoglutarate, derived from the tricarboxylic acid cycle, catalyzed by glutamate dehydrogenase. The second reaction, requiring ATP, is catalyzed by glutamine synthetase. Thus an increased ammonia load could in theory (1) deplete α-ketoglutarate, impairing oxidative metabolism; (2) decrease the amount of NADH available for oxidation in the electron transport chain, thereby decreasing oxygen consumption and energy production; and (3) increase energy demands by consuming ATP in the amidation of glutamate to glutamine. In humans, about half of the ammonia in the cerebral arterial blood is extracted in a single pass [109]. Most of a bolus of labeled ammonia injected into the carotid artery of rats is incorporated into glutamine within 5 s [183].

Rats subjected to acute loads of ammonium salts exhibit no change in brain α-ketoglutarate, but glutamine rises sharply and glutamate falls slightly; the cytoplasmic ratio of NADH to NAD$^+$ increases [184]. Brain phosphocreatine falls in all regions, probably indicating a pH-induced shift in the creatine phosphokinase equilibrium secondary to lactate accumulation. A slight reduction in brain ATP and an increase in ADP and AMP are seen, especially in the brainstem [185, 186]. Glycolysis is increased, thus compensating for the utilization of α-ketoglutarate.

In isolated perfused dog brain exposed to 0.2 mM ammonium acetate for 20 min, the uptake of ammonia is entirely accounted for by glutamine synthesis ($\frac{3}{4}$) and alanine synthesis ($\frac{1}{4}$) [187]. Brain α-ketoglutarate does not change, and no significant increase in oxygen uptake, adenine nucleotide or phosphocreatine concentrations occurs. Carbohydrate metabolism is activated, as evidenced by increased glucose uptake, glycogenolysis, and accelerated aerobic and anaerobic glycolysis. As a result, the Gibbs free energy is estimated to be substantially increased. The lactate/pyruvate ratio and the cytoplasmic $NADH/NAD^+$ ratio rise.

Intraperitoneal injections of ammonium acetate in mice decrease brain phosphocreatine and also GTP levels [188]. ATP levels fall only in the most severely intoxicated animals. Brain protein synthesis is depressed.

The conversion of ammonia to glutamine involves not only stimulation of glutamine synthetase activity but also inhibition by ammonium ions of glutaminase. This could reduce the content and release of glutamate and related transmitters from excited neurons [189]. In rat hippocampus, exposure to 3mM NH_4Cl abolishes the KCl-induced release of endogenous glutamate [190]. In cerebral cortex, ammonia at three times normal concentrations abolishes the suppression of action potential generated by postsynaptic inhibition [191], an effect which may explain neurotoxicity.

Pathologic changes are seen in the brain in experimental hyperammonemia. For example, astrocytes in culture respond to an increase in glutamine concentration in the medium by showing enlargement and distortion of nuclei [192]. Both Alzheimer type I and type II astrocytes appear in the brains of rats with portacaval anastomoses [193].

DIAGNOSIS OF UREA CYCLE ENZYMOPATHIES

Each of the urea cycle disorders presents with a distinct clinical picture, and for each, different techniques are available to establish the diagnosis, as noted in the sections that follow. One technique that should be avoided if possible is open liver biopsy. A number of children have died or nearly died during a hyperammonemic crisis brought on by the catabolic stress of this procedure [194–196].

Prenatal diagnosis is possible in deficiencies of the cytosolic but not the mitochondrial enzymes of the cycle. In fetuses at risk for OCT deficiency, prenatal sex determination will assist in determining the urgency of the situation that may or may not occur at birth.

Newborn screening for urea cycle disorders has not yet been widely practiced, partly because of the probability that irreversible brain damage will have already occurred in homozygotes or hemizygotes before the screening is performed or before the test results become available. Screening of newborns at risk is relatively straightforward. A plasma or urine amino acid analysis and blood ammonia determination performed within the first day or two of life generally will detect affected infants.

Screening all newborns for hyperammonemia, hyperglutaminemia, or hyperglutaminuria is not likely to be particularly helpful unless the test results can be made available within a day or two of birth, a practical impossibility in most settings. A method for detecting hyperammonemia that can be applied to one drop of blood and gives results in 15 min has been described [197].

The use of bacterial auxotrophs requiring arginine for growth, when applied to dried blood specimens, has been extensively studied during the past decade. ASA is added to an agar plate containing minimal media and the auxotroph. ASAL in a normal blood spot converts ASA or arginine, producing a measurable zone of growth [198]. Out of 900,000 newborns tested in several countries including the United States, only 3 cases of ASAL deficiency were detected. In Massachusetts, use of a similar paper chromatographic technique in 700,000 newborns detected 9 infants with ASAL deficiency, many of whom were asymptomatic carriers [199]. Naylor [200] has summarized these results of screening programs for urea cycle disorders.

A simple screening test for arginase deficiency has been described [201, 202]. Talbot et al. [203] have devised an improved screening method capable of detecting ASAS deficiency, ASAL deficiency, argininemia, and ornithinemia by using a multiple auxotroph that utilizes citrulline, arginine, or ornithine growth. The test yields a low false-positive rate, which is not a significant disadvantage.

PRINCIPLES OF THERAPY

Symptoms in the urea cycle enzymopathies are most commonly the result of impairment in the capacity for waste nitrogen excretion. The accumulated intermediate may also cause clinical disturbances, especially in argininemia and possibly in ASAS and ASAL deficiency. And finally, arginine deficiency caused by defective arginine synthesis and loss of the ornithine portion of the arginine molecule in the urine (as citrulline or as ASA) may itself cause symptoms. Treatment is therefore aimed at (1) reducing the circulating levels of urea precursors, including ammonia, as well as the levels of the accumulated intermediate, (2) reducing the requirement for ureagenesis, and (3) correcting arginine deficiency when necessary. Thoene and Nyhan [204] have recently reviewed the treatment of urea cycle disorders.

Extrarenal Removal of Urea Precursors

The cornerstone of therapy of hyperammonemic crisis has been the removal of ammonia and other urea precursors by extrarenal routes in conjunction with the administration of glucose with or without insulin. Exchange transfusion, peritoneal dialysis, and hemodialysis are the most commonly employed techniques. Charcoal hemoperfusion has also been employed successfully [205]. All of these techniques remove waste nitrogen not only as ammonium but also as glutamine, glutamate, alanine, and other amino acids [206]. Controlled comparisons of the efficacy of these techniques are not available. Based on retrospective comparison of outcomes in infants treated at 29 different hospitals by peritoneal dialysis, exchange transfusion, or both, Batshaw and Brusilow [206] concluded that peritoneal dialysis was the more effective of the two. Donn et al. [207] tried both of these measures and also hemodialysis in an OCT patient and found that hemodialysis removed ammonia more rapidly than either of the other techniques.

It is important to recognize the speed with which irreversible hyperammonemic coma can develop in infants with urea cycle defects. In at least two cases, a crisis that proved fatal has begun within hours after a normal checkup, including a normal blood ammonia determination [208]. A fall in plasma α-ketoglutarate may precede the rise in ammonia [209], but this determination is not generally available.

Accelerating Renal Excretion of Accumulated Intermediates

Since there is suggestive (though far from conclusive) evidence that citrulline, ASA, and arginine may impair neurodevelopment in neonates (see below), attempts to increase the renal clearance of citrulline and arginine in particular might be worthwhile. ASA is not reabsorbed by the renal tubules to any significant extent, and efforts to increase its clearance would probably be futile. Arginine is almost certainly neurotoxic at high levels, and inhibition of its tubular reabsorption should prove useful. So far, no agents that accomplish this goal have been described.

Another reason to increase the excretion of accumulated intermediates, based on an entirely different rationale, is to exploit the intermediate as a vehicle for the removal of waste nitrogen. Arginine supplementation, in both ASAS deficiency and ASAL deficiency, may augment the rate of excretion of citrulline and ASA, respectively (though, as noted below, this has not been conclusively demonstrated). Here the goal is to increase the circulating level of the accumulated intermediate rather than to decrease it. Stimulation of orotic acid and orotidine excretion by administration of allopurinol or azauridine may result in the excretion of significant amounts of nitrogen in these compounds [210].

Stimulating the Residual Urea Cycle Enzyme Capacity

AGA penetrates the mitochondrion from the cytosol poorly if at all. Hence it cannot be used to stimulate CPS I activity. N-Carbamoylglutamate activates CPS I and combats hyperammonemia when administered to intact rats [211]. Recently, a case of AGAS deficiency has been successfully treated with carbamoylglutamate, 1–3 mmol/kg/day [42]. In partial CPS I deficiency, this agent should also be useful. Whether it would be of any benefit in partial defects of the other enzymes of the cycle is conjectural.

Reducing the Requirement for Waste Nitrogen Production

Since protein intake (in developed countries) is usually in excess of the requirement for growth, restricting dietary protein to the minimum daily requirement is often an effective measure provided caloric intake remains adequate. More efficient retention of dietary nitrogen can be achieved by substituting essential amino acids for part or all of the dietary pro-

tein. Even more efficient retention can be achieved by replacing some of these amino acids by their α-keto or α-hydroxy analogues. Although one would expect that nonessential nitrogen might become limiting for growth under these circumstances, this in fact rarely occurs. In infants with complete CPS or OCT deficiency, normal physical growth has occurred on very low nitrogen intakes when essential amino acids or analogues are supplied (see below).

Design of the optimal mixture of amino, keto, and hydroxy acids for this purpose is a difficult problem, particularly because patients probably vary in their requirements for individual components of the mixture. The branched chain compounds are effective as amino acids or, in larger dosage, as keto-analogues. The keto-analogue of isoleucine, $S(+)$-α-keto-β-methylvalerate, should probably be used instead of the R,S mixture because isoleucine falls when the racemic mixture is given in substantial dosage [212]. Phenylalanine may be given as such or as its keto-analogue, phenylpyruvate. The latter compound causes a brown discoloration in the presence of iron, which is inconvenient in formulas. The hydroxy-analogue, L-phenyllactate, is fully effective in adults [213] but may not be so in infants. Methionine can be replaced by its D,L-α-hydroxy-analogue with no loss of efficiency [214]. The remaining analogues of essential amino acids are either prohibitively expensive or ineffective. The addition of nonessential amino acids such as tyrosine, cystine, and taurine may be advisable in neonates. Arginine should be added in all disorders except arginase deficiency. Greater amounts (2 to 4 mmol/kg/day) are required in ASAS and ASAL deficiency than in CPS or OCT deficiency.

Organic acidemia should be excluded before keto acids are used, because they may precipitate ketoacidosis in such patients [214a].

Sodium Benzoate

Oral or intravenous sodium benzoate rapidly reduces blood ammonia in acutely hyperammonemic infants [206, 215]. By conjugation with glycine, benzoate leads to the excretion of a nearly stoichiometric quantity of nitrogen as hippurate, with isonitrogenous reduction in urea nitrogen excretion [216]. The toxicity of benzoate at the usual doses employed (200 to 500 mg/kg/day) is low; only two instances of toxicity, one associated with glycine depletion, have been reported [217]. In the other, edema, respiratory insufficiency, and abdominal distension occurred on two occasions [217a]. In children given benzoate chronically, the serum benzoate level remains very low [217]. In hyperammonemic neonates given 125 mg/kg intravenously every 6 h, the steady-state serum benzoate level varied from 231 to 517 mg/liter. The onset of renal failure led to a level exceeding 1000 mg/liter, with substantial increase of the unbound fraction of serum bilirubin [218].

Chronic benzoate therapy may provide a useful mechanism for nitrogen excretion. In mutant mice with OCT deficiency (sparse for mice), chronic administration of sodium benzoate permits a higher protein intake and reduces orotic aciduria [219]. A recent report that benzoate at low concentrations inhibits OCT in vitro [42] suggests that it should be used with caution in partial CPS or OCT deficiency. Its use in hyperammonemia caused by organic acidemia has not been studied: Organic acidemia should be excluded first.

Phenylacetate has also been suggested as a useful agent for the treatment of hyperammonemia since it augments urinary nitrogen excretion as phenylacetylglutamine [215]. Long-term toxicity studies of this agent must necessarily precede its use for this purpose.

N-ACETYLGLUTAMATE SYNTHETASE DEFICIENCY

Bachmann et al. [42, 217a] have reported recently in preliminary form the first case of congenital *AGA deficiency*. A full-term male infant developed hyperammonemia on the third day of life and showed a nonspecific hyperaminoacidemia without orotic aciduria. A liver biopsy showed normal levels of CPS, but AGA synthetase was undetectable. Hyperammonemic episodes, with characteristic symptomatology, were treated initially by sodium benzoate. A liver biopsy was obtained during one such episode. OCT was 12 percent of normal on the first biopsy, but this same degree of inhibition of OCT was found to occur in normal liver homogenate incubated in the presence of therapeutic levels of benzoate (0.15 mM). Consequently benzoate therapy was discontinued. The patient has been maintained on carbamoylglutamate, 1–3 mmol/kg/day, arginine, 1 mmol/kg/day, and a diet containing 2 g per kilogram of protein. At age 9 months, he is ataxic and slightly retarded [217a].

CARBAMOYL PHOSPHATE SYNTHETASE DEFICIENCY

CPS I catalyzes the synthesis of CP from ammonia and bicarbonate and is the first committed step in urea synthesis. Deficiency of this enzyme was previously known as *congenital hyperammonemia type I*. The first probable case was reported in 1964 by Freeman et al. [195, 220]. At least 24 additional cases have now been reported [45, 221–240], and one more is reported briefly here, making a total of 26.

Clinical Features and Diagnosis

The neonatal form of CPS deficiency associated with complete or almost complete absence of the enzyme has been seen in 11 patients, all but 2 of whom died in the neonatal period (Table 20-3). These two patients whose condition is summarized briefly here, survived to ages 8 and 15 months (see below). In all 11 patients, characteristic symptoms of hyperammonemia appeared within the first few days after birth, including vomiting, lethargy, hypothermia, hypotonia or spasticity, irritability, and opisthotonus. Most patients have shown a nonspecific hyperaminoacidemia and aminoaciduria, elevated serum transaminase values, normal or low normal blood urea, normal blood electrolytes, pH, and calcium, and normal urinary orotic acid excretion. Hyperammonemia, in most cases, is pronounced. Pulmonary and gastrointestinal hemorrhages occur. Symptoms in seven neonates with partial deficiency have been similar but milder.

CPS deficiency should be suspected in any patient with

hyperammonemic symptoms in the neonatal period in whom elevations of citrulline, argininosuccinic acid, or arginine levels are not seen in the plasma and in whom orotic aciduria is absent. The differential diagnosis includes hyperammonemia caused by parenteral alimentation with amino acid solutions, transient hyperammonemia of infancy, whether associated with asphyxia or delayed development of urea cycle enzymes, *N*-acetylglutamate synthetase deficiency, Reye's syndrome [241], and organic acidemia (Chaps. 22, 23). Organic acidemia is associated with metabolic acidosis and an anion gap. It can generally be excluded by measurement of urinary organic acids, but two patients [224, 225, 242] excreted β-hydroxy-β-methyl glutaric acid in the neonatal period. One died; in the other, this organic acid later disappeared from the urine. Respiratory acidosis and hyperammonemia caused by amino acid infusions are readily diagnosed. The other disorders cannot be excluded without a liver biopsy for enzyme determinations, but it is doubtful whether a liver biopsy should be performed in neonates for this purpose. The diagnosis of CPS deficiency can be made by assaying the enzyme in biopsied rectal [243] or duodenal [232] tissue. Whether leukocytes can be used to assay CPS is controversial [244, 245]. Reduction in hepatic CPS activity may also occur in Reye's syndrome [241], nonketotic hyperglycinemia (Chap. 27), hyperornithinemia with hyperammonemia and homocitrullinuria (Chap. 19), and organic acidemia (Chap. 23).

The clinical picture of partial CPS deficiency is usually different, although seven patients have shown symptoms in the first weeks of life (Table 20-3). More typically, episodic symptoms of hyperammonemia develop on weaning from breast feeding or on changing from formula to cow's milk. Vomiting, low-grade fever with irritability, screaming episodes, or lethargy occurs. Usually recovery from these episodes occurs in about a week, sometimes with the aid of intravenous fluids but more often without treatment. Developmental retardation has been seen in all patients. Computerized axial tomography may show cortical atrophy or dilatation of the ventricles. Recurrent seizures may occur, and even when they do not, the EEG may be abnormal. Blood urea nitrogen levels are low or normal, and hyperammonemia between attacks is usually mild. Glutamine, alanine, glutamate, glycine, and lysine concentrations in plasma often are increased; citrulline is decreased or absent, and arginine and phenylalanine may be low. Orotic acid excretion is normal.

A history of migraine attacks in the mother of one patient [233] and of protein intolerance in the mother of another [232] is consistent with heterozygosity in these individuals and was confirmed by duodenal biopsy in one [232].

Partial CPS deficiency should be suspected in the presence of episodic hyperammonemia without orotic aciduria, organic acidemia, or a specific plasma amino acid abnormality. Needle biopsy of the liver is required to confirm the diagnosis.

Pathology

No consistent abnormalities have been found at autopsy, but several infants have shown pulmonary or gastrointestinal hemorrhages [40, 222–224, 232]. Changes in the liver such as those that occur in Reye's syndrome have not been observed [244], but diffuse fatty infiltration may occur [230] and one infant exhibited abnormal mitochondria and smooth endoplasmic reticulum [235].

Table 20-3 Reported cases of neonatal deficiency of CPS I

Sex	Age at onset	Liver enzyme % of control	Treatment	Outcome	Reference
F	10 d	22		Died at 5 mo	[196, 220]
F	7 d	13	PR	Well at 15 mo	[226]
M	6 wk	<25	PR	Well at 15 mo	[227]
M	2 d	0		Died at 4 d	[221]
M	2 d	0.2		Died at 5 d	[228]
M	5 d	16		Not reported	[234]
M	3 d	0		Died at 5 d	[40]
F	3 d	50	PR	Well at 4 yr	[232]
F	1 wk	0	Arg, KA	Died at 15 mo	[224, 225]
F	2 d	0	Arg, KA	Died at 5 mo	[249]
M	1 d	0		Died at 2 d	[237]
M	3 d	0.2		Died at 4 d	[223]
M	1 d	0		Died at 4 d	[230]
F	2 d	0		Died at 4 d	[222]
M	3 d	9		Died at 9 d	[229]
F	1 d	1		Died at 2 d	[236]
M	2 wk	21		Not reported	[235]
M	—	5	EAA, KA, Arg	Not reported	[238, 239]
M	1 d	10		Died at 5 d	[235]

Abbreviations: PR, protein restriction alone; Arg, arginine plus protein restriction; KA, keto-analogues plus protein restriction; EAA, essential amino acids plus protein restriction.

Biochemical Investigations

Few additional biochemical observations have been made. Urinary excretion of N-carbamoyl aspartate and N-carbamoyl-β-alanine was normal in one [222], and the pattern of urinary pyrimidines and purines was normal in another [236]. A vitamin K–responsive clotting defect was observed in two patients [232]. The hypophenylalaninemia observed in one older patient failed to respond to substantial doses of phenylpyruvate or phenylalanine [248].

Enzyme Defect

CPS activity has varied from 0 to 50 percent of controls in the neonatal onset cases and from 5 to 40 percent of controls in the later onset cases. In almost all of these assays, AGA was added in optimal amounts (2.5 to 10 mM), and the assay therefore includes both CPS I and CPS II activity. Since the activity of the latter enzyme is only a minute fraction of the former, most of the enzyme assayed must be CPS I except in those cases in which activity approaches zero. Omission of AGA probably does not give a reliable value for CPS II activity because traces of this substance are likely to be present in liver homogenate [33]. Kinetic variants have apparently not been identified.

Genetics

Autosomal recessive inheritance of CPS deficiency was suggested by the occurrence of both partial and complete deficiency in males and females, parental consanguinity in two families [229, 231], and the absence of protein intolerance in most parents of affected children. The disorder affects males and females with equal frequency. One neonatal female patient had had a male sib who died in coma on the fifth day of life [249]. Another had two female sibs who died within the first 2 weeks of life [229]. McReynolds et al. [45] recently analyzed hepatic tissue from all members of the immediate family of two girls with severe but partial CPS deficiency. The parents had CPS activities of 32 percent and 54 percent of controls, while a brother had normal activity. These data establish that the trait is inherited as an autosomal recessive trait.

Treatment

Complete or virtually complete deficiency has proven fatal in the neonatal period in almost all patients so far reported, including one in whom the diagnosis was suspected at delivery because of a previous sib with the disorder [222]. The condition of two who survived 15 and 5 months, respectively, is summarized briefly here.

A female infant with zero CPS activity who developed respiratory distress and seizures during the first week of life was treated for 4 months with protein restriction and arginine; she remained hyperammonemic and grew little. She was then given a supplement containing nitrogen-free analogues of five essential amino acids and six amino acids as such (including histidine, arginine, and taurine). She developed normally, both physically and mentally, until age 15 months, when she developed a hyperammonemic crisis, unresponsive to peritoneal dialysis and sodium benzoate therapy, following rubella vaccination [224, 225].

A female infant with 1.9 percent CPS activity (zero when assayed without AGA) developed symptoms on the second day of life. She was treated initially by peritoneal dialysis and then with a similar supplement plus 1.1 g/kg per day of protein from age 5 days until her death at age 5 months. She showed good weight gain (50th percentile) but a progressively abnormal head circumference (below the 3d percentile). Difficulty was experienced in regulating plasma arginine, and some hyperammonemic episodes occurred. She had cortical blindness, apparently caused by intracranial bleeding in the neonatal period [249].

A 6-month-old boy with 5 percent CPS activity was treated with essential amino acids including arginine and briefly with a supplement containing five keto-analogues in place of essential amino acids [238, 239]. Although ammonia levels fell, amino acid imbalance occurred, and he was subsequently given the essential amino acid supplement with good initial results.

A male infant with 43 percent CPS activity who developed symptoms at age 6 weeks did well initially on arginine, 0.6 mmol/kg/day, plus protein 2 g/kg/day. The authors suggest that arginine activation of AGAS, thereby stimulating residual CPS activity, accounted for these results [231].

A 13-year-old girl with 15 percent CPS activity who had symptoms from age 3 weeks was treated for several years with a similar supplement, with good biochemical control, improved growth, and reduction in the frequency of seizures [233, 248].

Whether benzoate should be used in partial CPS defects is open to question in view of the report [42] that benzoate inhibits OCT in vitro. The use of carbamoylglutamate [42, 53, 211] might be helpful in such patients since the activity of CPS is not stimulated maximally by normal AGA levels, at least in the absence of hyperammonemia [59].

ORNITHINE CARBAMOYL TRANSFERASE DEFICIENCY

OCT *deficiency* is the most common of the urea cycle enzyme defects, having been reported in more than 110 patients. It is inherited as an X-linked dominant trait and therefore causes virtually complete enzyme lack in hemizygous males. In most such patients, the condition is probably not diagnosed. Heterozygous females have varying degrees of partial deficiency.

Clinical Features and Diagnosis

Hemizygous Males In most of the 40 to 45 reported males [36, 209, 210, 217, 223, 234, 250–267], hyperammonemic symptoms have appeared within a few days of birth—sometimes within the first few hours. Lethargy, irritability, or poor feeding are usually the first symptoms detected. Grunting respiration, vomiting, and spasticity or hypotonia may occur. Convulsions, coma, apnea, and areflexia soon develop, proceeding to death in untreated patients. Apart from pronounced hyperammonemia and nonspecific hyperaminoacidemia, the most characteristic finding is orotic aciduria, usually of extreme degree (up to 9 mmol/g creatinine). Serum transaminase values are often elevated, and the liver may be enlarged. Hematemesis may occur. Blood urea is normal or low. Plasma citrulline is subnormal, and arginine may also be low.

The diagnosis is based upon the presence of neonatal hyperammonemia without a specific abnormality of the plasma amino acid pattern (other than hypocitrullinemia), plus severe orotic aciduria. Few other conditions yield this group of findings, and liver biopsy in the neonatal period is therefore not essential for diagnosis. In newborn males at risk for OCT deficiency, the low or absent plasma citrulline level should provide a useful diagnostic marker and permit therapy to be started before hyperammonemia or orotic aciduria develops [268]. Biopsy of rectal mucosa may be useful, since OCT activity in this tissue is half as great as in liver [243]. Duodenal biopsy may also be useful [232]. Organic acidemia can usually be excluded by the absence of metabolic acidosis with an anion

gap, but one patient had associated propionic acidemia [269].

Heterozygous Females In females the first symptoms may occur as early as the neonatal period or as late as 9 years of age, depending upon the residual enzyme activity [36, 46, 47, 234, 247, 252, 254, 256, 263, 269–288]. Typically, these symptoms include episodic feeding difficulties, vomiting, screaming, headache, slurred speech, and lethargy and may be precipitated by a change in protein intake, infections, vaccination, anesthesia, or surgery. During these episodes patients may develop muscular rigidity, opisthotonus, or hepatomegaly. Impaired neurodevelopment and physical growth usually appear, sometimes with recurrent seizures. Most patients develop an aversion to protein-rich foods.

The condition should be suspected in female infants with recurrent episodes of vomiting, especially if associated with the symptoms summarized above. Measurement of blood ammonia, urinary orotic acid, and plasma amino acid concentrations will reveal whether OCT deficiency is a likely cause. Needle biopsy of the liver should generally be performed to confirm the diagnosis, although rectal [243] or duodenal [232] biopsy may suffice. Recurrent Reye's syndrome exhibits normal OCT levels in the liver between attacks [289]. The use of serum levels of OCT and the ratio between these levels and transaminase activities has been suggested as an alternative to liver biopsy [275, 290] but has not been studied widely enough to justify its diagnostic use. Similarly, controversy exists as to whether leukocyte levels of OCT can be used for this purpose [244, 245, 272, 291, 292]

Late Onset Syndrome in Males At least 18 male infants have been clearly shown to have OCT deficiency without neonatal onset of symptoms. In some [43, 49, 252, 254, 256, 262, 266, 293–296], the deficiency has been less than complete, which may explain the late onset. In others [49, 297], the deficiency has been substantially complete, despite a normal neonatal course. While some workers [297] have inferred from this finding that virtually complete deficiency may cause only minor symptoms in infancy, a more plausible possibility, mentioned by the same authors [297], is that the in vitro assay of OCT fails to reflect the in vivo activity of the enzyme. This could be caused by the presence of an inhibitor of OCT activity. Nevertheless in one case, the addition of liver homogenate from the patient to normal rat liver homogenate did not inhibit OCT [49].

The clinical course in such patients is characterized by a normal neonatal period, followed by progressively severe hyperammonemic episodes during infancy or childhood. The diagnosis requires needle biopsy of the liver for confirmation and to exclude Reye's syndrome, which can cause a similar clinical picture and may be associated with low hepatic levels of OCT and CPS [241]. As noted below, the hepatic pathology is different.

Asymptomatic Carriers When female antecedents of known male cases are examined by measuring orotic acid excretion following protein loads, heterozygotes can be detected [46, 257, 298–300]. Duodenal mucosal biopsy can also be used, but false negatives occur [298]. In one pedigree, seven heterozygotes had slightly but significantly lower IQs and a wider discrepancy between verbal and performance IQs than an equal number of noncarriers in the same pedigree [299]. Thus, it is possible that even mild OCT deficiency may cause some impairment of brain development, presumably due to unrecognized episodes of hyperammonemia in infancy. This report does not indicate whether the heterozygotes identified in this study had an aversion to protein-rich foods, a history of cyclic vomiting in infancy, or complained of nausea, headache, and lethargy after eating protein-rich foods. All of these features have been previously described in otherwise asymptomatic OCT heterozygotes, identified by orotic aciduria after protein or ammonium loads [257, 298] or by other techniques [234, 236, 263].

Pathology

The liver has been reported to show no abnormalities in hemizygous male infants [49, 259, 301], but both heterozygous females and males exhibiting the delayed onset clinical syndrome show numerous pathologic abnormalities on liver biopsy, including steatosis and microvesicular fat accumulation, distorted endoplasmic reticulum, focal areas of inflammation or mononuclear cell infiltration, and stellate portal scarring [247].

Microvesicular fat accumulation can be induced in rats by repeated injections of urease, which induces hyperammonemia without orotic aciduria [302]. An arginine-free diet causes a similar lesion [303]. When the conversion of orotic acid to uridine monophosphate is blocked by azauridine in urease-treated animals, these fatty changes are reduced markedly [302]. Thus high production rates of uridine monophosphate may play a role in this lesion. The mitochondrial lesions characteristic of Reye's syndrome [247] are not seen, but morphologic changes can be seen on electron microscopy [262].

The brain pathology in OCT deficiency is described in detail in the previous edition [301]. In brief, dilated ventricles, cortical atrophy, and Alzheimer type II astrocytes are seen.

Biochemical Investigations

Apart from hyperammonemia, the characteristic biochemical abnormality of OCT deficiency is the accumulation of pyrimidine metabolites. CP synthesized intramitochondrially accumulates because its reaction with ornithine to produce citrulline is impeded. As a result, it passes into the cytosol [60, 118–121, 304], where it becomes available for conversion to carbamoyl aspartate and thence to pyrimidines (Fig. 20-1). Not only orotic acid but also uridine and uracil accumulate in plasma and are excreted in the urine in greatly increased quantities [234, 236, 276]. The renal clearances of these three substances are relatively high; orotic acid clearance in one patient was 226 ml/(min·1.73 m), indicating tubular secretion [276]. Orotidine excretion usually is not increased, nor is thymine or pseudouridine excretion [236, 276]. The latter compounds are derived from nucleotide breakdown, and increased excretion therefore would not be expected.

While orotic acid and uracil excretion tend to be correlated with blood ammonia levels in various types of hyperammonemia, Van Gennip et al. [236] reported that the increase in uridine excretion appears to be more specific for OCT deficiency and suggested that the accumulation of uridine monophosphate, not used for *de novo* nucleotide synthesis, may inhibit the orotidine-5-phosphate-orotate phosphoribosyltransferase enzyme complex, promoting orotic acid accumulation. The activity of this enzyme complex, when measured in the livers of mice with congenital OCT deficiency (sparse fur mice), is found to be less than in normal mice [305].

N-Carbamoyl-β-alanine excretion is increased, possibly as a result of the inhibition of ureidopropionase by high ammonia levels [236].

Urinary purine excretion also increases, which may be attributable to altered tubular transport since plasma levels of uric acid are not increased [276]. Uric aciduria does not always parallel plasma ammonia levels [236]. *N*-Carbamoylaspartate may also be excreted in abnormal quantities [237].

Enzyme Defect

By far the most common type of enzyme defect reported in OCT deficiency is a reduction in maximal enzyme activity, but many kinetic mutants have been reported. Abnormal pH dependency was first noted by Levin et al. [280] and has been reported several times [277, 301]. Decreased or, less commonly, increased affinity of the enzyme for ornithine [43, 256, 257, 301], decreased affinity for CP [256, 301, 306], and decreased inhibition of the enzyme by ornithine [275, 306] have been described. Recently, a patient was reported in whom the temperature dependence of activity, as well as the kinetic constants, was abnormal [257].

Briand et al. [307] have recently obtained monospecific antibodies against OCT from rabbits and have shown that hemizygous males, including the late onset variants, usually have deficient cross-reactive material but may in some cases have a normal amount. Results in heterozygotes were variable. Similarly, in one patient whose enzyme exhibited normal kinetic parameters but a maximal activity only 9 percent that of controls, Mori et al. [47] recently showed by isoelectric focusing techniques that an inactive form of enzyme also was present and constituted the major portion of immunoreactive material. Two phenotypic classes of cells have been demonstrated in the liver of a female heterozygote, one with normal activity and one with no activity [308]. In mutant mice bearing the X-chromosomal spf gene, the K_m for CP is significantly lower than in normal mice [305], and both normal and abnormal forms of the enzyme are present [309].

Genetics

It has been established that OCT deficiency is inherited as an X-linked dominant trait [36, 252, 264] (Fig. 20-10), as suggested by study of one of the first cases identified [310]. A review by Palmer et al. [263] of 20 families confirmed the generality of this observation. Indeed, it appears that no cases have been reported in which any other mode of inheritance is required to explain the family history. The late onset male variants have in general had no family history that could establish any specific mode of inheritance; several have had male sibs with similar clinical histories, and maternal OCT deficiency has been detected in a few.

Treatment

In the hemizygous male, death within the first week or two after birth was invariable until recently. Oral antibiotics, enemas, lactulose, peritoneal dialysis, exchange transfusions, a

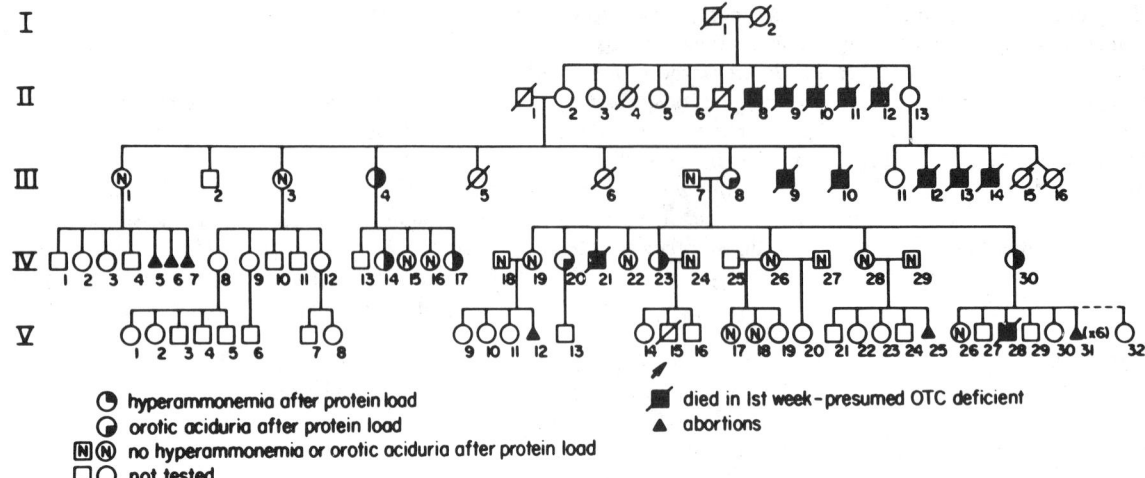

Figure 20-10 Pedigree of an OCT-deficient kindred. (*From Batshaw et al.* [299], *with permission.*)

diet containing arginine-rich protein [279], and the administration of *N*-carbamoylglutamate plus arginine [259] all proved of no avail. One male infant with complete enzyme deficiency survived 8 weeks on protein restriction plus essential amino acids, arginine, and aspartic acid [258].

McReynolds et al. [253] reported the first patient with complete deficiency to survive the neonatal period. A previous male sib had died on the third day of life with a clinical picture consistent with OCT deficiency, and a female sib had been identified by liver biopsy as having partial OCT deficiency. Consequently, preparations were made before delivery to treat the disorder. Amniocentesis had established that the fetus was a male, but the mother elected to continue the pregnancy, since there was a 50 percent chance that he would be unaffected. By 24 h of age, the infant was irritable, jittery, and mildly hypertonic, with a blood ammonia level at the upper limit of normal. A small protein feeding produced mild hyperammonemia. Treatment with 1.2 to 1.8 g/kg/day of a mixture of five nitrogen-free analogues plus the remaining essential amino acids as such (including histidine and arginine) and a low protein diet (0.5 g/kg initially, increased gradually to 1 g/kg) maintained normal growth and development to age 5 months, when an abrupt episode of hyperammonemia proved fatal. Four changes in the proportions and dosage of the supplement were made in response to growth and to abnormalities of plasma amino acid concentrations. An insufficient dosage of arginine may have been a factor in his demise, since plasma arginine fell below normal during the final illness. Autopsy findings were unremarkable. OCT activity was undetectable in a liver biopsy.

A second male infant with absent OCT activity was treated in a similar fashion and developed normally until age 6 months, when he died of sepsis [260]. Another boy treated in this manner developed normally until 8 weeks, when a hyperammonemic crisis unresponsive to benzoate proved fatal [209].

A fourth male lacking any OCT activity was in deep hyperammonemic coma by age 3 days. After peritoneal dialysis, he was treated with a similar supplement plus protein 0.5 g/kg/day, and grew normally except for head circumference, which became progressively subnormal, with severe mental retardation. He had six hyperammonemic episodes before a terminal episode unresponsive to benzoate at age 16 months. These episodes were apparently related to amino acid imbalances and led to many changes in the composition and dosage of the supplement. He also had an unexplained normochromic normocytic anemia [261].

A fifth male with no OCT activity [210, 311] has been treated in the same manner since age 2 weeks and is now 4 years old. He is severely retarded, presumably because of the prolonged period of deep coma in the first 2 weeks of life, as well as several hyperammonemic episodes during the first year of life. Height and weight are normal; head circumference is markedly subnormal. Low dose benzoate has now been added to his regimen.

A sixth male infant lacking OCT activity was lethargic at age 5 days, with a plasma ammonia level of 398 μM. At that point therapy was instituted, with a mixture of essential amino acids (plus arginine) at a dose of 1.1 g/kg/day and sodium benzoate, 2 mmol/kg/day. Protein intake was gradually increased to 1 g/kg/day. Neurodevelopment was normal at 8 months of age, weight was at the 25th percentile, and height was at the 3d percentile. Head circumference was not reported [217].

These results strongly suggest that normal growth and development are possible in the complete absence of OCT activity. Further work is necessary to establish whether nitrogen-free analogues, benzoate, or a combination of both is most effective. In addition, the detection and treatment of hyperammonemic crises remains largely an unsolved problem. It would appear that benzoate is effective, particularly during catabolic crises, whereas nitrogen-free analogues are not. Thus the treatment of crises in patients already on maximal doses of benzoate may pose a problem. Serial observations in two hemizygous males on keto acid treament indicated that a fall in plasma α-ketoglutarate preceded hyperammonemia [209]. Thus measurement of this substrate may become a useful guide to management.

In female heterozygotes, treatment by protein restriction alone usually will suffice. If the patient cannot tolerate the minimum daily requirement of protein for her age, then essential amino acids or nitrogen-free analogues plus arginine should be given and protein intake further restricted [46]. In view of the report [42] that benzoate inhibits OCT activity at concentrations as low as 0.15 mM, it should perhaps not be used, although the benefit derived by providing an alternate pathway for nitrogen excretion may in some cases outweigh the deleterious effect of inhibiting residual OCT. Study of sparse-fur mice with OCT deficiency may clarify this question [219].

In males with the delayed onset type of OCT deficiency, some promising results have been reported. One patient survived $2\frac{1}{2}$ years with only 4 percent of normal OCT activity on protein restriction and arginine supplementation. Growth and development were impaired [49]. Another male with 6 percent of control OCT activity was nearly normal in terms of growth and development at age 18 months when reported in preliminary form [293], on protein restriction alone. A complete report of this case has not yet appeared.

ARGININOSUCCINATE SYNTHETASE DEFICIENCY (CITRULLINEMIA)

ASAS deficiency, or citrullinemia, was first reported by McMurray et al. in 1962 [312]. It is characterized by pronounced accumulation of citrulline in body fluids. At least 53 symptomatic cases have been reported in whole or in part (Table 20-4). A unique form of the disorder occurs almost exclusively in Japan.

Clinical Features and Diagnosis

Neonatal Type Twenty cases of the severe neonatal form of citrullinemia have been reported in some detail (Table 20-4), and two others are summarized here. Irritability, lethargy,

poor feeding, grunting, and tachypnea appear within the first few days of life and usually proceed to rigidity, sometimes with opisthotonus, apnea, convulsion, coma, and death. Thirteen of the patients died in the neonatal period, but four survived for 7 or 8 months with treatment, one is still alive at 16 months [327], one at $2\frac{1}{2}$ years [217], one at 6 years [329], and one was well when reported at 4 years [319]. Hyperammonemia and orotic aciduria are pronounced, and metabolic acidosis may be present. One patient lacking ASAS activity died of brain damage without ever exhibiting hyperammonemia. This suggests that citrulline at high concentrations may be neurotoxic [317, 352]. The diagnosis is made by the finding of a plasma citrulline level 40 to 200 times normal.

Transient hyperammonemia in premature infants may possibly be attributable to developmental delay in ASAS (see below).

Subacute Type A few children with partial deficiencies have been reported in whom episodic hyperammonemia and physical and mental retardation were observed (Table 20-4). One infant with no ASAS in fibroblasts was asymptomatic until age 6 months and did well on protein restriction alone; presumably some residual enzyme was present in the liver [335].

Late Onset Type In Japan at least 22 cases of a distinct form of citrullinemia have been reported (Table 20-4). One similar case was reported from the United States [338, 339]. Only those cases have been included in the table in which citrullinemia was demonstrated, whether or not ASAS deficiency was documented. As noted below, a significant degree of citrullinemia (in the absence of argininosuccinic acidemia) is virtually pathognomonic for ASAS deficiency. The ages at onset listed in the table are somewhat arbitrary in that many of these

Table 20-4 Reported cases of symptomatic citrullinemia

Sex	Age at onset	ASAS activity % of control*		Homocitrul-linuria	Hyperam-monemia	Plasma (Cit) mM	Treatment†	Outcome	Reference
					NEONATAL CASES				
F	4 d	6(B),	0(L)	No	Yes	4.6	—	Died at 7 d	[313]
M	3 d	1(B),	1(L)	No	Yes	3.1	—	Died at 5 d	[314, 315]
M	3 d	50(F),	1(B), 0(L)	No	Yes	2.1	—	Died at 6 d	[314]
M	2 d	—	—	Yes	Yes	2.3	—	Died at 6 d	[316]
M	3 d	100(B),	0(L)	No	No	2.7	—	Died at 7 d	[317]M
M	2 m	100(K),	0(L)	Yes	Yes	2.3	—	Died at 8 m	[318]
F	10 d	1(F)	—	Yes	Yes	0.6–4.6	EAA, Arg	Normal at 32 m	[319, 320]
F	6 d	—	—	—	—	(11.3)‡	—	Died at 8 d	[321]
M	4 d	—	—	—	—	5.3	—	Died at 6 d	[322]
M	1 d	—	—	—	Yes	0.4–3.9	Arg	Well until death at 7 m	[323]
M	2 d	0(F)	—	No	Yes	1.5–3.9	KA, Arg	Well until death at 8 m	[324]
M	4 d	0(L)	—	No	Yes	1.4–3.7	KA, Arg	Well until death at 7 m	[325]
F	3 d	0(F)	—	—	—	3.8	—	Died at 8 d	[326]
F	5 d	—	—	—	Yes	0.9–4.4	KA, Arg, Benz, EAA	Retarded at 26 m	[217]
M	7 d	0(F)	—	—	Yes	0.8–3.9	KA, Arg, Benz	Sl. retarded at 16 m	[327]
M	2 d	~5(A)	—	—	Yes	0.3	—	Died at 3 d	[328]
M	1 d	0(L)	—	—	Yes	0.11	—	Died at 6 d	[328, 329]
F	2 d	0(L)	—	—	Yes	0.15	—	Died at 7 d	[328, 329]
M	8 d	0(L)	—	—	Yes	0.17	—	Died at 13 d	[328, 329]
M	2 d	0(L)	—	—	Yes	0.16	—	Died at 13 d	[329]
M	8 d	1(L)	—	—	Yes	—	—	Not reported	[329]
M	3 d	1(L)	—	—	Yes	0.17	—	Alive at 6 y	[329]

NOTE: See page 420 for footnotes.

Table 20-4 Reported cases of symptomatic citrullinemia (*Continued*)

Sex	Age at onset	ASAS activity % of control*	Homocitrul-linuria	Hyperam-monemia	Plasma (Cit) mM	Treatment†	Outcome	Reference
				SUBACUTE TYPE				
M	9 m	5	No	Yes	1.6–2.2	—	Retarded at 9 m	[312, 330–332]
F	5 m	Abn. kinetics	Yes	Yes	1.0–2.0	Arg	Retarded at 2 y	[320, 333, 334]
M	7 y	12(F)	No	Yes	2.0–2.3	—	Retarded at 7 y	[321]
M	6 m	—	—	—	—	PR	Well at 8 m	[335]
F	1 m	5(F)	No	Yes	0.5–0.8	PR	Well at 18 m	[336]
M	1 y	5.5(L)	Yes	—	—	—	—	[234]
M	4 m	~9(A)	—	Yes	0.1	—	Died at 10 m	[328]
				LATE ONSET VARIANT				
F	20 y	21(L)	—	Yes	1.0	—	—	[337]
M	1 y	1(F)	Yes	Yes	1.5	—	Retarded at 33 y	[338, 339]
M	14 y	36(L), 16(B)	No	Yes	0.16–0.60	—	Died at 22 y	[340, 341]
F	Child-hood	31(L)	No	Yes	0.1–0.2	—	Retarded at 18 y	[342, 343]
M	21 y	—	—	Yes	0.9	PR	Spastic at 24 y	[344]
F	Child-hood	Decr. (W)	No	Yes	0.1–0.2	—	Retarded at 23 y	[342, 345]
M	25 y	—	—	Yes	0.3	—	Retarded at 27 y	[346]
F	27 y	—	—	Yes	0.7	—	Retarded at 28 y	[346]
F	9 y	—	—	Yes	0.1–0.3	PR	Well at 20 y	[347]
F	18 y	20(L)	—	Yes	0.1–0.3	PR	Died at 31 y	[347]
F	22 y	—	—	Yes	0.1–0.3	PR	Well at 24 y	[347]
M	23 y	—	—	Yes	1.0	—	—	[348]
M	23 y	50(L), 100(W)	—	Yes	0.7	—	—	[348]
—	—	Abn. kinetics	—	—	—	—	—	—
F	—	Abn. kinetics	—	No	0.4	—	—	[349]
M	—	50(L)	—	Yes	0.6	—	—	[350]
M	23 y	—	—	Yes	0.3	—	Died at 23 y in coma	[351]
F	Child-hood	Abn. kinetics	No	Slight	0.4	—	Ill at 24 y	[35]
M	20 y	2(L)	—	Yes	0.16–0.6	—	Died at 46 y of infection	[44, 50], [341]
M	48 y	22(L)	—	Yes	0.15–0.4	—	Died of infection	[50, 341]
F	24 y	8(L)	—	Yes	2.0	PR	Well	[50, 341]
M	24 y	25(L)	—	Yes	0.6	PR	Well	[50, 341]
—	Adult	50(L)	—	Yes	0.09–0.13	—	—	[50]
—	Adult	37(L)	—	Yes	0.4	—	—	[50]

* ASAS, argininosuccinate synthetase; L, liver; F, fibroblasts; A, amniotic fluid cells; C, lymphocytes; B, brain; K, kidney; W, white blood cells.
† PR, protein restriction alone; EAA, protein restriction plus essential amino acids; Arg, protein restriction plus arginine; KA, protein restriction, essential amino acids, and nitrogen-free analogues; Benz: sodium benzoate.
‡ Urine citrulline, mmol/mmol creatinine

patients had some sort of difficulty during infancy or early childhood. The age of onset shown is the age at which a significant clinical abnormality, not readily explained in any other way, first appeared. The most characteristic feature of this variant is the late onset of serious and continuing symptomatology, varying from childhood to age 48 years. This is different from all other urea cycle enzymopathies and has never been adequately explained. Five of the patients have died under observation, but whether their deaths were directly related to the disease is uncertain except in one case [351]. Many have become incapacitated during adulthood.

In infancy or childhood, almost all the patients have exhibited some transient symptoms which varied in severity. These include enuresis, delayed menarche, insomnia, sleep reversal, nocturnal terrors and sweats, recurrent vomiting (especially at night), diarrhea, tremors, episodes of confusion following meals, lethargy, convulsions, delusions and hallucinations, and brief episodes of coma. Delayed mental or physical development has occurred in some.

In most of these patients, a peculiar fondness for beans, peas, and peanuts has been noted from early childhood, usually associated with a dislike for rice, other vegetables, and sweets. These preferred foods may contain relatively high amounts of arginine [353]. Thus the dietary predilections of these patients may reflect arginine deficiency. None have been alcoholics; in fact, several have shown intolerance for alcohol.

As the patients grow older, the episodic disturbances become more frequent and bizarre behavior begins to appear, including manic episodes, echolalia, and frank psychosis. At this stage motor weakness or frank paralysis of the limbs is often seen, as well as dysarthria. Patients become difficult to arouse. Muscle spasms, myoclonus, and hyperreflexia as well as pathologic reflexes occur.

Additional findings that have been seen at this stage include severe mental retardation and hepatomegaly, with mildly abnormal liver function tests. One patient became jaundiced. The hair is normal. Kayser-Fleischer rings have not been seen, and ceruloplasmin and copper levels in serum are normal.

Portal-systemic shunts have been excluded by angiography in several cases, and varices have not been reported except in one autopsied case. At this stage blood ammonia is almost always elevated, sometimes to very high levels (1.2 mg/dl).

Citrulline levels in plasma vary from 0.1 to 2.0 mM (Table 20-4). A lesser elevation of citrulline is seen in cerebrospinal fluid. Plasma arginine and ornithine are usually normal or somewhat elevated. Blood urea is normal. As little as 3 g NH_4Cl by mouth may induce a pronounced increase in blood ammonia [44, 351]. Homocitrulline was found in the urine in only one of five subjects.

A few patients have died in coma at this stage. Others have died of intercurrent illness. Some have improved on protein restriction.

Pathologic findings include fatty liver in all cases. Round-cell infiltration, focal necrosis, mild fibroblasts, and abnormal hepatocyte morphology may be seen. At autopsy, the brains of these patients have shown atrophy, Alzhiemer type II glia, and spongy degeneration.

In 15 of the 23 cases summarized in Table 20-4, ASAS activity has been measured and found to be deficient. Two patients showed kinetic abnormalities, but the kinetics of the deficient enzyme in the other patients have been normal [50, 341, 345]. Two patients [44, 50, 338, 339, 341] have had almost absent ASAS activity in fibroblast and liver, respectively, but nevertheless survived to adulthood. In one patient, kidney ASAS was normal [50]. Decrease in enzyme protein assayed immunologically has been demonstrated in several cases [44, 50, 341].

The genetics of this variant have not been elucidated. A few of the parents have been consanguine. Cases among sibs have occurred. One patient's mother and son both had mild asymptomatic citrullinemia. The occurrence of this unique variant almost exclusively in Japan suggests the possibility of a common ancestor among these patients. Studies of this possibility have apparently not been performed.

Asymptomatic Carriers   Wick et al. [314] reported one patient in whom citrullinemia was detected by routine hospital screening and whose growth and development were normal at age 4 years. Whelan et al. [336] also reported a patient in whom citrullinemia was detected by routine screening. Although hyperammonemia (473 µg/dl) occurred at 1 month of age, the child remained asymptomatic and was developing normally at age 18 months on a restricted protein diet. Plasma citrulline varied from 0.46 to 0.84 mM. Several instances of elevated citrulline levels in asymptomatic relatives of patients have been reported [321, 336, 354].

Diagnosis

The finding of markedly elevated plasma citrulline without elevated argininosuccinic acid is pathognomonic of ASAS deficiency and has not been reported to occur in any other disorder. Mild elevation (fivefold) is seen in saccharopinuria, evidently due to inhibition by saccharopine of ASAS [355], and a smaller increase is seen in renal failure [356] as a result of impaired renal uptake of citrulline. In cerebrospinal fluid, a pronounced elevation of citrulline may occur (up to 0.5 mM) in adults with hepatic coma [357], so that this fluid should not be used for diagnosis for ASAS deficiency.

On paper or thin-layer chromatograms, citrulline can be identified by applying Ehrlich's aldehyde reagent to the ninhydrin-position spot, a bright yellow or peach color appears. Amniotic fluid cells can be used for prenatal diagnosis [317, 322, 333, 358]. In diagnosing the disorder from study of cultured amniotic fluid cells, it should be borne in mind that ASAS activity is very low in epithelioidlike cells as compared with fibroblastlike cells [358a]. The use of two incubation times may help to overcome this difficulty [328].

Pathology

In neonatal citrullinemia, focal areas of hepatocellular necrosis have been described in several cases but have been absent in others. Fatty droplets in the cytoplasm of hepatocytes were noted in several cases [301, 315, 345]. Abnormal patterns of rough endoplasmic reticulum are seen on electron microscopy [315]. In the brain, widespread focal necrosis and edema are seen. The pathology of the late onset form of the disease reported from Japan is summarized above. Pulmonary hemorrhage may occur in citrullinemic infants [314, 359].

Biochemical Investigations

In citrullinemia, as distinct from CPS deficiency or OCT deficiency, the intermediate that accumulates proximal to the metabolic block is excreted in substantial quantities in the urine. Although the death of one neonate at age 7 days without ever developing hyperammonemia [317, 352] suggests that citrullinemia itself may have caused his demise, others have done well for months despite comparable degrees of citrullinemia [217, 323–325]. Thus the bulk of the evidence indicates that citrulline is not toxic.

Citrulline excretion may comprise more than half of the total urinary nitrogen [325]. Thus such patients have been said to be *citrullinotelic* [360]. Urea formation continues but contributes a smaller portion of urinary nitrogen. Furthermore, most if not all of the urea formed in neonatal cases may be derived from ingested arginine by the action of arginase. Thus urea excretion in such patients may not contribute to the removal of waste nitrogen from the body. This was shown indirectly in one neonatal case [325] by the demonstration of a linear relationship with an intercept on the abscissa rather than the ordinate between urea excretion (or plasma urea) and arginine intake (Fig. 20-11). The authors inferred that urea excretion and plasma urea would go to zero if arginine intake were zero. This hypothesis could not be verified because arginine intakes of less than 2 mmol/kg/day were associated with hypoargininemia and hyperammonemia. On the other hand, McMurray et al. [330] found that [^{14}C]ureido-citrulline injections in one patient led to the conversion of 31 percent of the dose to [^{14}C]urea. Thus their patient must have had an incomplete defect.

Because of the continued excretion of substantial amounts of citrulline, such patients must either receive a disproportionately large intake of arginine or must synthesize ornithine by the operation of ornithine aminotransferase in the reverse of the usual direction. They also need arginine for creatine synthesis (following conversion of arginine to guanidinoacetate and ornithine via arginine transamidinase), a requirement which cannot be met by ornithine synthesis. These considera-

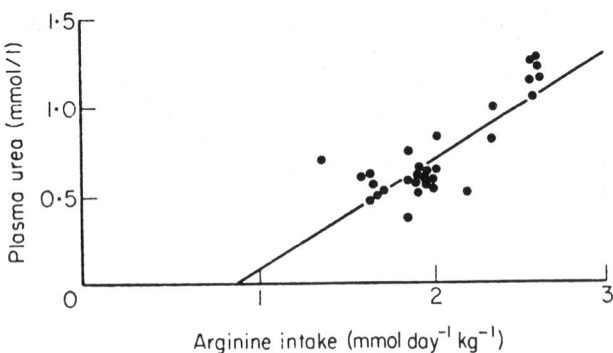

Figure 20-11 Plasma urea as a function of arginine intake in an infant with complete ASAS deficiency. A significant linear relationship is seen ($r = 0.15$, $p < 0.001$) with a negative intercept, suggesting that urea is formed exclusively from ingested arginine through the action of arginase. (*From Walser et al. [325], with permission.*)

tions probably explain the substantial intake of arginine required to prevent hypoargininemia in neonatal cases [314, 317, 321, 324, 325] but not in the subacute or adult onset forms [324]. Ornithine diversion via the OAT reaction was estimated to be 0.64 mmol/kg/day in one neonatal case [325]. Ornithine levels in plasma are usually normal.

Orotic aciduria, as well as increased excretion of uridine and uracil, is seen during hyperammonemic episodes [236]. N-Carbamoyl-β-alanine and N-carbamoylaspartate may also be excreted in abnormal amounts [237].

Hyperammonemia is not present consistently in citrullinemia, and when it occurs, it reflects either arginine deficiency or a rate of amino acid catabolism too great for the residual capacity of citrullinogenesis. Plasma lysine and urinary homocitrulline and homoarginine may be increased, especially after lysine loads, for unknown reasons. N-Acetylcitrulline may appear in the urine [321, 361].

Enzyme Defect

The enzyme defect in citrullinemia may exhibit several different forms, indicating genetic heterogeneity. In neonatal cases ASAS activity may be undetectable, or may be detected only when the citrulline concentration is enormously increased [333]. In addition, the affinity of the enzyme for aspartate may be reduced more than 200 times. The enzyme defect seen in the late onset of citrullinemia is summarized above.

The defect is readily demonstrable in cultured fibroblasts [335]. Enzyme levels in brain or kidney may be less subnormal than in liver, but in one case the reverse was seen [322]. Whether these data indicate differing genetic origins for ASAS in liver as compared with these other tissues is uncertain.

Citrullinemia secondary to ASAS deficiency has been described in dogs [362]. In a Chinese hamster cell line deficient in ASAS, citrulline was shown to be concentrated normally with respect to the medium, even though citrulline failed to support growth in the absence of arginine [363].

Genetics

Citrullinemia as seen outside of Japan is inherited as an autosomal recessive trait. The structural gene for ASAS expression is carried on chromosome 9 [364]. Sex distribution appears to be approximately equal (Table 20-4). Wick et al. [354] dem-

onstrated mild degrees of citrullinemia in both parents and five other family members in one neonatal case. By studies of polyethylene glycol–induced heterokaryons derived from paired combinations of fibroblasts from different citrullinemic patients, Kennaway and Curtis [365] and Cathelineau et al. [329] have demonstrated that interallelic, but not intergenic, complementation may occur.

Treatment

One neonatal patient survived to age 7 months with protein restriction plus arginine [323]. Another patient with neonatal symptoms was doing well on protein restriction plus essential amino acids (including arginine) when reported at age 4 years [319]. Thoene et al. [324] treated a neonatal patient with a mixture of five keto-analogues plus the remaining essential amino acids (including histidine and arginine) at a total dose of 1 g/kg/day from age 26 days until his death caused by type 5 adenovirus encephalitis at age 8 months. Arginine intake was progressively increased to 2 mmol/kg/day. He showed catch-up growth and developmental progress but was slightly retarded. ASAS was undetectable in fibroblasts. A second patient, lacking detectable ASAS activity in the liver, survived on the same regimen to age 7 months [325]. A third patient who also had neonatal symptoms but in whom no enzyme assay was available did well on the same regimen for 1 year and then on essential amino acids for the next year. Sodium benzoate, 1.75 mmol/kg/day, was added from the sixth month on. She is still developing normally except for moderate mental retardation at age 2½ years [217].

A male infant lacking ASAS activity in fibroblasts has been treated with keto-analogues and essential amino acids (including arginine, 3 mmol/kg/day) since age 2 weeks, plus benzoate during hyperammonemic episodes. Physical growth has been poor, but he now is only mildly developmentally retarded at age 16 months [327]. Chronic benzoate therapy has recently been added.

Thus long-term survival is possible in neonatal citrullinemia. Keto acid or essential amino acid supplements, including a substantial dose of arginine, should be given in conjunction with a low protein diet. Sodium benzoate may improve protein tolerance in infants with complete or nearly complete enzyme deficiency. In partial defects, its inhibitory effect on OCT [42] might outweigh its beneficial effect via hippurate excretion. Presumably protein restriction alone, with benzoate reserved for hyperammonemic crises, should suffice in patients with partial defects; arginine supplementation may also be useful.

ARGININOSUCCINATE LYASE DEFICIENCY (ARGININOSUCCINIC ACIDURIA)

ASAL deficiency was first described by Allan et al. in 1958 [366]. It is the second most commonly reported of the urea cycle disorders. Long-term survival without symptoms or treatment occurs in a significant fraction of cases (about 20 percent). Its incidence is reported as 1 in 70,000 live births in the United States but is lower in other countries [199]. It is characterized by the accumulation in body fluids and excretion into the urine of large amounts of argininosuccinic acid.

Clinical Features and Diagnosis

Neonatal Type Nine infants with symptoms in the neonatal period were discussed in the preceding edition [301]; at least 12 more have been reported in the interim [34, 51, 217, 359, 367–372]. About two-thirds of the patients were males. Symptoms begin within the first few days of life and include respiratory distress, feeding difficulties, vomiting, tachypnea, and lethargy. Hypotonia, periorbital edema, seizures, hypothermia, jaundice, hepatomegaly, and hyperchloremia due to metabolic acidosis or respiratory alkalosis may occur. One infant did not develop symptoms until the seventh week [51]. Most of these patients have died in the neonatal period, but three have survived with treatment and one without (see below).

Subacute and Delayed Onset Types Thirty-four patients who exhibited less severe symptoms or no symptoms in the neonatal period were discussed in the preceding edition [301]. A smaller number has been reported in the interim [234, 373–378]. In the subacute form, anorexia, vomiting, convulsions, and hepatomegaly appear in infancy, and mental and physical retardation is pronounced. In the late onset form, similar but less severe symptoms are seen beginning after the neonatal period. The predominant feature of these cases is the appearance of psychomotor retardation in the first or second year of life. The earlier symptoms include irritability and vomiting episodes in infancy. Seizures and EEG abnormalities are frequent, as well as intermittent unsteadiness or ataxia sometimes associated with fever and lethargy. These episodes presumably reflect hyperammonemia provoked by a change in protein intake or a catabolic insult. Serum transaminase levels are usually elevated. Shih [301] described 11 patients detected by neonatal screening who remained clinically well on protein restriction, arginine supplementation, or both. Whether they would have remained well without treatment is unknown.

The diagnosis of ASAL deficiency is based on the finding of enormously increased levels of ASA and its anhydrides in plasma and urine. Normally, these substances are scarcely detectable in these fluids [128, 129]. ASA is usually higher in cerebrospinal fluid than in plasma.

Trichorrhexis nodosa, a hair abnormality characterized grossly by dry, brittle hair and microscopically by nodular protrusions along the hairs (Fig. 20-12), occurs in a substantial fraction of cases. The cause is unknown. Although it was at first thought to represent arginine deficiency, since keratin is high in arginine, the absence of this disturbance in defects of the previous steps in the cycle or in lysinuric protein intolerance, all of which cause arginine deficiency, argues against this interpretation. An initial report that argininosuccinic acid could be found on hydrolysis of hair protein [380] has not been confirmed [381]. In two patients analysis of hair amino acid composition was normal [301]. In another child, the cystine content of the hair was about half normal but increased as the patient grew older; concomitant improvement in the strength of the hair occurred [382]. Improvement has also been noted in other cases.

Prenatal diagnosis can be made by studying the metabolism of labeled citrulline by amniotic fluid cells [373, 383, 384]. Care must be taken to rule out mycoplasma contamination, which may cause erroneous results [385]. It is also important to use fibroblast-type amniotic cells, which have much higher activity than epithelial-type cells [373]. Less well established techniques for prenatal diagnosis include measurement of

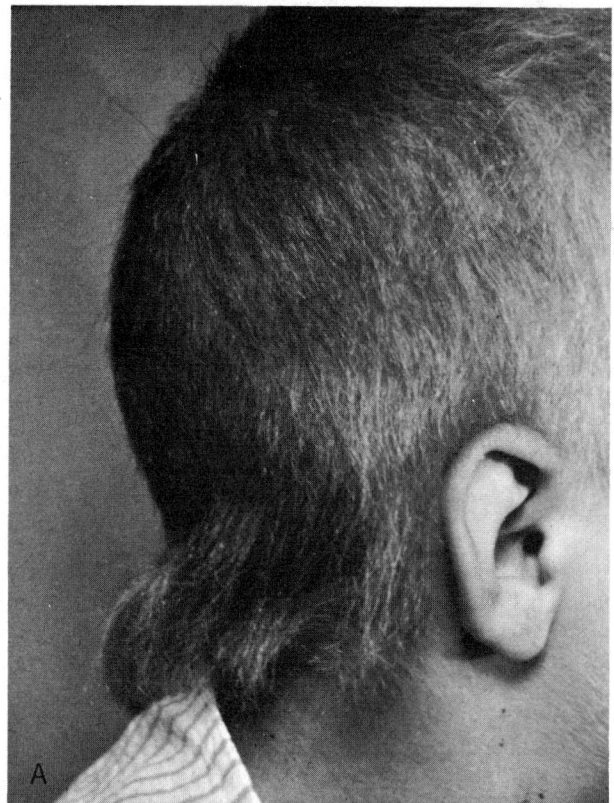

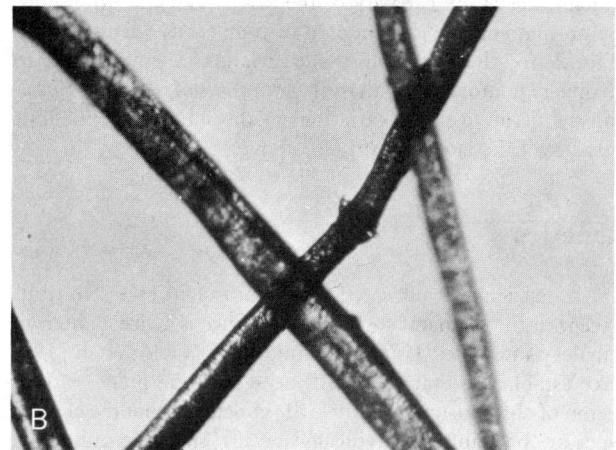

Figure 20-12 *A.* Patient with argininosuccinic aciduria, showing dry, breakable, and short hair *B.* Microscopic appearance of hair from a patient with argininosuccinic aciduria. This illustrates classic trichorrhexis nodosa, a condition in which minute nodes are formed in the hair shafts, causing the hair to split and break incompletely at these points. *(A. From Farrell et al. [379], with permission.)*

maternal argininosucciduria and its augmentation during pregnancy [373, 383, 384, 386] or measurement of ASA in amniotic fluid [358, 383–387].

Pathology

In neonatal cases, the brain usually shows focal necrosis, spongy degeneration, and Alzheimer type II astrocytes. The liver is usually normal but may show fatty deposits. Pulmonary hemorrhages may occur [359].

Biochemical Investigation

As in citrullinemia, the accumulated intermediate, argininosuccinic acid, is excreted in large quantities in the urine, along with some increase in citrulline excretion as well, thus tending to deplete ornithine and arginine stores. Plasma arginine and, to a lesser extent ornithine, are reduced. Because the renal clearance of argininosuccinic acid is approximately equal to the glomerular filtration rate [388, 389], the plasma level of this intermediate does not become as high as citrulline does in citrullinemia. Some increase in plasma citrulline as well as ASA is usually seen in ASAL deficiency and reflects the reversibility of the ASAL reaction. Exercise may aggravate hyperammonemia and provoke symptoms [390], probably because of the substantial release of ammonia from muscle which occurs during exercise [105, 107].

Enzyme Defect

The severity of the enzyme deficiency may vary considerably among tissues. Erythrocytes, brain, and kidney may exhibit normal or reduced activity in spite of severe hepatic deficiency [34, 217, 391]. Cultured fibroblasts may be less deficient in ASAL than is the liver [367] or may be more deficient [392]. The level of argininosuccinic acid is usually higher in cerebrospinal fluid and in the brain than in the blood [51, 301, 366, 369, 374, 393]. This may occur even when brain ASAL activity is normal [51] and perhaps reflects a rate of citrulline uptake which exceeds the capacity of the brain enzyme [301]. Since the normal enzyme is composed of four nearly identical subunits [2, 56], these tissue-to-tissue variations are more likely to involve regulatory genes than structural genes. Another possibility is tissue-to-tissue variations in the subunit proportions noted by Takada et al. [89] (see above).

Genetics

ASAL deficiency is inherited as an autosomal recessive trait. Except in the neonatal form, the incidence is twice as high in females as in males. Using bioautography, Naylor et al. [394] have established that the ASAL gene is in the pter → q22 region of chromosome 7. Shih [301] concluded that the clinical types are probably genotypically specific, since the same type has recurred in each family. In general, parents of affected infants are clinically well but have reduced ASAL activity in erythrocytes or fibroblasts, and may excrete small amounts of ASA, especially after citrulline loads [369].

Treatment

Ever since the earliest cases were diagnosed, the rationale of treatment has varied between restriction of protein or arginine intake, in hopes of reducing the level of the presumed toxic metabolite, argininosuccinic acid and arginine supplementation, with the aim of correcting arginine deficiency. Dent [395] gave arginine by mouth and by vein to an 8-year-old patient with no clinical effect. Westall [396] found that arginine supplementation did not increase argininosuccinic aciduria, but supplements of ornithine or citrulline did.

A neonatal patient treated by protein restriction alone showed normal physical growth and only moderate development mental delay when reported at 8 months of age [371]. Another neonatal patient with 10 percent ASAL activity in fibroblasts was treated by protein restriction alone (1.6 g/kg/day) and was developing normally when reported at 4 months of age [372]. A third neonatal patient was given arginine, 3 mmol/kg/day, from age 3 weeks on; later the dose was doubled [386]. She was normal when reported at age 6 months.

Shih [397] treated a neonatal patient with 1.4 to 1.6 g per day of protein plus 200 to 400 mg per day of arginine hydrochloride; physical and mental development were normal at 2 years. Farriaux et al. [369] treated a neonatal patient lacking ASAL activity with severe protein restriction plus a supplement of nine essential amino acids, arginine, glutamate, cystine, and tyrosine, at a total dose up to 1 g/kg/day. The patient did well for 3 months, then died suddenly following an episode of lethargy culminating in massive hematemesis without hyperammonemia. Brain pathology showed niether Alzheimer type II cells nor demyelination. Nutritional therapy may have prevented these changes [393]. Levin [381] initially treated his neonatal patient, who had zero hepatic ASAL activity, with an amino acid mixture devoid of arginine, on the assumption that ASA was toxic. Argininosuccinic aciduria fell markedly, but clinical deterioration occurred. The addition of about 3 mmol/kg/day arginine eliminated the symptoms and restored argininosuccinic aciduria to its initial level.

Böhles et al. [377] treated a 22-year-old patient with 10 percent of normal erythrocyte ASAL activity with a diet containing only 20 to 25 g protein per day (0.5 g/kg/day) supplemented with 14 g nitrogen-free analogues of amino acids and 2.2 g threonine, tryptophan, lysine, and histidine for 5 months. Arginine was not included. Seizures ceased immediately, plasma ammonia fell to normal concomitant with a return of plasma glutamine, glycine, and alanine to normal levels, and there was an increase in the subnormal levels of branched chain amino acids. Weight gain occurred and serum albumin rose. Argininosuccinic aciduria initially decreased and then rose again as protein intake was liberalized. Since the regimen involved a reduction in arginine intake, *de novo* ornithine synthesis via OAT must have increased to compensate for the loss of ornithine skeletons as argininosuccinic acid in the urine. Clinically significant arginine deficiency evidently did not occur, though plasma arginine values were not reported.

The suggestion to exploit argininosuccinic aciduria as a route of waste nitrogen excretion was made by Brusilow et al. [398]. Brusilow and Batshaw [399] treated two neonatal cases with arginine, 4 to 5 mmol/kg/day. One already had lethal brain damage but improved biochemically before death; a second, with 31 percent ASAL activity [400], was growing and developing normally when first reported at age 2 months [399]; by age 31 months mental retardation was apparent [217]. Plasma arginine and ornithine were maintained at three to four times normal. Another neonatal patient was treated successfully with about one-fourth as much arginine and was growing normally but was mentally retarded when reported at age 18 months [368]. A third neonatal patient received 5 mmol/kg/day and was doing well when reported at 1 month of age [370]. A fourth neonatal patient was doing well on 4 mmol/kg/day arginine plus 250 mg/kg/day sodium benzoate when reported in preliminary form at age 9 months [401]. A delayed onset patient with virtually zero ASAL activity treated by protein restriction (1.2 g/kg/day) and arginine (2 g/day), was only moderately retarded when reported at age $10\frac{1}{2}$ years [378].

These two approaches to treatment are diametrically opposite, but some information is now available to assess their relative merits. Hypoargininemia certainly occurs in neonatal cases, and arginine supplementation may well be life-saving. The long-term effect of such therapy should be to augment argininosuccinic acidemia, which may conceivably impair neurodevelopment. Hence, in older patients, it may be more rational to attempt to reduce argininosuccinic acidemia by protein restriction, by administration of essential amino acids or nitrogen-free analogues thereof, or by giving sodium benzoate.

ARGINASE DEFICIENCY (ARGININEMIA)

Argininemia is the least common of the urea cycle disorders (except for N-acetylglutamate synthetase deficiency), having been identified in only eight kindreds [29, 402–410] totaling 13 patients. Four kindreds including seven patients are of Spanish or Spanish-American origin [207, 405, 406, 408, 409]. Many cases may be unrecognized or may be erroneously diagnosed as cystinuria because of the urinary amino acid pattern.

Clinical Features and Diagnosis

The first probable case, reported by Peralta Serrano in 1965 [409], was a male who developed atypical convulsions on the sixth day of life recurring over 8 to 16 days thereafter. He exhibited hypertonicity, hyperreflexia, severe psychomotor retardation, curious discoloration of the scalp, hepatomegaly, and an abnormal EEG. Arginine was markedly elevated in blood and even more so in the cerebrospinal fluid. Argininuria was noted except during two symptom-free intervals. Although arginase was not assayed, the observation that 2 g arginine administered daily for 5 days at age 20 months induced status epilepticus strongly suggests that the patient did indeed have arginase deficiency.

The clinical picture of argininemia in the other 11 cases reported in detail has been remarkably uniform and unlike that seen in any of the other urea cycle enzymopathies. In early infancy, no symptoms other than irritability and marginally delayed development are seen. Motor difficulties are first noted at ages varying from 2 months to 4 years. The most characteristic feature is a scissoring or "tiptoe" gait, reflecting spasticity of the lower extremities, which usually progresses to spastic diplegia with signs of an upper motor neuron lesion. Irritability, hyperactivity, vomiting, tremors, clumsiness, ataxia, and choreoathetosis progress to seizures, psychosis, and severe mental retardation, sometimes with microcephaly. Drooling and dysphagia may occur. EEG abnormalities and cerebral atrophy are seen. The liver may be enlarged.

Serum transaminase levels are elevated. Moderate hyperammonemia with pronounced orotic aciduria occurs only intermittently. Except during hyperammonemic episodes, the only abnormality of plasma amino acids is the four- to twentyfold increase in arginine concentration. Urinary excretion of arginine, lysine, cystine, citrulline, β-aminoisobutyric acid, and ornithine is increased. Arginine levels in cerebrospinal fluid may be as abnormal as in plasma. Serum urea nitrogen is normal or low; urinary urea excretion may be less than normal. A vitamin K–resistant clotting defect may occur.

The diagnosis can be made by assaying arginase in erythrocytes. It has been reported to be virtually absent in all cases in which it has been measured. White blood cells [406, 411] and stratum corneum [405] also show the enzyme defect. Arginase activity is barely detectable in the liver [405, 406]. In fibroblasts, arginase activity is reportedly normal [412], so that these cells cannot be used for diagnosis.

Heterozygotes can be diagnosed by measuring arginine levels in leukocytes; arginine is as high as in leukocytes of homozygotes [411].

Prenatal diagnosis can be made by measuring enzyme activity in fetal erythrocytes obtained during amniocentesis and amnioscopy. The fetal enzyme appears to be identical to the enzyme in red cells of normal children [413].

Pathology

Severe multifocal hydropic changes may be seen on liver biopsy. The mitochondria appear normal [406]. No autopsied cases appear to have been reported.

Biochemical Investigations

Accumulation of arginine, the substrate proximal to the metabolic block, is the hallmark of the disease. More proximal urea cycle substrates, including argininosuccinic acid and citrulline [405], may also accumulate to some degree and appear in the urine, although this is not always the case [408]. One would expect that ornithine deficiency might be a prominent feature of the disorder, due to the loss of the ornithine skeleton in these three forms in the urine. Ornithine levels in plasma are usually normal [404, 406–408], however, or only moderately reduced [411, 414]. The ratio of erythrocyte arginine to plasma arginine is greater than normal [411]. Following loads of protein [404], arginine [408, 414], or ornithine [415], plasma arginine rises sharply and falls slowly. In contrast to normal subjects, little or no increase in ornithine is seen following arginine or protein loads. Ammonia may rise [407]. While this is explained readily by the absence of arginase, it is difficult to explain why loads of alanine or glycine do not increase plasma arginine [408].

Continued urea excretion in argininemia cannot be attributed to arginase action on dietary arginine, as it can in complete defects of other urea cycle enzymes. More probably, urea formation in argininemia is attributable to the presence of arginase in extrahepatic tissues such as the kidney (see below).

The orotic aciduria is puzzling, especially since it sometimes occurs in the absence of hyperammonemia [407, 415, 416]. Not only orotic acid but also uridine and uracil may be excreted in extremely large amounts [416]. Orotic acid appears in increased amounts following protein [416] or arginine [408] loads, but uracil excretion is more stable [416]. Bachmann and Colombo [234] have suggested that the cause of increased pyrimidine synthesis in argininemia is the stimulatory effect of arginine on ASA synthetase [60] in conjunction with a relative or absolute deficiency of ornithine. CP would thus accumulate and be channeled into pyrimidine synthesis. There is in fact little evidence for ornithine deficiency in this disorder, except in one patient [29]. Furthermore, ornithine loading failed to eliminate the increased pyrimidine excretion in two patients [415].

The urinary excretion of other monosubstituted guanidines is markedly increased, including guanidinoacetic acetic acid, N-α-acetylarginine, γ-guanidinobutyric acid, argininic acid, and α-ketoguanidinovaleric acid [414, 416, 417]. Guanidinosuccinic acid excretion is scarcely increased [414, 418]. Yet this compound, as well as α-guanidinoglutaric acid and glycocyamine, appears in the urine of normal subjects or animals following arginine loads [418–420]. Evidently arginase plays some role in their production.

Enzyme Defect

The deficiency of arginase is demonstrable in liver, erythrocytes, leukocytes, and stratum corneum. In kidney, arginase activity was found greater than normal [421] but failed to react with rabbit antihuman liver arginase. An enzymatically inactive protein that did react with this antibody was present in this kidney biopsy. The authors conclude that there are two arginase genes, one expressed in liver (named *A I*) and two expressed in kidney (*A I* and *A II*). In argininemia, A II is normally expressed, accounting for, a residual urea-synthesizing capacity, but A I is abnormal. These data have not yet been reconciled with multiple forms of arginase identified by various workers [422], such as the three isoenzymes, designated A_1, A_3, and A_4, found by Porembska et al. [423]; A_1 and A_3 were found in the liver of several species, while A_1 and A_4 were found in the kidney. Normal fibroblasts show either pattern or a mixture of both [424], which may explain why they do not exhibit the enzyme defect [412]. Fibroblasts from one argininemic patient exhibited the A_1, A_4 pattern, and a sib exhibited the A_1, A_3, A_4 pattern [412]. In erythrocytes of the heterozygotes of one family, the kinetics of arginase were normal [407]. OCT activity was normal in one of the liver biopsies [405].

Genetics

Argininemia is inherited as an autosomal recessive trait [408] (Fig. 20-13). It has been reported with nearly equal frequency in males and females (eight females, five males). Sibs, parents, and grandparents of affected children usually have subnormal erythrocyte and leukocyte arginase activity but normal [404–406, 408] or slightly increased [407, 411, 425] plasma arginine. Sometimes blood cells of heterozygotes show normal arginase activity, but leukocyte arginine is nevertheless high [411].

Treatment

Protein restriction alone is unsatisfactory [408, 414]. Lysine supplementation has been tried not only to augment argininuria but also in the hope that lysine might compete effectively with arginine for uptake into the brain, thus lowering brain arginine levels and possibly correcting brain lysine deficiency [405, 426]. No improvement was seen.

An attempt at gene replacement by intravenous injection of the Shope papilloma virus was unsuccessful [425], as were attempts to introduce arginase into patients' erythrocytes

[427] or to reduce argininemia by transfusing normal erythrocytes [405].

The first successful therapy was reported by Snyderman et al. [408], who were able to institute dietary therapy shortly after birth in a sib of two previous patients. A mixture of nine essential or semiessential amino acids, excluding arginine but including cystine and tyrosine, was fed at a dose of 2 g/kg as the only source of amino acids for the first 4 months of life. Thereafter small amounts of proteins were allowed (up to 5 g/day). Plasma arginine has remained normal, and physical and neurologic development were normal when reported at age 32 months. In two other patients from the same kindred, treated in the same manner from age 4 years on, plasma arginine fell to a value two to three times normal and the growth rate became normal. An older patient, previously reported [405], has been treated in the same manner for the past year; plasma arginine has fallen to the upper limit of normal [428]. Two older patients were also treated in the same way by Cederbaum and colleagues [415, 429]. Plasma arginine and cerebrospinal fluid arginine remained three to four times normal. Only when five nitrogen-free analogues were substituted for five essential amino acids in the formula in one patient did plasma and the cerebrospinal fluid arginine concentration become normal. Unfortunately, the child could not tolerate this formula.

Qureshi et al. [407, 430] treated their patient with sodium benzoate, 250 mg/kg/day, plus 0.5 g protein per kilogram, and achieved successful biochemical control. Orotic aciduria disappeared. Hippurate comprised 27 percent of urinary nitrogen.

MULTIPLE UREA CYCLE ENZYME DEFECTS

When a single enzyme of the urea cycle is grossly deficient, it is not uncommon to find that the activities of other enzymes further down the metabolic path to urea are also somewhat reduced. This could be explained by enzyme repression resulting from diminished flux through the urea synthetic pathway. The rate of urea formation commonly exceeds the flux through the cycle because of urea production from dietary arginine via arginase. In patients on protein restriction, especially when supplemented with essential amino acids or keto analogues, flux would be expected to be low.

Several patients appear to have had deficiencies of more than one enzyme, including CPS I and OCT in three patients [431, 432]. One of these has only 2.5 percent of normal CPS activity and 5 percent of normal OCT activity but has responded unusually well to treatment with amino acids and a low protein diet. She exhibited normal psychomotor development when reported at age 7 years [432].

An unusual case was reported by Sogawa et al. [433, 434] of an 18-year-old mentally and physically retarded male with 22 percent of normal hepatic ASAS activity and 29 percent of normal hepatic arginase activity. Other urea cycle enzymes as well as lysine NAD oxidoreductase were within normal limits. He exhibited moderate citrullinemia, argininemia, lysinemia, and homocitrullinemia, all aggravated by increasing protein intake. Lysine and citrulline loads were disposed at a subnormal rate. Lysine inhibited residual arginase to an abnormal degree and increased citrullinemia.

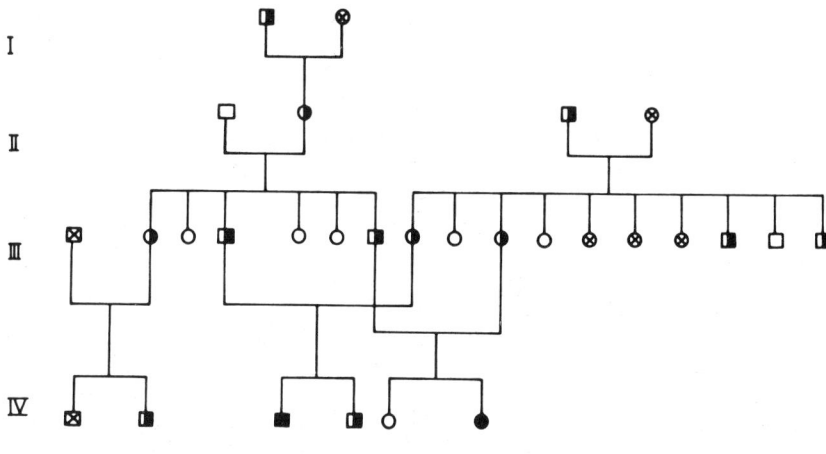

I

II

III

IV

Figure 20-13 Pedigree of a family affected by argininemia. (*From Snyderman et al. [408], with permission.*)

☐ Male Normal
⊠ Male Not Examined
◧ Male, Reduced Activity
■ Male Affected

○ Female Normal
⊗ Female Not Examined
◑ Female, Reduced Activity
● Female Affected

Raijman [431] has pointed out that the probability of double mutations is so low (about 1 in 10^{10}) that a single mutation at another locus, affecting two enzymes, is a more likely explanation of such occurrences. Other possible explanations include acquired defects or an inherited abnormality of mitochondria.

LYSINURIC PROTEIN INTOLERANCE (HYPERDIBASIC AMINOACIDURIA)

In 1965, Perheentupa and Visakorpi [435] described a syndrome of *protein intolerance and defective transport of basic amino acids.* At least 80 cases have now been described, of whom more than half are Finnish. The incidence of the disease is estimated to be 1 in 60,000 to 80,000 live births in Finland [436]. Cases have been identified in Canadians [437], Japanese [438–440], Turks [441], black and white Americans [442, 443], Moroccans [444], Irish [445], Italians [446, 447], Dutch [236], and Swedes [448]. The underlying defect appears to be an impairment in transport of dibasic amino acids in the basolateral membranes of intestinal and renal tubular cells, but many aspects of the disease remain unexplained.

Clinical Features and Diagnosis

In most cases, protein intolerance, manifested by feeding difficulties, vomiting, diarrhea, and poor growth, appears in infancy, usually on ingestion of cow's milk or formula. Aversion to protein-rich foods develops, and episodes of lethargy, convulsions, or coma, associated with hyperammonemia, may occur. Mental retardation is usual. Hepatosplenomegaly, short stature, muscular weakness, osteoporosis, and lens opacities are common. The skin may be hyperelastic and the joints hyperextensible. The hair is often sparse and brittle. Normochromic anemia, neutropenia, and thrombocytopenia are seen in some patients. Blood urea is usually low normal. Hyperammonemia occurs after protein-containing meals; a protein

challenge in one 3-year-old patient produced an episode of coma with an isoelectric EEG from which he nevertheless recovered [443]. Serum levels of transaminases, lactic dehydrogenase, aldolase, and alkaline phosphatase are often elevated. The characteristic plasma amino acid pattern includes subnormal levels of lysine, arginine, ornithine, leucine, and tyrosine. Serine and citrulline are normal or slightly increased, and glutamine and alanine may be considerably increased. Urinary excretion of lysine and to a lesser extent ornithine, arginine, and citrulline is increased. Cystinuria is slight or absent. Orotic aciduria is sometimes seen, along with increased excretion of uracil and uridine. Serum concentrations of ferritin, thyroxine, and thyroid-binding globulin are often increased. Despite ferritinemia, tissue iron is low [449].

The diagnosis is based upon the finding of dibasic aminoaciduria without cystinuria, impaired intestinal absorption of basic amino acids, and protein intolerance.

Pathology

Liver biopsies may be normal on electron microscopy, [450] or may show increased smooth endoplasmic reticulum, vesicles filled with fibrogranular material, and abundant glycogen particles [436]. In older patients fatty infiltration [451, 452] and hepatocytes with pyknotic nuclei may be seen. Jejunal biopsies usually show no abnormalities [436]. In one sibship, bone marrow showed autophagy of erythroblasts by granuloblasts and clusters of degenerated erythroblast nuclei [446].

Biochemical Investigations

In addition to reduced renal tubular reabsorption of dibasic amino acids, patients with this disorder show a markedly attenuated rise in plasma levels of ornithine, arginine, or lysine after oral loads of these substances [435, 441, 442, 450, 453, 454], indicating defective absorption. Protein loads fail to increase plasma concentrations of ornithine, lysine, and arginine as the concentrations of most other amino acids rise [445]. In contrast, intestinal absorption of citrulline is normal

[442, 454]. Study of lysine fluxes in jejunal biopsy specimens indicates a marked reduction in Na-dependent efflux from cells to serosa across the basolateral membranes [444]. Hence, lysine accumulation within cells occurred. These findings clearly differentiate this disorder from cystinuria, in which the transport defect is located at the luminal membrane and Na-dependent lysine accumulation is subnormal (Chap. 80). Not only free dibasic amino acids but also lysylglycine is poorly absorbed [455].

Loading with basic amino acids shows that the renal tubular reabsorptive capacity can be increased to normal values at high plasma concentrations [456]. Citrulline loading leads to citrullinuria, massive argininuria, and moderate ornithinuria, but lysine excretion scarcely changes [457]. The authors suggest that the normal conversion of citrulline to arginine in tubular cells is impeded by high intracellular arginine concentrations as a result of impairment of basolateral efflux, and infused citrulline is largely excreted because conversion to arginine is impeded. Nevertheless, some conversion to arginine (and then ornithine) occurs and accounts for the increase in excretion of these amino acids (Fig. 20-14). Lysinuria remains unaffected by citrulline loads because it is not interconverted to these other amino acids.

Simell [458] has also studied dibasic amino acid transport in leukocytes and in liver slices obtained at laporotomy from affected patients. No abnormalities could be detected in leukocytes, but some impairment of liver uptake of homoarginine, a nonmetabolizable analogue, was demonstrable. This observation provided indirect support for the view that hepatic ornithine deficiency may be present, as originally suggested by Kekomäki [459], and may account for protein intolerance. Ornithine concentration in the liver was increased in one patient [440, 450] despite hypoornithinemia. Lysine and arginine concentrations in the liver were high normal.

Urea cycle enzyme activities are reported to be normal [460]. OAT was low in the one subject in whom it was measured [461]. This may explain the fact that the metabolic clearance rate of intravenously infused arginine or ornithine is subnormal [462], since OAT is the only known enzyme capable of metabolizing ornithine at a substantial rate (Chap. 19).

The impairment of arginine metabolism that lysine infusion induces by inhibiting arginase is no different in this disorder from the impairment seen in normal subjects [462].

Thus the mechanism for the hyperammonemia and protein intolerance in these patients remains uncertain. Probably it is a reflection of arginine or ornithine deficiency at some critical site, but the only site identified where these amino acids are deficient is the plasma. Nevertheless, the addition of ornithine [436, 448, 451, 459] or arginine [441, 448, 450] to an intravenous alanine load prevents the hyperammonemia that occurs following alanine alone.

Some variants have been reported. One patient had normal or increased plasma lysine, despite abnormal intestinal absorption of lysine and increased renal excretion [441]. The authors inferred that a defect in lysine catabolism must have been present. Another patient had normal plasma lysine, arginine, and ornithine [447].

Genetics

Lysinuric protein intolerance is inherited as an autosomal trait. It affects females about twice as often as males. The proportion of affected sibs, corrected by Apert's a priori method, is about 0.26. Consanguine parents are common. The heterozygous trait may be undetectable [463, 464] or may be expressed as a partial impairment in intestinal absorption of dibasic amino acids after oral loads [454]. Thus the pattern is one of a recessive trait.

Whelan and Scriver [437] identified 13 of 33 members of a French-Canadian pedigree who exhibited dibasic aminoaciduria but no decrease in plasma concentrations of dibasic amino acids and no protein intolerance. They also showed impairment in intestinal absorption of lysine after a lysine load. They concluded that the disorder in this family was inherited as an autosomal dominant; no homozygotes were identified.

Treatment

Arginine supplementation with a low protein diet corrects hypoargininemia and hypoornithinemia and improves growth and physical performance as well as protein tolerance [436, 445, 463], but it may cause diarrhea because of defective absorption [436], tends to aggravate hypolysinemia and lysinuria [442], and increase orotic acidura [452]. Citrulline supplementation improves hypolysinemia [442]. A supplement of citrulline plus lysine was most effective in correcting the abnormal amino acid pattern [442]. During long-term use of citrulline, liver histology and catch-up growth occurs, protein intolerance improves, and the hair becomes normal. Hepatosplenomegaly, osteoporosis, and elevated serum enzyme levels

Figure 20-14 Diagrammatic representation of the renal tubular defect in lysinuric protein intolerance (LPI), as proposed by Rajantie et al. [457]. Efflux from the cell of arginine and ornithine is impaired (dotted lines), but luminal uptake is not. Hence cellular concentrations and backflux into the lumen increase, as indicated by enlarged type and arrows. As a result, the normal conversion of a portion of reabsorbed citrulline to arginine is impeded, and citrulline is also accumulated intracellularly and appears in increased quantities in the urine. (*From Rajantie et al. [457], with permission.*)

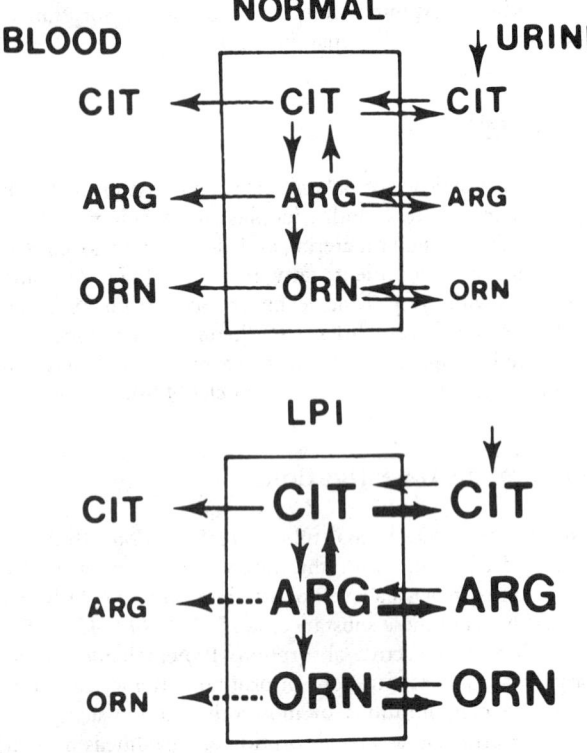

and thyroxine levels persist [452]. Some of these abnormalities may reflect lysine deficiency, but attempts to correct this problem by oral lysine supplementation may induce diarrhea or cramps.

TRANSIENT HYPERAMMONEMIA IN INFANCY NOT CAUSED BY CONGENITAL DEFECTS OF THE UREA CYCLE

The differential diagnosis of *congenital hyperammonemia* includes urea cycle disorders and lysinuric protein intolerance, as well as other inherited metabolic defects, including organic acidemia (Chaps. 22, 23), hyperlysinemia (Chap. 21), and nonketotic hyperglycinemia (Chap. 27). In addition, hyperammonemia in infancy may be caused by Reye's syndrome, by portal-systemic shunting, or by excessive dosage of salicylates [465]. There remains a group of patients who exhibit hyperammonemia of a reversible form, not explained by any of the above disorders. No clear-cut clinical entity has been delineated, but several factors have been identified that may contribute to transient hyperammonemia in infants.

First, delayed development of the urea cycle enzymes could account for protein intolerance in the neonatal period, especially in preterm infants. Several authors [466–468] have described the development of the urea cycle enzymes during fetal and neonatal life. CPS, OCT, ASAS, ASAL, and arginase are all present in fetuses as early as 12 weeks of age and increase progressively in specific activity during gestation and early infancy.

In rats, normal birth or cesarean section on day 21.5 causes a sharp increase within a few hours in CPS and OCT activities. Premature delivery (1 day early) provokes similar increases. The increase was not prevented by actinomycin D but was abolished by administering glucose every 2 h after birth [469, 470]. This observation suggests that parenteral glucose infusions in neonates might retard the normal development of these enzymes. Cathelineau et al. [471] have recently measured AGA synthetase activity in developing rat liver and have shown that, in contrast to the other urea cycle enzymes, this enzyme is very low until birth occurs.

Oyanagi et al. [468] observed no unusual depression of urea cycle enzymes in premature infants, with the exception of ASAS. Activity of this enzyme in premature infant liver was one-fourth that in full-term infants and lower than in any fetuses examined.

Clinically, transient hyperammonemia in infancy is seen in association with prematurity, respiratory distress, and parenteral nutrition, all three of which tend to occur together. In premature infants it is often asymptomatic. According to Batshaw [472], 89 percent of infants with birth weights of 2500 g or less, but only 4 percent of infants with birth weights over 2500 g have asymptomatic hyperammonemia. Orotic aciduria and subnormal plasma α-ketoglutarate levels were also observed in the low birth weight infants, but no differences were noted in plasma glutamine, alanine, or glutamate concentrations between the two groups.

A severe form of neonatal hyperammonemia was described by Ballard et al. [37] in five preterm infants. All had mild respiratory distress and lethargy within a few hours of birth that progressed within 48 h to deep coma requiring ventilatory assistance. Plasma ammonia was markedly elevated. Orotic aciduria was absent in the two cases in which it was looked for. Plasma amino acid analysis in two patients showed increased glutamine in one, increased alanine in another, and slightly elevated citrulline in both. Urinary amino acids were unremarkable. Urea cycle enzymes were normal when assayed at age 2 months in two patients and at post mortem in a third who died in hyperammonemic coma; ASA synthetase was not measured.

Goldberg et al. [473] described 12 infants, including two premature and five postmature, who had severe perinatal hyperammonemia associated with asphyxia. Five of seven survivors had severe neurologic dysfunction. Urea cycle enzymes were not assayed, nor was orotic acid. The authors suggest that the hyperammonemia was caused by the catabolic effect of asphyxia plus hypoxic liver dysfunction.

Pollack et al. [474] described three infants (one preterm) who had severe hyperammonemia, seizures, and apnea but recovered and showed no evidence of urea cycle deficiency. Evidence has been presented that hypercapnia induces hyperammonemia in dogs by opening portal-systemic shunts [475]. The same mechanism could explain hyperammonemia in association with asphyxia in neonates.

Donn et al. [476] described a 2.5-kg infant delivered at 35 weeks' gestation who went into hyperammonemic coma by 24 h of age. Plasma citrulline was moderately elevated (109 μM), as was urine orotic acid (46 μg/mg creatinine). Despite arginine infusion sufficient to raise plasma arginine and ornithine above 2 mM, hyperammonemia persisted during exchange transfusions. Three hours of hemodialysis brought blood ammonia from 2184 to 275 μg/dl, and the infant recovered completely. In a patient with a similar presentation who died, analysis of the urea cycle enzymes in the liver revealed 12.5 percent of control ASAS activity [477, 478]. The authors suggest that developmental delay of ASAS was the cause. Two other preterm infants with hyperammonemic coma and apnea who recovered completely have been reported [479, 480].

The possibility that developmental delay in AGA synthetase is responsible for this syndrome appears to have been excluded by the recent report that levels of this enzyme were normal during transient hyperammonemia in three premature infants [42].

While the effect of parenteral infusions of amino acid solutions on blood ammonia in neonates is well known [481], the fact that salt-poor albumin, platelet preparations, and other blood products may contain significant quantities of ammonium is not well recognized. According to Sanchez et al. [482], these exogenous sources of ammonia can cause hyperammonemia in low birth weight infants.

The general problem of the differential diagnosis of asphyxia versus heritable metabolic disease has been reviewed recently by Nyhan [483].

Supported by a grant from the National Institutes of Health (AM 18020). I am greatly indebted to Jean Stallings and Tessie Ferkany for bibliographic assistance, to Yoko Ohashi for translating Japanese articles, and to Drs. L. E. Rosenberg and C. Bachmann for reviewing the manuscript. I would also like to thank the many workers who sent me preprints of their forthcoming papers.

REFERENCES

1. BRADFORD NM, McGIVAN JD: Evidence for the existence of an ornithine/citrulline antiporter in rat liver mitochondria. *FEBS Lett* 113:294, 1980

1a. GAMBLE JG, LEHNINGER AL: Transport of ornithine and citrulline across the mitochondrial membrane. *J Biol Chem* 248:610, 1973

2. RATNER S: Enzymes of arginine and urea synthesis. *Adv Enzymol* 39:3, 1973

3. RATNER S: Enzymes of arginine and urea synthesis, in Grisolia S, Báguena R, Mayor F (eds): *The Urea Cycle*. New York, John Wiley & Sons, Inc, 1976, p 181

4. HALL LM, JOHNSON RC, COHEN PP: The presence of carbamyl phosphate synthetase in intestinal mucosa. *Biochim Biophys Acta* 37:144, 1960

5. JONES ME, ANDERSON AD, ANDERSON C, HODES S: Citrulline synthesis in rat tissues. *Arch Biochem Biophys* 95:499, 1961

6. RAIJMAN L: Citrulline synthesis in rat tissues and liver content of carbamoyl phosphate and ornithine. *Biochem J* 138:225, 1974

7. WINDMUELLER HG, SPAETH AE: Uptake and metabolism of plasma glutamine in the small intestine. *J Biol Chem* 249:5070, 1974

8. WINDMUELLER HG, SPAETH AE: Respiratory fuels and nitrogen metabolism *in vivo* in small intestine of fed rats: Quantitative importance of glutamine, glutamate, and aspartate. *J Biol Chem* 255:107, 1980

9. WEBER FL, MADDREY WC, WALSER M: Amino acid metabolism of dog jejunum before and during absorption of ketoanalogues. *Am J Physiol* 232:E263, 1977

10. ROSS G, DUNN D, JONES ME: Ornithine synthesis from glutamate in rat intestinal mucosa homogenates: Evidence for the reduction of glutamate to gamma-glutamyl semialdehyde. *Biochem Biophys Res Commun* 85:140, 1978

11. HENSLEE JG, JONES ME: Ornithine synthesis from glutamate in mitochondria from rat small intestinal mucosa. *Fed Proc* 40:1683, 1981

12. WAKABAYASHI Y: Pyrroline-5-carboxylate synthesis in intestinal mucosa mitochondria. *Fed Proc* 40:1683, 1981

13. TIZIANELLO A, DE FERRARI G, GARIBOTTO G, GURRERI G, ROBAUDO C: Renal metabolism of amino acids and ammonia in subjects with normal renal function and in patients with chronic renal insufficiency. *J Clin Invest* 65:1162, 1980

14. BORSOOK H, DUBNOFF JW: The conversion of citrulline to arginine in kidney. *J Biol Chem* 141:717, 1941

15. RATNER S, PETRACK B: The mechanism of arginine synthesis from citrulline in kidney. *J Biol Chem* 200:175, 1953

16. FEATHERSTON WR, ROGERS QR, FREEDLAND RA: Relative importance of kidney and liver in synthesis of arginine by the rat. *Am J Phys* 224:127, 1973

17. KAYSEN GA, STRECKER HJ: Purification and properties of arginase of rat kidney. *Biochem J* 133:779, 1973

18. HERZFELD A, RAPER SM: The heterogeneity of arginases in rat tissues. *Biochem J* 153:469, 1976

19. SADASIVUDU B, RAO TI: Studies on functional and metabolic role of urea cycle intermediates in brain. *J Neurochem* 27:785, 1976

20. SPORN MB, DINGMAN W, DEFALCO A, DAVIES RK: The synthesis of urea in the living rat brain. *J Neurochem* 5:62, 1959

21. STEWART JA, CARON H: Arginases of mouse brain and liver. *J Neurochem* 29:657, 1977

22. SATO Y, ERIKSSON S, HAGENFELDT L, WAHREN J: Influence of branched chain amino acid infusion on arterial concentrations and brain exchange of amino acids in patients with hepatic cirrhosis. *Clin Physiol* 1:151, 1981

23. DE FERRARI G, GHIGGERI GM, GARIBOTTO G, ROBAUDO C, LUTMAN M: Brain metabolism of amino acids and ammonia in patients with chronic renal insufficiency. *Kidney Int* 20:505, 1981

24. STEWART JA: Metabolite alterations in the genetically spastic mouse. *J Neurochem* 36:780, 1981

25. BUNIATIAN HC, DAVTIAN MA: Urea synthesis in brain. *J Neurochem* 13:743, 1966

26. PAUSCH J, GEROK W: Studies on carbamoyl phosphate metabolism in hyperammonemia. *Verh Dtsch Ges Inn Med* 85:655, 1979

27. CRIST RD, PARELLADA PP: Carbamyl phosphate—cyanate and CNS toxicity, in Grisolia S, Báguena R, Mayor F (eds): *The Urea Cycle*. New York, John Wiley & Sons, Inc, 1976, p 491

28. TOMLINSON S, WESTALL RG: Argininosuccinic aciduria, argininosuccinase and arginase in human blood cells. *Clin Sci* 26:261, 1964

29. COLOMBO JP, BACHMANN C, TERHEGGEN HG, LAVINHA F, LOWENTHAL A: Argininemia, in Grisolia S, Báguena R, Mayor S (eds): *The Urea Cycle*. New York, John Wiley & Sons, Inc, 1976, p 415

30. SHIH VE, JONES TC, LEVY HL, MADIGAN PM: Arginase deficiency in *Macaca fascicularis*. I. Arginase activity and arginine concentration in erythrocytes and in liver. *Pediatr Res* 6:548, 1972

31. PISARENKO SI, MINKOVSKII EB, STUDNEVA IM: Urea synthesis in heart muscle. *Bull Exp Biol Med* 89:138, 1980

32. NUZUM CT, SNODGRASS PJ: Urea cycle enzyme adaptation to dietary protein in primates. *Science* 172:1042, 1971

33. NUZUM CT, SNODGRASS PJ: Multiple assays of the five urea-cycle enzymes in human liver homogenates, in Grisolia S, Báguena R, Mayor F (eds): *The Urea Cycle*. New York, John Wiley & Sons, Inc, 1976, p 325

34. GLICK NR, SNODGRASS PJ, SCHAFER IA: Neonatal argininosuccinic aciduria with normal brain and kidney but absent liver argininosuccinate lyase activity. *Am J Hum Genet* 28:22, 1976

35. MATSUDA Y, TSUJI A, KATUNUMA N, HAYASHI M, TAKAHASHI Y: Studies on liver argininosuccinate synthetase in a patient with citrullinemia and in normal subjects. *J Biochem (Tokyo)* 85:191, 1979

36. SHORT EM, CONN HO, SNODGRASS PJ, CAMPBELL AGM, ROSENBERG LE: Evidence for X-linked dominant inheritance of ornithine transcarbamylase deficiency. *N Engl J Med* 288:7, 1973

37. BALLARD RA, VINOCUR B, REYNOLDS JW, WENNBERG RP, MERRITT A, SWEETMAN L, NYHAN WL: Transient hyperammonemia of the preterm infant. *N Engl J Med* 299:920, 1978

38. MAIER K-P, VOLK B, HOPPE-SEYLER G, GEROK W: Urea-cycle enzymes in normal liver and in patients with alcoholic hepatitis. *Eur J Clin Invest* 4:193, 1974

39. HAAG G, HOLLDORF AW, GEROK W: Veränderungen der argininosuccinat-synthetaseaktivität in der Leber bei chronischen Lebererkrankungen. *Klin Wschr* 50:887, 1972

40. FARRIAUX JP, PONTE CL, POLLITT RJ, LEQUIEN P, FORMSTECHER P, DHONDT JL: Carbamyl phosphate synthetase deficiency with neonatal onset of symptoms, *Acta Paediatr Scand* 66:529, 1977

41. KHATRA RS, SMITH RB III, MILLIKAN WJ, SEWALL CW, RUDMAN D: Activities of Krebs-Henseleit enzymes in normal and cirrhotic liver. *J Lab Clin Med* 84:708, 1974

42. BACHMANN C, KRÄHENBÜHL S, COLOMBO JP, SCHUBIGER G, JAGGI KH, TÖNZ O: N-Acetylglutamate synthetase deficiency: A disorder of ammonia detoxification. *N Engl J Med* 304:543, 1981

42a. COUDÉ FX, GRIMBER G, PARVY P, KAMOUN P: N-acetyl glutamate synthetase in human liver: Regulation of activity by L-arginine and N-acetylglutamate. *Biochem Biophys Res Comm* 102:1016, 1981

43. CATHELINEAU L, BRIAND P, PETIT F, NUYTS J-P, FARRIAUX J-P, KAMOUN PP: Kinetic analysis of a new human ornithine carbamoyltransferase variant. *Biochim Biophys Acta* 614:40, 1980

44. YAMAUCHI M, KITAHARA T, FUJISAWA K, KAMEDA H, TAKASAKI S, KOMORI R, SAHEKI T, KATSUNUMA T, KATURUMA N: An autopsied case of hypercitrullinemia in an adult caused by partial deficiency of liver argininosuccinate synthetase. *Acta Hepatol Jap* 21:326, 1980

45. McREYNOLDS JW, CROWLEY B, MAHONEY MJ, ROSENBERG LE: Autosomal recessive inheritance of human mitochondrial carbamyl phosphate synthetase deficiency. *Am J Hum Genet* 33:345, 1981

46. GLASGOW AM, KRAEGEL JH, SCHULMAN JD: Studies of the cause and treatment of hyperammonemia in females with ornithine transcarbamylase deficiency. *Pediatrics* 62:30, 1978

47. MORI M, UCHIYAMA C, MIURA S, TATIBANA M, NAGAYAMA E: Ornithine carbamoyltransferase deficiency: Coexistence of active and inactive forms of enzyme. *Clin Chim Acta* 104:291, 1980

48. SHAPIRO JM, SCHAFFNER F, TALLAN HH, GAULL GE: Mitochondrial abnormalities of liver in primary ornithine transcarbamylase deficiency. *Pediatr Res* 14:735, 1980

49. VAN DER HEIDEN C, BAKKER HD, DESPLANQUE J, BRINK M, DE BREE PK, WADMAN SK: Attempted dietary treatment of a boy with hyperammonemia due to ornithine transferase deficiency. *Eur J Pediatr* 128:261, 1978

50. SAHEKI T, TSUDA M, TAKADA S, KUSUMI K, KATSUNUMA T: Role of argininosuccinate synthetase in the regulation of urea synthesis in the rat and argininosuccinate synthetase-associated metabolic disorder in man. *Adv Enzymol* 18:221, 1980

51. PERRY TL, WIRTZ MLK, KENNAWAY NG, HSIA YE, ATIENZA FC, UEMURA HS: Amino acid and enzyme studies of brain and other tissues in an infant with argininosuccinic aciduria. *Clin Chim Acta* 105:257, 1980

52. PIERSON DL, BRIEN JM: Human carbamylphosphate synthetase I: Stabilization, purification, and partial characterization of the enzyme from human liver. *J Biol Chem* 255:7891, 1980

53. RUBIO V, RAMPONI G, GRISOLIA S: Carbamoyl phosphate synthetase I of human liver: Purification, some properties and immunological cross-reactivity with the rat liver enzyme. *Biochim Biophys Acta* 659:150, 1981

54. PIERSON DL, COX SL, GILBERT BE: Human ornithine transcarbamylase. Purification and characterization of the enzyme from normal liver and the liver of a Reye's syndrome patient. *J Biol Chem* 252:6464, 1977

55. KALOUSEK F, FRANCOIS B, ROSENBERG LE: Isolation and characterization of ornithine transcarbamylase from normal human liver. *J Biol Chem* 253:3939, 1978

56. O'BRIEN WE, BARR RH: Argininosuccinate lyase: Purification and characterization from human liver. *Biochemistry* 20:2056, 1981

57. BERÜTER J, COLOMBO JP, BACHMANN C: Purification and properties of arginase from human liver and erythrocytes. *Biochem J* 175:449, 1978

58. MEIJER AJ, HENSGENS HESJ: Ureogenesis, in Sies H (ed): *Metabolic Compartmentation*. New York, Academic Press, Inc, in press

59. STEWART PM, WALSER M: Short term regulation of ureagenesis. *J Biol Chem* 255:5270, 1980

60. TATIBANA M, SHIGESADA K: Regulation of urea biosynthesis by the acetylglutamate-arginine system, in Grisolia S, Báguena R, Mayor F (eds): *The Urea Cycle.* New York, John Wiley & Sons, Inc, 1976, p 301

61. COUDE FX, SWEETMAN L, NYHAN WL: Inhibition by propionyl-coenzyme A of N-acetylglutamate synthetase in rat liver mitochondria: A possible explanation for hyperammonemia in propionic and methylmalonic acidemia. *J Clin Invest* 64:1544, 1979

62. STEWART PM, WALSER M: Failure of the normal ureagenic response to amino acids in organic acid-loaded rats: Proposed mechanism for the hyperammonemia of propionic and methylmalonic acidemia. *J Clin Invest* 66:484, 1980

63. AOYAGI K, MORI M, TATIBANA M: Inhibition of urea synthesis by pent-4-enoate associated with decrease in N-acetylglutamate concentration in isolated rat hepatocytes. *Biochim Biophys Acta* 587:515, 1979

64. GRUSKAY J, ROSENBERG LE: Inhibition of hepatic mitochondrial carbamyl phosphate synthetase by acyl CoA esters: Possible mechanism of hyperammonemia in the organic acidemias. *Pediatr Res* 13:475, 1978

64a. BACHMANN C, COLOMBO JP: Computer simulation of the urea cycle: Trials for an appropriate model. *Enzyme* 26:259, 1981

64b. BRITTON HG, RUBIO V, GRISOLIA S: Mechanism of carbamoyl-phosphate synthetase: Properties of the two binding sites for ATP. *Eur J Biochem* 102:521, 1979

65. MARSHALL M, METZENBERG RL, COHEN PP: Physical and kinetic properties of carbamyl phosphate synthetase from frog liver. *J Biol Chem* 236:2229, 1961

66. FAHIEN L, SCHOOLER JM, GEHRED GA, COHEN PP: Studies on the mechanism of action of acetylglutamate as an activator of carbamyl phosphate synthetase. *J Biol Chem* 239:1935, 1964

67. GUTHÖHRLEIN G, KNAPPE J: Structure and function of carbamoyl phosphate synthetase. I. Transitions between two catalytically inactive forms. *Eur J Biochem* 7:119, 1968

68. CHABAS A, GRISOLIA S, SILVERSTEIN R: On the mechanism of carbamoylphosphate synthetase. *Eur J Biochem* 29:333, 1972

69. LUSTY CJ: Catalytically active monomer and dimer forms of rat liver carbamyl phosphate synthetase. *Biochemistry* 20:3665, 1981

70. COHEN NS, RAIJMAN L: The apparent K_m of ATPMg for carbamyl phosphate synthetase (ammonia) *in situ*. *J Biol Chem* 255:3352, 1980

70a. POWERS SG: Regulation of rat liver carbamyl phosphate synthetase I. Inhibition by metal ions and activation by amino acids and other chelating agents. *J Biol Chem* 256:11160, 1981

71. LUSTY CJ: Carbamoylphosphate synthetase I of rat-liver mitochondria. *Eur J Biochem* 85:373, 1978

72. SHORE GC, CARIGNAN P, RAYMOND Y: *In vitro* synthesis of a putative precursor to the mitochondrial enzyme carbamyl phosphate synthetase EC-2.7.2.5. *J Biol Chem* 254:3141, 1979

73. RAYMOND Y, SHORE GC: The precursor for carbamyl phosphate synthetase is transported to mitochondria via a cytosolic route. *J Biol Chem* 254:9335, 1979

74. CLARKE S: A major polypeptide component of rat liver mitochondria: Carbamyl phosphate synthetase. *J Biol Chem* 251:950, 1976

75. RAIJMAN L, JONES ME: Purification, composition, and some properties of rat liver carbamyl phosphate synthetase. *Arch Biochem Biophys* 175:270, 1976

76. CHARLES R, DE GRAAF A, MOORMAN AFM: Radioimmunochemical determination of carbamoyl phosphate synthetase (ammonia) content of adult rat liver. *Biochim Biophys Acta* 629:36, 1980

77. ELLIOTT KRF: Kinetic studies on mammalian liver carbamyl phosphate synthetase, in Grisolia S, Báguena R, Mayor F (eds): *The Urea Cycle.* New York, John Wiley & Sons, Inc, 1976, p 123

78. MEIJER AJ: Regulation of carbamoyl phosphate synthetase (ammonia) in liver in relation to urea cycle activity. *Trends Biochem Sci* 4:83, 1979

79. MEIJER AJ, VAN WOERKOM GM, STEINMAN R, WILLIAMSON JR: Inhibition by Ca^{2+} of carbamoylphosphate synthetase (ammonia). *J Biol Chem* 256:3443, 1981

80. MARSHALL M, COHEN PP: Ornithine transcarbamylase from *Streptococcus faecalis* and bovine liver: II. Multiple binding sites for carbamyl-P and L-norvaline, correlation with steady state kinetics. *J Biol Chem* 247:1654, 1972

81. LUSTY CJ, JILKA RL, NIETSCH EH: Ornithine transcarbamylase of rat liver: Kinetic, physical, and chemical properties. *J Biol Chem* 254:10030, 1979

81a. JOSEPH RL, BALDWIN E, WATTS DC: Studies on carbamoyl phosphate-L-ornithine carbamoyltransferase from ox liver. *Biochem J* 87:409, 1963

82. CLARKE S: The polypeptides of rat liver mitochondria: Identification of a 36,000 dalton polypeptide as the subunit of ornithine transcarbamylase. *Biochem Biophys Res Commun* 71:1118, 1976

83. MARSHALL M, COHEN PP: Ornithine transcarbamylase from *Streptococcus faecalis* and bovine liver: I. Isolation and subunit structure. *J Biol Chem* 247:1641, 1972

84. CONBOY JG, KALOUSEK F, ROSENBERG LE: *In vitro* synthesis of a putative precursor of mitochondrial ornithine transcarbamylase. *Proc Natl Acad Sci USA* 76:5724, 1979

84a. MORI M, MORITA T, IKEDA F, AMAYA Y, TATIBANA M, COHEN PP: Synthesis, intracellular transport, and processing of the precursors for mitochondrial ornithine transcarbamylase and carbamoylphosphate synthetase I in isolated hepatocytes. *Proc Natl Acad Sci USA* 78:6056, 1981

85. MARSHALL M: Ornithine transcarbamylase from bovine liver, in Grisolia S, Báguena R, Mayor F (eds): *The Urea Cycle.* New York, John Wiley & Sons, Inc, 1976, p 169

86. NORDLIE RC, LARDY HA: Subcellular distribution of rat-liver inorganic pyrophosphatase activity. *Biochim Biophys Acta* 50:189, 1961

87. ROCHOVANSKY O, RATNER S: Biosynthesis of urea: Further studies on argininosuccinate synthetase: Substrate affinity and mechanism of action. *J Biol Chem* 242:3839, 1967

88. ROCHOVANSKY O, KODOWAKI H, RATNER S: Biosynthesis of urea: Molecular and regulatory properties of crystalline argininosuccinate synthetase. *J Biol Chem* 252:5287, 1977

89. TAKADA S, KUSUMI T, SAHEKI T, TSUDA M, KATSUNUMA T: Studies of rat liver argininosuccinate synthetase. The presence of three forms, and their physicochemical, catalytic and immunochemical properties. *J Biochem (Tokyo)* 86:1353, 1979

90. TAKADA S, SAHEKI T, IGARASHI Y, KATSUNUMA T: Studies on rat liver argininosuccinate synthetase. Inhibition by various amino acids. *J Biochem (Tokyo)* 85:1309, 1979

91. HENSGENS HESJ, MEIJER AJ: Inhibition of urea cycle activity by high concentrations of alanine. *Biochem J* 186:1, 1980

92. AMEEN M, PHILIP MA, PALMER T: Inhibition of urea cycle metabolism by lysine metabolites, and of lysine metabolism by urea cycle metabolites. *IRCS Med Sci: Biochem* 7:428, 1979

93. KIMBALL ME, JACOBY LB: Purification and properties of argininosuccinate synthetase from normal and canavanine-resistant human lymphoplasts. *Biochemistry* 19:705, 1980

94. CHEUNG C-W, RAIJMAN L: Arginine, mitochondrial arginase, and the control of carbamyl phosphate synthesis. *Arch Biochem Biophys* 209:643, 1981

95. CARVAJAL N, VENEGAS A, OESTREICHER G, PLAZA M: Effect of manganese on the quaternary structure of human liver arginase. *Biochim Biophys Acta* 250:437, 1971

96. SAHEKI T, SATO Y, TAKADA S, KATSUNUMA T: Regulation of urea synthesis in rat liver: Inhibition of urea synthesis by L-norvaline. *J Biochem* 86:745, 1979

97. PAIK WK, NOCHUMSON S, KIM S: Effect of modification of inhibitory amino acids on arginase activity. *Biochem Med* 19:39, 1978

98. COHEN NS, CHEUNG CW, RAIJMAN L: The effects of ornithine on mitochondrial carbamyl phosphate synthesis. *J Biol Chem* 255:10248, 1980

99. ZUURENDONK PF, TISCHLER ME, AKERBOOM TPM, VAN DER MEER R, WILLIAMSON JR, TAGER JM: Rapid separation of particulate and soluble fractions from isolated cell preparations (digitonin and cell cavitation procedures), in Fleischer S, Packer L (eds): *Methods in Enzymology.* New York, Academic Press, Inc, 1979, vol 55, p 207

100. ZUURENDONK PF, REISS PD, VEECH RL: Distribution of metabolites in ultra-fast frozen hepatocytes. *Fed Proc* 40:1620, 1981

101. BROSNAN JT: Factors affecting intracellular ammonia concentration in liver, in Grisolia A, Báguena R, Mayor F (eds): *The Urea Cycle.* New York, John Wiley & Sons, Inc, 1976, p 443

102. SAINSBURY, GM: The distribution of ammonia between hepatocytes and extracellular fluid. *Biochim Biophys Acta* 631:305, 1980

103. WANDERS RJA, HOEK JB, TAGER JM: Origin of the ammonia found in protein-free extracts of rat liver mitochondria and rat hepatocytes. *Eur J Biochem* 110:197, 1980

104. ONSTAD GR, ZIEVE L: What determines blood ammonia? *Gastroenterology* 77:803, 1979

105. DAWSON AM: Regulation of blood ammonia. *Gut* 19:504, 1978

106. VISEK WJ: Ammonia metabolism, urea cycle capacity and their biochemical assessment. *Nutr Rev* 37:273, 1979

107. LOWENSTEIN JM: Ammonia production in muscle and other tissues: The purine nucleotide cycle. *Physiol Rev* 52:382, 1972

108. OWEN EE, TYOR MP, FLANAGAN JF, BERRY JN: The kidney as a source of blood ammonia in patients with liver disease: The effect of acetazolamide. *J Clin Invest* 39:288, 1960

109. LOCKWOOD AH, MCDONALD JM, REIMAN RE, GELBARD AS, LAUGHLIN JS, DUFFY TE, PLUM F: The dynamics of ammonia metabolism in man: Effects of liver disease and hyperammonemia. *J Clin Invest* 63:449, 1979

110. KREBS HA, HEMS R, LUND P: Some regulatory mechanisms in the synthesis of urea in the mammalian liver. *Adv Enzyme Regul* 11:361, 1973

111. MCGIVAN JD, BRADFORD NH, MENDES-MOURÃO J: The regulation of carbamoyl phosphate synthase activity in rat liver mitochondria. *Biochem J* 154:415, 1976

112. REGLERO A, RIVAS J, MENDELSON J, WALLACE R, GRISOLIA S: Deacylation and transacetylation of acetyl glutamate and acetyl ornithine in rat liver. *FEBS Lett* 81:13, 1977

113. MEIJER AJ, VAN WOERKOM GM: Control of the rate of citrulline synthesis by short-term changes in N-acetylglutamate levels in isolated rat liver mitochondria. *FEBS Lett* 86:117, 1978

114. SHIGESADA K, AOYAGI K, TATIBANA M: Role of acetylglutamate in ureotelism. *Eur J Biochem* 85:383, 1976

115. MEIJER AJ, VAN WOERKOM GM: Transport of N-acetylglutamate across the liver mitochondrial membrane, in Quagliariello E, et al (eds): *Function and Molecular Aspects of Biomembrane Transport*. Amsterdam, Elsevier/North-Holland Biomedical Press, 1979, p 365

116. KESNER L: The effect of ammonia administration on orotic acid excretion in rats. *J Biol Chem* 240:1722, 1965

117. HENSGENS HESJ: *Regulation of Urea Cycle Activity in Rat Liver*, Ph.D. Thesis. University of Amsterdam, Rodopi, 1980

118. PAUSCH JG, KEPPLER DOR, GEROK W: Increased de novo pyrimidine nucleotide synthesis in liver induced by ammonium ions in amounts surpassing the urea cycle capacity. *Eur J Biochem* 76:157, 1977

119. NATALE PJ, TREMBLAY GC: Studies on the availability of intramitochondrial carbamoylphosphate for utilization in extramitochondrial reactions in rat liver. *Arch Biochem Biophys* 162:357, 1976

120. TREMBLAY GC, CRANDALL DE, KNOTT CE, ALFANT M: Orotic acid biosynthesis in rat liver: Studies on the source of carbamoylphosphate. *Arch Biochem Biophys* 178:264, 1977

121. HASSAN AS, MILNER JA: Orotic acid biosynthesis in arginine-deficient rats. *Arch Biochem Biophys* 194:24, 1979

122. KUCHEL PW, ROBERTS DV, NICHOL LW: The simulation of the urea cycle: Correlation of effects due to inborn errors in the catalytic properties of the enzymes with clinical-biochemical observations. *Aust J Exp Biol Med Sci* 55:309, 1977

123. RAMPONI G: Carbamylphosphate phosphatase, in Grisolia S, Báguena R, Mayor F (eds): *The Urea Cycle*. New York, John Wiley & Sons, Inc, 1976, p 157

124. REMESY C, DEMIGNE C, AUFRERE J: Inter-organ relationships between glucose, lactate and amino acids in rats fed on high-carbohydrate or high-protein diets. *Biochem J* 170:321, 1978

125. FELIG P, WAHREN J: Amino acid metabolism in exercising man. *J Clin Invest* 50:2703, 1971

126. VOLPE P, SAWAMURA R, STRECKER HJ: Control of ornithine delta-transaminase in rat liver and kidney. *J Biol Chem* 244:719, 1969

127. STUMPF DA, PARKS JK: Urea cycle regulation: I. Coupling of ornithine metabolism to mitochondrial oxidative phosphorylation. *Neurology* 30:178, 1980

128. RATNER S: Determination of argininosuccinate in normal blood serum and liver. *Anal Biochem* 63:141, 1975

129. PALMER T, OBERHOLZER VG, LEVIN B, BURGESS EA: Urinary excretion of argininosuccinic acid. *Clin Chim Acta* 47:443, 1973

130. KENNEDY J: Properties and chemistry of urea and related intermediates, in Grisolia S, Báguena R, Mayor F (eds): *The Urea Cycle*. New York, John Wiley & Sons, Inc, 1976, p 39

131. HORNER WH, SIEGEL I, BRUTON J: The synthesis of arginine from guanidinoacetic acid. *J Biol Chem* 220:861, 1956

132. COCKROFT DW, GAULT MH: Prediction of creatinine clearance from serum creatinine. *Nephron* 16:31, 1975

133. CHEEK DB, HOLT AB, HILL DE, TALBERT JL: Skeletal muscle cell mass and growth: The concept of the deoxyribonucleic acid unit. *Pediatr Res* 5:312, 1971

134. SNYDERMAN SE, BOYER A, HOLT LE Jr: The arginine requirement of the infant. *Am J Dis Child* 97:192, 1959

135. ANON: Evidence for liver damage in subjects fed amino acid diets lacking arginine and histidine. *Nutr Rev* 28:170, 1970

136. MILNER JA, VISEK WJ: Urinary metabolites characteristic of urea-cycle amino acid deficiencies. *Metabolism* 24:643, 1975

137. MORRIS JG, ROGERS QR: Ammonia intoxication in the near-adult cat as a result of dietary deficiency of arginine. *Science* 199:431, 1978

138. STEWART PM, BATSHAW M, VALLE D, WALSER M: Effects of arginine-free meals on ureagenesis in cats. *Am J Physiol* 241:E310, 1981

139. WILLIAMSON DH, LUND P, KREBS HA: The redox state of free nicotinamide-adenine dinucleotide in the cytoplasm and mitochondria of rat liver. *Biochem J* 103:514, 1967

140. WALSER M, BODENLOS LJ: Urea metabolism in man. *J Clin Invest* 38:1617, 1959

141. WALSER M: Determinants of ureagenesis, with particular reference to renal failure. *Kidney Int* 17:709, 1980

142. HAYASE K, YOKOGOSHI H, YOSHIDA A: Effect of dietary proteins and amino acid deficiencies on urinary excretion of nitrogen and the urea synthesizing system in rats. *J Nutr* 110:1327, 1980

143. RAIJMAN L, BARTULIS T: Effect of ATP translocation on citrulline and oxaloacetate synthesis by isolated rat liver mitochondria. *Arch Biochem Biophys* 195:188, 1979

144. WANDERS RJA, VAN WOERKOM GM, NOOTEBOOM RF, MEIJER AJ, TAGER JM: Relationship between the rate of citrulline synthesis and bulk changes in the intramitochondrial ATP/ADP ratio in rat-liver mitochondria. *Eur J Biochem* 113:295, 1981

145. ZOLLNER H, ESTERBAUER H: Regulation of urea synthesis by the ammonia concentration in rat liver. *IRCS Med Sci: Biochem* 8:574, 1980

146. HENSGENS HESJ, VERHOEVEN AJ, MEIJER AJ: The relationship between intramitochondrial N-acetylglutamate and activity of carbamoyl phosphate synthetase (ammonia). *Eur J Biochem* 107:197, 1980

147. SAHEKI T, OHKUBO T, KATSUNUMA T: Regulation of urea synthesis in rat liver. Increase in the concentrations of ornithine and acetylglutamate in rat liver in response to urea synthesis stimulated by the injection of an ammonium salt. *J Biochem (Tokyo)* 84:1423, 1978

148. WALSER M, STEWART PM: Organic acidemia and hyperammonemia. *J Inher Metab Dis* 4:177, 1981

149. RAFOTH RJ, ONSTAD GR: Urea synthesis after oral protein ingestion in man. *J Clin Invest* 56:1170, 1975

150. RUDMAN D, DIFULCO TJ, GALAMBOS JT, SMITH RB, SALAM AA, WARREN WD: Maximal rates of urea synthesis in normal and cirrhotic subjects. *J Clin Invest* 52:2241, 1973

151. RYPINS EB, HENDERSON JM, FULENWIDER JT, MOFFITT S, GALAMBOS JT, WARREN WD, RUDMAN D: A tracer method for measuring rate of urea synthesis in normal and cirrhotic subjects. *Gastroenterology* 78:1419, 1980

152. ROGNSTAD R: Rate-limiting steps in metabolic pathways. *J Biol Chem* 254:1875, 1979

153. SAHEKI T, KATUNUMA N: Analysis of regulatory factors for urea synthesis by isolated perfused rat liver. I. Urea synthesis with ammonia and glutamine as nitrogen sources. *J Biochem (Tokyo)* 77:659, 1975

154. SCHIMKE RT: Differential effects of fasting and protein-free diets on levels of urea cycle enzymes in rat liver. *J Biol Chem* 237:1921, 1962

155. SCHIMKE RT: Adaptive characteristics of urea cycle enzymes in the rat. *J Biol Chem* 237:459, 1962

156. SCHIMKE RT: Studies on factors affecting levels of urea cycle enzymes in rat liver. *J Biol Chem* 238:1012, 1963

157. DAS TK, WATERLOW JC: The rate of adaptation of urea cycle enzymes, aminotransferases and glutamic dehydrogenase to changes in dietary protein intake. *Br J Nutr* 32:353, 1974

158. NICOLETTI M, GUERRI C, GRISOLIA S: Turnover of carbamyl-phosphate synthetase, of other mitochondrial enzymes and of rat tissues: Effect of diet and of thyroidectomy. *Eur J Biochem* 75:583, 1977

159. SAHEKI T, OHBUKO T, KATSUNUMA T: Regulation of urea synthesis in rat liver: Changes of ornithine and acetylglutamate concentrations in livers of rats subjected to dietary transitions. *J Biochem* 82:551, 1977

160. COHEN PP: Regulation of the ornithine-urea cycle enzymes, in Waterlow JC (ed): *Nitrogen Metabolism in Man*. London, Applied Science Publishers, in press

161. MCLEAN P, GURNEY MW: Effect of adrenalectomy and of growth hormone on enzymes concerned with urea synthesis in rat liver. *Biochem J* 87:96, 1963

162. RÄIHÄ NCR: Developmental changes of urea-cycle enzymes in mammalian liver, in Grisolia S, Báguena R, Mayor F (eds): *The Urea Cycle*. New York, John Wiley & Sons, Inc, 1976, p 261

163. EDKINS E, RÄIHÄ NCR: Changes in activities of enzymes of urea synthesis caused by dexamethasone and dibutyryladenosine 3'-5'-cyclic monophosphate in fetal rat-liver maintained in organ-culture. *Biochem J* 160:159, 1976

164. GAUTIER C, VAILLANT R: Effects of administration of hydrocortisone, actinomycin-D, and puromycin on carbamoylphosphate synthetase-I and ornithine carbamoyltransferase activities in fetal rat-liver. *Biol Neonate* 33:289, 1978

165. GEBHARDT R, MECKE D: Permissive effect of dexamethasone on glucagon induction of urea-cycle enzymes in perfused primary monolayer-cultures of rat hepatocytes. *Eur J Biochem* 97:29, 1979

166. LAMERS WH, MOOREN PG: Role of glucocorticosteroid hormones on the levels of rat liver carbamoylphosphate synthase (ammonia) and arginase activity during ontogenesis. *Biol Neonate* 37:113, 1980

167. YAMAZAKI RK, GRAETZ GS: Glucagon stimulation of citrulline formation in isolated hepatic mitochondria. *Arch Biochem Biophys* 178:19, 1977

168. TRIEBWASSER KC, FREEDLAND RA: The effect of glucagon on ureagenesis from ammonia by isolated rat hepatocytes. *Biochem Biophys Res Commun* 76:1159, 1977

169. SNODGRASS PJ, LIN RC, MULLER WA, AOKI TT: Induction of urea cycle enzymes of rat liver by glucagon. *J Biol Chem* 253:2748, 1978

170. HALESTRAP AP, SCOTT RD, THOMAS AP: Mitochondrial pyruvate transport and its hormonal regulation. *Int J Biochem* 11:97, 1980

171. TITHERADGE MA, HAYNES RC Jr: The hormonal stimulation of ureagenesis in isolated hepatocytes through increases in mitochondrial ATP production. *Arch Biochem Biophys* 201:44, 1980

172. CATHELINEAU L, RABIER D, PETIT F, KAMOUN P: Role of acetylglutamate in the stimulation of citrullinogenesis by glucagon. *C R Acad Sci Paris* 291:625, 1980

173. COHEN PP: Biochemical differentiation during amphibian metamorphosis. *Science* 168:533, 1970

174. COHEN PP, BRUCKER RF, MORRIS SM: Cellular and molecular aspects of thyroid-hormone action during amphibian metamorphosis, in Li CH (ed):

Hormonal Proteins and Peptides, vol 6: *Thyroid Hormones*. New York, Academic Press, Inc, 1978, p 273

175. RYAN WL, WELLS IC: Homocitrulline and homoarginine synthesis from lysine. *Science* 144:122, 1964

176. RYAN WL, BARAK AJ, JOHNSON RJ: Lysine, homocitrulline, and homoarginine metabolism by the isolated perfused rat liver. *Arch Biochem Biophys* 123:294, 1968

177. SCOTT-EMUAKPOR AB, KOHRMAN AF: New evidence for the existence of lysine transcarbamylation and its possible role in ammonia disposal. *Niger J Sci* 6:47, 1972

178. GATES SC, DENDRAMIS N, WILSON RW, KOHRMAN AF: Identification of a new metabolite of L-homocitrulline. *Biochem Med* 18:87, 1977

179. STRANDHOLM JJ, BUIST NRM, KENNAWAY NG: Homoargininosuccinic acid synthesis by an enzyme from pig kidney. *Biochim Biophys Acta* 237:293, 1971

180. PAIK WK, PEARSON E, NOCHUMSON S, KIM S: Replacement of L-ornithine with L-lysine for urea cycle enzymes. *Int J Biochem* 8:317, 1977

181. CATHELINEAU L: Hyperammonemia in pediatric disease. *Arch Fr Pediatr* 36:724, 1980

182. WEIL-MALHERBE H: Ammonia metabolism in the brain, in Elliott KAC, Page IH, Quastel JH (eds): *Neurochemistry*. Springfield, Ill, Charles C Thomas, Publisher, 1962, p 321

183. COOPER AJL, McDONALD JM, GELBARD AD, GLEDHILL RF, DUFFY TE: The metabolism fate of 13-N labeled ammonia in rat brain. *J Biol Chem* 254:4982, 1979

184. HINDFELT B: On mechanisms of hyperammonemic coma—with particular reference to hepatic encephalopathy. *Ann NY Acad Sci* 252:116, 1975

185. HINDFELT B, SIESJO BK: Cerebral effects of acute ammonia intoxication: II. The effect upon energy metabolism. *Scand J Clin Lab Invest* 28:365, 1971

186. SCHENKER S, McCANDLESS DW, BROPHY E, LEWIS MS: Studies on the intracerebral toxicity of ammonia. *J Clin Invest* 46:838, 1967

187. BENZI G, ARRIGONI E, STRADA P, PASTORIS O, VILLA RF, AGNOLI A: Metabolism and cerebral energy state: Effect of acute hyperammonemia in beagle dog. *Biochem Pharmacol* 26:2397, 1977

188. BESSMAN SP, PAL N: Ammonia intoxication—energy metabolism in brain protein synthesis. Magnes Memorial Issue, *Israel J Med Sci,* in press

189. BENJAMIN AM: Control of glutaminase activity in rat brain cortex *in vitro*: Influence of glutamate, phosphate, ammonium, calcium and hydrogen ions. *Brain Res* 208:363, 1981

190. HAMBERGER A, HEDQUIST B, LUNDBORG H, NYSTROM B: Hippocampal glutamate release after porta cava anastomosis: Reduced sensitivity to ammonia inhibition. *J Neurosci Res* 5:313, 1980

191. RAABE WA: Ammonia and disinhibition in cat motor cortex by ammonium acetate, monofluoroacetate and insulin-induced hypoglycemia. *Brain Res* 210:311, 1981

192. LUMSDEN CE: Nervous tissue in culture, in Bourne GH (ed): *Structure and Function of Nervous Tissue*. New York, Academic Press, Inc, 1968, vol 1, p 67

193. CAVANAGH JB, KYU MH: Colchicine-like effect on astrocytes after portacaval shunt in rats. *Lancet* 2:620, 1969

194. HOPKINS IJ, CONNELLY JF, HOCKING B, MADDISON TG: Neurological abnormalities in primary hyperammonaemia. *Proc Aust Assoc Neurol* 5:183, 1968

195. FREEMAN JM, NICHOLSON JF, MASLAND WS, ROWLAND LP, CARTER S: Ammonia intoxication due to a congenital defect in urea synthesis. *J Pediatr* 65:1039, 1964

196. YASUOKA M, KOKUBO A: Anesthetic management of a patient with ornithine transcarbamylase deficiency associated with hyperammonemia. *Anesthesia (Japan)* 27:526, 1978

197. TADA K, OKUDA K, WATANABE K, LIMURA Y, YAMADA S: A new method for screening for hyperammonemia. *Eur J Pediatr* 130:105, 1979

198. MURPHEY WH, PATCHEN L, GUTHRIE R: Screening tests for argininosuccinic aciduria, orotic aciduria, and other inherited enzyme deficiencies using dried blood specimens. *Biochem Genet* 6:51, 1972

199. LEVY HL, COULOMBE JT, SHIH VE: Newborn urine screening, in Bickel H, Guthrie R, Hammersen G (eds): *Neonatal Screening for Inborn Errors of Metabolism*. Berlin, Springer-Verlag, 1980, p 89

200. NAYLOR EW: Newborn screening for urea cycle disorders. *Pediatrics* 68:453, 1981

201. ORFANOS AP, NAYLOR EW, GUTHRIE R: Fluorometric micromethod for determination of arginase activity in dried blood spots on filter paper. *Clin Chem* 26:1198, 1980

202. NAYLOR EM, ORFANOS AP, GUTHRIE R: A simple screening test for arginase deficiency (hyperargininemia). *J Lab Clin Med* 89:876, 1977

203. TALBOT HW, SUMLIN AB, NAYLOR EW, GUTHRIE R: A neonatal screening test for argininosuccinic acid lyase deficiency and other urea cycle disorders. *Pediatrics,* in press

204. THOENE JG, NYHAN WL: Therapy of urea cycle disorders, in *Diet Therapy for MSUD and Organic Acidurias*, Subcommittee on Amino Acids of the Nutrition Committee of the American Academy of Pediatrics under contract with the FDA. Evanston, Ill, 1978, p 15

205. CHAVERS BM, KJELLSTRAND CM, WIEGAND C, EBBEN J, MAUER SM: Techniques for use of charcoal hemoperfusion in infants: Experience in two patients. *Kidney Int* 18:386, 1980

206. BATSHAW ML, BRUSILOW SW: Treatment of hyperammonemic coma caused by inborn errors of urea synthesis. *J Pediatr* 97:893, 1980

207. DONN DM, SWARTZ RD, THOENE JG: Comparison of exchange transfusion, peritoneal dialysis, and hemodialysis for the treatment of hyperammonemia in an anuric newborn infant. *J Pediatr* 95:67, 1979

208. SHERWOOD G: Personal communication, 1981

209. BATSHAW ML, WALSER M BRUSILOW SW: Plasma alpha-ketoglutarate in urea cycle enzymopathies and its role as a harbinger of hyperammonemic coma. *Pediatr Res* 14:1316, 1980

210. BEAUDET AL, MICHELS VV, O'BRIEN WE: Drug-induced orotic aciduria for treatment of ornithine transcarbamylase deficiency. *Am J Hum Genet* 30:21A, 1978

211. KIM S, PAIK WK, COHEN PP: Ammonia intoxication in rats: Protection by N-carbamoyl-L-glutamate plus L-arginine. *Proc Natl Acad Sci USA* 69:3530, 1972

212. WALSER M, SAPIR DG, MITCH WE, CHAN W: Effects of branched chain ketoacids in normal subjects and patients, in Walser M, Williamson JR (eds): *Metabolism and Clinical Implications of Branched Chain Amino and Ketoacids*. New York, Elsevier/North-Holland Medical Press, 1981, p 291

213. MITCH WE, WALSER M: Utilization of calcium l-phenyllactate as a substitute for phenylalanine by uremic patients. *Metabolism* 26:1041, 1977

214. MITCH WE, WALSER M: Nitrogen balance of uremic patients receiving branched chain ketoacids and the hydroxyanalogue of methionine as substitutes for the respective amino acids. *Clin Nephrol* 8:341, 1977

214a. HARRIS DJ, YANG BIY, WOLF B, SNODGRASS PJ: Dysautonia in an infant with secondary hyperammonemia due to propionyl coenzyme A carboxylase deficiency. *Pediatrics* 65:107, 1980

215. BRUSILOW SW, TINKER J, BATSHAW ML: Amino acid acylation: A mechanism of nitrogen excretion in inborn errors of urea synthesis. *Science* 207:659, 1980

216. LEWIS HB: Studies in the synthesis of hippuric acid in the animal organism. II. The synthesis and rate of elimination of hippuric acid after benzoate ingestion in man. *J Biol Chem* 18:225, 1914

217. BATSHAW ML, PAINTER MJ, SPROUL GT, SCHAFER IA, THOMAS GH, BRUSILOW S: Therapy of urea cycle enzymopathies: Three case studies. *Johns Hopkins Med J* 148:34, 1981

217a. BACHMANN C, COLOMBO JP, JAGGI K: N-acetylglutamate synthetase (NAGS) deficiency: Diagnosis, clinical observations and treatment, in Mori A, Lowenthal A (eds): *The Urea Cycle*. New York, Plenum Publishing Corp, in press

218. GREEN TP: Sodium benzoate in the treatment of hyperammonemia in newborns. *Pediatr Res* 15:630, 1981

219. QURESHI IA, LETARTE J, OUELLET R: Effet protecteur du benzoate de sodium (BS) sur la tolérance aux protéines des souris hyperammoniémiques, abstract ed. Twenty-second Meeting of Club de Récherche Clinique du Quebec, La Nolliaie, 1980, p 40

220. FREEMAN JM, NICHOLSON JF, SCHIMKE RT, ROWLAND LP, CARTER S: Congenital hyperammonemia: Association with hyperglycemia and decreased levels of carbamyl phosphate synthetase. *Arch Neurol* 23:430, 1970

221. GELEHRTER TD, SNODGRASS PJ: Lethal neonatal deficiency of carbamyl phosphate synthetase. *N Engl J Med* 290:430, 1974

222. MANTAGOS S, TSAGARAKI S, BURGESS EA, OBERHOLZER V, PALMER T, SACKS J, BAIBAS S, VALAES T: Neonatal hyperammonemia with complete absence of liver carbamyl phosphate synthetase activity. *Arch Dis Child* 53:230, 1978

223. SHEFFIELD LJ, DANKS DM, HAMMOND JW, HOOGENRAAD NJ: Massive pulmonary hemorrhage as a presenting feature in congenital hyperammonemia. *J Pediatr* 88:450, 1976

224. MACLEOD PM, APPLEGARTH D, BATSHAW M, BRUSILOW S, TOONE JR, KIRBY LT, MACLEAN JR, MAMER OA, MONTGOMERY JA, WALSER M: Unpublished observations

225. APPLEGARTH DA, MACLEOD PM, TOONE JR, KIRBY LT, MACLEAN R, MAMER OA, MONTGOMERY JA: Organic acids and Reye's syndrome. *Lancet* 1:1147, 1979

226. ARASHIMA S, MATSUDA I: A case of carbamyl phosphate synthetase deficiency. *Tohoku J Exp Med* 107:143, 1972

227. ODIEVRE M, CHARPENTIER C, CATHELINEAU L, VEDRENNE J, DELACOUX F, MERCIE C: Hyperammoniémie constitutionelle avec déficit en carbamylphosphate-synthetase. *Arch Fr Pediatr* 30:5, 1973

228. FARRIAUX JP: *Le cycle de l'urée et ses anomalies*. Paris, Doin, Deren Cie Editions, 1978

229. LAMBOTTE C, ADAM A, VAN DER HOFSTADT J, DODINVAL-VERSIE J, GIELEN J: Severe neonatal deficiency of carbamyl phosphate synthetase. *Acta Paediatr Belg* 30:151, 1977

230. WILSON RG, MASTERS PL: Neonatal death due to carbamyl phosphate synthetase deficiency. *Aust Paediatr J* 13:119, 1977

231. GLASGOW AM, ORLOFF S, MUKHERJEE A, BUTLER EJ, SCHULMAN JD:

Hyperammonemia with partial carbamyl phosphate synthetase deficiency responsive to arginine therapy. *Pediatr Res* 11:456, 1977

232. HOOGENRAAD NJ, MITCHELL JD, DON NA, SUTHERLAND TM, McLEAY AC: Detection of carbamyl phosphate synthetase I deficiency using duodenal biopsy samples. *Arch Dis Child* 55:292, 1980

233. BATSHAW M, BRUSILOW S, WALSER M: Treatment of carbamyl phosphate synthetase deficiency with keto analogues of essential amino acids. *N Engl J Med* 292:1085, 1975

234. BACHMANN C, COLOMBO JP: Diagnostic value of orotic acid excretion in heritable disorders of the urea cycle and in hyperammonemia due to organic acidurias. *Eur J Pediatr* 134:109, 1980

235. ZIMMERMANN A, BACHMANN C, COLOMBO JP: Ultrastructural pathology in congenital defects of the urea cycle: Ornithine transcarbamylase and carbamylphosphate synthetase deficiency. *Virchows Arch A* 393:321, 1981

236. VAN GENNIP AH, VAN BREE-BLOM EJ, GRIFT J, DEBREE PK, WADMAN SK: Urinary purines and pyrimidines in patients with hyperammonemia of various origins. *Clin Chim Acta* 104:227, 1980

237. OBERHOLZER VG, PALMER T: Increased excretion of N-carbamoyl compounds in patients with urea cycle defects. *Clin Chim Acta* 68:73, 1976

238. KLINE JJ, HUG G, SCHUBERT WK, BROWN T, BERRY HK: Treatment of an infant boy with carbamyl phosphate synthetase deficiency with alpha keto analogs of essential amino acids. *Pediatr Res* 10:355, 1976

239. KLINE JJ, HUG G, SCHUBERT WK, BERRY H: Arginine deficiency syndrome—its occurrence in carbamyl phosphate synthetase deficiency. *Am J Dis Child* 135:437, 1981

240. HOMMES FA, DE GROOT CJ, WILMINK CW, JONXIS JHP: Carbamylphosphate synthetase deficiency in an infant with severe cerebral damage. *Arch Dis Child* 44:688, 1969

241. SINATRA F, YOSHIDA T, APPLEBAUM M, MASON W, HOOGENRAAD NJ, SUNSHINE P: Abnormalities of carbamyl phosphate synthetase and ornithine transcarbamylase in liver of patients with Reye's syndrome. *Pediatr Res* 9:829, 1975

242. WYSOCKI SJ, HAHNEL R, TRUSCOTT RJW, HALPERN B, WILCKEN B: Hyperammonemia and urinary organic acids. *Lancet* 2:371, 1979

243. MATSUSHIMA A, ORII T: The activity of carbamylphosphate synthetase I (CPS I) and ornithine transcarbamylase (OTC) in the intestine and the screening of OTC deficiency in the rectal mucosa. *J Inher Metab Dis* 4:83, 1981

244. WOLFE DM, GATFIELD PD: Leukocyte urea cycle enzymes in hyperammonemia. *Pediatr Res* 9:531, 1975

245. RABIER D, CATHELINEAU L, KAMOUN P: Letter to the editor: Lack of mitochondrial enzymes of the urea cycle in human white blood cells. *Pediatr Res* 13:207, 1979

246. SNODGRASS PJ, DELONG GR: Urea-cycle enzyme deficiencies and an increased nitrogen load producing hyperammonemia in Reye's syndrome. *N Engl J Med* 294:855, 1976

247. LABRECQUE DR, LATHAM PS, RIELY CA, HSIA YE, KLATSKIN G: Heritable urea cycle enzyme deficiency—liver disease in 16 patients. *J Pediatr* 94:580, 1979

248. BATSHAW ML, BRUSILOW S, WALSER M: Long-term management of a case of carbamyl phosphate synthetase deficiency using ketoanalogues and hydroxyanalogues of essential amino acids. *Pediatrics* 58:227, 1976

249. CLOW C, CUMMINGS CC, SCRIVER C, BRUSILOW S, BATSHAW ML, SNODGRASS PJ, WALSER M: Unpublished observations

250. GOLDSTEIN AS, HOOGENRAAD NJ, JOHNSON JD, FUKANAGA K, SWIERCZEWSKI E, CANN HM, SUNSHINE P: Metabolic and genetic studies of a family with ornithine transcarbamylase (OTC) deficiency. *Pediatr Res* 8:5, 1974

251. CAMPBELL AGM, ROSENBERG LE, SNODGRASS PJ, NUZUM CT: Lethal neonatal hyperammonaemia due to complete ornithine-transcarbamylase deficiency. *Lancet* 2:217, 1971

252. CATHELINEAU L, NAVARRO J, POLONOVSKI C, SAUDUBRAY J-M: X-linked transmission of structural gene mutations responsible for ornithine-transcarbamylase deficiencies. *Lancet* 1:261, 1973

253. McREYNOLDS JW, MANTAGOS S, BRUSILOW S, ROSENBERG LE: Treatment of complete ornithine transcarbamylase deficiency with nitrogen-free analogues of essential amino acids. *J Pediatr* 93:421, 1978

254. HAAN EA, DANKS DM, HOOGENRAAD NJ, ROGERS JG: Hereditary hyperammonaemic syndromes—a six year experience. *Aust Pediatr J* 15:142, 1979

255. SCHUCHMANN L, COLOMBO JP, FISCHER H: Hyperammonemia due to ornithine transcarbamylase deficiency—a cause of lethal metabolic crisis during the newborn period and infancy. *Klin Paediatr* 192:281, 1980

256. CATHELINEAU L, BRIAND P: Human OTC deficiencies. Abstract from a Symposium on Hyperammonemia, Dec. 12, 1980, Paris, unpublished

257. STOLL C, BIETH R, DREYFUS J, FLORI E, LUTZ P, LEVY J-M: Une nouvelle famille avec mutation du gène de structure de l'ornithine carbamyltransferase humaine. *Arch Fr Pediatr* 35:512, 1978

258. SNYDERMAN SE, SANSARICQ C, PHANSALKAR SV, SCHACHT RG, NORTON PM: The therapy of hyperammonemia due to ornithine transcarbamylase deficiency in a male neonate. *Pediatrics* 56:65, 1975

259. GELEHRTER TD, ROSENBERG LE: Ornithine transcarbamylase deficiency: Unsuccessful therapy of neonatal hyperammonemia with N-carbamyl-L-glutamate and L-arginine. *N Engl J Med* 292:351, 1975

260. WIEGAND C, THOMPSON T, BOCK GH, MATHIS RK, KJELLSTRAND CM, MAUER SM: The management of life-threatening hyperammonemia: A comparison of several therapeutic modalities. *J Pediatr* 96:142, 1980

261. GLASGOW AM, SCHULMAN J, BATSHAW MB, WALSER M: Unpublished observations

262. LONGHI R, BUTTE C, VALSASINA R, ROSSI L, BORZANI M: Mitochondrial abnormalities in a male with ornithine transcarbamylase deficiency. *Pediatr Res* 15:634, 1981

263. PALMER T, OBERHOLZER VG, BURGESS EA, BUTLER LJ, LEVIN B: Hyperammonemia in 20 families: Biochemical and genetical survey, including investigations in 3 new families. *Arch Dis Child* 49:443, 1974

264. SCOTT CR, TENG CC, GOODMAN SI, GREENSHER A, MACE JW: X-linked transmission of ornithine-transcarbamylase deficiency. *Lancet* 2:1148, 1972

265. KANG ES, SNODGRASS PJ, GERALD PS: Ornithine transcarbamylase deficiency in the newborn infant. *J Pediatr* 82:642, 1973

266. SAUDUBRAY JM, CATHELINEAU L, CHARPENTIER C, BOISSE J, ALLANEAU C, LE BONT H, LESAGE B: Déficit héréditaire en ornithine-carbamly-transferase avec anomalie enzymatique qualitative. *Arch Fr Pediatr* 30:15, 1973

267. MACLEOD P, MACKENZIE S, SCRIVER CR: Partial ornithine carbamyl transferase deficiency: An inborn error of the urea cycle presenting as orotic aciduria in a male infant. *Can Med Assoc J* 107:405, 1972

268. BEAUDET A: Personal communication

269. KRIEGER I, BACHMANN C, GRONEMEYER WH, CEJKA J: Propionic acidemia and hyperlysinemia in a case with ornithine transcarbamylase (OTC) deficiency. *J clin Endocrinol Metab* 43:796, 1976

270. SEBASTIO G, VAJRO P, STRIANO S, ANDRIA G: Sindrome iperammoniemica in bambina con grave compromissione neurologica. *Riv Ital Pediatria*, in press

271. YOKOYAMA S, FUJIWARA T, OYANAGI K, KIMURA, ORII T, YASUDA I, MOTOMURA S, HOSODA O, KARUBE K, TOGAWA H: A case of hyperammonemia due to ornithine transcarbamylase deficiency. *J Clin Pediatr (Japan)* 25:31, 1977

272. BEAUDREY MA, LETARTE J, COLLU R, LEBOEUF G, DUCHARME JL, MELANCON SB, DALLAIRE L: Chronic hyperammonemia with orotic aciduria—evidence of pyrimidine pathway stimulation. *Diabet Metab* 1:29, 1975

273. HERRIN JT, McCREDIE DA: Peritoneal dialysis in the reduction of blood ammonia levels in a case of hyperammonaemia. *Arch Dis Child* 44:149, 1969

274. SCHNEIDER S, NICHOLSON JF, CHUTORIAN AB: Sex-linked hyperammonemia: Response to reduced dietary protein. *Trans Am Neurol Assoc* 95:86, 1970

275. GRAY RFG, BLACK JA, LYONS VH, POLLITT RJ: Ornithine transcarbamylase deficiency: Enzyme studies on a further case and a method of diagnosis using plasma enzyme ratios. *Pediatr Res* 10:918, 1976

276. WEBSTER DR, SIMMONDS HA, BARRY DMJ, BECROFT DMO: Pyrimidine and purine metabolites in ornithine carbamoyl transferase deficiency. *J Inher Metab Dis* 4:27, 1981

277. QURESHI IA, LETARTE J, OUELLET R: Study of enzyme defect in a case of ornithine transcarbamylase deficiency. *Diabet Metab* 4:239, 1978

278. MORLEY C, SARDHARWALLA IB: Case of hyperammonemia due to ornithine transcarbamylase deficiency. *Arch Dis Child* 49:747, 1974

279. KREBS HA, HEMS R, LUND P: Regulatory mechanisms in the synthesis of urea, in Hommes FA, Van Den Berg C (eds): *Inborn Errors of Metabolism.* New York, Academic Press, Inc, 1973, p 201

280. LEVIN B, ABRAHAM JM, OBERHOLZER VG, BURGESS EA: Hyperammonaemia: A deficiency of liver ornithine transcarbamylase. Occurrence in mother and child. *Arch Dis Child* 44:152, 1969

281. HOPKINS IA, CONNELLY JF, DAWSON AG, HIRD FJR, MADDISON TG: Hyperammonemia due to ornithine transcarbamylase deficiency. *Arch Dis Child* 44:143, 1969

282. SUNSHINE P, LINDENBAUM JE, LEVY HL, FREEMAN JM: Hyperammonemia due to a defect in hepatic ornithine transcarbamylase. *Pediatrics* 50:100, 1972

283. CORBEEL LM, COLOMBO JP, VAN SANDE M, WEBER A: Periodic attacks of lethargy in a baby with ammonia intoxication due to a congenital defect in ureogenesis. *Arch Dis Child* 44:681, 1969

284. NAGAYAMA E, KITAYAMA T, OGUCHI H: Hyperammonemia: A deficiency of liver ornithine transcarbamylase. *Paediatr Univ Tokyo* 18:167, 1970

285. MATSUDA I, ARASHIMA S, NAMBRU H, TAKEKOSHI Y, ANAKURA M: Hyperammonemia due to a mutant enzyme of ornithine transcarbamylase. *Pediatrics* 48:595, 1971

286. RUSSELL A, LEVIN B, OBERHOLZER VG, SINCLAIR L: Hyperammonaemia. A new instance of an inborn enzymatic defect of the biosynthesis of urea. *Lancet* 2:699, 1962

287. LEVIN B, RUSSELL A: Treatment of hyperammonaemia. *Am J Dis Child* 113:142, 1967

288. SALLE B, LEVIN B, LONGIN B, RICHARD P, ANDRE M, GAUTHIER J: Hyperammoniémie congénitale par déficit en ornithine carbamyl transferase et carbamyl phosphate synthetase. *Arch Fr Pediatr* 29:493, 1972

289. MORIN CL, WEBER M, QURESHI I, LETARTE J: Reye's syndrome in infancy. Studies on ammonia metabolism, in Crocker JFS, Bagnell PC, Lee SH, Ozere RL, Renton KW, Rozee KR (eds): *Reye's Syndrome II*. New York, Grune & Stratton, 1979, p 101

290. VAN DER HEIDEN C, DESPLANQUE J, BAKKER HD: A simple approach to predict residual liver ornithine carbamoyltransferase (OTC) activity from serum enzyme ratios. *Clin Chim Acta* 84:259, 1978

291. SNODGRASS PJ, WAPPNER RS, BRANDT IK: Letter to the editor. *Pediatr Res* 12:873, 1978

292. NAGATA N, AKABOSHI I, YAMAMOTO J, MATSUDA I, OHTSUKA H, KATSUKI T: Ornithine transcarbamylase (OTC) in white blood cells. *Pediatr Res* 14:1370, 1980

293. QURESHI IA, LETARTE J, OUELLET R: Biochemical evaluation and dietary control of ornithine transcarbamylase (OTC) deficiency in a male child. *Clin Res* 26:865A, 1978

294. AYLSWORTH AS, SWISHER CN, KIRKMAN HN: Lethal hyperammonemia due to partial ornithine transcarbamylase deficiency in a 6 year old male. *Am J Hum Genet* 27:15A, 1975

295. MATSUSHIMA A: Ornithine transcarbamylase (OTC). *Clin Pediatr (Japan)* 27:381, 1979

296. LEVIN B, DOBBS RH, BURGESS EA, PALMER T: Hyperammonaemia. A variant type of deficiency of liver ornithine transcarbamylase. *Arch Dis Child* 44:162, 1969

297. KRIEGER I, SNODGRASS PJ, ROSKAMO J: Atypical clinical course of ornithine transcarbamylase deficiency due to a new mutant (comparison with Reye's disease) *J Clin Endocrinol Metab* 48:338, 1979

298. HAAN EA, DANKS DM, GRIMES A, HOOGENRAAD NJ: Carrier detection in ornithine transcarbamylase deficiency. *J Inher Metab Dis*, in press

299. Batshaw M, Roan Y, Jung AI, Rosenberg LA, Brusilow SW: Cerebral dysfunction in asymptomatic carriers of ornithine transcarbamylase deficiency. *N Engl J Med* 302:482, 1980

300. HOKANSON JT, O'BRIEN WE, IDEMOTO J, SCHAFER IA: Carrier detection in ornithine transcarbamylase deficiency. *J Pediatr* 93:75, 1978

301. SHIH VE: Urea cycle disorders and other congenital hyperammonemic syndromes, in Stanbury JB, Wyngaarden JB, Fredrickson DS (eds): *The Metabolic Basis of Inherited Disease*, ed 4. New York, McGraw-Hill Book Co, 1978, p 362

302. STATTER M, SAGI E, RUSSELL A, LIVNI N, DECKELBAUM R: Experimental models of microvesicular fatty changes in rat liver, abstract ed. First International Congress of Pediatric Laboratory Medicine, October 1980, Jerusalem,

303. AOYAMA Y, ASHIDA K: Prevention by urea cycle intermediates and adenine on the lipid accumulation in the liver induced by refeeding an arginine-devoid diet in rats. *Nutr Rep Int* 20:483, 1979

304. NATALE PJ, TREMBLAY GC: On the availability of intramitochondrial carbamoylphosphate for the extramitochondrial biosynthesis of pyrimidines. *Biochem Biophys Res Commun* 37:512, 1969

305. QURESHI IA, LETARTE J, OUELLET R: Activity of orotate metabolizing enzyme complex and various urea-cycle enzymes in mutant mice with ornithine transcarbamylase deficiency. *Experientia*, in press

306. VAN DER HEIDEN C, DESPLANQUE J, BAKKER HD: Some kinetic properties of liver ornithine carbamoyl transferase (OCT). *Clin Chim Acta* 80:519, 1977

307. BRIAND P, FRANCOIS B, CATHELINEAU L: Human male ornithine carbamoyl transferase deficiencies: Kinetics, immunochemical classification and comparison with deficiencies in mouse. *Biochim Biophys Acta*, in press

308. RICCIUTTI FC, GELEHRTER TD, ROSENBERG LE: X-chromosome inactivation in human liver: Confirmation of X-linkage of ornithine transcarbamylase. *Am J Hum Genet* 28:332, 1976

309. DEMARS R, LEVAN SL, TREND BL, RUSSELL LB: Abnormal ornithine carbamyltransferase in mice having the sparse-fur mutation. *Proc Natl Acad Sci USA* 73:1693, 1976

310. LEVIN B, OBERHOLZER VG, SINCLAIR L: Biochemical investigations of hyperammonaemia. *Lancet* 2:170, 1969

311. MICHELS VV, BEAUDET A, BATSHAW M, WALSER M: Dietary therapy of ornithine transcarbamylase (OTC) deficiency. *Pediatr Res* 12:454, 1978

312. MCMURRAY WC, MOHYUDDIN F, ROSSITER RJ, RATHBUN JC, VALENTINE GH, KOEGLER SJ, ZARFAS DE: Citrullinuria: A new aminoaciduria associated with mental retardation. *Lancet* 1:138, 1962

313. VAN DER ZEE SPM, TRIJBELS JMF, MONNENS LAH, HOMMES FA, SCHRETLEN EDAM: Citrullinaemia with a rapidly fatal neonatal course. *Arch Dis Child* 48:847, 1971

314. WICK H, BACHMANN C, BAUMGARTNER R, BRECHBUHLER T, COLOMBO JP, WIESMANN U, MIHATSCH MJ, ORNACKER H: Variants of citrullinaemia. *Arch Dis Child* 48:636, 1973

315. MIHATSCH NJ, RIEDE UN, OHNACKER H, WICK H, BACHMANN C: Liver morphology in a case of citrullinemia (a light and electron microscopic study). *Beitr Path Bd* 151:200, 1974

316. GHISOLFI J, AUGIER D, MARTINEZ J, BARTHE PH, ANDRIEU P, BESSE P, REGNIER CL: Forme néonatale de citrullinémie à évolution mortelle rapide. *Pediatrie* 27:55, 1972

317. ROERDINK FH, GOUW WLM: Citrullinemia. Report of a case, with studies on antenatal diagnosis. *Pediatr Res* 7:863, 1973

318. VIDAILHET M, LEVIN B, DAUTREVAUX M, PAYSANT P, GELOT S, BADONNEL Y, PIERSON M, NEIMANN N: Citrullinémie. *Arch Fr Pediatr* 28:521, 1971

319. BUIST NRM, KENNAWAY NG, HEPBURN CA, STRANDHOLM J, RAMBERG DA: Citrullinemia: Investigation and treatment over a four-year period. *J Pediatr* 85:208, 1974

320. KENNAWAY NG, HARWOOD PJ, RAMBERG DA, KOLER RD, BUIST NMR: Citrullinemia: Enzymatic evidence for genetic heterogeneity. *Pediatr Res* 9:554, 1975

321. BURGESS EA, OBERHOLZER VG, SEMMENS JM, STERN J: Acute neonatal and benign citrullinaemia in one sibship. *Arch Dis Child* 53:179, 1978

322. CHRISTENSEN E, BRANDT NJ, PHILIP J, KENNAWAY NG: Citrullinaemia: The possibility of prenatal diagnosis. *J Inher Metab Dis* 3:73, 1980

323. DANKS DM, TIPPETT P, ZENTNER G: Severe neonatal citrullinemia. *Arch Dis Child* 49:579, 1974

324. THOENE J, BATSHAW M, SPECTOR E, KULOVICH S, BRUSILOW S, WALSER M, NYHAN W: Neonatal citrullinemia: Treatment with ketoanalogues of essential amino acids. *J Pediatr* 90:218, 1977

325. WALSER M, BATSHAW M, SHERWOOD G, ROBINSON B, BRUSILOW S: Nitrogen metabolism in neonatal citrullinaemia. *Clin Sci Mol Med* 53:173, 1977

326. LEIBOWITZ J, THOENE J, SPECTOR E, NYHAN W: Citrullinemia. *Virchows Arch (Pathol Anat Histol)* 377:249, 1978

327. PACKMAN S, THALER M, LARKINS J, NEWTON TH, SNODGRASS PJ, WALSER M: Unpublished observations.

328. CATHELINEAU L, PHAM DINH D, BOUE J, SAUDUBRAY JM, FARRIAUX JP, KAMOUN P: Improved method for the antenatal diagnosis of citrullinemia. *Clin Chim Acta* 116:111, 1981

329. CATHELINEAU L, PHAM DINH D, BRIAND P, KAMOUN P: Complementation in argininosuccinate synthetase and argininosuccinate lyase deficiencies in human fibroblasts. Unpublished

330. MCMURRAY WC, MOHYUDDIN F, BAYER SM, RATHBUN JD: Citrullinuria: A disorder of amino acid metabolism associated with mental retardation. International Copenhagen Congress on the Scientific Study of Mental Retardation, Denmark, Aug. 7–14, 1964

331. MOHYUDDIN F, RATHBUN JC, MCMURRAY WC: Studies on amino acid metabolism in citrullinemia. *Am J Dis Child* 113:152, 1967

332. MCMURRAY WC, RATHBUN JC, MOHYUDDIN F, KOEGLER SJ: Citrullinuria. *Pediatrics* 3:347, 1963

333. TEDESCO TA, MELLMAN WJ: Argininosuccinate synthetase activity and citrulline metabolism in cells cultured from a citrullinemic subject. *Proc Natl Acad Sci USA* 57:829, 1967

334. MORROW G, BARNESS LA, EFRON ML: Citrullinemia with defective urea production. *Pediatrics* 40:565, 1967

335. SPECTOR E, KENNAWAY N, PUNNETT H, GREENE AE, CORIELL LL: Citrullinemia, argininosuccinate synthetase deficiency: Repository identification no GM-1044. *Cytogenet Cell Genet* 19:51, 1977

336. WHELAN DT, BRUSSO T, SPATE M: Citrullinemia: Phenotypic variations. *Pediatrics* 57:935, 1976

337. OGASAWARA T: Special type of liver-brain syndrome. Monograph, *Modern Psychiatric Medicine Series*, vol 13B. Inose S (ed). Tokyo, Nakayama Shotem, 1975, p 23. Cited by ref 44

338. SCOTT-EMUAKPOR A, HIGGINS JV, KOHRMAN AF: Citrullinemia: A new case, with implications concerning adaptation to defective urea synthesis. *Pediatr Res* 6:626, 1972

339. SPECTOR EB, BLOOM AD: Citrullinemic lymphocytes in long term culture. *Pediatr Res* 7:700, 1973

340. TAKAMIZAWA M, TORU M, KOJIMA T, WATANABE A, HIROKAWA K: An autopsy case of juvenile hepatocerebral degeneration (non-Wilsonian Inose-type) with mental retardation with special reference to amino acids metabolism. *Psychiatr Neurol Jap* 75:370, 1973

341. SAHEKI T, UEDA A, HOSOYA M, KUSUMI K, TAKADA S, TSUDA M, KATSUNUMA T: Qualitative and quantitative abnormalities of argininosuccinate synthetase in citrullinemia. *Clin Chim Acta* 109:325, 1981

342. MATSUDA I, ARASHIMA S, IMANISHI Y, YAMAMOTO J, AKABOSHI I, SHINOZUKA S, NAGATA N: Lysine intolerance in a variant form of citrullinemia. *Pediatr Res* 13:1134, 1979

343. IMANISHI K, OKAJIMA T, IDETA T, UENO H, MATSUMOTO Y: Juvenile hepatocerebral disease with citrullinemia. *Clin Neurol (Tokyo)* 16:389, 1976

344. MIYAZAKI M, FUKUDA S, AKI M, EZAWA T, KITAMURA M, TAMURA Z: A case of hepatic encephalomyelopathy associated with citrullinemia. *Brain Nerv* 23:19, 1971

345. MATSUDA I, ANAKURA M, ARASHIMA S, SAITO Y, OKA Y: Variant form of citrullinemia. *J Pediatr* 88:824, 1976

346. TSUJII T, MORITA T, MATSUYAMA Y, MATSUI T, TAMURA M, MATSUOKA Y: Sibling cases of chronic recurrent hepatocerebral disease with hypercitrullinemia. *Gastroenterol J* 11:328, 1976

347. SAITO Y, TAKAHATA N, SUWA N, NISHI N, NISHIOKA N: Hepato-cerebral

diseases caused by abnormal amino acid metabolism—clinical observation in 3 cases of citrullinemia. *Brain Nerv* 28:263, 1976

348. KOOKA T, HIGASHI Y, UEBAYASHI Y, KOBAYASHI R: A special form of hepatocerebral degeneration with citrullinemia. *Neurol Med* 6:47, 1977

349. HAYASHI S: A case of hypercitrullinemia caused by abnormal argininosuccinate synthetase. *Metabolism (Japan)* 15:9, 1978. Cited by ref 44

350. AKAMATSU K: A case of adult type hypercitrullinemia probably caused by genetic abnormality in argininosuccinic acid synthetase. Lecture, 14th meeting of Japanese Society for Hepatic Diseases, 1978. Cited by ref 44

351. MURAWAKI Y, YOSHIDA K, HIRAYAMA C, NAKAO T, NAKAYA Y: Inherited hyperammonemia in adults. *Acta Hepatol Jap* 18:856, 1977

352. OKKEN A, VAN DER BLIJ JF, HOMMES FA: Citrullinaemia and brain damage. *Pediatr Res* 7:52, 1973

353. PAUL AA, FOSGATE DAT: *McCance and Widdowson's The Composition of Foods*, ed 4. New York, Elsevier/North-Holland Medical Press, 1978

354. WICK HT, BRECHBUHLER, GIRARD J: Citrullinemia: Elevated serum citrulline levels in healthy siblings. *Experientia* 26:823, 1970

355. PALMER T, AMEEN M: Enzyme inhibition as a possible cause of secondary increases in metabolite levels in patients with inborn errors of metabolism. *J Inher Metab Dis* 3:79, 1980

356. WALSER M: Conservative management of the uremic patient, in Brenner BM, Rector FC (eds): *The Kidney*, ed 2. Philadelphia, WB Saunders Co, 1981, vol 2, p 2383

357. ALSHAMAONY FTAA, ALMALLAH Z, SHIKARA I, ALSAYED M: Citrulline as a diagnostic parameter and a major amino acid constituent of cerebrospinal fluid. *J Clin Chem Clin Biochem* 15:221, 1977

358. SHIH VE, LITTLEFIELD JW: Argininosuccinase activity in amniotic-fluid cells. *Lancet* 2:45, 1970

358a. JACOBY LB, SHIH VE, STRUCKMEYER C, NIERMEIJER MF, BOUE J: Variation in argininosuccinate synthetase activity in amniotic fluid cell cultures: Implications for prenatal diagnosis of citrullinemia. *Clin Chem Acta* 116:1, 1981

359. ANON: Familial neonatal pulmonary hemorrhage associated with defects of the urea cycle. *Pediatr Res* 13:81, 1979

360. WALSER M, BATSHAW M, BRUSILOW S: Citrullinotelism. *Clin Res* 25:524A, 1977

361. STRANDHOLM JJ, BUIST NRM, KENNAWAY NC, CURTIS HT: Excretion of alpha-N-acetylcitrulline in citrullinemia. *Biochim Biophys Acta* 244:214, 1971

362. STROMBECK DR, MEYER DJ, FREEDLAND RA: Hyperammonemia due to a urea cycle enzyme deficiency in two dogs. *J Am Vet Med Assoc* 166:1109, 1975

363. GONZALEZ-NORIEGA A, VERDUZCO J, PRIETO E, VELAZQUEZ A: Argininosuccinic acid synthetase deficiency in a hamster cell line and its complementation of argininosuccinic aciduria human fibroblasts. *J Inher Metab Dis* 3:45, 1980

364. CARRITT B: Somatic cell genetic evidence for the presence of a gene for citrullinemia on human chromosome 9. *Cytogenet Cell Genet* 19:44, 1977

365. KENNAWAY NG, CURTIS HC: Complementation analysis in fibroblasts from eight patients with clinically different forms of citrullinaemia. *J Inher Metab Dis* 4:23, 1981

366. ALLAN JD, CUSWORTH DC, DENT CE, WILSON VK: A disease, probably hereditary, characterized by severe mental deficiency and a constant gross abnormality of amino acid metabolism. *Lancet* 1:182, 1958

367. VAN DER HEIDEN C, GERARDS LJ, VAN BIERVLIET JPGM, DESPLANQUE J, DE BREE PK, VAN SPRANG FJ, WADMAN SK: Lethal neonatal argininosuccinate lyase deficiency in four children from one sibship. *Helv Paediatr Acta* 31:407, 1976

368. COLLINS FS, SUMMER GK, SCHWARTZ RP, PARKE JC: Neonatal argininosuccinic aciduria: Survival after early diagnosis and dietary management. *J Pediatr* 96:429, 1980

369. FARRIAUX JP, CARTIGNY B, DHONDT JL, KINT J, LOUIS J, DELATTRE P, FONTAINE G: Á propos d'une observation d'argino-succinylurie néonatale: essai de traitement diététique. *Acta Paediatr Belg* 28:193, 1974

370. JOHN EG, BHAT R, VIDYASAGAR D: Neonatal survival after early diagnosis and treatment of argininosuccinic aciduria. *J Pediatr* 97:867, 1980

371. CARTON D: Disorders of urea cycle and related diseases, in Vinken PJ, Bruyn GW, Klawans HL (eds): *Metabolic and Deficiency Diseases of the Nervous System*, part 3, *Handbook of Clinical Neurology 29*, Amsterdam, North-Holland Publishing Company, 1977, p 87

372. RATHBUN MA, BRYSON MF, MEYERS GJ, SHIH V: Argininosuccinic aciduria: A survivor of the neonatal variant. *Pediatr Res* 11:462, 1977

373. FLEISHER LD, RASSIN DK, DESNICK RH, SALWEN HR, ROGERS P, BEAN M, GAULL GE: Argininosuccinic aciduria: Prenatal studies in a family at risk. *Am J Hum Genet* 31:439, 1979

374. HAMBRAEUS L, HARDELL LI, WESTPHAL O, LORENTSEN R, HJORTH G: Argininosuccinic aciduria: Report of three cases and the effect of high and reduced protein intake on the clinical state. *Acta Paediatr Scand* 63:525, 1974

375. ANDRIA G, VAIRO P, STRISCIUGLIO P, SANNOLO N, KOSOVA P: Argino-succinico-aciduria subacuta con insolita presentazione. *Riv Ital Pediatria* 6:495, 1980

376. QURESHI IA, LETARTE J, OUELLET R, LEMIEUX B. Enzymologic and metabolic studies in two families affected by argininosuccinic aciduria. *Pediatr Res* 12:256, 1978

377. BÖHLES H, HEID H, HARMS D, SCHMID D, FEKL W: Argininosuccinic aciduria: Metabolic studies and effects of treatment with keto-analogues of essential amino acids. *Eur J Pediatr* 128:225, 1978

378. SCHUTGENS RBH, BEEMER FA, TEGELAERS WHH, DE GROOT WP: Mild variant of argininosuccinic aciduria. *J Inher Metab Dis* 2:13, 1979

379. FARRELL G, RAUSCHKOLB EW, MOURE J, HEADLEE RE, MOSER I: Argininosuccinic aciduria. *Tex Med* 65:90, 1969

380. SHELLEY WB, RAWNSLEY HM: Aminogenic alopecia loss of hair associated with argininosuccinic aciduria. *Lancet* 2:1327, 1965

381. LEVIN B: Argininosuccinic aciduria. *Am J Dis Child* 113:162, 1967

382. POTTER JL, TIMMONS GD, SILVIDI AA: Argininosuccinic aciduria—the hair abnormality revisited. *Am J Dis Child* 134:1095, 1980

383. DHONDT JL, FARRIAUX JP, POLLITT RJ, VAMOS E, RICHARD P, BLANCK-AERT C, DELECOUR M, MONNIER JC, FONTAINE G: Attempt at antenatal diagnosis of argininosuccinic acidura. *Ann Genet (Paris)* 19:23, 1976

384. GOODMAN SI, MACE JW, TURNER B, GARRETT WJ: Antenatal diagnosis of argininosuccinic aciduria. *Clin Genet* 4:236, 1973

385. FENSOM A-H, BENSON PF, BAKER JE, MUTTON DE: Prenatal diagnosis of argininosuccinic aciduria: Effect of mycoplasma contamination on the indirect assay for argininosuccinate lyase. *Am J Hum Genet* 32:761, 1980

386. HARTLAGE PL, CORYELL ME, HALL WK, HAHN DA: Argininosuccinic aciduria: Perinatal diagnosis and early dietary management. *J Pediatr* 85:86, 1974

387. JACOBY LB, LITTLEFIELD JW, MILUNSKY A, SHIH VE, WILROY RS JR: A microassay for argininosuccinase in cultured cells. *Am J Hum Genet* 24:321, 1972

388. CUSWORTH DC, DENT CE: Renal clearances of amino acids in normal adults and in patients with aminoaciduria. *Biochem J* 74:550, 1960

389. LEVIN B, MACKAY HMM, OBERHOLZER VG: Argininosuccinic aciduria: An inborn error of amino acid metabolism. *Arch Dis Child* 36:622, 1961

390. HAMBRAEUS L, HARDELL LI, ELLINGSEN E: Effect of dietary protein and physical exercise on patients with argininosuccinic aciduria. *Nutr Metab* 21(suppl) 1:75, 1977

391. COLOMBO JP, BAUMGARTNER R: Argininosuccinate cleavage enzyme of the kidney in AS aciduria, in *Proceedings of the 6th Symposium of the Society for the Study of Inborn Errors of Metabolism, Zurich, June 24–25, 1968.* Edinburgh: Churchill Livingstone, 1969, p 119

392. POLLITT RJ: Argininosuccinate lyase levels in blood, liver, and cultured fibroblasts of a patient with argininosuccinic aciduria. *Clin Chim Acta* 46:33, 1973

393. FARRIAUX JP, DHONDT JL, FORMSTECHER P, MARTIN JJ, POLLITT RJ, KNIT J, LAGROU A, MARDENS Y, FONTAINE G: Pathological and biochemical studies on a neonatal case of argininosuccinic aciduria. *Acta Neurol Belg* 76:26, 1976

394. NAYLOR SL, KLEBE RJ, SHOWS TB: Argininosuccinic aciduria assignment of the argininosuccinate lyase Ec-4.3.2.1. gene to the P-TER to Q-22 region of human chromosome 7 by bioautography. *Proc Natl Acad Sci USA* 75:6159, 1978

395. DENT CE: Argininosuccinic aciduria and maple syrup urine disease. *Bull Schweiz Akad Med Wiss* 17:329, 1961

396. WESTALL RG: Argininosuccinic aciduria: Identification and reactions of the abnormal metabolite in a newly described form of mental disease, with some preliminary metabolic studies. *Biochem J* 77:135, 1960.

397. SHIH VE: Early dietary management in an infant with argininosuccinase deficiency: Preliminary report. *J Pediatr* 80:645, 1972

398. BRUSILOW S, BATSHAW M, WALSER M: Use of ketoacids in inborn errors of urea synthesis, in Winick M (ed): *Nutritional Management of Genetic Disorders*. New York, John Wiley & Sons, Inc, 1979, p 65

399. BRUSILOW SW, BATSHAW ML: Arginine therapy of argininosuccinase deficiency. *Lancet* 1:124, 1979

400. SNODGRASS, PM: Personal communication

401. MATALON RK, MICHALS K, GROSS S, BATSHAW ML, BRUSILOW SW: Diagnosis, treatment and follow up of neonatal argininosuccinic acidemia. *Pediatr Res* 15:636, 1981

402. TERHEGGEN HG, SCHWENK A, LOWENTHAL A, VAN SANDE M, COLOMBO JP: Argininaemia with arginase deficiency. *Lancet* 2:748, 1969

403. COLOMBO JP, TERHEGGEN HG, LOWENTHAL A, VAN SANDE M, ROGERS S: Argininaemia, in Hommes FA, Van den Berg A (eds): *Report of a Symposium on the Relation Between Developmental Biochemistry and Inborn Errors of Metabolism*. New York, Academic Press, Inc, 1973, p 239

404. CEDERBAUM SD, SHAW KNF, VALENTE M: Hyperargininemia. *J Pediatr* 90:569, 1977

405. MICHELS VV, BEAUDET AL: Arginase deficiency in multiple tissues in argininemia. *Clin Genet* 13:61, 1978

406. CEDERBAUM SD, SHAW KNF, SPECTOR EB, VERITY MA, SNODGRASS PJ, SUGARMAN GI: Hyperargininemia with arginase deficiency. *Pediatr Res* 13:827, 1979

407. QURESHI IA, LETARTE J, OUELLET R, LELIEVRE M, LABERGE C: Ammonia metabolism in a family affected by hyperargininemia. *Diabet Metabol* 7:5, 1981

408. SNYDERMAN SE, SANSARICQ C, CHEN WJ, NORTON PM, PHANSALKAR SV: Argininemia. *J Pediatr* 90:563, 1977

409. PERALTA SERRANO A: Argininuria, convulsiones y oligofrenia; un nuevo error innato del metabolismo? *Rev Clin Esp* 97:176, 1965

410. YASHINO M: Personal communication to R Guthrie

411. MARESCAU B, PINTENS J, LOWENTHAL A, TERHEGGEN HG, ADRIANSSENS K: Arginase and free amino acids in hyperargininemia: Leukocyte arginine as a diagnostic parameter for heterozygotes. *J Clin Chem Clin Biochem* 17:211, 1979

412. VAN ELSEN A, LEROY JG: Human hyperargininemia: A mutation not expressed in skin fibroblasts? *Am J Hum Genet* 29:350, 1977

413. SPECTOR EB, KIERNAN M, BERNARD B, CEDERBAUM SD: Properties of fetal and adult red blood cell arginase deficiency. *Am J Hum Genet* 32:79, 1980

414. TERHEGGEN HG, LOWENTHAL A, LAVINHA F, COLOMBO JP: Familial hyperargininaemia. *Arch Dis Child* 50:57, 1975

415. CEDERBAUM SD, MOEDJONO SJ, SHAW KNF, NAYLOR E, WALSER M, CARTER M: Treatment of hyperargininemia due to arginase deficiency with a chemically defined diet. *J Inher Metab Dis*, in press

416. NAYLOR EW, CEDERBAUM SD: Urinary pyrimidine excretion in arginase deficiency. *J Inher Metab Dis* 4:207, 1981

417. MARESCAU B, PINTENS J, LOWENTHAL A, TERHEGGEN HG: Excretion of alpha-keto-gamma-guanidinovaleric acid and its cyclic form in patients with hyperargininemia. *Clin Chim Acta* 98:35, 1979

418. WIECHERT P, MORTELMANS J, LAVINHA F, CLARA R, TERHEGGEN HG, LOWENTHAL A: Excretion of guanidino-derivatives in urine of hyperargininemic patients. *J Genet Hum* 24:61, 1976

419. MORI A, MATSUMOTO M, HIRAMATSU C: Alpha-guanidinoglutaric acid in urine of arginine-loaded rabbits. *IRCS Med Sci: Biochem* 8:75, 1980

420. STEIN IM, COHEN BD, KORNHAUSER RS: Guanidinosuccinic acid in renal failure, experimental azotemia and inborn errors of the urea cycle. *N Engl J Med* 280:926, 1969

421. SPECTOR EB, RICE SCH, CEDERBAUM SD: Evidence for two genes encoding human arginase. *Am J Hum Genet* 32:55A, 1980

422. SOBERON G, PALACIOS R: Arginase, in Grisolia S, Báguena R, Mayor F (eds): *The Urea Cycle*. New York, John Wiley & Sons, Inc, 1976, p 221

423. POREMBSKA Z, BARANCZYK A, JACHIMOWICZ J: Arginase isoenzymes in liver and kidney of some mammals. *Acta Biochim Polon* 18:77, 1971

424. VAN ELSEN A: Krebs-Henseleit urea cycle in cultured human diploid fibroblasts. *Arch Int Physiol Biochim* 83:204, 1975

425. TERHEGGEN HG, LOWENTHAL A, LAVINHA F, COLOMBO JP, ROGERS S: Unsuccessful trial of gene replacement in arginase deficiency. *Z Kinderheilk* 119:1, 1975

426. PARDRIDGE WM: Lysine supplementation in hyperargininemia. *J Pediatr* 91:1032, 1977

427. ADRIAENSSENS K, KARCHER D, LOWENTHAL A, TERHEGGEN HG: Use of enzyme-loaded erythrocytes in in-vitro correction of arginase-deficient erythrocytes in familial hyperargininemia. *Clin Chem* 22:323, 1976

428. BEAUDET AJ: Personal communication

429. MOEDJONO SJ, SHAW KN, CEDERBAUM SD: A chemically defined diet for the treatment of hyperargininemia due to arginase deficiency. *Pediatr Res* 13:432, 1979

430. QURESHI IA, LETARTE J, OUELLET R, LELIEVRE M: Sodium benzoate therapy and dietary control in hyperargininemia. *Pediatr Res* 15:638, 1981

431. RAIJMAN L: Double deficiencies of urea cycle enzymes in human liver. *Biochem Med* 24:226, 1979

432. MATSUSHIMA A, TAGA T, ORII T, MATSUDA Y, TSUJI A, KATSUNUMA N: Hyperammonemia due to ornithine transcarbamylase deficiency accompanied by decreased activity of carbamylphosphate synthetase. *Brain Dev (Japan)* 11:343, 1979

433. SOGAWA H, OYANAGI K, NAKAO T: Periodic hyperammonemia, hyperlysinemia, and homocitrullinemia associated with decreased argininosuccinate synthetase and arginase activities. *Pediatr Res* 11:949, 1977

434. SOGAWA H: Studies on the etiology of hyperammonemia associated with inborn errors of amino acid metabolism, part 1: Etiology of hyperammonemia associated with disorder of lysine metabolism. *Sapporo Med J* 47:204, 1978

435. PERHEENTUPA J, VISAKORPI JK: Protein intolerance with deficient transport of basic amino acids. *Lancet* 2:813, 1965

436. SIMELL O, PERHEENTUPA J, RAPOLA J, VISAKORPI JK, ESKELIN L-E: Lysinuric protein intolerance. *Am J Med* 59:229, 1975

437. WHELAN DT, SCRIVER CR: Hyperdibasicaminoaciduria: An inherited disorder of amino acid transport. *Pediatr Res* 2:525, 1968

438. OYANAGI K, MIURA R, YAMANOUCHI T: Congenital lysinuria: A new inherited transport disorder of dibasic amino acids. *J Pediatr* 77:259, 1970

439. KATO T, TANAKA E, HORISAWA S: Hyperdibasicaminoaciduria and hyperammonemia in familial protein intolerance. *Am J Dis Child* 130:1340, 1976

440. SOGAWA H: Studies on the etiology of hyperammonemia associated with inborn errors of amino acid metabolism, part 2: Etiology of hyperammonemia associated with hyperdibasic aminoaciduria. *Sapporo Med J* 47:215, 1978

441. ENDRES W, ZCULEK G, SCHAUB J: Hyperdibasicaminoaciduria in a Turkish infant without evident protein intolerance. *Eur J Pediatr* 131:33, 1979

442. AWRICH AE, STACKHOUSE WJ, CANTRELL JE, PATTERSON JH, RUDMAN D: Hyperdibasic aminoaciduria, hyperammonemia and growth retardation: Treatment with arginine, lysine and citrulline. *J Pediatr* 87:731, 1975

443. CHAN H, BILLMEIER GJ JR, MOLINARY SV, TUCKER HN, SHIN BC, SCHAFFER A, CAVALLO K: Prolonged coma and isoelectric electroencephalogram in a child with lysinuric protein intoleracnce. *J Pediatr* 91:79, 1977

444. DESJEUX J-F, RAJANTIE J, SIMELL O, DUMONTIER A-M, PERHEENTUPA J: Lysine fluxes across the jejunal epithelium in lysinuric protein intolerance. *J Clin Invest* 65:1382, 1980

445. CARSON NA, REDMOND OA: Lysinuric protein intolerance. *Ann Clin Biochem* 14:135, 1977

446. ANDRIA G, SEBASTIO G, STRISCIUGLIO P, DEL GIUDICE E: Lysinuric protein intolerance: Possible genetic heterogeneity? *J Inher Metab Dis* 4:151, 1981

447. KIHARA H, VALENTE M, PORTER MT, FLUHARTY AL: Hyperdibasicaminoaciduria in a mentally retarded homozygote with a peculiar response to phenothiazines. *Pediatrics* 51:223, 1973

448. MALMQUIST J, JAGENBURG R, LANDSTEDT G: Familial protein intolerance: Possible nature of enzyme defect. *N Engl J Med* 284:997, 1971

449. RAJANTIE J, RAPOLA J, SIIMES MA: Ferritinemia with subnormal iron stores in lysinuric protein intolerance. *Metabolism* 30:3, 1981

450. OYANAGI K, SOGAWA H, MINAMI R, NAKAO T, CHIBA T: Mechanism of hyperammonemia in congenital lysinuria. *J Pediatr* 94:255, 1979

451. KEKOMÄKI M, TOIVAKKA E, HÄKKINEN V, SALASPURO M: Familial protein intolerance with deficient transport of basic amino acids: report on an adult patient with chronic hyperammonemia. *Acta Med Scand* 183:357, 1968

452. RAJANTIE J, SIMELL O, RAPOLA J, PERHEENTUPA J: Lysinuric protein intolerance—a 2-year trial of dietary supplementation therapy with citrulline and lysine. *J Pediatr* 97:927, 1980

453. BROWN JH, FABRE IF JR, FARRELL GL, ADAMS ED: Hyperlysinuria with hyperammonemia. *Am J Dis Child* 124:127, 1972

454. RAJANTIE J, SIMELL O, PERHEENTUPA J: Intestinal absorption in lysinuric protein intolerance. *J Br Soc Gastroenterol—Gut* 21:519, 1980

455. RAJANTIE J, SIMELL O, PERHEENTUPA J: Basolateral-membrane transport defect for lysine in lysinuric protein intolerance. *Lancet* 1:1219, 1980

456. SIMELL O, PERHEENTUPA J: Renal handling of diamino acids in lysinuric protein intolerance. *J Clin Invest* 54:9, 1974

457. RAJANTIE J, SIMELL O, PERHEENTUPA J: Lysinuric protein intolerance: Basolateral transport defect in renal tubuli. *J Clin Invest* 67:1078, 1981

458. SIMELL O: Diamino acid transport into granulocytes and liver slices of patients with lysinuric protein intolerance. *Pediatr Res* 9:504, 1975

459. KEKOMÄKI M: *Familial Protein Intolerance: Studies on an Inborn Error of Metabolism and Related Biochemical Problems*, thesis. University of Helsinki, 1969

460. KEKOMÄKI M: Enzymes of urea synthesis in familial protein intolerance with deficient transport of basic amino acids. *Acta Paediatr Scand* 56:631, 1967

461. KEKOMÄKI MP, RÄIHÄ NCR, BICKEL H: Ornithine-ketoacid aminotransferase in human liver with reference to patients with hyperornithinemia and familial protein intolerance. *Clin Chim Acta* 23:203, 1969

462. SIMELL O, PERHEENTUPA J: Defective metabolic clearance of plasma arginine and ornithine in lysinuric protein intolerance. *Metabolism* 23:691, 1974

463. KEKOMÄKI M, VISAKORPI JK, PERHEENTUPA J, SAXEN L: Familial protein intolerance with deficient transport of basic amino acids. An analysis of 10 patients. *Acta Paediatr Scand* 56:617, 1967

464. NORIO R, PERHEENTUPA J, KEKOMÄKI M, VISAKORPI JK: Lysinuric protein intolerance, an autosomal recessive disease: A genetic study of 10 Finnish families. *Clin Genet* 2:214, 1971

465. MÄKELÄ AL, LANG H, KORPELA P: Toxic encephalopathy with hyperammonemia during high dose salicylate therapy. *Acta Neurol Scand* 61:146, 1980

466. RÄIHÄ NCR, KEKOMÄKI M: Development of the ornithine-urea cycle, in Stave U (ed): *Perinatal Physiology*. New York, Plenum Publishing Corp, 1978, p 547

467. NAKAMURA K: Studies on urea cycle enzyme in human fetal livers. *Sapporo Med J* 47:127, 1978

468. OYANAGI K, NAKAMURA K, SOGAWA H, TSUKAZAKI H, MINAMI R, NAKAO

T: Study of urea synthesizing enzymes in prenatal and postnatal human liver. *Pediatr Res* 14:236, 1980

469. GAUTIER C, VAILLANT R: Post natal changes in carbamyl phosphate synthetase I and ornithine transcarbamylase activities after normal birth, premature delivery and prolonged gestation in rat liver: Effects of actinomycin D and glucose. *Biol Neonate* 35:298, 1979

470. GAUTIER C, VAILLANT R: Regulation of ornithine transcarbamylase activity in neonatal rat liver. *Biochem Biophys Res Commun* 98:51, 1981

471. CATHELINEAU L, RABIER D, PETIT F, KAMOUN P: Physiological and hormonal variations of acetylglutamate and citrullinogenesis in rat liver mitochondria: Development of foetus and neonates; variation in pregnant and post partum females; rapid effect of glucagon in adult males. *Enzyme* 26:245, 1981

472. BATSHAW ML, BRUSILOW SW: Asymptomatic hyperammonemia in low birth weight infants. *Pediatr Res* 12:221, 1978

473. GOLDBERG RN, CABAL LA, SINATRA FR, PLAJSTEK CE, HODGMAN JE: Hyperammonemia associated with perinatal asphyxia. *Pediatrics* 64:336, 1979

474. POLLACK L, HANSEN T, ADAMS J JR, BEAUDET A: Transient hyperammonemia in term and preterm infants. *Pediatr Res* 12:532, 1978

475. STEPANEK J: Hypercapnic hyperammonemia. *Lung* 154:149, 1977

476. DONN SM, SWARTZ RD, THOENE JG: Transient hyperammonemia of prematurity (THP): Response to hemodialysis (HD). *Pediatr Res* 15:658, 1981

477. LEGUENNEC JC, QURESHI IA, BARD H, SIRIEZ JY, LETARTE J: Transient hyperammonemia in an early preterm infant. *J Pediatr* 96:470, 1980

478. QURESHI IA, LETARTE J, OUELLET R, BARD H: The cause of transient hyperammonemia in an early preterm infant. *Biol Neonate,* in press

479. ROSENTHAL P, VINOCUR B: Neonatal hyperammonemia letter. *J Pediatr* 94:847, 1979

480. TOLLEFSEN SE, McCABE ER, GOODMAN SI: Neonatal hyperammonemia letter. *Pediatrics* 65:1197, 1980

481. HEIRD WC, WINTERS RW: Total parenteral nutrition: The state of the art. *J Pediatr* 86:2, 1975

482. SANCHEZ R, UKRAINSKI C, PERLIN B, FARBER S, GOLDFINGER D, POMERANCE J: Hyperammonemia in low birth weight infants. *Pediatr Res* 12:534, 1978

483. NYHAN WL: Heritable metabolic disease in the differential diagnosis of asphyxia, in Gluck L (ed): *Intrauterine Asphyxia and the Developing Fetal Brain.* Chicago, Year Book Medical Publishers, Inc, 1977, p 421

21

THE HYPERLYSINEMIAS

This summary is adapted from a summary written by H. Ghadimi for the fourth edition of this book [1].

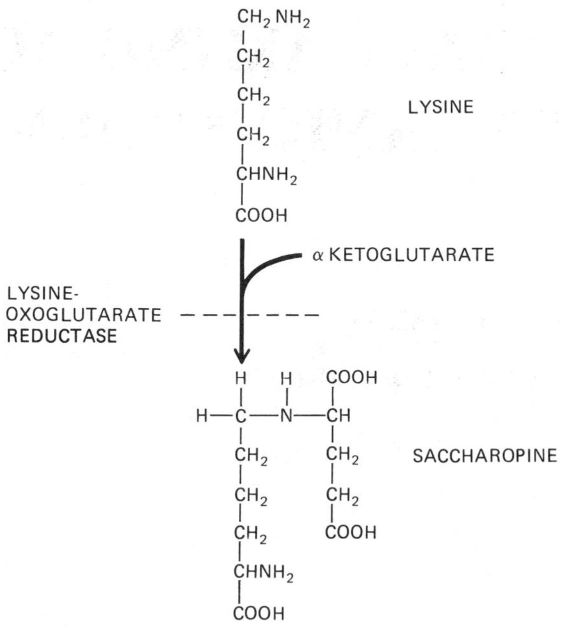

Figure 21-1 The metabolic block in one form of hyperlysinemia, persistent hyperlysinemia, involves a deficiency of the enzyme that converts lysine and α-ketoglutarate to saccharopine.

1. *Two types of hyperlysinemia have been described: (1) periodic hyperlysinemia associated with hyperammonemia, and (2) persistent hyperlysinemia without hyperammonemia. Both of these rare disorders are believed to result from defects in enzymes that participate in the catabolic pathway by which lysine is converted to acetoacetyl CoA.*

2. *In periodic hyperlysinemia, normal protein intake results in hyperlysinemia within a short time. The elevated level of lysine, in turn, inhibits the last step of urea formation by competitive inhibition of arginase. Hyperammonemia ensues. The hyperammonemia and its clinical manifestations are reversed by fluid therapy and dietary restriction of protein. On the other hand, high protein intake or administration of a lysine load will precipitate severe crises and coma. A partial deficiency (25 percent) of L-lysine dehydrogenase, the enzyme that converts lysine to a α-keto-ε-aminocaproic acid, has been demonstrated in a liver biopsy from a single patient (a 3-month-old girl). No information is available on the genetics of this rare disorder.*

3. *Approximately 12 cases of persistent hyperlysinemia have been reported. The clinical and biochemical abnormalities in these patients have varied widely, and there is no firm evidence that the hyperlysinemia is responsible for the clinical disturbances. Some patients have been severely retarded, while others have had normal intelligence. The salient biochemical feature of all patients is the persistence of hyperlysinemia and hyperlysinuria without hyperammonemia. When patients are given an oral load of lysine, metabolites of*

the catabolic pathway of lysine metabolism may appear in biologic fluids, but hyperammonemia does not occur.

4. *Persistent hyperlysinemia is believed to be inherited as an autosomal recessive trait, as judged by a high frequency of consanguinity among the parents of affected children. Isotopic studies of lysine metabolism in vivo and in cultured fibroblasts suggest that the basic defect is a deficiency of the activity of the first enzyme responsible for the degradation of lysine, i.e., lysine: α-ketoglutarate reductase, which converts lysine and α-ketoglutarate to saccharopine. Several patients have been reported to have an additional deficiency in the activity of the enzyme responsible for the second step in the degradation of lysine, i.e., saccharopine dehydrogenase, which converts saccharopine to α-amino-adipic-6-semialdehyde and glutamate. The genetic basis for a defect in these two sequential enzymes has not been defined.*

REFERENCES

1. Ghadimi H: The hyperlysinemias, in Stanbury JB, Wyngaarden JB, Fredrickson DS (eds): *The Metabolic Basis of Inherited Disease,* ed 4. New York, McGraw-Hill Book Co, 1978, p 387
2. Dancis J, Hutzler J, Cox RP: Familial hyperlysinemia: Enzyme studies, diagnostic methods, comments on terminology. *Am J Hum Genet* 31:290, 1979

22

DISORDERS OF BRANCHED CHAIN AMINO ACID AND ORGANIC ACID METABOLISM

KAY TANAKA

LEON E. ROSENBERG

1. *The branched chain amino acids (BCAAs), leucine, isoleucine, and valine, are neutral aliphatic amino acids with a 4- or 5-carbon skeleton and a branched methyl group at the 3 or 4 position. They are catabolized by analogous mechanisms for the first three steps: transamination of the parent amino acid, oxidative decarboxylation of the branched chain 2-keto acid (BCKA), and dehydrogenation of the resulting branched chain acyl CoA to enoyl CoA.*

2. *Transamination of BCAAs is catalyzed by one or more enzymes in the cytosol of extrahepatic tissue cells. Oxidative decarboxylation of the resultant BCKAs is catalyzed by an enzyme complex, the branched chain 2-keto acid dehydrogenase (BCKADH) complex, which is localized mainly in liver and kidney. This enzyme complex is composed of three component enzymes: BCKA decarboxylase (E_{1b}); dihydrolipoyl transacylase (E_{2b}), and dihydrolipoyl dehydrogenase (E_3). The third step in metabolism of BCAAs is catalyzed by two distinct branched chain acyl CoA dehydrogenases; one oxidizes isovaleryl CoA exclusively and the other oxidizes both isobutyryl CoA and 2-methylbutyryl CoA.*

3. *Because of the peculiar tissue distribution patterns of the first two enzymes, the catabolism of the BCAAs plays an important role in the regulation of body fuel metabolism, as conceptualized in the modified glucose-alanine cycle.*

4. *Nine known inherited metabolic disorders are due to deficiencies of enzymes in the pathway of BCAA metabolism. These are hypervalinemia, hyperleucine-isoleucinemia, maple syrup urine disease (MSUD), isovaleric acidemia, glutaric aciduria type II, ethylmalonic-adipic aciduria, 3-methylcrotonyl CoA carboxylase deficiency, 3-hydroxy-3-methylglutaryl CoA lyase deficiency, and 3-ketothiolase deficiency. Jamaican vomiting sickness, an acquired metabolic disorder, also involves a defect in the metabolic pathways of the three BCKAs. Many of these disorders share a clinical picture highlighted by metabolic acidosis, hypoglycemia, and developmental retardation. All appear to be inherited as autosomal recessive traits except for glutaric aciduria type II. Diagnosis of four conditions is aided by the presence of peculiar and specific odors of the patient or urine: "maple syrup" in MSUD, "sweaty feet" in isovaleric acidemia and glutaric aciduria type II, and "tomcat's urine" in 3-methylcrotonyl CoA carboxylase deficiency.*

5. *Hypervalinemia, hyperleucine-isoleucinemia, and MSUD can be diagnosed by amino acid analysis since the parent amino acid(s) accumulate in these disor-*

ders. In patients with the remaining diseases of BCAA catabolism, the enzyme deficiency is located at an intermediary step, resulting in the accumulation of organic acids (organic acidemias) which can be detected and identified by gas chromatography or gas chromatography–mass spectrometry.

6. Hypervalinemia (one case reported) and hyperleucine-isoleucinemia (two sibs reported) are both characterized by developmental retardation. The separate occurrence of these two defects suggests the existence of at least two substrate-specific BCAA transaminases, one for valine and the other for leucine-isoleucine.

7. MSUD is characterized by ketoacidosis and in some cases by developmental retardation. Five distinct clinical phenotypes have been recognized: classic, intermittent, intermediate, thiamine-responsive, and E3 deficiency. Each of these is due to deficient activity of the BCKADH complex. In classic MSUD two genetic complementation groups have been identified, at least one of which results from deficiency of the decarboxylase (E1). Some patients with the intermittent type appear to be compound heterozygotes, having inherited two different mutant alleles at the same locus.

8. Isovaleric acidemia is characterized by episodic ketoacidosis and, in some cases, developmental delay. Neutropenia and thrombocytopenia are often observed in severe ketoacidotic episodes. Severity in the neonatal period differs greatly from patient to patient. While 50 percent of the patients with this disease die in the neonatal period, those who survive subsequently follow a mild intermittent course. The disease is caused by deficiency of isovaleryl CoA dehydrogenase, which results in the excessive urinary excretion of isovalerylglycine (glycine conjugate of isovaleryl CoA) and episodic accumulation of isovaleric acid causing acute attacks. Despite the wide range of clinical severity, no convincing evidence for biochemical or genetic heterogeneity exists. The clinical variability appears to be due to differences in environment.

9. Glutaric aciduria type II (GA II) and ethylmalonic-adipic aciduria (EMA) are characterized by severe hypoglycemia and acidosis without ketosis. Several metabolic pathways, including those for BCAAs, fatty acids, lysine, hydroxylysine, and tryptophan, are blocked at an acyl CoA dehydrogenase step, causing a complex organic aciduria. Numerous short-chain fatty acids, hydroxy acids, and aliphatic dicarboxylic acids with C_4 to C_{10} carbon chains accumulate. Despite the deficiency of several acyl CoA dehydrogenase activities in vivo, the acyl CoA dehydrogenase enzymes are normal in vitro in patients with GA II. The activity of the electron-transferring flavoprotein (ETF), which accepts electrons from several acyl CoA dehydrogenases, is also normal. Thus, the precise enzyme defect remains obscure. A block in electron flow from ETF to coenzyme Q is likely.

10. Jamaican vomiting sickness is a lethal metabolic disorder caused by ingestion of an unripe local fruit, ackee. Extreme hypoglycemia and severe metabolic acidosis without ketosis are the main clinical fea-

tures. The same acyl CoA dehydrogenase activities which are deficient in patients with GA II and EMA are inhibited by methylenecyclopropylacetyl CoA, which is derived from a toxin, hypoglycin, contained in the fruit. This results in accumulation of the same organic acids as those detected in patients with GA II and EMA.

11. 3-Methylcrotonyl CoA carboxylase deficiency is usually observed as part of multiple carboxylase deficiency (Chap. 23). Only two patients suspected of having isolated 3-methylcrotonyl CoA carboxylase deficiency have been described. Clinical manifestations in these two children differed considerably: one had neurodegenerative symptoms similar to those of Werdnig-Hoffmann disease; the other presented with profound infantile metabolic acidosis.

12. 3-Hydroxy-3-methylglutaryl CoA lyase deficiency is characterized by episodes of extreme hypoglycemia and metabolic acidosis. Patients with this disease excrete 3-methylglutaconic and 3-methylglutaric acids, in addition to 3-hydroxy-3-methylglutaric acid.

13. Patients with 3-ketothiolase deficiency suffer attacks of metabolic ketoacidosis. Patients excrete increased amounts of several intermediates in the isoleucine pathway: 2-methylacetoacetic acid; its by-product, butanone; and its precursor, 2-methyl-3-hydroxybutyric acid. Some patients with this disorder constantly excrete the abnormal metabolites regardless of the presence or absence of ketosis. Others excrete the abnormal metabolites only when they are ketotic. While the metabolic basis for the former remains obscure, the latter is due to a deficiency of K^+-dependent acetoacetyl CoA 3-ketothiolase.

OVERVIEW

In 1954, Menkes, Hurst, and Craig described a family in which four of six infants died during the first weeks of life [1]. The prominent findings in these children were vomiting, muscular hypertonicity, and a maple syrup odor to the urine. In 1957, Westall, Dancis, and Miller reported an infant with brain damage, a similar odor to the urine, and increased levels of the branched chain amino acids (BCAAs) leucine, isoleucine, and valine in the blood and urine [2]. Since these initial observations on maple syrup urine disease (MSUD), eight additional enzymatic deficiencies concerned with the degradation of BCAAs have been identified, excluding disorders of propionate metabolism which are discussed in Chap. 23. These disorders are hypervalinemia [3], hyperleucine-isoleucinemia [4], isovaleric acidemia [5, 6], glutaric aciduria type II [7], ethylmalonic-adipic aciduria [8], 3-methylcrotonyl CoA carboxylase deficiency [9], 3-ketothiolase deficiency [10], and 3-hydroxy-3-methylglutaryl CoA (HMG CoA) lyase deficiency [11]. Jamaican vomiting sickness, an acquired disturbance, is also due to a metabolic block affecting, among other things, the pathway of BCAA metabolism [12]. The study of these metabolic disorders has provided considerable information relevant to the care of patients with these diseases; moreover, such study has contributed valuable insight into the reaction mechanisms and the nature of enzymes involved in BCAA metabolism.

The amino acids included in the category of BCAAs are leucine, isoleucine, and valine. All are essential, neutral, aliphatic amino acids with a 4- or 5-carbon skeleton and a branched methyl function at either the 3 or 4 position. Biochemically they are metabolized by analogous mechanisms for the first three steps of metabolism: transamination of the parent amino acids; oxidative decarboxylation of the 2-keto acids; and dehydrogenation of the resulting branched chain acyl CoAs (Fig. 22-1). Their degradative pathways then diverge.

The BCAAs play a unique role in metabolic regulation that

Figure 22-1 Metabolic pathways for the branched chain amino acids (leucine, isoleucine, valine). Wavy lines and circled numbers indicate sites 1 hypervalinemia; 2 hyperleucine-isoleucinemia; 3 maple syrup urine disease; 4 isovaleric acidemia; 5 glutaric aciduria type II, ethylmalonic-adipic aciduria, and Jamaican vomiting sickness; 6 3-methylcrotonyl CoA carboxylase deficiency; 7 3-hydroxy-3-methylglutaryl CoA lyase deficiency; and 8 3-ketothiolase deficiency.

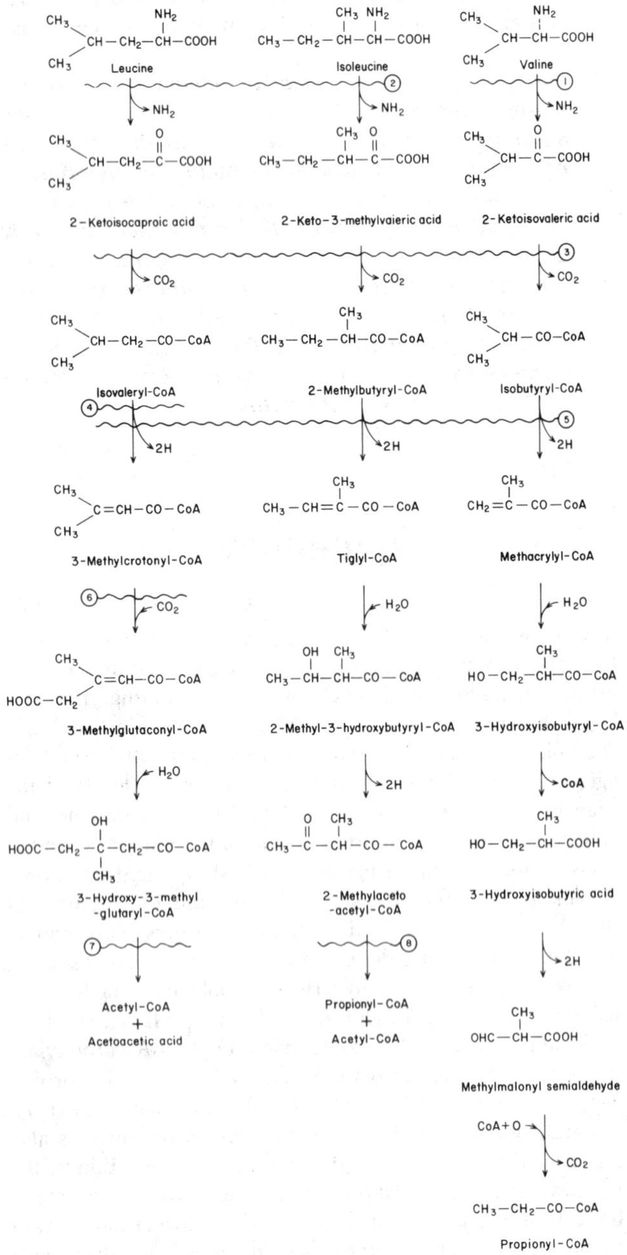

has become increasingly well understood since 1961. At that time Miller demonstrated that, while most amino acids were oxidized in the liver, the BCAAs were primarily oxidized in extrahepatic tissues [13]. It was subsequently shown that the first enzyme in the pathway, BCAA transaminase, is much more active in such extrahepatic tissues as kidney, heart, and skeletal muscle than in liver [14]. In contrast, the enzyme which catalyzes the oxidative decarboxylation of branched chain 2-keto acids (BCKAs) has much greater activity in liver and kidney than in other tissues [15–17]. Because of these peculiar patterns of tissue distribution, the transaminase step is rate-limiting in the metabolism of BCAAs in liver, while the 2-keto acid decarboxylation step is rate-limiting in heart and skeletal muscle [18–21]. Furthermore, BCKA decarboxylation is modulated by nutritional and endocrine stimuli [19–23] which affect the concentrations of glucose, pyruvate, glucagon, and epinephrine. Other factors also contribute to the key role of BCAAs in metabolic regulation. For instance, the transamination of BCAAs in muscle generates amino groups. Skeletal muscle, unlike liver, cannot synthesize urea from these amino groups because of a lack of the urea cycle enzymes. On the other hand, skeletal muscle is a major site of anaerobic and aerobic glycolysis, producing large amounts of pyruvic and 2-ketoglutaric acids which are converted to alanine and glutamic acid, respectively, by transamination that utilizes the amino groups from the BCAAs. The latter amino acids are then exported from muscle and utilized in liver as substrates for further oxidation or for gluconeogenesis, depending on the metabolic state of the individual. Thus, alanine production in muscle (via transamination with BCAAs) plays an important role in the maintenance of blood glucose. This mechanism has been called the "glucose-alanine cycle" [24] (Fig. 22-2). More recently, the importance of glutamate formation has been noted and a modification of the original glucose-alanine cycle has been proposed [25, 26]. This modification has been necessitated by the observation that pyruvic acid is a poor amino acceptor for BCAA transaminase [14]. Therefore, alanine formation in muscle must be mediated by two steps: first glutamate formation catalyzed by BCAA transaminase, then amino transfer from glutamate to pyruvate by the action of alanine transaminase [25] (Fig. 22-2).

Concurrently, important progress has been made in the study of inherited disorders of BCAAs. MSUD and hypervalinemia were discovered using amino acid chromatographic and dinitrophenylhydrazine (DNPH) precipitation methods [27]. However, discovery of inborn errors that affect reactions distal to keto acid formation was hampered because the organic acids that are produced by such reactions cannot be detected by the methods just mentioned. Patients with these "organic acidemias" were not identified until a reliable method for the detection of these organic acids became available [28], namely gas chromatography (GC) and mass spectrometry coupled with GC (GC/MS). In 1966, the first two sibs with an inborn error of organic acid metabolism, isovaleric acidemia, were identified by Tanaka et al. using this methodology [5, 6, 29]. Since then, many other inborn errors of organic acid metabolism have been similarly discovered [7–11, 30, 31]. These techniques also facilitated studies on BCAA metabolism using compounds labeled with stable isotopes. The recent studies on the mechanisms of several steps in the valine pathway [32–35] and on those of the R pathway of isoleucine metabolism [36–38] are examples of such applications.

The study of disorders of BCAA metabolism has also pro-

Figure 22-1 (chemical pathway diagram)

Leucine pathway:
Leucine → 2-Ketoisocaproic acid → Isovaleryl-CoA → 3-Methylcrotonyl-CoA → 3-Methylglutaconyl-CoA → 3-Hydroxy-3-methyl-glutaryl-CoA → Acetyl-CoA + Acetoacetic acid

Isoleucine pathway:
Isoleucine → 2-Keto-3-methylvaleric acid → 2-Methylbutyryl-CoA → Tiglyl-CoA → 2-Methyl-3-hydroxybutyryl-CoA → 2-Methylaceto-acetyl-CoA → Propionyl-CoA + Acetyl-CoA

Valine pathway:
Valine → 2-Ketoisovaleric acid → Isobutyryl-CoA → Methacrylyl-CoA → 3-Hydroxyisobutyryl-CoA → 3-Hydroxyisobutyric acid → Methylmalonyl semialdehyde → Propionyl-CoA

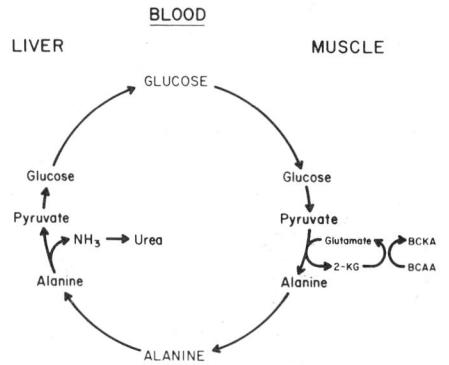

BLOOD

LIVER   MUSCLE

Figure 22-2 The modified glucose-alanine cycle. Abbreviations are as follows: BCAA, branched chain amino acid; BCKA, branched chain keto acid; 2-KG, 2-ketoglutaric acid. (*Adapted from Felig [24].*)

vided important information on the nature of some enzymes in these pathways. For example, results from studies on MSUD led Petit et al. [39] to isolate branched chain 2-keto acid dehydrogenase (BCKADH), and those from studies on isovaleric acidemia enabled Tanaka and associates to identify and purify isovaleryl CoA dehydrogenase [40, 41].

Finally, considerable progress has been made in recent years in clinically relevant areas. These include clarification of the molecular basis of the heterogeneity noted in MSUD [42, 43] and in 3-methylcrotonyl CoA carboxylase deficiency [44, 45]. They include new modes of therapy as well, such as the use of thiamine in MSUD [46], of biotin in biotin-responsive 3-methylcrotonyl CoA carboxylase deficiency (multiple carboxylase deficiency) [44], and of glycine in isovaleric acidemia [47].

METABOLISM OF THE BCAAs

Three Common Steps (Transamination, Oxidative Decarboxylation, and Acyl CoA Dehydrogenation)

The three BCAAs are metabolized in an analogous manner for the first three steps. These steps are the transamination to 2-keto analogues, the oxidative decarboxylation of the 2-keto acids to the saturated branched chain acyl CoAs, and the dehydrogenation of the saturated acyl CoAs to 2,3-unsaturated acyl CoAs (enoyl CoAs), as illustrated in Fig. 22-1. Because the BCAAs have similar chemical characteristics and are metabolized by analogous mechanisms at each of these three steps, investigators have long asked whether each of these steps is catalyzed by a single enzyme or by multiple enzymes specific for only one amino acid. This question is of particular importance for an understanding of the enzymatic basis of four inborn errors of metabolism: hypervalinemia, hyperleucine-isoleucinemia, MSUD, and isovaleric acidemia. The enzyme deficiencies in patients with MSUD and isovaleric acidemia appeared to be more specific than the substrate specificities of the pertinent enzymes isolated in the 1950s and 1960s. Studies on patients with these diseases provided biochemists with valuable guidelines for the purification of BCKADH and of isovaleryl CoA dehydrogenase.

Transamination

The finding that only valine accumulated in the single reported patient with hypervalinemia [3, 48] suggested that specific transaminases exist for individual BCAAs [49]. Biochemical data on BCAA transaminase(s) from experimental animals have not been in accord with this concept, however. Transaminases for BCAAs from the hearts of rats and pigs have been studied extensively by Ichihara and associates [14, 50–52] and by Taylor and Jenkins [53–55]. The transaminases from both species showed a shared specificity for leucine, valine, isoleucine, and glutamic acid as amino donors; no activity was found when alanine, phenylalanine, methionine, and other natural amino acids were used as amino donors [14, 54]. As an amino acceptor, 2-ketoglutarate was preferred and could not be replaced by either pyruvic or oxalacetic acid [54]. Therefore, the production of alanine from pyruvate and an amino group from BCAAs must proceed via glutamate formation and subsequent glutamate-pyruvate transamination [56]. The 2-keto analogues of leucine, isoleucine, and valine (2-ketoisocaproic, 2-keto-3-methylvaleric, and 2-ketoisovaleric acids, respectively) were almost as effective amino acceptors as 2-ketoglutarate, indicating that BCAA transamination is not only reversible but can occur among the BCAAs themselves via their 2-keto analogues.

Transaminase activity is high in heart, kidney, and skeletal muscle, but very low in liver [14, 55]. The specific activity in rat liver is only 0.5 to 1 percent of that in heart muscle [14]. In heart, most activity (65 percent and 80 percent in rat and pig, respectively) is found in the soluble fraction, but a significant amount of activity is also detectable in mitochondria [14, 55]. The enzyme from the cytoplasmic fraction of pig heart has been purified 440-fold to near homogeneity. Its molecular weight is 75,000 and 1 mol of the enzyme contains 1 mol of pyridoxal 5′-phosphate, which appears to be bound to an ε-amino group of a lysine residue. During the purification process the ratios of the relative specific activities for leucine, isoleucine, and valine remained constant, indicating that a single enzyme may be catalyzing transamination of the three BCAAs [54]. The K_m values of pig heart enzyme for leucine, isoleucine, and valine are 11.0, 3.8, and 3.8 mM, respectively. These are considerably higher than the known concentrations of these amino acids in human plasma (Leu, ~0.13 mM; Ile, ~0.07 mM; Val, ~0.25 mM) [5] and in rat heart (Leu, 0.14; Ile, 0.09; Val, 0.15 μmol per gram wet weight) [57]. It is not known whether more specific enzymes with lower K_m values exist.

Ichihara and associates also examined the mitochondrial transaminases from pig heart and other tissues. Transaminase from pig heart mitochondria was purified 250-fold. Its substrate specificity was similar to that of the pig heart cytoplasmic enzyme but it differed considerably in chromatographic and electrophoretic behavior. Its K_m values were approximately ten times higher and its V_{max} ten times lower than those of the cytosolic enzyme [51]. This suggests that its role in vivo is limited. More recently, a transaminase that utilizes leucine as an amino donor and glyoxylate as an amino acceptor has been isolated from rat liver peroxisomes [58, 59].

The existence of multiple transaminases is supported by recent somatic cell genetic studies by Naylor and associates using mutagenized Chinese hamster cells deficient in BCAA transaminases [60, 61]. These cells cannot grow in media in which BCAAs are replaced by their corresponding BCKAs [60, 62]. By selecting for somatic cell hybrids formed between these

Chinese hamster cells and several human lines, they obtained evidence for the existence of at least two human transaminase loci, one coded on chromosome 12 and the other on chromosome 19, each capable of catalyzing the transamination of the three BCAAs [62].

Oxidative Decarboxylation of the BCKAs

General Mechanisms: Pyruvate Dehydrogenase Complex as a Model   BCKAs produced from leucine, isoleucine, and valine are oxidatively decarboxylated through a sequence of complicated reactions, as illustrated in Fig. 22-3. This is the step at which the metabolism of the three BCAAs is blocked in patients with MSUD. Since this reaction is analogous to that of the pyruvate dehydrogenase (PDH) complex and that of the 2-ketoglutarate dehydrogenase (KGDH) complex which catalyze the conversion of pyruvate and 2-ketoglutarate to acetyl CoA and succinyl CoA, respectively, the structure and reaction mechanisms of BCKADH have been assumed to be similar to those of the PDH and KGDH complexes. This assumption has finally been substantiated by the isolation and characterization of the BCKADH [39]. Although knowledge about this enzyme

is not as detailed as that for the PDH complex (due, in part, to low BCKADH activity [63]), their similarity in structure and function is now clear [39]. Therefore, the structure and reaction mechanisms of the PDH complex are briefly summarized here as a model for the BCKADH complex.

The PDH complex has been purified and studied extensively in both bacteria and in mammalian tissues by Reed and associates as summarized in Chap. 9 and elsewhere [64, 65]. It catalyzes the conversion of pyruvate to acetyl CoA and consists of three tightly complexed enzymes. The PDH complex is located in the inner membrane of mitochondria. Thiamine pyrophosphate (TPP) and lipoamide are the essential prosthetic groups bound to the first (E_{1p}, pyruvate decarboxylase) and second (E_{2p}, dihydrolipoyl transacetylase) enzymes of the complex, respectively. CoA is also a required cofactor for the transacetylase. The initial step of the reaction is the transfer of the acetaldehyde unit from pyruvate to the TPP bound to E_{1p} (Fig. 22-3). This step removes CO_2 from the carboxyl group of pyruvate. In the second step, the "active acetaldehyde" thus

Figure 22-3   Sequence of reactions catalyzed by the branched chain keto acid dehydrogenase complex. Abbreviations are as follows: E_{1b}, BCKA decarboxylase; R, acyl chain; TPP, thiamine pyrophosphate; E_{2b}, dihydrolipoyl transacylase; Lip, lipoic acid; E_3, dihydrolipoyl dehydrogenase; and FAD, flavin adenine dinucleotide.

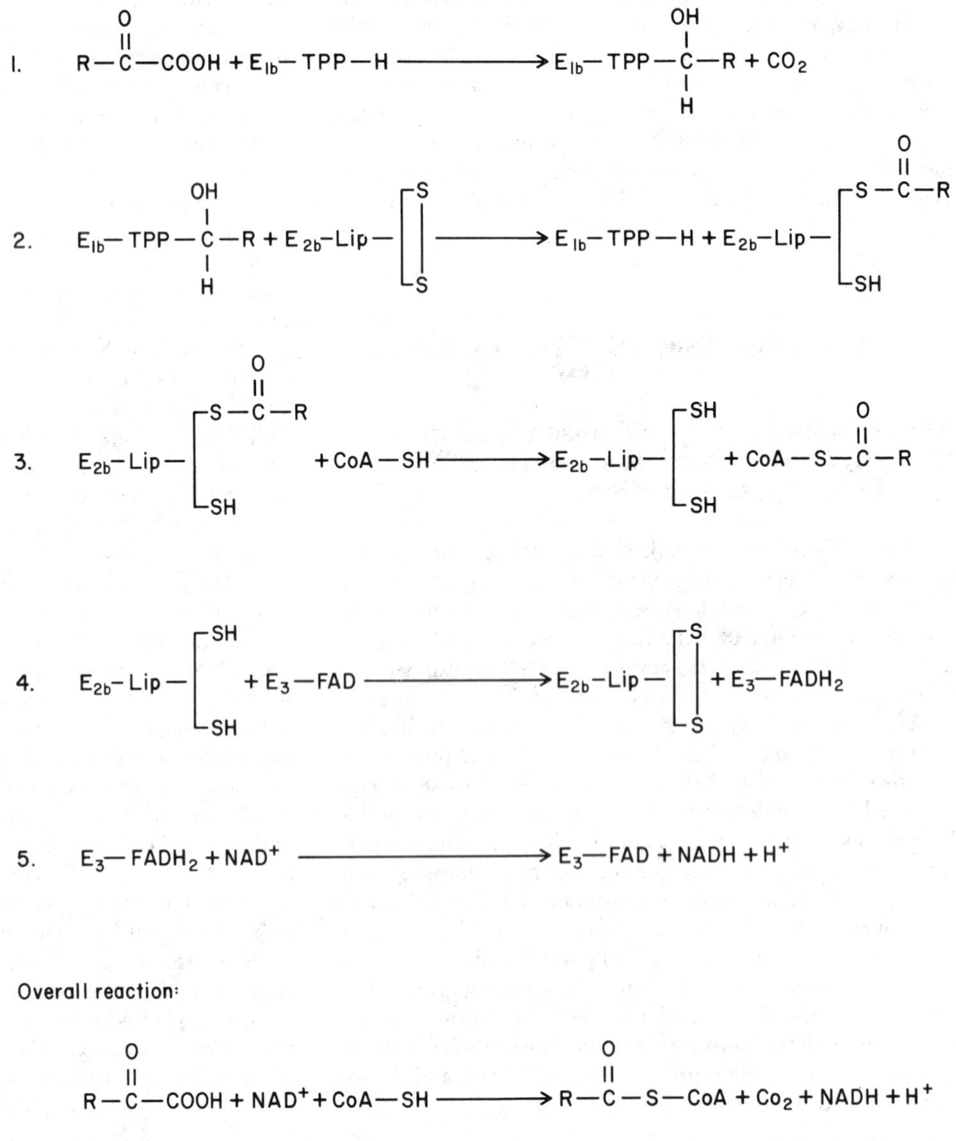

Overall reaction:

formed is transferred to a sulfhydryl (SH) group of a lipoamide unit that is linked to E_{2p}, thus forming acetyllipoamide. Finally, the acetyl group is transferred to an SH group of CoA, resulting in the formation of acetyl CoA. This reaction liberates the disulfhydryl form of lipoamide, which is subsequently reoxidized to the disulfide form by dihydrolipoyl dehydrogenase (E_3) [64, 65]. A single E_3 appears to serve both PDH and KGDH [66].

In addition to E_{1p}, E_{2p}, and E_3, two other enzymes are known to be components of the PDH complex. These are Mg^{2+} ATP-dependent pyruvate dehydrogenase kinase (PDH$_a$ kinase) and pyruvate dehydrogenase phosphatase (PDH$_b$ phosphatase). These two enzymes catalyze phosphorylation and dephosphorylation, respectively, of E_{1p}, thus comprising a regulatory system for the activity of the PDH complex [64].

Mammalian E_{1p} is an $\alpha_2\beta_2$ tetramer [67]. The α subunit (mol wt 40,000) catalyzes the first step of pyruvate decarboxylation, the formation of α-hydroxyethylthiamine pyrophosphate, and is the subunit that undergoes an inactivation-activation cycle by the phosphorylation-dephosphorylation process mentioned above. The β subunit (mol wt 30,000) catalyzes the second step, i.e., the reductive acetylation of the lipoyl moiety of E_{2p}. Mammalian E_2 is a monomer with a molecular weight of about 50,000. There are 60 E_{2p} molecules comprising the core of the PDH complex. The kinase is known to be attached to E_{2p}, but the site of attachment is not known. Although there is a disagreement concerning the number of other enzyme components, it has been generally agreed that up to 60 units each of E_{1p}, E_3, and E_{1p} kinase and phosphatase are organized in an ordered fashion with E_{2p} to form a functional unit. The molecular weight of the whole mammalian PDH complex is estimated to be 7.4 to 8.0 million [67–70], and one bovine kidney mitochondrion is said to contain about 15 molecules of this macromolecular complex [64].

The activity of the PDH complex is intricately and decisively regulated by tissue concentrations of substrates and products through the kinase-phosphatase cycle. PDH$_a$ kinase is stimulated by NADH, ATP, and acetyl CoA, the net result being formation of the inactive form (PDH$_b$). Conversely, ADP, NAD^+, free CoA, and TPP inhibit PDH$_a$ kinase activity. In addition, the response of PDH$_a$ kinase to the aforenamed effectors may be influenced by fluctuations in the levels of free Mg^{2+} and K^+. Thus, the PDH$_a$ kinase activity is modulated by changes in the intramitochondrial ATP/ADP ratio, NADH/NAD^+ ratio, and acetyl CoA/CoA ratio. Moreover, PDH is under substrate control, pyruvate being stimulatory, acetyl CoA being inhibitory [71, 72]. The overall activity of the complex can be assayed by measuring the formation of NADH spectrophotometrically in the presence of NAD^+, TPP, and CoA-SH as shown in Fig. 22-3. The first reaction (decarboxylation) can be measured separately using ferricyanide as the electron acceptor [73].

The BCKADH Complex Since 2-ketoisocaproic (KIC), 2-keto-3-methylvaleric (KMV), and 2-ketoisovaleric acid (KIV) accumulate in urine of patients with MSUD [27], it had long been speculated that these three keto acids are decarboxylated commonly by a single enzyme. This assumption was supported by the experimental observation that the enzyme activities which decarboxylate these three keto acids in rat liver were coinduced linearly and in constant proportion to each other by casein feeding [74]. Early attempts to purify and characterize this enzyme met with difficulties, however, and the

enigma—a single common enzyme or multiple specific enzymes—remained to be solved. Some of the observations which seemed to lend support to the multiple enzyme hypothesis, and which will be discussed in some detail to forestall confusion, may now be either discarded as insignificant or explained in the light of the new information.

Snyderman argued that the much greater elevation of plasma leucine concentration in patients with MSUD over that of isoleucine and valine could not be explained by the single common enzyme hypothesis [75]. The ratios of plasma valine vs. leucine and of isoleucine vs. leucine in 11 MSUD patients were 0.23 ± 0.19 (SD) and 0.47 ± 0.16 (SD), respectively. However, relative BCAA accumulation could reflect different intakes of these essential amino acids. Moreover, the relatively small accumulation of isoleucine could be explained in part by its conversion to alloisoleucine [76, 77], and that of valine by the fact that, unlike KIC and KMV, KIV is converted to 2-hydroxyisovaleric acid and excreted in the urine. The amount of urinary KIV in patients with MSUD is only 10 to 30 percent of that of 2-hydroxyisovaleric acid [78–80]. In contrast, the amounts of the hydroxyl analogues of KIC and KMV are very small.

Connelly, Danner, and Bowden [16, 81] isolated an enzyme complex capable of catalyzing the oxidative decarboxylation of both KIC and KMV from bovine liver, with an overall purification of 67-fold over crude homogenates. The K_m values of this enzyme for KIC and KMV were 3.5 mM and 2.5 mM, respectively, but the enzyme was totally inactive with KIV. Retrospectively, the K_m values of this enzyme for KIC and KMV are more than 50 times higher than those of the enzyme purified by Petit et al. [39] and almost 200 times higher than the KIC concentration in rat liver [82]. Therefore, it is unlikely that the enzyme purified by Connelly and associates plays any significant role in BCKA metabolism under physiologic conditions.

Other efforts to purify BCKADH were initially unsuccessful. Parker and Randle [83, 84] and Danner et al. [63, 85] were unable to achieve more than a 25-fold enrichment of BCKADH activity from rat and bovine livers, but the pattern of the enrichment and the kinetic parameters obtained from their studies were consistent with the single enzyme hypothesis. Danner et al. [63] isolated BCKADH from bovine liver mitochondria in two forms; one a 275,000-dalton unit, and the other a 2×10^6-dalton component. Both showed a characteristic flavin spectrum and catalyzed all functions of the complex; this suggested that ten small units aggregated into the large unit, as in the case of PDH. The large complex was visible under electron microscopy and had a diameter ranging from 12 to 24 nm, corresponding to a molecular weight of 2×10^6.

BCKADH was finally purified 280-fold in 1978 from bovine kidney mitochondria by Petit et al. [39] using a simple, elegant procedure. The most important observation made in this study was that, unlike PDH and KGDH, E_3 was readily dissociated from the rest of the complex and it was necessary to add E_3 from PDH to the assay mix to obtain maximal activity. (Loss of E_3 may have been the problem which plagued other investigators.) This observation indicated that BCKADH shares a common E_3 with PDH and KGDH, a conclusion supported by genetic evidence from a study on a patient with dihydrolipoyl dehydrogenase deficiency [43, 86]. The existence of three subunits with molecular weights of 46,000, 35,000, and 52,000, respectively, was demonstrated. The first two are the subunits of the decarboxylase (or dehydrogenase; E_{1b}) and the third was E_{2b}. These results indicate that BCKADH has a structure very similar to that of PDH (Fig. 22-3, Table 22-1). The activity of this complex was totally dependent on the availability of CoA-SH, thiamine pyrophosphate (TPP), and NAD^+. A lipoyl moiety appears to be covalently attached to the transacylase. The complex exhibited marked product inhibition by isobutyryl CoA, isovaleryl CoA, and NADH.

The BCKADH studied by Petit et al. [39] was not inactivated under conditions that resulted in the relatively rapid phosphorylation-inactivation of the bovine kidney PDH complex, namely incubation with PDH kinase and ATP. More recent studies indicate that in heart and skeletal muscle mitochondria, BCKADH activity can be activated as much as twentyfold by depleting ATP [87–89], and the activated enzyme can be inhibited by incubation with ATP. Direct evidence for the phosphorylated enzyme has also been presented [90]. There is controversy as to whether BCKADH is activated in liver and kidney as well [87, 88]. It is also not known whether a specific kinase is necessary for phosphorylation of this enzyme. In summary, BCKADH is controlled by two basic mechanisms, namely product inhibition and phosphorylation-dephosphorylation. In addition, this enzyme complex can be stabilized against thermal and chymotryptic inactivation via a conformational change conferred by adding saturating amounts of TPP [91]. It has been postulated that TPP can increase the biologic half-life of BCKADH in vivo by this mechanism [85, 92, 93].

In general, the activity of BCKADH is high in the liver and kidney, but until recently its activity was believed to be quite low in heart and skeletal muscle [15–17]. This distribution is in sharp contrast to that of the BCAA transaminase. The different tissue distributions of the first two enzymes in the BCAA pathway caused speculation that 2-keto acids produced in extrahepatic tissues are transported to the liver for futher oxidation. Recent evidence indicates that the amount of BCKADH in the extrahepatic tissues may have been grossly underestimated for two reasons: first, the BCKADH in heart and skeletal muscle is present primarily in an inactive phosphorylated form the activity of which is only one-twentieth that of the active form [87–89]; second, the methods of cell disruption that were utilized in the preparation of muscle homogenates were destructive of the enzyme [56, 94]. Thus, BCKADH activity in heart and skeletal muscle may, in fact, be much higher than previously believed. Even after careful reexamination and consideration of all of these factors, BCKADH

still appears to be the rate-limiting step in BCAA metabolism in muscle [56, 95]. Considerable amounts of BCKAs are released into the incubation media after muscle homogenates or mitochondria are incubated with leucine [56] or into perfusion media from perfused rat hind limbs [76].

BCKADH is located almost exclusively in mitochondria [56, 93, 96]. It was initially believed to be localized on the outer surface of the inner mitochondrial membrane [96]. More recent evidence indicates its localization on the inner surface of the inner membrane since the addition of NAD^+, ATP, and CoA does not enhance oxidative decarboxylation by intact mitochondria [97–100]. Concurrently, a number of branched chain acylcarnitines such as isovalerylcarnitine, 2-methylbutyrylcarnitine, and isobutyrylcarnitine were identified [101–103]; their biosynthesis in mitochondria [103] and the enhancement of BCAA and BCKA oxidation by carnitine were observed [98, 104]. This effect of carnitine was pronounced in muscle but was less noticeable in liver [99, 100, 104]. These observations initially led some investigators to hypothesize that carnitine stimulated BCKA oxidation by enhancing the transport of acyl CoAs into the mitochondrial matrix [101, 103, 104]. More recent evidence indicates that carnitine exerts this effect by converting isovaleryl CoA and other acyl CoAs to carnitine esters, thereby preventing their product inhibition of BCKADH. The significance of the effect of carnitine in vivo and the ultimate fate of acylcarnitine are not yet known. In patients with isovaleric acidemia in vivo [29] and in rat liver slices treated with hypoglycin in vitro [105], conjugation with glycine is the major system for removing excessive isovaleryl CoA via a glycine N-acylase present in mitochondria of liver and kidney [106–108]. It is possible that the branched chain acylcarnitines serve as vehicles for the interorgan transport of excessive acyl moieties or for conjugation with glycine in liver or kidney.

Keto-Enol Tautomerization: Formation of Alloisoleucine

Isoleucine is unique among the BCAAs; unlike leucine and valine, which contain only one chiral center (asymmetric carbon) at the α position, isoleucine contains two chiral centers at the α and β positions. Therefore there are four enantiomeric forms of isoleucine, as shown in Fig. 22-4 [109], but only L-isoleucine (2S,3S) is known to be present in normal humans [110, 111].

Early reports on plasma amino acids in patients with MSUD described a large unknown peak which was initially identified as methionine [2]. This peak was later identified as alloisoleucine (2S,3R) by Norton et al. [76, 77]. They proposed that L-alloisoleucine was formed in patients with MSUD via keto-enol tautomerization of 2-KMV ($3S \rightarrow 3R$) and subsequent transamination as illustrated in Fig. 22-5. The existence of this mechanism had previously been proposed from physicochemical and nutritional studies [112, 113]. More recently, the occurrence of KMV tautomerization was directly demonstrated by infusing a large amount of S(+)-2-KMV into normal dogs and following the relatively slow time course of change in optical rotation [114]. Matthews et al. also identified [^{15}N]alloisoleucine after infusion of [^{15}N]leucine into patients with MSUD [111]. Thus, it has now been shown unequivocally that accumulated S(+)-KMV can be converted to alloisoleucine via R(−)-KMV, but it is not known whether enolization in vivo

Table 22-1   Component enzymes of BCKADH complex

Enzymes	Molecular weight	Prosthetic group (P) and cofactors (C)
BCKA decarboxylase (E_{1b})		
α subunit	46,500	Thiamine pyrophosphate (P)
β subunit	35,000	
Dihydrolipoyl transacylase (E_{2b})	52,000	Lipoic acid (P), CoA (C)
Dihydrolipoyl dehydrogenase (E_3)	55,000	FAD (P), NAD^+ (C)
BCKADH kinase*		ATP (C), Mg^{2+} (C)
BCKADH phosphatase*		Ca^{2+} (C)

* BCKADH kinase and phosphatase have not been isolated but results of kinetic studies suggest their existence [90].

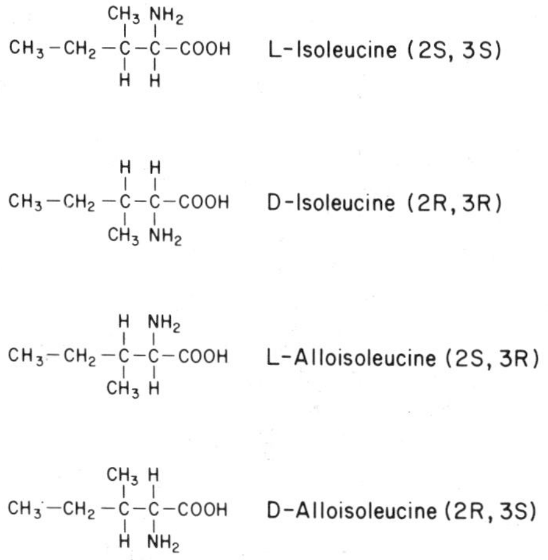

CH₃—CH₂—C—C—COOH   L-Isoleucine (2S, 3S)

CH₃—CH₂—C—C—COOH   D-Isoleucine (2R, 3R)

CH₃—CH₂—C—C—COOH   L-Alloisoleucine (2S, 3R)

CH₃—CH₂—C—C—COOH   D-Alloisoleucine (2R, 3S)

Figure 22-4 Four enantiomers of isoleucine.

occurs nonenzymatically or enzymatically [114] or whether it occurs under physiologic conditions. The R-series intermediates of isoleucine have been shown to be catabolized by a pathway (R pathway) which is different from that for the S-series intermediates [36–38]. Since there is no L-alloisoleucine in normal human tissues, the amount of R-series intermediates which might be produced depends totally on the rate of keto-enol tautomerization. Tanaka et al. [35] have shown, using valine chirally labeled with ^{13}C {(2RS,3S)[4-^{13}C]valine}, that keto-enol tautomerization does not occur to an appreciable degree in the metabolism of valine in rats in vivo when there is no accumulation of KIV. Thus the rate of enolization is too slow to occur under physiologic conditions in general. A similar study must be carried out using chirally labeled isoleucine.

Dehydrogenation of Branched Chain Acyl CoAs

Three branched chain acyl CoAs are produced from the corresponding 2-keto acids by the action of the BCKADH complex (Fig. 22-3). These are isovaleryl CoA (from leucine), 2-methylbutyryl CoA (from isoleucine), and isobutyryl CoA (from valine). These branched chain acyl CoAs had long been assumed to be dehydrogenated at the α and β carbons by a mechanism similar to that for straight-chain acyl CoAs such as butyryl CoA (see Fig. 22-6). The identity of the enzymes which catalyze the dehydrogenation of branched chain acyl CoAs were not known until recently.

In the early 1950s, Green, Mahler, and associates showed that there are three acyl CoA dehydrogenases. These are butyryl CoA dehydrogenase (BDH), general acyl CoA dehydrogenase (GADH), and long-chain acyl CoA dehydrogenase (LADH). BDH catalyzes the dehydrogenation of straight-chain acyl CoAs with 4 to 6 carbons; GADH those with 8 to 14 carbons; and LADH those with 8 to 16 carbons [115, 116]. Each of these acyl CoA dehydrogenases is a flavin-dependent enzyme with molecular weight of 155,000 to 166,000 comprising four identical subunits ($M_r = 38,500$ to 42,000), each containing one molecule of flavin adenine dinucleotide (FAD) [115, 116]. In the natural state, electron-transferring flavoprotein (ETF), another flavoprotein with a molecular weight of 58,000, is required to accept electrons from the dehydrogenase [115, 117] (Fig. 22-6). There is biochemical evidence for a sin-

gle ETF serving more than one dehydrogenase [117–119]. More recently, a sulfur-iron–containing flavoprotein (Fe-S-flavoprotein) has been identified from beef heart mitochondria [120, 121]. Fe-S-flavoprotein transmits electrons from the reduced ETF to coenzyme Q (Fig. 22-7). The Fe-S-flavoprotein is also called ETF dehydrogenase.

The branched chain acyl CoAs were initially believed to be dehydrogenated by BDH [122–124], but when the first two cases of isovaleric acidemia were discovered, only isovaleric acid [5] and its glycine conjugate (isovalerylglycine) [29] accumulated. Since other short-chain fatty acids such as n-butyric, isobutyric, and n-hexanoic acids and their conjugates did not accumulate in these patients, Tanaka et al. proposed that isovaleryl CoA was dehydrogenated by a specific enzyme, isovaleryl CoA dehydrogenase, and the patients with isovaleric acidemia were deficient in the activity of this enzyme [5, 29, 125]. This hypothesis was not substantiated by biochemical evidence until 1980. The delay was due partly to difficulties in assaying acyl CoA dehydrogenases in crude homogenates by the dye-reduction method [123]. It was also due to the far lower activity of isovaleryl CoA dehydrogenase than that of other acyl CoA dehydrogenases.

Rhead and Tanaka [126, 127] developed a new sensitive, specific tritium-release assay for acyl CoA dehydrogenases which utilizes appropriate [2,3-^{3}H]acyl CoAs (isovaleryl or butyryl CoAs) as substrates. The activity of acyl CoA dehydrogenases can then be assayed by measuring the amount of ^{3}H$_2$O released into the medium. Using this method, it was conclusively shown that isovaleryl CoA dehydrogenase in rat liver mitochondria can be separated from BDH and GADH by isoelectric focusing and DEAE-cellulose column chromatography [40], and that patients with isovaleric acidemia are deficient in this enzyme [126]. Furthermore, isovaleryl CoA dehydrogenase has recently been purified from rat liver mitochondria by Ikeda, Noda, and Tanaka [41]. This enzyme is an FAD enzyme with a molecular weight of 170,000. It consists of four subunits of equal size (42,500 daltons). It oxidizes isovaleryl CoA with a high specific activity, and n-valeryl CoA at much slower rates, but does not oxidize other acyl CoAs, including isobutyryl CoA, 2-methylbutyryl CoA, n-butyryl CoA, and n-hexanoyl CoA, and straight-chain acyl CoAs with longer chain lengths, at appreciable rates [41, 128]. The K_m for isovaleryl CoA is 30 μM. It is almost 100 percent inhibited by 10 μM methylenecyclopropylacetyl CoA (MCPA CoA), the toxic metabolite of hypoglycin. It is also inhibited by N-ethylmaleimide and p-hydroxychloromercuribenzoate, which indicates that SH group(s) participate at the active site [128]. Strong isovaleryl CoA dehydrogenase activity is found in heart, liver, kidney, and skeletal muscle in decreasing order [129, 130]. It is almost exclusively found in the matrix or inner face of the inner membrane of mitochondria [130]. A similar enzyme has also been isolated from pig liver mitochondria [131].

An enzyme fraction which dehydrogenates both 2-methylbutyryl CoA and isobutyryl CoA has recently been separated from isovaleryl CoA dehydrogenase, BDH, medium-chain acyl

Figure 22-5 Keto-enol tautomerization of isoleucine.

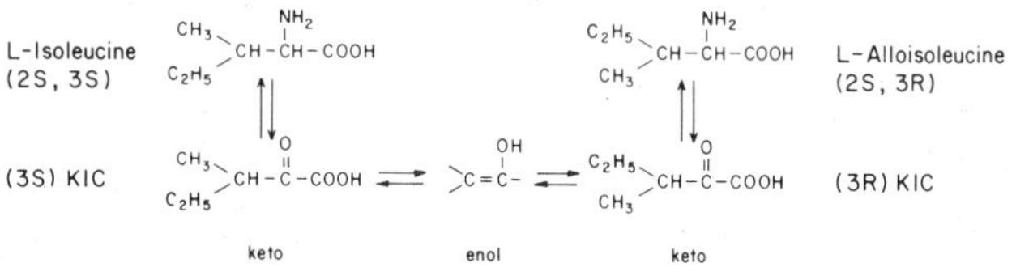

L-Isoleucine (2S, 3S)   L-Alloisoleucine (2S, 3R)   (3S) KIC   keto   enol   keto   (3R) KIC

$$R-CH_2-CH_2-CO-CoA+ETF \xrightarrow[\text{DEHYDROGENASE}]{\text{ACYL CoA}} R-CH=CH-CO-CoA+H_2-ETF$$

ETF: ELECTRON-TRANSFERRING FLAVOPROTEIN

Figure 22-6 General mechanism of acyl CoA dehydrogenase reactions.

CoA dehydrogenase, and LADH by hydroxylapatite column chromatography; this indicates the existence of at least one additional branched chain acyl CoA dehydrogenase [132].

The stereochemical mechanisms of acyl CoA dehydrogenation have recently been studied. In rats, isobutyryl CoA dehydrogenation occurs by abstracting one hydrogen each from the 2-proS-methyl and the α-methine groups, respectively [34]. Isovaleryl CoA dehydrogenation is accomplished by elimination of one hydrogen each from the β-methine and 2-proR hydrogen at the α position [133]. In butyryl CoA dehydrogenation, the 2-proR and 3-proS hydrogens are eliminated [134, 135]. These results indicate that acyl CoA dehydrogenase reactions in general proceed by an antiplanar elimination of hydrogens at the α and β carbons [133]. From this general rule, it can be predicted that the dehydrogenation of the 2 enantiomers of 2-methylbutyryl CoA would yield two different products: tiglyl CoA (2-methylcrotonyl CoA) from S-2-methylbutyryl CoA and ethylhydracrylyl CoA (2-ethyl-3-hydroxypropionyl CoA) from R-2-methylbutyryl CoA. This prediction is in line with current hypotheses [37, 38], but remains to be proved experimentally.

Hypoglycin

Hypoglycin is described here for two reasons. First, it is an unusual neutral BCAA isolated from natural sources and is metabolized to an acyl CoA by mechanisms similar to those for leucine, isoleucine, and valine. Second, its acyl analogue is a very potent inhibitor of short-chain acyl CoA dehydrogenation, including that for the three BCAAs and causes a complex but striking organic aciduria when ingested in vivo.

Hypoglycin is a plant toxin extracted from unripe ackee fruit grown in Jamaica. Ingestion of unripe ackee fruit had been assumed since the turn of this century to be the cause of Jamaican vomiting sickness, a lethal disease resulting in severe hypoglycemia and acidosis; this assumption has been confirmed only recently [12]. Hassal and Reyle isolated hypoglycin A and B from the unripe fruit and seeds of ackee in 1956 [137], and the structure of these hypoglycins was determined by six groups of scientists in subsequent years [136]. Hypoglycin A (now called hypoglycin) is a 7-carbon L-amino acid with an unusual structure: L-amino-3-(methylenecyclopropyl)propionic acid (Fig. 22-8). Hypoglycin B is γ-glutamyl hypoglycin. After a single sublethal dose of hypoglycin, cats, dogs, and monkeys are incapacitated for several days. It induces acute symptoms such as severe hypoglycemia, vomiting, prostration, coma, and death in laboratory animals [138, 139]. Severe histologic changes such as depletion of hepatic glycogen and fatty infiltration of the viscera are also observed [139]. These clinical manifestations and histologic changes are very similar to those observed in patients with Jamaican vomiting sickness. Hypoglycin is metabolized by a sequence of transamination and oxidative decarboxylation reactions to its acyl CoA analogue, methylenecyclopropylacetyl CoA (MCPA CoA) (Fig. 22-8) [140]. MCPA CoA is the true toxin [141]. It is not

metabolized further in mammals but is excreted mainly as a glycine conjugate in rats [142]. In early biochemical studies it was shown that hypoglycin inhibits fatty acid oxidation [141, 143–145], thereby inhibiting gluconeogenesis and causing severe hypoglycemia [146]. The mechanism of action remained to be elucidated [146, 147].

In 1967, Posner and Raben [148] showed that hypoglycin inhibited leucine oxidation in rat liver slices but the site of inhibition was not pinpointed. Tanaka and associates demonstrated subsequently that oxidation of [2-^{14}C]leucine by rat liver slices is 90 percent inhibited by the 2-keto analogue of hypoglycin and that [^{14}C]isovalerylglycine accumulates in the incubation medium [105]. Since isovaleryl CoA is the substrate for glycine N-acylase, their data indicated that the hypoglycin metabolite inhibited isovaleryl CoA dehydrogenase rather than sequestering free CoA and carnitine. Subsequent studies in rats and cats in vivo revealed that hypoglycin inhibited other short-chain acyl CoA dehydrogenases as well, causing a pronounced organic aciduria. This consisted of the excretion of dicarboxylic acids such as glutaric, adipic, octenedioic, decenedioic, and decadienedioic acids in extremely large quantities. In addition, large amounts of isovalerylglycine, butyrylglycine, and MCPA-glycine were also excreted in the urine of rats and cats treated with hypoglycin. This organic aciduria persisted for more than 2 days after a single sublethal dose [142, 149]. Large amounts of isovaleric and 2-methylbutyric acids (47 mg/dl) and MCPA (4.3 mg/dl) accumulated in the blood of these animals [149, 150]. The inhibition of isovaleryl CoA dehydrogenase and BDH by hypoglycin metabolites was later confirmed by experiments in vitro using rat liver mitochondria as an enzyme source [151–153]. In recent studies using individual enzymes purified from rat liver mitochondria, Ikeda and Tanaka [154] revealed that 10 μM MCPA CoA almost completely inhibited the activities of the purified isovaleryl CoA, butyryl CoA, and medium-chain acyl CoA dehydrogenases, but did not inhibit the activity of the LADH. Thus, it is now clear that the inhibition of the oxidation of leucine and fatty acids by hypoglycin is due to the inhibition of these acyl CoA dehydrogenases by MCPA CoA. The occurrence of C_6 to C_{10} dicarboxylic acids in urine of hypoglycin-treated rats is due to the blockade of fatty acid β oxidation at the C_6 to C_{10} monocarboxylic acid stage. The C_6 to C_{10} monocarboxylic acids are then alternatively oxidized by the ω-oxidation system.

It should be noted that, in the course of hypoglycin research, pent-4-enoic acid was believed to have the same inhibitory effect on fatty acid oxidation and was, therefore, widely used experimentally in vitro because of the difficulty in obtaining hypoglycin. This rationale is unfounded. Although pent-4-enoic acid appears to cause inhibition of fatty acid oxidation

Figure 22-7 Flow of electrons from acyl CoAs to molecular oxygen in mitochondria. Sites of electron entry from sarcosine, pyruvate, and succinate are also shown.

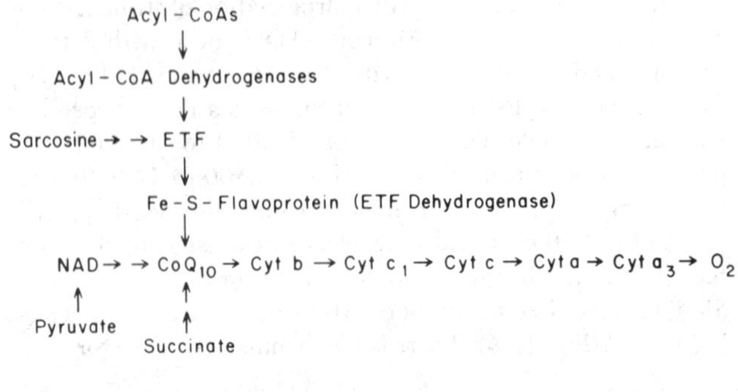

Acyl − CoAs
↓
Acyl − CoA Dehydrogenases
↓
Sarcosine → → ETF
↓
Fe − S − Flavoprotein (ETF Dehydrogenase)
↓
NAD → → CoQ$_{10}$ → Cyt b → Cyt c$_1$ → Cyt c → Cyt a → Cyt a$_3$ → O$_2$
↑   ↑
Pyruvate   Succinate

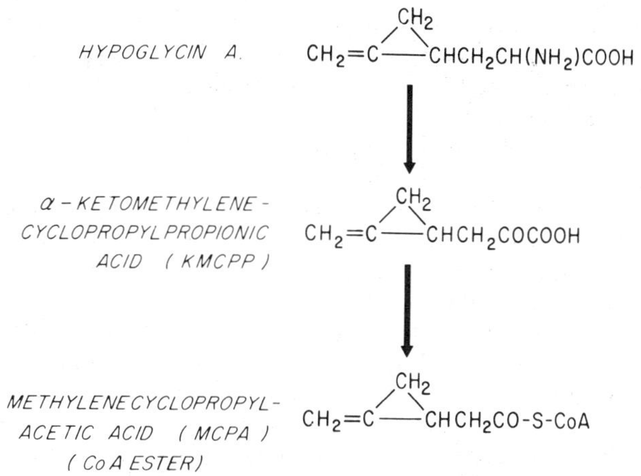

Figure 22-8 The structure and metabolism of hypoglycin. Transamination and oxidative decarboxylation convert the amino acid to its acyl CoA analogue.

and to induce hypoglycemia to some degree, the effects of pent-4-enoic acid are much weaker and of shorter duration than those of hypoglycin [155]. Unlike hypoglycin, it does not inhibit acyl CoA dehydrogenases in vitro and in vivo [105, 154] and does not induce organic aciduria [142]. Despite the extensive studies by Sherratt and associates, the enzymatic mechanisms of pent-4-enoic acid action remained unclear until recently [147]. It appears to be a rather nonspecific cytotoxin, oxidized by the β-oxidation system via acroyl CoA [146]. Fong and Schultz recently concluded that the effect of pent-4-enoic acid is due mainly to inhibition of 3-ketothiolase [156].

Further Catabolism of Leucine

3-Methylcrotonyl CoA, produced by isovaleryl CoA dehydrogenation, is carboxylated at the β carbon by 3-methylcrotonyl CoA carboxylase to form 3-methylglutaconyl CoA, which is then hydrated to 3-hydroxy-3-methylglutaryl CoA (HMG CoA) by the action of 3-methylglutaconase. HMG CoA is then cleaved by HMG CoA lyase to acetoacetic acid and acetyl CoA (Fig. 22-1).

3-Methylcrotonyl CoA carboxylase was first identified and isolated from bacterial sources by Lynen and associates in the early 1960s [157, 158], and its molecular structure and mechanism of action were extensively studied [159, 160]. This bacterial enzyme has a molecular weight of 760,000 and is tetrameric; 1 mol of the enzyme contains 4 mol of biotin, which are covalently bound to an ε-amino group of a lysine residue [159, 160]. This enzyme can also catalyze the carboxylation of free biotin, a feature important for the detailed characterization of its reaction mechanism [157, 158]. The carboxylation of 3-methylcrotonyl CoA proceeds in two steps: carboxylation of the covalently bound biotin and transfer of the carboxyl group to the β carbon of the substrate [159, 160]. More recently, Schiele et al. [161] demonstrated that 3-methylcrotonyl CoA carboxylase from *Achromobacter* is composed of two nonidentical subunits (A and B) of 78,000 and 96,000 daltons, respectively. The entire enzyme is composed of four protomers, each of which consists of A and B subunits. Only the B subunit contains biotin. It can catalyze the carboxylation of biotin but is not capable of catalyzing the overall reaction. The A subunit is inactive in itself. When these subunits are combined, the ability to catalyze the overall reaction is restored. Mammalian 3-methylcrotonyl CoA carboxylase has been characterized only recently [162–164]. When isolated from bovine kidney this enzyme has a molecular weight of 835,000 and like the bacterial enzyme, each protomer is composed of a biotin-free A subunit (M_r = 61,000) and a biotin-containing B subunit (M_r = 73,500). The enzyme is localized exclusively on the inner mitochondrial membrane and may be composed of six protomers.

The hydration of 3-methylglutaconyl CoA to HMG CoA is catalyzed by a specific hydratase, 3-methylglutaconase [165]. This enzyme does not catalyze the hydration of either crotonyl CoA or 3-methylcrotonyl CoA. 3-Methylglutaconase has been purified fiftyfold from sheep liver. The HMG CoA formed by the action of this enzyme is then cleaved to acetoacetic acid and acetyl CoA by the action of HMG CoA lyase [166]. This catalytic action appears to be stereospecific and requires divalent cations [167]. Strong activity of HMG CoA lyase is found in liver, kidney, and heart, but only weak activity is detectable in muscle and brain. It is primarily localized in mitochondria [168]. HMG CoA lyase has been purified 2000-fold from beef liver. It is a monomer with a molecular weight of 48,000 [167].

Further Catabolism of Isoleucine

The S Pathway Tiglyl CoA (2-methylcrotonyl CoA) produced by dehydrogenation of S-2-methylbutyryl CoA is hydrated by the action of crotonase to form 2-methyl-3-hydroxybutyryl CoA, which is then dehydrogenated to 2-methylacetoacetyl CoA (Fig. 22-1). The α,β cleavage of 2-methylacetoacetyl CoA by the action of 3-ketothiolase then produces propionyl CoA and acetyl CoA [169]. These three steps in the pathway of isoleucine are analogous to those of the β-oxidation pathway for straight-chain fatty acids. This is the primary, natural pathway of isoleucine catabolism. Since another pathway (R pathway) of isoleucine catabolism has been proposed, the pathway described here may be designated the S pathway to avoid confusion [37]. This name is based on the **S** configuration of 2-methylbutyryl CoA which occurs in this pathway.

Crotonase has been purified in crystalline form from several sources [170–175]. It hydrates branched chain enoyl CoAs such as tiglyl CoA and 3-methylcrotonyl CoA with efficiencies lower than that for crotonyl CoA [171]. Hydration of longer chain enoyl CoAs is catalyzed by another hydratase [175]. Crotonases from beef liver [172] and porcine heart [174] have molecular weights of 164,000 and 155,000, respectively, and both are hexamers of identical subunits.

3-Ketothiolases have also been studied extensively [176–179]. Three thiolases are known to be present in mammalian tissues. Two of these are mitochondrial enzymes which catalyze the cleavage of 3-ketoacyl CoAs. The third is a cytoplasmic enzyme which catalyzes the biosynthesis of 3-ketoacyl CoAs from smaller analogues by the reverse reaction [179]. One of the mitochondrial enzymes is highly specific for acetoacetyl CoA [178] and its activity is enhanced by K^+ ions [180], whereas the other mitochondrial enzyme mainly cleaves 3-ketoacyl CoAs with longer acyl chains [178]. The action of the latter enzyme is not enhanced by K^+ ions. 2-Methylacetoacetyl CoA has not been tested as a substrate for acetoacetyl CoA thiolase but recent evidence from a study on a patient with ketothiolase deficiency is consistent with the hypothesis that

2-methylacetoacetyl CoA is cleaved by this enzyme [181]. The existence of a 3-ketothiolase which is specific for 2-methylacetoacetyl CoA has also been suggested from the study on other patients with 3-ketothiolase deficiency [182]. Acetoacetyl CoA thiolase has been purified 700-fold from pig heart extract to a crystalline form and has a molecular weight of 170,000. It consists of four subunits of similar size [178].

The R Pathway Prior to the study by Robinson et al., which established that isoleucine was catabolized through the oxidation of it longer acyl chain [169] (S pathway), there was controversy concerning whether it was oxidized on its longer chain or shorter one [183]. This controversy has been revived recently in a somewhat different form. In 1959, Stalder identified 2-ethylmalonic acid in small quantities in normal human and rat urines and proposed that the ethylmalonic acid was produced by the oxidation of the shorter chain of isoleucine via 2-methylbutyric, 2-ethylacrylic, and 2-ethylhydracrylic (2-ethyl-3-hydroxyproionic) acids [184] (Fig. 22-9). This pathway is analogous to the valine pathway with a single difference: The side chain is an ethyl group. Subsequently, Mamer and Tjoa detected ethylhydroacrylic acid in small amounts in normal human urine [185]. They also demonstrated that, after administration of a racemic mixture of deuterated 2-methylbutyric acid to rats in vivo, urinary ethylhydracrylic acid was labeled; this indicates that the pathway proposed by Stalder was indeed operative under these conditions [36, 37]. They proposed that the R enantiomer of 2-methylbutyric acid was metabolized by this pathway (R pathway). However, the find-

ing that the isotope enrichment in urinary ethylmalonic acid from these rats was far lower than that in ethylhydracrylic acid indicated that ethylmalonic acid was not produced directly from ethylhydracrylate.

Concurrently, ethylmalonic acid was identified in large quantities in the urine of patients with Jamaican vomiting sickness [12, 186] and that of a patient with glutaric aciduria type II [7]. The carboxylation of butyryl CoA was a more likely mechanism of formation of ethylmalonic acid than the direct oxidation of ethylhydracrylic acid. Baretz, Lollo, and Tanaka investigated this problem using n-butyric acid and (RS)-2-methylbutyric acid labeled with ^{13}C at various positions as precursors, and hypoglycin to trap the butyrate intermediate [38]. They showed that, as in the case of methylmalonyl semialdehyde in valine metabolism, ethylmalonyl semialdehyde from ethylhydracrylic acid is first oxidatively decarboxylated to butyryl CoA, which then enters the butyryl CoA pool along with long-chain fatty acid oxidation products [38] (Fig. 22-9). Normally butyryl CoA is then oxidized further by β oxidation. When BDH is inhibited, it is carboxylated, forming ethylmalonyl CoA [38]. Furthermore, it has been shown that butyryl CoA can be carboxylated by purified propionyl CoA carboxylase at a rate one-eighth of that with propionyl CoA as substrate [187].

Further Metabolism of Valine

Methacrylyl CoA, produced via isobutyryl CoA, is hydrated to 3-hydroxyisobutyryl CoA [188] and then deacylated to 3-hydroxyisobutyric acid by a specific deacylase [189] (Fig. 22-1). The hydration step is a stereospecific reaction with water addition on the re face, producing S(+)-3-hydroxyisobutyryl-CoA [190]. 3-Hydroxyisobutyric acid is dehydrogenated by a specific 3-hydroxyisobutyrate dehydrogenase which requires NAD$^+$ as a cofactor, forming 2-methylmalonyl semialdehyde [191]. Previously, Coon proposed that methylmalonyl semialdehyde is oxidized at the aldehyde group, directly producing methylmalonyl CoA [192], but this proposal was made without experimental evidence. Tanaka and associates recently reinvestigated this step by administering precursors labeled with ^{13}C at various positions to a patient with methylmalonic acidemia [32], and to normal rats [33]. They showed unequivocally that methylmalonyl semialdehyde undergoes oxidative decarboxylation, losing its carboxyl group while the aldehyde group is oxidized, thus producing propionate as an obligate intermediate [32, 33].

DISEASE STATES

Disorders of Transamination

Hypervalinemia Only a single female patient with hypervalinemia has been reported from Japan [3]. The parents were not related to each other and the results of their valine loading tests were normal [48, 193]. A few additional patients are said to have been found recently in the United States and Japan [194, 195], but detailed reports have not yet been published.

Shortly after birth the patient was noted to suck poorly and

Figure 22-9 The R pathway of L-alloisoleucine metabolism.

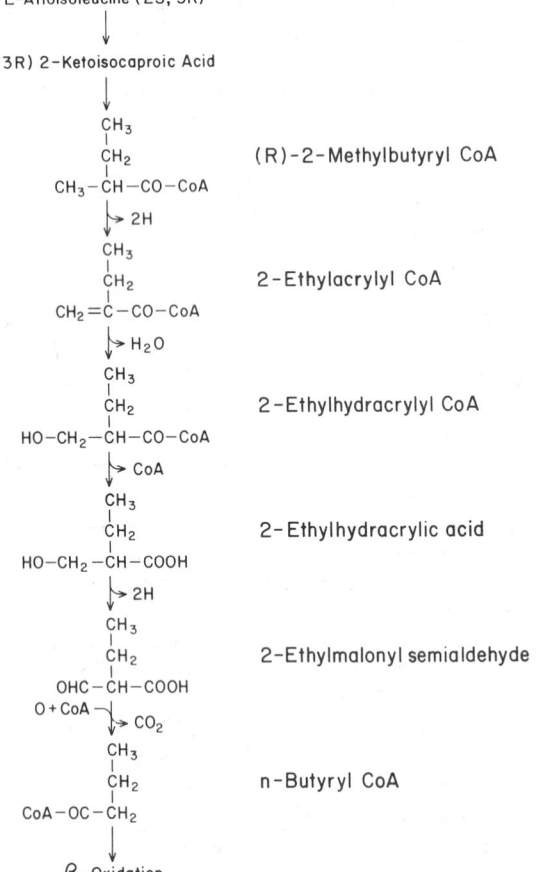

to vomit frequently. She failed to thrive and had frequent episodes of fever. She was hypotonic and hyperkinetic [48]. Following the introduction of a low valine diet at 9 months of age, the vomiting ceased, weight gain improved, and hyperactivity decreased. Concomitantly, the serum valine concentration fell to the normal range [48, 193]. Treatment with pyridoxal phosphate (30 to 60 mg/day) for 3 weeks caused no significant change in blood valine.

Five- to tenfold elevations of valine concentrations in blood and urine and the absence of 2-ketoisovaleric acid accumulation were suggestive of a defect in the transamination of valine (Fig. 22-1). This defect appeared to be specific for valine since the blood concentrations of leucine and isoleucine were within the normal range. This hypothesis appears to have been confirmed by transaminase assays using peripheral leukocytes as the enzyme source. The transaminating activity using 2 mM valine as an amino donor was undetectable, while the corresponding activities using leucine and isoleucine were normal [49] (Table 22-2).

At present, it is difficult to reconcile the data concerning this patient with current knowledge on BCAA transaminases. As discussed earlier, the cytosolic transaminase from extrahepatic tissues appears to be the dominant enzyme in mammals since it has high activity and relatively low K_m values for amino donors. This enzyme is equally active for the three BCAAs. Two general explanations for the apparent discrepancy between the clinical and experimental findings should be mentioned. First, a mutation could lead to the synthesis of a variant common transaminase capable of catalyzing the transamination of leucine and isoleucine but incapable of transaminating valine. Second, specific transaminases for valine, leucine, and isoleucine which have a high affinity (low K_m) for the specific substrate may yet await identification (see page 443).

This diagnosis rests on the demonstration of selective hypervalinemia in the absence of ketoaciduria. If another such patient is found, extensive studies to characterize the enzyme deficiency further would be important, paying special attention to the conditions used for transaminase assay. In particular, a wide range of concentrations of amino donors and acceptors would be critical.

Hyperleucine-Isoleucinemia Only two young French sibs (male and female) with this biochemical abnormality have been reported [4]. These children had similar clinical manifestations, which first appeared at 2 to 3 months of age. They included seizures, failure to thrive, and mental retardation. The affected girl had retinal degeneration and sensorineuronal hearing loss as well. Analysis of plasma amino acids revealed increased concentrations of leucine (2 to 5 times normal), isoleucine (2 to 9 times normal), and proline (3 to 7 times normal). The concentration of valine was not significantly elevated. Urinary excretion of glycine and of Δ'-pyrroline-5-carboxylic acid was increased, but that of leucine and isoleucine was normal. Results from loading tests in both parents indicated that the defects in leucine and proline metabolism were probably independent.

The accumulation of leucine and isoleucine suggested a deficiency of transaminase activity specific for leucine and isoleucine. When BCAA transaminase activity was measured in leukocyte extracts at substrate concentrations less than 0.25 mM, less than half-normal activity was found in the patient's extracts with leucine and isoleucine as substrates but normal

Table 22-2 Transamination of amino acids by intact leukocytes of a patient with hypervalinemia and control subjects

Amino acid	Hypervalinemia	Control A	Control B
Valine	0	134	71
Isoleucine	346	268	222
Leucine	387	183	143
Methionine	198	98	55
Phenylalanine	48	32	42

NOTE: Leukocytes isolated from 2 ml blood were incubated with one of the following substrates: 4 μmol (0.4 μCi) of DL-[1-^{14}C]valine, DL-[1-^{14}C]leucine, DL-[1-^{14}C]phenylalanine, or 2 μmol (0.2 μCi) of L-[U-^{14}C]isoleucine or L-[methyl-^{14}C]methionine. Each flask also contained 1 μmol of the respective unlabeled keto acid, 10 μg pyridoxamine and Krebs-Ringer phosphate buffer in a total of 1 ml. The radioactive keto acids are reported in disintegrations per minute. SOURCE: From Dancis et al. [49].

activity was found with valine as substrate. These findings, plus those in the child with hypervalinemia, suggest strongly the existence of two BCAA transaminases with different substrate specificities.

Treatment with a low protein [2 g/(kg·day)] diet and the selective restriction of leucine and isoleucine reduced plasma amino acid concentrations to normal, but no clinical improvement was observed. The affected male sib died at the age of 3 years due to hyperthermia and coma; the female sib was alive at $2\frac{1}{2}$ years.

Maple Syrup Urine Disease (Branched Chain Ketoaciduria)

Introduction Maple syrup urine disease (MSUD) has been recognized for more than 20 years. The existence of several different clinical forms and sites of biochemical abnormality in MSUD has been demonstrated. Such clinical and biochemical characterizations have been achieved largely with two techniques: quantitative amino acid analyses of body fluids and measurements of the $^{14}CO_2$ evolved from intact leukocytes or cultured skin fibroblasts incubated with [^{14}C]amino or [^{14}C]keto acids. Despite the many publications in this area, our knowledge of the fundamental biochemical and genetic mechanisms responsible for MSUD remains limited. Further exploration of the mechanisms underlying the heterogeneity in MSUD is needed, using more powerful biochemical and cell biologic techniques.

Clinical Manifestations Currently, five different phenotypes are generally recognized. These have been designated as follows: (1) classic, (2) intermittent, (3) intermediate, (4) thiamine-responsive, and (5) E_3 deficiency (Table 22-3). Two additional "variant" types have been claimed on the basis of single case reports [197, 198], but these cannot yet be accepted as conclusive.

CLASSIC TYPE The infant appears to be normal at birth. By the end of the first week, and as early as the fourth day of life, the typical patient fails to thrive, feeds poorly, and vomits. Neurologic signs such as convulsions and generalized rigidity soon appear. Stupor, hypotonia, and irregular respirations follow. An odor, described as that of maple syrup or curry, is often noted, particularly in the urine. The untreated patient becomes progressively more lethargic, falls into a coma, and

Table 22-3 Classification of maple syrup urine disease (MSUD) phenotypes

Phenotypic designation	Major clinical features	Constant or intermittent	BCAA* accumulation, mM in plasma			Substrate oxidation by intact cells,[†] % of normal
			Leu	Ile	Val	
Classic	Onset of severe ketoacidosis soon after birth; seizures, coma, and death in many patients; high likelihood of mental retardation in survivors	Constant	~5.0	~1.0	~1.0	0–2
Intermittent	Ketoacidotic episodes triggered by infection, vaccination, or protein surfeit; occasionally fatal; well between episodes; usually normal psychomotor development	Intermittent	~5.0 (only during acute episodes)	~1.0	~1.0	2–40
Intermediate	Mental retardation, no obvious ketoacidotic episodes	Constant	~2.0	~1.0	~1.2	5–25
Thiamine-responsive	Similar to those in Intermediate	Constant	Variable			~40
Dihydrolipoyl dehydrogenase (E$_3$) deficiency	Floppiness and lethargy accompanied by ketoacidosis. Downhill course over 7 months	Constant	~0.6	~0.3	~0.5	~10

*Branched chain amino acids
† Usually assessed in peripheral blood leukocytes or cultured fibroblasts with [1-^{14}C]-labeled branched chain amino or keto acids.

dies. Wide variation in age at onset and in the rapidity of clinical deterioration is noteworthy, even in affected sibs [1, 199, 200]. Infections often hasten the terminal event. Plasma concentrations of BCAAs are persistently elevated more than tenfold.

If the untreated patient survives the first weeks, EEG abnormalities, severe psychomotor retardation, generalized dystonic posturing, and other evidences of severe brain dysfunction are the rule. Bilateral ptosis, ophthalmoplegia, and facial diplegia have been observed in several patients [201–203], as has moderate to severe hypoglycemia [204–206].

INTERMITTENT AND INTERMEDIATE TYPES   In 1961, Morris et al. described a patient with a variant form of MSUD characterized by episodic and milder clinical manifestations [207]. Numerous patients of this type have since been reported [208–216]. Typically, the postnatal course is uneventful. The first clinical signs are usually seen at 12 to 24 months of age, generally triggered by infections of the middle ear or upper respiratory tract, vaccination, operation, or sudden increase in dietary protein. The patient becomes irritable, ataxic, and progressively lethargic. With good supportive care, the child recovers, only to experience repeated similar episodes until diagnosed and treated. The maple syrup odor is typically noted during these episodes, as is elevation of BCAAs and BCKAs in blood and urine. During remission the BCAA and BCKA concentrations in body fluids are normal. Despite the generally mild and intermittent course, the long-term outcome is occasionally fatal; among 20 cases reviewed, 5 died due to a severe acidotic episode [208–210, 216]. Psychomotor development tends to be normal in the remainder.

In 1970 Schulman et al. diagnosed MSUD in a 19-month-old female infant because the odor of maple syrup was noted during evaluation for mental retardation [217]. Her postnatal course was unremarkable except for a substantial delay in developmental milestones. Neither seizures, ataxia, excessive vomiting, nor episodic drowsiness were ever noted. The patient had tolerated several immunizations and mild febrile illnesses without becoming acutely ill. She eagerly consumed large quantities of milk, eggs, and meat during infancy. There were no focal neurologic abnormalities although mild general-

ized hypotonia was present. Unlike typical patients with the intermittent type of MSUD, the BCAA and BCKA levels in the blood and urine were consistently elevated on an unrestricted diet. Moderate anemia, hyperuricemia, and mild systemic acidosis were also noteworthy. With restriction of dietary protein to 1.5 g/(kg·day), the concentrations of BCAAs and BCKAs in the blood and urine dramatically decreased. The administration of 100 mg thiamine per day for a week while the patient was on a low protein diet produced no significant biochemical changes. Several additional cases that fall into this intermediate category have since been reported [218–222]. Although such patients have been considered clinically distinct from the intermittent type, enzymatic differences remain to be demonstrated.

THIAMINE-RESPONSIVE TYPE   Scriver et al. [46] described an 11-month-old female infant with significant developmental retardation. Excessive amounts of BCAAs and BCKAs were detected in blood and urine. When 10 mg/day of thiamine hydrochloride was given while the patient was on a low protein diet [2 g/(kg·day)], plasma BCAA concentrations abruptly fell within a few days. With the withdrawal of thiamine hydrochloride, plasma BCKA concentrations rose to pre-thiamine-treatment values within 5 days; a second trial with thiamine hydrochloride was followed by the same response.

Thiamine responsiveness has since been observed in several additional patients with MSUD [219–224]. Clinically, all of these children were of the intermittent type and the responses to thiamine were not as dramatic as that seen in the case reported by Scriver et al. [46]. In the five patients reported by Elsas, Danner, and associates, biochemical improvement required up to 3 weeks of vitamin supplementation [223, 225]. In one patient correction was only partial [222]; in another, 1 g thiamine hydrochloride per day was required for a distinct chemical response [220, 221].

VALIDITY OF THE CLINICAL CLASSIFICATION   There is little doubt that there are at least three clinical types of MSUD, namely a severe (classic) type, a mild form(s), and a thiamine-responsive one. The apparent distinction between the intermittent type and the intermediate type could reflect environmental differences such as quantity of protein ingested. The term intermediate is unsatisfactory because it suggests that the severity of the enzyme deficiency is between that found in classic and intermittent types. In fact, the extent of enzyme deficiency in the intermediate type is similar to or less severe than that found in the intermittent type. The frequency of thiamine responsiveness in the milder types of MSUD is unknown. It is also not known whether any patients with the classic type are thiamine-responsive.

Incidence   Previous experience in nine European countries [226] and in Massachusetts [228] indicates an overall incidence of MSUD of between 1:120,000 (12 cases in 1.5 million tests) and 1:290,000 (3 classic cases in 873,000 newborns), respectively. The most extensive survey was compiled by Naylor and Guthrie [228]. In this collaborative survey of five screening laboratories, 13 confirmed cases of MSUD were detected in 2.8 million newborns screened (1:216,000). Of these, 10 were of the classic type and 3 were of the intermittent type.

MSUD has a panethnic distribution, having been reported in Japanese [222, 229], Blacks [224], Jews [230], and Indians [218, 231], in addition to Caucasians.

Biochemical Abnormalities

ABNORMAL METABOLITES   Accumulation of the three BCAAs in blood and urine of affected patients was first reported by Westall and associates in 1957 [2]. Subsequently, Menkes documented the accumulation of the corresponding BCKAs [27]. These data suggested that the degradation of the three BCAAs was blocked at the 2-keto acid stage. The accumulation of the BCAAs was considered to be due to the reversibility of BCAA transaminase. In patients with classic MSUD, persistent and dramatic increases in plasma and urinary BCAAs and BCKAs are observed in the untreated patient. Plasma BCAA concentrations as high as 5.0 mM for leucine and 1.0 mM for both isoleucine and valine, and plasma BCKA concentrations as high as 0.6 to 4.6 mM for KIC, 0.2 to 1.5 mM for KMV, and 0.02 to 0.35 mM for KIV have been observed (Table 22-3). A strong correlation between plasma concentrations of BCKAs and those of the corresponding BCAAs reflects effective reversibility of the transaminase reaction [232]. These results are consistent with the hypothesis that a single common enzyme which catalyzes the oxidative decarboxylation of the three BCKAs is deficient in patients with MSUD.

Additional important information has been obtained from metabolite analysis. First, L-alloisoleucine, which is not normally detectable, also accumulates in patients with MSUD. This compound is produced from L-isoleucine via keto-enol tautomerizaton and transamination of KMV, as discussed on pages 446 and 447. Second, 2-hydroxyisovaleric acid, the hydroxy analogue of KIV, is the major metabolite from valine and its amount is much greater than that of KIV [78–80], whereas the hydroxy analogues of KIC and KMV are found in much smaller amounts. Third, neither analysis of cord blood nor of early postnatal urine is likely to reveal significant abnormalities in BCAAs or BCKAs, because concentrations of these metabolites in the fetus are well regulated by the placenta and maternal circulation.

In patients with intermittent MSUD, BCAAs and BCKAs do not accumulate during remission. During acute episodes of ketoacidosis, BCAA and BCKA concentrations in blood and urine may be as high as those observed in patients with classic MSUD. In patients with the intermediate type, persistent increases in BCAAs and BCKAs are the rule. In such patients, the reported ranges for plasma BCAAs are 1.14 to 1.97 mM for leucine, 0.50 to 0.85 mM for isoleucine, and 0.82 to 1.24 mM for valine (Table 22-3) [217, 221, 222].

SUBSTRATE OXIDATION BY INTACT CELLS   Dancis and coworkers demonstrated that the ability of isolated leukocytes [233] and cultured fibroblasts [234] from patients with classic MSUD to produce $^{14}CO_2$ from [1-^{14}C]Leu, [1-^{14}C]Ile, and [1-^{14}C]Val was only 0 to 2 percent of that of controls, while the ability of the cells to produce the corresponding keto acids was normal. These results, consistent with those from metabolite analysis in vivo, support the contention that the three BCKAs are decarboxylated by a single enzyme and that patients with MSUD are deficient in this enzyme. This concept was further supported by similar experiments in vitro in which [1-^{14}C]BCKAs were used as substrates.

Dancis and associates went on to compare $^{14}CO_2$ formation from [1-^{14}C]BCAAs by intact fibroblasts from six patients with classic MSUD and six with the milder variant forms [235]. In general, the activities of cells from patients with the milder variant types were deficient, but the magnitude of deficiency was distinctly less than that found in cells from classic patients. They classified the MSUD lines according to the degree of residual activity as follows: grade 1, 0 to 2 percent of normal; grade 2, 2 to 8 percent of normal; grade 3, greater than 8 percent of normal. The highest residual activity observed was 40 percent of normal [209, 217]. All classic MSUD cell lines fell into the grade 1 category. The six cell lines of the variant types were in either grade 2 or grade 3. They pointed out that there was not always a consistent relationship between residual activity and clinical course. For instance, a cell line with an activity of 3 percent of normal was from a clinically normal teenage girl, whereas another with an activity of 3 to 4 percent of normal was from a mentally retarded patient. They attributed this discrepancy primarily to the diet followed by these patients. No consistent difference in residual activity was noted between those with the intermittent type and those with the intermediate type.

Wendel et al. [236] studied the kinetics of $^{14}CO_2$ production from [1-^{14}C]BCKAs in cultured skin fibroblasts. They observed biphasic degradation kinetics with regard to substrate concentration for each BCKA in normal cells. The component with the higher substrate affinity (apparent K_m ~1.5 mM) was either altered or not detectable in MSUD cells. They surmised that the activity of the lower affinity component (apparent K_m ~15 mM) is probably not physiologically significant.

CHARACTERIZATION OF ENZYME DEFICIENCY   Only two reports have addressed the question of which component enzyme of the BCKADH complex is deficient in patients with MSUD. Rudiger et al. assayed the activity of E_{1b} and E_3 using partially purified enzyme preparations from kidney and liver of a patient with classic MSUD and of a control [237]. The preparations from the control had two components with E_1 activity, one with low K_m values (3.4 to 6.4 mM) for substrates and the other with high K_m values (16 to 22 mM). The preparations from the patient were specifically deficient in the low K_m component; E_3 activity was normal. Recently, Chuang et al. studied activities of E_{1b}, E_{2b}, and E_3 in disrupted preparations of cultured skin fibroblasts from two classic MSUD patients [238]. In both MSUD cell lines the E_{2b} and E_3 activities were normal, but the activity of E_{1b} exhibited sigmoidal kinetics as a function of substrate concentration, with an estimated K_m of 1.0 mM for substrate. E_{1b} activity from normal cell lines showed hyperbolic kinetics with a substrate K_m of 0.1 mM. V_{max} was similar for the normal and these two MSUD lines. These data indicate that the activity of the high affinity component of E_{1b} is deficient in classic MSUD. There are, however, other data which suggest that classic MSUD type may not be a single entity biochemically and genetically. Singh et al. studied the effects of cofactor addition in a reconstituted, cell-free BCKADH system using ten normal, five classic MSUD, and one intermittent MSUD fibroblast lines [239]. The BCKADH activity was partially restored (15 to 70 percent) by the addition of CoASH and NAD$^+$ in each normal line. This partial restoration was also observed in the intermittent and two classic MSUD lines, but not in three other classic MSUD lines. In these three, all four cofactors, (CoASH, NAD$^+$, TPP, and Mg^{2+}), had to be added for any restoration of activity.

The enzymatic basis for the intermittent and the intermediate types has not been studied further. Three children with E_3 deficiency have been described by Robinson and associates [43, 86, 240, 241] and will be described in a subsequent section.

BIOCHEMICAL BASIS FOR THIAMINE RESPONSIVENESS In the thiamine-responsive patient reported by Scriver et al., the capacity of intact leukocytes to produce $^{14}CO_2$ from [1-^{14}C]leucine was 40 percent of normal when the leucine concentration was 0.1 mM. At 5 mM leucine the activity was normal, indicating the possibility of a K_m mutant [46]. Danner et al. isolated the mitochondrial inner membrane from cultured skin fibroblasts from a thiamine-responsive MSUD patient to study the cofactor requirements and other kinetic parameters [223]. The most significant difference found between the normal and the thiamine-responsive MSUD preparations was that, while the BCKADH activity in the normal preparations could be enhanced about twentyfold over the basal level by the addition of NAD$^+$, CoASH, and Mg^{2+} (omitting TPP), there was no augmentation of activity in the thiamine-responsive MSUD preparation under these conditions. When TPP was added in addition to the three other cofactors, there was a threefold enhancement of the activity for both the mutant and normal preparations. The apparent K_m for TPP in the MSUD preparation was essentially the same as that in the control. Also, addition of TPP had a significant protective effect against heat inactivation for both normal and MSUD preparations. From these observations, Danner et al. suggested that the defect in this patient lies in either E_2 or E_3 and attributed the effect of thiamine to its stabilizing effect on the enzyme complex. Their data are equally consistent with deficiency of E_1, if one assumes that in the mutant line E_1 is rate-limiting and that TPP specifically enhances E_1 activity. According to this interpretation, addition of NAD$^+$, CoASH, and Mg^{2+} would not be expected to effect overall BCKADH activity in the mutant extract because these three cofactors are required by E_2 and E_3.

Genetics

AUTOSOMAL RECESSIVE INHERITANCE The classic type of MSUD is inherited as an autosomal recessive trait. Family history data reveal multiple examples of this type in sibs of both sexes [1, 232, 242]. Further, in several families, the ability of leukocytes or cultured fibroblasts from both parents to produce $^{14}CO_2$ from [1-^{14}C]BCKA or [1-^{14}C]BCAA is approximately 50 percent of normal values [204, 242–246].

GENETIC HETEROGENEITY Results of studies measuring [1-^{14}C]KIC oxidation by intact leukocytes from parents of children with the intermittent type of MSUD have yielded particularly interesting results. Goedde et al. observed that, in each of two Scandinavian families, one parent's cells demonstrated normal KIC oxidation, whereas those of the other showed about 50 percent of normal activity [247]. Similar results were obtained by others in three additional families [215, 216, 244]. These data suggest that the affected probands in these families are compound heterozygotes, i.e., that they are heterozygous for each of two different mutant alleles at the same locus. In two other families cells of both parents showed normal KIC oxidation [217, 247], consistent with the notion that the affected patients therein are homozygous for a mutant allele distinct from that leading to classic MSUD.

The nature of the genetic heterogeneity observed in MSUD has been explored further in two studies employing genetic complementation analyses. In both studies Sendai virus–mediated heterokaryons were formed from pairwise crosses of fibroblast lines from patients with MSUD. The first study, by Lyons and colleagues, used four mutant lines—two classic and two intermittent [42]; the second, by Singh et al., used five mutant lines—four classic and one intermittent [239]. Both studies obtained evidence for the existence of two complementation groups among patients with classic MSUD. It is not yet clear whether such complementation is intergenic (implying defects at two different loci) or interallelic (implying two different defects at the same locus). Significantly, Lyons et al. showed no complementation between their two intermittent MSUD lines and a classic one. Thus, at least in these lines, it seems likely that different defects at a single locus can lead to the clinical heterogeneity known for so long.

Diagnosis Since a large number of disorders can produce the clinical hallmarks of MSUD, diagnosis must be made by specific laboratory tests. The distinctive odor of the urine (or the patient) is often the first clue. The substance responsible for the maple syrup odor is unknown at present; the odor is not due to BCKAs.

Two general types of diagnostic tests can be used: measurements of BCAAs and BCKAs in blood and urine using chromatographic and chemical procedures and determination of $^{14}CO_2$ released from [1-^{14}C]BCAAs or [1-^{14}C]BCKAs by leukocytes or cultured skin fibroblasts.

ANALYTICAL PROCEDURES Some simple chemical tests may be utilized for preliminary screening. Yellow precipitates will be observed by the dinitrophenylhydrazine (DNPH) test when BCKAs are present [248]. A color which is described as gray with greenish tinge may be observed in the ferric-chloride test [248]. Although these tests are useful, they are by no means sensitive or specific. Thin-layer chromatographic determination of DNPHs of BCAAs was previously employed for identification and quantitation [249], but resolution and sensitivity were unsatisfactory.

For GC analysis, BCKAs must be derived at both the carboxyl and the keto groups. The carboxyl group is usually converted to its trimethylsylyl (TMS) ester. The keto group is converted to either oxime-TMS [78–80] or quinoxalinol derivatives [250, 251]. An extensive list of retention indexes of organic acids, including BCKAs, has been provided so that identification of the BCKAs can be accomplished by GC (thereby obviating the need for mass spectrometry) [252]. One of the features of the oxime-TMS method is that the two isomers of KMV can be separated from each other but one overlaps with the KIC peak on most of the GC systems [78–80]. In contrast, the two isomers of KMV are not separable as quanoxalinol-TMS derivatives but they are separated from KIC [250, 251]. Therefore, for the purpose of separate quantitation of KIC, KMV, and KIV, the latter method is preferred. A typical chromatogram of urinary organic acids in MSUD is shown in Fig. 22-10A. It should be noted that while KIC and KMV are essentially excreted as they are, most of the KIV is excreted as its hydroxy analogue [78–80]. Therefore, if the extract of MSUD urine is derived with TMS without the protection of keto groups with oxime or quinoxalinol, the only unusual compound detectable is 2-hydroxyisovaleric acid. Mass spectral data are also available for both types of derivatives [253, 254].

The diagnosis of MSUD can also be made by finding elevated concentrations of leucine, isoleucine, valine, and alloisoleucine in plasma and urine using an amino acid analyzer. Preliminary amino acid analysis may be accomplished by paper electrophoresis [255] or thin-layer chromatography [256].

CELL STUDIES   BCKADH assays in cell-free systems are subject to many variables such as the method of cell disruption [56, 94] and the addition of cofactors [76, 83–85, 239]; they are not suitable for routine assay. For diagnostic pruposes, the use of whole cells is preferred. Such studies have varied considerably with regard to cell types (leukocytes [233, 242, 243] or cultured skin fibroblasts [234, 257]), substrate, and buffers. Studies with cultured fibroblasts appear to give more consistent results than do those using leukocytes [235, 249, 257]. Less test variability has been obtained with labeled amino acids than with labeled keto acids [257] because the latter are unstable and give a high background. A micromethod which utilizes as few as 50,000 cultured fibroblasts or 50 μl blood has been described [259, 260].

PRENATAL DIAGNOSIS   Several fetuses affected with MSUD have been diagnosed prenatally by oxidation studies using cultured amniotic fluid cells [260–262]. Significantly, concentrations of BCAAs and BCKAs in amniotic fluid of an affected pregnancy between the sixteenth and twentieth weeks of gestation were not different from controls, excluding the possibility of prenatal diagnosis by BCAA and BCKA determinations [263].

Secondary Changes

HYPOGLYCEMIA   A severe to moderate fasting hypoglycemia (17 to 60 mg/dl) is often observed in both the classic and mild variant types [201, 204–207, 213, 219]. Initially this hypoglycemia was attributed to leucine-induced hypoglycemia. Haymond et al. studied glucose and amino acid metabolism in several children with MSUD and fasting hypoglycemia [205, 206]. Plasma concentrations of gluconeogenic amino acids, with the exception of glutamic acid, were markedly reduced. Plasma insulin was undetectable (<5 μU/ml) in the face of hypoglycemia. When concentrations of BCAAs fell following initiation of a diet free of BCAAs, glutamine and ala-

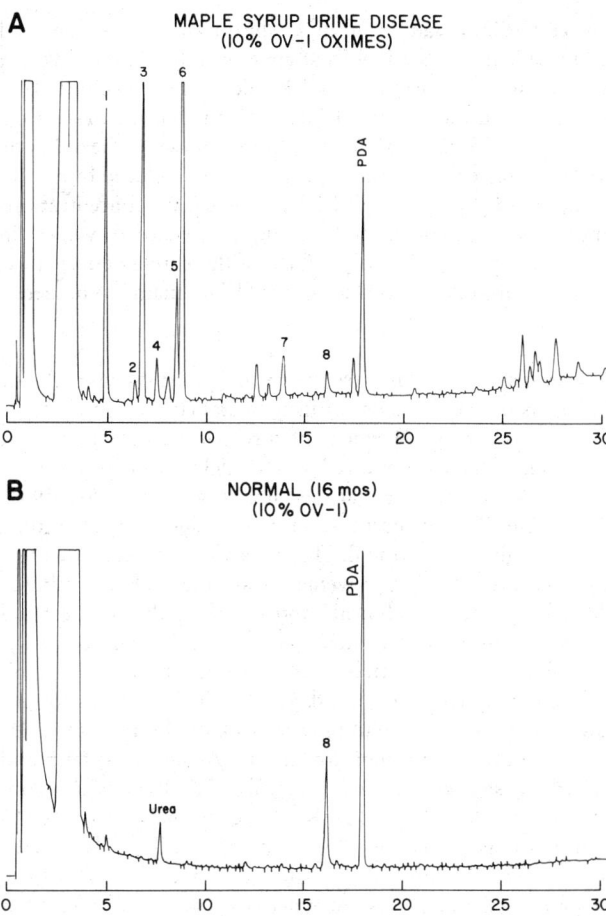

Figure 22-10 Urinary organic acids from a patient with maple syrup urine disease (A) and a normal child (B). Elution was from a 10% OV-1 column. The acids noted in the figure are: 1, lactic; 2, pyruvic-oxime; 3, 2-hydroxyisovaleric; 4, 2-ketoisovaleric-oxime; 5, 2-keto-3-methylvaleric-oxime; 6, 2-ketoisocaproic-oxime, 7, 2-ketoglutaricoxime; and 8, hippuric. n-Pentadecanoic acid (PDA), 1 mg per milligram creatinine, was added as an internal standard. (*From Tanaka et al.* [80].)

nine concentrations rapidly increased. These data indicate that the hypoglycemia associated with MSUD is due to defective gluconeogenesis from amino acids and not to inhibition of gluconeogenic enzymes or hyperinsulinemia [205]. A reduced availability of glucogenic substrates in the liver appears to be the cause of decreased gluconeogenesis.

EFFECTS OF BCAAS AND BCKAS ON CENTRAL NERVOUS SYSTEM STRUCTURE AND FUNCTION   Due to the cerebral dysfunction and histologic changes seen in patients with MSUD, effects of BCAAs and BCKAs on a number of biochemical and cell biologic factors have been tested. A diet containing 8 percent leucine caused a 22 percent reduction in serotonin content in rat brain [264]. BCAAs and BCKAs inhibited glutamate decarboxylase in rat brain, reducing the amount of formation of 4-aminobutyric acid [265]. Oxygen uptake by rat brain slices or homogenates was not inhibited by any of the BCAAs but was slightly (10 to 27 percent) inhibited by 10 mM KIC [266]. KIC (5 mM) also inhibited mitochondrial pyruvate and 3-hydroxybutyrate oxidation by inhibiting the transport of these compounds into mitochondria [267, 268]; PDH and 3-hydroxybutyrate dehydrogenase were not inhibited. Addition of 1 to 2 mM KIC to cultures containing myelinating newborn rat cerebellum caused a delay in myelin formation and decreased numbers of normal-appearing myelinated axons; with higher concentrations of KIC, degeneration of neuroglia was observed [269]. KIC (15 mM) also induced marked prolongation of G_1 and, to a lesser degree, S phases in the cell cycle of C6 glioma cultures. Similar changes were induced by a combination of BCAAs and BCKAs added in concentrations approximately similar to the highest recorded values in patients with MSUD [270]. Which of these many effects bear on the neurologic dysfunction in MSUD remains to be determined.

Treatment Dietary treatment of patients with classic MSUD is difficult because of its neonatal clinical onset, acute course, and the involvement of three essential amino acids. Dent and Westall pioneered in this field by treating an 8-month-old infant with various diets low in BCAAs. Blood BCAA and BCKA concentrations were reduced to values only slightly higher than normal. The patient gained weight on these diets but no clinical improvement was noted. They attributed the failure to achieve clinical improvement to the late start and the short duration of dietary treatment [271]. Subsequently, Westall treated an affected sib in the same family with a semisynthetic diet from the sixth day of life. This diet was formulated from an amino acid mixture lacking the three BCAAs, natural sources of proteins low in BCAAs such as gelatin and baker's yeast, sucrose, and arachis oil [272]. Blood BCAA concentrations were kept slightly above normal levels. At 13 months of age, when the report was written, the child's development was judged normal. One important conclusion from this study was that it was essential to include a small amount of natural protein to promote growth. Snyderman et al. subsequently reported extensive data on dietary management of seven patients with classic MSUD [77]. Since then new dietary formulations for the treatment of MSUD patients have been described [273–275]. Commercial products for the treatment of MSUD are now available; these are MSUD-AID (Milner Scientific and Medical Research Co., Liverpool, England) and GIBCO Amino Acid Mixture for Treatment of MSUD (Grand Island Biological Co., Grand Island, NY) [276].

A few cautions have been voiced concerning dietary treatment. Levy et al. [277] called attention to the risk of folic acid deficiency if proprietary multivitamin preparations are substituted for the vitamins suggested in the Snyderman diet. Foreman et al. recently reported the occurrence of hyperchloremic acidosis during the management of an affected newborn infant, the evident cause of which was the high amount of chloride-containing amino acid salts (lysine, arginine, and histidine), in an infant unable to excrete the acid load because of immature renal function [278].

In making decisions on dietary treatment, the clinical severity and the residual BCKADH activity should be taken into consideration. Dancis et al. [235] suggested that for patients with grade 1 deficiency (0 to 2 percent of normal, classic type) much of the dietary nitrogen must be provided as low BCAA mixture. Patients with grade 2 deficiency (2 to 8 percent normal) tolerate the intake of 1.5 to 2 g protein per kilogram per day in infancy, an amount sufficient to satisfy the amino acid requirements for maintenance and growth. Such patients can be raised on breast milk or proprietary milks patterned after breast milk, but introduction of whole milk and other high protein foods may cause symptoms. Patients with grade 3 deficiency (8 to 15 percent normal) should tolerate an unrestricted diet safely. Some patients with the so-called intermediate form who have 5 to 15 percent of normal activity have developmental retardation and require dietary restriction [217].

In addition to dietary treatment, thiamine treatment (10 to 1000 mg/day) must be tried on symptomatic patients. To one classic MSUD patient and four children with grade 3 deficiency, Elsas et al. administered 150 to 200 mg thiamine per day and observed significant reduction in blood BCAA and BCKA concentrations in each mildly affected patient, but not in the one with classic MSUD. It is important to note that in their experience the response to thiamine was not immediate and required 3 weeks for expression [225]. Duran et al. increased the amount of thiamine to 1 g/day before lowering the amount of urinary BCKA in a single patient [221].

Gaull used peritoneal dialysis in the management of an acute ketoacidotic episode in a patient with classic MSUD [279]. Clear-cut neurologic improvement occurred during the dialysis without concomitant improvement in the metabolic acidosis. BCAAs and BCKAs were removed into the dialysate with only modest decreases in their plasma values. Apparently, the plasma pool of BCAAs was continuously replenished by a large intracellular pool. Since then this therapy has been utilized in several additional patients. Recently Wendel et al. reported that peritoneal BCAA clearance was about 40 to 50 percent of that for urea [280]. Finally, Hammersen et al. treated three newborns with MSUD with multiple exchange transfusions [281]. This procedure was satisfactory, achieving rapid clinical and biochemical improvement during acute episodes.

Pathology In two classic MSUD patients who died at 11 and 14 days of age, respectively, the main finding was failure of myelinization. There were no signs of demyelinization, glial reaction, or neuronal degeneration [1]. Silberman et al. described detailed autopsy findings on two additional cases. Both died at 9 months of age. They observed, in addition to deficient myelinization, a spongy change and a decrease in the number of oligodendroglia and astrocytes in the white matter; again there was no sign of myelin breakdown [282]. In a patient with intermittent MSUD who died at 8 years of age due to a fulminant episode, considerable spongy degeneration of the deep layers of the cortex was observed. The nerve cells were fairly well preserved [209]. The most impressive changes were found in the cerebellum where pannecrosis of the entire granular cell layer with preservation of the molecular and Purkinje cell layers was noted. There was also considerable nerve cell loss in the pontine nuclei and substantia nigra. Prior to the catastrophic episode which led to his death, his psychomotor development was normal and he was regarded as the brightest boy in his class. Hence, it is not clear whether the neuropathologic changes were acute or chronic.

Chemical analyses of the brain of patients with MSUD have been reported by several investigators. In general, a reduction in the total lipids, particularly in proteolipids and cerebrosides, has been observed [283–285]. These chemical changes are consistent with the loss of myelin. In contrast, the brain of a patient who was treated with a low BCAA diet at an early age had a normal cerebral lipid composition [285, 286].

E_3 Deficiency In the process of purifying the BCKADH from pig kidney mitochondria, Petit et al. demonstrated that the BCKADH complex has the same E_3 as do the PDH and KGDH complexes [39]. Thus, one might expect a deficiency of E_3 to result in the accumulation of BCKAs and BCAAs, in addition to lactic acidosis and 2-ketoglutaric aciduria. In 1978 Robinson and associates reported a patient with lactic acidosis due to E₃ deficiency [43] (discussed further in Chap. 9). They reported that BCKADH activity in tissues (kidney, liver, and brain) of this patient was much reduced while 2-ketoisocaproate decarboxylase (E₁b) activity was normal. Significantly, plasma BCKA concentrations were regularly elevated during the 8 months of this patient's life [86]. Thus, E_3 deficiency may be regarded as a variant form of MSUD. Since then, two additional cases of E_3 deficiency have been reported [240, 241].

Isovaleric Acidemia

Incidence   No reliable data on large-scale screening for isovaleric acidemia are currently available because of the lack of a simple reliable assay for this disease. Therefore, the incidence of this disease in large populations is currently unknown. Since the first two sibs with isovaleric acidemia were described in 1966 by Tanaka et al. [5, 6], at least 27 confirmed cases have been reported [29, 47, 287–306]. If to this number are added those sibs of affected probands who died of symptoms similar to those of the probands, the number of affected patients reaches at least 37. We have also detected three additional patients who have not been reported and are aware of a number of other unreported cases from other laboratories. Thus, isovaleric acidemia is not an extremely rare inherited metabolic disease; it has been detected among Caucasians, blacks [47, 303], Jews [295], and Japanese [301].

Clinical Manifestations   In general, two different types of clinical courses have been observed: the acute severe type and the chronic intermittent type. Based on these clinical observations, genetic heterogeneity in isovaleric acidemia has long been proposed [288, 295]. Nevertheless, careful review of the family history and clinical course of the 27 reported patients reveals that these two clinical phenotypes may not reflect genetic heterogeneity. Moreover, no recognizable heterogeneity has been observed by biochemical and genetic studies.

ACUTE FORM   Typically, patients with the acute type are normal at birth but, within a few days, begin to vomit and refuse to feed. They become listless and increasingly lethargic; sometimes they are tremulous. They are often hypothermic. In most cases a strong "sweaty feet" odor is noted. They become cyanotic, lapse into coma, and death often ensues [288, 291, 292, 295, 297]. Among the 37 patients reviewed in the literature, 20 fell into this category. Within 3 weeks of birth 16 died. In many fatal cases severe ketoacidosis, a hemorrhagic diathesis, or infection appeared to be the cause of death [288, 289, 291, 292, 295, 297, 306]. Because of severe vomiting 4 patients were operated on in the neonatal period. In 3 of these, hypertrophic pyloric stenosis was purportedly found and corrected [6, 301, 305], and in the fourth, duodenal obstruction due to an abnormal peritoneal band was noted [288]. If the patients with this form survive the fulminant neonatal period with appropriate treatment, their subsequent course is that of the chronic intermittent form [6, 300] and they may develop normally [300] (Table 22-4).

CHRONIC INTERMITTENT FORM   Clinical features in this type encompass recurrent episodes of vomiting, lethargy, and coma accompanied by ketoacidosis and sweaty feet odor. These episodes are usually triggered by upper respiratory infection or the overeating of protein foods. Symptoms subside several days after treatment with glucose infusion. The first episode may start as early as 2 weeks of age or as late as 1 year. Ketoacidotic episodes tend to occur frequently in early infancy and young childhood, but their frequency diminishes as the patient grows older. Such children often show a natural aversion to protein foods, even at a young age. In spite of the repeated ketoacidotic episodes, approximately 70 percent of the patients with this type achieve normal psychomotor development [287, 297–304, 305], while the remainder have been described as being low average to severely retarded [6, 47, 292, 294, 296] (Table 22-4). Most of the patients who have achieved normal development were detected after 1970 and were treated with a low protein diet or with glycine supplements. Two retarded patients were microcephalic [47, 292].

Biochemical Abnormalities

ABNORMAL METABOLITES   When the first two sibs were studied, an analysis of serum short-chain fatty acids were carried out because the patients' odor was similar to that of short-chain fatty acids [5, 6]. A large single peak of isovaleric acid was identified by GC/MS (Fig. 22-11). The concentration of isovaleric acid in serum ranged from 6 to 30 mg/dl (100 to 500 times normal) when the children were lethargic or in coma [5, 6]. Values as high as 35 to 50 mg/dl have since been observed in children during acute episodes [288, 294, 300, 301]. The serum isovaleric acid concentration drops to 3 to 4 times normal as the acute symptoms dissipate [5, 6]. 3-Methylcrotonic acid, which follows isovaleric acid in the degradation of leucine (Fig. 22-12), did not increase in the serum when isovaleric acid was increased. Therefore it was postulated that the metabolic block was located at the step of isovaleryl CoA dehydro-

Table 22-4   Clinical and laboratory features of patients with isovaleric acidemia

Features	Patients detected
Clinical	
Sex	
Male	18/37*
Female	19/37
Age of onset	
Birth–2 wk	28/37
2 wk–1 yr	7/37
Later than 1 yr	2/37
Outcome	
Dead	16/37
Alive	21/37
Development in surviving cases	
Retarded	4/21
Mildly retarded to low average	3/21
Normal	14/21
Laboratory	
Hematology	
Neutropenia and thrombocytopenia	22/29
Plasma glycine	
Elevated	2/20
Normal	16/20
Decreased (during acute episode)	2/20

* Of 37 patients, 27 are confirmed cases; 10 are sibs of the confirmed cases who died in the neonatal period due to ketoacidosis.

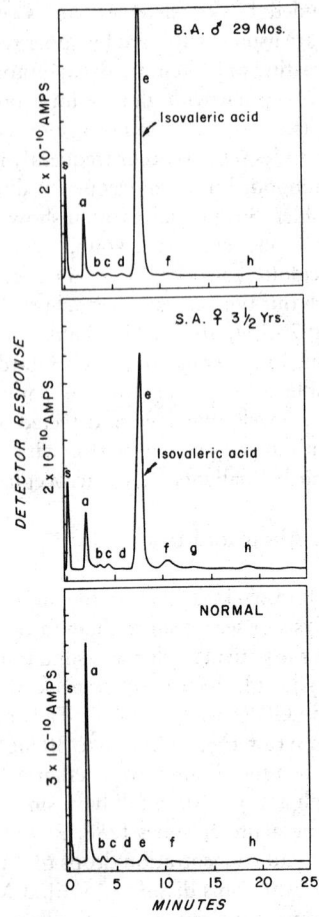

Figure 22-11 Gas chromatograms of serum short-chain fatty acids from two sibs with isovaleric acidemia and a control (*bottom*). The short-chain fatty acids noted in the figure are: a, acetic; b, propionic; c, isobutyric; d, *n*-butyric; e, isovaleric; f, crotonic; g, 3-methylcrotonic; and h, *n*-hexanoic. S stands for solvent. (*From Tanaka et al.* [5].)

genation. This concept was further supported by the following evidence (1) when L-leucine (100 mg/kg) was given orally to these patients during remission, a prompt and sustained increase in concentration of serum isovaleric acid was observed; (2) administration of the same amount of isoleucine or valine did not increase the concentration of the corresponding short-chain fatty acids in the patients' serum; and (3) the ability of the patients' white blood cells to oxidize [1-^{14}C]isovaleric acid in vitro was only one-sixth to one-eighth that of the controls [5, 6]. Also, since other short-chain fatty acids such as isobutyric, *n*-butyric, 2-methylbutyric, and *n*-hexanoic acids did not accumulate during ketoacidotic episodes, Tanaka and associates hypothesized that the dehydrogenation of isovaleryl CoA must be carried out by a specific enzyme, isovaleryl CoA dehydrogenase, and that patients with isovaleric acidemia were deficient in the activity of this enzyme [5, 6]. It was earlier believed that the dehydrogenation of isovaleryl CoA was carried out by a common enzyme, butyryl CoA dehydrogenase, which oxidized CoA esters of butyric and hexanoic acids [123, 124].

Subsequently, two major abnormal metabolites, isovalerylglycine [29] and 3-hydroxyisovaleric acid [307] were identified in the urine of patients with isovaleric acidemia by Tanaka and associates. Isovalerylglycine was continuously excreted in large amounts in both acute episodes and in remission [29]. In contrast, 3-hydroxyisovaleric acid was excreted in large amounts

only during acute attacks when free isovaleric acid accumulated [307]. From these studies it appears that unoxidized isovaleryl CoA can be conjugated with glycine (Fig. 22-12), since it is known that acyl CoAs are substrates for the glycine acylation reaction [107, 108]. In affected patients, this glycine conjugation system is efficient enough to handle the amount of isovaleryl CoA ordinarily produced during periods of remission; hence, free isovalerate does not accumulate. When the leucine load exceeds the capacity of the glycine conjugation system, an excess of isovaleryl CoA is hydrolyzed, resulting in the release and accumulation of free isovaleric acid in the blood. Free isovaleric acid is then hydroxylated by ω − 1 oxidation to form 3-hydroxyisovaleric acid, which is efficiently excreted in urine (Fig. 22-12) [125, 307]. This scheme may explain the clinically episodic nature of isovaleric acidemia.

Recently 4-hydroxyisovaleric acid, methaconic acid, and methylsuccinic acid have been detected in large amounts in two children with isovaleric acidemia during acute episodes [306, 308], providing evidence for the long suspected ω oxidation of isovaleric acid [307, 311]. It follows that while 3-hydroxyisovaleric acid is not subject to further oxidation because it is a secondary alcohol, 4-hydroxyisovaleric acid is further oxidized to methylsuccinic and methaconic acids.

The possibility that KIC might also accumulate in patients with isovaleric acidemia was tested initially using thin-layer chromatography for DNPHs. KIC was not detected in a significant amount even in acute episodes [5]. This matter was explored further by GC with oxime-TMS derivatives [80], but again KIC was not detected [312]. The lack of KIC accumulation is probably due to the irreversibility of the BCKA dehydrogenation reaction, although this reaction is considerably inhibited in patients with isovaleric acidemia, as discussed below.

SUBSTRATE OXIDATION STUDIES   The biochemical mechanisms underlying isovaleric acidemia were further studied by Tanaka, Mandel, and Shih using cultured skin fibroblasts [245]. They showed that $^{14}CO_2$ production from [2-^{14}C]leucine by three isovaleric acidemia cell lines was 0.2, 1.1, and 1.5 percent, respectively, that of controls (Table 22-5). Further, labeled isovaleric acid accumulated in the medium used to

Figure 22-12 The altered metabolism of leucine in isovaleric acidemia (heavy solid arrows) and 3-methylcrotonyl CoA carboxylase deficiency (broken arrows). (*From Tanaka* [28].)

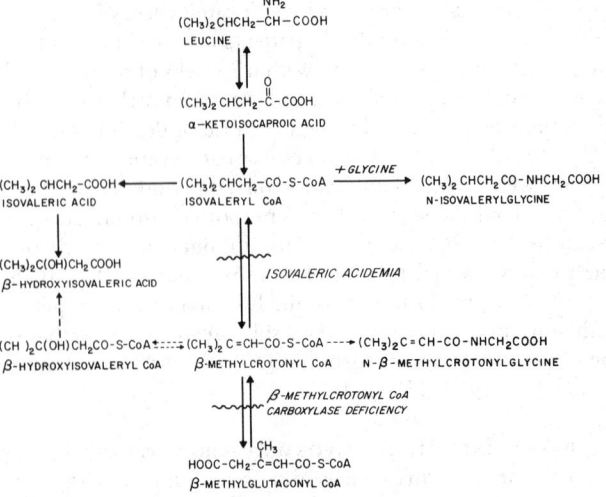

Table 22-5 Production of $^{14}CO_2$ from [1-^{14}C]- and [2-^{14}C]leucine by cultured skin fibroblasts from patients with isovaleric acidemia and MSUD

	Substrates, picomoles per 10^6 cells per hour	
	[1-^{14}C]leucine	[2-^{14}C]leucine
Controls (6)	2140 ± 870	453 ± 199
Isovaleric acidemia		
Homozygotes		
B.A.	362	5
S.A.	412	7
K.Fa.	516	1
Heterozygote		
Mrs. A.	879	177
Maple syrup urine disease		
Homozygotes		
C.C.	3	17
S.Fo.	27	12
Heterozygotes		
Mr. Fo.	408	—*
Mrs. Fo.	439	—*

* Not measured.

NOTE: Control values represent mean ± SD. Number of cell lines tested is presented in parentheses. All experiments were done in duplicate.
SOURCE: From Tanaka, Mandell, and Shih [245].

assay patients' cells. These data are consistent with the earlier observation on the reduced ability of the patients' leukocytes to oxidize [1-^{14}C]isovaleric acid [5, 6] (see page 458). Unexpectedly, $^{14}CO_2$ release from [1-^{14}C]leucine was also depressed to 20 percent of normal, though not nearly to values as low as those (0.2 to 1.3 percent of control) found in two lines from classic MSUD patients [245] (Table 22-5). The depression of $^{14}CO_2$ release from [1-^{14}C]leucine was thought to be due to product inhibition of BCKADH by isovaleryl CoA, a thesis supported by the observation that addition of 5 mM isovaleric acid to the assay medium inhibited [1-^{14}C]leucine oxidation in control cells by 32 percent. This hypothesis has been confirmed by recent evidence that BCKADH purified from pig kidney was markedly inhibited by isovaleryl CoA [39] (for details see page 446). Tanaka and associates [245] also showed that the same pattern of inhibition—a marked (95 percent) inhibition of $^{14}CO_2$ release from [2-^{14}C]leucine and a lesser (66 percent) inhibition from [1-^{14}C]leucine—was induced by the addition of methylenecyclopropylacetic acid, a toxic metabolite of hypoglycin and a known inhibitor of isovaleryl CoA dehydrogenase [105] (see pages 448 to 449).

IDENTIFICATION OF ENZYME DEFICIENCY   The above data from metabolite analyses and substrate-oxidation studies were consistent with the hypothesis that isovaleric acidemia is due to a deficiency of an isovaleryl CoA–specific dehydrogenase. Direct experimental support for this idea was not available until 1980 because of technical difficulties in assaying this enzyme activity in crude cell homogenates using a dye reduction assay [123]. Rhead and Tanaka devised a new method for acyl CoA dehydrogenase assay which utilized [2,3-^{3}H]acyl CoA as substrate [126, 127]. Using this new assay method and mitochondria isolated from cultured skin fibroblasts as an enzyme source, they showed that mitochondrial isovaleryl CoA dehydrogenase activities in five cell lines from patients

with isovaleric acidemia was 13 percent of the mean of four normal controls, while BDH activity in affected cells was normal [126] (Table 22-6). Subsequently, an isovaleryl CoA–specific dehydrogenase was demonstrated [40] and isolated [41] by Tanaka and colleagues (for details see page 447).

PHYSIOLOGIC EFFECTS OF ISOVALERIC ACID   The accumulation of isovaleric acid has been considered directly responsible for the presence of acute symptoms such as vomiting, lethargy, and coma [5]. Short-chain fatty acids caused electroencephalographic changes such as slow waves [313, 314]. These changes in central nervous system function are caused by depression of the activating system in the reticular formation of midbrain neocortex [315]. Biochemically it is known that short-chain fatty acids lead to uncoupling of oxidative phosphorylation [316, 317], mitochondrial swelling [318], and inhibition of Na-K-ATPase in the brain [319]. It was thought previously that neurotoxicity of short-chain fatty acid was related to these actions. However, Walker et al. have suggested that coma induced by short-chain fatty acids may not be the result of impaired cerebral energy transformation, since they observed that energy transformation in the brain is unaltered by the administration of short-chain fatty acids in vivo [320]. They proposed that short-chain fatty acids probably induce coma by interfering with neuronal membrane function. It is interesting to note that oleic acid induces mitochondrial swelling and causes the uncoupling of oxidative phosphorylation, but it does not cause electroencephalographic changes [314]. It is reasonable to assume, therefore, that the uncoupling of oxidative phosphorylation induced by short-chain fatty acids may not be the cause of coma.

GLYCINE METABOLISM   The glycine concentration in blood and urine has been normal in most patients [6, 47, 288], although modest hyperglycinemia (~0.55 mM) has been noted in two patients [290, 297] (Table 22-4). Ando et al. administered [1-^{14}C]glycine and [2-^{14}C]glycine to a patient with isovaleric acidemia with mild hyperglycinemia and observed that conversion to serine was normal. Most of the radioactivity in the urine was recovered as isovalerylglycine. Bartlett and Gompertz examined the substrate specificity of glycine N-acylase and found that the velocity of the reaction was very fast when isovaleryl CoA and tiglyl CoA were used as substrates but very slow with propionyl CoA. No reaction occurred with methylmalonyl CoA [108]. This specificity of glycine N-acylase may account, in part, for the relatively low plasma glycine concentrations in patients with isovaleric acidemia. In contrast, plasma glycine concentrations are often high in patients with propionic and methylmalonic acidemias, as discussed in Chap. 23. Also, it should be noted that low glycine concentrations were occasionally observed during acute episodes in patients with isovaleric acidemia (Table 22-4). This suggests that the glycine supply is insufficient when the isovaleryl CoA load is increased [6, 47]. This observation and due consideration of the kinetics of glycine N-acylase led Krieger and Tanaka to initiate glycine therapy.

Genetics   More than one affected sib has been found in a number of families [5, 6, 289, 292, 294, 297]. Approximately equal numbers of male and female patients with this disease have been found (Table 22-4). [2-^{14}C]Leucine oxidation by fibroblasts from obligate heterozygotes is about 50 percent of control values [245, 297, 303] (Table 22-5) although more

Table 22-6   Isovaleryl CoA and butyryl CoA dehydrogenase activities in mitochondria from fibroblasts of controls and patients with isovaleric acidemia

	Specific activity, picomoles product per minute per milligram protein*			
	Tritium-release assay		Dye-reduction assay	
Origin of mitochondria	Isovaleryl CoA dehydrogenase	Butyryl CoA dehydrogenase	Isovaleryl CoA dehydrogenase	Butyryl CoA dehydrogenase
Control cells (4)†	310 ± 42	440 ± 91	1310 ± 208	738 ± 4
Isovaleric acidemia cells (5)	39 ± 3	475 ± 80	163 ± 68	714 ± 142
Percent normal	13 percent	108 percent	12 percent	97 percent

* All results are expressed as mean ± S.E.
† Number of cell lines of each type is shown in parentheses.
SOURCE: From Rhead and Tanaka [126].

extensive studies are needed to confirm this observation. These findings are consistent with autosomal recessive inheritance.

As discussed above, while two clinical presentations have been observed, further clinical perusal of individual families containing more than one affected sib and results from biochemical and genetic complementation studies have failed to provide evidence for genetic heterogeneity. In some families with a patient who died after a fulminant course in the neonatal period, other sibs have survived following a mild episodic course [289, 292, 297]. Moreover, some patients who survived the acute, severe course in the neonatal period did well and lead a relatively uneventful life, as do patients with the mild episodic form [6, 300]. These clinical findings indicate that there is no basic difference between the two clinical phenotypes.

Biochemically, the ability to oxidize [2-^{14}C]leucine has been tested in cell lines from five patients. One died after a fulminant neonatal course [297], the second patient is a sib of two patients who died after severe neonatal bouts [289], the third survived a severe neonatal episode [6], and the other two patients have the mild episodic form [6, 303]. The activities of these five lines were all 0.2 to 1.3 percent of control values [245, 297, 303].

Recently Dubiel, Wetts, and Tanaka [321] devised a simple macromolecular labeling test (MLT) to assay the ability of cultured fibroblasts to oxidize [1-^{14}C]isovaleric acid in situ. With this assay, all ten isovaleric acidemia cell lines, including the five lines mentioned above, had activities approximately 10 percent (10 ± 2.0 percent) of normal. Of these ten cell lines, four are from patients with the severe form; while the other six are from patients with the mild episodic form. Further, they utilized this method in polyethylene glycol–induced heterokaryons to study genetic complementation. No complementation was observed in any combination of the ten lines tested [321]. This failure to detect genetic heterogeneity is in line with the recent finding that isovaleryl CoA dehydrogenase is composed of four identical subunits [41, 128] (for detail, see page 447). The results do not exclude the possibility that more than one mutant allele for the isovaleryl CoA dehydrogenase gene exists, and produces distinct but equally deficient mutant enzymes.

Secondary Findings   Moderate to severe hematologic abnormalities such as leukopenia and thrombocytopenia have been observed in 75 percent of patients. These changes are particularly severe in the newborn period or during acute episodes (Table 22-4). Blood hemoglobin content may also be

depressed in severe episodes [300]. A detailed hematologic study of two severely affected newborns has been reported by Kelleher et al. [322]. Pancytopenia due to arrested maturation of hemopoietic precursors was observed during acute life-threatening crises in both. These children were successfully treated with transfusions of packed red cells and platelets. Their hematologic status during remission was normal.

In some cases serum Ca^{2+} concentrations as low as 4 mg/dl have been reported [288, 294, 296, 300], with increased neuromuscular irritability. Moderate hyperammonemia (up to 400 μg/dl) has also been observed [296, 298], as has total transient alopecia [47, 298].

Diagnosis   Isovaleric acidemia should be most reliably detected by the GC identification of urinary isovalerylglycine, because this compound is always excreted in large amounts [29, 125]. Its daily excretion ranges from 50 to 250 mg for affected newborns [300] and 400 to 2000 mg for 3- to 5-year-old children [29, 47, 297]. These values represent 2 to 10 mg per milligram creatinine [47, 297, 300, 301]. MS was previously needed for chemical identification [29]. With currently available GC retention indexes of organic acids, identification of isovalerylglycine can be achieved readily by GC alone [80, 252]. During remission, isovalerylglycine is the only major abnormal compound detectable in urine (Fig. 22-13A) [29]. In acute episodes 3-hydroxyisovaleric [307], 4-hydroxyisovaleric [306, 308], methylsuccinic acids [306, 311] plus lactic, 3-hydroxybutyric, and acetoacetic acids are excreted in large amounts as well (Fig 22-13B). The amount of free isovaleric acid in urine is small [28, 125].

Determination of serum isovaleric acid is necessary to follow the course of an acute episode. It can be as high as 30 to 50 mg/dl [5, 294, 300]. Special precautions must be undertaken for the quantitative analysis of isovaleric acid because of its volatile nature [323]. Serum extracts must be distilled prior to GC analysis [5, 290, 294]. Short-chain fatty acids thus prepared should be analyzed as free acids using a GC column with packings doubly coated with a stationary phase and phosphoric acid [5, 294] (doubly coated packings are now available from commercial sources). Complete resolution of isovaleric acid and 2-methylbutyric acid is not possible by GC. MS has been utilized for separate quantitation of these two isomers [5, 324]. Alternatively, short-chain fatty acids can be analyzed as TMS derivatives [325], but the quantitative accuracy of this method is not known.

Diagnosis using intact cultured skin fibroblasts can readily be accomplished measuring $^{14}CO_2$ release from [2-^{14}C]leucine

[245, 326] or the [1-^{14}C]isovaleric acid MLT [319]. Direct assay of isovaleryl CoA dehydrogenase activity in isolated mitochondria of these cells using the tritium-release assay is even more definitive [126, 127]. Use of the dye-reduction assay to measure isovaleryl CoA dehydrogenase activity in crude tissue homogenates should be avoided because of strong interference by thioesterase and other nonspecific endogenous reductants [116, 123].

Prenatal diagnosis has not been reported. Release of ^{14}CO$_2$ from [2-^{14}C]leucine [326] or the [1-^{14}C]isovalerate MLT assay [321] using amniotic fluid cells would be useful for this purpose.

Identification of heterozygotes has not been extensively studied. The activity of heterozygote cells to oxidize [2-^{14}C]leucine is approximately 50 percent of normal but because of the wide range of control values, heterozygote detection cannot be reliably accomplished using this method (Table 22-5). Guibaud et al., using thin-layer chromatography for chemical identification, claimed that obligate heterozygotes excreted increased amounts of isovalerylglycine after leucine loading [296]. On the other hand, Malan et al. found no increase in urinary isovalerylglycine in obligate heterozygotes after leucine loading using GC for isovalerylglycine identification [298].

Figure 22-13 Urinary organic acids from a patient with isovaleric acidemia: (*A*), during remission (*B*), during a ketoacidotic episode. A 10% OV-1 column was used for analysis of both samples. The compounds noted in these figures are as follows: 1, lactic; 2, 3-hydroxybutyric; 3, acetoacetic (peak 1); 4, 3-hydroxyisovaleric; 5, acetoacetic (peak 2); 6, isovalerylglycine, monotrimethylsilyl (TMS) derivative; and 7, isovalerylglycine, di-TMS. *n*-Pentadecanoic acid (PDA), 1 mg/mg creatinine, was added as an internal standard. 3-Keto acids such as acetoacetic acid are detected as two peaks of di-TMS of the enol forms (cis and trans). (*From Tanaka et al. [80].*)

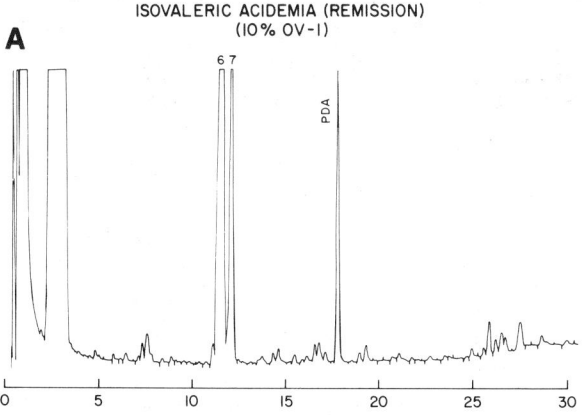

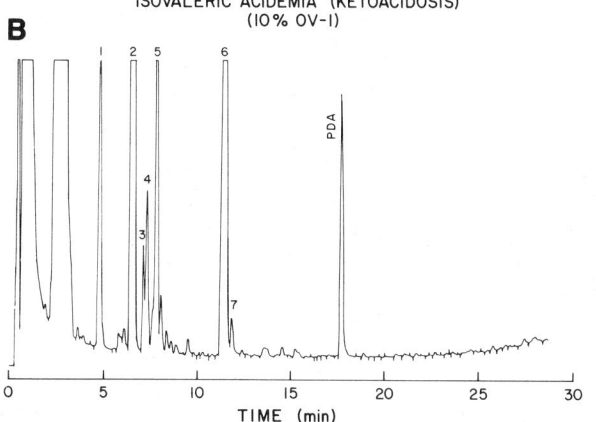

Treatment Ketotic attacks have been treated nonspecifically with the parenteral infusion of glucose and sodium bicarbonate. In two patients restriction of dietary leucine to a level of 115 to 120 mg per kilogram body weight per day appeared to reduce the frequency of acute episodes [293, 294]. Several other patients have been treated with a low protein diet [1.5 to 2 g/(kg·day)] with excellent results. This amount of protein provides approximately that content of leucine which can be handled by the glycine conjugation system under normal circumstances.

Krieger and Tanaka [47] tested the therapeutic effects of glycine administration based on the following observations. Plasma glycine values are usually not elevated in patients with isovaleric acidemia; rather, plasma glycine tends to be lower during ketoacidotic attacks than in remission [6, 47]. The latter finding suggests that, during acute attacks, there is an inadequate supply of glycine to conjugate the increased amounts of isovaleryl CoA produced. This rationale is supported by consideration of the kinetics of glycine *N*-acylase activity in tissues which suggests that acylation of glycine by isovaleryl CoA may be enhanced if the glycine concentration in liver tissue is raised.

Krieger and Tanaka administered leucine (125 mg/kg) to a patient with isovaleric acidemia both with and without simultaneous oral glycine (250 mg/kg). When the leucine was given with glycine, serum isovaleric acid concentrations were much lower and the amount of urinary isovalerylglycine was more than twice that observed with leucine loading alone [47]. Similar effects of glycine administration were observed in other patients with isovaleric acidemia as well [299, 301]. Cohn et al. subsequently treated two severely affected neonates with glycine [250 mg/(kg·day)] via nasogastric tube [300]. The biochemical response to glycine therapy in both patients was dramatic. Serum and urine isovalerate concentration declined to less than 1 mg/dl within 3 days. Concomitant with this fall was a rise of urinary isovalerylglycine excretion, which increased nearly twofold in patient 1 and more than threefold in patient 2. This brisk biochemical response to glycine therapy was not accompanied by as dramatic a clinical response. Both infants remained extremely hypotonic and in profound coma for 3 to 4 days after initiation of treatment, but then improved. Both have been treated with oral glycine (800 mg/day) since discharge. The psychomotor development of these children now 6 months and 13 months of age, respectively, is entirely normal on a diet providing approximately 1.5 g protein per kilogram per day and 80 kcal/(kg·day). Both children have had several intercurrent respiratory and enteric infections without suffering recurrence of metabolic acidemia. These workers concluded that glycine supplementation may permit some liberalization of dietary protein restriction in affected patients.

Pathology Several autopsied cases have been reported [288, 291, 295, 306]. Major findings have included hemorrhages in the lung, brain, and kidney; extensive fatty liver has also been observed.

Glutaric Aciduria Type II and Ethylmalonic-Adipic Aciduria

In six reported patients [7, 327–330] with glutaric aciduria type II (GA II) and in a single documented [8] patient with ethylmalonic-adipic aciduria (EMA), several metabolic pathways including those of BCAAs, fatty acids, lysine, hydroxylysine, and tryptophan are blocked at an acyl CoA dehydrogenase step (Fig. 22-14).

Clinical Manifestations In 1976, Przyrembel et al. [7] described a male newborn who was normal at birth but developed metabolic acidosis and hypoglycemia (24 mg/dl) by age 16 h. In spite of treatment with glucose and bicarbonate infusions, blood glucose fell to 5 mg/dl and metabolic acidosis worsened. A strong odor of sweaty feet was noted. The patient became hypothermic (32° C), had seizures, and died at the age of 70 h. Dicarboxylic acids, including ethylmalonic, glutaric, adipic, suberic, and sebacic acids, were noted in urine, as were unsaturated dicarboxylic acids with 8 or 10 carbons. Short-chain fatty acids such as isobutyric, isovaleric, and butyric acids were also found in abundance. Quantitatively, glutarate was by far the largest single component (85.7 μmol per milligram creatinine), the other dicarboxylic acids being present at about one-tenth its value (Table 22-7). Therefore, this disease was named glutaric aciduria type II (GA II) to distinguish it from patients with glutaric aciduria type I, who excreted mainly glutaric, glutaconic, and 3-hydroxyglutaric acids [331]. The abnormality in the latter patients is confined to the glutarate pathway and appears to be due to a deficiency of glutaconyl CoA decarboxylase. In contrast, patients with glutaric aciduria type II seem to have metabolic blocks in several metabolic pathways. One of the two patients subsequently reported by Sweetman et al. [327] and the patient reported by Gregersen et al. [330] had a clinical course very similar to that noted by Przyrembel et al.

In 1979 Mantagos et al. reported a 5-year-old girl who had had repeated episodes of vomiting, lethargy, and coma accompanied by acidosis and hypoglycemia [8]. Symptoms were first noted at 7 weeks of age when, after a period of poor oral

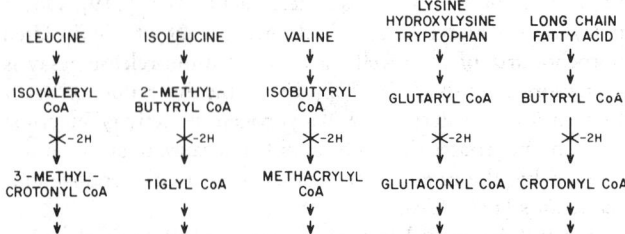

Figure 22-14 Multiple pathways blocked in glutaric aciduria type II, ethylmalonic-adipic aciduria, and Jamaican vomiting sickness.

intake, she presented with a brief episode of tonic seizures. She recovered spontaneously and on evaluation a few hours later was normal. During the following 4 years, the patient had two episodes of coma and convulsions associated with hypoglycemia and acidosis. The first occurred at 1 year of age during a mild attack of gastroenteritis and was highlighted by lethargy, seizures, and hypoglycemia (30 mg/dl). At 4 years of age the second episode of vomiting, convulsions, and coma with severe hypoglycemia (12 mg/dl) occurred. Ketotic hypoglycemia was suspected, but all tests for this condition and for other causes of infantile hypoglycemia were unrevealing. Analysis of urinary organic acids revealed the accumulation of ethylmalonic and adipic acids, and hexanoylglycine. The amount of glutaric acid was small and often not detectable. Therefore, this disease was named ethylmalonic-adipic aciduria (EMA). Goodman et al. [328] reported a similar case, but referred to it as GA II.

Biochemical Abnormalities

METABOLITE ANALYSIS Results of urinary organic acid analyses in two patients with severe GA II and representative data for the child with EMA are presented in Table 22-7. Isobutyric, isovaleric, and 2-methylbutyric acids are metabolites

Table 22-7 Urinary excretion of organic acids in two patients with glutaric aciduria type II and a patient with ethylmalonic-adipic aciduria

Acids	Glutaric aciduria type II		Ethylmalonic-adipic aciduria patient‡	Normal
	Patient 1*	Patient 2† μmol per mg creatinine		
Short-chain fatty acids				
Isobutyric	13.6	21.1	0.4	<0.01
n-Butyric	3.5	6.8	0.2	<0.01
2-Methylbutyric	14.3	11.1	0.2	<0.04
Isovaleric				
n-Hexanoic	0.8	23.0	1.9	0
Dicarboxylic acids				
Ethylmalonic	5.1	0.4	2.7	<0.01
Glutaric	85.7	48.9	0.2	<0.01
Adipic	8.4	6.2	5.8	<0.6
C_8	2.5	2.7	<0.2	<0.01
C_{10}	4.6	2.8	<0.2	<0.01
Hydroxyacids				
Lactic	91.5	0.5	nd	<2.0
2-Hydroxybutyric	0.4	0.2	nd	<0.01
3-Hydroxybutyric	0.2	nd	nd	<0.64
2-Hydroxyisovaleric	0.9	0.9	nd	<0.01
2-Hydroxyglutaric	1.2	5.5	nd	<0.50

* From Przyrembel et al. [7]
† From Sweetman et al. [327]
‡ From Mantagos, Genel, and Tanaka [8]
NOTE: nd = not detectable

of valine, leucine, and isoleucine, respectively. Glutarate is a known metabolite from lysine, hydroxylysine, and tryptophan. Ethylmalonic acid is known to be produced by the carboxylation of butyryl CoA when BDH is inhibited [38, 186]. Hexanoylglycine and adipate are produced presumably by glycine conjugation of hexanoyl CoA [332] and ω oxidation of hexanoic acid, respectively. The pattern of urinary organic acids in GA II is very similar to that seen in hypoglycin-treated rats [142, 149] (see pages 448 and 449) and in patients with Jamaican vomiting sickness [12]. The accumulation of these organic acids suggested that the metabolism of BCAAs, fatty acids, lysine, hydroxylysine, and tryptophan were blocked at a particular acyl CoA dehydrogenase step (Fig. 22-14).

In the EMA patient ethylmalonic and adipic acids and hexanoylglycine were the major urinary metabolites. Since these are alternate metabolites of butyryl CoA and hexanoyl CoA, specific deficiency of BDH was initially hypothesized [333], but loading tests with medium-chain triglycerides (MCT), leucine, and lysine indicated that in addition to fatty acid oxidation, leucine metabolism was also blocked in this patient [8].

SUBSTRATE OXIDATION STUDY   Przyrembel et al. [7] studied the oxidation of several substrates by cultured fibroblasts from their patient with GA II. These included, [1,5-^{14}C]glutaric acid (14 percent of normal), [U-^{14}C]valine (15 percent of normal), [U-^{14}C]leucine (53 percent of normal), [U-^{14}C]isoleucine (27 percent of normal), [U-^{14}C]KIV (1 percent of normal), [U-^{14}C]KIC (27 percent of normal), and [1-^{14}C]pyruvate (normal).

Mantagos, Gentel, and Tanaka [8] carried out a substrate oxidation study using fibroblasts from the EMA patient and from the GA II patient (reported by Przyrembel et al. [7]) as well (Table 22-8). Unexpectedly, the oxidation of [1-^{14}C]butyrate, [2-^{14}C]leucine, and [2-^{14}C]lysine were all impaired (15 to 25 percent of normal) in EMA cells as in GA II cells, although the magnitude of impairment was significantly greater in the latter (Table 22-8).

ENZYME STUDIES   The enzymatic reactions that are impaired in these patients are all dehydrogenases for different acyl CoAs. Przyrembel et al. [7] speculated that these several dehydrogenases might have a common protein component essential for their function and that this component is deficient in GA II. Since it is now known that BDH [122], isovaleryl CoA dehydrogenase [41, 128], and GADH [116] consist of four identical subunits, this mechanism became unlikely. Lack of a common flavin coenzyme due to impaired vitamin transport or impaired coenzyme synthesis was also possible. Since a single electron-transferring flavoprotein (ETF) functions for all these acyl CoA dehydrogenases, ETF could be deficient in patients with GA II and EMA [8, 328] (Figs. 22-7 and 22-14). This hypothesis was supported by the detection of urinary sarcosine in the case reported by Goodman et al. [328] and that reported by Gregersen et al. [330], since sarcosine dehydrogenase requires the same ETF [119].

To study this possibility, Rhead, Mantagos, and Tanaka isolated mitochondria from GA II fibroblasts. As expected, the activities of mitochondrial BDH and isovaleryl CoA dehydrogenase as measured by the tritium-release assay were normal in GA II cells and indicated that these dehydrogenases per se are intact [334]. Normal glutaryl CoA dehydrogenase activity has also been found in the case reported by Gregersen et al. [330]. Rhead et al. further assayed the ETF activity using a modified dye-reduction method in which an excessive amount of purified pig liver GADH was added to make ETF activity rate-limiting. Unexpectedly, the mitochondrial ETF activity in GA II cells was normal [334]. Thus, the precise enzymatic defect in GA II and EMA remains obscure. A metabolic block in the electron transport from ETF to coenzyme Q is likely.

MECHANISM OF HYPOGLYCEMIA   The most important clinical manifestation in these patients has been life-threatening hypoglycemia. Impaired oxidation of fatty acid results in decreased production of acetyl CoA and reducing equivalents. Since acetyl CoA and reducing equivalents are required for pyruvate carboxylase activation [335] and 3-phosphoglycerate dehydrogenase activity (reversed reaction) [336], respectively, and since these reactions are the key steps in the gluconeogenic pathway, inhibition of fatty acid oxidation is likely to be one of the causes of the hypoglycemia [337]. Futhermore, glutaryl CoA and ethylmalonic acid are inhibitors of the mitochondrial transport of malate in vitro, a rate-limiting step in gluconeogenesis [155]. Therefore, the accumulation of ethylmalonic acid and glutaryl CoA may also contribute to the hypoglycemia.

Genetics   Biochemically, GA II and EMA are distinct in the urinary metabolite patterns. They also differ in that cellular butyrate oxidation was more distinctly impaired in GA II than in EMA ($p < 0.001$). It is not yet known whether this heterogeneity reflects mutations of two different genes or two different mutant alleles of the same gene. Studies of family members of the proband with EMA are consistent with autosomal recessive inheritance. Intact cultured cells from the father, mother, and two clinically unaffected sibs demonstrated values for [1-^{14}C]butyrate oxidation between those of the proband and controls. These findings are consistent with the notion that the proband is homozygous for a mutant allele while the other family members studied are heterozygous. Considerable variation in butyrate oxidation was observed among these putative heterozygotes. This could mean that the proband is a compound heterozygote. It could also mean that the study of intact cells is too crude an index with which to define precisely the genetics of EMA or of GA II.

The heterogeneous nature of the diseases in this category was further emphasized by the detection of a 19-year-old woman who had repeated episodes of hypoglycemia accompanied by elevated serum concentrations of free fatty acids, fatty infiltration of the liver, hepatic dysfunction, and proximal myopathy [329]. Increased quantities of glutaric acid, ethylmalonic acid, dicarboxylic acids with 6 to 10 carbons, and isovalerylglycine were consistently found in her urine. Since glutaric acid was always the dominating urinary metabolite, this patient was diagnosed as having GA II. The ability of cultured skin fibroblasts from the patient to oxidize [1-^{14}C]butyrate and [2-^{14}C]lysine was 26 percent and 41 percent of control, respectively [329]. This patient appears to differ clinically as well as biochemically from those with the severe type of GA II and from the patient with EMA.

Sweetman et al. [327] noted that, in the families of two patients with severe GA II, all four affected patients were male while all female sibs were normal. They suggested, therefore, that GA II might be inherited as an X-linked recessive trait, but a female newborn, who died at the age of 3 days due to severe GA II, has since been reported [330], thereby weakening the argument for X-linkage.

Table 22-8   Oxidation of [1-^{14}C]butyrate, [2-^{14}C]lysine, [2-^{14}C]leucine, and [1,4-^{14}C]succinate by cultured skin fibroblasts from a patient with glutaric aciduria type II and a patient with ethylmalonic-adipic aciduria

	Substrates, nanomoles $^{14}CO_2$ produced per 10^6 cells per hour			
Cells	[1-^{14}C]butyrate	[2-^{14}C]lysine	[2-^{14}C]leucine	[1,4-^{14}C]succinate
Control (6)	2.57 ± 0.39	0.53 ± 0.08	0.47 ± 0.03	0.89 ± 0.20
Glutaric aciduria type II (1)	0.08, 0.08	0.05, 0.05	0.04, 0.04	0.60, 1.22
Ethylmalonic-adipic aciduria (1)	0.35 ± 0.04*	0.15 ± 0.03*	0.11 ± 0.04*	0.89 ± 0.18*

* Mean of 4 to 6 experiments ± SE. Each experiment was done in duplicate.
NOTE: Data are expressed as mean ± SE unless otherwise mentioned.
SOURCE: From Mantagos, Genel, and Tanaka [8].

Diagnosis   Severe hypoglycemia of unknown etiology accompanied by acidosis without concomitant ketosis is suggestive of this disease. The absence of ketosis in the face of severe acidosis is a peculiar finding for diseases in this group, as it is in Jamaican vomiting sickness (see below), because pathways for the two major sources of ketone bodies, namely the catabolism of leucine and fatty acids, are blocked in these diseases. Definitive diagnosis should be readily accomplished by GC analysis of urine [80, 252] (Fig. 22-15). Definitive identification of the organic acids by GC/MS is desirable.

Figure 22-15   Urinary organic acids from a patient with glutaric aciduria type II (acute stage) (top) and a patient with ethylmalonic aciduria (remission) (bottom). A 10 percent OV-1 column was used for analyses of both samples. The acids noted in these figures are: 1, ethylmalonic; 2, succinic; 3, methylsuccinic; 4, glutaric; 5, adipic; 6, octanedioic (suberic); 7, hippuric; 8, decenedioic; 9, decanedioic (sebacic) and 10, palmitic. n-Pentadecanoic acid (PDA), 1 mg/per milligram creatinine, was added as an internal standard. (From Tanaka et al. [80].)

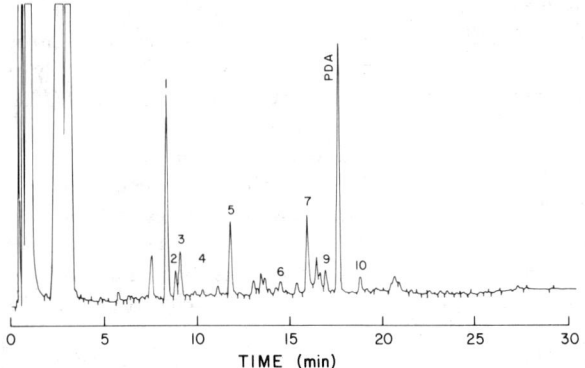

GLUTARIC ACIDURIA TYPE II (ACUTE STAGE)
(10% OV-1)

ETHYLMALONIC ACIDURIA (REMISSION)
(10% OV-1)

TIME (min)

Treatment   In spite of intensive treatment with glucose and sodium bicarbonate infusions, three neonates with GA II died within 3 days of birth. The EMA patient has been treated with a low fat–high carbohydrate diet. Urinary ethylmalonic acid remained essentially unchanged, but excretion of other organic acids was greatly decreased [8]. On dietary treatment she has had four episodes of vomiting and lethargy but in none of these episodes has she become hypoglycemic or acidotic.

Pathology   Diffuse fatty liver was found in two autopsied patients. Cerebral edema, patchy destruction of the cerebral white matter, and some reactive gliosis were also noted [327, 330].

Jamaican Vomiting Sickness

This disease is not an inherited metabolic disorder, but it is described here briefly because the biochemical findings of this disease are very similar to those of GA II and EMA [12].

Incidence and Clinical Manifestations   Jamaican vomiting sickness has been known to occur endemically in Jamaica since as early as 1875 [338]. The major clinical features are acute onset and severe vomiting, which are usually followed by convulsions, coma, and death. Severe hypoglycemia, with blood glucose levels as low as 3 mg/dl, is observed in most patients [339, 340]. Children between 2 and 10 years of age represent the largest proportion of reported cases, but older people are also known to have been affected. The mortality rate was about 80 percent before 1952 because the etiology and mechanism of the disease were not understood. The most prominent findings in autopsied cases have been depletion of liver glycogen and a peculiar type of diffuse fatty infiltration with small lipid droplets in the liver, kidney, and other organs [340].

Biochemical Mechanisms   Ingestion of the arillus of unripe ackee, a local fruit, had been identified as a source of this disease in popular folklore and medical literature from the beginning of this century [338]. Ripe ackee fruit was believed to be nontoxic and has been a main staple in the diet in Jamaica. The association of unripe ackee with this disease was not substantiated scientifically until the isolation of two toxins, hypoglycins A and B, from arilli and seeds of unripe ackee by Hassal and Reyle in 1955 [137]. Hypoglycin A in a single dose induces acute severe hypoglycemia, vomiting, prostration, coma, and death in laboratory animals [138, 139]. Severe histologic changes such as depletion of hepatic glycogen and fatty infiltration of viscera, very much like the changes seen in patients with Jamaican vomiting sickness, are also observed. The chemistry and biochemistry of hypoglycins were described earlier (pages 448 and 449).

In spite of the substantial progress in understanding the mode of actions of hypoglycin, biochemical investigation of patients with Jamaican vomiting sickness had been reported rarely until recently. Tanaka, Kean, and Johnson recently analyzed blood and urine specimens from two sibs who died on the same day after a sudden onset and short fulminant course typical of Jamaican vomiting sickness [12]. They identified methylenecyclopropylacetic acid, a known metabolite of hypoglycin A, in the urine of two patients with Jamaican vomiting sickness. Excretion of unusual dicarboxylic acids such as ethylmalonic, methylsuccinic, glutaric, adipic, and dicarboxylic acids with 8- and 10-carbon chains were also detected in both patients. The amounts of these dicarboxylic acids were 70 to 1000 times higher than normal. These metabolites had previously been identified in urine of hypoglycin-treated rats [142]. Urinary excretion of short-chain fatty acids was also increased up to 300 times normal. This evidence strongly implicates hypoglycin A as the etiologic agent in Jamaican vomiting sickness.

3-Methylcrotonyl CoA Carboxylase Deficiency

Only two patients suspected of having isolated deficiency of 3-methylcrotonyl CoA carboxylase have been reported. The first was a 4½-month-old Norwegian girl of consanguine parents reported by Eldjarn et al. in 1970 [9, 341]. Her first week of life was unremarkable, but feeding difficulties, including choking, were experienced from the second week. Her growth was not retarded, but her motor development was far behind that expected for her age. Major clinical manifestations included severe hypotonia, atrophy of skeletal muscles, absence of the deep tendon reflexes, and fibrillation of the tongue. She could not raise her head or hold objects in her hands, but she was mentally alert. Sensation and sphincter function were normal. This clinical picture was similar to that of infantile spinal muscular atrophy (Werdnig-Hoffmann disease). She was neither ketotic nor acidotic. A peculiar odor, which was likened to that of "tomcat's urine," was noted.

Two unusual organic acids, 3-hydroxyisovaleric acid and 3-methylcrotonylglycine, were detected in large amounts in her urine (430 to 490 mg/day and 60 to 90 mg/day, respectively). Coon and associates had previously shown that 3-hydroxyisovalerate may be produced in vitro via hydration of 3-methylcrotonyl CoA by enoyl hydrase (crotonase), although this is not an obligate metabolic step. 3-Methylcrotonylglycine is a glycine conjugate of 3-methylcrotonyl CoA. Therefore, excretion of these two compounds is apparently the result of a defect of 3-methylcrotonyl CoA carboxylase. Significantly, 3-methylcrotonic acid did not accumulate in the blood (less than 0.5 mg/dl) (Fig. 22-12). The patient was fed a low leucine diet with supplements of 0.25 mg biotin daily. Although the amount of urinary 3-hydroxyisovalerate and 3-methylcrotonylglycine decreased to 20 to 100 mg/day and 30 to 100 mg/day, respectively, her clinical condition did not improve and she died 3 months later.

Finnie et al. subsequently described a female infant who died at 3 months of age due to a profound metabolic acidosis [342].

She, too, had a neonatal history of feeding difficulty and failure to thrive. Large amounts of 3-hydroxisovaleric, lactic, and 2-ketoglutaric acids were detected in her urine. A mitochondrial preparation obtained from her liver had no detectable activity of 3-methylcrotonyl CoA carboxylase, but the propionyl CoA carboxylase activity in this preparation was comparable to that found in rat liver [342].

Since then at least 13 additional patients who excreted increased amounts of 3-hydroxyisovaleric acid and 3-methylcrotonylglycine have been reported. It has become clear from urinary metabolite analysis, enzyme studies, and clinical biotin responsiveness that most of these were, in fact, patients with multiple-carboxylase deficiency (see Chap. 23). In the latter group, the main clinical manifestations were metabolic acidosis and dermatitis. Increased amounts of lactic and pyruvic acids, and metabolites typical of propionic acidemia were excreted in urine in addition to the compounds characteristic of 3-methylcrotonyl CoA carboxylase deficiency. At present, then it is not certain that the patients reported by Eldjarn [9, 341], Finnie [342] and colleagues represent examples of isolated deficiency of 3-methylcrotonyl CoA carboxylase.

HMG CoA Lyase Deficiency

Incidence and Clinical Manifestations Since the first report of this disease by Faull and associates in 1976 [11], four additional patients have been reported [343–346]. Affected patients are normal at birth. Three of these five patients began having severe episodes of vomiting, cyanosis, hypotonia, lethargy, and metabolic acidosis a few days after birth. Extreme hypoglycemia, ranging from 1.8 to 7.2 mg/dl, was observed in these infants. The other two patients had their first episode at 6 to 9 months of age. Two of the five patients died during such an episode [343–345]. Two others recovered from a severe episode after correction of the hypoglycemia and subsequently achieved normal development when treated with a protein-restricted diet. During remission, mild compensated metabolic acidosis has been observed in these children. In the fifth child, severe brain damage occurred during an episode, causing hemiplegia and choreoathetoid movement [345].

Biochemical Abnormalities HMG, 3-methylglutaconic, 3-hydroxyisovaleric, and 3-methylglutaric acids are excreted in large amounts in the urine of these patients [347–349]. From this metabolite pattern, patients with this disease were considered to have a metabolic block at the last step in leucine catabolism, namely HMG CoA lyase. This could cause the accumulation of HMG CoA and the more proximal intermediates, such as 3-methylglutaconyl CoA and 3-methylcrotonyl CoA. HMG and 3-methylglutaconic acid would accordingly be produced from the corresponding CoA esters by hydrolysis. Finally, 3-methylglutaric and 3-hydroxyisovaleric acids would presumably be produced by hydrogenation of 3-methylglutaconyl CoA and hydration of 3-methylcrotonyl CoA, respectively, followed by thioester cleavage.

Severe HMG CoA lyase deficiency (0 to 3 percent of control) has, in fact, been demonstrated in tissues and cells from three of these patients [343, 344, 350]. In the child with delayed clinical onset reported by Truscott et al. [345], HMG CoA lyase activity in fibroblasts was 60 percent of the control value. Although the combined total of the three major urinary metabolites (HMG, 3-methylglutaconic, and 3-methylglutaric acids) in this child was at least seven times the highest normal value, it was less than 5 percent of that observed in severely affected patients. It is conceivable that this child may be a heterozygote who excreted increased amounts of urinary metabolites under severe metabolic stress (see below).

Finally, Greter and associates reported two sibs with progressive encephalopathy consisting of spastic paraphareses, dementia, and optic atrophy, who excreted increased amounts of 3-methylglutaconic acid in the urine [351]. The amount of 3-methylglutaconic acid excreted was relatively small, and corresponded to no more than 2 percent of the daily leucine intake. A preliminary report on a similar case had been presented previously [352], but this patient was later found to have HMG CoA lyase deficiency [353]. Since 3-methylglutaconic acid is one of the major urinary metabolites found in patients with HMG CoA lyase deficiency [347], the patients described by Greter et al. [351] must be further defined by enzymatic study.

Genetics Although the mode of inheritance of this disease is not precisely known, it appears to be autosomal recessive. Two of the five patients were female, but one had intermediate values for both enzyme activity and urinary metabolites [345]. The other affected female has not been well characterized [346]. The parents of two severely affected sibs each had intermediate enzyme activities: the activity in leukocytes from the mother and from the father were 5.1 and 10.8 nmol/min per milligram protein, respectively (normal value: 16.4 to 27.5 nmol/min per milligram protein). Interestingly, the mother excreted small but increased amounts of the metabolites characteristic of this disorder, but the father did not [344].

3-Ketothiolase Deficiency

This condition involves an enzyme catalyzing the last step of isoleucine catabolism, i.e., that leading to propionyl CoA formation (Fig. 22-1). Its deficiency thus forms a bridge between those conditions discussed here and those described in Chap. 23.

Clinical Manifestations In 1971 Daum et al. [10] described a 6-year-old boy with a history of episodic ketoacidosis dating from age 17 months. Several of these episodes had required hospital admission and parenteral fluid and alkali therapy; others had abated spontaneously. Despite these recurrent setbacks he was physically and intellectually intact. Subsequently, this group [182] described a second family with three affected sibs. One, a 5-year-old girl, also had recurrent ketoacidosis and normal psychomotor development. Her two sibs fared much worse. One died at age 1 year during an episode of fever, vomiting, hyperventilation, and seizures; the second was alive at age 8 but with distinct psychomotor retardation subsequent to repeated ketoacidotic attacks. Two children from two other families have similar, although not identical, clinical findings. The girl described by Keating et al. [354, 355] began having attacks of lethargy and vomiting as early as age 12 weeks, which left her with residual developmental delay. She also demonstrated neutropenia, thrombocytopenia, hyperglycinemia, hyperglycinuria, and hyperammonemia. These manifestations abated as her episodes of ketoacidosis were controlled. In contrast, the patient reported by Gompertz et al. [356] had experienced only one episode of acidosis following an appendectomy. He, too, had hyperglycinuria but not hyperglycinemia. The marked differences in age of onset, frequency of attacks, and ultimate outcome among these six patients may reflect different degrees of enzymatic impairment, but could also depend on such factors as dietary protein content and frequency of intercurrent bacterial or viral infections. More recently, Robinson et al. [181] described a 1-year-old girl who developed severe ketoacidosis and vomiting. This patient had an apparent salicylate level of 11 mg/dl, leading initially to the clinical diagnosis of salicylism, but further investigation by GC/MS analysis of blood revealed that this patient did not have salicylate intoxication. Rather, the increased concentrations of acetoacetate in blood and urine were responsible for the falsely high salicylate concentration.

Biochemical Abnormalities Of the seven children described above, five have been studied chemically. In each, GC study of urinary organic acids has revealed large amounts of 2-methyl-3-hydroxybutyrate, 2-methylacetoacetate, and butanone. Although quantitative data are sparse, it is clear that excretion of these metabolites was much greater during attacks than in intercritical periods. These unusual metabolites, found in only trace amounts in normal subjects, led to the current understanding of this entity.

As shown in Fig. 22-1, each of the metabolites excreted by these patients appears in the pathway of isoleucine catabolism, thereby suggesting a block in one of the distal steps in this metabolic sequence. This view is supported by several observations: augmentation of 2-methyl-3-hydroxybutyrate and 2-methylacetoacetate excretion by protein or isoleucine loading [182, 354, 356]; excretion of N-tiglylglycine, another isoleucine intermediate, by several of these patients [182, 354–356]; absence of abnormal amounts of propionate or methylmalonate in body fluids [182, 355, 356]; and impaired oxidation of [^{14}C]isoleucine by the patients' intact, cultured fibroblasts [182, 354, 356]. All these findings are consistent with a defect in the cleavage of 2-methylacetoacetyl CoA to propionyl CoA and acetyl CoA. This reaction has been characterized in animal tissues [166] but the enzyme which catalyzes it has not been well defined (see page 449).

There may be two different types of this disease. In three children reported by Daum et al. [182], a large excess of 2-methyl-3-hydroxybutyric acid and a smaller excess of 2-methylacetoacetic acid were present at all times regardless of the presence or absence of the ketone bodies (3-hydroxybutyric and acetoacetic acids). This finding plus the observation that acetoacetate metabolism was normal, led Daum et al. to propose that 2-methylacetoacetyl CoA 3-ketothiolase is a specific enzyme acting on 2-methylacetoacetyl CoA, but no enzyme assays were carried out on this patient. In contrast, in the patient reported by Robinson et al. 2-methyl-3-hydroxybutyric and 2-methylacetoacetic acids appeared only when the ketone bodies accumulated under metabolic stress [181]. Importantly, K$^+$-dependent acetoacetyl CoA 3-ketothiolase was deficient in fibroblasts from their patients when acetoacetyl CoA was used as substrate. It is not clear whether the patients reported by Keating [354, 356] and Gompertz [356] and colleagues belong to either of these putative types, or whether one or more ketothiolases exist. Gompertz et al. [356] showed that leukocyte extracts from their patient incorporated only 10 percent as much tritiated water into propionate when incubated with tiglyl CoA as did control extracts. This result is consistent with a defect between tiglyl CoA and propionyl CoA but does not identify the specific step and enzyme involved.

Pathologic Physiology Although a block at the 3-keto-thiolase step adequately explains the urinary accumulation of organic acids and ketones in this disorder, it cannot account for the distinct hyperglycinemia or hyperglycinuria seen in some patients [352, 354, 355]. Hillman and colleagues [354, 355] have made some observations relevant to propionic acidemia and methylmalonic acidemia as well as to 3-ketothiolase deficiency. They reported that cultured cells from their 3-keto-thiolase–deficient patient accumulated glycine when incubated with isoleucine. Such cells or extracts thereof also demonstrated impaired oxidation of [^{14}C]glycine to $^{14}CO_2$ and impaired conversion of glycine to serine. Since tiglic acid, 2-methyl-3-hydroxybutyrate, 2-methylacetoacetate, and butanone also accumulated in the culture medium under these conditions, it was reasoned that one or more of these intermediates was responsible for the observed defects in glycine utilization and presumably for hyperglycinemia in vivo.

Genetics Although few patients have been reported, considerable evidence already suggests that 3-ketothiolase deficiency is inherited as an autosomal recessive trait: (1) the sex ratio among affected children is approximately 1:1 (3 males, 4 females), (2) parental consanguinity was present in one of the four families reported [182], (3) no instance of both affected parents and children has been noted, and (4) all the parents who have been tested [182, 355, 356] exhibit increased amounts of 2-methyl-3-hydroxybutyrate in their urine, although not nearly to the extent observed in their affected offspring. All these findings imply that affected children are homozygous for a mutant allele passed on by heterozygous parents.

Diagnosis and Management Since the clinical findings in this condition are observed in many other disease states, diagnosis depends on GC analysis of the urine. Urinary findings may be unremarkable when the child is well, thereby mandating chemical analysis during episodes of ketoacidosis or after challenge with protein or isoleucine. Experience thus far suggests that moderate dietary protein restriction and effective management of acute episodes may be sufficient to allow normal somatic and intellectual development in most (and perhaps all) of these children.

REFERENCES

1. MENKES JH, HURST PL, CRAIG JM: New syndrome: Progressive familial infantile dysfunction associated with an unusual urinary substance. *Pediatrics* 14:462, 1954
2. WESTALL RG, DANCIS J, MILLER S: Maple sugar urine disease. *Am J Dis Child* 94:571, 1957
3. WADA Y, TADA K, MINAGAWA A, YOSHIDA T, MORIKAWA T, OKAMURA T: Idiopathic hypervalinemia. *Tohoku J Exp Med* 81:46, 1963
4. JEUNE M, COLLOMBEL C, MICHEL M, DAVID M, GUIBAUD P, GUERRIER G, ALBERT J: Hyperleucinisoleucinemie par defaut partiel de transamination associee a une hyperprolinemie de type 2. Observation familale d'une double aminoacidopathie. *Ann Pediat* 17:85, 1970
5. TANAKA K, BUDD MA, EFRON ME, ISSELBACHER KJ: Isovaleric acidemia: A new genetic defect of leucine metabolism. *Proc Nat Acad Sci USA* 56:236, 1966
6. BUDD MA, TANAKA K, HOLMES LB, EFRON ML, CRAWFORD JD, ISSELBACHER KJ: Isovaleric acidemia: Clinical features of a new genetic defect of leucine metabolism. *N Engl J Med* 277:321, 1967
7. PRZYREMBEL H, WENDEL U, BECKER K, BREMER HJ, BRUINVIS L, KETTING D, WADMAN SK: Glutaric aciduria type II: Report of a previously undescribed metabolic disorder. *Clin Chim Acta* 66:227, 1976
8. MANTAGOS S, GENEL M, TANAKA K: Ethylmalonic-adipic aciduria: In vivo

9. ELDJARN L, JELLUM E, STOKKE O, PANDE H, WAHLER PE: β-Hydroxyisovaleric aciduria and β-methylcrotonylglycinuria. A new error of metabolism. *Lancet* 2:521, 1970
10. DAUM RS, LAMM PH, MAMER OA, SCRIVER CR: A "new" disorder of isoleucine catabolism. *Lancet* 2:1289, 1971
11. FAULL K, BOLTON P, HALPERN B, HAMMOND J, DANKS DM, HAHNEL R, WILKINSON SP, WYSOCKI SJ, MASTERS PL: Patient with defect in leucine metabolism. *N Engl J Med* 294:1013, 1976
12. TANAKA K, KEAN EA, JOHNSON B: Vomiting sickness of Jamaica: Biochemical investigation of two cases. *N Engl J Med* 295:461, 1976
13. MILLER LL: The role of the liver and non-hepatic tissues in the regulation of free amino acid levels in the blood, in Holden JT (ed): *Amino Acid Pools.* Amsterdam, Elsevier, 1961
14. ICHIHARA A, KOYAMA E: Transaminase of branched chain amino acids. I. Branched chain amino acids—α-ketoglutarate transaminase. *J Biochem* 59:160, 1966
15. DANCIS J, HUTZLER J, LEVITZ M: Tissue distribution of branched chain ketoacid decarboxylase. *Biochim Biophys Acta* 52:60, 1961
16. CONNELLY JL, DANNER DJ, BOWDEN JA: Branched chain α-keto acid metabolism. I. Isolation, purification and partial characterization of bovine liver α-ketoisocaproic α-keto-β-methylvaleric acid dehydrogenase. *J Biol Chem* 243:1198, 1968
17. KHATRA BS, CHAWLA RK, SEWELL CW, RUDMAN D: Distribution of branched chain α-keto acid dehydrogenases in primate tissues. *J Clin Invest* 59:558, 1977
18. BUSE MG, BIGGERS JF, FREDERICI KH, BUSE JF: Oxidation of branched chain amino acids by isolated hearts and diaphragms of the rat. *J Biol Chem* 247:8085, 1972
19. BUSE MG, BIGGERS JF, DRIER C, BUSE JF: The effect of ephedrine, glucagon and the nutritional state on the oxidation of branched chain amino acids and pyruvate by isolated hearts and diaphragms of the rat. *J Biol Chem* 248:697, 1973
20. BUSE M, JURSINIC S, REID SS: Regulation of branched chain amino acid oxidation in isolated muscles, nerves and aorta of rats. *Biochem J* 148:363, 1975
21. SHINNICK FL, HARPER AE: Branched chain amino acid oxidation by isolated rat tissue preparations. *Biochim Biophys Acta* 437:477, 1976
22. MANCHESTER KL: Oxidation of amino acids by isolated rat diaphragm and the influence of insulin. *Biochim Biophys Acta* 100:295, 1965
23. ODESSEY R, GOLDBERG AL: Oxidation of leucine by rat skeletal muscle. *Am J Physiol* 223:1376, 1972
24. FELIG P: Amino acid metabolism in man. *Ann Rev Biochem* 44:933, 1975
25. GOLDBERG AL, CHANG TW: Regulation and significance of amino acid metabolism in skeletal muscle. *Fed Proc* 37:2301, 1978
26. ADIBI SA: Roles of branched chain amino acids in metabolic regulation. *J Lab Clin Med* 95:475, 1980
27. MENKES JH: Maple syrup urine disease: Isolation and identification of organic acids in the urine. *Pediatrics* 23:348, 1959
28. TANAKA K: Disorders of organic acid metabolism, in Gaull GE (ed): *Biology of Brain Dysfunction.* New York, Plenum Press, 1975, vol 3, p 145
29. TANAKA K, ISSELBACHER KJ: The isolation and identification of N-isovalerylglycine from urine of patients with isovaleric acidemia. *J Biol Chem* 242:2966, 1967
30. TANAKA K: Studies on organic acid metabolism and its disorders using gas chromatography-mass spectrometry and stable isotopes, in *Proceedings of the Annual Meeting of the Japanese Biomed Mass Spec Society.* Tokyo, 1978, p 13
31. GOODMAN SI: An introduction to gas chromatography–mass spectrometry and the inherited organic acidemias. *Am J Human Genet* 32:781, 1980
32. TANAKA K, ARMITAGE IM, RAMSDELL HS, HSIA YE, LIPSKY SR, ROSENBERG LE: [^{13}C]Valine metabolism in methylmalonic acidemia using nuclear magnetic resonance: Identification of propionate as an obligate intermediate. *Proc Nat Acad Sci USA* 72:3692, 1975
33. BARETZ BH, TANAKA K: Metabolism in rats *in vivo* of isobutyrates labeled with stable isotopes: Identification of propionate as an obligate intermediate. *J Biol Chem* 253:4203, 1978
34. AMSTER J, TANAKA K: Metabolism in rats *in vivo* of (2S)[3,3,3-^{2}H$_3$] isobutyrate: Identification of (2proS) methyl group as the source of a proton in dehydrogenation. *J Biol Chem* 255:7763, 1980
35. TANAKA K, ABERHART J, AMSTER JI, JENKINS EE, HSU CT: Metabolism of valine chirally labeled with carbon 13 and deuterium in vitamin B$_{12}$-folate deficient rats *in vivo*: Studies on the physiological role of keto-enol tautomerization. *J Biol Chem* 255:7763, 1980
36. MAMER OA, TJOA SS: 2-Ethyl-3-deuterohydracrylic acid, the major urinary metabolite of 2-trideuteromethylbutyric acid by a new metabolic pathway. *Biomed Mass Spec* 2:133, 1975
37. MAMER OA, TJOA SS, SCRIVER CR, KLASSEN GA: Demonstration of a new

mammalian isoleucine catabolic pathway yielding an R series of metabolites. *Biochem J* 160:417, 1976

38. BARETZ BH, LOLLO CP, TANAKA K: Metabolism in rats *in vivo* of RS-2-methylbutyrate and *n*-butyrate labeled with stable isotopes at various positions: Mechanism of biosynthesis and degradation of ethylmalonyl semialdehyde and ethylmalonic acid. *J Biol Chem* 254:3468, 1979

39. PETIT FH, YEAMAN SJ, REED LJ: Purification and characterization of branched chain α-ketoacid dehydrogenase complex of bovine kidney. *Proc Nat Acad Sci USA* 75:4881, 1978

40. NODA C, RHEAD WJ, TANAKA K: Isovaleryl-CoA dehydrogenase: Demonstration in rat liver mitochondria by ion exchange chromatography and isoelectric focusing. *Proc Nat Acad Sci USA* 77:2646, 1980

41. IKEDA Y, NODA C, TANAKA K: Purification and characterization of isovaleryl CoA dehydrogenase from rat liver mitochondria, in Walser M, Williamson JR (eds): *Metabolism and Clinical Implications of Branched Chain Amino and Ketoacids*. New York, Elsevier/North Holland, 1981, p 41

42. LYONS LB, COX RP, DANCIS J: Complementation analysis of MSUD in heterokaryons derived from cultured human fibroblasts. *Nature* 243:533, 1973

43. ROBINSON BH, TAYLOR J, SHERWOOD WG: Deficiency of dihydrolipoyl dehydrogenase (a component of the pyruvate and α-keto-glutarate dehydrogenase complex): A cause of congenital chronic lactic acidosis in infancy. *Pediatr Res* 11:1198, 1977

44. GOMPERTZ D, DRAFFAN GH, WATTS JL, HULL D: Biotin-responsive β-methylcrotonylglycinuria. *Lancet* 2:22, 1971

45. BARTLETT K, GOMPERTZ D: Combined carboxylase defect: Biotin-responsiveness in cultured fibroblasts. *Lancet* 2:804, 1976

46. SCRIVER CR, MACKENZIE S, CLOW CL, DELUIN E: Thiamin responsive maple syrup urine disease. *Lancet* 1:310, 1971

47. KRIEGER I, TANAKA K: Therapeutic effects of glycine in isovaleric acidemia. *Pediatr Res* 10:25, 1976

48. TADA K, WADA Y, ARAKAWA T: Hypervalinemia: Its metabolic lesion and therapeutic approach. *Am J Dis Child* 113:64, 1967

49. DANCIS J, HUTZLER J, TADA K, WADA Y, MORIKAWA T, ARAKAWA T: Hypervalinemia: A defect in valine transamination. *Pediatrics* 39:813, 1967

50. ICHIHARA A, TAKAHASHI H, AKI H, SHIRAI A: Transaminase of branched chain amino acids. II. Physiological change in enzyme activity in rat liver and kidney. *Biochem Biophys Res Commun* 26:674, 1967

51. AKI K, OGAWA K, SHIRAI A, ICHIHARA A: Transaminase of branched chain amino acids. III. Purification and properties of the mitochondrial enzyme from hog heart and comparison with the supernatant enzyme. *J Biochem* 62:610, 1967

52. AKI K, OGAWA K, ICHIHARA A: Transaminase of branched chain amino acids. IV. Purification and properties of two enzymes from rat liver. *Biochim Biophys Acta* 159:276, 1968

53. TAYLOR RT, JENKINS WT: Leucine aminotransferase: I. Colorimetric assays. *J Biol Chem* 241:4391, 1966

54. TAYLOR RT, JENKINS WT: Leucine aminotransferase: II. Purification and characterization. *J Biol Chem* 241:4396, 1966

55. TAYLOR RT, JENKINS WT: Leucine aminotransferase: III. Activation by β-mercaptoethanol. *J Biol Chem* 241:4406, 1966

56. ODESSEY R, GOLDBERG AL: Leucine degradation in cell free extracts of skeletal muscle. *Biochem J* 178:475, 1979

57. ADIBI S: Interrelationships between level of amino acids in plasma and tissues during starvation. *Am J Physiol* 221:829, 1971

58. HSIEH B, TOLBERT NE: Glyoxylate aminotransferase in peroxisomes from rat liver and kidney. *J Biol Chem* 251:4408, 1976

59. COOPER AJL: Asparagine transaminase from rat liver. *J Biol Chem* 252:2032, 1977

60. JONES C, MOORE EE: Isolation of mutants lacking branched chain amino acid transaminase. *Somatic Cell Genet* 2:235, 1976

61. NAYLOR SL, BUSBY LL, KLEBE RJ: Biochemical selection systems for mammalian cells: The essential amino acids. *Somatic Cell Genet* 2:93, 1976

62. NAYLOR SL, SHOWS TB: Branched chain aminotransferase deficiency in Chinese hamster cells complemented by two independent genes on human chromosomes 12 and 19. *Somatic Cell Genet* 6:641, 1980

63. DANNER DJ, LEMMON SK, BESHARSE JC, ELSAS LJ: Purification and characterization of branched chain α-ketoacid dehydrogenase from bovine liver mitochondria. *J Biol Chem* 254:5522, 1979

64. REED LJ, LINN TC, PETIT FH, OLIVER RM, HUCHO F, PELLEY JW, RANDALL DD, ROCHE TE: Pyruvate dehydrogenase complex: Structure, function and regulation, in Mehlman MA, Hanson RW (eds): *Energy Metabolism and the Regulation of Metabolic Processes in Mitochondria*. New York, Academic Press, 1972, p 253

65. TANAKA K, ROSENBERG LE: Inborn errors of pyruvic acid metabolism, in Freinkel N (ed): *Contemporary Metabolism*. New York, Plenum Press, 1979, vol 1, p 461

66. SAKURAI Y, FUKUYOSHI Y, HAMADA M, HAYAKAWA T, KOIKE M: Mammalian α-keto acid dehydrogenase complexes. VI. Nature of the multiple

67. forms of pig heart lipoamide dehydrogenase. *J Biol Chem* 245:4452, 1970

67. BARRERA CR, NAMIHARA G, HAMILTON L, MUNK P, ELEY MH, LYNN TC, REED L: α-Keto acid dehydrogenase complex. XVI. Studies on the subunit structure of the pyruvate dehydrogenase complexes from bovine kidney and heart. *Arch Biochem Biophys* 148:343, 1972

68. ROCHE TE, REED LJ: Function of the nonidentical subunits of mammalian pyruvate dehydrogenase. *Biochem Biophys Res Commun* 48:840, 1972

69. HUBNER G, NEEF H, SCHELLENBERGER A, BERNHARDT R, KHAILOVA L: Two-center mechanism for the oxidative decarboxylation of pyruvate by the pyruvate decarboxylating component of the pyruvate dehydrogenase complex of pigeon breast muscle. *FEBS Lett* 86:6, 1978

70. HAYAKAWA T, KANZAKI T, KITAMURA T, FUKUYOSHI Y, SAKURAI Y, KOIKE K, SUEMATSU T, KOIKE M: Mammalian α-keto acid dehydrogenase complexes. V. Resolution and reconstitution studies of the pig heart pyruvate dehydrogenase complex. *J Biol Chem* 244:3660, 1969

71. WIELAND OH, SIESS EA, WEISS L, LOFFLER G, PATZELT C, POSTENHAUSER R, HARTMANN U, SCHIRMANN A: Regulation of the mammalian pyruvate dehydrogenase complex by covalent modification. *Symp Soc Exp Biol* 27:381, 1973

72. CATE RL, ROCHE TE: A unifying mechanism for stimulation of mammalian pyruvate dehydrogenase kinase by reduced nicotinamide adenine dinucleotide dihydrolipoamide, acetyl coenzyme A or pyruvate. *J Biol Chem* 253:496, 1978

73. REED LJ, WILMS CR: Purification and resolution of the pyruvate dehydrogenase complex, in Wood WA (ed): *Methods in Enzymology*. New York, Academic Press, 1966, vol 9, p 247

74. WOHLHUETER RM, HARPER AE: Coinduction of rat liver branched chain α-keto acid dehydrogenase activities. *J Biol Chem* 245:2391, 1970

75. SNYDERMAN SE: Maple syrup urine disease, in Nyhan WL (ed): *Amino Acid Metabolism and Genetic Variation*. New York, McGraw-Hill, 1967, p 171

76. NORTON PM, ROITMAN E, SNYDERMAN SE, HOLT LE JR: A new finding in maple syrup urine disease. *Lancet* 1:26, 1962

77. SNYDERMAN SE, NORTON PM, ROITMAN E, HOLT JE JR: Maple syrup urine disease with particular reference to dietotherapy. *Pediatrics* 34:454, 1964

78. LANCASTER G, MAMER OA, SCRIVER CR: Branched chain alpha-keto acids isolated as oxime derivatives—relationship to the corresponding hydroxy acids and amino acids in maple syrup urine disease. *Metabolism* 23:257, 1974

79. JAKOBS C, SOLEM E, EK J, HALVORSEN K, JELLUM E: Investigation of the metabolic pattern in maple syrup urine disease by means of glass capillary gas chromatography and mass spectroscopy. *J Chromatogr* 143:31, 1977

80. TANAKA K, WEST-DULL A, HINE DG, LYNN TB: A gas chromatographic method for analysis of urinary organic acids. II. Description of procedures and its application for diagnosis of patients with organic acidurias. *Clin Chem* 26:1847, 1980

81. BOWDEN JA, CONNELLY JL: Branched chain α-keto acid metabolism. II. Evidence for the common identity of α-ketoisocaproic acid and α-keto-β-methylvaleric acid dehydrogenases. *J Biol Chem* 243:3526, 1968

82. HUTSON SM, CREE TC, HARPER AE: Regulation of leucine and α-ketoisocaproate metabolism in skeletal muscle. *J Biol Chem* 253:8126, 1978

83. PARKER PJ, RANDLE PL: Branched chain 2-oxo-acid dehydrogenase complex of rat liver. *FEBS Lett* 90:183, 1978

84. PARKER PJ, RANDLE PL: Partial purification and properties of branched chain 2-oxo-acid dehydrogenase of ox liver. *Biochem J* 171:751, 1978

85. DANNER DJ, LEMMON SK, ELSAS LJ: Substrate specificity and stabilization by thiamine pyrophosphate of rat liver branched chain α-keto acid dehydrogenase. *Biochem Med* 19:27, 1978

86. TAYLOR J, ROBINSON BH, SHERWOOD G: A defect in branched chain amino acid metabolism in a patient with congenital lactic acidosis due to dihydrolipoyl dehydrogenase deficiency. *Pediat Res* 12:60, 1978

87. PARKER PJ, PRANDLE PL: Active and inactive forms of branched chain 2-oxoacid dehydrogenase complex in rat heart and skeletal muscle. *FEBS Lett* 112:186, 1980

88. ODESSEY R: Reversible ATP-induced inactivation of branched chain 2-oxoacid dehydrogenase. *Biochem J* 192:155, 1980

89. SANS RM, JOLLY WW, HARRIS RA: Studies on the regulation of leucine metabolism: Mechanism responsible for oxidizable substrate inhibition and dichloroacetate stimulation by the heart. *Arch Biochem Biophys* 200:336, 1980

90. OSESIEY R: Direct evidence for the inactivation of the branched chain oxoacid dehydrogenase by enzyme phosphorylation. *FEBS Lett* 121:306, 1980

91. DANNER DJ, LEMMON SK, ELSAS LJ; Stabilization of mammalian liver branched chain α-keto acid dehydrogenase by thiamine pyrophosphate. *Arch Biochem Biophys* 202:23, 1980

92. DANNER DJ, DAVIDSON ED, ELSAS LJ: Thiamine increases the specific activity of human liver branched chain α-keto acid dehydrogenase. *Nature* 254:529, 1975

93. DANNER DJ, ELSAS LJ: Subcellular distribution and cofactor function of human branched chain α-keto acid dehydrogenase in normal and mutant cultured skin fibroblasts. *Biochem Med* 13:7, 1975

94. SKETCHER RD, FERN EB, JAMES WPT: The adaptation in muscle oxidation of leucine to dietary protein and energy metabolism. *Br J Nutr* 31:333, 1974

95. WAYMACK PP, DEBUYSERE MS, OLSEN MS: Studies on the activation and inactivation of the branched chain α-keto acid dehydrogenase in the perfused rat heart. *J Biol Chem* 255:9773, 1980

96. JOHNSON WA, CONNELLY JL: Cellular localization and characterization of bovine liver branched chain α-keto acid dehydrogenase. *Biochemistry* 11:1967, 1972

97. NODA C, ICHIHARA A: Control of ketogenesis from amino acids. II. Ketone bodies formation from α-ketoisocaproate, the keto-analog of leucine, by rat liver mitochondria. *J Biochem* 76:1123, 1974

98. VAN HINSBERGH VW, VEERKAMP JH, ENGELEN PJM, GHIJSEN WJ: Effect of L-carnitine on the oxidation of leucine and valine by rat skeletal muscle. *Biochem Med* 20:115, 1978

99. VAN HINSBERGH VWM, VEERKAMP JH, ZUURVELD JGEM: Role of carnitine in leucine oxidation by mitochondria of rat muscle. *FEBS Lett* 92:100, 1978

100. MAY ME, AFTRING RP, BUSE MG: Mechanism of the stimulation of branched chain oxoacid oxidation in liver by carnitine. *J Biol Chem* 255:8394, 1980

101. BIEBER LL, CHOI YR: Isolation and identification of aliphatic short-chain acylcarnitines from beef heart: Possible role for carnitine in branched chain amino acid metabolism. *Proc Nat Acad Sci USA* 74:2795, 1977

102. CHOI YR, FOGLE PJ, CLARKE PRH, BIEBER LL: Quantitation of water soluble acylcarnitines and carnitine acyltransferases in rat tissues. *J Biol Chem* 252:7930, 1977

103. BREMER J, DAVID EJ: The effect of acylcarnitines on the oxidation of branched chain α-keto acids in mitochondria. *Biochim Biophys Acta* 528:269, 1978

104. PAUL HS, ADIBI SA: Effect of carnitine on branched chain amino acid oxidation by liver and skeletal muscle. *Am J Physiol* 234:E494, 1978

105. TANAKA K, MILLER EM, ISSELBACHER KH: Hypoglycin A: A specific inhibitor of isovaleryl CoA dehydrogenase. *Proc Nat Acad Sci USA* 68:20, 1971

106. KIELLEY RK, SCHNEIDER WC: Synthesis of p-aminohippuric acid by mitochondria of mouse liver homogenates. *J Biol Chem* 185:869, 1950

107. SCHACHTER D, TAGGART JV: Glycine N-acylase: Purification and properties. *J Biol Chem* 208:263, 1954

108. BARTLETT K, GOMPERTZ D: The specificity of glycine N-acylase and acylglycine excretion in the organic aciduria. *Biochem Med* 10:15, 1974

109. GREENSTEIN JP, LEVINTOW L, BAKER CG, WHITE J: Preparation of the four isomers of isoleucine. *J Biol Chem* 188:647, 1951

110. HALPERN B, POLLACK GE: The configuration of the alloisoleucine present in maple syrup urine disease plasma. *Biochem Med* 4:352, 1970

111. MATTHEWS DE, BEN-GALIM E, HAYMOND MW, BIER DM: Alloisoleucine formation in maple syrup urine disease: Isotopic evidence for the mechanism. *Pediatr Res* 14:858, 1980

112. MEISTER A: Studies on d- and l-α-keto-β-methylvaleric acids. *J Biol Chem* 190:269, 1951

113. MEISTER A, WHITE A: Growth response of the rat to the ketoanalogues of leucine and isoleucine. *J Biol Chem* 191:211, 1951

114. WEINBERG RB, WALSER M: Racemization of the keto-analog of isoleucine in the intact dog. *Biochem Med* 17:164, 1977

115. GREEN DE, ALLMAN DW: Fatty acid oxidation, in Greenberg DM (ed): *Metabolic Pathways.* 3d ed. New York, Academic Press, 1968, vol II, p 1

116. HALL C: Acyl CoA dehydrogenase and electron transferring flavoprotein, in Fleisher S, Packer L (eds): *Methods in Enzymology.* New York, Academic Press, 1978, vol 53, p 502

117. HOSKINS DD, BJUR RA: The oxidation of N-methylglycines by primate liver mitochondria. *J Biol Chem* 239:1856, 1964

118. HOSKINS DD, BJUR RA: The electron transferring flavoprotein of primate liver mitochondria. *J Biol Chem* 240:2201, 1965

119. HOSKINS DD: The electron transferring flavoprotein as a common intermediate in the mitochondrial oxidation of butyryl Co A and sarcosine. *J Biol Chem* 241:4472, 1966

120. RUZICKA FJ, BEINERT H: A new membrane iron-sulfur flavoprotein of the mitochondrial transfer system. The entrance point of the fatty acyl dehydrogenation pathway. *Biochem Biophys Res Commun* 66:622, 1975

121. RUZICKA FJ, BEINERT H: A new iron-sulfur flavoprotein of the respiratory chain. A component of the fatty acid β-oxidation pathway. *J Biol Chem* 252:8440, 1977

122. GREEN DE, MII S, MAHLER HR: Studies on the fatty acid oxidizing system of animal tissues. III. Butyryl coenzyme A dehydrogenase. *J Biol Chem* 206:1, 1954

123. BEINERT H: Acyl dehydrogenases from pig and beef liver and beef heart, in *Methods in Enzymology.* New York, Academic Press, 1962, vol V p 546

124. BACHHAWAT BK, ROBINSON WG, COON MJ: Enzymatic carboxylation of β-hydroxyisovaleryl coenzyme A. *J Biol Chem* 219:539, 1956

125. TANAKA K: Isovaleric acidemia and its induction in experimental animals by hypoglycin, in Hommes FA, CJ van den Berg (eds): *Inborn Errors of Metabolism.* London, Academic Press, 1973, p 269

126. RHEAD WR, TANAKA K: Demonstration of a specific mitochondrial isovaleryl CoA dehydrogenase deficiency in fibroblasts from patients with isovaleric acidemia. *Proc Nat Acad Sci USA* 77:580, 1980

127. RHEAD WJ, HALL CL, TANAKA K: Novel tritium release assays for isovaleryl CoA dehydrogenases. *J Biol Chem* 256:1616, 1981

128. IKEDA Y, TANAKA K: Purification and characterization of isovaleryl CoA dehydrogenase from rat liver mitochondria. *Fed Proc* 40:1583, 1981

129. RHEAD WJ, DUBIEL B, TANAKA K: The tissue distribution of isovaleryl CoA dehydrogenase in the rat, in Walser M, Williamson JR (eds): *Metabolism and Clinical Implications of Branched Chain Amino and Keto Acids.* New York, Elsevier/North Holland, 1981, p 47

130. RHEAD WJ, TANAKA K: Manuscript in preparation

131. HALL C: Isovaleryl CoA dehydrogenase from pig liver mitochondria, in Walser M, Williamson JR (eds): *Metabolism and Clinical Implications of Branched Chain Amino and Keto Acids.* New York, Elsevier/North Holland, 1981, p 35

132. IKEDA Y, TANAKA K: Isolation of 2-methyl-branched chain acyl-CoA dehydrogenase from rat liver mitochondria. *Fed Proc* in press, 1982

133. ABERHART DJ, TANN CH: Substrate stereochemistry of isovaleryl CoA dehydrogenase: Elimination of the 2-pro-R hydrogen in biotin-deficient rats. *Bioorg Chem* 10:200, 1981

134. HIRTH CG, BIELMANN JF: Stereochemistry of the oxidation at the β-carbon of butyryl Coa. *FEBS Lett* 8:55, 1970

135. BUCKLERS L, UMANI-RONCHI A, RETEY J, ARIGONI D: Zur Stereochemie der enzymatischen Dehydrierung von Butyryl CoA. *Experientia* 15:931, 1970

136. TANAKA K: Jamaican vomiting sickness, in Vinken PJ, Bruyn GW (eds): *Handbook of Clinical Neurology (Intoxications of the Nervous System).* Amsterdam, Elsevier/North Holland, 1979, vol 37 p 511

137. HASSAL CH, REYLE K: Hypoglycin A and B, two biological active polypeptides from *Blighis sapida. Biochem J* 60:334, 1955

138. CHEN KK, ANDERSON RC, McCOWEN MC, HARRIS PN: Pharmacologic action of hypoglycin A and B. *J Pharmacol Exp Ther* 121:272, 1957

139. FENG PC, PATRICK SJ: Studies of the action of hypoglycin A, a hypoglycaemic substance. *Br J Pharmacol* 13:125, 1958

140. VON HOLT C: Methylenecyclopropylacetic acid, a metabolite of hypoglycin. *Biochim Biophys Acta* 125:1, 1966

141. VON HOLT C, VON HOLT M, BOHM H: Metabolic effects of hypoglycin and methylenecyclopropylacetic acid. *Biochim Biophys Acta* 125:11, 1966

142. TANAKA K: Mode of action of hypoglycin A (III): Isolation and identification of cis-4-decene-1,10-dioate, cis,-cis-4,7-decadiene,cis-4-octene-1, 8-dioate, glutarate, adipate, N-methylene-cyclopropyl)acetylglycine, and N-isovalerylglycine from urine of hypoglycin A administered rats. *J Biol Chem* 247:7465, 1972

143. VON HOLT C, BENEDICT I: Biochemie des hypoglycins A. II. Der Einflus des Hypoglycins auf die Oxydation von Glucose und Fettsauren. *Biochem Z* 331:430, 1959

144. McKERNS KW, BIRD HH, KALEITA E, COULOMB BS, DE RENZO EC: Effects of hypoglycin on certain aspects of glucose and fatty acid metabolism in the rat. *Biochem Pharmacol* 3:305, 1960

145. ENTEMAN M, BRESSLER R: The mechanism of action of hypoglycin on long chain fatty acid oxidation. *Mol Pharmacol* 3:333, 1967

146. BRESSLER R, CORREDOR C, BRENDEL K: Hypoglycin and hypoglycin-like compounds. *Pharmacol Rev* 21:105, 1969

147. SHERRATT HSA, HOLLAND PC, OSMUNDSEN H, SENIOR AE: On the mechanism of inhibition of fatty acid oxidation by hypoglycin and by pent-4-enoic acid, in Kean EA (ed): *Hypoglycin.* New York, Academic Press, 1975, p 127

148. POSNER BI, BABEN MS: Inhibition of the oxidation of leucine by hypoglycin. *Biochim Biophys Acta* 136:179, 1967

149. TANAKA K: Branched pentanoic acidemia and medium chain decarboxylic aciduria induced by hypoglycin: A: Inhibition of several short chain acyl CoA dehydrogenases, in Kean EA (ed): *Hypoglycin.* New York, Academic Press, 1975, p 67

150. TANAKA K, ISSELBACHER KJ, SHIH V: Isovaleric and α-methylbutyric acidemias induced by hypoglycin A: Mechanism of Jamaican vomiting sickness. *Science* 175:69, 1972

151. BILLINGTON D, KEAN EA, OSMUNDSEN H, SHERRATT HSA: Inhibition of butyryl CoA dehydrogenase and isovaleryl CoA dehydrogenase in rat liver mitochondria by hypoglycin metabolites. *Int Res Commun Syst (Biochem Pharmacol)* 2:1712, 1974

152. OSMUNDSEN H, SHERRATT HSA: A novel mechanism for inhibition of β-oxidation by methylenecyclopropylacetyl CoA, a metabolite of hypoglycin. *FEBS Lett* 55:38, 1975

153. KEAN EA: Selective inhibition of acyl-CoA dehydrogenases by a metabolite of hypoglycin. *Biochim Biophys Acta* 422:8, 1976

154. IKEDA Y, TANAKA K: Unpublished observations
155. TANAKA K, KERLEY R: Synergistic hypoglycemic effects of lysine and tryptophan with hypoglycin A: Interrelationship between the inhibition of glutaryl CoA dehydrogenase and gluconeogenesis, in Kean EA (ed): *Hypoglycin*. New York, Academic Press, 1975, p 163
156. FONG JC, SCHULZ H: On the rate-determining step of fatty acid oxidation in heart: Inhibition of fatty acid oxidation by 4-pentenoic acid. *J Biol Chem* 253:6917, 1978
157. KNAPPE J, SCHLEGEL HG, LYNEN F: Zur biochemischen Funktion des Biotins: 1, Die Beteiligung der β-Methylcrotonyl Carboxylase un der Bildung von β-hydroxy-β-methylglutaryl CoA aus β-Hydroxyisovaleryl CoA. *Biochem Z* 335:101, 1961
158. LYNEN F, KNAPPE J, LORCH E, JUTTING G, RINGELMAN E, LACHANCE JP: Zur biochemischen Function des Biotins: II, Reinigung und Wirkungsweise der β-Methylcrotonyl-carboxylase. *Biochem Z* 335:123, 1961
159. HIMES RH, YOUNG DL, RINGELMAN E, LYNEN F: The biochemical function of biotin. *Biochem Z* 337:48, 1963
160. APITZ-CASTRO R, REHN K, LYNEN F: β-Methylcrotonyl-CoA-Carboxylase: Krystallization und einige physikalische Eigenschaften. *Eur J Biochem* 16:71, 1970
161. SCHIELE U, NIEDERMEIER R, STURZER M, LYNEN F: Investigation of the structure of 3-methylcrotonyl-CoA carboxylase from Achromobacter. *Eur J Biochem* 60:259, 1975
162. LAU EP, COCHRAN BC, MUNSON L, FALL RR: Bovine kidney 3-methylcrotonyl CoA and propionyl CoA carboxylases: Each enzyme contains non-identical subunits. *Proc Nat Acad Sci USA* 76:214, 1979
163. LAU E, COCHRAN BC, FALL RR: Isolation of 3-methylcrotonyl-coenzyme A carboxylase from bovine kidney. *Arch Biochem Biophys* 205:352, 1980
164. HECTOR M, COCHRAN BC, LOGUE EA, FALL RR: Subcellular localization of 3-methylcrotonyl-coenzyme A carboxylase in bovine kidney. *Arch Biochem Biophys* 199:28, 1980
165. HILZ H, KNAPPE J, RINGELMAN E, LYNEN F: Methylglutaconase, eine neue Hydratase, die am Stoffwechsel verzweigter Carbonsauren beteiligt ibt. *Biochem Z* 329:476, 1958
166. BACHHAWAT BK, ROBINSON WG, COON MJ: The enzymatic cleavage of β-hydroxy-β-methylglutaryl coenzyme A to acetoacetate and acetyl CoA. *J Biol Chem* 216:727, 1955
167. STEGNIK LD, COON MJ: Stereospecificity and other properties of highly purified β-hydroxy-β-methylglutaryl coenzyme A cleavage enzyme from bovine liver. *J Biol Chem* 243:5272, 1968
168. CLINKENBREAD KD, REED WD, MOONEY RA, LANE MD: Intracellular localization of the 3-hydroxy-3-methylglutaryl coenzyme A cycle enzymes in liver. *J Biol Chem* 250:3108, 1975
169. ROBINSON WG, BACHHAWAT BK, COON MJ: Tiglyl coenzyme A and α-methylacetoacetyl coenzyme A, intermediates in the enzymatic degradation of isoleucine. *J Biol Chem* 218:391, 1956
170. STERN JR, DEL CAMPILLO A, RAW I: Enzymes of fatty acid metabolism. I. General introduction: Crystalline crotonase. *J Biol Chem* 218:971, 1956
171. STERN JR, DEL CAMPILLO A: Enzymes of fatty acid metabolism. II. Properties of crystalline crotonase. *J Biol Chem* 218:985, 1956
172. HASS GM, HILL RL: The subunit structure of crotonase. *J Biol Chem* 244:6080, 1969
173. DOUNCE AL, LEGGE G, VOLKMAN D, CHANDA SK: A simple method for the crystallization of beef liver crotonase. *Biochim Biophys Acta* 342:81, 1974
174. WILLADSEN P, EGGERER H: Substrate stereochemistry of the enoyl-CoA hydratase reaction. *Eur J Biochem* 54:247, 1975
175. FONG JD, SCHULZ H: Purification and properties of pig heart crotonase and presence of short chain and long chain enoyl coenzyme A hydratases in pig and guinea pig tissues. *J Biol Chem* 252:542, 1977
176. GEHRING U, LYNEN U: Thiolase, in Boyer PD (ed): *The Enzymes*. 3d ed. New York, Academic Press, 1972, vol 7, p 391
177. STERN JH, OCHOA S: Studies on enzymes of fatty acid metabolism, crystalline crotonyl hydrase (crotonase) and purified heart thiolase, in Popjak G, Le Breton E (eds): *Biochemical Problems of Lipids*. London, Butterworths, 1956
178. GEHRING U, RIEPERTINGER C, LYNEN F: Reinigung und kristallization der Thiolase, Untersuchungen zum Wirkungsmechanisms. *Eur J Biochem* 6:264, 1968
179. SEUBERT W, LAMBERTS I, KRAMER R, OHLY B: On the mechanism of malonyl CoA-independent fatty acid synthesis: I. The mechanism of elongation of long-chain fatty acids by acetyl CoA. *Biochim Biophys Acta* 164:498, 1968
180. MIDDLETON B: The oxoacyl-coenzyme A thioesters of animal tissues. *Biochem J* 132:717, 1973
181. ROBINSON BH, SHERWOOD G, TAYLOR J, BALFE JW, MAMER OA: Acetoacetyl CoA thiolase deficiency. A cause of severe ketoacidosis in infancy simulating salicylism. *J Pediatr* 95:228, 1979
182. DAUM RS, SCRIVER CR, MAMER OA, DEVLIN E, LAMM P, GOODMAN H: An inherited disorder of isoleucine catabolism causing accumulation of

α-methylacetoacetate and α-methyl-β-hydroxybutyrate, and intermittent metabolic acidosis. *Pediatr Res* 7:149, 1973
183. CARTER HE: The oxidation of branched chain fatty acids. *Biol Symposia* 5:47, 1941
184. STALDER K: Uber das vorkommen von Äthylmalonsäure im Harn. *Hoppe-Seylers Z Physiol Chem* 314:205, 1959
185. MAMER OA, TJOA SS: 2-Ethylhydracrylic acid: A newly described urinary organic acid. *Clin Chim Acta* 55:199, 1974
186. TANAKA K, RAMSDELL HS, BARETZ BH, KEEFE MB, KEAN EA, JOHNSON B: Identification of ethylmalonic acid in urine of two patients with the vomiting sickness of Jamaica. *Clin Chim Acta* 69:105, 1976
187. KAZIRO Y, OCHOA S, WARNER RC, CHEN JY: Metabolism of propionic acid in animal tissues. VIII. Crystalline propionyl carboxylase. *J Biol Chem* 236:1917, 1961
188. ROBINSON WG, NAGLE R, BACHHAWAT BK, KUPIECKI FP, COON MJ: Coenzyme A thiol esters of isobutyric, methacrylic and β-hydroxyisobutyric acids as intermediates in the enzymatic degradation of valine. *J Biol Chem* 224:1, 1957
189. RENDINA G, COON MJ: Enzymatic hydrolysis of the coenzyme A thiol esters of β-hydroxypropionic and β-hydroxyisobutyric acid. *J Biol Chem* 225:523, 1957
190. AMSTER J, TANAKA K: Isolation and identification of S(+)-3-hydroxyisobutyric acid in the urine of rats loaded with isobutyric acid. *Biochim Biophys Acta* 585:643, 1979
191. ROBINSON WG, COON MJ: The purification and properties of β-hydroxyisobutyric dehydrogenase. *J Biol Chem* 225:511, 1957
192. COON MJ: Enzymatic synthesis of branched chain acids from amino acids. *Fed Proc* 14:762, 1955
193. WADA Y: Idiopathic hypervalinemia: Valine and α-keto-acids in blood following an oral dose of valine. *Tohoku J Exp Med* 87:322, 1965
194. TADA K: Personal communication
195. HILLMAN R: Personal communication
196. DANCIS J, HUTZLER J, ROKKONES T: Intermittent branched-chain ketonuria: Variant of maple syrup urine disease. *N Engl J Med* 276:84, 1967
197. ZIPF W, HIEBER VC, ALLEN RC: Valine-toxic intermittent maple syrup urine disease: A previously unrecognized variant. *Pediatrics* 63:286, 1979
198. HARKNESS RA, COCKBURN F, GRANT M, GILES MM, TURNER TL: A new variety of maple syrup urine disease. *Ann Clin Biochem* 14:146, 1977
199. DANCIS J, LEVITZ M, MILLER S, WESTALL RG: Maple sugar urine disease. *Br Med J* 1:91, 1959
200. MACKENZIE DY, WOOLF LI: Maple syrup urine disease: An inborn error of metabolism of valine, leucine, and isoleucine associated with gross mental deficiency. *Br Med J* 1:90, 1959
201. ZEE DS, FREEMAN JM, HOLTZMAN NA: Ophthalmoplegia in maple syrup urine disease. *J Pediatr* 84:113, 1974
202. MACDONALD JT, SHER PK: Ophthalmoplegia as a sign of metabolic disease in the newborn. *Neurology* 27:970, 1977
203. CHHABRIA S, TOMASI LG, WONG PWK: Ophthalmoplegia and bulbar palsy in variant form of maple syrup urine disease. *Ann Neurol* 6:71, 1979
204. ELSAS LJ, PASK BA, WHEELER FB, PERL DP, TRUSTER S: Classical maple syrup urine disease: Cofactor resistance. *Metabolism* 21:929, 1972
205. HAYMOND MW, KARL IE, FEIGIN RD, DEVIVO D, PAGLIARA AS: Hypoglycemia and maple syrup urine disease—defective gluconeogenesis. *Pediatr Res* 7:500, 1973
206. HAYMOND MW, BEN-GALIM E, STROBEL KS: Glucose and alanine metabolism in children with maple syrup urine disease. *J Clin Invest* 62:398, 1978
207. MORRIS MD, LEWIS BD, DOOLAN PD, HARPER HA: Clinical and biochemical observations on an apparently non-fatal variant of branched-chain ketoaciduria (maple syrup urine disease). *Pediatrics* 28:918, 1961
208. LONSDALE D, MERCER RD, FAULKNER WR: Maple syrup urine disease: Report of two cases. *Am J Dis Chid* 106:258, 1963
209. KIIL R, ROKKONES T: Late manifesting variant of branched-chain ketoaciduria (maple syrup urine disease). *Acta Paediat Scand* 53:356, 1964
210. MORRIS MD, FISHER DA, FISER R: Late-onset branched-chain ketoaciduria (maple syrup urine disease). *J Lancet* 86:149, 1966
211. STEEN-JOHNSEN J, VELLAN EJ, GJESSING LR: Maple syrup urine disease variant amino acid patterns and problems of treatment during acute attacks. *Acta Paediat Scand* 59:71, 1970
212. IRWIN WC, MARTEL SB, GOLUBOFF N: Intermittent branched-chain ketonuria (variant of maple syrup urine disease). *Clin Biochem* 4:52, 1971
213. HAMBRAEUS L, WESTPHAL O, HAGBERG B: Ketotic hypoglycemia associated with transient branched-chain amino acidemia. *Acta Paediatr Scand* 61:81, 1972
214. GHODSI A, AJUNDANI TS, GHARAVI M, HATEFI GV: Intermittent maple syrup urine disease. *S Afr Med J* 51:758, 1977
215. ZALESKI LA, DANCIS J, COX RP, HUTZLER J, ZALESKI WA, HILL A: Variant maple syrup urine disease in mother and daughter. *Can Med Assoc J* 109:299, 1973

216. VALMAN HB, PATRICK AD, SEAKINS JWT, PLATT JW, GOMPERTZ D: Family with intermittent maple syrup urine disease. *Arch Dis Child* 48:255, 1973

217. SCHULMAN JD, LUSTBERG TJ, KENNEDY JL, MUSCLES M, SEEGMILLER JE: A new variant of maple syrup urine disease (branched chain ketoaciduria). *Am J Med* 49:118, 1970

218. KALYANARAMAN K, CHAMUKUTTAN S, ARJUNDAS G, GAJANAN N, RAMAMURTHI B: Maple syrup urine disease (branched-chain keto-aciduria) variant type manifesting as hyperkinetic behaviour and mental retardation. Report of two cases. *J Neurol sci* 15:209, 1972

219. FISCHER MH, GERRITSEN T: Biochemical studies on a variant of branched-chain ketoaciduria in a 19-year-old female. *Pediatrics* 48:795, 1971

220. VAN DER HORST JL, WADMAN SK: A variant form of branched-chain ketoaciduria. *Acta Paediatr Scand* 60:594, 1971

221. DURAN M, TIELENS GM, WADMAN SK, STIGTER JCM, KLEIJER WJ: Effects of thiamine in a patient with a variant form of branched chain ketoaciduria. *Acta Paediatr Scand* 67:367, 1978

222. KODAMA S, SEKI A, HANABUSA M, MORISITA Y, SAKURAI T, MATSUO T: Mild variant of maple syrup urine disease. *Eur J Pediatr* 124:31, 1976

223. DANNER JD, WHEELER FB, LEMMON SK, ELSAS LJ: *In vivo* and *in vitro* response of human branched chain α-ketoacid dehydrogenase to thiamine and thiamine pyrophosphate. *Pediatr Res* 12:235, 1978

224. PUESCHEL SM, BRESNAN MJ, SHIH VE, LEVY SM: Thiamine-responsive intermittent branched chain ketoaciduria. *J Pediatr* 94:628, 1979

225. ELSAS L, DANNER D, LUBITZ D, FERNHOFF P, DEMBURE P: Metabolic consequence in inherited defects in branched chain α-ketoacid dehydrogenase: Mechanism of thiamine action, in Walser M, Williamson JR (eds): *Metabolism and Clinical Implications of Branched Chain Amino and Ketoacids*. New York, Elsevier/North-Holland, 1981, p 369

226. Collective results of mass screening for inborn metabolic errors in eight European countries. *Acta Paediatr Scand* 62:413, 1973

227. LEVY HL: Genetic screening, in Harris H, Hirschhorn K (eds): *Advances in Human Genetics*. New York, Plenum Press, 1973, vol 4, p 389

228. NAYLOR EW, GUTHRIE R: Newborn screening for maple syrup urine disease (branched chain ketoaciduria). *Pediatrics* 61:262, 1978

229. TADA K, WADA Y, OKAMURA T: A case of maple syrup urine disease. *Tohoku J Exp Med* 79:142, 1963

230. CHEMKE J, LEVIN S: Maple syrup urine disease. Two cases in Israel. *Israel J Med Sci* 11:809, 1975

231. RAO GP, RAMANAMURTHY PS, GHAFOORUNNIS A, RAFEEQ MR, PATHAK R: Maple syrup urine disease: Report of a case. *Indian Pediatr* 11:585, 1974

232. LANGENBECK U, WENDEL U, MENSCH-HOINOWSKI A, KUSCHEL D, BECKER K, PRZYREMBEL H, BREMER HJ: Correlations between branched-chain amino acids and branched chain α-keto acids in blood in maple syrup urine disease. *Clin Chim Acta* 88:283, 1978

233. DANCIS J, HUTZLER J, LEVITZ M: Metabolism of the white blood cells in maple syrup urine disease. *Biochim Biophys Acta* 43:342, 1960

234. DANCIS J, JANSEN V, HUTZLER J, LEVITZ M: The metabolism of leucine in tissue culture of skin fibroblasts of maple syrup urine disease. *Biochim Biophys Acta* 77:523, 1963

235. DANCIS J, HUTZLER J, SNYDERMAN SE, COX RP: Enzyme activity in classical and variant forms of maple syrup urine disease. *J Pediatr* 81:312, 1972

236. WENDEL U, WENTRUP H, RUDIGER HW: Maple syrup urine disease: Analysis of branched chain ketoacid decarboxylation in cultured fibroblasts. *Pediatr Res* 9:709, 1975

237. RUDIGER HW, LANGENBECK U, SCHULZE-SCHENCKING M, GOEDDE HW: Defective decarboxylase in branched chain ketoacid oxidase multienzyme complex in classic type of maple syrup urine disease. *Humangenetik* 14:257, 1972

238. CHUANG DT, NIU WL, COX RP: Activities of branched-chain 2-oxo-acid dehydrogenase and its component in skin fibroblasts from normal and classical maple syrup urine disease subjects. *Biochem J*, in press

239. SINGH S, WILLERS I, GOEDDE HW: Heterogeneity in maple syrup urine disease: Aspects of cofactor requirement and complementation in cultured fibroblasts. *Clin Genet* 11:277, 1977

240. ROBINSON BH, TAYLOR J, SHERWOOD WG: The genetic heterogeneity of lactic acidosis: Occurrence of recognizable inborn errors of metabolism in a pediatric population with lactic acidosis. *Pediatr Res* 14:956, 1980

241. ROBINSON BH, TAYLOR J, KAHLER SG, KIRKMAN HN: Lactic acidemia, neurologic deterioration and carbohydrate dependence in a girl with dihydrolipoyl dehydrogenase deficiency. *Eur J Pediatr* 136:35, 1981

242. GOEDDE HW, RICHTER E, HUFNER M, VON ZUR MUHLEN A: Untersuchungen zur Ahornsirupkrankheit im zwei Familien. *Humangenetik* 1:163, 1964

243. GOEDDE HW, RICHTER E, HUFNER M, SIXEL B: Arbeitsvorschrift eines vereinfachten Heterozygotenteates fur die Ahornsirup-krankheit. *Klin Wschc* 42:818, 1964

244. LANGENBECK U, RUDIGER HW, SCHULZE-SCHENCKING M, KELLER W, BRACKERTZ D, GOEDDE HW: Evaluation of a heterozygote test for maple syrup urine disease in leucocytes and cultured fibroblasts. *Humangenetik* 11:304, 1971

245. TANAKA K, MANDELL R, SHIH VE: Metabolism of [1-^{14}C] and [2-^{14}C] leucine in cultured skin fibroblasts from patients with isovaleric acidemia. Characterization of metabolic defects. *J Clin Invest* 58:164, 1976

246. SHIH V, MANDELL R, SCHOLL ML: Historical observation in maple syrup urine disease. *J Pediatr* 85:868, 1974

247. GOEDDE HW, LANGENBECK U, BRACKERTZ D, KELLER W, ROKKONES T, HALVORSEN SK, KIIL R, MORTON B: Clinical and biochemical-genetic aspects of intermittent branched-chain ketoaciduria. *Acta Paediatr Scand* 59:83, 1970

248. THOMAS GH, HOWELL RR: *Selected Screening Tests for Genetic Metabolic Diseases*. Chicago, Year Book, 1973, p 9

249. DANCIS J, HUTZLER J, LEVITZ M: Thin-layer chromatography and spectrophotometry of α-keto acid hydrazones. *Biochim Biophys Acta* 78:85, 1963

250. LANGENBECK U, HOINOWSKI A, MANTEL K, MOHRING HU: Quantitative gas chromatography and single-ion detection of aliphatic ketoacids from urine as their O-trimethylsilylquinoxalinol derivatives. *J Chromatogr* 14:339, 1977

251. LANGENBECK U, MOHRING HU, DIECKMANN KP: Gas chromatography of α-keto acids as their O-trimethylsilylquinoxalinol derivatives. *J Chromatogr* 115:65, 1975

252. TANAKA K, HINE DG, WEST-DULL A, LYNN TB: A gas-chromatographic method for analysis of urinary organic acids: Retention indices of 155 metabolically important compounds. *Clin Chem* 26:1839, 1980

253. *Mass Spectra of Compounds of Biological Interest*. Technical Information Center, U.S. Department of Commerce, Springfield, VA

254. LANGENBEC U, MOHRING HU, HINNEY B, SPITELLER M: Quinoxalinol derivatives of aliphatic 2-oxocarboxylic acids. *Biomed Mass Spec* 4:197, 1977

255. SHIH VE: *Laboratory Techniques for the Detection of Hereditary Metabolic Disorders*. Cleveland: CRC Press, 1973, p 11

256. WADMAN SK, DE JONGE HJ, DE BREE PK: Rapid, high resolution two-dimensional amino acid chromatography on micro scale chromatograms. *Clin Chim Acta* 25:87, 1969

257. DANCIS J, HUTZLER J, COX RP: Maple syrup urine disease: Branched chain keto acid decarboxylation in fibroblasts as measured with amino acids and keto acids. *Am J Human Genet* 29:272, 1977

258. WENDEL U, WOHLER W, GOEDDE HW, LANGENBECK U, PASSARGE E, RUDIGER, HW: Rapid diagnosis of maple syrup urine disease (branched chain ketoaciduria) by micro-enzyme assay in leucocytes and fibroblasts. *Clin Chim Acta* 45:433, 1973

259. FENSOM AH, BENSON PF, BAKER J: A rapid method for assay of branched-chain keto acid decarboxylation in cultured cells and its application to prenatal diagnosis of maple syrup urine disease. *Clin Chim Acta* 87:169, 1978

260. WENDEL U, RUDIGER HW, PASSARGE E, MIKKELSEN M: Maple syrup urine disease: Rapid prenatal diagnosis by enzyme assay. *Humangenetik* 19:127, 1973

261. COX R, HUTZLER J, DANCIS J: Antenatal diagnosis of maple syrup urine disease. *Lancet* 2:212, 1978

262. WENDEL U, CLAUSSEN U: Antenatal diagnosis of maple syrup urine disease. *Lancet* 1:161, 1979

263. WENDEL U, CLAUSSEN U, LANGENBECK, U: Pattern of branched-chain α-keto acids in amniotic fluid. *Clin Chim Acta* 120:267, 1980

264. YUWILER A, GELLER E: Serotonin depletion by dietary leucine. *Nature* 208:83, 1965

265. TASHIAN RE: Inhibition of brain-glutamic decarboxylase by phenylalanine, leucine, and valine derivatives: A suggestion concerning the neurological defect in phenylketonuria and branched-chain keto aciduria. *Metabolism* 10:393, 1961

266. HOWELL RK, LEE M: Influence of α-keto acids on the respiration of brain in vitro. *Proc Soc Exp Biol Med* 113:660, 1963

267. HALESTRAP AP, BRAND MD, DENTON RM: Inhibition of mitochondrial pyruvate transport by phenylpyruvate and alpha-ketoisocaproate. *Biochim Biophys Acta* 367:102, 1974

268. LAND JM, MOWBRAY J, CLARK JB: Control of pyruvate and beta-hydroxybutyrate utilization in rat brain mitochondria and its relevance to phenylketonuria and maple syrup urine disease. *J Neurochem* 26:823, 1976

269. SILBERBERG DH: Maple syrup urine disease metabolites studied in cerebellum cultures. *J Neurochem* 16:1141, 1969

270. LIAO CL, HERMAN MM, BENSCH KG: Prolongation of G_1 and S phase in C-6 glioma cells treated with maple syrup urine disease metabolites: Morphologic and cell cycle studies. *Lab Invest* 38: 122, 1978

271. DENT CE, WESTALL RG: Studies in maple syrup urine disease. *Arch Dis Child* 36:259, 1961

272. WESTALL RG: Dietary treatment of a child with maple syrup urine disease (branched chain keto-aciduria). *Arch Dis Child* 38:485, 1963

273. ACOSTA PB, ELSAS LJ, II: Dietary treatment of branched chain ketoaciduria (MSUD), in *Dietary Management of Inherited Metabolic Disease: Phenyl-*

ketonuria, Galactosemia, Tyrosinemia, Homocystinuria, Maple Syrup Urine Disease. Atlanta, ACELMU Publishers, 1976

274. BELL L, CHAO E, MILNE J: Dietary management of maple-syrup-urine disease: An evaluation based on equivalency systems. *J Am Diet Assoc* 74:357, 1979

275. KINDT E, SVERIC HALVORSEN: The need of essential amino acids in children: An evaluation based on the intake of phenylalanine tyrosine, leucine, isoleucine and valine in children with phenylketonuria, tryosine amino transferase defect, and maple syrup urine disease. *Am J Clin Nutr* 33:279, 1980

276. American Academy of Pediatrics: Special diets for infants with inborn errors of amino acid metabolism. *Pediatrics* 57:783, 1976

277. LEVY HL, TRUMAN JT, GANZ RN, LITTLEFIELD JW: Folic acid deficiency secondary to a diet for maple syrup urine disease. *J Pediatr* 77:294, 1970

278. FOREMAN, JW, YUDKOFF M, BERRY G, SEGAL S: Acidosis associated with dietotherapy of maple syrup urine disease. *J Pediatr* 96:62, 1980

279. GAULL GE: Pathogenesis of maple syrup urine disease: Observation during dietary management and treatment of coma by peritoneal dialysis. *Biochem Med* 3:130, 1969

280. WENDEL U, BECKER K, PRZYREMBEL H, BULLA M, MANEGOLD C, MENCH-HIONOWSKI A, LANGENBECK U: Peritoneal dialysis in maple-syrup-urine disease: Studies on branched-chain amino and ketoacids. *Eur J Pediatr* 134:57, 1980

281. HAMMERSEN G, WILLIE L, SCHMITT H, LUTZ P, BICKEL H: Maple syrup urine disease: Treatment of the acutely ill newborn. *Eur J Pediatr* 129:157, 1978

282. SILBERMAN J, DANCIS J, FEIGIN IH: Neuropathological observations in maple syrup urine disease: Branched chain ketoaciduria. *Arch Neurol* 5:351, 1961

283. MENKES JH, PHILIPPORT M, FIOL RE: Cerebral lipids in maple syrup disease. *J Pediatr* 66:584, 1965

284. PRENSKY AL, MOSER HW: Brain lipids, proteolipids, and free amino acids in maple syrup urine disease. *J Neurochem* 13:863, 1966

285. MENKES JH, SOLCHER H: Maple syrup urine disease: Effects of diet therapy on cerebral lipids. *Arch Neurol* 16:486, 1967

286. PRENSKY AL, CARR S, MOSER HW: Development of myelin in inherited disorders of amino acid metabolism. *Arch Neurol* 19:552, 1968

287. ULSTROM RA: Commentary. *J Pediatr* 69:961, 1966

288. NEWMAN CGH, WILSON BDR, CALLAGHAN P, YOUNG L: Neonatal death associated with isovaleric acidemia. *Lancet* 2:439, 1967

289. ALLEN PM, NECHELES TF, RICKER R, SENIOR B: Reversible neonatal pancytopenia due to isovaleric acidemia. *Soc Pediatr Res* p 156, 1969 (abstract)

290. ANDO T, KLINGBERG WG, WARD AN, RASMUSSEN K, NYHAN WL: Isovaleric acidemia presenting with altered metabolism of glycine. *Pediatr Res* 5:478, 1971

291. SIDBURY JB, SMITH EK, HARLAN W: An inborn error of short chain fatty acid metabolism. *J Pediatr* 70:8, 1967

292. ANDO T, NYHAN WL, BACHMANN C, RASMUSSEN K, SCOTT R, SMITH EK: Isovaleric acidemia: Identification of isovalerate, isovalerylglycine and 3-hydroxyisovalerate in urine of a patient previously reported as having butyric and hexanoic acidemia. *J Pediatr* 82:243, 1973

293. LOTT IT, ERICKSON AM, LEVY H: Dietary treatment of an infant with isovaleric acidemia. *Pediatrics* 49:617, 1972

294. LEVY HL, ERICKSON AM, LOTT IT, KURTZ DJ: Isovaleric acidemia: Results of family study and dietary treatment. *Pediatrics* 52:83, 1973

295. SPIRER Z, SWIRSKY-FEIN S, ZAKUT V, LEGUM C, BOGAR N, CHARLES R, GIL-AV, E: Acute neonatal isovaleric acidemia. A report of two cases. *Israel J Med Sci* 11:1005, 1975

296. GUIBAUD P, DIVRY P, DUBOIS Y, COLLOMBEL C, LARBRE F: Une observation d'acidemie isovalerique. *Arch Franc Ped* 30:633, 1973

297. SAUDUBRAY J-M, SORIN M, DEPONDT E, HEROUIN C, CHARPENTIER C, POUSSET JL: Acidemie isovalerique. Etude et traitement chez trois freres. *Arch Franc Ped* 33:795, 1976

298. MALAN C, NEETHLING AC, SHANLEY BC, GOMPERTZ D, BARLETT K, SCHRAADER EB: Isovaleric acidemia in two South African children. *S Afr Med J* 52:980, 1977

299. YUDKOFF M, COHN RM, PUSCHAK R, ROTHMAN R, SEGAL S: Glycine therapy in isovaleric acidemia. *J Pediatr* 92:813, 1978

300. COHN RM, YUDKOFF M, ROTHMAN R, SEGAL S: Isovaleric acidemia: Use of glycine therapy in neonates. *N Engl J Med* 299:996, 1978

301. ICHIBA Y, SATO K, YUASA S: Report of a case of isovaleric acidemia. *J Japanese Pediatr Soc* 83:480, 1979

302. DURAN M, VAN SPRANG FJ, DREWES JG, BRUINVIS L, KETTING D, WADMAN SK: Two sisters with isovaleric acidemia, multiple attacks of ketoacidosis and normal development *Eur J Pediatr* 131:205, 1979

303. BLASKOVICS ME, NG WG, DONNELL GN: Prenatal diagnosis and a case report of isovaleric acidemia. *J Inher Metab Dis* 1:9, 1978

304. WINOKUR PA, VASHISTHA K, SESHAMANI R: Isovaleric acidemia: A case report. *Pediatrics* 61:902, 1978

305. LEHNERT W, SCHENCK W, NIEDERHOF H: Isovalerianacidamia kombiniert mit hypertrophisher Pylorusstenose. *Klin Padiat* 191:477, 1979

306. TRUSCOTT RJW, MALEGAN D, MC CAIRNS E, BURKE D, HICK L, TANAKA K, SWEETMAN L, NYHAN WL, HAMMOND J, BUMACK C, DANKS DM: New metabolites in isovaleric acidemia. *Clin Chim Acta* 110:187, 1981

307. TANAKA K, ORR JC, ISSELBACHER KJ: Identification of β-hydroxyisovaleric acid in the urine of a patient with isovaleric acidemia. *Biochim Biophys Acta* 15:638, 1968

308. LEHNERT W, NIEDERHOF H: 4-Hydroxyisovaleric acid: A new metabolite in isovaleric acidemia. *Eur J Pediatr,* in press

309. DEN H: The biological oxidation of 2,2-dimethyloctanoic acid. *Biochim Biophys Acta* 98:462, 1965

310. PREISS B, BLOCH K: ω-Oxidation of long chain fatty acids in rat liver. *J Biol Chem* 239:85, 1964

311. NAKAMURA E, ROSENBERG LE, TANAKA K: Microdetermination of methylmalonic acid and other short chain dicarboxylic acids by gas chromatography: Use in prenatal diagnosis of methylmalonic acidemia and in studies of isovaleric acidemia. *Clin Chim Acta* 68:127, 1976

312. TANAKA K, HINE D: Unpublished observations

313. WHITE RP, SAMSON FE: Effects of fatty acid anions on the electroencephalogram of unanesthesized rabbits. *Am J Physiol* 196:271, 1956

314. HOLMQUIST B, INGVAR DH: Effects of short chain fatty acid anions upon cortical blood flow and EEG in cats. *Experientia* 13:331, 1957

315. MUTO Y, TAKAHASHI Y, KAWAMURA H: Effects of short chain fatty acid anions on the electrical activity of neo-, paleo- and archicortical system. *No to Shinkei* 16:61, 1964

316. HIRD FJR, WEIDMANN MJ: Oxidative phosphorylation accompanying oxidation of short chain fatty acids by rat-liver mitochondria. *Biochem J* 98:378, 1966

317. AHMED K, SCHOLEFIELD PG: Studies on fatty acid oxidation. 8. The effects of fatty acids on metabolism of rat-brain cortex *in vitro. Biochem J* 81:45, 1961

318. ZBOROWSKI J, WOJICZAK L: Induction of swelling of liver mitochondria by fatty acids of various chain lengths. *Biochim Biophys Acta* 70:596, 1963

319. DAHL DR: Short chain fatty acid inhibition of rat brain Na-K-adenosine triphosphatase. *J Neurochem* 15:815, 1968

320. WALKER CO, MC CANDLESS DW, MC GARRY JD, SHENKER S: Cerebral energy metabolism in short chain fatty acid induced coma. *J Lab Clin Med* 76L:569, 1970

321. DUBIEL B, WETTS R, TAKAKA K: Heterogeneity in diseases of leucine metabolism: Complementation studies using cultured skin fibroblasts. *Pediatr Res* 14:521, 1980

322. KELLEHER JF, YUDKOFF M, HUTCHINSON R, AUGUST CS, COHN RM: The pancytopenia of isovaleric acidemia. *Pediatrics* 65:1023, 1980

323. TANAKA K: Problems in the gas chromatographic analysis of short chain fatty acids, in Mamer OA, Mitchell WJ, Scriver CR (eds): *Application of Gas Chromatography and Mass Spectrometry to the Investigation of Human Disease.* Montreal, 1973, p 129

324. TANAKA K, YU G: A method for the separate determination of isovalerate and α-methylbutyrate by use of GLC-mass spectrometer. *Clin Chim Acta* 43:151, 1973

325. MAMER OA, GIBBS BJ: Simplified gas chromatography of trimethylsilyl esters of C_1 through C_5 fatty acids in serum and urine. *Clin Chem* 19:1006, 1973

326. SHIH VE, MANDELL R, TANAKA K: Diagnosis of isovaleric acidemia in cultured fibroblasts. *Clin Chim Acta* 48:437, 1973

327. SWEETMAN L, NYHAN WL, TRAUNER DA, MERRITT TA, SINGH M: Glutaric aciduria type II. *J Pediatr* 96:1020, 1980

328. GOODMAN SI, MC CABE ERB, FENNESSEY PV, MACE JW: Multiple acyl-CoA dehydrogenase deficiency (glutaric aciduria type II) with transient hypersarcosinemia and sarcosinuria; possible inherited deficiency of an electron transfer flavoprotein. *Pediatr Res* 14:12, 1980

329. DUSHEIKO G, KEW MC, JOFFE BI, LEWIN JR, MANTAGOS S, TANAKA K: Glutaric aciduria type II: A cause of recurrent hypoglycemia in an adult. *N Engl J Med* 301:1405, 1979

330. GREGERSEN N, KOLVERAA S, RASMUSSEN K, CHRISTENSEN E, BRANDT NJ, EBBESEN F, HANSE FH: Biochemical studies in a patient with defects in metabolism of acyl CoA and sarcosine: Another possible case of glutaric aciduria type II. *J Inher Metab Dis* 3:67, 1980

331. GOODMAN SI, KOHLHOFF JG: Glutaric aciduria: Inherited deficiency of glutaryl CoA dehydrogenase activity. *Biochem Med* 13:138, 1975

332. BARETZ BH, RAMSDELL HS, TANAKA K: Identification of n-hexanoylglycine in urines from two patients with Jamaican vomiting sickness. *Clin Chim Acta* 73:199, 1976

333. TANAKA K, MANTAGOS S, GENEL M, SEASHORE M, BILLINGS BA, BARETZ BH: New defect in fatty acid metabolism with hypoglycemia and organic aciduria. *Lancet* 2:986, 1977

334. RHEAD W, MANTAGOS S, TANAKA K: Glutaric aciduria type II: In vitro studies on substrate oxidation, acyl CoA dehydrogenases and electron

transferring flavoprotein in cultured skin fibroblasts. *Pediatr Res* 14:1339, 1980

335. UTTER M, KEECH DB, SCRUTTON MC: A possible role for acetyl CoA in the control of gluconeogenesis. Adv. Enzyme Regul 2:49, 1964

336. WILLIAMSON JR, ROSTAND SG, PETERSON MJ: Control factors affecting gluconeogenesis in perfused rat liver. Effect of 4-pentenoic acid. *J Biol Chem* 245:3242, 1970

337. SÖLING HD, KLEINECKE J, WILMS B, JASON G, KULIZE A: Relationship between intracellular distribution of phospho-enol pyruvate carboxykinase, regulation of gluconeogenesis, and energy cost of glucose formation. *Eur J Biochem* 37P:233, 1973

338. HILL KR: The vomiting sickness of Jamaica: A review. *West Indian Med J* 1:243, 1952

339. JELLIFFE DB, STUART KL: Acute toxic hypoglycaemia in the vomiting sickness of Jamaica. *Br Med J* 1:75, 1954

340. HILL KR, BRAS G, CLEARKIN KP: Acute toxic hypoglycemia occurring in the vomiting sickness of Jamaica. *West Indian Med J* 4:91, 1955

341. STOKKE O, ELDJARN L, JELLUM E, PANDE H, WAALER PE: β-Methylcrotonyl CoA carboxylase deficiency: A new metabolic error in leucine degradation. *Pediatrics* 49:726, 1972

342. FINNIE MDA, COTTRALL K, SEAKINS JWT, SNEDDEN W: Massive excretion of 2-oxoglutaric acid and 3-hydroxyisovaleric acid in a patient with a deficiency of 3-methylcrotonyl-CoA carboxylase. *Clin Chim Acta* 73:513, 1976

343. SCHUTGENS RBH, HYMANS H, KETEL A, VEDER HA: Lethal hypoglycemia in a child with a deficiency of 3-hydroxy-3-methylglutaryl coenzyme A lyase. *J Pediatr* 94:89, 1979

344. DURAN M, SCHUTGENS RBH, KETEL A, HEYMANS H, BERNTSSEN MWJ, KETTING D, WADMAN SK: 3-Hydroxy-3-methylglutaryl coenzyme A lyase deficiency: Postnatal management following prenatal diagnosis by analysis of maternal urine. *J Pediatr* 95:1004, 1979

345. TRUSCOTT RJW, HALPERN B, WYSOCKI SJ, HAHNEL R, WILCKEN B: Studies on a child suspected of having a deficiency in 3-hydroxy-3-methylglutaryl CoA lyase. *Clin Chim Acta* 95:11, 1979

346. LEONARD JV, SEAKINS JW, GRIFFIN NK: β-Hydroxy-β-methylglutaricaciduria presenting as Reye's syndrome. *Lancet* 1:680, 1979

347. FAULL KF, BOLTON PD, HALPERN B, HAMMOND J, DANKS DM: The urinary organic acid profile associated with 3-hydroxy-3-methylglutaricaciduria. *Clin Chim Acta* 73:553, 1976

348. DURAN M, KETTING D, WADMAN SK, JAKOBS C, SCHUTGENS RBH, VEDER HA: Organic acid excretion in a patient with 3-hydroxy-3-methylglutaryl CoA lyase deficiency: Facts and artefacts. *Clin Chim Acta* 90:187, 1978

349. WYSOCKI SJ, WILKINSON SP, HAHNEL R, WONG CYB, PANEGYERS PK: 3-Hydroxy-3-methylglutaric aciduria, combined with 3-methylglutaconic aciduria. *Clin Chim Acta* 70:399, 1976

350. WYSOCKI SJ, HAHNEL R: 3-Hydroxy-3-methylglutaric aciduria: Deficiency of 3-hydroxy-3-methylglutaryl coenzyme A lyase. *Clin Chim Acta* 71:349, 1976

351. GRETER J, HAGBERG B, STEEN G, SODERHJELM U: β-Methylglutaconic 3-aciduria: A new disorder of leucine metabolism. *Pediatr Res* 10:371, 1976 (abstract)

352. ROBINSON BH, SHERWOOD WG, LAMPTY M, LOWDEN JA: β-Methylglutaconic aciduria: A new disorder of leucine metabolism. *Pediatr Res* 10:371, 1976 (abstract)

353. ROBINSON JP, FEIGIN RD, TENEBAUM SM, HILLMAN RE: Hyperglyceinemia with ketosis due to a defect in isoleucine catabolism. *Pediatrics* 50:890, 1972

354. ROBINSON BH: Personal communication

355. HILLMAN RE, KEATING JP: β-Ketothiolase deficiency as a cause of the "ketotic hyperglycinemia syndrome." *Pediatrics* 53:221, 1974

356. GOMPERTZ D, SAUDUBRAY JM, CHARPENTIER C, BARTLETT K, GOODEY PA, DRAFFAN GH: A defect in isoleucine metabolism associated with α-methyl-β-hydroxybutyric and α-methylacetoacetic aciduria: Quantitative in vivo and in vitro studies. *Clin Chim Acta* 57:269, 1974

23

DISORDERS OF PROPIONATE AND METHYLMALONATE METABOLISM

LEON E. ROSENBERG

1. *Propionyl CoA, formed in the catabolism of several essential amino acids (isoleucine, valine, methionine, threonine), odd-chain fatty acids, and cholesterol, is metabolized primarily by enzymatic conversion to methylmalonyl CoA, which is subsequently isomerized to succinyl CoA. This sequence depends on the activity of several enzymes (Fig. 23-2): propionyl CoA carboxylase, methylmalonyl CoA racemase, and methylmalonyl CoA mutase. Propionyl CoA carboxylase requires biotin as a cofactor, while methylmalonyl CoA mutase requires a cobalamin (vitamin B_{12}) coenzyme, adenosylcobalamin (AdoCbl).*

2. *Four enzymatic carboxylation reactions in mammalian cells require biotin as a cofactor: the cytosolic enzyme, acetyl CoA carboxylase; and three mitochondrial matrix enzymes, propionyl CoA carboxylase, β-methylcrotonyl CoA carboxylase, and pyruvate carboxylase. Biotin is covalently bound to these apoproteins in a reaction catalyzed by one or more holocarboxylase synthetases found in the cytosol and mitochondrion. Little is known about the transmembrane transport or intracellular distribution of biotin.*

3. *Only two enzymatic reactions in mammalian cells are known to require cobalamin coenzymes, each depending on a different coenzyme: the adenosylcobalamin-dependent mutase mentioned above and the*

methylcobalamin (MeCbl)-dependent homocysteine-N^5-methyltetrahydrofolate methyltransferase. These cobalamin coenzymes are formed intracellularly from the precursor vitamin by a complex process which involves numerous steps: receptor-mediated binding of the transcobalamin II-cobalamin complex to the cell surface; adsorptive endocytosis of the complex; intralysosomal degradation of transcobalamin II with coordinate release of cobalamin; and enzyme-catalyzed reduction, methylation, and adenosylation.

4. *Nine different inherited defects impair this pathway of propionate utilization in humans. Three of these alter propionyl CoA carboxylase activity, while six affect methylmalonyl CoA mutase (Fig. 23-17).*

5. *Propionyl CoA carboxylase deficiency, a major cause of the ketotic hyperglycinemia syndrome, results in the accumulation of propionate in blood and urine. Two complementation groups, pcc A and pcc BC, have been defined among propionyl CoA carboxylase-deficient patients. These groups probably correspond to mutations affecting the two nonidentical subunits of the carboxylase apoprotein. Other metabolites which accumulate in urine of these children include propionylglycine, β-hydroxypropionate, methylcitrate, tiglate, and long-chain ketones (butanone, pentanone, and hexanone). Clinically, the disorder leads to*

severe metabolic ketoacidosis, which often appears in the neonatal period and which requires vigorous alkali therapy and protein restriction.

6. *Multiple carboxylase deficiency is a disorder that leads to impaired activity of three biotin-dependent enzymes: propionyl CoA carboxylase, β-methylcrotonyl CoA carboxylase, and pyruvate carboxylase. This condition results from one or more defects in cellular biotin transport or metabolism. The clinical hallmarks of this disorder include ketoacidosis, a diffuse erythematous skin rash, alopecia, and developmental retardation.*

7. *Neonatal or infantile metabolic ketoacidosis is also the clinical hallmark of defects involving the methylmalonyl CoA mutase apoenzyme. Cells from some of these children have no functional mutase (designated mut°); cells from others contain a structurally altered mutase with reduced affinity for AdoCbl and with reduced stability (mut⁻). Such children exhibit methylmalonic acidemia and methylmalonic aciduria that do not respond to cobalamin supplementation but can sometimes be treated effectively with dietary protein restriction.*

8. *Two abnormalities in adenosylcobalamin synthesis only (designated cbl A and cbl B) lead to impaired methylmalonyl CoA mutase activity and result in methylmalonic acidemia. In most but not all patients with these defects, pharmacologic supplements of cyanocobalamin or hydroxocobalamin produce distinct reduction in methylmalonate accumulation and offer a valuable therapeutic adjunct to dietary protein limitation.*

9. *Two other distinct mutations, designated cbl C and cbl D, lead to impaired synthesis of AdoCbl and MeCbl, and, accordingly to deficient activity of methylmalonyl CoA mutase and homocysteine: N^5-methyltetrahydrofolate methyltransferase. Such children have methylmalonic aciduria and homocystinuria. Those children with the cbl C mutation appear to be more severely affected clinically than the two known sibs in the cbl D group. Major clinical problems in cbl C patients include failure to thrive, developmental retardation, and such hematologic abnormalities as megaloblastic anemia and hemolysis. The precise defect in the cbl C and cbl D patients is not yet known, but it involves an early step in the intracellular metabolism of cobalamins.*

10. *The discriminating biochemical features of the six known forms of inherited methylmalonic acidemia are shown in Table 23-5.*

11. *All of the disorders of propionate and methylmalonate metabolism for which there are adequate data are inherited as autosomal recessive traits. Heterozygotes for the following mutations can be detected: pcc A; mut°, mut⁻; and cbl B. Genetic complementation analyses with somatic cell heterokaryons have been particularly useful in demonstrating genetic heterogeneity and in confirming the existence of autosomal recessive inheritance among the propionic acidemias and the methylmalonic acidemias.*

12. *Prenatal detection of fetuses with propionyl CoA carboxylase deficiency, methylmalonyl CoA mutase deficiency, and defective synthesis of adenosylcobalamin*

has been accomplished using cultured amniotic cells and chemical determinations on amniotic fluid or maternal urine.

Methylmalonic acid and its immediate precursor, propionic acid, are detectable in normal human blood, urine, and cerebrospinal fluid only in trace amounts. The minuscule quantities of these compounds in extracellular fluids have obscured, until recently, the key role that these acids play in human metabolism. Biochemists investigating animal nutrition have been interested in propionate metabolism for more than 20 years, because ruminants derive most of their energy requirements from the oxidation of propionate and acetate produced by bacterial fermentation in their rumens [1]. Although propionate and methylmalonate are of little quantitative importance in human beings as direct sources of energy, these acids, found intracellularly largely as their coenzyme A (CoA) esters, are vital intermediates in the catabolism of fat and protein.

Several independent, and seemingly unrelated, lines of evidence drew the attention of the physician and the clinical investigator to the study of propionate and methylmalonate metabolism. In 1959 and 1960, several groups reported that adenosylcobalamin (AdoCbl), one of the coenzyme forms of cobalamin (vitamin B_{12}), is an essential cofactor in the enzymatic conversion of L-methylmalonyl CoA to succinyl CoA [2–4]. Shortly thereafter, patients with acquired cobalamin deficiency were shown to excrete large amounts of methylmalonic acid in the urine [5, 6]. The methylmalonic aciduria was rapidly reversed by administration of physiologic doses of cobalamin and was attributed to an acquired block in methylmalonate catabolism caused by inadequate amounts of the needed cobalamin coenzyme.

In 1961, Childs and associates [7] described a young boy with recurrent attacks of severe ketoacidosis who had elevated concentrations of glycine and several other amino acids in his blood and urine. A series of detailed metabolic studies demonstrated that the attacks were precipitated by protein feeding and more specifically by ingestion of the branched chain amino acids, methionine and threonine. Since elevation in plasma glycine level was the most striking biochemical abnormality, the disorder was called *ketotic hyperglycinemia*. Recent evidence indicates that this disorder is caused by an inherited defect in the catabolism of propionate, not by a primary abnormality in glycine utilization or biosynthesis [8, 9].

Since 1967, a number of critically ill children have been described who draw these seemingly disparate observations together and focus attention on the enzymes and coenzymes that regulate the pathway responsible for the formation of propionate and its conversion to succinate. Oberholzer [10], Stokke [11], and their colleagues described infants with profound metabolic acidosis and hyperglycinemia (or hyperglycinuria) who excreted huge amounts of methylmalonic acid in the urine but who were not cobalamin-deficient. Subsequently, Rosenberg and his colleagues [8] reported that urine from the index patient with ketotic hyperglycinemia and from his affected sister contained no methylmalonic acid. This observation indicated that primary methylmalonic acidemia and ketotic hyperglycinemia were different disorders with identical clinical manifestations [8].

The latter group and Lindblad et al. [12, 13] also described children with ketoacidosis and methylmalonic acidemia who were not cobalamin-deficient but who responded to administration of pharmacologic doses of cyanocobalamin or its coenzyme with a marked fall in concentration of urinary methylmalonic acid. The index patient [8] was subsequently shown to suffer from a primary defect in AdoCbl synthesis [14, 15], not from a defect of the apoenzyme which catalyzes the conversion of methylmalonyl CoA to succinyl CoA.

These observations, and others which will be discussed in detail subsequently, emphasize that numerous inherited abnormalities in the metabolic pathway for propionate and methylmalonate occur, and that these defects lead to profound illness and, in many cases, death due to a disturbed acid-base balance or developmental failure. The study of these disorders has led to important insights in our understanding of the role of this pathway in human beings and has illustrated, once again, that a group of clinically identical disorders can be produced by several different mutations affecting the synthesis of related apoenzymes and coenzymes. Several reviews of this subject matter have appeared recently [16–18].

BIOCHEMICAL PATHWAYS

Propionate Metabolism

Formation of Propionate and Methylmalonate Most of the propionic acid utilized by ruminant animals is formed by bacterial fermentation in the rumen [1]. By contrast, nonruminant mammals derive nearly all their propionate from the catabolism of lipid and protein. As noted in Fig. 23-1, catabolism of the branched chain amino acid isoleucine leads to the formation of propionyl CoA, as does the degradation of methionine and threonine [19]. Recent studies with [13C]valine in a patient with methylmalonic acidemia [20], and with the valine catabolite, [13C]isobutyrate, in rats [21] indicate that valine is also a propionate precursor and is not catabolized directly to methylmalonyl CoA, as suggested earlier. Catabolism of these amino acids accounts for much of the propionate formed in humans, but other sources are known. Beta oxidation of fatty acids with an odd number of carbon atoms ultimately leads to the formation of 1 mol of propionyl CoA per mole of fatty acid [22]. Degradation of the side chain of cholesterol also leads to the synthesis of propionyl CoA, but this pathway appears to be of little quantitative significance [23].

Methylmalonyl CoA is synthesized from two sources (Fig. 23-1). Catabolism of thymine accounts for only a small amount of the intracellular methylmalonyl CoA compared to that formed from the carboxylation of propionyl CoA. Propi-

onate has long been known to be glycogenic in animals [24], but the pathway by which propionate is converted to carbohydrate became clear only when Lardy and Adler demonstrated that liver mitochondria contain enzymes which synthesize succinate from propionate [24]. The discovery in 1955 that methylmalonate is an intermediate in the formation of succinate from propionate (Fig. 23-1) provided an important further step in the characterization of this pathway [25, 26].

Kaziro and Ochoa first defined the individual steps of propionate catabolism in animal tissues and characterized the enzymes involved [22]. Propionyl CoA, formed either by the degradative reactions discussed above or by the enzymatic esterification of propionate itself [27], may be considered the precursor of this reaction sequence (Fig. 23-2). Three enzymatic reactions are responsible for the conversion of propionyl CoA to succinyl CoA. The first involves the carboxylation of propionyl CoA to methylmalonyl CoA [27, 28], a reaction catalyzed by propionyl CoA carboxylase (EC 6.4.1.3). Although two diastereoisomers of methylmalonyl CoA are known, only the D form is produced in the carboxylation reaction [29, 30]. This isomer is not a substrate for the subsequent mutase reaction and must be racemized to the L configuration by another enzyme, methylmalonyl CoA racemase (EC 5.1.99.1) [31]. The third reaction, catalyzed by methylmalonyl CoA mutase (EC 5.4.99.2), isomerizes L-methylmalonyl CoA to succinyl CoA [32]. The latter compound enters the tricarboxylic acid cycle and is ultimately glycogenic because of its conversion to pyruvate by way of oxaloacetate. The sum of all these reactions may be written as follows:

$$\text{Propionate} + \text{ATP} \longrightarrow \text{pyruvate} + 4\text{H} + \text{ADP} + \text{P}_i \qquad (1)$$

In bacteria, propionate is formed from pyruvate by reversal of the reaction sequence just described [22], but in mammalian systems the equilibrium of the system is far in the direction of propionate catabolism rather than biosynthesis.

Apoenzymes

Propionyl CoA Carboxylase This enzyme, first crystallized from pig heart [33], has been purified to homogeneity from bovine kidney [34] and human liver [35]. The latter two reports [34, 35] both conclude that the enzyme is composed of nonidentical subunits and that the required cofactor, biotin, is bound exclusively to the larger (or α) subunit. The native human enzyme has a molecular weight of ~540,000 and its subunits (α and β) of 72,000 and 56,000, respectively. Each mole of enzyme contains 4 moles of biotin. This is consistent with other evidence that the native enzyme is a tetramer of protomers, each protomer containing a single α and a single β subunit. The native enzyme thus appears to have an $(\alpha\beta)_4$ quaternary structure. Several groups have shown that the carboxylation of propionyl CoA is a two-step reaction [22]. In the first step, which requires ATP and Mg^{2+} and is stimulated by K^+, bicarbonate is attached to the ureido nitrogen of the apoenzyme-biotin complex (Fig. 23-3), forming a carboxybiotin-apoenzyme intermediate. This complex, in turn, reacts with

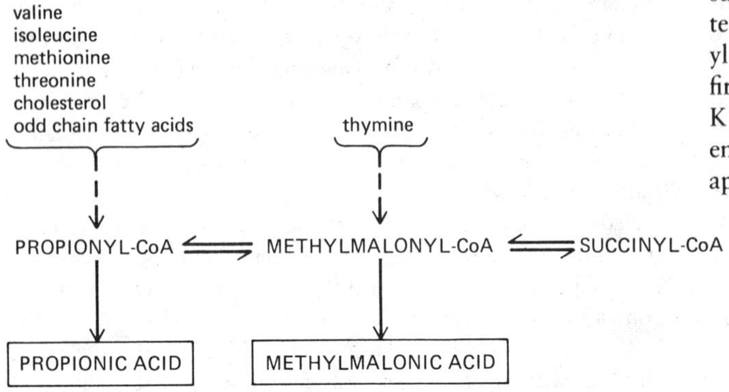

valine
isoleucine
methionine
threonine
cholesterol
odd chain fatty acids   thymine

PROPIONYL-CoA ⇌ METHYLMALONYL-CoA ⇌ SUCCINYL-CoA

PROPIONIC ACID   METHYLMALONIC ACID

Figure 23-1 Precursors of and major catabolic pathway for propionate and methylmalonate. The free acids are derived from their CoA esters by hydrolysis. A number of clinical disorders arise from errors at various steps in these pathways. Broken arrows indicate the presence of several reactions.

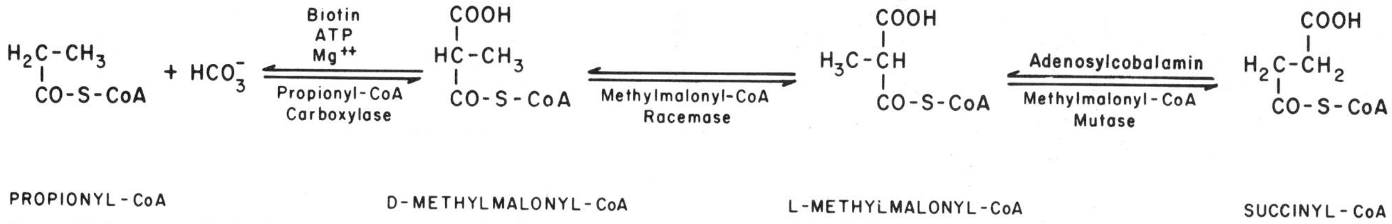

$$H_2C-CH_3 \atop | \atop CO-S-CoA \quad + \quad HCO_3^- \quad \underset{\substack{Propionyl-CoA \\ Carboxylase}}{\overset{\substack{Biotin \\ ATP \\ Mg^{++}}}{\rightleftharpoons}} \quad {COOH \atop | \atop HC-CH_3 \atop | \atop CO-S-CoA} \quad \underset{\substack{Methylmalonyl-CoA \\ Racemase}}{\rightleftharpoons} \quad {COOH \atop | \atop H_3C-CH \atop | \atop CO-S-CoA} \quad \underset{\substack{Methylmalonyl-CoA \\ Mutase}}{\overset{\substack{Adenosylcobalamin}}{\rightleftharpoons}} \quad {COOH \atop | \atop H_2C-CH_2 \atop | \atop CO-S-CoA}$$

PROPIONYL-CoA   D-METHYLMALONYL-CoA   L-METHYLMALONYL-CoA   SUCCINYL-CoA

Figure 23-2 Enzymatic details of major catabolic pathway for propionyl CoA and methylmalonyl CoA. Succinyl CoA has several metabolic fates, including oxidation through the tricarboxylic acid cycle and condensation with glycine to form δ-aminolevulinic acid. Two coenzymes act in the reaction sequence: biotin in the carboxylation of propionyl CoA, and adenosylcobalamin (AdoCbl) in the isomerization of L-methylmalonyl CoA to succinyl CoA.

propionyl CoA and transfers the carboxyl group from biotin to the second carbon of propionyl CoA, forming D-methylmalonyl CoA. As with several other biotin-catalyzed, carbon dioxide fixation reactions, the biotin molecule is directly responsible for the transfer of the carboxyl group [36].

Methylmalonyl CoA Racemase This enzyme owes its discovery to the observation that methylmalonyl CoA synthesized chemically is a substrate for the mutase reaction (Fig. 23-2), whereas methylmalonyl CoA formed enzymatically from the carboxylation of propionyl CoA will not react with the mutase unless it is first heated. Ultimately the demonstration that heating converts D-methylmalonyl CoA to DL-methylmalonyl CoA led to the conclusion that only the L form of the ester will react with the mutase enzyme. This interpretation was confirmed by separating mutase activity from racemase activity using Sephadex chromatography [22, 31, 37]. The racemase has been purified extensively from sheep liver [31]. It has no known cofactor requirements and catalyzes the conversion of D- to L-methylmalonyl CoA by inducing a shift in the α-hydrogen atom [31, 37].

Methylmalonyl CoA Mutase In 1955, Flavin et al. [25] and Katz and Chaikoff [26] observed independently that the isomerization of methylmalonyl CoA to succinyl CoA was catalyzed by an enzyme found in sheep kidney and rat liver. The chemical analogy between this isomerization reaction and the isomerization of glutamate to β-methylaspartate in bacteria [38], along with the demonstration by Barker and his colleagues [39, 40] that a coenzyme form of cobalamin was needed for the latter reaction, led to the finding in several laboratories that a cobalamin coenzyme is also required for the isomerization of methylmalonyl CoA [2–4]. This enzyme, originally called *methylmalonyl CoA isomerase*, but now designated *methylmalonyl CoA mutase*, was first crystallized from sheep kidney [41] and bacteria [42, 43]. More recently, it has been purified to homogeneity from human placenta [44] and human liver [45]. From both human sources, the enzyme appears to be a dimer (MW ~145,000 to 150,000) of identical subunits (MW ~72,000 to 77,000). The holoenzyme contains 1 mol of adenosylcobalamin (AdoCbl) per mol of subunit, the cobalamin cofactor being very tightly bound to the apoenzyme (estimated K_m of the sheep kidney enzyme for AdoCbl ~2 × $10^{-8}M$). The human enzyme displays complex kinetics with regard to the binding of methylmalonyl CoA [45] and AdoCbl [46], leading to the thesis that the active sites of the dimeric enzyme are not equivalent [46]. In this regard it is significant that hydroxocobalamin (OH-Cbl) appears to act as both a competitive and an irreversible inhibitor of human mutase [36, 47].

Figure 23-2 shows that the isomerization reaction could occur by transfer of either the free carboxyl group or the A carboxyl radical. Studies using isotopically labeled methylmalonyl CoA demonstrated convincingly that it is the CoA carboxyl group that is transferred [48] through an intramolecular isomerization [49, 50]. The exact role of the cobalamin coenzyme in the isomerization reaction remains undefined, but the mechanism surely involves cleavage of the carbon-cobalt bond, followed by transfer of hydrogen from the substrate to the 5'-deoxyadenosyl fragment produced by the cleavage reaction [51].

Alternative Pathways of Propionate Metabolism

Although the catabolism of propionate to succinate through methylmalonate is the major pathway for propionate utilization in mammalian systems, alternative pathways exist. Propionyl CoA can replace acetyl CoA as a "primer" for long-chain fatty acid synthesis [52] and lead to the formation of odd-chain fatty acids, notably heptanoate, nannanoate, and undecanoate. There are also alternative catabolic mechanisms, one of which is described in Fig. 23-4 [22]. The first step in this sequence involves the formation of the α,β-unsaturated fatty acid acrylyl CoA, which may be subsequently hydrated, leading to the formation of either lactyl CoA or β-OH-propionyl CoA. The former compound is hydrolyzed to lactate, thus providing a second means by which propionate may be converted to pyruvate. Catabolism of β-OH-propionyl CoA leads ultimately to the synthesis of acetyl CoA or β-alanine, compounds discussed elsewhere in this volume. In addition, propionyl CoA may condense with oxaloacetate to form methylcitrate in a reaction

Figure 23-3 A proposed model of the mammalian propionyl CoA carboxylase protomer containing two nonidentical subunits (α and β), a biotin carrier site, and multiple substrate and effector sites. See text for details.

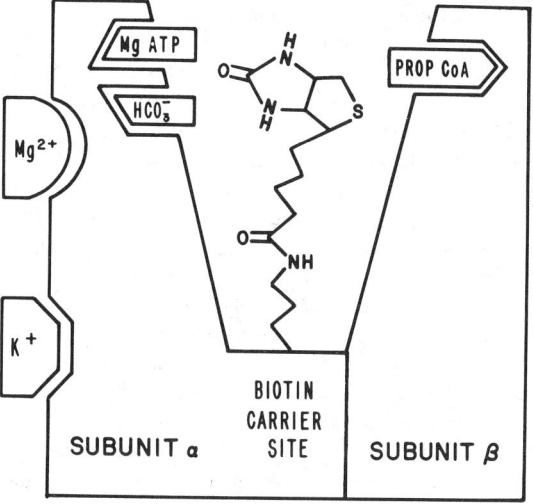

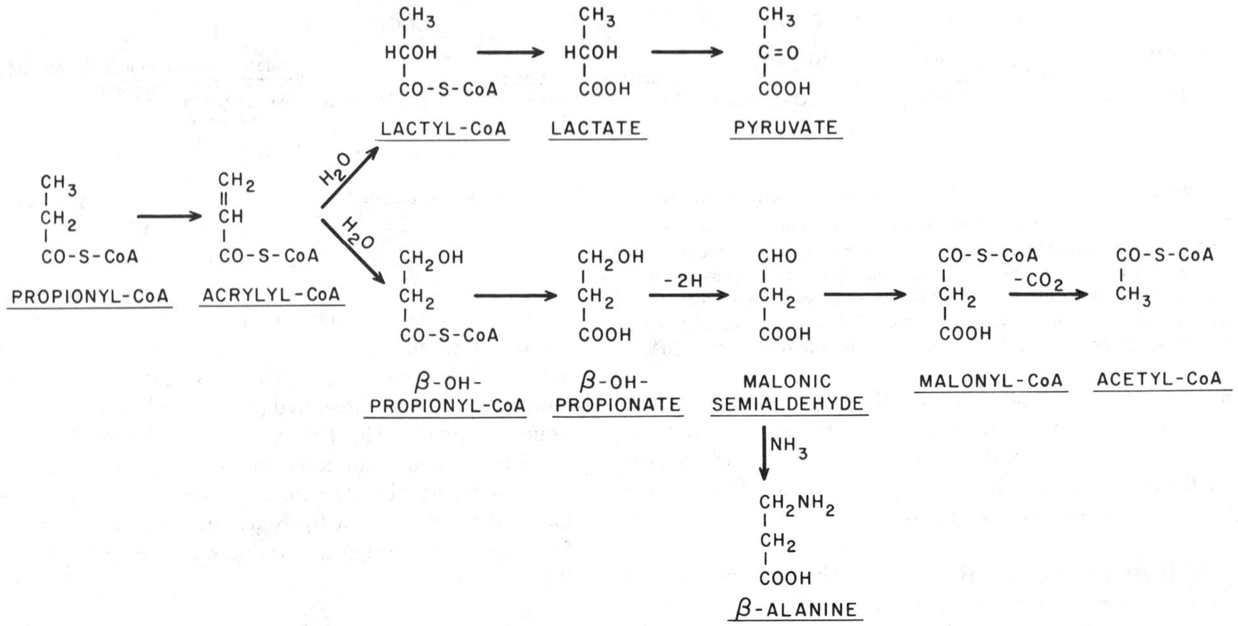

Figure 23-4 Minor pathways of propionate catabolism. Note that both pathways can ultimately generate acetyl CoA. The significance of these minor pathways is discussed in the text.

analogous to the biosynthesis of citric acid from acetyl CoA and oxaloacetate [53]. These alternative pathways are of little quantitative significance in normal subjects but become much more prominent in patients with blocks in the major pathway of propionate metabolism [54, 55].

Coenzymes

Biotin Biotin is widely distributed in plants and animal tissues and is readily synthesized by a variety of microorganisms. It was first isolated from egg yolk in 1936 by the Dutch biochemist, Kögl, and its structure was defined soon thereafter by duVigneaud and colleagues. Our understanding of this water-soluble cofactor is inextricably linked with the evolution of our knowledge concerning avidin, an egg white protein which binds biotin most tightly. Comprehensive reviews on biotin [56] and on biotin-dependent enzymes [57] exist.

STRUCTURE AND FUNCTION Biotin (Fig. 23-3) is a relatively simple molecule, being composed of fused imidazole and thiophene rings to which is attached an *n*-valeric acid side chain. It has a molecular weight of 244. Like many other water-soluble vitamins, biotin functions as a cofactor in enzyme-catalyzed reactions. Specifically, biotin is a prosthetic group for four mammalian enzymes, each of which catalyzes the carboxylation of its substrate. One of these biotin-dependent carboxylases, acetyl CoA carboxylase, is cytosolic and catalyzes the key step in long-chain fatty acid biosynthesis—the formation of malonyl CoA from acetyl CoA. The three other biotin-dependent carboxylases are found in the mitochondrial matrix, where they catalyze critical steps in amino acid degradation (β-methylcrotonyl CoA carboxylase), organic acid rearrangement (propionyl CoA carboxylase), or gluconeogenesis (pyruvate carboxylase). The sequence of partial reactions by which these biotin-requiring enzymes carry out their functions appears to be similar (Fig. 23-3). First, biotin is covalently attached to an epsilon amino group of a lysine residue on the apoprotein [57]; this reaction is catalyzed by an enzyme(s) called *holocarboxylase synthetase* found in the cytosol and

mitochondria of animal cells [57, 58]. Next, an activated carboxyl group (bound to one of the carboxylase subunits) is transferred to a ureido nitrogen group of biotin, forming carboxybiotin. Finally, the carboxyl is shuttled to the substrate bound to the other carboxylase subunit, thereby completing the carboxylation and regenerating the cofactor. It seems likely that the several biotin-dependent carboxylases owe their substrate specificity to their respective substrate-binding subunits. As will be discussed subsequently, it is likely that each carboxylase contains a unique bicarbonate-binding subunit as well.

ABSORPTION AND DISTRIBUTION Surprisingly little information exists about the intestinal absorption and distribution of biotin in humans or other mammals. Presumably, free biotin is formed in the intestinal lumen, either by enzymatic hydrolysis of ingested, tissue-bound biotin or by release from microorganisms. A saturable, sodium-dependent system for biotin absorption has been demonstrated in hamster small intestine [59, 60] but the physiologic importance of this process has not been defined. Even less is known about the transport of biotin in plasma or about its uptake by tissue cells. As depicted schematically in Fig. 23-5, however, it is certain that intracellular biotin must be compartmentalized in cytosol and mitochondria because the apocarboxylases which require it are found in these two subcellular fractions.

BIOTIN DEFICIENCY Spontaneous biotin deficiency has almost never been reported in humans, probably because the daily requirement is very small (estimated at ~20 μg/day) and because intestinal microorganisms synthesize sufficient amounts of the cofactor even in the absence of nutritional sources. Biotin deficiency has been reported recently, however, in a patient with the "short bowel syndrome" being fed exclusively by parenteral alimentation [61]. Experimental biotin deficiency has been produced in animals and humans by ingestion of large amounts of egg white, which contains the potent biotin binder avidin [62]. Under these conditions, four experimental human subjects developed cutaneous pallor, dermatitis, depression, lassitude, muscle pains, hyperesthesia, and finally anemia and electrocardiographic changes. All these symptoms and signs were reversed rapidly by administration of 150 to 300 μg biotin daily for several days. In animals, experimental biotin deficiency has been shown to produce decreased activity of biotin-dependent carboxylases in tissues [56, 57].

Cobalamin (Vitamin B$_{12}$)   The structure and function of this compound have intrigued students of human biology since 1926, when Minot and Murphy demonstrated that oral administration of crude liver extract was effective in the treatment of pernicious anemia [63]. In 1948, this "anti-pernicious anemia factor" was isolated from liver and kidney [64, 65] and was named *vitamin B$_{12}$*. Administration of as little as 1 μg of the vitamin daily was shown to prevent relapse of pernicious anemia. Although the vitamin is widely distributed in animal tissues, there is strong evidence that it is synthesized only in microorganisms found in soil, water, or the rumen and intestine of animals.

STRUCTURAL FEATURES   The isolation of vitamin B$_{12}$ culminated in the elucidation of its three-dimensional structure by Hodgkin and coworkers using x-ray crystallographic techniques [66]. Vitamin B$_{12}$ or, as it is now officially designated, *cobalamin,* is composed of a central cobalt atom (Co) surrounded by a planar corrin ring and a complex side chain extending down from the corrin plane consisting of a 5,6-dimethylbenzimidazole group, a ribose molecule, and a phosphate moiety (Fig. 23-6). The benzimidazole is linked to the cobalt atom through one of its nitrogens, while the phosphate is bonded to the D member of the corrin ring. The molecule is completed by coordinate linkage from the corrin plane of one of several different radicals to the cobalt nucleus. Thus, cyanocobalamin or, more strictly, α-(5,6-benzimidazolyl)-cobamide cyanide is formed by the attachment of a cyanide radical to the cobalt atom. Although this compound is the most common commercial form of the vitamin, it is an artifact of isolation and does not occur naturally in microorganisms, plants, or animal tissues. Many other cobalamins have been formed by replacement of the cyanide radical, but only three have been isolated from mammalian tissue: hydroxocobalamin, methyl-

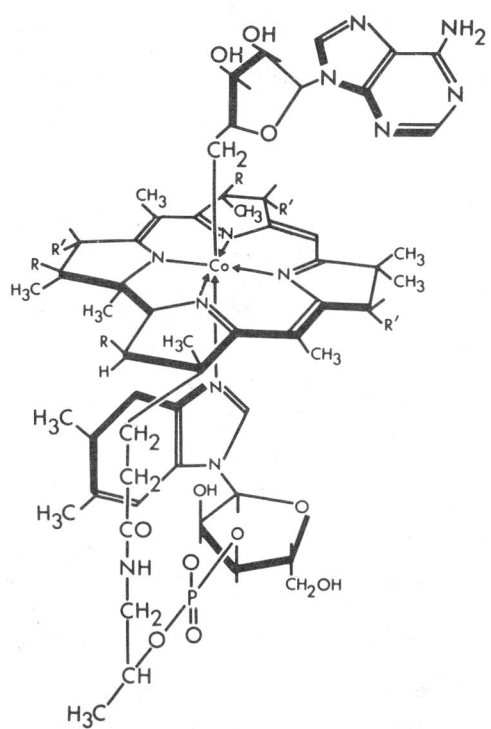

Figure 23-6   Structure of adenosylcobalamin (AdoCbl). R = CH$_2$CONH$_2$; R′ = CH$_2$CH$_2$CONH$_2$. Other radicals which may be coordinately linked to the cobalt atom include CH$_3$ (methylcobalamin), OH$^-$ (hydroxocobalamin), and CN$^-$ (cyanocobalamin). (*Reproduced from Babior [51], with permission of the author and publisher.*)

cobalamin, and adenosylcobalamin. The latter two compounds are unique for two reasons: They are the only two compounds in nature known to have a direct carbon-cobalt bond, and they are the only two forms of cobalamin known to act as specific coenzymes in mammalian systems.

The structure and nomenclature of the cobalamins are further complicated by oxidation and reduction of the cobalt atom. In hydroxocobalamin the cobalt atom is trivalent [cob(III)alamin], and this compound has been called *vitamin B$_{12a}$*. When the cobalt is reduced to a divalent state [cob(II)alamin], the molecule is called vitamin B$_{12r}$, and in the monovalent state cob(I)alamin it is called *vitamin B$_{12s}$*. These oxidation-reduction states are important, since there appear to

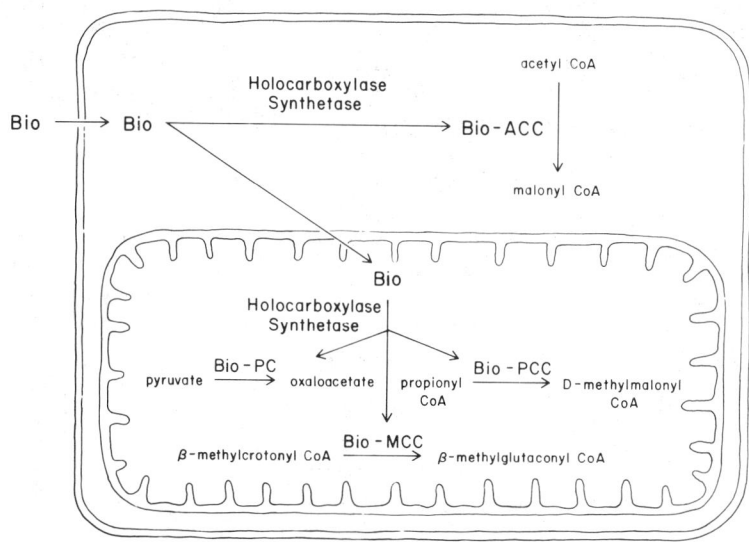

Figure 23-5   Schematic representation of biotin uptake and metabolism by tissue cells. Neither the mechanism by which biotin is transported across the plasma membrane nor that by which it enters the mitochondrion is understood. Abbreviations: bio, biotin; ACC, acetyl CoA carboxylase; PC, pyruvate carboxylase; MCC, β-methylcrotonyl CoA carboxylase; PCC, propionyl CoA carboxylase.

be specific reductase enzymes which sequentially convert cob(III)alamin to cob(I)alamin, with cob(II)alamin acting as an intermediate [67]. The cobalt atom must be reduced to its monovalent state prior to formation of methylcobalamin or adenosylcobalamin.

COBALAMIN COENZYMES   In 1958, Barker and his colleagues demonstrated that the glutamate mutase reaction in *Clostridium tetanomorphum* required vitamin B_{12} [38] and, more specifically, that the active coenzyme form of the vitamin was adenosylcobalamin [39, 40]. One year later, Smith and Monty reported that the analogous isomerization of methylmalonyl CoA to succinyl CoA was defective in the liver of cobalamin-deficient rats [2]. They suggested that cobalamin is a cofactor for the latter isomerization system, a thesis born out by Gurnani et al. [3] and Stern and Friedmann [4], who showed in vitro that the activity of methylmalonyl CoA mutase in liver from cobalamin-deficient animals could be restored to normal by addition of adenosylcobalamin, but not by cyanocobalamin or other vitamin B_{12} analogues. For several years, because adenosylcobalamin was the only known coenzyme form of vitamin B_{12}, it was designated *coenzyme* B_{12}. This is no longer valid.

In 1966 Weissbach and his colleagues [68] demonstrated that methylcobalamin (MeCbl) is a cofactor in the complex series of reactions by which homocysteine is remethylated to methionine (Fig. 23-7). This reaction requires *S*-adenosylmethionine and N^5-methyltetrahydrofolate (Me-H_4folate), as well as the methyltransferase apoenzyme and methylcobalamin. The exact mechanism of homocysteine remethylation remains obscure but probably involves the following sequence: Me-H_4folate is converted to tetrahydrofolate (H_4folate) by transferring its methyl group to a cobalamin prosthetic group of the methyltransferase apoenzyme; in turn, the methyl group is transferred from MeCbl to homocysteine, leading to the formation of methionine [69, 70]. This sequence of reactions, which is relevant to the manifestations of cobalamin deficiency and to the interrelationships between folate and cobalamins, will be discussed in more detail subsequently.

The conversion of methylmalonyl CoA to succinyl CoA and the methylation of homocysteine to methionine are the only cobalamin-dependent reactions that have been demonstrated conclusively in mammalian systems. Poston has reported that AdoCbl acts as a cofactor in the enzymatic reaction by which α-leucine is isomerized to β-leucine [71], but this has not yet been confirmed in other laboratories. In microorganisms several other apoenzymes require adenosylcobalamin [51, 72]: glutamate mutase; diol dehydrase; glycerol dehydrase; ethanolamine ammonia-lyase; and oligonucleotide reductase. In addition, MeCbl catalyzes the formation of methane and acetic acid and the fermentation of lysine in bacteria, but the specific enzymes that catalyze these reactions are not known.

COBALAMIN ABSORPTION AND DISTRIBUTION   The cobalamin vitamins have a unique and highly specialized mechanism of intestinal absorption that has been reviewed in detail recently [73, 74]. The ability to transport physiologic quantities of the vitamin depends on the combined action of gastric, ileal, and pancreatic components. The gastric substance, called *intrinsic factor (IF)* by Castle, who first demonstrated its existence, is a glycoprotein that binds cobalamins in the intestinal lumen. IF, which has been isolated and characterized extensively [73], is synthesized by gastric parietal cells. Evidence obtained in vitro [75, 76] and in vivo [77] suggests that three events precede the formation of IF-cobalamin (Cbl) in the gut lumen. First, cobalamins are released from dietary protein in the acid environment of the stomach. Second, cobalamins bind to "R" proteins of salivary and gastric origin; these R proteins are members of a family of glycoproteins with high affinity for cobalamins. Third, pancreatic proteases digest the R proteins, thereby liberating cobalamins in the upper small intestine, where they are complexed to IF. Subsequently, the IF-Cbl complex interacts through its protein moiety with specific ileal receptor sites in the presence of calcium ions. In this process the IF-Cbl complex is dissociated and the vitamin is transported across the ileal membrane into the portal blood. Once in the bloodstream, the free vitamin is bound by at least three different globulins, designated *transcobalamin I (TC I)*, *transcobalamin II (TC II)*, and *transcobalamin III (TC III)* (see Refs. 73, 78, and 79 for reviews). TC I and TC III are glycoproteins of the R family which carry the majority of cobalamin found in plasma; their physiologic role, however is still unclear. TC II, a β-globulin, is the transport protein for newly absorbed vitamin. When labeled cobalamin is administered intravenously or orally, most of the labeled vitamin is immediately bound to TC II and disappears from the plasma in a few hours [80, 81]. Only a small fraction binds to TC I, and this component turns over very slowly. Surprisingly, MeCbl is the major circulating cobalamin species, accounting for 60 to 80 percent of total plasma cobalamin; OH-Cbl and AdoCbl make up the remainder [82]. Since >90 percent of total plasma cobalamin is bound to TC I, it is clear that most of the circulating MeCbl travels with this R binder. This unusual cobalamin distribution pattern is puzzling, particularly in the face of evidence indicating that AdoCbl accounts for ~70 percent of total hepatic cobalamins, whereas MeCbl constitutes a mere 1 to 3 percent [82]. This preponderance of AdoCbl is also present in such other tissues as erythrocytes, kidney, and brain. The physiologic significance of these widely different fractional cobalamin breakdown products in extracellular and intracellular compartments remains obscure.

TC II also facilitates cobalamin uptake by mammalian tissues. Finkler and Hall [83] showed that CN-Cbl bound to TC II was accumulated by HeLa cells much more rapidly than free

Figure 23-7 Reactions catalyzed by cobalamin coenzymes in mammalian tissues. Note the specificity of adenosylcobalamin for the isomerization of methylmalonyl CoA and of methylcobalamin for the methylation of homocysteine. Me-H_4folate = N^5-methyltetrahydrofolate; H_4folate = tetrahydrofolate.

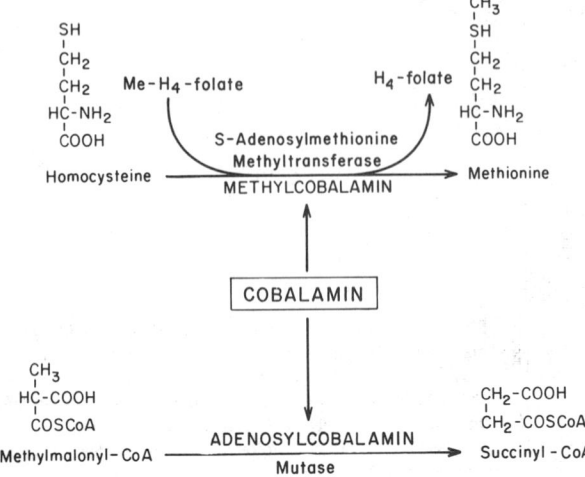

CN-Cbl or CN-Cbl bound to TC I, IF, or other binding proteins. Such TC II-mediated uptake was subsequently confirmed in a variety of cell types, both in vivo and in culture (liver, kidney, heart, spleen, lung, small intestine; cultured fibroblasts, Chinese hamster ovary cells, mouse L cells, lymphoma cells, and phytohemagglutinin-stimulated lymphocytes) (see Ref. 74 for a review). These findings, coupled with the observations in vivo that TC II disappeared from plasma as TC II-cobalamin was absorbed [84], and appeared in lysosomal fractions of hepatic [85] and kidney cells [86], led to the proposal that the circulating TC II-Cbl complex is recognized by a specific, widely distributed plasma membrane receptor. This notion is now supported by considerable experimental evidence (Fig. 23-8). Using ^{125}I-labeled TC II-Cbl complexes, Youngdahl-Turner and associates [87] showed that the complex binds to a specific, high-affinity ($K_a \sim 10^{10}\ M^{-1}$) cell surface receptor on cultured skin fibroblasts through a membrane site which recognizes TC II, and by a mechanism dependent on Ca^{2+}. They showed further that the TC II-Cbl complex is then internalized intact via adsorptive endocytosis [88], and that the degradation of TC II and release of Cbl from the complex occur as a result of lysosomal protease activity [87, 88]. Cobalamin then exits from the lysosome by processes poorly understood, and is either converted to MeCbl and bound to the methyltransferase in the cytosol or enters the mitochondrion, where, after reduction and adenosylation, it is bound to methylmalonyl CoA mutase [89, 90].

The intricate process just described is surely the most widely distributed physiologic means by which mammalian cells obtain cobalamins, but it is not the only means. Hepatocytes, for instance, contain a surface receptor for asialoglycoproteins, and this receptor interacts with TC I-Cbl (and perhaps TC III-Cbl) complexes, thereby providing a second potential means by which this particular tissue obtains cobalamins [91]. Finally, there is growing evidence that at least some tissues are capable of taking up free (unbound) cobalamin if the concentration of unbound vitamin is raised to sufficiently high concentrations. In cultured fibroblasts this uptake process for free cobalamin is saturable, Ca^{2+} independent, and sensitive to inhibitors of protein synthesis and sulfhydryl reagents [92]. Its functional role, under most circumstances, is probably negligible.

COENZYME BIOSYNTHESIS AND COMPARTMENTATION   Since methylmalonyl CoA mutase, the mammalian enzyme dependent on AdoCbl, is a mitochondrial protein [93], whereas the MeCbl-dependent methyltransferase is cytoplasmic [94], it becomes important to relate the cellular biology of the vitamin to its cellular and molecular chemistry. Significant progress in this direction is being made. The chemical pathway of AdoCbl synthesis was defined initially in bacteria [67, 95]. Three enzymes were required for coenzyme synthesis, two reductases and an adenosyltransferase. The reductases are flavoproteins which require NAD as a cofactor. The first (EC 1.6.99.8) is responsible for converting cob(III)alamin, i.e., hydroxocobalamin, to cob(II)alamin and the second (EC 1.6.99.9) for catalyzing the further reduction to cob(I)alamin. The latter compound and ATP are substrates for an adenosyltransferase (EC 2.5.1.17) which completes the synthesis of AdoCbl. Neither of the reductases has been purified extensively, but the adenosyltransferase has. It has a pH optimum of 8, requires Mn^{2+}, and has a K_m of $1 \times 10^{-5}\ M$ for cob(I)alamin and $1.6 \times 10^{-5}\ M$ for ATP [95]. The biosynthetic steps leading to MeCbl formation are not as clear. They may involve a concerted reduction-methylation sequence on or around the methyltransferase apoenzyme [96, 97].

Evidence is accumulating which indicates that mammalian cell metabolism of cobalamin may proceed by a very similar set of reactions (see Fig. 23-8). In 1964, Pawalkiewicz et al. [98] showed that human liver and kidney homogenates could convert CN-Cbl to AdoCbl. Several years later, AdoCbl synthesis from OH-Cbl was observed in HeLa cell extracts incubated with ATP and a reducing system which presumably bypassed the enzymatic reduction of OH-Cbl [cob(III)alamin] to cob(II)alamin [99]. Subsequently, Mahoney and Rosenberg [100] demonstrated the synthesis of both AdoCbl and MeCbl by intact human fibroblasts growing in a tissue culture medium containing ^{57}Co-OH-Cbl. This system was subsequently characterized in cell extracts [101, 102]. As with the HeLa cell system, chemical reductants were employed to bypass both cobalamin reductases [102]. Such extracts synthesized AdoCbl, thereby demonstrating that the adenosyltransferase found in bacteria also exists in normal human cells. These experiments also revealed that the adenosyltransferase was mitochondrial in location, implying that both the synthesis and

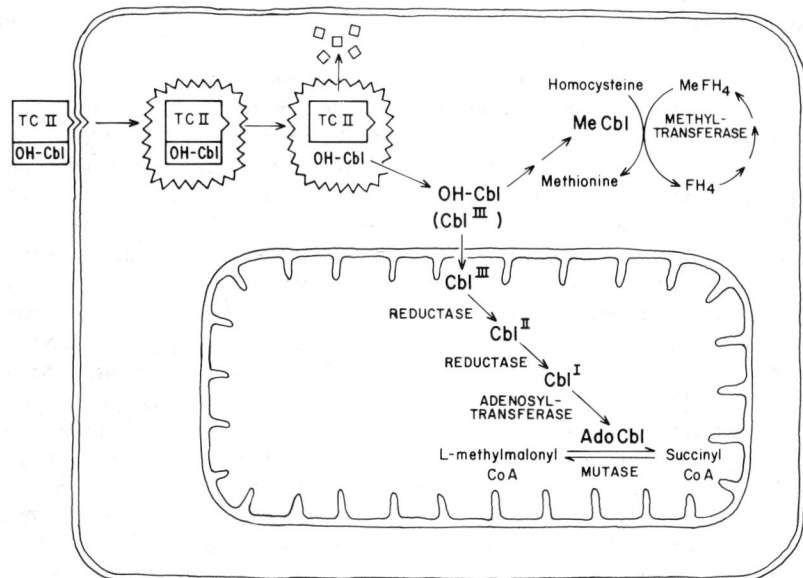

Figure 23-8 General pathway of the cellular uptake and subcellular compartmentation of cobalamins, and of the intracellular distribution and enzymatic synthesis of cobalamin coenzymes. Abbreviations: TC II, transcobalamin II; OH-Cbl, hydroxocobalamin; MeCbl, methylcobalamin; AdoCbl, adenosylcobalamin; Cbl^{III}, Cbl^{II}, Cbl^{I}, cobalamins with cobalt valence of 3$^+$, 2$^+$, and 1$^+$, respectively.

cofactor activity of AdoCbl take place in this organelle. It seems almost certain, as shown in Fig. 23-8, that MeCbl synthesis takes place in the cytosol.

METABOLIC ABNORMALITIES IN COBALAMIN DEFICIENCY The biochemical abnormalities in plasma and urine of patients with cobalamin deficiency reflect the dysfunction of the enzymes dependent on cobalamin coenzymes. The first relevant observation in this context was the demonstration by Cox and White [5] and by Barness and his colleagues [6] that methylmalonic acid excretion in the urine was distinctly increased in cobalamin-deficient patients with classic pernicious anemia. The methylmalonic aciduria in these patients was reversed rapidly by administration of physiologic doses of cobalamin, indicating that repletion of cobalamin stores restored the methylmalonyl CoA mutase reaction to normal. Later, Cox et al. reported that patients with cobalamin deficiency also have distinctly increased amounts of propionic acid in the urine, this abnormality again being reversed by treatment [103]. Interestingly, they also found excessive amounts of acetic acid in the urine of cobalamin-deficient subjects. The mechanism of this abnormality is not clear, since acetate does not participate in the major pathway of propionate catabolism. The finding could, of course, reflect increased utilization of the alternative pathways of propionate metabolism in the face of a block in the major pathway, since each of the alternative routes leads eventually to the formation of acetyl CoA (Fig. 23-4). Excessive excretion of homocystine has also been documented in cobalamin-deficient patients [104, 105], as has combined methylmalonic aciduria and homocystinuria [106]. The latter report is particularly interesting since it documents congenital but not hereditary cobalamin deficiency due, in this instance, to acquired cobalamin deficiency in the offspring of a strict vegetarian mother also deficient in the vitamin.

Biochemical studies in an animal model, the cobalamin-deficient pig, have yielded other significant biochemical findings. Cardinale and his colleagues [107] noted that, as expected, the concentrations of total cobalamin and of adenosylcobalamin were markedly reduced in the liver, kidney, and brain of cobalamin-deficient pigs. They also observed that the methylmalonyl CoA mutase apoenzyme content appeared to be increased. The latter finding suggests the possibility of a feedback control system between apoenzyme and coenzyme that must be explored further.

COBALAMINS AND FOLIC ACID   An interesting, important, and still puzzling aspect of cobalamin function concerns its relationship to folic acid [108]. Several lines of evidence bear out this relationship: the appearance of megaloblastic anemia in either cobalamin or folate deficiency; the reversal of megaloblastic anemia in cobalamin deficiency by large doses of folate; the amelioration of megaloblastic changes in folic acid deficiency by pharmacologic doses of cyanocobalamin; the increased plasma concentrations of N^5-methyltetrahydrofolate in patients with cobalamin deficiency; the excretion of excessive amounts of formiminoglutamic acid (FIGLU) after histidine loading in patients with either cobalamin or folate deficiency; and the reduced amounts of total cobalamin in the liver of patients with folate deficiency. A plausible explanation for most of these effects was proposed independently by Herbert [109], Noronha [110], Larrabee [111], and their colleagues and has been referred to as the *folate trap hypothesis*. This thesis rests on the evidence that the conversion of N^5-methyltetrahydrofolate to tetrahydrofolate depends on the MeCbl-dependent reaction, in which homocysteine is methylated to methionine. If methionine biosynthesis is the only quantitatively significant reaction using N^5-methyltetrahydrofolate, cobalamin deficiency will interfere with the folate cycle and, barring other control mechanisms, will lead to the accumulation of N^5-methyltetrahydrofolate and the depletion of other folate derivatives. This depletion could become severe enough to interfere with other reactions requiring tetrahydrofolate, such as the synthesis of purines or pyrimidines and the conversion of formiminoglutamate to glutamate. Under these circumstances tetrahydrofolate deficiency could be relieved by administration of either folate or cobalamin, but only the latter would complete the folate cycle. This scheme, if totally correct, would obviate the need for additional cobalamin-dependent mechanisms to explain the megaloblastic changes observed in cobalamin deficiency and would account for the specific disorders of folate metabolism observed in cobalamin-deficient human beings. It does not explain the low cobalamin content of livers from folate-deficient subjects or the hematologic response of folate-deficient patients to cobalamin. These relationships between folate and cobalamins are discussed further in Chap. 24.

DISEASE STATES

Several different inborn errors of metabolism may lead to metabolic ketoacidosis or protein intolerance during the neonatal period or infancy or both. Designations such as *idiopathic acidosis of infancy* and *idiopathic lactic acidosis* are giving way to specific etiologic diagnoses. The following inborn errors of carbohydrate, amino acid, or organic acid metabolism must now be considered in the differential diagnosis of infantile metabolic ketoacidosis: glycogen storage disease (type I) (see Chap. 6); pyruvate carboxylase or pyruvate dehydrogenase deficiency; branched chain ketonuria (maple syrup urine disease) (see Chap. 22); isovaleric acidemia (see Chap. 22); β-ketothiolase deficiency (see Chap. 22); propionic acidemia; and methylmalonic acidemia.

The present discussion will concern only the last two conditions. Some patients with β-ketothiolase deficiency, propionic acidemia, methylmalonic acidemia demonstrate ketosis and hyperglycinemia in addition to the primary chemical abnormalities which identify and differentiate them. Such patients can be said to have the *ketotic hyperglycinemia* syndrome [7], a widely used but increasingly nonspecific designation. More interesting than the name, however, is the question of the mechanism of hyperglycinemia and hyperglycinuria observed in these several closely related disorders. This is only one of a large number of puzzling questions about these conditions that remain to be answered.

The disorders to be discussed herein will be grouped according to their most prominent and specific biochemical abnormalities, with full recognition that this classification may require modification in the light of future clinical or biochemical investigation.

The Propionic Acidemias

In 1961, Childs et al. [7] described a male infant with episodic metabolic ketoacidosis, protein intolerance, and remarkably elevated plasma glycine concentration. More than 100 children with similar clinical and biochemical findings have since been described. Many of these children were subsequently found to have methylmalonic acidemia [112]; a few had β-ketothiolase deficiency (see Chap. 22). However, the patient described by Childs et al. [7] and many reported subsequently have propionic acidemia due to a primary and specific deficiency of propionyl CoA carboxylase activity (Fig. 23-2). This conclusion was derived independently from the description of a patient with massive propionate accumulation in blood [113], from another with impaired propionate oxidation in leukocytes [9] and defective carboxylase activity in fibroblast extracts [114], and from a third with both propionic acidemia and defective carboxylase activity [115]. We now recognize that propionyl CoA carboxylase deficiency also occurs in children with inherited abnormalities in biotin metabolism leading to deficiency of multiple biotin-dependent carboxylases. Hence, we must now use the term *propionic acidemias* to refer to this heterogeneous group of related inborn errors. As will be discussed subsequently, a similar kind of heterogeneity exists among the *methylmalonic acidemias*.

Propionyl CoA Carboxylase Deficiency

CLINICAL MANIFESTATIONS   E.G., the patient described by Childs, Nyhan et al. [7, 116, 117] presented with dehydration, lethargy, and coma on the first day of life. He was found to be severely ketoacidotic and responded slowly to massive alkali replacement. The clinical course was characterized by recurrent attacks of ketoacidosis, precipitated by infections or protein ingestion, and by developmental retardation, electroencephalographic abnormalities, and osteoporosis. The patient had episodic neutropenia and thrombocytopenia prior to death at age 7. A sister (A.G.) also became ketotic and acidotic during the first 4 days of life, but the course of her condition has been modified dramatically because of the extensive experience gained in studying her brother. Although she has had mild attacks of ketoacidosis during intercurrent infections, maintenance on a low protein diet has resulted in little need for hospital care and normal somatic and mental development up to age 15 years [118].

In 1968, Hommes and his colleagues [113] described a male infant with hyperventilation, areflexia, and grunting at age 60 h. There was a profound metabolic acidosis (arterial pH 6.98), and in spite of administration of massive amounts of sodium bicarbonate and trishydroxyaminomethane (THAM), the infant died on the fifth day of life. Leukocytes and platelets were normal. Postmortem examination showed only a fatty liver and degeneration of Purkinje cells and the granular layer of the cerebellum.

Subsequent descriptions of patients with this form of propionic acidemia have confirmed that most patients present in the newborn period with severe metabolic acidosis leading to dehydration, lethargy, and coma [115, 119]. It should be emphasized that other patients have presented later, either with episodic ketoacidosis or with developmental retardation uncomplicated by attacks of ketosis or acidosis [120]. Interestingly, still other children with almost complete deficiency of propionyl CoA carboxylase activity in cultured fibroblast extracts have had no clinical abnormalities whatever and have been identified during family studies [121]. No satisfactory explanation for this striking lack of clinical-enzymatic correlation exists at present.

BIOCHEMICAL ABNORMALITIES   Childs and Nyhan [7, 116, 117, 122] studied their index patient extensively. Because of the hyperglycinemia, they focused their attention on the pathways of glycine formation and utilization but found no consistent abnormalities. Normal hemoglobin concentration in the peripheral blood indicated that the pathway from glycine to δ-aminolevulinic acid was not blocked. Slices of the patient's liver incorporated [14C]glycine into protein and carbon dioxide as well as rat liver slices did. Salicylate and benzoate were normally conjugated with glycine, and the glutathione concentration of whole blood was normal. Although the rate of conversion of tritiated glycine to serine in vivo was slower than in controls, this difference may have reflected the enlarged glycine pool rather than a specific block in the conversion of glycine to serine [122].

Several observations suggested an abnormality in the catabolism of the branched chain amino acids, methionine and threonine: Plasma concentrations of valine, isoleucine, and leucine were elevated intermittently; administration of leucine, valine, isoleucine, threonine, and methionine each precipitated attacks of ketoacidosis, but no other amino acids were toxic. Menkes [123] reported that the urine contained large amounts of butanone (a 4-carbon ketone which is a by-product of isoleucine catabolism) and the longer-chain ketones, pentanone and hexanone. These long-chain ketones were not detected in the urine of patients with ketosis due to diabetes, starvation, or ketogenic diets. Since isoleucine, valine, threonine, and methionine are all precursors of propionate, a defect in propionate metabolism seemed likely, but patient E.G. died before any other studies of propionate catabolism could be performed. Subsequently, Hsia et al. [9] demonstrated a striking defect in propionate catabolism in A.G., the affected sister of E.G. When leukocytes isolated from her peripheral blood were incubated with [3-14C] propionate, negligible quantities of 14CO2 were evolved compared to values in controls (Fig. 23-9), but her cells oxidized methylmalonate and succinate normally. Identi-

Figure 23-9 Oxidation of radioisotopically labeled propionate, methylmalonate, and succinate by leukocytes from patient A.G. and from healthy controls. Cells were incubated for 3 h at 37° C in Krebs bicarbonate buffer. See discussion of defective propionate carboxylation for details. (*From Hsia et al.* [9].)

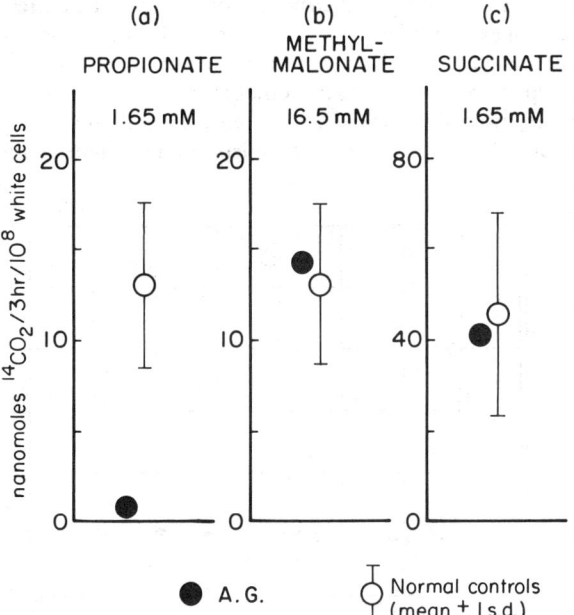

cal findings were obtained using fibroblasts grown in tissue culture. These data showed that the primary metabolic defect in E.G. and A.G. was in the conversion of propionyl CoA to D-methylmalonyl CoA, a reaction catalyzed by propionyl CoA carboxylase. This conclusion was confirmed subsequently by assay of carboxylase activity in fibroblast extracts [114].

In their child with lethal neonatal acidosis, Hommes et al. [113] found that the serum propionic acid concentration was 400 mg/dl (5.4 mM), a value more than 100 times that reported in normal infants (Fig. 23-10). The liver contained fatty acids with 15 and 17 carbon atoms in addition to the even-chain fatty acids found in control livers (Fig. 23-11). From these data, Hommes et al. also postulated a defect in propionyl CoA carboxylation in their patient.

Subsequent investigations have confirmed and extended these early findings. Analysis of body fluids in several additional patients [53–55, 115] showed that propionate accumulation in blood and urine occurs regularly, its magnitude being related to the severity of the clinical course and the time at which sampling is performed. Ando and colleagues have stressed that other propionate derivatives also accumulate in urine. These include methylcitrate, which is probably formed from the intramitochondrial condensation of propionyl CoA with oxalacetate [53]; propionylglycine, which results from the conjugation of propionate with glycine [54]; β-hydroxypropionate, an intermediate in one of the alternative pathways of propionate catabolism [55] (Fig. 23-4); and tiglic acid [124], an isoleucine catabolite several steps proximal to the block. Although the exact amounts of these compounds in urine have not been determined, they appear to account for a small fraction of the propionate pool that accumulates in vivo in this disease. Their presence may be important in mitigating the toxic effects of propionate excess.

Other compounds, not directly concerned with the propionate pathway, have also been found in significantly increased amounts. In addition to hyperglycinemia and hyperglycinuria, which were discussed earlier, marked hyperammonemia has been documented in several patients [125], and a distinct correlation between plasma propionate and blood ammonia has been noted in two patients [126].

THE ENZYMATIC DEFECT   The molecular pathology in propionyl CoA carboxylase deficiency is both complex and interesting. Cell extracts from a number of affected patients share a common finding, namely, reduction in propionyl CoA carboxylase activity to 1 to 5 percent of that in controls [127–129]. Such enzymatic dysfunction reflects different mutations at a minimum of two loci, because complementation studies with heterokaryons formed between pairs of affected cell lines demonstrate the existence of two major complementation groups (designated *pcc A* and *pcc BC*) [130, 131]. The *pcc BC* class, too, is heterogeneous, being subdivided into *pcc B* and *pcc C* mutants. These findings are supported by independent biochemical observations which show that *pcc A* and *pcc BC* mutants can be distinguished by differences in thermostability, affinity for the effector K$^+$, and their responses to avidin addition [128]. Moreover, cell extracts from obligate heterozygotes of the *pcc A* class have about 50 percent of control propionyl CoA carboxylase activity, while those of heterozygotes of the *pcc BC* class have carboxylase activity indistinguishable from that in controls [129]. The simplest and most attractive way to account for this biochemical and genetic heterogeneity is to propose that the two major classes of *pcc* mutants correspond to structural alterations of the two nonidentical subunits of the carboxylase molecule (see Fig. 23-2 and related discussion), i.e., that the *pcc A* class reflects abnormalities in the α (or β) subunit, while the *pcc BC* class reflects defects in the other subunit. Since antibodies to the native enzyme and subunits exist, it should soon be possible to test this thesis directly. Such studies should also help explain why all cell lines from affected patients retain a few percent of residual propionyl CoA carboxylase activity.

PATHOLOGIC PHYSIOLOGY   A defect in the carboxylation of propionate provides a satisfactory explanation for many of the findings reported in this disorder. This defect would be expected to lead to an elevated concentration of propionate in the blood and an inability of leukocytes to catabolize propionate to carbon dioxide. Since isoleucine, valine, threonine, and methionine are precursors of propionate, such a block should also lead to the observed protein and specific amino acid intolerance. The appearance of long, odd-chain fatty acids in the liver suggests that when propionyl CoA carboxylation is blocked, odd-chain fatty acid biosynthesis may be augmented because propionyl CoA is the "primer" for such compounds. Finally, the presence of such compounds as butanone, methylcitrate, β-hydroxypropionate, propionylglycine, and tiglic acid very likely results from reversal of reactions proximal to the primary carboxylase block or from increased utilization of alternative pathways. It is not at all clear from the foregoing why some patients have a severe and often life-threatening course and others are mildly affected clinically. Major differences in dietary protein or in alternate mechanisms for propi-

Figure 23-10 Gas-liquid chromatograms of serum short-chain fatty acids from a control (*A*) and from a patient with propionic acidemia (*B*). 1 = solvent; 2 = formic acid; 3 = propionic acid. (*Reproduced from Hommes et al.* [113], with permission of the authors and publisher.)

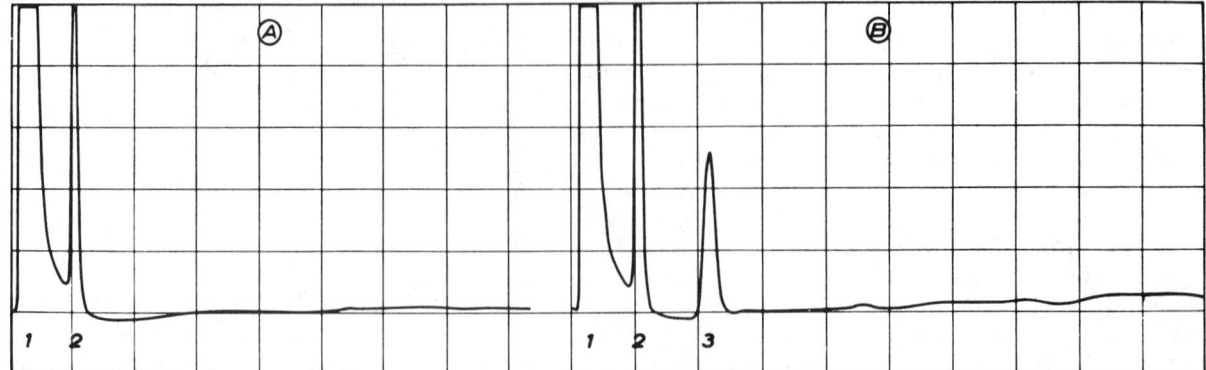

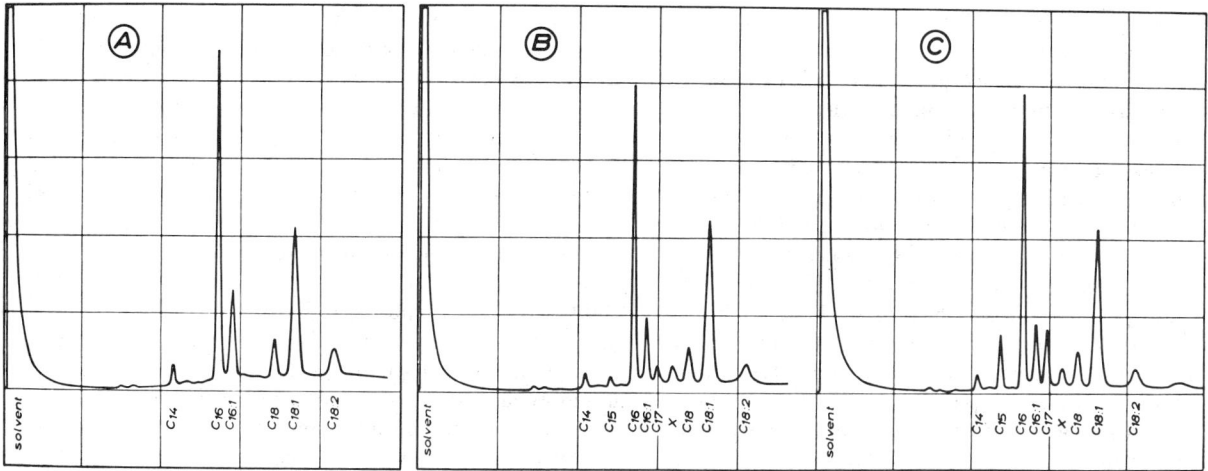

Figure 23-11 Gas-liquid chromatograms of methyl esters of fatty acids extracted from liver of a control (*A*); a patient with propionic acidemia (*B*); and a patient with propionic acidemia plus added methyl esters of C_{15} and C_{17} fatty acids (*C*). C_{14}, C_{15}, etc. = chain length of fatty acids. (*Reproduced from Hommes et al. [113], with permission of the authors and publisher.*)

onate disposal are possible explanations for the wide clinical spectrum, but the prominent intrafamilial differences in severity are not easily explained this way [121]. Further, several other features of the disease are not adequately explained by the block in propionate catabolism. The ketosis produced in E.G. by leucine is not understood, since this amino acid is not catabolized to propionate. It is, however, ketogenic in normal subjects, suggesting that its effect in E.G. was nonspecific. The cause for the hyperglycinemia seen in many, but not all, of these patients has not been adequately defined. Since the infant described by Hommes et al. [113] with massive propionic acidemia never showed hyperglycinemia, the latter cannot be ascribed simply to the acidosis or ketosis. Numerous theses have been put forth. One or more products of isoleucine catabolism may interfere with glycine cleavage or glycine-serine interconversion [122, 132, 133]. Ando et al. [53] speculated that methylcitrate cleavage in the cytosol may yield propionate and glyoxylate, the latter being used as a substrate for glycine overproduction. Impaired glycine conjugation systems have been suggested, but no data in support of this notion have been forthcoming. Since plasma glycine concentration may rise in sick children with negative nitrogen balance of many causes [134], the hyperglycinemia may be nonspecific. The hyperammonemia often observed in this disorder has been the subject of considerable recent investigation. It appears very likely that this secondary but clinically important finding results from inhibition of the first enzyme of the urea cycle, mitochondrial carbamyl phosphate synthetase (CPS I), by the organic acids and CoA esters which accumulate intramitochondrially behind the block in propionyl CoA carboxylation. This conclusion rests on the following data from studies with experimental animals and animal tissues: Propionate inhibits ureagenesis in rat liver slices when ammonia, but not citrulline or aspartate, is the nitrogen-donating substrate [135]; administration of sufficiently large amounts of propionate or methylmalonate to produce hyperammonemia in rats is associated with a marked fall in hepatic concentration of *N*-acetyl glutamate (NAG) [136], the required allosteric effector of CPS I, probably by competitively inhibiting NAG synthetase [136a]; and propionyl CoA and methylmalonyl CoA inhibit CPS I activity markedly when measured in rat and human liver homogenates, in

isolated mitochondria, or with pure rat liver enzyme [137]. These results suggest that there are two discrete mechanisms of CPS I inhibition in patients with propionyl CoA carboxylase (and β-ketothiolase or methylmalonyl CoA mutase) deficiency: a direct effect of the accumulated CoA esters on the enzyme [137], and an indirect effect on CPS I activity via impaired formation of NAG [136, 136a]. That such CPS I inhibition occurs in vivo as well as in vitro is supported by case reports that describe selective impairment of CPS I activity in the livers of patients with propionic acidemia [138] or methylmalonic acidemia [139].

GENETICS The presence of two affected sibs, one of each sex, in the index family with this condition suggested autosomal recessive inheritance. This suggestion has been amply supported for both the *pcc A* and *pcc BC* classes. (1) Several families in each class with two or more affected sibs have been described. (2) Propionyl CoA-carboxylase activity in cultured skin fibroblast extracts from both parents of affected children in the *pcc A* class have about 50 percent of normal propionyl CoA carboxylase activity [114, 129]. (3) Complementation testing with heterokaryons formed between cell lines of several carboxylase-deficient patients has revealed that the enzyme defect behaves as a recessive in culture [130].

DIAGNOSIS AND TREATMENT A defect in propionate carboxylation must be considered in any child who develops ketosis or acidosis in the neonatal period. Other inborn errors of metabolism must be ruled out, as must the more common causes of acidosis in the newborn period. Determinations of propionic acid in blood or urine and studies of propionyl CoA carboxylase activity in leukocyte or fibroblast extracts are required for such definitive diagnosis. The latter test is, in fact, the only absolutely specific one, since propionate accumulation can occur in patients with defects of methylmalonate metabolism as well as in those with propionyl CoA carboxylase deficiency. Such assays on cord blood leukocytes should allow immediate diagnosis in a high-risk newborn. Prenatal diagnosis has been accomplished by measuring carboxylase activity in cultured amniotic fluid cells [140].

A low protein diet [0.5 to 1.5 g/(kg·day)] or one selectively reduced in the content of propionate precursors appears to be the best treatment for the disorder at this time. Such diets will minimize the number of attacks of ketoacidosis but will not necessarily prevent them or allow normal development in all patients. Attacks of ketoacidosis should be treated vigorously by withdrawing all dietary protein and administering sodium bicarbonate parenterally. Since propionyl CoA carboxylase requires biotin as a coenzyme, it is possible that some patients may improve when given supplementary biotin. Only one biotin-responsive patient with presumably specific propionyl CoA carboxylase deficiency has been reported [141]. In this child, administration of 5 mg biotin daily blunted the isoleucine-induced rise in plasma propionate concentrations and minimized the ketosis produced by challenge with isoleucine. Whereas most patients with specific propionyl CoA carboxylase deficiency do not so respond to biotin supplements, their cells often show some increase in enzyme activity [142], indicating that a trial of biotin supplementation is in order in all patients with this disorder. Dramatic biotin responsiveness has been described in several children in whom propionyl CoA carboxylase deficiency was part of the constellation now called *multiple carboxylase deficiency*. This entity will be discussed separately since its etiology and pathogenesis differ markedly from those of the aforementioned abnormalities in the structure and function of apo-propionyl CoA carboxylase.

Multiple Carboxylase Deficiency   In 1971 Gompertz et al. [143] reported a male infant (J.R.) thought to have specific deficiency of the mitochondrial, biotin-dependent enzyme β-methylcrotonyl CoA carboxylase (see Chap. 22 and Fig. 23-5). This infant developed a diffuse, erythematous skin rash at age 5 weeks and was admitted to the hospital at age 5 months because of a worsening rash, recurrent vomiting, irritability, and a mild metabolic acidosis. His urine, which smelled like "tom cats' urine," was analyzed for organic acids and was found to contain large excesses of β-methylcrotonylglycine, tiglylglycine, and β-hydroxyisovaleric acid. When he was given 10 mg biotin (about 100 times the estimated human requirement) by mouth daily for several days, the rash, vomiting, irritability and abnormal urine metabolites all disappeared dramatically. Several years later, it became clear that J.R. had multiple—not specific—carboxylase deficiency: His reanalyzed urine contained metabolites characteristic of propionyl CoA carboxylase deficiency as well as β-methylcrotonyl CoA carboxylase deficiency [144]; his cultured fibroblast extracts were deficient in pyruvate carboxylase [145] as well as propionyl CoA and β-methylcrotonyl CoA carboxylase [146, 147]; and supplementation of the fibroblast growth medium with biotin led to complete correction of the deficiency of all three biotin-dependent enzymes [145–147]. Subsequently, at least seven additional children have been described with features consistent with multiple carboxylase deficiency [148–152]. Five of these children (three in one sibship, see Ref. 148) have developed a skin rash, as well as metabolic acidosis within the first 3 months of life [148–150]; in the other two, the rash was first noted at 10 [151] and 14 months [152], respectively. All have responded dramatically, both clinically and chemically, to oral biotin supplements (5 to 10 mg/day). Other features described in some, but not all, affected patients include alopecia [148, 151, 152], seizures [148, 149, 152], hypotonia [149, 151], abnormal urinary odor [149, 150], and defective T-cell and B-cell immunity [148].

The absence of a reproducible clinical phenotype has been associated as well with major differences in studies with cultured cells. As with J.R.'s cells, those of several other patients have shown deficient activity of the mitochondrial biotin-dependent enzymes in cells grown in basal or biotin-depleted medium, such deficiencies being corrected by supplementing the growth medium, but not the cell extracts, with biotin [145]. A defect in holocarboxylase synthetase activity (Fig. 23-5) has been proposed but not documented in such cells [145–147]. A defect in transmembrane or intracellular transport of biotin could account for the observations as well. Significantly, cultured cells from the two patients with the latest clinical onset [151, 152] showed no abnormality in carboxylase activity, regardless of whether the cells were grown in biotin-depleted or -supplemented medium. Since one of these children has been reported to have distinctly reduced plasma and urinary concentrations of biotin under basal conditions [152], it has been proposed that this child suffers from a defect in intestinal absorption of biotin rather than from a defect in other tissue cells. This intriguing notion must now be tested. The available data are most consistent with the idea that at least two different biochemical bases for biotin-responsive multiple carboxylase deficiency exist, each of which leads to an eminently treatable metabolic disorder.

The Methylmalonic Acidemias

In 1967 Oberholzer [10], Stokke [11], and their colleagues described critically ill infants with profound metabolic ketoacidosis and developmental retardation who accumulated huge amounts of methylmalonate in their blood and urine. These children had none of the hematologic or neurologic stigmata of cobalamin deficiency, failed to respond to cobalamin supplements, and excreted much larger amounts of methylmalonate than those observed in patients with pernicious anemia [6, 7]. They were presumed to have a congenital defect of methylmalonyl CoA racemase or of the methylmalonyl CoA mutase apoenzyme (Fig. 23-2). Shortly thereafter, Rosenberg [8, 153], Lindblad [12, 13], and their coworkers reported children with similar clinical presentations whose methylmalonic aciduria responded dramatically to pharmacologic but not physiologic amounts of cyanocobalamin or adenosylcobalamin (AdoCbl). Such children were found subsequently to have a primary defect of AdoCbl synthesis which resulted in impaired mutase activity [14, 15]. The array of different biochemical and clinical disturbances of methylmalonate metabolism was broadened still further in 1969 and 1970, when Mudd [154], Goodman [155], and their associates described children with methylmalonic aciduria whose clinical and chemical findings differed from those described above: Ketoacidosis was not present, and the increased methylmalonate excretion was accompanied by homocystinuria, cystathioninuria, and hypomethioninemia. This biochemical constellation was interpreted as evidence for defective synthesis of both cobalamin coenzymes, with secondary impairment of AdoCbl-dependent methylmalonyl CoA mutase and MeCbl-dependent homocysteine-N^5-methyltetrahydrofolate methyltransferase (Fig. 23-7). These early descriptions, coupled with a growing body of data to be discussed subsequently, have demonstrated at least six discrete biochemical bases for inherited forms of methylmalonic acidemia (shown with their currently employed genetic designations; see Ref. 17): two distinct defects of the mutase apoenzyme—one producing complete mutase deficiency (*mut°*), the other partial deficiency (*mut−*); two distinct defects of AdoCbl synthesis only—one probably due to deficiency of a mitochondrial Cbl reductase (*cbl A*), the other to deficiency of mitochondrial cob(I)alamin adenosyltransferase *(cbl B)*; and two distinct defects of AdoCbl and MeCbl synthesis due to abnormal cytosolic metabolism of cobalamins *(cbl C* and *cbl D)*. Those patients with lesions producing methylmalonic acidemia only *(mut°, mut−, cbl A, cbl B)* share many clinical features and will be discussed as a group; discussion of the much smaller group of patients whose lesions produce methylmalonic acidemia and homocystinuria *(cbl C* and *cbl D)* will follow.

Methylmalonyl CoA Mutase Deficiency

CLINICAL AND LABORATORY PRESENTATION   Nearly 100 children with isolated mutase deficiency have been documented. Although, as mentioned above, there are four known etiologies for such deficiency, the clinical findings in affected patients from the four etiologic groups are remarkable more for their similarities than for their differences. We have surveyed recently the natural history in 45 such patients; 15 were *mut°*; 5 were *mut−*; 14 were *cbl A*, and 11 were *cbl B*. There were approximately equal numbers of males and females in each group. Information was obtained from questionnaires completed by the patients' physicians, published reports, unpublished communications, and personal experience. The most common signs and symptoms at the onset of clinical difficulty were lethargy, failure to thrive, recurrent vomiting, dehydration, respiratory distress, and muscular hypotonia (Table 23-1). Little interclass difference was observed for these major clinical manifestations or for such less common ones as developmental retardation, hepatomegaly, or coma. Patients in the *mut°* class, however, presented earlier than those in the other groups (Fig. 23-12). Whereas 80 percent of children in the *mut°* class became ill during the first week of life, less than half of the children in the three other groups presented during this interval. Furthermore, clinical onset occurred in ~90 percent of *mut°* patients before the end of the first month, whereas onset beyond the first month was observed in an appreciable fraction of patients in each of the other groups.

The laboratory findings in affected patients at the time that methylmalonic acidemia (with or without aciduria) were first documented are shown in Table 23-2. As expected, serum cobalamin concentrations were routinely normal. Metabolic acidosis, with blood pH values as low as 6.9 and serum bicarbonate concentrations as low as 5 meq/liter, was observed in the majority of patients in all four groups. Ketonemia or ketonuria was found in ~80 percent of patients, with hyperam-

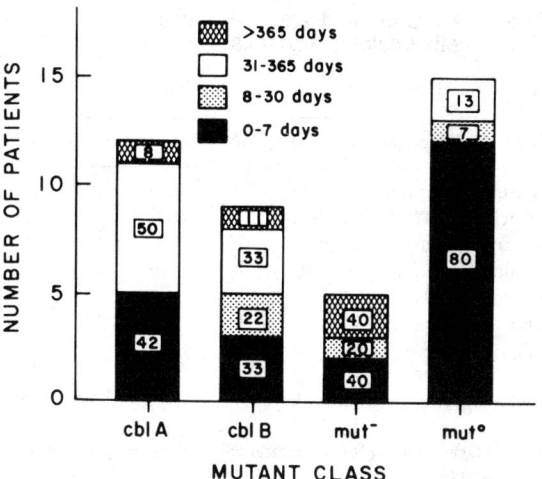

Figure 23-12 Age at clinical onset in 45 patients with methylmalonic acidemia. Inset numbers denote percentages of patients in each group. (*From Matsui et al.* [156].)

monemia being only slightly less common—occurring in ~70 percent. Hyperglycinemia or hyperglycinuria was also observed in ~70 percent of affected patients. Leukopenia, thrombocytopenia, and anemia were the only other manifestations that were noted in 50 percent or more of this group of patients. Earlier case reports (reviewed in Ref. 157) reported that hypoglycemia occurs in about 40 percent of affected patients. Inadvertently, this parameter was not assessed in the recent survey.

CHEMICAL ABNORMALITIES IN VIVO   Large amounts of methylmalonic acid have appeared in the urine or blood of all reported patients. Whereas normal children and adults excrete less than 5 mg methylmalonate daily, children with isolated methylmalonic acidemia have excreted from 240 to 5700 mg in a 24-h period. Their plasma concentrations of methylmalonate, which is undetectable in normal subjects, have ranged from 2.6 to 34 mg/dl. In those few patients in whom it was measured, the cerebrospinal fluid concentration of methylmalonate equaled that of plasma (see Ref. 157 for references to early case reports). No relationship between the quantities of methylmalonate accumulated in body fluids and the etiology of mutase deficiency (i.e., apoenzyme versus coenzyme deficiency) has been reported. Methylmalonate is surely the major, but not the only, abnormal metabolite found in body fluids of these patients. Since propionyl CoA carboxylation is reversible, propionate and some of its precursors (butanone) or metabolites (β-hydroxypropionate and methylcitrate) also accumulate in blood and urine [8, 53, 54, 158, 159], their amounts being small compared to that of methylmalonate.

Several groups have studied the relationship between protein or amino acid loading and methylmalonate accumulation in these patients. Without exception, administration of protein or those amino acids known to be precursors of propionate and methylmalonate, such as methionine, threonine, valine, or isoleucine, has resulted in augmented methylmalonate accumulation and, in some instances, ketosis or acidosis [8, 10–12]. When cobalamin-responsive patients are given supplements of this vitamin, such augmentation by methylmalonate precursors is lessened considerably [160]. All these findings suggest that patients with discrete defects at the mutase step have a major block in the utilization of methylmalonyl CoA which is expressed as methylmalonate accumulation.

Table 23-1 Clinical presentation in 45 patients with methylmalonic acidemia

Signs and symptoms at onset	cbl A	cbl B	mut−	mut°	Total
Lethargy	78	83	100	85	84
Failure to thrive	75	86	40	77	73
Recurrent vomiting	58	86	80	77	73
Dehydration	64	86	100	62	71
Respiratory distress	89	67	50	55	67
Muscular hypotonia	44	57	33	91	63
Developmental retardation	36	33	25	65	47
Hepatomegaly	11	67	0	57	41
Coma	50	29	40	38	40

SOURCE: From Matsui et al. [156]. Numerical values represent percentages of patients in each group.

Table 23-2 Laboratory findings in 45 patients with methylmalonic acidemia

Finding at clinical onset	Mutant class				
	cbl A	cbl B	mut⁻	mut°	Total
Normal serum cobalamin	100	100	100	100	100
Metabolic acidosis	100	88	100	85	92
Ketonemia and/or ketonuria	78	67	100	85	81
Hyperammonemia	50	83	80	75	71
Hyperglycinemia and/or -glycinuria	70	83	40	70	68
Leukopenia	70	45	60	62	60
Anemia	10	45	0	58	55
Thrombocytopenia	75	45	40	40	50

SOURCE: From Matsui et al. [156]. Numerical values represent percentages of patients in each group.

LOCALIZATION OF ENZYMATIC DEFECTS Since the conversion of propionate to succinate is blocked in each of the methylmalonic acidemias, an early screening test for these disorders measured the ability of intact peripheral blood leukocytes or cultured fibroblasts to oxidize [14C]propionate to 14CO2 and compared this with the oxidation of [14C]succinate to 14CO2 [9, 153]. By including estimation of [14C]methylmalonate oxidation as well, this test can distinguish between deficiency of propionyl CoA carboxylase and that of methylmalonyl CoA mutase. More recently, incorporation of [14C]propionate into trichloroacetic acid-precipitable material by intact cultured cells has replaced the more cumbersome 14CO2 evolution technique [161, 162]. Further discrimination among the methylmalonic acidemias has depended on studies of cobalamin uptake and AdoCbl formation by intact cultured fibroblasts, on assays of mutase activity in cell extracts, and on genetic complementation studies with cultured cell heterokaryons.

Mutase apoenzyme deficiency Morrow and colleagues [163] provided the first evidence in vitro for apoenzyme abnormalities and for biochemical heterogeneity among the methylmalonic acidemias. In four patients who had died, they studied mutase activity in liver homogenates by measuring the conversion of DL-[3H]methylmalonyl CoA to [3H]succinyl CoA (Table 23-3). Activity was barely detectable in three and showed no response when AdoCbl was added at concentrations sufficient to saturate the normal enzyme. In the fourth, mutase activity was restored to control values by AdoCbl. These findings were interpreted as evidence for a mutase apoenzyme defect in the first three patients and for defective AdoCbl synthesis in the fourth. These findings were confirmed subsequently in studies with cultured fibroblasts [164]. Cells from the first three patients synthesized AdoCbl normally but had much reduced mutase activity in extracts regardless of the amount of AdoCbl added; cells from the fourth had a distinct defect in AdoCbl synthesis.

Subsequently, it has become clear that two general types of apomutase defects exist. In one type, designated *mut°* and constituting about two-thirds of the *mut* group, mutase activity in extracts of cultured fibroblasts is undetectable (<0.1 percent of control), even when assayed in the presence of AdoCbl concentrations greatly in excess of that normally required to saturate the enzyme [164–166]. When cross-reacting material (CRM) was sought in cell lines from 21 such patients by radioimmunoassay, 12 had no immunologically identifiable mutase

protein (CRM⁻), while 9 had reduced amounts of CRM ranging from 1 to 40 percent of that found in control extracts [167].

The second type, designated *mut−*, involves a structurally abnormal mutase apoenzyme. Thus far, lines from seven patients fall into this group. The mutant apoenzymes in these cell extracts retain maximally 2 to 75 percent of control activity, have a K_m for AdoCbl approximately 200 to 5000 times normal, show a normal K_m for methylmalonyl CoA, and exhibit increased thermolability relative to control enzyme [165, 166, 168]. By radioimmunoassay, the amount of immunologically reactive mutase protein in these extracts ranges from 20 to 100 percent of control [167]. Since pairwise crosses between *mut°* and *mut−* yield noncomplementing heterokaryons, it seems likely that both mutant types reflect abnormalities of the locus coding for the apomutase structural gene [165, 166]. This conclusion is further supported by the identification of affected individuals who appear to be *mut°/mut−* compound heterozygotes—a finding expected for allelic mutations [166]. Finally, it should be mentioned that the only patient thus far reported to have methylmalonyl CoA racemase deficiency [169] has been restudied subsequently and shown conclusively to be a *mut−* mutant biochemically and genetically [16].

Defective synthesis of adenosylcobalamin A series of observations by Rosenberg [14], Mahoney [15], and their colleagues on the fibroblasts of the index patient with cobalamin-responsive methylmalonic acidemia led to the demonstration of a primary defect in AdoCbl synthesis (Fig. 23-13): (1) Such cells were unable to oxidize propionate or methylmalonate in a medium containing 25 to 50 pg/ml cobalamin and under these conditions, the cell content of adenosylcobalamin was only 10 percent of normal [14]. (2) Supplementation of the medium to 250,000 pg/ml raised the AdoCbl content to that of controls and led to a distinct increase in propionate oxidation [14]. (3) Such intact cells were unable to convert 57Co-OH-Cbl to 57Co-AdoCbl, although they took up the labeled vitamin normally and had no abnormality in synthesizing the other cobalamin coenzyme, MeCbl [15]. (4) Mutase activity in cell-free extracts supplemented with AdoCbl was normal [14]. (5) Cell-free extracts from this line synthesized AdoCbl normally when incubated with 57Co-OH-Cbl, ATP, and a reducing system designed to bypass cob(III)alamin reductase and cob(II)alamin reductase and to measure only cob(I)alamin adenosyltransfer-

Table 23-3 Methylmalonyl CoA mutase activity in liver homogenates from patients with methylmalonic acidemia

Subjects	Enzymatic activity*	
	Without added AdoCbl	With added AdoCbl (4 × 10⁻⁵ M)
Controls (3)	535–866	799–1058
Patients		
1	1	3
2	8	33
3	3	7
4	80	1368

* Assayed by measuring conversion of DL-[3H]methylmalonyl CoA to [3H]succinyl CoA. Values expressed as picomoles of succinate formed per milligram protein per 30 min.
SOURCE: Adapted from Morrow et al. [163].

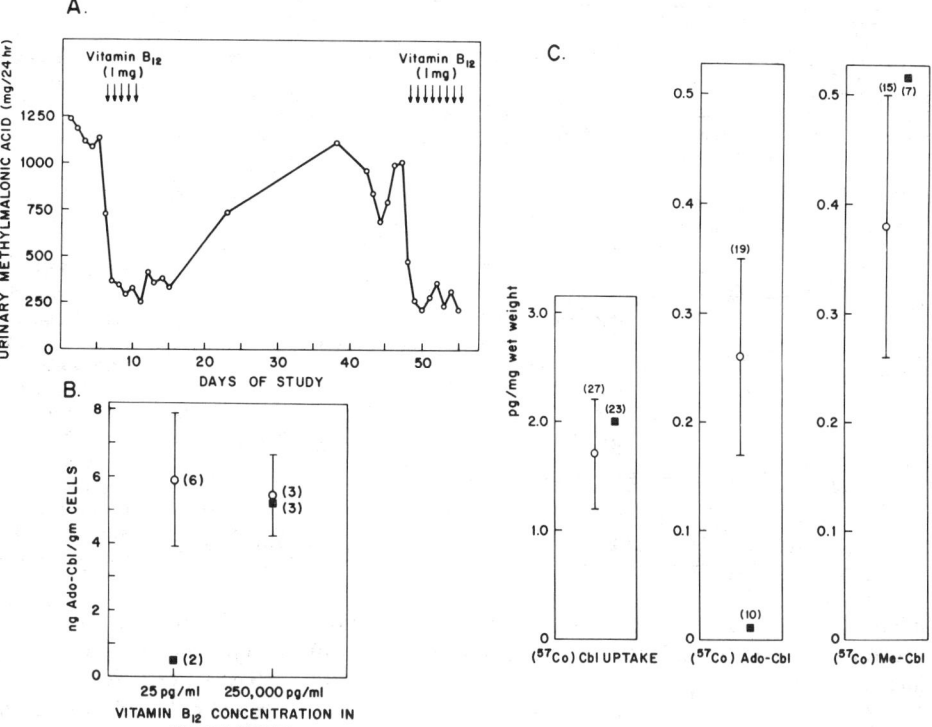

Figure 23-13 The trail of evidence in the index patient with cobalamin-responsive methylmalonic acidemia. *(A).* Fall in urinary methylmalonate excretion after intramuscular administration of 1 mg cyanocobalamin daily. Treatment with smaller quantities of cyanocobalamin (50 to 250 μg daily) produced no response in methylmalonate excretion. *(B).* Reduced content of adenosylcobalamin (AdoCbl) in the patient's cultured skin fibroblasts (■) compared to controls (○) when propagated in medium containing 25 pg/ml cobalamin, and restoration to normal AdoCbl content when cells were grown in a medium containing 250,000 pg/ml cobalamin. *(C).* Defective accumulation of [57]Co-AdoCbl by the patient's intact fibroblasts (■) grown in a medium containing [57]Co-OH-Cbl. Note that uptake of [57]Co-Cbl and formation of MeCbl are normal (○). *(Figures adapted from Rosenberg [14], Mahoney [15], and colleagues.)*

ase (Fig. 23-8) [*101*]. Subsequent biochemical [*101*] and genetic complementation [*170–172*] studies again showed two distinct mutant classes among patients whose intact cells are unable to synthesize AdoCbl normally, thereby leading to deficient holomutase activity. One class, which contains the index-responsive patient just described and is designated *cbl A*, is very likely characterized by deficiency of one of the mitochondrial cobalamin reductases. The second, designated *cbl B*, has been shown to result from a specific deficiency of cob(I)alamin adenosyltransferase [*17, 102*].

PATHOPHYSIOLOGY All studies in vivo and in vitro in patients with methylmalonic acidemia due to specific methylmalonyl CoA mutase deficiency indicate that the primary block in the conversion of methylmalonyl CoA to succinyl CoA explains admirably the accumulation of methylmalonate in blood and urine, the augmentation of methylmalonate excretion and the precipitation of ketosis by protein, amino acids, or propionate, and the excretion of long-chain ketones formed in the catabolism of branched chain amino acids. The primary block does not explain several important physiologic disturbances: the acidosis, hypoglycemia, hyperglycinemia, and hyperammonemia. Oberholzer et al. [*10*] pointed out that the concentration of methylmalonate in the blood (no more than 2 m*M*) could not alone explain the acidosis, and suggested other possibilities. They proposed that an accumulation of coenzyme A "trapped" intracellularly as methylmalonyl CoA could lead to an insufficiency of this widely utilized coenzyme and secondarily to impaired carbohydrate metabolism and subsequent acidosis. Alternatively, they suggested that methylmalonyl CoA, a known inhibitor of pyruvate carboxylase [*173*], could interfere with gluconeogenesis and lead directly to hypoglycemia and indirectly to excessive catabolism of lipid, with ketosis and acidosis. Halperin et al. [*174*] showed that methylmalonate inhibited the transmitochondrial shuttle of malate and argued that impairment of this key step in glu-

coneogenesis could lead to hypoglycemia. As discussed earlier for deficiencies of β-ketothiolase (see Chap. 22) and propionyl CoA carboxylase, the mechanism of the hyperglycinemia and hyperammonemia so often observed in children with any one of these disorders probably reflects inhibition of the intramitochondrial glycine cleavage enzyme and of CPS I, respectively, by the accumulated organic acids or their CoA esters [*132, 133, 135–137*]. Thus, as shown in Fig. 23-14, each of the major secondary abnormalities in the propionic and methylmalonic acidemias can be explained satisfactorily by inhibition of specific intramitochondrial processes by the accumulated organic acids and esters.

By comparing and contrasting the findings in patients with isolated mutase deficiency with those in patients with cobalamin deficiency (as in classic pernicious anemia), it should be possible to shed some light on the mechanism responsible for the hematologic and neurologic abnormalities in the latter disorder. Thus, the absence of megaloblastic anemia in any patient with isolated mutase deficiency militates against any involvement of this enzyme in the typical megaloblastosis seen in cobalamin deficiency. Similarly, the cerebellar and posterior column abnormalities so often encountered in cobalamin-deficient patients have never been observed in patients with methylmalonic acidemia due to specific mutase dysfunction. Therefore, the notion that neurologic dysfunction in pernicious anemia reflects aberrant incorporation of odd-chain or branched chain fatty acids into myelin because of a block in the propionate pathway has little to recommend it. It appears likely, then, that abnormalities in the cobalamin-dependent methyltransferase account for the hematologic and neurologic abnormalities in cobalamin-deficient patients. This matter will be discussed further when we consider that group of patients with methylmalonic acidemia and homocystinuria.

As mentioned earlier, however, about half of the reported patients with isolated methylmalonic acidemia show pancytopenia [*156*]. A recent report suggests that methylmalonate

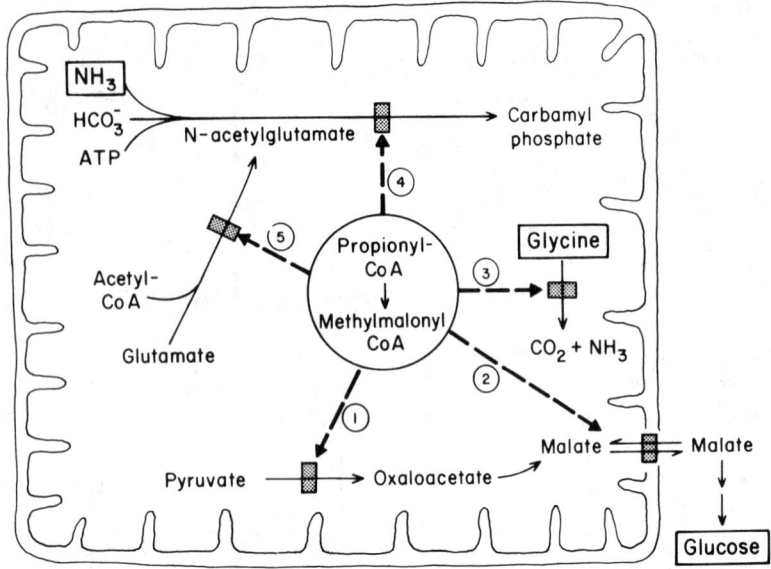

Figure 23-14 Proposed mechanisms of hypoglycemia, hyperglycinemia, and hyperammonemia in patients with inherited deficiencies of β-ketothiolase (see Chap. 22), propionyl CoA carboxylase, or methylmalonyl CoA mutase. Inhibitory effects of the enlarged intramitochondrial pools of acyl CoA esters (such as propionyl CoA) or their respective free acids on selected mitochondrial functions are shown by the numbered dashed lines corresponding to the following enzymatic or shuttle-mediated reactions: (1) pyruvate carboxylase; (2) the transmitochondrial malate shuttle; (3) the glycine cleavage enzyme; (4) carbamyl phosphate synthetase I; and (5) N-acetylglutamate synthetase. See text for discussion.

inhibited growth of marrow stem cells in a concentration-dependent fashion [175]. Further studies of this sort will be of interest.

GENETIC CONSIDERATIONS   Each of the four etiologic bases for specific methylmalonyl CoA mutase deficiency (mut°, mut−, cbl A, and cbl B) is almost certainly inherited as an autosomal recessive trait. This conclusion is based on the following findings. First, approximately equal numbers of affected males and females are encountered in each group [156]. Second, no instance of vertical transmission from affected parent to affected child has been reported. Third, interclass heterokaryons formed between cell lines from different etiologic groups (i.e., mut° × cbl A) complement each other, whereas intraclass heterokaryons (i.e., mut° × mut°) do not; thus, each mutant class behaves as a recessive in culture [170–172]. Fourth, cell lines from heterozygotes for the mut°, mut−, and cbl B mutations show partial mutase apoenzyme deficiency [166] and partial adenosyltransferase deficiency [102], respectively. And fifth, among a large group of mut mutants studied, some have inherited a genetically different mutant allele from each parent—thereby being compound heterozygotes (i.e., mut°/mut−) rather than true homozygotes (i.e., mut°/mut°) [166].

It is not yet possible to define with any precision the prevalence of these disorders in the general population. A recent survey of newborns in Massachusetts has suggested that methylmalonic acidemia may occur in 1:48,000 infants [176]. Since this study screened urines from infants ages 3 to 4 weeks, and since it is known that many children with methylmalonic acidemia die in the first week of life from ketoacidosis or hyperammonemia or both, the true prevalence must be considerably greater.

DIAGNOSIS, TREATMENT, AND PROGNOSIS   Since simple colorimetric assays for urinary methylmalonate and more complex gas-liquid chromatographic assays for serum and urinary methylmalonate are now available, it should no longer be difficult to make a diagnosis of methylmalonic acidemia, once this condition is considered. Other sources of neonatal or infantile ketoacidosis must be ruled out. If excessive amounts of methylmalonate are found in the urine, cobalamin defi-

ciency can be excluded by direct measurement of serum cobalamin concentration. Confirmation and etiologic designation (i.e., mut or cbl) depend on more laborious studies with cultured cells and extracts therefrom [16]; such laboratory confirmation should and can be regionalized. Prenatal detection of methylmalonic acidemia has been accomplished on several occasions in two different ways: by measurement of methylmalonate in amniotic fluid and maternal urine at midtrimester [177, 178] and by studies of mutase activity and cobalamin metabolism in cultured amniotic fluid cells [161, 178, 179]. Mutase apoenzyme [161, 177] and AdoCbl synthesis [178, 179] deficiences have been identified in these ways.

Two treatment regimens for children with methylmalonic acidemia exist and should be employed in tandem. A diet restricted in protein (or a special formula restricted in amino acid precursors of methylmalonate) should be instituted as soon as such life-threatening problems as ketoacidosis, hypoglycemia, or hyperammonemia have been addressed; and supplementary cobalamin [1 to 2 mg cyanocobalamin (CN-Cbl) or hydroxocobalamin (OH-Cbl) intramuscularly daily for several days] should be given as soon as the diagnosis of methylmalonic acidemia is made (or even seriously considered). Such measures should decrease the circulating concentrations of methylmalonate and propionate. Even cobalamin-unresponsive children with delayed development have been shown to improve markedly when treated with careful dietary protein restriction [180].

Our previously mentioned survey [156] suggests that both the response to cobalamin supplements and the long-term outcome in affected patients depend considerably on the nature of the biochemical lesion causing the methylmalonic acidemia. As shown in Fig. 23-15, essentially none of the children designated mut° or mut− responded to cobalamin supplements with a distinct fall in blood or urinary methylmalonate, whereas >90 percent of the cbl A and ~40 percent of the cbl B patients showed such a response. Given the complete absence of mutase activity in cells from the mut° group, it is not surprising that they were regularly cobalamin-unresponsive in vivo. The disappointing absence of response in four mut− patients presumably means that even parenteral cobalamin supplements could not drive tissue concentrations of AdoCbl sufficiently high to increase significantly their mutase holoenzyme activity. That fraction (~60 percent) of *cbl B* patients unresponsive to cobalamin supplements presumably have such complete adenosyltransferase deficiency that AdoCbl synthesis cannot be augmented by cobalamin supplements, as apparently it can in the *cbl B* patients with "leaky" mutations that permit responsiveness in vivo. Patients in the *cbl A* group were uniformly responsive, suggesting either that the responsible mutations are leaky, thereby allowing mass action to result in more AdoCbl synthesis, or that alternative pathways of cobalamin reduction which require high substrate concentrations exist in cells. It should be emphasized that responsiveness in vivo does not mean complete correction of mutase deficiency. Studies with cultured cells from a variety of patients with methylmalonic acidemia [16, 172] suggest that raising holomutase activity to only ~10 percent of normal values by supplementing the growth medium with OH-Cbl results in distinct augmentation of propionate pathway activity (or, conversely, in a distinct decrease in the magnitude of the metabolic block). Some patients, unresponsive to CN-Cbl or OH-Cbl in vivo, might be expected to respond to AdoCbl itself, but no published reports documenting the efficacy of this logical alternative exist at present.

The long-term outlook for affected patients is revealing. As noted in Fig. 23-16, the *mut°* group has the poorest prognosis, with 60 percent decreased and 40 percent distinctly impaired developmentally at the time of the survey. In sharp contrast, the *cbl A* patients (i.e., that group biochemically most responsive to cobalamin supplements) had the best outcome—~70 percent were alive and well at ages up to 14 years. The *cbl B* and *mut−* groups were intermediate, with about equal fractions in each group being found in the alive and well, the alive and impaired, or the deceased category. It is interesting, albeit anecdotal, that the index patient in the *cbl A* group (now 14 years old) discontinued cobalamin supplements at age 9 years in spite of our advice to the contrary. In the ensuing 5 years, his development and general health have remained excellent despite the accumulation of very large amounts of methylmalonate in the blood and urine. Perhaps, as in some other inherited metabolic disorders, treatment of methylmalonic acidemia is most critical during the early years of life. If this experience is borne out by others, it makes expert clinical management in the early weeks or months of life most important. Finally, the

Figure 23-15 Biochemical response to cobalamin supplementation in 45 patients with methylmalonic acidemia. *MMA* refers to the concentration of methylmalonate. The supplementation protocol generally employed 1 mg CN-Cbl parenterally daily for 7 to 14 days. Inset numbers denote the percentage of patients in each group. (*From Matsui et al. [156].*)

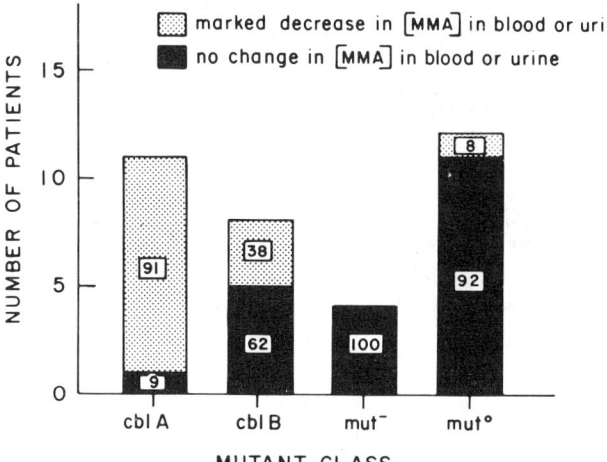

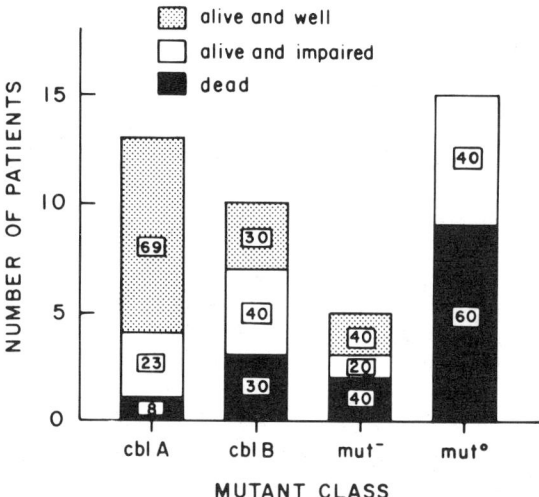

Figure 23-16 Long-term outcome in 45 patients with methylmalonic acidemia. The ages of the patients surveyed ranged from a few weeks to 14 years. (*From Matsui et al. [156].*)

feasibility of prenatal therapy with cobalamin supplements has also been demonstrated. Ampola et al. [178] showed that administration of cobalamin supplements to a woman carrying a cobalamin-responsive, affected fetus resulted in significant reduction in maternal excretion of methylmalonate. The utility of this provocative observation must await the demonstration that prenatal damage occurs if therapy is withheld.

Combined Deficiency of Methylmalonyl CoA Mutase and Homocysteine: Methyltetrahydrofolate Methyltransferase

CLINICAL AND LABORATORY PRESENTATIONS   Ten children with inherited methylmalonic acidemia and homocystinuria are known to this author. Seven of these children have been the subject of individual case reports [155, 181–185]; three have not yet been formally reported. Cells from these children comprise two biochemically and genetically distinct complementation groups, designated *cbl* C and *cbl* D [101, 170, 171]. The clinical findings in the two male sibs who constitute the *cbl D* group [155] are so different from those in the larger number of *cbl C* patients [181–185] as to predict that these groups will also be biochemically distinct.

As noted in Table 23-4, detailed clinical information is available on six children in the *cbl C* group. Three are male and three are female. Five of these six presented in the first 2 months of life because of failure to thrive and developmental retardation. Other prominent findings included seizures and feeding difficulties. When initially evaluated, five of these children had significant anemia; in four, the marrow was megaloblastic. Hypersegmented polymorphonuclear leukocytes and thrombocytopenia were noted in two. Significantly, serum cobalamin and folate concentrations were normal in each child. In sharp contrast, neither of the brothers in the *cbl D* group had any clinically significant problems until much later in life. The older brother came to medical attention because of severe behavioral pathology and moderate mental retardation at 14 years of age. He had, as well, a poorly defined neuromuscular problem involving his lower extremities. His then 2-year-old brother was asymptomatic, although biochemically affected. No hematalogic abnormalities have been noted in either sib.

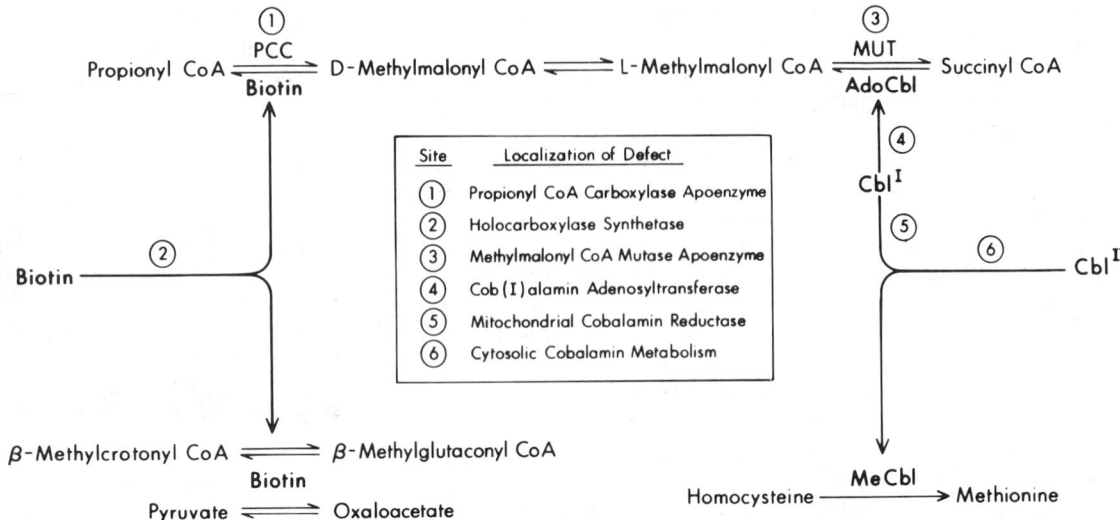

Figure 23-17 Summary scheme of inherited defects of propionate and methylmalonate metabolism. The circled numbers and their key signify the six general sites at which abnormalities have been identified. Abbreviations: PCC, propionyl CoA carboxylase; MUT, methylmalonyl CoA mutase; Cbl^{III}, cob(III)alamin (e.g., OH-Cbl); Cbl^{I}, cob(I)alamin; AdoCbl, adenosylcobalamin; MeCbl, methylcobalamin.

CHEMICAL ABNORMALITIES IN VIVO   In addition to the methylmalonic aciduria and homocystinuria which characterize this group of patients, they have shown hypomethioninemia and, in some instances, cystathioninuria. This constellation of chemical abnormalities, plus the normal serum cobalamin values, led to the proposal [154, 181], which will be discussed in detail subsequently, that these children suffered from a defect in cellular metabolism of cobalamins such that both cobalamin-dependent enzyme activities (mutase and methyltransferase, see Fig. 23-7) were deficient. The methylmalonic aciduria in these children was distinctly less severe than that encountered in children with isolated mutase deficiency (see above). Moreover, neither hyperglycinemia nor hyperammonemia has been reported in any of the *cbl C* or *cbl D* patients (Fig. 23-17).

LOCALIZATION OF DEFECTIVE CELLULAR METABOLISM OF COBALAMINS   It has long been clear that patients in the *cbl C* and *cbl D* groups have a defect in cellular metabolism of cobalamins. This conclusion is based on the following data: Total cobalamin content of liver, kidney, and cultured fibroblasts is markedly reduced [154, 182, 186, 187]; the ability of cultured cells to retain ^{57}Co-labeled CN-Cbl [188] or to convert ^{57}Co-labeled CN-Cbl or OH-Cbl to AdoCbl and MeCbl is markedly impaired [15, 171]; activity of methylmalonyl CoA mutase and of homocysteine:N^5-methyltetrahydrofolate methyltransferase in cultured cells is deficient, such deficiency being improved by supplementation of the growth medium with OH-Cbl [171, 172, 189]; and the mutase and methyltransferase apoenzymes in cells from affected patients appear to be normal [154, 155, 171, 172, 190]. The precise nature of the metabolic defect in the *cbl C* and *cbl D* classes remains elusive, but considerable progress has been made. Since these mutant cells demonstrate normal receptor-mediated adsorptive endocytosis of the TC II-Cbl complex and normal intralysosomal hydrolysis of TC II [16, 87, 88, 171], perusal of Fig. 23-8 makes it clear that the defects in the *cbl C* and *cbl D* cells must affect some step or steps subsequent to cellular uptake, common to the synthesis of both coenzymes and prior to the binding of the cobalamin coenzymes to their respective apoproteins. Significantly, *cbl C* (and, to a lesser extent, *cbl D*) cells use CN-Cbl less well than OH-Cbl [189, 191] and are unable to convert CN-Cbl to OH-Cbl, a step shown in normal cells to

be a metabolic prerequisite for the synthesis of both AdoCbl and MeCbl [191]. The latter results have been interpreted as evidence for a defect in a cytosolic cob(III)alamin reductase, which is required for reducing cobalamin's trivalent cobalt prior to alkylation [191]. More direct assays of such a putative reductase in extracts of *cbl C* and *cbl D* cells will be necessary to confirm or deny this thesis. Finally, it should be mentioned that the distinction between the *cbl C* and *cbl D* classes is based

Table 23-4   Clinical and laboratory features of patients with methylmalonic acidemia and homocystinuria

	Mutant class	
Finding	*cbl C*	*cbl D*
Clinical		
Sex (male/female)	3/3	2/0
Neonatal onset	5/6	0/2
Failure to thrive	5/6	0/2
Developmental retardation	5/6	1/2
Seizures	4/6	0/2
Feeding difficulties	3/6	0/2
Laboratory		
Normal serum cobalamin	6/6	2/2
Anemia	5/6	0/2
Megaloblastic marrow	4/6	0/2
Hypersegmented PMN	2/6	0/2
Thrombocytopenia	2/6	0/2
Complications		
Hemolytic episodes	4/6	0/2
Congestive failure	3/6	0/2
Thromboemboli	0/6	1/2
Current status		
Living and well	0/6	1/2
Living and impaired	2/6	1/2
Deceased	4/6	0/2

SOURCE: Information obtained from published case reports [155, 181–185] and personal communications. Numerical ratios denote patients showing particular finding/total number of patients in each mutant class.

Table 23-5 Salient biochemical features of cultured fibroblasts from patients with the various methylmalonic acidemias

Biochemical parameter	Mutant class*					
	mut°	mut⁻	cbl A	cbl B	cbl C	cbl D
Studies with intact cells						
[^{14}C]propionate oxidation	−	−	−	−	−	−
[^{14}C]MeTHF fixation	+	+	+	+	−	−
MeCbl synthesis	+	+	+	+	−	−
AdoCbl synthesis	+	+	−	−	−	−
Conversion of CN-Cbl to OH-Cbl	+	+	+	+	−	±
Enzyme activities in cell extracts†						
Mutase holoenzyme	−	−	−	−	−	−
Mutase total enzyme	−	±	+	+	+	+
Methyltransferase holoenzyme	+	+	+	+	−	−
Methyltransferase total enzyme	+	+	+	+	±	±
Cob(I)alamin adenosyltransferase	+	+	+	−	+	+

* + = normal; − = markedly deficient or undetectable; ± = partially deficient.

† *Holoenzyme* is defined as that enzyme activity measured in the absence of added cofactor; *total enzyme* is that activity measured in the presence of saturating concentrations of cofactor.

Abbreviations: MeTHF, N^5-methyltetrahydrofolate; MeCbl, methylcobalamin; AdoCbl, adenosylcobalamin; CN-Cbl, cyanocobalamin; OH-Cbl, hydroxocobalamin.

first and foremost on complementation studies which define the two classes as unique [171]. Their biochemical differences appear to be quantitative rather than qualitative, with the *cbl* C group having more severe metabolic derangements (and, pari passu, more severe clinical involvement) than the sibs designated *cbl* D [171] (Table 23-5).

PATHOPHYSIOLOGY The megaloblastic anemia so commonly observed in the *cbl* C patients almost surely reflects the enzymatic disturbance of the homocysteine:N^5-methyltetrahydrofolate methyltransferase. This can be stated with some assurance since patients with isolated methylmalonyl CoA mutase deficiency (*mut°, mut⁻, cbl A, cbl B*) more severe than that encountered in the *cbl* C patients exhibit no such hematologic dysfunction. The early and severe CNS abnormalities encountered in the *cbl* C group probably reflect the methyltransferase abnormality as well, in that such patients do not have the severe metabolic ketoacidosis that probably accounts for the CNS problems in patients with mutase deficiency only. Thus, patients with severe, inherited dysfunction in the synthesis of both cobalamin coenzymes resemble closely patients with exogenous cobalamin deficiency—both groups having prominent hematologic and neurologic manifestations resulting from the blocked methyltransferase system.

GENETIC CONSIDERATIONS Because equal numbers of affected males and affected females exist in the *cbl* C group (Table 23-4), because females have been as seriously affected as males, and because cells from affected patients behave as recessives in complementation studies [170], it seems safe to predict that this disorder is inherited as an autosomal recessive trait. The mode of inheritance of the *cbl* D mutation cannot yet be defined, because of the paucity of known patients and because both affected patients in the only family yet described are males. Identification of heterozygotes for either the *cbl* C or the *cbl* D group has not yet been accomplished. One additional contribution of the somatic cell genetic studies used to characterize these disorders deserves mention. The locus coding for the human methyltransferase structural gene has been mapped

to chromosome 1 using human hamster hybrids [190]. This assignment is the first for any known enzyme or protein concerned with cobalamin metabolism.

DIAGNOSIS, TREATMENT, AND PROGNOSIS The combination of methylmalonic aciduria, homocystinuria, and normal serum cobalamin concentrations is the triad needed to distinguish patients in the *cbl* C or *cbl* D groups from those with isolated mutase deficiency, with such other causes of homocystinuria as cystathionine synthase deficiency or $N^{5,10}$-methylenetetrahydrofolate reductase deficiency, or with cobalamin deficiency. Such distinctions, easily confirmed by cell studies, are critical because appropriate therapy depends on making them. Whereas exogenous cobalamin deficiency will respond dramatically to physiologic amounts of cobalamin and certain forms of homocystinuria will respond to supplements of pyridoxine or folate (see Chaps. 24 and 25), successful management of *cbl* C and *cbl* D patients probably demands administration of very large amounts (up to 1 mg daily) of OH-Cbl [155, 183, 185]. Such treatment has resulted in dramatic decreases in urinary methylmalonate (and less dramatic decreases in urinary homocystine) in those patients who have received it. In fact, early diagnosis and prompt institution of therapy with cobalamin supplements may be the only way to change the outcome of these patients which, in the case of the *cbl* C group, has been dismal thus far. As shown in Table 23-4, four of the six reported *cbl* C patients have died at ages 7 weeks [181], 3 months (personal communication), 4 months [184], and 7 years [182], respectively; the other two are alive but distinctly retarded at ages 3 years [185] and 11 years [183]. Severe hemolytic anemia has been a major complication in the deceased *cbl* C patients, as has congestive heart failure. Thromboemboli, so often encountered in patients with homocystinuria due to cystathionine synthase deficiency have, thus far, been documented only in the older of the two *cbl* D brothers, and this complication was not noted until he reached 18 years of age. Until patients in the *cbl* C group are diagnosed before birth or soon thereafter, and treated immediately with cobalamin supplements, we will not know whether the poor outcome in this group can be modified significantly. Documentation of such experience will be particularly important in assessing the clinician's ability to modify the natural history of this disorder.

REFERENCES

1. MARSTON HR, ALLEN SH, SMITH RM: Primary metabolic defect supervening on vitamin B_{12} deficiency in the sheep. *Nature (Lond)* 190:1085, 1961

2. SMITH RM, MONTY KJ: Vitamin B_{12} and propionate metabolism. *Biochem Biophys Res Commun* 1:105, 1959

3. GURNANI S, MISTRY SP, JOHNSON BC: Function of vitamin B_{12} in methylmalonate metabolism. I. Effect of a cofactor form of B_{12} on the activity of methylmalonyl-CoA isomerase. *Biochim Biophys Acta* 38:187, 1960

4. STERN JR, FRIEDMANN DC: Vitamin B_{12} and methylmalonyl-CoA isomerase I. Vitamin B_{12} and propionate metabolism. *Biochem Biophys Res Commun* 2:82, 1960

5. COX EV, WHITE AM: Methylmalonic acid excretion: Index of vitamin-B_{12} deficiency. *Lancet* 2:853, 1962

6. BARNESS LA, YOUNG D, MELLMAN WJ, KAHN SB, WILLIAMS WJ: Methylmalonate excretion in patient with pernicious anemia. *N Engl J Med* 268:144, 1963

7. CHILDS B, NYHAN WL, BORDEN M, BARD L, COOKE RE: Idiopathic hyperglycinemia and hyperglycinuria: New disorder of amino acid metabolism. I. *Pediatrics* 27:522, 1961

8. ROSENBERG LE, LILLJEQVIST A-C, HSIA YE: Methylmalonic aciduria: An inborn error leading to metabolic acidosis, long-chain ketonuria and intermittent hyperglycinemia. *N Engl J Med* 278:1319, 1968

9. HSIA YE, SCULLY KJ, ROSENBERG LE: Defective propionate carboxylation in ketotic hyperglycinaemia. *Lancet* 1:757, 1969

10. OBERHOLZER VC, LEVIN B, BURGESS EA, YOUNG WF: Methylmalonic aciduria: An inborn error of metabolism leading to chronic metabolic acidosis. *Arch Dis Child* 42:492, 1967

11. STOKKE O, ELDJARN L, NORUM KR, STEEN-JOHNSEN J, HALVORSEN S: Methylmalonic aciduria: A new inborn error of metabolism which may cause fatal acidosis in the neonatal period. *Scand J Clin Lab Invest* 20:313, 1967

12. LINDBLAD B, OLIN P, SVANBERG B, ZETTERSTRÖM R: Methylmalonic acidemia. *Acta Paediatr Scand* 57:417, 1968

13. LINDBLAD B, LINDSTRAND K, SVANBERG B, ZETTERSTRÖM R: The effect of cobamide coenzyme in methylmalonic acidemia. *Acta Paediatr Scand* 58:178, 1969

14. ROSENBERG LE, LILLJEQVIST A-C, HSIA YE, ROSENBLOOM FM: Vitamin B_{12} dependent methylmalonicaciduria: Defective B_{12} metabolism in cultured fibroblasts. *Biochem Biophys Res Commun* 37:607, 1969

15. MAHONEY MJ, ROSENBERG LE, MUDD SH, UHLENDORF BW: Defective metabolism of vitamin B_{12} in fibroblasts from patients with methylmalonicaciduria. *Biochem Biophys Res Commun* 44:375, 1971

16. WILLARD HF, ROSENBERG LE: Inherited deficiencies of methylmalonyl CoA mutase activity: Biochemical and genetic studies in cultured skin fibroblasts, in Hommes FA (ed): *Models for the Study of Inborn Errors of Metabolism.* Amsterdam, Elsevier North-Holland Biomedical Press, 1979, p 297

17. FENTON WA, ROSENBERG LE: Genetic and biochemical analysis of human cobalamin mutants in cell culture. *Ann Rev Genet* 12:223, 1978

18. ROSENBERG LE: The inherited methylmalonic acidemias: A model system for the study of vitamin metabolism and apoenzyme-coenzyme interactions (Milner Lecture), in Belton, NR, Toothill C (eds): *Transport and Inherited Disease.* Lancaster, England, MTP Press Ltd, in press

19. MEISTER A: *Biochemistry of the Amino Acids.* New York, Academic Press, Inc, 1965, pp 674, 729, 735

20. TANAKA K, ARMITAGE IM, RAMSDELL HS, HSIA YE, LIPSKY SR, ROSENBERG, LE: [^{13}C]Valine metabolism in methylmalonic acidemia using nuclear magnetic resonance: Propionate as an obligate intermediate. *Proc Natl Acad Sci USA* 72:3692, 1975

21. BARETZ BH, TANAKA, K: Metabolism in rats *in vivo* of isobutyrates labeled with stable isotopes at various positions: Identification of propionate as an obigate intermediate. *J Biol Chem* 253:4203, 1978

22. KAZIRO Y, OCHOA S: The metabolism of propionic acid. *Adv Enzymol* 26:283, 1964

23. DANIELSSON H: Present status of research on catabolism and excretion of cholesterol. *Adv Lipid Res* 1:335, 1963

24. LARDY HA, ADLER J: Synthesis of succinate from propionate and bicarbonate by soluble enzymes from liver mitochondria. *J Biol Chem* 219:935, 1956

25. FLAVIN M, ORTIZ PJ, OCHOA S: Metabolism of propionic acid in animal tissues. *Nature (Lond)* 176:823, 1955

26. KATZ J, CHAIKOFF IL: The metabolism of propionate by rat liver slices and the formaton of isosuccinic acid. *J Am Chem Soc* 77:2659, 1955

27. FLAVIN M, OCHOA S: Metabolism of propionic acid in animal tissues. I. Enzymatic conversion of propionate to succinate. *J Biol Chem* 229:965, 1957

28. TIETZ A, OCHOA S: Metabolism of propionic acid in animal tissues. V. Purification and properties of propionyl carboxylase. *J Biol Chem* 234:1394, 1959

29. SPRECHER M, CLARK MJ, SPRINSON DB: The absolute configuration of methylmalonyl-CoA and stereochemistry of the methylmalonyl-CoA mutase reaction. *Biochem Biophys Res Commun* 15:581, 1964

30. RETEY J, LYNEN F: The absolute configuration of methylmalonyl-CoA. *Biochem Biophys Res Commun* 16:358, 1964

31. MAZUMDER R, SASAKAWA T, KAZIRO Y, OCHOA S: Metabolism of propionic acid in animal tissues. IX. Methylmalonyl coenzyme A racemase. *J Biol Chem* 237:3065, 1962

32. BECK WS, FLAVIN M, OCHOA S: Metabolism of propionic acid in animal tissues. III. Formation of succinate. *J Biol Chem* 229:997, 1957

33. KAZIRO Y, OCHOA S, WARNER RC, CHEN J: Metabolism of propionic acid in animal tissues. VIII. Crystalline propionyl carboxylase. *J Biol Chem* 236:1917, 1961

34. LAU EP, COCHRAN BC, MUNSON L, FALL RR: Bovine kidney 3-methylcrotonyl-CoA and propionyl-CoA carboxylases: Each enzyme contains nonidentical subunits. *Proc Natl Acad Sci USA* 76:214, 1979

35. KALOUSEK F, DARIGO MD, ROSENBERG LE: Isolation and characterization of propionyl-CoA carboxylase from normal human liver: Evidence for a protomeric tetramer of nonidentical subunits. *J Biol Chem* 255:60, 1980

36. MISTRY SP, DAKSHINAMURTI K: Biochemistry of biotin. *Vitam Horm* 22:1, 1964

37. OVERATH P, KELLERMAN GM, LYNEN F, FRITZ HP, KELLER HJ: Zum Mechanismus der Umlagerung von Methylmalonyl-CoA in Succinyl-CoA. II. Versuche zur Wirkungweise von Methylmalonyl-CoA-Isomerase und Methylmalonyl-CoA-Racemase. *Biochem Z* 335:500, 1962

38. BARKER HA, SMYTH RD, WAWSZKIEWICZ EJ, LEE MN, WILSON RM: Enzymatic preparation and characterization of an α-L-β-methylaspartic acid. *Arch Biochem Biophys* 78:468, 1958

39. BARKER HA, WEISSBACH H, SMYTH RD: A coenzyme containing pseudo-vitamin B_{12}. *Proc Natl Acad Sci USA* 44:1093, 1958

40. WEISSBACH H, TOOHEY J, BARKER HA: Isolation and properties of B_{12} coenzymes containing benzimidazole or dimethylbenzimidazole. *Proc Natl Acad Sci USA* 45:521, 1959

41. CANNATA JJB, FOCESI A Jr, MAZUMDER R, WARNER RC, OCHOA S: Metabolism of propionic acid in animal tissues. XII. Properties of mammalian methylmalonyl coenzyme A mutase. *J Biol Chem* 240:3249, 1965

42. OVERATH P, STADTMAN ER, KELLERMAN GM, LYNEN F: Zum Mechanismus der Umlagerung von Methylmalonyl-CoA in Succinyl-CoA. III. Reinigung und Eigenschaften der Methylmalonyl-CoA-Isomerase. *Biochem Z* 336:77, 1962

43. KELLERMEYER RW, ALLEN SHG, STJERNHOLM R, WOOD HG: Methylmalonyl isomerase. IV. Purification and properties of the enzyme from propionibacteria. *J Biol Chem* 239:2562, 1964

44. KOLHOUSE JF, UTLEY C, ALLEN RH: Isolation and characterization of methylmalonyl-CoA mutase from human placenta. *J Biol Chem* 255:2708, 1980

45. FENTON WA, HACK AM, WILLARD HF, GERTLER A, ROSENBERG LE: Purification and properties of methylmalonyl CoA mutase from human liver. Submitted to *Arch Biochem Biophys*

46. WILLARD HF, ROSENBERG LE: Interactions of methylmalonyl CoA mutase from normal human fibroblasts with adenosylcobalamin and methylmalonyl CoA: Evidence for nonequivalent active sites. *Arch Biochem Biophys* 200:130, 1980

47. WILLARD HF, ROSENBERG LE: Effect of cobalamin supplementation in culture on methylmalonyl CoA mutase activity in normal and mutant human fibroblasts: Inhibition of apoenzyme and holoenzyme by hydroxocobalamin. Submitted to *J Clin Invest*

48. EGGERER H, STADTMAN ER, OVERATH P, LYNEN F: Zum Mechanismus der durch Cobalamin-Coenzym katalysierten Umlagerung von Methylmalonyl-CoA in Succinyl-CoA. *Biochem Z* 333:1, 1960

49. KELLERMEYER RW, WOOD HG: Methylmalonyl isomerase: A study of the mechanism of isomerization. *Biochemistry* 1:1124, 1962

50. PHARES EF, LONG MV, CARSON SF: An intramolecular rearrangement in the methylmalonyl isomerase reacton as demonstrated by positive and negative mass analysis of succinic acid. *Biochem Biophys Res Commun* 8:142, 1962

51. BABIOR BM: Cobamides as cofactors: Adenosylcobamide dependent reactions, in Babior BM (ed): *Cobalamin Biochemistry and Pathophysiology.* New York, John Wiley & Sons, Inc, 1975, p 141

52. LYNEN F: Biosynthesis of saturated fatty acids. *Fed Proc* 20:941, 1961

53. ANDO T, RASMUSSEN K, WRIGHT JM, NYHAN WL: Isolation and identifi-

cation of methylcitrate, a major metabolic product of propionate in patients with propionic acidemia. *J Biol Chem* 247:2200, 1972

54. RASMUSSEN K, ANDO T, NYHAN WL, HULL D, COTTOM D, WADLINGTON W, KILROY AW: Excretion of propionylglycine in propionic acidemia. *Clin Sci* 42:665, 1972

55. ANDO T, RASMUSSEN K, NYHAN WL, HULL D: 3-Hydroxypropionate: Significance of β-oxidation of propionate in patients with propionic acidemia and methylmalonic acidemia. *Proc Natl Acad Sci USA* 69:2807, 1972

56. SEBRELL WH, HARRIS RS: Biotin, in *The Vitamins: Chemistry, Physiology, Pathology Methods*. New York, Academic Press, Inc, 1978, p 261

57. MOSS J, LANE MD: The biotin-dependent enzymes. *Adv Enzymol* 35:321, 1971

58. MURTHY PNA, MISTRY SP: *In vitro* synthesis of propionyl-CoA holocarboxylase by a partially purified mitochondrial preparation from biotin-deficient chicken liver. *Can J Biochem* 52:800, 1974

59. SPENCER RP, BRODY KR: Biotin transport by small intestine of rat, hamster, and other species. *Am J Physiol* 206:633, 1964

60. BERGER E, LONG E, SEMENZA G: The sodium activation of biotin absorption in hamster small intestine in vitro. *Biochim Biophys Acta* 255:873, 1972

61. MOCK DM, DELORIMER AA, LIEBMAN WM, SWEETMAN L, BAKER H: Biotin deficiency: An unusual complication of parenteral alimentation. *N Engl J Med* 304:820, 1981

62. SYDENSTRICKER VP, SINGAL SA, BRIGGS AP, DEVAUGHN NM: Preliminary observations on "egg white injury" in man and its cure with a biotin concentrate. *Science* 95:176, 1942

63. MINOT GR, MURPHY LP: Treatment of pernicious anemia by a special diet. *JAMA* 87:470, 1926

64. SMITH EL: Purification of anti-pernicious anemia factors from liver. *Nature (Lond)* 161:638, 1948

65. RICKES EL, BRINK NG, KONIUSZY FR, WOOD TR, FOLKERS K: Crystalline vitamin B$_{12}$. *Science* 107:396, 1948

66. HODGKIN DC, KAMPER J, MACKAY M, PICKWORTH J, TRUEBLOOD KN, WHITE JG: Structure of vitamin B$_{12}$. *Nature (Lond)* 178:64, 1956

67. WALKER GA, MURPHY S, HEUNNEKENS FH: Enzymatic conversion of vitamin B$_{12}$ to adenosyl-B$_{12}$: Evidence for the existence of two separate reducing systems. *Arch Biochem Biophys* 134:95, 1969

68. WEISSBACH H, TAYLOR R: Role of vitamin B$_{12}$ in methionine biosynthesis. *Fed Proc* 25:1649, 1966

69. TAYLOR RT, WEISSBACH H: Enzymatic synthesis of methionine: Formation of a radioactive cobamide enzyme with N^5methyl-^{14}C-tetrahydrofolate. *Arch Biochem Biophys* 119:572, 1967

70. TAYLOR RT, WEISSBACH H: *Escherichia coli* B N^5-methyltetrahydrofolate-homocysteine vitamin-B$_{12}$ transmethylase: Formation and photolability of a methylcobalamin enzyme. *Arch Biochem Biophys* 123:109, 1968

71. POSTON JM: Leucine 2,3-aminomutase, an enzyme of leucine catabolism. *J Biol Chem* 251:1859, 1976

72. POSTON JM, STADTMAN TC: Cobamides as cofactors: Methylcobamides and the synthesis of methionine, methane and acetate, in Babior BM (ed): *Cobalamin Biochemistry and Pathophysiology*. New York, John Wiley & Sons, Inc, 1975, p 111

73. DONALDSON RM JR: Intrinsic factor and the transport of cobalamin, in Johnson LR (ed): *Physiology of the Gastrointestinal Tract*. New York, Raven Press, 1981, in press

74. SENNETT C, MELLMAN IS, ROSENBERG LE: Transmembrane transport of cobalamin in prokaryotic and eukaryotic cells. *Ann Rev Biochem* 1981, in press

75. ALLEN RH, SEETHARAM B, PODELL E, ALPERS DH: Effect of proteolytic enzymes on the binding of cobalamin to R protein and intrinsic factor. In vitro evidence that a failure to partially degrade R protein is responsible for cobalamin malabsorption in pancreatic insufficiency. *J Clin Invest* 61:47, 1978

76. ALLEN RH, SEETHARAM B, ALLEN NC, PODELL ER, ALPERS DH: Correction of cobalamin malabsorption in pancreatic insufficiency with a cobalamin analogue that binds with high affinity to R protein but not to intrinsic factor. In vivo evidence that a failure to partially degrade R protein is responsible for cobalamin malabsorption in pancreatic insufficiency. *J Clin Invest* 61:1628, 1978

77. MARCOULLIS G, PARMENTIER Y, NICOLAS J-P, JIMENEZ M, GERARD P: Cobalamin malabsorption due to nondegradation of R proteins in the human intestine: Inhibited cobalamin absorption in exocrine pancreatic dysfunction. *J Clin Invest* 66:430, 1980

78. ALLEN RH: Human vitamin B$_{12}$-transport proteins. *Prog Hematol* 9:57, 1975

79. ELLENBOGEN LE: Uptake and transport of cobalamins. *Int Rev Biochem* 27:45, 1979

80. HALL CA, FINKLER AE: The dynamics of transcobalamin. II. A vitamin B$_{12}$ binding substance in plasma. *J Lab Clin Med* 65:459, 1965

81. HOM BL: Plasma turnover of ^{57}cobalt-vitamin B$_{12}$ bound to transcobalamin I and II. *Scand J Haematol* 4:321, 1967

82. LINNELL JC: The fate of cobalamins *in vivo*, in Babior BM (ed): *Cobalamin: Biochemistry and Pathophysiology*. New York, John Wiley & Sons, Inc, 1975, p 287

83. FINKLER AE, HALL CA: Nature of the relationship between vitamin B$_{12}$ binding and cell uptake. *Arch Biochem Biophys* 120:79, 1967

84. TAN CH, HANSEN HJ: Studies on the site of synthesis of transcobalamin II. *Proc Soc Exp Biol Med* 127:740, 1968

85. PLETSCH QA, COFFEY JW: Properties of the proteins that bind vitamin B$_{12}$ in subcellular fractions of rat liver. *Arch Biochem Biophys* 151:157, 1972

86. NEWMARK P, NEWMAN GE, O'BRIEN JRP: Vitamin B$_{12}$ in the rat kidney: Evidence for an association with lysosomes. *Arch Biochem Biophys* 141:121, 1970

87. YOUNGDAHL-TURNER P, ROSENBERG LE, ALLEN RH: Binding and uptake of transcobalamin II by human fibroblasts. *J Clin Invest* 61:133, 1978

88. YOUNGDAHL-TURNER P, MELLMAN IS, ALLEN RH, ROSENBERG LE: Protein mediated vitamin uptake: Adsorptive endocytosis of the transcobalamin II-cobalamin complex by cultured human fibroblasts. *Exp Cell Res* 118:127, 1979

89. MELLMAN IS, YOUNGDAHL-TURNER P, WILLARD HF, ROSENBERG LE: Intracellular binding of radioactive hydroxocobalamin to cobalamin-dependent apoenzymes in rat liver. *Proc Natl Acad Sci USA* 74:916, 1977

90. KOLHOUSE JF, ALLEN RH: Recognition of two intracellular cobalamin binding proteins and their identification as methylmalonyl-CoA mutase and methionine synthetase. *Proc Natl Acad Sci USA* 74:921, 1977

91. BURGER RL, SCHNEIDER RJ, MEHLMAN CS, ALLEN RH: Human plasma R-type vitamin B$_{12}$ binding protein. II. The role of transcobalamin I, transcobalamin III and the normal granulocyte vitamin B$_{12}$-binding protein in the plasma transport of vitamin B$_{12}$. *J Biol Chem* 250:7707, 1975

92. BERLINER N, ROSENBERG LE: Uptake and metabolism of free cyanocobalamin by cultured human fibroblasts from controls and a patient with transcobalamin II deficiency. *Metabolism* 30:230, 1981

93. FRENKEL EP, KITCHENS RL: Intracellular localization of hepatic propionyl-CoA carboxylase and methylmalonyl-CoA mutase in humans and normal and vitamin B$_{12}$ deficient rats. *Br J Haematol* 31:501, 1975

94. WANG FK, KOCH J, STOKSTAD EL: Folate coenzyme pattern, folate linked enzymes and methionine biosynthesis in rat liver mitochondria. *Biochem Z* 246:458, 1967

95. VITOLS E, WALKER GA, HUENNEKENS FM: Enzymatic conversion of vitamin B$_{12}$ to a cobamide coenzyme, α(5,6-dimethylbenzimidazolyl) deoxyadenosylcobamide (adenosyl-B$_{12}$). *J Biol Chem* 241:1455, 1966

96. ERTEL R, BROT N, TAYLOR R, WEISSBACH H: Studies on the nature of the bound cobamide in *E. coli* N^5-methyltetrahydrofolate-homocysteine transmethylase. *Arch Biochem Biophys* 126:353, 1968

97. TAYLOR RT, WEISSBACH H: *E. coli* B N^5-methyltetrahydrofolate-homocysteine methyltransferase: Sequential formation of bound methylcobalamin with S-adenosyl-L-methionine and N^5-methyltetrahydrofolate. *Arch Biochem Biophys* 129:728, 1969

98. PAWALKIEWICZ J, GORNA M, FENRYCH W, MAGAS S: Conversion of cyanocobalamin in vivo and in vitro into its coenzyme form in humans and animals. *Ann NY Acad Sci* 112:641, 1964

99. KERWAR SS, SPEARS C, MCAUSLAN B, WEISSBACH H: Studies on vitamin B$_{12}$ metabolism in HeLa cells. *Arch Biochem Biophys* 142:231, 1971

100. MAHONEY MJ, ROSENBERG LE: Synthesis of cobalamin coenzymes by human cells in tissue culture. *J Lab Clin Med* 78:302, 1971

101. MAHONEY MJ, HART AC, STEEN VD, ROSENBERG LE: Methylmalonicacidemia: Biochemical heterogeneity in defects of 5'-deoxyadenosylcobalamin synthesis. *Proc Natl Acad Sci USA* 72:2799, 1975

102. FENTON WA, ROSENBERG LE: The defect in the *cbl B* class of human methylmalonic acidemia: Deficiency of cob(I)alamin adenosyltransferase activity in extracts of cultured fibroblasts. *Biochem Biophys Res Commun* 98:283, 1981

103. COX EV, ROBERTSON-SMITH D, SMALL M, WHITE AM: The excretion of propionate and acetate in vitamin B$_{12}$ deficiency. *Clin Sci* 35:123, 1968

104. SHIPMAN RT, TOWNLEY RRW, DANKS DM: Homocystinuria, Addisonian pernicious anaemia, and partial deletion of a G chromosome. *Lancet* 2:693, 1969

105. HOLLOWELL JG JR, HALL WK, CORYELL ME, MCPHERSON J JR, HAHN DA: Homocystinuria and organic aciduria in a patient with vitamin-B$_{12}$ deficiency. *Lancet* 2:1428, 1969

106. HIGGINBOTTOM MC, SWEETMAN L, NYHAN WL: A syndrome of methylmalonic aciduria, homocystinuria, megaloblastic anemia and neurologic abnormalities in a vitamin B$_{12}$-deficient breast-fed infant of a strict vegetarian. *N. Engl J Med* 299:317, 1978

107. CARDINALE GJ, DREYFUS PM, AULD P, ABELES RH: Experimental vitamin B$_{12}$ deficiency: Its effect on tissue vitamin B$_{12}$-coenzyme levels and on the metabolism of methylmalonyl-CoA. *Arch Biochem Biophys* 131:92, 1969

108. BECK WS: Metabolic features of cobalamin deficiency in man, in Babior BM (ed): *Cobalamin: Biochemistry and Pathophysiology*. New York, John Wiley & Sons, Inc, 1975, p 403

109. HERBERT V, ZALUSKY R: Interrelations of vitamin B₁₂ and folic acid metabolism: Folic acid clearance studies. *J Clin Invest* 41:1263, 1962

110. NORONHA JM, SILVERMAN M: On folic acid, vitamin B₁₂, methionine and formiminoglutamic acid metabolism, in Heinrich HC (ed): *Vitamin B₁₂ and Intrinsic Factor*. Stuttgart, Verlag, 1962

111. LARRABEE AR, ROSENTHAL S, CATHOW RE, BUCHANAN JM: Enzymatic synthesis of the methyl group of methionine. IV. Isolation, characterization, and role of 5-methyl tetrahydrofolate. *J Biol Chem* 238:1025, 1963

112. MORROW G, BARNESS LA, AUERBACH VH, DI GEORGE AM, ANDO T, NYHAN WL: Observations on the coexistence of methylmalonic acidemia and glycinemia. *J Pediatr* 74:680, 1969

113. HOMMES FA, KUIPERS JRG, ELEMA JD, JANSE JF, JONXIS JJP: Propionic-acidemia, a new inborn error of metabolism. *Pediatr Res* 2:519, 1968

114. HSIA YE, SCULLY KJ, ROSENBERG LE: Inherited propionyl-CoA carboxylase deficiency in "ketotic hyperglycinemia." *J Clin Invest* 50:127, 1971

115. GOMPERTZ D, STORRS CN, BAU DCK, PETERS TJ, HUGHES EA: Localization of enzyme defect in propionicacidemia. *Lancet* 1:1140, 1970

116. NYHAN WL, BORDEN M, CHILDS B: Idiopathic hyperglycinemia: A new disorder of amino acid metabolism. II. The concentrations of other amino acids in the plasma and their modification by the administration of leucine. *Pediatrics* 27:539, 1961

117. CHILDS B, NYHAN WL: Further observations of a patient with hyperglycinemia. *Pediatrics* 33:403, 1964

118. BRANDT IK, HSIA YE, CLEMENT DH, PROVENCE SA: Propionicacidemia (ketotic hyperglycinemia): Dietary treatment results in normal growth and development. *Pediatrics* 53:391, 1974

119. NYHAN WL, ANDO T, RASMUSSEN K: Ketotic hyperglycinemia, in Stern J, Toothill C (eds): *Organic Acidurias*. London, Churchill Livingstone, Ltd, 1972, p 1

120. MAHONEY MJ, HSIA YE, ROSENBERG LE: Propionyl-CoA carboxylase deficiency (propionicacidemia): A cause of non-ketotic hyperglycinemia, abstracted. *Pediatr Res* 5:395, 1971

121. WOLF B, PAULSEN EP, HSIA YE: Asymptomatic propionyl CoA carboxylase deficiency in a 13-year-old girl. *J Pediatr* 95:563, 1979

122. NYHAN WL, CHILDS B: Hyperglycinemia. V. The miscible pool and turnover rate of glycine and the formation of serine. *J Clin Invest* 43:2404, 1964

123. MENKES JH: Idiopathic hyperglycinemia: Isolation and identification of three previously undescribed urinary ketones. *J Pediatr* 69:413, 1966

124. NYHAN WL, ANDO T, RASMUSSEN K, WADLINGTON W, KILROY AW, COTTOM D, HULL D: Tiglic aciduria in propionicacidemia. *Biochem J* 126:1035, 1972

125. HSIA YE: Inherited hyperammonemic syndromes. *Gastroenterology* 67:347, 1974

126. WOLF B, HSIA YE, TANAKA K, ROSENBERG LE: Correlation between serum propionate and blood ammonia concentrations in propionic acidemia. *J Pediatr* 93:471, 1978

127. HSIA YE, SCULLY KJ, ROSENBERG LE: Human propionyl CoA carboxylase: Some properties of the partially purified enzyme in fibroblasts from controls and patients with propionic acidemia. *Pediatr Res* 13:746, 1979

128. WOLF B, HSIA YE, ROSENBERG LE: Biochemical differences between mutant propionyl-CoA carboxylases from two complementation groups. *Am J Hum Genet* 30:455, 1978

129. WOLF B, ROSENBERG LE: Heterozygote expression in propionyl coenzyme A carboxylase deficiency: Differences between major complementation groups. *J Clin Invest* 62:931, 1978

130. GRAVEL RA, LAM K-F, SCULLY KJ, HSIA YE: Genetic complementation of propionyl-CoA carboxylase deficiency in cultured human fibroblasts. *Am J Hum Genet* 29:378, 1977

131. WOLF B, WILLARD HF, ROSENBERG LE: Kinetic analysis of genetic complementation in heterokaryons of propionyl CoA carboxylase-deficient human fibroblasts. *Am J Hum Genet* 32:16, 1980

132. HILLMAN RE, SOWERS LH, COHEN JL: Inhibition of glycine oxidation in cultured fibroblasts by isoleucine. *Pediatr Res* 7:945, 1973

133. HILLMAN RE, OTTO EF: Inhibition of glycine-serine interconversion in cultured human fibroblasts by products of isoleucine catabolism. *Pediatr Res* 8:941, 1974

134. SNYDERMAN SE, HOLT CE, NORTON PM, ROITMAN E, PHANSALKAR SV: The plasma aminogram. I. Influence of the level of protein intake and a comparison of whole protein and amino acid diets. *Pediatr Res* 2:131, 1968

135. GLASGOW AM, CHASE HP: Effect of propionic acid on fatty acid oxidation and ureagenesis. *Pediatr Res* 10:683, 1976

136. STEWART PM, WALSER M: Failure of the normal ureagenic response to amino acids in organic acid loaded rats: A proposed mechanism for the hyperammonemia of propionic and methylmalonic acidemia. *J Clin Invest* 66:484, 1989

136a. COUDE FX, SWEETMAN L, NYHAN WL: Inhibition by propionyl CoA of N-acetylglutamate synthetase in rat liver mitochondria. *J Clin Invest* 64:1544, 1979

137. GRUSKAY JA, ROSENBERG LE: Inhibition of mitochondrial carbamyl phosphate synthetase in rat and human liver by acyl CoA esters: A possible mechanism for hyperammonemia in the inherited organic acidemias. Submitted to *J Biol Chem*

138. KIRKMAN HN, KIESEL JL: Congenital hyperammonemia, abstracted. *Pediatr Res* 3:358, 1969

139. HARRIS DJ, YANG BJ-Y, SNODGRASS PJ: Carbamyl phosphate synthetase deficiency: A possible transient phenocopy of dysautonomia. *Am J Hum Genet* 29:52A, 1977

140. GOMPERTZ D, GOODEY PA, THOM H, RUSSELL G, JOHNSTON AW, MELLOR DH, MACLEAN MW, FERGUSON-SMITH ME, FERGUSON-SMITH MA: Prenatal diagnosis and family studies in case of propionicacidemia. *Clin Genet* 8:244, 1975

141. BARNES ND, HULL D, BALGOBIN L, GOMPERTZ D: Biotin-responsive propionicacidemia. *Lancet* 2:244, 1970

142. WOLF B: Reassessment of biotin-responsiveness in "unresponsive" propionyl CoA carboxylase deficiency. *J Pediatr* 97:964, 1980

143. GOMPERTZ D, DRAFFAN GH, WATTS JL, HULL D: Biotin-responsive β-methylcrotonyl-glycinuria. *Lancet* 2:22, 1971

144. SWEETMAN L, BATES SP, HULL D, NYHAN WL: Propionyl-CoA carboxylase deficiency in a patient with biotin-responsive 3-methylcrotonyl-glycinuria. *Pediatr Res* 11:1144, 1977

145. SAUNDERS M, SWEETMAN L, ROBINSON B, ROTH K, COHN, R, GRAVEL RA: Biotin-response organicaciduria. Multiple carboxylase defects and complementation studies with propionicacidemia in cultured fibroblasts. *J Clin Invest* 64:1695, 1979

146. BARTLETT K, GOMPERTZ D: Combined carboxylase defect: Biotin-responsiveness in cultured fibroblasts. *Lancet* 2:804, 1976

147. WEYLER W, SWEETMAN L, MAGGIO DC, NYHAN WL: Deficiency of propionyl-CoA carboxylase and methylcrotonyl-CoA carboxylase in a patient with methylcrotonylglycinuria. *Clin Chim Acta* 76:321, 1977

148. COWAN MJ, WARA DW, PACKMAN S, AMMANN AJ, YOSHINO M, SWEETMAN L, NYHAN W: Multiple biotin-dependent carboxylase deficiencies associated with defects in T-cell and B-cell immunity. *Lancet* 2:115, 1979

149. LEHNERT W, NIEDERHOFF H, JUNKER A, SAULE H, FRASCH W: A case of biotin-responsive 3-methylcrotonylglycin- and 3-hydroxyisovaleric aciduria. *Eur J Pediatr* 132:107, 1979

150. ROTH KS, YANG W, FOREMAN JW, ROTHMAN R, SEGAL S: Holocarboxylase synthetase deficiency: A biotin-responsive organic acidemia. *J Pediatr* 96:845, 1980

151. CHARLES BM, HOSKING G, GREEN A, POLLITT R, BARTLETT K, TAITZ LE: Biotin-responsive alopecia and developmental regression. *Lancet* 2:118, 1979

152. THEONE J, BAKER H, YOSHINO M, SWEETMAN L: Biotin-responsive carboxylase deficiency associated with subnormal plasma and urinary biotin. *N Engl J Med* 304:817, 1981

153. ROSENBERG LE, LILLJEQVIST A, HSIA YE: Methylmalonicaciduria: Metabolic block localization and vitamin B₁₂ dependency. *Science* 162:805, 1968

154. MUDD SH, LEVY HL, ABELES RH: A derangement in B₁₂ metabolism leading to homocystinemia, cystathioninemia and methylmalonicaciduria. *Biochem Biophys Res Commun* 35:121, 1969

155. GOODMAN SI, MOE PG, HAMMOND KB, MUDD SH, UHLENDORF BW: Homocystinuria with methylmalonic aciduria: Two cases in a sibship. *Biochem Med* 4:500, 1970

156. MATSUI SM, MAHONEY MJ, ROSENBERG LE: The natural history of the inherited methylmalonic acidemias. Submitted to *N Engl J Med*

157. ROSENBERG LE: Disorders of propionate, methylmalonate and cobalamin metabolism, in Stanbury JB, Wyngaarden JB, Fredrickson DS (eds): *The Metabolic Basis of Inherited Disease*, 4th ed. New York, McGraw-Hill Book Co, 1978, p 411

158. ANDO T, RASMUSSEN K, NYHAN WL, DONNELL GN, BARNES, ND: Propionicacidemia in patients with ketotic hyperglycinemia. *J Pediatr* 78:827, 1971

159. STOKKE O, JELLUM E, ELDJARN L, SCHNITLER R: The occurrence of β-hydroxy-n-valeric acid in a patient with propionic and methylmalonic acidemia. *Clin Chim Acta* 45:391, 1973

160. HSIA YE, SCULLY K, LILLJEQVIST A-CH, ROSENBERG LE: Vitamin B₁₂ dependent methylmalonicaciduria. *Pediatrics* 46:497, 1970

161. WILLARD HF, AMBANI LM, HART AC, MAHONEY MJ, ROSENBERG LE: Rapid prenatal and postnatal detection of inborn errors of propionate, methylmalonate, and cobalamin metabolism: A sensitive assay using cultured cells. *Hum Genet* 34:277, 1976

162. MORROW G, REVSIN B, MATHEWS C, GILES H: A simple rapid method for prenatal detection of defects in propionate metabolism. *Clin Genet* 10:218, 1976

163. MORROW G, BARNESS LA, CARDINALE GJ, ABELES RH, FLAKS JG: Congenital methylmalonic acidemia: Enzymatic evidence for two forms of the disease. *Proc Natl Acad Sci USA* 63:191, 1969

164. MORROW G, MAHONEY MJ, MATHEWS C, LEBOWITZ J: Studies of methylmalonyl coenzyme A carbonylmutase activity in methylmalonic acide-

mia. I. Correlation of clinical, hepatic and fibroblast data. *Pediatr Res* 9:641, 1975

165. WILLARD HF, ROSENBERG LE: Inherited deficiencies of human methylmalonyl CoA mutase activity: Reduced affinity of mutant apoenzyme for adenosylcobalamin. *Biochem Biophys Res Commun* 78:927, 1977

166. WILLARD HF, ROSENBERG LE: Inherited methylmalonyl CoA mutase apoenzyme deficiency in human fibroblasts: Evidence for allelic heterogeneity, genetic compounds, and codominant expression. *J Clin Invest* 65:690, 1980

167. KOLHOUSE JF, UTLEY C, FENTON W, ROSENBERG LE: Determination of methylmalonyl CoA mutase by radioimmunoassay in fibroblasts of patients with congenital methylmalonic acidemia, *Proc Nat Acad Sci, USA*, 1981, in press

168. MORROW G III, REVSIN B, CLARK R, LEBOWITZ J, WHELAN DT: A new variant of methylmalonic acidemia: Defective coenzyme-apoenzyme binding in cultured fibroblasts. *Clin Chim Acta* 85:67, 1978

169. KANG ES, SNODGRASS PJ, GERALD PS: Methylmalonyl-CoA racemase defect: Another cause of methylmalonicaciduria. *Pediatr Res* 6:875, 1972

170. GRAVEL RA, MAHONEY MJ, RUDDLE FH, ROSENBERG LE: Genetic complementation in heterokaryons of human fibroblasts defective in cobalamin metabolism. *Proc Natl Acad Sci USA* 72:3181, 1975

171. WILLARD HF, MELLMAN IS, ROSENBERG LE: Genetic complementation among inherited deficiencies of methylmalonyl-CoA mutase activity: Evidence for a new class of human cobalamin mutant. *Am J Hum Genet* 30:1, 1978

172. WILLARD HF, ROSENBERG LE: Inborn errors of cobalamin metabolism: Effect of cobalamin supplementation in culture on methylmalonyl CoA mutase activity in normal and mutant human fibroblasts. *Biochem Genet* 17:57, 1979

173. UTTER MF, KEECH DB, SCRUTTEN ML: A possible role for acetyl-CoA in the control of gluconeogenesis, in Webber G (ed): *Advances in Enzyme Regulation*. New York, Pergamon Press, Inc, 1964, vol 2, p 49

174. HALPERIN ML, SCHILLER CM, FRITZ IB: The inhibition by methylmalonic acid of malate transport by the dicarboxylate carrier in rat liver mitochondria. *J Clin Invest* 50:2276, 1971

175. INOUE S, KREIGER I, SARNAIK A, RAVINDRANATH Y, FRACASSA M, OTTENBREIT MJ: Inhibition of bone marrow stem cell growth *in vitro* by methylmalonic acid: A mechanism for pancytopenia in a patient with methylmalonic acidemia. *Pediatr Res* 15:95, 1981

176. COULOMBE JT, SHIH VE, LEVY HL: Massachusetts metabolic disorders screening program. II. Methylmalonic aciduria. *Pediatrics* 67:26, 1981

177. MORROW G, SCHWARTZ RH, HALLOCK JA, BARNESS LA: Prenatal detection of methylmalonic acidemia. *J Pediatr* 77:120, 1970

178. AMPOLA MG, MAHONEY MJ, NAKAMURA E, TANAKA K: Prenatal therapy of a patient with vitamin B_{12} responsive methylmalonic acidemia. *N Engl J Med* 293:313, 1975

179. MAHONEY MJ, ROSENBERG LE, LINDBLAD B, WALDENSTROM J, ZETTERSTROM, R: Prenatal diagnosis of methylmalonic aciduria. *Acta Paediatr Scand* 64:44, 1975

180. NYHAN WL, FAWCETT N, ANDO T, RENNERT OM, JULIUS RL: Response to dietary therapy in B_{12} unresponsive methylmalonic acidemia. *Pediatrics* 51:539, 1973

181. LEVY HL, MUDD SH, SCHULMAN JD, DREYFUSS PM, ABELES RH: A derangement in B_{12} metabolism associated with homocystinemia, cystathioninemia, hypomethioninemia and methylmalonic aciduria. *Am J Med* 48:390, 1970

182. DILLON MJ, ENGLAND JM, GOMPERTZ D, GOODEY PA, GRANT DB, HUSSEIN HA, LINNELL JC, MATHEWS DM, MUDD SH, NEWNS GH, SEAKINS JWT, UHLENDORF BW, WISE IJ: Mental retardation, megaloblastic anemia, methylmalonic aciduria and abnormal homocysteine metabolism due to an error in vitamin B_{12} metabolism. *Clin Sci Mol Med* 47:43, 1974

183. ANTHONY M, MCLEAY AC: A unique case of derangement of vitamin B_{12} metabolism. *Proc Aust Assoc Neurol* 13:61, 1976

184. BAUMGARTNER ER, WICK H, MAURER R, EGLI N, STEINMANN B: Congenital defect in intracellular cobalamin metabolism resulting in homocystinuria and methylmalonic aciduria. *Helv Paediatr Acta* 34:465, 1979

185. CARMEL R, BEDROS AA, MACE JW, GOODMAN SI: Congenital methylmalonic aciduria-homocystinuria with megaloblastic anemia: Observations on response to hydroxocobalamin and on the effect of homocysteine and methionine on the deoxyuridine suppression test. *Blood* 55:570, 1980

186. LINNELL JC, MATTHEWS DM, MUDD SH, UHLENDORF BW, WISE IJ: Cobalamins in fibroblasts cultured from normal control subjects and patients with methylmalonic aciduria. *Pediatr Res* 10:179, 1976

187. BAUMGARTNER ER, WICK H, LINNELL JC, GAULL GE, BACHMANN C, STEINMANN B: Congenital defect in intracellular cobalamin metabolism resulting in homocystinuria and methylmalonic aciduria. *Helv Paediatr Acta* 34:483, 1979

188. ROSENBERG LE, PATEL L, LILLJEQVIST A: Absence of an intracellular cobalamin binding protein in cultured fibroblasts from patients with defective synthesis of 5'-deoxyadenosylcobalamin and methylcobalamin. *Proc Natl Acad Sci USA* 72:4617, 1975

189. MUDD SH, UHLENDORF BW, HINDS KR, LEVY HL: Deranged B_{12} metabolism: Studies of fibroblasts grown in tissue culture. *Biochem Med* 4:215, 1970

190. MELLMAN IS, LIN P-F, RUDDLE FH, ROSENBERG LE: Genetic control of cobalamin binding in normal and mutant cells: Assignment of the gene for 5-methyltetrahydrofolate:L-homocysteine S-methyltransferase to human chromosome 1. *Proc Natl Acad Sci USA* 76:405, 1979

191. MELLMAN I, WILLARD HF, YOUNGDAHL-TURNER P, ROSENBERG LE: Cobalamin coenzyme synthesis in normal and mutant human fibroblasts: Evidence for a processing enzyme activity deficient in *cb1* C cells. *J Biol Chem* 254:11847, 1979

24

INHERITED DISORDERS OF FOLATE METABOLISM

PETER B. ROWE

1. In order to provide a background for an understanding of inborn errors of folate metabolism, this chapter examines normal folate metabolism with a special emphasis on human beings. The structure of folates and the chemical and biochemical mechanisms for their synthesis are reviewed. A brief discussion of the major enzymes of folate metabolism and of the possible mechanisms for their regulation is included. The most recent data available on the physiologic handling of folate by the mammal are presented, followed by a discussion of the biochemical and clinical sequelae of folate deficiency in humans. The critical relationship between folate and cobalamin metabolism is examined, since the interaction between these two cofactors is the key to our understanding of 1-carbon metabolism and consequently of defects in folate metabolism.

2. Each of the five groups of inborn errors of folate metabolism in humans so far described is discussed in detail. They consist of (1) congenital defects of folate absorption; (2) dihydrofolate reductase deficiency; (3) "formiminotransferase" deficiency syndromes; (4) methylene THF reductase deficiency; and (5) THF methyltransferase deficiency.

3. Congenital defect of folate absorption from the small intestine has resulted in three somewhat different clinical syndromes, which might possibly be the result of the variable therapeutic regimens employed. All patients have appeared in infancy with failure to thrive and a folate-responsive megaloblastic anemia. Severe central nervous system dysfunction may be a prominent feature if therapy is inadequate or if there is an associated defect in folate transport across the blood-brain barrier.

4. Dihydrofolate reductase deficiency also presents in infancy and may result in stillbirth or abortion, depending upon the degree of enzyme deficiency, which appears to be quite variable. Surviving infants fail to thrive and have a severe megaloblastic anemia. Therapy with folinic acid (leucovorin) bypasses the enzyme block and corrects the defect.

5. The formiminotransferase deficiency syndromes consist, clinically and biochemically, of two different types of defect. The initial patients described could represent a double enzyme defect in the histidine catabolic pathway, with the deficiency of formiminotransferase being of secondary importance to that of the associated enzyme cyclodeaminase. This is a severe disorder, and it is doubtful whether any therapy would be effective in these children, who appear in early childhood with failure to thrive and extensive changes in the central nervous system. Patients in the second group probably have single enzyme defects, although the deficiency of formiminotransferase may be due to different alleles. It is not clear whether these children are significantly

affected by the enzyme defect, but they are not normal clinically, and therapy with large doses of folic acid might be justifiable.

6. *Methylene THF reductase deficiency, the most common and widely studied of the inherited disorders of folate metabolism, is a condition in which the clinical severity correlates with the degree of enzyme deficiency. The clinical features largely reflect damage to the central nervous system. Biochemically, the key findings are homocystinuria with normal plasma methionine levels. No effective therapy has yet been found.*

7. *Tetrahydrofolate methyltransferase deficiency is mentioned only briefly because most of the patients have had disorders of cobalamin metabolism. The initial patient described by Arakawa and his colleagues was severely affected, with gross disturbance of the bone marrow and central nervous system. The diagnosis in this case has been questioned. It is not likely that available therapy will modify the course of this particular disorder.*

The large group of pteridine compounds referred to collectively as *folic acid* (Fig. 24-1) has a fundamental role in cell growth and division throughout the phylogenetic spectrum. A number of critical 1-carbon transfer reactions are dependent upon folic acid coenzymes, including those involved in the biosynthesis of methionine, serine, deoxythymidylic acid (dTMP), and purines and in the degradation of histidine and purines. There are almost certainly a number of other important reactions as yet unidentified.

At the time when the European chemists were isolating and characterizing the pteridine pigments from butterflies, a series of remarkable nutritional studies by Lucy Wills and her colleagues [1, 2] on pregnant women and on monkeys led to the isolation of a number of factors from foodstuffs which possessed the same basic chemical structure, N-(4-{(2-amino-4-hydroxy-6-pteridinyl) methyl) amino}benzoyl) glutamic acid, or pteroylglutamic acid (Fig. 24-2). The removal of these factors from the diet of primates resulted in a macrocytic, megaloblastic anemia. The chemists who, in 1946, accomplished the synthesis of the basic parent compound [3] also demonstrated that much of the structural variation among the different factors resulted from linkage of variable numbers of glutamic acid residues to the free gamma carboxyl group of pteroylglutamic acid (Fig. 24-2).

The term *folic acid* was introduced in 1940 to designate a nutritional factor isolated from spinach leaves which was essential for the growth of *Streptococcus fecalis* R [4]. Although this term is still used loosely to embrace the entire range of related chemical structures with similar nutritional effects, it should be reserved for pteroylglutamic acid, while the related compounds should be referred to as *folic acid derivatives* or *folates*.

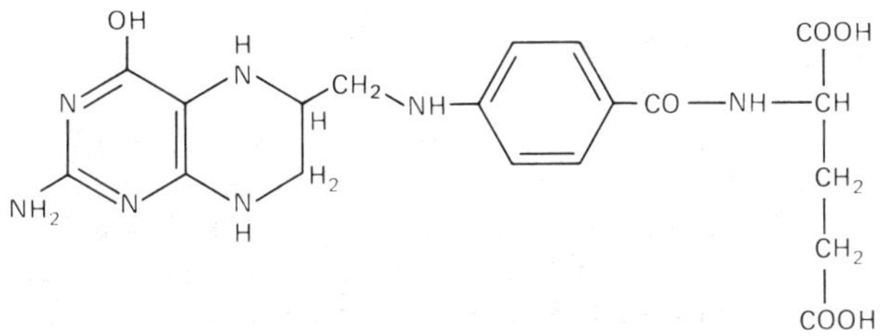

The period 1948 to 1968 saw an enormous amount of painstaking and often ingenious experimentation undertaken to elucidate the biochemistry of folic acid and its derivatives. Blakley's superb monograph [5] has provided us with a most comprehensive review up to 1968.

The introduction of chemical techniques of peptide synthesis [6, 7] made available a range of natural folate derivatives containing gamma glutamyl peptides of defined chain length. This has resulted in a thorough reinvestigation of many aspects of folate metabolism, as well as opening up new avenues for research. This account will be based primarily on mammalian folate metabolism, with special emphasis on human beings and the small number of inherited enzymatic defects so far described.

THE CHEMISTRY OF FOLIC ACID AND ITS DERIVATIVES

The folates consist of a large group of natural molecules derived from the reduction of and addition to the parent compound, folic acid.[1] As summarized in Fig. 24-2, there are (1) at least three states of reduction of the pyrazine ring of the pteridine moiety, (2) at least six different 1-carbon groups substituted at position N^5 or N^{10} or both, and (3) gamma glutamyl peptide chains of varying length linked to the gamma carboxyl group of the glutamic acid residue.

The gamma glutamyl peptide chain of the natural folate derivatives has a linear series of free α-carboxyl groups. The pK_a values for the α- and γ-carboxyl groups of glutamic acid are 2.19 and 4.25, respectively [8]. Accordingly, at pH levels above 2.19 the polyglutamate is a polyanion and assumes the structure of an extended rod [9]. This structure affects the binding of these compounds to intracellular organelles and to enzymes, as well as their behavior on both gel filtration and ion-exchange chromatography. These effects are directly related to the peptide chain length, the 1-carbon substitutions, and the state of reduction of the pteridine moiety [10, 11].

In spite of the obvious difficulties in dealing with such a large family of compounds, present in low concentrations in nature, the problems of their variable instability on exposure to oxygen and light, and their rapid degeneration or modification by enzymes associated with them in biologic samples, the structures of the major derivatives have been conclusively established. It does not appear that folic acid exists as such in nature. Only the reduced derivatives normally serve any biologic role. Apart from the enzyme that reduces folic acid and dihydrofolic acid (DHF) to tetrahydrofolic acid (THF), all other folate-dependent enzymes can use only fully reduced (tetrahydro) derivatives.

The chemical and physical properties of folic acid are largely predictable based on the fact that it is essentially a 6-alkylpterin. The limited water solubility of the un-ionized form is

Figure 24-1 The structure of 5,6,7,8-tetrahydrofolic acid.

---

[1] All folates are referred to as *derivatives* of folic acid. The abbreviations for dihydrofolic acid and tetrahydrofolic acid are *DHF* and *THF*, respectively. The polyglutamyl peptides are all gamma-bonded. *Folic acid* (or *folyl*) *diglutamate* designates pteroylglutamyl-γ-glutamyl glutamic acid, i.e., a derivative containing three glutamate residues.

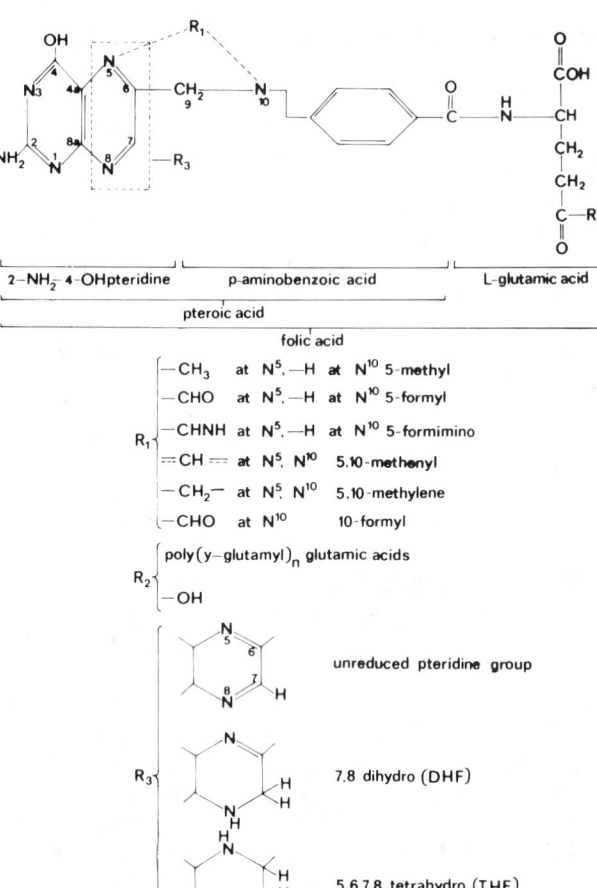

Figure 24-2 Schematic representation of the structure of folic acid and its derivatives. (*Based on Baugh and Krumdieck [11]*).

increased a thousandfold (to 15 g/liter at 0°C) by the formation of the disodium salt. Under anaerobic conditions folic acid is alkali stable, but it is cleaved aerobically to *p*-aminobenzoylglutamic acid and pterin-6-carboxylic acid. Aerobic hydrolysis in acid yields 6-methylpterin [12]. Polyglutamate derivatives are hydrolyzed by alkali anaerobically to folic acid and glutamic acid [12]. Photodecomposition of folic acid occurs in sunlight, producing *p*-aminobenzoylglutamic acid and an unidentified pterin [13]. The two folic acid analogues, aminopterin (4-amino-4-deoxyfolic acid) and methotrexate (10-methyl-4-deoxy-4-aminofolic acid), have broadly similar chemical properties.

Folic acid and many of its analogues can be readily reduced. The end product is either the 7,8 dihydro derivative or the 5, 6, 7,8 tetrahydro derivative, depending upon the conditions used. The progressive reduction of the pyrazine ring of the pteridine is associated with increasing water solubility and with characteristic changes in the absorbance and fluorescence spectra [14]. The reduced derivatives, DHF and THF, are readily oxidized in air, and the mechanism of these reactions and their end products have been extensively studied [14]. The only effective method of ensuring long-term stability is storage of the dried material in vacuo over phosphorus pentoxide in the dark at −20°C.

Reduction of folic acid to THF introduces an asymmetric center into the molecule at carbon 6, in addition to the asymmetric center already present in the glutamic acid moiety. The x-ray crystallographic and nuclear magnetic resonance analy-

ses of the absolute configuration about C-6 of THF and the 1-carbon derivatives showed inaccuracies in the chemical designation of the natural and unnatural diastereoisomers [15]. The absolute configuration of C-6 in the reduced pyrazine ring for all of the natural folate derivatives is R, which corresponds to the *S* configuration of THF itself [16].

5,10-Methylene THF

Pterins, folic acid, and various folic acid analogues and polyglutamate derivatives react nonenzymatically with formaldehyde. The most stable of the resultant compounds is formed from THF, and the product is 5,10-methylene THF. This derivative is far more stable to oxidation than THF, particularly in the presence of excess formaldehyde [17]. The diastereoisomers of methylene THF are readily separated by anion-exchange chromatography [18–20]. This is the only folic acid derivative whose biologically active and inactive isomers are readily isolated from one another.

5-Formyl THF, 10-Formyl THF, and 5,10-Methenyl THF

10-Formylfolic acid can be readily formed from folic acid by treatment with 98 percent formic acid [21]. 10-Formyl THF can then be generated by the platinum-catalyzed reduction of this derivative [22]. On being heated at pH 12, 10-formyl THF is partly converted to 5-formyl THF (also known as *folinic acid* or *leucovorin*). Though the former compound is sensitive to oxidizing agents, the introduction of the 5-formyl group results in stabilization [23]. Furthermore, the 5-formyl group is removed only with difficulty by alkaline hydrolysis, in contrast to the easy cleavage of the 10-formyl group [22–24]. The chemical stability of 5-formyl THF is the reason for its widespread clinical use.

At acid pH, both 5-formyl and 10-formyl THF lose a molecule of water to form, 5,10-methenyl THF (also known as *anhydroleucovorin*). This provides an efficient method for its synthesis [25]. While the acid-catalyzed conversion of 10-formyl THF is rapid, occurring within minutes, the dehydration of 5-formyl THF takes several hours to reach equilibrium. This has a significant bearing on the absorption of the intact 5-formyl derivative from the gut.

5,10-Methenyl THF is rapidly hydrolyzed at neutral or alkaline pH to 10-formyl THF, a reaction which is markedly dependent on the nature of the buffer ions in the solution [26, 27]. 5,10-Methenyl THF can be irreversibly reduced by borohydride [28] to 5,10-methylene THF. 5-Formyl THF and 10-formyl THF cannot be similarly reduced. The interconversions between the different derivatives are associated with specific changes in ultraviolet and fluorescence absorbance spectrums, as summarized by Blakley [29].

5-Methyl THF

This important derivative has been synthesized by a variety of chemical techniques, the best features of which are combined in the method of Blair and Saunders [30]. At alkaline pH, 5-methyl THF is reversibly oxidized to 5,6-dihydro-5-methyl folate. The dihydrofolate derivative is relatively stable to further oxidation [31], although at acid pH levels under anaerobic conditions, the C-9–N-10 bond is cleaved to produce a tetrahydropteridine and p-aminobenzoylglutamic acid [32]. This is extremely important in the design of chemical methods for the analysis of tissue folates (see below).

5-Formimino THF

Only the enzymatic synthesis of this derivative has been described. In aqueous solution it is rapidly hydrolyzed with loss of ammonia from the formimino group, and in acid solution it is converted to 5,10-methenyl THF [33].

THE BIOCHEMISTRY OF FOLIC ACID AND ITS DERIVATIVES

The major metabolic pathways of folic acid and its reduced derivatives have been established in a variety of prokaryotic and eukaryotic cells [34]. In the mammal, the major reactions (Fig. 24-3) constitute a series of interlocking pathways in which (1) folic acid is reduced to DHF and then to THF (re-

actions 1 and 2); (2) THF is then converted to a series of 1-carbon carrier derivatives, viz., 10-formyl THF (reaction 3), 5,10-methylene THF (reaction 4), and 5-formimino THF (reaction 10), all of which can potentially be converted to 5,10-methenyl THF (reactions 5, 6, and 11, respectively); (3) these derivatives can be used either directly in purine biosynthesis *de novo* (reactions 14 and 15) or in the synthesis of dTMP (reaction 9) or, following the reduction of 5,10-methylene THF to 5-methyl THF (reaction 7), in the methylation of homocysteine to methionine (reaction 8). In each case, reduced folate is recycled into the intracellular pool. The enzymatic synthesis of 5-formyl THF (reaction 12) has not yet been fully clarified in the mammal [35], although an enzyme has been partially purified from hog liver [36] and from rat liver [37] which catalyzed this reaction. The ATP-dependent conversion of 5-formyl to 5,10-methenyl THF (reaction 13) by the enzyme 5-formyl THF cyclodehydrase [38] has been demonstrated in many tissues. There is no evidence of the direct participation of 5-formyl THF in 1-carbon donor reactions.

Reactions 14 and 15 are responsible for the introduction of carbon atoms 2 and 8 into the purine ring. Reactions 10 and 11, which constitute a 1-carbon salvage pathway in the course of histidine catabolism, will be discussed in some detail, since they are related to a major folate pathway defect. The glycine-cleavage system (reaction 16) is located within the mitochondrion and involves the NAD-dependent generation of 5,10-methylene THF. The role of the system in overall folate metabolism has not yet been resolved [39].

Early studies by Du Vigneaud and Rachele led most investigators to believe that the synthesis of methionine from homocysteine and betaine by the enzyme betaine-homocysteine methyltransferase (EC 2.1.1.5) was of primary importance in mammals [40]. More recent studies on the rat have demonstrated that this reaction is confined to the liver [41] and that the prime mechanism for the methylation of homocysteine is mediated by THF methyltransferase (reaction 8).

The overall folate pathway is largely confined to the cytosol, although individual enzymes have been isolated from different organelles. The enzyme catalyzing reaction 4, serine transhydroxymethylase, for example, has been isolated from rabbit and rat liver mitochondria [42]. Genetic studies have shown that the cytosol and mitochondrial species are distinct [43].

The folate substrates for each of the reactions shown in Fig. 24-3 have been designated as the *monoglutamate derivatives*. Most tissue folates are in the form of polyglutamate derivatives [44], although the relative proportion of these may be modulated by the amount of folic acid available to the cell [45] or by the changes in the steady state of 1-carbon metabolism [46].

Most of the folate pathway enzymes studied prefer the polyglutamate derivatives [47, 48], and these may provide a form of regulatory control, as exemplified by the increasing relative specific activities (Vm:Km) of AICAR formyltransferase (EC 2.1.2.3) as a function of polyglutamate chain length [49].

Biosynthesis of Folate Polyglutamates

Several years ago, Griffin and Brown [50] demonstrated the synthesis of polyglutamate derivatives of THF in cell-free extracts of *Escherichia coli*. The reaction required glutamic acid, ATP, and divalent cations. Neither DHF nor folic acid could substitute for THF.

Sakami et al. [51] described a THF-dependent system in

Figure 24-3 Major metabolic pathways of folic acid and its derivatives in the mammal. Additional abbreviations used are 5-aminoimidazole-4-carboxamide ribonucleotide (AICAR), 5-formimidoimidazole-4-carboxamide ribonucleotide (FAICAR), β-glycinamide ribonucleotide (GAR), and α-N-formylglycinamide ribonucleotide (FGAR). (*Based on Rowe and Lewis [27].*)

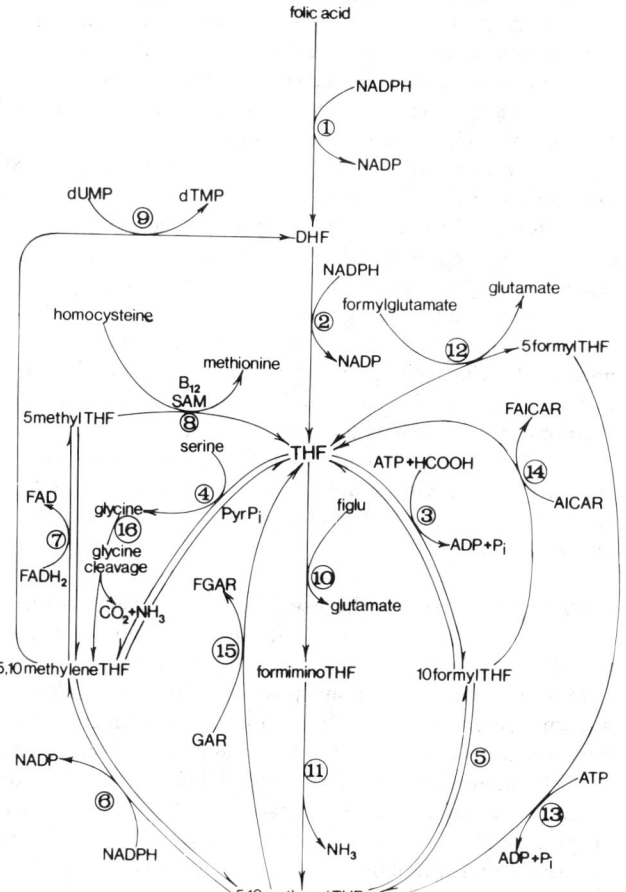

Neurospora in which two enzymes were involved, one for diglutamate synthesis and another for higher-order derivatives. McGuire et al. [52] have recently described a rat liver folylpolyglutamate synthetase with a limited capacity for the synthesis of derivatives beyond diglutamates. All naturally occurring folates apparently served as substrates.

Human cell experiments have been carried out by Lavoie et al. [53] on phytohemagglutinin (PHA)-stimulated lymphocytes incubated with [^{3}H]folic acid and 5-[^{14}C]methyl THF. The same proportion of tritium-labeled folic acid was incorporated into folate polyglutamates in both normal and cobalamin-deficient lymphocytes, while no radiolabel could be detected in the polyglutamates from normal cells supplied with the 5-methyl THF. These experiments suggest that lymphocytes cannot utilize 5-methyl THF as a substrate for polyglutamate derivative synthesis.

The biologic importance of the polyglutamates has been emphasized by the observations of McBurney and Whitmore [54] on cultured Chinese hamster cells. They have shown that the multiple auxotrophy of a mutant cell line (AUXB1) for glycine, adenosine, and thymidine results from low intracellular levels of folate coenzymes. Those derivatives that were present were primarily monoglutamates, whereas the folates from wild-type cells were predominantly pentaglutamyl peptides. They have proposed that the polyglutamyl synthetase enzyme is defective in the mutant cells, and they support this view with their studies on a similar, but temperature-sensitive, multiple auxotroph (*ts* AUXB1) [55]. Their proposal has been supported by studies by Taylor and Hanna [56]. As a result of the failure of polyglutamate synthesis, it was proposed that the cells cannot retain folate derivatives, implying a role for polyglutamyl peptides in limiting transmembrane movement.

Degradation of Folate Polyglutamates   The gamma bonds of the polyglutamate peptide chain are cleaved by a group of peptidases referred to collectively as *conjugases* or, more specifically, as gammaglutamyl hydrolase (EC 3.4.22.12). These enzymes are distributed throughout the phylogenetic spectrum and are present in high levels in pancreas, liver, intestine, kidney, spleen, and brain. The mammalian enzymes are acid hydrolases, consistent with their lysosomal localization [57].

Using a sensitive assay based on the release of [^{14}C]glutamic acid from synthetic polyglutamate derivatives, Baugh and his colleagues studied a partly purified human liver enzyme [58]. This enzyme was similar to a bovine liver enzyme purified 25,000-fold [59]. The bovine enzyme, a thermostable glycoprotein of MW 100,000, requires Zn^{2+} ion for stability, and highly reactive sulfhydryl groups are essential for activity. While the enzyme specifically cleaves gamma bonds, a carboxyl terminal gamma bond is essential. Cleavage is independent of the presence or nature of the N-terminal pteroyl moiety. Longer-chain polyglutamates are preferentially attacked. While intestinal conjugases are required for the digestion of dietary polyglutamate derivatives, the general biologic role of these enzymes is still unclear. They may be concerned with the cleavage of natural folates, with the release ultimately of *p*-aminobenzoylglutamate as part of the process of folate catabolism [60].

The interesting and significant observations [61] on mammalian intestinal conjugases, a group of enzymes with varying substrate specificity, have not been carried further.

Folate Pathway Enzymes

In any discussion of the individual enzymes of the pathway, the implications of multienzyme complexes must be considered. A single polypeptide chain containing 10-formyl THF synthetase (EC 6.3.4.3), 5,10-methenyl THF cyclohydrolase (EC 3.5.4.9), and 5,10-methylene THF dehydrogenase (EC 1.5.1.5) has been isolated from both sheep [62] and pig [63] liver. The ad3 mutants of the yeast *Saccharomyces cerevisiae* have reduced levels of all three of these enzyme activities [64].

A complex has now been purified from chicken liver containing not only these three enzyme activities, but also those of serine transhydroxymethylase (EC 2.1.2.1), GAR transformylase (EC 2.1.2.2), and AICAR transformylase (EC 2.1.2.3) [65]. Formimino-THF cyclodeaminase (EC 4.3.1.4) and glutamate formiminotransferase (EC 2.1.2.5), long known to copurify from avian liver, have been shown to constitute an octomeric enzyme containing bifunctional polypeptides [66]. These observations have important genetic and biochemical implications particularly in terms of the conservation of labile biologic intermediates and of the regulatory systems involved in pathway control.

The activity of the various folate pathway enzymes may vary considerably with the stage of the cell cycle [47]. This is extremely important given the increasing use of cultured cells.

Dihydrofolate Reductase   Reactions 1 and 2 are catalyzed by dihydrofolate reductase [5,6,7,8 THF:NAD(P) oxidoreductase (EC 1.5.1.3)]. This key enzyme in 1-carbon metabolism has been extensively studied over the past 20 years. The enzyme consists, in all species, of a single nonaggregating polypeptide chain of MW 20,000. The amino acid sequences of enzyme from a number of bacterial and animal cells are known [15]. This, combined with recent x-ray diffraction studies, has resulted in a reasonably detailed understanding of the enzyme mechanism [67]. Many other studies have recently been reported on various properties of the mammalian enzyme [68]. One of these studies [69] demonstrated that the enzyme from a methotrexate-resistant subline of human KB cells did not preferentially utilize polyglutamate substrates, in contrast to the findings of earlier studies from Bertino's group [70].

One of the major developments has been the demonstration of dihydrofolate reductase gene amplification as the mechanism underlying cellular resistance to the potent inhibitor methotrexate [71]. This observation has many implications for chemotherapy as well as for the field of molecular biology in general. Unstable gene amplification resistance to methotrexate is associated with double minute chromosomes, while in stably amplified cells the genes are associated with large chromosomes [72].

10-Formyl THF Synthetase   Reaction 3, the ATP-dependent formylation of THF to 10-formyl THF, will need to be reevaluated from the point of view of its kinetic properties within a single multifunctional protein, particularly with polyglutamate derivatives of THF as substrate. The kinetics of the enzymes apparently are not altered significantly [62, 63], but only the monoglutamate derivative of THF was used in the assays. A relatively crude preparation of the bovine liver enzyme utilizes the pentaglutamate derivative of THF more effectively than the monoglutamate, with a fall in K_m from

1.4×10^{-4} to 2×10^{-5} M and an associated decrease in the K_m for formate from 7.0 to 0.1 mM [73]. This latter observation is significant, as intracellular formate levels are supposedly very low in mammals.

In humans, the greatest quantity of enzyme is found in the liver, but it is almost certainly present in all cell types. While most of the available information came from studies on the purified clostridial enzyme, which apparently does not have the multifunctional properties of the liver enzymes, the gross kinetic parameters are similar. An excellent review was published in 1973 [74], and several studies on the mammalian enzyme have recently appeared [68].

The extent to which this enzyme is involved in synthesis of 1-carbon derivatives of THF in the mammal is uncertain. Rabinowitz and Tabor [75] demonstrated that formate derived from the 2 position of the indole ring of tryptophan was the major source of urinary formate in the rat and that this formate was increased in folate deficiency. More recently, Henderson's laboratory [76] has shown that formate derived in this way is extensively utilized for 1-carbon donor reactions in purine biosynthesis in the rat, although the contribution from tryptophan would appear to be much less than that from the 3 carbon of serine.

Serine Transhydroxymethylase   Reaction 4, in which the β carbon of serine is transferred to THF with the formation of 5,10-methylene THF and glycine, is catalyzed by serine transhydroxymethylase, a pyridoxal phosphate enzyme. This enzyme has been detected in tissues from many species, and especially high levels are found in vertebrate livers.

In rat liver approximately 71 percent of the β carbon of serine is catabolized by this reaction, and it is accordingly a major source of 1-carbon units [77]. Alternative degradation pathways via pyruvate or 3-phosphoglyceric acid would appear to be limited under normal physiologic conditions [39]. The bulk of enzyme activity is in the cytosol, but a genetically distinct enzyme is found in mitochondria. The importance of the mitochondrial species has been emphasized by the gly$^-$ A class of CHO cells which as a result of the loss of mitochondrial activity has become a glycine auxotroph [43].

The rabbit liver enzyme catalyzes the following reactions [78]:

$$\text{L-Serine} + \text{THF} \rightleftharpoons \text{glycine} + \text{5,10-methylene THF} \quad (1)$$
$$\alpha\text{-Methylserine} + \text{THF} \rightleftharpoons \text{D-alanine} + \text{5,10-methylene THF} \quad (2)$$
$$\text{L-Threonine (L-allothreonine)} \rightleftharpoons \text{glycine} + \text{acetaldehyde} \quad (3)$$
$$\beta\text{-Phenylserine} \rightleftharpoons \text{glycine} + \text{benzaldehyde} \quad (4)$$
$$\text{Aminomalonate} \rightleftharpoons \text{glycine} + \text{CO}_2 \quad (5)$$
$$\text{D-Alanine} + \text{holoenzyme} \; (E\text{-pyridoxal Pi})$$
$$\rightleftharpoons \text{pyruvate} + E\text{-pyridoxamine Pi} \quad (6)$$

Reaction 1 appears to be the major biochemical function of the protein in mammals. The K_m values for serine range from 5 to 7×10^{-4} M and for THF between 7.2×10^{-4} and 7×10^{-5} M.

The proposed reaction mechanism, based primarily on the work of Schirch and his colleagues, has been recently reviewed [15], and a number of recent reports emphasize the interest in this protein [68].

Cyclohydrolase   Reaction 5, the reversible formation of the N^5-N^{10} methenyl bridge, is catalyzed by the enzyme 5,10-methenyl THF cyclohydrolase, commonly known as *cyclohydrolase*. The nonenzymatic pH-mediated interconversion of the two THF derivatives, 5,10-methenyl THF and 10-formyl THF, has been referred to earlier (see "The Chemistry of Folic Acid and Its Derivatives"). Above pH 6, ring cleavage is favored, with formation of 10-formyl THF, a reaction which becomes almost instantaneous above pH 8. Below pH 6, cyclization of the N^5-N^{10} ring is favored.

Because of its instability, little information is available about the enzyme, even though it is widely distributed throughout mammalian tissues. The bovine liver enzyme has been partially purified by different groups, with some variance in results.

This is not surprising in view of the subsequent demonstration that activity is associated with a trifunctional protein [62, 63] which is also part of an enzyme complex [65]. The K_m values for the natural isomers of 5,10-methenyl THF and 10-formyl THF of 2.5×10^{-4} M and 4.7×10^{-4} M, respectively, have been reported for the enzyme activity in the sheep liver trifunctional enzyme [62].

Within the physiologic pH range, the ring cleavage reaction is the only one detectable. This raises a serious question about the role of the enzyme in maintaining an equilibrium between two THF derivatives which are critical 1-carbon donors in different reactions in purine biosynthesis *de novo*.

The reaction mechanism has been recently reviewed [15], but further studies with the enzyme complex are required.

Methylene THF Dehydrogenase   Reaction 6, the NADP-dependent oxidation of 5,10-methylene THF to 5,10-methenyl THF, is catalyzed by the enzyme 5,10-methylene THF dehydrogenase. The enzyme has widespread species and tissue distribution, and the liver and kidneys of vertebrates, including humans, have extremely high levels of activity.

Although a moderate amount of research has been carried out on the bacterial enzyme, little information is available concerning the highly unstable mammalian enzyme. The kinetic parameters observed for the enzyme as part of the multifunctional protein isolated from liver are similar to those demonstrated for the crude enzyme from calf thymus [20] and bovine liver [27]. The K_m for NADP was 2×10^{-5} M, while that of the natural isomer of 5,10-methylene THF was 2×10^{-5} [62, 63], a little lower than that reported earlier [20, 27].

NAD does not serve as an electron acceptor. The mammalian and yeast enzymes are activated by monovalent cations such as Na$^+$ and K$^+$ but are inhibited by Ca^{2+}, Ba^{2+}, and Mg^{2+}. No investigations have been reported on the ability of the enzymes to utilize polyglutamate derivative substrates.

Methylene THF Reductase   Reaction 7, the enzymatic reduction of 5,10-methylene THF to 5-methyl THF, is the first committed step in the biosynthesis of methyl groups. The enzyme catalyzing the reaction, methylene THF reductase 5-methyltetrahydrofolate:NAD$^+$ oxidoreductase (EC 1.1.1.58), was first isolated from horse liver by Donaldson and Keresztesy. There has been relatively little study of this key enzyme, which is present in the livers of a number of vertebrates, including humans, as well as in bacteria [79].

The *E. coli* enzyme has somewhat different properties from those of the highly purified enzyme from rat and pig liver [80]. The mammalian enzyme is a flavoprotein specific for FAD, and NADPH is the obligatory electron donor. The reaction catalyzed:

$$\text{5,10-Methylene THF} + \text{NADPH} + \text{H}^+$$
$$\xrightarrow{\text{FAD}} \text{5-methyl THF} + \text{NADP} \quad (7)$$

is virtually irreversible. Apparent K_m values for the pig liver enzyme were 33×10^{-6} M for NADPH and 10^{-5} M for 5,10-methylene THF (natural isomer).

Recent kinetic studies of the purified pig liver enzyme with polyglutamate derivatives have been difficult to interpret [81]. With increasing γ-polyglutamate chain lengths of 5,10-methylene THF, the relative V_{max} increases by a factor of 1.74 up to four glutamate residues and then decreases by a factor of 0.6. The K_m for the folate derivative falls progressively from 7.1 to 0.1 μM as the chain length increases to six residues and then rises to 0.51 μM. The K_m for NADPH actually increases from 16 to 185 μM over the one to six glutamate residue range. Dihydrofolate is an inhibitor, with a K_i of 6.5 μM, while dihydropteroylhexaglutamate has a K_i of 0.013 μM. These studies emphasize the need for detailed kinetic studies with the natural polyglutamate derivatives of THF for all folate pathway enzymes.

THF Methyltransferase   The methylation of homocysteine to methionine is catalyzed, in mammals, by the cobalamin-containing enzyme 5-methyl-tetrahydrofolate-homocysteine methyltransferase (EC 2.1.1.13) and requires catalytic levels of a reducing system and S-adenosylmethionine (SAM). Polyglutamates are effective substrates [82]. Given the complexity of the overall methyl transfer reaction, it is not surprising that knowledge of the detailed enzyme mechanism has not proceeded beyond the earlier hypotheses [83].

The tissue distribution has been well defined [82], but the overall activity is relatively low in most cell types when compared with that of other folate pathway enzymes involved in 1-carbon metabolism. This low activity is the reason most cell lines in culture require methionine for maximum growth rates. Methylation reactions involved, for example, in phospholipid biosynthesis, RNA and DNA modification, and creatine biosynthesis are mediated via SAM. The extent to which methionine supplied in the diet or the culture medium, compared with that synthesized via the intracellular 1-carbon pool utilized for SAM synthesis, requires clarification for each cell type.

Thymidylate Synthetase   Because of the unique position of dTMP and its triphosphate dTTP in DNA synthesis, the enzyme involved in reaction 9, thymidylate synthetase [5,10-methylene THF:dUMP C-methyl-transferase (EC 2.1.1.6)], has been the subject of intensive research by scientists involved in development of antibiotics and chemotherapeutic agents.

The uniqueness of dTTP biosynthesis lies in its relatively circuitous route of biosynthesis particularly in the methylation of dUMP to dTMP, with the oxidation of the tetrahydrofolate donor to dihydrofolate. Both prokaryotic and eukaryotic cells have low levels of enzyme activity except during cell division. This probably accounts in part for the relatively high levels in neoplastic tissue. The most extensive reviews [84] are concerned with the properties of the enzyme from a strain of Lacto-bacillus casei resistant to methotrexate which contains high levels of stable activity [85].

The isolation of a homogeneous enzyme preparation from human leukemic cells has further stimulated work on the mechanism of action of the enzyme, particularly in relation to the binding of potent inhibitors such as 5'-fluoro-2'-deoxyuridylate [86]. The general properties of the human enzyme are similar to those of the bacterial enzyme in terms of the MW of 66,000, the two identical subunits, and the substrate kinetic parameters. The amino acid composition is somewhat different.

Studies with the bacterial enzyme have confirmed that polyglutamate derivatives of methylene THF are more effective substrates than the monoglutamate [87] and that, more significantly, folate and methotrexate polyglutamates and their corresponding dihydro and tetrahydro forms are potent inhibitors [87, 88]. It is evident that the γ-polyglutamate peptide is a critical factor in the enzyme-substrate interaction [89], and much of the data acquired from the vast number of studies with enzyme inhibitors will have to be reevaluated.

Formiminotransferase-cyclodeaminase   The last two steps in the salvage of the 1-carbon unit in histidine catabolism are reactions 8 and 9:

$$\text{THF + formiminoglutamic acid (figlu)} \longrightarrow$$
$$\text{5-formimino THF + glutamic acid} \quad (8)$$
$$\text{5-formimino THF} \longrightarrow \text{5,10-methenyl THF + NH}_3 \quad (9)$$

Reaction 8 is catalyzed by formiminotransferase [(N-formimino-L-glutamate:THF 5-formiminotransferase (EC 2.1.2.5)] and reaction 9 by cyclodeaminase [5-formimino THF ammonia lyase (cyclizing) (EC 4.3.1.4)]. These two enzymes exist in mammalian tissues as a large octomeric protein made up of bifunctional peptides of MW 64,000 arranged in a circular structure [90]. The two active sites are clearly in different domains of the peptide and can be selectively destroyed or modified by a variety of techniques.

Studies with THF polyglutamates have revealed no change in the V_{max} but K_m values of 48, 31, and 3.5 μM for one, three, and five glutamate residues, respectively. There was no apparent accumulation of the intermediate 5-formimino THF with time when the pentaglutamate derivative was the substrate [90].

Liver tissues contain high levels of activity, but cultured human lymphoblasts, fibroblasts, amniotic fluid cells [91], and human lymphocytes [92] have no detectable activity.

Folate Derivative Flux and Enzyme Regulation

The folate pathway is a complex series of interlocking enzymatic reactions which generate a number of relatively unstable folate coenzymes critical for several important biosynthetic reactions. The overall pathway appears to be confined to the cytoplasm, and control mechanisms must be available to regulate metabolite flux through the various reactions. One study on extracts of bovine liver has reported the relative maximal activities of a number of the pathway enzymes in vitro [93] which may not be relevant to the intracellular conditions. As mentioned earlier, the relative activity of different enzymes may vary with the stage of the cell cycle [47], the availability of folate [45], and the 1-carbon balance within the cell [46].

Studies with murine lymphoma cells using the radioactively double-labeled folate derivative 5[^{14}C]methyl-3', 5', 9-^{3}H THF showed that 81 to 85 percent of the total [^{14}C]methyl groups were transferred to nonfolate compounds within 5 min and that the transfer was, initially, presumably to methionine but later to insoluble cellular materials [94]. After 60 min, over 80 percent of the tritium label was identified as 5-methyl THF. This demonstrated a high turnover of folate coenzymes, with 5-methyl THF being the only derivative accumulating. As an extension of this, cell lines L1210 and L1210R (a subline resistant to methotrexate) were incubated with 5-formyl (6-

[3]H) THF and methotrexate. Within 60 min, 28 percent of the tritium label had been transferred to dTMP by the L1210 cells and 52 percent by the L1210R cells. This indicated a high rate of folate flux through this section of the pathway. The difference in the two cell lines resulted from the block of DHF reductase by methotrexate in the L1210 cells. This suggested product inhibition of thymidylate synthetase (see reaction 9). This was confirmed by the accumulation of 23 percent of 5-methyl(3′, 5′, 9-^{3}H) THF by methotrexate-treated L1210 cells as (3′, 5′, 9-^{3}H) DHF, while the methotrexate-resistant L1210R line showed no such accumulation. The differential of incorporation into dTMP by the two cell lines of 5-formyl (6-^{3}H) THF cannot be explained solely by a block in the recycling of folate derivatives, since the synthesis of dTMP results in the removal of the ^{3}H label from the carbon 6 position of the folate molecule (see reaction 9).

A number of the folate enzymes are subject to feedback inhibition and also to induction and repression in a wide variety of bacterial and in some mammalian cells [95]. The data available on mammalian enzyme regulation are still limited, and no overall study has been undertaken on a whole series of these enzymes within one tissue or cell type.

Definitive experiments will require the use of natural polyglutamate derivatives and must recognize the existence of multifunctional protein and multienzyme complexes. This has been emphasized by the studies on methylene THF reductase [81] and thymidylate synthetase [87, 88]. While it is evident that many of the folate pathway enzymes are subject to regulation by a variety of mechanisms, including substrate levels, the presence of other folate derivatives, and cation concentrations, the bulk of these studies (summarized in the previous edition) were performed using monoglutamate derivatives and will need to be reevaluated.

DIETARY AND TISSUE FOLATES

Human beings are entirely dependent upon dietary sources for their supply of folates. An adult requires 50 to 100 μg folate per day [96]. A normal infant probably needs 20 to 50 μg per day [97]. Requirements also increase during pregnancy. Willoughby has estimated a minimal daily requirement of 350 μg [98]. Most normal Western diets contain adequate folic acid, but it has been suggested that consumption of processed foods leads to a borderline intake. Human nutritional requirements and recommended daily allowances have recently been reviewed [99]. This discussion also pointed up the continuing conflict concerning the folate content of foods related to methodologic inadequacies.

Both quantitative and qualitative analyses of the various tissue folate derivatives have relied heavily on microbiologic assays with bacteria which are folate auxotrophs. These were summarized in the previous edition.

The relatively low cellular folate content, together with the relatively crude extraction and analytic procedures, makes data relating to the differential quantitation of the various 1-carbon natural folate derivatives difficult to interpret [100]. Shin et al. determined that 85 to 90 percent of rat liver folate consists of fully reduced tetraglutamate derivatives of folic acid, with 5-methyl THF as the major component [101]. Studies with L1210 cells suggested that, in logarithmic growth, folate derivatives were present as polyglutamates. These consisted predominantly of THF (29.7 percent), 5-formyl THF (23.9 percent), 10-formyl THF (23 percent), and 5-formyl THF (10.2 percent), although there was variation between different batches of cells [44]. Again, the stage of the cell cycle and the contents of the culture medium may affect the relative distribution and polyglutamate chain lengths of the various cellular folates [45, 46]. In studies with phytohemagglutinin-activated human peripheral blood lymphocytes, virtually all the folate present was in the form of the pentaglutamate of THF [102].

In a study on human liver in which due precautions were taken for the protection of the natural derivatives [103], over 85 percent of the folate derivatives contained more than three glutamate residues. Again, no real attempt was made to identify the pteridine groups. In an earlier study using frozen liver, Chanarin et al. [104] found that 5-methyl THF was the only significant folate derivative present.

5-Methyl THF polyglutamates are virtually the only folate derivatives present in the red cells of most species, including humans. In the rat [105], erythrocyte folates are almost exclusively 5-methyl THF polyglutamates containing four (6 percent), five (54 percent), and six (30 percent) glutamate residues. These folates appear to be strongly protein bound and are not exchangeable with the general body pool. In light of the virtual absence of any THF methyltransferase activity in the human red cells [106], it is not clear what biochemical role is played by these folate stores. Human serum contains 5-methyl THF predominantly [107], and this appears to be the case for the serums of other mammals as well. No polyglutamate derivatives are present. Cow's milk contains monoglutamates (60 percent) and polyglutamates (ranging from di- to heptaglutamates), and 90 to 95 percent is in the 5-methyl THF form [108]. The high monoglutamate content may result from polyglutamate digestion by conjugase during the process of apocrine secretion. This provides the newborn intestine with predigested folate derivatives, an advantage while intestinal digestive mechanisms are still developing. Samuel et al. [109] have reported that relatively large oral doses of both mono- and polyglutamate derivatives of folic acid are adequately absorbed by infants of low birth weight.

It is evident that the range of folate derivatives is extremely variable from tissue to tissue and in different species. In mammalian tissues, especially liver, which has the bulk of the body folate stores and in which the greatest metabolic activity related to folate metabolism takes place, polyglutamate derivatives of 5-methyl THF are the major folates.

FOLATE ABSORPTION, TRANSPORT, EXCRETION, AND PHYSIOLOGIC DISTRIBUTION

Absorption

Dietary folates consist primarily of methyl and formyl derivatives of reduced folate polyglutamates. Most of the current concepts of handling of folates by the digestive tract have been developed from studies with synthetic crystalline folic acid, which is not a physiologically significant compound. Rosenberg has provided the most recent review of the gastrointestinal physiology of folates [110].

Digestion of the gammaglutamyl peptides of dietary folates

is necessary prior to their transport from the intestinal lumen to the portal circulation. This transport process entails the movement of folate molecules across the plasma membrane, and the polyanionic nature of the peptide would almost certainly preclude this in the physiologic pH range. The digestive process is carried out by the enzyme gammaglutamyl carboxypeptidase or conjugase, which is present in high concentrations in the mucosal cells of the small intestine. However, studies on rats [110] and guinea pigs [111] indicate that the enzyme is lysosomal and is not located within the brush border. This would imply a pinocytotic mechanism for folate polyglutamate uptake, which may not be available to the mature mammalian intestinal cell. The evidence for conjugase activity in the fluid of the small intestine and in the bile is by no means conclusive, and at any rate, the pH conditions are not suitable for conjugase action.

An alternative explanation might be provided by the studies of Blair [112]. They have demonstrated a pH of 5.5 in the middle of the glycocalyx of the rat jejunal cell. They have proposed that folates cannot be taken up by these cells unless they are largely non-ionized. This would require a pH of about 3 for folate molecules, which they consider to be the pH at the external surface of the plasma membrane. It is possible that conjugase is present within this relatively acid glycocalyx. The pH conditions would be ideal for conjugase action, and this would provide an explanation of the variable conjugase content of intestinal fluid. It would also account for the failure to detect conjugase in more peripheral parts of the cell, since the glycocalyx is readily lost during the processing of intestinal tissue. Recent studies have suggested the existence of an Mg^{2+}-activated ATPase located on the brush border which has properties suited for the generation of acidic microenvironment [113]. The chicken intestinal "conjugase," a complex of three enzymes [61], has a neutral pH optimum, but the site of action is unknown.

The vast majority of the intestinal folate absorption studies have been carried out on the rat and a few on humans. Few studies have used the reduced natural folate derivatives, and Blair [112] has critically reviewed many of these experiments.

A folate absorptive defect which has been described in humans suggests the existence of a specific protein or carrier system involved in the absorption mechanism. Nevertheless, the experiments concerned with demonstrating the existence of such a carrier system capable of transporting folate against a concentration gradient have led to conflicting results, with no clear-cut picture emerging [112, 114]. Leslie and Rowe [115] isolated a brush border membrane protein from the small intestine of the rat, with binding specificity for folic acid which was altered by 1-carbon substitution of the molecule but not by its state of reduction. 5-Methyl THF, however, did not bind to this protein. This implies the existence of a second (and more physiologic) carrier. Other studies have confirmed the presence of a folate-binding protein (FABP) in the intestinal mucosal cells, but again it was difficult to envisage its role in the natural folate uptake system [113, 116]. Strum et al. [114] have presented data indicating that the biologically active isomer of 5-methyl THF is transferred unchanged across the entire length of the small intestine of the rat by a passive transfer mechanism.

It is quite clear, from a large number of different experiments in humans and other mammals, that folic acid and its natural derivatives (other than 5-methyl THF) are modified significantly within the intestinal cell. The degree of modification is limited by the capacity of the cellular enzymes to handle the experimental load and is probably related to the folate status of the cell. This applies particularly to folic acid, which is relatively slowly reduced to the biochemically active derivatives and, depending upon the dose, a significant fraction of which is absorbed unaltered into the portal circulation. In this context, the observations on the distribution of folates in monkey tissue are relevant [117]. The intestinal cells contain large amounts of folate polyglutamates, although the state of reduction and 1-carbon substitution of the pteridine moieties were not determined. The pattern of folates obtained on anion-exchange chromatography was far more complex than that of kidney or liver. The presence of large amounts of 5-methyl THF polyglutamate raises the question of a storage role for the intestinal cell, particularly if no THF methyltransferase is present in the monkey intestine, as is the case in the rat [41]. This possibility has also been raised by Olinger et al. [118].

Reduced folates and their derivatives are readily absorbed and metabolized, largely to 5-methyl THF, prior to their transfer to the portal circulation. Depending upon the load or the dose administered, a significant fraction may be transferred without enzymatic modification. The efficient absorption of 5-formyl THF by humans, either as such or as the 5-methyl derivative, is therapeutically extremely important, since this derivative is widely used for "leucovorin rescue" in methotrexate chemotherapy [119].

The various factors involved in the processes of digestion and absorption of folic acid and its derivatives are shown diagrammatically in Fig. 24-4. A more detailed knowledge of the

Figure 24-4 Diagrammatic summary of digestion and absorption of folic acid and dietary folate derivatives by the small intestinal cell. The major points are as follows. (1) The site of action of the digestive enzyme conjugase is still not clear, but only monoglutamate or, at most, diglutamate derivatives are incorporated into the cell. (2) The derivatives are fully reduced by dihydrofolate reductase and, depending upon the load, are (a) transported directly into the portal blood, (b) converted to 5-methyl THF and thence transferred to the portal system, or (c) converted directly (or perhaps via THF) into folate polyglutamate stores. It is not clear to what extent 5-methyl THF can act as a substrate for polyglutamate synthetase. The possible absence of THF methyltransferase from the human intestine (as appears to be the case in the rat) might suggest that it is. (3) These folate stores can be degraded by intracellular conjugase for release into the circulation. (4) Folic acid can be transferred directly into the portal blood or reduced and incorporated into the general folate pool. The relative flux into each of these alternatives is dependent upon the load presented to the cell.

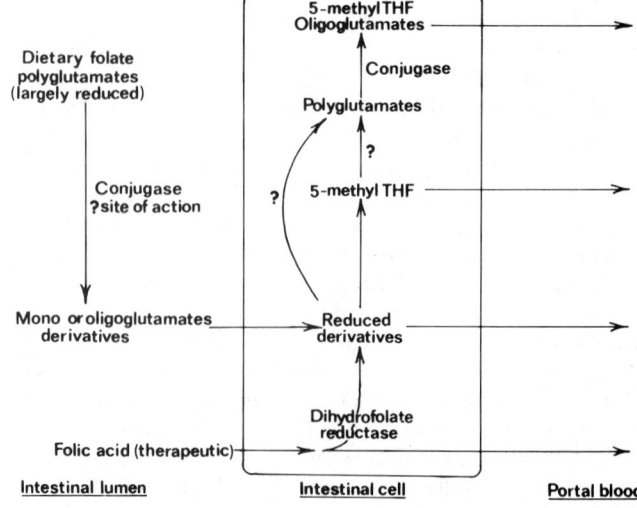

metabolism of folates within the intestinal cells of humans is required before we can interpret the mass of physiologic data that has been accumulated. Any realistic hypotheses explaining the changes in folate absorption that occur in certain disease states and in response to the administration of certain drugs will demand this basic information.

Transport

For many years, it has been generally accepted that folates are transported in the serum and other body fluids of mammals, either in the free form or in a loose association with albumin. Experiments by Johns et al. [120] indicated that over a range of plasma folate concentrations from 5 ng/ml to 3 μg/ml, approximately two-thirds of the folate is loosely bound to protein. Early attempts to identify a specific folate-binding protein (FABP) were unsuccessful. In 1967 Ghitis [121] isolated a specific FABP in cow's milk, which others have shown to be a minor component of the β-lactoglobulin fraction [122]. Since then, a human serum FABP has been identified. It is normally present at very low levels but increases markedly in severe folate deficiency, although it does not change in cobalamin deficiency [123]. Kamen and Caston [124] have demonstrated the presence of large quantities of folate-binding protein (MW 40,000) with a high affinity for 5-methyl THF in human umbilical cord serum. This observation is consistent with the hypothesis proposed for the preferential uptake of folate derivatives by the fetus.

Waxman [125] has summarized the current views on the status of FABP in human beings. The protein, which has a molecular weight of approximately 25,000, is present in much higher levels in human milk than in serum. It has been proposed that it is a glycoprotein containing sialic acid and is membrane bound. This results in the high concentration in milk, which is an apocrine secretion. The binding of folic acid depends on pH and ionic strength. Folic acid bound to the protein is not available for uptake by HeLa cells or by bacteria such as *L. casei*. Furthermore, protein-bound folic acid polyglutamates are not hydrolyzed by conjugase. Goat's milk has approximately 10 times as much FABP as human milk (700 pg folic acid bound per milligram of protein) and about 3 times as much as bovine milk. This may well account for the relatively low estimates, based on bioassays, of folic acid in goat's milk and for the occasional development of folate deficiency in certain infants fed on goat's milk.

Unfortunately, data for the binding of natural folate derivatives by FABP are still sparse, although the derivatives do not appear to have as high an affinity for the protein. FABP does, however, strongly bind polyglutamates of folic acid. It is still not clear what role FABP serves in overall folate metabolism; Colman and Herbert have suggested that there is in fact a heterogeneous group of serum FABPs [126].

Tissue Uptake

Parenterally and orally administered radiolabeled folates are rapidly cleared from the serum to the tissues. The mechanisms for this rapid clearance are still obscure. The high concentration of folate derivatives in human bile suggests an enterohepatic circulation [127]. Studies in the rat using both folic acid and 5-methyl THF confirmed that both oral and parenteral

folates are rapidly taken up initially by the liver and participate in an enterohepatic cycle [128]. The interpretations of the data from these latter experiments should be regarded with caution.

Two classes of cellular FABPs have been isolated. One group, the membrane-associated proteins, are presumably involved in transport. They have been isolated from the small intestine [115, 116] and the choroid plexus [129]. Another group of three FABPs, one of which is dihydrofolate reductase, has been detected in rat liver cytosol [130], while another, identified as dimethylglycine dehydrogenase, has been purified from rat liver mitochondria [131]. The role played by any of these molecules in cellular folate uptake is unknown.

Goldman [132, 133] has performed extensive studies on the transport of methotrexate and the natural folates by L1210 murine leukemia cells, Ehrlich ascites tumor cells, and rabbit reticulocytes. Both types of tumor cell have a special active transport carrier system for methotrexate. This transport system is shared, at least in part, by the natural folate derivatives and has a high affinity for the principal serum folate, 5-methyl THF. The affinity is lowest for folic acid. The analysis of the transport of folates is complicated by their incorporation into metabolic pathways. Methotrexate is not significantly metabolized, and its highly specific binding to dihydrofolate reductase makes it an ideal agent for short-term unidirectional influx studies.

Henderson et al. have isolated a binding component on the external surface of L1210 cells which has a high affinity for 5-methyl THF ($K_D = 0.11$ μM) [134]. There are approximately 8×10^4 binding sites per cell, and they participate in the high-affinity transport system for both 5-methyl THF and methotrexate.

A high-affinity, saturable, energy-dependent mechanism for the uptake of 5-methyl THF has also been demonstrated in mitogen-stimulated lymphocytes [135], human bone marrow cells [136], human erythrocytes [137], and rat hepatocytes [138]. This mechanism appears to differ from a carrier-mediated system for the transport of folic acid and from a low-affinity, passive "diffusion" system available to various folate derivatives.

The higher concentrations of 5-methyl THF in the cerebrospinal fluid compared with those in serum [139], the selective conservation of folates by the central nervous system [140], and the association of neuropsychiatric disorders with disturbances of folate coenzyme metabolism [141, 142] indicate an essential role for these compounds in neural metabolism. The first two of these observations suggest a homeostatic mechanism for the maintenance of cerebrospinal fluid concentration, perhaps involving a selective transport mechanism at the blood-brain barrier.

Levitt et al. [143], using intravenous injections of radioactive, double-labeled 5-methyl THF and 5-formyl THF, studied their equilibrium between serum and cerebrospinal fluid and identified the derivatives accumulated in the spinal fluid. They concluded that 5-methyl THF is preferentially absorbed into the spinal fluid and that other folate derivatives are converted to this derivative prior to their uptake. Their failure to demonstrate a transfer of folic acid was consistent with very low levels of the enzyme dihydrofolate reductase in the central nervous system, which would preclude the utilization of nonreduced derivatives.

The choroid plexus of the rabbit [144] and the hog [145] has a mechanism for the transport of folates. The process is energy dependent, and its existence has been supported by the isolation of an FABP from the cell membranes of the choroid plexus of the rabbit [129].

Folate Excretion

Folate derivatives are removed primarily by renal excretion. Nixon and Bertino [146], in a series of experiments with radio-labeled 5-formyl and 5-methyl THF on a human subject, showed that the urinary excretion of 5-methyl THF was directly related to the serum level, while 5-formyl THF was excreted even when it could not be detected in the serum. The excretion of compounds identified as either 10-formyl THF or 5,10-methenyl THF appeared to be fairly constant and again unrelated to serum levels.

Studies on urinary folate excretion in the rat [105] showed that these were largely 5-methyl THF, with a significant proportion of 5-formyl THF. This latter derivative was not a significant folate in either liver or kidney tissues, and the data therefore indicated its preferential excretion. Both these studies suggested that the kidney serves both a regulatory and metabolic role in folate excretion.

The preferential uptake of folate by the fetus, even in the face of folate depletion of the mother, is probably related to a selective transport system or to a high-capacity, high-affinity fetal FABP. No data are available to clarify this phenomenon, the implications of which will be discussed in the next section. Studies in the rat have shown that folate derivatives are catabolized initially by cleaveage of the C-9—N-10 bond to yield a group of pteridines which are retained by the liver and p-aminobenzoyl-1 glutamate, which is ultimately excreted in the urine as acetamidobenzoyl glutamate [60].

FOLATE DEFICIENCY

The causes, effects, and detection of folate deficiency in human beings and experimental animals have been extensively reviewed [147, 148]. Only primates and the guinea pig develop megaloblastic anemia following the exclusion of folate from the diet. Other mammals, such as the rat, require the administration of an intestinal antiseptic or a folate antagonist such as methotrexate to produce symptoms of folate deficiency, and then they usually do not develop megaloblastosis, even when they develop severe leukopenia [148]. Herbert [149] has summarized the causes of folate deficiency in humans in terms of the five basic reasons for nutrient deficiency—inadequate ingestion, absorption, or utilization and increased excretion or requirements.

The progressive clinical effects of dietary folate deficiency in an otherwise healthy adult male have been described in Herbert's classic study [150]. In this study, the peripheral blood and bone marrow changes which occurred after 4 months were preceded much earlier by a fall in serum folate and a rise in urinary formiminoglutamic acid levels. Psychological and mental changes followed but were rapidly reversed by folic acid supplementation.

The basic problem in the diagnosis of folate deficiency is that there is no adequate single test for body folate depletion. Whereas the pathologic findings referred to above are usually clear-cut in persons with severe folate depletion, the data are not as readily interpretable in early or borderline cases. Certain clinical situations, such as chronic alcoholism, should alert the clinician to the possibility of folate deficiency, but it is difficult to detect in the otherwise well patient. This applies particularly to the problem of folate deficiency in pregnancy, which not only is important in tropical countries but is becoming increasingly prevalent in highly industrialized Western societies. An incidence of 50 percent has been estimated in pregnant women from groups whose diets consist exclusively of finely divided, well-boiled foods. The worldwide incidence of folate deficiency approaches one-third of all pregnant women [151].

Reynolds et al. [152] have suggested that organic brain disease, more severe than the reversible behavioral disturbances described above, may result from folate deficiency secondary to drug administration and that these disturbances are independent of the degree of anemia or the presence of alcoholism. The major problem in assessing data of this type procured from hospital in-patients with severe neurologic disorders is that the sequence of cause and effect is often difficult to establish. Nevertheless, the possible production, by long-term anticonvulsant therapy, of folate deficiency and secondary intellectual damage demands the careful evaluation of such therapy, particularly in young children and during pregnancy.

Apart from anticonvulsants such as diphenylhydantoin and the barbiturates, a number of other drugs, such as the oral contraceptive agents and cycloserine, have been associated with impaired absorption or utilization of folates. The mechanism for their action is obscure, although it does not appear that they inhibit the enzyme conjugase in the intestine. Widespread use of these drugs and others which are specific "antifolates," i.e., which exert their pharmacologic effects by the inhibition of the enzyme dihydrofolate reductase (methotrexate, trimethoprim, and triamterene), increases the incidence of iatrogenic folate deficiency [153].

The folate deficiency of pregnancy is multifactorial in origin. It results from an inadequate diet compounded by anorexia and attempts to avoid weight gain and the demands of the growing fetus, particularly in the third trimester. In the last trimester, the quantity of folates required for growth is maximal, not ony because of the size of the fetus but also because the fetus accumulates folate stores for early postnatal life. Nelson and her colleagues [154] have shown that fetal development in the rat is severely affected by brief periods of folate deficiency in the second week of gestation and that such deficiency may result in multiple congenital anomalies or death. It is not clear that maternal folate deficiency will produce any overt effects on the human fetus. The fetus appears to be able to acquire folate at maternal expense, even though maternal stores may be limited. The report of Stone et al. [155] of excessive formiminoglutamic acid excretion in five infants born to folate-deficient mothers and in one infant born with folate-responsive megaloblastosis indicates that a more thorough examination should be made of this clinical situation.

Hibbard and Hibbard [156] have suggested that congenital malformations, particularly facial clefts and neural tube defects, are twice as common in the children of women with impaired folate metabolism compared with the general population. This has been disputed by Hall [157], who studied the folate status of the mothers in early pregnancy when organogenesis was occurring. There is adequate evidence that the antifolate drugs referred to above should be avoided during early pregnancy. The potent drugs, such as methotrexate, can produce either abortion or severe congenital malformation, both in humans [158] and in experimental animals [159]. Shaw [160] has published a follow-up on a child born to a mother who had ingested aminopterin from day 55 to day 58 of her pregnancy [161]. At birth, this infant had numerous skeletal defects similar to those in a patient reported by Warkany et al. [162] and was given a poor prognosis for physical and mental development. At the age of 9 years she still had some growth retardation and skeletal deformation, particularly of the skull, but her mental and social development was normal.

Serum and red cell folate levels are high in full-term newborn infants but fall rapidly to adult levels over the first 3 months of life. In premature babies, the initial levels are low and drop to folate-deficient adult levels within 4 to 6 weeks. This is presumed to be the result of a relatively accelerated growth rate and consequent depletion of maternally derived folate stores normally acquired in the last trimester. Premature infants also appear to have a failure of the renal tubular conservation of folate, and their urinary folate loss, on a surface area basis, is eight times that of an adult [163]. This precarious folate status may be exacerbated by problems such as respiratory distress syndrome. Accordingly, routine dietary folate supplementation has been recommended by some authorities [164]. Studies on folate-deficient infants have demonstrated structural and functional abnormalities of the small intestine, confirming studies previously performed on adults [165]. These abnormalities resulted in chronic diarrhea and failure to thrive.

INTERACTION OF COBALAMIN AND FOLATES

Although cobalamin metabolism is covered extensively in Chap. 23 (which see), no discussion of folate metabolism can be complete without a consideration of the interaction of cobalamin and folates. The intensive research in this area, particularly over the past 20 years, has resulted in a significant understanding of the metabolism of folates, cobalamin, amino acids (especially homocysteine and methionine), and nucleic acids in mammals. The single known point of interaction

between folates and cobalamin is shown in Fig. 24-5 and is the transfer of the 5-methyl group from 5-methyl THF to homocysteine to produce methionine (reaction 8, Fig. 24-3), a transfer catalyzed by the cobalamin enzyme tetrahydrofolate methyltransferase.

Many years ago, it was observed that the megaloblastic anemia resulting from cobalamin deficiency secondary to intrinsic factor deficiency in humans could be corrected by pharmacologic doses of folic acid. The *methyl trap hypothesis* was put forward to account for this observation [166, 167]. The neurologic disturbances produced by cobalamin deficiency and often exacerbated by folic acid therapy indicated the existence of a different cobalamin-mediated reaction essential for nervous system metabolism which could perhaps be secondarily influenced by large amounts of folic acid. The basis for the hypothesis was that the demethylation of the predominant natural derivative 5-methyl THF is the only known mechanism available for the supply of the other reduced cell folates necessary for purine and pyrimidine biosynthesis, since the methylene THF reductase reaction is essentially irreversible. A defect in the function of the methyltransferase would result initially in an accumulation of 5-methyl THF in serum and tissues, i.e., reduced folates are trapped as a functionally "dead-end" derivative, and the individual becomes effectively folate deficient. Megaloblastosis was considered to result primarily from a consequent failure of dTMP synthesis. Large doses of folic acid or 5-formyl THF (folinic acid) could overcome the trapping effect by supplying the other reduced natural folates, thereby relieving the megaloblastosis.

This hypothesis was reviewed by Nixon and Bertino in 1970 [168] and more recently by Nixon [169]. Since then, a number of other significant observations have been made which justify another review. Not only are the data acquired in attempts to prove or disprove the hypothesis important to our understanding of the pathogenesis of the megaloblastic anemias, but they have contributed significantly to our understanding of mammalian 1-carbon metabolism.

A number of points need to be made preliminary to any discussion of the methyl trap hypothesis. The hypothesis was initially invoked to explain the folate deficiency of human cobalamin deficiency. Unfortunately, there is no animal model equivalent to the human disease. Two mammals, the rat and the sheep, have been generally used in studies on folic acid and

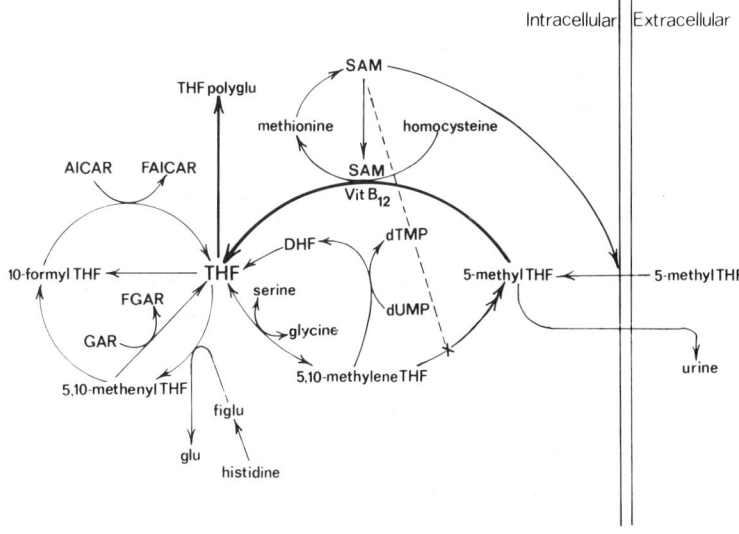

Figure 24-5 Interconversion of the folate coenzymes, emphasizing (1) the critical role served by the cobalamin-dependent demethylation of the predominant tissue fluid folate, 5-methyl THF, in controlling the flux of reduced folate derivatives into the folate pathways; (2) the limitation of folate polyglutamate synthesis if this critical mechanism is disturbed and THF is the required substrate for polyglutamate synthetase; (3) the possible regulatory role of SAM in facilitating cell membrane transport for a wide variety of metabolites, including 5-methyl THF; (4) the regulatory role of SAM in (a) maintaining activity of THF methyltransferase and (b) regulating its own synthesis via methionine by allosteric inhibition of methylene THF reductase.

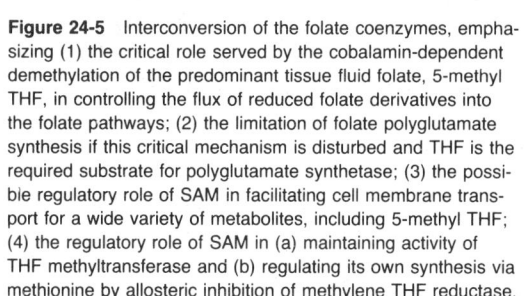

cobalamin metabolism. Cobalamin deficiency can be produced in rats by feeding them vegetable protein diets, but no hematologic changes are observed unless the dams of the experimental animals have also been maintained on a deficient diet. Even then megaloblastosis does not occur, but only anemia and leukopenia [148]. The major effect on the weanling offspring is reduced growth rate.

Cobalamin deficiency occurs in sheep maintained on cobalt-deficient diets. This results in a loss of appetite and a reduced growth rate, with eventual weight loss, severe anemia, and death. The anemia is not megaloblastic and does not respond to large doses of folic acid. It appears that sheep have a much higher cobalamin requirement than other animals [148].

The other major feature of cobalamin deficiency in humans is demyelination of the central nervous system, affecting predominantly the posterior and lateral columns of the spinal cord. Primates had been reported as developing "cage paralysis" on cobalamin-deficient diets [170], but more recent studies have failed to confirm this [171, 172]. No other mammals develop specific neurologic damage as a result of cobalamin deficiency. The cobalamin-deficient Egyptian fruit bat has been shown to develop spinal cord changes similar to those in humans [173], but no hematologic abnormalities were observed.

It appears that human metabolism may be significantly different in cobalamin–folic acid biochemistry than that of the widely used experimental animals. Accordingly, the application of animal data to the human situation may not be entirely relevant. Another consideration in assessing animal data is that the specific dietary deprivation has often been instituted at a very early age through the phases of rapid growth and maturation. The response in the developing animal may be quite different from that of the mature adult.

Many of the physiologic studies that have been performed on both humans and animals in order to gain information on events at a cellular level have utilized pharmacologic rather than physiologic doses of folic acid and its derivatives. In addition, the use of folic acid, an unnatural compound which is not efficiently handled by metabolic pathways, makes the data even more difficult to interpret. These problems are compounded by those of isotope purity, since most of the supposedly pure commercial folate preparations contain at least 10 to 15 percent of radiochemical impurities, which are often impossible to identify, and even purified materials deteriorate rapidly unless stored dry below $-60°C$. Furthermore, isotope exchange takes place from the highly specific-radioactivity tritium-labeled folates such as $(3',5',9-^3H)$ folic acid.

According to the methyl trap hypothesis, (1) 5-methyl THF is converted to other folate derivatives only by the cobalamin-dependent methyltransferase reaction, and the activity of the enzyme is significantly decreased in cobalamin deficiency; (2) the utilization of 5-methyl THF for methionine biosynthesis is decreased secondary to this loss of activity; (3) the total body pool of folates becomes predominantly 5-methyl THF; (4) the decreased availability of the other reduced folate derivatives slows the rates of the reactions for which they are essential cofactors, i.e., the rates of purine, pyrimidine, and consequently nucleic acid synthesis; and (5) the impairment of DNA synthesis results in megaloblastosis.

Studies by Taylor et al. [174] on extracts of human bone marrow have illustrated that the synthesis of methionine from 5-methyl THF and homocysteine is a reaction which requires both a flavin-reducing system and S-adenosyl methionine. No requirement for added cobalamin was found in normal bone marrow extracts in vitro. In cobalamin-deficient megaloblastic bone marrow extracts, the very low rate of methionine synthesis was stimulated eightfold by added cobalamin, reaching a level identical to that obtained in assays of the bone marrow taken from the same patient after 2 weeks of parenteral cobalamin therapy. These data do not preclude the existence of a noncobalamin pathway, as in bacteria, but they suggest that if present, it must be a subordinate reaction.

Lavoie et al. [53] demonstrated that the transfer of the methyl group from 5-[^{14}C]methyl THF to nonfolate compounds was greatly reduced in PHA-stimulated lymphocytes from patients with pernicious anemia. The addition of cobalamin to the incubation medium restored the rate of transfer of the methyl group to normal. A mixture of the active and inactive diastereoisomers of 5-methyl THF was used in these experiments, but the possibility of cobalamin's acting by selectively influencing the transport of the active isomer was discounted on the basis that the absolute radioactivity, recovered from the cells as folate, fell in response to cobalamin. Nixon and Bertino [175] undertook similar studies on nucleated bone marrow cells from a patient with pernicious anemia before and after therapy but employed the double-labeled natural isomer of 5-[^{14}C]methyl-^{3}H THF. The uptake of the isotope was considerably decreased, and no transfer of the methyl group to nonfolate compounds was detected in the megaloblastic cells. Analysis of the intracellular folates confirmed that no other labeled folate derivatives were present. In contrast, normal cells showed a 22 percent transfer of the methyl group to nonfolate compounds over 15 min, while 50-min incubations showed a significant (10 percent) content of labeled 10-formyl or 5,10-methenyl THF. A similar result was obtained with the patient's marrow cells following cobalamin therapy.

In summary, with respect to the first requirement of the hypothesis, it appears that cobalamin deficiency produces a decrease in the methyltransferase activity of a number of species, including humans. This activity can be restored by the addition of cobalamin to the assay in vitro and by cobalamin therapy of the affected patient. No firm evidence has been produced that a cobalamin-independent reaction takes place in mammals, although this has not been fully examined in humans.

In the studies by Lavoie et al. [53] and Nixon and Bertino [175], attention was given to the utilization of the methyl groups of 5-methyl THF in cobalamin-deficient human cells. No direct measurements of the incorporation into methionine were made, but the incorporation of methyl groups into protein (presumably via methionine) was significantly reduced in cobalamin-deficient lymphocytes [53]. Further direct studies are required to established this point fully.

The prediction that a methyltransferase block should lead to an expanded body pool of 5-methyl THF, both absolutely and relative to the other reduced folate derivatives, is difficult to prove because the bulk of the body folates is already largely 5-methyl THF (as polyglutamate derivatives). Admittedly, serum folate is almost entirely in monoglutamate form, but this level can be regulated by renal mechanisms. The supposed intracellular "accumulation" of 5-methyl THF was presumed to result in a decreased clearance of this derivative from the serum; this has been convincingly confirmed by Nixon and Bertino [175] using physiologic doses of the active isomer in cobalamin-deficient patients. The interpretation of the data, however, is not so simple, because it may be that both cobalamin and methionine (or more likely, the derivative S-adenosylmethionine) have a direct or indirect role in cell transport mechanisms for folate. SAM has been shown to be important for the transport of certain amino acids and sugars into E. coli [176] and may serve a similar role in mammalian cell transport. The rapid clearance of folic acid from the serum in both normal and cobalamin-deficient patients emphasizes that it is a nonphysiologic compound.

Furthermore, mature red cells from pernicious anemia patients contain an increased ratio of short-chain to long-chain folate polyglutamates [177]. This implies a failure of polyglutamate biosynthesis, and this could reflect a failure of demethylation, as a result of which the true substrate of polyglutamate biosynthesis, THF, is no longer available. Accordingly, a short-term accumulation of 5-methyl THF inside the cell may result in its combining with or its delayed release from the membrane carrier, causing a decreased rate of uptake. As mammalian cells appear to contain very small quantities of folate monoglutamates, it is likely that they are cleared from the cell if not incorporated into polyglutamates. These experiments have not been done.

The net result of all these processes will be a decreased tissue folate level, as has been shown in the livers of experimental animals [178, 179]. Although decreased intracellular folate levels have been reported in human erythrocytes [180], no studies have been reported on human liver. The animal studies also demonstrated an excess of methylated compared with formylated folate derivatives. The sheep studies [179] were later modified [181] to avoid effects due to severe protein-calorie malnutrition, and a more complex pattern of the tissue folate profile emerged. These results did not really alter our current analysis of the methyl trap hypothesis.

The decreased availability of other essential folate coenzymes and the consequent slowing of the various associated enzyme reactions have been studied indirectly in human beings. Formiminoglutamic acid (FIGLU) excretion in the urine is increased in folate deficiency (particularly following a histidine load), reflecting a decreased availability of THF as a 1-carbon trap in histidine catabolism. Similar observations have been made in cobalamin deficiency states in humans and animals. The high rate of FIGLU excretion in cobalamin deficiency has been reduced by the administration of folate, methionine, or glycine, but the effect is variable [182].

De Grazia et al. [183] have shown that the oxidation of the β carbon of serine to carbon dioxide is reduced both in folate deficiency and in pernicious anemia. This release of carbon dioxide is dependent upon the function of serine transhydroxymethylase and the availability of THF. Similarly, the incorporation of formate into serine by lymphocytes of cobalamin-deficient patients is significantly diminished [184].

Thymidylate (dTMP) biosynthesis does not take place to any significant extent in normal liver but may be studied in bone marrow aspirates and PHA-stimulated lymphocytes by measuring the incorporation of radioactive dUMP into dTMP. Synthesis of dTMP is greatly decreased in folate- or cobalamin-deficient cells [185, 187]. In folate-deficient cells, dTMP synthesis is increased by the addition of folic acid, 5-methyl THF, and homocysteine (but not cobalamin) to the incubation medium. Correction of the defect in cobalamin-deficient cells was achieved with methylcobalamin; partial correction was produced by folic acid, cobalamin, and homocysteine, but not by 5-methyl THF. Methionine significantly decreased dTMP synthesis even further in both deficiency states [185, 188]. These studies indicated a deficiency of 5,10-methylene THF in both bone marrow cells and lymphocytes of folate-deficient and cobalamin-deficient patients. As a consequence, synthesis of dTMP and secondarily of DNA is impaired, with the result that megaloblastic cells are produced which do not mature normally, although the DNA base composition is normal [189].

One of the inconsistencies of these studies relates to the effect of methionine in cobalamin deficiency. In cobalamin-deficient rats [178] and sheep [181], methionine restored the depleted liver folates and also increased the short-term uptake of folates [181]. One of the effects of methionine may well result from its conversion to S-adenosylmethionine, an allosteric inhibitor of 5,10-methylene THF reductase, which would modify the diversion of folates into 5-methyl THF. SAM is important for transport functions in E. coli, and many of the effects of methionine could be explained by a similar effect on mammalian cells. Methionine depresses the dTMP synthesis in pernicious anemia patients while exacerbating the megaloblastosis [190] and reducing urinary FIGLU excretion [191].

The role of methionine in cell growth and metabolism is complex. It is an essential requirement for many mammalian cells in culture, but it can be replaced in baby hamster kidney cells by homocysteine and cobalamin provided the folic acid concentration of the culture medium is raised to 100 μM [192].

In recent years, the nitrous oxide-treated animal has been used extensively as a model for human vitamin B_{12} deficiency. Data acquired from extensive studies on these animals have been combined with other data derived from both human and animal studies in an attempt to refute the methyl trap hypothesis [193]. The extent of the metabolic effects of exposure of these animals to nitrous oxide is unknown. They may not be valid model systems, since the biochemical pathology of human vitamin B_{12} deficiency is apparently unique.

The data relating to the methyl trap hypothesis are summarized in Fig. 24-6. The original hypothesis has had to be greatly expanded. A major stumbling block to acceptance of the hypothesis in humans has been the identification of a hereditary deficiency of methyltransferase activity. In the first patient described [194], the activity of the hepatic enzyme was reduced to one-third of control levels and was associated with high serum and red cell folate levels and megaloblastosis. Three patients were later described [195, 196] with defective cobalamin metabolism [197]. As expected, these patients had widespread metabolic defects but were not anemic or megaloblastic, despite significant reduction in methyltransferase activity. In a more recent instance, a child suffered from an unusual relapsing megaloblastic anemia, which was found on autopsy to be associated with subacute combined degeneration of the spinal cord [198]. These findings indicate that the trap hypothesis is insufficient to explain cobalamin-deficient megaloblastosis and that there are other as yet unknown functions of cobalamin coenzymes in mammalian tissues.

INBORN ERRORS OF FOLATE METABOLISM

Although a number of defects of folate metabolism have been described in bacteria, yeast, and cultured mammalian cells, this discussion will be concerned with those disorders described in

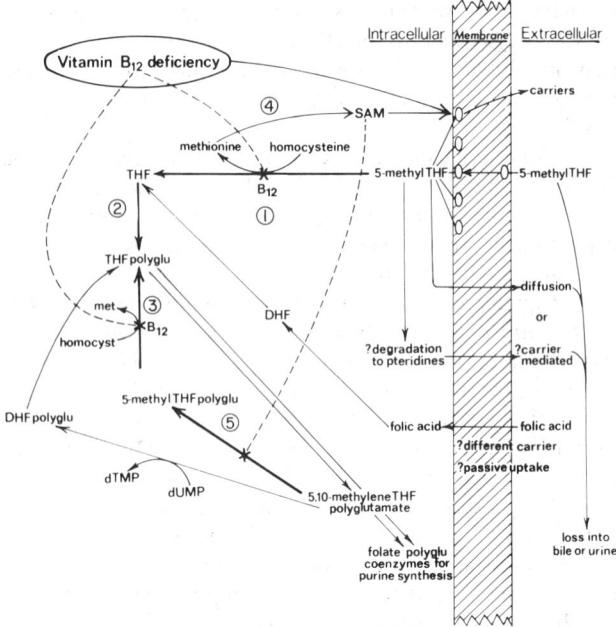

Figure 24-6 Diagrammatic representation of the extended implications of the methyl trap hypothesis. Cobalamin deficiency results in (1) a decreased rate of demethylation of 5-methyl THF (reaction 1), the predominant tissue fluid folate. This results in decreased availability of THF for polyglu biosynthesis (reaction 2) and, consequently, in reduced amounts of other essential folate derivatives. In addition, failure of demethylation at the polyglutamate level (reaction 3) results in an accumulation of 5-methyl THF polyglu. (2) The initial rise in the cellular concentration of 5-methyl THF, producing a reduced rate of uptake of this derivative by preventing the release of carriers from the internal surface of the cell membrane. The 5-methyl THF level reaches an equilibrium level in the cell which is maintained by exchange with the extracellular fluids or by degradation and removal of pteridine products (3), SAM levels falling secondary to the decreased rate of methionine synthesis (reactions 1 and 4). This results in a loss of feedback inhibition of methylene THF reductase (reaction 5), a decreased activation of THF methyltransferase (reactions 1 and 3), and possibly a direct effect on cellular transport systems (which may also be mediated via another effect of cobalamin deficiency, viz., abnormal membrane lipids). Folic acid uptake is not affected, but its potential effect is limited by the enzymatic reducing capacity of the cell. Only pharmacologic doses effectively reach such organs as the liver and bone marrow, since physiologic doses are probably converted to 5-methyl THF in the intestine.

human beings. They will be considered under the following headings:

1. Congenital defect of folate absorption
2. Dihydrofolate reductase deficiency
3. "Formiminotransferase" deficiency syndromes
4. Methylene THF reductase deficiency
5. Tetrahydrofolate methyltransferase deficiency

Congenital Defects of Folate Absorption

Three clinical syndromes have been reported resulting from intestinal defects in absorption of folate. In 1961 Luhby and colleagues [199] described a child suffering from megaloblastic anemia at age 3 months. After an initial hematologic response to parenteral folic acid, she relapsed at age 9 months and again at 15 months because of a failure to continue large oral doses of folic acid. Absorption studies at 3 years of age demonstrated a specific defect in uptake of folate from the intestine, with no abnormalities in absorption of fat, glucose, or vitamin A. Later, these authors described a female sib with the same dis-

order; at this time, both children had megaloblastic anemia, increased urinary formiminoglutamic acid, moderate physical and mental retardation, ataxia, and convulsions [200, 201]. Further investigation confirmed a specific defect in folate transport both across the intestinal wall and into the cerebrospinal fluid. Oral folic acid, 10 mg/day, produced a hematologic response in both children but failed to prevent progressive central nervous system deterioration.

The next patient, reported by Lanzkowsky et al. [142, 202], again presented at age 3 months with failure to thrive and a macrocytic megaloblastic anemia. After an initial blood transfusion and parenterally administered folic acid had produced a hematologic remission, the patient followed a relapsing course for several years, during which time a normal blood picture could be maintained only by 40 mg oral folic acid per day. At age 9 years she developed petit mal and occasional grand mal seizures. At age 20 years she presented with athetoid movements of the upper limbs without evidence of tremor, ataxia, or cerebellar disorder. She was profoundly retarded mentally. Investigation revealed punctate calcification of the basal ganglia and normal gastrointestinal structure and function as disclosed by radiologic studies, jejunal biopsy, and studies of absorption of fat, glucose, vitamin A, and cobalamin.

On withdrawal of folic acid supplements, this patient became sluggish and developed anorexia and ulceration of the buccal mucosa. Seizures became less frequent, with some improvement in electroencephalograms. The classic peripheral blood and bone marrow picture of severe megaloblastic anemia developed rapidly, and folates could not be detected in plasma, erythrocytes, or cerebrospinal fluid. Small (250-mg) oral doses of folic acid failed to produce a hematologic response, but this was achieved when the same dose was given intramuscularly. There was a marked rise in serum folate levels, but folate could not be detected in spinal fluid. The di- and triglutamate derivatives of folic acid, 5-methyl THF, and 5-formyl THF were not absorbed orally, although serum folate clearance after intravenous injection was normal. This patient was considered to have a specific defect of folate transport across the small intestine. Following the restoration of normal serum folate levels there was marked deterioration of the electroencephalogram, with increased seizure frequency. Seizure frequency had been reduced by folic acid therapy in Luhby's patients. This suggested a different clinical disorder.

The fourth patient was different from the others [203]. This child, born to first cousins, was apparently normal at birth but developed increasingly severe diarrhea from the age of 1 week. At age 3 months, she was failing to thrive and had a severe megaloblastic anemia. Oral folic acid, 15 mg/day, failed to produce clinical improvement, but a prompt hematologic and gastrointestinal response was obtained with the same dose given intramuscularly for 1 week. The growth rate remained satisfactory on this dose, given every 3 to 4 weeks, but cessation of therapy resulted in the development of anorexia, stomatitis, glossitis, and vulvovaginitis. Her mental development appeared to be normal, although she subsequently had some schooling difficulties.

She was fully investigated at the age of 11 years after being maintained on regular parenteral therapy since the age of 3 months. Oral therapy in doses up to 40 mg folic acid per day had proved ineffective. She was normal physically, and psychometric testing indicated an IQ of 90 with difficulties in abstract thinking. Results of biochemical and radiologic studies were normal, as was the electroencephalogram. Serum folate concentrations measured immediately prior to her routine therapy were 1.0 to 2.5 ng/ml; serum cobalamin levels and absorption of α-xylose and vitamin A were normal.

Folate absorption studies, using 5-mg doses of folic acid and 5-formyl THF and a 10-g dose of brewer's yeast, showed that minimal uptake occurred from the intestine. Increasing the dose of folic acid to 100 mg failed to produce a significant rise in serum folate levels. Similar studies on members of her family showed that her mother and her two brothers were normal, but results on her father, who was clinically well, fell into an intermediate range.

Plasma clearance of folic acid was normal following intravenous injection, although peak serum levels and urinary excretion were lower than in normal controls. These results may have reflected depleted body stores. This child is different from other patients reported, her failure to respond to very large oral doses of folic acid probably indicating a more severe absorptive defect.

These inborn errors of folate transport support the existence of specific carrier mechanisms both in small intestine and at the blood-brain barrier. The requirements for oral pharmacologic doses in the first two types and for parenteral therapy in the third suggest a degree of specificity for folic acid uptake and argue against the passive diffusion mechanism.

Dihydrofolate Reductase Deficiency

Three cases of this disorder have been reported, with the diagnosis based primarily on low hepatic levels of the key enzyme dihydrofolate reductase. Activity levels vary enormously in different mammalian tissues (see above) and although, in general terms, the highest levels are seen in actively dividing cells, this does not apply to lymphoblasts. The subsequent clinical course of all of these patients and later studies performed on cultured cells cast some doubt on the diagnosis of the basic enzyme defect.

In 1967 Walters [204] described a child, 6 weeks of age, with megaloblastic anemia. At age 3 years this patient had normal bone marrow. At age 7 years he had pancytopenia and megaloblastosis, with an elevated urinary FIGLU excretion. A Schilling test showed normal results but produced a hematologic response, followed by a relapse 3 months later. This patient responded to orally administered folic acid, 5 mg/day, and relapsed on cessation of therapy. Low (100-μg) doses of folic acid, given both orally and parenterally, did not induce a remission, but 100 μg 5-formyl THF was effective. Serum folate levels in relapse were normal, but a liver biopsy showed a reduction of dihydrofolate reductase activity to 35 percent of control values. The only clinical symptom was glossitis. Radiologic, biopsy, and absorption studies of the small intestine were normal. Erbe has discussed further studies on this patient [47], then 19 years old. He was only mildly retarded mentally but was incarcerated in a penitentiary because of "repeated episodes of sociopathic behavior." He was still folate dependent. Fibroblasts derived from skin biopsy specimens taken from this patient showed normal levels of dihydrofolate reductase activity and required normal levels of folic acid for growth. Enzyme kinetics were also normal.

Subsequently, Tauro et al. [205] described two patients with dihydrofolate reductase deficiency from two different families. The mutations appear to be different in each instance. The first patient was a female Caucasian infant delivered at 36 weeks'

gestation following an induced labor. The first child born to these healthy, unrelated parents had died at birth following a prolonged 43 weeks' gestation. The child had been pale and hydropic, but not jaundiced, and had a large spleen. The placenta was enlarged. No necropsy was performed.

The propositus weighed 2.36 kg, was pale, and had a large spleen. The placenta was enlarged (675 g). There was no jaundice, although the amniotic fluid had contained 15 mg per 100 ml bilirubin a week previously. Hemoglobin in cord blood was 9.8 g per 100 ml. The blood film showed a mixture of normochromic macrocytes and hypochromic microcytes. Serum folic acid, cobalamin, and iron levels were normal. No cause for a hemolytic anemia was detected, but the hemoglobin fell to 5.5 g per 100 ml by day 12, necessitating transfusion. By day 60, she was again severely anemic (2.4 g per 100 ml), with megaloblastosis. Treatment with oral folic acid, 2.5 mg/day, and cobalamin, 1000 ng/day, produced no effect, and she was again transfused. The hemoglobin level fell once more, and on day 97 a deoxyuridine suppression test indicated a severe folate deficiency which could be corrected only with reduced folate derivatives. The response clinically and hematologically to parenteral 5-formyl THF, 3 mg/day, was immediate. On day 130, a liver biopsy was performed. No dihydrofolate reductase activity was detectable in the routine assay, but normal levels (1.0 to 1.7 nmol dihydrofolate reduced per minute per milligram of protein) were found in the presence of 0.6 M KCl. Further studies were performed on the bone marrow at age 3 years. The specific activity of dihydrofolate reductase was reduced to 10 percent of control levels. The kinetic parameters and activation by KCl were identical to those of normal enzyme. The enzyme was extremely heat labile and had a molecular weight of 58,000, which was significantly different from that of normal enzyme [206].

Growth rate and hematologic status were normal with 5-formyl THF, 6 mg three times a week intramuscularly. Relapse followed a reduction in dosage and one attempt at oral therapy. At age $3\frac{1}{2}$ years the patient was normal physically but was mildly retarded mentally, extremely irritable, and subject to severe temper tantrums. This child is now 9 years old. She is severely intellectually retarded, although no specific neurologic deficit is present. For the past 2 years, she has been maintained on oral folic acid, 30 mg/day. At 15 mg/day, macrocytic changes appeared in the peripheral blood film. There is reportedly no defect in folate uptake in the intestine [207]. The definitive diagnosis has not yet been obtained.

The second patient was a male Caucasian infant, the fourth child of healthy, unrelated parents. Their first child, also a male, had died at age 6 months with pancytopenia and megaloblastosis. He had presented at the age of 10 days with oral moniliasis and megaloblastosis unrelieved by treatment with folic acid and cobalamin. A partial remission was achieved with four intramuscular doses of 5-formyl THF, but the child died following a smallpox vaccination. Two other sibs were healthy and hematologically normal.

The propositus was first seen at age 26 days because of oral and anal moniliasis and poor feeding. Investigation revealed a normal hemoglobin level but a low neutrophil count (480 per cubic millimeter) and low platelet count (45,000 per cubic millimeter). Over the following two weeks, the hemoglobin level fell to 7.4 g per 100 ml and the bone marrow became megaloblastic. The serum folate level, at 9.5 ng/ml, was borderline normal for his age; the serum cobalamin level was normal. A deoxyuridine suppression test showed a folate deficiency correctable with reduced folates, although correction was not attempted by normal serum with added cobalamin. Assay of liver biopsy material disclosed dihydrofolate reductase activity of 0.27 nmol/min per milligram of protein, which increased to only 0.49 with the addition of 0.6 M KCl. The child responded to daily intramuscular doses of 6 mg 5-formyl THF. At age 1 year he was physically, mentally, and hematologically normal. The subsequent course of this child has been discussed by Erbe [47]. Based on the clinical observations, the response during a hematologic relapse to high-dose cobalamin therapy, and the presence of normal enzyme levels in cultured fibroblasts, a diagnosis of transcobalamin II deficiency has been proposed. Publication of the details of the later studies would be helpful. The immunologic studies necessary for a diagnosis such as transcobalamin II deficiency would be of interest.

The enzyme assays indicated that the defect was different in these two children. The first child had no activity in the usual assay system but normal activity in the presence of high potassium concentrations. The second child demonstrated an activity equivalent to that in the case described by Walters but showed some cation activation.

These findings, together with the different modes of clinical presentation, suggest that all three patients represent different mutations. The efficacy of 5-formyl THF therapy is to be expected, as it bypasses the site of the enzyme block. The therapy is in effect a permanent leucovorin rescue as applied to methotrexate chemotherapy. It is difficult to understand why oral therapy was not effective initially in the latter two patients, since 5-formyl THF is normally effectively absorbed by the intestine [146]. It is possible that this outcome was related to fairly specific problems in the folate transport system secondary to the primary disorder and that these were corrected by overcoming the primary reduced folate deficiency.

The defect in the first child described by Tauro et al. [205] is probably the most severe, as indicated by early presentation and the stillbirth of her sib. The occurrence of two probable cases in each of two families suggests autosomal recessive inheritance.

It is most important that these cases be studied in more detail. They could provide key information concerning the role of dihydrofolate reductase in human biology.

"Formiminotransferase" Deficiency Syndromes

The patients reported as having formiminotransferase deficiency almost certainly have defects in two different enzymes in the histidine catabolic pathway and represent two contrasting clinical syndromes. There is good reason to suspect that the first patients described have defects in the associated enzyme cyclodeaminase.

Since 1963, Arakawa and his associates [208, 209] have described five definite instances of a disorder characterized by mental and physical retardation, cortical atrophy with dilatation of the cerebral ventricles, abnormal electroencephalograms, and increased urinary FIGLU excretion after an oral histidine load in spite of abnormally high serum folate and normal serum cobalamin levels. All but one, identified in an adult psychiatric institution (and who, incidentally, had normal serum folate levels) at the age of 21 years, had had signs and symptoms in the first 18 months of life. Only one child had evidence of definite folate-responsive megaloblastic anemia.

Enzyme assays carried out on liver biopsy material from each patient indicated a significant reduction in formiminotransferase activity ranging from 14 to 50 percent of control values. There was no correlation between the levels of enzyme activity and urinary FIGLU excretion. This group reported another patient [210] who appeared to be clinically similar to the others but in whom reduced enzyme activity was demonstrated only in erythrocytes.

Three other groups have reported patients who are clinically and biochemically distinct from the first group but excreted huge quantities of FIGLU in the urine. No hepatic enzyme assays have been performed, but the patients of these two groups are presumed to have deficiencies of formiminotransferase.

Niederwieser et al. [211] described two sisters who excreted approximately 0.5 g FIGLU in the urine per day (normal, 0 to 7.5 mg) on ordinary diets. Both children were physically normal. The elder sister, who was initially investigated at age 5 years because of slow speech development, had an IQ (Kramer) of 0.58, which had increased, with the aid of special schooling, to 0.83 at age 7 years. Her sister, younger by 2 years, is intellectually normal. Extensive biochemical studies failed to detect any condition known to be associated with excessive FIGLU excretion. Serum folate and cobalamin levels were normal, and the excretion of FIGLU was not affected by large doses of folic acid or cobalamin or by serine or glycine loading. FIGLU excretion was reduced by a low histidine diet; it increased markedly with histidine loading. Hematologic findings were normal. FIGLU excretion with and without a histidine load was normal in both parents and three sibs.

Two similar patients, brother and sister, were described by Perry et al. [212]. These children excreted similar quantities of FIGLU in the urine. The younger child, a 3¼-year-old male, was one SD below the mean for height and weight; his head circumference was one SD above the mean. His IQ evaluation was normal. He exhibited generalized hypotonia, clumsiness, a wide-based gait, and delayed speech development. The electroencephalogram was normal. An 8-year-old sister was also hypotonic and clumsy, with delayed speech and reading development which had affected her progress at school, but she was not considered to be mentally retarded. The electroencephalogram was diffusely abnormal.

Serum folate levels and hematologic studies were normal. Unlike the previous two children, these patients showed a 75 percent decrease in FIGLU excretion resulting from folate loading: in one child, oral folic acid, 5 mg every 8 h for 3 days; and in the other, 6 mg 5-formyl THF intramuscularly for 3 days. A younger, otherwise normal sister demonstrated mild microcephaly. The mother had had delayed speech development, while a maternal aunt was profoundly mentally retarded. FIGLU excretion, with and without a histidine load, was normal in both parents. Perry et al. doubted any connection between the metabolic disorders and what they considered to be mild cerebral dysfunction, but in the light of Niederwieser's findings, this conclusion may not be justified.

Another patient studied by Russell et al. [213] appears to be similar to although more severely affected than these latter cases. This 7-year-old boy exhibited hyperkinetic behavior associated with a diffusely abnormal electroencephalogram and retarded speech development. The biochemical findings were significantly different. Apart from massive FIGLU excretion, histidinemia, hypomethioninemia, and moderate histidinuria were found together with the urinary excretion of the histidine dipeptides carnosine and anserine. Hepatic formimi-notransferase activity was completely absent. Serum folate and vitamin B_{12} levels were normal. Short-term treatment with oral methionine in doses of 6 to 9 g/day resulted in a 50 percent decrease in FIGLU excretion, although no observations were made on the effect on the low serum methionine. Long-term treatment (6 months) led to improvement in the neurologic signs, but no assessment of the electroencephalogram was reported.

The patients described by Niederwieser et al., Perry et al., and Russell et al. represent closely related genetic defects and result from a severe deficiency of formiminotransferase activity which causes the excretion of massive quantities of FIGLU. The disorder of formiminotransferase deficiency, as exempli-fied by these patients, is best considered as a histidine catabolic defect without any serious secondary effects on folate metab-olism. The response of Perry's patients to folate loading with a decrease in FIGLU excretion suggests that the enzyme muta-tion has resulted in a high K_m for its substrate THF. Nieder-wieser's patients suggest a different type of mutation.

The case of Russell et al. may be yet another variant in that the different biochemical sequelae appear to result from *total* loss of enzyme activity. None of the proposals [213] for a mechanism of production of (1) the low serum methionine lev-els and (2) the lowered urinary FIGLU excretion by oral methi-onine is consistent with our current understanding of human 1-carbon metabolism.

The patients described by Arakawa's group are different, both clinically and biochemically. These patients have a se-verely disabling disease with a probable disruption of folate metabolism reflected in (1) high serum folate concentrations and abnormal FIGLU excretion, and (2) a cerebral disorder resembling that observed in the offspring of pregnant rats ren-dered folate deficient or treated with dihydrofolate reductase inhibitors such as methotrexate. FIGLU excretion was rela-tively low compared with that of the other patients and reached significantly abnormal levels only with a histidine load. Although direct assays established the partial loss of for-miminotransferase activity, there was sufficient residual activ-ity to handle the bulk of the FIGLU arising from histidine catabolism.

A possible explanation for the defect in these children can be offered by considering the relation between the two enzymes responsible for the 1-carbon salvage, i.e., formiminotransfer-ase and cyclodeaminase. As discussed earlier, both activities are associated with a single protein, and it is likely that a muta-tion has occurred which, while slightly reducing the activity of the first enzyme, had produced a considerable loss of cyclode-aminase activity. The assay method used by Arakawa's and Russell's groups measures both activities simultaneously and would not selectively detect a relative loss of activity of the second enzyme.

A cyclodeaminase defect would lead to an accumulation of 5-formimino THF (or a derivative thereof), the level of which would be related to the rate of histidine catabolism. This folate compound, while not itself acting as a 1-carbon donor, might exert regulatory effects on critical folate interconversion enzymes. The rise in serum folate concentration may reflect an accumulation of this compound which should be utilized by *L. casei* in the assay employed by Arakawa et al. Whatever the prime enzyme defect, it does not produce the classic effects of human folate deficiency, since only mild megaloblastosis was detected in one child.

The proposed correlation between the two basic types of defect discussed here, the true formiminotransferase deficiency and the formiminotransferase-cyclodeaminase deficiency, are represented diagrammatically in Fig. 24-7. Though there were no selective enzyme assays to support this proposal, the model does account for the data so far provided and for the outstand-ing features of the patients of Arakawa et al., viz., the high and variable serum folate levels (which would reflect concurrent histidine catabolism) and the severe central nervous system lesions in the absence of megaloblastosis.

Arakawa and his associates consider that the morbid changes result from a deficiency of 1-carbon folate derivatives normally supplied by histidine catabolism. That this is not the underlying pathologic mechanism is clear from those patients described by Niederwieser et al., Perry et al., and Russell et al. in whom the formiminotransferase block is more severe. In spite of the considerable FIGLU excretion in these latter patients, it is not clear what is the normal flux through the pathway and to what extent it is responsible for maintaining the 1-carbon folate derivative pool. Serine transhydroxymeth-ylase, cyclohydrolase, formyl THF synthetase, and 5,10-meth-ylene THF dehydrogenase activities were normal in the liver of patient 4 reported by Arakawa et al. [214], and these should provide an adequate supply of folate derivatives. Folate com-pounds such as formimino THF that would accumulate behind a cyclodeaminase block may exert as yet unknown controls on these enzymes and on the various folate transport systems.

Herman et al. [215] have reported formiminotransferase deficiency (as measured in the red cells and jejunum) in a 42-year-old, intelligent, physically normal white woman. The level of urinary FIGLU excretion was one-tenth that in the patients described by Niederwieser et al. and Perry et al. and was responsive to oral folate administration. Her clinical symptoms were related to carbohydrate intolerance.

Figure 24-7 Proposed mechanisms for enzyme defects underlying for-miminotransferase deficiency syndromes.

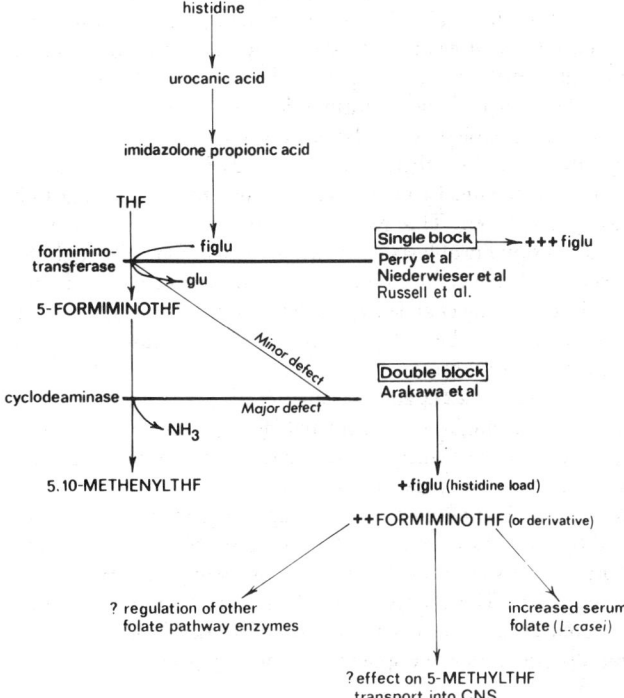

Methylene THF Reductase Deficiency

This condition is the most clearly defined disorder of folate metabolism and was reviewed in 1979 [47]. First described in 1972, at least 14 cases have been reported. Extensive observations, including studies on cultured fibroblasts, have been made on several cases. While the essential clinical feature consists of varying degrees of neurologic abnormality associated with mental retardation, the characteristic biochemical changes are moderate homocystinuria with homocystinemia and relatively normal levels of plasma methionine. The severity of the clinical manifestations and the extent of the biochemical derangement parallel the degree of enzyme deficit, which can be readily assessed in liver, fibroblasts, lymphocytes, and leukocytes.

The cases can be divided into three clinical groups. The first of these presents in the neonatal period, and affected individuals die in infancy. A second group develops symptoms in early childhood and death often occurs suddenly, at the end of the first decade or in the early teens. A third group, with milder symptoms, tends to survive into adult life.

The cases described by Narisawa et al. [216] are representative of the first group. Both cases were characterized by the onset of recurrent apneic episodes and generalized convulsions, with a rapid downhill course leading to death in infancy. Apart from homocystinuria and homocystinemia with normal plasma methionine levels, folate levels were low in both serum and cerebrospinal fluid. Based on differential bacterial assays, the low folate level was associated with low levels of 5-methyl THF. Methylene THF reductase activity was virtually absent in the liver, brain, kidney, and peripheral leukocytes. Intermediate levels of enzyme activity were observed in obligate heterozygotes, the parents of one of these children.

The four affected children in the family described by Wong et al. [217] are typical of the second group of cases. These children suffered from an essentially identical disorder consisting of the early onset of delayed psychomotor development, severe mental retardation, and generalized hyperactivity associated with spasticity. Three of the children died relatively suddenly at the ages of 9, 10, and 13 years, respectively. Autopsies on two of the three deceased showed generalized intravascular thromboses. Detailed autopsy studies on one of these cases revealed morphologic abnormalities closely resembling those observed in patients with classic homocystinuria secondary to cystathionine-β-synthetase deficiency [218].

The biochemical changes were similar to those in the first group. Methylene THF reductase activity could be detected in cultured skin fibroblasts from two of the children, although the levels were reduced to 6 and 12 percent, respectively, of control levels. Wong et al. [219] and Baumgartner et al. [220] have described and Erbe [47] has referred to other cases which fit into this second group.

Mudd et al. [221] and Freeman et al. [222] described two sisters who might be considered as representing the third group. These were mentally retarded, homocystinuric teenagers, one of whom presented with symptoms that were consistent with schizophrenia. These symptoms were initially modified by large doses of oral folic acid. Fibroblast cultures from both patients confirmed low levels of methylene THF reductase activity. These were higher than in the two more severely affected groups. Both girls subsequently developed a severe, rapidly progressive peripheral neuropathy [47].

These case groupings are not clear-cut. Erbe [47] refers to a case intermediate in severity between the second and third groups, while the original case described by Shih et al. [223] is perhaps the least affected of all.

Rosenblatt et al. [224], in an elegant study on cultured fibroblasts derived from a range of cases of varying severity, demonstrated that in most of the mutant cells, not only was the absolute concentration of 5-methyl THF reduced, but there was a reduction in the proportion of total cell folate which was 5-methyl THF. There was a direct correlation between the reduced proportion of methyl THF, the clinical severity of the disease, and the loss of enzyme activity. The studies showed that: (1) methylene THF reductase is the only significant pathway for the synthesis of methyl THF in the mutant control cells under the conditions of culture employed; (2) the level of methyl THF is regulated by the enzyme activity; (3) the bulk of the intracellular folate is in the form of polyglutamates; and (4) the relative distribution of folates may be the controlling factor in the overall folate metabolic pathway [27].

The inheritance pattern appears to be autosomal recessive, but thermal stability studies have suggested possible allelic variations. Detailed kinetic studies would be valuable to support this. Studies on a patient with disease of intermediate severity demonstrated that extracts from liver and peripheral blood lymphocytes were devoid of enzyme activity using menadione as an electron acceptor but possessed low levels of FAD-mediated activity [225]. This was consistent with a reaction mechanism for the synthesis of methyl THF which involved the irreversible reduction of enzyme-bound FAD by NAD(P)H followed by reversible oxidation of reduced FAD by methylene THF. The mutant enzyme retained some ability to bind FAD and to catalyze the reversible step but was unable to catalyze the irreversible reaction.

There is no effective treatment for this condition. The initial response of one of the patients [222] to large doses of oral folic acid has not been sustained [47]. The vulnerability of the central nervous system highlights the significance of methyl THF and, probably more importantly, of endogenously synthesized methionine in the synthesis of neurotransmitters such as dopamine and serotonin and its precursors. The schizophrenic patient referred to above [222] went into a sudden unexplained coma which was associated with a pronounced disturbance of serotonin and dopamine metabolites in the cerebrospinal fluid [47].

The continued exploration of the metabolic derangement associated with this disease will lead to a clearer understanding not only of overall folate and sulfur metabolism but also of the methylation reactions involving S-adenosyl methionine.

Tetrahydrofolate Methyltransferase Deficiency

Defects involving this enzyme were discussed briefly in the section on folate-cobalamin interrelationships and have also been discussed by Rosenberg in Chap. 23 from a different point of view. They also represent a range of clinical disorders that have not yet been fully clarified.

The first patient, described by Arakawa et al. [194], presented at the age of 5 months with diarrhea, vomiting, and pallor. She had a mild megaloblastic anemia which responded to oral therapy with a multivitamin preparation, from which she received 750 ng folic acid and 500 ng cobalamin per day. This was continued for 1 month. After a 1-month lapse of therapy, she was admitted to the hospital with myoclonic seizures. There was mild delay of physical development and moderate hepatosplenomegaly, with severe failure of central nervous system development. The electroencephalogram displayed hypsarrhythmia, and pneumoencephalography showed pronounced cerebral ventricular dilatation. The serum and red cell folates (*L. casei*) were very high: 63 ng/ml and 1989 ng/ml, respectively, while cobalamin was normal. Methylmalonic acid was not detected in the urine. Intense macrocytosis and bone marrow megaloblastosis were present. This blood picture was unaltered by cobalamin therapy. Oral folic acid produced a reticulocytosis, although the hemoglobin concentration did not change significantly. The megaloblastosis persisted despite 15 mg folic acid per day for 16 days.

Enzyme assays on a liver biopsy sample showed that THF methyltransferase activity was reduced to one-third of control levels, while serine transhydroxymethylase and cyclohydrolase levels were normal. Formyl THF synthetase and methylene THF dehydrogenase levels were normal in erythrocyte lysates. Urinary FIGLU excretion after an oral histidine load was normal initially but increased several months later. This excessive response was abolished by orally administered folic acid, 5 mg/day for 7 days.

The biochemical data obtained from this patient were consistent with the methyl trap hypothesis. The effects of much larger doses of folic acid or of 5-methyl THF on the bone marrow and on the electroencephalogram would have been interesting. Erbe [47] has reviewed the biochemical data derived from this case, and he considers that in the absence of homocystinuria and the presence of reportedly normal levels of enzyme activity in cultured skin fibroblasts, the original diagnosis is unwarranted.

The other patients described with deficiencies of this enzyme have primarily disorders of cobalamin metabolism [195, 196, 197]. However, the patient described by Dillon et al. [198] differed from the others in that severe mental retardation and megaloblastosis were present, together with clinical and autopsy findings characteristic of subacute combined degeneration of the spinal cord. The findings were consistent with the methyl trap hypothesis, although the clinical and biochemical pictures were different from those of the patient of Arakawa et al.

The author was supported by the Australian Department of Health and by grants from the National Health and Medical Council Research and the University of Sydney Cancer Research Fund during the preparation of this chapter and in his research into mammalian folate metabolism. Grateful acknowledgment is made to Drs. Martin Silink, Garth Leslie, Paul Russell, and Roger Reddel for their contributions to this research, and especially to Mr. Garry Lewis, not only for his research efforts but also for many hours of valuable discussion.

REFERENCES

1. Wills L: Treatment of "pernicious anaemia of pregnancy" and "tropical anaemia." *Br Med J* 1:1059, 1931
2. Wills L, Stewart A: Experimental anemia in monkeys with special reference to macrocytic nutritional anemia. *Br J Exp Pathol* 16:444, 1935
3. Angier RB, Booth JH, Hutchings BL, Mowat JH, Semb J, Stokstad ELR, Subbarow Y, Waller CW, Cosulich DB, Fahrenbach MJ, Hultquist ME, Kun E, Northey EH, Seeger DR, Sickels JP, Smith JM Jr: The structure and synthesis of the liver *L. casei* factor. *Science* 103:667, 1946
4. Mitchell HK, Snell EE, Williams RJ: Concentrations of folic acid. *J Am Chem Soc* 63:2284, 1941
5. Blakley RL: in Neuberger A, Tatum EL (eds): *The Biochemistry of Folic Acid and Related Pteridines.* North Holland Research Monographs, Frontiers of Biology. Amsterdam and London, Elsevier North Holland, 1969, vol 13
6. Krumdieck CL, Baugh CM: The solid phase synthesis of polyglutamates of folic acid. *Biochemistry* 8:1562, 1969
7. Godwin HA, Rosenberg IH, Ferenz CR, Jacobs PM, Meienhofer J: The synthesis of biologically active pteroyloligo-γ-glutamates (folic acid conjugates). *J Biol Chem* 247:2266, 1972
8. Meister A: *The Biochemistry of the Amino Acids.* New York, Academic Press, Inc, 1965, vol 1, p 28
9. Kovacs J, Kapoor A, Ghatack UR, Mayers GL, Giannasio VR, Giannoti R, Senyk G, Nitecki DE, Goodman JW: Synthesis of poly-γ-glutamyl-γ-aminobutyric acids and their reactivity against *Bacillus* anthracic polypeptide. *Chemistry* 2:1953, 1972
10. Shin YS, Buehring KU, Stokstad ELR: Separation of folic acid compounds by gel chromatography on Sephadex G-15 and G-25. *J Biol Chem* 247:7266, 1972
11. Baugh CM, Krumdieck CL: Naturally occurring folates. *Ann NY Acad Sci* 186:7, 1971
12. Stokstad ELH, Hutchings BL, Mowat JH, Boothe JH, Waller CW, Angier AB, Semb J, Subbarow Y: The degradation of the fermentation *Lactobacillus casei* factor. *J Am Chem Soc* 70:5, 1948
13. Stokstad ELR, Fordham D, DeGruningen A: The inactivation of pteroyl glutamic acid (liver *Lactobacillus casei* factor) by light. *J Biol Chem* 167:877, 1947
14. Blakley RL: in Neuberger A, Tatum EL (eds): *The Biochemistry of Folic Acid and Related Pteridines.* North-Holland Research Monographs. Amsterdam and London, Elsevier North Holland, 1969, p 80
15. Benkovic S: On the mechanism of action of folate and biopterin requiring enzymes. *Ann Rev Biochem* 49:227, 1980
16. Poe M, Jackman LM, Benkovic S: 5, 10-Methylene 5, 6, 7, 8 tetrahydrofolate. Conformation of the tetrahydropyropyrazine and imidazolidine rings. *Biochemistry* 18:5527, 1979
17. Blakely RL: Spectrophotometric studies on the combination of formaldehyde with tetrahydropteroylglutamic acid and other hydropteridines. *Biochem J* 74:71, 1960
18. Kaufman BT, Donaldson KO, Keresztesy JC: Chromatographic separation of the diastereoisomers of *dl*, L-5, 10-methylenetetrahydrofolate. *J Biol Chem* 238:1498, 1963
19. Ramasastri BV, Blakley RL: Optical rotations of the diastereoisomers of *dl*, L-methylenetetrahydrofolate. *Biochem Biophys Res Commun* 12:478, 1963
20. Yeh YC, Greenberg DM: Purification and properties of N^5, N^{10} methylenetetrahydrofolate dehydrogenase of calf thymus. *Biochim Biophys Acta* 105:279, 1965
21. Gordon M, Ravel JM, Eakin RE, Sheave WJ: Formylfolic acid, a functional derivative of folic acid. *J Am Chem Soc* 70:878, 1948
22. May M, Bardos TJ, Barger FL, Lansford M, Ravel JM, Sutherland GL, Shive W: Synthetic and degradative investigations of the structure of folinic acid-SF: *J Am Chem Soc* 73:3067, 1951
23. Roth B, Hultquist ME, Fahrenbach MJ, Cosulich DB, Broquist HP, Brockman JA Jr, Smith JM Jr, Parker RP, Stokstad ELR, Jukes TH: Synthetic of leucovorin. *J Am Chem Soc* 74:3247, 1952
24. Cosulich DB, Roth B, Smith JM Jr, Hultquist ME, Parker RP: Chemistry of leucovorin. *J Am Chem Soc* 74:3252, 1952
25. Rowe PB: A simple method for the synthesis of N^5, N^{10} methenyltetrahydrofolic acid. *Anal Biochem* 22:166, 1968
26. Rabinowitz JC: Folic acid, in Boyer PB, Lardy H, Myback K (eds): *The Enzymes,* ed 2. New York, Academic Press, Inc, 1960, vol 2, p 185
27. Rowe PB, Lewis GP: Mammalian folate metabolism: Regulation of folate interconversion enzyme. *Biochemistry* 12:1962, 1973
28. Osborn JJ, Talbert PT, Heunnekens FM: The structure of "active formaldehyde" (N^5, N^{10} methylenetetrahydrofolic acid). *J Am Chem Soc* 82:4921, 1960
29. Blakley RL: in Neuberger A, Tatum EL (eds): *The Biochemistry of Folic Acid and Related Pteridines.* North Holland Research Monographs, Frontiers of Biology. Amsterdam and London, Elsevier North Holland, 1969, vol 13, p 92
30. Blair JA, Saunders KJ: A convenient method for the preparation of *dl*-5-methylenetetrahydrofolic acid (*dl*-5-methyl-5, 6, 7, 8-tetrahydropteroyl-L-monoglutamic acid). *Anal Biochem* 34:376, 1970
31. Blakley RL: in Neuberger A, Tatum EL (eds): *The Biochemistry of Folic Acid and Related Pteridines.* North Holland Research Monographs, Fron-

tiers of Biology. Amsterdam and London, Elsevier North Holland, 1969, vol 13, p 91

32. DEITS TL, RUSSELL A, FUJII K, WHITELEY JM: Synthesis and properties of 5-methyldihydrofolate, in Pfleiderer W (ed): *The Chemistry and Biology of Pteridines.* Berlin, W. de Gruyter, 1975, p 525

33. RABINOWITZ JC: Colowick SP, Kaplan NO (eds): *Methods in Enzymology,* New York, Academic Press, Inc, 1963, vol 6, p 812

34. BLAKLEY RL: in Neuberger A, Tatum EL (eds): *The Biochemistry of Folic Acid and Related Pteridines.* North Holland Research Monographs, Frontiers of Biology. Amsterdam and London, Elsevier North Holland, 1969, vol 13, p 188

35. BLAKLEY RL: *The Biochemistry of Folic Acid and Related Pteridines,* North Holland Research Monographs, Frontiers of Biology. Amsterdam and London, Elsevier North Holland, 1969, vol 13, p 203

36. SILVERMAN M, KERESZTESY JC, KOVAL GJ, GARDINER R: Citrovorum factor and the synthesis of formylglutamic acid. *J Biol Chem* 226:83, 1957

37. WANG FK, KOCH J, STOKSTAD ELR: Folate coenzyme pattern folate linked enzymes and methionine biosynthesis in rat liver mitochondria. *Biochem Z* 346:458, 1967

38. GREENBERG DM, WYNSTON LK, NAGABHUSHANAM A: Further studies on N^5-formyltetrahydrofolic acid cyclodehydrase. *Biochemistry* 4:1872, 1965

39. KIKUCHI G: The glycine-cleavage system: Composition, reaction, mechanism, and physiological significance. *Mol Cell Biochem* 1:169, 1973

40. DU VIGNEAUD V, RACHELE JR: The concept of transmethylation in mammalian metabolism, and its establishment by isotopic labelling through in-vivo experimentation, in Shapiro SK, Schlenck (eds): *Transmethylation and Methionine Biosynthesis.* Chicago, University of Chicago Press, 1965, p 1

41. FINKELSTEIN JD, KYLE WE, HARRIS BJ: Methionine metabolism in mammals. Regulation of homocysteine methyltransferases in rat tissue. *Arch Biochem Biophys* 146:84, 1971

42. FUJIOKA M: Purification and properties of serine hydroxymethylase from soluble and mitrochondrial fractions of rabbit liver. *Biochim Biophys Acta* 185:338, 1969

43. CHASIN LA, FELDMAN A, KONSTAM M, URLAUB G: Reversion of a Chinese hamster cell auxotrophic mutant. *Proc Natl Acad Sci USA* 71:718, 1974

44. MORAN RG, WERKHEISER WC, ZAKREWSKI SF: Folate metabolism in mammalian cells in culture. *J Biol Chem* 251:3569, 1976

45. HILTON JG, COOPER BA, ROSENBLATT DS: Folate polyglutamate synthesis and turnover in cultured human fibroblasts. *J Biol Chem* 254:8398, 1979

46. THOMSON RW, LEICHTER J, CORNWELL PE, KRUMDIECK CL: Alterations in the chain length of pteroly poly-γ-glutamates and in the activity of pteroyl-γ-glutamate hydrolase in response to changes in the steady state of one-carbon metabolism. *Am J Clin Nutr* 30:1583, 1977

47. ERBE RW: Genetic aspects of folate metabolism, in Harris H, Hirschorn K (eds): *Advances in Human Genetics.* New York, Plenum Publishing Corp, 1979

48. LEWIS GP, ROWE PB: The regulation of methyltetrahydrofolate methyltransferase by folates, abstracted. *Proc Aust Biochem Soc* 7:45, 1974

49. BAGGOT JE, KRUMDIECK CL: Folylpoly-γ-glutamates as cosubstrates of 10-formyltetrahydrofolate-5'-phosphoribosyl-5-amino-4-imidazole carboxamide formyltransferase. *Biochemistry* 18:1036, 1979

50. GRIFFIN MJ, BROWN GM: The biosynthesis of folic acid III. Enzymatic formation and dihydrofolic acid from dihydropteroic acid and of tetrahydropteroylpolyglutamic acid compounds from tetrahydrofolic acid. *J Biol Chem* 239:310, 1964

51. SAKAMI W, RITARI SJ, BLACK CW, RZEPKA J: Polyglutamate synthesis by *Neurospora crassa,* abstracted. *Fed Proc* 32:471, 1973

52. McGUIRE JJ, HSIEH P, COWARD JK, BERTINO J: Enzymic synthesis of folylpolyglutamates. *J Biol Chem* 255:5776, 1980

53. LAVOIE A, TRIPP E, HOFFBRAND AV: The effect of vitamin B_{12} deficiency on methyl folate metabolism and pteroyl-polyglutamate synthesis in human cells. *Clin Sci Mol Med* 47:617, 1974

54. McBURNEY MW, WHITMORE FG: Isolation and biochemical characterization of folate deficient mutants of Chinese hamster cells. *Cell* 2:173, 1974

55. McBURNEY MW, WHITMORE FG: Characterization of a Chinese hamster cell with a temperature-sensitive mutation in folate metabolism. *Cell* 2:183, 1974

56. TAYLOR RT, HANNA ML: Folate-dependent enzymes in cultured Chinese hamster cells. *Arch Biochem Biophys* 181:331, 1977

57. SILINK M, ROWE PB: The localisation of glutamate carboxypeptidase in rat liver lysosomes. *Biochim Biophys Acta* 381:28, 1975

58. BAUGH CM, STEVENS JC, KRUMDIECK CL: Studies on γ-glutamyl carboxypeptidase 1. The solid-phase synthesis of analogues of polyglutamates of folic acid and their effects on human liver γ-glutamyl carboxypeptidase. *Biochim Biophys Acta* 212:116, 1970

59. SILINK M, REDDEL RR, BETHEL M, ROWE PB: Gamma glutamyl hydrolase (conjugase): Purification and properties of the bovine hepatic enzyme. *J Biol Chem* 250:5982, 1975

60. REED B, WEIR D, SCOTT J: The occurrence of folate-derived pteridines in rat liver. *Clin Sci Mol Med* 54:355, 1978

61. ROSENBERG IH, NEUMANN H: Multistep mechanism in the hydrolysis of pteroyl polyglutamates by chicken intestine. *J Biol Chem* 249:5125, 1974

62. PAUKERT JL, STRAUS LD, RABINOWITZ JC: Formyl-methenylmethylene tetrahydrofolate synthetase (combined). *J Biol Chem* 251:5104, 1976

63. TAN LUL, DRURY EJ, MacKENZIE RE: Methylase-tetrahydrofolate dehydrogenase-methenyltetrahydrofolate cyclohydrolase—formyltetrahydrofolate synthetase. *J Biol Chem* 252:1117, 1977

64. LAZOWSKA J, LUZZATTI M: Biochemical deficiency associated with ad3 mutation in *Saccharomyces cerevisiae. Biochem Biophys Res Commun* 39:34, 1970

65. CAPARELLI CA, BENKOVIC PA, CHETTUR G, BENKOVIC SJ: Purification of a complex catalyzing folate cofactor synthesis and transformylation in de novo purine biosynthesis. *J Biol Chem* 255:1885, 1980

66. BEAUDET R, MacKENZIE RL: Formiminotransferase-cyclodeaminase form porcine liver: An octomeric enzyme containing biofunctional polypeptides. *Biochim Biophys Acta* 453:151, 1976

67. GREADY JE: Dihydrofolate reductase: The current story. *Nature (Lond)* 282:674, 1979

68. Selected papers in *Chemistry and Biology of Pteridines,* Kisliuk RL, Brown GM (eds). New York, Elsevier North-Holland, 1979

69. DOMIN BA, CHENG Y-C, HAKALA MT: Properties of dihydrofolate reductase from a methotrexate resistant sublime of human KB cells and its interaction with polyglutamates, in Kisliuk RL, Brown GM (eds): *Chemistry and Biology of Pteridines.* New York, Elsevier North-Holland, 1979, p 295

70. COWARD JK, PARAMESWARAN KN, CASHMORE AR, BERTINO JR: 7, 8 Dihydropterolyoligo-γ-L-glutamates: Synthesis and kinetic studies with purified dihydrofolate reductase from mammalian sources. *Biochemistry* 13:3899, 1974

71. SCHIMKE RT, KAUFMAN RJ, ALT FW, KELLEMS RF: Gene amplifications and drug resistance in cultured murine cells. *Science* 202:1051, 1978

72. KAUFMAN RJ, BROWN PC, SCHIMKE RT: Amplified dihydrofolate reductase genes in unstably methotrexate resistant cells are associated with double minute chromosomes. *Proc Natl Acad Sci USA* 76:5669, 1979

73. LEWIS GP, SALEM M, ROWE PB: Substrate specificity of 10-formyltetrahydrofolate synthetase, abstracted. *Proc Aust Biochem Soc* 9:9, 1976

74. HIMES RH, HARMONY JAK: Formyltetrahydrofolate synthetase. *CRC Crit Rev Biochem* 1:501, 1973

75. RABINOWITZ JC, TABOR H: The urinary excretion of formic acid and formiminoglutamic acid in folic acid deficiency. *J Biol Chem* 233:252, 1958

76. LETTER AA, ZOMBOR G, HENDERSON JF: Tryptophan as a source of one-carbon units for purine biosynthesis de novo. *Can J Biochem* 51:486, 1973

77. KRETCHMAR AL, PRICE EJ: Use of respiration pattern analysis for study of serine metabolism in vivo. *Metabolism* 18:684, 1969

78. WANG E, KALLEN R, WALSH G: D-Fluoroaniline: A suicide inhibitor for serine transhydroxymethylase, in Kisliuk RL, Brown GM (eds): *Chemistry and Biology of Pteridines.* New York, Elsevier North-Holland, 1979, p 507

79. DONALDSON KO, KERESZTESY JC: Naturally occurring forms of folic acid II. Enzymatic conversion of methylene THF to prefolic A-methyl THF. *J Biol Chem* 237:1298, 1962

80. KUTZBACH C, STOKSTAD ELR: Mammalian methylene THF reductase. Partial purification properties and inhibition by S-adenosylmethionine. *Biochim Biophys Acta* 250:459, 1971

81. MATTHEWS RG, BAUGH CM: Interactions of pig liver methylenetetrahydrofolate reductase with methylenetetrahydropteroyl polyglutamate substrates and with dihydropteroylpolyglutamate inhibitors. *Biochemistry* 19:2040, 1980

82. TAYLOR RT, WEISSBACH H: N^5 Methyl THF-homocysteine methyltransferase, in Boyer PD (ed): *The Enzymes,* ed 3. New York, Academic Press, Inc, 1973, vol 9, p 121

83. TAYLOR RT, WEISSBACH H: *Escherichia coli* B. N^5-Methyltetrahydrofolate-homocysteine methyltransferase: Activation with S-adenosyl-L-methionine and the mechanism for methyl group transfer. *Arch Biochem Biophys* 129:745, 1969

84. FRIEDKIN M: Thymidylate synthetase. *Adv Enzymol* 38:235, 1973

85. DUNLAP RB, HARDING NGL, HEUNNEKENS FM: Thymidylate synthetase and its relationship to dihydrofolate reductase: *Ann NY Acad Sci* 186:153, 1971

86. LOCKSHIN A, MORAN RG, DANENBERG PV: Thymidylate synthetase purified to homogeneity from human leukaemic cells. *Proc Natl Acad Sci USA* 76:750, 1979

87. KISLIUK RL, GAUMONT Y, BAUGH CM: Polyglutamyl derivatives of folate as substrates and inhibitors of thymidylate synthetase. *J Biol Chem* 249:4100, 1974

88. KISLIUK RL, GAUMONT Y: Inhibition of thymidylate synthetase by poly-γ-glutamyl derivatives of folate and methotrexate, in Kisliuk RL, Brown

GM (eds): *Chemistry and Biology of Pteridines*. New York, Elsevier North-Holland, 1979, p 431

89. LOCKSHIN A, DANENBERG PV: Thymidylate synthetase and 2^1-deoxyuridylate form a tight complex in the presence of pteroyltriglutamate. *J Biol Chem* 254:12285, 1979
90. MACKENZIE RE: Formiminotransferase-cyclodeaminase, a bifunctional protein from pig liver, in Kisliuk RL, Brown GM (eds): *Chemistry and Biology of Pteridines*. New York, Elsevier North-Holland, 1979, p 443
91. ERBE RW: Inborn errors of folate metabolism. *N Engl J Med* 293:753, 807, 1975
92. ROWE PB, TRIPP E, CRAIG GC: Folate metabolism in lectin activated human peripheral blood lymphocytes, in Kisliuk RL, Brown GM (eds): *Chemistry and Biology of Pteridines*. New York, Elsevier North-Holland, 1979, p 587
93. ROWE PB: Inborn errors of folic acid metabolism: Regulation of the interconversion of active derivatives of folic acid. *Minn Med* 54:391, 1971
94. NIXON PF, SLUTSKY G, NAHAS A, BERTINO JR: The turnover of folate coenzymes in murine lymphoma cells. *J Biol Chem* 248:5932, 1973
95. SILBER R, MANSOURI A: Regulation of folate-dependent enzymes. *Ann NY Acad Sci* 186:55, 1971
96. SULLIVAN LW, HERBERT V: Suppression of hematopoesis by ethanol. *J Clin Invest* 43:2048, 1964
97. SULLIVAN LW, LUHBY AL, STREIFF RR: Studies of daily requirement of folic acid in infants and the etiology of folate deficiency in goat's milk megaloblastic anemia, abstracted. *Am J Clin Nutr* 18:311, 1966
98. WILLOUGHBY MNL: An investigation of folic acid requirements in pregnancy. II. *Br J Haematol* 13:503, 1967
99. COLEMAN N: Folate deficiency in humans, in Draper HH (ed): *Advances in Nutritional Research*. New York, Plenum Publishing Corp, 1977, vol 1, p 80
100. LEWIS GP, ROWE PB: Oxidative and reductive cleavage of folates—a critical appraisal. *Anal Biochem* 93:91, 1979
101. SHIN YS, WILLIAMS MA, STOKSTAD ELR: Identification of folic acid compounds in rat liver. *Biochem Biophys Res Commun* 47:35, 1972
102. ROWE PB: Unpublished data
103. WHITEHEAD VM: Polygammaglutamyl metabolites of folic acid in human liver. *Lancet* 1:743, 1973
104. CHANARIN L, HUTCHISON M, McLEAN A, MOULE M: Hepatic folate in man. *Br Med J* 1:396, 1966
105. SHIN YS, BUEHRING KU, STOKSTAD ELR: Studies of folate compounds in nature. Folate compounds in rat kidney and red blood cells. *Arch Biochem Biophys* 162:211, 1974
106. WAGNER C, LEVICH M: The utilisation of formate by human erythrocytes. *Biochim Biophys Acta* 304:623, 1973
107. HERBERT V, LARRABEE AR, BUCHANAN JM: Studies on the identification of a folate compound of human serum. *J Clin Invest* 41:1134, 1962
108. SHIN YS, KIM ES, WATSON JE, STOKSTAD ELR: Studies of folic acid compounds in nature IV. Folic acid compounds in soy beans and cow's milk. *Can J Biochem* 53:338, 1975
109. SAMUEL PD, BURLAND WL, SIMPSON K: Response to oral administration of pteroylmonoglutamic acid or pteroylpolyglutamate in newborn infants of low birth weights. *Br J Nutr* 30:165, 1973
110. ROSENBERG IH: Absorption and malabsorption of folates. *Clin Haematol* 5:589, 1976
111. HOFFBRAND AV, PETERS TJ: The subcellular localization of pterolypolyglutamate hydrolase and folate in guinea pgi intestinal mucosa. *Biochim Biophys Acta* 192:479, 1969
112. BLAIR JA: The handling and metabolism of folates in rat and man with especial relationship to disease, in Pfleiderer W (ed): *Chemistry and Biology of Pteridines*. Berlin, W de Gruyter, 1975, p 373
113. NORONHA JM, KEVASAN V: Studies on the mechanism of intestinal folate absorption, in Kisliuk RL, Brown GM (eds): *Chemistry and Biology of Pteridines*. New York, Elsevier North-Holland, 1979, p 571
114. STRUM W, NIXON PF, BERTINO JR, BINDER HJ: Intestinal folate absorption. I. 5-Methyltetrahydrofolate. *J Clin Invest* 50:1910, 1971
115. LESLIE GL, ROWE PB: Folate binding by the brush border membrane proteins of small intestinal epithelial cells. *Biochemistry* 11:1696, 1972
116. SELHUB J, GAY AC, ROSENBERG IH: Folate binding activity in epithelial brush border membranes in Kisliuk RL, Brown GM (eds): *Chemistry and Biology of Pteridines*. New York, Elsevier North-Holland, 1979, p 593
117. BROWN JP, DAVIDSON GE, SCOTT JM: The identification of the forms of folate found in the liver, kidney and intestine of the monkey and their biosynthesis from exogenous pteroyglutamic acid (folic acid). *Biochim Biophys Acta* 343:78, 1974
118. OLINGER EJ, BERTINO JR, BINDER HJ: Intestinal folate absorption. II. Conversion and retention of pteroylmonoglutamates by jejunum. *J Clin Invest* 52:2138, 1973
119. WHITEHEAD VM, PRATT R, VIALLET A, COOPER BA: Intestinal conversion of folinic acid to 5-methyltetrahydrofolate in man. *Br J Haematol* 22:63, 1972

120. JOHNS DG, SPERTI S, BERGIN ASV: The metabolism of tritiated folic acid in man. *J Clin Invest* 40:1684, 1961
121. GHITIS J: The folate-binding in milk. *Am J Clin Nutr* 20:1, 1967
122. FORD JE, SALTER DN, SCOTT KJ: The folate binding protein in milk. *J Dairy Res* 26:435, 1969
123. WAXMAN S, SCHREIBER C: Measurement of serum folate levels and folic acid binding protein by ^{3}H PGA radioassay. *Blood* 42:281, 1973
124. KAMEN BA, CASTON JD: Purification of folate binding factor in normal umbilical cord serum. *Proc Natl Acad Sci USA* 72:4261, 1975
125. WAXMAN S: Folate binding protein. *Br J Haematol* 29:23, 1975
126. COLMAN N, HERBERT V: Kinetic and chromatographic evidence for heterogeneity of the high affinity folate binding proteins in serum, in Kisliuk RL, Brown GM (eds): *Chemistry and Biology of Pteridines*. New York, Elsevier North-Holland, 1979, p 525
127. PRATT RF, COOPER BA: Folates in plasma and bile of man after feeding folic acid-^{3}H and 5-formyltetrahydrofolate (folinic acid). *J Clin Invest* 50:455, 1971
128. STEINBERG SE, CAMPBELL CL, HILLMAN RS: Kinetics of the normal folate enterohepatic cycle. *J Clin Invest* 64:83, 1979
129. SPECTOR R: Identification of folate binding macromolecule in rabbit choroid plexus. *J Biol Chem* 252:3364, 1977
130. ZAMIEROSKI MM, WAGNER C: Identification of folate binding protein in rat liver. *J Biol Chem* 252:933, 1977
131. WITTWER AJ, WAGNER C: Identification of folate binding protein of mitochondria as dimethylglycine dehydrogenase. *Proc Natl Acad Sci USA* 77:4484, 1980
132. GOLDMAN ID: The characteristics of the membrane transport of amethopterin and the naturally occurring folates. *Ann NY Acad Sci* 186:400, 1971
133. BOBZIEN WF III, GOLDMAN ID: The mechanism of folate transport in rabbit reticulocytes. *J Clin Invest* 51:1688, 1972
134. HENDERSON GB, GRZELAKOWSKA-SZTABERT B, EVELY EM, HUENNEKENS FM: Binding properties of the 5-methyltetrahydrofolate/methotrexate transport system in L1210 cells. *Arch Biochem Biophys* 202:144, 1980
135. DAS KC, HOFFBRAND AV: Studies of folate uptake by phytohaemagglutinin-stimulated lymphocytes. *Br J Haematol* 19:581, 1970
136. CORCINO JJ, WAXMAN S, HERBERT V: Uptake of tritiated folates by human bone marrow cells in vitro. *Br J Haematol* 20:503, 1971
137. BRANDA RF, ANTHONY BK, JACOBS HS: The mechanism of 5-methyl tetrahydrofolate transport by human erythrocytes. *J Clin Invest* 61:1270, 1978
138. HORNE DW, BRIGGS WT, WAGNER C: Transport of 5-methyltetrahydrofolic acid and folic acid in freshly isolated hypatocytes. *J Biol Chem* 253:3529, 1978
139. HERBERT V, ZALUSKY R: Selective concentration of folic acid activity in cerebrospinal fluid. *Proc Soc Exp Biol Med* 20:453, 1961
140. ALLEN CD, KLIPSTEIN FA: Brain folate concentration in rats receiving diphenylhydantoin, abstracted. *Neurology* 4:403, 1970
141. REYNOLDS EH: Mental effects of anticonvulsants and folic acid metabolism. *Brain* 91:197, 1968
142. LANZKOWSKY P, ERLANDSON ME, BEZAN AI: Isolated defects of folic acid absorption associated with mental retardation and cerebral calcification. *Blood* 34:452, 1969
143. LEVITT M, NIXON PF, PINCUS JH, BERTINO JR: Transport of folates in cerebrospinal fluid: A study utilizing doubly labelled 5-methyltetrahydrofolate and 5-formyltetrahydrofolate. *J Clin Invest* 50:1301, 1971
144. SPECTOR R, LORENZO AV: Folate transport by the choroid plexus in vitro. *Science* 187:540, 1975
145. CHEN CP, WAGNER C: Folate transport in the choroid plexus. *Life Sci* 16:1571, 1975
146. NIXON PF, BERTINO JR: Effecive absorption and utilization of oral formyltetrahydrofolate in man. *N Engl J Med* 286:175, 1972
147. BLAKLEY RL: in Neuberger A, Tatum EL (eds): *The Biochemistry of Folic Acid and Related Pteridines*. North-Holland Research Monographs, Frontiers of Biology. Amsterdam and London, Elsevier North-Holland, 1969, vol 13, p 389
148. STOKSTAD ELR: Experimental anemias in animals resulting from folic acid and vitamin B$_{12}$ deficiencies, in Harris RS, Wool IG, Lorrinae JA (eds): *Vitamins and Hormones*. New York, Academic Press, Inc, 1968, vol 26, p 443
149. HERBERT V: The five possible causes of all nutrient deficiency: Illustrated by deficiency of vitamin B$_{12}$ and folic acid. *Aust NZ Med* 1:69, 1972
150. HERBERT V: Experimental nutritional folate deficiency in man. *Trans Assoc Am Physicians* 75:307, 1962
151. JOINT FAO/WHO EXPERT GROUP: Requirements of ascorbic acid, vitamin D, vitamin B$_{12}$ folate and iron. *WHO Technical Report, Series No 452*, Geneva, 1970
152. REYNOLDS FH, ROTHFELD P, PINCUS JH: Neurological disease associated with folate deficiency. *Br Med J* 3:398, 1973
153. WAXMAN S, CORCINO JJ, HERBERT V: Drugs, toxins and dietary aminoacids affecting vitamin B$_{12}$ and folic acid absorption or utilization. *Am J Med* 48:599, 1970

154. Nelson MM, Wright HV, Baird CDC, Evans HM: Effect of 36 hour period of pteroylglutamic acid deficiency on fetal development in the rat. *Proc Soc Exp Biol Med* 92:554, 1956

155. Stone ML, Luhby AL, Feldman R, Gordon M, Cooperman JM: Folic acid metabolism in pregnancy. *Am J Obstet Gynecol* 99:638, 1967

156. Hibbard BM, Hibbard ED: Folate metabolism and reproduction. *Br Med Bull* 24:10, 1968

157. Hall MM: Folic acid deficiency and congenital malformation. *J Obstet Gynecol Br Commonw* 79:159, 1972

158. Thiersch JB: Therapeutic abortions with a folic acid antagonist, 4-aminopteroylglutamic acid (4-amino P.G.A.) administered by the oral route, *Am J Obstet Gynecol* 63:1298, 1952

159. Blakley RL: in Neuberger A, Tatum EL (eds): *The Biochemistry of Folic Acid and Related Pteridines.* North-Holland Research Monographs, Frontiers of Biology. Amsterdam and London, North-Holland, 1969, vol 13, p 468

160. Shaw EB: Fetal damage due to maternal aminopterin ingestion. *Am J Dis Child* 124:93, 1972

161. Shaw EB, Steinbach HL: Aminopterin-induced fetal malformations. Survival of infant after attempted abortion. *Am J Dis Child* 115:477, 1968

162. Warkany J, Beaudry PH, Hornstein S: Attempted abortion with aminopterin. *Am J Dis Child* 97:274, 1959

163. Landon MJ, Hey FN: Renal loss of folate in the newborn infant. *Arch Dis Child* 49:292, 1974

164. Dallman PR: Iron, vitamin E and folate in the preterm infant. *J Pediatr* 6:742, 1974

165. Davidson GP, Townley RRW: Structural and functional abnormalities of the small intestine due to nutritional folic acid deficiency in infancy. *J Pediatr* 90:590, 1977

166. Noronha JM, Silverman MJ: On folic acid, vitamin B$_{12}$, methionine and formiminoglutamic acid metabolism, in Henrich HC (ed): *Vitamin B$_{12}$ and Intrinsic Factor.* Second European Symposium, Hamburg, 1961, Stuttgart, Enke Verlag, 1962, p 728

167. Herbert V, Zalusky R: Interrelationships of vitamin B$_{12}$ and folic acid metabolism: Folic acid clearance studies. *J Clin Invest* 41:1263, 1962

168. Nixon PF, Bertino JR: Interrelationships of vitamin B$_{12}$ and folate in man. *Am J Med* 48:555, 1970

169. Nixon PF: *Studies on the Utilization of Folate Coenzymes,* thesis. University of Sydney, 1974

170. Oxnard CE, Smith WT: Neurological degeneration and reduced serum vitamin B$_{12}$ levels in captive monkeys. *Nature (Lond)* 210:507, 1966

171. Kark JA, Victor M, Hines JD, Harris JW: Nutritional vitamin B$_{12}$ deficiency in Rhesus monkeys. *Am J Clin Nutr* 27:470, 1974

172. Siddons RC: The experimental production of vitamin B$_{12}$ deficiency in the Baboon (Papio cynocephalus): A 2-year study. *Br J Nutr* 32:219, 1974

173. Green R, Vantonder SV, Oettle GJ, Cole G, Metz J: Neorological changes in fruit bats deficient in vitamin B$_{12}$. *Nature (Lond)* 254:148, 1975

174. Taylor RT, Hanna ML, Hutton JJ: 5-Methyl THF-homocysteine cobalamin methyltransferase in human bone marrows and its relationship to pernicious anemia. *Arch Biochem Biophys* 165:787, 1974

175. Nixon PF, Bertino JR: Impaired utilisation of serum folate in pernicious anemia: A study with radiolabeled 5-methylTHF. *J Clin Ivest* 51:1431, 1972

176. Cox GS, Kaback HR, Weissbach H: Defective transport in *S*-adenosylmethionine synthetase mutants of *Escherichia coli. Arch Biochem Biophys* 161:610, 1974

177. Chanarin I, Perry J, Lumb M: Biochemical lesion in vitamin B$_{12}$ deficiency in man. *Lancet* 1:1251, 1974

178. Thenen SW, Stokstad ELR: Effect of methionine on specific folate coenzyme pools in vitamin B$_{12}$ deficient and supplemented rats. *J Nutr* 103:363, 1973

179. Smith RM, Osborne-White WS: Folic acid metabolism in vitamin B$_{12}$ deficient sheep: Depletion of liver folates. *Biochem J* 136:229, 1973

180. Cooper BA, Lowenstein L: Relative folate deficiency of erythrocytes in pernicious anemia and its correction with cyanocobalamin. *Blood* 24:502, 1964

181. Smith RM, Osborne-White WS, Gawthorne JM: Folic acid metabolism in vitamin B$_{12}$ deficient sheep: Effects of injected methionine on liver constituents associated with folate metabolism. *Biochem J* 142:105, 1974

182. Blakley RL: in Neuberger A, Tatum EL (eds): *The Biochemistry of Folic Acid and Related Pteridines.* North-Holland Research Monographs, Frontiers of Biology. Amsterdam and London, Elsevier North-Holland, 1969, vol 13, p 446

183. DeGrazia JA, Fish MB, Pollycove M, Wallerstein RO, Hollander L: The oxidation of the beta carbon of serine in human folate and vitamin B$_{12}$ deficiency. *J Lab Clin Med* 80:395, 1972

184. Ellegard J, Essman V: Folate deficiency in pernicious anemia measured by determination of decreased serine synthesis in lymphocytes. *Br J Haematol* 24:571, 1973

185. Metz J, Kelly A, Swett VC, Waxman S, Herbert V: Deranged DNA synthesis by bone marrow from vitamin B$_{12}$ deficient humans. *Br J Haematol* 14:575, 1968

186. Das KC, Hoffbrand AV: Lymphocyte transformation in megaloblastic anaemia: Morphology and DNA synthesis. *Br J Haematol* 19:459, 1970

187. Van der Weyden MB, Cooper M, Firkin BG: Defective DNA synthesis in human megaloblastic bone marrow. Effects of hydroxy B$_{12}$ 5'-deoxyadenosyl B$_{12}$ and methyl B$_{12}$. *Blood* 41:299, 1973

188. Waxman S, Metz J, Herbert V: Defective DNA synthesis in human megaloblastic marrow: Effects of homocysteine and methionine. *J Clin Invest* 48:284, 1969

189. Hoffbrand AV, Pegg AE: Base composition of normal and megaloblastic bone marrow DNA. *Nature (New Biol)* 235:187, 1972

190. Rundles WB, Brewer SS: Hematologic responses in pernicious anemia to orotic acid. *Blood* 13:99, 1958

191. Herbert V, Sullivan LR: Formiminoglutamicaciduria in humans with magalonlastic anemia: Diminution by methionine or glycine. *Proc Soc Exp Biol Med* 112:304, 1963

192. Kamely D, Littlefield JB, Erbe RW: Regulation of 5-methyl THF homocysteine methyltransferase activity by methionine, vitamin B$_{12}$ and folate in cultured baby hamster kidney cells. *Proc Natl Acad Sci USA* 70:2585, 1973

193. Chanarin I, Deacon R, Lumb M, Perry J: Vitamin B$_{12}$ regulates folate metabolism by the supply of formate. *Lancet* 2:505, 1980

194. Arakawa TS, Narisawa K, Tanno K, Ohara K, Higashi O, Honda Y, Tamura T, Wada Y, Mizuno T, Hayashi T, Hirooka Y, Ohno T, Ikeda M: Megaloblastic anemia and mental retardation associated with hyperfolicacidaemia. Probably due to N^5-methyltetrahydrofolate transferase deficiency. *Tohoku J Exp Med* 93:1, 1967

195. Levy HL, Mudd SH, Schulman JD, Dreyfus PM, Ables RH: A derangement in B$_{12}$ metabolism associated with homocysteinemia, cystathioninemia, hypomethioninemia and methylmalonicaciduria. *Am J Med* 48:390, 1970

196. Goodman SI, Moe PG, Hammond KB, Mudd SH, Uhlendorf BW: Homocystinuria and methylmalonicacidura: Two cases in a sibship. *Biochem Med* 4:505, 1970

197. Mahoney MJ, Rosenberg LE, Mudd SH, Uhlendorf BW: Defective metabolism of vitamin B$_{12}$ in fibroblasts from children with methylmalonicacidura. *Biochem Biophys Res Commun* 44:375, 1971

198. Dillon MJ, England JM, Gompertz D, Goodey PA, Grant DB, Hussein Ha-A, Linnell JC, Matthews DM, Mudd SH, Newns GH, Seakins JWT, Uhlendorf BW, Wise UK: Mental retardation, megaloblastic anaemia, methylmalonicaciduria, and abnormal homocysteine metabolism due to an error in vitamin B$_{12}$ metabolism. *Clin Sci Mol Med* 47:43, 1974

199. Luhby AL, Eagle FJ, Roth E, Cooperman JM: Relapsing megaloblastic anemia in an infant due to a specific defect in gastrointestinal absorption of folic acid. *Am J Dis Child* 102:482, 1961

200. Luhby AL, Cooperman JM, Pesci-Bouret A: A new inborn error of metabolism. Folic acid-responsive megaloblastic anemia, ataxia, mental retardation and convulsions. American Pediatric Society, Annual Meeting, May 1965

201. Luhby AL, Cooperman JM: Congenital megaloblastic anemia and progressive central nervous system degeneration. Further clinical and physiological characterisation and therapy of syndrome due to inborn error of folate transport. American Pediatric Society, Annual Meeting, April 1968

202. Lanzkowsky P: Congenital malabsorption of folate. *Am J Med* 48:580, 1970

203. Santiago-Borrero PJ, Santini R Jr, Perez-Santiago E, Maldonado N: Congenital isolated defect of folic acid absorption. *J Pediatr* 82:450, 1973

204. Walters TR: Congenital megaloblastic anemia responsible to N^5-formyltetrahydrofolic acid administration, abstracted. *J Pediatr* 70:686, 1967

205. Tauro GP, Danks DM, Rowe PB, Van der Weyden MB, Schwarz MA, Collins VL, Neal BW: Dihydrofolate reductase deficiency causing megaloblastic anemia in two families. *N Engl J Med* 294:466, 1976

206. McGready RK, Tauro GP, Van der Weyden M: Physical and kinetic characteristics of a mutant dihydrofolate reductase. *Proc Aust Biochem Soc* 9:9, 1976

207. Tauro GP: Personal communication

208. Arakawa TS: Congenital defects in folate utilisation. *Am J Med* 48:594, 1970

209. Arakawa TS: Congenital and acquired disturbances of histidine metabolism. *Clin Endocrinol Metab* 3:17, 1974

210. Arakawa TS, Fuii M, Ohara E: Erythrocyte formiminotransferase activity in formiminotransferase deficiency syndrome. *Tohoku J Exp Med* 88:195, 1966

211. Niederwieser A, Giliberti P, Matasovic A, Pluznik S, Steinmann B, Baerlocher K: Folic acid non-dependent formiminoglutamicaciduria in two siblings. *Clin Chim Acta* 54:293, 1974

212. PERRY TL, APPLEGARTH DE, EVANS ME, HANSEN S, JELLUM E: Metabolic studies of a family with massive formiminoglutamicaciduria. *Pediatr Res* 9:117, 1975

213. RUSSELL A, STATTER M, ABZUG-HOROWITZ S: Methionine dependent glutamic acid formiminotransferase deficiency, in Sperling O, de Vries H (eds): *Inborn Errors of Metabolism in Man.* Basel, S Karger, 1978, p 65

214. ARAKAWA TS, TUMURA TS, OHARA K, NARISAWA K, TANNO K, HONDA Y, HIGASHI O: Familial occurrence of formiminotransferase deficiency syndrome. *Tohoku J Exp med* 96:211, 1968

215. HERMAN RH, ROSENWEIG NS, STIFEL FB, HERMAN YF: Adult formiminotransferase deficiency: A new entity, abstracted. *Clin Res* 17:304, 1969

216. NARISAWA K, WADA Y, SAITO T, SUZUKI H, KUDO M, ARAKAWA TS, KATSUSHIMA N, TSUBOI R: Infantile type of homocystinuria with $N^{5,10}$-methylenetetrahydrofolate reductase defect. *Tohoku J Exp Med* 121:185, 1977

217. WONG P WK, JUSTICE P, HRUBY M, WEISS EB, DIAMOND E: Folic acid nonresponsive homocystinuria due to methylenetetrahydrofolate reductase deficiency. *Pediatrics* 59:749, 1977

218. KANWAR YS, MANALIGOD JR, WONG PWK: Morphologic studies in a patient with homocystinuria due to 5, 10-methylenetetrahydrofolate reductase deficiency. *Pediatr Res* 10:598, 1976

219. WONG PWK, JUSTICE P, BEROW S: Detection of homozygotes and heterozygotes with methylene tetrahydrofolate reductase deficiency. *J Lab Clin Med* 90:283, 1977

220. BAUMGARTNER ER, SCHWEIZER K, WICK H: Different congenital forms of defective remethylation in homocystinuria. Clinical, biochemical and morphologic studies. *Pediatr Res* 11:1015, 1977

221. MUDD SH, UHLENDORF BW, FREEMAN JM, FINKLESTEIN JD, SHIH VE: Homocystinuria associated with decreased methylenetetrahydrofolate reductase activity. *Biochem Biophys Res Commun* 46:905, 1972

222. FREEMAN JM, FINKLESTEIN JD, MUDD SH: Folate-responsive homocystinuria and "schizophrenia." a defect in methylation due to deficient 5, 10-methylenetetrahydrofolate reductase activity. *N Engl J Med* 292:491, 1975

223. SHIH VE, SALAM MZ, MUDD SH, UHLENDORF BW, ADAMS RD: A new form of homocystinuria due to $N^{5,10}$-methylenetetrahydrofolate reductase deficiency, abstracted. *Pediatr Res* 6:135, 1972

224. ROSENBLATT DS, COOPER BA, LUE-SHING S, WONG PWK, BERLOW S, NARISAWA K, BAUMGARTNER R: Folate distribution in cultured human cells. *J Clin Invest* 63:1019, 1979

225. LEWIS GP, ROWE PB: Properties of bovine and human methylenetetrahydrofolate reductase, abstracted. *Proc Aust Biochem Soc* 13:64, 1980

25

DISORDERS OF TRANSSULFURATION

S. HARVEY MUDD

HARVEY L. LEVY

1. *Five patients have been described with deficiencies of hepatic methionine adenosyltransferase. These children were ascertained during routine screening of newborns for hypermethioninemia and were clinically well up to 6 years of age. Each possesses some residual activity of hepatic methionine adenosyltransferase. Methionine adenosyltransferase activities in tissues other than liver were normal, suggesting isoenzymes under separate genetic control. The residual activity of methionine adenosyltransferase in liver, as well as the normal activities in nonhepatic tissues, together provide for synthesis of some S-adenosylmethionine.*

2. *Cystathionine β-synthase deficiency is the most frequently encountered cause of homocystinuria. In addition to homocyst(e)ine, methionine and a variety of other metabolites of homocysteine accumulate in the body or are excreted in the urine of patients with this deficiency. More than 350 cases of proved or presumptive cystathionine β-synthase deficiency have been described. Dislocation of the optic lens, osteoporosis, thinning and lengthening of the long bones, mental retardation, and thromboembolism affecting large and small arteries and veins are the most common clinical features, although affected patients vary widely in the extent to which they manifest these abnormalities.*

3. *Cystathionine β-synthase deficiency is inherited as a Mendelian recessive trait, but available evidence suggests considerable genetic heterogeneity in known patients. Some patients have small residual activities of cystathionine β-synthase; others have no such activities detected by the most sensitive methods. The presence of some residual activity of cystathionine β-synthase may well be a necessary, but not sufficient, condition for clinical responsiveness of patients to vitamin B$_6$ administration.*

4. *Newborns with cystathionine β-synthase deficiency in which hypermethioninemia is the initial diagnostic criterion, are currently being detected by routine screening programs, with a frequency worldwide of approximately 1 in 200,000 live births.*

5. *Management of cystathionine β-synthase-deficient patients emphasizes amelioration of the characteristic biochemical abnormalities by use of low methionine, cystine-supplemented diets for patients not responsive to vitamin B$_6$ administration, and by pyridoxine treatment, perhaps accompanied by less stringent methionine dietary restriction, for vitamin B$_6$-responsive patients. Limited experience with patients treated from early infancy suggests that such management may prevent or retard the development of major clinical manifestations of cystathionine β-synthase deficiency.*

6. *γ-Cystathionase deficiency leads to persistent excretion of large amounts of cystathionine in the urine, as well as to accumulation of cystathionine in body tis-*

sues and fluids. N-Acetylcystathionine and a variety of additional cystathionine metabolites are excreted as well. The clinical status of proved or presumptive γ-cystathionase-deficient patients suggests that there are no clinical abnormalities characteristically associated with this enzyme deficiency. The deficiency is inherited as an autosomal Mendelian trait. Considerable genetic heterogeneity is likely to exist among known patients. One manifestation of genetic heterogeneity is responsiveness of the cystathioninuria associated with γ-cystathionase deficiency to vitamin B_6 administration.

The transsulfuration pathway converts the sulfur atom of methionine into the sulfur atom of cysteine. This pathway is the chief route of disposal of methionine and explains why cysteine is not an essential amino acid in normal human beings. Intimately related are two additional metabolic sequences: the transmethylation reactions whereby the methyl group of methionine is ultimately transferred to form any of a host of methylated compounds; and the re-formation of methionine by methylation of homocysteine.

METABOLISM OF METHIONINE, HOMOCYSTEINE, AND CYSTATHIONINE

The pertinent reactions of the transsulfuration pathway and related areas of metabolism are summarized in Fig. 25-1. At least nine specific genetic disorders have been recognized which affect one of the reactions shown. In the present chapter primary coverage will be given to three disorders involving reactions 1, 4, and 5, which are steps in the transsulfuration pathway.

S-Adenosylmethionine Formation

The gateway to all these interconversions is reaction 1, the formation of S-adenosylmethionine, catalyzed by methionine adenosyltransferase (EC 2.5.1.6.). In this unusual reaction, the adenosyl moiety of ATP is transferred to methionine, forming a sulfonium bond between the 5' carbon atom of the ribose and the sulfur atom of the amino acid. The tripolyphosphate which results from transfer of the adenosyl portion of ATP remains bound to the enzyme, which, by virtue of a second catalytic activity, cleaves this compound to inorganic phosphate and pyrophosphate. This tripolyphosphatase activity is specifically and markedly stimulated by S-adenosylmethionine [1, 2]. Removal of tripolyphosphate assists in making the synthesis of S-adenosylmethionine essentially irreversible under physiologic conditions [1]. Mammalian methionine adenosyltransferase has been partially purified from pig [3], rabbit [4], and rat [5, 6] liver. Activity of the liver enzyme requires both divalent [7, 8] and monovalent [8] cations. The animal enzyme has a rather strict substrate specificity for ATP [9] and a somewhat broader specificity for methionine [3, 10–13].

It has been found that mammalian livers contain as many as three chromatographically separable forms of methionine adenosyltransferase [14–17]. These isoenzymes have widely differing K_m's for methionine [16]. The dominant enzyme in rat liver is a "high K_m" form [14, 16], the activity of which is totally dependent upon the presence of a sulfhydryl compound [14] and which, at nonsaturating substrate concentrations, can be stimulated markedly by dimethylsulfoxide [15, 17]. The isoenzyme pattern in human liver has not been as well characterized. The dominant adenosyltransferase in human liver is said to be stimulated [18] or not to be stimulated [19] by dimethylsulfoxide.

Adenosyltransferase activities in mammalian tissues other than liver are not stimulated by dimethylsulfoxide [17, 18]. Human erythrocytes, cultured fibroblasts, and cultured lymphocytes each contain tissue-specific mixtures of at least two adenosyltransferase isoenzymes separable by chromatography

Figure 25-1 The metabolism of methionine, homocysteine, and cystathionine. (*From Mudd and Poole [23], with permission.*)

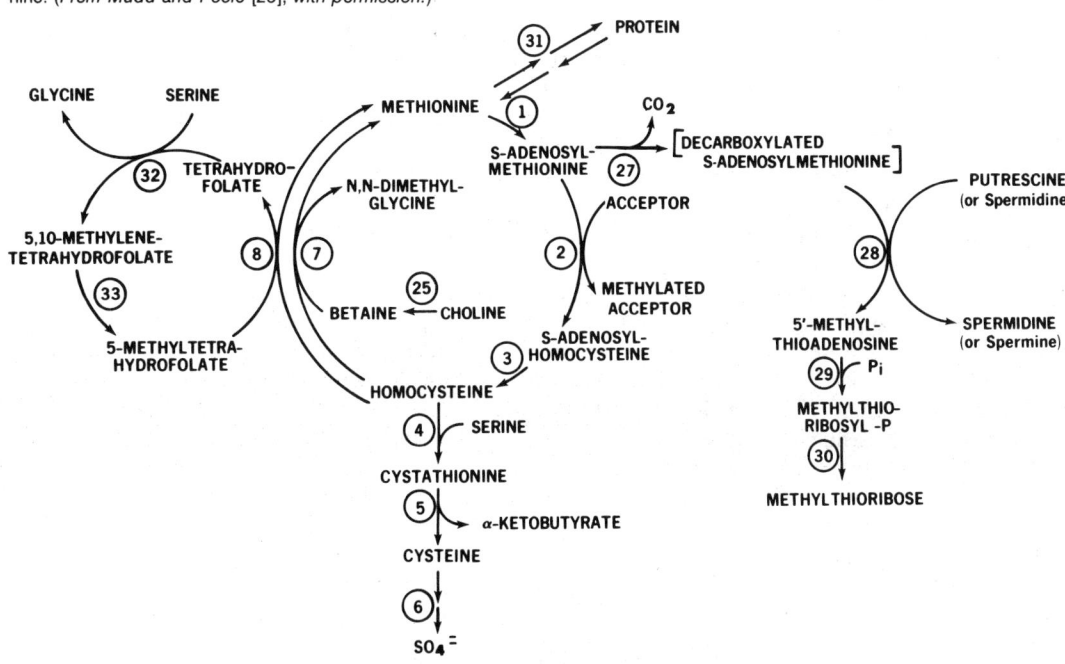

from each other and from human liver adenosyltransferase [19]. The relationships of these various forms to one another remain to be clarified.

Transmethylation

Because of its sulfonium bonds, S-adenosylmethionine may be regarded as a "high-energy" compound [20]. Each substituent of the sulfonium atom of this compound is energetically capable of participating in one or more transfer reactions. Many methyl transfers originate from S-adenosylmethionine. In addition, this compound, after decarboxylation, is the source of the 3-carbon moieties of the polyamines, spermidine and spermine [21]. Details of the biochemical mechanisms involved in methyl group transfer have been reviewed elsewhere [22]. The transmethylation reactions likely to occur in normal humans have been compiled, and an assessment made of the relative quantitative demands of each upon the available supply of S-adenosylmethionine [23, 24]. All these reactions produce a common sulfur-containing product, S-adenosylhomocysteine. In contrast to the earlier impression that this thioether is present in vertebrate livers at concentrations close to those of S-adenosylmethionine, measurements carried out with precautions to avoid postmortem artifacts indicate that in normal adult rat liver S-adenosylhomocysteine is present at 0.013 μmol/g, whereas S-adenosylmethionine is present at 0.06 to 0.09 μmol/g [25, 26]. Many S-adenosylmethionine-dependent methyltransferases are strongly inhibited by S-adenosylhomocysteine [27], and it has been calculated that when S-adenosylhomocysteine is present at a ratio of 1:4 with respect to S-adenosylmethionine, a variety of methyltransferases will decrease their activities by 10 to 60 percent [27]. S-Adenosylhomocysteine is further metabolized by a hydrolase (EC 3.3.1.1.) which cleaves the thioether to homocysteine and adenosine [28]. This enzyme is widely distributed in mammalian tissues [29, 30]. Although the equilibrium of the reaction favors S-adenosylhomocysteine accumulation, the reaction may be driven in the hydrolytic direction by removal of one or both of its products [28]. In vivo, homocysteine is normally rapidly removed, so that S-adenosylhomocysteine hydrolase presumably functions chiefly in the cleavage direction, generating adenosine and homocysteine.

Homocysteine Methylation

Homocysteine lies at an important metabolic branch point. It may be either converted to cystathionine through the transsulfuration pathway (reaction 4) or methylated to form methionine (reactions 7 and 8), thus completing the sulfur conservation cycle. At least two alternative mechanisms exist in humans for homocysteine methylation. In one, the methyl group originates in betaine. Betaine-dependent methylation of homocysteine is catalyzed by the enzyme betaine-homocysteine methyltransferase (EC 2.1.1.5). The reaction is essentially irreversible [31]. In rat and horse liver, two separable enzymes possess this catalytic activity [32].

The second mechanism for homocysteine methylation utilizes 5-methyltetrahydrofolic acid as methyl donor. The reaction is catalyzed by a cobalamin (vitamin B_{12})-containing enzyme, 5-methyltetrahydrofolate-homocysteine methyltransferase [33]. Again, the reaction favors methionine formation,

with an equilibrium constant of 1.4×10^5 in this direction [34]. This complex methyl transfer reaction involves the intermediate formation of an enzyme-bound methylcobalamin [33]. Several patients have been described who are unable to carry out the 5-methyltetrahydrofolate-dependent methylation of homocysteine because of a primary inability to form or accumulate methylcobalamin [35]. Certain other patients are unable to form the cosubstrate, 5-methyltetrahydrofolate, because of lack of activity of 5,10-methylenetetrahydrofolate reductase (EC 1.1.1.68; reaction 33, Fig. 25-1) [35]. Patients in both these groups excrete excess homocystine in their urine (i.e., are homocystinuric) and suffer from other abnormalities of sulfur amino acid metabolism [35]. They are discussed in Chaps. 23 and 24, which deal with disorders in the metabolism of vitamin B_{12} (i.e., cobalamin) and folic acid, respectively.

Cystathionine Synthesis

In the metabolism of homocysteine, the major alternative to methylation is condensation with serine to form the thioether cystathionine. The reaction is catalyzed by cystathionine β-synthase (EC 4.2.1.22), an enzyme which has been highly purified from several vertebrate livers (see Ref. 36). The purified enzyme contains firmly bound pyridoxal phosphate, upon which it depends for activity [36–38]. The homogeneous enzyme from human liver has an estimated molecular weight of 94,000 and is composed of two apparently identical subunits of molecular weight of 48,000 [36]. Earlier reports of higher molecular weights for the human liver enzyme [39–42] and of an $\alpha2\beta2$ subunit structure [41–43] are now thought to be due to the tendency of cystathionine β-synthase to form complexes with other proteins during purification [36]. Mammalian cystathionine β-synthase, including the human form, can catalyze an alternative reaction, cysteine sulfhydration, in which sulfide, rather than homocysteine, is combined with serine: H_2S + serine $\rightarrow$ cysteine + H_2O [36, 44, 45]. Although the condensation of homocysteine and serine catalyzed by cystathionine β-synthase can be reversed if homocysteine is rapidly removed [38], the equilibrium of the reaction is very much toward cystathionine formation under physiologic conditions. Formation of this thioether therefore serves to remove sulfur from the homocysteine-methionine cycle [46]. Deficiency of cystathionine β-synthase activity is the most frequently encountered genetic disorder of transsulfuration and will be described in a subsequent section.

Cystathionine Cleavage

The transsulfuration sequence is completed by cleavage of cystathionine to cysteine and α-ketobutyrate (reaction 5), catalyzed by the enzyme γ-cystathionase (EC 4.4.1.1). Molecular weights reported for γ-cystathionase from rat liver have been 170,000 to 210,000 [47] and 160,000 [48, 49]; from mouse liver, 160,000 [50]; and from human cultured lymphoid cells, 190,000 [51]. The rat liver enzyme is thought to consist of eight like subunits [48]; the mouse liver enzyme, of four like subunits [50]. The crystalline enzyme contains pyridoxal phosphate [52], upon which it depends for activity [53]. Dissociation constants of 1.4×10^{-6} and 4.6×10^{-6} have been reported for the γ-cystathionase-pyridoxal phosphate complex, based, respectively, upon fluorimetric titration [54] and measurement of catalytic activity [55]. Mammalian γ-cystathionase has several catalytic activities in addition to cystathionine cleavage, including the ability to catalyze cysteine desulfhydration: cysteine + H_2O → pyruvate + NH_3 + H_2S [56] (other activities are summarized in Ref. 57). Mammalian γ-cystathionase will catalyze the formation of cystathionine if incubated with cysteine in the presence of either homoserine [58–60] or homocysteine [61]. The role of such reverse reactions at physiologic concentrations of homoserine or homocysteine is questionable [61], and reversal in the presence of α-ketobutyrate, the physiologic product, has not been reported. Thus, it appears that γ-cystathionase normally functions almost entirely in the direction of cystathionine cleavage to produce, rather than to consume, cysteine. Patients with genetically determined defects of γ-cystathionase activity will be discussed below.

Quantitative Relationships among Transmethylation, Transsulfuration, and Homocysteine Methylation

Some information about the quantitative relationships among methyl transfer reactions, transsulfuration, and homocysteine methylation has been provided by studies of normal young adults maintained in metabolic steady states on varying defined intakes of methionine and choline. These studies showed that utilization of methyl groups is normally accounted for chiefly by creatine-creatinine formation. This reaction consumes more S-adenosylmethionine than all other transmethylations together. Male subjects utilize more methyl groups for methyl transfer reactions than they consume in a normal diet in the form of methionine and choline. The difference presumably is made up by de novo formation of methyl groups through the tetrahydrofolate-dependent pathway. Such methyl groups, as well as methyls equivalent to the main portion of ingested dietary choline, are used to methylate homocysteine. To the extent that homocysteine is methylated, the fraction of this compound diverted at any given moment to cystathionine is decreased. In male subjects on normal diets, at least 47 percent of the available homocysteine is methylated. Nevertheless, in the steady state metabolic condition, the intake of methionine sulfur is balanced by metabolism of an equivalent amount of homocysteine sulfur through the transsulfuration pathway. These observations indicate that during its passage through the body, the average homocysteinyl moiety cycles more than once between methionine and homocysteine. For males on normal diets, the calculated mean of such cycles is at least 1.9. For females there is less demand for methyl groups; a minimum of 33 percent of homocysteine is methylated, and the average homocysteinyl moiety cycles at least 1.5 times. If dietary intakes of labile methyls decrease, methylneogenesis increases accordingly. For example, males receiving daily only 4.7 mmol labile methyl in the form of methionine and choline (normal, 13.5 mmol) form at least 13.0 mmol methyl groups daily, and methylate at least 74 percent of the available homocysteine, so that the average homocysteinyl moiety cycles a minimum of 3.9 times [23]. This type of study has been extended to a subject unable to remove sarcosine metabolically because of a genetic defect in her sarcosine-oxidizing system. The results obtained permit a slight upward revision of the minimal estimates for homocysteine methylation to 50 percent, and of the number of times the average homocysteinyl moiety cycles to two times, respectively, in the human female. The results also suggest that when the dietary intake of labile methyl moieties exceeds the amount required for creatine formation, for other ongoing methyl transfer reactions, and for polyamine biosynthesis, the excess is disposed of by methylation of glycine, forming sarcosine, which, in the normal human, is then converted to a 1-carbon fragment at the formaldehyde oxidation level, with regeneration of the glycine [24]

Tissue Variations in Enzyme Patterns

The patterns just described apply only to the total body metabolism of the young adult. The distributions and the specific activities of the pertinent enzymes are such that the bulk of this metabolism must occur in the liver. It is likely that gross departures from the specified patterns occur locally in other tissues. In the rat and other mammals, methionine adenosyltransferase and S-adenosylhomocysteine hydrolase are present in almost all tissues [5, 29, 30, 62–66]. Analogous surveys with human tissues have not been extensive, and extrapolation of the animal data is not entirely safe, since striking differences in enzyme patterns have been described [65, 67]. Nevertheless, the available results suggest that almost all human tissues have some capacity to convert methionine to homocysteine. By contrast, the apportionment of homocysteine to the transsulfuration or remethylation pathways may vary markedly from tissue to tissue [35]. Among human tissues other than liver, brain has a comparatively high concentration of cystathionine β-synthase [63] and 5-methyltetrahydrofolate-homocysteine methyltransferase [68] but is low in γ-cystathionase and betaine-homocysteine methyltransferase activities [63, 64, 68]. Brain homocysteine may flow to both cystathionine and methionine. By contrast, human kidney is low in cystathionine β-synthase activity [64] but is rich in both betaine- and 5-methyltetrahydrofolate-homocysteine methyltransferase [67, 68]. It appears that in this tissue virtually all homocysteine will be remethylated, and transsulfuration will be minimal. This pattern (homocysteine remethylation in the absence of transsulfuration) may be widespread, since it recurs in a variety of tissues in the rat [35].

Age-dependent Variations in Enzyme Patterns

The enzyme activities under discussion are quantitatively different in fetuses than in adults. The specific activity of methionine adenosyltransferase is lower in the liver of the human fetus [69] and in a number of animal fetuses [9, 70, 71] than in adults of these species. Betaine-homocysteine methyltransferase-specific activities are lower in human fetal liver, brain, and kidney than in the corresponding adult tissues, whereas 5-methyltetrahydrofolate-homocysteine methyltransferase activities are higher in the fetal tissues [68]. Specific activities of cystathionine β-synthase in fetal liver are one-fifth those in the adult [69]. Together, these changes should serve in the fetus to direct a larger proportion of available homocysteine through the 5-methyltetrahydrofolate-dependent methylation cycle than in the direction of cystathionine synthesis, with concomitant increases in methylneogenesis and conservation of the homocysteine moiety.

γ-Cystathionase activity is virtually absent from human fetal liver and brain [69, 72–74]. Second-trimester fetal kidney possesses two-thirds the mean specific activity of mature kidney [68]. The placenta lacks each of the enzymes of transsulfuration [64, 69]. γ-Cystathionase activity appears in the liver during the first few days of the neonatal period [69]. The apparent block in the fetus at the cystathionine cleavage step led to the suggestion that cyst(e)ine may be an essential amino acid at this stage of life [72]. The limited capacity of infants to convert methionine to cysteine is supported by the observations that urinary excretion of cystathionine is elevated in low-birth-weight [75] or term [76] neonates fed protein intakes higher than those provided by human milk. The possible importance of these findings for maternal and newborn nutrition has been discussed elsewhere [69, 72, 77, 78]. Cysteine supplementation did not alter nitrogen retention or growth of newborn infants maintained on cysteine-free feeding [78a].

HYPERMETHIONINEMIA, HOMOCYSTINURIA, CYSTATHIONINURIA: DIFFERENTIAL DIAGNOSES

The terms *hypermethioninemia*, *homocystinuria* (or *-emia*), and *cystathioninuria* (or *-emia*) designate biochemical abnormalities, not specific disease entities. Each of these abnormalities may be the result of more than one specific and distinct genetic lesion. For example, four different genetic abnormalities are now known to lead to the excretion of excessive urinary homocystine (i.e., homocystinuria). The demonstation of one or more biochemical abnormalities in a given patient is often the starting point for a specific diagnosis of the underlying genetic lesion. In this section we will present brief differential diagnoses of hypermethioninemia, homocystinuria, and cystathioninuria, including both genetic and nongenetic causes. This discussion is summarized in Table 25-1.

Hypermethioninemia

Aside from protein synthesis, almost all known major pathways for methionine metabolism are initiated by conversion of methionine to S-adenosylmethionine (Fig. 25-1). Impairment of this conversion leads to abnormal methionine accumulation and hypermethioninemia, as borne out by studies of patients with methionine adenosyltransferase deficiency (to be discussed below). A different type of hypermethioninemia accompanies virtually all cases of cystathionine β-synthase deficiency. Presumably, the homocysteine accumulation which is the primary result of this enzymatic lesion leads secondarily to enhanced rates of remethylation by way of reactions 7 and 8. Hypermethioninemia in patients with cystathionine β-synthase deficiency is due to overproduction of this amino acid, rather than to underutilization. The homocystinuria which accompanies this particular hypermethioninemia serves to distinguish it from most of the other hypermethioninemias discussed here.

Serum concentrations of methionine, as well as other amino

Table 25-1 Hypermethioninemia, homocystinuria, cystathioninuria: Differential diagnoses

I. Hypermethioninemia (-uria)
   A. Methionine adenosyltransferase deficiency
   B. Cystathionine β-synthase deficiency
   C. Severe generalized liver disease
   D. In association with hereditary tyrosinemia
   E. Transient hypermethioninemia of infants
   F. 6-Azauridine triacetate administration
   G. D-Methioninuria due to DL-methionine ingestion
   H. Persistent and specific, associated with myopathy
   I. Persistent and specific, not associated with myopathy

II. Homocystinuria (-emia)
   A. Cystathionine β-synthase deficiency
   B. Impaired activity of 5-methyltetrahydrofolate-homocysteine methyltransferase
      1. Failure to form or accumulate methylcobalamin
      2. 5,10-Methylenetetrahydrofolate reductase deficiency
      3. Defective absorption of vitamin B_{12}
      4. Nutritional vitamin B_{12} deficiency
   C. 6-Azauridine triacetate administration
   D. Artifactual, due to bacterial metabolism of urinary cystathionine

III. Cystathioninuria
   A. Transient cystathioninuria of (usually premature) infants
   B. γ-Cystathionase deficiency
   C. Impaired activity of 5-methyltetrahydrofolate-homocysteine methyltransferase
      1. Failure to form or accumulate methylcobalamin
      2. 5,10-Methylenetetrahydrofolate reductase deficiency
      3. Nutritional vitamin B_{12} deficiency
   D. Vitamin B_6 deficiency
   E. Thyrotoxicosis
   F. Liver disease
   G. Neuroblastoma, ganglioblastoma, hepatoblastoma
   H. Defective renal transport

acids, may be elevated in patients with generalized liver disease. The methionine elevation tends to be more striking and more specific in patients with advanced disease, especially those in hepatic coma. In the latter situation, there is also often a disproportionate rise in serum tyrosine concentration [79, 80a].

A possibly similar but poorly understood form of hypermethioninemia often accompanies the syndrome of hereditary tyrosinemia. The nature of the primary genetic lesion which leads to this heritable syndrome is still a matter of discussion (see Chap. 13). The accompanying hypermethioninemia has been attributed by some to the generalized hepatic cirrhosis which is part of this syndrome [81, 82], and by others to a primary defect in methionine metabolism [83]. In two patients, partial deficiencies of hepatic methionine adenosyltransferase and cystathionine β-synthase activities were found [84]. As just described, each of these deficiencies can lead to hypermethioninemia. Nevertheless, patients with other types of cirrhosis with similar decreases of these two enzymes activities did not have hypermethioninemia. To account for these observations, it was postulated that patients with hereditary tyrosinemia have yet a third factor leading toward methionine accumulation, viz., a generalized failure to utilize amino acids because of the failure of protein synthesis [84]. Such generalized failure might help to explain the many-fold manifestations of this puzzling syndrome. Measurements of tissue S-adenosylmethionine concentrations might be helpful in assessing the relative contributions of decreases in protein synthesis, cystathionine β-synthase, and methionine adenosyltransferase to this form of methionine accumulation. In the liver of the patient reported by Perry and coworkers [83], the S-adenosylmethionine concentration was more than 20 times the mean control value, a finding which precluded a primary deficiency of methionine adenosyltransferase activity as the sole cause of the syndrome in this patient [85].

A transient hypermethioninemia has been observed in many infants given diets rich in protein—usually 7 g/(kg·day) or more [75, 86–89]. These observations may possibly be explained by "immaturity" of methionine adenosyltransferase and cystathionine β-synthase. The mean specific activities of these enzymes in livers of several premature infants were 31 percent and 19 percent of the mean adult hepatic specific activities [69]. Nevertheless, the hypermethioninemia in question has not been strikingly associated with prematurity and, indeed, has usually developed after several weeks of extrauterine life [86, 88, 89]. Information on the activities of the pertinent enzymes is not available for this period, but this time sequence suggests that the correct explanation of this form of hypermethioninemia may be complex.

6-Azauridine triacetate treatment brings about significant rises in methionine serum concentrations [90], accompanied by abnormal homocystine excretion [91], a pattern suggestive of decreased cystathionine β-synthase activity. It has been proposed that 6-azauridine triacetate or one of its metabolites may act as an inhibitor of cystathionine β-synthase as well as a number of other pyridoxal phosphate-dependent enzymes [90].

Urinary excretion of D-methionine has been observed in infants fed diets supplemented with DL-methionine. Inefficient metabolism and ineffective renal tubular reabsorption of the D-enantiomorph are presumed to explain the abnormal methionine excretion [92].

Gaull and colleagues [93] have described several patients with hypermethioninemia which they suggest may be due to none of the above causes. One child at age $7\frac{1}{2}$ was discovered to have specific hypermethioninemia accompanied by myopathy and mental deficiency. Methionine adenosyltransferase activity, measured with saturating concentrations of substrates, was normal or increased in the liver, muscle, erythrocytes, and cultured fibroblasts. Cystathionine β-synthase activities in liver and cultured fibroblasts were normal. S-Adenosylmethionine in whole blood was above normal (3.3 and 5.9 nmol/ml; normal, 1.0 ± 0.3 SD) at times when the patient was taking a normal diet and when her plasma methionine concentration was elevated to 0.55 to 0.70 μmol/ml (normal, 0.02 to 0.04). A second patient with hypermethioninemia and myopathy was mentioned in the same publication but not described in further detail [94]. Gaull and associates [93] additionally mention unpublished studies of three patients with specific and persistent hypermethioninemia without myopathy. In each instance, methionine adenosyltransferase activities (apparently measured at saturating substrate concentrations) were stated to be normal in the liver, erythrocytes, cultured fibroblasts, and lymphoid cell lines [95, 96]. For the moment, the cause of the hypermethioninemia in these patients, with or without myopathy, remains obscure. Gaull et al. [93] suggest that methionine adenosyltransferase deficiency is not the underlying cause. Studies of the isoenzyme forms of this enzyme, both in normal humans and in these patients, determination of hepatic methionine adenosyltransferase activities as functions of the concentration of substrates, and measurement of liver S-adenosylmethionine concentrations would all help to evaluate this suggestion.

Benevenga and associates have published evidence that rat liver can catalyze an S-adenoyslmethionine-independent series of reactions in which methionine is transaminated to α-keto-γ-methiolbutyrate, which is then oxidatively decarboxylated to CO_2 and 3-methylthiopropionate [96a, 96b, 96c]. 3-Methylthiopropionate may be further degraded to CO_2, sulfate, methanethiol, and H_2S [96d]. The presence of this complete series of reactions in humans, and the quantitative contribution of this pathway to degradation of methionine under normal physiologic conditions, remain to be established. Genetic lesions affecting one of the first two steps in such a pathway offer conceivable explanations of hypermethioninemia in subjects without methionine adenosyltransferase deficiency. No experimental evidence relevant to these possibilities appears to have been reported.

Homocystinuria

Decreased rates of metabolism of homocysteine through either the transsulfuration (reaction 4) or the 5-methyltetrahydrofolate-dependent sulfur conservation (reaction 8) pathways lead to accumulation of homocysteine with resultant homocyst(e)inemia and homocystinuria. These two forms of homocystinuria are readily distinguished by several chemical criteria: Serum methionine concentrations are usually elevated in cystathionine β-synthase deficiency, but low, or low normal, when 5-methyltetrahydrofolate-dependent homocysteine methylation is severely decreased. Excretion of inorganic urinary sulfate after a methionine load proceeds at an abnormally low rate in the former condition, but not in the latter.

Three genetic lesions are presently known to lead to decreases in 5-methyltetrahydrofolate-dependent homocysteine methylation sufficiently severe to cause homocystinuria: (1) inability to form or accumulate methylcobalamin, to date always encountered in patients also unable to form or accumulate adenosylcobalamin (see Chap. 23); (2) decreased 5, 10-methylenetetrahydrofolate reductase activity (see Chap. 24); and (3) Imerslund's syndrome (familial proteinuria and pernicious anemia, due to defective absorption of vitamin B_{12} in the presence of intrinsic factor) [35, 97]. The first two conditions are best distinguished from each other on the basis of direct enzyme assays, which may be performed on extracts of fibroblasts cultured from skin. Measurements of serum folate concentrations may also be useful in this regard [35].

Homocystinuria, accompanied by cystathioninuria and methylmalonic aciduria, was observed in a 6-month-old infant with severe megaloblastic anemia and coma. All three manifestations were secondary to nutritional vitamin B_{12} deficiency brought about because the child was exclusively breast-fed by a strictly vegetarian mother [98]. For reasons which are not clear, homocystinuria has not been reported in adults with vitamin B_{12} deficiency.

The homocystinuria due to 6-azauridine triacetate administration was mentioned above.

Finally, an artifactual form of homocystinuria has been caused by bacterial conversion of cystathionine to homocyst(e)ine. This conversion occurred in contaminated urine specimens from an infant with massive cystathioninuria [46, 99]. Whether similar phenomena account for the homocystinuria reported in occasional additional patients with cystathioninuria [100–104] remains to be clarified. Demonstration of homocystinemia is a useful means of proving that homocystinuria is not artifactual.

Cystathioninuria

In an extensive study, Endres and Seibold found that only 17 percent of clinically normal individuals, aged 3 days to 56 years, had no cystathionine in their urine [105]. The amounts ranged up to 146 μmol/g creatinine. Expressed on the basis of body surface area, mean cystathionine excretion did not change with age, but expressed on the basis of urinary creatinine, cystathionine excretion was lower in adults (23 to 56 years of age; median, 7 μmol/g creatinine) than in children (3 days to 14 years; median, 28 μmol/g).

Cystathionine is an almost constant constituent of the urine of premature infants [76, 105]. Such premature infants excrete more cystathionine than term infants of similar postgestational ages [105]. Premature infants fed protein- [76] or methionine-enriched [105, 106] diets excreted increased amounts of cystathionine, and low-birth-weight infants fed increased protein intakes had mild elevations of cystathionine in plasma and urine [75]. Transient cystathioninuria (amount unspecified) was detected in 13 of 35,809 apparently normal infants screened in Australia at age 6 weeks. By the time these 13 children were age 5 months, cystathionine was not detected in the urine of 11 and was present only in trace amounts in the other two [103]. These findings may be explained by the observations of Gaull and coworkers (described above) that γ-cystathionase is absent in fetal liver tissue but appears in the liver of newborns. Apparently the capacity to cleave cystathionine is marginal in premature infants but matures in almost all children within a few weeks of birth.

Persistent cystathioninuria of genetic origin may be due either to underutilization or to overproduction of cystathionine. Underutilization accounts for the persistent, often massive cystathioninuria encountered in patients with genetically determined impairment of γ-cystathionase activity. Overproduction occurs when a normal amount of cystathionine β-synthase is provided with abnormally elevated concentrations of its substrate, homocysteine. This situation occurs, for example, when 5-methyltetrahydrofolate-homocysteine methyltransferase activity is impaired by lack of methylcobalamin or by lack of 5-methyltetrahydrofolate. Abnormal cystathionine excretion has been noted in some [98, 107, 108] but not all [109, 110] patients with such defects and when present, has been less than the cystathionine excretion of patients with γ-cystathionase deficiency. This difference and the accompanying homocystinuria provide means of distinguishing patients with decreased homocysteine methylation from those with γ-cystathionase deficiency.

A number of nongenetic conditions lead to excessive cystathionine excretion. Vitamin B_6 deficiency produces cystathioninuria in animals [111] and humans [112, 113]. The cystathioninuria of premature infants is decreased by large oral doses of vitamin B_6 [106]. Both cystathionine β-synthase and γ-cystathionase activities are pyridoxal phosphate-dependent, but studies of vitamin B_6-deficient rats have shown that the γ-cystathionase holoenzyme contents of the liver, kidney, and pancreas of such animals are much more decreased than are the cystathionine β-synthase holoenzyme contents [114, 115]. In vitamin B_6 deficiency, cystathionine synthesis continues at a rate such that homocystine may be absent from the urine, or present only in trace amounts, whereas cystathionine excretion may become quite marked [113].

Abnormal cystathionine excretion has also been reported in thyrotoxic patients [116]. Animal studies have shown that thyroxine treatment reduces hepatic γ-cystathionase activity [70, 117] but not the activity of cystathionine β-synthase [70]. The cystathioninuria occurring in many instances of severe generalized liver damage [118–121] may also be due to an impaired capacity to cleave cystathionine.

An unusual type of moderate familial cystathioninuria was suggested by Frimpter to be due to a renal defect affecting the transport of this amino acid. The patient in question excreted virtually all the cystathionine filtered at the glomerulus [122], whereas normal subjects reabsorb a maximum of approximately 1 μmol/min per 1.73 m² body surface area [123].

Many functional neural tumors contain relatively high concentrations of cystathionine [124], and patients with these tumors are cystathioninuric [125–127]. Since nervous tissue contains relatively more cystathionine β-synthase than γ-cystathionase activity [63, 128], this form of cystathioninuria may represent a local imbalance between production and utilization. Similar imbalances could account for the cystathioninuria reported in some cases of hepatoblastoma [119, 129–131].

The majority of these nongenetic causes of cystathioninuria lead to excretion of abnormal amounts of this amino acid in the absence of striking abnormalities of the other sulfur amino acids. Confusion with γ-cystathionase deficiency might therefore be possible, and these nongenetic conditions should be carefully excluded by the usual diagnostic criteria before it is concluded that any particular case of cystathioninuria is due to genetically determined γ-cystathionase deficiency.

HEPATIC METHIONINE ADENOSYLTRANSFERASE DEFICIENCY

Since 1974, five children (two males and three females) have been reported with specific and persistent hypermethioninemia associated with deficient methionine adenosyltransferase activity in the liver [132–137]. Hypermethioninemia was discovered in each during the perinatal period as a result of routine screening procedures, originally introduced as a means of detecting the hypermethioninemia associated with cystathionine β-synthase deficiency. When last reported [136, 137], two of these children were 6 years of age; the others ranged down to less than 1 year. At ascertainment, plasma methionine concentrations were 0.25 to 1.27 μmol/ml. Hypermethioninemia of approximately 0.40 μmol/ml has generally persisted when the patients were placed on diets with methionine intakes reduced as low as 55 mg/(kg·day). The plasma of these patients also contains abnormally high concentrations of methionine sulfoxides, but not of homocystine or tyrosine. The urine contains increased amounts of methionine [136, 137] and an "abnormal quantity" (amount not specified) of α-keto-γ-methylthiolbutyric acid [136].

Activity of methionine adenosyltransferase in extracts of liver was between 8 and 18 percent of mean control values when assayed at high (1 to 20 mM) methionine concentrations [135, 137]. For one patient, a more complete kinetic analysis of hepatic adenosyltransferase was performed. As the methionine concentration in the assay mixture was decreased, the patient's activity approached the mean control value more closely, reaching 30 percent of control when the reaction mixture contained 0.006 mM methionine [135]. For this patient, adenosyltransferase activities in tissues other than liver have not been reported. The four additional patients each had activities in erythrocytes, cultured skin fibroblasts, and long-term lymphoid cell lines no different from control values [137]. The activities in fibroblasts and lymphoid cells had the same chromatographic properties as control activities [19]. Although genetic heterogeneity among the individuals within this group is certainly possible, even likely, for the moment the weight of evidence appears compatible with the hypothesis that these patients have genetic defects affecting the dominant hepatic form of methionine adenosyltransferase. Studies of animal [14, 16] and (perhaps) human [18] hepatic adenosyltransferase make it likely that this is a high K_m isoenzyme. The form or forms of methionine adenosyltransferase present in nonhepatic tissues are apparently unaffected, and are therefore strongly suggested to be under separate genetic control.

In these patients hepatic activities of S-adenosylhomocysteine hydrolase, γ-cystathionase, betaine-homocysteine methyltransferase, and 5-methyltetrahydrofolate-homocysteine methyltransferase have been normal [135, 137]. Hepatic cystathionine β-synthase has been moderately low in two of the three cases for whom it was reported [135, 137].

S-Adenosylmethionine concentrations, measured in whole blood of two patients at times when they were hypermethioninemic, were at least as high as control values. S-Adenosylmethionine in a liver biopsy from a single patient was comparable to the mean for human liver samples (obtained post mortem). These findings are in accord with expectations that (1) a complete lack of S-adenosylmethionine might be lethal and that (2) given elevated methionine concentrations, residual adenosyltransferases in liver and peripheral tissues might combine to provide a near-normal supply of S-adenosylmethionine [57, 135].

In general, these patients with proven partial defects in hepatic methionine adenosyltransferase activity have not been severely affected clinically. However, nonspecific ultrastructural abnormalities in the endoplasmic reticulum and outer mitochondrial membranes of liver have been reported [137]. Taken together with the facts that each of these patients was identified in neonatal screening programs and none is currently over 6 years of age, these considerations suggest that these children may yet develop clinical difficulties.

The pattern of inheritance of hepatic methionine adenosyltransferase deficiency remains obscure. Of the two parents for whom liver adenosyltransferase assays were performed, one father had a value of 55 percent of the mean control value, whereas one mother had normal activity [137]. One additional father and one mother had moderately impaired plasma methionine tolerance curves following oral loads of methionine [137]. The presence of isoenzymes under different genetic control and the possibility that human females may have higher hepatic adenosyltransferase activities than do males (as is the case in rats; see Ref. 138) may confound the interpretation of any of these results.

CYSTATHIONINE β-SYNTHASE DEFICIENCY

The disease entity which is now recognized as cystathionine β-synthase deficiency was first reported in 1962. During screening tests of mentally retarded patients in Northern Ireland, two sisters were found to be excreting homocystine, an amino acid not detected in normal urine [139, 140]. Independent investigation of children in Wisconsin with mental retardation and failure to thrive revealed a single male infant with homocystinuria [141]. Within a short time, these initial cases, as well as others discovered subsequently by the same workers, had been studied sufficiently to outline the pattern of clinical and biochemical abnormalities which characterize the patients in question [142, 143]. Meanwhile, a third team of investigators had discovered homocystine in the urine of a 7-year-old girl who presented with dislocated optic lenses. The abnormalities in this patient were similar to those reported from Ireland and Wisconsin [144], and in 1964, assay of enzyme activities in an extract of a percutaneous liver biopsy showed that she had a specific defect in cystathionine β-synthase activity [145]. Thus, within 2 years the genetic disorder of cystathionine β-synthase deficiency had been established and its chief clinical manifestations outlined. These observations will be discussed in more detail in the following sections.

The Genetic Defect and Genetic Heterogeneity

To date, deficient activity of cystathionine β-synthase has been reported in extracts of liver from at least 30 homocystinuric patients [128, 145–154] and in extracts of fibroblasts cultured from skin from close to 100 homocystinuric patients [45, 155–166]. (Undoubtedly there is a great deal of overlap between the two groups of patients.) When examined, cystathionine β-synthase activity was also found to be abnormally low in the brain [128], in phytohemagglutinin-stimulated lymphocytes [167, 168], and in long-term cultures of lymphocytes [169] from such patients. A single report [170] suggests that cystathionine β-synthase activity (measured indirectly) may not have been deficient in the optic lens from one homocystinuric patient with clinical findings otherwise typical of cystathionine β-synthase deficiency [57].

Several additional enzymes involved in sulfur amino acid metabolism generally overlap the normal range in tissue extracts of cystathionine β-synthase-deficient patients. These include methionine adenosyltransferase [145, 147, 155, 165], γ-cystathionase [63, 147, 165], betaine-homocysteine methyltransferase, thetin-homocysteine methyltransferase, glutathione-homocysteine transhydrogenase [171], 5-methyltetrahydrofolate-homocysteine methyltransferase [65, 172], and 5,10-methylenetetrahydrofolate reductase [173].

A number of studies have provided some insight into the properties of residual cystathionine β-synthases (or immunologically related molecules) in individual patients with deficiencies of this enzyme. There appear to be numerous differences both between residual activities and normal cystathionine β-synthase and between the residual activities in different affected individuals. The following has been shown: (1) Among affected individuals, residual cystathionine β-synthase activities in cultured fibroblasts differ significantly, ranging from no detectable activitiy up to 10 percent or more of mean control activity [156, 160, 161, 164–166]. In one large series of patients, Uhlendorf et al. [156] noted that there was less variation in residual activities between members of single sibships than between members of different sibships. (2) The stimulation of cystathionine β-synthase activities in crude extracts by addition of pyridoxal phosphate in vitro often differs between patients and control subjects and differs widely among affected patients [156, 160, 174]. (3) Affinities of residual cystathionine β-synthases for pyridoxal phosphate, measured with partially purified enzymes [175], crude enzymes from which cofactor had been removed chemically [160], or enzymes depleted of cofactor by prior growth of cells in pyridoxal-free medium [176], have usually been lower than control affinity and have differed markedly among affected patients. (4) Less extensive measurements have shown that the affinities of residual cystathionine β-synthase for serine may be slightly lower than normal [175], and that affinities for homocysteine may be lower than normal [175], or that the effect of homocysteine concentration upon residual synthase activities may be qualitatively different from the effect upon control synthase [161]. (5) During heat inactivation, residual cystathionine β-synthase activities may be more labile than control activity [159, 160, 175, 177], less labile than control activity [159], or display other differences [154]. (6) Immunologic studies (reported to date only in abstract; see Ref. 163) have shown that cells from cystathionine β-synthase-deficient patients may, or may not, have material which cross-reacts with monospecific antibody to normal human hepatic cystathionine β-synthase. In those cells which had both residual synthase activity and cross-reacting material, there was no obvious quantitative correlation between these two parameters. (7) The residual cystathionine β-synthase from a single patient examined differed in both isoelectric point and electrophoretic mobility from control synthase [41, 42]. Although falling short of absolute proof, such as would be provided by amino acid sequence determinations, taken together these results strongly indicate that there is much genetic heterogeneity among the lesions which produce cystathionine β-synthase deficiency in different individuals (or, more probably, in different sibships). Indeed, when sufficient studies have been carried out, it may turn out that members of any one cystathionine β-synthase-deficient sibship differ from the members of most other such sibships with respect to the genetic determinants which affect cystathionine β-synthase activity. The available results virtually prove, also, that in at least a few individuals the lesion affecting cystathionine β-synthase resides in the structural gene for this enzyme, rather than in a regulatory gene. Again, this seems likely to be true for the majority of affected patients. Although an occasional case of cystathionine β-synthase deficiency has been suggested to be due to a regulatory gene mutation [178], the evidence in support of this conclusion cannot presently be regarded as compelling in any single case.

Mode of Inheritance

Cystathionine β-synthase deficiency is inherited as an autosomal recessive trait, as shown both by pedigree studies [179, 180] and by studies of enzymes in parents of affected children. A combination of data from several studies [57] showed that parents have 22 to 47 (mean, 34) percent of mean control cystathionine β-synthase-specific activities in extracts of liver [146, 148, 150], 21 to 45 percent in extracts of cultured fibroblasts [156, 158, 165, 181], and a mean of 17 percent in phytohemagglutinin-stimulated lymphocytes [168]. Thus, in each tissue obligate heterozygotes have less than 50 percent of the mean control specific activity of the affected enzyme. Human cystathionine β-synthase is normally composed of two apparently identical subunits [36], and it has been suggested that the decrease below 50 percent activity in heterozygotes may be due to negative interaction between mutant and normal subunits combined in "hybrid" molecules of cystathionine β-synthase [57].

Metabolic Sequelae

One of the most characteristic biochemical features of cystathionine β-synthase deficiency is the presence of abnormal accumulations of both homocystine and methionine in plasma. Normally, fasting human plasma contains less than 0.03 μmol/ml methionine, and homocystine is not detected by methods of the usual sensitivity. Untreated cystathionine β-synthase-deficient patients have been reported with fasting plasma concentrations up to 2 μmol/ml for methionine and 0.2 μmol/ml for homocystine [182–184]. The metabolically active form of homocystine is the sulfhydryl, homocysteine. The presence in tissues of relatively large concentrations of reduced glutathione [185], as well as an enzyme which catalyzes a disulfide interchange between glutathione and homocyst(e)ine [186], ensures that intracellularly homocysteine will predominate over homocystine. By appropriate techniques it has been shown that freshly drawn blood or freshly voided urine contains homocysteine as well as homocystine [182, 184], although with customary amino acid analyzer techniques the total of these two compounds is recovered almost entirely as homocystine, possibly accompanied by mixed disulfides, such as that formed between homocysteine and cysteine.

Abnormal accumulations of methionine and homocystine may occur in other body fluids, such as cerebrospinal fluid [187–190] and aqueous humor [191].

Renal tubular reabsorption of methionine is very efficient, and even at moderate elevations of plasma methionine the urinary excretion of this amino acid may be within normal limits [142, 183, 190]. Homocystine is reabsorbed less well [142, 183], and in patients with severe untreated cystathionine β-synthase deficiency more than 1 mmol of this disulfide may be excreted in each day's urine [182, 183].

Few analyses of tissue amino acids have been reported for cystathionine β-synthase–deficient patients. Homocystine was not detected in five liver specimens examined in Maryland or New York [192, 193] but was detected in abnormal amounts in three specimens examined in Japan [190, 194]. In most of these specimens, methionine concentrations were abnormally high [190, 193, 194]. No homocystine was found in either of two brain samples [171, 195], one of which contained a moderate increase of methionine [195]. Homocystine was detected in red blood cells from only one of four patients, of which the three most severely affected had elevated methionine concentrations [196]. Neither homocystine nor an abnormal concentration of methionine was found in cultured skin fibroblasts from a cystathionine β-synthase patient [197], although each of three such lines examined elsewhere was reported to have abnormally high homocystine concentrations [161].

Failure to detect homocystine more consistently in tissues from cystathionine β-synthase-deficient patients may possibly be due to the equilibrium of the reversible condensation between homocysteine and adenosine, which strongly favors S-adenosylhomocysteine formation [28]. Indeed, the three liver specimens from cystathionine β-synthase-deficient patients examined in Maryland, in which no (i.e., less than 0.1 μmol per g wet weight liver) homocystine was detected, each contained abnormally large amounts of S-adenosylhomocysteine (0.23 to 0.97 µmol/g) [192].

The abnormal methionine elevations in cystathionine β-synthase deficiency are presumably due to enhanced rates of homocysteine methylation brought about by increased concentrations of the latter compound. Factors affecting the rate of homocysteine methylation affect the balance between the accumulation of methionine and homocyst(e)ine. For example, there is evidence suggesting that some cystathionine β-synthase-deficient patients in the newborn period may accumulate relatively more methionine and less homocystine than do most adult patients [198]. Perhaps such observations will be explained by a carryover of the relatively high activities of 5-methyltetrahydrofolate-homocysteine methyltransferase found in the fetus [68] into the first weeks or months of extrauterine life [67]. Conversely, a few untreated older cystathionine β-synthase-deficient patients have been described who were homocystinemic and homocystinuric, but who did not have plasma methionine concentrations above the normal range [199–201]. Enhanced methionine-homocystine ratios may be brought about by administration of betaine or its metabolic precursor, choline [202], thus providing more substrate for betaine-homocysteine methyltransferase. Treatment with folic acid leads to similar shifts in the methionine-homocystine balance, probably by increasing the rate of 5-methyltetrahydrofolate-dependent homocysteine methylation [203, 204].

A number of derivatives of homocysteine and methionine are also present in abnormally elevated amounts in plasma or urine of cystathionine β-synthase-deficient patients. These compounds are listed in Table 25-2. A detailed discussion of their likely origins, and the amounts excreted, has been presented elsewhere [57].

Compounds metabolically distal to the block at cystathionine β-synthase would be expected to form at abnormally slow rates in patients with deficiency of this enzyme. Evidence compatible with this expectation has emerged from studies of cystathionine, cyst(e)ine, and sulfate:

1. *Cystathionine.* This product of the cystathionine β-synthase reaction is present in human brain at concentrations which are high compared with those in other tissues or with those in the brains of nonprimates [205, 206]. Brains from three cystathionine β-synthase-deficient children had very low concentrations of cystathionine, ranging from 0 to 0.4 mg per 100 g wet weight, whereas in comparable control specimens the concentrations were 4.8 to 93.3 mg per 100 g [171, 195].

2. *Cyst(e)ine.* Early studies of cystathionine β-synthase-deficient patients revealed that plasma cystine concentrations, as well as urinary excretions, were low or low normal [142, 143]. Subsequent studies have confirmed that plasma and urine cystine of untreated patients may be so low as to be undetectable by the usual methods [174, 207, 208]. Several lines of evidence suggest that the low plasma cyst(e)ine concentrations may at least partially be the result of removal of cyst(e)ine by oxidation or disulfide exchange in the presence of an excess of homocyst(e)ine [57]. Thus measurements of plasma cyst(e)ine concentrations in homocystinemic patients may not furnish reliable indications of either the availability of cysteine to cells or the rates of metabolic formation of cysteine from methionine. In agreement, Rassin and coworkers have reported that at least normal concentrations of cystine were present in liver biopsy specimens obtained from two cystathionine β-synthase-deficient patients at times when their plasma cystine concentrations were below normal [193].

Evidence of the inability of some cystathionine β-synthase-deficient patients to form cysteine at normal rates has resulted from studies with tracer doses of ^{35}S-L-methionine [209] or by use of the technique of nitrogen balance [157, 210]. The latter studies clearly show that some cystathionine β-synthase-deficient patients (chiefly those with no detectable residual activity of cystathionine β-synthase) are able to convert methionine to cysteine only at abnormally low rates. Other cystathionine β-synthase-deficient patients (those with small residual enzyme activities) are able to carry out this conversion at rates sufficient to maintain nitrogen balance even when exogenous cyst(e)ine is withheld from the diet, and are thus forming at least 2.5 to 4.0 mmol cysteine from methionine each day [57].

3. *Sulfate.* In the normal adult human, 80 to 90 percent of the total excretory sulfur is in the form of sulfate, either inorganic sulfate or lesser amounts of sulfate "esters" derived metabolically from inorganic sulfate. Thus, the bulk of the dietary sulfur, ingested chiefly as methionine or cystine, is normally converted to sulfate. Studies with tracer doses of ^{35}S-L-methionine [209], as well as methionine loading studies [153, 211], have provided evidence that cystathionine β-synthase-deficient patients have a specific deficit in their ability to convert methionine sulfur to sulfate. Whereas normal humans have the capacity to convert at least 84 mmol/day of methionine sulfur to sulfate, the three cystathionine β-synthase-deficient patients studied by Mudd et al. [153] could convert a maximum amount of about 8 mmol/day (when they were receiving a normal dietary intake of vitamin B$_6$). In spite of this deficit, since the normal daily dietary intake of methionine may be 8 to 12 mmol [212], it is reasonable to suppose that these patients might dispose of almost all the methionine in a normal diet by conversion to sulfate. This would explain the repeated observations that sulfate is the chief sulfur-containing compound in

Table 25-2 Homocyst(e)ine and methionine derivatives found in abnormal amounts in plasma or urine of cystathionine β-synthase-deficient subjects*

I. Homocysteine derivatives
  A. Oxidation products: homocysteic acid and homocysteine sulfinic acid
  B. S-Adenosylhomocysteine
  C. 5-Amino-4-imidazolecarboxamide-5′-S-homocysteinylribonucleoside
  D. Mixed disulfide of homocysteine and cysteine
  E. Peptides containing homocysteine bound to cysteine in disulfide linkage
  F. Homolanthionine
  G. A variety of compounds formed from homocystine, mixed disulfide of homocysteine and cysteine, or homolanthionine by transamination followed by either reduction or decarboxylation
  H. Other thio ethers likely to be derived from homocyst(e)ine: S-(1,2-dicarboxyethyl)-homocysteine and S-carboxymethyl-homocysteine
  I. Mixed disulfide of homocysteine and cysteinylglycine [204a]
II. Methionine derivatives
  A. Methionine sulfoxide
  B. "Bound" methionine

*See Ref. 57.

the urine of cystathionine β-synthase-deficient patients [157, 196, 210, 211], whereas homocystine contributes only a relatively minor portion of the total sulfur [142, 157, 211].

In summary, the metabolic sequelae of severe cystathionine β-synthase deficiency include accumulation of abnormal amounts of homocyst(e)ine, methionine, and a variety of metabolites derived from these compounds. Intracellularly, accumulation of S-adenosylhomocysteine may predominate over that of homocysteine. Under conditions of methionine loading, homocystine accounts for only a very small portion of the abnormal urinary sulfur [212]. For untreated patients on relatively normal diets (8 to 12 mmol methionine), the available data [57] suggest that together homocystine, homocysteine-cysteine mixed disulfide, S-adenosylhomocysteine, 5-amino-4-imidazole carboxamide-5'-S-homocysteinylribonucleoside, methionine, methionine sulfoxide, and homolanthionine may account (very approximately) for 2 to 3 mmol of daily urinary sulfur. Other compounds are known to be present in the urine in abnormal amounts, but these account for relatively very minor amounts of sulfur. The major portion of methionine sulfur is converted to sulfate. In patients with residual activities of cystathionine β-synthase, at least 2.5 to 4.0 mmol methionine sulfur is converted to cysteine daily, and this pathway would explain formation of an almost equivalent amount of sulfate. For patients without residual activities of cystathionine β-synthase, less, if any, cysteine is formed, and some conversion of methionine sulfur to sulfate probably occurs by alternative metabolic routes [57].

The Pyridoxine Effect and Its Mechanism

In 1967 Barber and Spaeth reported for the first time that three cystathionine β-synthase-deficient patients responded to very high doses (250 to 500 mg daily) of pyridoxine with decreases of plasma methionine levels to normal, and virtual elimination of homocystine from plasma and urine [213]. This observation has since been extended to many additional patients by many authors. During the response to pyridoxine, there are decreases in a number of additional compounds formed proximal to the metabolic block at cystathionine β-synthase and increases in compounds distal to the block [57]. Some cystathionine β-synthase-deficient patients are not responsive to vitamin B_6—they show little or no change in plasma or urine sulfur amino acids when given comparably large doses of this vitamin. In a review of patients with cystathionine β-synthase deficiency, both published [57, 160, 162, 178, 214–231] and known to us but unpublished [57], we found that among 272 classified with respect to vitamin B_6 responsiveness, 110 (40.5 percent) were considered responsive, 129 (47.4 percent) were considered nonresponsive, and 33 (12.1 percent) were considered to have intermediate or questionable responses.

There is ample evidence that the vitamin B_6 induced response of those cystathionine β-synthase-deficient patients who do respond is not due to correction of a preexisting vitamin B_6 deficiency or to alleviation of a defect in vitamin B_6 metabolism which renders these patients unable to form pyridoxal-5'-phosphate, the form of vitamin B_6 active as a cofactor for cystathionine β-synthase [57]. Some untreated cystathionine β-synthase-deficient patients have abnormally low serum folate concentrations [203, 204], and this tendency may be exacerbated by treatment with pyridoxine [232, 233]. The bio-

chemical response to pyridoxine may not be manifest in folate-depleted patients until after folate replenishment [204, 233]. Thus, folate depletion may explain the apparent failure of some patients to respond to pyridoxine treatment, and studies of the effect of pyridoxine are interpretable only in the presence of adequate folate.

When different patients are compared, it is apparent that "pyridoxine-responsive" patients are not uniform. Some patients in response continue to have slight elevations of homocystine in plasma or urine [153, 232, 234], although others do not [147, 196, 234]. On the basis of the clinical responses of their patients to pyridoxine, Brenton and Cusworth defined three classes of vitamin B_6 responsiveness, including a group intermediate between those who display little or no response and those with very clear responses [234]. Even those patients who respond most favorably are clearly not restored to biochemical normality. Such patients in response have markedly abnormal rises in concentrations of plasma and urinary homocystine after methionine loads [147, 153], and restoration of plasma methionine to basal concentrations is delayed [147]. Their maximal capacities for transsulfuration in vivo continue to be far below the maximal capacities of normal subjects, as measured by sulfate excretion following oral methionine loads [153].

Classification of increasing numbers of cystathionine β-synthase-deficient patients as to their pyridoxine responsiveness has provided unequivocal evidence that pyridoxine responsiveness is constant within sibships: All cystathionine β-synthase-deficient members of a particular sibship are either responsive to vitamin B_6 or unresponsive. If the sibships reviewed by Mudd and Levy [57] are combined with those more recently reported [154, 162, 164, 166, 221, 226, 235, 236], it is found that constancy of responsiveness within sibships prevailed among at least 38 sibships with a total of at least 86 patients. A few possible exceptions do not appear to be sufficiently compelling to challenge seriously this generalization [57]. This constancy indicates not only that the capacity to respond to vitamin B_6 is genetically determined, but also that the genetic determinant governing responsiveness is closely linked with, or identical to, that determining cystathionine β-synthase deficiency itself. If the two genetic factors were unlinked and segregated separately, variation of responsiveness within cystathionine β-synthase-deficient members of the same sibship might be expected. The simplest interpretation is that the same mutation which makes an individual cystathionine β-synthase deficient also determines whether he or she will be vitamin B_6 responsive. A single alteration of apoenzyme structure might well determine both properties.

Studies of cystathionine β-synthase activities support the hypothesis that responsiveness or nonresponsiveness may be determined by the specific properties of the mutant enzyme molecule. There is a strong correlation between the presence of detected residual activity of cystathionine β-synthase and clinical responsiveness to vitamin B_6 and between absence of detected residual activity and nonresponsiveness. Residual activities have been detected in liver extracts from each of seven vitamin B_6-responsive patients but not in extracts from any of three vitamin B_6-nonresponders [57]. More extensive data with cultured fibroblasts [156, 160, 164–166] show (1) that the presence or absence of detected residual cystathionine β-synthase activity is constant within sibships, and (2) that among sibships responsive to vitamin B_6, 31 had residual activities of cystathionine β-synthase in cultured fibroblasts; only eight lacked such activity. In contrast, among sibships not responsive to vitamin B$_6$, only six had detected residual activity of cystathionine β-synthase, whereas 20 had no detected activity.

Quantitatively, the residual activities of cystathionine β-synthase in extracts of fibroblasts cultured from vitamin B$_6$-responsive patients have varied from about 0.1 to 10 percent of mean control values [156, 160, 165]. When potentially vitamin B$_6$-responsive patients were receiving normal vitamin B$_6$ intakes, their liver extracts, assayed in the presence of ample pyridoxal phosphate, have had residual activities of 1 to 2 percent of mean control values [153], 3.7 to 9.4 percent [146], or, in one case, 31 percent [152]. When the same patients were receiving large dietary intakes of pyridoxine, the cystathionine β-synthase specific activities in their liver extracts were enhanced 1.5- to 3.0-fold [153] or 1.3- to 4.5-fold [146].

Taken together, these results suggest that, in most patients, vitamin B$_6$-responsiveness is based upon the presence of a small amount of residual mutant cystathionine β-synthase, the steady-state activity of which is enhanced somewhat when the patient is taking large doses of vitamin B$_6$. Although the enhanced activity does not attain control levels, it does become sufficient to metabolize the homocysteine arising from a normal methionine intake without an accumulation severe enough to produce homocyst(e)inemia or homocystinuria. A number of quantitative considerations which support this formulation have been reviewed in more detail elsewhere [57, 237, 238]. This formulation leaves unexplained the mechanism of response in those responsive patients for whom cystathionine β-synthase activity has not been detected in cultured fibroblasts. If these negative findings for fibroblasts accurately reflect the situation in the livers of such patients, presumably some other basis will have to be found for their vitamin B$_6$ responsiveness.

The molecular properties of mutant cystathionine β-synthases crucial in conferring vitamin B$_6$ responsiveness remain obscure. The mere presence of some residual cystathionine β-synthase activity is not sufficient, as proven by the finding of clinically nonresponsive patients with readily detectable residual activities. With enzymes from responsive patients, restoration of near-normal activity by high concentrations of pyridoxal phosphate in vitro such as would take place if the mutations affected only the K_m for this cofactor, has usually not occurred [57, 156, 159, 160]. Some of the largest observed enhancements of activity by addition of pyridoxal phosphate in vitro have occurred with enzymes from clinically nonresponsive patients [156, 160]. Indeed, Lipson and coworkers [176] have suggested that for a patient to be vitamin B$_6$ responsive, not only must some residual cystathionine β-synthase activity be present, but the affinity of this mutant enzyme for cofactor must not be too severely impaired. Further studies of mutant enzymes resolved from cofactor by the growth of fibroblasts in pyridoxine-free medium [176], and of the factors determining the rates of turnover of mutant forms of cystathionine β-synthase in liver and other tissues [238], may be expected to throw additional light upon this question.

Clinical Manifestations

For purposes of the discussion to follow, we have reviewed the literature and found at least 350 reported cases in which sufficient evidence is available to support a diagnosis of cystathi-

onine β-synthase deficiency [57, 162, 178, 214–226]. These are cases of homocystinuria accompanied by either demonstrated abnormally low cystathionine β-synthase activity (which we regard as "proved") or by hypermethioninemia or dislocated optic lenses, or both (which we regard as "presumed") cystathionine β-synthase deficiency. To these reported cases have been added 21 unreported cases with which we are familiar [57]. As a result of a recent survey, we are aware of at least 100 additional cases which, to our knowledge, are unreported [239], but which are not included in this review because we lack knowledge of clinical details. Also excluded from consideration in determination of specific clinical manifestations are those individuals identified in the neonatal period who received therapy designed to prevent clinical complications.

Four organ systems show major involvement in patients with cystathionine β-synthase deficiency: the eye, the skeletal system, the central nervous system, and the vascular system. Other organs, including the liver, hair, and skin, may also show changes. The abnormalities in question are listed in Table 25-3. Most of them will be discussed in greater detail below. Individuals with cystathionine β-synthase deficiency are almost always normal at birth and have been born after normal pregnancies. Thus, the clinical abnormalities noted in association with this disorder develop after birth. That they are very likely related to the disorder itself is suggested by the similarity of major abnormalities among known affected individuals and by the fact that the abnormalities are progressive at least throughout childhood and adolescence.

Ocular Probably the most consistent finding in patients

Table 25-3 Clinical abnormalities in cystathionine β-synthase deficiency

I. Ocular	3. Retarded lunate development
A. Very frequent	4. Pectus carinatum or excavatum
1. Ectopia lentis	
2. Iridodonesis	III. Central nervous system
3. Myopia	A. Frequent: mental retardation
B. Less frequent	B. Less frequent
1. Glaucoma	1. Seizures
2. Optic atrophy	2. Abnormal EEG
3. Retinal degeneration	3. Spasticity
4. Retinal detachment	4. Focal neurologic signs
5. Cataracts	5. Psychiatric disturbances
II. Skeletal	IV. Vascular
A. Very frequent	A. Frequent
1. Osteoporosis	1. Arterial and venous thromboemboli
2. Dolichostenomelia	2. Malar flush
3. Biconcave ("fish") vertebrae	3. Livedo reticularis
4. Scoliosis	V. Other involvement
5. Genu valgum	A. Fair, brittle hair
6. Widened femoral/tibial condyles	B. Thin skin
7. Pes cavus	C. High-arched palate
8. Growth arrest line	D. Crowded and protruding upper teeth
9. Metaphyseal spicules	E. Fatty change in liver
B. Less frequent	F. Inguinal hernia
1. Arachnodactyly	G. Myopathy
2. Enlarged carpal bones	

with cystathionine β-synthase deficiency is ectopia lentis (dislocation of the lens) (Fig. 25-2). The lenticular dislocation rarely, if ever, occurs before age 3 years but generally has taken place by age 10 years [179]. Exceptional individuals may develop ectopia lentis later in life [162, 179, 219, 221, 240]. One author has stated (but without providing supporting details) that dislocation occurs ultimately in over 90 percent of affected individuals [241, 242]. The dislocation is usually downward, although it may occur in any direction [179, 241–243].

The ectopia lentis is secondary to disruption of the zonular fibers that connect the lens to the ciliary body. In cystathionine β-synthase deficiency these fibers are thickened and broken and may be contrasted to the zonular fibers in Marfan's syndrome, which are thin and elongated and appear to be decreased in number [244]. Careful examination of cystathionine β-synthase-deficient patients may reveal the thickened white zonular remnants undulating freely at the equatorial region of the dislocated lens [245] (Fig. 25-2).

Several abnormalities occur as a secondary result of the loosening and subsequent subluxation of the lenses. The most common is iridodonesis (quivering of the iris), which occurs when the iris no longer lies on a stationary lens. Iridodonesis is particularly evident when the head is moved. A marked myopia and astigmatism are always associated with ectopia lentis. Although the myopia may to some extent be due to an excessively long globe [179], myopia and astigmatism worsen when subluxation occurs. The lens may dislocate anteriorly, where it can obstruct the pupil and cause acute pupillary block glaucoma [227]. This produces severe ocular pain and may be the presenting clinical problem [246–249]. Staphyloma may also result from this increased intraocular pressure in younger children. Cataracts have been noted in a number of the dislocated lenses [250, 251], possibly occurring as a result of trauma to the lens associated with dislocation. A notable exception to the sequence of cataracts preceded by ectopia lentis occurred in one of the first patients described, who at the age of 1 month had bilateral zonular cataracts without evidence of ectopia len-

tis [143]. Perhaps in this patient the cataracts were coincidental with the cystathionine β-synthase deficiency.

Ocular abnormalities other than ectopia lentis and its complications are frequently seen in patients with cystathionine β-synthase deficiency. Among these are light irides, optic atrophy, and retinal changes such as degeneration and detachment. [250–252]. In two patients optic atrophy was apparently secondary to occlusion of the central retinal artery [253, 254].

Skeletal

OSTEOPOROSIS   Among the most striking changes in persons with cystathionine β-synthase deficiency are those of the skeleton. Some of these changes are illustrated in Figs. 25-3 and 25-4. The most consistent skeletal abnormality is osteoporosis. In a large series of cases ascertained on the basis of ectopia lentis, osteoporosis was present in all [251]. Subsequent studies have confirmed the very frequent, though not constant, presence of osteoporosis [162, 231, 255–257]. As is true for ectopia lentis, osteoporosis has rarely been noted in early childhood. However, osteoporosis of the spine was present in a child at age 6 years [256], and generalized osteoporosis has been reported in children 4 to 10 years of age [231, 249]. The spine is the most common site for osteoporosis [256–259], followed by the long bones [256, 257, 259]. Perhaps as a result of spinal osteoporosis, scoliosis occurs in many affected individuals [231, 256, 257, 259], although scoliosis has been reported in the absence of osteoporosis [257]. Osteoporosis of the spine may lead to vertebral collapse [251], while osteoporosis of the long bones predisposes to pathologic fractures that heal slowly [251, 260].

OTHER SKELETAL MANIFESTATIONS   Biconcavity of the vertebrae (usually referred to as *codfish* or *fish* vertebrae) is a frequent finding [231, 251, 261] (Fig. 25-3). Although it has usually been attributed to spinal osteoporosis, Brenton et al. [260] pointed out that unlike the biconcavity typical of osteoporosis, the biconcavity in cystathionine β-synthase deficiency is posteriorly placed in the vertebral body. Westerman et al. [261] noted that the biconcavity is identical to that in chronic hemolytic disease and postulated that, as in the hemolytic diatheses, it results from occlusion of long branches of the vertebral nutrient arteries. Flattening and anterior wedging of the vertebrae are present in many affected individuals and are believed to cause the kyphosis that is sometimes seen [231].

Individuals with cystathionine β-synthase deficiency usually are tall and thin by the time they reach later childhood. The long bones are thin and excessively lengthened, a situation known as *dolichostenomelia* [231, 256, 258, 259, 261a] (Fig. 25-4). The distal extremities are often also elongated, although arachnodactyly as determined by a metacarpal index of greater than 8.5 [262] has been reported in fewer than half the patients [162, 179, 257, 261a]. The metaphyses and epiphyses of the long bones are often widened, an abnormality most easily recognized in the knees (Fig. 25-4). Genu valgum and humerus valgum, as well as bowing of the long bones, are frequent concomitants of this widening. Prominent growth arrest lines are often present in the distal tibia [231, 257].

Radiographic changes may also be present in the hands and feet. Most frequent are metaphyseal spicules; enlargement of the carpal bones and elongation of the talus may also occur [231, 256, 257, 259, 261a]. Curiously, development of the lunate has been selectively retarded in a number of patients

Figure 25-2 Inferonasal dislocation of the optic lens in a 9-year-old girl with cystathionine β-synthase deficiency. A fringe of zonular remnants is present at the equator of the lens. (*From Ramsey et al.* [243], *with permission.*)

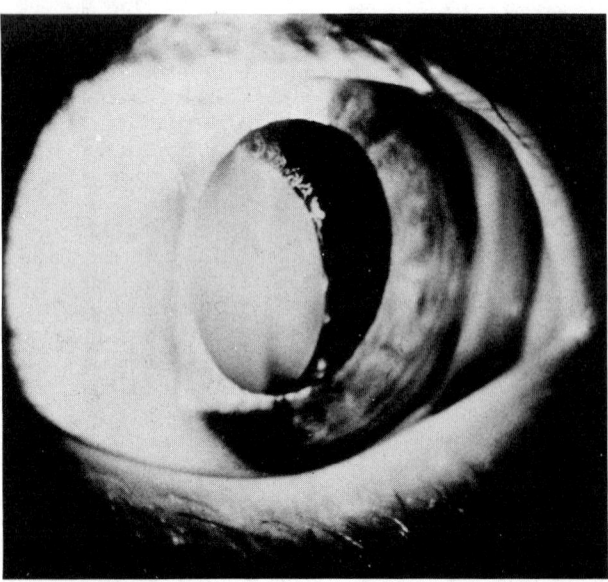

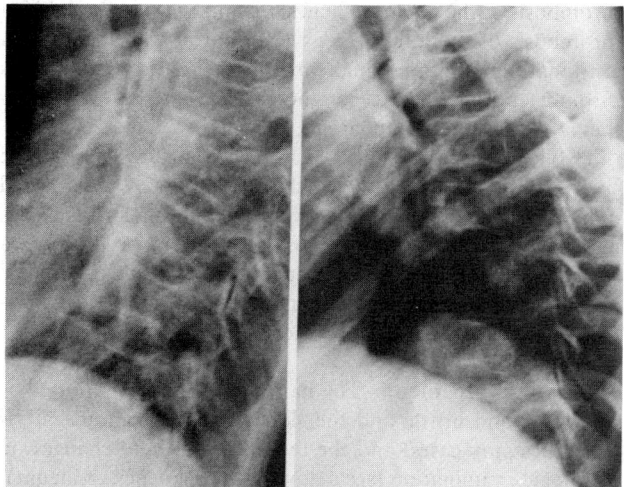

Figure 25-3 Roentgenograms of the spine in two patients with cystathionine β-synthase deficiency. *Left:* 18-year-old girl. *Right:* 11-year-old girl. The characteristic findings of osteoporosis and biconcavity or "codfish" deformity of the vertebrae are considerably more marked in the latter patient.

[256, 259, 263]. Bone age is usually normal, although on occasion it is advanced or retarded [255, 256, 259, 264].

The appearance of the chest may be striking because of pectus carinatum or excavatum. The former is the more frequent [260]. The facial appearance may be altered by protrusion of the upper teeth. The palate is almost always high-arched [260]. The feet usually have a pronounced pes cavus, although pes planus is occasionally seen [260].

Central Nervous System

MENTAL RETARDATION   The most frequent abnormality of the central nervous system is mental retardation. Often this is the first recognized sign of cystathionine β-synthase deficiency, presenting as developmental delay during the first or second year of life [226, 265, 266]. Developmental delay has been noted as early as the first weeks [143]. The lag in development is similar to that in patients with other inborn errors of metabolism. The infant may not sit unsupported or crawl until 1 year of age, may not walk until age 2 years or later, and may not begin speaking until well beyond 2 years of age. When walking begins, the gait is usually waddling or "Charlie Chaplin-like" [267]. These children are often seen by orthopedic surgeons because of the late walking and peculiar gait [268].

Mental retardation, when present, becomes obvious in middle childhood. The IQs reported among those who are retarded have varied from less than 30 to 75 [142, 190, 226, 260, 269, 270]. This wide range in IQ may to some degree depend upon the age when the test was performed. Thus, among sibs, the older often has had the lower IQ [152, 271]. Mental retardation, however, undoubtedly varies in extent among affected individuals, as illustrated by sibships in which IQ differences were independent of age [208, 265, 272–275]. In general, the mental retardation is less severe than in phenylketonuria. This is perhaps one factor in the apparent low incidence of cystathionine β-synthase–deficient individuals among those institutionalized for mental retardation.

About 20 percent of reported patients have had normal or near-normal intelligence. This frequency is almost certainly too low, reflecting the greater likelihood that patients with

mental retardation will be diagnosed and reported in the literature. In a review by McKusick et al. [179], ascertainment was largely based on ectopia lentis, and about 50 percent of 84 cases had at least average intelligence. Similarly, in an Australian series [221], 12 of 25 cases over the age of 1 year were not mentally retarded, although many of these individuals were considered to be less clever than their unaffected sibs.

CONVULSIONS   Convulsions, often severe, have been noted in 10 to 15 percent of all cases. The seizures may begin in infancy, be focal in type, and be followed by specific neurologic signs such as hemiparesis, suggesting the occurrence of a cerebrovascular occlusion [273, 276]. On the other hand, the seizures have often been generalized, occurring with or without fever, and have been severe, with prolonged apnea and postictal unconsciousness [142, 189, 265, 277]. In one child, the first seizure followed poliomyelitis immunization [267]. In another, diencephalic seizures characterized by attacks of abdominal pain were reported [188], although these seizures may well have been unrelated to the cystathionine β-synthase

Figure 25-4 Roentgenogram of the lower femur and knee of a cystathionine β-synthase-deficient patient. In addition to osteoporosis, there is widening of the distal metaphysis and epiphysis of the femur.

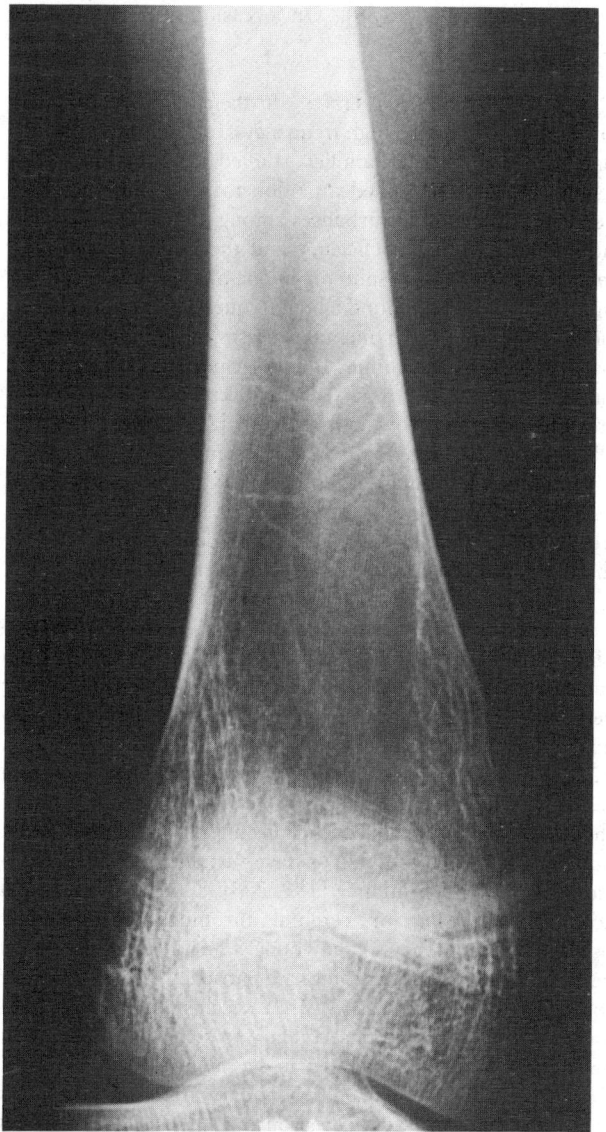

deficiency. Myoclonic seizures were noted in one case [278], and minor motor seizures have been reported in at least two affected individuals [146, 279].

ELECTROENCEPHALOGRAPHY   A number of patients have had electroencephalographic abnormalities, although these have not been constant features of cystathionine β-synthase deficiency. Excessive slow wave activity has been common [179, 199, 265, 273, 280]. Spikes and sharp wave discharges have also been reported [146, 273]. While these abnormalities have often been present in individuals with a history of seizures, individuals with similar histories have had normal electroencephalograms [142, 189, 267]. Abnormal electroencephalograms have been reported in individuals without seizures [146, 179, 199, 265, 273, 274, 281]. In one case, electroencephalographic abnormalities were present only at times shortly after generalized seizures [280].

NEUROLOGIC ABNORMALITIES   Specific neurologic findings have generally not been striking and have usually been associated with obvious cerebrovascular disease. Thus unilateral weakness and spasticity have accompanied unilateral cerebral thrombosis [189, 273]. Deep-tendon reflexes have been increased in association with other evidence of cerebrovascular brain damage [142, 189]. On occasion they have been decreased [264, 267].

PSYCHIATRIC ABNORMALITIES   In their initial report, Carson et al. [142] noted a high frequency of schizophrenia on the maternal side of the families studied. Shortly thereafter, Schimke et al [251] called attention to a possibly increased frequency of mental disturbances among individuals with cystathionine β-synthase deficiency and their families and later described chronic schizophrenia in one of their patients [282]. Dunn et al [273] also found a high frequency of serious behavior disorders and other mental illnesses among those on the maternal side of two families and on the paternal side of a third family. Others have reported the occurrence of "nervous breakdowns" [246] or schizophrenia [204, 248, 266, 274, 280, 283, 284] among patients or in members of their immediate families. It is not clear whether there is truly an increased frequency of such derangement among homozygotes and heterozygotes for cystathionine β-synthase deficiency or whether these reports reflect merely chance associations.

Vascular   The life-threatening complication of cystathionine β-synthase deficiency is thromboembolism. Large and small arteries and veins may be affected. Involvement of large vessels has resulted in death or disability from carotid or coronary thrombosis or pulmonary emboli [146, 179, 189, 220, 221, 267, 273]. In one infant, seizures and death occurred as a result of a massive thrombosis of the superior lateral sinus of the brain [276]. Vascular occlusions may occur at any age. A number of affected individuals have sustained major cerebrovascular thrombi in infancy [189, 273]. Sudden death due to coronary occlusion or cerebral thrombosis has usually occurred after infancy in the young adult or even childhood years [220, 221, 274]. Thrombi are particularly likely to occur following surgery [179, 267, 283]. Occlusions may occur in any vessel. Renal infarcts secondary to small and large renal arterial thrombi have resulted in severe hypertension [240]. Cor pulmonale secondary to pulmonary artery occlusion has also been reported [240]. Brenton et al [260] have reported

thrombosis of the common iliac vein, and Schimke et al. [251] thrombosis of the inferior vena cava. In fact, at postmortem examination, multiple small and large arterial and venous thrombi and emboli are commonly encountered even when they were clinically inapparent.

Two features presumably of vascular origin are visible in the skin. One is a malar flush which is striking in some affected individuals. The second is livedo reticularis, an erythematous mottling of the extremities, most marked on the legs. From reported cases it appears that at least 50 percent of affected individuals have these features. In our experience these cutaneous signs generally occur together.

Other Involvement   The hair has often been reported as being fair and brittle and the skin as thin. Hepatomegaly is noted in many cases, and the liver has had fatty changes on histologic examination (see below). The frequency of inguinal hernia seems to be increased among affected individuals [179]. Electromyographic evidence of myopathy has been reported [270]. Hyperinsulinemia with pathologic glucose tolerance and increased levels of growth hormone have also been reported [229, 285].

Reproductive Fitness   A search of the literature reveals reports summarizing the outcomes of 44 pregnancies in 16 cystathionine β-synthase–deficient women [57, 162, 286, 287]. Of these pregnancies, 36 occurred in vitamin B₆-responsive patients. Seventeen of the latter pregnancies occurred before homocystinuria had been discovered, and the mother was therefore untreated; 15 ended in fetal loss, and two produced normal children. One pregnancy in a vitamin B₆-responsive patient who had discontinued treatment was terminated by therapeutic abortion at 22 weeks [236]. Of 18 pregnancies in responders who received vitamin B₆ during pregnancy, one ended in spontaneous abortion, 15 produced normal children (including one premature), one, a child with brain damage presumably secondary to a precipitous delivery, and one, a child with trisomy 21. Five pregnancies in untreated vitamin B₆-nonresponsive patients produced one spontaneous abortion and four normal children [286, 288]. Three pregnancies in patients not classified with respect to their vitamin B₆-responsiveness [179] produced two normal children and one hydrocephalic stillbirth.

Absence of chorionic vessels [289] and placental infarcts [290] have been reported in the unsuccessful pregnancies. The fetus studied after therapeutic abortion [236], genetically and by enzyme assay of cultured amniotic fluid cells determined to be a heterozygote for cystathionine β-synthase deficiency, had abnormally high concentrations of methionine in the liver and brain, and of cystathionine in the liver, brain, and kidney. Homocystine was not detected in any tissue [193].

It is difficult to judge the extent to which these published results are biased by a tendency not to report normal pregnancies with normal outcomes. Nevertheless, it appears that untreated cystathionine β-synthase–deficient patients may have a high rate of fetal loss, and that vitamin B₆ responders treated with vitamin B₆ may have a considerably reduced risk.

Men with cystathionine β-synthase deficiency have fathered phenotypically normal children [179, 287]. The data reported are insufficient to permit an assessment of whether the obligate heterozygous fetuses sired by such fathers and who are carried by normal women are at increased risk during gestation.

Variation in Clinical Manifestations The number of clinical complications and their severity vary markedly among different individuals with cystathionine β-synthase deficiency. At one end of the spectrum are those afflicted with most of the major complications, including ectopia lentis, severe skeletal abnormalities, mental retardation, and vascular occlusions, and with many of the minor complications, including malar flushing, livedo reticularis, and others. At the other are those with only ectopia lentis or with virtually no discernible clinical complications [144, 162, 221, 291]. Between them are individuals who may have ectopia lentis and mild skeletal abnormalities but who have normal mentality and no evidence of thromboembolic diathesis [162, 179, 221, 292]. The reason (or reasons) for these variations in clinical manifestations is (are) as yet obscure, but two generalizations appear to be warranted: (1) the clinical severity is generally similar among sibs whose disease has not been altered by therapy [221, 265, 273]; (2) generally, but not invariably, those individuals who have relatively mild clinical disease respond biochemically to vitamin B₆ supplementation [162, 179, 221, 233]. Both these generalizations suggest that some of the clinical variation is determined genetically.

It is not yet certain whether ascertainment bias has influenced our present picture of the clinical manifestations of cystathionine β-synthase deficiency. Testing for this disorder has generally been conducted among individuals known to have one or more of the typical clinical complications [179]. Are there many affected individuals who are clinically normal but who have never been detected because they have not come to medical attention? Study of patients ascertained during routine neonatal screening programs is not likely to produce an accurate picture of the natural history of this disease, since individuals diagnosed in this manner are currently given treatment. A potential alternative means of determining the clinical spectrum of cystathionine β-synthase deficiency is to study individuals ascertained by the screening of all available family members after identification of a propositus in the family. Unfortunately, most reports of sibships or kindreds with this disorder do not specify either the completeness of the family screening or whether biochemical testing of affected family members was performed because of observable clinical abnormalities. However, we have been able to find at least 18 families in which 25 additional cases of cystathionine β-synthase deficiency have been discovered as a result of complete family screening [146, 180, 201, 217, 221, 226, 247, 292–295]. Of these 25 individuals, 19 had one or more of the known clinical manifestations. The six exceptions are as follows: three individuals from Australia, ages up to 24 years, clinically normal, although possibly less intelligent than their unaffected sib [221]; one girl, clinically normal (except for severe myopia) at age 19 years [180]; a child, entirely normal at age 8 years, but who has been treated with pyridoxine and has been in biochemical remission since 5 years of age [146, 293]; and a 6-year-old boy, normal, but increasingly hyperactive since age 5 years [226]. In spite of these possible exceptions, on the whole the findings described suggest that clinical normality is unusual among individuals with cystathionine β-synthase deficiency who have not received treatment from early infancy.

Not included in the above are two additional clinically normal homocystinuric individuals whose genetic status is not clearly defined by the evidence available [156, 165]. One woman, the cousin of a proven cystathionine β-synthase–deficient patient [144], was clinically normal at age 28 [196]. She had mild homocystinuria and hypermethioninemia. Enzyme activity was 12 percent of the mean control value in an extract of her liver [148] but was 67 percent of the mean control value in fibroblast extracts [156]. The second such patient, a boy, is free of severe clinical stigmata at age 14. Untreated, he excreted relatively little homocystine. His plasma had mildly elevated homocystine, methionine at the upper limit of normal, and slightly depressed cystine. Cystathionine β-synthase activity in fibroblast extracts was approximately 48 percent of the mean control value and 119 percent of the mean heterozygote value. Two homocystinuric, clinically affected sibs of this boy had no detected cystathionine β-synthase activity in extracts of fibroblasts [165]. The two patients under discussion could be either very mildly affected homozygotes or, somewhat more likely in our view, heterozygotes with hepatic cystathionine β-synthase activities so unusually low for heterozygotes (for unknown reasons) as to lead to homocystinemia and homocystinuria.

Pathology

Underlying many of the clinical features characteristic of cystathionine β-synthase deficiency are equally characteristic pathologic findings.

Ocular The most common findings noted on pathologic examination (and also visible clinically) are fraying and disruption of the zonular fibers (Fig. 25-2). The ocular lens, which is held in place by these fibers, becomes subluxated when they break. The zonular fibers often recoil to the surface of the ciliary body, there lying matted and fused with the thickened basement membrane of the unpigmented ciliary epithelium [296], then assuming the appearance of a thickened PAS-positive amorphous layer that becomes more obvious with age [297]. Zonular remnants have also been observed on the lens, where they acquire the electron-microscopic appearance of masses of short, disorganized filaments similar to that of the fibers attached to the ciliary body [245].

Other histopathologic changes in the eye include peripheral retinal degeneration, which is common, as is atrophy of the nonpigmented ciliary epithelium [297]. Pigmentation of the retinal periphery and a whitish membrane covering the ciliary processes have also been described [298]. Occlusion of the greater arterial circle of the iris has been reported [297]. The posterior sclera may be thin and the choroid atrophic [296].

Skeletal The gross changes in the spine are consistent with the radiographic findings. Thus, the vertebral bodies reveal rarefaction of spongy bone within the intact bony margin and the codfish configuration [259]. Within the long bones there is an enlarged zone of bradytrophic vacuolated cartilage in the epimetaphyseal areas [259]. Histopathologic studies suggest that there is a defect of bone formation preferentially involving endochondral epimetaphyseal ossification [259].

Central Nervous System Within the central nervous system lesions in the brain are the most striking. Infarcts, secondary to cerebrovascular occlusions, are common [189, 220, 273, 276, 280, 299]. These infarcts may contain cystic changes. Chou and Waisman [300] described a single patient with extensive spongy degeneration and demyelination in the white matter of the cerebrum, cerebellum, basal ganglions, brainstem, and cervical spinal cord. These changes have not been noted in other studies, and Dunn et al. [273] specifically reported the absence of these changes in one of their patients. Gaull et al. [250] reported neuronal loss in the cerebral cortex and hippocampus. The lipid composition of the brain has been analyzed in one patient and was normal [230].

Vascular The striking vascular lesions associated with cystathionine β-synthase deficiency have attracted much attention at postmortem examination. Thrombi and emboli have been reported in almost every major artery or vein and in many smaller vessels. Involvement of major cerebral vessels has resulted in infarcts in the cerebrum, cerebellum, midbrain, and thalamus [189, 220, 250, 273, 276, 280, 299]. Thrombi in the dural sinuses have also been reported [276, 299]. Other vascular involvement has resulted in coronary occlusions [251, 274], pulmonary infarcts [301], renal infarcts [189, 273], and thrombophlebitis with pulmonary emboli [251].

Arterial walls have been the sites of the most unusual changes. Marked fibrous thickening of the intima is found even in children and young adults [180, 189, 299]. Intimal fibrosis of the aorta was so extensive in one patient that a mild degree of coarctation was produced [302]. The thickening may be symmetrical, with resulting severe luminal narrowing, or patchy with formation of pads [299]. Within the media the muscle fibers are frayed and split, with increased interstitial collagen [251, 299]. The elastic fibers in the media of large arteries may be frayed and fragmented [180, 250, 251], and there may be changes in the internal elastic lamella [180, 274, 299]. Advanced atherosclerotic degenerative changes were found in a large abdominal aortic aneurysm from a 36-year-old man [218]. Virtually any large- or medium-sized artery may be affected [180, 299].

Changes in the walls of veins have been noted only by Gibson et al. [299], who reported fibrous endophlebitis in a renal vein of one patient. Gaull [302] found no lesions in veins.

Other Organs Fatty change of the liver has been found in virtually all patients studied post mortem or by liver biopsy [179]. Based upon their light- and electron-microscopic studies [146, 279], Gaull and his group reported that fat accumulation was largely in the centrolobular hepatocytes. Mitochondria were abnormally shaped, with fingerlike projections and tapered ends, and the smooth endoplasmic reticulum was hypertrophic. Endocardial fibroelastosis of the left atrium has also been reported [251, 299]. Structural abnormalities of collagen and elastic fibers of skin have been described [302a].

Pathophysiology

Perhaps no aspect of cystathionine β-synthase deficiency has remained so obscure as the analysis of the intermediate steps by which the enzyme deficiency leads to the specific clinical manifestations associated with it. On the one hand, the clinical manifestations themselves are variable from patient to patient and in time of onset. On the other, the array of abnormally accumulated metabolites formed proximal to the enzyme block complicates attribution of any given clinical abnormality to a specific metabolite. In addition, there is the possibility of deficiencies of cystathionine, cysteine, or even sulfate distal to the block. Finally, the lack of experimental animals with cys-

tathionine β-synthase deficiency has severely limited empirical exploration of this aspect of the problem.

Evidence relevant to the pathophysiology of cystathionine β-synthase deficiency and available up to 1975 has been reviewed in detail [57]. In this chapter, therefore, summary statements only will be presented, with elaboration of more recent experimental work bearing on these matters.

Methionine and Homocysteine Toxicity It has been known for many years that an excessive intake of either methionine [303] or homocystine retards growth of the rat [304]. Many accompanying metabolic and morphologic changes have been noted [57]. However, cystathionine β-synthase-deficient patients do not develop the specific anatomic changes manifested by rats fed excessive methionine or homocystine, nor, conversely, has mention been made in these experimental animals of dislocated optic lenses, bony changes, or the thromboembolic tendencies characteristic of cystathionine β-synthase deficiency. Thus the animal studies appear to offer little hope of clarifying the sequence of metabolic events responsible for these particular clinical phenomena [57].

Homocystinemia, Thrombosis, and Atherosclerosis Many investigations have been carried out with the aim of defining the cause of the abnormal clotting and atherosclerotic tendencies of cystathionine β-synthase-deficient patients. An early report by McDonald et al. [305] that the platelets from homocystinemic, presumed cystathionine β-synthase-deficient patients were abnormally adhesive drew attention to the possibility that abnormalities of the platelets themselves might underlie these tendencies. The finding of McDonald et al. has since been confirmed by workers using similar methods [306] in at least three other laboratories [196, 210, 232, 240, 307]. By this technique, which measures the adherence of platelets to a relatively small glass surface during relatively long times of exposure, abnormally elevated adhesiveness has been found for the platelets from at least 26 homocystinemic patients; the platelets from four such patients were reported to be normal [232, 269]. Homocystine added to normal blood at concentrations such as might be found in samples from cystathionine β-synthase-deficient patients was reported to bring about increased adhesiveness of normal platelets [196, 305, 307]. Similar effects were achieved by the addition of methionine [307]. Administration of pyridoxine to responsive patients has often (but not always) led to restoration of platelet adhesiveness to, or toward, normal [196, 232, 240]. On the other hand, when platelet adhesiveness has been measured by a technique involving exposure of the platelets to relatively large glass surfaces for relatively brief times [308], the platelets from at least 17 patients have been reported to be normal [251, 269, 272, 290, 294, 309, 310]; platelets from only four patients were abnormally adhesive by this method [272, 311]. To our knowledge, only one side-by-side measurement of platelet adhesiveness from the same patient by both techniques has been reported. Both measurements were normal [269]. Such studies might be useful in evaluating whether there are truly abnormalities in the adhesiveness of platelets from homocystinemic patients demonstrable by one technique [306] but not by another [308], or whether the results to date merely reflect difficulties in controlling all the pertinent experimental variables [307].

Reported morphologic abnormalities detected by electron

microscopy of platelets from cystathionine β-synthase-deficient patients [312, 313] have not been confirmed by other workers [314]. Abnormalities affecting platelet aggregation, found in occasional patients [315, 316], have not been present in larger numbers of additional patients [57]. A single report of a clotting abnormality due to activation of the Hageman factor (factor XII) by homocystine [317] has not been followed up by later workers.

A different, and important, line of investigation was initiated by McCully, who found that the vascular pathology in a child dying at 7½ weeks with homocystinemia, cystathioninemia, and hypomethioninemia secondary to deranged cobalamin metabolism [318] was similar in many important respects to that found in an 8-year-old patient with presumed cystathionine β-synthase deficiency. In each case numerous focal lesions involved large, medium, and small arteries in many organs. Focal intimal and medial fibrosis caused luminal narrowing. Proliferation of perivascular connective tissue, thickening of the media, and prominence of the internal elastic membranes were present. Both patients had homocystinemia, but the first had abnormally low methionine and high cystathionine, whereas the other had abnormally high methionine and low cystathionine. It was suggested that the vascular damage was produced specifically as an effect of elevated homocyst(e)ine or its derivatives [318].

Subsequently, detailed morphologic observations have been reported for four additional patients who died from genetic defects producing homocystinemia with low or normal plasma methionine concentrations. Two patients with deficiencies of 5,10-methylenetetrahydrofolate reductase activity, dying at ages 10 years and 3½ years, each had vascular lesions very similar to those found in cystathionine β-synthase-deficient patients [319, 320]. Of two patients with deranged cobalamin metabolism, one, dying at age 4 months, also had similar vascular lesions [320, 321], whereas the other, dying at 7 years [322], had vascular lesions judged to be unlike those reported by McCully [318] both by virtue of their restriction to the brain and their histologic nature [323, 324]. On the whole, these findings strongly support the hypothesis that homocyst(e)ine, or its derivatives other than methionine, may be the principal contributor to the vascular damage of cystathionine β-synthase deficiency.

Additional evidence on the role of homocystine has been provided by animal experiments. McCully and Ragsdale gave homocysteine thiolactone to rabbits and reported the production of arteriosclerotic lesions which reproduced "the essential features of the vascular lesions found in individuals with homocystinemia" [325], although other workers were unable to find differences between the vascular lesions present in rabbits treated with homocysteine thiolactone and in controls [326]. Monkeys fed high-methionine, high-fat diets for 14 months did not develop atherosclerosis, even when superimposition of vitamin B6 deficiency decreased hepatic cystathionine β-synthase activities by 55 percent. The relevance of these studies to the possible production of atherosclerosis by homocysteine is uncertain because homocyst(e)ine concentrations in the plasma of these monkeys were not reported [327]. Harker and his colleagues produced arteriosclerotic and prearteriosclerotic intimal lesions by continuous infusion of baboons with homocystine for as long as 3 months [309, 328]. The infusions also led to decreases in platelet survival times, which became more marked as homocystine plasma levels increased.

Platelet turnover increased also, but other platelet function tests showed no change. Patchy areas of de-endothelialization of the walls of major arteries were noted in these experimental animals, and it was concluded that "the underlying process in homocystinemic thrombosis probably involves formation of platelet thrombus on altered, nonendothelialized endarterial surfaces" [328].

In accord with this formulation, it has further been shown that single intravenous injections of homocystine led to increased numbers of circulating endothelial cells in the blood of rats, accompanied by other signs of endothelial damage and by decreases in circulating platelets [329]. In vitro, homocysteine produced cytotoxic effects on cultured human [330, 331] or bovine [331] endothelial cells at concentrations such as are likely to occur in the plasma of untreated cystathionine β-synthase-deficient patients. Comparable concentrations of methionine or homocystine were much less cytotoxic.

In four cystathionine β-synthase-deficient patients, Harker and coworkers also observed decreased platelet survival times of 4.3 ± 0.6 days, as compared to normal times of 9.5 ± 0.6 days, with corresponding increases in platelet turnovers. Treatment of vitamin B6-responsive patients with pyridoxine, or of any of the patients with dipyridamole, restored platelet survival times and turnovers virtually to normal [309]. Other workers found normal platelet survival times in six cystathionine β-synthase-deficient patients [314], two of whom had also been studied by Harker et al. [309]. Methodologic differences have been proposed as an explanation of the discordant findings [332]. On the whole, the combined weight of these several lines of evidence seems to indicate that homocysteine toxicity to endothelial cells, leading to patchy endothelial desquamation followed by platelet-mediated intimal proliferation of smooth muscle cells and development of typical atherosclerotic lesions, as proposed by Harker and coworkers [328], provides the most promising formulation of the genesis of the vascular lesions in cystathionine β-synthase deficiency.

The possible relevance of homocyst(e)ine toxicity to a wider clinical group has recently been suggested by Wilcken and Wilcken [333]. These workers found that 4 h following a standard methionine load, the plasma concentrations of homocysteine-cysteine mixed disulfide in 25 patients under age 50 with angiographically proved ischemic heart disease tended to be significantly higher than in 22 control subjects (17 with normal coronary arteries at angiography and five healthy volunteers). Seven patients had concentrations of mixed disulfide between 10 and 30 μmol/liter, whereas only one value for the control group was in this range. These values are comparable to those found after similar loading of obligate heterozygotes for cystathionine β-synthase deficiency [334]. One interpretation of these findings is that even the mild homocystinemia which occurs in heterozygotes for cystathionine β-synthase deficiency might produce a very significant (at least sevenfold, possibly much greater) increase in the risk of developing ischemic heart disease by age 50. In that case, mild homocystinemia might be an important cause of much of the early heart disease currently unassociated with known risk factors. To evaluate these possibilities, a study has recently been completed of the cardiovascular risk in parents and grandparents in 203 families with cystathionine β-synthase-deficient children [239]. No statistically significant increases in the incidence of heart attacks or strokes were consistently detected in these relatives. The data available are sufficient virtually to exclude an increase in the cardiovascular risk for heterozygotes for cystathionine β-synthase deficiency of as much as fivefold compared to controls, and to make improbable a relative risk of as much as threefold. Less than 5 percent of such heterozygotes are likely to have a fatal or nonfatal heart attack by age 50. These results fail to support the possibility that mild homocyst(e)inemia is an important contributory factor in the overall incidence of cardiovascular disease.

The Collagen Structural Abnormality Considerable experimental support exists for the possibility that homocysteine interferes with the normal cross-linking of collagen. Most collagen molecules are composed of three polypeptide chains which are bound together by inter- and (possibly) intramolecular cross-links. An essential step in cross-linking is the formation of aldehydic groups by the oxidation of the terminal amino groups of several of the lysyl or hydroxylysyl residues in collagen monomers. These aldehydes form cross-links both by Schiff-base formation with amino groups of lysine or hydroxylysine on other chains and by aldol condensation between two aldehydes. These bifunctional cross-links undergo further, as yet poorly characterized, reactions, which produce polyfunctional, nonreducible cross-links of unknown structure [335–340]. Following a suggestion by McKusick that this sequence might be disrupted in homocystinuric patients [341], Harris and Sjoerdsma demonstrated that an increased fraction of the collagen in skin specimens from two patients with "classical manifestations of homocystinuria" was soluble in acidic solution, and that there was an abnormally high ratio of single polypeptide chains to double-chain components. No abnormalities were demonstrated in the collagen of two homocystinurics who were not mentally retarded [342, 343]. The two patients subsequently studied by Kang and Trelstad [344] also had increased portions of collagen soluble in nondenaturing solvents (7.8 and 10.2 percent, as compared to 2.4 and 2.9 percent for two control subjects). These authors in addition found decreased contents of precursor aldehyde and cross-link compounds in the patients' collagen. The latter abnormalities were more marked in specimens from two vitamin B_6-nonresponsive patients than in a vitamin B_6-responsive subject studied while in response [344]. Several young patients with presumed cystathionine β-synthase deficiency have been reported to excrete increased amounts of urinary glycosaminoglycans and hydroxyproline [345]. It is uncertain whether this increased output of hydroxyproline reflects a structural abnormality of collagen or an increased growth rate of the patients, as is presently thought to be the case with the hydroxyprolinuria of young subjects with Marfan's syndrome [346].

Several mechanisms have been proposed to account for the apparent abnormality of cross-linking of collagen from homocystinurics [57]. Because of the similarity in the structures of D-penicillamine (β,β-dimethylcysteine) and homocysteine, Jackson suggested that these two aminothiols might affect connective tissue in the same manner [347]. Depending upon the dose employed, D-penicillamine is known to affect cross-linking in collagen and elastin of various tissues and to operate by a variety of mechanisms [340, 348]. In agreement, at high concentrations (10^{-1} to 10^{-3} M) in vitro homocysteine inhibited lysyl oxidase [349] and prevented formation of insoluble fibrils and bifunctional cross-links when purified rat skin collagen was undergoing polymerization [344]. Lower concentrations of homocysteine (10^{-4} to 10^{-5} M), such as are more likely to occur in cystathionine β-synthase-deficient patients,

did not inhibit lysyl oxidase activity but did affect collagen cross-linking by another mechanism. These concentrations of homocysteine, as well as D-penicillamine, increased the number of bifunctional collagen cross-links formed from hydroxylysine and the hydroxylysine-derived aldehyde by delaying the synthesis of more complex polyfunctional cross-links [348, 350, 351]. In all these actions homocysteine was much more effective than homocystine or methionine, suggesting that the sulfhydryl compound may be the major cause of the collagen abnormality of cystathionine β-synthase deficiency, as it may also be of the thrombotic abnormality. These indications of the preferential toxicity of homocysteine are consistent, too, with the fact that injection of rats with homocystine plus methionine for as long as 41 days produced only minor, and apparently inconsistent, changes in the solubility and cross-link content of collagen and elastin [352].

Which of the particular clinical abnormalities in cystathionine β-synthase-deficient patients will ultimately be found to be secondary effects of the collagen (and probably elastin) structural abnormalities is also a matter of conjecture. Rats given β-aminopropionitrile, an irreversible inhibitor of lysyl oxidase [340], develop the soft tissue abnormalities of skin, bony abnormalities, kyphoscoliosis, hernias, and dissection of the aorta together known as *osteolathyrism* [353, 354]. Animals fed D-penicillamine in low doses develop similar abnormalities of the skin but do not develop the skeletal abnormalities of osteolathyrism unless very large, toxic doses are administered [348]. These model systems suggest that the thin skin, the restricted mobility of joints, and perhaps the spinal scoliosis, deformities of long bones, and hernias of homocystinuric patients may eventually be ascribed to connective tissue abnormalities. Although collagen plays a role in promoting the platelet aggregation which is a step in the normal hemostatic sequence initiated by endothelial injury, available evidence indicates that the structural alterations which may be present in the collagen of cystathionine β-synthase-deficient patients are not likely to explain the thrombotic tendency of these patients [57, 354a].

Dislocation of the Optic Lenses A number of authors have considered dislocation of the optic lens as a manifestation of an underlying structural defect in the collagen of cystathionine β-synthase-deficient patients. Direct evidence for this supposition is lacking, and indeed chemical analyses suggest that the degenerative changes in the zonular fibers which are the probable cause of ectopia lentis are not likely to be due to abnormalities of collagen. The zonular fibers supporting the optic lens of the ox are composed of a collagenase-resistant fibrous protein [355]. The chemical composition of this material does not indicate a close relationship to either collagen or elastin. Unlike either of these proteins, the zonular fibers contain a significant amount of cyst(e)ine [356, 357]. These findings, which have been at least partially confirmed in the rabbit [144, 358], permit postulation of the alternative possibility that zonular degeneration is due to some interference with cystine cross-linking. The three known patients with sulfite oxidase deficiency each suffered dislocated optic lenses at early ages [359–363]. Irreverre et al. suggested that a feature common to both cystathionine β-synthase deficiency and sulfite oxidase deficiency might be disruption of disulfide bonds due to disulfide exchange (with homocysteine) or sulfonation (by sulfite) [359]. The pathogenesis of ectopia lentis and the other ocular abnormalities in cystathionine β-synthase-deficient patients has been discussed extensively by Spaeth and Barber [252].

Does Homocyst(e)ine Replace Cyst(e)ine in Metabolic Reactions?
Several investigations, previously reviewed in detail [57], have produced no evidence to support the hypothetical possibility that homocysteine might cause damage by acting as a structural analogue of cysteine and participating in metabolic reactions for which cysteine is normally the sole substrate, either in protein synthesis or in the reactions leading from cysteine to taurine.

Neurologic Abnormalities and Mental Retardation
Several investigators have considered the possibility that one or another chemical abnormality of the central nervous system might contribute to the neurologic difficulties and mental retardation found in some cystathionine β-synthase-deficient subjects: (1) Cystathionine. This immediate product of the cystathionine β-synthase reaction is present in unusually high concentrations in normal human brain as compared with the concentrations either in brains of other species or in other human tissues [205]. Investigations of a possible neurotransmitter role for cystathionine have yielded inconclusive results (reviewed elsewhere; see Ref. 364). Cystathionine β-synthase activity was not detected in brain tissue of the two cystathionine β-synthase-deficient patients examined post mortem, although this enzyme activity is present in control human brain [128]. The three autopsy brain specimens examined from cystathionine β-synthase-deficient patients were grossly deficient in cystathionine [171, 195]. The latter results cannot be extrapolated to all cystathionine β-synthase-deficient patients since those with some residual activity of this enzyme may well accumulate significant amounts of cystathionine in brain tissue, and since alternative routes exist for cystathionine formation, not dependent upon cystathionine β-synthase and operative under unusual dietary conditions [57]. A reasonably convincing indication that cystathionine is not needed for physiologic brain function would be provided by the discovery of individuals lacking any residual cystathionine β-synthase activity, yet of normal intelligence. Several well-documented descriptions of vitamin B_6-nonresponsive patients with normal IQ values [202, 221, 228, 234, 281] are strong evidence in this regard, and together make it unlikely that gross mental deficiency or neurologic malfunction necessarily results from a virtual absence of cystathionine from the brain. (2) Homocyst(e)ine and methionine. Very high intraperitoneal doses of DL-homocysteine induce tonic-clonic seizures of the grand mal type in rats [365–367] and mice [368]. Inhibition of glutamate decarboxylase, either directly by the keto analogue of homocysteine [369] or by removal of pyridoxal phosphate through complex formation with homocysteine [370], has been suggested as a possible cause of these convulsions. Lower doses of homocysteine, which did not produce seizures, led to rises in brain ammonia concentration [367]. Intraperitoneal injections of homocystine, or homocystine and methionine, produced decreases in the concentrations in brain of several amino acids and of dopa, dopamine, and noradrenaline. These effects could be due to decreased amino acid transport into brain [371], but their implications for the central nervous system dysfunction in cystathionine β-synthase-deficient patients remain to be clarified. (3) S-Adenosylhomocysteine. In view of the likelihood that in cystathionine β-synthase deficiency the intracellular accumulation of homocysteine is outweighed by the accumulation of S-adenosylhomocysteine, the possible functional effects of the latter compound merit consideration. Intraperitoneal administration of S-adenosylhomocysteine to experimental animals has sleep-inductive and anticonvulsant effects [372, 373]. S-Adenosylhomocysteine binds tightly in vitro to membranes from rat cerebral cortex [374]. Mouse lymphocytes, preincubated under conditions leading to intracellular accumulation of S-adenosylhomocysteine, had five- to fortyfold enhancements in the accumulation of cyclic AMP in response to various adenylate cyclase activators [375]. S-Adenosylhomocysteine is known to inhibit a variety of transmethylation reactions [27], and evidence has been produced that the effects of this compound on transmethylation may produce toxic effects in certain lines of cultured human cells [376]. Inactivation of S-adenosylhomocysteine hydrolase, the enzyme which acts to remove S-adenosylhomocysteine, has been observed in children with adenosine deaminase deficiency, in the red blood cells of patients treated with 2'-deoxycoformycin, and in subjects treated with adenine arabinoside [376]. Observation of such individuals may provide some insight into at least the acute effects of S-adenosylhomocysteine accumulation on central nervous system function.

An alternative view of the cause of central nervous system dysfunction in cystathionine β-synthase deficiency is that repeated cerebral vascular thromboses produce many infarctions of the brain, too small individually to come to clinical attention, but together sufficient to produce the abnormalities in question [202]. If this hypothesis were true, an increased frequency of focal neurologic signs would be expected among patients with mental retardation. Cerebrovascular occlusions in infancy and early childhood do result in mental retardation [273], but most patients with mental retardation have no focal neurologic signs.

Diagnosis

The presence of one or more of the typical clinical signs may lead to a suspicion of cystathionine β-synthase deficiency, but definitive diagnosis is based on the presence of certain characteristic biochemical abnormalities. These abnormalities were mentioned earlier in this chapter and are included in Table 25-1.

The most consistent biochemical finding is homocystinuria. No patient in the untreated state and beyond the period of early infancy has yet been described who did not have this abnormality. The presence of homocyst(e)ine is most easily suspected when the urinary cyanide-nitroprusside reaction is positive [377].[1] Since the urinary cyanide-nitroprusside test detects most disulfides, it may be positive in other disulfidurias (e.g., cystinuria, β-mercaptolactatecysteinuria). Consequently, homocyst(e)ine must be specifically identified. Spaeth and Barber have described a modified nitroprusside colorimetric reagent which does not react with cystine in concentrations as high as 100 mg/dl and therefore drastically reduces the number of false positives when screening for homocystinuria [378].

---

[1] This test is performed by adding 1 ml of a 5 percent aqueous solution of sodium cyanide to 1 ml urine, mixing well, and allowing the mixture to remain at room temperature for 5 min. Three to five drops of a 5 percent aqueous solution of sodium nitroferricyanide (nitroprusside) are then added, and the mixture is observed for an immediate color change. In the presence of homocystinuria the color reaction is usually deep red to magenta, although a dilute urine specimen, or one containing less than the usual amount of homocystine, may yield only a deep pink or slightly red color reaction.

Paper or thin-layer chromatography, using either the cyanide-nitroprusside sequence [379] or a modification of the iodoplatinate solution [295], high-voltage paper electrophoresis [180], two-way sequential paper chromatography [380], and, finally, quantitation of amino acids in urine by a sensitive and accurate system of column chromatography [379], may each be useful in assessing a possible case of homocystinuria [57]. In cystathionine β-synthase-deficient individuals the last procedure may reveal the presence of abnormal amounts of other sulfur-containing compounds, including homocysteic acid, homocysteine sulfinic acid, S-adenosylhomocysteine, 5-amino-4-imidazole-carboxamide-5'-S-homocysteinylribonucleoside, homolanthionine, and the mixed cysteine-homocysteine disulfide (Table 25-2).

False negative results can be encountered in testing for homocystinuria by the cyanide-nitroprusside test and by paper or thin-layer chromatography. Some individuals with the pyridoxine-responsive form of cystathionine β-synthase deficiency may show marked responses to relatively low intakes of pyridoxine. For example, three patients studied at the National Institutes of Health while maintained on supplemental folate, 2 mg twice weekly, decreased their homocystine excretions almost as much upon daily doses of 5 to 10 mg pyridoxine hydrochloride as upon doses of up to 300 mg daily. In one of these patients, even 2 mg pyridoxine daily decreased homocystine excretion by 95 percent [381]. Thus an affected individual with this type of responsiveness who ingests as little as one vitamin tablet daily[2] for reasons of general health might have negative reactions to screening tests for homocystinuria. Valle [382] has encountered this situation. Two sibs with ectopia lentis and chronic psychiatric problems were screened for cystathionine β-synthase deficiency. The sister had homocystinuria and hypermethioninemia, whereas the brother had normal findings; the brother was ingesting large amounts of vitamins, including pyridoxine. Homocystine was readily detectable in his urine 2 weeks after he discontinued the supplementary vitamin ingestion. Drayer et al. [162] also encountered negative urinary cyanide-nitroprusside reactions in two of seven pyridoxine-responsive patients. These two patients might have been ingesting vitamin supplements when they were initially tested, although there is no information relevant to this in the published report. In light of the possibility of false negative screening results, all individuals with a clinical problem that strongly suggests the diagnosis of cystathionine β-synthase deficiency (e.g., ectopia lentis) but whose results on screening for homocystinuria are negative should be questioned about dietary intake with particular attention to supplemental vitamin ingestion. Any source of supplementary pyridoxine should be discontinued, and the patient should be retested in 2 to 4 weeks. In addition, at least one of these urine specimens should be analyzed by column chromatography so that the presence of a small amount of homocystine will not be overlooked.

The presence of homocystinuria is not sufficient to establish unequivocally the diagnosis of cystathionine β-synthase deficiency. Not only is homocystinuria noted in other disorders, such as 5,10-methylenetetrahydrofolate reductase deficiency (see Chap. 24 and Table 25-1), but it may be seen as an artifact of bacterial contamination of urine in cystathioninuria [46, 99]. Consequently, amino acids in the plasma or serum should be measured in all suspected individuals.

In cystathionine β-synthase deficiency this measurement should reveal homocystine, usually accompanied by a markedly reduced concentration or even absence of cystine. Furthermore, an increased concentration of methionine is found in most patients (Table 25-1). Hypermethioninemia is an important finding since in other metabolic disorders accompanied by homocystinuria, such as defects in homocysteine methylation, the blood methionine concentration is low or low normal (see Chaps. 23 and 24). The semiquantitative Guthrie bacterial assay for methionine, often used in newborn screening for hypermethioninemia [383], offers a relatively simple means of assaying for this abnormality in patients with homocystinuria. A "normal" blood methionine concentration by this method usually indicates a concentration of approximately 0.1 μmol/dl or less. Since this lower limit of sensitivity is still about three times the normal blood methionine concentration, it is important to measure the blood amino acids of all homocystinuric patients by a more quantitative method when the bacterial assay appears normal. When the bacterial assay indicates an increased blood methionine concentration, cystathionine β-synthase deficiency is the likely diagnosis when homocystinuria is also present.

The demonstration of markedly reduced activity of cystathionine β-synthase confirms the diagnosis of cystathionine β-synthase deficiency. This activity can be assayed with liver biopsy specimens [148], cultured phytohemagglutinin-stimulated lymphocytes [167], or cultured skin fibroblasts [155]. Cystathionine β-synthase activities in extracts of cultured fibroblasts below the established control range have invariably been correlated with other indications of cystathionine β-synthase deficiency [156, 158, 160, 174, 181]. An occasional homocystinuric patient, however, may have a specific activity of cystathionine β-synthase in fibroblast extracts that is within the control range and yet may have no other apparent cause for homocystinuria. Uhlendorf et al. [156] encountered two such cases in their series of 40 cystathionine β-synthase-deficient subjects. One of these unusual patients has dislocated lenses, homocystinuria, and hypermethioninemia. The enzyme activity in her cultured fibroblasts barely overlapped the low end of the control range. The second such patient is the clinically normal 28-year-old woman discussed above in the section "Variation in Clinical Manifestations." A third such patient, reported by Bittles and Carson [165], was also discussed in the same section. Although the genetic status of the latter two patients is uncertain, their mild homocystinurias are presumably caused by low hepatic activities of cystathionine β-synthase. In the absence of additional knowledge, conclusions based solely upon fibroblast assays might have led to erroneous conclusions regarding the cause of the homocystinuria of these two patients.

Management

The management of cystathionine β-synthase deficiency can be divided into two general approaches: (1) control or elimination of biochemical abnormalities with the goal of preventing clinical disease, preventing the progression of existing clinical defects, or ameliorating clinical manifestations that may be reversible; and (2) the medical treatment of complications.

It is reasonable to assume that one or more of the biochemical abnormalities is responsible for the clinical complications in cystathionine β-synthase deficiency and that treatment

---

[2] Most general vitamin preparations contain 2 to 5 mg pyridoxine hydrochloride in each tablet or capsule.

should aim to control or reverse these biochemical abnormalities. In certain patients the administration of large amounts of pyridoxine accomplishes this (see "The Pyridoxine Effect and its Mechanism" earlier in this chapter). In other patients even massive amounts of pyridoxine do not produce biochemical changes. In the latter patients, biochemical control may be accomplished with a diet that contains methionine and is supplemented with cystine. Certain additional dietary measures may also be helpful for optimal biochemical control in both pyridoxine responders and nonresponders. Whenever possible, therapy to achieve biochemical control should begin before clinical complications occur, since many of these complications are irreversible. Even before clinical effects are recognizable, tissue damage may occur. Thus maximal benefit from therapy may be possible only when the disorder is detected in the newborn period, either as a result of known disease in the family or through routine neonatal screening programs.

Diet   Diets used in treating patients with cystathionine β-synthase deficiency are specifically low in methionine. This is designed to reduce the accumulation of methionine, homocysteine, and their metabolites. The diets are supplemented with L-cystine to provide at least some cyst(e)ine, which may be an essential amino acid for certain patients with this disorder.

Three types of low methionine diet have been used [57]. Two of these, the gelatin- and the soybean-based, have largely been supplanted by diets based on a partially or completely synthetic mixture that is free or almost free of methionine. This mixture, available as a proprietary formula,[3] consists of amino acids, minerals, and other nutrients. Carbohydrate and fat as well as fat-soluble vitamins must be added to this formula [384, 385]. Similar mixtures can be prepared by addition of free amino acids other than methionine to a proprietary nutrient base[4] or by mixing these ingredients from individual sources [384]. The methionine requirement is met by addition of small amounts of milk to the formula during infancy and later by allowing ingestion of low protein foods in carefully controlled quantities [386]. The desired amount of dietary methionine is judged by maintenance of blood methionine levels within or near the normal range (<0.04 μmol/ml) and by the presence of little or no homocystine in blood and urine [386]. It is often impossible to eliminate urinary homocystine while maintaining a methionine intake sufficient for normal growth. Even when free homocystine is undetectable in blood, the concentration of protein-bound homocyst(e)ine may be above normal [387]. Supplementation with L-cystine may be desirable. The amount of L-cystine required to maintain detectable levels of cystine in blood is 150 to 200 mg/kg body weight per day. It is usually impossible to achieve normal levels of cystine in the blood of affected individuals [202].

The effectiveness of a low methionine diet when given from early infancy in preventing the clinical complications of cystathionine β-synthase deficiency was surveyed by Pullon [228]. Among 21 individuals classified as nonresponders to pyridoxine, two developed ectopia lentis at 7 and 8 years of age despite dietary control and cystine supplementation. The IQs of these patients were 75 to 80 and 103. Another pyridoxine nonresponder had an IQ of 74 at 12 years of age, but there was no mention of the eye status or of whether cystine supplementation was given. All other patients who were nonresponsive to

pyridoxine were clinically normal, but were no older than 6 years of age at the time of the survey. Consequently, the efficacy of dietary therapy, even when begun in the neonatal period, is as yet unproven, although affected individuals so treated seem to have less severe complications than their untreated sibs [202, 388].

Certain of the progressive complications of cystathionine β-synthase deficiency may possibly be prevented, or at least ameliorated, by therapy begun after clinical disease is present. Low methionine diets with supplemental cystine have been given to a number of patients with preexisting clinical complications [202, 207, 208, 388–392]. Amelioration of the biochemical findings was generally noted. One patient who had developed slowly until age 14 months thereafter developed normally on the restricted diet, although ectopia lentis occurred at age 3 years [392]. A second patient showed "striking improvement in school performances" during such therapy [392]. In other cases there was no reversal of major clinical abnormalities. Normal physical growth was maintained [202, 390] and in one patient no thromboembolic episodes occurred in 5 years of dietary treatment, whereas there had been two such occurrences in the 6 months prior to institution of the diet [202]. Acceptance of the restrictive and unpalatable low methionine diet by an older child may be very difficult to achieve [391, 393, 394].

Pyridoxine   The administration of relatively large amounts of pyridoxine (vitamine B₆), usually orally in the form of pyridoxine hydrochloride, has been effective in reducing or eliminating the biochemical abnormalities in many patients with cystathionine β-synthase deficiency [213]. The probable dependence of this response upon residual cystathionine β-synthase activity has already been discussed (see "The Pyridoxine Effect and its Mechanism" earlier in this chapter). The doses of pyridoxine administered have varied considerably in various studies. Barber and Spaeth [213] utilized doses of 250 to 500 mg/day; Gaull et al. [395], 800 to 1200 mg/day. Some patients who have a biochemical response at one level of pyridoxine supplementation will have a greater response with a larger amount of pyridoxine [232]. In general, for older children a dose of at least 150 mg pyridoxine per day has been used [232], although an occasional patient has responded to doses as low as 25 mg/day [151], or even less, as exemplified by the three patients studied at the National Institutes of Health and discussed in the earlier section on "Diagnosis." According to Perry [202], a patient should not be considered unresponsive to pyridoxine until a dose of 500 to 1000 mg/day has been given for a period of several weeks. As was noted (under "The Pyridoxine Effect and Its Mechanism"), a biochemical response to pyridoxine may not be manifest in a potentially responsive patient if that patient is folate depleted [204].

Has pyridoxine therapy in pyridoxine-responsive cystathionine β-synthase-deficient individuals been effective in preventing the clinical complications of this disease? In Pullon's survey of affected infants detected by newborn screening and treated from early infancy [228], only four were classified as pyridoxine responders. All were treated with pyridoxine and none had developed clinical abnormalities at the time of reporting, when the oldest of these children was 13 years of age. Since some pyridoxine-responsive individuals do not develop complications (e.g., ectopia lentis) until their adult years [179, 240], the question of whether pyridoxine therapy protects pyridoxine-responsive cystathionine β-synthase-deficient individuals from

---

[3] Methionaid, Milner Scientific and Medical Research Co., Ltd., Liverpool, England.

[4] Product 80056, Mead Johnson Laboratories, Evansville, Indiana 47721.

clinical complications cannot at present be considered as fully answered. There are preliminary indications that pyridoxine therapy may retard or prevent the progression of clinical complications in pyridoxine-responsive patients who already have clinical disease [392, 396]. Improvement in behavior and in IQ scores has been observed in several pyridoxine-responsive patients in whom pyridoxine therapy began after clinical complications developed [392].

Should pyridoxine therapy alone be considered adequate treatment for patients who are pyridoxine responsive, or should such therapy be combined with a low methionine diet and possibly cystine supplementation? An empirical answer to this question is not provided by existing studies, so judgment must be based on a priori considerations. For patients incompletely responsive to pyridoxine, methionine restriction is desirable since additional therapy may further correct the biochemical abnormalities. Even patients with maximum pyridoxine responsiveness have reduced tolerance to methionine as measured by methionine loading tests [147, 153, 234], so that such patients may in theory experience abnormal episodic increases in methionine and homocyste(e)ine concentrations following methionine ingestion. Some methionine restriction or the use of small, frequent feedings might be prudent [153].

Additional Dietary Measures   Administration of choline [207], a precursor of the methyl donor betaine, or of betaine itself [388] has resulted in lower homocystine and higher methionine concentrations in patients with cystathionine β-synthase deficiency. The mechanism of this effect is presumed to be an increase in the rate of homocysteine methylation through betaine-homocysteine methyltransferase (Fig. 25-1). This redistribution of metabolites may be desirable to the extent that one considers the evidence compelling that methionine and its derivatives make lesser contributions to the pathophysiology of cystathionine β-synthase deficiency than do homocysteine and its metabolites (see "Pathophysiology" earlier in this chapter). Treatment of two patients with betaine for more than 2 years was accompanied by clinical improvement without apparent ill effects [396a].

Folic acid depletion has been noted in a number of cystathionine β-synthase-deficient patients [203, 204]. In two of these patients, therapy with folate alone produced reductions in the excretion of homocystine and increases in the excretion of methionine [203]. In other patients, therapy with folate in combination with vitamin B$_{12}$ and pyridoxine resulted in a lower concentration of homocystine, with little or no increase in the methionine concentration [204]. As already noted, folate repletion may be necessary to permit a pyridoxine response. As in therapy with choline or betaine, methionine accumulation should be watched for in patients given high doses of folate.

Several authors have considered means for replenishing cystathionine in cystathionine β-synthase-deficient patients [59, 397, 398]. The possibility that cystathionine plays an essential role in brain function, and reasons for doubting this possibility, have been discussed previously (see "Pathophysiology" earlier in this chapter). To our knowledge, direct replacement of cystathionine has not been attempted. Cystathionine is rapidly cleared by the kidney, may not penetrate into brain cells, and is so costly that any therapeutic trial would be expensive. Replenishment of cystathionine through reversal of the γ-cystathionase reaction is likely to require frequent administration

of very large doses of both homoserine and cysteine [59, 398, 399]. Such a regimen has not been attempted in patients, and the chance that it would be beneficial appears remote.

Treatment of cystathionine β-synthase deficiency has been attempted by increasing the renal excretion of homocystine. Cusworth and Dent [240] suggested that homocystine might be "accidentally" reabsorbed by the same mechanism that is responsible for cystine, lysine, arginine, and ornithine reabsorption (see Chap. 80). A marked increase in homocystinuria following the infusion of arginine was demonstrated in one patient [240, 400]. α-Aminoisobutyric acid, a competitive inhibitor of dibasic amino acid transport in the kidney, has also been shown to increase homocystinuria [401]. This mode of therapy has not resulted in reduction of plasma homocystine concentrations, so it would appear that this type of treatment has limited, if any, use in this disorder.

Specific Drug Therapy   Other than treatment to reverse the basic biochemical abnormalities, no medical therapy has been attempted or suggested for any of the clinical complications except the thrombotic tendency. As previously discussed (see "Pathophysiology" earlier in this chapter), Harker et al. [309] found decreased platelet survivals in several patients and were able to correct this abnormality almost completely with dipyridamole, with no reduction in the plasma homocystine concentration. The therapeutic regimen used was 100 mg four times a day in oral doses. A similar response was achieved with an alternate regimen of dipyridamole, 100 mg once daily, plus acetylsalicylic acid (aspirin), 1 g once daily. No thromboembolic phenomena were observed during a 3-year follow-up of two pyridoxine-unresponsive patients receiving the latter regimen. These patients had suffered at least five thrombotic episodes during the year prior to the onset of medication. Schulman et al. [288, 402] reported two patients who experienced thromboembolic problems while on similar therapies. One was a 13-year-old boy who developed thrombophlebitis and bilateral pulmonary emboli while receiving 100 mg dipyridamole and 900 mg aspirin per day. The second was a 20-year-old woman who developed femoral thrombophlebitis post partum while receiving even larger doses of dipyridamole and aspirin. Further evidence is required to permit an evaluation of the efficacy of antithrombotic therapy. Certain authors have suggested that it may be wise to avoid factors associated with an increased risk of thromboembolism, e.g., oral contraceptives [180, 202, 219] and perhaps even pregnancy [202].

Complications   The treatment of clinical complications is essentially the same as the treatment of these complications when due to other causes. Pathologic fractures resulting from osteoporosis are treated by conventional orthopedic procedures, and the effects of thrombi and emboli are treated by the appropriate medical supportive measures. An important exception to conventional treatment is the avoidance of surgery whenever possible, since in cystathionine β-synthase deficiency the danger of thromboemboli may be greatly increased postoperatively [241, 298], presumably as a result of the propensity of clotting to increase postoperatively superimposed on the predisposition for thrombosis in this disorder [180]. A number of patients have died from thromboembolic disease following ocular surgery [187, 252, 267, 296]. Furthermore, ocular complications of such surgery, including marked and prolonged vitreous hemorrhage, vitreous loss, and retinal detachment, seem to be particularly frequent in cystathionine β-synthase deficiency [241, 248, 253]. Should surgery be unavoidable, the risk of thromboemboli may be lessened by increasing hydration via intravenous fluids preoperatively and postoperatively [224, 225].

Acute glaucoma due to pupillary block by the dislocated lens can usually be treated medically [246, 248]. Initially, the pupil should be fully dilated with any suitable mydriatic and the lens repositioned from the anterior chamber by pressure on the cornea. Should this fail, a peripheral iridectomy may be performed. Following any of these procedures, miosis should be constantly maintained so as to prevent the lens from again dislocating anteriorly [248].

Prevalence and Screening

Homocystinuria proved or presumed to be due to cystathionine β-synthase deficiency has been discovered in virtually every part of the world in which it has been sought, including not only North America and Europe but also many Asiatic nations such as Japan [190], India [201, 271, 277], and Thailand [249]. Jews [146] as well as blacks [247] have been identified with the disorder.

The prevalence of cystathionine β-synthase deficiency has yet to be finally established. Among individuals in institutions for the mentally retarded, the reported frequencies have varied widely. Carson et al. [187] detected 10 in 2920 screened patients in Northern Ireland (1:292). Chase et al. [294] found two individuals among 1700 screened in Colorado (1:850); Coffey et al. [403] identified four in 5966 screened in Ireland (1:1492); and Spaeth and Barber [378] found only two among 9488 patients (1:4744). Among more than 3500 individuals in institutions for the mentally retarded and mentally ill screened in Massachusetts, only one case was discovered [404]. As many as five percent of individuals with nontraumatic dislocation of the optic lens may have cystathionine β-synthase deficiency [251]. None of these data include all cases in the general population, since the screening programs in question would have failed to identify cystathionine β-synthase-deficient individuals lacking the particular clinical manifestation(s) necessary for inclusion in the screened populations.

Questionnaires sent to 103 institutions in central Europe revealed 32 recognized cases among centers serving a population of 104 million (frequency about 1:3 million) [405]. This frequency is far lower than the estimated prevalence of 1:24,000 for Northern Ireland [227], based on 27 cases identified among 650,000 individuals born between 1955 and 1975 [406]. It is also much lower than the frequency of 1:58,000 for New South Wales in Australia, calculated from 14 cases ascertained among the 820,797 individuals born during 1960 to 1969 [221].

In theory, a better estimate of prevalence might result from routine screening of the general population. Such screening among newborn infants has been conducted in several centers for a number of years [407]. In programs which use an elevation of the blood methionine concentration as the identifying criterion, 97 cases have been detected among 19.3 million infants screened in the United States, Europe, Australia, New Zealand, and Japan [228, 408]. The apparent prevalence from these data is approximately 1:200,000 and, interestingly, is unchanged from that based on results from the first 5 million infants screened [57]. The prevalence may be relatively high in Ireland, where 10 cases have been detected among 573,206 newborns [409], and in Northern Ireland, where three cases were discovered among 218,729 routinely screened newborns [385]. The resulting frequencies of 1:57,000 and 1:73,000 may be compared to frequencies of 1:100,000 in Manchester, England [228], 1:146,000 in Japan [410], and 1:160,000 in West Germany [411]. No cases have been found among 945,566 screened newborns in Belgium [412] or among 634,060 newborns in the state of Oregon [413]; and only single cases were discovered among 824,198 screened neonates in Scotland [414] and among 745,475 newborns screened in Austria [415]. In Italy, two cases were discovered among 116,000 newborns screened [415a].

There are several reasons for supposing that at least some of these figures are underestimates of the true prevalence [180]. Five cases are known to have been missed by neonatal blood screening for hypermethioninemia [198, 228, 385, 416, 417]. A few older patients with cystathionine β-synthase deficiency do not have hypermethioninemia [200, 201, 208]. Others may have only mild hypermethioninemia, and the methods commonly used to detect elevations of methionine in newborn blood are not sensitive to levels less than three times normal (see "Diagnosis" earlier in this chapter). There is now evidence that some cystathionine β-synthase-deficient individuals destined later to have hypermethioninemia have normal concentrations of blood methionine during the first week of life, when routine newborn screening is usually performed [198, 417]. Whiteman et al. [418] reported that in England, subsequent to changes in infant feeding practices which led to decreased protein intake, there was an apparent decrease in the rate at which cystathionine β-synthase deficiency was detected by newborn screening for hypermethioninemia. If cases are being missed by this technique, lower protein intake may have been a critical factor [418]. Breast milk contains only 50 to 60 percent as high a methionine concentration as infant formulas commonly used in the United States [419, 420]. Deficient vitamin B_{12} or folic acid, low betaine or choline intake, high vitamin B_6 intake, or some combination thereof [180] are all possible contributing factors in false negative tests for cystathionine β-synthase deficiency as indicated by hypermethioninemia. The impact of each of these factors, as well as of the recent increase in the prevalence of breast-feeding, clearly requires further evaluation.

Alternative screening programs utilizing the criterion of homocystine detectable in neonatal urine have been conducted in Massachusetts [421] and Australia [422]. Among more than 700,000 infants tested in this manner, only one case of cystathionine β-synthase deficiency has been discovered [221]. As with hypermethioninemia, however, homocystinuria might be absent in the neonate with cystathionine β-synthase deficiency, or present at such low concentrations as to be undetectable by urine screening methods [198]. In Australia one case is known to have been missed by neonatal urine screening [221].

McKusick has suggested that the prevalence in newborns of cystathionine β-synthase deficiency should be, very roughly, 1:45,000 [180]. The limits for this estimate have been placed at 1:450,000 and 1:9000 [57]. The lower prevalence rather than the higher one may be more representative of typical values for the human genome [423]. Nevertheless, McKusick's estimate emphasizes the possibility that many cystathionine β-synthase-deficient individuals may have been missed in the mass screening programs conducted so far and underlines the need for continuing evaluation to ensure that the maximal benefit is being derived from such programs.

Identification of Heterozygotes

Techniques are now available which permit tentative identification of individuals heterozygous for cystathionine β-synthase deficiency. Three of these methods involve enzyme assays of tissue extracts:

1. *Liver.* Of the eight obligate heterozygotes for whom specific activities of hepatic cystathionine β-synthase have been determined, seven had values below the control range [146, 148, 150], whereas one barely overlapped the low end of the control range [146].

2. *Cultured fibroblasts.* Extracts of fibroblasts cultured from obligate heterozygotes have been assayed for cystathionine β-synthase activity in three laboratories. Uhlendorf et al. studied nine patients. The specific enzyme activities of eight of these patients overlapped the control range [156]. No case of overlap occurred in the five obligate heterozygotes studied by Fleisher et al. [181]. Overlap also occurred for four of the six heterozygotes reported by Bittles and Carson [158, 165].

3. *Phytohemagglutinin-stimulated lymphocytes.* Goldstein et al. measured cystathionine β-synthase activities in extracts of phytohemagglutinin-stimulated lymphocytes grown from 17 obligate heterozygotes. The specific activities for three overlapped the control range [168].

In each of these experimental series, although the mean specific activity of cystathionine β-synthase for obligate heterozygotes was less than 50 percent of the mean control specific activity, the activities in tissue extracts of a significant portion of the individual obligate heterozygotes have overlapped with the control ranges. The implication is that at present each of these methods will identify some, perhaps most, heterozygotes, but that other heterozygotes will fail to be identified with certainty. Whether this situation reflects real variations in cystathionine β-synthase activities, or whether it reflects merely inadequate control of all the pertinent experimental variables [181] will be established only by additional work.

Alternative approaches to the identification of heterozygous individuals take advantage of the presence of abnormal concentrations of sulfur-containing metabolites in such individuals under certain experimental conditions. A number of early studies of methionine or homocystine, or both, in urine or in plasma, and of urinary sulfate excretion of obligate heterozygotes after oral L-methionine loads failed to develop criteria which could conclusively distinguish these subjects from normal persons with sufficient reliability to be of practical use [182, 188, 211, 273, 294, 424]. In 1974, Sardharwalla and coworkers [334] reported that after administration of methionine loads under strictly standardized conditions, several criteria served to distinguish heterozygotes from normals. Plasma homocystine concentrations 6 and 9 hours postloading, homocysteine-cysteine mixed disulfide plasma concentrations up to 24 hours postload, and the ratios of urinary homocystine/ cystine appeared most useful. Subsequent reports of the use of these techniques are lacking.

Another promising approach was reported by Kang and collaborators [387], who found that treatment of plasma proteins with 2-mercaptoethanol could liberate small amounts of bound homocyst(e)ine which otherwise would have gone undetected. Eight normal subjects had bound homocysteine concentrations from 0.5 to 2.2 nmol/ml plasma; two obligate heterozygotes for cystathionine β-synthase deficiency had values of 3.5 and 4.8 nmol/ml; and one untreated homozygote, 59 nmol/ml. Further experience with this technique may be expected to determine its usefulness in identification of heterozygotes for cystathionine β-synthase deficiency.

Prenatal Diagnosis

To our knowledge, no case of cystathionine β-synthase deficiency has yet been diagnosed in utero. Several studies suggest that such a diagnosis should be feasible by assay of cystathionine β-synthase activity in extracts of cultured amniotic cells. Uhlendorf and Mudd studied 13 lines of control cells grown in culture from amniotic fluid and found readily detectable activities of cystathionine β-synthase in extracts of each [155, 425]. Cells from two fetuses known to be at risk because of affected older sibs were also studied. In each case, the presence of cystathionine β-synthase activity led to the correct prediction that the children in question would not be so deficient in cystathionine β-synthase as to be homocystinuric. Similar findings were reported by Fleisher and colleagues, who also correctly predicted that a fetus at risk would be unaffected [426]. Bittles and Carson [158] and Rassin et al. [193] studied amniotic cells cultured from fetuses carried by cystathionine β-synthase-deficient mothers. The specific activities of cystathionine β-synthase in extracts of these cells were compatible with the likely possibility that these children were heterozygotes.

Whether measurements of homocystine or methionine or both in amniotic fluid will be useful in antenatal diagnosis will be determined only when appropriate specimens from an affected fetus have been studied. Homocystine has specifically been excluded as a detected constituent of normal human amniotic fluid at 14 to 18 weeks of pregnancy [236, 427] and at full term [427], nor was homocystine mentioned in numerous studies of normal amniotic fluids obtained over somewhat wider ranges of gestation [428–433].

γ-CYSTATHIONASE DEFICIENCY

In 1959 Harris and his colleagues described a 64-year-old, mentally retarded woman who excreted more than 2 mmol cystathionine daily in her urine [434]. The amino acid was rigorously identified. An oral load of methionine increased the cystathionine excretion. Postmortem examination revealed abnormally high concentrations of cystathionine in the liver, kidney, and brain [171, 434]. Two relatives excreted about one-tenth as much cystathionine as did the patient. On the basis of these findings, Harris et al. suggested a genetically determined defect in the activity of the γ-cystathionase, the enzyme which cleaves cystathionine to cysteine and α-ketobutyrate. This suggestion has been confirmed by direct enzymatic assays performed subsequently on patients with similar biochemical findings (as described in the next section). In a search for the same amino acid abnormality among more than 1000 severely mentally retarded persons, Harris and coworkers failed to discover a single additional case. They warned that the association of the metabolic disorder with the mental defect in their patient might be fortuitous, a warning which subsequent experience has shown to be well taken. As more cases of γ-cystathionase deficiency have been discovered, it has become clear that as yet no specific clinical manifestations may unequivocally be attributed to this biochemical abnormality.

The Genetic Defect and Genetic Heterogeneity

Deficient γ-cystathionase activity in cystathioninuric subjects was first demonstrated by Frimpter in a study of extracts of liver from two such individuals [435]. Subsequent studies have brought to seven the total cases of γ-cystathionase deficiency proven by assay of the hepatic enzyme [101, 436–438].

Long-term lymphoid cell lines established from peripheral blood leukocytes after stimulation of lymphocytes with phytohemagglutinin have been employed to demonstrate deficient activity of γ-cystathionase in four cystathioninuric subjects [439–441], one of whom had previously also been shown to have deficient hepatic activity [101]. The deficiency was most marked when cell extracts were assayed without added pyridoxal phosphate [439, 440].

Bittles and Carson [165, 442] reported that γ-cystathionase activity was readily detected in eight lines of fibroblasts grown in tissue culture from skin biopsy specimens of control subjects. The γ-cystathionase specific activity in an extract of fibroblasts grown from a cystathioninuric individual was 15 percent of the mean control specific activity and 31 percent of the lowest control value [442]. Workers in two other laboratories have found either "absent or minimal" [425] or variable, and in some cases undetected [439, 440], activity of this enzyme in control cultured fibroblasts. The reasons for these differences in the γ-cystathionase activities of control fibroblast lines have not been clarified, and until this is done the cultured fibroblast system cannot be regarded as reliable for the study of normal human γ-cystathionase or for demonstration of the lack of this enzyme in cystathioninuric individuals.

Finkelstein et al. showed that the homoserine dehydratase activity of the liver of their γ-cystathionase-deficient patient was also very low [436]. Similar results were obtained by Kint and Carton with liver samples from three additional γ-cystathionase-deficient children [443]. These findings indicate that human γ-cystathionase also possesses homoserine dehydratase activity, as is true of the analogous enzyme from rat liver [58, 444], and that the genetic mutation, or mutations, in the patients studied had affected both activities. No reports have appeared of measurements in γ-cystathionase-deficient patients of the further alternative activities catalyzed by this enzyme, including cysteine desulfhydrase [56], homocysteine desulfhydrase [445], and L-diaminopropionate ammonia lyase [49].

Several additional enzyme activities involved in sulfur amino acid metabolism have been normal in tissues of cystathioninuric individuals. Methionine adenosyltransferase and cystathionine β-synthase activities were studied in extracts of a single γ-cystathionase-deficient liver [436]. Activities of S-adenosylmethionine decarboxylase and of N^5-methyltetrahydrofolate-homocysteine methyltransferase were within the normal ranges in extracts of four lines of γ-cystathionase-deficient, long-term lymphoid cells [440].

As the foregoing summary indicates, enzyme studies have been carried out in relatively few γ-cystathionase-deficient subjects. Nevertheless, the data available indicate differences between the residual activities of γ-cystathionase (when present) and normal γ-cystathionase, and between the residual γ-cystathionase activities of different affected individuals: (1) Residual γ-cystathionase activities have in some cases been stimulated more by the addition of pyridoxal phosphate to the assay reaction mixture than was control γ-cystathionase activity [435, 439, 440]; in other cases such high stimulations did not occur [436–438]. (2) Residual γ-cystathionase activities from two deficient individuals were sensitized to heat inactivation by pyridoxal phosphate, whereas normal γ-cystathionase was stabilized to such inactivation by pyridoxal phosphate [441]. (3) Immunologic studies of long-term lymphoid lines have shown the absence in one line of γ-cystathionase-deficient cells of material which cross-reacted with rabbit antibody to control human hepatic γ-cystathionase, whereas three such lines did have cross-reacting material. These cross-reacting materials had weak γ-cystathionase activities in the presence of pyridoxal phosphate. More detailed immunologic studies suggested that there might be differences between the cross-reacting materials of these three lines [439, 440]. As with cystathionine β-synthase deficiency, these results strongly suggest genetic heterogeneity among the lesions which produce γ-cystathionase deficiency and a mutation in the structural gene for γ-cystathionase.

Additional Patients

Some observations made on the 10 cystathioninuric patients in whom γ-cystathionase deficiency has been directly demonstrated by enzyme assay are summarized in Table 25-4 (patients 1 to 9 and 46). Without pyridoxine treatment, and on unrestricted diets, these patients excreted from 1000 to 5800 μmol cystathionine daily in their urine. Cystathionine excretion tends to increase with age as dietary methionine intake increases. Based upon urinary creatinine, cystathionine excretion ranged from 1400 to 16,300 μmol/g creatinine, being highest in the youngest children.

Also summarized in Table 25-4 are the findings with several additional cystathioninuric patients (patients 10 to 45 and 47). Although enzyme assays have not been reported for these patients, their cystathionine excretions are comparable to the excretions of those proven to be γ-cystathionase deficient. Together with the lack of alternative explanations for the cystathioninuria and, in some cases, the familial incidence of this aminoaciduria, these cystathionine excretions are evidence that all the patients in question have γ-cystathionase deficiency. This conclusion is open to some doubt in at least two cases (patients 14 and 19; details discussed previously; see Ref. 57).

In this chapter, the 10 patients in Table 25-4 with proved γ-cystathionase deficiency, as well as the 37 additional patients with presumptive deficiency, will be referred to as the γ-cystathionase-deficient group. This group excludes a few additional cystathioninuric patients for whom quantitative data on the extent of the cystathioninuria have not been presented [465], who had cystathioninuria not permitting clear classification as homozygotes rather than heterozygotes [461], or for whom more complicated explanations of cystathioninuria have been proposed [102, 104].

Also excluded from Table 25-4 are the two cystathioninuric brothers described by Schneiderman [466]. During studies 3 years apart, these patients had cystathioninuria barely detectable during routine chromatography of basal urine samples,

Table 25-4 Cystathioninuric patients with proved or probable primary deficiency of γ-cystathionase

Patient*	Age†	(Sex)	Urinary cystathionine excretion μmol/24 h	Urinary cystathionine excretion μmol/g creatinine	Clinical status	Vitamin B_6 responsive	References
1	44	(M)	4300–5800	2200–4300	Acromegaly, congenital defects, mental aberrations	Yes	[435, 446, 447]
2	2	(M)	1100–1400	8500–12,200	Thrombocytopenic purpura, renal calculi	Yes	[435, 448]
3	12	(M)	2100–3300	—	Motor and mental retardation, frequent convulsions	Yes	[436, 449]
4	0.8	(M)	1000	16,300	Mild developmental retardation	No	[101]
5	8	(M)	1100	—	Mental retardation	Yes	[437]
6	6	(F)	1500	—	Sister of patient 5, clinically normal	Yes	[437]
7	6	(F)	1600	—	Dizygotic twin of patient 6, clinically normal	Yes	[437]
8	2.5	(M)	Not specified	—	Repeated chest infections, otherwise normal	Yes	[442]
9	15	(F)	1900	1600–1900	Normal at age 22 years	Yes	[440, 450]
10	64	(F)	2200	—	Imbecile	Not specified	[434]
11	49	(F)	500–5800	2700	Sister of patient 1; died, age 48 years, of cerebrovascular accident probably due to rheumatic heart disease	Not specified	[447, 451]
12	13	(F)	2300–3400	—	Normal, except for electroencephalographic abnormality	Yes	[452]
13	2.5	(F)	2100	6300	Phenylketonuria and mental retardation	Yes	[118]
14	1.1	(M)	100–800	1000–10,800	Nephrogenic diabetes insipidus, vitamin B_6-responsive anemia	Yes	[453]
15	8	(F)	1000–1500	1600–2500	Normal at age 11 years	Yes	[454, 454a]
16	2	(M)	600	1800–2300	Brother of patient 15, normal at age 5 years	Yes	[454, 454a]
17	13	(F)	2300–5100	—	No clinical details published	No‡	[455]
18	9	(F)	2000–4000	—	Sister of patient 17, no clinical details published	Uncertain	[455]
19	18	(M)	2200	—	Goiter, poor hearing, retarded growth: all responsive to thyroxine (as was cystathioninuria); chromosomal abnormalities	Yes	[456]
20	18	(M)	1200	600	Normal at age 29 except for sequelae of automobile accident at age 25	Not specified	[457]
21	9	(M)	500	1700	Brother of patient 20, mild mental retardation	Yes	[457]
22	2	(F)	—	700	Sister of patient 20, normal at age 14 years	Not specified	[457]
23	0.4	(M)	—	8700	Normal at age 11 years	Yes	[103, 463]
24	0.4	(M)	—	8600	Normal at age 11 years	Yes	[103, 463]
25	33	(M)	3600–4000	—	Normal, except for renal calculi	Yes	[458]
26	7.5	(F)	—	2800	Normal at age 7 years	No	[292, 459]
27	12.5	(M)	1300	—	Mental retardation, juvenile diabetes mellitus	Yes	[460]
28	7	(M)	—	1300	Age 7 years; hyperactive, learning disorder	Yes	[292]
29	3	(M)	—	1300–2800	Normal at age 8 years	Yes	[292]
30	0.8	(M)	—	5800	Normal at age 4 years	Yes	[292]
31	6	(M)	—	6300	Normal at age 9 years	Yes	[292]
32	3	(M)	—	3500	Brother of patient 31; normal at age 6 years	Yes	[292]
33	17	(M)	—	1400	Normal at age 17 years	Yes	[292]
34	13	(M)	—	1400	Brother of patient 33; hyperactive; IQ 76; age 14 years	Yes	[292]
35	4	(F)	—	9000	Normal at age 4 years	Uncertain	[292]
36	14	(M)	—	800	Mental retardation (now age 25)	Not specified	[461a]
37	8	(F)	—	900	Sister of patient 36, mental retardation (now age 19)	Not specified	[461a]
38	7	(M)	—	1500	Brother of patient 36, mental retardation (now age 14)	Yes	[461a]
39	3.5	(F)	—	2600	Slow motor development, short, cataracts	Not specified	[461]
40	5	(F)	95–255	400–2300	Mental retardation	Yes	[462]
41	10	(F)	—	4700	Sister of patient 28; normal at age 10 years	Yes	[292]
42	4	(M)	—	1400	Normal at age 4 years	Yes	[292]
43	3	(M)	—	1600	Age three years; borderline hyperactive	Yes	[292]
44	5	(M)	—	430	Normal at age 6 years	Yes	[292]
45	0.5	(F)	—	12,600	Normal at age 1 year	No	[292]
46	15	(F)	—	1400–1900	Normal at age 22 years	Yes	[440, 450]
47	6	(M)	—	—	Normal at age 6 years	Not tested	[463]

* Each patient has been assigned the same number as was used in Table 23-4 (Ref. 57), except that former patient 9 has been removed because of an erroneous duplication and replaced by a new patient 9.
† Age in years at the time that cystathionine excretion was measured.
‡ Although it was originally stated that patients 17 and 18 were "successfully treated" with pyridoxine [455], a later report showed that cystathionine excretion of patient 17 increased during pyridoxine treatment [464].

but cystathionine excretions after oral loads of 5 g DL-methionine rose to approximately 2200 μmol/liter urine. The vast majority of control subjects showed no detectable cystathioninuria after similar methionine loads. Although the exclusive use of paper chromatographic methods for this study made quantitation inexact, the mother of the two propositi and a brother excreted approximately 20 percent as much cystathionine as did the propositi after methionine loads. The father was not available for study. These data suggest the presence in the two brothers of a γ-cystathionase activity intermediate between that of the severely deficient individuals described in Table 25-4 and that of heterozygotes for γ-cystathionase deficiency (summarized in Table 23-5 of Ref. 57). The existence of a γ-cystathionase gene contributing an intermediate amount of activity is implied. This interpretation of Schneiderman's results does not specify whether the mother and brother were heterozygous for the allele of intermediate activity or for an allele contributing little or no activity. Individuals with cystathioninuria after a methionine load similar to that observed in the mother and brother appear to be rather common, since Schneiderman found three such persons by screening 50 mentally retarded patients and one by screening 50 healthy subjects.

Mode of Inheritance

Enzyme studies indicate an autosomal recessive mode of inheritance for γ-cystathionase deficiency. No quantitative assays of the γ-cystathionase activity in the liver of obligate heterozygotes have been published. Pascal and coworkers [440] reported that γ-cystathionase-specific activities in extracts of long-term lymphoid lines cultured from five parents of γ-cystathionase-deficient children ranged from 11.2 to 18.9 nmol/mg protein per hour (assayed in the presence of 0.25 mM pyridoxal phosphate). The mean was 15.8 ± 1.5 (SE). Twenty-one control lymphocyte lines had a mean specific activity of 25.8 ± 1.7, with an approximate range of 12.5 to 47.5; and three cystathioninuric patients who were offspring of the parents in question had specific activities ranging from 3.6 to 7.3. Thus, the parents had intermediate values, but there was extensive overlap with the lower end of the control range.

Cystathionine excretions, measured in a number of parents of γ-cystathionase-deficient subjects under various experimental conditions, are not inconsistent with autosomal recessive inheritance. These results have been summarized elsewhere [57]. Thirty-four parents were studied while on normal diets. Of these, 12 excreted amounts of cystathionine judged by the investigators reporting the results to be abnormally elevated. The excretions ranged from 20 to 270 μmol/g creatinine, values which are small in comparison to those listed in Table 25-4 for affected γ-cystathionase-deficient individuals, and which overlap extensively the urinary cystathionine excretions subsequently reported by Endres and Siebold for "normal" adults [105]. Sixteen parents received oral methionine loads. Of these, 14 were judged to have abnormal postload increases in cystathionine excretion, suggesting that the heterozygous defect may be more readily identified under these conditions.

Metabolic Sequelae

γ-Cystathionase-deficient patients not only excrete abnormal

amounts of cystathionine in their urine but accumulate elevated concentrations of this amino acid in their body fluids and tissues. Plasma cystathionine concentrations have been presented for 17 of the vitamin B₆-responsive patients in Table 25-4. In 16, the concentrations were definitely elevated, ranging from 0.01 to 0.06 μmol/ml [103, 437, 447–449, 454, 457, 458, 460, 461], whereas in one patient none was detected [118]. Cystathionine is usually not detected in normal plasma. Two vitamin B₆-nonresponsive patients had plasma cystathionine concentrations of 0.06 and 0.08 μmol/ml [101, 459].

Cystathionine concentrations in cerebrospinal fluid have been 0.01 μmol/ml [449], 0.001 μmol/ml [446], 0.0005 μmol/ml [454], and "not detected." Control values were not listed, but only traces (i.e., <0.001 μmol/ml) of cystathionine are present in normal spinal fluid [467].

Tissues from patient 10 (Table 25-4), obtained post mortem, were examined for cystathionine. The concentrations were: liver, 1.3 to 2.0 μmol/g (control range, 0.05 to 0.9); kidney, 0.56 to 0.82 μol/g (none detected in control kidney); and frontal lobe of brain, 2.6 to 3.0 μmol/g (control range, 0.22 to 0.35) [171, 434]. A liver biopsy specimen from patient 4, who was not responsive to pyridoxine, contained 9.6 μmol/g [194].

In addition to cystathionine, γ-cystathionase-deficient patients excrete substantial amounts of N-acetylcystathionine. This compound was discovered and identified by Perry and coworkers [468]. Patient 15 (Table 25-4) excreted 443 to 474 μmol of this compound each day, and patient 16 excreted 134 to 246 μmol. Large amounts of N-acetylcystathionine were also detected in the urine of some of the other cystathioninuric patients in whom this compound was sought [46, 450, 464], but not in others [461]. N-Acetylcystathionine presumably arises by the acetylation in vivo of the α-amino group of the 3-carbon moiety of cystathionine [468].

A number of additional sulfur-containing compounds have been identified in urine from a cystathioninuric girl studied intensively by Kodama and associates [469]. These compounds fall into three groups:

1. Cystathionine sulfoxide. Small amounts of this oxidation product of cystathionine were isolated from a large pooled urine sample. It is not certain that the sulfoxide was formed in vivo or during the isolation procedure [469].

2. Compounds formed from either cystathionine or N-acetylcystathionine by transamination, followed by either reduction or decarboxylation. The structure of these compounds and the pathways proposed for their formation have been detailed previously [57]. Each of these compounds is present in minor amounts only, as compared to cystathionine and N-acetylcystathionine.

3. Very minor amounts of S-(3-hydroxy-3-carboxy-n-propylthio)-homocysteine and S-(β-carboxyethylthio)-homocysteine [464]. These compounds are present in homocystinuric urine and are thought to derive from homocystine (Table 25-3). Their presence in cystathioninuric urine is unexplained.

Little evidence has emerged to suggest that γ-cystathionase-deficient patients have functional lacks of sulfur-containing metabolites formed distal to the metabolic block. In contrast to the decreased plasma cyst(e)ine concentrations often found in cystathionine β-synthase-deficient patients, plasma cyst(e)ine concentrations have been reported as normal in γ-cystathionase-deficient subjects [435, 448, 449]. Possible explanations for this difference have been discussed [57], but there are ample reasons to believe that at least γ-cystathionase-deficient individuals with detected residual activities of this enzyme retain the capacity to metabolize to cysteine and α-ketobutyrate a major portion of the cystathionine formed from a normal dietary intake of methionine [57].

The Pyridoxine Effect and Its Mechanism

γ-Cystathionase deficiency provided the first instance in which, in a human, the major biochemical abnormality due to a defined enzyme defect was clearly shown to be alleviated by administration of large doses of pyridoxine [446]. As is shown in Table 25-4, the majority of γ-cystathionase-deficient patients encountered (33 of the 37 classified in this respect) respond to high intakes of vitamin B$_6$ with major decreases in urinary cystathionine excretion. Four patients have shown little or no response. The decrease in urinary cystathionine excretion may be accompanied by an increase in urinary sulfate [446] or by an increase in the ratio of urinary sufate to total urinary sulfur [470], although the increment in sulfate is small compared to the basal rate of sulfate excretion and has not been detected in all studies [457].

Although cystathioninuria is a prominent manifestation of vitamin B$_6$ deficiency [112, 113], the response in γ-cystathionase-deficient patients is not attributable to correction of a preexisting vitamin B$_6$ deficiency [57]. The factors affecting vitamin B$_6$ responsiveness or nonresponsiveness in γ-cystathionase-deficient patients are strongly reminiscent of the analogous situation in cystathionine β-synthase-deficient patients. Thus: (1) Responsiveness or nonresponsiveness in γ-cystathionase deficiency has so far been constant within sibships (Table 25-4). (2) There is a correlation between the presence of detected residual activity of γ-cystathionase and clinical responsiveness to vitamin B$_6$ and between the absence of detected residual activity and nonresponsiveness. Adequately sensitive assays have demonstrated low residual activities of γ-cystathionase in liver extracts of three out of three vitamin B$_6$-responsive subjects studied [435, 436] (although no activities were detected in three γ-cystathionase-deficient vitamin B$_6$-responsive sibs when assays were performed which required at least 6 percent of control activity for detection [437, 438]). With cultured cells, activities were detected in one fibroblast line [442] and three long-term lymphoid lines [439, 440] from four vitamin B$_6$-responsive individuals, but not in the single lymphoid line studied from a vitamin B$_6$-nonresponsive subject [439, 440]. (3) The residual γ-cystathionase activities in tissue extracts from vitamin B$_6$-responsive subjects have shown variable enhancements due to the addition of pyridoxal phosphate to enzyme assay mixtures. In one instance, 0.05×10^{-3} M pyridoxal phosphate enhanced activity by only 1.3-fold [436], whereas in other instances enhancements have been as much as fiftyfold [435, 440] when unspecified [435] or 0.25 to 1.0 mM pyridoxal phosphate [440] was added. In no instance has γ-cystathionase activity been restored to normal by even the highest concentration of pyridoxal phosphate.

A considerable body of evidence suggests that normal humans have a large reserve capacity of γ-cystathionase in comparison to the amount of cystathionine metabolized during intake of a normal diet [57]. As discussed above, vitamin B$_6$ responsiveness in γ-cystathionase deficiency is probably dependent upon a small residual activity of the deficient enzyme. The steady-state activity of this enzyme is presumably enhanced somewhat when the patient is taking large doses of vitamine B$_6$, and becomes sufficient to metabolize the cystathi-onine arising from a normal methionine intake without accumulation severe enough to produce cystathioninuria. The molecular mechanism (or mechanisms) of the enhancement requires further clarification.

Clinical Manifestations

Following the discovery of γ-cystathionase deficiency in a mentally retarded individual [434], the search for cystathioninuric patients was initially concentrated on the mentally retarded. The resulting ascertainment bias may have fostered the early impression that γ-cystathionase deficiency is a cause of mental abnormalities. In addition to mental retardation, a wide assortment of other clinical aberrations has been found in individuals with presumptive γ-cystathionase deficiency (Table 25-4). Among these are convulsions, hypoplastic genitalia, acromegaly, thrombocytopenia, urinary calculi, nephrogenic diabetes insipidus, and juvenile diabetes mellitus.

Nevertheless, it is doubtful that any clinical abnormalities result specifically from γ-cystathionase deficiency. Ascertainment bias may be minimized by selection from Table 25-4 of those patients discovered (1) during routine newborn screening (patients 23, 24, 26, 28–30, 32, 35, 42, 43, 45, 47); (2) as a result of family screening following the discovery of a cystathionine-excreting individual in a family (patients 6, 7, 11, 15, 20, 22, 31, 33, 34, 36, 37, 41); (3) as a result of screening all hospital admissions (patient 5); (4) because of fortuitous testing (patient 16). Of these 26 patients, only five (patients 5, 28, 34, 36, and 37) have clinical aberrations that could be related to the metabolic disorder. Patient 5 is mentally retarded. Patient 28 is hyperactive and has a learning disorder, but his cystathioninuric sib is normal. Patient 34 is also hyperactive and has an IQ of 76, but, again, his cystathioninuric sib is normal. Patients 36 and 37 are mentally retarded, but the fact that another sib in this family was mentally retarded but probably only heterozygous for γ-cystathionase deficiency [461] suggests that the mental retardation may be coincidental. Although several of the clinically normal cystathioninuric individuals described in Table 25-4 are children and may be too young for complications to have developed, this table also includes a number of older children, teenagers, and adults who might be expected to manifest any abnormality caused by γ-cystathionase deficiency.

Included in Table 25-4 are four individuals with pyridoxine-nonresponsive cystathioninuria, in whom the biochemical defect may be more complete than in those with pyridoxine-responsive cystathioninuria (see "The Pyridoxine Effect and Its Mechanism" earlier in this chapter). Of these, patient 4, who is mentally retarded, was ascertained in a screening program among the mentally retarded. Patients 26 and 45, who are normal, were ascertained during a routine neonatal urine screening program. No clinical information about patient 17 has been published.

Diagnosis

The characteristic finding in γ-cystathionase deficiency is a specific and easily detectable cystathioninuria. This is most readily demonstrable by amino acid paper chromatography of urine using a bidimensional technique and ninhydrin staining [379], or by unidimensional chromatography and a specific sulfur stain such as iodoplatinate reagent [295]. Unidimensional chromatography using ninhydrin staining lacks the sensitivity and the resolution necessary for specific identification. In γ-cystathionase deficiency, metabolites of cystathionine may be present, most notably N-acetylcystathionine (see the section on "Metabolic Sequelae" of γ-cystathionase deficiency), but sulfur amino acids such as homocystine will be absent. Should homocystine also be present, consideration should be given to the presence of a homocysteine methylation defect, rather than γ-cystathionase deficiency (Table 25-1).

It is important that the urine examined for cystathioninuria be clean and that it contain a preservative such as thymol or toluene that inhibits bacterial growth. Microorganisms contain β-cystathionase, an enzyme which cleaves cystathionine to homocysteine and pyruvate. Thus in a contaminated urine sample, cystathionine may be converted to homocyst(e)ine and the defect may be misdiagnosed [46].

Plasma or serum should be analyzed for amino acids using a suitable quantitative technique [379]. In γ-cystathionase deficiency this will almost always reveal cystathionine, an amino acid normally not detected in blood. The methionine concentration will be normal, in contrast to the hypermethioninemia usually seen in patients with cystathionine β-synthase deficiency and also in contrast to the hypomethioninemia which may be noted in association with a homocysteine methylation defect (Table 25-1). The plasma cystine concentration has usually been normal in γ-cystathionase deficiency, again in contrast to cystathionine β-synthase deficiency, in which plasma cystine is usually undetectable.

Cystathioninuria per se does not establish the diagnosis of inherited γ-cystathionase deficiency. Cystathioninuria may also occur transiently in the newborn or young infant, in association with liver disease, neuroblastoma, ganglioblastoma, or hepatoblastoma, in vitamin B6 deficiency, and perhaps even in an occasional individual with thyrotoxicosis (Table 25-1). In transient cystathioninuria of infancy, urinary cystathionine is usually quite small and disappears by age 3 months [103]. When cystathioninuria accompanies liver disease or the tumors noted above, the underlying disease is usually clinically apparent [119, 126, 127, 129]. Whenever cystathioninuria is discovered, it is important to rule out those disorders in which cystathioninuria may appear secondarily and which may be in need of specific therapy. When cystathioninuria has been established as persistent and of an apparently primary nature, a trial of supplemental pyridoxine should be given to establish whether or not the disorder is pyridoxine responsive. Initially, oral pyridoxine hydrochloride in amounts of 100 mg/day should be administered and the urine examined after 2 weeks. If there is no response, the dose of pyridoxine hydrochloride should be increased by 100 mg and the urine examined for cystathionine at the end of another 2 weeks.

While the diagnosis can be confirmed by measurement of γ-cystathionase activity in liver obtained by biopsy, the risk entailed in a liver biopsy militates against such confirmation of this probably benign disorder. Enzymatic analyses of cultured lymphoid cell lines [439, 440] or (perhaps) of fibroblasts cultured from skin [442] are alternative means of diagnosis.

Management

Since γ-cystathionase deficiency is probably a benign disorder, no specific management is indicated. In those individuals responsive to pyridoxine, oral pyridoxine hydrochloride can be given without known risk. The dose has usually been 100

mg or more daily [449]. The amount necessary can be judged only by titration. Conceivably, a low methionine diet could reduce the accumulation of cystathionine, and might be considered for pyridoxine-unresponsive patients if further experience indicates that such individuals are at risk for specific clinical complications.

Prevalence and Screening

Among 633,331 newborns screened in Massachusetts by paper chromatography of urine, followed by ninhydrin staining, nine children with persistent cystathioninuria severe enough to lead to the presumptive diagnosis of γ-cystathionase deficiency have been discovered. This is a prevalence of 1:70,000 [471]. In Australia, screening of 1,000,000 infants disclosed three subjects with comparably persistent and severe cystathioninuria, a prevalence of 1:333,000 [422].

REFERENCES

1. MUDD SH: The adenosyltransferases, in Boyer PD (ed): *The Enzymes*, ed 3. New York, Academic Press, Inc, 1973, vol 8, part A, p 121
2. LOMBARDINI JB, CHOU T-C, TALALAY P: Regulatory properties of adenosine triphosphate-L-methionine S-adenosyltransferase of rat liver. *Biochem J* 135:43, 1973
3. CANTONI GL: Activation of methionine for transmethylation. *J Biol Chem* 189:745, 1951
4. CANTONI GL, DURELL J: Activation of methionine for transmethylation. II. The methionine-activating enzyme: Studies on the mechanism of the reaction. *J Biol Chem* 225:1033, 1957
5. PAN F, TARVER H: Effects on diets and other factors on methionine adenosyltransferase levels in rat liver. *J Nutr* 92:274, 1967
6. LOMBARDINI JB, COULTER AW, TALALAY P: Analogues of methionine as substrates and inhibitors of the methionine adenosyltransferase reaction: Deductions concerning the conformation of methionine. *Mol Pharmacol* 6:481, 1970
7. CANTONI GL: Methylation of nicotinamide with a soluble enzyme system from rat liver. *J Biol Chem* 189:203, 1951
8. MUDD SH, CANTONI GL: Activation of methionine for transmethylation. III. The methionine-activating enzyme of bakers' yeast. *J Biol Chem* 231:481, 1958
9. HANCOCK RL: S-Adenosylmethionine-synthesizing activity of normal and neoplastic mouse tissues. *Cancer Res* 26:2425, 1966
10. STEKOL JA: Formation and metabolism of S-adenosyl derivatives of S-alkylhomocysteines in the rat and mouse, in Shapiro SK, Schlenk F (eds): *Transmethylation and Methionine Biosynthesis*. Chicago, University of Chicago Press, 1965, p 231
11. PAN F, TARVER H: Comparative studies on methionine, selenomethionine, and their ethyl analogues as substrates for methionine adenosyltransferase from rat liver. *Arch Biochem Biophys* 119:429, 1967
12. COX R, SMITH RC: Inhibition of S-adenosylmethionine formation by analogues of methionine. *Arch Biochem Biophys* 129:615, 1969
13. LOMBARDINI JB, TALALAY P: Formation, functions and regulatory importance of S-adenosyl-L-methionine, in Weber G (ed): *Advances in Enzyme Regulations*. Elmsford, NY, Pergamon Press, Inc, 1971, vol 9, p 349
14. LIAU MC, LIN GW, HURLBERT RB: Partial purification and characterization of tumor and liver S-adenosylmethionine synthetases. *Cancer Res* 37:427, 1977
15. HOFFMAN JL, KUNZ GL: Differential activation of rat liver methionine adenosyltransferase isozymes by dimethylsulfoxide. *Biochem Biophys Res Commun* 77:1231, 1977
16. LIAU MC, CHANG CF, BELANGER L, GRENIER A: Correlation of isozyme patterns of S-adenosylmethionine synthetase with fetal stages and pathological states of the liver. *Cancer Res* 39:162, 1979
17. KUNZ GL, HOFFMAN JL, CHIA CS, STREMEL B: Separation of rat liver methionine adenosyltransferase isozymes by hydrophobic chromatography. *Arch Biochem Biophys* 202:565, 1980
18. KUNZ GL: Fractionation and regulatory properties of rat methionine adenosyltransferase isozymes, thesis. University of Louisville, 1979
19. TALLAN HH: Methionine adenosyltransferase in man: Evidence for multiple forms. *Biochem Med* 21:129, 1979
20. MUDD SH, KLEE WA, ROSS PD: Enthalpy changes accompanying the

transfer of a methyl group from S-adenosylmethionine and other sulfonium compounds to homocysteine. *Biochemistry* 5:1653, 1966

21. TABOR H, ROSENTHAL SM, TABOR CW: The biosynthesis of spermidine and spermine from putrescine and methionine. *J Biol Chem* 233:907, 1958

22. MUDD SH: Biochemical mechanisms in methyl group transfer, in Fishman WH (ed): *Metabolic Conjugation and Metabolic Hydrolysis*. New York, Academic Press, Inc, 1973, vol 3, p 297

23. MUDD SH, POOLE JR: Labile methyl balances for normal humans on various dietary regimens. *Metabolism* 24:721, 1975

24. MUDD SH, EBERT MH, SCRIVER CR: Labile methyl group balances in the human: The role of sarcosine. *Metabolism* 29:707, 1980

25. HOFFMAN DR, CORNATZER WE, DUERRE JA: Relationship between tissue levels of S-adenosylmethionine, S-adenosylhomocysteine, and transmethylation reactions. *Can J Biochem* 57:56, 1979

26. HOFFMAN DR, MARION DW, CORNATZER WE, DUERRE JA: S-Adenosylhomocysteine metabolism in isolated rat liver: Effects of L-methionine, L-homocysteine, and adenosine. *J Biol Chem* 255:10822, 1980

27. CANTONI GL, RICHARDS HH, CHIANG PK: Inhibitors of S-adenosylhomocysteine hydrolase and their role in the regulation of biological methylation, in Usdin E, Borchardt RT, Creveling CR (eds): *Transmethylation*. New York, Elsevier North-Holland, Biomedical Press, 1979, p 155

28. DE LA HABA G, CANTONI GL: The enzymatic synthesis of S-adenosyl-L-homocysteine from adenosine and homocysteine. *J Biol Chem* 234:603, 1959

29. FINKELSTEIN JD, HARRIS B: Methionine metabolism in mammals: Synthesis of S-adenosylhomocysteine in rat tissues. *Arch Biochem Biophys* 159:160, 1973

30. WALKER RD, DUERRE JA: S-Adenosylhomocysteine metabolism in various species. *Can J Biochem* 53:312, 1975

31. DURELL J, ANDERSON DG, CANTONI GL: The synthesis of methionine by enzymic transmethylation. I. Purification and properties of thetin homocysteine methylpherase. *Biochim Biophys Acta* 26:270, 1957

32. KLEE WA, RICHARDS HH, CANTONI GL: The synthesis of methionine by enzymic transmethylation, VII. Existence of two separate homocysteine methylpherases on mammalian liver. *Biochim Biophys Acta* 54:157, 1961

33. TAYLOR RT, WEISSBACH H: N5-Methyltetrahydrofolate-homocysteine methyltransferases, in Boyer PD (ed): *The Enzymes*, 3d. New York, Academic Press, Inc, 1973, vol 9, part B, p 121

34. RUDIGER H, JAENICKE L: Methionine synthesis: Demonstration of the reversibility of the reaction. *FEBS Lett* 4:316, 1969

35. MUDD SH: Homocystinuria and homocysteine metabolism: Selected aspects, in Nyhan WL (ed): *Heritable Disorders of Amino Acid Metabolism*. New York, John Wyle & Sons, Inc, 1974, p 429

36. KRAUS S, PACKMAN S, FOWLER B, ROSENBERG LE: Purification and properties of cystathione β-synthase from human liver. *J Biol Chem* 253:6523, 1978

37. KIMURA H, NAKAGAWA H: Studies on cystathionine synthetase: Characteristics of purified rat liver enzyme. *J Biochem (Tokyo)* 69:711, 1971

38. BROWN FC, GORDON PH: Cystathionine synthase from rat liver: Partial purification and properties. *Can J Biochem* 49:484, 1971

39. TUDBALL N, REED MA: Purification and properties of cystathionine synthase from human liver. *Biochem Biophys Res Commun* 67:550, 1975

40. ANSELL PRJ, TUDBALL N: The existence of human liver cystathionine β-synthase in multiple molecular forms. *Biochim Biophys Acta* 483:443, 1977

41. GRIFFITHS R, TUDBALL N: The molecular defect in a case of (cystathionine β-synthase)-deficient homocystinuria. *Eur J Biochem* 74:269, 1977

42. GRIFFITHS R: Cystathionine β-synthase deficiency: Observations on the biochemical lesion in a vitamin B₆ non-responsive patient. *Monogr Hum Genet* 9:135, 1978

43. KASHIWAMATA S, KOTAKE Y, GREENBERG DM: Studies of cystathionine synthase of rat liver: Dissociation into two components by sodium dodecyl sulfate disc electrophoresis. *Biochim Biophys Acta* 212:501, 1970

44. BRAUNSTEIN AE, GORYACHENKOVA EV, TOLOSA EA, WILLHARDT IH, YEFREMOVA LL: Specificity and some other properties of liver serine sulphhydrase: Evidence for its identity with cystathionine β-synthase. *Biochim Biophys Acta* 242:247, 1971

45. PORTER PN, GRISHAVER MS, JONES OW: Characterization of human cystathionine β-synthase: Evidence for the identity of human L-serine dehydratase and cystathionine β-synthase. *Biochim Biophys Acta* 364:128, 1974

46. LEVY HL, MUDD SH, UHLENDORF BW, MADIGAN PM: Cystathioninuria and homocystinuria. *Clin Chim Acta* 58:51, 1975

47. MATSUO Y, GREENBERG DM: A crystalline enzyme that cleaves homoserine and cystathionine. I. Isolation procedure and some physiochemical properties. *J Biol Chem* 230:545, 1958

48. CHURCHICH JE, DUPOURQUE D: Dissociation of cystathionase. *Biochem Biophys Res Commun* 46:524, 1972

49. MUSHAHWAR IK, KOEPPE RE: Rat liver L-diaminopropionate ammonia lyase: Identification as cystathionase. *J Biol Chem* 248:7407, 1973

50. BIKEL I, PAVLATOS TN, LIVINGSTON DM: Purification and subunit structure of mouse liver cystathionase. *Arch Biochem Biophys* 186:168, 1978

51. IGLEHART JD, YORK RM, MODEST AP, LAZARUS H, LIVINGSTON DM: Cystine requirement of continuous human lymphoid cell lines of normal and leukemic origin. *J Biol Chem* 252:7184, 1977

52. MATSUO Y, GREENBERG DM: A crystalline enzyme that cleaves homoserine and crystathionine. II. Prosthetic group. *J Biol Chem* 230:561, 1958

53. MATSUO Y, GREENBERG DM: A crystalline enzyme that cleaves homoserine and cystathionine. III. Coenzyme resolution, activators, and inhibitors. *J Biol Chem* 234:507, 1959

54. OH K-J, CHURCHICH JE: Binding of pyridoxal 5-phosphate to cystathionase. *J Biol Chem* 248:7370, 1973

55. GORYACHENKOVA EV, POLYAKOVA LA, YEFREMOVA LL, FLORENTIEV VL: Interaction of pyridoxal phosphate analogues with apoenzymes of β-cystathionase and serine sulphhydrase. *Biochem Biophys Res Commun* 55:1021, 1973

56. LOISELET J, CHATAGNER F: Purification et etude de quelques proprietes de la cysteine desulfurase "soluble" (cystathionase) du foie de rat. *Bull Soc Chim Biol* 47:33, 1965

57. MUDD SH, LEVY HL: Disorders of transsulfuration, in Stanbury JB, Wyngaarden JB, Fredrickson DS (eds): *The Metabolic Basis of Inherited Disease*, ed. 4. New York, McGraw-Hill Book Co, 1978, p 458

58. MATSUO Y, GREENBERG DM: A crystalline enzyme that cleaves homoserine and cystathionine. IV. Mechanism of action, reversibility, and substrate specificity. *J Biol Chem* 234:516, 1959

59. WONG PWK, SCHWARZ V, KOMROWER GM: The biosynthesis of cystathionine in patients with homocystinuria. *Pediatr Res* 2:149, 1968

60. CHATAGNER F, TIXIER M, PORTEMER C: Biosynthesis of cystathionine from homoserine and cysteine by rat liver cystathionase. *FEBS Lett* 4:231, 1969

61. TALLAN HH, STURMAN JA, PASCAL TA, GAULL GE: Cystathionine γ-synthesis from homocysteine and cysteine by mammalian tissue. *Biochem Med* 9:90, 1974

62. PAN F, CHANG G, LEE S, TANG M: Induction of methionine adenosyltransferase in rat liver by corticosteroids. *Proc Soc Exp Biol Med* 128:611, 1968

63. MUDD SH, FINKELSTEIN JD, IRREVERRE F, LASTER L: Transsulfuration in mammals: Microassays and tissue distributions of three enzymes of the pathway. *J Biol Chem* 240:4382, 1965

64. STURMAN JA, RASSIN DK, GAULL GE: Distribution of transsulphuration enzymes in various organs and species. *Int J Biochem* 1:251, 1970

65. FINKELSTEIN JD, KYLE WE, HARRIS BJ: Methionine metabolism in mammals: Regulation of homocysteine methyltransferases in rat tissue. *Arch Biochem Biophys* 146:84, 1971

66. FINKELSTEIN JD, HARRIS B: Methionine metabolism in mammals: S-adenosylhomocysteine hydrolase in rat intestinal mucosa. *Arch Biochem Biophys* 171:282, 1975

67. MUDD SH, LEVY HL, MORROW G III: Deranged B₁₂ metabolism: Effects on sulfur amino acid metabolism. *Biochem Med* 4:193, 1970

68. GAULL GE, VON BERG W, RAIHA NCR, STURMAN JA: Development of methyltransferase activities of human fetal tissues. *Pediatr Res* 7:527, 1973

69. GAULL GE, STURMAN JA, RAIHA NCR: Development of mammalian sulfur metabolism: Absence of cystathionase in human fetal tissues. *Pediatr Res* 6:538, 1972

70. FINKELSTEIN JD: Methionine metabolism in mammals: Effects of age, diet, and hormones on three enzymes of the pathway in rat tissues. *Arch Biochem Biophys* 122:583, 1967

71. SHEID B, BILIK E: S-Adenosylmethionine synthetase activity in some normal rat tissues and transplantable hepatomas. *Cancer Res* 28:2512, 1968

72. STURMAN JA, GAULL GE, RAIHA NCR: Absence of cystathionase in human fetal liver: Is cystine essential? *Science* 169:74, 1970

73. PASCAL TA, GILLAM BM, GAULL GE: Cystathionase: Immunochemical evidence for absence from human fetal liver. *Pediatr Res* 6:773, 1972

74. HEINONEN K, RAIHA NCR: Induction of cystathionase in human foetal liver. *Biochem J* 144:607, 1974

75. GAULL GE, RASSIN DK, RAIHA NCR, HEINONEN K: Milk protein quantity and quality in low-birth-weight infants. III. Effects on sulfur amino acids in plasma and urine. *J Pediatr* 90:348, 1977

76. PRZYREMBEL H, BREMER HJ: Cystathioninuria in premature infants. *Clin Chim Acta* 41:95, 1972

77. GAULL GE, RAIHA NCR, SAARIKOSKI S, STURMAN JA: Transfer of cyst(e)ine and methionine across the human placenta. *Pediatr Res* 7:908, 1973

78. FLEISHER LD, GAULL GE: Methionine metabolism in man: Development and deficiencies. *Clin Endocrinol Metab* 3:37, 1974

78a. ZLOTKIN SH, BRYAN MH, ANDERSON GH: Cysteine supplementation to cysteine-free intravenous feeding regimens in newborn infants. *Am J Clin Nutr* 34:914, 1981

79. IBER FL, ROSEN H, LEVENSON SM, CHALMERS TC: The plasma amino acids in patients with liver failure. *J Lab Clin Med* 50:417, 1957

80. GEROK W: Quantitative Bestimmung der Aminosauren im Serum bei Erkrankungen der Leber. *Dtsch Med Wochenschr* 88:1188, 1963

80a. HOROWITZ JH, RYTINS EB, HENDERSON JM, HEYMSFIELD SB, MOFFITT SD, BAIN RP, CHAWLA RK, BLEIER JC, RUDMAN, D: Evidence for impairment of transsulfuration pathway in cirrhosis. *Gastroenterology* 81:668, 1981

81. GJESSING LR, HALVORSEN S: Hypermethioninaemia in acute tyrosinosis. *Lancet* 2:1132, 1965

82. SCRIVER CR, CLOW CL, SILVERBERG M: Hypermethioninaemia in acute tyrosinosis. *Lancet* 1:153, 1966

83. PERRY TL, HARDWICK DF, DIXON GH, DOLMAN CL, HANSEN S: Hypermethioninemia: A metabolic disorder associated with cirrhosis, islet cell hyperplasia and renal tubular degeneration. *Pediatics* 36:236, 1965

84. GAULL GE, RASSIN DK, SOLOMON GE, HARRIS RC, STURMAN JA: Biochemical observations on so-called hereditary tyrosinemia. *Pediatr Res* 4:337, 1970

85. MUDD SH: Errors of sulfur metabolism, in Muth OH, Oldfield JE (eds): *Symposium: Sulfur in Nutrition.* Westport, Conn, Avi Publishing Co, 1970, p 222

86. SNYDERMAN SE, HOLT LE Jr, NORTON PM, ROITMAN E, PHANSALKAR SV: The plasma aminogram. I. Influence of the level of protein intake and a comparison of whole protein and amino acid diets. *Pediatr Res* 2:131, 1968

87. LEVY HL, SHIH VE, MADIGAN PM, KAROLKEWICZ V, CARR JR, LUM A, RICHARDS AA, CRAWFORD JD, MacCREADY RA: Hypermethioninemia with other hyperaminoacidemias. Studies in infants on high-protein diets. *Am J Dis Child* 117:96, 1969

88. KOMROWER GM, ROBINS AJ: Plasma amino acid disturbance in infancy. I. Hypermethioninaemia and transient tyrosinaemia. *Arch Dis Child* 44:418, 1969

89. VALMAN HB, BROWN RJK, PALMER T, OBERHOLZER VG, LEVIN B: Protein intake and plasma amino-acids of infants of low birth weight. *Br Med J* 4:789, 1971

90. SLAVIK M, LOVENBERG W, KEISER HR: Changes in serum and urine amino acids in patients with progressive systemic sclerosis treated with 6-azauridine triacetate. *Biochem Pharmacol* 22:1295, 1973

91. HYANEK J, BREMER HJ, SLAVIK M: "Homocystinuria" and [urinary] excretion of β-amino acids in patients treated with 6-azauridine. *Clin Chim Acta* 25:288, 1969

92. EFRON ML, McPHERSON TC, SHIH VE, WELSH F, MacCREADY RA: D-Methioninuria due to DL-methionine ingestion. *Am J Dis Child* 117:104, 1969

93. GAULL GE, BENDER AN, VULOVIC D, TALLAN HH, SCHAFFNER F: Methioninemia and myopathy: A new disorder. *Ann Neurology* 9:423, 1981

94. BUIST NRM: Personal communication to GE Gaull, cited in [93], 1981

95. JHAVERI BM, BUIST NRM, GAULL GE: Unpublished observations cited in [93], 1981

96. PRZYREMBEL H, GAULL GE, TALLAN HH: Unpublished observations cited in [93], 1981

96a. CASE GL, BENEVENGA NJ: Evidence for S-adenosylmethionine independent catabolism of methionine in the rat. *J Nutr* 106:1721, 1976

96b. MITCHELL AD, BENEVENGA NJ: The role of transamination in methionine oxidation in the rat. *J Nutr* 108:67, 1978

96c. STEELE RD, BENEVENGA NJ: Identification of 3-methylthiopropionic acid as an intermediate in mammalian methionine metabolism *in vitro. J Biol Chem* 253:7844, 1978

96d. STEELE RD, BENEVENGA NJ: The metabolism of 3-methylthiopropionate in rat liver homogenates. *J Biol Chem* 254:8885, 1979

97. HOLLOWELL JG Jr, HALL WK, CORYELL ME, McPHERSON J Jr, HAHN DA: Homocystinuria and organic aciduria in a patient with vitamin-B$_{12}$ deficiency. *Lancet* 2:1428, 1969

98. HIGGINBOTTOM MC, SWEETMAN L, NYHAN WL: A syndrome of methylmalonic aciduria, homocystinuria, megaloblastic anemia and neurologic abnormalities in a vitamin B$_{12}$-deficient breast-fed infant of a strict vegetarian. *N Engl J Med* 299:317, 1978

99. LEVY HL, MUDD SH: Homocystinuria due to bacterial contamination in pyridoxine-unresponsive cystathioninemia. *Pediatr Res* 7:162, 1973

100. HARAGUCHI H, IWATANI E, HIROSAWA M, YAMASHITA F, NAGAYAMA T: Cystathioninuria. *Igakunoayumi (Jap)* 61:72, 1967

101. TADA K, YOSHIDA T, YOKOYAMA Y, SATO T, NAKAGAWA H, ARAKAWA T: Cystathioninuria not associated with vitamin B$_6$ dependency: A probably new type of cystathioninuria. *Tohoku J Exp Med* 95:235, 1968

102. COIGNET J, PASSERON P, LAURENT B, ROUAULT F: A propos d'un cas de cystathionurie avec excretion d'homocystine. *Pediatrie* 26:317, 1971

103. LYON ICT, PROCOPIS PG, TURNER B: Cystathioninuria in a well baby population. *Acta Paediatr Scand* 60:324, 1971

104. LAURENT B, COIGNET J: Cystathioninurie: Trouble possible de regulation enzymatique. *Clin Chim Acta* 43:171, 1973

105. ENDRES W, SEIBOLD H: Renal excretion of cystathionine and creatinine in humans at different ages. *Clin Chim Acta* 87:425, 1978

106. ENDRES W, VOGT R, RIEGEL KP, BREMER HG: The influence of vitamin B$_6$ on cystathioninuria in premature infants. *Clin Chim Acta* 86:89, 1978

107. LEVY HL, MUDD SH, SCHULMAN JD, DREYFUS PM, ABELES RH: A derangement in B$_{12}$ metabolism associated with homocystinemia, cystathioninemia, hypomethioninemia, and methylmalonic aciduria. *Am J Med* 48:390, 1970

108. SHIH VE, SALAM MZ, MUDD SH, UHLENDORF BW, ADAMS RD: A new form of homocystinuria due to $N^{5,10}$-methylenetetrahydrofolate reductase deficiency. *Pediatr Res* 6:135, 1972

109. GOODMAN SI, MOE PG, HAMMOND KB, MUDD SH, UHLENDORF BW: Homocystinuria with methylmalonic aciduria: Two cases in a sibship. *Biochem Med* 4:500, 1970

110. FREEMAN JM, FINKELSTEIN JD, MUDD SH: Folate-responsive homocystinuria and "schizophrenia": A defect in methylation due to deficient 5,10-methylenetetrahydrofolate reductase activity. *N Engl J Med* 292:491, 1975

111. HOPE DB: L-Cystathionine in the urine of pyridoxine-deficient rats. *Biochem J* 66:486, 1957

112. SCRIVER CR, HUTCHISON JH: The vitamin B$_6$ deficiency syndrome in human infancy: Biochemical and clinical observations. *Pediatrics* 31:240, 1963

113. PARK YK, LINKSWILER H: Effect of vitamin B$_6$ depletion in adult man on the excretion of cystathionine and other methionine metabolites. *J Nutr* 100:110, 1970

114. STURMAN JA, COHEN PA, GAULL GE: Effects of deficiency of vitamin B$_6$ on transsulfuration. *Biochem Med* 3:244, 1969

115. FINKELSTEIN JD, CHALMERS FT: Pyridoxine effects on cystathionine synthase in rat liver. *J Nutr* 100:467, 1970

116. GJESSING LR: Cystathioninuria during a load of thyroxine. *Scand J Clin Lab Invest* 16:680, 1964

117. CHATAGNER F, JOLLES-BERGERET B, TRAUTMANN O: Hormones thyroidiennes et enzymes de desulfuration de la L-cysteine du foie du rat. *Biochim Biophys Acta* 59:744, 1962

118. SHAW KNF, LIEBERMAN E, KOCH R, DONNELL GN: Cystathioninuria. *Am J Dis Child* 113:119, 1967

119. LIEBERMAN E, SHAW KNF, DONNELL GN: Cystathioninuria in galactosemia and certain types of liver disease. *Pediatrics* 40:828, 1967

120. VON STUDNITZ, W: Secondary cystathioninuria. *Acta Paediatr Scand* 58:173, 1969

121. ENDRES W, WUTTAGE B: Occurrence of secondary cystathioninuria in children with inherited metabolic disorders, liver diseases, neoplasms, cystic fibrosis and celiac disease. *Eur J Pediatr* 129:29, 1978

122. FRIMPTER GW: Cystathioninuria in a patient with cystinuria. *Am J Med* 46:832, 1969

123. FRIMPTER GW, GREENBERG AJ: Renal clearance of cystathionine in homozygous and heterozygous cystathioninuria, cystinuria, and the normal state. *J Clin Invest* 46:975, 1967

124. GJESSING LR: Studies of functional neural tumors. III. Cystathionine in the tumor tissue. *Scand J Clin Lab Invest* 15:479, 1963

125. GJESSING LR: Studies of functional neural tumors. II. Cystathioninuria. *Scand J Clin Lab Invest* 15:474, 1963

126. Gjessing LR: Studies of functional neural tumors. IV. Isolation and identification of urinary cystathionine. *Scand J Clin Lab Invest* 15:601, 1963

127. VON STUDNITZ W: Sulfur-containing amino acids in the urine of patients with tumours from sympathetic nervous tissue. *Scand J Clin Lab Invest* 17(suppl):86, 190, 1965

128. MUDD SH, LASTER L, FINKELSTEIN JD, IRREVERRE F: Studies on homocystinuria, in Himwich HE, Kety SS, Smythies JR (eds): *Amines and Schizophrenia.* Elmsford, NY, Pergamon Press, Inc, 1967, p 247

129. GJESSING LR, MAURITZEN K: Cystathioninuria in hepatoblastoma. *Scand J Clin Lab Invest* 17:513, 1965

130. VOUTE PA Jr, WADMAN SK: Cystathioninuria in hepatoblastoma. *Clin Chim Acta* 22:373, 1968

131. GEISER CF, SHIH VE: Cystathioninuria and its origin in children with hepatoblastoma. *J Pediatr* 96:72, 1980

132. GAULL GE, TALLAN HH: Methionine adenosyltransferase deficiency: New enzymatic defect associated with hypermethioninemia. *Science* 186:59, 1974

133. GAULL GE: Deficiency of methionine adenosyltransferase: A new etiology for hypermethioninemia in infancy, in Salvatore F, Borek E, Zappia V, Williams-Ashman HG, Schlenk F (eds): *The Biochemistry of Adenosylmethionine.* New York, Columbia University Press, 1977, p 37

134. FINKELSTEIN JD: Enzyme defects in sulfur amino acid metabolism in man in Greenberg DM (ed): *Metabolism of Sulfur Compounds,* vol 7, *Metabolic Pathways,* ed 3. New York, Academic Press, Inc, 1975, p 547

135. FINKELSTEIN JD, KYLE WE, MARTIN JJ: Abnormal methionine adenosyl-

transferase in hypermethioninemia. *Biochem Biophys Res Commun* 66:1491, 1975

136. GOUT J-P, SERRE J-C DIETERLEN M, ANTENER I, FRAPPAT P, BOST M, BEAUDOING A: Une nouvelle cause d'hypermethioninemie de l'enfant: Le deficit en S-adenosyl-methionine-synthetase. *Arch Fr Pediatr* 34:416, 1977

137. GAULL GE, TALLAN HH, LONSDALE D, PRZYREMBEL H, SCHAFFNER F, von BASSEWITZ DB: Hypermethioninemia associated with methionine adenosyltransferase deficiency: Clinical, morphological and biochemical observations on four patients. *J Pediatr* 98:734, 1981

138. NATORI Y: Studies on ethionine. VI. Sex-dependent behavior of methionine and ethionine in rats. *J Biol Chem* 238:2075, 1963

139. FIELD CMB, CARSON NAJ, CUSWORTH DC, DENT CE, NEILL DW: Homocystinuria: A new disorder of metabolism. *Abstracts of the Tenth International Congress of Paediatricians (Lisbon)*, 1962, p 274

140. CARSON NAJ, NEILL DW: Metabolic abnormalities detected in a survey of mentally backward individuals in Northern Ireland. *Arch Dis Child* 37:505, 1962

141. GERRITSEN T, VAUGHN JG, WAISMAN HA: The identification of homocystine in the urine. *Biochem Biophys Res Commun* 9:493, 1962

142. CARSON NAJ, CUSWORTH DC, DENT CE, FIELD CMB, NEILL DW, WESTALL RG: Homocystinuria: A new inborn error of metabolism associated with mental deficiency. *Arch Dis Child* 38:425, 1963

143. GERRITSEN T, WAISMAN HA: Homocystinuria, an error in the metabolism of methionine. *Pediatrics* 33:413, 1964

144. SPAETH GL, BARBER GW: Homocystinuria: In a mentally retarded child and her normal cousin. *Trans Am Acad Ophthalmol Otolaryngol* 69:912, 1965

145. MUDD SH, FINKELSTEIN JD, IRREVERRE F, LASTER L: Homocystinuria: An enzymatic defect. *Science* 143:1443, 1964

146. GAULL GE, STURMAN JA, SCHAFFNER F: Homocystinuria due to cystathionine synthase deficiency: Enzymatic and ultrastructural studies. *J Pediatr* 84:381, 1974

147. GAULL GE, RASSIN DK, STURMAN JA: Enzymatic and metabolic studies of homocystinuria: Effects of pyridoxine. *Neuropadiatrie* 1:199, 1969

148. FINKELSTEIN JD, MUDD SH, IRREVERRE F, LASTER L: Homocystinuria due to cystathionine synthetase deficiency: The mode of inheritance. *Science* 146:785, 1964

149. MUDD SH, FINKELSTEIN JD, IRREVERRE F, LASTER L: Threonine dehydratase activity in humans lacking cystathionine synthase. *Biochem Biophys Res Commun* 19:665, 1965

150. LASTER L, SPAETH GL, MUDD SH, FINKELSTEIN JD: Homocystinuria due to cystathionine synthase deficiency. Combined clinical staff conference at the National Institutes of Health. *Ann Intern Med* 63:1117, 1965

151. HOLLOWELL JG JR, CORYELL ME, HALL WK, FINDLEY JK, THEVAOS TG: Homocystinuria as affected by pyridoxine, folic acid, and vitamin B₁₂. *Proc Soc Exp Biol Med* 129:237, 1968

152. YOSHIDA T, TADA K, YOKOYAMA Y, ARAKAWA T: Homocystinuria of vitamin B₆ dependent type. *Tohoku J Exp Med* 96:235, 1968

153. MUDD SH, EDWARDS WA, LOEB PM, BROWN MS, LASTER L: Homocystinuria due to cystathionine synthase deficiency: The effect of pyridoxine. *J Clin Invest* 49:1762, 1970

154. LONGHI, RC, FLEISHER LD, TALLAN HH, GAULL GE: Cystathionine β-synthase deficiency: A qualitative abnormality of the deficient enzyme modified by vitamin B₆ therapy. *Pediatr Res* 11:100, 1977

155. UHLENDORF BW, MUDD SH: Cystathionine synthase in tissue culture derived from human skin: Enzyme defect in homocystinuria. *Science* 160:1007, 1968

156. UHLENDORF BW, CONERLY EB, MUDD SH: Homocystinuria: Studies in tissue culture. *Pediatr Res* 7:645, 1973

157. POOLE JR, MUDD SH, CONERLY EB, EDWARDS WA: Homocystinuria due to cystathionine synthase deficiency: Studies of nitrogen balance and sulfur excretion. *J Clin Invest* 55:1033, 1975

158. BITTLES AH, CARSON NAJ: Tissue culture techniques as an aid to prenatal diagnosis and genetic counselling in homocystinuria. *J Med Genet* 10:120, 1973

159. FLEISHER LD, LONGHI RC, TALLAN HH, GAULL GE: Cystathionine β-synthase deficiency: Differences in thermostability between normal and abnormal enzymes from cultured human cells. *Pediatr Res* 12:293, 1978

160. FOWLER B, KRAUS J, PACKMAN S, ROSENBERG LE: Homocystinuria: Evidence for three distinct classes of cystathionine β-synthase mutants in cultured fibroblasts. *J Clin Invest* 61:645, 1978

161. HEMRAJ F, GRIFFITHS R: Enzyme studies in cystathionine-β-synthase deficiency: A possible effect of elevated intracellular levels of homocystine in kinetic studies. *J Inher Metab Dis* 1:171, 1978

162. DRAYER JIM, CLEOPHAS AJM, TRIJBELS JMF, SMALS AGH, KLOPPENBORG PWC: Symptoms, diagnostic pitfalls, and treatment of homocystinuria in seven adult patients. *Neth J Med* 23:89, 1980

163. SKOVBY F, KRAUS J, REDLICH C, ROSENBERG L: Immunochemical studies of cystathionine β-synthase deficiency. *Am J Hum Genet* 32:55A, 1980

164. FOWLER B, SARDHARWALLA IB: Homocystinuria: Cystathionine synthase activity in cultured skin fibroblasts, in *International Symposium on Inborn Errors of Metabolism in Humans.* Switzerland, 1980, p 20

165. BITTLES AH, CARSON NAJ: Homocystinuria: Studies on cystathionine β-synthase, S-adenosylmethionine synthase, and cystathionase activities in skin fibroblasts. *J Inher Metab Dis*, 1981, in press

166. FOWLER B, SARDHARWALLA IB: Personal communication, 1981

167. GOLDSTEIN JL, CAMPBELL BK, GARTLER SM: Cystathionine synthase activity in human lymphocytes: Induction by phytohemagglutinin. *J Clin Invest* 51:1034, 1972

168. GOLDSTEIN JL, CAMPBELL BK, GARTLER SM: Homocystinuria: Heterozygote detection using phytohemagglutinin-stimulated lymphocytes. *J Clin Invest* 52:218, 1973

169. FLEISHER LD, BERATIS NG, TALLAN HH, HIRSCHHORN K, GAULL GE: Homocystinuria due to cystathionine synthase (CS) deficiency: Investigations in cultured long-term lymphocytes, fetal skin fibroblasts and amniotic fluid cells. *Pediatr Res* 8:388, 1974

170. GAULL GE, GAITONDE MK: Homocystinuria: An observation on the inheritance of cystathionine synthase deficiency. *J Med Genet* 3:194, 1966

171. BRENTON DP, CUSWORTH DC, GAULL GE: Homocystinuria: Biochemical studies of tissues including a comparison with cystathioninuria. *Pediatrics* 35:50, 1965

172. MUDD SH, UHLENDORF BW, HINDS KR, LEVY HL: Deranged B₁₂ metabolism: Studies of fibroblasts grown in tissue culture. *Biochem Med* 4:215, 1970

173. MUDD SH, UHLENDORF BW, FREEMAN JM, FINKELSTEIN JD, SHIH VE: Homocystinuria associated with decreased methylenetetrahydrofolate reductase activity. *Biochem Biophys Res Commun* 46:905, 1972

174. SEASHORE MR, DURANT JL, ROSENBERG LE: Studies of the mechanism of pyridoxine-responsive homocystinuria. *Pediatr Res* 6:187, 1972

175. KIM YJ, ROSENBERG LE: On the mechanism of pyridoxine responsive homocystinuria. II. Properties of normal and mutant cystathionine β-synthase from cultured fibroblasts. *Proc Natl Acad Sci USA* 71:4821, 1974

176. LIPSON MH, KRAUS J, ROSENBERG LE: Affinity of cystathionine β-synthase for pyridoxal 5'-phosphate in cultured cells. *J Clin Invest* 66:188, 1980

177. GRIFFITHS R, TUDBALL N: Studies on the use of skin fibroblasts for the measurement of cystathionine synthase activity with respect to homocystinuria. *Clin Chim Acta* 73:157, 1976

178. ANDLAUER A-C, DAVID M, FEIT J-P, MACABEO V, VIBERT J, COLLOMBEL C, ROLLAND M-O, JEUNE M: Homocystinurie et insuffisance respiratoire chronique: A propos d'une observation. *Pediatrie* 33:669, 1978

179. McKUSICK VA, HALL JG, CHAR F: The clinical and genetic characteristics of homocystinuria, in Carson NAJ, Raine DN (eds): *Inherited Disorders of Sulphur Metabolism.* London, Churchill Livingstone, Ltd, 1971, p 179

180. McKUSICK VA: *Heritable Disorders of Connective Tissue,* ed 4. St Louis, CV Mosby Co, 1972, p 224

181. FLEISHER LD, TALLAN HH, BERATIS NG, HIRSHHORN K, GAULL GE: Cystathionine synthase deficiency: Heterozygote detection using cultured skin fibroblasts. *Biochem Biophys Res Commun,* 55:38, 1973

182. BRENTON DP, CUSWORTH DC, GAULL GE: Homocystinuria: Metabolic studies on 3 patients. *J Pediatr* 67:58, 1965

183. WERDER EA, CURTIUS H-CH, TANCREDI F, ANDERS PW, PRADER A: Homocystinurie. *Helv Paediat Acta* 21:1, 1966

184. PERRY TL, HANSEN S, MacDOUGALL L, WARRINGTON PD: Sulfur-containing amino acids in the plasma and urine of homocystinurics. *Clin Chim Acta* 15:409, 1967

185. JOCELYN PC: Glutathione metabolism in animals, in Crook EM (ed): *Glutathione.* Cambridge, Cambridge University Press, 1959, p 43

186. RACKER E: Glutathione-homocystine transhydrogenase. *J Biol Chem* 217:867, 1955

187. CARSON NAJ, DENT CE, FIELD CMB, GAULL GE: Homocystinuria: Clinical and pathological review of ten cases. *J Pediatr* 66:565, 1965

188. KENNEDY C, SHIH VE, ROWLAND LP: Homocystinuria: A report in two siblings. *Pediatrics* 36:736, 1965

189. WHITE, HH, ROWLAND LP, ARAKI S, THOMPSON HL, COWEN D: Homocystinuria. *Arch Neurol* 13:455, 1965

190. TADA K, YOSHIDA T, HIRONO H, ARAKAWA, T: Homocystinuria: Amino acid pattern of the liver. *Tohoku J Exp Med* 92:325, 1967

191. CURTIUS H-CH, MARTENET AC, ANDERS PW: Bestimmung von freien Aminosauren im Augenkammerwasser des Menschen bei Homocystinurie-patienten und Kontrollfallen. *Clin Chim Acta* 19:469, 1968

192. MUDD SH, EDWARDS WA: Unpublished results

193. RASSIN DK, LONGHI RC, GAULL GE: Free amino acids in liver of patients with homocystinuria due to cystathionine synthase deficiency: Effects of vitamin B₆. *J Pediatr* 91:574, 1977

194. TADA K, YOSHIDA T, ARAKAWA T: Free amino acid pattern in the liver from the patients with amino acid disorders: Postmortem diagnosis of inborn errors of amino acid metabolism. *Tohoku J Exp Med* 101:223, 1970

195. GERRITSEN T, WAISMAN HA: Homocystinuria: Absence of cystathionine in the brain. *Science* 145:588, 1964
196. BARBER GW, SPAETH GL: The successful treatment of homocystinuria with pyridoxine. *J Pediatr* 75:463, 1969
197. SHIH VE, MANDELL R, LEVY HL, LITTLEFIELD JW: Free amino acids in extracts of cultured skin fibroblasts from patients with various amino acid metabolic disorders. *Clin Genet* 7:421, 1975
198. LEVY HL, SHIH VE, MACCREADY RA: Screening for homocystinuria in the newborn and mentally retarded population, in Carson NAJ, Raine DN (eds): *Inherited Disorders of Sulphur Metabolism.* London, Churchill Livingstone, Ltd, 1971, p 235
199. SHIH VE, EFRON ML: Pyridoxine-unresponsive homocystinuria. *N Engl J Med* 283:1206, 1970
200. GROBE H: Homocystinurie: Klinisches Bild, Behandlung und Ergebnisse bei acht Patienten. *Dtsh Med Wochenschr* 98:1313, 1973
201. RAO BSSR, NARAYANAN HS, REDDY GNN: Homocystinuria in three Indian children. *Indian J Med Res* 59:569, 1971
202. PERRY TL: Homocystinuria, in Nyhan WL (ed): *Heritable Disorders of Amino Acid Metabolism.* New York, John Wiley & Sons, Inc, 1974, p 395
203. CAREY MC, FENNELLY JJ, FITZGERALD O: Homocystinuria. II. Subnormal serum folate levels, increased folate clearance and effects of folic acid therapy. *Am J Med* 45:26, 1968
204. MORROW G, III, BARNESS LA: Combined vitamin responsiveness in homocystinuria. *J Pediatr* 81:946, 1972
204a. PERRY TL, HANSEN S: Cystinylglycine in plasma: Diagnostic relevance for pyroglutamic acidemia, homocystinuria, and phenylketonuria. *Clin Chim Acta,* in press
205. TALLAN HH, MOORE S, STEIN WH: L-Cystathionine in human brain. *J Biol Chem* 230:707, 1958
206. OKUMURA N, OTSUKI S, KAMEYAMA A: Studies on free amino acids in human brain. *J Biochem* 47:315, 1960
207. PERRY TL, HANSEN S, LOVE DL, CRAWFORD LE, TISCHLER B: Treatment of homocystinuria with a low-methionine diet, supplemental cystine, and a methyl donor. *Lancet* 2:474, 1968
208. SARDHARWALLA IB, JACKSON SH, HAWKE HD, SASS-KORTSAK A: Homocystinuria: A study with low-methionine diet in three patients. *Can Med Assoc J* 99:731, 1968
209. BRENTON DP, CUSWORTH DC: Homocystinuria: Metabolism of [³⁵S]methionine. *Clin Sci* 31:197, 1966
210. BRENTON DP, CUSWORTH DC, DENT CE, JONES EE: Homocystinuria: Clinical and dietary studies. *Q J Med* 35:325, 1966
211. LASTER L, MUDD SH, FINKELSTEIN JD, IRREVERRE F: Homocystinuria due to cystathionine synthase deficiency: The metabolism of L-methionine. *J Clin Invest* 44:1708, 1965
212. MUDD SH: Homocystinuria: The known causes, in Carson NAJ, Raine DN (eds): *Inherited Disorders of Sulphur Metabolism.* London, Churchill Livingstone, Ltd, 1971, p 204
213. BARBER GW, SPAETH GL: Pyridoxine therapy in homocystinuria. *Lancet* 1:337, 1967
214. BERIO A: Considerazioni su di un nuovo caso di omocistinuria identificato con il metodo di Scriver e coll. *Minerva Pediatr* 29:2381, 1977
215. BERIO A, CAVALLO V, COTTAFAVA C, DI STEFANO A, DRAGO G, CAMOZZI C, CAPINERI A: Su di un caso di omocistinuria individuato con i metodi di depistaggio. *Minerva Pediatr* 29:2479, 1977
216. KOSSOWICZ H: Surgical treatment of dislocated lenses in homocystinuria. *Metab Ophthalmol* 1:121, 1977
217. SHULMAN D: Homocystinuria in two South African Negro siblings. *S Afr Med J* 52:127, 1977
218. ALMGREN B, ERIKSSON I, HEMMINGSSON A, HILLERDAL G, LARSSON E, ABERG H: Abdominal aortic aneurysm in homocystinuria. *Acta Chir Scand* 144:545, 1978
219. GROBE H: Homocystinuria and oral contraceptives. *Lancet* 1:158, 1978
220. VANDRESSE, JH, DE SAINT HUBERT E, EVRARD P: Homocystinuria and carotid arteriography. *Neuroradiology* 17:57, 1978
221. WILCKEN B, TURNER G: Homocystinuria in New South Wales. *Arch Dis Child* 53:242, 1978
222. AGARWAL MB, MEHTA BC: Homocystinuria and response to pyridoxine. *Indian Pediatr* 16:1049, 1979
223. BARASHNEV YI, GOLIKOVA TM, SEMYACHKINA AN, BARYSHNIKOVA SS, GUSEVA NK: Cerebral disturbances in homocystinuria. *Vopr Okhr Materin Det* 24:35, 1979
224. FROST PM: Anaesthesia and homocystinuria. *Anaesthesia* 35:918, 1980
225. FUKS AB, KAUFMAN E, GALILI D, GARFUNKEL A: Comprehensive dental treatment under general anesthesia for patients with homocystinuria. *J Dent Child* 47:340, 1980
226. VALLE D, PAI GS, THOMAS GH, PYERITZ RE: Homocystinuria due to cystathionine β-synthase deficiency: Clinical manifestations and therapy. *Johns Hopkins Med J* 146:110, 1980
227. JOHNSTON SS: Homocystinuria. *Ophthalmologica* 176:282, 1978
228. PULLON DHH: Homocystinuria and other methioninemias, in Bickel H,

Guthrie R, Hammersen G (eds): *Neonatal Screening for Inborn Errors of Metabolism.* Berlin, Springer Verlag, 1980, p 29
229. SCHEDEWIE HK, LIPINSKI C, SCHMIDT H: Elevated growth hormone levels in untreated homocystinuria: Mechanism of tall stature? *Clin Res* 25:69A, 1977
230. SAITO S, TAMAI Y, MATSUSHITA M: Lipid composition of brain in a patient with mental retardation due to encephalopathy in an infantile period and one due to homocystinuria. *Jpn J Exp Med* 49:257, 1979
231. THOMAS PS, CARSON NAJ: Homocystinuria: The evolution of skeletal changes in relation to treatment. *Ann Radiol* 21:95, 1978
232. CARSON NAJ, CARRE IJ: Treatment of homocystinuria with pyridoxine: A preliminary study. *Arch Dis Child* 44:387, 1969
233. WILCKEN B, TURNER B: Homocystinuria: Reduced folate levels during pyridoxine treatment. *Arch Dis Child* 48:58, 1973
234. BRENTON DP, CUSWORTH DC: The response of patients with cystathionine synthase deficiency to pyridoxine, in Carson NAJ, Raine DN (eds): *Inherited Disorders of Sulphur Metabolism.* London, Churchill Livingstone, Ltd, 1971, p 264
235. SCHMIDT H, LUTZ P, KRAUS-MACKIW E: Course studies in homocystinuria cases. *Metab Ophthalmol* 1:189, 1977
236. KURCZYNSKI TW, MUIR WA, FLEISHER LD, PALOMAKI JF, GAULL GE, RASSIN DK, ABRAMOWSKY C: Maternal homocystinuria: Studies of an untreated mother and fetus. *Arch Dis Child* 55:721, 1980
237. MUDD, SH: Diseases of sulphur metabolism: Implications for the methionine-homocysteine cycle, and vitamin responsiveness, in *Sulphur in Biology,* Ciba Foundation Symposium. New York, Elsevier North-Holland Biomedical Press, 1980, vol 72 (new series), p 239
238. MUDD SH: Vitamin-responsive genetic abnormalities. *Adv Nutri Res* 1981, in press
239. MUDD SH, HAVLIK R, LEVY HL, McKUSICK VA, FEINLEIB M: A study of cardiovascular risk in heterozygotes for homocystinuria. *Am J Human Genet,* in press
240. CUSWORTH DC, DENT CE: Homocystinuria. *Br Med Bull* 25:42, 1969
241. FRANCOIS J: Homocystinuria, in Winkelman JE, Crone RA (eds): *Perspectives in Ophthalmology.* Amsterdam, Excerpta Medica, 1970, vol 2, p 81
242. FRANCOIS J: Ocular manifestations in aminoacidopathies. *Adv Ophthalmol* 25:28, 1972
243. RAMSEY MS, DAITZ LD, BEATON JW: Lens fringe in homocystinuria. *Arch Ophthalmol* 93:318, 1975
244. WALTON D: Personal communication, 1975
245. RAMSEY MS, DICKSON DH: Lens fringes in homocystinuria. *Br J Ophthalmol* 59:338, 1975
246. LIEBERMAN TW, PODOS SM, HARTSTEIN J: Acute glaucoma, ectopia lentis and homocystinuria. *Am J Ophthalmol* 61:252, 1966
247. THOMAS RP, HOLLOWELL JG, PETERS HJ, CORYELL ME, LESTER RH: Homocystinuria and ectopia lentis in Negro family *JAMA* 198:560, 1966
248. ELKINGTON AR, FREEDMAN SS, JAY B, WRIGHT P: Anterior dislocation of the lens in homocystinuria. *Br J Ophthalmol* 57:235, 1973
249. TUCHINDA C, BEDAVANIJA A, MEKANANDHA V: Homocystinuria: The first report in Thailand. *J Med Assoc Thailand* 56:541, 1973
250. GAULL GE, CARSON NAJ, DENT CE, FIELD CMB: Homocystinuria: Clinical and pathological description of 10 cases, in Oster J (ed): *Proceedings of the International Copenhagen Congress on the Scientific Study of Mental Retardation.* Copenhagen, 1964, vol 1, p 91
251. SCHIMKE RN, McKUSICK VA, HUANG T, POLLACK AD: Homocystinuria. *JAMA* 193:711, 1965
252. SPAETH GL, BARBER GW: Homocystinuria—its ocular manifestations. *J Pediatr Ophthalmol* 3:42, 1966
253. WILSON RS, RUIZ RS: Bilateral central retinal artery occlusion in homocystinuria. *Arch Ophthalmol* 82:267, 1969
254. SCHULMAN JD: Personal communication, 1975
255. GAUDIER B, FRANCOIS P, BISERTE G, DAUTREVAUX M, NUYTS J-P, BOMBART E: L'Homocystinurie: A propos de trois observations. *Arch Fr Pediatr* 25:541, 1968
256. MORREELS CL JR, FLETCHER BD, WEILBAECHER RG, DORST JP: The roentgenographic features of homocystinuria. *Radiology* 90:1150, 1968
257. BRILL PW, MITTY HA, GAULL GE: Homocystinuria due to cystathionine synthase deficiency: Clinical-roentgenologic correlations. *Am J Roentgenol Radium Ther Nucl Med* 121:45, 1974
258. SMITH SW: Roentgen findings in homocystinuria. *Am J Roentgenol Radium Ther Nucl Med* 100:147, 1967
259. SCHEDEWIE H, WILLICH E, GROBE H, SCHMIDT H, MULLER KM: Skeletal findings in homocystinuria: A collaborative study. *Pediatr Radiol* 1:12, 1973
260. BRENTON DP, DOW CJ, JAMES JIP, HAY RL, WYNNE-DAVIES R: Homocystinuria and Marfan's syndrome: A comparison. *J Bone Joint Surg* 54B:277, 1972
261. WESTERMAN MP, GREENFIELD GB, WONG PWK: "Fish vertebrae," homocystinuria, and sickle cell anemia. *JAMA* 230:261, 1974

261a. MacCarthy JMT, Carey MC: Bone changes in homocystinuria. *Clin Radiol* 19:128, 1968

262. Sinclair RJG, Kitchin AH, Turner RWD: The Marfan syndrome. *Q J Med* 29:19, 1960

263. Gfeller J, Budliger H: Homocystinuria and os lunatum. *Lancet* 2:548, 1966

264. Arnott EJ, Greaves DP: Ocular involvement in homocystinuria. *Br J Ophthalmol* 48:688, 1964

265. Turner G, Dey J, Turner B: Homocystinuria: A report of two Australian families. *Aust Pediatr J* 3:48, 1967

266. Beals RK: Homocystinuria: A report of two cases and review of the literature. *J Bone Joint Surg* 51A:1564, 1969

267. Komrower GM, Wilson VK: Homocystinuria. *Proc R Soc Med* 56:996, 1963

268. Garston JB, Gordon RR, Hart CT, Pollitt RJ: An unusual case of homocystinuria. *Br J Ophthalmol* 54:248, 1970

269. Brett EM: Homocystinuria with epilepsy. *Proc R Soc Med* 59:484, 1966

270. Hurwitz LJ, Chopra JS, Carson NAJ: Electromyographic evidence of a muscle lesion in homocystinuria. *Acta Paediatr Scand* 57:401, 1968

271. Verma JC, Sinclair S: Homocystinuria: Report of two cases in siblings. *Indian J Pediatr* 37:263, 1970

272. Holmgren G, Hambraeus L, Lestrup E, Tangen O: The effect of pyridoxine on platelet adhesiveness in homocystinuria. *Neuropadiatrie* 5:402, 1974

273. Dunn HG, Perry TL, Dolman CL: Homocystinuria. *Neurology* 16:407, 1966

274. Carey MC, Donovan DE, Fitzgerald O, McAuley FD: Homocystinuria, I. A clinical and pathological study of nine subjects in six families. *Am J Med* 45:7, 1968

275. Hagberg B, Hambraeus L: Some aspects of the diagnosis and treatment of homocystinuria. *Dev Med Child Neurol* 10:479, 1968

276. Hopkins I, Townley RRW, Shipman RT: Cerebral thrombosis in a patient with homocystinuria. *J Pediatr* 75:1082, 1969

277. Verma IC, Sud N, Manerikar S: Homocystinuria: Report of two cases in siblings. *Indian Pediatr* 11:753, 1974

278. Kang ES, Byers RK, Gerald PS: Homocystinuria: Response to pyridoxine. *Neurology* 20:503, 1970

279. Gaull GE, Schaffner F: Electron microscopic changes in hepatocytes of patients with homocystinuria. *Pediatr Res* 5:23, 1971

280. Kaeser AC, Rodnight R, Ellis BA: Psychiatric and biochemical aspects of a case of homocystinuria. *J Neurol Neurosurg Psychiatry* 32:88, 1969

281. Shih VE: Personal communication

282. Spiro HR, Schimke RN, Welch JP: Schizophrenia in a patient with a defect in methionine metabolism. *J Nerv Ment Dis* 141:285, 1965

283. Price J, Vickers CFH, Brooker BK: A case of homocystinuria with noteworthy dermatological features. *J Ment Defic Res* 12:111, 1968

284. Rahman M: Homocystinuria: Review of four cases. *Br J Ophthalmol* 55:338, 1971

285. Holmgren G, Falkmer S, Hambraeus L: Plasma insulin content and glucose tolerance in homocystinuria. *Upsala J Med Sci* 78:215, 1973

286. Lamon JM, Lenke RR, Levy HL, Schulman JD, Shih VE: Selected metabolic disease, in Schulman JD, Simpson JL (eds): *Selected Metabolic Diseases*. New York, Academic Press, Inc, 1981, p 1

287. Brenton DP, Cusworth DC, Biddle SA, Garrod PJ, Lasley L: Pregnancy and homocystinuria. *Ann Clin Biochem* 14:161, 1977

288. Schulman JD, Mudd SH, Shulman NR, Landvater L: Pregnancy and thrombophlebitis in homocystinuria. *Blood* 56:326, 1980

289. Van Sprang FJ: General discussion on the treatment of homocystinuria, in Carson NAJ, Raine DN (eds): *Inherited Disorders of Sulphur Metabolism*. London, Churchill Livingstone, Ltd, 1971, p 303

290. Hilden M, Brandt NJ, Nilsson IM, Schonheyder F: Investigations of coagulation and fibrinolysis in homocystinuria. *Acta Med Scand* 195:533, 1974

291. Ritchie JWK, Carson NAJ: Pregnancy and homocystinuria. *J Obstet Gynaecol Br Commonw* 80:664, 1973

292. Levy HL, Shih VE: Unpublished observations

293. Gaull GE: Personal communication, 1975

294. Chase HP, Goodman SI, O'Brien D: Treatment of homocystinuria. *Arch Dis Child* 42:514, 1967

295. Wilcken B, Turner B, Brown DA: Detection of abnormal sulphur-containing amino acid excretion in a mass urine-screening programme. *Med J Aust* 1:1193, 1972

296. Henkind P, Ashton N: Ocular pathology in homocystinuria. *Trans Ophthalmol Soc UK* 85:21, 1965

297. Ramsey MS, Yanoff M, Fine BS: The ocular histopathology of homocystinuria: A light and electron microscopic study. *Am J Ophthalmol* 74:377, 1972

298. Martenet AC, Witmer R, Speiser P: Alterations oculaires dans l'homocystinurie. *Ophthalmologica* 154:318, 1967

299. Gibson JB, Carson NAJ, Neill DW: Pathological findings in homocystinuria. *J Clin Pathol* 17:427, 1964

300. Chou S-M, Waisman HA: Spongy degeneration of the central nervous system: Case of homocystinuria. *Arch Pathol* 79:357, 1965

301. Waisman HA, Gerritsen T: Homocystinuria: A metabolic defect associated with mental retardation, in Oster J (ed): *Proceedings of the International Copenhagen Congress on the Scientific Study of Mental Retardation*. Copenhagen, 1964, vol 1, p 507

302. Gaull GE: Homocystinuria. *Adv Teratol* 2:101, 1967

302a. Meynadier J, Guilhou JJ, Thorel M, Barneon G: Homocystinurie. Etude histologique et ultrastructurale. *Dermatologica* (Basel) 163:34, 1981

303. Brown JH, Allison JB: Effects of excess dietary dl-methionine and/or l-arginine on rats. *Proc Soc Exp Biol Med* 69:196, 1948

304. Cohen HP, Choitz HC, Berg CP: Response of rats to diets high in methionine and related compounds. *J Nutr* 64:555, 1958

305. McDonald L, Bray C, Field C, Love F, Davies B: Homocystinuria, thrombosis, and the blood-platelets. *Lancet* 1:745, 1964

306. Wright HP: The adhesiveness of blood platelets in normal subjects with varying concentrations of anti-coagulants. *J Pathol Bacteriol* 53:255, 1941

307. Bray CL: Discussion, in Brett EM: Homocystinuria with epilepsy. *Proc R Soc Med* 59:484, 1966

308. Hellem AJ: The adhesiveness of human blood platelets *in vitro*. *Scand J Clin Lab Invest* 12: (suppl) 51, 1, 1960

309. Harker LA, Slichter SJ, Scott CR, Ross R: Homocystinemia: Vascular injury and arterial thrombosis. *N Engl J Med* 291:537, 1974

310. Efron ML: In discussion of GE Gaull, The pathogenesis of homocystinuria. *Am J Dis Child* 113:103, 1967

311. Cline JW, Goyer RA, Lipton J, Mason RG: Adult homocystinuria with ectopia lentis. *South Med J* 64:613, 1971

312. Grobe H, von Bassewitz DB: Thromboembolische Komplikationen und Thrombocytenanomalien bei Homocystinurie. *Z Kinderheilkd* 112:309, 1972

313. Grobe H, Balleisen L, Stahl K: Platelet function and morphology in homocystinuria. *Pediatr Res* 13:72, 1979

314. Uhlemann ER, TenPas JH, Lucky AW, Schulman JD, Mudd SH, Shulman NR: Platelet survival and morphology in homocystinuria due to cystathionine synthase deficiency. *N Engl J Med* 295:1283, 1976

315. Zweifler AJ, Allen RJ: An intrinsic blood platelet abnormality in an homocystinuric boy, corrected by pyridoxine administration. *Thromb Diath Haemorrh* 26:15, 1971

316. Hampton JR, Mitchell JRA: A transferable factor causing abnormal platelet behaviour in vascular disease. *Lancet* 2:764, 1966

317. Ratnoff OD: Activation of Hageman factor by L-homocystine. *Science* 162:1007, 1968

318. McCully KS: Vascular pathology of homocysteinemia: Implications for the pathogenesis of arteriosclerosis. *Am J Pathol* 56:111, 1969

319. Kanwar YS, Manaligod JR, Wong PWK: Morphologic studies in a patient with homocystinuria due to 5,10-methylenetetrahydrofolate reductase deficiency. *Pediatr Res* 10:598, 1976

320. Baumgartner R, Wick H, Ohnacker H, Probst A, Maurer R: Vascular lesions in two patients with congenital homocystinuria due to different defects of remethylation. *J Inher Metab Dis* 3:101, 1980

321. Baumgartner ER, Wick H, Maurer R, Egli N, Steinmann B: Congenital defect in intracellular cobalamin metabolism resulting in homocystinuria and methylmalonic aciduria. I. Case report and histopathology. *Helv Paediatr Acta* 34:465, 1979

322. Dillon MJ, England JM, Gompertz D, Goodey PA, Grant DB, Hassein HA-A, Linnell JC, Matthews DM, Mudd SH, Newns GH, Seakins JWT, Uhlendorf BW, Wise IJ: Mental retardation, megaloblastic anaemia, methylmalonic aciduria, and abnormal homocysteine metabolism due to an error in B₁₂ metabolism. *Clin Sci Molec Med* 47:43, 1974

323. Dayan AD, Ramsey RB: An inborn error of vitamin B₁₂ metabolism associated with cellular deficiency of coenzyme forms of the vitamin: Pathological and neurochemical findings in one case. *J Neurol Sci* 23:117, 1974

324. Dayan AD: Personal communication, 1975

325. McCully KS, Ragsdale BD: Production of arteriosclerosis by homocysteinemia. *Am J Pathol* 61:1, 1970

326. Donahue S, Sturman JA, Gaull GE: Arteriosclerosis due to homocyst(e)inemia: Failure to reproduce the model in weanling rabbits. *Am J Pathol* 77:167, 1974

327. Krishnaswamy K, Rao SB: Failure to produce atherosclerosis in *Macaca radiata* on a high-methionine, high-fat, pyridoxine-deficient diet. *Atherosclerosis* 27:253, 1977

328. Harker LA, Ross R, Slichter SJ, Scott CR: Homocystine-induced arteriosclerosis: The role of endothelial cell injury and platelet response in its genesis. *J Clin Invest* 58:731, 1976

329. Hladovec J: Experimental homocystinemia, endothelial lesions and thrombosis. *Blood Vessels* 16:202, 1979

330. WALL RT, HARLAN JM, HARKER LA, STRIKER GE: Homocysteine-induced endothelial cell injury *in vitro:* A model for the study of vascular injury. *Thromb Res* 18:113, 1980

331. WEIMANN BJ, KUHN H, BAUMGARTNER HR: Effect of homocysteine (Ho) on cultured bovine (BEC) and human (HEC) endothelial cells. *Experientia (Basel)* 36:762, 1980

332. HARKER LA, SCOTT CR: Platelets in homocystinuria. *N Engl J Med* 296:818, 1977

333. WILCKEN DEL, WILCKEN B: The pathogenesis of coronary artery disease: A possible role for methionine metabolism. *J Clin Invest* 57:1079, 1976

334. SARDHARWALLA IB, FOWLER B, ROBINS AJ, KOMROWER GM: Detection of heterozygotes for homocystinuria: Study of sulphur-containing amino acids in plasma and urine after L-methionine loading. *Arch Dis Child* 49:553, 1974

335. TRAUB W, PIEZ KA: The chemistry and structure of collagen. *Adv Protein Chem* 25:243, 1971

336. GRANT ME, PROCKOP DJ: The biosynthesis of collagen: Third of three parts. *N Engl J Med* 286:291, 1972

337. GALLOP PM, BLUMENFELD OO, SEIFTER S: Structure and metabolism of connective tissue proteins. *Ann Rev Biochem* 41:617, 1972.

338. TANZER ML: Cross-linking of collagen. *Science* 180:561, 1973

339. GALLOP PM, PAZ MA: Posttranslational protein modifications, with special attention to collagen and elastin. *Physiol Rev* 55:418, 1975

340. SIEGEL RC: Lysyl oxidase. *Int Rev Connect Tissue Res* 8:73, 1979

341. McKUSICK VA: *Heritable Disorders of Connective Tissue,* ed 3. St Louis, CV Mosby Co, 1966, p 150

342. HARRIS ED JR, SJOERDSMA A: Collagen profile in various clinical conditions. *Lancet* 2:707, 1966

343. HARRIS ED JR, SJOERDSMA A: Effect of penicillamine on human collagen and its possible application to treatment of scleroderma. *Lancet* 2:996, 1966

344. KANG AH, TRELSTAD RL: A collagen defect in homocystinuria. *J Clin Invest* 52:2571, 1973

345. BARASHNEV YI, SEMYACHKINA AN: The status of connective tissue in homocystinuria. *Vop Med Khim* 25:238, 1979

346. McKUSICK VA: *Heritable Disorders of Connective Tissue,* ed 4. St Louis, CV Mosby Co, 1972, p 61

347. JACKSON SH: The reaction of homocysteine with aldehyde: An explanation of the collagen defects in homocystinuria. *Clin Chim Acta* 45:215, 1973

348. SIEGEL RC: Collagen cross-linking: Effect of D-penicillamine on cross-linking *in vitro. J Biol Chem* 252:254, 1977

349. LINDBERG KA, HASSETT A, PINNELL SR: Inhibition of lysyl oxidase by homocysteine: A proposed connective tissue defect in homocystinuria. *J Clin Res* 24:265A, 1976

350. SIEGEL RC: The connective tissue defect in homocystinuria (HS). *Clin Res* 23:263a, 1975

351. SIEGEL RC: The connective tissue defect in homocystinuria (HS). *Arthritis Rheum* 18:425, 1975

352. GRIFFITHS R, TUDBALL N, THOMAS J: Effect of induced elevated plasma levels of homocystine and methionine in rats on collagen and elastin structures. *Connect Tissue Res* 4:101, 1976

353. PONSETI IV, SHEPARD RS: Lesions of the skeleton and other mesodermal tissues in rats fed sweet-pea (*Lathyrus odoratus*) seeds. *J Bone Joint Surg* 36A:1031, 1954

354. SELYE H: Lathyrism. *Rev Can Biol* 16:1, 1957

354a. RIVARD GE, LAZERSON J, IZADI P, KIM YJ: Collagen in homocystinuria. *N Engl J Med* 291:1364, 1974

355. PIRIE A, VAN HEYNINGEN R: *Biochemistry of the Eye.* Springfield, Ill, Charles C Thomas, Publisher, 1956, pp 251–252

356. BUDDECKE E, WOLLENSAK J: Zur Biochemie der Zonulafaser des Rinderauges. *Z Naturforsch* 21B:337, 1965

357. WOLLENSAK J: Zonula Zinnii. *Fortschr Augenheilkd* 16:240, 1965.

358. BARBER GW: Personal communication, 1975

359. IRREVERRE F, MUDD SH, HEIZER WD, LASTER L: Sulfite oxidase deficiency: Studies of a patient with mental retardation, dislocated ocular lenses, and abnormal urinary excretion of *S*-sulfo-L-cysteine, sulfite, and thiosulfate. *Biochem Med* 1:187, 1967

360. SHIH VE, ABROMS IF, JOHNSON JL, CARNEY M, MANDELL R, ROBB RM, CLOHERTY JP, RAJAGOPALAN KV: Sulfite oxidase deficiency: Biochemical and clinical investigations of a hereditary metabolic disorder in sulfur metabolism. *N Engl J Med* 297:1022, 1977

361. VAN DER HEIDEN C, BEEMER FA, BRINK W, WADMAN SK, DURAN M: Simultaneous occurrence of xanthine oxidase and sulfite oxidase deficiency: A molybdenum dependent inborn error of metabolism? *Clin Biochem* 12:206, 1979

362. JOHNSON JL, WAUD WR, RAJAGOPALAN KV, DURAN M, BEEMER FA, WADMAN SK: Inborn errors of molybdenum metabolism: Combined deficiencies of sulfite oxidase and xanthine dehydrogenase in a patient lacking the molybdenum cofactor. *Proc Natl Acad Sci USA* 77:3715, 1980

363. BEEMER FA, DELLEMAN JW: Combined deficiency of xanthine oxidase and sulfite oxidase; ophthalmological findings in a 3-week-old girl. *Metab Pediatr Ophthalmol* 4:49, 1980

364. TUDBALL N, BEAUMONT A: Studies on the neurochemical properties of cystathionine. *Biochim Biophys Acta* 588:285, 1979

365. SPRINCE H, PARKER CM, JOSEPHS JA JR: Homocysteine-induced convulsions in the rat: Protection by homoserine, serine, betaine, glycine and glucose. *Agents Actions* 1:9, 1969

366. SPRINCE H, PARKER CM, JOSEPHS JA JR, MAGAZINO J: Convulsant activity of homocysteine and other short-chain mercaptoacids: Protection therefrom. *Ann NY Acad Sci* 166:323, 1969

367. BLENNOW G, FOLBERGROVA J, NILSSON B, SIESJO BK: Cerebral metabolic and circulatory changes in the rat during sustained seizures induced by DL-homocysteine. *Brain Res* 179:129, 1979

368. FOLBERGROVA J: Energy metabolism of mouse cerebral cortex during homocysteine convulsions. *Brain Res* 81:443, 1974

369. REINGOLD DF, ORLOWSKI M: Inhibition of human and mouse brain glutamate decarboxylase by the α-keto analogs of cysteine and homocysteine. *Chem Pharmacol* 27:2567, 1978

370. DEWHURST I, GRIFFITHS R: Inhibition of glutamate decarboxylase by homocysteine: The reason for convulsive episodes in cystathionine synthase deficiency? in *International Symposium on Inborn Errors of Metabolism in Humans,* Switzerland, 1980, p 14

371. TUDBALL N, GRIFFITHS R: Biochemical changes in the brain of experimental animals in response to elevated plasma homocystine and methionine. *J Neurochem* 26:1149, 1976

372. FONLUPT P, ROCHE M, CRONENBERGER L, PACHECO H: La *S*-adenosyl-L-homocysteine: 1. Inductrice de sommeil. *Can J Physiol Pharmacol* 58, 160, 1980

373. FONLUPT P, ROCHE M, ANDRE A-C, CRONENBERGER L, PACHECO H: La *S*-adenosyl-L-homocysteine: 2. Anticonvulsivante. *Can J Physiol Pharmacol* 58:493, 1980

374. FONLUPT P, REY C, PACHECO H: *In vitro* and *in vivo* binding of *S*-adenosyl-L-homocysteine to membranes from rat cerebral cortex. *J Neurochem* 36:165, 1981

375. ZIMMERMAN TP, SCHMITGES CJ, WOLBERG G, DEEPROSE RD, DUNCAN GS, CUATRECASAS P, ELION GB: Modulation of cyclic AMP metabolism by *S*-adenosylhomocysteine and *S*-3-deazaadenosylhomocysteine in mouse lymphocytes. *Proc Natl Acad Sci USA* 77:5639, 1980

376. KREDICH NM, HERSHFIELD MS: Perturbations in *S*-adenosyl-homocysteine and *S*-adenosyl-methionine metabolism: Effects on transmethylation. *Adv Enzyme Regul* 18:181, 1980

377. BRAND E, HARRIS MM, BILOON S: Cystinuria: The excretion of a cystine complex which decomposes in the urine with the liberation of free cystine. *J Biol Chem* 86:315, 1930

378. SPAETH GL, BARBER GW: Prevalence of homocystinuria among the mentally retarded: Evaluation of a specific screening test. *Pediatrics* 40:586, 1967

379. SHIH VE: *Laboratory Techniques for the Detection of Hereditary Metabolic Disorders.* Cleveland, CRC Press, Inc, 1973

380. EFRON ML: Two-way separation of amino acids and other ninhydrin-reacting substances by high-voltage electrophoresis followed by paper chromatography. *Biochem J* 72:691, 1959

381. MUDD SH, POOLE JR, SIGGERS DC: Unpublished observations

382. VALLE D: Personal communication, 1981

383. GUTHRIE R: Screening for "inborn errors of metabolism" in the newborn infant—a multiple test program. *Birth Defects Original Article Series* 4:92, 1968

384. Committee on Nutrition, Subcommittee on Amino Acid Modified Diets, American Academy of Pediatrics: Special diets for infants with inborn errors of amino acid metabolism. *Pediatrics* 57:783, 1976

385. CARSON NAJ: Personal communication, 1980

386. ACOSTA PB, ELSAS LJ II: *Dietary Management of Inherited Metabolic Disease: Phenylketonuria, Galactosemia, Tyrosinemia, Homocystinuria, Maple Syrup Urine Disease.* Atlanta, ACELMU Publishers, 1976, p 52

387. KANG S-S, WONG PWK, BECKER N: Protein-bound homocyst(e)ine in normal subjects and in patients with homocystinuria. *Pediatr Res* 13:1141, 1979

388. KOMROWER GM, SARDHARWALLA IB: The dietary treatment of homocystinuria, in Carson NAJ, Raine DN (eds): *Inherited Disorders of Sulphur Metabolism.* London, Churchill Livingstone, Ltd, 1971, p 254

389. CARSON NAJ: Homocystinuria: Trial treatment of a 5-year-old severely retarded child with a natural diet low in methionine. *Am J Dis Child* 113:95, 1967

390. PERRY TL: Treatment of homocystinuria with a low-methionine diet and supplemental L-cystine, in Carson NAJ, Raine DN (eds): *Inherited Disorders of Sulphur Metabolism.* London, Churchill Livingstone, Ltd, 1971, p 245

391. VAN SPRANG FJ, WADMAN SK: Treatment of homocystinuria, in Carson NAJ, Raine DN (eds): *Inherited Disorders of Sulphur Metabolism.* London, Churchill Livingstone, Ltd, 1971, p 275

392. GROBE H: Homocystinuria (cystathionine synthase deficiency): Results of treatment in late-diagnosed patients. *Eur J Pediatr* 135:199, 1980.

392a. BERIO A: Trattamento dietetico prolungato di un caso di omocistinuria. *Min Ped* 32:1167, 1980

393. PARKINSON MS: Therapeutic problems of adolescent homocystinuria. *Proc R Soc Med* 62:909, 1969

394. SCHULMAN JD: Approaches to the treatment of inborn errors of sulphur amino acid and peptide metabolism, in Papadatos CJ, Bartsocas CS (eds): *The Management of Genetic Disorders*. New York, Alan R Liss, Inc, 1979, p 201

395. GAULL GE, RASSIN DK, STURMAN JA: Pyridoxine-dependency in homocystinuria. *Lancet* 2:1302, 1968

396. SCHMIDT H, LUTZ P, KRAUS-MACKIW E: Course studies in homocystinuria cases. *Metab Ophthalmol* 1:189, 1977

396a. SMOLIN LA, BENEVENGA J, BERLOW S: The use of betaine for the treatment of homocystinuria. *J Pediatr* 99:467, 1981

397. WAISMAN HA: Some theoretical considerations in the treatment of homocystinuria. *Am J Dis Child* 113:101, 1967

398. WONG PWK, FRESCO R: Tissue cystathionine in mice treated with cysteine and homoserine. *Pediatr Res* 6:172, 1972

399. GAULL GE, WADA Y, SCHNEIDMAN K, RASSIN DK, TALLAN HH, STURMAN JA: Homocystinuria: Observations on the biosynthesis of cystathionine and homolanthionine. *Pediatr Res* 5:265, 1971

400. CUSWORTH DC, GATTEREAU A: Inhibition of renal tubular reabsorption of homocystine by lysine and arginine. *Lancet* 2:916, 1968

401. FALCHUK ZM, EDWARDS WA, LASTER L: Effects of alpha-amino-isobutyric acid on urinary excretion of homocystine in patients with homocystinuria. *Metabolism* 22:605, 1973

402. SCHULMAN JD, AGARWAL B, MUDD SH, SHULMAN NR: Pulmonary embolism in a homocystinuric patient during treatment with dipyridamole and acetylsalicylic acid. *N Engl J Med* 299:661, 1978

403. COFFEY VP, MOORE PT, MARTIN M: A survey of inborn errors of metabolism in Ireland 1965–1976. *J Ir Med Assoc* 70:132, 1977.

404. LEVY HL: Unpublished observations

405. SCHMIDT H, LUTZ P: Homocystinurie in Mitteleuropa. *Deut Mediz Wochenscht* 45:1737, 1971

406. JOHNSTON SS: Personal communication, 1978

407. LEVY HL: Genetic screening, in Harris H, Hirschhorn K (eds): *Advances in Human Genetics*. New York, Plenum Publishing Corp, 1973, vol 4, p 1

408. GUTHRIE R, BLOOM S: Personal communication, 1981

409. CAHALANE S: Personal communication, 1981

410. NARUSE H, KITAGAWA T, OVRA T, YAMASHITA F: Personal communication, 1981

411. BICKEL H, SANDER J, GRUTTNER P, MENNE F, WITZENHAUSEN R: Personal communication, 1981

412. SCHIMPFESSEL L: Personal communication, 1981

413. MURPHEY WB: Personal communication, 1981

414. KENNEDY R, STEVENSON J: Personal communication, 1981

415. THALHAMMER O: Personal communication, 1981

415a. ANTONOZZI I, DOMINICI R, ANDREOLI M, MONACO F: Neonatal screening in Italy for congenital hypothyroidism and metabolic disorders: Hyperphenylalaninemia, maple syrup urine disease and homocystinuria. *J Endocrinol Invest* 4:357, 1980

416. ALM J, LARSSON A: A follow up of a nationwide neonatal metabolic screening program in Sweden. *Pediatr Res* 13:79, 1979

417. SARDHARWALLA IB: Comment in Whiteman PD, Clayton BE, Ersser RS, Lilly P, Seakins JWT: Changing incidence of neonatal hypermethioninaemia: Implications for the detection of homocystinuria. *Arch Dis Child* 54:593, 1979

418. WHITEMAN PD, CLAYTON BE, ERSSER RS, LILLY P, SEAKINS JWT: Changing incidence of neonatal hypermethioninaemia: Implications for the detection of homocystinuria. *Arch Dis Child* 54:593, 1979

419. INFANT FORMULA PRODUCTS: *Nutrient Information*. Evansville, Ind. Mead Johnson and Co, 1979, p 4

420. ROSS LABORATORIES: *Product Handbook*. Columbus, Ohio, Ross Laboratories, 1977, p 46

421. LEVY HL, MADIGAN PM, SHIH VE: Massachusetts metabolic disorders screening program. I. Technics and results of urine screening. *Pediatrics* 49:825, 1972

422. WILCKEN B, SMITH A, BROWN DA: Urine screening for aminoacidopathies: Is it beneficial? *J Pediatr* 97:492, 1980

423. VOGEL F: Spontaneous mutation in man, in Vogel F, Rohrborn G (eds): *Chemical Mutagenesis in Mammals and Man*. New York, Springer-Verlag, 1970, p 16

424. WHITE HH, THOMPSON HL, ROWLAND LP, COWEN D, ARAKI S: Homocystinuria. *Trans Am Neurol Assoc* 89:24, 1964

425. MUDD SH: Discussion, in Carson NAJ, Raine DN (eds): *Inherited Disorders of Sulphur Metabolism*. London, Churchill Livingstone, Ltd, 1971, p 311

426. FLEISHER LD, LONGHI RC, TALLAN HH, BERATIS NG, HIRSCHHORN K, GAULL GE: Homocystinuria: Investigations of cystathionine synthase in cultured fetal cells and the prenatal determination of genetic status. *J Pediatr* 85:677, 1974

427. LEVY HL, EASTERDAY CL, MONTAG PP, LITTLEFIELD JW: Amino acids in amniotic fluid, in Dorfman A (ed): *Antenatal Diagnosis*. Chicago, University of Chicago Press, 1972, p 109

428. EMERY AEH, BURT D, NELSON MM, SCRIMGEOUR JB: Antenatal diagnosis and aminoacid composition of amniotic fluid. *Lancet* 1:1307, 1970

429. SAIFER A, A'ZARY E, VALENTI C, SCHNECK L: Quantitative cation-exchange chromatographic analysis of free amino acids in human amniotic fluid collected during early pregnancy. *Clin Chem* 16:891, 1970

430. O'NEILL RT, MORROW G III, HAMMEL D, AUERBACH VH, BARNES LA: Diagnostic significance of amniotic fluid amino acids. *Obstet Gynecol* 37:550, 1971

431. THOMAS GH, PARMLEY TH, STEVENSON RE, HOWELL RR: Developmental changes in amino acid concentrations in human amniotic fluid: Abnormal findings in maternal phenylketonuria. *Am J Obstet Gynecol* 111:38, 1971

432. REID DWJ, CAMPBELL DJ, YAKYMYSHYN LY: Quantitative amino acids in amniotic fluid and maternal plasma in early and late pregnancy. *Am J Obstet Gynecol* 111:251, 1971

433. SCOTT CR, TENG C, NELSON T: Free amino acids in human amniotic fluid during early pregnancy, in Dorfman A (ed): *Antenatal Diagnosis*. Chicago, University of Chicago Press, 1972, p 115

434. HARRIS H, PENROSE LS, THOMAS DHH: Cystathioninuria. *Ann Hum Genet* 23:442, 1959

435. FRIMPTER GW: Cystathioninuria: Nature of the defect. *Science* 149:1095, 1965

436. FINKELSTEIN JD, MUDD SH, IRREVERRE F, LASTER L: Deficiencies of cystathionase and homoserine dehydratase activities in cystathioninuria. *Proc Natl Acad Sci USA* 55:865, 1966

437. HOOFT C, CARTON D, DESCHRYVER F: Cystathioninemia in three siblings, in Allan JD, Holt KS, Ireland JT, Pollitt RJ (eds): *Enzymopenic Anaemias, Lysosomes and Other Papers*. London, Churchill Livingstone, Ltd, 1969, p 200

438. HOOFT C: Personal communication, 1975

439. PASCAL TA, GAULL GE, BERATIS NG, GILLAM BM, TALLAN HH, HIRSCHHORN K: Vitamin B$_6$-responsive and -unresponsive cystathioninuria: Two variant molecular forms. *Science* 190:1209, 1975

440. PASCAL TA, GAULL GE, BERATIS NG, GILLAM BM, TALLAN HH: Cystathionase deficiency: Evidence for genetic heterogeneity in primary cystathioninuria. *Pediatr Res* 12:125, 1978

441. PASCAL TA, BERATIS NG, TALLAN HH, GAULL GE: Cystathionase deficiency: The effect of cofactor on the stability of normal and abnormal enzyme from lymphoid cell lines. *Enzyme* 24:265, 1979

442. BITTLES AH, CARSON NAJ: Cystathionase deficiency in fibroblast cultures from a patient with primary cystathioninuria. *J Med Genet* 11:121, 1974

443. KINT JA, CARTON D: New evidence for the identity of homoserine deaminase and cystathionase in human liver. *Arch Int Physiol Biochem* 79:202, 1971

444. PASCAL TA, TALLAN HH, GILLAM BM: Hepatic cystathionase: Immunochemical and electrophoretic studies of the human and rat forms. *Biochim Biophys Acta* 285:48, 1972

445. ROISIN M-P, CHATAGNER F: Purification et etude de quelques proprietes de l'homocysteine desulfhydrase du foie de rat. Identification a la cystathionase. *Bull Soc Chim Biol* 51:481, 1969

446. FRIMPTER GW, HAYMOVITZ A, HORWITH M: Cystathioninuria. *N Engl J Med* 268:333, 1963

447. FRIMPTER GW: Cystathioninuria, in Stanbury JB, Wyngaarden JB, Fredrickson DS (eds): *The Metabolic Basis of Inherited Disease*, ed 2. New York, McGraw-Hill Book Co, 1966, p 409

448. MONGEAU J-G, HILGARTNER M, WORTHEN HG, FRIMPTER GW: Cystathioninuria: Study of an infant with normal mentality, thrombocytopenia, and renal calculi. *J Pediatr* 69:1113, 1966

449. BERLOW S: Studies in cystathioninemia. *Am J Dis Child* 112:135, 1966

450. STEINMANN B: Personal communication, 1981

451. FRIMPTER GW: Personal communication, 1981

452. HARAGUCHI H, IWATANI E, HIROSAWA M, YAMASHITA F, NAGAYAMA T: Studies on cystathioninuria. *Igakunoayumi (Jap)* 61:72, 1967

453. PERRY TL, ROBINSON GC, TEASDALE JM, HANSEN S: Concurrence of cystathioninuria, nephrogenic diabetes insipidus and severe anemia. *N Engl J Med* 276:721, 1967

454. PERRY TL, HARDWICK DF, HANSEN S, LOVE DL, ISRAELS S: Cystathioninuria in two healthy siblings. *N Engl J Med* 278:590, 1968

454a. PERRY TL: Personal communication, 1981

455. KODAMA H, YAO I, KOBAYASHI K, HIRAYAMA K, FUJII Y, MIZUHARA S, HARAGUCHI H, HIROSAWA M: New sulfur-containing amino acids in the urine of cystathioninuric patients. *Physiol Chem Phys* 1:72, 1969

456. NISHIKAWA M, ITO S, SANO K, NISHIOEDA Y, NASAKO Y, FUJISAWA T, MORI T, SEO K: A case of familial cystathioninuria with goiter and some anomalies. *Endocrinol Jap* 17:57, 1970

457. SCOTT CR, DASSELL SW, CLARK SH, CHIANG-TENG C, SWEDBERG KR: Cystathioninemia: A benign genetic condition. *J Pediatr* 76:571, 1970

458. FRIMPTER GW: Recurrent urinary tract calculi possibly due to inherited cystathioninuria. *Aerosp Med* 44:1300, 1973

459. LEVY HL, MUDD SH, MADIGAN PM: Pyridoxine-unresponsive cystathioninemia. *Pediatr Res* 7:162, 1973

460. AVRUSKIN TW, KANG ES: Cystathioninuria, mental retardation, and juvenile diabetes mellitus. *Am J Dis Child* 127:250, 1974

461. WADMAN SK, HEIDEN CVD, VAN SPRANG FJ, VOUTE PA: Primary cystathioninuria and cystathioninuria in patients with neurogenic turmors. Analytical results, in Carson NAJ, Raine DN (eds): *Inherited Disorders of Sulphur Metabolism.* London, Churchill Livingstone, Ltd, 1971, p 56

461a. WADMAN SK: Personal communication, 1981

462. BREMER HJ, ENDRES W: Primary cystathioninuria: Methionine load tests and response to pyridoxine. *Helv Paediatr Acta* 27:525, 1972

463. WILCKEN B: Personal communication, 1981

464. KODAMA H, IKEGAMI T, HIRAYAMA K, MIZUHARA S: Effect of pyridoxine treatment of a cystathioninuric patient on the urinary excretion of some unusual sulfur-containing amino acids. *Clin Chim Acta* 51:29, 1974

465. FERRANTE E, BRUNI L, GRIMALDI S: Rottura paracentromerica del braccio longo di un cromosoma 2 in una bambina di 9 mesi affetta da cistationuria, ritardo psicomotorio e cataratta. *Riv Clin Pediatr* 81:612, 1968

466. SCHNEIDERMAN LJ: Latent cystathioninuria. *J Med Genet* 4:260, 1967

467. PERRY TL, JONES RT: The amino acid content of human cerebrospinal fluid in normal individuals and in mental defectives. *J Clin Invest* 40:1363, 1961

468. PERRY TL, HANSEN S, LOVE D, FINCH CA.: N-Acetylcystathione: A new urinary amino-acid in congenital cystathioninuria. *Nature (Lond)* 219:178, 1968

469. KODAMA H, ISHIMOTO Y, SHIMOMURA M, HIROTA T, OHMORI S: Isolation of two new sulfur-containing amino acids from the urine of a cystathioninuric patient. *Physiol Chem Phys* 7:147, 1975

470. FRIMPTER GW, KOZLOWSKI KK, HORWITH M: distribution of sulfur in urine of patients with cystathioninuria before and during administration of pyridoxine. *Metabolism* 25:355, 1976

471. LEVY HL, COULOMBE JT, SHIH VE: Newborn urine screening, in Bickel H, Guthrie R, Hammersen G (eds): *Neonatal Screening for Inborn Errors of Metabolism.* Heidelberg, Springer-Verlag, 1980, p 89

26

HYPERSARCOSINEMIA

This summary is adapted from a summary written by Theo Gerritsen and Harry A. Waisman for the fourth edition of this book [1].

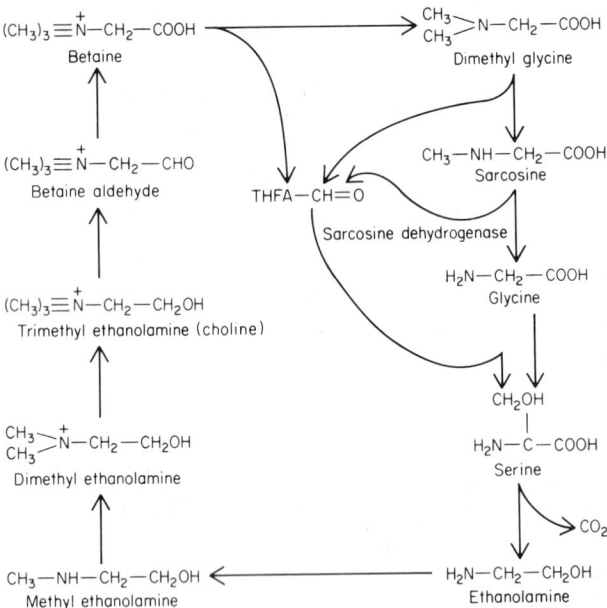

The 1-carbon cycle, illustrating the site of action of sarcosine dehydrogenase, which converts sarcosine to glycine and a 1-carbon unit. A deficiency of this enzyme is responsible for hypersarcosinemia.

1. Hypersarcosinemia *with sarcosinuria is a rare disorder that has been reported in a few individuals of both sexes, including two pairs of sibs and at least four unrelated patients. One of the isolated patients was a product of a consanguine marriage. Considerable variation exists in the mental and physical symptoms of the individuals, and no specific clinical features can yet be assigned.*

2. *The metabolic defect in hypersarcosinemia is in the activity of the sarcosine dehydrogenase complex, an enzyme system that converts sarcosine into glycine and a 1-carbon unit. Sarcosine is derived from dimethylglycine, which in turn is derived from betaine. This series of reactions constitutes part of the 1-carbon cycle. Sarcosine dehydrogenase does not appear to be an essential enzyme activity in humans.*

3. *The inheritance pattern of hypersarcosinemia is presumably autosomal recessive. Loading tests with sarcosine in patients and their relatives have suggested that a distinction is possible between homozygotes, heterozygotes, and normal subjects. Skin fibroblasts from normal subjects do not contain sarcosine dehydrogenase activity, and it is thus improbable that hypersarcosinemia can be detected prenatally using cultured amniotic fluid cells.*

REFERENCE

1. GERRITSEN T, WAISMAN HA: Hypersarcosinemia, in Stanbury JB, Wyngaarden JB, Fredrickson DS (eds): *The Metabolic Basis of Inherited Disease,* ed 4. New York, McGraw-Hill Book Co, 1978, p 514

27

NONKETOTIC HYPERGLYCINEMIA

WILLIAM L. NYHAN

1. *Nonketotic hyperglycinemia is an inborn error of amino acid metabolism in which large amounts of glycine accumulate in body fluids.*
2. *Most patients are severely mentally retarded and have seizure disorders. The disease may be life-threatening early in the postnatal period.*
3. *The concentration of glycine in the cerebrospinal fluid (CSF) is particularly high. The ratio of the concentration in the CSF to that of the plasma may distinguish this condition from others in which there is hyperglycinemia.*
4. *The site of the metabolic block is the glycine cleavage reaction, which converts glycine to CO_2, NH_3, and a single-carbon tetrahydrofolate derivative.*

Nonketotic hyperglycinemia is an inborn error of metabolism in which large amounts of glycine are found in body fluids and in which organic acids cannot be demonstrated in the blood or urine [1]. It is distinguished in this way from the ketotic hyperglycinemia syndrome which occurs in propionic acidemia and other disorders of organic acid metabolism. Nonketotic hyperglycinemia is a relatively frequent metabolic cause of overwhelming illness in the first year of life.

Nonketotic hyperglycinemia was first described in detail by Gerritsen et al. [2]. The disorder is probably heterogeneous. While patients with relatively mild mental retardation have

been seen, the classic presentation is of a very young infant with overwhelming illness. Survivors often have intractable seizures, usually with myoclonus, and little or no evidence of cerebral development. The fundamental defect is in the glycine cleavage reaction (Fig. 27-1).

GLYCINE METABOLISM

Glycine is the simplest of the amino acids, but it has a complex pattern of metabolism. It is a nonessential amino acid that can be synthesized in humans. It is present in high concentrations in collagen and gelatin and is abundant in most animal proteins. The daily intake for the average adult in the United States is 3 to 5 g.

Glycine originally received a name reminiscent of sugar because it has a sweet taste. It is also a glycogenic amino acid. If one feeds a starved animal large quantities of glycine, glycogen is laid down in the liver.

Synthetic Reactions Involving Glycine

The metabolism of glycine is concerned largely with its role in synthetic processes, of which there are a number in addition to

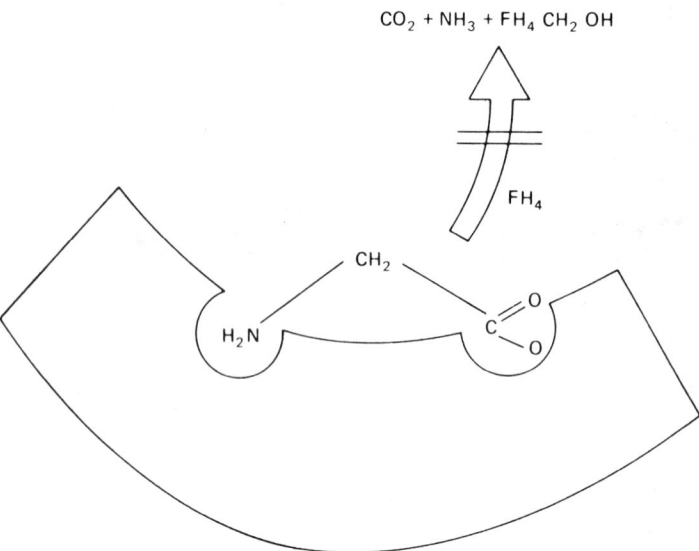

$$CO_2 + NH_3 + FH_4 CH_2 OH$$

Figure 27-1   The glycine cleavage reaction, site of the defect in nonketotic hyperglycinemia.

the synthesis of proteins (Fig. 27-2). Its important role in the synthesis of proteins may be its ability to permit the construction of proteins with minimal steric restraint. This would facilitate such things as the helical structure of collagen. Approximately 50 percent of dietary glycine is employed for the synthesis of protein [1]. Approximately 10 percent is found in the body in nonprotein nitrogen. Forty percent is excreted directly in the urine and 2 to 3 percent in the feces. In experiments using ^{14}C- or ^{15}N-labeled glycine, most of the label found in proteins is in glycine and serine. Some is in glutamate and aspartate. The extent of conversion to protein serine is about four times that of direct incorporation into protein [1]. These observations indicate the importance of the glycine-serine interconversion.

When labeled glycine is fed, there is a lag of 6 to 8 h before glycogen is formed. The peak is at about 12 h. This suggests that glycine must first be converted to other molecules, which are subsequently converted to glucose. Furthermore, there appears in glycogen twice as much of the α carbon of glycine as of the carboxyl carbon. This suggests that there is first a conversion to serine. There is also a lag of 6 to 8 h before the nitrogen of glycine appears in the urine as urea. This indicates further that glycine is to a considerable extent involved in synthetic reactions which tie up the molecule.

Glycine plays an important role in the synthesis of purines. It

is incorporated *in toto* into what become the 4, 5, and 7 positions of the purine ring, and it provides a source of 1-carbon units for *de novo* purine synthesis. This pathway accounts for about a tenth of a percent of metabolized glycine.

Glycine undergoes a series of reactions in which acyl derivatives are formed. The most prominent of these is hippuric acid, in which an amide bond is formed between benzoic acid and glycine which is like the peptide bonds in proteins. The acylation of glycine proceeds after formation of a CoA derivative of the carboxyl group of benzoic acid. A similar reaction serves in the detoxification of salicylates through the formation of salicyluric acid, and bile acids are excreted into the intestine in the form of glycine conjugates. Large amounts of isovalerylglycine are found in the urine of patients with isovaleric acidemia [3].

Catabolism of Glycine

Many of the catabolic reactions may be in fact primarily synthetic in character. For example, the glycine-succinate reaction is primarily concerned with the synthesis of porphyrins and probably plays no significant part in the degradation of glycine. Similarly, some reversible reactions may be more concerned with the synthesis of glycine itself than with its catabolism.

The Glycine-Serine Interconversion   The interconversion of glycine and serine (Fig. 27-3) is the most important pathway in the catabolism of glycine. Definitive evidence for conversion of serine to glycine was provided by experiment in which rats were fed serine labeled with ^{15}N and ^{13}C [1]. The ratio of ^{15}N to ^{13}C was the same in hippurate isolated from the urine as in the precursor. This was a strong indication that the conversion was direct. Similarly, when ^{14}C-labeled glycine was fed to rats, the protein of the liver was found to contain labeled serine [1]. The formation of serine from ^{13}C-labeled glycine and ^{14}C-labeled formate was demonstrated in the rat. Moreover, in human beings labeled serine appears in the blood promptly after the injection of labeled glycine [1]. All these observations indicate that glycine can be converted to serine and that serine can be converted to glycine.

In studies in which glycine was labeled in the 2 position with

Figure 27-2   Metabolic pathways of glycine concerned particularly with the synthesis of other molecules.

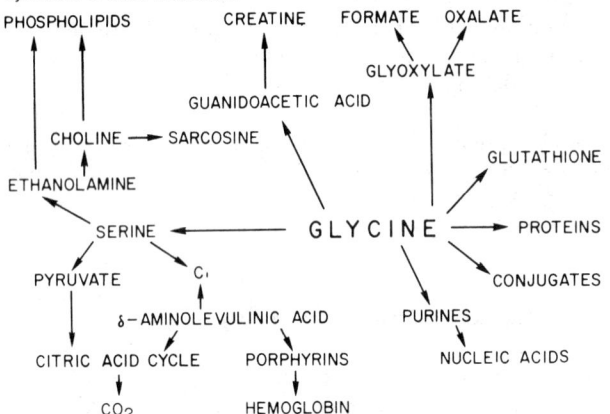

^{14}C, the label was found in the 2 and 3 positions of serine [1]. One enzyme involved in this transformation is serine hydroxymethyl transferase (L-serine:tetrahydrofolate-5,-10-hydroxymethyl transferase, EC 2.1.2.1) [1]. The proportions of carbon 2 of glycine converted to carbon 2 and carbon 3 of serine have generally been found to be about equal, but this labeling pattern may obtain only when relatively large amounts of glycine are administered. In experiments in which labeled amino acids were fed for 20 to 40 days until a steady-state pattern was developed, this labeling pattern was found when glycine constituted 2 percent of the diet, but with 0.5 percent glycine the specific activity of carbon 3 of serine was only 20 percent of that of carbon 2 [1]. Thus, experiments in which large loads of substrate are employed may demonstrate pathways which are operative only under those conditions. In these experiments the turnover of serine was 35 mmol/kg in rats; that of glycine was 25 mmol/kg. These data were interpreted to indicate that serine is generally the precursor of glycine and that glycine is converted to serine under conditions in which there is need for catabolizing large quantities of glycine. Nevertheless, under all conditions studied there was conversion of glycine to serine. One might interpret the glycine-to-serine conversion as an important physiologic pathway which is subject to stimulation by large amounts of glycine when there is need for glycine catabolism. Similarly, the enzyme system which converts glycine to single-carbon units in *Escherichia coli* is adaptive. It is induced by glycine and repressed by single-carbon units derived from other sources.

The system involved in the conversion of glycine to serine was extensively studied in avian liver and in *Peptococcus glycinophilus* [1]. A close relationship was observed between the production of CO_2 and NH_3 and the synthesis of serine. Pyridoxal phosphate, NAD, and tetrahydrofolic acid were stimulatory. These observations are consistent with the following pathway (FH_4 indicates tetrahydrofolic acid and FH_4CH_2OH, its hydroxymethyl derivative):

$$NH_2CH_2COOH + FH_4 + H_2O \longrightarrow FH_4CH_2OH + NH_3 \quad (1)$$

$$FH_4CH_2OH + NH_2CH_2COOH \longrightarrow$$
$$HOCH_2CHNH_2COOH + FH_4 \quad (2)$$

The overall reaction for the synthesis of serine from glycine by this pathway is as follows:

$$2NH_2CH_2COOH + H_2O \longrightarrow$$
$$HOCH_2CHNH_2COOH + CO_2 + HN_3 \quad (3)$$

As suggested in Fig. 27-3, there are many sources of the CH_2OH group of FH_4CH_2OH other than glycine. It derives from the so-called 1-carbon pool. Reaction 1, therefore, is not required for the conversion of glycine to serine by way of reaction 2. It is reaction 2 that is catalyzed by serine hydroxymethyl transferase [1]. Reaction 1 requires NAD and pyridoxal phosphate as cofactors.

The mechanisms of these reactions are complex. The enzymes involved were first studied in *P. glycinophilus* [1]. Four protein fractions, originally called P_1, P_2, P_3, and P_4 and sometimes designated E_1, E_2, E_3, and E_4, have been separated. The enzyme catalyzing the decarboxylation of glycine has been purified, and the reaction is reversible [1]. All four proteins are required to catalyze the overall conversion of glycine to CO_2, NH_3, and an FH_4 derivative. E_1 contains a bound pyridoxal phosphate. E_2 is a heat-stable protein. E_1 and E_2 are required for the formation of CO_2 from glycine. E_3 is a flavoprotein which is reduced in the presence of E_2 and glycine and which transfers electrons to NAD. E_4 functions in the presence of the rest of the system to transfer carbon 2 of glycine to FH_4.

The glycine-serine interconversion in mammalian systems has been clarified largely through the work of Kikuchi and colleagues [1, 4–6]. It was first found that rat liver mitochondria can synthesize glycine by a CO_2-fixation reaction in which serine and ammonia yield two molecules of glycine. The β carbon of serine and bicarbonate carbon were incorporated in a 1:1 ratio into the α and carboxyl carbons of glycine. Methylene-FH_4 was effective in replacing serine in the synthesis of glycine. The enzyme preparation also catalyzed the decarboxylation of glycine; the glycine cleavage required FH_4. The extracts also catalyzed an exchange between the carboxyl carbon of glycine and CO_2. Pyridoxal phosphate is a component of the enzyme complex. These observations indicated the presence in mammalian liver of a system similar to that in *P. glycinophilus*.

The glycine cleavage system is entirely mitochondrial. The four protein components have now been designated P, H, T, and L (Fig. 27-4) [4–6]. P protein is the pyridoxal phosphate-dependent glycine decarboxylase. H protein is a lipoic acid-

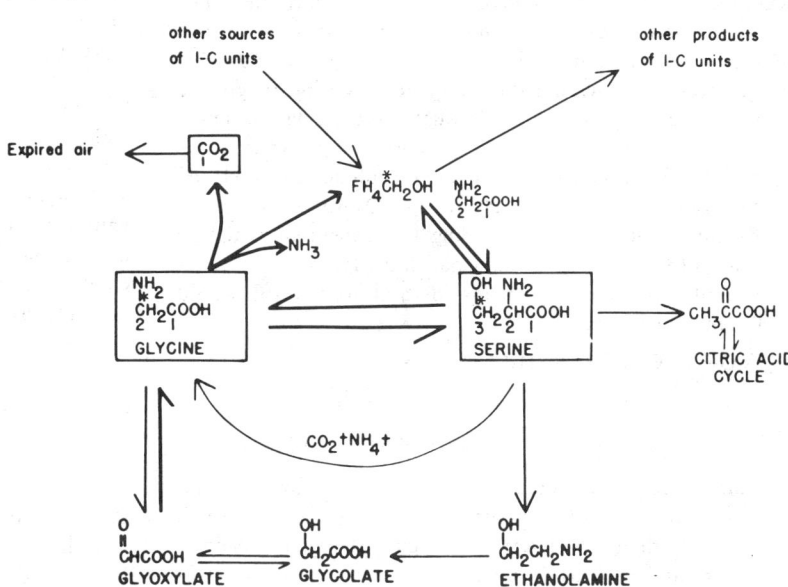

Figure 27-3 The metabolic interconversion of glycine and serine. The two arrows in the center connecting the glycine and serine boxes indicate that the two molecules are interconvertible, and by a number of pathways, without specification as to type. The two carbons of glycine are numbered 1 and 2; in this way, it is possible to see that carbon 1 and carbon 2 are incorporated directly into the corresponding 1 and 2 carbons of serine. Carbon 2 is also convertible to a tetrahydrofolate derivative, which then becomes carbon 3 of serine. The asterisk has been employed to follow this carbon through this reaction sequence. The sequence is reversible. The CO_2-fixation reaction which produces two molecules of glycine from one molecule of serine is drawn with the curved arrow below for clarity. FH_4, tetrahydrofolic acid; 1-C unit, single-carbon unit. (*By permission from Ando T, et al, Pediatr Res 2:254, 1968.*)

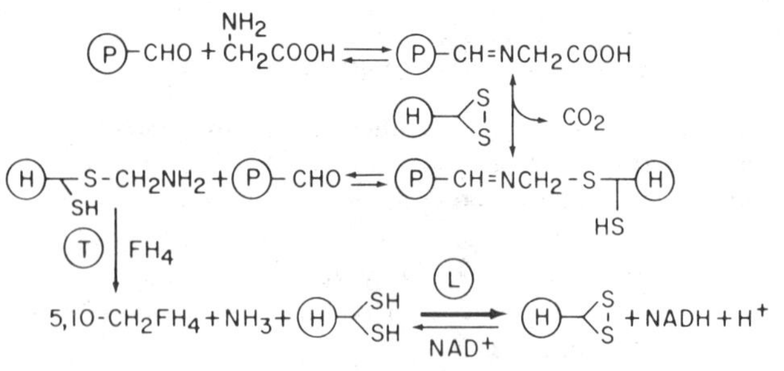

Figure 27-4 The glycine cleavage system.

containing protein originally labeled as a hydrogen carrier protein. This protein has now been established as the aminomethyl carrier protein. T protein is a tetrahydrofolate-requiring enzyme. L protein is the lipoamide dehydrogenase.

The H protein is small. It undergoes a protein-protein interaction with the P protein, which appears to make a conformational change in the latter, resulting in activation and enhanced affinity for substrate and leading to the decarboxylation of glycine.

Glycine Oxidase and Transaminases   The conversion of glycine to glyoxylate and NH_3 is catalyzed by an enzyme which is the same as D-amino acid oxidase [1]. It has a high K_m and is therefore thought not to play a major role in the degradation of glycine. Glyoxylate may also be formed from glycine by transamination [1], but it is unlikely that these pathways serve significantly in the degradation of glycine because thermodynamic considerations strongly favor the synthesis of glycine rather than its catabolism [1].

Amino Ketone Formation   δ-Aminolevulinic acid is formed by the condensation of glycine and succinyl CoA, an essential step in the biosynthesis of porphyrins and heme [1].

$$HOOCCH_2CH_2CO - S - CoA + CH_2NH_2COOH \longrightarrow$$
$$[HOOCCH_2CH_2COCHNH_2COOH]$$
$$\downarrow CO_2$$
$$HOOCH_2CH_2COCH_2NH_2 \quad (4)$$

The α carbon of glycine becomes the δ carbon of δ-aminolevulinic acid, and is a precursor of a 1-carbon unit. The rest of the compound yields α-ketoglutaraldehyde, which can be converted to α-ketoglutaric acid. Thus, this pathway could operate as a cycle, providing the complete oxidation of glycine while regenerating succinate. Although this cycle has been proposed as a major route for the degradation of glycine, studies using ^{14}C-labeled glycine and δ-aminolevulinic acid disclosed that the rate of conversion of glycine to CO_2 was 25 times that of δ-aminolevulinic acid, a finding not consistent with the function of the cycle as a major pathway [1].

A similar condensation of glycine and acetyl CoA would yield aminoacetone:

$$CH_3CO-S-CoA + CH_2NH_2COOH \longrightarrow$$
$$CO_2$$
$$[CH_3COCH_2NH_2COOH] \xrightarrow{\qquad} CH_3COCH_2NH_2 \quad (5)$$

The aminoacetone synthesized can be converted by transamination or by action of monoamine oxidase to methylglyoxal, which could then be converted through a glyoxalase reaction to lactate and then to pyruvate. Thus, the synthesis of this

amino ketone could also lead to the complete metabolism of glycine, and this pathway could operate as a cycle.

Aminoacetone is readily formed from acetyl CoA and glycine in guinea pig liver mitochondria. It has been calculated that conversion to aminoacetone could account for as much as one-quarter of the glycine metabolized each day [1], but our studies indicate that this is not a major route for the catabolism of glycine in human beings [1]. Following the administration of ^{14}C-labeled glycine, there was no evidence of incorporation of label into aminoacetone. By contrast, there was significant conversion of the label of administered threonine to aminoacetone. Thus in humans the source of urinary aminoacetone is threonine, not glycine.

Synthesis of Glycine

Glycine is a nonessential amino acid which can be synthesized in a number of ways, including transamination of glyoxylate and conversion from serine. The CO_2-fixation reaction is considered to be the major route for the formation of glycine. Glycine could also be synthesized from serine by way of ethanolamine:

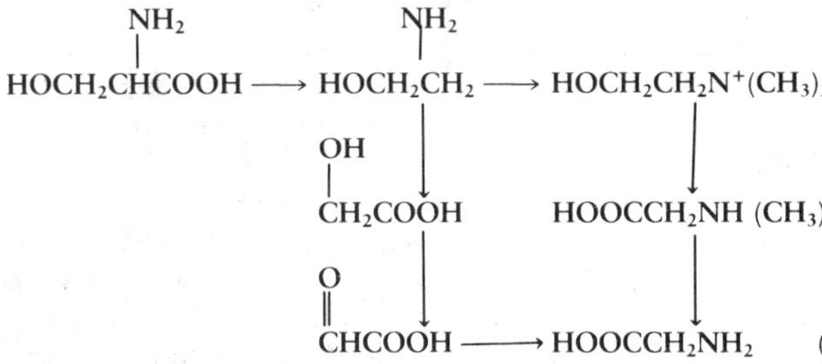

$$HOCH_2CHCOOH \longrightarrow HOCH_2CH_2 \longrightarrow HOCH_2CH_2N^+(CH_3)_3$$

(with NH_2 group on the first carbon chain; branches:)

OH → CH_2COOH → O‖CHCOOH → $HOOCCH_2NH_2$; and $HOOCCH_2NH(CH_3)$ (6)

Glycine may also derive from threonine. In this process threonine is degraded to glycine and acetaldehyde [1]. In the rat, one-third to one-fifth of ingested threonine may be converted to glycine [1].

Turnover of Glycine

The rate of turnover of glycine has been measured in human beings and animals. In the rat glycine is synthesized at the rate of about 2 g/(kg·day). In human beings a glycine turnover of 1 g/(kg·day) was found.

The normal concentration of glycine in plasma as measured by column chromatography is approximately 1 mg/dl [1]. In children 5 to 14 years of age, the mean value was 0.65 mg/dl. The average adult excretes glycine at the rate of approximately 100 mg/24 h, with a range of 50 to 200 mg/24 h [1]. These values amount to 0.1 to 0.2 mg glycine per milligram creatinine. Similar values have been found in children [1]. The concentration of glycine in cerebrospinal fluid (CSF) is approximately 0.1 g/dl [1].

CLINICAL FEATURES

Patients with this disease in general have had severe mental retardation. The child reported by Gerritsen et al. [2] was listless, lacked spontaneous movements even in the neonatal period, failed to thrive physically, and failed to develop mentally. He did not sit up, roll over, or respond to his mother at 5 months of age. At 5 years of age, he could only lie in a hyper-extended position. There was no adaptive or social behavior. The patient we first studied [1] was similarly lethargic from the third day of life. By 33 months he was diffusely hypotonic, had severe developmental retardation, and was unaware of his environment. He was unresponsive to social stimulation.

In the patient we studied with Baumgartner et al. [1], the diagnosis was made on the fourth day of life. By that time, he was so overwhelmingly ill that a respirator was required. Except for myoclonic jerks, generalized seizures, and persistent hiccuping, there was no movement or spontaneous respiration. Exchange transfusion reversed most of these findings, but the patient promptly relapsed and his condition continued to deteriorate. At 7 months of age he was unaware of his surroundings, had only a few spontaneous movements, and showed no head control. Tendon reflexes were exaggerated. He died shortly thereafter.

A similar early course was reported in the majority of the patients [7–9]. This is now considered the classic phenotype of the disease. Onset is after a period of hours or days in which the patient appears well, but following the first symptoms, progression to deep coma is rapid. Apnea requiring a respirator is the rule. A fulminant course may lead to death as early as 3 weeks despite heroic measures [9].

Different degrees of involvement may be seen in the same kindred. For instance, one infant [10] had an overwhelming illness and died on the sixth day in spite of exchange transfusion and artificial respiration. His older brother had been referred at 1 year of age for mental retardation [11]. On the other hand, there does appear to be a different phenotype in which all members of the family have a mild degree of mental retardation. We have studied a family of three affected girls whose developmental retardation was much less severe [12]. Two sets of sibs from each of two other families had a similar more benign clinical picture [13, 14].

More recently, we have reported [15] a very different phenotype in which the patient developed relatively normally for the first months of life and then had a rapid degenerative course similar to that of a neurolipidosis, leading rapidly to death. At autopsy the brain was similar to that of other patients with nonketotic hyperglycinemia.

Convulsive seizures have been prominent in virtually all reported patients with nonketotic hyperglycinemia [1]. These range in severity from myoclonic seizures to grand mal convulsions. Hiccuping is frequent. The electroencephalogram is usually diffusely abnormal, and the pattern may be that of hypsarrhythmia. A pseudoperiodic or burst suppression pattern has been described as more typical [16, 17]. Most of the patients have had clinical evidence of spastic cerebral palsy. Opisthotonos is common.

Neutropenia may be found in patients with nonketotic hyperglycinemia. In one patient [1] the percentage of neutrophils in smears of peripheral blood seldom exceeded 20, and the total neutrophil count was often under 2000 per cubic millimeter and sometimes well under 1000.

The neuropathology of this disorder consists of diffuse alterations in myelination that take place after birth [18–20]. The earliest changes are vacuolation in the myelin, followed by loss of myelin and gliosis. Similar changes have been seen in other aminoacidopathies, including propionic acidemia, phenylketonuria, and maple syrup urine disease. Crystals have been reported [19, 20] in vacuoles in brain and liver. On the other hand, Reploh et al. [21] reported the light-microscopic examination of the liver to be normal, but they observed crystalline osmiophobic inclusions on electron microscopy.

BIOCHEMICAL CHARACTERISTICS

Plasma Concentrations

The concentration of glycine in the blood is elevated [1, 14]. In the patient of Gerritsen et al. [2] the plasma concentration averaged 8.1 mg/dl, with a range of 6.9 to 9.3 mg/dl. In a series of 31 patients collected from the literature, the mean was 7.5 mg/dl [14]. The plasma concentration of glycine may be lowered by rigid restriction of protein intake and by the administration of sodium benzoate.

Glycine in Urine and Cerebrospinal Fluid

The excretion of glycine in the urine by these patients may be enormous. The patient of Gerritsen et al. [2] excreted between 1 and 3 g glycine per day at 5 years of age. A normal adult excretes about 0.1 g glycine per day, or 0.1 to 0.2 mg per milligram creatinine. In a series of 31 patients of various ages from the literature, the range was from 1.112 to 2.00 g/day. In spite of the large amounts of glycine found in the urine, it is possible to miss a patient with hyperglycinemia when screening the urine for amino acids by paper chromatography or electrophoresis. The normal glycine spot is prominent. Also, patients are often studied when acutely ill, not eating, and being maintained on parenterally administered fluids. Under these circumstances the excretion of glycine in hyperglycinemic patients may be normal. In general, it is better to screen for hyperglycinemia using blood rather than urine, because the blood concentration is seldom brought into the normal range by treatment.

Elevated excretion of proline and hydroxyproline has not been observed in hyperglycinemia. There is a common transport system for proline, hydroxyproline, and glycine in the human kidney. This was elucidated when patients with hyperprolinemia were found to have increased excretion of glycine and hydroxyproline as a consequence of a primary elevation of proline concentration in blood and urine [22].

The concentration of glycine in the CSF is elevated in patients with nonketotic hyperglycinemia. In reported patients, it has varied from 1.0 to 1.7 mg/dl [1]. In control subjects the concentration has generally been less than 0.1 mg/dl.

Perry [23] has pointed out that glycine concentrations in CSF are particularly elevated in nonketotic hyperglycinemia. The ratio of the CSF concentration to that of the plasma is substantially higher in patients with nonketotic hyperglycinemia than in hyperglycinemic patients with organic acidemia [23, 24]. In a series of 12 patients from the literature, the mean ratio was 0.17 ± 0.09, while in control individuals the ratio was 0.02 [14, 23].

We have observed patients with milder degrees of clinical expression in whom the ratios were abnormal, but less elevated than in the classic severe phenotype. This may be one way in which to characterize heterogeneity of expression. In two sibs in whom the degree of retardation was mild, the ratios were said to be typical of nonketotic hyperglycinemia [13]. As we calculated their ratios according to the method of Perry [23], values of 0.065 and 0.086 were found and were considerably lower than Perry's lowest value of 0.200. In fact, we found values as high as 0.040 in propionic acidemia.

Hypooxaluria was initially described as a feature of this syndrome [2]. It is not clear that a diminished excretion of oxalate is not characteristic. Oxalate excretion was not decreased in a number of patients, including the original patient restudied [1]. Glyoxylate excretion was also normal. These observations provided evidence against the hypothesis of a defect in glycine oxidase, as originally postulated.

Glycine Metabolism

Delayed disappearance of glycine from plasma has been observed in the course of loading tests [1]. During loading there was no appreciable increase in the plasma concentration of serine. By contrast, there is abundant evidence of ready conversion of serine to glycine. The prompt rise and fall in the concentration of serine after a serine load indicated its normal metabolism, but the glycine concentration rose steadily over a 4-h period. These data are consistent with a defect in the utilization of glycine.

Defective glycine utilization was first assessed in studies in vivo of metabolism of glycine designed to evaluate separately the fates of carbon 1 and carbon 2, using [1-^{14}C]glycine or [2-^{14}C]glycine injected separately intravenously [1]. Collection of expired air permitted measurement of the kinetics of conversion of glycine to CO_2. Blood was also drawn at intervals, and the glycine was isolated. In this way the specific activity of the glycine pool was known. The serine of the plasma was also isolated, and after the specific activity was measured, the molecule was degraded and the β carbon trapped. Control subjects were studied in the control state and during constant infusion of glycine at a rate which increased the pool to a level comparable to that of patients.

The formation of $^{14}CO_2$ from glycine is shown in Fig. 27-5. A defect in the conversion of carbon 1 of glycine to CO_2 was demonstrated in three patients with nonketotic hyperglycinemia. The curves obtained were virtually identical.

The kinetics of the conversion of glycine to plasma serine were similar whether the glycine administered was [1-^{14}C]glycine or [2-^{14}C]glycine. The specific activities of serine in the patients were considerably lower than those of control subjects for at least 30 min, and the curves of the patients were so flat that it appeared again that a different process was under study in patient and control. The process was elucidated through degradation of the isolated serine with periodate. This permitted the selective trapping of carbon 3 as the dimedon derivative. The specific activities of this β carbon are shown in Fig. 27-6. In this experiment, patients and control subjects had similar concentrations of glycine in the plasma. There was virtually no conversion of carbon 2 of glycine to carbon 3 of serine in the patients.

These data indicate a defect in the metabolism of glycine in nonketotic hyperglycinemia. The formation of CO_2 from carbon 1 of glycine and the formation of carbon 3 of serine from carbon 2 of glycine were both strikingly defective. These findings are consistent with a block in the glycine cleavage system.

We postulated from this work that the glycine cleavage system prior to that time reported in avian liver and in bacteria was present in human beings and that it was defective in nonketotic hyperglycinemia. These conclusions were supported by the work of others [1, 11], using liver homogenates. The rates of conversion of [2-^{14}C]glycine to serine were about equal to those of [1-^{14}C]glycine. In contrast, in control liver the rate of incorporation of [2-^{14}C]glycine to serine was 1.6 times that of [1-^{14}C]glycine. These data indicate that normally carbon 2 of glycine is converted to carbons 2 and 3 of serine, while in the patients carbon 2 of glycine is converted only to carbon 2 of serine.

Yoshida and Kikuchi [25] discovered that the glycine cleavage reaction is the major pathway of glycine catabolism in mammalian liver. Defective in vitro cleavage of glycine in liver has now been shown in a number of patients with nonketotic hyperglycinemia [26, 27], including one who also had hyperammonemia [27]. A similar abnormality was reported in a patient with methylmalonic acidemia [26]. We have also studied glycine metabolism in vivo using [^{13}C]glycine as a tracer

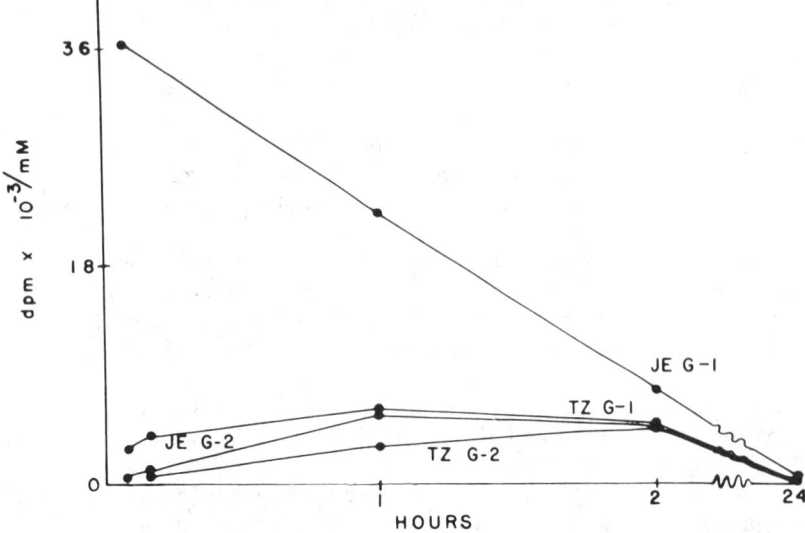

Figure 27-5 The conversion of glycine to CO_2. The data plotted are the specific activities of respiratory CO_2 collected following the intravenous injection of glycine. The curves are labeled with the initials of the subject, T.Z., and of a control, J.E., and with G-1 for [1-^{14}C]glycine and G-2 for [2-^{14}C]glycine. (*By permission from Nyhan WL, Ando T, Gerritsen T, in Amino Acid Metabolism and Genetic Variation, New York, McGraw-Hill Book Co, 1967, pp 255–265.*)

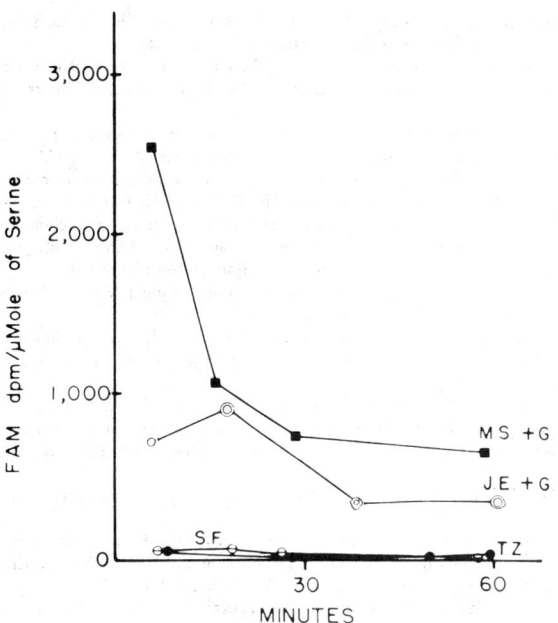

Figure 27-6 Conversion of [2-^{14}C]glycine to carbon 3 of serine. T.Z. and S.F. were patients; J.E. and M.S. were controls. The designation +G indicates the creation of an artificially elevated glycine pool. (*By permission from Ando T, et al, Pediatr Res 2:254, 1968.*)

compound; the patient with nonketotic hyperglycinemia may be distinguished from control subjects by defective glycine decarboxylation to respiratory CO_2 [28].

Perry and colleagues [29] have reported that the concentration of glycine in brain is elevated in this condition, in contrast to findings in patients with ketotic hyperglycinemia. Consistent with this, they have found that the activity of the glycine cleavage system, as measured by the exchange of $^{14}CO_2$ with glycine, is active in brain and is virtually absent in the brain of patients with nonketotic hyperglycinemia.

The glycine cleavage system has been studied in detail in liver specimens of patients with hyperglycinemia and organic acidemia [30] due to propionyl CoA carboxylase and methylmalonyl CoA mutase deficiency. As compared with controls, the activity of the entire system was reduced. Each component enzyme was assayed separately and was reduced. The data suggest an inhibition in the synthesis or assembly of the system. In nonketotic hyperglycinemia the activity of the glycine cleavage reaction, as measured by the conversion [1-^{14}C]glycine to $^{14}CO_2$ in liver specimens was about 2 to 4 percent of the normal level [31]. Since the affinity of the enzyme for glycine was not abnormal, the problem was in the synthesis of the enzyme.

The molecular nature of the defect in nonketotic hyperglycinemia has been studied using the sophisticated methods now available [32] in only the patient with the phenotype of cerebral degenerative disease [15]. The defect in the glycine cleavage system in autopsied liver and brain involved reduction in the activity of both P protein and H protein. The overall activity of glycine cleavage in liver was 2 to 7 percent that of controls [31]. The activity of the T protein and of lipoamide dehydrogenase was normal. Immunochemical studies using antibody specific to P protein showed that the amount of enzyme protein was normal, as were its kinetic properties. H protein, the aminomethyl carrier, appeared to be the site of mutant gene action. Its content was reduced to about 35 per-

cent that of controls and had only two instead of the normal four thiol groups. This suggested that it was devoid of lipoic acid. The purified protein was incapable of reacting with lipoamide dehydrogenase, but it reacted with P protein to stimulate some exchange of carbon 1 of glycine with CO_2. However, its activity in this activation of P protein was only about 4 percent of normal.

Similar secondary reductions of the activity of P protein have been reported by these investigators in the ketotic hyperglycinemia syndrome [30] and in the livers of dipropylacetic acid treated rats [33].

Diagnosis

In many patients, careful assessment of the clinical picture permits one to distinguish patients with nonketotic hyperglycinemia from those with the ketotic hyperglycinemia syndrome. Even so, we prefer to investigate all hyperglycinemic patients for the accumulation of organic acids, especially propionic and methylmalonic acids. This may be done by examination of the urine for methylcitrate, isovalerylglycine, and other organic acids. Those who do not have organic acidemia or organic aciduria are considered to have nonketotic hyperglycinemia. The importance of this was highlighted by a patient who had propionic acidemia but presented with hyperglycinemia and overwhelming illness in the absence of ketosis [34]. The distinction is far from academic. Excellent results can be obtained using dietary therapy for patients with propionic acidemia and methylmalonic acidemia, but there is no effective treatment for nonketotic hyperglycinemia.

The activity of propionyl CoA carboxylase and methylmalonyl CoA mutase has been found normal in the liver and fibroblasts of patients with acute neonatal nonketotic hyperglycinemia [35].

A syndrome has been described [36] in which nonketotic hyperglycinemia is associated with D-glyceric acidemia. A 2-year-old boy had hypotonia from birth that was severe enough to suggest a diagnosis of myasthenia gravis. He developed seizures and choreiform movements. Mental retardation was severe. Elevated concentrations of glycine were found in blood, urine, and CSF. The excretion of glyceric acid in the urine ranged from 1.5 to 2.5 g/day. The concentration in the serum was 1200 µmol/liter. Assay of D-glyceric acid dehydrogenase in leukocytes was significantly lower in the patient than in controls [37].

Free benzoic acid was found in the urine of a patient with nonketotic hyperglycinemia [38] but proved to be a consequence of a urinary tract infection, with hydrolysis of hippuric acid. It was eliminated by treatment of the infection.

The Valine Effect

A variety of approaches have been used to attempt to understand the pathogenesis of this disorder. Among the most provocative is the effect of valine. Levy and associates [39] found that most amino acids were without clinical effect in a patient with nonketotic hyperglycinemia, but valine induced a comatose state that lasted 6 h. Smaller doses were followed by somnolence and ataxia. We and others [40] have observed similar effects. We have also studied patients in whom valine was without effect. Valine-responsive patients with nonketotic hyperglycinemia regularly develop abnormalities of the electroencephalogram along with changes in consciousness following administration of the amino acid.

GENETICS

Nonketotic hyperglycinemia appears to be a rare autosomal recessive condition. Most instances have been sporadic. Consanguinity has been reported in two families [7, 11]. Two involved patients have been reported in two families [7, 11].

TREATMENT

Effective treatment has not been found. Exchange transfusion or peritoneal dialysis may be lifesaving in the neonatal period, but the improvement is only temporary. The plasma concentrations of glycine may be lowered by dietary restriction or by the administration of sodium benzoate [1, 40], but these measures have not appreciably altered the course of the disease. A temporary decrease in glycine concentration in serum was observed following the infusion of N^5-formyltetrahydrofolate (leucovorin) [1], and treatment with methionine in order to provide 1-carbon groups [11] may reduce the glycine concentration of plasma, but the course of the disease does not appear to be altered by these approaches. Bachmann and colleagues [9] have pointed out the potential toxicity of methionine treatment. The content of methionine in the brain of their patient was quite high. Very high levels of methionine in the plasma were reported by others following treatment with methionine [19, 41]. Treatment with pyridoxine does not result in improvement of the chemical hyperglycemia [41].

Glycine itself is a neurotransmitter whose action is inhibitory. Glycine has been reported to cause acute inhibition in cultured neurons but to lead to insensitivity to glycine continuously present [42]. The cells remained responsive to γ-aminobutyric acid. Postsynaptic potentials were also reduced by glycine. Although the postsynaptic inhibitory effects of glycine occur predominantly in the spinal cord and brainstem rather than in the cortex [43], they have been considered potentially similar to those of strychnine, and strychnine blocks glycinergic inhibition [44].

Others have reasoned that strychnine might, for this latter reason, be therapeutic in nonketotic hyperglycinemia, and a number of patients have now been treated. Two reports of modest success have been reported [45, 46]. It is also true that we and others have treated patients who have failed to respond, and the consensus is now that the majority of the patients, those with the classic forms of the disease, do not respond [47, 48]. Those who respond appear to be much less severely incapacitated. It is possible that the effects of this agent may serve to define heterogeneity in this condition.

REFERENCES

1. NYHAN WL: Nonketotic hyperglycinemia, in Stanbury JB, Wyngaarden JB, Fredrickson DS (eds): *The Metabolic Basis of Inherited Disease*, ed 4. New York, McGraw-Hill Book Co, 1978, pp 518–527

2. GERRITSEN T, KAVEGGIA E, WAISMAN HA: A new type of idiopathic hyperglycinemia with hypo-oxaluria. *Pediatrics* 36:882, 1965

3. ANDO T, KLINGBERG WG, WARD AN, RASMUSSEN K, NYHAN WL: Isovaleric acidemia presenting with altered metabolism of glycine. *Pediatr Res* 5:478, 1971

4. YOSHIDA T, KIKUCHI G: Comparative study on major pathways of glycine and serine catabolism in vertebrate livers. *J Biochem* 72:1503, 1972

5. KIKUCHI G: The glycine cleavage system: Composition, reaction mechanism, and physiological significance. *Mol Cell Biochem* 1:169, 1973

6. MOTOKAWA Y, KIKUCHI G: Glycine metabolism by rat liver mitochondria. Reconstitution of the reversible glycine cleavage system with partially purified protein components. *Arch Biochem Biophys* 164:624, 1974

7. SIMILA S, VISAKORPI JK: Clinical findings in three patients with nonketotic hyperglycinaemia. *Ann Clin Res* 2:151, 1970

8. FERDINAND W, GORDON RR, OWEN G: Nonketotic hyperglycinaemia: Clinical findings and amino acid analyses on the plasma of a new case. *Clin Chim Acta* 30:745, 1970

9. BACHMANN C, MIHATSCH MJ, BAUMGARTNER RE, BRECHBUHLER T, BUHLER UK, OLAFSSON A, OHNACKER H, WICK H: Nicht-ketotische hyperglyzinämie: Perakuter verlauf im Neugeborenenalten. *Helv Paediatr Acta* 26:228, 1971

10. OKKEN A, DEGROOT CJ, HOMMES FA: Nonketotic hyperglycinemia. *J Pediatr* 77:164, 1970

11. DEGROOT CJ, TROELSTRA HA, HOMMES FA: Nonketotic hyperglycinemia: An in vitro study of the glycine-serine conversion in liver of three patients and the effect of dietary methionine. *Pediatr Res* 4:238, 1970

12. ANDO T, NYHAN WL, BICKNELL WL, HARRIS R, STERN J: Non-ketotic hyperglycinaemia in a family with an unusual phenotype. *J Inher Metab Dis* 1:79, 1978

13. FRAZIER DM, SUMMER GK, CHAMBERLIN HR: Hyperglycinuria and hyperglycinemia in two siblings with mild developmental delays. *Am J Dis Child* 132:777, 1978

14. HOLMGREN G, BLOMQUIST HK: Non-ketotic hyperglycinemia in 2 sibs with mild psycho-neurological symptoms. *Neuropaediatrie* 8:67, 1977

15. TRAUNER DA, PAGE T, GRECO C, SWEETMAN L, KULOVICH S, NYHAN WL: Progressive neurodegenerative disorder in a patient with nonketotic hyperglycinemia. *J Pediatr* 98:272, 1981

16. AICARDI J, GOUTIERES F: Encéphalopathie myoclonique néonatale. *Rev E E G Neurophysiol* 8:99, 1978

17. MISES J, MOUSSALLI-SALEFRANQUE F, PLOUIN P, TEMAM G, SAUDUBRAY JM: l'E.E.G. dans les hyperglycinémies sans cétose. *Rev Electroencephalogr Neurophysiol* 8:102, 1978

18. SHUMAN RM, LEECH RW, SCOTT CR: The neuropathology of the nonketotic and ketonic hyperglycinemias: Three cases. *Neurology* 28:139, 1978

19. DIEZEL PB, MARTIN K: Hyperglycinämie (Glycinose) mit familiärer idiopathischer Hyperglycinurie, Erste Biobachtung in Deutschland. *Dtsch Med Wochenschr* 50:2249, 1966

20. DIEZEL PB: Hyperglycinaemie (Glycinose) mit familiärer Idiopathischer Hyperglycinurie. *Dtsch Gesel Pathol* 48:155, 1964

21. REPLOH H, GRÖBE L, DIEKMANN D, PALM DB, BASSEWITZ V, JENNETT W: The clinical findings in a patient with nonketotic hyperglycinemia. *Z Kinderheilk* 114:191, 1973

22. SCRIVER CR, BERGERON M: Amino acid transport in kidney. The use of mutation to dissect membrane and transepithelial transport, in Nyhan WL (ed): *Heritable Disorders of Amino Acid Metabolism*. New York, John Wiley & Sons, Inc, 1974, pp 515–592

23. PERRY TL, URQUHART N, MACLEAN J, EVANS ME, HANSEN S, DAVIDSON AGF, APPLEGARTH DA, MACLEOD PJ, LOCK JE: Nonketotic hyperglycinemia. *N Engl J Med* 292:1269, 1975

24. LEVY HL, NISHIMURA RN, ERICKSON AM, JANOWSKA SE: Hyperclycinemia: In vivo comparison of nonketotic and ketotic (propionic acidemic) forms, I. CSF glycine concentrations and blood/CSF glycine, *Pediatr Res* 6:400, 1972 (abstract)

25. YOSHIDA T, KIKUCHI G: Major pathways of glycine and serine catabolism in rat liver. *Arch Biochem Biophys* 139:380, 1970

26. TADA K, CORBEEL LM, EECKELS R, EGGERMONT E: A block in glycine cleavage reaction as a common mechanism in ketotic and nonketotic hyperglycemia. *Pediatr Res* 8:721, 1974

27. WADA Y, TADA K, TAKADA G, OMURA K, YOSHIDA T, KUNIYA T, AOYAMA T, HAKUI T, HARADA S: Hyperglycinemia associated with hyperammonemia: In vitro glycine cleavage in liver. *Pediatr Res* 6:622, 1972

28. SWEETMAN L, NYHAN WL, KLEIN PD, SZCZEPANIK PA: Glycine-1, 2-^{13}C in the investigation of children with inborn errors of metabolism, in Klein PD, Peterson SV (eds): *Proceedings of the 1st International Conference on Stable Isotopes in Chemistry, Biology, and Medicine*. Argonne, Ill, Argonne National Laboratory, May 9–11, 1973. Springfield, Va, US Atomic Energy Commission, National Technical Information Service, US Dept of Commerce, 1973, pp 404–409

29. PERRY TL, URQUHART N, HANSEN S: Studies of the glycine cleavage enzyme system in brain from infants with glycine encephalopathy. *Pediatr Res* 11:1192, 1977

30. MOTOKAWA Y, KIKUCHI G, NARISAWA K, ARAKAWA T: Reduced level of glycine cleavage system in the liver of hyperglycinemia patients. *Clin Chim Acta* 79:173, 1977

31. HIRAGA K, KOCHIH H, HOWASAKA K, KIKUCHI G, NYHAN WL: Defective glycine cleavage system in nonketotic hyperglycinemia: Occurrence of a less active glycine decarboxylase and an abnormal aminomethyl carrier protein. *J Clin Invest* 68:525, 1981

32. HIRAGA K, KIKUCHI G: The mitochondrial glycine cleavage system. *J Biol Chem* 255:1161, 1980

33. KOCHI H, HAWASAKA K, HIRAGA J, KIKUCHI G: Reduction of the level of glycine cleavage system in the rat liver resulting from administration of dipropylacetic acid: An experimental approach to hyperglycinemia. *Arch Biochem Biophys* 198:589, 1979

34. WALDLINGTON WB, KILROY A, ANDO T, SWEETMAN L, NYHAN WL: Hyperglycinemia and propionyl-CoA carboxylase deficiency and episodic severe illness without consistent ketosis. *J Pediatr* 86:707, 1975

35. BAUMGARTNER ER, BACHMANN C, BRECHBÜHLER T, WICK H: Acute neonatal nonketotic hyperglycinemia: Normal propionate and methylmalonate metabolism. *Pediatr Res* 9:559, 1975

36. BRANDT NJ, RASMUSSEN K, BRANDT S, KØLVRAA S, SCHØNHEYDER F: D-Glyceric-acidaemia and non-ketotic hyperglycinaemia. *Acta Paediatr Scand* 65:17, 1976

37. KØLVRRA S, RASMUSSEN K, BRANDT NJ: D-Glyceric acidemia: Biochemical studies of a new syndrome. *Pediatr Res* 10:825, 1976

38. VISAKORPI JK, DONNER M, NORIO R: Hyperglycinuria with severe neurological manifestations. *Ann Paediatr Fenn* 11:114, 1965

39. LEVY HL, NISHIMURA RN, ERICKSON AM, JANOWSKA SE: Hyperglycinemia: In vivo comparison of nonketotic and ketotic (propionic acidemic) forms. II. Valine response in nonketotic hyperglycinemia. *Pediatr Res* 6:395, 1972

40. KRIEGER I, HART ZH: Valine-sensitive nonketotic hyperglycinemia. *J Pediatr* 85:43, 1974

41. TRIJBELS JMF, MONNENS LAH, VAN DER ZEE, SPM, VRENKEN JATH, SENGERS RCA, SCHRETLEN EDAM: A patient with nonketotic hyperglycinemia: Biochemical findings and therapeutic approaches. *Pediatr Res* 8:598, 1974

42. RANSOM BR: Possible pathophysiology of neurologic abnormalities associated with nonketotic hyperglycinemia. *N Engl J Med* 294:1295, 1976

43. KELLY JS, KRNJEVIC K: The action of glycine on cortical neurones. *Exp Brain Res* 9:155, 1969

44. KRNJEVIC K: Chemical nature of synaptic transmission in vertebrates. *Physiol Rev* 54:418, 1974

45. GITZELMANN R, STEINMANN B, OTTEN A, DUMERMUTH G, HERDAN M, REUBI JC, CUENOD M: Nonketotic hyperglycinemia treated with strychnine, a glycine receptor antagonist. *Helv Paediat Acta* 32:517, 1977

46. ARNESON D, CH'IEN LT, CHANCE P, WILROY RS: Strychnine therapy in nonketotic hyperglycinemia. *Pediatrics* 63:369, 1979

47. MACDERMOT KD, NELSON W, REICHERT CM, SCHULMAN JD: Attempts at use of strychnine sulfate in the treatment of nonketotic hyperglycinemia. *Pediatrics* 65:61, 1980

48. VON WENDT L: Nonketotic hyperglycinaemia. A clinical and experimental study. *Acta Univ Ouluenis*, Series D, Medica 53 *(Med Interna Paediatr)* no 8, 1980

28

DISORDERS OF β-ALANINE, CARNOSINE, AND HOMOCARNOSINE METABOLISM

CHARLES R. SCRIVER

THOMAS L. PERRY

WALTER NUTZENADEL

1. Free β-alanine is found only in very small amounts in mammalian tissues and body fluids; the amino acid is normally oxidized very rapidly. Peptide-bound β-alanine is 500-fold more prominent, appearing as carnosine (β-alanyl-L-histidine) in human tissues (skeletal muscle primarily) and also as anserine (β-alanyl-l-methyl-L-histidine) in many nonhuman species. β-Alanine and carnosine are taken up by tissues on independent β-amino acid and β-alanyl peptide-preferring membrane transport systems. Cleavage of carnosine by carnosinase precedes oxidation of the β-alanine residue. Two forms of carnosinase are present in human tissues, only one of which occurs in serum.

2. Two disorders of β-alanine metabolism have been identified in humans. One involves free β-alanine catabolism (hyper-β-alaninemia); the other, the degradation of carnosine in serum.

3. Hyper-β-alaninemia has been reported in only one proband, who was affected from birth with severe depression of the central nervous system punctuated by uncontrollable seizures. He died in his fifth month; three sibs who died in utero or at birth may also have had the same presumably autosomal recessive trait.

4. Abnormal accumulation of β-alanine and γ-aminobutyric acid occurred in plasma, cerebrospinal fluid, and urine. A deficiency in β-alanine-α-ketoglutarate amino transferase was the presumed enzymatic abnormality.

5. Excretion of the two natural β-amino metabolites, β-aminoisobutyric acid and taurine, is increased in hyper-β-alaninemia. Hyper-β-aminoaciduria, which is directly proportional to the plasma concentration of β-alanine, reflects a combined saturation and competitive inhibition of the tubular transport system, with selective preference for β-amino compounds.

6. Tissue concentrations of β-alanine, γ-aminobutyric acid, and carnosine are elevated. Dipeptide accumulation presumably reflects increased endogenous synthesis in the presence of an expanded free β-alanine pool. The absence of carnosine from the urine distinguishes hyper-β-alaninemia from serum carnosinase deficiency.

7. Serum carnosinase deficiency is a rare trait (probably autosomal recessive, but X linkage has not been excluded). Probands have all presented with profoundly abnormal neurologic findings, but there are carnosinuric sibs without clinical signs.

8. Serum carnosinase deficiency is accompanied by persistent endogenous hypercarnosinuria (at least 25-fold increased above normal), even when dietary intake of carnosine (in meat and fowl) is eliminated. Dietary exposure to anserine does not yield the normal brisk 1-methylhistidinuria, which indicates

defective anserine cleavage by carnosinase. Carnosinemia is not a consistent finding in persons with the trait, since the dipeptide is rapidly cleared into urine and taken up into tissues. Tissue carnosine (and homocarnosine) levels are not elevated.

9. *Two forms of tissue carnosinase activity have been identified: the negatively charged form is deficient in patients with the trait; the residual positively charged activity is apparently able to maintain tissue carnosine pools within the normal range. Serum carnosinase activity is almost totally lacking in persons with the trait; absence of the positively charged form in normal serum is implied.*

10. *No treatment has been identified for hyper-β-alaninemia or serum carnosine deficiency. Pyridoxine (vitamin B₆) may be of benefit in future patients with hyper-β-alaninemia, and carnosinase replacement by serum infusions might have a place in the treatment of CRM⁺ subjects with serum carnosinase deficiency.*

11. *Homocarnisosis involves excessive accumulation of homocarnosine (γ-aminobutyryl-L-histidine) only in cerebrospinal fluid (CSF) and brain. Homocarnosinase activity in brain is severely deficient. The relationship between the biochemical phenotype and clinical symptoms is unclear. In the single known pedigree, one patient is asymptomatic in her seventh decade; three of her offspring (34 to 41 years old) have elevated CSF homocarnosine and progressive neurologic disease, with late onset spastic paraplegia, loss of intelligence, and retinal pigmentation. Treatment, if it were available, might be irrelevant. It is possible that homocarnosinase deficiency and the neurologic disorder are separate entities that segregate independently in the index Norwegian pedigree.*

Hyper-β-alaninemia is a metabolic disorder characterized by an elevated concentration of free β-alanine in plasma, cerebrospinal fluid, and urine, and in tissues such as brain, kidney, liver, and skeletal muscle [1]. Taurine and β-aminoisobutyric acid, two ubiquitous β-amino acids in human metabolism, are also present in elevated amounts in urine. Interaction on a β-amino-preferring transport system in the renal tubule accounts for the complex hyper-β-aminoaciduria in hyper-β-alaninemia. γ-Aminobutyric acid (GABA) is also present in excess in urine, plasma, and cerebrospinal fluid (CSF); its concentration is elevated in brain and kidney, where it is synthesized. A proposed deficiency of β-alanine:α-keto glutarate amino transferase is the most logical but still unproved explanation for these unique findings. An excess of tissue carnosine (β-alanyl-L-histidine), without accumulation in urine, blood, or CSF, suggests enhanced disposal of β-alanine into the peptide pool in hyper-β-alaninemia. The disorder has been described, so far, in only one infant proband, who presented with seizures and somnolence and who subsequently died.

Serum carnosinase deficiency with persistent carnosinuria is usually, but not always, accompanied by *carnosinemia;* it is a disorder of peptide-bound β-alanine which does not affect free β-alanine metabolism [2, 3]. Carnosinuria persists even when dietary foods containing carnosine are excluded. Two forms of carnosinase, the enzyme which hydrolyzes carnosine to its free constituents, are present in tissues; one form is lacking in the

trait, along with a near-total absence of serum carnosinase (Fig. 28-1). Studies in four pedigrees suggest autosomal recessive inheritance of the trait, which has usually been ascertained in probands with a profound deteriorative convulsive disorder; the presence of a symptom-free carnosinuric subject in one of these pedigrees raises the possibility that serum carnosinase deficiency may not be the cause of the neurologic abnormalities.

Homocarnosinosis, associated with deficiency of homocarnosinase activity, has been found in a single pedigree containing members with a neurologic disorder. Homocarnosine is elevated in CSF and brain but not in plasma or urine. The relationship between biochemical and clinical findings is unclear.

METABOLISM OF β-ALANINE, CARNOSINE, AND OTHER DIPEPTIDES

β-Alanine Metabolism

β-alanine forms an insignificant fraction of the free amino acid pool in human body fluids [4–6]. Liver, kidney, and brain, unlike other mammalian tissues which have been examined, contain a small amount of free β-alanine [7–9].

Synthesis The principal endogenous sources of β-alanine in mammalian tissues are found in the metabolism of the pyrimidine uracil and in the dipeptides carnosine (β-alanyl-L-histidine) and anserine (β-alanine-1-methyl-L-histidine) (Fig. 28-2).

Microorganisms can form β-alanine by alpha decarboxylation of aspartic acid, but this reaction does not occur in mammalian tissue. It is possible that the contents of the large intestine might serve as an exogenous source of β-alanine under appropriate conditions. Hydrolysis of dietary dipeptides which contain β-alanine will release β-alanine into the free pool.

β-Alanine can be removed from the free pool by two reactions in the mammalian tissues. It may be degraded first to malonic semialdehyde by the action of β-alanine-α-ketoglutarate amino transferase, an enzyme which has been well characterized in microorganisms [10]. Impairment of this enzyme as

Figure 28-1 The blocked cleavage of carnosine in carnosinemia.

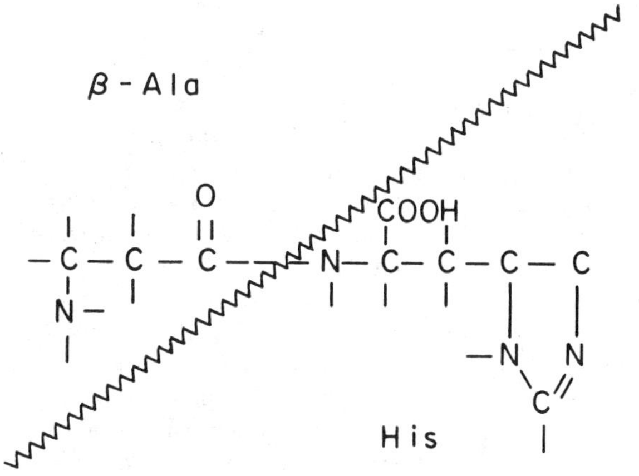

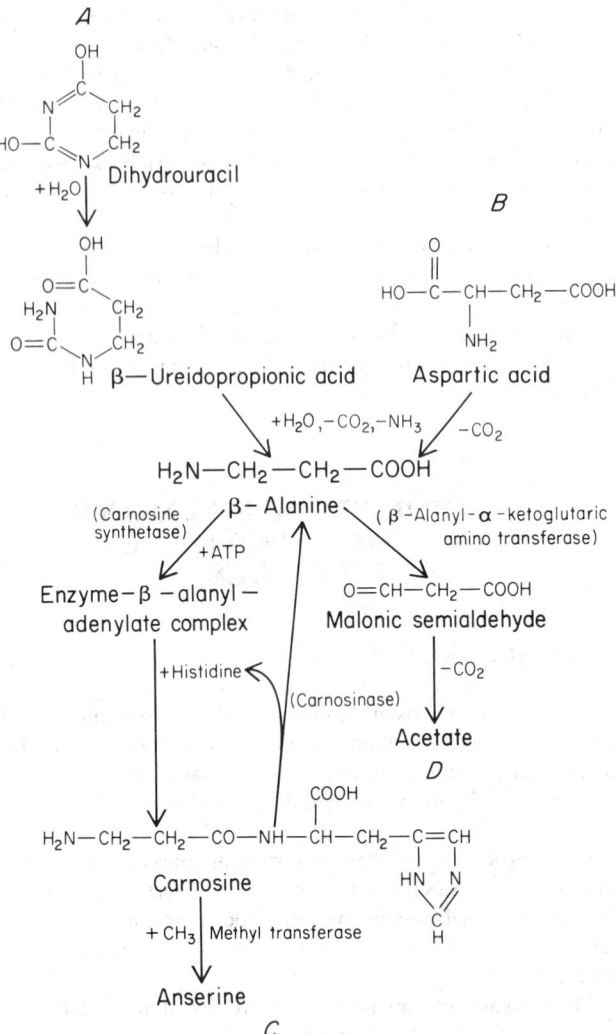

Figure 28-2 Simplified metabolic scheme for β-alanine and carnosine.

the result of mutation completely blocks oxidative catabolism of β-alanine in *Pseudomonas* [11, 12]. Little is known about the characteristics of this initial step of β-alanine oxidation in human or other mammalian tissues. It has been suggested [13] that β-alanine, γ-aminobutyric acid, and β-aminoisobutyric acid may utilize the same transaminase. Decarboxylation of malonic semialdehyde to form acetate [10] presumably occurs in human tissues as the next step toward complete oxidation to CO_2. β-Alanine oxidation is particularly vigorous in mammalian kidney cortex (Table 28-1).

Incorporation

β-ALANYL-IMIDAZOLE DIPEPTIDES The majority of β-alanine in the human body is bound in the dipeptide carnosine [14]. The bound concentration in skeletal muscle may be 500 times greater than the free form. Incorporation of β-alanine into carnosine (Figs. 28-2 and 28-3) is an important reaction which has been studied intensively in the skeletal muscles of mammals and birds. Carnosine is not present in cardiac muscle [15, 16]. It is present in brain, particularly in the primary olfactory pathways; its concentration in olfactory bulbs and olfactory epithelium is maintained by intact olfactory pathways. This suggests that it may play a role as a possible neurotransmitter [17]. It is synthesized by carnosine synthetase (EC

6.3.2.11), an enzyme which requires ATP during the formation of an enzyme-β-alanyl-adenylate complex [18–20]. L-Histidine is then united with β-alanine, and the dipeptide (β-alanyl-L-histidine) is released from the enzyme.

Skeletal muscle of birds and certain species of mammals, notably the rabbit, rat, and whale [21, 22], can also form anserine (β-alanyl-1-methyl-L-histidine) (Figs. 27-3 and 27-4). Anserine is absent from human skeletal muscle [2, 23]. The methyl group of anserine is added to the peptide after formation of carnosine by the enzyme S-adenosyl methionine: carnosine N-methyl transferase [20, 24]. Vitamin E deficiency causes impaired synthesis of anserine [25], and the dipeptide is lost from muscle.

The physiologic function of β-alanyl-imidazole dipeptides is not completely understood. Davey [22] has suggested that they may serve as buffers in stabilizing the pH of muscle contracting anaerobically. Avena and Bowen [26] have shown that carnosine and anserine serve in vitro as potent activators of myosin ATPase in concentrations comparable to those found in skeletal muscle. The dipeptides chelate copper [26a]. When transported into tissues, they enhance copper uptake and thus may participate in the pathogenesis of Wilson's disease. Anserine is most prominent in muscles of species where rapid contractile activity is a function of successful adaptation and survival (e.g., limb muscle of the rabbit and pectoral muscle of the bird, Fig. 28-4). Apparently anserine has some particular function apart from carnosine, which is worthy of the burden of the additional genetic and enzymatic apparatus in the cell.

COENZYME A β-Alanine is a constituent of coenzyme A in its pantothenate moiety (Fig. 28-3). Incorporation into pantothenic acid does not occur in mammalian tissues. Pantothenate is thus an essential human nutrient [27].

β-Alanyl-Dipeptide Catabolism Carnosine is hydrolyzed to β-alanine and histidine by the enzyme carnosinase,

Table 28-1 Distribution of β-alanine and carnosine (0.11 mM) after uptake by various tissues

	Kidney*	Intestine*	Skeletal Muscle*
Carnosine			
Total uptake rate (μmol per liter intracellular H_2O · min)	56.0	15.4	0.4
Percent of substrate:			
In original form	7.4	8.0	38.4
As alternative form†	4.9	83.7	61.6
As CO_2	87.7	8.3	0
β-ALANINE			
Total uptake rate (μmol per liter intracellular H_2O · min)	40.7	28.2	0.9
Percent of substrate:			
In original form	9.0	95.6	95.0
As alternative form†	0	0	5.0
As CO_2	91.0	4.4	0

* Period of incubation in minutes: kidney, 30 min for β-alanine and 60 min for carnosine; intestine, 15 min for both substrates; muscle, 60 min for both substrates.
† Alternative forms are carnosine for β-alanine, and β-alanine for carnosine.
SOURCE: Nutzenadel and Scriver [42].

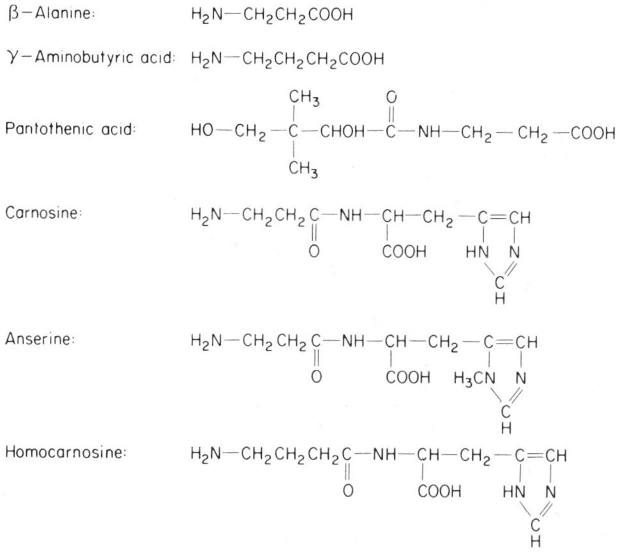

β-Alanine: $H_2N-CH_2CH_2COOH$

γ-Aminobutyric acid: $H_2N-CH_2CH_2CH_2COOH$

Pantothenic acid:

Carnosine:

Anserine:

Homocarnosine:

Figure 28-3 β-alanine and related compounds of interest in hyper-β-alaninemia and carnosinemia.

which has been found in the liver, spleen, and kidney of the rat [28], and has been isolated and purified from the kidney of swine [28, 29]. It is a metalloprotein, and although it is activated in vitro by both manganese and zinc ions, it is probable that zinc is the metal which occurs naturally in the enzyme of tissues [29]. Tissue carnosinase also hydrolyzes anserine to β-alanine and 1-methylhistidine [28]. The same enzyme, or at least one which is similar to that which hydrolyzes carnosine and anserine but not other imidazole dipeptides, is present in human serum [30].

Related Imidazole Dipeptides Cetasine, or β-alanyl-3-methyl-L-histidine, as well as anserine, occurs in the muscle of fin and sei whales [31]. homocarnosine, or γ-aminobutyryl-L-histidine (Fig. 28-3), was first isolated from bovine brain [32]; later it was also found in the brains of a number of other species of mammals, including humans [33]. Several workers [7, 34, 35] have investigated the regional distribution of homocarnosine in human brain. The concentration varies in different areas from 20 to 110 μmol per 100 g.

Homocarnosine, like its precursor, γ-aminobutyric acid, is found in the central nervous system. To date, it has not been found in other tissues. Human brain content of homocarnosine varies according to region [123]. Homocarnosine and carnosine are both synthesized in mammalian brain by the same enzyme, although this enzyme may not be identical with that which forms carnosine in muscle [36]. Homocarnosine is not hydrolyzed by the carnosinase present in human serum [30] but is hydrolyzed by tissue carnosinase from pig kidney [32]. The finding implies two forms of carnosinase with different specificity (see the section "Carnosinase Activity" under "Serum Carnosinase Deficiency"). The physiologic role of homocarnosine in human brain remains unknown.

Homocarnosine is found in normal brain in much larger amounts than carnosine [1, 33, 37, 38, 123]. Related dipeptides also found in mammalian tissues are homoanserine (γ-aminobutyryl-L-methylhistidine) in bovine brain [39], α-(γ-aminobutyryl)-lysine in the brain of a number of mammalian species [40], and α-(β-alanyl)-lysine in rabbit muscle [41]. The physiologic roles of these peptides are unknown.

Transport and Metabolism of β-Alanine and Carnosine

The uptake and metabolic fate of the dipeptide, and its β-amino acid constituent, have been studied in isolated enterocytes of jejunum, kidney cortex, and intact hemidiaphragm muscle in the rat [42]. These preparations expose different types of plasma membranes and also provide an opportunity to examine tissues which play different roles in β-alanine and carnosine metabolism (absorption by intestine, oxidation by kidney, and storage of dipeptide in striated skeletal muscle).

Amino nitrogen absorption from the diet in humans occurs largely in the form of oligopeptides [43–45]. Transport systems have been identified for oligopeptides with specificities which exclude significant interaction with free amino acids [46–48]. Because carnosine is quite slowly hydrolyzed inside the cell [43, 49–50], the characteristics of its uptake can be examined and compared with those of β-alanine. Furthermore, (amino) oxyacetic acid, an inhibitor of β-alanine transamination [42, 51], effectively blocks β-alanine metabolism after uptake, and provides an advantage equivalent to that gained in the blocked catabolic state in microbial mutants [12, 14] for the study of β-alanine and carnosine uptake.

Kidney takes up carnosine and β-alanine by membrane carriers which discriminate one substrate from the other and both from α-amino acids and other dipeptides (Fig. 28-4). Over 90 percent of the carnosine and β-alanine taken up is oxidized to CO_2 at concentrations that could be encountered in vivo (about 0.1 mM) (Table 18-1). Uptake by kidney cortex slices is achieved predominantly across the basilar membranes [52] and kinetic analysis of concentrations-dependent uptake reveals "low-K_m" (<0.2 mM) and "high-K_m" (>2.0 mM) carriers for β-alanine and carnosine. Taurine, another β-amino compound, metabolically inert in kidney and yet present at appreciable intracellular concentrations (10 to 20 mM), is taken up by the kidney at the same sites which serve β-alanine [53].

Intestinal enterocytes transport both substrates by their high-K_m systems only; the latter discriminate β-alanine and carnosine from each other and from the α-amino acids and other dipeptides. Intracellular hydrolysis, however, reduces the internal concentration of carnosine, so that uptake is not likely to occur against a chemical gradient in vivo although uptake against an isotopic gradient is achieved (Fig. 28-4). β-Alanine is readily taken up against a chemical gradient. Neither substance is oxidized efficiently by intestine (Table 28-1).

Striated muscle neither transports nor oxidizes β-alanine or carnosine vigorously. Uptake of the ^{14}C-labeled substrates, though mediated by discriminating membrane carriers, does not occur against an isotopic gradient (Fig. 27-4). However, the endogenous content of muscle carnosine is high enough [16] that uptake of the peptide could occur against a chemical gradient at 0.1 mM external concentration. The rate of peptide hydrolysis by carnosinase is low in muscle relative to intestine and kidney (Table 28-1).

These combined observations clearly indicate that plasma membranes of absorbing epithelium and internally oriented organs are endowed with reactive sites which specifically serve the uptake of β-amino acids and β-amino-N-terminal oligopeptides such as carnosine. The internal fate of the substrates depends on the tissue into which they enter.

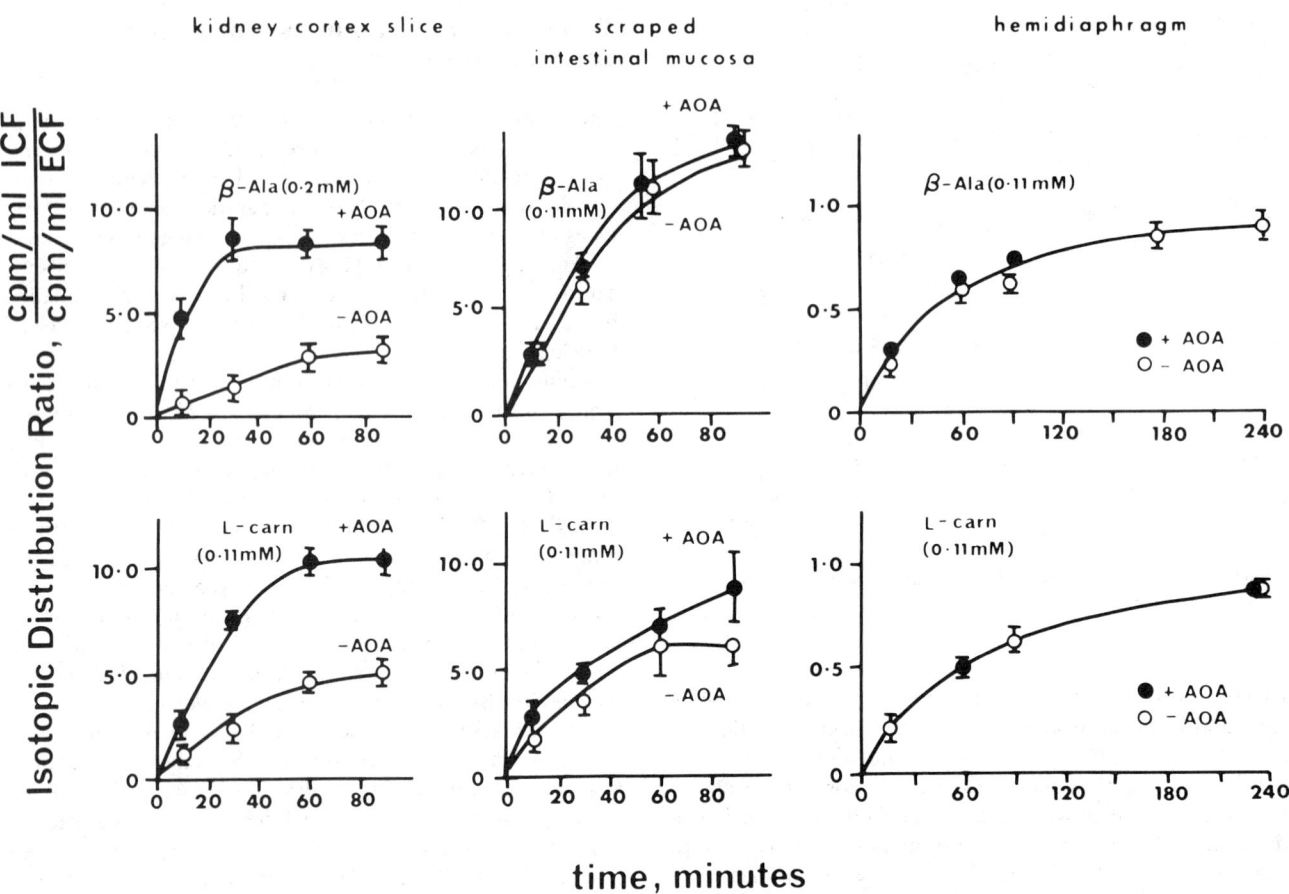

time, minutes

Figure 28-4 Uptake of ^{14}C-labeled β-alanine and carnosine ([1-^{14}C]β-alanyl-L-histidine) by intestinal enterocytes, kidney cortex slices, and intact hemidiaphragm preparations from the rat [42]. Other experiments shown that β-alanine is taken up by a system which discriminates β-amino compound from α-amino acids and from β-alanyl oligopeptides. As shown here uptake is concentrative (for both chemical and isotopic ratios) in kidney. Only β-alanine is concentrated against a chemical gradient in the enterocyte; carnosinase acts on the dipeptide in this tissue. Uptake will occur against a chemical gradient in vivo in muscle because of its endogenous concentration. AOA [(amino) oxyacetic acid] is an inhibitor of β-alanine transaminase and prevents oxidation to CO_2 with loss of label into gaseous phase.

Transport of β-Alanine and Carnosine in the Hartnup Trait

The segregation of β-alanine transport from carnosine uptake has been put to advantage in defining the nature of the intestinal transport defect in the Hartnup trait, a hereditary disorder in the transport of certain neutral α-amino acids [54] (Chap. 66). In the normal subject, constituent amino acids are released from carnosine more slowly into the systemic circulation than if equimolar amounts of free β-alanine and histidine are instilled into the intestinal lumen [49]; slow intracellular hydrolysis is believed to be the limiting step in the series of mechanisms that transfer substrate first across the brush border (luminal) membrane, through the intracellular pool, and finally out across the basilar membrane. In the patient with Hartnup's trait the blood histidine response is normal following carnosine feeding, but it is attenuated following L-histidine feeding [55]. Whether intracellular histidine in the enterocyte is derived from free extracellular histidine or from carnosine is of no concern to the efflux mechanism at the basilar membrane. Therefore, a normal blood response after carnosine loading indicates that efflux integrity is intact in patients with the Hartnup trait. The transport defect must, therefore, be confined to the luminal membrane. The transport defect itself is highly selective, affecting free amino acids and not the dipeptide and affecting only an α-amino acid-binding site and not the β-amino-preferring system [55]. The Hartnup trait thus corroborates the above-mentioned delineation of β-amino acid and β-alanyl peptide transport systems.

Imidazole Dipeptides in Physiologic Fluids and Relation to Diet

Carnosine and anserine are not detectable in the fasting plasma of normal persons, nor are they usually found in significant amounts in the urine of normal subjects who are consuming diets low in meat. Normal urine contains scores of unidentified ninhydrin-reacting compounds, some of which include β-alanine and imidazole in peptide linkage [56]. For this reason, qualitative identification of carnosine or anserine in the urine should first be made with paper chromatography or electrophoresis. If a large amount of either dipeptide is present, then the amino acid analyzer can properly be employed for quantitation.

Normal persons consuming considerable carnosine or anserine in their diet, as they do if they eat chicken or turkey [2, 23, 57–59], excrete these dipeptides in the urine, presumably because they escape complete hydrolysis in the intestine. After absorption they will then appear in blood, from which they can be cleared by glomerular filtration into urine without efficient reclamation by the renal tubule. Under these conditions a person may have carnosine in the plasma 2 h after a heavy meal of meat [2]. Since renal clearance of dipeptides is high, the urine reflects the endogenous appearance of these compounds better than plasma. All forms of meat and poultry, including soup stocks made from meat, contain carnosine. The most common dietary sources of anserine are chicken, turkey, duck, and rabbit. White meat of chicken or turkey seems to be one of the richest dietary sources of anserine [23, 57] (Fig. 28-5).

Subjects fed large amounts of carnosine or anserine may also excrete small amounts of free β-alanine in the urine [2, 23, 56]. The consumption of even modest amounts of anserine in the diet regularly leads to the appearance of 1-methylhistidine in the urine [23, 58, 59], except in patients with carnosinemia [2]. 1-Methylhistidine is irregularly detectable when fasting human plasma is chromatographed on the amino acid analyzer; its appearance probably indicates recent consumption of anserine-containing foods. Since renal clearance of 1-methylhistidine is rapid [60, 61], the urine is more likely to reflect its presence than plasma. Large amounts of 1-methylhistidine in urine may give a green ferric chloride reaction when the reagent is added dropwise to the urine [23]. Dietary carnosinuria is found more frequently in young children than in adults, and presumably reflects a relatively lower level of serum carnosinase activity in children than in adults [30].

Homocarnosine is not detectable in the plasma or urine of normal subjects, but this dipeptide is routinely found in the gray matter of the brain [62] and in the CSF of normal children [63]. It can usually be detected in the CSF of normal adults and in neurologically diseased adults. In 27 neurologically normal infants and children under the age of $3\frac{1}{2}$ years, the mean homocarnosine concentration in the CSF was 8 μmol/liter. The mean concentration in the CSF of 43 adults with a variety of neurologic disorders was 1.8 μmol/liter [64].

HYPER-β-ALANINEMIA

A more detailed version of the clinical features is found in the third and fourth editions of this text and the original report [1]. A résumé is provided here.

> The only reported patient was a 2-month-old male at diagnosis; he died in the 5th month of life with an uncontrolled seizure disorder punctuated by extreme somnolence. Persistent lethargy was observed from birth after a normal delivery in the 38th week of gestation. Intrauterine movements had been obtunded. Seizures appeared at the 7th week of life. The moro and sucking reflexes were impaired. The infant was continuously somnolent and hypotonic. All anticonvulsant medications were ineffective.
>
> At autopsy, performed 2h postmortem, the brain was small (470 g vs 620 ± 71 g); body length and weight were below the 3d percentile for age. Cerebral ventricles were enlarged, the white matter demarcation was blurred and diffuse edema was present. Beading of myelin sheaths was the only significant abnormality observed by microscopy.

Laboratory Findings in Hyper-β-alaninemia

The most important finding was made initially on a urine specimen. Although results of a number of simple chemical screening tests [65, 66] were normal, a partition filter paper chromatogram of the urine revealed a striking abnormality in amino acid excretion (Fig. 28-6). A large amount of β-alanine was present; this substance is normally detected in human urine only in very small amounts [6, 56] during urinary putrefaction. The excretion of β-aminoisobutyric acid and of taurine was particularly prominent. Another unusual ninhydrin-reactive component was found (Fig. 28-5) and identified as GABA [1].

The concentrations of β-alanine and GABA were also increased in the plasma and in cerebrospinal fluid (Table 27-2). Neither substance is detected normally in CSF [63, 64, 67], and only β-alanine is present, in very small amounts, in normal plasma [4, 5, 61]. With the exception of the β-amino acids and GABA, the concentrations of all other free amino acids in plasma and urine were normal. The concentrations in body fluids of the dipeptides carnosine and anserine, and of pantothenic acid, were also normal at all times.

Family History and Inheritance

The patient was the fourth child of the second marriage of an Anglo-Canadian mother to a French Canadian (Fig. 28-7). A half-brother (II-1) and half-sister (II-2) of the patient are

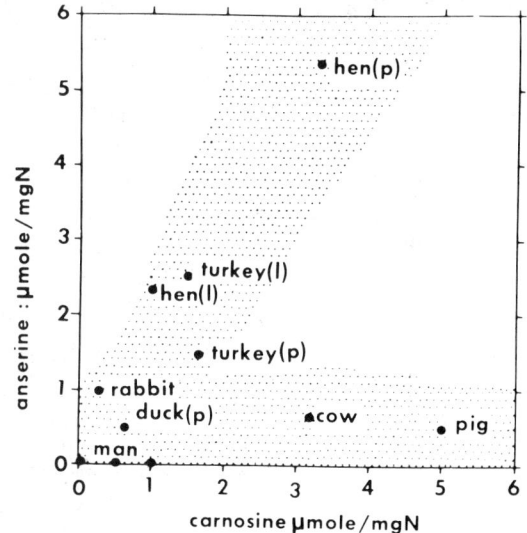

Figure 28-5 Carnosine and anserine content of muscle in various species. In all cases, skeletal muscle was analyzed [16]. p, pectoral muscle; l, leg muscle. Limb muscles examined where type not specified.

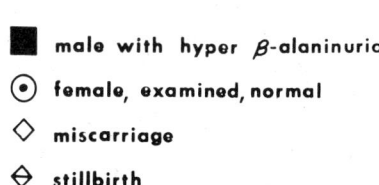

■ male with hyper β-alaninuria

⊙ female, examined, normal

◇ miscarriage

⬦ stillbirth

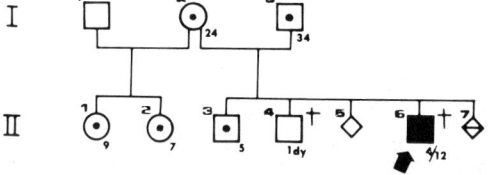

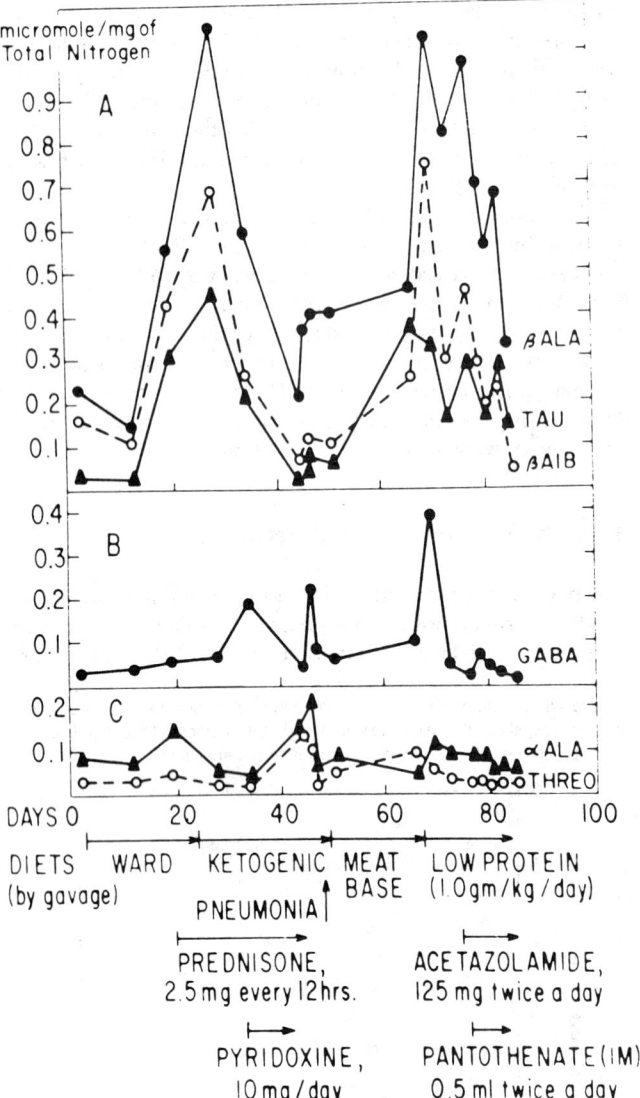

Figure 28-6 Excretion of β-amino compounds, β-alanine, taurine, and β-aminoisobutyric acid in urine of a patient with hyper-β-alaninemia under various conditions of diet and medication. Excretion of GABA, which is independent of the excretion of β-amino acids, is also shown. Excretion of two α-amino acids, threonine and α-alanine, is shown to indicate specificity of hyper-β-aminoaciduria. (*Reproduced from Scriver et al. [1], with permission.*)

healthy. Four children were conceived by the second father; only the eldest (II-3) is alive and well. The second child (II-4) died with "breathing trouble" 4 h after birth. The third pregnancy (II-5) terminated in a miscarriage at the third month. The mother had one further pregnancy in 1966 after the proband died; this child (II-7) was stillborn at term. There is no consanguinity between the parents, and they have no relatives with convulsive disorders, mental retardation, or chronic diseases. The available living members of the immediate family were investigated for β-alaninuria before and after a meat-containing meal, but the amino acid content of the urine was normal. The information is not sufficient for any definite statement concerning the presumed inheritance of hyper-β-alaninemia, but the circumstances of the pedigree suggest that the trait, if it is inherited, is autosomal recessive.

Hyper-β-alaninemia in liveborn infants is apparently a rare disease. Although many thousands of patients with manifestations of disordered function of the nervous system have been examined with reliable chromatographic methods throughout the world, only one additional proband with a fatal neurologic condition resembling that described here, and accompanied by presumed hyper-β-alaninuria, on at least one occasion, has been discussed with the authors; additional information is not available.

Proposed Site of Metabolic Defect in Hyper-β-alaninemia

The normal distribution of certain free amino acids in hyper-β-alaninemia (Table 28-2) is only part of the story. Tissues obtained within 2 h of death [1] revealed another aspect of this disease. The concentration of carnosine in the tissues was six times greater than in the postmortem tissues of age-matched controls (Table 28-3). The increase of carnosine paralleled the excess of free β-alanine. The accumulation of carnosine cannot be attributed to deficient carnosinase activity, for when this occurs, as in carnosinemia [2, 30], carnosine is present in plasma and is also excreted in urine, yet the concentration of free β-alanine is normal. The accumulation of carnosine in tissues in hyper-β-alaninemia can therefore be attributed to overproduction of the dipeptide in the presence of an expanded free β-alanine pool.

Accumulation of homocarnosine was not recognized if it was present, but it is possible that it could occur as a result of the increased amount of GABA available for synthesis by a mechanism analogous to that proposed for the augmentation of brain carnosine in hyper-β-alaninemia.

There is no evidence that intestinal overproduction of β-alanine accounted for the disorder. Fecal amino acid content was normal, particularly with respect to β-alanine and aspartic acid [1]. Overproduction from uracil was not specifically investigated, but it seems an unlikely cause of hyper-β-alaninemia in humans.

Impaired oxidation of β-alanine is the most probable cause of the abnormality. Malonic semialdehyde was not found in urine extracted with 2,4-dinitrophenylhydrazine [10, 68] and examined chromatographically. Furthermore, hydrogenation of the phenylhydrazine derivatives [69] did not produce detectable amounts of β-alanine. Thus, though these studies involved an unstable compound and were performed on acidified urine which had been frozen at −20°C for 4 months, there appeared to be no accumulation of malonic semialdehyde. A block in decarboxylation, accordingly, is unlikely.

Figure 28-7 Pedigree of a proband with hyper-β-alaninuria.

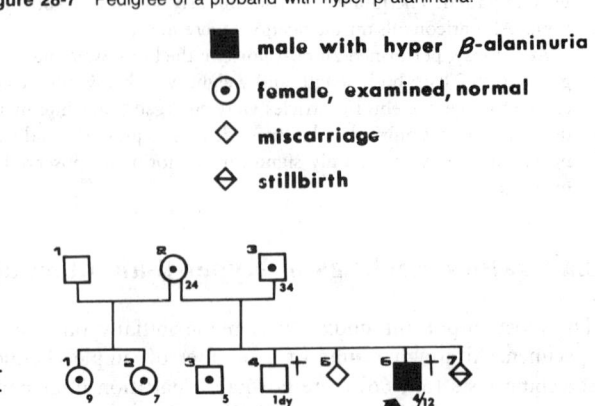

Table 28-2   Concentration of β-alanine and γ-aminobutyric acid in body fluids

Amino acid	Source*	Plasma μmol/liter		Urine, μmol/g total nitrogen		Cerebrospinal fluid, μmol/liter
		Mean	Range	Mean	Range	
β-Alanine	Normal	—	14	—	10	0
	Patient	33.0	20–51	564	140–1060	45
GABA	Normal	0	—	0	—	0
	Patient	4.4	1–7	81	25–400	1–2

* Normal values from Dickinson et al. [5], and from data cited and compiled elsewhere [4].

If β-alanine oxidation was indeed impaired in the disorder, it is more likely that the defect was at the stage of transamination. Two features point to this possibility:

1. The transaminase requires pyridoxal-5-phosphate as coenzyme. One trial of pyridoxine (10 mg/day) during the lifetime of the patient was accompanied by an abrupt fall in β-alanine excretion (Fig. 28-6). When administration of pyridoxine was stopped, β-alanine excretion rose sharply. The specificity of the response may be questioned, since fluctuation in β-alanine excretion occurred at times when pyridoxine intake did not vary. Unfortunately, because no clinical improvement accompanied it, this interesting biochemical response to the vitamin was recognized only when analyses were completed after the infant had died.

2. The concentration of GABA, which is a presynaptic neuroinhibitor substance [72, 73], was elevated in postmortem samples of brain and kidney (Table 28-3), and GABA was also detected in plasma, CSF, and urine (Table 28-3). Therefore, the metabolism of GABA also seems to have been impaired. Glutamic acid decarboxylase (GAD) and its product, GABA, which were once thought to be present only in brain [75–76], have now been identified in nonneural tissues, including kidney [70, 71, 77–80]. This may explain the accumulation of GABA in the kidney. Free GABA in brain is either bound to membrane sites [76] or degraded by transamination; GABA and β-alanine probably share the same transaminase [3, 8]. Loss of this transaminase might thus cause accumulation of β-alanine and GABA. On the other hand, there is evidence [82] that β-alanine is not the natural substrate for GABA transaminase in brain, and that β-alanine is an inhibitor of its activity [71, 82]. Thus GABA accumulation might have reflected only a secondary effect of a deficiency in a specific β-alanine transaminase, which caused β-alanine accumulation and competitive inhibition of GABA transaminase.

Mechanism for β-Aminoaciduria in Hyper-β-alaninemia

A combined mechanism underlies the excretion of β-amino acids in hyper-β-alaninemia. β-Alanine concentration in plasma is elevated. Its own high excretion rate, which is directly proportional to the plasma concentration (Fig. 28-8A), can therefore be attributed to increasing occupancy of the membrane site at which it is transported in the tubule. This form of hyperaminoaciduria is the result of a saturation mechanism.[1] However, the urinary excretion of β-aminoisobutyric

acid (βAIB), which may occur by secretion as well as by filtration [87], was not proportional to its plasma concentration in the patient. Instead, βAIB excretion varied in direct proportion to the concentration of β-alanine in the plasma (Fig. 28-8B). Similarly, taurine excretion in urine varied more in relation to β-alanine in plasma than to its own plasma concentration (Fig. 28-8C). Therefore, βAIB and taurine were excreted in excess because of impaired tubular conservation of these two compounds. The determinant of this relationship presumably was the degree of hyper-β-alaninemia.

If one postulates that β-amino compounds are transported at a common site with preference for these solutes over α-amino acids, then the mechanism of the hyper-β-aminoaciduria becomes apparent. At the high concentrations of β-alanine found in the patient the amino acid behaved as a competitive inhibitor at the membrane site shared by the other two substrates. The latter were displaced, appearing in the urine as if by a "renal" mechanism [84–86]. The selective hyperaminoaciduria involving β-amino acids was therefore the result of combined overflow and renal mechanisms [87]. A similar mechanism accounts for the selective hyperaminoaciduria (iminoglycinuria) of hyperprolinemia [88] (see Chap. 18).

Evidence for a membrane site with preference for β-amino acid transport has been found under other circumstances. Gilbert et al. [89] studied interactions between β-amino compounds in mouse kidney in vivo and found indications of a

Table 28-3   Concentration of β-alanine, carnosine, and GABA in postmortem tissues of a patient with hyper-β-alaninemia

Tissue	Source*	β-Alanine, μmol/g wet wt	Carnosine, μmol/g wet wt	GABA, μmol/g wet wt
Brain	Patient	0.20	0.39	3.83†
	Control	0	<0.02	0.8†
Muscle‡	Patient	0.07–0.11	36.1–45.0	<0.02
	Control	<0.01	6.62–6.84	0
Liver	Patient	0.36	0	<0.02
	Control	0.16	0	0
Kidney	Patient	1.12	0	0.24
	Control	—	—	0.03–0.45§

* Postmortem control is an age-matched, male patient with Werdnig-Hoffmann disease. Tissues from patient and control were obtained 2 and 3 h, respectively, after death.

† Values indicate total (bound and free) GABA in occipital cortex, deproteinized with picric acid [1]. The patient's value is high for his age when compared with control and published data on infants and children [83]. The wide range of published control values [38, 62, 83] reflects techniques of tissue preparation and an age effect, since GABA content of brain increases during human infancy [83].

‡ Deltoid and rectus abdominis.

§ Values obtained from Whelan et al. [70] and Zachmann et al. [71].

---

[1] The terms *overflow* and *prerenal* are often used to describe the hyperaminoaciduria occurring by a saturation mechanism; they suggest the catalytic nature of membrane transport of amino acids [84–86].

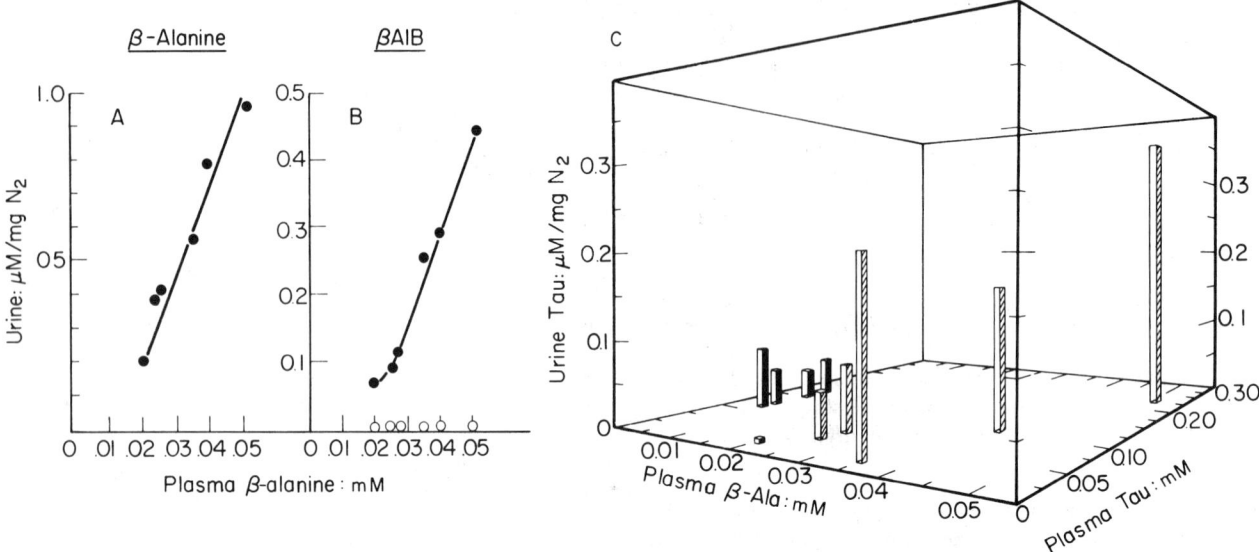

Figure 28-8 Excretion of β-amino compounds (A, β-alanine; B, β-amino-isobutyric acid; C, taurine) in relation to plasma concentration of β-alanine in the patient with hyper-β-alaninuria. The direct relationship indicates that hyper-β-aminoaciduria reflects interaction at a tubular transport site selective for these compounds. This specific aminoaciduria is of the "combined" type, representing overflow (β-alanine) and renal (βAIB and taurine) mechanisms, the latter by virtue of competitive inhibition by β-alanine. (*Reproduced from Scriver et al.* [1], *with permission.*)

tubular absorptive system with preference for β-amino acids. Wilson and Scriver [90] and Goldman and Scriver [91] studied interactions between β-amino compounds in the rat in vivo and found that β-amino acids interacted with one another but not with α-amino acids during tubular absorption. Christensen [92] and Nutzenadel and Scriver [42] found evidence for β-amino–preferring membrane transport systems in a variety of mammalian tissues, including the ascites tumor cell, intestinal enterocytes, kidney tubule epithelium, and striated muscle. Rozen et al. [93] found β-amino acid recognition sites that determine reclamation of β-alanine and taurine from urine, located in the brush border membrane in the mammalian nephron.

GABAuria

GABA and other ω-amino acids are poorly transported across plasma cell membranes [94]. In the patient, the GABAuria varied independently of the β-alanine concentration in urine (Fig. 28-6) but in direct proportion to its own plasma level [1]. GABAuria was accordingly related to the initial impairment of GABA metabolism and apparently not to any modulation in tubular transport. Because metabolism by the GABA pathway in mammalian kidney cortex is significant, supporting at least one-quarter of glutamate oxidation [78], it is possible that a transamination defect affecting GABA oxidation would cause intrarenal GABA to accumulate and appear in urine by a mechanism of efflux from tubular cells into urine. The intensity of GABA excretion in urine relative to its level in plasma in hyper-β-alaninemia is compatible with that interpretation of GABAuria in this disease.

Interpretation of Clinical Symptoms

β-alanine is a neuroinhibitory substance in cortex, brainstem, and spinal cord [95]. The depressed activity of the central nervous system could have been one manifestation of hyper-β-alaninemia.

GABA, too, is a neuroinhibitory substance [74, 96], and depletion of GABA in brain produces seizures [75]. GABA acts

as a neuroinhibitor following a presynaptic binding, and β-alanine inhibits binding of GABA by brain [97]. Thus, although the total amount of GABA was elevated in the brain of the patient with hyper-β-alaninemia, it is possible that the amount bound to the sites which mediate its neurochemical effect was actually decreased. The seizures may have reflected this postulated imbalance.

GABA also participates in an "oxidative shunt" which has quantitative significance in brain metabolism [98]. Any inhibition of GABA oxidation would depress the activity of this shunt and contribute to the pathogenesis of seizures in hyper-β-alaninemia by a metabolic, rather than a neurochemical, mechanism.

The significance of an elevated level of carnosine (and possibly of homocarnosine) in brain must also be considered [99, 100]. Carnosinemia [2] and hyper-β-alaninemia are both accompanied by retarded development of the nervous system and a severe convulsive disorder. Only the latter has impaired metabolism of β-alanine and GABA; in both carnosinemia and hyper-β-alaninemia there is some abnormality of imidazole dipeptide metabolism. Thus, one might ask: Is too much carnosine (and homocarnosine) harmful to the central nervous system? Allen et al. [100] have found that homocarnosine is present in excess in phenylketonuric brain fluid and CSF. Further study of this facet of dipeptide metabolism is required before the question can be answered.

Diagnosis

The color of β-alanine on a partition chromatogram developed in Dent's system [101] and stained with ninhydrin is so unmistakable that diagnosis should not be missed in a simple preliminary chromatographic investigation. Urine is the preferred source of material for diagnosis, since it also contains the other β-amino compounds and GABA. The latter substance is not found in normal human urine [6, 56]. Since the plasma concentrations of β-alanine and GABA are low even if abnormally elevated, one cannot expect detection of the trait in the newborn by the simple screening methods which have been used to discover amino acidopathies in blood and plasma [102, 103]. These screening methods permit detection of β-alanine only when the concentration in plasma exceeds 0.1 mM; the concentration in the patient did not exceed 0.05mM.

Acquired causes of β-alaninuria should be excluded and confirmatory investigations should be performed when the patient is not on a diet rich in foods containing carnosine or anserine. Certain drugs may also cause hyper-β-alaninuria; they include isoniazid, amino oxyacetic acid [104], and γ-vinyl GABA [105]. We have studied one patient treated with isoniazid for a granulomatous disease. Prominent hyper-β-alaninuria was observed, and the plasma β-alanine concentration was 0.025 mM. The abnormality of β-alanine metabolism disappeared when pyridoxine was added. This form of β-alaninuria is probably caused by the inhibition of β-alanine transaminase following depletion of pyridoxine by isoniazid.

Treatment

No effective therapy was discovered during the lifetime of the patient (Fig. 28-6). Only one agent showed therapeutic promise. Pyridoxine appeared to restore some degree of biochemical order in the patient; pyridoxal-5-phosphate is the coenzyme for β-alanine transaminase. Although no clinical improvement accompanied the temporary reduction of β-alanine accumulation, it is possible that the biochemical disorder would respond to vitamin B_6 therapy, as have other inborn errors of amino acid metabolism [106].

SERUM CARNOSINASE DEFICIENCY

Patients have been reported with a biochemical phenotype (Table 28-4) characterized by persistent carnosinuria and serum and tissue carnosinase deficiency; the associated clinical features, although striking, do not consistently accompany the biochemical phenotype and thus may not be a primary feature of the trait.

Current reports [2, 3, 107, 109] indicate that probands with serum carnosinase deficiency come to medical attention because of neurologic symptoms (Table 28-4), usually myoclonic seizures and psychomotor retardation, apparent in the first year of life. Overt manifestations are accompanied by nonspecific electroencephalographic abnormalities. If the clinical course permits survival, severe mental retardation and spasticity declare themselves in later infancy and childhood. Where pathology findings are available [108, 111], axonal degeneration in peripheral nerves, demyelination of pyrimidal and spinal cerebellar tracts, Purkinje cell loss, cerebellar gliosis, and neuronal loss in the cerebral cortex are reported, as well as deteriorative findings in muscle cells.

Severe neurologic disease associated with serum carnosinase deficiency has been observed in probands (patients A1, B1, C1, and D1, Table 28-4) and sibs (patient D3). Evidence against a consistent clinical deficit in serum carnosinase deficiency consists of observations of one female sib (patient D2), who in her fifth year of life was "developing normally, [with] normal intelligence and no apparent physical abnormalities" [109];

and of a proband [110] detected by newborn screening who is healthy at 20 months despite evidence for tissue carnosinase deficiency.

Biochemical Features

Carnosinuria Carnosine excretion by normal children and adults on standard diets is negligible (<20 μmol/g creatinine [112]); but it will occur readily when carnosine-containing diets are ingested during infancy [23], presumably because serum carnosinase activity is low in infancy. Persistence of excessive carnosinuria, even when dietary sources of carnosine (meat and fowl, Fig. 28-5) are excluded, is a consistent finding in persons with serum carnosinase deficiency. When carnosinuria occurs under conditions of strict dietary control, it is assumed that the origin of the dipeptide is endogenous. The quantity of carnosine excreted during ingestion of meat-free diets varies between 0.5 and 1 mmol per gram creatinine; the amount is two- to threefold higher on a regular diet [2, 107, 109]. Anserine is not excreted by patients with serum carnosinase deficiency, unless an exogenous source of anserine exists since human tissues contain no anserine (Fig. 28-5).

Urinary carnosine and anserine excretions can be sharply increased by feeding meat or fowl to subjects with serum carnosinase deficiency [2, 107, 109]. The normal subject responds to the anserine challenge by excreting large amounts of 1-methylhistidine [23, 109], which is otherwise without an endogenous source in humans; patients with serum carnosinase deficiency excrete either no 1-methylhistidine [2] or only small amounts upon exposure to anserine [107, 109].

Serum Carnosine Levels Carnosinemia is absent in normal subjects; it was present in the first-reported proband (patient A1, Table 28-4), and it was this finding which led to use of the term *carnosinemia* to describe the trait [2, 3, 30]. However, serum carnosine levels may not be consistently elevated in a given patient [2, 30, 107, 110]. The customary serum carnosine levels in the probands of two pedigrees (B and C) were lower than in the probands of the A and D pedigrees (Table 28-4). Therefore reliance on "carnosinemia" as a diagnostic feature may be unwise. Some authors [107] have recommended that the term *carnosinemia* be replaced by *serum carnosinase deficiency*.

Carnosine and Homocarnosine in Cerebrospinal Fluid Homocarnosine was present at normal levels (11 μmol/liter) in the CSF of patient A1; carnosine was absent from CSF in the same patient [2, 30], which is a normal finding and suggests that the level of brain carnosine was not elevated in the patient. The observation has not been reported in other patients.

Carnosine and Homocarnosine in Tissues Skeletal muscle and brain were examined at autopsy in patient B1 [2]. Neither carnosine (0.67 to 0.81 μmol per gram wet weight) nor homocarnosine (0.14 μmol per gram wet weight) was elevated in concentration when compared with concentrations in control subjects of various ages, implying adequate tissue dipeptidase activity.

Carnosinase Activity An assay for carnosinase in serum was developed by Perry et al. [30]. The amounts of histidine and β-alanine produced by the enzymatic hydrolysis of carnosine are estimated quantitatively on an amino acid analyzer.

Table 28-4 Serum carnosinase activity: controls, patients, and parents

Pedigree	Case no.	Sex	Age at dx. yr.	Carnosin-uria*	Serum carnosine µM†	Serum carnosinase activity (per age)‡	1-methyl histidine formed in vivo§	Neurologic symptoms	Ref.
						METHOD A (µmol/ml · 16 h)			
A	1	M	11/12	+	0–53	2.3 (8³/₁₂)	0	+	2,30
B	1	M	4/12	+	0–3	0.7 (9/12 yr)	0	+	2,30
C	1	M	3⁸/₁₂	+	<0.5	0.5–1.1 (3⁸/₁₂)	+	+	105
	2¶	M	2/12	+		0 (2/12)	—	0	—
						METHOD B (µmol/ml · h)			
D	1	M	7	+	30	<0.03 (7)	+	+	106,107
	2	F	4⁸/₁₂	+	—	<0.03 (4⁸/₁₂)	—	+	—
	3	M	3⁶/₁₂	+	—	<0.03 (3⁶/₁₂)	—	0	—
E	1	M	1/12	+	+	"Normal"	?	0	107
F	1	M	12	+	0	(1 (14% of control)	+	+	107

* Carnosinuria is of endogenous origin and >20 µmol per gram creatinine on meat-free diet; levels in phenotype >500 µmol per gram creatinine.
† Carnosinemia is an inconsistent occurence in phenotype.
‡ Method A [30, 107], normal values (µmol/ml · 16 h): 1–12 yr, 10 ± 6.2 SD; adults 20.1 ± 7.6 SD. Method B [109, 113], normal values (µmol/ml · h): children 0.1–5.2; adults, 2–7. Van Munster assay [114], normal value (µmol/liter per minute): infants 0.82 (n = 19); adults, 44.2 ± 14 SD.
§ After feeding anserine.
¶ Follow-up data not available. Validity of diagnosis open to question.

The peptidase in normal human serum readily hydrolyzes L-carnosine and L-anserine but shows no activity toward three other imidazole dipeptides, L-homocarnosine, β-L-aspartyl-L-histidine, and L-histidyl-L-proline [30]. The assay has been modified slightly [107] to increase its sensitivity, by increasing the serum volume threefold. Another version of the assay [113] carries out the reaction in 0.3 M tris HCl buffer pH 8 and measures histidine released by a fluorimetric method. Yet another version [114] carries out the reaction under comparable conditions of incubation for 1 h but uses labeled β-alanine in the substrate, which, after cleavage and separation from the reaction mixture by partition chromatography, is measured by scintillation spectrometry.

Serum Carnosinase Levels Serum carnosinase activity is age-dependent in normal subject (Fig. 28-9); the level of activity is low during infancy and rises during childhood to reach adult levels by early adolescence. Low serum carnosinase activity may account for the prominent carnosinuria and anserinuria which follows the ingestion of chicken during infancy.

Serum carnosinase activity is depressed in most patients (Table 28-4). Two probands have a variant pattern: One, (case E [110], has normal serum activity with carnosinuria, implying deficient tissue activity; the other, case F [111], has partial deficiency of tissue and serum carnosinase and has neurologic symptoms. Carnosinuric patients usually have deficient anserine cleavage activity [107]. Some parents (pedigrees A, C, D, and F) but not all (pedigrees B and E) have partial deficiency of serum carnosinase activity compatible with heterozygosity for an autosomal allele.

Serum carnosinase activity can be raised in the affected proband by infusion of normal plasma [107]. The exogenous carnosinase activity is cleared from plasma within about 24 h. In vitro mixing experiments, using serum from normal subjects and patients, yield the expected combined activity [30, 109].

This indicates that a circulating inhibitor of serum carnosinase activity is not the cause of its deficiency in the trait.

Tissue Carnosinase Significant carnosinase activity was first reported by Perry et al. [2] in liver, kidney, and heart of one patient at autopsy, despite demonstrable serum carnosinase deficiency in life (patient B1, Table 28-4). Moreover, postmortem blood in the patient contained 30 times the carnosinase activity measured in serum before death. This obser-

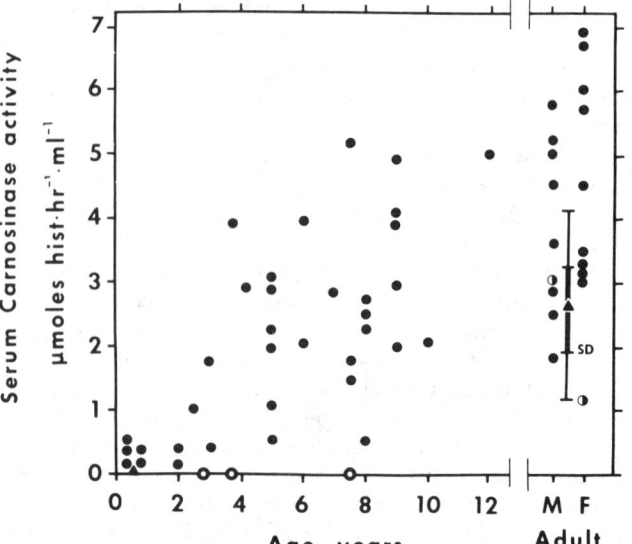

Figure 28-9 Serum carnosinase activity according to age in normal subjects (●), from the data of Murphey et al. [109]. Additional data from Van Munster et al. (▲) showing mean values (and ± 1 SD and range in adults) for infants and adults [114] are added to show that age-dependent relationships are not altered by the assay method. Data for three probands with serum carnosinase deficiency in the D pedigree (O) are shown [109]; data on the parents of these patients are also given (◑).

vation suggests that tissues may contain a form of carnosinase activity that is different from that normally present in serum; evidence in support of this hypothesis is now at hand.

Murphey and colleagues [109, 113] have described two forms of carnosinase activity in postmortem human tissues which can be separated by starch-block electrophoresis (Fig. 28-10). The two forms exhibit no differences in their substrate specificity or in their relative cleavage activity against various dipeptides [113]. Carnosinase specific activity is highest in kidney (cortical and medullary activity being about equal), least in liver, and intermediate in spleen; the range of activity in these tissues varied between about 0.1 and 0.6 μmol histidine released per hour per milligram of protein. Intestine was not assayed, and skeletal muscle contained no carnosinase activity. Postmortem tissues from patient D1 (Table 28-4) contained only one form of carnosinase activity (Fig. 28-10); the more negatively charged form of the enzyme was deficient in the subject with serum carnosinase deficiency. Total carnosinase activity was most deficient in the postmortem liver of this patient, and relatively more activity was retained in kidney; this observation is in keeping with a relative predominance of the positively charged form of carnosinase in normal kidney and a more equal distribution between the two forms in normal liver (Fig. 28-10).

At present it is unknown whether the retention of slight but significant cleavage activity, as reflected in the modest capacity for 1-methylhistidine formation from anserine in serum carnosinase-deficient subjects (e.g. patients C1 [107] and D1 [109]), indicates the action of a small residual serum activity or the effect of tissue carnosinase on dipeptide that enters kidney and liver, for example [42], then to be cleaved. The retention of one form of carnosinase in the tissues is the likely explanation for the normal tissue carnosine content observed in proband B1 post mortem [2]. Dipeptide leaking from tissues is apparently not hydrolyzed rapidly enough in the presence of serum carnosinase deficiency to prevent rapid dipeptide clearance into urine.

Diagnosis

The diagnosis of carnosinuria is suspected when two-dimensional paper chromatography of urine discloses carnosine or anserine. When pyridine:acetone:ammonium hydroxide:water (45:30:5:20) is used as the first solvent, followed by isopropanol:formic acid:water (75:12.5:12.5) as the second solvent, and the sheets are sprayed with ninhydrin-lutidine [115], carnosine and anserine appear as yellow or tan-yellow spots close to and partially overlapping histidine. The two dipeptides can be conveniently identified if the chromatogram is countersprayed with diazotized sulfanilic acid. When this is done, histidine turns from purple to orange-brown, carnosine turns red, anserine turns grayish-blue, and all other ninhydrin-positive spots on the chromatogram are decolorized [2]. Carnosine and anserine can also be identified by their characteristic positions and colors with the same staining reagents, when the chromatogram is developed in a phenollutidine system [101].

To distinguish between true carnosinemia and the relatively common carnosinuria that follows consumption of large amounts of meat or poultry, the patient can be fed white meat of chicken or turkey as a source of anserine. If urine collected after such a meal contains easily detectable 1-methylhistidine, the possibility of serum carnosinase deficiency is excluded. 1-

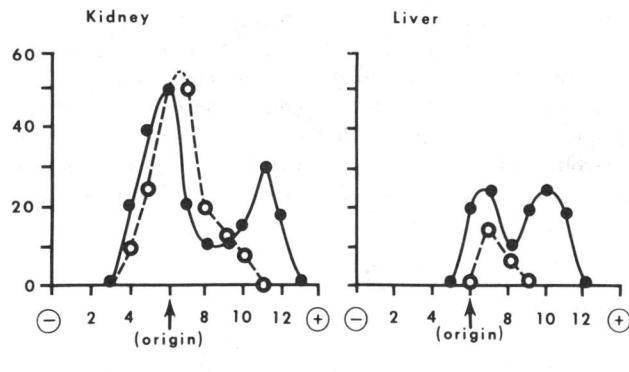

Figure 28-10 Evidence for more than one form of carnosinase activity in human tissues. The carnosinase assay [113] has been applied to 1-cm sections of starch block after electrophoresis of the 2000 × g × 20-min supernatant from a 200-mM sucrose homogenate of tissues. Electrophoresis was performed at 4°C in phosphate-citrate buffer, pH 7.0, at 7.5 mA/cm × 4 h. Elution for assay performed directly in a 1 to 8-ml carnosinase assay mixture. Normal tissue (●—●) yields positively and negatively charged carnosinase activities; the latter fraction is largely absent in patients with serum carnosinase deficiency (O—O). Application of the technique to serum has not yet been reported.

Methylhistidine is conveniently identified by two-dimensional paper chromatography of urine.[2] If 1-methylhistidine is absent from the urine at a time when the urine contains anserine, determination of serum carnosinase is indicated; the finding of little or no carnosinase activity in blood confirms the diagnosis of carnosinemia. The absence of 1-methylhistidine from the urine, if it contains anserine and carnosine, also differentiates "carnosinemia" from the imidazoluria reported by Bessman and Baldwin [116], Levenson et al. [117], and Tocci and Bessman [112] in children with juvenile amaurotic idiocy (Spielmeyer-Vogt syndrome).

Confirmation of serum carnosinase deficiency can be obtained by any of the existing assays [30, 107, 109, 113, 114]. Caution is required in the interpretation of low activity in the postnatal period and during infancy (Fig. 28-9). Demonstration of a deficiency of the negatively charged component of tissue carnosinase would be desirable, but at present no data on the ontogeny of tissue activity, for comparison with serum activity, have been published to our knowledge.

Therapy

Unlike the tissue carnosine accumulation which characterizes hyper-β-alaninemia, tissue carnosine levels are not significantly perturbed in serum carnosinase deficiency; nor are brain homocarnosine levels elevated [2]. Thus one cannot defend any attempt during treatment to modulate tissue dipeptide levels.

Since there is at least one reported subject (patient D2) in whom the phenotype of persistent carnosinuria with serum carnosinase deficiency was not yet accompanied by declared neurologic disease, even in the fifth year of life, it is equally hard to defend a regimen that would replace serum carnosinase activity by enzyme infusion; since carnosine is excreted into urine from endogenous pools by patients with the trait, there is

---

[2] Described by Dent [101] as compounds 51 and 53 on his map. 1-Methylhistidine gives a characteristic green color after the paper chromatogram is stained with ninhydrin and heated to 105°C for a few minutes.

little that dietary therapy can offer except to avoid the addition of exogenous carnosine to the endogenous burden. Should enzyme replacement eventually prove to be of value it will be necessary to study the immunologic specificity of the mutant phenotype to determine whether the proband forms cross-reaction material (CRM$^+$ phenotype) or not (CRM$^-$ phenotype). CRM$^-$ subjects should not be exposed to unmodified serum carnosinase from donors [118].

Genetics

It is reasonable to suspect that serum carnosinase deficiency is an inherited disorder. Moreover the data on serum and tissue carnosinase activities suggest that more than one gene locus may be responsble for the different forms of the enzyme. Different genes may code for different polypeptides which aggregate to form the observed molecular forms of the enzyme; or one gene may instruct synthesis of a polypeptide chain, while a second gene may code for an enzyme which modifies the protein product of the first gene, e.g., by glycosylation. These are merely speculations in the absence of any substantive investigation on the problem to our knowledge.

The inheritance pattern of serum carnosinase deficiency is still unclear. Two pedigrees (A and C, Table 28-4) reveal parental consanguinity, and two contain affected sibs (C and D, Table 28-4), findings which suggest autosomal recessive inheritance. However, the five subjects with associated neurologic disease are all male, while the one subject with serum carnosinase deficiency and a benign clinical history is female; this observation is compatible with X-linked inheritance. Partial deficiency of serum carnosinase activity in three mothers (in pedigrees A, C, and D, Table 28-5) is also favorable to an X-linked hypothesis. Partial deficiency of serum carnosinase activity in both parents of the C pedigree favors autosomal recessive inheritance.

In the absence of a definitive Mendelian inheritance pattern and without unequivocal evidence that the trait is harmful there can be no informed genetic counseling for affected families.

HOMOCARNOSINOSIS (HOMOCARNOSINASE DEFICIENCY)

Homocarnosinosis has been identified in a single Norwegian pedigree [119–121]. A 69-year-old woman (patient 1) and three of her four children (patients 2 to 4; ages 34 to 41 years) have concentrations of homocarnosine in their CSF that are 20 to 40 times the normal level. These patients do not have detectable homocarnosine in plasma, nor do they excrete abnormal amounts of the dipeptide in their urine. The three affected offspring have a progressive spastic paraplegia with onset between 6 and 29 years of age, mental deterioration, and retinal pigmentation; the mother has normal neurologic and mental function, despite her metabolic abnormality. A brain biopsy was obtained from the nondominant frontal cortex of patient 2 when she was age 40 years. Marked atrophy of the cortical gyri was observed, and there was enlargement of the subarachnoid space; histologic examination of the brain biopsy specimen was unremarkable. Two sisters of patient 1, the father of patients 2 to 4, and a sister of patients 2 to 4 are clinically normal and exhibit normal CSF homocarnosine levels [120]. Patient 3 has two children, aged 8 and 6 years, who are clinically normal but whose CSF homocarnosine levels have not been determined [121].

Biochemical Features

An elevated level of homocarnosine (40 to 75 μmol/liter; normal <10.2 μmol/liter) [64, 122] was detected in the CSF of all four patients. In particular, carnosine levels were normal. Only CSF, not plasma or urine, had an elevated homocarnosine content.

Amino acid analysis of the quick-frozen frontal cortex biopsy from patient 2, and of frontal or temporal cortex biopsy specimens from patients with underlying brain tumors or with focal epilepsy, revealed the homocarnosine content in the patient to be four times higher than that of controls [121, 122]. Brain GABA and histidine were similar in patients and controls (Table 28-5). The elevated homocarnosine content of the frontal cortex in patient 2 makes it unlikely that the high levels of the dipeptide in CSF are a failure to transport homocarnosine back into brain from CSF.

Homocarnosine-carnosine synthetase [L-histidine:β-alanine ligase (AMP) (EC 6.3.2.11)] activity was assayed in the brain biopsy specimen from patient 2 by a radiochemical method [119]. Synthetase activity was 2 nmol per gram wet weight per hour in the patient (normal range for 12 control adults, 1 to 10 nmole per gram per wet weight per hour). Activity of homocarnosinase (EC number not assigned), the cobalt-dependent brain enzyme that hydrolyzes the dipeptide, was undetectable in the patient's brain. The assay [123] employed homocarnosine labelled with ^{14}C in the GABA moiety, with subsequent measurement of radioactive GABA freed during incubation. It showed considerable homocarnosinease activity in cortical biopsy speciments from 15 control subjects (normal range for 15 control adults, 69 to 287 nmol per gram per wet weight per 25 min).

Table 28-5 Homocarnosine in human cortex

Subjects	Cortical area biopsied	Homocarnosine content*	GABA content*	Histidine content*
Patient 2	Frontal	1.29	0.76	0.07
13 nonepileptic adults	Frontal (majority)	0.28 ± 0.14	0.62 ± 0.14	0.09 ± 0.03
25 epileptic patients	Temporal (majority)	0.34 ± 0.14	0.80 ± 0.18	0.11 ± 0.03

* Content of amino compounds expressed in μmol per gram wet weight, with means ± SD shown for control subjects.

Genetics

It is likely that two different hereditary disorders are present in the Norwegian homocarnosinosis pedigree. One of them, a progressive neurologic disease of unknown etiology, probably has been inherited as an autosomal recessive disorder. Three of four children in the sibship are affected, and the parents are presumably clinically unaffected heterozygotes. The second, homocarnosinosis, may be asymptomatic, since one patient is in good health at 69 years of age. Although there is no known consanguinity between the parents in this pedigree [120], one can propose that the father is heterozygous for homocarnosinase deficiency, the mother is homozygous for the mutant gene, and the disorder in their offspring was inherited as an autosomal recessive trait. Homocarnosinase concentration has not been reported in any other adults, out of many hundreds of individuals whose CSF has been subjected to amino acid analysis [123]. The abnormality was not found in 14 patients with familial spastic paraplegias when a specific attempt was made to detect it [124].

Therapy

Inasmuch as there is no convincing evidence that an excessive amount of homocarnosine in brain *by itself* produces neurologic disease or intellectual deterioration, no specific therapy for homocarnosinosis is indicated. In addition, it is difficult at this time to envisage how one might lessen the synthesis of homocarnosine in human brain or introduce homocarnosinase enzyme activity.

Addendum

Leininger et al. [126] described a 7-year-old male patient with persistent carnosinuria and elevated serum carnosine (13.3 μmol/liter) during a meat-free regimen. Carnosine loading increased serum and urine carnosine. A convulsive encephalopathy began at 14 months coincidental with meat feeding. Serum carnosine activity was not measured. Three healthy older sibs are described; their carnosine excretion was not reported. There was no parental consanguinity.

This work was supported in part by grants from the Medical Research Council of Canada to C.R.S. and T.I.P. and from Deutsche Forschungsgemeinschaft to W.N.

REFERENCES

1. SCRIVER CB, PUESCHEL S, DAVIES E: Hyper-β-alaninemia associated with β-aminoaciduria and γ-aminobutyricaciduria, somnolence and seizures. *N Engl J Med* 274:636, 1966
2. PERRY TL, HANSEN S, TISCHLER B, BUNTING R, BERRY K: Carnosinemia: A new metabolic disorder associated with neurologic disease and mental defect. *N Engl J Med* 277:1219, 1967
3. PERRY TL: Carnosinemia, in Nyhan WH (ed): *Heritable Disorders of Amino Acid Metabolism.* New York, John Wiley & Sons, Inc, 1974, pp 293–305
4. SCRIVER CR, ROSENBERG LE: *Amino Acid Metabolism and Its Disorders.* Philadelphia, WB Saunders Co, 1973
5. DICKINSON JC, ROSENBLUM H, HAMILTON PB: Ion exchange chromatography of the free amino acids in the plasma of the newborn infant. *Pediatrics* 36:2, 1965

6. SOUPART P: Free amino acids of blood and urine in the human, in Holden JT (ed): *Amino Acid Pools: Distribution, Formation and Function of Free Amino Acids.* Amsterdam, Elsevier/North-Holland Publishing Co, 1962, p 220
7. ROBERTS E, SIMONSEN DG: Free amino acids in animal tissues, in Holden JT (ed): *Amino Acid Pools: Distribution, Formation and Function of Free Amino Acids.* Amsterdam, Elsevier/North-Holland Publishing Co, 1962, p 285
8. PERRY TL, BERRY K, HANSEN S, DIAMOND S, MOK C: Regional distribution of amino acids in human brain obtained at autopsy. *J Neurochem* 18:513, 1971
9. PERRY TL, HANSEN S: Sustained drug-induced elevation of brain GABA in the rat. *J Neurochem* 21:1167, 1973
10. HAYAISHI O, NISHIZUKA Y, TATIBANA M, TAKESHITA M, KUNO S: Enzymatic studies on the metabolism of β-alanine. *J Biol Chem* 236:781, 1961
11. HECHTMAN P, SCRIVER CR, MIDDLETON RB: Isolation and properties of a β-alanine transaminaseless mutant of *Pseudomonas fluorescens. J Bacteriol* 104:851, 1970
12. HECHTMAN P, SCRIVER CR: The isolation and properties of a β-alanine permeaseless mutant of *Pseudomonas fluorescens. Biochim Biophys Acta* 219:428, 1970
13. ROBERTS E, BREGOFF HM: Transamination of γ-aminobutyric acid and β-alanine in brain and liver. *J Biol Chem* 201:393, 1953
14. CRUSH KC: Carnosine and related substances in animal studies. *Comp Biochem Physiol* 34:3, 1970
15. SCHMIDT G, CUBILES R: Comparative studies on occurrence of carnosine-anserine fraction in skeletal muscle and heart. *Arch Biochem Biophys* 58:227, 1955
16. REDDY WJ, HEGSTED DM: Measurement and distribution of carnosine in rat. *J Biol Chem* 237:705, 1962
17. MARGOLIS FL: Carnosine in the primary olfactory pathway. *Science* 184:909, 1974
18. KALYANKAR GD, MEISTER A: Enzymatic synthesis of carnosine and related β-alanyl and γ-aminobutyryl peptides. *J Biol Chem* 234:3210, 1959
19. STENESH JJ, WINNICK T: Carnosine-anserine synthetase of muscle. 4. Partial purification of the enzyme and further studies of β-alanyl peptide synthesis. *Biochem J* 77:575, 1960
20. McMANUS IR, BENSON MS: Studies on the formation of carnosine and anserine in pectoral muscle of the developing chick. *Arch Biochem Biophys* 119:444, 1967
21. DuVIGNEAUD V, BEHRENS O: Carnosine and anserine. *Ergebn Physiol* 41:917, 1939
22. DAVEY CL: Significance of carnosine and anserine in straited skeletal muscle. *Arch Biochem Biophys* 89:303, 1960
23. DAVIES E, SCRIVER CR: l-Methylhistidinuria in man: A festive index. *Proceedings of the Society for Pediatric Research,* N.J., Atlantic City, 1967, p 134
24. McMANUS IR: Enzymatic synthesis of anserine in skeletal muscle by N-methylation of carnosine. *J Biol Chem* 237:1207, 1962
25. McMANUS IR: Metabolism of anserine and carnosine in normal and vitamin E-deficient rabbits. *J Biol Chem* 235: 1398, 1960
26. AVENA RM, BOWEN WJ: Effects of carnosine and anserine on muscle adenosine triphosphatases. *J Biol Chem* 244:1600, 1969
26a. BROWN CE, ANTHOLINE WE: Evidence that carnosine and anserine may participate in Wilson's disease. *Biochem Biophys Res Comm* 92:470–477, 1980
27. Report of the Food and Nutrition Board, of the National Academy of Science & Natural Research Council on Recommended Daily Allowances, 7th rev ed. Publication 1694, Washington, 1968
28. HANSON IT, SMITH EL: Carnosinase: Enzyme of swine kidney. *J Biol Chem* 179:789, 1949
29. ROSENBERG A: Purification and some properties of carnosinase of swine kidney. *Arch Biochem Biophys* 88:83, 1960
30. PERRY TL, HANSEN S, LOVE DL: Serum-carnosinase deficiency in carnosinaemia. *Lancet* I:1229, 1968
31. NAKAI T, TSUJIGADO N: β-Alanyl dipeptide preparations from whale muscles made by several workers, *J Biochem* 57:812, 1965
32. PISANO JJ, WILSON JD, COHEN L, ABRAHAM D, UDENFRIEND S: Isolation of γ-aminobutyrylhistidine (homocarnosine) from brain. *J Biol Chem* 236:499, 1961
33. ABRAHAM D, PISANO JJ, UDENFRIEND S: The distribution of homocarnosine in mammals. *Arch Biochem Biophys* 99:210, 1962
34. KANAZAWA A, SANO I: Method of determination of homocarnosine and its distribution in mammalian tissues. *J Neurochem* 14:211, 1967
35. URQUHART N, PERRY TL, HANSEN S, KENNEDY J: GABA content and glutamic acid decarboxylase activity in brain of Huntington's chorea patients and control subjects. *J Neurochem* 24:1071, 1975
36. SKAFER SD, DAS S, MARSHALL FD: Some properties of a homocarnosine-carnosine synthetase isolated from rat brain. *J Neurochem* 21:1429, 1973

37. HOSEIN EA, SMART M: The presence of anserine and carnosine in brain tissue. *Can J Biochem Physiol* 38:569, 1960

38. TALLAN HH: A survey of the amino acids and related compounds in nervous tissue, in Holden JT (ed): *Amino Acid Pools: Distribution, Formation and Function of Free Amino Acids.* Amsterdam, Elsevier/North-Holland Publishing Co, 1962, p 471

39. NAKAJIMA T, WOLFGRAM F, CLARK WG: The isolation of homoanserine from bovine brain. *J Neurochem* 14:1107, 1967

40. NAKAJIMA T, KAKIMOTO Y, KUMON A, MATSUOKA M, SANO I: α-(γ-Aminobutyryl)-lysine in mammalian brain: Its identification and distribution. *J Neurochem* 16:417, 1969

41. MATSUOKA M, NAKAJIMA T, SANO I: Identification of α-(β-alanyl)-lysine in rabbit muscle, *Biochim Biophys Acta* 177:169, 1969

42. NUTZENADEL W, SCRIVER CR: Transport and metabolism of β-alanine and β-alanyl-L-histidine (L-carnosine) by rat intestinal enterocytes, kidney cortex and striated muscle in vitro. Role in nutrition. *Am J Physiol* 230:643, 1976

43. ADIBI, SA, MORSE EL: Intestinal transport of dipeptides in man: Relative importance of hydrolysis and intact absorption. *J Clin Invest* 50:2266, 1971

44. ADIBI SA, MERCER DW: Protein digestion in human intestine as reflected in luminal, mucosal and plasma amino acid concentration after meals. *J Clin Invest* 52:1586, 1973

45. ADIBI SA, SOLEIMANAW MR: Functional characterization of dipeptide transport system in human jejunum. *J Clin Invest* 53:1368, 1974

46. MATTHEWS DM: Absorption of amino acids and peptides from the intestine, in *Clinics in Endocrinology and Metabolism.* London, WB Saunders Co, 1974, vol 3, pp 3–16

47. SILK DBA: Peptide absorption in man. *Gut* 15:494, 1974

48. ADDISON JM, BURSTON D, PAYNE JW, WILKINSON S, MATTHEW DM: Evidence for active transport of tripeptides by hamster jejunum *in vitro. Clin Sci Molec Med* 49:305, 1975

49. ASATOOR AM, BARDON JK, LANT AF, MILNE MD, NAVAB F: Intestinal absorption of carnosine and its constituent amino acids in man. *Gut* 11:250, 1970

50. MATTHEWS DM, ADDISON JM, BURSTON D: Evidence for active transport of the dipeptide carnosine (β-alanyl-L-histidine) by hamster jejunum in vitro. *Clin Sci Molec Med* 46:693, 1974

51. BAXTER CF, ROBERTS E: Elevation of γ-aminobutyric acid in brain: Selective inhibition of γ-aminobutyric-α-ketoglutaric acid transaminase. *J Biol Chem* 236:3287, 1961

52. WEDEEN RP, WEINER B: The distribution of ρ-aminohippuric acid in rat kidney slices. 1:Tubular localization. *Kidney Int* 3:205, 1973

53. CHESNEY RW, SCRIVER CR, MOHYUDDIN F: Aminoaciduria caused by mutation localization of the membrane defect in transepithelial transport by parallel studies in vivo and in vitro *J Clin Invest* 57:183, 1976

54. SCRIVER CR: Hartnup disease: A genetic modification of intestinal and renal transport of certain neutral alpha-amino acids. *N Engl J Med* 273:530, 1965

55. NAVAB F, ASATOOR AM: Studies on intestinal absorption of amino acids and a dipeptide in a case of Hartnup disease. *Gut* 11:373, 1970

56. WESTALL RG: The amino acids and other ampholytes of urine. 3. Unidentified substances expected in normal human urine. *Biochem J* 60:247, 1955

57. BLOCK WD, HUBBARD RW, STEELE BF: Excretion of histidine and histidine derivatives by human subjects ingesting protein from different sources. *J Nutr* 85:419, 1965

58. HUBBARD RW, BLOCK WD: Urinary excretion of 1-methylhistidine and histidine in human subjects on low and high protein intake. *Fed Proc* 22:320, 1963

59. BUTTS JH, FLESHLER B: Anserine, a source of 1-methylhistidine in urine of man. *Proc Soc Exp Biol Med* 118:722, 1965

60. CUSWORTH DC, DENT CE: Renal clearances of amino acids in normal adults and in patients with aminoaciduria. *Biochem J* 74:550, 1960

61. SCRIVER CR, DAVIES E: Endogenous renal clearance rates of free amino acids in pre-pubertal children. *Pediatrics* 32:592, 1965

62. PALO J, SAIFER A, MAZELIS F: Free amino acids in Tay-Sachs and normal human brain gray matter. *Clin Chim Acta* 22:327, 1968

63. PERRY TL, HANSEN S, STEDMAN D, LOVE D: Homocarnosine in human cerebrospinal fluid: An age-dependent phenomenon. *J Neurochem* 15:1203, 1968

64. PERRY TL, HANSEN S, KENNEDY J: CSF amino acids and plasma-CSF amino acid ratios in adults. *J Neurochem* 24:587, 1975

65. PERRY TL, HANSEN, MacDOUGALL L: Urinary screening tests in the prevention of mental deficiency. *Can Med Assoc J* 95:89, 1966

66. TOCCI PM: The biochemical diagnosis of metabolic disorders by urinalysis and paper chromatography, in Nyhan WL (ed): *Amino Acid Metabolism and Genetic Variation.* New York, McGraw-Hill Book Co, 1967, p 461

67. PERRY TL, JONES RT: The amino acid content of human cerebrospinal fluid in normal individuals and in mental defectives. *J Clin Invest* 40:1363, 1961

68. McARDLE B: Quantitative estimation of pyruvic and α-oxoglutaric acids by paper chromatography in blood, urine and cerebrospinal fluid. *Biochem J* 66:144, 1957

69. SMITH I, SMITH MJ: Keto acids, in Smith I (ed): *Chromatographic and Electrophoretic Techniques.* New York, Wiley-Interscience, 1960, vol 1, p 261

70. WHELAN DT, SCRIVER CR, MOHYUDDIN F: Glutamic acid decarboxylase and gamma-aminobutyric acid in mammalian kidney. *Nature (Lond)*, 224:916, 1969

71. ZACHMANN M, TOCCI P, NYHAN WL: The occurrence of γ-aminobutyric acid in human tissues other than brain. *J Biol Chem* 241:1355, 1966

72. ROBERTS E, FRANKEL S: Glutamic acid decarboxylase in brain. *J Biol Chem* 188:789, 1951

73. WINGO WJ, AWAPARA J: Decarboxylation of L-glutamic acid by brain. *J Biol Chem* 187:267, 1950

74. ROBERTS E (ed): *Inhibition of the Nervous System and γ-Aminobutyric Acid.* New York, Pergamon Press, Inc, 1960

75. ROBERTS E, WEIN J, SIMONSEN DG: γ-Aminobutyric acid (γABA), vitamin B₆ and neuronal function—a speculative synthesis. *Vitam Horm* 22:503, 1964

76. ELLIOTT KAC: γ-Aminobutyric acid and other inhibitory substances. *Br Med Bull* 21:70, 1965

77. SCRIVER CR, WHELAN DT: Glutamic acid decarboxylase in mammalian tissue outside the central nervous system, and its possible relevance to hereditary vitamin B₆ dependency with seizures. *Proc NY Acad Sci* 166:83, 1969

78. LANCASTER G, MOHYUDDIN F, SCRIVER CR, WHELAN DT: A γ-aminobutyrate pathway in mammalian kidney cortex. *Biochim Biophys Acta* 297:229, 1973

79. HABER B, KURIYAMA K, ROBERTS E: An anion stimulated L-glutamic acid decarboxylase in non-neural tissues. Occurrence and subcellular localization in mouse kidney and developing chick brain. *Biochem Pharmacol* 19:119, 1970

80. VON SEILER N, WIECHMANN M: Zum Vorkommen der γ-Aminobuttersäure und der γ-Amino-β-hydroxy-buttersäure in tierischem Gewebe. *Hoppe-Seylers Z Physiol Chem* 350:1493, 1969

81. BAXTER CF, ROBERTS E: Elevation of γ-aminobutyric acid in brain: Selective inhibition of γ-aminobutyric-α-ketoglutaric acid transaminase. *J Biol Chem* 236:3287, 1961

82. VAN GELDER NM: The histochemical demonstration of γ-aminobutyric acid metabolism by reduction of a tetrazolium salt. *J Neurochem* 12:231, 1965

83. OKAMURA N, OTSUKI S, KAMEYAMA A: Studies on free amino acids in human brain. *J Biochem (Tokyo)* 47:315, 1960

84. DENT CE, WALSHE JM: Amino acid metabolism. *Br Med Bull* 10:249, 1954

85. SCRIVER CR, BERGERON M: Amino acid transport in kidney. The use of mutation to dissect membrane and transepithelial transport, in Nyhan WH (ed): *Heritable Disorders of Amino Acid Metabolism.* New York, John Wiley & Sons, Inc, 1974, p 515

86. SCRIVER CR: The use of human genetic variation to study membrane transport of amino acids in kidney. *Am J Dis Child* 117:4, 1969

87. ARMSTRONG MD, YATES K, KAKIMOTO Y, TANIGUCHI K, KAPPE T: Excretion of β-aminoisobutyric acid by man. *J Biol Chem* 238:1447, 1963

88. SCRIVER CR, EFRON ML, SCHAFER IA: Renal tubular transport of proline, hydroxyproline and glycine in health and in familial hyperprolinemia. *J Clin Invest* 43:374, 1964

89. GILBERT JB, KU Y, ROGERS LL, WILLIAMS RL: The increase in urinary taurine after intraperitoneal administration of amino acids to the mouse. *J Biol Chem* 235:1055, 1960

90. WILSON OH, SCRIVER CR: Specificity of transport of neutral and basic amino acids in rat kidney. *Am J Physiol* 213:185, 1967

91. GOLDMAN H, SCRIVER CR: A transport system in mammalian kidney with preference for β-amino compounds. *Pediatr Res* 1:212, 1967

92. CHRISTENSEN HN: Relations in the transport of β-alanine and α-amino acids in the Ehrlich cell. *J Biol Chem* 239:3584, 1964

93. ROZEN R, TENENHOUSE MS, SCRIVER CR: Taurine transport in renal brush-border membrane vesicles. *Biochem J* 180:245, 1979

94. CHRISTENSEN HN: Reactive sites and biological transport. *Adv Protein Chem* 15:239, 1960

95. KRNJEVIĆ K: Action of drugs on single neurones in the cerebral cortex. *Br Med Bull* 21:10, 1965

96. STEINER FA: L-Glutamic acid, GABA and pyridoxal-5-phosphate at single unit level in brain. *Proc NY Acad Sci* 166:199, 1969

97. TSUKADA Y, NAGATA Y, HIRANO S, MATSUTANI T: Active transport of amino acids into cerebral cortex slices. *J Neurochem* 10:241, 1963

98. McKHANN GM, LABERS RW, SOKOLOFF L, MICKELSEN O, TOWER DB: The quantitative significance of the gamma-aminobutyric acid pathway in cerebral oxidative metabolism, in Roberts E, et al. (eds): *Inhibitions of the Nervous System and γ-Aminobutyric Acid.* London, Pergamon Press, Inc, 1960, p 169

99. Scriver CR: Carnosinaemia (letter to the editor) *Lancet* 1:1249, 1968
100. Allen RJ, Tourtellotte WW, Adriaessens K, Lowenthal A, Mardens Y: Letter to the editor. *Lancet* 1:1249, 1968
101. Dent CE: A study of the behaviour of some sixty amino acids and other ninhydrin reacting substances on phenol-"collidine" filter paper chromatograms with notes as to the occurrence of some of them in biological fluids. *Biochem J* 43:169, 1948
102. Efron ML, Young D, Moser HW, MacCready RA: A simple chromatographic screening test for the detection of disorders of amino acid metabolism: A technique using blood or urine collected on filter paper. *N Engl J Med* 270:1378, 1964
103. Scriver CR, Davies E, Cullen AM: Application of a simple method to the screening of plasma for a variety of aminoacidopathies. *Lancet* 2:230, 1964
104. Perry TL, Hansen S: Biochemical effects in man and rat of three drugs which can increase brain GABA content. *J Neurochem* 30:679, 1978
105. Perry TL, Kish SJ, Hansen S: γ-vinyl GABA: Effects of chronic administration of the metabolism of GABA and no other amino compounds in rat brain. *J Neurochem* 32:1641, 1979
106. Scriver CR: Vitamin B$_6$ deficiency and dependency in man. *Am J Dis Child* 113:109, 1967
107. van Heeswijk PJ, Trijbels JMF, Schretlen EDAM, van Munster PJJ, Monnens LAH: A patient with a deficiency of serum carnosinase activity. *Acta Paediatr Scand* 58:584, 1969
108. Terplan KL, Cares HL: Histopathology of the nervous system in carnosinase enzyme deficiency with mental retardation. *Neurology* 22:644, 1972
109. Murphey WH, Lindmark DG, Patchen LI, Housler ME, Harrod EK, Mosovich L: Serum carnosinase deficiency concomitant with mental retardation. *Pediatr Res* 7:601, 1973
110. Gordon EF Jr, Coulombe JT, Sepe SJ, Levy HL: A variant of carnosinemia with normal serum carnosinase activity in an infant. *Pediatr Res* 11:456, 1977
111. Fleisher LD, Rassin DK, Wisniewski K, Salwen HR: Carnosinase deficiency: a new variant with high residual activity. *Pediatr Res* 14:269, 1980
112. Tocci PM, Bessman SP: Histidine peptiduria, in Nyhan WL (ed): *Amino Acid Metabolism and Genetic Variation*. New York, McGraw-Hill Book Co, 1967, p 161
113. Murphey WH, Patchen LI, Lindmark DG: Carnosinase. A fluorometric assay and demonstration of two electrophoretic forms in human tissue extracts. *Clin Chim Acta* 42:309, 1972
114. van Munster PJJ, Trijbels JMF, van Heeswijk PJ, Schmit-Jansen B, Moerkerk C: A new sensitive method for the determination of serum carnosinase activity using L-carnosine (l-^{14}C)-β-alanyl as substrate. *Clin Chim Acta* 29:243, 1970
115. Perry TL, Shaw KNF, Walker D, Redlich D: Urinary excretion of amines in normal children. *Pediatrics* 30:576, 1962
116. Bessman SP, Baldwin R: Imidazole aminoaciduria in cerebromacular degeneration. *Science* 135:789, 1962
117. Levenson J, Lindahl-Kiessling K, Rayner S: Carnosine excretion in juvenile amaurotic idiocy. *Lancet* 2:756, 1964
118. Boyer SM, Siggers DC, Krueger LJ: Caveat to protein replacement therapy for genetic disease. Immunological implication of accurate molecular diagnosis. *Lancet* 2:654, 1973
119. Gjessing LR, Sjaastad O: Homocarnosinosis: A new metabolic disorder associated with spasticity and mental retardation. *Lancet* 2:1028, 1974
120. Sjaastad O, Berstad J, Gjesdahl P, Gjessing L: Homocarnosinosis: 2. A familial disorder associated with spastic paraplegia, progressive mental deficiency, and retinal pigmentation. *Acta Neurol Scand* 53:275, 1976
121. Perry TL, Kish SJ, Sjaastad O, Gjessing LR, Nesbakken R, Schrader H, Loken AC: Homocarnosinosis: Increased content of homocarnosine and deficiency of homocarnosinase in brain. *J Neurochem* 32:1637, 1979
122. Gjessing LR, Gjesdahl P, Sjaastad O: The free amino acids in human cerebrospinal fluid. *J Neurochem* 19:1807, 1972
123. Kish SJ, Perry TL, Hansen S: Regional distribution of homocarnosine, homocarnosine-carnosine synthetase and homocarnosinase in human brain. *J Neurochem* 32:1629, 1979
124. Sjaastad O, Gjessing L, Berstad JR, Gjesdahl P: Homocarnosinosis: 3. Spinal fluid amino acids in familial spastic paraplegia. *Acta Neurol Scand* 55, 158, 1977
125. Perry TL: Unpublished results
126. Leininger ML, Chapoy P, Charvet J, Vovan L, Louchet E: La Carnosinémie. Première Observation française. *Pédiatrie* 35:341, 1980

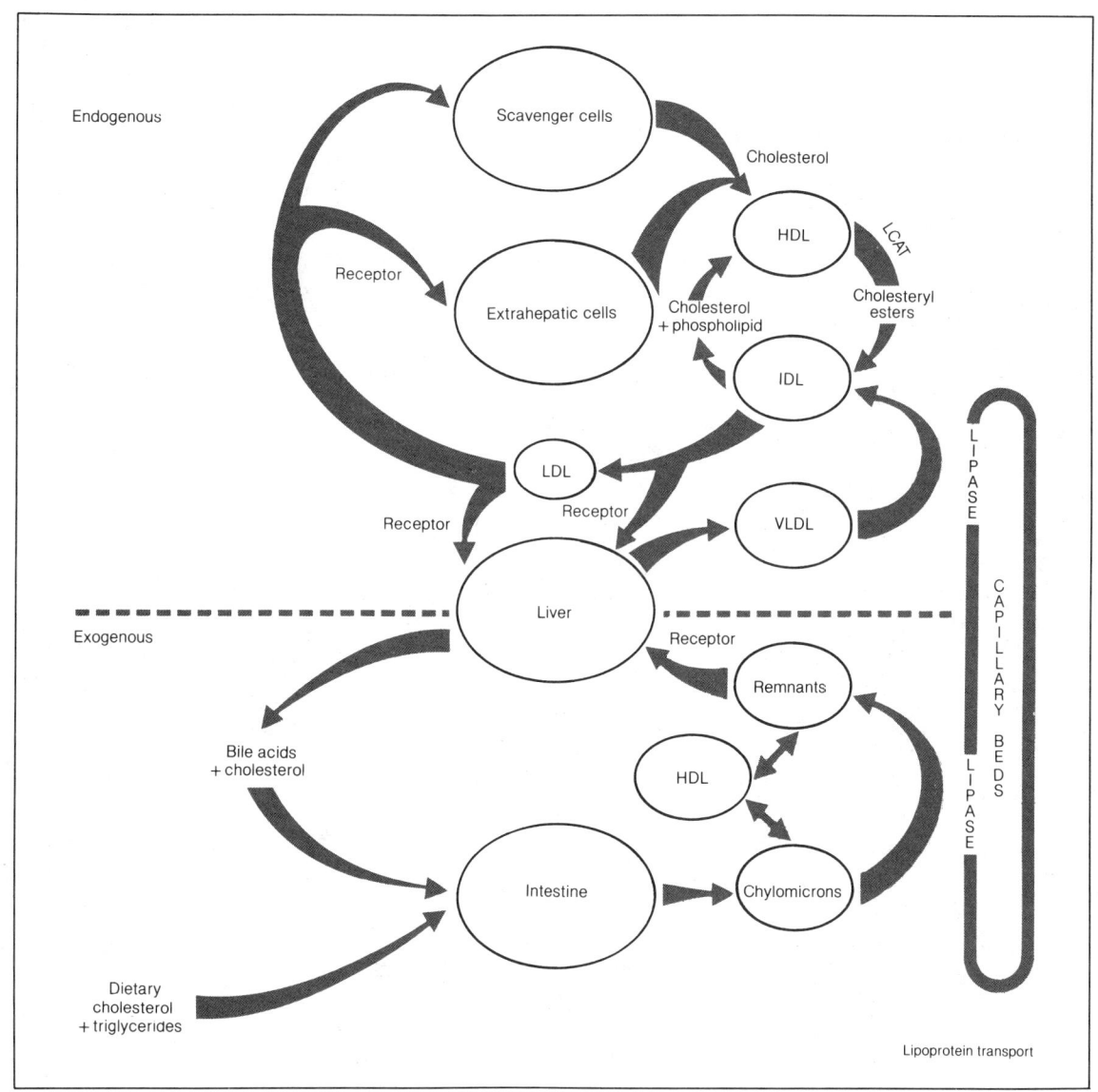

PART 4

Lipoprotein transport

DISORDERS OF LIPOPROTEIN AND LIPID METABOLISM

29

FAMILIAL LIPOPROTEIN DEFICIENCY: Abetalipoproteinemia, Hypobetalipoproteinemia, and Tangier Disease

PETER N. HERBERT

GERD ASSMANN

ANTONIO M. GOTTO, JR.

DONALD S. FREDRICKSON

1. *The inherited lipoprotein deficiency states are of two major types. One type, exemplified by* abetalipoproteinemia *and* familial hypobetalipoproteinemia, *primarily affects the plasma lipoproteins that contain a protein called apolipoprotein B (apo B). These lipoproteins include chylomicrons and very low density lipoproteins (VLDL), which are transporters of triglycerides, and low density lipoproteins (LDL), which are end products of VLDL catabolism and which are transporters of cholesterol. Another deficiency state, exemplified by* Tangier disease, *involves primarily the lipoproteins containing A apolipoproteins, A-I and A-II (apo A-I and apo A-II). These are the high density lipoproteins (HDL), the functions of which are not established but may include the transport of cholesterol from peripheral cells to the liver.*

2. *Abetalipoproteinemia is characterized clinically by fat malabsorption, ataxic neuropathy, retinitis pigmentosa, and acanthocytosis. The usual mechanisms for transport of triglyceride from the intestine and liver are abolished, and chylomicrons, VLDL, and LDL are absent from the plasma. The defect is presumed (without direct proof) to involve the synthesis of apo B or intracellular assembly of apo B with lipid. The disorder is rare and is inherited as an autosomal recessive trait. A high proportion of cases (~ 50 percent) have resulted from consanguine matings. Obligate heterozy-*

gotes show no clinical manifestations and typically have normal levels of plasma cholesterol and LDL. Vitamin E may prevent many of the morbid consequences in the homozygote.

3. *Familial hypobetalipoproteinemia is a rare disorder that is distinguished from abetalipoproteinemia on genetic grounds: heterozygotes for familial hypobetalipoproteinemia have low plasma levels of cholesterol and LDL, whereas heterozygotes for abetalipoproteinemia have normal levels. Homozygotes with familial hypobetalipoproteinemia are phenotypically indistinguishable from patients with abetalipoproteinemia except for possibly milder neuromuscular impairment. A high proportion of homozygotes (~ 70 percent) have resulted from consanguine matings. In at least some heterozygotes, the abnormality appears to involve a decrease in LDL (and presumably VLDL) synthesis. Several variant forms of hypobetalipoproteinemia have been described; these may be due to defective synthesis of apo B–containing lipoproteins by either the liver or intestinal mucosa.*

4. *Tangier disease is characterized clinically by hyperplastic orange tonsils, storage of cholesteryl esters in other reticuloendothelial tissues, corneal opacities, and relapsing neuropathy. This rare disorder is inherited as an autosomal recessive trait. Approximately 25 percent of cases have resulted from consanguine mat-*

ings. Heterozygotes have plasma HDL levels approximately half normal but do not develop neuropathy or cholesteryl ester storage. Homozygotes accumulate cholesteryl esters in tonsils, spleen, lymph nodes, bone marrow, skin, thymus, intestinal mucosa, and probably Schwann cells and cornea. The profound HDL deficiency results in the generation of abnormal chylomicron remnants, and these, after phagocytosis, may account for the accumulation of cholesteryl esters in histiocytes. Histiocyte phagocytosis of the cell membranes of effete blood and parenchymal cells, with loss of normal clearance of histiocyte cholesterol by HDL, may also promote cholesterol accumulation. Apo A-I and apo A-II are found in Tangier plasma, and neither has yet been shown to be abnormal. The disease may involve a defect in the regulation of HDL synthesis or catabolism.

Table 29-1 Total plasma cholesterol levels in white men and women*†

Age, years	Males, mg/dl		Females, mg/dl	
	Mean	5th to 95th Percentile	Mean	5th to 95th Percentile
<10	155	125–190	165	130–195
10–19	155	120–200	160	120–210
20–29	175	125–230	175	130–230
30–39	195	145–265	185	135–240
40–49	210	155–270	200	145–265
50–59	215	160–280	225	165–290
60–69	220	165–290	235	170–300
70+	210	145–270	225	175–280

* Lipid Research Clinics visit I data from white North American males and females. Samples taken after a 12-h fast. Means and 5th and 95th percentiles rounded to nearest 5 mg/dl.
† The numbers of black persons surveyed were not great enough to warrant generalization. Compared to whites, blacks of either sex have lower mean values in all age strata.
SOURCE: The Lipid Research Clinics, Population Studies Data Book, vol. 1, 1980. Recalculation of data by 10-year age strata courtesy of Dr. Basil Rifkind, NHLBI.

Many metabolic diseases are associated with abnormal plasma lipid and lipoprotein patterns. Most of these are secondary or incidental. Chapters 29 to 35 deal with primary disorders in the metabolism of lipids or lipoproteins. Clinically, they are most often first detected by abnormal concentrations of one or both of the most frequently measured plasma lipids, cholesterol and triglycerides. Most of these known monogenic disorders of lipid metabolism are associated with extreme changes in cholesterol or triglyceride concentrations. This chapter is concerned with heritable lipoprotein deficiency states or hypolipoproteinemias.

LIPID AND LIPOPROTEIN LEVELS

Hypo- and hyperlipoproteinemia are traditionally defined by fiducial cutoff points, respectively the 5th and 95th percentiles of lipid and lipoprotein distributions in the general population. Specialized laboratories now commonly use precipitation and ultracentrifugation methods to quantify the cholesterol content of a specific lipoprotein class as an estimate of lipoprotein mass. Simpler methods, such as quantitative lipoprotein electrophoresis, present great problems in standardization. Techniques which may be more specific, such as apolipoprotein quantitation, are still research tools.

The National Institutes of Health (NIH) Lipid Research Clinics have made available, for the first time, summary statistics of lipid and lipoprotein cholesterol distributions in the United States population [1–4]. Their data (Tables 29-1 to 29–4) confirmed earlier impressions of age-related changes in serum cholesterol levels but demonstrated clearly different trends in males and females. Triglyceride values (Table 29-2) are strikingly higher than those previously reported for North America, and levels in men are particularly skewed toward higher concentrations.

Lipoprotein cholesterol concentrations (Tables 29-3 and 29-4) provide information that is basic to traditional definitions of types [5] or patterns of hyperlipoproteinemia (Table 29-5). Direct estimation of very low density lipoprotein (VLDL) cholesterol levels, to document cholesterol enrichment of VLDL, is still an important marker of type 3 hyperlipoproteinemia and requires preparative ultracentrifugation (Chap.

32). In subjects with normal triglyceride levels or other forms of hyperlipoproteinemia, the VLDL cholesterol concentration can be approximated as the quotient of plasma triglycerides (mg/dl) divided by 5 [6]. VLDL cholesterol is always elevated in hypertriglyceridemic states, unless chylomicrons account for most of the plasma triglycerides.

Measurement of high density lipoprotein (HDL) cholesterol concentrations is widely performed since low HDL levels have been convincingly associated with augmented risk for cardiovascular disease. Conversely, abnormally high HDL concentrations appear to portend longevity [7]. HDL cholesterol is usually equated with the cholesterol remaining in plasma after precipitation of VLDL and low density lipoproteins (LDL) with polyanions and divalent cations [8]. Prepubertal boys and girls have very similar HDL cholesterol values (Tables 29-3 and 29-4), but HDL cholesterol levels in boys decline from a mean of around 56 mg/dl to 46 mg/dl after puberty. It is noteworthy that there is no decline in the HDL cholesterol concentration in postmenopausal women.

LDL cholesterol levels can be estimated by subtracting from the total plasma cholesterol that measured in the HDL fraction and that determined or approximated to be in VLDL. Hypercholesterolemia, in the absence of hypertriglyceridemia or hyperalphalipoproteinemia, is synonymous with elevated LDL concentrations. The largest age-related increases in LDL occur in men between the third and fifth decades (Table 29-3) and in women after the menopause (Table 29-4).

The Hypolipoproteinemias

The inherited lipoprotein deficiency states are of two major kinds. One primarily affects the plasma lipoproteins which contain a protein called apolipoprotein B (apo B). These lipoproteins include chylomicrons and VLDL, which carry most of the triglyceride transported in plasma, and LDL. LDL are end products of VLDL catabolism, contain about 70 percent of the plasma cholesterol in normal individuals (Tables 29-3 and 29-4), and may be the source of most cholesterol utilized by extrahepatic tissues.

The other major lipoprotein deficiency state primarily

involves lipoproteins containing the A apolipoproteins, apo A-I and apo A-II. These are the HDL, which have functions interrelated with those of LDL in cholesterol transport and homeostasis. HDL, moreover, interact extensively with the triglyceride-rich lipoproteins and contribute to the modulation of VLDL and chylomicron metabolism.

Hypoalphalipoproteinemia is considered present in any adult man or woman with HDL cholesterol levels, respectively, of 27 mg/dl and 33 mg/dl or less. The LDL cholesterol value defining hypobetalipoproteinemia is about 65 mg/dl in both men and women (Tables 29-3 and 29-4). As is true for the total serum cholesterol concentration, the contribution of genetic and other factors to the variance in lipoprotein cholesterol levels between individuals is not well delineated. Similarly, the percentage of subjects with monogenic hypobeta- and hypoalphalipoproteinemia among subjects in the lower 5th percentile of LDL and HDL cholesterol levels is not known. The disorders discussed in this chapter, however, appear quite rare and constitute a distinct minority of even those hypolipoproteinemias attributable mainly to genetic control.

The Plasma Lipoproteins

Four major classes of plasma lipoproteins are defined (Table 29-6) and subclasses within these undoubtedly exist [9]. All lipoproteins have their origin in the intestine or liver, or both [10] and appear to have a pseudomicellar structure [11]. Neutral lipids, in particular, cholesteryl esters and triglycerides, are maintained in the lipoproteins in a soluble and stable form through interactions with the apolipoproteins and phospholipids, which are more polar. Unesterified cholesterol is also present in these complexes. Its polarity lies between that of cholesteryl esters and triglycerides and that of the apolipoproteins and phospholipids [12–14]. An outer surface consisting of apolipoproteins, unesterified cholesterol, and phospholipids surrounds a water-insoluble core of cholesteryl esters and triglycerides, protecting the apolar lipids from the aqueous environment. This general structural concept has been supported by low-angle x-ray scattering studies and by other physical methods in which a variety of probes have been used to explore the structure of the lipoproteins [15–19]. The most obvious important function of the plasma lipoproteins is the solubilization and transport of the neutral plasma lipids [20].

Table 29-2 Total plasma triglyceride levels in white men and women*

Age, years	White Males, mg/dl		White Females, mg/dl	
	Mean	5th to 95th Percentile	Mean	5th to 95th Percentile
<10	50	30–90	65	30–130
10–19	70	35–135	70	40–125
20–29	100	45–185	85	40–165
30–39	130	50–285	90	40–185
40–49	150	55–310	105	45–205
50–59	145	65–295	125	55–255
60–69	135	55–255	135	55–265
70+	135	65–260	130	60–325

* Lipid Research Clinics visit I data from white North American males and females. Samples taken after a 12-h fast. Means and 5th and 95th percentiles rounded to nearest 5 mg/dl.
SOURCE: The Lipid Research Clinics, Population Studies Data Book, vol. 1, 1980. Recalculation of data by 10-year age strata courtesy of Dr. Basil Rifkind, NHLBI.

Chylomicrons The largest of the lipoproteins, chylomicrons have been defined by a variety of operational criteria [21–23] but the term is appropriately applied to both large and small triglyceride-rich lipoproteins elaborated by the intestinal mucosa [24, 25]. Use of the appellation "intestinal VLDL" creates confusion with VLDL of hepatic origin. No categorical chemical or metabolic distinction between large and small chylomicrons has yet been made [26], although separate compartmentalization within intestinal cell Golgi secretory vesicles has been suggested [27].

Most of the small intestine is probably capable of secreting chylomicrons into intestinal lymph, and the bulk are produced by the jejunum [25]. The precise steps involved in all phases of chylomicron synthesis are not yet known. Digested dietary fat is presented to the brush border membrane as fatty acids and 2-monoglycerides in micellar form through the action of bile acids. Uptake is a passive but highly efficient process, and transfer of fatty acids through the cytosol may be mediated by specific binding proteins [28]. The fatty acids and monoglycerides are resynthesized to triglycerides in the smooth endoplasmic reticulum [24] in the apical portion of the absorptive cell. Phospholipids are formed from reacylation of absorbed lysolecithin or de novo synthesis. Cholesterol is derived from at least three sources: absorption of sterol from the intestinal lumen, synthesis in the mucosal cell, and from circulating lipoproteins. The last may be a major source [29] after nascent chylomicrons are secreted from the cell. Chylomicrons accumulate in the Golgi zone before secretion, and some glycosylation of the apolipoproteins probably takes place during transit through the Golgi apparatus [30–32]. Unlike intestinal HDL, which are secreted into both lymph and the circulation, chylomicrons are only released into the mesenteric lymph.

Protein synthesis is required for chylomicron secretion [33], and immunochemical methods have demonstrated a marked increase in the apo B, apo A-I, and apo A-IV content of intestinal epithelium during active fat absorption [34–38]. As detailed later in this chapter, apo B is thought essential for chylomicron structure, intracellular transport, or transcellular release. It is not known if other apolipoproteins are also critical to this process.

Apolipoproteins account for only about 1 percent of the mass of chylomicrons (Table 29-6) found in mesenteric lymph. Uncertainty exists concerning their possible structural roles, the extent to which they are derived from plasma lipoproteins, and their eventual contribution to total plasma apolipoprotein. The C apolipoproteins comprise about 30 percent of mesenteric lymph chylomicron apoprotein, but little if any of the C apolipoproteins is synthesized by the intestine [10, 39–42]. Additional C apoproteins are acquired on exposure to plasma and they may eventually account for 60–70 percent of the chylomicron apoprotein. The apo E present in chylomicrons does not appear to be made by the intestine [36, 37, 40–42] and is acquired from the plasma or its ultrafiltrate in the lymph.

Apoproteins A-I, A-II, and A-IV are all associated with chylomicrons [38, 43–46], and intestinal synthesis of these A apoproteins has been documented [10, 36–38, 40–42, 47]. Much of the chylomicron complement of A apoproteins is lost, and C and E apoproteins are acquired when chylomicrons are exposed to plasma or HDL [46]. Intestinal production of the A apoproteins may be regulated by factors other than fat absorption and chylomicron formation [42].

Very Low Density Lipoproteins The liver secretes triglyceride into the circulation primarily in VLDL, and the con-

Table 29-3 Plasma lipoprotein cholesterol levels in white men*

Age, years	VLDL, mg/dl		LDL, mg/dl		HDL, mg/dl	
	Mean	5th to 95th Percentile	Mean	5th to 95th Percentile	Mean	5th to 95th Percentile
<10	10	0–20	95	65–135	50	40–75
10–19	10	0–25	95	65–130	50	35–75
20–29	15	5–35	110	70–165	45	30–65
30–39	25	5–55	130	80–190	45	30–65
40–49	25	5–55	140	90–195	45	30–65
50–59	25	5–60	145	90–200	45	30–65
60–69	20	0–45	150	95–210	50	30–80
70+	20	0–40	145	90–195	50	30–80

* Data from Lipid Research Clinics Study of white North American males. The means and 5th and 95th percentiles from the original data have been rounded to the nearest 5 mg/dl.
SOURCE: The Lipid Research Clinics, Population Studies Data Book, vol. 1, visit II, 1980. Recalculation of data by 10-year age strata courtesy of Dr. Basil Rifkind, NHLBI.

trol of this process is complex. The channeling of available fatty acids to triglyceride synthesis and secretion is affected not only by the availabilty of alternate energy sources but also by a variety of hormonal and other factors [48–58]. Enzymes of both the rough and smooth endoplasmic reticulum can synthesize triglycerides and phospholipids; and particles of VLDL size are first visualized by electron microscopy in the transition zone between these two regions of the endoplasmic reticulum [59]. VLDL have acquired at least the B apoprotein by the time they accumulate in the Golgi bodies [60–63]. Agents that inhibit protein synthesis or disrupt the microtubular systems block VLDL secretion from the liver [55, 64, 65]. VLDL are within membrane-bound vacuoles when they reach the sinusoidal cell border, and the final step in the secretory process may involve the fusion of secretory granule and plasma membranes before release into the space of Disse [59].

The extensive exchange and net transfer of apolipoproteins known to occur in the circulation contributes considerably to the apolipoprotein content of serum VLDL (Table 29-6). VLDL isolated from rat liver Golgi bodies have been studied to determine which apoproteins are present in nascent VLDL. Earlier studies demonstrated that Golgi VLDL and VLDL from a liver perfused with plasma-free media were deficient in C apoproteins [61], while apo B was unequivocally present. More recent studies have confirmed these observations and provided evidence that apo B and apo E are the major newly synthesized apoproteins in Golgi VLDL [63]. Only small quantities of apo A-I and C apoproteins could be demonstrated in these particles thought representative of nascent VLDL.

Intermediate Density and Low Density Lipoproteins Studies of the disappearance from plasma of radiolabeled VLDL suggest that lipoproteins of so-called intermediate density (IDL, buoyant density 1.006 to 1.019 g/ml) are generated through progressive catabolism of the core triglycerides of VLDL [11, 66, 67]. IDL are of size [68], composition, and electrophoretic mobility [69] intermediate between VLDL and LDL. IDL contain 85 percent lipid by weight, and cholesteryl esters and triglycerides are the most abundant lipid components. Apo B is the major protein in IDL, but small quantities of apo E and the C apoproteins are also present [70]. Increased plasma quantities of IDL typify type 3 hyperlipoproteinemia and are often observed in other hypertriglyceridemic states following interventions such as drastic caloric restriction [71].

LDL in humans also appear to be derived largely from VLDL through the catabolic cascade that first generates IDL. In normal subjects the turnover of apo B in VLDL and LDL is identical, implying that all LDL originates in VLDL and that both VLDL and IDL are quantitatively converted to LDL [67, 72]. There is evidence that VLDL and IDL may be cleared from plasma without conversion to LDL in certain hypertriglyceridemic states [67, 73, 74]. Kinetic studies in patients with either homozygous familial hypercholesterolemia or type 3 hyperlipoprteinemia, moreover, have suggested independent secretion of IDL and LDL [67, 75, 76]. Direct secretion of LDL by isolated perfused rat [77] and pig [78] livers has also been demonstrated.

LDL contains about 75 percent lipid and 25 percent protein by weight [79]. Apo B comprises over 90 percent of the total protein. The core neutral lipid composition of LDL (Table 29-6) is not invariate, and triglyceride may replace cholesteryl ester as the major lipid in severe hypertriglyceridemia. LDL have electrophoretic mobility approximating that of β-globulins in most zonal electrophoresis systems.

High Density Lipoproteins The major proteins of HDL are synthesized by both liver and intestine, but details of the intracellular assembly and transcellular secretion of HDL are not known. When rat livers are perfused with a medium containing inhibitors of lecithin:cholesterol acyltransferase (LCAT), HDL released into the perfusate appear to be discoidal bilayer particles [80]. Similarly, when LCAT inhibitors are added to rat mesenteric lymph, about half of the HDL visualized are disk-shaped (190 × 5.5 nm). This suggests that these lipoproteins are typical of newly secreted (nascent) HDL [81]. Nascent HDL from rat liver, like the discoidal HDL of familial LCAT deficiency, contain primarily apo E rather than apo A-I [80]. Apo A-I, in contrast, is the major apoprotein of the disk-shaped HDL in mesenteric lymph. Compared to plasma HDL, both forms of putative nascent HDL are very enriched in phospholipid and unesterified cholesterol. Equivalent discoidal particles have not yet been described in primate lymph or plasma, nor in the perfusates of subhuman primate livers. HDL₂ from human hepatic venous blood may contain particles representing modified disks [82].

HDL contain more protein (45 to 55 percent by weight) and less lipid than the other classes of plasma lipoproteins (Table 29-6). They have α_1-electrophoretic mobility and are often subdivided into fractions of density 1.063 to 1.120 (HDL₂) and 1.120 to 1.210 (HDL₃) g/ml. This subclassification of

HDL has received considerable attention because variation in HDL$_2$ levels accounts for much of the interindividual variance in HDL cholesterol levels [83, 84]. HDL$_2$ particles are larger (9.5 to 10 nm vs. 7 to 7.5 nm) and contain more unesterified cholesterol and triglyceride than HDL$_3$ [9]. While published reports of HDL subfraction apoprotein content vary considerably [85–89], findings in two laboratories [88, 90] indicate an apo A-I/apo A-II weight ratio of about 6 in HDL$_2$ and 3 in HDL$_3$. HDL$_2$ also contain proportionately more C apoproteins than do HDL$_3$ [91, 92].

The Apolipoproteins

Apolipoproteins are the lipid-free protein components of the plasma lipoproteins obtained by treating intact lipoproteins with organic solvents, detergents, or chaotropic agents. The ABC nomenclature system suggested by Alaupovic [93] is now widely employed. It should be viewed as noncommittal with respect to evolutionary origin or metabolic interrelationships of these proteins. Nomenclature will undoubtedly be revised when specific functions in lipid transport are identified for each putative apolipoprotein. Not all proteins captured with lipoproteins necessarily have a role in lipid transport. A pertinent example is the recent recognition that the serum amyloid A proteins, acute phase reactants, are transported in plasma bound to HDL [94]. These low molecular weight proteins may comprise up to 30 percent of apo HDL in inflammatory states [95], but it is doubtful that they have specific lipid transport roles.

We consider here only the better characterized apolipoproteins, apo A through E (Fig. 29-1). Current knowledge of their distribution, molecular weights, polymorphism, origins, concentrations, and functions is summarized in Table 29-7. The primary structures of five of the apolipoproteins—A-I, A-II, C-I, C-II, and C-III—have been reported [96]. These proteins contain about the same proportion of polar and nonpolar amino acids as do other soluble proteins; this fact and the finding that the sequences of the apolipoproteins do not contain long stretches of hydrophobic amino acids led to the hypothesis that there are specific and specialized lipid-binding regions within these molecules [12]. Such regions have been identified and are called amphipathic helices.

The amphipathic helix has been shown by model building to occur in the five apolipoproteins of known primary structure

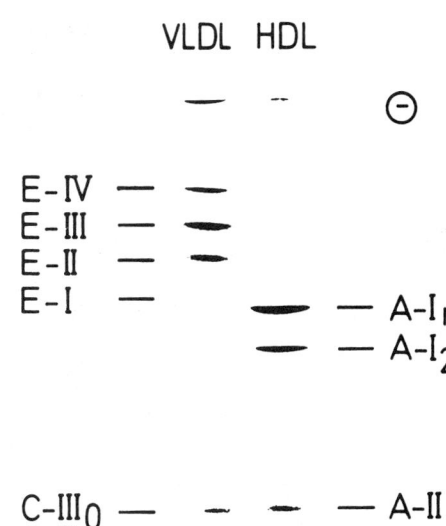

Figure 29-1 The apolipoproteins of normal VLDL and HDL visualized after isoelectric focusing in polyacrylamide gel.

[97]. In the amphipathic helical structure the polar, water-soluble amino acids are situated on one face of the helix, while the nonpolar, water-insoluble amino acids are located on the opposite face of the helix. These helices are believed to permit the apolipoproteins to form soluble stable structures with the polar phospholipids approximating a monolayer at the surface of the plasma lipoproteins.

Table 29-4 Plasma lipoprotein cholesterol levels in white women*

Age, years	VLDL, mg/dl Mean	VLDL, mg/dl 5th to 95th Percentile	LDL, mg/dl Mean	LDL, mg/dl 5th to 95th Percentile	HDL, mg/dl Mean	HDL, mg/dl 5th to 95th Percentile
<10	10	0–25	100	70–140	55	30–75
10–19	10	0–25	95	65–140	50	35–75
20–29	15	0–30	110	65–165	55	35–80
30–39	15	0–30	115	70–165	55	35–80
40–49	15	0–35	125	75–180	60	35–90
50–59	20	0–45	140	90–210	60	35–95
60–69	15	0–40	150	95–225	65	35–95
70+	15	0–50	150	95–205	60	35–95

* Data from Lipid Research Clinics Study of white North American females. The means and 5th and 95th percentiles from the original data have been rounded to the nearest 5 mg/dl.
SOURCE: The Lipid Research Clinics, Population Studies Data Book, vol. 1, visit II, 1980. Recalculation of data by 10-year strata courtesy of Dr. Basil Rifkind, NHLBI.

Table 29-5   Abnormal lipoprotein patterns in familial hyperlipoproteinemia

Type*		Lipoprotein abnormalities	Appearance of plasma†	Usual changes in lipid concentrations
1	(1)	Chylomicrons present and markedly increased	Cream layer on top, clear below	C ↑, TG ↑
	(2)	VLDL, LDL, HDL normal or decreased		
2a	(1)	LDL increased	Clear	C ↑, TG normal
	(2)	VLDL normal		
2b	(1)	LDL increased	Usually clear, may be slightly turbid	C ↑, TG ↑
	(2)	VLDL increased		
3	(1)	Presence of β-VLDL ("floating beta," LDL of abnormal lipid composition)	Usually turbid, often with faint cream layer	C ↑, TG ↑
4	(1)	VLDL increased	Usually turbid, no cream layer	C normal, TG ↑
	(2)	Chylomicrons "absent"		
	(3)	LDL not increased		
5	(1)	Chylomicrons present	Cream layer on top, turbid below	C ↑, TG ↑
	(2)	VLDL increased		

* Adapted from [5].
† After standing at 4 °C for 18 h or more.
NOTE: C, cholesterol; TG, triglycerides.

Apolipoprotein A-I   Apo A-I is the major protein component of all primate HDL. It consists of a single chain of 243 to 245 residues; does not contain cystine, cysteine, leucine, or carbohydrate; and exists in several isoforms (Fig. 29-1). Primary structural analyses of apo A-I, which differ in amino acid assignment at about 25 positions, have been described [98, 99]. Mutant forms of apo A-I have recently been recognized and are considered later in this chapter. Apo A-I has an α-helical content of about 55 percent in the lipid-free state, which increases to about 75 percent upon binding phospholipid. Repeating cycles of 11 helical residues have been identified in this apolipoprotein [100]. It has been suggested that these units represent a single ancestral chain which, by gene duplication, has generated a 22-residue repeat unit. These units have close sequence homology and are believed to represent the lipid-binding regions of the protein.

Apo A-I is a potent activator of LCAT, a plasma enzyme catalyzing the conversion of cholesterol and phosphatidylcholine to cholesteryl esters and lysophosphatidylcholine [101–103]. Specific lipid-binding regions of apo A-I have been found to activate LCAT, and this activity has been associated with the property of lipid binding [104]. As already noted, liver and intestine synthesize apo A-I, but their relative contributions to the total plasma content and the factors modulating apo A-I production are not well defined (see Ref. 105 for a recent review). More than 90 percent of plasma apo A-I is associated with HDL, less than 1 percent with VLDL and LDL, and no more than 10 percent with the lipoprotein-free fraction of plasma [88].

Apolipoprotein A-II   Apo A-II is also a major constituent of human HDL, accounting for about a third of the total protein and 15 percent of HDL mass. It exists as a dimer of two identical chains of 77 residues, which are linked covalently at cysteine 6 by a disulfide bond, and its primary structure is known [106]. Both the monomeric and dimeric forms of apo A-II are capable of reassembling with phospholipid. The α helix content of apo A-II increases from about 40 to 65 percent

on interaction with egg lecithin [107], and specific lipid binding segments have been identified and synthesized [108].

The specific role of apo A-II in lipid transport has not been identified, and it is a quantitatively minor HDL apoprotein in most lower species. The bulk of plasma apo A-II is found in HDL, with less than 5 percent in other density classes.

Minor HDL Apolipoproteins   The designation apo A-III [109] or apo D [110] has been applied to a protein of about 32,000 molecular weight which comprises less than 5 percent of the HDL apoprotein. Apo D was originally thought to stimulate LCAT [111], but this activity was not apparent in later studies [103, 112].

Another protein of about 46,000 molecular weight, first recognized as a major component of rat HDL [113], has been identified in human plasma and lymph [45, 114]. This so-called A-IV apoprotein is found predominantly in the lipoprotein-free fraction of plasma [114], synthesized by both intestine and liver [10], and may be cyclically reincorporated into chylomicrons [115]. An acidic apolipoprotein of 26,000 to 32,000 molecular weight, termed apolipoprotein F, has also been purified from human plasma HDL [116], as has another, provisionally called "D-2" [117]. Functions have not been found for any of these proteins.

Apolipoprotein B   Apo B is an obligatory constituent of chylomicrons, VLDL, and LDL. It comprises more than 90 percent of the protein of LDL and is also a major protein of VLDL and chylomicrons. Because of the difficulty in solubilizing and dissociating apo B, knowledge about its structure is still scant. Nevertheless, evidence for apo B heterogeneity has been emerging, particularly from studies in the rat. Rat liver has been shown to produce variants of apo B with apparent molecular weights of 335,000 and 240,000 [118]. The small intestine, in contrast, produces primarily, if not exclusively, the smaller form of apo B. Moreover, the circulating half-life of the larger form of apo B is much longer than the lower molecular weight species [118–120]. This suggests that they are not incorporated into the same lipoprotein particles. Thus a structural basis for the rapid turnover of chylomicron apo B relative to that in VLDL and LDL may soon be elucidated. The liver, moreover, may synthesize apo B–containing lipoproteins with different metabolic fates.

Evidence has also been provided for heterogeneity of human apo B. One series of proteins found in plasma LDL is represented by species of molecular weight 549,000 (B-100), 407,000 (B-74), and 126,000 (B-26) [121]. Based on their size and amino acid composition, the B-74 and B-26 subspecies appear derived from the predominant B-100 form [121]. A distinct second type of apo B that is a major component of chylomicrons and which is not found in LDL has a molecular weight of about 265,000. This presumably is analogous to the 240,000 mol wt protein elaborated by the rat intestine. Immunological differences between the large and small varieties of apo B probably also exist. These findings, together with evidence for structural and chemical differences, suggest that they are products of different genes.

The role of apo B in the synthesis of chylomicrons and VLDL has already been discussed. Apo B also appears critical to receptor-mediated uptake of LDL since chemical modification of its arginine or lysine residues may abolish binding and uptake by both fibroblasts [121a] and hepatocytes [121b] in vitro. Moreover, alteration of apo B arginine residues with cyclohexanedione prolongs the life of LDL in the circulation of humans, providing further evidence for a role of apo B in LDL clearance [121c, 121d] as well as formation.

More than 90 percent of the apo B in plasma of normal subjects and most hypercholesterolemic patients is in the LDL. The apo B in VLDL and chylomicrons may account for 20 to 50 percent of the total in moderate to severe hypertriglyceridemia [122, 123]. The Lp(a) lipoprotein [124], which also contains apo B, is found in the HDL density region and only rarely contributes significantly to the total serum apo B concentration [125].

Apolipoprotein C-I   Apo C-I makes up approximately 10 percent of the protein of VLDL and 2 percent of HDL. It binds phospholipid and can activate LCAT. The protein is a single chain of 57 residues, the amino acid sequence of which has been established [126, 127]. The α-helical content of apo C-I, determined by circular dichroism, is about 56 percent, increasing to 73 percent when combined with vesicles of phosphatidylcholine [14]. Phospholipid binding based on the amphipathic helix model has been predicted for three regions of apo C-I. A peptide corresponding to residues 32 to 57, containing one of the predicted binding regions, has been synthesized in the laboratory and shown to form a stable complex with phospholipid [14].

The capacity of apo C-I to activate LCAT in vitro is less than that of apo A-I when unsaturated acyl donors [102, 103] like those in plasma phosphatidylcholine are used. Apo C-I has been completely synthesized by solid phase techniques, and the synthetic protein also activates LCAT [14]. Unresolved is the relative importance of apo A-I and apo C-I in the physiologic activation of LCAT.

Apolipoprotein C-II   Apo C-II, the activator of lipoprotein lipase, accounts for about 10 percent of the protein of VLDL, 1 to 2 percent of that in HDL$_2$, and less than 1 percent in HDL$_3$ [128]. It is a single-chain protein of 78 to 79 residues [129, 130] whose sequence has been reported [129]. Isoelectric heterogeneity of apo C-II has been noted [131], but the chemical basis of this polymorphism is not known. Lipid-free apo C-II contains about 30 percent α helix, increasing to 45 percent α-helical content when reassembled with phospholipid [132, 133].

This apoprotein is a potent activator of lipoprotein lipase, the enzyme catalyzing the hydrolysis of triglyceride in chylomicrons and VLDL. Studies performed with synthetic peptides indicate that, unlike LCAT activation by apo A-I, lipid binding and lipase activation by apo C-II occur in separate domains of

Table 29-6 Chemical and apolipoprotein composition of the lipoprotein classes, percent of dry weight

	Chylomicrons	VLDL	LDL	HDL
Lipoprotein constituents				
Unesterified cholesterol	1–2	4–7	5–8	3–5
Phospholipid	4–6	15–22	16–25	26–32
Protein	1–2	6–10	18–22	45–55
Esterified cholesterol	1–2	15–22	45–50	15–20
Triglyceride	85–95	45–65	3–9	2–7
Apolipoprotein components*				
A-I	Major	Minor	Trace	Major
A-II	Major	Minor	Trace	Major
A-IV	Major	Trace	Absent	Minor
B	Major	Major	Major	Minor
C-I	Major	Major	Trace	Minor
C-II	Major	Major	Trace	Minor
C-III	Major	Major	Trace	Minor
D	Unknown	Minor, if present	Trace	Minor
E	Minor	Major	Minor	Minor

* "Major" refers to proteins comprising 5 percent or more of the total protein in mesenteric lymph chylomicrons and plasma VLDL, LDL, and HDL.

Table 29-7 Human plasma apolipoproteins

Apolipoprotein	Molecular weight	Plasma concentration, mg/dl	Origin	Function
A-I	28,300	90–130	Intestine, liver	LCAT activator
A-II	17,000	30–50	Intestine, liver	Unknown
B-100	~549,000	80–100	Liver	Neutral lipid transport
B-48	~264,000	<5	Intestine, liver	
C-I	6,500	4–7	Liver	LCAT activator
C-II	8,800	3–8	Liver	LPL activator
C-III	8,750	8–15	Liver	Unknown
E	35–39,000	3–6	Liver	?Receptor-mediated lipoprotein remnant catabolism

the protein [134]. The physiologic importance of lipase activation was unequivocally documented when one form of severe familial hypertriglyceridemia was shown to be secondary to an absolute deficiency of apo C-II [135] (discussed in detail in Chap. 30). Normally, the quantity of apo C-II in plasma considerably exceeds that required for lipoprotein lipase activation.

Apolipoprotein C-III Apo C-III is the most abundant of the C apoproteins, accounting for about 50 percent of the protein in VLDL [136] and about 2 percent of that in HDL. It is a single-chain, 79-amino-acid protein of known sequence [137, 138] with galactose and galactosamine attached together in glycosidic linkage at residue 74. Apo C-III exists in at least three polymorphic forms containing, respectively, two (apo C-III-2), one (apo C-III-1), or no (apo C-III-0) sialic acid residues at the end of the carbohydrate chain.

Apo C-III has primarily a disordered structure in aqueous solutions, but the addition of phosphatidylcholine causes the content of the α helix to increase from 22 to 54 percent [139]. Thrombin cleaves apo C-III into two peptides of equal size. The amino-terminal fragment of 40 residues does not bind phospholipid, whereas the carboxyl-terminal 39-residue peptide does [140].

About 25 percent of the apo C-III in normal plasma is associated with VLDL, whereas 60 percent is in HDL. Greater than 50 percent of total apo C-III may be in VLDL in hypertriglyceridemic serum [141]. Under appropriate in vitro conditions apo C-III can diminish lipoprotein lipase activity [142, 143], but this property is not unique to apo C-III and is of doubtful physiologic significance.

Apolipoprotein E Apoprotein E comprises 10 to 20 percent of VLDL protein and can be detected immunochemically in all lipoprotein classes. Reported molecular weights range from 33,000 to 38,000 [144, 145]. The protein usually occurs as a single chain but may form a mixed disulfide with apo A-II [146]. Extensive heterogeneity of apo E has been defined by isoelectric focusing (Fig. 29-1) [145, 147–149]. Differences in sialic acid content may account for some but not all of the isoelectric species [150, 151]. The three major isoforms of apo E (termed E-2, E-3, and E-4, the latter being most basic) are thought to be products of three alleles at a single locus [151]. Preliminary data suggest that the isoforms differ in their cysteine content, and it has been suggested that cysteine-arginine substitutions account for the heterogeneity [152].

When apo E forms stable complexes with phospholipid, the α helicity of the protein increases from 45 to 65 percent [153].

Certain apo E–containing lipoproteins from cholesterol-fed dogs bind with higher affinity to cell surface receptors of cultured fibroblasts than do LDL [154]. Hepatic uptake and catabolism of apo E appear preferentially to involve the more basic isoforms (E-3 and E-4), and their recognition by hepatocyte receptors may provide a link in the normal conversion of VLDL remnants to LDL [155, 156].

Apo E is synthesized by the liver, and intestinal production has not been demonstrated [10]. Diet does not have a pronounced effect on apo E concentrations in plasma [157]. Serum levels correlate highly with triglyceride concentrations [158], and highest levels are observed in type 3 hyperlipoproteinemia [159, 160]. As discussed in Chap. 32, the latter disorder is associated with an abnormal complement of E isoproteins [161], which appear to be slowly catabolized [162].

Lipoprotein Interactions

It has long been recognized that the surface components of lipoproteins, including free fatty acids, unesterified cholesterol, partial glycerides, and phospholipids, readily exchange among all circulating lipoprotein classes and with cell membranes of most if not all tissues. Dynamic equilibrium with membrane-like surfaces is probably generally affected by random molecular collision, although phopholipid exchange may be facilitated by plasma transfer factor(s) [163–165].

Some but not all of the apolipoproteins, which are located primarily on the particle surface, readily exchange among lipoproteins. The C apoproteins preferentially associate with triglyceride-rich lipoproteins but return to HDL when triglyceride is hydrolyzed in muscle and adipose tissue [166]. The A-IV apoprotein too may be cyclically reincorporated into chylomicrons while circulating in a lipid-free form in the postabsorptive state [115]. A-I and A-II show no affinity for plasma VLDL and chylomicrons but exchange readily among HDL subclasses [167, 168]. Only apo B has never been shown to exchange within or between lipoprotein classes.

The apolar lipids, which comprise the bulk of the lipoprotein core, also undergo extensive exchange and sometimes net transfer between lipoproteins. The cholesteryl ester exchange protein [169], identified in the serums of all species but the rat [170] and pig [171], promotes rapid equilibration between cholesteryl esters in all lipoprotein fractions [165, 169–174]. Facilitated exchange and net transfer of triglycerides between lipoprotein classes has also been shown, a process which may be mediated by a separate transfer protein [175]. Net transfer of cholesteryl esters from HDL to VLDL, and reciprocal transfer of triglyceride to HDL has been noted in vitro [176] and appears to take place in vivo [177].

The extent and rate of these exchange and transfer processes leave little doubt that lipoprotein core lipid is not hermetically sealed within a phospholipid-protein casing, awaiting scavenger or receptor-mediated clearance of the lipoprotein particle. The possibility that these recently discovered transfer and exchange proteins mediate net lipid transfer to tissues is intriguing and as yet unexplored.

Lipoprotein Interconversions and Catabolism

Catabolism of chylomicrons and VLDL is initiated by lipoprotein lipase at the endothelial surface. The triglycerides are hydrolyzed, producing a smaller remnant particle relatively depleted of triglyceride and containing an excess of surface components. Unesterified cholesterol, phospholipids, and C apoproteins may be transferred to HDL$_3$ [178–180], thereby generating the larger HDL$_2$ particle (Fig. 29-2). Consistent with this postulated mechanism of HDL$_2$ formation is the observation that VLDL and HDL$_2$ plasma levels are inversely correlated [180, 181].

Remnants produced by hydrolysis of chylomicron triglycerides are rapidly removed by the liver, at least in lower species [182, 185]. Even in humans very little if any of the B apoprotein in chylomicrons later appears in LDL [186]. Liver plasma membranes have a much greater affinity for chylomicron remnants than chylomicrons themselves [187], and the uptake appears to be inhibited by C apoproteins and enhanced by apo E [188, 189]. Cholesterol derived from chylomicrons is a very effective inhibitor of hepatic cholesterol synthesis, an effect that reflects the much higher rate of transport of chylomicron cholesterol into the hepatocyte than the cholesterol carried in LDL or HDL [190].

Progressive hydrolysis of VLDL triglyceride, as already noted, leads eventually to the formation of LDL. Metabolic studies in normal subjects have demonstrated that during this conversion virtually all of the apo B in VLDL is converted to LDL apo B [72]. This contrasts with the rat, whose VLDL remnants are mostly cleared directly by the liver and not catabolized to

LDL [192]. This probably accounts for the low plasma concentrations of LDL in this species as compared to humans.

Studies in the rat have also suggested that direct hepatic degradation accounts for only a small proportion of the LDL cleared from plasma [193]. Most LDL is thought to be catabolized by extrahepatic tissues, approximately one-third by a highly specific receptor-mediated process and the remainder by a receptor-independent pathway [194]. The regulation of LDL uptake by tissues and its role in both body and cellular cholesterol homeostasis is considered in detail in Chap. 33.

Perfusion of isolated rat livers with radiolabeled HDL has, as with LDL, demonstrated that direct uptake by the liver accounts for only a small fraction of total HDL degradation [195]. Moreover, with the exception of a minor HDL population containing apo E [196], HDL are not bound, internalized, and degraded by the LDL-receptor system. It is therefore presumed that HDL are cleared from plasma by extrahepatic tissues, but details concerning the modulation of this process are not yet available.

ABETALIPOPROTEINEMIA

History

The association of atypical retinitis pigmentosa, malformed erythrocytes, and a "form of Friedreich's ataxia" was first described in 1950 in an 18-year-old Jewish girl [198]. Bassen and Kornzweig noted childhood "celiac-disease" in this patient, an abnormality which was more accurately described in the second reported case as fat malabsorption [199]. Profound hypocholesterolemia was added to the syndrome complex [200], and in 1960, three laboratories independently demonstrated the total absence of LDL from the plasma of similar patients [201–203]. The potential etiologic implications of this finding were reflected in the rapid substitution of "abetalipoproteinemia" for the eponymic designation "Bassen-Kornzweig syndrome." This focus is appropriate since no feature of "abetalipoproteinemia" is unique to the disorder except the

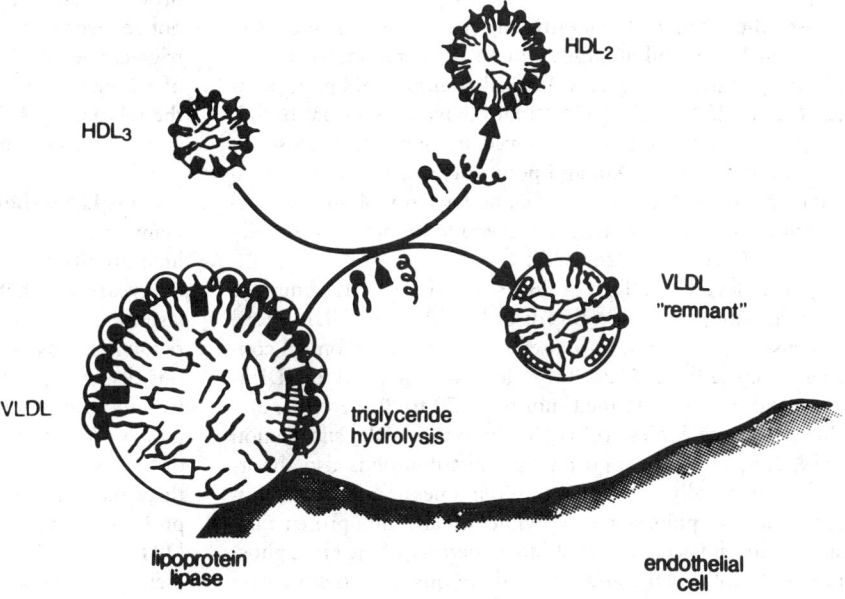

Figure 29-2 Proposed model of HDL$_3$ transformation to HDL$_2$ through the assimilation of phospholipid, cholesterol, and the proteins released from VLDL during its lipolysis. (*From Mahley et al. [197]. Used by permission.*)

absence of detectable plasma apoprotein B. More than 50 examples of abetalipoproteinemia have now been recorded [204–211].

Plasma Lipids, Lipoproteins, and Apolipoproteins

Lipids   Concentrations of all the major plasma lipids are reduced to less than 50 percent of normal in abetalipoproteinemia (see Ref. 212 for detailed discussion). Triglyceride concentrations, particularly, are usually below levels which can be confidently measured by conventional laboratory procedures. This reflects the total absence of chylomicrons and VLDL. In several subjects, evaluated by identical techniques [213, 214], total plasma phospholipid concentrations were reduced by approximately 75 percent. This reduction, moreover, is selective; phosphatidylcholine levels are only 15 to 20 percent of controls, while sphingomyelin concentrations approach 50 percent of normal. This accounts for the widely recognized alteration of the plasma phosphatidylcholine/sphingomyelin ratio in this disorder (5:4 versus 3:1 in the normal person).

About 70 percent of the plasma cholesterol in normal subjects is carried in the LDL and the absence of these lipoproteins results in striking hypocholesterolemia. Virtually all the plasma cholesterol in abetalipoproteinemia is associated with HDL. HDL concentrations are highly variable, however, and occasional patients have been reported with plasma cholesterol concentrations within the accepted normal range [215–217]. The average plasma cholesterol level is below 50 mg/dl, and concentrations lower than 25 mg/dl have frequently been recorded [213, 218–220].

β-Lipoproteins   Lipoprotein electrophoresis demonstrates the absence of chylomicrons, pre-β-, and β-lipoproteins even after fat feeding or the addition of excess free cholesterol and phosphatidylcholine to the plasma [221]. Reports to the contrary [222, 223] notwithstanding, most workers have been unable to find traces of any proteins in plasma that react with antiserums specific for apo B. These findings presumably reflect the inability of intestine or liver in this disorder to elaborate B protein–containing lipoproteins.

α-Lipoproteins   Preparative ultracentrifugation at density less than 1.063 g/ml of large amounts of abetalipoproteinemic plasma permits the recovery of small quantities of lipoproteins [214, 216, 224–226]. These "LDL" have an unusual barrel-shaped configuration when viewed by electron microscopy [227], are rich in protein and poor in cholesteryl esters when compared to normal LDL [225], and have α mobility on electrophoresis. They contain all the apolipoproteins usually found in HDL [225, 226, 228].

Plasma levels of HDL_2 (1.063 < density < 1.12 g/ml) are approximately normal in this disorder, while the HDL_3 (1.12 < density < 1.21 g/ml) are present in a third of control concentrations [214, 226, 229]. Cholesterol contained in HDL is about 50 percent esterified (normally 70 to 80 percent), and the excess free cholesterol is largely in the HDL_2 subfraction [214, 226]. The HDL phospholipid distribution is also abnormal. HDL usually contain six to seven times as much phosphoglyceride as sphingomyelin, while in abetalipoproteinemia sphingomyelin accounts for 37 to 45 percent of the HDL phospholipid. Both HDL_2 and HDL_3 share this threefold increase

in sphingomyelin [214]. The sphingomyelin enrichment of HDL may be a secondary abnormality since tissue sphingomyelin is selectively transferred to HDL [230] and then exchanged with lower density lipoproteins.

The apoproteins A-I and A-II from HDL in abetalipoproteinemia are identical to their normal counterparts, as judged by immunochemical [223, 225, 226] and electrophoretic [225, 226] criteria and by amino acid analysis [226]. Plasma apo A-I levels are reduced by 50 to 70 percent [231, 232], while apo A-II concentrations are depressed only 30 to 40 percent [232]. HDL metabolism has been studied in a single patient. It was concluded that apo A-I synthesis was 33 percent lower than normal, while the apo A-I catabolic rate was not increased [208]. The plasma HDL cholesterol and apo A-I levels in this subject were within the normal range.

The three C apolipoproteins, isolated from the HDL of abetalipoproteinemic patients, have the expected amino acid composition [223]. The monosialylated apo C-III-1 is absent or present in only trace quantities [204, 223, 226]. This defect may be comparable to that seen in the rat when orotic acid has been administered to block VLDL release from the liver. It has been argued from these findings that the sialic acid–rich form of apo C-III, apo C-III-2, that is present in abetalipoproteinemic plasma is normally elaborated with HDL. The less sialylated apo C-III-1 that is absent from plasma in this disease may be secreted only in combination with VLDL [223].

Apoproteins D [225] and E [232] are present in HDL in abetalipoproteinemia. The relative proportion of E appears greater than normal [232], and much of the apo E is present as a mixed disulfide [232], presumably in combination with apo A-II [234].

Lipase and LCAT Activities   The plasma postheparin lipolytic activity in two patients with abetalipoproteinemia has been very low [235, 236]. It cannot be inferred, however, that any absolute deficiency of postheparin lipases (see Chap. 30) exists, because of the well-known depression of their activity when dietary fat (or chylomicron formation) is restricted.

Deficient LCAT activity has also been shown in several studies of affected subjects [221, 225, 226]. This, too, may be secondary since partially purified LCAT has very little activity against HDL_2 [237], the dominant HDL species in abetalipoproteinemia. The mass of plasma LCAT in this disorder has not yet been quantitated, and it has been suggested that hepatic triglyceride and LCAT secretion are linked [238]. Irrespective of whether substrate or enzyme concentrations are limiting, the relative LCAT deficiency in this disease is probably of no clinical consequence.

Sterol Metabolism   Sterol metabolism in abetalipoproteinemia has been studied to assess in vivo the importance of high-affinity cell surface receptors for LDL. It was noted several years ago that activity of the rate-limiting enzyme in cholesterol biosynthesis, 3-hydroxy-3-methylglutaryl-coenzyme A reductase, was normal in scalp hair roots from a patient with this disorder [239]. Acetate incorporation into cholesterol by freshly isolated lymphocytes appeared increased in two patients [205] but normal in a third [240]. Moreover, studies of LDL surface binding and catabolism by lymphocytes from three patients revealed no high-affinity binding sites. There is probably some increase in whole-body cholesterol synthesis [241–243], but this can be attributed to malabsorption of dietary and biliary cholesterol [243].

It may be unrealistic to anticipate that expression of the LDL receptor in tissues freshly obtained would be comparable to that in rapidly dividing cells in culture. The expectation that cholesterol synthesis would be increased in vivo in abetalipoproteinemia derives from the assumption that circulating lipoproteins in this disease cannot fill tissue cholesterol requirements. The prominence of apo E in abetalipoproteinemia HDL [232] may be important, since lipoproteins containing apo E show high-affinity binding to the LDL receptor [224]. Such lipoproteins are a minority population in normal HDL, but this may not be the case in abetalipoproteinemia.

Clinical and Pathophysiologic Correlates

Gastrointestinal System The gastrointestinal problems of patients with abetalipoproteinemia are stereotypic. Fat malabsorption is present from birth, and the neonatal period is characterized by poor appetite, vomiting, loose voluminous stools, and little weight gain. Symptoms have led to the correct diagnosis as early as age 4 to 6 weeks [213, 245]. The syndrome is consistent with a number of other disorders affecting either the intraluminal or mucosal phases of digestion. Roentgenographic examination of the upper gastrointestinal tract is rarely normal [246, 247] and may show striking clumping and segmentation of contrast material (see Fig. 29-3) [202, 248, 249]. The diagnoses of cystic fibrosis and celiac disease typically are entertained and later excluded by laboratory tests and failure to respond to appropriate therapy.

MUCOSAL CHANGES Endoscopy, not routinely undertaken in children, has revealed yellow discoloration of the duodenum [207] which may be similar to that seen in Tangier disease [250]. The jejunal biopsy of patients with abetalipoproteinemia is generally pathognomonic. Light microscopy excludes the diagnosis of celiac disease with the demonstration of unblunted, well-formed villi. The mucosal cells, particularly those near the villus tip, are extensively vacuolated [215, 249, 250], and conventional stains show that the "vacuoles" are lipid droplets [246, 251–253]. The lipid content is 1.5 to 3.5 times normal [246], with triglyceride accounting for virtually all the increase.

Although the dietary origin of the mucosal lipid droplets in abetalipoproteinemia is not disputed, their relationship to such droplets visualized during normal fat digestion is less clear. The lipid droplets which appear during normal fat absorption are quite clearly bound by the membranes of the endoplasmic reticulum, with an additional ring of increased density surrounding the lipid drop. Moreover, the Golgi vacuoles in the normal cell become distended with small lipid droplets, and lipophilic particles of chylomicron size are visualized in the intercellular "peg" areas and the lacteals in the lamina propria [250]. In abetalipoproteinemia, it is difficult to demonstrate membranous envelopes around the larger lipid droplets, the continuity of these lipid droplets with the endoplasmic reticulum is less clear (Fig. 29-4), and the Golgi zone never accumulates lipoprotein-sized droplets. The lipid droplets in the mucosa in abetalipoproteinemia lack the ring of increased density around the lipid droplet [250]. Thus, the triglyceride in the affected cell does not appear to receive the normal apoprotein coating, is not normally transported to the Golgi zone through the endoplasmic reticulum, and does not serve as a lipoprotein precursor. The missing protein presumably is apoprotein B,

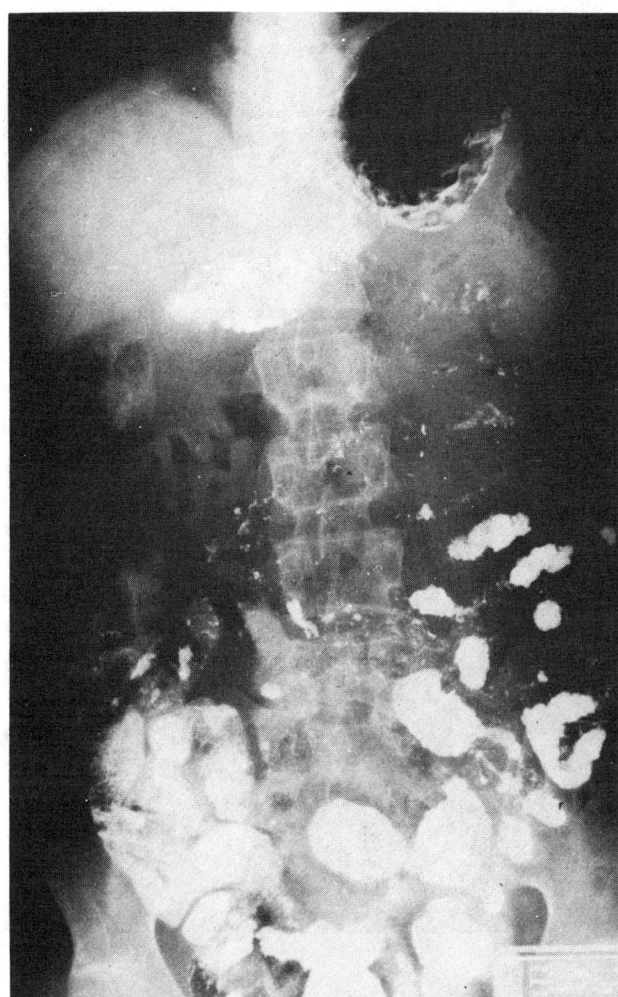

Figure 29-3 Upper gastrointestinal series from the patient with familial homozygous hypobetalipoproteinemia described by Biemer and McCammon [326]. Flocculation and segmentation of contrast material are like those frequently seen in patients with abetalipoproteinemia.

which is not detectable in the intestinal mucosa in abetalipoproteinemia [254].

INTESTINAL ABSORPTIVE FUNCTIONS The morphological changes notwithstanding, the mucosal cell in abetalipoproteinemia does absorb long-chain fatty acids and normally reesterifies them with glycerol [251, 253, 255]. In the affected mucosal cell the lysosomes increase in number and have an unusual appearance [250] which suggests that they may provide an auxiliary mechanism to clear the accumulating triglycerides. The triglycerides are presumably hydrolyzed and the fatty acids transported into the portal venous system bound to albumin. Such a mechanism must account for the fact that steatorrhea in abetalipoproteinemia is relatively mild. Adult patients challenged with diets containing 100 g fat per day complain of bloating, flatulence, and diarrhea but excrete only 15 to 20 percent of the ingested fat in their stools.

Fat-soluble vitamins that are transported in chylomicrons are also poorly absorbed. Vitamin A in foodstuffs is hydrolyzed to retinol before absorption from the intestinal lumen [256]. In transit through the mucosal cell it is reesterified, usually with palmitic acid, and is secreted into the intestinal lymph in chylomicrons [257]. Vitamin A absorption curves in abetalipoproteinemia are characteristically flat [251, 258, 259], and

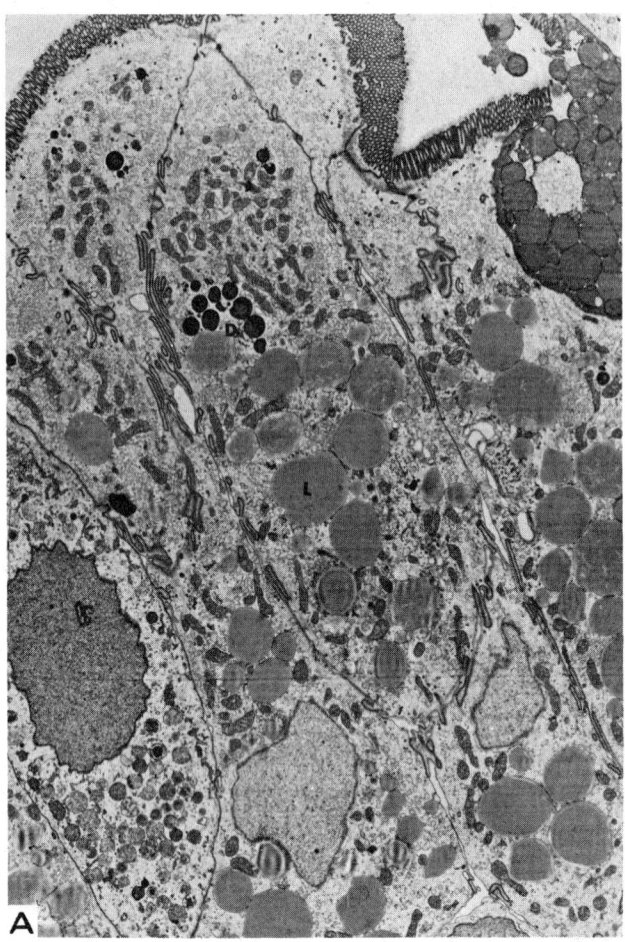

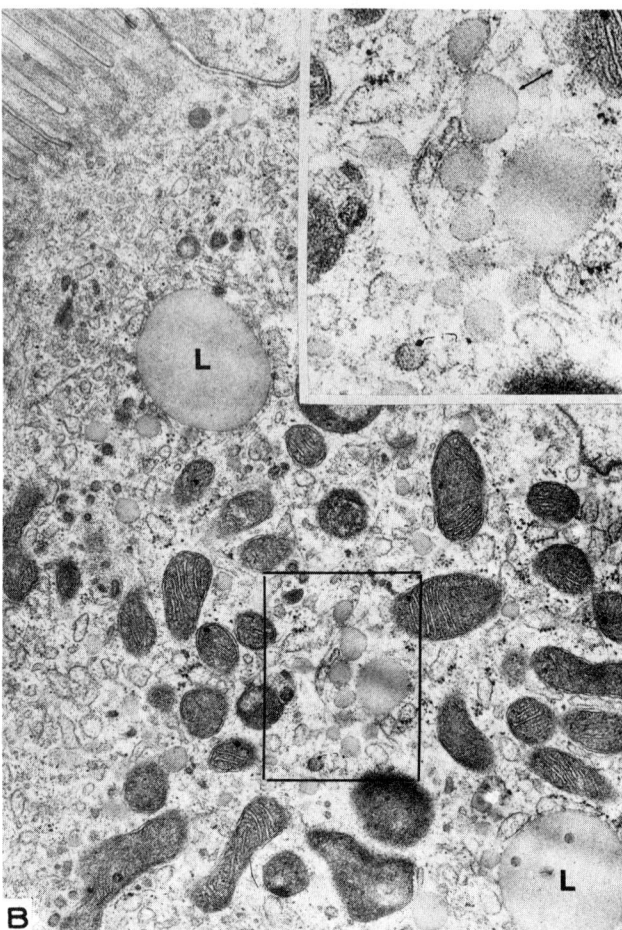

Figure 29-4 Duodenojejunal biopsies from a patient with abetalipoproteinemia. *A.* Electron micrograph of intestinal absorptive cells containing massive amounts of lipid (L). Portions of a goblet cell (right upper corner) and an argentaffin cell (left lower corner) are seen. There are numerous dense bodies (D). Biopsy obtained while fasting, but during a period of normal diet with corn oil supplementation. Bicarbonate-buffered osmium; magnification, ×5500. *B.* Patient consumed a low fat diet for 34 days. Thirty minutes before the biopsy 1.5 ml/kg of corn oil was instilled into the upper duodenum. Two large lipid droplets (L) presumably were present before fat instillation. Recently absorbed lipid is seen within profiles of the endoplasmic reticulum (outlined area). S-Collidine–buffered osmium: magnification, ×30,500. *Inset:* Enlargement of outlined area on figure demonstrating endoplasmic reticulum (arrows) around lipid droplets. Magnification, ×62,200. (*Photograph kindly provided by Dr. W. O. Dobbins, III. Reprinted from* [250] *with permission.*)

low plasma concentrations are typical in untreated patients [215, 219, 252, 260]. When large supplements are given, levels rise to the normal range. The mechanism of this increase is unclear. Possibly the vitamin is transported in HDL secreted by the intestine, or some unesterified vitamin may gain access to the circulation through direct uptake by the retinol-binding protein.

The lowest serum levels of vitamin E recorded in humans have been found in abetalipoproteinemia [224, 261]. The possible clinical significance of this fact is discussed later. Tocopherol absorption normally is greatest when it is administered with dietary fat, but the vitamin is also absorbed from food containing no lipids [262]. Vitamin E in the latter circumstance is probably transported to the circulation in small chylomicrons continuously formed in the absence of fat absorption. Single oral loads of large amounts of water-miscible vitamin E to abetalipoproteinemic subjects do not induce detectable blood levels during the ensuing 24 h [263]. Moreover, the importance of LDL in vitamin E transport after absorption [262] is reflected by the relatively low blood levels achieved after parenteral administration [263]. Enteric absorption of vitamin E, perhaps through the portal venous system [264], and detectable blood levels can be achieved in abetalipoproteinemia when very large quantities of fat or water-miscible preparations are ingested for prolonged periods [263, 265].

Hypoprothrombinemia, secondary to vitamin K malabsorption, is also well documented in this disorder [220, 222, 246, 266]. Natural vitamins K_1 and K_2, which physically are oils,

are absorbed almost exclusively in the lymph. Signs of abnormal hemostasis have been described in only two children [210, 251].

Other intestinal absorptive functions in this disorder are normal or minimally impaired [202, 215, 218, 219, 246, 251–253].

Liver Detectable liver abnormalities are not common. Gross hepatic enlargement has been described in only one child with abetalipoproteinemia [267], and elevated levels of the serum transaminase in two subjects [255, 267]. Light-microscopic studies have demonstrated that most hepatocytes are extensively vacuolated and lipid-laden, but gross disturbances of lobule architecture are not observed [253, 255]. The usual hepatic steatosis of this condition progressed to micronodular cirrhosis in at least one case [267]. The infant described was unusual in that elevated transaminase levels in association with hepatomegaly were recorded throughout the period of observation. The Golgi zones were devoid of VLDL-containing saccules, and the smooth endoplasmic reticulum adjacent to the Golgi zone was vestigial. The development of hyalin degeneration and frank cirrhosis in this patient was linked by the authors to treatment with medium-chain triglycerides. Recently another child was found to have fibrosis in addition to fatty transformation after only 1.5 years of medium-chain triglyceride treatment [211].

Hepatic triglyceride accumulation is presumably due to absent VLDL synthesis or secretion. As in the intestine, it is clear that triglyceride synthesis is not defective. Auxiliary pathways for triglyceride hydrolysis, perhaps by lysosomal enzymes, may operate to release fatty acids for oxidation or plasma transport to peripheral tissues. Teleologically, one might argue that such mechanisms could normally mediate fat transport from the liver and might question any *a priori* necessity for VLDL synthesis or secretion.

Neuromuscular Manifestations The neuromuscular manifestations of abetalipoproteinemia are devastating (Fig. 29-5). Neonatal psychomotor development is usually slow, but the relationship of the motor retardation to the invariable nutritional problems is unclear. The majority of infants and children remain below the 3d percentile for height and weight. At least one-third of affected children have symptomatic neuromuscular problems in the first decade of life, and many have demonstrated moderate to severe ataxia before age 20. Only occasional patients are able to stand unassisted by their fourth decade.

The neurologic syndrome of abetalipoproteinemia has been nosologically considered one of the heredofamilial spinocerebellar degenerative disorders. The disease selectively involves the pathways of the large, heavily myelinated sensory neurons whose cell bodies are in the spinal ganglions and whose fibers enter the spinal cord most medially in the dorsal root zone, adjacent to the lateral aspect of the posterior funiculus.

The earliest neurologic finding is the loss of stretch reflexes. Diminution of deep-tendon reflexes at age 17 months has been reported [218], with complete absence as early as age 3 to 5 years [202, 258, 268]. Preservation of any deep-tendon reflexes into the second decade has been described in only two instances [152, 198]. The loss of stretch reflexes has been attributed to the posterior column degeneration and interruption of spinocerebellar pathways. The unusual severity and lack of sparing of the upper extremities warrants investigation of other possible causes, particularly selective loss of cell bodies in the spinal ganglions.

Disturbances of proprioceptive pathways to the brain also occur early. As in the case of the stretch reflexes, the degree of impairment is much greater than that characterizing the other forms of spinocerebellar degeneration. Position and vibratory sensation are lost, and a positive Romberg sign typical of sensory ataxia can be elicited in most subjects. Pathologically, these findings are correlated with extensive demyelinization of the fasciculi gracilis and cuneatus in the posterior spinal columns [220, 266].

Pyramidal tract involvement has been suggested by the presence of extensor plantar responses in several patients [198, 215, 255, 266], and mild loss of anterior horn nuclei has been found at autopsy [266]. Spasticity does not occur.

OTHER NEUROLOGIC PATHWAYS Signs of nonspecific or mixed peripheral neuropathy in abetalipoproteinemia are rare. Mild hypesthesia to pain, temperature, and touch sometimes is present, usually in a stocking-glove distribution [202, 215, 269]. There is little published evidence of actual peripheral axon degeneration, and the observed peripheral nerve demyelinization is patchy or segmental in nature.

Well-defined cerebral cortical disease is not a feature of abe-

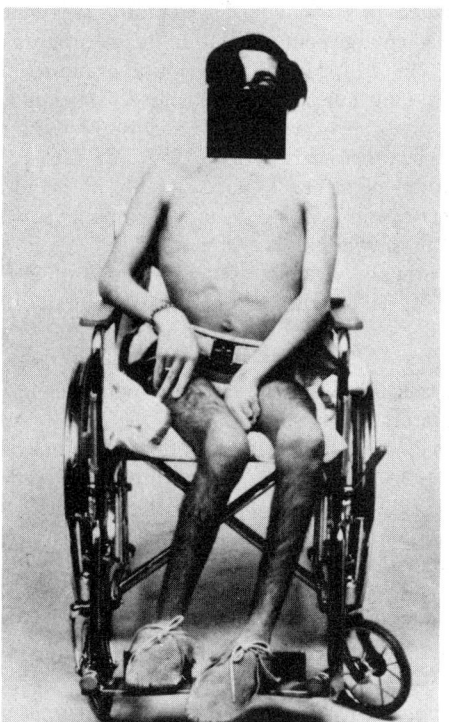
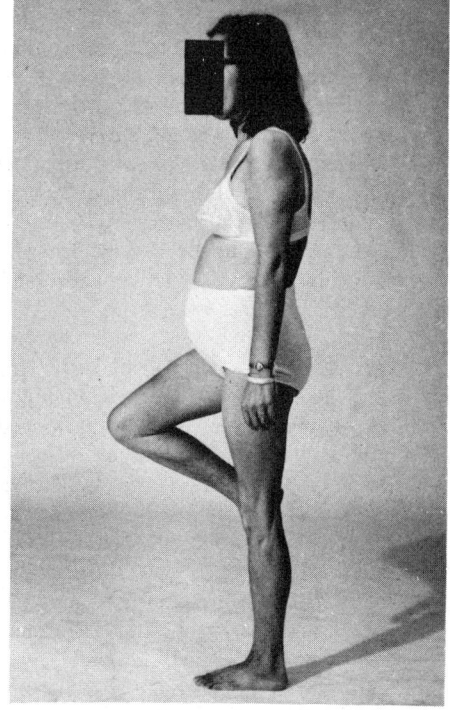

Figure 29-5 The patient with abetalipoproteinemia is a 17-year-old man with severe generalized weakness, kyphoscoliosis, and lordosis. The 43-year-old woman with familial homozygous hypobetalipoproteinemia has minimal neuromuscular defects.

ABETALIPOPROTEINEMIA   HOMOZYGOUS HYPOBETALIPOPROTEINEMIA

talipoproteinemia. Electroencephalographic findings have been abnormal in only a few patients, and the irregularities have been mild and nonspecific [247, 248, 251]. Mental retardation as measured by formal intelligence testing and performance in school has been apparent in about a third of reported patients, and all but two of these patients [248, 252] have been the product of consanguine relationships [202, 247, 270–272].

CEREBELLUM   The spinocerebellar axis is interrupted in abetalipoproteinemia, and because both the anterior and posterior spinocerebellar pathways undergo demyelination, the degree of primary cerebellar disease is difficult to appraise. Dysdiadochokinesia, dysmetria, scanning of speech, hypotonia, asthenia, and intention tremor have all been described. At postmortem examination, the cerebellum was normal in one patient [220] while showing some loss of molecular and Purkinje cell nuclei in another [266]. It seems likely that in most instances the "cerebellar signs" are primarily of spinal and brainstem origin.

MUSCLE   Weakness and muscle atrophy are usually attributed to disuse and spinocerebellar degeneration. A patient with rapidly progressive and severe weakness thought secondary to primary muscle disease has been reported [206]. Electromyography showed polyphasic, short-duration action potentials in the deltoid muscle. Serum transaminases, aldolase, and creatine phosphokinase were elevated without myoglobinuria. Striated muscle biopsy showed accumulation of ceroid pigment in interstitial fibroblasts and macrophages. While most muscle fibers appeared normal, some contained electron-dense bodies (presumed ceroid). The relationship of the profound weakness to the mild pathologic changes was uncertain.

Cardiac disturbances occur in abetalipoproteinemia, but their prevalence is difficult to judge from the published literature. Electrocardiographic findings have been reported in 11 patients, and 3 have demonstrated T-wave changes or premature ventricular beats [220, 266, 273]. Cardiac enlargement and murmurs have been noted in four subjects [198, 215, 218, 220]. The hearts of two patients have been examined at autopsy. In one there were no abnormalities of valves, myocardium, epicardium, or coronary arteries [266]. The other heart [220] had extensive interstitial fibrosis, lipochrome pigmentation of the myocardium, and thick, fibrous pericardium and epicardium. These changes are reminiscent of those typifying Friedreich's ataxia, but the high incidence of early and severe cardiac involvement in the latter syndrome [274] renders the parallelism uncertain.

NEUROMUSCULAR PATHOPHYSIOLOGY   It is speculated that abnormal lipid peroxidation of the highly unsaturated phosphatides of myelin, secondary to prolonged vitamin E deficiency, underlies the neuromuscular degeneration. Since the last edition of this book, vitamin E deficiency has been convincingly linked with neuromuscular pathology in other malabsorption states, including cholestasis and cystic fibrosis [275–277]. The resemblance of the neurologic findings to those in abetalipoproteinemia is striking. Moreover, there is evidence that myopathy [278] and neuropathy [279] in vitamin E deficiency are partially reversible.

Less attractive is the postulate that plasma lipoproteins help maintain the structural integrity of the central nervous system. While it is likely that lipoproteins exchange free cholesterol,

lecithin, and sphingomyelin with neuronal tissue as they do with other plasma membranes, there is no *a priori* reason to presume this function is essential.

Skeletal Involvement   Skeletal abnormalities in abetalipoproteinemia are similar to those in other heredofamilial spinocerebellar degenerations; they include pes cavus and equinovarus, kyphoscoliosis, and hyperlordosis (Fig. 29-5). These probably result from muscle imbalance during skeletal maturation and do not reflect primary bone disease.

Ocular Manifestations   As the neuromuscular abnormalities in abetalipoproteinemia appear to be a forme fruste of Friedreich's ataxia, so the ophthalmic findings bear a striking resemblance to other heredofamilial retinal pigmentary degenerations. Retinitis pigmentosa, in fact, occurs on rare occasions in Friedreich's ataxia, but it has been a constant finding in abetalipoproteinemia.

The age of onset of the signs and symptoms of ocular abnormalities in this disorder is highly variable. Night blindness, secondary to rod degeneration, has been a complaint, particularly in younger children with rapidly progressing retinal disease [198, 252]. Dark adaptometry shows delayed responses and elevated thresholds in the majority of patients. Loss of visual acuity has been documented as early as age 7 to 9 years [215, 271] and has been delayed to as late as age 30 years [266]. This reflects the degree of "macular sparing" and other individual differences in the rate of progression of retinal degeneration. It is perhaps noteworthy that those patients with evidence of the most severe macular degeneration and blindness have also had severe neuromuscular dysfunction [198, 199, 215, 273].

Nystagmus is common in abetalipoproteinemia. This could be secondary to lesions in the upper spinal cord or cerebellum, but the available data suggest that it is of ocular origin, with impaired fixation from loss of central vision and macular degeneration. This contention is supported by an obvious association between pronounced loss of visual acuity and the description of more florid oscillating, vertical, horizontal, and dissociated nystagmus [198, 199, 202].

The cause of the frequently noted ophthalmoplegia [200, 248, 252, 258, 269, 272] is not known. The ptosis which is occasionally observed [215, 258] is presumed to be neurogenic. Two patients with mild pupillary inequality have been described [207, 266]. In one, the finding was stationary over several years of observation, and pupil reactivity to light was preserved bilaterally. Lenticular opacities, presumably posterior polar cataracts, were noted during life in one patient [200]. The infrequency of cataracts in abetalipoproteinemia contrasts with their prevalence in typical retinitis pigmentosa [280].

There are no data bearing directly on the molecular defect responsible for the retinal pigmentary degeneration. The neuroepithelium of the retina, like the posterior columns and spinocerebellar tracts, appears unusually vulnerable to a variety of heredofamilial and metabolic defects [281]. In contrast to the central nervous system the ocular defects do not appear to involve neuronal demyelinization [282]. The retinitis pigmentosa is somewhat atypical in its indiscriminate destruction of cones in addition to rods, but in the majority of patients it is clinically indistinguishable from the more common forms of pigmentary degeneration of the retina.

Much attention has been directed to the deficiency of vitamin A in abetalipoproteinemia. Two patients in their twenties have been treated with massive doses of vitamin A with partial or complete reversal of abnormalities of the electroretinogram and of dark adaptation [283]. Less dramatic improvement was noted in two younger patients who received similar treatment [284]. Overall, it is evident that some of the ocular symptoms and signs in this condition are probably related to vitamin A deficiency.

Several other lines of evidence suggest that this is not the basic defect. Efforts to relate vitamin A deficiency to the classic form of retinitis pigmentosa have been unconvincing [285, 286]. The ocular effects of natural vitamin A deficiency in humans [287] and that induced by nutritional deficiency in animals [288, 289] are not characterized by retinal pigmentary degeneration. Also, patients with abetalipoproteinemia do not exhibit typical manifestations of vitamin A deficiency. Finally, pharmacologic doses of water-miscible vitamin A administered for 3 years to a child with abetalipoproteinemia raised the serum levels of vitamin A to normal but failed to prevent the development of retinal degeneration [290].

Photoreceptor and pigment epithelial changes have been demonstrated in vitamin E–deficient rats [291, 292], and vitamin E deficiency secondary to short bowel syndrome has been linked to the development of both neurologic changes and retinitis pigmentosa [279]. The possibility that vitamin E may prevent the development of retinopathy in abetalipoproteinemia has been suggested [265] and supporting evidence should soon be available.

Hematologic Manifestations

THE ACANTHOCYTE The striking malformation of the erythrocyte in abetalipoproteinemia led to the initial differentiation of this syndrome from other forms of retinitis pigmentosa [198] and for 10 years was considered the diagnostic countermark [199, 269, 270, 273]. The acanthocyte is not unique to abetalipoproteinemia, but it has appropriately received considerable attention as a signal reflection of the effects of the plasma lipoprotein abnormality on plasma membrane structure and function.

The proportion of red cells in the peripheral blood transformed into acanthocytes is at least 50 to 70 percent. The thorny projections of typical cells (Fig. 29-6) [293] prevent normal rouleau formation and, in the absence of plasma LDL, result in very low erythrocyte sedimentation rates. The life span of the red corpuscle, determined by the isotopic ^{51}Cr method, is usually shortened [248, 258, 273] but may be normal [215]. Increased red cell turnover in the patients is reflected in low or absent haptoglobins [294], hyperbilirubinemia [248, 255, 273], reticulocytosis [215, 246], and bone marrow erythroid hyperplasia [255, 259, 266, 273].

Acanthocytes are not found in the bone marrow in patients with abetalipoproteinemia, and the membrane distortion is presumed to be acquired after release into the peripheral circulation. The total red cell lipid and phospholipid levels are normal, but the distribution of the phospholipids is distinctly abnormal and appears unique to this disorder. Specifically, the usual ratio of phosphatidylcholine to sphingomyelin (1:3) is reversed in the acanthocyte (1:0.6). The red cell phospholipid distribution qualitatively mirrors that in the plasma. It has been suggested that sphingomyelin enrichment reduces the fluidity of the acanthocyte plasma membrane and contributes to its "remodeling" during circulation. Cow red blood cells con-

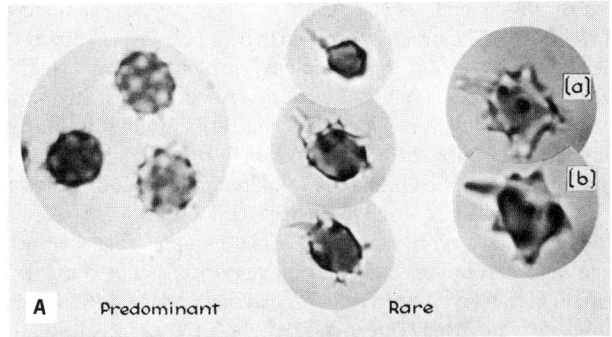

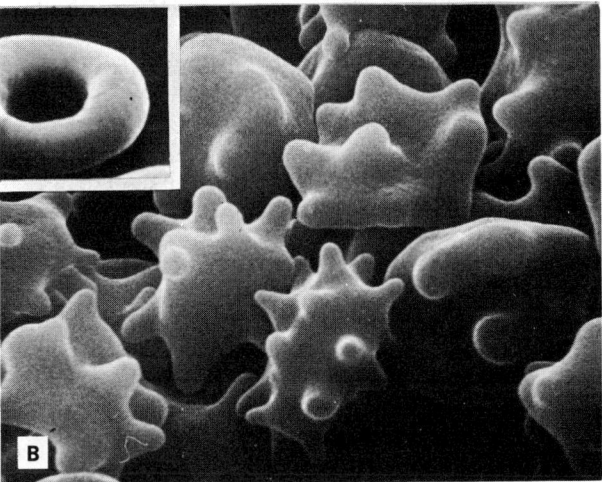

Figure 29-6 Acanthocytes in abetalipoproteinemia as visualized with the scanning electron microscope. A normal erythrocyte is presented in the inset (*upper left*). Magnification, ×5000. (*Photographs supplied by Dr. Herbert Kayden. From Kayden and Bessis [293]. Used by permission.*)

tain proportionately more sphingomyelins rich in saturated fatty acids and do not exhibit acanthocytic transformation.

Autohemolysis of red cells incubated in vitro is five- to tenfold greater than normal in abetalipoproteinemia [222, 246, 251, 294]. This may be related to vitamin E deficiency. Autohemolysis was reduced from 90 percent to 10 percent by the addition of small quantities of tocopherol phosphate in vitro. Comparable changes were achieved by the intramuscular administration of vitamin E to patients [224].

ANEMIA AND ABNORMAL HEMOSTASIS Severe anemia with hemoglobin levels as low as 4 to 8 g/dl is not uncommon in young children with abetalipoproteinemia [220, 248, 270, 295] and in several instances has required transfusion. Most adult patients do not have significant anemia, and that described in children is probably secondary to broad nutritional deficiencies attending malabsorption. Correction of the anemia with parenteral iron or folate therapy is usually possible [218, 246, 271]. Vitamin B_{12} absorption and plasma concentrations are normal [248, 255], and serum iron levels are maintained without specific supplements [219, 258]. Prolongation of the prothrombin time secondary to vitamin K malabsorption is readily treated, and excessive bleeding does not contribute to the anemia. Platelet content of free cholesterol is increased, but in vitro platelet aggregation is not abnormal [296].

Other Clinical Findings Developmental abnormalities associated with abetalipoproteinemia have usually been limited to the skeletal system. Annular deformities of the fingers [198, 272, 273], brachymesophalangia [247, 248], supernumerary digits [200], microcephaly, prognathia, and high-arched palate [247] have all been described. Other "stigmata of degeneration" have included epicanthal folds and early Dupuytren's contracture [198], webbing of fingers [200], and small, tightly applied pinnae [248]. Ureterovesicle obstruction has been noted in a single patient [295].

Patients have widely been described as appearing younger than their chronologic age, and the majority, as noted earlier, remain in the lowest percentile for height and weight. Bone age and density are usually normal [198, 247, 251, 258], although transient "osteomalacia" has been described [202, 271]. Rickets secondary to deficiency of the fat-soluble vitamin D is not a feature of this disease, since the luminal phase of fat absorption is normal and the vitamin is probably transported from the intestinal mucosal cell by an α_2-globulin [297]. The growth hormone status of abetalipoproteinemic patients has not been extensively investigated, but in two patients of short stature the growth hormone rise to arginine infusion was normal [252]. Abnormalities of thyroid function have not been reported.

Information on steroid hormone metabolism in abetalipoproteinemia is sparse but of interest since circulating lipoproteins may be a major source of cholesterol for synthesis of corticosteroid [298–302] and gonadal hormones [303]. Symptoms of adrenocorticoid insufficiency have not been noted. Normal urinary excretion of 17-keto and ketogenic steroids have been found in unstimulated patients [200, 246, 271], one of whom reportedly had a normal response to ACTH administration [246]. Two other patients, in contrast, had a blunted rise in plasma [304] and urinary steroids [200, 304] after ACTH. If confirmed, the latter observations would complement the in vitro finding that the human adrenal preferentially utilizes LDL rather than HDL cholesterol [302].

In contrast to patients with Friedreich's ataxia, patients with abetalipoproteinemia rarely have diabetes mellitus [266, 273]. Other unusual and probably unrelated abnormalities have included acrodermatitis enteropathica [217], nonspecific aminoaciduria [218], normal ceruloplasmin with increased copper excretion, schizophrenia [266], hypoalbuminemia [252], and diminished plasma γ-globulin levels [219, 251]. Recurrent infections, usually respiratory, have received comment in several reports [211, 218, 252, 260, 271].

Genetics

Abetalipoproteinemia has been reported from twelve countries. Patients have included Caucasians, blacks, Arabs, Orientals, and a Maori. Of all known affected subjects, 25 percent have been Ashkenazic Jews.

The familial nature of the disease is proven. Two or more cases have been documented in eight sibships [209, 211, 216, 247, 252, 259, 269], and it seems likely that two or more will be found in a ninth [295]. Males have constituted 68 percent of the cases. In the 20 families in which all sibs have been examined, 46 percent of the males as opposed to 24 percent of the females had the disorder. The predominance of affected males has not been explained, and it is possible that the clinical expression of the disease is sex-influenced.

Available data are consistent with an autosomal recessive mode of inheritance. Fourteen affected subjects from eleven kindreds have been the product of consanguine matings. Con-

sanguinity has been found in almost 50 percent of pedigrees when any effort was made to establish the degree of parental relatedness. This finding attests to the rarity of the trait. Vertical transmission of the disease has never been described, and an X-linked trait is rendered unlikely, not only by the fact that 32 percent of cases have been female, but also by the observation that both sexes have been affected in six of the seven instances in which more than one sib had the disease. Chromosomal analyses have been infrequently reported, but in at least two instances normal karyotypes were found [219, 271].

Obligate heterozygotes for classic abetalipoproteinemia cannot presently be identified in the absence of an affected child. Detailed descriptions of plasma lipid and lipoprotein levels in clinically normal family members have been presented for less than a third of known cases. Nevertheless, the plasma cholesterol, triglyceride, and phospholipid levels do not distinguish heterozygotes from normal persons in the apparently more commom form (as opposed to kindred with "homozygous hypobetalipoproteinemia," described below). Mild to moderate hypercholesterolemia has, in fact, been found in five parents [225, 271, 272, 305].

Diagnosis

As indicated earlier, acanthocytosis, retinal degeneration, neuromuscular disorders (particularly involving the posterior spinocerebellar tracts), and malabsorption all require consideration of abetalipoproteinemia. A highly suggestive finding is the simultaneous presence of very low plasma concentrations of cholesterol (less than 100 mg/dl), and triglycerides (less than 30 mg/dl). The diagnosis depends upon confirmation of the absence of apolipoprotein B in plasma. This is accomplished by using anti-LDL (antibetalipoprotein) serum in a variety of immunochemical tests now available. If the diagnosis is established, it is further important to measure the concentration of LDL in all obligate heterozygotes. The heterozygote is not abnormal in classic abetalipoproteinemia. In familial hypobetalipoproteinemia, described below, the heterozygote has lower than normal concentrations of LDL and apoprotein B.

Treatment

Recognition of abetalipoproteinemia in the affected neonate may reduce some morbid consequences and make it possible to prevent the early death which may result from this disorder. Correct early diagnosis is the exception rather than the rule because the disease is so rare and the symptoms are not unique.

Restricting the intake of triglycerides containing long-chain fatty acids (C_{16} to C_{24}) is important in relieving the gastrointestinal manifestations in the infant and child. Whether the prescribed diet should simply provide for isocaloric substitution of fat by protein and carbohydrate, or whether medium-chain triglycerides (MCT; C_8 to C_{14}) should be recommended in place of long-chain triglycerides is unresolved. The question is important, for it is difficult to maintain caloric balance, let alone weight gain, on severely fat restricted diets.

MCT are absorbed into the portal system and do not require chylomicron formation for transport. The liver oxidizes most MCT to two-carbon fragments with little or no chain elongation. MCT treatment does not appear to aggravate hepatic steatosis [253, 267], but two children have been observed to develop hepatic fibrosis during the course of MCT supplementation. It seems reasonable to use MCT feeding only in those infants who are very malnourished and then to monitor liver function carefully.

Supplements of the fat-soluble vitamins A and K should be provided to prevent abnormalities of scotopic vision and coagulation. The adequacy of supplementation is easily evaluated by measuring serum levels of vitamin A and the thrombin time.

The importance and efficacy of treatment with pharmacologic doses of vitamin E are not proved, but this method of treatment may have great significance. The correction of in vitro and possibly in vivo autohemolysis in abetalipoproteinemia by vitamin E has been reported [224, 246, 314], and it was suggested that vitamin E may retard the progression or even induce clinical improvement in the retinal and neuromuscular abnormalities in this disorder [261]. Doses of 100 mg/(kg·day) of either the water-miscible or fat-soluble preparations are necessary to maintain detectable serum levels of the vitamin. Muller and Lloyd have followed the course of eight patients for 3 to 16 years on regimens that include fat restriction and supplements of vitamins A, E, and K [265]. In their three patients between 11 and 17 years of age vitamin E therapy apparently prevented or stopped the neuromuscular and retinal degeneration. Other reports appear to confirm this effect [204, 211, 315]. It is advisable to begin high-dose vitamin E therapy as soon as the diagnosis is established. Unfortunately, routine monitoring of the serum levels achieved is not possible.

FAMILIAL HYPOBETALIPOPROTEINEMIA

History

Familial hypobetalipoproteinemia is a genetic disorder distinct from classic abetalipoproteinemia. Three diagnostic criteria have been proposed [316]: "(1) LDL abnormally low but present and identifiable immunochemically, while concentrations of HDL are normal; (2) absence of diseases to which hypobetalipoproteinemia may be secondary; and (3) detection of a similar pattern in a first-degree relative." It is now known that these criteria pertain only to subjects heterozygous for the abnormal gene. Matings of such heterozygotes have produced progeny who have abetalipoproteinemia with clinical features that may be identical to the classic form of this disease.

One of the earliest reports of a patient with abetalipoproteinemia may have been the first description of familial hypobetalipoproteinemia in both heterozygous and homozygous form. A child with a syndrome indistinguishable from typical abetalipoproteinemia was born to parents who both had low plasma cholesterol and LDL concentrations [201]. Six years later three brothers were described who had hypocholesterolemia and hypotriglyceridemia without acanthocytosis, fat malabsorption, or neuromuscular disease. They were described as having "congenital β-lipoprotein deficiency" [317]. The parents of the proband were not tested, and his two children had normal plasma lipid concentrations. In 1969 investi-

gators in America and France reported the appearance of hypobetalipoproteinemia in three and two successive generations, respectively [318, 319], establishing both the familial nature of the disorder and an apparent autosomal dominant mode of inheritance. At least five other kindreds with affected heterozygotes have been identified [320–324]. In the last 6 years, four kindreds have been reported in which abetalipoproteinemia has occurred in six apparently homozygous abnormal subjects [325–328]. It seems likely that this disorder, though chemically indistinguishable from typical abetalipoproteinemia, represents a different mutation or mutations.

Plasma Lipids and Lipoproteins

The Heterozygote   Mild to moderate hypolipemia is usually present in heterozygotes, but sometimes the concentrations overlap the normal range. Plasma cholesterol levels in subjects identified as affected have ranged from 42 to 182 mg/dl, plasma phospholipids from 74 to 190 mg/dl, and triglycerides from 15 to 125 mg/dl. The majority of heterozygotes, even adults, rarely have plasma triglyceride concentrations in excess of 100 mg/dl, and many have had concentrations of 50 mg/dl or less. The fatty acid contents of phospholipids and cholesteryl esters and the degree of esterification of the plasma cholesterol are normal in heterozygotes [317–319, 324].

Concentrations of VLDL and LDL are typically low in heterozygotes [324]. As determined by analytic ultracentrifugation, 13 affected subjects in one large kindred had LDL levels approximately 25 percent of those found in their normal relatives [318]. When LDL concentrations are estimated by methods employing preparative ultracentrifugation or polyanionic precipitation, the concentrations have been 10 to 50 percent [319], 16 to 30 percent [320], and 20 to 60 percent [322] of the means for normal subjects. The LDL have a normal ratio of lipid to protein, as well as unremarkable ultracentrifugal and optical properties [320]. The apoprotein content of the LDL also had an amino acid composition and immunochemical reactivity indistinguishable from those of controls.

Plasma HDL concentrations in heterozygotes have been reported to be high [324, 325], normal [318, 322], or low [319, 321]. The HDL levels affect the sensitivity of the simple plasma cholesterol determination in screening for this disorder, since large quantities of cholesterol carried in HDL will obscure the anticipated hypocholesterolemia. The available data [319, 319, 322] suggest no gross alterations of HDL composition in heterozygous familial hypobetalipoproteinemia, although the HDL apolipoproteins in heterozygotes have not been characterized.

The Homozygote   Profound hypocholesterolemia and hypotriglyceridemia are typical in homozygous hypobetalipoproteinemia. Fat feeding does not induce chylomicronemia [201, 325, 326], and lipoproteins of β mobility (LDL) and pre-β mobility (VLDL) are absent from the plasma in the homozygote. The B apolipoprotein has not been found in plasma when conventional immunochemical methods for its detection have been employed. Small quantities of "LDL" can be recovered by preparative ultracentrifugation. These particles are indistinguishable by electron microscopy from those already described in abetalipoproteinemia [204, 329]. They contain primarily the A-I apolipoprotein, but immunochemical traces of the A-II and C apolipoproteins are found. Apo B is not detectable.

The plasma HDL concentrations have been reduced in all seven homozygotes. All the A and C apolipoproteins have been identified in the HDL, with the possible exception of the monosialylated apo C-III [232]. Qualitative or quantitative differences in plasma lipids, lipoproteins, or apolipoproteins, therefore, do not serve to distinguish abetalipoproteinemia and hypobetalipoproteinemia.

Clinical and Pathophysiologic Correlates

Gastrointestinal System Fatty food intolerance has been cited in some presumed heterozygotes [318] but is either not mentioned or denied in most cases [316, 317, 319–321, 324]. Fat absorption [319, 325] and the intestinal mucosa [317, 318] are probably normal in heterozygotes. It is interesting that fasting chylomicronemia was observed in several members of one kindred after an overnight fast when high fat meals had been consumed the preceding day [316]. One of several interpretations of this observation is that the capacity to synthesize chylomicrons may have been limited, with chylomicron release extending an unusually long time into the postabsorptive period. The only observations reflecting a possible comparable defect in VLDL release by the liver in heterozygotes is their usual low plasma triglyceride concentrations and the mild hepatic steatosis found in the one reported liver biopsy [317].

In homozygous hypobetalipoproteinemia the gastrointestinal findings mimic those of abetalipoproteinemia (Fig. 29-3). No homozygote has chylomicronemia after fat ingestion [201, 325–327] and 30 to 40 percent of the fat consumed is not absorbed [325, 327]. Plasma vitamin A and E levels are low in untreated patients [201, 325, 326], although one adult woman had a plasma α-tocopherol of 101 µg/dl (normal, 500 to 1000 µg/dl) while receiving no vitamin E supplements [204].

Extensive neutral fat accumulation in the intestinal columnar absorptive epithelium is found in homozygotes [201, 325, 327]. Hepatic steatosis has been documented in two children [325]. As in abetalipoproteinemia, the accumulation of triglyceride in intestinal mucosa and liver is presumably due to failure to elaborate chylomicrons and VLDL. Intracellular apo B has not been sought in small-bowel biopsy specimens, and inability to synthesize apo B in this mutant remains to be demonstrated.

Neuromuscular Manifestation It is unlikely that neuromuscular disease is a feature of uncomplicated heterozygous hypobetalipoproteinemia [316, 317, 319, 322]. Several subjects have been described with neurologic disorders and hypobetalipoproteinemia with and without documented familial involvement [318, 321, 324, 325, 330]. Ascertainment of these cases may be related to awareness of the association between hypolipoproteinemia and neurologic disease.

The oldest homozygous hypobetalipoproteinemic patient (Fig. 29-5) [326], now 48 years of age, had no deep-tendon reflexes and an equivocal Romberg test when first examined. Ataxia, weakness, and skeletal abnormalities were absent. Neuromuscular symptoms were not noted at 14 [328] and 17 [265] years in two girls without deep-tendon reflexes, one of whom was a member of her school track team [328]. Abnormal neurologic findings have also been absent from the four prepubertal children reported thus far [325, 327]. The degree of neuromuscular sparing demonstrated by the three older

patients with homozygous hypobetalipoproteinemia contrasts strikingly with the rapidly progressive disease typical of abetalipoproteinemia. Two unanswerable questions are raised. Is the paucity of identified cases related to the benign clinical course of this disorder? Conversely, did the capacity of one patient to absorb some vitamin E [204] or the early institution of vitamin E supplementation [265, 328] in others retard or prevent the neuromuscular degeneration?

Ocular Manifestations Atypical retinitis pigmentosa has not developed in any patient heterozygous for familial hypobetalipoproteinemia. Normal corrected and twilight vision was found in one 46-year-old man whose fundi showed "bilateral fine shining dots" [317]. Funduscopic examination in another heterozygote revealed slight irregularity and clumping of pigment at the equator in the inferonasal quadrants of both eyes. The electroretinogram was normal bilaterally, and cone thresholds were elevated by 0.5 log unit only in the right eye [331].

The oldest homozygote with this disorder had florid pigmentary degeneration when first examined at age 37 years. A 17-year-old girl had slight pigmentary retinopathy at 5 years despite vitamin A supplementation [290]. The appearance of the retina remained stable over the next 12 years when vitamin E supplements were provided [265]. The youngest children [325, 328] did not have retinitis pigmentosa at the time of detection, and it will be of great interest to learn if vitamin E therapy can prevent retinal degeneration.

Hematologic Changes The heterozygotes rarely have acanthocytes in their peripheral blood. One heterozygotic child was felt to have approximately 5 percent acanthocytes when she was examined at age 11 months; LDL was then "undetectable" in the plasma. By age 26 months, LDL was definitely present and only "rare" acanthocytes were observed [326].

All homozygotes reported to date have had typical acanthocytes. Red cell chemical abnormalities, including increased cholesterol and sphingomyelin content and reduced linoleic acid and increased oleic acid esterified to phosphatidylcholine, were indistinguishable from the abnormalities in abetalipoproteinemia [213]. In addition, hypoprothrombinemia has been found in two of the homozygotes [325, 326].

Other Clinical Findings Growth is probably normal when nutritional problems related to steatorrhea are corrected [265, 327, 328]. As in abetalipoproteinemic patients, those with homozygous hypobetalipoproteinemia appear to have diminished adrenal reserve after ACTH or metyrapone challenge [327].

Pathogenesis

The outstanding difference between familial hypobetalipoproteinemia and abetalipoproteinemia is the inability of the bearers of a single allele for the former disorder to maintain a normal concentration of LDL [316]. Studies of LDL metabolism in heterozygous hypobetalipoproteinemia have shown reduced synthesis and normal catabolic rates [320, 332]. The homozygous abnormal subjects for either disease appear unable to elaborate chylomicrons or VLDL and have no trace of LDL or apoprotein B in plasma.

Available information is insufficient to determine if these two disorders are allelic. Any one of a number of possible events in the intracellular assembly and intracellular and transcellular transport of chylomicrons and VLDL may be involved. Further, knowledge of the structure of apo B and the number of loci and alleles coding its synthesis is rudimentary. Earlier in this chapter the identification and possible significance of two molecular species of apo B was discussed. Whatever the basis of this apo B heterogeneity, it is noteworthy that no form of this protein, including components of the Lp and Ag systems [333], is found in the serum of affected homozygotes.

Genetics

Definite or probable kindreds with familial hypobetalipoproteinemia have been reported in the Netherlands, France, Japan, Israel, England, and the United States. Male-to-male transmission of the trait in heterozygotes has been documented in seven instances, and an autosomal recessive mode of inheritance with limited expression in the heterozygote is consistent with available data [316].

The prevalence of familial hypobetalipoproteinemia is difficult to judge because the heterozygous condition is usually asymptomatic. Nevertheless, the observation that five of seven reported homozygotes were the issue of consanguine matings [325–327] indicates that the disorder is rare.

Diagnosis

The diagnosis of familial hypobetalipoproteinemia is suspected when plasma cholesterol concentrations are below 100 mg/dl and triglyceride levels are below 50 mg/dl. Quantitative measurements of LDL with immunochemical tests or ultracentrifugation reveal the concentration of these lipoproteins in heterozygotes to be not more than about half the mean for age- and sex-matched control subjects. Familial studies reveal a distribution of the abnormality consistent with autosomal dominant inheritance. Diagnostic criteria for the homozygous abnormal condition are the same as in abetalipoproteinemia, plus demonstration of hypobetalipoproteinemia in obligate heterozygotes. It is necessary to exclude a number of conditions which can mimic some of the features of primary LDL deficiency. Malnutrition, liver, and gastrointestinal disease have been associated with profound hypobetalipoproteinemia, and acanthocytosis has been observed without an acompanying lipoprotein deficiency (reviewed elsewhere [204, 212]).

Variant Forms of Hypobetalipoproteinemia

Two other forms of hypobetalipoproteinemia, each probably representing different mutants, have recently been described [333a, 333b]. A man of 67 years was found to have LDL cholesterol levels of 4 to 8 mg/dl, normal triglyceride concentrations, hypoalphalipoproteinemia, mild steatorrhea, and prolonged chylomicron plasma residence times [333a]. His VLDL apoproteins appeared totally devoid of apo C-III-1, a defect formerly noted only in abetalipoproteinemia and homozygous hypobetalipoproteinemia. Characterization of his B apoproteins has not yet been described, but it is noteworthy that his serum triglycerides fell instead of rising when he ate a high

carbohydrate, low fat diet. It is possible that this mutation represents defective secretion of a specific VLDL subpopulation (e.g., that containing the B-100 apoprotein), which normally also contains apo C-III-1. The familial nature of the disorder was well documented. Two sibs had LDL levels as low as the proband, and his mother, three other sibs, and two children had LDL levels that were half-normal. It is possible that the proband, and his brother and sister with LDL cholesterol concentrations of 3 to 8 mg/dl, may indeed be homozygous for a dominant allelic mutation [333a].

A phenotypically different abnormality was noted in an 8-year-old girl found to have serum cholesterol and triglyceride levels of 25 and 30 mg/dl, respectively [333b]. Serum vitamin E levels were low and gait was ataxic, but retinal studies were normal and there was minimal if any acanthocytosis. The ataxia appeared to improve after vitamin E supplementation. Fat absorption and jejunal biopsy 16 h after a fat load were normal. HDL levels were low, and, in contrast to abetalipoproteinemia, HDL$_3$ rather than HDL$_2$ was the predominant HDL species. Phospholipids of all density classes, including VLDL and chylomicrons, were enriched in sphingomyelin.

While diminished, reactivity with anti–apo B was present in both the HDL and VLDL/chylomicron fractions from this patient's plasma [333b]. The A, C, and E apolipoproteins were present, but the relative amount of apo C-III-1 was considered reduced. Of particular note was the total absence of the B-100, B-74 and B-26 forms of apo B. By analogy with findings in the rat [118–120], this observation suggests defective production of a B apoprotein synthesized only by liver. This patient, unlike the subject described by Steinberg et al. [333a], approximately doubled her serum triglyceride concentration when provided with a high carbohydrate diet. This may reflect augmented hepatic secretion of VLDL containing only the B-48 form of apo B.

Treatment

There is no specific therapy for familial hypobetalipoproteinemia. None is indicated in the heterozygotes. For homozygotes with low plasma concentrations of the fat-soluble vitamins, supplementation is recommended (see earlier, under "Abetalipoproteinemia").

FAMILIAL HDL DEFICIENCY: TANGIER DISEASE

Tangier disease is a rare disorder named after the Chesapeake Bay island home of the first two patients recognized. It is characterized by severe deficiency or absence of normal HDL in plasma and by the accumulation of cholesteryl esters in many tissues throughout the body. These include the liver, spleen, lymph nodes, thymus, intestinal mucosa, skin, and probably the cornea. A combination of two features is pathognomonic: a low plasma cholesterol concentration in combination with normal or elevated triglyceride levels, and hyperplastic orange-yellow tonsils and adenoidal tissue. Of the 26 patients known to have the disease [204], 12 have also had peripheral neuropathy. The small amounts of HDL in Tangier plasma differ qualitatively and quantitatively from normal HDL, particularly with respect to apolipoprotein content. The disorder appears to be due to an autosomal recessive gene affecting HDL synthesis or catabolism. Heterozygotes in families with known homozygotes can usually be identified by low HDL concentrations.

History

The history of the discovery of Tangier disease has been recounted elsewhere [334]. Unusual tonsils were removed from a 5-year-old boy from Tangier Island, Virginia, and when many foam cells were observed on microscopic examination, he was referred to the National Institutes of Health with tentative diagnostic alternatives of histiocytosis or lipid-storage disease. The initial biochemical abnormality observed was a marked increase in cholesteryl ester content of a cervical lymph node. Eventually it was discovered that the level of plasma HDL was very low. An exhaustive search of Tangier Island for similarly affected subjects uncovered a single additional case, the 6-year-old sister of the index patient. Two more sibs from an unrelated kindred in Missouri were soon found [335], and examination of these two kindreds established that the obligate heterozygotes and other putative heterozygous relatives had abnormally low serum HDL concentrations [336].

Tangier disease has since been reported from England, New Zealand, Australia, Switzerland, Germany, and Poland. One-third of the patients were identified because of large, yellow-orange tonsils and another third because of symptoms of neuropathy. Identification in the remaining cases was related to splenomegaly, hypocholesterolemia, and family screening in relatives of affected subjects. The incidental finding at autopsy of abnormal tonsils prompted the diagnosis in one subject [337].

Lipoprotein and Apolipoprotein Abnormalities

Plasma Lipids Among the lipoprotein deficiency states, and indeed, among all known diseases, the combination of very low cholesterol and elevated triglyceride concentrations gives Tangier disease a unique signature. Some patients may have normal triglyceride levels in the postabsorptive state and may superficially resemble those with LDL deficiency. The total plasma cholesterol level ranges from about 40 to 125 mg/dl, within the range also observed in abetalipoproteinemia and hypobetalipoproteinemia. Values under 20 mg/dl have been recorded in one patient on many occasions. The average percentage of plasma cholesterol esterified was 75 percent in eight samples from five patients (range, 67 to 86 percent).

Individual variation in the plasma triglyceride levels is considerable and is highly contingent on diet. Plasma phospholipid concentrations in Tangier disease are typically 30 to 50 percent lower than normal [316, 338]. The quantitative distribution of the various phospholipid classes has not been fully investigated, but a preponderance of phosphatidylcholine relative to sphingomyelin has been noted in several instances [213, 338]. This may reflect the HDL deficiency since, as already noted, tissue sphingomyelin preferentially transfers to HDL. Analysis of the glycosphingolipid content of one subject's serum showed the total concentrations to be slightly lower than normal, with greatest reductions in lactosyl ceramide and galactosylgalactosylglucosyl ceramide [333].

Plasma Lipoproteins and Apolipoproteins The plasma lipoprotein pattern which attends Tangier disease is distinctive [204]. Lipoprotein electrophoresis demonstrates no lipoproteins of α mobility and a distinct pre-β band is rarely visualized (Fig. 29-7). Preparative and analytic ultracentrifugation confirm that HDL are absent or present in only trace quantities. Unconcentrated Tangier plasma only occasionally generates faint precipitin lines of α mobility on immunoelectrophoresis against low-titer anti-HDL serums [340, 341]. Antigen-antibody–crossed electrophoresis has demonstrated precipitation against anti-α-lipoprotein serum [341].

LOWER DENSITY LIPOPROTEINS IN TANGIER DISEASE Patients with Tangier disease often exhibit chylomicronemia after a 12- to 14-h abstinence from food. Plasma concentrations of VLDL (S_f 20 to 400) are normal or modestly elevated. The gross protein and phospholipid contents of Tangier VLDL are normal, but the cholesteryl ester content is a third less than in control VLDL [342].

Lipoproteins of intermediate density (1.006 to 1.019 g/ml) do not accumulate in Tangier plasma. Tangier LDL are slightly smaller [341, 342] than normal LDL, and their chemical composition is very different. Triglyceride accounts for approximately 30 percent of Tangier LDL mass (6 percent in controls) and the cholesteryl ester content is 50 percent less than normal [342]. It is likely that the reduced cholesteryl ester content of Tangier VLDL and LDL reflects the fact that these lipoproteins normally derive a significant proportion of their cholesteryl esters from HDL.

TANGIER HDL Approximately 0.5 to 6 mg of protein can be isolated in the HDL fraction from 100 ml of Tangier plasma. The lipid content of Tangier HDL varies not only among patients but also in the same patient studied on more than one occasion [204]. Lipoprotein electrophoresis and electron microscopy reveal striking heterogeneity in the Tangier HDL. Large bizarre translucent forms, greater than 100 nm diameter (Fig. 29-8), appear to represent chylomicron remnants since they disappear from the HDL when dietary fat is withdrawn [343]. Round particles, 20 to 25 nm diameter, appear identical

Figure 29-7 Lipoprotein electrophoresis of plasma from a normal subject and from a patient with Tangier disease. In this system, employing 0.5 percent agarose, pre-β-lipoproteins are visualized. The LDL in Tangier plasma have greater than normal mobility. (*Lipoprotein electrophoretograms kindly provided by Dr. N. Papadopoulos.*)

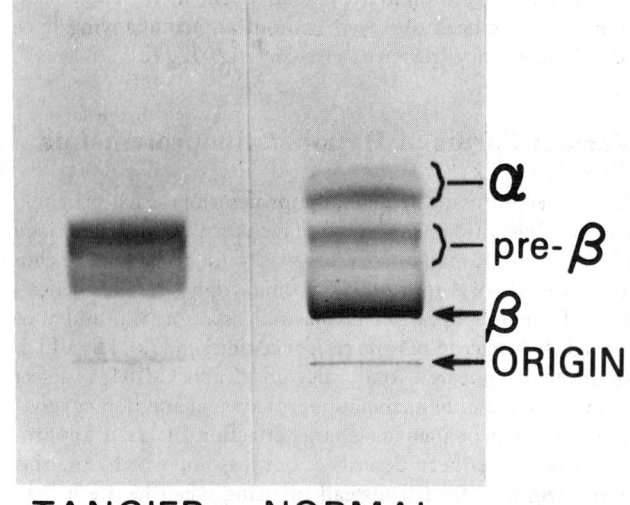

TANGIER   NORMAL

TANGIER HDL

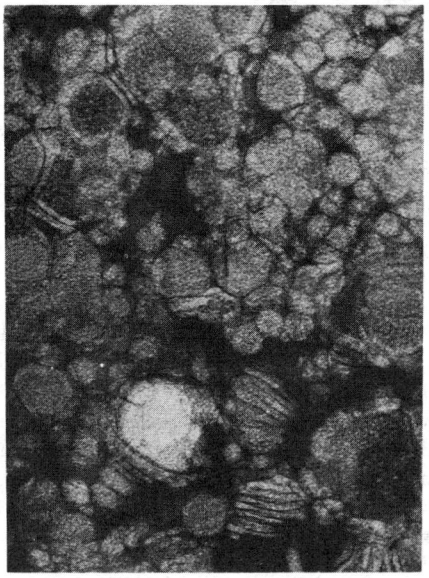

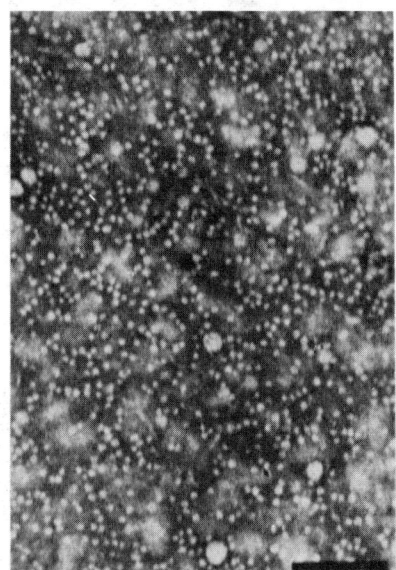

Figure 29-8 HDL in Tangier disease. The chylomicron remnants in the unfractionated HDL obscure all other morphological forms. The A-II particles were isolated from the plasma HDL by agarose column chromatography [328]. They are chemically similar to normal HDL but contain only the A-II apoprotein. (*The bar in the right panel indicates 100 nm; photomicrographs courtesy of Dr. Trudy Forte.*)

"Chylomicron Remnants"   "A-II Particles"

to the Lp(a) lipoproteins. A third species of particles, isolated by molecular sieve chromatography, is 5.5 to 7.5 nm in diameter and has α mobility on electrophoresis [338]. The chemical composition of these particles is similar to that of normal HDL, but only apo A-II is present in significant quantity. Apo A-I and the C apolipoproteins are nearly or completely absent. Thus normal HDL, as defined by protein composition and morphology, has not yet been detected in the plasma of any patient with Tangier disease.

A APOLIPOPROTEINS IN TANGIER DISEASE   The apo A-I content of Tangier plasma is typically less than 1 percent of normal, and apo A-II levels are about 5 to 7 percent of those in control plasma [344–347]. About 95 percent of the apo A-II can be recovered with the plasma lipoproteins after ultracentrifugation, and this apo A-II has α mobility on electrophoresis [345]. After ultracentrifugation, most of the apo A-I is found in the lipoprotein-free fraction of plasma [345, 346]. Moreover, the apo A-I in Tangier plasma has an abnormal pre-β electrophoretic mobility [345], providing further evidence that Tangier apo A-I and apo A-II are not associated with the same lipoprotein particles.

The apo A-II in Tangier plasma comigrates with its normal counterpart in a variety of electrophoretic systems, has the same amino acid composition [340, 341, 344], and yields tryptic peptides with normal mobility in anionic urea polyacrylamide gels. It produces a precipitin line of identity with normal apo A-II on immunodiffusion, and combines in vitro with sphingomyelin, producing particles indistinguishable from those formed by normal apo A-II [344].

Tangier apo A-I is not as well characterized. It has mobility similar to normal apo A-I on anionic urea [340] and sodium dodecylsulfate polyacrylamide gel electrophoresis [341], and a similar isoelectric focusing pattern [345]. Very homogeneous preparations are difficult to obtain, but the amino acid composition of Tangier apo A-I closely resembles normal apo A-I [340]. Studies of the capacity of Tangier apo A-I to recombine

with phospholipid and HDL are still incomplete [348], but association with detergents, as judged by charge shift electrophoresis [348], is not abnormal.

Current evidence, therefore, does not conclusively exclude structural alterations in either of the A apolipoproteins in Tangier disease, particularly in apo A-I. Adequate quantities of Tangier apo A-I for detailed structure and function studies must be obtained to resolve this issue.

OTHER APOLIPOPROTEINS IN TANGIER DISEASE   Apo B in Tangier VLDL and LDL has amino acid composition and immunochemical properties identical to those in normal lipoproteins [342]. The apo E in Tangier VLDL also does not differ from its normal counterpart as judged by sodium dodecylsulfate polyacrylamide gel electrophoresis and amino acid analysis [342]. All of the C apolipoproteins have been identified in Tangier VLDL [342], but, in contrast to normal plasma, they are present in only trace amounts in Tangier HDL [342, 344]. The C apoproteins usually comprise about 40 percent of the total VLDL protein but may account for less than 20 percent of Tangier VLDL protein under certain dietary conditions [342, 350]. These observations are consistent with the concept that HDL provide a reservoir of C apolipoproteins for cyclic reincorporation into chylomicrons and VLDL. Conservation of the C apoproteins in HDL appears to depend on the availability of normal HDL to complex with the C apoproteins. The latter apoproteins do not appear to be capable of independent HDL formation in vivo.

Lipoprotein Metabolism in Tangier Disease   The administration of normal HDL or partial plasma exchange in Tangier homozygotes produces an immediate increase in the VLDL cholesteryl ester content, and the broad-β band visualized on agarose electrophoresis is resolved into distinct β and pre-β bands (Fig. 29-9) [351, 352]. These changes probably reflect transfer of both cholesteryl esters and C apolipoproteins from the administered HDL. An increase in the electrophoretic

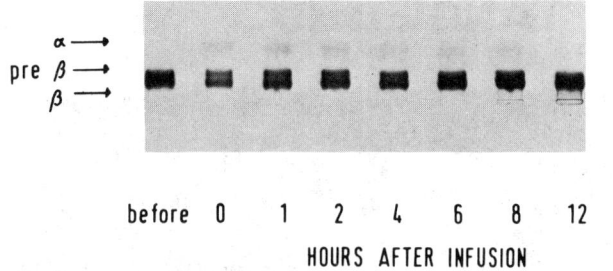

before 0   1   2   4   6   8   12
HOURS AFTER INFUSION

Figure 29-9 Agarose electrophoresis of serum obtained before and after a patient with Tangier disease received sufficient normal HDL intravenously to raise the serum HDL cholesterol concentration to 25 mg/dl (0 = immediately after infusion). (*From Assmann and Smootz* [357]. *Used by permission.*)

mobility of Tangier VLDL, in fact, can be induced in vitro by adding HDL in concentrations as low as 10 mg/dl.

Rapid disappearance of normal HDL from the plasma of patients with Tangier disease has been shown in several studies [340, 351–355]. The plasma residence times of autologous HDL in two obligate heterozygotes appeared half as long as normal, while calculated synthetic rates were similar to controls. The mean plasma residence time in two homozygotes given tracer quantities of homologous HDL was only 0.52 days (normal, 8 days) and the computed synthetic rates of HDL apoproteins were about half normal [353]. Interpretation of these tracer studies in homozygotes is confounded by possible effects of a negligible HDL pool size and the observation that only 10 percent of the apo A-I and apo A-II actually decayed from the HDL density class [353, 356].

The infusion of large quantities of HDL either as isolated lipoprotein or homologous plasma has confirmed augmented catabolism in homozygotes [357, 358]. These studies have also shown that apo A-I catabolic rates greatly exceeded those of apo A-II. The preferential loss of apo A-I from the plasma compartment resulted in the generation of an abnormal β migrating lipoprotein (Fig. 29-10) which contained apo A-II as the major if not sole protein constituent. Studies in one laboratory have suggested that newly synthesized apo A-II, but not apo A-I, appeared in the HDL density region after administration of normal HDL to Tangier homozygotes [358]. Contradictory findings were reported from another laboratory [355]. Resolution of these discrepant conclusions is critical to

determining whether Tangier disease is caused by a defect in HDL synthesis or catabolism.

SYNTHESIS OF A APOPROTEINS   Two lines of evidence indicate that at least the intestinal mucosa elaborates A apoproteins in Tangier disease. Apo A-I can be identified in Tangier chylomicrons and some (but not all) workers have observed an increase in the plasma apo A-I concentration after fat ingestion in homozygotes [359]. Immunofluorescence has also demonstrated the presence of both A apolipoproteins in intestinal mucosa of homozygotes [358]. The pattern of fluorescence in jejunal epithelial cells (Fig. 29-11) and the collecting lymph vessels was indistinguishable from that in controls [358–360]. Comparable information regarding the hepatic A apoproteins is not yet available.

A apoproteins that reach the circulation in chylomicrons are usually rapidly transferred to circulating HDL. This transfer does not proceed normally in Tangier homozygotes [361], but this probably reflects the absence of HDL from Tangier plasma. Administration of HDL to Tangier homozygotes results in normal chylomicron metabolism [362].

LIPOLYTIC ENZYMES   It might be anticipated that the absence of normal HDL and the profound deficiency of apo A-I in Tangier disease could be associated with an impairment of LCAT activity. Nevertheless, measurements of LCAT activity in Tangier plasma have established that significant cholesterol esterification occurs [363–365] and that the fractional rate of cholesterol esterification equals that in control plasma. The ratio of cholesterol to cholesteryl esters in the plasma of Tangier patients is approximately normal, and linoleic acid is the predominent fatty acid constituent of plasma cholesteryl esters [366]. The molar rate of cholesterol esterification [nmol/(ml·h)] in normal plasma is significantly correlated with the concentration of free cholesterol [367]. Therefore, low molar esterification rates in Tangier plasma as measured in vitro [341, 368, 369] presumably reflect the low cholesterol concentrations rather than a deficiency or diminished activity of the LCAT enzyme itself.

Postheparin lipolytic activity in Tangier plasma has been determined in only a few cases. Lipoprotein lipase and triglyceride lipase of hepatic origin have been partially purified from

0   6   20   25   30   44

Anti HDL

Anti Apo A·I

Anti Apo A·II

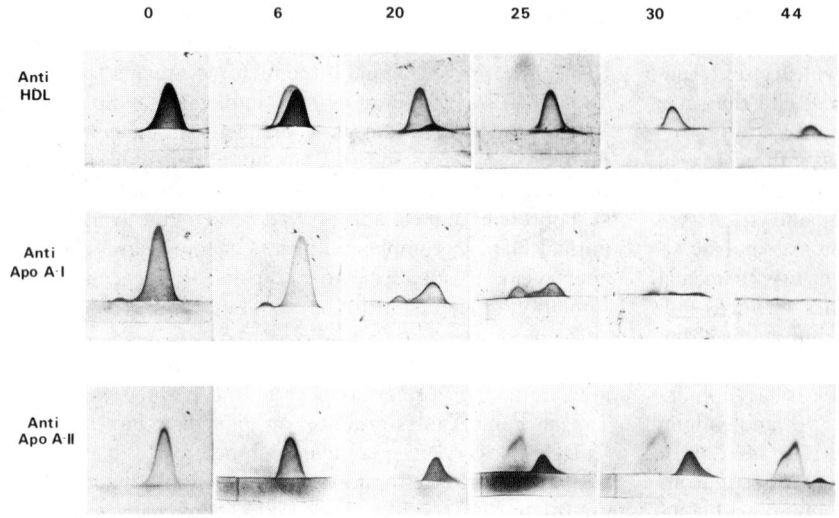

Figure 29-10 Two-dimensional immunoelectrophoresis of serum from two patients with Tangier disease after administration of normal HDL. An antiserum to HDL was used for immunoprecipitation in the second (vertical) dimension. During the course of HDL catabolism it is seen that a second immunoprecipitin line is generated which corresponds to an apo A-II–containing lipoprotein. (*From Assmann and Smootz* [357]. *Used by permission.*)

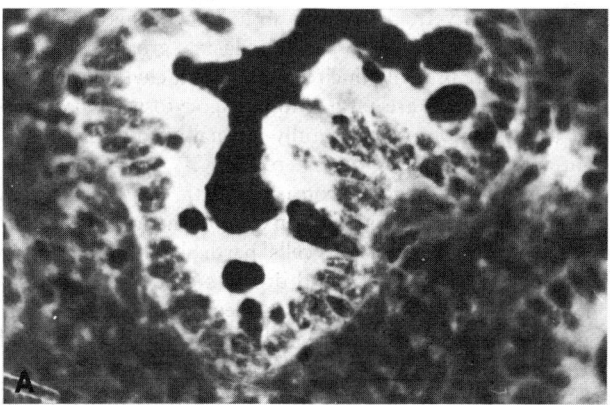

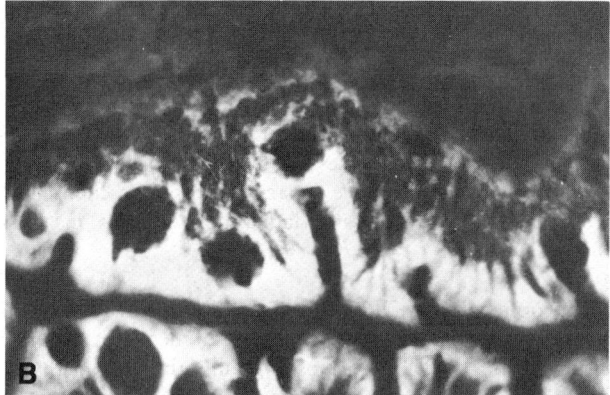

Figure 29-11 Immunofluorescence of the A apolipoproteins in jejunal mucosa from a patient with Tangier disease. Cryostat sections were treated with FITC-labeled apo A-I (A) and apo A-II (B) antiserums. Fluorescence is mainly confined to the apex of the mucosal epithelial cells. (*From Assmann et al. [358]. Used by permission.*)

postheparin Tangier plasma, and no deficiency in activity of either of these enzymes has been detected [363].

Clinical and Pathophysiologic Correlates

Cholesteryl ester accumulation in histiocytes of many organs is the dominant pathologic finding in Tangier homozygotes. Lipid deposition also occurs in other tissues including the cornea, Schwann cells, and nonvascular smooth-muscle cells (Table 29-8) [370–376]. Involvement of histiocytes regularly causes distinctive tonsillar hyperplasia, mild lymphadenopathy, and splenomegaly. Hepatomegaly and hypersplenism are much less common. Corneal infiltrates do not impair vision, but Schwann cell involvement appears to underlie the neuropathy which may be asymptomatic or devastating. The functional significance, if any, of lipid deposits in nonvascular smooth-muscle cells is not known. Quite obviously, the mechanisms by which cholesteryl ester accumulates in these various tissues must be intimately related to the still poorly defined physiologic roles of HDL. Therein resides the great interest in this rare mutant.

Clinical Findings The unique appearance of the tonsils makes it possible to diagnose the disorder through examination of the oropharynx. The tonsils are large and lobulated and have a distinctive orange or yellowish-gray overlay of coloration on the normal red mucosa (Fig. 29-12). When the tonsils

have been removed, small plaques or tags of mucosa having the same appearance will usually betray the diagnosis if one examines carefully. Several patients have had a history of recurrent "tonsillitis" or symptoms of obstruction which have led to tonsillectomy.

Splenomegaly is accompanied by mild thrombocytopenia and reticulocytosis in many patients. Splenectomy was necessary in one patient because of progressive anemia and thrombocytopenia. The pulp of the excised spleen was filled with intracytoplasmic liquid droplets and scattered clusters of cholesterol crystals [335].

Physical examination does not usually reveal striking lymphadenopathy, but enlarged or normal-sized lymph nodes have exhibited bright yellow streaks and morphological characteristics like those found in the tonsils [334, 337, 338]; and the cholesteryl ester content has been more than 100-fold greater than in control lymph nodes [338]. Lipid deposition in the thymus has been most extreme [337, 338], with almost complete replacement of the lobule cortex by large, pale macrophages.

Enlargement of the liver has been noted at some time in about one-third of patients, but this may be a transient finding. Lipid infiltration of hepatic parenchymal cells has not been observed, and abnormal liver function tests are unusual [335, 377]. Histologic examination of the liver has revealed only occasional clusters of intralobular foam cells [335, 337, 377], identified as histiocytes. Moderate numbers of foam cells have also been identified in the gallbladder mucosa [337].

The gross appearance of the rectal mucosa has been abnormal in every case examined and may be the most reliable physical finding when palatine and pharyngeal tonsils have earlier been completely removed. Proctoscopy demonstrates a mucosa studded with 1- to 2-mm discrete orange-brown spots. Biopsy

Table 29-8 Cholesteryl ester storage in Tangier Disease

Histiocytes
    Bone marrow, thymus, spleen, mucosa of the rectum and large and small intestine, pulmonary artery, renal pelvis and ureters, mitral and tricuspid valves, skin; with inflammation in gall bladder and bile ducts, uterine cervical mucosa, and blood vessel adventitia
Schwann cells
    Nerves of skin and colon submucosa
Nevus cells
    Pigmented nevi
Smooth-muscle cells
    Muscularis mucosa, peritoneal soft tissue (inguinal hernia)
Mast cells
    Colonic mucosa
Fibroblasts
    Subepidermis, gingiva, cornea, colonic mucosa

UNAFFECTED CELL TYPES IN TANGIER DISEASE

Endothelial cells—arteries and veins
Smooth-muscle cells—arteries and veins, myoepithelial cells of apocrine and exocrine glands
Fibroblasts—adventitia of arteries and veins
White blood cells
Epidermal cells—keratinocytes, squamous epithelial cells
Bone marrow mesenchymal (reticulum) cells
Peritoneal mesothelial cells
Parenchymal cells—hepatocytes, intestinal mucosa, bile duct epithelium

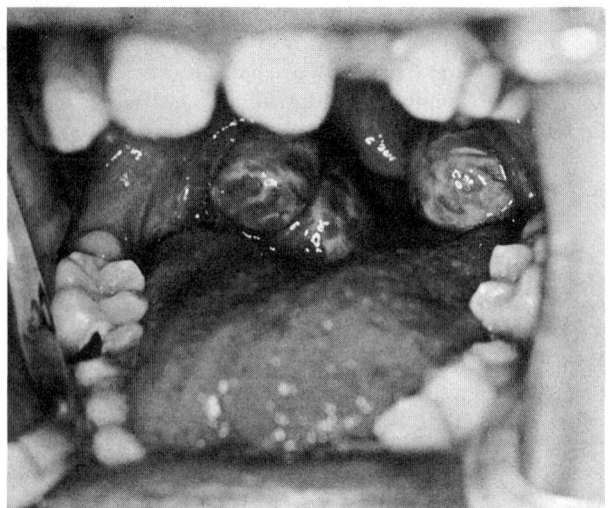

Figure 29-12 Tonsils in Tangier disease. The patient is from the original sibship [334]. The lighter bands on the tonsils appeared orange *in situ* and yellow-white after removal.

shows foamy histiocytes throughout the mucosa and submucosa. The ileum and colon have also had numerous mucosal elevations, but the jejunum has been grossly normal [337], and the jejunal mucosal villi have been free of foam cells [371], the latter being found only below the muscularis mucosa. Bowel habits and food tolerance are usually normal in Tangier disease, though complaints of frequent loose stools and intermittent diarrhea and abdominal pain have received comment [335, 378]. One patient had severe ulcerative colitis and underwent colectomy [379]. The gastrointestinal series is without distinctive finding, although mild uniform thickening of the mucosal folds has been observed throughout the jejunum. The pattern was not unlike that found in amyloidosis, giardiasis, and intestinal lymphangiectasia.

Focal collections of foamy histiocytes have even been seen in normal skin [337, 371, 372, 377], ureters and renal pelves, tunica albuginea of testicles, mitral and tricuspid valves [337], and pulmonary artery [338]. Bone marrow foam cells have been found in 9 of 13 patients examined [371]. Corneal infiltration, evident only on slit-lamp examination, has been present in every patient who has reached the fifth decade and in two women in their third decade [204]. The opacities and fine dots involve all layers of the corneal stroma.

Pathology and Pathophysiology   The histiocytic foam cells contain sudanophilic lipid droplets and occasionally crystalline material. The major part of the droplets within the cytoplasm is not bound by membranes and consists of deposits of cholesteryl esters (mostly cholesteryl oleate). Contrasting with similar storage phenomena in primary lysosomal deficiency states, the lipids in Tangier disease accumulate largely outside of lysosomes.

The distribution of lipid-storing histiocytes within different organs may reflect the source of the accumulated material. Histiocytes occur in all tissues which are engaged in the breakdown of cells under physiologic or pathologic conditions. Lipid-laden macrophages in the bone marrow and in the spleen pulp are known to degrade phagocytized red blood cells and senescent granulocytes. A similar cell phagocytosis occurs in chronically inflamed areas. It is likely, therefore, that at least part of the histiocytic lipid content derives from phagocytosis of cell

debris. Alternatively, tissues rich in histiocytes may also take up lipoprotein remnants. In Tangier plasma, grossly abnormal lipoproteins are present which may represent chylomicron surface remnants that are targets for phagocytosis [343]. Similarly, sequestration of structurally normal or abnormal HDL might account for tissue cholesterolosis.

Ultrastructural data are consistent with the concept that abnormal products of chylomicron catabolism are components of the lipid deposits in various cells, particularly histiocytes. In the spleen, gray-appearing lipid droplets that fuse with lysosomal granules can be visualized by electron microscopy (Fig. 29-13). Their size is compatible with that of chylomicrons, and their content is osmiophilic, indicative of the presence of polyunsaturated fatty acids. By contrast, cholesteryl oleate, which is a product of cellular cholesterol reesterification, has a low binding capacity for osmium tetroxide and is extracted by solvents applied in the procedure for tissue embedding.

It is tempting to speculate that removal of ingested cholesterol from histiocytes requires the extracellular presence of HDL and that the depletion of HDL from the plasma of Tangier patients specifically causes cholesterol storage within these cells. HDL, indeed, have the capacity to promote cholesterol egress from cholesteryl ester–laden macrophages in vitro [380].

Neuropathology   The neurologic abnormalities of the 26 Tangier homozygotes were discussed in detail in the last edition of this book [204]. Nosologically, the neuropathy of Tangier disease may be considered a form of mononeuritis multiplex. The clinical manifestations may be subtle or overt; sensory, motor, or mixed; and transient or permanent. Most, if not all, patients eventually have some degree of neuromuscular dysfunction, but careful examination may be necessary to demonstrate the abnormalities. Symptoms have included weakness, paresthesias, dysesthesias, increased sweating, and diplopia. Objectively, reduced strength, ptosis, ocular muscle palsies, diminished or absent deep-tendon reflexes, muscle atrophy, and loss of pain and temperature sensibilities may be found. Abnormalities of proprioception are not common.

Progressive debilitating neuropathy has characterized the clinical course of three patients [378, 381–384]. The diagnosis in one was confused with syringomyelia [381]. Symptoms were present for more than 20 years before the correct diagnosis was made in another case [378, 382].

Figure 29-13 Electron micrograph of cytoplasm of a spleen macrophage containing lipoprotein-derived osmiophilic lipid surrounded by dense lysosomal bodies. Magnification, ×40,000.

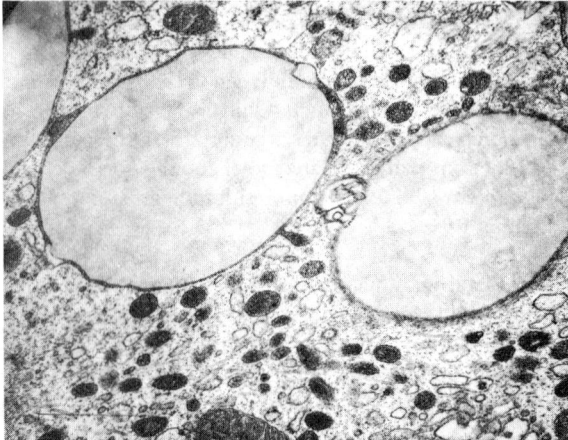

A syringomyelia-like syndrome was also observed in a woman with the onset of symptoms at 51 years [383, 384]. She suffered progressive facial diplegia, hand muscle wasting, and sensation loss in brachial, cervical, and cranial dermatomes over the next 17 years. Biopsied fascicles of cutaneous nerves demonstrated selective vulnerability of unmyelinated and small myelinated fibers [383], consonant with the clinical findings of severe impairment of nociperception and thermal sensitivity.

An interesting unresolved question is the relationship of the HDL deficiency to lipid storage in neurons, and whether lipid storage precedes or follows axonal degeneration. A sural nerve biopsy from one patient with symptomatic neuropathy showed no gross changes evident by light microscopy [379], and lipid storage was not found in neurons or macrophages of the central nervous system of a necropsied patient [337]. Others have found extensive sudanophilic inclusions [385], even in small nerves obtained from clinically normal skin [371]. Phagocytosis of lipoproteins or effete cell membranes is not a known activity of Schwann and smooth-muscle cells, and the observed lipid deposits are probably of intracellular origin. The lipid appears to be cholesterol [384]. It remains tempting to speculate that its accumulation is due to inadequate transport away from Schwann cells by HDL and that the cholesterol deposition precedes and perhaps causes the axonal degeneration.

HDL, Atherosclerosis, and Tangier Disease

As recently reviewed, the amount of clinically evident vascular disease in homozygous Tangier patients is not striking [386]. No coronary heart disease or evidence of vascular disease has been found in homozygotes of 40 years or less. Documented evidence of coronary heart disease exists in three older patients. One man developed significant chest pain on exertion at age 59; coronary angiography at ages 60 and 61 revealed total occlusion of the left circumflex artery beyond its origin [386]. His affected brother had the onset of moderate angina pectoris at age 43 years [387]. Electrocardiogram at 48 years of age showed nonspecific repolarization abnormalities. He was hypertensive, obese, and also a heavy cigarette smoker. He died suddenly outside the hospital and no autopsy was performed. Another hypertensive homozygote had characteristic angina pectoris by age 43. Cerebrovascular disease resulted in stroke and the eventual death of one 69-year-old woman with Tangier disease.

Findings in homozygotes cannot be considered at variance with compelling epidemiologic evidence relating low HDL levels to risk for atherosclerosis. Tangier homozygotes typically have quite low serum cholesterol concentrations. Hypocholesterolemia is related not only to the absence of HDL but to reduced LDL concentrations and substitution of triglycerides for cholesteryl esters as the major LDL neutral lipid. Thus, the necessity for HDL to inhibit uptake or promote egress of cholesterol from the arterial wall may not be as important in Tangier homozygotes as it is postulated to be in normal persons. The thrombocytopenia and hyporeactive platelets [388] typical of this disorder could also limit the atherosclerotic reaction [389, 390]. Finally, it must be recognized that the very small number of involved patients and the paucity of objective data obviate any generalizations regarding atherosclerosis in Tangier disease.

Findings in Heterozygotes

No consistent pattern of clinical abnormalities has emerged with extended observation of obligate heterozygotes and other presumably affected first-degree relatives. Neither abnormal tonsils nor neuropathic changes have been seen. The lipid content of the tonsils of one heterozygote has been determined and the tissue subjected to histochemical analysis. There was no evidence of cholesteryl ester storage [338]. Foam cells were found in the bone marrow of three of six obligate heterozygotes. Lipid-laden histiocytes have also been identified in rectal biopsies of several heterozygous patients [391].

Symptoms or signs of atherosclerosis have not been observed in heterozygotes before 40 years of age. Approximately half of the known obligate heterozygotes older than 45 years were reported to have symptoms of coronary heart disease [386], but apparently none have died of any cause before age 60. Since the biochemical defect in Tangier disease has not been precisely defined, "carriers" of the gene in an unselected population cannot be identified with certainty. HDL concentrations in obligate heterozygous patients are usually below the normal range [336]. Studied in a German kindred revealed that the concentrations of HDL cholesterol, apo A-I, and apo A-II in obligate heterozygotes, while quite variable among individuals, were decreased by approximately 50 percent [391]. The molar ratio of apo A-I to apo A-II contained in HDL was not significantly different from that of normal subjects, and the morphological appearance of HDL, as ascertained by electron microscopy, was similar to control preparations [391]. Others have reported that apo A-I levels were decreased to 50 percent or less of the control values, even when estimates of HDL cholesterol concentrations were normal [346].

The fact that the serum concentrations of both A apolipoproteins in heterozygous patients are decreased by 50 percent does not necessarily imply a defect in two separate structural genes or one controlling gene. It is certainly possible, although currently speculative, that the availability of normal amounts of one of the A apolipoproteins limits the formation of HDL. This may be apo A-I, the major HDL apo protein in lower species and the activator of LCAT.

Genetics

Tangier disease has not yet been described in blacks or Orientals, and it has been found in only one Jewish patient [378, 382]. Evidence of consanguinity has been sought in most of the published kindreds and has been documented in five [334, 336, 378, 391, 392]. Several families were extensively investigated to determine the mode of inheritance [335, 336, 391]. These indicated that full expression of Tangier disease occurs in subjects homozygous for a mutant autosomal allele. The absence of recently identified cases, in spite of the enormous popularity of HDL cholesterol measurements, appears to attest to the rarity of this mutant.

Other Familial HDL Deficiencies

A woman with diffuse planar xanthomatosis, corneal opacities, hepatosplenomegaly, but normal tonsils, has been described [352, 393]. She may represent the twenty-seventh case of Tangier disease [386]. She had virtually no HDL and normal liver function. The plasma lipoprotein pattern differed from other subjects with Tangier disease in that elevated levels of intermediate density lipoproteins were found. The familial nature of her HDL deficiency was not well defined, but she conceivably may have Tangier disease in combination with type 3 hyperlipoproteinemia or another dyslipoproteinemia.

An Italian family with very low HDL cholesterol levels (7 to 14 mg/dl) in three members with mild hypertriglyceridemia was recently reported [347]. No tonsillar abnormalities, splenomegaly, corneal opacities, neuropathy, or vascular disease were noted. Analysis of the apolipoprotein content of the HDL isolate from these patients revealed proteins with relative molecular weights of 55,000, 35,000, and 28,000 [345]. The $M_r = 28,000$ apolipoprotein coelectrophoresed with authentic apo A-I on SDS polyacrylamide gels and showed immunochemical identity with apo A-I on double diffusion against an apo A-I antiserum. It contained two amino acid residues, cysteine and isoleucine, which are not present in normal apo A-I. This variant form of apolipoprotein A-I was designated the A-I Milano apolipoprotein. By virtue of the presence of cysteine, the A-I Milano apolipoprotein was capable of forming intermolecular disulfide bonds. Thus, the 55,000-dalton apolipoprotein was formed as a dimer of A-I Milano. The 35,000-dalton apolipoprotein was composed of two different subunits, apo A-I Milano and apo A-II [394].

Recent studies employing isoelectric focusing and two-dimensional gel electrophoresis suggest the presence of normal apo A-I in the plasma of patients with apo A-I Milano [367]. Vertical transmission of apo A-I Milano has been shown [347] and the patients described thus appear heterozygous at the apo A-I allele. This mutant appears to constitute the first documented example of A apoprotein allelism. Preliminary studies in a German family with low HDL cholesterols suggest that at least one other variant (apo A-I Marburg) may exist [395].

Low HDL cholesterol concentrations together with hypertriglyceridemia have been noted in a familial disorder that has been termed "fish-eye disease" [351, 396]. The disease is characterized by corneal opacities that impair vision, but the relationship of the ocular abnormality to the HDL deficiency is uncertain.

Diagnosis

In any patient with unexplained hepatic or splenic enlargement, corneal deposits, or neuropathy, a close examination of the oropharynx and rectal mucosa and a plasma cholesterol determination are indicated. A cholesterol level below 125 mg/dl must lead directly to triglyceride determination and lipoprotein electrophoresis. Triglyceride levels will be high or normal in Tangier disease and low in most of the LDL deficiency states. Lipoprotein electrophoresis, irrespective of the supporting media employed, should demonstrate no trace of lipoproteins of α_1 mobility. The HDL cholesterol concentration, as routinely determined using precipitation techniques, should be below 5 mg/dl.

Other diseases that should be considered in the differential diagnosis of Tangier disease include: (1) Familial deficiency of lecithin:cholesterol acyltransferase (LCAT) (Chap. 31). Here HDL is very low, but the plasma cholesterol level is normal or high and most of the cholesterol is unesterified. (2) Obstructive liver disease, in which the plasma HDL and A apoproteins may be reduced to levels as low as those seen in Tangier disease. In

this disorder the cholesterol level is not low, but high; and most of the cholesterol is not esterified. (3) Severe malnutrition or hepatic parenchymal disease. Transient infections, presumed viral, and hepatic infiltration by lymphoma have produced plasma lipoprotein patterns indistinguishable from that in Tangier disease. Similar consequences have been noted in malnourished patients receiving total parenteral nutrition [397]. (4) Acquired HDL deficiency due to dysglobulinemia, including possible development of antibodies to HDL [398]. (5) Other storage diseases associated with foam cells and hepatosplenomegaly: in these conditions HDL levels are higher than those seen in Tangier disease, and typical tonsillar abnormalities are absent.

Treatment

There is no treatment for Tangier disease. Consideration might be given to reducing the fat content of the diet, since remnants of triglyceride-bearing lipoproteins appear to accumulate in the plasma in association with fat intake. However, lack of certainty that blood vessel or other tissue changes are a function of abnormal chylomicrons, VLDL, or LDL generates little enthusiasm for prescriptions of radical diet changes.

The critical advice and assistance of Dr. William A. Bradley in the preparation of this manuscript is gratefully acknowledged.

REFERENCES

1. THE LIPID RESEARCH CLINICS PROGRAM EPIDEMIOLOGY COMMITTEE: Plasma lipid distributions in selected North American populations. The Lipid Research Clinics Program Prevalence Study. *Circulation* 60:427, 1979
2. HEISS G, TAMIR I, DAVIS CE, TYROLER HA, RIFKIND BM, SCHONFELD G, JACOBS D, FRANTZ ID JR: Lipoprotein-cholesterol distributions in selected North American populations. The Lipid Research Clinics Program Prevalence Study. *Circulation* 61:302, 1980
3. BEAGLEHOLE R, TROST DC, TAMIR I, KWITEROVICH P, GLUECK CJ, INSULL W, CHRISTENSEN B: Plasma high-density lipoprotein cholesterol in children and young adults. The Lipid Research Clinics Program Prevalance Study. *Circulation* 62(IV):83, 1980
4. TYROLER HA, GLUECK CJ, CHRISTENSEN B, KWITEROVICH PO JR: Plasma high-density lipoprotein cholesterol comparisons in black and white populations. The Lipid Research Clinics Program Prevalence Study. *Circulation* 62(IV):99, 1980
5. BEAUMONT JL, CARLSON LA, COOPER GR, FEJFAR Z, FREDRICKSON DS, STRASSER T: Classification of hyperlipidaemias and hyperlipoproteinaemias. *Bull WHO* 43:891, 1970
6. FRIEDEWALD WT, LEVY RI, FREDRICKSON DS: Estimation of the concentration of low-density lipoprotein cholesterol in plasma, without use of the preparative ultracentrifuge. *Clin Chem* 18:499, 1972
7. GLUECK CJ, GARTSIDE P, FALLAT RW, STEINER PM: Longevity syndromes: Familial hypobeta and familial hyperalpha lipoproteinemia. *J Lab Clin Med* 88:941, 1976
8. ALBERS JJ, WARNICK GR, CHEUNG MC: Quantitation of high density lipoproteins. *Lipids* 13:926, 1978
9. NELSON G: *Blood Lipids and Lipoproteins: Quantitation, Composition, and Metabolism.* New York, Wiley-Interscience, 1972
10. WU A-L, WINDMUELLER HG: Relative contributions by liver and intestine to individual plasma apolipoproteins in the rat. *J Biol Chem* 254:7316, 1979
11. SATA T, HAVEL RJ, JONES AL: Characterization of subfractions of triglyceride-rich lipoproteins separated by gel chromatography from blood plasma of normolipemic and hyperlipemic humans. *J Lipid Res* 13:757, 1972
12. SEGREST JP, JACKSON RL, MORRISETT JD, GOTTO AM JR: A molecular theory of lipid protein interactions in the plasma lipoproteins. *FEBS Lett* 38:247, 1974

13. JACKSON RL, MORRISETT JD, GOTTO AM JR, SEGREST JP: The mechanism of lipid-binding by plasma lipoproteins. *Mol Cell Biochem* 6:43, 1975

14. JACKSON RL, MORRISETT JD, SPARROW JT, SEGREST JP, POWNALL HJ, SMITH LC, HOFF HF, GOTTO AM JR: The interaction of apolipoprotein-serine with phosphatidylcholine. *J Biol Chem* 249:5314, 1974

15. ATKINSON D, DAVIS MAF, LESLIE RB: The structure of a high density lipoprotein (HDL₃) from porcine plasma. *Proc R Soc Lond B* 186:165, 1974

16. LAGGNER P, KRATKY O, KOSTNER G, SATTLER J, HOLASEK A: Small angle x-ray scattering of LpA, the major lipoprotein family of human plasma lipoprotein HDL₃. *FEBS Lett* 27:53, 1972

17. LAGGNER P, MÜLLER K, KRATKY O, KOSTNER G, HOLASEK A: Studies on the structure of lipoprotein A of human high density lipoprotein HDL₃. The spherically averaged electron density distribution. *FEBS Lett* 33:77, 1973

18. MÜLLER K, LAGGNER P, KRATKY O, KOSTNER G, HOLASEK A, GLATTER O: X-ray small angle scattering of human plasma high density lipoprotein LpA from HDL₂. Application of a new evaluation method. *FEBS Lett* 40:213, 1974

19. SHIPLEY CG, ATKINSON D, SCANU AM: Small-angle x-ray scattering of human serum high-density lipoproteins. *J Supramol Struc I* 98:1972

20. MORRISETT JD, JACKSON RL, GOTTO AM JR: Lipoproteins: Structure and function. *Ann Rev Biochem* 44:183, 1975

21. GAGE S II: The free granules (chylomicrons) of the blood as shown by the dark-field microscope *Cornell Vet* 10:154, 1920

22. LOSSOW WJ, LINDGREN FT, MURCHIO JC, STEVENS GR, JENSEN LC: Particle size and protein content of six fractions of the S_f > 20 plasma lipoproteins isolated by density gradient centrifugation. *J Lipid Res* 10:68, 1969

23. YOKOYAMA A, ZILVERSMIT DB: Particle size and composition of dog lymph chylomicrons. *J Lipid Res* 6:241, 1965

24. CARDELL RR JR, BADENHAUSEN S, PORTER KR: Intestinal triglyceride absorption in the rat: An electron microscopical study *J Cell Biol* 34:123, 1967

25. TYTGAT GN, RUBIN CE SAUNDERS DR: Synthesis and transport of lipoprotein particles by intestinal absorptive cells in man. *J Clin Invest* 50:2065, 1971

26. GLICKMAN RM, KIRSCH K: The apoproteins of various size classes of human chylous fluid lipoproteins. *Biochim Biophys Acta* 371:255, 1974

27. MAHLEY RW, BENNETT BD, MORRE DJ, GRAY ME, THISTLETHWAITE W, LEQUIRE VS: Lipoproteins associated with the Golgi apparatus isolated from epithelial cells of rat small intestine. *Lab Invest* 25:435, 1971

28. OCKNER RK, MANNING JA: Fatty acid binding proteins. Role in esterification of absorbed long chain fat in rat intestine. *J Clin Invest* 58:632, 1976

29. QUINTAO ECR, DREWIACKI A, STECHHAHN K, DE FARIA EC, SIPAHI AM: Origin of cholesterol transported in intestinal lymph: Studies in patients with filarial chyluria. *J Lipid Res* 20:941, 1979

30. BIZZI A, MARSH JB: Further observations on the attachment of carbohydrate to lipoproteins by rat liver Golgi membranes. *Proc Soc Exp Biol Med* 144:762, 1973

31. LO CH, MARSH JB: The synthesis of plasma lipoproteins: Incorporation of ¹⁴C-glucosamine by cells and subcellular fractions of rat liver. *J Biol Chem* 245:5001, 1970

32. WETMORE S, MAHLEY RW, BROWN WV, SCHACHTER H: Incorporation of sialic acid into sialidase-treated apolipoprotein of human very low density lipoprotein by a pork liver sialyltransferase. *Can J Biochem* 52:655, 1974

33. GLICKMAN RM, KIRSCH K, ISSELBACHER KJ: Fat absorption during inhibition of protein synthesis: Studies of lymph chylomicrons. *J Clin Invest* 51:356, 1972

34. GLICKMAN RM, KHORANA J, KILGORE A: Localization of apolipoprotein B in intestinal epithelial cells. *Science* 193:1254, 1976

35. GLICKMAN RM, GREEN PHR: The intestine as a source of apolipoprotein A₁. *Proc Nat Acad Sci USA* 74:2569, 1977

36. RACHMILEWITZ D, ALBERS JJ, SAUNDERS DR, FAINARU M: Apoprotein synthesis by human duodenojejunal mucosa. *Gastroenterology* 75:677, 1978

37. SCHONFELD G, BELL E, ALPERS DH: Intestinal apoproteins during fat absorption. *J Clin Invest* 61:1539, 1978

38. GREEN PHR, GLICKMAN RM, RILEY JW, QUINET E: Human apolipoprotein A-IV. Intestinal origin and distribution in plasma. *J Clin Invest* 65:911, 1980

39. WINDMUELLER HG, HERBERT PN, LEVY RI: Biosynthesis of lymph and plasma lipoprotein apoproteins by isolated perfused rat liver and intestine. *J Lipid Res* 14:215, 1973

40. IMAIZUMI K, HAVEL RJ, FAINARU M, VIGNE J-L: Origin and transport of the A-I and argine-rich apolipoproteins in mesenteric lymph of rats. *J Lipid Res* 19:1038, 1978

41. WU A-L, WINDMUELLER HG: Identification of circulating apolipoproteins synthesized by rat small intestine *in vivo*. *J Biol Chem* 253:2525, 1978

42. WINDMUELLER HG, WU A-L: Biosynthesis of plasma apolipoproteins by rat small intestine without dietary or biliary fat. *J Biol Chem* 256:3012, 1981

43. KOSTNER G: Studien über die Zusammensetzung der Lipoproteine der menschlichen Lymphe. *Hoppe-Seylers Z Physiol Chem* 353:1863, 1972

44. KOSTNER G, HOLASEK A: Characterization and quantitation of the apolipoprotein from human chyle chylomicrons. *Biochemistry* 11:1217, 1972

45. WEISGRABER KH, BERSOT TP, MAHLEY RW: Isolation and characterization of an apoprotein from the d<1.006 lipoproteins of human and canine lymph homologous with the rat A-IV apoprotein. *Biochem Biophys Res Commun* 85:287, 1978

46. GREEN PHR, GLICKMAN RM, SAUDER CD, BLUM CB, TALL AR: Human intestinal lipoproteins. Studies in chyluric subjects. *J Clin Invest* 64:233, 1979

47. HOLT PR, WU A-L, CLARK SB: Apoprotein composition and turnover in rat intestinal lymph during steady-state triglyceride absorption. *J Lipid Res* 20:494, 1979

48. HAVEL RJ, KANE JP, BALASSE EO, SEGEL N, BASSO LV: Splanchnic metabolism of free fatty acids and production of triglycerides of very low density lipoproteins in normotriglyceridemic and hypertriglyceridemic humans. *J Clin Invest* 49:2017, 1970

49. NIKKILA EA, KEKKI M: Plasma triglyceride metabolism in thyroid disease. *J Clin Invest* 51:2103, 1972

50. BARTER PJ, NESTEL PJ, CARROLL KF: Precursors of plasma triglyceride fatty acid in humans. Effects of glucose consumption, chlofibrate administration, and alcoholic fatty liver. *Metabolism* 21:117, 1972

51. REAVEN EP, KILTERMAN OG, REAVEN GM: Ultrastructural and physiological evidence for corticosteroid-induced alterations in hepatic production of very low density lipoprotein particles. *J Lipid Res* 15:74, 1974

52. LUSKEY KL, BROWN MS, GOLDSTEIN JL: Stimulation of the synthesis of very low density lipoproteins in rooster liver by estradiol. *J Biol Chem* 249:5939, 1974

53. ZECH LA, GRUNDY SM, STEINBERG D, BERMAN M: Kinetic model for production and metabolism of very low density lipoprotein triglycerides. Evidence for a slow production pathway and results for normolipidemic subjects. *J Clin Invest* 63:1262, 1979

54. GRUNDY SM, MOK HYI, ZECH L, STEINBERG D, BERMAN M: Transport of very low density lipoprotein triglycerides in varying degrees of obesity and hypertriglyceridemia. *J Clin Invest* 63:1274, 1979

55. DAVIS RA, ENGELHORN SC, PANGBURN SH, WEINSTEIN DB, STEINBERG D: Very low density lipoprotein synthesis and secretion by cultured rat hepatocytes. *J Biol Chem* 254:2010, 1979

56. DAVIS RA, ENGELHORN SC, WEINSTEIN DB, STEINBERG D: Very low density lipoprotein secretion by cultured rat hepatocytes. Inhibition by albumin and other macromolecules. *J Biol Chem* 255:2039, 1980

57. HOWARD BV, ZECH L, DAVIS M, BENNION LJ, SAVAGE PJ, NAGULESPARAN M, BILHEIMER D, BENNETT PH, GRUNDY SM: Studies of very low density lipoprotein triglyceride metabolism in an obese population with low plasma lipids: Lack of influence of body weight or plasma insulin. *J Lipid Res* 21:1032, 1980

58. MURTHY VK, SHIPP JC: Regulation of hepatic triglyceride synthesis in diabetic rats. *J Clin Invest* 67:923, 1981

59. STEIN O, STEIN Y: Synthesis and intracellular degradation of serum lipoproteins, in Schettler G, Greten H, Schlierf G, Seidel D (eds): *Fettstoffwechsel*. New York, Springer-Verlag, 1976, p 197

60. CHAPMAN MJ, MILLS GL, TAYLAUR CE: The effect of a lipid-rich diet on the properties and composition of lipoprotein particles from the Golgi apparatus of guinea pig liver. *Biochem J* 131:177, 1973

61. MAHLEY RW, BERSOT TP, LEQUIRE VS, LEVY RI, WINDMUELLER HG, BROWN WV: Identity of very low density lipoprotein apoproteins of plasma and liver Golgi apparatus. *Science* 168:380, 1970

62. MAHLEY RW, HAMILTON RL, LEQUIRE VS: Characterization of lipoprotein particles isolated from the Golgi apparatus of rat liver. *J Lipid Res* 10:433, 1969

63. SWIFT LL, MANOWITZ NR, DUNN GD, LEQUIRE VS: Isolation and characterization of hepatic Golgi lipoproteins from hypercholesterolemic rats. *J Clin Invest* 66:415, 1980

64. LE MARCHAND Y, SINGH A, ASSIMACOPOULOS-JEANNET F, ORCI L, ROUILLER C, JEANRENAUD B: A role for the microtubular system in the release of very low density lipoprotein by perfused mouse livers. *J Biol Chem* 248:6862, 1973

65. STEIN O, RACHMILEWITZ D, SANGER L, EISENBERG S, STEIN Y: Metabolism of iodinated very low density lipoprotein in the rat: Autoradiographic localization in the liver. *Biochim Biophys Acta* 360:205, 1974

66. PHAIR RD, HAMMOND MG, BOWDEN JA, FRIED M FISHER WR, BERMAN M: A preliminary model for human lipoprotein metabolism in hyperlipoproteinemia. *Fed Proc* 34:2263, 1975

67. BERMAN M, HALL M III, LEVY RI, EISENBERG S, BILHEIMER DW, PHAIR RD, GOEBEL RH: Metabolism of apoB and apoC lipoproteins in man: Kinetic studies in normal and hyperlipoproteinemic subjects. *J Lipid Res* 19:38, 1978

68. PATSCH JR, SAILER S, BRAUNSTEINER H, FORTE T: Electron microscopic characterization of lipoproteins from patients with familial type III hyperlipoproteinemia. *Eur J Clin Invest* 6:307, 1976

69. PATSCH JR, SAILER S, BRAUNSTEINER H: Lipoprotein of the density 1.006–1.020 in the plasma of patients with type III hyperlipoproteinemia in the postabsorptive state. *Eur J Clin Invest* 5:45, 1975

70. SHORE VG, SHORE G: Heterogeneity of human plasma very low density lipoproteins: Separation of species differing in protein components. *Biochemistry* 12:502, 1973

71. PATSCH JR: Type III hyperlipoproteinemia, in Day CE (ed): *Low Density Lipoproteins.* Plenum, New York, 1976, p 197

72. SIGURDSSON G., NICOLL A, LEWIS B: Conversion of very low density lipoprotein to low density lipoprotein. A metabolic study of apolipoprotein B kinetics in human subjects. *J Clin Invest* 56:1481, 1975

73. SIGURDSSON G, NICOLL A, LEWIS B: The metabolism of low density lipoprotein in endogenous hypertriglyceridaemia. *J Clin Invest* 6:151, 1976

74. GINSBERG HN, LE N-A, MELISH J, STEINBERG D, BROWN WV: Effect of a high carbohydrate diet on apoprotein-B catabolism in man. *Metabolism* 30:347, 1981

75. SOUTAR AK, MYANT NB, THOMPSON GR: Simultaneous measurement of apolipoprotein B turnover in very low and low density lipoproteins in familial hypercholesterolaemia. *Atherosclerosis* 28:247, 1977

76. SOUTAR AK, MYANT NB, THOMPSON GR: Metabolism of apolipoprotein B-containing lipoproteins in familial hypercholesterolaemia. *Atherosclerosis* 32:315, 1979

77. FAINARU M, FELKER TE, HAMILTON RL, HAVEL RJ: Evidence that a separate particle containing B-apoprotein is present in high-density lipoproteins from perfused rat liver. *Metabolism* 26:999, 1977

78. NAKAYA N, CHUNG BH, PATSCH JR, TAUNTON OD: Synthesis and release of low density lipoproteins by the isolated perfused pig liver. *J Biol Chem* 252:7530, 1977

79. SKIPSKI VP: Lipid composition of lipoproteins in normal and diseased states, in Nelson GJ (ed): *Blood Lipids and Lipoproteins: Quantitation, Composition and Metabolism.* New York, Wiley-Interscience, 1972, p 471

80. HAMILTON RL, WILLIAMS MC, FIELDING CJ, HAVEL RJ: Discoidal bilayer structure of nascent high density lipoproteins from perfused rat liver. *J Clin Invest* 58:667, 1976

81. GREEN PHR, TALL AR, GLICKMAN RM: Rat intestine secretes discoid high density lipoprotein. *J Clin Invest* 61:528, 1978

82. TURNER P, MILLER N, CHRYSTIE I, COLTART J, MISTRY P, NICOLL A, LEWIS B: Splanchnic production of discoidal plasma high-density lipoprotein in man. *Lancet* 1:645, 1979

83. ANDERSON DW, NICHOLS AV, FORTE TM, LINDGREN FT: Particle distribution of human serum high density lipoproteins. *Biochim Biophys Acta* 493:55, 1977

84. ANDERSON DW, NICHOLS AV, PAN SS, LINDGREN FT: High density lipoprotein distribution. Resolution and determination of three major components in a normal population study. *Atherosclerosis* 29:161, 1978

85. KOSTNER GM, PATSCH JR, SALIER G, BRAUNSTEINER H, HOLASEK A: Polypeptide distribution of the main lipoprotein density classes separated from human plasma by rate zonal ultracentrifugation. *Eur J Biochem* 45:611, 1974

86. FRIEDBERG SJ, REYNOLDS JA: The molar ratio of the two major polypeptide components of human high density lipoprotein. *J Biol Chem* 251:4005, 1976

87. CURRY MD, ALAUPOVIC P, SUENRAM CA: Determination of apolipoprotein A and its constitutive A-I and A-II polypeptides by separate electroimmunoassays. *Clin Chem* 22:315, 1976

88. CHEUNG MC, ALBERS JJ: The measurement of apolipoprotein A-I and A-II levels in men and women by immunoassay. *J Clin Invest* 60:43, 1977

89. SCHONFELD G, CHEN J-S, McDONNELL WF, JENG I: Apolipoprotein A-II content of human plasma high density lipoproteins measured by radioimmunoassay. *J Lipid Res* 18:645, 1977

90. HENDERSON LO, MUSLINER TA, CAMPBELL J, GARNER P, HERBERT PN: Unpublished observations

91. SCHAEFER EJ, FOSTER DM, JENKINS LL, LINDGREN FT, BERMAN M, LEVY RI, BREWER, HB JR: The composition and metabolism of high density lipoprotein subfractions. *Lipids* 14:511, 1979

92. HAVEL RJ, KANE JP, KASHYAP ML: Interchange of apolipoproteins between chylomicrons and high density lipoproteins during alimentary lipemia in man. *J Clin Invest* 52:32, 1973

93. ALAUPOVIC P: Conceptual development of the classification systems of plasma lipoproteins, in Peeters H (ed): *Protides of the Biological Fluids.* Oxford, England, Pergamon, 1971, p 9

94. BENDITT EP, ERIKSEN N: Amyloid protein SAA is associated with high density lipoprotein from human serum. *Proc Natl Acad Sci USA* 74:4025, 1977

95. BAUSSERMAN LL, HERBERT PN, McADAM KPWJ: Heterogeneity of human serum amyloid A proteins. *J Exp Med* 152:641, 1980

96. JACKSON RL, MORRISETT JD, GOTTO AM JR: Lipoproteins and lipid transport: Structural and functional concepts, in Levy RI, Rifkind BM (eds): *Hyperlipidemia, Diagnosis and Therapy.* New York, Grune and Stratton, 1977, p 1

97. SPARROW JT, MORRISETT JD, POWNALL HJ, JACKSON RL, GOTTO AM JR: The mechanism of lipid binding by the plasma lipoproteins: Synthesis of model peptides, in Walter R, Meinhofer J (eds): *Peptides: Chemistry, Structure and Biology.* Ann Arbor, Michigan, Ann Arbor Science, 1975, p 597

98. BAKER HN, DELAHUNTY T, GOTTO AM JR, JACKSON RL: The primary structure of high density apolipoprotein-glutamine-I. *Proc Nat Acad Sci USA* 71:3631, 1974

99. BREWER HB JR, FAIRWELL T, LARUE A, ROMAN R, HOUSER A, BRONZERT TJ: The amino acid sequence of human apo-I, an apolipoprotein isolated from high density lipoproteins. *Biochem Biophys Res Commun* 80:623, 1978

100. McLACHLIN AD: Repeated helical pattern in apolipoprotein A-I. *Nature* 267:465, 1977

101. FIELDING CJ, SHORE VG, FIELDING PE: A protein cofactor of lecithin:cholesterol acyltransferase. *Biochem Biophys Res Commun* 46:1493, 1972

102. SOUTAR AK, GARNER CW, BAKER HN, SPARROW JT, JACKSON RL, GOTTO AM, SMITH LC: Effect of the human plasma apolipoproteins and phosphatidylcholine acyl donor on the activity of lecithin:cholesterol acyltransferase. *Biochemistry* 14:3057, 1975

103. ALBERS JJ: Lecithin:cholesterol acyltransferase. *Artery* 5:61, 1979

104. SOUTAR AK, GARNER CW, BAKER HN, SPARROW JT, JACKSON RL, GOTTO AM JR, SMITH LC: The effects of plasma apolipoproteins in lecithin:cholesterol acyltransferase, *Biochemistry* 14:3057, 1975

105. NICOLL A, MILLER NE, LEWIS B: High-density lipoprotein metabolism. *Adv Lipid Res* 17:53, 1980

106. BREWER HB JR, LUX SE, RONAN R, JOHN KM: Amino acid sequence of human apoLp-Gln-II (ApoA-II), an apolipoprotein isolated from the high density lipoprotein complex. *Proc Natl Acad Sci USA* 69:1304, 1972

107. JACKSON RL, MAO SJT, GOTTO AM JR: Effects of maleylation on the lipid-binding and immunochemical properties of human plasma high density apolipoprotein A-II. *Biochem Biophys Res Commun* 61:1317, 1974

108. MAO SJT, SPARROW JT, GILLIAM EB, GOTTO AM JR, JACKSON RL: Mechanism of lipid-protein interaction in the plasma lipoproteins: Lipid-binding properties of synthetic fragments of apolipoprotein A-II. *Biochemistry* 16:4150, 1977

109. KOSTNER GM: Studies of the composition and structure of human serum lipoproteins: Isolation and partial characterization of apolipoprotein A-III. *Biochim Biophys Acta* 336:383, 1974

110. McCONATHY WJ, ALAUPOVIC P: Isolation and partial characterization of apolipoprotein D: A new protein moiety of the human plasma lipoprotein system. *FEBS Lett* 37:178, 1973

111. KOSTNER G: Studies on the cofactor requirement for lecithin:cholesterol acyltransferase. *Scand J Clin Lab Invest* 33(suppl 137):19, 1974

112. OLOFSSON SO, GUSTAFSON A: Degradation of high density lipoproteins (IIDL) *in vitro. Scand J Clin Lab Invest* 33(suppl 137):57, 1974

113. SWANEY JB, REESE H, EDER HA: Polypeptide composition of rat high density lipoprotein: characterization by SDS-gel electrophoresis. *Biochem Biophys Res Commun* 59:513, 1974

114. BEISIEGEL U, UTERMANN G: An apolipoprotein homolog of rat apolipoprotein A-IV in human plasma. *Eur J Biochem* 93:601, 1979

115. FIDGE NH: The redistribution and metabolism of iodinated apolipoprotein A-IV in rats. *Biochim Biophys Acta* 619:129, 1980

116. OLOFSSON SO, McCONATHY WJ, ALAUPOVIC P: Isolation and partial characterization of a new acidic apolipoprotein (apolipoprotein F) from high density lipoproteins of human plasma. *Biochemistry* 17:1032, 1978

117. LIM CT, CHUNG J, KAYDEN HJ, SCANU AM: Apoproteins of human serum high density lipoproteins. Isolation and characterization of the peptides of Sephadex fraction V from normal subjects and patients with abetalipoproteinemia. *Biochim Biophys Acta* 420:332, 1976

118. WU A-L, WINDMUELLER HG: Variant forms of plasma apolipoprotein B. Hepatic and intestinal biosynthesis and heterogeneous metabolism in the rat. *J Biol Chem* 256:3615, 1981

119. ELOVSON J, HUANG YO, BAKER N, KANNAN R: Apolipoprotein B is structurally and metabolically heterogeneous in the rat. *Proc Nat Acad Sci USA* 78:157, 1981

120. SPARKS CE, MARSH JB: Metabolic heterogeneity of apolipoprotein B in the rat. *J Lipid Res* 22:519, 1981

121. KANE JP, HARDMAN DA, PAULUS HE: Heterogeneity of apolipoprotein B: Isolation of a new species from human chylomicrons. *Proc Nat Acad Sci USA* 77:2465, 1980

121a. MAHLEY RW, WEISGRABER KH, MELCHIOR GW, INNERARITY TL, HOLCOMBE KS: Inhibition of receptor-mediated clearance of lysine and arginine-modified lipoproteins from the plasma of rats and monkeys. *Proc Nat Acad Sci USA* 77:5923, 1980

121b. ATTIE AD, PITTMAN RC, STEINBERG D: Metabolism of native and of lactosylated human low density lipoprotein: Evidence for two pathways for catabolism of exogenous proteins in rat hepatocytes. *Proc Nat Acad Sci USA* 77:5923, 1980

121c. SHEPHERD J, BICKER S, LORIMER AR, PACKARD CJ: Receptor mediated low density lipoprotein catabolism in man. *J Lipid Res* 20:999, 1979

121d. SHEPHERD J, PACKARD CJ, BICKER S, LAWRIE TDV, MORGAN HG: Cholestyramine promotes receptor-mediated low-density-lipoprotein catabolism. *N Engl J Med* 302:1219, 1980

122. SCHONFELD G, LEES RS, GEORGE PK, PFLEGER B: Assay of total plasma apolipoprotein B concentration in human subjects. *J Clin Invest* 53:1458, 1974

123. ALBERS JJ, CABANA VG, HAZZARD WR: Immunoassay of human plasma apolipoprotein B. *Metabolism* 24:1339, 1975

124. UTERMANN G, LIPP K, WIEGANDT H: Studies on the Lp(a)-lipoprotein of human serum. IV. The disaggregation of the Lp(a)-lipoprotein. *Humangenetik* 14:142, 1972

125. ALBERS JJ, ADOLPHSON JL, HAZZARD WR: Radioimmunoassay of human plasma Lp(a) lipoprotein. *J Lipid Res* 18:331, 1977

126. SHULMAN RS, HERBERT PN, WEHRLY K, FREDRICKSON DS: The complete amino acid sequence of C-I (ApoLp-Ser), an apolipoprotein from human very low density lipoproteins. *J Biol Chem* 250:182, 1975

127. JACKSON RL, SPARROW JT, BAKER HN, MORRISETT J, TAUNTON OD, GOTTO AM JR: The primary structure of apolipoprotein-serine. *J Biol Chem* 249:5308, 1974

128. KASHYAP ML, SRIVASTAVA LS, CHEN CY, PERISUTTI G, CAMPBELL M, LUTMER RF, GLUECK CJ: Radioimmunoassay of human apolipoprotein C-II. A study in normal and hypertriglyceridemic subjects. *J Clin Invest* 60:171, 1977

129. JACKSON RL, BAKER HN, GILLIAM EB, GOTTO AM JR: Primary structure of very low density apolipoprotein C-II of human plasma. *Proc Nat Acad Sci USA* 74:1942, 1977

130. MUSLINER TA, HERBERT PN, CHURCH EC: Activation of lipoprotein lipase by native and acylated peptides of apolipoprotein C-II. *Biochim Biophys Acta* 573:501, 1979

131. HAVEL RJ, KOTITE L, KANE JP: Isoelectric heterogeneity of the cofactor protein for lipoprotein lipase in human blood plasma. *Biochem Med* 21:121, 1979

132. MORRISETT JD, JACKSON RL, GOTTO AM JR: Lipid-protein interactions in the plasma lipoproteins. *Biochim Biophys Acta* 472:93, 1977

133. MANTULIN WW, ROHDE MF, GOTTO AM JR, POWNALL HJ: The conformational properties of human plasma apolipoprotein C-II. *J Biol Chem* 255:8185, 1980

134. SMITH LC, VOYTA JC, CATAPANO AL, KINNUNEN PKJ, GOTTO AM JR, SPARROW JT: Activation of lipoprotein lipase by synthetic fragments of apoC-II, in Gotto AM Jr, Smith LC, Allen B (eds): *Atherosclerosis V*, New York, Springer-Verlag, 1980, p 397

135. BRECKENRIDGE WC, LITTLE JA, STEINER G, CHOW A, POAPST M: Hypertriglyceridemia associated with deficiency of apolipoprotein C-II. *N Engl J Med* 298:1265, 1978

136. CATAPANO AL: The distribution of apo C-II and apo C-III in very low density lipoproteins of normal and type IV subjects. *Atherosclerosis* 35:419, 1980

137. BREWER HB JR, SHULMAN R, HERBERT P, RONAN R, WEHRLY K: The complete amino acid sequence of alanine apolipoprotein (apo C-III), an apolipoprotein from human plasma very low density lipoproteins. *J Biol Chem* 249:4975, 1974

138. SHULMAN RS, HERBERT PN, FREDRICKSON DS, WEHRLY K, BREWER HB JR: Isolation and alignment of the tryptic peptides of alanine apolipoprotein, an apolipoprotein from human plasma very low density lipoprotein. *J Biol Chem* 249:4969, 1974

139. MORRISETT JD, POWNALL HJ, SPARROW JT, JACKSON RL, GOTTO AM JR: The interaction of apolipoprotein alanine (apo C-III) with lipids: Study of structural features required for binding. *Adv Exp Med Biol* 63:7, 1974

140. SPARROW JT, POWNALL HJ, HSU F-J, BLUMENTHAL LE, CULWELL AR, GOTTO AM: Lipid binding by fragments of apolipoprotein C-III-1 obtained by thrombin cleavage. *Biochemistry* 16:5427, 1977

141. CURRY MD, MCCONATHY WJ, FESMIRE JD, ALAUPOVIC P: Quantitative determination of human apolipoprotein C-III by electroimmunoassay. *Biochim Biophys Acta* 617:503, 1980

142. BROWN WV, BAGINSKY ML: Inhibition of lipoprotein lipase by an apoprotein of human very low density lipoprotein. *Biochem Biophys Res Commun* 46:375, 1972

143. KRAUSS RM, HERBERT PN, LEVY RI, FREDRICKSON DS: Further observations on the activation and inhibition of lipoprotein lipase by apolipoproteins. *Circ Res* 33:403, 1973

144. SHELBURNE FA, QUARFORDT SH: A new apoprotein of human plasma very low density lipoproteins. *J Biol Chem* 249:1428, 1974

145. ZANNIS VI, BRESLOW JL: Characterization of a unique human apolipoprotein E variant associated with Type III hyperlipoproteinemia. *J Biol Chem* 255:1759, 1980

146. WEISGRABER KH, MAHLEY RW: Apoprotein (E-A-II) complex of human plasma lipoproteins. I. Characterization of this mixed disulfide and its identification in a high density lipoprotein subfraction. *J Biol Chem* 253:6281, 1978

147. UTERMANN G: Isolation and partial characterization of an arginine-rich apolipoprotein from human plasma very low density lipoproteins: apolipoprotein E. *Hoppe-Seylers Z Physiol Chem* 356:1113, 1975

148. UTERMANN G, ALBRECHT G, STEINMETZ A: Polymorphism of apolipoprotein E. I. Methodological aspects and diagnosis of hyperlipoproteinemia type III without ultracentrifugation. *Clin Genet* 14:351, 1978

149. UTERMANN G, WEBER W, BEISIEGEL U: Different mobility in SDS-polyacrylamide gel electrophoresis or apolipoprotein E from phenotypes apoE-N and apoE-D. *FEBS Lett* 101:21, 1979

150. JAIN RS, QUARFORDT SH: The carbohydrate content of apolipoprotein E from human very low density lipoproteins. *Life Sciences* 25:1315, 1979

151. ZANNIS VI, BRESLOW JL: Human very low density lipoprotein apolipoprotein E isoprotein polymorphism is explained by genetic variation and post-translational modification. *Biochemistry* 20:1033, 1981

152. WEISGRABER KH, RALL SC JR, MAHLEY RW: Human E apoprotein heterogeneity: Cysteine-arginine interchanges in the amino acid sequence of the apoE isoforms. *J Biol Chem* 256:9077, 1981

153. ROTH RI, JACKSON RL, POWNALL HJ, GOTTO AM JR: Interaction of plasma "arginine-rich" apoprotein with dimyristoylphosphatidylcholine. *Biochemistry* 16:5030, 1977

154. INNERARITY TL, MAHLEY RW: Enhanced binding by cultured human fibroblasts of apo E–containing lipoproteins as compared with low density lipoproteins. *Biochemistry* 17:1440, 1978

155. CHAO Y-S, WINDLER EE, CHEN GC, HAVEL RJ: Hepatic catabolism of rat and human lipoproteins in rats treated with 17α-ethinyl estradiol. *J Biol Chem* 254:11360, 1979

156. HAVEL RJ, CHAO Y-S, WINDLER EE, KOTITE L, GUO LSS: Isoprotein specificity in the hepatic uptake of apolipoprotein E and the pathogenesis of familial dysbetalipoproteinemia. *Proc Nat Acad Sci USA* 77:4349, 1980

157. FALKO JM, SCHONFELD G, WITZTUM JL, KOLAR JB, WEIDMAN SW, STEELMAN R: Effects of diet on apoprotein E levels and on the apoprotein E subspecies in human plasma lipoproteins. *J Clin Endocrinol Metab* 50:521, 1980

158. BLUM CB, ARON L, SCIACCA R: Radioimmunoassay studies of human apolipoprotein E. *J Clin Invest* 66:1240, 1980

159. KUSHWAHA RS, HAZZARD WR, WAHL PW, HOOVER JJ: Type III hyperlipoproteinemia: Diagnosis in whole plasma by apolipoprotein E immunoassay. *Ann Intern Med* 87:509, 1977

160. HAVEL RJ, KOTITE L, VIGNE J-L, KANE JP, TUN P, PHILLIPS N, CHEN GC: Radioimmunoassay of human arginine-rich apoprotein, apoprotein E. Concentration in blood plasma and lipoproteins as affected by apoprotein E-3 deficiency. *J Clin Invest* 66:1351, 1980

161. UTERMANN G, CANZLER H, HEES M, JAESCHKE M, MUHFELLNER G, SCHOENBORN W, VOGELBERG KH: Studies on the metabolic defect in broad-β disease (hyperlipoproteinaemia type III). *Clin Genet* 12:139, 1977

162. GREGG RE, ZECH LA, SCHAEFER EJ, BREWER HB JR: Type III hyperlipoproteinemia: Defective metabolism of an abnormal apolipoprotein E. *Science* 211:584, 1981

163. BREWSTER ME, IHM J, BRAINARD JR, HARMONY JAK: Transfer of phosphatidylcholine facilitated by a component of human plasma. *Biochim Biophys Acta* 529:147, 1978

164. JACKSON RL, WESTERMAN J, WIRTZ KWA: Complete exchange of phospholipids between microsomes and plasma lipoproteins mediated by liver phospholipid-exchange proteins. *FEBS Lett* 94:38, 1978

165. IHM J, HARMONY JAK, ELLSWORTH J, JACKSON RL: Simultaneous transfer of cholesteryl ester and phospholipid by protein(s) isolated from human lipoprotein-free plasma. *Biochem Biophys Res Commun* 93:1114, 1980

166. HAVEL RJ, KANE JP, KASHYAP ML: Interchange of apolipoproteins between chylomicrons and high density lipoproteins during alimentary lipemia in man. *J Clin Invest* 52:32, 1973

167. SHEPHERD J, PATSCH JR, PACKARD CJ, GOTTO AM JR, TAUNTON OD: Dynamic properties of human high density lipoprotein apoproteins. *J Lipid Res* 19:383, 1978

168. GROW TE, FRIED M: Interchange of apoprotein components between the human plasma high density lipoprotein subclasses HDL₂ and HDL₃ *in vitro*. *J Biol Chem* 253:8034, 1978

169. ZILVERSMIT DB, HUGHES LB, BALMER J: Stimulation of cholesterol ester exchange by lipoprotein-free rabbit plasma. *Biochim Biophys Acta* 409:393, 1975

170. BARTER PJ, LALLY JI: The activity of an esterified cholesterol transferring factor in human and rat serum. *Biochim Biophys Acta* 531:233, 1978

171. HA YC, CALVERT GD, MCINTOSH GH, BARTER PJ: A physiologic role for the esterified cholesterol transfer protein: *In vivo* studies in rabbits and pigs. *Metabolism* 30:380, 1981

172. BARTER PJ, JONES ME: Rate of exchange of esterified cholesterol between human plasma low and high density lipoproteins. *Atherosclerosis* 34:67, 1979

173. BARTER PM, JONES ME: Kinetic studies of the transfer of esterified cholesterol between human plasma low and high density lipoproteins. *J Lipid Res* 21:238, 1980

174. BARTER PJ, HA YC, CALVERT GD: Studies of esterified cholesterol in subfractions of plasma high density lipoproteins. *Atherosclerosis* 38:165, 1981

175. RAJARAM OV, WHITE GH, BARTER PJ: Partial purification and characterization of a triacylglycerol-transfer protein from rabbit serum. *Biochim Biophys Acta* 617:383, 1980

176. HOPKINS GJ, BARTER PJ: Transfers of esterified cholesterol and triglyceride between high density and very low density lipoproteins: In vitro studies of rabbits and humans. *Metabolism* 29:546, 1980

177. NESTEL PJ, REARDON M, BILLINGTON T: In vivo transfer of cholesteryl esters from high density lipoproteins to very low density lipoproteins in man. *Biochim Biophys Acta* 573:403, 1979

178. REDGRAVE TG, SMALL DM: Quantitation of the transfer of surface phospholipid of chylomicrons to the high density lipoprotein fraction during the catabolism of chylomicrons in the rat. *J Clin Invest* 64:162, 1979

179. TALL AR, GREEN PHR, GLICKMAN RM, RILEY JW: Metabolic fate of chylomicron phospholipids and apoproteins in the rat. *J Clin Invest* 64:977, 1979

180. PATSCH JR, GOTTO AM Jr, OLIVECRONA T, EISENBERG S: Formation of high density lipoprotein2-like particles during lipolysis of very low density lipoproteins in vitro. *Proc Nat Acad Sci* 75:4519, 1978

180a. PATSCH JR, GOTTO AM Jr: Die rolle von "high-density" lipoproteine (HDL) im katabolismus triglyceridreicher lipoproteine, in *Lipoproteine und Herzinfarkt*. New York, Verlag Gerhard Witzstrock, 1979, p 17

181. PATSCH JR, GOTTO AM Jr: Separation and analysis of HDL subclasses by zonal ultracentrifugation, in Kippel K (ed): *Report of the High Density Lipoproteins Workshop*. Department of Health, Education and Welfare, National Institutes of Health, 79-1661, 1979, p 310

182. QUARFORDT SH, GOODMAN DS: Metabolism of doubly-labeled chylomicron cholesteryl esters in the rat. *J Lipid Res* 8:264, 1967

183. REDGRAVE TG: Formation of cholesteryl ester–rich particulate lipid during metabolism of chylomicrons. *J Clin Invest* 49:465, 1970

184. MJOS OD, FAERGMAN O, HAMILTON RL, HAVEL RJ: Characterization of remnants produced during the metabolism of triglyceride-rich lipoproteins of blood plasma and intestinal lymph in the rat. *J Clin Invest* 56:603, 1975

185. COOPER AD, YU PYS: Rates of removal and degradation of chylomicron remnants by isolated perfused rat liver. *J Lipid Res* 19:635, 1978

186. SCHAEFER EJ, JENKINS LL, BREWER HB Jr: Human chylomicron apolipoprotein metabolism. *Biochem Biophys Res Commun* 80:405, 1978

187. CARRELLA M, COOPER AD: High affinity binding of chylomicron remnants to rat liver plasma membranes. *Proc Nat Acad Sci USA* 76:338, 1979

188. WINDLER E, CHAO Y-S, HAVEL RJ: Regulation of the hepatic uptake of triglyceride-rich lipoproteins in the rat. *J Biol Chem* 255:8303, 1980

189. PATTNAIK NM, ZILVERSMIT DB: Effect of size and competition by lipoproteins and apolipoproteins on the uptake of chylomicrons and chylomicron remnants by hepatoma cells in culture. *Biochim Biophys Acta* 617:335, 1980

190. ANDERSEN JM, TURLEY SD, DIETSCHY JM: Low and high density lipoproteins and chylomicrons as regulators of rate of cholesterol synthesis in rat liver in vivo. *Proc Nat Acad Sci USA* 76:165, 1979

191. EISENBERG S. BILHEIMER DW, LEVY RI, LINDGREN FT: On the metabolic conversion of human plasma very low density lipoprotein to low density lipoprotein. *Biochim Biophys Acta* 326:361, 1973

192. FAERGEMAN O, SATA T, KANE JP, HAVEL RJ: Metabolism of apoprotein B of plasma very low density lipoproteins in the rat. *J Clin Invest* 56:1396, 1975

193. SIGURDSSON G, NOEL S-P, HAVEL RJ: Catabolism of the apoprotein of low density lipoproteins by the isolated perfused rat liver. *J Lipid Res* 19:628, 1978

194. SHEPHERD J, BICKER S, LORIMER AR, PACKARD CJ: Receptor-mediated low density lipoprotein catabolism in man. *J Lipid Res* 20:999, 1979

195. SIGURDSSON G, NOEL S-P, HAVEL RJ: Quantification of the hepatic contribution to the catabolism of high density lipoproteins in rats. *J Lipid Res* 20:316, 1979

196. MAHLEY RW: Alterations in plasma lipoproteins induced by cholesterol feeding in animals including man, in Dietschy JM, Gotto AM Jr, Ontko JA (eds): *Disturbances in Lipoprotein Metabolism*. Bethesda, Maryland, American Physiological Society, 1978, p 181

197. MAHLEY RW, INNERARITY T, BERSOT TP, LIPSON A, MARGOLIS S: Alterations in human high-density lipoproteins, with or without increased plasma cholesterol, induced by diets high in cholesterol. *Lancet* 2:807, 1978

198. BASSEN FA, KORNZWEIG AL: Malformation of the erythrocytes in a case of atypical retinitis pigmentosa. *Blood* 5:381, 1950

199. JAMPEL RS, FALLS HF: Atypical retinitis pigmentosa, acanthocytosis, and heredodegenerative neuromuscular disease. *Arch Ophthalmol* 59:818, 1958

200. FRIEDMAN IS, COHN H, ZYMORIS M, GOLDMAN MG: Hypocholesterolemia in idiopathic steatorrhea. *Arch Intern Med* 105:112, 1960

201. SALT HB, WOLFF OH, LLOYD JK, FOSBROOKE AS, CAMERON AH, HUBBLE DV: On having no beta-lipoprotein: A syndrome comprising abetalipoproteinemia, acanthocytosis, and steatorrhea. *Lancet* 2:325, 1960

202. LAMY M, FREZAL J, POLONOVSKI J, REY J: L'Absence congénitale de beta-lipoprotéines. *C R Soc Biol (Paris)* 154:1974, 1960

203. MABRY CC, DI GEORGE AM, AUERBACH VH: Studies concerning the defect in a patient with acanthocytosis. *Clin Res* 8:371, 1960

204. HERBERT PN, GOTTO AM, FREDRICKSON DS: Familial lipoprotein deficiency (abetalipoproteinemia, hypobetalipoproteinemia and Tangier disease), in Stanbury JB, Wyngaarden JB, Fredrickson DS (eds): *The Metabolic Basis of Inherited Disease*, 3d ed. New York, McGraw-Hill, 1978, pp 544, chap 28

205. HO YK, FAUST JR, BILHEIMER DW, BROWN MS, GOLDSTEIN JL: Regulation of cholesterol synthesis by low density lipoprotein in isolated human lymphocytes. *J Exp Med* 145:1531, 1977

206. KOTT E, DELPRE G, KADISH U, DZIATELOVSKY M, SANDBANK U: Abetalipoproteinemia (Bassen-Kornzweig Syndrome). *Acta Neuropathol (Berlin)*, 37:255, 1977

207. DELPRE G, KADISH U, GLANTZ I, AVIDOR I: Endoscopic assessment in abetalipoproteinemia (Bassen-Kornzweig Syndrome). *Endoscopy* 10:59, 1978

208. SHEPHERD J, CASLAKE M, FARISH E, FLECK A: Chemical and kinetic study of the lipoproteins in abetalipoproteinaemic plasma. *J Clin Pathol* 31:382, 1978

209. KAYDEN HJ: Is essential fatty acid deficiency part of the syndrome of abetalipoproteinemia? *Nutr Rev* 38:244, 1980

210. CABALLERO FM, BUCHANAN GR: Abetalipoproteinemia presenting as severe vitamin K deficiency. *Pediatrics* 65:161, 1980

211. ILLINGWORTH DR, CONNOR WE, MILLER RG: Abetalipoproteinemia. Report of two cases and review of therapy. *Arch Neurol* 37:659, 1980

212. HERBERT PN, FREDRICKSON DS: The hypobetalipoproteinemias, in Schettler G, Greten H, Schlierf G, Seidel D (eds): *Handbuch der Inneren Medizin, VII/4:Fettstoffwechsel*. Heidelberg, Springer-Verlag, 1976, p 485

213. SHACKLADY MM, DJARDJOURAS EM, LLOYD JK: Red cell lipids in familial alpha-lipoprotein deficiency (Tangier disease). *Lancet* 2:151, 1968

214. JONES JW, WAYS P: Abnormalities of high density lipoproteins in abetalipoproteinemia. *J Clin Invest* 46:1151, 1967

215. SCHWARTZ JF, ROWLAND LP, EDER H, MARKS PA, OSSERMAN EF, HIRSCHBERG E, ANDERSON H: Bassen-Kornzweig syndrome: Deficiency of serum beta-lipoprotein. *Arch Neurol* 8:438, 1963

216. LEVY RI, FREDRICKSON DS, LASTER L: The lipoproteins and lipid transport in abetalipoproteinemia. *J Clin Invest* 45:531, 1966

217. AZIZI E: Abetalipoproteinemia in acrodermatitis enteropathica. *N Engl J Med* 284:1387, 1971

218. BECROFT DMO, COSTELLO JM, SCOTT PJ: Abetalipoproteinemia (Bassen-Kornzweig syndrome). *Arch Dis Child* 40:40, 1965

219. BELANGER M, TREMBLAY M, LAPOINTE JR: Absence congenitale des bêta-lipoproteines; Syndrome rare et bizarre. Nouvelle observation. *Laval Med* 42:332, 1971

220. DISCHE MR, PORRO RS: The cardiac lesions in Bassen-Kornzweig syndrome. *Am J Med* 49:568, 1970

221. COOPER RA, GULBRANDSEN CL: The relationship between serum lipoproteins and red cell membranes in abetalipoproteinemia: Deficiency of lecithin:cholesterol acyltransferase. *J Lab Clin Med* 78:323, 1971

222. LEES RS: Immunological evidence for the presence of B protein (apoprotein of β-lipoprotein) in normal and abetalipoproteinemic plasma. *J Lipid Res* 8:396, 1967

223. GOTTO AM, LEVY RI, JOHN K, FREDRICKSON DS: On the nature of the protein defect in abetalipoproteinemia. *N Engl J Med* 284:813, 1971

224. KAYDEN HJ, SILBER R: The role of vitamin E deficiency in the abnormal autohemolysis of acanthocytosis. *Trans Assoc Am Phys* 78:334, 1965

225. KOSTNER G, HOLASEK A, BOHLMANN HG, THIEDE H: Investigation of serum lipoproteins and apoproteins in abetalipoproteinemia. *Clin Sci Mol Med* 46:457, 1974

226. SCANU AM, AGGERBECK LP, KRUSKI AW, LIM CT, KAYDEN HJ: A study of the abnormal lipoproteins in abetalipoproteinemia. *J Clin Invest* 53:440, 1974

227. FORTE T, NICHOLS AV: Application of electron microscopy to the study of plasma lipoprotein structure. *Adv Lipid Res* 10:1, 1972

228. HERBERT P, HEINEN R, FREDRICKSON DS: Unpublished observations

229. FREDRICKSON DS, LEVY RI, LINDGREN FT: A comparison of heritable abnormal lipoprotein patterns as defined by two different techniques. *J Clin Invest* 47:2446, 1968

230. BLUMENFELD OO, SCHWARTZ E, ADAMANY AM: Efflux of phospholipids from cultured aortic smooth muscle cells. *J Biol Chem* 254:7183, 1979

231. KARLIN JB, JUHN DJ, STARR JI, SCANU AM, RUBENSTEIN AH: Measurement of human high density lipoprotein apolipoprotein A-I in serum by radioimmunoassay. *J Lipid Res* 17:30, 1976

232. HERBERT PN, HEINEN RJ, BAUSSERMAN LL, HENDERSON LO, MUSLINER TA: Abetalipoproteinemia and hypobetalipoproteinemia: Questions still exceed insights, in Gotto AM Jr, Smith LC, Allen B, (eds): *Atherosclerosis V*. Proceedings of the Fifth International Symposium on Atherosclerosis. New York, Springer-Verlag, 1980, p 684

233. HENDERSON L, HERBERT P, WINDMUELLER H, KRAUSS R: The C apolipoproteins of the orotic acid rat: A model for abetalipoproteinemia. *Circulation* 50(III):114, 1974

234. WEISGRABER KH, MAHLEY RW: Apoprotein (E-A-II) complex of human plasma lipoproteins. *J Biol Chem* 253:6281, 1978

235. BARNARD G, FOSBROOKE AS, LLOYD JK: Neutral lipids of plasma and adipose tissue in abetalipoproteinemia. *Clin Chim Acta* 28:417, 1970

236. KUO PT, BASSETT DR, DI GEORGE AM, CARPENTER GG: Lipolytic activity of post-heparin plasma in hyperlipemia and hypolipemia. *Circ Res* 16:221, 1965

237. FIELDING CJ, FIELDING PE: Purification and substrate specificity of lecithin-cholesterol acyltransferase from human plasma. *FEBS Lett* 15:355, 1971

238. ALBERS JJ, ADOLPHSON JL, CHEN CH: Radioimmunoassay of human plasma lecithin-cholesterol acyltransferase. *J Clin Invest* 67:141, 1981

239. BRANNAN PG, GOLDSTEIN JL, BROWN MS: 3-hydroxy-3-methylglutaryl coenzyme A reductase activity in human hair roots. *J Lipid Res* 16:7, 1975

240. REICHL D, MYANT NB, LLOYD JK: Surface binding and catabolism of low-density lipoprotein by circulating lymphocytes from patients with abetalipoproteinaemia, with observations on sterol synthesis in lymphocytes from one patient. *Biochim Biophys Acta* 530:124, 1978

241. MYANT NB, REICHL D, LLOYD JK: Sterol balance in a patient with abetalipoproteinemia. *Atherosclerosis* 29:509, 1978

242. KAYDEN HJ: Abetalipoproteinemia—Abnormalities of serum lipoproteins, in Peeters H (ed), *Protides of the Biological Fluids* (proceedings of the 25th Coll., Bruges, 1977). Oxford, Pergamon Press, 1978, p 271

243. ILLINGWORTH DR, CONNOR WE, LIN DS, DI LIBERTI J: Lipid metabolism in abetalipoproteinemia: A study of cholesterol absorption and sterol balance in two patients. *Gastroenterology* 78:68, 1980

244. INNERARITY TL, MAHLEY RW: Enhanced binding by cultured human fibroblasts of apo-E-containing lipoproteins as compared with low density lipoproteins. *Biochemistry* 17:1440, 1978

245. LLOYD JK: Disorders of the serum lipoproteins. I. Lipoprotein deficiency states. *Arch Dis Child* 43:393, 1968

246. WAYS PO, PARMENTIER CM, KAYDEN HJ, JONES JW, SAUNDERS DR, RUBIN CE: Studies on the absorptive defect for triglyceride in abetalipoproteinemia. *J Clin Invest* 46:35, 1967

247. BOHLMANN HG, THIEDE H, ROSENSTIEL K, HERDEMERTEN S, PANITZ D, TACKMANN W: A-B-Lipoproteinämie bei drei Geschwistern. *Dtsch Med Wochenschr* 97:892, 1972

248. MIER M, SCHWARTZ SO, BOSHES B: Acanthocytosis, pigmentary degeneration of the retina and ataxic neuropathy: A genetically determined syndrome with associated metabolic disorder. *Blood* 5:1586, 1960

249. WEINSTEIN MA, PEARSON KD, AGUS SG: Abetalipoproteinemia. *Radiology* 108:269, 1973

250. DOBBINS WO III: An ultrastructural study of the intestinal mucosa in congenital betalipoprotein deficiency with particular emphasis upon the intestinal absorptive cell. *Gastroenterology* 50:195, 1966

251. BACH C, POLONOVSKI J, POLONOVSKI C, LELUC R, JOLLY G, MOSZER M: L'absence congenitale de B-lipoproteines: Une nouvelle observation. *Arch Fr Pediatr* 24:1093, 1967

252. SPERLING MA, HENGSTENBERG F, YUNIS E, KENNY FM, DRASH AL: Abetalipoproteinemia: Metabolic, endocrine, and electron-microscopic investigations. *Pediatrics* 48:91, 1971

253. ISSELBACHER KJ, SCHEIG R, PLOTKIN GR, CAUFIELD JB: Congenital beta-lipoprotein deficiency: An hereditary disorder involving a defect in the absorption and transport of lipids. *Medicine* 43:347, 1964

254. GLICKMAN RM, GREEN PHR, LEES RS, LUX SE, KILGORE A: Immunofluorescence studies of apolipoprotein B in intestinal mucosa. *Gastroenterology* 76:288, 1979

255. HOOGHWINKEL GJM, BRUYN GW: Congenital lack of serum β-lipoproteins: A study of blood phospholipids in a patient and his family. *J Neurol Sci* 3:374, 1966

256. GLOVER J, WALKER RJ: Absorption and transport of vitamin A. *Exp Eye Res* 3:327, 1964

257. HUANG HS, GOODMAN DS: Vitamin A and carotenoids. I. Intestinal absorption and metabolism of ^{14}C-labeled vitamin A alcohol and beta-carotene in the rat. *J Biol Chem* 240:2839, 1965

258. WAYS P, REED CF, HANAHAN DJ (technical assistance of DONG D, PALMER S, MURPHY M, ROBERTS G): Red cell and plasma lipids in acanthocytosis. *J Clin Invest* 42:1248, 1963

259. FARQUHAR JW, WAYS P: Abetalipoproteinemia, in Stanbury JB, Wyngaarden JB, Fredrickson DS (eds): *The Metabolic Basis of Inherited Disease*, 2d ed. New York, McGraw-Hill, 1966, p 509

260. WALLIS K, GROSS M, ZAIDMAN JL, JULSARY A, SZEINBERG A, KOOK A: Tocopherol therapy in acanthocytosis. *Pediatrics* 48:669, 1971

261. MULLER DPR, HARRIES JT, LLOYD JK: Vitamin E therapy in a-beta-lipoproteinemia. *Arch Dis Child* 45:715, 1970

262. MCCORMICK EC, CORNWELL DG, BROWN JB: Studies on the distribution of tocopherol in human serum lipoproteins. *J Lipid Res* 1:221, 1960

263. MULLER DPR, HARRIES JT, LLOYD JK: The relative importance of the factors involved in the absorption of vitamin E in children. *Gut* 15:966, 1974

264. MACMAHON MT, NEALE G, THOMPSON GR: Lymphatic and portal venous transport of α-tocopherol and cholesterol. *Eur J Clin Invest* 1:288, 1971

265. MULLER DPR, LLOYD JK, BIRD AC: Long-term management of abetalipoproteinemia. *Arch Dis Child* 52:209, 1977

266. SOBREVILLA LA, GOODMAN ML, KANE CA: Demyelinating central nervous system disease, macular atrophy and acanthocytosis (Bassen-Kornzweig syndrome). *Am J Med* 37:821, 1964

267. PARTIN JS, PARTIN JC, SCHUBERT WK, MCADAMS AJ: Liver ultrastructure in abetalipoproteinemia: Evolution of micronodular cirrhosis. *Gastroenterology* 67:107, 1974

268. WOLFF JA, BAUMAN WA: Studies concerning acanthocytosis: A new genetic syndrome with absent beta lipoprotein. *J Dis Child* 102:478, 1961

269. KORNZWEIG AL, BASSEN FA: Retinitis pigmentosa, acanthocytosis, and heredodegenerative neuromuscular disease. *Arch Opthalmol* 58:183, 1957

270. SINGER K, FISHER B, PERLSTEIN MA: Acanthocytosis: A genetic erythrocyte malformation. *Blood* 7:577, 1952

271. FORSYTH CC, LLOYD JK, FOSBROOKE AS: A-beta-lipoproteinaemia. *Arch Dis Child* 40:47, 1965

272. KHACHADURIAN AK, FREYHA R, SHAMMA'A MM, BAGHDASSARIAN SA: A-beta-lipoproteinemia and colour blindness. *Arch Dis Child* 46:871, 1971

273. DRUEZ G: Un noveau cas d'acanthocytose; Dysmorphie erythrocytaire congéntale avec rétinite, troubles nerveux et stigmates dégénératifs. *Rev Hematol* 14:3, 1959

274. BOYER SH, CHISHOLM AW, MCKUSICK VA: Cardiac aspects of Friedreich's ataxia. *Circulation* 25:493, 1962

275. GELLER A, GILLES F, SCHWACHMAN H: Degeneration of fasciculus gracilis in cystic fibrosis. *Neurology (Minneapolis)* 27:185, 1977

276. SUNG JH, PARK SW, MASTRI AR, WARWICK WJ: Axonal dystrophy in the gracile nucleus in congenital biliary atresia and cystic fibrosis (mucoviscidosis): Beneficial effect of vitamin E therapy. *J Neuropathol Exp Neurol* 39:584, 1980

277. ROSENBLUM JL, KEATING JP, PRENSKY AL, NELSON JS: A progressive neurologic syndrome in children with chronic liver disease. *N Engl J Med* 304:503, 1981

278. TOMASI LG: Reversibility of human myopathy caused by vitamin E deficiency. *Neurology (Minneapolis)* 29:1182, 1979

279. OVESEN L, SATYA-MURTI S, CHU R, HOWARD L: Reversible neurological symptoms caused by vitamin E deficiency in a patient with short bowel syndrome. *Am J Clin Nutr*. In press

280. WALSH FB, HOYT E: *Clinical Neuro-ophthalmology*, 3d ed. Baltimore, Williams & Wilkins, 1969

281. LEVY IS: Pigmentary retinopathy associated with metabolic defects. *Trans Opthalmal Soc UK* 92:285, 1972

282. VON SALLMANN L, GELDERMAN AH, LASTER L: Ocular histopathologic changes in a case of a-beta-lipoproteinemia (Bassen-Kornzweig syndrome). *Doc Ophthalmol* 26:451, 1969

283. GOURAS P, CARR RE, GUNKEL RD: Retinitis pigmentosa in abetalipoproteinemia: Effects of vitamin A. *Invest Ophthalmol* 10:784, 1971

284. SPERLING MA, HILES DA, KENNERDELL JS: Electroretinographic responses following vitamin A therapy in a-beta-lipoproteinemia. *Am J Ophthalmol* 73:342, 1972

285. SHEARER ACI: Absorption of β-carotene in human retinitis pigmentosa. *Exp Eye Res* 3:427, 1964

286. CAMPBELL DA, HARRISON R, TONKS EL: Retinitis pigmentosa. Vitamin A levels in relation to clinical findings. *Exp Eye Res* 3:412, 1964

287. RODGER FC: The ocular effects of vitamin A deficiency in man in the tropics. *Exp Eye Res* 3:367, 1964

288. DOWLING JE: Nutritional and inherited blindness in the rat. *Exp Eye Res* 3:348, 1964

289. SCOTT PP, GREAVES JP, SCOTT MG: Nutritional blindness in the cat. *Exp Eye Res* 3:357, 1964

290. WOLFF OH, LLOYD JK, TONKS EL: A-beta-lipoproteinaemia with special reference to the visual defect. *Exp Eye Res* 3:439, 1964

291. ROBISON WG JR, KUWABARA T, BIERI JG: Vitamin E deficiency and the retina: Photoreceptor and pigment epithelial changes. *Invest Ophthalmol Vis Sci* 18:683, 1979

292. ROBISON WG JR, KUWABARA T, BIERI JG: Deficiencies of vitamin E and A in the rat: Retinal damage and lipofuscin accumulation. *Invest Ophthalmol Vis Sci* 19:1030, 1980

293. KAYDEN HJ, BESSIS M: Morphology of normal erythrocyte and acanthocyte using Nomarski optics and the scanning electron microscope. *Blood* 35:427, 1970

294. SIMON ER, WAYS P: Incubation hemolysis and red cell metabolism in acanthocytosis. *J Clin Invest* 43:1311, 1964

295. LEYLAND FC, FOSBROOKE AS, LLOYD JK, SEGALL MM, TAMIR I, TOMKINS R, WOLFF OH: Use of medium-chain triglyceride diets in children with malabsorption. *Arch Dis Child* 44:170, 1969

296. SHASTRI KM, CARVALHO ACA, LEES RS: Platelet function and platelet lipid composition in the dyslipoproteinemias. *J Lipid Res* 21:467, 1980

297. AVIOLI LV: Absorption and metabolism of vitamin D₃ in man. *Am J Clin Nutr* 22:437, 1969

298. GWYNNE JT, MAHAFFEE D, BREWER HB JR, NEY RL: Adrenal cholesterol uptake from plasma lipoproteins: Regulation by corticotropin. *Proc Nat Acad Sci USA* 73:4329, 1976

299. FAUST JR, GOLDSTEIN JL, BROWN MS: Receptor-mediated uptake of low density lipoprotein and utilization of its cholesterol for steroid synthesis in cultured mouse adrenal cells. *J Biol Chem* 252:4861, 1977

300. KOVANEN PT, FAUST JR, BROWN MS, GOLDSTEIN JL: Low density lipoprotein receptors in bovine adrenal cortex. I. Receptor-mediated uptake of low density lipoprotein and utilization of its cholesterol for steroid synthesis in cultured adrenocortical cells. *Endocrinology* 104:599, 1979

301. HALL PF, NAKAMURA M: The influence of adrenocorticotropin on transport of a cholesteryl linoleate–low density lipoprotein complex into adrenal tumor cells. *J Biol Chem* 254:12547, 1979

302. BROWN MS, KOVANEN PT, GOLDSTEIN JL: Receptor-mediated uptake of lipoprotein-cholesterol and its utilization for steroid synthesis in the adrenal cortex. *Rec Prog Horm Res* 35:215, 1979

303. ANDERSEN JM, DIETSCHY JM: Relative importance of high and low density lipoproteins in the regulation of cholesterol synthesis in the adrenal gland, ovary, and testis of the rat. *J Biol Chem* 253:9024, 1978

304. ILLINGWORTH DR, ORWOLL ES, CONNOR WE: Impaired cortisol secretion in abetalipoproteinemia. *J Clin Endocrinol Metab* 50:977, 1980

305. HERBERT PN, FREDRICKSON DS: Unpublished observations

306. BIERMAN EL, PORTE D, O'HARA DD, SCHWARTZ M, WOOD FC: Characterization of fat particles in plasma of hyperlipemic subjects maintained on fat-free high carbohydrate diets. *J Clin Invest* 44:261, 1965

307. O'HARA DD, PORTE D, WILLIAMS RH: Use of constant composition polyvinylpyrrolidone columns to study the interaction of fat particles with plasma. *J Lipid Res* 7:264, 1966

308. ZILVERSMIT DB: The composition and structure of lymph chylomicrons in dog, rat and man. *J Clin Invest* 44:1610, 1965

309. AVIGAN J: Modification of human serum lipoprotein fractions by lipid extraction. *J Biol Chem* 226:957, 1957

310. ALAUPOVIC P, SANBAR SS, FURMAN RH, SULLIVAN ML, WALRAVEN SL: Studies of the composition and structure of serum lipoproteins: Isolation and characterization of very high density lipoproteins of human serum. *Biochemistry* 5:4044, 1966

311. GLICKMAN RM, KIRSCH K: The apoproteins of various size classes of human chylous fluid lipoproteins. *Biochim Biophys Acta* 371:255, 1974

312. SCANU AM, EDELSTEIN C, KEIM P: Serum lipoproteins, in Putnam FW (ed): *The Plasma Proteins.* New York, Academic, 1975, p 317

313. GAGE SH, FISH PA: Fat digestion and assimilation in man and animals as determined by dark-field microscope, and fat-soluble dye. *Am J Anat* 34:1, 1924

314. DODGE JT, COHEN G, KAYDEN HJ, PHILLIPS GB: Peroxidative hemolysis of red blood cells from patients with abetalipoproteinemia (acanthocytosis). *J Clin Invest* 46:357, 1967

315. AZIZI E, ZAIDMAN JL, ESCHAR J, SZEINBERG A: Abetalipoproteinemia treated with parenteral and oral vitamins A and E, and with medium chain triglycerides. *Acta Paediatr Scand* 67:797, 1978

316. FREDRICKSON DS, GOTTO AM, LEVY RI: Familial lipoprotein deficiency, in Stanbury JB, Wyngaarden JB, Fredrickson DS (eds): *The Metabolic Basis of Inherited Disease,* 3d ed. New York, McGraw-Hill, 1972, p 493

317. VAN BUCHEM FSP, POL G, DE GIER J, BÖTTCHER CJF, PRIES C: Congenital β-lipoprotein deficiency. *Am J Med* 40:794, 1966

318. MARS H, LEWIS LA, ROBERTSON AL JR, BUTKUS A, WILLIAMS GH JR: Familial hypo-β-lipoproteinemia: A genetic disorder of lipid metabolism with nervous system involvement. *Am J Med* 46:886, 1969

319. RICHET G, DUREPAIRE H, HARTMANN L, OLLIER M-P, POLONOVSKI J, MAITROT B: Hypolipoprotéinémie familiale asymptomatique prédominant sur les bêta-lipoprotéines. *Presse Med* 77:2045, 1969

320. LEVY RI, LANGER T, GOTTO AM, FREDRICKSON DS: Familial hypobetalipoproteinemia, a defect in lipoprotein synthesis. *Clin Res* 18:539, 1970

321. MAWATARI S, IWASHITA H, KUROIWA Y: Familial hypo-β-lipoproteinemia. *J Neurol Sci* 16:93, 1972

322. FOSBROOKE A, CHOKSEY S, WHARTON B: Familial hypo-β-lipoproteinemia. *Arch Dis Child* 48:729, 1973

323. BROWN BJ, LEWIS LA, MERCER RD: Familial hypobetalipoproteinemia: Report of a case with psychomotor retardation. *Pediatrics* 54:111, 1974

324. TAMIR I, LEVTOW O, LOTAN D, LEQUIN C, HELDENBERG D, WERBIN B: Further observations on familial hypobetalipoproteinemia. *Clin Genet* 9:149, 1976

325. COTTRILL C, GLUECK CJ, LEUBA V, MILLET F, PUPPIONE D, BROWN WV: Familial homozygous hypobetalipoproteinemia. *Metabolism* 23:779, 1974

326. BIEMER JJ, MCCAMMON RE: The genetic relationship of abetalipoproteinemia and hypobetalipoproteinemia: A report of the occurrence of both diseases within the same family. *J Lab Clin Med* 85:556, 1975

327. FEIT J-P, DAVID M, MACABÉO V, DIVRY P, BERNARD J-C, LAMBERT D, BEUCLER I, JEUNE M: L'Abêtalipoprotéinémie. Etude clinique, génétique, endocrinienne et métabolique d'une nouvelle observation familiale. *Pediatrie* 32:753, 1977

328. ILLINGWORTH DR, CONNOR WE, BUIST NRM, JHAVERI BM, LIN DS, MCMURRY MP: Sterol balance in abetalipoproteinemia: Studies in a patient with homozygous familial hypobetalipoproteinemia. *Metabolism* 28:1152, 1979

329. FORTE T, HERBERT PN, HEINEN R: Unpublished observations

330. SCOTT BB, MILLER JP, LOSOWSKY MS: Hypobetalipoproteinaemia—A variant of the Bassen-Kornzweig syndrome. *Gut* 20:163, 1979

331. YEE RD, HERBERT PN, BERGSMA DR, BIEMER JJ: A typical retinitis pigmentosa in familial hypobetalipoproteinemia. *Am J Ophthalmol* 82:64, 1976

332. SIGURDSSON G, NICOLL A, LEWIS B: Turnover of apolipoprotein-B in two subjects with familial hypobetalipoproteinemia. *Metabolism* 26:25, 1977

333. GIBLETT ER: Beta lipoprotein allotypes: The Ag and Lp systems. In *Genetic Markers in Human Blood,* Oxford, Blackwell Scientific Publications, 1969, p 176

333a. STEINBERG D, GRUNDY SM, MOK HYI, TURNER JD, WEINSTEIN JB, BROWN WV, ALBERS JJ: Metabolic studies in an unusual case of asymptomatic familial hypobetalipoproteinemia with hypoalphalipoproteinemia and fasting chylomicronemia. *J Clin Invest* 64:292, 1979

333b. MALLOY MJ, KANE JP, HARDMAN DA, HAMILTON RL, DALAL KB: Normotriglyceridemic abetalipoproteinemia. Absence of the B-100 apolipoprotein. *J Clin Invest* 67:1441, 1981

334. FREDRICKSON DS, ALTROCCHI PH, AVIOLI LV, GOODMAN DS, GOODMAN HC: Tangier disease. *Ann Intern Med* 55:1016, 1961

335. HOFFMANN HN, FREDRICKSON DS: Tangier disease (familial high density lipoprotein deficiency): Clinical and genetic features in two adults. *Am J Med* 39:582, 1965

336. FREDRICKSON DS: The inheritance of high density lipoprotein deficiency (Tangier disease). *J Clin Invest* 43:228, 1964

337. BALE PM, CLIFTON-BLIGH P, BENJAMIN BN, WHYTE HM: Pathology of Tangier disease. *J Clin Pathol* 24:609, 1971

338. FREDRICKSON DS: Familial high density lipoprotein deficiency: Tangier disease, in Stanbury JB, Wyngaarden JB, Fredrickson DS (eds): *The Metabolic Basis of Inherited Disease,* 2d ed. New York, McGraw-Hill, 1966, p 486

339. DAWSON G, KRUSKI AW, SCANU AM: Distribution of glycosphingolipids in the serum lipoproteins of normal human subjects and patients with hypo- and hyperlipidemias. *J Lipid Res* 17:125, 1976

340. LUX SE, LEVY RI, GOTTO AM, FREDRICKSON DS: Studies on the protein defect in Tangier disease: Isolation and characterization of an abnormal high density lipoprotein. *J Clin Invest* 51:2505, 1972

341. UTERMANN G, MENZEL HJ, SCHOENBORN W: Plasma lipoprotein abnormalities in a case of primary high density lipoprotein (HDL) deficiency. *Clin Genet* 8:258, 1975

342. HEINEN RS, HERBERT PN, FREDRICKSON DS, FORTE T, LINDGREN FT: Properties of the plasma very low and low density lipoproteins in Tangier disease. *J Clin Invest* 61:120, 1978.

343. HERBERT PN, FORTE T, HEINEN RJ, FREDRICKSON DS: Tangier Disease. One explanation for lipid storage. *N Engl J Med* 299:519, 1978

344. ASSMANN G, HERBERT PN, FREDRICKSON DS, FORTE T: Isolation and characterization of an abnormal high density lipoprotein in Tangier disease. *J Clin Invest* 60:242, 1977

345. ASSMANN G, SMOOTZ E, ADLER K, CAPURSO A, OETTE K: The lipoprotein abnormality in Tangier disease. Quantitation of A apoproteins. *J Clin Invest* 59:565, 1977

346. HENDERSON LO, HERBERT PN, FREDRICKSON DS, HEINEN RJ, EASTERLING JC: Abnormal concentration and anomalous distribution of apolipoprotein A-I in Tangier disease. *Metabolism* 27:165, 1978

347. FRANCESCHINI G, SIRTORI CR, CAPURSO A, WEISGRABER KH, MAHLEY RW: A-I-Milano Apoprotein. Decreased high density lipoprotein cholesterol levels with significant lipoprotein modifications and without clinical atherosclerosis in an Italian family. *J Clin Invest* 66:892, 1980

348. SCHMITZ G, ASSMANN G: Tangier Apoprotein A-I fails to interact with normal HDL. In preparation

349. UTERMANN G, BEISIEGEL U: Charge-shift electrophoresis of apolipoproteins from normal humans and patients with Tangier disease. *FEBS Lett* 97:245, 1979

349a. ZANNIS VI, BRESLOW JL: Accumulation of precursor apo A-I isoproteins in the plasma of a Tangier disease patient. *Circulation* 4:159, 1981

350. ASSMANN G, SCHMITZ G, MENZEL HJ: Characterization of Tangier lipoproteins. In preparation.

351. CARLSON LA, PHILIPSON B: Fish-eye disease. A new familial condition with massive corneal opacities and dyslipoproteinemia. *Lancet* 2:921, 1979

352. GUSTAFSON A, MCCONATHY WJ, ALAUPOVIC P, CURRY MD, PERSSON B: Identification of lipoprotein families in a variant of human plasma apolipoprotein A deficiency. *Scand J Clin Lab Invest* 39:377, 1979

353. SCHAEFER EJ, BLUM CB, LEVY RI, JENKINS LL, ALAUPOVIC P, FOSTER DM, BREWER HB: Metabolism of high-density lipoprotein apolipoproteins in Tangier disease. *N Engl J Med* 299:905, 1978

354. BREWER HB JR, SCHAEFER EJ, ZECH LA BRONZERT TM: Tangier disease, Gotto AM Jr, Smith LC, Allen B (eds): *Athercosclerosis V*, New York, Springer-Verlag 1980, p 680

355. SCHAEFER EJ, ANDERSON DW, ZECH LA, LINGREN FT, BRONZERT TB, RUBALCABA EA, BREWER HB JR: Metabolism of high density lipoprotein subfractions and constituents in Tangier disease following the infusion of high density lipoproteins. *J Lipid Res* 22:217, 1981

356. HERBERT P: The metabolic defect in Tangier disease. *N Engl J Med* 300:432, 1979

357. ASSMANN G, SMOOTZ E: High density lipoprotein infusion and partial plasma exchange in Tangier disease. *Eur J Clin Invest* 8:131, 1978

358. ASSMANN G, CAPURSO A, SMOOTZ E, WELLNER U: Apoprotein A metabolism in Tangier disease. *Atherosclerosis* 30:321, 1978

359. GLICKMAN RM, GREEN PHR, LEES RS, TALL A: Apoprotein A-I synthesis in normal and intestinal mucosa and in Tangier disease. *N Engl J Med* 299:1424, 1978

360. SCHWARTZ DE, LIOTTA L, SCHAEFER EJ, BREWER HB JR: Localization of apoprotein A-I, A-II, and B in normal, Tangier, and abetalipoproteinemia intestinal mucosa. *Circulation* 58 (suppl 2, II): 90, 1978

361. SCHAEFER EJ, BREWER HB JR: Tangier disease: A defect in the conversion of chylomicrons to high density lipoproteins. *Clin Res* 26:4974A, 1978

362. ASSMANN G: The metabolic role of high density lipoproteins: perspectives from Tangier disease, in Gotto AM Jr, Miller NE, Oliver MF (eds): *High Density Lipoproteins and Atherosclerosis*. New York, Elsevier North-Holland, 1978, p 77

363. GRETEN H, HANNEMANN T, GUSEK W, VIVELL O: Lipoproteins and lipolytic plasma enzymes in a case of Tangier disease. *N Engl J Med* 291:548, 1974

364. ASSMANN G, SCMITZ G, HECKERS H: Lecithincholesterol acyltransferase in Tangier disease. *Scand J Clin Lab Invest* (suppl 150) 38:98, 1978

365. ASSMANN G: Structure-function relationship of lipoproteins in Tangier disease, in Greten H (ed): *Lipoprotein Metabolism*. Berlin, Springer-Verlag, 1976, p 106

366. YAO JK, DYCK PJ: In vitro cholesterol esterification in human serum. *Clin Chem* 23:447, 1977

367. UTERMANN G, STEINMETZ A, FRANCESCHINI G, HAAS J, FEUSSNER G: Submitted for publication, 1981

368. CLIFTON-BLIGH P, NESTEL PJ, WHYTE HM: Tangier disease: Report of a case and studies of lipid metabolism. *N Engl J Med* 286:567, 1972

369. SCHERER R, RUKENSTROTH-BAUER G: Untersuchung der lecithin-cholesterincyltransferase-aktivität im Serum von drei Patienten mit Tangier-krankheit (Hyp-alpha-lipoproteinamie). *Klin Wochenschr* 51:1059, 1973

370. SCHAEFER HE, ASSMANN G: Morphological findings in Tangier disease. In preparation.

371. FERRANS VJ, FREDRICKSON DS: The pathology of Tangier disease: A light and electron microscopic study. *Am J Pathol* 78:101, 1975

372. WALDORF DS, LEVY RI, FREDRICKSON DS: Cutaneous cholesteryl ester deposition in Tangier disease. *Arch Dermatol* 95:161, 1967

373. DYCK PM, ELLEFSON RD, YAO JK, HERBERT PN: Adult-onset Tangier disease. I. Morphometric and pathologic studies suggesting delayed degradation of neutral lipids after fiber degeneration. *J Neuropathol Exp Neurol* 37:119, 1978

374. ASSMANN G, SCHAEFER HE: Possible mechanisms of lipid storage in Tangier disease, in Gotto AM Jr, Smith LC, Allen B (eds): *Atherosclerosis V*, New York, Springer-Verlag, 1980, p 666

375. ASSMANN G, SCHAEFER HE: High density lipoprotein deficiency and lipid deposition in Tangier disease, in Carlson LA, et al. (eds): *International Conference on Atherosclerosis*. New York, Raven Press, 1978, p 97

376. CHU FC, KUWABARA T, COGAN DG, SCHAEFER EJ, BREWER HB JR: Ocular manifestations of familial high-density lipoprotein deficiency (Tangier disease). *Arch Ophthalmol* 97:1926, 1979

377. KUMMER H, LAISSUR J, SPIESS H, PFLUGSHAUPT R, BUCHER U: Familiäre Analphalipoproteinämie (Tangier-krankheit). *Schweiz Med Wochenschr* 98:406, 1968

378. HAAS LF, AUSTAD WI, BERGIN JD: Tangier disease. *Brain* 97:351, 1974

379. ENGEL WK, DORMAN JD, LEVY RI, FREDRICKSON DS: Neuropathy in Tangier disease: α-Lipoprotein deficiency manifesting as familial recurrent neuropathy and intestinal lipid storage. *Arch Neurol* 17:1, 1967

380. BROWN MS, HO YK, GOLDSTEIN JL: The cholesteryl ester cycle in macrophage foam cells. *J Biol Chem* 255:9344, 1980

381. KOCEN RS, LLOYD JK, LASCELLES PT, FOSBROOKE AS, WILLIAMS D: Familial α-lipoprotein deficiency (Tangier disease) with neurological abnormalities. *Lancet* 1:1341, 1967

382. HAAS LF, BERGIN JD: Alpha lipoprotein deficiency with neurological features. *Aust Ann Med* 19:76, 1970

383. DYCK PJ, ELLEFSON RD, YAO JK, HERBERT PN: Adult-onset of Tangier disease. 1. Morphometric and pathologic studies suggesting delayed degradation of neutral lipids after fiber degeneration. *J Neuropathol Exp Neurol* 37:119, 1978

384. YAO JK, HERBERT PN, FREDRICKSON DS, ELLEFSON RD, HEINEN RJ, FORTE T, DYCK PJ: Biochemical studies in a patient with a Tangier syndrome. *J Neuropathol Exp Neurol* 37:138, 1978

385. KOCEN RS, KING RHM, THOMAS PK, HAAS LF: Nerve biopsy findings in two cases of Tangier disease. *Acta Neuropathol* 26:317, 1973

386. SCHAEFER EJ, ZECH LA, SCHWARTZ DE, BREWER HB JR: Coronary heart disease prevalence and other clinical features in familial high-density lipoprotein deficiency (Tangier disease). *Ann Intern Med* 93:261, 1980

387. ASSMANN G: Tangier-Krankheit, in Schettler G, Greten H, Schlierf G, Seidel D (eds): *Handbuch der Inneren Medizin, VII/4: Fettstoffwechsel*. Heidelberg, Springer-Verlag, 1976, p 461

388. SHASTRI K, CARVALHO ACA, LEES RS: Platelet function and platelet lipid composition in the dyslipoproteinemias. *J Lipid Res* 21:47, 1980

389. ROSS R, GLOMSET JA: Atherosclerosis and the arterial smooth muscle cell. *Science* 180:1332, 1973

390. ROSS R, GLOMSET JA, KARIYA B, HARKER L: A platelet-dependent serum factor that stimulates the proliferation of arterial smooth muscle cells in vitro. *Proc Nat Acad Sci USA* 71:1207, 1974

391. ASSMANN G, SIMANTKE O, SCHAEFER HE, SMOOTZ E: Characterization of high density lipoproteins in patients heterozygous for Tangier disease. *J Clin Invest* 60:1025, 1977

392. HUTH K, KRACHT J, SCHOENBORN W, FUHRMANN W: Tangier-krankheit (hypo-α-lipoproteinämie). *Dtsch Med Wochenschr* 95:2357, 1970

393. LINDESKOG GR, GUSTAFSON A, ENERBACH L: Serum lipoprotein deficiency in diffuse "normolipidemic" plane xanthoma. *Arch Dermatol* 106:592, 1972

394. WEISGRABER KH, BERSOT TP, MAHLEY RW, FRANCESCHINI G, SIRTORI CR: A-I-MIlano Apoprotein. Isolation and characterization of a cysteine-containing variant of the A-I-apoprotein from human high density lipoproteins. *J Clin Invest* 66:901, 1980

395. UTTERMAN G: Personal communication

396. CARLSON LA: A further case of fish-eye disease. *Lancet* 2:1376, 1979

397. FRIEDLAND ML, HERBERT PN, HENDERSON LO: Unpublished observations

398. NOSEDA G, RIESEN W, MORELL A, SCHLUMPF E: Hyperkatabole Hypo-β-lipoproteinämie infolge Autoanitkörper. *Kongr Inn Med* 78:1313, 1972.

30

FAMILIAL LIPOPROTEIN LIPASE DEFICIENCY AND RELATED DISORDERS OF CHYLOMICRON METABOLISM

ESKO A. NIKKILÄ

1. This chapter discusses three inherited disorders in which chylomicrons accumulate in plasma: familial lipoprotein lipase deficiency, familial apolipoprotein C-II deficiency, and familial type 5 hyperlipoproteinemia.

2. Familial lipoprotein lipase deficiency is a rare autosomal recessive disorder characterized by a massive accumulation of chylomicrons in plasma and a corresponding increase of plasma triglyceride concentration (type 1 lipoprotein pattern). The concentration of very low density lipoprotein (VLDL) is normal. The disease is usually detected in childhood on the basis of repeated episodes of abdominal pain, recurrent attacks of pancreatitis, eruptive cutaneous xanthomatosis, and hepatosplenomegaly. The severity of symptoms is proportional to the degree of chylomicronemia, which in turn is dependent on dietary fat intake. The disorder is caused by a deficiency of lipoprotein lipase, a lipolytic enzyme that is present in vascular endothelial cells of extrahepatic tissues. This enzyme is normally responsible for hydrolysis and removal of chylomicron and VLDL triglycerides. The enzyme is released into the blood by heparin and can be assayed in postheparin plasma or directly in biopsies of adipose tissue. Diagnosis is based on low or absent enzyme activity in an assay system that excludes other lipolytic enzymes and contains normal human plasma or apoprotein C-II, a

necessary cofactor of the enzyme. Heterozygotes exhibit a 50 percent decrease of lipoprotein lipase activity but have normal or only slightly elevated plasma triglyceride levels. The disorder is not associated with atherosclerotic vascular disease, but recurrent pancreatitis may threaten the patient's life. Restriction of dietary fat to 20 g/day or less is usually sufficient to reduce plasma triglyceride levels and keep the patient free of symptoms. Available lipid-lowering drugs are not effective.

3. Familial apolipoprotein C-II deficiency is a rare autosomal recessive disorder in which the clearance of chylomicrons and VLDL from the blood is greatly impaired and both lipoproteins accumulate in plasma, causing hypertriglyceridemia and a mild to moderate increase of plasma cholesterol (type 1 or type 5 lipoprotein pattern). The disorder is diagnosed in children or adults on the basis of recurrent attacks of pancreatitis or by milky fasting plasma detected by chance. The underlying biochemical defect is a deficiency of apolipoprotein C-II, a cofactor for lipoprotein lipase. Absence of this peptide creates a functional enzyme deficiency with accumulation of the substrate lipoproteins in the blood. The diagnosis is based on assay of lipoprotein lipase activity in postheparin plasma and on gel electrophoresis of VLDL apoproteins. Transfusion of normal plasma into the patient is followed by a

dramatic fall of plasma triglyceride level. Heterozygotes have a 50 percent reduction in apo C-II levels and may exhibit slightly elevated triglyceride concentrations. Treatment involves use of a moderately fat restricted diet throughout life. In case of severe pancreatitis, transfusion of 1 or 2 units of normal plasma is helpful.

4. *Familial type 5 hyperlipoproteinemia is characterized by fasting chylomicronemia and an increased concentration of plasma VLDL. The plasma triglyceride level is markedly elevated, while cholesterol is only slightly above normal. Clinical symptoms include abdominal pain, pancreatitis, eruptive xanthomas, and peripheral polyneuropathy. Symptoms may appear in childhood, but usually the disorder is expressed at a later age, earlier in males than in females. The risk of developing atherosclerotic vascular disease may be increased. The underlying biochemical defect is unknown. Catabolism of VLDL and chylomicrons is impaired, but lipoprotein lipase activity varies from low to normal in different families. The mode of inheritance is not clear, but it is likely to be autosomal dominant. About half of the affected subjects have a type 4 lipoprotein pattern with increased VLDL and normal chylomicrons. Other biochemical abnormalities, including hyperglycemia, hyperinsulinemia, and hyperuricemia, are common among affected family members. Treatment consists of weight reduction and avoidance of excess fat and alcohol. Nicotinic acid, clofibrate, and anabolic or progestational steroids have been used with variable success.*

Lipoprotein lipase (LPL) is an enzyme that hydrolyzes the triglycerides of chylomicrons and very low density lipoprotein (VLDL). The functional enzyme is present in the capillary endothelium of certain tissues and can be released by heparin. It is responsible for removal of the exogenous and endogenous triglycerides from the circulation. Deficiency of LPL is typically manifested by the development of gross hyperlipemia, caused mainly by an excessive accumulation of chylomicrons in the blood. The common clinical symptoms include eruptive skin xanthomas, periodic abdominal pains, and recurrent attacks of pancreatitis, but the patient may also remain asymptomatic and be detected on the basis of the milky appearance of fasting plasma. Characteristically, the lipemia is abolished and the symptoms disappear upon elimination of fat from the diet.

In the WHO classification system [1] of hyperlipoproteinemia, most patients with LPL deficiency are classified as having type 1 hyperlipoproteinemia (pure hyperchylomicronemia), but occasional patients may also have elevated VLDL levels and belong to the type 5 category (see Chap. 29). Indeed, the primary type 1 hyperlipoproteinemia is often held synonymous with LPL deficiency, and the majority of published cases show a selective increase of chylomicrons associated with low levels of other lipoproteins. In the absence of lipoprotein analysis this pattern can be inferred from a combination of massive hypertriglyceridemia with normal or slightly elevated serum cholesterol levels (low cholesterol/triglyceride ratio).

Among the diverse hyperlipoproteinemias, the familial type 1 disorder is one of the few in which the underlying biochem-

ical defect is relatively well characterized. Two separate molecular forms of the disease have been identified, but it is possible that even more will be found in the future. The defined traits include a deficiency of the enzyme LPL itself and a defect of apolipoprotein C-II, a cofactor of LPL. Both defects are expressed as an insufficient or absent function of LPL, and they give rise to a similar but not completely identical clinical syndrome, the hallmark of which is type 1 hyperlipoproteinemia.

In addition to the above two disorders of the LPL system, there is a third familial disorder, termed familial type 5 hyperlipoproteinemia, in which chylomicrons also accumulate in the plasma. Although the basic defect in familial type 5 hyperlipoproteinemia has not been clearly defined, the disorder is included in this chapter because it shares many biochemical and clinical features in common with familial lipoprotein lipase deficiency and familial apolipoprotein C-II deficiency.

FAMILIAL LIPOPROTEIN LIPASE (LPL) DEFICIENCY

Historical Aspects

The first recorded case of obvious primary hyperchylomicronemia was published by Bürger and Grütz in 1932 [2]. The patient was an 11-year-old boy with extensive cutaneous xanthomatosis, hepatosplenomegaly, and creamy fasting plasma. The lipemia cleared and all symptoms disappeared after switching to a fat-free diet. The familial nature of the disorder was suggested by the fact that the patient's parents were first cousins. This view was confirmed in a detailed description of two affected sibs by Holt et al. in 1939 [3]. The proband was an 11-year-old girl with gross hyperlipemia and severe attacks of abdominal pain, the latter always related to excessive levels of blood fat and probably caused by pancreatitis. The symptoms disappeared and remained absent during periods of low-fat diet. Interestingly, the authors performed a number of therapeutic trials, including testing the effect of transfusion of normal blood in order to determine whether a defect of some plasma factor might have been the cause of the lipemia. In retrospect, it is unfortunate that this patient apparently did not happen to have a deficiency of apo C-II.

Visible hyperlipemia, i.e., a milky or creamy appearance of fasting serum, was well known even before the above case reports, and its association with cutaneous xanthomatosis has been frequently recognized. However, many of the earlier patients were adults who had uncontrolled diabetes, and it is unlikely that the lipemia was based on an inherited defect. After the introduction of the term *idiopathic* or *essential hyperlipemia*, a large number of cases were reported under this diagnosis. In 1954 Malmros et al. [4] compiled 27 cases of "essential hyperlipemia" from the literature but could find evidence for a familial background in only 3 of these. It is obvious that primary type 1 hyperlipoproteinemia or LPL deficiency comprises only a small proportion of the adults diagnosed as having idiopathic hyperlipemia, the major part belonging to the more common WHO phenotype of type 5 hyperlipoproteinemia and some having a type 3 lipoprotein pattern. In contrast, the cases appearing in early childhood probably have true LPL deficiency.

Before the 1960s there were few possibilities for subdivision of idiopathic hyperlipemia into definite entities, even though the etiological heterogeneity of the syndrome, as well as the rather specific clinical picture of the "juvenile-onset" variant described by Bürger and Grütz [2] and by Holt et al. [3], was well recognized. Attempts to measure the lipolytic activity in postheparin plasma were made. In one case the activity was also measured in adipose tissue [5], but no defect was detected until Havel and Gordon [6] reported three sibs who had fasting chylomicronemia and were all shown to possess very low lipolytic activity against chylomicrons in their postheparin plasma and a slow clearance of chylomicrons in vivo. These subjects were contrasted with two unrelated patients who also had increased amounts of chylomicrons in their fasting plasma, but whose postheparin plasma lipase activity was normal. This classic work thus provided the first evidence for the presence of a genetic defect in the enzyme lipoprotein lipase and indicated a heterogeneous etiology of hyperchylomicronemia. This was verified in 1978 when a patient with typical type 1 hyperlipoproteinemia and apparent LPL deficiency was shown to have a complete deficiency of apoprotein C-II [7], an essential cofactor for normal expression of LPL activity.

A specific diagnosis of LPL deficiency and apoprotein C-II deficiency is relatively easy at present, inasmuch as selective techniques are available for the assay of lipoprotein lipase activity from postheparin plasma and for quantitation of individual apolipoproteins. This was not the case a few years ago when total postheparin plasma lipolytic activity (so-called PHLA) was generally used in assessing the activity of lipoprotein lipase. It is now well recognized that the latter method is highly nonspecific, measuring hepatic lipase, phospholipase, and monoglyceride lipase activities in addition to that of lipoprotein lipase. All of these lipolytic enzymes are present in postheparin plasma, contribute to a variable extent to lipolytic activity depending on the substrate used, and are likely to be normal in patients with LPL deficiency. Many cases of LPL deficiency may have been overlooked or misdiagnosed in the past due to the use of PHLA as a measure of LPL. Moreover, the possibility of an LPL cofactor defect has not been tested systematically and therefore cases with apo C-II deficiency may have been misclassified as primary defects of the enzyme itself. For all these reasons, it is difficult to determine in retrospect how many of the reported cases of familial type 1 hyperlipoproteinemia may have been caused by the LPL deficiency or apo C-II deficiency or possibly by some other, yet unidentified molecular defect. It is likely that most cases represent a true LPL deficiency (see below).

Clinical Characteristics

Familial LPL deficiency (including apoprotein C-II deficiency) is a rare disease, even though one must consider the possibility that some cases remain undetected. Fredrickson, Goldstein, and Brown have estimated that severe forms of type 1 hyperlipoproteinemia occur less frequently than 1 in 1 million [8]. The clinical features of the published cases may be learned from selected collections of case reports made by Fredrickson and Lees in 1966 [9], Fredrickson and Levy in 1972 [10], and Lees et al. [11] in 1973. The last review compiled the data of 43 patients, but many additional cases have been published since then. Excellent additional reviews on type 1 hyperlipoproteinemia have been published by Brown and Greten [12] and by Brown, Baginsky, and Ehnholm [13].

The disease is usually manifested in childhood. Of the 43 patients, 35 had been detected before the age of 10 years, and only 4 were adults at diagnosis [11]. One-third of the cases were diagnosed during the first year of life. It is assumed that the enzyme defect is present at birth, but the appearance of symptoms may be delayed until adolescence or adulthood in patients who are accustomed to a diet with low or moderate fat content. The age at onset of symptoms seems to be related to the plasma triglyceride concentration at diagnosis. Infection and pregnancy may be precipitating factors. In some cases the symptoms appeared early in life, but the diagnosis was delayed. On the other hand, family screenings have disclosed affected individuals who have been asymptomatic in spite of the presence of marked hyperchylomicronemia. It is possible that these patients fail to develop the most severe degrees of hyperlipemia, either by some unknown mechanism or by learned aversion to fatty foods with subsequent spontaneous restriction of fat intake.

The disease has been described among whites, blacks, and Japanese people, and it affects both sexes with equal frequency [10, 11].

Skin Xanthomas The only xanthomatous lesion of skin that is associated with type 1 hyperlipoproteinemia is *eruptive xanthoma*. Its presence was recorded in 23 of the 43 patients listed by Lees et al. [11], but it is likely that the lesions often go unnoticed both by patient and physician, and the true prevalence is thus higher. Eruptive xanthomas are white to yellow cutaneous nodules raised on a slightly erythematous base. The diameter of a single lesion varies from 1 to 4 mm, but they are often clustered and may coalesce to form larger plaques that may even simulate tuberous xanthomas (see Chap. 32). The eruptive xanthomas are preferentially localized over the buttocks, shoulders, and on extensor surfaces of extremities, but they may be found at any site including the face and even on mucous membranes. The lesions are neither painful nor pruritic (except on regression), and the patient often mistakes them for acne.

The eruptive xanthomas usually appear within a few days after plasma triglyceride levels have begun to increase. They are seldom seen in patients with fasting chylomicron-triglyceride concentrations below 2000 mg/dl; on the other hand, some patients with triglyceride levels above 5000 mg/dl do not develop xanthomas. The number of nodules varies from a few single, scattered ones up to hundreds. When the lipemia starts to vanish, the xanthomas rapidly begin to decrease in size, first loosing their central yellow area and then the erythema, leaving finally a slight pigmentation. The lesions may fade as rapidly as they appeared but usually it takes 1 to 3 weeks.

The eruptive skin xanthomas contain a yellowish, greasy material and sometimes milky fluid. Microscopy reveals chylomicronlike particles and macrophages filled with large fat droplets. Ultrastructural studies suggest that in massive hyperchylomicronemia the large fat particles present in blood penetrate the walls of cutaneous capillaries and appear in perivascular macrophages, forming the xanthomatous lesions [14]. The chemical composition of these xanthomas resembles that of chylomicrons and of dietary fatty acids.

Abdominal Pain and Pancreatitis The most common clinical manifestation of hyperchylomicronemia is episodic abdominal pain. Its intensity, duration, and localization are variable, but only a few patients with LPL deficiency fail to have this symptom. The attacks may be mild, resembling dyspepsia, but in typical cases the pain increases in intensity during a few days and may end in severe acute abdominal crisis with intense colic and diffuse or local tenderness of the peritoneum. Many subjects have undergone exploratory abdominal surgery, in which the only findings have been signs of slight serosal inflammation and small amounts of milky peritoneal fluid. In some cases pancreatic inflammation or hemorrhagic pancreatitis with mesenteric fat necroses has been observed at operation.

The abdominal pain does not have any definite localization. It may be diffuse or epigastric or localized to the middle abdomen with occasional radiation to the back or shoulders (pancreatitis), or it may be felt in the region of the left (splenic enlargement) or right costal margin, mimicking a gallstone attack (hepatomegaly). The attacks may be preceded or associated with anorexia, nausea, vomiting, abdominal distension, fever, and diarrhea, i.e., symptoms which may mislead the physician to almost any gastrointestinal diagnosis. Physical examination during the attack may reveal only diffuse peritoneal tenderness, or there may be enlargement of liver and spleen. The abdominal episodes are rather similar in a given patient, although they are variable among different subjects.

The onset of abdominal symptoms is evidently related to a rise of blood lipid levels following increased fat intake, use of alcohol, or a stressful situation such as an upper respiratory infection. On recovery from the attack the plasma triglycerides have been observed to fall remarkably, but this may be related to the decreased food intake during the attack. In exceptional cases the abdominal complaints may also appear in an individual on a low-fat diet and without any known exogenous cause.

Recurrent attacks of acute pancreatitis are a known complication of hyperchylomicronemia [9–13, 15]. However, recognition of the causal association between these two disorders has been confused by the suspicion that elevation of plasma triglyceride levels may occur as a consequence of pancreatitis and that both conditions may have common etiological factors, such as alcoholism and diabetes. The precise incidence of pancreatitis in patients with familial LPL deficiency is not known. Among 32 subjects reviewed by Fredrickson and Levy [10], 12 had some evidence of acute pancreatic involvement; but this may be an underestimate, since the routine diagnostic methods may fail to detect pancreatitis in the presence of hyperlipemia [16, 17]. Pancreatitis has been described in several affected sibs with probable LPL deficiency [18, 19]. The pancreatic damage may ultimately result in secondary diabetes and pancreatogenic steatorrhea with partial amelioration of the lipemia [20]. Several deaths due to pancreatitis have been recorded [10].

Additional cases of primary hyperchylomicronemia may be detected by lipid-screening of patients with acute or recurrent pancreatitis. In a careful prospective study, Cameron et al. [21] found that 21 percent of patients with acute pancreatitis have lactescent serum and heavy elevation of plasma triglycerides on admission. On a restudy of the patients during asymptomatic periods, 6 of 22 patients had persistent hyperlipemia, 2 having a type 1 and 6 a type 5 pattern [22].

The pathogenesis of the pancreatic involvement in hyperchylomicronemia is speculative. The pancreatic involvement is related to plasma triglyceride levels, the symptoms appearing only above 1000 mg/dl [23]. One possibility suggested by Havel [24] is that pancreatic lipase hydrolyzes the extravasated chylomicrons, resulting in an unphysiologically high local concentration of free fatty acids, which are toxic to the pancreatic tissue. It has also been suggested that clusters of chylomicrons could cause pancreatic capillaries to form microembolisms [15].

Hepato- and Splenomegaly Enlargement of the liver and spleen occurs particularly in infants and children with LPL deficiency. The size of these organs varies, often in parallel with the fat content of the diet. The increase is probably caused by an accumulation of chylomicron fat in histiocytes, macrophages, and Kupffer cells, rather than in parenchymal cells. Large foam cells, measuring 10 to 90 μm and containing lipid droplets and ceroid pigment, have been identified in the spleen of a patient with type 1 hyperlipoproteinemia [25]. It is likely that these cells represent macrophages that have taken up chylomicrons by phagocytosis and metabolized them to ceroid [25]. Similar cells are found in bone marrow aspirates [26] (Fig. 30-1).

Retinopathy (Lipemia Retinalis) In the presence of intense hyperlipemia the arteries and veins in peripheral parts of the retina have a milky or tomato juice appearance. The whole ocular fundus may have an altered pale pink, salmonlike color. The change is related to the degree of lipemia and is caused by a laminar flow of red cell–poor creamy plasma along the periphery of the smallest vessels. The retina may contain white lipid deposits. The retinal circulation may also become disturbed, and vascular changes with microaneurysms and hemorrhages have been described [27, 28].

Figure 30-1 Foam cell in bone marrow from a patient with familial LPL deficiency. Nomarski interference contrast micrograph ×1700. *(From Ferrans et al. [26]. Used by permission.)*

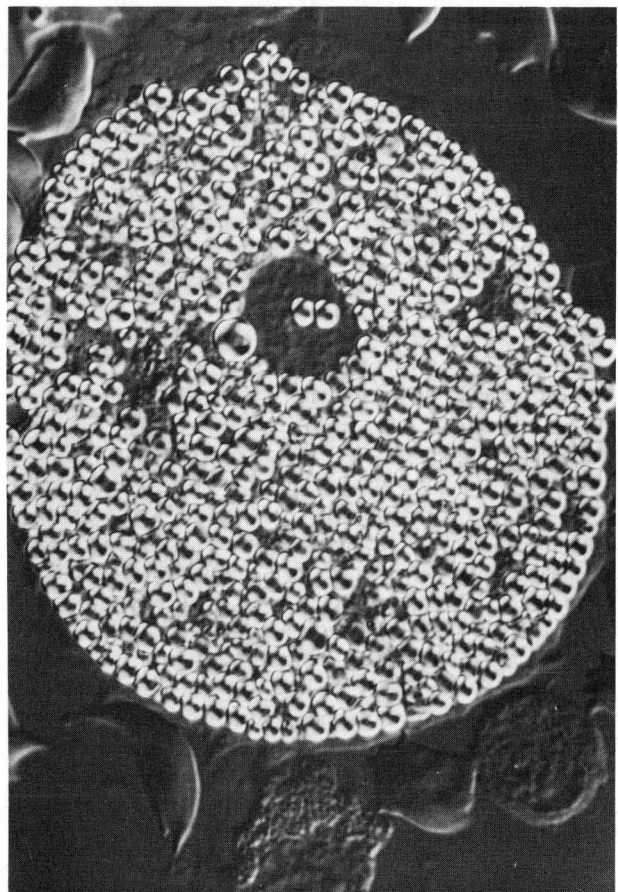

Atherosclerotic Vascular Disease and Life Expectancy
Since from birth, patients with LPL deficiency have very high triglycerides and often moderately elevated cholesterol levels in the plasma, they have been expected to be predisposed to premature cardiovascular disease. On the other hand, hyperchylomicronemia in combination with low levels of the other lipoproteins is not believed to be particularly atherogenic. Unfortunately, neither of these views is supported by any systematic clinical or autopsy studies. The small number of patients and their young average age at diagnosis render these studies difficult to perform. The author knows of reports on only five autopsied cases with type 1 disease, and none of these showed significant atherosclerotic changes of the major arteries or evidence of myocardial infarction. Three of the patients were women, aged 24, 28, and 42 years [8, 29], and two were men, aged 31 and 38 years [8, 29]. The early literature contains reports of patients with "idiopathic hyperlipemia" dying from premature vascular disease [30, 31], but a closer examination of the data indicated that these patients had type 2 or 3 hyperlipoproteinemia.

The major threat to the life of patients with LPL deficiency is acute pancreatitis. Most of the recorded deaths of the type 1 cases have been due to severe pancreatitis or its complications. Few data are available on the long-term prognosis of the disease, but there are no reasons to suspect a shortened life span in patients who avoid the pancreatic catastrophe. One female patient has undergone two normal pregnancies without complications [10].

Other Symptoms   Other clinical features have occasionally been observed in patients with type 1 disease, but it is uncertain whether these have any relationship to the basic metabolic abnormality. The index patient described by Holt et al. [3] suffered from chronic leg ulcers, and, curiously enough, all three brothers of the first identified LPL-deficient family [3] had ulcers in their lower extremities since early childhood. It may be that the excessive hyperlipemia increases blood viscosity and impairs the capillary circulation.

Some patients have been reported to have anemia, but neither this nor signs of hypersplenism are typical [8]. One infant presented with sudden bruising in association with abdominal symptoms [32]. A few children with type 1 have been noted to have growth retardation, but this is not a characteristic feature. Unexplained bone changes may occur [29].

Lipids and Lipoproteins

The patients with familial LPL deficiency usually have a type 1 hyperlipoproteinemia, but occasionally a type 5 pattern may be found. The abnormality is so striking and specific that by using the routine modern laboratory methods there are seldom any diagnostic problems. In patients eating an average diet the serum taken after an overnight fast is always turbid, the appearance varying from that of skim milk to heavy cream. On standing over night at 4°C a creamy layer separates to the top of the tube, leaving a clear or slightly turbid infranatant. This simple test usually distinguishes type 1 hyperlipoproteinemia from the other forms of hyperlipemia associated with lactescent serum. In the latter instances the infranatant serum remains turbid even after separation of the largest fat particles to the surface.

The plasma triglyceride concentrations of type 1 patients are very high, typically ranging from 1500 to 4500 mg/dl, but values up to 25,000 mg/dl have been recorded. Conversely, the plasma cholesterol levels are either quite normal or moderately elevated, the common range being from 160 to 400 mg/dl. Only in cases with extreme hypertriglyceridemia does the cholesterol concentration go up to 1000 mg/dl. A diagnostic feature of type 1 disorder is a low plasma cholesterol/triglyceride ratio, reflecting the composition of chylomicrons. Expressed in weight units, the cholesterol/triglyceride ratio in type 1 is always less than 0.2, usually being close to 0.1 (in molar units the ratio may rise up to 0.5) [11]. This contrasts with the situation in other forms of hyperlipoproteinemia where the cholesterol/triglyceride ratio is usually greater than 0.2. However, there is a certain overlapping with type 5 patients, who may also have cholesterol/triglyceride ratios of 0.2 or less. The diagnosis of LPL deficiency (or type 1) is questionable in cases where this ratio is clearly above 0.2, and it is highly unlikely when the ratio approaches 0.5.

The lipoprotein pattern is characteristic (Fig. 30-2). Both lipoprotein electrophoresis and ultracentrifugation reveal the presence of excessive amounts of chylomicrons in the fasting serum. The concentration of VLDL is either normal or slightly elevated, but the low density lipoprotein (LDL) and high density lipoprotein (HDL) levels are always markedly depressed. Thus, LDL cholesterol concentration in type 1 varies from 20 to 40 mg/dl (normal, 100 to 160 mg/dl) and HDL cholesterol from 5 to 20 mg/dl (normal, 40 to 70 mg/dl) [6, 10, 33, 34]. The rise of VLDL above the normal range may be seen particularly in patients who habitually eat a diet that is relatively low in fat and high in carbohydrate. Such a rise is regularly observed during the treatment of type 1 patients on an isocaloric fat-free diet [10]. When present, the increase of VLDL levels is moderate compared to that of chylomicrons, and there are therefore seldom difficulties in distinguishing the type 1 pattern from that of type 5 hyperlipoproteinemia. However, the lipoprotein distribution in both types may vary according

Figure 30-2 Electrophoretic *(top)* and ultracentrifugal *(bottom)* patterns of plasma lipoproteins in type 1 hyperlipoproteinemia as compared to normal. The chylomicrons are much increased, while the concentrations of small VLDL (pre-β) and of LDL (β) and HDL (α) are subnormal.

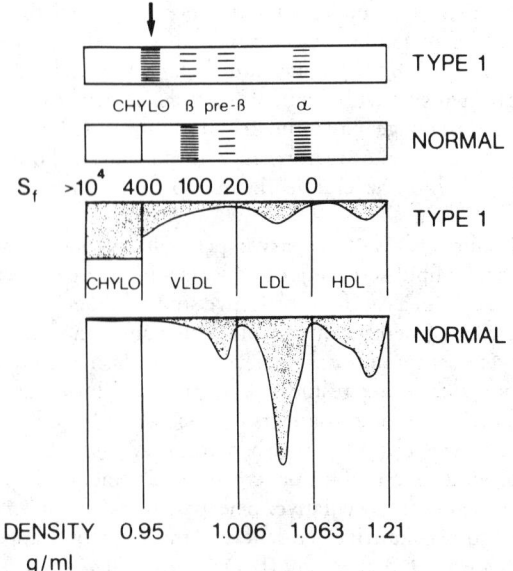

to diet, and therefore diagnosis of LPL deficiency must be based on enzyme assays rather than on lipoprotein phenotype.

There are also alterations in the apolipoprotein concentrations and in the chemical composition of lipoproteins. The plasma apolipoprotein C-II levels in patients with true LPL enzyme deficiency are four- to sixfold higher than in normal patients (but absent by definition in patients with apo C-II deficiency), most of the C-II peptide being found in triglyceride-rich lipoproteins and not in HDL as in normal subjects [35]. In spite of this increase, the molar ratio of triglyceride to apo C-II in chylomicrons and VLDL is higher in the LPL-deficient patients than in normal patients or in subjects with type 4 or 5 hyperlipoproteinemia [35]. Also the LDL of type 1 patients has abnormal composition, since in spite of markedly decreased total LDL and LDL-cholesterol concentrations the LDL-triglyceride levels have been found to be normal [36] or high [36a], and the LDL apo B concentrations are either normal [37] or low [36, 36a]. Both subfractions of HDL, i.e., HDL$_2$ and HDL$_3$, are depressed in type 1 patients, and the apoprotein A-I content is also reduced [36, 36a].

The diagnosis of type 1 hyperlipoproteinemia is confirmed by a characteristic response of serum lipids and lipoproteins to diet. Upon eliminating dietary fat (< 10 g daily) and substituting for it isocalorically with carbohydrate and protein, the chylomicrons virtually disappear within a few days and plasma triglyceride levels fall to a range of 200 to 500 mg/dl in 4 to 7 days. At the same time that the plasma lipoprotein pattern changes so that there are few if any chylomicrons left, the VLDL is increased two- to threefold above normal and the LDL increases toward normal range, but the HDL remains low [10, 13].

Other Laboratory Findings

In contrast to other familial forms of primary hypertriglyceridemia, the patients with LPL deficiency generally have normal glucose tolerance. A secondary diabetes may develop following repeated attacks of acute pancreatitis or a silent chronic pancreatic insufficiency [20]. Such a history was present in the first reported patient with apo C-II deficiency [7].

The excessively high serum fat content can secondarily influence the results of many laboratory tests. The intense serum turbidity interferes with photometric or fluorometric assays. The increase in the volume of the plasma lipid phase restricts the aqueous phase, and because many solutes are partitioned only in the latter phase, their concentration in whole plasma is decreased in the presence of massive hyperlipemia. This is mainly seen as a reduced serum sodium concentration [13]. High triglyceride levels interfere with serum amylase assays, giving rise to falsely low values and subsequent eventual overlooking of the presence of pancreatitis [16]. This error can be partly eliminated by doing the amylase assays from diluted serum [16] or by using the urinary amylase/creatinine clearance ratio [17].

Some patients with type 1 have mild anemia, but usually there are no major signs of increased hemolysis. In association with the abdominal pains there may be leukocytosis and an increased sedimentation rate. Hyperlipemia as such can elevate the sedimentation rate to some extent. The bone marrow is usually normal, apart from the presence of large foam cells

similar to those seen in the spleen [26]. The cytoplasm of the foam cells is filled with vacuoles containing either lipid droplets, chylomicronlike particles, or ceroid granules [26].

Pathogenesis

The hyperchylomicronemia and abnormally low levels of LDL and HDL exhibited by patients with LPL deficiency are all consistent with current knowledge of the central role of LPL in plasma lipoprotein metabolism. The occurrence of these lipoprotein abnormalities in LPL deficiency constitutes the most convincing evidence for the key position of LPL in the removal of plasma triglyceride–rich lipoproteins and in the formation of the other lipoproteins. The only biochemical finding in LPL-deficient patients that is not completely understood is the disproportionately small accumulation of plasma VLDL particles.

Chylomicron Metabolism   Chylomicrons are the largest lipoprotein particles of blood. These particles normally begin to enter the plasma within 1 h after ingestion of fat and are completely removed 5 to 8 h after the last meal. In normal individuals eating an average diet the plasma chylomicrons originate entirely from dietary fat, but in some hyperlipemic states and during a high carbohydrate intake, particles of similar size and composition may be synthesized from endogenous precursors [38, 39]. The normal chylomicrons are produced in intestinal absorptive cells and transported to the blood through mesenteric lymph capillaries and thoracic duct, whereas the "endogenous" chylomicrons may have a hepatic origin.

Defined by their physical and chemical properties, chylomicrons form a highly heterogeneous population of particles, ranging from 75 to 1000 nm (750 to 10,000 Å) in diameter, from 0.90 to 0.95 g/ml in density, and from $S_f = 400$ to 40,000 in ultracentrifugal flotation rates. The particle consists of a large core of triglycerides and esterified cholesterol and of a monomolecular surface film containing phospholipids, free cholesterol, and apoproteins A, B, C, and E. The largest chylomicrons contain up to 95 percent triglyceride, while in the smallest particles triglyceride content is only 80 to 85 percent, with a correspondingly higher amount of phospholipids.

Chylomicrons are formed mainly in the absorptive cells of jejunal villi [40], where resynthesized dietary triglycerides are coated by apoproteins A-I, A-IV, and B and phospholipids. The particles are then secreted from the Golgi vacuoles into intracellular spaces, moving thereafter into lymphatic channels [40, 41]. In thoracic duct lymph and ultimately in plasma the chylomicrons receive C apoproteins from HDL, increasing their protein content from 1 to 3 percent [42]. The size and composition of intestinal lipoprotein particles and of circulating chylomicrons is essentially dependent on the fat content of the meal. In the fasting state lipoprotein particles found in jejunal mucosa are mainly VLDL, but after intake of fat, chylomicrons of various sizes appear in addition to VLDL [40]. After ingestion of small quantities of fat or only phospholipids, the particles appearing in blood are small chylomicrons and large VLDL ($S_f = 100$ to 400) [43, 44], while after fat-rich meals most dietary triglyceride is transported as chylomicrons [43].

Chylomicrons are normally removed from the circulation with a half-life of a few minutes. The removal occurs primarily in extrahepatic tissues, and it involves hydrolysis of chylomicron triglycerides by endothelial LPL as an obligatory step. Removal is almost completely inhibited in the absence of LPL from the tissue [45] or of apoprotein C-II from the surface of the chylomicrons [46]. During the hydrolysis the surface materials, including phospholipids, free cholesterol, and C apoproteins, are transferred to HDL. The fate of the core remnant in human beings is still obscure, but it is likely to form LDL [47].

Lipoprotein Lipase   Lipoprotein lipase (glycerol-ester hydrolase) is an enzyme (or a group of enzymes) that hydrolyzes circulating chylomicron and VLDL triglycerides at the vascular endothelial surface. The enzyme is released by heparin from its tissue binding sites in vivo and in vitro. It is dependent on the presence of a specific plasma cofactor, apoprotein C-II, for activity and is inhibited by a high salt concentration and by protamine. The enzyme shows its highest activity toward chylomicron and VLDL triglycerides, which constitute its physiological substrate, but in the presence of added apo C-II it also hydrolyzes triglycerides artificially dispersed with emulsifiers, detergents, or phospholipids. The latter substrates are generally used for quantitation of LPL activity, although the kinetics may not be fully comparable with those obtained with natural substrate. The LPL specifically cleaves the 1, 3-ester bonds of the triglyceride molecule, producing 2-monoglyceride, which is further broken down to glycerol and free fatty acids (FFA).

The major sites of LPL activity in human beings and other mammalian species are adipose tissue, skeletal muscle, myocardium, mammary gland, and lung. These tissues are known to take up triglycerides for storage (adipose tissue), oxidation (muscles), or secretion (milk).

The functionally active part of the enzyme is present on the luminal surface of vascular endothelium, where it is probably attached by a membrane-bound glycosaminoglycan chain [48] (Fig. 30-3), which is broken by heparin [48a]. Another part of tissue LPL is localized intracellularly in parenchymal cells. In adipose tissue this enzyme is found in fat cells [49]; in heart it probably lies in myocytes and mesenchymal cells [50]. The endothelial and parenchymal forms of LPL have not been isolated separately, and little is therefore known of their possible structural and functional identity. It is thought that all LPL is synthesized in parenchymal cells and transported from there to the site of action in capillary endothelium. The intracellular part might thus represent a storage pool of a LPL "proenzyme," which continuously supplies the membrane-bound pool with new molecules of active enzyme [51].

The lipoprotein lipases of different tissues are probably not identical proteins, although they share antigenic determinants [45, 52, 53] and many basic enzymatic characteristics. The heparin-releasable LPL of rat heart, for example, shows a much higher substrate affinity than the corresponding enzyme in adipose tissue [54]. The high affinity and low affinity LPL species isolated from rat postheparin plasma have molecular weights of 34,000 and 69,000, respectively [55]. The different substrate affinity of the heart and adipose tissue lipoprotein lipases clearly has an important physiologic role in the diversion of triglycerides to the proper tissues. Thus, in the fasting state with low plasma triglyceride concentration, the myocardium utilizes lipids at a much higher rate than adipose tissue, whereas in the postprandial state the rising plasma triglyceride concentration turns the excess flux to adipose tissue, the heart enzyme already being saturated [56].

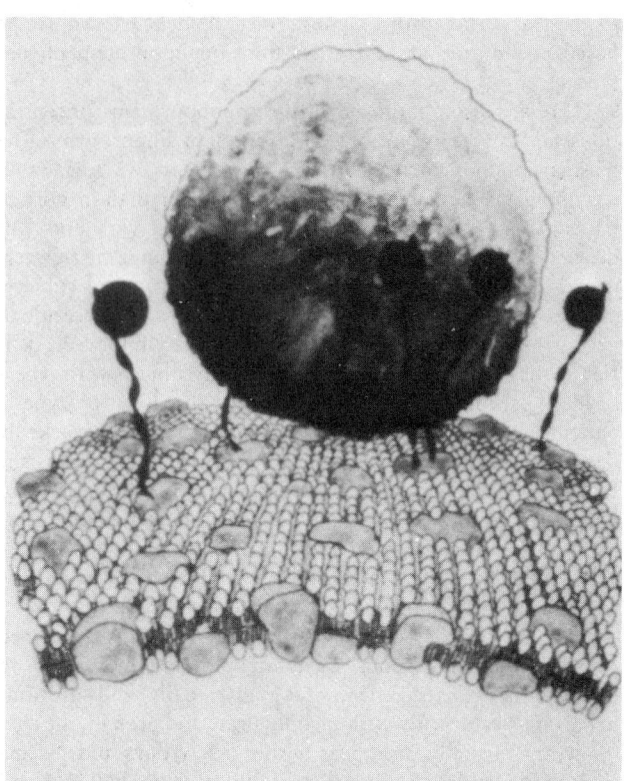

Figure 30-3   A schematic model of the action of lipoprotein lipase at the capillary endothelium as outlined by Olivecrona et al. [48]. The LPL molecules (black balls) are attached to the plasma membrane of endothelial cell by a proteoglycan chain and can interact with the substrate lipoprotein particle at a distance from the endothelial surface. (Used by permission.)

The activity of LPL is sensitively regulated by nutrients and hormones. The enzyme activity in adipose tissue rises rapidly after intake of carbohydrate [57–59] or fats [60] and falls again upon fasting. These effects are likely to be mediated by insulin [61] or by gastrointestinal hormones such as GIP [62, 62a], and they reflect changes in the activity of the membrane-bound functional LPL, although the exact mechanism of this regulation is not known [51]. Also glucagon, epinephrine, and prolactin can modulate LPL activity. The LPL in mammary gland is fully dependent on stimulation by prolactin [63], increasing several fold during lactation. This enables the direct utilization of blood triglycerides for milk production and serves as an excellent example of a physiologically meaningful regulation of fat metabolism.

Function of LPL in Lipoprotein Metabolism   The primary physiologic function of LPL is the transfer of triglyceride fatty acids from blood to tissues for oxidation, storage, or secretion. This enzyme not only determines the overall rate by which chylomicron and VLDL triglycerides are removed from the circulation, but it also directs their relative distribution between different tissues. Moreover, LPL has a key role in the metabolism of LDL and HDL, which arise as end products during the catabolism of triglyceride-rich lipoproteins and have important functions in plasma cholesterol and phospholipid transport. Thus, LPL is indeed located at the crossroad of the metabolic pathways of all plasma lipoproteins.

The removal of chylomicrons and VLDL from the blood is almost completely dependent on their degradation by LPL at the endothelial surface. Inactivation of the enzyme by a specific antiserum in vivo [45, 64] or depletion by heparin perfusion in vitro [65, 66] results in a complete loss of the ability of tissues to assimilate chylomicron or VLDL triglycerides. Prior to hydrolysis the chylomicrons become attached to the endothelial membrane by binding directly to the lipase or to specific membrane receptors recognizing some apolipoprotein structures [67]. Subsequently, the particle is partly enveloped by fingerlike processes extending from the endothelial cells into the capillary lumen [68] (Fig. 30-4). A similar process is also likely to initiate the degradation of VLDL, although this has not been documented. The exact nature and fate of the products of the LPL reaction are still incompletely known. The liberated fatty acids are partly returned to the circulation as albuminbound FFA, but part is directly taken up into the respective tissue by "lateral diffusion" within cell membranes [68]. The surface coat of chylomicrons and VLDL, containing unesterified cholesterol, phospholipids, and C apoproteins, becomes fused with HDL [69–74], converting HDL$_3$ partly to HDL$_2$ [75, 76]. The core lipids of VLDL, i.e., some unhydrolyzed triglyceride and esterified cholesterol together with apolipoprotein B, are reassembled and ultimately form an LDL-like particle [47, 77]. A major part of plasma HDL (HDL$_2$) and the LDL originate at the lipolytic process, and the concentration of HDL (HDL$_2$) is to a large extent controlled by the activity of LPL [78–81], whereas the LDL levels are not.

In spite of the fact that both chylomicrons and VLDL serve as ideal substrates for LPL, it is not certain that the catabolism of the two types of particles is completely identical. There is morphological evidence that chylomicrons become trapped in the endothelium [68, 82] and may remain at the site where they were originally attached until the hydrolysis has proceeded to a certain advanced stage, the remnants then being released into circulation. On the other hand, heart perfusion studies suggest that chylomicron hydrolysis takes place in a stepwise fashion, with repeated release of smaller intermediate particles before the formation of a final remnant particle [83]. For VLDL the latter mechanism of degradation seems very likely on the basis of both biochemical and kinetic data [37, 67, 84, 85]. Thus, VLDL probably undergoes a stepwise delipidation at multiple endothelial binding sites, giving rise to a spectrum of partially degraded plasma VLDL particles with progressively higher density and smaller size, ranging from S$_f$ =100–400 particles to S$_f$ = 10–20 intermediate density lipoproteins (IDL) [85a]. Since both chylomicrons and VLDL are secreted into plasma as particles with greatly variable size [85b], it is difficult to prove that the stepwise degradation process really occurs in human

beings. In roosters the average size of VLDL particles is increased by 50 percent after inhibition of LPL by LPL antiserum, suggesting that part of circulating VLDL is indeed a product of partial lipolysis [64].

Even though chylomicrons and VLDL share common removal sites at the LPL molecule, the triglycerides carried in chylomicrons are cleared from plasma at much greater velocity than those in VLDL. Thus, the plasma half-life is only 4 to 6 min for chylomicron triglycerides but amounts to 2 to 4 h for the VLDL [86–89]. Moreover, the clearance of chylomicrons is inversely related to the concentration of VLDL [38, 86, 89], whereas interference with the removal of VLDL by chylomicrons has never been demonstrated. These differences are best explained by assuming that the rate-limiting factor in triglyceride removal is not the actual hydrolytic activity but the number of available particle binding sites on the LPL or endothelial receptor [89]. Almost 30 VLDL particles are needed to transport the amount of triglyceride contained in one chylomicron [67], and, thus, the VLDL may occupy many more enzyme loci than chylomicrons for hydrolysis of an equivalent amount of triglyceride.

Effect of LPL Deficiency on Lipoprotein Metabolism

Havel and Gordon clearly demonstrated the insufficient clearance of chylomicrons from the blood in the first family with verified familial LPL deficiency [6]. The authors took chylomicrons from one patient and infused them into his LPL-deficient brother; the latter patient was kept on a fat-free diet to eliminate his own chylomicrons, which could have secondarily impaired the clearance of the infused chylomicrons. Under these conditions the half-life of the infused chylomicrons was much longer in the patient than in a healthy control subject. Furthermore, the removal of chylomicrons was not accelerated after injection of heparin, as occurs in normal subjects, because the LPL released into the blood causes intravascular lipolysis. The slow clearance of chylomicrons during a fat-free diet has been confirmed in another patient with LPL deficiency [90].

In contrast to the expected defect in chylomicron catabolism, the removal of VLDL seems not to be impaired in LPL-deficient patients. Three separate studies using either apoprotein-labeled [37, 91] or triglyceride-labeled [90] VLDL have uniformly shown that the fractional removal rate of this lipoprotein in LPL-deficient patients is not impaired when compared to subjects who have similar VLDL concentrations but a normal LPL activity. Thus, the VLDL removal (delipidation) rate may be reduced in LPL-deficient patients but only to an extent predicted by their VLDL concentration. Moreover, the VLDL apo B seems to be converted to LDL apo B at an almost normal rate in patients with LPL deficiency [91]. Even though the results of all of these studies may have been influenced by the obligatory use of a highly abnormal diet (very low in fat and high in carbohydrate) which increases VLDL concentration, they nevertheless show that subjects with LPL deficiency can clear VLDL from their blood and must therefore possess some alternative routes for catabolism of this lipoprotein. Uptake of intact unhydrolyzed VLDL has been observed in isolated cells [92, 93]. The possibility that VLDL is hydrolyzed by the other heparin-releasable endothelial lipase, the hepatic lipase, has been suggested [91] and seems to be a most plausible explanation for the nearly normal VLDL levels in LPL deficiency. This enzyme hydrolyzes VLDL and LDL triglycerides more readily than those of chylomicrons [91], and its activity is usually near normal in type 1 patients (see below).

Figure 30-4 Detail of a capillary endothelium in lactating rat mammary gland taken 10 min after intravenous injection of chylomicrons. The endothelium (E) contains vesicles (V) and has fingerlike processes (LP) which project into the capillary lumen (L). One of the processes enmeshes a chylomicron (C). ×67,000. *(From Scow et al. [68]. Used by permission.)*

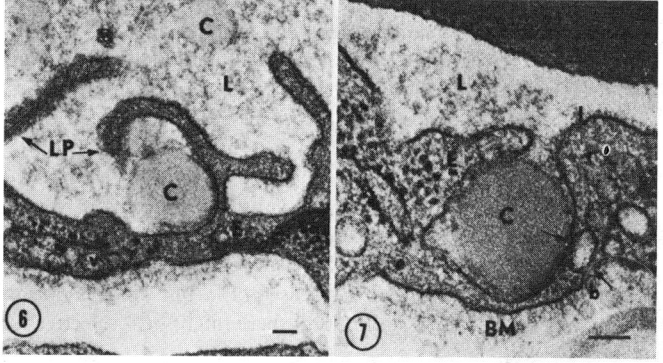

The abnormally low LDL and HDL levels observed in LPL-deficient patients are consistent with the view that these lipoproteins are products of lipoprotein lipase–mediated catabolism of triglyceride-rich lipoproteins. During treatment of the patients with a low fat diet the LDL is increased [6, 10] in spite of the continuously low chylomicron catabolism. The new LDL is possibly derived from VLDL metabolism, which is increased by high dietary carbohydrates.

Diagnosis of Familial LPL Deficiency

The diagnosis of familial LPL deficiency must be confirmed by specific assays of LPL activity from either postheparin plasma or adipose tissue or preferably from both. The currently available methods are relatively simple and specific, but they are only in use in laboratories with a special interest in lipid metabolism. Adipose tissue has the advantage over postheparin plasma in that it does not contain hepatic lipase, and the recently developed methods are sufficiently sensitive for measuring the activity from minimal amounts of tissue which can be easily obtained by a single-needle aspiration biopsy [94–98].

Measurements of lipolytic activity in postheparin plasma have been used extensively over the years. Besides LPL, heparin also releases hepatic lipase into plasma from endothelial cells surrounding the liver sinusoids [99]. The latter enzyme has a relatively low activity against chylomicron triglycerides, but it readily degrades triglycerides in artificial emulsions and also contains a high phospholipase A activity [100]. The presence of hepatic lipase activity in postheparin plasma seriously invalidates the assay of LPL with most nonnatural substrates, and, therefore, a total lipolytic activity of postheparin plasma cannot be used as a measure of lipoprotein lipase without separation of the two activities. Prior to 1974 most clinical studies did not distinguish between LPL and hepatic lipase, and therefore the data are of uncertain significance. It is fortunate that chylomicrons were used as substrate in the discovery of the first family with LPL deficiency [6], since with the use of fat emulsions the correct diagnosis could have been missed.

A reliable index of the presence of LPL deficiency can be obtained by methods that selectively measure LPL activity in postheparin plasma. Three basic techniques are currently available. In the method of Krauss et al. [101, 102] protamine sulfate is used for inhibition of LPL activity; LPL activity is then calculated as the difference between total lipolytic activity and the protamine-resistant (hepatic lipase) activity. A similar method using 1 M sodium chloride for inhibition of LPL has been described and successfully applied to the diagnosis of LPL deficiency [103]. In the second method the hepatic lipase activity is inhibited by an antiserum prepared against purified human postheparin plasma hepatic lipase [104–106]. The results obtained with this assay compare relatively well with those of the protamine inhibition method [104]. The third method is more arduous since it is based on chromatographic separation of the two lipolytic activities [107]. All of the selective postheparin lipase assay methods use a pure radioactive triolein substrate, which is dispersed by sonication with inert colloid or detergent. The LPL activity varies according to the average particle size of the emulsion, and therefore the sonication procedure must be strictly standardized with known enzyme standards included in each assay series. Variations in

enzyme activity are further reduced by using a large heparin dose (100 IU = 1 mg per kilogram body weight) and by sampling the plasma 15 min after the injection of heparin [104, 105].

The LPL and hepatic lipase activities of healthy normolipemic human subjects measured by protamine inhibition [102] and by immunochemical methods [105] are given in Table 30-1. The activities obtained by the former method are on average lower than those of the immunochemical assay, and the relative contribution of LPL to total lipolytic activity is very low in the protamine method. In spite of this difference both methods show consistently that women have higher LPL, but lower hepatic lipase activity, than men. Also, in adipose tissue the LPL activity is higher in women than in men [79, 108], whereas in skeletal muscle the activities are similar in the two sexes [79]. Physically highly active people exhibit greater LPL activities in both muscle and adipose tissue than sedentary subjects [109].

Postheparin plasma LPL activities of less than 10 percent of the mean level of normolipemic controls of similar age and sex are usually diagnostic for LPL deficiency, while values between 10 and 20 percent of the control mean are suspect. Low values should be further checked by adding normal serum (or apo C-II) to the assay mixture in order to exclude the possible apoprotein C-II deficiency. If the activity is significantly increased by the addition of normal serum, the latter diagnosis is likely, and it can be confirmed by testing the ability of the patient's plasma to activate LPL in guinea pig postheparin plasma [110] or in skim milk, both of which lack apo C-II. It may also be advisable to confirm the diagnosis of a true primary LPL deficiency by making additional assays of LPL activity from adipose tissue and skeletal muscle.

Nature of the Enzyme Defect

It is recognized that primary type 1 hyperlipoproteinemia has a heterogeneous etiology. Yet, after a few years of using selective LPL assay methods, it appears that only a few patients with a typical type 1 disorder do not have a defect either of LPL or of the cofactor, apoprotein C-II. Table 30-2 is a compilation of published cases of type 1 disease in which LPL has been assayed by a selective method from postheparin plasma (using either chylomicrons as substrate or excluding the hepatic lipase activity) or from adipose tissue and where there is no evidence for apo C-II deficiency.

Among almost 60 reported cases, only two patients had postheparin plasma LPL activity within the normal range, one of these having a very low activity in adipose tissue [111]. Moreover, in one unusual case the patient did not show any activity in postheparin plasma but had a normal LPL in his adipose tissue [111]. It is thus obvious that in most patients with the type 1 syndrome there is either a true deficiency of LPL or a deficiency of apoprotein C-II (= functional LPL deficiency). The molecular nature of the enzyme defect is unknown so far. The enzyme deficiency may be due to a true absence of the enzyme, caused by an inability to synthesize the enzyme protein, or it may represent a structurally abnormal enzyme with insufficient ability to bind with substrate or to hydrolyze the triglyceride ester bonds. A defective activation by apoprotein C-I of one subtype of LPL has been postulated to be present in patients with type 1 disease [112], but this has not been confirmed. The possibility that there might be a selective

Table 30-1 Lipoprotein lipase and hepatic lipase activities in postheparin plasma of normal human subjects

| | Krauss et al. [102] | | Huttunen et al. [105] | |
	Protamine-inactivated*	Protamine-resistant†	Lipoprotein lipase	Hepatic lipase
Males				
5–16 years	6.7 ± 1.5	11.0 ± 3.1		
19–70 years	4.2 ± 1.5	15.0 ± 5.4	18.6 ± 6.2	26.8 ± 9.9
Females				
7–16 years	3.8 ± 1.1	11.1 ± 3.8		
19–70 years	4.9 ± 2.3	10.5 ± 3.3	25.8 ± 9.3	18.6 ± 7.5

* Approximately identical with lipoprotein lipase.
† Approximately identical with hepatic lipase.
NOTE: Measured in micromoles of free fatty acid per hour per milliliter, plus or minus the standard deviation.

deficiency of either high affinity (heart) or low affinity (adipose tissue) forms of LPL [113] is exciting, but its presence has not been established so far.

Genetics

The occurrence of LPL deficiency in sibs has been repeatedly documented. There is also a high frequency of consanguine marriages among the parents of the LPL-deficient patients. On the other hand, there are no examples of vertical transmission of the syndrome, and the data are most compatible with an autosomal recessive pattern of inheritance. Thus, two mutant alleles are required for expression of the disease as type 1 hyperlipoproteinemia. In the 1972 edition of this book Fredrickson and Levy [10] reported on eight families in which one or more affected sibs of the proband were found. Among a total of 29 sibs including the probands, 12 had type 1 syndrome, while 17 had normal plasma lipids. The distribution of values for postheparin plasma lipolytic activity (= PHLA, not equivalent to lipoprotein lipase) in these sibs was bimodal, the healthy sibs being intermediate between normal subjects and the affected patients. The adipose tissue LPL activity is also depressed to about 50 percent of normal in the parents and healthy sibs of type 1 subjects [114]. In spite of this partial LPL defect, heterozygotes usually have completely normal fasting plasma triglyceride levels [103, 114], but the triglyceride response to fatty meals may be exaggerated and prolonged [114], indicating a mild impairment of chylomicron clearance. Some family members of LPL-deficient patients have elevated VLDL and triglyceride levels (type 4 pattern), but they usually have normal or near normal postheparin plasma LPL activities [32, 103].

One family has been described in which type 1 hyperlipoproteinemia was associated with thyroxine-binding globulin (TBG) deficiency [115]. This is likely to be a coincidental defect, especially since the locus for TBG is X-linked.

The frequency of the abnormal gene causing LPL deficiency is unknown but is probably extremely low in all populations.

Diagnostic Problems

Usually the clinical picture of LPL deficiency is so unique that diagnostic difficulties do not arise. A secondary hypertriglycer-idemia with milky serum may occur in association with pancreatitis, uncontrolled juvenile- or adult-onset diabetes, or severe alcoholism. The LPL activity may be low in these conditions, particularly in the diabetic patients, who in addition to chylomicronemia almost always have a concomitant increase in plasma VLDL resulting in a type 5 lipoprotein pattern.

A typical fat-induced type 1 hyperlipoproteinemia with recurrent bouts of pancreatitis and with low postheparin plasma lipolytic activity has been described in two patients with increased immunoglobulin levels and with systemic lupus erythematosus [116, 117]. In distinction from patients with familial LPL deficiency, these patients exhibited a normal lipolytic response to larger doses (1 mg/kg) of heparin, and it was shown that IgG isolated from the plasma of the patients actually bound heparin and therefore inhibited its releasing effect on LPL from adipose tissue. The patients were thus not actually LPL deficient; rather, their enzyme was inactivated by the binding of endogenous heparin or glycosaminoglycans by the circulating immunoglobulins. In patients exhibiting type 1 hyperlipoproteinemia, the presence of immunoglobulin dyscrasias should be excluded by protein electrophoresis.

A rare form of massive hyperlipemia, presumably of type 1, has been reported in infants with malignant histiocytic proliferation [118–120]. This is an interesting disorder that needs more detailed investigation.

In practice the most common problem is the distinction between familial LPL deficiency and the familial form of type 5 hyperlipoproteinemia (chylomicronemia and elevation of VLDL). Indeed, the demarcation between the two disorders may not be sharp since the patients with familial LPL deficiency may have elevated VLDL levels in addition to chylomicronemia, i.e., they may express a type 5 pattern, while, on the other hand, patients with type 5 may have LPL activity clearly below the normal range [105, 121]. Inasmuch as patients with the type 5 disorder may have symptoms that are characteristic of the primary LPL deficiency, it may be difficult to distinguish between the two at times. The presence of type 5 or type 4 hyperlipoproteinemia in patients, or in several other close relatives, favors the diagnosis of familial type 5 disease. Patients with low LPL activity exhibiting a type 5 pattern should be carefully screened for the presence of apo C-II deficiency since the latter condition is often expressed as type 5 rather than type 1 phenotype (see below). Postheparin plasma histaminase activity, which is depressed in familial LPL deficiency [122], has been normal in at least some kindreds with type 5 [121, 122] and may thus serve as a promising discriminator between

Table 30-2 Patients with type 1 hyperlipoproteinemia studied for lipoprotein lipase activity with selective assay methods

Authors (reference)	Number of patients	Number of families	LPL assay from	LPL activity
Havel & Gordon [6]	3	1	Postheparin plasma	None against chylomicrons
Harlan et al. [114]	2	1	Adipose tissue	Less than 20%*
Ford et al. [90]	1	1	Adipose tissue	20%*
Damgaard-Pedersen & Dyerberg [136]	6	2	Adipose tissue	Absent (data not given)
Schreibman et al. [137]	2	1	Postheparin plasma	None against chylomicrons
Krauss et al. [102]	12	?	Postheparin plasma	0 to 15%*
Greten et al. [106]	8	Familial	Postheparin plasma	2 to 15%*
Berger & Abraham [138]	8	4	Postheparin plasma	0 to 20%*
Burton & Nadler [139]	1	1	Postheparin plasma	High
Gagné et al. [103]	4	1	Postheparin plasma	Absent
Kashyap et al. [35]	2	1	Postheparin plasma	0 and 19%*
Brunzell et al. [111]	3	?	Postheparin plasma and adipose tissue	Both less than 10%
Brunzell et al. [111]	1	1	Postheparin plasma and adipose tissue	Low in postheparin plasma, normal in adipose tissue
Brunzell et al. [111]	1	1	Postheparin plasma and adipose tissue	Low in adipose tissue, normal in postheparin plasma
Crepaldi et al. [36]	4	2	Adipose tissue	Absent

* Compared to the mean of control subjects.

the two lipid disorders. Glucose intolerance is common in type 5 but rare in type 1 patients.

Treatment

One of the characteristic features of familial LPL deficiency is the dramatic response of hypertriglyceridemia to restriction of dietary fat. Because of the potential danger of pancreatitis, such a regimen should be instituted immediately and carefully maintained in all patients. The risk of pancreatitis is essentially eliminated at triglyceride levels of less than 1000 mg/dl, these usually being achieved with a moderate reduction of fat intake. Most adults can readily adapt to diets containing less than 50 g of fat per day, but if this is not adequate in reducing the triglyceride levels below the above value, a further restriction must be attempted. It is important to note that the above maximal permissible triglyceride limit applies not only to fasting plasma but should also be maintained in the postprandial state. Therefore, the triglyceride levels should also be monitored from nonfasting plasma samples taken in the afternoon or evening. The amount of fat eaten with one meal should never exceed 20 g. It is not important whether the fat is saturated or polyunsaturated, but an adequate intake of essential fatty acids must be guaranteed.

Since most of the type 1 patients are not obese, a reduction of fat intake must be compensated by a carbohydrate or protein increase. A marked decrease of dietary fat usually means a corresponding increase of carbohydrate intake, and this in turn may result in a considerable increase of VLDL concentration. Thus, normal triglyceride levels are seldom reached even though the chylomicrons disappear (conversion of type 1 pattern to type 5 or 4). In order to improve the therapeutic response without giving excessive amounts of carbohydrates, part of the fat calories can be supplied in the form of medium-chain triglycerides (MCT). These are absorbed directly into the portal circulation and their hydrolysis is not dependent on LPL. The drawbacks of MCT are their limited tolerance by many patients and the relatively high price.

Additional measures in the prevention of excessive hyperlipemia are avoidance of the use of alcohol [123] and of drugs, such as estrogens, which are known to increase endogenous triglyceride synthesis. During pregnancy the patients need strict dietary control and monitoring of triglyceride levels.

None of the lipid-lowering drugs has been shown to be effective in the treatment of familial LPL deficiency.

FAMILIAL APOLIPOPROTEIN C-II DEFICIENCY

An essential step in the removal of triglyceride-rich lipoproteins, i.e., chylomicrons and VLDL, from the circulation is their prior hydrolysis by LPL at the endothelial surface. To be active this enzyme requires the presence of a plasma cofactor [124], which has been shown to be apolipoprotein C-II (apo C-II) [70, 125, 126], or actually only a carboxy-terminal peptide fragment of apo C-II [127, 128]. The cofactor peptide binds to LPL [129], increasing the maximal rate of triglyceride hydrolysis [56, 130]. In the absence of exogenously added apo C-II, the enzyme has a low activity when tested with synthetic substrates and a normal activity when tested with chylomicrons or VLDL, each of which normally contains apo C-II in excess of that required for maximal hydrolysis. The C apoproteins are secreted into plasma with HDL from the liver, but they equilibrate rapidly with chylomicrons and VLDL and are returned to HDL in the course of hydrolysis of triglycerides by LPL. Thus, normal chylomicrons and VLDL serve as an ideal substrate for the enzyme without the need for an additional cofactor.

In 1978 Breckenridge and coworkers [7] described an adult patient from Toronto who had gross hyperlipemia and absent postheparin plasma lipolytic activity. Blood transfusion given for anemia was followed by a dramatic fall of plasma triglycerides. This suggested that the patient's lipid disorder was caused by a deficiency of some plasma factor. Closer examination revealed that the patient actually had a normal LPL activity in his postheparin plasma but that he completely lacked apo C-II, so that his own triglyceride-rich lipoproteins were not hydrolyzed by the enzyme without addition of normal plasma. Screening of the relatives of the patient showed that the defect had a definite familial basis. The apo C-II deficiency thus is a newly recognized inherited disease of lipoprotein metabolism, expressed as an inability to clear triglycerides from the plasma. Discovery of this disorder has confirmed the essential role of apo C-II in chylomicron and VLDL metabolism of human beings.

Genetics

Since the discovery of apo C-II deficiency in 1978, data have been obtained from 19 affected patients and from 35 relatives derived from 4 separate families. The kindred of the first apo C-II–deficient patient (reported from Toronto) originated from a highly inbred, isolated Caribbean population of British ancestry [131].

In 1980 there were 14 homozygotes and 23 obligate heterozygotes identified in that particular family [7, 132]. Another family, from Japan, with two affected sibs, their healthy parents, and one additional sib, has been described [133]. Consanguinity of the parents was also present in this case. A third family, from Italy, with two affected sibs and their four relatives [36] and another from England, with proband and five examined relatives [36a], have been reported. The pedigree data are consistent with transmission of the defect as an autosomal recessive trait, which is confirmed by the results of biochemical analyses. The mutant gene is responsible for synthesis of apolipoprotein C-II. The gene frequency in populations is presumably low but not yet known.

Clinical Characteristics

Since the apo C-II deficiency results in functional deficiency of LPL, the biochemical disturbance should, in theory, be similar to that of the primary LPL deficiency. The clinical and laboratory data reported thus far have revealed, however, that there are some exciting differences between the manifestations of the two disorders. Understanding these differences may possibly help to explain the pathogenesis of symptoms in familial LPL deficiency.

Compared to the patients with familial LPL deficiency, the homozygous apo C-II–deficient subjects have generally been detected at a relatively late age. The first proband was 59 years old at diagnosis, and the age of the reported cases has varied from 13 to 60 years. Yet the symptoms have often been traced back to childhood or adolescence, but they have apparently not been as severe as in many patients with familial LPL deficiency. In the original family, reported from Toronto, the mean age at onset of symptoms was 10 years [132], but the Japanese patients were free of all symptoms at the ages of 13 and 15 [133] and the proband of the English family was symptomless at 30 years [36a].

The leading symptom in the reported C-II-deficient patients has been recurrent abdominal pain, apparently caused by repeated attacks of acute pancreatitis. The prevalence of pancreatitis in the Canadian kindred was found to be as high as 64 percent [132], which is clearly more than the reported frequency of pancreatitis in familial LPL–deficient patients [134].

One presumed homozygote had died of acute pancreatitis. The index patient of the Canadian family had suffered repeated attacks of pancreatitis, as a result of which he developed chronic pancreatic insufficiency with insulin-dependent diabetes, peripheral neuropathy, diabetic retinopathy, and steatorrhea [7].

In view of the high risk of acute pancreatitis in homozygous apo C-II deficiency, it is remarkable that these patients suffer few of the other clinical manifestations which are common in patients with familial LPL deficiency. Thus, apo C-II–deficient patients do not show xanthomas or hepatomegaly, and only 3 of 14 had splenomegaly. In contrast, anemia, which is infrequent in primary LPL deficiency, was found in 8 of the 14 patients in the Canadian family [132]. The type and pathogenesis of the anemia is not clear; increased polychromatophilia of red cells has been reported as suggestive evidence of hemolysis [132]. There is no evidence for premature atherosclerosis in these patients.

The striking differences observed between the clinical manifestations of apo C-II deficiency and familial LPL deficiency so far have no adequate explanation. Apart from pancreatitis, the former condition shows milder symptoms, which might be related either to a less severe defect in the clearance of chylomicrons and VLDL or to a habitual low-fat diet eaten by the Japanese and Canadian families. The biochemical findings point to the former possibility.

Lipids and Lipoproteins

The homozygous apo C-II–deficient subjects have markedly elevated fasting plasma triglyceride levels when eating an unrestricted diet. The reported values range from 500 to 9500 mg/dl, but most patients have triglyceride levels between 1000 and 3000 mg/dl. A major portion of the excess triglyceride is in the chylomicron fraction, but there is also a regular increase of VLDL. Furthermore, the chylomicrons are principally of the small-sized variety, possessing flotation rates of 400 to 5000 S_f units and pre-β mobility on electrophoresis [7]. The VLDL cholesterol concentrations are regularly above the normal range, while the LDL and HDL cholesterol levels are very low [36, 36a, 133, 135], as in familial LPL deficiency. The relative triglyceride content of the LDL and HDL fractions is increased above normal [36a, 135]. Both HDL_2 and HDL_3 subfractions are reduced, as is also total plasma apoprotein A-1 concentration [36, 36a]. The characteristic lipoprotein pattern of apo C-II–deficient patients is thus intermediate between types 1 and 5, even though by strict criteria it should be classified as type 5.

The obligate heterozygotes for apo C-II deficiency usually have normal plasma lipid and lipoprotein concentrations [36, 131, 133]. However, when compared as a group with a normal population of similar age and sex, the heterozygotes appear to have significantly increased average levels of total triglycerides and VLDL cholesterol and decreased HDL cholesterol [132]. An occasional case of hyperchylomicronemia in a heterozygote has been detected [132], and it is possible that a delayed clearance of alimentary fat is present in heterozygote subjects, although it is not reflected as elevated levels in blood taken after an overnight fast.

Why then do patients with apo C-II deficiency and those with primary LPL deficiency show a partially different lipoprotein pattern in spite of a similar functional enzyme defect? There is no straightforward answer to this question, but a likely possibility is that the ability to degrade chylomicrons is partially retained in patients with apo C-II deficiency but is virtually absent in primary LPL deficiency. Since apo C-II is not necessary for binding LPL to its substrate and the enzyme has some (although low) activity in the absence of apo C-II, a normal catabolism of triglyceride-rich lipoproteins might continue at a slow rate in apo C-II–deficient patients but not in those with LPL deficiency. The small-sized chylomicrons and VLDL might arise as intermediate products of this slow catabolism, but accumulate in plasma because of the severely insufficient removal capacity.

Diagnosis

A deficiency of apo C-II may be verified either directly by electrophoresis of the tetramethylurea-soluble VLDL apoproteins (see Chap. 29) or indirectly by assay of LPL activity in postheparin plasma, with and without the addition of normal plasma or apo C-II. The amount of lipase activator can be titrated by adding increasing volumes of the plasma to guinea pig postheparin plasma [110] or to skim milk, both of which contain LPL but no apo C-II or other cofactors. No apo C-II has been detected in any of the affected members of the apo C-II-deficient families [36, 131, 133, 135] (Fig. 30-5). In accordance with this, plasma of the patients is totally devoid of the LPL cofactor activity, but there is a small amount of LPL activity present in postheparin plasma [7, 133]. Obligate heterozygotes have VLDL apo C-II concentrations of about 30 to 50 percent of normal values. As a result, the apo C-II/C-III ratio is reduced to about one-half of normal, and the ability to activate milk lipoprotein lipase is approximately 50 percent of the corresponding normal value, even though some overlapping exists between heterozygotes and normals [133, 135].

Treatment

The hypertriglyceridemia of apo C-II–deficient patients responds to moderate restriction of dietary fat, which remains the treatment of choice in prevention of the recurrent attacks of pancreatitis. In a symptomatic patient with excessive hyperlipemia an acute remission may be obtained by transfusion of 1 or 2 units of normal human plasma, which raises the plasma apo C-II levels to only 5 to 10 percent of the normal range, but this is enough for reducing the plasma triglyceride concentrations to near normal levels. The synthetic peptide fragments (residues 55 to 78) of apo C-II, which possess the cofactor activity, may become a useful replacement therapy in the future [128] and serve then as a good example of a successful correction of an identified molecular defect.

FAMILIAL TYPE 5 HYPERLIPOPROTEINEMIA

Type 5 hyperlipoproteinemia is defined as a disorder of lipoprotein metabolism with fasting chylomicronemia and elevated levels of VLDL [1]. This lipoprotein abnormality may be a primary familial disease, or it may be secondary to a variety of conditions, such as diabetes, alcoholism, nephrotic syn-

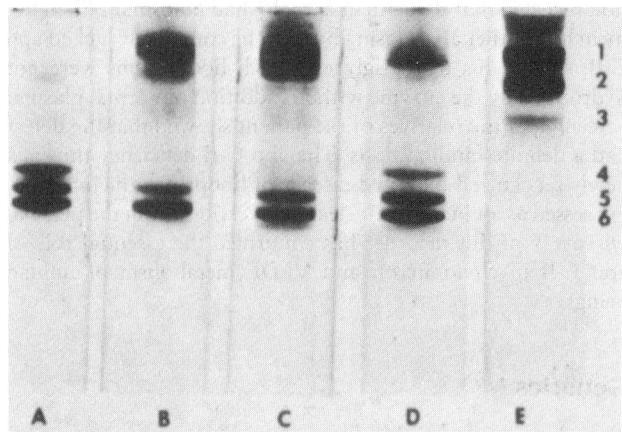

Figure 30-5 Apoprotein pattern of a patient with apo C-II deficiency. Polyacrylamide gel electrophoresis of tetramethylurea-soluble apoproteins. Gel A represents VLDL from a normal subject; gel B shows chylomicrons; and gel C, VLDL from the patient with apolipoprotein C-II deficiency; gel D shows a mixture of VLDL from the patient and a normal subject; and gel E shows HDL from the patient.

Band 1 denotes apolipoprotein E; band 2, apolipoprotein A-I; band 3, apolipoprotein A-II; band 4, apolipoprotein C-II; band 5, apolipoprotein C-III₁; and band 6, apolipoprotein C-III₂. *(From Breckenridge et al. [7]. Used by permission.)*

drome, or hypothyroidism. Depending on the degree of hypertriglyceridemia, the fasting plasma appears opalescent to milky, and the clinical picture shows many similarities to familial LPL deficiency. Biochemically, the type 5 disease seems to be closely related to type 4 hyperlipoproteinemia and by an appropriate treatment a type 5 pattern can be converted to type 4. Yet there are a number of arguments suggesting that primary type 5 hyperlipoproteinemia is a genetic syndrome (certainly not a single disease) separate from familial type 4 hypertriglyceridemia.

Type 5 is a relatively uncommon disorder but not as rare as familial LPL deficiency. In population screenings of small scale, it is often not found at all, since the prevalence among males is 0.2 to 0.3 percent [140–142] and among females, still smaller. A higher frequency is found among populations that are selected on the basis of ischemic heart disease [143].

Historical Aspects

Obvious cases with primary type 5 hyperlipoproteinemia were described over the years under different names, including idiopathic hyperlipemia, essential hyperlipemia, primary xanthomatous hyperlipemia, mixed hyperlipemia, or fat- and carbohydrate-induced hyperlipemia. These were not clearly distinguished from type 1 hyperlipoproteinemia, and some may have been mixed with type 3 hyperlipoproteinemia before the introduction of the lipoprotein classification system. There was also some confusion in the separation of primary and secondary forms of type 5. Such separation is not feasible without family screening and may remain ambiguous even after that because factors causing secondary hyperlipemia can be superimposed on a primary genetic trait.

The first three kindreds with defined familial type 5 hyperlipoproteinemia were presented by Fredrickson and Lees in 1966 [9]. Up to the 1972 edition of this book the number of type 5 families studied at the National Institutes of Health (NIH) had increased to 22, and in 1977 Greenberg et al. published a detailed analysis of 32 kindreds identified by a type 5 proband at the NIH [144]. The latter study provides the best review thus far of clinical manifestations of the type 5 disorder in probands and their families. Other extensive compilations of primary type 5 patients have been reported by Lees et al. (24 patients) [11] and by Fallat and Glueck (17 patients) [145]. In addition, a number of published single case histories are documented by lipoprotein data and family screenings [106, 121, 146–151]. Other reported series of type 5 patients have not attempted to distinguish between the familial and acquired forms [152, 153].

Clinical Features

The presenting symptoms of type 5 are related to excessive chylomicronemia and are thus similar to those seen in patients with familial LPL deficiency, including eruptive xanthomatosis and episodic abdominal pains, with or without established pancreatitis. The two disorders differ in many respects, which may give important clues for diagnosis. In contrast to type 1, the onset of symptoms in type 5 patients dates to adulthood and even to middle age. Occasionally children with familial type 5 have been reported [10, 121, 151], but usually the disease is manifested between 20 and 50 years of age, males presenting earlier than females [11, 144]. The onset of clinical symptoms may be associated with some factor which in itself causes hypertriglyceridemia, such as pregnancy [154], use of estrogenic hormones [155], excessive alcohol consumption, rapid gain in body weight, or appearance of uncontrolled diabetes [145]. The increased risk of males to have symptoms at an earlier age may also be related to their physiologically higher triglyceride levels compared with those of females. Overweight is also a predisposing factor [11, 156], obviously because of the basic abnormality of triglyceride metabolism in obese people. Alcoholism, on the other hand, is not a characteristic feature of the type 5 families [144], but there seems to be a curious and so far unexplained clustering of diabetes, gout, and hypertension in these kindreds [11, 144]. The frequency of typical clinical manifestations in type 5 patients is shown in Table 30-3.

Pancreatitis Recurrent abdominal pain is the leading symptom in 50 to 75 percent of patients [10, 11]. It varies from

Table 30-3 Prevalence of symptoms and signs in patients with familial type 5 hyperlipoproteinemia

	Percent affected		
	Lees et al. [11]	Fallat & Glueck [145]	Greenberg et al. [144]
Abdominal pain	48	70	—
Pancreatitis	—	50	38
Eruptive xanthomatosis	41	33	34
Hepatosplenomegaly	24	57	—
Abnormal glucose tolerance	69	70	28
Hyperuricemia	52	47	40
Ischemic heart disease	24*	23	15

* = all atherosclerotic vascular disease.

mild to severe and may be a sign of acute pancreatitis or of hepatic or splenic distension or it may remain unexplained. The frequency of verified pancreatitis varies from 40 to 60 percent [144, 145] among the probands but is curiously low among the relatives, even in the presence of hyperlipoproteinemia [144]. The subjects with a history of pancreatitis have much higher average triglyceride levels than those without such a history, even when the former are studied between the attacks [144]. The pains may be severe enough to lead to surgical intervention, particularly since preoperative diagnosis of pancreatitis is often missed due to falsely normal amylase values [16]. Chronic pancreatitis or steatorrhea has not been found among type 5 subjects [144].

Xanthomas Occurrence of eruptive xanthomas is reported by one-third to one-half of the probands with familial type 5 disease [10, 157]. The lesions usually appear when triglyceride concentration exceeds 2000 mg/dl and fade rapidly upon correction of hyperlipemia [144, 156]. Tuberoeruptive xanthomatosis is rare in type 5 patients [11, 156], and such patients should be carefully screened for the possible presence of type 3 hyperlipoproteinemia (Chap. 32). Planar palmar xanthomas characteristic of type 3 are not found in type 5 patients [156].

Diabetes One of the typical features of the type 5 syndrome is a high prevalence of decreased glucose tolerance and of mild to moderate non-insulin-requiring diabetes. Abnormal glucose tolerance may be present in 80 percent of patients with type 5 [158], but usually the frequency is lower [11, 144, 145] (see Table 30-3). The impaired glucose tolerance is most common among women after 50 years of age but appears less frequently in men and in younger age groups [144]. The poor glucose tolerance is associated with hyperinsulinism and indicates the presence of insulin resistance [158]. The frequency of an exaggerated insulin response is much higher in type 5 than in type 4 patients and is not solely accounted for by associated obesity [158]. The mechanism of the development of insulin resistance in connection with greatly elevated triglyceride levels is obscure but may relate to the observed stimulation of insulin release by fat [159].

Since the type 5 pattern may also occur as a secondary phenomenon in uncontrolled diabetes, it is sometimes difficult to distinguish between the primary and secondary forms of type 5 in a diabetic patient. In fact, it has been suggested that diabetic patients with a triglyceride level consistently in excess of 400 mg/dl are likely to have a familial hyperlipoproteinemia [160]. A heavy family history of diabetes is often present in type 5 patients, even when the proband is not diabetic.

Hyperuricemia Elevated serum uric acid levels are present in 40 to 50 percent of type 5 probands, but these levels are also prevalent among relatives without hyperlipemia or in those with a type 4 pattern [144]. Symptoms of gout are reported by 10 to 20 percent of members of type 5 families, but gouty arthritis is rare.

Polyneuropathy Symptoms of peripheral polyneuropathy consisting of paresthesias, burning sensations, and mild to severe periodic aching pains in arms and legs are noted by many subjects with type 5 (or type 4) hyperlipemia [10, 11, 150, 160, 161]. In some patients the neurogenic pains in the extremities have been the prominent symptom, their intensity fluctuating in parallel with the degree of hypertriglycidemia [150]. The exact prevalence of neurologic symptoms is unknown, but obviously they are not uncommon. Because of the common occurrence of mild or moderate diabetes in these patients, it has been difficult to determine whether the neurologic disease represents diabetic neuropathy or a specific "hyperlipemic neuropathy," a term coined by Sandbank et al. [163]. Arguments for the latter view are as follows: (1) occurrence of neuropathy in nondiabetic patients also [162, 164], (2) demonstration of specific neural lesions by electron miscroscopy [163], and (3) duplication of similar abnormalities in peripheral nerves of rats with dietary fat-induced hyperlipemia [165]. A case of transient dementia in association with type 5 hyperlipoproteinemia has been recorded [166], but the etiological relationship remains doubtful.

Other Clinical Findings Other clinical abnormalities observed in patients with type 5 include general retinal lipemia (see above), patchy accumulation of lipids in the retina ("xanthomatous retinopathy" [150]), and occurrence of foam cells in bone marrow. Fatty infiltration of the parotid glands, leading to their bilateral enlargement, has been described in a type 5 patient, but this finding is probably more common in other forms of hypertriglyceridemia [167]. Enlarged parotid glands in type 5 patients may also occur combined with arthritic symptoms and dryness of eyes and mouth, making up a sicca-like syndrome which can be distinguished from a true Sjögren's syndrome by a normal histology of minor salivary glands [168]. The presence of decreased salivary flow and abnormal salivary scintiscan suggests that the condition arises by a mechanism similar to that of pancreatitis [168].

Lipids and Lipoproteins

During Unrestricted Diet The presence of chylomicrons in fasting blood makes the serum opalescent or turbid, the appearance varying from that of skim milk to cream. When the serum tube is kept overnight at +4°C, part of the chylomicrons float to the top; but in contrast to type 1 serum the infranatant remains more or less opaque, and no sharp boundary is formed between the top and bottom layers. Both chylomicron and VLDL concentrations vary widely according to the diet, but usually most of the excess triglycerides are in chylomicrons, with the VLDL level being relatively less elevated.

The plasma total triglyceride concentration in type 5 patients living on a free diet usually ranges from 600 to 3000 mg/dl, but values above 10,000 mg/dl are possible. There is no sharp, discriminating triglyceride limit between types 1 and 5. On the other hand, an elevation of total cholesterol level above the normal range is the rule in type 5 patients but is rare in type 1. Calculation of the cholesterol/triglyceride ratio for total plasma may be helpful in a preliminary differentiation of type 5 from the other hypertriglyceridemias. In mass units this ratio is usually between 0.2 and 0.5 [11, 169], but in cases with very high triglyceride levels the ratio may be less than 0.2, overlapping with values of type 1. Plasma cholesterol/triglyceride ratios exceeding 0.5 during an unmodified diet suggest the presence of type 4, 3, or 2b hypertriglyceridemia rather than type 5 (see Chap. 29).

The lipoprotein pattern in familial type 5 patients includes, besides chylomicronemia, an excess VLDL level and subnormal concentrations of LDL and HDL (Fig. 30-6). Chylomicrons of all size (density) classes are present, but there is a shift toward the smaller particles approaching the size and density of VLDL. As the increase within VLDL occurs predominantly in the least dense particles with $S_f = 100$ to 400 [34, 170], there is actually an accumulation of a continuum of particles ranging from largest VLDL to smaller and medium-sized chylomicrons without sharp separation of the two fractions. In lipoprotein electrophoresis of whole plasma or of an isolated, $d < 1.006$ g/ml fraction, this population of particles often gives rise to a broad, continuous fraction extending from the origin to the pre-β region [34, 169]. The concentrations of LDL and HDL in type 5 patients vary from very low to normal, being roughly reciprocally related to the degree of the triglyceride abnormality. The LDL cholesterol values range from 10 to 180 mg/dl and the HDL cholesterol from 10 to 50 mg/dl, the average for both being approximately 50 percent of the mean of healthy control subjects [8]. The LDL apo B levels are also decreased but to a lesser extent than the LDL cholesterol levels [171, 172]. On the other hand, the apo C-II levels are high [173].

Changes with Diet The lipoprotein pattern of type 5 patients can be altered by changing the intake of either fat or carbohydrate or of total calories, but the responses are much less dramatic than those seen in type 1 patients. During deprivation of all food the chylomicrons disappear and the VLDL concentrations are reduced, there being a simultaneous shift from large ($S_f = 100$ to 400) to smaller ($S_f = 20$ to 100) VLDL particles and an increase of LDL [170]. A similar response can be obtained by a reduction of either fat or carbohydrate intake without replacement [38] or by giving medium-chain fatty acids in the form coconut oil [170]. With these manipulations chylomicronemia is greatly decreased; but if calories are balanced by substituting carbohydrate for fat, the VLDL level is

Figure 30-6 Electrophoretic *(top)* and ultracentrifugal *(bottom)* pattern of plasma lipoproteins in type 5 hyperlipoproteinemia as compared to normal. The chylomicron and VLDL (pre-β) levels are increased, while the LDL (β) and HDL (α) levels are subnormal.

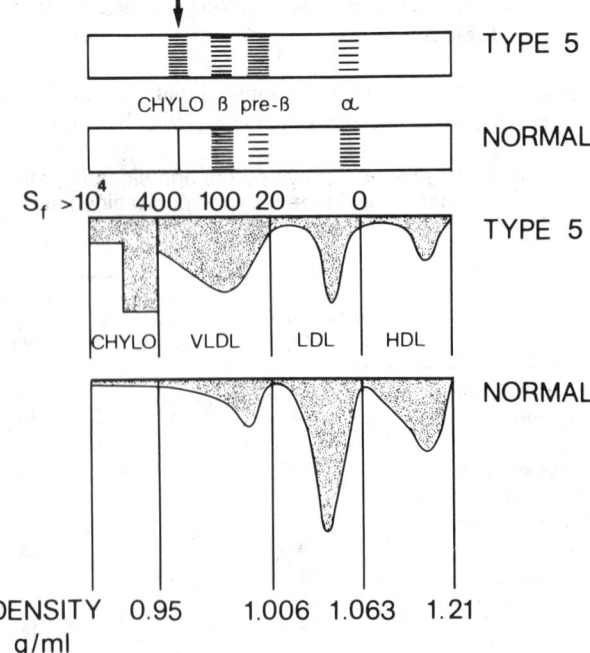

increased and chylomicrons will reappear [38]. Thus, the lipoprotein abnormalities of type 5 respond favorably to caloric restriction, but some reversal occurs as soon as an isocaloric diet is reinstituted, irrespective of whether it is made up of fat or carbohydrate. The low HDL concentrations in type 5 are relatively resistant to dietary changes [170, 174].

Arterial Disease

A typical type 5 syndrome is associated with a number of abnormalities that are known to predispose to premature atherosclerotic vascular disease. These include elevated VLDL and decreased HDL levels, hyperglycemia, hyperinsulinemia, hyperuricemia, and hypertension. It is thus likely that these patients carry a particularly high risk of coronary heart disease and peripheral vascular disease. Evidence for this remains controversial, and the relative rarity of the disorder prevents collection of sufficient epidemiologic data. Many type 5 patients are detected at middle age on the basis of symptoms of coronary heart disease, and several cases with extensive coronary atherosclerosis have been described [149, 150, 153, 175, 176]. A high prevalence of peripheral arterial disease [177] or coronary heart disease [145] has been recorded among type 5 probands, but in the families registered at NIH arterial disease was not a prominent feature [144]. Among patients with verified ischemic heart disease, type 5 is also rare, but the reported rates of 1 to 2 percent [143, 178] are many times higher than the frequency of type 5 in the general population.

Genetics

The familial nature of primary type 5 hyperlipoproteinemia is well documented [10, 121, 144, 145]. Hypertriglyceridemia is commonly found in parents, sibs, and children of type 5 probands, but many of the affected relatives have "only" a type 4 pattern. Among 181 first-degree relatives of 32 type 5 probands registered at NIH, 16 percent had a type 5 abnormality and 15 to 30 percent showed the type 4 pattern, the overall frequency of hypertriglyceridemia in the kindreds being around 50 percent [144]. In another study, 44 percent of sibs and offspring of type 5 probands had hypertriglyceridemia, usually of type 4 and in only a few cases type 5 [145]. There is thus a definite aggregation of severe hypertriglyceridemia in the families of type 5 patients. Another peculiar feature is the unusually high prevalence of adult-onset diabetes among many type 5 kindreds.

The pattern of inheritance of the type 5 disorder is not clear. The published data are most consistent with autosomal dominant transmission, but it is unclear why the abnormal trait is variably expressed as type 4 or type 5, which remains the same if no intervention is made [144]. That the type 5 pattern is more common in males and adults than in females and adolescents suggests that some physiologic mechanisms may interfere with the genetic factor and determine the phenotype to be either 4 or 5. The presence of individuals with type 5 lipoprotein phenotype is the hallmark for type 5 disorder, distinguishing it from familial hypertriglyceridemia, in which all affected family members show a type 4 pattern. Yet type 5 disease is likely to be heterogeneous, and some forms may be close to that of familial hypertriglyceridemia.

Biochemical Defect

The possible biochemical defect(s) underlying primary type 5 disorder has not been identified and is therefore a matter of speculation only. It seems likely that the primary abnormality involves an increase of VLDL, which secondarily leads to an accumulation of chylomicrons. Since the latter particles have catabolic pathways in common with VLDL (at least those involving lipoprotein lipase), the expanding VLDL mass and particle number progressively restrict the clearance of chylomicrons [89], until it is slow enough to retain in morning plasma chylomicrons formed during the preceding day. Upon reduction of fat intake the chylomicrons can temporarily disappear (phenotype is converted from 5 to 4), but if the VLDL is simultaneously increased by replacing the dietary fat with carbohydrate, the chylomicrons may soon reappear. Thus, the chylomicronemia could be only a consequence of an extreme rise in VLDL level, saturating the LPL (or possible other removal pathway) by its large number of particles. Subtypes may exist among type 5 patients (families) whose defect affects the clearance of chylomicrons more than of VLDL.

Kinetic studies using radiolabeled VLDL are not very useful in assessing the nature of the metabolic defect, since they are by necessity carried out in patients having very high concentrations and a greatly expanded pool size of VLDL, which secondarily overloads the catabolic pathways. Indeed, type 5 subjects have been shown to have extremely low fractional catabolic rates of VLDL apo B or triglyceride [179, 180]. They also exhibit a moderate increase of VLDL production (= total catabolic rate), but this is not essentially different from that of type 4 patients, who show much smaller elevations of VLDL [179]. Thus, in relation to their VLDL synthetic rates, the type 5 patients have disproportionally high VLDL concentrations, which suggests a defect in the clearance of VLDL. This pathogenetic mechanism could also explain the low LDL and HDL levels. The increased VLDL production seen in these patients may simply be a consequence of obesity, which is known to stimulate VLDL synthesis [181]. The fractional conversion of VLDL apo B to LDL apo B is normal in type 5 [180], as is the synthetic rate of LDL apo B [171, 172, 182]. The fractional catabolic rate of LDL apo B is increased [171, 180, 182], but it is not known whether this is a primary abnormality or reflects only the diminished LDL pool.

The reasons for the poor clearance of VLDL in type 5 remain obscure. There is little evidence for any structural anomalies of the lipoprotein, even though such defects may be difficult to prove. It has been postulated that type 5 VLDL is abnormal [183] and stimulates LPL much less than normal VLDL [184], but these findings have not been confirmed. LPL activity in postheparin plasma of type 5 patients is reported to be normal with few exceptions [102, 144, 145, 151]. Also, the postheparin plasma histaminase activity, which is low in type 1 patients, exhibits normal values in type 5 subjects [122]. However, low values of LPL have been observed in several patients with type 5 using a specific antiserum assay for postheparin plasma [105, 106] or performing assays from adipose tissue [108]. As an example of the heterogeneity of the syndrome Kwiterowich et al. have reported two families with type 5 disease, one of which had about 50 percent deficiency of LPL, while the other had values within the normal range [121]. We have assayed LPL from heparin eluates of adipose tissue and skeletal muscle of five patients with familial type 5 and found consistently subnormal values (Table 30-4) [76]. It is thus possible that in type 5 patients the LPL is deficient selectively in some tissues but not in all, and therefore the defect is not reflected in postheparin plasma. Why then do patients with total LPL deficiency accumulate chylomicrons and not VLDL, while subjects with partial deficiency behave in an opposite way? This crucial question cannot be answered presently, but it is probably relevant that apo C-II deficiency with normal but nonfunctional LPL gives rise to a type 5 and not to a type 1 pattern.

Diagnosis

Severe hypertriglyceridemia with the type 5 lipoprotein pattern is often secondary to other conditions, of which heavy drinking is probably the most common [185–187]. Diagnosis of familial type 5 hyperlipoproteinemia cannot be made by exclusion of other causes only; it must be based on lipid and lipoprotein analyses of first-degree relatives, preferably of adults. Differentiation between types 1 and 5 may sometimes be conjectural for several reasons: (1) LPL-deficient type 1 subjects may have increased levels of VLDL, and (2) type 5 subjects may exhibit low LPL activities. Particularly, the patients with apo C-II deficiency exhibit a type 5 rather than a type 1 pattern [7, 133, 135]. Difficulties may also be encountered in distinguishing familial hypertriglyceridemia (type 4) from familial type 5. On the other hand, type 5 is seldom confused with type 3 or with familial combined hyperlipemia. In the latter disorder, different affected relatives in the same family can have one of several lipoprotein patterns (e.g., types 2a, 2b, or 4) (see Chap. 33).

Treatment

Treatment of type 5 hyperlipoproteinemia by diet alone or in combination with drugs is usually not very successful in bringing plasma lipoprotein levels to within a normal range. It will, however, considerably reduce the excessive hypertriglyceridemia, which is usually enough to prevent attacks of pancreatitis and to keep the patient free of symptoms. Thus, long-term treatment of type 5 should be instituted and continued. Even though the response of type 5 hyperlipemia to diet is much less dramatic than that of type 1, dietary management forms the basis of treatment and only selected cases are further benefited from the combination of drugs.

The choice of the initial diet depends on the body weight and degree of hypertriglyceridemia. In obese patients with excessive chylomicronemia (triglyceride levels >1000 mg/dl), it is important to reduce fat intake to less than 50 g/day without substituting the calories from any other nutrient. A simultaneous reduction of carbohydrate intake with restriction of calories to 1000 to 1200/day is desirable. Alcohol intake should also be minimized, with particular attention being paid to elimination of drinking bouts. These interventions usually abolish chylomicronemia and reduce serum VLDL levels, keeping the total triglyceride level between 250 to 750 mg/dl, as long as the weight reduction continues. In nonobese patients the proportion of calories derived from fat is reduced to about 30 percent, leaving 50 percent to carbohydrate and 20 percent for protein. Alcohol and large single meals are avoided. Careful dietary control of triglycerides is needed in women during pregnancy [154] and during use of estrogens [155].

Table 30-4 Lipoprotein lipase activity in adipose tissue, skeletal muscle, and postheparin plasma in males with type 5 hyperlipoproteinemia and in weight-matched normolipemic males (mean ± SEM)

LPL activity in	Type 5 (n = 8)	Controls (n = 28)
Adipose tissue*	0.92 ± 0.20‡	2.16 ± 0.26
Skeletal muscle*	0.30 ± 0.04‡	0.85 ± 0.10
Postheparin plasma†	15.2 ± 0.90§	21.6 ± 1.02

* μmol FFA per hour per gram.
† μmol FFA per hour per milliliter.
‡ $p < 0.001$.
§ $p < 0.05$ for the difference from controls.
SOURCE: Taskinen and Nikkilä [60].

Use of polyunsaturated fats with an increased dietary P/S ratio does not seem to offer any advantages in treating type 5 hyperlipoproteinemia. In contrast, medium-chain fatty acids given either as an artificial mixture (MCT) or as natural fat (coconut oil) seem to be effective in reducing the raised VLDL levels and abolishing chylomicronemia [121, 170].

The average response of plasma lipoprotein abnormalities of type 5 to currently available drugs is far from excellent, and some cases may be completely resistant or the effect is transient. The result is unpredictable, and, therefore, all patients who are not adequately controlled with diet should be given a trial of medical treatment. The first choice is nicotinic acid, which, if tolerated, may lead to a dramatic fall in triglycerides and to a rise in LDL and HDL levels [188, 189]. The increase in HDL particularly adds to the merits of using nicotinic acid as the first drug, since this change is not achieved by diet [170, 174] or other drugs [190]. The effect of nicotinic acid on VLDL and HDL may be based on the induction of lipoprotein lipase activity [191] or of fatty acid esterification in adipose tissue ("FIAT") [189]. Clofibrate and related drugs are not particularly effective in reducing the triglyceride levels of type 5 patients [192]. A few cases do respond favorably, and a trial of 4 to 6 weeks' duration is therefore worthwhile in cases where nicotinic acid has failed.

Steroid hormones with androgenic, anabolic, or progestational activity have been found to reduce type 5 hyperlipoproteinemia [190, 193]. Norethindrone acetate may strikingly reduce triglyceride levels in women but is not very effective in men [193]. Oxandrolone, an anabolic steroid with androgenic activity, decreases triglyceride and cholesterol levels in both sexes but fails to increase HDL cholesterol [190]. Even normal lipid levels may be attained by the latter drug [190]. The mechanism of suppression of elevated VLDL levels by androgenic steroids is not understood, but these steroids are known to increase dramatically the postheparin plasma hepatic lipase activity [194]. Since this lipase has some activity against VLDL triglycerides [91], it may be speculated that the androgens open up the alternative hepatic lipolytic pathway for VLDL when it is not adequately catabolized through the normal lipoprotein lipase route.

REFERENCES

1. BEAUMONT J, CARLSON LA, COOPER G, FEJAR Z, FREDRICKSON DS, STRASSER T: Classification of hyperlipidemias and hyperlipoproteinemias. *Bull WHO* 43:891, 1970

2. BÜRGER M, GRÜTZ O: Über hepatosplenomegale Lipoidose mit xanthomatösen Veränderungen in Haut und Schleimhaut. *Arch Dermatol Syph* 166:542, 1932

3. HOLT LE JR, AYLWARD FX, TIMBRES HG: Idiopathic familial lipemia. *Bull Johns Hopkins Hosp* 64:279, 1939

4. MALMROS H, SWAHN B, TRUEDSSON E: Essential hyperlipaemia. *Acta Med Scand* 149:91, 1954

5. NIKKILÄ EA, OJALA K, TURUNEN M: Adipose tissue metabolism and enzymes in idiopathic hyperlipemia. *Circulation* 26:664, 1962

6. HAVEL RJ, GORDON RS JR: Idiopathic hyperlipemia: Metabolic studies in an affected family. *J Clin Invest* 39:1777, 1960

7. BRECKENRIDGE WC, LITTLE JA, STEINER, G, CHOW A, POAPST M: Hypertriglyceridemia associated with deficiency of apolipoprotein C-II. *N Engl J Med* 298:1265, 1978

8. FREDRICKSON DS, GOLDSTEIN JL, BROWN MS: The familial hyperlipoproteinemias, in Stanbury JB, Wyngaarden JB, Fredrickson DS (eds): *The Metabolic Basis of Inherited Disease*, 4th ed. New York, McGraw-Hill, 1978, p 604

9. FREDRICKSON DS, LEES RS: Familial hyperlipoproteinemia, in Stanbury JB, Wyngaarden JB, Fredrickson DS (eds): *The Metabolic Basis of Inherited Disease*, 2nd ed. New York, McGraw-Hill, 1966, p 429

10. FREDRICKSON DS, LEVY RI: Familial hyperlipoproteinemia, in Stanbury, JB, Wyngaarden JB, Fredrickson DS (eds): *The Metabolic Basis of Inherited Disease*, 3rd ed. New York, McGraw-Hill, 1972, p 545

11. LEES RS, WILSON DE, SCHONFELD G, FLEET S: The familial dyslipoproteinemias, in Steinberg AG, Bearn AG (eds): *Progress in Medical Genetics*. New York, Grune & Stratton, 1973, vol 9, p 237

12. BROWN WV, GRETEN H: Type I hyperlipoproteinaemia, in Rifkind BM (ed): *Clinics in Endocrinology and Metabolism*, vol 2, *Disorders of Lipid Metabolism*. London, Saunders, 1973, p 73

13. BROWN WV, BAGINSKY ML, EHNHOLM C: Primary type I and type V hyperlipoproteinemia, in Rifkind BM, Levy RI (eds): *Hyperlipidemia: Diagnosis and Therapy*. New York/San Francisco/London, Grune & Stratton, 1977, p 93

14. PARKER F, BAGDADE JD, ODLAND GF, BIERMAN EL: Evidence for the chylomicron origin of lipids accumulating in diabetic eruptive xanthomas: A correlative lipid biochemical, histochemical, and electron microscopic study. *J Clin Invest* 49:2172, 1970

15. KLATSKIN G, GORDON MD: Relationship between relapsing pancreatitis and essential hyperlipemia. *Am J Med* 12:3, 1952

16. FALLAT RW, VESTER JW, GLUECK CJ: Suppression of amylase activity by hypertriglyceridemia. *J Am Med Assoc* 225:1331, 1973

17. LESSER PB, WARSHAW AL: Diagnosis of pancreatitis masked by hyperlipemia. *Ann Intern Med* 82:795, 1975

18. POULSEN HM: Familial lipemia, a new form of lipoidosis showing increase in neutral fats combined with attacks of acute pancreatitis. *Acta Med Scand* 138:413, 1950

19. LÖFFLER A, FILIPPINI L, PULVER W: Exokrine Pankreasinsuffizienz bei familiärer Hyperlipoproteinämie. *Schweiz Med Wochenschr* 101:634, 1971

20. KRAUSS RM, LEVY AG: Subclinical chronic pancreatitis in type I hyperlipoproteinemia. *Am J Med* 62:144, 1977

21. CAMERON JL, CAPUZZI DM, ZUIDEMA GD, MARGOLIS S: Acute pancreatitis with hyperlipemia: The incidence of lipid abnormalities in acute pancreatitis. *Ann Surg* 177:483, 1973

22. CAMERON JL, CAPUZZI DM, ZUIDEMA GD, MARGOLIS S: Acute pancreatitis with hyperlipemia. Evidence for a persistent defect in lipid metabolism. *Am J Med* 56:482, 1974

23. FARMER RG, WINKELMAN EI, BROWN HB, LEWIS LA: Hyperlipoproteinemia and pancreatitis. *Am J Med* 54:161, 1973

24. HAVEL RJ: Pathogenesis, differentiation and management of hypertriglyceridemia. *Adv Intern Med* 15:117, 1969

25. FERRANS VJ, BUJA LM, ROBERTS WC, FREDRICKSON DS: The spleen in type I hyperlipoproteinemia. Histochemical, biochemical, microfluorometric and electron microscopic observations. *Am J Pathol* 64:67, 1971

26. FERRANS VJ, ROBERTS WC, LEVY RI, FREDRICKSON DS: Chylomicrons and the formation of foam cells in type I hyperlipoproteinemia. A morphologic study. *Am J Pathol* 70:253, 1973

27. MOREAU PG, PICHON P, RIFLE G: Manifestations choriorétiniennes des hyperlipidémies. La rétinopathie hyperlipidémique. A propos de 44 observations. *Sem Hop* 46:3467, 1970

28. HENKENS HE, HOUTSMULLER AJ, BOS PJM, CRONE RA: Fundus changes in primary hyperlipaemia. *Ophthalmologica* 173:190, 1976

29. DE GENNES J-L, MÉNAGÉ J-J, TRUFFERT J: Hyperglycéridémie exogène (hyperchylomicronémie) essentielle de type I. Etude clinique et évolutive de cinq observations. *Nouv Presse Med* 1:1835, 1972

30. BOGGS JD: The genetic mechanism of idiopathic hyperlipemia. *N Engl J Med* 257:1101, 1957

31. KRAMER A: Essentielle Hyperlipaemie und Myokardinfarkt im jugendlichen Alter. *Z Kreisl Forsch* 49:497, 1960

32. POTTER JM, MACDONALD WB: Primary type I hyperlipoproteinaemia—A metabolic and family study. *Aust NZ J Med* 9:688, 1979

33. FURMAN RH, HOWARD RP, BRUSCO OJ, ALAUPOVIC P: Effects of medium chain length triglyceride (MCT) on serum lipids and lipoproteins in familial hyperchylomicronemia (dietary fat-induced lipemia) and dietary carbohydrate-accentuated lipemia. *J Lab Clin Med* 66:912, 1965

34. FREDRICKSON DS, LEVY RI, LINDGREN FT: A comparison of heritable abnormal lipoprotein patterns as defined by two different techniques. *J Clin Invest* 47:2446, 1968

35. KASHYAP ML, SRIVASTAVA LS, TSANG RC, TASKINEN MR, HYND BA, PERISUTTI G, BRADY DW, GLUECK CJ, AHUMADA CA, MCCARTHY JA, SOSA RA, REEDS TO: Apolipoprotein CII in type I hyperlipoproteinemia. *J Lab Clin Med* 95:180, 1980

36. CREPALDI G, FELLIN R, BAGGIO G, AUGUSTIN J, GRETEN H: Lipoprotein and apoprotein, adipose tissue and hepatic lipoprotein lipase levels in patients with familial hyperchylomicronemia and their immediate family members, in Gotto AM Jr, Smith LC, Allen B (eds): *Atherosclerosis V*. New York, Springer-Verlag, 1980, p 250

36a. MILLER NE, RAO SN, ALAUPOVIC P, NOBLE N, SLACK J, BRUNZELL JD, LEWIS B: Familial apolipoprotein C II deficiency: Plasma lipoproteins and apolipoproteins in heterozygous and homozygous subjects and the effects of plasma infusion. *Eur J Clin Invest* 11:69, 1981

37. BERMAN M, HALL M III, LEVY RI, EISENBERG S, BILHEIMER DW, PHAIR RD, GOEBEL RH: Metabolism of apoB and apoC lipoproteins in man: Kinetic studies in normal and hyperlipoproteinemic subjects. *J Lipid Res* 19:38, 1978

38. BRUNZELL JD, HAZZARD WR, PORTE D JR, BIERMAN EL: Evidence for a common saturable, triglyceride removal mechanism for chylomicrons and very low density lipoproteins in man. *J Clin Invest* 52:1578, 1973

39. MANCINI M, MATTOCK M, RABAYA E, CHAIT A, LEWIS B: Studies of the mechanisms of carbohydrate-induced lipaemia in normal man. *Atherosclerosis* 17:445, 1973

40. TYTGAT GN, RUBIN CE, SAUNDERS DR: Synthesis and transport of lipoprotein particles by intestinal absorptive cells in man. *J Clin Invest* 50:2065, 1971

41. FRIEDMAN HI, CARDELL RR JR: Morphological evidence for the release of chylomicra from intestinal absorptive cells. *Exp Cell Res* 75:57, 1972

42. GREEN PHR, GLICKMAN RM, SAUDEK CD, BLUM CB, TALL AR: Human intestinal lipoproteins—Studies in chyluric subjects. *J Clin Invest* 64:233, 1979

43. LEWIS B, CHAIT A, FEBRUARY AW, MATTOCK M: Functional overlap between "chylomicra" and "very low density lipoproteins" of human plasma during alimentary lipaemia. *Atherosclerosis* 17:455, 1973

44. BEIL FU, GRUNDY SM: Studies on plasma lipoproteins during absorption of exogenous lecithin in man. *J Lipid Res* 21:525, 1980

45. KOMPIANG, IP, BENSADOUN A, YAN MWW: Effect of an antilipoprotein lipase serum on plasma triglyceride removal. *J Lipid Res* 17:498, 1976

46. LUKENS TW, BORENSZTAJN J: Effects of C apoproteins on the activity of endothelium-bound lipoprotein lipase. *Biochem J* 175:1143, 1978

47. DECKELBAUM RJ, EISENBERG S, FAINARU M, BARENHOLZ Y, OLIVECRONA T: In vitro production of human plasma low density lipoprotein-like particles. *J Biol Chem* 254:6079, 1979

48. OLIVECRONA T, BENGTSSON G, MARKLUND S-E, LINDAHL U, HÖÖK M: Heparin-lipoprotein lipase interactions. *Fed Proc* 36:60, 1977

48a. SHIMADA K, GILL PJ, SILBERT JE, DOUGLAS WHJ, FANBURG BL: Involvement of cell surface heparin sulfate in the binding of lipoprotein lipase to cultured bovine endothelial cells. *J Clin Invest* 68:995, 1981

49. CUNNINGHAM VJ, ROBINSON DS: Clearing-factor lipase in adipose tissue. Distinction of different states of the enzyme and the possible role of the fat cell in the maintenance of tissue activity. *Biochem J* 112:203, 1969

50. CHAJEK T, STEIN O, STEIN Y: Rat heart in culture as a tool to elucidate the cellular origin of lipoprotein lipase. *Biochim Biophys Acta* 488:140, 1977

51. NILSSON-EHLE P, GARFINKEL AS, SCHOTZ MC: Lipolytic enzymes and plasma lipoprotein metabolism. *Ann Rev Biochem* 49:667, 1980

52. SCHOTZ MC, TWU J-S, PEDERSEN ME, CHEN C-H, GARFINKEL AS, BORENSZTAJN J: Antibodies to lipoprotein lipase. Application of perfused heart. *Biochim Biophys Acta* 489:214, 1977

53. HERNELL O, EGELRUD T, OLIVECRONA T: Serum-stimulated lipases (lipoprotein lipases). Immunological crossreaction between the bovine and the human enzymes. *Biochim Biophys Acta* 381:233, 1975

54. FIELDING CJ: Lipoprotein lipase: Evidence for high- and low-affinity enzyme sites. *Biochemistry* 15:879, 1976

55. FIELDING PE, SHORE VG, FIELDING CJ: Lipoprotein lipase, isolation and characterization of a second enzyme species from postheparin plasma. *Biochemistry* 16:1896, 1977

56. FIELDING CJ, HAVEL RJ: Lipoprotein lipase. *Arch Pathol Lab Med* 101:225, 1977

57. NILSSON-EHLE P, CARLSTRÖM S, BELFRAGE P: Rapid effects on lipoprotein lipase activity in adipose tissue of humans after carbohydrate and lipid

intake. Time course and relation to plasma glycerol, triglyceride and insulin levels. *Scand J Clin Lab Invest* 35:373, 1975

58. PYKÄLISTÖ OJ, SMITH PH, BRUNZELL JD: Determinants of human adipose tissue lipoprotein lipase. Effect of diabetes and obesity on basal- and diet-induced activity. *J Clin Invest* 56:1108, 1975

59. LITHELL H, BOBERG J, HELLSING K, LUNDQVIST G, VESSBY B: Lipoprotein-lipase activity in human skeletal muscle and adipose tissue in the fasting and the fed states. *Atherosclerosis* 30:89, 1978

60. TASKINEN M-R, NIKKILÄ EA: Unpublished observations

61. ROBINSON DS; The function of the plasma triglycerides in fatty acid transport, in Florkin M, Stotz EH (eds): *Comprehensive Biochemistry*, vol 18, *Lipid Metabolism*. Amsterdam, Elsevier, 1970, p 51

62. ECKEL RH, FUJIMOTO WY, BRUNZELL JD: Gastric inhibitory polypeptide enhanced lipoprotein lipase activity in cultured preadipocytes. *Diabetes* 28:1141, 1979

62a. WASADA T, MCCORKLE K, HARRIS V, KAWAI K, HOWARD B, UNGER RH: Effect of gastric inhibitory polypeptide on plasma levels of chylomicron triglycerides in dogs. *J Clin Invest* 68:1106, 1981

63. ZINDER O, HAMOSH M, FLECK TRC, SCOW RO: Effect of prolactin on lipoprotein lipase in mammary gland and adipose tissue of rats. *Am J Physiol* 226:744, 1974

64. BENSADOUN A, KOMPIANG IP: Role of lipoprotein lipase in plasma triglyceride removal. *Fed Proc* 38:2622, 1979

65. SCOW RO, HAMOSH M, BLANCHETTE-MACKIE EJ, EVANS AJ: Uptake of blood triglyceride by various tissues. *Lipids* 7:497, 1972

66. FIELDING CJ, HIGGINS JM: Lipoprotein lipase: Comparative properties of the membrane-supported and solubilized enzyme species. *Biochemistry* 13:4324, 1974

67. STEIN Y, STEIN O: Metabolism of plasma lipoproteins, in Gotto AM Jr, Smith LC, Allen B (eds): *Atherosclerosis V*. New York, Springer-Verlag, 1980, p 653

68. SCOW RO, BLANCHETTE-MACKIE EJ, SMITH LC: Role of capillary endothelium in the clearance of chylomicrons. A model for lipid transport from blood by lateral diffusion in cell membranes. *Circ Res* 39:149, 1976

69. NESTEL PJ, HAVEL RJ, BEZMAN A: Metabolism of constituent lipids of dog chylomicrons. *J Clin Invest* 42:1313, 1963

70. HAVEL RJ, KANE JP, KASHYAP ML: Interchange of apolipoproteins between chylomicrons and high density lipoproteins during alimentary lipemia in man. *J Clin Invest* 52:32, 1973

71. MJØS OD, FAERGEMAN O, HAMILTON RL, HAVEL RJ: Characterization of remnants produced during the metabolism of triglyceride-rich lipoproteins of blood plasma and intestinal lymph in the rat. *J Clin Invest* 56:603, 1975

72. TALL AR, GREEN PHR, GLICKMAN RM, RILEY JW: Metabolic fate of chylomicron phospholipids and apoproteins in the rat. *J Clin Invest* 64:977, 1979

73. REDGRAVE TG, SMALL DM: Quantitation of the transfer of surface phospholipid of chylomicrons to the high density lipoprotein fraction during the catabolism of chylomicrons in the rat. *J Clin Invest* 64:162, 1979

74. CHAJEK T, EISENBERG S: Very low density lipoprotein. Metabolism of phospholipids, cholesterol, and apolipoprotein C in the isolated perfused rat heart. *J Clin Invest* 61:1654, 1978

75. PATSCH JR, GOTTO AM JR, OLIVECRONA T, EISENBERG S: Formation of high density lipoprotein$_2$-like particles during lipolysis of very low density lipoproteins in vitro. *Proc Nat Acad Sci USA* 75:4519, 1978

76. TASKINEN M-R, NIKKILÄ EA: High density lipoprotein subfractions in relation to lipoprotein lipase activity in man—Evidence for reciprocal regulation of HDL$_2$ and HDL$_3$ levels by lipoprotein lipase. *Clin Chim Acta* 112:325, 1981

77. EISENBERG S: Origin in plasma of low density and high density lipoproteins, in Gotto AM Jr, Smith LC, Allen B (eds): *Atherosclerosis V*. New York, Springer-Verlag, 1980, p 146

78. NIKKILÄ EA: Metabolic and endocrine control of plasma high density lipoprotein concentrations. Relation to catabolism of triglyceride-rich lipoproteins, in Gotto AM Jr, Miller NE, Oliver MF (eds): *High Density Lipoproteins and Atherosclerosis*. Amsterdam, Elsevier, 1978, p 177

79. NIKKILÄ EA, TASKINEN M-R, KEKKI M: Relation of plasma high-density lipoprotein cholesterol to lipoprotein-lipase activity in adipose tissue and skeletal muscle of man. *Atherosclerosis* 29:497, 1978

80. NIKKILÄ EA: Dynamic regulation of plasma high-density lipoprotein concentrations: A concept of the function of HDL, in Hayase S, Murao S (eds): Proceedings of the VIII Congress of Cardiology, International Congress Series No. 470. Amsterdam, Excerpta Medica, 1979, p 198

81. NIKKILÄ EA, KUUSI T, HARNO K, TIKKANEN M, TASKINEN M-R: Lipoprotein lipase and hepatic endothelial lipase are key enzymes in the metabolism of plasma high density lipoproteins, particularly of HDL$_2$, in Gotto AM Jr, Smith LC, Allen B (eds): *Atherosclerosis V*. New York, Springer-Verlag, 1980, p 387

82. SCOW RO, BLANCHETTE-MACKIE EJ, SMITH LC: Transport of lipid across capillary endothelium. *Fed Proc* 39:2610, 1980

83. HIGGINS JM, FIELDING CJ: Lipoprotein lipase. Mechanism of formation

of triglyceride-rich remnant particles from very low density lipoproteins and chylomicrons. *Biochemistry* 14:2288, 1975

84. BARTER PJ, NESTEL PJ: Precursor-product relationship between pools of very low density lipoprotein triglyceride. *J Clin Invest* 51:174, 1972

85. EISENBERG S, BILHEIMER DW, LEVY RI, LINDGREN FT: On the metabolic conversion of human plasma very low density lipoprotein to low density lipoprotein. *Biochim Biophys Acta* 326:361, 1973

85a. STREJA D, KALLAI MA, STEINER G: The metabolic heterogeneity of human very low density lipoprotein triglyceride. *Metabolism* 26:1333, 1977

85b. STEINER G, ILSE WK: Heterogeneity of VLDL triglyceride production by the liver and intestine. *Can J Biochem* 59:637, 1981

86. NESTEL PJ: Relationship between plasma triglycerides and removal of chylomicrons. *J Clin Invest* 43:943, 1964

87. REAVEN GM, HILL DB, GROSS RC, FARQUHAR JW: Kinetics of triglyceride turnover of very low density lipoproteins of human plasma. *J Clin Invest* 44:1826, 1965

88. NIKKILÄ EA, KEKKI M: Measurement of plasma triglyceride turnover in the study of hyperglyceridemia. *Scand J Clin Lab Invest* 27:97, 1971

89. GRUNDY SM, MOK HYI: Chylomicron clearance in normal and hyperlipidemic man. *Metabolism* 25:1225, 1976

90. FORD S JR, SCHUBERT WK, GLUECK CJ, BOZIAN RC: Familial hyperchylomicronemia. Enzymatic and physiologic studies. *Am J Med* 50:536, 1971

91. NICOLL A, LEWIS B: Evaluation of the role of lipoprotein lipase and hepatic lipase in lipoprotein metabolism: In vivo and vitro studies in man. *Eur J Clin Invest* 10:487, 1980

92. BRENNEMAN DE, SPECTOR AA: Utilization of ascites plasma very low density lipoprotein triglycerides by Ehrlich cells. *J Lipid Res* 15:309, 1974

93. HOWARD BV: Uptake of very low density lipoprotein triglyceride by bovine aortic endothelial cell in culture. *J Lipid Res* 18:561, 1977

94. NILSSON-EHLE P: Human lipoprotein lipase activity: Comparison of assay methods. *Clin Chim Acta* 54:283, 1974

95. PERSSON B, SMITH U, LARSSON B: A study of different methods for the assay of lipoprotein lipase activity in human adipose tissue. *Atherosclerosis* 22:425, 1975

96. PYKÄLISTÖ OJ, SMITH PH, BRUNZELL JD: Human adipose tissue lipoprotein lipase: Comparison of assay methods and expressions of activity. *Proc Soc Exp Biol Med* 148:297, 1975

97. LITHELL H, BOBERG J: A method of determining lipoprotein-lipase activity in human adipose tissue. *Scand J Clin Lab Invest* 37:551, 1977

98. TASKINEN M-R, NIKKILÄ EA, HUTTUNEN JK, HILDEN H: A micro-method for assay of lipoprotein lipase activity in needle biopsy samples of human adipose tissue and skeletal muscle. *Clin Chim Acta* 104:107, 1980

99. KUUSI T, NIKKILÄ EA, VIRTANEN I, KINNUNEN PKJ: Localization of the heparin-releasable lipase in situ in the rat liver. *Biochem J* 181:245, 1979

100. EHNHOLM C, SHAW W, GRETEN H, BROWN WV: Purification from human plasma of a heparin-released lipase with activity against triglyceride and phospholipids. *J Biol Chem* 250:6756, 1975

101. KRAUSS RM, WINDMUELLER HG, LEVY RI, FREDRICKSON DS: Selective measurement of two different triglyceride lipase activities in rat postheparin plasma. *J Lipid Res* 14:286, 1973

102. KRAUSS RM, LEVY RI, FREDRICKSON DS: Selective measurement of two lipase activities in postheparin plasma from normal subjects and patients with hyperlipoproteinemia. *J Clin Invest* 54:1107, 1974

103. GAGNÉ C, BRUN D, MOORJANI S, LUPIEN P-J: Hyperchylomicronémie familiale: Étude de láctivité lipolytique dans une famille. *Union Med Can* 106:333, 1977

104. HUTTUNEN JK, EHNHOLM C, KINNUNEN PKJ, NIKKILÄ EA: An immunochemical method for selective measurement of two triglyceride lipases in human postheparin plasma. *Clin Chim Acta* 63:335, 1975

105. HUTTUNEN JK, EHNHOLM C, KEKKI M, NIKKILÄ EA: Post-heparin plasma lipoprotein lipase and hepatic lipase in normal subjects and in patients with hypertriglyceridaemia: Correlations to sex, age and various parameters of triglyceride metabolism. *Clin Sci Mol Med* 50:249, 1976

106. GRETEN H, DEGRELLA R, KLOSE G, RASCHER W, DE GENNES JL, GJONE E: Measurement of two plasma triglyceride lipases by an immunochemical method: Studies in patients with hypertriglyceridemia. *J Lipid Res* 17:203, 1976

107. BOBERG J, AUGUSTIN J, BAGINSKY ML, TEJADA P, BROWN WV: Quantitative determination of hepatic and lipoprotein lipase activities from human postheparin plasma. *J Lipid Res* 18:544, 1977

108. PERSSON B: Lipoprotein lipase activity of human adipose tissue in health and in some diseases with hyperlipidemia as a common feature. *Acta Med Scand* 193:457, 1973

109. NIKKILÄ EA, TASKINEN M-R, REHUNEN S, HÄRKÖNEN M: Lipoprotein lipase activity in adipose tissue and skeletal muscle of runners: Relation to serum lipoproteins. *Metabolism* 27:1661, 1978

110. CHU P, MILLER AL, MILLS GL: Assay of an activator for lipoprotein lipase. *Clin Chim Acta* 66:281, 1976

111. BRUNZELL JD, CHAIT A, NIKKILÄ EA, EHNHOLM C, HUTTUNEN JK,

STEINER G: Heterogeneity of primary lipoprotein lipase deficiency. *Metabolism* 29:624, 1980

112. GANESAN D, BRADFORD RH, GANESAN G, McCONATHY WJ, ALAUPOVIC P, BASS HB: Purified postheparin plasma lipoprotein lipase in primary hyperlipoproteinemias. *J Appl Physiol* 39:1022, 1975

113. FIELDING PE, SHORE VG, FIELDING CJ: Lipoprotein lipase, isolation and characterization of a second enzyme species from postheparin plasma. *Biochemistry* 16:1896, 1977

114. HARLAN WR JR, WINESETT PS, WASSERMAN AJ: Tissue lipoprotein lipase in normal individuals and in individuals with exogenous hypertriglyceridemia and the relationship of this enzyme to assimilation of fat. *J Clin Invest* 46:239, 1967

115. LAMBERTS SWJ, CASPARIE AF, MIEDEMA K, HENNEMANN G, HULSMANS HAM: Thyroxine binding globulin deficiency in a family with type I hyperlipoproteinaemia. *Clin Endocrinol* 6:197, 1977

116. GLUECK CJ, KAPLAN AP, LEVY RI, GRETEN H, GRALNICK H, FREDRICKSON DS: A new mechanism of exogenous hyperglyceridemia. *Ann Intern Med* 71:1051, 1969

117. GLUECK CJ, LEVY RI, GLUECK HI, GRALNICK HR, GRETEN H, FREDRICKSON DS: Acquired type I hyperlipoproteinemia with systemic lupus erythematosus, dysglobulinemia and heparin resistance. *Am J Med* 47:318, 1969

118. HAGBERG B, HULTQUIST G, SVENNERHOLM L, VOSS H: Malignant hyperlipemia in infancy. *Am J Dis Child* 107:267, 1964

119. STAUFFER UG, HITZIG WH, ZAHLER P: Hyperlipämie bei malignen Erkrankungen. *Klin Wochenschr* 48:111, 1970

120. JAEKEN J, CASTEELS-VAN DAELE M, HARVENGT L, CORBEEL L, BROECKAERT-VAN ORSHOVEN A, VAN DAMME B, KENIS H, RECKELS R: A hyperlipemia syndrome in infancy with rapidly fatal evolution. *Helv Paediat Acta* 28:67, 1973

121. KWITEROVICH PO, FARAH JR, BROWN WV, BACHORIK PS, BAYLIN SB, NEILL CA: The clinical, biochemical, and familial presentation of type V hyperlipoproteinemia in childhood. *Pediatrics* 59:513, 1977

122. BAYLIN SB, BEAVEN MA, KRAUSS RM, KEISER HR: Response of plasma histaminase activity to small doses of heparin in normal subjects and patients with hyperlipoproteinemia. *J Clin Invest* 52:1985, 1973

123. LITTLE JA, WHAYNE TF, BHAGWAT AG, BUCKLEY GC, KALLOS A: A case of type I hyperlipoproteinemia unusually sensitive to dietary alcohol and fat with induction of lipemia. *Clin Res* 18:736, 1970

124. KORN ED: Clearing factor, a heparin-activated lipoprotein lipase. Substrate specificity and activation of coconut oil. *J Biol Chem* 215:15, 1955

125. LaROSA JC, LEVY RI, HERBERT P, LUX SE, FREDRICKSON DS: A specific apoprotein activator for lipoprotein lipase. *Biochem Biophys Res Commun* 41:57, 1970

126. BIER DM, HAVEL RJ: Activation of lipoprotein lipase by lipoprotein fractions of human serum. *J Lipid Res* 11:565, 1970

127. KINNUNEN PKJ, JACKSON RL, SMITH LC, GOTTO AM JR, SPARROW JT: Activation of lipoprotein lipase by native and synthetic fragments of human plasma apolipoprotein C-II. *Proc Nat Acad Sci USA* 74:4848, 1977

128. CATAPANO AL, KINNUNEN PKJ, BRECKENRIDGE WC, GOTTO AM JR, JACKSON RL, LITTLE JA, SMITH LC, SPARROW JT: Lipolysis of apoC-II deficient very low density lipoproteins: Enhancement of lipoprotein lipase action by synthetic fragments of apoC-II. *Biochem Biophys Res Commun* 89:951, 1979

129. MILLER AL, SMITH LC: Activation of lipoprotein lipase by apolipoprotein glutamic acid. Formation of a stable surface film. *J Biol Chem* 248:3359, 1973

130. FIELDING CJ: Kinetics of lipoprotein lipase activity: Effects of the substrate apoprotein on reaction velocity. *Biochem Biophys Acta* 316:66, 1973

131. COX DW, BRECKENRIDGE WC, LITTLE JA: Inheritance of apolipoprotein C-II deficiency with hypertriglyceridemia and pancreatitis. *N Engl J Med* 299:1421, 1978

132. LITTLE JA, COX D, BRECKENRIDGE WC, McGUIRE VM: Introduction to deficiencies of apolipoproteins CII and EIII with some associated clinical findings, in Gotto AM Jr, Smith LC, Allen B (eds): *Atherosclerosis V.* New York, Springer-Verlag, 1980, p 671

133. YAMAMURA T, SUDO H, ISHIKAWA K, YAMAMOTO A: Familial type I hyperlipoproteinemia caused by apolipoprotein C-II deficiency. *Atherosclerosis* 34:53, 1979

134. FREDRICKSON DS, LEVY RI: Familial hyperlipoproteinemia, in Stanbury JB, Wyngaarden, JB, Fredrickson DS (eds): *The Metabolic Basis of Inherited Disease,* 3d ed. New York, McGraw-Hill, 1972, p 545

135. BRECKENRIDGE WC, COX D, LITTLE JA: Apolipoprotein CII deficiency, in Gotto AM Jr, Smith LC, Allen B (eds): *Atherosclerosis V.* New York, Springer-Verlag, 1980, p 675

136. DAMGAARD-PEDERSEN K, DYERBERG J: Observation implicating that familial type I hyperlipoproteinemia is not a lipoprotein-lipase deficient condition, in Schettler G, Weizel A (eds): *Atherosclerosis III.* Berlin, Springer-Verlag, 1974, p 553

137. SCHREIBMAN PH, ARONS DL, SAUDEK CD, ARKY RA: Abnormal lipoprotein lipase in familial exogenous hypertriglyceridemia. *J Clin Invest* 52:2075, 1973

138. BERGER GMB, ABRAHAM PR: Selective protamine sulphate inactivation of lipoprotein lipase and hepatic lipase in human post-heparin plasma: Specific lipase levels in normals and in type I hyperlipoproteinaemia. *Clin Chim Acta* 81:219, 1977

139. BURTON BK, NADLER HL: Primary type-I hyperlipoproteinemia with normal lipoprotein lipase activity. *J Pediat* 90: 777, 1977

140. WOOD PDS, STERN MP, SILVERS A, REAVEN GM, VON DER GROEBEN J: Prevalence of plasma lipoprotein abnormalities in a free-living population of the Central Valley, California. *Circulation* 45:114, 1972

141. FULLER JH, PINNEY S, JARRETT RJ, KILBOURN K, KEEN H: Plasma lipids in a London population and their relation to other risk factors for coronary heart disease. *Brit Heart J* 40:170, 1978

142. JONES GJL, HEWITT D, GODIN GJ, BRECKENRIDGE WC, BIRD J, MISHKEL MA, STEINER G, LITTLE JA: Plasma lipoprotein levels and the prevalence of hyperlipoproteinemia in a Canadian working population. *Can Med Assoc J* 122:37, 1980

143. LEWIS B, CHAIT A, WOOTOM IDP, OAKLEY CM, KRIKLER DM, SIGURDSSON G, FEBRUARY A, MAURER B, BIRKHEAD J: Frequency of risk factors for ischaemic heart-disease in a healthy British population with particular reference to serum-lipoprotein levels. *Lancet* 1:141, 1974

144. GREENBERG BH, BLACKWELDER WC, LEVY RI: Primary type V hyperlipoproteinemia. A descriptive study in 32 families. *Ann Intern Med* 87:526, 1977

145. FALLAT RW, GLUECK CJ: Familial and acquired type V hyperlipoproteinemia. *Atherosclerosis* 23:41, 1976

146. NIXON JC, MARTIN WG, KALAB M, MONAHAN GJ: Type V hyperlipoproteinemia. A study of a patient and family. *Clin Biochem* 2:389, 1969

147. LOSSOW WJ, LINDGREN FT, WEIZEL A, WOOD PD: A study of a type V hyperlipoproteinemia patient. *Clin Chim Acta* 36:33, 1972

148. KALOFOUTIS A, SIMONS M, JULLIEN GL: Hyperlipoproteinemia type V: Biochemical observations in two cases. *Clin Chim Acta* 52:361, 1974

149. RALEIGH J, REDDY J, FRIEDLANDER D, HOPE R: Type V hyperlipoproteinaemia: A family study. *NZ Med J* 82:300, 1975

150. HECKERS H, OEHLER G: Typ-V-Hyperlipoproteinämie. *Med Welt* 26:1766, 1975

151. YESHURUN D, CHUNG H, GOTTO AM JR, TAUNTON DO: Primary type V hyperlipoproteinemia in childhood. *J Am Med Assoc* 238:2518, 1977

152. SIMONS LA, WILLIAMS PF, TURTLE JR: Type V hyperlipoproteinaemia re-visited: Findings in a Sydney population. *Aust NZ J Med* 5:210, 1975

153. SCHLESINGER M, JACOTOT B, BEAUMONT V, BUXTORF J-C: Hyperlipoprotéinémie de type V. 54 observations. *Nouv Presse Med* 8:833, 1979

154. GLUECK CJ, CHRISTOPHER C, MISHKEL MA, TSANG RC, MELLIES MJ: Pancreatitis, familial hypertriglyceridemia, and pregnancy. *Am J Obstet Gynecol* 136:755, 1980

155. GLUECK CJ, SCHEEL D, FISHBACK J, STEINER P: Estrogen-induced pancreatitis in patients with previously covert familial type V hyperlipoproteinemia. *Metabolism* 21:657, 1972

156. BORRIE P, SLACK J: A clinical syndrome characteristic of primary Type IV-V hyperlipoproteinaemia. *Brit J Dermatol* 90:245, 1974

157. LEES RS, WILSON DE, SCHONFELD G, FLEET S: The familial dyslipoproteinemias, in Steinberg AG, Bearn AG (eds): *Progress in Medical Genetics.* New York, Grune & Stratton, 1973, vol 9, p 237

158. GLUECK CJ, LEVY RI, FREDRICKSON DS: Immunoreactive insulin, glucose tolerance, and carbohydrate inducibility in types II, III, IV and V hyperlipoproteinemia. *Diabetes* 18:739, 1969

159. TASKINEN M-R: Effect of free fatty acids and exogenous triglycerides upon the action and secretion of insulin. Dissertation, University of Helsinki, 1969

160. BRUNZELL JD, PORTE D JR, BIERMAN EL: Abnormal lipoprotein-lipase-mediated plasma triglyceride removal in untreated diabetes mellitus associated with hypertriglyceridemia. *Metabolism* 28:901, 1979

161. CHRISTENSEN S, DOLLERUP E, ESKJAER JENSEN S: Idiopathic hyperlipemia, latent diabetes mellitus, and severe neuropathy. *Acta Med Scand* 159:57, 1958

162. FESSEL WJ: Fat disorders and peripheral neuropathy. *Brain* 94:531, 1971

163. SANDBANK U, BECHAR M, BORNSTEIN B: Hyperlipemic neuropathy. *Acta Neuropathol* 19:290, 1971

164. NAUSIEDA PA: Hyperlipemic neuropathy, in Vinken PJ, Bruyn GW (eds): *Handbook of Clinical Neurology.* Amsterdam, Elsevier, 1977, vol 29, p 429

165. SANDBANK U, BUBIS J: Hyperlipemic neuropathy. Experimental study. *Brain* 96:355, 1973

166. HEILMAN KM, FISHER WR: Hyperlipidemic dementia. *Arch Neurol* 31:67, 1974

167. KALTREIDER HB, TALAL N: Bilateral parotid gland enlargement and hyperlipoproteinemia. *J Am Med Assoc* 210:2067, 1969

168. REINERTSEN JL, SCHAEFER EJ, BREWER HB, MOUTSOPOULOS HM: Sicca-like syndrome in type V hyperlipoproteinemia. *Arthr Rheum* 23:114, 1980

169. GOTTO AM JR: Type V hyperlipoproteinaemia, in Rifkind BM (ed): *Clinics in Endocrinology and Metabolism*, vol 2, *Disorders of Lipid Metabolism*. London, Saunders, 1973, p 11

170. LOSSOW WJ, LINDGREN FT, WEIZEL A, WOOD PD: A study of a type V hyperlipoproteinemic patient. *Clin Chim Acta* 36:33, 1972

171. SIGURDSSON S, NICOLL A, LEWIS B: The metabolism of low density lipoprotein in endogenous hypertriglyceridaemia. *Eur J Clin Invest* 6:151, 1976

172. BROOK JG, TORSVIK H, LEES RS, McCLUSKEY MA, FELDMAN HA: Low density lipoprotein metabolism in type IV and type V hyperlipoproteinemia. *Metabolism* 28:4, 1979

173. KASHYAP ML, SRIVASTAVA LS, CHEN CY, PERISUTTI G, CAMPBELL M, LUTMER RF, GLUECK CJ: Radioimmunoassay of human apolipoprotein CII. A study in normal and hypertriglyceridemic subjects. *J Clin Invest* 60:171, 1977

174. FALKO JM, WITZTUM JL, SCHONFELD G, BATEMAN J: Dietary treatment of type V hyperlipoproteinemia fails to normalize low levels of high-density lipoprotein cholesterol. *Ann Intern Med* 91:750, 1979

175. STEINER G, ADELMAN AG, SILVER MD: Early coronary atherosclerosis in primary type V hyperlipoproteinemia. *Can Med Assoc J* 105:1172, 1971

176. MIDDELHOFF G, MORDASINI R, ZEBE H, GRETEN H: Koronare Herzkrankheit bei Patienten mit Hyperlipoproteinämie Type V. *Klin Wochenschr* 56:457, 1978

177. SLACK J: Risks of ischaemic heart-disease in familial hyperlipoproteinaemic states. *Lancet* 2:1380, 1969

178. LEWIS B: Type V hyperlipoproteinaemia, in *The Hyperlipidaemias. Clinical and Laboratory Practice*. Oxford, Blackwell, 1976, p 258

179. SIGURDSSON G, NICOLL A, LEWIS B: Metabolism of very low density lipoproteins in hyperlipidaemia: Studies of apolipoprotein B kinetics in man. *Eur J Clin Invest* 6:167, 1976

180. PACKARD CJ, SHEPHERD J, JOERNS S, GOTTO AM, TAUNTON OD: Apolipoprotein B metabolism in normal, type IV, and type V hyperlipoproteinemic subjects. *Metabolism* 29:213, 1980

181. GRUNDY SM, MOK HYI, ZECH L, STEINBERG D, BERMAN M: Transport of very low density lipoprotein triglycerides in varying degrees of obesity and hypertriglyceridemia. *J Clin Invest* 63:1274, 1979

182. SIMONS LA, WILLIAMS PF: The biochemical composition and metabolism of lipoproteins in type V hyperlipoproteinaemia. *Clin Chim Acta* 61:341, 1975

183. BEUCLER I, SALMON S, AYRAULT M, RAYMOND J-P, ETIENNE J, POLONOVSKI J: Anomalie des lipoprotéines de faible densité et de leurs apolipoprotéines chez un sujet atteint d'une hyperlipémie de type V. *Pathol Biol* 25:95, 1977

184. LISCH H-J, PATSCH W, RIEDLER L, SAILER S, BRAUNSTEINER H: Activation of adipose tissue lipoprotein lipase by lipoprotein fractions from normals and patients with type V hyperlipoproteinemia. *Klin Wochenschr* 56:1067, 1978

185. AMATUZIO DS, HAY LJ: Dietary control of essential hyperlipemia. Effect of dairy foods, phospholipid, coconut oil, and alcohol. *Arch Intern Med* 102:173, 1958

186. CHAIT A, MANCINI M, FEBRUARY AW, LEWIS B: Clinical and metabolic study of alcoholic hyperlipidaemia. *Lancet* 2:62, 1972

187. BAUMGARTNER HP, FILIPPINI L: Alkoholinduzierte Hyperlipoproteinämien. *Schweiz Med Wochenschr* 107:1406, 1977

188. CARLSON LA, ERIKSSON I, WALLDIUS G: A case of massive hypertriglyceridaemia and impaired fatty acid incorporation into adipose tissue glycerides (FIAT), both corrected by nicotinic acid. *Acta Med Scand* 194:363, 1973

189. CARLSON LA, OLSSON AG, BALLANTYNE D: On the rise in low density and high density lipoproteins in response to the treatment of hypertriglyceridaemia in type IV and type V hyperlipoproteinaemias. *Atherosclerosis* 26:603, 1977

190. GLUECK CJ, STEIN EA, KASHYAP ML: Persistent hypoalphalipoproteinemia during therapy of familial type 5 hyperlipoproteinemia. *Artery* 5:463, 1979

191. NIKKILÄ EA, PYKÄLISTÖ O: Induction of adipose tissue lipoprotein lipase by nicotinic acid. *Biochim Biophys Acta* 152:421, 1968

192. KISSEBAH AH, ADAMS PW, HARRIGAN P, WYNN V: The mechanism of action of clofibrate and tetranicotinoylfructose (Bradilan) on the kinetics of plasma free fatty acid and triglyceride transport in type IV and type V hypertriglyceridaemia. *Eur J Clin Invest* 4:163, 1974

193. GLUECK CJ, LEVY RI, FREDRICKSON DS: Norethindrone acetate, postheparin lipolytic activity, and plasma triglycerides in familial types I, III, IV, and V hyperlipoproteinemia. Studies in 26 patients and 5 normal persons. *Ann Intern Med* 75:345, 1971

194. EHNHOLM C, HUTTUNEN JK, KINNUNEN PJ, MIETTINEN TA, NIKKILÄ EA: Effect of oxandrolone treatment on the activity of lipoprotein lipase, hepatic lipase and phospholipase A 1 of human postheparin plasma. *N Engl J Med* 292:1314, 1975

31

FAMILIAL LECITHIN:CHOLESTEROL ACYLTRANSFERASE DEFICIENCY

JOHN A. GLOMSET

KAARE R. NORUM

EGIL GJONE

1. Familial lecithin:cholesterol acyltransferase (LCAT) deficiency *is characterized by a combination of clinical, tissue, and plasma lipoprotein abnormalities that result from a failure of LCAT to esterify cholesterol in the plasma.*

2. *The clinical abnormalities include corneal opacities, anemia, and frequently, though not invariably, proteinuria. Renal failure can be a life-threatening complication.*

3. *The disease is inherited as a rare autosomal recessive trait. A total of 26 patients from 12 families have been described. The defect has been localized to chromosome 16.*

4. *The tissue abnormalities include foam cells in the bone marrow and glomerular tufts, lamellar inclusions in cells of the spleen, and target-shaped erythrocytes that contain abnormally high amounts of unesterified cholesterol and phosphatidylcholine.*

5. *The plasma lipoprotein abnormalities involve all lipoprotein classes and affect composition, shape, distribution, and concentration. Unusual particles, rich in unesterified cholesterol and phosphatidylcholine, are particularly striking.*

6. *Active LCAT is absent from the plasma since, in contrast to normal, little or no esterification of cholesterol occurs when the plasma is incubated in vitro. Nevertheless, immunochemical techniques have revealed*

LCAT protein in the plasma of several patients. Apparently, mutation of the LCAT gene on chromosome 16 can lead to synthesis and secretion of an inactive enzyme. As a result, unesterified cholesterol and phosphatidylcholine accumulate in the plasma, and there is a plasma cholesteryl ester deficit. Unesterified cholesterol and phoshatidylcholine accumulate in tissues as well, and this may ultimately give rise to tissue dysfunction.

HISTORY

In 1966, a 33-year-old woman (patient A.R.) from western Norway was admitted to Rikshospitalet, the National Hospital of Norway, in Oslo. She had diffuse grayish corneal opacities, anemia, proteinuria, and hyperlipemia, and was presumed to have chronic nephritis. Renal function proved to be normal, and the serum albumin level was only slightly reduced. Both plasma triglyceride (TG) and cholesterol levels were increased, but most of the cholesterol was unesterified. Plasma PC (phosphatidylcholine or lecithin) level was increased, but the level of plasma lysolecithin was decreased, and no pre-β- or α-lipoproteins could be detected on electrophoresis. A kidney biopsy was most unusual, in that it showed foam cells in the glomerular tufts. Subsequently, the same clinical features and the same relative abnormalities in plasma cholesterol and phospholipid were found in two of the patient's sisters, and further studies of all three sibs disclosed the absence of lecithin:cholesterol acyltransferase (LCAT) activity in plasma (Fig. 31-1). Because all three were afflicted and because none had a history of liver or kidney disease which could account for the abnormalities, it appeared that they suffered from a previously undiscovered inborn error of metabolism [1–3].

In 1969, a Swedish family with this condition was described [4]. A 47-year-old woman had corneal opacities, anemia, proteinuria, hyperlipemia, and the same plasma lipid and lipoprotein abnormalities as the three Norwegian sisters. The level of plasma LCAT activity was very low. The patient's brother had developed the same symptoms and died of uremia at the age of 40 years. Three additional Norwegian families have been found since 1970 [5–8]. They live in the same general area of Norway as the first family. One of the patients is of special interest; though nearly 70 years of age, she has no proteinuria. Other patients have been discovered in Germany [9], the United Kingdom [10, 11], France [12, 13], Canada [14, 15], and Japan [16]. Altogether, 26 patients from 12 different families are now known (Table 31-1).

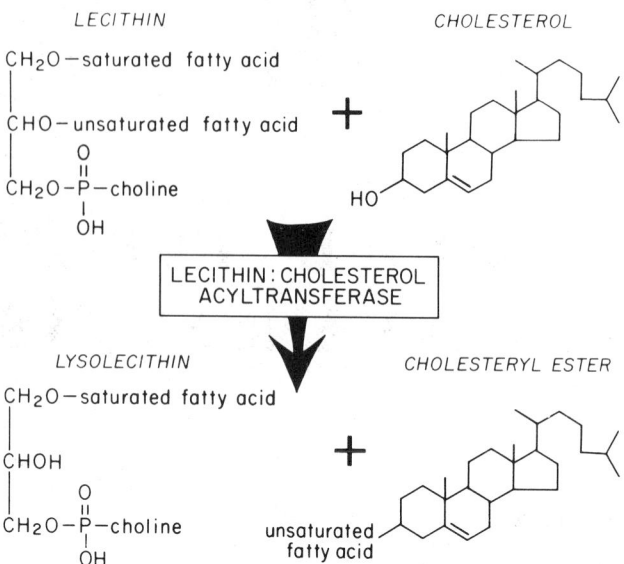

Figure 31-1 Principal lipid reactants in the plasma lecithin:cholesterol acyltransferase (EC 2.3.1.43) reaction.

CHARACTERISTICS

Present information about familial LCAT deficiency is largely derived from studies of the Scandinavian patients. These patients show significant heterogeneity, even within families, and the possibility cannot be ruled out that still greater heterogeneity will be found among patients from other parts of the world.

Clinical and Tissue Abnormalities

Ocular Features   Corneal opacities are present in all patients from early childhood and are easily detectable. They consist of numerous minute, grayish dots in the entire corneal stroma that give the cornea a cloudy to misty appearance (Fig. 31-2). Near the limbal area the dots increase in number, forming a grayish, circular band resembling an arcus lipoides senilis [17]. The material in the dots has not yet been identified, but ultrastructural examination of sections obtained by superficial keratectomy [10, 14] has revealed the presence of numerous vacuoles, many of which contain electron-dense, or "membranous," deposits. These vacuoles occur in both Bowman's layer and the anterior stroma.

Fundus changes have been observed in two patients. Angioid streaks were found in one, whereas the other developed papilledema and impaired ocular blood supply with functional loss, presumably caused by arterial obstruction and leakage of lipid material into the nervous tissue of the optic disk [18]. Although the presence of excess lipids has not been verified chemically or morphologically, crystals that may be cholesterol have been seen by polarized light in both the cornea and the fundus.

Hematologic Features   Anemia with a hemoglobin concentration of about 10 g/dl is seen in most patients and is of the normochromic type [19]. Hematologic data (Table 31-2) and bone marrow studies suggest that the anemia is due to moderate hemolysis combined with reduced compensatory erythropoiesis. Radioisotope studies of the erythrocyte life span have shown half-lives of 16 to 17 days in two patients (normal half-life, 23 to 35 days). The patients' spleens have not been particularly active in erythrocyte destruction.

The erythrocytes show abnormalities in appearance and lipid composition [20]. "Target cells" are found in increased numbers in dry smears of both peripheral blood and bone marrow. Measurements of whole erythrocytes from Scandinavian patients revealed up to twice the normal amount of unesterified cholesterol (UC) and PC, but decreased amounts of sphingomyelin and phosphatidylethanolamine (PE), and normal amounts of total phospholipid. Measurements of erythrocyte membrane preparations from Canadian and Japanese patients [16, 21] revealed similar abnormalities in content of UC, PC, and PE, although the content of sphingomyelin was normal. It is not yet clear whether other blood cells show related abnormalities, but platelet function and lipid composition are normal [23].

Foam cells have been found in the bone marrow of several patients. Giemsa stain has revealed "sea-blue histiocytes" (Fig. 31-3) in both bone marrow and spleen of all patients studied [19, 23], and ultrastructural studies [24] have shown that the histiocyte granules are composed of membranes in a lamellar arrangement (Fig. 31-4). These membranes presumably contain UC and PC since both lipids are present in increased amounts in the spleen as well as in the liver [25].

Renal Manifestations   In most patients the urine contains protein, erythrocytes, and hyaline casts. Most of the urinary protein migrates in the position of albumin on electrophoresis; α_1- and α_2-migrating proteins are also present. Proteinuria is detected early in life, and remains moderate (about 0.5 to 1.5 mg protein per milliliter of urine) for many years, but increases with the onset of renal insufficiency. Thus, when first studied, all but one of the Scandinavian patients had moderate proteinuria. (The exception, patient D.J., has always had normal urine.) In many patients, proteinuria increased markedly in the fourth and fifth decades of life as renal function deteriorated.

The concentration of albumin in the serum is usually only slightly reduced, but it decreases considerably in association with the increased proteinuria that accompanies renal failure. Serum creatinine and urea concentrations, as well as clearance of creatinine, inulin, and *para*-aminohippuric acid (PAH), remain normal for many years, as does the blood pressure. Renal insufficiency and hypertension may develop rapidly and without warning [19].

Light microscopic examination of renal biopsies has revealed foam cells in the glomerular tufts in all patients examined so far. Arterioles have thickened intima and narrow lumen. Subendothelial deposits of lipid material have been found in the renal arteries and arterioles. Lipid analysis of isolated glomeruli has shown that the amounts of UC and phospholipid are markedly higher than normal (Table 31-3) [25]. Electron microscopic studies [24, 26] have demonstrated capillary lumens that are partly filled with a meshwork of membranes and particles with an amorphous mottled structure. The capillary walls appear to be abnormal. Endothelial cells are frequently absent, the basal lamina is of irregular thickness, endothelial foot processes are fused, and membrane-surrounded particles are present in both the subendothelial and subepithelial regions.

Atherosclerosis   Early atherosclerosis has developed in many patients with familial LCAT deficiency. Calcification in the aorta has been demonstrated before the age of 40 (patient A.R.), and postmortem examinations have revealed atherosclerosis of the aorta and large arteries (patients D.B. and A.R.)

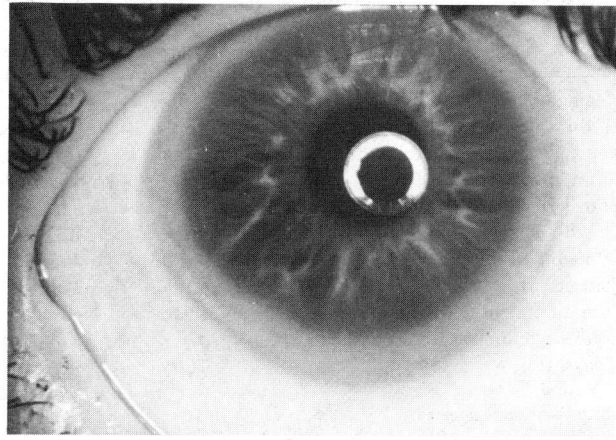

Figure 31-2 Corneal infiltrate in patient A.R. It is localized to the parenchyma, is composed of numerous minute dots, and is most prominent in the periphery, where it resembles a corneal arcus. (*From Gjone and Bergaust* [17].)

[19, 25]. Renal arteries and arterioles also show early atherosclerotic changes. Histologic examination shows fibrosis and hyalinization of renal arterial walls, with marked narrowing of the vessel lumens [24].

Electron microscopic studies of sections from renal and iliac arteries and from the aorta have revealed accumulation of lipidlike material of the same type observed in the other organs. This material is present in the different layers of the vessel wall. Foam cells are present as well, and there is sometimes smooth-muscle-cell proliferation in the intimal layer [25].

Lipid analysis of an atheroma from a renal artery revealed

Table 31-1 Known patients with familial LCAT deficiency (as of January 1981)

Family	Patient	Sex	Born	Age at diagnosis, years	National origin	Corneal opacity	Anemia	Proteinuria	Uremia	Cholesterol total mg%	CE%	TG mg%	Reference
1	1	F	1936	34	Norwegian	+	+	+	+	300	3	400	1, 2, 3
	2	F	1934	32	Norwegian	+	+	+	+	500	8	570	
	3	F	1946	20	Norwegian	+	+	+	−	140	5	130	
2	4	F	1921	48	Swedish	+	+	+	+	369	27	533	4
	5	M	1935	—	Swedish	+	+	+	+	137	?	?	
3	6	F	1926	44	Norwegian	+	+	+	−	215	14	900	5
	7	M	1932	38	Norwegian	+	+	+	+	235	13	630	
4	8	M	1918	55	Norwegian	+	+	+	+	135	3	251	6, 7
	9	F	1913	60	Norwegian	+	+	−	−	107	2	105	
5	10	M	1942	30	Italian	+	+	+	+	131	13	190	9
	11	M	1942	28	Italian	+	+	+	−	64	31	169	
6	12	M	1955	20	East Indian	+	−	−	−	83	10	107	10
7	13	M	1944	30	Engl-Canadian	+	+	+	−	125	13	128	14
	14	M	1939	35	Engl-Canadian	+	+	−	−	86	17	169	
8	15	F	1934	40	French	+	+	+	−	175	8	250	12, 13
	16	F			French	+	+	+	−				
9	17	M	1959	16	Ital-Swedish	+	+	+	−	162	3	340	15, 16
	18	F	1954	21	Ital-Swedish	+	+	min	−	120	25	278	
10	19	F	1946	30	Japanese	+	+	min	−	42	0	110	16
	20	M	1948	28	Japanese	+	+	+	−	94	20	222	
	21	M	1950	26	Japanese	+	+	+	−	163	29	346	
11	22	F	1924	56	Irish	+	+	−	−	213	16	218	11
	23	F	1931	49	Irish	+	+	−	−	194	12	226	
	24	F	1932	48	Irish	+	+	+	+	194	9	507	
	25	M	1932	—	Irish	+	+	+	+				
12	26	F	1954	26	Norwegian	+	+	+	−	142	8	192	8

Table 31-2 Hematologic data on eight patients with LCAT deficiency

	A.R.	I.S.	M.R.	A.A.	L.G.	M.L.	K.Å.	D.J.
Hemoglobin, g/dl	8.7–10.5	9.5	10.5–11.5	8.9–10.9	11.2–12.2	10.5	6.1	11.0
Erythrocytes, $10^6/\mu l$	2.9–3.7	3.88	3.58–3.47	3.13	3.89–4.51	3.8	2.2	4.6
Reticulocytes (per 1000 erythrocytes)	0.1–16	18	14	—	—	12–74	73	28
Serum iron ($\mu g/dl$)	30–90	85	170	138	115	159	55	178
Transferrin (iron-binding capacity, $\mu g/dl$)	140	240	270	—	—	252	200	305
White blood cells per μl	4500–7000	4100–5300	3700–4500	4600	4700	4400	5800	4900
Platelets, $10^3/\mu l$	113–148	132–179	143	220	320	140	205	382
Osmotic fragility	Normal	Normal	Normal	—	—	Normal	—	—
Erythrocyte life-span (chromium) (days, t½)	16	—	—	—	—	17	—	—

NOTE: — = not examined.

that only 35 percent of total cholesterol was esterified (Table 31-4). This contrasts with findings of about 75 percent cholesteryl ester (CE) in the atheroma of patients dying with other diseases [27]. The fatty acid pattern of atheroma CE was distinctly different from that usually seen in atherosclerotic lesions. The ratio of oleic to linoleic acid was about 4:1, whereas this ratio in plaques usually varies between 2:1 and 1:1. Thus, the CE fatty acid composition of the atheroma resembles the abnormal pattern found in plasma (see below) as well as the intracellular pattern normally formed by acyl coenzyme A:cholesterol acyltransferase (see Chap. 33).

Plasma Lipoprotein Abnormalities

Patients who have familial LCAT deficiency show multiple plasma lipoprotein abnormalities, some readily detectable by analysis of the whole plasma. All patients have high concentrations of plasma UC and PC, and all have low concentrations of plasma CE and lysolecithin [28]. The CE contain abnormally high proportions of palmitic and oleic acids and an abnormally low proportion of linoleic acid. Upon electrophoresis of the plasma on paper or agarose gel, no pre-β-lipoprotein band is seen, although hypertriglyceridemia may be present, and an α_1-lipoprotein band, if visible, is very faint.

Many additional abnormalities become apparent when the plasma lipoproteins are isolated and examined by special techniques such as ultracentrifugation, gel filtration, electron microscopy, and apolipoprotein analysis. Very low density lipoproteins (VLDL), i.e., lipoproteins of $d<1.006$ g/ml, show abnormal β mobility on electrophoresis and are frequently elevated in concentration. Whether elevated or not, they contain high amounts of UC compared with PC, low amounts of total protein, and particularly low amounts of apolipoproteins C-II and C-III (apo C-II, apo C-III) [31]. Since these apolipoproteins are normally the most electronegative components of VLDL, their low content in VLDL from patients probably accounts for the unusually slow electrophoretic mobility of these lipoproteins.

When patient VLDL of different sizes are examined by gel filtration and electron microscopy, those that are 60 nm in diameter or larger can be seen to include notched particles. The same sized VLDL contains an unusually high proportion of surface components (Table 31-5), *high* amounts of CE and apolipoproteins C-I and E (apo C-I, apo E), and two major tetramethylurea-insoluble proteins. One of the proteins insoluble in tetramethylurea is similar in size to apolipoprotein B (apo B); the other appears to be somewhat smaller than apo B. It has been suggested that the notched particles are chylomicron remnants [29]. When the concentration of plasma TG is high the lipoproteins of $d<1.006$ g/ml include a high proportion of particles that are greater than 90 nm in diameter. These particles are present in the plasma of patients who have fasted overnight, but disappear or decrease markedly in concentration when the patients consume fat-free diets for several days [30], and hence they are believed to be chylomicrons. Patient

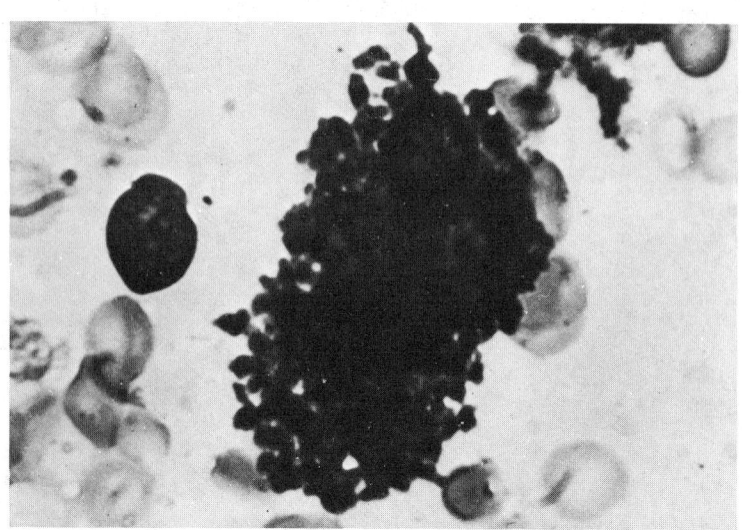

Figure 31-3 Sea-blue histiocyte in a spleen aspirate from a patient with LCAT deficiency.

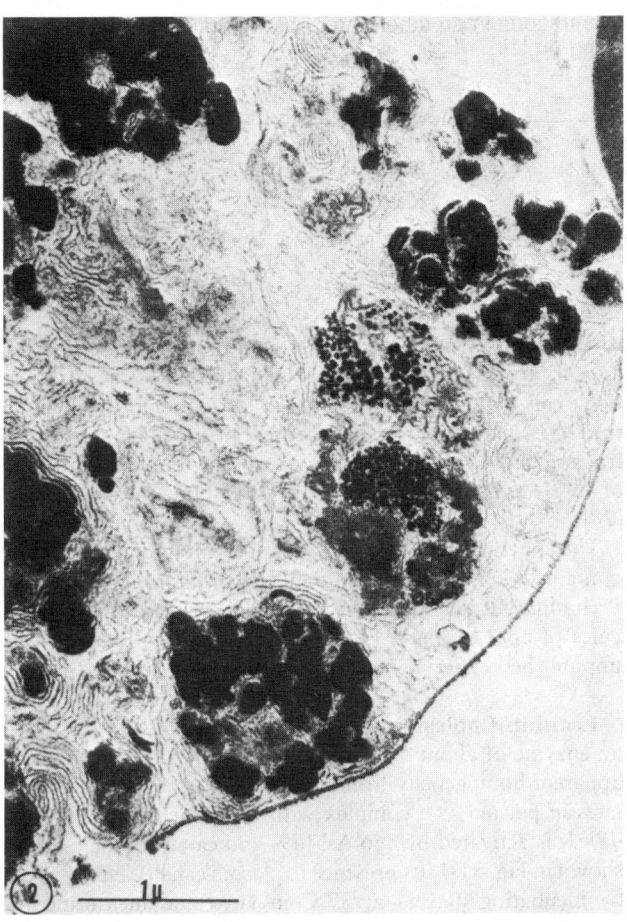

Figure 31-4 Sea-blue histiocyte from spleen with inclusions and cytoplasmic membranes. Note the plasma membrane, which is about three times thicker than normal. (*From Jacobsen et al. [23].*)

VLDL that are 40 nm in diameter or smaller are probably of hepatic origin. They contain low amounts of CE, normal amounts of apo C-I and apo E, and a single protein insoluble in tetramethylurea that cannot be distinguished from apo B.

Less is known about the patients' intermediate density lipoproteins (IDL, LDL$_1$), i.e., lipoproteins of $d<1.006$ to 1.019 g/ml. These include both normal-sized and unusually large particles, as demonstrated by gel filtration on 2 percent agarose [31]. The composition of the large and normal-sized particles is intermediate between that of corresponding sized VLDL and low density lipoproteins of density 1.019 to 1.063 g/ml (LDL$_2$).

The LDL$_2$ also frequently include unusually large particles. After filtration through 2 percent agarose, the LDL$_2$ usually yield three relatively well defined subfractions, whereas normal LDL$_2$ yield only one (Fig. 31-5). These three fractions of LDL$_2$ are believed to be formed from the action of lipoprotein lipase on TG-rich lipoproteins (Fig. 31-6). One of the LDL$_2$ subfractions not found in normal plasma emerges in the void volume of the 2 percent agarose column (Fig. 31-5). It is comprised of particles 90 nm in diameter that have a multilamellar structure and that contain UC and PC in the unusually high molar ratio of 2:1 (Table 31-6). The two types of "surface" lipid no doubt account for the lamellar structure of the particles, since the width of the lamella, measured by electron microscopy, is identical to that of UC-PC bilayers formed in vitro. The very small amount of protein present in the particles is largely albumin. The total concentration of these particles in

the plasma of different patients varies from 0 to 48 mg cholesterol per deciliter plasma, and appears to be roughly proportional to the concentration of chylomicrons. Moreover, the concentrations of the large LDL and of chylomicrons both decrease when the patients consume fat-free diets [30].

A second subfraction of patient LDL$_2$ is made up of particles 30 to 80 nm in diameter that emerge just after the void volume. These particles also have no obvious counterparts in normal plasma, although similar particles (Lp X) are found in cholestasis [32]. The particles have a disk-shaped appearance when examined by electron microscopy and often form stacks (Fig. 31-6). They largely contain UC, PC, and apo C. Preliminary studies of the quantitative distribution of individual apo C suggest that the relative content of apo C-I is very high [Glomset, unpublished experiments]. The total concentration of Lp X-like particles in patient plasma has been estimated after isolation of the Lp X by an electrophoretic technique [33]. It ranges from about 10 to 60 mg cholesterol per deciliter plasma.

Other LDL$_2$ in the second subfraction that emerges from 2 percent agarose are spherical and resemble normal remnants of chylomicrons and VLDL metabolism (Fig. 31-6). They can be separated from the Lp X-like particles by adsorption on heparin-agarose and appear to contain TG, CE, and both apo B and apo E [Glomset, unpublished experiments].

A third subfraction of patient LDL$_2$ contains spherical particles that, like normal LDL$_2$, are 20 to 22 nm in diameter (Fig. 31-6). Unlike normal LDL$_2$, the spherical particles of patient LDL$_2$ contain large amounts of TG, but the content of CE is correspondingly reduced; thus both the content of total "core" lipid and the proportion of core lipid to surface lipid and protein are normal [28, 31]. Furthermore, the protein is apo B, as in normal LDL$_2$. The concentration of the normal-sized LDL$_2$ appears to be quite low, however, since the concentration of apo B in patient plasma is only one-half to one-third that in normal persons [28].

Patient HDL also include particles of unusual shape and composition [34–38]. Some of the particles are disk-shaped, while others are spherical as in normal HDL, but unusually small. The disk-shaped particles mainly contain UC, PC, and apo E or apolipoprotein A-I and A-II (apo A-I, apo A-II) [39]. Patient disk-shaped HDL that contain apo E have recently

Table 31-3 Lipid concentrations in kidneys, liver, and spleen of LCAT-deficient patient A.R., nmol lipid/mg protein

Organ	TC	UC	PL	TG	UC/PL
Kidneys:					
Cortex, A.R., Jan. 1973		170	257	9	0.7
Cortex, A.R., July 1973*		80	207	12	0.4
Cortex, control		50	109	4	0.5
Glomeruli, A.R., Jan. 1973		416	455	9	0.9
Glomeruli, A.R., July 1973*		153	229	21	0.7
Glomeruli, control		57	103	14	0.6
Liver:					
A.R., Jan. 1973	90	83	273	21	0.3
Control	20	18	185	9	0.1
Spleen:					
A.R., Jan. 1973	284	268	372	12	0.7
Control	3	3	—	14	—

* In kidney from normal donor transplanted 6 months earlier.
NOTE: TC, total cholesterol; UC, unesterified cholesterol; PL, total phospholipids; TG, triglyceride; —, not determined.
SOURCE: From Stokke et al. [25].

Table 31-4 Lipid concentrations in an atheroma of LCAT-deficient patient A.R., nmol lipid/mg protein

	TC	UC	PL	TG	UC/PL	CE/TC
Atheroma, A.R., Jan. 1973	749	485	371	21	1.31	0.35
Plaque material from controls*					1.12	0.75

* Smith [27].
NOTE: TC = total cholesterol, UC = unesterified cholesterol, PL = total phospholipids, TG = triglyceride, CE = cholesteryl esters.
SOURCE: From Stokke et al. [25].

been isolated and characterized sufficiently to allow calculation of their composition and structure [40] (Table 31-7). The particles show many similarities to disk-shaped "nascent HDL" that have been isolated from rat liver perfusates [41, 42]. A notable feature of both types of particle is that the disk thickness corresponds to that of a phospholipid bilayer, while just enough apolipoprotein is present to form a three-tiered rim of amphipathic helix that defines the disk perimeter (Fig. 31-7). Perhaps for this reason the linkage of apo E to the particle is unusually stable [41].

The disk-shaped HDL that contain apo A-I are similar in shape and lipid composition to the disk-shaped HDL that contain apo E. Several types of these apo A-I-rich particles can be separated by gradient gel electrophoresis, but pure particles rich in apo A-I have not yet been characterized sufficiently to permit calculation of their structure. Characterization of the particles may never be complete because the linkage of apo A-I

Figure 31-5 Subfractions of LDL of density 1.019 to 1.063 g/ml from patients M.R. and L.G., obtained by filtration through 2% agarose columns. L, I, and S = subfractions comprised of large, intermediate, and small particles, respectively. Normal LDL will emerge from the columns where the S subfraction emerges. (*From Glomset et al. [31].*)

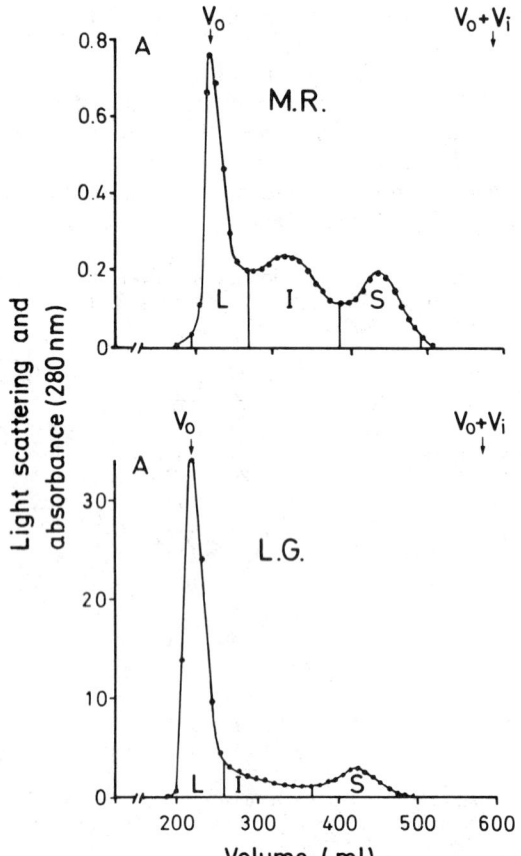

to the particles is unusually labile and much of the apo A-I appears to dissociate from the HDL during ultracentrifugation. This may partially explain the low content of protein in the HDL fraction and the high content of apo A-I in the protein fraction of $d > 1.25$ g/ml [43]. Even so, the total concentration of apo A-I in patient plasma is only about one-third of normal [28].

The spherical HDL are only about 6 nm in diameter. They contain UC, PC, a small amount of core lipid, and apo A-I. Preliminary calculations suggest that there may be two molecules of apo A-I per 94,600-dalton particle [Glomset et al., unpublished experiments].

Lecithin:Cholesterol Acyltransferase (LCAT) LCAT is an enzyme of about 59,000 daltons that has been purified to apparent homogeneity from human plasma [44–46]. It circulates in plasma as a complex with components of HDL [47, 48]. It is activated by apo A-I [49] and catalyzes the reaction shown in Fig. 31-1. Its presence in plasma can be demonstrated by incubating plasma at 37°C in vitro and measuring the decrease in concentration of plasma UC. Alternatively, radioactive UC can be incubated with plasma and the amount of radioactive CE formed can be determined [50]. Little or no activity is demonstrable in patient plasma by either method [1].

Absence of LCAT activity is not due to the presence of inhibitors, since addition of patient plasma to normal plasma does not inhibit LCAT activity [1]. Moreover, incubation of patient plasma with LCAT that has been purified from normal plasma leads to formation of substantial amounts of CE [51].

Recent measurements of the mass of LCAT protein present in patient plasma by immunochemical techniques [52, 53] have shown that some plasma samples contain no LCAT protein, whereas samples from other patients contain very small amounts of an apparently inactive enzyme.

In vivo studies have yielded results that are consistent with the in vitro data [1]. The plasma UC of patient I.S. rapidly became labeled when she was injected with radioactive mevalonate whereas no label appeared in the plasma CE. Plasma UC and CE both are labeled when normal subjects are treated similarly.

Other Findings The lipoprotein lipase level was low in several of the Norwegian patients, whereas the hepatic lipase level was normal [54].

Serum uric acid concentrations were elevated in three of the hyperlipidemic patients (A.R., A.A., L.G.), and one of the patients has developed gout. Slightly elevated serum acid phosphatase levels also have been observed.

Usually, the liver and spleen are not enlarged, and there is no evidence of generalized hepatic dysfunction. No symptoms suggestive of central nervous system dysfunction are found.

Xanthomatous deposits of the skin are not observed, and lymph nodes and tonsils are not enlarged. The tonsils are normal in color.

PATHOPHYSIOLOGY

A simple working hypothesis concerning familial LCAT deficiency is that primary failure to synthesize or secrete active LCAT into the plasma causes abnormalities in the structure and function of HDL, and that these abnormalities give rise to other lipoprotein and tissue abnormalities that ultimately lead to clinical complications. This hypothesis is largely based on results of in vitro and in vivo experiments with patient lipoproteins and erythrocytes.

There are several reasons for believing that the abnormalities in patient HDL depend on the LCAT deficiency. First, incubation experiments with mixtures of normal LCAT and patient lipoproteins have shown that the enzyme reacts directly with patient HDL, but minimally if at all with other patient lipoproteins [35]. Second, early studies showed that incubation with LCAT converts the disk-shaped HDL into spherical particles that resemble normal HDL [28], and more recent kinetic studies have shown that the HDL are initially converted into particles that are similar in size to normal HDL_2 and HDL_3 [51]. These changes are probably direct effects of the conversion of HDL UC and PC to CE. The latter are thought to penetrate between the surface layers of the disk-shaped HDL to form a spherical interior core. The LCAT reaction presumably continues until just enough surface lipid remains to form a tightly packed monolayer surrounding the newly formed CE core. This disk-to-sphere transition is not yet completely understood. The kinetic studies mentioned above showed that formation of HDL_2- and HDL_3-sized particles continues for some time after HDL CE have ceased to accumulate, which

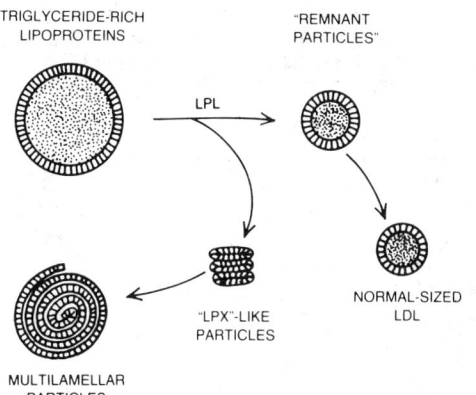

Figure 31-6 Proposed mechanism of formation of patient large-, intermediate-, and small-molecular-weight LDL_2 by action of lipoprotein lipase (LPL) on triglyceride-rich lipoproteins. LPL produces two direct products: "remnant particles" that contain both core and surface material, and which float in the VLDL and IDL range; and Lp X-like particles that contain surface materials and float in the LDL_2 range. The remnant particles give rise to normal-sized LDL_2. The Lp X-like particles, which are equivalent to the intermediate-sized LPL_2 (Fig. 31-5), are converted to multilamellar particles, which are equivalent to the large-sized LDL_2 (Fig. 31-5).

suggests that extensive particle rearrangements are taking place.

Reaction of patient HDL with LCAT alters not only the shape, distribution, and lipid composition of the HDL, but also the content of apo E, apo A-I, and apo C. The content of apo E decreases whether the HDL are incubated in the absence or presence of other lipoproteins [51]. As mentioned earlier, the linkage of apo E to native HDL from a patient appears to be unusually stable. Apo E dissociates readily from patient HDL that have been incubated with LCAT, as it does from normal HDL. This effect may depend directly on the disk-to-sphere transition. If three tiers of apo E amphipathic helix form a rim that defines the perimeter of patient disk-shaped HDL (Fig. 31-6), then hydrophobic interactions between the helices and

Table 31-5 Comparison of patient and control VLDL of two different diameters*

	40-nm particles		60-nm particles	
	Patients	*Controls*	*Patients*	*Controls*
Total protein, gram × 10^{-19}/particle	30§	52	55§	93
Apoproteins, molecules/particle				
E	6.0	7.4	25.5§	9.4
C-I	9.5	6.4	21.7†	13.1
C-II	6.1§	12.2	13.3§	37.4
C-III$_1$	12.4§	49.4	25.1§	124.0
C-III$_2$	14.9§	42.5	33.4§	110.0
Lipids, 10^3 molecules/particle				
PL	4.9	4.7	15.8§	12.0
UC	4.4§	2.7	15.5§	6.3
CE	0.9§	2.3	4.6‡	2.8
TG	13.8†	12.2	47.1§	53.0

* Values for patient and control lipoproteins predicted from analyses of subfractions obtained by gel filtration
† $P < 0.05$.
‡ $P < 0.01$.
§ $P < 0.001$.
SOURCE: From Glomset et al. [29].

Table 31-6 Lipid/lipoprotein ratios of normal LDL and large, intermediate, and small LDL$_2$ particles from two patients with familial LCAT deficiency, μmole lipid/mg protein

	PC	UC	CE	TG
Normal* LDL	0.48	1.4	1.8	0.11
Large LDL$_2$				
Patient L.G.	21.5	39.8	0.40	1.72
Patient M.R.	12.0	20.9	0.50	1.23
Intermediate LDL$_2$				
Patient L.G.	5.05	8.64	0.19	0.95
Patient M.R.	5.54	8.24	0.32	0.58
Small LDL$_2$				
Patient L.G.	1.01	1.0	0.19	1.53
Patient M.R.	0.78	0.83	0.47	0.95

* The mean from six normal females.
NOTE: The subfractions correspond to those shown in Fig. 31-5.
SOURCE: From Glomset et al. [31].

phospholipid acyl chains, coupled with electrostatic interactions among the helices, might account for the unusual stability of the apo E–disk linkage. The LCAT-dependent conversion of the disks to spheres might then substantially weaken the apo E–HDL linkage by changing the orientation of the acyl chains.

Incubation of patient HDL with LCAT *promotes* the binding of apo A-I. The mechanism that underlies this normalizing effect is not clear, but it must be very different from that affecting the binding of apo E. Binding of apo A-I to CE may be involved since the conformation of apo A-I appears to be affected by CE [55], and direct evidence for binding of apo A-I to CE has recently been obtained [56].

Incubation of patient HDL with LCAT also appears to promote the binding of apo C. Thus, when patient HDL are incubated with patient VLDL in the presence of LCAT, transfer of apo C occurs from the VLDL to the HDL, while transfer of apo E occurs in the opposite direction [51]. Additional studies will be required to determine whether the change in apo C also tends to normalize the apolipoprotein content of patient HDL.

To summarize, reaction of patient HDL with LCAT alters their shape, distribution, and lipid and apolipoprotein composition. This strongly suggests that the native HDL from patients are not abnormal in the strict sense, but are nascent particles that have been secreted by the liver [41] or intestine [57] or formed by interaction of apo A-I with TG-rich lipoproteins [58]. In other words, patient HDL may be unusual only because they have not reacted with LCAT. Even the abnormally low content of apo A-I in patient plasma may depend directly on the LCAT deficiency if apo A-I dissociates from patient HDL as readily in vivo as it does in vitro, and if free apo A-I is rapidly removed from the circulation.

If incubation studies with LCAT and patient HDL support the idea that absence of LCAT from the plasma leads directly to the HDL abnormalities that characterize familial LCAT deficiency, what evidence is there that the HDL abnormalities affect other plasma lipoproteins? Evidence derived from in vitro studies indicates that action of LCAT on patient HDL indirectly affects both LDL and VLDL [43]. Most of the UC and PC consumed when patient whole plasma is incubated with LCAT is in fact contributed by LDL and VLDL, and most of the CE produced is recovered in these lipoproteins. The UC and PC are mainly derived from the large- and intermediate-

sized LDL (Fig. 31-6) and from the large VLDL, whereas the CE are recovered in normal-sized particles. Thus, it appears that UC and PC, associated with the large LDL and VLDL, either transfer to or are converted to HDL, that the latter subsequently react with LCAT, and that the CE formed is subsequently transferred to normal-sized LDL and VLDL by the plasma CE exchange protein [59–61]. The combined effect of these transfer reactions is to normalize the LDL, since the concentrations of the large- and intermediate-sized LDL decrease and the content of CE in the normal-sized LDL increases by as much as fivefold. The transfer reactions also appear to have a normalizing effect on the VLDL since, as mentioned earlier, VLDL that are 60 nm in diameter or larger contain excess surface lipid, whereas those that are 40 nm in diameter or smaller contain abnormally low amounts of CE. The transfer of apo E from HDL to VLDL and the transfer of apo C from VLDL to HDL (see above) exaggerate rather than ameliorate abnormalities in the native VLDL. Both these abnormalities and the abnormalities in concentration of the VLDL and LDL thus remain to be explained.

In vivo studies of patient lipoproteins have provided insight into the origin of the large- and the intermediate-sized LDL$_2$. When patients consumed fat-free diets for several days, the concentrations of both the large VLDL, i.e., the putative chylomicrons, and the large- and intermediate-sized LDL$_2$ decreased markedly [30]. In one case, the concentration of the small spherical HDL decreased as well. In contrast, changing the intake of dietary cholesterol influenced only the content of CE in the VLDL, and substitution of a medium-chain TG diet for a fat-free diet had no effect. This suggests that the large- and intermediate-sized LDL$_2$, and possibly the small spherical HDL, may be derived from chylomicrons. In vitro studies by others [62] support the possibility that unusual particles, rich in UC and PC, are formed when TG-rich lipoproteins are attacked by lipoprotein lipase. Furthermore, the possibility that action in vivo of lipoprotein lipase on patient chylomicrons might have a similar effect is consistent with the sugges-

Table 31-7 Comparison of patient apolipoprotein E–rich HDL with "nascent HDL" from rat liver perfusates*

	Patient HDL	Nascent HDL†
Dimensions, nm		
Diameter	19.5	19.1
Thickness	4.4	4.5
ΔR‡	1.5	1.5
Particle weight, daltons	892,000	843,000
Apolipoproteins, molecules/particle		
Apo E	7.4	9.0
Apo A-I	0.6	1.0
Lipids, molecules/particle		
Phospholipid	569	401
Unesterified cholesterol	441	261
Cholesteryl ester	n.d.	55
Triglyceride	n.d.	52

* Values predicted from a disk-shaped model.
† Data from Hamilton et al. [41].
‡ ΔR is protein rim width chosen to approximate diameter of amphipathic helix ($d = 1.5$ nm).
NOTE: n.d. = not detected
SOURCE: From Mitchell et al. [40].

HDL disc

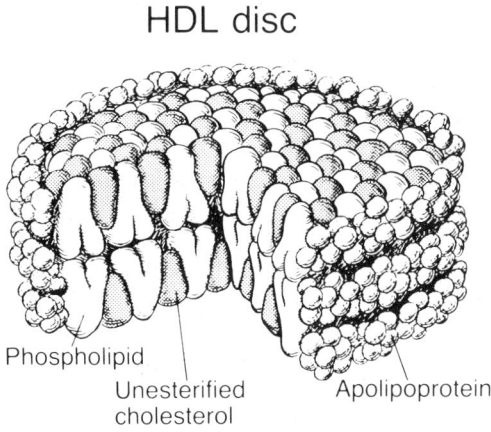

Phospholipid

Unesterified
cholesterol

Apolipoprotein

Figure 31-7 Model of patient disk-shaped apo E–rich HDL. (*Based on data from Mitchell et al. [40].*)

tion of Schumaker and Adams [63] that LCAT normally plays a role in the catabolism of TG-rich lipoproteins. These authors pointed out that an excess of surface lipid would be expected to develop as the TG-rich interior of chylomicrons or VLDL is removed by the hydrolytic action of lipoprotein lipase. They suggested that the role of the LCAT reaction might be to correct the resulting imbalance between surface lipid and core lipid by converting surface UC and PC to CE. Although they envisaged that LCAT might act directly on remnants of chylomicrons and VLDL, present evidence favors the possibility that segments of the remnant surface pinch off to form particles that float in the density range of LDL$_2$, and that these particles subsequently contribute lipid substrates for the LCAT reaction, as mentioned earlier. The CE formed might then be transferred to lipoproteins such as VLDL, IDL, or LDL that have a core of nonpolar lipid that can act as an acceptor.

Thus, studies of familial LCAT deficiency support the possibility that two types of remnant particle are formed from TG-rich lipoproteins (Fig. 31-6). One type has flotation properties similar to VLDL. It contains residual core lipid, i.e., TG and CE, and is spherical, though notched. The CE is probably derived from the intestinal mucosa. As mentioned previously, it increases in concentration following ingestion of cholesterol-rich diets. It has a fatty acid composition similar to that of normal human thoracic duct lipoproteins, and it becomes labeled following the ingestion of radioactive cholesterol, but not following the injection of radioactive mevalonate [1].

The second type of remnant particle has a density similar to LDL$_2$, contains surface lipid, i.e., UC and PC, but no core lipid, and has a bilayered or lamellar character. This type of surface remnant may give rise to the large- and intermediate-sized LDL$_2$ observed in patient plasma. Why core remnant accumulate in patient plasma is not yet known, but surface remnants presumably accumulate because the UC and PC are not converted into CE in the absence of LCAT. Formation of HDL CE from surface remnant UC and PC would normally prevent accumulation of the particles. The CE would be transferred to VLDL, IDL, and LDL, and then be removed from the plasma by receptor-dependent mechanisms.

A question of considerable interest is whether the accumulation of putative surface remnants in patient plasma ultimately causes tissue abnormalities. For example, removal of the large LDL$_2$ by reticuloendothelial cells may account for the lamellar inclusions observed in sea-blue histiocytes in the spleen. Moreover, the unusually high content of UC in the

large LDL$_2$ may tend to increase the content of UC in erythrocytes and other cells.

Results of incubation studies with patient erythrocytes clearly indicate that the abnormally high content of UC in the erythrocyte membranes is related to the high content of this lipid in patient plasma. Patient erythrocytes lose UC when incubated in normal plasma, whereas normal erythrocytes gain UC when exposed to patient plasma [64]. Similar effects can be anticipated in relation to erythrocyte PC, although this phospholipid is thought to exchange only slowly with plasma phospholipids [65].

A question not yet answered is whether the abnormal lipid composition of patient erythrocytes and the high content of lipid in the spleen and bone marrow account for the anemia that accompanies familial LCAT deficiency. Anemia is seen in other conditions associated with high relative contents of UC in the plasma [28], but the basis for the anemia is not yet clear. The basis for the corneal and renal abnormalities also remains to be established. The possibility that normal pathways of lipoprotein uptake may be altered in several critical tissues and that this eventually leads to tissue dysfunction merits exploration, especially in relation to the atherosclerotic changes that occur in familial LCAT deficiency.

A different question relates to patient heterogeneity. Even the Scandinavian patients show marked differences in the concentrations of plasma TG and large- and intermediate-sized LDL$_2$. Furthermore, patients of Sardinian origin, studied in Germany [9], show other differences. Their plasma may lack disk-shaped HDL, which are rich in apolipoprotein E. No LCAT-dependent changes in distribution of this apolipoprotein have been observed in incubation studies [66]. In addition, some Canadian patients show abnormalities in endocrine glands not seen in other patients [67]. These differences presumably depend on the action of genes that are not immediately related to LCAT. The possibility that different primary abnormalities are involved remains to be excluded.

GENETICS

Knowledge of the genetics of familial LCAT deficiency was initially derived from studies of four Scandinavian families, three Norwegian and one Swedish [68]. A fourth Norwegian family has now been described [8]. The Norwegian families come from the same geographically isolated area of Norway. In the four sibships there are eight affected members, while nine brothers and sisters are healthy. Genetic studies of families from other parts of the world have revealed a similar pattern [16], which strongly suggests an autosomal recessive mode of inheritance (Fig. 31-8).

The cluster of cases in Norway is especially interesting. The epidemiology of the disease indicates that the genetic basis of the Norwegian form of LCAT deficiency is one mutational event. The family studies show that this must have occurred before approximately the year 1700. Because of inbreeding and chance, the defective gene has acquired a surprisingly high frequency in the part of Norway where these four families live. From the number of patients and the population size, a gene frequency of about 2 percent can be estimated in this region of the country. This gives a frequency of heterozygous carriers of approximately 4 percent.

Fam. 1:

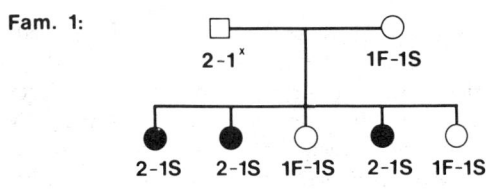

Fam. 2:

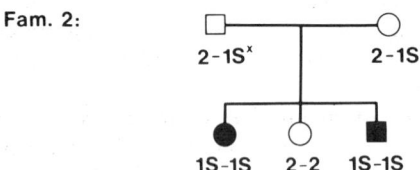

Fam. 3:

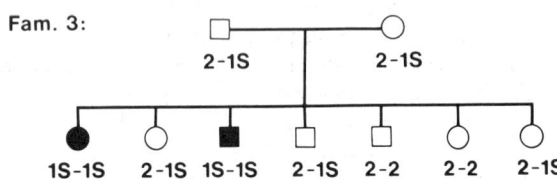

Figure 31-8 Haptoglobin (Hp) subtypes in the members of three families where LCAT deficiency has been found. Hp types marked with an X have been deduced from the types of the other family members. Filled symbols: patients with LCAT deficiency. Open symbols: family members with no signs of disease. (*From Teisberg et al. [68].*)

Linkage studies in the three Norwegian families first described revealed nonrandom distribution between LCAT deficiency and serum haptoglobin (Hp) types. After Hp subtyping, a combined lod (log odds) score of 3.41 at a recombination fraction of 0.00 was obtained (Table 31-8). Association was revealed between the LCAT-deficiency gene and the Hp^{15} gene. It is therefore proposed that the LCAT gene is located in close proximity to the α-haptoglobin locus, which is situated between the middle and terminal point of the long arm of chromosome 16 [69]. The linkage to Hp has been confirmed in a recently described Japanese family [16]. The fourth Norwegian family also confirms the association between the LCAT-deficient Norwegian gene and the Hp^{15} gene.

Lately, important information with regard to LCAT mass and LCAT activity in the plasma of homozygous LCAT-deficient patients, heterozygotes, and normal persons has appeared [52, 53]. This information convincingly indicates that different LCAT-deficient genes vary with regard to LCAT activity and LCAT mass in plasma. Thus, the plasma of the homozygous Norwegian LCAT-deficient patients contains 10 to 20 percent of the LCAT mass found in plasma, whereas the plasma of the Sardinian patients contains only about 5 to 10 percent of the normal amount, and patients from one of the Canadian families have no detectable LCAT mass in plasma. A recent, expanded study (to be published) of three of the four Norwegian families has revealed that the plasma of heterozygotes contains less than the normal amount of LCAT activity. This finding is consistent with observations made on families living in other parts of the world [52, 53].

The observed heterogeneity in what appears to be a clinical entity is not surprising. Model studies, especially of the hemoglobins, indicate that such heterogeneity is the rule rather than the exception in genetic disease. Each mutation may be expected to produce its own biochemical pattern with regard to amount and functional activity of the protein produced.

TREATMENT

Blood Transfusion

Since at present it is not possible to treat the disease by intravenous LCAT replacement, whole plasma or blood transfusions have been employed. In one instance, patient A.R. was given 450 ml blood and 500 ml plasma in a single transfusion [70]. This caused an immediate rise in plasma CE, followed by a slower increase to a peak level at 6 days. The peak level considerably exceeded that attributable to CE of the transfused plasma, the plasma CE composition shifted toward that of normal plasma, and the plasma lysolecithin increased. Therefore, the changes in CE were probably caused by the transfused LCAT. The plasma CE had again diminished to the pretreatment level 2 weeks later. This diminution probably reflected the half-life of the transfused LCAT, which was 4.6 days on another occasion.

In another instance the same patient was treated with several successive plasma transfusions. The plasma CE increased from 35 to 310 mg/dl, while the UC concentration decreased moderately. The lesser change in UC may have been due to an influx from plasma membranes, because erythrocyte cholesterol (all unesterified) decreased from 1.8 to 1.3 mg per 10^{10} cells. The relative concentration of plasma PC increased from 1.8 to 3.4 percent. No other changes in plasma phospholipid pattern were observed, nor did α_1-lipoproteins appear. Furthermore, the plasma TG concentration did not change significantly, although some lipoproteins of pre-β mobility appeared. The edema cleared, but there was no apparent change in the anemia or proteinuria. Similar effects of transfusion obtained in patient M.L. suggested that treatment would have to be continued for much longer periods if plasma lipoprotein and plasma membrane defects, or anemia and proteinuria, were to be corrected.

Dietary Treatment

Dietary treatment has been tried, with particular interest focused on the large LDL$_2$ and their possible association with the kidney damage. Since the large LDL may be diminished by dietary change, we advise our patients with LCAT deficiency to restrict the intake of fat. Whether this can delay or prevent the serious kidney complications is so far unknown.

Kidney Transplantation

Kidney transplants have been performed in four patients. Transplantation does not reverse the lipid or lipoprotein abnormalities in plasma or increase the LCAT activity, but the concentration of TG in the plasma of patient A.R. was much lower after transplantation than before, when she had a nephrotic syndrome.

There is evidence that early deposition of lipid occurs in the transplanted kidneys. The renal graft of patient A.R. showed morphological changes six months after transplantation consistent with lipid deposition both in the mesangium and in the basement membrane. Similar changes were found after 14 months in the renal graft of patient K.A.

Table 31-8 LCAT-Hp linkage relations

	Scorable matings	Scorable offspring	Lod scores at recombination fraction						Probability of linkage (prior 0.045)
			0.00	0.05	0.10	0.20	0.30	0.40	
Males	3	12	1.83	1.62	1.40	0.95	0.51	0.15	0.404
Females	3	10	1.58	1.39	1.20	0.80	0.42	0.12	0.298
Both sexes*	4	18	3.41	3.01	2.60	1.75	0.93	0.27	0.935

* Family 1 is scored as Z2 from both sexes. Families 2 and 3 as Z4.
SOURCE: From Teisberg et al. [68].

Nevertheless, the clinical course after renal transplantation has generally been successful, and good renal function has been maintained [71, 72].

The studies described in this chapter were partially supported by the Howard Hughes Medical Institute, U.S. Public Health Service grant RR00166, The R. J. Reynolds Industries, Incorporated, the Anders Jahre Foundation, and the Norwegian Research Council for Science and the Humanities.

REFERENCES

1. NORUM KR, and GJONE E: Familial plasma lecithin:cholesterol acyltransferase deficiency. Biochemical study of a new inborn error of metabolism. *Scand J Clin Lab Invest* 20:231, 1967

2. GJONE E, NORUM KR: Familial serum-cholesterol ester deficiency: Clinical study of a patient with a new syndrome. *Acta Med Scand* 183:107, 1968

3. TORSVIK H, GJONE E, NORUM KR: Familial plasma cholesteryl ester deficiency: Clinical studies in a family. *Acta Med Scand* 183:387, 1968

4. HAMNSTRØM B, GJONE E, NORUM KR: Familial plasma lecithin:cholesterol acyltransferase deficiency: Report of a Swedish family. *Br Med J* 2:283, 1979

5. NORUM KR, BØRSTING S, GRUNDT I: Familial lecithin:cholesterol acyltransferase deficiency. *Acta Med Scand* 188:323, 1970

6. GJONE E, SKARBØVIK AJ, BLOMHOFF JP, TEISBERG P: Familial lecithin:cholesterol acyltransferase deficiency: Report of a third Norwegian family with two afflicted members. *Scand J Clin Lab Invest* 33:suppl. 137, 101, 1974

7. GJONE E, BLOMHOFF JP, SKARBØVIK AJ: Possible association between an abnormal low density lipoprotein and nephropathy in lecithin:cholesterol acyltransferase deficiency. *Clin Chim Acta* 54:11, 1974

8. GJONE E, BLOMHOFF JP, HOLME R, HOVIG T, OLAISEN B, SKARBØVIK AJ, TEISBERG P: Familial LCAT deficiency: Report of a fourth family from Northwestern Norway. *Acta Med Scand*. In press

9. UTERMANN G, SCHOENBORN W, LANGER KH, DICKER P: Lipoproteins in LCAT deficiency. *Humangenetik* 16:295, 1972

10. BRON AF, LLOYD JK, FOSBROOKE AS, WINDER AF, TRIPATHI RC: Primary lecithin:cholesterol acyltransferase deficiency disease. *Lancet* 1:928, 1975

11. THOMPSON G, SOUTAR A: To be published

12. CHEVET D, RAMEE PL, THOMAS R, GARRE M, ALCINDOR LG: Hereditary lecithin:cholesterol acyltransferase deficiency: Report of a new family with two affected sisters. *Kidney Inter* 10:185, 1976

13. SALMON S, ALCINDOR LG, BEUCLER I, AYRAULT-JARRIER M, INFANTE R, CHEVET D, POLONOVSKI J: Etude-immunoelectrophoretique des lipoproteines plasmatiques dans un cas de deficience familiale en lecithine-cholesterol acyltransferase. *Clin Chim Acta* 66:311, 1976

14. BETHELL W, McCULLOCH C, GHOSH M: Lecithin:cholesterol acyltransferase deficiency. Light and electron microscopic findings from two corneas. *Can J Ophthalmol* 10:494, 1975

15. FROHLICH J, GODOLPHIN WJ, REEVE CE, EVELYN K: Familial LCAT deficiency. Report of two patients from a Canadian family of Italian and Swedish descent. *Scand J Clin Lab Invest* 38:suppl. 150, 156, 1978

16. IWAMOTO A, NAITO C, TERAMOTO T, KATU H, KAKA M, KARIYA T, SHIMUZU T, OKA H, ODA T: Familial lecithin:cholesterol acyltransferase deficiency complicated with unconjugated hyperbilirubinemia and peripheral neuropathy. The first reported case in the Far East. *Acta Med Scand* 204:219, 1978

17. GJONE E, BERGAUST B: Corneal opacity in familial plasma cholesterol ester deficiency. *Acta Ophthalmol* 47:222, 1969

18. HØRVEN I, GJONE E, EGGE K: Ocular manifestations in familial LCAT deficiency. *National Foundation—March of Dimes* 12:271, 1976

19. GJONE E: Familial lecithin:cholesterol acyltransferase deficiency: A clinical survey. *Scand J Clin Lab Invest* 33:suppl. 137, 73, 1974

20. GJONE E, TORSVIK H, NORUM KR: Familial plasma cholesterol ester deficiency: A study of the erythrocytes. *Scand J Clin Lab Invest* 21:327, 1968

21. GODIN DV, GRAY GR, FROHLICH J: Erythrocyte membrane alterations in lecithin:cholesterol acyltransferase deficiency: *Scand J Clin Lab Invest* 38:150, 162–167, 1978

22. NORDØY A, GJONE E: Familial plasma lecithin:cholesterol acyltransferase deficiency: A study of the platelets. *Scand J Clin Lab Invest* 27:263, 1965

23. JACOBSEN CD, GJONE E, HOVIG T: Sea-blue histiocytes in familial lecithin:cholesterol acyltransferase deficiency. *Scand J Haematol* 9:106, 1972

24. HOVIG T, GJONE E: Familial lecithin:cholesterol acyltransferase deficiency: Ultrastructural aspects of a new syndrome with particular reference to lesions in the kidneys and the spleen. *Acta Pathol Microbiol Scand* 81:681, 1973

25. STOKKE KT, BJERVE KS, BLOMHOFF JP, ØYSTESE B, FLATMARK A, NORUM KR, GJONE E: Familial lecithin:cholesterol acyltransferase deficiency: Studies on lipid composition and morphology of tissues. *Scand J Clin Lab Invest* 33:suppl 137, 93, 1974

26. HOVIG T, GJONE E: Familial lecithin:cholesterol acyltransferase deficiency: Ultrastructural studies on lipid deposition and tissue reactions. *Scand J Clin Lab Invest* 33:suppl 137, 135, 1974

27. SMITH EB: The influence of age and atherosclerosis on the chemistry of aortic intima. *J Atheroscler Res* 5:224, 1965

28. GLOMSET JA, NORUM KR: The metabolic role of lecithin:cholesterol acyltransferase: Perspectives from pathology. *Adv Lipid Res* 2:1, 1973

29. GLOMSET JA, APPLEGATE K, FORTE T, KING WC, MITCHELL CD, NORUM KR, GJONE E: Abnormalities in lipoproteins of $d < 1.006$ g/ml in familial lecithin:cholesterol acyltransferase deficiency. *J Lipid Res* 21:1116, 1980

30. GLOMSET JA, NORUM KR, NICHOLS AV, KING WC, MITCHELL CD, APPLEGATE KR, GONG EL, GJONE E: Plasma lipoproteins in familial lecithin:cholesterol acyltransferase deficiency: Effects of dietary manipulation. *Scand J Clin Lab Invest* 35:suppl 142, 3, 1975

31. GLOMSET JA, NICHOLS AV, NORUM KR, KING W, FORTE T: Plasma lipoproteins in familial lecithin:cholesterol acyltransferase deficiency: Further studies of very low and low density lipoprotein abnormalities. *J Clin Invest* 52:1078, 1973

32. HAMILTON RL, HAVEL RJ, KANE JP, BLAUROCK AE, SATA T: Cholestasis: Lamellar structure of the abnormal human serum lipoprotein. *Science* 172:475, 1971

33. RITLAND S, GJONE E: Quantitative studies of LP-X in familial lecithin:cholesterol acyltransferase deficiency and during cholesterol esterification. *Clin Chim Acta* 59:109, 1975

34. TORSVIK H: Presence of α_1-lipoprotein in patients with familial plasma lecithin:cholesterol acyltransferase deficiency. *Scand J Clin Lab Invest* 24:187, 1969

35. GLOMSET JA, NORUM KR, KING W: Plasma lipoproteins in familial lecithin:cholesterol acyltransferase deficiency; lipid composition and reactivity *in vitro*. *J Clin Invest* 49:1827, 1970

36. NORUM KR, GLOMSET JA, NICHOLS AV, FORTE T: Plasma lipoproteins in familial lecithin:cholesterol acyltransferase deficiency: Physical and chemical studies of low and high density lipoproteins. *J Clin Invest* 50:1131, 1971

37. TORSVIK H, SOLAAS MH, GJONE E: Serum lipoproteins in plasma lecithin:cholesterol acyltransferase deficiency studied by electron microscopy. *Clin Genet* 1:139, 1970

38. FORTE T, NORUM KR, GLOMSET JA, NICHOLS AV: Plasma lipoproteins in familial lecithin:cholesterol acyltransferase deficiency: Structure of low and high density lipoproteins as revealed by electron microscopy. *J Clin Invest* 50:1141, 1971

39. TORSVIK H: Studies on the protein moiety of serum high density lipoprotein from patients with familial lecithin:cholesterol acyltransferase deficiency. *Clin Genet* 3:188, 1972

40. MITCHELL CD, KING WC, APPLEGATE KR, FORTE T, GLOMSET JA, NORUM KR, GJONE E: Characterization of apolipoprotein E-rich high density lipoproteins in familial lecithin:cholesterol acyltransferase deficiency. *J Lipid Res* 21:625, 1980

41. HAMILTON RL, WILLIAMS MC, FIELDING CJ, HAVEL RJ: Discoidal bilayer structure of nascent high density lipoproteins from perfused rat livers. *J Clin Invest* 58:667, 1976

42. FELKER TE, FAINARU M, HAMILTON RL, HAVEL RJ: Secretion of the arginine-rich and A-I apolipoproteins by the isolated perfused rat liver. *J Lipid Res* 18:465, 1977

43. NORUM KR, GLOMSET JA, NICHOLS AV, FORTE T, ALBERS JJ, KING WC, MITCHELL CD, APPLEGATE KR, GONG EL, CABANA V, GJONE E: Plasma lipoproteins in familial lecithin:cholesterol acyltransferase deficiency. Effects of incubation with lecithin:cholesterol acyltransferase deficiency *in vitro*. *Scand J Clin Lab Invest* 35:suppl 142, 31, 1975.

44. ALBERS JJ, CABANA VG, STAHL YDB: Purification and characterization of human plasma lecithin:cholesterol acyltransferase. *Biochemistry* 15:1084, 1976.

45. ARON L, JONES S, FIELDING CJ: Human plasma lecithin:cholesterol phospholipase activity. *J Biol Chem* 253:7220, 1978

46. CHUNG J, ABANO DA, FLESS GM, SCANU AM: Isolation, properties, and mechanism of *in vitro* action of lecithin:cholesterol acyltransferase from human plasma. *J Biol Chem* 254:7459, 1979

47. GLOMSET JA: The plasma lecithin:cholesterol acyltransferase reaction. *J Lipid Res* 9:155, 1968

48. FIELDING PE, FIELDING CJ: A cholesteryl ester transfer complex in human plasma. *Proc Nat Acad Sci USA* 77:3327, 1980

49. FIELDING CJ, SHORE VG, FIELDING PE: A protein cofactor of lecithin:cholesterol acyltransferase. *Biochem Biophys Res Commun* 46:1493, 1972

50. STOKKE KT, NORUM KR: Determination of lecithin:cholesterol acyltransfer in human blood plasma. *Scand J Clin Lab Invest* 27:21, 1971

51. GLOMSET JA, MITCHELL CD, KING WC, APPLEGATE KR, FORTE T, NORUM KR, GJONE E: In vitro effects of lecithin:cholesterol acyltransferase on apolipoprotein distribution in familial lecithin:cholesterol acyltransferase deficiency. *Ann NY Acad Sci* 348:224, 1980

52. ALBERS JJ, ADOLPHSON JL, CHEN CH: Radioimmunoassay of human plasma lecithin:cholesterol acyltransferase. *J Clin Invest.* 67:141, 1981

53. ALBERS JJ, UTERMANN G: Genetic control of lecithin:cholesterol acyltransferase: Measurement of LCAT mass in a large kindred with LCAT deficiency. *Am J Hum Genet.* 33:702, 1981

54. BLOMHOFF JP, HOLME R, SAUAR J, GJONE E: Familial lecithin:cholesterol acyltransferase deficiency. Further studies on plasma lipoproteins and plasma postheparin lipase activity of a patient with normal renal function. *Scand J Clin Lab Invest* 38:suppl 150, 177, 1978

55. LUX SE, HIRZ R, SHRAGER RI, GOTTO AM: The influence of lipid on the conformation of human plasma high density apolipoproteins. *J Biol Chem* 247:2598, 1972

56. STOFFEL: Personal communication

57. GREEN PHR, TALL AR, GLICKMAN RM: Rat intestine secretes discoid high density lipoprotein. *J Clin Invest* 61:528, 1978

58. CHEN CH, ALBERS JJ: To be published

59. PATTNAIK NM, ZILVERSMIT DB: Interaction of cholesteryl ester exchange protein with human plasma lipoproteins and phospholipid vesicles. *J Biol Chem* 254:2782, 1979

60. CHAJEK T, FIELDING CJ: Isolation and characterization of human serum cholesteryl ester transfer protein. *Proc Nat Acad Sci USA* 75:2445, 1978

61. ALBERS JJ, CHEUNG MC, EWENS SL, TOLLEFSON JH: Characterization and immunoassay of apolipoprotein D. *Atherosclerosis.* 39:395, 1981

62. DECKELBAUM RJ, EISENBERG S, FAINARU M, BARENHOLZ Y, OLIVECRONA T: *In vitro* production of human plasma low density lipoprotein-like particles. A model for very low density lipoprotein catabolism. *J Biol Chem* 254:6079, 1979

63. SCHUMAKER VN, ADAMS GH: Very low density lipoproteins: Surface-volume changes during metabolism. *J Theor Biol* 26:89, 1970

64. NORUM KR, GJONE E: The influence of plasma from patients with familial plasma lecithin:cholesterol acyltransferase deficiency on the lipid pattern of erythrocytes. *Scand J Clin Lab Invest* 22:94, 1968

65. NELSON GJ: Lipid composition and metabolism of erythrocytes, in Nelson GJ (ed): *Blood Lipids and Lipoproteins: Quantitation, Composition, and Metabolism.* New York, Wiley-Interscience, 1972

66. UNTERMANN G, MENZEL HJ, ADLER G, DIEKER P, WEBER W: Substitution *in vitro* of lecithin:cholesterol acyltransferase, analysis of changes in plasma lipoproteins. *Eur J Biochem* 107:225, 1980

67. ANGEL A, EPSTEIN D, DALE R, BRECKENRIDGE WC, KUKSIS A: Familial lecithin:cholesterol acyltransferase (LCAT) deficiency. To be published

68. TEISBERG P, GJONE E, OLAISEN B: Genetics of lecithin:cholesterol acyltransferase deficiency. *Ann Hum Genet* 38:327, 1975

69. TEISBERG P, GJONE E: The lecithin:cholesterol acyltransferase deficiency locus in man: Probable linkage to the alpha-haptoglobin locus on chromosome no. 16. *Nature* 249:550, 1974

70. NORUM KR, GJONE E: The effect of plasma transfusion on the plasma cholesteryl esters in patients with familial plasma lecithin:cholesterol acyltransferase deficiency. *Scand J Clin Lab Invest* 22:339, 1968

71. FLATMARK AL, HOVIG T, MYHRE E, GJONE E: Renal transplantation in patients with familial lecithin:cholesterol acyltransferase deficiency. *Transplantation Proc* 9:1665, 1977

72. MYHRE E, GJONE E, FLATMARK A, HOVIG T: Renal failure in familial lecithin–cholesterol acyltransferase deficiency. *Nephron* 18:239, 1977

32

FAMILIAL TYPE 3 HYPERLIPOPROTEINEMIA (Dysbetalipoproteinemia)

MICHAEL S. BROWN

JOSEPH L. GOLDSTEIN

DONALD S. FREDRICKSON

1. Patients with familial type 3 hyperlipoproteinemia (also called familial dysbetalipoproteinemia) have elevated plasma concentrations of cholesterol and triglycerides, owing to the accumulation in plasma of remnant particles derived from the partial catabolism of very low density lipoproteins (VLDL) and chylomicrons.

2. Affected individuals typically do not manifest hyperlipidemia or any clinical features of the disease until after age 20. Thereafter, they frequently develop two types of cutaneous xanthomas: xanthoma striata palmaris (yellow discolorations of the palmar and digital creases) and tuberous or tuberoeruptive xanthomas (bulbous cutaneous xanthomas). Severe atherosclerosis involving the coronary arteries, internal carotids, and abdominal aorta is also prominent.

3. The defect involves a polymorphic genetic locus that specifies the structure of apoprotein E, a component of remnant lipoproteins derived from chylomicrons and VLDL. Apoprotein E is believed to bind to hepatic surface receptors, thereby promoting the uptake of remnant lipoproteins into the liver. All clinically affected individuals are homozygous for the E^d allele. The protein specified by this allele can be distinguished from the product of the normal (E^n) allele by isoelectric focusing of the apoproteins extracted from plasma VLDL. Remnant particles containing the abnormal E^d

apoprotein are not cleared normally from the circulation and they accumulate to high levels in plasma. The remnants are deposited in scavenger cells and other cell types, producing xanthomas and atheromas.

4. Homozygosity for the E^d allele is common, involving about 1 in 100 Europeans and Americans. Yet, the full-blown clinical expression of the type 3 disease is relatively rare, involving about 1 in 10,000 persons. Thus, most individuals who inherit the mutant apoprotein E have normal lipid levels. Expression of the clinical disease requires the interaction of the E^d/E^d genotype with other genetic or environmental factors or both. Predisposing factors include hypothyroidism, obesity, and the independent inheritance of diabetes mellitus or familial multiple lipoprotein-type hyperlipidemia (combined hyperlipidemia).

5. Diagnosis of type 3 disease is suggested by the finding of palmar or tuberous xanthomas in a patient with elevated lipid levels. A definitive diagnosis can be made by finding the E^d/E^d pattern on isoelectric focusing of the apoproteins of plasma VLDL.

6. The hyperlipidemia in affected patients is remarkably responsive to diet (low calories, 300 mg cholesterol per day, low saturated fat) and drugs (clofibrate alone or in combination with nicotinic acid). On this regimen, plasma lipid levels can be returned to normal and xanthomas usually disappear.

In patients with familial type 3 hyperlipoproteinemia, the plasma concentrations of cholesterol and triglycerides are both elevated because of the accumulation of cholesterol-rich remnant lipoproteins derived from the partial catabolism of chylomicrons and very low density lipoproteins (VLDL) [1]. All individuals with the type 3 disease are homozygous for the E^d allele at a polymorphic genetic locus that specifies the structure of apoprotein E, a normal component of remnants derived from chylomicrons and VLDL [2]. Remnants containing the abnormal apoprotein E are not cleared normally from the circulation and they accumulate to high levels in plasma. Although the full-blown clinical expression of the type 3 disease is relatively rare (about 1 in 10,000 persons), homozygosity for the E^d allele is common (about 1 in 100). Hence, most individuals who inherit the mutant apoprotein have normal lipid levels. Expression of the clinical disease requires the interaction of the appropriate apoprotein E genotype with other genetic or environmental factors or both.

The interest in familial type 3 hyperlipoproteinemia as an inborn error stems from several of its features: (1) patients have an extremely high propensity for atherosclerosis, (2) the hyperlipidemia is unusually responsive to diet and drug therapy, and (3) the cholesterol-rich remnants that accumulate in the plasma of affected individuals are the human counterparts of the cholesterol-rich particles that accumulate in the plasma of cholesterol-fed animals that develop fulminant atherosclerosis. Hence, insights into the pathogenesis of type 3 hyperlipoproteinemia may yield general information about the role of specific lipoprotein particles in atherosclerosis.

HISTORICAL ASPECTS

Clinically, the variable hypercholesterolemia and hypertriglyceridemia in the type 3 disorder overlap some of the other inherited forms of hyperlipidemia. Prior to about 1970, patients with the disease were doubtless included among individuals reported as having "essential hypercholesterolemia," "mixed hyperlipidemia," or other nonspecific terms. At one time some of these patients were referred to as having "xanthoma tuberosum" [3].

The distinctness of the type 3 disorder from other forms of genetic hyperlipidemia was established in 1967 by Fredrickson et al. [4]. Classifying hyperlipidemic patients by a combination of ultracentrifugation and lipoprotein electrophoresis, they found one group whose VLDL showed β mobility on electrophoresis rather than the usual pre-β mobility (Fig. 32-1). These so-called β-VLDL particles [5] or "floating beta lipoproteins" [4] also caused a "broad-beta" band to appear on electrophoresis of whole plasma (Fig. 32-2). This disorder was given the designation type 3 hyperlipoproteinemia in the typing system of Fredrickson et al. and is also called broad-beta or floating beta disease [4] or dysbetalipoproteinemia [6].

As comparisons later proved [5], type 3 hyperlipoproteinemia is identical with the xanthoma tuberosum studied 20 years earlier by Gofman et al. [3]. Using analytical ultracentrifugation, Gofman found that patients with xanthoma tuberosum had a distinctive lipoprotein pattern [3] with the following abnormalities: an *increase* in plasma lipoproteins with flotation rates of $S_f = 12$ to 20, which includes small VLDL and

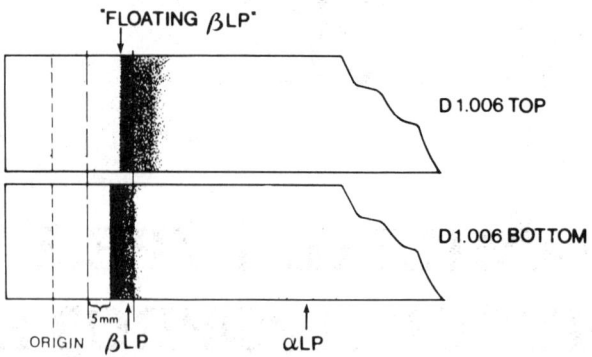

Figure 32-1   Diagram illustrating the "floating beta" of β-VLDL. Paper electrophoresis was performed on the supernatant ($d < 1.006$ g/ml, *top*) and infranatant ($d > 1.006$ g/ml, *bottom*) fractions obtained by preparative ultracentrifugation of plasma without adjustment of density. The strips were stained with a lipid-binding dye (oil red 0), dried, and the origins aligned. The LDL (β-LP) and HDL (α-LP) are found in the bottom fractions. Normally, VLDL (pre-β mobility) is present in the top fraction and migrates such that its tailing edge is beyond the leading edge of the β-LP band. The presence of a band in the top fraction that begins between the indicated lines shows the presence of β-VLDL. *(From Fredrickson et al. [12]. Used by permission.)*

intermediate density lipoproteins (IDL) of density 1.006 to 1.019 g/ml; an *increase* in lipoproteins with flotation rates of $S_f = 20$ to 400 (VLDL); and a *decrease* in lipoproteins with flotation rates of $S_f = 0$ to 12, which includes low density lipoprotein (LDL, density 1.019 to 1.063 g/ml) (Fig. 32-2).

It was established in the early studies of xanthoma tuberosum [3] and type 3 hyperlipoproteinemia [4, 7–9] that the chylomicrons, β-VLDL, and IDL of these patients contained an abnormally high content of cholesterol relative to triglyceride. Initial findings of apoprotein abnormalities in the β-VLDL [10] were extended in 1973 by Havel and Kane, who showed that the β-VLDL of affected individuals contained an absolute increase in apoprotein E [11]. This finding was soon followed in 1975 by the important genetic studies of Utermann, who discovered that the primary genetic defect in this disorder results from homozygosity for a mutant allele at the apoprotein E locus [2].

CLINICAL FEATURES

Blood Lipids and Lipoproteins

Although the abnormal lipoproteins that characterize familial type 3 hyperlipoproteinemia can be detected even when the plasma triglyceride and cholesterol concentrations are normal [12, 13], their detection requires sophisticated techniques that are not usually applied to persons with normal lipid levels. As a result, most probands who have been detected so far have exhibited hyperlipidemia. Because of this bias to selection, the mean lipid concentrations compiled in untreated patients tend to be greatly above normal (Table 32-1) and may be much above those in many affected but unrecognized subjects. The plasma cholesterol level in such patients is usually over 300 mg/dl and may occasionally exceed 1000 mg/dl [14]. The absolute triglyceride concentrations are usually in the range of 200 to 800 mg/dl and tend to exceed those of cholesterol. Occasionally, the triglyceride level may exceed 2000 mg/dl [14, 15]. Perhaps because of the sensitivity of the lipid levels to caloric intake [14, 16], the variability of cholesterol and triglyceride concentrations in a given patient is greater in the type 3 disorder than in any other form of genetic hyperlipidemia, with the possible exception of familial lipoprotein lipase deficiency (Chap. 30).

The results obtained from conventional fractionation of plasma lipoproteins in the preparative ultracentrifuge, with quantification based on the cholesterol content of the fractions, are shown in Table 32-2. The VLDL fraction, defined as all lipoproteins of density less than 1.006 g/ml, is increased in type 3 patients. The concentration of the fraction with densities of 1.006 to 1.063, which includes IDL plus LDL, is modestly decreased. This change is caused by a marked decrease in LDL and an increase in IDL. The HDL concentration is reduced. When the VLDL concentration is reduced by treatment, the HDL tend to rise to normal, but the LDL concentrations tend to remain depressed [14].

The pattern in the analytical ultracentrifuge (Fig. 32-2) is more revealing of the abnormality [3, 5]. The expected increase in lipoproteins of $S_f = 20$ to 400 is accompanied by a most unusual pattern in the LDL region. Here there is an abnormally low quantity of lipoprotein having S_f values of 0 to 12, which in normal subjects is the most abundant LDL subclass, and there is a marked increase in lipoproteins of $S_f = 12$ to 20. As mentioned above, the former correspond to the LDL fraction of density 1.019 to 1.063 g/ml in the preparative ultracentrifuge, and the latter to the IDL fraction of density 1.006 to 1.019 g/ml.

Electrophoresis of plasma on paper, agarose, or cellulose acetate, followed by staining for lipids, reveals an increase in pre-β-lipoproteins (VLDL), and frequently there is a broadbeta band extending between and appearing to combine the β- and pre-β-lipoproteins (Fig. 32-2). The marked decrease in conventional LDL is detectable on polyacrylamide gel, where a band in the usual β position is rarely visible [17]. As mentioned above and as illustrated is Fig. 32-1, electrophoresis of the ultracentrifuge fraction of density less than 1.006 g/ml usually reveals a β-migrating band, the "floating beta" of the original diagnostic test for type 3.

Figure 32-2 Plasma lipoprotein pattern in type 3 hyperlipoproteinemia. The *upper* illustration shows an analytical ultracentrifugal pattern of plasma run at $d = 1.063$ g/ml. The dotted line shows the pattern observed in normal plasma, and the hatched area shows the pattern in type 3 plasma. $S_f = 0$ to 12 denotes LDL; $S_f = 12$ to 20 denotes IDL; $S_f = 20$ to 400 denotes VLDL. The *lower* illustration shows the broad-beta band of type 3 plasma that was subjected to paper electrophoresis.

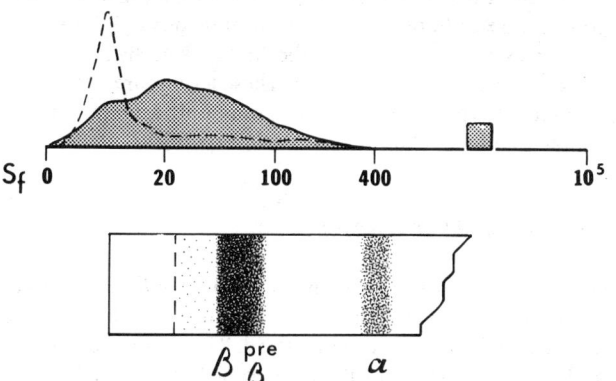

Table 32-1 Plasma lipid concentrations in subjects with untreated type 3 hyperlipoproteinemia*

Subjects	Number	Cholesterol, mg/dl	Triglycerides, mg/dl
Type 3 hyperlipoproteinemia			
All subjects	47	453 ± 21	699 ± 77
Men, mean age 40	27	440 ± 25	694 ± 104
Women, mean age 49	20	470 ± 36	705 ± 117
Control			
Men, age 30–39	50	210 ± 5	78 ± 6
Women, age 40–49	44	217 ± 5	80 ± 6

* Values cited are mean ± SEM; control values are derived from Fredrickson et al. [4].
SOURCE: Adopted from Morganroth et al. [14].

Abnormal Lipoproteins

In familial type 3 hyperlipoproteinemia the plasma contains normal lipoproteins as well as certain abnormal populations that are not detected in significant amounts in normal subjects. Some of these lipoproteins may appear inconsistently in patients with other forms of hyperlipidemia. The normal lipoproteins present in type 3 plasma include chylomicrons derived from dietary fat, VLDL having conventional mobility on electrophoresis (and called α-VLDL, after their mobility on starch [7]), LDL of density 1.019 to 1.063 g/ml, and HDL.

The abnormal lipoproteins include some unusual large particles that appear to be remnants of chylomicrons, the pathognomonic β-VLDL, and intermediate particles in the IDL region having density of 1.006 to 1.019 g/ml [18, 19].

The definitions of the abnormal forms, like those of their normal neighbors in the lipoprotein continuum, are partly operational. The separation of β-VLDL and IDL, for example, is critically dependent upon the length of time the plasma is exposed to the ultracentrifugal fields conventionally used for separating VLDL and LDL [18]. The amounts of β-VLDL and IDL, their aggregate compositions, and, indeed, the question of whether they are distinct metabolic entities, remain subject to some uncertainty. Some of the current knowledge of the aberrant lipoproteins in type 3 hyperlipoproteinemia is summarized in Tables 32-3, 32-4, and 32-5. The data are adapted primarily from the work of Sata, Havel, and Jones [20], Havel and Kane [11], Patsch, Sailer, and Braunsteiner [18], and Havel et al. [21].

Compared to the usual α-VLDL, the β-VLDL of type 3 hyperlipoproteinemia tend to be slightly smaller particles (a mean diameter about 35 nm instead of about 40 nm) and occupy the lower S_f region (20 to 60) of the entire $S_f = 20$ to 400 spectrum of VLDL. There are two features of the composition of β-VLDL that distinguish it from normal VLDL. One is the increase in cholesterol (mainly cholesteryl esters) relative to triglyceride content [20]. The other is an apoprotein content that is both quantitatively and qualitatively different from normal VLDL. There is a deficiency in C apoproteins relative to apoprotein B [10, 11], and an absolute increase in the total amount of apoprotein E [11, 21]. In addition, the usual types of apoprotein E in VLDL are replaced by a nonfunctional type (the product of the E^d allele, which is discussed below) [2]. It is believed that the difference in surface charge resulting from the change in apoprotein complement, and possibly also the dif-

Table 32-2 Plasma lipoprotein concentrations in subjects with untreated type 3 hyperlipoproteinemia*

Subjects	Number	Cholesterol content, mg/dl		
		VLDL	LDL + IDL	HDL
Type 3				
All subjects	47	287 ± 25	121 ± 8	38 ± 3
Men, mean age 40	27	268 ± 32	131 ± 14	37 ± 3
Women, mean age 49	20	307 ± 39	131 ± 9	39 ± 5
Controls				
Men, age 30–39	50	21 ± 2	143 ± 4	48 ± 2
Women, age 40–49	44	14 ± 1	130 ± 4	62 ± 2

* Values cited are mean ± SEM; control values are derived from Fredrickson et al. [4].
SOURCE: Adopted from Morganroth et al. [14].

ference in cholesterol content, causes these particles to migrate more slowly on electrophoresis than normal [22].

The IDL, which have an S_f = 12 to 20, are presumed to represent a transition form from VLDL to LDL [19]. They have a higher content of triglyceride than the bulk of normal LDL, which have an S_f = 0 to 12. The IDL contain apoproteins C and E, in addition to apoprotein B, while normal LDL contains B apoprotein almost exclusively. Patsch et al. have concluded that these IDL and β-VLDL are discrete populations rather than a spectrum of abnormal particles that extend across the 1.006 g/ml density boundary used for defining normal families of lipoproteins [18]. This interpretation tends to be supported by kinetic data [23].

Frequently, plasma withdrawn from patients with type 3 hyperlipoproteinemia some 12 h after the last meal will have a faint cream layer at the top, or material at the origin of electrophoretograms indicative of chylomicrons. These particles represent not so much a delay in fat assimilation as abnormal metabolism of chylomicrons. Chylomicrons isolated from plasma during the period immediately after ingestion of fat loads appear to be normal in lipid composition [11, 24]. Some hours later, smaller particles (about 80 nm in mean diameter) are recoverable, and these become progressively richer in cholesteryl esters [24]. It is believed that these particles also contain more free cholesterol than their complement of phospholipid can accommodate at the surface, and that some of the excess sterol is probably packed in the particle core [20]. It has been suggested that these postabsorptive particles are remnants of chylomicrons that are accumulating either because of the same processing defect that gives rise to the β-VLDL [22] or because the normal clearing mechanism is saturated by the excess of other triglyceride-rich particles.

Age of Onset

Eight publications over the past decade have described 200 well-documented cases of familial type 3 hyperlipoproteinemia [14, 21, 25–29], including 9 in one large kindred [25, 30]. Among these patients the age of detection has varied from 16 to 95 years. In addition to these cases, at least 50 other patients with well-documented type 3 disease have been described. Only seven affected individuals under the age of 20 have been reported to date [6]. Of these, the youngest is a 12-year-old boy [31]. The disorder has also occurred in a set of 16-year-old female monozygotic twins with hypothyroidism secondary to autoimmune thyroiditis [15]. In most series men tend to

present earlier than women, and there is some correlation between obesity and earlier appearance of hyperlipidemia or xanthomas. The disease has been described largely in Caucasians thus far, although at least one black patient has been seen [1].

Xanthomas

The most striking clinical feature of familial type 3 hyperlipoproteinemia is the occurrence of yellowish lipid deposits in the creases of the palm (Fig. 32-3). In a total of 115 patients reported from four clinics [14, 25–27], about one-half of untreated probands have had these lesions. A smaller percentage of affected subjects detected through family screening were also noted [14]. Popularized as "planar xanthomas" in the first descriptions [4], these lesions are more specifically termed xanthoma striata palmaris (or xanthochromia striata palmaris when they are not elevated) [32]. In one series of more than 1000 patients with primary hyperlipidemia, only those with type 3 were observed to have such lesions [1, 4]. Palmar xanthomas, having a similar appearance but located elsewhere than in the creases and usually in a vertical position between the bases of the fingers, also occur in familial hypercholesterolemia, especially in homozygotes (Chap. 33). Xanthoma striata palmaris can occur in patients with hyperlipidemia secondary to paraproteinemia.

Other kinds of xanthomas also appear in patients with type 3 (Table 32-6 and Fig. 32-3). Among these the most common are elevated tuberous lesions on the elbows, frequently surrounded by satellite lesions with an erythematous base ("tuberoeruptive xanthomas"). Flesh-colored periosteal xanthomas on the tibial tuberosities are also common. Much less frequent are xanthomas in the calcaneal tendons (Achilles tendons) or extensor tendons of the hands. Xanthelasmas and corneal arcus are sometimes seen. These lesions are not pathognomonic of type 3 and are most commonly seen in patients with familial hypercholesterolemia (Chap. 33).

Premature Atherosclerosis

In the series of nearly 50 patients described by Morganroth et al. [14], 43 percent had detectable vascular disease. Ischemic heart disease was present in one-third. The mean age of onset was 38 years in males and about a decade later in females [14]. Peripheral vascular disease was also found in about one-third, again appearing earlier in males than in females. In comparison with a large collection of patients with familial hypercholesterolemia, the authors obtained convincing evidence that claudication is much more common in type 3 [14]. Cerebrovascular disease occurred in 5 of their 47 patients [14]. In the screening of 500 survivors of myocardial infarction and their families for hyperlipidemia in Seattle, Goldstein et al. found one unequivocal and three other possible cases of type 3 [33].

The observed prevalence of vascular disease in type 3 hyperlipoproteinemia depends somewhat upon the manner in which the patients have presented. Borrie, a dermatologist, found less evidence of this complication in his patients [26] than did either Morganroth et al. [14] or Mischkel [27]. Nevertheless, type 3 hyperlipoproteinemia probably affords as high a risk of

premature vascular disease (Table 32-6) as any form of hyperlipidemia except for homozygotes for familial hypercholesterolemia. A patient who has hyperlipidemia and peripheral vascular disease should always raise the suspicion of type 3.

Other Clinical Abnormalities

Asymptomatic hyperuricemia is present in up to half of patients with type 3 [14], but only about 5 percent have clinical gout (Table 32-6). An even more frequent abnormality is glucose intolerance, appearing in 55 percent in one series [14]. However, only 4 percent of subjects have clinical diabetes (Table 32-6). Most hyperlipidemic individuals with type 3 are obese [4], and this may account for their insulin resistance.

Patients with type 3 hyperlipoproteinemia tend to be unusually well-studied, and it is notable that, with the possible

Figure 32-3 Xanthomas commonly seen in type 3 hyperlipoproteinemia. *A,B,C,D* include tuberoeruptive xanthomas on elbows, buttocks, and knees; *D* displays subperiosteal xanthomas over the tibial tuberosities. *A, E,* and *F* demonstrate xanthomas striata palmaris.

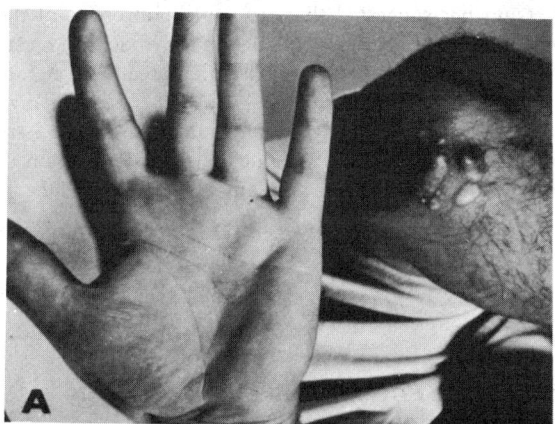
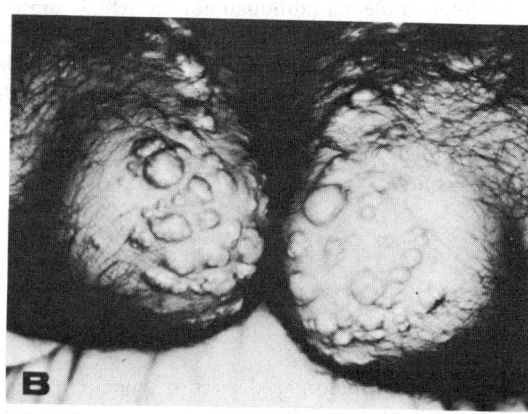
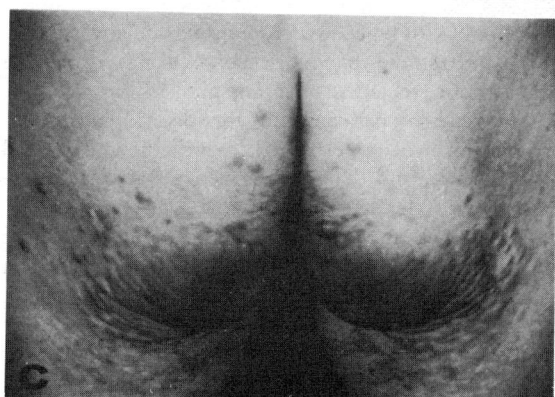
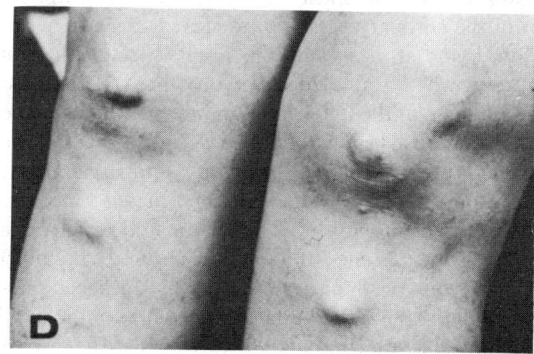
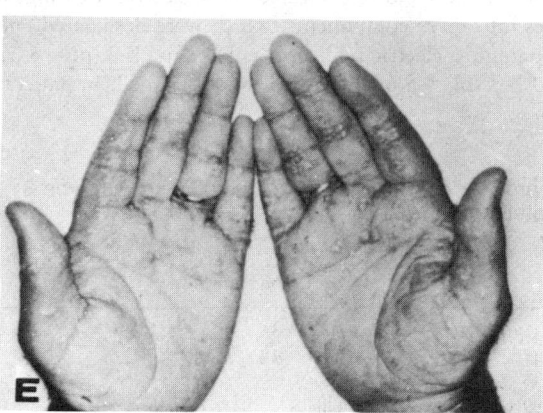
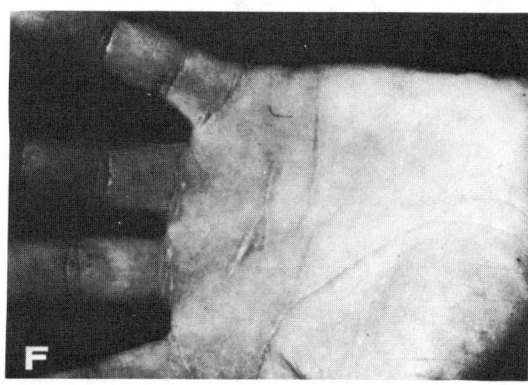

Table 32-3 Plasma lipoproteins of $d < 1.006$ g/ml in subjects with type 3 hyperlipoproteinemia

Lipoprotein	Mean diameter, mm	C/TG	Protein, %	Apoprotein content
Chylomicron remnants	80	0.5	2	B 30% E > C's
α-VLDL	40	0.3	10	B 45% C's > E
β-VLDL	35	2	9	B 55% E > C's

NOTE: C = cholesterol; TG = triglycerides; C's = apoproteins C-I, C-II, C-III.
SOURCE: Adapted from data of Sata et al. [20], and Havel and Kane [11].

exception of cholelithiasis, none of the many associated diseases found in some patients [14] has consistently appeared in others. Thyroid function has a marked effect on the expression of the disease [1, 34]. Hyperthyroidism can completely eliminate the hyperlipidemia (although not the telltale presence of β-VLDL), while hypothyroidism markedly exaggerates all the lipid and lipoprotein abnormalities. Low levels of thyroid-binding globulin have been reported in two patients [14, 35], but at least three others have had normal levels [14]. About 4 percent of patients have clinical hypothyroidism at some point during the course of their disease (Table 32-6).

PATHOLOGIC ASPECTS

Information about the organ defects of type 3 hyperlipoproteinemia is rather scanty. There have been four reported autopsies [36–39]. The first [36] and fourth [39] patients examined post mortem had the most interesting abnormalities. The lumens of the coronary vessels of the first patient were severely narrowed, and at many sites this resulted from collections of foam cells, which stained deeply with oil red 0. On the endocardial surface of the left atrium and the ventricular aspect of the anterior mitral leaflet, there also were grossly visible yellow deposits, which contained numerous similar-staining foam cells. In some parts of the endocardium these formed a single layer under the intima [36]. The unique finding in the fourth patient was the presence of foam cells in the renal glomerulus [39]. Foam cells were also present in the thickened endocardium overlying the healed infarcts, as well as in the intima of vessels affected with coronary atherosclerosis. The second [37] and third [38] patients had no such foam cell lesions, and their coronary artery disease resembled the usual plaques seen in normolipidemic individuals and in subjects with other types of hyperlipoproteinemia.

The spleen and bone marrow in patients with familial type 3 hyperlipoproteinemia are also laden with foam cells [36]. The macrophages contain ceroid pigment along with birefringent lipid droplets. Observations in Tangier disease and lecithin:cholesterol acyltransferase (LCAT) deficiency have laid emphasis on the propensity of the reticuloendothelial system for removing abnormal lipoproteins by phagocytosis, with resulting accumulation of masses of foam cells in the tissues. Different kinds of lipoproteins appear to be handled differently, in terms of both organ sites of deposition and types of tissue lesions.

Recently, it was shown that mouse peritoneal macrophages and other macrophages have receptors on their surfaces that bind β-VLDL and mediate their uptake and degradation within the cell. This leads to massive cellular cholesteryl ester accumulation (see below and Refs. 94 and 95). The β-VLDL particles used in these studies were obtained from plasma of cholesterol-fed animals. Whether β-VLDL particles from type 3 patients bind to these receptors is unknown.

Zilversmit has suggested that remnant lipoproteins of the kind seen in type 3 hyperlipoproteinemia are toxic to the vascular wall with formation of foam cells that greatly accelerate the development of atherosclerosis [40]. If this is so, it may prove that efforts to control hyperlipidemia per se in type 3 are less important than specifically reducing the concentration of one or all of the chylomicron remnants, β-VLDL, or IDL.

GENETICS

Apoprotein E Polymorphism: One Locus with Three Alleles

The familial nature of type 3 hyperlipoproteinemia was recognized in the early studies of Fredrickson et al. [1, 4], but the mode of inheritance remained uncertain until 1975 when Utermann discovered that patients with this disease had a deficiency of one form of apoprotein E, which they designated apoprotein E-3 [2], and that this deficiency state was transmitted as a simple Mendelian trait [28, 41–44].

This discovery was made possible by the application of the technique of isoelectric focusing to the study of the proteins in VLDL of type 3 patients. In normal subjects, the apoprotein E of VLDL appears as a single broad band on sodium dodecyl sulfate polyacrylamide gel electrophoresis, a technique that separates proteins according to size (Fig. 32-4, left panel). When this single band is subjected to isoelectric focusing, it separates into three components, which were designated apo E-1 [apparent isoelectric point (pI) = 5.3], apo E-2 (pI = 5.5), and apo E-3 (pI = 5.6) (Fig. 32-4, middle panel). In patients

Table 32-4 Plasma lipoproteins of $d > 1.006$ g/ml in subjects with type 3 hyperlipoproteinemia

Mobility	S_f	C, %	TG, %	PL, %	Protein, %
IDL (intermediates)	β to pre-β	12 to 20	36	19	24	20
LDL	β	0 to 12	42	8	22	28

NOTE: C = cholesterol; TG = triglycerides; PL = phospholipids

Table 32-5 Concentration of lipoprotein lipids and apoprotein E in patients with familial type 3 hyperlipoproteinemia and their relatives*

Genotype	Number	VLDL (d < 1.006 g/ml), mg/dl			IDL + LDL (d = 1.006–1.063 g/ml), mg/dl			HDL (d = 1.063–1.210 g/ml), mg/dl		
		Cholesterol	Triglycerides	Apoprotein E	Cholesterol	Triglycerides	Apoprotein E	Cholesterol	Triglycerides	Apoprotein E
Probands E^d/E^d	10	148 ± 106	256 ± 169	11 ± 7.9	102 ± 51	67 ± 83	6.2 ± 3.0	39 ± 12	14 ± 4	6.2 ± 2.6
Heterozygotes E^n/E^d E^4/E^d	19	26 ± 28	77 ± 80	2.0 ± 1.8	104 ± 36	36 ± 17	2.3 ± 1.6	50 ± 15	17 ± 9	4.8 ± 2.3
Normals E^n/E^n E^4/E^4 E^n/E^4	11	10 ± 7	44 ± 25	0.9 ± 0.4	106 ± 40	23 ± 9	1.3 ± 1.2	48 ± 10	13 ± 6	3.8 ± 1.9

* Values cited are mean ± SD.
SOURCE: Adapted from Havel et al. [21]

with classic type 3 hyperlipoproteinemia, the E-3 band is missing and the E-2 band is increased in amount (Fig. 32-4, right panel) [2, 41–44]. The increase in E-2 more than balances the decrease in E-3, thus explaining the increase in total apoprotein E in VLDL that had been noted earlier by Havel and Kane [11] (see Table 32-5). The E-1 band is the same in all individuals and does not appear to be related to the type 3 disease.

Utermann's observations on the lack of apo E-3 in the VLDL from patients with type 3 hyperlipoproteinemia have been confirmed by a number of investigators, including Havel [21, 45], Hazzard [46, 47], and Schonfeld [48, 49] and their coworkers. Virtually every type 3 patient studied to date has shown a complete or near complete deficiency of apo E-3 [6].

In family studies, Utermann showed that patients with apo E-3 deficiency were apparently homozygous for a gene that prevented its normal expression [28, 42–44]. Parents of apo E-3–deficient individuals, who were obligate heterozygotes, had levels of E-3 that were between those of normal subjects and the homozygous-deficient subjects. These intermediate values could be assessed most conveniently by densitometric scanning of isoelectric focusing gels performed on heparin-magnesium–precipitated VLDL with calculation of the ratio of apoprotein E-2 to apoprotein E-3. Normal subjects had a ratio less than 0.52; heterozygotes had a ratio of 0.62 to 2.5; and homozygotes had a ratio greater than 3.4 [28, 43]. On the basis of these data, Utermann originally proposed that the genetic locus specifying apoprotein E be called the *apo E–N/D* locus (*N* for *normal* and *D* for *deficient*) and that the polymorphism of apoprotein E was controlled by two codominant alleles, *apo E^n* and *apo E^d*, giving the three genotypes of E^n/E^n (ratio of E-2/E-3, <0.52), E^n/E^d (ratio of E-2/E-3, 0.62 to 2.5), and E^d/E^d (ratio of E-2/E-3, >3.4).

A survey of nearly 500 asymptomatic blood donors showed that apo E-3 deficiency was extremely common in the German population [42–44]. About 1 percent were apo E-3–deficient, 16 percent were heterozygous for apo E-3 deficiency, and 83 percent were normal. These are the relative frequencies expected from the Hardy-Weinberg law if the E-3–deficient state represents homozygosity at a single genetic locus.

In subsequent population and family studies, Utermann detected the presence of a fourth apo E component in the VLDL, present in about 25 to 30 percent of the German population. This component, which had an apparent isoelectric

point of 5.75, was designated the apo E-4 variant [44]. Although Utermann originally believed that the locus specifying apo E-4 was distinct from that specifying E-2 and E-3, he observed that all individuals who were deficient in E-3 (genotype, E^d/E^d) were always lacking E-4 [44].

Although 1 percent of unselected asymptomatic individuals are homozygous for E-3 deficiency, most of these subjects have normal lipid levels and do not have the classic type 3 disease [43, 50]. All of these individuals can be shown to possess an abnormal VLDL as judged by the presence of elevated ratios of VLDL-cholesterol to total triglyceride or by the presence of β-VLDL on electrophoresis [50]. Even though β-VLDL is present, the concentration of total plasma cholesterol is low in these apo E-3–deficient subjects because there is an overall reduction in the plasma concentration of LDL [50].

These seminal findings of Utermann gave a new focus to research in type 3 hyperlipoproteinemia and pointed out that a polymorphism at the apoprotein E locus may have profound effects on lipid metabolism in humans. These studies have stimulated much subsequent research, and the details of Utermann's scheme have had to be refined, but the overall concept

Figure 32-4 *Left:* Sodium dodecyl sulfate polyacrylamide gel electrophoresis in 10% gels of apo-VLDL *(A)* and purified apo E *(B)* from a normal subject. *Middle:* Analytical isoelectric focusing in polyacrylamide gels at pH 3.5 to 10 of urea-soluble apo-VLDL *(A)* and apo E *(B)* from a normal subject. *Right:* Analytical isoelectric focusing in 7.5% polyacrylamide gels of apo-VLDL from a patient with familial type 3 hyperlipoproteinemia *(A)* and a normal subject *(B)*. All gels were stained with Coomassie brilliant blue. *(Photographs provided by Dr. Gerd Utermann.)*

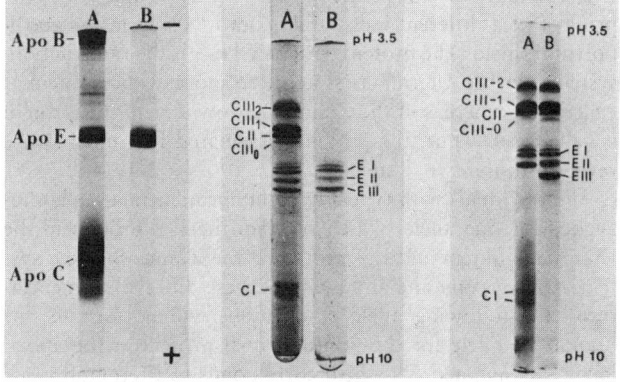

Table 32-6 Clinical data on 115 patients with type 3 hyperlipoproteinemia

No. of patients	115
Age range, years	16 to 95
Mean cholesterol, mg/dl	410
Mean triglyceride, mg/dl	576

	Percent of patients
Xanthomas	
Striata palmaris	47
Tendon	13
Tuberous and tuberoeruptive	57
Xanthelasma	9
Corneal arcus	11
Coronary heart disease	28
Peripheral vascular disease	19
Cerebrovascular disease	7
Gout	5
Diabetes mellitus (clinical)	4
Hypothyroidism	4

SOURCE: From the pooled date of Morganroth et al. [*14*], Borrie [*26*], Mishkel [*27*], and Hazzard [*25*].

of a polymorphism at the apoprotein E locus has been substantiated.

Zannis and Breslow have recently applied the technique of two-dimensional gel electrophoresis to the study of the apoprotein E polymorphism [*51–53*]. In this technique the proteins are first subjected to isoelectric focusing, which separates the proteins by charge, and they are then subjected to sodium dodecyl sulfate–polyacrylamide gel electrophoresis in the second dimension, which separates the proteins according to size. When this procedure was performed on the VLDL from normal individuals, large numbers of apoprotein E spots were observed [*51–53*]. Much of this heterogeneity was due to the presence of varying amounts of sialic acid on the apo E glycoproteins, a posttranslational modification that creates differences in size and charge. When the VLDL apoproteins were first treated with neuraminidase to remove the sialic acid residues and then subjected to two-dimensional electrophoresis, the complex patterns of the apo E proteins were more easily resolved [*53*].

Using the above method, Zannis and Breslow have shown that the apoprotein E locus is a single polymorphic locus, with three common alleles segregating in the population [*52, 53*]. Correlating the Zannis-Breslow findings with the Utermann findings is complicated because the same proteins are assigned different numerals in the two systems. In both systems, the protein components specified by the E locus are designated E-2, E-3, and E-4. The protein designated E-1 is likely to be the product of a different locus and is not involved in the apo E polymorphism. The protein designated E-3 is the same in both systems. In the Utermann system the most acidic protein is called E-2, whereas in the Zannis-Breslow system this protein is called E-4. Thus, the proteins designated E-2 and E-4 are reversed in the two systems.

All individuals with type 3 hyperlipoproteinemia are homozygous for one allele, which specifies the E-2 protein in the Utermann system and E-4 protein in the Zannis-Breslow system. To overcome the ambiguity of these different nomenclatures, the following allele designations will be used in this book. The allele for the nonfunctional protein at the apo E locus is designated E^d, which corresponds to Utermann's ear-

lier "deficiency" allele [*43*]. This E^d allele denotes the most acidic apoprotein, which is designated E-2 by Utermann and E-4 by Zannis and Breslow. The allele specifying E-3 (both systems) is designated E^n. The allele specifying the most basic apoprotein, which is designated E-4 by Utermann and E-2 by Zannis and Breslow, is here designated E^4. Individuals with type 3 disease have genotype E^d/E^d. Heterozygotes for this defect can have one of two genotypes: E^n/E^d or E^4/E^d. Normal individuals can possess one of three genotypes: E^n/E^n, E^4/E^4, or E^n/E^4.

The allele frequencies and the genotype frequencies of the various combinations of alleles according to the data of Utermann and of Zannis and Breslow are summarized in Tables 32-7 and 32-8.

Mode of Inheritance as Defined by Clinical Genetic Studies

All patients with symptomatic type 3 hyperlipoproteinemia are homozygous for the E^d allele [*28, 43, 52*]. Moreover, all patients with the E^d/E^d genotype have detectable β-VLDL on electrophoresis. Nevertheless, no more than 1 in 50 of these latter individuals ever develops clinical signs of the type 3 disease. Probably no more than 1 in 5,000 people among the general population show the typical clinical features of familial type 3 hyperlipoproteinemia. On the other hand, 1 to 3 percent of people are of genotype E^d/E^d (Table 32-8). Thus, the presence of the E^d/E^d genotype is a necessary but not a sufficient condition for the development of the clinical syndrome of familial type 3 [*54*].

In 1979 Utermann made the surprising observation that those homozygous E^d/E^d individuals who were not hypercholesterolemic were actually hypocholesterolemic [*28*]. The mean cholesterol level in such E^d/E^d homozygotes was 161 mg/dl, as opposed to a mean value of 202 mg/dl in age and sex-matched subjects who did not possess the E^d allele. This reduction was present even though the E^d/E^d subjects had an increased VLDL-cholesterol of 42 mg/dl (normal = 16 mg/dl). Moreover, an intermediate value for total plasma cholesterol (185 mg/dl) could be demonstrated in heterozygotes for the E^d allele. On the basis of these findings, a schematic diagram for the distribution of plasma cholesterol in these genotypes was proposed (Fig. 32-5). It was also proposed that in individuals with the E^d/E^d genotype the plasma cholesterol could be raised above normal by the simultaneous but independent inheritance of other defects that produce hyperlipidemia [*50*]. Among

Table 32-7 Apo E gene frequencies in German and American populations

	Gene frequency	
Apo E allele	Germans (n = 489)	Americans (n = 61)
E^n	0.77	0.72
E^4	0.15	0.11
E^d	0.08	0.17

SOURCE: The German and American data were obtained by Utermann [*42, 44*] and by Zannis and Breslow [*52, 53*], respectively.

Table 32-8   Frequency of apo E genotypes in German and American populations*

Genotype	Germans (n = 489) Observed %	Germans (n = 489) Expected %	Americans (n = 61) Observed %	Americans (n = 61) Expected %
E^n/E^n	59	59	49	52
E^n/E^4	22	22	15	16
E^4/E^4	3	2	2	1
E^n/E^d	13	13	31	25
E^4/E^d	2	3	3	4
E^d/E^d	1	1	0	3

* The German population studied by Utermann consisted of 489 consecutive normal blood donors [42, 44]. The American population studied by Zannis and Breslow consisted of 61 unrelated volunteers, excluding individuals with known hyperlipidemia and those with a family history of premature coronary heart disease [52, 53].

The *expected* apo E genotypes were calculated assuming a Hardy-Weinberg distribution of alleles whose frequencies correspond to those given in Table 32-7.

these was the inheritance of the gene for familial multiple-lipoprotein-type hyperlipoproteinemia (also called familial combined hyperlipoproteinemia) [55] and perhaps familial hypercholesterolemia. When E^d/E^d individuals inherited one of these other diseases, they exhibited large amounts of β-VLDL and the classic type 3 syndrome.

Direct support for this two-factor hypothesis was obtained by Utermann in a study of 19 kindreds ascertained through a proband with an E^d/E^d genotype [28]. Those subjects who

Figure 32-5   Schematic representation demonstrating the presence of three overlapping distributions of plasma cholesterol levels in the population as determined by apo E genotype. Note the interaction of genotype apo E-D and "hyperlipidemia genes" in producing clinical type 3 hyperlipoproteinemia. Apo E-D denotes E^d/E^d; apo E-ND denotes E^n/E^d; apo E-N denotes E^n/E^n; HLP denotes hyperlipidemia. (From Utermann et al. [50]. Used by permission.)

showed classic type 3 disease came from families in which other relatives had "hyperlipidemic" genes. Some of these families showed evidence of multiple-lipoprotein-type hyperlipoproteinemia. On the other hand, if an individual with an E^d/E^d genotype was normolipidemic, hyperlipidemic relatives were not found [28].

Figure 32-6 shows a large pedigree, the O'D. family of Seattle [13, 47], that nicely illustrates the concept that the type 3 disease results from the independent inheritance of at least two factors: the E^d/E^d genotype and the presence of another gene causing hyperlipidemia. This kindred has been studied extensively by Hazzard and coworkers. Inspection of the pedigree shows that the apo E alleles and the gene for multiple-lipoprotein-type hyperlipidemia are segregating independently. When the hyperlipidemia gene and the E^d/E^d genotype coincided in an individual, clinical type 3 hyperlipoproteinemia resulted; when the hyperlipidemia gene coincided with any other genotype at the E locus, the patients exhibited lipoprotein types 2a, 2b, or 4, but never type 3. These multiple lipoprotein patterns in the O'D. pedigree are distributed in a manner consistent with autosomal dominant transmission, thus suggesting that, in addition to dysbetalipoproteinemia, this family exhibits familial multiple lipoprotein-type hyperlipidemia [55].

Another factor that produces symptomatic hyperlipidemia in individuals with the E^d/E^d genotype is thyroid deficiency [25]. When the hypothyroidism is treated, the hyperlipidemia is relieved, but β-VLDL particles can still be detected in small amounts in plasma. In addition to hypothyroidism and familial multiple-lipoprotein-type hyperlipidemia, it is likely that other genetic and nongenetic factors modify the expression of hyperlipidemia in individuals with the E^d/E^d genotype. Heterozygous familial hypercholesterolemia is one of these factors [47]. Among the other factors may be obesity and glucose intolerance, two conditions that are found in a large proportion of E^d/E^d homozygotes who manifest the type 3 disease (see

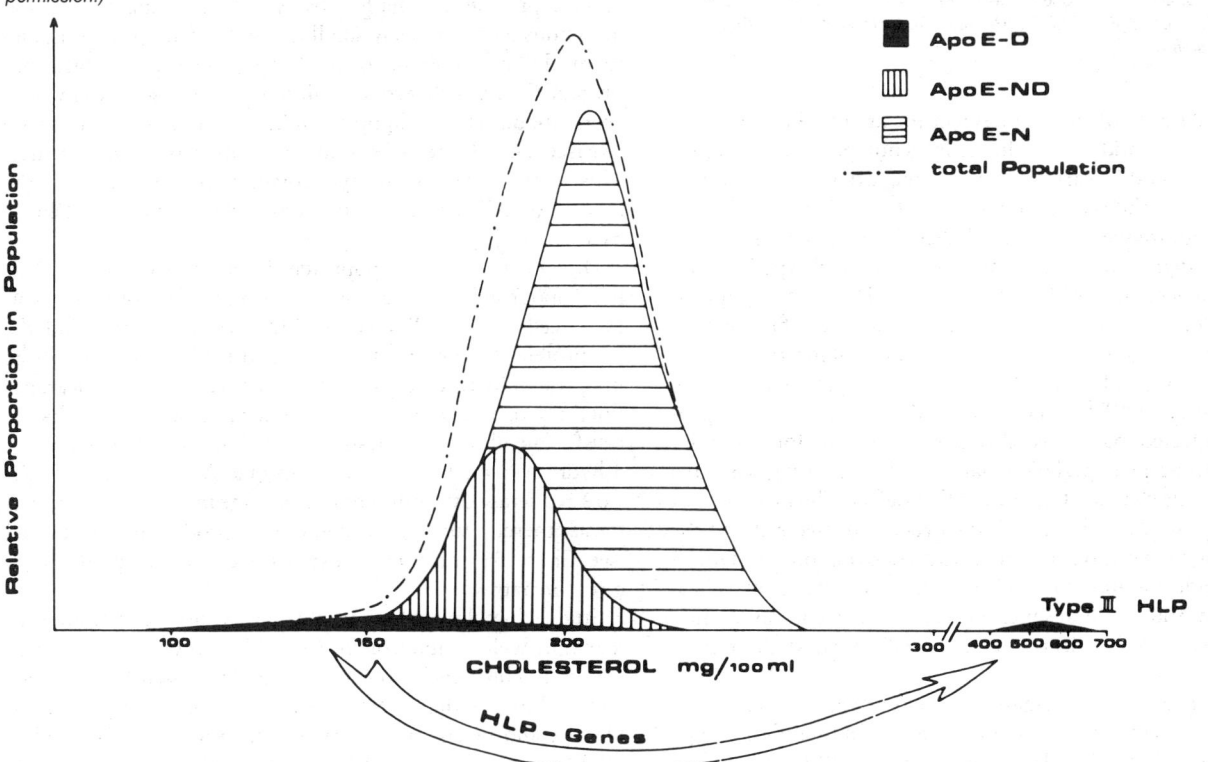

Apo E-D
Apo E-ND
Apo E-N
total Population

Type III HLP

CHOLESTEROL mg/100 ml

HLP-Genes

Relative Proportion in Population

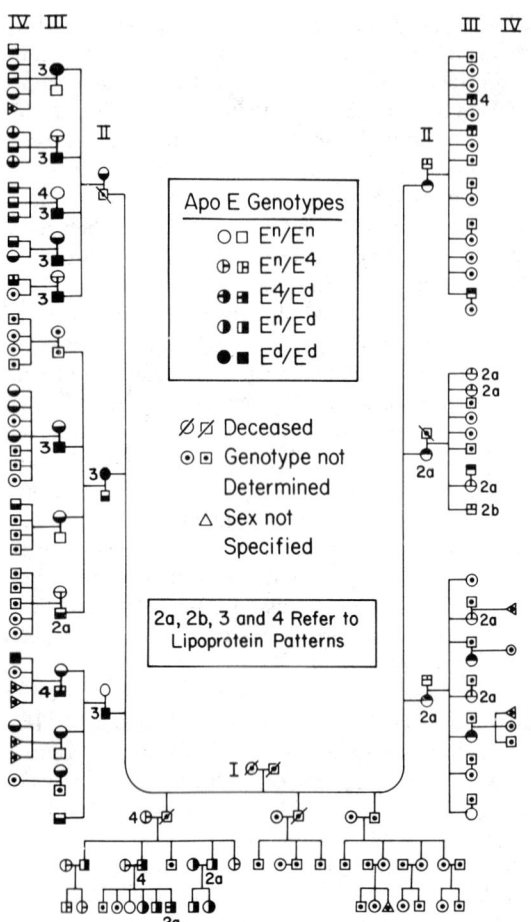

Figure 32-6 Pedigree of a large family, the O'D. kindred, in which nine members show the typical clinical signs of familial type 3 hyperlipoproteinemia and the E^d/E^d genotype. There is one young member with the E^d/E^d genotype who has not yet expressed clinical signs of type 3 (see generation IV). Family members with forms of hyperlipidemia other than type 3 (i.e., types 2a, 2b, and 4) have one of the following genotypes at the apo E locus: E^n/E^n, E^n/E^4, E^n/E^d, or E^4/E^d. (Redrawn from Hazzard et al. [30]. Used by permission.)

above). Because of the requirement for an additional precipitating event in addition to the E^d/E^d genotype, this model predicts considerable variation in the phenotypic expression of patients with the type 3 disease.

The high frequency of the E^d allele in the population gives rise to pedigrees in which symptomatic familial type 3 occurs in several generations of the same family. This is an example of pseudodominant inheritance. It is caused by the fact that an E^d/E^d homozygote has a 15 percent chance of marrying a person heterozygous for the E^d allele. In such a mating, half of the offspring are E^d/E^d homozygotes. Moreover, if the symptomatic affected parent is also a heterozygote for multiple-lipoprotein-type hyperlipidemia, his or her offspring will have a 50 percent chance of inheriting that defect. Thus $\frac{1}{2} \times \frac{1}{2}$ or $\frac{1}{4}$ of the offspring will inherit both the hyperlipidemic trait and the E^d/E^d homozygosity, and thus express symptomatic type 3 hyperlipidemia. In such families the disease will appear to be a dominant trait, with the exception that 25 percent, rather than 50 percent, of first-degree relatives will manifest the type 3 disease.

These new genetic insights may help to explain many puzzling findings that turned up in the early family studies of type 3 disease [13, 14, 29]. For example, in the 29 kindreds analyzed by Morganroth et al., vertical transmission of the type 3

disease was noted, yet only 25 percent of the first-degree relatives of affected probands showed a type 3 lipoprotein pattern with typical β-VLDL. An additional 25 percent of the first-degree relatives were hyperlipidemic, but they manifested type 2a, 2b, and 4 patterns without evidence of β-VLDL. In retrospect, these families illustrate the pseudodominant inheritance pattern of the dysbetalipoproteinemia and the interplay of the apo E polymorphism with other hyperlipidemia disorders, such as familial multiple-lipoprotein-type hyperlipidemia or familial hypercholesterolemia.

PATHOGENESIS

Normal Metabolism of VLDL and Chylomicron Remnants

Role of Apoprotein E The action of lipoprotein lipase (see Chap. 31) upon the two triglyceride-carrying lipoproteins, chylomicrons and VLDL, generates triglyceride-depleted, cholesterol-enriched remnant particles that are analogous to the IDL and β-VLDL lipoproteins that accumulate in type 3 patients. Early studies in animals indicated that chylomicrons were not taken up immediately and directly by the liver. It was only after the circulating chylomicrons had been exposed to lipoprotein lipase that the resultant remnant particles were rapidly cleared by the liver [6, 56, 57]. These findings suggested that the liver possesses a specific mechanism for taking up cholesterol-rich lipoproteins and that this mechanism can somehow distinguish between chylomicrons and remnants. The nature of this mechanism remained obscure until the existence of receptor-mediated endocytosis of lipoproteins was discovered in cultured cells [58].

Apoprotein E appears to play an important role in the hepatic uptake process and may be one factor that allows lipoprotein receptors in the liver to selectively bind remnants [6]. Chylomicrons have relatively small amounts of apoprotein E, and relatively large amounts of the C apoproteins, including apoprotein C-2, which activates lipoprotein lipase. As chylomicrons are digested by lipoprotein lipase, the C apoproteins are released and the relative amount of apoprotein E increases. This relative increase in apoprotein E content parallels the increased ability of the chylomicron remnants to be taken up by the liver [6].

Direct evidence that apoprotein E might be involved in cellular lipoprotein uptake came from studies performed in cultured cells. Such cells express LDL receptors that bind the apoprotein B component of LDL and facilitate uptake of the lipoprotein by receptor-mediated endocytosis and its degradation in lysosomes [58]. The liberated cholesterol is used by the cell for membrane synthesis. It also suppresses the activity of 3-hydroxy-3-methylglutaryl coenzyme A reductase (HMG-CoA reductase), the rate-limiting enzyme in cholesterol biosynthesis, thereby turning off cholesterol production by the cell (see Chap. 33 for a more extensive discussion of the LDL receptor pathway).

Studies in cultured human fibroblasts showed that apoprotein E as well as apoprotein B can bind to the LDL receptor [59, 60]. This conclusion was originally drawn from experiments showing that HMG-CoA reductase activity in fibroblasts could be suppressed by a unique form of HDL called HDL$_c$, which was isolated from the plasma of cholesterol-fed dogs [59]. HDL$_c$ does not contain apoprotein B, but it does contain large amounts of apoprotein E. HDL$_c$ did not suppress HMG-CoA reductase in cells from a familial hypercholesterolemia homozygote that lacked LDL receptors, thereby suggesting that this particle entered fibroblasts by virtue of its ability to bind to the LDL receptor [60]. Inasmuch as A-I, the only other protein in HDL$_c$, was known not to bind to the LDL receptor, the fibroblast data suggested that apo E must have the ability to bind this receptor [60].

Subsequent extensive studies by Mahley and coworkers demonstrated directly that synthetic complexes of ^{125}I-labeled apoprotein E and phospholipid could bind to the LDL receptor of fibroblasts [61–63]. In fact, the affinity of the receptor for apoprotein E–containing particles was 10 to 20 times higher than its affinity for apoprotein B–containing particles [64].

The relevance of these observations to remnant uptake in liver was established by the observation that the livers of all experimental animal species tested so far, including rats [65–68], rabbits [69], and dogs [70], possess a lipoprotein receptor that resembles the fibroblast LDL receptor. Like the fibroblast LDL receptor, the hepatic lipoprotein receptor has a much higher affinity for apoprotein E–containing particles than for apoprotein B–containing particles. When apoprotein E–containing lipoproteins are perfused through a rat liver they are taken up with extreme rapidity by this receptor mechanism [66–68]. The presence of the C apoproteins interferes with uptake; therefore the fastest uptake rates are observed for particles like remnant particles that are rich in apo E and depleted in apo C [71, 71a].

The above studies suggest that one physiologic role for apoprotein E may be to bind to hepatic receptors and to facilitate the uptake and degradation of remnant lipoproteins that are enriched in apoprotein E. In isolated hepatocytes, apoprotein E–containing particles suppress HMG-CoA reductase, apparently owing to their uptake through this hepatic receptor mechanism [72]. From these data, it seems reasonable to suppose that the genetically abnormal form of apoprotein E that is present in patients with type 3 hyperlipoproteinemia has a diminished ability to bind to hepatic lipoprotein receptors, thereby causing the lipoprotein to accumulate in plasma.

This hypothesis was originally tested by Havel and coworkers [73]. As an experimental model, these workers used rats treated with pharmacologic doses of 17α-ethinyl estradiol. Such estrogen-treated rats develop a tenfold or greater increase in the number of hepatic lipoprotein receptors [65, 67]. When ^{125}I-labeled lipoproteins containing apoprotein B or E from rats or humans are perfused into the liver of an estradiol-treated rat, the particles are taken up and degraded with extreme efficiency. Havel applied this system to the analysis of type 3 hyperlipoproteinemia by isolating apoprotein E from normal VLDL and from β-VLDL of patients with type 3. The apoproteins were iodinated and incorporated into phospholipid vesicles. When perfused into the liver of an estradiol-treated rat, the vesicles containing normal apo E were taken up several times faster than those containing apo E from patients with type 3 hyperlipoproteinemia [73]. Havel et al. also purified the individual proteins of apoprotein E and incorporated them into phospholipid vesicles. When vesicles containing apo E-2 (the product of the E^d allele) were infused into an estradiol-treated rat, the rate of uptake was low in comparison with the vesicles containing apo E-3 or E-4 (products of the E^n and E^4 alleles, respectively) [73]. These data suggested that the E^d allele produces a mutant E protein that does not bind to hepatic lipoprotein receptors normally. Individuals homozygous for the E^d allele express hyperlipemia because their chylomicron or VLDL remnants cannot be taken up normally by the liver.

A retarded clearance from the circulation of lipoproteins containing apo E^d has been demonstrated recently in humans [73a]. Simultaneous intravenous infusion of apo E^d and apo E^n labeled with ^{125}I and ^{131}I has demonstrated a twofold more rapid clearance of apo E^n from the circulation of normal subjects as well as patients with type 3 hyperlipoproteinemia (Fig. 32-7).

Direct studies of the binding of normal and abnormal apo E to lipoprotein receptors have recently been conducted, with surprising results [73b]. In these experiments apo E was isolated from VLDL by several different methods, and the isolated apoprotein was incorporated into phospholipid vesicles or disks. The apo E-phospholipid complexes were tested for their ability to bind to LDL receptors from a variety of sources. Binding was assessed by measurement of the ability of the apo E-phospholipid complexes to compete with ^{125}I-LDL or with ^{125}I-labeled β-VLDL for binding to LDL receptors in four assay systems: cultured human fibroblasts, solubilized LDL receptors from bovine adrenal cortex, liver membranes from rats treated with 17α-ethinyl estradiol, and liver membranes

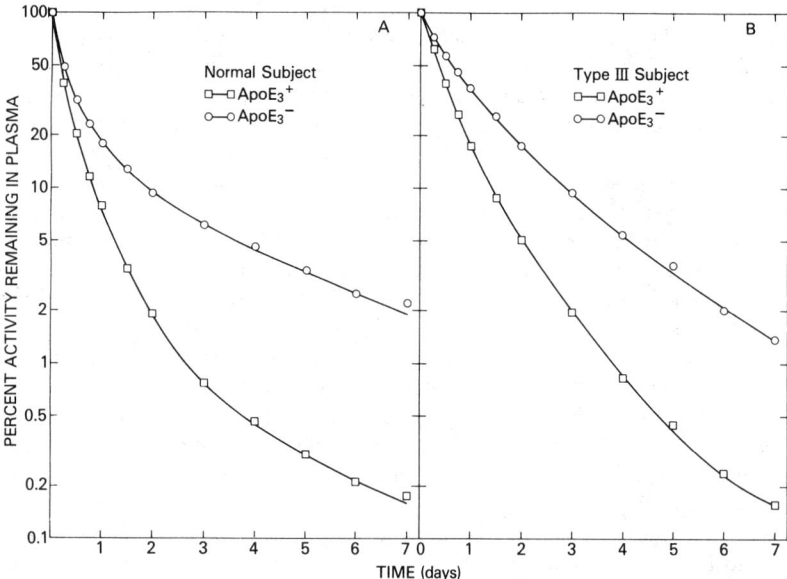

Figure 32-7 Clearance of simultaneously injected apo E^n (□) and apo E^d (○) from the plasma of a normal subject (A) and a patient with type 3 hyperlipoproteinemia (B). All values were normalized to 100 percent at day 0. *(From Gregg et al. [73a]. Used by permission.)*

from normal rabbits. Apo E^d protein was obtained from nine patients with classic symptomatic type 3 hyperlipoproteinemia and the apo E^n protein was obtained from eight control subjects. The apo E^d from six of the nine type 3 patients showed binding affinities for LDL receptors that were reduced by more than 98 percent in all receptor assays. These patients were designated group 1. The apo E^d from the three other type 3 patients showed a near-normal binding ability in all four of the receptor assays (group 2 patients). All of the group 1 patients were unequivocally of genotype E^d/E^d by the criterion of isoelectric focussing. One of the group 2 patients was also of the E^d/E^d genotype by the same criterion. Determination of the genotype in the other two group 2 patients was more complex in that they both showed traces of a protein that corresponded in isoelectric point to apo E^n as well as to a major protein that corresponded to apo E^d. The difference between group 1 and group 2 patients was also apparent when the apo E was radioiodinated and tested directly for its ability to bind to liver membranes from rats treated with 17α-ethinyl estradiol (which induces high levels of LDL receptor activity). The ^{125}I-labeled apo E from a group 2 patient, but not a group 1 patient, was taken up rapidly when perfused through the liver of an estradiol-treated rat, indicating that the receptor binding ability of apo E in vitro correlated with uptake in the intact liver in vivo [73b].

This study raises a great many questions about the relation between the receptor binding defect of the apo E^d protein and the hyperlipoproteinemia of type 3 patients. In the group 1 patients the binding defect clearly correlates with the observed elevation in plasma β-VLDL levels. On the other hand, group 2 patients also have elevated β-VLDL levels, even though their apo E seemed able to bind to receptors in vivo and to be taken up rapidly by rat liver in vivo. It is possible that the protein designated apo E^d in the group 2 patients is in reality the product of a different allele than the one in the group 1 patients, even though both have the same isoelectric point. Alternatively, the apo E^d protein may be the same in the two groups of patients, but there may be some posttranslational modification that differs in the two groups. Presumably, the apo E^d protein in the group 2 patients is defective in binding to the receptors of these patients in vivo, but the mechanism for this failure in vivo, but not in vitro, is unknown.

Conversion of VLDL Remnants to LDL In rats the majority of remnants derived from both chylomicrons and VLDL are taken up by the liver and degraded [74]. In humans the remnants derived from VLDL are not degraded in the liver [6, 75–77]. Rather, they undergo a further modification in which nearly all of the remaining triglycerides are removed and in which all of the apoproteins other than apo B are removed. During this process the particles become progressively smaller and more dense and pass through a stage designated as intermediate density lipoproteins, or IDL ($d=1.006$ to 1.019 g/ml). The end result of this process of reduction is a particle that contains apo B as the sole apoprotein and cholesteryl ester as the predominant core component—namely, LDL ($d=1.019$ to 1.063 g/ml). Direct plasma turnover studies have documented the conversion of VLDL particles containing ^{125}I-labeled apo B to ^{125}I-labeled LDL [75–77]. In normal humans the calculated amount of apo B derived from VLDL is sufficient to account for all of the apo B that appears in plasma. No direct secretion of LDL appears to occur [75–77].

The body sites at which the IDL undergoes the final conversion to LDL are not known. Incubation of VLDL with lipoprotein lipase in vitro gives rise to a triglyceride-depleted particle that has some features of LDL but is not identical to the lipoprotein that is formed in vivo. The size of the in vitro particle is larger (diameter 27 nm) as compared with native LDL (diameter 21.5 nm) [78]. Moreover, much of the C and E apoproteins, which leave the particle in vivo cannot be removed by lipolysis in vitro. Thus, there is reason to believe that the final conversion of IDL to LDL may require the participation of tissue factors and may occur in the liver. If this conversion requires the binding of apo E to hepatic receptors, then the inability of the mutant E^d protein to bind to these receptors might lead to a deficient generation of LDL. Whether chylomicron remnants are also converted to LDL in normal humans is not known, and hence it is not yet possible to tell whether there is an important lack of this conversion in type 3 patients.

Defective Remnant Metabolism in Patients with Type 3

The mechanism for the hyperlipidemia in type 3 hyperlipoproteinemia as postulated above predicts that the clearance of VLDL and IDL particles and their conversion to LDL should be retarded in type 3 patients as compared with normal subjects. The turnover of VLDL in patients with type 3 has been studied by three groups [23, 79–81]. In all of these studies, VLDL particles were radioiodinated, a procedure that labels all of their apoproteins, including apo B, apo E, and the apo C proteins. The labeled VLDL was injected into patients with type 3 and the specific radioactivity of the apo B protein in VLDL was measured at intervals. In addition, the appearance of the ^{125}I-labeled apoprotein B in the LDL fraction was monitored. All three groups of investigators observed a marked retardation in the turnover of VLDL apo B in type 3 patients as compared with controls [23, 79, 81] or patients with endogenous hypertriglyceridemia [80]. The fractional catabolic rate (FRC) was reduced by two- to sevenfold, with the normal value being about 0.29 per hour [81]. In addition, all three groups observed a marked reduction in the conversion of VLDL apo B to LDL apo B. The FCR for LDL apo B was normal or somewhat increased in the type 3 patients (0.31 to 0.45 per day) [23, 79–81].

Figure 32-8 shows a typical study of the plasma turnover of ^{125}I-VLDL in a type 3 patient (panel B) as compared to a patient with endogenous hypertriglyceridemia (panel A). This study illustrates the delayed conversion of VLDL to IDL and LDL in the type 3 subject. These data were obtained by the injection of VLDL from a hypertriglyceridemic patient into a patient with type 3 hyperlipoproteinemia [80]. Presumably the normal apoprotein E of the injected particle exchanged rapidly with the apoprotein E of the patient's own abnormal particle, and this accounted for the failure of the normal ^{125}I-VLDL to leave the plasma at its normal rate. Similar results have been obtained when type 3 patients are injected with their own β-VLDL particles [81].

In addition to reporting a similar block in VLDL catabolism, Berman et al. reported that the production rate of VLDL was increased in patients with type 3 hyperlipoproteinemia [23]. This abnormality has not been observed by the other two groups, both of whom found the VLDL apo B production rate to be at the upper limits of normal [79–81]. Berman and coworkers also attempted to reach mechanistic conclusions about detailed abnormalities in VLDL and IDL metabolism in these patients through extensive multicompartmental comput-

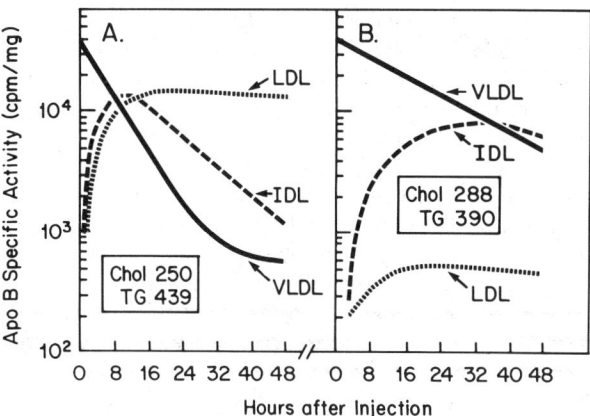

Figure 32-8 Apoprotein B–specific activity curves following the intravenous injection of ^{125}I-labeled VLDL into the plasma of a subject with endogenous hypertriglyceridemia *(A)* and a subject with type 3 hyperlipoproteinemia *(B)*. The plasma lipid levels in milligrams per deciliter at the time of the study are shown in the boxes. *(From Chait et al. [80]. Used by permission.)*

er modeling of the plasma radioactivity die-away curves [23]. The results were interpreted to indicate direct input of apo B into β-VLDL and IDL and direct catabolism of β-VLDL and IDL without passage through LDL in these patients. These conclusions, which were derived from kinetic modeling, require substantiation by an independent technique.

Considered together, the data from the in vivo studies of VLDL turnover in type 3 patients are consistent with the hypothesis that the primary reason for the elevation of β-VLDL and IDL levels relates to a block in the degradation of chylomicrons or VLDL or both and in their conversion to LDL. How much of the β-VLDL originates from chylomicrons and how much originates from VLDL is not known.

If the mutant apo E protein in type 3 patients (apo E^d) is unable to bind to the hepatic lipoprotein receptors, it remains unclear as to why most patients with homozygous E^d/E^d fail to show clinical hyperlipidemia. Although small amounts of β-VLDL are usually detectable in these patients [28], these amounts are much below the levels to be expected if there were a total block in β-VLDL catabolism. Moreover, although the LDL level is low on average, some patients homozygous for the E^d gene have LDL levels within the normal range.

From these observations, it seems likely that many E^d/E^d individuals are somehow able to metabolize their chylomicron and VLDL remnant particles at a normal or near-normal rate. If the E^d apoprotein retains some ability to bind to the receptor, then a normal hepatic uptake might be achieved by a compensatory increase in the number of hepatic lipoprotein receptors. Such an increase in receptors might occur as a consequence of any one of several factors that are known to improve the clinical status of type 3 patients, such as weight loss, change in diet, or thyroid hormone (see below). Alternatively, normal uptake may occur because the E^d apoprotein as well as the E^n and the E^4 apoproteins can exist in both active and inactive states. Studies in a variety of systems have suggested that normal apoprotein E is not always active. The most striking example of this was demonstrated by Mahley and coworkers in in vivo experiments with apo E HDL_c isolated from plasma of cholesterol-fed dogs [82]. This cholesteryl ester–rich lipoprotein has apparently normal apoprotein E as its sole protein. When the particles were iodinated and injected into normal dogs, the apo E HDL_c initially disappeared from the plasma at an extremely rapid rate [82]. However, after about 60 percent of the labeled apoprotein had disappeared,

the remainder disappeared with a much longer half-life. Presumably the iodinated apoprotein E had transferred to other particles in which it was not as active in binding to hepatic receptors, and thus it remained in the plasma.

Several potential mechanisms for the activation and inactivation of apoprotein E are known. One of these mechanisms, referred to above, relates to the apparent opposite effects of apoproteins C and E in binding of lipoproteins to hepatic receptors. The presence of C apoproteins on VLDL particles retards their binding, uptake, and degradation in the perfused rat liver [71, 71a]. Moreover, apoprotein C-enriched particles also show a diminished ability to bind to rat hepatic lipoprotein receptors as measured by in vitro membrane-binding assays [67]. Along the same line, there is evidence to indicate that large VLDL particles ($S_f = 100$ to 400) and chylomicrons, both of which contain abundant apoprotein E, do not show high affinity binding to the LDL receptor of human fibroblasts. After these particles are incubated in vitro with lipoprotein lipase and have had their content of apo E reduced relative to that of apo B, they acquire the ability to bind to the LDL receptor and to deliver cholesterol to cells [83–86].

In addition to being masked by C proteins, the activity of apo E can be affected by its interaction with apoprotein A-II. Mahley and coworkers showed that some of the apo E isolated from human plasma is present in the form of a disulfide-linked dimer with A-II [87]. Particles containing this dimer are not fully active in binding to fibroblast LDL receptors [88], but when the particles are subjected to reduction and alkylation (i.e., splitting the disulfide bond), they become fully active in binding to fibroblast receptors. If such dimers are formed and broken reversibly in vivo, they may modulate the ability of apo E to bind to hepatic receptors. Finally, normal apo E is known to exist in a variety of modified forms bearing different numbers of sialic acid residues [53]. It is possible that the activity of apo E is modulated by the insertion or removal of these residues.

Given this complexity in apoprotein E structure and function and given the evidence that its activity may be modulated, it seems likely that the mutant E^d apoprotein, as well as the normal E^n and E^4 apoproteins, may exist in active and inactive forms. The apo E^d may differ from the apo E^n and E^4 in that the E^d protein is relatively resistant to conversion to the active form, albeit some such activation may nevertheless be possible. When the E^d protein is in the active form, patients might have normal clearance of remnant particles. When it is inactive, these clearance mechanisms may be ineffective. In this regard it is of interest that estrogen therapy may restore plasma lipid levels to normal in type 3 patients, although detectable amounts of β-VLDL are still present [79, 79a]. This apparent improvement in β-VLDL clearance can occur even though normal apoprotein E is not produced [79, 79a]. Further experiments are necessary to determine whether any of the above-postulated mechanisms actually operate in vivo and whether the apo E^d protein can, in fact, exist in both active and inactive forms.

Familial Type 3 as a Human Counterpart of Hyperlipidemia in Cholesterol-Fed Animals

Of all the diseases producing hyperlipidemia in humans, type 3 hyperlipoproteinemia most closely resembles the condition that results when animals are placed on a high-cholesterol diet. The animals that develop the most profound hypercholesterolemia, and the ones that develop the most fulminant atherosclerosis, are the ones that develop β-VLDL particles in plasma. This is true of cholesterol-fed rabbits [89] and cholesterol-fed dogs [90]. In addition, monkeys, swine, and rats develop elevated β-VLDL levels when fed a high-cholesterol diet [91].

The studies of Mahley have demonstrated a correlation between the appearance of β-VLDL in the plasma and the occurrence of atherosclerosis in dogs [90]. When dogs are fed cholesterol, there is initially an elevation in levels of plasma LDL and in HDL$_c$. Even though these animals have cholesterol levels as high as 700 mg/dl, they do not develop significant atherosclerosis. In those dogs in which the plasma cholesterol rises above 750 mg/dl, β-VLDL particles appear, and there is a concomitant massive deposition of cholesterol in foam cells throughout the body, including the arterial wall [91]. The foam cell accumulation in these animals is similar to that occurring in patients with type 3 hyperlipoproteinemia. Moreover, the β-VLDL particles that accumulate in these animals also resemble those that accumulate in patients with type 3 hyperlipoproteinemia. Like the patient's particles, the animal lipoproteins are rich in apoprotein E, poor in apoprotein C, and abundant in apoprotein B [90, 91]. Moreover, the animal particles show a high cholesterol/protein ratio similar to that of the β-VLDL from type 3 patients.

Zilversmit and coworkers showed that most of the β-VLDL particles that accumulate in cholesterol-fed rabbits are derived from dietary chylomicrons [40, 92]. These particles presumably accumulate because the normal hepatic clearance mechanism for remnants is overloaded [92, 93]. In rabbits this hepatic clearance system is easily saturated as a result of the high affinity but low capacity of the hepatic lipoprotein receptors [69]. Thus, when a rabbit is fed cholesterol, the removal rate for β-VLDL fails to increase commensurate with the increased production, and the particles accumulate in plasma. It seems likely that this failure of hepatic clearance is analogous to the failure of hepatic clearance that occurs in patients with type 3 hyperlipoproteinemia. The difference is that in the case of the animals this clearance defect requires an extremely high-cholesterol diet to overload the normal clearance mechanism. In type 3 patients, the abnormal β-VLDL particles are not cleared normally even when the patients are on a normal diet.

Of considerable interest to the pathogenesis of type 3 is the recent demonstration that β-VLDL particles, but no other naturally occurring lipoproteins, have a selective ability to produce marked cholesteryl ester deposition in macrophages [94]. The deposition is produced by a receptor on the surfaces of macrophages that recognizes β-VLDL particles. This receptor has been studied most intensively on mouse peritoneal macrophages, but it also occurs on human monocytes as well [95].

When mouse peritoneal macrophages are incubated with β-VLDL isolated from the plasma of cholesterol-fed rabbits, dogs, monkeys, and rats, the macrophages bind the lipoprotein at this high affinity site, internalize it by adsorptive endocytosis, and degrade it in lysosomes [94, 95]. The liberated cholesterol is reesterified in the cytoplasm and accumulates within the cell as cholesteryl ester droplets. These droplets give the cell an appearance similar to that of the foam cells seen in tissues of cholesterol-fed animals.

The macrophage binding site for β-VLDL does not recognize normal VLDL, LDL, or HDL, nor does it recognize apo E HDL$_c$, another cholesterol-rich lipoprotein that accumulates in cholesterol-fed animals but whose presence is not necessarily accompanied by atherosclerosis [90]. The apoproteins responsible for the binding of β-VLDL to the macrophage receptor are not known. All of the apoproteins known to be present on β-VLDL are also present on other particles that do not bind to this receptor. (See Chap. 33 for a more extensive discussion of lipoprotein metabolism in macrophages.) It is not known as yet whether the β-VLDL particles from type 3 patients bind to macrophage receptors, but it is noteworthy that the tissues of these patients display cholesterol-overloaded macrophage foam cells that appear identical to those that occur in cholesterol-fed animals (discussed above).

Several years ago Zilversmit formulated the hypothesis that cholesterol-rich chylomicron remnant particles are major contributors to atherosclerosis in humans as well as experimental animals [40, 96]. The severe atherosclerosis seen in type 3 patients supports this hypothesis. Moreover, as stated by Zilversmit, these considerations raise the possibility that the common forms of atherosclerosis that occur in patients who do not have fasting hyperlipidemia may be caused, in large part, by cholesterol-rich chylomicron remnant particles that are present in the plasma transiently after high-fat, high-cholesterol meals. Little information is available regarding the extent to which the postprandial levels of these lipoproteins vary among different subjects.

DIAGNOSIS

In the absence of any apparent cause of secondary hyperlipidemia, the probability that a given adult patient with elevated concentrations of both cholesterol and triglyceride has familial type 3 hyperlipoproteinemia is between 1 in 100 and 1 in 1000. The probability increases if peripheral vascular disease is present and jumps markedly if lipid deposits are visible in palmar creases. A fairly dramatic disappearance of both hyperlipidemia and xanthomas upon treatment is also highly suggestive of the diagnosis (discussed below).

Many laboratory tests have been proposed for the diagnosis of type 3. The simplest one, electrophoresis of whole plasma, has not proved to be reliable since the broad-beta band in the electrophoretograms is present in only one-half of type 3 patients [17] and may be present in other subjects with other forms of primary hyperlipidemia [97] as well as in patients with rare disorders such as LCAT deficiency (Chap. 31) and Tangier disease (Chap. 29). The subsequent application of electrophoresis to the $d < 1.006$ g/ml fraction of ultracentrifuged plasma yielded a more practical definition based on the occurrence of β-migrating lipoproteins in the VLDL density class [1, 4]. This marker has proved not to be completely satisfactory inasmuch as it is present in patients with other forms of genetic and secondary hyperlipidemia [12, 15].

Various quantitative indexes related to the presence of cholesterol-rich VLDL have been used with somewhat greater success. These include the ratio of cholesterol to triglyceride in VLDL [98, 15], of cholesterol in VLDL to plasma triglycerides [12, 15], and the quotient of this ratio in VLDL to that in LDL [99]. One problem with these ratios is that they depend on the relative amounts of β-VLDL to pre-β-VLDL. Not only does the proportion vary in patients with type 3, but many normal subjects or those with other forms of hyperlipidemia have two ("fast" and "slow") components of VLDL, the latter of which represent remnant-like particles rich in cholesterol [45].

Although the above tests were of considerable help in the early stages of the understanding of the type 3 disorder, none has proved specific in the sense that it is a valid marker for the underlying genetic defect. The discovery of the specific abnormality in apoprotein E in 1975 overcame this problem and provided the diagnostic test that had been badly needed [2]. As discussed earlier in the chapter, isoelectric focusing of VLDL can be carried out to demonstrate the presence of E^d/E^d genotype that underlies type 3. The isoelectric focusing can be accurately performed without the need for preparative ultracentrifugation by using a combined VLDL-IDL-LDL fraction that is separated from plasma by precipitation with heparin in the presence of magnesium ion [96]. This approach is already proving invaluable in elucidation of the genetics and epidemiology of the type 3 disease. In this regard, it is important to note that the apo E genotype, unlike earlier markers, persists in the face of a variety of metabolic perturbations, including lowering of plasma lipid levels after treatment with diet, clofibrate, and nicotinic acid [28, 49, 100].

Current attention is now being directed at the identification of the factors that predispose to hyperlipidemia in individuals with the E^d/E^d genotype. This will require careful attention to diet, gonadal function, body weight, and related diseases such as diabetes mellitus, hypothyroidism, and other forms of genetic hyperlipidemia. An important unresolved question is whether heterozygous individuals with the E^n/E^d or E^4/E^d genotypes are predisposed to hyperlipidemia or premature atherosclerosis or both. In a recent preliminary study of 328 individuals with myocardial infarction, Utermann found that 12.5 percent were E^d heterozygotes, a frequency that was not significantly different from that found in 490 normal blood donors (15 percent) [54]. If confirmed by additional studies, this result suggests that the E^n/E^d or E^4/E^d genotype per se (i.e., primary dysbetalipoproteinemia without hyperlipidemia) is not a risk factor for atherosclerosis.

The importance of determining the apo E genotype in patients with xanthomatosis of unknown etiology has recently been emphasized by a striking case report published by Grundy, Kane, and coworkers [101]. The patient was a 43-year-old man who had extensive tuberous xanthomas, especially involving the elbows, and marked palmar xanthomatosis associated with a normal concentration of plasma cholesterol (200 mg/dl) and triglyceride (115 mg/dl). The patient's plasma VLDL showed β-mobility on electrophoresis, a high cholesterol/triglyceride ratio, and an increased content of apoprotein B. In contrast to patients with type 3, the content of apoprotein E in VLDL was normal. Nevertheless, the isoelectric focusing pattern of the VLDL indicated that the patient's genotype at the apo E locus was E^d/E^d. This unique patient represents an example of xanthomatosis associated with abnormal lipoprotein structure without excess circulating cholesterol. These findings support the notion that the existence of abnormal lipoproteins, especially β-VLDL, may be sufficient to produce xanthomatosis without an elevation in plasma total cholesterol levels.

TREATMENT

The therapy of type 3 leads to the most gratifying response of plasma lipids seen in any form of familial hyperlipoproteinemia. Such therapy always involves diet control and usually the addition of one of several medications. The success of therapy is currently measured by the ability to maintain plasma cholesterol and triglyceride concentrations within normal limits.

Diet

If necessary, caloric intake is restricted until ideal body weight is achieved. The maintenance diet usually used today contains about 40 percent of calories from carbohydrate and 40 percent from fats. In selecting the latter, the amount of saturated fat is decreased and fats high in polyunsaturated fatty acids are increased. Cholesterol is kept to about 300 mg/day, and alcohol intake is restricted [16].

Drugs

Additional lowering of lipid levels is virtually always achieved by adding clofibrate, 2.0 g/day, to the regimen [16]. In view of the recent demonstration of serious but poorly understood effects of clofibrate on mortality [102, 103], this drug should be used cautiously. Nicotinic acid, 1.0 to 3.0 g/day, has a similar effect on hyperlipidemia, but has more immediate side effects such as flushing and gastrointestinal distress. Cholestyramine does not lower blood lipid levels in type 3 and may indeed increase triglyceride concentrations.

The cutaneous xanthomas disappear within a few weeks or months concomitant with the decline in lipid concentrations. Detectable β-VLDL and the mutant E^d apoprotein always remain. Zelis and colleagues [104] have described improvement in plethysmographic measurements of peripheral blood flow in type 3 patients after several months of therapy.

Schonfeld and coworkers recently reported the results of a study in which seven men and six women with familial type 3 were treated with diet and clofibrate over periods of 2 to 8 months [105]. The mean plasma total cholesterol and triglyceride levels declined by 51 and 74 percent, respectively, from the pretreatment values of 498 and 685 mg/dl. Despite the fall in total plasma cholesterol, the mean levels of HDL-cholesterol rose from 34 to 50 mg/dl. Visible regression of cutaneous xanthomas was noted in six of six patients. In addition a subjective diminution or disappearance of symptoms of intermittent claudication was noted in five patients with peripheral vascular disease and of angina pectoris in two patients with coronary heart disease [105]. Objective evidence of improvement or retardation in progression of vascular disease due to treatment of the lipoprotein abnormality is still insufficient.

REFERENCES

1. FREDRICKSON DS, LEVY RI: Familial hyperlipoproteinemia, in Stanbury, JB, Wyngaarden, JB, Fredrickson DS (eds): *The Metabolic Basis of Inherited Disease*, chap. 28, 3d ed. New York, McGraw-Hill, 1972, p 545

2. UTERMANN G, JAESCHKE M, MENZEL J: Familial hyperlipoproteinemia type III: Deficiency of a specific apolipoprotein (apo E-III) in very low density lipoproteins. *FEBS Lett* 56:352, 1975

3. GOFMAN JW, DELALLA O, GLAZIER F, FREEMAN NK, LINDGREN FT, NICHOLS AV, STRISOWER B, TAMPLIN AR: The serum lipoprotein transport system in health, metabolic disorders, atherosclerosis and coronary heart disease. *Plasmatiche* 2:413, 1954

4. FREDRICKSON DS, LEVY RI, LEES RS: Fat transport in lipoproteins—An integrated approach to mechanisms and disorders. *N Engl J Med* 276:32, 94, 148, 215, 273, 1967

5. FREDRICKSON DS, LEVY RI, LINDGREN FT: A comparison of heritable abnormal lipoprotein patterns as defined by two different techniques. *J Clin Invest* 47:2446, 1968

6. HAVEL RJ, GOLDSTEIN JL, BROWN MS: Lipoproteins and lipid transport, in Bondy PK, Rosenberg LE (eds): *Metabolic Control and Disease*, chap. 7, 8th ed. Philadelphia, WB Saunders, 1980, p 393

7. QUARFORDT SH, LEVY RI, FREDRICKSON DS: On the lipoprotein abnormality in type III hyperlipoproteinemia. *J Clin Invest* 50:754, 1971

8. HAZZARD WR, PORTE D, JR, BIERMAN EL: Abnormal lipid composition of

chylomicrons in broad-beta disease (type III hyperlipoproteinemia). *J Clin Invest* 49:1853, 1970

9. HAZZARD WR, LINDGREN FT, BIERMAN EL: Very low density lipoprotein subfractions in a subject with broad-beta disease (type III hyperlipoproteinemia), and a subject with endogenous lipemia (type IV); chemical composition and electrophoretic mobility. *Biochim Biophys Acta* 202:517, 1970

10. BROWN, WV, LEVY RI, FREDRICKSON DS: A comparative study of the very low density lipoproteins in normal subjects and patients with types III, IV, and V hyperlipoproteinemia. *Circulation* suppl 39:III-4, 1969

11. HAVEL RJ, KANE RJ: Primary dysbetalipoproteinemia; predominance of a specific apoprotein species in triglyceride-rich lipoproteins. *Proc Nat Acad Sci USA* 70:2015, 1973

12. FREDRICKSON DS, MORGANROTH J, LEVY RI: Type III hyperlipoproteinemia: An analysis of two contemporary definitions. *Ann Int Med* 82:150, 1975

13. HAZZARD WR, O'DONNELL TF, LEE YL: Broad-β-disease (type III hyperlipoproteinemia) in a large kindred. *Ann Intern Med* 82:141, 1975

14. MORGANROTH J, LEVY RI, FREDRICKSON DS: The biochemical, clinical, and genetic features of type III hyperlipoproteinemia. *Ann Intern Med* 82:158, 1975

15. MISHKEL M, NAZIR DJ, CROTHER S: A longitudinal assessment of lipid ratios in the diagnosis of type III hyperlipoproteinemia. *Clin Chem Acta* 58:121, 1975

16. LEVY RI, FREDRICKSON DS, SHULMAN R, BILHEIMER DW, BRESLOW JL, STONE NJ, LUX SE, SLOAN HR, KRAUS RM, HERBERT PN: Dietary and drug treatment of primary hyperlipoproteinemia. *Ann Intern Med* 77:267, 1972

17. MASKET BH, LEVY RI, FREDRICKSON DS: The use of polyacrylamide gel electrophoresis in differentiating type III hyperlipoproteinemia. *J Lab Clin Med* 81:794, 1973

18. PATSCH JR, SAILER S, BRAUNSTEINER H: Lipoprotein of the density 1.006–1.020 in the plasma of patients with type III hyperlipoproteinemia in the postabsorptive state. *Eur J Clin Invest* 5:45, 1975

19. LEVY RI, BILHEIMER DW, EISENBERG S: The structure and metabolism of chylomicrons and very low density lipoproteins (VLDL), in Smellie RMS (ed): *Plasma Lipoproteins*. New York, Academic Press, 1971, p 3

20. SATA G, HAVEL RJ, JONES AL: Characterization of subfractions of triglyceride-rich lipoproteins separated by gel chromatography from blood plasma of normolipidemic and hyperlipidemic humans. *J Lipid Res* 13:757, 1972

21. HAVEL RJ, KOTITE L, VIGNE J-L, KANE JP, TUN P, PHILLIPS N, CHEN GC: Radioimmunoassay of human arginine-rich apolipoprotein (apoprotein E): Concentration in blood plasma and lipoproteins as affected by apoprotein E-3 deficiency. *J Clin Invest* 66:1351, 1980

22. HAVEL RJ: Hyperlipoproteinemia: Problems in diagnosis and challenges posed by the "type III" disorder. (Editorial) *Ann Intern Med* 82:273, 1975

23. BERMAN M, HALL M, III, LEVY RI, EISENBERG S, BILHEIMER DW, PHAIR RD, GOEBEL RH: Metabolism of apo B and apo C lipoproteins in man: Kinetic studies in normal and hyperlipoproteinemic subjects. *J Lipid Res* 19:37, 1978

24. HAZZARD WR, BIERMAN EL: Broad-β disease versus endogenous hypertriglyceridemia: Levels and lipid composition of chylomicrons and very low density lipoproteins during fat-free feeding and alimentary lipemia. *Metabolism* 24:817, 1975

25. HAZZARD WR: Primary type III hyperlipoproteinemia, in Rifkind BM, Levy RI (eds): *Hyperlipidemia Diagnosis and Therapy*, New York, Grune and Stratton, 1977, p 137

26. BORRIE P: Type III hyperlipoproteinaemia. *Br Med J* 2:665, 1969

27. MISCHKEL MA: Type III hyperlipoproteinemia with xanthomatosis, in Peeters H (ed): *Protides of the Biological Fluids*, New York: Pergamon Press, 1971, p 283

28. UTERMANN G, VOGELBERG KH, STEINMETZ A, SCHOENBORN W, PRUIN N, JAESCHKE M, HEES M, CANZLER H: Polymorphism of apolipoprotein E. II. Genetics of hyperlipoproteinemia type III. *Clin Genet* 15:37, 1979

29. VESSBY B, HEDSTRAND H, LUNDIN L-G, OLSSON U: Inheritance of type-III hyperlipoproteinemia. Lipoprotein patterns in first-degree relatives. *Metabolism* 26:225, 1977

30. HAZZARD WR, WARNICK GR, UTERMANN G, ALBERS JJ: Genetic transmission of isoapolipoprotein E phenotypes in a large kindred: Relationship to dysbetalipoproteinemia and hyperlipidemia. *Metabolism* 30:79, 1981

31. GODOLPHIN WJ, CONRADI G, CAMPBELL DJ: Type 3 hyperlipoproteinemia in a child. *Lancet* 1:209, 1972

32. POLANO MK: Xanthomatosis and hyperlipoproteinemia. *Dermatologica* 149:1, 1974

33. HAZZARD WR, GOLDSTEIN JL, SCHROTT HG, MOTULSKY AG, BIERMAN EL: Hyperlipidemia in coronary heart disease. III. Evaluation of lipoprotein phenotypes of 156 genetically defined survivors of myocardial infarction. *J Clin Invest* 52:1569, 1973.

34. HAZZARD WR, BIERMAN EL: Aggravation of broad-β disease (type III hyperlipoproteinemia) by hypothyroidism. *Arch Intern Med* 130:822, 1972

35. DYERBERG J: Type III hyperlipoproteinemia with low plasma thyroxine binding globulin. *Metabolism* 18:50, 1969

36. ROBERTS WC, LEVY RI, FREDRICKSON DS: Hyperlipoproteinemia—a review of the five types with the first report of necropsy findings in type III. *Arch Pathol* 90:46, 1970

37. HOLIMON JL, WASSERMAN AJ: Autopsy findings in type III hyperlipoproteinemia. *Arch Pathol* 92:415, 1971

38. ROBERTS WC, FARRANS VJ, LEVY RI, FREDRICKSON DS: Cardiovascular pathology in hyperlipoproteinemia. *Am J Cardiol* 31:557, 1973

39. AMATRUDE JM, MARGOLIS S, HUTCHINS GM: Type III hyperlipoproteinemia with mesangial foam cells in renal glomeruli. *Arch Pathol* 98:51, 1974

40. ZILVERSMIT DB: Atherogenesis: A postprandial phenomenon. *Circulation* 60:473, 1979

41. UTERMANN G, CANZLER H, HEES M, JAESCHKE M, MÜHLFELLNER G, SCHOENBORN W, VOGELBERG KH: Studies on the metabolic defect in broad-β disease (hyperlipoproteinaemia type III). *Clin Genet* 12:139, 1977

42. UTERMANN G, HESS M, VOGELBERG KH: Broad-beta disease (hyperlipoproteinaemia type III): Genetics, gene frequency and diagnosis without ultracentrifugation, in *Electrofocusing and Isotachophoresis*. Berlin, Walter de Gruyter, 1977, p 281

43. UTERMANN G, HEES M, STEINMETZ A: Polymorphism of apolipoprotein E and occurrence of dysbetalipoproteinaemia in man. *Nature* 269:604, 1977

44. UTERMANN G, LANGENBECK U, BEISIEGEL U, WEBER W: Genetics of the apolipoprotein E system in man. *Am J Hum Genet* 32:339, 1980

45. PAGNAN A, HAVEL RJ, KANE JP, KOTITE L: Characterization of human very low density lipoproteins containing two electrophoretic populations: Double pre-beta lipoproteinemia and primary dysbetalipoproteinemia. *J Lipid Res* 18:613, 1977

46. WARNICK GR, MAYFIELD C, ALBERS JJ, HAZZARD WR: Gel isoelectric focusing method for specific diagnosis of familial hyperlipoproteinemia type 3. *Clin Chem* 25:279, 1979

47. HAZZARD WR, WARNICK GR, UTERMANN G, ALBERS JJ, LEWIS B: The complex genetics of type III hyperlipoproteinemia: Influence of co-inherited monogenic hyperlipidemia upon the phenotypic expression of apolipoprotein E3 deficiency, in Gotto AM, Jr, Smith LC, Allen B (eds): *Atherosclerosis V*. New York, Springer-Verlag, 1980, p 260

48. WEIDMAN SW, SUAREZ B, FALKO JM, WITZTUM JL, KOLAR J, RABEN M, SCHONFELD G: Type III hyperlipoproteinemia: Development of a VLDL apo E gel isoelectric focusing technique and application in family studies. *J Lab Clin Med* 93:549, 1979

49. FALKO JM, SCHONFELD G, WITZTUM JL, KOLAR JB, WEIDMAN SW, STEELMAN R: Effects of diet on apoprotein E levels and on the apoprotein E subspecies in human plasma lipoproteins. *J Clin Endocrinol Metab* 50:521, 1980

50. UTERMANN G, PRUIN N, STEINMETZ A: Polymorphism of apolipoprotein E. III. Effect of a single polymorphic gene locus on plasma lipid levels in man. *Clin Genet* 15:63, 1979

51. ZANNIS VI, BRESLOW JL: Characterization of a unique human apolipoprotein E variant associated with type III hyperlipoproteinemia. *J Biol Chem* 255:1759, 1980.

52. ZANNIS VI, JUST PW, BRESLOW JL: Human apolipoprotein E isoprotein subclasses are genetically determined. *Am J Hum Genet* 33:11, 1981

53. ZANNIS VI, BRESLOW JL: Human very low density lipoprotein apolipoprotein E isoprotein polymorphism is explained by genetic variation and post-translational modification. *Biochemistry* 20:1033, 1981

54. UTERMANN G: Polymorphism of apolipoprotein E, in Gotto AM, Jr, Smith LC, Allen B (eds): *Atherosclerosis V*. New York, Springer-Verlag, 1980, p 689

55. GOLDSTEIN JL, SCHROTT HG, HAZZARD WR, BIERMAN EL, MOTULSKY AG: Hyperlipidemia in coronary heart disease. II. Genetic analysis of lipid levels in 176 families and delineation of a new inherited disorder, combined hyperlipidemia. *J Clin Invest* 52:1544, 1973

56. GOODMAN DeWS: The metabolism of chylomicron cholesterol ester in the rat. *J Clin Invest* 41:1886, 1962

57. REDGRAVE TG: Formation of cholesteryl ester-rich particulate lipid during metabolism of chylomicrons. *J Clin Invest* 49:465, 1970

58. BROWN MS, GOLDSTEIN JL: Receptor-mediated control of cholesterol metabolism. *Science* 191:150, 1976

59. ASSMANN G, BROWN BG, MAHLEY RW: Regulation of 3-hydroxy-3-methylglutaryl coenzyme A reductase activity in cultured swine aortic smooth muscle cells by plasma lipoproteins. *Biochemistry* 14:3996, 1975

60. BERSOT TP, MAHLEY RW, BROWN MS, GOLDSTEIN JL: Interaction of swine lipoproteins with the low density lipoprotein receptor in human fibroblasts. *J Biol Chem* 251:2395, 1976

61. INNERARITY TL, PITAS RE, MAHLEY RW: Binding of arginine-rich (E) apo-

protein after recombination with phospholipid vesicles to the low density lipoprotein receptors of fibroblasts. *J Biol Chem* 254:4186, 1979

62. PITAS RE, INNERARITY TL, MAHLEY RW: Cell surface receptor binding of phospholipid:protein complexes containing different ratios of receptor-active and -inactive E apoprotein. *J Biol Chem* 255:5454, 1980

63. INNERARITY TL, PITAS RE, MAHLEY RW: Receptor binding of cholesterol-induced high-density lipoproteins containing predominantly apoprotein E to cultured fibroblasts with mutations at the low-density lipoprotein receptor locus. *Biochemistry* 19:4359, 1980

64. PITAS RE, INNERARITY TL, ARNOLD KS, MAHLEY RW: Rate and equilibrium constants for binding of apo-E HDL$_c$ and low density lipoproteins to human fibroblasts: Evidence for multiple receptor binding of apo-E HDL$_c$. *Proc Nat Acad Sci USA* 76:2311, 1979

65. KOVANEN PT, BROWN MS, GOLDSTEIN JL: Increased binding of low density lipoprotein to liver membranes from rats treated with 17α-ethinyl estradiol. *J Biol Chem* 254:11367, 1979

66. CHAO Y-S, WINDLER EE, CHEN GC, HAVEL RJ: Hepatic catabolism of rat and human lipoproteins in rats treated with 17α-ethinyl estradiol. *J Biol Chem* 254:11360, 1979

67. WINDLER EET, KOVANEN PT, CHAO Y-S, BROWN MS, HAVEL RJ, GOLDSTEIN JL: The estradiol-stimulated lipoprotein receptor of rat liver: A binding site that mediates the uptake of rat lipoproteins containing apoproteins B and E. *J Biol Chem* 255:10464, 1980

68. CHAO Y-S, JONES AL, HRADEK GT, WINDLER EET, HAVEL RJ: Autoradiographic localization of the sites of uptake, cellular transport and catabolism of low density lipoproteins in the liver of normal and estrogen-treated rats. *Proc Nat Acad Sci USA*, 78:597, 1981

69. KOVANEN PT, BROWN MS, BASU SK, BILHEIMER DW, GOLDSTEIN JL: Saturation and suppression of hepatic lipoprotein receptors: A mechanism for the hypercholesterolemia of cholesterol-fed rabbits. *Proc Nat Acad Sci USA*, 78:1396, 1981

70. KOVANEN PT, BILHEIMER DW, GOLDSTEIN JL, JARAMILLO JJ, BROWN MS: A regulatory role for hepatic low density lipoprotein receptors *in vivo* in the dog. *Proc Nat Acad Sci USA*, 78:1194, 1981

71. WINDLER E, CHAO Y-S, HAVEL RJ: Determinants of hepatic uptake of triglyceride-rich lipoproteins and their remnants in the rat. *J Biol Chem* 255:5475, 1980

71a. SHELBURNE F, HANKS J, MEYERS W, QUARFORDT S: Effect of apoproteins on hepatic uptake of triglyceride emulsions in the rat. *J Clin Invest* 65:652, 1980

72. BRESLOW JL, LOTHROP DA, CLOWES AW, LUX SE: Lipoprotein regulation of 3-hydroxy-3-methylglutaryl coenzyme A reductase activity in rat liver cell cultures. *J Biol Chem* 252:2726, 1977

73. HAVEL RJ, CHAO Y-S, WINDLER EE, KOTITE L, GUO LSS: Isoprotein specificity in the hepatic uptake of apolipoprotein E and the pathogenesis of familial dysbetalipoproteinemia. *Proc Nat Acad Sci USA* 77:4349, 1980

73a. GREGG RG, ZECH LA, SCHAEFER EJ, BREWER HB: Type III hyperlipoproteinemia: Defective metabolism of an abnormal apolipoprotein E. *Science* 211:584, 1981

73b. SCHNEIDER WJ, KOVANEN PT, BROWN MS, GOLDSTEIN JL, UTERMANN G, WEBER W, HAVEL RJ, KOTITE L, KANE JP, INNERARITY TL, MAHLEY RW: Familial dysbetalipoproteinemia: Abnormal binding of mutant apoprotein E to LDL receptors of human fibroblasts and membranes from liver and adrenal of rats, rabbits, and cows. *J Clin Invest* 68:1075, 1981

74. FAEGEMAN O, SATA T, KANE JP, HAVEL RJ: Metabolism of apoprotein B of plasma very low density lipoproteins in the rat. *J Clin Invest* 56:1396, 1975

75. EISENBERG S, BILHEIMER DW, LINDGREN FT, LEVY RI: On the metabolic conversion of human plasma very low density lipoprotein. *Biochim Biophys Acta* 326:361, 1973

76. SIGURDSSON G, NOEL S-P, HAVEL RJ: Catabolism of the apoprotein of low density lipoproteins by the isolated perfused rat liver. *J Lipid Res* 19:628, 1978

77. REARDON MF, FIDGE NH, NESTEL PJ: Catabolism of very low density lipoprotein B apoprotein in man. *J Clin Invest* 61:850, 1978

78. DECKELBAUM RJ, EISENBERG S, FAINARU M, BARENHOLZ Y, OLIVECRONA T: *In vitro* production of human plasma low density lipoprotein-like particles. A model for very low density lipoprotein catabolism. *J Biol Chem* 254:6079, 1979

79. CHAIT A, ALBERS JJ, BRUNZELL JD, HAZZARD WR: Type-III hyperlipoproteinaemia ("remnant removal disease"). *Lancet* 1:1176, 1977

79a. KUSHWAHA RS, HAZZARD WR, GAGNE C, CHAIT A, ALBERS JJ: Type III hyperlipoproteinemia: Paradoxical hypolipidemic response to estrogen. *Ann Intern Med* 87:517, 1977

80. CHAIT A, HAZZARD WR, ALBERS JJ, KUSHWAHA RP, BRUNZELL JD: Impaired very low density lipoprotein and triglyceride removal in broad beta disease: Comparison with endogenous hypertriglyceridemia. *Metabolism* 27:1055, 1978

81. JANUS ED, NICOLL AM, TURNER PR, MAGILL P, LEWIS B: Kinetic bases of the primary hyperlipidaemias: Studies of apolipoprotein B turnover in genetically defined subjects. *Eur J Clin Invest* 10:161, 1980

82. MAHLEY RW, INNERARITY TL, WEISGRABER KH, OH SY: Altered metabolism (*in vivo* and *in vitro*) of plasma lipoproteins after selective chemical modification of lysine residues of the apoproteins. *J Clin Invest* 64:743, 1979

83. SCHONFELD G, PATSCH W, PFLEGER B, WITZTUM JL, WEIDMAN SW: Lipolysis produces changes in the immunoreactivity and cell reactivity of very low density lipoproteins. *J Clin Invest* 64:1288, 1979

84. CATAPANO AL, GIANTURCO SH, KINNUNEN PKJ, EISENBERG S, GOTTO AM, JR, SMITH LC: Suppression of 3-hydroxy-3-methylglutaryl-CoA reductase by low density lipoproteins produced *in vitro* by lipoprotein lipase action on nonsuppressive very low density lipoproteins. *J Biol Chem* 254:1007, 1979

85. GIANTURCO SH, PACKARD CJ, SHEPHERD J, SMITH LC, CATAPANO AL, SYBERS HD, GOTTO AM, JR: Abnormal suppression of 3-hydroxy-methylglutaryl-CoA reductase activity in cultured human fibroblasts by hypertriglyceridemic very low density lipoprotein subclasses. *Lipids* 15:456, 1980

86. FLORÉN C-H, ALBERS JJ, KUDCHODKAR B, BIERMAN EL: Receptor-dependent uptake of human chylomicron remnants by cultured skin fibroblasts. *J Biol Chem* 256:425, 1981

87. WEISGRABER KH, MAHLEY RW: Apoprotein (E-A-II) complex of human plasma lipoproteins. I. Characterization of this mixed disulfide and its identification in a high density lipoprotein subfraction. *J Biol Chem* 253:6281, 1978

88. INNERARITY TL, MAHLEY TW, WEISGRABER KH, BERSOT TP: Apoprotein (E—A-II) complex of human plasma lipoproteins. II. Receptor binding activity of a high density lipoprotein subfraction modulated by the apo (E—A-II) complex. *J Biol Chem* 253:6289, 1978

89. SHORE VG, SHORE B, HART RG: Changes in apolipoproteins and properties of rabbit very low density lipoproteins on induction of cholesterolemia. *Biochemistry* 13:1579, 1974

90. MAHLEY RW, WEISGRABER KH, INNERARITY T: Canine lipoproteins and atherosclerosis. II. Characterization of the plasma lipoproteins associated with atherogenic and nonatherogenic hyperlipidemia. *Circ Res* 35:722, 1974

91. MAHLEY RW: Dietary fat, cholesterol, and accelerated atherosclerosis. *Athero Rev* 5:1, 1979

92. ROSS AC, ZILVERSMIT DB: Chylomicron remnant cholesteryl esters as the major constituent of very low density lipoproteins in plasma of cholesterol-fed rabbits. *J Lipid Res* 18:169, 1977

93. KUSHWAHA RP, HAZZARD WR: Catabolism of very low density lipoproteins in the rabbit: Effect of changing composition and pool size. *Biochim Biophys Acta* 528:176, 1978

94. GOLDSTEIN JL, HO YK, BROWN MS, INNERARITY TL, MAHLEY RW: Cholesteryl ester accumulation in macrophages resulting from receptor-mediated uptake and degradation of hypercholesterolemic canine β-very low density lipoproteins. *J Biol Chem* 255:1839, 1980

95. MAHLEY RW, INNERARITY TL, BROWN MS, HO YK, GOLDSTEIN JL: Cholesteryl ester synthesis in macrophages: stimulation by β-very low density lipoproteins from cholesterol-fed animals of several species. *J Lipid Res* 21:970, 1980

96. ZILVERSMIT DB: A proposal linking atherogenesis to the interaction of endothelial lipoprotein lipase with triglyceride-rich lipoproteins. *Circ Res* 33:633, 1973

97. SCHNEIDER J, MAURER M, KAFFARNIK H: Haufigkeit der Hyperlipoproteinamie Typ III bei elektrophoretisch nachweisbarer breiter β-bande. *Klin Wschr* 52:941, 1974

98. HAZZARD WR, PORTE D, JR, BIERMAN EL: Abnormal lipid composition of very low density lipoproteins in diagnosis of broad beta disease (type III hyperlipoproteinemia). *Metabolism* 21:1009, 1972

99. VESSBY B: Studies on the serum lipoprotein composition in 50-year-old men. A suggestion of chemical criteria for diagnosis of hyperlipoproteinemia type III (broad-beta disease). *Clin Chim Acta* 69:29, 1976

100. UTERMANN G, ALBRECHT G, STEINMETZ A: Polymorphism of apolipoprotein E. I. Methodological aspects and diagnosis of hyperlipoproteinemia type III without ultracentrifugation. *Clin Genet* 14:351, 1978

101. ABRAMS JJ, GRUNDY SM, KANE JP, CHANG C-M: Normocholesterolemic dysbetalipoproteinemia with xanthomatosis. *Metabolism* 28:113, 1979

102. OLIVER MF, HEADY JA, MORRIS JN, COOPER J: A cooperative trial in the primary prevention of ischaemic heart disease using clofibrate. Report from the committee of principal investigators. *Br Heart J* 40:1069, 1978

103. OLIVER MF, HEADY JA, MORRIS JN, COOPER J: The World Health Organization cooperative trial on primary prevention of ischaemic heart disease using clofibrate to lower serum cholesterol: mortality follow-up. Report of the committee of principal investigators. *Lancet* 2:379, 1980

104. ZELIS R, MASON DT, BRAUNWALD E, LEVY RI: Effects of hyperlipoproteinemias and their treatment on the peripheral circulation. *J Clin Invest* 49:1007, 1970

105. FALKO JM, WITZTUM JL, SCHONFELD G, WEIDMAN SW, KOLAR JB: Type III hyperlipoproteinemia. Rise in high-density lipoprotein levels in response to therapy. *Am J Med* 66:303, 1979

33

FAMILIAL HYPERCHOLESTEROLEMIA

JOSEPH L. GOLDSTEIN

MICHAEL S. BROWN

1. Familial hypercholesterolemia *is characterized clinically by (1) a selective elevation in the plasma level of low density lipoprotein (LDL), the major cholesterol-transport protein in human plasma; (2) deposition of LDL-derived cholesterol in tendons (xanthomas) and in arteries (atheromas); and (3) inheritance as an autosomal dominant trait with a gene dosage effect, i.e., homozygotes are more severely affected than are heterozygotes.*

2. *The prevalence of heterozygotes among European, American, and Japanese populations is about 1 in 500 persons, placing this disease among the most common inborn errors of metabolism. Heterozygotes have moderate hypercholesterolemia (350 to 550 mg/dl) from birth. Tendon xanthomas and coronary atherosclerosis develop after age 30.*

3. *Homozygotes number 1 in 1 million persons in the United States. They have severe hypercholesterolemia (650 to 1000 mg/dl). Cutaneous xanthomas appear within the first 4 years of life. Coronary heart disease begins in childhood and frequently causes death from myocardial infarction before age 20.*

4. *The primary genetic defect in familial hypercholesterolemia results from one of several mutations in the gene specifying the receptor for plasma LDL. Located on the surfaces of most body cells, the LDL receptor normally binds LDL and facilitates its cellular uptake and delivery to lysosomes, where the LDL is degraded* and its cholesterol is released for use in the synthesis of cell membranes (most cell types), steroid hormones (adrenocortical cells), and bile acids (liver cells). The deficiency of LDL receptors in patients leads to a decreased rate of removal of LDL from plasma, the plasma level of LDL rising in inverse proportion to the reduction in LDL receptors. The excess plasma LDL is deposited in scavenger cells and other cell types, producing xanthomas and atheromas.

5. *Three classes of mutant alleles at the LDL receptor locus have been identified in cultured fibroblasts. The most common allele, designated receptor-negative or $R^{b°}$, specifies a gene product that is nonfunctional. The second most frequent allele, designated receptor-defective or R^{b-}, produces a receptor that has detectable, but reduced LDL binding activity. The third allele, designated $R^{b+,i°}$, produces a receptor that binds LDL normally but is unable to transport the lipoprotein into the cell. This very rare allele produces the so-called internalization defect. Phenotypic homozygotes possess two mutant alleles at the LDL receptor locus, and hence their cells show a total or near-total inability to bind or take up LDL. Heterozygotes have one normal allele and one of the three mutant alleles at the LDL receptor locus, and hence their cells are able to bind and take up LDL at approximately half the normal rate.*

6. *Prenatal diagnosis of receptor-negative homozygotes (genotype, $R^{b°}/R^{b°}$) can be performed by quantitative*

assays of LDL receptor activity in cultured amniotic fluid cells.

7. *Treatment for heterozygotes and homozygotes is directed at lowering the plasma level of LDL. In heterozygotes the most effective therapy is the combined administration of a bile acid–binding resin (which removes sterol from the body and enhances LDL receptor activity in the liver) and nicotinic acid. Homozygotes are resistant to drug therapy. Their plasma LDL levels can be lowered by: (1) the use of a continuous-flow blood cell separator to perform repeated plasma exchange, or (2) the surgical creation of a portacaval shunt. Evidence that lowering LDL levels by any of these procedures prolongs the life of heterozygotes or homozygotes is not available.*

Familial hypercholesterolemia results from one of several genetic defects in a cell surface receptor that normally controls the degradation of plasma LDL. The disorder is characterized clinically by a lifelong elevation in the concentration of LDL-bound cholesterol in blood; pathologically by xanthomas, arcus corneae, and premature coronary heart disease; and genetically by autosomal dominant inheritance. Familial hypercholesterolemia was the first genetic disorder recognized to cause myocardial infarction [1, 2]. To this day, it remains the most cogent illustration of the causal relation between high blood cholesterol levels and coronary atherosclerosis. But above and beyond its traditional place among diseases of lipid metabolism, familial hypercholesterolemia has recently acquired importance as a prototype for a class of diseases caused by defects in receptor molecules [3].

Patients with familial hypercholesterolemia manifest two distinct clinical syndromes, depending on whether the gene is present in the heterozygous or homozygous form. Heterozygotes, who have one normal gene and one mutant gene at the LDL receptor locus, occur in the general population at a frequency of about 1 in 500, placing familial hypercholesterolemia among the most common single gene–determined diseases in human beings. As expected, homozygotes, who inherit two mutant genes at the LDL receptor locus, are much less numerous than heterozygotes, occurring with a prevalence of 1 in 1 million in the general population. Homozygotes exhibit a syndrome that is more severe than the disease in heterozygotes.

In considering familial hypercholesterolemia, one should note that this disease is only one of several disorders that are included in the designation *familial type 2 hyperlipoproteinemia*. Thus, simply finding an elevated LDL cholesterol level in a patient does not mean that the patient has familial hypercholesterolemia. Ascertainment requires either the demonstration of a decrease in LDL receptors or the presence of ancillary clinical findings such as tendon xanthomas, autosomal dominant transmission, and expression in childhood.

HISTORICAL ASPECTS

The simultaneous occurrence in a single patient of xanthomas in tendons and atheromas in arteries was repeatedly described

before 1900 [4–7]. In the 1930s both Muller [1, 2] and Thannhauser [8, 9] recognized the familial clustering of patients exhibiting xanthomas, premature coronary artery disease, and hypercholesterolemia. Their suggestion of a genetic basis for hypercholesterolemia was substantiated in the 1940s and 1950s by the family studies of Wilkinson [10, 11], Adlersberg [12–14], and others [15–20]. Understanding the genetics of familial hypercholesterolemia was greatly advanced by the extensive observations of Khachadurian, whose studies in Lebanon in the early 1960s clearly delineated both clinical and genetic differences between heterozygotes and homozygotes [21]. These studies of Khachadurian provided the first unequivocal evidence for the single gene inheritance of this disorder.

Using their technique of analytical ultracentrifugation, Gofman and coworkers in the mid 1950s showed that the hypercholesterolemia in familial hypercholesterolemia was due to a selective increase in the plasma concentration of one lipoprotein, now referred to as LDL [22, 23]. Fredrickson, Levy, and coworkers in the 1960s developed the concept that familial hypercholesterolemia is a disorder involving the metabolism of both the apoprotein and cholesterol components of LDL [24]. The most recent developments relate to the use of cultured fibroblasts from homozygotes to define the basic biochemical defect. The studies of Brown and Goldstein disclosed the existence of the cell surface LDL receptor and demonstrated that familial hypercholesterolemia is caused by a mutation in the gene specifying this receptor [3, 25].

CLINICAL FEATURES

The most informative data on the natural history of heterozygous familial hypercholesterolemia have been derived from studies in which the frequency of various clinical findings has been determined in affected relatives of different ages from the same large family [17, 18, 26, 27]. The results of one such analysis are shown in Fig. 33-1. The earliest detectable manifestation of the gene is hypercholesterolemia, which is present

Figure 33-1 Prevalence of clinical manifestations at different ages in the affected heterozygotes from a single large family with familial hypercholesterolemia. (*Data redrawn from Schrott et al. [27].*)

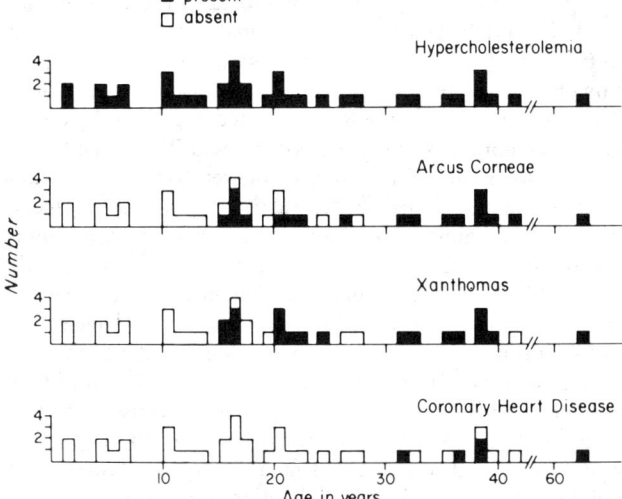

at birth in virtually all affected subjects [28] and remains the only clinical finding throughout the first decade of life [29]. Arcus corneae and tendon xanthomas begin to appear in the latter part of the second decade, and by the third decade each is present in about half of all adult heterozygotes. By the time of death, 80 percent of heterozygotes have xanthomas [27]. Clinical symptoms of coronary heart disease begin to appear in the fourth decade.

In homozygotes the natural history has been defined by the long-term follow-up studies of Khachadurian [21, 30, 32] and by the clinical studies of Fredrickson and Levy [31]. The clinical picture in these patients is remarkably uniform and distinctly different from that in heterozygotes. Marked hypercholesterolemia, present at birth, persists throughout life. Unique yellow-orange cutaneous xanthomas are frequently present at birth and develop in all homozygotes by 4 years of age [30–32]. Homozygotes inevitably develop tendon xanthomas and arcus corneae in childhood, as well as very early evidence of generalized atherosclerosis. Death from myocardial infarction typically occurs before 30 years of age [30–32]. In addition to atherosclerosis of the coronary, cerebral, and peripheral vessels, homozygotes also develop a characteristic form of xanthomatous infiltration of the aortic valve that is clinically and hemodynamically indistinguishable from rheumatic or calcific aortic valvular stenosis [21, 33].

Blood Lipids and Lipoproteins

When large numbers of heterozygotes with familial hypercholesterolemia are studied, a remarkable uniformity in their mean plasma cholesterol levels is observed [34]. For example, plasma cholesterol levels averaged 340 mg/dl in the 56 obligate Lebanese heterozygotes studied by Khachadurian [30]; 350 mg/dl in the 36 affected members of the large Aleutian kindred reported by Schrott et al. [27]; 341 mg/dl in 73 affected first-degree relatives in 55 British families studied by Nevin and Slack [35]; 366 mg/dl in 262 U.S. Caucasian heterozygotes followed by Fredrickson and Levy [31]; and 358 mg/dl in 40 Japanese heterozygotes described by Habh et al. [36]. Despite this uniformity in mean cholesterol levels among large numbers of heterozygotes, the cholesterol levels in individual patients, even within the same family, may vary as much as twofold (i.e., from about 270 to 550 mg/dl). In homozygotes the plasma cholesterol concentration is uniformly higher than in heterozygotes, ranging from 600 to 1200 mg/dl [30–32].

Cholesteryl esters, which normally make up 70 to 75 percent of the total plasma cholesterol fraction, form a similar proportion of the cholesterol in both heterozygotes and homozygotes. Total plasma phospholipids are elevated slightly in heterozygotes and more strikingly in homozygotes [37]. Although some heterozygotes with familial hypercholesterolemia have a slight elevation of the plasma triglyceride concentration, the mean value and distribution of plasma triglycerides are not significantly different from those of the general population (Table 33-1) [27, 29, 31]. In homozygotes the mean level of plasma triglycerides is slightly elevated, but many patients have values in the normal range [30–32]. These findings indicate that the mutation in the LDL receptor gene does not affect directly the metabolism of triglyceride-carrying very low density lipoproteins (VLDL). Occasionally, however, a heterozygote or a homozygote with documented familial hypercholesterolemia will have a plasma triglyceride level of more than 250 mg/dl. The reason for this infrequent occurrence is unknown.

The excess cholesterol in the plasma of heterozygotes and homozygotes is found entirely in the lipoprotein fraction of density 1.006 to 1.063 g/ml, that is, the LDL [22, 23, 31]. The mean LDL cholesterol concentration in heterozygotes at all ages is roughly two to three times the mean of normal subjects of similar age. The mean LDL cholesterol concentration in homozygotes is about two to three times that of heterozygotes and about six times that of normal subjects (Table 33-1). A number of studies have indicated that LDL particles are increased in number in the plasma of patients with familial hypercholesterolemia and that each particle is of nearly normal composition and structure with regard to lipid and protein content, amino acid composition, flotation properties, and immunochemical reactivity [38–40]. In comparison to normal LDL, LDL from these patients may show a small decrease in triglyceride content [37, 41], a small difference in hydrated density [42], and a slight increase in the ratio of cholesterol to phospholipid [40]. It is likely that these changes in LDL composition in familial hypercholesterolemia patients represent minor secondary alterations in LDL structure that result from excessively prolonged circulation of the lipoprotein due to the LDL receptor defect [40]. The minor structural changes in LDL of familial hypercholesterolemia patients do not affect the metabolism of the particles. Thus, when LDL from a homozygote was injected into the circulation of a normal subject, the LDL was metabolized normally [43]. Moreover, LDL from homozygotes binds to LDL receptors [44] and suppresses 3-hydroxy-3-methylglutaryl coenzyme A reductase activity in normal fibroblasts in the same manner as LDL from normal subjects [45].

The HDL cholesterol levels in familial hypercholesterolemia patients are slightly lower, on average, than in normal subjects [29, 46, 47]. This decrease is seen in heterozygotes as well as in homozygotes at all ages (Table 33-1). The mechanism of this reduction in HDL is not known.

Xanthomas

Accompanying the increase of LDL cholesterol concentration in plasma, there is deposition of LDL-derived cholesterol in several tissues of the body, especially in tendons (xanthomas) and in arterial plaques (atheromas). The occurrence of xanthomas in familial hypercholesterolemia is a function of age and genotype [21, 31]. The major determinants are severity and duration of the elevation in LDL, but local trauma and some unknown factors also dictate differences in the rate and location of tissue deposition. The types of xanthomas seen in familial hypercholesterolemia are illustrated in Figs. 33-2 (A to K) and 33-3 (A to H). Homozygotes and heterozygotes both may have tendon xanthomas (especially in the Achilles tendons and in the extensor tendons of the hand) (Fig. 33-2F to H), tuberous xanthomas (especially over the elbows), and subperiosteal xanthomas (commonly below the knee and over the olecranon process) (Fig. 33-2D, E). Palpebral xanthomas (xanthelasma) occur commonly in heterozygotes (Fig. 33-2A, B), but for some reason they are rare in homozygotes. Unlike tendon xanthomas, which are virtually specific for familial hypercholesterolemia, xanthelasma can occur in subjects with normal lipid levels [22, 23] and may be transmitted in some families as a genetic trait in the absence of hypercholesterolemia. Elevated orange-yellow planar xanthomas lying superficially in the skin over the extremities, buttocks, and hands (especially in the interdigital web between the first and second fingers) (Fig.

Table 33-1   Plasma lipids and lipoproteins in familial hypercholesterolemia

Genotype	Age, years	Number of patients	Plasma cholesterol, mg/dl				Plasma triglyceride, mg/dl
			Total	VLDL	LDL	HDL	
Normal	1–19	128	175 ± 28	13 ± 8	110 ± 25	53 ± 13	60 ± 25
Heterozygotes	1–19	105	299 ± 63	15 ± 11	241 ± 60	43 ± 12	82 ± 51
Homozygotes	1–19	10	678 ± 170	19 ± 8	625 ± 160	34 ± 10	101 ± 51
Normal	≥20	76	194 ± 34	16 ± 10	123 ± 31	53 ± 16	83 ± 31
Heterozygotes	≥20	88	368 ± 78	27 ± 17	298 ± 78	44 ± 13	148 ± 75

Mean ±1 SD.
SOURCE: Data from Kwiterovich et al. [29].

33-3B, C, E, F) are unique to homozygotes [30–32]. Xanthomas of the tongue and the buccal mucosa occur occasionally in homozygotes.

The frequency of xanthomas in heterozygotes as a function of age is shown in Table 33-2. These data illustrate the long lag period in heterozygotes before xanthomas appear.

Patients with cerebrotendinous xanthomatosis, an extremely rare autosomal recessive disorder (Chap. 34), may develop tendon xanthomas that are clinically indistinguishable from those in familial hypercholesterolemia [48, 49]. Other clinical features such as cataracts, mental deterioration, and normal plasma LDL cholesterol levels are sufficient to distinguish these patients from familial hypercholesterolemia heterozygotes (see Chap. 34).

Arcus Corneae

Arcus corneae (Fig. 33-2B) appears in about 10 percent of heterozygotes before 30 years of age and is present in about 50 percent of heterozygotes above age 30 [31]. It usually occurs before age 10 in homozygotes (Fig. 33-3A). Like xanthelasma, arcus corneae can also be observed in patients with normal lipid levels [22, 23] and may appear in several members of the same family. It is frequently seen in otherwise healthy black subjects [50].

Premature Atherosclerosis

Familial hypercholesterolemia is the outstanding example of a single-gene mutation that produces both hypercholesterolemia and atherosclerosis. In homozygotes the cardiac disease is rapidly progressive, and the clinical findings in these patients are remarkably uniform. Angina pectoris, myocardial infarction, or sudden death—three of the cardinal features of adult ischemic heart disease—occur commonly in homozygotes between the ages of 5 and 30 [30–32]. One homozygote is even recorded as having had an acute myocardial infarction as early as 18 months of age [31], and another is known to have died of an acute myocardial infarction at 3 years of age [51]. In homozygotes, severe atherosclerosis occurs in the thoracic and abdominal aorta as well as in the major pulmonary arteries [21, 52, 53]. Very few homozygotes survive past age 30 [32, 47].

Figure 33-4 and Table 33-3 show the prevalence of coronary heart disease in a group of 54 homozygotes, whose fibroblasts have been analyzed for LDL receptor activity (discussed below). These homozygotes are subdivided into two groups, according to whether or not their cells exhibit any detectable LDL receptor activity. The two most noteworthy findings are: (1) the earlier onset of clinical signs of coronary heart disease,

and (2) the higher frequency of coronary deaths in homozygotes in whom no LDL receptor activity is detectable (receptor-negative homozygotes) as compared to those in whom some residual receptor activity (2 to 25 percent of normal) can be detected (receptor-defective homozygotes).

Xanthomatous plaquing and thickening of the endocardial surfaces of the mitral valve and endocardium have also been observed in homozygotes and may explain the clinical findings of mitral regurgitation and mitral stenosis that are occasionally reported [9, 54, 55]. Since the homozygote often has painful joints [56], a persistently elevated sedimentation rate [57], and cardiac murmurs, a misdiagnosis of acute rheumatic fever may easily be made [56].

Unlike the homozygote in whom clinical evidence of severe atherosclerosis occurs characteristically before age 30, the pattern of cardiac disease in the heterozygote is much more variable. In a study of 104 heterozygotes derived from 46 different families, Slack documented the occurrence of premature coronary artery disease and found that the mean age of its onset was 43 years for men and 53 years for women [58]. For heterozygous men, the chance of having a myocardial infarction was 5 percent by age 30, 51 percent by age 50, and 85 percent by age 60. For affected women the risks at comparable ages were 0, 12, and 58 percent. In a 20-year follow-up of 331 members of 11 Danish families, Jensen et al. found that the prevalence of coronary heart disease among heterozygotes with familial hypercholesterolemia (32 percent) was 25 times greater than among unaffected relatives (1.3 percent) [59]. In studies from Norway, Heiberg found that the mean age at death for 32 male heterozygotes and 25 female heterozygotes was 55 and 64 years, respectively [60].

In a study of 116 families involving over 1000 relatives, Stone et al. found that the cumulative probability of developing nonfatal or fatal coronary heart disease by age 40 in male heterozygotes was 16 percent, and by age 60 the expectation of a coronary event had risen to 52 percent [61]. In female heterozygotes, the risk of developing nonfatal or fatal coronary artery disease by age 60 was 32.8 percent as compared with only 9.1 percent in unaffected females. Thus, in spite of the presence of the same genetic abnormality and similarly elevated plasma LDL levels, heterozygous women manifest coronary heart disease less often and at a later age than do heterozygous men. Interestingly, this sex difference, which is also a characteristic feature of the usual form of normolipidemic atherosclerotic heart disease, does not seem to be operative in homozygotes ([52] and Fig. 33-4).

Table 33-4 shows the percentage of heterozygotes who exhibit symptoms of coronary artery disease or death from myocardial infarction at different ages. These values represent estimates compiled from the data of five large studies involving over 1000 heterozygotes [58–62].

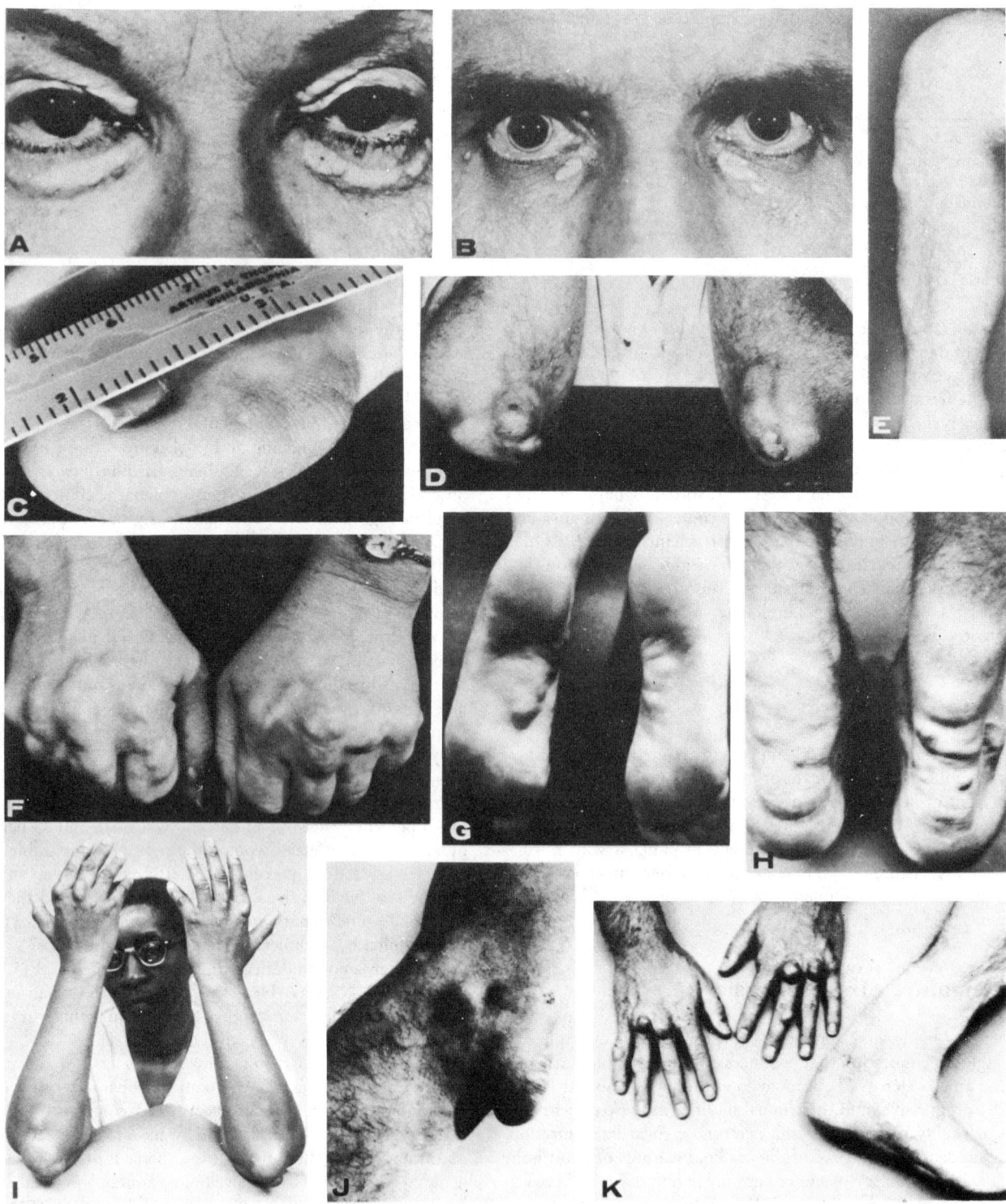

Figure 33-2   Forms of xanthomas and other lipid deposits seen in heterozygotes with familial hypercholesterolemia. *A.* Xanthelasma. *B.* Arcus corneae and xanthelasma. *E.* Subperiosteal xanthoma over tibial tuberosity. *C., D.,* and *F.* to *K.* Either tendon xanthomas or a combination of tendon and tuberous xanthomas.

An increased frequency of hypertension and of premature cerebrovascular disease is not generally observed in heterozygotes [31]. Peripheral vascular disease probably does occur at a slightly increased frequency in familial hypercholesterolemia [31], although it is considerably less prevalent than premature coronary heart disease. Symptomatic atherosclerosis of peripheral vessels appears to be much more common in patients with familial type 3 hyperlipoproteinemia than in heterozygotes with familial hypercholesterolemia [63].

Migratory Polyarthritis

Patients with familial hypercholesterolemia, either heterozygotes or homozygotes, may have recurrent attacks of polyarthritis and tenosynovitis, especially in the ankles, knees, wrists,

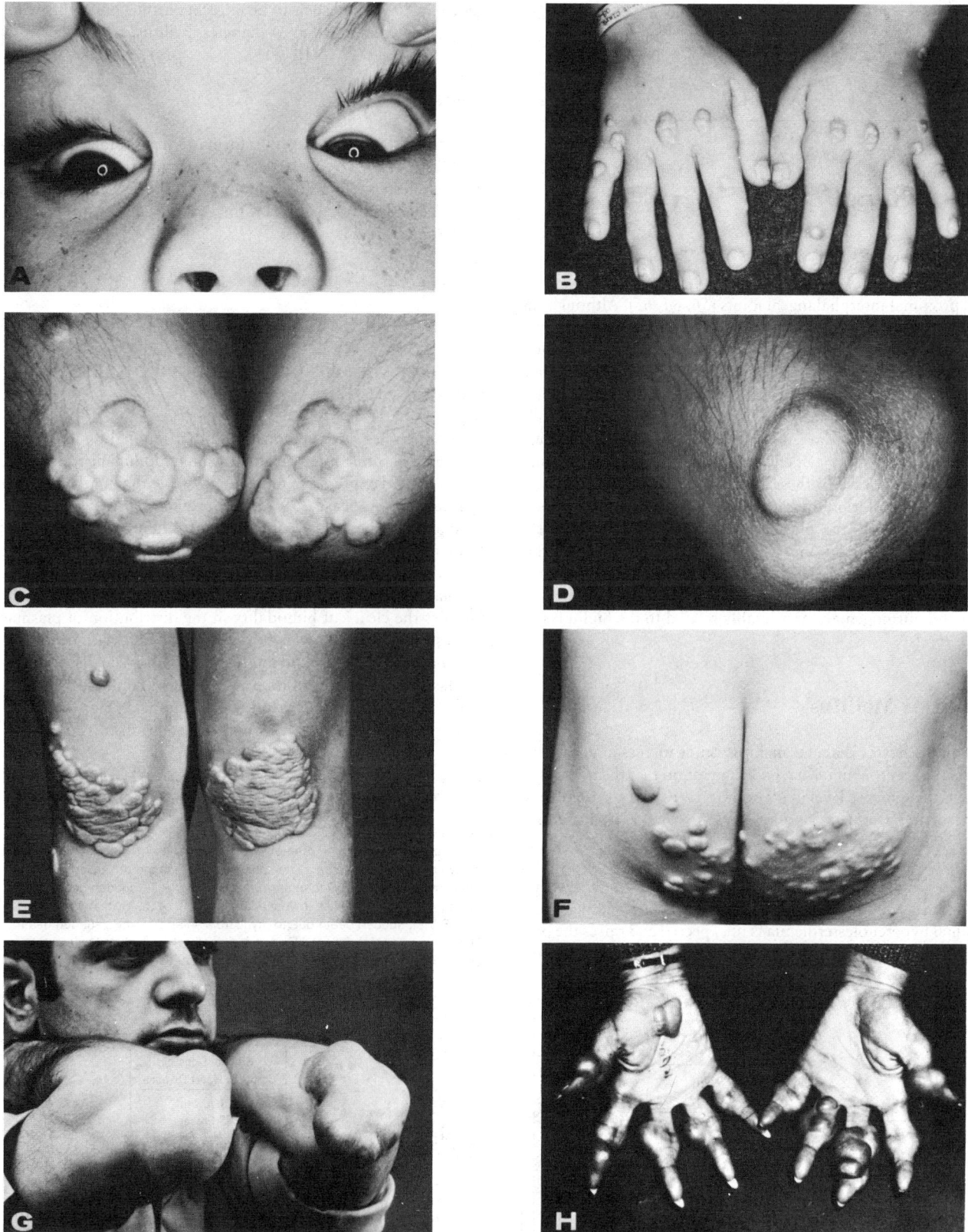

Figure 33-3   Forms of xanthomas and other lipid deposits frequently seen in homozygotes with familial hypercholesterolemia. *A*. Arcus corneae. *B., C., E.,* and *F*. Cutaneous planar xanthomas, usually having a bright orange hue. *C.* and *D.* Tuberous xanthomas on the elbows. *H*. Tendon and tuberous xanthomas. (*H reproduced through the courtesy of A. Khachadurian.*)

Table 33-2 Frequency of xanthomas as a function of age in heterozygotes with familial hypercholesterolemia

Age, years	Number of heterozygotes	Percentage with xanthomas
1–9	38	2.6%
10–19	32	12.5%
20–29	13	69.2%
30–39	30	90.0%
40–59	29	70.3%

SOURCE: Data from Kwiterovich et al. [29].

and proximal interphalangeal joints [56, 64, 65]. Although the joints may be painful and inflamed, fever, leukocytosis, and elevated sedimentation rate occur infrequently. The typical attack begins quickly, with joint symptoms becoming maximal within 24 h of onset. Multiple peripheral joints are involved, but back pain is not a feature. The signs and symptoms usually persist for 3 to 12 days, after which a complete resolution occurs. There is no evidence that anti-inflammatory drugs influence the course of these attacks [65].

The sedimentation rate may be elevated about fourfold above normal in the plasma of homozygotes, even in the absence of joint symptoms [57]. Plasma fibrinogen levels may also show a twofold elevation in homozygotes as compared with normal persons [57]. These elevations in sedimentation rate and fibrinogen are presumably related to the high plasma LDL levels.

Diabetes Mellitus

The frequency of diabetes mellitus is not increased in familial hypercholesterolemia. Khachadurian found that the mean fasting plasma glucose level in 49 homozygotes was 81 mg/dl, and none of these subjects had an elevated value [32]. Heterozygotes have normal fasting plasma glucose levels as well as normal responses to oral glucose tolerance tests [66]. Since diabetes mellitus occurs in at least 2 percent of the general population, the absence of reports of coincident diabetes and familial hypercholesterolemia is unexpected and raises the possibility that the expression of the familial hypercholesterolemia

gene may be altered so as to be unrecognizable in patients who also have a genetic form of diabetes mellitus.

Obesity

In contrast to most of the other forms of hyperlipidemia associated with coronary heart disease, the expression of familial hypercholesterolemia does not appear to be related to obesity [67]. A slender body habitus is the general rule in both heterozygotes and homozygotes.

GENETICS

Mode of Inheritance as Defined by Clinical Genetic Studies

Clinical studies have demonstrated that familial hypercholesterolemia is transmitted as an autosomal dominant trait, with more marked expression in the homozygote than in the heterozygote [68]. At least 2500 heterozygotes representing more than 350 families with well-documented familial hypercholesterolemia have been described. In two kindreds, the number of relatives studied in each family was large enough so that a clinical genetic analysis could be carried out [26, 27]. In both families the clear-cut bimodality in the distribution of plasma cholesterol values allowed an unbiased classification of family members into affected and unaffected groups. The distribution of plasma cholesterol values in one of these families, the Aleutian family reported by Schrott et al., is shown in Fig. 33-5. The pedigree of this family, illustrating vertical transmission of the

Figure 33-4 Prevalence of clinical signs of coronary heart disease at different ages in homozygotes with the receptor-negative (A) and receptor-defective (B) forms of familial hypercholesterolemia. See Table 33-3 for additional information on these patients. The initials of each patient are shown at the bottom of each bar; the sex of the patient (M = male, F = female) is shown at the top of the bar. The causes of death in the deceased homozygotes were as follows: *Receptor-negative group:* R.T., sudden death due to myocardial infarction; N.D., myocardial infarction; M.C., myocardial infarction; P.V.L., sudden death due to myocardial infarction; J.P., sudden death; D.A., myocardial infarction; J.S., sudden death; P.A., ruptured spleen due to surgical complication. *Receptor-defective group:* M.Y., acute myocardial infarction. (From Goldstein and Brown [262].)

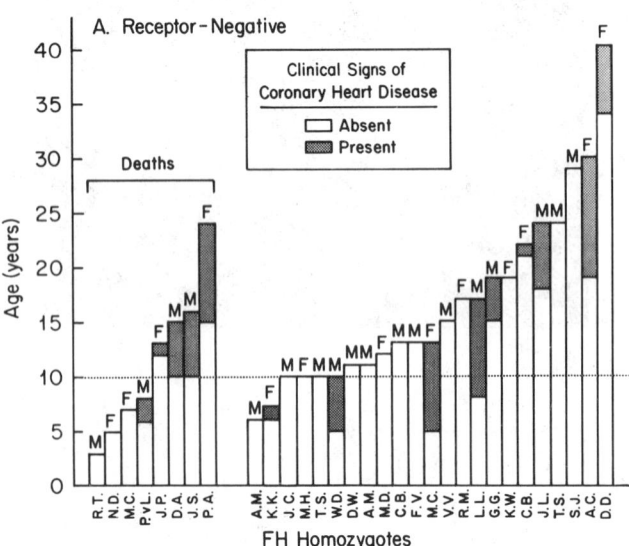

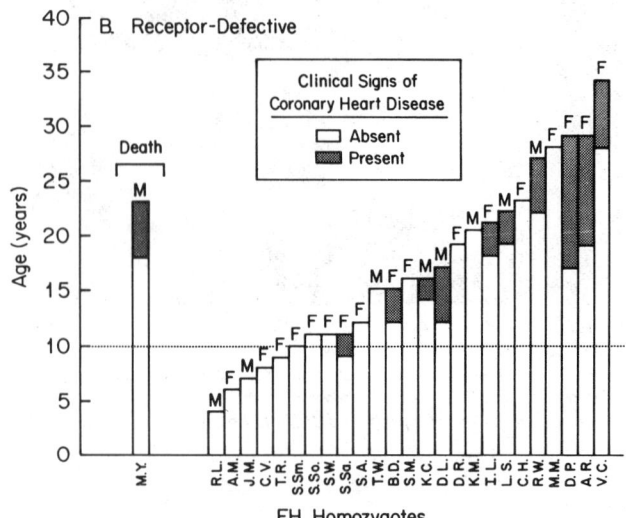

Table 33-3 Coronary heart disease (CHD) in homozygotes subdivided according to genotype at the LDL receptor locus

	Receptor-negative			Receptor-defective		
	Males	Females	Total Group	Males	Females	Total Group
Number of patients	18	13	31	9	17	26
Mean age, years	15	17	16	17	17	17
Prevalence of CHD*						
Age, 0–10 years	3/6‡	3/4	6/10 (60%)	0/2‡	0/4	0/6 (0%)
Age, 10–20 years	4/9	3/6	7/15 (47%)	2/4	2/7	4/11 (36%)
Age, >20 years	1/3	3/3	4/6 (67%)	3/3	4/6	7/9 (78%)
All ages	8/18	9/13	17/31 (55%)	5/9	6/17	11/26 (42%)
Deaths from CHD†	4/18‡	4/13	8/31 (26%)	1/9‡	0/17	1/26 (4%)
Mean age at death, years	10	12	11	23		23

* CHD, coronary heart disease. Clinical signs of coronary heart disease were considered to be present if the patient had any one of the following: classic angina pectoris, evidence of atherosclerosis on coronary arteriography, myocardial infarction, or sudden death.

† Deaths occurring during the follow-up period after the diagnostic skin biopsy was obtained. The mean duration of follow-up was 3.9 years and 3.7 years for the receptor-negative and receptor-defective patients, respectively.

‡ Number affected/total number in group.

NOTE: The data in this table and Fig. 33-4 were obtained from clinical summaries of 57 of the 64 homozygotes whose cultured skin fibroblasts have been analyzed by Goldstein and Brown (see Tables 33-6 and 33-8). Four of the 64 homozygotes (patients of R. S. Lees) are not included in this table because up-to-date clinical information could not be obtained. One receptor-negative homozygote who was diagnosed prenatally [86] and the two homozygotes with the internalization defect are also not included.

SOURCE: From Goldstein and Brown [262].

gene between heterozygotes, is shown in Fig. 33-6. Segregation analysis of all mating types produced results that were consistent with transmission of a Mendelian autosomal dominant gene [27]. Similar conclusions have also been reached in studies in which data from a large number of small families were pooled and subjected to genetic analysis [29, 31, 35].

The earliest clinical proof that severely affected individuals from some families with familial hypercholesterolemia are homozygotes rather than severely affected heterozygotes came from the population studies of Khachadurian in Lebanon [21, 32]. He studied 49 young individuals with juvenile xanthomatosis and rapidly developing atherosclerosis. Three lines of evidence suggested that they were homozygous for the familial hypercholesterolemia gene:

1. Their mean cholesterol level (740 mg/dl) was approximately twice that of their parents, which in turn was twofold greater than that of normal Lebanese control subjects. As shown in Fig. 33-7, these cholesterol values could be segregated into three discrete groups. This strongly supported the hypothesis that these presumed homozygotes did in fact possess two abnormal alleles and that each of their parents possessed one abnormal allele.

2. Of these homozygotes, 58 percent were born to consanguine parents, but the frequency of parental consanguinity in the general Lebanese population was only 10 percent. This finding was consistent with inheritance of the same mutant allele from each parent, thus suggesting true homozygosity rather than a genetic compound state.

3. Sibship analysis of the Lebanese data using the Leng-Hogben formula yielded the number of homozygotes, heterozygotes, and normals expected for a single gene–determined trait.

In addition to the 49 Lebanese homozygotes, more than 100 other homozygotes from at least 40 families throughout the world have been reported [47, 52, 69, 70]. In virtually all cases, these children have resulted from the marriage of two clinically identifiable heterozygotes.

Clinical Manifestations of the Familial Hypercholesterolemia Gene

Analysis of available family data on heterozygotes leads to the following conclusions regarding the clinical expression of the familial hypercholesterolemia gene:

1. When either the plasma total cholesterol or LDL cholesterol level is used as a genetic marker for analyzing known affected families, the familial hypercholesterolemia gene is seen to be highly penetrant at all ages. The calculated penetrance value in heterozygotes is about 90 percent (i.e., 90 percent of persons carrying the gene have a plasma cholesterol value greater than the 95th percentile value of the general population [34]). The LDL cholesterol level appears to be a slightly better marker for the gene than is the total plasma cholesterol level [29]. However, as discussed below, an elevation in neither of these measurements is specific for familial hypercholesterolemia.

2. Although heterozygotes have a reduced life expectancy, symptoms do not usually appear until after the childbearing years. Hence, the gene does not cause a diminution of reproductive fitness [68]. In contrast, homozygotes almost never reproduce. There is only one report in the literature document-

Table 33-4 Estimated risk of heterozygotes having symptoms of coronary heart disease and dying of myocardial infarction at different ages

	Male heterozygotes		Female heterozygotes	
Age	Coronary symptoms	Coronary death	Coronary symptoms	Coronary death
40 years	20%	—	3%	0%
50 years	45%	25%	20%	2%
60 years	75%	50%	45%	15%
70 years	—	80%	75%	30%

SOURCE: These estimates were compiled from the data of Slack [58], Jensen et al. [59], Stone et al. [61], Heiberg [60], and Beaumont et al. [62].

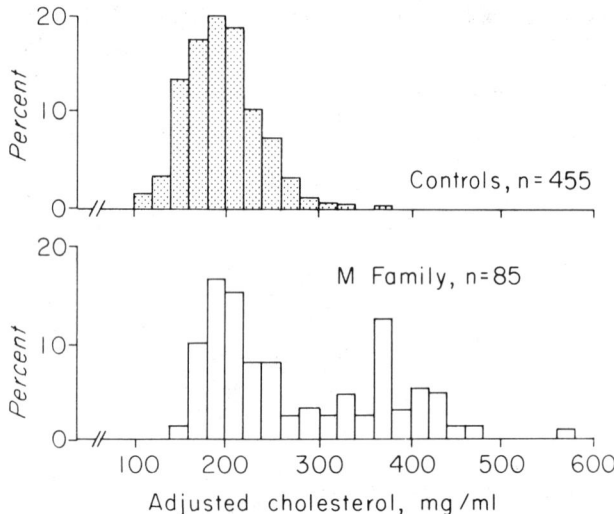

Figure 33-5 Comparison of the distribution of age- and sex-adjusted total plasma cholesterol levels in control subjects (upper histogram) and in members of a single large family with familial hypercholesterolemia. (*From Schrott, et al. [27]. Used by permission.*)

ing the occurrence of a normal pregnancy, parturition, and lactation in a 28-year-old female homozygote [71]. Studies of the skin fibroblasts of this patient showed that she has the receptor-defective phenotype with 10 to 15 percent of normal LDL receptor activity [51].

3. Expression of the familial hypercholesterolemia gene does not appear to be influenced by other genetically determined factors, such as obesity or diabetes mellitus, that affect plasma lipid levels.

4. Evidence from three separate family studies suggests that the gene responsible for familial hypercholesterolemia is linked to the gene specifying the third component of complement (C3) [72–74]. The recombination fraction between these two loci is estimated to be about 0.25. The chromosomal location of these loci is not known.

5. Biochemical studies in fibroblasts cultured from the skin of patients with the homozygous phenotype have disclosed the existence of at least three different classes of mutations affecting the cell surface LDL receptor (discussed below). Thus, familial hypercholesterolemia, like most inherited disorders of metabolism, is genetically heterogeneous, and a similar clinical picture may result from distinct, but related, mutations at a single genetic locus [68].

Population Prevalence

The prevalence of heterozygotes with familial hypercholesterolemia among patients with coronary heart disease has been determined by detailed family analysis of consecutively studied hyperlipidemia survivors of myocardial infarction. The data, which have been collected by three groups of investigators, have yielded remarkably similar estimates. Three percent of 193 survivors in London (Patterson and Slack [75]), 4 percent of 366 survivors in Seattle (Goldstein et al. [76]), and 6 percent of 101 survivors in Helsinki (Nikkilä and Aro [77]) appeared to have the heterozygous form of familial hypercholesterolemia.

Considerable information on the prevalence of heterozygotes in the general population is now available. Using the data

from their population-genetic analysis of hyperlipidemia in survivors of myocardial infarction, Goldstein et al. estimated a minimal heterozygote frequency for familial hypercholesterolemia of 1 in 500 Caucasian individuals with a range of 1 in 200 to 1 in 1000 [76]. This figure is in reasonably close agreement with the estimate of Carter, Slack, and Myant, who used the prevalence of homozygotes in London (about 10 in 10 million persons) to derive a heterozygote frequency of about 1 in 200 persons [78]. A more recent revised estimate by Slack, which was based on the Hardy-Weinberg equation and on the identification of 7 living homozygotes in England and Wales, suggests a heterozygote frequency of 1 in 500 [79]. This estimate agrees with the observations of Leonard et al., who found three asymptomatic heterozygotes among 1391 children admitted to a London hospital [80]. Similar population frequencies for heterozygotes have been reported from Norway [81], Denmark [82], Japan [69, 83], and Lebanon [79].

A remarkably high prevalence of familial hypercholesterolemia has been noted among white Afrikaaners in the Johannesburg area of South Africa [47, 84]. The estimated prevalence of homozygotes and heterozygotes in this African population is 1 in 30,000 and 1 in 100, respectively [47]. This high frequency is believed to be due to a founder effect. The current Afrikaaner population of 2.7 million stems from a few Dutch, German, and French founder families (about 1000 individuals) who settled in the Cape during the latter part of the seventeenth century [47]. If more than 2 of these original 1000 founders possessed the familial hypercholesterolemia gene, this could explain the present high frequency.

Families with familial hypercholesterolemia have been reported from most countries throughout the world [31]. If the disorder is as frequent in other countries as it appears to be in America, Europe, and Japan, it is probably the most common single-gene disorder affecting humans.

PATHOLOGIC ASPECTS

Comprehensive studies of the pathology of homozygous familial hypercholesterolemia have been carried out by L. M. Buja and his colleagues at the University of Texas Health Science Center at Dallas. These workers reported morphological findings in 1 aborted 20-week-old fetus and 3 patients with homozygous familial hypercholesterolemia and have reviewed the pathologic findings in 21 other homozygotes who have been reported in the literature [70]. These data are summarized in Table 33-5. Only limited pathologic data are available for patients who are clearly identified as heterozygotes [85].

Initial Pathologic Manifestations: Autopsy Findings in a Homozygote Fetus

A 20-week-old fetus, whose cultured amniotic fluid cells were shown to lack LDL receptors at the time of prenatal diagnosis, was examined at autopsy after therapeutic abortion [86]. Only one minute focus of intimal lipid accumulation was found in the aorta and coronary arteries of the homozygote fetus (Fig. 33-8A). The fetus, however, exhibited multifocal lipid deposition of a mild degree in stromal macrophages in the thy-

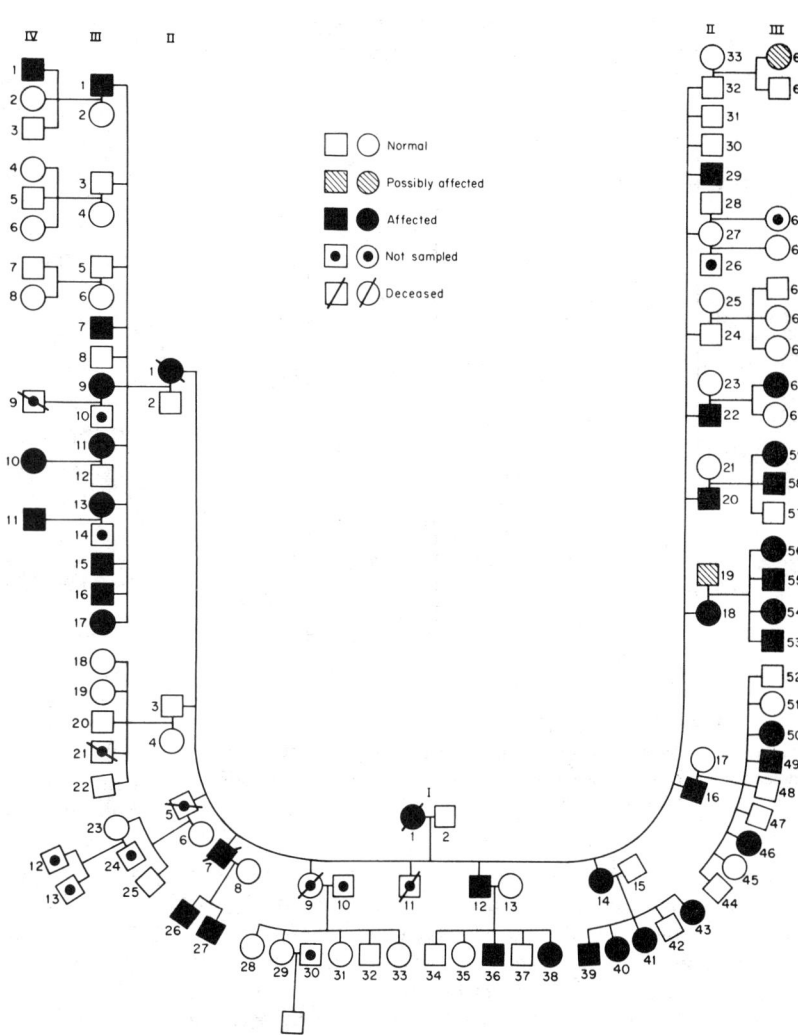

Figure 33-6 Pedigree of a family with familial hypercholesterolemia. All affected persons are heterozygotes. I-1, II-1, and II-7 each had hypercholesterolemia and tendon xanthomas and died as a result of coronary heart disease. (*From Schrott et al. [27]. Used by permission.*)

mus, spleen (Fig. 33-8*B, C*), skin, and other organs and in both stromal and parenchymal cells of the kidneys. The lipid deposits were uniformly oil red O–positive, and some foci showed marked birefringence by polarization microscopy, indicating a high cholesteryl ester content. Electron microscopy showed that most lipid deposits in the stromal cells were round, moderately electron dense, non-membrane-bound, cytoplasmic droplets. Similar lipid deposits in stromal cells were not observed in three control fetuses. Although the hepatocytes of the homozygote fetus showed prominent lipid accumulation, the control fetuses also had hepatic lipid deposits, suggesting that the hepatocellular lipid accumulation in the homozygote fetus may have represented a nonspecific fatty metamorphosis, possibly induced by intrauterine hypoxia [70].

Cord-blood cholesterol in the homozygote fetus was 279 mg/dl, as compared with an average of 31 mg/dl in control fetuses of similar gestational age [86]. Esterified cholesterol content of the thymus of the fetus was four times that of one control fetus (0.51 mg sterol per gram of tissue versus 0.12 mg sterol per gram), and the esterified cholesterol content of most other tissues was 1.5 times that of the control fetus. The findings in the 20-week-old homozygote fetus suggest that homozygous familial hypercholesterolemia leads to an early cholesteryl ester accumulation in stromal macrophages and that atherosclerosis in homozygotes does not commence in a major way during preterm fetal development.

Atherosclerosis of Aorta and Coronary Arteries

Homozygous children exhibit severe atherosclerosis of the aorta and coronary arteries (Figs. 33-9 to 33-11), myocardial infarcts or related forms of ischemic myocardial damage, sclerosis, and lipid deposition in aortic and mitral valves, arcus corneae, and cutaneous and tendinous xanthomas (Fig. 33-12) [70]. Lipid deposition in stromal macrophages of lymph nodes, spleen, and other organs has been reported in a few homozygotes [70]. However, the degree to which lipid is deposited in extravascular sites other than in xanthomas is not well defined in familial hypercholesterolemia since most reports have emphasized examination of the cardiovascular system.

Comparison of findings in the homozygote fetus and young homozygotes indicates a very rapid postnatal progression of atherosclerosis in familial hypercholesterolemia (Figs. 33-9 to 33-11). The atherosclerotic process appears to involve major arteries selectively and to spare veins, in spite of severe hypercholesterolemia [70]. Atherosclerosis of the aorta in homozygotes typically has a generalized distribution, but it also frequently shows a distinctive, unusually severe involvement of the thoracic aorta, particularly the ascending portion with extension into the coronary ostia [70]. Severe atherosclerosis also occurs in the abdominal aorta and in the major pulmonary arteries [52].

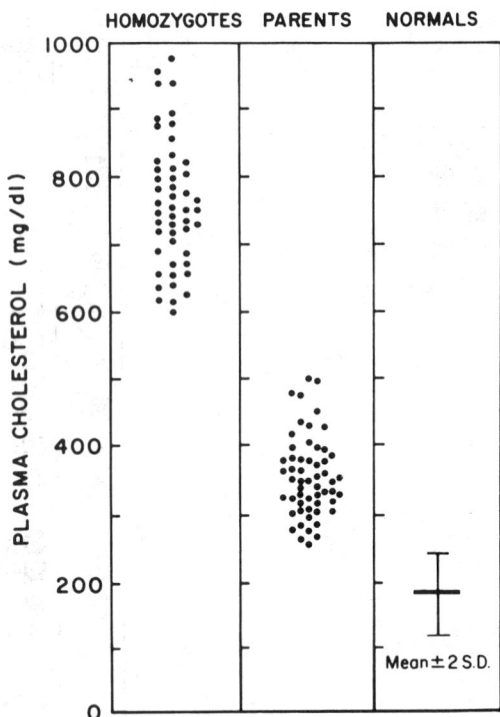

Figure 33-7 Distribution of total plasma cholesterol levels in 49 homozygotes, their parents (obligate heterozygotes), and normal controls. (*Data redrawn from Khachadurian [30, 32].*)

Figures 33-10 and 33-11 illustrate the histologic and ultrastructural features of aortic atherosclerotic lesions in a 9-year-old homozygote. A segment of ascending aorta from this patient showed: (1) foam cell transformation of many medial smooth-muscle cells, (2) abnormal vascularization of the inner media and intima, and (3) intimal involvement by a typical atherosclerotic plaque with fibrous capsule and central atheromatous core. Cells of the plaque capsule close to the luminal surface were devoid of lipid deposits, whereas oil red O–positive cellular lipid deposits were present in the deeper portions of the plaque in elongated cells of the plaque capsule and in elongated and ovoid foam cells adjacent to the plaque core. This core was composed of lipid-rich debris and numerous cholesterol clefts. The fibrous cap of the atherosclerotic plaque contained abundant collagen but only a few small elastic fibers. The cells of the capsule had features previously described as those of altered smooth-muscle cells or myointimal cells (Fig. 33-11A). These features included a thin elongated shape, prominent rough-surfaced endoplasmic reticulum, a basement membrane, and numerous pinocytotic vesicles and cytoplasmic filaments. The foam cells adjacent to the core of the plaque (Fig. 33-11B) usually had an ovoid shape, lacked basement membranes, had relatively sparse cytoplasmic filaments, generally lacked identifiable features of smooth-muscle cells, and actually resembled histiocytic foam cells found in the cardiac valves and in xanthomas in the homozygotes. Cellular lipid deposits in plaque cells (Fig. 33-11), medial smooth-muscle cells, and xanthomas occurred predominantly in the form of round, neutral, lipid droplets which showed variable electron density and were not membrane-bound. Some lipid deposits were located in bodies which were lined by trilaminar membranes and had features of lysosomes. The membrane-bound lipid included round droplets as well as elongated acic-

ular forms with the appearance of free cholesterol crystals [70].

In accord with the findings in the 9-year-old homozygote, similar descriptions of several morphologically distinguishable cell types in human and experimental atherosclerotic plaques have previously appeared [70]. These findings suggest that plaque cells may originate from multiple sources, including smooth-muscle cells, endothelial cells, intimal histiocytes, and circulating monocytes. In this regard, recent studies indicate that a significant proportion of cells in human and experimental atherosclerotic plaques have functional characteristics of macrophages, including Fc receptors and lysozyme activity [86a]. Since lipid-laden foam cells have not been identified in the blood of homozygotes or patients with other conditions predisposing to severe atherosclerosis, it seems likely that macrophages acquire their lipids after the cells have entered the atherosclerotic lesions.

Aortic and Mitral Valve Involvement

Atheromatous and xanthomatous involvement of the aortic valve is another characteristic cardiac manifestation in the homozygote. Clinically significant aortic stenosis is more frequent than aortic regurgitation as a cause of congestive heart failure in these patients [52]. Changes consistent with significant aortic stenosis were reported in 12 (55 percent) of 21 homozygotes and evidence of mitral insufficiency in 2 (9.5 percent) of these 21 patients [70]. One 12-year-old homozygote is reported to have undergone successful surgical correction of her severely deformed and atherosclerotic aortic valve [33], and another 7-year-old homozygote had successful replacement of both the aortic and mitral valves [70].

The distinctive nature of prominent lipid deposits in the aortic valves of homozygotes has been emphasized [52]. In several cases, histologic studies have demonstrated cholesterol clefts and foam cells in the aortic valve cusps [52]. Buja et al. considered aortic valvular involvement in homozygotes to represent a greatly accelerated form of degenerative (atherosclerotic) aortic valve disease of the type associated with calcific aortic stenosis in the general adult population [70]. Aortic valvular sclerosis and lipid deposition appear to be primarily responsible for aortic stenosis in some homozygotes. Other

Figure 33-8 Histologic findings in a 20-week-old fetus with homozygous familial hypercholesterolemia. *A.* Coronary artery is normal. *B.* Thymocytes contain oil red O–positive (dark) lipid droplets. *C.* Oil red O–positive lipid deposits are also present in the splenic capsule. (*Used by permission of L. M. Buja.*)

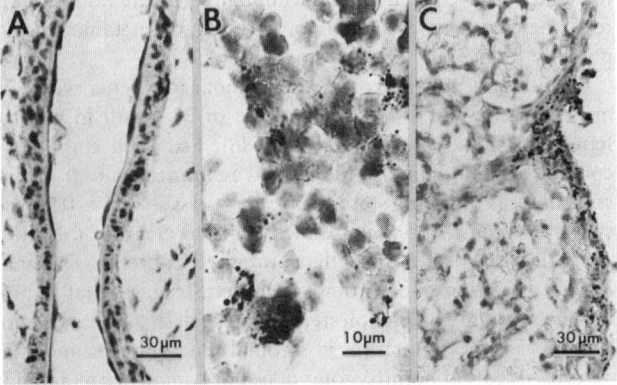

Table 33-5 Clinicopathologic findings in patients with homozygous familial hypercholesterolemia

Report	Age (sex)	Atherosclerosis of aorta and coronaries	Heart pathology	Xanthomas	Other extravascular lipid deposits
Bloom et al., 1942	23 (F)	+	Myocardial degeneration	+	Lipid plaques, renal medullary pyramids; microscopic description limited to the aorta
Cook et al., 1947	13 (M)	+	AV sclerosis (AS) MV mild sclerosis with gross lipid deposits Early infarct	+	Lipid deposits, renal medullary papillae; other lipid deposits not described on microscopic examination
Rigdon & Willeford, 1950	12 (M)	+	AV sclerosis (?AS) MV few gross lipid plaques Myocardial degeneration	+	None identified on microscopic examination
Barr et al., 1954	20 (M)	+	AV sclerosis with gross lipid deposits (foam cells and cholesterol clefts) (AS), also seen in adjacent mural endocardium MV extensive gross lipid deposits PV mild gross lipid deposits	+	None identified, but only cardiac findings emphasized
Maher et al., 1958	16 (F)	+	AV ring sclerosis with gross lipid deposits (AS) MV sclerosis with gross lipid deposits	+	Cholesterolosis of gallbladder; other lipid deposits not described on microscopic examination
	13 (M)	+	AV sclerosis with gross lipid deposits (foam cells) MV sclerosis with gross lipid deposits (foam cells)	+	Moderate lipidosis, liver Some foam cells, lymph nodes
McCleary et al., 1959	6 (M)	+	MV gross lipid deposits	+	Lipid plaques, renal medullary papillae
	7½ (M)	+	AV sclerosis (AS) Healed infarct	+	None identified, but microscopic examination not described
	21 (F)	+	AV sclerosis with gross lipid deposits (?AS) Recent infarct	+	None identified, but microscopic examination not described
Stanley, 1965	12 (F)	+	Aortic root atherosclerosis (supravalvular AS)	+	Only heart examined at operation
Mishkel & Freeman, 1966	21 (F)	+	Valves normal Myocardial necrosis, fibrosis	+	None identified on microscopic examination
Miettinen, 1967	10 (F)	+	AV sclerosis with gross lipid deposits Myocardial fibrosis	+	Foam cells, lymph nodes, and spleen
Rothbard et al., 1967	17 (F)	+	AV sclerosis (AS) with gross lipid deposits (foam cells) MV sclerosis with gross lipid deposits (foam cells and cholesterol clefts)	+	Cholesterolosis, gallbladder; other lipid deposits not identified on microscopic examination
Watanabe et al., 1968	4 (M)	+	AV gross lipid deposits (foam cells), also seen in adjacent mural endocardium MV gross lipid deposits (foam cells) Healed and recent infarcts	+	Lipid deposits including foam cells—left renal medullary papillae, thymus, lymph nodes, lungs, endosternum, and marrow of sternum, brain (Virchow-Robin spaces)
Chomette et al., 1971	11 (M)	+	AV ring sclerosis with lipid deposits Healed and recent infarcts	+	Lipid deposits, including foam cells—choroid plexus and Virchow-Robin spaces of brain; glomeruli, loops of Henle and medullary pyramids of kidneys; histiocytes and alveolar lining cells of lungs; spleen (red pulp); Kupffer cells and hepatocytes (rare) of liver

(continued on page 684)

Table 33-5 Clinicopathologic findings in patients with homozygous familial hypercholesterolemia (*Continued*)

Report	Age (sex)	Atherosclerosis of aorta and coronaries	Heart pathology	Xanthomas	Other extravascular lipid deposits
	22 (F)	+	Healed infarct	+	Lipid droplets in Kupffer cells (rare) and marked lipidosis of hepatocytes of liver; lipid droplets, loops of Henle, kidneys; lipid deposits and inflammation, mastoid region
Sanguinetti & Picchio, 1971	19 (M)	+	AV sclerosis with lipid deposits (AS) MV sclerosis with lipid deposits (MR)	+	None identified on microscopic examination
Wennevold & Jacobsen, 1971	22 (F)	+	Aortic root atherosclerosis and AV sclerosis (supravalvular AS) Healed infarcts	+	Only cardiovascular finding reported
Roberts et al., 1973	28 (M)	+	AV sclerosis with lipid deposits (AS) MV sclerosis with lipid deposits (foam cells and cholesterol clefts) Healed infarct	+	No obvious foam cells, some cells with weakly autofluorescent lipofuscin—spleen
Taketomi et al., 1975	4 (F)	+		+	Lipoid pneumonia LDL (immunofluorescence) in hepatocytes and capillaries and glomeruli of kidneys
Buja et al., 1979	9 (F)	+	AV sclerosis (AS) with lipid deposits (foam cells) MV sclerosis (MR) with lipid deposits (foam cells) Papillary muscle fibrosis and myocytolysis	+	Other sites not examined

NOTE: AS = aortic stenosis; AV = aortic valve; LDL = low density lipoprotein; MR = mitral regurgitation; MV = mitral valve; PV = pulmonic valve. Clinicopathologic evidence of valvular dysfunction is indicated by the designation of AS or MR.
SOURCE: Buja et al. [70].

homozygotes with left ventricular outflow tract obstruction, however, have a major contributory component of supravalvular aortic stenosis due to bulky atherosclerotic plaques in the ascending aorta [70].

Cutaneous and Tendon Xanthomas

Cutaneous xanthomas are a prominent pathologic feature of homozygous familial hypercholesterolemia. Detailed histologic and ultrastructural features of four xanthomas from three homozygotes have been reported [70, 87]. The lesions are composed of large numbers of histiocytic foam cells in a fibrovascular stroma (Fig. 33-12). The large ovoid foam cells contain inclusions consisting predominantly of large, non-membrane-bound, round droplets as well as some lipid-containing membrane-bound structures, including multivesicular bodies, bodies with round or crystalloid deposits, concentric lamellar bodies (myelin figures), and lipofuscin (ceroid) granules. Lipid droplets are rarely observed in extracellular regions. It is noteworthy that endothelial cells of small blood vessels in the lesions are devoid of lipid deposits, suggesting selective lipid accumulation in tissue histiocytes of the xanthomas [70, 87].

As discussed above, cellular lipid accumulation in vascular and extravascular lesions of homozygotes occurs predomi-

nantly in the form of cytoplasmic neutral lipid droplets that lack discrete trilaminar membranes, although some membrane-bound lipid deposits are consistently found in the lipid-containing cells. These findings suggest that the cytoplasm is the major site of intracellular lipid storage in this disease. The production of foam cells in homozygotes could, theoretically, involve the following mechanisms: (1) excessive endocytosis of LDL by an LDL receptor–independent pathway in response to chronic hypercholesterolemia, with subsequent lysosomal processing of the LDL and cytoplasmic accumulation of cholesteryl esters; and (2) increased cellular cholesterol synthesis and accumulation of cholesteryl esters due to impaired feedback regulation resulting from an absence of LDL receptors. As discussed below, current evidence from metabolic studies indicates that lipid accumulation in homozygotes results primarily from overloading with plasma LDL via an LDL receptor–independent pathway in macrophages and other cells that perform a scavenger function [88–90].

The pattern of intracellular lipid deposition in familial hypercholesterolemia patients is distinctly different from that seen in Wolman's disease and cholesteryl ester storage disease. In these two disorders, which are caused by a deficiency in lysosomal cholesteryl ester hydrolase, cholesterol deposits are found within lysosomes of stromal histiocytes as well as parenchymal cells (see Chap. 39).

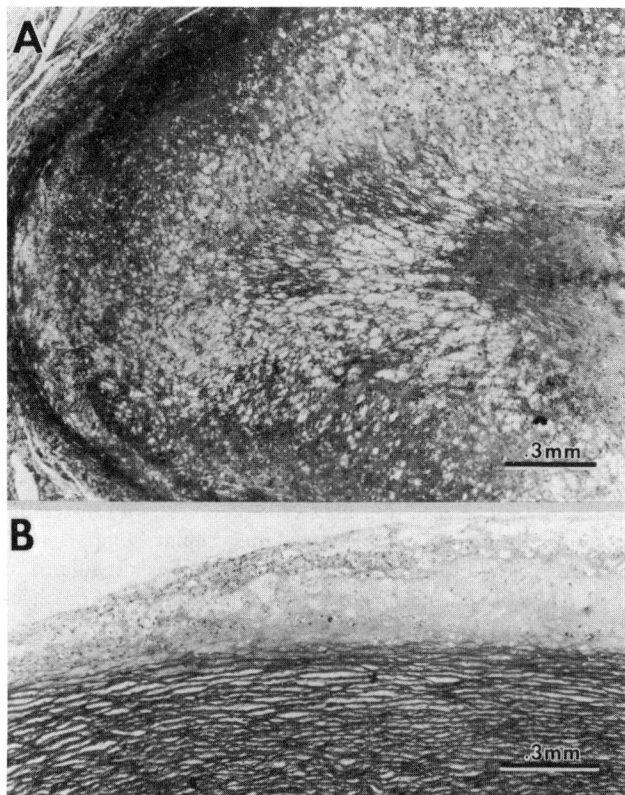

Figure 33-9 Coronary artery (*A*) and aorta (*B*) from a 4-year-old boy with homozygous familial hypercholesterolemia reported by Watanabe et al. [*180*]. These photomicrographs were made by L. M. Buja from histologic sections submitted by K. Tanaka of Kyushu University, Fukuoka, Japan. *A*. The lumen of the coronary artery is markedly narrowed by an atherosclerotic plaque containing numerous foam cells. (The lipid has been removed in the preparation of the paraffin sections.) *B*. The aortic intima is thickened by an atherosclerotic plaque. (*Used by permission of L. M. Buja.*)

PATHOGENESIS AT THE CELLULAR LEVEL

The LDL Receptor Pathway in Cultured Cells

The nature of the genetic defect in familial hypercholesterolemia was deduced from studies of cholesterol metabolism in human fibroblasts in tissue culture [*2, 25*]. Mammalian cells in tissue culture cannot survive unless they acquire cholesterol, either from a usable exogenous source or as a result of *de novo* synthesis within the cell [*91, 92*]. The cholesterol plays a required structural role in the plasma membrane of the cell, where it serves to modulate the fluidity of the phospholipid bilayer. Any cholesterol that accumulates within the cell above the amount that can be inserted into the phospholipid bilayer is esterified with a long-chain fatty acid and stored within the cytoplasm as cholesteryl ester droplets [*93*].

Sequential Biochemical Steps and Their Ultrastructural Counterparts
When mammalian cells are grown in the presence of animal or human serum, they do not produce their own cholesterol but preferentially utilize the cholesterol of the LDL that is present in the serum of the culture medium

[*92, 93*]. Figure 33-13 shows the pathway by which these cells acquire cholesterol from LDL. The key to the uptake is a cell surface receptor that binds LDL by interacting with its apoprotein B component [*93–96*]. Human fibroblasts produce a maximum of about 20,000 to 50,000 LDL receptors per cell [*97*], the number varying according to cellular cholesterol requirements (discussed below) [*98*]. Experiments with intact cells suggested originally that the receptor is a protein molecule. Its binding activity was exquisitely sensitive to destruction by proteases (pronase, trypsin, or chymotrypsin) but was resistant to the action of glycosidases and other hydrolytic enzymes [*92*]. Binding activity of the receptor was also destroyed by protein modification reactions, such as acetylation and treatment with glutaraldehyde [*93*].

Recently the LDL receptor has been solubilized from bovine adrenocortical membranes [*99*] and purified to homogeneity [*99a, 99b*]. The receptor is an acidic protein. When maintained in solution in the presence of the detergent octyl-β-D-glucoside, the receptor activity has a sedimentation coefficient, $s_{20,w}$, of 7.3 and a Stokes radius of 5.35 nm. The purified receptor has a molecular weight of 164,000, as determined by

Figure 33-10 Ascending aorta with atherosclerotic plaque from a 9-year-old girl with homozygous familial hypercholesterolemia. Light micrographs of thin sections from epoxy-embedded tissue (*A* to *C*) and of a frozen section stained with oil red O (*D*). *A*. The plaque core adjacent to the media contains abundant extracellular lipid deposits (clear spaces due to lipid extraction during tissue processing). *B*. Some elongated cells of the fibrous capsule of the plaque contain lipid deposits. *C*. Ovoid foam cells adjacent to the plaque core contain numerous lipid vacuoles. *D*. Frozen section stained with oil red O confirms the presence of neutral lipid in the foam cells. (*Used by permission of L. M. Buja.*)

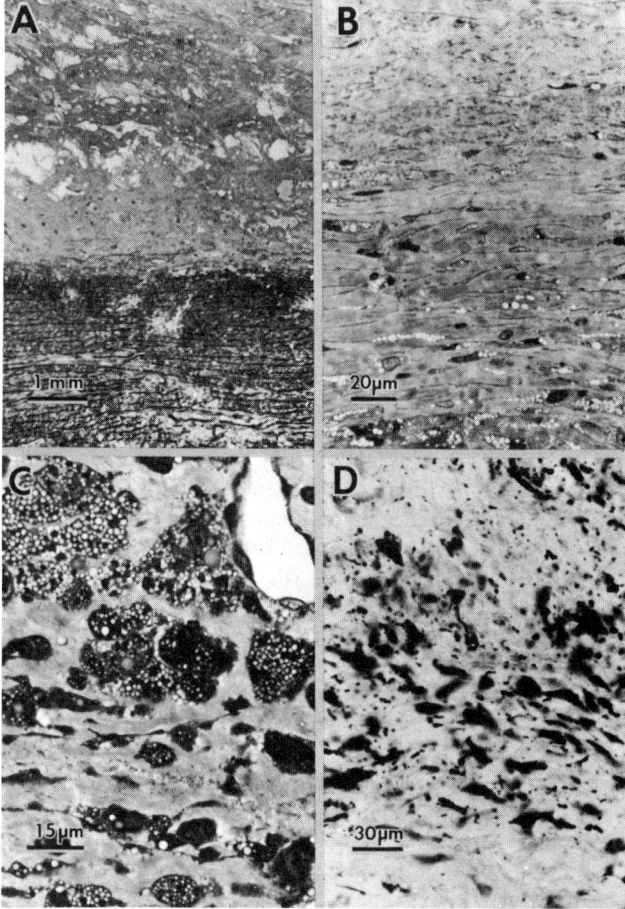

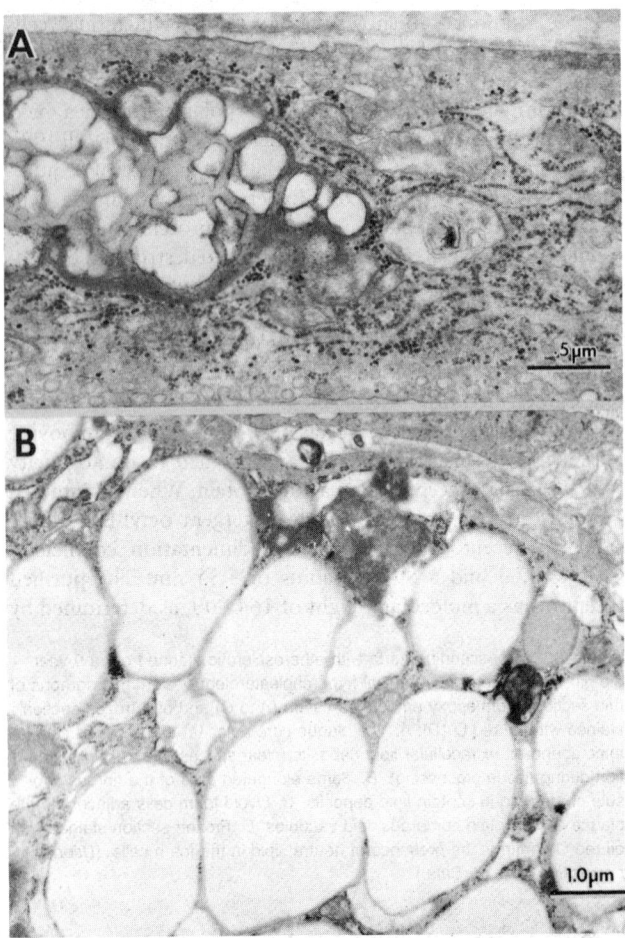

Figure 33-11 Atherosclerotic plaque from a 9-year-old girl with homozygous familial hypercholesterolemia. *A.* Elongated cell of the plaque capsule exhibits a basement membrane, pinocytotic vesicles, cytoplasmic filaments, rough-surfaced endoplasmic reticulum, and a large lipid inclusion. *B.* Ovoid foam cell contains numerous non-membrane-bound lipid deposits. (*Used by permission of L. M. Buja.*)

sodium dodecyl sulfate polyacrylamide gel electrophoresis [99b].

The LDL receptor binds lipoproteins that contain apoprotein E with even higher affinity than those that contain apoprotein B [93, 100]. In fibroblasts the affinity for lipoproteins containing solely apoprotein E (such as apo E HDL$_c$, which appears in the plasma of cholesterol-fed dogs) is about twentyfold higher than the affinity for apoproteins containing only apoprotein B (such as LDL) [100]. However, at saturation, four times as many LDL particles as apo E HDL$_c$ particles are bound. A model to explain these findings has been proposed by Mahley and coworkers who postulate that a single particle of apo E HDL$_c$ may bind to four LDL receptors, whereas a single LDL particle binds to one receptor [101]. The abilities of apo E HDL$_c$ and LDL to bind to the LDL receptor are abolished when the lysine residues of the lipoproteins are modified by reaction with acetic anhydride [102] or diketene [103], or when the arginine residues are blocked by reaction with cyclohexanedione [96]. The latter observation has provided a powerful tool by which to quantify receptor-mediated removal of LDL from human plasma in vivo (see below).

Electron microscopy has shown that the LDL receptors in cultured fibroblasts are clustered in specialized regions, called *coated pits,* of the plasma membrane [104–106]. Coated pits are regions where the plasma membrane is indented and its

cytoplasmic surface is coated by a fuzzy material [107] (Fig. 33-14A). The fuzzy coat is composed of a 180,000-dalton protein called *clathrin,* which is attached noncovalently to the cytoplasmic surface of the membrane [108, 109]. In human fibroblasts, the coated pits cover only 2 percent of the cell surface, yet they contain 50 to 80 percent of the LDL receptors [104–106].

When fibroblasts are incubated with LDL at 4°C, binding to the receptors occurs, but internalization does not take place. When the cells are warmed to 37°C, the coated pits containing the receptor-bound LDL invaginate and pinch off to form endocytic vesicles (coated vesicles), which subsequently shed their coats and migrate through the cytoplasm until they fuse with lysosomes [105]. Within the lysosomes the bound lipoprotein is degraded by acid hydrolytic enzymes. The apoprotein of LDL is hydrolyzed by proteases to amino acids, and the cholesteryl esters are hydrolyzed by a lysosomal acid lipase [110, 111]. The resulting unesterified cholesterol crosses the lysosomal membrane and enters the cellular compartment, where it is used for membrane synthesis and as a regulator of intracellular cholesterol homeostasis [112]. The internalization of LDL is remarkably rapid; half of the surface-bound LDL is internalized every 5 min. The rapid uptake of LDL is due to the clustering of the LDL receptors in coated pits that invaginate immediately after they are formed [105].

The localization of LDL receptors in coated pits on the surface of human fibroblasts was demonstrated originally by thin-section electron microscopy with the use of LDL coupled to the iron-containing, electron-dense protein ferritin [104, 105] and subsequently by ^{125}I-labeled LDL autoradiography [113]. Figure 33-14 shows the visual sequence of events by which LDL-ferritin is bound, internalized, and delivered to lysosomes in human fibroblasts. Using the technique of freeze-etching and rotary shadowing, Heuser et al. have been able to visualize native LDL bound to the LDL receptor on the true surface of human fibroblasts. In the freeze-etch micrograph shown in Fig. 33-15, numerous particles of LDL are seen entering the cell through coated pits.

Regulatory Actions of LDL-derived Cholesterol   The cholesterol derived from the lysosomal hydrolysis of LDL cho-

Figure 33-12 Electron micrograph showing a typical foam cell (scavenger cell) filled with numerous lipid droplets. This mature histiocytic foam cell was observed in a tuberous xanthoma excised from a 17-year-old girl with homozygous familial hypercholesterolemia. (*From Bulkey et al.* [87]. *Used by permission.*)

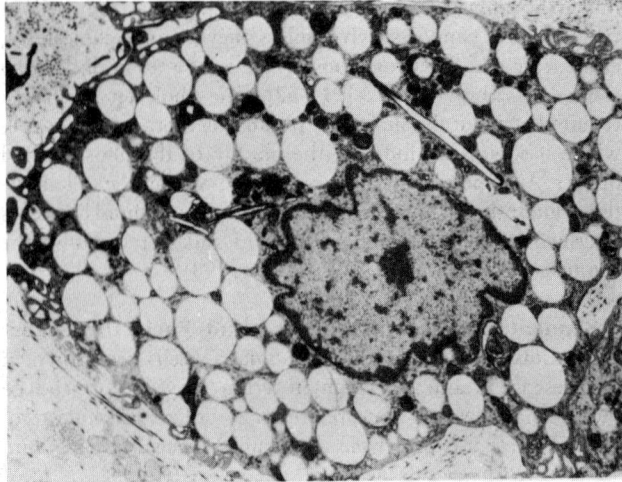

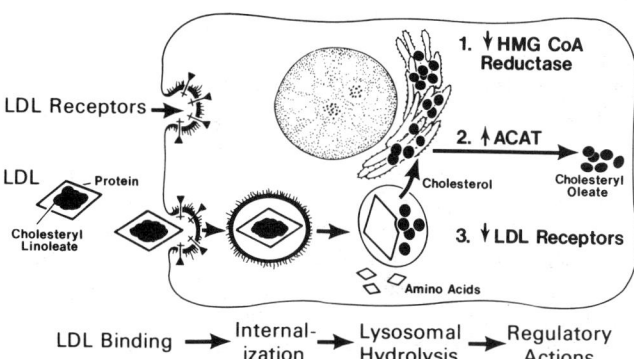

Figure 33-13 Sequential steps in the LDL receptor pathway in cultured mammalian cells. LDL denotes low density lipoprotein; HMG-CoA reductase denotes 3-hydroxy-3-methylglutaryl CoA reductase; and ACAT denotes acyl CoA:cholesterol acyltransferase. (*From Brown and Goldstein [260].*)

lesteryl esters mediates a sophisticated system of feedback control that stabilizes the intracellular cholesterol concentration [114]. First, this cholesterol suppresses the activity of 3-hydroxy-3-methylglutaryl CoA reductase (HMG-CoA reductase), the rate-controlling enzyme in cholesterol biosynthesis, thereby turning off cholesterol synthesis in the cell [115]. Second, the cholesterol activates a cholesterol-esterifying enzyme called acyl CoA:cholesterol acyltransferase (ACAT) so that excess cholesterol can be stored as cholesteryl esters [116]. Third, the cholesterol turns off the synthesis of the LDL receptor, preventing further entry of LDL and thereby protecting cells against an overaccumulation of cholesterol [98] (Fig. 33-13).

The overall effect of this regulatory system is to coordinate the intracellular and extracellular sources of cholesterol so as to maintain a constant level of cholesterol within the cell in the face of fluctuations in the external supply of lipoproteins. Human fibroblasts and other mammalian cells grow in the absence of lipoproteins because they can synthesize cholesterol from acetyl CoA. On the other hand, when LDL is available, the cells preferentially use the receptor to take up LDL and keep their own cholesterol synthesis suppressed [92, 93, 114].

Figure 33-16 summarizes the pattern of regulation of the LDL pathway in cultured human fibroblasts. When the cells are grown in the presence of normal plasma containing LDL, they establish a steady state in which HMG-CoA reductase activity (and hence cholesterol synthesis) is low and the cells derive the small amounts of cholesterol that they need by means of a small number of LDL receptors. Under these conditions, the activity of ACAT is held at an intermediate level so that the rate of synthesis of cholesteryl esters equals their rate of hydrolysis (Fig. 33-16, "steady state with LDL present"). The delicate balance inherent in this regulated steady state is disclosed only when LDL is removed from the culture medium (Fig. 33-16, "no LDL present"). Under these conditions, the number of LDL receptors and the activity of HMG-CoA reductase greatly increase, while cholesterol esterifying activity declines. Since LDL is absent from the culture medium, the LDL receptors are not able to supply the cell with cholesterol and hence the cholesterol required for membrane formation is derived both from accelerated *de novo* synthesis and from a net hydrolysis of cholesteryl esters stored within the cell. When LDL is added back to the culture medium (Fig. 33-16, "initial response to LDL"), the lipoprotein is bound at the receptor site, internalized, and degraded to yield free cholesterol. The

liberated sterol, in turn, suppresses *de novo* cholesterol synthesis and stimulates the esterifying system so that excess cholesterol can be reesterified and stored as cholesteryl esters. When sufficient cellular cholesterol has accumulated, the number of LDL receptors becomes suppressed and the cells return to their original steady state (Fig. 33-16, "steady state with LDL present"), thus completing a metabolic cycle. This "steady state with LDL present" duplicates the condition of most cells in the body [25, 117, 118].

Figure 33-14 Electron micrographs showing representative stages in the receptor-mediated endocytosis of LDL-ferritin and its subsequent delivery to lysosomes. Normal human fibroblasts were incubated with 47.5 μg protein per milliliter of LDL-ferritin for 2 h at 4°C, washed extensively, and then warmed to 37°C for various times. Scale bar = 100 nm. *A.* A typical coated pit (time at 37°C, 1 min). ×67,900. *B.* A coated pit being transformed into an endocytic vesicle with LDL-ferritin included (time at 37°C, 1 min). ×56,700. *C.* Formation of a coated vesicle. As the plasma membrane begins to fuse to form the vesicle, some of the LDL-ferritin is excluded from the interior and is left on the surface of the cell (arrow) (time at 37°C, 1 min). ×38,150. *D.* A fully formed coated vesicle that appears to be losing its cytoplasmic coat on the right side (time at 37°C, 2 min). ×52,500. *E.* An endocytic vesicle that has completely lost its cytoplasmic coat. Note the irregular shape of this vesicle (time at 37°C, 2 min). ×52,500. *F.* An irregularly shaped endocytic vesicle that contains more LDL-ferritin than a typical coated vesicle and also has a region of increased electron density within the lumen (time at 37°C, 6 min). ×52,500. *G.* An endocytic vesicle similar to that in *F* with more electron-dense material in the lumen (time at 37°C, 6 min). ×48,300. *H.* A secondary lysosome that contains LDL-ferritin (time at 37°C, 8 min). ×52,500. (*From Anderson et al. [105]. Used by permission.*) All electron micrograph reduced to 54 percent original size.

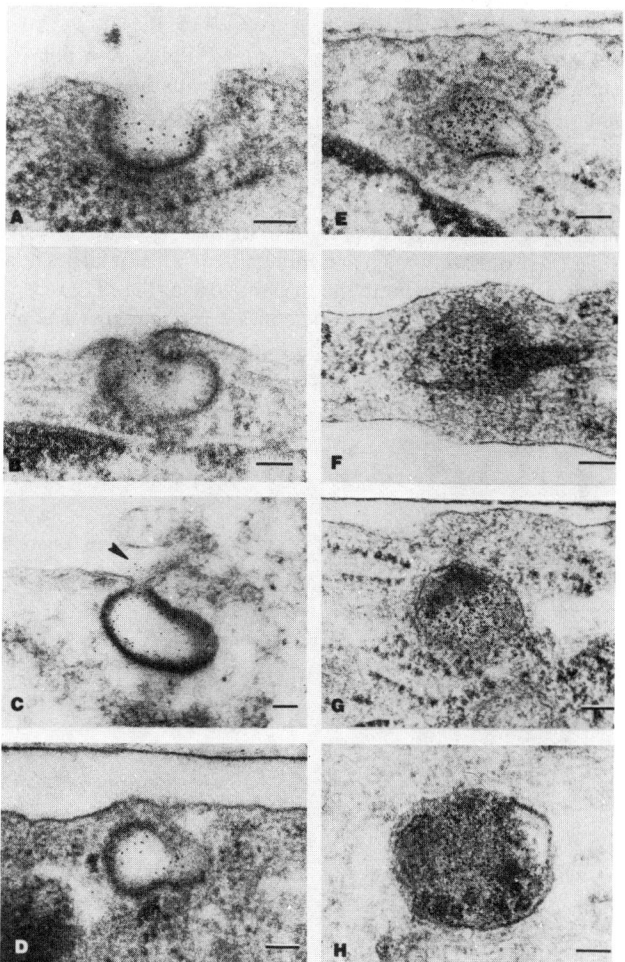

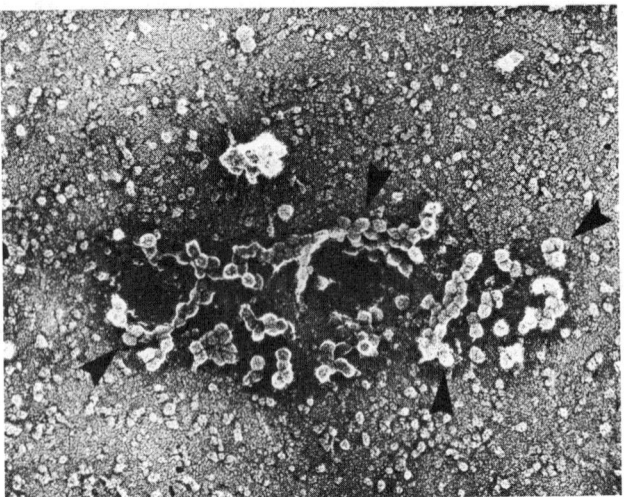

Figure 33-15 Visualization of LDL bound to receptors on the surface of human fibroblasts. Normal human fibroblasts were incubated with 15 μg protein per milliliter of native LDL at 4°C for 2 h, after which the cells were washed extensively, warmed to 37°C for 3 min, and then fixed with glutaraldehyde. The cells were then processed by the rapid-freezing, replica technique of Heuser [261]. This picture shows the appearance of native LDL bound to LDL receptors that are clustered around coated pits. The arrows point to typical LDL particles. ×112,000 (reduced to 69 percent original size).

Biochemical Genetics of LDL Receptor Mutations

One Locus with Multiple Mutant Alleles Fibroblasts cultured from a large number of patients with the typical phenotype of homozygous familial hypercholesterolemia have displayed evidence of a primary abnormality in the function of the LDL receptor. To date, three different classes of mutations have been identified [68, 119, 120]. Although definitive genetic proof is lacking, at present it seems reasonable to consider these mutations as representing three different alleles at a single genetic locus specifying the structure of the LDL receptor. One class of alleles, $R^{b°}$, specifies a receptor that has no detectable binding activity. The second class of alleles, R^{b-}, specifies a receptor that has detectable but markedly reduced

binding activity [119]. The third mutant allele, $R^{b+,i°}$, specifies a receptor that can bind LDL normally but that cannot mediate the internalization of the receptor-bound lipoprotein [120, 121].

$R^{b°}$ ALLELE   The distribution of the three types of mutant alleles in fibroblast strains derived from 64 homozygotes is summarized in Table 33-6. The strains can be divided into three classes based on their ability to bind ^{125}I-labeled LDL in vitro. The receptor-negative class comprises 34 of the 64 fibroblast strains. These cells exhibit no functional LDL receptors within the limits of the current assays, which permit detection of 2 percent of the normal amount of high affinity LDL binding. As a result of this lack of LDL receptor activity, the receptor-negative cells cannot take up and degrade LDL at a normal rate. In these cells LDL does not suppress HMG-CoA reductase activity or cholesterol synthesis, nor does it activate cholesteryl ester formation [45, 110, 115, 116]. Figure 33-17A shows the striking biochemical differences in these LDL-mediated processes in fibroblasts derived from a normal subject and from a receptor-negative homozygote. Ultrastructural studies using ferritin-labeled LDL have confirmed the absence of LDL receptors in the mutant cells [104, 106].

The defect in regulation of cholesterol metabolism in fibroblasts from the receptor-negative homozygotes can be overcome if cholestrol is delivered to the cells in an artificial nonlipoprotein form that permits the sterol to enter the cell without a requirement for the LDL receptor [25]. For example, the cholesterol content of the homozygotes' fibroblasts can be raised by adding cholesterol dissolved in ethanol to the culture medium. When this occurs, HMG-CoA reductase activity and cholesterol synthesis are suppressed and cholesteryl ester formation is activated in the same manner as in normal cells [25]. These findings indicate that the homozygote cells possess all of the intracellular factors necessary to respond to cholesterol, provided that the sterol can be delivered to the proper intracellular site. Certain oxygenated derivatives of cholesterol, such as 7-ketocholesterol and 25-hydroxycholesterol, are up to 100 times more potent on a molar basis than is cholesterol itself in suppressing HMG-CoA reductase and in activating cholesterol esterification in cultured cells [122–124]. These oxygenated sterols, like cholesterol, are equally effective in cells from homozygotes and normals.

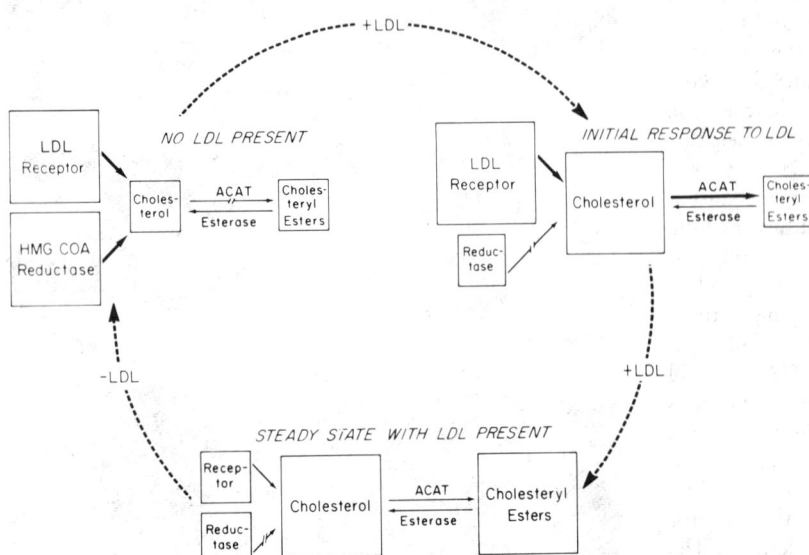

Figure 33-16 Cyclic changes in cholesterol metabolism that occur in cultured human fibroblasts when LDL is removed from the culture medium (− LDL) and is subsequently returned to the medium (+ LDL). The relative level of each constituent is indicated by the size of the square. HMG-CoA reductase denotes 3-hydroxy-3-methylglutaryl CoA reductase; ACAT denotes acyl CoA:cholesterol acyltransferase. (*From Brown and Goldstein* [25]. *Used by permission.*)

Table 33-6 Genetic analysis of fibroblasts cultured from 64 individuals with the clinical phenotype of homozygous familial hypercholesterolemia

Number of subjects	Genotype at LDL receptor locus	Cellular phenotype
34	$R^{b°}/R^{b°}$	Receptor-negative
28	R^{b-}/R^{b-} or $R^{b°}/R^{b-}$	Receptor-defective
2	$R^{b°}/R^{b+,i°}$	Internalization-defective

SOURCE: Modified from Goldstein and Brown [68].

Genetic and biochemical studies suggest that the receptor-negative patients are homozygous for the $R^{b°}$ allele (genotype, $R^{b°}/R^{b°}$) [68, 120, 125]. Fibroblasts from the parents of these subjects express about one-half of the normal number of LDL receptors and are presumed to have the genotype $+/R^{b°}$ [125]. As expected from genetic considerations, the receptors that are functional in heterozygotes show a normal affinity for LDL and thus appear to represent the product of the normal allele at the LDL receptor locus [125, 126]. Under assay conditions in which the concentration of LDL is saturating, fibroblasts from heterozygotes bind half as many LDL particles as do normal cells, and thus they degrade the lipoprotein and form cholesteryl esters at half the rate of normal cells [125, 126].

R^{b-} ALLELE   The second class of familial hypercholesterolemia homozygotes, designated receptor-defective, comprises 28 of the 64 fibroblast strains [68, 127] (Table 33-6). Cells from these individuals show a detectable but markedly reduced number of LDL receptors. In each case the relative amount of receptor binding correlates with the relative ability of LDL to suppress partially HMG-CoA reductase activity and to produce a limited activation of cholesteryl ester formation [119, 127]. This class of homozygotes is likely to be highly heterogeneous in that the range of LDL receptor activity among the various cell strains varies from as low as 2 percent of normal (which is the lower limit of accurate detection using current biochemical assays) to as high as 25 percent of normal. In most cases, the decreased receptor activity is due to a decrease in the number of receptors without an alteration in their affinity for LDL. However, in several cell strains a decreased affinity (apparent K_d, two- or threefold above normal) as well as a reduced number of binding sites have been noted [51, 127].

Figure 33-17B shows the biochemical differences in the LDL-mediated processes in fibroblasts derived from a normal subject and from a homozygote whose cells have about 20 percent of the normal number of LDL receptors. In this particular mutant strain, the amount of residual LDL binding was sufficient to allow detailed studies of the binding reaction. No qualitative alterations were detected in that (1) receptor binding in the mutant cells, like that in the normal cells, showed an absolute requirement for divalent cation [128]; (2) the binding affinity for LDL in the mutant cells was five- to tenfold higher at 4°C than at 37°C, as in normal cells [97]; (3) the mutant receptors showed normal metabolic regulation in that their binding activity was suppressed when the intact fibroblasts were incubated with cholesterol (dissolved in ethanol) or one of its oxygenated derivatives [98]; and (4) the rate of turnover of the mutant receptors, as estimated after cycloheximide

treatment of intact cells, was the same as that observed in normal fibroblasts (half-life of about 20 h) [98].

The following lines of evidence indicate that patients with the receptor-defective cellular phenotype have inherited one mutant allele from each parent and that at least one of the two mutant alleles is different from the functionless $R^{b°}$ allele:

1. Like receptor-negative homozygotes, each receptor-defective individual is the offspring of two hypercholesterolemic parents who show the typical clinical features of heterozygous familial hypercholesterolemia and whose fibroblasts show about one-half of the normal number of LDL receptors.

Figure 33-17 LDL receptor actions in normal fibroblasts (●) and fibroblasts from homozygotes of the three genotypes (△): A. Receptor-negative; B. receptor-defective; C. internalization-defective. Cells were incubated with ^{125}I-labeled LDL or unlabeled LDL at 37°C for 5 h. Assays were performed in growing cells in monolayers as described [260]. All data are normalized to 1 mg of total cell protein. The units for each assay are as follows: *Binding*, micrograms of ^{125}I-labeled LDL bound to cell surface; *internalization*, micrograms of ^{125}I-labeled LDL contained within the cell; *hydrolysis of apoprotein B*, micrograms of ^{125}I-labeled LDL degraded to mono-[^{125}I]iodotyrosine per hour; *hydrolysis of cholesteryl esters*, nanomoles of [^{3}H]cholesterol formed per hour from the hydrolysis of [^{3}H]cholesteryl linoleate–labeled LDL; *cholesterol synthesis*, nanomoles of [^{14}C]acetate incorporated into [^{14}C]cholesterol per hour by intact cells; *cholesterol esterification*, nanomoles of [^{14}C]oleate incorporated into cholesteryl[^{14}C]oleate per hour by intact cells. (*Redrawn from Goldstein and Brown [68].*)

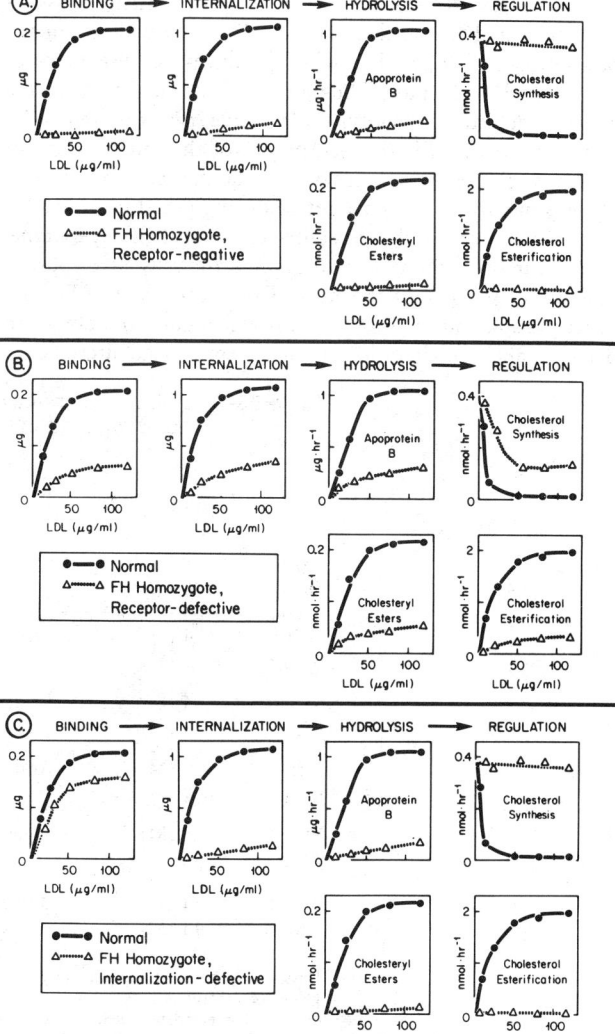

2. Each receptor-defective individual has a clinical syndrome that is distinctly worse than in either parent.

3. Both the receptor-defective and the receptor-negative cellular phenotypes breed true in a given family. Analyses have been performed on fibroblasts from five pairs of sibs, who exhibit the typical clinical features of homozygous familial hypercholesterolemia (Table 33-7). In three of these sib pairs (N.D. and W.D., M.S. and J.S., and A.M. and R.M. in Table 33-7), the cells of both members had virtually no detectable LDL receptor activity in all essays (< 2 percent of normal on average), a finding that is consistent with a genotype assignment of $R^{b°}/R^{b°}$. In contrast, the cells of both members of two sib pairs (Y.Y. and K.M., and A.M. and S.M. in Table 33-7) showed detectable but markedly reduced LDL receptor activity in all assays (5 to 15 percent of normal), suggesting that each member of a sib pair has inherited the same alleles.

Many of the "homozygotes" in the receptor-defective class are likely to represent genetic compounds (also known as "mixed heterozygotes," "compound heterozygotes," or "allozygotes"). They are likely to possess two different mutant alleles at the LDL receptor locus in a manner analogous to other genetic compounds, such as SC hemoglobinopathy [129]. One mutant allele may be the same as the functionless allele that is present in receptor-negative individuals ($R^{b°}$) and the other allele may be one of those that specifies a receptor with a low level of activty (R^{b-}). In this case the genotype would be $R^{b-}/R^{b°}$ [3, 68, 119]. As more sensitive assays become available, it is likely that the R^{b-} allele will turn out to be a series of alleles, each of which produces a different type of defective LDL receptor. Thus, many of the subjects with the receptor-defective phenotype may have two different R^{b-} alleles (genotype, R^{b-}/R^{b-}). Analysis of this situation is not now possible because heterozygotes for the receptor-negative allele (genotype, $+/R^{b°}$) cannot be distinguished from heterozygotes for any of the receptor-defective alleles (genotype, $+/R^{b-}$). In both types of heterozygotes, the cells have approximately 50 percent of the normal receptor activity. Further genetic dissection of the R^{b-} class will require the ability to detect qualitative alterations in the receptor (e.g., altered electrophoretic mobility), in addition to the quantitative deficiency in the number of binding sites.

$R^{b+, i°}$ ALLELE   A third type of mutation has been identified in fibroblasts from two patients with the typical clinical and pedigree features of homozygous familial hypercholesterolemia [3, 68, 120, 121]. The LDL receptors in these unique cell strains, designated J.D. and B.H., show a normal ability to bind LDL (Fig. 33-17C). However, once bound to the receptor the LDL is not taken up into the cell. As a result, cells from these patients are unable to degrade LDL or utilize its cholesterol, and hence they display secondary abnormalities in the regulation of cholesterol metabolism that are the same as those in cells from receptor-negative homozygotes (compare Fig. 33-17A with Fig. 33-17C). Ultrastructural studies using ferritin-labeled LDL [130] and ^{125}I-labeled LDL autoradiography [113] indicate that the failure of these cells to internalize receptor-bound LDL results from an abnormality in the location of the LDL receptor on the cell membrane. Whereas in normal cells the receptor is concentrated in coated pits, in the internalization-defective cells the receptors are located at random along the membrane. Thus, even though a normal number of coated pits is present, these cells fail to internalize LDL because they are unable to cluster their receptors in the coated pits [130].

The defect in the internalization of LDL in the cells of patients J.D. and B.H. is highly specific. Their fibroblasts show normal endocytosis of inert molecules such as [^{14}C]sucrose, [^{14}C]inulin, and ^{125}I-labeled gamma globulin [3, 121]. They also show a normal ability to take up and degrade ^{125}I-labeled epidermal growth factor [3, 131] and ^{125}I-labeled α-2-macroglobulin [132], two molecules that are bound to surface receptors, internalized, and degraded in a manner similar to LDL [133].

A model to explain the genetic defect in the internalization-defective cells has been advanced on the basis of studies of fibroblasts from the parents of J.D. [3, 120]. The two parents exhibit hypercholesterolemia and other clinical features typical of heterozygous familial hypercholesterolemia. However, the

Table 33-7 LDL receptor activity in five pairs of sibs with the clinical phenotype of homozygous familial hypercholesterolemia

			LDL receptor activity (percentage of normal value)		
Sib pair	Age (sex)	Ethnic origin	Receptor-bound ^{125}I-labeled LDL	Degraded ^{125}I-labeled LDL	LDL-mediated stimulation of cholesteryl ester formation
N.D.*	4 (F)	French	0.0	1.1	0.4
W.D.*	7 (M)		0.0	1.0	0.0
M.S.	4 (F)	Japanese	0.0	0.0	ND
J.S.	5 (M)		0.0	1.6	ND
A.M.	9 (M)	Arab	2.0	2.5	0.1
R.M.	12 (F)		1.1	3.5	0.1
Y.Y.	25 (M)	Japanese	11	7.2	ND
K.M.	39 (F)		6.8	2.5	ND
A.M.†	11 (F)	Italian	21	12	7.9
S.M.†	11 (M)		18	13	13.3

*First-cousin parental consanguinity
†Nonidentical twins
NOTE: ND = not determined
SOURCE: Data obtained from Goldstein and Brown [68] and Haba et al. [36].

fibroblast studies revealed that the two parents exhibited different mutations at the receptor locus. When the fibroblasts from J.D.'s mother were incubated with ^{125}I-labeled LDL, they bound half the normal amount of lipoprotein [120]. Studies with LDL-ferritin showed that a normal proportion of her receptors were in coated pits [130]. When her cells were warmed to 37°C, all of the receptor-bound ^{125}I-labeled LDL entered the cell within 10 min [120]. Thus, the mother's cells were biochemically identical to those of the usual heterozygote for the receptor-negative allele (genotype, $+/R^{b°}$). Since the product of the $R^{b°}$ allele does not bind LDL, this allele is silent. All of the functional receptors expressed in the mother's cells were the product of the normal allele, and thus they functioned normally. However, since she had only one functional allele, the mother made only one-half the normal number of receptors.

The situation was strikingly different in the father of J.D. [120]. Although the father had the clinical phenotype of heterozygous familial hypercholesterolemia, his cells bound about 1.5-fold more ^{125}I-labeled LDL than normal cells [120]. Studies with LDL-ferritin demonstrated that his cells had two populations of LDL receptors. One of these populations was located in coated pits, and the other population was located along noncoated segments of membrane [130]. Both populations of receptors bound LDL-ferritin, but when the cells were warmed, only the LDL-ferritin that was bound to receptors in the coated pits entered the cell. The LDL-ferritin bound to receptors in the noncoated portions of membrane remained on the cell surface. Quantitative studies with ^{125}I-labeled LDL showed that half of the receptor-bound ^{125}I-labeled LDL in the father's cells was internalized within 10 min and the other half remained on the surface for more than 30 min [120].

Finding two populations of receptors in the father's cells suggested that he also had one normal allele and one mutant allele at the receptor locus. The receptors produced by the normal allele were located in coated pits and carried their bound LDL into the cell. The receptors specified by the mutant allele were able to bind LDL but were unable to become incorporated into coated pits. As a result, the LDL bound to these receptors was not internalized by the cells. This allele was designated $R^{b+,i°}$ (binding, positive; internalization, negative), and the genotype of the father was designated $+/R^{b+,i°}$ [120].

The pedigree of the J.D. family is shown in Fig. 33-18. Study of the offspring of this marriage supported the notion that the $R^{b°}$ mutation in the mother and the $R^{b+,i°}$ mutation in the father are allelic [3, 120]. Their marriage produced three offspring. The proband, who had severe hypercholesterolemia and the homozygous phenotype, is designated by his initials, J.D. The sister of J.D. was clinically normal (Fig. 33-18). Her fibroblasts had a normal number of LDL receptors and internalized the bound LDL normally. Presumably she inherited the normal allele from both parents. The brother of J.D. had a moderately elevated plasma cholesterol level and clinically appeared to be a heterozygote. His fibroblasts behaved identically to the father's. They bound a somewhat higher than normal amount of LDL, but only half the bound lipoprotein was internalized. Moreover, by electron microscopy, his cells, like the father's, had only half the normal number of receptors in coated pits. Thus, the brother of J.D. appeared to have inherited the normal allele from the mother and the $R^{b+,i°}$ allele from the father (Fig. 33-18).

As described above, J.D.'s cells bound slightly less LDL than

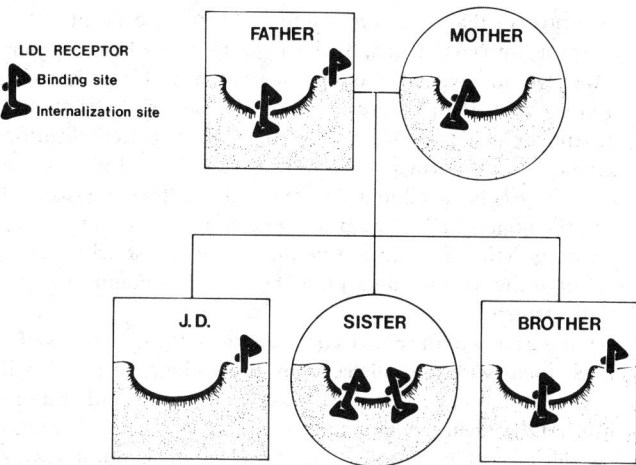

Figure 33-18 Family pedigree of an individual with the internalization-defective form of homozygous familial hypercholesterolemia. The proband is designated by his initials J.D. The diagram illustrates the genetic basis of the internalization defect in this family. A normal cell (genotype, $+/+$) is exemplified by the sister of J.D. and is shown as having two functional LDL receptors. The proposed genotypes of the other family members are as follows: father, $+/R^{b+,i°}$; mother, $+/R^{b°}$; J.D., $R^{b°}/R^{b+,i°}$; and brother, $+/R^{b+,i°}$. (From Brown and Goldstein [260].)

normal. None of the receptors were located in coated pits and none of the bound LDL was internalized. This pattern would be explained if this subject were a genetic compound. From his mother, he inherited the silent allele, $R^{b°}$. From his father, he inherited the internalization-defective allele, $R^{b+,i°}$. All of the receptors that can bind LDL are of the $R^{b+,i°}$ type, and hence none of the bound LDL is internalized (Fig. 33-18).

Virtually identical biochemical and genetic results have been obtained recently from the study of the family of B.H., the other individual with the internalization-defective form of homozygous familial hypercholesterolemia. In this case, B.H. inherited the $R^{b°}$ allele from his father and the $R^{b+,i°}$ allele from his mother [134].

The mechanism stated above implies that the binding mutation and the internalization mutation are alternate alleles at a single locus specifying the LDL receptor. Other more complex mechanisms might be invoked to account for the findings in the J.D. pedigree. For example, the LDL receptor might have multiple subunits encoded by independent genes. The mother might be heterozygous for a mutation in the gene for the binding subunit, and the father might be heterozygous for a mutation in another gene specifying the internalization subunit. In this case the severely affected offspring would be a double heterozygote; that is, he would carry single mutant alleles at two genetic loci. If each receptor is composed of a single binding subunit and a single internalization subunit, the double heterozygote should have a half-normal number of binding sites, but half of these should be associated with normal internalization subunits. As a result, half of the bound LDL in J.D. should be internalized normally. Moreover, the absolute rate of internalization of ^{125}I-labeled LDL in the J.D. cells should be one-fourth that of normal (half-normal binding × half-normal internalization). However, direct measurements show that ^{125}I-labeled LDL internalization in these cells is less than 2 percent of the normal rate [3, 120, 121, 135]. This finding tends to exclude the possibility that the two mutations involve genes for different subunits.

A second alternative hypothesis is that the internalization defect is due not to a defect in the receptor itself, but to a defect in a protein that functions catalytically to incorporate LDL receptors into coated pits. By this hypothesis, the heterozygous father would have half the normal amount of this internalization enzyme. If this were the case, the father's cells should internalize all of the bound LDL, but the rate of internalization should be half-normal. However, as summarized above, the father's cells behaved in a different fashion; they internalized half the bound LDL at a normal rate and failed to internalize the other half [120]. Such a finding suggests a stoichiometric defect in the receptor and not a half-normal amount of a catalytic protein.

On the basis of the above considerations, the hypothesis of a single locus with two alleles seems most likely. Its proof will require isolation of the allelic receptor proteins and demonstration that their primary amino acid sequences are altered as a result of both mutations. The above genetic hypothesis was strongly supported recently when Miyake et al. described a homozygote for the internalization defect (genotype $R^{b+,i^\circ}/R^{b+,i^\circ}$) [134a]. This patient was the product of a consanguine mating. Fibroblasts from both parents appeared to be of genotype $+/R^{b+,i^\circ}$.

Table 33-8 shows the ethnic origin of 64 familial hypercholesterolemia homozygotes whose fibroblasts have been studied in one laboratory. Among the 19 Americans, the receptor-negative and receptor-defective cellular phenotypes are equally frequent. A similar equal distribution was found among the 11 Italians who have been studied. On the other hand, 11 of 14 French homozygotes showed the receptor-negative phenotype, whereas all 5 English homozygotes were receptor-defective. Whether these differences prove to be statistically significant and whether they represent different relative gene frequencies for the $R^{b\circ}$ and R^{b-} alleles in these various ethnic groups is not yet known.

The R^{b+,i° allele, which is responsible for the internalization defect, has so far been observed in only three families. The heterozygous father $(+/R^{b+,i^\circ})$ in the J.D. family was born in southern Italy near Naples, and the heterozygous mother $(+/R^{b+,i^\circ})$ in the B.H. family was born in the United States in Minnesota. Analysis of the fibroblasts from four nonrelated individuals from the Naples area who have the clinical features of homozygous familial hypercholesterolemia failed to turn up any evidence for an internalization defect. One of these homozygotes was receptor-negative and three were receptor-defective [68]. These findings suggest that this allele is extremely rare and is considerably less frequent than the $R^{b\circ}$ and R^{b-} alleles.

Use of the R^{b+,i° Allele to Formulate a Model for the Assembly of LDL Receptors   The mechanistic explanation for the internalization mutation has suggested a working model for the assembly of LDL receptors in coated pits [3, 130, 133] (Fig. 33-19). This model is based on analogies between the genetic studies of the LDL receptor and studies of the assembly of lipid envelope viruses in mammalian cells [136, 137]. According to this formulation the LDL receptor is a transmembrane protein that is made on membrane-bound ribosomes. By analogy with viral transmembrane proteins, the LDL receptor is presumably glycosylated in the Golgi complex and then inserted into the plasma membrane at random. The genetic data on the internalization defect suggest that the receptor has two active sites. One of these, the binding site for LDL, must be on the external surface of the membrane. The second site is postulated to contain a specific amino acid sequence that allows the receptor to be recognized as a component of coated pits. It seems likely that this internalization site is on the cytoplasmic surface of the membrane. Receptors that contain a functional internalization site gather together by lateral movement in the plane of the membrane and are incorporated in coated pits. This clustering of receptors in coated pits is postulated to occur as a result of an interaction of the internalization site of the receptor with the coat protein clathrin or with some other protein that is itself bound to clathrin. The clustering of receptors does not appear to be induced by the binding of LDL. Available data indicate that the sequence of receptor insertion into the plasma membrane, clustering into coated pits, and internalization proceeds continuously, whether or not LDL is present [130].

Once clustered into coated pits, the LDL receptors are quickly internalized when the coated pits pinch off to form coated vesicles. Kinetic evidence indicates that the receptors are recycled; that is, after they deposit their LDL in lysosomes, the receptors return to the cell surface where they again cluster together in coated pits [97]. When the LDL receptor carries a mutation in the internalization site, as in the patient with the internalization defect, the receptor is inserted into the membrane, but it is unable to become incorporated into the coated pits. As a result, the receptor remains randomly distributed in noncoated segments of the plasma membrane.

Regulation of the LDL Receptor Locus in Heterozygotes   In normal fibroblasts, the synthesis of the LDL receptor is regulated by a sensitive system of feedback suppression. As discussed above, the number of functional receptors declines by about tenfold when cellular cholesterol stores are increased by prolonged incubation of cells with a usable exogenous source of cholesterol, such as LDL or cholesterol dissolved in ethanol [98]. The number of receptors increases again

Table 33-8 Relation of cellular phenotype to ethnic origin in 64 individuals with the clinical phenotype of homozygous familial hypercholesterolemia

Ethnic origin	Total number of individuals	Cellular phenotype		
		Receptor-negative	Receptor-defective	Internalization-defective
American	19	9*	9†	1
French	14	11§	3	0
Italian	11	4	6‡	1
English	5	0	5	0
Arab	3	2	1	0
Belgian	2	2	0	0
Greek Cypriot	1	1	0	0
Lebanese	1	1	0	0
Norwegian	1	1	0	0
Colombian	1	1	0	0
Mexican	1	1	0	0
Japanese	1 (6)	1 (3)	0 (3)	0
Hawaiian	1	0	1	0
Algerian	1	0	1	0
American Indian	1	0	1	0
Guyanan	1	0	1	0

*Seven white individuals and two black individuals
†Nine white individuals
‡Includes two Sicilians
§Includes three French Canadians
NOTE: Numbers in parentheses represent homozygotes who were studied by Haba et al. [36].
SOURCE: Modified from Goldstein and Brown [68].

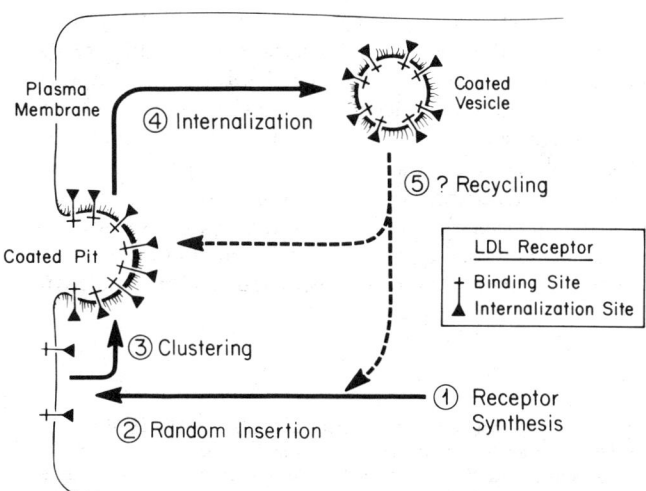

Figure 33-19 Diagram illustrating the proposed mechanism by which LDL receptors become localized in coated pits on the plasma membrane of human fibroblasts. The sequential steps are as follows: (1) synthesis of LDL receptors on polyribosomes; (2) insertion of LDL receptors at random sites along noncoated segments of plasma membrane; (3) clustering together of LDL receptors in coated pits; (4) internalization of LDL receptors as coated pits invaginate to form coated endocytic vesicles; and (5) recycling of internalized LDL receptors to the plasma membrane. (*From Anderson et al.* [130]. *Used by permission.*)

when the exogenous cholesterol is removed and cellular cholesterol levels fall. In the steady state, the number of receptors is adjusted to allow just enough LDL uptake to provide sufficient cholesterol for cell growth and to balance cholesterol losses [25, 92].

The existence of this regulatory mechanism raised the question as to whether the single functional allele at the LDL receptor locus in familial hypercholesterolemia heterozygotes could be stimulated to produce twice its normal number of LDL receptors and thus compensate for the nonfunctional partner allele. Subsequent studies showed that under growth conditions that induced a maximal rate of receptor synthesis (i.e., growth in the absence of an exogenous source of cholesterol), the heterozygote cells produced about one-half as many functional receptors as did normal cells [138]. More important, when grown in the presence of increasing amounts of exogenous cholesterol, the heterozygote and normal cells suppressed their LDL receptor activities in parallel. Over a ten- to twentyfold range of LDL receptor activities, at any given level of cellular cholesterol stores the heterozygote cells expressed about one-half as many receptors as did normal cells [138]. This relationship was evident even in the range of LDL receptor levels in which the heterozygote cells clearly had the capacity to produce as many active LDL receptors as did the normal cells, i.e., when the appropriate number of receptors was less than half the maximal number [138]. These findings indicate that in the heterozygote cells the regulatory mechanism dictates that the normal allele produce only the amount of gene product that it would normally produce at a given level of cellular cholesterol.

The failure of the regulatory mechanism to stimulate the normal allele at the LDL receptor locus to produce twice its normal amount of gene product leaves the heterozygote cells with a persistent 50 percent deficiency in LDL receptors under all conditions of cell growth. The most likely explanation for this finding is that the $R^{b°}$ allele actually produces a gene product, but the product is inactive. The cellular machinery somehow senses that this product is being made, and so the system adjusts to synthesize the normal number of receptors on each chromosome, even though only one set of the receptors is active.

PATHOGENESIS AT THE WHOLE BODY LEVEL

The demonstration of the LDL receptor pathway in cultured human fibroblasts was followed by its demonstration in virtually all animal cells that grow in culture [93]. These cells have been obtained from humans [smooth-muscle cells, endothelial cells, lymphoblasts, Burkitt lymphoma (Raji) cells, acute myelogenous leukemia cells, HeLa cells, SV40 transformed fibroblasts]; mice (teratocarcinoma cells, adrenal Y-1 cells, L cells, L 1210 leukemia cells); hamsters (Chinese hamster ovary cells, fibroblasts); cows (adult adrenocortical cells, endothelial cells); dogs (fibroblasts, smooth-muscle cells); rabbits (fibroblasts); and swine (fibroblasts, smooth-muscle cells). In each of these cell types, LDL cholesterol is used for membrane synthesis and for the regulation of cholesterol homeostasis. In cultured mouse and bovine adrenal cells, the LDL serves an additional function—its cholesterol is a precursor for steroid hormone formation [139–141].

Normal Expression of the LDL Receptor Pathway in Vivo

LDL Metabolism in Freshly Isolated Human Blood Cells   The ubiquitous occurrence of the LDL receptor in cultured cells and the demonstration that its absence causes the syndrome of familial hypercholesterolemia provided the initial evidence that the LDL receptor was expressed on cells in the body. Recently, this hypothesis has been confirmed [142]. When circulating mononuclear cells from normal individuals were isolated and incubated immediately thereafter with ^{125}I-labeled LDL, they degraded the lipoprotein by a process that was competitively inhibited by an excess of unlabeled LDL, indicating that a specific surface receptor was involved [143, 144]. When this degradation assay was used to measure the number of receptors on freshly isolated cells, normal subjects had detectable LDL receptor activity, cells from heterozygotes had a half-normal number of receptors, and cells from homozygotes had no detectable LDL receptor activity [144].

Blood lymphocytes are nondividing cells that are exposed chronically to high levels of plasma LDL. The studies with fibroblasts predicted that if lymphocytes were deprived of lipoproteins, they should develop a cholesterol deficit and an enhanced LDL receptor activity. This prediction was verified experimentally, as shown in Fig. 33-20. When freshly isolated blood lymphocytes from normal subjects were incubated in the absence of LDL, the number of lipoprotein receptors increased markedly. Under the same conditions of receptor induction, the receptors remained undetectable in homozygotes, and the lymphocytes from heterozygotes expressed half the normal number of LDL receptors [144].

The LDL receptor defect in lymphocytes from homozygotes has also been demonstrated by a novel visual approach. Krieger et al. devised a method to remove the cholesteryl esters

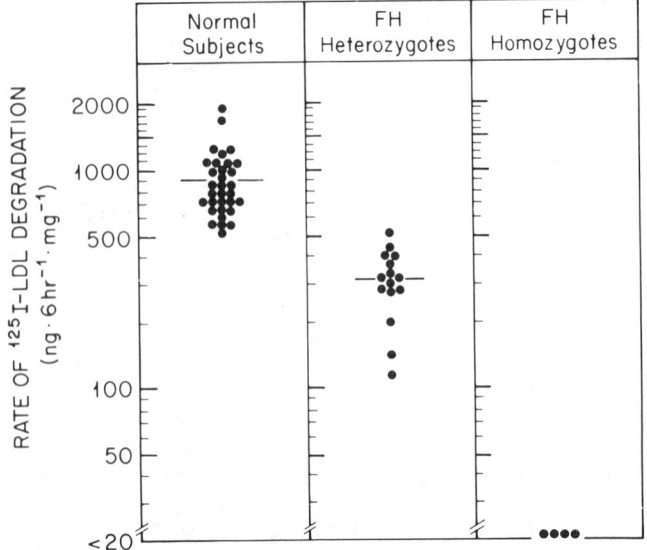

Figure 33-20 LDL receptor activity in normal, heterozygote, and homozygote lymphocytes that were subjected to prior incubation in the absence of lipoproteins. Lymphocytes were isolated from venous blood and the cells were incubated for 67 h at 37°C in a medium containing 10% human lipoprotein-deficient serum, after which LDL receptor activity was assessed by measurement of the high affinity degradation of ^{125}I-labeled LDL at 37°C, as described by Bilheimer et al. [144].

patients with chronic myelogenous leukemia or acute lymphocytic leukemia did not show a marked elevation in LDL receptor number. In addition to their high levels of LDL receptors, the acute myelogenous leukemia cells also showed a high rate of cholesterol synthesis from [^{14}C]acetate and a low content of cholesterol when compared to normal lymphocytes [149]. These data suggest that the acute myelogenous leukemia cells have an enhanced turnover of cholesterol, perhaps associated with some abnormality of the plasma membrane, or perhaps owing to a more rapid rate of growth and new membrane synthesis.

Figure 33-21 Receptor-mediated uptake of fluorescent LDL by freshly isolated lymphocytes from a normal subject (A and B) and from a subject with homozygous familial hypercholesterolemia (C and D). Nonadherent lymphocytes were prepared from blood mononuclear cells as described [144]. The cells were incubated for 93 h at 37°C in a 5% CO_2 incubator in RPMI 1640 medium containing 10% human lipoprotein-deficient serum and 20 μg protein per milliliter of LDL reconstituted with the fluorescent cholesteryl ester probe, 3-pyrenemethyl-23,24-*dinor*-5-cholen-22-oate-β-yl oleate (PMCA oleate) [146]. After incubation, the cells were washed, mounted on glass coverslips, and photographed. Panels A and C were visualized by phase contrast microscopy and panels B and D were visualized by fluorescence microscopy. ×500 (reproduced at 133 percent original size). (*From Goldstein and Brown* [90].)

from the core of LDL and to replace them with fluorescent cholesteryl esters [145]. With this method about 1000 fluorescent molecules can be incorporated into each LDL particle. Cells that take up this reconstituted LDL become intensely fluorescent, whereas cells that lack LDL receptors fail to become fluorescent [146]. The upper left panel of Fig. 33-21 shows a phase contrast view of normal human lymphocytes that were isolated from the bloodstream and then incubated with fluorescent LDL. The upper right panel shows the same field under the fluorescence microscope. More than 90 percent of the normal lymphocytes have taken up fluorescent LDL. The bottom two panels show lymphocytes from a homozygote studied in the same experiment. There is no fluorescence in these mutant cells.

The LDL receptors on incubated lymphocytes are functional in a physiologic sense, i.e., they deliver cholesterol to the cells and allow suppression of cholesterol synthesis [147]. Thus, when fresh lymphocytes were incubated for 72 h in the absence of LDL, they developed a maximal number of LDL receptors and a high rate of cholesterol synthesis. When increasing amounts of LDL were added back to the cells, the lipoprotein completely suppressed cholesterol synthesis in cells from normal subjects. On the other hand, in cells from homozygotes, the lack of LDL receptors prevented LDL from suppressing cholesterol synthesis [147]. In cells from heterozygotes, a 2.5-times higher concentration of LDL was required to produce the same degree of suppression as in normal cells [148]. This pattern of response in freshly isolated lymphocytes is the same as in cultured fibroblasts.

Studies in tissue culture have demonstrated that rapidly dividing cells express more LDL receptors than nondividing cells [110, 121]. This phenomenon may also occur in vivo. Circulating malignant mononuclear cells from patients with acute myelogenous leukemia were reported to express three- to a hundredfold more LDL receptors than did normal blood mononuclear cells [149]. On the other hand, cells from

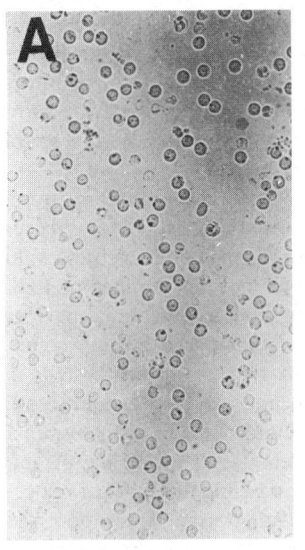
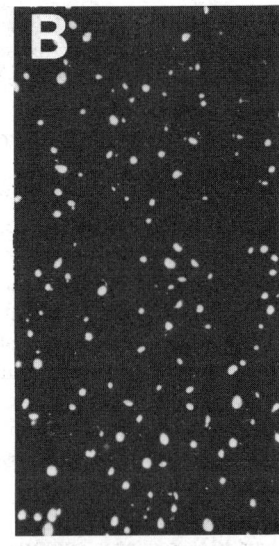
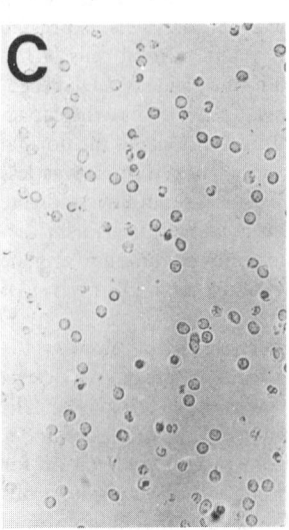

LDL Binding to Membranes from Tissues A second approach to the demonstration of LDL receptors in vivo involves the use of membrane binding assays. For this purpose, human or animal organs are homogenized, the membranes are isolated, and their ability to bind ^{125}I-labeled LDL with high affinity is assayed. When this assay was applied to cultured fibroblasts, it could be shown that the receptor that binds ^{125}I-labeled LDL in isolated membranes is the same as the one that functions physiologically to carry LDL into cells [150]. This assay has recently been used to survey LDL receptor activity in membranes prepared from homogenates of 16 tissues of the cow [151]. The results of this survey are shown in Fig. 33-22. Membranes from nearly all of these fresh tissues showed high affinity LDL binding activity. The number of ^{125}I-labeled LDL binding sites was highest in the membranes of the adrenal cortex and the ovarian corpus luteum, the two tissues that secrete steroids and thus have the highest requirements for cholesterol. In contrast, the adrenal medulla and the ovarian interstitium, which do not produce large amounts of steroid, showed much lower ^{125}I-labeled LDL binding activity. High affinity binding was also detected in many other tissues, including adipose tissue, myocardium, and skeletal muscle. No high affinity binding of ^{125}I-labeled LDL was detected in mature red cells. A similar tissue distribution of LDL receptors has also been found in a study of ^{125}I-labeled LDL binding to membranes from different organs of a human fetus [141].

The finding that the number of LDL receptors in the cow and human fetus in vivo is highest in tissues that actively secrete steroids correlates with the earlier demonstration that cultured mouse and bovine adrenal cells have large numbers of LDL receptors and use these receptors as one source of cholesterol for steroid hormone synthesis [139, 140].

Uptake of LDL by Organs of Lipoprotein-deficient Animals Studies in rats and mice have supported the notion that one function of lipoprotein receptors is to supply cholesterol to extrahepatic tissues. Quantitative studies have shown that the liver and intestine together account for about 75 percent of the cholesterol synthesized in the body of a rat on a low cholesterol diet and that the remaining 25 percent is synthesized in a variety of other tissues, each of which synthesizes cholesterol at a rate that is less than one-tenth of the rate in intestine and liver [117, 152]. When cholesterol is fed to the animal, the rate of cholesterol synthesis in liver is markedly reduced, owing to a reduction in HMG-CoA reductase activity. Rates of sterol synthesis in other tissues remain low [117, 152].

The low rates of sterol synthesis in extrahepatic tissues of the rat appear to be mediated by lipoprotein delivery systems analogous to the LDL receptor system of lymphocytes and cultured cells. This conclusion was first suggested on the basis of studies performed with the drug 4-aminopyrazolopyrimidine (4-APP) [153–156]. This drug blocks the secretion of lipoproteins from the liver of rats, which, in turn, leads to a profound drop in the plasma cholesterol level [157]. This drop in plasma cholesterol is accompanied by a marked increase in the activity of HMG-CoA reductase in the kidney and the lung [153]. The increase in the activity of this rate-limiting enzyme is accompanied by the expected increase in cholesterol biosynthesis in tissue slices as measured from [14C]acetate and [14C]octonoate. Increases of cholesterol synthesis are also observed in most other extrahepatic tissues [154, 156].

In rats and mice the tissue that shows the most dramatic

changes in cholesterol metabolism when the plasma cholesterol level is lowered by 4-APP is the adrenal gland [141, 155, 156]. The drop in plasma cholesterol level is accompanied by a drastic fall in the content of stored cholesteryl esters within the adrenal gland. At the same time, there is a two-hundredfold rise in adrenal HMG-CoA reductase activity. When human LDL is infused intravenously into the 4-APP-treated rat or mouse, all of the above changes are reversed. The plasma cholesterol level rises, the level of adrenal cholesteryl esters is restored, and adrenal HMG-CoA reductase becomes suppressed [155]. Similar changes are produced by the infusion of HDL. The most recent studies indicate that the adrenal gland of the mouse and rat possess two different lipoprotein receptor systems [158, 159]. One is specific for LDL and is indistinguishable from the fibroblast LDL receptor. The other is a receptor that recognizes human HDL and rat HDL particles that are devoid of apoprotein E. How this latter receptor delivers cholesterol to the adrenal gland is not known.

The testis and ovary of the rat also appear to have receptor-mediated uptake mechanisms for both HDL and LDL [141, 151, 156]. On the other hand, in other tissues, such as the intestine and the kidney, cholesterol synthesis in the 4-APP-treated rat is suppressed by infusion of LDL, but not HDL [153, 156]. Thus, these tissues, like lymphocytes and cultured cells, may express only one type of lipoprotein receptor—the LDL receptor. On the other hand, steroid-secreting tissues may exhibit two types of receptors—one for LDL and one for HDL.

Considered together, the data from tissue cultures, blood mononuclear cells, tissue homogenates, and intact animals all point to a role for the LDL receptor in delivering cholesterol to extrahepatic cells and thereby keeping extrahepatic cholesterol synthesis suppressed. At the same time, the LDL receptor–mediated uptake process accounts for the degradation of a portion of LDL in extrahepatic tissues.

Role of the Liver in LDL Metabolism Recent studies have begun to resolve a series of crucial questions regarding the role of the liver in LDL metabolism—namely, does the liver produce LDL receptors under normal circumstances, and if so, what functions do these receptors perform and how are they regulated? These questions have been impossible to answer directly in human beings. Although some answers have begun to emerge from animal studies, the quantitative aspects of lipoprotein metabolism in other animal species are so different from those in human beings that observations made in lower animals, especially rodents, can be related to humans only with reservation.

The one undisputed role of the liver in lipoprotein clearance is its role in removing chylomicron remnants from plasma [118]. Studies performed on dogs and rats indicate that the liver takes up native chylomicrons only at a slow rate. However, after the chylomicrons have been perfused through peripheral tissues and have been acted upon by lipoprotein lipase, the chylomicron remnants are cleared by the liver at a rapid rate [118]. Direct hepatic perfusion studies in the rat show that the initial step in this uptake process is saturable [160], suggesting binding to specific receptors. Lipoproteins containing apoproteins E and B are cleared by the same mechanism, but the apoprotein E–containing lipoproteins are cleared at a much higher efficiency than the B–containing lipoproteins [161]. As discussed above, the LDL receptor of fibroblasts, adrenal cells, and other extrahepatic tissues also recog-

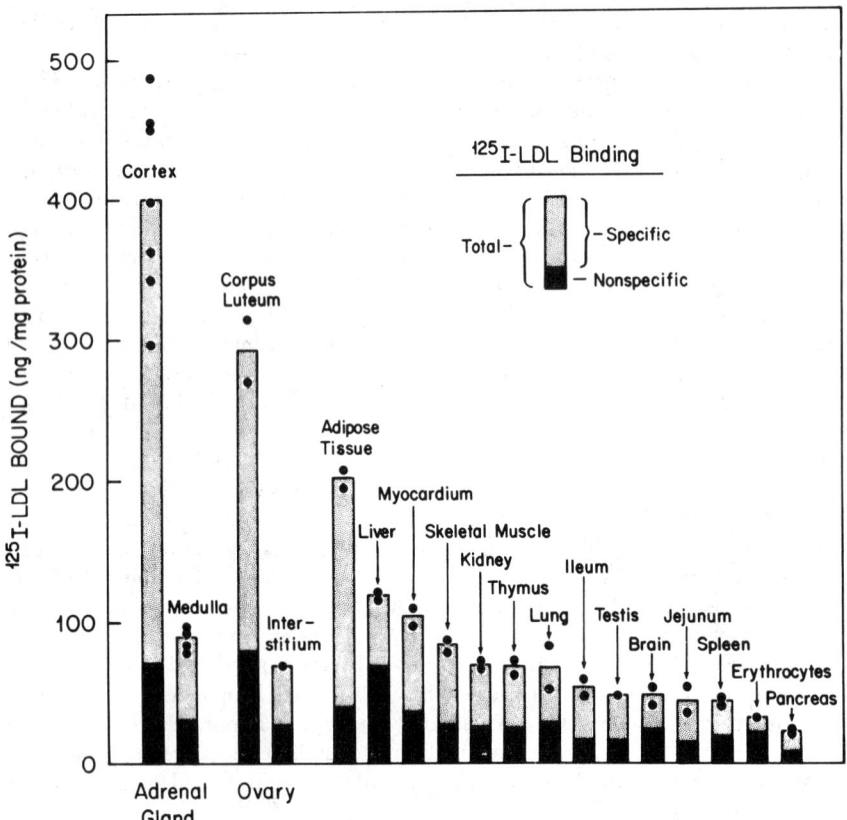

Figure 33-22 Measurement of ^{125}I-labeled LDL binding to membranes prepared from 18 bovine tissues. Fresh tissues were homogenized, the 8000- to 100,000-g membrane pellets were isolated, and ^{125}I-labeled LDL binding assays were performed at 4°C as described [151]. Total binding represents the amount of ^{125}I-labeled LDL bound to the membranes in the absence of excess unlabeled LDL. Specific (high affinity) binding and nonspecific binding are those components of the total binding that were, respectively, inhibited and not inhibited competitively by the presence of the excess unlabeled LDL. Each point represents the average of duplicate assays performed on the membranes contained from one animal. (*Data redrawn from Kovanen et al.* [151].)

nizes apoprotein E—containing lipoproteins with higher affinity than those that contain apoprotein B. Thus, the findings in the perfused liver raise the possibility that the liver does, in fact, use a receptor whose properties are similar to those of the classic LDL receptor of extrahepatic tissues.

The most direct evidence demonstrating the existence of a hepatic lipoprotein receptor has come from a series of in vitro and in vivo studies conducted in rats treated with pharmacologic doses of 17α-ethinylestradiol [162–164]. In these animals the rate of removal of LDL from plasma is enhanced dramatically, owing to a marked increase in the number of lipoprotein binding sites on liver cell membranes. In vitro studies of ^{125}I-labeled LDL binding to membranes of liver homogenates from estradiol-treated rats show that these binding sites bear a remarkable resemblance to the LDL receptor [162, 164]. Thus, they bind apoprotein E—containing lipoproteins with higher affinity than those containing apoprotein B; binding is prevented by lysine- and arginine-modifying agents; binding requires calcium; and the binding sites are exquisitely sensitive to protease digestion. Electron-microscopic autoradiography studies of estradiol-treated rat livers perfused with ^{125}I-labeled LDL show that the receptors are clustered on the plasma membrane of hepatocytes [165]. The bound ligand is internalized rapidly in endocytic vesicles, a sequence that is similar to that of the LDL receptors of extrahepatic tissues.

A binding site with properties identical to those of the estradiol-treated rat liver has also been identified in liver membranes from untreated rats [164], and in liver membranes from normal rabbits [166], dogs [167], and human fetuses [141].

Considered together, the available data suggest that the liver may well synthesize an LDL receptor, at least in the rat, dog, and rabbit, and possibly in humans. It is likely that this receptor contributes to the clearance of LDL from plasma. Support

for this hypothesis has come from studies of the metabolism of LDL labeled with [14C]sucrose in pigs [168] and rats [169]. When LDL is taken up by a tissue and delivered to lysosomes, the [14C]sucrose is liberated but remains trapped within the lysosome. Thus, the amount of [14C]sucrose in a tissue provides an indication of the total amount of LDL that has been degraded in that tissue [168]. With the use of this technique, Steinberg and coworkers concluded that about 40 percent of LDL degradation occurred in the liver in the pig and rat. The LDL receptor in liver appears to play a role in the normal clearance of apo E—containing particles such as chylomicron and VLDL remnants, as well as LDL [164–167].

From the standpoint of familial hypercholesterolemia, the important question to resolve is whether this hepatic lipoprotein receptor is the product of the same gene as is the LDL receptor of extrahepatic tissues. In homozygotes who lack the genetic capacity to produce LDL receptors, there is no clinical evidence of delayed clearance of chylomicron or VLDL remnants from the plasma. The simplest explanation is that these remnants are taken up by a hepatic receptor that is genetically different from the LDL receptor of extrahepatic tissues, although it may share many of its properties. Alternatively, remnant particles might be normally cleared through an LDL receptor in liver that is the product of the same gene as the LDL receptor in extrahepatic tissues. If this is the case, it would be necessary to postulate that when this receptor is genetically absent, alternate pathways for converting the VLDL and chylomicron remnants into LDL are so active that the end result is an increase in the synthetic rate for LDL, with no accumulation of VLDL or chylomicron remnants in the circulation. Whether either of these two mechanisms applies to human beings is not known at present.

Three other lipoprotein binding sites that differ from the

LDL receptor have been found in the liver of animals. One, identified in rat liver, is a binding site that recognizes chylomicron remnants and HDL, but not native chylomicrons, VLDL, or LDL [170]. In addition to a different specificity, this binding site differs from the LDL receptor in that it is not inhibited by EDTA and the binding occurs at 37°C, but not at 4°C [170]. There is as yet no direct evidence that this binding site is involved in the hepatic clearance of chylomicron remnants or HDL. Another lipoprotein binding site has been identified in membrane homogenates from swine liver [171]. This binding site appears to bind all lipoproteins as well as phospholipid vesicles that are devoid of apoproteins [171]. A third high affinity binding site that has been identified in rat liver membranes recognizes HDL particles that are devoid of apoproteins B and E [162]. It does not recognize human or rat LDL. Whether either of these two latter binding sites functions as a receptor in vivo is also not known.

The role of the liver in LDL metabolism and the regulation of hepatic LDL receptors have recently been reviewed in Ref. 171a.

Mechanisms for the High Plasma LDL Level in Heterozygotes and Homozygotes

Turnover studies using ^{125}I-labeled lipoproteins have begun to shed some light on the mechanism by which the LDL receptor deficiency produces an increased plasma LDL level in heterozygotes and homozygotes with familial hypercholesterolemia. The earliest such study, conducted by Langer, Strober, and Levy [172], showed that heterozygotes exhibited a normal production rate and a diminished fractional catabolic rate for LDL. The fractional catabolic rate (FCR) is an expression of the fraction of the total pool of LDL that is degraded daily. More recent studies, carried out in several laboratories, have confirmed the low FCR for LDL in heterozygotes but have suggested a slight-to-moderate overproduction of LDL as well [173–175]. Both of these abnormalities are more pronounced in homozygotes than in heterozygotes; that is, there is a more marked reduction in the FCR for LDL as well as more greatly enhanced production of LDL [173,174, 176–179].

An extensive series of ^{125}I-labeled LDL turnover studies in familial hypercholesterolemia heterozygotes and homozygotes has been conducted by Bilheimer and associates [173, 174] and by Myant, Thompson, Soutar, and coworkers [176–179]. The correlation of these results with the results of LDL receptor assays in fibroblasts from the same subjects is shown in Fig. 33-23. Normal subjects, whose fibroblasts can produce about 10,000 receptors per cell, catabolize about 45 percent of their LDL pool per day under the conditions of these ^{125}I-labeled LDL turnover studies in vivo. Heterozygotes, whose cells produce on average 4500 receptors per cell, catabolize 25 to 30 percent of their LDL pool daily; and homozygotes, whose cells produce few to no detectable LDL receptors, degrade about 15 percent of their LDL pool daily.

The line relating the LDL fractional catabolic rate to the number of LDL receptors in Fig. 33-23 does not go through zero. Thus, homozygotes, whose cells produce little to no LDL receptors, can nevertheless degrade 15 percent of their plasma LDL daily. The percentage of LDL degraded daily in homozygotes does not change when the pool size of LDL is lowered by the creation of a portacaval shunt [173] or by the performance

of plasmaphoresis [178]. This indicates that the fixed FCR is due to the loss of LDL receptors and not to the saturation of some other LDL removal mechanism [178].

On the basis of these findings, Goldstein and Brown suggested several years ago that in normal humans there are at least two mechanisms for the removal of LDL from plasma, one mediated by the LDL receptor and the other mediated by a receptor-independent process [88]. The receptor-independent pathway was postulated to account for the removal of 15 percent of the LDL pool daily in all individuals, irrespective of the number of LDL receptors. If the total clearance of LDL in normal subjects is 45 percent per day and if 15 percent is removed by receptor-independent pathways, then the remaining 30 percent must be removed by the LDL receptor [88]. By this reasoning, in heterozygotes the total LDL clearance rate is 25 to 30 percent per day, 10 to 15 percent being receptor-mediated and 15 percent receptor-independent; and in homozygotes the total clearance is 15 percent per day, all receptor-independent (Fig. 33-23).

As a further working hypothesis, it was proposed that much of the receptor-independent clearance of LDL occurred in macrophages and histiocytes of the reticuloendothelial system, which were referred to collectively as "scavenger cells" [88, 89]. These cells were implicated in the receptor-independent LDL clearance for two reasons: (1) the generally accepted notion that these cells participate in the clearance of proteins from plasma; and (2) the observation that homozygotes, in whom the largest amounts of LDL are removed by receptor-independent pathways, accumulate considerable cholesterol in splenic macrophages, hepatic Kupffer cells, bone marrow histiocytes, and similar scavenger cells in many organs. Thus these cells appear to be taking up and degrading large amounts of LDL [70, 180–182].

In the discussion below, the terms *scavenger cell pathway* and *receptor-independent pathway* are used interchangeably. However, it should not be construed that scavenger cells are

Figure 33-23 Relation between the fractional catabolic rate (FCR) for plasma LDL and the number of LDL receptors on fibroblasts in patients with familial hypercholesterolemia (FH). The values for the fractional catabolic rate were derived from studies of the turnover of ^{125}I-labeled apo-LDL in the plasma of 6 normal subjects, 6 FH heterozygotes, and 11 FH homozygotes. These turnover studies were performed by Bilheimer et al. [173, 174] and by Myant, Thompson, and coworkers [176, 178]. The number of LDL receptors per cell was calculated from experiments in which maximal ^{125}I-labeled LDL binding was measured at 4°C in actively growing fibroblasts that were deprived of LDL for 48 h [93].

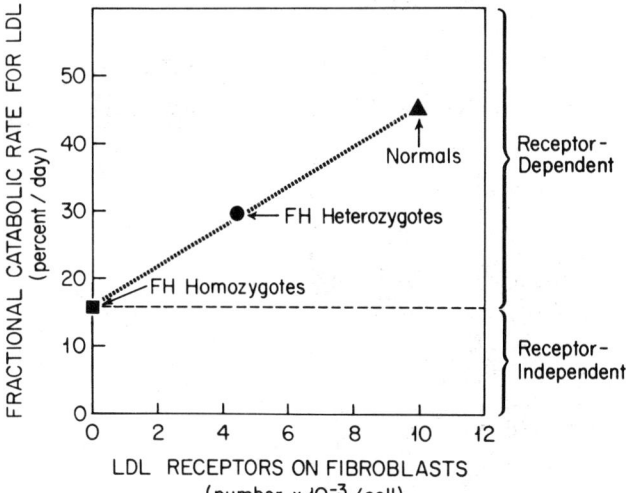

the only cells that degrade LDL by receptor-independent mechanisms. Rather, the above two terms should be thought of as representing the sum of all LDL that is degraded by routes that do not involve the LDL receptor.

By multiplying the measured FCR by the measured plasma pool size of LDL, it is possible to calculate the total amount of LDL degraded daily in homozygotes, heterozygotes, and normal individuals. Moreover, based on the theoretical reasoning outlined above, one can then assign an estimate of the absolute amount of LDL degraded daily in tissue parenchymal cells through the receptor pathway and in scavenger cells through the receptor-independent scavenger cell pathway [88, 89]. It should be emphasized that the calculations of absolute rates of receptor-dependent and receptor-independent LDL catabolism are indirect estimates that emerge from a working hypothesis and are not proven facts. The results of these calculations are shown schematically in Fig. 33-24. In normal individuals, who have a plasma LDL cholesterol level of 120 mg/dl, a total of 1500 mg of LDL cholesterol is removed from the plasma daily in association with the degradation of the protein. Two-thirds of this amount (1000 mg cholesterol per day) was postulated to be taken up by parenchymal cells through the physiologic LDL receptor, and one-third (500 mg cholesterol per day) was postulated to be removed in scavenger cells [88]. In heterozygotes, the plasma LDL cholesterol level on average is increased 2.5 times to about 300 mg/dl. Even though only 10 to 15 percent of the LDL pool is degraded through the receptor pathway daily in heterozygotes, as opposed to 30 percent in normal individuals, the expanded LDL pool size in the heterozygotes partially compensates for the decreased FCR so that a nearly normal absolute amount of LDL is degraded through the receptor pathway daily (800 mg/day in heterozygotes as compared with 1000 mg/day in normal individuals). However, since the amount of LDL degraded in scavenger cells is a linear 15 percent function of the LDL pool size, the expanded LDL pool size in heterozygotes dictates that the amount of LDL degraded in scavenger cells is 2.5 times above normal, or about 1200 mg/day [88]. In homozygotes this situation is carried to the extreme. The LDL cholesterol level rises to 700 mg/dl, and 15 percent of this expanded LDL pool is cleared by the scavenger cells daily, which means that the scavenger cells must remove 6 times more LDL-cholesterol from plasma than normal, or about 3000 mg/day (Fig. 33-24).

A corollary of the above model, and one that has been demonstrated directly by the ^{125}I-labeled LDL turnover studies, is the large degree of overproduction of LDL in homozygotes

(twofold above normal) and the lesser overproduction in heterozygotes (30 percent above normal) [173–179]. While the LDL receptor deficiency offers a direct explanation for the reduced FCR for LDL, it does not offer an obvious explanation for the LDL overproduction. One clue to the nature of this overproduction comes from the recent work of Soutar et al. [179, 183] and of Lewis and associates [184]. The original studies of Bilheimer, Eisenberg, and Levy had shown that in normal individuals, all of the apoprotein B in LDL can be accounted for by conversion from VLDL [184a]. Soutar et al. found that in homozygotes, this was not true [179, 183]. Simultaneous studies of the turnover of ^{125}I-labeled VLDL and ^{131}I-labeled LDL showed that in homozygotes, but not in normal subjects, up to 50 percent of the LDL entered plasma directly, presumably due to direct secretion from the liver. Based on these findings, Brown and Goldstein suggested that perhaps the liver normally synthesizes LDL receptors and that when normal amounts of LDL are binding to these receptors, this somehow serves as a signal to the liver that prevents it from secreting LDL directly into plasma [185]. By this hypothetical formulation, the lack of LDL receptors in the liver of homozygotes would disrupt this regulatory mechanism and cause the liver to secrete LDL directly into plasma. To date there is no direct evidence in support of this formulation, but the recent finding of LDL receptors in animal livers (discussed above) constitutes indirect support of at least one aspect of the model.

The suggestion of receptor-dependent and receptor-independent pathways for LDL catabolism, with a reduction in the former in familial hypercholesterolemia patients, has received strong support from the recent pioneering studies of Shepherd and coworkers in Glasgow [186, 187] and of Thompson et al. in London [188, 189]. These workers capitalized upon the observation that treatment of LDL with cyclohexanedione, which couples with arginine residues, blocks the ability of the lipoprotein to bind to the LDL receptor [96]. Shepherd et al. infused mixtures of ^{131}I-labeled cyclohexanedione-treated

Figure 33-24 Proposed model for the clearance of plasma LDL cholesterol. The quantitative estimates are based on studies of the turnover of ^{125}I-labeled apo LDL in the plasma of human subjects [88]. In general, these turnover studies show that in normal subjects a total of about 45 percent of the plasma LDL pool is removed from the plasma daily, whereas in familial hypercholesterolemia (FH) heterozygotes this value is 25 to 30 percent and in homozygotes it is about 15 percent. In using these data to develop the above model, two assumptions were made: (1) that the 15 percent clearance in the FH homozygote represents LDL cleared by LDL receptor-independent pathways (i.e., in "scavenger cells"); and (2) that this same 15 percent clearance through the scavenger cell pathway occurs in all subjects and is independent of the plasma level of LDL. The daily degradation of LDL cholesterol (i.e., the sum of the absolute values for the clearance through the LDL receptor and scavenger cell pathways) is highest in the FH homozygote (3000 mg cholesterol), intermediate in the FH heterozygote (2000 mg cholesterol), and lowest in the normal subjects (1500 mg cholesterol). These numbers are within the range of the respective synthetic rates for apo LDL as measured in steady state turnover studies. (*From Goldstein and Brown [88]. Used by permission.*)

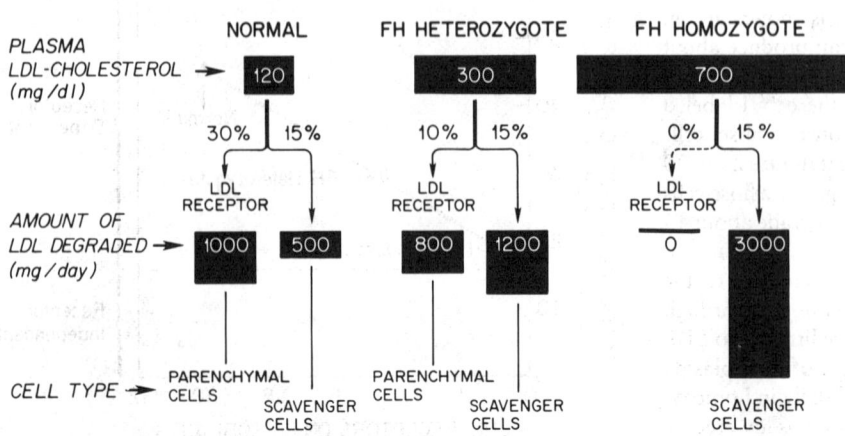

LDL and ^{125}I-labeled native LDL into normal subjects and heterozygotes [186]. The rationale for these studies lies in the theory that the ^{125}I-labeled LDL will be cleared from the plasma by receptor-dependent as well as receptor-independent pathways, whereas the ^{131}I-labeled cyclohexanedione-LDL will be cleared only by receptor-independent routes. The difference between the rates of clearance of ^{131}I-labeled cyclohexanedione-LDL and ^{125}I-labeled LDL gives an estimate of the fraction of LDL that is being cleared by the receptor route.

Investigators in Glasgow and London place their subjects on a different diet than do American researchers (ad-lib diet versus low cholesterol diet), and therefore their values for the normal clearance of LDL in subjects of all genotypes are lower than those obtained by Bilheimer et al. [173, 174]. For example, the FCR for ^{125}I-labeled LDL is 0.33 per day in the Shepherd studies in normal individuals [186] and 0.45 per day in the Bilheimer studies [173, 174]. Nevertheless, the estimates of the rates of receptor-dependent and receptor-independent clearance are in relatively close agreement with the predictions made from the indirect reasoning as outlined above and as shown in Fig. 33-24.

In normal individuals the comparison of the decay rates for ^{125}I-labeled LDL and ^{131}I-labeled cyclohexanedione-LDL indicated that about 33 percent of the LDL that left the plasma daily was removed by the receptor mechanism [186]. In heterozygotes only 16 percent of the LDL that left the plasma was removed by the receptor. When this reduced FCR was multiplied by the expanded LDL pool size in heterozygotes, the result was that the absolute rate of receptor-mediated clearance in heterozygotes was 83 percent of the normal value, and the receptor independent clearance was twofold greater than normal. These calculated values are in remarkable agreement with the corresponding figures of 80 percent and 2.5 times that were predicted on the basis of the indirect method [88], as outlined above (see Fig. 33-24).

The most striking findings to emerge from the double-isotope technique have been made by Thompson et al., who applied the method to homozygotes. These researchers found that simultaneously administered ^{125}I-labeled LDL and ^{131}I-labeled cyclohexanedione-LDL were cleared at similar low rates in two such patients, thereby confirming directly the severe reduction in functional LDL receptors in homozygotes [188, 189]. One of the turnover studies of Thompson et al. is reproduced in Fig. 33-25.

The cyclohexanedione-LDL turnover technique has also been used to document two new findings about the biology of the LDL receptor. First, the administration of the bile acid sequestrant cholestyramine to normal subjects was shown to enhance the rate of removal of ^{125}I-labeled LDL from the circulation without affecting the removal rate for ^{131}I-labeled cyclohexanedione-LDL, suggesting that cholestyramine lowers LDL cholesterol levels in humans primarily by enhancing the receptor-mediated removal of the lipoprotein from the circulation, presumably in the liver [187]. Second, when a patient with a high plasma LDL level secondary to severe hypothyroidism was treated with thyroxine, the diminished FCR for ^{125}I-labeled LDL rose to normal without a change in the FCR for ^{131}I-labeled cyclohexanedione-LDL (Fig. 33-26). These in vivo findings complement earlier in vitro studies which showed that LDL receptors were increased in thyroxine-treated fibroblasts [190] and suggest a role for thyroid hormone in modulating LDL receptor activity in vivo. The cylohexanedione-treated

LDL turnover technique shows great promise for permitting the dissection of the genetic and environmental factors that govern the receptor-mediated removal of LDL from the circulation of human beings.

On the basis of the above studies, it seems reasonable to conclude that in normal Europeans one-third to two-thirds of the LDL that is removed from the circulation is removed by the LDL receptor and that this fraction may vary with dietary and hormonal changes. Moreover, the elevation of LDL levels in familial hypercholesterolemic heterozygotes and homozygotes is due in large part to the reduced fractional rate of clearance of LDL from the circulation, owing to the reduced number of functional LDL receptors. The next step is to determine which tissues normally express the most LDL receptors and to ascertain whether the liver normally uses this mechanism. The tissues that remove LDL by receptor-independent pathways must also be identified, and the nature of these removal mechanisms must be explored. Finally, it must be realized that despite these advances in knowledge of the fundamental mechanism for the LDL elevation in familial hypercholesterolemia, the pathogenesis of the disease will not be fully understood until insight is gained into the mechanisms by which the elevated LDL level leads to accelerated atherosclerosis.

The Scavenger Cell Pathway for Lipoprotein Degradation

Recent studies have begun to explore the mechanisms by which scavenger cells degrade LDL [191, 192]. The most informative model system has been one that uses monolayers of freshly isolated macrophages obtained from the peritoneal cavity of mice. These cells are allowed to adhere to plastic, whereupon they form monolayers that can be maintained in a functionally active, nonproliferative state for several days [193].

When such macrophages are incubated with human ^{125}I-labeled LDL, they fail to take up or degrade the lipoprotein with high affinity [191, 192]. This is in contrast to cultured mouse fibroblasts and adrenal cells, which express large numbers of receptors for human LDL [139, 140]. Despite the fact that macrophages are known to take up denatured proteins, the macrophages did not take up most forms of denatured LDL. Indeed, when LDL was denatured by a variety of drastic techniques—including heat treatment; repeated freeze-thawing; or exposure to strong acids, bases, or oxidants—the lipoprotein was still not degraded by the macrophages. Several modifications of LDL did enhance its uptake, however. The first one that was studied in detail was chemical acetylation [191, 192]. Treatment of LDL with acetic anhydride had earlier been shown to destroy the ability of the lipoprotein to interact with the fibroblast LDL receptor [102]. By this treatment acetyl groups are attached to several structures on the lipoprotein, most notably the ϵ-amino groups of lysine. Since these acetyl residues neutralize the positive charge of the lysine residues, they enhance the net negative charge of the lipoprotein.

Although they do not recognize native LDL, mouse peritoneal macrophages have surface binding sites that recognize acetyl-LDL [191, 192, 194]. These binding sites are of high affinity and saturability and they are trypsin-sensitive. Immediately after the acetyl-LDL binds to these receptor sites, the lipoprotein is internalized by the cells, apparently through

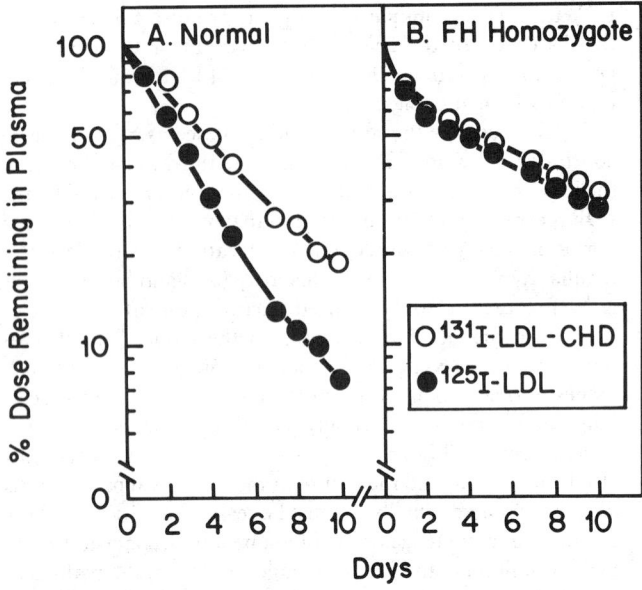

Figure 33-25 Plasma die-away curves in a normal subject (*A*) and a patient with homozygous familial hypercholesterolemia (*B*) after the simultaneous intravenous injection of 30 μCi of ^{125}I-labeled LDL (●) and 30 μCi of cyclohexanedione-modified ^{131}I-labeled LDL (O). (*Redrawn from Thompson et al.* [188].)

endocytosis, and delivered to lysosomes where it is quickly digested. The protein component of acetyl-LDL is digested completely into amino acids. When the protein component of the acetyl-LDL is labeled with ^{125}I, the liberated mono[^{125}I]iodotyrosine is immediately excreted from the cell.

Figure 33-27 shows the striking difference in the way in which macrophages and fibroblasts metabolize ^{125}I-labeled LDL and acetyl-LDL. The fibroblasts bind, take up, and degrade with high affinity ^{125}I-labeled LDL, but not ^{125}I-labeled acetyl-LDL. On the other hand, the macrophages bind, take up, and degrade with high affinity ^{125}I-labeled acetyl-LDL, but not ^{125}I-labeled LDL. In general, the expression of LDL receptors and acetyl-LDL receptors by a given cell type tends to be mutually exclusive; with few exceptions, cells express high levels of either the native LDL receptor or the acetyl-LDL receptor. Nonmacrophage cells, such as fibroblasts, smooth-muscle cells, adrenocortical cells, circulating blood lymphocytes, malignant lymphocytes, and teratocarcinoma cells, express native LDL receptors but not acetyl-LDL receptors [191, 194, 195]. On the other hand, all macrophage-type cells so far studied, including peritoneal macrophages and hepatic Kupffer cells, have abundant receptors for acetyl-LDL but very few receptors for LDL. Of interest is the finding that macrophages derived from blood monocytes express receptors for both acetyl-LDL and native LDL [194, 196].

The cholesteryl esters of the internalized acetyl-LDL are hydrolyzed efficiently in the lysosomes, but only half of the liberated cholesterol is excreted from the cell [192]. The remaining cholesterol is transferred from the lysosome to the cytoplasmic compartment where it is then reesterified by a membrane-bound acyl CoA:cholesterol acyltransferase (ACAT) enzyme. By electron microscopy the reesterified cholesterol is seen to accumulate in the form of homogeneous, cytoplasmic, neutral lipid droplets that are not surrounded by a membrane [192]. These droplets are birefringent and stain with the fat stain oil red O, further identifying them as cholesteryl ester droplets. When macrophages are incubated with acetyl-LDL for several days in vitro, the cellular cholesteryl ester content can exceed 300 μg sterol per milligram of protein (six times the level of unesterified cholesterol in the cell), and the cells become so vacuolated that they resemble the foam cells of the atheromas and xanthomas of patients with familial hypercholesterolemia [192].

The cholesteryl ester droplets of these artificially created macrophage foam cells are not inert. The cholesteryl esters are continually being hydrolyzed and reesterified (Fig. 33-28).

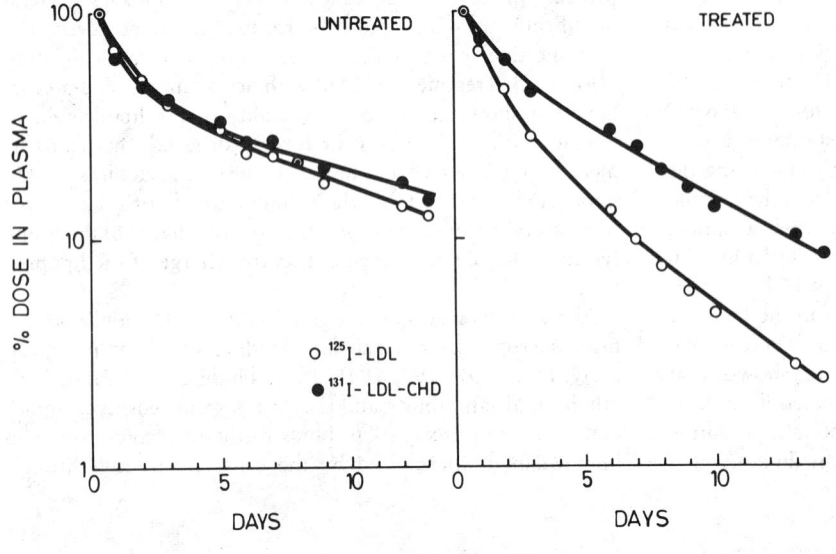

Figure 33-26 Plasma die-away curves in a hypothyroid patient before (*left* panel) and after treatment with L-thyroxine 0.2 mg/day for 6 weeks (*right* panel). For each turnover study, the patient received simultaneous injections of 30 μCi of ^{125}I-labeled LDL (O) and 30 μCi of cyclohexanedione-modified ^{131}I-labeled LDL (●). (*From Thompson et al.* [188].)

Hydrolysis of the cytoplasmic cholesteryl esters is not interrupted when the cell's lysosomal acid lipase is inhibited by chloroquine and other lysosomal enzyme inhibitors. This suggests that the hydrolytic reaction is catalyzed by a nonlysosomal cholesteryl esterase [197]. Reesterification is mediated by a microsomal ACAT whose activity can be inhibited by progesterone. Inasmuch as the ACAT enzyme uses fatty acyl CoA derivatives whose synthesis requires ATP, the continual hydrolysis and reesterification of cytoplasmic cholesteryl esters constitutes a futile cycle that wastes energy (Fig. 33-28) [197].

When macrophages that have accumulated cholesteryl esters are incubated in serum-free medium, the cholesteryl ester cycle operates continuously at such a rate that one-half of the stored cholesteryl esters are hydrolyzed and reesterified each day. The addition of serum to the culture medium interrupts this cycle by removing free cholesterol from this cell. The cholesterol that is liberated from the hydrolyzed cholesteryl esters is now excreted instead of being reesterified. Thus, in the presence of serum the macrophages exhibit a net excretion of 50 percent of the stored cholesterol per day [197].

In the absence of serum or a serum substitute, macrophages and other cultured cells cannot excrete cholesterol. Serum exerts its cholesterol-removing effect by virtue of its ability to bind cholesterol. Several of the components of serum contribute to its cholesterol-removing activity [198–200]. Among the lipoproteins, HDL is many times more effective as a cholesterol-removing agent than is LDL, which has little activity in this regard. The nonlipoprotein fraction of serum (density > 1.215 g/ml) also has cholesterol-removing activity [200]. However, the two major components of this fraction, albumin and gamma globulin, are inactive in the mouse peritoneal macrophage system.

Intact red blood cells were extremely potent in their ability to remove cholesterol from cholesterol-overloaded macrophages [200]. On the other hand, artificial lecithin liposomes were not active, perhaps because they became toxic to the cells at concentrations below which their cholesterol-removing activity was manifested [200]. In other cell types that can tolerate higher concentrations of phospholipids in their environment, phospholipids are effective removers of cholesterol [201].

At the present time, the relevance of the in vitro macrophage studies to the accumulation of cholesteryl esters in scavenger cells of patients with familial hypercholesterolemia is not yet established. It has been shown, however, that foam cells from humans with other forms of atherosclerosis, as well as from atheromas of cholesterol-fed animals, incorporate radiolabeled fatty acids into cholesteryl esters at an accelerated rate [202]. These findings, coupled with the observation that the cholesteryl esters that accumulate in vivo like those in vitro, are stored as non-membrane-bound cytoplasmic droplets suggests that the cholesteryl ester cycle may operate in these cells in vivo.

The modification of LDL that is responsible for its uptake by arterial wall scavenger cells in vivo is not yet known. Acetylation of LDL requires an activated form of acetate as a donor and is not known to occur in extracellular fluid. However, other modification reactions such as oxidation of the ε-amino groups of lysine are known to occur in vivo. One such type of lysine-modifying reaction consists of the formation of Schiff bases with aldehydes. Fogelman and coworkers showed that incubation of LDL in vitro with high concentrations of malondialdehyde converts the lipoprotein into a form that is taken up and degraded by macrophages [196]. The malondialdehyde-

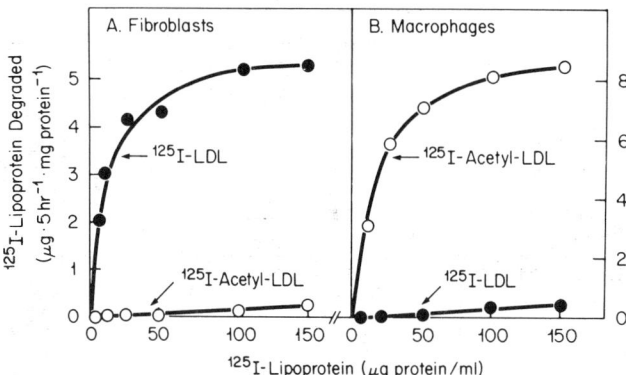

Figure 33-27 Differences in the metabolism of ^{125}I-labeled LDL and ^{125}I-labeled acetyl-LDL by monolayers of human fibroblasts (*A*) and mouse peritoneal macrophages (*B*). Monolayers of growing fibroblasts were incubated in lipoprotein-deficient serum for 48 h prior to the experiment in order to induce maximal LDL receptors [260]. Monolayers of freshly isolated macrophages were studied without prior incubation in lipoprotein-deficient serum [191]. For degradation assays, each monolayer received medium containing 10% lipoprotein-deficient serum and the indicated concentration of either human ^{125}I-labeled LDL (●) or ^{125}I-labeled acetyl-LDL (0). After incubation for 5 h at 37°C, the amount of ^{125}I-labeled acid-soluble material in the medium was determined.

treated LDL binds to the same surface binding site that recognizes acetyl-LDL [194]. The provocative feature of the malondialdehyde reaction is that the reactant malondialdehyde is known to be released from cells that are actively synthesizing prostaglandins, most notably platelets [203]. It is tempting to postulate that the local release of malondialdehyde at sites of mural thrombosis modifies the LDL that is trapped in the clot, thereby allowing it to be taken up and degraded by macrophages. Unfortunately the malondialdehyde reaction in vitro requires concentrations of malondialdehyde that are at least two orders of magnitude higher than those known to be produced by platelets during the clotting reaction in vivo [194, 196]. It is possible that some other factor exists in vivo to enhance the efficiency of the malondialdehyde reaction, but until it can be demonstrated in vitro, the role of malondialdehyde in macrophage foam cell function must be considered speculative.

The acetyl-LDL binding site is not the only mechanism that macrophages can use for taking up LDL in vitro. Two other mechanisms have been demonstrated, one involving the uptake of human LDL that is bound to dextran sulfate [204] and the other involving the uptake of β-migrating very low density lipoproteins (β-VLDL) obtained from cholesterol-fed animals, including dogs, rats, rabbits, and monkeys [205, 206]. Macrophages internalize the LDL–dextran sulfate complex and β-VLDL by absorptive endocytosis, each lipoprotein being recognized by a different surface binding site that is distinct from the acetyl-LDL receptor. In each case, the lipoprotein is delivered to lysosomes, where its cholesteryl esters are hydrolyzed and reesterified.

Cholesterol Synthetic Rates in Heterozygotes and Homozygotes

In cultured fibroblasts from familial hypercholesterolemia patients, the deficiency of LDL receptors creates a situation in which the rate of cholesterol synthesis is higher in cells from heterozygotes and homozygotes than in cells from normal subjects when all are exposed to the same level of LDL in the

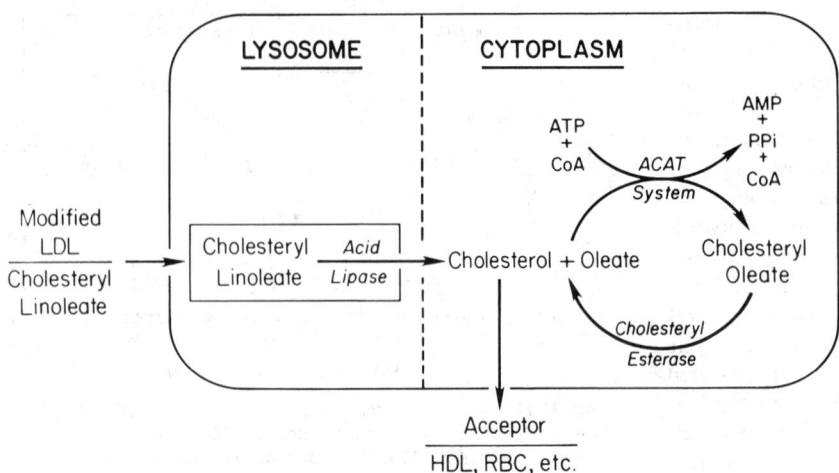

Figure 33-28 The macrophage cholesteryl ester cycle. The salient features of this model are discussed in the text. (*Brown et al.* [197]. *Used by permission.*)

incubation medium [45, 115]. It has been pointed out, however, that these in vitro findings do not imply that the total-body cholesterol synthesis rate would be elevated in these patients [173]. This is because in vivo the patients do not have normal levels of LDL cholesterol. Heterozygotes, for example, maintain a two- to threefold elevation of plasma LDL levels. In tissue culture, such an increase is sufficient to reduce cholesterol synthesis to the same levels that are seen in cells from normal subjects [138]. This type of compensation also seems to take place in vivo. Total-body sterol synthetic rates have been measured in heterozygotes using the sterol balance technique. These studies have shown normal rates of total-body cholesterol synthesis [173, 207–209].

It is not clear whether this type of LDL-related compensation can occur in homozygotes. In actively growing fibroblasts from receptor-negative homozygotes, cholesterol synthesis cannot be fully suppressed, even when very high levels of LDL are present in the culture medium [45, 115, 210]. However, when fibroblasts become confluent and cease to grow, the rate of cholesterol synthesis falls in homozygote cells as well as in normal cells [115]. Thus, it might be expected that in vivo cholesterol synthesis in homozygotes might be higher than normal in rapidly growing cells and perhaps in cells that use LDL for the production of steroid hormones. Whether this increase would be sufficient to produce a detectable increase in overall total-body cholesterol synthesis is not known.

Studies of cholesterol synthetic rates in homozygotes with the use of sterol balance [173, 174, 207, 211, 212] or isotopic turnover [213] techniques have shown an interesting dichotomy of results. Younger subjects in general appear to have total-body rates of cholesterol synthesis that are two- to threefold above normal, as reflected by an enhanced excretion of cholesterol from the body as compared with normal subjects of the same age. However, in homozygotes who have been studied after the age of 10, the cholesterol synthetic rates are generally at the upper limits of normal. Bile acid synthetic rates are generally normal [173, 174, 207, 211–213]. Although the number of subjects studied by these techniques is small, the results nevertheless suggest that young familial hypercholesterolemic homozygotes may have a total-body overproduction of cholesterol, whereas older homozygotes may not show such overproduction. The tissues in which such overproduction occurs are not known.

DIAGNOSIS

Clinical Diagnosis: Differentiation from Other Disorders Producing Type 2 Hyperlipoproteinemia

Homozygotes   The clinical diagnosis of familial hypercholesterolemia in the homozygote usually causes no difficulty. Not only is the clinical picture of cutaneous xanthomas and juvenile atherosclerosis distinct, but finding a plasma cholesterol level exceeding 650 mg/dl in a nonjaundiced child is virtually pathognomonic.

The one disorder that may occasionally be confused clinically with homozygous familial hypercholesterolemia is the even less frequent entity called *pseudohomozygous type 2 familial hypercholesterolemia*. This disorder was first described in 1974 [214], and to date six affected individuals from six unrelated families have been identified [51, 214–217]. The clinical picture is that of a child with the following abnormalities: (1) severe hypercholesterolemia (total plasma cholesterol level of about 350 to 600 mg/dl) due to a selective elevation in plasma LDL; (2) a normal plasma triglyceride level; (3) cutaneous planar xanthomas of the type seen in homozygous familial hypercholesterolemia; (4) normal plasma cholesterol levels in both parents; and (5) a striking response to dietary restriction of cholesterol, with plasma cholesterol levels falling as much as 40 percent, accompanied by regression of the xanthomas [214, 215].

Although pseudohomozygous type 2 familial hypercholesterolemia superficially resembles homozygous familial hypercholesterolemia, it can be distinguished clinically from the latter disorder by the following features: (1) the absence of heterozygous familial hypercholesterolemia in the parents and in other first-degree relatives; (2) the apparent absence of juvenile atherosclerosis, at least in the few cases so far described; and (3) the remarkable sensitivity to dietary manipulation. The combination of a low cholesterol diet (<200 mg/day) and oral cholestyramine (12 g/day) lowers plasma LDL cholesterol levels well into the normal range [214, 215], a completely different result from that obtained with homozygous familial hypercholesterolemia.

Studies of the cultured fibroblasts of one of the two originally described patients with pseudohomozygous type 2 familial hypercholesterolemia (case 2, B.H.) [51] and one other patient showed no abnormality in any of the steps in the LDL receptor pathway [51]. This finding suggests that the elevation in LDL cholesterol levels is not caused by an abnormality in the receptor-mediated catabolism of LDL. In addition, LDL isolated from the plasma of affected patients was taken up, degraded, and metabolized normally by normal human fibroblasts [51]. Studies of total-body cholesterol and bile acid production and of ^{125}I-labeled apo-LDL turnover in plasma performed while the patients are ingesting low and high amounts of dietary cholesterol should be especially informative in identifying the biochemical lesion in this disorder.

Heterozygotes   In order to diagnose the heterozygote with familial hypercholesterolemia, it is first necessary to document an elevation in the plasma level of LDL. In most cases the finding of hypercholesterolemia is sufficient to establish that the LDL cholesterol level is elevated, since in the absence of extreme elevation of VLDL (as indicated by a plasma triglyceride level greater than 600 mg/dl), the total plasma cholesterol level directly reflects the LDL cholesterol concentration in nearly all individuals [118]. In rare cases when the total cholesterol level is at the upper limits of normal (i.e., at or near the 95th percentile cutoff), the measurement of LDL cholesterol by ultracentrifugation may help to clarify whether the concentration of LDL is elevated [29, 118].

Having documented the presence of hypercholesterolemia (hyperbetalipoproteinemia), the physician then must determine whether the cause of the elevation is the heterozygous form of familial hypercholesterolemia. This distinction is of crucial importance because most patients with an elevation in total plasma cholesterol or LDL cholesterol (i.e., a type 2a or type 2b lipoprotein pattern) do *not* have familial hypercholesterolemia [76]. It has been estimated that probably no more than 1 in 20 individuals in the general population with hypercholesterolemia and a type 2 lipoprotein pattern has this genetic defect [76]. Most persons with a type 2 lipoprotein pattern appear to have a form of hypercholesterolemia that is multifactorial in origin and probably derives from a combination of environmental and poorly understood polygenic factors [76, 218]. Moreover, in addition to familial hypercholesterolemia, there is at least one other monogenic cause of type 2 hyperlipoproteinemia, *familial combined hyperlipidemia* [76, 77, 219]. Thus, the term familial hypercholesterolemia should not be considered genetically equivalent to, or synonymous with, the term familial type 2 hyperlipoproteinemia.

The diagnosis of familial hypercholesterolemia can be made on clinical grounds if the hypercholesterolemic patient has tendon xanthomas or a pedigree in which one of the parents and about one-half of the first-degree relatives have hypercholesterolemia in association with tendon xanthomas. However, many heterozygotes, including most below age 20 and approximately 25 percent of those above age 20, have only hypercholesterolemia without tendon xanthomas [76, 218]. Without family analysis, familial hypercholesterolemia in these latter subjects is especially difficult to separate on clinical grounds from other causes of an elevated plasma level of LDL cholesterol.

In individual patients with a primary type 2 lipoprotein pattern and no tendon xanthomas, there are several useful clinical clues to help distinguish between familial hypercholesterol-

emia and the other monogenic cause of high LDL levels, familial combined hyperlipidemia. These are:

1. Heterozygotes with familial hypercholesterolemia tend to have, on the average, higher cholesterol levels. The finding of a total plasma cholesterol level about 400 mg/dl is highly suggestive of this diagnosis.

2. Heterozygotes with familial hypercholesterolemia do not usually have relatives with lipoprotein abnormalities of multiple types (i.e., types 2a, 2b, 4, and 5), but this is characteristic of familial combined hyperlipidemia [76, 77, 219].

3. Hypercholesterolemic individuals with familial combined hyperlipidemia rarely, if ever, have tendon xanthomas [76, 219].

4. Hypercholesterolemia does not appear to express itself in children with familial combined hyperlipidemia, as it does in those with familial hypercholesterolemia [76, 118]; hence the finding of a hypercholesterolemic child in the family is strongly suggestive of familial hypercholesterolemia.

A variety of nongenetic disturbances can also cause the plasma LDL cholesterol level to be elevated. For example, a type 2a lipoprotein pattern may be observed in patients with hypothyroidism, nephrotic syndrome, hepatoma, Cushing's syndrome, acute intermittent porphyria, anorexia nervosa, and Werner's syndrome [118]. Patients with primary biliary cirrhosis and other forms of obstructive jaundice may also manifest a type 2a lipoprotein pattern, but their plasma will also contain elevated amounts of lipoprotein X [118].

Laboratory Diagnosis: Measurements of LDL Receptors

It is now possible to measure LDL receptor function in cultured skin fibroblasts and thus to confirm directly a 50 percent deficiency of LDL receptors in a heterozygote and a complete or near-complete deficiency of LDL receptor activity in the three types of homozygotes [68]. Six tests are available for quantitation of LDL receptor function in monolayers of fibroblasts cultured from the skin of patients: (1) measurement of the cell surface binding and intracellular uptake of ^{125}I-labeled LDL [97]; (2) measurement of the rate of proteolytic degradation of ^{125}I-labeled LDL [110]; (3) measurement of the hydrolysis of [^{3}H]cholesteryl linoleate contained within LDL [111]; (4) measurement of the LDL-mediated increase in cellular cholesteryl esters by gas-liquid chromatography [112]; (5) measurement of LDL-mediated suppression of the synthesis of [^{14}C]cholesterol from [^{14}C]acetate or of HMG-CoA reductase activity as assayed in cell-free extracts [45, 115]; and (6) measurement of LDL-mediated stimulation of the incorporation of [^{14}C]oleate into cellular cholesteryl[^{14}C]oleate [116].

The LDL receptor defect in familial hypercholesterolemia can also be demonstrated in circulating blood mononuclear cells, thus obviating the necessity for long-term culture [143, 144]. Immediately after mononuclear cells are isolated from the bloodstream of normal subjects, they express a small but detectable number of LDL receptors, as estimated by the rate of high affinity degradation of ^{125}I-labeled LDL; cells from heterozygotes express, on average, half the normal number of receptors; and cells from homozygotes show no receptor activity by this assay [143, 144]. It should be noted that the performance of these analyses on freshly isolated mononuclear cells is technically difficult, because the amount of trichloroacetic acid–soluble ^{125}I-radioactivity that is generated from the degradation of ^{125}I-labeled LDL is only several-fold above the background level of trichloroacetic acid–soluble radioactivity that is present in all but the best preparations of ^{125}I-labeled LDL [144].

To improve the precision and sensitivity of the ^{125}I-labeled LDL degradation assay, the blood mononuclear cells are fractionated into lymphocytes and monocytes by differential adherence to plastic, which removes essentially all of the monocytes. The lymphocytes, which do not adhere to the plastic, are then incubated in suspension for 48 to 72 h in a medium containing serum from which the lipoproteins have been removed by ultracentrifugation (so-called lipoprotein-deficient serum). During this incubation the lymphocytes are deprived of LDL, which is their normal source of cholesterol. As a result, the feedback system is activated and the cells synthesize an increased number of LDL receptors [143, 144]. The number of receptors attained is proportional to the number of functional genes at the receptor locus, i.e., cells from heterozygotes express a half-normal number of receptors and cells from receptor-negative homozygotes have virtually no detectable LDL receptors (see Fig. 33-20).

While this type of assay has been used to confirm the nature of the genetic defect in familial hypercholesterolemia, it has not been proved to be useful for diagnostic purposes in the general population. The one large study that has been reported dealt with 10 heterozygotes and 7 unaffected individuals from a single large family with familial hypercholesterolemia [144]. The heterozygotes, as a group, were clearly separable from the unaffected individuals on the basis of a mean LDL receptor level that was 50 percent of normal. However, even in this one family there was a small degree of overlap between the two groups. It is anticipated that this degree of overlap might be troublesome if this test were to be applied to the general population [144]. Since unaffected subjects outnumber familial hypercholesterolemic heterozygotes by 500 to 1 in the general population, an individual with a borderline low LDL receptor activity is more likely to represent the small population of normal individuals that fall into the heterozygote range rather than a true heterozygote.

A new method for analysis of LDL receptors, which shows promise in reducing the scatter among the normal subjects and thus allowing a more precise identification of heterozygotes, has recently become available [220]. This technique makes use of reconstituted LDL particles in which the cholesteryl ester core of LDL is extracted with heptane and replaced with a synthetic cholesteryl ester that contains a fluorescein derivative as a part of its structure [145, 146]. In this way approximately 1000 fluorescein molecules are incorporated into each LDL particle, which retains its ability to bind to the LDL receptor and thereby to enter cells. In the diagnostic test, lymphocytes are isolated from the bloodstream and incubated for 48 h in lipoprotein-deficient serum to induce high levels of LDL receptors. The cells are then incubated for an additional 24 h with the fluorescein-containing reconstituted LDL [220]. At the end of this incubation the cells are washed several times by centrifugation and then passed through a fluorescence-activated cell sorter. This instrument incorporates each lymphocyte into a single droplet. The droplets are passed in a stream through a laser light beam, and the amount of fluorescence in each cell is measured and recorded at a rate that approaches 5000 cells per second. The data are fed into a microprocessor that calculates the median fluorescence intensity per cell for the entire population. This median value is remarkably constant from one normal individual to the next. Cells from familial hypercholesterolemic heterozygotes are also tightly grouped at a value that is one-half of normal. Although this test has yet to be applied to a large population, it offers promise for permitting the assignment of an unequivocal diagnosis of heterozygous familial hypercholesterolemia based on screening of unselected individuals in the population.

Prenatal Diagnosis of Receptor-Negative Homozygotes

The development of assay methods for the quantitative assessment of LDL receptor activity in cultured cells allowed Brown, Goldstein, and coworkers in 1978 to make a prenatal diagnosis of homozygous familial hypercholesterolemia [86]. Amniotic cells were obtained at the sixteenth week of pregnancy from the uterus of a woman who had already borne one child with the receptor-negative form of homozygous familial hypercholesterolemia and who was therefore at 25 percent genetic risk for producing another affected offspring. The amniotic cells were grown in culture and their LDL receptor activity was assessed. Cells cultured simultaneously from two other women who were not at risk for homozygous familial hypercholesterolemia were also studied as controls. The cultured amniotic fluid cells from the fetus were found to have less than 5 percent of the LDL receptor activity of the control cells as revealed by assays of the binding, uptake, and degradation of ^{125}I-labeled LDL and of the LDL-mediated suppression of HMG-CoA reductase and stimulation of cholesteryl ester synthesis. The woman elected to have a therapeutic abortion after 20 weeks gestation, and the diagnosis of homozygous familial hypercholesterolemia was confirmed when the blood cholesterol level of the aborted fetus was found to be 279 mg/dl, a value that was ninefold higher than the plasma cholesterol level of control fetuses of similar gestational age [86].

More recently, amniotic cells from a second at-risk pregnancy were analyzed and found to have LDL receptor activity that was about 50 percent of the values in simultaneously studied control cells [221]. The mother allowed her pregnancy to proceed, and at term the infant had a cord-blood cholesterol level of 69 mg/dl, with an LDL cholesterol level of 42 mg/dl and an HDL cholesterol level of 24 mg/dl [221]. These values are compatible with the diagnosis of heterozygous familial hypercholesterolemia [28].

Analysis of the cultured amniotic fluid cells from a third pregnancy at genetic risk for homozygous familial hypercholesterolemia indicated that the fetus was unaffected [222]. This diagnosis was confirmed by repeated determinations of plasma cholesterol levels during the first 11 months of life.

From the above experience it would appear that the feasibility of making the prenatal diagnosis of receptor-negative homozygous familial hypercholesterolemia has been established. It has not yet been established, however, that cells from receptor-defective homozygotes, which possess detectable but reduced LDL receptor activity, can be distinguished from heterozygote cells with sufficient certainty to justify the performance of a therapeutic abortion. This question may be rendered moot by the recent data suggesting that the clinical sequelae of familial hypercholesterolemia are less severe in the receptor-defective homozygotes than in receptor-negative ones (see Table 33-3 and Fig. 33-4). Because of their severe symptoms, the receptor-negative homozygotes may be the only ones for whom therapeutic abortion will be considered.

Neonatal Diagnosis of Heterozygotes

By measuring the level of LDL cholesterol in the cord blood of babies born to a parent who is already known to carry the familial hypercholesterolemia gene, it is possible to diagnose heterozygotes at the time of birth [28]. Neonatal cord-blood screening is not a reliable means for identification of heterozygotes in the general population, because, just as with adults, the vast majority of newborns with elevations of LDL cholesterol do not have familial hypercholesterolemia [223, 224]. The earliest age at which heterozygotes can be accurately identified in the general population is probably 1 year, and even then a family analysis is required to confirm that the elevated LDL cholesterol level is due to familial hypercholesterolemia.

TREATMENT

Heterozygotes

Because of their frequency in the population and because of their poor prognosis, familial hypercholesterolemia heterozygotes constitute an important therapeutic problem in American medicine. The ideal cholesterol-lowering agent in this disease would be one that caused an enhanced production of LDL receptors in those tissues that normally use this receptor to take up and degrade LDL. Inasmuch as heterozygotes have one normal LDL receptor gene that is known to be under feedback regulation [138], it may be possible to induce body cells to produce an increased number of receptors by stimulating the transcription and translation of this normal gene. One way to do this has been suggested by results in cultured cells [114]. When the demand for cholesterol is elevated, cells produce an increased number of LDL receptors. This increase is even more pronounced when intracellular cholesterol synthesis is inhibited, thus forcing cells to rely entirely on LDL cholesterol [225, 226].

One class of drugs that may act by stimulating the production of LDL receptors are the bile acid–binding resins, cholestyramine and colestipol. These agents have been used extensively for two decades in the treatment of heterozygous familial hypercholesterolemia and other hypercholesterolemic states [227–230a]. In general, they produce a 15 to 30 percent lowering of LDL cholesterol levels.

Cholestyramine and colestipol are nonabsorbable, anion-exchange resins that bind bile acids in the intestinal lumen and thus prevent their absorption from the ileum (reviewed in Ref. 229). This leads to increased fecal excretion of bile acids, which elicits an increased conversion of cholesterol to bile acids in the liver [228]. The mechanism by which the enhanced bile acid synthesis leads to a specific lowering of plasma LDL cholesterol levels has recently been disclosed by double-label LDL turnover studies in human beings. As discussed above (see page 698), treatment of heterozygotes with cholestyramine leads to an enhanced fractional catabolic rate (FCR) for plasma ^{125}I-labeled LDL but not ^{131}I-labeled cyclohexane-dione-treated LDL, which cannot bind to the LDL receptor [187]. This important finding suggests that the liver can be made to produce a larger number of LDL receptors if its demand for cholesterol is enhanced. This suggestion has been supported by two studies in animals. When rabbits were given cholestyramine, the uptake of intravenously administered ^{125}I-labeled LDL by the liver was enhanced by several-fold, whereas the hepatic uptake of ^{131}I-labeled cyclohexanedione-LDL was not increased [231]. Similarly, in dogs treated with colestipol the number of LDL receptors in liver membranes increased and the FCR for intravenously administered ^{125}I-labeled LDL increased proportionately [167]. Thus, in the dog, as well as in humans, the bile acid sequestrants lower plasma LDL levels by enhancing the efficiency of receptor-mediated removal of LDL from the plasma without changing the synthetic rate for the lipoprotein.

The effectiveness of bile acid sequestrants has long been known to be blunted because the liver responds by developing an enhanced rate of cholesterol synthesis [207, 232]. The enhanced rate of cholesterol synthesis would be expected to allow continued lipoprotein synthesis to occur despite the external removal of cholesterol in the form of bile acids. Moreover, by helping to replace the drained intracellular cholesterol pool, the increased hepatic cholesterol synthesis would blunt the rise in hepatic LDL receptors. Therefore, on theoretical grounds, it would be expected that an inhibitor of cholesterol synthesis should act synergistically with a bile acid sequestrant in lowering plasma LDL levels [114, 167].

The recent development of a new class of cholesterol synthesis inhibitors has allowed this hypothesis to be confirmed in animals. The prototype for this class of drug is compactin (ML-236B), a fungal metabolite that was isolated from *Penicillium citrinum* in 1976 by Endo and associates at the Sankyo Drug Company in Japan [233]. Compactin is a bicyclic diene with a side chain that contains a β-hydroxy-δ-lactone which resembles mevalonate. Compactin is a potent reversible inhibitor of HMG-CoA reductase that acts competitively with HMG-CoA [233, 234]. The K_i for compactin is on the order of 1 nM, which is 10,000-fold lower than the K_m for the natural substrate HMG-CoA (about 10 μM). More recently, a similar compound, mevinolin, was discovered in a strain of *Aspergillus* [235]. Mevinolin consists of compactin plus an additional methyl group. It is even more potent than compactin in inhibiting HMG-CoA reductase.

When administered to dogs [167, 235, 236], monkeys [237], rabbits [238], and human beings [239], compactin and mevinolin lower the plasma level of LDL cholesterol, without significantly affecting HDL cholesterol levels. Compactin and mevinolin do not lower the plasma cholesterol level in mice or rats [240].

Studies of ^{125}I-labeled LDL turnover in young beagle dogs indicate that mevinolin lowers the plasma LDL level by two mechanisms: (1) it inhibits LDL synthesis by about 50 percent; and (2) it enhances the FCR for LDL by twofold [167]. The increase in FCR is associated with a parallel increase in the number of LDL receptors in liver membranes. Consistent with the hypothesis presented above, the combination of a bile acid sequestrant (colestipol) and mevinolin was synergistic in increasing hepatic LDL receptors and lowering plasma LDL levels in normal young beagle dogs. This combination also produced a synergistic twofold increase in the FCR for LDL [167]. Figure 33-29 shows a plot of the FCR for LDL versus the amount of LDL receptor activity in liver membranes in the

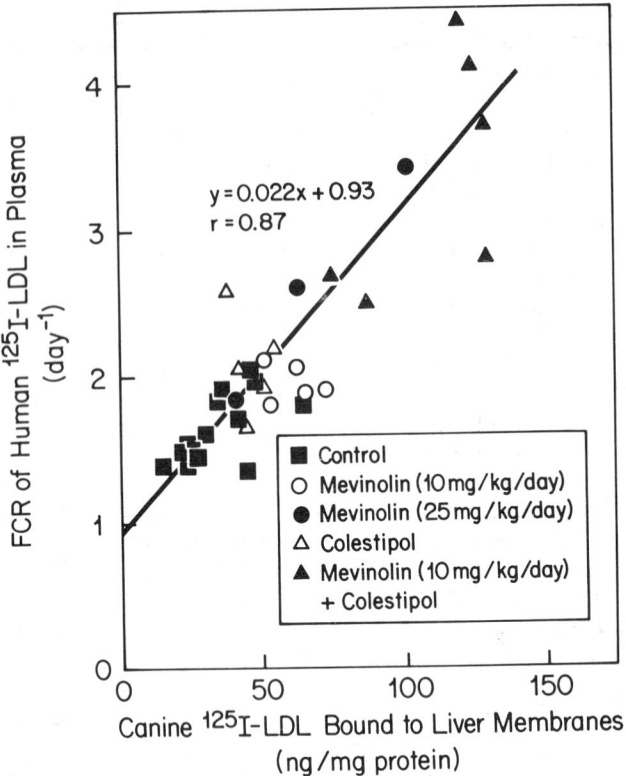

Figure 33-29 Relation between canine ¹²⁵I-labeled LDL binding to canine liver membranes and the FCR for human ¹²⁵I-labeled LDL in the plasma of intact young male beagle dogs subjected to various treatments: ■, none; 0, mevinolin [10 mg/(kg·day)] given orally for 17 days; ●, mevinolin [25 mg/(kg·day)] given orally for 23 days; △, colestipol [700 mg/(kg·day)] given orally for 17 days; or ▲, mevinolin [10 mg/(kg·day)] plus colestipol for 17 days. Three days before the end of the treatment period, each dog received an intravenous injection of 20 μCi of human ¹²⁵I-labeled LDL, and the FCR was measured. At the end of the treatment period, each dog was killed and liver membranes were prepared for ¹²⁵I-labeled LDL binding studies. Each data point for specific membrane binding and plasma FCR was obtained on the same dog. (*From Kovanen et al.* [*167*].)

variously treated dogs, illustrating the synergistic actions of mevinolin and colestipol.

These data raise the possibility of a truly effective drug therapy for heterozygotes with familial hypercholesterolemia. Since these individuals have the genetic capacity to produce LDL receptors, it is postulated that they may show a response to compactin or mevinolin, and they may respond even more profoundly to the combination of mevinolin or compactin plus colestipol. At the time of this writing, large-scale clinical trials with compactin and mevinolin were just beginning.

Among the established forms of therapy, the most impressive results in heterozygotes have been achieved with the use of a combination of a bile acid sequestrant and nicotinic acid [230]. The mechanism of action of nicotinic acid has not been established. A surgically created partial ileal bypass prevents bile salt reabsorption and produces the same therapeutic effect in heterozygotes as does cholestyramine [241–243].

Dietary discretion is generally recommended for every person with hypercholesterolemia, including those with familial hypercholesterolemia. In general, the diet should be altered in a reasonable manner such that total cholesterol intake is limited to no more than 300 mg/day for adults (roughly equivalent to the cholesterol content of one egg yolk) and no more than 150 mg/day for children. In addition, the intake of saturated fat

should be reduced and the intake of polyunsaturated fat increased [229, 230].

A discussion of the drug therapy for children with heterozygous familial hypercholesterolemia is beyond the scope of this chapter. This subject is discussed in several recent articles [244–247]. The reader is also referred to a recent review article by Levy, who discusses the doses and side effects of the various drugs used for the treatment of heterozygotes [229].

Homozygotes

Homozygotes are generally more resistant to treatment. There is little response in plasma cholesterol levels to either dietary changes or cholestyramine administration [230, 248]. Nevertheless, several investigators have observed that skin xanthomas soften or regress during cholestyramine therapy, even when plasma cholesterol levels do not decrease [230, 248]. Recent studies suggest that the use of cholestyramine in combination with nicotinic acid may be more effective in homozygotes than either drug given alone [230].

Several new approaches to therapy for homozygotes have recently been introduced, each of which is partially successful, and all of which open up new avenues for investigation into the mechanism underlying the hypercholesterolemia in this disorder. First, Starzl and coworkers observed that intravenous hyperalimentation caused a profound reduction in the plasma cholesterol level of one homozygote [249]. Similar results were subsequently obtained in other homozygotes [250, 251]. The mechanism for this effect is unknown. As a second therapeutic approach, Starzl and coworkers also observed that following the performance of an end-to-side portacaval anastomosis in a homozygote patient, the plasma cholesterol level declined from 772 mg/dl to 240 mg/dl [249]. Associated with this reduction was a disappearance of angina pectoris and an improvement in the patency of the coronary arteries as determined by angiography. This improvement notwithstanding, the patient died suddenly of an apparent cardiac arrhythmia about 18 months following the operation [252, 253].

At least 20 homozygotes have now been reported to have undergone portacaval shunt surgery, and in most of them the plasma cholesterol level was reduced about 50 percent [253–255]. Detailed metabolic studies in one of these homozygotes showed that the portacaval anastomosis reduced total-body cholesterol synthesis by 62 percent and lowered the synthetic rate for plasma LDL by 48 percent. The plasma LDL level in this patient was reduced by 39 percent, despite a 17 percent reduction in the fractional catabolic rate for the lipoprotein [173]. Despite the effects of the portacaval shunt on hepatic LDL and cholesterol synthesis in homozygotes, plasma albumin levels have remained unaltered and no significant changes in other liver functions have been observed [173, 253].

Perhaps the most successful new therapeutic approach consists of the use of a continuous-flow blood cell separator to perform repeated plasma exchange in homozygotes [256]. As practiced most extensively by Thompson and Myant, plasma exchange can lower the plasma cholesterol by about 300 mg/dl [255]. However, the plasma cholesterol quickly increases again. To be maximally effective, plasma exchange must be repeated at 2- to 3-week intervals, and it should be accompanied by dietary and drug therapy including maximal doses of nicotinic acid and cholestyramine [254]. While xanthomas have been reported to regress under this therapy, it is not yet known whether the atherosclerotic process can be altered or even reversed [258].

Homozygotes rarely if ever respond to cholestyramine therapy or to the performance of an ileal bypass [242]. Considered together with the data reviewed above, this suggests that response to these treatments requires the capacity to produce significant numbers of LDL receptors. In one Japanese homozygote, treatment with compactin did not affect the plasma LDL level, but cutaneous xanthomas were said to regress under this therapy [239]. The resistance of homozygotes to therapy is illustrated most poignantly by a series of experiments in which a bile fistula was created so that all biliary cholesterol and bile acids were drained to the exterior for periods up to 1 year. Although many grams of cholesterol were directly removed from the body by this route, there was no significant change in the plasma LDL cholesterol level [259].

It is usually assumed that a sustained lowering of plasma LDL cholesterol levels will prevent or retard the only life-threatening complication of familial hypercholesterolemia, atherosclerosis. However, since the hypercholesterolemia is present from birth, at what age must the plasma cholesterol level be lowered to prevent atherosclerosis? Can the atherosclerotic lesions be made to regress? Answers to these questions await a better understanding of the cellular metabolism of cholesterol and lipoproteins and of how these biochemical processes relate to the pathogenesis of the atherosclerotic lesion itself.

REFERENCES

1. MULLER C: Xanthomata, hypercholesterolemia, angina pectoris. *Acta Med Scand* suppl 89:75, 1938
2. MULLER C: Angina pectoris in hereditary xanthomatosis. *Arch Intern Med* 64:675, 1939
3. BROWN MS, GOLDSTEIN JL: Familial hypercholesterolemia: Model for genetic receptor disease. *Harvey Lect Ser* 73:163, 1979
4. FOGGE CH: General xanthelasma or vitiligoidea. *Trans Pathol Soc,* London 24:242, 1872
5. FOX TC: A case of xanthelasma multiplex. *Lancet* 2:688, 1879
6. POENSGEN A: Mittheilung eines seltenen Falles von Xanthelasma multiplex. *Arch Pathol Anat Physiol* 91:350, 1883
7. LEHZEN G, KNAUSS K: Uber Xanthoma multiplex planum, tuberosum, mollusciforme. *Arch Pathol Anat Physiol* 116:85, 1889
8. THANNHAUSER SJ, MAGENDANTZ H: The different clinical groups of xanthomatous diseases: A clinical physiological study of 22 cases. *Ann Intern Med* 11:1662, 1938
9. THANNHAUSER SJ: *Lipiodoses.* Oxford, New York, 1950
10. WILKINSON CF, HAND EA, FLIEGELMAN MT: Essential familial hypercholesterolemia. *Ann Intern Med* 29:671, 1948
11. WILKINSON CF: Essential familial hypercholesterolemia: Cutaneous metabolic and hereditary aspects. *Bull NY Acad Med* 26:670, 1950
12. ADLERSBERG D, PARETS AD, BOAS EP: Genetics of atherosclerosis. Studies of families with xanthomas and unselected patients with coronary artery disease under the age of fifty years. *JAMA* 141:246, 1949
13. ADLERSBERG D: Hypercholesterolemia with predisposition to atherosclerosis: An inborn error of lipid metabolism. *Am J Med* 11:600, 1951
14. ADLERSBERG D: Inborn errors of lipid metabolism. *Arch Pathol* 60:481, 1955
15. BLOOM D, KAUFMAN SR, STEVENS RA: Hereditary xanthomatosis: Familial incidence of xanthoma tuberosum associated with hypercholesterolemia and cardiovascular involvement with report of several cases of sudden death. *Arch Derm Syph* 45:1, 1942
16. ALVORD RM: Coronary heart disease and xanthoma tuberosum associated with hereditary hyperlipemia. *Arch Intern Med* 84:1002, 1949
17. PIPER J, ORRILD L: Essential familial hypercholesterolemia and xanthomatosis. *Am J Med* 21:34, 1956
18. EPSTEIN FH, BLOCK WD, HAND EA, FRANCIS T, JR: Familial hypercholesterolemia, xanthomatosis and coronary heart disease. *Am J Med* 26:39, 1959
19. HIRSCHHORN K, WILKINSON CF: The mode of inheritance in essential familial hypercholesterolemia. *Am J Med* 26:60, 1959
20. GURAVICH JL: Familial hypercholesterolemic xanthomatosis: A preliminary report. *Am J Med* 24:8, 1959
21. KHACHADURIAN AK: The inheritance of essential familial hypercholesterolemia. *Am J Med* 37:402, 1964
22. GOFMAN JW, DELALLA O, GLAZIER F, FREEMAN NK, LINDGREN FT, NICHOLAS AV, STRISHOWER EH, TAMPLIN AR: The serum lipoprotein transport system in health metabolic disorders, atherosclerosis and coronary artery disease. *Plasma* 2:413, 1954
23. GOFMAN JW, RUBIN L, McGINLEY JP, JONES HB: Hyperlipoproteinemia. *Am J Med* 17:514, 1954
24. FREDERICKSON DS, LEVY RI, LEES RS: Fat transport in lipoproteins—An integrated approach to mechanisms and disorders. *N Engl J Med* 276:32, 94, 148, 215, 273, 1967
25. BROWN MS, GOLDSTEIN JL: Receptor-mediated control of cholesterol metabolism. *Science* 181:150, 1976
26. HARLAN WR, JR, GRAHAM JB, ESTES EH: Familial hypercholesterolemia: A genetic and metabolic study. *Medicine* 45:77, 1966
27. SCHROTT HG, GOLDSTEIN JL, HAZZARD WR, McGOODWIN MM, MOTULSKY AG: Familial hypercholesterolemia in a large kindred. Evidence for a monogenic mechanism. *Ann Intern Med* 76:711, 1972
28. KWITEROVICH PO, JR, LEVY RI, FREDERICKSON DS: Neonatal diagnosis of familial type II hyperlipoproteinaemia. *Lancet* 1:118, 1973
29. KWITEROVICH PO, JR, FREDERICKSON DS, LEVY RI: Familial hypercholesterolemia (one form of familial type II hyperlipoproteinaemia). A study of its biochemical, genetic, and clinical presentation in childhood. *J Clin Invest* 53:1237, 1974
30. KHACHADURIAN AK: A general view of clinical and laboratory features of familial hypercholesterolemia (type II hyperbetalipoproteinemia). *Protides Biological Fluids* 19:315, 1971
31. FREDERICKSON DS, LEVY RI: Familial hyperlipoproteinemia, in Stanbury JB, Wyngaarden JB, Frederickson DS (eds): *The Metabolic Basis of Inherited Disease,* 3d ed. New York: McGraw-Hill, 1972, p 545
32. KHACHADURIAN AK, UTHMAN SM: Experiences with the homozygous cases of familial hypercholesterolemia. A report of 52 patients. *Nutr Metab* 15:132, 1973
33. STANLEY P, CHARTRAND C, D'AVIGNON A: Acquired aortic stenosis in a twelve-year-old girl with xanthomatosis. *N Engl J Med* 273:1378, 1965
34. BROWN MS, GOLDSTEIN JL: Familial hypercholesterolemia: Genetic, biochemical and pathophysiologic considerations. *Adv Intern Med* 20:273, 1975
35. NEVIN NC, SLACK J: Hyperlipidaemic xanthomatosis. II. Mode of inheritance in 55 families with essential hyperlipidaemia and xanthomatosis. *J Med Genet* 5:9, 1968
36. HABA T, MABUCHI H, YOSHIMURA A, WATANABE A, WAKASUGI T, TATAMI T, UEDA K, UEDA R, KAMETANI T, KOIZUMI J, MIYAMOTO S, TAKEDA R, TAKESHITA H: Effects of ML-236B (compactin) on sterol synthesis and low density lipoprotein receptor activities in fibroblasts of patients with homozygous familial hypercholesterolemia. *J Clin Invest* 67:1532, 1981
37. SLACK J, MILLS GL: Anomalous low density lipoproteins in familial hyperbetalipoproteinaemia. *Clin Chim Acta* 29:15, 1970
38. GOTTO AM, BROWN WV, LEVY RI, BIRNBAUMER ME, FREDERICKSON DS: Evidence for the identity of the major apoprotein in low density and very low density lipoprotein in normal subjects and patients with familial hyperlipoproteinemia. *J Clin Invest* 51:1486, 1972
39. FISHER WR, HAMMOND MG, WARMKE GL: Measurements of the molecular weight variability of plasma low density lipoproteins among normals and subjects with hyper-β-lipoproteinemia. Demonstration of macromolecular heterogeneity. *Biochemistry* 11:519, 1972
40. JADHAV AV, THOMPSON GR: Reversible abnormalities of low density lipoprotein composition in familial hypercholesterolaemia. *Eur J Clin Invest* 9:63, 1979
41. BAGNALL TF, LLOYD JK: Composition of low-density lipoprotein in children with hyperlipoproteinaemia. *Clin Chim Acta* 59:271, 1975
42. GRANT EH, SHEPPARD RJ, MILLS GL, SLACK J: A dielectric investigation of the water of hydration of low-density lipoproteins in familial hyperbetalipoproteinaemia. *Lancet* 1:1159, 1972
43. REICHL D, SIMONS LA, MYANT NB: The metabolism of low-density lipoprotein in a patient with familial hyperbetalipoproteinaemia. *Clin Sci Mol Med* 47:635, 1974
44. PATSCH W, WITZTUM JL, OSTLUND R, SCHONFELD G: Structure, immunology, and cell reactivity of low density lipoprotein from umbilical vein of a newborn type II homozygote. *J Clin Invest* 66:123, 1980
45. GOLDSTEIN JL, BROWN MS: Familial hypercholesterolemia: Identification of a defect in the regulation of 3-hydroxy-3-methylglutaryl coenzyme A reductase activity associated with overproduction of cholesterol. *Proc Nat Acad Sci USA* 70:2804, 1973
46. STREJA D, STEINER G, KWITEROVICH PO, JR: Plasma high-density lipoproteins and ischemic heart disease: Studies in a large kindred with familial hypercholesterolemia. *Ann Intern Med* 89:871, 1978

47. SEFTEL HC, BAKER SG, SANDLER MP, FORMAN MB, JOFFE BI, MENDELSOHN D, JENKINS T, MIENY CJ: A host of hypercholesterolaemic homozygotes in South Africa. *Brit Med J* 281:633, 1980

48. MENKES JH, SCHIMSCHOCK JR, SWANSON PD: Cerebrotendinous xanthomatosis. *Arch Neurol* 19:47, 1968

49. PHILIPPART M, VAN BOGAERT L: Cholestanolosis (cerebrotendinous xanthomatosis). *Arch Neurol* 21:603, 1969

50. MACAREG PVJ, JR, LASAGNA L, SNYDER B: Arcus not so senilis. *Ann Intern Med* 68:345, 1968

51. GOLDSTEIN JL, BROWN MS: Unpublished observations

52. GOLDSTEIN JL: The cardiac manifestations of homozygous and heterozygous forms of familial type II hyperbetalipoproteinemia. *Birth Defects: Original Article Series* 8:202, 1972

53. MISHKEL MA, FREEMAN Z: Hypercholesterolemic xanthomatosis: A case studied for three years. *Med J Aust* 1:794, 1966

54. MAHER JA, EPSTEIN FH, HAND EA: Xanthomatosis and coronary heart disease: Necropsy study of two affected siblings. *Arch Intern Med* 102:437, 1958

55. SCHETTLER FG: Essential familial hypercholesterolemia, in Schettler FG, Boyd GS (eds): *Atherosclerosis.* Amsterdam, Elsevier, 1969, p 543

56. KHACHADURIAN AK: Migratory polyarthritis in familial hypercholesterolemia (type II hyperlipoproteinemia). *Arthr Rheum* 11:385, 1968

57. KHACHADURIAN AK: Persistent elevation of the erythrocyte sedimentation rate (ESR) in familial hypercholesterolemia. *J Med Liban* 20:31, 1967

58. SLACK J: Risks of ischaemic heart-disease in familial hyperlipoproteinaemic states. *Lancet* 2:1380, 1969

59. JENSEN J, BLANKENHORN DH, KORNERUP V: Coronary disease in familial hypercholesterolemia. *Circulation* 36:77, 1967

60. HEIBERG A: The risk of atherosclerotic vascular disease in subjects with xanthomatosis. *Acta Med Scand* 198:249, 1975

61. STONE NJ, LEVY RI, FREDERICKSON DS, VERTER J: Coronary artery disease in 116 kindred with familial type II hyperlipoproteinemia. *Circulation* 49:476, 1974

62. BEAUMONT V, JACOTOT B, BEAUMONT JL: Ischaemic disease in men and women with familial hypercholesterolaemia and xanthomatosis. A comparative study of genetic and environmental factors in 274 heterozygous cases. *Atherosclerosis* 24:441, 1976

63. MORGANROTH J, LEVY RI, FREDERICKSON DS: The biochemical, clinical, and genetic features of type III hyperlipoproteinemia. *Ann Intern Med* 82:158, 1975

64. GLUECK CJ, LEVY RI, FREDERICKSON DS: Acute tendinitis and arthritis. A presenting symptom of familial type II hyperlipoproteinemia. *JAMA* 206:2895, 1968

65. ROONEY PJ, THIRD J, MADKOUR MM, SPENCER D, DICK WC: Transient polyarthritis associated with familial hyperbetalipoproteinaemia. *Quart J Med* (new series) 47:249, 1978

66. GLUECK CJ, LEVY RI, FREDERICKSON DS: Immunoreactive insulin, glucose tolerance and carbohydrate inducibility in types II, III, IV and V hyperlipoproteinemia. *Diabetes* 18:739, 1969

67. MIETTINEN TA, ARO A: Comparison of clinical findings in patients with hyperglyceridaemia and familial hypercholesterolaemia. *Ann Clin Res* 5:1, 1973

68. GOLDSTEIN JL, BROWN MS: The LDL receptor locus and the genetics of familial hypercholesterolemia. *Ann Rev Genet* 13:259, 1979

69. MABUCHI H, TATAMI R, HABA T, UEDA K, UEDA R, KAMETANI T, ITOH S, KOIZUMI J, OOTA M, MIYAMOTO S, TAKEDA R, TAKESHITA H: Homozygous familial hypercholesterolemia in Japan. *Am J Med* 65:290, 1978

70. BUJA LM, KOVANEN PT, BILHEIMER DW: Cellular pathology of homozygous familial hypercholesterolemia. *Am J Pathol* 97:327, 1979

71. TSANG RC, GLUECK CJ, MCLAIN C, RUSSELL P, JOYCE T, BOVE K, MELLIES M, STEINER PM: Pregnancy, parturition, and lactation in familial homozygous hypercholesterolemia. *Metabolism* 27:823, 1978

72. OTT J, SCHROTT HG, GOLDSTEIN JL, HAZZARD WR, ALLEN FH JR, FALK CT, MOTULSKY AG: Linkage studies in a large kindred with familial hypercholesterolemia. *Am J Hum Genet* 26:598, 1974

73. BERG K, HEIBERG A: Linkage studies on familial hyperlipoproteinemia with xanthomatosis: Normal lipoprotein markers and the C3 polymorphism. *Cytogenet Cell Genet* 16:266, 1976

74. ELSTON RC, NAMBOODIRI KK, GO RCP, SIERVOGEL RM, GLUECK CJ: Probable linkage between essential familial hypercholesterolemia and third complement component (C3). *Cytogenet Cell Genet* 16:294, 1976

75. PATTERSON D, SLACK J: Lipid abnormalities in male and female survivors of myocardial infarction and their first-degree relatives. *Lancet* 1:393, 1972

76. GOLDSTEIN JL, SCHROTT HG, HAZZARD WR, BIERMAN EL, MOTULSKY AG: Hyperlipidemia in coronary heart disease. II. Genetic analysis of lipid levels in 176 families and delineation of a new inherited disorder, combined hyperlipidemia. *J Clin Invest* 52:1544, 1973

77. NIKKILA EA, ARO A: Family study of serum lipids and lipoproteins in coronary heart disease. *Lancet* 1:954, 1973

78. CARTER CO, SLACK J, MYANT NB: Genetics of hyperlipoproteinaemias. *Lancet* 1:400, 1971

79. SLACK J: Inheritance of familial hypercholesterolemia. *Atherosclerosis Rev* 5:35, 1979

80. LEONARD JV, FOSBROOKE AS, LLOYD JK, WOLFF OH: Screening for familial hyper-β-lipoproteinaemia in children in hospital. *Arch Dis Child* 51:842, 1976

81. HEIBERG A, BERG K: The inheritance of hyperlipoproteinaemia with xanthomatosis. *Clin Genet* 9:203, 1976

82. ANDERSEN GE, LOUS P, FRIIS-HANSEN B: Screening for hyperlipoproteinemia in 10,000 Danish newborns. Follow-up studies in 522 children with elevated cord serum VLDL-LDL-cholesterol. *Acta Paediatr Scand* 68:541, 1979

83. MABUCHI H, TATAMI R, UEDA K, UEDA R, HABA T, KAMETANI T, WATANABE A, WAKASUGI T, ITO S, KOIZUMI J, OHTA M, MIYAMOTO S, TAKEDA R: Serum lipid and lipoprotein levels in Japanese patients with familial hypercholesterolemia. *Atherosclerosis* 32:435, 1979

84. JENKINS T, NICHOLLS E, GORDON E, MENDELSOHN D, SEFTEL HC, ANDREW MJA: Familial hypercholesterolaemia—A common genetic disorder in the Afrikaans population. *S Afr Med J* 57:943, 1980

85. ROBERTS WC, FERRANS VJ, LEVY RI, FREDERICKSON DS: Cardiovascular pathology in hyperlipoproteinemia. Anatomic observations in 42 necropsy patients with normal or abnormal serum lipoprotein patterns. *Am J Cardiol* 31:557, 1973

86. BROWN MS, KOVANEN PT, GOLDSTEIN JL, EECKELS R, VANDENBERGHE K, VAN DEN BERGH H, FRYNS JP, CASSIMAN JJ: Prenatal diagnosis of homozygous familial hypercholesterolaemia: Expression of a genetic receptor disease in utero. *Lancet* 1:526, 1978

86a. SCHAFFNER T, TAYLOR K, BARTUCCI EJ, FISCHER-DZOGA K, BEESON JH, GLAGOV S, WISSLER RW: Arterial foam cells with distinctive immunomorphologic and histochemical features of macrophages. *Am J Pathol* 100:57, 1980

87. BULKLEY BH, BUJA LM, FERRANS VJ, BULKLEY GB, ROBERTS WC: Tuberous xanthoma in homozygous type II hyperlipoproteinemia. *Arch Pathol* 99:293, 1975

88. GOLDSTEIN JL, BROWN MS: Atherosclerosis: The low-density lipoprotein receptor hypothesis. *Metabolism* 26:1257, 1977

89. GOLDSTEIN JL, BROWN MS: Familial hypercholesterolemia: Pathogenesis of a receptor disease. *Johns Hopkins Med J* 143:8, 1978

90. GOLDSTEIN JL, BROWN MS: Insights into the pathogenesis of atherosclerosis derived from studies in familial hypercholesterolemia, in Carlson LA, Pernow B (eds): *Metabolic Risk Factors in Atherosclerosis.* New York, Raven, 1981, pp 17–34

91. BAILEY JM: Regulation of cell cholesterol content, in *Atherogenesis: Initiating Factors,* Ciba Foundation Symposium, 12(NS):63, 1973

92. GOLDSTEIN JL, BROWN MS: The LDL pathway in human fibroblasts: A receptor-mediated mechanism for the regulation of cholesterol metabolism. *Curr Top Cell Regul* 11:147, 1976

93. GOLDSTEIN JL, BROWN MS: The low-density lipoprotein pathway and its relation to atherosclerosis. *Ann Rev Biochem* 46:897, 1977

94. BROWN MS, GOLDSTEIN JL: Familial hypercholesterolemia: Defective binding of lipoproteins to cultured fibroblasts associated with impaired regulation of 3-hydroxy-3-methylglutaryl coenzyme A reductase activity. *Proc Nat Acad Sci USA* 71:788, 1974

95. STEINBERG D: Lipoprotein metabolism—New insights from cell biology, in Kritschevsky D, Paoletti R, Holmes WL (eds): *Drugs, Lipid Metabolism, and Atherosclerosis.* New York, Plenum, 1978, p 3

96. MAHLEY RW, INNERARITY TL, PITAS RE, WEISGRABER KH, BROWN JH, GROSS E: Inhibition of lipoprotein binding to cell surface receptors of fibroblasts following selective modification of arginyl residues in arginine-rich and B-apoproteins. *J Biol Chem* 252:7279, 1977

97. GOLDSTEIN JL, BASU SK, BRUNSCHEDE GY, BROWN MS: Release of low density lipoprotein from its cell surface receptor by sulfated glycosaminoglycans. *Cell* 7:85, 1976

98. BROWN MS, GOLDSTEIN JL: Regulation of the activity of the low density lipoprotein receptor in human fibroblasts. *Cell* 6:307, 1975

99. SCHNEIDER WJ, BASU SK, MCPHAUL MJ, GOLDSTEIN JL, BROWN MS: Solubilization of the low density lipoprotein receptor. *Proc Nat Acad Sci USA* 76:5577, 1979

99a. SCHNEIDER WJ, GOLDSTEIN JL, BROWN MS: Partial purification and characterization of the low density lipoprotein receptor from bovine adrenal cortex. *J Biol Chem* 255:11442, 1980

99b. SCHNEIDER WJ, BEISIEGEL U, GOLDSTEIN JL, BROWN MS: Purification of the low density lipoprotein receptor, an acidic glycoprotein of 164,000 molecular weight. *J Biol Chem* 257:2664, 1982

100. PITAS RE, INNERARITY TL, ARNOLD KS, MAHLEY RW: Rate and equilibrium constants for binding of apo-E HDL_c and low density lipoproteins to human fibroblasts: Evidence for multiple receptor binding of apo-E HDL_c. *Proc Nat Acad Sci USA* 76:2311, 1979

101. PITAS RE, INNERARITY TL, MAHLEY RW: Cell surface receptor binding of

phospholipid protein complexes containing different ratios of receptor-active and -inactive E apoprotein. *J Biol Chem* 255:5454, 1980

102. BASU SK, GOLDSTEIN JL, ANDERSON RGW, BROWN MS; Degradation of cationized low density lipoprotein and regulation of cholesterol metabolism in homozygous familial hypercholesterolemia fibroblasts. *Proc Nat Acad Sci USA* 73:3178, 1976

103. WEISGRABER KH, INNERARITY TL, MAHLEY RW: Role of the lysine residues of plasma lipoproteins in high affinity binding to cell surface receptors on human fibroblasts. *J Biol Chem* 253:9053, 1978

104. ANDERSON RGW, GOLDSTEIN JL, BROWN MS: Localization of low density lipoprotein receptors on plasma membrane of normal human fibroblasts and their absence in cells from a familial hypercholesterolemia homozygote. *Proc Nat Acad Sci USA* 73:2434, 1976

105. ANDERSON RGW, BROWN MS, GOLDSTEIN JL: Role of the coated endocytic vesicle in the uptake of receptor-bound low density lipoprotein in human fibroblasts. *Cell* 10:351, 1977

106. ORCI L, CARPENTER J-L, PERRELET A, ANDERSON RGW, GOLDSTEIN JL, BROWN MS: Occurrence of low density lipoprotein receptors within large pits on the surface of human fibroblasts as demonstrated by freeze-etching. *Exp Cell Res* 113:1, 1978

107. ROTH TF, PORTER KR: Yolk protein uptake in the oocyte of the mosquito *Aedes Aegypti L. J Cell Biol* 20:313, 1964

108. PEARSE BMF: Coated vesicles from pig brain: Purification and biochemical characterization. *J Mol Biol* 97:93, 1975

109. ANDERSON RGW, VASILE E, MELLO RJ, BROWN MS, GOLDSTEIN JL: Immunocytochemical visualization of coated pits and vesicles in human fibroblasts: Relation to low density lipoprotein receptor distribution. *Cell* 15:919, 1978

110. GOLDSTEIN JL, BROWN MS: Binding and degradation of low density lipoproteins by cultured human fibroblasts: Comparison of cells from a normal subject and from a patient with homozygous familial hypercholesterolemia. *J Biol Chem* 249:5153, 1974

111. GOLDSTEIN JL, DANA SE, FAUST JR, BEAUDET AL, BROWN MS: Role of lysosomal acid lipase in the metabolism of plasma low density lipoprotein: Observations in cultured fibroblasts from a patient with cholesteryl ester storage disease. *J Biol Chem* 250:8487, 1975

112. BROWN MS, FAUST JR, GOLDSTEIN JL: Role of the low density lipoprotein receptor in regulating the content of free and esterified cholesterol in human fibroblasts. *J Clin Invest* 55:783, 1975

113. CARPENTER J-L, GORDEN P, GOLDSTEIN JL, ANDERSON RGW, BROWN MS, ORCI L: Binding and internalization of ^{125}I-LDL in normal and mutant human fibroblasts: A quantitative autoradiographic study. *Exp Cell Res* 121:135, 1979

114. BROWN MS, GOLDSTEIN JL: A general scheme for the regulation of cholesterol metabolism in mammalian cells, in Dietschy JM, Gotto AM, Ontko J (eds): *Disturbances in Lipid and Lipoprotein Metabolism*, American Physiological Society, Bethesda, Md, 1978, p 173

115. BROWN MS, DANA SE, GOLDSTEIN JL: Regulation of 3-hydroxy-3-methylglutaryl coenzyme A reductase activity in cultured human fibroblasts: Comparison of cells from a normal subject and from a patient with homozygous familial hypercholesterolemia. *J Biol Chem* 249:789, 1974

116. GOLDSTEIN JL, DANA SE, BROWN MS: Esterification of low density lipoprotein in human fibroblasts and its absence in homozygous familial hypercholesterolemia. *Proc Nat Acad Sci USA* 71:4288, 1974

117. DIETSCHY JM, WILSON JD: Regulation of cholesterol metabolism. *N Engl J Med* 282:1128, 1970

118. HAVEL RJ, GOLDSTEIN JL, BROWN MS: Lipoproteins and lipid transport, in Bondy PK, Rosenberg LE (eds): *Metabolic Control and Disease*, 8th ed. Philadelphia, Saunders, 1980, p 393

119. GOLDSTEIN JL, DANA SE, BRUNSCHEDE GY, BROWN MS: Genetic heterogeneity in familial hypercholesterolemia: Evidence for two different mutations affecting functions of low-density lipoprotein receptor. *Proc Nat Acad Sci USA* 72:1092, 1975

120. GOLDSTEIN JL, BROWN MS, STONE NJ: Genetics of the LDL receptor: Evidence that the mutations affecting binding and internalization are allelic. *Cell* 12:629, 1977

121. BROWN MS, GOLDSTEIN JL: Analysis of mutant strain of human fibroblasts with a defect in the internalization of receptor-bound low density lipoprotein. *Cell* 9:663, 1976

122. KANDUTSCH AA, CHEN HW; Inhibition of sterol synthesis in cultured mouse cells by 7α-hydroxycholesterol, 7β-hydroxycholesterol, and 7-ketocholesterol. *J Biol Chem* 248:8408, 1973

123. BROWN MS, GOLDSTEIN JL: Suppression of 3-hydroxy-3-methylglutaryl coenzyme A reductase activity and inhibition of growth of human fibroblasts by 7-ketocholesterol. *J Biol Chem* 249:7306, 1974

124. BROWN MS, DANA SE, GOLDSTEIN JL: Cholesterol ester formation in cultured human fibroblasts: Stimulation by oxygenated sterols. *J Biol Chem* 250:4025, 1975

125. BROWN MS, GOLDSTEIN JL: Expression of the familial hypercholesterolemia gene in heterozygotes: Mechanism for a dominant disorder in man. *Science* 185:61, 1974

126. GOLDSTEIN JL, BROWN MS: Expression of the familial hypercholesterolemia gene in heterozygotes: Model for a dominant disorder in man. *Trans Assoc Am Physicians* 87:120, 1974

127. BROWN MS, GOLDSTEIN JL: Familial hypercholesterolemia: A genetic defect in the low-density lipoprotein receptor. *N Engl J Med* 294:1386, 1976

128. GOLDSTEIN JL, BROWN MS, ANDERSON RGW: The LDL pathway in human fibroblasts: Biochemical and ultrastructural correlations, in Brinkley BR, Porter KR (eds): *International Cell Biology 1976–1977*. New York, Rockefeller University Press, 1977, p 639

129. MCKUSICK VA: Analytic review: Phenotypic diversity of human diseases resulting from allelic series. *Am J Hum Genet* 25:446, 1973

130. ANDERSON RGW, GOLDSTEIN JL, BROWN MS: A mutation that impairs the ability of lipoprotein receptors to localize in coated pits on the cell surface of human fibroblasts. *Nature* 270:659, 1977

131. GOLDSTEIN JL, BUJA LM, ANDERSON RGW, BROWN MS: Receptor-mediated uptake of macromolecules and their delivery to lysosomes in human fibroblasts, in Segal HL, Doyle DF (eds): *Protein Turnover and Lysosome Function*. New York, Academic, 1978, p 455

132. VAN LEUVEN F: Personal communication, 1980

133. GOLDSTEIN JL, ANDERSON RGW, BROWN MS: Coated pits, coated vesicles, and receptor-mediated endocytosis. *Nature* 279:679, 1979

134. GOLDSTEIN JL, KOTTKE B, BROWN MS: Biochemical genetics of LDL receptor mutations in familial hypercholesterolemia, in *Proceeding of 5th International Congress of Human Genetics*, 1982, in press

134a. MIYAKE Y, TAJINA S, YAMAMURA T, YAMAMOTO A: Homozygous familial hypercholesterolemia mutant with a defect in internalization of low density lipoprotein. *Proc Nat Acad Sci USA* 78:5151, 1981

135. INNERARITY TL, PITAS RE, MAHLEY RW: Receptor binding of cholesterol-induced high-density lipoproteins containing predominantly apoprotein E to cultured fibroblasts with mutations at the low-density lipoprotein receptor locus. *Biochemistry* 19:4359, 1980

136. LENARD J, COMPANS RW: The membrane structure of lipid-containing viruses. *Biochim Biophys Acta* 344:51, 1974

137. KNIPE DM, BALTIMORE D, LODISH HF: Separate pathways of maturation of the major structural proteins of vesicular stomatitis virus. *J Virol* 21:1128, 1977

138. GOLDSTEIN JL, SOBHANI MK, FAUST JR, BROWN MS: Heterozygous familial hypercholesterolemia: Failure of normal allele to compensate for mutant allele at a regulated genetic locus. *Cell* 9:195, 1976

139. FAUST JR, GOLDSTEIN JL, BROWN MS: Receptor-mediated uptake of low density lipoprotein and utilization of its cholesterol for steroid synthesis in cultured mouse adrenal cells. *J Biol Chem* 252:4861, 1977

140. KOVANEN PT, FAUST JR, BROWN MS, GOLDSTEIN JL: Low density lipoprotein receptors in bovine adrenal cortex. I. Receptor-mediated uptake of low density lipoprotein and utilization of its cholesterol for steroid synthesis in cultured adrenocortical cells. *Endocrinology* 104:599, 1979

141. BROWN MS, KOVANEN PT, GOLDSTEIN JL: Receptor-mediated uptake of lipoprotein-cholesterol and its utilization for steroid synthesis in the adrenal cortex. *Recent Prog Hormone Res* 35:215, 1979

142. BROWN MS, KOVANEN PT, GOLDSTEIN JL: Evolution of the LDL receptor concept—from cultured cells to intact animals. *Ann NY Acad Sci* 348:48, 1980

143. HO YK, BROWN MS, BILHEIMER DW, GOLDSTEIN JL: Regulation of low density lipoprotein receptor activity in freshly isolated human lymphocytes. *J Clin Invest* 58:1465, 1976

144. BILHEIMER DW, HO YK, BROWN MS, ANDERSON RGW, GOLDSTEIN JL: Genetics of the low density lipoprotein receptor: Diminished receptor activity in lymphocytes from heterozygotes with familial hypercholesterolemia. *J Clin Invest* 61:678, 1978

145. KRIEGER M, BROWN MS, FAUST JR, GOLDSTEIN JL: Replacement of endogenous cholesteryl esters of low density lipoprotein with exogenous cholesteryl linoleate: Reconstitution of a biologically active lipoprotein particle. *J Biol Chem* 253:4093, 1978

146. KRIEGER M, SMITH LC, ANDERSON RGW, GOLDSTEIN JL, KAO YJ, POWNALL HJ, GOTTO AM, JR, BROWN MS: Reconstituted low density lipoprotein: A vehicle for the delivery of hydrophobic fluorescent probes to cells. *J Supra Struct* 10:467, 1979

147. HO YK, FAUST JR, BILHEIMER DW, BROWN MS, GOLDSTEIN JL: Regulation of cholesterol synthesis by low density lipoprotein in isolated human lymphocytes: Comparison of cells from normal subjects and patients with homozygous familial hypercholesterolemia and abetalipoproteinemia. *J Exp Med* 145:1531, 1977

148. BROWN MS, GOLDSTEIN JL: Familial hypercholesterolemia: Unraveling a genetic receptor disease. *Trans Assoc Am Phys* 90:91, 1977

149. HO YK, SMITH G, BROWN MS, GOLDSTEIN JL: Low-density lipoprotein (LDL) receptor activity in human acute myelogenous leukemia cells. *Blood* 52:1099, 1978

150. BASU SK, GOLDSTEIN JL, BROWN MS: Characterization of the low density lipoprotein receptor in membranes prepared from human fibroblasts. *J Biol Chem* 253:3852, 1978

151. KOVANEN PT, BASU SK, GOLDSTEIN JL, BROWN MS: Low density lipoprotein receptors in bovine adrenal cortex. II. Low density lipoprotein binding to membranes prepared from fresh tissue. *Endocrinology* 104:610, 1979

152. JESKE DJ, DIETSCHY JM: Regulation of rates of cholesterol synthesis in vivo in the liver and carcass of the rat measured using [³H]water. *J Lipid Res* 21:364, 1980

153. BALASUBRAMANIAM S, GOLDSTEIN JL, FAUST JR, BROWN MS: Evidence for regulation of 3-hydroxy-3-methylglutaryl coenzyme A reductase activity and cholesterol synthesis in nonhepatic tissues of rat. *Proc Nat Acad Sci USA* 73:2564, 1976

154. ANDERSON JM, DIETSCHY JM: Cholesterogenesis: Depression in extrahepatic tissues with 4-aminopyrazolo[3,4-d]pyrimidine. *Science* 193:903, 1976

155. BALASUBRAMANIAM S, GOLDSTEIN JL, FAUST JR, BRUNSCHEDE GY, BROWN MS: Lipoprotein-mediated regulation of 3-hydroxy-3-methylglutaryl coenzyme A reductase activity and cholesteryl ester metabolism in the adrenal gland of the rat. *J Biol Chem* 252:1771, 1977

156. ANDERSON JM, DIETSCHY JM: Regulation of sterol synthesis in 15 tissues of rat. II. Role of rat and human high and low density plasma lipoproteins and of rat chylomicron remnants. *J Biol Chem* 252:3652, 1977

157. SHIFF TS, ROHEIM PS, EDER HA: Effects of high sucrose diets and 4-aminopyrazolopyrimidine on serum lipids and lipoproteins in the rat. *J Lipid Res* 12:596, 1971

158. KOVANEN PT, SCHNEIDER WJ, HILLMAN GM, GOLDSTEIN JL, BROWN MS: Separate mechanisms for the uptake of high and low density lipoproteins by mouse adrenal gland *in vivo*. *J Biol Chem* 254:5498, 1979

159. KOVANEN PT, GOLDSTEIN JL, CHAPPELL DA, BROWN MS: Regulation of low density lipoprotein receptors by adrenocorticotropin in the adrenal gland of mice and rats *in vivo*. *J Biol Chem* 255:5591, 1980

160. SHERRILL BC, DIETSCHY JM: Characterization of the sinusoidal transport process responsible for uptake of chylomicrons by the liver. *J Biol Chem* 253:1859, 1978

161. SHERRILL BC, INNERARITY TL, MAHLEY RW: Rapid hepatic clearance of the canine lipoproteins containing only the E apoprotein by a high affinity receptor. *J Biol Chem* 255:1804, 1980

162. KOVANEN PT, BROWN MS, GOLDSTEIN JL: Increased binding of low density lipoprotein to liver membranes from rats treated with 17α-ethinyl estradiol. *J Biol Chem* 254:11367, 1979

163. CHAO Y-S, WINDLER EE, CHEN GC, HAVEL RJ: Hepatic catabolism of rat and human lipoproteins in rats treated with 17α-ethinyl estradiol. *J Biol Chem* 254:11360, 1979

164. WINDLER EET, KOVANEN PT, CHAO Y-S, BROWN MS, HAVEL RJ, GOLDSTEIN JL: The estradiol-stimulated lipoprotein receptor of rat liver: A binding site that mediates the uptake of rat lipoprotein containing apoproteins B and E. *J Biol Chem* 255:10464, 1980

165. CHAO Y-S, JONES AL, HRADEK GT, WINDLER EET, HAVEL RJ: Autoradiographic localization of the sites of uptake, cellular transport and catabolism of low density lipoproteins in the liver of normal and estrogen-treated rats. *Proc Nat Acad Sci USA*, 78:597, 1981

166. KOVANEN PT, BROWN MS, BASU SK, BILHEIMER DW, GOLDSTEIN JL: Saturation and suppression of hepatic lipoprotein receptors: A mechanism for the hypercholesterolemia of cholesterol-fed rabbits. *Proc Nat Acad Sci USA*, 78:1396, 1981

167. KOVANEN PT, BILHEIMER DW, GOLDSTEIN JL, JARAMILLO J, BROWN MS: A regulatory role for hepatic low density lipoprotein receptors *in vivo* in the dog. *Proc Nat Acad Sci USA*, 78:1194, 1981

168. PITTMAN RC, ATTIE AD, CAREW TE, STEINBERG D: Tissue sites of degradation of low density lipoprotein: Application of a method for determining the fate of plasma proteins. *Proc Nat Acad Sci* 76:5345, 1979

169. CAREW TE, FORAN WA, STEINBERG D: Tissue sites of degradation of unmodified and reductively methylated low density lipoprotein in the rat. *Circulation* 62(part II):(III)17, 1980

170. CARRELLA M, COOPER AD: High affinity binding of chylomicron remnants to rat liver plasma membranes. *Proc Nat Acad Sci USA*, 76:338, 1979

171. BACHORIK PS, KWITEROVICH PO, COOKE JC: Isolation of a porcine liver plasma membrane fraction that binds low density lipoproteins. *Biochemistry* 17:5287, 1978

171a. BROWN MS, KOVANEN PT, GOLDSTEIN JL: Regulation of plasma cholesterol by lipoprotein receptors. *Science* 212:628, 1981

172. LANGER T, STROBER W, LEVY RI: The metabolism of low density lipoprotein in familial type II hyperlipoproteinemia. *J Clin Invest* 51:1528, 1972

173. BILHEIMER DW, GOLDSTEIN JL, GRUNDY SM, BROWN MS: Reduction in cholesterol and low density lipoprotein synthesis after portacaval shunt surgery in a patient with homozygous familial hypercholesterolemia. *J Clin Invest* 56:1420, 1975

174. BILHEIMER DW, STONE NJ, GRUNDY SM: Metabolic studies in familial hypercholesterolemia: Evidence for a gene-dosage effect *in vivo*. *J Clin Invest* 64:524, 1979

175. PACKARD CJ, THIRD JLHC, SHEPHERD J, LORIMER AR, MORGAN HG, LAWRIE TDV: Low density lipoprotein metabolism in a family of familial hypercholesterolemic patients. *Metabolism* 25:995, 1976

176. SIMONS LA, REICHL D, MYANT NB, MANCINI M: The metabolism of the apoprotein of plasma low density lipoprotein in familial hyperbetalipoproteinaemia in the homozygous form. *Atherosclerosis* 21:283, 1975

177. THOMPSON GR, MYANT NB: Low density lipoprotein turnover in familial hypercholesterolaemia after plasma exchange. *Atherosclerosis* 23:371, 1976

178. THOMPSON GR, SPINKS T, RANICAR A, MYANT NB: Non-steady-state studies of low-density lipoprotein turnover in familial hypercholesterolaemia. *Clin Sci Mol Med* 52:361, 1977

179. SOUTAR AK, MYANT NB, THOMPSON GR: Simultaneous measurement of apolipoprotein B turnover in very-low- and low-density lipoproteins in familial hypercholesterolaemia. *Atherosclerosis* 28:247, 1977

180. WATANABE T, TANAKA K, YANAI N: Essential familial hypercholesterolemic xanthomatosis—An autopsy case with special reference to the pathogenesis of its cardiovascular lipidosis. *Acta Pathol Jap* 18:319, 1968

181. MIETTINEN M: Familial hypercholesterolaemic xanthomatosis and coronary heart disease in a ten-year old girl. *Ann Paediat Fenn* 13:35, 1967

182. CHOMETTE G, DEGENNES JL, DELCOURT A, HAMMOU JC, PERIE G: La xanthomatose cutanéo-tendineuse hypercholestérolémique familiale: Etude anatomo-clinique *Annales d'Anatomie Pathologique* 16:233, 1971

183. SOUTAR AK, MYANT NB, THOMPSON GR: Metabolism of apolipoprotein B—containing lipoproteins in familial hypercholesterolaemia. *Atherosclerosis* 32:315, 1979

184. JANUS ED, NICOLL A, WOOTTON R, TURNER PR, MAGILL PJ, LEWIS B: Quantitative studies of very low density lipoprotein: conversion to low density lipoprotein in normal controls and primary hyperlipidaemic states and the role of direct secretion of low density lipoprotein in heterozygous familial hypercholesterolaemia. *Eur J Clin Invest* 10:149, 1980

184a. Bilheimer DW, Eisenberg S, Levy RI: The metabolism of very low density lipoprotein proteins. I. Preliminary *in vitro* and *in vivo* observations. *Biochim Biophys Acta* 260:212, 1972

185. BROWN MS, GOLDSTEIN JL: Familial hypercholesterolemia: A genetic defect in the low-density lipoprotein receptor. *N Engl J Med* 294:1386, 1976

186. SHEPHERD J, BICKER S, LORIMER AR, PACKARD CJ: Receptor mediated low density lipoprotein catabolism in man. *J Lipid Res* 20:999, 1979

187. SHEPHERD J, PACKARD CJ, BICKER S, LAWRIE TDV, MORGAN HG: Cholestyramine promotes receptor-mediated low-density-lipoprotein catabolism. *N Engl J Med* 302:1219, 1980

188. THOMPSON GR, SOUTAR AK, KNIGHT BL, GAVIGAN S, MYANT NB, SHEPHERD J: Evidence for defect of receptor-mediated low-density lipoprotein catabolism in familial hypercholesterolaemia *in vivo*. *Clin Sci* 58:2p, 1980

189. THOMPSON GR, SOUTAR AK, SPENGEL FA, JADHAV A, GAVIGAN SJP, MYANT NB: Defects of receptor-mediated low density lipoprotein catabolism in homozygous familial hypercholesterolemia and hypothyroidism *in vivo*. *Proc Nat Acad Sci USA* 78:2591, 1981

190. CHAIT A, BIERMAN EL, ALBERS JJ: Regulatory role of triiodothyronine in the degradation of low density lipoprotein by cultured human skin fibroblasts. *J Clin Endocrinol Met* 48:887, 1979

191. GOLDSTEIN JL, HO YK, BASU SK, BROWN MS: Binding site on macrophages that mediates uptake and degradation of acetylated low density lipoprotein, producing massive cholesterol deposition. *Proc Nat Acad Sci USA* 76:333, 1979

192. BROWN MS, GOLDSTEIN JL, KRIEGER M, HO YK, ANDERSON RGW: Reversible accumulation of cholesteryl esters in macrophages incubated with acetylated lipoproteins. *J Cell Biol* 82:597, 1979

193. EDELSON PJ, COHN ZA: Purification and cultivation of monocytes and macrophages, in Bloom BR, David JR (eds): *In Vitro Methods in Cell-Mediated and Tumor Immunity*. New York, Academic Press, 1976, p 333

194. BROWN MS, BASU SK, FALCK JR, HO YK, GOLDSTEIN JL: The scavenger cell pathway for lipoprotein degradation: Specificity of the binding site that mediates the uptake of negatively-charged LDL by macrophages. *J Supra Struct*, 13:67, 1980

195. GOLDSTEIN JL, BROWN MS, KRIEGER M, ANDERSON RGW, MINTZ B: Demonstration of low density lipoprotein receptors in mouse teratocarcinoma stem cells and description of a method for producing receptor-deficient mutant mice. *Proc Nat Acad Sci USA* 76:2843, 1979

196. FOGELMAN AM, SCHECHTER I, SEAGER J, HOKOM M, CHILD JS, EDWARDS PA: Malondialdehyde alteration of low density lipoproteins leads to cholesteryl ester accumulation in human monocyte-macrophages. *Proc Nat Acad Sci USA* 77:2214, 1980

197. BROWN MS, HO YK, GOLDSTEIN JL: The cholesteryl ester cycle in macrophage foam cells: Continual hydrolysis and re-esterification of cytoplasmic cholesteryl esters. *J Biol Chem* 255:9344, 1980

198. Bailey JM: Lipid metabolism in cultured cells. IV. Serum alpha globulins and cellular cholesterol exchange. *Exp Cell Res* 37:175, 1965

199. Stein O, Stein Y: The removal of cholesterol from Landschutz ascites cells by high-density apolipoprotein. *Biochim Biophys Acta* 326:232, 1973

200. Ho YK, Brown MS, Goldstein JL: Hydrolysis and excretion of cytoplasmic cholesteryl esters by macrophages: Stimulation by high density lipoprotein and other agents. *J Lipid Res* 21:391, 1980

201. Phillips MC, McLean LR, Stoudt GW, Rothblat GH: Mechanism of cholesterol efflux from cells. *Atherosclerosis* 36:409, 1980

202. St Clair RW: Metabolism of the arterial wall and atherosclerosis. *Athero Rev* 1:61, 1976

203. Smith JB, Ingerman CM, Silver MJ: Malondialdehyde formation as an indicator of prostaglandin production by human platelets. *J Lab Clin Med* 88:167, 1976

204. Basu SK, Brown MS, Ho YK, Goldstein JL: Degradation of low density lipoprotein/dextran sulfate complexes associated with deposition of cholesteryl esters in mouse macrophages. *J Biol Chem* 254:7141, 1979

205. Goldstein JL, Ho YK, Brown MS, Innerarity TL, Mahley RW: Cholesteryl ester metabolism in macrophages resulting from receptor-mediated uptake and degradation of hypercholesterolemia canine β-very low density lipoproteins. *J Biol Chem* 255:1839, 1980

206. Mahley RW, Innerarity TL, Brown MS, Ho YK, Goldstein JL: Stimulation by β-very low density lipoproteins from cholesterol-fed animals of several species. *J Lipid Res* 21:970, 1980

207. Grundy SM, Ahrens EH Jr, Salen G: Interruption of the enterohepatic circulation of bile acids in man: Comparative effects of cholestyramine and ileal exclusion on cholesterol metabolism. *J Lab Clin Med* 78:94, 1971

208. Grundy SM, Ahrens EH Jr, Davignon J: The interaction of cholesterol absorption and cholesterol synthesis in man. *J Lipid Res* 10:304, 1969

209. Quintao E, Grundy SM, Ahrens EH Jr: Effects of dietary cholesterol on the regulation of total body cholesterol in man. *J Lipid Res* 12:233, 1971

210. Khachadurian AK, Kawahara FS: Cholesterol synthesis by cultured fibroblasts: Decreased feedback inhibition in familial hypercholesterolemia. *J Lab Clin Med* 83:7, 1974

211. Lewis B, Myant NB: Studies in the metabolism of cholesterol in subjects with normal plasma cholesterol levels and in patients with essential hypercholesterolaemia. *Clin Sci* 32:201, 1967

212. Schwarz KB, Witzum J, Schonfeld G, Grundy SM, Connor WE: Elevated cholesterol and bile acid synthesis in a young patient with homozygous familial hypercholesterolemia. *J Clin Invest* 64:756, 1979

213. Samuel P, Perl W, Holtzman CM, Rochman ND, Lieberman S: Long-term kinetics of serum xanthoma cholesterol radioactivity in patients with hypercholesterolemia. *J Clin Invest* 51:266, 1972

214. Morganroth J, Levy RI, McMahon AE, Gotto AM Jr: Pseudohomozygous type II hyperlipoproteinemia. *J Pediatr* 85:639, 1974

215. Mishkel MA: Pseudohomozygous and pseudoheterozygous type II hyperlipoproteinemia. *Am J Dis Child* 130:991, 1976

216. Breslow JL: Personal communication, 1977

217. Kayden HJ: Personal communication, 1977

218. Goldstein JL: Genetic aspects of hyperlipidemia in coronary heart disease. *Hosp Prac* 8:53, 1973

219. Rose HG, Kranz P, Weinstock M, Juliano J, Haft JI: Inheritance of combined hyperlipoproteinemia: Evidence for a new lipoprotein phenotype. *Am J Med* 148:160, 1973

220. Krieger M, Brown MS, Goldstein JL: Unpublished observations

221. Goldstein JL, Brown MS, Rose V, Hughes HE, Steiner G: Unpublished observations

222. Weinker TF, Utermann G, Ropers H-H: Prenatal diagnosis of homozygous familial hypercholesterolemia: Investigation of a case at risk. *Clin Genet* 9:545, 1976

223. Darmady JM, Fosbrooke AS, Lloyd JK: Prospective study of serum cholesterol levels during first year of life. *Brit Med J* 2:685, 1972

224. Goldstein JL, Albers JJ, Schrott HG, Hazard WR, Bierman EL, Motulsky AR: Plasma lipid levels and coronary heart disease in adult relatives of newborns with normal and elevated cord blood lipids. *Am J Hum Genet* 26:727, 1974

225. Goldstein JL, Helgeson JAS, Brown MS: Inhibition of cholesterol synthesis with compactin renders growth of cultured cells dependent on the low density lipoprotein receptor. *J Biol Chem* 254:5403, 1979

226. Brown MS, Goldstein JL: Multivalent feedback regulation of HMG CoA reductase, a control mechanism coordinating isoprenoid synthesis and cell growth. *J Lipid Res* 21:505, 1980

227. Hashim SA, Van Itallie TB: Cholestyramine resin therapy for hypercholesterolemia. *JAMA* 192:289, 1965

228. Grundy SM: Treatment of hypercholesterolemia by interference with bile acid metabolism. *Arch Intern Med* 130:638, 1972

229. Levy RI: Drugs used in the treatment of hyperlipoproteinemias, in Gilman AG, Goodman LS, Gilman A (eds): *The Pharmacological Basis of Therapeutics*, 6th ed. New York: Macmillan, 1980, p 834

230. Levy RI, Fredrickson DS, Stone NJ, Bilheimer DW, Brown WV, Glueck CJ, Gotto AM, Herbert PN, Kwiterovich PO, Langer T, LaRosa J, Lux SE, Rider AK, Shulman RS, Sloan HR: Cholestyramine in type II hyperlipoproteinemia. A double-blind trial. *Ann Intern Med* 79:51, 1973

230a. Kuo PT, Hayase K, Kostis JB, Moreyra AE: Use of combined diet and cholestipol in long-term (7–7-½ years) treatment of patients with type II hyperlipoproteinemia. *Circulation* 59:199, 1979

231. Slater HR, Packard CJ, Bicker S, Shepherd J: Effects of cholestyramine on receptor mediated plasma clearance and tissue uptake of human low density lipoproteins in the rabbit. *J Biol Chem* 255:10210, 1980

232. Moutafis CD, Simons LA, Myant NB, Adams PW, Wynn V: The effect of cholestyramine on the faecal excretion of bile acids and neutral steroids in familial hypercholesterolaemia. *Atherosclerosis* 26:329, 1977

233. Endo A, Kuroda M, Tanzawa K: Competitive inhibition of 3-hydroxy-3-methylglutaryl coenzyme A reductase by ML-236A and ML-236B fungal metabolites, having hypocholesterolemic activity. *FEBS Lett* 72:323, 1976

234. Brown MS, Faust JR, Goldstein JL, Kaneko I, Endo A: Induction of 3-hydroxy-3-methylglutaryl coenzyme A reductase activity in human fibroblasts incubated with compactin (ML-236B), a competitive inhibitor of the reductase. *J Biol Chem* 253:1121, 1978

235. Alberts AW, Chen J, Kuron G, Hunt V, Huff J, Hoffman C, Rothrock J, Lopez M, Joshua H, Harris E, Patchett A, Monaghan R, Currie S, Stapley E, Albers-Schonberg G, Hensens O, Hirschfield J, Hoogsteen K, Liesch J, Springer J: Mevinolin, a highly potent competitive inhibitor of HMG-CoA reductase and cholesterol lowering agent. *Proc Nat Acad Sci USA* 77:3957, 1980

236. Tsujita Y, Kuroda M, Tanzawa K, Kitano N, Endo A: Hypolipidemic effects in dogs of ML-236B, a competitive inhibitor of 3-hydroxy-3-methylglutaryl coenzyme A reductase. *Atherosclerosis* 32:307, 1979

237. Kuroda M, Tsujita Y, Tanzawa K, Endo A: Hypolipidemic effects in monkeys of ML-236B, a competitive inhibitor of 3-hydroxy-3-methylglutaryl coenzyme A reductase. *Lipids* 14:585, 1979

238. Endo A: Personal communication, 1979

239. Yamamoto A, Sudo H, Endo A: Therapeutic effects of ML-236B in primary hypercholesterolemia. *Atherosclerosis* 35:259, 1980

240. Endo A, Tsujita Y, Kuroda M, Tanzawa K: Effects of ML-236B on cholesterol metabolism in mice and rats: Lack of hypocholesterolemic activity in normal animals. *Biochim Biophys Acta* 575:266, 1979

241. Buchwald H, Moore RB, Varco RL: Ten years clinical experience with partial ileal bypass in management of the hyperlipidemias. *Ann Surg* 180:384, 1974

242. Thompson GR, Gotto AM Jr: Ileal bypass in the treatment of hyperlipoproteinaemia. *Lancet* 2:35, 1973

243. Miettinen TA, Lempinen M: Cholestyramine and ileal by-pass in the treatment of familial hypercholesterolaemia. *Eur J Clin Invest* 7:509, 1977

244. Glueck CJ, Tsang RC, Fallat RW, Mellies M: Therapy of familial hypercholesterolemia in childhood: Diet and cholestyramine resin for 24 to 36 months. *Pediatr* 60:433, 1977

245. Farah JR, Kwiterovich PO Jr, Neill CA: Dose-effect relation of cholestyramine in children and young adults with familial hypercholesterolaemia. *Lancet* 1:59, 1977

246. Glueck CJ, Tsang RC, Fallat RW, Mellies MJ: Diet in children heterozygous for familial hypercholesterolemia. *Am J Dis Child* 131:162, 1977

247. Malloy MJ, Kane JP, Rowe JS: Familial hypercholesterolemia in children: Treatment with p-aminosalicylic acid. *Pediatrics* 61:365, 1978

248. Khachadurian AK: Cholestyramine therapy in patients homozygous for familial hypercholesterolemia (familial hypercholesterolemic xanthomatosis). *J Athero Res* 8:177, 1968

249. Starzl TE, Putnam CW, Chase HP, Porter KA: Portacaval shunt in hyperlipoproteinaemia. *Lancet* 2:94, 1973

250. Torsvik H, Fischer JE, Feldman HA, Lees RS: Effects of intravenous hyperalimentation on plasma-lipoproteins in severe familial hypercholesterolaemia. *Lancet* 1:601, 1975

251. King MEE, Breslow JL, Lees RS: Plasma-exchange therapy of homozygous familial hypercholesterolemia. *N Engl J Med* 302:1457, 1980

252. Starzl TE, Chase HP, Putnam CW, Nora JJ: Follow-up of patient with portacaval shunt for the treatment of hyperlipidaemia. *Lancet* 2:714, 1974

253. Starzl TE, Putnam CW, Koep LJ: Portacaval shunt and hyperlipidemia. *Arch Surg* 113:71, 1978

254. Stein EA, Mieny C, Spitz L, Saaron I, Pettifor J, Heimann KW, Bersohn I, Dinner M: Portacaval shunt in four patients with homozygous hypercholesterolaemia. *Lancet* 1:832, 1975

255. McMillian GC: Personal communication, 1978

256. Thompson GR, Lowenthal R, Myant NB: Plasma exchange in the management of homozygous familial hypercholesterolaemia. *Lancet* 1:1208, 1975

257. THOMPSON GR: Management of familial hypercholesterolemia and new approaches to the treatment of atherosclerosis. *Athero Rev* 5:67, 1979

258. THOMPSON GR, MYANT NB, KILPATRICK D, OAKLEY CM, RAPHAEL MJ, STEINER RE: Assessment of long-term plasma exchange for familial hypercholesterolaemia. *Brit Heart J* 43:680, 1980

259. DECKELBAUM RJ, LEES RS, SMALL DM, HEDBERG SE, GRUNDY SM: Failure of complete bile diversion and oral bile acid therapy in the treatment of homozygous familial hypercholesterolemia. *N Engl J Med* 296:465, 1977

260. BROWN MS, GOLDSTEIN JL: Receptor-mediated endocytosis: Insights from the lipoprotein receptor system. *Proc Nat Acad Sci USA* 76:3330, 1979

261. HEUSER J: Three-dimensional visualization of coated vesicle formation in fibroblasts. *J Cell Biol* 84:560, 1980

262. GOLDSTEIN JL, BROWN MS: The LDL receptor defect in familial hypercholesterolemia: Implications for pathogenesis and therapy. *Med Clin N Amer* 1982, in press

34

FAMILIAL DISEASES WITH STORAGE OF STEROLS OTHER THAN CHOLESTEROL: Cerebrotendinous Xanthomatosis and Sitosterolemia with Xanthomatosis

GERALD SALEN

SARAH SHEFER

VLADIMIR M. BERGINER

1. This chapter describes two lipid storage diseases, cerebrotendinous xanthomatosis and sitosterolemia with xanthomatosis, both of which are characterized by the accumulation of unusual sterols and cholesterol in the blood and tissues.

2. Cerebrotendinous xanthomatosis (CTX) is a rare familial sterol storage disease characterized by progressive neurologic dysfunction (dementia, spinal cord paresis, and cerebellar ataxia), tendon xanthomas, cataracts, and premature atherosclerosis. Cholestanol and cholesterol accumulate in every tissue, with particularly large deposits in nervous tissue, xanthomas, and bile. Fifty-three patients with the classic syndrome have been reported to date.

3. CTX is inherited as an autosomal recessive trait. The underlying biochemical defect involves a deficiency of a hepatic enzyme that catalyzes the 24S hydroxylation of 5β-cholestane-3α,7α,12α,25-tetrol, an intermediate on the bile acid synthetic pathway. The defective enzyme causes a block in bile acid synthesis, resulting in a marked deficiency of cholic acid and chenodeoxycholic acid and the excretion of bile acid precursors (bile alcohol glucuronides) in bile. The excessive tissue deposits of cholesterol and cholestanol are believed to be due to the increased hepatic synthesis of cholesterol and cholestanol, which results from the deficiency of bile acids (particularly chenodeoxycholic acid) in the enterohepatic circulation.

4. Treatment of patients with CTX with chenodeoxycholic acid inhibits abnormal bile acid synthesis, reduces plasma cholestanol concentrations, and offers the promise of preventing the further progression of the disease.

5. Sitosterolemia with xanthomatosis is a rare familial sterol storage disease characterized by tendon and tuberous xanthomas, premature atherosclerosis, and abnormal red blood cells. Increased amounts of the plant sterols campesterol and sitosterol, as well as cholesterol, are present in the plasma, red blood cells, xanthomas, and other tissues of affected individuals. Sixteen patients with the classic syndrome have been reported to date.

6. Sitosterolemia with xanthomatosis is inherited as an autosomal recessive trait. The basic biochemical defect is not known, but increased intestinal absorption coupled with decreased removal of plant sterols plays a role.

7. Treatment of patients with sitosterolemia consists of limiting the dietary absorption of plant sterols and cholesterol. This is accomplished with a diet low in plant sterol content along with using the resin cholestyramine to promote tissue sterol excretion.

This chapter describes two lipid storage diseases characterized by the accumulation of unusual sterols in the blood and tissues. In cerebrotendinous xanthomatosis (CTX), cholestanol (5α-cholestan-3β-ol) accumulates in blood and tissues, with disproportionately high amounts in the brain, tendons, lungs, and bile. The second disease, sitosterolemia with xanthomatosis, was first described in 1973 and involves the deposition of plant sterols, particularly sitosterol, in blood and tissues, notably as xanthomas. CTX is a progressive disorder that if untreated, results in the eventual death of the patient because of neurologic impairment or progressive atherosclerosis, or both. The prognosis in sitosterolemia may also be serious. Patients with this disorder may develop hemolytic anemia and atherosclerosis. In this chapter we describe both the clinical and pathologic features of these two syndromes and present evidence that administration of bile acids (chenodeoxycholic acid) may be an effective treatment for CTX, whereas the removal of bile acids (binding resins such as cholestyramine) may be an effective treatment for sitosterolemia.

CEREBROTENDINOUS XANTHOMATOSIS

Cerebrotendinous xanthomatosis (CTX) is a rare inherited disease characterized by xanthomas in tendons, lungs, and brain that develop in the presence of low plasma cholesterol levels. Principal clinical manifestations include progressive neurologic dysfunction, cerebellar ataxia, and spinal cord paresis, dementia, subnormal intelligence, cataracts, coronary atherosclerosis, and endocrine abnormalities [1]. In 1968, large amounts of cholestanol (5α-cholestan-3β-ol) were demonstrated within the central nervous system [2] and in xanthomas [3]. Subsequent studies showed that the cholestanol deposition was distributed throughout the body [4]. Extensive myelin destruction, foam cells, and gliosis were found in the brain stem and cerebellum, and increased amounts of both cholestanol and cholesterol were present in these tissues [4]. The excessive neutral sterol deposits develop in the presence of low normal plasma cholesterol and low density lipoprotein (LDL) concentrations. Plasma cholestanol levels are high, and bile acid synthesis is abnormal [4]. There is a defect in the oxidation of the cholesterol side chain in the formation of cholic and chenodeoxycholic acids, with low levels of biliary chenodeoxycholic acid [5]. Replacement therapy with chenodeoxycholic acid has normalized the plasma cholestanol levels and halted progression of the disease [6].

Historical Aspects

Credit for the description of CTX is given to van Bogaert, who in 1937 with Scherer and Epstein published the clinical and pathologic findings in a patient with dementia, ataxia, and cataracts, and xanthomas in the tendons and nervous system [1]. One year earlier, Schneider had described xanthomatous lesions in the nervous system of a mentally retarded and epileptic patient who died at age 36 [7]. Histopathologic studies showed lipid deposits in the dentate nucleus, substantia nigra, and basal ganglia, as well as partial demyelination, neuron dysfunction, and gliosis, but tendon xanthomas were not

described, and, therefore, it was not possible to establish conclusively that this patient had the same disorder as that described by van Bogaert. Later van Bogaert reported similar findings in a paternal cousin of his first patient [8, 9]. Although tendon xanthomas were not present, postmortem examination showed central nervous system lesions comparable to those of the first patient. Subsequently, Epstein and Lorenz [10] and Epstein and Kreitner [11] described patients with similar symptoms under the eponym "van Bogaert's disease." Since then, 48 additional patients, making a total of 53, have been reported [2, 3, 4, 7–40].

In 1968, Menkes and colleagues made the key discovery that the cerebrum and cerebellum of two patients with CTX contained greatly increased concentrations of cholestanol [2]. Since then, cholestanol has been demonstrated in increased amounts in blood and other tissues, particularly in xanthomas (tendon, tuberous, and pulmonary) and bile [3, 4, 28, 29, 32, 33, 36–40]. In addition, tissue cholesterol concentrations are elevated and the biliary bile acid pattern is distinctly abnormal, with low levels of chenodeoxycholic acid [4]. In 1974, Setoguchi et al. discovered a block in bile acid synthesis, which resulted in incomplete oxidation of the cholesterol side chain to a carboxylic acid [5]. More recent studies demonstrated the partial deletion of the enzyme that catalyzes the 24(S)-hydroxylation of 5β-cholestane-3α,7α,12α,25-tetrol to form 5β-cholestane-3α,7α,12α,24(S),25-pentol on the path to cholic acid. As a result, total bile acid production and pool size are diminished and hepatic sterol production is enhanced, presumably due to decreased feedback regulation by the lowered bile acid pool. Replacement therapy with chenodeoxycholic acid has resulted in reduced rates of cholesterol and cholestanol synthesis, diminished plasma cholestanol concentrations, and, importantly, has halted the progression of the disease.

Clinical Manifestations

Of the 53 patients reported to have CTX [1, 4, 7, 40], the diagnosis appears to be established in 46. Neuropathologic or chemical confirmation of the diagnosis is not available for 7 patients [10, 11, 13, 14, 15, 26], although they had many of the features typical of the disease. The major clinical features are listed in Table 34-1. They include Achilles tendon xanthomas (Fig. 34-1), neurologic dysfunction, subnormal intelli-

Table 34-1 Clinical findings in CTX

	No. of patients		
	Documented	Absent	Not mentioned
Tendon xanthomas			
Achilles	49	4	—
Other	16	33	4
Xanthelasma	6	15	32
Neurologic dysfunction			
Motor paresis	34	8	11
Ataxia	34	8	11
Speech	15	8	30
Cataracts	35	7	11
Low intelligence	38	5	10
Cardiovascular disease	4	21	28
Respiratory insufficiency	4	18	31
Endocrine abnormalities	3	2	49

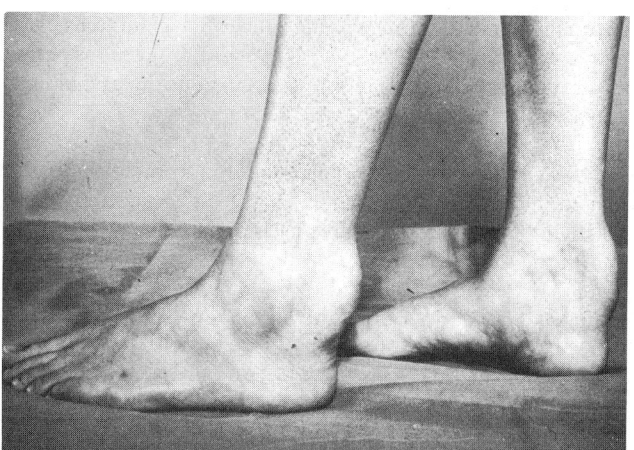

Figure 34-1 Achilles tendon xanthomas in CTX. (*Courtesy of Drs. M. Swartz and K. Burman.*)

gence, and cataracts (Fig. 34-2). Abnormalities have also been recorded in the cardiovascular, pulmonary, and endocrine systems. In one patient, severe hypothyroidism and adrenal insufficiency [4] were noted, while increased urinary adrenal steroids were detected in several individuals [28, 33]. Gallstones have been found in four patients with CTX.

The onset of symptoms is often insidious and unpredictable. Tendon xanthomas have been demonstrated by age 15 [13, 14], dementia at age 10 [1, 3], cataracts at age 15, and ataxia by age 18 [10, 11]. Van Bogaert et al. divided the course of this disease into several time phases [1]. The initial stage begins in childhood and is characterized by dementia. Mental retardation, mental deterioration, and borderline intelligence have often been described [1, 2, 7–15, 17, 19–30, 32–40]; but in some patients mental retardation was not present in childhood and did not affect the individual until the third or fourth decade of life. A few patients in the sixth decade of life have had normal intellectual function in spite of neurologic impairment (ataxia and spinal cord paresis) [4, 17].

Spasticity often associated with ataxia develops during adolescence and young adulthood and becomes progressively more severe. Juvenile cataracts and tendon xanthomas are seen in this second stage of the disease. With advancing age, spasticity becomes more severe, and usually by the fourth or fifth decade, the patient becomes incapacitated [1, 3, 10, 11, 13, 14]. Ataxia is usually associated with spasticity, but it may be absent [12, 13]. By young adulthood, the cataracts are well developed and require excision [1, 2, 8, 9, 13, 14, 22–28], but they are not always present [4, 10–12, 39, 40].

Tendon xanthomas have been observed in the second decade [2, 4, 10, 11, 13, 14, 21, 29, 30, 32, 38–40] but usually are not noticed until the third or fourth decade [1, 4, 8–11, 17, 22, 24–28, 39, 40]. The Achilles tendon is the most common site. Tendon xanthomas may occur on the tibial tuberosities [1, 10, 11, 17, 39, 40], the extensor tendons of the fingers, and in the triceps [4, 10, 11, 13, 14, 22, 24, 25, 27, 28, 37, 39, 40]. They are superficially similar to those seen in familial hypercholesterolemia (Chap. 33). These xanthomas are indistinguishable histologically from the xanthomas found in the hyperlipoproteinemic patients. Tuberous xanthomas and xanthelasma (palpebral xanthomas) may also be present [1, 8, 10, 11, 39, 40]. Achilles tendon xanthomas are not invariable. They were not found [4, 40] in two chemically documented CTX subjects.

In the third and final stage of CTX, enlargement of the xanthomas and neurologic deterioration are severe. As spasticity

and ataxia worsen, speech becomes difficult, and tremors and muscular atrophy, particularly of the distal musculature, become noticeable [1, 4, 8, 10, 12, 17, 22–24, 26, 28, 29, 32, 37, 39, 40]. Swallowing becomes impaired, and bladder and bowel incontenance develop [40]. Bilateral Babinski signs are present [1, 4, 12, 23, 28, 37, 39, 40], and pain and vibratory sensation may be lost [1, 8, 9, 37, 40]. Death usually results from progressive neurologic deterioration and pseudobulbar paralysis. Four of ten deaths reported so far have resulted from acute myocardial infarctions [4, 21, 23]. Death usually occurs between the fourth and sixth decades, but two sisters who were observed at age 44 and 46, respectively, had tendon xanthomas and spastic gait but were otherwise functioning normally [4]. A similar patient with tendon xanthomas, cataracts, and spastic walk was functioning well at age 44 [17].

Pathology

The most striking pathologic changes in CTX occur in the nervous system and in the tendons.

Nervous System The clinicopathologic description of the brain and spinal cord pathology has been provided by van Bogaert et al. [1, 3, 8, 9].

CEREBELLUM The most striking and consistent abnormalities of the nervous system occur in the cerebellum. Yellow, granulomatous deposits (xanthomas), which are present in the white matter of the lateral hemispheres, may reach 1.5 cm in diameter and may eventually extend to replace most of the white matter [1, 3, 8, 10, 22–24]. There may also be some atrophy of the adjacent folia [1, 23]; and there is extensive demyelination of the cerebellar white matter lateral to the dentate nucleus and superior cerebellar peduncles. The white matter adjacent to and medial to the dentate nucleus is spared [1, 7, 23]. Many cystic spaces and needle-shaped clefts (Fig. 34-3) are seen in these areas of demyelination. These cysts contain large mononuclear cells with foamy, vacuolated cytoplasm [1, 11, 12, 23]. Similar macrophages and multinucleated giant cells may surround the clefts and cysts [1, 23].

Frozen sections of the cerebellum stained with oil red O show neutral fat around the blood vessels and cystic spaces [1, 23]. The needle-shaped clefts do not stain with oil red O but are birefringent [1, 23]. In the cerebellar cortex adjacent to the

Figure 34-2 Zonular cortical lens cataracts in CTX. (*Courtesy of Drs. M. Swartz and K. Burman.*)

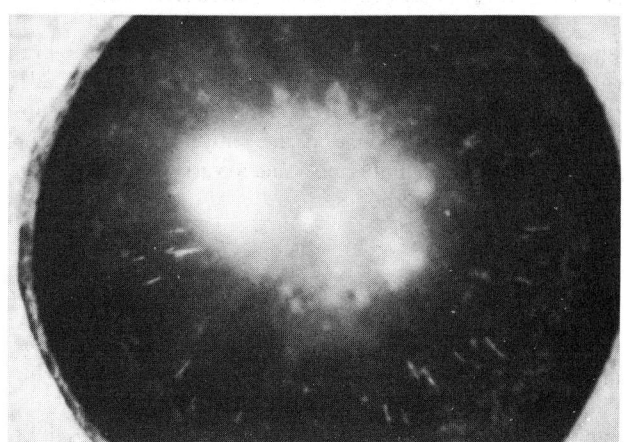

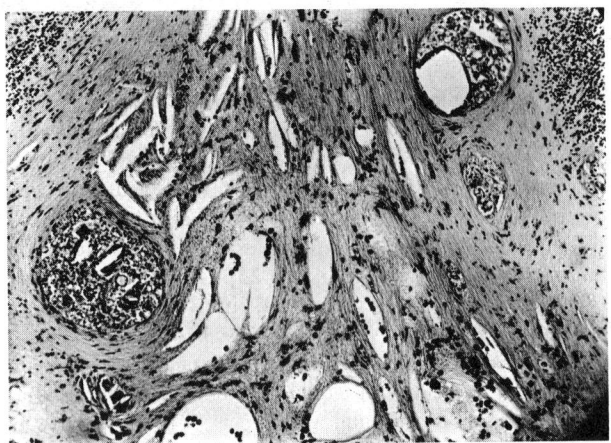

Figure 34-3 Section of cerebellum from a patient with CTX. Clefts and cystic areas of necrosis are surrounded by macrophages with foamy cytoplasm and multinucleated giant cells. ×104. (*Courtesy of Dr. P.D. Swanson* [23]. *Used by permission.*)

areas of demyelination, there is excessive loss of Purkinje cells and granule cells [1, 3, 23]. Philippart and van Bogaert noted almost complete destruction of the dentate and fastigial nuclei in one subject [3, 8]. Degeneration of olivocerebellar fibers has also been observed [1, 8].

FOREBRAIN   Xanthomas have also been observed in the cerebral peduncles and globus pallidus [1, 8]. Perivascular collections of large mononuclear cells with foamy cytoplasm may be found in the globus pallidus, caudate nucleus, and basal ganglia [1, 3, 8, 10, 22]. Foam cells may be scattered in the thalamus [1] and in the white matter adjacent to the lateral ventricles [1, 8, 22, 24]. Extensive demyelination occurs in the cerebral peduncles and in the fibers of the ansa lenticularis [1, 3, 23], as well as in areas of dense gliosis in the globus pallidus and in the central part of the corona radiata [3]. Marked atrophy of the entire optic pathway has been observed [1, 12]. The cerebral cortex is virtually free of the pathologic abnormalities, despite the presence of dementia and mental retardation in many patients.

BRAINSTEM   Gliosis and demyelination may be scattered thoughout the brainstem [1, 3, 8]. Van Bogaert et al. [1, 3, 8] have described the pathology of the lesions of the midbrain.

SPINAL CORD AND PERIPHERAL NERVES   As in the other parts of the nervous system, perivascular cuffing by large mononuclear cells may occur in the spinal cord [1, 23]. There may be extensive demyelination of the posterior and lateral columns [1, 3, 8] and of the pyramidal tracts from the cerebral peduncles to the interior extremes of the spinal cord [1, 3, 23]. Recent examination of several nerve biopsies from CTX subjects have shown demyelination and remyelination, with the production of onion bulbs and much variability in myelin thickness between internodes [36].

Other Tissues

TENDONS   An almost essential feature of CTX is the presence of large tendon xanthomas (Fig. 34-1). The gross appearance of the xanthomas is similar to that observed in patients with familial hypercholesterolemia (Chap. 33). Light microscopy reveals a dense accumulation of birefringent, crystalline

clefts surrounded by many multinucleated giant cells with foamy cytoplasm [1, 10, 12, 23] (Fig. 34-4). Collections of free fat around the blood vessels and throughout the granulomatous areas stain brightly with oil red O.

LUNG AND BONE   Granulomatous lesions containing needle-shaped birefringent crystalline clefts, multinucleated giant cells, and large foam cells have been observed in the lung [1, 23], in the femur [1, 8], and in the bodies of the lumbar vertebrae [1]. The lung lesions also contain extracellular deposits of lipid, particularly around the blood vessels [23].

CARDIOVASCULAR SYSTEM   Four patients with CTX have died (at ages 60, 46, 48, and 36 years) following myocardial infarction [4, 22–24]. The aorta and the atheromatous plaque obtained at autopsy of one patient contained cholestanol as 2 and 2.8 percent, respectively, of the total sterols [4]. Thus, premature atherosclerosis may be a common feature in this disease.

LENS   Zonular cortical lens opacities have been well documented as a part of CTX [1, 3, 5] (Fig. 34-2). Using electron microscopy, Seland and Slagsvold found electron-lucent areas in the anterior cortex and vacuoles in the epithelial cells of the lens of a patient [42].

LIVER   Recently, liver specimens from two patients were examined by light and electron microscopy [43]. Under low magnification (Fig. 34-5A), the hepatocytes contained a light golden pigment which at high magnification appeared in two forms: either as diffuse, amorphous electron-dense material enveloped by the smooth endoplasmic reticulum (Fig. 34-5B) or as free-floating bodies in the cytosol. In addition, the cytosol also contained free rhomboid-shaped crystals.

Lipid Metabolism

In most patients plasma cholesterol concentrations have been within the normal range, i.e., 117 to 220 mg/dl [1, 8, 13, 14, 27]. Elevated plasma cholesterol levels 240 to 400 mg/dl have been reported in a few patients, but normal values have also been observed in these same subjects [1, 10, 11, 39, 40].

Figure 34-4 Section of Achilles tendon from a patient with CTX. Large clefts are surrounded by evidence of cellular reaction, including a few darkly stained multinucleated giant cells. ×104. (*Courtesy of Dr. P. D. Swanson* [23]. *Used by permission.*)

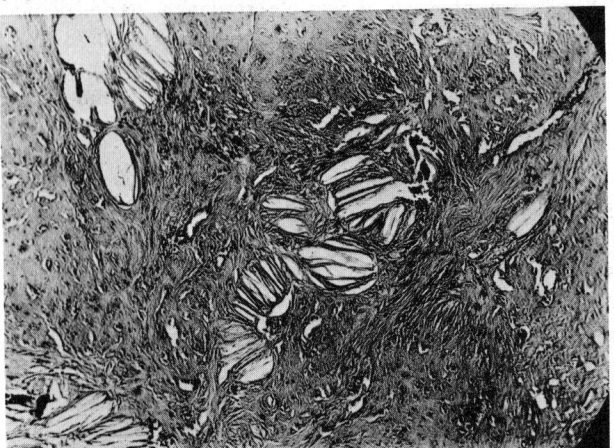

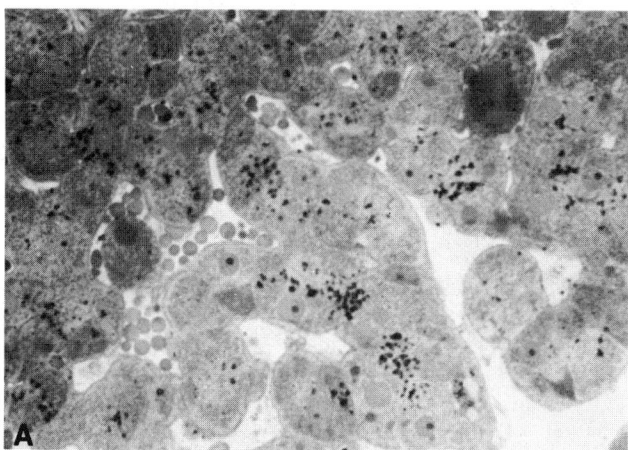

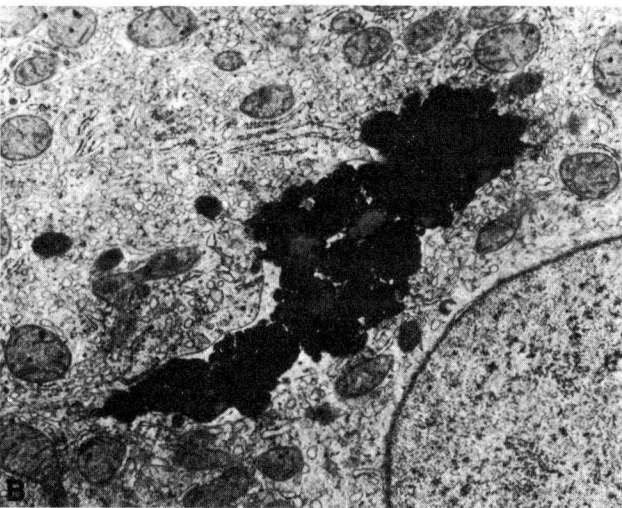

Figure 34-5 *A.* Toluidine blue–stained histologic section showing marked deposition of pigment granules in the hepatocytes of CTX liver cells. ×950. [43] (*From Salen et al.* [43]). *B.* Membrane-bound agglomerate of fatty pigmented material near the nucleus. ×6000. (*From Salen et al.* [43].)

Plasma triglyceride concentrations have also been normal [4, 27, 28], except in two patients who exhibited hyperprebetali-poproteinemia at levels of 345 mg/dl and 273 mg/dl [27, 39]. Plasma phospholipid concentrations are normal [27]. A major diagnostic feature of this disorder is the elevated plasma cholestanol concentration. Values range from 1.3 to 15 mg/dl and are between 3 and 20 times higher than mean values in normal plasma [2, 4, 27, 29, 32, 33, 27–40].

Chemistry and Metabolism of Cholestanol 5α-Cholestan-3β-ol, or cholestanol (Fig. 34-6), is the 5,6-dihydro derivative of cholesterol and differs from cholesterol by the reduction of the double bond at C-5,6 with a hydrogen atom in the 5α position. The 5α refers to the stereochemistry at the junction between rings A and B, and the 3β refers to the position and configuration of the hydroxyl group at carbon atom 3. The sterol is digitonin-precipitable, like cholesterol. Most commonly, cholestanol is separated from cholesterol by argentation thin-layer chromatography and quantified by gas-liquid chromatography [4]. Direct gas chromatographic and mass fragmentographic methods for the measurement of cholestanol in the presence of large amounts of cholesterol have been developed [35, 44, 45].

Small amounts of cholestanol accompany cholesterol in virtually every mammalian tissue [4, 6]. Like cholesterol, choles-

tanol appears both free and as the fatty acyl ester. Convincing evidence from both normal and CTX subjects has been presented that cholestanol is derived solely from cholesterol [7, 48]. According to current views [49–55] (Fig. 34-7), the first step involves the enzymatic oxidation of the 3β-hydroxy of cholesterol to a ketone, to yield cholest-5-en-3-one, followed by an enzyme catalyzed isomerization which converts cholest-5-en-3-one to cholest-4-en-3-one. This compound then is reduced by a reductase to 5α-cholestan-3-one, which then undergoes reduction of the ketone by another reductase to give cholestanol. Recently, liver biopsies from two CTX subjects showed four times more activity in converting cholesterol to cholest-4-en-3-one than control liver specimens. Both normal and CTX individuals show equal ability to reduce cholest-4-en-3-one to cholestanol [56].

Although an alternative pathway for the formation of cholestanol that does not involve cholesterol has been proposed by Kandutsch and Russell [57], two lines of evidence demonstrate that cholestanol arises solely from cholesterol in CTX [48]. After [4-14C]cholesterol was injected intravenously into a CTX subject, the cholestanol isolated from the plasma became radioactive. The falling specific activity curve of cholesterol intersected with the rising specific activity curve of cholestanol as in a precursor-product relationship [48]. In a second study in a patient, a mixture of stereospecifically labeled [2-14C]-mevalonate and 3R,4R[4-3H]mevalonate was injected intravenously as a pulse label, and the 3H/14C ratios were measured in cholesterol, cholestanol, 24-dihydrolanosterol, and lanosterol. These ratios were compared to the 3H/14C ratio of biosynthetic squalene that was prepared from the same mevalonate mixture. The results are given in Table 34-2 and Fig. 34-8. Note that both cholestanol and cholesterol had the same 3H/14C ratios; whereas lanosterol, 24-dihydrolanosterol, and 7-cholesten-3β-ol, which are the 5α-dihydro precursors of cholesterol, showed 3H/14C ratios at least 20 percent higher. These experiments show that cholestanol is derived from cholesterol and not directly via 5α-saturated cholesterol precursors such as lanosterol [49, 55].

The metabolism of cholestanol has not been investigated thoroughly. There is some evidence that rats, rabbits, chickens, and monkeys can absorb cholestanol and that in the rabbit and to a lesser extent in the rat, cholestanol is converted to allobile acids [46]. In the case of the rabbit, increased amounts of the glycine conjugate of allodeoxycholic acid are formed after cholestanol feeding and precipitate in the gallbladder to form gallstones [59–61].

In humans less than 0.1 percent of the cholesterol that is present in food is cholestanol. Thus, virtually all of the body cholestanol is produced endogenously. Bhattacharyya and Connor reported that only 3 to 5 percent of a test dose of [4-14C]cholestanol was absorbed in two CTX subjects [28]. After an injection of [1,2-3H]cholestanol, turnover was observed to conform to a two-pool model [62]. Quantitatively,

Figure 34-6 The structures of cholesterol and cholestanol.

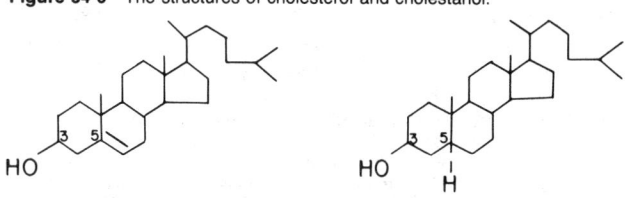

Cholesterol   Cholestanol

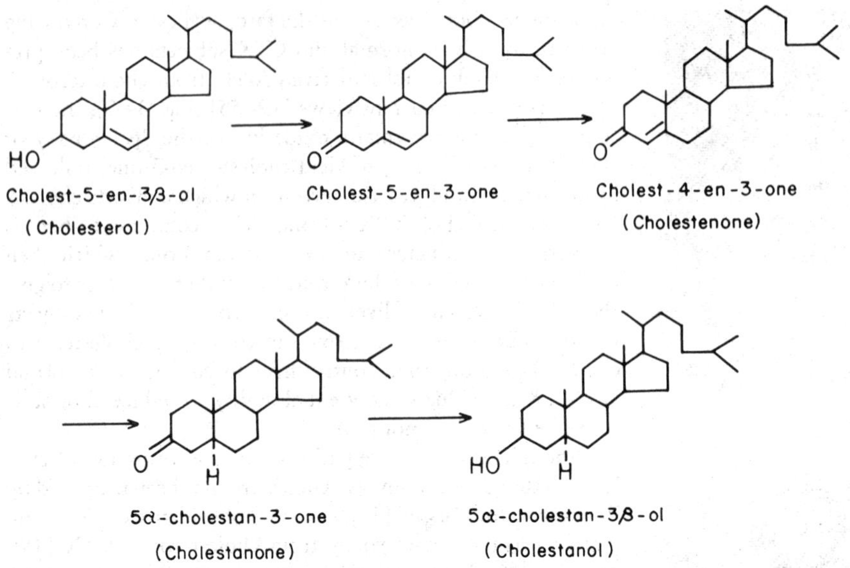

Cholest-5-en-3β-ol
(Cholesterol)

→

Cholest-5-en-3-one

→

Cholest-4-en-3-one
(Cholestenone)

→

5α-cholestan-3-one
(Cholestanone)

→

5α-cholestan-3β-ol
(Cholestanol)

Figure 34-7 The biosynthetic pathway of cholestanol from cholesterol.

cholestanol turnover (PR_A) ranged from 6 to 18.6 mg/day (mean, 11.8 ± 6.0 mg) in five control subjects, of whom one was normal and four were hyperlipidemic. The rapidly miscible pool (pool A, M_A) in these subjects varied from 22 to 83 mg (mean, 48 ± 23 mg). The daily fecal excretion of cholestanol and neutral sterols ranged between 7 to 13 mg/day, and fecal output of acidic steroids derived from cholestanol (allobile acid) ranged from 2 to 5 mg/day. In all subjects, cholestanol was rapidly excreted in the bile [62]. The pathway of cholesterol biosynthesis has also been investigated in patients with CTX. Substantial quantities of lanosterol, 24-dihydrolanosterol and 7-cholesten-3β-ol, in addition to cholesterol and cholestanol, have been found in the bile. After the injection of [2-^{14}C]mevalonate, all sterols became labeled and specific activity decay curves intersected, revealing precursor-product relationships between lanosterol, 24-dihydrolanosterol, 7-cholesten-3β-ol, cholesterol, and cholestanol. This experiment suggests that the pathway for the conversion of lanosterol to cholesterol involves intermediates with saturated side chains [58].

Chemical Abnormalities

BRAIN   Normally, only small amounts of free and esterified cholestanol are detected in the brain. In 1968, Menkes et al. first reported abnormally high concentrations of free and ester-

Table 34-2   Isotope ratios (^{3}H/^{14}C) of sterols isolated from feces of a CTX subject[*]

Sterol	$^3H/^{14}C$	
	Experimental[†]	Theoretical
Lanosterol	0.83 ± 0.01 (8)	0.83 (5/6)
24,25-Dihydrolanosterol	0.80 ± 0.03 (6)	0.83 (5/6)
7-Cholesten-3β-ol	0.78 ± 0.01 (7)	0.80 (4/5)
Cholesterol	0.63 ± 0.01 (16)	0.60 (3/5)
Cholestanol	0.63 ± 0.01 (11)	0.60 (3/5)

[*] Sterols extracted after intravenous administration of [2-^{14}C]mevalonate and 3R,4R[4-^{3}H]mevalonate.
[†] Experimental values shown above have been divided by the ^{3}H/^{14}C ratio of the squalene standard. Values are given as the mean $\pm$ SEM(N). Squalene (^{3}H/^{14}C was 4.79) was prepared biosynthetically by G. Popják and A. Polito from original mevalonate mixtures [48].

ified cholestanol in the brain of a patient with CTX [2]. Cholestanol comprised 25 percent of the total free sterols in histologically abnormal portions of the cerebellum and 20 percent of the total free sterols in normal-appearing gray and white matter of the cerebrum. Cholestanol esters accounted for 49 percent of the total esterified sterols in the histologically abnormal sections of the cerebellum. Philippart and van Bogaert confirmed these observations in a second patient with CTX [3]. Although the two brains had been stored in formaldehyde, the large accumulation of cholestanol that was present was not related to formaldehyde storage because frozen-stored brain from another CTX subject also contained large amounts of cholestanol [4, 22, 24]. In addition, in histologically normal frontal lobe and abnormal cerebellum from a third CTX subject, cholestanol comprised 20 and 34 percent, respectively, of total sterols [4]. In addition, the cholesterol content of both normal and abnormal brain tissue was significantly increased due almost entirely to the deposition of cholesteryl esters [4, 16].

PERIPHERAL NERVES   Both the free and esterified cholestanol are increased in peripheral nerves in patients with CTX [28]. Bhattacharyya and Connor reported that 20 percent of the total sterols was cholestanol, of which 59 percent was in the esterified form. This is consistent with the functional neuropathy reported by Kuritzy et al. [37] and the myelination and demyelination changes noted by Ohnishi et al. [36].

TENDONS   Menkes found only trace amounts of free or esterified cholestanol in the histologically abnormal sections in tendons from two patients with CTX [2], but Philippart and van Bogaert demonstrated the accumulation of free cholestanol in the tendon xanthoma (about 3 percent of total sterols) in this same patient and one other [3]. We found that cholestanol accounted for 11 percent of the total sterols in an Achilles tendon xanthoma and 7.3 percent of the sterols in a tuberous xanthoma. Bhattacharyya and Connor have also found that cholestanol constituted 11 percent of the total sterols of three tendon xanthomas biopsied from a CTX patient and that 49 to 86 percent of the cholestanol was esterified [28]. Despite the high content of xanthoma cholestanol, cholesterol remains the major sterol in the xanthomas, accounting for about 90 percent of the total sterols [2, 3, 4, 28].

PLASMA Elevated plasma cholestanol levels have become a constant and diagnostic feature of this disease. Philippart and van Bogaert found that cholestanol accounted for 6 percent of their patient's total plasma sterols (normal, <1 percent) [3]. Since 1971, plasma cholestanol has been measured in 26 patients and has been found in increased levels in all. The range has been between 1.3 and 15 mg/dl [4, 25, 27–29, 32, 33, 37–40], compared to normal plasma cholestanol levels of between 0.1 and 0.6 mg/dl [4, 25, 28]. Cholestanol is transported primarily in the low density lipoprotein (LDL) fraction of plasma. Very low density (VLDL) and high density lipoproteins (HDL) also transport smaller amounts [62]. No special lipoprotein that preferentially transports cholestanol has been found. Plasma cholestanol is also present in an esterified form. Esterification of cholestanol presumably results from the activity of plasma lecithin:cholesterol acyltransferase (LCAT), the enzyme responsible for the esterification of plasma cholesterol (Chap. 31). LCAT activity in CTX is normal [62, 63].

Recently, defective HDL metabolism was suspected in CTX subjects because of a finding of abnormal lipid and apolipoprotein composition [39]. The mean HDL cholesterol concentration in 8 CTX subjects was 14.5 ± 3.2 mg/dl (normal, 48.0 ± 9.0 mg/dl) (Table 34-3). The decreased HDL cholesterol content reflected a low level of plasma HDL, particularly the HDL_2 subfraction, as determined by analytical ultracentrifugation and an abnormal lipid composition. Relative to normal HDL lipids, the proportion of cholesteryl esters, particularly cholesteryl linoleate, was decreased. Free cholesterol and phospholipid levels were normal and triglyceride levels were increased. The ratio of apoprotein to total cholesterol in the HDL of patients with CTX was two to three times greater than normal, while the ratio of apo A-I to apo A-II was increased and the proportions of apo C proteins was decreased. A minor form of apo A-I (apo A-I_x) was present in increased amounts in the HDL of CTX patients. These abnormalities may reflect a disordered physiologic function of HDL in CTX, including the

postulated removal of excess cholesterol and cholestanol from peripheral tissues [39].

BILE Normally, bile contains small amounts of cholestanol (less than 1 percent) and a trace amount of lanosterol (0.02 percent) and other methylated sterols which are cholesterol precursors. In the CTX subjects, substantial amounts of cholestanol are excreted in the bile and range from 4 to 11 percent of the total biliary neutral sterols [4, 28]. In addition, large amounts of lanosterol, 24-dihydrolanosterol, and 7-cholesten-3β-ol are also excreted in the bile of CTX patients (about 3 percent) [4].

In normal patients 80 percent of biliary bile acid is almost equally divided between cholic and chenodeoxycholic acid (Fig. 34-9). The remaining bile acids, deoxycholic acid (20 percent) and lithocholic acid (2 to 4 percent,) are bacterial intermediates and secondary bile acids. In 1971, we discovered exceedingly low levels of chenodeoxycholic acid in the bile of CTX patients. Thus, the proportion of cholic acid was increased to about 80 percent of the total bile acids. In addition, about 2 percent of the total bile acids in the CTX patients was allocholic (i.e., 5α-saturated bile acids derived from cholestanol) [64]. Similar findings have been reported by Bhattacharyya and Connor [28]. A major discovery was the demonstration of appreciable amounts of C_{27} bile alcohols in the bile and feces of CTX subjects [51]. These compounds contain four or five hydroxyl groups, and most are hydroxylated at C-25 [65–68] (Fig. 34-10). Recently, Hoshita et al. discovered that these bile alcohols (tetrols and pentols) are excreted in the bile as conjugates of glucuronic acid but are found free in the feces [69]. We have confirmed this important observation [70].

OTHER TISSUES Increased amounts of cholestanol (1.1 to 2.7 percent of the total sterols) were found in virtually every tissue, including the spleen, liver, kidney, adipose tissue, and muscle and other tissues, in a patient with CTX [4]. The cho-

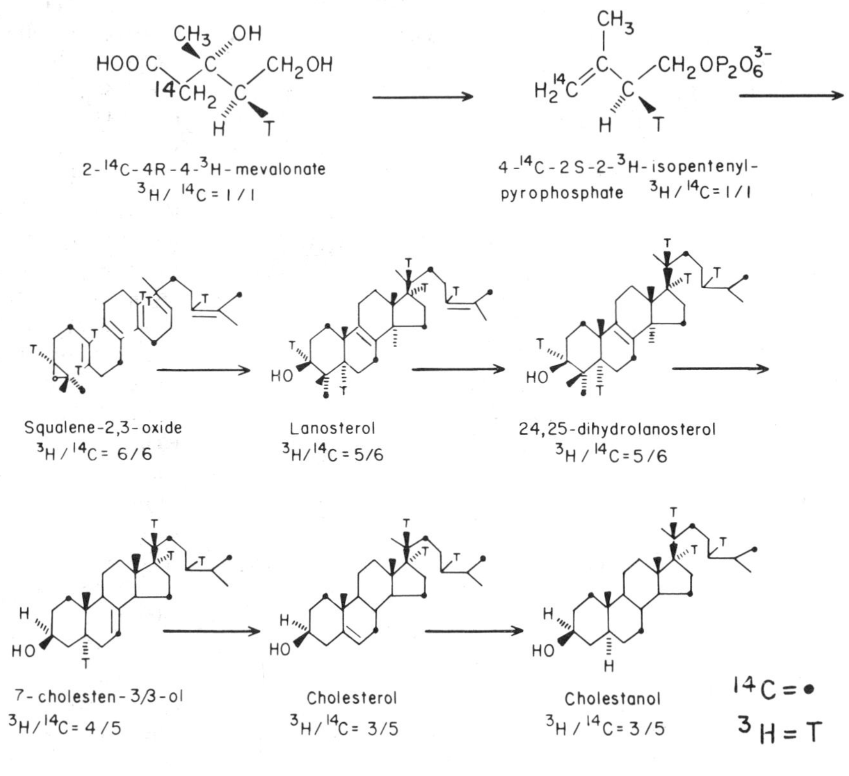

Figure 34-8 Stereospecific labeling of squalene, lanosterol, 24, 25-dihydrolanosterol, 7-cholesten-3β-ol, and cholesterol after administration of mevalonate[2-^{14}C-4R-4-^{3}H], and postulated distribution of radioactive atoms in 5α-cholestanol. The experimental finding of a 3:5 ratio of ^{3}H:^{14}C in 5α-cholestanol relative to squalene indicates that cholesterol (^{3}H^{14}C = 3:5) served as the direct precursor. (From Salen and Polito [48].)

Table 34-3 Plasma triglyceride, cholesterol, cholestanol, and HDL-cholesterol levels in CTX and normal subjects, mg/dl

Subjects	Triglyceride	Cholesterol	Cholestanol	HLD Cholesterol
Normolipemic	115 ± 33[*]	230 ± 25.0	0.6 ± 0.02	48.0 ± 9.0
CTX	123 ± 64[†]	165 ± 25	2.9 ± 0.9	14.5 ± 3.2

[*] Mean ± SD of 7 male and 3 female subjects.
[†] Mean ± SD of 3 male and 5 female patients.

lestanol content of a pulmonary xanthoma was 8 percent. Bhattacharyya and Connor found that the sterols from the skin and adipose tissue of a patient contained between 5 and 11 percent cholestanol [28]. Previously, Menkes et al. [3] failed to detect cholestanol in the liver, lung, adrenal gland, and kidneys of one patient [2].

The Metabolic Defect(s)

The generalized accumulation of cholestanol and cholesterol in the nervous system, tendons, and virtually every tissue suggests a combined defect in both cholesterol and cholestanol metabolism in this disorder. Obviously, the accumulation of both sterols represents an imbalance in either influx or efflux of the sterols from the tissues. The origin of tissue cholestanol could involve local biosynthesis, influx from the blood after synthesis elsewhere, or perhaps absorption from the diet. Cholestanol, like cholesterol, is not catabolized locally. HDL may play a role in the removal of both sterols.

By analogy with other storage diseases, Philippart and van Bogaert have suggested that CTX may be due to a defect in the tissue catabolism of cholestanol [3, 71]. On the other hand, Menkes et al. have postulated a defect in the transport of tissue cholesterol across the cell membrane, with the result that some of the excess tissue cholesterol may be converted to cholestanol and stored as either free or esterified sterol [2]. The data of Gardner-Medwin et al. [72] and Derby et al. [21], derived from the in vivo labeling of cerebral and cerebellar sterols, support the concept of a deficiency in the mechanism of removal of cholesterol and cholestanol from the tissues. It is noteworthy that when grown in a cholesterol-free medium, fibroblasts

Figure 34-9 Structures of cholic acid, chenodeoxycholic acid, and ursodeoxycholic acid.

Cholic acid

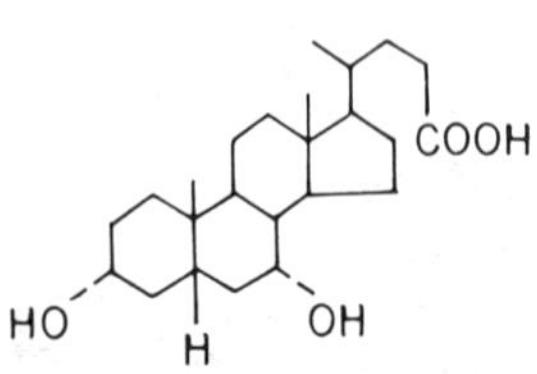

Chenodeoxycholic acid

Ursodeoxycholic acid

from CTX patients synthesize cholesterol but not cholestanol. Furthermore, these fibroblasts respond normally to the addition of LDL by suppressing 3-hydroxy-3-methylglutaryl coenzyme A reductase (HMG-CoA reductase) and stimulating cholesteryl oleate synthesis [73]. These findings argue against the local formation of cholestanol by peripheral tissues.

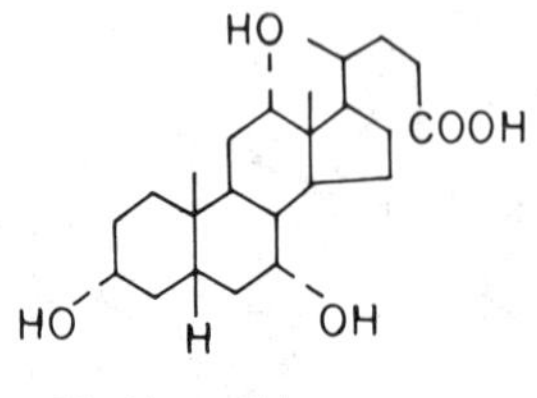

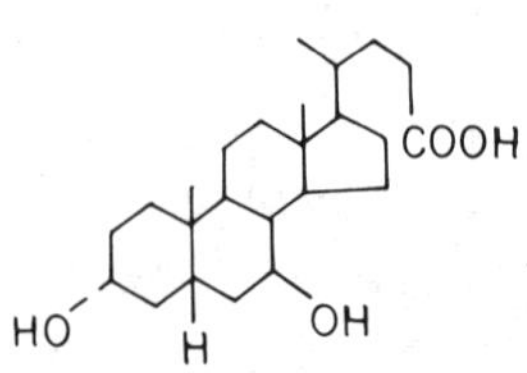

Recently we have suggested that the excessive tissue sterol deposits of cholesterol and cholestanol in CTX are related to hyperactive hepatic neutral sterol synthesis (see Table 34-5), which is secondary to a deficiency of bile acids (particularly chenodeoxycholic acid) in the enterohepatic circulation [4, 62]. Further, we believe that cholestanol and cholesterol are produced principally in the liver and are transported by blood lipoproteins for deposit in other tissues. Because HDL lipid and apoprotein compositions are abnormal, removal of both sterols from peripheral tissue by this lipoprotein may be limited [39]. Using isotope kinetic techniques, measurements of cholesterol and cholestanol synthesis in CTX subjects have been made and compared with the activity of hepatic HMG-CoA reductase, the rate-determining enzyme for cholesterol biosynthesis. This method demonstrates that sterol synthesis is high in CTX subjects and that the rate-controlling step in cholesterol biosynthesis is elevated (Tables 34-4 and 34-5) [62, 74].

In spite of the finding of increased sterol synthesis [62], we believe that a major biochemical, and perhaps the basic genetic, abnormality in CTX involves a defect in bile acid synthesis [5]. The evidence in favor of this hypothesis can be summarized as follows. In sharp contrast to the elevation of cholesterol biosynthesis in CTX, bile acid production as measured by the sterol balance technique was subnormal [62]. In two CTX subjects, bile acid excretion averaged 114 mg/day, which is about 50 percent of the mean value of 214 mg/day found in five control subjects. Paradoxically, the activity of cholesterol 7α-hydroxylase, the rate-determining enzyme for bile acid synthesis, was significantly elevated in two CTX subjects: 240 units compared to a mean value of 190 units in a group of control subjects and 90 units in subjects with gallstones (Table 34-4) [75, 76]. Therefore, CTX subjects should be able to produce adequate amounts of 7α-hydroxycholesterol, the first committed precursor in bile acid synthesis. However, bile acid production, as measured by the sterol balance technique, was abnormally low. Therefore, we postulated an enzymatic defect that was responsible for the incomplete transformation of 7α-hydroxycholesterol into bile acids. This postulate proved correct.

More than 10 percent, or about 100 mg/day, of the neutral sterol fraction isolated from the feces of CTX subjects was composed of compounds more polar than cholesterol [5]. These polar neutral sterols could be divided into two groups. The first group consisted almost entirely of a tetrahydroxy bile alcohol, 5β-cholestane-3α,7α,12α,25-tetrol (see Fig. 34-10). The second was a complex mixture of pentahydroxy bile alco-

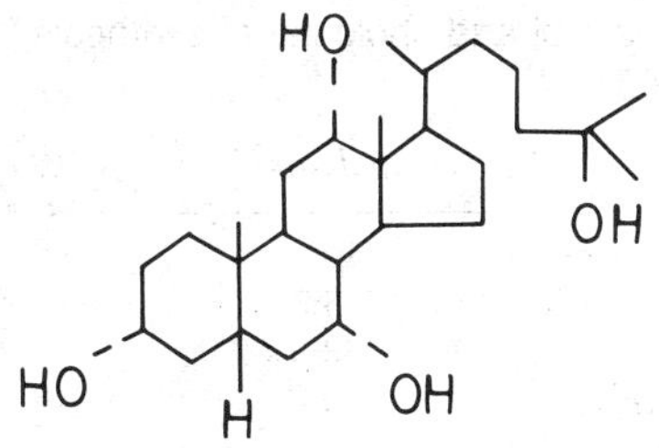

5β-cholestane-3α,7α,12α,25-tetrol

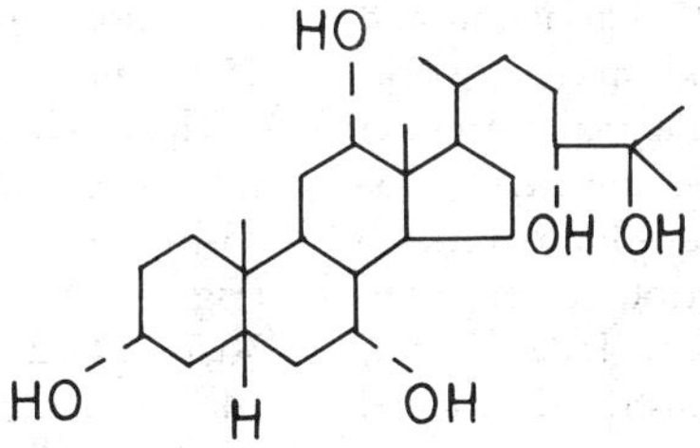

5β-cholestane-
3α,7α,12α,24R,25-pentol

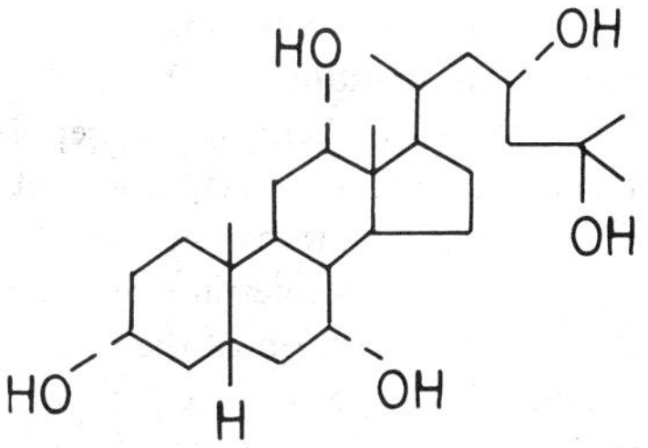

5β-cholestane-
3α,7α,12α,23R,25-pentol

Figure 34-10 Structures of bile alcohols excreted in feces of CTX subjects (neither 5β-cholestane-3α, 7α, 12α, 23R, 25-pentol nor 5β-cholestane-3α, 7α, 12α, 24R, and 25-pentol is a precursor of cholic acid). (*From Shefer et al. [81].*)

hols in which 5β-cholestane-3α,7α,12α,24R,25-pentol and 5β-cholestane-3α,7α,12α,23R,25-pentol predominated [5, 65–68] (Fig. 34-10). The discovery of a family of C-25 hydroxylated bile alcohols was surprising. We had expected to find C-26 hydroxylated intermediates, since the known pathway of bile acid synthesis involves 26-hydroxylation of bile alcohols (Fig. 34-11). For example, in the biosynthesis of cholic acid (step XI), 5β-cholestane-3α,7α,12α-triol (step V) is presumably transformed into 5β-cholestane-3α,7α,12α,26-tetrol (step VI). We therefore considered the possibility that in CTX, there is an alternate pathway of cholic acid biosynthesis. This pathway follows the known steps from cholesterol (step

I), to 5β-cholestane-3α,7α,12α-triol (step V), and then continues via 5β-cholestane-3α,7α,12α,25-tetrol (step VIII) and 5β-cholestane-3α,7α,12α, 24S,25-pentol (step IX) to yield cholic acid (step XI).

To substantiate the existence of this alternate pathway, we studied the metabolism of tritium-labeled 5β-cholestane-3α,7α,12α,25-tetrol in CTX subjects. When tracer doses of this tetrol were injected intravenously, the resulting specific activity curves of 5β-cholestane-3α,7α,12α,25-tetrol and cholic acid revealed a precursor-product relationship [77] (Fig. 34-12). When tritium-labeled tetrol was administered to two normal subjects, radioactivity was rapidly incorporated into cholic acid. The resulting curve decayed exponentially and more rapidly than in the CTX subjects (in whom bile acid synthesis was impaired). On the basis of these findings, we conclude that in human beings there is a pathway of bile acid synthesis that involves C-25 hydroxy intermediates. In the case of the CTX subjects, cholic acid is derived almost entirely from the 25-hydroxytetrol, whereas in normal subjects the quantitative significance of the 25-hydroxy pathway remains to be established. In this regard Hanson et al. have recently compared the transformation of tracer doses of 5β-cholestane-3α,7α,12α,25-tetrol and 5β-cholestane-3α,7α,12α,26-tetrol to cholic acid in two normal subjects [78]. More 26-hydroxytetrol was converted to cholic acid than 25-hydroxytetrol, suggesting that the 26-hydroxytetrol was the preferred substrate. It should be noted that the 25-hydroxy pathway is microsomal (see below), and, accordingly, injected precursors must be taken up by the liver cells and carried through the cell cytoplasm in order to reach the microsomes and must be incorporated for conversion to cholic acid. Further, 25-hydroxy bile alcohols are excreted in bile as glucuronides. This suggests that the 25-hydroxy bile alcohols may be diverted from bile acid synthesis when they are converted to glucuronides [69]. In contrast, 26-

Table 34-4 Key enzymes in hepatic bile acid synthesis

Enzyme	*Rate of product formation, pmol per milligram of protein per 10 min*	
	Control	*CTX*
HMG-CoA reductase	590[*]	2080[†]
Cholesterol 7α-hydroxylase	190[*]	240[†]
7α-hydroxy-4-cholest-3-one-12α-hydroxylase	480[*]	1620[†]
5β-cholestane-3α,7α,12α,25-hydroxylase	5480[†]	7110[†]
5β-cholestane-3α,7α,12α,25-24S-hydroxylase[‡]	636[†]	151[†]
Cleavage enzyme[§]	9160[†]	7310

[*] Determined in 9 patients.
[†] Determined in 2 patients.
[‡] We believe that the deficiency of this enzyme in CTX is the key biochemical and genetic defect [41].
[§] Enzyme(s) catalyzing the conversion of 5β-cholestane-3α,7α,12α,24S,25-pentol to cholic acid.

Table 34-5 Cholesterol and cholestanol synthesis,*
mg/(kg·day)

Subject	Cholesterol	Cholestanol
Control (2)	10.0	0.17
CTX (2)	18.2	0.94
CTX treated with chenodeoxycholic acid†	8.2	0.27

* Isotope kinetic method [6, 62].
† 0.75g/day for 42 days.

hydroxy intermediates are oxidized by mitochondria to 5β-cholestanoic acids.

Recent in vitro work in other laboratories has also suggested that the degradation of the cholesterol side chain to cholic acid involves intermediates hydroxylated at C-25. Cronholm and Johansson (working with rats) [79] and Björkhem et al. (working with human beings) [80] reported that the major product formed during the incubation of 5β-cholestane-3α,7α,12α-triol with liver microsomes was 5β-cholestane-3α,7α,12α,25-tetrol, not 5β-cholestane-3α,7α,12α,26-tetrol, as expected from a consideration of the "classic" pathway. Indeed, mitochondrial 26-hydroxylase activity was demonstrated in only 4 of 10 normal subjects tested, and when present, this activity was one-fourth as great as microsomal 25-hydroxylase activity that was found in every liver preparation [80].

We have recently demonstrated that 5β-cholestane-3α,7α,12α-triol can be converted to cholic acid in human and rat liver in vitro via a 25 hydroxylation pathway (Fig. 34-10) without the participation of 26-oxygenated derivatives [81, 82]. Incubation of 5β-cholestane-3α,7α,12α,25-tetrol with the hepatic microsomal fraction from normolipidemic controls or CTX patients yielded 5β-cholestane-3α,7α,12α,24S,25-pentol as the major product [83]. At the same time the rate of formation of 5β-cholestane-3α,7α,12α,24S,25-pentol by CTX hepatic microsomes was only one-fourth as great as by control microsomes [41] (Table 34-4). The reduced rate of 24S hydroxylation in CTX subjects may explain the accumulation of 5β-cholestane-3α,7α,12α,25-tetrol in bile and feces and also is probably responsible for the reduced rate of bile acid synthesis in CTX.

The enzyme catabolizing the transformation of 5β-cholestane-3α,7α,12α,24S,25-pentol to cholic acid was located predominantly in the 100,000-g supernatant fraction (Table 34-4). This transformation proceeded at approximately equal rates in both normal and CTX liver fractions. In both groups the reaction appeared to be stereospecific in that only the 24S epimer was transformed to cholic acid at appreciable rates. This stereospecificity and rapid metabolism might explain the fact that only the 24R epimers of 5β-cholestane-3α,7α,12α,23,25-pentol and 5β-cholestane-3α,7α,12α,24,25-pentol could be detected in the bile and feces of CTX subjects [66, 67]. We were unable to find 5β-cholestane-3α,7α,12α,24S,25-pentol, presumably because it was rapidly transformed.

The soluble enzyme system required NAD for the formation of cholic acid [66]. The reaction most probably involves a 24-ketone intermediate, which has been isolated from in vitro incubations of human and rat liver and identified by chemical ionization–mass spectroscopy as 5β-cholestane-3α,7α,12α,25-tetrahydroxy-24-one (Fig. 34-11) [83].

The results of the above studies suggest that there is a pathway of cholic acid biosynthesis in human beings involving 25-hydroxylation of 5β-cholestane-3α,7α,12α-triol (step V) (Fig. 34-11). This pathway proceeds via 5β-cholestane-3α,7α,12α,25-tretol (step VIII), 5β-cholestane-3α,7α,12α,24S,25-pentol (step IX), and probably 5β-cholestane-3α,7α,12α,25-tetrahydroxy-24-one (step X), and does not involve 5β-cholestanoic acids as intermediates. Virtually all the cholic acid in CTX subjects is formed via this route. The accumulation of 5β-cholestane-3α,7α,12α,25-tetrol, the absence of 5β-cholestane-3α,7α,12α,24S,25-pentol, and the low activity of the microsomal 24S-hydroxylase (Table 34-4) point to defective 24 hydroxylation as the primary enzymatic defect in CTX.

An alternative view has been put forth by Oftebro et al. [84]. These investigators examined hepatic microsomal and mitochondrial hydroxylation in one CTX and one control subject. They could demonstrate no mitochondrial 26 hydroxylation of 5β-cholestane-3α,7α,12α-triol in the CTX subject, whereas activity was present in the control. In addition, small amounts of 5β-cholestane-3α,7α,12α-triol and 5β-cholestane-3α,7α,12α,25-tetrol were measured in the hepatic homogenate and microsomes of the CTX liver. Oftebro et al. concluded that absent mitochondrial 26-hydroxylase activity was the primary enzymatic defect in CTX, and accordingly that cholic acid biosynthesis proceeds by the less efficient alternative, the micro-

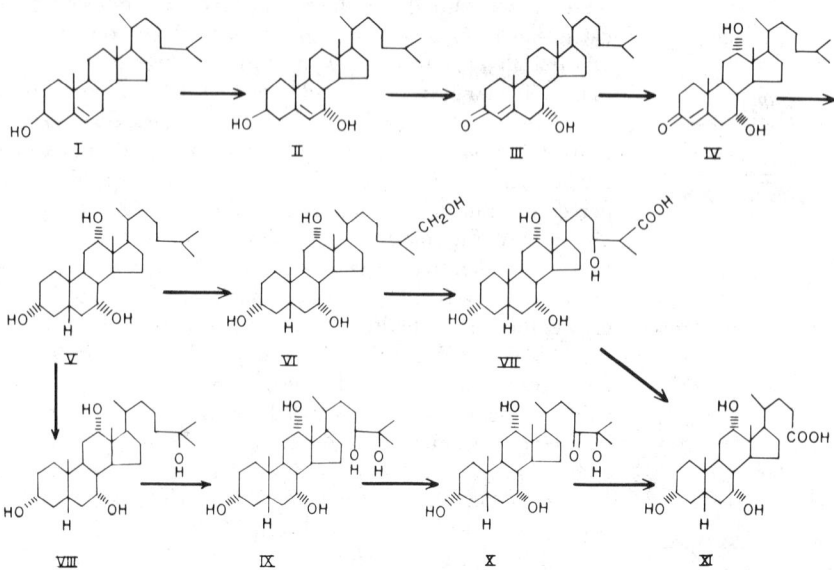

Figure 34-11 Pathway of cholic acid biosynthesis showing side chain degradation via both 26-hydroxylated and, alternatively, 25-hydroxylated intermediates. I. cholesterol; II. cholest-5-en-3β, 7α-diol; III. 7α-hydroxycholest-4-en-3-one; IV. 7α, 12α-dihydroxycholest-4-en-3-one; V. 5β-cholestane-3α, 7α, 12α-triol; VI. 5β-cholestane-3α, 7α, 12α, 26-tetrol; VII. 3α, 7α, 12α, 24ξ-tetrahydroxy-5β-cholestanoic acid; VIII. 5β-cholestane-3α, 7α, 12α, 25-tetrol; IX. 5β-cholestane-3α, 7α, 12α, 24S, 25-pentol; X. 3α, 7α, 12α, 25-tetrahydroxy-5β-cholestan-24-one; XI. cholic acid.

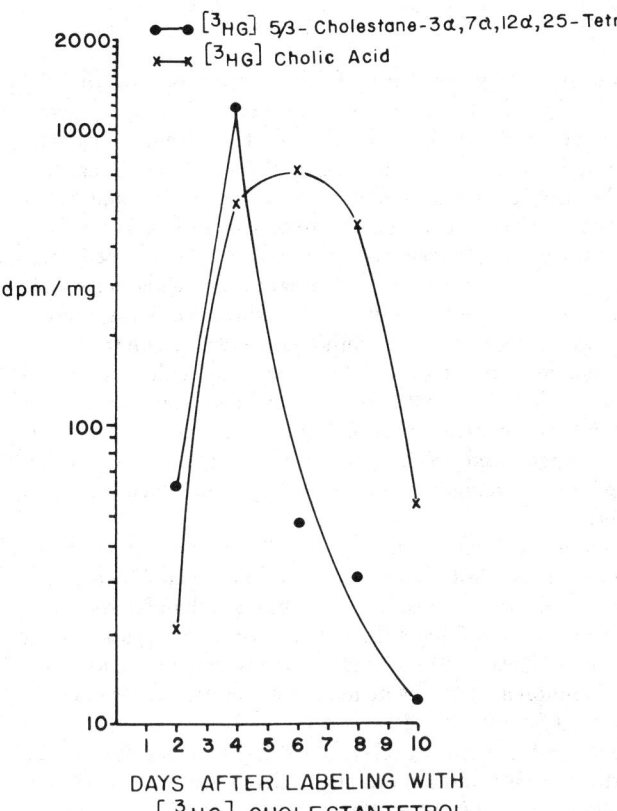

Figure 34-12 Specific activity versus time decay curves of 5β-cholestane-3α, 7α, 12α, 25-tetrol and cholic acid isolated from a CTX subject after intravenous pulse labeling with [G-³H]5β-cholestane-3α, 7α, 12α, 25-tetrol.

somal 25 hydroxylation side chain pathway [81]. It may be noted that 26 mitochondrial hydroxylation cannot be demonstrated in most normal livers [80] and further that microsomal 26-hydroxylase activity has been found in both control and CTX livers [85].

The deficiency of chenodeoxycholic acid in the bile of CTX subjects has also been investigated [86]. Three potential radioactive chenodeoxycholic acid precursors—7α-hydroxy-4-cholesten-3-one; 5β-cholestane-3α,7α,25-triol; and 5β-cholestane-3α,7α,26-triol—were injected intravenously as a pulse label in two CTX subjects and two controls. The three precursors were actively 12α-hydroxylated and diverted into the cholic acid biosynthetic pathway in the CTX patients. Further, both the 26- and 25-hydroxylated intermediates were hindered in their conversion into chenodeoxycholic acid. Thus, the relative absence of chenodeoxycholic acid in the bile of CTX individuals may be related to active 12α hydroxylation and preferential diversion of these precursors into the cholic acid synthetic pathway. In vitro measurements of 12α-hydroxylase activity show that CTX microsomes have more than three times the normal activity (Table 34-4) [76].

Diagnosis

The diagnosis of CTX may be difficult during the first decade of life because the classic symptoms (neurologic dysfunction, cataracts, xanthomas) may be absent or vague in the early stages of the disease. Time is required for the accumulation of both cholesterol and cholestanol. The characteristic features may not appear until the late teens or early twenties. The dis-

ease should be considered if tendon xanthomas or cataracts are present in young subjects. These features may precede the appearance of the neurologic dysfunction. The demonstration of low or normal plasma cholesterol levels in combination with the above-mentioned clinical features mandates that plasma cholestanol also be measured. In normal or hyperlipidemic patients plasma cholestanol does not exceed 1 mg/dl. Values in excess should suggest the diagnosis of CTX. In order to establish the diagnosis more definitively, analysis of bile is often helpful. Biliary cholestanol concentrations are high in CTX (between 6 and 11 percent of total sterols are cholestanol), and the cholesterol precursors lanosterol, 24-dihydrolanosterol, and 7-cholesten-3β-ol may also be present. Further, the biliary bile acid pattern is distinctive, with low levels of chenodeoxycholic acid (less than 10 percent of total bile acid). In addition, bile alcohols, which may be precursors of cholic acid, i.e., 5β-cholestane-3α,7α,12α,25-tetrol and 5β-cholestane-3α,7α,12α,24R, 25-pentol, are found in abundant amounts (in bile these alcohols are present as glucuronides [69, 70].

Another helpful diagnostic feature is high levels of cholestanol in xanthomas. Hepatic morphology is unusual and the demonstration of intrahepatic pigment and crystal forms may be sought [43]. The diagnosis of CTX is not difficult when the neurologic dysfunction is far advanced, cataracts are present, tendon xanthomas are large, and the plasma and biliary steroids are abnormal. Since therapy is available (see below), the earlier the diagnosis can be made and treatment instituted, the greater the possibility of preventing the devastating neurologic manifestations. Thus, plasma cholestanol should be measured in every subject in whom tendon xanthomas appear in the presence of normal or slightly elevated cholesterol levels or when unexplained juvenile cataracts are detected.

Treatment

The treatment of CTX is based upon the hypothesis that the disease results from a block in bile acid synthesis. As a result of reduced synthesis, the enterohepatic circulation of cholic acid and chenodeoxycholic acid is low; cholesterol and cholestanol production become overactive; and the HDL transport of both sterols is abnormal. Treatment with chenodeoxycholic acid was begun in 1972 and was designed to expand the deficient bile acid pool [4]. Preliminary data from three patients fed 750 mg/day showed that plasma cholestanol dropped 50 percent after 6 weeks of treatment and that cholesterol and cholestanol production rates as measured by the isotope kinetic method were substantially suppressed during bile acid therapy (see Fig. 34-13 and Table 34-5). In addition, HMG-CoA reductase, the rate-controlling enzyme of cholesterol biosynthesis, was inhibited fourfold during chenodeoxycholic acid therapy [6, 87]. Other changes included the disappearance of bile alcohols from the bile. This indicated that endogenous cholic acid formation and the defective pathway were being suppressed. Of interest was the finding that ursodeoxycholic acid, the 7β epimer of chenodeoxycholic acid (Fig. 34-9), increased substantially in the bile during treatment [88].

The number of CTX subjects treated with chenodeoxycholic acid has recently increased to 13. After 6 months, mean plasma cholestanol levels have decreased from 5.0 mg/dl to 1.6 mg/dl. In addition, a number of these patients have shown reversal of their neurologic disability, with clearing of the dementia, better orientation, a rise in IQ, and improved strength and inde-

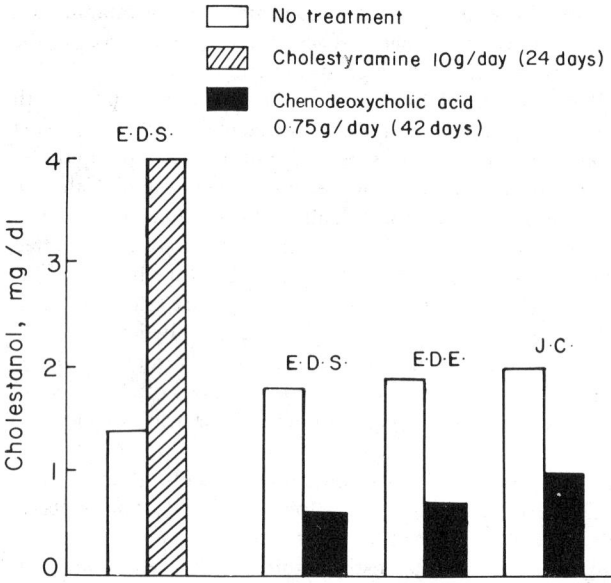

Figure 34-13 The effect of treatment on plasma cholestanol concentrations in CTX.

pendence. Cholestyramine, a drug which binds bile acids in the intestine and promotes their excretion, would be expected to aggravate the bile acid synthetic defect in CTX. One CTX subject so treated (Fig. 34-13) showed a fourfold rise in plasma cholestanol [6]. This finding supports the hypothesis that suppression of bile acid synthesis may be an effective treatment.

Genetics

All evidence to date indicates that CTX is transmitted as an autosomal recessive trait [1, 3, 4, 8, 9, 18, 27, 32, 33, 39, 40]. Not only is there a high incidence of consanguinity with repeated marriages of first cousins, but also both brothers and sisters are affected with the disease. Parents and children of affected individuals show no evidence of neurologic disease and have normal cholestanol levels [4].

SITOSTEROLEMIA AND XANTHOMATOSIS

This rare familial disorder was reported first by Bhattacharyya and Connor [90, 91]. In the original report the condition was characterized by the accumulation of the plant sterols campesterol, stigmasterol, and sitosterol in blood and tissues of two sisters, and the major clinical manifestations included tendon and subcutaneous xanthomas which developed in childhood. Plasma cholesterol concentrations were normal or only slightly elevated. The metabolic defect in this disorder has not been established. Bhattacharyya and Connor have suggested that the intestinal absorption of sitosterol[1] and other plant sterols is increased, while the excretion of these sterols from the body is impaired. The disease is inherited as an autosomal recessive trait.

[1] Throughout this chapter the term *sitosterol* is used instead of β-*sitosterol* when referring to 24-ethyl cholesterol. The β prefix is unnecessary, since it has no configurational meaning.

Clinical History

The first two reported cases of this disorder appeared in 1973 [90, 91]. One of two sisters, who were university students, complained of pain in the knees and heels. Xanthomas were present in the extensor tendons of both hands from the age of 8 and subsequently appeared in the patellar, plantar, and Achilles tendons of both sisters. The third patient is a 31-year-old woman with xanthomatosis, hypercholesterolemia, and hyperbetalipoproteinemia [92]. Her initial plasma cholesterol concentration was 300 mg/dl. Small xanthomas were present beneath the right eye, and xanthomas were noted on the extensor tendon of the right middle finger along with very prominent xanthomas in both Achilles tendons. Xanthomas were present in other areas of her body as early as age 1½. The patient had experienced repeated episodes of arthritis which responded to analgesics, and recently an abdominal bruit was detected.

A fourth patient was a 29-year-old man in whom extensive xanthomatosis was associated with normocholesterolemia, hemolysis, hypersplenism, and premature atherosclerotic vascular disease requiring a three-vessel coronary bypass [93]. A fifth patient was a 20-year-old woman with tendon and tuberous xanthomas [94]. Severe hypecholesterolemia was noted at age 12 (650 mg/dl).

The sixth patient is a 12-year-old girl with xanthomatosis, aortic stenosis, and abnormal platelet function [95]. Hypercholesterolemia (750 mg/dl) was found at age 3, and at age 12 angina developed. A 90-mm pressure gradient was measured across the aortic valve, but the coronary arteries were normal.

The C. family, studied by Khachadurian and Salen [96], consists of four children (three girls aged 22, 20, and 17 and one boy, age 16), three of whom show tendon and tuberous xanthomas and normal plasma cholesterol levels. No other clinical or hematologic abnormalities have been noted.

The tenth subject is a 42-year-old Chinese male with tendon and tuberous xanthomas and severe atheromatous changes in the coronary arteries [97]. In addition, chronic hemolytic anemia with spherostomatocytic erythrocytes and an enlarged spleen are present. The eleventh patient is a 12-year-old girl with hypercholesterolemia and xanthomatosis, repeated hemolytic episodes, and platelet abnormalities [98].

Recently, Kwiterovich et al. [98a] reported five subjects from an Amish kindred who had tendon and tuberous xanthomas. A 13-year-old boy died from coronary atherosclerosis. Hyperapobetalipoproteinemia was found in the five affected subjects, as well as in the two sisters originally reported by Bhattacharyya and Connor [91].

The clinical findings in these subjects are summarized in Table 34-6. Tendon xanthomas involving the Achilles tendon and extensor tendons of the hand are consistently found. Less frequently, xanthelasma and arcus corneae are noted. Cataracts are not present. Premature atherosclerosis affecting the coronary vessels and the aorta has been found in four subjects. In addition, hemolysis with an enlarged spleen and platelet abnormalities have been observed in four individuals. Hypercholesterolemia was also detected at some stage of the disease in four patients.

In the course of these investigations the plant sterols—sitosterol, campesterol, and stigmasterol—were discovered in high concentrations in the blood (Table 34-7). Other sterols such as cholestanol, sitostanol, and campesterol (the 5α-dihydro deriv-

Table 34-6 Clinical manifestations in sitosterolemia with xanthomatosis

	No. of patients		
	Documented	Absent	Not mentioned
Tendon xanthomas			
Achilles	16	—	—
Other	16	—	—
Xanthelasma	2	6	8
Arcus corneae	2	6	8
Atherosclerosis			
Coronary	2	7	7
Large vessel	3	8	5
Hemolysis	3	7	6
Hypersplenism	3	7	6
Platelet abnormalities	4	3	9
Arthralgia-arthritis	3	3	10
Hypercholesterolemia	9	7	—

atives of cholesterol, sitosterol, and campesterol) were also present in large amounts in some subjects. One patient showed increased plasma levels of avenosterol. Substantial quantities of bile alcohols (5β-cholestane-3α,7α,12α,25-tetrol; 27-nor-5β-cholestane-3α,7α,12α,24,25-pentol; and 5β-cholestane-3α,7α,12α,25,26-pentol), which may be related to cholic acid biosynthesis, were found in the feces [99]. The presence of bile alcohols suggests that a partial block in cholic acid synthesis may exist in these subjects. The structures of all sterols were identified by gas chromatography and mass spectroscopy [100].

Chemistry, Absorption, and Metabolism of Plant Sterols in Humans

The three plant sterols—sitosterol, campesterol, and stigmasterol—are usually found in the lipids of plants and are particularly plentiful in vegetable oils, nuts, and fat-rich vegetables and fruits. In chemical structure the plant sterols resemble cholesterol except for minor differences in the side chain (Fig. 34-14). Sitosterol and stigmasterol have C_{29} moieties and contain an ethyl substituent at the C-24 position. Stigmasterol, in addi-

tion, has a double bond at the C-22 position. Campesterol is a C_{28} sterol with a methyl substituent at the C-24 position. Their respective 5α-dihydro derivatives resemble cholestanol. These sterols are digitonin-precipitable. The unsaturated sterols react similarly to cholesterol in the colorimetric assays. They can be separated and quantitated by gas-liquid chromatography (Fig. 34-15). Like cholestanol, the 5α-dihydro derivatives of the plant sterols can be isolated by argentation thin-layer chromatography, but under normal circumstances they are present in only trace quantities.

Plant sterols are present in most human diets. About 250 mg is consumed each day [101]. Generally, sitosterol makes up 65 percent of the total sterols, with campesterol (about 30 percent) next in abundance; the remainder, about 5 percent, is stigmasterol [102].

In most humans, the intestinal absorption of plant sterols is quite limited. Only about 5 percent of the amount in the diet is absorbed [102, 103, 104]. The unabsorbed sterols pass through the intestine and are metabolized by intestinal bacteria similarly to cholesterol. Under special circumstances (such as formula diets), sitosterol, like cholesterol, may be degraded and lost in the feces [105]. Normally, only small amounts of plant sterols are present in the blood of human beings. The plasma concentration of sitosterol ranges from 0.3 to 1.7 mg/dl in humans consuming a typical U.S. diet [102]. During infancy, considerable amounts of sitosterol can be found in the blood (up to 9 mg/dl) and have also been detected in the aorta of infants fed vegetable oil–rich formulas [106, 107]. Large quantities of plant sterols inhibit cholesterol absorption. Cytellin, a drug rich in plant sterols, has been used to treat hypercholesterolemia by interfering with intestinal cholesterol absorption [108, 109].

Sitosterol turnover was found to conform to a two-pool model when the human subjects were fed a regular diet. The half-lives of the two exponentials of the sitosterol decay curves were much shorter than for cholesterol, and pool sizes of sitosterol were also smaller than those of cholesterol. On the basis of isotopic turnover studies, we have concluded that sitosterol is not synthesized in human beings [102]. Further, humans fed diets free of sitosterol for periods of 4 weeks or longer do not excrete sitosterol, or its bacterial transformation products, in the feces [102]. Thus, sitosterol is not produced in human tis-

Table 34-7 Plasma sterol concentrations in patients with sitosterolemia, mg/dl (% esterified)

Patients (with refs.)	Cholesterol	Cholestanol	Sitosterol	Sitostanol	Campesterol
I.[90, 91]	193 (71)	—	2.7 (56)	—	9.7 (59)
R.[90, 91]	206 (76)	—	17.1 (61)	—	8.2 (61)
P.[92]	242 (71)	—	12.3 (69)	—	6.1 (72)
D.*[93]	164 (70)	—	25.0	—	13.0
W.[94]	248	4.5	26.4	—	14.0
K.†[95]					
Ki.C.[96]	172	3.0	9.8	1.4	5.1
Ke.C.[96]	142	2.7	13.0	1.9	6.2
R.C.[96]	186	4.0	18.0	2.8	10.0
L.[97]	134	10.3	22.4	—	12.6
E.D.‡[98]	105	1.8	27.0	2.5	10.0
A family[98a]	269 (225–324)§	—	27.0 (21–34)	—	12.0 (8–16)

* Avenosterol, 5.0 mg/dl, was found in addition to above sterols.
† Only total plant sterols, 72.0 mg/dl, were determined.
‡ Campestanol, 1.5 mg/dl, was also found.
§ Numbers in these parentheses denote a range for five subjects [98a].

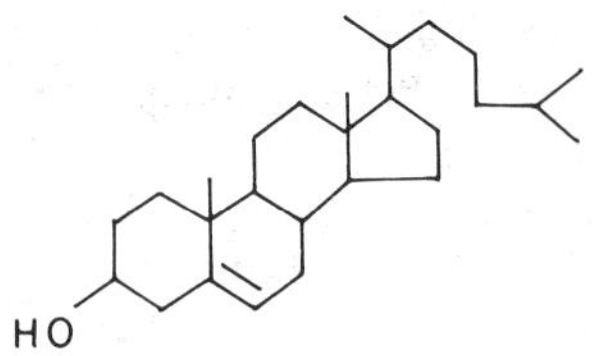

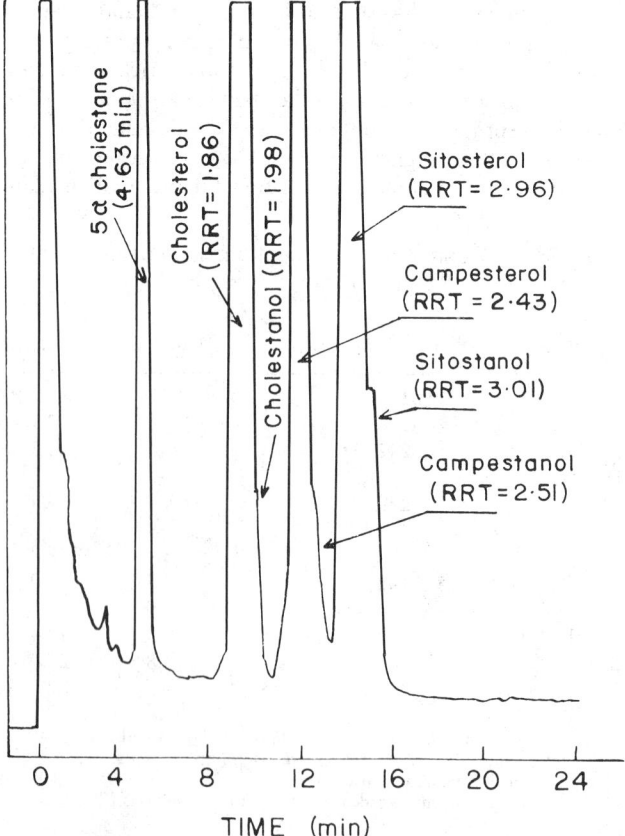

Cholesterol ($C_{27}H_{46}O$)

M·W· 386·6

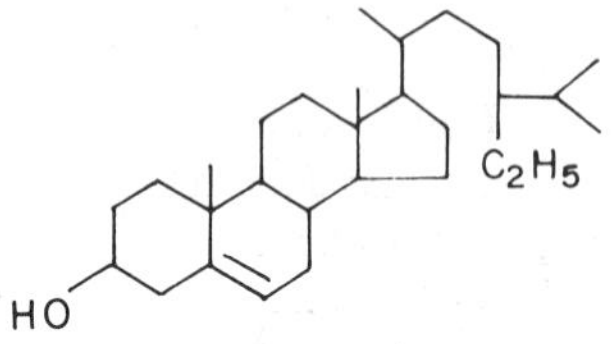

Sitosterol ($C_{29}H_{50}O$)

M·W· 414·7

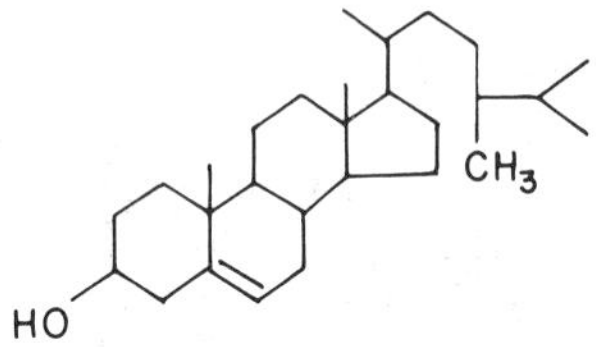

Campesterol ($C_{28}H_{48}O$)

M·W· 400·7

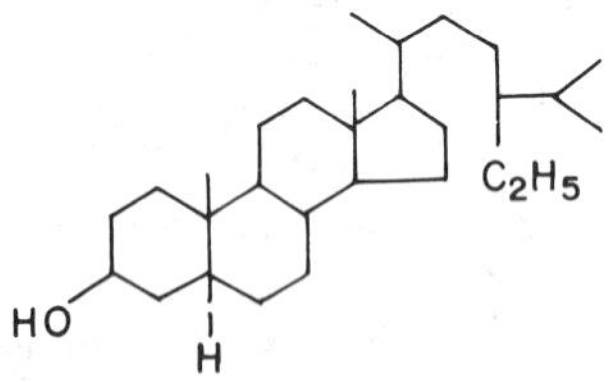

Sitostanol ($C_{29}H_{52}O$)

M·W· 416·7

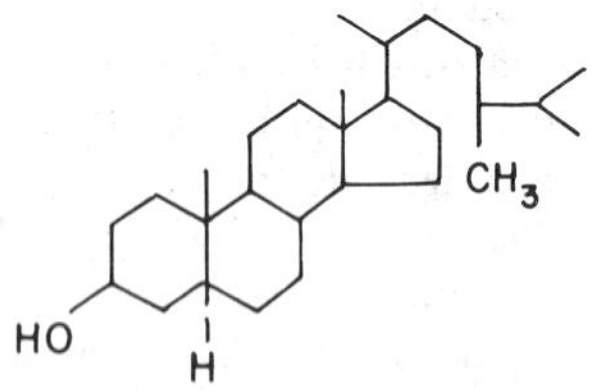

Campestanol ($C_{28}H_{50}O$)

M·W· 402·7

Figure 34-14 The chemical structures of cholesterol; two plant sterols, sitosterol and campesterol; and their respective 5α-dihydro derivatives, sitostanol and campestanol.

sues, and indeed there is no evidence that any animal tissue can synthesize plant sterols [110]. The capacity resides entirely in plants, in which these sterols serve as necessary components of membranes.

We have found that about 20 percent of the absorbed dietary sitosterol is converted to bile acids and the remainder is excreted as the free sterol in the bile [102]. The excretion is more rapid than that of cholesterol [102]. Sitosterol and the other two plant sterols are also excreted through the skin. As much as 33 percent of the absorbed sitosterol may be eliminated from the skin surface [111, 112].

The bile acids that are formed from sitosterol in human beings are cholic acid and chenodeoxycholic acid and are similar to those formed from cholesterol [102]. Similar findings regarding bile acid synthesis have been reported by Bhattacharyya and Connor [113]. In contrast, Subbiah has suggested that C_{26} and C_{29} bile acids are formed from sitosterol in the rat [114, 115]. Although the pathway of bile acid synthesis from sitosterol has not been elucidated, the ability to form bile acids from sitosterol may depend upon the animal's capacity to dealkylate sitosterol to cholesterol, perhaps via demosterol [116]. It would thus appear that humans may have the ability to dealkylate sitosterol.

Chemical Abnormalities

Blood High concentrations of sitosterol and campesterol (Figs. 34-14 and 34-15) are the characteristic features of sitosterolemia with xanthomatosis (Table 34-7). From 13 to 37 mg/dl, or from 7 to 16 percent, of the total plasma sterols are plant sterols. Sitosterol predominates with concentrations from 8 to 27 mg/dl. The campesterol and stigmasterol concentrations are much lower. About 67 percent of the plasma sitosterol and 72 percent of the cholesterol is esterified [91]. Lecithin:cholesterol acyltransferase (LCAT) is responsible for the esterification of plant sterols, as for cholesterol. Recently, increased amounts of the 5α-dihydro derivatives of sitosterol (sitostanol), campesterol (campestanol), and cholesterol (cholestanol) have been discovered in the plasma of six patients with this syndrome [94, 96, 97, 98].

The plasma plant sterols are distributed between LDL (70 percent of the total) and HDL. The VLDL carry only trace amounts of plant sterols [91, 93]. No specific lipoprotein or apoprotein has been found that transports plant sterols.

Erythrocytes from these subjects contain plant sterols. All sterols are in the free form [91]. Since the ratio of cholesterol to sitosterol in the red blood cells is similar to that in plasma, there presumably is free exchange across the red cell membrane [91].

Tendons Plant sterols, principally sitosterol, in tendons account for 12 to 27 percent of the total sterols found [91, 97].

Figure 34-15 Gas chromatogram of the plasma sterols of a subject (C.L.) with sitosterolemia and xanthomatosis. GLC on 3 percent QF-1 column, 240°C, N_2 = 40 ml/min. It is important to note the presence not only of the unsaturated plant sterols (sitosterol and campesterol) but also of their respective 5-dihydro derivatives (sitostanol and campestanol), which are seen as shoulder peaks.

5α cholestane (4·63 min)

Cholesterol (RRT= 1·86)

Cholestanol (RRT= 1·98)

Sitosterol (RRT= 2·96)

Campesterol (RRT = 2·43)

Sitostanol (RRT= 3·01)

Campestanol (RRT= 2·51)

TIME (min)

Virtually all the plant sterols are unesterified [91]. Cholesterol is the predominant sterol in the xanthomas and accounts for 70 to 88 percent of the total [91, 97]. Cholesteryl ester constitutes only 8 percent of the total cholesterol. Histologically, these lesions are similar to the tendon xanthomas found in familial hypercholesterolemia and in cerebrotendinous xanthomatosis.

Adipose Tissue and Skin Bhattacharyya and Connor measured the adipose tissue and skin sterol content of three patients [91]. They found increased amounts of plant sterols, ranging from 15 to 18 percent of total sterols.

Bile The concentration of plant sterols is much lower in bile than in plasma and tissues. Bhattacharyya and Connor found trace amounts of plant sterols in the bile of one subject, while two others showed the same ratio of sitosterol to cholesterol in bile as plasma [28]. We have confirmed the relatively low sitosterol/cholesterol ratios in our patients and believe, as do Bhattacharyya and Connor [91] and Miettinen [93], that reduced secretion of plant sterols from the liver represents one mechanism for their accumulation. The biliary bile acid pattern appears to be normal [28, 93].

Feces Examination of the feces from three subjects showed cholesterol, sitosterol, campesterol, and their 5β-saturated derivatives, as well as substantial amounts of the following bile alcohols: 5β-cholestane-3α,7α,12α,25-tetrol; 27-nor-5β-cholestane-3α,7α,12α,24,25-pentol; and 5β-cholestane-3α,7α,12α,25,26-pentol [96, 99]. The fecal bile acid pattern was also unusual in that it showed only deoxycholic acid, the 7-dehydroxy derivative of cholic acid. Chenodeoxycholic acid and its 7-dehydroxy bacterial by-product, lithocholic acid, which are normally present in the stools, were not detected. These findings suggest some alteration in the formation and excretion of bile acids in this disease.

Pathophysiology and the Metabolic Defect(s)

The studies of Bhattacharyya and Connor [92] and Miettinen [93] indicate that the absorption of dietary sitosterol is greatly increased. Normally, only about 5 percent of the sitosterol in the diet is absorbed [102]. Bhattacharyya and Connor [91] found that 18 to 35 percent and Miettinen [93] that 19 percent of the dietary sitosterol was absorbed. Although the exact mechanism enhancing the absorption of plant sterols is not known, a number of hypotheses have been suggested. The intestinal esterification of plant sterols during absorption may be increased. Since esterification is important in regulating cholesterol absorption, the mechanism whereby sitosterol limits intestinal absorption is believed to be related to less effective intestinal esterification. Thus, if the intestinal mucosa has lost its specificity to discriminate between sitosterol and cholesterol, the absorption of the plant sterol would be enhanced.

Alternatively, it has been suggested that the biliary secretion of sitosterol and cholesterol is limited [28, 93]. Thus, both sitosterol and cholesterol could accumulate because of defective removal. We have previously shown that the liver preferentially discriminates against sitosterol and increases the biliary excretion of this plant sterol relative to cholesterol [102]. Also, the excretion of bile alcohols in the feces of these subjects indicates some impairment of bile acid formation [96, 99].

Thus, increased absorption of plant sterols coupled with defective excretion and perhaps conversion to bile acid may cause tissue accumulation. In addition, since cholesterol also accumulates in the plasma and in xanthomas, the same defect may apply to cholesterol metabolism as well. Obviously, more studies are needed to explore these possibilities.

The accumulation of plant sterols sitosterol and campesterol in the plasma suggests that these abnormal sterols may play a role in promoting the development of the xanthomas in this disease. As in CTX, the major sterol that deposits in the tissue is cholesterol. Furthermore, the minor sterols, cholestanol, and the respective 5α-dihydro plant sterols may also play a role in accelerating tissue sterol deposition. It has been postulated that the presence of plant sterols in lipoproteins may affect their stability and, therefore, promote the deposition of cholesterol and sitosterol into the tissue [28]. Alternatively, these sterols may affect lipoprotein removal of sterols from the tissues. Miettinen has shown that HDL cholesterol levels are low in this disorder [93]. It has also been postulated that plant sterols may initiate xanthoma formation either by promoting net transfer or by stimulating local biosynthesis of cholesterol [117].

It is also postulated that plant sterols may play a role in the development of the atherosclerotic vascular disease seen in these patients. It is possible that plant sterols may favor the deposition of cholesterol into specific tissues such as the arterial wall and tendon, which in the former case leads to premature atherosclerosis. The development of an aortic bruit in one patient and coronary atherosclerosis in two other subjects is evidence in support of this view [92, 95, 97].

Diagnosis

Sitosterolemia with xanthomatosis should be considered in every patient who develops xanthomas in childhood and who does not have familial hypercholesterolemia or the CTX syndrome. Since some individuals with this syndrome present with high plasma cholesterol levels, measurement of plasma sterols by gas-liquid chromatography may be necessary to distinguish the true nature of the lipid disorder. The demonstration of increased amounts of sitosterol, campesterol, stigmasterol, or unusual plant sterols such as avenosterol by gas-liquid chromatography establishes the diagnosis.

Normally less than 1 percent of the total plasma sterols is sitosterol. In addition to plasma, erythrocyte sterols also have increased plant sterol levels. Thus, subjects with unexplained hemolytic anemia should be examined for xanthomas. In addition, 5α-saturated sterols should be sought in plasma and the excretion of bile alcohols in feces should be measured. If available, xanthoma, adipose tissue, and skin should be analyzed for sterols.

Treatment

The treatment of sitosterolemia with xanthomatosis is a diet low or devoid of plant sterols. In the study reported by Bhattacharyya and Connor, the plasma sitosterol concentration decreased 44 percent after 58 days on a sitosterol-free diet, or plant sterol–free diet [28]. In a second patient who received the diet for only 25 days, the plasma sitosterol level decreased 29 percent [117]. Plasma cholesterol levels also were reduced in these two patients.

As Bhattacharyya and Connor pointed out, planning a diet low in plant sterols is diametrically opposed to the low cholesterol diet used in the treatment of hypercholesterolemia. The guiding purpose of the diet is to remove vegetable fats, such as vegetable oils, shortening, and margarine; to eliminate all plant foods with high fat content, such as nuts, seeds, chocolate, olives, and avocado; and to use only refined cereal products in which the germ has been removed [28]. The removal of plant sterols from the diet should be in one phase of the program and should be supplemented, as suggested by Whitington et al. [94] and Kottke et al. [95], with cholestyramine. This drug binds bile acids in the intestinal tract and promotes their excretion. As a result, hepatic bile acid synthesis is accelerated, and cholesterol and presumably sitosterol are transformed more rapidly into bile acid. A low plant sterol diet supplemented with cholestyramine may result in the more rapid depletion of the increased body pool of sitosterol. Miettinen suggested the use of neomycin, a nonabsorbable antibiotic which also promotes the intestinal loss of cholesterol and plant sterols [93].

Genetics

Limited information about the inheritance of sitosterolemia with xanthomatosis is available. Based on the report of Bhattacharrya and Connor, the disorder seems to be inherited as an autosomal recessive trait. They observed that the parents of affected individuals are normal (no xanthomas) and that the children of one subject showed no defect [28, 91, 92, 98a].

REFERENCES

1. VAN BOGAERT L, SCHERER HJ, EPSTEIN E: *Une Forme cerebrale de la cholestérinose généralisée*. Masson et Cie, Paris, 1937
2. MENKES J, SCHIMSHOCK JR, SWANSON PD: Cerebrotendinous xanthomatosis: The storage of cholestanol within the nervous system. *Arch Neurol* 19:47, 1968
3. PHILIPPART M, VAN BOGAERT L: Cholestanolosis (cerebrotendinous xanthomatosis): A follow-up study on the original family. *Arch Neurol* 21:603, 1969
4. SALEN G: Cholestanol deposition in cerebrotendinous xanthomatosis: A possible mechanism. *Ann Intern Med* 75:843, 1971
5. SETOGUCHI T, SALEN G, TINT GS, MOSBACH EH: A biochemical abnormality in cerebrotendinous xanthomatosis: Impairment of bile acid biosynthesis associated with incomplete degradation of the cholesterol side chain. *J Clin Invest* 531:1395, 1974
6. SALEN G, MERIWETHER TW, NICOLAU G: Chenodeoxycholic acid inhibits increased cholesterol and cholestanol synthesis in patients with cerebrotendinous xanthomatosis. *Biochem Med* 14:57, 1975
7. SCHNEIDER C: Uber eine eigenartige Hirnerkrankung (vaskulare Lipoidose). *Allg Z Psychiatr* 104:144, 1936
8. VAN BOGAERT L, SCHERER HJ, FROELICH A, EPSTEIN E: Une deuxième Observation de cholestérinose tendineuse symétrique avec symptomes cérébraux. *Ann Med* 42:69, 1937
9. VAN BOGAERT L: Les Aspects neurologiques des cholestérinoses généralisées. *Prog Med (Paris)* 22:785, 1938
10. EPSTEIN E, LORENZ K: Beitrag zur Pathologie und Pathochemie der cholesterinigen Lipidose vom Typus van Bogaert-Scherer. *Klin Wochenschr* 16:1320, 1937
11. EPSTEIN E, KREITNER H: Beitrag zu einer vergleichnden Pathologie und Pathochemie der allgemeinen Cholesterinlipoidoses. *Virchows Arch (Zellpathol)* 306:53, 1940
12. GUILAIN G, BERTRAND I, GODET-GUILLAIN M: Etude anatomoclinique d'un cas de cholestérinose cérébrale. *Rev Neurol (Paris)* 74:249, 1942
13. GIAMPALMO A: Uber einen Fall von cholesterinlipidose vom Typus van Bogaert-Scherer. *Verh Dtsch Ges Pathol* 34:227, 1950
14. VINDITTI D: Una rara Lipidosi di interesse ortopedico: Forma cerebrotendinea della cholesterinosi generalizzata. *Chir Organi Mov* 34:429, 1950
15. GIAMPALMO A: Les Lipoidoses cholestériniques du système nerveaux. *Rev Neurol (Paris)* 89:322, 1953
16. GIAMPALMO A: Les Lipoidoses cholesteriniques due système nerveaux. *Acta Neurol Belg* 54:786, 1954
17. STEIN W, CZUCZWAR S: W. sprawie cholesterozy mosgowosciengnowej v. Bogaerta-Scherera-Epsteina. *Neurol Neurochir Pol* 9:599, 1959
18. VAN BOGAERT L: Le Cadre des xanthomatoses et leurs differents types: Xanthomatoses secondaires. *Rev Med (Liege)* 17:433, 1972
19. MENKES JH, PHILIPPART M: Cholestanol storage in the nervous system of two patients with cerebrotendinous xanthomatosis. *Trans Am Neurol Assoc* 93:66, 1968
20. MUCKENHAUSEN C, DERBY BM, MOSER HW: Conversion of C^{14} cholesterol to cholestanol in cerebrotendinous xanthomatosis. *Fed Proc* 28:882, 1968 (abstract)
21. DERBY BM, POGACAR S, MUCKENHAUSEN C, MOSER HW, RICHARDSON EP: Cerebrotendinous xanthomatosis: A clinicopathological, biochemical and metabolic study. *J Neuropathol Exp Neurol* 29:139, 1970 (abstract)
22. NAARDEN A: In discussion of Ref. 19
23. SCHIMSCHOCK JR, ALVORD EC JR, SWANSON PD: Cerebrotendinous xanthomatosis: Clinical and pathological studies. *Arch Neurol* 18:688, 1968
24. STAHL WL, SUMI SM, SWANSON PD: Subcellular distribution of cerebral cholestanol in cerebrotendinous xanthomatosis. *J Neurochem* 18:403, 1971
25. PASTERSHANK SP, YIP S, SODHI HS: Cerebrotendinous xanthomatosis. *J Assoc Can Radiol* 25:282, 1974
26. TRUSWELL AS, PFISTER PJ: Cerebrotendinous xanthomatosis. *Brit Med J* 1:353, 1972
27. SCHREINER A, HOPEN G, SKREDE S: Cerebrotendinous xanthomatosis (cholestanolosis): Investigations on two sisters and their family. *Acta Neurol Scand* 51:405, 1975
28. BHATTACHARYYA AK, CONNOR WE: Familial diseases with storage of sterols other than cholesterol: Cerebrotendinous xanthomatosis, and β-sitosterolemia and xanthomatosis, in Stanbury JB, Wyngaarden JB, Fredrickson DS (eds): *The Metabolic Basis of Inherited Diseases*, 3d ed. New York, McGraw-Hill, 1978, p 656
29. FARPOUR H, MAHLOUDJI M: Familial cerebrotendinous xanthomatosis. *Arch Neurol* 32:223, 1975
30. KEARNS W, WOOD WS: Cerebrotendinous xanthomatosis. *Arch Ophthalmol* 94:148, 1976
31. HAYE C, ROUFFY J, DUFIER JL: Une Cause rare de cataracte juvenile, la xanthomatosis cerebrotendineuse de van Bogaert-Scherer-Epstein. *Ann el 'Oculist* 209:501, 1976
32. BERGINER V, KORCZYN AP, MAYERSDORF A: Cerebrotendinous xanthomatosis. *Harefuah* 92:537, 1977
33. DE JONG JGY, VAN GENT CM, DELLMAN JW: Cerebrotendinous cholestanolosis in relation to other cerebral xanthomatosis. *Clin Neurol Neurosurg* 79:253, 1977
34. BRASSEUR G, MARX P, LANGLOIS J, HOUDENT G: Cerebrotendinous xanthomatosis. *Bull Soc Ophthalmol Fr* 78:913, 1978
35. SEYAMA Y, ICHIKAWA K, YAMAKAWA T: Quantitative determination of cholestanol in plasma with mass fragmentography. Biochemical diagnosis of cerebrotendinous xanthomatosis. *J Biochem* 80:223, 1976
36. OHNISHI A, YAMASHITA Y, GOTO I, KUROIWA Y, MURAKAMI S, IKEDA M: De- and remyelination and onion bulb in cerebrotendinous xanthomatosis. *Acta Neuropathol* 45:43, 1979
37. KURITZY A, BERGINER VM, KORCZYN AD: Peripheral neuropathy in cerebrotendinous xanthomatosis. *Neurology* 29:880, 1979
38. SWARTZ M, BURMAN KD, SALEN G: Cerebrotendinous xanthomatosis. *Am J Med Sci* 1982, in press
39. SHORE V, SALEN G, CHENG FW, FORTE T, SHEFER S, TINT GS, LINGREN F: Abnormal high density lipoproteins in cerebrotendinous xanthomatosis. *J Clin Invest* 68:1295, 1981
40. SALEN G: Unpublished observations
41. SALEN G, SHEFER S, CHENG FW, DAYAL B, BATTA AK, TINT GS: Cholic acid biosynthesis: The enzymatic defect in cerebrotendinous xanthomatosis. *J Clin Invest* 63:38, 1979
42. SELAND JH, SLAGSVOLD JE: The ultrastructure of lens and iris in cerebrotendinous xanthomatosis. *Acta Ophthalmol* 55:201, 1977
43. SALEN G, ZAKI FG, SABESIN S, BOEHME D, SHEFER S, MOSBACH EH: Intrahepatic pigment and crystal forms in patients with cerebrotendinous xanthomatosis (CTX). *Gastroenterology* 74:82, 1978
44. KLAUSE KA, SUBBIAH MTR: Improved resolution of cholestanol and cholesterol by gas-liquid chromatography: Application to pigeon testicular sterols. *J Chromatog* 103:170, 1975
45. ISHIKAWA TT, BRAZIER JB, STEWART LF, FALLOT RW, GLUECK CJ: Direct quantification of cholestanol in plasma by gas-liquid chromatography. *J Lab Clin Med* 87:345, 1976
46. COOK RP (ed): Cholesterol: *Chemistry, Biochemistry and Pathology*. New York, Academic, 1958

47. ROSENFELD RS, ZUMOFF B, HELLMAN L: Conversion of cholesterol injected into man to cholesterol via a 3-ketonic intermediate. *J Lipid Res* 8:16, 1967

48. SALEN G, POLITO A: Biosynthesis of 5α-cholestan-3β-ol in cerebrotendinous xanthomatosis. *J Clin Invest* 51:134, 1972

49. SHEFER S, MILCH S, MOSBACH EH: Biosynthesis of 5α-cholestan-3β-ol in the rabbit and guinea pig. *J Biol Chem* 239:1731, 1964

50. SHEFER S, MILCH S, MOSBACH EH: Biosynthesis of 5α-cholestan-3β-ol in rat and guinea pig liver in vitro. *J Lipid Res* 6:33, 1965

51. SHEFER S, HAUSER S, MOSBACH EH: Biosynthesis of cholestanol: 5α-Cholestan-3-one reductase of rat liver. *J Lipid Res* 7:763, 1966

52. WERBIN H, CHAIKOFF IL, IMADA NR: 5α-cholestan-3β-ol: Its distribution in tissues and its synthesis from cholesterol in the guinea pig. *J Biol Chem* 237:2072, 1962

53. WERBIN H, CHAIKOFF IL, PHILLIPS BP: Conversion of cholesterol to 5α-cholestan-3β-ol in germ free guinea pigs. *Biochemistry* 3:1558, 1964

54. BJÖRKHEM I, KARLMAR KE: Biosynthesis of cholestanol: Conversion of cholesterol into 4-cholesten-3-one by rat liver microsomes. *Biochim Biophys Acta* 337:129, 1974

55. TINT GS, SALEN G: Transformation of 5α-cholest-7-en-3β-ol to cholesterol and cholestanol in cerebrotendinous xanthomatosis. *J Lipid Res* 15:256, 1974

56. SHEFER S, SALEN G: Unpublished observations

57. KANDUTSCH AA, RUSSELL AE: Preputial gland tumor sterols. III. A metabolic pathway from lanosterol to cholesterol. *J Biol Chem* 235:2256, 1960

58. TINT GS, SALEN G: Evidence for the early reduction of the 24,25 double bond in the conversion of lanosterol to cholesterol in cerebrotendinous xanthomatosis. *Metabolism* 26:721, 1977

59. MOSBACH EH, BEVANS M: Formation of gallstones in rabbits fed 3β-cholestanol. *Arch Biochem Biophys* 63:258, 1958

60. BEVANS M, MOSBACH EH: Biological studies of dihydrocholesterol: Production of biliary concrements and inflammatory lesions of the biliary tract in rabbits. *Arch Pathol* 62:112, 1956

61. HOFMANN AF, BOKKENHEUSER V, HIRSCH RL, MOSBACH EH: Experimental cholelithiasis in the rabbit induced by cholestanol feeding. Effect of neomycin treatment on bile composition and gallstone formation. *J Lipid Res* 9:244, 1968

62. SALEN G, GRUNDY SM: The metabolism of cholestanol, cholesterol, and bile acids in cerebrotendinous xanthomatosis. *J Clin Invest* 52:2822, 1973

63. SKREDE S, STOKKE KT: Plasma esterification of cholestanol, normally and in cerebrotendinous xanthomatosis. *Scand J Clin Lab Invest* 33:97, 1974

64. ELLIOT WH: Allo-bile acids, in Nair PP, Kritchevsky D (eds): *The Bile Acids: Chemistry, Physiology and Metabolism*. New York, Plenum, 1971, p 47

65. SHEFER S, DAYAL B, TINT GS, SALEN G, MOSBACH EH: Identification of pentahydroxy bile alcohols in cerebrotendinous xanthomatosis: Characterization of 5β-cholestane-3α,7α,12α,24ε,25-pentol and 5β-cholestane-3α,7α,12α,23ε,25-pentol. *J Lipid Res* 16:280, 1975

66. DAYAL B, SALEN G, TINT GS, TOOME V, SHEFER S, MOSBACH EH: Absolute configuration of pentahydroxy bile alcohols excreted by patients with cerebrotendinous xanthomatosis: A circular dichroism study. *J Lipid Res* 19, 187, 1978

67. HOSHITA T, YASUHARA M, KIHIRA K, KURAMOTO T: Identification of (23S)-5β-cholestane-3α,7α,12α,23,25-pentol excreted by patients with cerebrotendinous xanthomatosis. *Steroids* 27:657, 1976

68. DAYAL B, TINT GS, SHEFER S, SALEN G: Configurational assignment of 5β-cholestane-3α,7α,12α,23,25-pentol excreted by patients with cerebrotendinous xanthomatosis (a circular dichroism study). *Steroids* 33:327, 1979

69. HOSHITA T, YASUHARA M, UNE M, KIBE A, ITOGA E, KITO S, KURAMOTO T: Occurrence of bile alcohol glucuronides in bile of patients with cerebrotendinous xanthomatosis. *J Lipid Res* 21:1015, 1980

70. DAYAL B, TINT GS, SALEN G, BOSE AK, PRAKASH O: Excretion of bile alcohol glucuronides. A diagnostic sign for cerebrotendinous xanthomatosis (CTX). 28th Congress International Union of Pure and Applied Chemistry (IUPAC), Vancouver, BC, Canada, August 1981. Abstract OR 242)

71. PHILIPPART M, VAN BOGAERT L: Cerebrotendinous xanthomatosis: A generalized disorder of cholestanol metabolism. *Trans Am Neurol Assoc* 94:322, 1969

72. GARDNER-MEDWIN D, KISHIMOTO Y, DERBY BM, MOSER HW: Cerebrotendinous xanthomatosis: In vivo labelling of cerebral sterols and sterol esters. *Trans Am Neurol Assoc* 96:241, 1971

73. TINT GS, SALEN G: Synthesis of cholesterol and its precursors but not cholestanol in cultured fibroblasts from patients with cerebrotendinous xanthomatosis. Submitted for publication.

74. NICOLAU G, SHEFER S, SALEN G, MOSBACH EH: Determination of hepatic 3-hydroxy-3-methylglutaryl CoA reductase activity in man. *J Lipid Res* 15:94, 1974

75. NICOLAU G, SHEFER S, SALEN G, MOSBACH EH: Determination of hepatic cholesterol 7α-hydroxylase activity in man. *J Lipid Res* 15:146, 1974

76. MOSBACH EH, SALEN G: Defective side-chain oxidation of cholesterol in patients with cerebrotendinous xanthomatosis, in Matern S, Hackenschmidt J, Back P, Gerok W (eds): *Advances in Bile Acid Research*. III Bile Acid Meeting, 1974. Stuttgart, New York, PK Schataner, p 111

77. SALEN G, SHEFER S, SETOGUCHI T, MOSBACH EH: Bile acid metabolism in man. Conversion of 5β-cholestane-3α,7α,12α,25-tetrol to cholic acid. *J Clin Invest* 54:226, 1975

78. HANSON RF, STAPLES AB, WILLIAMS GC: Metabolism of 5β-cholestane-3α,7α,12α,26-tetrol and 5β-cholestane-3α,7α,12α,25-tetrol into cholic acid in normal subjects. *J Lipid Res* 20:489, 1979

79. CROHNHOLM T, JOHANSSON G: Oxidation of 5β-cholestane-3α,7α,12α-triol by rat liver microsomes. *Eur J Biochem* 16:373, 1970

80. BJÖRKHEM I, GUSTAFSSON J, JOHANSSON G, PERSSIN B: Biosynthesis of bile acids in man: Hydroxylation of the C₂₇-steroid side chain. *J Clin Invest* 55:178, 1975

81. SHEFER S, CHENG FW, DAYAL B, HAUSER S, TINT GS, SALEN G, MOSBACH EH: A 25-hydroxylation pathway of cholic acid biosynthesis in man and rat. *J Clin Invest* 57:897, 1976

82. CHENG FW, SHEFER S, DAYAL B, TINT GS, SETOGUCHI T, SALEN G, MOSBACH EH: Cholic acid biosynthesis: Conversion of 5β-cholestane-3α,7α,12α,25-tetrol into 5β-cholestane-3α,7α,12α,24β,25-pentol by human and rat liver microsomes. *J Lipid Res* 18:6, 1977

83. SHEFER S, SALEN G, CHENG FW, DAYAL B, BATTA AK, TINT GS, BOSE AK, PRAMANIK BN: Chemical ionization-mass spectrometric approach to structure determination of an intermediate in bile acid biosynthesis. *Anal Biochem* 1982, in press

84. OFTEBRO H, BJÖRKHEM I, SKREDE S, SCHREINER A, PEDERSON J: Cerebrotendinous xanthomatosis: A defect in mitochondrial 26-hydroxylase required for normal biosynthesis of cholic acid. *J Clin Invest* 65:1418, 1980

85. SALEN G, MOSBACH EH: The metabolism of sterols and bile acids in cerebrotendinous xanthomatosis, in Nair PP, Kritchevsky D (eds): *The Bile Acids: Chemistry, Physiology and Metabolism*. New York, Plenum, 1976, p 115

86. SALEN G, SHEFER S, MOSBACH EH, HAUSER S, COHEN BI, NICOLAU G: Metabolism of potential precursors of chenodeoxycholic acid in cerebrotendinous xanthomatosis (CTX). *J Lipid Res* 20:22, 1979

87. SALEN G, MERIWETHER T: Chenodeoxycholic acid (CDCA) inhibits sterol biosynthesis in cerebrotendinous xanthomatosis. *Clin Res* 20:465, 1972 (abstract)

88. SALEN G, TINT GS, ELIAV B, DEERING N, MOSBACH EH: Increased formation of ursodeoxycholic acid in patients treated with chenodeoxycholic acid. *J Clin Invest* 53:612, 1974

89. BHATTACHARYYA AK, CONNOR WE: Effects of diet and drugs on plasma cholestanol and biliary bile acid composition in cerebrotendinous xanthomatosis. *Clin Res* 24:356, 1976 (abstract)

90. BHATTACHARYYA AK, CONNOR WE: β-Sitosterolemia and xanthomatosis. A newly described lipid storage disease in two sisters. *J Clin Invest* 52:9a, 1973 (abstract)

91. BHATTACHARYYA AK, CONNOR WE: β-Sitosterolemia and xanthomatosis. A newly described lipid storage disease in two sisters. *J Clin Invest* 53:1033, 1974

92. SHULMAN RS, BHATTACHARYYA AK, CONNOR WE, FREDERICKSON DS: β-Sitosterolemia and xanthomatosis. *N Engl J Med* 294:482, 1976

93. MIETTINEN T: Phytosterolemia, xanthomatosis and premature atherosclerotic disease: A case with high plant sterol absorption, impaired sterol elimination and low cholesterol synthesis. *Eur J Clin Invest* 10:27, 1980

94. WHITINGTON GL, RAGLAND JB, SABESIN SM, KUIKEN LB: Neutral sterolemia and xanthomatosis. *Circulation* 60:(II)33, 1979 (abstract)

95. KOTTKE BA, CORNICELLI JA, DIDISHEIM P, KAZMIER FJ, BARHAM SS, WEIDMAN WH: Phytosterolemia, xanthomatosis and acquired aortic valve stenosis. *Circulation* 62:(II)24, 1980 (abstract)

96. KHACHADURIAN AK, SALEN G: Familial phytosterolemia, cholestanolemia and abnormal bile salt composition. *Clin Res* 28(3):397A, 1980 (abstract)

97. WANG CCL, LIN HJ, CHAN TK, SALEN G, CHAN WC, TSE FF: A unique patient with coexisting cerebrotendinous xanthomatosis and β-sitosterolemia. *Am J Med* 71:313, 1981

98. KAYDEN HJ, SALEN G: Unpublished observations

98a. KWITEROVITCH PO, BACHORIK PS, SMITH HS, McKUSICK VA, CONNOR WE, TENG B, SNIDERMAN AD: Hyperapobetalipoproteinemia in two families with xanthomas and phytosterolemia. *Lancet* 1:466, 1981

99. DAYAL B, TINT GS, TOOME V, SALEN G: Structure and stereochemistry of a new C₂₆ sterol excreted by patients with neutral sterolemia and xanthomatosis: A circular dichroism study. 181st American Chemical Society Meeting (Organic Division), Atlanta, Georgia, March 1981 (abstract)

100. RAO MKG, PERKINS EG, CONNOR WE, BHATTACHARYYA AK: Identification of β-sitosterol, campesterol and stigmasterol in human serum. *Lipids* 10:566, 1975

101. CONNOR WE: Dietary sterols: Their relationship to athersclerosis. *J Am Diet Assoc* 52:202, 1968

102. SALEN G, AHRENS EH JR, GRUNDY SM: Metabolism of β-sitosterol in man. *J Clin Invest* 49:952, 1970

103. GOULD RG: Absorbability of beta-sitosterol. *Trans NY Acad Sci* 18:129, 1955

104. GOULD RG, JONES RJ, LEROY GV, WISSLER RW, TAYLOR CB: Absorbability of β-sitosterol in humans. *Metabolism* 18:652, 1969

105. GRUNDY SM, AHRENS EH JR: Dietary β-sitosterol as an internal standard to correct for cholesterol losses in sterol balance studies. *J Lipid Res* 9:374, 1968

106. MELLIES M, GLUECK CJ, SWEENEY C, FALLAT RW, TSANG RC, ISHIKAWA TT: Plasma and dietary phytosterols in children. *Pediatrics* 57:60, 1976

107. MELLIES MJ, ISHIKAWA TT, GLUECK CJ, BOVE K, MORRISON J: Phytosterols in aortic tissue in adults and infants. *J Lab Clin Med* 88:914, 1976

108. SHIPLEY RE, PFEIFFER RR, MARCH MM, ANDERSON RC: Sitosterol feeding: Chronic animal and clinical toxicology and tissue analysis. *Circ Res* 6:373, 1958

109. GRUNDY SM, AHRENS EH JR, DAVIGNON J: The interaction of cholesterol absorption and cholesterol synthesis in man. *J Lipid Res* 10:304, 1969

110. NICHOLAS HJ: The biogenesis of terpenes in plants, in Bernfeld P (ed): *Biogenesis of natural compounds*, 2d ed. New York, Pergamon, 1967, chap 14, p 829

111. BHATTACHARYYA AK, CONNOR WE, SPECTOR AA: Excretion of sterols from the skin of normal and hypercholesterolemic humans: Implications for sterol balance studies. *J Clin Invest* 51:2060, 1972

112. NIKKARI T, SCHREIBMAN PH, AHRENS EH JR: In vivo studies of sterol and squalene secretion by human skin. *J Lipid Res* 15:563, 1974

113. BHATTACHARYYA AK, CONNOR WE: Metabolic studies in the new lipid storage disease, β-sitosterolemia and xanthomatosis. *Circulation* 52:(II)5, 1975 (abstract)

114. SUBBIAH MTR, KUKSIS A, MOOKHERJEA S: Secretion of bile salts by intact and isolated rat liver. *Can J Biochem* 47:847, 1969

115. SUBBIAH MTR, KUKSIS A: Metabolism of β-sitosterol-4-^{14}C in the rat liver. *Proc Can Fed Biol Soc* 12:69, 1969

116. CLAYTON RB: The utilization of sterols by insects. *J Lipid Res* 5:3, 1964

117. BHATTACHARYYA AK: The pathogenesis of xanthomata: The role of sterols. *Artery* 2:2, 1976

35

PHYTANIC ACID STORAGE DISEASE (REFSUM'S DISEASE)

DANIEL STEINBERG

1. *Phytanic acid storage disease is a rare inborn disorder of lipid metabolism inherited as an autosomal recessive trait and recognized clinically as a predominantly neurologic syndrome. As first described by Sigvald Refsum in 1946, the cardinal manifestations are retinitis pigmentosa, peripheral neuropathy, cerebellar ataxia, and elevated cerebrospinal fluid protein concentration. Less constant features include nerve deafness, anosmia, skeletal abnormalities, ichthyosis, and nonspecific electrocardiographic abnormalities.*

2. *Almost without exception, the typical neurologic syndrome is associated with the accumulation in blood and tissues of an unusual 20-carbon, branched chain fatty acid—phytanic acid (3,7,11,15-tetramethylhexadecanoic acid). It can account for 5 to 30 percent of total fatty acids in plasma and up to 50 percent of total fatty acids in liver and kidneys of patients; only trace amounts are found in normal tissues and normal plasma (less than 0.5 percent of total fatty acids).*

3. *The phytanic acid that accumulates is exclusively exogenous in origin; endogenous biosynthesis has not been demonstrated. Dietary phytanic acid itself is the major source; dairy products and ruminant fats are especially rich sources, but small amounts are found in many dietary fats. Free phytol is readily converted to phytanic acid, but the phytol in chlorophyll (the major dietary source of phytol) is poorly absorbed.*

4. *The major mechanism for phytanic acid degradation is via a novel α-oxidative pathway, involving an initial α hydroxylation followed by decarboxylation to generate the 19-carbon lower homologue, pristanic acid. The further degradation of pristanic acid occurs by a series of β-oxidative steps analogous to those involved in oxidation of straight-chain fatty acids.*

5. *The rate of oxidation of phytanic acid in patients is less than 5 percent of that in normal subjects. The site of the defect has been localized to the initial step, catalyzed by phytanic acid α-hydroxylase.*

6. *Skin fibroblasts from patients oxidize phytanic acid at less than 5 percent the normal rate; fibroblasts from obligate heterozygotes oxidize phytanic acid at about 50 percent of the normal rate. Heterozygotes do not accumulate phytanic acid and remain asymptomatic. The carrier state can be demonstrated in fibroblast cultures.*

7. *Treatment with diets low in phytanic acid reduces plasma phytanic acid levels and brings about significant improvement in peripheral nerve function, in skin abnormalities, and in electrocardiographic patterns. However, full restoration of function is seldom achieved and cranial nerve dysfunction is not affected. Plasmapheresis combined with diet can be used to effect more rapid decreases in phytanic acid stores. Treatment that keeps plasma phytanate levels low arrests progress of the disease and prevents relapses. It should be instituted as early as possible and continued for life.*

HISTORY

In 1946 Sigvald Refsum published his definitive monograph identifying a new familial neurologic syndrome, which he designated heredopathia atactica polyneuritiformis [1]. The primary clinical features, almost all of them seen in Refsum's original cases, are listed in Table 35-1. Individually, none of the findings was unique, but Refsum astutely concluded that the pattern in his five original cases, occurring in two inbred Norwegian families, could be distinguished from those seen in the many clinically similar heredoataxic syndromes previously described.

The first direct evidence that the syndrome described by Refsum stemmed from a specific biochemical defect was published by Klenk and Kahlke in 1963 [2]. They analyzed postmortem tissues from a 7-year-old girl diagnosed as an example of Refsum's syndrome by Richterich and coworders in Berne. [3]. Liver and kidney were grossly infiltrated with lipid, mostly neutral lipid, but no unusual complex lipids were detected. Gas chromatographic analysis revealed a large, abnormal peak which accounted for over 50 percent of the total fatty acids in liver lipids. This component was isolated in pure form and fully characterized as phytanic acid, a 20-carbon, branched chain acid not previously reported in human tissues (Fig. 35-1). In the plasma of patients with Refsum's syndrome, phytanic acid was found in amounts corresponding to 5 to 30 percent of the total fatty acids [4]. Normal human plasma contains only traces of phytanic acid (less than 0.3 mg/dl), amounts so small that they are generally undetectable in routine analyses [5, 6].

Two general hypotheses suggested themselves concerning the origin of the accumulated phytanic acid [7, 8]. The polyisoprenoid structure of phytanic acid suggested a biosynthetic origin by pathways related to that for sterol synthesis. However, studies in patients with Refsum's syndrome [9, 10] and in experimental animals [11] failed to demonstrate any endogenous synthesis. These results pointed to an exogenous origin for the accumulated phytanic acid and a defect in catabolism as the basis for its accumulation. Phytol, a component of the chlorophyll molecule, was shown to be readily convertible to phytanic acid, and both phytol and phytanic acid itself were shown to be potential dietary sources since they accumulated when fed in large doses to experimental animals [9–17].

A series of studies by Steinberg and coworkers established the major pathway for phytanic acid oxidation in humans and experimental animals (Fig. 35-2) [18–22]. It involves (1) an unusual initial α oxidation to yield α-hydroxyphytanic acid, and then, by decarboxylation, the $(n - 1)$ fatty acid, pristanic acid; and (2) a series of successive β-oxidation steps for the further degradation of pristanic acid. Rates of phytanic acid

Table 35-1 Clinical features in phytanic acid storage disease

Retinitis pigmentosa: failing night vision,* progressive constriction of visual field, lenticular opacities
Peripheral polyneuropathy: generally symmetrical, motor and sensory losses, absent or diminished deep tendon reflexes
Cerebellar ataxia: dyscoordination out of proportion to the degree of peripheral neuropathy, unsteady gait, positive Romberg sign, intention tremor, nystagmus
Elevated cerebrospinal fluid protein level without pleocytosis.
Familial incidence with autosomal recessive pattern of inheritance.
Nerve deafness, anosmia, pupillary abnormalities, nystagmus
Nonspecific ECG changes.
Ichthyosislike changes ranging from mild hyperkeratosis of palms and soles to florid ichthyosis on trunk
Epiphyseal dysplasia: short fourth metatarsal, syndactyly, hammer toe, pes cavus, osteochondritis dissecans

* Some authors have used the term hemeralopia to designate poor vision in dim light, whereas medical dictionaries define the term to mean "day blindness." We shall use the less ambiguous term *night blindness*.

oxidation in patients were shown to be less than 5 percent of normal [9, 10, 23, 24], and the defect was shown to persist in fibroblast cell cultures [25]. The latter finding greatly facilitated further studies, which led to identification of the site of the metabolic block. Evidence from clinical observations [24] and cell culture studies [25–27] indicated that the primary enzyme defect lies at the first step in the new metabolic pathway, i.e., in the conversion of phytanic acid to α-hydroxyphytanic acid. Results of studies with model substrates structurally related to phytanic acid were compatible with this conclusion [28, 29].

As soon as it was established that phytanic acid had an exogenous origin, the possibility of therapeutic intervention by eliminating dietary sources of phytanate and its precursors was investigated. It was clearly shown that dietary modification reduces levels of phytanic acid in plasma and tissue [23, 30–32]. Experience to date shows that dietary treatment with reduction of phytanate levels arrests progress and leads to partial remission (see "Treatment" in this chapter).

Several reviews are available that include extensive discussion of clinical aspects, differential diagnosis, and pathologic findings [23, 33–35]. Cammermeyer has reviewed and synthesized the findings in 16 cases in which autopsies were performed [36]. Emphasis in this chapter will be placed primarily on the metabolic pathway for phytanic acid oxidation, the nature of the enzymatic deficiency, genetic aspects, and pathogenesis. Space limitations preclude reference to all of the approximately 400 papers dealing with this disease. Readers are referred to the previous edition of this book [37] and to other reviews for more complete documentation.

Figure 35-1 Structure of phytanic acid, a 20-carbon, fully saturated fatty acid. The branched chain structure is that characteristic of terpenes, presumably derived from four 5-carbon isoprenoid precursors.

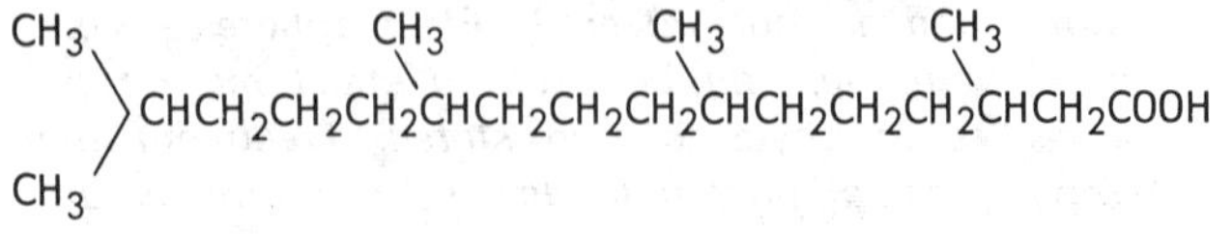

PHYTANIC ACID

(3, 7, 11, 15 - tetramethylhexadecanoic acid)

CLINICAL FINDINGS AND DIFFERENTIAL DIAGNOSIS

The diagnostic tetrad of retinitis pigmentosa, peripheral polyneuropathy, cerebellar ataxia, and high cerebrospinal fluid protein concentration in the absence of pleocytosis has been found in virtually every patient with phytanic acid storage disease. Additional clinical findings are listed in Table 35-1. The various clinical features may appear sequentially as the disease progresses; thus, incomplete syndromes early in the course are to be expected and have been described in patients already showing storage of phytanic acid.

The onset of the disease has been detected in early childhood in some patients, but not until the fifth decade in others. Most patients have clear-cut manifestations before age 20. Presenting complaints relate to failing vision and weakness in extremities or unsteadiness of gait. The earliest symptom is almost always night blindness, although it may require careful questioning to elicit this history and establish the true date of onset.

The course of the disease is one of gradually progressive deterioration, interrupted in over half of the patients by unexplained and sometimes lengthy periods of remission. Dramatic exacerbation associated with a poorly defined febrile illness, a surgical procedure, or pregnancy has been noted, as in Friedreich's ataxia. Gradual recovery of function following such episodes is the rule, but residual neurologic deficits remain.

A number of deaths have occurred suddenly and without obvious cause. In view of the ECG changes that accompany the disease, which are nonspecific in most cases but include a few examples of impaired AV conduction and bundle branch block, a cardiac arrhythmia is suspected as the cause of sudden death. Two deaths were attributed to respiratory paralysis and two to bacterial pneumonia, respiratory insufficiency not being mentioned explicitly as a factor.

Much increased levels of phytanic acid have been demonstrated in the serum of virtually every patient with Refsum's syndrome examined for them. Conversely, no increases in phytanic acid levels have been found in any of a wide variety of other neurologic syndromes, some of them closely related clinically to Refsum's syndrome. Some of the more important disorders with negative results for phytanic acid acccumulation are Dejerine-Sottas hypertrophic peripheral neuropathy, Friedreich's ataxia, multiple sclerosis, retinitis pigmentosa of both the recessive and dominant types, a larger number of nonspecific heredoataxias, peroneal muscular atrophy (Charcot-Marie-Tooth syndrome), abetalipoproteinemia, high-density lipoprotein deficiency (Tangier disease), amyotrophic lateral sclerosis, Sjogren-Larsson syndrome, Spielmeyer-Vogt disease, and Tay-Sachs disease. Kahlke, Goerlich, and Feist [38] described an infant with cerebral damage, arrested development, icterus, and hepatomegaly in whom phytanate was unequivocally elevated in the serum and in a liver biopsy but the clinical picture was decidedly not that of Refsum's syndrome. A female sib born 6 years later developed a similar neurologic disorder but no phytanate was found in the plasma (Dr. W. Kahlke, personal communication).

Concordance between clinical diagnosis and phytanic acid storage has been established in 75 cases, but there are some exceptions. Several patients with clinical features difficult to distinguish from those typically found in Refsum's syndrome have been described in whom there was no demonstrable accu-

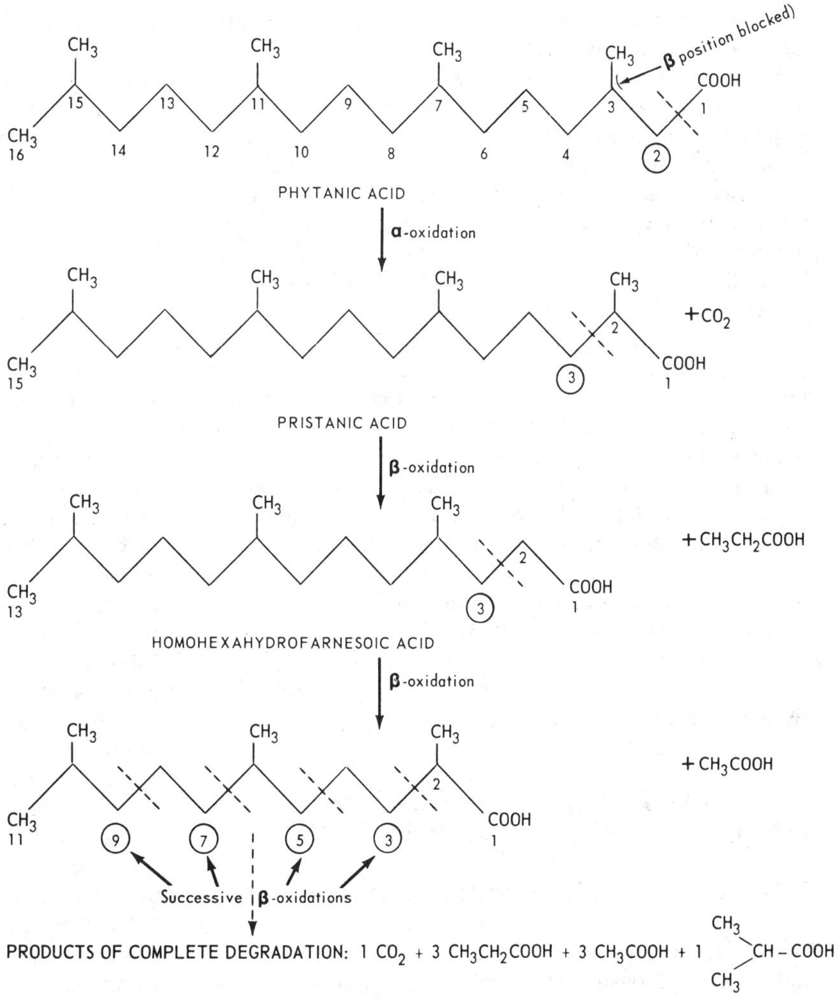

Figure 35-2 The major pathyway for oxidation of phytanic acid in mammals. The first step, introduction of an hydroxyl function at the α position, is the site of the metabolic block in phytanic acid storage disease. This is followed by decarboxylation to yield the (n−1) lower homologue, pristanic acid, and then a series of successive β oxidations.

PRODUCTS OF COMPLETE DEGRADATION: 1 CO_2 + 3 CH_3CH_2COOH + 3 CH_3COOH + 1

mulation of phytanate. [32, 39–44]. In one of these, metabolic studies and cell culture studies showed that the patient oxidized phytanate normally, and autopsy failed to show the findings characteristic of Refsum's disease [44]. Further work may clarify the relationship between pathogenesis in cases *without* phytanate and that of the more usual cases *with* phytanate. At present it is preferable to designate as examples of phytanic acid storage disease only those patients with both (1) the typical clinical syndrome, and (2) demonstrated accumulation of phytanic acid or demonstrated reduction in capacity to oxidize phytanic acid. The latter stipulation is included since even patients with drastically reduced capacity to metabolize phytanate may, when kept on the appropriate diet, all but free themselves of the stored acid [31, 32]. Their capacity to oxidize phytanate, however, remains deficient [24].

An even narrower definition at the biochemical level can be proposed. In 14 clinically typical patients studied in vivo or in cell culture, or both, the oxidation of pristanic acid, the α-oxidation product of phytanic acid, was normal. This established that the metabolic error is a phytanic acid α-oxidase deficiency [45]. In 8 of the 14 patients thus far tested, oxidation of α-hydroxyphytanate was also normal [24, 27, 46]. Thus these patients, and perhaps most or all others with phytanic acid storage disease, are examples of *phytanic acid α-hydroxylase deficiency*.

Presumed heterozygotes (parents or sibs of clinical cases) have occasionally shown phytanate accumulation without evidence of neurologic involvement [47, 48]. Since heterozygotes have about a 50 percent reduction in capacity to oxidize phytanate [45], it is understandable that these individuals may tend to accumulate phytanic acid but to a much more limited extent than homozygotes. The normal level of oxidative capacity is far in excess of that needed to dissimilate the usual intake of phytanate and precursors in the diet. On the other hand, it is conceivable that under the appropriate circumstances (excessive dietary load or imposition of extrinsic factors accentuating the metabolic defect) these heterozygotes may store phytanic acid to a limited degree (and possibly even develop clinical disease). Heterozygotes may be designated as examples of *phytanic acid storage trait*.

A definitive diagnosis of phytanic acid storage disease requires demonstration of abnormal levels of phytanic acid in blood or tissues accompanying the typical clinical syndrome. Gas-liquid chromatography of the fatty acid methyl esters is the method of choice [49]. Because of its branched structure, methyl phytanate behaves like a straight-chain, 17-carbon fatty acid on gas-liquid chromatography. Mass spectroscopy may be needed for unequivocal identification. A satisfactory preliminary screening tool is provided by thin-layer chromatography, which is based on the greater mobility of triglycerides that contain phytanate [50–52]. Even when phytanate accounts for only 10 percent of total serum fatty acids, the phytanate-containing glycerides can be identified. Verification can then be made by gas-liquid chromatography.

METABOLIC BASIS FOR ACCUMULATION OF PHYTANATE

Evidence against Endogenous Synthesis

The polyisoprenoid structure of phytanic acid suggested that it might be endogenously synthesized by a pathway such as that

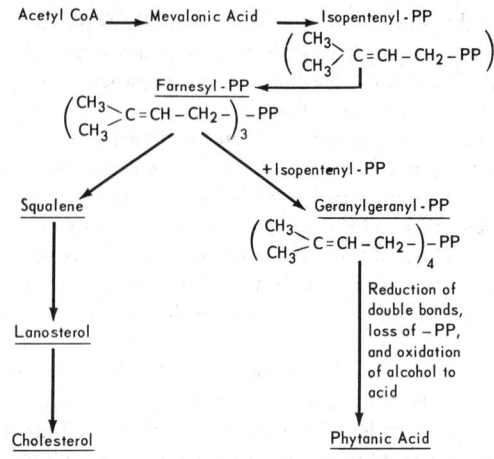

Figure 35-3 Postulated scheme for endogenous biosynthesis of phytanic acid by a pathway branching from that for sterol biosynthesis. While this pathway may operate in plants and bacteria, no evidence for the pathway shown on the right has been obtained in animals or humans.

outlined in Fig. 35-3 [7, 8]. Geranylgeranyl pyrophosphate is a normal intermediate in carotene biosynthesis in plants, and its synthesis has been reported in mammalian liver. In plants, phytol is formed from mevalonic acid by such a pathway and thus there is precedent for the reduction of double bonds in the polyisoprenoid series. The postulated conversion of the alcohol to a carboxylic acid would be analogous to the demonstrated oxidation of farnesol to farnesoic acid.

Attempts to demonstrate biosynthesis of phytanic acid from [2-^{14}C] mevalonic acid in a patient with phytanic acid storage disease were negative, and neither labeled acetate nor mevalonate was incorporated into phytanate in experimental animals [9–11]. To rule out the possibility of a very slow rate of endogenous synthesis and to test for alternative pathways of biosynthesis from small molecules, clinical studies were carried out in two patients using D_2O as a precursor [10, 31]. The patients' body water levels were held at a constant level of enrichment over 4 to 5 months. Plasma cholesterol levels showed the expected progressive enrichment in deuterium, but plasma phytanate levels showed minimal enrichment, corresponding to replacement of only two to four hydrogen atoms. Some enrichment would be expected as a result of the conversion of dietary phytol to phytanic acid (see below). The results make it unlikely that much if any of the phytanate that accumulates in this disease arises from endogenous *de novo* biosynthesis. The fact that elimination of phytanate from the diet reduces body stores of the compound (see below) clearly establishes the quantitative importance of exogenous sources. Nevertheless, the postulated pathway via geranylgeranyl pyrophosphate may operate at a low level and may be induced by environmental or genetic factors.

Dulaney et al. [53] recently reported the occurrence of small amounts of a triunsaturated form of phytanic acid in the serum and urinary lipids of patients (but not of normal subjects). This compound could represent a metabolite of geranylgeranyl pyrophosphate with only one of the four double bonds reduced, the pyrophosphate cleaved, and the alcohol function oxidized (Fig. 35-3). Further metabolic studies are awaited with interest.

Origin from Dietary Phytanic Acid

Addition of phytanic acid to the diet of rats or mice leads to its accumulation in blood and tissues [9, 16, 17]. Large amounts must be fed to exceed the large capacity of the normal animal to catabolize phytanate. In mice fed diets containing 2 percent by weight phytanate for 2 weeks, the phytanate levels in liver and serum reached values of 20 to 30 percent of total fatty acids, levels approaching those seen in affected patients. It should be noted that daily dietary intake of phytanate in humans is less than 100 mg/day or about 1 mg/kg/day; the intake needed to cause significant accumulation in mice and rats is about 1000 mg/kg/day! Since phytanic acid is efficiently absorbed by way of the lymph—as efficiently as palmitic acid [54]—these feeding experiments indicate that the compound is rapidly metabolized. This is confirmed by the rapid disappearance of stored phytanate (within a week or two) when the animals are returned to a normal diet.

Dairy products and ruminant fats in the human diet are probably the major sources of phytanic acid [55, 56]. Ruminants ingest large quantities of chlorophyll and the resident bacteria in the rumen effectively degrade it, liberating the phytol from its linkage to the propionic acid side chain of the porphyrin. Free phytol is then readily converted to phytanic acid, as discussed below. Some conversion occurs even within the rumen [57]. Phytanic acid can account for as much as 5 to 10 percent of the total fatty acids in bovine plasma, whereas plasma of nonruminant animals and of normal humans contains only traces. Butterfat can contain more than 100 mg phytanate per 100 g wet weight [56]. Only limited data are available on the phytanate content of individual foodstuffs [23, 56, 58–61] (see below, Table 35-2). Estimates based on analyses of pooled aliquots of an ordinary diet yield values of 56 to 89 mg/day [23, 62].

In the rat, orally administered phytanic acid is well absorbed even when fed in large doses, and most of the absorption occurs by way of the lymph [54]. Direct studies of phytanic acid absorption in humans are not available. Since phytol absorption in humans is similar to that in the rat [9, 13–15], it may be reasonable to assume that at least 50 to 75 percent of the phytanic acid in the daily diet is in fact absorbed.

Origin From Dietary Phytol

Free Phytol   Phytol, differing in structure from phytanic acid only in having a Δ^2 double bond and an alcohol rather than a carboxylic acid function at the 1 carbon (Fig. 35-4), is readily converted to phytanic acid [9–15]. Two pathways are possible, depending on the sequence in which the double bond reduction and the oxidation of the alcohol function occur. Both the 2,3-unsaturated acid (phytenic acid; Δ^2-3,7,11,15-tetramethylhexadecenoic acid) and the saturated alcohol (dihydrophytol) can be converted to phytanic acid, so that both pathways are potentially available [11, 14]. After administration of phytol to experimental animals, large amounts of phytenic acid are found but little or no dihydrophytol. This suggests that oxidation of the alcohol function is normally the initial step [11, 54]. Nevertheless, the possibility that there is a rapid turnover of dihydrophytol remains. Further studies are needed before the alternative pathways can be properly evaluated.

Orally administered phytol is efficiently absorbed by normal human subjects (61 to 94 percent of a tracer dose) and similar values have been found in two patients with phytanic acid storage disease [10]. Studies in rats show that absorption is mainly by way of the thoracic duct [54], and in the course of absorption about 10 to 20 percent of the dose is converted to phytanic acid. Since similar values were found in a germ-free rat, it is unlikely that the intestinal flora play any major role in the phytol–phytanic acid conversion.

Klenk and Kremer, on examining the liver fatty acids of phytol-fed rats, noted the presence of three or four different isomeric forms of phytenic acid, but these were not further characterized [14]. Baxter and Milne developed chromatographic methods that improved resolution of these isomers and made possible their individual isolation on a preparative scale [63]. They showed that the usual saponification procedures lead to isomerization but that transesterification under acid conditions does not. Five isomers were demonstrated in the lymph of phytol-fed rats: the cis and trans forms of Δ^2-phytenic acid, the cis and trans forms of Δ-phytenic acid, and the 3-methylene isomer. The trans-Δ^2 form predominated (70 percent of total phytenic acid). These findings are interesting in relation to the question of the mechanism of the phytol-phytanate conversion and may also be relevant to the question of the variable ratios of phytanic acid diastereoisomers found in different animal species and different patients with phytanic acid storage disease [55, 64, 65].

Chlorophyll-Bound Phytol   The ubiquitous presence of chlorophyll in green vegetables suggested that this might be an important dietary precursor since it contains 1 mol phytol per

Table 35-2   Examples of phytanic acid content of foodstuffs [23,56,61]

	mg per 100 g wet weight
Butter	50–500
Margarines	6–130
Cheeses	5–50
Herring	11.2
Palm oil	11.2
Beef liver	2.6
Lard	1.8
Calves liver	1.5
Veal	0.75
Skim milk powder	0.5–0.6
Codfish	0.32
Milk	0.26
Egg yolk	0.22
Tomato	0.13
Pork	0.04
Squash	0.04
Chicken legs	0.01

The values given represent in many cases analyses of only a single sample and should not be generalized. The wide variations in phytanate content of dairy products in part reflect seasonal differences in cattle feeding practices, in part differences in total fat content (cheeses). The wide variations in margarines reflects the different sources of fat used in their manufacture, especially differences in use of oils of marine origin. Margarine of exclusively vegetable oil origin tends to have the lowest phytanate content.

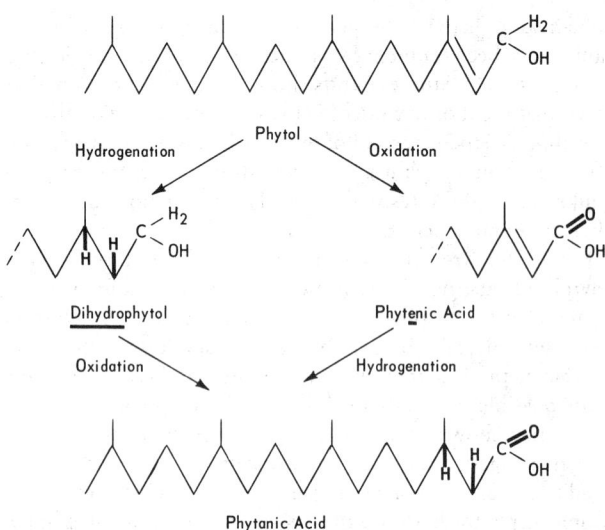

Figure 35-4 Two alternative pathways for the conversion of phytol to phytanic acid. The operation of the pathway shown on the right has been demonstrated. Conversion of dihydrophytol to phytanic acid has been demonstrated, but the overall pathway shown at the left has not yet been verified experimentally.

mole, bound in ester linkage to a propionic acid side chain of one of the pyrrole rings. However, Baxter and Steinberg, using high-specific-activity [14C]pheophytin *a* (Mg^{2+}-free chlorophyll *a*), showed that in the thoracic duct–cannulated rat not more than 2 percent of bound phytol was absorbed [66]. Baxter's clinical balance studies showed that 95 percent of the phytol administered orally as [14C]pheophytin was recovered in the feces, both in normal control subjects and in two patients with phytanic acid storage disease [98]. He also fed 180 g spinach to a human subject with the thoracic duct cannulated and recovered only 2 percent of the spinach phytol in a 24-h lymph collection. From these results it is clear that, while free phytol is an excellent precursor of phytanic acid, the bound phytol in the chorophyll molecule cannot be a quantitatively important dietary source of stored phytanate. In the course of preparing vegetables for the table some of the phytol may be released from ester form and become available. However, even the total amount of phytol in the usual diet is less than 10 percent of the amount of preformed phytanic acid [31, 56].

Other Precursors

Billeter et al. [67], studying the metabolism in pigeons of orally administered phylloquinone labeled both in the nucleus and in the phytyl side chain, found that the latter was split off by intestinal bacteria. The fate of the side chain was further studied using a side chain–labeled phylloquinone. It was possible to isolate an acidic lipid with the properties of phytanic acid from breast muscle. Data are not available to assess the quantitative importance of this pathway.

It is possible that the intestinal flora contribute to the stored phytanate in patients. Some bacteria can synthesize phytanate itself and others may synthesize related isoprenoid compounds convertible to phytanate [68, 69]. If such synthesis occurs *de novo* in the bacteria (from acetate by way of mevalonate), the clinical studies with D$_2$O described above should have detected it, since the total body water, including that in the intestine, was presumably at the same level of enrichment with deuterium. On the other hand, if the bacteria were to modify the structure of higher molecular weight branched chain compounds in the diet, such structural modification might not necessarily entail incorporation of hydrogen from water and would go undetected. Additional evidence against a quantitatively important contribution by intestinal bacteria comes from clinical studies of phytanic acid excretion in feces. After 10 days on a phytanic acid–low formula diet, fecal excretion of phytanate fell to about 2 mg/day [31].

There is some reason to suspect that not all of the dietary precursors are known. The amounts of phytanic acid accumulated in the tissues of patients, as estimated from biopsies and postmortem analysis, are considerable—up to 200 to 400 g. Even assuming a dietary intake of 100 mg/day and no degradation or excretion at all, it would take 5 to 10 years to accumulate such large stores. While this is by no means unfeasible, the possibility must be considered that there are additional sources of phytanate. The possibility that there is endogenous biosynthesis in infants and children should be tested, other branched chain dietary constituents should be considered as precursors, and production by unusual intestinal flora should be explored.

DEFECTIVE OXIDATION OF PHYTANIC ACID

Normal Oxidative Capacity

A number of lines of evidence indicate that normal animals, including human beings, have a large capacity to dissimilate phytanic acid and prevent its accumulation even at high levels of intake. [U-14C]phytanic acid injected intravenously into normal humans as the albumin complex is converted to $^{14}CO_2$ at a rate comparable to that for [1-14C]palmitic acid [24]. This is so even though the initial rate of disappearance of the labeled free phytanic acid from the plasma is distinctly lower than that of palmitic acid. Orally administered [U-14C]phytol, which is probably oxidized to $^{14}CO_2$ in large part only after prior conversion to phytanic acid, is also efficiently oxidized—about 21 percent of the absorbed dose in the first 12 h [10].

The capacity of experimental animals to oxidize and excrete phytanate can be exceeded, but this requires the addition of relatively large amounts of phytanic acid or phytol to the diet, as discussed above. In humans, according to Avigan, even after ingestion of 9.5 g of phytol in a single dose by a normal subject, plasma phytanate had risen only to 2.4 mg/dl after 18 h [5]. In a heroic study this same volunteer ate 3.5 kg of boiled spinach over a 60-h interval; his plasma phytanic acid level did not change perceptibly! Further evidence comes from studies showing that the fractional rate of oxidation of phytol to CO$_2$ in normal volunteers is the same whether only a tracer dose is given or whether a full 1-g dose of carrier phytol is given with it [10].

Defective Oxidation in Patients

Clinical Studies   The first demonstration of the reduced capacity of patients to oxidize phytanic acid utilized [U-14C]phytol as a precursor [9]. Observed rates of $^{14}CO_2$ production in two patients were only about one-fifth those in normal volunteers. Subsequent studies in three additional cases using intravenously injected [U-^{14}C]phytanic acid itself showed an even more striking defect, initial rates of $^{14}CO_2$ production being less than 5 percent of those in control subjects [24]. The apparent difference in the degree of block suggested by the clinical studies using these two different precursors probably does not reflect basic differences in the degree of enzyme block in the patients studied. Later cell culture studies using fibroblasts derived from skin biopsies showed that all five patients had comparably severe deficits, phytanic acid being oxidized at rates less than 5 percent of those observed in normal fibroblast cultures [45]. The results suggest the possibility that phytol can be oxidized to a significant degree by a pathway not involving phytanate as an intermediate.

After intravenous injection of labeled phytanic acid, less than 0.001 percent of the dose was recovered in the feces of either controls or patients, showing that biliary excretion or other mechanisms of excretion by way of the intestinal tract are quantitatively unimportant [24]. Less than 6 percent of the injected radioactivity appeared in the urine, 95 percent of it in nonlipid forms.

Eldjarn and coworkers compared controls and patients with regard to oxidation of model compounds [70–72] but not phytanic acid itself. These model compounds (3,6-dimethyloctanoic acid and 4,14,14-trimethylpentadecanoic acid) resemble phytanate in having a methyl substituent on the 3 carbon and, like phytanate itself, are not susceptible to ordinary β oxidation. Moreover, the substituents at the ω ends of these molecules should prevent β oxidation from that end also. The former compound, labeled in the ω terminus (carbon 8), was oxidized to a limited extent by normal controls—2 to 3 percent in 10 h—but in two patients with phytanic acid storage disease no $^{14}CO_2$ could be detected above background. One of these patients was restudied after plasma phytanate levels had been drastically reduced by dietary means [72]. At that time there was a small but significant yield of $^{14}CO_2$—0.5 to 1 percent of the administered dose. The oxidation of the other model compound, 3,14,14-trimethylpentadecanoic acid, which was labeled with tritium by catalytic exchange, was determined by measuring the release of tritium to body water. In control subjects, 31 to 37 percent of the dose was found in body water at the maximum but in two patients, only 8 and 17 percent, respectively [72]. The metabolic pathway by which the trimethylpentadecanoic acid was degraded was not established and the cumulative yield of labeled metabolites in the urine was apparently no different in patients and controls. The other model compound, 3,6-dimethyloctanoic acid, is largely degraded by ω oxidation, a small fraction undergoing α oxidation as discussed below.

Fibroblast Cell Culture Studies   As in a growing list of inherited diseases of metabolism, the defect in phytanic acid storage disease persists in cultured fibroblasts [25]. Normal human fibroblasts derived from skin biopsies oxidize added phytanate at rates comparable to those for added palmitate. Cells derived from patients with phytanic acid storage disease, on the other hand, while oxidizing palmitate at a normal rate, oxidize phytanate at only about 1 percent of the normal rate. The low rate of phytanate oxidation is not due to a defect in uptake; the rate of incorporation of phytanate into cell lipids was in fact greater in the patients' cells than in the controls' cells, but the sum of [^{14}C]phytanate in cell lipids and in $^{14}CO_2$

was almost exactly the same. This indicated a normal uptake mechanism [27].

Another interpretation of the observed low rate of $^{14}CO_2$ production was that phytanate incorporated into ester linkages might be released at a low rate in the cells of patients and thus not be as readily available for subsequent oxidation. In other words, the defect might lie in a modified or deleted hydrolytic system(s) rather than in the oxidizing system per se. Direct studies of the rate of release of phytanate previously incorporated into cultured cells during incubation in unlabeled medium showed no difference in this regard between the cells of patients and control cells [27]. Laurell has shown that the phytanyl ester bonds in glyceryl triphytanate are extremely resistant to hydrolysis by lipoprotein lipase [73]. Since the plasma of patients contains diphytanyl and monophytanyl triglycerides but no detectable triphytanyl triglycerides [50–52, 74], this finding leaves undecided the question of whether the phytanyl ester bonds in the naturally occurring mixed glycerides also are resistant to hydrolysis. Studies by Avigan and Steinberg, using the serum of a patient with phytanic acid storage disease or chyle from a phytanic acid–fed rat as substrate, indicated that even in mixed glycerides the phytanyl ester bond is resistant to the action of lipoprotein lipase [75]. Ellingboe, using synthetic mixed glycerides containing phytanate, showed that the phytanyl ester bond is relatively resistant to hydrolysis by pancreatic lipase as well as by lipoprotein lipase from rat adipose tissue [76]. These findings may explain the fact that phytanic acid in the depot fat of patients or phytanic acid–fed rats accounts for a much lower percentage of the total than it does in the plasma. No difference has thus far been reported between control subjects and patients in their ability to hydrolyze phytanyl ester bonds.

The studies summarized to this point establish that there is little or no endogenous biosynthesis of phytanic acid, that phytol and phytanic acid are potential dietary precursors (and perhaps other compounds), and that the metabolic error lies in a degradative pathway (Fig. 35-5).

PATHWAY FOR PHYTANIC ACID OXIDATION IN RELATION TO PREVIOUSLY DESCRIBED PATHWAYS FOR FATTY ACID OXIDATION

Based on the present knowledge of fatty acid oxidizing mechanisms, the theoretically possible modes of initial attack on the phytanic acid molecule are indicated in Fig. 35-6, and each will be discussed in turn.

β Oxidation

This ubiquitous mitochondrial system for successive cleavage of two carbon fragments from the carboxyl end of the chain is quantitatively the most important pathway for fatty acid oxidation. Five basic steps, repeated in cyclic fashion, are involved:

Activation (acylthiokinase, long chain):
$$RCH_2CH_2COOH + CoASH + ATP \longrightarrow$$
$$RCH_2CH_2COSCoA + AMP + PP_i \quad (1)$$

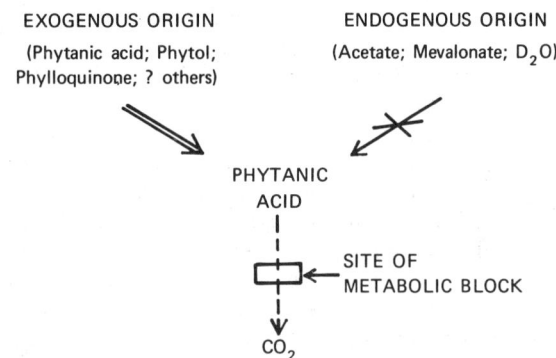

Figure 35-5 The metabolic error in phytanic acid storage disease.

Dehydrogenation (acyl CoA dehydrogenase):
$$RCH_2CH_2COSCoA + \text{flavoprotein} \longrightarrow$$
$$RCH{=}CHCOSCoA + \text{reduced flavoprotein} \quad (2)$$

Hydration (enoyl hydrase):
$$RCH{=}CHCOSCoA + H_2O \longrightarrow RCHOHCH_2COSCoA \quad (3)$$

Dehydrogenation (L(+)-β-hydroxyacyl-CoA dehydrogenase):
$$RCHOHCH_2COSCoA + NAD^+ \longrightarrow$$
$$R\overset{O}{\overset{\|}{C}}CH_2COSCoA + NADH + H^+ \quad (4)$$

Thiolytic cleavage (β-ketoacyl-CoA thiolase):
$$R\overset{O}{\overset{\|}{C}}CH_2COSCoA + CoASH \quad R\overset{O}{\overset{\|}{C}}SCoA + CH_3\overset{O}{\overset{\|}{C}}SCoA \quad (5)$$

Phytanic acid could undergo metabolism by way of this pathway only through Eq. 3. Because of the 3-methyl substituent, it could not be dehydrogenated at this stage to yield the β-keto intermediate.

Fatty acids with 2-methyl substituents can be oxidized by the classic β-oxidation system. The reactions are presumably entirely analogous except that Eq. 5 generates not acetyl CoA but rather propionyl CoA, as in the oxidation of α-methylbutyrate:

$$CH_3\overset{O}{\overset{\|}{C}} - \overset{CH_3}{\underset{|}{C}}H_2COSCoA + CoASH \longrightarrow$$
$$CH_3\overset{O}{\overset{\|}{C}}SCoA + CH_3CH_2\overset{O}{\overset{\|}{C}}SCoA \quad (6)$$

There are two ways in which phytanate could be modified initially that would bring it under the jurisdiction of the β-oxidation system. First, it could undergo an α-oxidative decarboxylation:

$$\overset{CH_3}{\underset{|}{R}CHCH_2COOH} \longrightarrow \overset{CH_3}{\underset{|}{R}CHCOOH} \quad (7)$$

(Phytanate; 20 carbons)   (Pristanate; 19 carbons)

This reaction converts a β-methyl fatty acid to an α-methyl fatty acid. It effects a "frame shift" such that the branch methyl groups no longer impede normal β oxidation. The first β-oxidation cycle would release propionyl CoA (see Eq. 6). A second cycle of β oxidation would then yield acetyl CoA and an α-methyl fatty acid, whereupon the full cycle could repeat itself. As discussed below, this is in fact probably the major pathway after formation of the (n − 1) acid, pristanic acid.

Second, the molecule could undergo an initial oxidation at the terminal carbon, i.e., ω oxidation:

$$\overset{CH_3}{\underset{\|}{C}H_3}\overset{CH_3}{\underset{|}{C}HCH}CH_2CH_2(CH_2\overset{CH_3}{\underset{|}{C}HCH}_2CH_2)_2CH_2\overset{CH_3}{\underset{|}{C}HCH}_2COOH \longrightarrow$$
$$HOOC\overset{CH_3}{\underset{|}{C}HCH}_2CH_2(CH_2\overset{CH_3}{\underset{|}{C}HCH}_2CH_2)_2CH_2\overset{CH_3}{\underset{|}{C}HCH}_2COOH \quad (8)$$

Note that at the ω-carboxyl end of the molecule, the branch-methyl substituent is in the α position. Thus oxidation could, after activation, proceed from this end of the molecule by β oxidation, yielding propionyl CoA and acetyl CoA, alternately.

α Oxidation [77]

Straight-Chain Fatty Acids Oxidation of long-chain, straight-chain fatty acids, including the common fatty acids such as palmitate and stearate, appears to be an important pathway in plants, but in mammalian systems only brain and nerve oxidize straight-chain fatty acids by attack at the α position. The longer-chain fatty acids, C_{20} and above, appear to be preferred substrates. The uniquely high concentrations of α-hydroxy acids in nerve tissue are probably due to the operation of this pathway. Similarly, the significant levels of odd-numbered, long-chain acids (e.g., 21:0, 23:0, 25:0) in nerve tissue reflect in part one-carbon shortening of even-numbered acids by this mechanism while some may arise from additions of two carbon units to propionate. The α-hydroxy and α-keto acids are believed to be intermediates, free or enzyme-bound. The overall sequence from even-numbered acid to (n − 1) acid has been difficult to demonstrate in cell-free systems, particularly the initial α hydroxylation. In any case, as discussed below, it appears that the system for α oxidation of phytanate is *not* identical with the system for α oxidation in nerve.

Phytanic Acid—Conversion to Pristanic Acid Conversion of labeled phytanic acid to its (n − 1) lower homologue, pristanic acid, was first demonstrated by Avigan and coworkers in 1966 [18]. The rate and extent of this conversion strongly suggested that this is the major normal pathway for phytanate oxidation, and subsequent studies in vivo and in vitro bear this out [18–22]. Unambiguous proof of direct conversion was provided by studies in which phytanic acid labeled with deuterium at the 2 and 3 positions was injected into rats. Pristanic acid was recovered from the liver and identified by mass spectrometry; one-half of the deuterium was lost, as expected, as a result of oxidation of the 2 carbon, but the enrichment at position 3 was nearly the same as that of the injected phytanate [18]. This result also served to rule out the possibility that phytanate might first be dehydrogenated to phytenic acid (3,7,11,15-tetramethylhexadec-2-enoic acid) and then hydrated to form the α-hydroxy acid (see the section which follows).

Net accumulation of pristanic acid has been demonstrated in mice and rats fed phytanic acid [19, 20, 78, 79], and trace amounts have been found in normal human tissues, including plasma [5], and in butterfat [80] and ruminant depot fat [81]. No systematic surveys of the relative capacities of different tissues to oxidize phytanate have been reported, but it seems likely that the system will prove to be widely distributed.

Phytanic Acid—Role of α-Hydroxyphytanate as an Intermediate α-Hydroxyphytanic acid was first isolated from incubations of phytanic acid with rat liver mitochondria, which contain all of the enzymes necessary for the complete oxidation of phytanic acid [21, 22]. That it is an obligatory intermediate was suggested by the following: (1) the rate of its formation relative to the rate of appearance of pristanic acid was consistent with such a role, (2) when labeled α-hydroxyphytanate was added as substrate it was converted to pristanic acid and further degradation products identical to those formed from labeled phytanate itself, (3) unlabeled α-hydroxyphytanate reduced the yield of labeled CO_2 from labeled phytanate. In the latter connection, the radioactivity recovered in the form of α-hydroxyphytanate was too small to account adequately for the reduced yield of labeled CO_2. Thus, the hydroxy intermediate may not ordinarily be released from the enzyme surface during the phytanate-pristanate conversion.

Studies on the mechanism of the hydroxylation in subcellular fractions of rat liver have shown that the activity is confined to the mitochondria [22]. The reaction is stimulated by NADPH and requires molecular oxygen. In these respects it resembles the several NADPH-dependent mixed-function oxygenase reactions linked to the cytochrome P_{450} system in liver microsomes, but the distinctly different subcellular localization distinguishes it clearly from them. Another unique property, not fully understood, is the marked stimulation of the hydroxylation due to the addition of ferric iron, whereas ferrous iron inhibits the reaction. These properties further distinguish the phytanate oxidizing system in the liver from the straight-chain α-oxidation system in the brain. The latter is primarily microsomal and is stimulated by ferrous iron [82, 83]. As noted above, the evidence for the conversion of long-chain, straight-chain fatty acids to the α-hydroxy form in subcellular preparations of mammalian brain is mostly indirect. The hydroxy acid may remain tightly bound as proposed for hydroxyphytanate; the latter, however, is to some extent dissociable and can be readily demonstrated as a major product.

Phytanic Acid—Further Oxidation of Pristanic Acid
The pathway for degradation beyond pristanic acid was first established by studies in mice fed phytanic acid [19]. This species, for reasons not fully understood, accumulates much larger quantities of pristanic acid when fed phytanic acid and, also, significant quantities of lower degradation products. The latter were clearly demonstrable by gas-liquid chromatography of liver fatty acids and could be completely characterized by the use of combined gas-liquid chromatography–mass spectrometry [20]. Confirmation of their direct formation from phytanic acid was obtained by injecting [U-14C]phytanic acid and demonstrating the presence of radioactivity in the relevant gas-liquid chromatography peaks. The compounds shown in Fig. 35-2 have all been characterized as products of phytanic acid either in vivo or in vitro or both. The products obviously form the series that would be expected from successive β oxidation of pristanic acid.

When labeled pristanic acid was incubated with rat liver

mitochondria, a new component with a retention time on gas-liquid chromatography greater than that of the starting material was detected. This was identified as the 2.3-unsaturated form of pristanic acid, Δ^2-pristenic acid [22]. This would be the expected dehydrogenation product in the classical β-oxidation sequence. The demonstrated formation of the α,β-unsaturated derivative supports the interpretation that further degradation of pristanic acid occurs by way of a β-oxidation pathway.

If the scheme shown in Fig. 35-2 is correct, 3 mol of propionic acid should be formed during the degradation of each mole of phytanic acid. Direct evidence for propionate as a degradation product was provided by studies in rat liver homogenates and, most convincingly, in studies utilizing mutant human skin fibroblasts [84, 85]. [U-14C]phytanic acid was incubated with cell lines from patients with inherited disorders blocking propionate degradation (propionic acidemia and methylmalonic acidemia). In both cell lines there was a striking accumulation of [14C]propionate and a decrease in the rate of $^{14}CO_2$ generation relative to that in normal fibroblasts. The latter would be anticipated since the degradation scheme predicts that almost half of the carbon atoms in phytanate reach CO_2 by way of propionate. Thus, the results considerably strengthen the case for the postulated major pathway.

ω Oxidation

ω Oxidation is initiated by oxygen attack at the ω carbon or at the penultimate (ω − 1) carbon of straight-chain fatty acids. The reaction requires NADPH and molecular oxygen and is catalyzed by a microsomal mixed-function oxygenase. The major product is a dicarboxylic acid of the same number of carbon atoms as the substrate. While straight-chain fatty acids can readily be shown to undergo this form of oxidation in an isolated microsomal system, there is evidence that the mitochondrial β-oxidation system is quantitatively much more important, at least for the long-chain, straight-chain fatty acids. When shorter-chain fatty acids are administered (C_6 to C_{10}), significant quantities of the dicarboxylic acid resulting from ω oxidation are excreted in the urine. After injection of straight-chain, long-chain fatty acids (C_{16} to C_{18}), only traces of radioactivity appear in the urine. If oxidation from the carboxyl end is inhibited by dimethyl substitution at the α position, significant ω oxidation takes place [86].

Using a novel experimental design, Antony and Landau have shown that ω oxidation of stearic acid by rat liver slices cannot account for more than 1 or 2 percent of the total amount oxi-

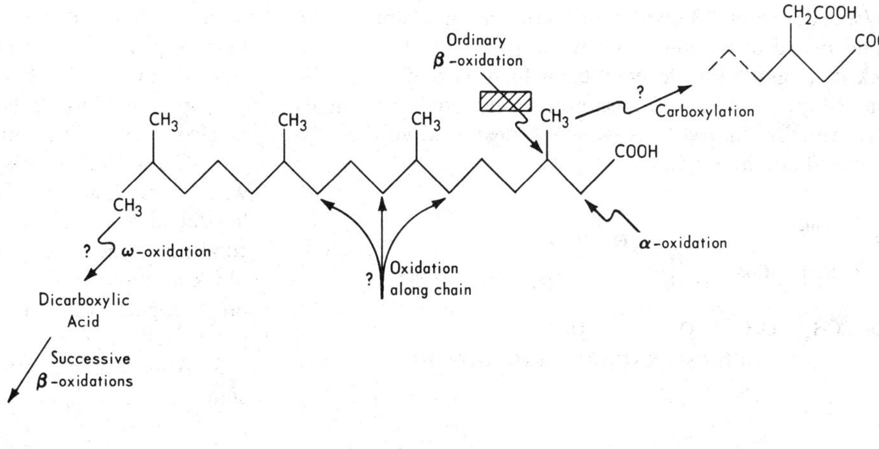

Figure 35-6 Schematic representation of the theoretically possible initial modes of oxidative attack on the phytanic acid molecule.

dized [87]. They incubated stearic acid labeled with ^{14}C at the 18 carbon so that acetate derived from that end of the molecule by ω oxidation would contain radioactivity in the carboxyl carbon, whereas acetate derived as a result of β oxidation would contain radioactivity in the methyl carbon. The distribution of ^{14}C in glucose (from glycogen) allowed an estimate of the relative contribution of [1-^{14}C]acetate and [2-^{14}C]acetate. The results gave no positive evidence for any ω oxidation although, because of limitations in methodology, a small amount of ω oxidation could not be completely ruled out.

As discussed above, initial ω oxidation of phytanic acid would make it possible for β oxidation to proceed from the ω end without interference by the branch methyl groups. Try has presented evidence suggesting ω oxidation of phytanic acid in rat liver homogenates [88]. Proof of structure was not presented, the conclusion being based mainly on the finding of radioactivity in fatty acids with properties similar to those of dicarboxylic acids. In any case, it was concluded that ω oxidation proceeded at best at a low rate. In the course of studies of phytanate oxidation by the mouse, which allowed the isolation of a large number of degradation products, and in studies of phytanic acid oxidation in isolated rat liver mitochondria, where many of the same degradation products could be identified, careful search was made for the formation of dicarboxylic acids but none was found [20, 22]. The evidence available suggests that under ordinary conditions ω oxidation is probably a minor pathway. However, in patients lacking the α-oxidation pathway, ω oxidation might become significant and account for the limited rate of phytanate oxidation that has been observed [23, 24]. Brenton et al. [89] have identified 3-methyl adipic acid in the urine of a patient with phytanic acid storage disease. This compound would be the predicted intermediate generated after five successive β-oxidative steps beginning at the ω end of ω-carboxy phytanic acid. It was estimated that the daily excretion of 3-methyl adipic acid corresponded to degradation of 26 mg phytanate. Interestingly, it appears that in order to effect a significant lowering of plasma phytanate levels it is necessary to reduce dietary intake to below 26 mg/day [31, 90, 91].

Removal of Methyl Groups after Fixation of CO_2

A β-substituted fatty acid (β-methylbutyric acid) is formed in the course of the oxidative degradation of leucine. This fatty acid (as the acyl CoA) could undergo the second and third steps of the usual β-oxidation cycle, namely, α,β-dehydrogenation and hydration to form the β-hydroxyacyl CoA derivative (see subsection "β Oxidation" earlier in this chapter). The second dehydrogenation to form the β-keto acid would be blocked. Degradation depends upon fixation of CO_2 to the β-methyl group of the α,β-unsaturated acid. Hydration yields hydroxymethylglutaryl CoA, which is cleaved to yield acetoacetic acid and acetyl CoA:

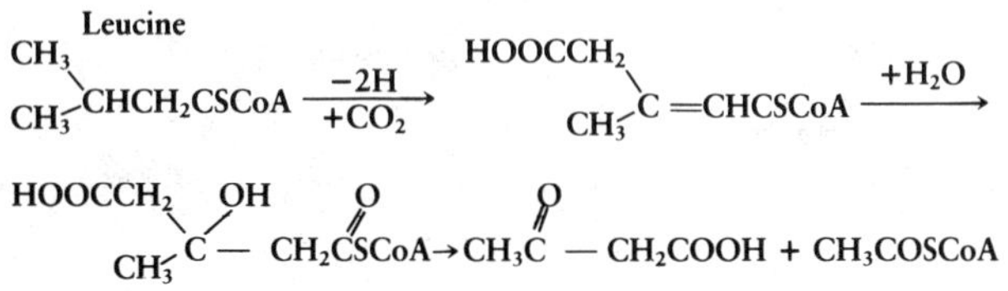

A similar CO_2-fixation "trick" has been shown by Seubert and Remberger [92] to function in bacteria in the oxidation of geranoic acid and farnesoic acid, β-methyl–substituted branched chain acids. The only difference in this case is that after fixation of CO_2 to the branch methyl group, free acetic acid is cleaved instead of acetyl CoA. This leaves a β-keto acyl CoA derivative, which can then be β oxidized in the usual fashion. The general similarity in structure of these unsaturated polyisoprenoid fatty acids and phytanic acid (cf. Fig. 35-2) suggested the possibility that phytanic acid might undergo an analogous oxidation. Eldjarn and coworkers [70] initially reported a CO_2 requirement for the oxidation of a model compound structurally related to phytanic acid (3,6-dimethyloctanoic acid) but were unable to confirm this in later studies [93, 94]. Tsai and coworkers [22] were unable to demonstrate a CO_2 dependency for the oxidation of phytanic acid itself in rat liver mitochondria. Moreover, in none of the systems in which the oxidation of phytanic acid itself has been studied has there been evidence for the appearance of the expected 20-carbon dicarboxylic acid intermediate, the 19-carbon 3-keto derivative, or the 17-carbon lower homologue that would be expected in such a pathway.

LOCALIZATION OF THE SITE OF THE ENZYMATIC ERROR

The site of the enzymatic block in phytanic acid oxidation in the patients has been localized to the initial α oxidation, probably in the α-hydroxylation step itself. This conclusion is based on studies of the rates of oxidation of phytanic acid and of its degradation products in cell cultures and is supported by studies in vivo in patients. The evidence can be summarized as follows:

1. While the rate of phytanic acid oxidation in cell cultures derived from patients is only 1 percent of that seen in control cell cultures, the rates of oxidation of labeled pristanic acid (Fig. 35-7) are comparable to the rates in control cells [25–27, 45]. The rate of oxidation of α-hydroxyphytanic acid has been found to be normal also [27], implying that the mutation involves the α-hydroxylation step.

2. The rate of oxidation of intravenously injected phytanic acid is depressed in patients, but the rate of oxidation of pristanic acid or of α-hydroxyphytanic acid is comparable to that seen in normal subjects [23, 24].

3. After incubation of normal fibroblasts with labeled phytanic acid the cell lipids can be shown to contain labeled α-hydroxyphytanic acid and labeled pristanic acid as well as labeled 4,8,12-trimethyltridecanoic acid [27]. In contrast, the cell lipids in fibroblasts derived from patients contain only labeled phytanic acid and no degradation products.

4. Careful study of serum and tissue lipids from patients with phytanic acid storage disease and of postmortem tissues has failed to reveal the accumulation of any branched chain congeners other than phytanic acid itself. Were the metabolic block at some lower point in the degradation pathway, one might expect to find at least some concentrations of accumulated intermediates [25].

5. After administration to normal subjects of a branched chain model compound related to phytanic acid in having a

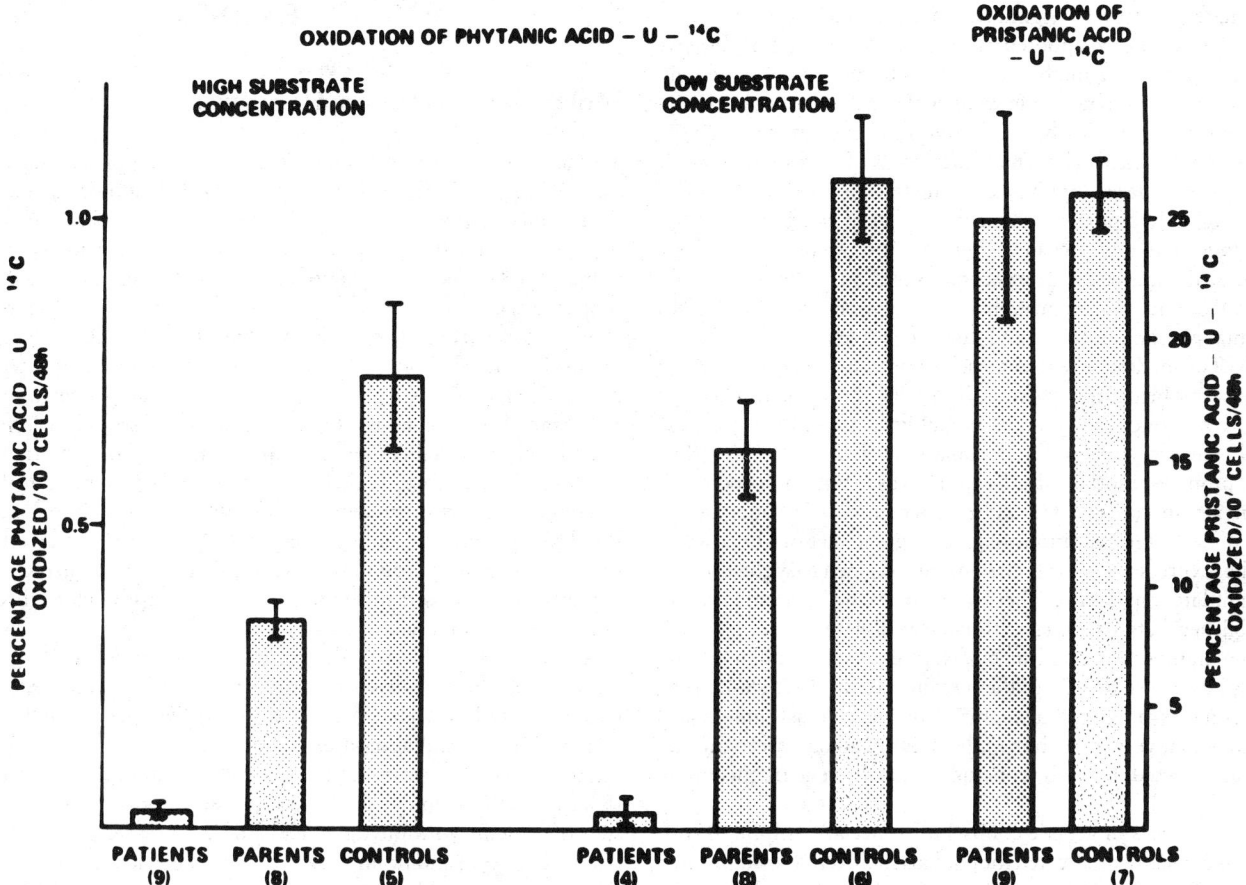

OXIDATION OF PHYTANIC ACID – U – ^{14}C

HIGH SUBSTRATE CONCENTRATION

LOW SUBSTRATE CONCENTRATION

OXIDATION OF PRISTANIC ACID – U – ^{14}C

PERCENTAGE PHYTANIC ACID – U – ^{14}C OXIDIZED / 10^7 CELLS/48h

PERCENTAGE PRISTANIC ACID – U – ^{14}C OXIDIZED/10^7 CELLS/48h

PATIENTS (9)   PARENTS (8)   CONTROLS (5)   PATIENTS (4)   PARENTS (8)   CONTROLS (6)   PATIENTS (9)   CONTROLS (7)

Figure 35-7   Rates of phytanic acid and pristanic acid oxidation in fibroblast cell cultures. The almost complete deletion of the phytanic acid oxidizing activity in homozygous patients is shown, as well as the normal rates of pristanic acid oxidation in patients. The rates of oxidation of phytanic acid in the obligate heterozygotes (parents) is approximately 50 percent of control values.

β-methyl substitution ([8-^{14}C]3,6-dimethyloctanoic acid), a small fraction of the administered dose of radioactivity is recovered in the urine in the form of the α-oxidation product (2,5-dimethylheptanoic acid) [71]. In contrast, patients failed to show any α-oxidation product in the urine. Normal subjects oxidized a small percentage of the administered radioactivity to CO_2, but patients oxidized none [70, 71]. If it is assumed that the model compound is metabolized by the same systems that oxidize phytanic acid itself, which is supported by the results in patients, these results support the conclusion that there is a defect in α oxidation.

On the basis of indirect evidence obtained by using model compounds, it was proposed that the accumulation of phytanic acid reflected a defect in ω oxidation [95]. However, studies showed that other compounds subject to ω oxidation were handled normally [96], and even the oxidation of the model compound used originally (tricaprin) returned toward normal in the patients after they had been maintained on a phytanate-low diet [97]. Possibly the stores of phytanate secondarily affect some ω-oxidation systems. As discussed above, there is no evidence for a major role of ω oxidation in the metabolism of phytanic acid in normal animals or in normal humans. On the other hand, the residual capacity of patients with phytanic acid storage disease to catabolize phytanate may be due to ω oxidation rather than a "leaky" mutation involving α hydroxylation [53].

GENETICS

The observed inheritance pattern is that expected for autosomal recessive transmission. The classic criteria appear to be well satisfied, viz., (1) parents of cases and children of cases are clinically unaffected, (2) the prevalence of consanguinity between parents of affected children is high, (3) prevalence in males and females is approximately equal, (4) the proportion of cases in affected sibships approximates the theoretical 25 percent. The demonstration of a partial defect in phytanic acid oxidation in cell cultures derived from presumed heterozygotes firmly established the recessive mode of inheritance [45]. Cultures derived from affected children were shown to oxidize phytanic acid at less than 3 percent of the rate seen in control cultures. Cultures from the parents, on the other hand, oxidized phytanic acid at 46 to 59 percent of the normal rate. There was no overlap between results in controls and results in the presumed heterozygotes when oxidation was measured at a high concentration of substrate (Fig. 35-7). None of the parents had clinically manifested neurologic disease, but one had been reported to have some elevation of phytanic acid in plasma. This exceptional case was chosen for study particularly in view of the report of phytanic acid accumulation.

Serum phytanic acid analyses have been reported in about 20 obligate heterozygotes. None showed clinical stigmata of Refsum's syndrome and, with three exceptions, phytanic acid levels were within normal limits. Thus, it appears that one-half the normal capacity for oxidation of phytanic acid is ordinarily adequate to prevent significant accumulation on ordinary diets. One of the exceptional parents was the mother of patient E.H., and was originally reported by Kahlke and Richterich [47] to have a phytanate level as high as that of her affected son. A serum sample obtained from this same patient in 1967 showed only the usual normal trace levels of phytanate (Herndon and Steinberg, unpublished results). Unless the single analysis originally reported represents analytical error, one has to conclude that this presumed heterozygote accumulated phytanic acid transiently. The second exception is the mother of cases E.S. and J.S., reported by Nevin et al. in 1967 [48]. Her plasma phytanate accounted for 2.6 percent of total fatty acids. The fact that she was herself symptom-free seems to rule against her being homozygous. The cell culture results classify her as a heterozygote rather unambiguously. Gibberd et al. [119] recently reported a phytanate level of 4 mg/dl in the asymptomatic mother of a bona fide case. With a 50 percent reduction in capacity to oxidize phytanate, it is conceivable that under some conditions (e.g., changes in diet or alterations in the expression of the enzyme defect) heterozygotes may accumulate phytanate. There are no recorded examples of established heterozygotes with clinical disease.

The number of confirmed cases reported through 1980 totals just under 100, 21 of them reported since 1975. Since the syndrome is now well recognized by neurologists, it seems unlikely that very many bona fide cases are going unrecognized and unreported. It can be concluded that the gene frequency is very low.

For purposes of genetic counseling, especially helpful in the case of clinically unaffected individuals in affected sibships, the carrier state can be diagnosed using the fibroblast cell culture method. It may be possible to design a simpler and more direct clinical "loading" test. A preliminary report suggests that plasma phytanate levels in a heterozygote may reach higher levels after ingestion of 10 g phytol than are reached in a control subject, but more extensive studies are needed to establish the usefulness of such a test [99]. The cell culture method is becoming increasingly accessible. Normal amniotic cells have been shown to have the capacity to oxidize phytanic acid [100], and so it should be possible to make a diagnosis of the homozygous or heterozygous state antepartum.

The biochemical evidence available is compatible with the postulate of a single mutation leading to the loss of a functional phytanic acid hydroxylase (Fig. 35-2). It is possible that the primary defect might lie in a system necessary for phytanic acid hydroxylation (e.g., a cofactor regenerating system), but not in the phytanic acid α-hydroxylase itself. Defective phytanate oxidation due to generation of a metabolic inhibitor has been tested by hydridizing a fibroblast line from a patient with a normal cell line (D 98); the cloned hybrid cells oxidized added [^{14}C]phytanate at a rate equal to or greater than that of the normal parent line (D. Hutton and D. Steinberg, unpublished observations). The possibility of multiple gene defects is always difficult to rule out, but thus far no biochemical errors have been established beyond the defect in phytanic acid α oxidation. While much insight has been gained into the biochemical basis for phytanic acid accumulation, it remains to be established how the accumulation of phytanic acid leads to the clinical manifestations of the disease. Indeed, it is not firmly established whether or not phytanic acid accumulation per se is the necessary and sufficient basis for all of the clinical signs and symptoms of Refsum's disease.

PATHOGENESIS

Molecular Distortion Hypothesis

The simplest hypothesis is that the incorporation of the multiple-branched, "thorny" phytanic acid molecule into tissue lipids in place of the normal straight-chain fatty acids interferes with myelin function or at least increases its susceptibility to damage [23]. The cross-sectional area of the phytanic acid molecule is at least 50 percent greater than that of the straight-chain fatty acids [101] and the binding forces at close range would be considerably less than those of straight-chain fatty acids. Thus, in highly ordered structures like that of myelin or membrane lipids generally, the displacement of straight-chain acids by phytanic acid might in itself lay the basis for evolution of the clinical disease. If this is the case, then elimination of phytanic acid and its precursors from the diet should prevent the development of lesions in very young patients and arrest the progress or even lead to some reversal of symptoms in older patients. As discussed in the next section in more detail, this appears to be the case.

Attempts to produce the disease in animals by feeding large amounts of phytanic acid or its precursors have yielded negative results [12–14, 16, 19, 20, 93]. In the five species studied (rat, rabbit, chinchilla, mouse, and polecat), it has been possible to increase the phytanic acid levels in serum and in most tissues to values similar to those reported in postmortem tissues of patients with phytanic acid storage disease. The levels reached in nerve and brain, however, have been low relative to those reported in the human disease. Consequently, the negative experimental results do not militate strongly against the hypothesis that phytanic acid storage in the nervous system is pathogenetic. Higher levels could not be attained because increasing the levels of intake still further caused serious toxic effects, including the arrest of growth and the death of the test animals. The mechanism of this marked toxicity of phytol or phytanic acid remains unknown. The administration of large doses of fat-soluble vitamins and polyunsaturated fats afforded no protection ([17] and unpublished results).

Dubois-Dalcq et al. [17, 102, 103] observed degenerative changes in explant cultures of mouse spinal ganglia exposed for several weeks to phytanic acid (60 to 100 mg/liter) complexed to albumin. There were similar changes, although less intense and slower to develop, in cultures exposed to equimolar concentrations of palmitic acid. Because phytanic acid binds less tightly to albumin than palmitic acid [104], the concentration of unbound phytanate was probably somewhat higher than that of palmitate. Thus, the observed changes may represent general responses to long-chain fatty acids rather than any specific response to phytanic acid per se.

Antimetabolite Hypothesis

The close structural similarity between phytanic acid and the isoprenoid side chains of the fat-soluble vitamins, particularly vitamins E and K, led to the suggestion that phytanic acid might be toxic by interfering with the function of these fat-soluble vitamins. However, the arrest in the growth of rats or mice fed large doses of phytanate was not prevented by the simultaneous administration of large doses of fat-soluble vitamins. These negative results do not completely rule out the hypothesis. Phytanic acid might be competing successfully, even noncompetitively, at the site of vitamin function. One reason this hypothesis has received attention follows from the resemblance between some of the clinical features of abetalipoproteinemia (in which fat-soluble-vitamin transport may be deficient) and the clinical features of phytanic acid storage disease. Other possibilities, such as interference with the function of coenzyme Q or other polyisoprenoid compounds can be mentioned speculatively, but no relevant data are as yet available.

Another hypothesis, not strictly in this "antimetabolite" category, is that advanced by Laurell [51]. He noted the low levels of linoleate in the patients' glycerides and speculated that there may be an induced relative linoleate deficiency. Displacement of linoleate and arachidonate has been noted in the phospholipids of liver, kidney, heart, and skin [105, 106]. Since ichthyosis is also seen in essential fatty acid deficiency it was suggested that phytanate might be pathogenetic in a related fashion [106]. It has also been proposed that the high concentrations of phytanate in skin, some of it in cholesterol esters, may induce ichthyosis by reducing the amount of free cholesterol available [107].

"Double-Function" Hypothesis

It could be proposed that the α-oxidation system necessary for the metabolism of phytanic acid (and deleted in patients) plays a physiologically important role in one or more other biochemical pathways. One specific hypothesis along these lines relates to the possibility of a generalized deficiency in α hydroxylation. α Hydroxylation of fatty acids in animals has only been observed in nerve tissue, as discussed in "α Oxidation" in this chapter; thus, a deficiency in this system might understandably manifest itself primarily in nervous system disease. Studies on the properties of the phytanic acid oxidizing system show clearly that it is distinct from the long-chain, straight-chain fatty acid α-oxidation system. Moreover, analyses of postmortem tissues failed to show any abnormality in concentration or composition of the straight-chain α-hydroxy fatty acids in brain or nerve [108, 109]. Analysis of skin biopsies in two cases showed an α-hydroxy fatty acid concentration at the lower limits of normal and with a normal distribution [110]. Finally, rats fed a phytanic acid–rich diet have shown no abnormality in α-hydroxy fatty acid concentration or composition in brain. Thus, there is no evidence that patients with phytanic acid storage disease have any difficulty in making α-hydroxy acids in the straight-chain fatty acid series.

Multiple-Gene Defects

Thus far there is no evidence of a consistent defect in any other biochemical pathway. The karyotype, when reported, has been normal. Nevertheless, the possibility of still undiscovered biochemical defects always remains open. One can ask whether the clinical features reported are all reasonably attributed to nerve damage or in some other way to phytanic acid accumulation. Certainly most of the clinical features are readily attributed to nerve damage, but not all. The electrocardiographic abnormalities may be caused by damage to the conduction system, but there are reports also of myocardial fibrosis. Patients have been reported to have shortening of the metacarpal and metatarsal bones, pes cavus, epiphyseal dysplasia, and ichthyosis. These are not readily attributable to nerve damage. They may be due to incorporation of phytanic acid into and distortion of the membranes of other cells.

TREATMENT

If the conclusion drawn from biochemical and clinical studies is correct—that the stored phytanate is exclusively of exogenous origin—then elimination of phytanate and its precursors from the diet should prevent further accumulation. To the extent that the patients retain some capacity to degrade phytanate (or excrete it unchanged), it should be possible to deplete body stores. In fact, reduction of plasma phytanate levels by dietary treatment has how been reported in at least 17 cases [23, 33, 34, 37, 90, 91, 111–120]. The fall can be quite dramatic, e.g., from 174 mg/dl to 13.5 mg/dl [115]. In a few cases normal levels have been achieved but in most the plasma level plateaus at about 10 to 30 mg/dl. As long as phytanic acid intake is kept at a suitably low level the plasma concentration stays down although there can be a temporary partial "escape." Two of the patients first treated with a rigorous dietary regimen [31, 90] have now been followed for 14 years with overall satisfactory control of plasma phytanate levels.

The response in plasma levels may be delayed for months after initiating the diet. This suggests that tissue stores are mobilized when intake is reduced. Adipose tissue biopsies taken before and after diet treatment show that this storage site shows the expected fall in concentration [31].

Evaluation of plasma phytanate levels is more complex than in the case of water-soluble compounds such as galactose. Almost all of the phytanate is present in the phospholipids and triglycerides of the plasma lipoproteins. The lipoproteins are synthesized and secreted primarily by the liver (very low density and high density lipoproteins) and to a lesser extent by the intestine. Precursors for the fatty acids in the lipoproteins include not only fatty acids synthesized de novo but also free fatty acids mobilized from adipose tissue and fatty acids stored in liver phospholipids and triglyceride. Phytanate can account for as much as 50 percent of the fatty acids in liver lipids, i.e., a higher concentration than that found in plasma. Thus if liver lipids are mobilized, the percentage of phytanate in plasma will tend to rise and may do so quite rapidly. In adipose tissue the percentage of phytanate is relatively low (1 to 5 percent of total fatty acids). Thus if adipose tissue lipids are rapidly mobilized the percentage of phytanate in plasma may not increase immediately and may even fall while the absolute concentration rises (especially if the patient develops significant hyperlipidemia). However, the normal straight-chain fatty acids can go on to be oxidized while the phytanate, because of the metabolic block, will tend to accumulate and increase both in absolute and relative concentration. For these reasons it is best to follow responses to diet both in terms of absolute phytanate levels (mg/dl) and in terms of relative phytanate content (percentage of total fatty acids).

A potential hazard of dietary treatment arises if the patient, in attempting to adapt to a new and rigorous diet, reduces his or her calorie intake and begins to lose weight. In several cases this has been associated with a paradoxical *rise* in plasma phytanate levels and an accompanying clinical relapse, which at times has been quite drastic [113, 115, 117, 119]. While not proved, this may well be explained by the mobilization of phytanate from lipids stored in the liver and in the adipose tissue, as discussed above. The total mass of phytanate stored in adipose tissue is enormous, even though phytanate accounts for only 5 percent or less of adipose tissue fatty acids.

In one patient in whom total tissue analyses were carried out, 286 out of 381 g of stored phytanic acid were found in adipose tissue [105]. To put this in perspective, consider that the average daily intake of phytanate in the diet is less than 100 mg/day. Thus, 286 g of phytanic acid corresponds to over 7 years of daily dietary phytanic acid intake! Turning the proposition around, phytanic acid accounts for only approximately 0.1 percent of the fatty acids taken in daily (100 mg or less phytanic acid vs. a total daily fat intake of approximately 100 g). Thus, the phytanic acid in the adipose tissue stores is present at a concentration 10 to 50 times that in the diet. Thus, mobilization of stored depot fat provides an "input" 10 to 50 times that provided by the usual diet on a gram for gram basis.

Several reports of relapses in patients experiencing weight loss *not* associated with an intercurrent illness suggest a possible reinterpretation of the relapses reported in patients experiencing various stresses such as surgery, pregnancy, viral infections, or other intercurrent illnesses. Is it possible that the common denominator in all of these instances is the loss of weight and the mobilization of depot fat? One case report in particular is strongly suggestive [121]. This patient experienced a progressive and rapid neurologic deterioration associated with marked weight loss following the development of hyperthyroidism together with diabetes mellitus. It is possible that neural function is adversely affected during intercurrent illnesses by mechanisms *not* related to weight loss and the accompanying increases in plasma phytanic acid. Patients with other neurologic syndromes, such as Friedreich's ataxia, have also been noted to suffer relapses associated with intercurrent illnesses. The biochemical basis remains unclear. At any rate, the association between weight loss and relapse in patients with phytanic acid storage disease is strong enough that rapid weight loss at any time should be avoided in patients with the established disease state.

Dietary Prescription

Management consists in eliminating from the diet as rigorously as possible all sources of phytanic acid. Unfortunately, data are not yet available on all foodstuffs. Dairy products of all kinds, ruminant fats, and ruminant meats are the major sources and these must be absolutey proscribed. Green vegetables were originally excluded from the diet because of the possibility that the phytate in chlorophyll might be absorbed and converted to phytanate [31]. However, chlorophyll-phytol is very poorly absorbed [98] and this exclusion may be unnecessary (although cooking may release some bound phytol). In any case phytol is relatively unimportant compared to phytanic acid itself as a dietary component. Some values for phytanate content of foods are presented in Table 35-2 and more information on dietary management is available in several publications [23, 31, 61, 91, 116, 119].

The magnitude and rate of fall in plasma phytanate levels depend on the rigor with which sources of phytanic acid are eliminated from the diet. Reducing intake from that in the usual diet—about 60 mg/day—to 21 mg/day caused less of a response and a slower response than was obtained on a drastically modified diet (mostly liquid formula) that contained less than 3 mg/day [31, 90]. Because phytanic acid is widely distributed (Table 35-2), it is difficult to reduce intake much below 20 mg/day using generally available foods. A regimen of a liquid formula as a major source of calories—supplemented with solid foods poor in phytanate—may be the best approach.

Periodic plasmapheresis or plasma exchange has been used in several clinics to reduce body stores [113, 117, 119, 120] of phytanate and, combined with dietary management, has helped keep plasma levels low. A lifetime program of such treatment may be unreasonably burdensome, but repeated plasmapheresis or plasma exchange during the early stages of management appears to be a rational way to obtain a good initial response. It cannot be regarded as a substitute for dietary management, only as a supplement.

Response to Diet

In those patients responding with a good fall in plasma phytanate levels there has been an arrest in the progress of the peripheral neuropathy and objectively documented regression. Improvement in nerve conduction velocity has been demonstrated in nine cases [31, 90, 91, 113, 114, 116, 118], returning to normal in some. In some instances unobtainable nerve response has given way to velocities above 25 to 30 m/s and previously unobtainable reflexes have been restored. Muscle strength and gait have improved and sensory deficits have receded. Ichthyotic changes can regress early after start of treatment. It may be particularly significant that the nonspecific electrocardiographic abnormalities have been corrected in some cases. There have been no reported deaths in the patients responding to dietary treatment. Indeed, in the patients maintaining low plasma phytanate there have been no relapses, some of them now under treatment for 5 to 14 years. No convincing regression has been noted in auditory or visual deficits, however.

The now much expanded experience with diet treatment supports the conclusion that exogenously derived phytanic acid is the source of the storage lipid in this disease and that it is pathogenetic, directly or indirectly. It is reasonable to expect that any therapeutic benefits will be more significant if treatment is initiated early. Once demyelination is extensive, restoration of function is unlikely even if progression is arrested. Every effort should be made to establish the diagnosis at an early age and institute treatment.

REFERENCES

1. REFSUM S: Heredopathia atactica polyneuritiformis. *Acta Psychiatr Scand* (suppl) 38:9, 1946
2. KLENK E, KAHLKE W: Uber das Vorkommen der 3,7,11,15-Tetramethylhexadecansaure (Phytansaure) in den Cholesterinestern und anderen Lipoidfraktionen der Organe bei einem Krankheitsfall unbekannter Genese (Verdacht auf Heredopathia actactica polyneuritiformis, Refsum's syndrome). *Hoppe Seyler Z Physiol Chem* 333:133, 1963
3. RICHTERICH R, VAN MECHELEN P, ROSSI E: Refsum's disease (heredopa-

thia atactica polyneuritiformis): An inborn error of lipid metabolism with storage of 3,7,11,15-tetramethylhexadecanoic acid. *Am J Med* 39:230, 1963

4. KAHLKE W: Refsum-Syndrome—Lipoidchemische Untersuchungen bei 9 Fallen *Klin Wochenschr* 42:1011, 1964

5. AVIGAN J: The presence of phytanic acid in normal human and animal plasma. *Biochim Biophys Acta* 116:391, 1966

6. KREMER GJ: Uber das Vorkommen der 3,7,11,15-Tetramethylhexadecansaure in den Lipoiden von Normalseren. *Klin Wochenschr* 43:517, 1965

7. STEINBERG D: Remarks on the biochemical basis of Refsum's disease. *Nord Med* 73:570, 1965

8. ELDJARN L: Biokjemiske synspunkter pa phytanasurens opprinnelse. *Nord Med* 73:569, 1965

9. STEINBERG D, AVIGAN J, MIZE C, ELDJARN L, TRY K, REFSUM S: Conversion of U-C14-phytol to phytanic acid and its oxidation in heredopathia atactica polyneuritiformis. *Biochem Biophys Res Commun* 19:783, 1965

10. STEINBERG D, MIZE CE, AVIGAN J, FALES HM, ELDJARN K, STOKKE O, REFSUM S: Studies on the metabolic error in Refsum's disease. *J Clin Invest* 45:1076, 1966; 46:313, 1967

11. MIZE CE, AVIGAN J, BAXTER JH, FALES HM, STEINBERG D: Metabolism of phytol-U-14C and phytanic acid-U-14C in the rat. *J Lipid Res* 7:692, 1966

12. STEINBERG D, AVIGAN J, MIZE, C, BAXTER JH: Phytanic acid formation and accumulation in phytol-fed rats. *Fed Proc* 24:290, 1965

13. STEINBERG D, AVIGAN J, MIZE C, BAXTER J: Phytanic acid formation and accumulation in phytol fed-rats. *Biochem Biophys Res Commun* 19:412, 1965

14. KLENK E, KREMER GJ: Untersuchungen zum stoffwechsel des phytols, dihydrophytols, und der phytansaure. *Hoppe Seyler Z Physiol Chem* 343:39, 1965

15. STOFFEL W, KAHLKE W: The transformation of phytol into 3,7,11,15-tetramethylhexadecanoic (phytanic) acid in heredopathia atactica polyneuritiformis (Refsum's syndrome). *Biochem Biophys Res Commun* 19:33, 1965

16. HANSEN RP, SHORLAND FB, PRIOR IAM: The fate of phytanic acid when administered to rats. *Biochim Biophys Acta* 116:178, 1966

17. STEINBERG D, AVIGAN J, MIZE CE, BAXTER JH, CAMMERMEYER J; FALES HM, HIGHET PF: Effects of dietary phytol and phytanic acid in animals. *J Lipid Res* 7:684, 1966

18. AVIGAN J, STEINBERG D, GUTMAN A, MIZE CE, MILNE GWA: Alpha-decarboxylation, an important pathway for degradation of phytanic acid in animals. *Biochem Biophys Res Commun* 24:838, 1966

19. MIZE CG, STEINBERG D, AVIGAN J, FALES HM: A pathway for oxidative degradation of phytanic acid in mammals. *Biochem Biophys Res Commun* 25:359, 1966

20. MIZE CE, AVIGAN J, STEINBERG D, PITTMAN RC, FALES HM, MILNE GWA: A major pathway for the mammalian oxidative degradation of phytanic acid. *Biochim Biophys Acta* 176:720, 1969

21. TSAI S-C, HERNDON JH JR, UHLENDORF BW, FALES HM, MIZE CE: The formation of alpha-hydroxyphytanic acid from phytanic acid in mammalian tissues. *Biochem Biophys Res Commun* 28:571, 1967

22. TSAI S-C, AVIGAN J, STEINBERG D: Studies on the alpha-oxidation of phytanic acid by rat liver mitochondria. *J Biol Chem* 244:2682, 1969

23. STEINBERG D, VROOM FQ, ENGEL WK, CAMMERMEYER J, MIZE CE, AVIGAN J: Refsum's disease—a recently characterized lipidosis involving the nervous system. *Ann Intern Med* 66:365, 1967

24. MIZE CE, HERNDON JH JR, BLASS JP, MILNE GWA, FOLLANSBEE C, LAUDAT P. STEINBERG D: Localization of the oxidative defect in phytanic acid degradation in patients with Refsum's disease. *J Clin Invest* 48:1033, 1969

25. STEINBERG D. HERNDON JH JR, UHLENDORF BW, MIZE CE, AVIGAN J, MILNE GWA: Refsum's disease: Nature of the enzyme defect. *Science* 156:1740, 1967

26. STEINBERG D, AVIGAN J, MIZE CE, HERNDON JH JR, FALES HM, MILNE GWA: The nature of the metabolic defect in Refsum's disease. *Pathol Eur* 3:450, 1968

27. HERNDON JH JR, STEINBERG D, UHLENDORF BW, FALES HM: Refsum's disease: Characterization of the enzyme defect in cell culture. *J Clin Invest* 48:1017, 1969

28. ELDJARN L, STOKKE O, TRY K: Alpha-oxidation of branched-chain fatty acids in man and its failure in patients with Refsum's disease showing phytanic acid accumulation. *Scand J Clin Lab Invest* 18:694, 1966

29. STOKKE O, TRY K, ELDJARN L: Alpha-oxidation as an alternative pathway for the degradation of branched-chain fatty acids in man, and its failure in patients with Refsum's disease. *Biochim Biophys Acta* 144:271, 1967

30. ELDJARN L, TRY K, STOKKE O, MUNTHE-KAAS AW, REFSUM S, STEINBERG D, AVIGAN J, MIZE C: Dietary effects on serum-phytanic-acid levels and on clinical manifestations in heredopathia atactica polyneuritiformis. *Lancet* 1:691, 1966

31. STEINBERG D, MIZE CE, HERNDON JH JR, FALES HM, ENGEL WK, VROOM FQ: Phytanic acid in patients with Refsum's syndrome and response to dietary treatment. *Arch Intern Med* 125:75, 1970

32. REFSUM S, ELDJARN L: Heredopathia atactica polyneuritiformis—an inborn defect in the metabolism of branched-chain fatty acids, in Banner HG (ed): *Future of Neurology*, Stuttgart, Thieme, 1967, p 36

33. REFSUM S: Heredopathia atactica polyneuritiformis (Refsum's disease), in Dyck PJ, Thomas PK, Lambert EH (eds): *Peripheral Neuropathy*. Philadelphia, Saunders, 1975, vol II, chap 42

34. STEINBERG D, HERNDON JH JR: Refsum's disease: Phytanic acid storage disease, in Goldenshon ES, Appel SH (eds): *Scientific Approaches to Clinical Neurology*. Philadelphia, Lea and Febiger, 1977, p 994

35. TRY K: Heredopathia atactica polyneuritiformis (Refsum's disease): The diagnostic value of phytanic acid determination in serum lipids. *Eur Neurol* 2:296, 1969

36. CAMMERMEYER J: Neuropathological changes in hereditary neuropathies: Manifestation of the syndrome heredopathia atactica polyneuritiformis in the presence of interstitial hypertrophic polyneuropathy. *J Neuropathol Exp Neurol* 15:340, 1956

37. STEINBERG D: Phytanic acid storage disease: Refsum's syndrome, in Stanbury JB, Wyngaarden JB, Fredrickson DS (eds): *The Metabolic Basis of Inherited Disease*. New York, McGraw-Hill, 1978, 4th ed, chap 33

38. KAHLKE W, GOERLICH R, FEIST D: Erhohte Phytansaurespiegel in Plasma und Leber bei einem Kleinkind mit unklarem Hirnschaden. *Klin Wochenschr* 52:651, 1974

39. KOLODNY EH, HASS WK, LANE B, DRUCKER WD: Refsum's syndrome: Report of a case including electron microscopic studies of the liver. *Arch Neurol* 12:583, 1965

40. SHY GM, SILBERBERG DH, APPEL SH, MISHKIN MM, GODFREY EH: A generalized disorder of nervous system, skeletal muscle, and heart resembling Refsum's disease and Hurler's syndrome. *Am J Med* 42:163, 1967

41. SOLCHER H: Uber Hirnveranderungen bei Heredopathia atactica polyneuritiformis (Refsum). *Acta Neuropathol (berl)* 24:92, 1973

42. RON MA, PEARCE J: Refsum's syndrome with normal phytate metabolism. *Acta Neurol Scand* 47:646, 1971

43. BRYNIARSKA D, GOLDSZTAJN M: A degenerative syndrome resembling Refsum's disease. *Neurol Neurochir Pol* 6:895, 1972

44. KAYDEN HJ, REAGAN TJ, MIZE CE, HERNDON JH JR, STEINBERG D: Diffuse cerebral sclerosis. *Arch Neurol* 28:304, 1973

45. HERNDON JH, STEINBERG D, UHLENDORF BW: Refsum's disease: Defective oxidation of phytanic acid in tissue cultures derived from homozygotes and heterozygotes. *N Engl J Med* 281:1034, 1969

46. HUTTON D, STEINBERG D: Localization of the enzymatic defect in phytanic acid storage disease (Refsum's disease). *Neurology (Minneap)* 23:1333, 1973

47. KAHLKE W, RICHTERICH R: Refsum's disease (heredopathia atactica polyneuritiformis), an inborn error of lipid metabolism with storage of 3,7,11,15-tetramethyl hexadecanoic acid. II. Isolation and identification of the storage product. *Am J Med* 39:237, 1965

48. NEVIN NC, CUMINGS JN, MCKEOWN F: Refsum's syndrome, heredopathia atactica polyneuritiformis. *Brain* 90:419, 1967

49. PITTMAN R, STEINBERG D: Isolation and measurement of phytanic acid and related isoprenoid compounds by gas chromatography, in Olson RE (ed): *Methods in Medical Research*. Chicago, Year Book Medical Publishers, 1970, vol 12, p 84

50. KARLSSON KA, NORRBY A, SAMUELSSON B: Use of thin-layer chromatography for the preliminary diagnosis of Refsum's disease (heredopathia atactica polyneuritiformis). *Biochim Biophys Acta* 144:162, 1967

51. LAURELL S: Separation and characterization of phytanic acid-containing plasma triglycerides from a patient with Refsum's disease. *Biochim Biophys Acta* 152:75, 1968

52. MOLZER B, BERNHEIMER H, BARLOLIN GS, HOFINGER E, LENZ H: Di-, mono- and nonphytanyl triglycerides in the serum: A sensitive parameter of the phytanic acid accumulation in Refsum's disease. *Clin Chim Acta* 91:133, 1979

53. DULANEY JT, WILLIAMS M, EVANS JE, COSTELLO CE, KOLODNY EH: Occurrence of novel branched-chain fatty acids in Refsum's disease. *Biochim Biophys Acta* 529:1, 1978

54. BAXTER JH, STEINBERG D, MIZE CE, AVIGAN J: Absorption and metabolism of uniformly 14C-labeled phytol and phytanic acid by the intestine of the rat studied with thoracic duct cannulation. *Biochim Biophys Acta* 137:277, 1967

55. ACKMAN RG, HANEN RP: The occurrence of diastereoisomers of phytanic and pristanic acids and their determination by gas-liquid chromatography. *Lipids* 2:357, 1967

56. GOERLICH R: Phytol und phytansaure in Nahrungstoffen. Ihre Bedeutung bei der Refsum-Krankheit. Doctoral dissertation. Ruprecht Karl Universitat, Heidelberg, 1974

57. PATTON S, BENSON AA: Phytol metabolism in the bovine. *Biochim Biophys Acta* 125:22, 1966

58. Ackman RG, Sipos JC: Isolation of the saturated fatty acids and branched-chain fatty acids. *Comp Biochem Physiol* 15:445, 1965

59. Peters H, Wieske TH: Detection of traces of polybranched fatty acids. *Fette Seifen Anstrichmittel* 68:947, 1966

60. Sen Gupta AK, Peters H: Isolation and structure determination of polybranched-chain fatty acids from fish oil. *Fette Seifen Anstrichmittel* 68:349, 1966

61. Ackman RG, Hooper SN: Isoprenoid fatty acids in the human diet: Distinctive geographical features in butterfats and importance in margarines based on marine oils. *Can Inst Food Technol J* 6:159, 1973

62. Prior, IAM, Alexander WE, Steinberg D, Mize CE, Herndon JH Jr: Unpublished results

63. Baxter JH, Milne GWA: Phytenic acid: Identification of five isomers in chemical and biological products of phytol. *Biochim Biophys Acta* 176:265, 1969

64. Eldjarn L, Try K: Different ratios of the LDD and DDD diastereoisomers of phytanic acid in patients with Refsum's disease. *Biochim Biophys Acta* 164:94, 1968

65. Lough AK: The stereochemistry of phytanic acid in Refsum's syndrome. *Lipids* 5:201, 1969

66. Baxter JH, Steinberg D: Absorption of phytol from dietary chlorophyll in the rat. *J Lipid Res* 8:615, 1967

67. Billeter M, Bolliger W, Maritius C: Unterschungen uber die Umwandlung von verfutterten K-Vitaminen durch Austausch der Seitenkette und die Rolle der Darmbakterien hierbei. *Biochem Z* 340:290, 1964

68. Velick SK, Anderson RJ: The chemistry of phytomonas tumefaciens. III. Phytomonic acid, a new branched-chain fatty acid. *J Biol Chem* 152:523, 1944

69. Kates M, Yengoyan LW, Sastry PS: A diether analog of phosphatidyl glycerophosphate in Halobacterium cutirubrum. *Biochim Biophys Acta* 98:252, 1965

70. Eldjarn L, Try K, Stokke O: The existence of an alternative pathway for the degradation of branched-chain fatty acids, and its failure in heredopathia atactica polyneuritiformis (Refsum's disease). *Biochim Biophys Acta* 116:395, 1966

71. Stokke O, Try K, Eldjarn L: α-Oxidation as an alternative pathway for the degradation of branched-chain fatty acids in man, and its failure in patients with Refsum's disease. *Biochim Biophys Acta* 144:271, 1967

72. Try K: Indications of only a partial defect in the alpha-oxidation mechanism in Refsum's disease. *Scand J Clin Lab Invest* 20:255, 1967

73. Laurell S: The action of lipoprotein lipase on glyceryl triphytanate. *Biochim Biophys Acta* 152:80, 1968

74. Laudat P, Wolf L-M: Repartition des esters phytaniques parmi les triglycerides plasmatiques de cinq patients atteints de maladie de Refsum: Etude per chromatographie en couche mince. *Biochim Biophys Acta* 176:425, 1969

75. Avigan J. Steinberg D: Unpublished results

76. Ellingboe J, Steinberg D: Differential susceptibility of phytanyl and palmityl ester bonds to enzymatic hydrolysis. *Biochim Biophys Acta* 270:92, 1972

77. Bowen DM, Radin NS: Hydroxy fatty acid metabolism in brain. *Adv Lipid Res* 6:255, 1968

78. Shorland FB, Hansen RP, Prior IAM: The effect of phytanic acid on the fatty acid composition of the lipids of the rat with further observations on its metabolism, in *Proceedings of the Seventh International Congress of Nutrition*. West Germany, Verlag Friedr, Vieweg & Sohn GmbH, 1966, vol V, p 399

79. Hansen RP, Shorland FB, Prior IAM: The occurrence of 4,8,12-trimethyltridecanoic acid in the tissues of rats fed high levels of phytanic acid. *Biochim Biophys Acta* 152:642, 1968

80. Hansen RP, Morrison JD: The isolation and identification of 2,6,10,14-tetramethylpentadecanoic acid from butter fat. *Biochem J* 93:225, 1964

81. Hansen RP: Occurrence of 2,6,10,14-tetramethylpentadecanoic acid in sheep fat. *Chem Industr*, p 1258, 1964

82. Levis GM, Mead JF: An α-hydroxy acid decarboxylase in brain microsomes. *J Biol Chem* 239:77, 1964

83. Davies WE, Hajra AK, Parmar SS, Radin NS, Mead JF: Decarboxylation of 2-keto fatty acids by brain. *J Lipid Res* 7:270, 1966

84. Hutton D, Steinberg D: Identification of propionate as a degradation production of phytanic acid oxidation in rat and human tissues. *J Biol Chem* 248:6871, 1973

85. Steinberg D, Hutton D: Phytanic acid storage disease, in Volk BW, Aronson SM (eds): *Sphingolipids, sphingolipidoses, and Allied Disorders*. New York, Plenum, 1972, p 515

86. Bergstrom S, Borgstrom B, Tryding N, Westoo G: Intestinal absorption and metabolism of 2,2-dimethylstearic acid in the rat. *Biochem J* 58:604, 1954

87. Anthony GJ, Landau BR: Relative contributions of alpha, beta, and omega-oxidative pathways to in vitro fatty acid oxidation in rat liver. *J Lipid Res* 9:267, 1968

88. Try K: The in vitro omega-oxidation of phytanic acid and other branched chain fatty acids by mammalian liver. *Scand J Clin Lab Invest* 22:224, 1968

89. Brenton DP, Duran M, Gale A, Krywawych S, Stern GM, Wadman SK: Refsum's disease—excretion of 3-methyladipate. *Proc Intl Symp on IEM in Humans*, Switzerland, 1980, p 11

90. Kark RAP, Engel WK, Blass JP, Steinberg D, Walsh GO: Heredopathia atactica polyneuritiformis (Refsum's disease): A second trial of dietary therapy in two patients, in *Nervous System, Birth Defects*, Original article series. New York, The National Foundation, 1971, vol VII, no 1, p 53

91. Laudat PH: Intolerance au phytol: Maladie de Refsum. *Biochimie* 54:735, 1972

92. Seubert W, Remberger U: Untersuchungen uber den bakteriellen Abbau von Isoprenoiden. II. Die Rolle der Kohlensaure. *Biochem Z* 338:245, 1963

93. Stokke O: Alpha-oxidation of fatty acids in various mammals, and a phytanic acid feeding experiment in an animal with a low alpha-oxidation capacity. *Scand J Clin Lab Invest* 20:305, 1967

94. Stokke O: Evidence against a CO_2-fixation mechanism in the degradation of a beta-methyl-substituted fatty acid in mammals. *Biochim Biophys Acta* 176:230, 1969

95. Eldjarn L: Heredopathia atactica polyneuritiformis (Refsum's disease)—a defect in the omega-oxidation mechanism of fatty acids. *Scand J Clin Lab Invest* 17:178, 1965

96. Eldjarn L, Try K, Stokke O: The ability of patients with heredopathia atactica polyneuritiformis to omega-oxidize and degrade several isoprenoid branch-chained fatty structures. *Scand J Clin Lab Invest* 18:141, 1966

97. Try K, Eldjarn L: Normalization of the tricaprin test for omega-oxidation in Refsum's disease upon lowering of serum phytanic acid. *Scand J Clin Lab Invest* 20:294, 1967

98. Baxter JH: Absorption of chlorophyll phytol in normal man and in patients with Refsum's disease. *J Lipid Res* 9:636, 1968

99. Gautier JC, Laudat PH, Rosa A, Gray F, Lhermitte F: Maladie de Refsum: Test de charge en phytol chez un descendant. *Nouv Presse Med* 2:2029, 1973

100. Uhlendorf BW, Jacobson CB, Sloan HR, Mudd SH, Herndon JH, Brady RO, Seegmiller JE, Fujimoto W: Cell cultures derived from human amniotic fluid: The possible application in the intrauterine diagnosis of heritable metabolic disease. *In Vitro* 4:158, 1969

101. O'Brien JB: Cell membranes—composition, structure, function. *J Theor Biol* 15:307, 1967

102. DuBois-Dalcq M, Gorge F: Neurocytologie—Action de l'acide phytanique sur le systeme nerveux peripherique in vitro. *C R Acad Sci[D]* (Paris), 270:2325, 1970

103. DuBois-Dalcq M, Menu R, Buyse M: Influence of fatty acids on fine structure of cultured neurons. *J Neuropathol Exp Neurol* 31:645, 1972

104. Arvidsson EO, Green FA, Laurell S: Branching and hydrophobic bonding: Partition equilibria and serum albumin binding of palmitic and phytanic acids. *J Biol Chem* 246:5373, 1971

105. Malmendier CL, Jonniaux G, Voet W, Van den Bergen CJ: Fatty acid composition of tissues in Refsum's disease (heredopathia atactica polyneuritiformis). Estimation of total phytanic acid accumulation. *Biomedicine* 20:398, 1974

106. Reynolds DJ, Marks R, Davies MG, Dykes PJ: The fatty acid composition of skin and plasma lipids in Refsum's disease. *Clin Chim Acta* 90:171, 1978

107. Anton-Lamprecht I, Kahlke W: Zur Ultrastruktur hereditarer Verhornungsstorungen. V. Ichthyosis beim Refsum-syndrom (heredopathia atactica polyneuritiformis). *Arch Derm Forsch* 250:185, 1974

108. Kishimoto Y, Radin NS, Steinberg D: Cited in [69]

109. MacBrinn MC, O'Brien JS: Lipid composition of the nervous system in Refsum's disease. *J Lipid Res* 9:552, 1968

110. Blass JP, Avigan J, Clark RG: Effects of phytol feeding and experimental allergic encephalomyelitis on myelin synthesis. *Fed Proc* 28:838, 1969

111. Wolf LM, Laudat PH, Chaumont P, Bonduelle M: Maladie de Refsum: Evolution clinique et bio-chimique sous regime sans phytol: investigations bio-chimiques complementaires. *Rev Neurol* (Paris) 120:89, 1969

112. Quinlan CD, Martin EA: Refsum's syndrome: Report of three cases. *J Neurol Neurosurg Psychiat* 33:817, 1970

113. Lundberg A, Lilja LG, Lundberg PO, Try K: Heredopathia atactica polyneuritiformis (Refsum's disease): Experiences of dietary treatment and plasmapheresis. *Eur Neurol* 8:309, 1972

114. Sahgal V, Olsen WO: Heredopathia atactica polyneuritiformis (phytanic acid storage disease): A new case with special reference to dietary treatment. *Arch Intern Med* 135:585, 1975

115. Dry J, Pradalier A, Delporte M-P, Leynadier F: A propos de deux nouveaux cas de maladie de Refsum. Evolution sous regime. *Sem Hoop Paris* 52:1675, 1976

116. THUMLER R, ATZPODIEN W, KREMER GJ, HAFERKAMP G: Refsum-syndrom (Heredopathia atactica polyneuritiformis). Klinik, Diagnostik und Diatetische Behandlung. *Dtsch Med Wochenscher* 102:1454, 1977

117. PENOVICH PE, HOLLANDER J, NUSBACHER JA, GRIGGS RC, MACPHERSON J: Note on plasma exchange therapy in Refsum's disease. *Adv Neurol* 21:151, 1978

118. BAROLIN GS, HODKEWITSCH E, HOFINGER E, SCHOLZ H, BERNHEIMER H, MOLZER B: Klinisch-biochemische Velaufsuntersuchungen bei Heredopathia atactica polyneuritiformis (Morbis Refsum). *Fortschr Neurol Psychiat* 47:53, 1979

119. GIBBERD FB: BILLIMORIA JD, PAGE NGR, RETSAS S: Heredopathia atactica polyneuritiformis (Refsum's disease) treated by diet and plasma-exchange. *Lancet* 1:575, 1979

120. MOSER HW, BATSHAW ML, MURRAY C, BRAINE H, BRUSILOW SW: Management of heritable disorders of the urea cycle and of Refsum's and Fabry's diseases, in Papadatos C, Eartsocas C (eds): *The Management of Genetic Disorders*. New York, Alan R Liss, 1979, p 183

121. FRYER DG, WINCKELMAN AL, WAYS PO, SWANSON AG: Refsum's disease. A clinical and pathological report. *Neurology* 21:162, 1971

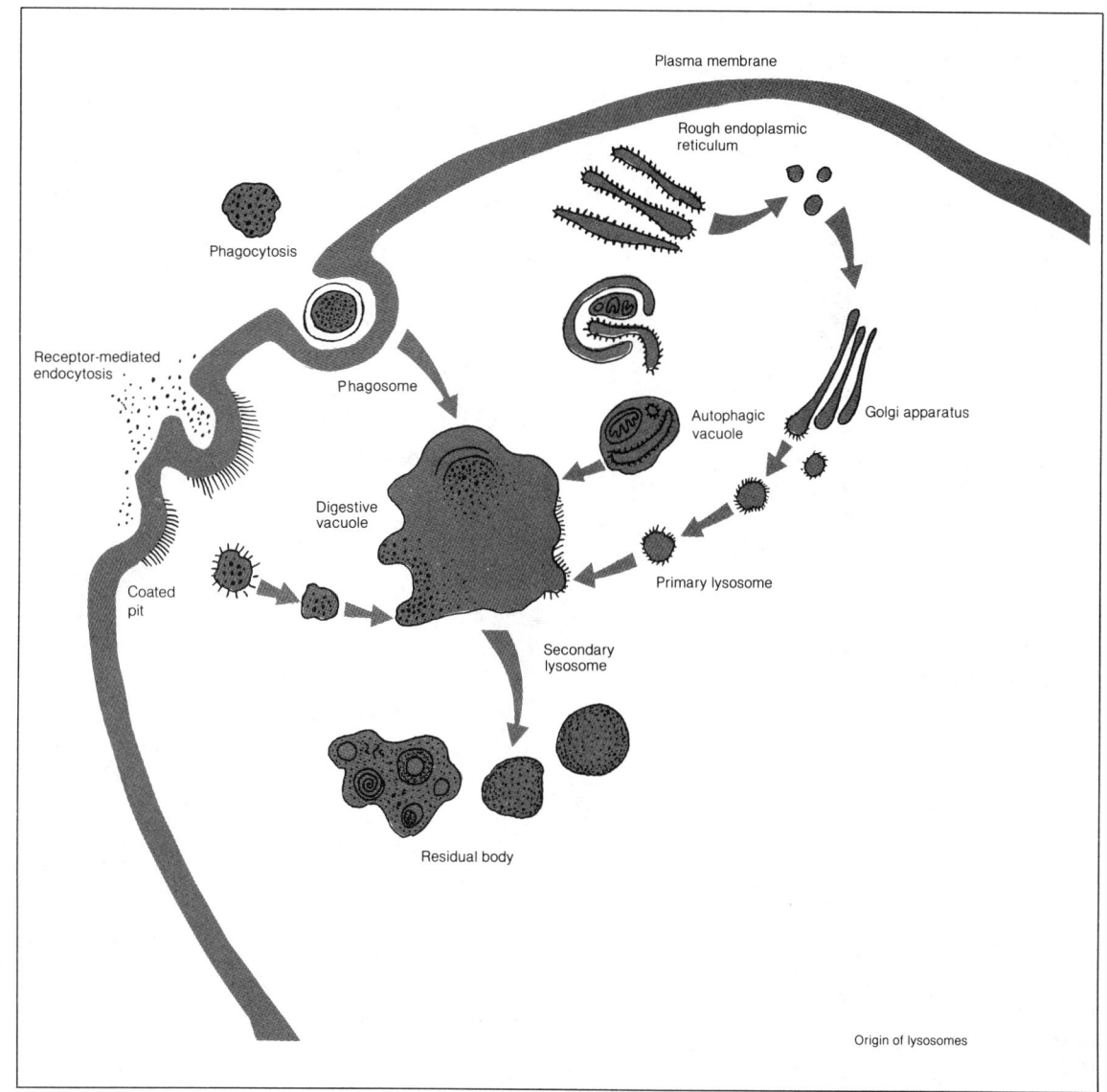

PART 5

Plasma membrane

Rough endoplasmic reticulum

Phagocytosis

Receptor-mediated endocytosis

Phagosome

Autophagic vacuole

Golgi apparatus

Digestive vacuole

Primary lysosome

Coated pit

Secondary lysosome

Residual body

Origin of lysosomes

DISORDERS OF LYSOSOMAL ENZYMES

36

THE MUCOPOLYSACCHARIDE STORAGE DISEASES

VICTOR A. McKUSICK

ELIZABETH F. NEUFELD

1. The mucopolysaccharidoses are lysosomal storage diseases. They result from deficiency of specific lysosomal enzymes involved in the degradation of dermatan sulfate, heparan sulfate, or keratan sulfate, singly or in combination. Incompletely degraded mucopolysaccharides accumulate in tissues and are excreted in the urine. The clinical, genetic, and biochemical characteristics of the well-studied forms of the disorder are summarized in Table 36-1.

2. The several mucopolysaccharidoses show clinical features in common. The particular combination of manifestations permits provisional clinical diagnosis in many instances; laboratory confirmation by specific enzyme assay is now available for all.

3. As in all lysosomal storage diseases, the mucopolysaccharidoses are progressive in nature and involve multiple tissues and organs. The clinical features relate to the following organs and tissues:

   a. Osseous skeleton: *All the disorders except the Morquio syndrome (MPS IV) show changes known generically as dysostosis multiplex. (The changes in the Morquio syndrome have both similarities to and differences from those of the Hurler syndrome, the prototype mucopolysaccharidosis. Striking platyspondyly and genu valgum are unique to the Morquio syndrome.) Short stature occurs in all except the Scheie syndrome. Hypoplasia or apla-* sia of the odontoid with atlantoaxial subluxation is a usual finding in the Morquio syndrome and an occasional finding in the others, e.g., Hurler syndrome (MPS I H) and the severe form of the Maroteaux-Lamy syndrome (MPS VI).

   b. Joints are stiff in all except the Morquio syndrome, with claw hand and limitations of motion, although this feature is mild in the Sanfilippo syndrome (MPS III). Nerve entrapment (e.g., carpal tunnel syndrome) and tendon entrapment (e.g., trigger finger) are, like stiff joints, the consequence of the secondary collagenosis.

   c. Eye: Corneal clouding occurs to some degree in most; the exceptions are the Hunter syndrome and the Sanfilippo syndrome. Indeed, even in the Hunter syndrome, corneal clouding is occasionally detectable late and in severe cases, although usually only with the slit lamp. Retinal pigmentary changes occur in some, e.g., the Scheie, Hunter, and Sanfilippo syndromes, but not in the Morquio and Maroteaux-Lamy syndromes. Glaucoma is a complication of several of the mucopolysaccharidoses, e.g., Scheie syndrome (MPS I S).

   d. Ear: Deafness of mixed or sensorineural type is frequent in all.

   e. Skin and teeth: Hirsutism is a feature of most, particularly of the Sanfilippo syndrome. Specific pebbly lesions over the scapula occur in the Hunter syndrome. In Morquio A syndrome (MPS IV A), the teeth are widely spaced with thin enamel. Dentigerous cysts occur in most of the forms of mucopolysaccharidosis except Morquio syndrome.

f. Cardiovascular: Arteriosclerosis develops in most of the mucopolysaccharidoses, in the aorta and coronary arteries, for example. Deposition of mucopolysaccharides in arterial smooth-muscle cells, comparable to the deposition of lipid in standard atherosclerosis, leads to proliferation of these cells and excessive production of collagen and elastin. Angina pectoris results. Involvement of the heart valves leads to stenosis and regurgitation.

g. Respiratory system: Stiffening of the thoracic cage, narrowing of the tracheobronchial airways by mucopolysaccharide deposition, and obstruction of the upper airways as part of the cramped nasopharynx (further compromised by enlarged adenoids) lead to respiratory insufficiency and cor pulmonale. In the Morquio syndrome, severe scoliosis can be a contributing factor in the cardiorespiratory complications.

h. Liver and spleen are enlarged in most mucopolysaccharidoses as a result of accumulation of incompletely degraded mucopolysaccharides in parenchymal and reticuloendothelial cells.

i. Central nervous system: Thickening of the meninges leads to communicating hydrocephalus in the Hurler syndrome and some of the other mucopolysaccharidoses. In the cervical area the same process, known as pachymeningitis cervicalis, results in myelopathy and spinal nerve root compression. Cervical myelopathy also is produced by atlantoaxial subluxation in the Morquio syndrome and less often in other mucopolysaccharidoses. Deposition of lipid as well as mucopolysaccharide in the cells of the brain leads to mental and neurologic deterioration.

j. Other cells: Metachromatic and vacuolar inclusions are found in circulating leukocytes and in bone marrow cells. These are particularly striking in the Maroteaux-Lamy syndrome and in β-glucuronidase deficiency (MPS VII).

4. The course in all the mucopolysaccharidoses is one of apparent normal development in the first years of life and progressive deterioration beginning at some time thereafter. Death occurs before age 10 in the prototype disorder, the Hurler syndrome, which is also the prognostically gravest of the mucopolysaccharidoses. On the other hand patients with the Scheie syndrome and a mild form of the Hunter syndrome have survived to their sixties or even later.

5. Keratansulfaturia characterizes the Morquio syndrome, heparansulfaturia the Sanfilippo syndrome, and dermatansulfaturia the Maroteaux-Lamy syndrome. In the others the urine contains an excess of dermatan sulfate and heparan sulfate in varying ratios.

6. Deficiency of 10 specific lysosomal enzymes has been demonstrated in various mucopolysaccharidoses, as indicated in Table 36-1. (These deficiencies are usefully studied in cultured fibroblasts.) All but one of these enzymes are acid hydrolases. The exception, deficient in Sanfilippo syndrome C, is an acetyltransferase, which catalyzes a change necessary for degradation of heparan sulfate. Each of the enzymes catalyzes cleavage at a specific site. Degradation of the mucopolysaccharide chains occurs sequentially and a defect at a given linkage prevents cleavage at subsequent linkages in the chain even though the enzyme catalyzing that cleavage is present. (A limited amount of degradation can result from endoglycosidases in some tissues such as liver.)

7. All 10 mucopolysaccharidoses are recessively inherited. The Hunter syndrome is X-linked; the others are autosomal.

8. The mucopolysaccharidoses illustrate genetic heterogeneity, pleiotropism, and variability—three main principles of clinical genetics. Fundamental heterogeneity is illustrated by the four forms of the Sanfilippo syndrome, which cannot be distinguished clinically in the individual case. Also, deficiency of either of two enzymes can produce the same or nearly the same clinical picture, the mild form of the Morquio syndrome. Extensive pleiotropism is illustrated by each mucopolysaccharidosis, as outlined earlier and in Table 36-1.

9. Variability resulting probably from different genetic changes in the same lysosomal enzyme ("allelic variants") is illustrated by each of the following classes: MPS I, MPS II, MPS III B, MPS IV A, MPS VI, and MPS VII. In each of these categories homozygotes for different alleles exist, with differing clinical severity. In addition, some affected persons are presumably compound heterozygotes (genetic compounds), not homozygotes, but with the present methods these cases cannot be identified as such with certainty. Even the previously presumed Hurler-Scheie genetic compound may in fact represent homozygosity for another allele at the MPS I locus. Intrafamilial variability presumably results from differences in the rest of the genome and in the environment of the individuals.

10. Prenatal diagnosis has been demonstrated, or is theoretically possible, in each of the mucopolysaccharidoses. Heterozygote identification is particularly important (but difficult) in the case of the Hunter syndrome (MPS II). Cloning of cultured fibroblasts and testing hair roots can be used to identify carriers but are labor-intensive and therefore prohibitively costly. Furthermore, the failure to find deficient clones or hair roots may only represent sampling or selection for normal cells in vivo, so that a normal genotype cannot be inferred with certainty.

11. No definitive therapy is available, although enzyme replacement by various methods has been attempted.

12. Several animal models (feline MPS I and MPS IV, murine β-glucuronidase deficiency, and drug-induced mucopolysaccharidosis) have been reported and should be useful for testing new therapeutic approaches.

The mucopolysaccharide storage diseases are clinically progressive, hereditary disorders characterized by the accumulation of mucopolysaccharides (glycosaminoglycans) in various tissues. The known disorders result from deficiency of a specific enzyme involved in the degradation of dermatan sulfate, heparan sulfate, and keratan sulfate, singly or in combination. Presently 10 enzymes are known, deficiency of any one of which can result in a specific mucopolysaccharide storage disease (Table 36-1). The storage occurs in lysosomes (Fig. 36-1), which normally are the site of degradation of mucopolysaccharides.

Reference is made to reviews elsewhere [1, 2] of the fascinating story of the nosography and biochemical elucidation of the mucopolysaccharide storage diseases. Schematic diagrams for the normal degradation of heparan sulfate, dermatan sulfate, and keratan sulfate are presented in Figs. 36-2, 36-3, and 36-4, respectively. The chemistry, synthesis, and degradation of mucopolysaccharides have been recently reviewed [3].

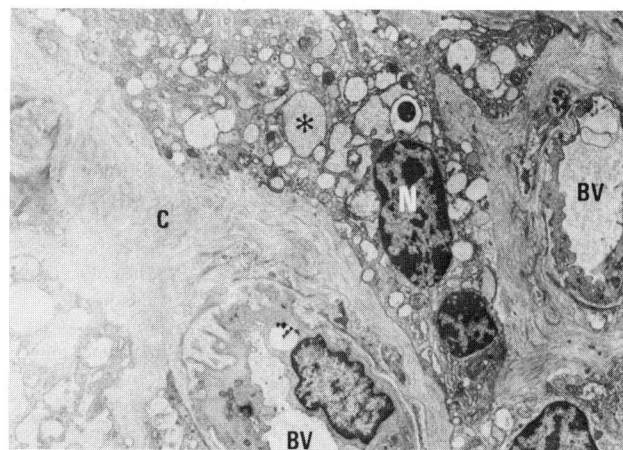

Figure 36-1 Characteristic appearance of cells in mucopolysaccharide storage diseases: electronmicrograph of conjunctival biopsy from patient with α-L-iduronidase deficiency, probably of the MPS I H/S type. The much enlarged lysosomes preempt most of the cytoplasmic space. One such lysosome filled with fibrillogranular material is labeled with an asterisk. BV, N, and C refer to blood vessel, nucleus, and collagen, respectively. The dense globular inclusion in the lysosome immediately above the large nucleus is of lipid nature. Some of the lysosomes appear empty because of the solubility of the mucopolysaccharide in the glutaraldehyde fixative. Magnification × 6200. (*Supplied by Dr. W. R. Green, Johns Hopkins Hospital, Baltimore.*)

TYPE I MUCOPOLYSACCHARIDOSES: THE α-L-IDURONIDASE DEFICIENCIES

There are at least three, and probably four, clinically and genetically distinct forms of α-L-iduronidase deficiency. The three best characterized are the Hurler and Scheie syndromes and the syndrome phenotypically intermediate between the Hurler and Scheie syndromes previously referred to as the Hurler-Scheie compound. At least one other form of α-L-iduronidase deficiency appears to exist. The genetic interrelationship of these forms will be discussed later.

Mucopolysaccharidosis I H (MPS I H; Hurler Syndrome; α-L-Iduronidase Deficiency, Hurler Type)

The Hurler syndrome (Fig. 36-5) is the prototype for all the mucopolysaccharide storage diseases. It is a severe, progressive disorder leading to death usually before the age of 10 years. Clouding of the cornea develops in all cases. These are the two characteristics that classically differentiate the Hurler form of MPS I from the Hunter syndrome (MPS II): early death and corneal clouding.

Patients with the Hurler syndrome are clinically normal in infancy. Indeed, they may be unusually large in the first year of life, but thereafter they progressively deteriorate, both mentally and physically. Lumbar lordosis, stiff joints, chest deformity, enlargement of the liver and spleen, or rhinorrhea with stertorous breathing may first prompt medical consultation. Dwarfing becomes evident by 2 or 3 years of age, after which growth seems practically to cease. Progressive clouding of the cornea takes place during the same period. (An exception [4] was in a case that probably represented a form of α-L-iduronidase deficiency other than the Hurler syndrome; see later.) Some patients develop glaucoma from interference with the drainage of the eye at the angle. The facies becomes coarse. The abdomen is prominent, with an enlarged liver and spleen, and often with umbilical and other hernias. The head is unusu-

ally large, often with a ridge along the sagittal suture. Stiff joints are an impressive feature and are evident, for example, at the elbows, in the fingers as claw hand, and in the hips as flexion contractures. Deafness, usually of combined conductive and neurosensory origin, is a finding in most of these patients. It is due in part to frequent middle ear infections, in part to deformity of the ossicles, and in part probably to abnormality of the inner ear. Angina pectoris and murmurs due to involvement of the coronary arteries and heart valves develop. The usual causes of death are respiratory infection and heart failure.

The radiographic changes in the Hurler syndrome represent the prototype for the entire group of mucopolysaccharidoses. (Unique features of one, the Morquio syndrome, or MPS IV, will be described later.) The most consistent skeletal abnormality revealed by roentgenograms is widening of the medial end of the clavicle [5]. The lateral portion of the clavicles may, on the other hand, be hypoplastic, curved, or absent. Skull sutures close early, the sagittal suture closing first, resulting in the scaphocephalic shape of the head. The orbits are shallow, accounting for proptosis. The sella turcica is often enlarged, the optic chiasm being particularly long, creating the so-called J-shaped or omega sella. Hydrocephalus of communicating type is usually present. This is thought to be caused by fibrous thickening of the meninges as a result of mucopolysaccharide disposition. The thickening may also damp normal pulsations and thereby account for the lack of the normal digital marking of the calvaria. In the first year of life the vertebral bodies appear more rounded and immature than usual on lateral roentgenograms. One or two of the upper lumbar or lower thoracic vertebral bodies are usually slightly smaller than the others and recessed, causing mild gibbus. By age 18 months the characteristic broad-hook appearance of the hypoplastic vertebra at the apex of the thoracic-lumbar gibbus has developed, the anterosuperior portion of this vertebral body being particularly poorly developed.

Table 36-1 The genetic mucopolysaccharidoses

Number	Eponym	Clinical	Genetics	Urinary MPS	Enzyme deficient
MPS I H	Hurler	Clouding of cornea, grave manifestations, death usually before age 10	Homozygous for MPS IH gene	Dermatan sulfate, heparan sulfate	α-L-iduronidase
MSP I S	Scheie	Stiff joints, cloudy cornea, aortic valve disease, normal intelligence and (?) life span	Homozygosity for MPS IS gene	Dermatan sulfate, heparan sulfate	α-L-iduronidase
MPS I H/S	Hurler-Scheie	Intermediate phenotype	Genetic compound of MPS I H and MPS I S genes	Dermatan sulfate, heparan sulfate	α-L-iduronidase
MPS II-XR, severe	Hunter, severe	No corneal clouding, milder course than in MPS IH, death before 15 years	Hemizygous for X-linked gene	Dermatan sulfate, heparan sulfate	Iduronate sulfatase
MSP II-XR, mild	Hunter, mild	Survival to thirties–sixties+, fair intelligence	Hemizygous for X-linked allele	Dermatan sulfate, heparan sulfate	Iduronate sulfatase
?MPS II-AR	?Autosomal Hunter	Same as mild or severe MPS II-XR	?Homozygous for autosomal gene; ?form of multiple sulfatase deficiency	Dermatan sulfate heparan sulfate	Iduronate sulfatase
MPS III A	Sanfilippo A	Indistinguishable phenotype: Mild somatic, severe central nervous system effects	Homozygous for Sanfilippo A gene	Heparan sulfate	Heparan N-sulfatase (sulfamidase)
MPS III BV	Sanfilippo B		Homozygous for Sanfilippo B gene	Heparan sulfate	N-acetyl-α-D-glucosaminidase
MPS III C	Sanfilippo C		Homozygous for Sanfilippo C gene	Heparan sulfate	Acetyl CoA: α-glucosaminide-N-acetyltransferase
MPS III D	Sanfilippo D		Homozygous for Sanfilippo D gene	Heparan sulfate	N-acetyl-α-D-glucosaminide-6-sulfatase
MPS IV A	Morquio A	Severe, distinctive bone changes, cloudy cornea, aortic regurgitation, thin enamel	Homozygous for Morquio A gene	Keratan sulfate	Galactosamine-6-sulfate sulfatase
MPS IV B	Morquio B	Mild bone changes, cloudy cornea, hypoplastic odontoid, normal enamel	Homozygous for Morquio B gene ?allele of mutant gene in G_{M1} gangliosidosis (on chromosome 3)	Keratan sulfate	β-galactosidase
MPS V	No longer used	—	—	—	—
MSP VI, severe	Maroteaux-Lamy, classic severe	Severe osseous and corneal changes, valvular heart disease, striking WBC inclusions, normal intellect; survival to twenties	Homozygous for Maroteaux-Lamy (M-L) gene (on chromosome 5)	Dermatan sulfate	Arylsulfatase B (N-acetylgalactosamine-4-sulfatase)

Table 36-1   The genetic mucopolysaccharidoses (*Continued*)

Number	Eponym	Clinical	Genetics	Urinary MPS	Enzyme deficient
MPS VI	Maroteaux-Lamy, intermediate	Moderately severe changes	Homozygous for allele at M-L locus or genetic compound	Dermatan sulfate	Arylsulfatase B (*N*-acetylgalac-tosamine-4-sulfatase)
MPS VI, mild	Maroteaux-Lamy, mild	Mild osseous and corneal change, normal intellect	Homozygous for allele at M-L locus	Dermatan sulfate	Arylsulfatase B (*N*-acetylgalac-tosamine-4-sulfatase)
MPS VII	Sly	Hepatosplenomeg-aly, dysostosis multiplex	Homozygous for mutant gene at β-glucuronidase locus (on chromosome 7)	Dermatan sulfate, heparan sulfate	β-glucuronidase

The pelvis shows excessive flaring of the iliac wings and a small body of the ilium. The acetabulum is very shallow and has an oblique roof. The hips show coxa valga. The ribs develop a width exceeding that of the intercostal spaces, yet their vertebral ends remain narrow, giving them the shape of oars.

The metacarpals lack diaphyseal constriction, and all except the first metacarpal are pointed proximally. The shafts of the long bones of the upper limb, particularly the humerus and proximal radius, may be wider than the metaphyses. The humeral neck shows severe varus deformity. The semilunar notch of the ulnar is shallow. At all ages the changes in the lower limbs below the lesser trochanters are considerably milder than those in the upper limbs—a characteristic of all the mucopolysaccharidoses.

Hypoplasia of the odontoid with atlantoaxial subluxation, spinal cord compression, and spastic quadriplegia is a more familiar feature of other mucopolysaccharidoses, especially MPS IV. This complication was also observed in a brother and sister, aged $4\frac{1}{2}$ and $6\frac{3}{4}$ years [6], who were reported as having the Hurler syndrome, but in fact had either the Hurler-Scheie syndrome or a variant form of iduronidase deficiency (personal observations).

Morbid Anatomy   Accumulation of material in parenchymal and mesenchymal cells characterizes Hurler syndrome. Electron microscopy shows that the inclusion material, primarily mucopolysaccharide, is situated in lysosomes, where it has a finely granular appearance (unless it is lost during fixation). In neurons the lysosomal inclusions are reminiscent of the zebra bodies seen in Tay-Sachs disease and are believed to contain lipid rather than mucopolysaccharide, although these fragile structures have thus far defied attempts at isolation and chemical analysis [7]. To accommodate the storage bodies, cortical neurons may develop large processes ("meganeurites") interposed between the axons and perikarya [8].

Mucopolysaccharides are deposited in the lining of arteries, including the coronary arteries [9], resulting in a "pseudo atheromatosis" or MPS atheromatosis. By electron microscopy the sclerotic lesions are found to consist of greatly proliferated smooth-muscle cells with distended lysosomes [10]. This is true in both the intima and the media of the aorta and coronary arteries. Massive proliferation of elastic fibers and collagen takes place. An overproduction of collagen at other sites may accompany the mucopolysaccharide disturbance and may be responsible in part for the joint stiffness, the carpal tunnel syn-

drome, and the thickening of the leptomeninges with hydrocephalus. Dermatan sulfate normally, plays a role in the extracellular organization of collagen, and an excess of dermatan sulfate may induce abnormally extensive collagen deposition. Indeed, precipitation of collagen may occur at inappropriate sites, e.g., within cells [11]. In addition to the so-called Hurler, balloon, gargoyle, or clear cells, which are connective tissue cells laden with large amounts of dermatan sulfate and heparan sulfate, a second type of abnormal connective tissue cell, small granular cells containing collagen fibrils, is thought to represent fibroblasts in an advanced state of degeneration [11].

Basic Defect   The activity of a specific lysosomal hydrolase, α-L-iduronidase, is essentially absent in the Hurler syndrome [12, 13]. This enzyme is required for the cleavage of L-iduronic acid residues, which are present in both heparan sulfate and dermatan sulfate (reaction 2 in Figs. 36-2 and 36-3), so that the degradation of both polymers is blocked in the Hurler syndrome. In certain tissues, such as liver, but apparently not in fibroblasts, there is limited degradation by endoglycosidases, (hyaluronidase for dermatan sulfate and several heparanases for heparan sulfate [3]). This gives rise to fragments which may escape from tissues and be excreted in urine.

α-L-Iduronidase has been purified to homogeneity from human kidney [14]. It was found to have a molecular weight of about 60,000 and to be composed of two chains of 30,000. These are probably not true subunits, but rather cleavage products of a single polypeptide chain [15].

The "Hurler corrective factor," previously identified as lacking in MPS I [16], is a form of α-L-iduronidase which is selectively taken up by fibroblasts [17]. It has a higher molecular weight than the purified kidney enzyme, which is not taken up, and contains the mannose-6-phosphate recognition marker (see Chapter 37). "Correction" of the defect of Hurler fibroblasts is the restoration of the normal pathway for degradation of dermatan sulfate and heparan sulfate as a result of the uptake of α-L-iduronidase [12].

Diagnosis   The earliest diagnostic tests were based on the mucopolysacchariduria which consistently accompanies the Hurler syndrome. Dermatan sulfate and heparan sulfate are usually present in the ratio of 7:3, but deviations from this ratio are frequent. The mucopolysacchariduria is so marked that it is readily detected in rapid screening procedures based

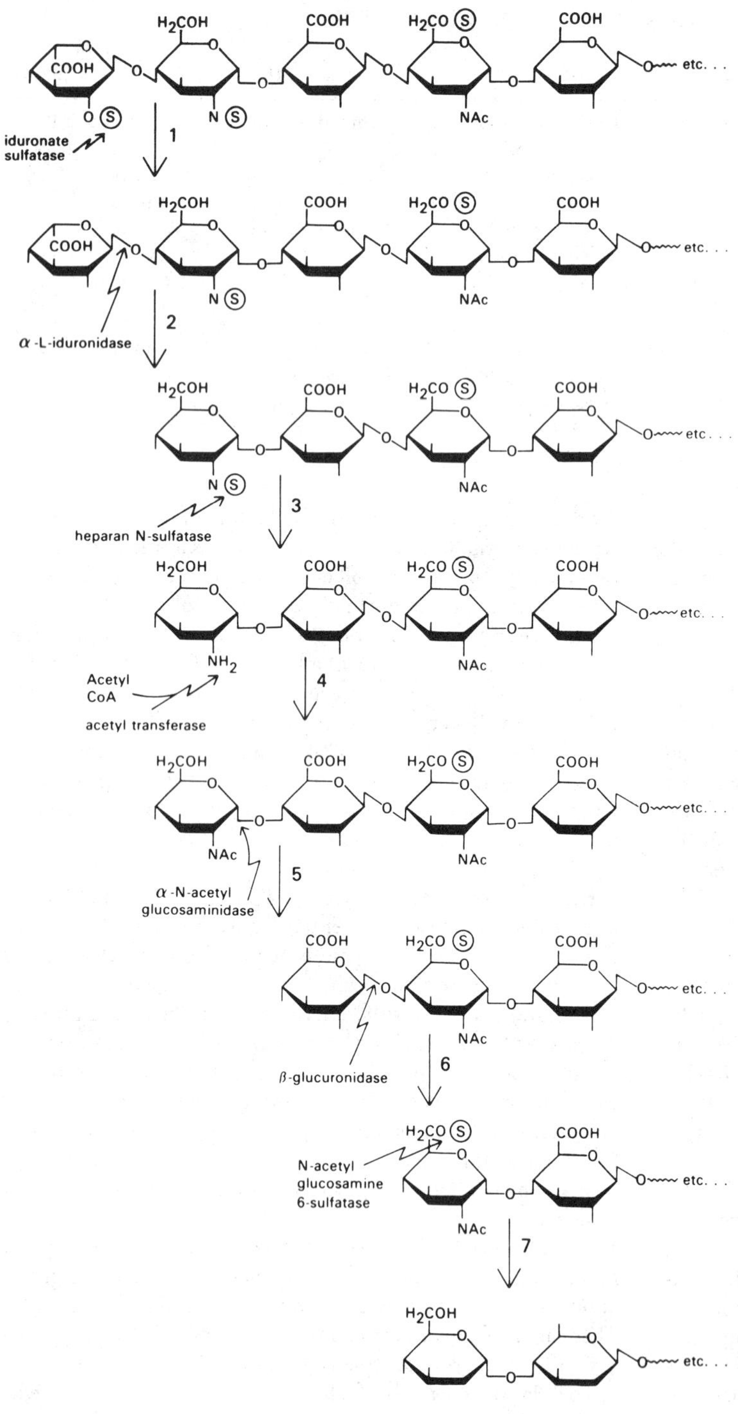

Figure 36-2 Schematic representation of steps in the degradation of heparan sulfate. Chains of heparan sulfate have alternative uronic acid and glucosamine residues. The former may be glucuronic acid, or else sulfated or unsulfated L-iduronic acid; the latter may be sulfated or acetylated on the amino nitrogen as well as sulfated on the 6 hydroxyl. Each of these residues is included in the diagram, without implying that they necessarily occur in the order or frequency shown. Every reaction catalyzed by a glycosidase, sulfatase or transferase has been assigned a number (seen over the arrow). The corresponding deficiency diseases are: 1- Hunter syndrome; 2- Hurler, Scheie, Hurler-Scheie syndromes; 3- Sanfilippo syndrome, type A, 4- Sanfilippo syndrome, type C; 5- Sanfilippo syndrome, type B; 6- β-glucuronidase deficiency; 7- Sanfilippo syndrome, type D.

on the appearance of a metachromatic spot on paper impregnated with toluidine blue, turbidity with acid-albumin, or a precipitate with cetylpyridinium salts.

Discrimination between MPS I and other mucopolysaccharidoses was first based on the finding of excessive [35S]mucopolysaccharide accumulation by cultured fibroblasts, and the reduction of this accumulation ("correction") by mixing with reference cell lines of another genotype, or by addition of purified Hurler correction factor [18]. These specific but cumbersome tests have largely been superseded by assays of α-L-iduronidase activity in leukocytes or cultured fibroblasts [19]. Substrates used for the purpose include phenyl and 4-methylumbelliferyl iduronides [20] as well as radioactive disaccharides containing iduronic acid in the nonreducing position [21–23].

The mean level of α-L-iduronidase of heterozygote fibroblasts or leukocytes is half that of normal cells [24, 25]. Unfortunately, the range of activity in both normal and carrier populations is great, and although the overlap is less in leukocytes than in cultured fibroblasts, it is difficult to ascertain the carrier status of a particular individual [26].

The Hurler syndrome is readily detected in second-trimester pregnancies by examination of cells cultured from amniotic fluid. These cells behave exactly as do skin fibroblasts with respect to [35S]mucopolysaccharide accumulation: excessive for Hurler cells but normal for heterozygous cells. The actual level of α-L-iduronidase activity is much lower in amniotic fluid cells than in skin fibroblasts; this may cause problems in the case of a heterozygous fetus, and special precautions have been recommended for assays that use phenyliduronide as substrate [19]. Use of 4-methylumbelliferyl iduronide (of good grade, free of β-glucuronide impurities) is recommended for prenatal diagnosis, because of the greater sensitivity of the assay with this fluorogenic substrate (Hall and Neufeld, unpublished results).

In one case of prenatal diagnosis of twins, one was found affected and the other normal; selective abortion of the affected twin was performed [27].

Genetics   The Hurler syndrome is inherited as an autosomal recessive disorder. It is caused by homozygosity for a mutant gene presumably at the structural locus for α-L-iduronidase.

The incidence of the Hurler syndrome in British Columbia was placed at about 1 in 100,000 births [28]. Extrapolating from this figure, one can estimate that about 30 new patients are born annually in the United States. The frequency of carriers is about 1 in 160 persons.

Management   No specific treatment is available. In 1971, DiFerrante et al. [29] introduced infusion of normal plasma as a possible means of replacing the missing enzyme. Transient improvement of some patients receiving such infusions was reported, but it is unlikely that the effect was due to true enzyme replacement, since the level of circulating α-L-iduronidase is vanishingly low. Leukocyte transfusion [30] and fibroblast transplantation [31] have also been tried. Although all these procedures are reported to result in qualitative changes in mucopolysaccharide excretion, there appears to be no significant clinical amelioration.

Mucopolysaccharidosis I S (MPS I S; Formerly MPS V; Scheie Syndrome; α-L-Iduronidase Deficiency, Scheie Type)

Although presumed cases can be found in the earlier literature, this condition was first clearly described by Scheie and colleagues in 1962 as a "forme fruste of Hurler's disease," which further studies showed it indeed to be. The same enzyme, α-L-iduronidase, is deficient in the Hurler and Scheie syndromes.

Clinical Manifestations   MPS I S (Fig. 36-6) is characterized by severe clouding of the cornea, deformity of the hands, and involvement of the aortic valve, with few other somatic effects and with normal intelligence. Stature is normal in this mucopolysaccharidosis. The facies is characteristically coarse, with a broad mouth. Stiff joints are particularly striking in the hands, where the claw-hand deformity is aggravated by development of the carpal tunnel syndrome. Acute angulation at the distal interphalangeal joint is probably the end stage of trigger finger [32]. Patients have genu valgum and pes cavus, with a stiff, painful foot. Large bone cysts in the head of the femur with consequent pathologic fracture and degenerative arthritis of the hip have been recorded [33], but they are probably exceptional. Deafness develops in some patients. Cardiac abnormality consists particularly of involvement of the aortic valve with aortic stenosis or regurgitation or both. Sleep apnea, relieved by tracheostomy, was described in two brothers, aged 18 and 25 years [34].

Corneal clouding, which is most dense in the periphery of the cornea, pigmentary degeneration of the retina, and glaucoma lead to major visual disability.

Psychiatric disturbance has been observed, but to what extent it is fundamentally related to the metabolic defect is unclear. Myelopathy due to compression of the cervical cord by thickened dura was reported [35, 36] in patients presumed, but not enzymatically proved, to have the Scheie syndrome. In these reported cases, because of the short stature and striking cytoplasmic inclusions in circulating leukocytes, it may be that in fact the disorder was MPS VI. "Pachymeningitis cervicalis" has many causes, a leading one of which is the group of mucopolysaccharidoses, particularly MPS II and MPS VI, but perhaps also MPS I S.

Patients reported earlier [37] as having a "new mucopolysaccharidosis" were subsequently found to have α-L-iduronidase deficiency and to satisfy the clinical characteristics of the Scheie syndrome. These patients developed signs of functionally significant mitral and aortic valve disease [38]. A brother had prosthetic aortic valve replacement for aortic stenosis at age 22 years and mitral valve replacement for mitral regurgitation at age 26.

Morbid Anatomy   The skin, cornea, and conjunctiva, as well as tissue from the region of the carpal tunnel, show qualitatively the same histologic changes, including electron microscopic changes, as in MPS I H. Brain autopsy shows that the

Figure 36-3 Schematic representation of steps in the degradation of dermatan sulfate. Dermatan sulfate is composed of alternating uronic acid and sulfated N-acetylgalactosamine residues. The uronic acid may be unsulfated or sulfated L-iduronic acid, or glucuronic acid. The deficiency diseases corresponding to the numbered reactions are: 1- Hunter syndrome; 2- Hurler, Scheie, Hurler-Scheie syndrome; 8- Maroteaux-Lamy syndrome; 9- uncertain, perhaps Sandhoff disease; 6- β-glucuronidase deficiency.

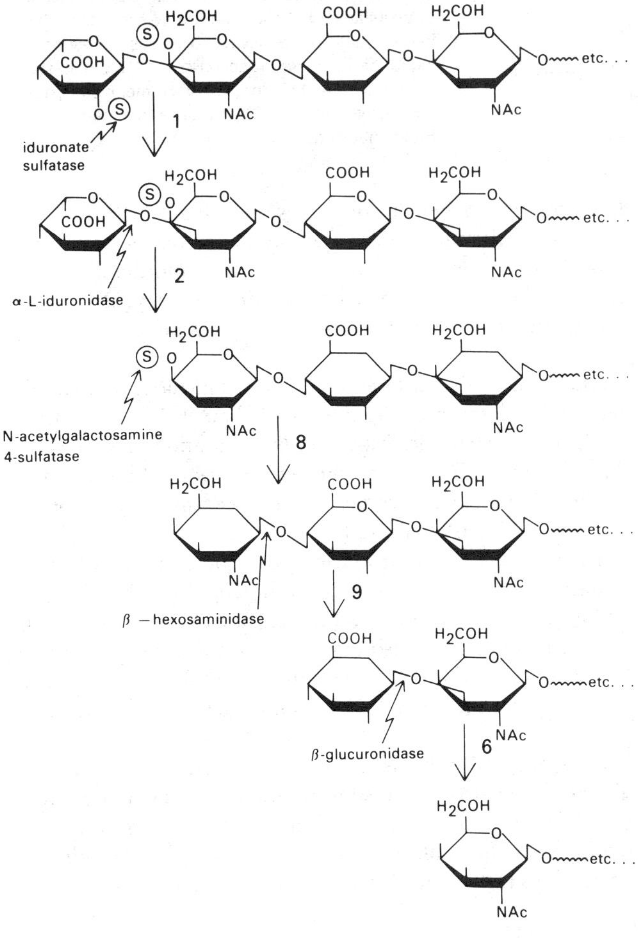

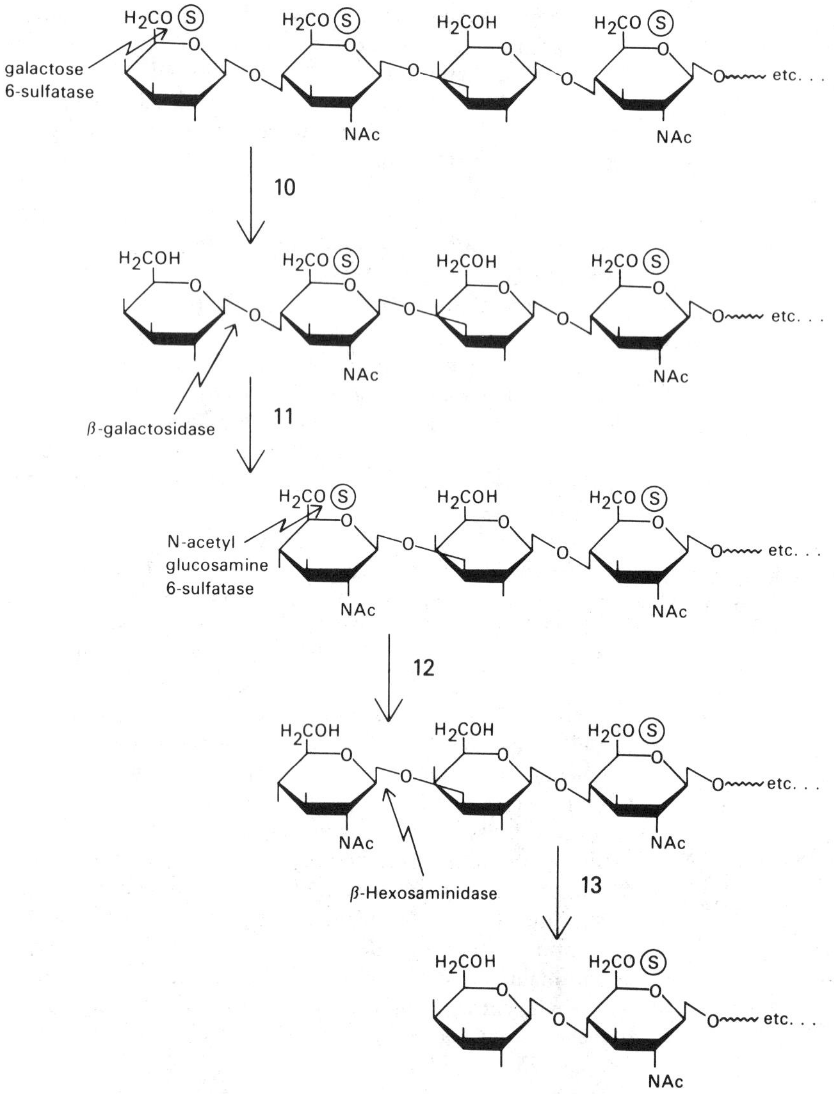

Figure 36-4 Schematic representation of steps in the degradation of keratan sulfate. This polymer contains galactose residues, which may be sulfated or unsulfated, that alternate with *N*-acetylglucosamine residues. The deficiency diseases corresponding to the numbered reaction are: 10- Morquio syndrome, type A; 11- Morquio syndrome, type B; 12- unclassified disorder (?); 13- uncertain, perhaps Sandhoff disease.

cortical neurons are histologically normal, in contradistinction to the findings in MPS I H. At the ultrastructural level the neurons in MPS I S show only a small number of lipofuscinlike inclusions and typical lipofuscin granules. Periadventitial mesenchymal tissues of the white matter show lesions similar to those of MPS I H. The brain glycosaminoglycan content is only slightly increased in MPS I S, as contrasted to a threefold increase in MPS I H. The lesions in liver, spleen, kidneys, lymph nodes, heart, and arteries in MPS I S are similar to those in MPS I H.

Basic Defect   As in the Hurler syndrome, a deficiency of α-L-iduronidase is found in the Scheie syndrome [12]. Some residual enzyme would be expected to function in vivo to explain the mild clinical picture. The search for such residual activity in cultured fibroblasts has led to variable results. Some investigators have failed to find significant residual activity using phenyl- or methylumbelliferyl iduronide, or iduronosyl anhydromannitol [19, 21]. On the other hand, Hopwood and Muller [39] reported some residual activity in both Hurler and Scheie fibroblasts using a radioactive disaccharide, iduronosyl anhydromannitol-6-sulfate. The mutant enzymes differed from each other and from the normal enzyme in kinetic constants and stability. Yet others [40] have found some iduroni-

dase activity in Scheie fibroblasts when using desulfated heparan (but not desulfated dermatan) as substrate. At present it is difficult to reconcile these diverse findings, and the difference between the Hurler and Scheie syndromes may have to be investigated by the methods of molecular genetics.

Diagnosis   The differential diagnosis includes particularly mild MPS VI and mucolipidosis III (Chapter 37). Aside from the specific enzymatic tests, the differentiation can be made clinically on the basis of height, which is normal or near normal in the Scheie syndrome, and reduced moderately or severely in both MPS VI and ML III.

The tests described for Hurler's syndrome (measurement of urinary mucopolysaccharides, [³⁵S]mucopolysaccharide accumulation and correction, and direct measurement of α-L-iduronidase activity) are also diagnostic of the Scheie syndrome. Differentiation of the two variants of MPS I can presently be made only on the basis of the clinical picture and course.

Genetics   MPS I S is inherited as an autosomal recessive disorder. The affected persons are thought to be homozygous for a mutation at the structural locus for α-L-iduronidase different from the mutation underlying the Hurler syndrome. Thus, the Hurler and Scheie syndromes appear to be allelic disorders. The failure of genetic complementation in heterokaryons prepared by fusion of Hurler and Scheie fibroblasts [40] supports allelism.

Offspring of affected individuals of either sex have been normal. The frequency of the Scheie syndrome in British Columbia was estimated to be about 1 in 500,000 births [28].

Management Because of the normal intelligence and satisfactory life span of patients with the Scheie syndrome, surgical and other measures for corrections of carpal tunnel syndrome, glaucoma, and aortic valve disease are worthwhile and have been performed with at least partial success in relieving disability.

Mucopolysaccharidosis I H/S (MPS I H/S; MPS I, Intermediate Type; Hurler-Scheie Syndrome; Hurler-Scheie "Compound"; α-L-Iduronidase Deficiency, Hurler-Scheie Type)

Clinical Features MPS I H/S (Fig. 36-7) is characterized by clinical features intermediate between those of the Hurler and Scheie syndromes. The patients are less severely affected than the Hurler patients and survive into the late teens or twenties. (The oldest patient known to us is now 29 years old, and pregnancy has been reported [42] in a patient with this mucopolysaccharidosis.) On the other hand, the patients are much

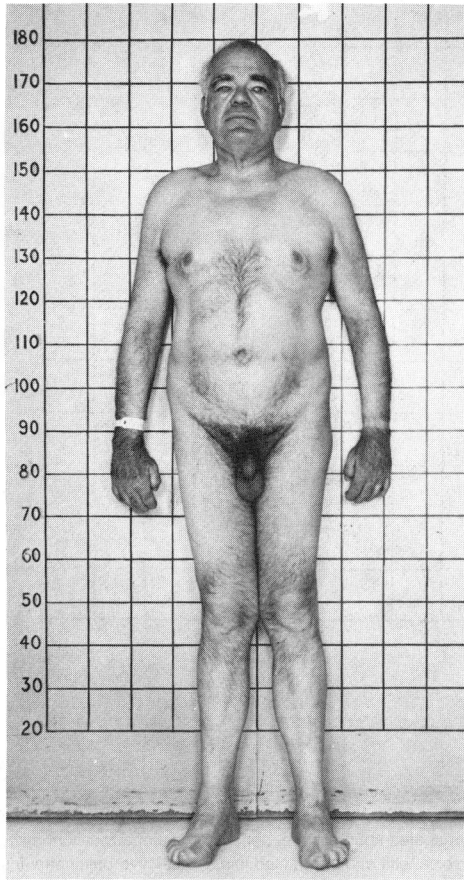

Figure 36-6 MPS I S (Scheie syndrome) in a 54-year-old practicing attorney. Stiff joints, particularly claw hands, and visual impairment due to corneal clouding, pigmentary retinal change, and glaucoma have been the incapacitating features. He also has or has had carpal tunnel syndrome, genu valgum, hypertrichosis, misshapen feet, inguinal hernia, deafness, "broadmouth" facies, and aortic regurgitation. Deformed feet and stiff fingers were noted at age 7 years; corneal clouding was first documented at age 13. The normal stature is noteworthy.

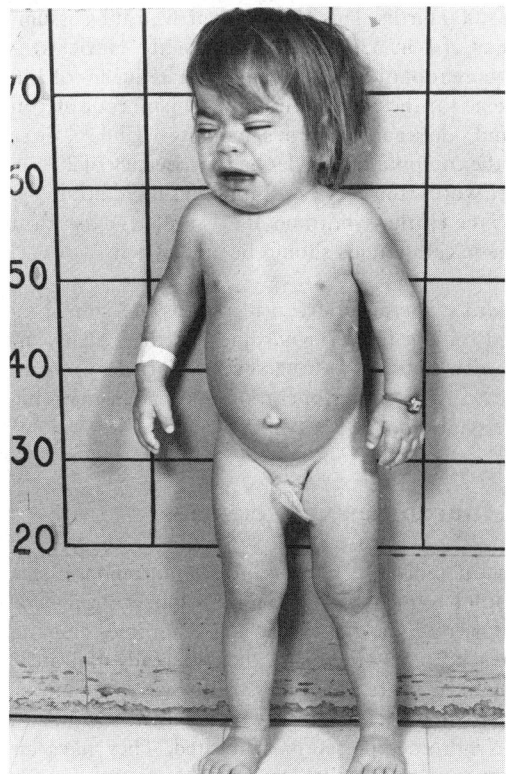

Figure 36-5 MPS I H (Hurler syndrome) in a 30-month-old female. The diagnosis was made when the child was 9 months old by an ophthalmologist, who was consulted for photophobia. At the time of the picture the patient showed irritability; cloudy corneas; coarse facies; prominent abdomen with hepatosplenomegaly and umbilical hernia; restricted motion in the shoulders, elbows, and fingers; mild hirsutism; upper lumbar kyphos; and mental retardation. The patient died at the age of 7 years.

more severely affected than those with the Scheie syndrome: They are short and mentally retarded and have severe dysostosis multiplex.

Clouding of the cornea occurs, as in other forms of α-L-iduronidase deficiency (with the rare exception noted later), and the patients become deaf. Hernia, stiff joints (including striking claw hand), and valvular heart disease also occur.

One feature of the Hurler-Scheie syndrome appears to be distinctive: the patients have consistently shown a receding chin (micrognathism), creating a characteristic facies (evident in published photographs, e.g., [43]).

The oldest patient with this disorder known to us, aged 29 years in 1981, has marked destruction in the region of the sella turcica and cribriform plate, presumably caused by an arachnoid cyst. She has had intermittent spinal fluid rhinorrhea for about 15 years and is blind from effects of arachnoid cysts on the optic nerves. These severe manifestations of arachnoid cysts may be unique to MPS I H/S. Such cysts occur in persons with the Hurler syndrome but never reach the proportions of those seen in the Hurler-Scheie intermediate, perhaps because of the shorter survival in the Hurler syndrome. One reported patient presented with acute paranoia [44]. She had significant basilar impression, an arachnoid cyst of the sella turcica, and partial spinal fluid block at the level of C2 and C5. Thus "pa-

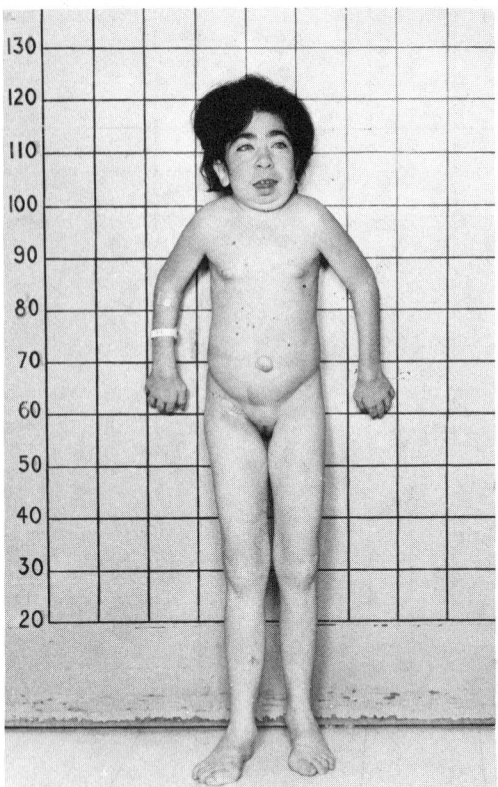

Figure 36-7 MPS I H/S (Hurler-Scheie compound) in a 17-year-old-girl, who demonstrated short stature, dense corneal opacification, micrognathia, a hoarse voice, stiff and contracted joints, restrictive pulmonary insufficiency, and hepatosplenomegaly. Moderate mitral stenosis and trivial mitral regurgitation and aortic regurgitation were suspected by auscultation and established by cardiac characterization. This patient also had glaucoma, treated with acetazolamide (Diamox). A similarly affected sister died at the age of 22 years [42]. Autopsy showed severe calcific mitral stenosis and somewhat less marked calcific diseases of the aortic valve.

chymeningitis cervicalis" occurs in the Hurler-Scheie syndrome, as in some other mucopolysaccharidoses.

Morbid Anatomy   Gross and microscopic evidence of mucopolysaccharide storage is found at autopsy in connective tissues throughout the body, as well as in parenchymal cells of liver and brain [44]. The dura is thickened and contains infiltrates of foamy macrophages and increased amounts of collagen. The anterior horn motor neurons of the spinal cord show massive accumulation of cytoplasmic granules with concentric and lamellar arrays of the ultrastructural level. These changes are less frequent in the neurons of the cerebral cortex, cerebellum, brain stem, and spinal cord. The mitral valve and chordae tendineae are thickened; fibroblasts contain cytoplasmic vacuoles, and collagen and PAS-positive ground substance are increased.

Basic Defect   As in patients with the Hurler and Scheie syndromes, deficiency of α-L-iduronidase is found in cultured fibroblasts, leukocytes, and tissues.

Diagnosis   A form of MPS I is diagnosed by the same methods described for the Hurler and Scheie syndromes. Specific identification of the Hurler-Scheie syndrome can be made only on the basis of clinical criteria. The characteristic receding chin, in combination with the severe manifestations described earlier, support the presumptive diagnosis.

Genetics   When the Hurler and Scheie syndromes were found to have deficiency of the same enzyme, raising the likelihood that they represent homozygosity for two different alleles at the structural locus for α-L-iduronidase, the existence of genetic compounds was predicted [45]. The situation was recognized as possibly analogous to the hemoglobinopathies SS, CC, and SC. The Hurler syndrome was compared to SS disease (sickle-cell anemia), a severe disorder; the Scheie syndrome was compared to CC disease, a mild disorder resulting from mutation at the same locus, indeed, in the same codon and nucleotide site as in SS disease. By analogy to hemoglobin SC disease (the genetic compound condition), a phenotype intermediate in severity and perhaps in some ways unique was anticipated and sought among the mucopolysaccharidoses. A number of patients were found who fulfilled the predictions for the genetic compound. These patients were, therefore, labeled as the "Hurler-Scheie compound" with the clinical characteristics described above. They were presumed to have derived a gene for the Hurler syndrome from one parent and a gene for the Scheie syndrome from the other parent. Parental consanguinity is not expected in this situation, and none was found in the first group of cases. Now, however, instances of consanguine parents of offspring with the Hurler-Scheie phenotype have been described [46, 47]. Thus, one is forced to conclude that the Hurler-Scheie phenotype is produced in some and perhaps all instances by homozygosity for yet another allele at the α-L-iduronidase structural locus. There is no evidence of heteromeric structure of the α-L-iduronidase protein, and failure of complementation in cell fusion studies [41] supports the hypothesis of allelism of cases in this category. Genetic compounds must exist but have not been yet identified with certainty (and perhaps cannot be until the defect at the DNA level is known for the several forms of α-L-iduronidase deficiency).

The frequency of occurrence of persons with one Hurler gene and one Scheie gene, whatever the phenotype, should be about 1 in 115,000 births. This estimate is arrived at by assuming a frequency of 1 in 330 for the gene for the Hurler syndrome (the square root of 1 in 100,000) and a frequency of 1 in 700 for the gene for the Scheie syndrome (square root of 1 in 500,000), and disregarding consanguinity. Under these assumptions the compound disorder has a frequency of $2 \times \frac{1}{330} \times \frac{1}{700}$. In other words, the genetic compound should be almost as frequent as the Hurler syndrome. If other alleles exist, then yet other genetic compounds should be anticipated.

Management   Therapeutic considerations are similar to those outlined for the Hurler syndrome and the Scheie syndrome. A lamellar corneal graft has been reported to remain clear for at least 4 years after operation in a patient with the Hurler-Scheie syndrome [48].

Other α-L-Iduronidase Deficiencies?

There are undoubtedly other forms of α-L-iduronidase deficiency. In addition to the three apparently homozygous phenotypes—the Hurler syndrome, the Scheie syndrome, and the Hurler-Scheie syndrome—there must be, as already indicated, genetic compounds. There are some patients with α-L-iduronidase deficiency who have a phenotype not consistent with any of the three syndromes presently delineated. They have an intermediate phenotype but differ from the Hurler-Scheie syndrome by the lack of the receding chin and otherwise characteristic facies which we have come to consider an invariable feature of that disorder.

It is likely that the patient with α-L-iduronidase deficiency but absent clouding of the cornea reported by Gardner and Hay [4] had a different defect in that enzyme than occurs in any of the three standard forms of MPS I. The patient was a 14-year-old retarded boy with severe joint contractures, dysostosis multiplex, and total absence of the enzyme in cultured fibroblasts. He apparently did not show the facies typical of the Hurler-Scheie syndrome.

MUCOPOLYSACCHARIDOSIS II (MPS II; HUNTER SYNDROME; IDURONATE SULFATASE DEFICIENCY)

The Hunter syndrome is clinically distinguished from the Hurler syndrome by the lack of corneal clouding and by longer survival. It is distinctive among the mucopolysaccharidoses in being inherited as an X-linked recessive (albeit a very rare autosomal recessive form may exist). Biochemically the pattern of mucopolysaccharide excretion in the urine is somewhat different from that in Hurler's syndrome, and a different lysosomal acid hydrolase is deficient. The occurrence of a wide range of severity, with severity tending to "breed true" within families (however, see [49]) suggests that two and probably more separate forms of MPS II exist; these may be allelic.

Clinical Features

As in MPS I H, leading features of the Hunter syndrome (Figs. 36-8, 36-9) are stiff joints, dwarfing, and coarse facial features. Mental deterioration usually occurs at a slower rate. Lumbar gibbus is a less striking feature but occasionally is severe [50]. Progressive deafness is demonstrated by essentially all patients. For practical purposes, corneal clouding does not occur in the Hunter syndrome, although in older patients slight clouding may be evident on slit-lamp examination. (All statements about the disease in comparison to the Hurler syndrome must recognize the wide range of severity and the existence of some unusually severely affected patients who show early and profound mental deterioration and even clouding of the cornea [51]. Such cases are the exception.) A feature distinctive for this mucopolysaccharidosis, and noted by Hunter in his original report in 1917, is the occurrence of pebbly ivory-colored skin lesions of the back usually overlying the inferior angle of the scapulae [52] and less often in the pectoral regions, nape of neck, and lateral aspects of the upper arms and thighs.

Adults with the Hunter syndrome tend to have "high coloration," rosy cheeks, or a plethoric appearance. The voice is hoarse. Airway obstruction, relieved by tracheostomy, has been reported. Heart disease, resulting from a combination of valvular, myocardial, and ischemic factors, is the usual cause of death. Diarrhea (due perhaps to involvement of the autonomic nervous control of the intestine) is a troublesome problem in some patients [53]. Degenerative arthritis in the hips is a problem in older patients. Pachymeningitis cervicalis can result

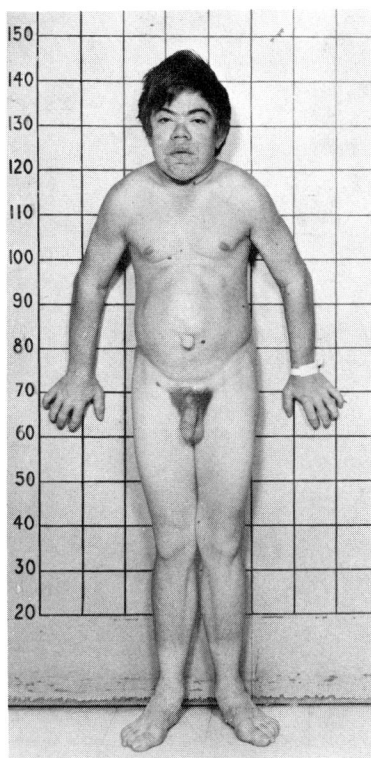

Figure 36-8 A relatively mild form of MPS II (Hunter syndrome) in a 17-year-old. This patient is a member of a kindred reported several times [192]. (The pedigree is presented in Fig. 11-15 of McKusick's *Heritable Disorders of Connective Tissue* fourth edition [4]. Affected males had died at ages 58, 60, and 61; one living at age 61 at the time the pedigree was constructed has since died at age 63. The patient showed short stature, claw hands and restricted motion in other joints, median nerve entrapment (carpal tunnel syndrome), coarse facies, hepatosplenomegaly, and umbilical hernia. Failing vision was accompanied by papilledema and elevated spinal fluid protein level. Section of the sclerooptic sheath produced little benefit. He was rated as "an A student."

in spastic quadraplegia or in less pronounced neurologic deficit from impingement on the cervical spinal cord [54].

The patients demonstrate an atypical retinitis pigmentosa which probably occurs in others of the mucopolysaccharidoses but is not easily studied in them because of clouding of the cornea. Chronic papilledema is also a frequent finding [55]. Although, as in the Hurler syndrome, hydrocephalus occurs due to pachymeningitis [56], the papilledema is probably most often due mainly to involvement of the optic nerve sheath. Progressive loss of vision occurs on the basis of either papilledema or retinitis pigmentosa or both.

In the jaws radiographs may show large radiolucent areas surrounding the crowns of unerupted permanent teeth [57]. These are typical dentigerous cysts and do not contain mucopolysaccharides. Smaller radiolucent lesions of the jaw are collagenous connective tissues lesions [57].

The longest known survival in MPS II is to age 87 years [58]; a few affected males have survived to their sixties (e.g., Fig. 36-8 and [2]). There are, on the other hand, severely affected patients with MPS II who die before age 15 years (Fig. 36-9). Death in these patients is preceded by progressive neurologic deterioration. Clinically these patients may be difficult to distinguish from those with the Sanfilippo syndrome (MPS III).

Mild instances of the Hunter syndrome are illustrated by the family [59] in which one member was a successful marine architect surviving to age 57 years, and by a remarkable family [60] in which three brothers suffered mainly from multiple

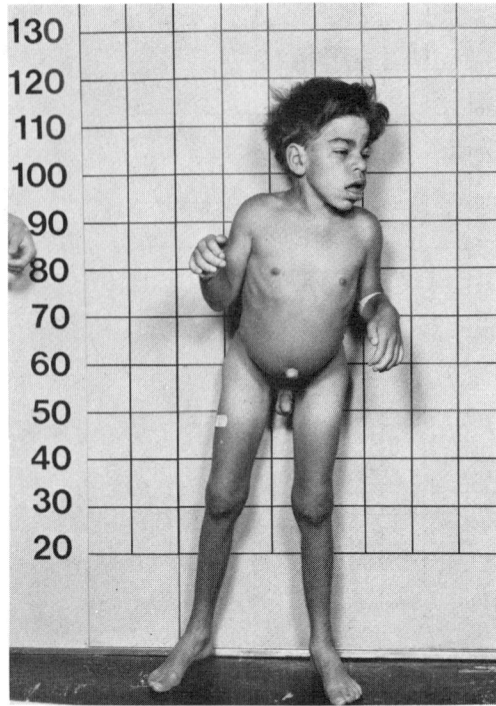

Figure 36-9 MPS II (Hunter syndrome), severe, in a 13½-year-old. He was considered normal until about age 5 (he could write his name), when he was noted to be clumsy and to have exaggerated lumbar lordosis and joint stiffness. His IQ at age 6 was 62. He deteriorated steadily thereafter, lost intelligible speech, forgot his toilet training, and displayed marked hyperactivity. Subcutaneous nodules over the scapulas and diarrhea showed diminution with plasma infusions at age 10 years. At the time of this picture he had hepatosplenomegaly, umbilical hernia, joint stiffness, marked lordosis, and atrophy of the leg muscles with toe walking. EMI scan showed marked hydrocephalus.

peripheral nerve entrapments, particularly of the median nerves at the carpal tunnel and the ulnar nerves at the cubital tunnel. One of the brothers, "about 5 feet in height," was "a 31-year-old army sergeant (who) had never sought medical advice and had passed his yearly checkups without problems."

Appreciable intrafamilial variability in severity has been reported [49], with brothers, for example, differing rather strikingly, although in our extensive experience we have not been impressed with intrafamilial variability. Presumably, differences in the genetic background or in environmental factors or in both account for variability within families. Although it is inescapable that more than one form of the Hunter syndrome exists and although the presumption is strong that these forms are allelic, a sharp differentiation into only two forms is presently not justified, and even within the same sibship variability may make prognostication difficult.

Pathology [61, 62]

In two patients with cutaneous papules over the scapula, Freeman [63] reported that, whereas fibrocytes from all areas of the skin contained metachromatic cytoplasmic material and vacuoles, only the papules contained extracellular accumulation of metachromatic material and evidence of coalescence and rupture of vacuoles. Elsner [53] found membranous cytoplasmic bodies in the ganglion and satellite cells of rectal intramural plexi and proposed this involvement as an explanation for the diarrhea.

Basic Defect

The deficiency in the Hunter syndrome involves iduronate sulfatase [64–66]. This enzyme is needed in the sequential degradation of heparan sulfate and dermatan sulfate (reaction 1 in Figs. 36-2 and 36-3). Sulfated iduronic acid residues are numerous in heparan sulfate and occasional in dermatan sulfate [3], but a single sulfated iduronic acid will, in the absence of the sulfatase, block the degradation of that portion of the chain which is to its reducing side. The consistent clinical differences between MPS I and MPS II (viz., presence or absence of corneal clouding in the two groups of diseases, respectively) can probably be explained by tissue-specific differences in the structure of the mucopolysaccharides. The dermatan sulfate of corneal stroma is unusual in that it occurs in a mixed chondroitin–dermatan sulfate proteoglycan [67]. Its degradation may be less dependent on iduronate sulfatase, either because of undersulfation or because of an easier bypass of the block by hyaluronidase.

Iduronate sulfatase has been purified extensively from human plasma, although not to homogeneity. It appears to have one polypeptide chain of molecular weight around 80,000 [68]. The substance previously isolated from urine as "Hunter corrective factor" [18] is iduronate sulfatase with the correct structure for receptor-mediated endocytosis (see Chapter 37). The plasma enzyme is not corrective [68].

The clinically mild and severe forms of the Hunter syndrome are deficient in iduronate sulfatase to the same degree—nearly total deficiency [69]. There is always a very slight degradation of the substrate (≤ 0.5 percent of normal values) but it is not known whether this is due to true residual activity of iduronate sulfatase or to the action of other sulfatases.

Diagnosis

Marked mucopolysacchariduria is detectable by screening tests. Most patients with the Hunter syndrome excrete approximately equal amounts of dermatan sulfate and heparan sulfate, but a higher ratio (even 100 percent) of heparan sulfate is not unusual. For a number of years the only specific test was accumulation of [^{35}S]mucopolysaccharide in cultured fibroblasts, correctible by mixing with cells other than Hunter cells, or by addition of purified Hunter corrective factor [18]. These are indirect demonstrations of deficiency of the enzyme iduronate sulfatase, which now can be assayed directly in serum, cells, and tissues [19].

As in all X-linked disorders, the female relatives of the affected individual have a high probability of being heterozygotes. A reliable test that would distinguish between the heterozygous state and the homozygous normal state would be of immense service to these women. Assays based on measurement of iduronate sulfatase in lymphocytes show a statistical difference between normals and heterozygotes, but the variability and overlap generally make it impossible to classify any particular individual [69]. Tests based on the mosaicism of heterozygotes are more reliable, but they are labor-intensive and therefore prohibitively costly. This applies both to the analysis of cloned cultures of skin fibroblasts for [^{35}S]mucopolysaccharide accumulation [70] and to the determination of iduronate sulfatase activity in individual hair roots. (Although hair roots are not truly clonal, as they are derived from several cells, a mosaic pattern of iduronate sulfatase is clearly discernible in Hunter heterozygotes [71, 72].) But since all available techniques would show a normal phenotype for heterozygotes if there had been selection of the normal cell population in vivo, a normal genotpye cannot be inferred with certainty. Indeed, the current data base is too small to assign a probability to such in vivo selection.

The prenatal diagnosis of the Hunter syndrome is now a routine procedure. It can be performed by analysis of iduronate sulfatase activity in amniotic fluid [73]. The Hunter syndrome is, in our experience, the only mucopolysaccharidosis for which analysis of the fluid is a reliable diagnostic approach. The benefit to the patient of obtaining a preliminary result within a few days of amniocentesis is obvious, but the results should be examined carefully because of the considerable maternal contribution to the iduronate sulfatase activity in amniotic fluid (Neufeld and Hall, unpublished results) and should be confirmed by analysis of cultured cells. A unique problem may arise in the case of female fetuses. The iduronate sulfatase activity in the fluid surrounding a heterozygous fetus may be almost as low as for an affected Hunter fetus, and the clonal growth of amniotic fluid cells may give rise to cultures with the Hunter phenotype. Thus, in the case of abnormal biochemical results for a 46,XX fetus, the probability of the rare Hunter syndrome in females (see below) must be weighed against the probability of in vitro selection for the abnormal cells of an X-linked heterozygote [74].

Genetics

The Hunter syndrome is inherited as an X-linked recessive. As indicated earlier, several mutations at the same X–linked structural locus probably account for differences of severity seen in different families. On the other hand, the variability occasionally seen within families must find its explanation in differences in the genetic background or environmental experience of the individuals or both.

Known to us are two affected males who had children [59, 75]. One [59] had a son who was normal and a daughter (who proved herself a carrier by having two affected sons). A second affected male [75] had two daughters who have not yet reached reproductive age. On the basis of Haldane's rule, one would predict that, since reproductive fitness of the Hunter gene is almost zero, about one-third of Hunter patients would be the result of a new mutation, if the mutation rate is the same in males and females. Studies for heterozygosity in mothers of affected males suggest, however, that the proportion of cases that represent new mutation may in fact be appreciably less than one-third. The same phenomenon has been observed in some other X-linked recessives that are genetic lethals, e.g., the Lesch-Nyhan syndrome [76]. The discrepancy between theory and nature may result from a greater rate of mutation in male gametogenesis than in female gametogenesis.

One would also predict that if the mutation rate for MPS II is equal to that for MPS I, the birth rate of persons with MPS II should be 1.5 times that of persons with MPS I, all the forms taken together [77]. In fact, available statistics [77] suggest that the reverse is true, indicating a lower mutation rate for MPS II. Schaap and Bach [78] estimated that the Hunter syndrome has a frequency of 1 in 67,500 births in Israel, as contrasted with 1 in 150,000 in British Columbia [28]. It has been postulated that the precise timing of intercourse in relation to ovulation affects sex ratio. "If the Hunter gene in carriers somehow affects the menstrual cycle so that a carrier observing the Jewish purity laws has a higher probability of conceiving a daughter, then an excess of heterozygous daughters would be born at the expense of hemizygous sons" [78]. The postulated heterozygous effect would apply anywhere that the Jewish law was followed; the apparent high frequency of the Hunter syndrome was found in all Jewish groups.

In agreement with the Lyon hypothesis, the Hunter heterozygote has two populations of cells, those with the maternal (MPS II–bearing) X-chromosome active and those with the paternal (normal) X-chromosome active. Clones derived from heterozygotes display either the normal or the Hunter phenotype, demonstrable by several biochemical techniques. The normal phenotype of heterozygotes is explained by the corrective effect of normal cells, which presumably supply the deficient cells with the enzyme iduronate sulfatase in vivo.

The possibility of an autosomal recessive form of iduronate sulfatase deficiency was raised by Neufeld et al. [79], who described two families, each with a girl clinically affected with the Hunter syndrome and with profound deficiency of iduronate sulfatase. The patients were karyotypically normal and had normal fathers. Cloning of the mothers' fibroblasts did not show the mosaicism expected of the carrier status of the X-linked disease. Homozygosity for a previously unsuspected autosomal recessive gene for iduronate sulfatase was considered the most likely explanation, although heterozygosity for the X-linked gene and subsequent selection for cells with the mutant-bearing X chromosome as the active one could not be completely excluded. (An alternative possibility might be an unusual form of multiple sulfatase deficiency [see Chapter 44], in which iduronate sulfatase was more profoundly affected than other sulfatases.) Studies of iduronate sulfatase at the molecular level and of complementation in somatic cell hybrids might distinguish between these possibilities. The mutation in the two families was presumably different (although perhaps allelic because it took the severe form in one family and the mild form in the other). Strong support for autosomal recessive inheritance came from the fact that the parents were first cousins in one family, and had ancestors from the same ethnic group and same small town in the other family.

A marked increase of iduronate sulfatase activity has been observed upon fusion of cells from Hunter patients and cells from patients with multiple sulfatase deficiency [80, 81]. This was anticipated, since multiple sulfatase deficiency is an autosomal recessive disorder, probably due to altered regulation of sulfatase synthesis or activity [82].

Management

There is no specific treatment. Evaluations of the effectiveness of plasma and lymphocyte infusions have varied widely [29, 83–86]. Since normal plasma contains significant iduronate sulfatase activity, some enzyme replacement may occur with plasma infusions, in contrast to the situation in patients with Hurler syndrome. Plasma exchange has been used to maximize the amount of circulating iduronate sulfatase administered to Hunter patients [87, 88]. Mucopolysaccharide was increased in the urine and the level of enzyme activity in the plasma reached about one-half the normal. Clinical improvement did not occur [87]. Corrective factor has been demonstrated in the urine of a patient with the Hunter syndrome given a skin graft from a histocompatible sib [89]. Fibroblast transplantation has also been used [90]; an increase in enzyme activity and in catabolism of heparan and dermatan sulfates could be demonstrated [90]. The long-term effects (if any) of plasma exchange or fibroblast transplantation are not yet known.

Carpal tunnel decompression can afford dramatic relief of hand symptoms [91]. Decompression of the optic nerve in a case (Fig. 36-8) of chronic papilledema in a teenager had no benefit (personal observation).

MUCOPOLYSACCHARIDOSIS III (MPS III; SANFILIPPO SYNDROME) TYPES A, B, C, AND D

The Sanfilippo syndrome (Fig. 36-10A,B) is clinically and biochemically distinct from the other mucopolysaccharidoses. It is itself heterogeneous; four biochemically distinct forms have been identified. The four forms of the Sanfilippo syndrome are not clinically distinguishable. In general, the four forms are characterized clinically by severe progressive mental deteriora-

Figure 36-10   MPS III (Sanfilippo syndrome) A. Type A in a 16-year-old girl. The parents were not concerned about her until she was about 42 months, when she was not toilet-trained and speech was delayed. At age 5, the IQ was estimated at 55. During the next year she deteriorated in speech and in her ability to use crayons and put puzzles together. At age 6½ years she was a large child with heavy facies, thick lips and hirsutism. She was institutionalized at age 7. She had occasional grand mal seizures. After age 11 she walked only with assistance. At the time of the picture she demonstrated spastic quadriparesis and pigmentary degeneration of the retina, but no hepatosplenomegaly or corneal clouding and little joint stiffness. The patient died at the age of 20 years. B. Type B in a 15-year-old girl. The patient began school at age 6 years and for 2 years apparently performed satisfactorily. In her third year she became inattentive and restless and refused to sit still in class. Progressive hearing loss was first noted at age 7. Limitations in motion of the elbows and fingers were noted first at age 10 or 11. Hepatomegaly, hirsutism, thick patulous lips, and clear corneas were found. At age 28, the patient lived at home, and largely cared for herself. Her brother, with the same disorder, died at age 20 years. Studying autopsy-obtained tissues of the brother, O'Brien [110] demonstrated deficiency of α-N-acetylglucosaminidase.

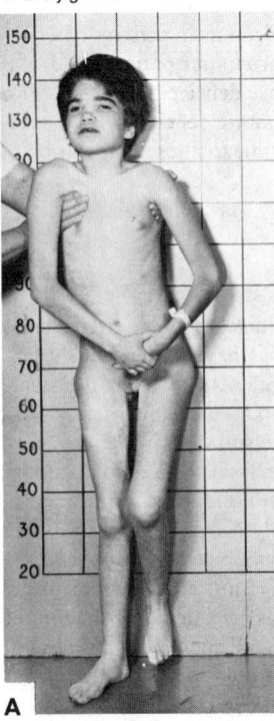
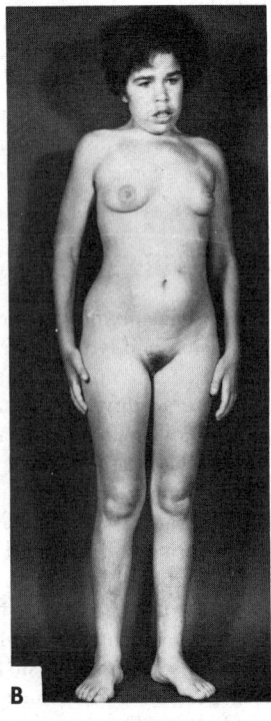

tion and relatively mild somatic manifestations of mucopolysaccharidosis, and biochemically by the excretion of heparan sulfate in the urine. Each has deficiency of a specific enzyme involved in the degradation of heparan sulfate (Fig. 36-2).

Clinical Features

Although variability in severity is observed, the usual clinical picture is one of severe progressive mental retardation having its onset in clearly evident form in the first few years of life and accompanied by relatively mild somatic features of mucopolysaccharidosis. Hyperactivity and sleep disorder usually start after 2 or 3 years of seemingly normal development. The patient may start regular school, but thereafter becomes a "behavior problem" and loses the capacity to speak. Severe behavioral disturbances combined with great unimpaired physical strength and increasing mental retardation often necessitate institutionalization. Most patients in a Dutch study [92] were admitted to an institution before age 11 years. Death occurs in most cases before age 20, although one patient with type B Sanfilippo syndrome is still living at age 33 (Fig. 36-10B). Generalized hirsutism is fairly marked. The facies is coarse and synophrys is usual. Especially in adults, the facies may not impress one as unusual [92]. Clouding of the cornea does not occur in the Sanfilippo syndrome. Hepatosplenomegaly is usually only slight, and stiffness of the joints is less severe than in the Hurler or Hunter syndrome. Dwarfing is also only moderate in degree, and radiologically the skeleton shows only a mild degree of dysostosis multiplex. The calvaria tend to be unusually dense, and the thoracolumbar vertebral bodies show an ovoid dysplasia, i.e., a biconvex configuration. Involvement of the heart is also usually more mild than in other mucopolysaccharidoses, but severe involvement of the mitral valve, requiring valve replacement at age 3 years, has been reported in a case of Sanfilippo syndrome B [93].

As the clinical and radiographic findings may be minimal and the usual screening tests for mucopolysacchariduria may be negative (see later), this disorder may be the most frequently undiagnosed of the mucopolysaccharidoses. In the individual patient the four forms of Sanfilippo syndrome cannot be clinically distinguished [94], although as a group type A tends to be most severe. Thus, in an extensive study of 73 patients from 41 sibships in the Netherlands, van de Kamp [92] found that two-thirds of MPS III A patients, but only a quarter of the B and C types, had severe manifestations before age 4 years. Types B and C patients survived longer; the oldest patient, type B, was 43 years old. A patient with type B, now aged 33 years, is shown in Fig. 36-10B. A particularly severe form of MPS III A is found in the Cayman Islands [95].

Within each of the four enzymatically distinct forms, both interfamilial and intrafamilial variability might be expected. Andria et al. [96] described mild and severe forms of MPS III B in the same sibship. Van de Kamp [97] found intrafamilial variability mainly in MPS III B.

Morbid Anatomy

Histopathologic studies of the MPS III show no differences among types A, B, and C [98–102]. In the viscera, light microscopy shows severe vacuolation in liver cells, Kupffer cells, cells lining the biliary ducts and splenic sinusoids, renal tubule cells, lymph nodes, and chondrocytes. Foam cells infiltrate thickened heart valves, arterial walls, and intima. Indeed, almost no cells or tissues are spared. The severe storage phenomenon is also seen in both the central and the peripheral nervous system. Electron microscopy shows zebra bodies and membranogranulovacuolar inclusions in both the viscera and the nervous system.

Very little histologic change was detectable in a 24-week-old fetus with MPS III A [103].

Basic Defect [104]

Four enzymatic steps are necessary for removal of N-sulfated or N-acetylated α-linked glucosamine residues from heparan sulfate chains (Fig. 36-2). Since these residues are unique to heparan sulfate (and to the closely related polymer, heparin [3]), individuals deficient in any one of the four enzymes could be expected to accumulate and excrete heparan sulfate only.

The disease arbitrarily designated as the A subtype of Sanfilippo syndrome is associated with a deficiency of the enzyme heparan N-sulfatase, also called heparan sulfamidase or sulfamatase [105-107]. This enzyme, which catalyzes the removal of sulfate from the terminal N-sulfated glucosamine (reaction 3 in Fig. 36-2), had originally been purified as the Sanfilippo A corrective factor [105] and has since been purified from placenta.

Removal of the N-sulfate exposes terminal glucosamine residues with a free amino group. It had been thought that glucosamines would be removed by an α-glucosaminidase, but a long search for such an enzyme proved unsuccessful. Instead of being cleaved directly, the glucosamine residues are acetylated by transfer of acetyl from acetyl CoA to the amino group, catalyzed by a specific N-acetyltransferase (reaction 4, Fig. 36-2). This enzymatic activity is deficient in patients with the C subtype of Sanfilippo syndrome [108, 109]. The reaction is so far unique in lysosomal pathways in that it is not hydrolytic, and in that it requires a cofactor, acetyl CoA. We must presume that there exists a mechanism for the transport of the cofactor into lysosomes, and that a defect in such transport would result in another biochemical form of Sanfilippo syndrome.

The acetylated glucosamines (or N-acetylglucosamine residues initially present in heparan sulfate) are cleaved by α-N-acetylglucosaminidase [110, 111] (reaction 5 in Fig. 36-2). This enzyme was originally identified as Sanfilippo B corrective factor [111] and has been purified to apparent homogeneity [112]. It was the first enzyme for which the saturation kinetics of uptake were demonstrated [113]. Cross-reactive material has been found in Sanfilippo B patients [114].

The fourth known subtype of Sanfilippo syndrome (type D) is a deficiency of the sulfatase for α-N-acetylglucosamine-6-sulfate residues [115] (reaction 7, Fig. 36-2). This enzyme has recently been purified [116] and shown to be distinct from the sulfatase for the β-linked N-acetylglucosamine-6-sulfate residues in keratan sulfate (Fig. 36-4, reaction 12).

Endoglycosidases present in many tissues cleave heparan sulfate at both glucuronide and hexosaminide linkages [3]. These are no doubt responsible for very small fragments of heparan sulfate that are excreted in urine.

In heparan sulfate, some glucosamine residues are both N-sulfated and O-sulfated. It has been proposed that there exists an O-sulfatase specific for such bis-sulfated glucosamine, distinct from the 6-O-sulfatase that requires N-acetylated glucos-

amine [117]. Thus another form of Sanfilippo syndrome caused by deficiency of such a bis-sulfatase is anticipated.

Diagnosis

Urinary excretion of heparan sulfate is strong presumptive evidence for the Sanfilippo syndrome. However, occasional Hunter patients also excrete heparan sulfate exclusively. The mucopolysacchariduria of Sanfilippo patients may be missed by certain procedures, such as the toluidine blue paper test, because it is in the form of small fragments of heparan sulfate, presumably generated by endoglycosidases (see above).

Earlier measures of [^{35}S]mucopolysaccharide accumulation and correction in cultured fibroblasts [18] have been largely superseded by the simpler assays of enzyme activity in fibroblasts and leukocytes, for the Sanfilippo syndromes A and B, or in the case of type B, by assays of α-N-acetylglucosaminidase in serum [19]. Enzyme assays for types C and D may be performed on fibroblasts and leukocytes [118]. They require the preparation of specific oligosaccharide substrates. Accumulation ^{35}S may continue to be useful as a screening test for all four types of MPS III, when one has no clue as to which type is present and perhaps in cases of borderline heparansulfaturia.

Prenatal diagnosis for the A [103] and B subtypes has been performed by analysis of cells cultured from amniotic fluid. Measurement of [^{35}S]mucopolysaccharide accumulation is recommended as a useful adjunct to the enzymatic tests, particularly for distinguishing heterozygotes from affected cells. The activity of enzymes in cells derived from heterozygous fetuses may be very low (Neufeld and Hall, unpublished results).

Serum assays of α-N-acetylglucosaminidase have been recommended for the identification of Sanfilippo B heterozygotes, but the identification of genetic polymorphism of this enzyme, with the presence of alleles for both high and low activity, makes this approach hazardous [119].

Genetics

All four types of the Sanfilippo syndrome are inherited as autosomal recessive disorders. In the Netherlands, van de Kamp [92] estimated that the mean inbreeding coefficient of Sanfilippo sibships was about 15 times those in the general population. Of 40 sibships studied, 19 were demonstrably related and had a common origin in a few small villages near Rotterdam. Most of these were type A.

Van de Kamp [92] estimated the collective frequency of MPS III to be about 1 in 24,000 in the Netherlands. This is a frequency 4 to 8 times greater than earlier estimated (e.g., [1]). Thus, although the Sanfilippo syndrome is perhaps the most undiagnosed of the mucopolysaccharidoses because it easily passes as nonspecific mental retardation, it may be the most frequent mucopolysaccharidosis. The proportions of the different types vary from series to series and the total frequency probably varies in different populations, possibly as a result of founder effect.

In the Netherlands, van de Kamp [92] studied 75 patients with the Sanfilippo syndrome: 32, III A; 20, III B; 14, III C; 9, unspecified. Klein et al. [109], who first described the enzyme defect in Sanfilippo syndrome type C, demonstrated the defect in 11 cases, indicating that this is a relatively frequent form.

Sanfilippo syndrome D has thus far been identified in only 2 patients, a 7-year-old East Indian boy and a 4-year-old Sardinian girl [115]. Curiously, only type A was found among 28 patients in the United Kingdom [120] and among 13 patients in Canada [121].

N-Acetylglucosaminidase is an addition to the rather lengthy list of enzymes [119] that occur both in "normal" polymorphic form and in rare disease-producing form.

Allelic forms of each of the Sanfilippo subtypes may exist and explain interfamilial variability. Wide intrafamilial variability in MPS IIIB [97] makes conclusions concerning allelic forms tentative at best.

Management

As with the other mucopolysaccharidoses, definitive therapy is not available. Management is difficult because of the aggressive hyperactivity and intellectual impairment in children who are strong and healthy until the late onset of physical and neurologic deterioration. Psychotropic drugs help little [99]. Behavior modification with use of positive reinforcement is to some extent effective in management. The availability in the home of a "childproof" room, i.e., room with nothing breakable or damageable, to which a child can be relegated for short periods, is useful. Limits on his or her behavior must be clear to the patient. In later stages, institutionalization is necessary for most patients.

MUCOPOLYSACCHARIDOSIS IV (MPS IV; MORQUIO SYNDROME; KERATANSULFATURIA), TYPES A AND B

MPS IV is unique among the mucopolysaccharidoses in the excretion of keratan sulfate in the urine and in certain of its clinical features. As with the Sanfilippo syndrome the same or nearly the same clinical picture can be produced by deficiency of either of two different enzymes.

The eponymic designation for MPS IV, the Morquio syndrome, is derived from the pediatrician in Montevideo, Uruguay, who in 1929 described a family of Swedish extraction in which the parents were first cousins and four sibs were affected. The earliest cases in the literature were probably those of the French-Canadian brother and sister reported by Osler in 1897 [122]. These were probably related to the numerous cases of the Morquio syndrome identified in recent years among French-Canadians of eastern Quebec Province [123].

During the 30 years after Morquio's description many skeletal dysplasias were mistakenly labeled Morquio syndrome. There was a tendency for any form of skeletal dysplasia with short limbs to be called achondroplasia and any short trunk dwarfism to be called the Morquio syndrome. About 1960 the Morquio syndrome became identified as a mucopolysaccharidosis and was separated definitively from other skeletal dysplasias [2].

Trojak et al. [124] made the following recommendations:

MPS IV A should be used to describe the classic Morquio syndrome when the enzymatic defect has been determined to be in galactos-

amine-6-sulfate sulfatase. MPS IV B should be used to designate the β-galactosidase-deficient mild Morquio-like syndrome. Mildly affected Morquio-like individuals in whom the enzyme defect is unknown but who have normal B-galactosidase activity should be described as having MPS IV mild. If the enzyme defect in these mildly affected individuals is known to be galactosamine-6-sulfate sulfatase, then the designation of MPS IV A mild is appropriate [124].

Clinical Features

The overwhelmingly predominant clinical features of the Morquio syndrome (Fig. 36-11A, B) are those related to the skeleton and its secondary effects on the nervous system, especially the spinal cord. A prominence of the lower ribs may first bring the patient to attention at the age of 12 to 18 months. The facies may be somewhat coarse at that stage. The finding of mucopolysacchariduria and identification of the excess mucopolysaccharide as keratan sulfate permit definitive diagnosis.

With growth during the first years of life, severe knock-knee (genu valgum) develops, as well as short trunk, prominence of the sternum (pectus carinatum), progressive platyspondyly, and short neck, so that the head appears to lie directly on the shoulders. The facies tends to be broad-mouthed, with spacing between the teeth. The dental enamel is abnormally thin. Growth seems virtually to stop after ages 6 to 7 years in severe cases.

As in most other mucopolysaccharidoses, clouding of the cornea occurs in the Morquio syndrome but is of only mild degree and rarely of functional significance. Progressive deafness is an almost invariable feature; by age 10 most patients show either a mixed or sensorineural hearing loss [125].

Many of the joints tend to be excessively loose, especially those of the wrist. Instability at the wrist contributes to disability in the hands. Claw hand with stiff finger joints does not occur in the Morquio syndrome.

An invariable feature of the Morquio syndrome is the absence or severe hypoplasia of the odontoid process of the second cervical vertebra [126]. With this is combined laxity, relative redundancy, and hyperplasia of the ligaments in that area such that atlantoaxial subluxation is a major complication. Acute, subacute, or chronic cervical myelopathy develops sooner or later in most patients with the severe form of the Morquio syndrome. It may be manifested in a small child as acute onset of quadriplegia after a fall. It may also be manifested as inability of the child to use his or her legs upon getting out of bed in the morning, by the child's asking to be picked up and carried, or by complaints of leg pains. Neurologic signs may be exceedingly subtle, and history is often more valuable than the physical examination in arriving at the diagnosis of cervical myelopathy. Unless the physician has a high index of suspicion based on familiarity with the natural history of the Morquio syndrome and this complication, the myelopathy is easily overlooked. The genu valgum may be surgically corrected on the mistaken impression that this is the basis of the complaints.

Intelligence is normal or minimally reduced. Aortic regurgitation develops in some patients. All patients with the Morquio syndrome show progressive dimunution in the amount of keratan sulfate excreted in the urine as they get older, so that by the late teens the absolute amount of mucopolysaccharide in the urine may not be outside the normal range. However, fractionation is likely to show excessive keratan sulfate in patients

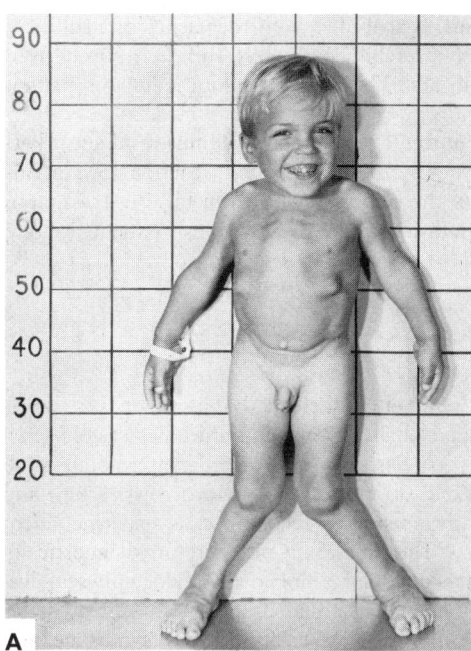

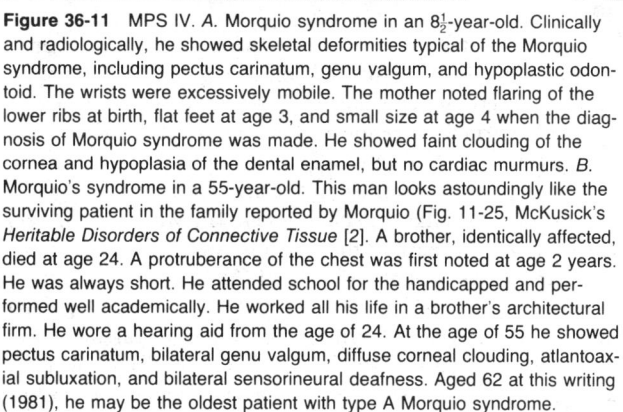

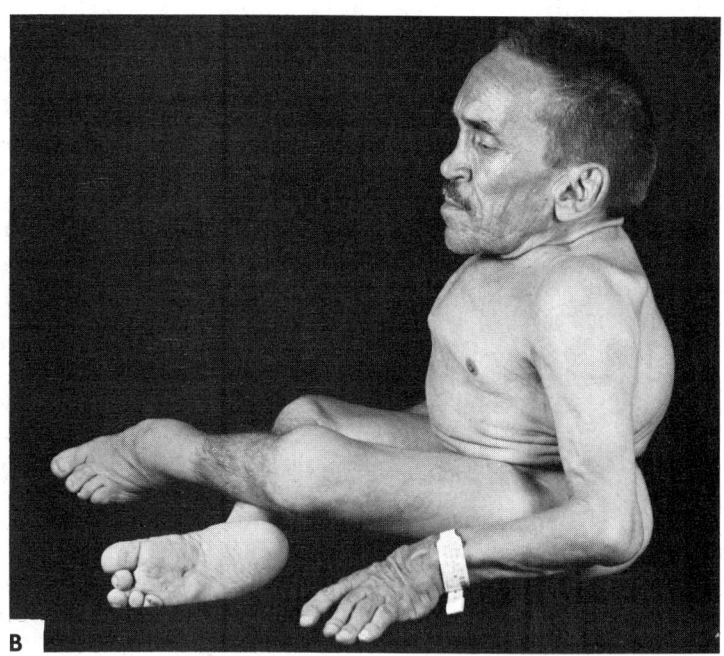

Figure 36-11 MPS IV. *A.* Morquio syndrome in an 8½-year-old. Clinically and radiologically, he showed skeletal deformities typical of the Morquio syndrome, including pectus carinatum, genu valgum, and hypoplastic odontoid. The wrists were excessively mobile. The mother noted flaring of the lower ribs at birth, flat feet at age 3, and small size at age 4 when the diagnosis of Morquio syndrome was made. He showed faint clouding of the cornea and hypoplasia of the dental enamel, but no cardiac murmurs. *B.* Morquio's syndrome in a 55-year-old. This man looks astoundingly like the surviving patient in the family reported by Morquio (Fig. 11-25, McKusick's *Heritable Disorders of Connective Tissue* [2]. A brother, identically affected, died at age 24. A protuberance of the chest was first noted at age 2 years. He was always short. He attended school for the handicapped and performed well academically. He worked all his life in a brother's architectural firm. He wore a hearing aid from the age of 24. At the age of 55 he showed pectus carinatum, bilateral genu valgum, diffuse corneal clouding, atlantoaxial subluxation, and bilateral sensorineural deafness. Aged 62 at this writing (1981), he may be the oldest patient with type A Morquio syndrome.

at all ages. Patients with a mild form of Morquio syndrome tend to excrete less keratan sulfate and to show a decline in keratan sulfate excretion toward the normal range at an earlier age. These patients were referred to earlier as the "non–keratan-sulfate-excreting form" of the Morquio syndrome.

Patients with the severe form of the Morquio syndrome may not survive beyond their twenties or thirties. This was particularly true in the past before the significance of atlantoaxial subluxation was recognized and measures adopted to correct it. Judging from observations in several affected brother-sister pairs, we conclude that males fare less well than females. Both sexes develop paralysis from the myelopathy, as well as serious cardiorespiratory insufficiency due to upper airway obstruction, restriction of the thoracic cage, paralysis of muscles of respiration, and valvular heart involvement. In the family which Morquio first described, three of the affected sibs died in their twenties of "pulmonary complications." The fourth was still living in 1971 at the age of 54 years. We are caring for a 62-year-old patient with the severe Morquio syndrome who looks strikingly like Morquio's surviving patient (Fig. 36-11*B*).

The above clinical description applies particularly to the classic Morquio syndrome (caused by N-acetylgalactosamine–6-sulfatase deficiency) which we would now designate MPS IV A, reserving the designation IV B for a generally milder form

which is due to β-galactosidase deficiency. Patients of the latter type have been reported by several groups of workers [124, 127, 128]. The dental enamel is normal in MPS IV B and is one way to distinguish mild MPS IV A from MPS IV B clinically. In addition to C1-C2 subluxation, C2-C3 subluxation has been observed in MPS IV B [114].

Pathology

The histology of brain [129], cartilage, and bone has been studied by light and electron microscopy. The cells of the basal and malpighian layers of the epidermis contain large single–membrane-bound vacuoles, whereas other cells of the skin are normal. (There may be a relation between thin dental enamel and involvement of the epidermis.) Chondrocytes are packed with similar vacuoles. The brain (which shows the enzyme deficiency present in other tissues such as liver) has only minimal changes of storage, consistent with the degree of mental and neurologic deficit [129]. Accumulation of keratan sulfate in the liver is demonstrable chemically [130]. Autopsy studies reveal marked thickening of the anterior longitudinal ligament in the first and second cervical area, a circumstance that undoubtedly aggravates the compression myelopathy in these patients. Factor et al. [131] found conspicuous intimal sclerosis of the coronary arteries at autopsy in a 15-year-old boy. Intimal smooth-muscle cells contained numerous storage vacuoles, and deposition of collagen and elastin was marked. A parallel to the role of lysosomal accumulation of cholesterol in the pathogenesis of conventional arteriosclerosis was drawn.

Basic Defect

The Morquio syndrome is due to defective degradation of keratan sulfate (Fig. 36-4). Since this mucopolysaccharide is found mainly in cartilage, nucleus pulposus, and cornea, it is not surprising to find these tissues specifically affected. The histologic studies cited earlier suggest that the abnormality in the Morquio syndrome may to some extent be cell-type specific. Cultured fibroblasts show essentially normal metabolism of the mucopolysaccharides, as indicated by studies with radiosulfate.

The deficient enzyme in the classic Morquio syndrome (MPS IV A) was found to be a sulfatase that hydrolyzes N-acetylgalactosamine-6-sulfate residues [132–134]. Such residues are present in chondroitin-6-sulfate (which is also excreted in Morquio syndrome) but not in keratan sulfate. This has led to the suggestion that because of the structural similarity between N-acetylgalactosamine and galactose, the enzyme also catalyzes the desulfation of galactose-6-sulfate residues in keratan sulfate (Fig. 36-4, reaction 10). The evidence for this suggestion is indirect [134]. A previous report [135] that the enzyme hydrolyzed galactitol-6-sulfate, the reduced form of galactose-6-sulfate, has been disputed [136]. Oligosaccharides derived from keratan sulfate appear not to have been tried as substrates. We therefore suggest that the defect in Morquio A syndrome be provisionally designated as N-acetylgalactosamine-6-sulfatase deficiency. It has been demonstrated in liver and brain [129], as well as in cultured fibroblasts.

The sulfatase has been extensively purified from human placenta [136]. Five patients with the A subtype of Morquio syndrome were shown to have no cross-reactive material [137].

The B subtype of the Morquio syndrome involves a deficiency of β-galactosidase [124, 127, 138, 139], which would cleave terminal galactose residues following their desulfation (reaction 11, Fig. 36-4). This deficiency presumably reflects a mutation of the β-galactosidase locus allelic to that which produces G_{M1} gangliosidosis. (The β-galactosidase gene deficient in the latter disorder has been assigned to chromosome 3 [140].) In MPS IV B, the mutation apparently primarily affects the ability of the enzyme to remove galactose residues from keratan sulfate, whereas in G_{M1} gangliosidosis the altered enzyme also fails to degrade the ganglioside. Cell fusion studies of complementation have not been done.

A mild form of the Morquio syndrome has been designated in the past as the Dale, non-keratansulfate-excreting [2], or long-legged variant. Some of these may have been examples of the β-galactosidase-deficient form; others have been examples of a mild, possibly allelic variant of N-acetylgalactosaminine-6-sulfatase deficiency (J. E. Trojak, personal communication). (Decline in the excessive keratansulfaturia may occur earlier in such cases, leading to the designation "non-keratansulfate–excreting.") Yet others may have a presently unidentified defect. Infants with G_{M1} gangliosiodsis have boney deformities, excrete excessive keratan sulfate in the urine [141], and store a keratan sulfate-like material, all of which may reflect an impairment in the hydrolysis of β-galactosyl residues of keratan sulfate in that disease also. The Kniest syndrome, an autosomal dominant skeletal dysplasia, was accompanied by keratansulfaturia in one family [142], but the biochemical basis is unknown.

The enzyme-cleaving sulfate from N-acetylglucosamine-6–sulfate residues (reaction 12, Fig. 36-4) was previously reported also to be involved in the degradation of heparan sulfate, and to be deficient in a patient who excreted both keratan sulfate and heparan sulfate in the urine [143]. This has since been found to be an error [144]. The hydrolysis of the 6-sulfate group on N-acetyloglucosamine requires a different enzyme for heparan sulfate and keratan sulfate (see sections on Sanfilippo syndrome, D subtype). Another patient with combined heparan and keratansulfaturia has now been reported [145] and his disease attributed to the deficiency of a sulfatase for the β-linked N-acetylglucosamine-6-sulfate groups derived from keratan sulfate. The heparansulfaturia in this patient awaits explanation.

The cleavage of the β-N-acetylglucosamine residues of keratan sulfate has not yet been elucidated (reaction 13, Fig. 36-4). In addition to the structures shown in Fig. 36-4), keratan sulfate may contain some fucose. Fucosidosis patients excrete keratan sulfate [146].

Diagnosis

A considerable number of skeletal dysplasias of the "short-trunk" variety were labeled Morquio syndrome between 1929 when Morquio first described the disorder and about 1960 when the extraskeletal features of the Morquio syndrome and the keratansulfaturia led to its recognition as a specific mucopolysaccharidosis. The simulating and therefore diagnostically confused disorders included X-linked spondyloepiphyseal dysplasia tarda, spondyloepiphyseal dysplasia congenita, metatropic dwarfism, diastrophic dwarfism, Kniest syndrome, and others [2].

Finding keratan sulfate in the urine is strong evidence for the Morquio syndrome, but this mucopolysaccharide may be missed in certain screening tests or in some older patients [141]. Abnormal excretion of keratan sulfate in Kniest syndrome [142, 147] and in G_{M1} gangliosidosis [141] need not occasion diagnostic confusion because the clinical and radiographic picture is likely to be different. (In MPS IV B the urine chromatographic pattern for gangliosides is qualitatively similar to that in G_{M1} gangliosidosis [139].

N-Acetylgalactosamine-6-sulfatase activity may be determined in cultured fibroblasts, leukocytes, or cultured amniotic fluid cells using a substrate derived from chondroitin-6-sulfate [118, 148]. β-galactosidase may be assayed in the same fashion as for G_{M1} gangliosidosis, using the p-nitrophenyl or 4-methylumbelliferyl β-galactosides.

Genetics

Both of the presently defined forms of the Morquio syndrome are inherited as autosomal recessive disorders. We know of a woman with the severe form of the disease (MPS IV A) who delivered two children by cesarean section, both normal.

Management

Orthopedic surgery is the main approach [149]. The genu valgum can be corrected by osteotomy. Surgery on the upper cervical spine can be lifesaving and is probably necessary at some stage in a majority of patients with the severe form of Morquio syndrome (MPS IV A). Simple decompression by spinal laminectomy is not beneficial because the compression is anterior, and indeed the procedure may be harmful. Posterior spinal fusion has been developed as a satisfactory procedure [150]. A special halo brace has been used for immobilization of the head before, during, and after surgery. Since, as pointed out earlier, the patients grow little after age 7 or 8 years, osteotomies of the lower limbs can be performed for genu valgum at about age 7 and reoperation will usually not be required. More than the usual hazards accompany any surgery requiring general anesthesia because of the C1/C2 instability and the impaired thoracic mechanics [151].

Hearing aids are necessary in many patients with MPS IV A (125).

MUCOPOLYSACCHARIDOSIS V (MPS V; THE SCHEIE SYNDROME)—NOW DESIGNATED MPS I S

When the Scheie syndrome was found to have deficiency of the same enzyme as the Hurler syndrome and, therefore, to represent in all probability an allelic variant, the numbering system for mucopolysaccharidoses, originally promulgated in 1965, was revised. To avoid confusion, number V has been left vacant, following the practice in the coagulation field of leaving the designation factor VI unused when it was found that the factor tentatively so designated was not a bona fide entity.

MUCOPOLYSACCHARIDOSIS VI (MPS VI; MAROTEAUX-LAMY SYNDROME; N-ACETYLGALACTOSAMINE-4-SULFATASE DEFICIENCY; ARYLSULFATASE B DEFICIENCY)

In 1963 Maroteaux, Lamy, and their colleagues [152] first recognized the existence of a Hurler-like condition characterized by severe somatic changes, but distinguishable from the Hurler syndrome clinically by a retention of normal intelligence and, in the laboratory, by the finding that the excess mucopolysacchariduria involved predominantly dermatan sulfate. Since description of the classic form of the Maroteaux-Lamy syndrome, milder, presumably allelic, variants have been described in which deficiency of the same lysosomal enzyme N-acetylgalactosamine-4-sulfatase is present.

Clinical Features

In the severe or classic form of MPS VI (Fig. 36-12), growth retardation usually brings the patient first to medical attention at the age of 2 or 3 years. Genu valgum, lumbar kyphosis, and anterior sternal protrusion are gradually progressive thereafter. The face shows the coarseness characteristic of the mucopolysaccharidoses, and articular movement is severely restricted with progressive development of claw hand. The corneas become clouded to a grossly obvious degree. Involvement of the heart valves is signaled by the development of murmurs and heart failure [153]. Hydrocephalus, sometimes requiring shunting, and neurologic complications resulting from hypoplasia of the odontoid process and consequent atlantoaxial subluxation also occur.

The hips, specifically the femoral heads, are involved in a severe manner. In general the skeletal changes in the severe form of MPS VI resemble rather closely those of the Hurler syndrome in both severity and type.

The longest survival of a patient with the severe form of

MPS VI is probably into the late twenties. After discovery of the existence of MPS VI on the basis of severe cases and after identification of the enzyme deficiency as involving N-acetylgalactosamine-4-sulfatase, milder, presumably allelic or genetic-compound varieties of the Maroteaux-Lamy syndrome came to light. For example, a mild case was that of a man (Fig. 36-13) with short stature (154 cm), dense corneal clouding, and minimal joint stiffness. He had had inguinal hernias repaired as well as treatment for bilateral "Legg-Perthes disease." He had signs of the carpal tunnel syndrome and the murmur of aortic stenosis had been known to be present from the age of 8 years. He was able to work regularly as an automobile mechanic and died at the age of 35 years from alchohol-related status epilepticus. Similar cases have been reported [154]. Other patients, who had aortic stenosis as a leading feature, probably had MPS VI [155]. Although the diagnosis was not well established in any of them, short stature, corneal clouding, and striking cytoplasmic inclusions suggest the diagnosis of MPS VI. The adult patient of Glober et al. [155], for example, had aortic stenosis with a mucopolysaccharidosis characterized by short stature, corneal clouding, normal intelligence, and striking cytoplasmic inclusions. Wilson et al. [156] described three brothers with MPS VI and aortic stenosis treated by aortic valve replacement. Their proband was 43 years old and 150 cm tall.

Some patients show a phenotype of intermediate severity (e.g., Fig. 36-14) resembling that of mucolipidosis III (pseudo-Hurler polydystrophy), as discussed in Chapter 37.

In a patient with the mild or intermediate form of MPS VI, myelopathy caused by compression of the cervical region of the spinal cord by thickened dura was observed [157]. The patient showed severe neurologic deterioration during the third trimester of pregnancy. Peterson et al. [158] also described myelopathy in MPS VI.

Three patients have been described—two sibs by Kennedy et al. [35] and a single patient reported by Paulson et al. [36]—as presumed instances of the Scheie syndrome complicated by pachymeningitis cervicalis. A diagnosis was not enzymatically proved in any of these patients, and because of the short stature and striking cytoplasmic inclusions of circulating leukocytes it is likely that they in fact had MPS VI. The carpal tunnel syndrome and other nerve entrapment syndromes occur in this as in several of the other mucopolysaccharidoses. Pachymeningitis cervicalis would be expected to aggravate the problem by interfering with axonal flow at sites near the spinal cord [159].

Pathology

Lysosomal inclusions similar to those found in MPS I and MPS II are seen in Kupffer cells, but the inclusions in hepatocytes are smaller [160]. Abnormal metachromatic inclusions in leukocytes are more striking in MPS VI than in any other mucopolysaccharide storage disorder (with the exception of MPS VII and multiple sulfatase deficiency). Inclusions are seen also in platelets [161] as well as in cells of the cornea, conjunctiva, and skin [162].

Basic Defect

The basic defect is an inability to hydrolyze the sulfate group from N-acetylgalactosamine-4-sulfate residues of dermatan

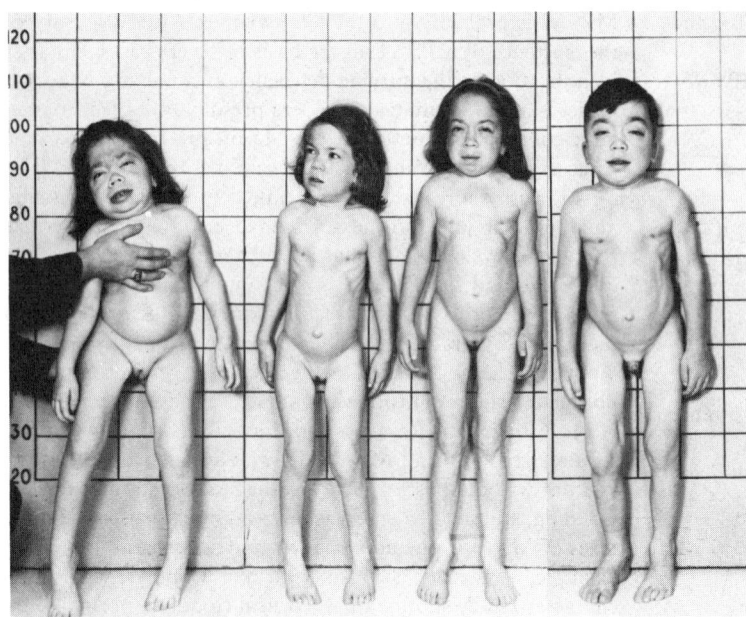

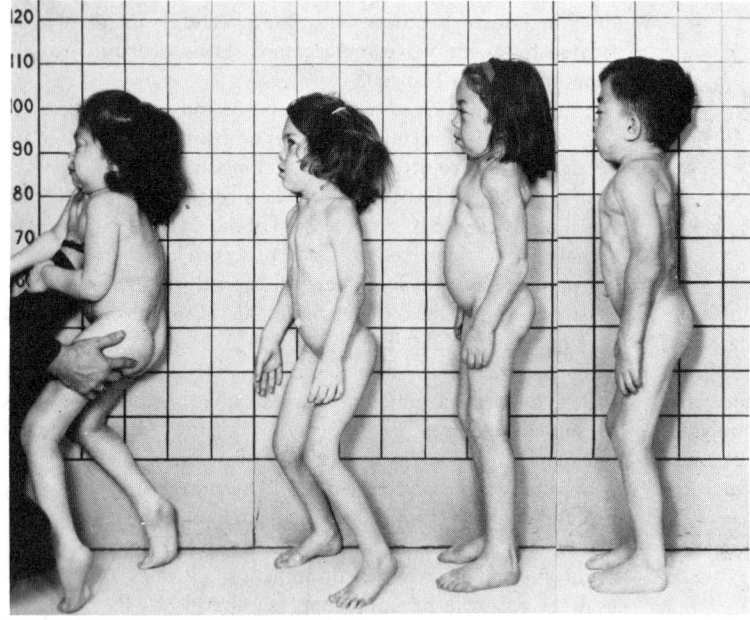

Figure 36-12 MPS VI (Maroteaux-Lamy syndrome), severe or classic form, in all of four sibs, aged (left to right) 14, 9, 13, and 11 years at the time of the picture. In the oldest, noisy breathing was noted at age 2 years, and mouth breathing and tongue protrusion at age 6 years. Flexion contractures at the knees began at about age 4. She was a good student; at the age of 9 she slowly developed generalized weakness to the point that she could not walk or feed herself, but she remained alert. She was incontinent. Myelogram was normal. At age 11 she was hospitalized for her first episode of congestive heart failure. At age 12, investigations, including cardiac catheterization, showed moderate aortic and mitral regurgitation. The patient showed corneal clouding and marked skeletal changes by x-ray, striking cytoplasmic inclusions, and heavy mucopolysacchariduria, almost exclusively dermatan sulfate. She died at the age of $15\frac{1}{2}$ years. The three other affected sibs have had a similar course. The brother died at age 21 years of heart failure. A second sister (second from left) died of pulmonary infection at age 11; she had required ventricular shunt. At this writing (1981) the third sister is living, at age 23 years, but is severely disabled.

sulfate (reaction 8, Fig. 36-3). The discovery of this enzymatic deficiency was preceded by the discovery of deficiency of arylsulfatase B [154, 163–165]). It is now clear that N-acetylgalactosamine-4-sulfatase and arylsulfatase B are the same enzyme, acting on natural and synthetic substrate, respectively [166]. These enzyme activities probably correspond to the Maroteaux-Lamy corrective factor [167].

Since N-acetylgalactosamine-4-sulfate residues are also components of chondroitin-4-sulfate, one might expect chondroitinsulfaturia in Maroteaux-Lamy patients. That it does not occur suggests that chondroitin-4-sulfate may be extensively degraded by hyaluronidase, to which it is readily susceptible. The oligosaccharide fragments that would result from hyaluronidase action would go undetected in measurements of excreted mucopolysaccharide.

Genetics

MPS VI is inherited as an autosomal recessive disorder, i.e., affected individuals are homozygous for a mutation presumably in the structural locus for N-acetylgalactosamine-4-sulfatase, which by somatic cell hybridization has been assigned to chromosome 5. There appear to be at least two alleles at the corresponding locus. Patients with the severe disease are homozygous for one allele and patients with mild disease are homozygous for a different allele. Genetic compounds, presumably in patients with intermediate severity, must exist. As indicated earlier, severe, mild, and intermediate phenotypes have been observed.

There are no data on the frequency of any of the forms of MPS VI. An unusually severe form of MPS VI has been observed in Australian aborigines [168].

Diagnosis

In addition to the clinical picture, urinary excretion of dermatan sulfate exclusively and very striking metachromatic inclusions in circulating leukocytes are strongly suggestive of the diagnosis of MPS VI. Measurement of arylsulfatase B activity is presently the simplest specific test. Prenatal diagnosis has been reported [169].

Clinically, the mild and intermediate forms of MPS VI are most easily confused with the Scheie syndrome and with mucolipidosis III, or pseudo-Hurler polydystrophy (Chapter 37). Short stature is a feature that probably distinguishes even the mildest forms of MPS VI from the Scheie syndrome. As far as we know, patients with MPS VI are always short, whereas patients with MPS I S are of average height. The striking inclusions in circulating leukocytes in MPS VI are another useful differential point. A brother and sister (L.S. and T.S.) reported in a radiologic study [170] of mucolipidosis III were shown to have fibroblasts with arylsulfatase B deficiency, accumulation of radioactive sulfate, and correction typical of MPS VI. This pair is of superior intelligence. The brother is a college graduate about to enter law school. The drastic changes that can occur in the hips in this form of MPS VI were demonstrated [170].

Management

Appropriate surgical procedures on the cornea, hips, and carpal tunnels are worthwhile, especially in the milder forms.

MUCOPOLYSACCHARIDOSIS VII (MPS VII; SLY SYNDROME; β-GLUCURONIDASE DEFICIENCY)

The basic defect, mode of inheritance, and potential therapy of this disorder were worked out at a time when only one case was known—a record probably matched previously only by a oroticaciduria.

Clinical Features

The first patient, discovered by Sly and his colleagues [171], was a black male, aged 7 weeks when first brought to medical attention (Fig. 36-15). He had unusual facies, metatarsus adductus, hepatosplenomegaly, umbilical hernia, diastasis recti, small thoracolumbar gibbus, and puffy hands and feet. Circulating and bone marrow granulocytes showed striking metachromatic granules. He subsequently developed bilateral inguinal hernias, which required repair, and anterior chest deformity. Between ages 2 and 3 years mental and physical development slowed, and his sister, a year younger, appeared to be catching up with him. Mucopolysaccharide levels in the urine were at that time minimally elevated.

Several other patients who appeared to have deficiency of the same enzyme, β-glucuronidase, were later described [172, 173]. The phenotype has differed somewhat in the several patients. For example, the patient of Gehler et al. [174] and patient K.B. of Beaudet et al. [175] had gross corneal clouding,

whereas the original patient of Sly et al. [171] had clear corneas at age 30 months. K.B. died at age 33 months. On the other hand, T.Y., the second patient of Beaudet et al. [175], was well at age 14 years except for hypertension and obstructive lesions of large blood vessels. The facies was somewhat coarse. He had normal stature and intelligence, and aortic regurgitation from at least age 8 years. A graft was placed in the abdominal aorta, which showed fibromuscular dysplasia with abundant intercellular mucopolysaccharides and large vacuolated cells.

All the patients have shown inclusions in circulating leukocytes. Several of them have suffered from repeated episodes of pneumonia in the first years of life.

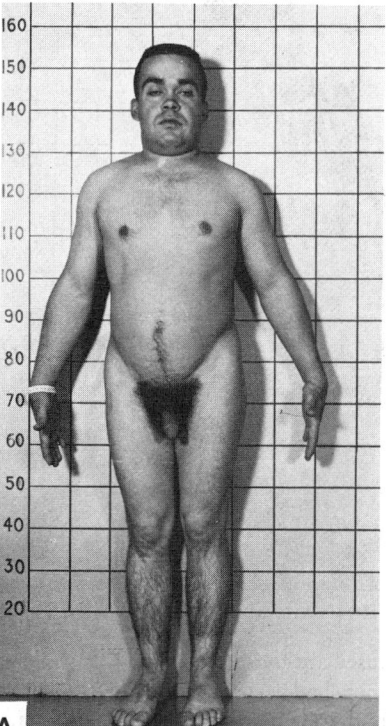

Figure 36-13 MPS VI (Maroteaux-Lamy syndrome), mild form, in a man 25 years old at the time of pictures. He had bilateral "Legg-Perthes disease" in childhood, and bilateral inguinal hernias were repaired at age 20 years. Mild stiffness of the hands and corneal clouding were first noted at age 20. At age 30 he had signs of carpal tunnel syndrome and the murmur of aortic stenosis, present since age 8 years. Leukocytes showed striking metachromatic inclusions, and excessive dermatan sulfate was demonstrated in the urine (see [2]). He is of average intelligence. *A.* Body view. Note the short stature and absence of gross skeletal deformity. *B.* Hand. Note the lack of contractures. Contrast both these pictures with those in Fig. 36-14.

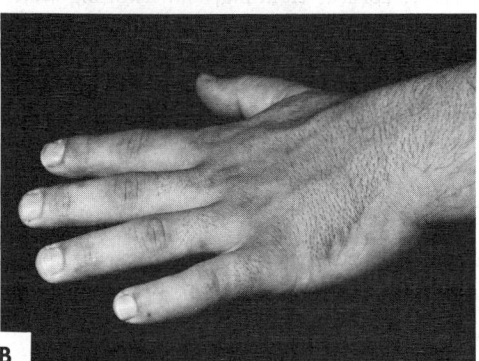

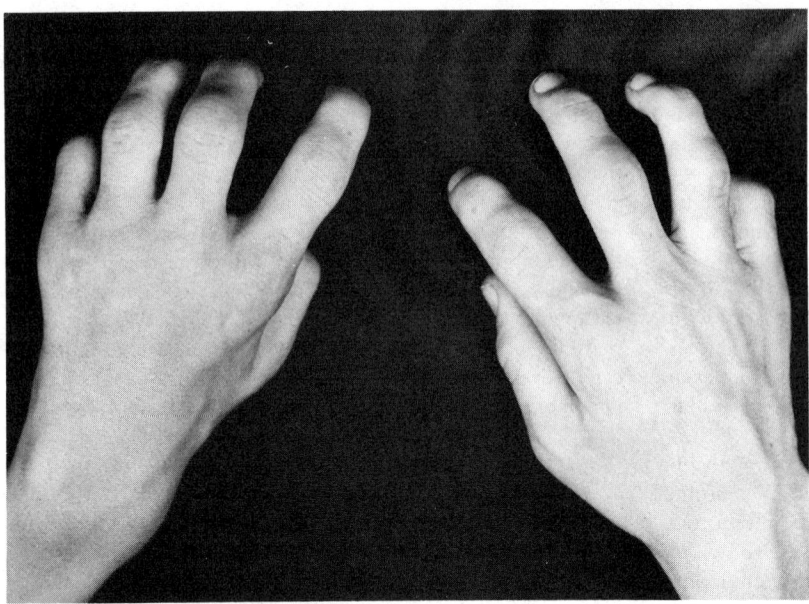

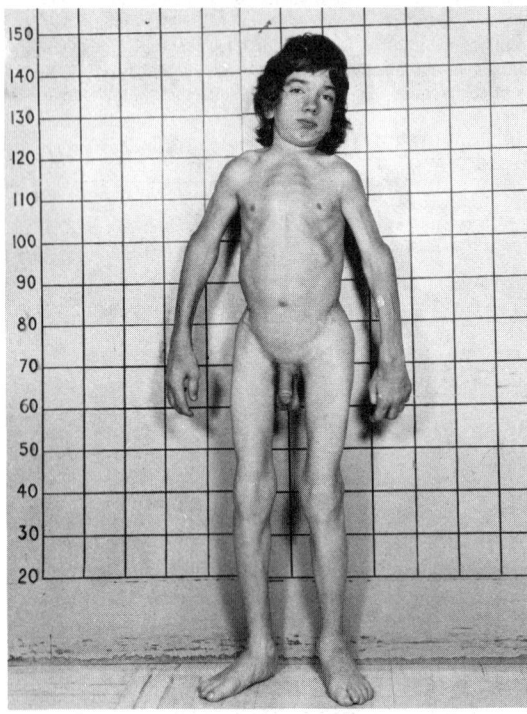

Figure 36-14 MPS VI (Maroteaux-Lamy syndrome), intermediate form, in a man 19 years old at the time of the pictures. Contractures of the fingers developed at age $4\frac{1}{2}$ years. Clouding of the corneas was detected by an optometrist when the patient was age 6 years. The joint contractures and corneal clouding progressed. He had frequent otitis media, requiring myringotomy. At age 13 years he had muscle release operations for treatment of flexion contractures of the hips. He walked with crutches from age 17 until age 19 (soon after these photographs), when successful bilateral total hip replacement was performed for pain as well as for limited mobility. The patient had aortic systolic and diastolic murmurs and signs of the carpal tunnel syndrome. He is a good student, attending college. This patient was thought to have mucolipidosis III (Chapter 37) until serum hexosaminidase was found to be normal, and fibroblasts arylsulfatase B was found to be absent [193].

The mildest cases are those reported by Gitzelmann et al. [176]. Two brothers had asymptomatic thoracic kyphosis and mild scoliosis as the main clinical features. Hernia, hepatosplenomegaly, corneal clouding, and dwarfing were absent. Both had striking Alder granulations in polymorphs and to a lesser degree in monocytes. Cultured skin fibroblasts also had metachromatic granules. Fibroblasts showed about 10 percent of normal β-glucuronidase activity.

Basic Defect

A deficiency of β-glucuronidase in fibroblasts, in leukocytes, and presumably in most tissues leads to a block in the degradation of dermatan sulfate and heparan sulfate (reaction 6 in Figs. 36-2 and 36-3). Since β-linked glucuronic acid comprises half the carbohydrate residues of chondroitin sulfate and of hyaluronic acid, one would expect the catabolism of these polymers to be similarly affected. However, careful analysis in two cases has shown urinary excretion of dermatan sulfate or heparan sulfate exclusively [175]. In another patient, the urinary mucopolysaccharide consisted primarily of partially degraded, unidentifiable fragments [174]. As discussed above for MPS VI, the explanation may lie in the susceptibility of chondroitin sulfate and hyaluronic acid to hyaluronidase, which would degrade these polymers to very small fragments. These would escape detection in the methods commonly used for measuring urinary mucopolysaccharides.

In four unrelated patients Bell et al. [177] demonstrated cross-reacting material on immunoassay of β-glucuronidase. Thus mutation in a structural gene for the enzyme is the likely defect. Titration patterns suggested genetic heterogeneity among the four cases [177].

Genetics

β-Glucuronidase deficiency is an autosomal recessive disorder. The mode of transmission was first deduced from the intermediate enzyme levels in parents and other relatives of the index patient [171]. Affected brothers have been reported [176]. MPS VII is very rare; only a dozen cases have been reported in the 10 years since its discovery.

The wide interfamilial variability in cases of β-glucuronidase deficiency suggests that there may be multiple allelic forms. The complexity of the genetic control of β-glucuronidase has been demonstrated in the mouse by the studies of Paigen and his associates. They have, for example, demonstrated regulatory loci [178]. Thus, some of the cases of human β-glucuronidase deficiency may have a mutation in a locus other than in the structural locus for β-glucuronidase.

By the study of somatic cell hybrids, several workers (e.g., [179]) assigned the structural locus for β-glucuronidase to chromosome 7.

Diagnosis

β-Glucuronidase activity is measured in fibroblasts, leukocytes, or serum with commercially available substrates [180]. An opportunity to use this test for prenatal diagnosis has been reported; the results were normal, indicating an unaffected fetus [181].

ANIMAL MODELS OF MUCOPOLYSACCHARIDOSES

α-L-Iduronidase deficiency has been found in a short-haired cat [182, 183], and a deficiency of arylsulfatase B in Siamese cats [184–186]. These feline disorders represent models for MPS I and MPS VI, respectively, and should be invaluable for the development and testing of therapeutic protocols.

β-Glucuronidase activity is markedly reduced in mice homozygous for the Gus^h allele at the β-glucuronidase locus. This enzyme activity is not so low as to be pathogenic, but low enough to allow the measurement of administered enzyme (e.g., [187, 188]). In addition, chimeric tetraparental mice, with cells of low and high β-glucuronidase concentrations, have been used to demonstrate intercellular transfer of the enzyme [189, 190].

A different kind of model has been developed by administration of suramin to rats [191]. The drug causes accumulation and urinary excretion of dermatan sulfate and heparan sulfate through inhibition of several enzymes of mucopolysaccharide degradation—particularly iduronate sulfatase, β-glucuronidase, and hyaluronidase [191].

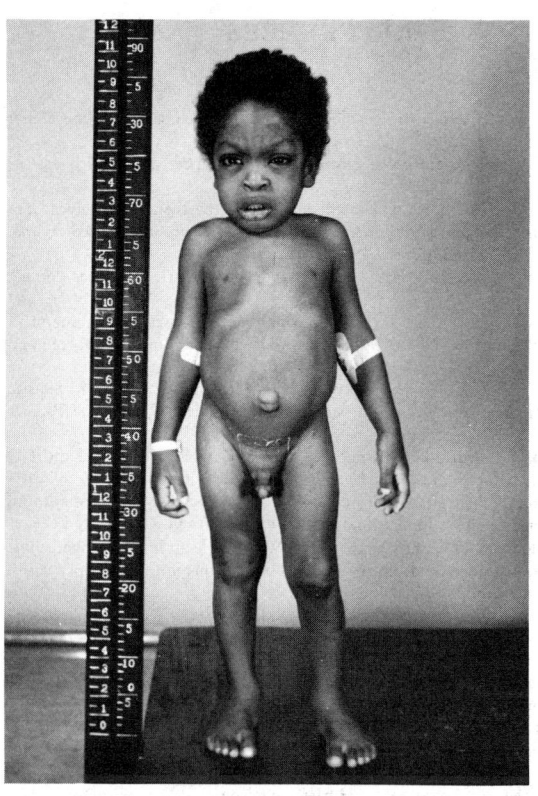

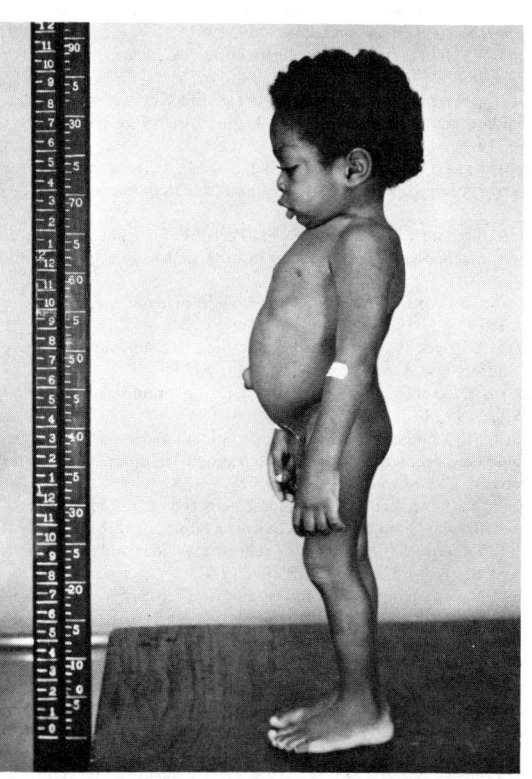

Figure 36-15 Mucopolysaccharidosis VII (β-glucuronidase deficiency disease) in the original patient of Sly and colleagues. Aged 3 years at the time of the photograph, the patient shows flare of the lower ribs, pigeon breast, prominent abdomen with hepatosplenomegaly and umbilical hernia, and a short trunk. He shows a cardiac murmur and striking leukocytic inclusions. (*Courtesy of Dr. William Sly, St. Louis*)

REFERENCES

1. McKusick VA: Genetic nosology—three approaches. *Am J Hum Genet* 30:105, 1978

2. McKusick VA: *Heritable Disorders of Connective Tissue*, 4th ed. St. Louis, Mosby, 1972

3. Roden L: Structure and metabolism of connective tissue proteoglycans, in Lennarz WJ (ed): *The Biochemistry of Glycoproteins and Proteoglycans*, New York, Plenum Press, 1980, p 267

4. Gardner RJM, Hay HR: Hurler's syndrome with clear corneas (letter). *Lancet* 2:845, 1974

5. Grossman H, Dorst JP: The mucopolysaccharidoses, in Kaufmann H (ed): *Progress in Pediatric Radiology*. Chicago, Year Book, 1973, vol IV, p 495

6. Brill CB, Rose JS, Godmilow L, Sklower S, Hirschhorn K: Spastic quadriparesis due to C_1—C_2 subluxation in Hurler syndrome. *J Pediatr* 92:441, 1978

7. Suzuki K: Neurological aspects of mucopolysaccharidoses, in Latjtha A (ed): *Handbook of Neurochemistry*. New York, Plenum, 1972, vol VII

8. Purpura DP, Suzuki K: Distortions of neural geometry and formation of aberrant synapses in neuronal storage disease. *Brain Res* 116:1, 1976

9. Renteria VG, Ferrans VJ, Roberts WC: The heart in Hurler syndrome. Gross, histologic and ultrastructural observations in five necropsy cases. *Am J Cardiol* 38:487, 1976

10. Goldfischer S, Coltoff-Schiller B, Biempica L, Wolinski H: Lysosomes and the sclerotic arterial lesion in Hurler's disease. *Hum Path* 6:633, 1975

11. Renteria VG, Ferrans VJ: Intracellular collagen fibrils in cardiac valves of patients with the Hurler syndrome. *Lab Invest* 34:263, 1976

12. Bach G, Friedman R, Weissmann B, Neufeld EF: The defect in the Hurler and Scheie syndromes: deficiency of α-L-iduronidase. *Proc Nat Acad Sci USA* 69:2048, 1972

13. Matalon R, Dorfman A: Hurler's syndrome, an α-L-iduronidase deficiency. *Biochem Biophys Res Commun* 47:959, 1972

14. Rome LH, Garvin AJ, Neufeld EF: Human kidney α-L-iduronidase; purification and characterization. *Arch Biochem Biophys* 189:344, 1978

15. Myerowitz R, Neufeld EF: Maturation of α-L-iduronidase in cultured human fibroblasts. *J Biol Chem*, 256:3044, 1981

16. Barton RW, Neufeld, EF: The Hurler corrective factor, *J Biol Chem* 246:7773, 1971

17. Shapiro LJ, Hall, CW, Leder IG, Neufeld EF: The relationship of α-L-iduronidase and Hurler corrective factor. *Arch Biochem Biophys* 172:156, 1976

18. Cantz M, Kreese H, Barton RW, Neufeld EF: Corrective factors for inborn errors of mucopolysaccharide metabolism. *Meth Enzymol* 28:884, 1972

19. Hall CW, Liebaers I, Dinatale P, Neufeld EF: Enzymic diagnosis of the genetic mucopolysaccharide storage disorders. *Meth Enzymol* 50:539, 1978

20. Weissmann B: Synthetic substrates for α-L-iduronidase. *Meth Enzymol* 50:141, 1978

21. Dinatale P, Leder IG, Neufeld EF: A radioactive substrate and assay for α-L-iduronidase. *Clin Chim Acta* 77:211, 1977

22. Thompson JN: Substrates for the assay of α-L-iduronidase. *Clin Chim Acta* 89:435, 1978

23. Hopwood JJ: α-L-iduronidase, β-D-glucuronidase and 2-sulfo-L-iduronate 2-sulfatase: preparation and characterization of radioactive substrates from heparin. *Carbohyd Res* 69:203, 1979

24. Hall CW, Neufeld EF: α-L-iduronidase activity in cultured skin fibroblasts and amniotic fluid cells. *Arch Biochem Biophys* 158:817, 1973

25. Kelly TE, Taylor HA Jr: Leukocyte values of α-L-iduronidase in mucopolysaccharidosis I. *J Med Genet* 13:149, 1976

26. Shapiro LJ: Current status and future direction for carrier detection in lysosomal storage diseases, in Callahan JW, Lowden JA (eds): *Lysosomes and Lysosomal Storage Diseases*. New York, Raven Press, 1981, p 343

27. Aberg A, Mitelman F, Cantz M, Gehler J: Cardiac puncture of fetus with Hurler's disease avoiding abortion of unaffected co-twin. (Letter). *Lancet* 2:990, 1978

28. Lowry RB, Renwick DHG: The relative frequency of the Hurler and Hunter syndromes. (Letter). *N Engl J Med* 284:221, 1971

29. Diferrante NM, Nichols BL Jr, Donnelly PV, Neri G, Hrgovcic R, Berglund RK: Induced degradation of glycosaminoglycans in Hurler's and Hunter's syndromes by plasma infusion. *Proc Nat Acad Sci USA* 68:303, 1971

30. Nishioka J, Mizushima T, Ono K: Treatment of mucopolysaccharidosis: clinical and biochemical aspects of leucocyte transfusion as compared with plasma infusion in patients with Hurler's and Scheie's syndromes. *Clin Orthop* 140:194, 1979

31. Gibbs DA, Spellacy E, Roberts AE, Watts RWE: The treatment of lysosomal storage diseases by fibroblast transplantation, in Desnick RJ (ed): *Enzyme Therapy in Genetic Diseases 2*, New York, March of Dimes Birth Defects Foundation, Alan Liss, 1980, p 457

32. MacDougal B, Weeks PM, Wray RC: Median nerve compression and trigger finger in the mucopolysaccharidoses and related diseases. *Plast Reconstr Surg* 59:260, 1977

33. Lamon JM, Trojak JE, Abbott MH: Bone cysts in mucopolysaccharidosis I S (Scheie syndrome). *Johns Hopkins Med J* 146:73, 1980

34. Perks WH, Cooper RA, Bradbury S, Horrocks P, Baldock N, Allen A, Van't Hoff W, Weidman G, Prowse K: Sleep apnoea in Scheie's syndrome. *Thorax* 35:85, 1980

35. Kennedy P, Swash M, Dean MD: Cervical cord compression in mucopolysaccharidosis. *Dev Med Child Neurol* 15:194, 1973

36. Paulson GW, Meagler JN, Burkhart J: Spinal pachymeningitis secondary to mucopolysaccharidosis: case report. *J Neurosurg* 41:618, 1974

37. Horton WA, Schimke RN: A new mucopolysaccharidosis. *J Pediatr* 77:252, 1970

38. Schimke RN: Personal communication, 1981

39. Hopwood JJ, Muller V: Biochemical discrimination of Hurler and Scheie syndromes. *Clin Sci* 57:265, 1979

40. Matalon R, Deanching M: The enzymic basis for the phenotypic variation of Hurler and Scheie syndromes. *Pediat Res* 11:519, 1977

41. Fortuin JJH, Kleijer WJ: Hybridization studies of fibroblasts from Hurler, Scheie, and Hurler-Scheie compound patients: support for the hypothesis of allelic mutants. *Hum Genet* 53:155, 1980

42. Thompson JN, Finley SC, Lorincz AE, Finley WH: Absence of α-L-iduronidase activity in various tissues from two sibs affected with presumably the Hurler-Scheie syndrome, in Bergsma D (ed): *Disorders of Connective Tissue*. New York, National Foundation—March of Dimes, 1975, vol XI, no 6, p 341

43. Kajii T, Matsuda I, Oshaw AT, Katsunuma H, Ichida T, Arashima S: Hurler-Scheie genetic compound (mucopolysaccharidosis IH-IS) in Japanese brothers. *Clin Genet* 6:394, 1974

44. Winters PR, Harrod MJ, Molenich-Heetred SA, Kirkpatrick J, Rosenberg RN: α-L-iduronidase deficiency and possible Hurler-Scheie genetic compound: clinical, pathologic, and biochemical findings. *Neurology* 26:1003, 1976

45. McKusick VA, Howell RR, Hussels IE, Neufeld EF, Stevenson R: Allelism, non-allelism and genetic compounds among the mucopolysaccharidoses: hypothesis. *Lancet* 1:993, 1972

46. Jensen OA, Pedersen C, Schwartz M, Vestermark S, Warburg M: Hurler-Scheie phenotype: report of an inbred sibship with tapeto-retinal degeneration and electron-microscopic examination of the conjunctiva. *Ophthalmologica* 176:194, 1978

47. Kaibara H, Eguchi M, Shibata K, Takagishi K: Hurler-Scheie phenotype: a report of two pairs of inbred sibs: *Hum Genet* 53:37, 1979.

48. Kajii T, Matsuda I, Ohsaw AT, Katsunuma H, Ichida T, Arashima S: Hurler-Scheie genetic compound (mucopolysaccharidosis IH-IS) in Japanese brothers. *Clin Genet* 6:394, 1974

49. Yatziv S, Erickson RP, Epstein CJ: Mild and severe Hunter syndrome (MPS II) within the sibships. *Clin Genet* 11:319, 1977

50. Benson PF, Button LR, Fensom AH, Dean MF: Lumbar kyphosis in Hunter's disease (MPS II). *Clin Genet* 16:317, 1979

51. Spranger J, Cantz M, Gehler J, Liebaers I, Theiss W: Mucopolysaccharidosis II (Hunter disease) with corneal opacities: report of two patients at the extremes of a wide clinical spectrum. *Eur J Pediatr* 129:11, 1978

52. Prystowsky SD, Maumenee IH, Freeman RG, Herndon JH, Harrod MJ: A cutaneous marker in the Hunter syndrome: a report of four cases. *Arch Dermatol* 113:602, 1977

53. Elsner B: Ultrastructure of the rectal wall in Hunter's syndrome. *Gastroenterology* 58:856, 1970

54. Ballenger CE, Swift TR, Leshner RT, El Gammal TA, McDonald TF: Myelopathy in mucopolysaccharidosis type II (Hunter syndrome). *Ann Neurol* 7:382, 1980

55. Young ID, Harper PS: Long-term complications in Hunter's syndrome. *Clin Genet* 16:125, 1978

56. Yatziv S, Epstein CJ: Hunter syndrome presenting as macrocephaly and hydrocephalus. *J Med Genet* 14:445, 1977

57. Lustmann J, Bimstein E, Yatziv S: Dentigerous cysts and radiolucent lesions of the jaw associated with Hunter's syndrome. *J Oral Surg* 33:679, 1975

58. Hobolth N, Pedersen C: Six cases of a mild form of the Hunter syndrome in five generations: three affected males with progeny. (Abstract). *Clin Genet* 13:121, 1978

59. Diferrante NM, Nichols BL Jr: A case of the Hunter syndrome with progeny. *Johns Hopkins Med J* 130:325, 1972

60. Karpati G, Carpenter S, Eisan AA, Wolfe LS, Feindel W: Multiple peripheral nerve entrapments: an unusual phenotypic variant of the Hunter syndrome (mucopolysaccharidosis II) in a family. *Arch Neurol* 31:418, 1974

61. NAGASHIMA K, ENDO H, SAKAKIBARA K, KONISHI Y, MIYACHI K, WEY JJ, SUZUKI Y, ONISAWA J: Morphological and biochemical studies of a case of mucopolysaccharidosis II (Hunter's syndrome). *Acta Pathol Jpn* 26:115, 1976

62. MEIER C, WIESMANN U, HERSCHKOWITZ N, BISCHOFF A: Morphological observations in the nervous system of prenatal mucopolysaccharidosis II (M. Hunter). *Acta Neuropathol* 48:139, 1979

63. FREEMAN RG: A pathological basis for the cutaneous papules of mucopolysaccharidosis II (the Hunter syndrome). *J Cutan Pathol* 4:318, 1977

64. BACH G, EISENBERG F JR, CANTZ M, NEUFELD EF: The defect in the Hunter syndrome: deficiency of sulfoiduronate sulfatase. *Proc Nat Acad Sci USA* 70:2134, 1973

65. SJOBERG I, FRANSSON LA, MATALON R, DORFMAN A: Hunter's syndrome: a deficiency of L-idurono-sulfate sulfatase. *Biochem Biophys Res Commun* 54:1125, 1973

66. COPPA GV, SINGH J, NICHOLS BL, DIFERRANTE N: Urinary excretion of disulfated disaccharides in Hunter syndrome: correction by infusion of a serum fraction. *Anal Lett* 6:225, 1973

67. HASSELL JR, NEWSOME DA, HASCALL VC: Characterization and biosynthesis of proteoglycans of corneal stroma from rheusus monkey. *J Biol Chem* 254:12346, 1979

68. WASTESON A, NEUFELD EF: Iduronate sulfatase from human plasma. *Meth Enzymol*, in press

69. LIEBAERS I, NEUFELD EF: Iduronate sulfatase activity in serum, lymphocytes, and fibroblasts—simplified diagnosis of the Hunter syndrome. *Pediatr Res* 10:733, 1976

70. MIGEON BR, SPRENKLE JA, LIEBAERS I, SCOTT JF, NEUFELD EF: X-linked Hunter syndrome: the heterozygous phenotype in cell culture. *Am J Hum Genet* 29:448, 1977

71. YUTAKA T, FLUHARTY AL, STEVENS RL, KIHARA H: Iduronate sulfatase analysis of hair roots for identification of Hunter syndrome heterozygotes. *Am J Hum Genet* 30:575, 1978

72. NWOKORO N, NEUFELD EF: Detection of Hunter heterozygotes by enzymatic analysis of hair roots. *Am J Hum Genet* 31:42, 1979

73. LIEBAERS I, DINATALE P, NEUFELD EF: Iduronate sulfatase in amniotic fluid: an aid in the prenatal diagnosis of the Hunter syndrome. *J Pediatr* 90:423, 1977

74. KLEIJTER WJ, MOOY PD, LIEBAERS I, VAN DE KAMP JJP, NIERMEIJER MF: Prenatal monitoring for the Hunter syndrome: the heterozygous female fetus. *Clin Genet* 15:113, 1979

75. LICHTENSTEIN JR, BILBREY GI, MCKUSICK VA: Probable genetic heterogeneity within mucopolysaccharidosis II: report of a family with mild form. *Johns Hopkins Med J* 131:425, 1972

76. FRANCKE U, FELSENSTEIN J, GARTLER SM, MIGEON BR, DANCIS J, SEEGMILLER JE, BAKAY F, NYHAN WL: The occurrence of new mutants in the X-linked recessive Lesch-Nyhan disease. *Am J Hum Genet* 28:123, 1976

77. MCKUSICK VA: The relative frequency of the Hunter and Hurler syndromes. *N Engl J Med* 283:853, 1970

78. SCHAAP T, BACH G: Incidence of mucopolysaccharidoses in Israel: is Hunter disease a "Jewish disease"? *Hum Genet* 56:221, 1980

79. NEUFELD EF, LIEBAERS I, EPSTEIN CJ, YATSIV S, MILUNKSY A, MIGEON BR: The Hunter syndrome in females: is there an autosomal recessive form of iduronate sulfatase deficiency? *Am J Hum Genet* 29:455, 1977

80. EISENBERG LR, MIGEON BR: Enrichment of human heterokaryons by Ficoll gradient for complementation analysis of iduronate sulfatase deficiency. *Somat Cell Genet* 5:1079, 1979

81. HORWITZ AL: Genetic complementation of studies of multiple sulfatase deficiency. *Proc Nat Acad Sci USA* 75:6496, 1979

82. FLUHARTY AL, STEVENS RL, DE LA FLOR SD, SHAPIRO LJ, KIHARA H: Arylsulfatase A modulation with pH in multiple sulfatase deficiency disorder fibroblasts. *Am J Hum Genet* 31:574, 1979

83. DEKABAN AS, HOLDEN KP, CONSTANTOPOULOS G: Effects of fresh plasma or whole blood transfusions on patients with various types of mucopolysaccharidoses. *Pediatrics* 50:688, 1972

84. ERICKSON RP, SANDMAN R, VAN B ROBERTSON W, EPSTEIN CJ: Inefficacy of fresh frozen plasma therapy of mucopolysaccharidosis II. *Pediatrics* 50:693, 1972

85. KNUDSEN AG JR, DIFERRANTE N, CURTIS JE: The effect of leukocyte transfusion in a child with type II mucopolysaccharidosis. *Proc Nat Acad Sci USA* 68:1738, 1971

86. YATZIV S, STRATTER M, ABELIUK P, MESHULAM M, RUSSELL A: A therapeutic trial of fresh plasma infusions over a period of 22 months in two siblings with Hunter syndrome. *Isr J Med Sci* 11:802, 1975

87. BROWN F, NEUFELD EF, HALL CW, MUNOZ LL, BRAINE HG, MOSER HW: Enzyme replacement by plasma exchange in Hunter syndrome. (Abstract). *Pediat Res* 14:519, 1980

88. MURPHY JV, MATALON R, MENITORE JE, BARKLEY RA: Enzyme replacement therapy in Hunter syndrome using plasmapheresis. (Abstract). *Ann Neurol* 8:217, 1980

89. DEAN MF, MUIR H, BENSON PF, BUTTON LE, BATCHELOR JR, BEWICK M: Increased breakdown of glycosaminoglycans and appearance of corrective enzyme after skin transplants in Hunter syndrome. *Nature* 257:609, 1975

90. DEAN MF, STEVENS RL, MUIR H, BENSON PF, BUTTON LR, ANDERSON RL, BOYLSTON A, BENSON PF: Enzyme replacement therapy by fibroblast transplantation: long-term biochemical study in three cases of Hunter's syndrome. *J Clin Invest* 63:138, 1979

91. SWIFT TR, MCDONALD TF: Peripheral nerve involvement in Hunter syndrome (mucopolysaccharidosis II). *Arch Neurol* 33:845, 1976

92. VAN DE KAMP JJP: The Sanfilippo syndrome: a clinical and genetical study of 75 patients in the Netherlands. (Doctoral thesis). 'S-Gravenhage, JH Pasmans, 1979

93. HERD JK, SUBRAMANIAN S, ROBINSON H: Type III mucopolysaccharidosis: Report of a case with severe mitral valve involvement. *J Pediatr* 82:101, 1973

94. BARTSOCAS C, GROBE H, VAN DE KAMP JJP, VON FIGURA K, FRESSE H, KLEIN U, GIESBERTS MAH: Sanfilippo type C disease: clinical findings in four patients with a new variant of mucopolysaccharidosis III. *Eur J Pediatr* 130:251, 1979

95. MATALON R, DEANCHING M, NAKAMURA F, BLOOM A: A recessively inherited lethal disease in a Caribbean isolate—a sulfamidase deficiency. *Pediatr Res* 14:524, 1980

96. ANDRIA G, DI NATALE P, DEL GIUDICE E, STRISCIUGLIO P, MURINO P: Sanfilippo B syndrome (MPS III): mild and severe forms within the same sibship. *Clin Genet* 15:500, 1979

97. VAN DE KAMP JJP, VAN PELT JF, LIEM KO, GIESBERTS MAH, NIEPOTH LTM, STAALMAN CR: Clinical variability in Sanfilippo B disease: a report of six patients in two related sibships. *Clin Genet* 10:279, 1976

98. VAN DE KAMP JJP, NIERMEYER MF, VON FIGURA K, GIESBERTS MAH: Genetic heterogeneity and clinical variability in the Sanfilippo syndrome (types A, B, and C). *Clin Genet*, in press

99. KELLY TE: Personal communication, 1981

100. KRIEL RL, HAUSER WA, SUNG JH, POSALAKY Z: Neuroanatomical and electroencephalographic correlations in Sanfilippo syndrome, type A. *Arch Neurol* 35:838, 1978

101. MARTIN JJ, CEUTERICK C, VAN DESSEL G, LAGROU A, DIETRICK W: Two cases of mucopolysaccharidosis type III (Sanfilippo): an anatomopathological study. *Acta Neuropathol* 46:185, 1979

102. SHIMAMURA K, HAKOZAKI H, TOKAHASHI K, KIMURA A, FUJINO J, SUZUKI Y, NAKAMURA N: Sanfilippo B syndrome: a case report. *Acta Pathol Jpn* 26:739, 1976

103. GREENWOOD RS, HILLMAN RE, ALCALA H, SLY WS: Sanfilippo A syndrome in the fetus. *Clin Genet* 13:241, 1978

104. VON FIGURA K, KLEIN U: Defects in the degradation of heparan sulfate, in Callahan JW, Lowden JA (eds): *Lysosomes and Lysosomal Storage Diseases.* New York, Raven Press, 1981

105. KRESSE H, NEUFELD EF: The Sanfilippo A corrective factor: purification and mode of action. *J Biol Chem* 247:2164, 1972

106. KRESSE H: Mucopolysaccharidosis III A (Sanfilippo A disease): deficiency of heparin sulfamidase in skin fibroblasts and leucocytes. *Biochem Biophys Res Commun* 54:1111, 1973

107. MATALON R, DORFMAN A: Sanfilippo A syndrome: sulfamidase deficiency in cultured skin fibroblasts and liver. *J Clin Invest* 54:907, 1974

108. KRESSE H, VON FIGURA K, KLEIN U: New biochemical subtype of the Sanfilippo syndrome: characterization of the storage material in cultured fibroblasts of Sanfilippo C patients. *Eur J Biochem* 92:333, 1978

109. KLEIN U, KRESSE H, VON FIGURA K: Sanfilippo syndrome type C: deficiency of acetyl-CoA: α-glucosaminide N-acetyltransferase in skin fibroblasts. *Proc Nat Acad Sci USA* 75:5185, 1978

110. O'BRIEN JS: Sanfilippo syndrome: profound deficiency of α-acetylglucosaminidase activity in organs and skin fibroblasts from type B patients. *Proc Nat Acad Sci USA* 69:1720, 1972

111. VON FIGURA K, KRESSE H: The Sanfilippo B corrective factor: an N-acetyl-α-D-glucosaminidase. *Biochem Biophys Res Commun* 48:262, 1972

112. VON FIGURA K: Human α-N-acetylglucosaminidase. *Eur J Biochem* 80:525, 1977

113. VON FIGURA K, KRESSE H: Quantitative aspects of pinocytosis and intracellular fate of N-acetyl-α-D-glucosaminidase in Sanfilippo B fibroblasts. *J Clin Invest* 53:85, 1974

114. VON FIGURA K, KRESSE H: Sanfilippo disease type B: presence of material cross reacting with antibodies against α-N-acetylglucosaminidase. *Eur J Biochem* 61:581, 1976

115. KRESSE H, PASCHKE E, VON FIGURA K, GILBERG W, FUCHS W: Sanfilippo disease type D; deficiency of N-acetylglucosamine-6-sulfate sulfatase required for heparan sulfate degradation. *Proc Nat Acad Sci USA* 77:6622, 1980

116. BASNER R, KRESSE H, VON FIGURA K: N-acetylglucosamine-6-sulfate sulfatase from human urine. *J Biol Chem* 254:1151, 1979

117. WEISSMAN BN, CHAO H, CHOW P: A glucosamine O,N-disulfate O-sulfohydrolase with a probably role in mammalian catabolism of heparan sulfate. *Biochem Biophys Res Commun* 97:827, 1980

118. KRESSE H, VON FIGURA K, KLEIN U, GLOSSL J, PACHKE E, POHLMANN R: Enzymic diagnosis of the genetic mucopolysaccharide storage disorders—an extension. *Meth Enzymol*, in press

119. HARRIS H: *The Principles of Human Biochemical Genetics*. 3d ed. New York, Elsevier North Holland, 1981

120. WHITEMAN P, YOUNG E: The laboratory diagnosis of Sanfilippo disease. *Clin Chim Acta* 76:139, 1977

121. GORDON BA, FELEKI V, BUDREAU CH, TYLER L: Defective heparan sulfate metabolism in the Sanfilippo syndrome and assay of this defect in the assessment of the mucopolysaccharidosis patient. *Clin Biochem* 8:184, 1975

122. MCKUSICK VA: Osler as a medical geneticist. *Johns Hopkins Med J* 139:163, 1976

123. GADBOIS P, MOREAU J, LABERGE C: La maladie de Morquio dans la province de Quebec. *Union Med Can* 102:602, 1973

124. TROJAK JE, HO CH, ROESEL RA, LEVIN LS, KOPTIS SE, THOMAS GH, TOMA S: Morquio-like syndrome (MPS IV B) associated with deficiency of a β-galactosidase. *Johns Hopkins Med J* 146:75, 1980

125. RIEDNER ED, LEVIN LS: Hearing patterns in Morquio's syndrome (mucopolysaccharidosis IV). *Arch Otolaryngol* 103:518, 1977

126. LIPSON SJ: Dysplasia of the odontoid process in Morquio's syndrome causing quadriparesis. *J Bone Joint Surg* 59:340, 1977

127. ARBISSER AI, DONNELLY KA, SCOTT CI Jr, DIFERRANTE NM, SINGH J, STEVENSON RE, AYLESWORTH AS, HOWELL, RR: Morquio-like syndrome with beta-galactosidase deficiency and normal hexosamine sulfate activity: mucopolysaccharidosis IV B. *Am J Med Genet* 1:195, 1977

128. GROEBE H, KRINS M, SCHMIDBERGER H, VON FIGURA K, HARZER K, KRESSE H, PASCHKE E, SEWELL A, ULLRICH K: Morquio syndrome (mucopolysaccharidosis IV B) associated with beta-galactosidase deficiency. Report of two cases. *Am J Hum Genet* 32:258, 1980

129. KOTO A, HORWITZ AL, SUZUKI K, TIFFANY CW, SUSUKI K: The Morquio syndrome: neuropathology and biochemistry. *Ann Neurol* 4:26, 1978

130. MINAMI R, KATSUYUKI A, KUDOH T, TSUGAWA S, OYANAGI K, NAKAO T: Identification of keratan sulfate in liver affected by Morquio syndrome. *Clin Chim Acta* 93:207, 1979

131. FACTOR SM, BIEMPICA L, GOLDFISCHER S: Coronary intimal sclerosis in Morquio's syndrome. *Virchows Arch Pathol Anat* 379:1, 1978

132. MATALON R, ARBOGAST B, JUSTICE P, BRANDT EK, DORFMAN A: Morquio's syndrome: deficiency of a chondroitin sulfate N-acetylhexosamine sulfate sulfatase. *Biochem Biophys Res Commun* 61:759, 1974

133. SINGH J, DIFERRANTE NM, NIEBES P, TAVELLA D: N-acetylgalactosamine 6-sulfate sulfatase in man: absence of the enzyme in Morquio disease. *J Clin Invest* 57:1036, 1976

134. HORWITZ AL, DORFMAN A: The enzymatic defect in Morquio's disease: the specificity of N-acetylhexosamine sulfatases. *Biochem Biophys Res Commun* 80:819, 1978

135. DI FERRANTE N, GINSBERG LC, DONNELLY PV, DI FERRANTE DT, CASKEY CT: Deficiencies of glucosamine-6-sulfate or galactosamine-6-sulfate sulfatases are responsible for different mucopolysaccharidoses. *Science* 199:79, 1978

136. GLOSSL J, TRUPPE W, KRESSE H: Purification and properties of N-acetylgalactosamine 6-sulfate sulfatase from human placenta. *Biochem J* 181:37, 1979

137. GLOSSL J, LEMBECK K, GAMSE G, KRESSE H: Morquio's disease type A: absence of material cross reacting with antibodies against N-acetylgalactosamine-6-sulfate sulfatase. *Hum Genet* 54:87, 1980

138. O'BRIEN JS, GUGLER E, GIEDION A, WIESMANN R, HERSCHKOWITZ N, MEIER C, LEROY JG: Spondyloepiphyseal dysplasia, corneal clouding, normal intelligence and acid β-galactosidase deficiency. *Clin Genet* 9:495, 1976

139. GROEBE H, KRINS M, SCHMIDBERGER H, VON FIGURA K, HARZER K, KRESSE H, PASCHKE E, SEWELL A, ULLRICH K: Morquio syndrome (mucopolysaccharidosis IV B) associated with β-galactosidase deficiency: report of two cases. *Am J Hum Genet* 32:258, 1980

140. SHOWS TB, SCROFFORD-WOLF L, BROWN JA, MEISLER M: Gm₁-gangliosidosis: chromosome 3 assignment of the β-galactosidase-A gene (β GAL-A). *Somat Cell Genet* 5:147, 1979

141. LONGDON K, PENNOCK CA: Abnormal keratan sulphate excretion. *Ann Clin Biochem* 16:152, 1979

142. KIM HJ, BERATIS NG, BRILL P, RAAB E, HIRSCHHORN K, MATALON R: Kniest syndrome with dominant inheritance and mucopolysacchariduria. *Am J Hum Genet* 27:755, 1975

143. GINSBERG LC, DONNELLY PV, DI FERRANTE DT, DI FERRANTE N, CASKEY CT: N-Acetylglucosamine-6-sulfatase in man: deficiency of the enzyme in a new mucopolysaccharidosis. *Pediatr Res* 12:805, 1978

144. DI FERRANTE N: N-Acetylglucosamine-6-sulfate sulfatase deficiency reconsidered. *Science* 210:448, 1980

145. MATALON R, HORWITZ A, WAPPNER R, DEANCHING M, BRANDT IK: Keratan and heparan sulfaturia—a mucopolysaccharidosis with an enzyme defect not previously identified (Abstract). *Pediatr Res* 12:453, 1978

146. GREILING H, STUHLSATZ HW, CANTZ M, GEHLER J: Increased urinary excretion of keratan sulfate in fucosidosis. *J Clin Chem Clin Biochem* 16:329, 1978

147. NYAKO R, MATALON R, RIMOIN DL, ROSENTHAL IM: Gas liquid chomatography of keratan sulfate in the Kniest syndrome. (Abstract). *Pediatr Res* 12:517, 1978

148. GLOSSL J, KRESSE H: A sensitive procedure for the diagnosis of N-acetylgalactosamine 6-sulfate sulfatase deficiency in classical Morquio's disease. *Clin Chem Acta* 88:111, 1978

149. KOPITS SE: Orthopedic complications of dwarfism. *Clin Orthop* 116:153, 1976

150. KOPITS SR, PEROVIC MN, MCKUSICK VA, ROBINSON RA, BAILEY JA: Congenital atlantoaxial dislocations in various forms of dwarfism. *J Bone Joint Surg* 54A:1349, 1972.

151. JONES AEP, CROLEY TF: Morquio syndrome and anesthesia. *Anesthesiology* 51:261, 1979

152. MAROTEAUX P, LEVEQUE B, MARIE J, LAMY M: Une nouvelle dysostose avec elimination urinaire de chondroitine-sulfate B. *Presse Med* 71:1849, 1963

153. SCHIEKEN RM, KERBER RE, IONASESCU VV, ZELLWEGER H: Cardiac manifestations of the mucopolysaccharidoses. *Circulation* 52:700, 1975

154. DI FERRANTE N, HYMAN BH, KLISH W, DONNELLY PV, NICHOLS BL, DUTTON RG: Mucopolysaccharidosis VI (Maroteaux-Lamy disease): clinical and biochemical study of a mild variant case. *Johns Hopkins Med J* 135:42, 1974

155. GLOBER GA, TANAKA KR, TURNER JA, LIU CK: Mucopolysaccharidosis, an unusual case of cardiac valvular disease. *Am J Cardiol* 22:133, 1968

156. WILSON CS, MANKIN HT, PLUTH JR: Aortic stenosis and mucopolysaccharidosis. *Ann Intern Med* 92:496, 1980

157. SOSTRIN RD, HASSO AN, PETERSON DI, THOMPSON JR: Myelographic features of mucopolysaccharidosis: a new sign. *Radiology* 125:421, 1977

158. PETERSON DI, BUCCHUS A, SEAICH L, KELLY TE: Myelopathy associated with Maroteaux-Lamy syndrome. *Arch Neurol* 32:127, 1975

159. UPTON ARM, MCCOMAS AJ: The double crush in nerve-entrapment syndromes. *Lancet* 2:359, 1973

160. TONDEUR M, NEUFELD EF: The mucopolysaccharidoses: biochemistry and ultrastructure, in Good RA, Day SB, Yunis JJ (eds): *Molecular Pathology*. Springfield, Charles C Thomas, 1975, p 600

161. LEVY LA, LEWIS JC: Ultrastructures of Reilly bodies (metachromatic granules) in the Maroteaux-Lamy syndrome (mucopolysaccharidosis VI): a histochemical study. *Am J Clin Pathol* 73:416, 1980

162. QUIGLEY HA, KENYON KR: Ultrastructural and histochemical studies of a newly recognized form of systemic mucopolysaccharidosis (Maroteaux-Lamy syndrome, mild phenotype). *Am J Ophthalmo* 77:809, 1974

163. FLUHARTY AL, STEVENS RL, SANDER DL, KIHARA H: Arylsulfatase B deficiency in Maroteaux-Lamy syndrome cultured fibroblasts. *Biochem Biophys Res Commun* 59:455, 1974

164. SHAPIRA E, DE GREGORIO RP, MATALON R, NADLER HL: Reduced arylsulfatase B activity of the mutant enzyme protein in Maroteaux-Lamy syndrome. *Biochem Biophys Res Commun* 62:448, 1975

165. STUMPF DA, AUSTIN JH, CROCKER AC, LAFRANCE M: Mucopolysaccharidosis Type VI (Maroteaux-Lamy syndrome): arylsulfatase B deficiency in tissues. *Am J Dis Child* 126:747, 1973

166. FLUHARTY AL, STEVENS RL, FUNG D, PEAK S, KIHARA H: Uridine diphospho-N-acetylgalactosamine-4-sulfate sulfohydrolase activity of human arylsulfatase B and its deficiency in the Maroteaux-Lamy syndrome. *Biochem Biophys Res Commun* 64:955, 1975

167. BARTON RW, NEUFELD EF: A distinct biochemical deficit in the Maroteaux-Lamy syndrome (mucopolysaccharidosis VI). *J Pediatr* 80:114, 1972

168. TAYLOR HR, HOLLOWS FC, HOPWOOD JJ, ROBERTSON EF: Report of a mucopolysaccharidosis occurring in Australian aborigines. *J Med Genet* 15:455, 1978

169. VAN DYKE DL, FLUHARTY AL, SCHAFER IA, SHAPIRO LJ, KIHARA H, WEISS L: Prenatal diagnosis of Maroteaux-Lamy syndrome. *Am J Med Genet* 8:235, 1981

170. MELHEM R, DORST JP, SCOTT CI Jr, MCKUSICK VA: Roengten findings in mucolipidosis III (pseudo-Hurler polydystrophy). *Radiology* 106:153, 1973

171. SLY WS, QUINTON BA, MCALISTER WH, RIMOIN DL: β-Glucuronidase deficiency: report of clinical, radiologic and biochemical features of a new mucopolysaccharidosis. *J Pediatr* 82:249, 1973

172. GUIBAUD P, MAIRE I, GODDON R, TEYSSIER G, ZABOT MT, MANDON G: Mucopolysaccharidose type VII par deficit en β-glucuronidase: étude d'une famille. *J Genet Hum* 27:29, 1979

173. HALL CW, CANTZ M, NEUFELD EF: A β-glucuronidase deficiency mucopolysaccharidosis: studies in cultured fibroblasts. *Arch Biochem Biophys* 155:32, 1973

174. GEHLER J, CANTZ M, TOLKSDORF M, SPRANGER J, GILBERT E, DRUBE H: Mucopolysaccharidosis VII (beta-glucuronidase deficiency). *Humangenetik* 23:149, 1974

175. BEAUDET AL, DIFERRANTE NM, FERRY GD, NICHOLS BL, MULLINS CE: Variation in the phenotypic expression of β-glucuronidase deficiency. *J Pediatr* 86:388, 1978

176. GITZELMANN R, WIESMANN UN, SPYCHER MA, HERSCHKOWITZ N, GIEDION A: Unusually mild course of β-glucuronidase deficiency in two brothers (mucopolysaccharidosis VII). *Helv Paediatr Acta* 33:413, 1978

177. BELL CE JR, SLY WS, BROT FE: Human β-glucuronidase deficiency mucopolysaccharidosis: identification of cross-reactive antigen in cultured fibroblasts of deficient patients by enzyme immunoassay. *J Clin Invest* 59:97, 1977

178. PAIGEN K, LABORCA C, WATSON G: A regulatory locus for mouse beta-glucuronidase induction, *Gur,* controls messenger RNA activity. *Science* 203:554, 1979

179. FRANCKE U: The human gene for beta-glucuronidase is on chromosome 7. *Am J Hum Genet* 28:357, 1976

180. GLASER JH, SLY WS: β-Glucuronidase deficiency mucopolysaccharidosis; methods for enzymatic diagnosis. *J Lab Clin Med* 82:969, 1973

181. GALJAARD H: *Genetic Metabolic Diseases—Early Diagnosis and Prenatal Analysis.* Amsterdam, Elsevier, 1980

182. HASKINS ME, JEZYK PF, DESNICK RJ, MCDONOUGH SK, PATTERSON DF: Mucopolysaccharidosis in a domestic short-haired cat—a disease distinct from that seen in the Siamese cat. *J Am Vet Med Assoc* 175:384, 1979

183. HASKINS ME, JEZYK PF, DESNICK RJ, MCDONOUGH SK, PATTERSON DF: α-L-Iduronidase deficiency in a cat: a model of mucopolysaccharidosis I. *Pediatr Res* 13:1294, 1979

184. COWELL KR, JESYK PF, HASKINS ME, PATTERSON DF: Mucopolysaccharidosis in a cat. *J Am Vet Med Ass* 169:334, 1976

185. JEZYK PF, HASKINS ME, PATTERSON DF, MELLMAN WJ, GREENSTEIN M: Mucopolysaccharidosis in a cat with arylsulfatase B deficiency: a model of Maroteaux-Lamy syndrome. *Science* 198:834, 1977

186. HASKINS ME, JEZYK PF, PATTERSON DF: Mucopolysaccharide storage disease in three families of cats with arylsulfatase B deficiency: leukocyte studies and carrier identification. *Pediatr Res* 13:1203, 1979

187. THORPE SR, FIDDLER MB, DESNICK RJ: Enzyme therapy IV: a method for determining the in vivo fate of bovine β-glucuronidase in β-glucuronidase deficient mice. *Biochem Biophys Res Commun* 61:1464, 1974

188. HUDSON LDS, FIDDLER MB, DESNICK RJ: Immunologic aspects of enzyme replacement therapy, Desnick RJ (ed): *Enzyme Therapy in Genetic Diseases 2,* March of Dimes—Birth Defects Foundation, New York, Alan Liss, 1980, p 163

189. FEDER N: Solitary cells and enzyme exchange in tetraparental mice. *Nature* 263:67, 1976

190. HERRUP K, MULLEN RJ: Intercellular transfer of β-glucuronidase in chimeric mice. *J Cell Sci* 40:21, 1979

191. CONSTANTOPOULOS G, REES S, CRAGG BG, BARRANGER JA, BRADY RO: Experimental animal model for mucopolysaccharidosis: suramin-induced glycosaminoglycan and sphingolipid accumulation in the rat. *Proc Nat Acad Sci USA,* 77:3700, 1980

192. BEEBE RT, FORMAL PF: Gargoylism: sex-linked-transmission in nine males. *Trans Am Clin Climatol Assoc* 66:199, 1954

193. KELLY TE, THOMAS GH, TAYLOR HA JR, MCKUSICK VA, SLY WS, GLASER JH, ROBINOW M, LUZZATTI L, ESPIRITU C, FEINGOLD M, BULL MJ, ASHENHURST EM, IVES EJ: Mucolipidosis III (pseudo-Hurler polydystrophy); clinical and laboratory studies in a series of 12 patients. *Johns Hopkins Med J* 137:156, 1975

37

DISORDERS OF LYSOSOMAL ENZYME SYNTHESIS AND LOCALIZATION:
I-Cell Disease and Pseudo-Hurler Polydystrophy

ELIZABETH F. NEUFELD

VICTOR A. McKUSICK

1. I-cell disease (*mucolipidosis II, or ML II*) and pseudo-Hurler polydystrophy (*mucolipidosis III, or ML III*) are biochemically related disorders of lysosomal function, transmitted in autosomal recessive fashion. Since they affect primarily connective tissue, cultured skin fibroblasts have proved most useful for elucidating the biochemical defects.

2. A number of acid hydrolases (including glycosidases, sulfatases, and cathepsins) are partially or profoundly deficient in cultured fibroblasts of patients with ML II or III but present in excess in culture medium. The more stable of the enzymes affected are strikingly elevated in plasma and other body fluids. The disorders may therefore be viewed as involving inappropriate localization of acid hydrolases—extracellular rather than intralysosomal.

3. The basic defect is in the posttranslational modification of acid hydrolases. Normal hydrolases are glycoproteins equipped with mannose-6-phosphate residues that guide them to lysosomes by a receptor-mediated process. Acid hydrolases synthesized by ML II fibroblasts are not phosphorylated, and those synthesized by ML III fibroblasts are either not phosphorylated or have greatly reduced phosphate content. The basic defect in these disorders is in the enzymatic pathway that phosphorylates mannose residues in newly synthesized acid hydrolases.

4. In normal fibroblasts, the phosphate is transferred from UDP-N-acetylglucosamine together with the N-acetylglucosamine, resulting in the formation of a mannose-P-N-acetylglucosamine diester structure, which is subsequently cleaved to uncover mannose phosphate. This transfer of N-acetylglucosamine phosphate appears to be the step affected by the mutation in the two disorders.

5. The deficiency in phosphorylation has a number of consequences: (a) the hydrolases are secreted rather than translocated to lysosomes; (b) the absence of phosphate groups on mannose residues allows alternate processing of the carbohydrate chains, resulting in enzymes enriched in sialic acid; (c) the secreted hydrolases fail to undergo the limited proteolysis which is the usual fate of these enzymes within lysosomes. Enzymes isolated from fluids and tissue of patients with ML II and ML III may therefore have many physicochemical properties (altered stability, molecular weight, electrophoretic mobility, carbohydrate composition, and lectin binding) that distinguish them from normal enzymes but are secondary to the absence of phosphorylation.

6. It is not clear why some types of cells (e.g., neurons and hepatocytes) appear to be affected little, if at all, in ML II and III, as judged by the absence of pathologic inclusions or by the level of acid hydrolases.

7. *Not all lysosomal enzymes are affected, even in cultured fibroblasts. Acid phosphatase and β-glucosidase are normal in activity and distribution. The reason for these exceptions is not known.*

8. *The clinical manifestations of ML II resemble those of the Hurler syndrome (although ML II patients are affected earlier and more severely); those of ML III resemble the Maroteaux-Lamy syndrome of intermediate severity. The resemblance to mucopolysaccharidoses and not to glycosphingolipidoses (as might have been predicted from the enzyme deficiencies in cultured fibroblasts) may be a function of cell types affected.*

9. *Diagnosis is based on the demonstration of a large twentyfold excess of some enzymes (e.g., β-hexosaminidase or iduronate sulfatase) in plasma or of the simultaneous deficiency of selected enzymes (β-galactosidase, arylsulfatase A, β-hexosaminidase, α-L-iduronidase, among others) in cultured fibroblasts. ML II and ML III cannot yet be reliably distinguished from each other by biochemical methods, and differential diagnosis is based on the clinical picture and course.*

10. *Prenatal diagnosis is possible, but reliable heterozygote identification is not. No definitive treatment is available.*

11. *One should anticipate the existence of diseases with a similar phenotype but caused by an alteration of other steps in the pathway leading to synthesis of the phosphorylated oligosaccharide or by an alteration in the receptor which recognizes the mannose-6-phosphate marker and guides the enzymes to lysosomes.*

HISTORY

In 1967, DeMars and Leroy [1] described "remarkable cells" in cultures of skin fibroblasts from a patient thought to have the Hurler syndrome. The cells were filled with innumerable phase-dense, acid phosphatase–positive inclusions, which occupied almost the entire cytoplasmic space, save for the Golgi area (Fig. 37-1). These unusual fibroblasts were called "inclusion cells", or "I-cells" [2]. Later [3], when because of its earlier appearance and greater severity, the disease for which such cells were characteristic had been shown to be distinct from the Hurler syndrome, the disease was named for the phenotype of the cultured cells. It was called "I-cell disease."

Six years later, Taylor et al. [4] found that the I-cell phenotype of cultured cells were shared by another disorder, pseudo-Hurler polydystrophy. It was the first clue of a relationship between this relatively mild disorder and I-cell disease [5, 6]. Biochemical studies subsequently confirmed the close relationship of the defect underlying the two disorders.

Spranger and Wiedemann [7] classified disorders which appeared to share some features of mucopolysaccharidoses as well as of sphingolipidoses under the term *mucolipidoses*. In this classification, I-cell disease and pseudo-Hurler polydystrophy were assigned numbers II and III, respectively. Time has shown that the classification was premature, for the primary defect of mucolipidoses II and III is now understood to differ in a fundamental way from that of the other mucolipidoses and,

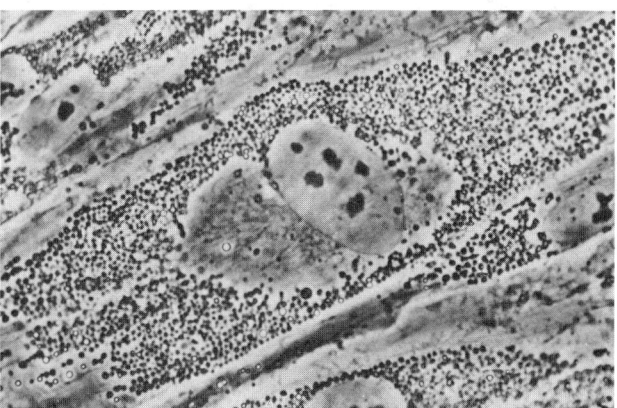

Figure 37-1 Cultured skin fibroblast from patient with I-cell disease, seen by phase contrast microscopy. The dense inclusions, which give the disease its name, are characteristically present throughout the cytoplasm, except for an area next to the nucleus. Magnification, ×740. (*Photograph kindly provided by Dr. Jules Leroy, University of Antwerp.*)

in fact, from that of all other known lysosomal storage diseases. But since the terms mucolipidosis II and mucolipidosis III (ML II and ML III) have become established in the literature as synonyms for I-cell disease and pseudo-Hurler polydystrophy, respectively, we will use them in this chapter.

CLINICAL MANIFESTATIONS

Mucolipidosis II

The patients demonstrate striking Hurler-like manifestations at an earlier age than are seen in the Hurler syndrome (Fig. 37-2). Indeed, cases described as neonatal Hurler syndrome [8] undoubtedly represented ML II. As in the Hurler syndrome (see Chap. 36), patients have coarse facial features and severe skeletal changes including kyphoscoliosis, lumbar gibbus, anterior beaking and wedging of vertebral bodies, widening of the ribs and proximal pointing of the metacarpi. Congenital dislocation of the hips occurs, and hernias and bilateral talipes equinovarus [9] may be present at birth. Retardation of growth and psychomotor development are progressive and severe. Marked joint contractures and frequent respiratory infections are major clinical problems. The skin is tight and thickened. The eyelids and skin around the eyes are puffy.

Striking gingival hyperplasia is a clinical feature that distinguishes ML II from the Hurler syndrome. Furthermore, corneal opacities, although present to a mild degree in later stages of the disorder or evident only by slit-lamp examination, are never as striking as in the Hurler syndrome. Increase in corneal diameter has been observed. Cardiomegaly may be evident from early in life [10]. Hepatosplenomegaly is often but not always present. Congestive heart failure is often present terminally. Death usually occurs before age 5.

The radiological changes of ML II are those of severe dysostosis multiplex. In addition, there are some distinctive features already evident at birth, such as periosteal cuffing of the shaft of the humerus and other long bones [8]. Premature cranial synostosis has been evident under 1 month of age [11].

In contrast to the Hurler syndrome, urinary excretion of mucopolysaccharides is within normal range.

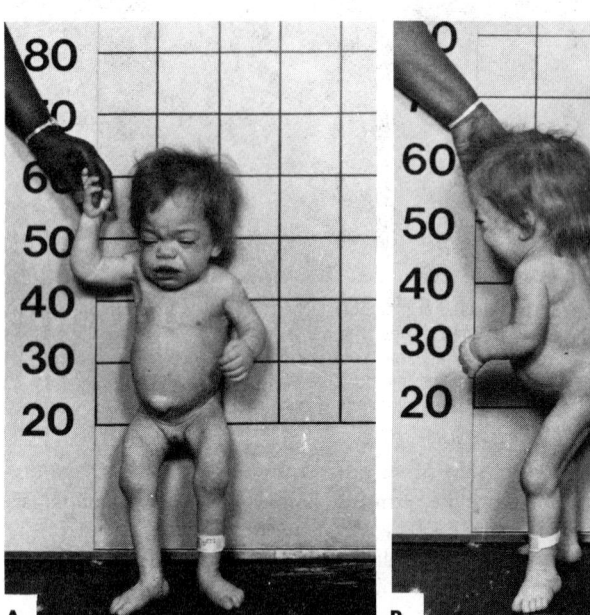

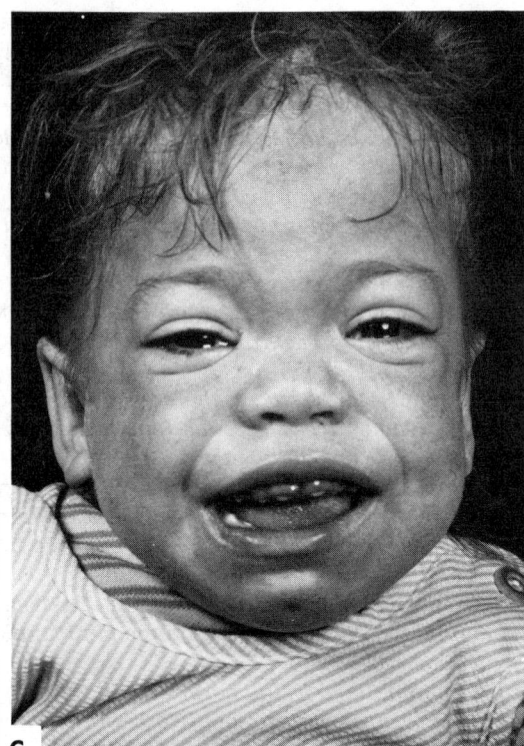

Figure 37-2 Mucolipidosis II (I-cell disease) in a 27-month-old child. Abnormality in appearance was noted by the parents when she was 2 months of age. Down syndrome and later Hurler syndrome were the diagnosis until she was 27 months old, when the correct diagnosis was suspected on clinical grounds and the serocellular paradox in level of lysosomal enzymes was demonstrated. The patient demonstrated severe dysostosis multiplex, mental retardation, hepatomegaly, cardiomegaly, recurrent upper respiratory infections, umbilical hernia, and diastasis recti abdominis—all progressive. Slit-lamp examination showed corneal clouding, which subsequently became grossly evident. The patient died of pneumonia at age 55 months. *A.*, *B.* Front and side views. Coarse facies, prominent abdomen, umbilical hernia, joint contractures, and upper lumbar kyphosis are evident. In the limbs the muscle mass was reduced and had a woody feel. *C.* Detail of facies, also showing gingival hyperplasia.

Mucolipidosis III

The patients usually present at age 4 or 5 years with stiff joints as a main feature. The stiffness is evident in the fingers, elbows, hips, and knees and may lead to a semicrouching stance (Fig. 37-3). Rheumatoid arthritis was suspected in a number of these patients at the time of onset of their joint stiffness. Growth is moderately retarded in the prepubertal period, and mental development may likewise be mildly impaired. A systolic murmur indicative of aortic valve involvement or the murmur of aortic regurgitation appears late in the first decade in some cases. Corneal clouding is grossly detectable by age 7 or 8 and is demonstrable by slit-lamp examination earlier.

The facial features are coarsened, suggesting a mild mucopolysaccharidosis, but there is no excess urinary excretion of acid mucopolysaccharides. The joint stiffness does not progress after puberty.

Carpal tunnel compression is a conspicuous feature by late childhood and contributes to the disability in the hands. Hypertrophic skin pads develop over the knuckles and at other pressure points. Drastic changes in the hips, specifically in the femoral heads, occur. Progressive destruction of the hip joints is a disabling feature in most ML III patients by their late teens.

The oldest patient known to us is in his thirties. In the older literature survival into the sixties has been described in cases that may represent ML III. Differentiation from a mild form of MPS VI (mucopolysaccharidosis VI) is difficult on the basis of clinical description (see Chap. 36).

Greatest diagnostic confusion occurs between ML III and the form of MPS VI that has intermediate severity. For example, three patients ascertained by Kelly et al. [5] as satisfying clinical criteria for ML III were found in fact to have a deficiency of aryltsulfatase B, as well as cell culture characteristics of MPS VI. (Two of these patients, brother and sister, had been reported by Melhem et al. [12] and by Quigley and Goldberg [13] from the radiographic and electronmicroscopic points of view, respectively, as cases of ML III.)

Severe pelvic and peculiar vertebral changes revealed by radiography are rather specific for ML III [14]. Spranger et al. [14] noted low iliac wings with hypoplastic bodies, flattened and irregular proximal femoral epiphyses with the femoral necks in valgus position, underdevelopment of the posterior parts of the vertebral bodies in the dorsal spine, and hypoplasia of the anterior third of the vertebral bodies in the lumbar spine. Kelly et al. [11] usefully contrasted the radiographic findings in ML III with those in the intermediate form of MPS VI, the mild form of MPS II, and the Hurler-Scheie variant of MPS I. In the brother-sister pairs that have been observed (see Ref. 11) clinical and radiographic changes have been rather consistently less severe in the female than in the male.

Relief of carpal tunnel compression and orthopedic procedures on the hips are worthwhile in these patients.

PATHOLOGY

Mucolipidosis II

Phase contrast microscropy of cultured fibroblasts shows the numerous and striking inclusions which have given this disease its name (Fig. 37-1). Electron microscopy shows that the inclusions are filled with osmophilic membranous material [15].

In the skin subepithelial connective tissue is hypercellular, and the numerous histiocytes and fibroblasts are extensively vacuolated [16]. Electron microscopy shows that the inclusions are single-membrane-limited and consist of fibrogranular and membranous lamellar material. Schwann cells and the axonal processes of peripheral nerves, as well as vascualr perithelial cells, show similar changes. Storage is relatively inconspicuous in parenchymal cells, for example, in the liver, and involves primarily connective tissue (mesenchymal) cells [17, 18]. Renal glomerular and tubular epithelium is markedly affected [17–19]. Pathologic changes have been seen in the

tissues of a 15-week-old fetus [20], and in placenta at the fourteenth week of pregnancy [21].

Postmortem examination of an 8-month-old infant showed thickening of the heart valves, infiltration of the myocardium by vacuolated fibroblasts, and subintimal proliferation of connective tissue in the aorta [18]. Myocardial cells also showed storage material.

Mucolipidosis III

To our knowledge, no autopsy studies of ML III patients have been reported. Histologic changes in corneal biopsies [22] are qualitatively identical to those seen in ML II [16, 23]. Cultured fibroblasts show phase-dense inclusions, though not always as prominently as in ML II fibroblasts [4, 6].

GENETICS

Mucolipidoses II and III are inherited as autosomal recessive disorders. Affected brothers and sisters have been reported, as well as parental consanguinity [5–7]. The precise genetic relationship between the two disorders is not known, but since ML III is likely to represent a case of residual activity of the phosphorylating enzyme that is totally lacking in ML II (see below), the diseases might be produced by different mutations at the same locus. Both disorders appear to be very rare in the United States and in Europe. A small Arab community with a high frequency of the ML II gene has been reported [24], and cases of ML II have been reported in Japan [25].

Figure 37-3 Mucolipidosis III (pseudo-Hurler polydystrophy) in A. a brother aged 11 and B. a sister aged 9¼ years. In this and other brother-sister pairs the male is more severely affected. In the boy, inability to raise his arms above the head and deformity of the hands were first noted at age 2 years. Growth was severely retarded after age 6 years. He performed at a "below age" level in an ungraded school. By age 11 he could not climb stairs. He showed stiff joints, claw hands, the murmur of aortic regurgitation, and extensive radiographic skeletal changes, including severe and characteristic changes in the hips. He had no hepatosplenomegaly and no corneal clouding, even by slit-lamp examination. At age 17 corneal clouding was clearly evident.

The mother observed that his sister had similar deformities when she was 3½ to 4 years old. She was held back in the first grade because of poor performance. Slit-lamp examination suggested a slight corneal haze. At age 13 the murmur of aortic regurgitation was demonstrated. In both ribs, attempts at surgical correction of severe bilateral hip disease were only partially successful. IQ was estimated to be about 70 in both.

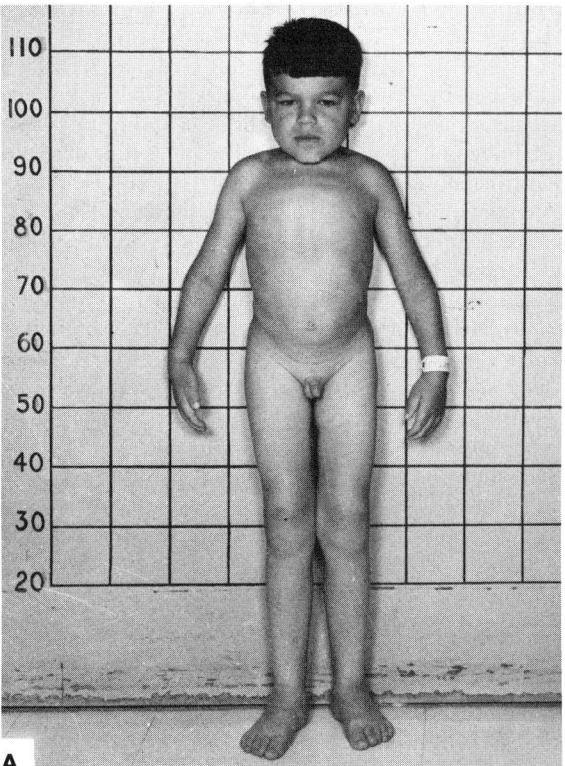
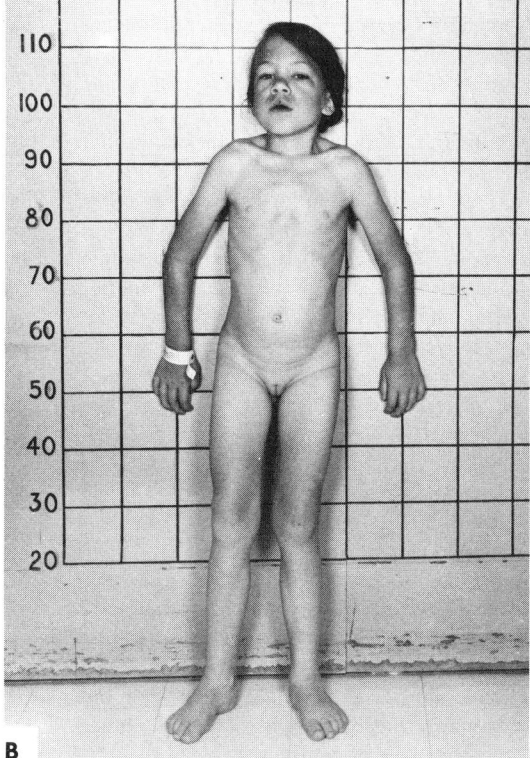

Prenatal diagnosis (see later) is possible, but heterozygotes cannot be reliably identified.

Mucolipidosis II fibroblasts fused with fibroblasts from patients with single lysosomal enzyme defects (e.g., Sandhoff disease, G_{M1} gangliosidosis, mannosidosis, and sialidosis) have resulted in each case in complementation [26–28]. The ML II fibroblasts are presumed to furnish the genetic information for a normal polypeptide and the other mutant cells for the posttranslational modification. Complementation was still observed when ML II fibroblasts were fused with enucleated cells of the other mutants, indicating that the posttranslational factor was stable and active in the cytoplasm for the 3-day duration of the experiment [29]. Hybrids of ML II and mouse fibroblasts have produced normal human acid hydrolases [30]. No complementation occurred upon fusion of fibroblasts from ML II and ML III patients, with the exception of one ML III line which must have been genetically distinct [31].

THE BIOCHEMICAL DEFECT

I-Cell Hydrolases Lack a Recognition Marker

Wiesmann and colleagues [32, 33] at the University of Bern were the first to note that fibroblasts from ML II patients were deficient in β-hexosaminidase, arylsulfatase A, and β-glucuronidase and that the culture medium contained these activities at an elevated level that approximately equaled the cellular deficit. These observations were confirmed in many laboratories [e.g., 34]; similar results were found for mucolipidosis III [5, 35, 36]. Wiesmann and coworkers [32] proposed that hydrolases leaked out of ML II fibroblasts because of some defect in the lysosomal or plasma membranes.

Hickman and Neufeld [37] tested the leakage hypothesis by taking advantage of the finding that even normal fibroblasts release small amounts of acid hydrolases into the medium and that these secreted enzymes can be endocytosed. It was shown that ML II cells take up and retain normal enzymes in normal fashion, thus ruling out lysosomal leakage. On the other hand, enzymes released by ML II fibroblasts fail to be endocytosed by other cells. This suggested that the defect is in the hydrolases themselves. The defect in ML II was postulated to be in some posttranslational modification that would produce a special structure, a "recognition marker," that would normally enable acid hydrolases to reach lysosomes. The hypothesis was subsequently extended to ML III cells [38, 39]. It took nearly a decade and the effort of several laboratories to understand the nature of that modification.

Chemistry of the Recognition Marker

The marker was postulated to be a carbohydrate, because it was possible to reduce the endocytosis of β-hexosaminidase by treating it with periodate (a reagent that selectively attacks carbohydrate residues) under conditions that did not destroy catalytic activity [38]. But direct chemical identification of the marker carbohydrate was not technically feasible at the time; ingenious indirect methods were therefore developed.

These methods were based on the proposition that the rec-

ognition marker would facilitate the endocytosis of proteins because it would allow them to bind to the cell surface. The Michaelis-Menten kinetics of uptake supported that prediction since such kinetics indicate binding to saturable sites [40, 41]. Therefore analogues of the recognition marker would be expected to act as competitive inhibitors of endocytosis and the closer the structural resemblance, the more effective the inhibition. Quantitative measurements of inhibition constants for uptake of a number of enzymes showed that of all simple sugars, mannose was the best inhibitor. Mannosides were better inhibitors than free mannose, and mannose-6-phosphate was most inhibitory [41–43]. In addition, phosphatase treatment of β-glucuronidase and of other enzymes prevented their subsequent endocytosis. On the basis of such evidence, Kaplan, Achord, and Sly [42] proposed that the recognition marker contains mannose-6-phosphate, a structure for which there was at the time no obvious precedent in mammalian glycoproteins.

With this clue to the nature of the marker, direct chemical analysis became feasible. It was realized that phosphorylated sugars in mammalian glycoproteins had probably not been observed because of the ubiquitous presence of phosphatases in enzyme preparations. With appropriate precautions to inhibit phosphatases and with the development of very sensitive micromethods, mannose-6-phosphate was demonstrated in a number of lysosomal enzymes [44–46].

Using [^{32}P]phosphate to label enzymes in lysosomal enzyme cultures, Bach et al. [47] and Hasilik and Neufeld [48] showed the presence of mannose-6-phosphate in enzymes elaborated by normal fibroblasts and its absence in enzymes made by cells from I-cell patients (Fig. 37-4). Enzymes synthesized by fibroblasts from several ML III patients had a markedly reduced but detectable level of phosphorylation [49].

The Probable Primary Defect in ML II and ML III

The mechanism by which lysosomal enzymes might become phosphorylated has emerged from the structure of the phosphorylated oligosaccharide [50–52]. The phosphate on the 6 position of mannose is also linked to the 1 position of α-N-acetylglucosamine. This diesterified form, shown in Fig. 37-5, appears to be a precursor of the recognition marker. A microsomal enzyme that releases the N-acetylglucosamine from the diester has been identified [53, 54]. It is distinct from lysosomal α-N-acetylglucosaminidase and is present in fibroblasts of I-cell patients.

The most likely precursor of such a structure would be a sugar nucleotide, such as UDP-N-acetylglucosamine, from which a phosphate would be transferred together with the N–acetylglucosamine. This would be analogous to the synthesis of mannose phosphate diesters in yeast. Evidence for such a reaction in normal fibroblasts and for its absence in I-cell fibroblasts has been recently presented [55, 55a–c]. The reaction proceeds at a very low rate in fibroblasts of ML III patients [55c].

Other Defects of Acid Hydrolases in ML II and ML III: Molecular Size

Absence of phosphorylation is not the only difference between

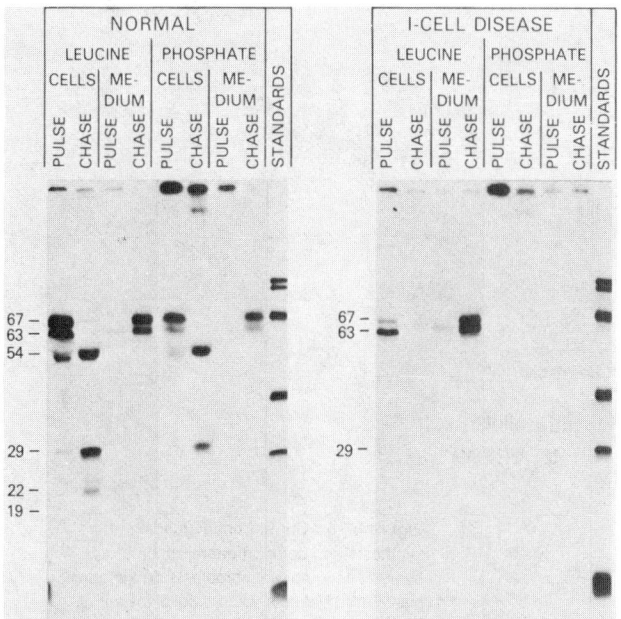

Figure 37-4 Biosynthesis of β-hexosaminidase in normal and I-cell fibroblasts. The numbers refer to molecular weight, in thousands, of enzyme subunits. The 67K band is the α precursor chain; 63K, β precursor; 54K, mature α; 29K and smaller fragments, mature β. The fibroblasts were exposed to [³H]leucine and [³²P]phosphate for a 3-h pulse, followed by a 20-h chase. β-Hexosaminidase was immunoprecipitated and the chains separated by polyacrylamide gel electrophoresis under reducing and denaturing conditions. Each isotopic label was visualized with minimal interference from the other. Note the absence of phosphorylation, as well as the lack of mature intracellular β-hexosaminidase in the I-cell fibroblasts [48].

enzymes from normal fibroblasts and enzymes from the fibroblasts of patients with ML II and ML III. Acid hydrolases (e.g., β-hexosaminidase, cathepsin D, and α-glucosidase) are synthesized in normal fibroblasts as precursors of higher molecular weight than the eventual size found in lysosomal enzymes [56]. The trimming occurs by limited proteolysis [57] and is presumed to occur in lysosomes. Secreted hydrolases are also of the larger precursor size, both in normal and abnormal fibroblasts. Thus, the bulk of ML II and ML III hydrolases (which are secreted) are of higher molecular weight than the bulk of normal hydrolases (which are intralysosomal). The size difference is merely a consequence of the inability of ML II hydrolases to reach their lysosomal destination where limited proteolysis would occur.

Sialic Acid and the Mucolipidosis Defect

Acid hydrolases secreted by ML II fibroblasts are more anionic

[58, 59] and bind differently to lectins [60, 61] than their normal counterparts. This has been attributed to an increased level of sialic acid. In addition, glycopeptides and oligosaccharides excreted in the urine [62, 63] or stored in fibroblasts [64] of ML II patients are very rich in sialic acid.

Since sialidase activity is very low in the fibroblasts of I-cell disease patients [64, 65], sialidase deficiency had been suggested as the primary defect [66]. However, a number of experimental results failed to substantiate this hypothesis. First, removal of sialic acid failed to restore the capacity for endocytosis to secreted ML II enzymes [67]. Second, infection of I-cell fibroblasts with influenza virus, which restored intracellular sialidase, had no effect on enzyme localization [68]. Third, in mucolipidosis I, where sialidase deficiency is clearly the primary defect, the pleiotropic manifestations of I-cell disease do not occur [69, 70].

It seems more useful to consider sialidase as one of the many acid hydrolases affected by the mutation in ML II and ML III. If sialidase deficiency is more profound than that of other hydrolases, it is perhaps because of the unusual lability of that enzyme in an inappropriate environment.

The excess of sialic acid in ML II enzymes can be attributed to the mode of synthesis of oligosaccharide chains in glycoproteins. The first steps in the synthesis of sialylated (or "complex") carbohydrate chains are the same as for the carbohydrate chains that contain predominantly mannose. Sialylation occurs after additional trimming of the high mannose-type chains and rebuilding into the complex type [71]. In normal fibroblasts phosphorylation of the high mannose-type chains would prevent further changes; in I-cell disease, absence of phosphorylation would allow these additional reactions to proceed.

An Explanation of the Multiple Defects of the ML II and ML III Mutations

The pleiotropic consequences of the primary defect can be readily understood from the sequence of events shown schematically in Fig. 37-6. In normal fibroblasts precursor acid hydrolases are glycosylated and phosphorylated. The mannose-6-phosphate termini are recognized by receptors present in the endoplasmic reticulum or Golgi region [72]. The receptor molecules bind the hydrolases and deliver them to lysosomes, where the hydrolases are trimmed by limited proteolysis to the mature form. The precise mechanism by which the hydrolases are translocated from the site of synthesis to the lysosomes is not clear. An earlier hypothesis considered the secretion and subsequent endocytosis of the hydrolases as obligatory to their insertion into lysosomes [37]. It has been shown, however, that this pathway carries only a small part of

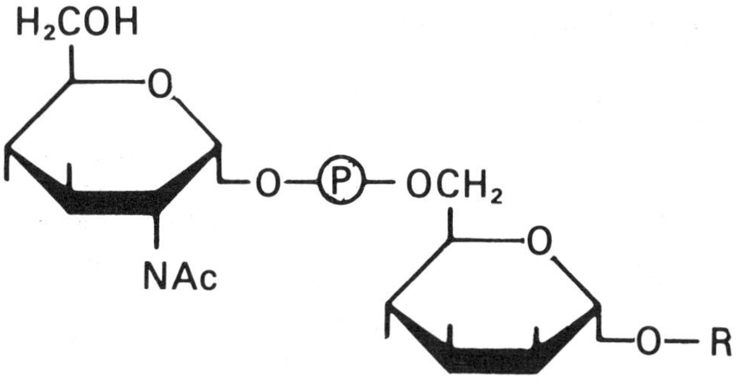

Figure 37-5 Structure of the phosphodiester N-acetylglucosamine-1-phosphate-6-mannose, the intermediate in the synthesis of the mannose-6-phosphate recognition marker. R represents the oligosaccharide, with 6 mannose to 8 mannose residues, on the newly synthesized acid hydrolases [50–52].

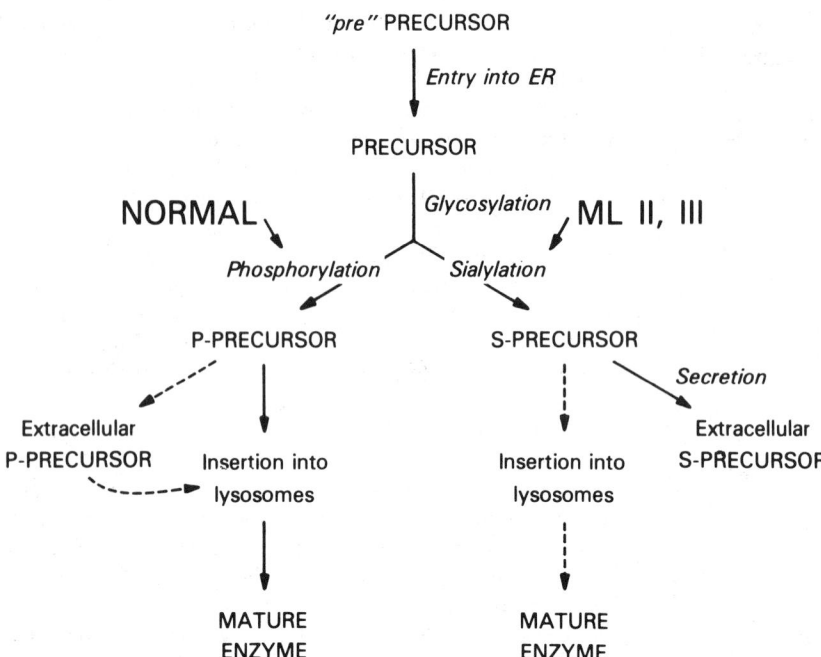

Figure 37-6 Current understanding of the synthesis and compartmentalization of acid hydrolases in normal fibroblasts and in fibroblasts from patients with mucolipidosis II or III. P-precursor = phosphorylated precursor; S-precursor = sialylated precursor.

newly synthesized hydrolases [73, 74]. Most hydrolases are transported to lysosomes without secretion as free enzyme into the medium. Whether that transport is purely intracellular or perhaps by way of the cell surface [75] is not known.

In mucolipidoses II and III, the complete or partial deficiency of the phosphorylating step deprives acid hydrolases of the recognition marker and hence of their key to entry into lysosomes. Instead, the hydrolases are secreted, perhaps after additional carbohydrate modifications (to give "complex" sialylated chains) have been introduced along the secretory route. The secreted hydrolases, devoid of mannose-6-phosphate recognition markers, cannot be taken up by endocytosis and thus remain in the medium. Since little or no proteolysis occurs extracellularly, the hydrolases remain in precursor form. The deficiency in intracellular hydrolase activity need not be precisely compensated by an equal level of extracellular enzyme, since the stability of the hydrolases may differ in the extracellular and lysosomal milieu (as may be the case for sialidase and β-galactosidase, which are low both intra- and extracellularly).

The intracellular deficiency of many lysosomal hydrolases has predictable consequences for lysosomal storage in affected cells. A variety of substances, including [^{35}S] mucopolysaccharide [76], lipids [77], and oligosaccharides [64], accumulate in fibroblasts in vitro and presumably in vivo.

Unexplained Biochemical Findings in Mucolipidoses II and III

Several conceptual problems remain. Acid phosphatase and β-glucosidase appear normal in amount and distribution in I-cell disease fibroblasts. Are they incorporated into lysosomes by a different recognition mechanism? Some kinds of cells appear to be little affected in I-cell disease (e.g., hepatocytes, neurons, Kupffer cells, granulocytes). Do these cells make use of a different gene encoding the phosphorylating enzyme or of a different recognition mechanism to target acid hydrolases to lysosomes? An alternative that should be seriously considered

is that enzymes secreted by fibroblasts might be taken up by other cells that have receptors for the endocytosis on nonphosphorylated oligosaccharides [78]. For example, it has been shown that enzymes secreted by I-cell fibroblasts are recognized and taken into nonparenchymal liver cells which have receptors for mannose residues [79]. Sialylated I-cell hydrolases could, if desialylated, be endocytosed into hepatocytes, which have receptors for asialoglycoproteins [80].

Are proteins other than lysosomal hydrolases affected in mucolipidoses II and III? It is known that fibroblasts from patients with I-cell disease are unusually sensitive to freezing, a property that can be transmitted to Sindbis or VSV virus grown in these fibroblasts [81, 82]. The sensitivity has been attributed to the glycoproteins or glycolipids of the plasma membrane. The activity of some glycosyltransferases on the surface of ML II fibroblasts is markedly altered, again pointing to changes in the plasma membrane [83]. On the other hand, circulating glycoproteins such as immunoglobulins have been shown to have a normal carbohydrate structure in I-cell disease [84].

Related Disorders to Be Anticipated

Examination of the pathway depicted in Fig. 37-6 allows a prediction of several genetic disorders that would affect different steps in the pathway. For instance, a defect in removal of the N-acetylglucosamine from the diester or in the synthesis of the oligosaccharide acceptor might be expected to have phenotypic consequences similar to those of ML II or ML III. Of great interest is the possibility of encountering individuals with a defective receptor for lysosomal enzymes. To date, no such patients have been reported, but mutant Chinese hamster ovary fibroblasts with defective mannose-6-phosphate receptors have been isolated and found to secrete a greater proportion of their newly synthesized enzymes than the parental line from which they were derived [85, 86].

Finally, the scheme in Fig. 37-6 predicts that the polypeptide portion of the hydrolase precursor should contain a sequence that would identify the molecule as a protein destined for lysosomes, and therefore an appropriate substrate for the phosphorylating enzyme. Mutation in such a sequence would cause a mislocation of the affected hydrolase but would probably not be pleiotropic, i.e., would not affect multiple enzymes.

DIAGNOSIS

Of the many acid hydrolases affected in ML II and ML III, for diagnostic purposes a laboratory should choose the ones that it can assay most easily and reliably. A ten- to twentyfold elevation of β-hexosaminidase, iduronate sulfatase, and aryl sulfatase A activity in serum is diagnostic of the two disorders [5, 87, 88]. When fibroblasts are available, the characteristic pattern of deficiencies may be used [5, 34, 89], as can the ratio of extracellular to intracellular levels of acid hydrolase activities, or even the detection of particular isoenzymes [90]. The same assays are not informative if performed on leukocytes, for the level of acid hydrolases is normal in granulocytes although somewhat reduced in lymphocytes [91, 92]. Measurement of [^{35}S]mucopolysaccharide accumulation in fibroblasts [93] is a useful auxiliary test, but an elevated level does not distinguish between ML II or III and the mucopolysaccharidoses. The differential diagnosis of ML II from ML III is based on clinical findings and generally cannot be performed on the basis of acid hydrolase activity and localization since these are similar in the two disorders (but significantly higher residual activities of β-galactosidase [94] and sialidase [95] have been reported for ML III).

The prenatal diagnosis of ML II has been made on the basis of elevated acid hydrolases in amniotic fluid [20, 96–98], different isoenzymes in the fluid [99], or multiple deficiency of acid hydrolases and elevated accumulation of [^{35}S]mucopolysaccharide in cells cultured from amniotic fluid [20, 96–98].

The acid hydrolases of ML II heterozygotes show some qualitative and quantitative differences from those of normal individuals [100–102]. There is considerable overlap, however, and the differences are not sufficiently reliable for genetic counseling. As the primary defect in the pathway of phosphorylation of the acid hydrolases is studied in depth, better tests for heterozygotes may be developed.

REFERENCES

1. DEMARS RI, LEROY JG: The remarkable cells cultured from a human with Hurler's syndrome: An approach to visual selection for *in vitro* genetic studies. *In Vitro* 2:107, 1967
2. LEROY, JG, DEMARS RI: Mutant enzymatic and cytological phenotypes in cultured human fibroblasts. *Science* 157:804, 1967
3. TONDEUR M, VAMOS-HURWITZ E, MOCKEL-POHL S, DEREUME JP, CREMER N, LOEB H: Clinical, biochemical, and ultrastructural studies in a case of chondrodystrophy presenting the I-cell phenotype in culture. *J Pediatr* 79:366, 1971
4. TAYLOR HA, THOMAS GH, MILLER CS, KELLY TE, SIGGERS D: Mucolipidosis III (pseudo-Hurler polydystrophy): Cytological and ultrastructural observations of cultured fibroblast cells. *Clin Genet* 4:388, 1973
5. KELLY TE, THOMAS GH, TAYLOR HA JR, MCKUSICK VA, SLY WS, GLASER JH, ROBINOW M, LUZZATTI L, ESPERITU C, FEINGOLD M, BULL MJ, ASHENHURST EM, IVES EJ: Mucolipidosis III (pseudo-Hurler polydystrophy): Clinical and laboratory studies in a series of 12 patients. *Johns Hopkins Med J* 137:156, 1975
6. STEIN H, BERMAN ER, LIONI N, MERIN S, SLESKIN J, COHEN T: Pseudo-Hurler polydystrophy (mucolipidosis III): A clinical biochemical, and ultrastructural study. *Isr J Med Sci* 10:463, 1974
7. SPRANGER JW, WIEDEMANN HR: The genetic mucolipidoses. *Humangenetik* 9:113, 1970
8. CAFFEY J: Gargoylism (Hunter-Hurler disease, dysostosis multiplex, lipochondrodystrophy): Prenatal and neonatal bone lesions and their early postnatal evolution. *Am J Roentgenol* 67:715, 1952
9. CIPOLLONI C, BOLDRINI A, DONTIEE, MAIORANA A, COPPA GB: Neonatal mucolipidosis II (I-cell disease): Clinical, radiological and biochemical studies in a case. *Helv Paediatr Acta* 35:85, 1980
10. SPRITZ RA, DOUGHTY RA, SPACKMAN TJ, MURNANE MJ, COATES PM, KOLDOVSKY O, ZACKAI EH: Neonatal presentation of I-cell disease. *J Pediatr* 93:954, 1978
11. PATRIQUIN HB, KAPLAN P, KIND HP, GIEDION A: Neonatal mucolipidosis II (I-cell disease): Clinical and radiologic features in three cases. *Am J Roentgenol* 129:37, 1977
12. MELHEM R, DORST JP, SCOTT CI JR, MCKUSICK VA: Roentgen findings in mucolipidosis III (pseudo-Hurler polydystrophy). *Radiology* 106:153, 1973
13. QUIGLEY HA, GOLDBERG MF: Conjunctival ultrastructure in mucolipidosis III (pseudo-Hurler polydystrophy). *Invest Ophthalmol* 10:568, 1971
14. SPRANGER JW, LANGER LO JR, WIEDEMANN HR: *Bone Dysplasias, an Atlas of Constitutional Disorders of Skeletal Development.* Philadelphia, Saunders, 1974
15. HANAI J, LEROY J, O'BRIEN JS: Ultrastructure of cultured fibroblasts in I-cell disease. *Am J Dis Child* 122:34, 1971
16. KENYON KR, SENSENBRENNER JA: Mucolipidosis II (I-cell disease): Ultrastructural observations of conjunctiva and skin. *Invest Ophthalmol* 10:555, 1971
17. GILBERT EF, DAWSON G, ZURHEIN GM, OPITZ JM, SPRANGER JW: I-cell disease, mucolipidosis II—Pathological, histochemical, ultrastructural and biochemical observation in four cases. *Z Kinderheiikd* 114:259, 1973
18. MARTIN JJ, LEROY JG, FARRIAUX JP, FONTAINE G, DESNICK RJ, CABELLO A: I-cell disease (mucolipidosis II)—A report on its pathology. *Acta Neuropathol* 33:285, 1975
19. SCOTT CR, LAGUNOFF D, PRITZL P: A mucopolysaccharide storage disease with involvement of the renal glomerular epithelium. *Am J Med* 54:549, 1973
20. AULA P, RAPOLA J, AUTIO S, RAIVIO K, KARJALAINEN O: Prenatal diagnosis and fetal pathology of I-cell disease (mucolipidosis type II). *J Pediatr* 87:221, 1975
21. RAPOLA J, AULA P: Morphology of the placenta in fetal I-cell disease. *Clin Genet* 11:107, 1977
22. LIBERT J, KENYON KR, MAUMENEE JH: Mucolipidosis III (pseudo-Hurler polydystrophy) ultrastructure of conjunctional biopsies. *Metab Ophthalmol* 1:145, 1977
23. LIBERT J, VAN HOOF F, FARRIAUX JP, TOUSSAINT D: Ocular findings in I-cell disease (mucolipidosis type II). *Am J Ophthalmol* 83:617, 1977
24. BACH G: Personal communication, 1980
25. OWADA M: Personal communication, 1981
26. OKADA S, KATO T, YABUUCHI H, OKADA, Y: The complementation of β-galactosidase in fused cells of mucolipidosis II with another variant of β-galactosidase deficiency using new single cell enzyme assay. *Biochem Biophys Res Commun* 88:559, 1979
27. D'AZZO A, HALLEY DJJ, HOOGEVEEN A, GALJAARD H: Correction of I-cell defect by hybridization with lysosomal enzyme deficient human fibroblasts. *Am J Hum Genet* 32:519, 1980
28. HOOGEVEEN AT, VERHEIJEN FW, D'AZZO A, GALJAARD A: Genetic heterogeneity in human neuraminidase deficiency. *Nature* 285:500, 1980
29. D'AZZO A, KONINGS A, VERKERK A, JONGKIND JO, GALJAARD H: Fusion with enucleated fibroblasts corrects "I-cell" defect. *Exptl Cell Res* 127:484, 1980
30. CHAMPION MJ, SHOWS TB: Correction of human mucolipidosis II enzyme abnormalities in somatic cell hybrids. *Nature* 270:64, 1977
31. GRAVEL RA, GRAVEL YL, MILLER AL, LOWDEN JA: Genetic complementation analysis of I-cell disease and pseudo-Hurler polydystrophy, in Callahan JW, Lowden JA (eds): *Lysosomes and Lysosomal Storage Diseases.* New York, Raven, 1981, p 289
32. WIESMANN UN, LIGHTBODY J, VASSELLA F, HERSCHKOWITZ NN: Multiple lysosomal enzyme deficiency due to enzyme leakage? *N Engl J Med* 284:109, 1971
33. WIESMANN UN, HERSCHKOWITZ NN: Studies on the pathogenetic mechanism of I-cell disease in cultured fibroblasts. *Pediatr Res* 8:865, 1974
34. LEROY JG, HO MW, MACBRINN MC, ZIELKE K, JACOB J, O'BRIEN JS: I-cell disease; biochemical studies. *Pediatr Res* 6:752, 1972
35. BERMAN E, KOHN G, YATSIV S, STEIN H: Acid hydrolase deficiencies and abnormal glycoproteins in mucolipidosis III (pseudo-Hurler polydystrophy). *Clin Chim Acta* 52:115, 1974
36. THOMAS GH, TAYLOR HA, REYNOLDS LW, MILLER CS: Mucolipidosis III (pseudo-Hurler polydystrophy): Multiple lysosomal enzyme abnormalities in serum and cultured fibroblast cells. *Pediatr Res* 7:751, 1973
37. HICKMAN S, NEUFELD EF: A hypothesis for I-cell disease: Defective hydrolases that do not enter lysosomes. *Biochem Biophys Res Commun* 49:992, 1972

38. HICKMAN S, SHAPIRO LJ, NEUFELD EF: A recognition marker required for uptake of a lysosomal enzyme by cultured fibroblasts. *Biochem Res Commun* 57:55, 1974

39. GLASER JH, McALISTER WH, SLY WS: Genetic heterogeneity in multiple lysosomal enzyme hydrolase deficiency. *J Pediatr* 85:192, 1974

40. VON FIGURA K, KRESSE H: Quantitative aspects of pinocytosis and the intracellular fate of N-acetyl-α-D-glucosaminidase in Sanfilippo B fibroblasts. *J Clin Invest* 53:85, 1974

41. SANDO GN, NEUFELD EF: Recognition and receptor-mediated uptake of a lysosomal enzyme, α-L-iduronidase, by cultured human fibroblasts. *Cell* 12:619, 1977

42. KAPLAN A, ACHORD DT, SLY WS: Phosphohexosyl components of a lysosomal enzyme are recognized by pinocytosis receptors on human fibroblasts. *Proc Nat Acad Sci USA* 74:2026, 1977

43. Ullrich K, Mersmann G, Weber E, Von Figura K: Evidence for lysosomal enzyme recognition by human fibroblasts via a phosphorylated carbohydrate moiety. *Biochem J* 170:643, 1978

44. NATOWIZC MR, CHI MM-Y, LOWRY OH, SLY WS: Enzymatic identification of mannose 6-phosphate on the recognition marker for receptor-mediated pinocytosis of β-glucuronidase by human fibroblasts. *Proc Nat Acad Sci USA* 76:4322, 1979

45. DISTLER J, HIEBER V, SAHAGIAN G, SCHMICKEL R, JOURDIAN GW: Identification of mannose 6-phosphate in glycoproteins that inhibit the assimilation of β-galactosidase by fibroblasts. *Proc Nat Acad Sci USA* 76:4235, 1979

46. VON FIGURA K, KLEIN U: Isolation and characterization of phosphorylated oligosaccharides from α-N-acetylglucosaminidase that are recognized by cell surface receptors. *Eur J Biochem* 94:347, 1979

47. BACH G, BARGAL R, CANTZ M: I-cell disease: Deficiency of extracellular hydrolase phosphorylation. *Biochem Biophys Res Commun* 91:476, 1979

48. HASILIK A, NEUFELD EF: Biosynthesis of lysosomal enzymes in fibroblasts; phosphorylation of mannose residues. *J Biol Chem* 255:4946, 1980

49. ROBEY PG, NEUFELD EF: Defective phosphorylation and processing of β-hexosaminidase by intact cultured fibroblasts from patients with mucolipidosis III. *Arch Biochem Biophys*, in press

50. TABAS I, KORNFELD S: Biosynthetic intermediates of β-glucuronidase contain high mannose oligosaccharides with blocked phosphate residues. *J Biol Chem* 255:6633, 1980

51. VARKI A, KORNFELD S: Structural studies of phosphorylated high mannose-type oligosaccharides. *J Biol Chem* 255:10847, 1980

52. HASILIK A, KLEIN U, WAHEED A, STRECKER G, VON FIGURA K: Phosphorylated oligosaccharides in lysosomal enzymes: Identification of α-N-acetylglucosaminyl(1)phospho(6)mannose diester groups. *Proc Nat Acad Sci USA* 77:7074, 1980

53. VARKI A, KORNFELD S: Identification of a rat liver α-N-acetylglucosaminyl phosphodiesterase capable of removing "blocking" α-N-acetylglucosamine residues from phosphorylated high mannose oligosaccharides of lysosomal enzymes. *J Biol Chem* 255:8398, 1980

54. WAHEED A, HASILIK A, VON FIGURA K: Processing of the phosphorylated recognition marker in lysosomal enzymes: Characterization and partial purification of a microsomal α-N-acetylglucosamine phosphodiesterase *J Biol Chem* 256:5717, 1981

55. HASILIK A, WAHEED A, VON FIGURA K: Enzymatic phosphorylation of lysosomal enzymes in the presence of UDP-N-acetylglucosamine. Absence of the activity in I-cell fibroblasts. *Biochem Biophys Res Commun* 98:761, 1981

55a. WAHEED A, POHLMANN R, HASILIK A, VON FIGURA K: Subcellular location of two enzymes involved in the synthesis of phosphorylated recognition markers in lysosomal enzymes. *J Biol Chem* 256:4150, 1981

55b. REITMAN ML, KORNFELD S: UDP-N-acetylglucosamine:glycoprotein N-acetyl-glucosamine-1-phosphotransferase. Proposed enzyme for the phosphorylation of the high mannose oligosaccharide units of lysosomal enzymes. *J Biol Chem* 256:4275, 1981

55c. REITMAN AL, VARKI A, KORNFELD S: Fibroblasts from patients with I-cell disease and pseudo-Hurler polydystrophy are deficient in uridine 5'-diphosphate-N-acetylglucosamine:glycoprotein N-acetylglucosaminylphosphotransferase activity. *J Clin Invest* 67:1574, 1981

56. HASILIK A, NEUFELD EF: Biosynthesis of lysosomal enzymes in fibroblasts; synthesis as precursors of higher molecular weight. *J Biol Chem* 255:4937, 1980

57. FRISCH A, NEUFELD EF: Limited proteolysis of the β-hexosaminidase precursor in a cell-free system. *J Biol Chem* 256:8242, 1981

58. VLADUTIU GD, RATTAZZI M: Abnormal lysosomal hydrolases excreted by cultured fibroblasts in I-cell disease (mucolipidosis II). *Biochem Biophys Res Commun* 67:956, 1975

59. MILLER A: I-cell disease: Isoelectric focusing, concanavalin A-sepharose 4B binding and kinetic properties of human liver β-D-galactosidase. *Biochem Biophys Acta* 522:174, 1978

60. KRESS BC, MILLER AL: Urinary lysosomal hydrolases in mucolipidosis II and mucolipidosis III. *Biochem J* 177:409, 1979

61. ROUSSON R, BEN-YOSEPH Y, FIDDLER MB, NADLER HL: Demonstration of altered acidic hydrolases from patients with mucolipidosis II by lectin titration. *Biochem J* 180:501, 1979

62. STRECKER G, PEERS MC, MICHALSKI JC, HONDI-ASSAH J, FOURNET B, SPIK G, MONTREUIL J, FARRIAUX JP, MAROTEAUX P, DURAND P: Structure of nine sialyl-oligosaccharides accumulated in urine of eleven patients with three different types of sialidosis. *Eur J Biochem* 35:391, 1977

63. OKADA S, KATO T, MIURA S, YABUUCHI H, NISHIGASKI M, KOBATA A, CHIYO H, FURUYAMA JI: Hyper-sialyloligosacchariduria in mucolipidoses: a method for diagnosis. *Clin Chim Acta* 86:159, 1978

64. THOMAS GH, TILLER JR GE, REYNOLDS LW, MILLER CS, BACE JW: Increased levels of sialic acid associated with sialidase deficiency in I-cell disease (mucolipidosis II) fibroblasts. *Biochem Biophys Res Commun* 71:188, 1976

65. STRECKER G, MICHALSKI JC, MONTREUIL J, FARRIAUX JP: Deficit in neuraminidase associated with mucolipidosis II (I-cell disease). *Biomedicine* 25:238, 1976

66. STRECKER G, MICHALSKI JC: Biochemical basis of six different types of sialidosis *FEBS Lett* 85:20, 1978

67. VLADUTIU GD, RATTAZZI MC: Desialylation of β-hexosaminidase and its effect on uptake by fibroblasts. *Biochim Biophys Acta* 539:31, 1978

68. SPRITZ RA, COATES PM, LIEF FS: I-cell disease: Intracellular desialylation of lysosomal enzymes using an influenza virus vector. *Biochim Biophys Acta* 582:164, 1979

69. CANTZ M, MESSER H: Oligosaccharide and ganglioside neuraminidase activities of mucolipidosis I (sialidosis) and mucolipidosis II (I-cell disease) fibroblasts. *Eur J Biochem* 97:113, 1979

70. LOWDEN JA, O'BRIEN JS: Sialidosis: A review of human neuraminidase deficiency. *Am J Hum Genet* 31:1, 1979

71. SCHACHTER H, ROSEMAN R: Mammalian glycosyltransferases. Their role in the synthesis and function of complex carbohydrates and glycolipids, in Lennarz WJ (ed): *The Biochemistry of Glycoproteins and Proteoglycans.* New York, Plenum, 1980, p 85

72. FISCHER HD, GONZALEZ-NORIEGA A, SLY WS, MORRE DJ: Phosphomannosyl-enzyme receptors in rat liver. Subcellular distribution and role in intracellular transport of lysosomal enzymes. *J Biol Chem* 255:9608, 1980

73. VLADUTIU GD, RATTAZZI MC: Excretion-reuptake route of β-hexosaminidase in normal and I-cell disease cultured fibroblasts. *J Clin Invest* 63:595, 1979

74. SLY WS, STAHL P: Receptor-mediated uptake of lysosomal enzymes in Silverstein SC (ed): *Transport of Macromolecules in Cellular Systems.* Berlin, Dahlem Konferenzen, 1978, p 229

75. VON FIGURA K, WEBER E: An alternative hypothesis of cellular transport of lysosomal enzymes in fibroblasts. *Biochem J* 176:943, 1978

76. HIEBER V, DISTLER J, JOURDIAN GW, SCHMICKEL R: Accumulation of ³⁵S-mucopolysaccharides in cultured mucolipidosis cells. *Birth Defects: Orig Art Ser* (no 6):307, National Foundation—March of Dimes, New York, 1975

77. DAWSON G, MATALON R, DORFMAN A: Glycosphingolipids in cultured human skin fibroblasts. *J Biol Chem* 247:5951, 1972

78. NEUFELD EF, ASHWELL G: Carbohydrate recognition systems for receptor-mediated pinocytosis, in Lennarz WJ (ed): *The Biochemistry of Glycoproteins and Proteoglycans.* New York, Plenum, 1980, p 241

79. ULLRICH K, VON FIGURA K: Endocytosis of β-N-acetylglucosaminidase from secretions of mucolipidosis II and III fibroblasts by non-parenchymal rat liver cells. *Biochem J* 182:245, 1979

80. ASHWELL G, MORELL HG: The role of surface carbohydrates in the hepatic recognition and transport of circulating glycoproteins. *Adv Enzymol* 41:99, 1974

81. SLY WS, LAGWINSKA E, SCHLESINGER S: Enveloped virus acquires membrane defect when passaged in fibroblasts from I-cell disease patients. *Proc Nat Acad Sci USA* 73:2443, 1976

82. SCHLESINGER S, SLY WS, SCHULZE IT: Effects of neuraminidase on the phenotype of Sindbis virus grown on fibroblasts obtained from patients with I-cell disease. *Virology* 89:409, 1976

83. DI DONATO S, WIESMANN UN, ROSSI E, HERSCHKOWITZ N: Multiple abnormalities of ectoglycosyltransferases in cultured fibroblasts from patients with mucolipidosis II: Possible indication for abnormal plasma membrane glycoprotein. *Pediatr Res* 11:1094, 1977

84. FREEZE H, KRESS BC, WILLIAMS JC, CERDA-RUIZ M, MILLER AL: Carbohydrate composition of purified serum glycoproteins in mucolipidosis II and mucolipidosis III. *Mol Cell Biochem* 21:17, 1978

85. ROBBINS AR, MYEROWITZ R, YOULE RJ, MURRAY GJ, NEVILLE DM JR.: The mannose 6-phosphate receptor of chinese hamster ovary cells. Isolation of mutants with altered receptors. *J Biol Chem* 256:10618, 1981

86. ROBBINS AR, MYEROWITZ R: The mannose 6-phosphate receptor of chinese hamster ovary cells. Compartmentalization of acid hydrolases in mutants with altered receptors. *J Biol Chem* 256:10623, 1981

87. HERD JK, DVORAK AD, WILTSE HE, EISEN JD, KRESS BC, MILLER AL: Mucolipidosis type III—Multiple elevated serum and urine enzyme activities. *Am J Dis Child* 132:1181, 1978

88. LIEBAERS I, NEUFELD EF: Iduronate sulfatase activity in serum, lymphocytes and fibroblasts—Simplified diagnosis of the Hunter syndrome. *Pediatr Res* 10:733, 1976

89. HALL CW, LIEBAERS I, DINATALE P, NEUFELD EF: Enzymic diagnosis of the genetic mucopolysaccharide storage disorders. *Methods Enzymol* 50:439, 1978

90. LIE KK, THOMAS GH, TAYLOR HA, SENSENBRENNER JA: Analysis of N-acetyl-β-D-glucosaminidase in mucolipidosis II (I-cell disease). *Clin Chim Acta* 45:243, 1978

91. KATO E, YOKOI T, TANIGUCHI N: Lysosomal acid hydrolases in lymphocytes of I-cell disease. *Clin Chim Acta* 95:285, 1979

92. TANAKA T, KOBAYASHI M, FUKUDA T, TSUZI Y, USUI T: I-cell disease: Nine lysosomal enzyme levels in lymphocytes and granulocytes. *Hiroshima J Med Sci* 28:190, 1979

93. CANTZ M, KRESSE H, BARTON RW, NEUFELD EF: Corrective factors for inborn errors of mucopolysaccharide metabolism. *Methods Enzymol* 28:884, 1972

94. LEROY JG, O'BRIEN JS: Mucolipidosis II and III: Different residual activity of beta galactosidase in cultured fibroblasts. *Clin Genet* 9:533, 1976

95. FRISCH A, NEUFELD EF: A rapid and sensitive assay for neuraminidase: Application to cultured fibroblasts. *Analyt Biochem* 95:222, 1979

96. HUIJING F, WARREN RJ, McLEOD AGW: Elevated activity of lysosomal enzymes in amniotic fluid of a fetus with mucolipidosis II (I-cell disease). *Clin Chim Acta* 44:453, 1973

97. MATSUDA I, ARASHUMA S, MITSUYAMA T, OKA Y, IKEUCHI T, KANEKO Y, ISHIKAWA M: Prenatal diagnosis of I-cell disease. *Hum Genet* 30:69, 1975

98. GEHLER J, CANTZ M, STOECKENIUS M, SPRANGER J: Prenatal diagnosis of mucolipidosis II (I-cell disease). *Eur J Pediat* 122:201, 1976

99. OWADA M, NISHIYA O, SAKIYAMA T, KITAGAWA T: Prenatal diagnosis of I-cell disease by measuring altered α-mannosidase activity in amniotic fluid. *J Inher Metabol Dis* 3:117, 1980

100. LEROY JG, VAN ELSEN AF: I-cell disease (mucolipidosis type II): Serum hydrolases in obligate heterozygotes. *Humangenetik* 20:119, 1973

101. VAN ELSEN AF, LEROY JG, VANNEUVILLE FJ, VERCRUYSSEN AL: Isoenzymes of serum N-acetyl-beta-D-glucosaminidase in the I-cell heterozygote. *Hum Genet* 31:75, 1976

102. VIDGOFF J, BUIST NRM: Serum hexosaminidase activity in I-cell disease carriers. *Hum Genet* 36:307, 1977

38

DISORDERS OF GLYCOPROTEIN DEGRADATION: Mannosidosis, Fucosidosis, Sialidosis, and Aspartylglycosaminuria

ARTHUR L. BEAUDET

1. *Glycoproteins are synthesized by two pathways. The glycosyltransferase pathway synthesizes oligosaccharides linked O-glycosidically to serine or threonine, while the dolicol, lipid-linked pathway synthesizes oligosaccharides linked N-glycosidically to asparagine. The oligosaccharides are degraded in the lysosome by (1) a group of exoglycosidases acting at the nonreducing termini, (2) an endo-β-N-acetylglucosaminidase, and (3) aspartylglycosaminidase. Specific deficiencies of these enzymes cause glycoprotein storage diseases.*

2. *The clinical phenotypes of the glycoprotein storage diseases generally resemble those of mild mucopolysaccharidosis. Mannosidosis is divided into types I and II for infantile and juvenile-adult disease, respectively. Fucosidosis type I patients show infantile onset and an abnormal sweat chloride test, while type II patients survive to adulthood and have angiokeratoma. Sialidosis type I patients have cherry-red spot-myoclonus syndrome without somatic features of mucopolysaccharidosis. Sialidosis type II includes juvenile, infantile, and congenital phenotypes with increasingly severe mucopolysaccharidosis-like phenotypes. Patients with aspartylglycosaminuria have a very mild mucopolysaccharidosis-like phenotype with progressive mental deterioration.*

3. *Pathologic studies in all four disorders show vacuolation of cells in most body tissues, with a reticulogranular pattern as the most frequent appearance of membrane-bound vacuoles on electron microscopy.*

4. *The biochemical accumulation in urine and tissues results primarily from incomplete degradation of N-glycosidically linked oligosaccharides. Multiple products are identified in all four disorders, but only oligosaccharides are found in mannosidosis and sialidosis, only glycoasparagines in aspartylglycosaminuria, and both oligosaccharides and glycoasparagines in fucosidosis. There is also accumulation of glycolipid in fucosidosis.*

5. *The lysosomal enzyme defects are as follows: α-D-mannosidase in mannosidosis, α-L-fucosidase in fucosidosis, glycoprotein specific α-neuraminidase in sialidosis (the ganglioside specific α-neuraminidase is normal), and aspartylglycosaminidase in aspartylglycosaminuria. The enzyme defects may be studied in cultured skin fibroblasts.*

6. *All of the disorders are established as autosomal recessive genetic defects. Ethnic predilections include fucosidosis in southern Italians, possibly sialidosis type I in Italians, juvenile type II sialidosis in Japanese, and aspartylglycosaminuria in Finns.*

7. *Although no definitive treatment of these disorders is*

available, prenatal diagnosis is possible and has been accomplished for three of the four diseases. Prenatal diagnosis of fucosidosis requires particular attention to procedural and interpretative pitfalls.

This chapter considers four lysosomal storage diseases that involve major defects in the degradation of glycoproteins. Glycoproteins are characterized by the presence of oligosaccharide chains covalently attached to the peptide backbone. Typical glycoproteins are peptides linked with oligosaccharides through the hydroxyl groups of serine or threonine or through the free amino group of asparagine. Proteoglycans and oligosaccharides linked to collagen and basement membrane proteins are considered separately in Chaps. 36 and 63, respectively. Genetic defects in degradation may be restricted to glycoproteins or may involve other macromolecules as well. This is because certain oligosaccharide linkages may be found in glycolipids and proteoglycans as well as in glycoproteins. Hence, a deficiency of a single lysosomal enzyme may result in accumulation of more than one class of oligosaccharide-containing macromolecules (Table 38-1).

The four glycoprotein storage diseases considered here all conform to the general conceptual framework of lysosomal storage diseases. They all demonstrate deficiency of a lysosomal hydrolase, accumulation of substrates ordinarily degraded by those enzymes, a progressive clinical course, and considerable variation of the phenotype within a single disorder. In addition, all four disorders have clinical manifestations that usually would be considered as part of the mucopolysaccharidosis phenotype, such as coarse facies and dysostosis multiplex.

SYNTHESIS AND STRUCTURE OF GLYCOPROTEINS

In addition to collagen and mucopolysaccharides, mammalian tissues contain two major groups of glycoproteins with distinct structural differences and separate synthetic pathways (Table 38-2). The discussion here is necessarily brief, but numerous chapters in recent books provide thorough reviews and a bib-

Table 38-1 Disorders of glycoprotein degradation

	Extent of degradative defect	
	Glycoproteins	*Glycolipids*
Mannosidosis	Major	None
Fucosidosis	Major	Present
Aspartylglycosaminuria	Major	None
Sialidosis	Major	Probably none
GM$_1$ Gangliosidosis*	Present	Major
GM$_2$ Gangliosidosis (Sandhoff)*	Present	Major
Mucolipidosis II and III†	Generalized degradative dysfunction	

* See Chap. 46.
† See Chap. 37.

Table 38-2 Synthesis and structure of glycoproteins

Sugar nucleotide pathway	*Dolichol pathway*
1. Sequential transfer of single sugars	1. Use of dolichol-linked intermediates
2. O-Glycosidic linkage of GalNAc to serine or threonine	2. N-Glycosidic linkage of GlcNAc to asparagine
3. Tunicamycin-resistant	3. Tunicamycin-sensitive
4. Blood group substance and submaxillary mucins are examples	4. Subtypes are high mannose and complex
	5. Thyroglobulin and IgM are examples

liography [1–5]. The oligosaccharides are synthesized as the proteins pass from the rough endoplasmic reticulum (ER) to the smooth ER and through the Golgi apparatus. The protein portions of the glycoproteins are synthesized on membrane-bound polysomes.

Sugar Nucleotide Pathway

The sugar nucleotide synthetic pathway involves the transfer to the growing oligosaccharide chain of single sugars from sugar nucleotides such as UDP-α-D-glucose, UDP-α-D-galactose, UDP-α-N-acetyl-D-glucosamine, GDP-α-N-acetyl-D-galactosamine, GDP-α-D-mannose, GDP-β-L-fucose, and CMP-sialic acid [3, 5]. Oligosaccharides synthesized by this pathway are found linked to protein through an O-glycosidic linkage of GalNAc (N-acetyl galactosamine) to serine or threonine. This synthetic pathway is resistant to inhibition by tunicamycin. Oligosaccharides of this type are found widely in animal proteins, including submaxillary mucins, human IgA, β subunit hCG (human chorionic gonadotropin), lymphocyte and RBC (red blood cell) membrane proteins, gastric mucin, and blood group substances. There is extensive diversity in the oligosaccharide structures within this category [1, 4]. A specific example of an O-glycosidic oligosaccharide is the blood group megalosaccharide shown in Fig. 38-1. The oligosaccharides of glycolipids which are synthesized by this pathway and related structures found on lipids are discussed in Chap. 15. Most of the degradative defects to be discussed involve structures of the N-glycosidic type discussed below, but defective degradation of the O-glycosidic oligosaccharides is involved in some instances.

Dolichol Pathway

The dolichol pathway for synthesis of oligosaccharides utilizes lipid-linked intermediates (Fig. 38-2) [2, 5]. The hydrophobic portion of the activated intermediates is a dolichol containing approximately 19 isoprene units. A first step in this pathway is the synthesis of Dol-P-P-GlcNAc (Dol-P, dolichol phosphate; GlcNAc, N-acetyl glucosamine) from Dol-P and UDP-GlcNAc. A second GlcNAc unit is added from UDP-GlcNAc. One mannose is then added from GDP-Man (GDP-mannose), followed by further mannose additions from Dol-P-Man. Glucose residues can then be donated, probably from Dol-P-Glc, to give the structure shown in Fig. 38-3. This structure is

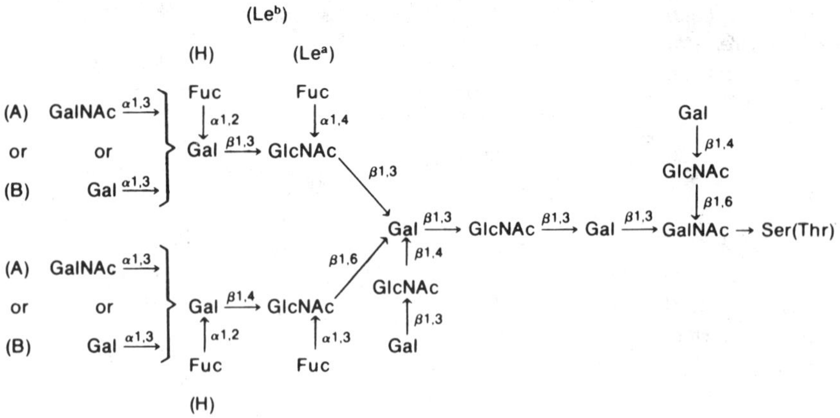

Figure 38-1 Composite megalosaccharide proposed for blood group substance. (*From Kornfeld and Kornfeld* [1], *as modified from Feizi et al.: J Immunol 106:1578, 1971.*)

Degradation of Glycoproteins

thought to be the common intermediate that is transferred to the peptide backbone. The entire oligosaccharide structure is linked to protein through an N-glycosidic linkage of GlcNAc to asparagine. Once transferred to the protein, the oligosaccharide structure undergoes a series of trimming and elongation steps, usually resulting in a final structure of the "high mannose" or "complex" type. These changes are summarized in Fig. 38-4, where structure A represents the final lipid intermediate, shown in detail in Fig. 38-3. Structure B represents a typical high mannose oligosaccharide unit, and structure C represents a typical complex oligosaccharide unit. Again, there is very extensive diversity in the detail of oligosaccharide structures [1, 4]. Tunicamycin specifically inhibits the lipid-linked pathway by selectively blocking the synthesis of Dol-P-P-GlcNAc from Dol-P and UDP-GlcNAc. The high mannose type structures occur widely, for example, in ovalbumin, bovine thyroglobulin, and human IgM. The complex structures usually include a trisaccharide attached to mannose in the outer chain, most often SA-Gal-GlcNAc (SA, sialic acid; Gal, galactose) (structure C, Fig. 38-4). The complex type of oligosaccharide unit is widely distributed and known to occur in many mammalian plasma proteins, including IgG, IgE, and transferrin, as well as in many membrane glycoproteins. The formation of high mannose and complex oligosaccharides involves a series of trimming and addition steps after transfer to the peptide backbone. These steps require a neutral α-mannosidase and many of the same glycosyltransferases used in the sugar nucleotide pathway. There is evidence that the Golgi apparatus is the major site of elongation of the terminal chains in the complex oligosaccharides.

Degradation of Glycoproteins

Since glycoproteins occur widely within cells, on the cell surface, and extracellularly, normal turnover results in a large amount of material requiring degradation. Glycoproteins are also abundant in nervous tissue [3], which is relevant to the neurologic involvement of some of the disorders for discussion. There is considerable evidence, not the least of which stems from study of the diseases considered here, suggesting that the bulk of this degradation occurs in lysosomes. The protein backbone must be degraded by a series of lysosomal peptidases. The major mechanism of oligosaccharide degradation appears to be through a sequence of hydrolytic steps whereby each unit is removed from the nonreducing ends of the oligosaccharide. The enzymes involved in these steps include α-

neuraminidase (sialidase), β-galactosidase, β-N-acetylhexosaminidase, α-mannosidase, and α-fucosidase. In addition, there is evidence for an important role for an endo-β-N-acetylglucosaminidase that hydrolyzes the chitobiose linkage (between the two GlcNAc residues) adjacent to the asparagine in oligosaccharides synthesized by the dolichol pathway. Lysosomal aspartylglycosaminidase is specifically required to hydrolyze the N-glycosidic linkage between GlcNAc and asparagine. Although the majority of mannose residues are α-linked, a Man $\xrightarrow{\beta\text{-}1,4}$ GlcNAc linkage occurs in the core region (Fig. 38-3). Studies of caprine β-mannosidosis provide strong evidence for a requirement for β-mannosidase in the degradation [5a]. A composite complex type N-glycosidic oligosaccharide and the proposed hydrolytic steps are shown in Fig. 38-5.

The deficiency of any of the required lysosomal enzymes results in products of partial degradation of the glycoproteins. Although these partial degradative products will be discussed further as stored materials under the specific disease sections, some of the findings are summarized in Fig. 38-6. It is satisfying that almost all of the stored materials in these lysosomal diseases can be viewed as expected products of incomplete degradation of known oligosaccharide structures resulting from specific enzyme deficiencies. These structures demonstrate the results of the three major types of hydrolysis: (1) single sugar removal from the nonreducing end, (2) endo-glycosidic hydrolysis at the chitobiose linkage, and (3) hydrolysis of the glycoasparagine linkage. Almost all of the storage disease structures in Fig. 38-6 can be found within typical high mannose or complex glycoproteins. Fucose can occur as a terminal residue on outer chains of complex structures. The Gal-GlcNAc-Asn (Asn, asparagine) structure found in aspartylglycosaminuria is an unusal one, as will be discussed below.

Some conclusions are implied from the data in Fig. 38-6. First, only oligosaccarides accumulate in mannosidosis and sialidosis. Only glycopeptides are found in aspartylglycosaminuria, while both oligosaccharides and glycopeptides accumulate in fucosidosis. The data from mannosidosis and sialidosis suggest the existence of an endo-β-N-acetylglucosaminidase, although its importance relative to β-N-acetylhexosaminidase in the nonpathologic state is unclear. The multiplicity of higher glycoasparagines suggest that the endo-β-N-acetylglucosaminidase and other glycosidases may be less effective if asparagine is still present. The chitobiose linkage is not found intact if asparagine is removed. Based on the findings in fucosidosis, the presence of fucose on the GlcNAc linked to Asn probably reduces the activity of the endoglycosidase and of aspartylglycosaminidase.

HISTORY

In the late 1960s a group of unusual patients with phenotypes resembling mucopolysaccharidosis were characterized clinically [6, 7] and biochemically [8]. These patients were described variously as having mucopolysaccharidosis, lipomucopolysaccharidosis, or mucolipidosis. A number of these patients were identified ultimately as having mannosidosis, which was first described by Öckerman in 1967 [9]. The same year, Jenner and Pollitt described a brother and sister with mental retardation and large quantities of aspartylglycosamine in the urine [10], and aspartylglycosaminidase deficiency was promptly demonstrated [11]. In 1968, fucosidosis was described by Durand et al. [12], and the enzyme defect was reported concomitantly by Van Hoof and Hers [13]. Sialidosis due to neuraminidase deficiency was not reported until 1977 [14, 15] in a patient who had been classified earlier as having lipomucopolysaccharidosis [6] and mucolipidosis I [7]. It was soon recognized that neuraminidase deficiency also was associated with the cherry-red spot-myoclonus syndrome. Other early reports are reviewed in a text on the lysosomal storage diseases [16].

MANNOSIDOSIS

Clinical Features

Clinical heterogeneity is evident for mannosidosis from the reports of at least 50 cases [9, 17-33]. A more severe infantile

phenotype is referred to as type I and a milder juvenile-adult phenotype as type II [25]. Virtually all patients have psychomotor retardation, facial coarsening, and some degree of dysostosis multiplex (Fig. 38-7, Table 38-3). Frequent findings include recurrent bacterial infections, deafness, hepatomegaly, hernias, and lenticular or corneal opacities. Susceptibility to infection may be related to a defect in leukocyte chemotaxis [34]. The ocular findings are distinctive and include posterior opacities in a spokelike pattern in the lens (Fig. 38-7) and superficial opacities in the cornea [26, 29, 35]. The skeletal dysplasia [27] includes thickening of the calvaria in the majority of patients. The vertebral bodies are prominently involved with ovoid configurations, flattening, and beak appearance, sometimes in association with gibbus deformity. The more severe infantile or type I phenotype includes rapid progression of mental deterioration, obvious hepatosplenomegaly, more severe dysostosis multiplex, and often death between 3 and 10 years of age. The milder juvenile-adult or type II phenotype is characterized by more normal early development but appearance of mental retardation during childhood and adolescence. Hearing loss is particularly prominent in type II patients. Dysostosis multiplex is milder, with survival into adulthood.

Laboratory findings include the presence of vacuolated lymphocytes in almost all cases. Most patients have been found not to have mucopolysacchariduria. Decreased serum IgG can occur, and a decreased PR interval on ECG has been reported [36].

Pathology

Pathologic studies of biopsy [37] and autopsy material [17, 38] are available. Light microscopy of the liver demonstrates a granular or foamy cytoplasm in the hepatocytes. PAS staining varies with the histochemical extraction procedure. Electron microscopy demonstrates multiple vacuoles in hepatocytes and

Figure 38-2 Postulated reaction scheme for lipid-mediated glycosyltransferases and possible steps in dolichol metabolism. (*From Waechter and Scher: Research Methods in Neurochemistry 1981, vol 5. Used by permission*)

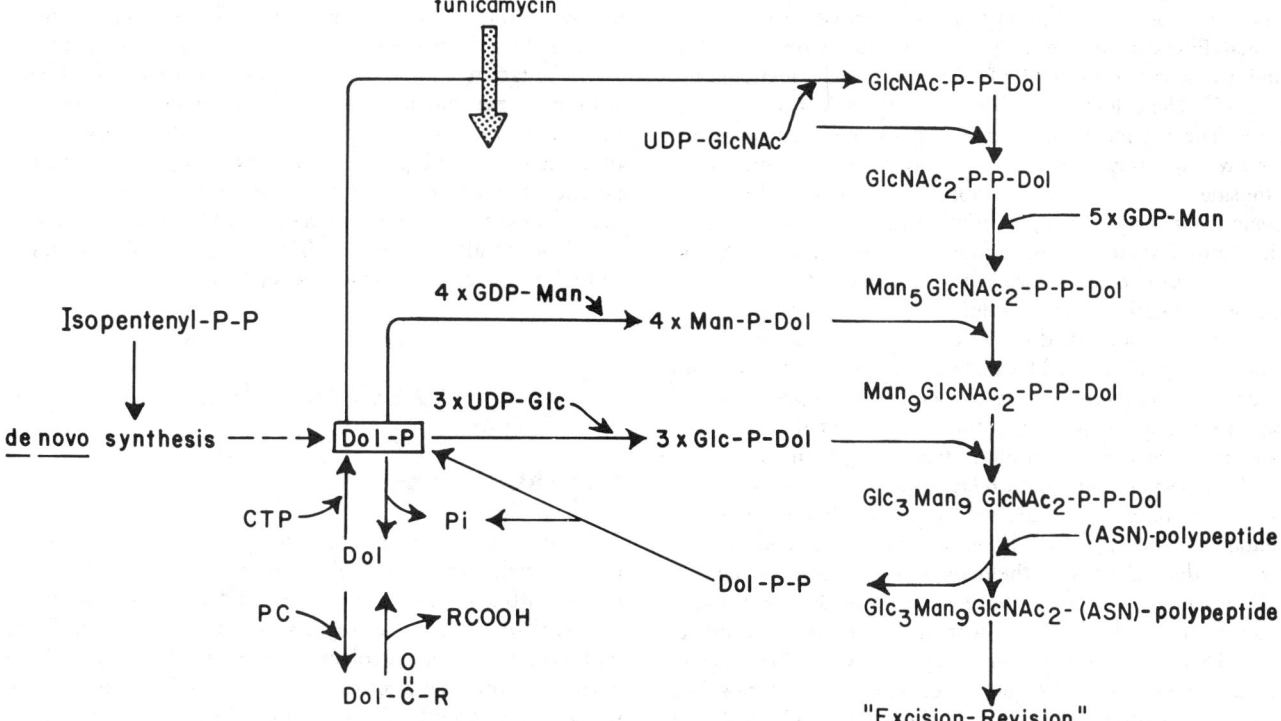

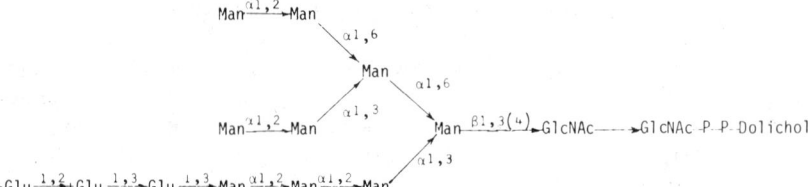

Figure 38-3 Proposed structure of the lipid-linked oligosaccharide precursor in glycoprotein synthesis. (*From S Kornfeld: J Biol Chem 253:7762, 1978. Used by permission.*)

Kupffer cells, often with a reticulogranular pattern, although many other types of inclusions are observed. Examination of the central nervous system reveals marked and widespread ballooning of the nerve cells. The cytoplasm has an empty or vacuolated appearance. Electron microscopy again demonstrates membrane-bound vacuoles with a predominantly reticulogranular pattern.

Biochemical Storage

The earliest reports indicated the presence of material containing mannose in the tissues of patients [9, 39]. The trisaccharide Man $\xrightarrow{\alpha\text{-}1,3}$ Man $\xrightarrow{\beta\text{-}1,4}$ GlcNAc was identified as the predominant material in the urine [40]. At least 16 oligosaccharides from the urine and tissues have been characterized [20, 40–44]. The more abundant urinary oligosaccharides are represented diagramatically in Fig. 38-6. The exact chemical linkages can be derived by integrating the data in Figs. 38-2 and 38-6. All of the oligosaccharides found in mannosidosis contain GlcNAc at the reducing end, with a variable number of mannose residues forming the remainder of the oligosaccharide. A recent analysis of the urinary oligosaccharides [42] appears relatively definitive, although it is at variance with some previous reports [41].

Enzyme Defect

The deficiency of α-mannosidase was noted in the original description of the condition [9]. Enzyme activity from normal human liver can be separated into two acidic forms (A and B) and one neutral form (C) by DEAE-cellulose chromatography [25, 45]. The acidic A and B forms are deficient in mannosidosis. The enzyme is studied routinely using 4-methylumbelliferyl-α-D-mannopyranoside or p-nitrophenyl-α-D-mannopyranoside as substrate. Multiple forms of the enzyme also can be demonstrated by electrophoresis [25]. Studies using cultured skin fibroblasts usually have found a single neutral form and either one or two acidic forms of the enzyme [33, 46–48]. The majority of patients have residual acidic β-mannosidase activity that shows a marked increase in the K_m for artificial substrates and has increased heat lability [25, 33, 48–51]. It is not clear why residual enzyme activity with these properties should be observed so frequently in this disease, but the data have been interpreted as indicating a structural gene mutation.

The molecular and genetic relationships of the various forms of mannosidase activity are not elucidated. Interestingly, the mutant enzyme appears to be activated by cobalt and variably by zinc, depending upon the tissue source of the enzyme [25, 52]. Immunologic studies have demonstrated cross-reacting immune material in some patients [50, 53] but not in others [54]. This may reflect genetic heterogeneity or differences in the antibodies and techniques used. Acidic α-D-mannosidase was purified 1400-fold from normal postmortem human liver

and was found to hydrolyze the trisaccharide Man $\xrightarrow{\alpha\text{-}1,3}$ Man $\xrightarrow{\beta\text{-}1,4}$ GlcNAc [55]. Studies of mannosidase in human serum demonstrate a deficiency in mannosidosis and indicate the presence of multiple forms with some differences in properties from the tissue enzymes [56–57].

Genetics

Mannosidosis is well established as an autosomal recessive genetic disorder. The majority of patients reported have been of European descent, although I have observed the disorder in an American black. The acidic mannosidase gene is mapped to chromosome 19 in human beings, using somatic cell hybridization [58]. Mutants of lysosomal β-mannosidase were isolated in Chinese hamster ovary cells using mutagenesis and replica plating techniques [59].

Other Observations

There is one report that α-mannosidase deficiency may occur with the human dermatologic condition ichthyosiform erythroderma bullosa [60]. There is a voluminous literature describing mannosidosis in Angus cattle [61, 62]. The bovine disorder is particularly common in New Zealand, where it is of economic importance, and heterozygote detection programs have been instituted. The occurrence of a chimeric calf with mannosidosis provided interesting data regarding the potential of enzyme replacement therapy [63]. Although the clinical condition was modified in the chimeric animal, the eventually unfavorable clinical outcome was interpreted to indicate that tissue transplantation as a therapy for lysosomal storage diseases with severe neurologic manifestations is unlikely to be successful. A phenocopy of mannosidosis occurs in livestock grazing on a legume of the genus *Swainsona*. The plant contains a potent inhibitor of lysosomal α-mannosidase [64]. A neurologic disorder in goats is associated with an accumulation of the trisaccharide Man $\xrightarrow{\beta\text{-}1,4}$ GlcNAc $\xrightarrow{\beta\text{-}1,4}$ GlcNAc and is caused by β-mannosidase deficiency [5a, 65].

FUCOSIDOSIS

Clinical Features

There is a report or personal knowledge of as many as 50 patients with fucosidosis [66]. A careful review indicates repetitive reporting of cases, but at least 30 definite cases are in the literature [67–88]. Other reports include an unclassified case with prominent bone involvement [89] and one with multiple partial enzyme deficiencies [83]. A fatal infantile form is referred to as type I, which accounts for about 60 percent of patients, while a milder phenotype with adult survival is designated type II. The type I phenotype has onset of psychomotor retardation recognizable at about 1 year of age. Coarse facies, growth retardation, dysostosis multiplex, and neurologic deterioration are present uniformly. Hepatosplenomegaly, cardiomegaly, seizures, and infections occur frequently but are variable. The sodium chloride content of sweat is increased markedly. The type II phenotype is associated with onset of psychomotor retardation between 1 and 2 years of age. The coarse facies, growth retardation, dysostosis multiplex, and neurologic signs are similar or slightly milder. The major distinguishing features of the type II phenotype are the presence of angiokeratoma (Fig. 38-7), longer survival often to adult years, and a more normal sweat sodium chloride value, although anhidrosis may be present.

The angiokeratomata that occur in fucosidosis are essentially indistinguishable from those seen in Fabry disease and the distribution is similar [69, 76, 90–93]. Telangiectatic lesions can occur in the mouth [94]. The ocular findings in fucosidosis are not prominent, but tortuosity of conjunctival vessels occurs and a pigmentary retinopathy has been described [92, 95]. The skeletal findings are those of a mild dysostosis multiplex [78, 96]. Changes in the vertebrae are prominent, with ovoid configuration and beaking. The acetabula are often deformed and sclerotic. The shaft of the long bones may be widened. Vacuolated lymphocytes have been present where examined.

Pathology

Postmortem examination of type I patients [67, 86] has revealed enlargement of the brain, heart, liver, spleen, and pancreas. The adrenal glands are atrophic. The gall bladder is described as strawberrylike. Biopsy studies from liver indicate the presence of foamy cytoplasm in some hepatocytes and Kupffer cells. Ultrastructural studies indicate the presence of vacuoles with heterogeneous content, some appearing empty, some with reticulum formation, and some with lamellar structures [68, 70]. Ultrastructural studies of biopsy material from brain indicate a similar heterogeneity in the appearance of storage vacuoles [68]. There is a striking vacuolization of the epithelial cells of the sweat glands [76, 79, 91] and of the conjunctiva [79].

Biochemical Storage

It was recognized from the earliest reports [12] that fucosidosis probably represented faulty degradation of both sphingolipids and polysaccharides. The major glycolipid accumulating is the H-antigen glycolipid Fuc $\xrightarrow{\alpha\text{-}1,2}$ Gal-β-GlcNAc-β-Gal-ceramide [97, 98]. There is a major accumulation of glycolipid in liver but only minor storage in brain. Studies of the oligosaccharides found in the tissues and urine of patients with fucosidosis have indicated the presence of a decasaccharide Fuc $\xrightarrow{\alpha\text{-}1,2}$ Gal $\xrightarrow{\beta\text{-}1,4}$ GlcNAc $\xrightarrow{\beta\text{-}1,2}$ Man[Fuc $\xrightarrow{\alpha\text{-}1,2}$ Gal $\xrightarrow{\beta\text{-}1,4}$ GlcNAc $\xrightarrow{\beta\text{-}1,2}$ Man] $\xrightarrow{\alpha\text{-}1,3/6}$ Man $\xrightarrow{\beta\text{-}1,4}$ GlcNAc, and a disaccharide, Fuc $\xrightarrow{\alpha\text{-}1,6}$ GlcNAc [98, 99] (see Fig. 38-6). Subsequent studies [100–103] identified numerous other oligosaccharides and glycoasparagines in the urine and tissues of fucosidosis patients. In one excellent study [104], 22 glycopeptides were identified in the urine of a patient, but the presence of the decasaccharide could not be confirmed. All of the glycopeptides contained a fucosyl residue on the GlcNAc which is linked to asparagine. Oligosaccharide accumulation predominates as the storage material in the brain of patients. The suggestion of increased keratan sulfate in the urine in fucosidosis requires further study [105].

The relationships to blood groups substances in fucosidosis deserve special mention. These substances are determined by oligosaccharide chains linked to proteins or lipids. The H, Le[a], and Le[b] antigens are determined by the presence of fucosyltransferases (see Chap. 45). On the one hand, the genotype at these loci may determine the exact nature of the stored material in fucosidosis patients. On the other hand, the presence of fucosidosis may increase the expression of these antigens [76, 106]. Data are insufficient at present to determine if blood type affects the clinical course of fucosidosis.

Enzyme Defect

Since fucosidase deficiency first was reported [13], the enzyme deficiency has been studied in serum leukocytes, fibroblasts, and body tissues [71, 77, 107–113]. The normal human enzyme has been purified from autopsy liver using affinity chromatography [114]. The properties of the enzyme have been reviewed in great detail [110, 114]. The native molecular weight is estimated to be 230,000, which is thought to repre-

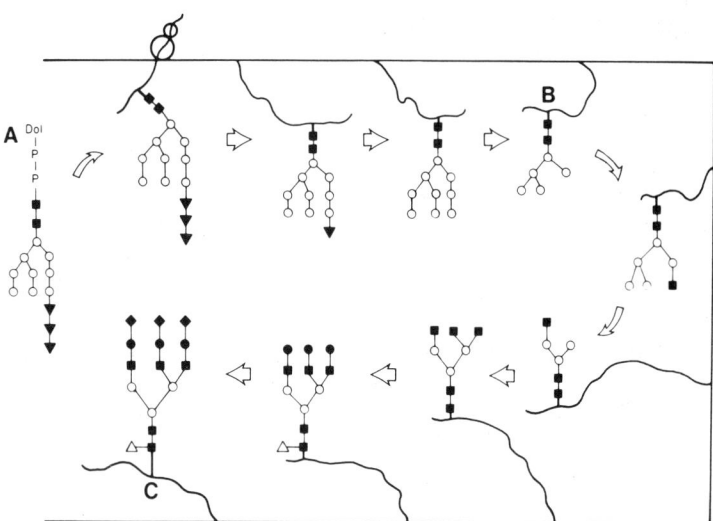

Figure 38-4 Proposed sequence for the synthesis of complex-type oligosaccharides. Dol = dolichol. The symbols are: ■, GlcNAc; ○, Man; ▼, Glc; ●, Gal; ◆, SA; △, Fuc. A. indicates the precursor shown in detail in Fig. 38-2; B. indicates a high mannose structure; and C. indicates a complex structure. (*With modification from S Kornfeld: J Biol Chem 253:7771, 1978. Used by permission.*)

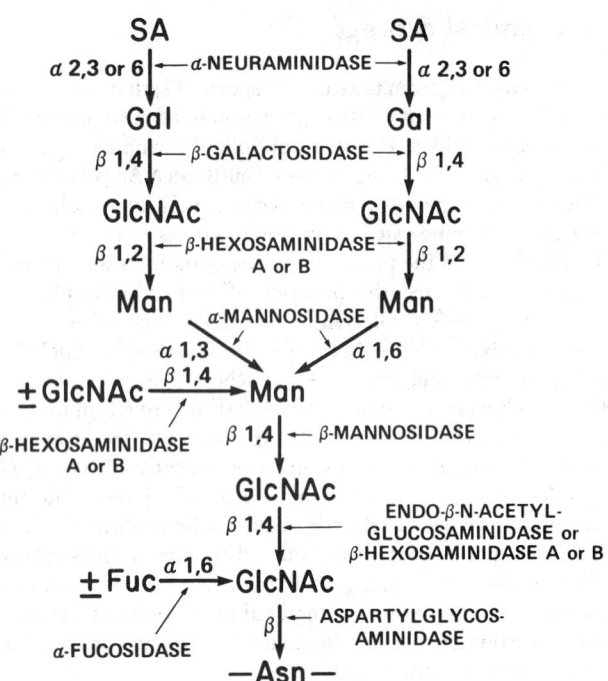

Figure 38-5 Probable steps for degradation of a complex-type oligosaccharide structure.

sent a tetramer of identical subunits. The enzyme has a pH optimum between 4 and 5 in most studies and is thought to be located in the lysosome [115].

Activity of the enzyme against natural oligosaccharide and glycosphingolipid substrates has been demonstrated [115]. The majority of studies are performed using 4-methylumbelliferyl-α-L-fucoside or p-nitrophenyl-α-L-fucoside as substrate. Marked deficiencies of enzyme activity have been noted in virtually all tissues tested using these substrates. Heterozygotes have intermediate levels of enzyme activity [66, 108]. Multiple isoenzymes of fucosidase can be demonstrated using starch-gel electrophoresis or isoelectric focusing [109–111]. Most investigators find four to seven forms of the enzyme [110]. This heterogeneity is related to sialic acid content and to high and low molecular weight forms [110]. Studies of residual enzyme acitivity in fucosidosis patients generally demonstrate low levels of activity but normal kinetic properties of the enzyme [111–113]. Immunologic studies demonstrate low to undetectable amounts of cross-reacting immune material [113, 114].

Genetics

Fucosidosis is established as an autosomal recessive disease with many instances of consanguinity and multiple affected sibs. The structural gene for the enzyme is mapped to human

Table 38-3 Clinical features of mannosidosis, fucosidosis, sialidosis, and aspartylglycosaminuria

Disorder	Age of onset	Facies	Dysostosis multiplex	Neurologic	Hepatospleno-megaly	Eye findings	Hematologic	Other
Mannosidosis:								
Type I	3–12 mo	Coarse	+++	Severe mental retardation	+++	Cataracts, corneal opacities	Vacuolated lymphocytes	Hearing loss
Type II	1–4 yr	Coarse	++	Mental retardation	++	Cataracts, corneal opacities	Vacuolated lymphocytes	Hearing loss prominent
Fucosidosis:								
Type I	3–18 mo	Mild coarsening	++	Mental retardation, seizures	++	Infrequent	Vacuolated lymphocytes	Sweat NaCl increased
Type II	1–2 yr	Mild coarsening	++	Mental retardation	++	Tortuous conjunctival vessels	Vacuolated lymphocytes	Angiokertoma, anhidrosis
Sialidosis:								
Type I	8–25 yr	Normal	– – –	Severe myoclonus, generalized seizures, neuropathy, ↓DTR	– – –	Blindness, cherry-red spot	Vacuolated lymphocytes rarely	
Type II:								
Juvenile	2–20 yr	Mild coarsening	++	Myoclonus, mental retardation	– – –	Reduced acuity, cherry-red spots	Vacuolated lymphocytes	Angiokeratoma
Infantile	0–12 mo	Coarse	+++	Mental retardation	+/–	Cherry-red spots	Vacuolated lymphocytes	Renal involvement
Congenital	In utero	Coarse	+++	Mental retardation	++	?	Vacuolated lymphocytes	Hydrops fetalis, stillbirth
Aspartylglycos-aminuria	1–5 yr	Coarse, sagging skin	+	Mental retardation	– – –	Lens opacities	Vacuolated lymphocytes	Acne, sun sensitivity

chromosome 1 [116]. The disease occurs in multiple ethnic groups but is found with increased frequency in the southern Italian region of Calabria [66]. Two instances of large pedigrees with type I and type II disease occurring in the same pedigree were reported [66]. Presence of consanguinity and common ancestors in the pedigrees would suggest that the type I and type II patients have the same genotype at the fucosidase locus, although compound heterozygotes cannot be ruled out. Various explanations have been discussed [66, 117, 118], including the possibility that variation in blood group genotype determines the clinical variation. The data might raise the possibility that the distinction between type I and type II phenotypes is artificial and based only on chance survival; however, to date the phenotype has been consistent within a sibship but not within a large pedigree.

Multiple forms of polymorphism exist for fucosidase. There is an electrophoretic polymorphism with three alleles, Fu^1, Fu^2, and Fu^0, the last being a silent allele causing fucosidosis [119, 120]. In addition, there is evidence for an inherited polymorphism affecting the level of fucosidase in plasma [77, 121, 122]. Individuals with this low plasma fucosidase polymorphism are healthy. The fucosidase activity of leukocytes in such individuals is reported to have altered kinetic properties [121], suggesting the possibility that both the electrophoretic polymorphism and the polymorphism for low plasma activity may involve the structural locus for fucosidase.

SIALIDOSIS

Clinical Features

Sialidosis was recognized as a distinct disorder rather belatedly, and a number of patients earlier reported as having β-galactosidase deficiency or the Goldberg syndrome are now known to have sialidosis with neuraminidase deficiency as the likely primary defect [123, 124]. The sialidosis phenotype without somatic involvement is designated type I and that with coarse facies and dysostosis multiplex as type II [123]. There are at least 11 confirmed and 9 probable cases of sialidosis type I with the cherry-red spot–myoclonus phenotype [123, 125–132]. The age of onset is variable but is usually in the second decade. The presenting complaint may be decreased visual acuity, myoclonus, or gait abnormalities. The visual handicap is progressive, often severe, and may be associated with impaired color vision [125, 132] or night blindness [128]. The ocular cherry-red spot is consistent but is sometimes atypical. Punctate lenticular opacities occur [125, 127, 131]. The myoclonus is generalized and frequently is debilitating and poorly controlled by medication. Exacerbation of the myoclonus is reported with stimuli, with smoking [131], and with the menstrual cycle [132]. Findings include painful neuropathy similar to Fabry disease [127], increased deep-tendon reflexes, and delayed nerve conduction [132]. Nystagmus, ataxia, and grand mal seizure are reported. Lupus nephritis in one patient [133] was presumed to be coincidental, although renal findings occur in type II sialidosis. Vacuolated lymphocytes are found in a minority of type I patients.

Sialidosis type II, the dysmorphic phenotype, has been divided into a juvenile form and an infantile form [123], and a congenital or hydropic form should be added. Eight patients with juvenile type II disease had onset between 2 and 20 years of age and were of Japanese background [134–140]; additional probable cases are known [123]. The somatic features include mild coarsening of the facies and dysostosis multiplex, which is most prominent in the lumbar vertebrae. Myoclonus similar to that in type I disease is frequent. Eye findings include progressive visual loss, cherry-red spots, punctate lenticular opacities, and occasional corneal opacities. Angiokeratomata similar to those found in Fabry disease and fucosidosis have been found in numerous patients [134, 135, 138, 139]. Additional neurologic findings include generalized seizures, nystagmus, ataxic gait, and delayed nerve conduction. Although mental function may be relatively normal in adolescence, the IQ is typically in the 60s and 70s later in life. Vacuolated lymphocytes are present consistently. These patients have survived to the fourth and fifth decade.

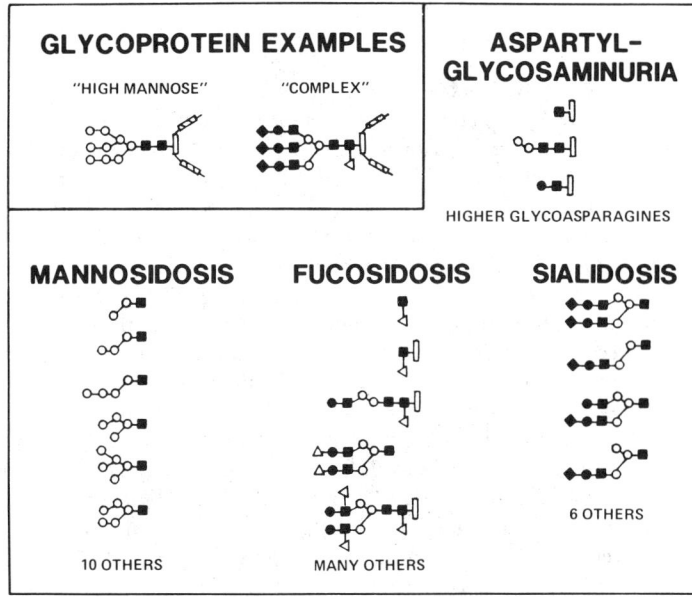

Figure 38-6 Graphic summary of storage products in four glycoprotein storage diseases. The symbols are as for Fig. 38-4, and the rectangle represents asparagine.

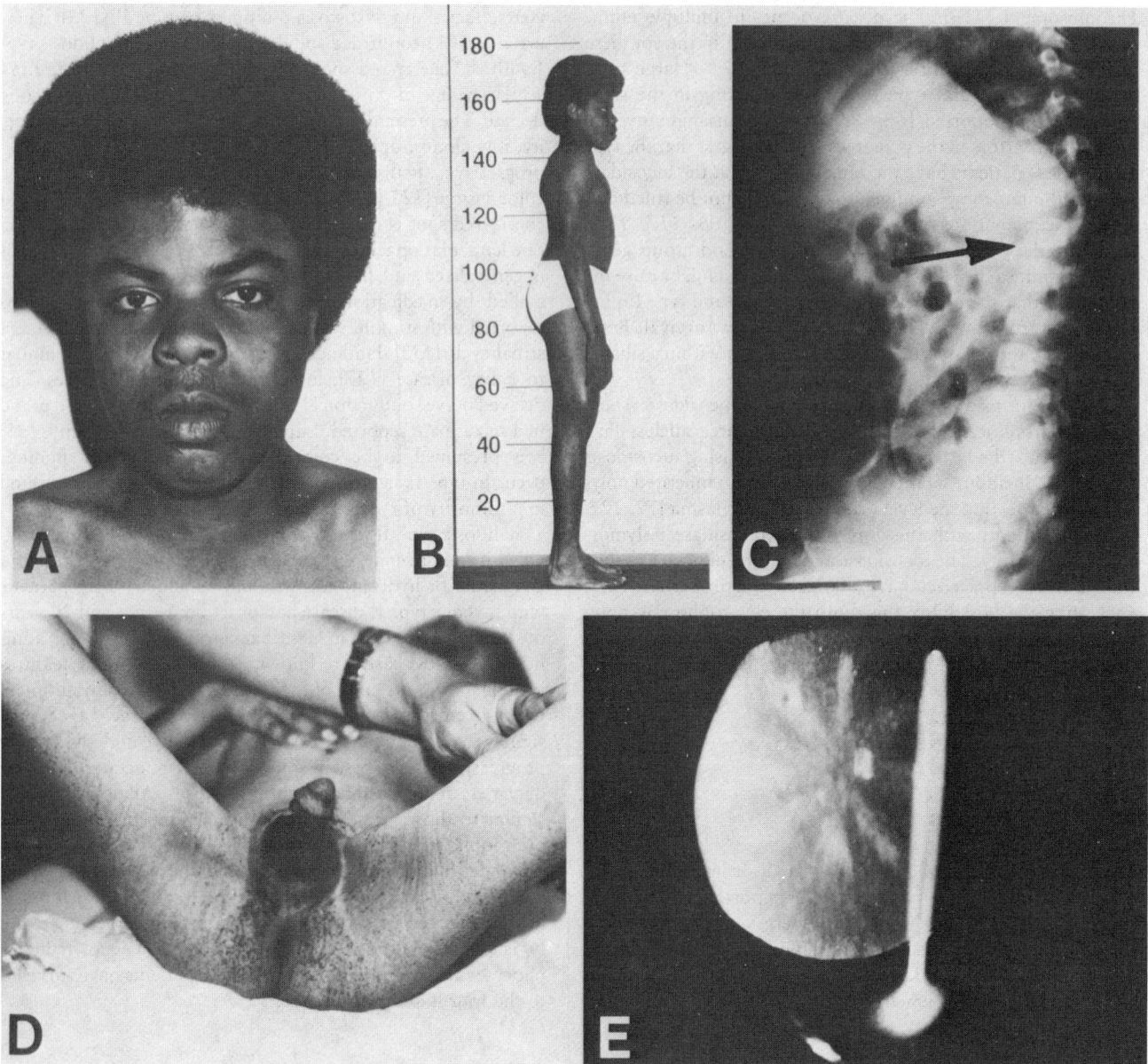

Figure 38-7 Clinical features of glycoprotein storage diseases. *A.* and *B.* Mannosidosis, type II, in a 15-year-old male; *C.* bone changes at 13 months of age in mannosidosis, type I; *D.* angiokeratoma in fucosidosis, type II; and *E.* cataract in a 5 year old with mannosidosis, type I. (*D and E from Snyder et al. [82] and Murphree et al. [26], respectively. Both used by permission.*)

The type II patients with infantile onset include those who were relatively normal or minimally abnormal at birth [*14, 15, 141–146*]. Another group has congenital involvement with ascites and hydrops fetalis [*147–150*]. There is a continuum of severity in this group, but they all develop a progressive, rather severe mucopolysaccharidosislike phenotype with visceromegaly, dysostosis multiplex, and mental retardation. Cherry-red spots, myoclonus, and other features of the type II juvenile disease are observed in older children, and survival to the second decade is reported for type II infantile patients. The type II congenital patients include at least three patients [*148, 150*] and perhaps a fourth [*149*] who were stillborn with hydrops fetalis. Many of the other patients have died at only a few months of age [*147, 149, 150*]. Facial edema, ascites, inguinal hernias, hepatosplenomegaly, stippling of the epiphyses, and periosteal cloaking may be present at birth. Significant renal involvement with proteinuria has occurred in two infantile cases [*144*] and one congenital case [*149*].

Pathology

Numerous clinical reports include pathologic descriptions and electron-microscopic findings [*125, 127, 132, 138, 139, 141, 144, 149*]; these have been reviewed [*123*]. Vacuolated lymphocytes and bone marrow foam cells are prominent in type II but lacking in type I. Liver biopsies demonstrate vacuolation that is prominent in Kupffer cells but is less in hepatocytes. Vacuolation was observed in nerve biopsies, tissue fibroblasts, myenteric plexus neurons, and in brain biopsy material. Electron-microscopic changes include membrane-bound vacuoles, which are variously described as containing reticulogranular material, electron-dense bodies, floccular material, lamellar inclusions, and lipofuscin.

Biochemical Storage

There has been little biochemical analysis of tissues of patients with sialidosis, but presumably accumulation of sialyloligosaccharides will be found. Lipid analysis of brain has shown minimal abnormalities [123]. Urinary excretion of sialic acid containing oligosaccharides is increased and is often elevated up to 100-fold with 5 to 150 mg/liter of individual oligosaccharides. Structural data originate largely from a single laboratory [151, 152], and all of the oligosaccharides described have a core structure which could be derived by partial degradation of a complex-type N-glycosidic–linked oligosaccharide chain. The structures of the four most abundant urinary oligosaccharides are shown schematically in Fig. 38-6. In all of these oligosaccharides the sialyl linkage is α-2, 6, but numerous other urinary oligosaccharides described [150, 151] include α-2, 3-sialyl linkages.

Enzyme Defect

Human lysosomal α-neuraminidase has not been characterized extensively, although the rat liver enzyme has been studied [153]. Studies of the enzyme in salidosis patients have focused almost exclusively on cultured skin fibroblasts [14, 126, 128, 129, 154–162] or rarely on leukocytes [154]. A wide variety of substrates have been used, including 2-(3′-methoxyphenyl)-N-acetyl-α-neuraminic acid (MPN), α-2,3- and α-2,6-neuramin-lactose, fetuin, α-L-N-acetylneuraminosyl-(2,6)-N-acetylgalactosaminitol, and urinary oligosaccharides. The conclusions are that all of the sialidosis phenotypes described above show a striking deficiency of α-neuraminidase in cultured skin fibroblasts. The enzyme activity is deficient against α-2,3 as well as against α-2,6 linkages. The data are compatible with the presence of a single neuraminidase that hydrolyzes both the linkages. Sensitivity is increased by using 4-methylumbelliferyl-α-D-N-acetylneuraminic acid (4-MU-NANA) as a substrate [157, 158, 161, 162], and studies using this substrate indicate that type I patients have greater residual enzyme activity than do type II patients [161]. Until the 4-MU-NANA is readily available, the MPN substrate provides a commercially available reagent for routine diagnostic procedures. The enzyme is unstable when frozen or exposed to excessive sonication and must be assayed in fresh fibroblast extracts. Multiple studies [129, 159, 160] have indicated that extracts of a patient's cells have normal neuraminidase activity when ganglioside substrates are used. These data suggest a genetically distinct lysosomal α-neuraminidase that hydrolyzes ganglioside substrates. There are now two reports that the ganglioside neuraminidase is deficient in mucolipidosis IV [163, 164].

The coexistence of α-neuraminidase deficiency and β-galactosidase deficiency in many patients is curious (see Ref. 123 for a review). The β-galactosidase deficiency can occur with any of the clinical phenotypes, but it is not present in all patients. Cultured cells from these sialidosis patients constituted a separate complementation group for β-galactosidase deficiency [165]. Mixing experiments do not suggest in vitro inhibition [123, 129]. It is thought that the β-galactosidase deficiency may be secondary to the neuraminidase deficiency since some heterozygotes have normal levels for β-galactosidase but intermediate levels for neuraminidase [129]. Based on complementation studies it was alternatively suggested that patients with both neuraminidase and β-galactosidase deficiency represent a separate genetic disorder [166]. If correct, the classification followed here will need revision in the future.

Genetics

Sialidosis can be accepted as an autosomal recessive disorder based on the occurrence of multiple affected sibs and the consanguine matings for multiple cases among all of the phenotypes. The type II juvenile disease has occurred predominantly in the Japanese population. Type I sialidosis has been found somewhat more frequently in Italians. While all of the forms of sialidosis may be allelic disorders involving the structural gene for the enzyme, there is no definitive evidence for this at the present time. The gene for sialidase has not been mapped. A partial deficiency of hepatic neuraminidase in mice has been mapped to chromosome 17, near the major histocompatibility complex [167].

ASPARTYLGLYCOSAMINURIA

Clinical Features

By 1974, seventy-one patients with aspartylglycosaminuria had been identified in Finland [168]. Other cases include eight Finnish patients in Norway [169, 170], the two original English cases [10], and a case in the United States [171]. The Finnish phenotype is quite consistent, as described in detail by Autio et al. [172]. The patients were healthy for the first few months of life. Recurrent infections, diarrhea, and hernias were noted during the first year of life. Head circumference and stature were decreased later in childhood in some patients, and hepatomegaly was found infrequently. Coarsening of the facies and sagging skin folds were subtle in the first decade and more obvious thereafter. Increased acne and sun sensitivity were found. Crystal-like lens opacities were observed in 8 of 17 patients more than 10 years of age. Joint laxity, macroglossia, hoarse voice, short stature, and brachycephaly were described in some patients. Mental development was relatively normal until about age 5, except for delayed speech. Mental deterioration occurred between the ages of 6 and 15 with IQ values usually below 40 in adults. Clumsiness and hypotonia were reported in some, and spasticity occurred in only a few older patients. Behavior frequently was uncontrolled, and the patients were excitable. Death was rarely directly attributable to the disease, and life expectancy was not grossly impaired, at least through the fourth decade. The English patients were mentally retarded. The single patient in the United States had more significant early developmental delay, although other factors were present. Hepatosplenomegaly was present early but disappeared; moderate mitral insufficiency was documented on cardiac catheterization. I am aware of two additional unreported cases in the United States.

Vacuolated lymphocytes were observed in 19 of 25 Finnish patients, while neutropenia was found in 13 of 25. The prothrombin time was decreased in 13 of 25, and the EEG was abnormal in 11 of 25. Marked aspartylglycosaminuria was

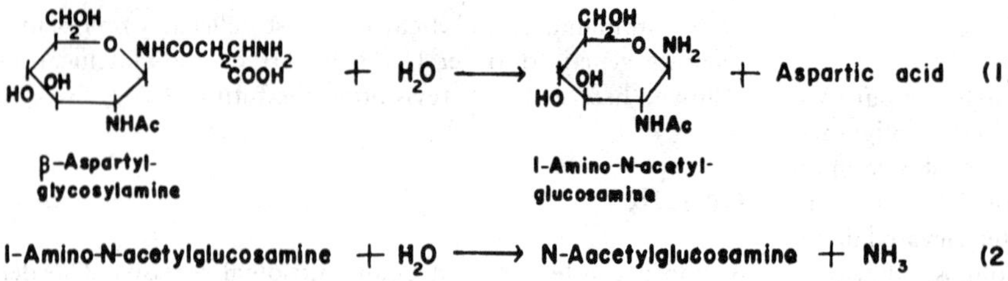

$$\text{β-Aspartyl-glycosylamine} + H_2O \longrightarrow \text{1-Amino-N-acetyl-glucosamine} + \text{Aspartic acid} \quad (1)$$

$$\text{1-Amino-N-acetylglucosamine} + H_2O \longrightarrow \text{N-Acetylglucosamine} + NH_3 \quad (2)$$

Figure 38-8 Aspartylglycosaminidase reaction. (*From Makino, Kojima, and Yamashina [183]. Used by permission.*)

present in all patients. Radiographic changes indicate a very mild dysostosis multiplex, with wedge-shaped vertebral bodies later in life and thickening of the cortex of the skull. Cerebral atrophy can be demonstrated.

Pathology

Pathologic studies of bone marrow, small intestine, skin, lymph node, kidney, and brain are available from biopsy specimens [173, 174], and one autopsy examination has been reported [175]. Light-microscopic examination of all tissues has demonstrated vacuolated cytoplasm with variable PAS staining. Hepatocytes may contain a large central vacuole and may superficially resemble advanced fatty metamorphosis. Electron-microscopic examination of all tissues has demonstrated small and huge vacuoles bounded by a single membrane. Much of the material is electonlucent, but electron-dense granular bodies occur, particularly in brain.

Biochemical Storage

The first biochemical insight into this disease was the discovery of aspartylglycosamine (GlcNAc-Asn) in the urine of the English sibs [10]. GlcNAc-Asn is the major abnormal compound in the urine of all patients studied, with 200 to 400 mg/day typically being excreted [10, 176–178]. A series of at least 13 other glycoasparagines is found in urine [176–181]. Two of the other more abundant compounds, Man $\xrightarrow{\alpha\text{-}1,6}$ Man $\xrightarrow{\beta\text{-}1,4}$ GlcNAc $\xrightarrow{\beta\text{-}1,4}$ GlcNAc-Asn and Gal $\xrightarrow{\beta\text{-}1,4}$ GlcNac-Asn, are shown in Fig. 38-6. Most of the reported structures could be derived by partial degradation of known N-glycosidically linked oligosaccharides in glycoproteins. The

structure Gal $\xrightarrow{\beta\text{-}1,4}$ GlcNAc-Asn is an unusual one which has not been found yet in glycoproteins. Some of the reported structures are sialylated [179–181]. Studies of liver and brain demonstrate that GlcNAc-Asn is again the predominant material, with higher glycoasparagines found in lesser amounts [176, 182]. In all storage compounds identified to date, the peptide portion is completely degraded to the asparagine linkage and diversity involves incomplete degradation of the carbohydrate portion.

Enzyme Defect

Before the identification of aspartylglycosamine in the urine of patients, an enzyme from mammalian sources capable of hydrolyzing the GlcNAc-Asn linkage was known [183]. The enzyme defect in aspartylglycosaminuria was quickly demonstrated [11]. The enzyme reaction occurs in two steps (Fig. 38-8), with the first hydrolysis yielding 1-amino-GlcNAc and aspartic acid. In a second step the 1-amino-GlcNAc is hydrolyzed to GlcNAc and NH_3. Enzyme activity is often measured by quantitation of the GlcNAc produced using the Morgan-Elson reaction [168, 183]. Enzyme activity is deficient in seminal fluid, plasma, leukocytes, liver, brain, spleen, and cultured skin fibroblasts [11, 168, 174, 184, 185]. There is evidence that aspartylglycosaminidase is enriched in the lysosomal fraction, and only a single band was observed on agarose-gel electrophoresis [186].

Genetics

Aspartylglycosaminuria is established as an autosomal genetic disorder. The majority of cases have been identified in Finland.

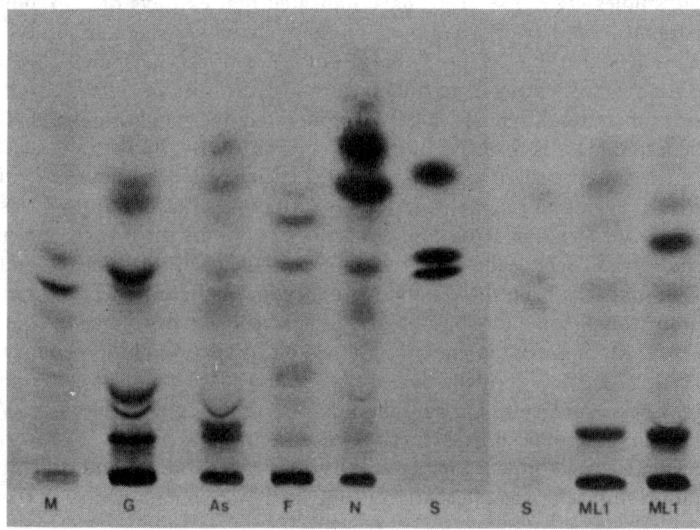

Figure 38-9 Thin-layer chromatogram of urines with orcinol detection. M, mannosidosis; G, GM_1, gangliosidosis; As, aspartylglycosaminuria; F, fucosidosis; N, normal control; S, standard mixture of fructose, lactose, and raffinose; ML1, sialidosis. (*From Sewell [187]. Used by permission.*)

The gene for the disorder has not been mapped to a specific human chromosome.

DIFFERENTIAL DIAGNOSIS AND MANAGEMENT

The diagnosis of the four disorders discussed here can be suspected on the basis of the clinical phenotypes described (Table 38-3). A mucopolysaccharidosis-like phenotype without mucopolysacchariduria is suggestive of these and related disorders such as β-galactosidase deficiency or mucolipidosis II and III. Skin biopsy or conjunctival biopsy should demonstrate membrane-bound vacuoles [29, 76, 79, 91, 174]. Analysis of urinary oligosaccharides and glycopeptides using thin-layer chromatography and orcinol staining is also a good screening procedure [187–189] (Fig. 38-9). Definitive diagnosis should be established using enzyme assay on leukocytes, fibroblasts, or other tissues as described for these disorders.

Successful prenatal diagnosis is reported for mannosidosis [50, 190, 191], fucosidosis [66, 80], and sialidosis [148, 150]. Prenatal diagnosis should be possible for aspartylglycosaminuria [168]. Prenatal diagnosis of fucosidosis requires particular care since there was a failure to detect affected twins [73] and since fucosidase activity is higher in epithelial cells than in fibroblastic cells in amniotic fluid cultures [192]. Use of techniques to demonstrate in vivo accumulation of fucose-containing compounds [193, 194] might improve reliability. A sizable heterozygote detection program has been carried out among relatives of fucosidosis patients in Calabria [66].

REFERENCES

1. KORNFELD R, KORNFELD S: Structure of glycoproteins and their oligosaccharide units, in Lennarz WJ (ed): *The Biochemistry of Glycoproteins and Proteoglycans.* New York, Plenum, 1980, p 1
2. STRUCK DK, LENNARZ WJ: The function of saccharide-lipids in synthesis of glycoproteins, in Lennarz WJ (ed): *The Biochemistry of Glycoproteins and Proteoglycans.* New York, Plenum, 1980, p 35
3. SCHACHTER H, ROSEMAN S: Mammalian glycosyltransferases: Their role in the synthesis and function of complex carbohydrates and glycolipids, in Lennarz WJ (ed): *The Biochemistry of Glycoproteins and Proteoglycans.* New York, Plenum, 1980, p 85
4. MARGOLIS RK, MARGOLIS RU: Structure and distribution of glycoproteins and glycosaminoglycans, in Margolis RU, Margolis RK (eds): *Complex Carbohydrates of Nervous Tissue.* New York, Plenum, 1979, p 45
5. WAECHTER CJ, SCHER MG: Biosynthesis of glycoproteins, in Margolis RU, Margolis RK (eds): *Complex carbohydrates of Nervous Tissue.* New York, Plenum, 1979, p 75
5a. JONES MZ, DAWSON G: Caprine β-mannosidosis: Inherited deficiency of β-D-mannosidase. *J Biol Chem* 256:5185, 1981
6. SPRANGER J, WIEDEMANN H-R, TOLKSDORF M, GRAUCOB E, CAESAR R: Lipomucopolysaccharidose: Eine neue speicherkrankheit. *Z Kinderheilk* 103:285, 1968
7. SPRANGER JW, WIEDERMANN H-R: The genetic mucolipidoses: Diagnosis and differential diagnosis. *Humangenetik* 9:113, 1970
8. VAN HOOF F, HERS HG: The abnormalities of lysosomal enzymes in mucopolysaccharidoses. *Eur J Biochem* 7:34, 1968
9. ÖCKERMAN P-A: A generalised storage disorder resembling Hurler's syndrome. *Lancet* 2:239, 1967
10. JENNER FA, POLLITT RJ: Large quantities of 2-acetamido-1(β-1-aspartamido)-1,2-dideoxyglucose in the urine of mentally retarded siblings. *Biochem J* 103:48p, 1967
11. POLLITT RJ, JENNER FA, MERSKEY H: Aspartylglycosaminuria: An inborn error of metabolism associated with mental defect. *Lancet* 2:253, 1968
12. DURAND P, BORRONE C, DELLA CELLA G, PHILIPPART M: Fucosidosis. *Lancet* 1:1198, 1968.
13. VAN HOFF F, HERS HG: Mucopolysaccharidosis by absence of α-fucosidase. *Lancet* 1:1198, 1968
14. CANTZ M, GEHLER J, SPRANGER J: Mucolipidosis I: Increased sialic acid content and deficiency of an α-N-acetylneuraminidase in cultured fibroblasts. *Biochem Biophys Res Commun* 74:732, 1977
15. SPRANGER J, GEHLER J, CANTZ M: Mucolipidosis I—A sialidosis. *Am J Med Genet* 1:21, 1977
16. HERS HG, VAN HOOF F: *Lysosomes and Storage Diseases.* New York, Academic, 1973
17. KJELLMAN B, GAMSTORP I, BRUN A, ÖCKERMAN P-A, PALMGREN B: Mannosidosis: A clinical and histopathologic study. *J Pediatr* 75:366, 1969
18. AUTIO S, NORDEN NE, ÖCKERMAN P-A, RIEKKINEN P, RAPOLA J, LOUHIMO T: Mannosidosis: Clinical, fine-structural and biochemical findings in three cases. *Acta Paediatr Scand* 62:555, 1973
19. NORDÉN NE, ÖCKERMAN P-A, SZABÓ L: Urinary mannose in mannosidosis. *J Pediatr* 82:686, 1973
20. TSAY GC, DAWSON G, MATALON R: Excretion of mannose-rich complex carbohydrates by a patient with α-mannosidase deficiency (mannosidosis). *J Pediatr* 84:865, 1974
21. FARRIAUX JP, LEGOUIS I, HUMBEL R, DHONDT JL, RICHARD P, STRECKER G, FOURMAINTRAUX A, RINGEL J, FONTAINE G: La mannosidose: A propos de 5 observations. *Nouv Presse Med* 4:1867, 1975
22. LOEB H, TONDEUR M, TOPPET M, CREMER N: Clinical, biochemical and ultrastructural studies of an atypical form of mucopolysaccharidosis. *Acta Paediatr Scand* 58:220, 1969
23. BOOTH CW, CHEN KK, NADLER HL: Mannosidosis: Clinical and biochemical studies in a family of affected adolescents and adults. *J Pediatr* 88:821, 1976
24. AYLSWORTH AS, TAYLOR HA, STUART CE, THOMAS GH: Mannosidosis: Phenotype of a severely affected child and characterization of α-mannosidase activity in cultured fibroblasts from the patient and his parents. *J Pediatr* 88:814, 1976
25. DESNICK RJ, SHARP HL, GRABOWSKI GA, BRUNNING RD, QUIE PG, SUNG JH, GORLIN RJ, IKONNE JU: Mannosidosis: Clinical, morphologic, immunologic, and biochemical studies. *Pediatr Res* 10:985, 1976
26. MURPHREE AL, BEAUDET AL, PALMER EA, NICHOLS BL: Cataract in mannosidosis. *Birth Defects* 12:319, 1976
27. SPRANGER J, GEHLER J, CANTZ M: The radiographic features of mannosidosis. *Radiology* 119:401, 1976
28. YUNIS JJ, LEWANDOWSKI RC, SANFILIPPO SJ, TSAI MY, FONI I, BRUHL HH: Clinical manifestations of mannosidosis—A longitudinal study. *Am J Med* 61:841, 1976
29. ARBISSER AI, MURPHREE AL, GARCIA CA, HOWELL RR: Ocular findings in mannosidosis. *Am J Opthalmol* 82:465, 1976
30. VIDGOFF J, LOVRIEN EW, BEALS RK, BUIST NRM: Mannosidosis in three brothers—A review of the literature. *Medicine (Baltimore)* 56:335, 1977
31. KISTLER JP, LOTT IT, KOLODNY EH, FRIEDMAN RB, NERSASIAN R, SCHNUR J, MIHM MC, DVORAK AM, DICKERSIN R: Mannosidosis: New clinical presentation, enzyme studies, and carbohydrate analysis. *Arch Neurol* 34:45, 1977
32. MILLA PJ, BLACK IE, PATRICK AD, HUGH-JONES K, OBERHOLZER V: Mannosidosis: Clinical and biochemical study. *Arch Dis Child* 52:937, 1977
33. BACH G, KOHN G, LASCH EE, EL MASSRI M, ORNOY A, SEKELES E, LEGUM C, COHEN MM: A new variant of mannosidosis with increased residual enzymatic activity and mild clinical manifestation. *Pediatr Res* 12:1010, 1978
34. QUIE PG, CATES KL: Clinical conditions associated with defective polymorphonuclear leukocyte chemotaxis. *Am J Pathol* 88:711, 1977
35. LETSON RD, DESNICK RJ: Punctate lenticular opacities in type II mannosidosis. *Am J Ophthalmol* 85:218, 1978
36. MEHTA J, DESNICK RJ: Abbreviated PR interval in mannosidosis. *J Pediatr* 92:599, 1978
37. MÓNUS Z, KONYAR E, SZABO L: Histomorphologic and histochemical investigations in mannosidosis. *Virchows Arch (Cell Pathol)* 26:159, 1977
38. SUNG JH, HAYANO M, DESNICK RJ: Mannosidosis: Pathology of the nervous system. *J Neuropathol Exp Neurol* 36:807, 1977
39. ÖCKERMAN P-A: Mannosidosis: Isolation of oligosaccharide storage material from brain. *J Pediatr* 75:360, 1969
40. NORDÉN NE, LUNDBLAD A, SVENSON S, AUTIO S: Characterization of two mannose-containing oligosaccharides isolated from the urine of patients with mannosidosis. *Biochemistry* 13:871, 1974
41. STRECKER G, FOURNET B, BOUQUELET S, MONTREUIL J, DHONDT JL, FARARIAUX JP: Etude chimique des mannosides urinairs excrétés au cours de la mannosidose. *Biochimie* 58:579, 1976
42. YAMASHITA K, TACHIBANA Y, MIHARA K, OKADA S, YABUUCHI H, KOBATA A: Urinary oligosaccharides of mannosidosis. *J Biol Chem* 255:5126, 1979
43. TSAY GC, DAWSON G, MATALON R: Glycopeptide storage in skin fibroblasts cultured from a patient with α-mannosidase deficiency. *J Clin Invest* 56:711, 1975

44. CHESTER MA, HULTBERG B, NORDÉN NE, SZABÓ L: The nature of mannose-containing material which accumulates in cultured fibroblasts from patients with mannosidosis. *Biochim Biophys Acta* 627:244, 1980

45. CARROLL M, DANCE N, MASSON PK, ROBINSON D, WINCHESTER BG: Human mannosidosis—The enzymatic defect. *Biochem Biophys Res Commun* 49:579, 1972

46. PHILLIPS NC, ROBINSON D, WINCHESTER BG: Immunological characterization of human α-D-mannosidases. *Biochem Soc Trans* 3:238, 1975

47. TAYLOR HA, THOMAS GH, AYLSWORTH A, STEVENSON RE, REYNOLDS LW: Mannosidosis: Deficiency of a specific α-mannosidase component in cultured fibroblasts. *Clin Chim Acta* 59:93, 1975

48. BURTON BK, NADLER HL: Mannosidosis: Separation and characterization of two acid α-mannosidase forms in mutant fibroblasts. *Enzyme* 23:29, 1978

49. BEAUDET AL, NICHOLS BL: Residual altered α-mannosidase in human mannosidosis. *Biochem Biophys Res Commun* 68:292, 1976

50. POENARU L, MIRANDA C, DREYFUS J-C: Residual mannosidase activity in human mannosidosis: Characterization of the mutant enzyme. *Am J Hum Genet* 32:354, 1980

51. BURDITT L, CHOTAI K, HALLEY D, WINCHESTER B: Comparison of the residual acidic α-D-mannosidase in three cases of mannosidosis. *Clin Chim Acta* 104:201, 1980

52. HULTBERG B, MASSON PK: Activation of residual acidic α-mannosidase activity in mannosidosis tissues by metal ions. *Biochem Biophys Res Commun* 67:1473, 1975

53. MERSMANN G, BUDDECKE E: Evidence for material from mannosidosis fibroblasts crossreacting with anti-acidic α-mannosidase antibodies. *FEBS Lett* 73:123, 1977

54. BURDITT LJ, CHOTAI KA, WINCHESTER BG: Evidence that the mutant enzyme in fibroblasts of a patient with mannosidosis does not crossreact with antiserum raised against normal acidic α-mannosidase. *FEBS Lett* 91:186, 1978

55. PHILLIPS NC, ROBINSON D, WINCHESTER BG: Characterization of human liver α-D-mannosidase purified by affinity chromatography. *Biochem J* 153:579, 1976

56. MASSON PK, LUNDBLAD A, AUTIO S: Mannosidosis: Detection of the disease and of heterozygotes using serum and leucocytes. *Biochem Biophys Res Commun* 56:296, 1974

57. HIRANI S, WINCHESTER B: The multiple forms of α-D-mannosidase in human plasma. *Biochem J* 179:583, 1979

58. CHAMPION MJ, SHOWS TB: Mannosidosis: Assignment of the lysosomal α-mannosidase B gene to chromosome 19 in man. *Proc Nat Acad Sci USA* 74:2968, 1977

59. ROBBINS AR: Isolation of lysosomal α-mannosidase mutants of Chinese hamster ovary cells. *Proc Nat Acad Sci USA* 76:1911, 1979

60. MALI JWH, BERGERS AMG, VAN DEN HURK JJMA, MIER PD, VAN DE STAAK WJBM: A lysosomal storage disorder of the epidermis characterized by a deficiency of α-mannosidase and an accumulation of mannose-rich materials. *Brit J Dermatol* 95:627, 1976

61. BURDITT LJ, PHILLIPS NC, ROBINSON D, WINCHESTER BG, VAN-DE-WATER NS, JOLLY RD: Characterization of the mutant α-mannosidase in bovine mannosidosis. *Biochem J* 175:1013, 1978

62. JOLLY RD: Mannosidosis of Angus cattle: A prototype control program for some genetic diseases. *Adv Vet Sci Comp Med* 19:1, 1975

63. JOLLY RD, THOMPSON KG, MURPHY CE, MANKTELOW BW, BRUERE AN, WINCHESTER BG: Enzyme replacement therapy—An experiment of nature in a chimeric mannosidosis calf. *Pediatr Res:* 10:219, 1976

64. DORLING PR, HUXTABLE CR, VOGEL P: Lysosomal storage in *Swainsona SPP* toxicosis: An induced mannosidosis. *Neuropathol Appl Neurobiol* 4:285, 1978

65. JONES MZ, LAINE RA: Caprine oligosaccharide storage disease: Accumulation of β-mannosyl(1→4)β-N-acetylglucosaminyl(1→4)β-N-acetylglucosamine in brain. *J Biol Chem* 256:5181, 1981

66. DURAND P GATTI R, BORRONE C, COSTANTINO G, CAVALIERI S, FILOCAMO M, ROMEO G: Detection of carriers and prenatal diagnosis for fucosidosis in Calabria. *Hum Genet* 51:195, 1979

67. DURAND P, BORRONE CX, DELLA CELLA G: Fucosidosis. *J Pediatr* 75:665, 1969

68. LOEB H, TONDEUR M, JONNIAUX G, MOCKEL-POHL S, VAMOS-HURWITZ E: Biochemical and ultrastructural studies in a case of mucopolysaccharidosis "F" (fucosidosis). *Helv Paediat Acta* 24:519, 1969

69. PATEL V, WATANABE I, ZEMAN W: Deficiency of α-L-fucosidase. *Science* 176:426, 1972

70. FREITAG F, KÜCHEMANN K, BLÜMCKE S: Hepatic ultrastructure in fucosidosis *Virchows Arch (Cell Pathol)* 7:99, 1971

71. ZIELKE K, OKADA S, O'BRIEN JS: Fucosidosis: Diagnosis by serum assay of α-L-fucosidase. *J Lab Clin Med* 79:164, 1972

72. MATSUDA I, ARASHIMA S, ANAKURA M, EGE A, HAYATA I: Fucosidosis. *Tohoku J Exp Med* 109:41, 1973

73. MATSUDA I, ARASHIMA S, OKA Y, MITSUYAMA T, ARIGA S, IKEUCHI T, ICHIDA T: Prenatal diagnosis of fucosidosis. *Clin Chim Acta* 63:55, 1975

74. BORRONE C, GATTI R, TRIAS X, DURAND P: Fucosidosis: Clinical, biochemical, immunologic, and genetic studies in two new cases. *J Pediatr* 84:727, 1974

75. KOUSSEFF BG, BERATIS NG, DANESINO C, HIRSCHHORN K: Genetic heterogeneity in fucosidosis. *Lancet* 2:1387, 1973

76. KOUSSEFF BG, BERATIS NG, STRAUSS L, BRILL PW, ROSENFIELD RE, KAPLAN B, HIRSCHHORN K: Fucosidosis type 2. *Pediatr* 57:205, 1976

77. NG WG, DONNELL GN, KOCH R, BERGREN WR: Biochemical and genetic studies of plasma and leukocyte α-L-fucosidase. *Am J Hum Genet* 28:42, 1976

78. TACONIS WK, VAN WIECHEN PJ, VAN GEMUND JJ: Radiological findings in a case of type II fucosidosis: A case report. *Radiol Clin (Basel)* 45:258, 1976

79. LIBERT J, VAN HOOF F, TONDEUR M: Fucosidosis: Ultrastructural study of conjunctiva and skin and enzyme analysis of tears. *Invest Ophthalmol* 15:626, 1976

80. POENARU L, DREYFUS J-C, BOUE J, NICOLESCO H, RAVISE N, BAMBERGER J: Prenatal diagnosis of fucosidosis, *Clin Genet* 10:260, 1976

81. MACPHEE GB, LOGAN RW: Fucosidosis in a native-born Briton. *J Clin Pathol* 30:278, 1977

82. SNYDER RD, CARLOW TJ, LEDMAN J, WENGER DA: Ocular findings in fucosidosis. *Birth Defects* 12(3):241, 1976

83. TROOST J, STAAL GEJ, WILLEMSE J, VAN DER HEIJDEN MCM: Fucosidosis; 1. Clinical and enzymological studies. *Neuropaediatrie* 8:155, 1977

84. ROMEO G, BORRONE C, GATTI R, DURAND P: Fucosidosis in Calabria: Founder effect or high gene frequency? *Lancet* 1:368, 1977

85. GIOVANNINI M, RIVA E, BELUFFI G, PEREGO O: Fucosidosis: Description of a clinical case. *Minerva Pediatr* 30:1307, 1978

86. LARBRISSEAU A, BROUCHU P, JASMIN G: Fucosidose de type 1: Etude anatomique. *Arch Fr Pediatr* 36:1013, 1979

87. SCHOONDEWALDT HC, LAMERS KJB, KLEIJNEN FM, VAN DEN BERG CJMG, DE BRUYN CHMM: Two patients with an unusual form of type II fucosidosis. *Clin Genet* 18:348, 1980

88. ALHADEFF JA, ANDREWS-SMITH GL, O'BRIEN JS: Biochemical studies on an unusual case of fucosidosis. *Clin Genet* 14:235, 1978

89. SCHAFER IA, POWELL DW, SULLIVAN JC: Lysosomal bone disease. *Pediatr Res* 5:391, 1971

90. EPINETTE WW, NORINS AL, DREW AL: Angiokeratoma corporis diffusum with α-L-fucosidase deficiency. *Arch Dermatol* 107:754, 1973

91. KORNFELD M, SNYDER RD, WENGER DA: Fucosidosis with angiokeratoma: Electron microscopic changes in the skin. *Arch Pathol Lab Med* 101:478, 1977

92. SMITH EB, GRAHAM JL, LEDMAN JA, SNYDER RD: Fucosidosis. *Cutis* 19:195, 1977

93. DVORETZKY I, FISHER BK: Fucosidosis. *Int J Dermatol* 18:213, 1979

94. PRINDIVILLE DE, STERN D: Oral lesions in fucosidosis. *J Oral Surg* 34:603, 1976

95. SNODGRASS MB: Ocular findings in a case of fucosidosis. *Brit J Ophthalmol* 60:508, 1976

96. BRILL PW, BERATIS NG, KOUSSEFF BG, HIRSCHHORN K: Roetgenographic findings in fucosidosis type 2. *Am J Roetgenol* 124:75, 1975

97. DAWSON G, SPRANGER JW: Fucosidosis: A glycosphingolipidosis. *N Engl J Med* 285:122, 1971

98. TSAY GC, DAWSON G: Oligosaccharide storage in brains from patients with fucosidosis, G_{M1}-gangliosidosis and G_{M2}-gangliosidosis (Sandhoff's disease) *J Neurochem* 27:733, 1976

99. TSAY GC, DAWSON G, SUNG S-SJ: Structure of the accumulating oligosaccharide in fucosidosis. *J Biol Chem* 251:5852, 1976

100. NISHIGAKI M, YAMASHITA K, MATSUDA I, ARASHIMA S, KOBATA A: Urinary oligosaccharides of fucosidosis: Evidence of the occurrence of X-antigenic determinant in serum-type sugar chains of glycoproteins. *J Biochem* 84:823, 1978

101. STRECKER G, FOURNET B, MONTREUIL J, DORLAND L, HAVERKAMP J, VLIEGENTHART JFG, DUBESSET D: Structure of the three major fucosylglycoasparagines accumulating in the urine of a patient with fucosidosis. *Biochimie* 60:725, 1978

102. NG YING KIN NMK, WOLFE LS: Urinary excretion of a novel hexasaccharide and a glycopeptide analogue in fucosidosis. *Biochem Biophys Res Commun* 88:696, 1979

103. LUNDBLAD A, LUNDSTEN J, NORDÉN NE, SJÖBLAD S, SVENSSON S, ÖCKERMAN P-A, GEHLHOFF M: Urinary abnormalities in fucosidosis: Characterization of a disaccharide and two glycoasparagines. *Eur J Biochem* 83:513, 1978

104. YAMASHITA K, TACHIBANA Y, TAKADA S, MATSUDA I, ARASHIMA S, KOBATA A: Urinary glycopeptides of fucosidosis. *J Biol Chem* 254:4820, 1979

105. GREILING H, STUHLSATZ HW, CANTZ M, GEHLER J: Increased urinary excretion of keratan sulfate in fucosidosis. *J Clin Chem Clin Biochem* 16:329, 1978

106. STAAL GEJ, VAN DER HEIJDEN MCM, TROOST J, MOES M, BORST-EILERS E: Fucosidosis and Lewis substances. *Clin Chim Acta* 76:155, 1977

107. ZIELKE K, VEATH M., O'BRIEN JS: Fucosidosis: Deficiency of alpha-L-fucosidase in cultured skin fibroblasts. *J Exp Med* 136:197, 1972
108. BERATIS NG, TURNER BM, HIRSCHHORN K: Fucosidosis: Detection of the carrier state in peripheral blood leukocytes. *J Pediatr* 87:1193, 1975
109. TROOST J, VAN DER HEIJDEN MCM, STAAL GEJ: Human leucocyte α-L-fucosidase. *Clin Chim Acta* 73:321, 1976
110. ALHADEFF JA, O'BRIEN JS: Fucosidosis, in Glew RH, Peters SP (eds): *Practical Enzymology of the Sphingolipidoses.* New York, Alan R Liss, 1977, p 247
111. DI MATTEO G, DURAND P, GATTI R, MARESCA A, ORFEO M, URBANO F, ROMEO G: Human α-fucosidase; Single residual enzymatic form in fucosidosis. *Biochim Biophys Acta* 429:538, 1976
112. BERATIS NG, TURNER BM, LABADIE G, HIRSCHHORN K: α-L-fucosidase in cultured skin fibroblasts from normal subjects and fucosidosis patients. *Pediatr Res* 11:862, 1977
113. THORPE R, ROBINSON D: Purification and serological studies of human α-fucosidase in the normal and fucosidosis states. *Clin Chim Acta* 86:21, 1978
114. ALHADEFF JA, MILLER AL, WENAAS H, VEDVICK T, O'BRIEN JS: Human liver α-L-fucosidase: Purification, characterization, and immunological studies. *J Biol Chem* 250:7106, 1975
115. DAWSON G, TSAY G: Substrate specificity of human α-L-fucosidase. *Arch Biochem Biophys* 184:12, 1977
116. GOSS SJ, HARRIS H: Gene transfer by means of cell fusion. II. The mapping of 8 loci on huyman chromosome 1 by statistical analysis of gene assortment in somatic cell hybrids. *J Cell Sci* 25:39, 1977
117. DURAND P, BORRONE C, GATTI R: On genetic variants in fucosidosis. *J Pediatr* 89:688, 1976
118. BERATIS NG, TURNER BM, HIRSCHHORN K: Reply, letter to the editor. *J Pediatr* 89:690, 1976
119. TURNER BM, TURNER VS, BERATIS NG, HIRSCHHORN K: Polymorphism of human α-fucosidase. *Am J Hum Genet* 27:651, 1975
120. TURNER BM, BERATIS NG, TURNER VS, HIRSCHHORN K: Silent allele as genetic basis of fucosidosis. *Nature* 257:391, 1975
121. WOOD S: Plasma alpha-L-fucosidase: Presence of a low activity variant in some normal individuals. *J Lab Clin Med* 88:469, 1976
122. PLAYFER JR, EVANS DAP: Enzyme activity in fucosidosis. *Lancet* 2:1415, 1976
123. LOWDEN JA, O'BRIEN JS: Sialidosis: A review of human neuraminidase deficiency. *Am J Hum Genet* 31:1, 1979
124. THOMAS GH, GOLDBERG MF, MILLER CS, REYNOLDS LW: Neuraminidase deficiency in the original patient with the Goldberg syndrome. *Clin Genet* 16:323, 1979
125. DURAND P, GATTI R, CAVALIERI S, BORRONE C, TOUNDEUR M, MICHALSKI J-C, STRECKER G: Sialidosis (mucolipidosis I). *Helv Paediatr Acta* 32:391, 1977
126. O'BRIEN JS: Neuraminidase deficiency in the cherry red spot—myoclonus syndrome. *Biochem Biophys Res Commun* 79:1136, 1977
127. RAPIN I, GOLDFISHER S, KATZMAN R, ENGEL J, O'BRIEN JS: The cherry red spot—myoclonus syndrome. *Ann Neurol* 3:234, 1978
128. THOMAS GH, TIPTON RE, CH'IEN LT, REYNOLDS LW, MILLER CS: Sialidase (α-N-acetyl neuraminic) deficiency: The enzyme defect in an adult with macular cherry-red spots and myoclonus without dementia. *Clin Genet* 13:369, 1978
129. WENGER DA, TARBY TJ, WHARTON C: Macular cherry-red spots and myoclonus with dementia: Coexistent neuraminidase and β-galactosidase deficiencies. *Biochem Biophys Res Commun* 82:589, 1978
130. GOLDSTEIN ML, KOLODNY EH, GASCON GG, GILLES FH: Macular cherry-red spot, myoclonic epilepsy, and neurovisceral storage in a 17-year-old girl. *Trans Am Neurol Assoc* 99:110, 1974
131. THOMAS PK, ABRAMS JD, SWALLOW D, STEWART G: Sialidosis type 1: Cherry red spots—myoclonus syndrome with sialidase deficiency and altered electrophoretic mobilities of some enzymes known to be glycoproteins. *J Neurol Neurosur Psychiatry* 42:873, 1979
132. STEINMAN L, THARP BR, DORFMAN LJ, FORNO LS, SOGG RL, KELTS KA, O'BRIEN JS: Peripheral neuropathy in the cherry-red spot—myoclonus syndrome (sialidosis type I). *Ann Neurol* 7:450, 1980
133. FEINFELD DA, SCHOLNICK HR, JANIS R: Lupus nephritis in a neuronal storage disease. *Arch Intern Med* 137:693, 1977
134. LOONEN MCB, VDLUGT L, FRANKE CL: Angiokeratoma corporis diffusum and lysosomal enzyme deficiency. *Lancet* 2:785, 1974
135. SUZUKI Y, NAKAMURA N, FUKUOKA K, SHIMADA Y, UONO M: β-Galactosidase deficiency in juvenile and adult patients. *Hum Genet* 36:219, 1977
136. OKADA S, KATO T, MIURA S, YABUUCHI H, NISHIGAKI M, KOBATA A, CHIYO H, FURUYAMA J-I: Hypersialyloligosachariduria in mucolipidoses: A method for diagnosis. *Clin Chim Acta* 86:159, 1978
137. OKADA S, YUTAKA T, KATO T, IKEHARA C, YABUUCHI H, OKAWA M, INUI M, CHIYO H: A case of neuraminidase deficiency associated with a partial β-galactosidase defect. *Eur J Pediatr* 130:239, 1979
138. MIYATAKE T, ATSUMI T, OBAYASHI T, MIZUNO Y, ANDO S, ARIGA T,

139. MATSUI-NAKAMURA K, YAMADA T: Adult type neuronal storage disease with neuraminidase deficiency. *Ann Neurol* 6:232, 1979
139. KOBAYASHI T, OHTA M, GOTO I, TANAKA Y, KUROIWA Y: Adult type mucolipidosis with β-galactosidase and sialidase deficiency: Histological and biochemical studies. *J Neurol* 221:137, 1979
140. KURIYAMA M, OKADA S, TANAKA Y, UMEZAKI H: Adult mucolipidosis with β-galactosidase and neuraminidase deficiencies. *J Neurol Sci* 46:245, 1980
141. KELLY TE, GRAETZ G: Isolated acid neuraminidase deficiency: A distinct lysosomal storage disease. *Am J Med Genet* 1:31, 1977
142. SPRANGER J, CANTZ M: Mucolipidosis I, the cherry-red spot—myoclonus syndrome and neuraminidase deficiency. *Birth Defects* 14(6B):105, 1978
143. BERARD M, TOGA M, BERNARD R, DUBOIS D, MARIANI R, HASSOUN J: Pathologic findings in one case of neuronal and mesenchymal storage disease: Its relationship to lipidoses and to mucopolysaccharidoses. *Pathol Europ* 3:172, 1968
144. MAROTEAUX P, POISSONNIER M, TONDEUR M, STRECKER G, LEMONNIER M: Sialidose par deficit en alpha (2-6) neuraminidase sans atteinte neurologique. *Arch Fr Pediatr* 35:280, 1978
145. MAROTEAUX P, HUMBEL R, STRECKER G, MICHALSKI J-C, MANDE R: Unnouveau type de sialidose avec atteinte renale: La nephrosialidose, 1. Etude clinique, radiologique et nosologique. *Arch Fr Pediatr* 35:819, 1978
146. WINTER RM, SWALLOW DM, BARAITSER M, PURKISS P: Sialidosis type 2 (acid neuraminidase deficiency): Clinical and biochemical features of a further case. *Clin Genet* 18:203, 1980
147. GRAVEL RA, LOWDEN JA, CALLAHAN JW, WOLFE LS, NG YIN KIN NMK: Infantile sialidosis: A phenocopy of type 1 G_{M1} gangliosidosis distinguished by genetic complementation and urinary oligosaccharides. *Am J Hum Genet* 31:669, 1979
148. KLEIJER WJ, HOOGEVEEN A, VERHEIJEN FW, NIERMEIJER MF, GALJAARD H, O'BRIEN JS, WARNER TG: Prenatal diagnosis of sialidosis with combined neuraminidase and β-galactosidase deficiency. *Clin Genet* 16:60, 1979
149. AYLSWORTH AS, THOMAS GH, HOOD JL, MALOUF N, LIBERT J: A severe infantile sialidosis: Clinical, biochemical, and microscopic features. *J Pediatr* 96:662, 1980
150. JOHNSON WG, THOMAS GH, MIRANDA AF, DRISCOLL JM, WIGGER JH, YEH MN, SCHWARTZ RC, COHEN CS, BERDON WE, KOENIGSBERGER MR: Congenital sialidosis: Biochemical studies: Clinical spectrum in four sibs; two successful prenatal diagnoses. *Am J Hum Genet* 32:43A, 1980
151. STRECKER G, PEERS M-C, MICHALSKI J-C, HONDI-ASSAH T, FOURNET B, SPIK G, MONTREUIL J, FARRIAUX J-P, MARTEAUX P, DURAND P: Structure of nine sialyl-oligosaccharides accumulated in urine of eleven patients with three different types of sialidosis. *Eur J Biochem* 75:391, 1977
152. DORLAND L, HAVERKAMP J, VLIEGENTHART JFG, STRECKER G, MICHALSKI J-C, FOURNET B, SPIK G, MONTREUIL J: 360-MHz ^{1}H nuclear-magnetic resonance spectroscopy of sialyl-oligosaccharides from patients with sialidosis (mucolipidosis I and II). *Eur J Biochem* 87:323, 1978
153. TULSIANI DRP, CARUBELLI R: Studies on the soluble and lysosomal neuraminidases of rat liver. *J Biol Chem* 245:1821, 1970
154. STRECKER G, MICHALSKI JC: Biochemical basis of six different types of sialidosis. *FEBS Lett* 85:20, 1978
155. O'BRIEN JS: The cherry red spot—myoclonus syndrome: A newly recognized inherited lysosomal storage disease due to acid neuraminidase deficiency. *Clin Genet* 14:55, 1978
156. FRISCH A, NEUFELD EF: A rapid and sensitive assay for neuraminidase: Application to cultured fibroblasts. *Anal Biochem* 95:222, 1979
157. POTIER M, BEAUREGARD G, BÉLISLE M, MAMELIA L, NGUYEN HONG V, MELANCON SB, DALLAIRE L: Neuraminidase activity in the mucolipidoses (types I, II, and III) and the cherry-red spot myoclonus syndrome. *Clin Chim Acta* 99:97, 1979
158. WARNER TG, O'BRIEN JS: Synthesis of 2'-(4-methylumbelliferyl)-α-D-N-acetylneuraminic acid and detection of skin fibroblast neuraminidase in normal humans and in sialidosis. *Biochemistry* 18:2783, 1979
159. MIYATAKE T, YAMADA T, SUZUKI M, PALLMANN B, SANDHOFF K, ARIGA T, ATSUMI T: Sialidase deficiency in adult-type neuronal storage disease. *FEBS Lett* 97:257, 1979
160. CANTZ M, MESSER H: Oligosaccharide and ganglioside neuraminidase activities of mucolipidosis I (sialidosis) and mucolipidosis II (I-cell disease) fibroblasts. *Eur J Biochem* 97:113, 1979.
161. O'BRIEN JS, WARNER TG: Sialidosis: Delineation of subtypes by neuraminidase assay. *Clin Genet* 17:35, 1980
162. DEN TANDT WR, LEROY JG: Deficiency of neuraminidase in the sialidoses and the mucolipidoses. *Hum Genet* 53:383, 1980
163. BACH G, ZEIGLER M, SCHAAP T, KOHN G: Mucolipidosis type IV: Gangliosidase sialidase deficiency. *Biochem Biophys Res Commun* 90:1341, 1979
164. HAHN LC, BEN-YOSEPH Y, NADLER HL: Glycoprotein and ganglioside α-N-acetylneuraminidases in sialidosis and mucolipidoses. *Am J Hum Genet* 32:41A, 1980

165. GALJAARD H, HOOGEVEEN A, KEIJZER W, WIT-VERBEEK HA, DE REUSER AJJ, HO MW, ROBINSON D: Genetic heterogeneity in G$_{M1}$ gangliosidosis. *Nature* 257:60, 1975

166. HOOGEVEEN AT, VERHEIJEN FW, D'AZZO A, GALJAARD H: Genetic heterogeneity in human neuraminidase deficiency. *Nature* 285:500, 1980

167. WOMACK JE, YAN DLS, POTIER M: Liver neuraminidase deficiency inherited as a single gene on mouse chromosome. *Am J Hum Genet* 32:59A, 1980

168. AULA P, AUTIO S, RAIVIO K, NÄNTÖ V: Detection of heterozygotes for aspartylglucosaminuria (AGU) in cultured fibroblasts. *Humangenetik* 25:307, 1974

169. BORUD O, TORP KH: Aspartylglycosaminuria in northern Norway. *Lancet* 1:1082, 1976

170. BORUD O, STRÖMME JH, LIE SO, TORP KH: Aspartylglycosaminuria in northern Norway in eight patients: Clinical heterogeneity and variations with the diet. *J Inher Metab Dis* 1:95, 1978

171. ISENBERG JN, SHARP HL: Aspartylglucosaminuria: Psychomotor retardation masquerading as a mucopolysaccharidosis. *J Pediatr* 86:713, 1975

172. AUTIO S: Aspartylglucosaminuria: Analysis of thirty-four patients. *J Ment Defic Res* Monogr Ser I:1, 1972

173. ARSTILA AU, PALO J, HALTIA M, RIEKKINEN P, AUTIO S: Aspartylglucosaminuria I: Fine structural studies on liver, kidney and brain. *Acta Neuropathol (Berlin)* 20:207, 1972

174. ISENBERG JN, SHARP HL: Aspartylglucosaminuria: Unique biochemical and ultrastructural characteristics. *Hum Pathol* 7:469, 1976

175. HALTIA M, PALO J, AUTIO S: Aspartylglucosaminuria: A generalized storage disease: Morphological and histochemical studies *Acta Neuropathol (Berlin)* 31:243, 1975

176. MAURY P: Accumulation of two glycoasparagines in the liver in aspartylglycosaminuria. *J Biol Chem* 254:1513, 1979

177. LUNDBLAD A, MASSON PK, NORDÉN NE, SVENSSON S, ÖCKERMAN P-A, PALO J: Structural determination of three glycoasparagines isolated from the urine of a patient with aspartylglycosaminuria. *Eur J Biochem* 67:209, 1976

178. MAURY P: Quantitative determination of 4-N-2-acetamido-2-deoxy-β-D-glucopyranosyl-L-asparagine in the urine of patients with aspartylglycosaminuria by gas-liquid chromatography. *J Lab Clin Med* 93:718, 1979

179. POLLITT RJ, PRETTY KM: The glycoasparagines in urine of a patient with aspartylglycosaminuria. *Biochem J* 141:141, 1974

180. AKASAKI M, SUGAHARA K, FUNAKOSHI I, AULA P, YAMASHINA I: Characterization of a mannose-containing glycoasparagine isolated from urine of a patient with aspartylglycosylaminuria (AGU). *FEBS Lett* 69:191, 1976

181. SUGAHARA K, FUNAKOSHI S, FUNAKOSHI I, AULA P, YAMASHINA I: Characterization of two glycoasparagines isolated from the urine of patients with aspartylglycosylaminuria (AGU). *J Biochem* 78:673, 1975

182. PALO J, POLLITT RJ, PRETTY KM, SAVOLAINEN H: Glycoasparagine metabolites in patients with aspartylglycosaminuria: Comparison between English and Finnish patients with special reference to storage materials. *Clin Chim Acta* 47:69, 1973

183. MAKINO M, KOJIMA T, YAMASHINA I: Enzymatic cleavage of glycopeptides. *Biochem Biophys Res Commun* 24:961, 1966

184. AULA P, RAIVIO K, AUTIO S: Enzymatic diagnosis and carrier detection of aspartylglucosaminuria using blood samples. *Pediatr Res* 10:625, 1976

185. PALO J, RIEKKINEN P, ARSTILA AU, AUTIO S, KIVIMÄKI T: Aspartylglucosaminuria II: Biochemical studies on brain, liver, kidney and spleen. *Acta Neuropathol (Berlin)* 20:217, 1972

186. SOMER H, PALO J, SAVOLAINEN H, KONTTINEN A: Studies on N-aspartyl-β-glucosaminidase in aspartylglycosaminuria. *Clin Chim Acta* 60:219, 1975

187. SEWELL AC: An improved thin-layer chromatographic method for urinary oligosaccharid screening. *Clin Chim Acta* 92:411, 1979

188. HOLMES EW, O'BRIEN JS: Separation of glycoprotein-derived oligosaccharides by thin-layer chromatography *Anal Biochem* 93:167, 1979

189. SEWELL AC: Urinary oligosaccharide excretion in disorders of glycolipid, glycoprotein and glycogen metabolism: A review of screening for differential diagnosis. *Eur J Pediatr* 134:183, 1980

190. MAIRE I, ZABOT MT, MATHIEU M, COTTE J: Mannosidosis: Tissue culture studies in relation to prenatal diagnosis. *J Inher Metab Dis* 1:19, 1978

191. POENARU L, GIRARD S, THEPOT F, MADELENAT P, HURAUZ-RENDU C, VINET M-C, DREYFUS J-C: Antenatal diagnosis in three pregnancies at risk for mannosidosis. *Clin Genet* 16:428, 1979

192. GERBIE AB, MELANCON SB, RYAN C, NADLER HL: Cultivated epithelial like cells and fibroblasts from amniotic fluid: Their relationship to enzymatic and cytologic analysis. *Am J Obstet Gynecol* 114:314, 1972

193. TURNER BM, TURNER VS, HIRSCHHORN K: Metabolic correction of fucosidosis fibroblasts by human α-L-fucosidase. *J Cell Physiol* 98:225, 1979

194. WOOD S: Cultured fucosidosis fibroblasts: A simple technique demonstrating storage of tritiated-fucose labeled material. *Clin Genet* 10:183, 1976

39

ACID LIPASE DEFICIENCY:
Wolman's Disease and Cholesteryl Ester Storage Disease

GERD ASSMANN

DONALD S. FREDRICKSON

1. *Deficient activity of lysosomal acid lipase results in massive accumulation of cholesteryl esters and triglycerides in most tissues of the body. Both of these lipids are substrates for the enzyme, one of the major functions of which is the hydrolysis of cholesteryl esters in low density lipoproteins as they are removed from plasma by tissues in the periphery. The deficiency state is expressed in two major phenotypes:* Wolman's disease *and* cholesteryl ester storage disease.

2. *Wolman's disease occurs in infancy and is nearly always fatal before the age of 1 year. Hepatosplenomegaly, steatorrhea, abdominal distension and other gastrointestinal symptoms, adrenal calcification demonstrable by x-rays, and failure to thrive are observed in the first few weeks of life.*

3. *Cholesteryl ester storage disease can be more benign. It may not be detected until adulthood. Lipid deposition is widespread although hepatomegaly may be the only clinical abnormality. Hyperbetalipoproteinemia is common, and premature atherosclerosis may be severe. Adrenal calcification is rare.*

4. *Diagnosis of both disorders is based on the clinical picture, combined with demonstration of acid lipase deficiency in cultured skin fibroblasts, lymphocytes, or other tissues. Both Wolman's disease and cholesteryl ester storage disease appear to be inherited in an autosomal recessive mode. The structural gene for the acid lipase enzyme is on chromosome 10. There is no specific therapy.*

Two diseases have been independently discovered in which prodigious amounts of cholesteryl esters and often triglycerides accumulate in lysosomes. Wolman's disease is the more severe form. It is associated with hepatosplenomegaly and adrenal calcification and is nearly always fatal in the first year of life. Cholesteryl ester storage disease (CESD) is more benign, usually compatible with adult life and very rarely associated with adrenal calcification [1, 2].

It appears that these disorders are allelic, involving mutations at loci controlling the activity of a hydrolase which cleaves cholesteryl esters and triglycerides under acidic conditions (Fig. 39-1). The enzyme has been variously called lysosomal acid lipase, acid lipase, or acid esterase, and the activities measured as acid cholesteryl ester hydrolase or acid lipase. Wolman's disease and CESD are here described in parallel and the findings then correlated in a discussion of the pathophysiology of acid lipase deficiency.

HISTORY

In 1956, Abramov, Schorr, and Wolman described an infant with abdominal distension, hepatosplenomegaly, and massive calcification of the adrenal glands [3]. In 1963, Wolman et al. reported two more affected sibs in this same family [4]. In the first report, Wolman and his colleagues [3] noted the accumulation of both cholesterol and triglycerides in the liver, adrenal

acid lipase deficiency

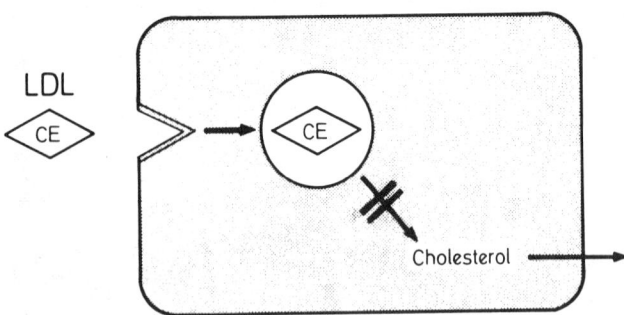

Figure 39-1 Schematic representation of the hydrolytic site affected by the enzyme deficiency underlying the disorders described in this chapter.

glands, spleen, and lymph nodes. The disorder was first called "generalized xanthomatosis with calcified adrenals" or "primary familial xanthomatosis with adrenal calcification" [3–5]. Later Crocker et al. [6] suggested the eponym *Wolman's disease*. In retrospect, a patient described by Alexander in 1946 [7] as having "Niemann-Pick disease" may have been the first example of this disorder to appear in the literature.

About 40 examples of Wolman's disease have been discovered. The clinical and morphological findings of the individual patients are described in patient reports [3, 4, 6, 8–50] and in previous editions of this book [1, 2]. In patients with Wolman's disease the abnormality of lipid metabolism becomes clinically evident in the first weeks of life. The most important clinical features include hepatosplenomegaly, digestive difficulties, steatorrhea, and enlargement and calcification of the adrenal glands. The condition is usually fatal by the age of 6 months.

In 1961, Wolman et al. demonstrated that most of the accumulated cholesterol was in the esterified form [5]. Later studies repeatedly confirmed these observations. In 1969, Patrick and Lake [23] demonstrated that activity of an acid hydrolase catalyzing the hydrolysis of both cholesteryl esters and triglycerides was severely deficient in the liver and spleen of patients with Wolman's disease. This has been confirmed in tissues [29, 51], including cultured fibroblasts [38, 52–54] and leukocytes [37, 50, 55] of other patients. In 1976, Cortner et al. demonstrated that lysosomal acid lipase activity of circulating lymphocytes and cultured fibroblasts can be separated by cellogel electrophoresis into isoenzymes A and B. Both Wolman's disease and CESD cells showed complete absence of the A isoenzyme [38, 56].

Brief published mention of CESD was first made by Fredrickson in 1963 in reference to a child with marked hyperlipemia, whose enlarged liver was found to contain 18 percent of its wet weight as cholesteryl esters. He called the disorder *hepatic cholesterol ester storage disease* [57]. In 1967, Lageron et al. [59] and Infante et al. [60] reported a 43-year-old man with apparently the same disease under the name *polycorie cholésterolique de l'adulte*. He had been known to have had hepatomegaly since age 14. At about the same time, Schiff et al. reported a brother and sister with similar clinical, morphological, and biochemical abnormalities [61]. Four of their five younger sibs also had hepatomegaly. Biopsy specimens of liver from three of these sibs were interpreted as showing minimal morphological abnormalities, suggesting a milder expression of the same inherited defect. These authors pointed out the presence of minimal cirrhosis in the liver, in addition to the fat loading of all hepatocytes seen in the other cases.

The following year Partin and Schubert [62] described detailed studies of jejunal and duodenal biopsy specimens in the two most severely affected children of the kindred of Schiff et al. [61]. The evidence they presented of cholesterol storage in the intestine first indicated that the involvement in CESD extends beyond the liver. This concept has been substantiated by necropsy studies in three patients with CESD [1, 58, 63]. The less limited term *cholesterol* (or *cholesteryl*) *ester storage disease* proposed by Partin and Schubert has subsequently been used for the disorder.

A total of 23 reported cases of this disease have been recognized [1, 2, 51, 59–79] (Table 39-1). As in Wolman's disease, the metabolic defect in CESD consists of severe deficiency in the activity of the acid cholesteryl ester hydrolase, or acid lipase, which catalyzes the hydrolysis of both cholesteryl esters and triglycerides [38, 51, 54, 58, 63, 70, 71, 76–79].

The enzymatic defect has been demonstrated in several types of cells and tissues, including liver, spleen, lymph nodes, aorta, peripheral blood leukocytes, and cultured skin fibroblasts. More recently the defect has been related to the sequence of events involved in catabolism of cholesteryl esters entering the cell during removal of plasma low density lipoproteins [80, 81] (see Chap. 33).

CLINICAL MANIFESTATIONS

Wolman's Disease

Most of the patients with Wolman's disease have had a remarkably similar clinical course. Increasing vomiting and diarrhea, hepatosplenomegaly, abdominal distension, anemia, and inanition are major clinical signs, and the child's general condition progresses rapidly downhill. Death usually occurs by age 3 to 6 months but has been protracted to as long as 14 months [21].

The disease usually has its onset in the first weeks of life. In most cases, the abnormality first noticed by the parents is persistent and forceful vomiting associated with marked abdominal distension. Several patients have also had frequent and watery stools in the first few weeks of life [18, 21, 26]. In a few patients jaundice [4, 6, 10, 33] or persistent low-grade fever has been observed [4, 6].

Anemia usually appears by the sixth week and becomes more severe as the disease progresses; the hemoglobin may fall to 6 g/dl. Thrombocytopenia has not been observed. Vacuolization of lymphocytes has been noted repeatedly. The vacuoles are both intracytoplasmic and intranuclear. Lipid-laden histiocytes, or foam cells, have been observed in bone marrow aspirates as early as 40 days of age. In the later stages of the illness the marrow almost invariably contains large numbers of foam cells. Similar cells have been observed in the peripheral blood [4]. Acanthocytosis has been reported in one patient [24]. Plasma lipids are usually at the low end of the normal range.

Hepatosplenomegaly has been observed as early as the fourth day of life [26]. It is an invariable feature of the disease and may be of massive proportions.

A most striking feature of Wolman's disease is calcification

Table 39-1 Patients with cholesteryl ester storage disease

Pat.	Ref.	S	D[A(y)]	R(D)[A(y)]	Hm	Sm	Ev	Hf	TC	TG	Other
1. L.Mc.	[1, 51]	F	3	(21)	+	+	0	+	402	150	Aortic stenosis, coronary arteriosclerosis
2. Mc.	[1, 51]	F	1/12	(1/12)	+	+	0	0	–	–	Respiratory distress
3. Lem.	[59, 60, 69]	M	14	43	+	0	0	+	275	140	Jaundice, polyposis coli
4. T.H.	[61, 62, 76, 77]	M	2	18	+	+	+	+	276	192	Early familial hepatic cirrhosis, serum bile acids elevated
5. W.H.T.	[61]	F	–	19	+	0	0	+	356	413	Eosinophilia
6. E.M.N.	[65]	F	7	17	+	0	+	+	400	353	Eosinophilia
7. Rad.	[67, 68, 69]	F	23	44	+	0	0	0	335	–	Recurrent abdominal pain
8. T.R.	[63]	F	6	(9)	+	+	+	+	–	–	Aortic arterial plaques, enlarged adrenal glands, hepatic coma
9. R.R.	[63]	F	–	(7)	+	+	0	+	–	–	Enlarged adrenal glands
10. J.R.	[38, 63, 78, 80, 81, 87]	F	2	13	+	+	0	+	230	69	Adrenal calcification, pulmonary hypertension
11. K.W.	[54, 63]	F	–	8	+	0	0	–	363	214	
12. A.L.	[64]	M	2	7	+	0	0	–	–	–	Eosinophilia
13. L.O.	[69, 70]	M	1	8	+	0	–	–	300	–	Recurrent abdominal pain
14. M.S.	[69, 70]	F	9	12	+	–	–	+	390	150	Febrile icterus
15. M.A.	[69]	F	6	9	+	–	–	+	285	160	Febrile icterus
16. C.N.	[69]	F	11	11	+	–	–	+	360	135	
17. K.N.	[72, 73]	M	2	8	+	0	–	+	301		
18. A.C.d.O.	[71]	M	4	6	+	0	0	–	380	122	Recurrent abdominal pain with fever
19. B.Z.	[74]	M	4	13	+	–	0	+	403	334	Vitamin D–resistant rickets
20. T.S.	[74]	M	3	12	+	0	–	+	247	121	Factor V deficiency
21. N.S.	[74]	F	7	11	+	0	–	+	252	187	Factor V deficiency, recurrent abdominal pain
22. J.M.	[74]	M	4	5	+	0	0	+	423	302	
23. B.U.	[75]	F	10	15	+	+	0	+	275	191	HDL₂ HDL₃
24. Le.M.	[66, 70]	F	1	12	+	0	–	0	385	310	Febrile icterus

NOTE: Pat. = patient; + = present; 0 = absent; – = not specifically mentioned; D = detection; R(D) = report or (death); A(y) = age (years); Hm = hepatomegaly; Sm = splenomegaly; Ev = esophageal varices; Hf = hepatic fibrosis; TC = total serum cholesterol; TG = serum triglycerides

of the adrenal glands (Fig. 39-2). This abnormality has been consistently demonstrated ante mortem by roentgenographic examination in all but four patients. The adrenals are markedly and symmetrically enlarged (up to 3.5 × 2.5 cm) and their normal pyramidal or semilunar shape is retained. They are extensively seeded with finely stippled or punctate calcific deposits. The enlarged adrenals may flatten the superior poles of the kidneys [6], but they do not deform the caliceal system or interfere with renal function.

Specific symptoms related to the central nervous system are uncommon in Wolman's disease, but neurologic development is not normal. Typically alert and active at birth, the infants show a progressive mental deterioration within a few weeks after the onset of symptoms. In several case reports mention has been made of the fact that the optic fundi were normal and that a cherry-red spot was not present. In one patient a Babinski sign was elicited [6]. Konno et al. described a patient who had exaggerated tendon reflexes, ankle clonus, and opisthotonus [10]. Paralysis and convulsions have not been observed.

There are no specific routine laboratory observations that suggest the diagnosis. Liver function tests are frequently abnormal. Laboratory studies support the clinical observations

of malabsorption and malnutrition. As determined by feeding ^{131}I-labeled triolein [24] or unlabeled fats [26], there appears to be a significant impairment of fat absorption. ACTH-stimulation studies have indicated depressed adrenal responsiveness [6, 26]. No gross abnormalities of the electroencephalogram have been observed in several patients [6, 10, 14, 24]. Chromosomal analyses in two patients were normal [10, 41].

Cholesteryl Ester Storage Disease

The history and clinical course of the original patients affected with CESD are extensively discussed in previous editions of this book [1, 2]. Table 39-1 summarizes some features of the 24 patients who are known to have CESD and 1 additional patient whom we regard as a probable case of CESD [64]. The principal and sometimes only sign, hepatomegaly, may be evident at birth or in early childhood. Occasionally it is delayed until the second decade of life (patients 3, 5, and 7). Hepatomegaly apparently increases with time and eventually leads to hepatic fibrosis. The spleen has been found to be enlarged in

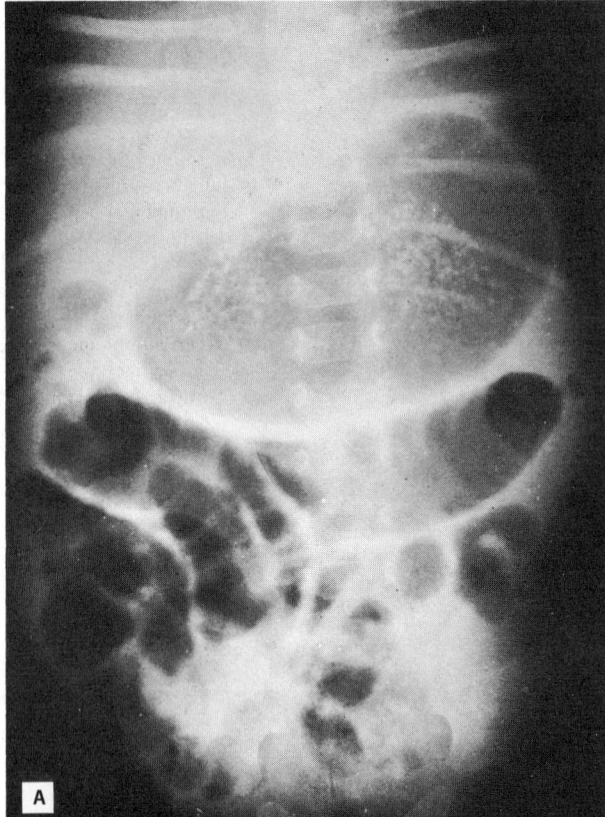

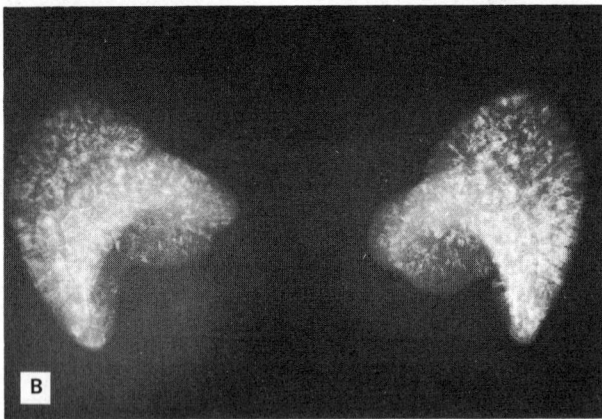

Figure 39-2 Roentgenogram showing the calcification of the enlarged adrenal glands in a patient with Wolman's disease. *A.* Patient in supine position. *B.* The adrenals after removal at autopsy. (*Photographs kindly supplied by Dr. Allen Crocker and reprinted from [6] with permission.*)

about a third of the patients. Esophageal varices have occasionally been detected. Patients 8 and 9 developed hepatitis with eventually fatal complications [63, 78] and in several other patients jaundice has been noted. Gallstones have not been found in any of the patients. A number of patients have had recurrent abdominal pain. Patient 4, a boy, and patients 6 and 22, two girls, had some delay in onset of puberty. Patients 1 and 10 had recurrent epistaxes, and several have had episodes of gastrointestinal bleeding. Patients 19 and 20 had a decreased concentration of blood clotting factor V, and patient 8, hypoprothrombinemia.

Malabsorption, malnutrition, or abnormalities involving the tonsils have not been described. The only neurologic changes have occurred in patient 3, who has had unexplained episodes

of headache, vertigo, hypersomnia, and loss of consciousness. One patient [10] has been found (at age 13) to have calcified adrenal glands detectable on abdominal roentgenograms. Patient 1 had roentgenographic evidence of calcification of the hepatic artery.

Exclusive of the plasma lipids, there are no other distinctive abnormalities in routine laboratory tests. Patient 3 is said to have had an indirect bilirubin of 6 mg but no jaundice [59]. Patients 6 and 11 had hyperglobulinemia. Total bile acids were grossly elevated in patient 4, and the ratio of cholic to chenodeoxycholic acid was low. Bone marrow aspirates in patients 1, 10, and 11 contained numerous large macrophages filled with birefringent droplets. Bone marrow appeared normal in patients 4 and 7.

PATHOLOGY

Liver

Hepatomegaly is a constant feature in Wolman's disease; the liver appears to increase in size throughout the course of the illness and by age 4 months may weigh 400 g, which is about twice the normal weight [14]. The liver has a firm consistency, and the cut surface is yellow and greasy.

The normal architecture of the liver is sometimes preserved [29] but may be so distorted that the portal spaces, even though infiltrated with lymphoid cells, provide the only readily recognizable landmarks [3, 4, 6, 21, 26]. The hepatic parenchymal cells are enlarged and vacuolated, and grossly enlarged and vacuolated Kupffer cells are prominent. Large numbers of foamy histiocytes are found in the portal and periportal areas and frequently in clusters between parencyhmal cells (Fig. 39-3). Portal and periportal fibrosis may be marked, and there may even be frank cirrhosis.

Under the electron microscope one sees that the organelles of the parenchymal cells have accumulated large osmiophilic lipid droplets. Most of these droplets are found within lysosomes [24]. The smooth and rough endoplasmic reticulum may appear dilated and distended [26]. It is not certain from histochemical studies whether both glycerides and cholesterol accumulate in the Kupffer and parenchymal cells [4, 6, 21, 26].

The liver in CESD also has an extraordinary orange or butter-yellow color and a smooth, soft texture. It is usually markedly enlarged, sometimes to twice the normal weight. Microscopic examination of the CESD liver reveals many of the same abnormalities as in Wolman's disease, with some possible differences related to a disease process of much longer standing. There are: (1) lipid droplets in hepatic parenchymal cells resembling those in ordinary fatty infiltration; (2) enlargement of Kupffer cells by smaller vacuoles and by PAS-positive granules; (3) variable amounts of septal fibrosis (Fig. 39-4), observed in 8 of the 10 patients in whom the liver has been examined and which has progressed in some patients to micronodular cirrhosis with esophageal varices; (4) focal periportal accumulations of lymphocytes, plasma cells, and foamy macrophages; and (5) massive storage of birefringent material, especially in hepatocytes. In sections embedded in paraffin or plastic the cytoplasm of the hepatocytes appears filled with vacuoles of various sizes and looks like lacework. The Kupffer cells are greatly enlarged; have several small, indented, darkly staining nuclei; and appear more finely and uniformly vacuolated than do hepatocytes. In frozen sections the lipid deposits in the hepatocytes are intensely birefringent and often exhibit elongated or irregularly shaped crystalline masses, whereas those in macrophages show little or no birefringence.

The deposits in the latter cells stain with various methods: oil red O, Sudan black B, Baker's acid hematin (for choline-containing lipids), periodic acid Schiff (PAS) and diastase-PAS (for periodic acid–reactive vicinal glycols), Schultz (for cholesterol), and Rinehart (for acidic substances); and they show yellowish autofluorescence [2]. Except for the Schultz reaction, these positive tests persist after extraction of the tissue with lipid solvents. Most of the deposits in the hepatocytes are not autofluorescent; they stain with the Schultz, oil red O, and Sudan black B methods, but not with the other methods cited above, and their positive reactions are abolished by pretreatment with lipid solvents. We interpret these findings to indicate that the deposits of cholesteryl esters and triglycerides in hepatocytes remain relatively stable. Those in macrophages, however, undergo extensive secondary changes, including peroxidation and polymerization of their fatty acids, which lead to the formation of insoluble masses of ceroid. Similar histochemical distinctions between two types of lipid deposits have been made in Wolman's disease, in which ceroid deposits also occur [27]. The gradual formation of ceroid deposits from accumulated neutral lipid has been observed in a variety of other disease states [83, 84]. In CESD the deposits in macrophages in bone marrow, spleen, lymph nodes, and other organs tend to resemble histochemically and ultrastructurally those in hepatic macrophages, while deposits in smooth-muscle cells, perivascular cells, and endothelial cells are more similar to those in hepatocytes.

Electron microscopy of liver tissue in CESD [2, 73] reveals: (1) Cytoplasmic inclusions in the hepatocytes, containing material which in part seems to solubilize during the preparation and tends to form crystals after formalin fixation and stor-

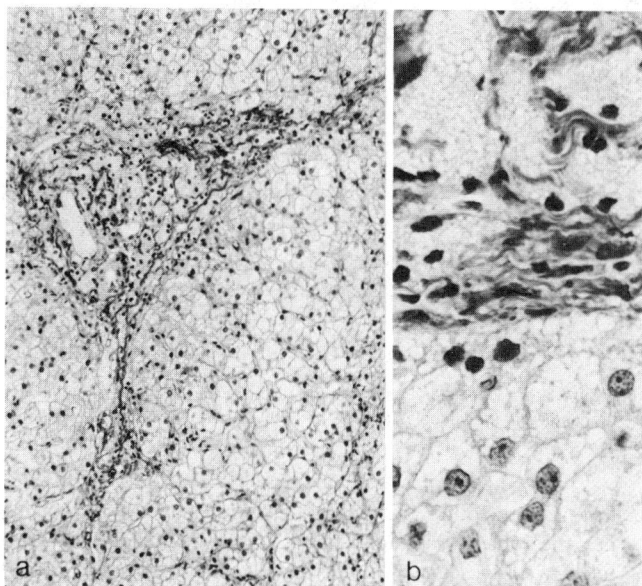

Figure 39-4 Cholesteryl ester storage disease. Light microscopy of paraffin section of liver. A. Septal pattern of fibrosis of moderate severity. Within the fibrous septum foamy histiocytes can be seen. Moderate lipid deposition in parenchymal cells. Magnification, X150. B. Area between foam cells in fibrous tissue (upper) and lipid-laden parenchymal cells (lower). Magnification, X600. (Courtesy of Prof. U. Pfeiffer.)

age at 4 C°. (2) These inclusions are limited by trilaminar membranes of 13 to 14 nm thickness (Fig. 39-5), consisting of a true vacuole membrane, a submembranous "halo" which is characteristic for lysosomes. There is also a thin, limiting layer which has also been described in Tangier disease (Chap. 29), in which the inclusions contain cholesteryl esters but are not limited by a membrane. (3) Heterogeneous storage material in Kupffer cells. (4) Membrane-limited vacuoles containing partly dissolved, partly osmiophilic lipid in the epithelial cells of small bile ducts as well as in endothelial cells (Fig. 39-6).

An animal model partly resembling the morphological findings in hepatocytes and Kupffer cells of CESD and Wolman's disease has been described by Drevon and Hovig [85]. These authors fed a semisynthetic diet containing 10 percent cottonseed oil and 1 percent cholesterol to guinea pigs and observed the accumulation of multivacuolated, secondary lysosomes, membrane-bound lipid vacuoles (lipolysosomes), and myelin figures in liver. These microscopic changes were due to a marked accumulation of cholesteryl esters.

Lipolysosomes (lysosomes containing large lipid droplets) can also be observed in livers of patients with various forms of hepatic injury [86]. Their numbers and sizes increase with the degree of fatty infiltration and probably represent a nonspecific finding.

Adrenal Glands

The adrenal glands in Wolman's disease are bright yellow and grossly and symmetrically enlarged; their configuration is, however, normal. Each gland may weigh as much as 13 g, compared with a normal weight of 5 g. The adrenals are usually quite firm, contain flecks of gritty calcified tissue, and are difficult to cut. In cut section, the outer rim of cortex is intensely yellow, and the central zone is gray or white.

Under microscopic examination it can be seen that the archi-

Figure 39-3 Wolman's disease. Electron microscopy of liver. A. Liver sinusoid lining cells distended by dropletlike crystal cleftlike lysosomes (Ly). Dropletlike lysosomes in liver parenchymal cell (P). Magnification, X4500. B. Membrane (arrows) of a dropletlike lysosome (Ly) in liver parenchymal cell. Glycogen granules (Gl). Magnification, X106,000. C. High resolution of crystal cleftlike lysosomes (Ly) in liver sinusoidal cells. Magnification, X30,000. (Courtesy of Dr. Dirk B. von Bassewitz.).

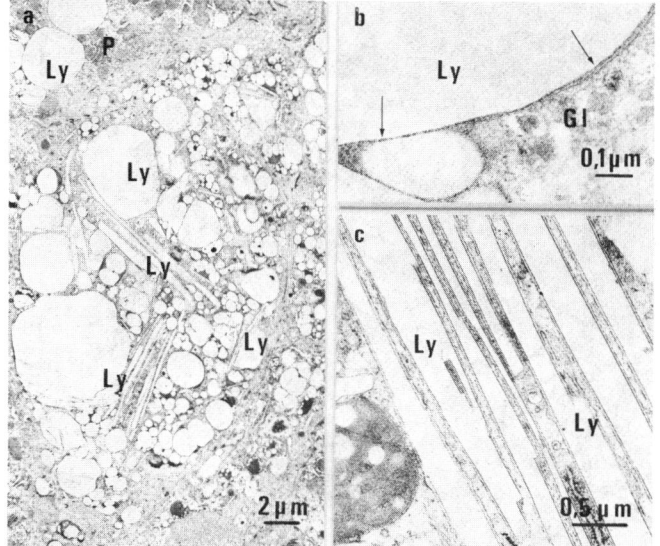

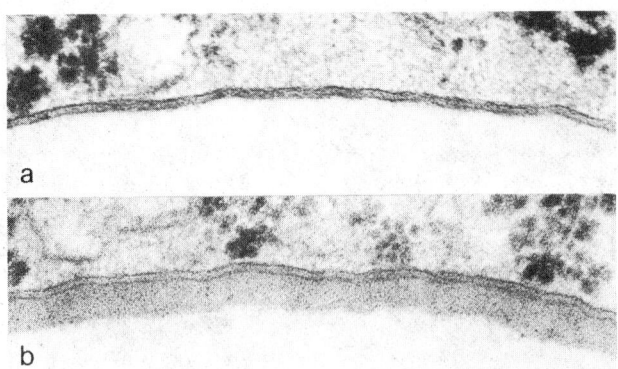

Figure 39-5 Cholesteryl ester storage disease. Ultrastructure of membranes of storage vacuoles in liver. X14,000. (*Courtesy of Prof. U. Pfeiffer.*)

tecture of the outer and part of the middle zones of the cortex, i.e., the zona glomerulosa and the zona fasciculata, are relatively well preserved. Many of the cells are swollen, vacuolated, and contain sudanophilic lipid [4, 21]. The areas corresponding to the inner fasciculata and the entire zona reticularis (the innermost portion of the cortex) are replaced by a broad zone of haphazardly arranged large cells with a vacuolated, foamy cytoplasm. Many of the cells contain anisotropic crystals or large clefts in the shape of cholesterol crystals [26]. Other foam cells seem necrotic, and their contents appear to have been released to form confluent lipid cysts. In the necrotic areas, calcification may be quite prominent. Most of the calcium occurs in finely granular deposits, but there may be areas in which it is condensed into dense lumps [21]. There is frequently extensive fibrosis in the inner half of the cortex [4, 21]. The adrenal medulla is usually very narrow but normal in appearance.

Electron micrographs of the adrenals show that the histiocytes contain lipid in both the crystalline and droplet forms [26]. In the severely affected portions of the cortex, histochemical techniques indicate the presence of large amounts of lipid with staining properties suggestive of cholesteryl esters and triglyceride [4, 6, 16, 26]. These include positive staining with oil red O, Sudan, and similar stains, as well as the Schultz stain for cholesterol. The histochemical findings in the large cells in the adrenals are also present in involved cells throughout other organs.

Adrenal calcification is not visually observed in CESD. Extensive chemical and histopathologic examination of the adrenals in CESD has not been done.

Intestines

The small intestine of patients affected with Wolman's disease is usually thickened and dilated, with a dull, opaque yellow serosa and a swollen yellow mucosa with thick, flattened, yellow villi. The changes are generally most marked in the proximal parts of the small intestine and least apparent in the terminal ileum. In the small intestine, and to some extent in the colon, the lamina propria of the mucosa is infiltrated by foamy histiocytes. Some of the mucosal cells are also foamy. The infiltration of the mucosa by foam cells converts the villi into thick, club-shaped structures [2]. Some foam cells extend through the muscularis mucosa to form small clusters in the submucosa, and similar cells are also present in the lymphoid tissue. Some

of the cells of the muscularis mucosa also stain positively for neutral lipid with Sudan stains. Sudanophilic staining may also be present in the myenteric plexus and in foamy endothelial cells within the intestinal adventitial layer.

Partin and Schubert orginally described changes in jejunal and duodenal biopsy specimens from patients 4 and 5 (Table 39-1) with CESD [77]. The epithelium was normal. Beneath the epithelium in the regions of the lacteals were collections of autofluorescent foam cells, which were especially densely packed in the villous tips. Large amounts of extracellular lipid were present throughout the lamina propria. This lipid appeared birefringent and stained similarly to the fat in the foam cells but was more nonpolar and gave only a weakly positive Schultz reaction. Under the electron microscope the lipid appeared electron-lucent with dense rims. Ultrastructural study of the lamina propria of the small intestine of patients 4 and 5 revealed several interesting features [62]. The lacteal endothelium was filled with round vacuoles that distended the smooth endoplasmic reticulum and looked as though they contained lipid taken up by pinocytosis. Many macrophages surrounded the lacteals and contained numerous vacuoles that were limited by membranes and were filled with material similar to those in hepatic macrophages. Lucent lipid droplets were present in adjacent smooth-muscle cells, vascular peri-

Figure 39-6 Cholesterol ester storage disease. Lipid storage vacuoles: *upper*, in endothelial cells of a blood vessel (X9000), *lower*, in epithelial cells of a small bile duct (X10,000). (*Courtesy Prof. U. Pfeiffer.*)

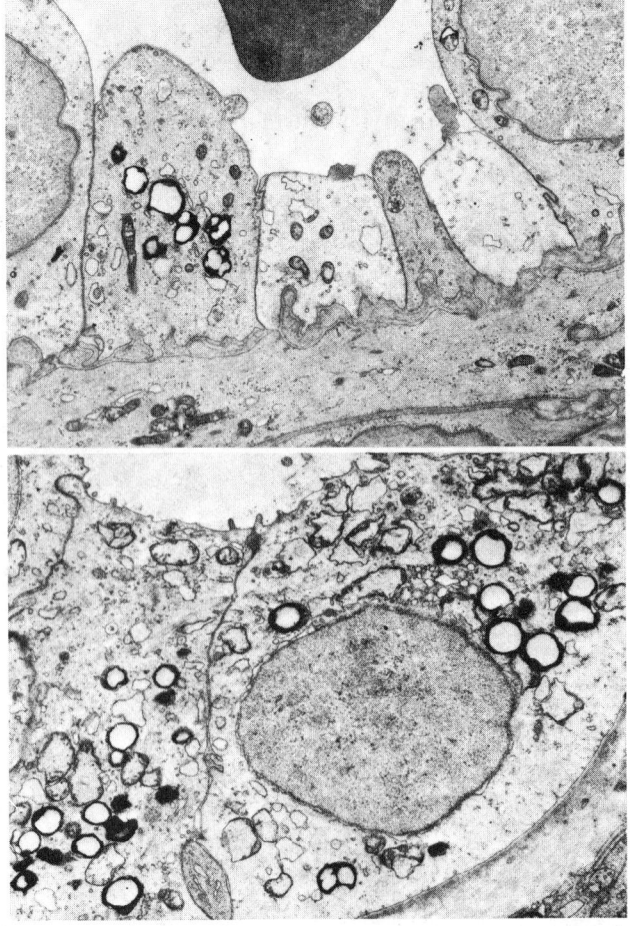

cytes, fibroblasts, and supporting cells of nerve fibers. The ultrastructural localization of membrane-limited lipid deposits in various cell types in intestinal mucosa and submucosa was similar in other patients. In patient 1, foam cells were few and small in the lamina propria of the colon and the esophagus.

Other Tissues

In Wolman's disease the spleen is always grossly enlarged and by age 3 months may weigh over 200 g, compared with the normal weight of 15 g [4]. The spleen is firm, and the cut surface is red or reddish-yellow; the surface may be mottled with yellow or brown flecks. The normal follicular architecture is replaced by a homogeneous appearance. Microscopically, only a small number of follicles are present, and they are small and compressed. Most of the reticulum cells are transformed into large foam cells, which make up the bulk of the organ. There is also swelling and vacuolization of the endothelial cells lining the sinusoids.

Lymph nodes throughout the body, particularly those in the mesentery, are enlarged, orange-yellow, firm, and elastic. Their cut surfaces are yellow and appear homogeneous. The microscopic and histochemical changes are quite similar to those found in the spleen. The bone marrow, thymus, and tonsils in Wolman's disease undergo changes that are almost identical to those in the spleen and lymph nodes. Vacuolization of lymphocytes in the blood and bone marrow has often been noted in Wolman's disease but is not specific. Excessive vacuolization of granulocytes has been reported in one case of Wolman's disease [50].

There are no gross kidney abnormalities in Wolman's disease. Under the light microscope, the tubules appear normal, but mesangial cells of the glomeruli may contain lipid droplets that are both sudanophilic and stain for cholesterol [14, 21]. There also may be foam cells in the interstitium. Foam cells have been observed in the thyroid [14], testes [6, 14, 21], and ovaries [21].

Wolman et al. observed sudanophilic droplets in the endothelium of capillaries of the gray matter and swollen neurons in the medulla oblongata and the retina [4]. Crocker et al. later described the presence of foamy histiocytes in the leptomeninges [6]. They also noted a moderate decrease in the number of cortical neurons and retarded myelination. Foam cells also occur in the interstitium of the choroid plexus [10]. Lipid storage in neurons, including Purkinje cells [16], and sudanophilic

granules within swollen microglia, periadventitial histiocytes, and, possibly, astrocytes have been observed in some patients [16, 20, 21]. One of the most extensive studies of the central nervous system in Wolman's disease was made by Guazzi et al. [14, 15]. These investigators found an abundance of sudanophilic material and diffuse isomorphic fibrillary gliosis of the white matter, which they interpreted as sudanophilic leukodystrophy directly related to abnormal lipid storage. The autopsy was delayed for 2 days after death, however, and some of the reported changes may have been artefactual. Byrd and Powers [48] examined ultrastructurally the peripheral and central nervous system following autopsy of a 4-month-old child affected with Wolman's disease. They demonstrated lipid storage in Schwann cells, perineural and endoneural cells. In the central nervous system, the oligodendrocytes were the principal sites of lipid accumulation, especially in areas of active myelination.

Kamoshita and Landing [17] first made the observation in Wolman's disease that ganglion cells of both Auerbach's and Meissner's plexuses were packed with sudanophilic granules. These changes were found in the stomach, duodenum, and small intestine and have been repeatedly confirmed. The storage of sudanophilic lipids in the sympathetic neurons has also been observed in one patient [16].

In CESD, lipid storage in most tissues is more discrete. In patient 1 foam cells were described in the interstitium in lung and renal glomeruli. Endothelial cells in numerous anatomic sites contained fine lipid droplets, as did smooth-muscle cells in certain arterioles, particularly in the spleen. Electron microscopy showed that the droplets in endothelium also were limited by single, trilaminar membranes. Histologic study of the central nervous system of patient 1 showed no evidence of lipid storage.

Abnormal lipid deposits can also be detected in lymphocytes (Fig. 39-7), monocytes, and cultured skin fibroblasts of CESD patients (Fig. 39-8) [63, 70, 77–79]. In lymphocytes (fresh, unstained preparations), secondary lysosomes storing cholesteryl esters can be visualized by birefringence in polarized light. These secondary lysosomes can be histochemically identified by acid phosphatase staining. α-Naphthylbutyrate esterase activity, normally present in lymphocytes, is completely absent from lymphocytes in CESD patients [79]. In electron microscopy, the storage lysosomes can be easily visualized through their typical trilaminar membranes. Except for lymphocytes and monocytes, all other blood cells are unaffected in CESD.

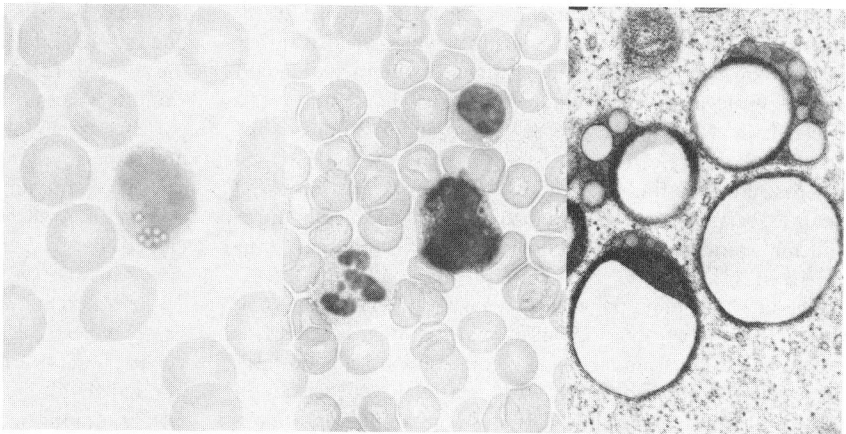

Figure 39-7 Cholesteryl ester storage disease. Lipid storage vacuoles in lymphocytes. *Left,* Histochemical staining for naphthylbutyrate esterase (−). *Middle,* Histochemical staining for lysosomal acid phosphatase (+ + +). *Right,* Electron microscopy of storage vacuoles X60,000. *(Courtesy of Prof. H. E. Schaefer.)*

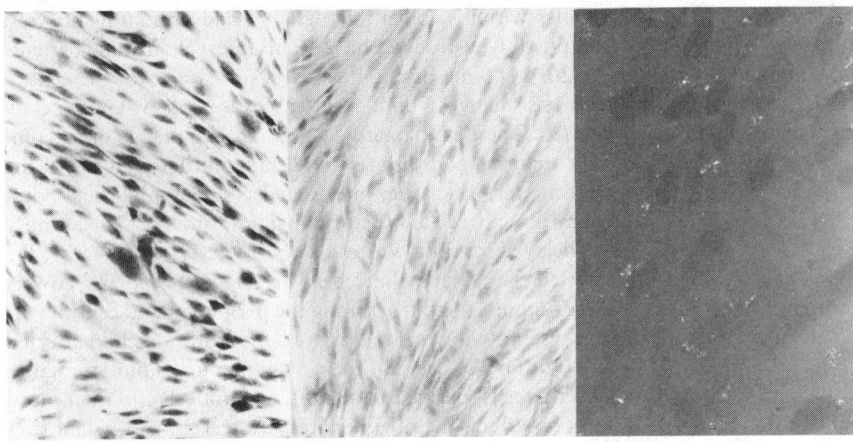

Figure 39-8 Cholesteryl ester storage disease. *Left,* Normal fibroblasts stained for naphthylbutyrate esterase (+ + +). *Middle,* CESD fibroblasts stained for napthylbutyrate esterase (− −). *Right,* CESD fibroblasts visualized in plane-polarized light birefringence (+ +). (*Courtesy Prof. H. E. Schaefer.*)

In cultured skin fibroblasts of CESD patients both birefringence in plane polarized light and the absence of α-naphthylbutyrate esterase staining permit the rapid identification of acid lipase deficiency.

Atherosclerosis

Upon gross examination, the heart and lungs of patients with Wolman's disease appear normal. Routine histologic examination of the heart also reveals no abnormalities, but in frozen sections many sudanophilic droplets may be found in the muscles [14] and vascular endothelium [6, 14]. Lipid deposition in the aorta may be extensive [27], but frank atherosclerosis has not been seen. Nevertheless, most patients affected with Wolman's disease in whom postmortem examination of the arteries was made showed some degree of fat accumulation [6, 21, 27, 29, 30, 34, 39]. The lungs contain variable numbers of foam cells in the alveoli and intestinal tissue [6, 14, 21].

With the exception of CESD patient 10, who developed obstructive pulmonary vascular disease at 15 years of age [87], none of the patients known to have CESD, including two who are in their fourth decade of life, have had clinical evidence of coronary or systemic atherosclerosis. Two of the three patients with CESD who came to necropsy, however, have had anatomic evidence of a much accelerated atherosclerotic process. Patient 1, who died at age 21, had severe (up to 75 percent) coronary arterial luminal narrowing by atheromatous plaques (Fig. 39-9), as well as striking, but functionally less severe, lesions in the circle of Willis, the abdominal aorta, and the common iliac arteries. This patient died a cardiac death, and at necropsy she also had recent cardiac necrosis, but her death appeared to be related to severe aortic valvular stenosis rather than to coronary artery disease. Patient 8, who died at age 9, had a few elevated yellow plaques in the ascending aorta. His affected sib, who died at age 8, had no abnormalities of the aorta or coronary arteries. It is not known how much of the atherosclerosis in these patients was directly related to CESD or to associated hypercholesterolemia and hyperbetalipoproteinemia. Patients with CESD do not develop xanthomas of the type seen in familial hypercholesterolemia (see Chap. 33).

The fact that most patients affected with CESD may be at increased risk of developing premature atherosclerosis is potentially of great importance. It could support a hypothesis of de Duve [90], who suggested that a relative deficiency of lysosomal acid lipase might lead to the accumulation of cholesteryl esters within lysosomes of arterial smooth-muscle cells [88, 89] and thus promote atheroma formation.

LIPID ABNORMALITIES

Wolman's Disease

The histologic evidence of generalized lipid storage in Wolman's disease is easy to confirm by qualitative lipid analyses such as thin-layer chromatograms of neutral lipid extracts from liver or spleen (Fig. 39-10). The principal lipids present in increased quantities are cholesteryl esters and triglycerides. Quantitative analyses of liver and spleen have been made in a number of patients [1, 2].

The triglyceride content of the liver may be 2 to 10 times the normal value. In the spleen, the triglycerides may be elevated from 8- to 100-fold. The triglyceride content of the adrenals has been reported in only one case [26] and was one-half the normal value. The concentrations of mono- and diglycerides were elevated 5- to 15-fold in the liver and spleen of the two patients in which they were measured [10, 26]; they were modestly, if at all, elevated in the adrenals of one patient [26].

The total cholesterol concentration of liver and spleen has been elevated in every case of Wolman's disease in which measurements have been reported. Although the free cholesterol concentration has frequently been greater than normal, the bulk of the increase in total cholesterol is due to the accumulation of cholesteryl esters. The cholesteryl ester content of the liver may be 5 to 160 times the normal value. It was shown in one case [26] that cholesteryl esters were elevated eightfold in the adrenals [2]. Analyses of the fatty acids of triglycerides and cholesteryl esters in the liver, spleen, and other tissues of patients with Wolman's disease revealed no consistent abnormality [2].

Upon examining chromatographs of published tissue analyses [21] as well as their own, Assmann and coworkers concluded that oxygenated steryl esters were also present in Wolman's disease [91]. They were identified as esters of 7α- and 7β-hydroxycholesterol, 7-ketocholesterol and 5,6β- and 5,6α-epoxycholesterol, in this order of preponderance. These oxygenated steryl esters were identified in liver, spleen, and adrenal glands. No such compounds were detectable in control tissues, among which were a number containing a very high content of cholesteryl esters, including normal brain and adrenals and tissues from patients with (CESD) and Tangier disease.

An increase in free fatty acid content of the liver and spleen has been reported in Wolman's disease [10, 23]. The phospholipid and glycolipid contents of the liver and spleen have not been abnormal. Lin and coworkers [92] have reported increased quantities in alkyl and alk-1-enyl glycerolipids in the liver, spleen, and adrenals of a patient with Wolman's disease. No consistent abnormalities have been detected in the neutral lipids, phospholipids, or glycolipids of the nervous systems.

Cholesteryl Ester Storage Disease

Chemical abnormalities in tissues in CESD are thus far known to be present in the liver, intestine, spleen, lymph node, aorta, and cultured skin fibroblasts.

Lipid analyses of liver of CESD patients are displayed in Table 39-5. The major abnormality of the patients investigated was an increase in cholesteryl esters, the concentration being 120 to 350 times normal.

In patient 1, 94 percent of the glyceride fraction was triglyceride, there being only small amounts of di- and monoglycerides as determined chromatographically [2]. The percentage distribution of hepatic phospholipids was phosphatidylcholine plus phosphatidylinositol, 49 percent; phosphatidylethanolamine, 31 percent; sphingomyelin, 11.5 percent; and lysophosphatidylcholine, 7 percent [2]. In patient 3, it was considered that the liver sphingomyelin might be increased and the phosphatidylethanolamine decreased [60]. Liver glycolipids or glyceryl esters have not been studied adequately in any patient with CESD.

In patient 1, the content of triglycerides and cholesteryl esters was increased in the spleen and aorta; in patients 8 and 9, cholesterol and triglyceride analyses of spleen, kidney, lung, and cerebral gray matter were reported as normal. In cultured skin fibroblasts of several patients (Table 39-6), the total concentration of cholesterol was close to that in controls, while the concentration of cholesteryl esters was markedly elevated.

The acyl groups in the cholesteryl esters in CESD liver have been reported to be predominantly oleic and linoleic acids [60, 61, 65, 73, 82], a pattern which is grossly similar to that seen in esters stored in Tangier disease, eosinophilic granuloma, or atheromas [93]. The fatty acid composition of cholesteryl esters in the intestinal mucosa of patient 4 did not differ markedly from that in controls or from the liver [61].

Plasma Lipids and Lipoproteins

Plasma cholesterol and triglycerides have been normal in most patients with Wolman's disease in whom such measurements have been made. Elevated triglycerides and VLDL (very low density lipoproteins) were reported in three patients [21, 50]. Four patients have had unquestionable decreases in plasma HDL (high density lipoproteins) as determined by electrophoresis or chemical tests [28, 29, 50]. The severely malnourished patient described by Eto and Kitagawa had a cholesterol level of 100 mg/dl, decreased LDL and HDL, and acanthocytosis [24].

All CESD patients in whom plasma lipid levels have been reported had hypercholesterolemia (Table 39-1). In some this has been associated with hypertriglyceridemia. The plasma lipoprotein pattern is either II A or II B. Patient 1 had a persistent, marked increase in LDL, in concentrations of about 330 mg LDL cholesterol per deciliter of plasma, and variable increases in VLDL. The LDL concentrations in patient 6 were elevated at both 11 and 17 years of age. Her father (age 50) and sister (age 22) both had hepatomegaly and hypercholesterolemia; the mother (age 50) had no clinical or lipid abnormalities.

The cholesterol ester/free cholesterol ratio and the pattern of cholesteryl ester fatty acid in serum is normal in CESD [1, 65, 82]. Direct investigation of the enzymatic activity of lecithin: cholesterol acyltransferase and of lipolytic enzymes contained in postheparin plasma has not been done.

The plasma lipoprotein abnormalities in CESD may include the HDL. Patient 1, observed over a long period of time, had extremely low levels of HDL, with concentrations varying

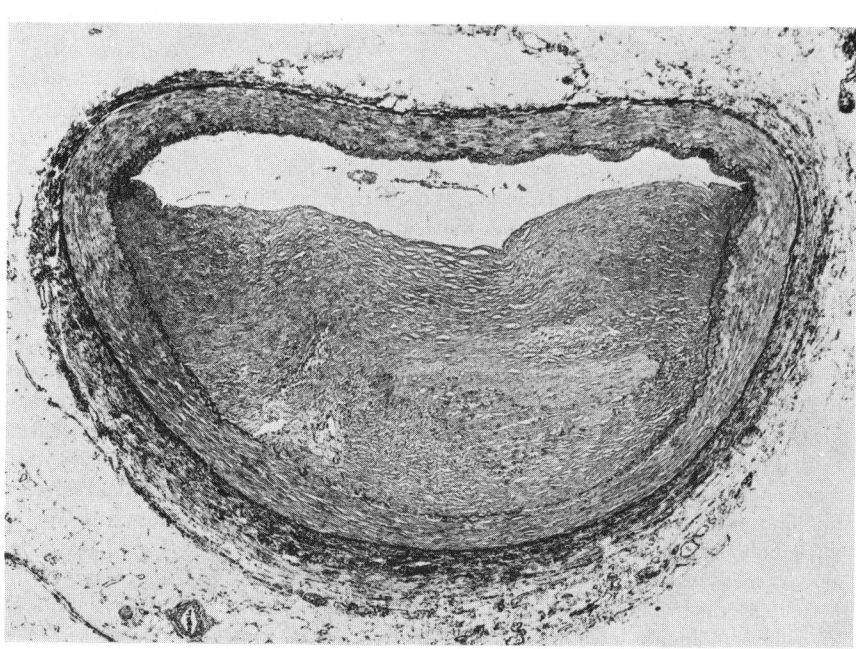

Figure 39-9 Atheromatous plaque in coronary artery of 21-year-old patient (no. 1 in Table 39-1) with CESD. Movat stain X35. (*From Fredrickson et al [58]. Used with permission.*)

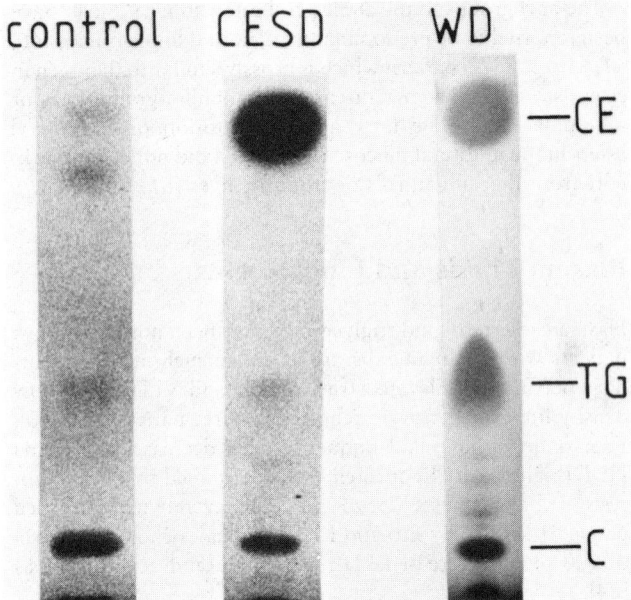

Figure 39-10 Thin-layer chromatography of liver lipids in CESD and Wolman's disease. CE, Cholesteryl esters; TG, triglycerides, C., cholesterol.

from 6 to 27 mg HDL cholesterol per deciliter of plasma, well below the 5 percent lower limit of normal and not explained by her modest hypertriglyceridemia. Patient 4 was also said to have low HDL (in terms of α-lipoproteins on the electrophoretic pattern). Patient 23 had low HDL cholesterol values on repeated determinations. A recent analysis of the distribution of the subfractions HDL_2 and HDL_3 in patient 23 by zonal centrifugation has revealed a remarkable discrepancy from normal: instead of the usual 1:10 ratio of HDL_2 and HDL_3, a 10:1 ratio was discovered in patient 23 [82]. The apoprotein composition of isolated lipoproteins was analyzed by SDS polyacrylamide electrophoresis and isoelectric focusing and found to be qualitatively normal [82].

PATHOPHYSIOLOGY

The Enzymatic Defect

The activity of lysosomal acid lipase activity of cultivated fibroblasts from patients affected with Wolman's disease and CESD has been characterized by various methods, including enzymatic analysis and histochemical and chemical procedures (Table 39-2). With native substrates the acid lipase activity is less than 10 percent of controls in homozygotes and about 50 percent in heterozygotes in both conditions. Similar results can be obtained with a variety of artificial substrates (Tables 39-3 and 39-4), such as synthetic derivatives of nitrophenol or 4-methylumbelliferone. The latter substrates can also be hydrolyzed by nonspecific esterases, and the residual activity measured with such compounds in general is higher compared to that obtained with native substrates. Acid lipase is distinct from phospholipase A, for there is no accumulation of phospholipids in patients affected with Wolman's disease or CESD. Phospholipase A may be responsible for some of the residual activity measured with artificial substrates in the patients.

Cellogel electrophoresis of normal fibroblast extracts followed by staining for lysosomal acid lipase using 4-methylum-

belliferyl oleate exhibits at least three acid lipase bands or isoenzymes, labeled A, B, and C [38]. The least anodal band, A, is the most prominent one in control fibroblasts but is reduced in heterozygotes (Wolman's disease) and is undetectable in both WD and CESD cells [38]. The acid lipase isoenzyme pattern observed in cultured skin fibroblasts is also present in amniotic fluid cells, lymphocytes, and several tissues (liver, spleen, lymph nodes, aorta) [38]. Prenatal diagnosis of Wolman's disease has been established by the combined recognition of deficiency of acid lipase and deficiency of the A band in electrophoresis of amniotic cell extracts [95].

The gene for the A band of acid lipase in humans has been localized to chromosome 10 [95a]. This assignment was based on electrophoretic analysis of the enzyme in hybrid cells formed from human and hamster fibroblasts (see Chap. 11). Koster et al. [96] compared the hydrolysis of 4-methylumbelliferyl oleate and cholesteryl oleate by acid ester hydrolase in human leukocytes, fibroblasts, and liver. They concluded, based upon differences in pH optima and behavior toward various inhibitory compounds, that acid lipase (measured using 4-methylumbelliferyl oleate as substrate) and acid cholesteryl esterase (measured using cholesteryl oleate as substrate) are either different enzymes or are one protein with a different active center for each substrate. These authors further hypothesized that these two catalytic activities might be separately involved in Wolman's disease and CESD.

Studies of acid lipase with native emulsified substrates have shown that in both Wolman's disease and CESD fibroblasts, cholesteryl ester hydrolase and triacylglycerol hydrolase activities are reduced proportionately [71]. Moreover, proportional deficiencies of the two activities have also been measured in fibroblasts from patients with I-cell disease or pseudo-Hurler polydystrophy [94]. The latter conditions are characterized by multiple lysosomal enzyme deficiencies due to a defect of posttransitional glycosylation (see Chap. 37).

These findings, taken together, suggest that cholesterol ester hydrolase and triacylglycerol hydrolase activities in fibroblasts reside in the same enzyme molecule (A isoenzyme). It is not clear at present to what extent the B and C isoenzymes which are retained in Wolman's disease and CESD fibroblasts may account for the residual enzyme activity measured in mutant cells with both artificial and radiolabeled native substrates. Wide variation in the reported residual acid lipase activities in Wolman's disease and CESD [38, 54, 71, 95] suggests that definite diagnosis rests on the use of native substrates.

In addition to cultured fibroblasts, leukocyte extracts can be used to establish the diagnosis of acid lipase deficiency (Table 39-4). The acid lipase activity assayed with 4-methylumbelliferyl esters is 10 to 15 times higher in mononuclear than polymorphonuclear leukocytes [56]. Studies performed by Patsch et al. [97] suggested that the acid glycerol ester hydrolase and acid cholesterol ester hydrolase in human mononuclear leukocytes are different proteins (or at least involve different catalytic sites on the same protein). These authors measured both enzyme activities in different subcellular leukocyte fractions and noted that cholesterol ester hydrolase activity is strongly associated with the lysosomal membrane and different from the main glycerol ester hydrolase activity in solubilization properties [97]. Nevertheless, in view of the isoenzyme pattern of acid lipase and the difficulties in the standardization of lipase assays, current data on the substrate specificity of acid lipases should be interpreted with caution. In three patients affected with Wolman's disease, in addition to the near absence of acid lipase activity, low leukocyte activity of β-galactosidase has been reported [50, 55]. The reason for this is not clear.

Goldstein et al. compared the relative rates of hydrolysis of [³H]cholesteryl linoleate–LDL in normal and mutant CESD cells. They compared fibroblast extracts incubated at acid pH and intact fibroblast monolayers [80]. While the cholesteryl esterase activity of mutant cell extracts was less than one-twentieth that of normal extracts, the intact mutant cells showed rates of cholesteryl ester hydrolysis that were nearly one-third that of normal cells. The origin of this discrepancy is not known, but it could be related to differences in the concentration or availability of substrate in the different conditions employed. The residual enzyme activity in intact CESD fibroblasts could be abolished by treatment of the cells with chloroquine, which suggested that the activity resided in the lysosomes.

Normally, cholesteryl esters bound to LDL demonstrate a strong regulatory effect on cholesterol metabolism in fibroblasts. When the fibroblasts are exposed to LDL, the activity of HMG CoA reductase falls and that of fatty acyl CoA: cholesteryl acyltransferase (EC 2.3.1.26) (ACAT) rises. In both CESD and Wolman's disease cells exposed to LDL, this effect of LDL is decreased. The reduced responsiveness to LDL in acid lipase–deficient fibroblasts can be restored when the mutant cells are cultured with normal fibroblasts [81]. It appears, therefore, that cholesteryl ester hydrolase is secreted by normal fibroblasts into the culture medium and can be taken up in an active form by the mutant cells. An alternative hypothesis is that there is a transfer factor which confers upon CESD cells the ability to synthesize new hydrolase. Studies in CESD fibroblasts have further revealed that hydrolysis of those cholesteryl esters synthesized within the cell is not impaired [81]. Thus, the lysosomal acid lipase is essential for the hydrolysis of cholesteryl esters entering the cell bound to lipoproteins.

It appears from the very different clinical course of CSD and Wolman's disease that the residual acid lipase activity directed against LDL cholesteryl esters is sufficient in CESD to keep the lysosomal accumulation of cholesteryl esters and subsequent cellular damage in most extrahepatic tissues to a level compatible with fairly normal life. In Wolman's disease the residual activity is insufficient to prevent overwhelming accumulation of cholesteryl esters and destruction of cell function.

Table 39-2 Documentation of enzyme deficiency in cholesteryl ester storage disease

Pat.	Ref.	Tissue	Cells	Enzyme analysis (see Tables 39-3, 39-4)	Lipid analysis (see Tables 39-5, 39-6)	Histochemical analysis
1. L.Mc.	[51]	Liver		+	+	
		Spleen		+		
		Lymph node		+		
		Aortic tissue		+		
			Fibroblasts	+		
2. Lem.	[69]	Liver			+	+
			Fibroblasts		+	
4. T.H.	[76, 77]	Liver		+	+	+
			Fibroblasts		+	
5. W.H.T.	[61]	Liver		+		+
6. E.M.N.	[38]		Fibroblasts	+		
7. Rad.	[69]	Liver				+
8. T.R.	[63]	Liver			+	
9. R.R	[63]	Liver			+	
10. J.R.	[38, 63, 78, 80, 81]		Leukocytes	+		
			Fibroblasts	+		
11. K.W.	[54]		Fibroblasts	+		
12. A.L.	[64]		Leukocytes	+		
13. L.O.	[69]	Liver			+	
	[70]		Fibroblasts		+	
14. M.S.	[70]		Fibroblasts		+	
	[69]	Liver				+
15. M.A.	[69]	Liver				+
16. C.N.	[69]	Liver				+
17. K.N.	[72]	Liver			+	+
18. A.C.d.O.	[71]	Liver		+	+	
			Fibroblasts	+		
			Leukocytes	+		
19. B.Z.	[74]		Fibroblasts	+		
20. T.S.	[74]		Fibroblasts	+		
21. N.S.	[74]	Liver			+	
22. J.M.	[74]		Fibroblasts	+	+	
23. B.U.	[82]	Liver		+	+	+
			Fibroblasts	+	+	+
			Leukocytes	+	+	+
24. Le.M.	[70]	Liver			+	

Table 39-3 Acid lipase activity in liver in cholesteryl ester storage disease

Pat.	Ref.	Activity expressed in	Substrates			
			[14C]Cholesteryl oleate	[14C]Cholesteryl palmitate	[14C]Trioleate	4-Muo
1. L.Mc.	[51]	pmol substrate/(mg wet tissue · h)	1	1.7	660	—
Control			107 ± 23	150 ± 32.8	5730 ± 3600	—
4. T.H.	[76]	µmol FFA liberated/(mg nitrogen · h)	—	—	—	—
Control			0.26–0.6			
5. W.H.T.	[61]	Reduced esterase activity	?	?	?	?
18. A.C.d.O.	[71]	nmol substrate/(g wet tissue · min)	1.7			
Control			5.6–15.4	—	—	—
23. B.U.	[82]	nmol substrate/(h · mg protein)	0.6	—	—	15
Control			3.5–10.4	—	—	105

NOTE: 4-Muo = 4-methylumbelliferyl oleate

Function of the Enzyme

Acid cholesteryl ester hydrolase activity is known to be widely distributed throughout the body and is also present in arterial wall cells. The latter localization gives rise to speculations concerning its possible role in atherogenesis [51, 88–90, 98–100]. The single most important demonstration of the crucial role of this enzyme is derived from the work of Brown and Goldstein and their coworkers concerning the uptake and catabolism of plasma LDL (see Chap. 33). On the basis of in vitro studies with cultured fibroblasts these investigators have demonstrated a process whereby LDL may be removed in peripheral body cells. This process involves a specific receptor on the plasma membrane of the cell which binds LDL. Binding of the lipoprotein to receptor initiates its endocytosis. The endocytotic vesicles fuse with lysosomes, after which the apolipoproteins, cholesteryl esters, and probably other lipid constituents, undergo hydrolysis by lysosomal enzymes.

The lysosomal degradation of LDL cholesteryl esters is catalyzed by the acid lipase activity that is deficient in CESD and Wolman's disease [80, 81]. The free sterol liberated is transferred from lysosomes to cellular membranes and initiates three important regulatory events. First, cellular synthesis of cholesterol is reduced through suppression of the activity of 3-hydroxy-3-methylglutaryl-CoA reductase, which controls the rate-limiting step in cholesterol metabolism. Second, coincident with the entry of LDL cholesterol into cells there is suppression of further transport of LDL into the cells through interference with LDL receptor synthesis. Third, cellular formation of cholesteryl esters is stimulated through activation of the membrane-bound ACAT. In the reaction catalyzed by this enzyme, the bulk of incoming plasma cholesteryl esters, which were mainly esterified to linoleic acid, now become esterified with oleic (C18:1) acid, or other C_{14} to C_{18} saturated or monounsaturated fatty acids. Under certain conditions, the reesterified cholesterol may accumulate as cytoplasmic liquid droplets that resemble the droplets seen in the foam cells of atherosclerotic lesions. The hydrolysis of cytoplasmic cholesteryl esters appears to be mediated by a cytoplasmic cholesteryl ester hydrolase whose activity is resistant to lysosomal inhibitors such as chloroquine or ammonium chloride [101, 102].

The latter enzyme has not been characterized and its functional role in Wolman's disease and CESD is not clear.

Plasma cholesteryl esters are derived from two main sources: (1) esterification of cholesterol in the intestine and transport of the esters into plasma by way of the lymph, in the company of dietary fat in chylomicrons, and (2) esterification of cholesterol by lecithin:cholesterol acyltransferase (see Chap. 31). Many details of the metabolism of chylomicrons are presented in Chaps. 29 and 30. Once in plasma these triglyceride-rich particles lose their triglycerides to extrahepatic tissues through the action of capillary-bound lipase (lipoprotein lipase, which has an alkaline pH optimum) and are reduced to "remnants" rich in cholesterol, phospholipids, and certain surface apoproteins. The remnants are removed by the liver at a rate which appears to be directly dependent upon the apolipoprotein composition in the remnant [103, 104]. Present data suggest that apo E fosters the hepatic uptake of the remnant, while other apolipoproteins, such as apo C-III, may inhibit this function [104, 105]. The cholesteryl esters taken up are hydrolyzed [106–109], a process which is inhibited by chloroquine [106, 110].

Therefore, the hydrolysis of cholesteryl esters in the liver appears to occur inside lysosomes in a manner similar to the fate of LDL cholesteryl esters taken up by fibroblasts. The liver uptake of lipoproteins is not confined to parenchymal cells. Both parenchymal and nonparenchymal liver cells are active in the binding and uptake of lipoproteins from the blood and contain the capacity to degrade protein and cholesteryl ester moieties of lipoproteins [111–114]. In rat liver cells about 50 percent of the total acid cholesterol esterase activity is present in nonparenchymal cells [114]. This is compatible with the observations that cholesteryl ester storage occurs in both hepatocytes and Kupffer cells in patients affected with lysosomal acid lipase deficiency.

In view of the extensive cholesteryl ester storage in the adrenals of patients affected with Wolman's disease, it is interesting to note that the adrenal glands possess receptors for lipoproteins and are able to take up and utilize cholesteryl esters carried in plasma LDL [115, 116] and HDL [117]. The steroids secreted by the adrenals are derived in large part from lipoprotein cholesterol. However, failure of lysosomal hydrolysis of lipoprotein cholesteryl esters in adrenal glands does not necessarily mean impairment of hormone production. Potentially, there are at least three major sources of cholesterol available to cells to meet their metabolic needs. These include cholesterol delivered directly from the uptake of lipoproteins into cells (involving lysosomal cholesteryl ester hydrolase), hydrolysis of stored cytoplasmic cholesteryl esters (involving neutral cholesteryl ester hydrolase), and cholesterol synthesized *de novo*. The study of patients with Wolman's disease and CESD might add information about the quantitative importance of these pathways in different tissues, but the steroidogenesis in these syndromes has not been investigated.

The precise origin of the elevation of plasma LDL and the decreased concentrations of plasma HDL in CESD are not yet understood. Of particular interest is the abnormal ratio of HDL_2 to HDL_3, so far investigated only in patient 23 [82]. Normally, HDL_2 concentrations show a highly significant negative correlation with postheparin hepatic lipase activity (see Chap. 30). Theoretically at least part of the observed HDL abnormality could be explained on the basis of a deficiency of the heparin-releasable liver lipase.

GENETICS

Mode of Inheritance

Wolman's disease is inherited as an autosomal recessive character. The sex of the patients has been found to be about equally distributed between male and female. In the original family reported by Wolman and his colleagues [3, 4] three sibs died of the disease, and numerous families since have had more than one affected child. The parents of the original patients and several subsequent pairs of parents were related [29, 32, 34, 36], although consanguinity has been denied in the majority of affected families [1, 2]. At least six cases, possibly seven [22], have been reported in Israel, and all but one of these have apparently been Jews of Iraqi or Iranian origin [29]. The other patients have been reported from North America, Western Europe, Pakistan, China, or Japan.

It seems probable that CESD is also inherited as an autosomal recessive character, but it is hazardous to construct a mode of inheritance from the aggregated data since it is not certain

Table 39-4 Acid lipase activity in cultured fibroblasts or circulating leukocytes in cholesteryl ester storage disease

Pat.	Ref.	Cells	Substrates	Activity		Expressed in
				Patient	Control	
1. L.Mc	[51]	Fibroblasts	4-Muo	1.4	25.8 ± 8.2	nmol substrate/ (min·mg protein)
			[^{14}C]Trioleate	0.1	36.5 ± 4.6	pmol substrate/ (h·mg protein)
			[^{14}C]C oleate	14.0	138.1 ± 53.9	
6. E.M.N.	[38]	Fibroblasts	Tridecanoate	0	0.403	nmol substrate/ (min·mg protein)
10. J.R.	[38, 63]	Leukocytes	P-Nitrophenyl laurate	0.88	8.39–20.17	nmol substrate/ (min·mg protein)
	[78, 80, 81]	Fibroblasts	[^{14}C]Trioleate	4.8	268 ± 39	pmol/(min·mg protein)
			[^{14}C]C oleate	0	40.2 ± 6.9	
			P-Nitrophenyl laurate	1.2	26.6 ± 5.1	nmol/(min·mg protein)
			[^{3}H]C linoleate	0.77	5.7	pmol[^{3}H]cholesterol/ (h·mg protein)
11. K.W.	[54]	Fibroblasts	[^{14}C]Trioleate	0.8	11.8 ± 1.7	
			[^{14}C]C oleate	0.4	3.8 ± 1.0	nmol/(h·mg protein)
			4-Muo	170.2	778.5 ± 123.2	
12. A.L.	[64]	Leukocytes	Substrate: P-nitrophenyl carboxylic esters			
			Result: deficiency of E-600 resistant acid esterase			
18. A.C.d.O	[71]	Fibroblasts	[^{14}C]C oleate	2.1	49–326	
		Leukocytes	[^{14}C]Triolate	15.6	236	nmol/(min·g protein)
			4-Muo	1000	2800	
			[^{14}C]C oleate	3.4	20–105	
19. B.Z.	[74]	Fibroblasts	Substrate: P-nitrophenyl palmitate			
			Result: deficiency of acid esterase			
20. T.S.	[74]	Fibroblasts	Substrate: 1. 4-Muo			
			2. [^{14}C]Trioleate			
			Result: 1. 10% of control activity			
			2. 4% of control activity			
22. J.M.	[74]	Fibroblasts	Substrate: ?			
			Result: reduced activity of acid esterase			
23. B.U.	[82]	Fibroblasts	[^{14}C] Trioleate	1.1	13.2 ± 1.4	nmol/(h·mg protein)
			[^{14}C] C oleate	0.6	5.1 ± 0.9	
			4-Muo	157.5	644 ± 142	

NOTE: 4-Muo = 4-methylumbelliferyl oleate; [^{14}C]Triolate = [^{14}C]Oleoyl triacylglycerol; [^{14}C]C oleate = [1–^{14}C]Cholesteryl oleate

that all families with CESD described here have an identical disease. Patients 4, 6, and 8 had esophageal varices and seemingly a more severe disorder than the others. Some patients have not been diagnosed by enzymatic assays or tissue analyses, and the presence of hepatomegaly in relatives cannot be entered at present as evidence of vertical transmission of CESD. No consanguinity in parents has yet been documented.

In general, Wolman's disease and CESD can be distinguished by their very different clinical courses. In Wolman's disease, there is marked accumulation of both triglycerides and cholesteryl esters, whereas in CESD storage of cholesteryl esters is much more pronounced. Enzymatic data are unable to explain why tissue triglycerides are not elevated in most cases with CESD. There is, however, a certain degree of phenotypic variation among the patients with acid lipase deficiency, a phenomenon common to most inborn lysosomal diseases. Besides the acute infantile form of Wolman's disease other forms may also exist which are of later onset and follow a less severe and more prolonged course [43]. Suzuki et al. described an atypical case of Wolman's disease with absence of splenomegaly and normal adrenal glands [37]. Lack of adrenal calcification was also emphasized in two further cases of Wolman's disease [21, 50]. On the other hand, adrenal calcification, considered pathognomonic for Wolman's disease, has also been observed in CESD (patient 10). The time of manifestation of liver cirrhosis and the severity of related symptoms differ considerably among the reported cases of CESD. Patients with acid lipase deficiency probably represent not only homozygous expression of different alleles but occasionally also genetic compounds.

Heterozygote Detection

It is now established that heterozygotes for acid lipase deficiency are detectable by enzyme assay. Young and Patrick [55] reported that leukocytes of the mother, father, and a sib of one patient with Wolman's disease contained about half the normal activity of the acid hydrolase. Lake [118] reported intermediate activity in lymphocytes on blood films prepared from obligate heterozygotes affected with Wolman's disease. Schaub

et al. [50] demonstrated subnormal levels of acid lipase activity with both the natural and synthetic substrates in the parents of one patient with Wolman's disease. These authors further noted that the patient's father and mother had elevated activity of other lysososmal hydrolases in their leukocytes. More recently, a fluorometric assay of acid lipase in human leukocytes has been described which requires only 1 ml of blood [119]. The test should be sensitive enough to distinguish subnormal levels of the enzyme in obligate carriers of Wolman's disease. In addition to leukocytes, cultured skin fibroblasts can be used to establish subnormal levels of acid lipase in heterozygous patients [52, 119].

In CESD, the parents and two sibs of patients 8, 9, and 10 had about 5 percent of the mean activity of acid lipase in control leukocytes and cultured fibroblasts [63]. Leukocytes from the mother of patient 11 contained about 40 percent of control acid lipase activity [64].

Thus, present data suggest that heterozygotes for both forms of acid ester hydrolase deficiency will have detectable abnormalities in enzyme assays, but that the two forms of the disease cannot be separated by such measurements alone. Vacuolation of peripheral lymphocytes does not permit heterozygote detection since this is also seen in homozygous abnormal patients and is also a common nonspecific finding in other lysosomal hydrolase deficiencies. Prenatal diagnosis of Wolman's disease has been established by quantitative assays and electrophoresis of lysosomal acid lipase in cultured amniotic fluid cells [95].

DIAGNOSIS

Wolman's disease must be considered in any infant with hepatosplenomegaly, gastrointestinal symptoms, and failure to thrive. The earliest examination should include careful attention to neurologic development. X-rays should be taken of the lungs and bones and of the abdomen to observe the calcification of the adrenals that is almost invariably present. Calcification of the adrenals may be observed in many other conditions such as Addison's disease [108], adrenal teratomas [120], hemorrhage [3, 18, 21], neuroblastoma, ganglioneuroma,

Table 39-5 Concentration of liver lipids in cholesteryl ester storage disease

Patient	Ref.	TC	FC	EC	TG	PL	Expressed in
1. L.Mc.	[51]		9	95–187	33–64	—	mg/g wet tissue
Control		—	—	1	19	—	
3. Lem.	[69]	—	11	174	36	21	mg/g wet tissue
4. T.H.	[76]	148.3	—	146.9	16.6	—	mg/g wet tissue
Control		4.8	—	1.1	10.1	—	
8. T.R.	[63]	—	3.6	—		—	mg/g wet tissue
9. R.R.	[63]	—	3.5	—		—	mg/g wet tissue
13. L.0	[70]	—	30	244	—	—	μg/mg protein
Control		—	30	20	—	—	
17. K.N.	[72]	—	Normal		Normal	—	
18. A.C.d.O.	[71]	259	—		Slightly elevated	—	mg/g wet tissue
21. N.S.	[74]	—	Normal		Slightly elevated	—	
23. B.U.	[82]	210	16	194	Normal	Double of control	mg/g wet tissue
Control		1.8	0.4	1.4	Normal	PS/SPM normal	
24. Le.M.	[70]	—	68	603	—	—	μg/mg protein
Control		—	30	20	—	—	

NOTE: TC = total cholesterol; FC = free cholesterol; EC = esterified cholesterol; TG = triglycerides; PL = phospholipids

Table 39-6 Lipid content of fibroblasts in cholesteryl ester storage disease

Patient	Ref.	Cell passage	TC	FC	EC	TG	PL	Expressed in
4. T.H.	[77]	15	0.2	—	0.33	0.14	1.17	mg/mg Kjeldahl nitrogen
Control		15	0.18	—	0.07	0.22	1.00	
13 L.O.	[70]	10–12	—	46–52	76–128	—	—	μg/mg protein
Control		6–13	—	25–39	9–14	—	—	
14. M.S.	[70]	11	—	17	25	—	—	μg/mg protein
Control		6–13	—	25–39	9–14	—	—	
22. J.M.	[74]	?	EC—10 times elevated 45% of TC			—	—	
23. B.U.	[82]	6–10	32–44	10–14	22–30			μg/mg protein
Control			40–52	32–40	8–12			

NOTE: TC = total cholesterol; FC = free cholesterol; EC = esterified cholesterol; TG = triglycerides; PL = phospholipids

adrenal cysts, cortical carcinoma, and pheochromocytoma [3, 18]. The presence of bilateral adrenal calcification associated with hepatosplenomegaly and gastrointestinal symptoms strongly supports the diagnosis of Wolman's disease. It is noteworthy that in Niemann-Pick disease, no adrenal calcification has ever been seen. The decreased adrenal responsiveness that has been observed in some cases of Wolman's disease must be differentiated from the syndrome of familial leukodystrophy with adrenal insufficiency and cutaneous melanosis [121]. This syndrome has a more protracted course, definite signs of central nervous system involvement, and is not easily confused with Wolman's disease. Moreover, acid lipase activity is normal in fibroblasts [122] and brain tissue homogenates [123] of patients affected with adrenoleukodystrophy.

Wolman's disease should be further distinguished from conditions in which triglycerides instead of cholesteryl esters accumulate in tissues [71, 124]. One patient with triglyceride accumulation in liver without cholesteryl ester storage has been described in association with acid lipase deficiency [71]. Numerous metabolic diseases (galactosemia, fructose intolerance, certain disorders of amino acid metabolism) may result in secondary triglyceride accumulation. "Triglyceride storage disease" is a separate biochemical and clinical entity accompanied by excessive extralysosomal triglyceride accumulation in various tissues due to a number of different metabolic defects in the pathways of triglyceride mobilization [124, 125].

CESD may be easily confused with glycogen storage disease (Chap. 6). In both disorders, marked hepatomegaly and hyperlipemia without splenic enlargement may appear in a child whose mental and physical development is otherwise unremarkable. Provocative tests for adequacy for glycogenolysis should be performed, and a survey of glycogen content, glucose-6-phosphatase, phosphorylase, and related enzymes may have to be made on liver removed by biopsy if enzymatic tests for CESD are equivocal. The absence of jaundice in any patient with CESD thus far suggests that the disorder need not be confused with congenital biliary cirrhosis. A normal proportion of esters in the total cholesterol in plasma should help exclude biliary obstruction. Vacuolation of hepatocytes can also be observed by light microscopy in Niemann-Pick disease, type B; several forms of mucopolysaccharidoses, and G_{M1} gangliosidosis. The latter disorders can be easily distinguished from CESD by examination of cryostat sections of liver under polarized light. In CESD, liver tissue reveals birefringence, which disappears upon heating the tissue to 50 to 60°C and reappears upon cooling. Heat-sensitive birefringence of liver tissue is highly suggestive for CESD or Wolman's disease and cannot be observed in other lysosomal deficiency states.

A child suspected of having CESD should have examination of bone marrow for foam cells and biochemical study of acid lipase activity in leukocytes and cultured skin fibroblasts.

Definitive diagnosis of acid lipase deficiency is feasible by analysis of the clinical picture and assay of acid ester hydrolase activity in cultured skin fibroblasts or peripheral leukocytes. Substrates for the determination of acid ester hydrolase include artificial compounds, such as nitrophenyl laurate and umbelliferyl oleate, as well as cholesteryl oleate solubilized by detergents or incorporated into LDL. Natural substrates are more specific for acid lipase determinations and should be preferred. Sufficient control data must be obtained, and the tissue from the patient with either Wolman's disease or cholesteryl ester storage disease should have only 1 to 10 percent of normal activity. It should rarely be necessary to employ open biopsy of the liver for confirmation of enzyme deficiency or abnormal storage of cholesteryl esters and triglycerides.

TREATMENT

There is no specific treatment for Wolman's disease and CESD. Replacement of the missing enzyme activity has not been attempted.

REFERENCES

1. SLOAN HR, FREDRICKSON DS: Rare familial diseases with neutral lipid storage: Wolman's disease, cholesteryl ester storage disease, and cerebrotendinous xanthomatosis, in Stanbury JB, Wyngaarden JB, Fredrickson DS (eds): *The Metabolic Basis of Inherited Disease*, 3d ed. McGraw-Hill, New York, 1972, p 808

2. FREDRICKSON DS, FERRANS VJ: Acid cholesteryl ester hydrolase deficiency (Wolman's disease and cholesteryl ester storage disease), in Stanbury JB, Wyngaarden JB, Fredrickson DS (eds): *The Metabolic Basis of Inherited Disease*, 4th ed. McGraw-Hill, New York, 1978, p 670

3. ABRAMOV A, SCHORR S, WOLMAN M: Generalized xanthomatosis with calcified adrenals. *J Dis Child* 91:282, 1956

4. WOLMAN M, STERK VV, GATT S, FRENKEL M: Primary familial xanthomatosis with involvement and calcification of the adrenals: Report of two more cases in siblings of a previously described infant. *Pediatrics* 28:742, 1961

5. WOLMAN M: Histochemistry of lipids in pathology, in Graumann W, Neumann K (eds): *Handbuch der Histochemie*. Stuttgart, Fischer-Verlag, 1964, vol 5, p 228

6. CROCKER AC, VAWTER GF, NEUHAUSER EBD, ROSOWSKY A: Wolman's disease: Three new patients with a recently described lipidosis. *Pediatrics* 35:627, 1965

7. ALEXANDER WS: Niemann-Pick-disease: Report of a case showing calcification in the adrenal glands. *NZ Med J* 45:43, 1946

8. NEUHAUSER EBD, KIRKPATRICK JA, WEINTRAUB H: Wolman's disease: A new lipidosis. *Ann Radiol* 8:175, 1965

9. ROSOWSKY A, CROCKER AC, TRITES DH, MODEST EJ: Gas-liquid chromatography analysis of the tissue sterol fraction in Wolman's disease and related lipidoses. *Biochim Biophys Acta* 98:617, 1965

10. KONNO T, FUJII M, WATANUKI T, KOIZUMI K: Wolman's disease: The first case in Japan. *Tohoku J Exp Med*, 90:375, 1966

11. SPIEGEL-ADOLF M, BAIRD HW, MCCAFFERTY M: Hematologic studies in Niemann-Pick and Wolman's disease (cytology and electrophoresis). *Confin Neurol* 28:399, 1966

12. CAFFEY J, SILVERMANN FN: *Pediatric X-ray Diagnosis*, 5th ed. Chicago, Year Book Medical Publishers, 1967, pp 672–674

13. SLOVITER HA, JANIC V, NAIMAN JL: Lipid synthesis by red blood cell preparations in Wolman's disease (a familial lipidosis). *Clin Chim Acta* 20:423, 1968

14. GUAZZI GC, MARTIN JJ, PHILIPPART M, ROELS H, VAN DER ERCKEN H, VRINTS L, DELBEKE MJ, HOOFT C: Wolman's disease. *Eur Neurol* 1:334, 1968

15. GUAZZI GC, MARTIN JJ, PHILIPPART M, ROELS H, HOOFT C, VAN DER ERCKEN H, DELBEKE MJ, VRINTS L: Wolman's disease: Distribution and significance of the central nervous system lesions. *Pathol Eur* 3:266, 1968

16. KAHANA D, BERANT M, WOLMAN M: Primary familial xanthomatosis with adrenal involvement (Wolman's disease): Report of a further case with nervous system involvement and pathogenetic considerations. *Pediatrics* 42:70, 1968

17. KAMOSHITA S, LANDING BH: Distribution of lesions in myenteric plexus and gastrointestinal mucosa in lipidoses and other neurological disorders of children. *Am J Clin Pathol* 49:312, 1968

18. MARKS M, MARCUS AJ: Wolman's disease. *Can Med Assoc J* 99:232, 1968

19. PARTIN JC, MEREU TR, SCHUBERT WK: Intestinal absorptive epithelium in Wolman's cholesterol lipidoses, in Arcenaux CJ (ed): *Proc. 26th Ann. Meeting Electron Microscope Soc. Am.* Baton Rouge, Claitor's, 1968, pp 194–195

20. WOLMAN M: Involvement of nervous tissue in primary familial xanthomatosis with adrenal calcification. *Pathol Eur* 3:259, 1968

21. MARSHALL WC, OCKENDEN BC, FOSBROOKE AS, CUMINGS JN: Wolman's disease: A rare lipidosis with adrenal calcification. *Arch Dis Child* 44:331, 1968

22. WERBIN BZ, WOLMAN M: Primary familial xanthomatosis with involvement and calcification of the adrenals (Wolman's disease). *Harefuah* 74:283, 1968

23. PATRICK AD, LAKE BD: Deficiency of an acid lipase in Wolman's disease. *Nature (London)* 222:1067, 1969

24. ETO Y, KITAGAWA T: Wolman's disease with hypolipoproteinemia and acanthocytosis: Clinical and biochemical observations. *J Pediatr* 77:862, 1970

25. LAKE BD, PATRICK AD: Wolman's disease: Deficiency of E600-resistant acid esterase activity with storage of lipids in lysosomes. *J Pediatr* 76:262, 1970

26. LOUGH J, FAWCETT J, WIEGENSBERG B: Wolman's disease: An electron microscopic, histochemical and biochemical study. *Arch Pathol (Chicago)* 89:103, 1970

27. LOWDEN JA, BARON AJ, WENTWORTH P: Wolman's disease: A microscopic and histochemical study showing accumulation of ceroid and esterified cholesterol. *Can Med Assoc J* 102:402, 1970

28. KYRIAKIDES EC, FILIPPONE N, PAUL B, GRATTAN W, BALINT JA: Lipid studies in Wolman's disease. *Pediatrics* 46:431, 1970

29. WALLIS K, GROSS M, KOHN R, ZAIDMAN J: A case of Wolman's disease. *Helv Paediat Acta* 26:98, 1971

30. LECLERC JL, HOULD F, LELIEVRE M, GAGNE F: Maladie de Wolman: Etude anatomo-clinique d'une nouvelle observation avec absence de calcifications radiologiques et macroscopiques des surrenales. *Laval Med* 42:461, 1971

31. PHILLIPPART M: Wolman's disease. *J Pediatr* 79:173, 1971

32. RAAFAT R, HASHEMIAN MP, ABRISHAMI MA: Wolman's disease: Report of two new cases with a review of the literature. *Am J Clin Pathol* 59:490, 1973

33. KAMALIAN N, DUDLEY AW, BEROUKHIM F: Wolman's disease with jaundice and subarachnoid hemorrhage. *Am J Dis Child* 126:671, 1973

34. UNO Y, TANIGUCHI A, TANAKA E: Histochemical studies in Wolman's disease: Report of an autopsy case accompanied with a large amount of milky ascites. *Acta Pathol Jap* 23:779, 1973

35. WOLF H, NOLTE K, NOLTE R: Das neue Syndrom: Wolman-Syndrom. *Mschr Kinderheilk* 121:697, 1973

36. LAJO A, GRACIA R, NAVARRO M, NISTAL M, ROBODAN B: Enfermede de Wolman en su forma aguda infantil. *An Esp Pediat* 7:438, 1974

37. SUZUKI Y, KAWAI S, KOBAYASHI A, OHBE Y, ENDO H: Partial deficiency of acid lipase with storage of triglycerides and cholesterol esters in liver. *Clin Chim Acta* 69:219, 1976

38. CORTNER JA, COATES PM, SWOBODA E, SCHNATZ JD: Genetic variation of lysosomal acid lipase. *Pediatr Res* 10:927, 1976

39. ELLIS JE, PATRICK D: Wolman disease in a Pakistani infant. *Am J Dis Child* 130:545, 1976

40. HARRISON RB, FRANCKE P JR: Radiographic findings in Wolman's disease. *Radiology* 124:188, 1977

41. OZSOYLU S, GÜRGERY A, KOCAK N, OZORAN Y, OZORAN A, KERSE I, CILIV G: Wolman's disease. A case report with lipid, chromosome and electronmicroscopic studies. *Turk J Pediatr* 19:57, 1977

42. VON BASSEWITZ DB, ROGGENKAMP K, STREHL H, OTTO H: Wolmansche Erkrankung. *Verh Dtsch Ges Path* 62:530, 1978

43. OZORAN Y, OZORAN A, KERSE I, GÜRGEY A, OZSOYLU S, KOCAK N, CILIV G: An ultrastructural study in a case of Wolman's disease (clinical, biochemical, light and electron microscopic study). *Turk J Pediatr* 20:100, 1978

44. HO FC, LIN HJ, CHAN WC: Wolman's disease: The first reported Chinese patient. *Mod Med Asia* 14:23, 1978

45. SCHAFFNER T, ELNER VM, BAUER M, WISSLER RW: Acid lipase: A histochemical and biochemical study using triton X 100-naphtyl palmitate micelles. *J Histochem Cytochem* 26:696, 1978

46. STY JR, STARSHAK RJ: Scintigraphy in Wolman's disease. *Clin Nucl Med* 3:397, 1978

47. YOUNG LW, STY JR, BABBITT JP: Wolman's disease. *Am J Dis Child* 133:959, 1979

48. BYRD JC, POWERS JM: Wolman's disease: Ultrastructural evidence of lipid accumulation in central nervous system. *Acta Neuropathol (Berlin)* 45:37, 1979

49. PERMANETTER W, MÜLLER-HÖCKER J, HÜBNER G, SCHAUB J: Wolman's disease. *Med Welt* 30:1783, 1979

50. SCHAUB J, JANKA GE, CHRISTOMANOU H, SANDHOFF K, PERMANETTER W, HÜBNER G, MEISTER P: Wolman's disease: Clinical, biochemical and ultrastructural studies in an unusual case without striking adrenal calcification. *Eur J Pediatr* 135:45, 1980

51. SLOAN HR, FREDRICKSON DS: Enzyme deficiency in cholesteryl ester storage disease. *J Clin Invest* 51:1923, 1972

52. KYRIAKIDES EC, PAUL B, BALIN JA: Lipid accumulation and acid lipase deficiency in fibroblasts from a family with Wolman's disease, and their apparent correction in vitro. *J Lab Clin Med* 80:810, 1972

53. GUY GJ, BUTTERWORTH J: Acid esterase activity in cultured skin fibroblasts and amniotic fluid cells using 4-methylumbelliferyl palmitate. *Clin Chim Acta* 84:361, 1978

54. BURTON BK, EMERY D, MUELLER HW: Lysosomal acid lipase in cultivated fibroblasts: Characterization of enzyme activity in normal and enzymatically deficient cell lines. *Clin Chim Acta* 101:25, 1980

55. YOUNG EP, PATRICK AD: Deficiency of acid esterase activity in Wolman's disease. *Arch Dis Child* 45:664, 1970

56. COATES PM, CORTNER JA, HOFFMAN GM, BROWN SA: Acid lipase activity of human lymphocytes. *Biochim Biophys Acta* 572:225, 1979

57. FREDRICKSON DS: Newly recognized disorders of cholesterol metabolism. *Ann Intern Med* 58:718, 1963

58. FREDRICKSON DS, SLOAN HR, FERRANS VJ, DEMOSKY SJ JR: Cholesteryl ester storage disease: A most unusual manifestation of deficiency of two lysosomal enzyme activities. *Trans Assoc Am Physicians* 85:109, 1972

59. LAGERON A, CAROLI J, STRALIN H, BARBIER P: Polycorie cholésterolique de l'adulte. I. Etude clinique, electronique, histochimique. *Presse Med (Paris)* 75:2785, 1967

60. INFANTE R, POLONOVSKI J, CAROLI J: Polycorie cholésterolique de l'adulte. II. Etude biochimique. *Presse Med (Paris)* 75:2829, 1967

61. SCHIFF L, SCHUBERT WK, MCADAMS AJ, SPIEGEL EL, O'DONNELL JF: Hepatic cholesterol ester storage disease, a familial disorder. I. Clinical aspects. *Am J Med* 44:538, 1968

62. PARTIN JC, SCHUBERT WK: Small intestinal mucosa in cholesterol ester storage disease: A light and electron microscope study. *Gastroenterology* 57:542, 1969

63. BEAUDET AL, FERRY GD, NICHOLS BL, ROSENBERG HS: Cholesterol ester storage disease: Clinical, biochemical and pathological studies. *J Pediatr* 90:910, 1977

64. ORME RLE: Wolman's disease: An unusual presentation. *Proc R Soc Med* 63:489, 1970

65. WOLF H, HUG G, MICHAELIS R, NOLTE K: Seltene angeborene Erkrankung mit Cholesterinester-Speicherung in der Leber. *Helv Paediatr Acta* 29:105, 1974

66. ALAGILLE D, COURTECUISSE V: Surcharge hepatique a esters du cholesterol (deux observations). *Jour Parisiennes Pediatr* 465, 1970

67. LAGERON A, LICHTENSTEIN H, BODIN F, CONTE M: Polycorie cholesterolique de l'adulte: A propos d'une nouvelle observation. *Nouv Presse Med* 3:1233, 1974

68. LAGERON A, LICHTENSTEIN H, BODIN F, CONTE M: Polycorie cholesterolique de l'adulte: Aspects cliniques et histochimiques. *Med Chir Dig* 4:9, 1975

69. LAGERON A: Histoenzymologie de la polycorie cholesterolique. *Med Chir Dig* 7:155, 1978

70. GAUTIER M, LAPONS D, RAULIN J: Maladie de surcharge a esters du cholesterol chez l'enfant. Etude biochimique comparative de cultures d'hepatocytes et de fibroblasts. *Arch Fr Pediatr* 35:38, (10 suppl): 1978

71. AUBERT-TULKENS G, VAN HOOF F: Acid Lipase deficiency: Clinical and biochemical heterogeneity. *Acta Paediatr Belg* 32:239, 1979

72. KELLER E, KÜNNERT B, BRAUN W: Cholesterinesterspeicherkrankheit der Leber im Kindesalter. *Dt Z Verdauungs Stoffwechselkr* 37:231, 1977

73. KÜNNERT B, COSSEL L, KELLER E: Zur Diagnostik und Morphologie der Leber bei Cholesterinester-Speicherkrankheit. *Zentralbl Allgem Pathol Pathol Anat* 123:71, 1979

74. PFEIFFER U, JESCHKE R: Cholesterylester-Speicherkrankheit. *Virchow Arch B Cell Path* 33:17, 1980

75. KUNTZ HD, MAY B, SCHEJBAL V, ASSMANN G: Cholesterinester-Speicherkrankheit der Leber. *Leber, Magen, Darm* 11:258, 1981

76. BURKE JA, SCHUBERT WK: Deficient activity of hepatic acid lipase in cholesterol ester storage disease. *Science* 176:309, 1972

77. PARTIN JC, SCHUBERT WK: The ultrastructure and lipid composition of cultured skin fibroblasts in cholesterol ester storage disease. *Pediatr Res* 6:393, 1972

78. BEAUDET AL, LIPSON MH, FERRY GD, NICHOLS BL JR: Acid lipase in cultured fibroblasts: Cholesterol ester storage disease. *J Lab Clin Med* 84:54, 1974

79. SCHAEFER HE, ASSMANN G, SCHMITZ G, MAY B: Histochemical and electron microscopic studies in cholesterol ester storage disease. In preparation.

80. GOLDSTEIN JL, DANA SE, FAUST JR, BEAUDET AL, BROWN MS: Role of lysosomal acid lipase in the metabolism of plasma low density lipoprotein: Observations in cultured fibroblasts from a patient with cholesteryl ester storage disease. *J Biol Chem* 250:8487, 1975

81. BROWN MS, SABHANI MK, BRUNSCHEDE GY, GOLDSTEIN JS: Restoration of a regulatory response to low density lipoprotein in acid lipase-deficient human fibroblasts. *J Biol Chem* 251:3277, 1976

82. SCHMITZ G, ASSMANN G, MAY B: Lipoprotein analysis in cholesterol ester storage disease. In preparation

83. FERRANS VJ, BUJA LM, ROBERTS WC, FREDRICKSON DS: The spleen in type I hyperlipoproteinemia: Histochemical, biochemical, microfluorimetric, and electron microscopic observations. *Am J Pathol* 64:67, 1971

84. FERRANS VJ, ROBERTS WC, LEVY RI, FREDRICKSON DS: Chylomicrons and the formation of foam cells in type I hyperlipoproteinemia: A morphologic study. *Am J Pathol* 70:253, 1973

85. DREVON CA, HOVIG T: The effects of cholesterol/fat feeding on lipid levels and morphological structures in liver, kidney and spleen in guinea pigs. *Acta Pathol Microbiol Scand* 85A:1, 1977

86. HAYASHI H, WINSHIP DH, STERNLIEB I: Lipolyosomes in human liver: Distribution in livers with fatty infiltration. *Gastroenterology* 73:651, 1977

87. MICHELS VV, DRISCOLL DJ, FERRY GD, DUFF DF, BEAUDET AL: Pulmonary vascular obstruction associated with cholesteryl ester storage disease. *J Pediatr* 94:621, 1979

88. GOLDFISCHER S, SCHILLER B, WOLINSKY H: Lipid accumulation in smooth muscle cell lysosomes in primate atherosclerosis. *Am J. Pathol* 78:497, 1975

89. PETERS, TT, TAKANO R, DE DUVE C: in Potter R, Knight J (eds): *Atherogenesis, Initiating Factors*, Ciba Foundation Symposium 12. Amsterdam, Elsevier 1973, p 197

90. DE DUVE C: Exploring cells with a centrifuge. *Science* 198:186, 1975

91. ASSMANN G, FREDRICKSON DS, SLOAN HR, FALES HM, HIGHET RJ: Accumulation of oxygenated steryl esters in Wolman's disease. *J Lipid Res* 16:28, 1975

92. LIN HJ, LIE KEN JIE MS, HO FC: Accumulation of glyceryl ether lipids in Wolman's disease. *J Lipid Res* 17:53, 1976

93. FREDRICKSON DS: Tangier disease, in Stanbury JB, Wyngaarden JB, Fredrickson DS (eds): *The Metabolic Basis of Inherited Disease*, 2d ed. New York, McGraw-Hill, 1966, p 486

94. PITTMAN RC, WILLIAMS JC, MILLER A, STEINBERG S: Acid acylhydrolase deficiency in I-cell disease and pseudo-Hurler polydystrophy. *Biochim Biophys Acta* 575:399, 1979

95. COATES, PM, CORTNER J: Acid lipase in cultured amniotic fluid cells. Implications for the prenatal diagnosis of Wolman's disease. *Pediatr Res* 12:450, 1978

95a. KOCH G, LALLEY PA, McAVOY M, SHOWS TB: Assignment of LIPA, associated with human lipase deficiency to human chromosome 10 and comparative assignment to mouse chromosome 19. *Som Cell Genet* 7:345, 1981

96. KOSTER JF, VAANDRAGER H, VAN BERKEL TJC: Study of the hydrolysis of 4-methylumbelliferyl oleate by acid lipase and cholesterol oleate by acid cholesteryl esterase in human leucocytes, fibroblasts and liver. *Biochim Biophys Acta* 618:98, 1980

97. PATSCH W, RINDLER-LUDWIG R, SAILER S, BRAUNSTEINER H: Acid cho-

98. TAKANO T, BLACK WJ, PETERS TJ, DE DUVE C: Assay, kinetics and lysosomal localization of an acid cholesteryl esterase in rabbit aortic smooth muscle cells. *J Biol Chem* 249:6732, 1974

99. PETERS TJ, DE DUVE C: Lysosomes of the arterial wall. II. Subcellular fractionation of aortic cells from rabbits with experimental atheroma. *Exp Mol Pathol* 20:228, 1974

100. SUKARADA T, ORIMO H, OKABE H, NOMA A, MURAKAMI M: Purification and properties of cholesterol ester hydrolase from human aortic intima and media. *Biochim Biophys Acta* 424:204, 1976

101. HO YK, BROWN MS, GOLDSTEIN JL: Hydrolysis and excretion of cytoplasmic cholesteryl esters by macrophages: Stimulation of high density lipoprotein and other agents. *J Lipid Res* 21:39, 1980

102. BROWN MS, HO YK, GOLDSTEIN JL: The cholesteryl ester cycle in macrophage foam cells. *J Biol Chem* 255:9344, 1980

103. FAERGEMAN O, HAVEL RJ: Metabolism of cholesteryl esters of rat very low density lipoproteins. *J Clin Invest* 55:1210, 1975

104. SHELBURNE FA, HANKS J, MEYERS W, QUARFORDT SH: Effect of apoproteins on hepatic uptake of triglyceride emulsions in the rat. *J Clin Invest* 65:652, 1980

105. QUARFORDT S, HANKS J, JONES RS, SHELBURNE F: The uptake of high density lipoprotein cholesteryl ester in the perfused rat liver. *J Biol Chem* 255:29, 1980

106. STEIN O, STEIN Y, GOODMAN DS, FIDGE NH: The metabolism of chylomicron cholesteryl esters in rat liver. A combined radioautographic-electron microscopic and biochemical study. *J Cell Biol* 418:410, 1969

107. FLOREN CH, NILSSON A: Degradation of chylomicron remnant cholesteryl ester by rat hepatocyte monolayers. Inhibition by chloroquine and colchicine. *Biochem Biophys Res Commun* 74:520, 1977

108. GOODMAN ZD, LEQUIRE VS: Transfer of esterified cholesterol from serum lipoproteins to the liver. *Biochim Biophys Acta* 398:325, 1975

109. COOPER AD, YU PYS: Rates of removal and degradation of chylomicron remnants by isolated perfused rat liver. *J Lipid Res* 19:635, 1978

110. FLOREN CH, NILSSON A: Binding, interiorization and degradation of cholesteryl ester–labeled chylomicron-remnant particles by rat hepatocyte monolayer. *Biochem J* 168:483, 1977

111. VAN BERKEL ThJC, VAN TOL A: In vivo uptake of human and rat low density and high density lipoprotein by parenchymal and nonparenchymal cells from rat liver. *Biochim Biophys Acta* 530:299, 1978

112. VAN BERKEL ThJC, VAN TOL A, KOSTER JF: Iodine labeled human and rat low-density and high density lipoprotein degradation by human liver and parenchymal and non-parenchymal cells from rat liver. *Biochim Biophys Acta* 529:138, 1978

113. VAN BERKEL ThJC, VAN TOL A: Role of parenchymal and non-parenchymal rat liver cells in the uptake of cholesterol ester-labeled serum lipoproteins. *Biochem Biophys Res Commun* 89:1097, 1979

114. VAN BERKEL ThJC, VAANDRAGER H, KRUYT JK, KOSTER JF: Characteristics of acid lipase and acid cholesteryl esterase in parenchymal and non-parenchymal rat liver cells. *Biochim Biophys Acta* 617:446, 1980

115. FAUST JR, GOLDSTEIN JL, BROWN MS: Receptor-mediated uptake of low density lipoprotein and utilization of its cholesterol for steroid synthesis in cultured mouse adrenal cells. *J Biol Chem* 252:4861, 1977

116. HALL PF, NAKAMARA M: The influence of adrenocorticotropin on transport of a cholesteryl linoleate-low density lipoprotein complex into adrenal tumor cells. *J Biol Chem* 254:12547, 1979

117. ANDERSON JM, DIETSCHY JM: Relative importance of high and low density lipoproteins in the regulation of cholesterol synthesis in the adrenal gland, ovary, and testis of the rat. *J Biol Chem* 253:9024, 1978

118. LAKE BD: Histochemical detection of the enzyme deficiency in blood films in Wolman's disease. *J Clin Pathol* 24:617, 1971

119. KELLY S, BAKHRU-KISHORE R: Fluorimetric assay of acid lipase in human leucocytes. *Clin Chim Acta* 97:239, 1979

120. MEYERS MA: Disease of the adrenal glands, in *Radiologic Diagnosis*. Springfield, Illinois, Charles C Thomas, 1963

121. AQUILAR MJ, O'BRIEN JS, TABER P: The syndrome of familial leucodystrophy, adrenal insufficiency, and cutaneous melanosis, in Aronson SM, Volk BW (eds): *Inborn Disorders of Sphingolipid Metabolism*. Third Int. Symp. Cerebral Sphingolipidoses. New York, Pergamon, 1967, p 149

122. MICHELS VV, BEAUDET AL: Cholesteryl lignocerate hydrolysis in adrenoleucodeptrophy. *Pediatr Res* 14:21, 1980

123. OGINO T, SCHAUMBURG HH, SUZUKI K, KISHIMOTO Y, MOSER AE: Metabolic studies of adrenoleucodeptrophy. *Adv Exp Med Biol* 100:601, 1978

124. GALTON DJ, GILBERT CH, LUCEY JJ, PATH MRC, WALKER-SMITH JA: Triglyceride storage disease: A defect in activation of lipolysis in adipose tissue. *Pediatr* 59:442, 1977

125. GALTON DJ, RECKLESS JPD, GILBERT CH: Triglyceride storage disease, in Collip PJ (ed): *Childhood Obesity*. Acton, Massachusetts, Publishing Sciences Group, 1975, p 149

lesterol ester and glycerol ester hydrolase activities. *Biochim Biophys Acta* 618:337, 1980

40

CERAMIDASE DEFICIENCY:
Farber's Lipogranulomatosis

HUGO W. MOSER

WINSTON W. CHEN

1. *Farber's disease is a genetically determined disorder of lipid metabolism, associated with deficiency of a lysosomal acid ceramidase and the tissue accumulation of ceramide.*
2. *The main clinical manifestations are painful and progressively deformed joints, subcutaneous nodules, particularly near the joints and over pressure points, and progressive hoarseness due to laryngeal involvement. These tissues show granulomas and the accumulation of lipid-laden macrophages. There may be moderate nervous system dysfunction related to the accumulation of ceramide and gangliosides in neurons. The lungs, heart, and lymph nodes may also be involved. The illness often leads to death within the first few years, but a more prolonged course has also been observed.*
3. *Specific diagnosis depends upon demonstration of a deficiency of acid ceramidase in cultured skin fibroblasts or in white blood cells. Acid ceramidase activity in heterozygotes is approximately half of that in normal individuals. Prenatal diagnosis has been accomplished by demonstrating acid ceramidase deficiency in cultured amniotic fluid cells.*
4. *The mode of inheritance is autosomal recessive. The disorder is rare.*
5. *There is no specific therapy.*

Farber's lipogranulomatosis is a rare progressive disorder characterized by hoarseness, painful and swollen joints, periarticular and subcutaneous nodules, pulmonary infiltrations, and the accumulation of lipids in the cytoplasm of neurons and certain other cells. Accumulation of ceramide or deficiency of a lysosomal acid ceramidase or both have been demonstrated in affected patients.

CLINICAL MANIFESTATIONS

A total of 27 patients have been described in some detail. Table 40-1 summarizes their main features. Eighteen of the twenty-seven were severely involved and either had died before 4 years of age (patients 1 to 16) or were terminally ill at the time of last report (patients 20, 21). Five patients had a more prolonged course and survived to the second decade or appeared relatively mildly involved at the time of last report (patients 18, 19, 25, 26, 27). Four additional patients (17, 22, 23, 24) appeared to be intermediate between the severe and the mild groups.

The clinical expression of the severe form of Farber's disease is so striking that diagnosis can almost be made at a glance. The characteristic features are painful swelling of joints (particularly the interphalangeal, metacarpal, ankle, wrist, knee,

820

and elbow), swelling and palpable nodules in relation to the affected joints and over pressure points, a hoarse cry which may progress to aphonia, feeding and respiratory difficulties, poor weight gain, and intermittent fever.

Symptoms usually first appear between ages 2 weeks and 4 months. The initial finding in most patients is painful and swollen joints, or hoarseness. Attention is first drawn to the limbs and joints by diffuse swelling and hyperesthesia. Later the generalized swelling of the extremities diminishes, and nodular thickenings around the joints and tendon sheaths indicate the articular involvements. The fingers are held flexed at the interphalangeal joints, and passive motion causes pain. Joint contractures develop. The older, more mildly affected patients have shown moderate flexion contractures of the knees, wrists, and fingers. The discrete, nodular, subcutaneous swellings increase in size and number as the disease advances (Figs. 40-1 and 40-2). They are found most often near the interphalangeal, ankle, wrist, and elbow joints. Other frequent locations are points subject to mechanical pressure, such as the occiput and the lumbosacral region of the spine (Fig. 40-1D). Nodules have also been observed in the conjunctiva, on the external ear, on the nostrils, and in the mouth (Fig. 40-2B). In a few instances they have regressed spontaneously.

Disturbances in swallowing, vomiting, and repeated episodes of pulmonary consolidation associated with fever occur frequently in the severely involved children, and pulmonary disease is the usual cause of death. The disturbances in swallowing and respiration often are due to swelling and granuloma formation in the epiglottis and larynx. Rib and sternal retraction and asthmatic breathing attest to the obstructive element of the respiratory disease and may require tracheostomy (Fig. 40-2). Other organs are also involved relatively frequently. Seven of the patients severely involved had moderate generalized lymphadenopathy. An enlarged tongue has been reported in six patients. Six have had cardiac involvement and patient 3 developed a grade 3/6 systolic murmur. The murmur was probably related to granulomatous lesions of the heart valves. Such lesions have been reported in three patients. Moderate enlargement of the liver has occurred in seven patients; a moderately enlarged spleen has been reported only once.

Evaluation of nervous system function in the severely affected young children is difficult because movement causes pain. Severe and progressive impairment of psychomotor development was reported in 10 cases; of these one was complicated by probably unrelated hydrocephalus severe enough to require a shunt (patient 3). Patients 17 and 18 had normal intelligence. Several other patients were thought to be mildly retarded or to have borderline intelligence. Salaam-type seizures, or infantile spasms, were reported in patients 10 and 16. Other signs of nervous system dysfunction arise mainly from the peripheral nerve involvement. Deep-tendon reflexes were diminished or absent in 12 patients. Hypotonia and muscular atrophy, which is observed frequently, may be related to the almost invariable lipid storage in the anterior horn cells or to peripheral nerve involvement [10] and to immobility and inanition. The electromyogram may show signs of denervation. In addition, patients 1 and 16 showed evidence of myopathy. The cerebrospinal fluid protein level was reported in 10 patients. In eight it was elevated, often markedly, and in two it was normal (Table 40-1).

Abnormalities of the eye have been detected in six patients. Cogan et al. [7] in their studies of patient 4 reported a diffuse grayish opacification of the retina about the foveola, with a cherry-red center, but without disturbance of visual function.

This abnormality, which resembles that seen in metachromatic leukodystrophy, is much more subtle than the cherry-red spot of Tay-Sachs disease. A second eye abnormality is a granulomatous lesion of the conjunctiva. This was particularly prominent in patient 18. Patients 15 and 24 showed corneal opacity and patient 13 lenticular opacity.

MORPHOLOGICAL CHANGES

Histopathology

Studies with the light microscope show granulomatous infiltrations in the subcutaneous tissues, joints, and many other organs. The earliest lesion appears to be the accumulation of macrophages or histiocytes, and in some areas this remains the principal pathologic feature. In other instances there are prominent foam cells. Although in certain tissues these foamy macrophages appear to have come from elsewhere, in other tissues (such as cartilage or in the heart valve) the storage material accumulates in the chondrocytes or endocardial cells which normally exist in these locations [14]. In some instances the lesions advance to an organized and full-blown granuloma, in which macrophages, lymphocytes, and multinucleated cells surround a core of foam cells. Older lesions show a prominent fibrotic reaction. In other lesions the most prominent feature is the accumulation of abnormal material with the histochemical properties of a glycolipid or glycoprotein, with relatively little cellular reaction [4].

The periarticular tissues, skin, and larynx have shown granulomatous lesions in all autopsied patients. Some of these lesions have invaded the joint capsule and on occasion the adjacent bone. The marrow in the diaphysis is much less involved.

The lungs have been involved in all the severely affected patients. They appear consolidated, and the interalveolar septums and the alveoli are infiltrated by massive numbers of macrophages. Granulomatous nodules are found on the parietal pleura. There is variability in respect to the degree of foam cell and granuloma formation. The heart has been involved in 6 of the 17 autopsied patients. In three there was thickening and nodule formation on the mitral and aortic valves and the chordae tendineae. Lesions are variably found in other sites, including lymph nodes, intestine, spleen, kidney, tongue, thymus, gallbladder, epithelium, and liver.

Histochemical studies of paraffin-fixed sections which had been dehydrated with lipid solvents showed material with the staining properties of mucopolysaccharides [14]. This, together with chemical assays in one patient [11], led to the supposition that Farber's disease is one of the mucopolysaccharidoses [11, 14]. However, when initial sample preparation avoided lipid solvents, two types of lipid-soluble storage materials were demonstrated: one of these had the tinctorial properties of ceramide [26], while the other was periodic acid Schiff (PAS)–positive and had the staining properties of a glycolipid [4, 6, 7] or ganglioside [26]. These findings are consistent with biochemical assays (see below).

Except in patients 9 and 18 the nervous system has been abnormal in all autopsied cases. The main change was the accumulation of storage material in neuronal cytoplasm. This accumulation has been particularly prominent in the anterior

Table 40-1   Farber's disease: Summary of 27 patients

Patient No.	Author(s)	Ref.	Sex	Age at death or last report	Origin	Sibs with Farber's	Unaffected sibs	Consan-guinity	Skin, joints, larynx	Tongue enlarged
1	Schonenberg	[2]	F	4 mo	German	0	4	No	+	0
2	Farber	[1]	M	6½ mo	Portuguese Azores	1 (patient 8)	4	No	+	+
3	Rampini	[3, 4, 5]	M	7 mo	Southern Italy	0	0	No	+	+
4	Moser, Prensky	[6, 7, 8]	F	9½ mo	French Canadian	0	3	No	+	−
5	Battin	[9]	F	1 yr	French	1 (patient 5)	?	No	+	+
6	Vital	[10]	F	14 mo	French	1 (patient 4)	?	No	+	+
7	Farber	[1]	F	14 mo	Scottish-Welsh	0	1 + 1 halfsib	No	+	+
8	Farber	[1]	M	14 mo	Portuguese Azores	1 (patient 2)	4	No	+	+
9	Bierman	[11, 12]	M	14 mo	Mexican-American	0	2	No	+	−
10	Becker	[13]	M	17 mo	Austria	−	−	−	+	−
11	Abul-Haj	[14, 15]	M	20 mo	Caucasian, USA	0	1	No	+	0
12	Toppet	[16, 17]	F	22 mo	Belgian	0	1	+	+	0
13	Hobolth	[18]	M	24 mo	Danish	0	3 + 1 halfsib	No	+	0
14	Moore	[19]	M	24 mo	Mexican	0	1	No	+	0
15	Ozaki	[20, 21]	M	25 mo	Japan	0	2	+	+	−
16	Neville, Turner	[22]	F	3½ yr	English	1	1	No	+	0
17	Pachman	[23]	F	5 9/12 yr	Irish-American	0	2	No	+	0
18	Zetterstrom	[24, 25, 26]	M	16 yr	Swedish	0	1	No	+	+
19	Pavone	[27]	F	17 yr	Sicily	1 (patient 25)	4	Possible	+	0
20	Amirhakimi	[28]	M	15 mo	Iran	2 (including patient 24)	2 + 2?	+	+	−
21	Schmoeckel	[29]	M	2 yr	Turkish	1	−	−	+	−
22	Horowitz	[30]	F	38 mo	Caucasian, USA	0	1 + 1 half brother	No	+	0
23	Coleman	[31]	F	5½ yr	Caucasian, USA	0	1 + 1 half brother	No	+	0
24	Amirhakimi	[28]	M	6 yr	Iran	2 (including patient 20)	2 + 2?	+	+	0
25	Pavone	[27]	F	9 yr	Sicily	1 (patient 19)	4	Possible	+	0
26	Barriere	[32]	F	13 yr	French	−	−	−	+	0
27	Pavone	[27]	F	17 yr	Sicily	0	1	Possible	+	0

NOTES: This table includes all of the 22 published cases of Farber's disease, as well as five cases (patients 18, 19, 22, 23, and 31) which so far are unpublished. All patient references in this article refer to this table. One case (Ref. 33), which had previously been diagnosed as mild Farber's disease, is not included here, because a subsequent fibroblast acid ceramidase assay was normal (see text).
Patients 1–19 are deceased. Patients 20–27 were alive at the time of last report.

Heart, lung	Liver, spleen, lymph nodes	Eyes	Mental function	Lower motor neuron involvement	Nerve cell storage	CSF protein, mg/dl	Tissue ceramide excess	Acid ceramidase activity, % control			Other
								Proband	Father	Mother	
Heart+ Lung+	Liver+ Lymph+	0	–	+	+	250–500	–	–	–	–	Myopathy
Lung+	Lymph+ Liver+	0	Impaired	+	+	130–418	–	–	–	–	
Heart+ Lung+	Liver+	–	Severe impaired	0	+	132–545	–	–	–	–	Shunted hydrocephalus
Lung+ Heart–	Lymph+	+ Retina	Intact	+	+	160	+	<1	44	73	
Heart+ Lung+	Lymph+	0	Intact	+	+	–	–	–	–	–	Enlarged ventricular system
Heart+ Lung+	Lymph+	0	–	+	+						
Heart+ Lung+	Lymph+	0	–	+							
Lung+	Spleen+ Lymph+	0	Impaired	+	+						
Heart+ Lung+	Lymph+	0	Impaired	–	–	Normal	–	–	–	–	Increased MPS in urine and tissues
Heart+ Lung+	0	–	Progressive impairment	+	+	Increased	+	–	–	–	Infantile spasm
Heart+ Lung+	Liver+	0	Impaired	+	+	70	–	–	–	–	
Lung+	Liver+ Spleen+ Lymph+	0	Normal	–	–	–	+	6	40	55	Congenital hypothyroid
–	–	+ (Cataract)	Probably normal	+	+	159–363	–	–	42	–	
Heart+ Lung+	Spleen+ Lymph+	0	–	–	–	–	–	–	–	–	
–	Liver±	+ (Cornea)	Impaired	+	–	150–300	+	–	–	–	
0	0	0	Impaired	+	+	–	+	4	29	36	Infantile spasm, myopathy
0	0	0	Normal	0	+	15	–	3	54	38	Father rheumatoid arthritis
0	0	0	Normal	0	0	–	+	<1	–	–	
0	0	0		0	–	–	–	–	–	–	
–	–	–	Normal	–	–	–	–	–	–	–	
–	–	–	Impaired	–	–	–	+	–	–	–	
0	0	0	Normal	–	–	–	–	3	18	–	
0	0	+ (Cornea)	Low-normal	+	–	–	–	5	–	64	
0	0	+ (Cornea)	Impaired	–	–	–	+	–	–	–	
0	0	0	IQ < 80	0	–	–	–	3	–	–	
0	0	0	IQ 60–65	–	–	–	–	–	–	–	
0	0	0	Slightly impaired	Possible	–	–	–	4	–	–	

All patients showed the triad of subcutaneous nodules, arthritis, and laryngeal involvement.
Notation of "possible" for consanguinity was made because members of both sides of the families lived in the same small communities.
Acid ceramidase activity was measured in cultured skin fibroblasts, except for patients 4 and 18 where measurements were made in postmortem tissues [56].
Symbols: +, feature present; 0, feature absent; –, no information.

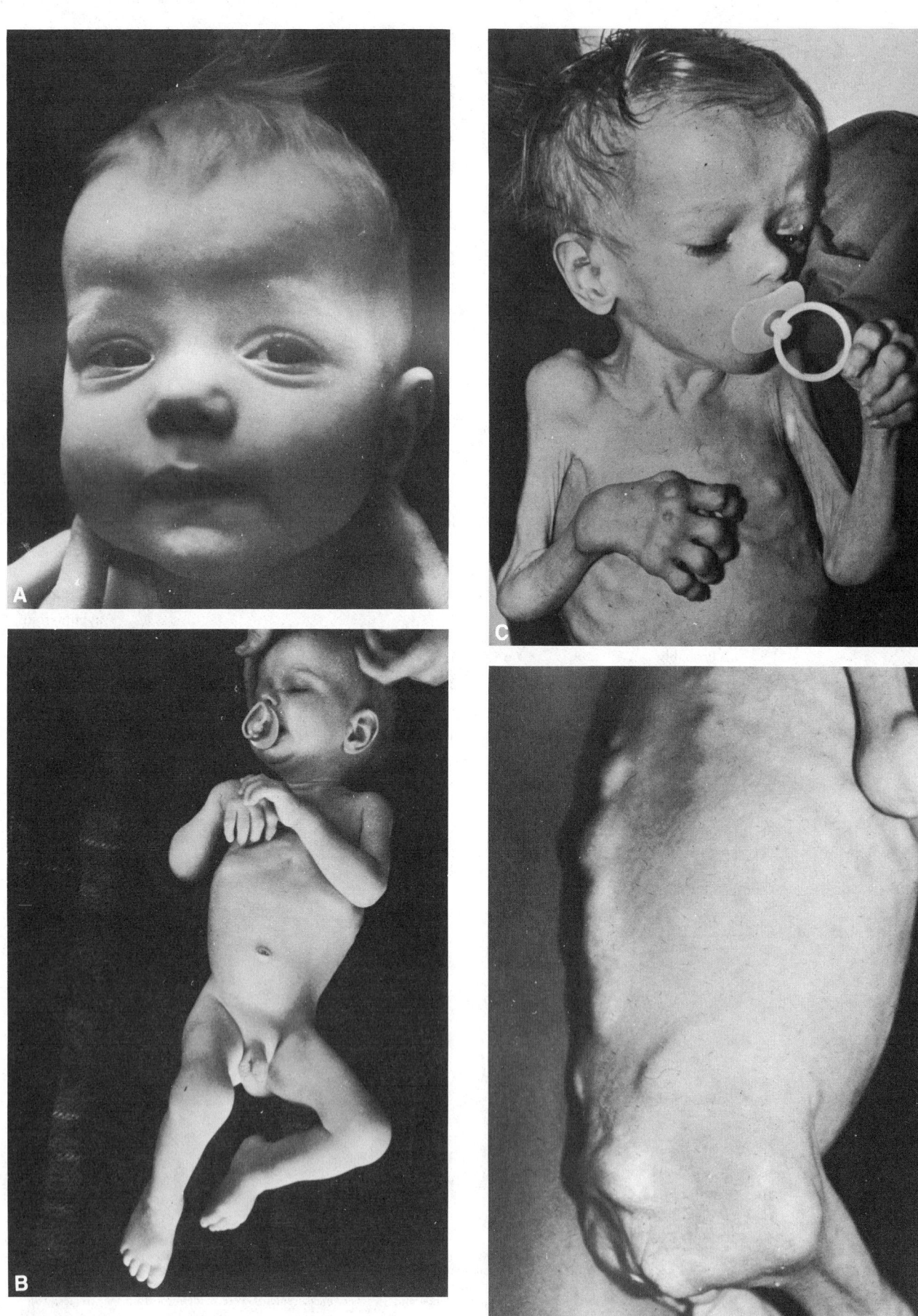

Figure 40-1   Patient 13 at 12 months (*A, B*) and at 21 months (*C, D*). (*Courtesy of Dr. Niels Hobolth.*)

horn cells in the spinal cord, but large nerve cells of the brainstem nuclei, basal ganglions, cerebellum, and retinal ganglion cells, and, to a lesser extent, the cortical neurons were also involved. Similar abnormalities occur in the peripheral nervous system, such as the autonomic ganglions, in posterior root cells, and, in some instances, in the Schwann cells. The storage material is PAS-positive, and much of it is extracted with lipid solvents, which suggests that it is glycolipid [4, 6, 7].

Ultrastructural Studies

Ultrastructural studies have been performed in seven individual patients (9, 10, 13, 16, 21, 29, and 34). These have shown cytoplasmic vacuoles of irregular shape up to 2 to 3 μm in size, which probably represent lysosomes since they have a single limiting membrane and show acid phosphatase activity. While these vacuoles contain a variety of materials, the most characteristic feature is comma-shaped curvilinear tubular structures. These consist of two dark lines separated by a clear space (Fig. 40-3). Although markedly variable, the diameter of the tubules is 14 nm on the average. It is likely that these tubular structures represent ceramide, since they can be produced in cultured fibroblasts from patients by adding ceramides containing nonhydroxy fatty acids to the growth medium [35]. Neurons and endothelial cells may also contain "zebra" bodies. These are often found in the neurons of patients with mucopolysaccharidoses or the gangliosidoses and are considered to be an ultrastructural expression of stored gangliosides. This is consistent with the increased ganglioside level of some Farber disease tissues, as has been demonstrated biochemically [6] and histochemically [26].

BIOCHEMICAL STUDIES

Alterations in Chemical Composition

Accumulation of Ceramide Accumulation of ceramide has been reported in all of the eight Farber's patients in whom the tissue level of this lipid has been analyzed (Table 40-2). High ceramide levels have been found in the subcutaneous nodules of the seven patients, and ceramide may make up 20 percent of total lipids. Ceramide levels are also increased in the kidney. For the other tissues the extent of ceramide excess appears to vary with the severity of the disease. The severely involved patients 6 and 16 showed high ceramide levels in the liver, as well as in the lungs and brain in patient 6, whereas in the more mildly affected patient 18, liver, lung, and brain ceramide levels were normal. Similarly, plasma ceramide levels were moderately increased in patient 6 and normal in patient 18.

Unlike those of normal subjects, the ceramides of patients with Farber's disease may contain significant proportions of 2-hydroxy fatty acids. In patient 6, 43 percent of kidney ceramides, 39 percent of those in the cerebellum, and 10 percent of those in the liver contained 2-hydroxy fatty acids [6, 37]. The 2-hydroxy acids in ceramide from Farber's disease consisted of cerebronic acid, which has a 24-carbon chain and lesser amounts of C_{22}, C_{20}, and C_{18} 2-hydroxy acids [25, 37]. This hydroxy–fatty acid pattern closely resembles that normally

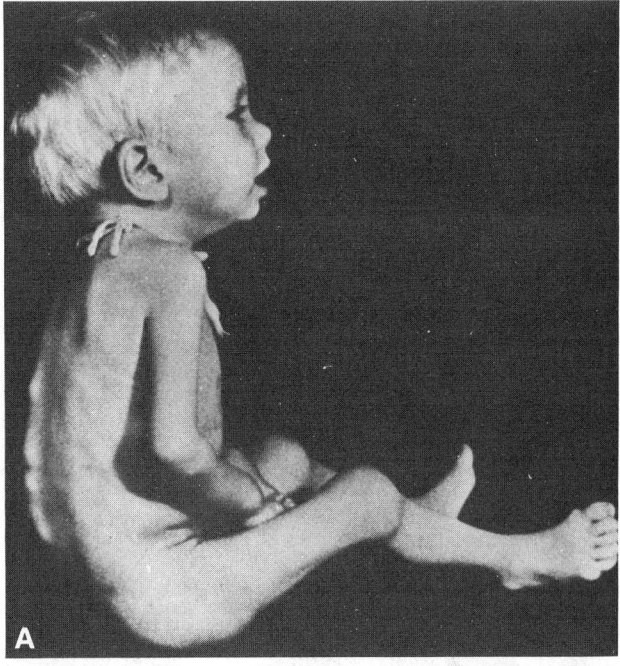

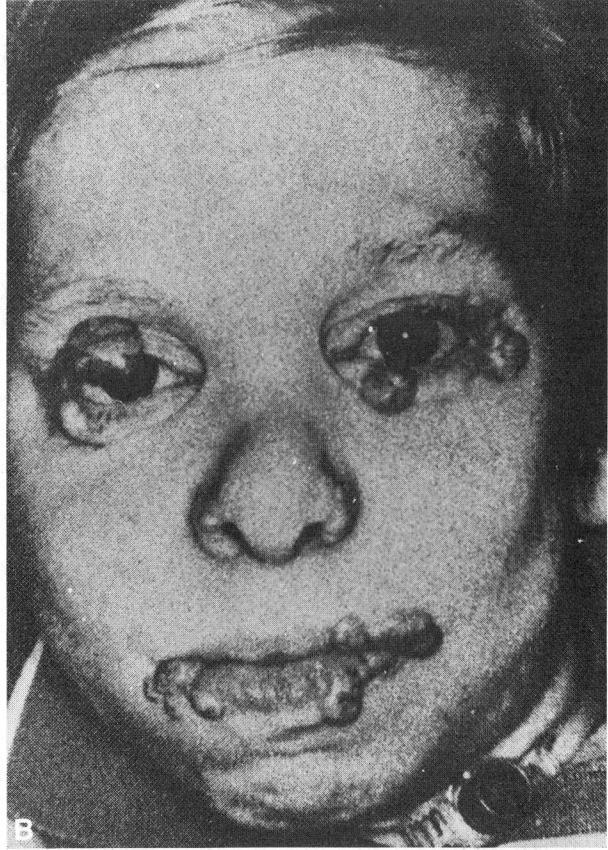

Figure 40-2 *A.* Patient 18 at 23 months. Note joint swelling and contractures and subcutaneous nodules over spinous processes. Tracheostomy was performed as a life-saving procedure at age 15 months. (*From Zetterstrom [24]. Used by permission.*) *B.* Patient 18 at 16 years. Granulomas over lips, nostrils, eyelids. Tracheostomy still in place. He was cachectic, weighed 20.3 kg, had atelectasis of the left lung and severe respiratory difficulties. Intelligence was normal, and he had learned to communicate well with the aid of an electric typewriter. He died 1 month later, due to cardiac arrest associated with the administration of a general anesthetic when granulomas were being removed from the eyelids. (*From Samuelsson, Zetterstrom, and Ivemark [26]. Used by permission.*)

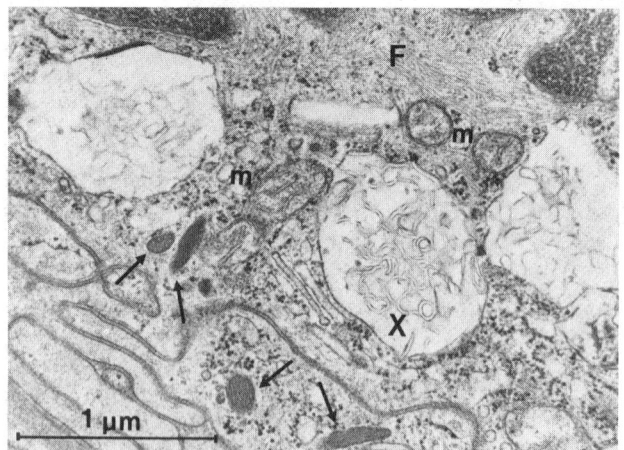

Figure 40-3 Farber's disease. Thin section of an endothelial cell with filaments (F), Wiebel-Palade bodies (arrows), mitochondria (m), and three vacuoles, one of which (x) contains "Farber bodies." Reduced from ×45,000. (*From Schmoeckel* [*65*].)

side. The liver glycolipid was unusual in that it contained glucose and galactosamine but not galactose [5]. Patient 6 had a three- to tenfold increase in ganglioside levels in the liver, kidney, lymph node, and subcutaneous nodule. The ganglioside consisted mainly of hematoside, and the extent of ganglioside accumulation correlated with the extent to which the tissue was infiltrated with foam cells containing PAS-positive material [6]. While all these studies suggest an accumulation of glycolipid, there is variation in the extent of accumulation and type of compound. Furthermore, the chemical structure of some of these materials has not been completely defined. Nevertheless, they probably contain ceramide, and, as will be discussed later, their accumulation could be secondary to a defect in ceramide degradation.

Accumulation of mucopolysaccharides was reported in patient 9 [*11*], but tissue and urinary polysaccharides were normal in patients 3, 6, 18, and 26.

seen in galactocerebrosides and sulfatides. No hydroxy fatty acids were demonstrable in the ceramides isolated from the subcutaneous nodule [25]. In other respects the composition of fatty acid and the long-chain bases in ceramide from patients with Farber's disease resembled those found in control tissues. The structural differences among the ceramides which accumulate in various tissues suggest that they are produced within these tissues [25].

Alterations in Other Tissue Components Farber et al. [1] isolated an abnormal "lipoglycoprotein complex" from the heart, liver, and lung of patients 2 and 8. This complex accounted for as much as 8 to 30 percent of total lipid but was not fully characterized. Patient 3 had a 30 percent increase in liver glycolipids and a comparable increase in brain ganglio-

Normal Ceramide Metabolism

Figure 40-4 shows the key role of ceramide in sphingolipid metabolism. It is an intermediate for the synthesis and degradation of gangliosides; myelin constituents, such as galactosylceramide and sulfatide; and membrane components such as sphingomyelin and the complex glycolipids.

Ceramide Biosynthesis Three biosynthetic pathways have been proposed: (1) microsomal synthesis from long-chain base and the fatty acid–CoA derivative, (2) the reverse ceramidase reaction, (3) a brain-specific ceramide synthetase. Reactions 2 and 3 utilize the free fatty acids rather than their CoA derivatives. The first pathway is probably the most significant one. The second pathway probably has a limited physiologic

Table 40-2 Ceramide levels in control and Farber's disease tissue

Tissue	Method	Control tissues mg/g ww	Control tissues %Total lipid	Patient 6 (Refs. 6, 36, 37) mg/g ww	Patient 6 (Refs. 6, 36, 37) %Total lipid	Patient 18 (Refs. 25, 26) mg/g ww	Patient 18 (Refs. 25, 26) %Total lipid	Patient 12 (Refs. 16, 17) mg/g ww	Patient 12 (Refs. 16, 17) %Total lipid	Patient 10 (Ref. 13)	Patient 15 (Ref. 20)	Patient 16 (Ref. 20)	Patient 21 (Ref. 29)	Patient 24 (Ref. 28)
Subcutaneous nodule	TLC			5920	12.9			9000	20		Qualitative increase		Qualitative increase	Qualitative increase
	GLC-MS					11,900								
Kidney	TLC	60	0.20	557	1.6					Qualitative increase				
	GLC-MS	128				966								
	HPLC	95		515										
Liver	TLC	123	0.32	8220	11.9							Qualitative increase		
	GLC-M	346				374								
Cerebral cortex	TLC	864	1.8	1238	2.6									
	GLC-MS	167				363								
Cerebral white matter	TLC	980	1.4	3530	4.5									
	GLC-MS	577				461								
	HPLC													
Cerebellum	TLC	63		311						Qualitative increase				
	GLC-MS													
	HPLC	54		167										
Plasma, µg/ml	GLC-MS	5.64 ±				6.21								
	HPLC	1.51 4.70		13.5										

NOTE: Ceramide levels were quantified: (1) by isolation of ceramides by thin-layer chromatography (TLC) [6] and spectrophotometric determination of sphingosine eluted from the TLC plate [*38*]; (2) by gas-liquid chromatography–mass spectometry (GLC-MS) [*25*]; or (3) by high-performance liquid chromatography (HPLC) [*36, 39, 40*]. In patient 6 [*6*] ceramide levels were also elevated in lung, but in patient 18 they were normal.

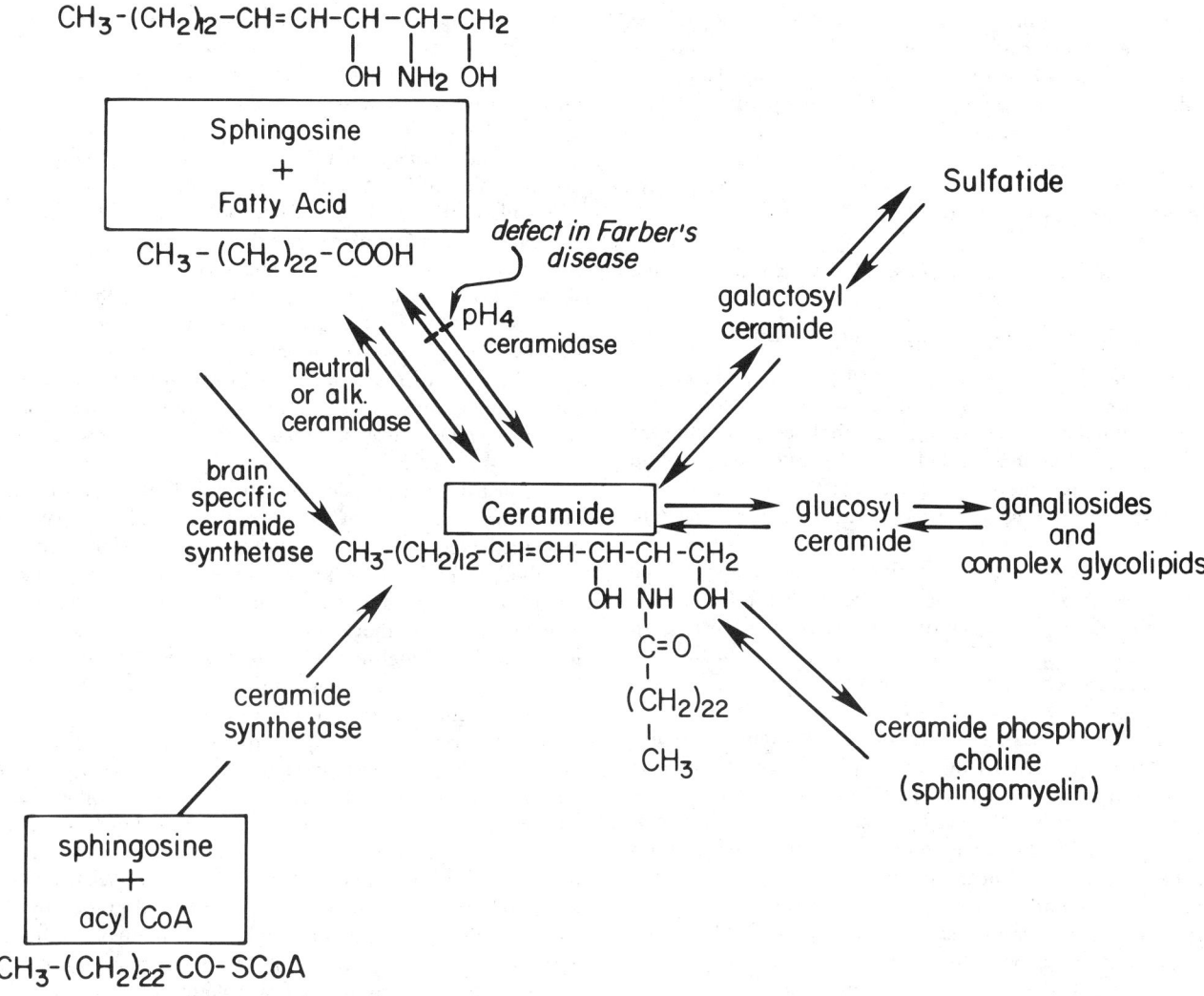

Figure 40-4 Ceramide metabolism and the metabolic defect in Farber's disease. The fatty acid shown in this figure is lignoceric acid, but a large variety of other fatty acids, including those with an α-hydroxy group, may be involved and there is also variability in respect to the long-chain bases shown here as sphingosine [25].

role, while the third pathway has been described only very recently and its role has not yet been fully assessed.

Synthesis of ceramide from sphingosine in vitro was first demonstrated by Scribney [41]:

Long-chain base + fatty acid–CoA ⟶ ceramide + CoA

This reaction is catalyzed by acyl-CoA:sphingosine N-acyltransferase (EC 2.3.1.24). The reaction has a pH optimum of 7.5 and occurs in the microsome. Free fatty acids are not reactive. The rates of conversion of stearoyl-, lignoceroyl-, palmitoyl-, and oleoyl-CoA were in approximate ratios of 60:12:3:1 [42]. These ratios resemble the distribution of these fatty acids in brain sphingolipids which suggests that the ceramide synthesis reaction determines the fatty acid composition of sphingolipids. There is much less specificity with respect to the long-chain base [43, 44].

There are several distinct acyl-CoA:sphingosine N-acyltransferases, which differ in respect to their specificity for the fatty acid–CoA moiety. Thus, in mouse brain preparations the enzyme which reacts with stearoyl-CoA differs in subcellular localization and maturational pattern from that which is most reactive with lignoceroyl-CoA (C₂₄) [45]. This conclusion is

also supported by results obtained in "quaking" mice, mutants with a deficiency of myelin. Brain microsomes from the "quaking" mouse have normal stearoyl-CoA:sphingosine N-acyltransferase activity, while the corresponding activity toward lignoceroyl-CoA is reduced by 55 percent [46]. There is suggestive evidence that the sphingosine acyltransferase for 2-hydroxy-stearoyl-CoA and that for cerebronoyl-CoA are also distinct [45].

Ceramidases are the enzymes responsible for degradation of ceramide. Acid, neutral, and alkaline ceramidases have been described. The acid and the alkaline ceramidases also appear to catalyze the reverse reaction, i.e., the synthesis of ceramide from sphingosine and free fatty acid [47–49]. The existence of this reverse reaction has recently been questioned, since it was reported that the reaction product was not ceramide but a condensation between long-chain fatty acids and ethanolamine, which formed part of the buffer system [50]. This question is not fully resolved, since the reverse reaction had been demonstrated in a variety of buffer systems which did not contain ethanolamine [49]. It seems likely that the reaction has limited physiologic significance [51].

Recently a novel pathway for ceramide synthesis has been

described in rat brain [52]. This pathway requires a pyridine nucleotide as well as a heat stable and a heat labile factor. As its substrates it utilizes sphingosine and very long chain fatty acids, such as lignoceric acid. This reaction appears to occur only in nervous tissue.

Ceramide Degradation

Acid Ceramidase   Ceramidase (EC 3.5.1.23) catalyzes the reaction:

$$\text{Ceramide} + H_2O \longrightarrow \text{long-chain base} + \text{fatty acid}$$

A ceramidase has been purified from rat brain. The enzyme has a pH optimum of 4.8, appears to be associated with the lysosome, is stimulated by cholate or taurocholate, and is inhibited by sphingosine and fatty acid [47, 48]. A greater than 200-fold purification was achieved by taking advantage of the fact that it withstands prolonged treatment with trypsin and chymotrypsin.

An acid ceramidase with analogous properties has been demonstrated in human kidney and cerebellum [49], and the enzyme has been partially purified from human placenta [53]. Recent studies in cultured skin fibroblasts provide further evidence that acid ceramidase is a lysosomal enzyme [54].

Neutral and Alkaline Ceramidases   Certain tissues also show ceramidase activity at alkaline pH. This is true at least for small intestine [54], cerebellum [40], cultured skin fibroblasts, and white blood cells. These neutral and alkaline ceramidases resemble the acid ceramidase in that the reactions appear reversible and in the synthetic reaction they act upon free fatty acids rather than their CoA derivatives. The small intestine alkaline ceramidase has a pH optimum of 7.6 and may be concentrated in the brush border [55]. The alkaline ceramidase in cerebellum has a pH optimum of 9.0 [49]. No systematic study has yet been reported on the normal distribution of the alkaline ceramidases or of their substrate specificities. Of the tissue studied so far, only kidney appears to lack the alkaline ceramidase [49].

Acid Ceramidase Deficiency and the Pathogenesis of Farber's Disease

A deficiency of acid ceramidase was first demonstrated in postmortem tissues of patients 6 and 18 [56] and subsequently in cultured skin fibroblasts of another seven patients ([57, 58] and Table 40-1), and in peripheral blood white cells [51]. The alkaline ceramidases appear to function normally in Farber's disease [49]. The defect in a degradative enzyme presumably accounts for the tissue accumulation of ceramide.

When Farber's disease cultured fibroblasts were incubated with [^{3}H]oleoylsphingosine (ceramide), the rate of uptake of ceramide was the same as in the control, but the rate of ceramide degradation was impaired, presumably secondary to the defect in acid ceramidase. The finding that retained radioactive ceramide was present in the lysosomal fraction provided further evidence that the defect involves a lysosomal enzyme [54]. These conclusions are reinforced by morphological studies. When ceramides are added to the culture medium in which Farber's disease fibroblasts are growing, these cells develop

large lysosomal inclusions that contain the curvilinear structures (Fig. 40-3) [35], which are considered characteristic of this disease. It is of interest, but so far unexplained, that these inclusions were produced by ceramides which contained nonhydroxy fatty acids, but not by those which contained the hydroxy fatty acids which normally occur in high concentration in brain and are found in Farber's disease tissues.

It is plausible that the deficiency of acid ceramidase leads to ceramide accumulation and that this is responsible in part for the cytoplasmic lipid storage. The accumulation of gangliosides and other glycolipids may be a secondary phenomenon, since ceramide is on the degradative pathway of these substances. The granuloma formation and histiocytic response may also be a consequence of ceramide accumulation, since subcutaneous injection of ceramide in rats produces lesions which resemble those observed in Farber's disease patients [6].

The distribution of lesions in Farber's disease and the variability of expression of the disease can only be partially explained. Neuronal storage is not unexpected, since ceramide metabolism in brain is known to be active. The striking involvement of subcutaneous tissues may be accounted for by recent observations that ceramide has an important role in normal skin. Ceramide makes up 16 to 20 percent of the total lipids in the stratum corneum [58] and forms an essential part of the intercellular barrier which preserves the water impermeability of normal skin [59]. The role of ceramide in synovial membranes has not been investigated. The absence of minimal involvement of the bone marrow and reticuloendothelial system in Farber's disease is surprising, since these tissues are known to have a very active ceramide metabolism and are involved so strikingly in Gaucher and Niemann-Pick disease. It is possible that in these tissues ceramide is degraded by the alkaline or neutral ceramidases which are uninvolved in Farber's disease or that the ceramide which cannot be degraded is reutilized for the synthesis of glycolipids or sphingomyelin (Fig. 40-4). The observed variation in severity of the disease is unexplained, but the enzyme defect in vitro appears the same in all cases (Table 40-1).

DIAGNOSIS

The Affected Patient

The diagnosis of Farber's disease can be easily made clinically, since the triad of subcutaneous nodules, arthritis, and laryngeal involvement is unique for this disease. Diagnostic concerns arise when one or more of these features are missing, such as in juvenile rheumatoid arthritis, in multicentric reticulohistiocytosis [60], or in disorders such as fibromatosis hyalinica multiplex juvenilis [61]. We have found normal acid ceramidase activities in patients with these disorders and in other persons who lacked the above triad, and, conversely, all nine patients with the triad studied so far showed essentially absent enzyme activity. Through the courtesy of Dr. Allan Crocker, we have also studied acid ceramidase activity in one of the previously reported mildly involved patients who had no demonstrable laryngeal abnormality [33]. At the time of the follow-up examination this 19-year-old patient was entirely well except for a slight limitation of finger movement, and cultured skin fibroblast acid ceramidase activity was 70 percent of control, far above that in the Farber's disease homozygotes.

The most significant laboratory test is the demonstration of defective acid ceramidase activity in cultured skin fibroblasts or in white blood cells. Activity in Farber's disease patients is less than 6 percent of control values. The technique for the assay is described in several publications [56, 57, 62].

Other diagnostic tests include demonstration of the characteristic morphological features on a biopsy specimen of a subcutaneous nodule or other tissue. These features include granuloma formation and the presence of macrophages with lipid cytoplasmic inclusions [1], which are PAS-positive and are extracted by lipid solvents [6] and which show curvilinear inclusions under the electron microscope [20, 29, 34, 35]. Sural nerve biopsy may also show a characteristic ultrastructural abnormality [10].

The third confirmatory approach involves the demonstration of ceramide accumulation in tissues or body fluids. Ceramide excess can easily be demonstrated qualitatively by thin-layer chromatography [6, 20], or quantitated by high-performance liquid chromatography [36, 39, 40], or by gas-liquid chromatography combined with mass spectrometry [25]. These techniques have been applied to biopsy specimens of subcutaneous nodules [13, 16, 17, 28, 29] and liver [22] and to postmortem tissues [6, 20, 25]. It is helpful to determine separately the ceramides containing α-hydroxy fatty acids. Most normal tissues contain only ceramides with non-hydroxy fatty acids, whereas both types are found in Farber's disease tissues [6, 25, 37, 38]. Ceramide levels in the subcutaneous nodule may make up 20 percent of total lipids. Although such a finding may be diagnostic of Farber's disease, this is not fully established, since at present there are no valid comparison samples and it has been shown that the outer layers of normal skin contain large quantities of ceramide [58, 59]. We demonstrated a 200-fold ceramide excess in the urine of patient 4 (Table 40-1) [63] but were unable to demonstrate such an excess in patient 23, and patients 12 and 15 also gave negative results.

Identification of the Heterozygote

Table 40-1 shows that all of the obligate heterozygotes tested so far had reduced acid ceramidase activity in cultured skin fibroblasts (see also Refs. 16, 27, 57, 62, 64).

Prenatal Diagnosis

Four pregnancies at risk for Farber's disease have been monitored in two mothers [62, 64]. In three instances acid ceramidase assays of cultured skin amniotic fluid cells led to the prediction that the fetus was either normal or heterozygous for Farber's disease. The pregnancies were continued, and the three children, now 2 to 8 years old, are normal. In the fourth pregnancy, acid ceramidase activity in cultured amniotic fluid cells was 8 percent of control, and the pregnancy was interrupted. The postmortem tissues showed elevated ceramide levels in kidney and liver, and greatly reduced acid ceramidase activity in brain and cultured skin fibroblasts [64].

GENETICS

The clinical genetic data strongly suggest an autosomal recessive mode of inheritance. Of the known cases, 14 have been female and 13 male. Table 40-1 shows the wide range of nationalities. So far no cases have been reported in black or Jewish families. Among the 21 families about whom some information is available, consanguinity was present in 3 and thought to be absent in 15. In 3 families parents or grandparents came from the same relatively small communities.

In 6 families more than one sib was affected. In 14 families the cases were isolated. When the index cases are omitted from enumeration, there were 7 Farber's disease sibs, 36 sibs who did not have Farber's disease, in addition to 4 unaffected half sibs and 2 sibs whose status was unknown. In no instances were parents involved, and no cases were reported in previous generations. The father of patient 17 had rheumatoid arthritis. The acid ceramidase in his cultured fibroblasts was 29 percent of control, compared to 4 percent in the child. A history of rheumatic fever or rheumatoid arthritis in previous generations was also reported for patients 4, 12, and 23.

This clinical evidence of an autosomal recessive mode of inheritance is supported further by the finding that the mean acid ceramidase activity in 11 obligate heterozygotes was 45 percent ± 16 percent SD of control.

The prevalence of Farber's disease is unknown. The fact that this unmistakable clinical picture has been reported in only 27 cases, coupled with the rather high frequency of consanguinity, suggest that it is a rare disorder.

THERAPY

There is no specific therapy. Corticosteroids may provide some relief. The laryngeal and pulmonary involvement require close supervision of respiratory function, and tracheostomy may be needed. Cosmetic surgery may be useful for some of the unsightly granulomas. Acid ceramidase is present in soluble form in human placenta, and it has been partially purified [54]. Enzyme replacement therapy may thus be considered eventually. This might be an attractive approach because Farber's disease affects visceral organs more severely than the nervous system and because many of the lesions are near the surface and the effectiveness of therapy could be readily evaluated.

REFERENCES

1. FARBER S, COHEN J, UZMAN, LL: Lipogranulomastosis. A new lipoglyco-protein "storage" disease. *J Mt Sinai Hosp* 24:816, 1957
2. SCHONENBERG H, LINDENFELSER R: Farber-Syndrom (disseminierte Lipogranulomatose). *Monatsschr Kinderheilkd* 122:153, 1974
3. RAMPINI S, CLAUSEN J: Farbersche Krankheit (disseminierte Lipogranulomatose) klinisches Bild und Zusammenfassung der chemischen Befunde. *Helv Paediatr Acta* 22:500, 1967
4. MOLZ G: Farbersche Krankheit: Pathologisch-anatomische Befunde. *Virchows Arch Pathol Anat* 344:86, 1966
5. CLAUSEN J, RAMPINI S: Chemical studies of Farber's disease. *Acta Neurol Scand* 46:313, 1970
6. MOSER HW, PRENSKY AL, WOLFE JH, ROSMAN NP, with technical assistance of CARR S, FERREIRA G: Farber's lipogranulomatosis: Report of a case and demonstration of an excess of free ceramide and ganglioside. *Am J Med* 47:869, 1969

7. COGAN DG, KUWABARA T, MOSER HW, HAZARD GW: Retinopathy in a case of Farber's lipogranulomatosis. *Arch Ophthalmol* 75:752, 1966

8. PRENSKY AL, FERREIRA G, CARR S, MOSER HW: Ceramide and ganglioside accumulation in Farber's lipogranulomatosis. *Proc Soc Exp Biol Med* 126:725, 1967

9. RIVEL J, VITAL C, BATTIN J, HEHEUNSTRE JP, LEGER H: La Lipogranulomatose disseminée de Farber. Etude anatomo-clinique et ultrastructurale, de deux observations. *Arch Anat Cytol Pathol* 25:37, 1977

10. VITAL C, BATTIN J, RIVEL J, HEHEUNSTRE JP: Aspects ultrastructuraux des lesions du nerf peripherique dans un cas de maladie de Farber. *Rev Neurol* 132:419, 1976

11. BIERMAN SM, EDGINGTON T, NEWCOMBER VD, PEARSON CM: Farber's disease: A disorder of mucopolysaccharide metabolism with articular, respiratory, and neurologic manifestations. *Arthr Rheum* 9:620, 1966

12. SCHANCHE AF, BIERMAN SM, SOPHER RL, O'LOUGHLIN BJ: Disseminated lipogranulomatosis: Early roentgenographic changes. *Radiology* 82:673, 1964

13. BECKER H, AUBOCK L, HAIDVOGL M, BERNHEIMER H: Disseminated lipogranulomatosis (Farber). Case report of the 16th case of a ceramidose. *Verh Dtsch Ges Pathol* 60:254, 1976

14. ABUL-HAJ SK, MARTZ DG, DOUGLAS WF, GEPPERT LJ: Farber's disease: Report of a case with observations on its histogenesis and notes on the nature of the stored material. *J Pediatr* 61:221, 1962

15. SCHULTZE G, LANG EK: Disseminated lipogranulomatosis: Report of a case. *Radiology* 74:428, 1960

16. TOPPET M, VAMOS-HURWITZ E, JONNIAUX G, CREMER N, TONDEUR M, PELC S: Farber's disease as a ceramidosis: Clinical, radiological and biochemical aspects. *Acta Paediatr Scand* 67:113, 1978

17. DUSTIN P, TONDEUR M, JONNIAUX G, VAMOS-HURWITZ E, PELC S: La Maladie de Farber: Etude anatomo-clinique et ultrastructurale. *Bull Acad Med Belg* 128:733, 1973

18. HOBOLTH N, RESKE-NIELSEN, E: To be published

19. MOORE, ROBERT: Personal communication

20. OZAKI H, MIZUTANI M, OKA E, OHTAHARA S, KIMOTO H, TANAKA T, HAKOZAKI H, TAKAHASHI K, SUZUKI Y: Farber's disease (disseminated lipogranulomatosis): The first case reported in Japan. *Acta Med Okayama* 32:69, 1978

21. TANAKA T, TAKAHASHI K, HAKOZAKI H, KIMOTO H, SUZUKI Y: Farber's disease (disseminated lipogranulomatosis). A pathological, histochemical and ultrastructural study. *Acta Pathol Jap* 29:135, 1979

22. NEVILLE BGR, TURNER DR: To be published

23. PACHMAN LM, FRANK J, LIU M, MOSER HW: Lipogranulomatosis (Farber's disease). *J Pediatr* 93:320, 1978

24. ZETTERSTROM R: Disseminated lipogranulomatosis (Farber's disease). *Acta Paediatr* 47:501, 1958

25. SAMUELSSON K, ZETTERSTROM R: Ceramides in a patient with lipogranulomatosis (Farber's disease) with chronic course. *Scand J Clin Lab Invest* 27:393, 1971

26. SAMUELSSON K, ZETTERSTROM R, IVEMARK BI: Studies on a case of lipogranulomatosis (Farber's disease) with protracted course, in Volk BW, Aronson SM (eds): *Sphingolipids, Sphingolipidoses and Allied Disorders*. New York, Plenum, 1972, p 533

27. PAVONE L, MOSER HW, MOLLICA F, REITANO C, DURAND P: Farber's lipogranulomatosis: Ceramide deficiency and prolonged survival in three relatives. *Johns Hopkins Med J* 147:193, 1980

28. AMIRHAKIMI GH, HAGHIGHI P, GHALAMBOR MA, HONARI S: Familial lipogranulomatosis (Farber's disease). *Clin Genet* 9:625, 1976

29. SCHMOECKEL C, HOHLFED M: A specific ultrastructural marker for disseminated lipogranulomatosis (Farber). *Arch Dermatol Res* 266:187, 1979

30. HOROWITZ S, ERICKSON C, STRUBLE R: Personal communication

31. COLEMAN RA: Personal communication

32. BARRIERE H, GILLOT F: La Lipogranulomatose de Farber. *Nouv Presse Med* 2:767, 1973

33. CROCKER AC, COHEN J, FARBER S: The "lipogranulomatosis" syndrome: Review, with report of patient showing milder involvement, in Aronson SM, Volk BW (eds): *Inborn Disorders of Sphingolipid Metabolism*. Oxford, Pergamon, 1967, p 485

34. VAN HOOF F, HERS HG: Farber's disease, in Hers HG, Van Hoof F (eds): *Lysosomes and Storage Diseases*. New York, Academic, 1973, p 559

35. RUTSAERT J, TONDEUR M, VAMOS-HURWITZ E, DUSTIN P: The cellular lesions of Farber's disease and their experimental reproduction in tissue culture. *Lab Invest* 36:474, 1977

36. SUGITA M, IWAMORI M, EVANS J, MCCLEUR RH, DULANEY JT, MOSER HW: High performance liquid chromatography of ceramides: Application to analysis in human tissues and demonstration of ceramide excess in Farber's disease. *J Lipid Res* 15:223, 1974

37. SUGITA M, CONNOLLY P, DULANEY JT, MOSER HW: Fatty acid composition of free ceramides of kidney and cerebellum from a patient with Farber's disease. *Lipids* 8:401, 1973

38. LAUTER CJ, TRAMS EG: A spectrophotometric determination of sphingosine. *J Lipid Res* 3:136, 1962

39. IWAMORI M, COSTELLO C, MOSER HW: Analysis and quantitation of free ceramide containing non-hydroxy and hydroxy fatty acids, and phytosphingosine by high performance liquid chromatography. *J Lipid Res* 20:86, 1979

40. YAHARA S, MOSER HW, KOLODNY EH, KISHIMOTO Y: Reverse phase high-performance liquid chromatography of cerebrosides, sulfatides and ceramides: Microanalysis of homolog composition without hydrolysis and application to cerebroside analysis in peripheral nerves of adrenoleukodystrophy patients. *J Neurochem* 34:694, 1980

41. SCRIBNEY M: Enzymatic synthesis of ceramide. *Biochim Biophys Acta* 125:542, 1966

42. MORELL P, RADIN NS: Specificity in ceramide biosynthesis from long chain bases and various fatty acyl coenzyme A's by brain microsomes. *J Biol Chem* 245:342, 1970

43. BRAUN, PE, MORELL P, RADIN NS: Synthesis of C18 and C20 dihydrosphingosines, ketodihydrosphingosines and ceramides by microsomal preparations from mouse brain. *J Biol Chem* 245:335, 1970

44. BORTZ WM: Specificity of the enzymatic synthesis of ceramide. *Biochim Biophys Acta* 152:627, 1968

45. ULLMAN MD, RADIN NS: Enzymatic formation of hydroxy ceramides and comparison with enzymes forming nonhydroxy ceramides. *Arch Biochem Biophys* 152:767, 1972

46. ZALC B, POLLET SA, HARPIN ML, BAUMANN NA: Ceramide biosynthesis in mouse brain microsomes: Comparison between C57 BL controls and quaking mutants. *Brain Res* 81:511, 1974

47. GATT S: Enzymatic hydrolysis of sphingolipids. I. Hydrolysis and synthesis of ceramides by an enzyme from rat brain. *J Biol Chem* 241:3724, 1966

48. YAVIN E, GATT S: Enzymatic hydrolysis of sphingolipids. VIII. Further purification and properties of rat brain ceramidase. *Biochemistry* 8:1692, 1969

49. SUGITA M, WILLIAMS M, DULANEY JT, MOSER HW: Ceramidase and ceramide synthesis in human kidney and cerebellum. Description of a new alkaline ceramidase. *Biochim Biophys Acta* 398:125, 1975

50. STOFFEL W, MELZNER I: Studies in vitro on the biosynthesis of ceramide and sphingomyelin. A reevaluation of proposed pathways. *Hoppe-Seyler's Z Physiol Chem* 361:755, 1980

51. MOSER HW: Ceramidase deficiency: Farber's lipogranulomatosis, in Stanbury JB, Wyngaarden JB, Fredrickson DS (eds): *The Metabolic Basis of Inherited Disease*, 4th ed. New York, McGraw Hill, 1978, p 707

52. SINGH I, KISHIMOTO Y: Ceramide synthesis in rat brain: Characterization of the synthesis requiring pyridine nucleotide. *Arch Biochem Biophys* 202:93, 1980

53. CHEN WW, MOSER HW: Purification of acid ceramidase from human placenta. *Fed Proc* 38:405, 1979

54. CHEN WW, MOSER AB, MOSER HW: Role of lysosomal acid ceramidase in the metabolism of ceramide in human skin fibroblasts. *Arch Biochem* 208:444, 1981

55. NILSSON A: The presence of sphingomyelin and ceramide cleaving enzymes in the small intestinal tract. *Biochim Biophys Acta* 176:339, 1969

56. SUGITA M, DULANEY JT, MOSER HW: Ceramidase deficiency in Farber's disease (lipogranulomatosis). *Science* 178:1100, 1972

57. DULANEY JT, MILUNSKY A, SIDBURY JB, HOBOLTH N, MOSER HW: Diagnosis of lipogranulomatosis (Farber's disease) by use of cultured fibroblasts. *J Pediatr* 89:59, 1976

58. GRAY GM, WHITE JR: Glycosphingolipids and ceramides in human and pig epidermis. *J Invest Derm* 70:336, 1978

59. ELIAS PM, BROWN BE, FRITSCH P, GOERKE J, GRAY GM, WHITE RJ: Localization and Composition of lipids in neonatal mouse stratum granulosum and stratum corneum. *J Invest Derm* 73:339, 1979

60. BARROW MV, HOLUBAR K: Multicentric reticulohistiocytosis. A review of 33 patients. *Medicine* 48:287, 1969

61. DRESCHER E, WOYKE S, MARKIEWICZ C, TEGI S: Juvenile fibromatosis in siblings (fibromatosis hyalinica multiplex juvenilis). *J Pediatr Surg* 2:427, 1967

62. DULANEY JT, MOSER HW: Farber's disease (lipogranulomatosis), in Glew RH, Peters SP (eds): *Practical Enzymology of the Sphingolipidoses*. New York, Alan R Liss, 1977, p 283

63. IWAMORI M, MOSER HW: Above normal urinary excretion of urinary ceramides in Farber's disease, and characterization of their components by high-performance liquid chromatography. *Clin Chem* 21:725, 1975

64. FENSOM AH, BENSON PF, NEVILLE BRG, MOSER HW, MOSER AB, DULANEY JT: Prenatal diagnosis of Farber's disease. *Lancet* 2:990, 1979

65. SCHMOECKEL C: Subtle clues to diagnosis of skin diseases by electron microscopy. "Farber bodies" in disseminated lipogranulomatosis (Farber's disease). *Am J Dermatopathol* 2:153, 1980

41

SPHINGOMYELIN LIPIDOSES:
Niemann-Pick Disease

ROSCOE O. BRADY

1. Sphingomyelin lipidoses (Niemann-Pick disease) *are characterized by accumulation of sphingomyelin (ceramide phosphorylcholine) in the organs and tissues of affected individuals. Sphingomyelin is normally catabolized by cleavage of phosphorylcholine from ceramide through the action of an acid hydrolase sphingomyelinase. Three distinct deficiency states of sphingomyelinase exist that are genetically determined. Constant features in each are hepatosplenomegaly and foam cells in the bone marrow. Pulmonary infiltration is common, and varying degrees of nervous system involvement, including a cherry-red spot in the retina, may also occur. In addition to the clear-cut sphingomyelinase deficiencies, there are instances of sphingomyelin lipidosis in which enzyme deficiency has not been identified.*

2. *The three clinical forms of sphingomyelinase deficiency are identified as types A, B, and C. Type A develops in infancy and is associated with severe central nervous system damage. The disorder is fatal by age 3 to 4. In type B, visceral involvement may be extensive and the manifestations may become apparent in infancy or childhood. Although occasional changes in the retina appear, function of the nervous system is normal. Except for organomegaly, the patients may attain adulthood in reasonably good health. Some patients with the so-called sea-blue histiocyte syndrome may*

have this form of Niemann-Pick disease. Patients with type C have both visceral and nervous system involvement. The course is subacute or chronic and usually fatal before age 20. A sphingomyelin lipidosis occurring in families with Nova Scotian ancestry, similar to type C but lacking evidence of sphingomyelinase deficiency, has been called type D Niemann-Pick disease. Adults found incidentally to have moderate sphingomyelin excess in one or more organs, but without evidence of familial involvement, have been considered to have "type E" Niemann-Pick disease. Reports of sphingomyelinase deficiency in some of these patients require confirmation.

3. *Types A, B, and C Niemann-Pick disease appear to be allelic disorders in which one of at least three different mutations affects the activity of sphingomyelinase. Affected siblings in a single family always manifest the same type of disorder. All three types are autosomal recessive in inheritance.*

4. *Only a presumptive diagnosis of Niemann-Pick disease may be made on the basis of hepatosplenomegaly and foam cells in the bone marrow. The diagnosis of types A, B, and C should be established by measuring sphingomyelinase activity in tissue samples, leukocyte extracts, or homogenates of cultured skin fibroblasts. ^{14}C-Labeled sphingomyelin or the chromogenic analogue of sphingomyelin, 2-hexadecanoyl-4-nitrophenyl*

phosphorylcholine (HNP), are equally useful substrates for this assay and both are commercially available. If sphingomyelinase activity is normal or equivocal, the quantity of sphingomyelin in a biopsy sample of liver or lymph node may assist in establishing the presence of another type of sphingomyelin lipidosis.

5. *Heterozygotes for type A and B may be identified by determining sphingomyelinase activity in fresh peripheral leukocyte preparations or extracts of cultured skin fibroblasts. HNP may be used as substrate for this purpose. Type C heterozygotes have not yet proved detectable.*

6. *Prenatal diagnosis of Niemann-Pick disease is an established procedure. Radioactive sphingomyelin or HNP can be used for these assays. Accurate genetic counseling is therefore available to prospective parents who are carriers of type A or B Niemann-Pick disease.*

7. *There is no specific therapy available at this time. Enzyme replacement trials are under investigation in animal models of the human disorder.*

Niemann-Pick disease consists of a group of disorders characterized by hepatosplenomegaly and accumulation of sphingomyelin and other lipids throughout the body. Most patients with this disorder exhibit organomegaly in the neonatal period along with severe progressive nervous and mental dysfunction. An increasing number of Niemann-Pick patients are being recognized who have delayed onset of these signs and symptoms. In some, central nervous system involvement is not evident at all. In others, the onset of organomegaly is delayed, and slowly progressing central nervous system damage becomes severe only in the terminal stage of the disease. The major identifiable forms of Niemann-Pick disease are designated types A, B, and C [1–3]. In all three there is deficient activity of the enzyme sphingomyelinase. The older classification also includes a type D for patients of Nova Scotian ancestry who have severe clinical manifestations comparable to type C but no measurable enzyme deficiency. There is also a type E, which is not clearly genetic in origin. A number of cases that do not fit readily into any of these categories have been described within the past several years [4–10].

HISTORY

In 1914, A. Niemann, a German pediatrician, described an 18-month-old Jewish child with hepatosplenomegaly, lymphadenopathy, edema, and pigmentation of the face. The child had central nervous system impairment and died before 2 years of age. Yellow deposits were found in the liver, spleen, lymph nodes, kidneys, and adrenals [11]. Large sudanophilic cells were present in these organs. There was some overlap between the pathologic findings in this patient and those previously reported in patients with Gaucher's disease. Niemann realized that the signs and symptoms and the rapid downhill course of the patient were significantly different from those that had been described in patients with Gaucher's disease. He therefore considered the condition an unknown illness. Between 1922

and 1927, L. Pick provided clear evidence of histologic differences between this disorder and Gaucher's disease and termed the condition Niemann-Pick disease [12, 13].

INCIDENCE AND GENETICS

The disorder is panethnic, but the majority of patients with the classic infantile form (type A) have Ashkenazic Jewish ancestry [2]. Patients with Niemann-Pick disease types B and C, and particularly those cases associated with sea-blue histiocytes in their bone marrow, do not have this racial predilection. An interesting group of Spanish-American children in the latter category has been described [6]. Patients with type D Niemann-Pick disease stem from an inbred group of Acadians in Yarmouth County in Nova Scotia whose ancestry is a mixture of French and Italian Catholics. Niemann-Pick disease is transmitted as an autosomal recessive trait. The gene frequency is not well established, although type A has been estimated to be about 1 in 100 for individuals of Ashkenazic Jewish ancestry [2].

CLINICAL MANIFESTATIONS

Type A (Acute Neuronopathic Form)

Most of the reported patients with Niemann-Pick disease have exhibited this form of the disorder. Visceral organs and the central nervous system are affected early in infancy, and the disease takes a rapidly fatal course. Spleen and liver enlargement is usually present by 6 months of age (Fig. 41-1). Because the infants have feeding difficulties, they become emaciated and have protuberant abdomens and thin extremities. Their skin may take on a brownish-yellow discoloration, and a cherry-red spot is found in the macular region of the eye in

Figure 41-1 A patient with type A Niemann-Pick disease. *A*. Six months of age. *B*. Same patient at 22 months. (*From Fredrickson and Sloan [2]. Used by permission.*)

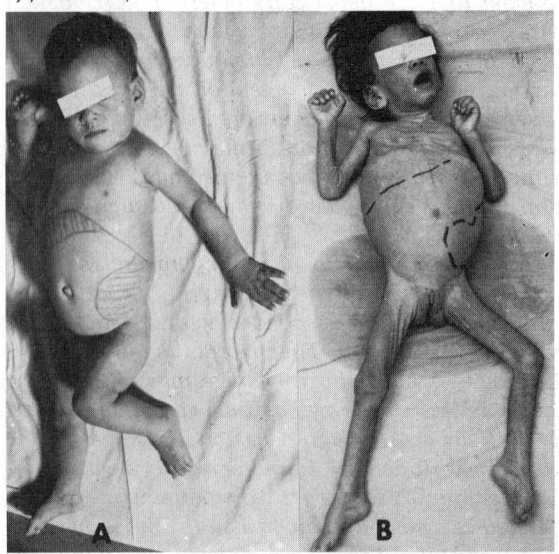

about 50 percent of patients. Corneal opacification, brownish discoloration of the anterior lens capsule, and retinal opacification have also been reported [14]. Enlarged foamy histiocytes appear in the bone marrow, splenic pulp, lymph nodes, adrenal medulla, and the alveoli of the lungs. The patients undergo general loss of motor function and progressive deterioration of intellectual capabilities. Previously learned skills are gradually lost, and hypotonia and flaccidity ensue. Death usually occurs by the third year.

Type B (Chronic Form without Nervous System Involvement)

Since the previous edition of this book [3], probably the greatest increase in the number of newly diagnosed Niemann-Pick patients has occurred in this category without neurologic damage. Patients with this form may develop visceral signs as early as those with type A, although a slightly later onset is more typical. There is no evidence of central nervous system impairment, and some have exceptionally high intellectual ability. Two patients have been reported with reduced peripheral nerve conduction velocity but no neurologic debility was apparent [15]. Enlargement of the spleen is usually the first manifestation of the disorder; hepatomegaly becomes evident later (Fig. 41-2). Not infrequently these patients are in the lowest percentiles for growth and height. The lung fields are often diffusely infiltrated, and dyspnea on exertion is a common complaint. There is little if any impairment of liver function, although abdominal distension due to the hepatomegaly becomes increasingly distressing with time. These patients are said to have increased susceptibility to respiratory infections and pneumonia because of the lung involvement. Birefringent foam cells are found in bone marrow aspirates.

Type C (Chronic Neuronopathic Form)

Patients with this form of Niemann-Pick disease usually appear normal for 1 to 2 years and sometimes even longer. They gradually develop neurologic abnormalities which are initially manifested by loss of speech previously learned, moderate ataxia, and grand mal seizures. The hepatosplenomegaly is less striking than in Niemann-Pick disease types A and B. The clinical course is characterized by progressive damage of the brain with failing mental and motor skills, loss of coordination, hypertonia, hyperactive reflexes, and increasingly frequent seizures (Fig. 41-3). Cholestasis has been observed in several patients [16, 17]. Foamy macrophages are present in marrow biopsy specimens. The majority of these patients die between 5 and 15 years of age.

Type D (Nova Scotia Variant)

Patients with this hereditary disorder, still apparently classified or misclassified [3] as a form of Niemann-Pick disease, share a common ancestry and live in a coastal area in western Nova Scotia. These cases have been traced to a couple born in Nova Scotia in the late 1600s. It has been speculated that the disease is the result of a single mutation in one of the ancestors. The heterozygote frequency in the district where most of the affected children live was estimated between 10 and 26 percent

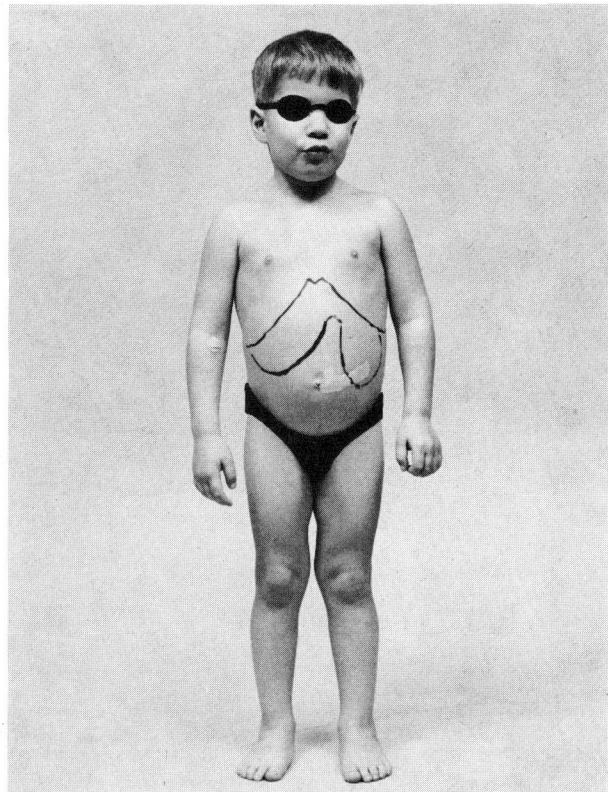

Figure 41-2 A patient with type B Niemann-Pick disease at age 4.7 years. (*From Fredrickson and Sloan [2]. Used by permission.*)

[18]. The condition resembles Niemann-Pick disease type C, with a protracted course and neurologic abnormalities that usually begin between the second and fourth years. The patients have hepatosplenomegaly, ataxia, impaired coordination, grand and petit mal seizures, and gradual deterioration of mental function that begins in early life (Fig. 41-4). Foam cells are present in the spleen and lymph nodes. Many of these patients are jaundiced.

Type E (Adult, Nonneuronopathic Form)

On the basis of an increase in the quantity of sphingomyelin in the liver and spleen, a small number of adults without neurologic difficulties but with moderate hepatosplenomegaly and foam cells in the marrow have been reported as having a variant form of Niemann-Pick disease [2, 19]. Some of these patients could represent a late-onset variant of Niemann-Pick type C [20].

PATHOLOGY

Niemann-Pick Cell

A large foamy, lipid-laden cell is present in the reticuloendothelial system of patients with Niemann-Pick disease. The cells are scattered throughout the spleen, bone marrow (Fig. 41-5), liver, lungs, and lymph nodes. Ganglion cells undergo similar pathologic alterations. These abnormal cells are readily distin-

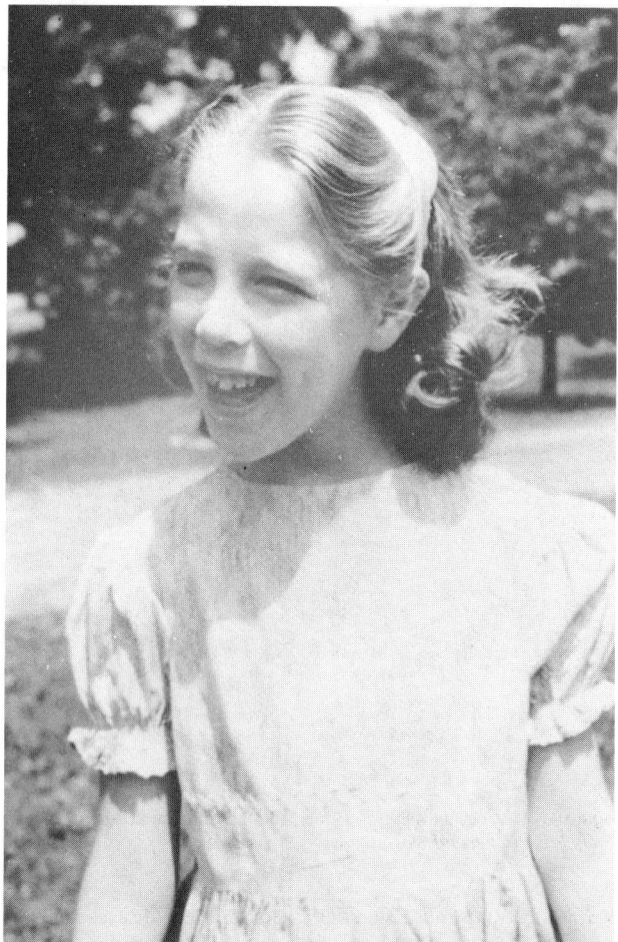

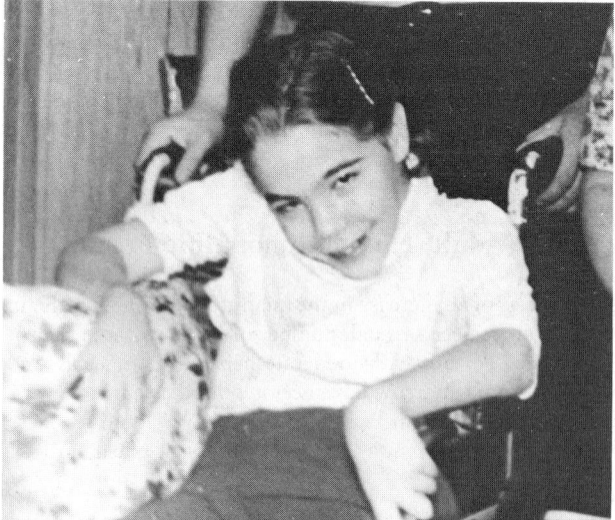

Figure 41-3 A patient with Niemann-Pick disease type C at ages 8 (*A*) and 10.5 years (*B*). (*From Fredrickson and Sloan [2]. Used by permission.*)

guished from the lipid-storing cells in Gaucher's disease by phase contrast microscopy or electron photomicroscopy. The size of the storage cell in Niemann-Pick disease ranges from 20 to 90 μm in diameter. The cytoplasm is filled with many droplets, which, in unstained preparations, impart a mulberry appearance to the cells (Fig. 41-6). The cells usually contain a single nucleus, although polynucleated cells have been reported. The cells may contain the brown pigment ceroid (lipo-

fuscin). Some cells are clear, some faintly yellow, and others dark brown or olive green. When tissue sections are stained with hematoxylin and eosin, there is considerable variation in the tinctorial quality of the cells, their color ranging from gray-yellow and greenish yellow to brownish yellow. The intracellular material, which appears in varying shades of blue or occasionally blue-green in bone marrow films, gives rise to the term *sea-blue histiocytes* [4–9], but such cells are not confined to Niemann-Pick disease. The cells stain red with oil red O and black with Sudan black B stains, depending on the amount of lipofuscin. The cells become blue-violet with Nile blue sulfate, violet with mercuric nitrate, blue-black with acid hematin, blue or blue-green with Giemsa, and variably positive with the periodic acid Schiff stain. The lipofuscin is autofluorescent in sections stained with hematoxylin and eosin and in unfrozen preparations. The accumulating lipid is easily removed from tissue sections with formaldehyde. The stain test for acid phosphatase is weakly positive, in contrast to the prominent reaction that occurs with Gaucher cells. The Schultz reaction is positive for cholesterol, a reaction that is negative in Gaucher cells.

Ultrastructure

The foam cells in Niemann-Pick disease have a normal histiocytic configuration, with a small typical nucleus eccentrically located in the cell. The cytoplasm contains lipid inclusions or lipid cytosomes (Fig. 41-7). The latter are generally polymorphic and range from 1 to 5 μm in diameter. The inclusions usually consist of concentrically laminated myelinlike figures with a periodicity of about 5 nm. There are occasional foci of electron-dense, black, granular nodules on the surface or incorporated into these inclusions. These granular nodules of Niemann-Pick disease are similar to those found in ceroid deposition in other lipid storage disorders, as well as in atheromas and aging cells. The cause of the ceroid deposition is unknown. Lipid cytosomes have been described in monocytes in peripheral blood of patients and carriers of type D Niemann-Pick disease [21], but these cells have not been found universally in the other forms of this disorder.

Organ and System Involvement in Niemann-Pick Disease

Spleen   The spleen is one of the most extensively altered organs in Niemann-Pick disease (Fig. 41-7). The splenic pulp may be almost completely replaced by masses of foam cells. The organ is enlarged and firm, and its margins are rounded. The color is lighter than normal, and the malpighian bodies appear as numerous reddish-yellow spots. The Niemann-Pick cells are usually distributed diffusely throughout the organ, especially in the pulp and around pulp arteries (Fig. 41-7A). In spite of the extensive involvement of the spleen, only moderate hematologic changes occur. These include a microcytic anemia and, in some patients, thrombocytopenia late in the course of the disease.

Liver and Lymph Nodes   The liver is usually about 1.5 times larger than normal, and hepatomegaly may exist before histologic changes can be recognized [3]. Certain patients with type B Niemann-Pick disease have much greater enlargement,

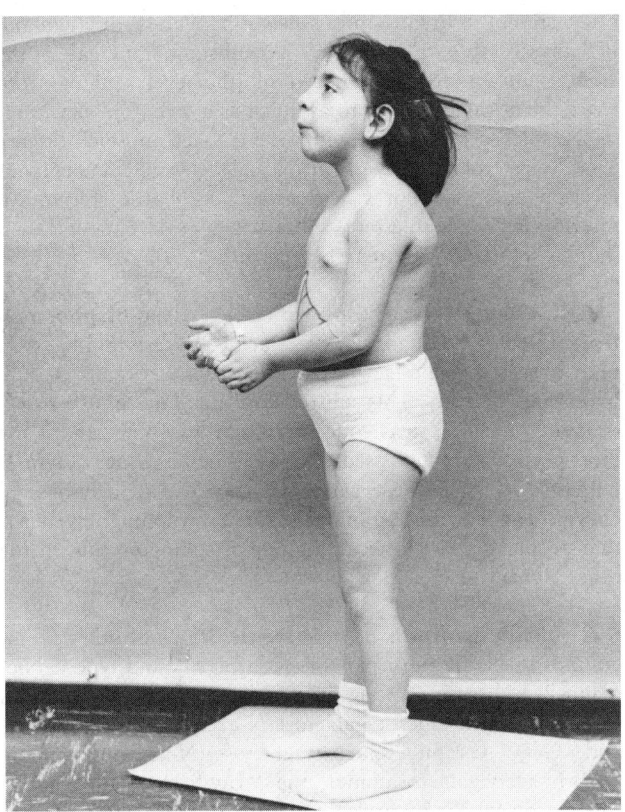

Figure 41-4 A patient with Niemann-Pick disease type D at age 5 years. (*From Fredrickson and Sloan* [2]. *Used by permission.*)

Other Organs The lamina propria and smooth-muscle cells of the intestine often contain foam cells. Foam cells in capillary loops of the glomeruli have been reported in approximately 50 percent of the patients with this disorder. The adrenals are enlarged, and Niemann-Pick cells may be abundant in the medulla without evidence of adrenal insufficiency. Other endocrine glands, such as the gonads, thyroid, and pituitary, and exocrine glands, such as the pancreas and salivary gland, may also show striking accumulations of lipid without evidence of functional impairment.

Nervous System The brain in patients with Niemann-Pick disease types A and C is atrophic, weighs between 50 and 90 percent of normal, and has an unusually firm consistency. Ganglion cells in the central nervous system are frequently swollen, and there is pale vacuolation of the cytoplasm. Membrane-bound inclusions are loosely arranged in concentric lamellar structures within these cells. The cortical architecture is disorganized because of loss of cells in the cerebral and cerebellar cortex, gliosis in both gray and white matter, and secondary demyelination in some portions of the white matter. Foam cells or lipid-laden glial cells are present in the leptomeninges, tela choroidea, endothelium, and perivascular spaces of the cerebral blood vessels. Other areas such as basal ganglia, brainstem, spinal cord, and spinal and autonomic ganglia may also undergo morphological changes similar to those seen in the cerebral cortex.

Figure 41-5 Foam cell in a bone marrow aspirate from a patient with Niemann-Pick disease.

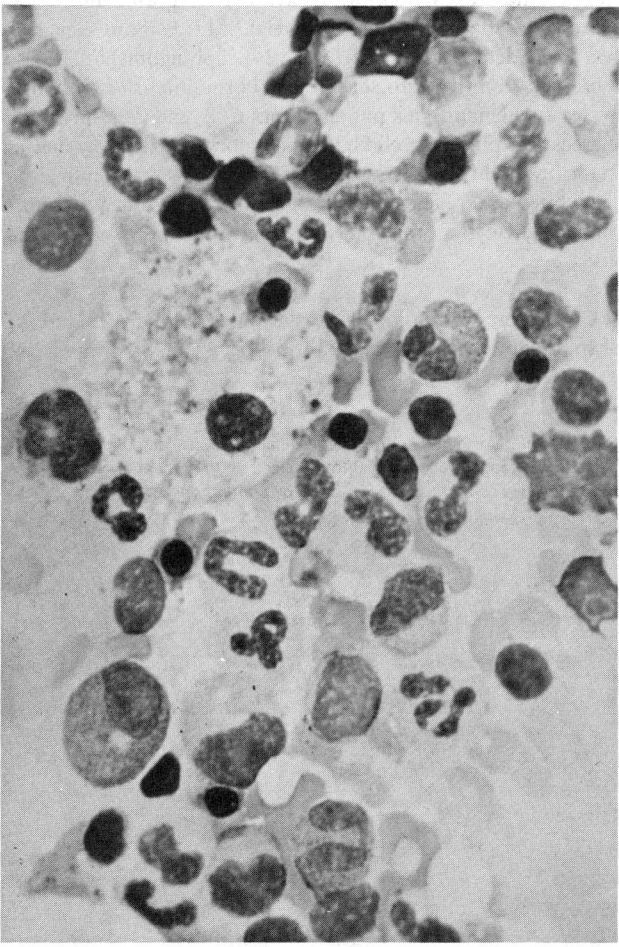

which can be the source of major cosmetic and physical difficulties. The distribution of lipid-storing cells is spotty in the early stages. Later massive infiltration of the sinuses occurs, and Kupffer cells and parenchymal cells become transformed into Niemann-Pick cells. The liver function tests are generally normal, although elevated activities of serum alkaline phosphatase, SGOT, and SGPT are not infrequent in type B Niemann-Pick disease.

Enlarged lymph nodes are found in the mesentery, hilus of the spleen, liver, and lungs. Although the etiology of type D Niemann-Pick disease has not been established, it has been suggested that enlargement of the lymph nodes in the region of the head of the pancreas may contribute to the jaundice. The thymus and tonsils may also become infiltrated with foam cells.

Bones The marrow is consistently invaded with foam cells, the degree of infiltration varying with the duration and clinical type. There is some osteoporosis, although it is generally not so extensive as in Gaucher patients. Coxa valga, long-bone expansion with modeling defects, and metacarpal widening have been reported in the various forms [22].

Lungs and Heart The lungs in most patients with Niemann-Pick disease usually have a diffuse reticular or finely nodular infiltration (Fig. 41-8). Foam cells are frequently present in the alveoli, lymphatic vessels, and branches of the pulmonary arteries but are rarely found in the sputum. Foam cells are frequently seen adjacent to myocardial fibers in the heart. Endocardial fibroelastosis has been reported in a Niemann-Pick infant [23].

PATHOPHYSIOLOGY

Accumulating Lipid(s)

Sphingomyelin The predominant accumulating substance in the organs and tissues of patients with Niemann-Pick disease is sphingomyelin (Fig. 41-9). This lipid comprises three portions. The first is the long-chain amino alcohol called sphingosine $[CH_3—(CH_2)_{12}—CH=CH—CH(OH)—CH(NH_2)—CH_2OH]$. Carbon atoms 1 and 2 are derived from the amino acid serine, and carbons 3 to 18 come from palmitic acid. A long-chain fatty acid is joined through an amide bond to the nitrogen atom on carbon 2 of sphingosine. This combination of a fatty acid and sphingosine is called *ceramide*. The third component of sphingomyelin is a molecule of phosphorylcholine linked by a phosphodiester bond to carbon atom 1 of the sphingosine moiety of ceramide.

The amount of sphingomyelin in the spleen of patients with type A Niemann-Pick disease can be increased from a normal value of 15 mg per gram dry weight to 370 mg per gram dry weight [2]. The quantity of this lipid in the spleens of two patients with type B disease was increased to 250 and 280 mg per gram dry weight [1, 2]. A wide range (25 to 255 mg/g) has been reported in type C patients. Patients with type D show only a moderate (~55 mg/g [2], 26 mg/g [24]) increase in splenic sphingomyelin. There is a striking increase of sphingomyelin in the liver of patients with type A and type B Niemann-Pick disease to as much as 270 and 338 mg per gram dry weight, respectively, over the normal level of ~10 mg per gram dry weight. Lesser quantities have been reported in type C patients (~80 mg per gram dry weight). Little if any elevation has been detected in type D [2, 24]. Sphingomyelin is also increased from three to seven times normal in affected lymph nodes in Niemann-Pick patients types A, B, and C. A moderate increase of sphingomyelin has been reported in the gray matter in the brain of type A patients; this increase is less prominent in the white matter. The quantity of sphingomyelin is not abnormally high in the brain of type B and type C Niemann-Pick disease.

Cholesterol In addition to the consistently large increase of sphingomyelin, elevated quantities of several other lipids are often present in organs and tissues of patients with Niemann-Pick disease. In particular, there is a substantial increase in the amount of unesterified cholesterol (the level ranging from twice the normal amount to as much as a sevenfold elevation) in the spleens of patients with type A Niemann-Pick disease [2]. Cholesterol in the liver is also usually elevated in Niemann-Pick patients, but not so extensively as in the spleen. An increase in liver cholesterol is seen in type D patients, even though sphingomyelin may be normal [2, 24].

Bis(monoacylglyceryl)phosphate [lyso-bisphosphatidic acid] The quantity of this acidic glycerolipid has also been observed to be elevated in the systemic organs of Niemann-Pick patients. This substance accumulates in other conditions as well [3]. It is concentrated in lysosomes and is the most prominently increased compound in the tissues of type D patients [24]. This observation is suggestive of a lysosomal enzyme defect distinct from the deficiency of sphingomyelinase that accounts for the accumulation of sphingomyelin in the other clinical forms.

Glycosphingolipids There are elevations of other sphingolipids in the brain of patients with type A and type C Niemann-Pick disease. Among these compounds are gangliosides G_{M3} (ceramide-glucose-galactose-N-acetylneuraminic acid) and G_{M2} [ceramide-glucose-galactose-(N-acetylneuraminic acid)-N-acetylgalactosamine], the "Tay-Sachs ganglioside." The reason for the increased quantities of these particular lipids is not established. It may be due to faulty degradation of membranes or membranelike structures in the ganglion cells (Fig. 41-7). Glucocerebroside may be increased in the spleen in type C Niemann-Pick disease [25]. A possible enzymatic explanation for this elevation is discussed below.

METABOLIC ABNORMALITY

The metabolic defect in Niemann-Pick disease is a deficiency of the enzyme that catalyzes the hydrolytic cleavage of phosphorylcholine from sphingomyelin, according to the following reaction:

$$\text{Sphingomyelin} + H_2O \xrightarrow{\text{sphingomyelinase}} \text{ceramide} + \text{phosphorylcholine}$$

The level of sphingomyelinase in liver tissue from patients with type A Niemann-Pick disease is less than 10 percent of normal [26]. Sphingomyelinase activity in leukocytes and cultured skin fibroblasts derived from these patients is in the neighborhood of 4 percent of controls [27, 28]. Patients with Niemann-Pick disease type B have only slightly more sphingomyelinase activity in these tissues [29]. The activity of this enzyme in fibroblasts from type C patients ranges from 38 to 63 percent of that in controls [30–32]. Sphingomyelinase activity in liver and spleen has been reported in the normal range in tissues obtained from type C patients [25, 33], but below normal in the brain and liver of a Niemann-Pick type C fetus [25]. Interestingly, glucocerebrosidase activity (the enzyme lacking in Gaucher's disease [34]) has been reported to be lower than normal in type C Niemann-Pick patients [25], an observation consistent with the increased quantity of glucocerebroside in

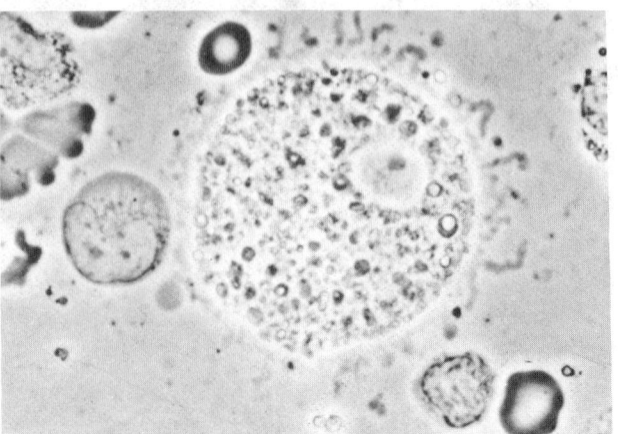

Figure 41-6 Unstained foam cell in Niemann-Pick disease under phase microscope. Magnification, ×430 (reproduced at 75 percent of original size). (*From Fredrickson and Sloan* [2]. *Used by permission.*)

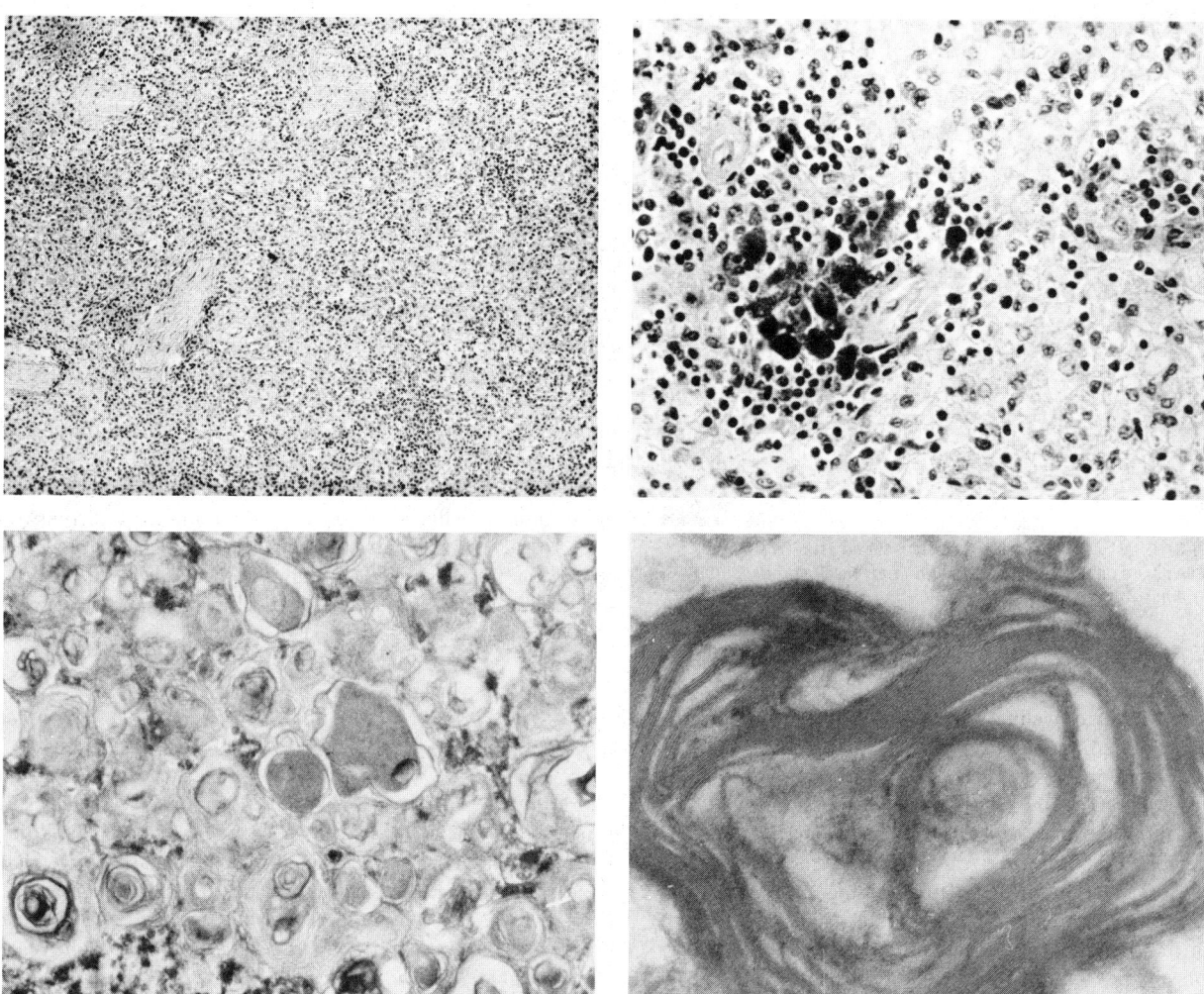

Figure 41-7 Foam cells in spleen from a patient with type C Niemann-Pick disease. *Upper left,* low power magnification showing compression of red pulp by white pulp filled with histiocytes. *Upper right,* higher magnification showing storage cells with pigment (ceroid) at left and without at right. *Lower left,* storage cells with myelin figures and overlying lipofuscin pigment. *Lower right,* electron-microscopic photograph showing periodicity. Magnification, ×100,000 (reproduced at 71 percent of original size). (*Courtesy of F. M. King,* A.F.I.P., neg. no. 81-10768 1-4.)

the gray matter of the brain [35] and in the liver and plasma of Niemann-Pick patients [36].

The enzymatic defect in patients with Niemann-Pick disease type D is unresolved. Extracts of liver tissue and cultured skin fibroblasts derived from these patients exhibit normal or even elevated sphingomyelinase activity [2, 28, 37]. Diminished splenic sphingomyelinase has been reported in one type D patient [33].

The etiology of type E Niemann-Pick disease is also unsettled. Total sphingomyelinase activity is normal or increased [20] in tissue extracts from patients with this variant of the disorder. When sphingomyelinase isoenzymes were separated by isoelectric focusing, three peaks of enzymatic activity were discerned in control fibroblasts extracts. Cells from patients with types C and E Niemann-Pick disease were said to lack the second isoenzyme [20, 37]. The validity of this technique has been questioned with regard to type C patients [25], and the specific loss in type E requires confirmation.

Sphingomyelin is a common lipid constituent of the plasma membrane, subcellular organelles, endoplasmic reticulum, and mitochondria of all mammalian cells. Sphingomyelin is also a major lipid of the myelin sheath and erythrocyte stroma. Thus, sphingomyelin that accumulates in various organs and tissues of patients with Niemann-Pick disease may arise from the turnover of any cell or cellular component in the body.

MOLECULAR BASIS OF NIEMANN-PICK DISEASE

It is logical to assume that the basic defect in Niemann-Pick disease lies in one or more alterations of the genetic code for sphingomyelinase with resultant change in the primary structure of the enzyme and thus in reduction of catalytic activity. The fact that patients with the various types of Niemann-Pick disease have some, although greatly attenuated, sphingomyelinase activity in their tissues is consistent with the presence of a protein with reduced efficiency. The actual amount of abnormal enzyme protein has not yet been determined in tissues from patients with the type A and B forms of this disorder, and an argument could be made for repressed production of the enyme.

Although the results of Callahan and Khalil [37] regarding losses of specific sphingomyelinase isoenzymes have been chal-

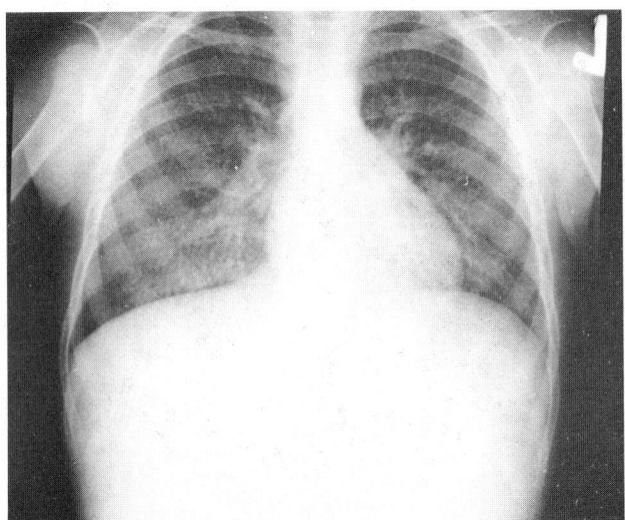

Figure 41-8   Chest x-ray of a patient with type B Niemann-Pick disease. The lung fields are diffusely infiltrated. (*From Fredrickson and Sloan* [2]. *Used by permission.*)

lenged, the fact that patients with type B Niemann-Pick disease have undetectable brain involvement coupled with such small total tissue sphingomyelinase activity seems to argue for the presence of more than one form of the enzyme. One obviously needs information concerning the forms and quantities of brain isoenzymes, their physiologic functions, and a critical comparison of these activities in Niemann-Pick patients. An interesting investigation along this line was carried out by Muller and Harzer, who concluded that sphingomyelinase from the brain of a type C patient had properties that were similar to those of the enzyme from a control tissue sample [38]. However, the specific activity of the most highly purified preparation was 59 percent of that in the control sample at a similar stage of purification.

A novel hypothesis of the pathogenesis of type C Niemann-Pick disease has been proposed by Baraton and Revol [39]. These authors assayed sphingomyelinase activity in liver, spleen, and fibroblasts in the presence of detergent to solubilize the labeled substrate or an "activator" from heated extracts of spleen or liver. They reported that decreased sphingomyelinase activity could be demonstrated only when the activator was used in place of detergent in the assay. These authors postulated that mutation(s) causing type A and type B disease involve the active site of sphingomyelinase, whereas in the type C patients there may be an alteration in the region where an allosteric activator interacts with the enzyme. Although this report has generated interest in the role of activators in the pathogenesis of lipid storage disorders such as Niemann-Pick disease, the finding of consistently decreased sphingomyelinase activity in cultured skin fibroblasts derived from type C patients, even when detergents are used in the assay for sphingomyelinase activity [30–32], lessens the plausibility of this explanation. The results obtained in mixing experiments carried out by Besley and coworkers [40] are consistent with this deduction. Potential functions of "activator specifiers," and detergents are discussed elsewhere [41].

Further understanding of the molecular basis of Niemann-Pick disease has been provided by cell hybridization experiments [40]. Fusion of fibroblasts derived from patients with types A and B Niemann-Pick disease did not result in an increase of sphingomyelinase activity, whereas definite augmentation was seen in heterokaryons formed by fusion of type A or type B with type C cells. The authors concluded that the component that is deficient in type C Niemann-Pick disease is under separate genetic control from that in type A or B. Thus mutations on different genes are involved in various forms of Niemann-Pick disease.

The cause of the accumulation of other lipids, such as bis(monoacylglyceryl)phosphate, and glycolipids, such as gangliosides G_{M3} and G_{M2}; and cholesterol remains uncertain. Because of the high concentration of bis(monoacylglyceryl)phosphate in lysosomes, it has been suggested that there is an increase in the quantity of these particles in storage cells [3]. The accumulation of gangliosides seems more difficult to reconcile, although increased quantities of these lipids are seen in a number of hereditary storage disorders [42]. These substances may arise from uncatabolized membranes that make up the multilamellar inclusions. Thus, diminution of activity of any critical enzyme may compromise the disposal of entire membrane fragments, which may also account for the extensive accumulation of cholesterol in all of the clinical forms of Niemann-Pick disease.

DIAGNOSIS

A presumptive diagnosis of type A Niemann-Pick disease can generally be made on the basis of hepatosplenomegaly, lipid-laden cells in the bone marrow, and mental retardation which appears early in life. It is more difficult to make a diagnosis of type B or C Niemann-Pick disease, but these conditions must be considered when lipid-storing cells are found in bone marrow aspirates. This supposition is strengthened by demonstration of increased quantities of sphingomyelin in tissue biopsy specimens. Procedures for the quantitation of sphingomyelin have been published [43, 44]. The diagnosis must be confirmed by enzymatic assays.

More frequently used diagnostic procedures are based on assays of sphingomyelinase activity in tissue extracts using radioactive sphingomyelin or the chromogenic analogue of sphingomyelin illustrated in Fig. 41-10. When the radioactive substrate is employed, sphingomyelin labeled in the choline portion of the molecule is preferred because of the relative ease in separating the water-soluble reaction product [^{14}C]phosphorylcholine from the water-insoluble sphingomyelin substrate [26, 45]. Sphingomyelin labeled in this portion of the molecule is available from several commercial sources.

The diagnosis of Niemann-Pick disease has been greatly facilitated by the development of the chromogenic analogue of sphingomyelin, 2-hexadecanoylamino-4-nitrophenyl phosphorylcholine hydroxine [29, 30, 46]. This substrate has the advantage of being soluble in water and its specificity for the

Figure 41-9   Structure of sphingomyelin. (*From Brady* [3]. *Used by permission.*)

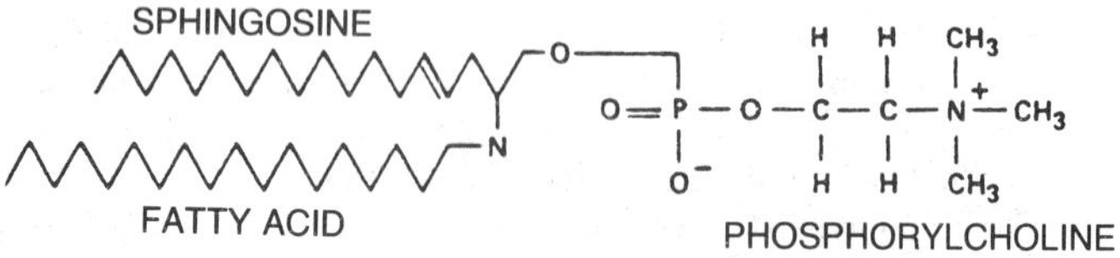

SPHINGOSINE

FATTY ACID

PHOSPHORYLCHOLINE

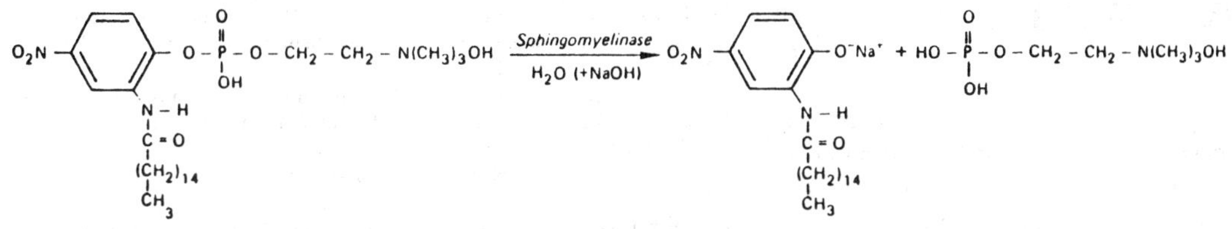

2-Hexadecanoylamino-4-Nitrophenylphosphorylcholine   (Yellow Product)   Phosphorylcholine

Figure 41-10 The chromogenic substrate 2-hexadecanoylamino-4-nitrophenyl phosphorylcholine (HNP) used for measurement of sphingomyelin activity. (*From Brady* [3]. *Used by permission.*)

enzyme is comparable to that of the natural lipid [29, 30]. It is commercially available. When using this substance, care should be exercised to ensure that the initial solution of the analogue is colorless. If the dissolved substrate is yellow, it may be possible to remove some of the undesired color by recrystallizing the compound from warm acetone. If the discoloration persists, substrate from a different source should be sought.

Type A and type B Niemann-Pick disease can be readily diagnosed by assaying sphingomyelinase activity in extracts of leukocytes obtained from small samples of venous blood. Labeled sphingomyelin [27] or the chromogenic analogue [29] may be used for these assays. The analogue may be superior to radioactive sphingomyelin in tissues such as leukocytes that contain comparatively little sphingomyelinase activity. There may be an appreciable amount of background radioactivity with the labeled substrate that tends to lessen the precision of the determination when only small quantities of product are produced by the activity of the enzyme. The facility with which leukocytes can be prepared and the rapidity with which reliable data can be obtained using the chromogenic analogue make this assay the diagnostic procedure of choice at this time.

Niemann-Pick disease types A, B, and C can also be diagnosed with sphingomyelinase assays performed on extracts of cultured skin fibroblasts using radioactive sphingomyelin [28] or the chromogenic analogue [30]. A 3- to 4-mm dermal biopsy is obtained under sterile conditions, placed into an appropriate culture medium, and allowed to grow until a convenient quantity of cells is available. Usually 20 to 30 million cells are adequate, but improvements in microassay techniques promise a significant reduction in the number of cells required and thus a diminution of the culturing time [47–50]. Fibroblasts have several advantages as source material. They have higher sphingomyelinase activity than most other cells, and the enzyme in harvested fibroblasts is comparatively stable on freezing. These benefits make it possible to grow these cells in various facilities throughout the world and to ship the frozen cell pellets to an appropriate laboratory for the enzyme analysis. Control cell cultures from various laboratories exhibit wide variation in sphingomyelinase activity [3]. It is therefore strongly recommended that at least two control fibroblast cultures be grown, harvested, and assayed simultaneously with cells derived from a suspected Niemann-Pick patient.

A number of additional diagnostic procedures have been proposed that include: (1) analysis of the lipid content of lymph nodes [51]; (2) high performance liquid chromatography to determine sphingomyelin and sphingomyelinase activity [52]; (3) measurement of sphingomyelinase in hair roots [53]; (4) use of tritiated [54], colored [55], and fluorescent [56] derivatives of sphingomyelin; (5) thin-layer chromatographic measurement of ceramide produced by the hydrolysis of sphingomyelin [57]; and (6) the use of bis(4-methylumbelliferyl)-phosphate [32], bis(4-methylumbelliferyl)pyrophosphate [58a], or [14C]phosphatidylcholine [58b] to monitor sphingomyelinase activity.

Detection of Heterozygotes

Identification of carriers of the Niemann-Pick trait is now well established. Sphingomyelinase assays with [14C]sphingomyelin in sonicated leukocyte extracts from heterozygotes revealed between 54 and 65 percent of that in control preparations [59]. The chromogenic analogue of sphingomyelin is also an excellent reagent for the detection of heterozygotes. Cultured skin fibroblasts are also frequently used for heterozygote detection [59]. The chromogenic analogue of sphingomyelin has been shown to be reliable for these tests [30]. Because of the greater sphingomyelinase activity and the fact that the enzyme in these cells is comparatively stable during freezing, fibroblasts are frequently used when shipment of specimens is required. Simultaneously grown control skin fibroblast cultures are mandatory. These should be derived from subjects without other lysosomal hydrolase defects in order to avoid the compensatory increases in sphingomyelinase and other lipid-hydrolyzing enzymes that may occur in such patients [60]. It is recommended that at least three control cell cultures be analyzed when heterozygosity is to be determined. No information is yet available concerning the detection of heterozygotes for Niemann-Pick type C patients. Sphingomyelinase activity in cultured skin fibroblasts from these homozygotes has an intermediate value, and it may not be possible to identify heterozygotes simply by measuring total sphingomyelinase activity. It has not been determined whether separation of sphingomyelinase isoenzymes is useful for the detection of the carriers of this form of the disorder. No information is available concerning the detection of type D or type E heterozygotes.

Prenatal Diagnosis of Niemann-Pick Disease

Cultured amniotic cells contain sphingomyelinase activity which approximates that found in cultured skin fibroblasts. Thus, amniocentesis and culture of fetal cells permits the monitoring of pregnancies at risk for type A [44] and probably type B Niemann-Pick disease. The chromogenic analogue of sphingomyelin may be used with confidence for prenatal diagnosis of type A Niemann-Pick disease [61, 62]. The limitation discussed in the preceding section concerning the intermediate level of activity, in type C fibroblasts makes the prenatal diagnosis of type C difficult, if not impossible [63].

TREATMENT

There is no specific therapy for Niemann-Pick disease at this time. Splenectomy is occasionally performed for mechanical reasons and for the rare Niemann-Pick patient with a hemorrhagic diathesis because of thrombocytopenia due to hypersplenism. Patients with lung infiltration appear to be prone to repeated upper respiratory infections and are said to be somewhat refractory to antibiotics used in the treatment of pneumonia.

It may be anticipated that attempts will be made to correct the metabolic defect through enzyme replacement in the future and that other potentially useful procedures will be explored [64, 65]. Sphingomyelinase has been isolated in highly purified form from human placental tissue, but the yield of pure enzyme has been too low to permit replacement trials in humans [66]. Furthermore, it must be borne in mind that the treatment of patients with types A and C Niemann-Pick disease will probably require the use of special techniques to deliver the exogenous enzyme to the brain [67]. This caveat is also applicable to considerations involving transplantation of organs such as the liver to correct the enzymatic deficiencies [68, 69].

The most reasonable way to predict the effectiveness of replacement procedures seems to be through the use of animal models. Pathologic and enzymatic resemblance to type A Niemann-Pick disease has been reported in a poodle dog [70] and Siamese cats [71]. A mouse model has been discovered that appears to be a close analogue of type C Niemann-Pick disease [72]. The latter animals are characterized by diminution of sphingomyelinase and glucocerebrosidase activities and the accumulation of sphingomyelin, glucocerebroside, lactosylceramide, cholesterol, gangliosides G_{M3} and G_{M2}, and bis(monoacylglyceryl)phosphate in various tissues. Pharmacologically induced sphingomyelinase-deficient rats have been produced by the administration of hypocholesterolemic agents [73–75]. These animal analogues of Niemann-Pick disease should be useful for investigation of therapeutic strategies that may eventually be applicable to humans.

REFERENCES

1. CROCKER AC: The cerebral defect in Tay-Sachs and Niemann-Pick disease. *J Neurochem* 7:69, 1961
2. FREDRICKSON DS, SLOAN HR: Sphingomyelin lipidoses: Niemann-Pick disease, in Stanbury JB, Wyngaarden JB, Fredrickson DS (eds): *The Metabolic Basis of Inherited Disease*, 3d ed. New York, McGraw-Hill, 1972, p 783
3. BRADY RO: Sphingomyelin lipidosis: Niemann-Pick disease, in Stanbury JB, Wyngaarden JB, Fredrickson DS (eds): *The Metabolic Basis of Inherited Disease*, 4th ed. New York, McGraw-Hill, 1978, p 718
4. GOLDE DW, SCHNEIDER EL, BAINTON DF, PENTCHEV PG, BRADY RO, EPSTEIN CJ, CLINE MJ: Pathogenesis of one variant of sea-blue histiocytosis. *Lab Invest* 33:371, 1975
5. LONG RG, LAKE BD, PETTIT JE, SCHEUER PJ, SHERLOCK S: Adult Niemann-Pick disease. Its relationship to the syndrome of sea-blue histiocytosis. *Am J Med* 62:627, 1977
6. WENGER DA, BARTH G, GITHENS JH: Nine cases of sphingomyelin lipidosis, a new variant in Spanish-American children. Juvenile variant of Niemann-Pick disease with foamy and sea-blue histiocyte. *Am J Dis Child* 131:955, 1977
7. SCHNEIDER EL, PENTCHEV PG, HIBBERT SR, SAWITSKY A, BRADY RO: A new form of Niemann-Pick disease characterized by temperature-labile sphingomyelinase. *J Med Genet* 15:370, 1978
8. FRIED K, BEER S, KREPIN HI, LEIBA H, DJALDETTI M, ZITMAN D, KLIBANSKY C: Biochemical, genetic and ultrastructural study of a family with the sea-blue histiocyte syndrome/chronic non-neuronopathic Niemann-Pick disease. *Eur J Clin Invest* 8:249, 1978

9. DEWHURST N, BESLEY GTN, FINLAYSON NDC, PARKER AC: Sea blue histiocytosis in a patient with chronic non-neuropathic Niemann-Pick disease. *J Clin Pathol* 32:1121, 1979
10. KUNISHITA K, TAKETOMI T: Sphingomyelin storage in a patient with myoclonus epilepsy as a main clinical symptom—A varient in Niemann-Pick disease Type C. *Jap J Exp Med* 49:151, 1979
11. NIEMANN A: Ein unbekanntes Krankheitsbild. *Jahrb kinderheilkd* 79:11, 1914
12. PICK L: Zur pathologischen Anatomie des Morbus Gaucher. *Med Klin* 18:1408, 1922
13. PICK L: Uber die lipoidzellige Splenohepatomegalie Typus Niemann-Pick als Stoffwechselerkrankung. *Med Klin* 23:1483, 1927
14. WALTON DS, ROBB RM, CROCKER AC: Ocular manifestations of group A Niemann-Pick disease. *Am J Ophthalmol* 85:174, 1978
15. PRISCU R, PANCU L, BALAN A, PETRESCU ThC, IACOB C: Die infantile chronisch-viszerale Form der Niemann-Pickschen Krankheit. *Klin Paediatr* 189:423, 1977
16. GUIBAUD P, VANIER MT, MALPUECH G, GAULME J, HOULLEMARE L, GODDON R, ROUSSON R: Early infantile, cholestatic, rapidly-fatal form of type C sphingomyelinosis. 2 cases. *Pediatrie* 34:103, 1979
17. JAEKEN J, PROESMAN W, EGGERMONT E, VAN HOOF F, DEN TANDT W, STANDAERT L, VAN HERCK G, CORBEEL L: Niemann-Pick Type C disease and early cholestasis in three brothers. *Acta Paediatr Belg* 33:43, 1980
18. WINSOR EJT, WELCH JP: Genetic and demographic aspects of Nova Scotia Niemann-Pick disease (Type D). *Am J Hum Genet* 30:530, 1978
19. CHAN WC, LAI KS, TODD D: Adult Niemann-Pick disease—A case report. *J Pathol* 121:177, 1977
20. CALLAHAN JW, KHALIL M: Sphingomyelinases in human tissues. III. Expression of Niemann-Pick disease in cultured skin fibroblasts. *Pediatr Res* 9:914, 1975
21. VETHAMANY VC, WELCH JP, VETHAMANY SK: Type D Niemann-Pick disease (Nova-Scotia variant): Ultrastructure of blood, skin fibroblasts, and bone marrow. *Arch Pathol* 93:537, 1972
22. LACHMAN R, CROCKER A, SCHULMAN J, STRAND R: Radiologic findings in Niemann-Pick disease. *Pediatr Radiol* 108:659, 1973
23. WESTWOOD M: Endocardial fibroelastosis and Niemann-Pick disease. *Brit Heart J* 39:1394, 1977
24. RAO BG, SPENCE MW: Niemann-Pick disease Type D: Lipid analyses and studies on sphingomyelinases. *Ann Neurol* 1:385, 1977
25. HARZER H, ANZIL ZP, SCHUSTER I: Resolution of tissue sphingomyelinase isoelectric profile in multiple components is extraction-dependent: Evidence for a component defect in Niemann-Pick disease type C is spurious. *J Neurochem* 29:1155, 1977
26. BRADY RO, KANFER JN, MOCK MB, FREDRICKSON DS: The metabolism of sphingomyelin. II. Evidence of an enzymatic defect in Niemann-Pick disease. *Proc Nat Acad Sci USA* 55:366, 1966
27. KAMPINE JP, BRADY RO, KANFER JN, FELD M, SHAPIRO D: Diagnosis of Gaucher's disease and Niemann-Pick disease with small samples of venous blood. *Science* 155:86, 1967
28. SLOAN HR, UHLENDORF BW, KANFER JN, BRADY RO, FREDRICKSON DS: Deficiency of sphingomyelin-cleaving enzyme in tissue cultures derived from patients with Niemann-Pick disease. *Biochem Biophys Res Commun* 34:582, 1969
29. GAL AE, BRADY RO, BARRANGER JA, PENTCHEV PG: The diagnosis of Type A and Type B Niemann-Pick disease and detection of carriers using leukocytes and a chromogenic analogue of sphingomyelin. *Clin Chim Acta* 104:129, 1980
30. GAL AE, BRADY RO, HIBBERT SR, PENTCHEV PG: A practical chromogenic procedure for the detection of homozygotes and heterozygous carriers of Niemann-Pick disease. *N Engl J Med* 293:632, 1975
31. BESLEY GTN: Sphingomyelinase defect in Niemann-Pick disease, Type C, fibroblasts. *FEBS Lett* 80:71, 1977
32. BESLEY GTN: Diagnosis of Niemann-Pick disease using a simple and sensitive fluorometric assay of sphingomyelinase activity. *Clin Chim Acta* 90:269, 1978
33. SCHNEIDER PB, KENNEDY EP: Sphingomyelinase in normal human spleens and in spleens from subjects with Niemann-Pick disease. *J Lipid Res* 8:202, 1967
34. BRADY RO, KANFER JN, SHAPIRO D: Metabolism of glucocerebrosides. II. Evidence of an enzymatic deficiency in Gaucher's disease. *Biochem Biophys Res Commun* 18:221, 1965
35. PHILIPPART M, MARTIN L, MARTIN JJ, MENKES JH: Niemann-Pick disease. Morphologic and biochemical studies in the visceral form with late central nervous system involvement (Crocker's Group C). *Arch Neurol* 20:227, 1969
36. DACREMONT G, KINT JA, CARTON D, COCQUYT G: Glucosylceramide in plasma of patients with Niemann-Pick disease. *Clin Chim Acta* 52:365, 1974
37. CALLAHAN JW, KHALIL M: Sphingomyelinase and the genetic defects in Niemann-Pick disease, in Volk BW, Schneck L (eds): *Current Trends in Sphingolipidoses and Allied Disorders*. New York, Plenum, 1976, p 367

38. MULLER H, HARZER K: Partial purification of acid sphingomyelinase from normal and pathological (M. Niemann-Pick Type C) human brain. *J Neurochem* 34:446, 1980

39. BARATON G, REVOL A: Activateur des sphingohydrolases et nature du deficit en sphingomyelinase dans la maladie de Niemann-Pick Type A, B et C. *Clin Chim Acta* 76:339, 1977

40. BESLEY GTN, HOOGEBOOM AJM, HOOGEVEEN AM, KLEIJER WJ, GALJAARD H: Somatic cell hybridization studies showing different gene mutations in Niemann-Pick variants. *Hum Genet* 54:409, 1980

41. BRADY RO: Sphingolipidoses. *Ann Rev Biochem* 47:687, 1978

42. CONSTANTOPOULOS G, DEKABAN AS: Neurochemistry of the mucopolysaccharidoses: Brain lipids and lysosomal enzymes in patients with four types of mucopolysaccharidosis and in normal controls. *J Neurochem* 30:965, 1978

43. UHLENDORF BW, HOLTZ AI, MOCK MB, FREDRICKSON DS: Persistence of a metabolic defect in tissue cultures derived from patients with Niemann-Pick disease, in Aronson SM, Volk BW (eds): *Inborn Disorders of Sphingolipid Metabolism.* New York, Pergamon, 1967, p 443

44. SCHNEIDER EL, ELLIS WG, BRADY RO, McCULLOCK JR, EPSTEIN CJ: Prenatal Niemann-Pick disease: Biochemical and histologic examination of a 19-gestational week fetus. *Pediatr Res* 6:720, 1972

45. KANFER JN, YOUNG OM, SHAPIRO D, BRADY RO: The metabolism of sphingomyelin. I. Purification and properties of a sphingomyelin-cleaving enzyme from rat liver tissue. *J Biol Chem* 240:1081, 1966

46. GAL AE, FASH FJ: Synthesis of 2-hexadecanoylamino-4-nitrophenyl phosphorylcholine-hydroxide, a chromogenic substrate for assaying sphingomyelinase activity. *Chem Phys Lipids* 16:71, 1976

47. MAZIERE JC, MAZIERE C, HÖSIL P: An ultramicrochemical assay for sphingomyelinase, in *Monographs in Human Genetics.* Basel, Karger, 1978, p 198

48. DEN TANDT WR, JAEKEN J, LEROY JG, EGGERMONT E: A micromethod for sphingomyelinase assay using a chromogenic artificial substrate. Its use in the diagnosis of Niemann-Pick disease. *Acta Paediatr Belg* 32:253, 1979

49. VANIER MT, REVOL A, FICHET M: Sphingomyelinase activities of various human tissues in control subjects and in Niemann-Pick disease—Development and evaluation of a microprocedure. *Clin Chim Acta* 106:257, 1980

50. GALJAARD H: Biochemical analysis of single cultured cells. *Trends Biochem Sci* August 1980, p 201

51. DEBUCH H, WIEDMANN H-R: Lymph node excision as simple diagnostic aid in rare lipidoses. *Eur J Pediatr* 129:99, 1978

52. JUNGAALWALA FB, MILUNSKY A: High performance liquid chromatogrphy for the detection of homozygotes and heterozygotes of Niemann-Pick disease. *Pediatr Res* 12:655, 1978

53. MAZIERE J-C, MAZIERE C, HOSLI P, POLONOVSKI J: Diagnosis of Niemann-Pick disease by analysis of hair-roots. *Biomedicine* 31:104, 1979

54. ZITMAN D, CHAZAN S, KLIBANSKY C: Sphingomyelinase activity levels in human peripheral blood leukocytes using [³H]-sphingomyelin as substrate: Study of heterozygotes and homozygotes for Niemann-Pick disease variants. *Clin Chim Acta* 86:37, 1978

55. GATT S, DINUR T, BARENHOLZ Y: A spectrophotometric method for determination of sphingomyelinase. *Biochim Biophys Acta* 530:503, 1978

56. GATT S, DINUR T, BARENHOLZ Y: A fluorometric determination of sphingomyelinase by use of fluorescent derivatives of sphingomyelin, and its application to diagnosis of Niemann-Pick disease. *Clin Chem* 26:93, 1980

57. HARZER K, BENZ HU: A simple sphingomyelinase determination for Niemann-Pick disease: Differential diagnosis of types A, B, and C. *J Neurochem* 21:999, 1973

58a. FENSOM AH, BENSON PF, BABARIK AW, GRANT AR, JACOBS L: Fibroblast phosphodiesterase deficiency in Niemann-Pick disease. *Biochem Biophys Res Commun* 74:877, 1977

58b. BEAUDET AL, HAMPTON MS, PATEL K, SPARROW JT: Acidic phospholipases in cultured human fibroblasts: Deficiency of phospholipase C in Niemann-Pick disease. *Clin Chim Acta* 108:403, 1980

59. BRADY RO, JOHNSON WG, UHLENDORF BW: Identification of heterozygous carriers of lipid storage diseases. *Am J Med* 51:423, 1971

60. BRADY RO, O'BRIEN JS, BRADLEY RM, GAL AE: Sphingolipid hydrolases in brain tissue of patients with generalized gangliosidosis. *Biochim Biophys Acta* 210:193, 1970

61. BRADY RO: Heritable catabolic and anabolic disorders of lipid metabolism. *Metabolism* 26:329, 1977

62. PATRICK AD, YOUNG E, KLEIJER WJ, NIERMEIJER MF: Prenatal diagnosis of Niemann-Pick disease Type A using chromogenic substrate. *Lancet* 2:144, 1977

63. HARZER K, SCHLOTE W, PEIFFER J, BENZ HU, ANZIL AP: Neurovisceral lipidosis compatible with Niemann-Pick disease Type C: Morphological and biochemical studies of a late infantile case and enzyme and lipid assays in a prenatal case of the same family. *Acta Neuropathol* 43:97, 1978

64. BRADY RO, BARRANGER JA, GAL AE, PENTCHEV PG, FURBISH FS, KUSIAK, JW: Treatment by lipidoses by enzyme infusion, in Lowden JA, Callahan JW (eds): *Lysosomes and Lysosomal Storage Disease.* New York, Raven, 1980, p 373

65. BRADY RO, BARRANGER JA, PENTCHEV PG, FURBISH FS, GAL AE: Prospects for enzyme replacement therapy in heritable metabolic disorders, in Aebi H, Herschkowitz NN (eds): *Inborn Errors of Metabolism in Humans.* London, MTP Press, 1981, in press

66. PENTCHEV PG, BRADY RO, GAL AE, HIBBERT SR: The isolation and characterization of sphingomyelinase from human placental tissue. *Biochim Biophys Acta* 488:312, 1977

67. BARRANGER JA, RAPOPORT SI, FREDERICKS WR, PENTCHEV PG, MacDERMOT KD, STREUSING JK, BRADY RO: Modification of the blood-brain barrier: Increased concentration and fate of enzymes entering the brain. *Proc Nat Acad Sci USA* 76:481, 1979

68. DALOZE P, DELVIN EE, GLORIEUX FH, CORMAN JL, BETTEZ P, TOUSSI T: Replacement therapy for inherited enzyme deficiency: Liver orthotopic transplantation in Niemann-Pick disease Type A. *Am J Med Genet* 1:229, 1977

69. BRADY RO: Genetic errors and enzyme replacement, in Kety SS (ed): *Genetics of Neurological and Psychiatric Disorders.* New York, Raven, 1981, in press

70. BUNDZA A, LOWDEN JA, CHARLTON KM: Niemann-Pick disease in a poodle dog. *Vet Pathol* 16:530, 1979

71. WENGER DA, SATTLER M, KUDOH T, SNYDER SP, KINGSTON RS: Niemann-Pick disease: A genetic model in Siamese cats. *Science* 208:1471, 1980

72. PENTCHEV PG, GAL AE, BOOTH AD, OMODEO-SALE F, FOUKS J, NEUMEYER BA, QUIRK JM, DAWSON G, BRADY RO: A lysosomal storage disorder in mice characterized by a dual deficiency of sphingomyelinase and glucocerebrosidase. *Biochim Biophys Acta* 619:669, 1980

73. SAKURAGAWA M: Niemann-Pick disease-like inclusions caused by a hypocholesteremic agent. *Invest Ophthalmol* 15:1022, 1976

74. SAKURAGAWA N, SAKURAGAWA M, KUWABARA T, PENTCHEV PG, BARRANGER JA, BRADY RO: Niemann-Pick disease experimental model: Sphingomyelinase reduction induced by AY-9944. *Science* 196:317, 1977

75. SAKURAGAWA N, WATANABE K, TAKADA K, NONAKA I, ARIMA M: The effects of a hypocholesterolemic agent (Boxidine) on developing rats, in Di Benedetta C, Balazs R, Gombos G, Porcellati G (eds): *Multidisciplinary Approach to Brain Development.* Amsterdam, Elsevier/North Holland, 1980, p 551

42

GLUCOSYLCERAMIDE LIPIDOSIS:
Gaucher's Disease

ROSCOE O. BRADY

JOHN A. BARRANGER

1. Gaucher's disease is the most common inherited metabolic disorder of glycolipid metabolism. Excessive quantities of glucocerebroside (glucosylceramide) accumulate in organs and tissues throughout the body of patients with this disorder. Glucocerebroside is composed of equimolar portions of the long-chain amino alcohol sphingosine, a long-chain fatty acid, and glucose. The lipid accumulates primarily in the cells of the reticuloendothelial system. The storage cells have distinctive histologic features and are called Gaucher cells. Clinical manifestations of the disorder include splenomegaly, hepatomegaly, hypersplenism, and osteoporotic erosion of the long bones, hip joints, and vertebral bodies.

2. The disorder has been detected in patients of all ages and has been divided into three clinical categories. Type 1, the adult, chronic, nonneuronopathic form, may be manifested at any time from birth to old age. The major signs are organomegaly, hematologic abnormalities attributable to hypersplenism, and bone lesions. The central nervous system is usually not affected. Type 2, the acute neuronopathic or infantile form, is usually apparent before 6 months of age and fatal by 2 years of age. In addition to the hepatosplenomegaly and Gaucher cells in the bone marrow, the cranial nerves and brainstem are heavily involved. There is minimal storage of glucocerebroside in ganglion cells, but there is loss of neurons, neuronophagia, and deposition of glycolipid in periadventitial cells. In type 3, the subacute neuronopathic or juvenile form, visceral organs and the central nervous system are involved, but the signs of neurologic damage appear later than in type 2 patients.

3. All three types of Gaucher's disease are caused by subnormal activity of the enzyme glucocerebrosidase, which catalyzes the hydrolytic cleavage of glucose from glucocerebroside. Each of the three types is inherited as an autosomal recessive trait.

4. The diagnosis of Gaucher's disease may be made on the basis of organomegaly and the presence of Gaucher cells in the bone marrow and other tissues. Confirmation may be obtained by measuring the quantity of glucocerebroside in tissues, e.g., by a needle biopsy of the liver. The diagnosis may also be readily made by measuring glucocerebrosidase activity in leukocytes or cultured skin fibroblasts. Radioactively labeled glucocerebroside is the most reliable substrate for these determinations, although the fluorogenic reagent 4-methylumbelliferyl-β-D-glucopyranoside may also be used with confidence under specified assay conditions. Hexadecanoylamino-4-dinitrophenyl-β-D-glucopyranoside has also been shown to be a useful substrate for the diagnosis of this disorder. The level of non-tartrate-inhibitable acid phosphatase is usually elevated in the plasma of Gaucher patients.

5. Gaucher heterozygotes, at least for type 1 and type 2,

may be identified using [^{14}C]glucocerebroside and fresh leukocyte preparations or extracts of cultured skin fibroblasts. 4-Methylumbelliferyl-β-D-glucopyranoside has also been used with fibroblast extracts for heterozygote detection.

6. *Fetuses at risk for Gaucher's disease (types 1 and 2) may be identified as deficient through measurement of glucocerebrosidase activity by assay of the enzyme in extracts of cultured amniotic cells using authentic, labeled lipid or the fluorogenic glucoside as substrate.*

7. *Enzyme replacement for Gaucher's disease is under intensive investigation in a number of laboratories. Although salutary effects have been reported in several patients, the ultimate effectiveness of this therapy remains to be established.*

The eponym Gaucher's disease is applied to heritable disorders of lipid metabolism in which glucosylceramide (also called glucocerebroside) accumulates in organs and tissues of afflicted individuals (Fig. 42-1). The most frequent manifestations of the disorder are hepatosplenomegaly and the presence of large, lipid-laden cells in the bone marrow. These signs may become apparent at any time. In some patients the signs may be present shortly after birth, while in others they may not occur until late in life. In the majority of Gaucher patients there is no central nervous system involvement. Infants with Gaucher's disease are encountered, however, in whom there is extensive brain damage and severe progressive mental retardation. Another comparatively small group of patients exhibits late onset of central nervous system involvement, usually manifested initially as seizures which become increasingly difficult to control. The variations in the clinical presentation of this disorder have led to the classification of patients with Gaucher's disease as types 1, 2, and 3 [1, 2]. This convention is widely used and is employed here.

HISTORY

In 1882, Phillippe C. E. Gaucher published a description of a patient with enlarged spleen and liver which he believed was caused by a primary epithelioma of the spleen [3]. Reports of additional patients with similar manifestations gradually appeared [1], and in 1924, Lieb isolated cerebroside from the spleen of patients with the disorder [4]. He realized that the stored material was a glycolipid but erroneously concluded that it was galactosylceramide. In 1933, Aghion reported that the accumulating substance was actually glucosylceramide [5]. This observation has been amply confirmed [1]. In 1965 Brady

and coworkers showed that the metabolic defect in Gaucher's disease is a deficiency of the enzyme glucocerebrosidase [6]. This observation has also been fully substantiated [1, 2].

PREVALENCE AND GENETICS

Gaucher's disease is the most frequently encountered sphingolipid storage disorder. There are more than 4000 patients with type 1 (adult form) in the United States alone. Patients with type 2 (infantile form) and type 3 (juvenile) Gaucher's disease are much less common. The disorder is panethnic, but type 1 Gaucher's disease is more frequent in Ashkenazic Jews than in all other groups. The incidence has been reported to be 1 in every 2500 births among the Ashkenazim [1, 2]. Type 2 patients are predominantly of non-Jewish extraction; this distribution also seems to be true for the type 3 individuals. No families have been reported in which more than one type of disorder occurs. This implies that the three types of Gaucher's disease are genetically distinct. Each of the three types is inherited as an autosomal dominant trait.

CLINICAL ASPECTS

The assignment of Gaucher patients, especially children, to a clinical subtype should be made only after careful examination for the presence or absence of neurologic signs. So far, no consistent biochemical feature has been useful in distinguishing these types.

Type 1: Chronic Nonneuronopathic Gaucher's Disease

This category was previously designated the "adult" form of Gaucher's disease, although it became increasingly apparent that many patients with onset of signs and symptoms comparatively soon after birth belonged to this group. The initial sign of this chronic form is usually splenomegaly, although exceptions have been noted [2, 9, 10]. Primary hypersplenism with thrombocytopenia, anemia, and leukopenia is frequently found. Patients may have platelet counts below 50,000 for a number of years before developing bleeding diatheses. Although hepatomegaly is often noted at the time the enlarged spleen is discovered, the liver may not be palpable until later in the course of the disease. Moderate hepatic dysfunction is generally signaled by elevation of liver enzymes in blood, reduced sulfobromophthalein clearance, and reduced and nonhomogeneous uptake of radionuclide tracers. Hepatic failure is an infrequent complication. Bone complications are frequently encountered in patients in this group. Bone scans reveal areas of decreased density in the proximal and distal regions of long bones, hip joints, knees, shoulders, and vertebrae. Aseptic necrosis of the proximal head of the femur is common, and the eroded long bones and vertebrae have a propensity to fracture. Severe episodic bone pain, usually in the long bones, occurs in a number of these patients and may be accompanied by fever and mistaken for osteomyelitis. Some patients with Gaucher's disease have significant pulmonary involvement; pulmonary

Figure 42-1 The defect in Gaucher's disease. The basic defect involves a glucocerebrosidase which catalyzes the cleavage of glucose (Glc) from the ceramide (Cer) portion of glucocerebroside. The site of hydrolytic cleavage is indicated by the wavy line.

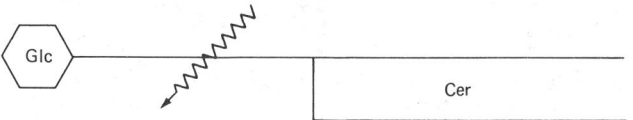

hypertension and cor pulmonale can occur. The lung involvement may predispose individuals to pneumonia, a major cause of death in young, severely affected patients.

Most patients have elevated serum acid phosphatase which is not inhibited by tartrate [11]. Some older patients have a yellow pallor and diffuse yellow-brown pigmentation on the face and lower legs. There may be limitation of physical growth, delayed menarche and dentition. No hormonal basis for these signs has been established, but the report of Gaucher cells in the pituitary of a patient with the chronic form of the disease is intriguing in this regard [12].

Age of Onset and Clinical Course   The age of onset and the severity of the disease process vary widely. Diagnosis may be made in a symptomatic infant as early as the first few months of life [13] or in an adult as late as the seventh or eighth decade. The course may be rapid in some children, but generally the prognosis is better. Even for patients diagnosed early in childhood, the course is usually slowly progressive with complications appearing or worsening over a period of years. Although individuals with type 1 typically do not develop neurologic complications, nervous system involvement has been reported in a small number of patients [14–20]. In some the nervous system involvement is not clearly related to the primary disease [16–19]. Others present a diagnostic dilemma between type 1 and type 3 [14, 15, 18, 20]. Operationally, a patient could be considered type 1 until some sign of neurologic damage appeared, then reclassified as type 3. More realistically, it would seem that nervous system changes can occur in some patients with type 1. Involvement of the nervous system may be limited and not result in overt clinical symptoms [21]. Whether a significant percentage of patients with type 1 Gaucher's disease actually have subclinical nervous system involvement can only be settled by additional pathologic observations.

Type 2: Acute Neuronopathic Gaucher's Disease

The average age of onset in patients with this form of the disorder is 3 months, with a range from birth to 18 months. Hepatosplenomegaly is invariably a presenting sign. Within a few months, or by the average age of 6 months, neurologic complications develop (Fig. 42-2). Signs of involvement of cranial nerve nuclei and extrapyramidal tracts appear in almost all patients. The triad of trismus, strabismus, and retroflexion of the head has been considered pathognomonic of type 2 Gaucher's disease, but it is not unique. Feeding problems and difficulty in handling secretions develop from uncoordinated movements of the oropharynx. Progressive spasticity, hyperreflexia, and pathologic reflexes develop. Seizures may occur but are not a frequent complication. Late in the course of the illness the child becomes hypotonic and apathetic. Death occurs between 1 month and 2 years of age with an average age of death at 9 months, usually from pulmonary infection or anoxia.

Type 3: Subacute Neuronopathic Gaucher's Disease

The subacute neuronopathic form of Gaucher's disease appears to be a syndrome distinct from type 1 and type 2, yet sharing some characteristics with these other forms. The clinical features, apart from those referrable to the nervous system, are common to all three types. Hepatosplenomegaly usually precedes neurologic disease. Involvement of other organ systems probably is as variable as in type 1, although generalizations are less reliably made in type 3 because of the heterogeneity of the reported cases [1, 22, 23]. Comparison of the neurologic involvement of type 3 patients with type 2 reveals that the former are less severely, although similarly, affected. Even though signs may appear moderately early in life, their course is much longer. The condition is associated with spasticity, ocular motor apraxia or paralysis, ataxia, retardation, and seizures [20, 24a, 24b].

PATHOLOGY

Gaucher Cell

One of the most striking features of Gaucher's disease is the presence of large lipid-laden cells in the tissues of patients with the disorder. These characteristic cells, called Gaucher cells, have been found in all parts of the reticuloendothelial system. The cytoplasm has a "wrinkled tissue paper" or "crumpled silk" appearance, the nucleus is eccentric, and the size ranges from 20 to 100 μm. The cells are particularly numerous in the red pulp of the spleen (Fig. 42-3), sinusoids of the liver, sinusoids and medullary portions of the lymph nodes, alveolar capillaries, and bone marrow (Fig. 42-4). They may also be found in the inner walls and adventitia of arterioles, veins, lymphatic vessels, and capillaries. These cells may appear in any organ and are derived from the histiocytes in the spleen, the Kupffer cells in the liver, the alveolar macrophages in the lung, and the periadventitial cells in the Virchow-Robin spaces in the brain (Fig. 42-5). They may also be seen in the pancreas, thyroid, and adrenals. In all locations the cell is in fact an altered macrophage and has been shown to have the same surface markers [25] and ultrastructure [26] as the monocyte-histiocyte series.

Microscopic Appearance   The histology of the Gaucher cell is sufficiently characteristic to permit its identification as a

Figure 42-2   A patient with type 2 Gaucher's disease at age 12 months. *(From Fredrickson and Sloan [1]. Used by permission.)*

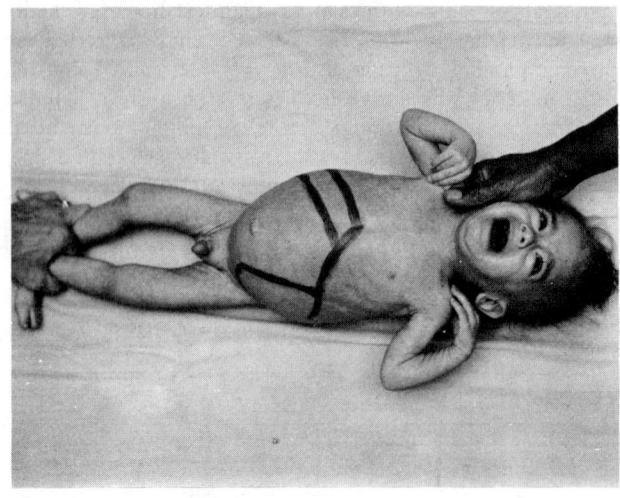

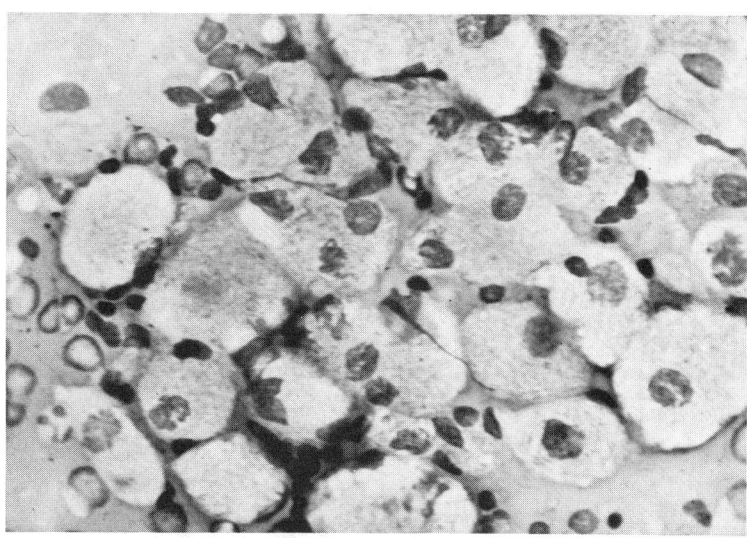

Figure 42-3 Lipid storage cells in the spleen of a patient with type 1 Gaucher's disease. *(From Brady [2]. Used by permission.)*

diagnostic criterion (Fig. 42-6). Foam cells, which are seen in other sphingolipidoses, are readily distinguished. Cells that have some resemblance to Gaucher cells, such as the "pseudo-Gaucher" cell found in multiple myeloma, have a completely different ultrastructure [27]. Gaucherlike cells are occasionally encountered in the leukemias [28–30], in thalassemia [31], and in congenital dyserythropoietic anemia [32]. Staining characteristics have been extensively reviewed [33]. The most useful stain for fixed preparations is periodic acid Schiff reagent (PAS). The cells are characteristically positive for acid phosphatase. Typical rodlike inclusions in the cytoplasm can be seen by Nomarski interference microscopy. Studies have suggested that the glycolipid which accumulates is aggregated with a protein to form tubular structures [34, 35]. Within the cytoplasm of the cells are spindle-shaped, membrane-delimited inclusion bodies (Gaucher bodies) ranging from 0.6 to 4 μm in diameter. These inclusions are filled with tubules twisted around each other (Fig. 42-7).

Spleen

Painless splenomegaly is nearly uniform among all types of Gaucher's disease. Occasional patients with type 1 and type 2 do not manifest a significant increase in organ size. In several type 1 patients the spleen is not palpable by physical examination but can be demonstrated to be larger than normal by radionuclide scan. The spleen is usually large, firm, pale, and less filled with blood than normal, which may explain why spontaneous rupture is uncommon [36]. The normal architecture is distorted, and considerable fibrosis is often seen. The red pulp contains numerous PAS-positive histiocytes (Fig. 42-3).

It has often been argued that the spleen serves as a reservoir for accumulating glucocerebroside and that removal of this organ accelerates the pathologic damage in other organs. Groth and coworkers investigated a patient with type 3 Gaucher's disease who had repeated liver biopsies before and subsequent to splenectomy. These investigators reported progressively rapid accumulation of lipid postoperatively [37]. We have followed one patient type 1 in whom glucocerebroside concentration did not increase over a 1-year period after splenectomy. The clinical status of the patient was commensurate with this observation.

Lymphatic System

Gaucher cells are frequently present in lymph nodes, thymus, Peyer's patches, and pharyngeal tonsils in type 2 and type 3 Gaucher's disease.

Liver

Although hepatomegaly is commonly found in Gaucher patients, clinical complications have rarely been reported. Bleeding from esophageal varices has been noted, as well as portal hypertension and ascites. Variable degrees of fibrosis and cirrhosis have been observed, and many patients have abnormalities of liver function tests [38]. Mildly affected patients have scattered foci of Gaucher cells in sinusoids, with little other involvement (Fig. 42-8). Other patients are more severely affected, and their livers may be markedly cirrhotic.

Kidney

Renal involvement in Gaucher's disease is uncommonly

Figure 42-4 Unstained lipid storage cell from the bone marrow of a patient with Gaucher's disease viewed under a phase microscope. *(From Fredrickson and Sloan [1]. Used by permission.)*

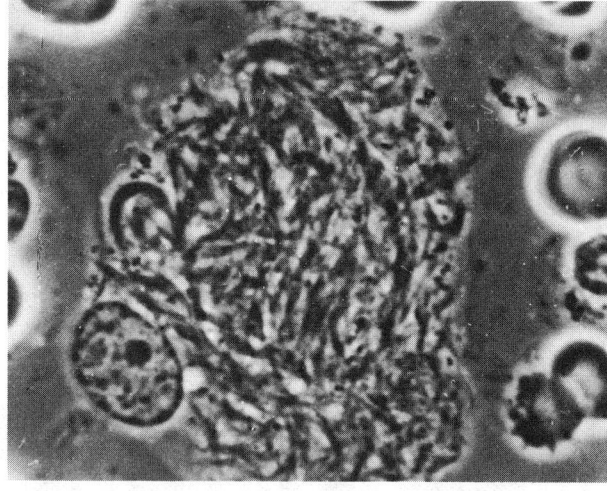

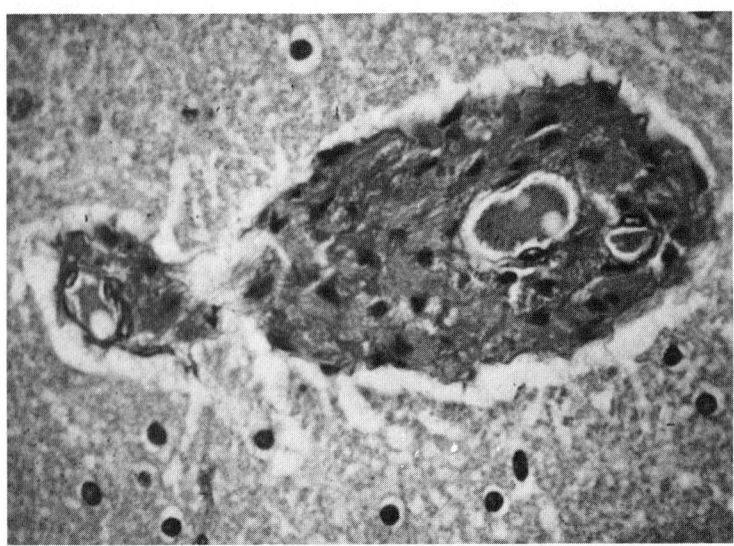

Figure 42-5 Lipid-laden cells in the Virchow-Robin spaces. *(From Brady [2]. Used by permission.)*

reported [39, 40]. It is not clear whether the alteration in renal function is the result of infiltration with storage material into tubule cells. Proteinuria may result from the invasion of Gaucher cells into the glomeruli and interstitial capillaries.

Cardiopulmonary System

Some children with Gaucher's disease have a productive cough, chest pain, recurrent pneumonia, and respiratory distress. A few have chronic pulmonary disease without cardiac lesions and with significant hypoxia, cyanosis, and clubbing [41]. The infiltration process seen in lung x-rays of other lipid storage diseases is not frequently seen in this disorder. Gaucher cells are present in the alveolar capillaries and lymphatic vessels and may be free in the alveoli (Fig. 42-9). Restrictive pericarditis has been reported in several cases. Interstitial infiltration of the myocardium, resulting in decreased left ventricular compliance and decreased cardiac output, has also been observed [39], as has pulmonary hypertension.

Bones

Skeletal involvement is frequent in patients with types 1 and 3 Gaucher's disease. As many as 50 to 75 percent of all patients may have osseous complications [42]. Joint pain and nonspecific bone pain is common. Acute, severe, episodic bone pain, usually in the femur, is often accompanied by fever, and the area is hot, tender, erythmatous, and swollen. Aseptic necrosis and collapse of the femoral head may occur in as many as half of these patients (Fig. 42-10). Vertebral collapse and pathologic fractures also occur frequently. Involvement of other long bones, skull, phalanges, and ribs is much less frequent. The expanded cortex of the distal femur (Erlenmeyer flask deformity) and bony erosion with cystlike cavities of various sizes comprise the typical roentgenographic findings. Cystlike lesions and root resorption of the mandible have been noted [43].

Eyes

Ocular motor apraxia, as described by Cogan [44], has been noted in type 1 and 3 patients and early in the course of type 2. This sign has been the only indication of neurologic involvement in five children with Gaucher's disease under our observation. Yellow-brown, wedge-shaped thickening of the cornea has been noted frequently in type 1 Gaucher's disease. These pingueculae have been reported to contain Gaucherlike foamy histiocytes. The cherry-red spot in the macula that occurs in several lipid storage diseases has not been reported in Gaucher's disease.

Figure 42-6 Electron photomicrograph of a Gaucher cell. Approximately ×4000. *(From Brady [2]. Used by permission.)*

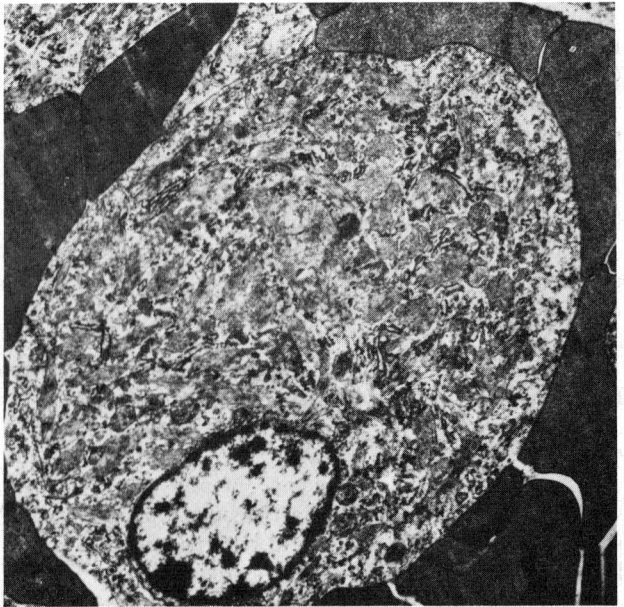

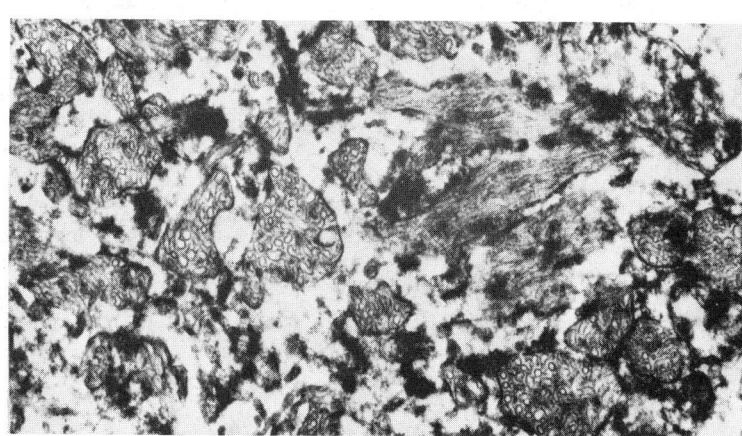

Figure 42-7 Electron photomicrograph of a Gaucher cell. Approximately ×15,000. *(From Brady [2]. Used by permission.)*

Skin

A number of patients have been reported with increased pigmentation, especially of the lower extremities. Gaucher cells are not found in the skin, but increased iron pigment and melanin are seen. The cause of the pigmentation is not known.

Immune System

Some patients appear to be susceptible to chronic infections. Monoclonal and polyclonal gammopathies have been reported in Gaucher patients [45–49], and concurrent amyloidosis has been noted [50, 51]. Multiple myeloma [52–54], leukemia [55–56], Hodgkin's disease [57–59], cerebral astrocytoma [60], and bronchogenic carcinoma [61] have been reported in association with Gaucher's disease. In addition, deficiency of T cells in spleen and peripheral blood has been observed [25]. The inference that a dysimmune diathesis occurs in Gaucher patients is supported by studies of cultured macrophages. These cells release lymphocyte-activating factors in response to the accumulation of glucocerebroside [62].

Plasma immunoglobulins and other proteins are elevated in Gaucher patients. Acid phosphatase [11, 63], angiotensin-converting enzyme [64, 65], several lysosomal hydrolases [66–68], and lysozyme [65, 69] are increased. Serum transcobalamin II, a protein frequently elevated in the plasma of patients with leukemia, is increased in Gaucher patients and has been thought to correlate with clinical severity [70]. Many patients have prolongation of partial thromboplastin time. A possible explanation of this observation is the demonstration of a deficiency of several coagulation factors in vitro, the most prominent being factor IX [71]. It has been postulated that the clotting abnormalities may be secondary to circulating glucocerebroside [72].

Nervous System

Surprisingly little is certain concerning the pathology of the brain in type 1 Gaucher's disease. Few patients with type 1 have had postmortem examinations that included the nervous system, and in only one has the periadventitial accumulation of the characteristic Gaucher cells been convincingly demon-

strated [19]. Reports of hypophyseal and leptomeningeal Gaucher cells in this form of Gaucher's disease require confirmation.

In type 2 the perivascular accumulation of Gaucher cells has been frequently noted. The arterioles in the subcortical white matter are surrounded by swollen adventitial cells which stain with PAS reagent. Typical Gaucher cells occur in the Virchow-Robin spaces (Fig. 42-5). Ultrastructural examination of cells in these locations reveal the typical rodlike inclusions. Neurons show various stages of degeneration. Some are swollen with eccentric nuclei, and the Nissl substance is displaced to the periphery. The cytoplasm is metachromatic and stains with PAS. Other cells are shrunken and have irregular, crumpled borders and demonstrate chromatolysis. Cell loss and neuronophagia may be prominent in certain areas. Neuronal storage of lipid and free Gaucher cells in the brain substance has been claimed but not confirmed ultrastructurally. Various regions of the brain, including the cranial nerve nuclei in the brainstem, basal ganglia, thalamus, Purkinje cell layer of the cerebellum, and pyramidal and ganglion cell layers of the cortex, are involved. Demyelination is a common, but irregular, feature of most cases.

Pathologic changes in type 3 are less well documented. Svennerholm has reported that there was no change in the glycolipid pattern in the brain of a type 3 patient [73]. A detailed pathologic report of additional type 3 patients is in preparation by Dreborg [74].

PATHOPHYSIOLOGY

Gaucher's disease is a lipid storage disorder resulting from the accumulation of glucocerebroside (glucosylceramide) in organs and tissues of afflicted individuals. Glucocerebroside comprises the long-chain amino alcohol sphingosine $[CH_3—(CH_2)_{12}—CH{=}CH—CH(OH)—CH(NH_2)—CH_2OH]$, a long-chain fatty acid, and a molecule of glucose (Fig. 42-11). The fatty acid is linked to the nitrogen atom on carbon 2 of sphingosine to form a complex called ceramide. The molecule of glucose is joined by a β-glycosidic bond to the carbon atom 1 of the sphingosine moiety of ceramide.

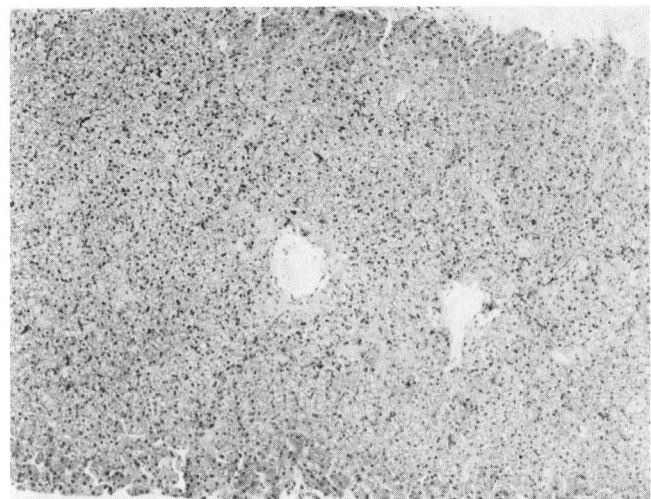

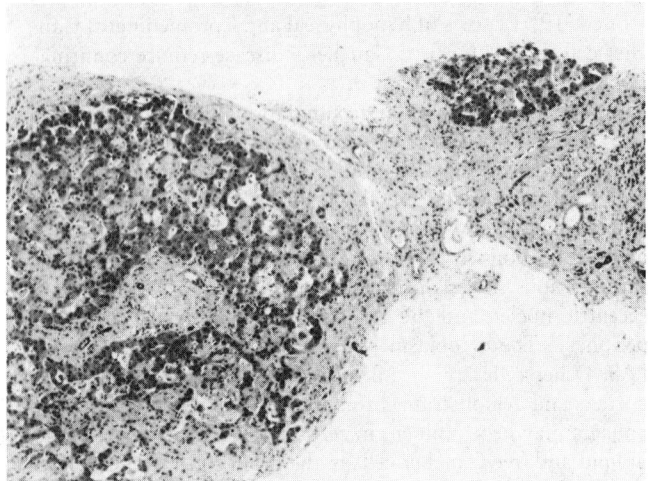

Figure 42-8 *Upper,* liver lobule showing Gaucher cells around the central vein and scattered throughout the parenchyma with minimal fibrosis. Magnification, ×80. *Lower,* liver with confluent patches of Gaucher cells, and scarring, degeneration and regeneration, and fibrosis typical of cirrhosis. Magnification, ×80.

Spleen

The quantity of glucocerebroside in normal human spleens ranges between 60 and 280 μg per gram wet weight with a mean value of 170 μg/g. The amount of glucocerebroside in the spleen of Gaucher patients is greatly increased. Values ranging from 3 to 40.5 mg per gram wet weight have been reported [1, 2]. These values represent an increase from 18 to 238 times above normal. Other sphingolipids are usually within the normal range. The mean chain length of the fatty acid moiety of spleen glucocerebrosides in Gaucher patients is 22 carbon atoms, and the calculated average molecular weight is 770.

Liver

Glucocerebroside is also increased manyfold above normal values of 31 μg per gram wet weight for males and 46 μg per gram wet weight for females. The levels in patients have ranged from 250 μg/g to 22.9 mg/g. There was no evidence of a correlation between the extent of lipid accumulation and the severity of the clinical manifestations.

Brain

Conflicting reports have appeared concerning the quantity of glucocerebroside in the brain of type 2 patients [1, 2]. Results of the most recently reported study indicate that glucocerebroside increased from 0.02 mg per gram wet weight to 0.21 mg/g in gray matter and from an undetectable level in the white matter of a control to 0.5 mg/g in the patient [75]. The author also reported the presence of sulfatide that contained glucose, a novel observation that requires substantiation. Accumulation of glucocerebroside in type 1 and type 3 patients has not been conclusively demonstrated.

Plasma and Erythrocytes

Glucocerebroside is only slightly elevated in the plasma of Gaucher patients over that in normal individuals [76]. Somewhat greater augmentation is seen in red blood cell glucocerebroside concentration, where increases between two- and threefold are common.

Pathogenetic Speculation

It may reasonably be concluded that most of the pathologic aspects of the disease result directly from the storage of glucocerebroside, but the lesser accumulation of certain related lipids and protein that occur in the storage granules [35] could contribute as well. The hypothesis that tissue pathology results from physical crowding in the cells or from compromise of blood flow is suggested by the histologic appearances. This explanation is not completely satisfactory for several reasons. First, the histology and numbers of Gaucher cells rarely correlate with clinical severity, especially with regard to the nervous system. Second, tissue levels of glucocerebroside do not correlate with either pathologic appearance or clinical complications. Third, although blood flow studies in liver and spleen may be abnormal, radionuclide scans of bone indicate increased blood flow. Correlations of blood flow in liver and

Figure 42-9 Gaucher cells occluding pulmonary alveolar capillaries. *(From Fredrickson and Sloan [1]. Used by permission.)*

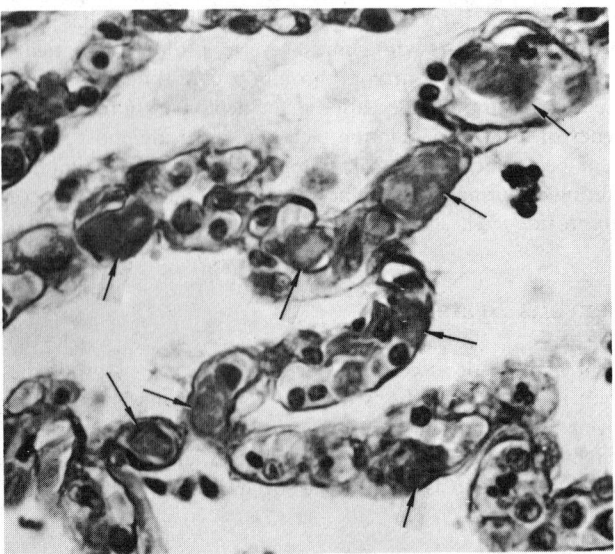

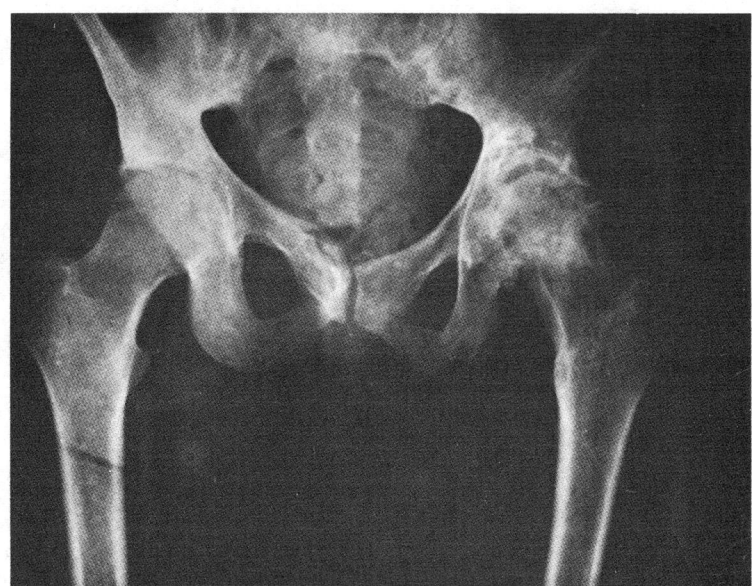

Figure 42-10 Collapse of the hip joint in a 39-year-old female with type 1 Gaucher's disease. *(From Brady [2]. Used by permission.)*

spleen do not accurately reflect clinical complications. Moreover, and this aspect appears especially significant, in Gaucher patients many tissue and plasma abnormalities have been described which may be the result of glucocerebroside storage within macrophages and may have no relationship to intracellular or extracellular crowding. The increased quantities of lysosomal hydrolases in tissues and plasma appear to be particularly significant in this regard. It has been repeatedly shown that these enzymes, fibroblast-stimulating factors, cytolytic factors, and lymphocyte-activating factors are released from macrophages in response to ingestion of toxic particles. Recent studies have shown that uptake of glucocerebroside by cultured macrophages causes the liberation of these enzymes and other macrophage-derived factors [62]. It is therefore not difficult to imagine that the Gaucher cells are directly involved in, and actually cause, injury or death of neighboring cells.

Another important aspect is the possibility of macrophage blockage. The damage that occurs in Kupffer cells may be an instructive model of a functional aberration that may occur in an organ when its macrophages are altered by accumulation of glucocerebroside. Injury of hepatocytes has been shown to occur when Kupffer cells take up large quantities of indigestible material, an effect that was postulated to be caused by a release of lysosomal enzymes [77]. Furthermore, during the period when Kupffer cells cannot actively phagocytose substances because the material within cannot be catabolized, hepatocytes are at risk from circulating toxins such as immune complexes and endotoxins. Thus, the Kupffer cells provide some degree of protection to the hepatocyte. If the Kupffer cell is continually accumulating glucocerebroside and the presence of this lipid impairs the protective function of the phagocyte, significant liver damage including cirrhosis may result. This complication has been observed in several patients with this disorder. The difficulty would be compounded in those patients with Gaucher's disease in whom myelophthisic marrows cannot replace the monocyte precursors of the tissue macrophages. Similar mechanisms might occur in the alveolar macrophages, bone osteoclasts, spleen histiocytes, or periadventitial Gaucher cells in any organ. Analogous pathogenetic mechanisms might be involved in patients with significant neurologic damage, but in whom little or no glucocerebroside accumulation can be demonstrated.

METABOLIC ABNORMALITY

Patients with all three forms of Gaucher's disease have subnormal activity of the enzyme glucocerebrosidase in their organs and tissues [6, 78]. This enzyme catalyzes the hydrolytic cleavage of glucose from glucocerebroside according to the following reaction:

$$\text{Glucocerebroside} + H_2O \xrightarrow{\text{glucocerebrosidase}} \text{ceramide} + \text{glucose}$$

On the basis of results obtained in an investigation of cerebroside synthesis in surviving human spleen tissue slices, the metabolic defect in Gaucher's disease was predicted several years before its demonstration. It was found that there was (1) no abnormality of galactose or glucose metabolism in tissues obtained from patients with Gaucher's disease, and (2) the rate of glucocerebroside synthesis was not accelerated. These observations led to the postulate that a deficiency of a glucocerebroside-catabolizing enzyme was the cause of lipid accumulation in this disorder [79]. This hypothesis was verified by investigating the metabolism of glucocerebroside that had been labeled in one preparation with ^{14}C in the glucose portion of the molecule and in another preparation with ^{14}C in the fatty acid moiety. All mammalian tissues that have been examined contain an enzyme which catalyzes the hydrolytic cleavage of glucose from glucocerebroside [80]. The activity of this enzyme in the organs and tissues of patients with Gaucher's disease is consistently less than that in normal individuals [6, 78]. This demonstration established the precedent of a deficiency of lipid-catabolizing enzyme, which has subsequently been shown to occur in all of the 10 known sphingolipid storage disorders. Although it has not been possible to demonstrate a consistent correlation between the degree of reduction of glucocerebrosidase activity with the severity of the clinical manifestations of the disorder [81], there are some indications that such a relationship may exist [78, 82]. More recent observations have shown that there are several isoenzymes of glucocerebrosidase in various tissues [83, 84]. Separation and measurement of the activities of the individual forms may provide a more consistent relationship between clinical status and enzymatic activity.

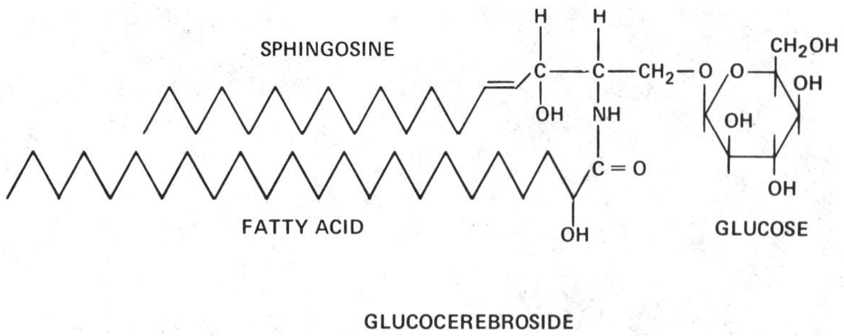

Figure 42-11   Structure of glucocerebroside (glucosylceramide). *(From Brady [2]. Used by permission.)*

Source of Accumulating Glucocerebroside

Erythrocytes normally contain some glucocerebroside, and some of the lipid accumulation in Gaucher's disease is derived from this material in senescent red blood cells. Erythrocytes contain other neutral sphingoglycolipids, such as ceramide lactoside (ceramide-glucose-galactose), ceramide trihexoside (ceramide-glucose-galactose-galactose), and globoside (ceramide-glucose-galactose-galactose-N-acetylgalactosamine). There are 3.4 nmol of glucocerebroside per milliliter of packed red blood cells, 14 nmol of ceramide lactoside, 11 nmol of ceramide trihexoside, and 64 nmol of globoside [85]. One molecule of glucocerebroside is derived from the catabolism of each molecule of the latter lipids. Other red cell lipids that give rise to glucocerebroside via erythrocytorrhexis and catabolism include paragloboside (ceramide-glucose-galactose-N-acetylglucosamine-galactose), A and B antigens, and sialic acid–containing lipids such as hematoside (ceramide-glucose-galactose-N-acetylneuraminic acid) and the major acidic glycolipid of red cells, ceramide-glucose-galactose-N-acetylglucosamine-galactose-N-acetylneuraminic acid [86].

The turnover of leukocytes constitutes another, and probably the major, source of accumulating glucocerebroside. Ceramide lactoside is the principal neutral glycolipid of white blood cells. It has been estimated that from 20 to 40 times more glucocerebroside arises during leukocyte turnover than from erythrocytes [87]. Some glucocerebroside probably also arises from the turnover of blood platelets. They contain the four major neutral glycolipids found in red cells as well as hematoside [88].

Because sphingolipids that contain glucosylceramide as a portion of their structure appear to be components of all mammalian cell membranes [2, 89–93], it seems likely that the accumulating glucocerebroside in Gaucher patients could arise from the normal turnover of cells in any tissue. It has been calculated that only a small fraction of the glucocerebroside catabolized each day actually accumulates in the organs of patients with Gaucher's disease [94]. Thus, it seems likely that there is a considerable excess of glucocerebrosidase activity in normal individuals. These deductions have important implications for enzyme replacement trials (see below).

A second aspect concerning glucocerebroside metabolism in Gaucher's disease is the extent of the liver and spleen enlargement in patients with this disorder. The extent of the hepatosplenomegaly seems disproportionately large in view of the fact that only a few milligrams of glucocerebroside accumulate per gram of tissue. Perhaps the organomegaly is due in part to an attempt by these tissues to compensate for the deficiency by providing additional enzyme resulting from the genetic defect. Creation of a hemolytic condition or the injection of lipids

from red cell stroma into normal animals elicits an effect of this type [95].

Another aspect that is difficult to resolve concerns the source of glucocerebroside in the brain of patients with type 2 and, presumably, type 3 Gaucher's disease. The major fatty acid in glucocerebroside isolated from the brain of Gaucher patients is stearic acid (C_{18}) rather than the normally predominant C_{24} fatty acids in cerebrosides [73, 75]. Because the fatty acid moiety in gangliosides is mainly stearic acid, Svennerholm [73] postulated that the accumulating glucocerebroside arose from the catabolism of gangliosides. Although Sudo [75] found less C_{18} fatty acid in cerebroside than Svennerholm, he also observed a considerable excess of this shorter-chain acid in the brain from Gaucher patients compared with that in control specimens. These observations appear to support the ganglioside origin of accumulating glucocerebroside. This deduction seems consistent with the rapid turnover of gangliosides in the neonatal period, followed by a dramatic reduction in ganglioside metabolism with maturation of the brain. The fact that there is no evidence of central nervous system involvement in most patients with type 1 Gaucher's disease has led to the supposition that these patients have sufficient residual glucocerebrosidase (or an appropriately active isoenzyme) in their brains to catalyze the hydrolysis of glucosylceramide that arises from ganglioside turnover [2].

A major difficulty in accepting the concept that gangliosides are the principal source of glucocerebroside in the nervous system is the fact that the Gaucherlike cells in the brain of patients with type 2 and type 3 Gaucher's disease (Fig. 42-5) have been convincingly demonstrated only in juxtavascular sites [1, 2, 19]. The possibility must be considered that these cells are caused by an accumulation of glucocerebroside which has been transported to this region from other organs by the circulation. The absence of a predominantly perivascular distribution of storage cells in other organs makes this hypothesis difficult to accept without invoking some special qualities of the storage cells in the Virchow-Robin spaces. It seems likely that this aspect of the pathogenesis of Gaucher's disease will be extraordinarily difficult to resolve until an authentic animal model of the disorder becomes available (see Ref. 96).

Gaucher Cells in Leukemia and Other Disorders

Gaucherlike cells have been reported in the spleen of as many as one-third of patients with chronic myelogenous leukemia [28–30, 87]. They have also been reported in multiple myeloma [27] and in dyserythropoietic anemia [32, 97]. It seems likely that the principal accumulating lipid in the leukemic patients may actually be lactosylceramide since the quantity of glucocerebroside in spleens from patients is only increased twofold over normal [87]. Furthermore, there are notable ultrastructural differences between the cells in these individuals compared with patients with Gaucher's disease [29]. The pathogenesis of the abnormal cells in the non-Gaucher conditions rests on a different basis from that in patients with a deficiency of glucocerebrosidase. Although the activity of this enzyme is known to be increased in circulating leukemic myelocytes [98], the ability of the engorged cells of the spleen to catabolize the excessive quantities of lipid that must be catabolized is presumably overwhelmed. This conclusion is still conjectural since the activity of these enzymes in the spleen of leukemic patients has apparently not been determined.

MOLECULAR BASIS OF GAUCHER'S DISEASE

The various clinical forms of Gaucher's disease are presumably due to structural alterations in the glucocerebrosidase molecule. Evidence in support of this hypothesis comes from a comparative study in which the enzymes from control human spleen tissue and from a patient with type 1 Gaucher's disease were co-purified through a 26,000-fold enrichment [99]. The most notable difference between the preparations was the reduction in the velocity of glucocerebroside hydrolysis (V_{max}) catalyzed by the enzyme from Gaucher spleen. Other parameters such as heat stability, K_m, and pH optimum were comparable to the control values. A further interesting finding was that the quantity of enzyme protein in normal and pathologic tissues appeared similar. The lack of increased cross-reacting material is consistent with similar observations in tissues from patients with other metabolic disorders [100–102].

Mutations at the same or different loci in the genetic code for glucocerebrosidase could result in varying degrees of catalytic activity. At present, there is no convincing evidence that different allelic or nonallelic mutations result in the various clinical types of Gaucher's disease. The failure to find examples of type 1 and type 2 disease in the same family suggests that they are different mutations. However, the occurrence of significantly different clinical severities in the same kindred or genetic group such as the Ashkenazim renders genetic conclusions premature. The fact that the amount of residual activity as measured in whole cell extracts does not correlate closely with clinical severity either between types or within types does not rule out this possibility. The assay of glucocerebrosidase using either natural or artificial substrates in vitro is clearly far removed from the milieu in which the membrane-bound lysosomal enzyme functions. In vitro conditions in which the highest specific activity of the enzyme is realized employ various detergents, buffers, and pH variations which may not reflect conditions in the intralysosomal environment of the enzyme that has been extracted from its hydrophobic surroundings. These circumstances, which are necessary in order to study the properties of the enzyme and to make its assay diagnostically useful, may so perturb the system that meaningful statements about its role in the pathogenesis in the various forms of Gaucher's disease cannot be made at our present level of sophistication. It is conceivable that a mutation could occur in the

enzyme that only partially affects the active site as measured in vitro but profoundly limits the accessibility of the poorly water-soluble glucosylceramide to the membrane-bound glucocerebrosidase. Even more simplistically, one could speculate that there are tissue-specific isoenzymes or posttranslational modifications of the enzyme protein [84] that result in decreased activity in one tissue more than another, thereby rendering assays performed on one tissue, such as leukocytes, inconclusive with respect to the activity in another, such as the brain. Moreover, there may be other factors, such as a heat-stable protein activator, whose presence in tissues may be variable. These speculations probably do not exhaust the list of possibilities that will eventually be shown to be involved in the molecular derangements in the various forms of this disorder. Solution of the genetic basis of Gaucher's disease and its clinical variations will likely be derived from studies on the primary structure of the enzyme and the isolation and characterization of the genes for this group of metabolic disorders.

DIAGNOSIS

The diagnosis of Gaucher's disease can be made on the basis of splenomegaly, and usually hepatomegaly, combined with the demonstration of Gaucher cells in bone marrow aspirates. The possibility of this disorder should always enter the differential diagnosis of infants with enlargement of the liver and spleen. Gaucher's disease should also be considered when patients present with thrombocytopenia or pathologic fractures, particularly if there is organomegaly. Elevation of serum nontartrate-inhibitable acid phosphatase is strongly suggestive of Gaucher's disease [11, 63, 103]. Substantiation of the diagnosis may be obtained by measuring the quantity of glucocerebroside in tissue samples. Needle biopsies of the liver are particularly useful in this regard. Although reliable procedures are available for the quantitation of glucocerebroside [75, 76, 78, 104, 105], the preferred method of making the diagnosis is by direct assay of glucocerebrosidase activity. This measurement has been greatly simplified by use of washed, sonicated leukocyte preparations obtained from small samples of venous blood [106]. Radioactively labeled glucocerebroside has characteristically been the most reliable substrate for this assay. Procedures for the chemical synthesis of [^{14}C]glucocerebroside [80] and [^{3}H]glucocerebroside [107] have been published; the latter compound is available from commercial sources. Considerable attention has been devoted to the use of the fluorogenic glycoside 4-methylumbelliferyl-β-D-glucopyranoside as substrate (Fig. 42-12) [108]. The principal difficulty encountered when using this material is that there are several β-glucosidases in mammalian tissues [83, 84, 109–111], and unless specific precautions are taken, unreliable results concerning glucocerebrosidase activity are obtained. Notable improvements in the method have been forthcoming following the original publication with the fluorogenic glucoside. These include the addition of sodium taurocholate [112, 113], sodium taurodeoxycholate [114], or sodium cholate and the detergent Cutscum [115] to the incubation medium to increase the specificity of the assay with regard to Gaucher's disease.

An even simpler procedure may be the separation of leukocyte homogenates into particulate and supernatant fractions.

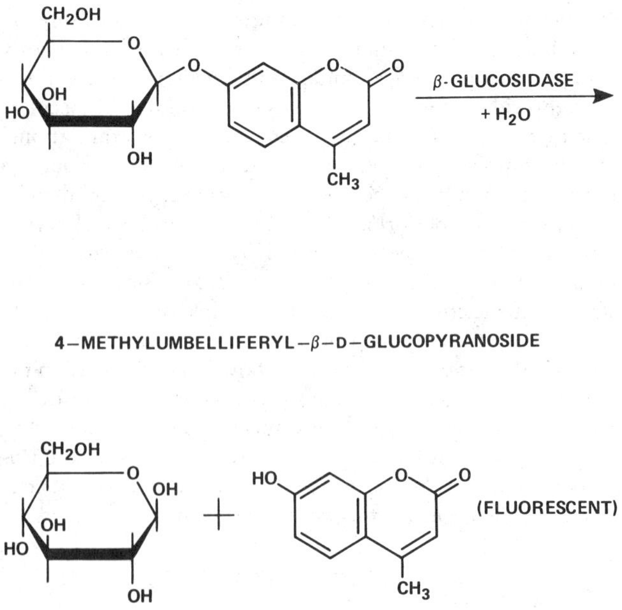

4−METHYLUMBELLIFERYL−β−D−GLUCOPYRANOSIDE

Figure 42-12 Structure of 4-methylumbelliferyl-β-D-glucopyranoside, a fluorogenic substrate for measuring β-glucosidase activity. *(From Brady [2]. Used by permission.)*

Because glucocerebrosidase is tightly bound to subcellular components, measuring β-glucosidase activity in particles may improve the diagnostic accuracy over that obtained in assays with whole homogenates [116].

Cultured skin fibroblasts are also a good source material for the diagnosis of Gaucher's disease. These cells contain a high level of glucocerebrosidase activity, and the enzyme in these cells is reasonably stable on freezing. Thus, they may be shipped in the frozen state to an appropriate laboratory for enzyme assay. [¹⁴C]Glucocerebroside has been used to validate the usefulness of these cells [117]. Many laboratories use the fluorogenic glucoside shown in Fig. 42-12 as substrate [118]. A number of modifications have been introduced to improve the specificity of the assay with this reagent [119–123].

The chromogenic substrate illustrated in Fig. 42-13 was synthesized and shown to be useful for the diagnosis of Gaucher's disease [124]. The procedure has been extended to assays with cultured skin fibroblasts, where its reliability has been demonstrated [125]. This chromogenic analogue of glucocerebroside is commercially available. Enzymatic estimation of the quantity of glucose released from nonlabeled glucocerebroside has been adapted for assays with fibroblast pellets [126].

Detection of Heterozygotes

Carriers of the Gaucher trait may be identified by assaying glucocerebrosidase activity in fresh peripheral leukocyte preparations using radioactively labeled glucocerebroside [8]. Heterozygote detection has also been reported using 4-methylumbelliferyl-β-D-glucopyranoside, although there was overlap between the enzymatic activity in specimens from obligatory heterozygotes and heterozygotes and that in noncarriers [108]. Improvements in the accuracy of carrier detection with the fluorogenic substrate are appearing [112–114].

Assay of glucocerebrosidase activity in cultured skin fibroblasts with labeled glucocerebroside as substrate is a reliable procedure for the detection of heterozygotes [8, 117]. The flu-

orogenic substrate has also been used for these assays [8, 108]. Proper selection of incubation conditions may be as essential with these cells as with leukocytes [119–123, 127]. Another critical factor for the detection of carriers is the mandatory use of a number of control cell cultures grown under identical conditions and harvested at the same time sufficient to provide statistically valid limits of normal. There is great variation in "normal" glucocerebrosidase activity in cultured cells obtained from different laboratories [128]. It seems likely that the chromogenic analogue of glucocerebroside (Fig. 42-13) also may become useful as a substrate for heterozygote identification with cultured fibroblasts [125].

Prenatal Diagnosis and Genetic Counseling

Gaucher's disease is an autosomal recessive disorder, and there is one chance in four that a child will be affected when both parents are carriers. The heterozygotes for types 1 and 2 can be collectively separated from normal individuals. Genetic counseling is available to such couples who are carriers, but no prediction as to phenotype (type 1 vs. type 2) can be made in the absence of prior typing of an affected child. The diagnosis of Gaucher's disease in utero was first demonstrated in 1972 using a radioactively labeled substrate to measure glucocerebrosidase activity in cultured aminocytes from a fetus at risk for type 2 Gaucher's disease [129]. The reliability of this procedure has been amply confirmed using glucocerebroside labeled with ¹⁴C in the fatty acid [130] or ³H in the sphingosine and fatty acid portions of the molecule [82]. Kitagawa and coworkers have also used enzymatic determination of glucose liberated from unlabeled glucocerebroside to monitor fetuses at risk for all three types of Gaucher's disease [131]. These investigators compared values with those obtained using 4-methylumbelliferyl-β-D-glucopyranoside as substrate. The flu-

Figure 42-13 Chromogenic substrate for measuring glucocerebrosidase activity. *(From Brady [2]. Used by permission.)*

2 - Hexadecanoylamino - 4 - Nitrophenyl - β - D - glucopyranoside

(Yellow Product)   Glucose

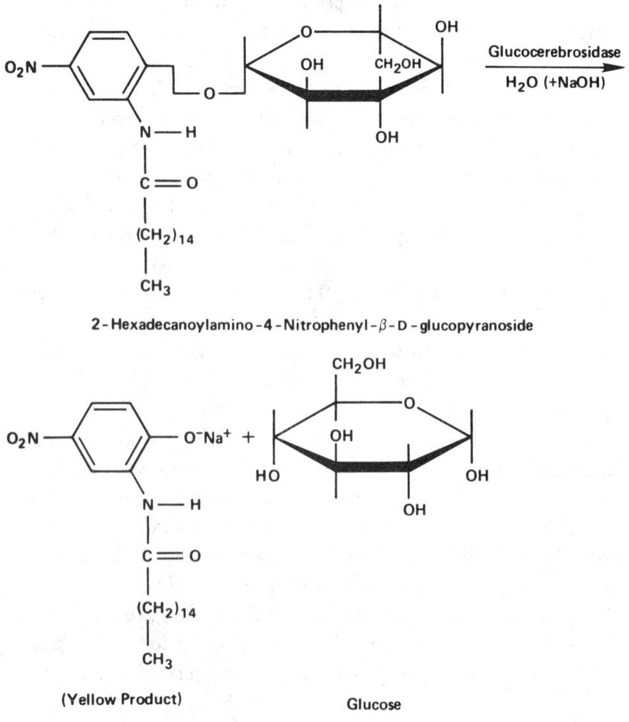

orogenic material could apparently be used to identify a type 3 Gaucher fetus correctly, although it did not seem to be as clear cut with cells from the fetus with type 1 Gaucher's disease. The fetus at risk for type 2 Gaucher's disease was judged to be normal based on glucosidase activity measured with the fluorogenic substrate. Confirmation of the reliability of artificial substrates for prenatal diagnosis of the various forms of Gaucher's disease is required. It is expected that the chromogenic analogue of glucocerebroside will also become useful for prenatal diagnosis of type 2 and type 3 Gaucher's disease.

TREATMENT

Supportive

Patients with Gaucher's disease require surveillance by hematologists throughout life. Attention must be directed to the number of platelets in the blood and to bleeding and clotting times. Many patients with Gaucher's disease require splenectomy because of thrombocytopenia and attendant hemorrhagic diathesis [1, 2, 36]. Some clinicians prefer to postpone splenectomy as long as possible because of potential acceleration of skeletal involvement following the operation, but this concept has been challenged [42]. Another aspect that requires the supervision of a hematologist is the anemia, which is usually improved by supplementation with vitamins, iron, or by splenectomy.

Pain in the bones and joints is a distressing problem for patients with Gaucher's disease and may require strong analgesics for relief. The progressive erosion of the hip, knee, and compression fractures of the vertebral bodies are common. Improved surgical techniques have led to increasing beneficial responses. It is difficult to guarantee success because of the progressive nature of the osteoporotic process and poor healing of involved bone.

Pulmonary involvement and pneumonia are frequent complications of Gaucher's disease and may be difficult to treat. An increasing number of patients have come to our attention with bleeding from esophageal varices due to cirrhotic changes in the liver.

Enzyme Replacement

Organ Allografts Knowledge of the enzymatic defect in Gaucher's disease and other storage disorders provided the conceptual basis for replacement strategies for the treatment of disorders of this type [132]. Early trials of spleen and kidney grafts were largely unsuccessful [2]. More recently a report has appeared regarding reduction of hepatic glucocerebroside in a type 3 patient following three renal transplants [133]. The clinical response was not encouraging and evidence of tissue rejection was apparent on autopsy. These results do not provide encouragement for the use of organ grafts as a source of enzymes. Since the amount of a particular catabolic enzyme appears to vary with the load of substrate that each tissue is required to degrade [95], we deduced that each tissue in the body synthesizes its own complement of biocatalysts [134]. Support for this hypothesis came from the results obtained by

van den Bergh and coworkers who found no evidence that α-galactosidase A had been transported from an apparently functioning kidney graft to the liver of a patient with Fabry's disease [135]. If enzyme replacement by tissue graft is to be pursued, it may be more reasonable to consider bone marrow replacement because enzymatically competent proliferating stem cells may be expected to migrate from the marrow to various organs, such as the spleen and liver, and may also be of help to the local bone problem [136].

Infusion of Purified Glucocerebrosidase The most extensive trials of enzyme replacement for a human metabolic disorder have been carried out in patients with Gaucher's disease. In the initial study intravenous injection of purified human placental glucocerebrosidase caused a reduction in the quantity of stored glucocerebroside in the liver and in the quantity of this material that was associated with circulating erythrocytes [76]. The fall in erythrocyte-associated glucocerebroside occurred progressively during the 3-day period following infusion of the enzyme. These kinetics are suggestive of a redistribution of the lipid from the circulation to recently cleared sites in tissues such as the liver. The reduction of red cell–associated glucocerebroside appeared to persist over a long period [137, 138]. A subsequent trial showed some, but proportionally less, reduction of hepatic glucocerebroside, and in this patient, no change in the elevated lipid in the blood was seen [139]. It appeared that considerably larger quantities of enzyme would be required to produce a significant reduction of the accumulated lipid in some patients with the disorder who store larger quantities of glucocerebroside than in the first two patients who received enzyme. Because the original method for isolation of the placental enzyme could not be scaled up sufficiently, another procedure was devised for purifying the enzyme in high yield [140]. Clinical trials with this enzyme have been made in four of six young males with type 1 Gaucher's disease who received the enzyme on a monthly or bimonthly schedule [134]. Various functions are being monitored to obtain firm information concerning the clinical responses in these recipients. The two individuals who did not appear to respond as satisfactorily had overt hepatic damage before the replacement trial was initiated.

It is clear that the ultimate benefit of enzyme replacement in Gaucher's disease, and in metabolic disorders in general, remains to be determined. A major problem is the highly preferential uptake of the exogenous placental enzyme by hepatocytes rather than by Kupffer cells where the lipid is stored [141]. This selectivity is probably due to the particular composition of the oligosaccharide portion of the glycoprotein enzyme. We have shown that sequential enzymatic removal of sugars leaving mannose as the terminal hexose results in a five-fold increase in Kupffer cell uptake of glucocerebrosidase [142]. An enzyme that has been altered in this fashion may be more clinically effective than the unmodified preparation. Trials with this product will be undertaken.

An alternative approach may be the chemical addition of mannose or mannose oligosaccharides [143] to placental glucocerebrosidase, and determination whether the Kupffer cell uptake of this modified enzyme is also enhanced. If these results are sufficiently encouraging, clinical trials with these preparations will be carried out. Although we [144] and others [145, 146] have convincingly demonstrated that infusion of unmodified placental glucocerebrosidase does not elicit antibody production, further careful monitoring of patients will be mandatory if the carbohydrate-modified preparations are used.

Finally, consideration must be given to the possibility of enzyme replacement for patients with type 2 and type 3 Gaucher's disease. Since most of the storage cells in patients with type 3 appear to be in the Virchow-Robin spaces, it is possible that combined intravenous and intrathecal injection of enzyme may be beneficial. With regard to type 2 patients, a similar approach may be helpful, but if the enzyme must be delivered to the interior of the brain, it will probably be necessary to resort to blood-brain barrier modification so that the exogenous enzyme can reach cells within the central nervous system [147].

REFERENCES

1. FREDRICKSON DS, SLOAN HR: Glucosyl ceramide lipidoses: Gaucher's disease, in Stanbury JB, Wyngaarden JB, Fredrickson DS (eds): *The Metabolic Basis of Inherited Disease*, 3d ed. New York, McGraw-Hill, 1972, p 730

2. BRADY RO: Glucosyl ceramide lipidosis: Gaucher's disease, in Stanbury JB, Wyngaarden JB, Fredrickson DS (eds): *The Metabolic Basis of Inherited Disease*, 4th ed. New York, McGraw-Hill, 1978, p 731

3. GAUCHER PCE: De l'Épithéliome primitif de la rate. *Thèse de Paris*, 1882

4. LIEB H: Cerebrosidespeicherung bei Morbus Gaucher. *Z Physiol Chem* 140:305, 1924

5. AGHION A: La Maladie de Gaucher dans l'enfance (forme cardiorénale). *Thèsis*, Paris, 1934

6. BRADY RO, KANFER JN, SHAPIRO D: Metabolism of glucocerebrosides. II. Evidence of an enzymatic deficiency in Gaucher's disease. *Biochem Biophys Res Commun* 18:221, 1965

7. KOLODNY EH, RAGHAVAN SS, TOPOL J, SPIELVOGEL C: Gaucher's disease: Estimate of gene frequency among Ashkenazim by leukocyte β-glucosidase assay. Seventh Meeting of the International Society for Neurochemistry, Sept. 2–6, 1979, Jerusalem, Abstract, p 425

8. BRADY RO, JOHNSON WG, UHLENDORF BW: Identification of heterozygous carriers of lipid storage diseases. *Am J Med* 51:423, 1971

9. BRINN L, GLAUBMAN S: Gaucher's disease without splenomegaly: Oldest patient on record, with review. *NY J Med* 62:2346, 1962

10. BLOCK M, JACOBSEN LO: The histiogenesis and diagnosis of the osseous type of Gaucher's disease. *Acta Haemat (Basel)* 1:165, 1948

11. TUCHMAN LR, SUNA H, CARR JJ: Elevation of serum acid phosphatase in Gaucher's disease. *J Mt Sinai Hosp* 23:277, 1956

12. TELIUM G: Die Gauschersche Krankheit mit der Beschreibung eines Falles, der Veranderungen in der Hypophyse und in Hypothalamus Zeigte. *Acta Med Scand* 116:170, 1944

13. HODSON P, GOLDBLATT J, BEIGHTON P: Non-neuronopathic Gaucher's disease presenting in infancy. *Arch Dis Child* 54:707, 1979

14. MILLER JD, MCCLUER R, KANFER JN: Gaucher's disease: Neurologic disorder in adult siblings. *Ann Intern Med* 78:833, 1973

15. KING TO: Progressive myoclonic epilepsy due to Gaucher's disease in an adult. *J Neurol Neurosurg Psychiatr* 38:849, 1975

16. MELAMED E, COHEN C, SOFFER D, LAVY S: Central nervous system complication in a patient with chronic Gaucher's disease. *Eur Neurol* 13:167, 1975

17. BENJAMIN D, DOUER D, PICK AI, ZER M, DINTSMAN M, PINKHAS J: Peripheral cryoglobulinemic neuropathy in a patient with Gaucher's disease. *Acta Haemat* 60:117, 1978

18. NEIL JF, GLEW RH, PETERS SP: Familial psychosis and diverse neurologic abnormalities in adult-onset Gaucher's disease. *Arch Neurol* 36:95, 1979

19. SOFFER D, YAMANAKA T, WENGER DA, SUZUKI K, SUZUKI K: Central nervous system involvement in adult-onset Gaucher's disease. *Acta Neuropathol* 49:1, 1980

20. NISHIMURA RN, OMOS-LAU C, AJAMONE-MARSAN C, BARRANGER JA: Electroencephalographic findings in Gaucher's disease. *Neurology* 30:152, 1980

21. DIEZEL PB: Histochemische Untersuchungen an den Globoidzellen der familiaren infantilen diffusen Sklerose vom Typus Krabbe (Zugleich eine differentialdiagnostiche Betrachtun der zentralnervosen Veranderungen beim Morbus Gaucher). *Virchow Arch (Pathol Anat)* 327:206, 1955

22. PETERS SP, LEE RE, GLEW RH: Gaucher's disease: A review and discussion of twenty cases. *Medicine* 56:424, 1977

23. SACK G: Clinical diversity in Gaucher's disease. *Johns Hopkins Med J* 146:166, 1980

24a. NEIL JF, MERIKANGAS JR, GLEW RH: EEG findings in adult neuronopathic Gaucher's disease. *Clin Electroencephalo* 10:198, 1979

24b. NISHIMURA RN, BARRANGER JA: Neurologic complications of Gaucher's disease Type 3. *Arch Neurol* 37:92, 1980

25. BURNS GF, CAWLEY JC, FLEMANS RJ, HIGGY KE, WORMAN CP, BARKER CR, ROBERTS BE, HAYHOE FGJ: Surface marker and other characteristics of Gaucher cells. *J Clin Pathol* 30:981, 1977

26. DJALDETTI M, FISHMAN P, BESSLER H: The surface ultrastructure of Gaucher cells. *Am J Clin Pathol* 71:146, 1979

27. SCULLIN DC, SHELBURNE JD, COHEN JD: Pseudo-Gaucher cells in multiple myeloma. *Am J Med* 67:347, 1979

28. ALBRECHT M: "Gaucher-Zellen" bei chronisch myeloidischer leukemie. *Blut* 13:169, 1966

29. LEE RE, ELLIS LD: The storage cells of chronic myelogenous leukemia. *Lab Invest* 24:261, 1971

30. HAYHOE FGJ, FLEMANS RJ, COWLING DC: Acquired lipidosis of marrow macrophages: Birefringent blue crystals and Gaucher-like cells, sea-blue histiocytes, and grey-green crystals. *J Clin Pathol* 32:420, 1979

31. ZAINO ED, ROSSI MB, PHAM TD, AZAR HA: Gaucher's cells in thalassaemia. *Blood* 38:457, 1971

32. ENQUIST RW, GOCKERMAN JP, JENIS MC, RAPHAEL ML, DILLON E: Type II congenital dyserythropoietic anemia. *Ann Intern Med* 77:371, 1972

33. BRADY RO, KING FM: Gaucher's disease, in Hers HG, van Hoof F (eds): *Lysosomes and Storage Diseases*. New York, Academic, 1973, p 381

34. LEE RE: The fine structure of the cerebroside occurring in Gaucher's disease. *Proc Nat Acad Sci USA* 61:484, 1968

35. ABE T, YAMAKAWA T, ENDOU H, NAGASHIMA K: Disc gel electrophoresis of proteins of membranous cytoplasmic inclusion bodies from the spleen of the patient with Gaucher's disease. *Jap J Exp Med* 48:177, 1978

36. SALKY B, KREEL I, GELERNT I, BAUER J, AUFSES AH JR: Splenectomy for Gaucher's disease. *Ann Surg* 190:592, 1979

37. GROTH CG, COLLSTE H, DREBORG S, HAKANSSON G, LUNDGREN G, SVENNERHOLM L: Attempt at enzyme replacement in Gaucher disease by renal transplantation, in Desnick RJ (ed): *Enzyme Therapy in Genetic Diseases 2*. New York, Alan R Liss, 1980, p 475

38. JAMES SP, STROMEYER FW, CHANG C, BARRANGER JA: Liver abnormalities in patients with Gaucher's disease. *Gastroenterology* 80:126, 1981

39. SMITH RRL, HUTCHINS GM, SACK GH JR, RIDOLFI RL: Unusual cardiac, renal, and pulmonary involvement in Gaucher's disease. Interstitial glucocerebroside accumulation, pulmonary hypertension, and fatal bone marrow embolization. *Am J Med* 65:352, 1978

40. CHANDER PN, NURSE HM, PIRANI CL: Renal involvement in adult Gaucher's disease after splenectomy. *Arch Pathol Lab Med* 103:440, 1979

41. SCHNEIDER EL, EPSTEIN CJ, KABACK MJ, BRANDES D: Severe pulmonary involvement in adult Gaucher's disease. Report of three cases and review of the literature. *Am J Med* 63:475, 1977

42. GOLDBLATT J, SACKS S, BEIGHTON P: The orthopedic aspects of Gaucher disease. *Clin Orthop* 137:208, 1978

43. BROWNE WG: Oral pigmentation and root resorption in Gaucher's disease. *J Oral Surg* 35:153, 1977

44. COGAN DG, ADAMS RD: A type of paralysis of conjugate gaze (ocular motor apraxia). *Arch Ophthalmol* 50:434, 1953

45. BLATTNER RJ: Gaucher's disease: Abnormalities in immunoglobulin. *J Pediatr* 73:626, 1968

46. PRATT PW, ESTREN S, KOCHWA S: Immunoglobulin abnormalities in Gaucher's disease. Report of 16 cases. *Blood* 31:633, 1968

47. MACDONALD M, MCCATHIE M, FAED MJW, PRINGLE R, GOODALL HB, BECK JS, TUDHOPE GR, MITCHELL PEG, WOOD AJJ, GUTHRIE W, SHAW D: Gaucher's disease with biclonal gammopathy. *J Clin Pathol* 28:757, 1975

48. WOLF P: Monoclonal gammopathy in Gaucher's disease. *Lab Med* 4:28, 1973

49. TURESSON I, RAUSING A: Gaucher's disease and benign monoclonal gammopathy. A case report with immonofluorescence study of bone marrow and spleen. *Acta Med Scand* 197:507, 1975

50. DIKMAN SH, GOLDSTEIN M, KAHN T, LEO MA, WEINREB N: Amyloidosis: An unusual complication of Gaucher's disease. *Arch Pathol Lab Med* 102:460, 1978

51. HANASH SM, RUCKNAGEL DL, HEIDELBERGER KP, RADIN NS: Primary amyloidosis associated with Gaucher's disease. *Ann Intern Med* 89:639, 1978

52. PINKHAS J, DJALDETTI M, YARON M: Coincidence of multiple myeloma with Gaucher's disease. *Israel J Med Sci* 1:537, 1965

53. BENJAMIN D, JOSHUA H, DJALDETTI M, HAZAZ B, PINKHAS J: Nonsecretory IgD-kappa multiple myeloma in a patient with Gaucher's disease. *Scand J Haematol* 22:179, 1979

54. RUESTOW PC, LEVINSON DJ, CATCHATOURIAN R, SREEKANTH S, COHEN H, ROSENFELD S: Coexistence of IgA myeloma and Gaucher's disease. *Arch Intern Med* 140:1115, 1980

55. GELFAND MI, GRIBOFF SI: Gaucher's disease and acute leukemia. *J Mt Sinai Hosp NY* 28:278, 1961

56. KRAUSE JR, BURES C, LEE RE: Acute leukemia and Gaucher's disease. *Scand J Haematol* 23:115, 1979

57. SHAVER LR, BRANDES JA, SILVER RT, GRAY GF: Association of Hodgkin's disease and Gaucher's disease. *Arch Pathol* 98:376, 1974

58. CHO SY, SASTRE M: Coexistence of Hodgkin's disease and Gaucher's disease. *Am J Clin Pathol* 65:103, 1976

59. BRUCKSTEIN AH, KARANAS A, DIRE JJ: Gaucher's disease associated with Hodgkin's disease. *Am J Med* 68:610, 1980

60. DAVIS M, DORFMAN J: Gaucher's disease associated with a cerebral astrocytoma. *Am Pract* 12:673, 1961

61. TSUNG SW, COTES E: Coexistence of bronchogenic carcinoma and Gaucher's disease. *Arch Pathol Lab Med* 101:56, 1977

62. GERY I, ZIGLER JS JR, BRADY RO, BARRANGER JA: Selective effects of glucocerebroside (Gaucher's storage material) on macrophage cultures. *J Clin Invest* 68:1182, 1981

63. ROBINSON DB, GLEW RH: Acid phosphatase in Gaucher's disease. *Clin Chem* 26:371, 1980

64. LIEBERMAN J, BEUTLER E: Elevation of serum angiotensin-converting enzyme in Gaucher's disease. *N Engl J Med* 294:1442, 1976

65. SILVERSTEIN E, FRIEDLAND J: Elevated serum and spleen angiotensin converting enzyme and serum lysozyme in Gaucher's disease. *Clin Chim Acta* 74:21, 1977

66. ÖCKERMAN PA, KAHLIN P: Acid hydrolases in plasma in Gaucher's disease. *Clin Chem* 15:61, 1969

67. MOFFITT KD, CHAMBERS JP, DIVEN WF, GLEW RH, WENGER DA, FARRELL DF: Characterization of lysosomal hydrolases that are elevated in Gaucher's disease. *Arch Biochem Biophys* 190:247, 1978

68. HULTBERG B, ISAKSSON A, SJOBLOD S, ÖCKERMAN PA: Acid hydrolases in serum from patients with lysosomal disorders. *Clin Chim Acta* 100:33, 1980

69. WEINREB NJ: Serum and splenic lysozyme in Gaucher's disease. *Clin Res* 24:295A, 1976

70. GILBERT HS, WEINREB NJ: Increased circulating levels of transcobalamin II in Gaucher's disease. *N Engl J Med* 295:1096, 1976

71. BOKLAN BF, SAWITSKY A: Factor IX deficiency in Gaucher's disease. An *in vitro* phenomenon. *Arch Intern Med* 136:489, 1976

72. BENJAMIN D, JOSHUA H, DOUER D, SHAKLAI M, KRUGLIAC Y, PINKHAS J: Circulating anticoagulant in patients with Gaucher's disease. *Acta Haemat* 61:233, 1979

73. SVENNERHOLM L: Metabolism of gangliosides in cerebral lipidoses, in Aronson SM, Volk BW (eds): *Inborn Disorders of Sphingolipid Metabolism*. New York, Pergamon, 1967, p 169

74. DREBORG S: Personal communication, 1980

75. SUDO M: Brain glycolipids in infantile Gaucher's disease. *J Neurochem* 29:379, 1977

76. BRADY RO, PENTCHEV PG, GAL AE, HIBBERT SR, DEKABAN AS: Replacement therapy for inherited enzyme deficiency: Use of purified glucocerebrosidase in Gaucher's disease. *N Engl J Med* 291:989, 1974

77. BRADFIELD JWB, SOUHAMI RL: Hepatocyte damage secondary to Kupffer cell phagocytosis, in Liehr H, Grun M (eds): *The Reticuloendothelial System and the Pathogenesis of Liver Disease*. New York, Elsevier, 1980, p 165

78. BRADY RO, KANFER JN, BRADLEY RM, SHAPIRO D: Demonstration of a deficiency of glucocerebroside-cleaving enzyme in Gaucher's disease. *J Clin Invest* 45:1112, 1966

79. TRAMS EG, BRADY RO: Cerebroside synthesis in Gaucher's disease. *J Clin Invest* 39:1546, 1960

80. BRADY RO, KANFER JN, SHAPIRO D: The metabolism of glucocerebrosides. I. Purification and properties of a glucocerebroside-cleaving enzyme from spleen tissue. *J Biol Chem* 240:39, 1965

81. PENTCHEV PG, BARRANGER JA, GAL AE, FURBISH FS, BRADY RO: Incorporation of exogenous enzymes into lysosomes. A theoretical and practical means for correcting lysosomal blockage, in Walborg EF Jr (ed): *Glycoproteins and Glycolipids in Disease Processes*. Washington, DC, American Chemical Society Symposium Series No. 80, 1978, p 150

82. HARZER K: Enzymic diagnosis in 27 cases with Gaucher's disease. *Clin Chim Acta* 106:9, 1980

83. MARET A, SALVAYRE R, NEGRE A, DOUSTEBLAZY L: Electrofocusing separation of molecular forms of splenic beta-glucosidase in normal subject and Gaucher's disease. *Biomedicine* 33:80, 1980

84. GINNS EI, BRADY RO, STOWENS DE, FURBISH FS, BARRANGER JA: A new group of glucocerebrosidase isozymes found in human white blood cells. *Biochem Biophys Res Commun* 97:1103, 1980

85. YAMAKAWA T, NAGAI Y: Glycolipids at the cell surface and their biological functions. *Trends in Biochem Sciences* 3:128, 1978

86. WHERRETT JR: Characterization of the major ganglioside in human red cells and of a related tetrahexosylceramide in white cells. *Biochim Biophys Acta* 326:63, 1973

87. KATTLOVE HE, WILLIAMS JC, GAYNOR E, SPIVACK M, BRADLEY RM, BRADY RO: Gaucher cells in chronic myelocytic leukemia: An acquired abnormality. *Blood* 33:379, 1969

88. SNYDER PD JR, DESNICK RJ, KRIVIT W: The glycosphingolipids and gly-

cosyl hydrolases of human blood platelets. *Biochem Biophys Res Commun* 46:1857, 1972

89. O'BRIEN JS: The gangliosidoses, in Stanbury JB, Wyngaarden JB, Fredrickson DS, Goldstein JL, Brown MS (eds): *The Metabolic Basis of Inherited Disease*, 5th ed. New York, McGraw-Hill, 1982

90. KWITEROVICH PO, SLOAN HR, FREDRICKSON DS: Glycolipids and other lipid constituents of normal human liver. *J Lipid Res* 11:322, 1970

91. MARTENSSON E: Neutral glycolipids of human kidney: Isolation, identification and fatty acid composition. *Biochim Biophys Acta* 116:196, 1966

92. MULLIN BR, PACUSZKA T, LEE G, KOHN L, BRADY RO, FISHMAN PH: Thyroid gangliosides with high affinity for tyrotropin: Potential role in thyroid regulation. *Science* 78:77, 1978

93. SWEELEY CC: *Cell Surface Glycolipids*, Washington DC, American Chemical Society Symposium Series No. 128, 1980

94. BRADY RO, PENTCHEV PG, GAL AE: Investigations in enzyme replacement therapy in lipid storage diseases. *Fed Proc* 34:1310, 1975

95. KAMPINE JP, KANFER JN, GAL AE, BRADLEY RM, BRADY RO: Response of sphingolipid hydrolases in spleen and liver to increased erythrocytorrhexis. *Biochim Biophys Acta* 137:135, 1967

96. VANDEWATER NS, JOLLY RD, FARROW BRH: Canine Gaucher disease— Enzymic defect. *Aust J Exp Biol Med Sci* 57:551, 1979

97. VAN DORPE A, BROECKAERT-VAN ORSHOVEN A, DESMET V, VERWILGHEN RL: Gaucher-like cells and congenital dyserythropoietic anaemia, type II (HEMPAS). *Brit J Haematol* 25:165, 1973

98. KAMPINE JP, BRADY RO, YANKEE RA, KANFER JN, SHAPIRO D, GAL AE: Sphingolipid hydrolases in leukemic leukocytes. *Cancer Res* 27:1312, 1967

99. PENTCHEV PG, BRADY RO, BLAIR HE, BRITTON DE, SORRELL SH: Gaucher disease: Isolation and comparison of normal and mutant glucocerebrosidase from human spleen tissue. *Proc Nat Acad Sci USA* 75:3970, 1978

100. STUMPF D, NEUWELT A, AUSTIN J, KOHLER P: Metachromatic leukodystrophy (MLD). X. Immunological studies of the abnormal sulfatase A. *Arch Neurol* 25:427, 1971

101. MEISLER M, RATTAZZI MC: Immunological studies of β-galactosidase in normal human liver and in G_{M1} gangliosidosis. *Am J Hum Genet* 26:683, 1974

102. SRIVASTAVA SK, ANSARI NH, HAWKINS LA, WIKTOROWICZ JE: Demonstration of cross-reacting material in Tay-Sachs disease. *Biochem J* 179:657, 1979

103. ROBINSON DB, GLEW RH: A tartrate-resistant acid phosphatase from Gaucher spleen: Purification and properties. *J Biol Chem* 255:5864, 1980

104. OSHIMA M, ARIGA T, MURATA T: Combined gas chromatography–chemical ionization mass spectrometry of sphingolipids. I. Glucosyl sphingosine, ceramides and cerebroside of the spleen in Gaucher's disease. *Chem Phys Lipids* 19:289, 1977

105. ULLMAN MD, PYERITZ RE, MOSER HW, WENGER DA, KOLODNY EH: Application of "high performance" liquid chromatography to the study of sphingolipidoses. *Clin Chem* 26:1499, 1980

106. KAMPINE JP, BRADY RO, KANFER JN, FELD M, SHAPIRO D: Diagnosis of Gaucher's disease and Niemann-Pick disease with small samples of venous blood. *Science* 155:86, 1967

107. McMASTER MC, RADIN NS: Preparation of 6-³H glucocerebroside. *J Label Comp Radiopharm* 8:353, 1977

108. BEUTLER E, KUHL W: Diagnosis of the adult type of Gaucher's disease and its carrier state by demonstration of a deficiency of glucosidase activity in peripheral blood leukocytes. *J Lab Clin Med* 76:747, 1970

109. PENTCHEV PG, BRADY RO, HIBBERT SR, GAL AE, SHAPIRO D: Isolation and characterization of glucocerebrosidase from human placental tissue. *J Biol Chem* 248:5256, 1973

110. FREESE A, BRADY RO, GAL AE: A β-glucosidase in feline kidney that hydrolyzes amygdalin (Laetrile). *Arch Biochem Biophys* 201:363, 1980

111. YAQOOB M, CARROLL M: Isoenzymes of membrane-bound β-glucosidase of human spleen. *Biochem J* 185:541, 1980

112. TURNER BM, BERATIS NG, HIRSCHHORN K: Cell-specific differences in membrane β-glucosidase from normal and Gaucher cells. *Biochim Biophys Acta* 480:442, 1977

113. WENGER DA, CLARK C, SATTLER M, WHARTON C: Synthetic substrate β-glucosidase activity in leukocytes: A reproducible method for the identification of patients and carriers of Gaucher's disease. *Clin Genet* 13:145, 1978

114. RAGHAVAN SS, TOPOL J, KOLODNY EH: Leukocyte β-glucosidase in homozygotes and heterozygotes for Gaucher's disease. *Am J Hum Genet* 32:158, 1980

115. SVENNERHOLM L, HAKANSSON G, DREBORG S: Assay of the β-glucosidase activity with natural labelled and artificial substrates in leukocytes from homozygotes and heterozygotes with the Norrbottnian type (Type 3) of Gaucher's disease. *Clin Chim Acta* 106:183, 1980

116. BRADY RO: Haematological aspects of lipid storage diseases. *Acta Haemat Pol* 8:103, 1977

117. HO MW, SECK J, SCHMIDT ML, JOHNSON W, BRADY RO, O'BRIEN JS:

Adult Gaucher's disease: Kindred studies and demonstration of a deficiency of acid β-glucosidase in cultured fibroblasts. *Am J Hum Genet* 24:37, 1972

118. BEUTLER E, KUHL W, TRINIDAD F, TEPLITZ R, NADLER H: β-Glucosidase activity in fibroblasts from homozygotes and heterozygotes for Gaucher's disease. *Am J Hum Genet* 23:62, 1971

119. CHOY FYM, DAVIDSON RG: Gaucher's disease. I. Solubilization and electrophoresis of β-glucosidase from leukocytes and cultured fibroblasts. *Pediatr Res* 12:1115, 1978

120. TURNER BM, HIRSCHHORN K: Properties of β-glucosidase in cultured skin fibroblasts from control and patients with Gaucher disease. *Am J Hum Genet* 30:346, 1978

121. BUTTERWORTH J, BROADHEAD DM: Gaucher's disease. Factors affecting the 4-methylumbelliferyl-β-D-glucosidase activity of cultured skin fibroblasts. *Clin Genet* 14:77, 1978

122. MUELLER OT, ROSENBERG A: Activation of membrane-bound glucosylceramide:β-glucosidase in fibroblasts cultured from normal and glucosylceramidotic human skin. *J Biol Chem* 254:3521, 1979

123. CHOY FYM, DAVIDSON RG: Gaucher's disease II. Studies on the kinetics of β-glucosidase and the effects of sodium taurocholate in normal and Gaucher tissues. *Pediatr Res* 14:54, 1980

124. GAL AE, PENTCHEV PG, FASH FJ: A novel chromogenic substrate for assaying glucocerebrosidase activity. *Proc Soc Exp Biol Med* 153:363, 1976

125. JOHNSON WG, GAL AE, MIRANDA AF, PENTCHEV PG: Diagnosis of adult Gaucher disease: Use of a new chromogenic substrate, 2-hexadecanoylamino-4-nitrophenyl-β-D-glucopyranoside, in cultured skin fibroblasts. *Clin Chim Acta* 102:91, 1980

126. CHOY FYM, DAVIDSON RG: Gaucher disease. III. Substrate specificity of glucocerebrosidase and the use of nonlabeled natural substrates for the investigation of patients. *Am J Hum Genet* 32:670, 1980

127. HAKANSSON G, DREBORG S, LINDSTEN J, SVENNERHOLM L: Assay of the β-glucosidase activity with natural labelled and artificial substrates in cultivated skin fibroblasts from homozygotes and heterozygotes with the Norrbottnian type of Gaucher disease. *Clin Genet* 18:268, 1980

128. GAL AE, BRADY RO, HIBBERT SR, PENTCHEV PG: A practical chromogenic procedure for the detection of homozygotes and heterozygous carriers of Niemann-Pick disease. *N Engl J Med* 293:632, 1975

129. SCHNEIDER EL, ELLIS WG, BRADY RO, MCCULLOCH JR, EPSTEIN CJ: Infantile (Type II) Gaucher's disease: In utero diagnosis and fetal pathology. *J Pediatr* 81:1134, 1972

130. CHAZAN S, ZITMAN D, KLIBANSKY C: Prenatal diagnosis of Gaucher's and Niemann-Pick diseases. Assays of glucocerebrosidase and sphingomyelinase in tissue cultures using natural substrates. *Clin Chim Acta* 86:45, 1978

131. KITAGAWA T, OWADA M, SAKIYAMA T, AOKI K, KAMOSHITA S, AMENOMORI Y, KOBAYASHI T: In utero diagnosis of Gaucher's disease. *Am J Hum Genet* 30:322, 1978

132. BRADY RO: The sphingolipidoses. *N Engl J Med* 275:312, 1966

133. GROTH SC, COLLSTE H, DREBORG S, HAKANSSON G, LUNDGREN G, SVENNERHOLM L: Attempt at enzyme replacement in Gaucher disease by renal transplantation. *Acta Paediatr Scand* 68:475, 1979

134. BRADY RO, BARRANGER JA, PENTCHEV PG, FURBISH FS, GAL AE: Prospects for enzyme replacement therapy in heritable metabolic disorders, in Aebi H, Herschkowitz NN (eds): *Inborn Errors of Metabolism in Humans.* London, MTP, 1981, in press

135. VAN DEN BERGH FAJTM, RIETRA PJGM, KOLK-VEGTER AJ, BOSCH E, TAGER JM: Therapeutic implications of renal transplantation in a patient with Fabry disease. *Acta Med Scand* 200:249, 1976

136. SLAVIN S, YATZIV S: Correction of enzyme deficiency in mice by allogenic bone marrow transplantation with total lymphoid irradiation. *Science* 210:1150, 1980

137. PENTCHEV PG, BRADY RO, GAL AE, HIBBERT SR: Replacement therapy for inherited enzyme deficiency: Sustained clearance of accumulated glucocerebroside in Gaucher's disease following infusion of purified glucocerebrosidase. *J Mol Med* 1:73, 1975

138. BRADY RO: Heritable catabolic and anabolic disorders of lipid metabolism. *Metabolism* 26:329, 1977

139. BRADY RO, PENTCHEV PG, GAL AE, HIBBERT SR, QUIRK JM, MOOK GE, KUSIAK JW, TALLMAN JF, DEKABAN AS: Enzyme replacement therapy for sphingolipidoses, in Volk BW, Schneck L (eds): *Current Trends in Sphingolipidoses and Allied Disorders.* New York, Plenum, 1976, p 532

140. FURBISH FS, BLAIR HE, SHILOACH J, PENTCHEV PG, BRADY RO: Enzyme replacement therapy in Gaucher's disease: Large-scale purification of glucocerebrosidase suitable for human administration. *Proc Nat Acad Sci USA* 74:3560, 1977

141. FURBISH FS, STEER CJ, BARRANGER JA, JONES EA, BRADY RO: The uptake of native and desialylated glucocerebrosidase by rat hepatocytes and Kupffer cells. *Biochem Biophys Res Commun* 81:1047, 1978

142. FURBISH FS, STEER CJ, KRETT NL, BARRANGER JA: Uptake and distribution of placental glucocerebrosidase in rat hepatic cells and effects of sequential deglycosylation. *Biochim Biophys Acta* 673:425, 1981

143. BRADY RO, BARRANGER JA, GAL AE, PENTCHEV PG, FURBISH FS: Status of enzyme replacement therapy for Gaucher's disease, in Desnick RJ (ed): *Enzyme Therapy in Genetic Diseases 2.* New York, Alan R Liss, 1980, p 361

144. BRITTON DE, LEINIKKI PO, BARRANGER JA, BRADY RO: Gaucher's disease: Lack of antibody response to intravenous glucocerebrosidase. *Life Sciences* 23:2517, 1978

145. BEUTLER E, DALE GL, KUHL W: Replacement therapy in Gaucher's disease, in Desnick RJ (ed): *Enzyme Therapy in Genetic Disease 2.* New York, Alan R Liss, 1980, p 369

146. GREGORIADIS G, NEERUNJUN D, MEADE TW, GOOLAMALI SK, WEERERATNE H, BULL G: Experiences after long-term treatment of a Type I Gaucher patient with liposome-entrapped glucocerebroside-β-glucosidase, in Desnick RJ (ed): *Enzyme Therapy in Genetic Diseases 2.* New York, Alan R Liss, 1980, p 383

147. BARRANGER JA, RAPOPORT SI, FREDERICKS WR, PENTCHEV PG, MACDERMOT KD, STEUSING JK, BRADY RO: Modification of the blood-brain barrier: Increased concentration and fate of enzymes entering the brain. *Proc Nat Acad Sci USA* 76:481, 1979

43

GALACTOSYLCERAMIDE LIPIDOSIS:
Globoid Cell Leukodystrophy (Krabbe's Disease)

KUNIHIKO SUZUKI

YOSHIYUKI SUZUKI

1. Krabbe's globoid cell leukodystrophy *is a rapidly progressive, invariably fatal disease of infants. The onset of symptoms is usually between ages 3 to 6 months. The disease usually begins with ambiguous symptoms such as irritability or hypersensitivity to external stimuli, but soon progresses to severe mental and motor deterioration. Long-tract signs are prominent. There is hypertonicity with hyperactive reflexes in the early stages, but patients later become flaccid and hypotonic. Blindness and deafness are common. Patients rarely survive the second year. There are clinical and laboratory signs of peripheral neuropathic change. Systemic manifestations are rare. The disease is transmitted as an autosomal recessive trait.*

2. *The presence of numerous multinucleated globoid cells in the white matter is the morphological basis for diagnosis. The globoid cells are macrophages of mesodermal origin that accumulate galactocerebroside. Severe myelin loss and astrocytic gliosis complete the pathologic picture in the white matter. Axonal degeneration, fibrosis, and histiocyte infiltration are also common in the peripheral nervous system.*

3. *Consistent with myelin loss, the white matter is depleted of all lipids, particularly glycolipids. The ratio of residual galactocerebroside to sulfatide is abnormally high. Galactocerebroside (Fig. 43-1) is a sphingoglycolipid containing sphingosine, fatty acid, and* galactose, normally found almost exclusively in the nervous system.

4. *The cause of Krabbe's disease is deficient activity of galactocerebroside β-galactosidase. This lysosomal enzyme normally cleaves galactocerebroside to ceramide and galactose. The defect is generalized and has been detected in brain, liver, spleen, kidney, peripheral leukocytes, serum, and cultured fibroblasts. It is postulated that accumulation of galactocerebroside and possibly of its deacylated derivative, psychosine, which is also a substrate for the missing enzyme, leads to destruction of oligodendroglia, the cells which produce myelin. The total brain content of galactocerebroside is thus not increased.*

5. *Assays of galactocerebroside β-galactosidase in white cells, serum, or cultured fibroblasts with the use of appropriate natural glycolipid substrates provide the means for definitive antemortem diagnosis of the disease.*

6. *There is no specific therapy for affected patients, but preventive measures are available through genetic counseling and intrauterine diagnosis of affected fetuses by galactocerebroside β-galactosidase assays on amniotic fluid cells.*

7. *Globoid cell leukodystrophy occurs in other mammalian species, most notably in certain strains of dogs and mice. Clinical and pathologic features are similar*

to those in the human disease. The animal diseases are also caused by a genetic deficiency of galactosylceramidase, thus providing invaluable tools for studies of globoid cell leukodystrophy.

In 1916 Krabbe described the clinical and histologic findings in two sibs who died of an "acute infantile familial diffuse sclerosis of the brain" [1]. He noted familial occurrence, early onset of spasticity, and a rapidly progressive course to death. He gave a detailed description of the globoid cells that are now considered the histologic hallmark of the disease. A retrospective search of the neuropathologic literature revealed two earlier descriptions of similar abnormal cells [2, 3]. Collier and Greenfield [4] were the first to coin the term *globoid* to describe the numerous abnormal cells in the white matter.

There was little progress in the understanding of the disease until the development of chemical and histochemical means of investigation. Hallervorden's earlier suggestion [5] that globoid cells might contain kerasin (a cerebroside) received the support of chemical [6, 7] and histochemical studies [8–10]. The experimental induction of the globoid cell reaction by intracerebral implantation of galactosylceramide, but not by any other lipids tested [11–13], further supported the close relationship between the globoid cells and cerebroside. Analytically, the most consistent abnormality in the white matter appeared to be the reduced ratio of sulfatide to cerebroside [14, 15]. In 1970 a profound deficiency of galactosylceramide β-galactosidase as the underlying genetic defect of the disease was demonstrated in the brain, liver, spleen, and kidney [16–18]. The same deficiency was then also found in peripheral leukocytes, serum, and cultured fibroblasts [19], and prenatal diagnosis of an affected fetus was first accomplished in 1971 [20].

INCIDENCE AND HEREDITY

Globoid cell leukodystrophy is a rare disease. The number of recognized cases has been increasing since the feasibility of enzymatic diagnosis on clinical samples was established in 1971 [19]. The incidence among the general population is not known. Hagberg et al. [21] reported 32 Swedish cases during the period from 1953 through 1967 and calculated the incidence as 1.9×10^{-5} per birth. This figure seems relatively high as compared to the number of cases reported in other countries. Metzke et al. [22] found 6 patients in 6 years in Germany, although they did not calculate the incidence of the disease there. One of the authors (Y.S.) encountered 13 Japanese cases between 1972 and 1980, including several reported patients

[23–26] and 2 fetuses aborted after prenatal diagnosis [27, 28].

In Japan, during an 8-year period at least 17 patients were found and the incidence can be calculated roughly as 2 to 3 per million births. Only 3 documented cases had been known in Japan before 1972 [29–31]. The geographic distribution is widespread. The incidence appears to be higher in the Scandanavian countries, but the disease has been recorded in England, Germany, France, Italy, Switzerland, the Netherlands, Poland, Russia, the United States, Canada, Japan, India, Spain, Thailand, and other countries.

The disease occurs equally in both sexes. It is hereditary, and more than one member of a family is often affected. Krabbe himself reported two instances in sibs (cases 1 and 2, 3 and 4). Jacob et al. [32] recently reported a Newfoundland family with three successive sibs affected by the disease, and the family reported by Metzke and Rath [33] also produced three affected children. Consanguinity of parents has been reported in some families [23, 30, 34, 35]. The mode of inheritance is autosomal recessive, and involvement of more than one generation has not been recorded.

CLINICAL MANIFESTATIONS

The clinical onset of the disease in most reported patients is between 3 and 6 months after birth, but some patients show clinical abnormalities sooner. The patient of Schochet et al. [36] was "stiff" from birth and had a tendency to keep her fists clenched and her arms and legs extended. The patient of Hagberg et al. [37] vomited from the first week of life, which, together with malnutrition, prompted the parents to bring the baby to the hospital at age $2\frac{1}{2}$ months. Some patients develop slowly for the first few months [7, 38, 39, 40], and it is possible that more may have earlier undetected symptoms.

Rarely, the clinical onset is delayed until late infancy [41]. Recently there have been increasing reports of even later onset of globoid cell leukodystrophy, either in childhood [2, 4, 34, 39, 42–45] or in adulthood [46–50]. In all these cases, pathologic diagnosis was made on the basis of globoid cells in the central nervous system. In a few instances, deficient activities of galactosylceramide β-galactosidase were demonstrated [51–53]. It is clear that globoid cell leukodystrophy as defined by a genetic defect in activity of galactosylceramide β-galactosidase can occur in older age groups. The patients with few or no globoid cells were neurologically abnormal in early infancy, but were characterized by a prolonged clinical course [40, 54]. Unlike the late-onset cases, peripheral neuropathy and elevated levels of cerebrospinal fluid (CSF) protein were demonstrated in these cases.

Krabbe's original report [1] of five patients is the classic description of the typical clinical course and manifestations of the disease. The course of the disease is steadily progressive, and Hagberg [55] has divided it into three stages. Stage I is characterized by generalized hyperirritability, hyperesthesia, episodic fever of unknown origin, and some stiffness of the limbs. The child, apparently normal for the first few months after birth, becomes hypersensitive to auditory, tactile, or visual stimuli and begins to cry frequently without apparent cause. Slight retardation or regression of psychomotor development, vomiting with feeding difficulty, and convulsive sei-

Figure 43-1 Galactosyl ceramide (galactocerebroside), and the defect in Krabbe's disease.

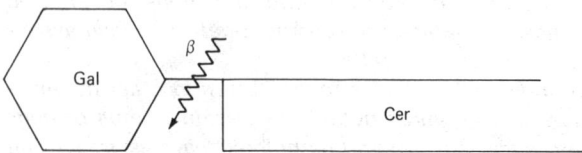

zures may occur as initial clinical symptoms. The CSF protein level is already increased. In stage II, rapid and severe motor and mental deterioration develop. There is marked hypertonicity, with extended and crossed legs, flexed arms, and the backward-bent head. Tendon reflexes are hyperactive. Minor tonic or clonic seizures occur. Optic atrophy and sluggish pupillary reactions to light may be observed. Stage III is the "burnt-out stage," attained often within a few weeks or months. The infant is decerebrate and blind and has no contact with the surroundings. Deafness may appear. The final stage may last for many years, although patients rarely survive for more than 2 years.

Head size is often small [56–59], but may be large [41, 60]. Hydrocephalus has occurred [61]. Convulsive seizures have often been observed, but infantile spasms are unusual [23, 54].

The symptoms and signs are confined almost exclusively to the nervous system. The viscera are not enlarged. Vomiting is sometimes prominent, resulting in progressive loss of weight. Musty ammoniacal breath was described in one patient [42], the origin of which was unknown. Bouts of hyperthermia, which might be ascribed to the involvement of hypothalamic system, have been reported in the absence of infection [1, 35, 37]. Obesity in one patient [56] was not explained by lesions in the hypothalamus. Generalized ichthyosis was present from early infancy in one patient [62].

Involvement of the peripheral nerves was once considered uncommon in globoid cell leukodystrophy, in contrast to metachromatic leukodystrophy [63]. Since the observations by Matsuyama et al. [29] of the pathologic changes in peripheral nerves in globoid cell leukodystrophy, however, these lesions have been intensively studied clinically and pathologically. Clinical examination does not always reveal neuropathy, especially in the early stages, because symptoms and signs of central nervous system involvement are overwhelming. Krabbe [1] pointed out originally that knee jerks could not be elicited in any of his five patients and also that stiffness passed into a flaccid state toward the end of the disease. Since then several authors have reported absent or depressed tendon reflexes in a single examination [54, 56, 59, 64–69] or disappearance of tendon reflexes in the course of the disease [40, 57, 69, 70]. There are descriptions of patients with normal [41] or hyperactive [71] tendon reflexes at age 15 months. Peripheral neuropathy can be a very early finding in Krabbe's disease, as demonstrated in a 7-week-old patient [72].

A Typical Clinical History

The patient [56], a male, was born after 40 weeks of gestation with a birth weight of 3460 g. The family history was noncontributory. Growth, development, and general health were unremarkable until age $4\frac{1}{2}$ months, when he had a generalized seizure associated with fever. At 5 months definite motor and developmental retardation as well as marked irritability were observed. Head control was poor. A "clasp-knife" response was present in all extremities. In contrast, the deep-tendon reflexes were decreased. Inspection of the fundi indicated loss of the foveal light reflex with equivocal pallor of the optic disc. Response to auditory stimuli was normal. An appropriate response to pain was demonstrated in all extremities. There was no enlargement of the viscera. Cerebral, muscle, and sural nerve biopsies at age 8 months established the diagnosis. At

age 1 year the infant required tube feedings and responded poorly to environmental stimuli. Occasional myoclonic seizures were observed. Spastic quadriparesis, prominent initially, later gave way to flaccidity with diminished deep-tendon reflexes. The head circumference at age 5 months was in the 25th percentile, and by age 9 months was below the third percentile. The patient's condition deteriorated steadily, and he died at age 14 months.

Atypical Cases

Some patients have atypical or misleading clinical histories. Wallace et al. [64] reported a patient who developed mental deterioration, apparently after mumps, at age 5 months. Convulsions started at age 7 months, and the disease progressed. The clinical diagnosis was mumps encephalitis, and the final diagnosis was established only at autopsy. A patient with a rapid course (total 3 months) was diagnosed as having encephalitis [65]. Another patient [61] was irritable from the neonatal period, and her psychomotor development was markedly retarded by age 4 months, with intermittent opisthotonus and increasing feeding difficulties. The head circumference increased progressively, with a bulging fontanel and a right abducens palsy 2 weeks after pneumoencephalography. The hydrocephalus persisted in spite of a ventriculoperitoneal shunting operation.

Late-Onset Globoid Cell Leukodystrophy

More than 10 patients have been reported whose disease had a significantly later onset and slower course than that of patients with typical globoid cell leukodystrophy. The diagnosis was established either by histopathology or enzymatic assays. Typical globoid cells were present in all autopsied patients. The morphological diagnosis of some patients with the so-called adult type of globoid cell leukodystrophy [46, 47] has been questioned [74, 75]. Enzymatic confirmation is not available for those cases reported prior to the biochemical definition of the disease.

Because of the unusual clinical course, patients with late-onset globoid cell leukodystrophy are commonly diagnosed as having diffuse sclerosis of other types, or Schilder's disease [73], and the correct diagnosis is made only by histologic or enzymatic examination. The late-onset form of the disease is probably genetically distinct from the more common infantile form. The clinical onset may be in late infancy, childhood, or even in adult life. The main clinical manifestations are visual impairment due to cortical blindness and optic atrophy, difficulty in walking, and generalized or unilateral spasticity with pyramidal signs. Peripheral neuropathy is not reported in most cases. In one patient decreased motor nerve conduction velocity and peripheral demyelination at autopsy were described, although the biopsied sural nerve had been reported as normal [43]. CSF protein levels are usually normal in the late-onset form [4, 39, 42, 43, 47]. Slight to moderate elevation of CSF protein levels was recorded in some patients [42, 75, 76].

While all patients with late-onset globoid cell leukodystrophy examined postmortem showed characteristic globoid cells in the CNS, a relatively small number of patients with the onset in the late infantile or later period have been examined for activity of galactosylceramidase and found deficient [51–53,

76]. The oldest case with enzymatic confirmation appears to be the patient reported by Kolodny et al. [76], who was 18 years old and was still alive at the time of the report. The three clinical types are summarized in Table 43-1.

CLINICAL DIAGNOSIS

In the infantile cases galactosylceramide lipidosis can be highly suspected from the following clinical features: early onset in infancy, irritability and muscle hypertonicity with progressive neurologic deterioration, signs of peripheral neuropathy, and elevation of CSF protein levels. The disease can be differentiated from nonprogressive CNS disorders of congenital or perinatal origin on the basis of the history of normal development for the first few months after birth, followed by psychomotor deterioration. Rarely, the disease may first be considered to be of traumatic, inflammatory, or neoplastic origin in atypical cases, but careful evaluation of the clinical picture and appropriate laboratory investigation usually exclude these possibilities.

Differentiation from other heredodegenerative diseases of infancy is often a major problem. Metachromatic leukodystrophy usually begins in the second year of life, with slowly progressive motor disturbance as the initial symptom. Spongy degeneration of white matter begins in early infancy and is characterized by an enlarged head, initial hypotonia, and normal CSF protein concentration. Alexander's disease includes megalocephaly as a characteristic symptom, but otherwise there are no specific clinical manifestations. Pelizaeus-Merzbacher disease may occur in the first year of life. The disease has a slowly progressive course, and abnormal involuntary eye movements, often described as nystagmus, are prominent and of diagnostic help. The CSF protein concentration is normal. Inheritance is generally considered to be X-linked recessive. Tay-Sachs disease (Chap. 46) is manifested in early infancy; the presence of cherry-red spots is characteristic. The initial clinical finding is sluggishness or apathy, rather than hyperirritability. G_{M1} gangliosidosis (Chap. 46) has an early onset and, both clinically and radiologically, more resembles Hurler's disease than it does Krabbe's disease. Gaucher's disease (Chap. 42) and Niemann-Pick disease (Chap. 41) can be differentiated from Krabbe's disease by enlarged viscera.

In patients with atypical symptoms or courses, and in patients with the late-onset form of the disease, it is practically impossible to make a clinical diagnosis of globoid cell leukodystrophy. Assays of serum, leukocytes, or cultured fibroblasts for activities of galactosylceramide β-galactosidase with one or more of its natural glycolipid substrates provide the most reliable means of antemortem diagnosis.

LABORATORY FINDINGS

No specific abnormalities have been recorded in blood chemistry test results.

The CSF protein concentration is usually high; the cell count is normal. The electrophoretic pattern of CSF protein may be diagnostically helpful, in that albumin and α_2-globulin levels are elevated and β_1- and γ-globulin levels are decreased [37, 69]. This pattern remains constant throughout the course of the disease and is found only in metachromatic leukodystrophy [77].

Allen and Reagan [78] found much-increased β-glucuronidase activity in the CSF in globoid cell leukodystrophy, as well as in diffuse meningeal dissemination of neoplasm and in acute necrotic myelopathy. The activity of this enzyme is normal in metachromatic leukodystrophy. They suggested that the increased β-glucuronidase activity has diagnostic value in globoid cell leukodystrophy if the clinical features are fully considered [79].

Radiologic examinations usually reveal only diffuse and symmetrical cerebral atrophy. Rarely is asymmetry demonstrated by pneumoencephalography or brain scan [60]. Computerized cranial tomography might show varying degrees of white matter abnormalities which, however, are not specific for the disease [80, 81].

The electroencephalogram (EEG) is normal in the initial stages, but the cerebral rhythms gradually become abnormal. Background activity becomes slow and disorganized [24, 25, 36, 41, 56, 58, 60, 71, 82–86] with changes that may be asymmetrical [60]. This is often accompanied by multifocal paroxysmal or epileptic discharges [23, 36, 38, 41, 52, 56, 83, 84, 87–89].

In accord with the clinical and pathologic observations of peripheral neuropathy, various abnormal results have been

Table 43-1 Clinical forms of globoid cell leukodystrophy

Clinical form	Age at onset, yr	Duration, yr	Clinical signs and symptoms	Peripheral neuropathy	CSF protein	Pathology	Galactosylceramide β-galactosidase
Infantile	$\frac{1}{4}$–$\frac{1}{2}$	<1	Psychomotor deterioration Irritability Pyramidal signs Optic atrophy Convulsion	+	Increased	Globoid cells	Deficient
Late-onset	2–6	1–5	Mental deterioration Pyramidal signs Visual impairment with optic atrophy	Variable	Variable	Globoid cells	Deficient
Adult	10–35	2–10	Mental deterioration Pyramidal signs Visual impairment with optic atrophy	Not described	Normal	Globoid cells	Deficient in one case

obtained by electrophysiologic procedures. These include a mild increase in polyphasic motor unit potentials [58], presence of high-amplitude NMU (neuromuscular unit) with a decrease in the number of units [23], and a few fibrillations [56, 58] in the routine electromyogram (EMG). Motor nerve conduction velocity has been low in all patients examined [23, 35, 36, 40, 56, 58, 62, 89–92]. Distal sensory latency of the median nerve was also prolonged in one patient [58].

PATHOLOGY

All important pathologic changes are confined to the nervous system. Austin found abnormal droplets in the renal tubular epithelial cells, which stained bluish with toluidine blue [68, 93]. Although its significance is uncertain, this is a noteworthy finding because the kidney is the only extraneural organ that normally contains significant amounts of galactocerebroside [94, 95]. Multinucleated giant cells have been occasionally observed outside the nervous system, but they differ morphologically and can be distinguished from typical globoid cells [82, 96]. In only one patient have giant cells similar to the globoid cells in white matter been observed in lung, lymph nodes, and spleen [97].

Central Nervous System

Gross Anatomy   The brain is usually markedly and uniformly reduced in size, but otherwise its external appearance is normal except for shrunken gyri and widened sulci. On cut section the white matter is seen to be extremely deficient and has a whitish-gray appearance and a firm, rubberlike consistency. This appearance is due to widespread diffuse demyelination with severe astrocytic gliosis. White matter changes are often more severe posterosuperiorly within the cerebral hemispheres, and the subcortical arcuate fibers tend to be spared. Phylogenetically newer tracts are usually more severely involved. In contrast to the grossly abnormal appearance of the white matter, the gray matter appears relatively normal, except for reduced cortical thickness.

Histology   Histologic involvement of the white matter is always much more severe than that of the gray matter. The major abnormalities are the presence of a large number of globoid cells, a severe lack of myelin, and astrocytic gliosis (Fig. 43-2).

GLOBOID CELLS   Conventionally, the characteristic abnormal cells, abundantly present in the white matter, are divided into two categories, epithelioid cells (globoid cells) and globoid bodies [98, 99]. The epithelioid cells are medium-sized round or oval mononuclear cells. The globoid bodies are large, irregular, multinucleated cells, ranging from 20 to 50 μm in diameter, with as many as 15 to 20 nuclei located near the plasma membrane. Aside from the number of nuclei, these cells are identical in staining characteristics, and among them are always cells which could be considered transitional. Experimental evidence strongly indicates that these two types of cells have the same origin [11–13].

The mononuclear globoid cells are scattered in white matter,

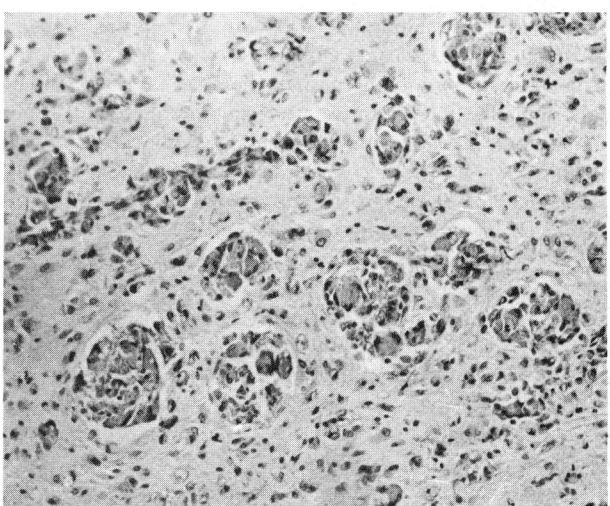

Figure 43-2   Typical light microscopic appearance of the white matter of globoid cell leukodystrophy. Conspicuous clusters of globoid cells occupy a considerable portion of whole white matter. Globoid cells are PAS-positive as shown here, and many contain multiple nuclei. The remainder of the tissue is mostly occupied by reactive astrocytes. PAS stain. Magnification ×120. *(Courtesy of Dr. Kinuko Suzuki.)*

most typically as perivascular packets of 10 to 20 cells. These cells are more common in recently affected areas than in the old lesions in the deep white matter. The globoid cells contain pale nuclei with prominent nucleoli. The cytoplasm is abundant and stains moderately positive with periodic acid Schiff (PAS) stain, and faintly positive with Sudan black B and Sudan IV. The cytoplasm is not metachromatic with the toluidine blue stain at acid pH. The globoid cells exhibit intense acid phosphatase activity [57, 64, 93, 100, 101]. The similarities in the morphological and histochemical characteristics between the globoid cells and the glucosylceramide-containing abnormal cells in Gaucher's disease have often been pointed out [5, 8].

A transient globoid cell reaction, virtually indistinguishable from the one in globoid cell leukodystrophy, can be produced experimentally in rats by intracerebral injection of solid galactocerebroside [11–13]. The experimental globoid cells are identical in appearance and staining properties with the globoid cells in Krabbe's disease. Galactocerebroside appears to be the only compound capable of inducing the histologic globoid cell reaction; sulfatide, glucocerebroside, ceramide, ganglioside, and acid mucopolysaccharides are all ineffective. Similar multinucleated cells also have been produced in tissue culture of the retina by the addition of cerebroside to the media [102].

The origin of the globoid cells in Krabbe's disease has been the subject of considerable controversy. They have been stated to be of glial origin [4], including microglia [7], microglia and astrocytes [103], astrocytes and adventitial cells [104], and oligodendroglia [105]. The experimental production of globoid cells provided strong evidence that globoid cells originate in nonneural, mesodermal cells. No transition from oligodendroglial cells or astrocytes to globoid cells was observed. The predominantly perivascular localization of globoid cells is difficult to explain on the basis of oligodendroglial or astrocytic origin. Recently, Oehmichen and Gruninger [106] suggested an interesting possibility. On the basis of DNA labeling with thymidine they concluded that globoid cells experimentally produced in animal brain by galactosylceramide implantation are derived from mesodermal cells. However, in the brains of patients the multinucleated globoid cells are of astrocytic origin and only the mononuclear epithelioid cells are of mesodermal origin. The interpretation was made on the basis of light microscopy. However, ultrastructural studies of affected human brains from other laboratories have failed to demonstrate glial fibers, leaving the suggestion of Oehmichen and Gruninger open to question. There is substantial morphological and biochemical evidence to support the view that globoid cells are derived from mesodermal cells, and that they are essentially macrophages. Although the globoid cells and most, if not all, microglia [107–109] now appear to be hematogenous in origin and histiocytic in nature, it does not follow that globoid cells necessarily arise through transformation of microglia. Globoid cells could be derived from other cells of mesodermal origin. Histochemical characteristics of the astrocytes, oligodendroglia, microglia, blood monocytes, and globoid cells have been reviewed in detail recently by Oehmichen [101].

LACK OF MYELIN   Myelin deficiency in the white matter of patients with globoid cell leukodystrophy is generally profound, but the subcortical U fibers tend to be spared, except in unusually severe cases, in which practically no myelin can be demonstrated within the cerebral hemispheres. Among the various white matter systems, phylogenetically newer areas tend to be more severely affected. Thus, fornix, hippocampus, mamillothalamic tract, and white matter of basal ganglia tend to be less involved than the centrum semiovale or cerebellar white matter [93, 110, 111]. In the spinal cord the pyramidal tracts are more severely affected than the dorsal columns. The areas with the most intense globoid cell infiltration are usually the areas with the least amount of preserved myelin, and vice versa. There is concomitant axonal degeneration, and generally no tendency to axonal preservation, such as that characteristically seen in multiple sclerosis. The oligodendroglial population is also severely diminished, and in the terminal state of some unusually severe cases they may be difficult to find. Generally, there are no inflammatory changes or deposits of amorphous sudanophilic material. In the areas of recent acute myelin breakdown, there may rarely be some indication of inflammation or a few sudanophilic droplets. The white matter is not spongy or edematous.

ASTROCYTIC GLIOSIS   Aside from the globoid cells, the areas of white matter previously occupied by axons, myelin, and oligodendroglial cells are filled with dense fibrous astrocytic proliferation. The astrocytes contain faintly PAS-positive cytoplasm and large pleomorphic nuclei. Although unusually severe, this appears to be fundamentally the same reactive astrocytic gliosis found in many other pathologic conditions.

CHANGES IN GRAY MATTER   In contrast to the devastated white matter, the gray matter is generally much less affected. Neurons do not show the "ballooned-out" appearance seen in many other lipid storage disorders. The cases reported by de Vries [112] and by Schenk et al. [113] are exceptional in that there were severe degenerative changes in the cerebral cortex. Typically, changes in the gray matter are limited to mild focal or laminar degenerative changes in the cerebral cortex and regressive changes in neurons of the pons, dentate nuclei, thalamus, and other areas [7, 65, 103, 112]. A recent study of the cerebral cortex with the Golgi technique also indicated remarkable preservation of the neuronal processes [114].

EVOLUTION OF MORPHOLOGICAL CHANGES   It is difficult to determine the chronological sequence of the various histologic changes described above, because it is rarely possible to follow morphological changes in the same patient during the course of the illness. Even if this were possible, there are always great regional variations. D'Agostino et al. [38] attempted to formulate the chronological evolution of the morphological changes through a study of multiple sections from three patients. Utilizing the degree of demyelination, they divided the course into four stages: (1) early, (2) advanced, (3) late, and (4) final. The early lesions are characterized by "the presence of both intracellular and extracellular PAS-positive material, with subsequent formation of mononuclear globoid cells and only a slight decrease in the intensity of myelin staining." In the advanced stage, the amount of myelin and axons are decreased and astrocytic gliosis becomes prominent. The globoid cells are more numerous and tend to cluster around blood vessels, and may become multinucleated. In the late stage, the globoid cells become fewer in number and are mostly clumped around blood vessels. The amounts of myelin and axons are markedly diminished at this stage. The final stage is characterized by predominant astrocytic gliosis, with remaining globoid cells and total loss of myelin and axons.

ULTRASTRUCTURE   For many years the report by Nelson et al. [41] was the only electron microscopic study of globoid cell leukodystrophy. Then in 1969 and 1970, 10 articles appeared [36, 43, 56, 60, 69, 115–119], describing the ultrastructure of both the central and peripheral nervous systems. The flow of such reports continues unabated [89, 90, 106, 120–124].

These reports are essentially in agreement. At the ultrastructural level, mononuclear and multinucleated globoid cells appear similar, except for the number of nuclei. They both contain numerous fine tortuous cytoplasmic processes (pseudopods) which are characteristic of macrophages; moderately electron-dense granular cytoplasm containing prominent rough endoplasmic reticulum; many free ribosomes, abundant fine filaments of approximately 9 to 10 nm, and scattered or clustered abnormal cytoplasmic inclusions (Fig. 43-3). The inclusions have moderately electron-dense straight or curved hollow tubular profiles in longitudinal section and appear irregularly crystalloid in cross section (Figs. 43-4 and 43-5). Often they are freely scattered among the normal cytoplasmic organelles, but sometimes they are packed in an electron-lucent space in the cytoplasm, with or without an outer limiting membrane. These tubules often have longitudinal striations of variable density, approximately 6 nm in width. Another type of abnormal tubular inclusion, first described by Yunis and Lee [60], has the structure of twisted tubules with 4- to 5-nm longitudinal striations and rectangular or irregularly round cross sections (Fig. 43-6). This second type of tubule is similar to those in Gaucher's disease, but the first larger tubules, with irregular, polygonal, or crystalloid cross sections, seem to be unique to globoid cell leukodystrophy. Yunis and Lee [119] pointed out the morphological similarities of these abnormal inclusions to negatively stained pure brain galactocerebroside. Ultrastructural study of the experimental globoid cells produced by the intracerebral injection into rats of pure galactocerebroside, prepared from the brain of a patient with Krabbe's disease, showed both types of tubules. This further supported their close relationship to galactocerebroside [125, 126]. In fact, the ultrastructure of the experimental globoid cells was essentially identical to that of human globoid cells (Figs. 43-7 and 43-8).

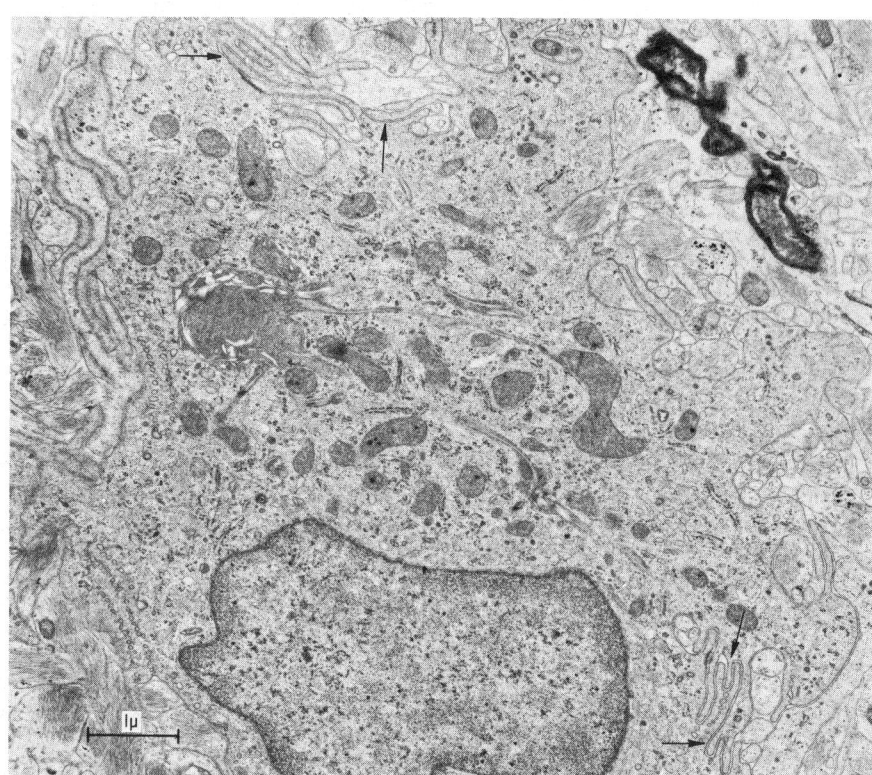

Figure 43-3 A low magnification electron micrograph showing a globoid cell. Only one nucleus is visible. There are numerous tortuous pseudopods (arrows) which characterize this cell as a macrophage. Within the cytoplasm, near the center of the picture, there are many abnormal tubular inclusions (for details see Figs. 43-4 and 43-5). The line indicates a scale of 1 μm. *(Courtesy of Dr. Kinuko Suzuki.)*

The ultrastructural appearance of human and experimental globoid cells, particularly the presence of numerous pseudopods, supports the view that these cells are macrophages. Astrocytes, identified by glial filaments, did not contain the abnormal tubular inclusions. The few remaining oligodendroglial cells, identifiable by their dense cytoplasm and microtubules, were also free of the tubules. On the other hand, endothelial and perithelial cells often contained cytoplasmic inclusions similar to those in globoid cells [56].

Degeneration of myelin, with or without associated axonal degeneration, is found in the white matter, but the remaining myelin has normal multilamellar configuration with normal periodicity. Cortical neurons appear normal ultrastructurally.

Figure 43-4 An electron micrograph showing the characteristic hollow, polygonal, or crystalloid cut sections of the abnormal inclusions in the cytoplasm of a globoid cell. Several longitudinal sections of tubules of the same type are seen on the right side of the picture. The line indicates 1 μm. *(Courtesy of Dr. Kinuko Suzuki.)*

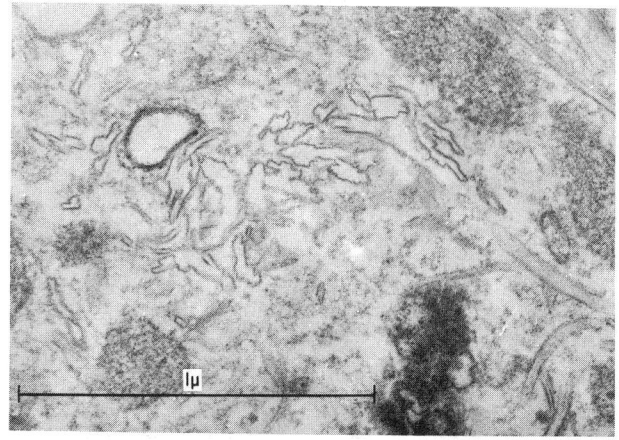

Peripheral Nervous System

Peripheral nerves, including the cranial nerves, usually do not show gross abnormalities. The optic nerve is an exception, but it is actually a white matter tract of the central nervous system, not a peripheral nerve. It shares the same gross and histologic abnormalities of CNS white matter [121, 122].

Earlier, pathologic changes in peripheral nerves had been reported rather sporadically [29, 57, 68]. Some investigators did not find morphological changes in peripheral nerves [10, 37, 70, 110]. More recent histologic and ultrastructural studies have shown that the peripheral nervous system is commonly affected [56, 58, 69, 117, 118, 127–131]. Dunn et al. [69] found peripheral nerve lesions in all of seven patients. Under light microscopy the peripheral nerve lesions consist of minimal to severe degenerative changes in axons and the myelin sheaths, associated with endoneural fibrosis and the accumulation of foamy histiocytes around endoneural blood vessels or trabeculae of the endoneurium. Segmental demyelination is common [56, 69, 117, 130]. Typical globoid cells are not found in peripheral nerves. Ultrastructurally, straight or curved tubular inclusions, similar to those in globoid cells in the brain, are found scattered or clustered in the cytoplasm of histiocytes, in the proliferated endoneural collagenous tissue, or around small blood vessels. These abnormal inclusions are often found in the Schwann cells also [118, 130].

BIOCHEMISTRY OF GALACTOSYLCERAMIDE

Chemistry of Galactosylceramide and Related Compounds

Galactocerebroside (galactosylceramide) belongs to the group

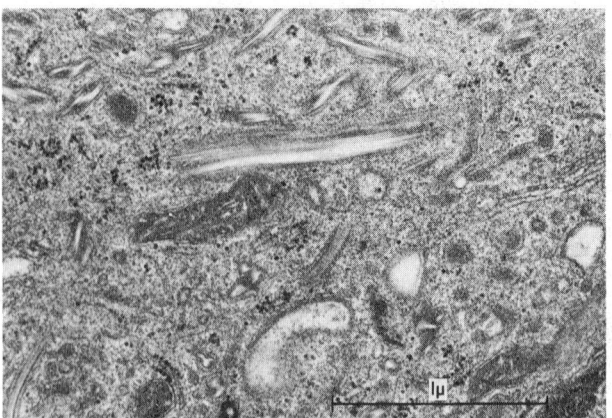

Figure 43-5 The abnormal hollow tubules show longitudinal striations approximately 6 nm wide. The line indicates a scale of 1 μm.

of lipids generically called sphingoglycolipids. This name indicates that the molecule contains a long-chain base, sphingosine, and a sugar moiety. Sphingosine is an unsaturated amino diol. The major sphingosine found in nature is C$_{18}$-sphingosine, having the structure D(+)-erythro-1,3-dihydroxy-2-amino-4-trans-octadecene [132–135]. Besides this major form, C$_{20}$-sphingosine (icosisphingosine) occurs in smaller amounts [136–138]. Small portions of these sphingosines are also present in saturated (dihydro) forms [139, 140]. In the galactocerebroside and sulfatide of normal adult human brains, C$_{18}$-sphingosine constitutes 95 percent or more of the total sphingosine, the remainder being C$_{18}$-dihydrosphingosine and much smaller amounts of a shorter-chain analogue, C$_{16}$-sphingosine. In immature human brains there are higher proportions of C$_{18}$-dihydrosphingosine, sometimes comprising 10 percent of the total [141]. C$_{20}$-sphingosine and its dihydro form do not appear to be components of brain galactocerebroside or sulfatide [139, 140].

Ceramide   The amino group of sphingosine is almost always acylated with long-chain fatty acid (C$_{14}$ to C$_{26}$). N-Acylsphingosine is generically called ceramide, the basic common building block of almost all sphingolipids. The fatty acid composition of galactocerebroside and sulfatide has been extensively studied both in normal adult brains and during development [142–146]. Generally, the fatty acids of galactocerebroside and sulfatide in the brain are characterized by the predominance of longer-chain fatty acids (C$_{20}$ to C$_{26}$), lack of polyunsaturated fatty acids, and the presence of α-hydroxy acids. Approximately two-thirds of the fatty acids in cerebrosides and one-third of those in sulfatides are α-hydroxy fatty acids. These are generally absent in other lipids of the brain, including glycerophospholipids, sphingomyelin, ceramide oligohexosides, and gangliosides. In galactocerebrosides and sulfatides, particularly those in white matter, 65 to 80 percent of the total unsubstituted fatty acids have chain lengths longer than 20 carbons. In the α-hydroxy fatty acids, the proportion of longer-chain fatty acids is even greater. Except for the sphingomyelins of white matter and myelin, the predominance of longer-chain fatty acid is unique for brain galactocerebrosides and sulfatides. Stearic acid (C$_{18:0}$) is the predominant fatty acid in brain gangliosides [15, 138, 147–149] and ceramide oligohexosides in the brain [150]. Lack of fatty acids with more than one double bond is a characteristic shared by all sphingolipids in the brain.

Galactocerebrosides and Related Compounds   The hydroxyl group at C-1 of ceramide can be substituted for by a variety of compounds. Cerebroside is defined as a monohexosyl ceramide, the hexose being linked to the C-1 of ceramide by a glycosidic linkage. The hexose is either D-glucose or D-galactose. Depending on the nature of the hexose, cerebroside is named glucocerebroside (glucosylceramide) or galactocerebroside (galactosylceramide). Both the glucose and galactose are in β configuration. Glucocerebrosides occur predominantly in systemic tissues other than the nervous system and are essentially absent in normal human brain after age 1 year. They are present in small amounts in brains of normal human fetuses and newborns [151] and in the brains of older children with certain diseases, notably ganglioside storage disorders [150, 152].

In contrast, galactocerebroside is characteristically a lipid of the nervous system. As indicated by the preceding descriptions, it has the structure shown in Fig. 43-9.

Brain sulfatide is derived from galactocerebroside, and it has an additional sulfate group, ester-linked to the C-3 of galactose [153, 154]. Like galactosylceramide, sulfatide is also present at high concentrations in the nervous system.

There are two other compounds chemically and metabolically related to galactosylceramide that are important biochemically and enzymologically in the pathogenesis of globoid cell leukodystrophy. Galactosylsphingosine (psychosine) is structurally galactosylceramide minus fatty acid. Although the compound is present in normal brain only in minute amounts [155–157], it has potential importance when the dynamic behavior of galactosylceramide is considered in relation to the pathogenesis of the disease. Another related compound important in globoid cell leukodystrophy is lactosylceramide, which has a lactose moiety, instead of galactose, at C-1 of ceramide. Lactosylceramide is distributed ubiquitously in most tissues, although its concentrations are generally low.

Though detailed structures of the individual moieties, such as fatty acids or sphingosines, differ among these glycosphingolipids, the simplified notations are convenient for purposes of most discussions in this chapter. Figure 43-10 depicts chemical, and to a large extent also metabolic, relationships among galactosylceramide and related compounds using such simplified notations.

METABOLSM OF GALACTOSYLCERAMIDE AND RELATED COMPOUNDS   Two alternate pathways have been proposed for

Figure 43-6 Another type of abnormal inclusions in globoid cells. They have the structure of twisted tubules with 4- to 5-nm striations (arrows). The line indicates a scale of 1 μm. *(Courtesy of Dr. Eduardo J. Yunis.)*

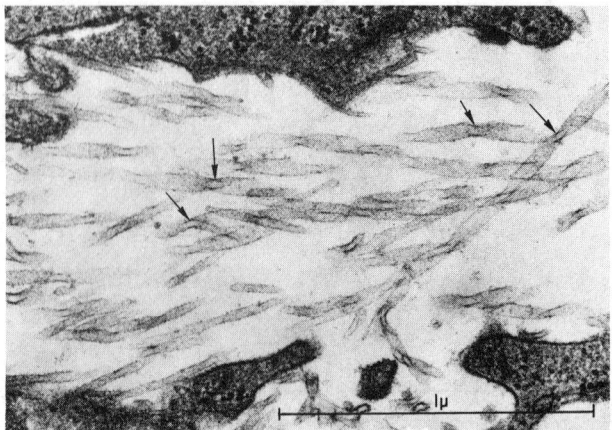

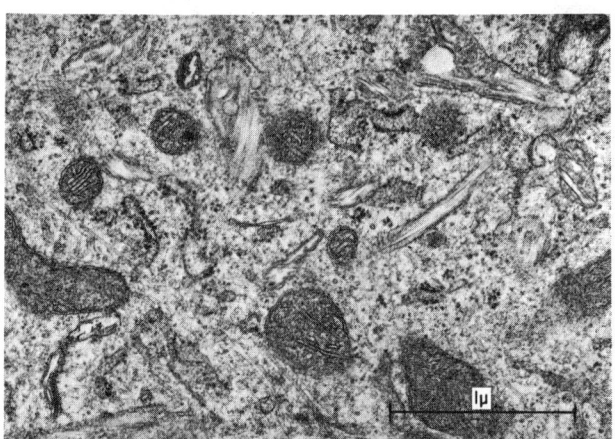

Figure 43-7 A high magnification electron micrograph of cytoplasm of a globoid cell, experimentally produced in rat brain by intracerebral injection of solid galactocerebroside. Abnormal hollow tubules, identical to those seen in human globoid cells (Figs. 43-4 and 43-5), are scattered within the cytoplasm. Note the similarities of the overall appearance to Fig. 43-5, which was taken from a human globoid cell. The line indicates a scale of 1 µm. *(Courtesy of Dr. Kinuko Suzuki.)*

biosynthesis of galactosylceramide (Fig. 43-10). One is through psychosine, which is formed from sphingosine and UDP-galactose [158, 159]. Psychosine, in turn, may be acylated by acyl-CoA to form galactosylceramide [160, 161]. Although the first step of psychosine synthesis has been confirmed on numerous occasions, acylation of psychosine has been difficult to reproduce [162]. Meanwhile, it has been conclusively demonstrated that galactosylceramide can be synthesized through ceramide [163, 164]. At this time, it appears that the major, if not exclusive, biosynthetic pathway for galactosylceramide is through ceramide. Biosynthesis of sulfatide occurs through cerebroside, with the "active sulfate," 3'-phosphoadenosine-5'-phosphosulfate (PAPS), as sulfate donor [165–170]. The actual biosynthetic process of sulfatide appears to be complex, involving participation of an intermediate lipid-protein complex [171, 172].

The initial step in degradation of sulfatide is removal of the sulfate group to convert it to galactocerebroside. This reaction is catalyzed by cerebroside sulfate sulfatase, which is present in the arylsulfatase A fraction [173]. Deficiency of this enzyme characterizes another inherited leukodystrophy, metachromatic leukodystrophy, in which abnormal accumulation of sulfatide occurs [174, 175; also Chap. 44].

Galactocerebroside is degraded to ceramide and galactose by a lysosomal hydrolytic enzyme, galactocerebroside β-galactosidase (galactosylceramidase), thus:

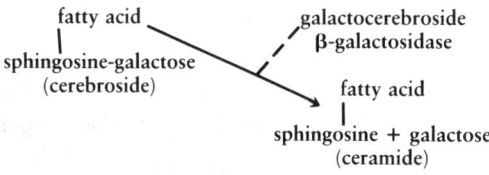

This enzyme in brain was first studied in detail by Radin and coworkers [176–179]. Ultracentrifugal fractionation indicated that it was associated with the lysosomal fraction. Approximately 300-fold purification was achieved by extraction with detergents, DEAE-Sephadex column chromatography, and differential precipitation at different pHs. The pH optimum of the enzyme is 4.5. Ceramide, sphingosine, lactosylceramide, galac-

tose, galactonolactone, and galactitol inhibit the enzyme in vitro. It is active on galactocerebroside with either unsubstituted or α-hydroxy fatty acids. In rat brain, galactocerebroside β-galactosidase is present before myelination when little galactocerebroside is present in the brain (at age 4 days), but the enzyme level then rises considerably (to three to four times the 4-day level) during active cerebroside deposition and myelination. The activity remains high in mature animals. In humans, galactocerebroside β-galactosidase activity in a 72-year-old brain was the same as that in a 21-year-old brain in gray matter, but was decreased to 60 percent of the activity of the young brain in white matter [16].

Intensive studies on purified galactosylceramidases from humans and other species have been undertaken in recent years [180–186]. The enzyme is hydrophobic and is exceedingly difficult to purify. Only one group of investigators has reported successful purification of human galactosylceramidase [187–189]. According to these authors, the monomer of human galactosylceramidase has a molecular weight of 125,000. The enzyme may exist as monomers, dimers, tetramers, or hexamers. They suggested that the forms of higher molecular weight might be the active forms in vivo. Relevant to the problems of globoid cell leukodystrophy, substrate specificity of the enzyme has been substantially clarified. While galactosylceramide is clearly the main natural substrate, the enzyme is also active in catalyzing hydrolysis of terminal galactose from galactosylsphingosine (psychosine) [190–193], monogalactosyldiglyceride [194], and under specific assay conditions, also from lactosylceramide [185, 195–205]. The information on the substrate specificity of the enzyme provides an important basis when we consider the pathogenetic mechanism, as well as enzymatic diagnosis of the disease. Galactosylceramidase can catalyze transgalactosylation reactions under appropriate assay conditions [206]. This is not surprising since galactosylceramide hydrolysis is a special case of galactose transfer to a water molecule. Attempts to replace the unnatural bile salt with a biologically more plausible component resulted in the demonstration that phosphatidylserine could specifically activate human brain galactosylceramidase [207, 208]. More recently, Wenger et al. [209] showed that a protein activator

Figure 43-8 Numerous slender, twisted tubules that were produced within experimental globoid cells in rat brain by the intracerebral injection of galactocerebroside purified from the brain of a human patient with globoid cell leukodystrophy. The twisted configurations of the tubules are clearly seen (arrows). The ultrastructural appearance of these tubules is identical to those described by Yunis and Lee [60] in human globoid cell leukodystrophy (Fig. 43-6). The line indicates a scale of 1 µm. *(Courtesy of Dr. Kinuko Suzuki.)*

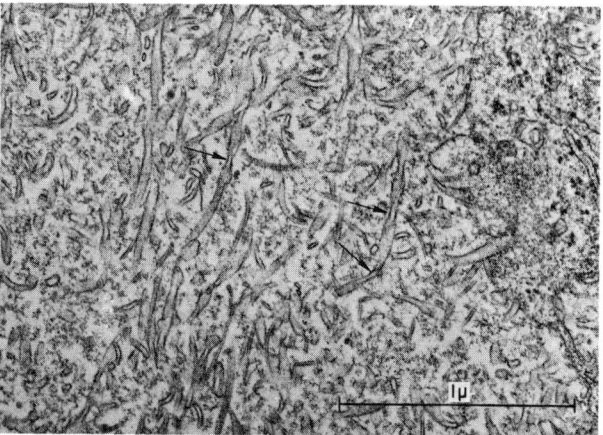

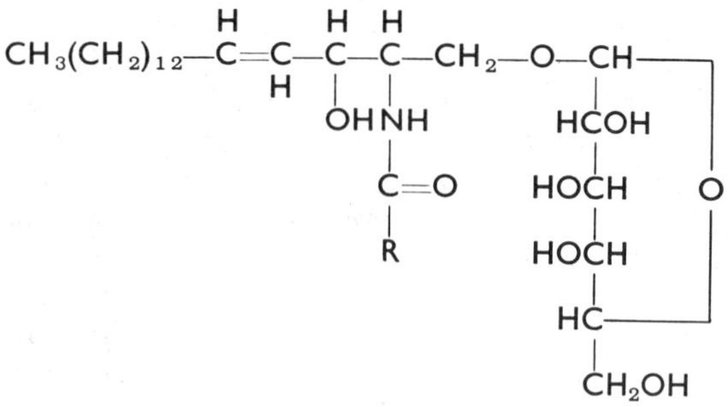

$$CH_3(CH_2)_{12}-\overset{H}{\underset{H}{C}}=C-\overset{H}{\underset{OH}{C}}-\overset{H}{\underset{NH}{C}}-CH_2-O-CH$$

Figure 43-9 Structure of galactocerebroside (galactosylceramide). The molecule consists of sphingosine, fatty acid, and galactose. R= $-(CH_2)_n CH_3$.

exists for galactosylceramidase. Activation of galactosylceramidase required this activator and phosphatidylserine.

GALACTOCEREBROSIDE, MYELIN, AND THEIR METABOLISM
The distribution of galactocerebrosides in mammalian organs is uniquely restricted. They are practically absent in systemic organs except in the kidney, which normally contains appreciable amounts of galactocerebroside, although much less than the brain [94, 95]. The brain, particularly white matter, is rich in galactocerebroside and its sulfate ester, sulfatide. Gray matter contains much smaller amounts of glycolipids. Galactocerebroside is mostly, if not exclusively, localized in the myelin sheath and, probably, oligodendroglial cells, since the myelin sheath is a specialized extension of the oligodendroglial cell membrane. This contention is supported (but not proved) by the virtual absence of galactocerebroside in the brain before myelination [210–212] and the similarly low cerebroside concentrations in pathologic conditions where almost total loss of myelin occurs [213, 214]. The sum of cerebroside and sulfatide is the most sensitive biochemical indicator of the mass of myelin present in the brain [215]. Increase in the brain cerebroside content coincides with the active myelination period. In fact, the amounts of total brain cerebroside correlate precisely with the amounts of myelin that can be isolated from the brain, whereas amounts of the other lipids do not [216].

Myelin of adult mammalian brains generally contains galactocerebroside at a concentration of 15 to 18 percent dry weight. The sum of galactocerebroside and sulfatide amounts to 20 percent of the dry weight of myelin. The content of galactocerebroside in myelin from the peripheral nerve is somewhat less than that of CNS myelin [217]. There are numerous original reports on the chemical composition of myelin iso-

lated from mammalian brains, and readers are referred to recent review articles on this subject [218–222]. In view of the unusually high concentration of galactocerebrosides and sulfatides in the myelin sheath, metabolic diseases involving these lipids would be expected to manifest themselves primarily in disturbances of white matter functions and peripheral neuropathy (globoid cell leukodystrophy and metachromatic leukodystrophy).

The metabolism of brain galactocerebroside is closely linked to the metabolism of myelin. This topic has been covered in recent review articles [223, 224]. The most significant metabolic features of CNS myelin are its high rate of formation and turnover during the relatively short period of active myelination, and its relative inertness in the adult. The period of active myelination in humans probably extends from the perinatal period to about age 18 months. Myelination does not stop after this period, and in the human brain may not be complete until age 20 years [225]. The amount of cerebroside in the immature brain is very low, and, compared to concentrations of cholesterol and phospholipids, is relatively far below that in mature brains. When measured by incorporation of labeled galactose administered in vivo, the rate of cerebroside synthesis in rat brain reaches a peak at 10 to 20 days, coinciding well with the most active period of myelination [158]. Synthesis of cerebroside occurs at a much lower rate in the adult. A series of long-term experiments by Davison and coworkers convincingly established the relative metabolic inertness of adult myelin. Their earlier studies, carried out on total white matter, were later confirmed by more refined experiments in which the incorporated labeled precursors were followed in isolated pure myelin fractions [226–229].

The half-life of cerebroside and sulfatide in the mature human brain is 1 year or longer. At any developmental stage, myelin is metabolically the most stable component of the subcellular fractions of the brain.

Let us summarize a few key features of galactocerebroside metabolism which will be crucial later in considering the pathophysiology of globoid cell leukodystrophy: (1) Galactocerebroside consists of a sphingosine, a fatty acid, and galactose. (2) Galactocerebroside is the precursor of sulfatide. (3) Both galactocerebroside and sulfatide are highly concentrated in the myelin sheath. (4) Sulfatide is normally degraded through galactocerebroside. (5) A lysosomal hydrolytic enzyme, galactocerebroside β-galactosidase, is responsible for the first step in normal degradation of cerebroside, in which galactocerebroside is cleaved to ceramide and galactose. A few

Figure 43-10 Chemical and metabolic relationship among galactosylceramide and related compounds.

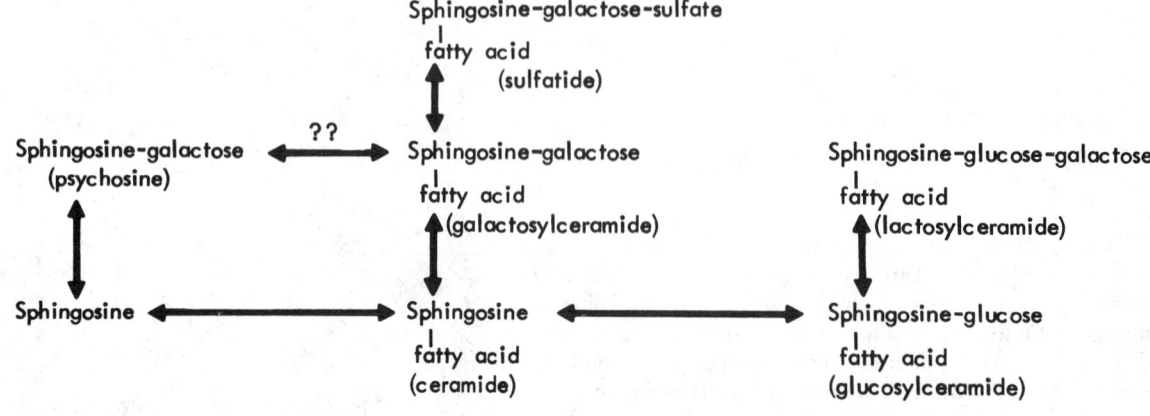

related galactolipids also serve as substrates for the same enzyme, including galactosylsphingosine (psychosine), monogalactosyl-diglyceride, and lactosylceramide. (6) Biosynthesis of galactocerebroside reaches a peak, coincident with the maximum myelination period (during the first year and a half in humans). (7) Galactocerebroside β-galactosidase activity is low before myelination and myelination increases sharply during the active myelination period, when myelin is turning over relatively rapidly. (8) Once formed, adult myelin is unusually stable metabolically, although by no means completely inert. (9) The high level of galactocerebroside β-galactosidase attained during the active myelination period is retained in the adult brain.

Chemical Pathology

Analytical Chemistry   Hallervorden was the first to point out the morphological similarities of the globoid cells to the storage cells in Gaucher's disease and to suggest that the globoid cells also might contain cerebroside in excess [5]. The strong tetrazonium reaction within the cytoplasm of the globoid cell is consistent with the presence of a protein cerebroside complex [96, 103, 230]. Austin [6] obtained fractions enriched in globoid cells from seven patients with globoid cell leukodystrophy. He found that globoid cells contain unusually large amounts of galactocerebroside but little sulfatide.

Earlier, Blackwood and Cumings found an abnormally high cerebroside concentration in white matter in one patient with globoid cell leukodystrophy [7]. They attributed this to the abnormal material in globoid cells, but increased total concentrations of cerebroside in the brains of patients with globoid cell leukodystrophy are now considered exceptional. In more recent analyses both galactocerebrosides and sulfatides are almost invariably much lower than normal in white matter [9, 14, 15, 37, 67, 71, 74, 157, 231–242]. Pilz reported that α-hydroxy fatty acid–containing cerebrosides were decreased more than were those with unsubstituted fatty acids [239].

The most consistent, although not necessarily invariable, finding in white matter of globoid cell leukodystrophy is the increased ratio of cerebroside to sulfatide [240]. In eight cases of globoid cell leukodystrophy, Austin [14, 231] found the cerebroside-sulfatide ratio to be between 5 to 10, whereas it is normally about 4. All his patients had reduced total glycolipids in white matter. In that series patients who showed more globoid cells histologically tended to have higher absolute and relative cerebroside values. The increased cerebroside-sulfatide ratio was also pointed out by others [15, 37]. To evaluate whether an abnormal ratio was due to increase of cerebroside concentrations or decrease of sulfatide concentrations, Austin related the values of these lipids to those of cholesterol and found in six patients that the average increase of levels of cerebroside was greater (plus 57 percent) than the average decrease of sulfatide concentrations (minus 30 percent) [99]. Suzuki et al. [16, 17] found that the sulfatide concentrations in white matter of patients with globoid cell leukodystrophy were generally similar to those in the white matter of patients with other devastating white matter diseases, such as Schilder's disease [214] or spongy degeneration of white matter [213], in which almost complete myelin loss also occurs. These authors concluded that the relative preservation of cerebroside is more impressive than the loss of sulfatide.

Besides the abnormalities of the major glycolipids of white

matter—galactocerebrosides and sulfatides—Menkes et al. [234] found an abnormal amount of dihexosyl ceramide and possibly a trihexosyl ceramide. The dihexosyl ceramide has been shown to be galactosylglucosyl ceramide [235, 243, 244]. In the brain of one patient, 16 percent of white matter cerebrosides was glucocerebroside, and two other sphingoglycolipids, digalactosylglucosyl ceramide and globoside (N-acetylgalactosaminyl-digalactosylglucosyl ceramide), were also present in significant amounts [235]. These "visceral-type" sphingoglycolipids in white matter were considered intrinsic lipids of globoid cells, which is consistent with the idea that the globoid cells are of mesodermal origin, a secondary phenomenon rather than a direct result of the primary enzymatic defect (Table 43-2). A more recent detailed study by Vanier and Svennerholm also demonstrated alteration of gangliosides in brains of patients [155]. Levels of gangliosides G_{D1a} and G_{M1} were reduced throughout, while G_{D1b} and G_{T1} levels were slightly decreased in cerebral cortex and increased in white matter. Amounts of normally minor gangliosides, G_{D2}, G_{D3}, and G_{M3}, which are metabolically related to G_{D1b} and G_{T1}, were increased throughout the brain. Similar results were reported by Berra et al. [245], who found no abnormalities in the composition of glycosaminoglycans and glycoproteins in the brain of patients. The fatty acid composition of sphingomyelin indicates contribution from mesodermal tissues [246].

The most important finding by Vanier and Svennerholm concerns psychosine. For the first time, they demonstrated that psychosine (galactosylsphingosine) is detectable in normal brain and that brains of patients with globoid cell leukodystrophy contain 10 to 100 times the normal amounts of psychosine [155–157]. Their finding provides strong support for the psychosine hypothesis concerning the pathogenesis of globoid cell leukodystrophy, which is described later.

Earlier, myelin isolated from patients with globoid cell leukodystrophy was reported to have a disproportionate lack of sulfatide [247], approximately half of normal when expressed as a percentage of the total concentration of sphingosine. These experiments did not refer the sulfatide content to the content of protein, total lipids, or sphingolipids of the myelin fraction, or distinguish between subcellular fractions which might contain abnormally low sulfatide and normal cerebroside levels or abnormally high cerebroside and normal sulfatide concentrations. Moreover, the technique of myelin isolation did not eliminate possible contamination with subcellular components of lighter density. The abnormal tubular or polygonal inclusions found in globoid cells are lighter than myelin and contain a high proportion of cerebroside but no sulfatide [248]. Therefore, the analytical values of the myelin fraction reported by these authors are likely to include the abnormal cerebroside-rich inclusions. In a more recent study [248], the abnormal tubular inclusions were present in an even larger amount than myelin. When they were carefully eliminated, the yield of the myelin was, as expected from histologic findings, only 0.4 percent of normal. The myelin had a normal ultrastructural configuration, and lipid composition was quite similar to that of normal myelin. Particularly, the amounts of glycolipids (cerebrosides and sulfatides) were normal. The cerebrosides were all galactocerebrosides, and none of the ceramide oligohexosides found in the whole white matter was present in the myelin (Table 43-3). Thus, in globoid cell leukodystrophy the brain is apparently capable of forming myelin with normal morphological appearance and normal chemical composition. The finding is in contrast to what occurs in meta-

Table 43-2 Analytical chemistry of globoid cell leukodystrophy

	Gray matter		White matter	
	Globoid	Normal	Globoid	Normal
Water content, % fresh wt	87.0	82.1	83.5	73.0
Chloroform-methanol				
insoluble residue	58.1	51.0	70.0	29.3
Total lipid	27.4	31.8	18.0	54.0
Proteolipid protein	0.7	3.2	0.5	8.6
Upper phase solids	13.6	14.0	11.5	8.0
Cholesterol	5.8	7.6	3.5	15.0
Phospholipid, total	21.4	22.1	12.9	23.9
Ethanolamine				
phospholipid	6.8	7.2	3.1	8.1
Lecithin	8.7	9.0	5.1	6.8
Sphingomyelin	2.5	1.8	2.3	4.3
Monophosphoinositide	0.8	0.7	0.5	0.4
Serine phospholipid	2.8	3.2	1.7	4.2
Glycolipids, total	0.44	0.92	1.6	14.6
Cerebroside*	0.25	0.50	0.99	12.5
Sulfatide	0.16	0.14	0.22	2.2
Ceramide dihexoside†	Trace	0.07	0.09	Trace
Ceramide trihexoside‡	. . .	. . .	0.04	
Globoside§	. . .	. . .	0.20	
Ceramide tetrahexoside¶	. . .	Trace	0.04	

* Glucocerebroside constituted 32 and 13 percent of total cerebroside in gray and white matter, respectively, in the brain of a patient with globoid cell leukodystrophy, whereas only galacto-cerebroside was present in the normal brain. This patient is somewhat atypical in that the cerebroside sulfatide ratio in white matter is normal.
† Galactosylglucosyl ceramide.
‡ Visceral-type trihexoside, i.e., digalactosylglucosyl ceramide.
§ N-Acetylgalactosaminyl-digalactosylglucosyl ceramide.
¶ Asialo G_{MI} ganglioside.
NOTE: Expressed as percent dry weight except for the water content.
SOURCE: Data from Eto and Suzuki [235].

chromatic leukodystrophy, in which myelin is formed with an excess sulfatide content [247, 249, 250].

Besides these specific chemical abnormalities, white matter in globoid cell leukodystrophy typically shows increased water content and drastic reduction of proteolipid protein and total lipid content, with consequent relative, but not absolute, increase of amounts of protein. Cholesterol, lecithin, sphingo-myelin, ethanolamine- and serine-phospholipids are all reduced in similar degrees. These findings are primarily the reflection of the devastating myelin loss. As expected from the histologic absence of sudanophilia, cholesteryl ester is not present in white matter (Table 43-2).

In contrast to the white matter, the chemical composition of the gray matter may be normal or only slightly abnormal (Table 43-2). Glycolipids in gray matter may be moderately low [15, 37, 235, 236] or normal [7, 231]. The ratio of cerebroside to sulfatide is often increased.

In keeping with the normal histologic appearance, nonneu-ral tissues do not show conspicuous compositional changes. Suzuki [251] examined galactosylceramide levels in the kid-neys of five patients and found them to be approximately 30 percent higher than normal. Since glucosylceramide level was also similarly high in patients' kidneys, it was concluded that there was a specific abnormal increase of galactosylceramide in the kidney. On the other hand, Dawson reported highly ele-vated levels of galactosylceramide in livers of three patients [252] although the actual amounts were still minute. This find-ing has been contradicted by a more recent report. [157]. Hof et al. [253] examined gangliosides in cultured fibroblasts and reported a moderate increase.

DEFICIENCY OF GALACTOSYLCERAMIDE β-GALACTOSIDASE

Specific experimental production of the globoid reactions by galactosylceramide, and the chemical and morphological evi-dence for the presence of galactosylceramide within the glo-boid cell, were strongly suggestive of an abnormality in the degradative pathway of galactosylceramide. The first step in galactocerebroside degradation is cleavage of the galactose moiety from the ceramide portion of cerebroside by the action of galactocerebroside β-galactosidase [176–179].

Profound deficiency of galactosylceramide β-galactosidase activity was first demonstrated in the gray and white matter, liver, and spleen of three patients with globoid cell leukodys-trophy [16, 17] (Table 43-4). The enzyme activity was assayed in tissue homogenates against the specific substrate, galacto-cerebroside. The labeled substrate was prepared from commer-cial bovine spinal cord galactocerebroside by oxidation with galactose oxidase and reduction by tritium-labeled sodium borohydride [254]. The label was located on C-6 of galactose, and the radioactivity of released galactose was determined as the measure of the enzyme activity. The activities of galacto-cerebroside β-galactosidase were generally in the range of 5 to 10 percent of that in tissues from normal controls and patients with a variety of other diseases. Postmortem handling and storage of the tissues were adequately controlled. Four other lysosomal hydrolytic enzymes were assayed with appropriate p-nitrophenyl compounds: β-glucosidase, β-galactosidase, N-acetyl-β-glucosaminidase, and N-acetyl-β-galactosaminidase. The high activities of these p-nitrophenyl glycosidases in tissue of patients with globoid cell leukodystrophy further indicated satisfactory preservation of tissue. It is noteworthy that β-galactosidase was not deficient when assayed with the synthetic substrate, in spite of the profound deficiency of galactocerebroside β-galactosidase. This indicated that only one specific β-galactosidase activity is deficient. This is in contrast to G_{M1} gangliosidosis, in which galactocerebroside β-galactosidase activity is normal or even higher than normal, while β-galactosidase activity assayed with p-nitrophenyl β-galactoside is extremely deficient [183, 197, 255; also Chap. 46].

The deficiency of galactocerebroside β-galactosidase was also not attributable to the extreme devastation of the white matter, because gray matter, much less involved histologically, and the histologically normal liver and spleen also showed the same deficiency. The galactocerebroside β-galactosidase activity was also normal in the white matter in Schilder's disease, in which there is almost complete loss of myelin and oligodendroglia. White matter in a patient with total hexosaminidase deficiency also exhibited severe loss of myelin but no decrease in galactocerebroside β-galactosidase activity. The presence of an enzyme inhibitor in the tissues of a patient with globoid cell leukodystrophy was ruled out by experiments showing no decrease of cerebroside cleavage by normal brain homogenates when brain homogenate with Krabbe's disease was added to the incubation. The deficiency in Krabbe's disease was also not due to a shift of the pH optimum of galactocerebroside β-galactosidase from its normal of about 4.5 [176]. The activity was uniformly deficient throughout the pH range of 4.1 to 8.1 [16].

The initial findings of Suzuki and Suzuki [16] were soon confirmed in a larger series in the brain, liver, and kidney of five additional patients [18]. The average activity of galactocerebroside β-galactosidase was less than 5 percent of that of the controls in all organs examined. The highest activities in the globoid cell leukodystrophy group were gray matter, 13.6 percent; white matter, 7.8 percent; liver, 30 percent; and kidney, 19 percent of the lowest activities among the controls, respectively.

Galactocerebroside β-galactosidase activity was soon found

Table 43-3 Chemical composition of isolated myelin

	Globoid cell leukodystrophy	Normal control*
Yield, mg/10 g wet wt	3.8	1000
Chloroform-methanol insoluble residue	25.7	12.4
Proteolipid protein	12.3	21.0
Total lipid	62.0	66.6
Cholesterol	12.2	15.6
Total phospholipid	30.3	30.1
Ethanolamine phospholipid	7.6	9.7
Lecithin	12.9	9.2
Sphingomyelin	5.0	5.1
Monophosphoinositide and serine phospholipid	4.2	5.8
Total galactolipid	17.0	17.4
Cerebroside	12.4	13.6
Sulfatide	4.6	3.8

* Average of two myelin preparations from normal brains, ages 2.5 and 5.5 years.
NOTE: Expressed as percent dry weight except for the yield.
SOURCE: Data from Eto et al. [248].

Table 43-4 Galactocerebroside β-galactosidase in globoid cell leukodystrophy

		Galactocerebroside β-galactosidase, nmol/(h·g)
Gray matter		
Krabbe's disease	1	12.1
	2	10.8
	3	5.7
Pathologic controls (n = 9)*		123 ± 32
Normal controls (n = 4)		123 ± 17
White matter		
Krabbe's disease	1	17.7
	2	21.8
	3	7.5
Pathologic controls (n = 9)*		197 ± 59
Normal controls (n = 4)		199 ± 55
Liver		
Krabbe's disease	3	6.4
Normal controls (n = 2)		125 and 113
Spleen		
Krabbe's disease	3	20.4
Normal controls (n = 2)		157 and 186

* Pathologic controls included metachromatic leukodystrophy, Schilder's disease, early and late-onset G_{M1} gangliosidosis, Tay-Sachs disease, G_{M2} gangliosidosis with total hexosaminidase deficiency, Hurler's syndrome, Gaucher's disease, and Niemann-Pick disease.
NOTE: Activities of four lysosomal p-nitrophenyl glycosidases were all normal in globoid cell leukodystrophy.
SOURCE: Data from Suzuki and Suzuki [16].

to be also extremely deficient in peripheral leukocytes [19, 256], serum [19], and cultured fibroblasts [19]. Both peripheral leukocytes and serum from patients with globoid cell leukodystrophy had galactocerebrosidase activities that were only a few percent of those obtained in normal or pathologic controls. Peripheral leukocytes and serum from parents of patients with Krabbe's disease, who are obligate heterozygous gene carriers, have galactocerebroside β-galactosidase activity that is intermediate between that of normal control individuals and that of patients [51, 258]. As in other organs, p-nitrophenyl β-galactosidase is normal in leukocytes and serum from patients with Krabbe's disease or their parents.

These findings are significant in two respects, one fundamental and the other practical: (1) the intermediate enzyme activities in heterozygous individuals strongly support the assumption that galactocerebrosidase deficiency is the genetically determined defect; (2) both leukocytes and serum provide the means of making definitive antemortem diagnosis of Krabbe's disease without resort to tissue biopsies; 1 ml of serum or leukocytes from 10 ml blood are sufficient for reliable assays, including the measurement of the activity of control enzymes such as p-nitrophenyl β-galactosidase.

Deficient activity of galactosylceramide β-galactosidase in globoid cell leukodystrophy can also be demonstrated with other natural substrates, galactosylsphingosine (psychosine) [191, 192], monogalactosyl-diglyceride [194], or lactosylceramide [195–205, 257]. Demonstration of the enzymatic deficiency with the use of lactosylceramide as the substrate requires a carefully standardized assay procedure, because another β-galactosidase, genetically distinct from galactosylceramide β-galactosidase, can also hydrolyze lactosylceramide under appropriate assay conditions [185, 197].

Globoid cell leukodystrophy is one of the two known human genetic disorders caused by a deficiency of β-galactosidase. The other disease is G_{M1} gangliosidosis, in which G_{M1} ganglioside β-galactosidase is deficient. Comparison of the enzymatic profiles of these two disorders is instructive (Table 43-5). Existence of these two diseases indicates that there are at least two genetically distinct lysosomal β-galactosidases with acidic pH optima that have largely different substrate specificities. Deficiencies of the respective enzymes result in entirely different disorders because of the different natural substrates involved. Both β-galactosidases share lactosylceramide as a common substrate, and consequently lactosylceramide accumulation does not occur to any significant degree in either globoid cell leukodystrophy or G_{M1} gangliosidosis. It can further be predicted that under these circumstances a specific disorder with accumulation of lactosylceramide probably does not occur in humans [259].

Nonspecific Enzyme Abnormalities

Austin et al. [260] earlier assayed brain, liver, and kidney tissue from patients with Krabbe's disease for a number of enzymatic activities. They found normal activities of acid and alkaline phosphatase, UDPG pyrophosphorylase, N-acetylglucosamine kinase, PAPS sulfatase, and arylsulfatase. In the brain, the activities of UDPG–glycogen transglucosylase and glucosamine-6-phosphate deaminase were somewhat increased.

In 1967, Austin and coworkers reported that the activity of PAPS:cerebroside sulfotransferase was deficient in the gray and white matter and in the kidneys of two patients with globoid cell leukodystrophy, compared with the activity of this enzyme in four matched control patients and one patient with metachromatic leukodystrophy [261, 262]. PAPS:cerebroside sulfotransferase is an anabolic enzyme that catalyzes the formation of sulfatide from cerebroside and active sulfate, phosphoadenosine phosphosulfate (PAPS), thus:

$$\text{Cerebroside} + \text{PAPS} \xrightarrow{\text{PAPS:cerebroside sulfotransferase}} \text{cerebroside sulfate (sulfatide)}$$

This deficiency of PAPS:cerebroside sulfotransferase once appeared to provide an enzymatic basis for the relative lack of sulfatide in white matter, but certain features in globoid cell leukodystrophy are difficult to explain on the basis of sulfotransferase deficiency. These include a relative excess of galactocerebroside in the white matter of patients with globoid cell leukodystrophy [16, 17], a normal glycolipid composition of residual myelin, the evidence that galactocerebroside is stored in the globoid cells, and the experimental production of globoid cells exclusively by intracerebral injection of galactocerebroside. Although questioned in at least one instance [263], the deficiency of sulfotransferase has been confirmed in additional cases by Austin [18], at least in gray and white matter, if not always in kidney.

One possible explanation for the deficiency of this enzyme is the abnormal histologic picture. Benjamins et al. [264] demonstrated that PAPS:galactosylceramide sulfotransferase is greatly enriched in oligodendroglial cells compared to neurons or astrocytes. This would be expected in view of the high concentration of sulfatide in the myelin sheath. The almost total loss of oligodendroglia in globoid cell leukodystrophy would result in a disproportionate loss of any enzymes enriched in the oligodendroglia. Another enzyme directly involved in galactosylceramide biosynthesis, UDP-galactose:ceramide galactosyltransferase, is also enriched in oligodendroglia [265], and it is likely that this enzyme is also reduced in the brain of patients with globoid cell leukodystrophy. It cannot yet be excluded that reduced activities of synthetic enzymes might be a result of metabolic regulation in the presence of a block in the degradative pathway.

Lees et al. [266] recently studied two enzymes localized in myelin, carbonic anhydrase and 2':3'-cyclic-nucleotide 3'-phosphohydrolase. Myelin isolated from white matter of a patient showed lower activities of these enzymes. While these abnormalities are not directly related to the genetic cause of the disease, they are of interest because they suggest that the myelin sheath in Krabbe's disease may be intrinsically abnormal. Myelin isolated from the brain of a metachromatic leukodystrophy patient was normal in the activities of these enzymes.

Pathophysiology If a genetic defect of galactosylceramide β-galactosidase is the underlying cause of globoid cell leukodystrophy, we should be able to explain the morphological and biochemical characteristics of the disease on the basis of this deficiency. These include (1) almost total loss of myelin and oligodendroglia, (2) normal chemical composition of remaining myelin [235], (3) morphological evidence of decrease in the amount of myelin during the illness [38], (4) massive infiltration by globoid cells, and (5) absence of excess accumulation of cerebroside in the brain despite a block in the degradative pathway.

Earlier Suzuki and Suzuki [16] formulated a plausible hypothesis based on the two apparently unique features of galactosylceramide. (1) Cerebroside is almost exclusively a constituent of myelin and oligodendroglia, as indicated by its virtual absence in the brain before myelination, and its almost complete loss in white matter of severely demyelinated brains [213, 213]. (2) Galactocerebroside appears to be unique among sphingoglycolipids in its ability to elicit the globoid cell reaction when injected into normal rat brain [11–13].

In accordance with this hypothesis, the following steps could occur in the brain of a patient with galactocerebroside β-galactosidase deficiency. Before myelination there is practically no cerebroside in the brain [210–212]. Therefore, lack of enzyme activity is of little consequence, although it is normally present at low concentrations even at this premyelination stage [179]. As soon as myelination begins, just before birth in humans, newly formed myelin begins to undergo normal turnover. This period coincides with a rapid rise of galactocerebroside β-galactosidase activity in normal brain [179]. In the brain of patients with Krabbe's disease, galactocerebroside from the

Table 43-5 β-Galactosidase profile of globoid cell leukodystrophy and G_{M1} gangliosidosis

Substrates	Globoid cell leukodystrophy	G_{M1} Gangliosidosis
4-methylumbelliferyl or ρ-nitrophenyl β-galactoside	Normal	Deficient
G_{M1} ganglioside	Normal	Deficient
Asialo G_{M1} ganglioside	Normal	Deficient
Lactosylceramide	Normal*	Deficient*
Lactosylceramide	Deficient†	Normal†
Galactosylceramide	Deficient	Normal
Galactosylsphingosine	Deficient	Normal
Monogalactosyl diglyceride	Deficient	Expected to be normal

* With the assay system of Tanaka and Suzuki [197].
† With the assay system of Wenger et al. [259].

catabolized myelin cannot be disposed of because of lack of the enzyme. This undegraded cerebroside elicits globoid cell infiltration. When globoid cells are produced experimentally by injection of cerebroside into normal brain, the globoid cell reaction subsides as excess cerebroside is digested. In Krabbe's disease, the globoid cells remain because galactocerebroside is not degraded. As myelination proceeds, galactocerebroside is formed, producing more globoid cells. However, myelination cannot proceed indefinitely, for ever-increasing globoid cells overwhelm the oligodendroglial cells, which soon die. When the stage of massive death of oligodendroglial cells is reached, rapid myelin breakdown occurs. Because myelin is an extension of oligodendroglial cell membranes, myelin breakdown contributes more cerebrosides, and these elicit further rapid increase of globoid cells. Finally, all the oligodendroglial cells die and all the myelin is broken down. The maximum globoid cell infiltration is achieved, for there is no further production of myelin cerebrosides. Therefore, the total amount of cerebroside that can accumulate in the brain during the short life-span of the patient is limited by the small amount of myelin produced before the death of all the oligodendroglial cells, and such total destruction usually takes place at what would have been normally a very early stage of myelination.

This hypothesis appears to explain the characteristic features of globoid cell leukodystrophy satisfactorily. The most crucial part of any hypothesis about the pathophysiology of this disease is the explanation of the lack of increase in the total galactocerebroside content in the brain. If galactocerebroside β-galactosidase deficiency is assumed to be present in vivo, the only logical explanation is that the production of galactocerebroside ceases at a stage of the disease when the total amount of cerebroside is still well below the concentration in normal brain. The almost exclusive localization of galactocerebroside in myelin and oligodendroglia and of UDP-galactose:ceramide galactosyltransferase in oligodendroglia, coupled with the almost total loss of these neural components in the terminal stage of the disease, supports the above hypothesis.

Critical to the hypothesis is the selective and almost complete loss of oligodendroglia. Perhaps the major weakness of the theory is its simple explanation of the loss of oligodendroglia. A competition between globoid cells and oligodendroglia as the possible mechanism of the oligodendroglial loss may seem contrived, because blockage of catabolism of the galactosylceramide within oligodendroglia would be likely to cause them to die before the globoid cell reaction. In an analogous genetic disorder, metachromatic leukodystrophy, the amount of sulfatide in white matter becomes excessive as a result of defective sulfatide degradation, but there is no massive oligodendroglial loss, and excess sulfatide accumulation does occur primarily within oligodendroglial cells (Chap. 44). Therefore, there must be something unique about the block of galactosylceramide catabolism.

These considerations led Miyatake and Suzuki to advance the psychosine hypothesis. Psychosine can be formed through UDP-galactose and sphingosine (Fig. 43-10). Although not firmly established, it is likely that UDP-galactose:ceramide galactosyltransferase also catalyzes galactosylation of sphingosine. Another potential route for psychosine formation—deacylation of galactosylceramide—could not be demonstrated in the author's laboratory or by Lin and Radin [267]. Psychosine with its free amino group is known to be highly cytotoxic [268]. Psychosine is also a substrate for galactosylceramide β-galactosidase, and patients with globoid cell leukodystrophy

are unable to degrade it. Thus, it is conceivable that psychosine generated within oligodendroglia during the period of active myelination might reach a toxic level, killing cells. Oligodendroglia are selectively destroyed because psychosine formation occurs primarily in these cells. This hypothesis seems to explain early destruction of oligodendroglial cells and the resultant cessation of myelination. Recently, Vanier, Svennerholm, and coworkers [155–157] provided strong support for this hypothesis by reporting up to 100-fold increases of psychosine in white matter of patients. Suzuki, Tanaka, and Suzuki [269] implanted psychosine into rat brain and found it to be highly toxic. When a mixture of 97 percent galactosylceramide and 3 percent psychosine was implanted, tissue degeneration was observed beyond the globoid cell proliferation expected from galactosylceramide alone. These findings are consistent with the psychosine hypothesis.

There is controversy whether Krabbe's disease represents early cessation of myelination or rapid breakdown of already formed myelin. On the basis of the above hypothesis, both processes are involved, and both occur as the result of the death of the oligodendroglia.

Malone et al. [270, 271] recently suggested formation of abnormal myelin on the basis of higher proportions of lighter, loosely compacted myelin. It is possible that their data reflect instead the early cessation of the normal myelination process. There is currently no solid evidence that the destruction of myelin is due to the formation of chemically abnormal myelin in Krabbe's disease.

Involvement of the peripheral nervous system is expected, for here the myelin also contains galactocerebroside. Histiocytes in peripheral nerves contain abnormal inclusions similar to those in the brain, but it is not clear why they are not transformed to the typical multinucleated globoid cells. The absence of discernible morphological and functional abnormalities outside the nervous system is understandable, because normally galactosylceramide is practically absent in most nonneural tissues. The residual activity of galactocerebroside β-galactosidase in these organs may be sufficient to maintain the normal turnover of minute amounts of galactocerebroside. Such appears to be the case in the kidney [251].

There is a fixed pattern of regional differences in susceptibility of the white matter to pathologic alterations. This question was approached recently by utilizing the canine globoid cell leukodystrophy model (see below) [272]. In normal dogs, no consistent regional differences were found in galactosylceramidase activity, but in vivo turnover of galactosylceramide appeared to be more rapid in those areas of the white matter which are consistently more severely affected by the disease. Therefore, such regional differences in the metabolic activity of galactosylceramide might be at least partially responsible for the regional differences in severity of the disease.

Krabbe's Disease as a Sphingolipidosis

Galactocerebroside β-galactosidase is a hydrolytic enzyme, normally localized in lysosomes. Therefore, the fundamental metabolic defect of Krabbe's disease corresponds to those in other inherited disorders of sphingolipid metabolism in which lysosomal hydrolytic enzymes involved in the degradation of particular sphingolipids are genetically defective. Of particular interest is the relationship of globoid cell leukodystrophy to Gaucher's disease. The sphingolipid involved in Gaucher's disease is glucocerebroside, and the missing enzyme is glucocerebrosidase. Glucocerebroside and galactocerebroside differ only in the sugar moiety, and the missing enzymes are those which cleave these sugars from the respective cerebrosides. The fundamental metabolic derangements in these diseases are quite similar, as are the morphological appearances of the globoid cells and Gaucher cells. Nevertheless, the clinical and overall pathologic features of the two diseases are entirely different. Galactocerebroside is almost exclusively localized in the nervous system, while glucocerebroside is normally present in visceral organs and is nearly absent in the normal brain except in the early developmental stages. Krabbe's disease is unique among the sphingolipidoses in that the total content of galactocerebroside is not elevated in spite of a metabolic block in its degradative pathway.

The two major criteria of Hers for an inborn lysosomal disease are (1) genetic deficiency of one of the acid hydrolases that is normally localized within the lysosome, and (2) consequent accumulation of undigested material within single membrane-bound organelles that are pathologically altered lysosomes [273]. Globoid cell leukodystrophy easily satisfies the first criterion, but not so clearly the second. At the stage of the disease in which brain tissues are usually examined very few oligodendroglia remain; the rare ones left contain no inclusions. Instead, numerous globoid cells are present that do contain abnormal inclusions, consisting of galactosylceramide. The abnormal inclusions appear, for the most part, to be scattered freely within the cytoplasm. Although they are occasionally found embedded within an electron-lucent or electron-dense matrix, only very rarely are they surrounded by a single limiting membrane. One could argue that the lack of the limiting membrane is seen in the terminal picture, similar to the typical full-fledged membranous cytoplasmic bodies in Tay-Sachs disease. However, the essentially identical ultrastructure of the experimental globoid cells, even at an early stage, appears to be against this explanation. Specimens from patients have not been studied for ultrastructural localization of the lysosomal marker enzyme acid phosphatase. In experimental globoid cells, acid phosphatase activity could not be demonstrated to be associated with the abnormal tubular inclusion or the surrounding matrix, although the enzyme was present within normal-appearing lysosomes that were occasionally found. Therefore, at present, there is no morphological, histochemical, or biochemical evidence for an association of the abnormal galactocerebroside-rich inclusions and lysosomes [274].

DIAGNOSIS AND TREATMENT

Brain biopsy had long been the final resort for the definitive antemortem diagnosis of globoid cell leukodystrophy since Blackwood and Cumings [7] emphasized the presence of the characteristic globoid cells. Because of the wide variations of morphological changes in different stages of the disease and in different areas of the brain, brain biopsy does not always establish the diagnosis. Giant cells, similar to globoid cells, may be encountered in other diseases, such as "the syndrome of familial leukodystrophy, adrenal insufficiency and cutaneous melanosis," in which half the patients showed globoidlike cells in cerebral white matter [275]. This disorder, now commonly called adrenoleukodystrophy [276], is characterized by

the presence of unusually long fatty acids in certain compounds in the brain and the adrenal system [277]. The diagnostic value of the peripheral nerve biopsy has not been fully explored, but, in view of consistent pathologic changes, particularly on the ultrastructural level, it may prove useful.

Assays of galactocerebroside β-galactosidase activity in readily available materials, such as serum, peripheral leukocytes, or cultured fibroblasts, unquestionably offer the best and most reliable means for definitive antemortem diagnosis of Krabbe's disease. The same assay is also useful for prenatal diagnosis of the affected fetus, using cultured amniotic fluid cells as the enzyme source. Since the first prenatal detection of the disease and confirmation of the diagnosis by histologic examination and by additional enzymatic assays on the fetal specimens (Table 43-6) [20, 278], a considerable number of affected fetuses have been detected. Although no comprehensive statistics exist, the following are the current summary of major centers: Göteborg-Lyon (10 affected out of 40 prenatal tests) [279], Denver (8 out of 33), New York (4 out of 18), Japan (2 out of 8). These cases add up to 24 affected cases in 107 pregnancies at risk. Other cases are sporadically reported in the literature [54, 280–285]. It is probably a reasonable estimate that 30 to 35 cases of globoid cell leukodystrophy have been diagnosed in utero.

Because of the broad specificity of galactosylceramidase, other natural substrates can, in principle, also be used for enzymatic diagnosis of globoid cell leukodystrophy. Galactosylsphingosine (psychosine) [190–193] or monogalactosyl-diglyceride [194] does not provide practical advantage, however, over the original assay for galactosylceramide hydrolysis. These substrates are more difficult to obtain and harder to label radioactively. The assay procedures are more complicated, and tissue activities may be lower than that toward galactosylceramide. The enzyme is more active toward lactosylceramide [257], but caution must attend use of this substrate for diagnosis of globoid cell leukodystrophy. There are two genetically distinct β-galactosidases in human tissues that are active toward lactosylceramide [197]. Lactosylceramidase I is probably identical to galactosylceramide β-galactosidase, and lactosylceramidase II is probably identical to G_{MI}-ganglioside β-galactosidase, which is deficient in G_{MI} gangliosidosis. For diagnosis of globoid cell leukodystrophy, therefore, one must use an assay system which determines lactosylceramidase I exclusively. The procedure developed by Wenger et al. [257] is excellent for this purpose. The important requirements are oleic acid, use of relatively small amounts of the substrate and pure sodium taurocholate, and absence of chloride ion. When these precautions are taken, G_{MI}-ganglioside β-galactosidase preparations free of galactosylceramidase activity are essentially inactive toward lactosylceramide [201, 286], thus making it possible to determine lactosylceramidase I in the presence of lactosylceramidase II. Lactosylceramidase II is not activated by taurocholate but is activated by sodium taurodeoxycholate, a major impurity in crude commercial taurocholate preparations [286]. If taurocholate is not pure, the lactosylceramidase I assay for diagnosis of globoid cell leukodystrophy may erroneously include activity due to lactosylceramidase II. The properties of the two lactosylceramidases and their distributions in tissues of patients with globoid cell leukodystrophy and G_{MI} gangliosidosis are compared in Table 43-7 and Fig. 43-11. A recent uptake and degradation study of lactosylceramide by cultured fibroblasts indicated that, not only in vitro, but in intact cells, both of the β-galactosidases are active

Table 43-6 Prenatal diagnosis of globoid cell leukodystrophy

Enzyme source	Galactosylceramide β-galactosidase, nmol/(h · mg protein)	4-Methylumbelliferyl β-galactosidase, nmol/(h · mg protein)
Cultured amniotic fluid cells		
Fetus at risk	0.09 and 0.10	698 and 542
Control 1	1.98 and 2.10	410 and 447
Control 2	1.80 and 1.56	485 and 467
Fetal brain		
Affected	0.03	70.0
Control 1	5.89	81.7
Control 2	6.28	84.7
Fetal liver		
Affected	0.03	265
Control 1	2.04	331
Control 2	2.77	337

NOTE: Amniocentesis was carried out at 14 gestational weeks, and the pregnancy was terminated at 20 weeks.
SOURCE: From Suzuki et al. [20].

toward lactosylceramide and that both globoid cell leukodystrophy and G_{M1} gangliosidosis fibroblasts, each lacking the respective lactosylceramidase, could degrade lactosylceramide at or near normal rate [287]. Conditions of assays with natural sphingolipid substrates have been carefully examined in several laboratories in recent years [288–293].

Assay of galactosylceramidase is also useful for detection of heterozygous carriers. Suzuki et al. [51] found fresh serum to be the most reliable enzyme source for carrier detection. The enzyme activity in serum is low and unstable, and loses activity in storage. Carrier detection is inherently less reliable than diagnosis of affected patients. Although average activity of herterozygotes always falls in the middle between that of the normal and of homozygous affected populations with high statistical significance, there is a range of overlap between the normal and carrier groups when sufficiently large numbers of individuals are tested [51, 293]. While a part of the reason for the overlap may be technical, the main reason appears to be the wide variation of the activity in the normal population. Since galactosylceramidase activity can easily vary over a threefold range in both normal and carrier populations, overlap is inevitable since the averages of the two populations differ only by a factor of 2.

One of the technical drawbacks of the enzymatic diagnosis of globoid cell leukodystrophy is the need for radioactively labeled natural substrates. Kato and Suzuki [294] developed a micromethod in which the galactosylceramidase reaction was coupled to the galactose dehydrogenase reaction with NAD as the acceptor. Although this procedure eliminates the need for the radioactive substrates and is highly sensitive, it is technically even more elaborate than the radioactivity assay. A chromogenic substrate developed by Gal et al. [295] (2-hexadecanoylamino-4-nitrophenyl-β-D-galactopyranoside) has become commercially available. A few reports indicated that this substrate is less specific for galactosylceramidase than the natural substrates and that its relatively low sensitivity could be a limitation [283, 285]. A new series of chromogenic and fluorogenic artificial substrates has been developed by Gatt [296]. These are essentially galactosylceramide chemically modified with an additional chromogenic or fluorogenic group at the ω end of the fatty acid. They appear to be as specific a substrate as the unmodified galactosylceramide. The fluorogenic substrate has an additional advantage of high sensitivity. Since the initial report was promising, confirmation with a larger number of samples is awaited.

Although profound deficiency of galactosylceramide β-galactosidase is almost always diagnostic of globoid cell leukodystrophy, the correspondence is not perfect. Wenger et al. [297] found a family in which some of the apparently healthy adult members showed levels of galactosylceramidase deficiency similar to those found in affected infants. Significance of this finding in relation to the pathogenetic mechanism of the disease is unclear, but it must be kept in mind when enzymatic diagnosis is attempted. None of the other laboratory diagnostic procedures advocated earlier for the diagnosis of globoid cell leukodystrophy, such as the pattern of CSF protein [37] or the elevated β-glucuronidase activity in CSF [78], is specific, and their usefulness is limited.

There is no specific treatment for patients with globoid cell leukodystrophy other than supportive care, nor is it expected that any effective specific treatment can be developed in the near future. Radin et al. [298] suggested the potential usefulness of synthetic compounds which stimulate galactosylceramide β-galactosidase activity in vitro. There are many fundamental obstacles to this approach or to enzyme replacement therapy. Any therapeutic attempt must deliver the agent or the enzyme to the brain across the blood-brain barrier. Furthermore, considerable neuropathologic changes are doubtless

Table 43-7 Comparison of two human lactosylceramidases

	Lactosylceramidase I	Lactosylceramidase II
Genetic relationship	Probably identical with galactocerebrosidase	May be identical with G_{M1} ganglioside β-galactosidase
Normal tissue distribution		
Brain	Major	Minor
Liver	Minor	Major
Krabbe's disease	Deficient	Normal or high
G_{M1} gangliosidosis	Normal or high	Deficient
Effect of assay system		
Pure taurocholate	+++	−
Crude taurocholate	+	+++
Pure taurodeoxycholate	+	++
Oleic acid	++	±
Chloride	±	+
Wenger assay system [257]	+++	−
Tanaka-Suzuki assay system [197]	+	+++

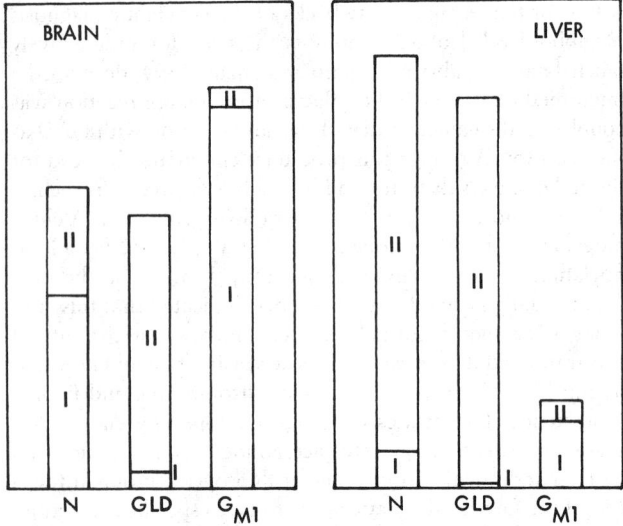

Figure 43-11 Distribution of lactosylceramidases in the brain and liver of normal individuals and in patients with globoid cell leukodystrophy or G_{M1} gangliosidosis. In normal brain, lactosylceramidase I is the major component while lactosylceramidase II is by far the major component in normal liver. Lactosylceramidase I is genetically deficient in globoid cell leukodystrophy, and lactosylceramidase II in G_{M1} gangliosidosis. Unaffected lactosylceramidases tend to be higher than normal in the respective disorders, as is often the case in genetic lysosomal disorders. The assay system of Wenger [257] exclusively determines the activity of lactosylceramidase I, and that of Tanaka and Suzuki [197] is optimal for lactosylceramidase I and less than optimal for lactosylceramidase II. If the assay system is poorly standardized, the determined activity of lactosylceramidase can include varying proportions of the two enzymes, thus making lactosylceramidase assays useless for diagnosis of either disease.

present at birth. Therapy must therefore start in utero, or ways must be found to overcome the essential irreversibility of once-damaged brain.

ANIMAL MODELS

Globoid cell leukodystrophy caused by genetic deficiency of galactosylceramidase also occurs in a few mammalian species other than humans. The disease in the cat was not characterized enzymatically [299]. In the single report of the disease in the sheep [300], galactosylceramidase activity in the brain was 6 percent of normal, and characteristic clinical and pathologic abnormalities were present. The best-characterized animal model is the canine form, and the newly discovered murine globoid cell leukodystrophy promises to be a useful tool for further research.

Canine Globoid Cell Leukodystrophy

In 1963, Fankhauser et al. [301] first reported that globoid cell leukodystrophy occurs in certain strains of dogs. The strains in which the disease is known are West Highland and Cairn terriers. The disease, which has been studied extensively from the clinical, morphological, and biochemical standpoints [302–319], appears to be transmitted as an autosomal recessive trait. The clinical picture is quite similar to that of the human disease. An example of clinical history is given here [303].

This male West Highland White Terrier seemed normal until three months of age when he gradually developed increasing difficulty in walking down stairs and in running on paved surfaces. He showed knuckling of digits while standing and began to fall on his hind limbs with bilateral extension of hock and stifle. On examination at 9 months of age, there was paraplegia with loss of placing and hopping reactions, hypoactive to absent deep reflexes of the posterior limbs, loss of sensation of the tail, and urinary incontinence.

Morphologically, there are remarkable similarities between the human and the canine forms of globoid cell leukodystrophy. The most conspicuous changes are the massive infiltration of globoid cells in the white matter, with morphological changes, distribution pattern, and staining characteristics identical to those in human globoid cells. There is severe loss of myelin, oligodendroglia, and axons, with concomitant marked astrocytic gliosis. Ultrastructurally, canine globoid cells are also quite similar to human globoid cells, containing the characteristic abnormal tubular inclusions. There are peripheral nerve lesions, again similar to those in human patients [311, 312]. Information regarding the lipid composition of the brain is still limited, but one author has reported decreased total lipid, decreased sulfatide, and slightly increased cerebroside [305].

Suzuki et al. [320] demonstrated that canine globoid cell leukodystrophy is also characterized by deficient galactocerebroside β-galactosidase activity. The enzyme was deficient in gray and white matter of the brain, liver, and kidney of two affected dogs (Table 43-8). As in human patients, there was no deficiency of p-nitrophenyl β-galactosidase activity. Moreover, one apparently healthy littermate of an affected dog had galactocerebrosidase activity intermediate between those of the affected dogs and another healthy littermate. The latter healthy littermate dog had the same high enzyme activities as a healthy mixed-breed dog. The littermate dog with intermediate enzyme values was probably a heterozygote. There was no PAPS:galactosylceramide sulfotransferase deficiency in the affected dogs [320]. As in human globoid cell leukodystrophy, peripheral leukocytes provide a convenient source for enzymatic diagnosis of affected and heterozygous carriers [321]. The enzymatic deficiency can also be demonstrated with psychosine [322] or lactosylceramide [323] as substrates.

Several pieces of evidence indicate that the canine disease is not identical with human globoid cell leukodystrophy. Serum is the most reliable enzyme source for diagnosis and carrier detection for human globoid cell leukodystrophy, but activities of galactosylceramide β-galactosidase are identical in sera of

Table 43-8 Galactocerebroside β-galactosidase in canine globoid cell leukodystrophy, nmol/(h · g)

	Gray matter	White matter	Liver	Kidney
Globoid cell leukodystrophy 1	14.1	13.0	16.7	12.3
2	15.1	15.0	37.6	
Normal 1	127		133	78.2
2	120	169	138	91.7
Heterozygous?*	76.2	108	75.6	29.5

* This dog was an asymptomatic littermate of the affected dog No. 1 and the normal dog No. 1
NOTE: There was no significant difference in the activities of p-nitrophenyl β-galactosidase in all specimens.
SOURCE: Data from Suzuki et al. [320].

affected, heterozygous, and normal control dogs [51]. This led to an observation that out of three electrofocusing peaks of hepatic galactosylceramidase, only the major peak is deficient in the canine globoid cell leukodystrophy, while all three peaks are essentially absent in the human disorder [322].

Recently, Constantino-Ceccarini et al. [324] used the canine model to investigate the biosynthetic activities of affected dog brains at various stages of the disease. Activity of UDP-galactose:ceramide galactosyltransferase was normal before the onset of clinical manifestations and then declined in white matter to approximately half normal as the disease progressed. When radioactive galactose was injected in vivo, the synthesis of important myelin components, such as galactosylceramide, cholesterol, or chloroform-methanol–soluble protein, was decreased, while synthesis of gangliosides and glycoproteins was unaffected.

A histologically similar disorder has also been described in blue-tick hound dogs [325] and in a beagle [326]. They were not characterized enzymatically.

Murine Globoid Cell Leukodystrophy (The Twitcher)

A new neurologic mutation was discovered recently in the mouse. It is a genetically and enzymatically authentic model of human globoid cell leukodystrophy. Like most of the known neurologic mouse mutants, this mutant, called twitcher, was first detected at the Jackson Laboratory, Bar Harbor, Maine. Affected mice develop clinical signs at approximately 20 days, with stunted growth, twitching, and hind leg weakness. By 40 days, they reach a near-terminal stage, and even with intensive maintenance care they die before 3 months. Histopathologic findings are similar to those of human and canine globoid cell leukodystrophy, both by light and electron microscopy [327, 328]. Enzymatic studies with galactosylceramide and lactosylceramide as the substrate unequivocally demonstrated that galactosylceramidase deficiency is the underlying lesion in this mutant [329, 330]. As a research tool, the canine and murine models offer complementary advantages and disadvantages. The canine model is more suitable for experiments which require relatively large amounts of tissue or dissection of different regions. On the other hand, the small size, rapid reproduction, and ease of maintenance make the mouse model far more convenient for experiments which require a large number of affected or heterozygous animals, or for in vivo injection of isotopes. The murine model has been utilized for peripheral nerve grafting experiments [331, 332]. The genetic status of individual mice can be conveniently and reliably determined by galactosylceramidase assays on homogenates of clipped tips of the tail within a few days of birth [333]. This permits morphological and biochemical studies of the disease process during the early critical period well before the clinical onset of the disease.

REFERENCES

1. KRABBE K: A new familial, infantile form of diffuse brain sclerosis. *Brain* 39:74, 1916
2. BULLARD WN, SOUTHARD EE: Diffuse gliosis of the cerebral white matter in a child. *J Nerv Ment Dis* 33:188, 1906
3. BENEKE R: Ein Fall hochgradigster ausgedehnter Sklerose des Centralnervensystems. *Arch Kinderheilkd* 47:420, 1908
4. COLLIER J, GREENFIELD JG: The encephalitis periaxialis of Schilder: A clinical and pathological study with an account of two cases, one of which was diagnosed during life. *Brain* 47:489, 1924
5. HALLERVORDEN J: Eine Speicherungshisticytose des kindlichen Gehirns (Gauchersche Krankheit?). *Verh Dtsch Ges Pathol* 32:96, 1948
6. AUSTIN JH: Studies in globoid (Krabbe) leukodystrophy. II. Controlled thin-layer chromatographic studies of globoid body fractions in seven patients. *J Neurochem* 10:921, 1963
7. BLACKWOOD W, CUMINGS JN: A histochemical and chemical study of three cases of diffuse cerebral sclerosis. *J Neurol Neurosurg Psychiat* 17:33, 1954
8. DIEZEL PB: Histochemische Untersuchungen an den Globoidzellen der familiären infantilen diffusen Sklerose vom Typus Krabbe. *Virchows Arch [Pathol Anat]* 327:206, 1955
9. DIEZEL PB: Histochemical investigations of degenerative diffuse sclerosis (leucodystrophy and diffuse sclerosis of the Krabbe type), in Cumings JN, Lowenthal A (eds): *Cerebral Lipidoses: A Symposium.* Springfield, Ill., Charles C Thomas, 1957, p 52
10. STAMMLER A: Klinik, Pathologie und Histochemie der infantilen diffusen Sklerose vom Typus Krabbe. *Dtsch Z Nervenheilkd* 174:505, 1956
11. AUSTIN J, LEHFELDT D, MAXWELL W: Experimental "globoid bodies" in white matter and chemical analysis in Krabbe's disease. *J Neuropathol Exp Neurol* 20:284, 1961
12. AUSTIN JH, LEHFELDT D: Studies in globoid (Krabbe) leucodystrophy. III. Significance of experimentally produced globoid-like elements in rat white matter and spleen. *J Neuropathol Exp Neurol* 24:265, 1965.
13. OLSSON R, SOURANDER P, SVENNERHOLM L: Experimental studies on the pathogenesis of leucodystrophies. I. The effect of intracerebrally injected sphingolipids in the rat brain. *Acta Neuropathol (Berl.)* 6:153, 1966
14. AUSTIN JH: Recent studies in the metachromatic and globoid body forms of diffuse sclerosis, in Folch-Pi J, Bauer H. (eds): *Brain Lipids and Lipoproteins, and the Leucodystrophies.* Amsterdam, Elsevier, 1963, p 120
15. SVENNERHOLM L: Some aspects of biochemical changes in leucodystrophy, in Folch-Pi J, Bauer H (eds): *Brain Lipids and Lipoproteins and the Leucodystrophies.* Amsterdam, Elsevier, 1963, p 104
16. SUZUKI K, SUZUKI Y: Globoid cell leucodystrophy (Krabbe's disease): Deficiency of galactocerebroside β-galactosidase. *Proc Nat Acad Sci USA* 66:302, 1970
17. SUZUKI K, SUZUKI Y, ETO Y: Deficiency of galactocerebroside β-galactosidase in Krabbe's globoid cell leucodystrophy, in Bersohn J, Grossman HJ (eds): *Lipid Storage Diseases: Enzymatic Defect and Clinical Implications.* New York, Academic, 1971, p 396
18. AUSTIN J, SUZUKI K, ARMSTRONG D, BRADY R, BACHHAWAT BK, SCHLENKER J, STUMPF D: Studies in globoid (Krabbe) leukodystrophy (GLD). V. Controlled enzymic studies in ten human cases. *Arch Neurol* 23:502, 1970
19. SUZUKI Y, SUZUKI K: Krabbe's globoid cell leukodystrophy: Deficiency of galactocerebrosidase in serum, leukocytes, and fibroblasts. *Science,* 171:73, 1971
20. SUZUKI K, SCHNEIDER EL, EPSTEIN CJ: In utero diagnosis of globoid cell leukodystrophy (Krabbe's disease). *Biochem Biophys Res Commun* 45:1363, 1971
21. HAGBERG B, KOLLBERG H, SOURANDER P, ÅKESSON HO: Infantile globoid cell leucodystrophy (Krabbe's disease): A clinical and genetic study of 32 Swedish cases 1953–1967. *Neuropädiatrie* 1:74, 1970
22. METZKE H, BERG U, ULRICH U: Zur Häufigkeit der diffusen infantilen familiären Hirnsklerose (Typ Krabbe). *Klin Pädiatr* 184:151, 1972
23. YOKOTA K, YUSA T, MITSUDOME A, TAKASHIMA S, KUROKAWA T, TAKESHITA K: An autopsy case of globoid cell leukodystrophy (Krabbe's disease). *Brain Dev. (Tokyo)* 5:296, 1973
24. OCHIAI Y, ARIMA M, TAKAHASHI K: A case of globoid cell leukodystrophy. *Jap J Pediat. (Tokyo)* 27:1092, 1974
25. WADA Y, ARAKAWA T, CHIDA N, ONUMA A, NAKAGAWA H, IINUMA K, YOSHIMURA Y, NAKAJIMA S, SUZUKI Y: Globoid cell leukodystrophy: The first case with antemortem diagnosis in Japan. *Tohoku J Exp Med* 115:53, 1975
26. WATANABE K, HARA K, YAMADA H, TAJIMA M, FUKUSHIMA M, IWASE K: A case of globoid cell leukodystrophy (Krabbe disease). *J Pediat Pract (Tokyo)* 40:461, 1977
27. SUKUZI Y, NAKAMURA N, JIMBO T, HORIGUCHI S, FUJII T: Prenatal diagnosis in twin pregnancy. *J Pediat* 93:293, 1978
28. OKEDA R, SUZUKI Y, HORIGUCHI S, FUJII T: Fetal globoid cell leukodystrophy in one of twins. *Acta Neuropathol* 47:151, 1979
29. MATSUYAMA H, MINOSHIMA I, WATANABE I: An autopsy case of leucodystrophy of Krabbe type. *Acta Pathol Jap* 13:195, 1963
30. OGATA J, KUME A, ITO Y, UZAWA N, YANAI N, KATSUKI S, TANAKA K: An autopsy case of Krabbe type leukodystrophy. *Adv Neurol Sci (Tokyo)* 13:318, 1969
31. KANEKO H, and UYEKUSA T: An autopsy case of Krabbe type leukodystrophy. *Adv Neurol Sci (Tokyo)* 13:435, 1969
32. JACOB JC, KUTTY KM, ISLAM M, DOMINIC RG, DAWSON G: Krabbe's

disease: Globoid cell leukodystrophy. *Can Med Assoc J* 108, 1398, 1973

33. METZKE H, and RATH FW: Über eine Familie mit diffuser familiärer infantiler Hirnsklerose. *Kinderaerztl Prax* 7:312, 1970

34. GEHUCHTEN P VAN: Sur l'origine des cellules globoides dans in cas de sclerose diffuse. *Rev Neurol (Paris)* 94:253, 1956

35. TAORI GM, SHALINI KCM, MARTIN KB, BHAKTAVIZIAM A, BACHHAWAT BK: Globoid leukodystrophy (Krabbe's disease). *Indian J Med Res* 58:993, 1970

36. SCHOCHET SS JR, HARDMAN JM, LAMPERT PW, EARLE KM: Krabbe's disease (globoid leukodystrophy): Electron microscopic observations. *Arch Pathol* 88:305, 1969

37. HAGBERG B, SOURANDER P, SVENNERHOLM L: Diagnosis of Krabbe's infantile leukodystrophy. *J Neurol Neurosurg Psychiat* 26:195, 1963

38. D'AGOSTINO AM, SAYRE GP, HAGLES AB: Krabbe's disease. *Arch Neurol* 8:82, 1963

39. CROME L, HANEFELD F, PATRICK D, WILSON J: Late onset globoid cell leukodystrophy. *Brain* 96:84, 1973

40. DUNN HG, DOLMAN CL, FARRELL DF, TISCHLER B, HASINOFF C, WOOLF LI: Krabbe's leukodystrophy without globoid cells. *Neurology* 26:1035, 1976

41. NELSON E, AUREBECK G, OSTERBERG K, BERRY J, JABBOUR JT, BORNHOFEN J: Ultrastructural and chemical studies on Krabbe's disease. *J Neuropathol Exp Neurol* 22:414, 1963

42. CHRISTENSEN E, MELCHIOR JC, ANDERSEN H: Diffuse infantile familial sclerosis (Krabbe-type). *Acta Psychiatr Neurol Scand* 35:431, 1960

43. LIU HM: Ultrastructure of globoid leukodystrophy (Krabbe's disease) with reference to the origin of globoid cells. *J Neuropathol Exp Neurol* 29:441, 1970

44. NEUBURGER K: Zur Histopathologie der multiplen Sklerose im Kindesalter *Z Neurol Psychiatr* 76:384, 1972

45. MCNAMARA ED: Encephalitis periaxilaris (Schilder). *Proc R Soc Med* 26:297, 1933

46. VERHAART WJC: A case of multiple sclerosis in an Indian in the Dutch East Indies. *Psychiatr Neurol Bladen (Amst)* 35:511, 1931

47. GUILLAIN G, BERTRAND I, GRUNER J: Sur un type anatomoclinique special de leucoencéphalite à nodules morulés gliogènes. *Rev Neurol (Paris)* 73:401, 1941

48. FERRARO A: Familial form of encephalitis periaxialis diffusa. *J Nerv Ment Dis* 66:329, 1927

49. FERRARO A: Familial form of encephalitis periaxialis diffusa. *J Nerv Ment Dis* 66:479, 1927

50. FERRARO A: Familial form of encephalitis periaxialis diffusa. *J Nerv Ment Dis* 66:616, 1927

51. SUZUKI K, SUZUKI Y, FLETCHER TF: Further studies of galactocerebroside β-galactosidase in globoid cell leukodystrophy, in Volk, BW Aronson SM (eds): *Sphingolipids, Sphingolipidoses and Allied Disorders.* New York, Plenum, 1972, p 487

52. YOUNG E, WILSON J, PATRICK AD, CROME L: Galactocerebrosidase deficiency in globoid cell leukodystrophy of late onset. *Arch Dis Child* 47:449, 1972

53. HANEFELD F, WILSON J, CROME L: Die juvenile Form der Globoidzell-Leukodystrophie. *Monatsschr Kinderheilkd* 121:293, 1973

54. GULLOTTA F, PAVONE L, MOLLICA F, GRASSO S, VALENTI C: Krabbe's disease with unusual clinical and morphological features. *Neuropädiatrie* 10:395, 1979

55. HAGBERG B: The clinical diagnosis of Krabbe's infantile leucodystrophy. *Acta Paediatr Scand* 52:213, 1963

56. SUZUKI K, GROVER WD: Krabbe's leukodystrophy (globoid cell leukodystrophy): An ultrastructural study. *Arch Neurol* 22:385, 1970

57. ALLEN N, DE VEYRA E: Microchemical and histochemical observations in a case of Krabbe's leukodystrophy. *J Neuropathol Exp Neurol* 26:456, 1967

58. HOGAN GR, GUTMANN L, CHOU SM: The peripheral neuropathy of Krabbe's (globoid) leukodystrophy. *Neurology (Minneapolis)* 19:1093, 1969

59. SCHOCHET SS, JR, McCORMICK WF, POWELL GF: Krabbe's disease. A light and electron microscopic study. *Acta Neuropath* 36:153, 1976

60. YUNIS EJ, LEE RE: The ultrastructure of globoid (Krabbe) leukodystrophy. *Lab Invest* 21:415, 1969

61. LAXDAL T, HALLGRIMSSON K: Krabbe's globoid cell leucodystrophy with hydrocephalus. *Arch Dis Child* 49:232, 1974

62. MOOSA A: Peripheral neuropathy and ichthyosis in Krabbe's leukodystrophy. *Arch Dis Child* 46:112, 1971

63. JACOBI M: Über Leukodystrophie und Pelizaeus-Merzbachersche Krankheit. *Virchows Arch [Pathol Anat]* 314:460, 1947

64. WALLACE BJ, ARONSON SM, VOLK BW: Histochemical and biochemical studies of globoid cell leucodystrophy (Krabbe's disease). *J Neurochem* 11:367, 1963

65. OSETOWSKA E, GAIL H, LUKASEWICZ D, KARCHER D, AND WISNIEWSKI H: Leucodystrophie infantile précoce (type Krabbe): (Remarques sur les pro-

liférations gliales et les atrophies de système quipeuvent s'y observer). *Rev Neurol (Paris)* 102:463, 1960

66. KASS A: Acute infantile sclerosis of the brain (Krabbe's disease). *Acta Paediatr* 42:70, 1953

67. BIGNAMI A, TINGEY AH, TORRE C: La sclerosi cerebrale diffusa tipo Krabbe. *Riv Neurol* 31:712, 1961

68. AUSTIN JH: Recent studies in the metachromatic and globoid forms of diffuse sclerosis. *Res Publ Assoc Res Nerv Ment Dis* 40:189, 1962

69. DUNN HG, LAKE BD, DOLMAN DL, WILSON J: The neuropathy of Krabbe's infantile cerebral sclerosis (globoid cell leucodystrophy). *Brain* 92:329, 1969

70. SACREZ R, LEVY JM, GRUNER JE, BILLUART J, CARLIER G: La leucodystrophie de Krabbe. *Arch Fr Pédiat* 22:641, 1965

71. CUMINGS JN, ROZDILSKY B: The cerebral lipid composition of the brain in six cases of Krabbe's disease. *Neurology (Minneapolis)* 15:177, 1965

72. LIEBERMAN JS, OSHTORY M, TAYLOR RG, DREYFUS PM: Perinatal neuropathy as an early manifestation of Krabbe's disease. *Arch Neurol* 37:446, 1980

73. POSER CM, VAN BOGAERT L: Natural history and evolution of the concept of Schilder's diffuse sclerosis. *Acta Psychiatr Scand* 31:285, 1956

74. NORMAN RM, OPPENHEIMER DR, TINGEY AH: Histological and chemical findings in Krabbe's leucodystrophy. *J Neurol Neurosurg Psychiat* 24:223, 1961

75. MALONE MJ, SZOKE MC, LOONEY GL: Globoid leukodystrophy. I. Clinical and enzymatic studies. *Arch Neurol* 32:606, 1975

76. KOLODNY EH, ADAMS RD, HALLER JS, JOSEPH J, CRUMRINE PK, and RAGHAVAN SS: Late-onset globoid cell leukodystrophy. *Ann Neurol* 8:219, 1980

77. HAGBERG B, SVENNERHOLM L: Metachromatic leucodystrophy—a generalized lipidosis: Determination of sulfatides in urine, blood plasma and cerebrospinal fluid. *Acta Paediatr* 49:690, 1960

78. ALLEN N, REAGAN E: Beta-glucuronidase activities in cerebrospinal fluid. *Arch Neurol* 11:144, 1964

79. ALLEN NE, SHUTTLEWORTH C, CLENDENON NR, GORDON WA: Cerebrospinal fluid β-glucuronidase activity in the diagnosis of Krabbe's leucodystrophy. *Int Congr Ser 193,* Amsterdam, Excerpta Medica, 1969, p 181

80. LANE B, CARROLL BA, PEDLEY TA: Computerized cranial tomography in cerebral diseases of white matter. *Neurology* 28:534, 1978

81. HEINZ ER, DRAYER BP, HAENGGELI CA, PAINTER MJ, CRUMRINE P: Computed tomography in white matter disease. *Radiology* 130:371, 1979

82. AUSTIN JH: Some newer findings in Krabbe (globoid) leucodystrophy. *Trans Am Neurol Assoc* 87:66, 1962

83. BLOM S, HAGBERG B: EEG findings in late infantile metachromatic and globoid cell leucodystrophy. *Electroencephalogr Clin Neurophysiol* 22:253, 1967

84. KLIEMANN FA, HARDEN A, PAMPIGLIONE G: Some EEG observations in patients with Krabbe's disease. *Dev Med Child Neurol* 11:475, 1969

85. IINUMA K, ONUMA A: Electroencephalographic findings in a case of globoid cell leukodystrophy. *Tohoku J Exp Med* 115:75, 1975

86. EGGERS C, LEDERER H, and SCHEFFNER D: EEG-Befunde im Verlaufe progredienter Hirnerkrankungen im Kindesalter. *Monatschr. Kinderheilkd.,* 125:8, 1977

87. BUGIANI O, MASTROPAOLO C, DE NEGRI M: Association d'une leucodystrophie à cellules globoides d'une gliomatose et d'une abiotrophie. *Acta Neurol Belg* 68:799, 1968

88. ANDREWS JM, CANCILLA PA, GRIPPO J, MENKES JH: Globoid cell leukodystrophy (Krabbe's disease): Morphological and biochemical studies. *Neurology* 21:337, 1971

89. ANZIL AP, BLINZINGER K, MEHRAEIN P, DORN G, NEUHAUSER G: Cytoplasmic inclusions in a child affected with Krabbe's disease (globoid leucodystrophy) and in the rabbit injected with galactocerebrosides. *J Neuropathol Exp Neurol* 31:370, 1972

90. LYON G, JARDIN L, AICARDI J: Étude au microscope électronique d'un nerf périphérique dans un cas de leucodystrophie de Krabbe. *J Neurol Sci* 12:263, 1971

91. WILSON J, LAKE BD, DUNN HG: Krabbe's leucodystrophy: Some clinical and pathogenetic considerations. *J Neurol Sci* 10:563, 1970

92. GUTMANN L, HOGAN G, CHOU SM: The peripheral neuropathy of Krabbe's (globoid) leucodystrophy. *Electroencephalogr Clin Neurophysiol* 27:715, 1969

93. AUSTIN JH: Histochemical and biochemical studies in diffuse cerebral sclerosis (metachromatic and globoid-body forms), IVth *Int Congr Neuropathol* vol 1, Stuggart, Thieme, 1962, p 35

94. MAKITA A: Biochemistry of organ glycolipids. II. Isolation of human kidney glycolipids. *J Biochem (Tokyo)* 55:269, 1964

95. MARTENSSON E: Neutral glycolipids of human kidney: Isolation, identification and fatty acid composition. *Biochim Biophys Acta* 116:296, 1966

96. DIEZEL PB: *Die Stoffwechselstörungen der Sphingolipoide.* Berlin, Springer-Verlag, 1957

97. HAGER H, OEHLERT W: Ist die diffuse Hirnsklerose des Typ krabbe eine entzündliche Allgemeinerkrankung? *Z Kinderheilkd* 80:82, 1957

98. GREENFIELD JG, NORMAN RM: Demyelinating diseases, in Blackwood W, McMenemy WH, Meyer A, Norman RM, Russel DS (eds): 2d ed. *Greenfield's Neuropathology.* Baltimore, Williams & Wilkins, 1963, p 475

99. AUSTIN JH: Globoid (Krabbe) leukodystrophy, in Minkler J (ed): *Pathology of the Nervous System.* New York, McGraw-Hill, 1968, p 843

100. OEHMICHEN M, WIETHÖLTER H, GENCIC M: Cytochemical markers for mononuclear phagocytes as demonstrated in reactive microglia and globoid cells. *Acta Histochem* 66:243, 1980

101. OEHMICHEN M: Enzyme-histochemical differentiation of neuroglia and microglia: A contribution to the cytogenesis of microglia and globoid cells. *Path Res Pract* 168:244, 1980

102. SOURANDER P, HANSSON HA, OLSSON Y, SVENNERHOLM L: Experimental studies on the pathogenesis of leucodystrophies. II. The effect of sphingolipids on various cell types in cultures from the nervous system. *Acta Neuropathol (Berlin)* 9:231, 1966

103. PFEIFFER J: Zur formalen Genese der Globoidzellen bei der diffusen Sklerose vom Typus Krabbe. *Arch Psychiatr Nervenkr* 195:446, 1957

104. EINARSON L, STRÖMGREN E: Diffuse progressive leucoencephalopathy (diffuse cerebral sclerosis) and its relationship to amaurotic idiocy: Histological and clinical aspects. *Acta Jutland* 33:5, 1961

105. CHRISTENSEN E, MELCHIOR JC, NEGRI S: A comparative study of 16 cases of diffuse sclerosis with special reference to the histopathological findings. *Acta Neurol Scand* 37:163, 1961

106. OEHMICHEN M, GRUNINGER H: The origin of multinucleated giant cells in experimentally induced and spontaneous Krabbe's disease (globoid cell leukodystrophy). *Beitr Pathol* 153:111, 1974

107. KONIGSMARK BW, SIDMAN RL: The origin of brain macrophages in the mouse. *J Neuropathol Exp Neurol* 22:643, 1963

108. HUNTINGTON HW, TERRY RD: The origin of reactive cells in cerebral stab wounds. *J Neuropathol Exp Neurol* 25:646, 1966

109. ROSEMANN U, FRIEDE RL: Entry of labeled donor cells from the blood stream into the CNS. *J Neuropathol Exp Neurol* 26:144, 1967

110. EINARSON L, NEEL AF, STRÖMGREN E: On the problem of diffuse brain sclerosis with special reference to the familial form. *Acta Jutland* 16:1, 1944

111. HALLERVORDEN J: Die degenerative diffuse Sklerose, in Lubarsch H, Rossle B (eds): *Handbuch der speziellen pathologischen Anatomie und Histologie.* Berlin, Springer-Verlag, 1956, vol XII, part 1, p 758

112. DE VRIES E: Gliomatous polio- and leucodystrophy in young child. *J Neuropathol Exp Neurol* 17:501, 1958

113. SCHENK VW, GLUSZCZ A, ZELMAN IB: Atypical form of Krabbe-type leucodystrophy in two siblings accompanied by poliodystrophic changes. *Neuropathol Pol* 11:117, 1973

114. WILLIAMS RS, FERRANTE RJ, CAVINESS VS JR: The isolated human cortex. A Golgi analysis of Krabbe's disease. *Arch Neurol* 36:134, 1979

115. ANDREWS JM, CANCILLA P: Cytoplasmic inclusions in human globoid cell leukodystrophy. *Arch Pathol* 89:53, 1970

116. SHAW C-M, CARLSON CB: Crystalline structures in globoid-epithelioid cells: An electron microscopic study of globoid leukodystrophy (Krabbe's disease). *J Neuropathol Exp Neurol* 29:306, 1970

117. LAKE BD: Segmental demyelination of peripheral nerves in Krabbe's disease. *Nature (London)* 217:171, 1968

118. BISCHOFF A, ULRICH J: Peripheral neuropathy in globoid cell leukodystrophy (Krabbe's disease): Ultrastructural and histochemical findings. *Brain* 92:861, 1969

119. YUNIS EJ, LEE RE: Tubules of globoid leukodystrophy: A right-handed helix. *Science* 169:64, 1970

120. BLINZINGER K, ANZIL AP: Non-membrane bound cytoplasmic deposits in Krabbe globoid leukodystrophy. Further evidence of a revised concept of lysosomal storage diseases. *Experientia* 18:780, 1972

121. YUNIS EJ, LEE RE: Further observations on the fine structure of globoid leukodystrophy: Peripheral neuropathy and optic nerve involvement. *Hum Pathol* 3:371, 1972

122. HARCOURT B, ASHTON N: Ultrastructure of the optic nerve in Krabbe's leukodystrophy. *Br J Ophthalmol* 57:885, 1973

123. BROWNSTEIN S, MEAGHER-VILLEMURE K, POLOMENO RC, LITTLE JM: Optic nerve in globoid leukodystrophy (Krabbe's disease). Ultrastructural changes. *Arch Ophthalmol* 96:864, 1978

124. YAJIMA K, FLETCHER TF, SUZUKI K: Sub-plasmalemmal linear density: A common structure in globoid cells and mesenchymal cells. *Acta Neuropath* 39:195, 1977

125. SUZUKI K: Ultrastructural study of experimental globoid cells. *Lab Invest* 23:612, 1970

126. ANDREWS JM, MENKES JH: Ultrastructure of experimentally produced globoid cells in the rat. *Exp Neurol* 29:483, 1970

127. SOURANDER P, OLSSON Y: Peripheral neuropathy in globoid cell leukodystrophy (Morbus Krabbe). *Acta Neuropathol (Berlin)* 11:69, 1968

128. SCHLAEPFER WW, PRENSKY AL: Quantitative and qualitative study of sural nerve biopsies in Krabbe's disease. *Acta Neuropathol (Berlin)* 20:55, 1972

129. JOOSTEN EM, KRIJGSMAN JB, GABREËLS-FESTEN AA, GABREËLS FJ, BAARS PEC: Infantile globoid cell leukodystrophy (Krabbe's disease): Some remarks on clinical and sural nerve biopsy findings. *Dev Med Child Neurol* 16:228, 1974

130. MARTIN JJ, CEUTERICK C, MARTIN L, LEROY JG, NUYTS JP, JORIS C: Globoid cell leukodystrophy (Krabbe's disease): Peripheral nerve lesion. *Acta Neurol Belg* 74:356, 1974

131. WATANABE K, HARA K, IWASE K: The evolution of neurological and neurophysiological features in a case of Krabbe's globoid cell leukodystrophy. *Brain Develop (Tokyo)* 8:432, 1976

132. CARTER HE, GLICK FJ, NORRIS WP, PHILLIPS GE: Biochemistry of the sphingolipids. III. Structure of sphingosine. *J Biol Chem* 170:285, 1947

133. CARTER HE: Sphingolipids, in Page IH (ed): *Chemistry of Lipids as Related to Atherosclerosis.* Springfield, Ill, Charles C Thomas, 1958, p 82

134. GROB CA, GADIENT F: Die Synthese des Sphingosins und seiner Steroisomeren. *Helv Chim Acta* 40:1145, 1957

135. SHAPIRO D, SEGEL H, FLOWERS HM: The total synthesis of sphingosine. *J Am Chem Soc* 80:1194, 1958

136. PROSTENIK M, MAJHDER-ORESCANIN B: Occurrence of a new sphingolipid base, C_{20}-sphingosine in horse and beef brain. *Naturwissenschaften* 47:399, 1960

137. STANACEV NZ, CHARGAFF E: Icosisphingosine, a long chain base constituent of mucolipids. *Biochim Biophys Acta* 59:733, 1963

138. SAMBASIVARAO K, MCCLUER RH: Lipid components of gangliosides. *J Lipid Res* 5:103, 1965

139. SWEELEY CC, MOSCATELLI EA: Qualitative microanalysis and estimation of sphingolipid bases. *J Lipid Res* 1:40, 1959

140. MOSCATELLI EA, MAYES JR: Sphingosine bases of normal human white matter. *Biochemistry* 4:1386, 1965

141. ISAACSON E, MOSCATELLI EA: Sphingolipids of developing human central nervous tissue: Changes in composition of sphingosine bases. *J Neurochem* 17:365, 1970

142. O'BRIEN JS, ROUSER G: The fatty acid composition of brain sphingolipids: Sphingomyelin, ceramide, cerebroside, and cerebroside sulfate. *J Lipid Res* 5:339, 1964

143. ENG LF, GERSTL B, HAYMAN RB, LEE YL, TIETSORT RW, SMITH JK: The 2-hydroxy fatty acids in white matter of infant and adult brains. *J Lipid Res* 6:135, 1965

144. STÄLLBERG-STENHAGEN S, SVENNERHOLM L: Fatty acid composition of human brain sphingomyelins: Normal variation with age and changes during myelin disorders. *J Lipid Res* 6:146, 1965

145. O'BRIEN JS, SAMPSON EL: Fatty acid and fatty aldehyde composition of the major brain lipids in normal human gray matter, white matter, and myelin. *J Lipid Res* 6:545, 1965

146. MENKES JH, PHILIPPART M, CONCONE MC: Concentration and fatty acid composition of cerebrosides and sulfatides in mature and immature human brain. *J Lipid Res* 7:479, 1966

147. KLENK E, GIELEN W: Untersuchungen über die Konstitution der Ganglioside aus Mesenchengehirn und die Trennung des Gemisches in die Komponenten. *Z Physiol Chem* 326:144, 1961

148. TRAMS EG, GUIFFRIDA LE, KARMEN A: Gas chromatographic analysis of long-chain fatty acids in gangliosides. *Nature (London)* 193:680, 1962

149. LEDEEN R, SALSMAN K, CABRERA M: Gangliosides in subacute sclerosing leukoencephalitis: Isolation and fatty acid composition of nine fractions. *J Lipid Res* 9:129, 1968

150. SUZUKI K, SUZUKI K, KAMOSHITA S: Chemical pathology of G_{M1}-gangliosidosis (generalized gangliosidosis). *J Neuropathol Exp Neurol* 28:25, 1969

151. SVENNERHOLM L: The distribution of lipids in the human nervous system. I. Analytical procedure: Lipids of foetal and newborn brain. *J Neurochem* 11:839, 1964

152. SUZUKI Y, JACOB JC, SUZUKI K, SUZUKI K: G_{M2}-gangliosidosis with total hexosaminidase deficiency. *Neurology (Minneapolis)* 21:313, 1971

153. YAMAKAWA T, KISO N, HANDA S, MAKITA A, YOKOYAMA S: On the structure of brain cerebroside sulfuric ester and ceramide dihexoside of erythrocytes. *J Biochem (Tokyo)* 52:226, 1962

154. STOFFYN P, STOFFYN A: Structure of sulfatides. *Biochim Biophys Acta* 70:218, 1963

155. VANIER M-T, SVENNERHOLM L: Chemical pathology of Krabbe's disease. III. Ceramide hexosides and gangliosides of brain. *Acta Paediatr Scand* 64:641, 1975

156. VANIER M, SVENNERHOLM L: Chemical pathology of Krabbe's disease: The occurrence of psychosine and other neutral sphingoglycolipids. *Adv Exp Med Biol* 68:115, 1976

157. SVENNERHOLM L, VANIER M-T, MANSSON JE: Krabbe disease: A galactosylsphingosine (psychosine) lipidosis. *J Lipid Res* 21:53, 1980

158. BURTON RM, SODD MA, BRADY RO: The incorporation of galactose into galactolipids. *J Biol Chem* 233:1053, 1958

159. CLELAND WW, KENNEDY EP: The enzymatic synthesis of psychosine. *J Biol Chem* 235:45, 1960

160. BRADY RO: Studies on the total enzymatic synthesis of cerebrosides. *J Biol Chem* 237:PC2416, 1962

161. BRADY RO: Biosynthesis of glycolipids, in Dawson RMC, Rhodes DN (eds): *Metabolism and Physiological Significance of Lipids*. London, Wiley, 1964, p 95

162. HAMMARSTRÖM S: On the biosynthesis of cerebrosides: Nonenzymatic N-acylation of psychosine by stearoyl coenzyme A. *FEBS Lett* 21:259, 1972

163. MORELL P, RADIN NS: Synthesis of cerebroside by brain from uridine diphosphate galactose and ceramide containing hydroxy fatty acid. *Biochemistry* 8:506, 1969

164. MORELL P, COSTANTINO-CECCARINI E, RADIN NS: The biosynthesis by brain microsomes of cerebrosides containing nonhydroxy fatty acids. *Arch Biochem Biophys* 141:738, 1970

165. GOLDBERG IH: The sulfolipids. *J Lipid Res* 2:103, 1961

166. RADIN NS, MARTIN FB, BROWN JR: Galactolipide metabolism. *J Biol Chem* 224:499, 1957

167. HAUSER G: Labelling of cerebroside and sulfatides in rat brain. *Biochim Biophys Acta* 84:212, 1964

168. MCKHANN G, LEVY R, HO W: Metabolism of sulfatides. I. The effect of galactocerebrosides on the synthesis of sulfatides. *Biochem Biophys Res Commun* 20:109, 1965

169. BALASUBRAMANIAN AS, BACHHAWAT BK: Studies on enzymic synthesis of cerebroside sulfate from 3'-phosphoadenosine-5'-phosphosulfate. *Indian J Biochem* 2:212, 1965

170. BALASUBRAMANIAN AS, BACHHAWAT BK: Formation of cerebroside sulfate from 3'-phosphoadenosine 5'-phosphosulfate in sheep brain. *Biochim Biophys Acta* 106:218, 1965

171. HERSCHKOWTIZ N, MCKHANN GM, SAXENA S, SHOOTER EM: Characterization of sulfatide-containing lipoproteins in rat brain. *J Neurochem* 15:1181, 1968

172. HERSCHKOWTIZ N, MCKHANN GM, SAXENA S: Synthesis of sulphatide-containing lipoproteins in rat brain. *J Neurochem* 16:1049, 1969

173. MEHL E, JATZKEWITZ H: Ein Cerebrosid Sulfatase aus Schweineniere. *Z Physiol Chem* 339, 260, 1964

174. AUSTIN JH, ARMSTRONG D, SHEARER L: Metachromatic form of diffuse cerebral sclerosis. V. The nature and significance of low sulfatase activity: A controlled study of brain, liver and kidney in four patients with metachromatic leucodystrophy (MLD). *Arch Neurol* 13:593, 1965

175. MEHL E, JATZKEWITZ H: Evidence for the genetic block in metachromatic leucodystrophy (ML). *Biochem Biophys Res Commun* 19:407, 1965

176. HAJRA AK, BOWEN DM, KISHIMOTO Y, RADIN NS: Cerebroside galactosidase of brain. *J Lipid Res* 7:379, 1966

177. BOWEN DM, RADIN NS: Purification of cerebroside galactosidase from rat brain. *Biochim Biophys Acta* 152:587, 1968

178. BOWEN DM, RADIN NS: Properties of cerebroside galactosidase. *Biochim Biophys Acta* 152:599, 1968

179. BOWEN DM, RADIN NS: Cerebroside galactosidase: A method for determination and a comparison with other lysosomal enzymes in developing rat brain. *J Neurochem* 16:501, 1969

180. SUZUKI K: Galactosylceramide galactosidase, in Ginsburg V (ed): *Methods in Enzymology. Complex Carbohydrates, part B*. New York, Academic, 1972, vol 28, p 839

181. SUZUKI Y, SUZUKI K: Glycosphingolipid β-galactosidases. I. Standard assay procedures, and characterization by electrofocusing and gel filtration of the enzymes in normal human liver. *J Biol Chem* 249:2098, 1974

182. SUZUKI Y, SUZUKI K: Glycosphingolipid β-galactosidases. II. Electrofocusing characterization of the enzymes in human globoid cell leukodystrophy (Krabbe's disease). *J Biol Chem* 249:2105, 1974

183. SUZUKI Y, SUZUKI K: Glycosphingolipid β-galactosidases. IV. Electrofocusing characterization in G_{M1}-gangliosidosis. *J Biol Chem* 249:2113, 1974

184. MIYATAKE T, SUZUKI K: Partial purification and characterization of β-galactosidase from rat brain hydrolyzing glycosphingolipids. *J Biol Chem* 250:585, 1975

185. WENGER DA, SATTLER M, CLARK C: Partial purification of galactosyl- and lactosylceramide β-galactosidase from human brain. *Trans Am Soc Neurochem* 6:151, 1975

186. AWASTHI YC, LUND HW, LO JT, SRIVASTAVA SK: Sphingolipid β-D-galactosidases in globoid cell leukodystrophy. *Birth Defects* 14:113, 1978

187. BEN-YOSEPH Y, HUNGERFORD M, NADLER HL: The nature of mutation in Krabbe disease. *Am J Hum Genet* 30:644, 1978

188. BEN-YOSEPH Y, HUNGERFORD M, NADLER HL: Galactosylceramide β-galactosidase in Krabbe disease: Partial purification and characterization of the mutant enzyme. *Arch Biochem Biophys* 196:93, 1979

189. BEN-YOSEPH Y, HUNGERFORD M, NADLER HL: The interrelationship between high- and low-molecular weight forms of normal and mutant (Krabbe disease) galactocerebrosidase. *Biochem J* 189:9, 1980

190. MIYATAKE T, SUZUKI K: Galactosylsphingosine galactosyl hydrolase: Partial purification and properties of the enzyme in rat brain. *J Biol Chem* 247:5398, 1972

191. MIYATAKE T, SUZUKI K: Globoid cell leukodystrophy: Additional deficiency of psychosine galactosidase. *Biochem Biophys Res Commun* 48:538, 1972

192. MIYATAKE T, SUZUKI K: Additional deficiency of psychosine galactosidase in globoid cell leukodystrophy: Implication to enzyme replacement therapy, in *Proceedings of Symposium on Enzyme Therapy in Genetic Diseases, Birth Defects*, 9(2):136, 1973

193. MIYATAKE T, SUZUKI K: Galactosylsphingosine galactosyl hydrolase in rat brain: Probable identity with galactosylceramide galactosyl hydrolase. *J Neurochem* 22:231, 1974

194. WENGER DA, SATTLER M, MARKEY SP: Deficiency of monogalactosyl diglyceride β-galactosidase activity in Krabbe's disease. *Biochem Biophys Res Commun* 53:680, 1973

195. WENGER DA, SATTLER M, HIATT W: Globoid cell leukodystrophy: Deficiency of lactosyl ceramide beta-galactosidase. *Proc Nat Acad Sci USA* 71:584, 1974

196. WEGNER DA: Studies on galactosylceramide and lactosylceramide β-galactosidase. *Chem Phys Lipids* 13:327, 1974

197. TANAKA H, SUZUKI K: Lactosylceramide β-galactosidase in human sphingolipidoses: Evidence for two genetically distinct enzymes. *J Biol Chem* 250:2324, 1975

198. SVENNERHOLM L, HÄKANSSON G, VANIER MT: Chemical pathology of Krabbe's disease. IV. Studies of galactosylceramide and lactosylceramide β-galactosidases in brain, white blood cells, and amniotic fluid cells. *Acta Paediat Scand* 64:649, 1975

199. WENGER DA, SATTLER M, CLARK C: Effect of bile salts on lactosylceramide β-galactosidase activities in human brain, liver, and cultured skin fibroblasts. *Biochim Biophys Acta* 409:297, 1975

200. TANAKA H, SUZUKI K: Specificities of the two genetically distinct β-galactosidases in human sphingolipidoses. *Arch Biochem Biophys* 175:332, 1976

201. TANAKA H, SUZUKI K: Substrate specificities of the two genetically distinct human brain β-galactosidases. *Brain Res* 122:325, 1977

202. TANAKA H, SUZUKI K: Lactosylceramidase assays for diagnosis of globoid cell leukodystrophy and G_{M1}-gangliosidosis. *Clin Chim Acta* 75:267, 1977

203. HARZER K: The two human lactosylceramidases and their respective enzyme activity deficiency disease: Inhibition studies using p-nitrophenyl β-D-galactoside. *Human Genet* 41:341, 1978

204. SUZUKI K, TANAKA H, YAMANAKA T, VAN DAMME O: The specificities of β-galactosidase in the degradation of gangliosides, in Svennerholm L, Mandel P, Dreyfus H, Urban P-F (eds): *Structure and Function of Gangliosides*. New York, Plenum, 1980, p 307

205. POULOS A, BECKMAN K: A comparison of the properties and bile salt specificities of galactosylceramide and lactosylceramide β-galactosidase activities in human leukocytes and fibroblasts. *Clin Chim Acta* 28:277, 1980

206. CARTER TP, BEBLOWSKI DW, SAVAGE MH, KANFER JN: Human brain cerebroside β-galactosidase: Deficiency of transgalactosidic activity in Krabbe's disease. *J Neurochem* 34:189, 1980

207. HANADA E, SUZUKI K: Activation of human brain galactosylceramidase by phosphatidylserine. *Biochim Biophys Acta* 575:410, 1979

208. HANADA E, SUZUKI K: Specificity of galactosylceramidase activation by phosphatidylserine. *Biochim Biophys Acta* 619:396, 1980

209. WENGER DA, SATTLER M, ROTH R: A protein activator of galactosylceramide β-galactosidase activity. *Trans Am Soc Neurochem* 12:210, 1981

210. FOLCH-PI J: Composition of the brain in relation to maturation, in Waelsch H (ed): *Biochemistry of the Developing Nervous System*. New York, Academic, 1955, p 121

211. CUZNER ML, DAVISON AN: The lipid composition of rat brain myelin and subcellular fractions during development. *Biochem J* 106:29, 1968

212. WELLS MA, DITTMER JC: A comprehensive study of the postnatal changes in the concentration of the lipids of developing rat brain. *Biochemistry* 6:3169, 1967

213. KAMOSHITA S, RAPIN I, SUZUKI K, SUZUKI K: Spongy degeneration of the brain: A chemical study of two cases including isolation and characterization of myelin. *Neurology (Minneapolis)* 18:975, 1968

214. SUZUKI Y, TUCKER SH, RORKE LB, SUZUKI K: Ultrastructural and biochemical studies of Schilder's disease. II. Biochemistry. *J Neuropathol Exp Neurol* 29:405, 1970

215. BASS NH, HESS HH: A comparison of cerebroside, proteolipid proteins, and cholesterol as indices of myelin in the architecture of rat cerebrum. *J Neurochem* 16:731, 1969

216. NORTON WT, PODUSLO SE: Myelination in rat brain: Changes in myelin composition during brain maturation. *J Neurochem* 21:759, 1973

217. O'BRIEN JS, SAMPSON EL, STERN MB: Lipid composition of myelin from the peripheral nervous system. *J Neurochem* 14:357, 1967

218. DICKERSON JWT: The composition of nervous tissues, in Davison AN, Dobbing J (eds): *Applied Neurochemistry*. Philadelphia, Davis, 1968, p 48

219. EICHBERG J, HAUSER G, KARNOVSKY ML: Lipids of nervous tissue, in Bourne GH (ed): *The Structure and Function of Nervous Tissue*. New York, Academic, 1969, vol III, p 185

220. MOKRASCH LC: Myelin, in Lajtha A (ed): *Handbook of Neurochemistry*. New York, Plenum, 1969, vol 1, p 171

221. NORTON WT: The myelin sheath, in Goldensohn ES, Appel SH (eds): *Scientific Approaches to Clinical Neurology.* Philadelphia, Lea & Febiger, 1977, p 259

222. NORTON WT: Isolation and characterization of myelin, in Morell P (ed): *Myelin.* New York, Plenum, 1977, p 161

223. SMITH ME: The metabolism of myelin lipids, in Paoletti R, Kritchevsky D (eds): *Advances in Lipid Research.* Vol 5, New York, Academic, 1967, p 241

224. BENJAMINS JA, SMITH ME: Metabolism of myelin, in Morell P (ed): *Myelin.* New York, Plenum, 1977, p 233

225. YAKOVLEV P, LECOURS AR: The myelogenetic cycles of regional maturation of the brain, in Minkowski A (ed): *Regional Development of the Brain in Early Life.* Oxford, Blackwell, 1967, p 3

226. AUGUST C, DAVISON AN, WILLIAMS FM: Phospholipid metabolism in nervous tissue. IV. Incorporation of ^{32}P into the lipids of subcellular fractions of the brain. *Biochem J* 81:8, 1961

227. CUZNER ML, DAVISON AN, GREGSON NA: Chemical and metabolic studies of rat myelin of the central nervous system. *Ann N.Y. Acad Sci* 122:86, 1965

228. DAVISON AN, GREGSON NA: Metabolism of cellular membrane sulpholipids in the rat brain. *Biochem J* 98:915, 1966

229. SMITH ME, ENG LF: The turnover of the lipid contents of myelin. *J Am Oil Chem Soc* 42:1013, 1965

230. RAPPAY G, POSALAKY Z: Beiträge zur Frage der Spezfität der Tetrazoniumreaktion. *Acta Histochem (Jena)* 7:212, 1959

231. AUSTIN J: Studies in globoid (Krabbe) leukodystrophy. I. The significance of lipid abnormalities in white matter in 8 globoid and 13 control patients. *Arch Neurol* 9:207, 1963

232. TINGEY AH, EDGAR GWF: A contribution to the chemistry of the leucodystrophies. *J Neurochem* 10:817, 1963

233. JATZKEWITZ H: Die Leukodystrophie, Typ Scholz (metachromatische form der diffusen Sklerose) als Sphingolipoidose (Cerebrosidschwefelsäureester-Speicherkrankheit). *Z Physiol Chem* 318:265, 1960

234. MENKES JH, DUNCAN C, MOOSSY J: Molecular composition of the major glycolipids in globoid cell leucodystrophy. *Neurology (Minneapolis)* 16:581, 1966

235. ETO Y, SUZUKI K: Brain sphingoglycolipids in Krabbe's globoid cell leucodystrophy. *J Neurochem* 18:503, 1971

236. LEES, MB: The chemical pathology of lipidoses and leukodystrophies. *Res Publ Assoc Res Nerv Ment Dis* 40:222, 1962

237. LEES MB, MOSER HW: The chemical pathology of Krabbe's disease and metachromatic leukodystrophy, in Aronson SM, Volk BW (eds): *Cerebral Sphingolipidosis.* New York, Academic, 1962, p 179

238. ROBINSON N, CUMINGS JN: Biochemical and histochemical observations on Krabbe's disease (globoid body diffuse sclerosis). *Acta Neuropathol (Berlin)* 9:280, 1967

239. PILZ H: Die Sphingolipoidveränderungen bei der Leukodystrophie Typ Krabbe im Vergleich zum akuten und chronischen sudanophilen Markzerfall. *Acta Neuropathol (Berlin)* 4:16, 1964

240. SVENNERHOLM L, VANIER MT: Brain gangliosides in Krabbe disease, in Volk BW, Aronson SM (eds): *Sphingolipids, Sphingolipidoses and Allied Disorders.* New York, Plenum, 1972, p 499

241. VANIER, MT, SVENNERHOLM L: Chemical pathology of Krabbe's disease. I. Lipid composition and fatty acid patterns of phosphoglycerides in brain. *Acta Paediatr Scand* 63:494, 1974

242. BRANTE G: Studies on lipids in the nervous system, with special reference to quantitative chemical determination and topical distribution. *Acta Physiol Scand* 18, suppl 63:164, 1949

243. EVANS JE, MCCLUER RH: The structure of brain dihexosylceramide in globoid cell leukodystrophy. *J Neurochem* 16:1393, 1969

244. NEIMANN N, MARCHAL C, VIDAILHET M, PHILIPPART M, FALL M, FLOQUET J: Étude clinique, anatomopathologique, ultrastructurale, biochimique et enzymatique de deux cas de maladie de Krabbe. *Ann Med de Nancy* 10:163, 1971

245. BERRA B, BRUNNGRABER EG, AGUILAR V: Gangliosides, glycoproteins, and glycosaminoglycans in Krabbe's disease. *Clin Chim Acta* 47:325, 1973

246. VANIER MT, SVENNERHOLM L: Chemical pathology of Krabbe's disease. II. Fatty acid composition of cerebrosides, sulfatides and sphingomyelins in brain. *Acta Paediatr Scand* 63:501, 1974

247. CUMINGS JN, THOMPSON EJ, GOODWIN H: Sphingolipids and phospholipids in microsomes and myelin from normal and pathological brains. *J Neurochem* 15:243, 1968

248. ETO Y, SUZUKI K, SUZUKI K: Globoid cell leucodystrophy (Krabbe's disease): Isolation of myelin with normal glycolipid composition. *J Lipid Res* 11:473, 1970

249. O'BRIEN JS, SAMPSON EL: Myelin membrane: A molecular abnormality. *Science* 150:1613, 1965

250. NORTON WT, PODUSLO SE: Metachromatic leucodystrophy: Chemically abnormal myelin and cerebral biopsy studies of three siblings, in Ansell GB, (ed): *Variations in the Chemical Composition of the Nervous System.* Oxford, Pergamon, 1966, p 82

251. SUZUKI K: Renal cerebroside in globoid cell leukodystrophy (Krabbe's disease). *Lipids* 6:433, 1971

252. DAWSON G: Hepatic galactosylceramide in globoid cell leukodystrophy (Krabbe's disease). *Lipids* 8:154, 1973

253. HOF L, MATALON R, DORFMAN A: Gangliosides in human skin fibroblasts and their enrichment in the "Hurler variant" and Krabbe's disease. *Z Physiol Chem* 352:1329, 1971

254. RADIN NS, HOF L, BRADLEY RM, BRADY RO: Lactosylceramide galactosidase: Comparison with other sphingolipid hydrolases in developing rat brain. *Brain Res* 14:497, 1969

255. OKADA S, O'BRIEN JS: Generalized gangliosidosis: Beta-galactosidase deficiency. *Science* 160:1002, 1968

256. MALONE MJ: Deficiency in a degradative enzyme system in globoid leucodystrophy. *Abstr 1st Conf Am Soc Neurochem* Albuquerque, 1970, p 56

257. WENGER DA, SATTLER M, CLARK C, MCKELVEY H: An improved method for the identification of patients and carriers of Krabbe's disease. *Clin Chim Acta* 56:199, 1974

258. FARRELL DF, PERCY AK, KABACK MM, MCKHANN GM: Globoid cell (Krabbe's) leukodystrophy: Heterozygote detection in cultured skin fibroblasts. *Am J Hum Genet* 25:604, 1973

259. WENGER DA, SATTLER M, CLARK C, TANAKA H, SUZUKI K, DAWSON G: Lactosylceramidosis: Normal activity for two lactosylceramide β-galactosidases. *Science* 188:1310, 1975.

260. AUSTIN JH, BALASUBRAMANIAN AS, PATTABIRAMAN TN, SARASWATHI S, BASU DK, BACHHAWAT BK: A controlled study of enzymic activities in three human disorders of glycolipid metabolism. *J Neurochem* 10:805, 1963

261. BACHHAWAT BK, AUSTIN J, ARMSTRONG D: A cerebroside sulphotransferase deficiency in a human disorder of myelin. *Biochem J* 104:15C, 1967

262. AUSTIN J, ARMSTRONG D, STUMPF D, KRETSCHMER L, MITCHELL C, VANZEE B, BACHHAWAT B: Defective sulfatide synthesis in Krabbe's disease (globoid leukodystrophy). *Trans Am Neurol Assoc* 175:179, 1967

263. PERCY AK, MCKHANN GM: The biochemistry of myelin and the leukodystrophies, in Vinken PJ, Bruyn GW (eds): *Handbook of Clinical Neurology.* Amsterdam, Elsevier, 1970, vol 10, p 134

264. BENJAMINS JA, GUARNIERI M, MILLER K, SONNEBORN M, MCKHANN GM: Sulfatide synthesis in isolated oligodendroglial and neuronal cells. *J Neurochem* 23:751, 1974

265. DESHMUKH DS, FLYNN TJ, PIERINGER RA: The biosynthesis and concentration of galactosyldiglyceride in glial and neuronal enriched fractions of actively myelinating rat brain. *J Neurochem* 22:479, 1974

266. LEES MB, SAPIRSTEIN VS, REISS DS, KOLODNY EH: Carbonic anhydrase and 2',3'-cyclic nucleotide 3'-phosphohydrolase activity in normal human brain and in demyelinating diseases. *Neurology* 30:719, 1980

267. LIN YN, RADIN NS: Alternate pathways of cerebroside catabolism. *Lipids* 8:732, 1973

268. TAKETOMI T, NISHIMURA K: Physiological activity of psychosine. *Jap J Exp Med* 34:255, 1964

269. SUZUKI K, TANAKA H, SUZUKI K: Studies on the pathogenesis of Krabbe's leukodystrophy: Cellular reaction of the brain to exogenous galactosylsphingosine, monogalactosyl diglyceride and lactosylceramide, in Volk BW, Schneck L (eds): *Current Trends in Sphingolipidoses and Allied Disorders.* New York, Plenum, 1976, p 99

270. MALONE MJ, SZOKE MC, DAVIS DA: Globoid leukodystrophy. II. Ultrastructure and chemical pathology. *Arch Neurol* 32:613, 1975

271. MALONE MJ, SAKURAGAWA N, SZOKE M: A comparative study of myelin fractions from metachromatic and globoid leukodystrophies. *Neurology* 25:827, 1975

272. YAMANAKA T, FLETCHER TF, TIFFANY CW, SUZUKI K: Galactosylceramide metabolism in different regions of the central nervous system: Possible correlation with regional susceptibility in genetic leukodystrophies, in Callahan JW, Lowden JA (eds): *Lysosomes and Lysosomal Storage Diseases.* New York, Raven, 1981, p 147

273. HERS HG: Inborn lysosomal diseases. *Gastroenterology* 48:625, 1965

274. SUZUKI K: Globoid cell leukodystrophy (Krabbe's disease), in Hers HG, van Hoof F (eds): *Lysosomes and Storage Diseases.* New York, Academic 1973, p 395

275. AGUILAR MH, O'BRIEN JS, TABER P: The syndrome of familial leukodystrophy, adrenal insufficiency and cutaneous melanosis, in Aronson SM, Volk BW (eds): *Inborn Disorders of Sphingolipid Metabolism.* Oxford, Pergamon, 1967, p 149

276. SCHAUMBURG HH, POWERS JM, RAINE CS, SUZUKI K, RICHARDSON EP: Adrenoleukodystrophy: A clinical and pathological study of 17 cases. *Arch Neurol* 32:577, 1975.

277. IGARASHI M, SCHAUMBURG H, POWERS J, KISHIMOTO Y, KOLODNY E, SUZUKI K: Fatty acid abnormality in adrenoleukodystrophy. *J Neurochem* 26:851, 1976

278. ELLIS WG, SCHNEIDER EL, MCCULLOUGH JR, SUZUKI K, EPSTEIN CJ: Fetal globoid cell leukodystrophy (Krabbe disease): Pathological and biochemical examination. *Arch Neurol* 29:253, 1973

279. VANIER MT, SVENNERHOLM L, MÄNSSON JE, HÄKANSSON G, BOUÉ A, LINDSTEN J: Prenatal diagnosis of Krabbe disease. *Clin Genet* 20:79, 1981

280. HARZER K, BENZ HU, KNÖRR-GÄRTNER H, JONATHA WD, KNÖRR K: Pränatale Diagnose der Globoidzell-Leukodystrophie (Morbus Krabbe). *Dtsch. Med. Wochenschr* 101:821, 1976

281. LARGET-PIET L, VANIER MT, BERTHELOT J, GUITTET J, LARGET-PIET A, BEUCHER A, OURY C: Maladie de Krabbe. *Pediatrie* 32:539, 1977

282. HARZER K: Prenatal diagnosis of globoid cell leukodystrophy (Krabbe's disease). Third documented case. *Human Genet* 35:193, 1977

283. BESLEY GT, BAIN AD: Use of a chromogenic substrate for the diagnosis of Krabbe's disease with special reference to its application in prenatal diagnosis. *Clin Chim Acta* 88:229, 1978

284. FARRELL DF, SUMI SM, SCOTT CR, RICE G: Antenatal diagnosis of Krabbe's leukodystrophy: Enzymatic and morphological confirmation in affected fetus. *J Neurol Neurosurg Psychiat* 41:76, 1978

285. BESLEY GT: The use of natural and artificial substrates in the prenatal diagnosis of Krabbe's disease. *J Inherited Metab Dis* 1:115, 1978

286. TANAKA H, MEISLER M, SUZUKI K: Activity of human hepatic β-galactosidase toward natural glycosphingolipid substrates. *Biochim Biophys Acta* 398:452, 1975

287. TANAKA H, SUZUKI K: Globoid cell leukodystrophy (Krabbe's disease): Metabolic studies with cultured fibroblasts. *J Neurol Sci* 38:409, 1978

288. BESLEY GT, BAIN AD: Krabbe's globoid cell leukodystrophy. Studies on galactosylceramide β-galactosidase and non-specific β-galactosidase of leukocytes, cultured skin fibroblasts, and amniotic fluid cells. *J Med Genet* 13:195, 1976

289. SUZUKI K: Globoid cell leukodystrophy (Krabbe's disease) and G$_{M1}$-gangliosidosis, in Glew RH, Peters, SP (eds): *Practical Enzymology of Sphingolipidoses*. New York, Alan Liss, 1977, p 101

290. SUZUKI K: Enzymatic diagnosis of sphingolipidoses. *Methods Enzymol* 50C:456, 1978

291. SVENNERHOLM L: Diagnosis of the sphingolipidoses with labelled natural substrates. *Adv Exp Med Biol* 101:689, 1978

292. SVENNERHOLM L, HÄKANSSON G, MAUNSSON JE, VANIER MT: The assay of sphingolipid hydrolases in white blood cells with labelled natural substrates. *Clin Chim Acta* 92:53, 1979

293. SVENNERHOLM L, VANIER MT, HÄKANSSON G, MÄNSSON JE: Use of leukocytes in diagnosis of Krabbe disease and detection of carriers. *Clin Chim Acta* 112:333, 1981

294. KATO T, SUZUKI Y: Enzymatic microdetermination method for galactocerebrosidase in tissue samples. *Proc Japan Acad* 55B:69, 1979

295. GAL AE, BRADY RO, PENTCHEV PG, FURBISH FS, SUZUKI K, TANAKA H, SCHNEIDER EL: A practical chromogenic procedure for the diagnosis of Krabbe's disease. *Clin Chim Acta* 77:53, 1977

296. BESLEY GTN, GATT S: Spectrophotometric and fluorimetric assays of galactocerebrosidase activity, their use in the diagnosis of Krabbe disease. *Clin Chim Acta* 110:19, 1981

297. WENGER DA, RICCARDI VM: Possible misdiagnosis of Krabbe disease. *J Pediatr* 88:76, 1976

298. RADIN NS, ARORA RC, ULLMAN MD, BRENKERT AL, AUSTIN J: A possible therapeutic approach to Krabbe's globoid leukodystrophy and the status of cerebroside synthesis in the disorder. *Res Commun Chem Pathol Pharmacol* 3:637, 1972

299. JOHNSON KH: Globoid leukodystrophy in the cat. *J Am Vet Med Assoc* 157:2057, 1970

300. PRITCHARD DH, NAPTHINE DV, SINCLAIR AJ: Globoid cell leukodystrophy in polled Dorset sheep. *Vet Path* 17:399, 1980

301. FANKHAUSER R, LUGINBÜHL H, HARTLEY WJ: Leukodystrophie vom Typus Krabbe beim Hund. *Schweiz Arch Tierheilkd* 105:198, 1963

302. FLETCHER TF, KURTZ HJ, LOW DG: Globoid cell leukodystrophy (Krabbe type) in the dog. *J Am Vet Med Assoc* 149:165, 1966

303. JORTNER BS, JONAS AM: The neuropathology of globoid cell leucodystrophy in the dog: A report of two cases. *Acta Neuropathol (Berlin)* 10:171, 1968

304. AUSTIN J, ARMSTRONG D, MARGOLIS G: Studies of globoid leukodystrophy in dogs. *Neurology (Minneapolis)* 18:300, 1968

305. AUSTIN J, ARMSTRONG D, MARGOLIS G: Canine globoid leukodystrophy: A model demyelinating disorder. *Trans Am Neurol Assoc* 93:181, 1968

306. FLETCHER T: Leukodystrophy in the dog. *Minn Vet* 9:19, 1969

307. AUSTIN J: Recent studies in two inborn errors of glycolipid metabolism, in Bogoch SE (ed): *The Future of the Brain Sciences*. New York, Plenum, 1969, p 397

308. McGRATH J, SCHUTTA H, YASEEN A, STEINBERG A: A morphology and biochemical study of canine globoid leukodystrophy. *J Neuropathol Exp Neurol* 28:171, 1969

309. HIRTH RS, NIELSEN SW: A familial canine globoid cell leukodystrophy ("Krabbe type"). *J Small Anim Pract* 8:569, 1967

310. FLETCHER TF, KURTZ HJ: Animal model: Globoid cell leukodystrophy in dog. *Am J Pathol* 66:375, 1972

311. KURTZ HJ, FLETCHER TF: The peripheral neuropathy of canine globoid cell leukodystrophy (Krabbe-type). *Acta Neuropathol (Berlin)* 16:226, 1970

312. FLETCHER TF, KURTZ HJ, STADLAN EM: Experimental Wallerian degeneration in peripheral nerves of dogs with globoid cell leukodystrophy. *J Neuropathol Exp Neurol* 30:593, 1971

313. FLETCHER TF: Electroencephalographic features of leukodystrophic disease in the dog. *J Am Vet Med Assoc* 157:190, 1970

314. FLETCHER TF, LEE DG, HAMMER RF: Ultrastructural features of globoid cell leukodystrophy in the dog. *Am J Vet Res* 32:177, 1971

315. YUNIS EJ, LEE RE: The morphologic similarities of human and canine globoid leukodystrophy. Thin section and freeze-fracture studies. *Am J Path* 85:99, 1976

316. YAJIMA K, FLETCHER TF, SUZUKI K: Canine globoid cell leukodystrophy. Part I. Further ultrastructural study of the typical lesion. *J Neurol Sci* 33:179, 1977

317. FLETCHER TF, JESSEN CR, BENDER AP: Quantitative evaluation of spinal cord lesions in canine globoid cell leukodystrophy. *J Neuropathol Exp Neurol* 36:84, 1977

318. YAJIMA K: Canine globoid cell leukodystrophy: Chronological neuropathological observation in the early lesions. *Brain and Develop* 12:153, 1980

319. ROSZEL JF, STEINBERG SA, McGRATH JT: Periodic acid-Schiff-positive cells in cerebrospinal fluid of dogs with globoid cell leukodystrophy. *Neurology* 22:738, 1972

320. SUZUKI Y, AUSTIN J, SUZUKI K, ARMSTRONG D, SCHLENKER J, FLETCHER T: Studies in globoid leukodystrophy: Enzymatic and lipid findings in the canine form. *Exp Neurol* 29:65, 1970

321. FLETCHER TF, SUZUKI K, MARTIN F: Galactocerebrosidase activities in canine globoid leukodystrophy. *Neurology* 27:758, 1977

322. SUZUKI Y, MIYATAKE T, FLETCHER TF, SUZUKI K: Glycosphingolipid β-galactosidases. III. Canine form of globoid cell leukodystrophy: Comparison with the human disease. *J Biol Chem* 249:2109, 1974

323. KURCZYNSKI TW, FLETCHER TF, SUZUKI K: Lactosylceramidases in canine globoid cell leukodystrophy. *J Neurochem* 29:37, 1977

324. CONSTANTINO-CECCARINE E, FLETCHER TF, SUZUKI K: Glycolipid metabolism in the canine form of globoid cell leukodystrophy, in Volk BW, Schneck L (eds): *Current Trends in Sphingolipidoses and Allied Disorders*. New York, Plenum, 1976, p 127

325. BOYSEN GB, TRYPHONAS L, HARRIES NW: Globoid cell leukodystrophy in the blue-tick hound dog. I. Clinical manifestations. *Can Vet J* 15:303, 1974

326. JOHNSON GR, OLIVER JE JR, SELCER R: Globoid cell leukodystrophy in a beagle. *J Am Vet Med Assoc* 167:380, 1975

327. DUCHEN LW, EICHER EM, JACOBS JM, SCARAVILLI F, TEIXEIRA F: A globoid cell type of leukodystrophy in the mouse: The mutant twitcher, in Baumann N (ed): *Neurological Mutations Affecting Myelination*. Amsterdam, Elsevier, 1980, p 107

328. DUCHEN LW, EICHER EM, JACOBS JM, SCARAVILLI F, TEIXEIRA F: Hereditary leucodystrophy in the mouse: The new mutant twitcher. *Brain* 103:695, 1980

329. KOBAYASHI T, SCARAVILLI F, SUZUKI K: Biochemistry of twitcher mouse: An authentic murine model of human globoid cell leukodystrophy, in Baumann N (ed): *Neurological Mutations Affecting Myelination*. Amsterdam, Elsevier, 1980, p 253

330. KOBAYASHI T, YAMANAKA T, JACOBS J, TEIXEIRA F, SUZUKI K: The twitcher mouse: An enzymatically authentic model of human globoid cell leukodystrophy (Krabbe disease). *Brain Res* 202:479, 1980

331. SCARAVILLI F, JACOBS JM, TEIXEIRA F: Quantitative and experimental studies on the twitcher mouse, in Baumann N (ed): *Neurological Mutations Affecting Myelination*. Amsterdam, Elsevier, 1980, p 115

332. SCARAVILLI F, JACOBS JM: Peripheral nerve grafting without immunological suppressive treatment in the twitcher mouse, a murine model of a human leucodystrophy. *Nature* 290:56, 1981

333. KOBAYASHI T, NAGARA H, SUZUKI K, SUZUKI K: The twitcher mouse: Determination of genetic status by galactosylceramidase assays on clipped tail. *Biochem Med*, 27:8, 1982

44

SULFATIDE LIPIDOSIS:
Metachromatic Leukodystrophy

EDWIN H. KOLODNY

HUGO W. MOSER

---

1. *Metachromatic leukodystrophy (MLD) is an inherited disorder of myelin metabolism. It is characterized by accumulation of galactosyl sulfatide (cerebroside sulfate) in the white matter of the central nervous system and in the peripheral nerves. Galactosyl sulfatide and to a smaller extent lactosyl sulfatide also accumulate within the kidney, gallbladder, and certain other visceral organs and are excreted in excessive amounts in the urine. In histological preparations, they form spherical granular masses that stain metachromatically.*

2. *The disease may appear at any age but is recognized most commonly in the second year of life. The child with this late-infantile form does not usually survive beyond the first decade. There is also a juvenile form presenting at age 5 to 7 and a more rare adult form that may begin at any time between the midteens and the seventh decade. In each of these variants the earliest signs are a gait disturbance, mental regression, and urinary incontinence. In the childhood variants, other common signs are blindness, loss of speech, quadriparesis, and peripheral neuropathy. In the adult, dementia is the major presenting sign and the disease may progress slowly over several decades.*

3. Multiple sulfatase deficiency, or mucosulfatidosis, is a rare form of MLD that resembles the late infantile variant but also includes features of a mucopolysaccharidosis. It presents at the same age as late infantile MLD but the affected child does not develop speech or the ability to walk. Additional findings are ichthyosis, coarse facial features, hepatosplenomegaly, abnormalities of the spine, and a mucopolysacchariduria.

4. *Cerebroside sulfate is normally metabolized by the hydrolysis of the 3-O-sulfate linkage to form galactocerebroside through the combined action of arylsulfatase A and a heat-stable nonenzymatic protein activator. The artificial compound p-nitrocatechol sulfate is the substrate most often employed to determine the level of arylsulfatase A activity. Deficiency of arylsulfatase A activity occurs in the late infantile, juvenile, and adult forms of MLD. In multiple sulfatase deficiency there is a deficiency not only of arylsulfatase A but also of other sulfatases including steroid sulfatase and the mucopolysaccharide sulfatases.*

5. *Several patients with many of the signs of juvenile MLD including a sulfatiduria have normal arylsulfatase A activity. These individuals are believed to be missing the activator necessary for in vivo hydrolysis of sulfatide.*

6. *Arylsulfatase A activity is occasionally deficient in some relatives of patients with MLD, in normal individuals, and in patients with other neurological diseases. In each of these circumstances, sulfatiduria does not occur and some cerebroside sulfate sulfatase activity can be found. In true MLD this particular activity is totally deficient.*

7. *MLD is transmitted as an autosomal recessive trait. Each form is probably genetically distinct, but a separate allele has only been demonstrated for multiple sulfatase deficiency. The locus that determines the expression of arylsulfatase A activity has been assigned to chromosome 22 on the basis of gene mapping experiments with human-rodent somatic cell hybrids.*

8. *The MLD heterozygote is identified by assaying leukocytes or cultured skin fibroblasts for their arylsulfatase A or cerebroside sulfate sulfatase activity. Similarly, prenatal diagnosis also can be performed by enzyme testing of cultured amniotic fluid cells provided that all cell pellets with arylsulfatase A deficiency are further checked with radioactively labelled sulfatide as substrate in in vitro or in situ tissue culture studies.*

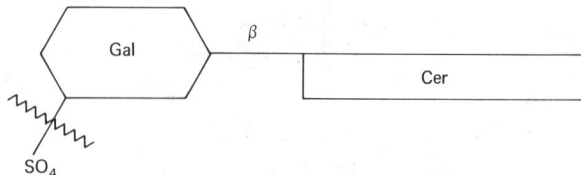

Figure 44-1   Galactosyl-3-sulfate ceramide, the major accumulating material in metachromatic leukodystrophy, and the site of the primary defect, a deficiency in arylsulfatase A.

HISTORICAL ASPECTS

Metachromatic staining [1] of the nervous system was first reported by Alzheimer [2] in 1910 in an adult patient with a clinical picture resembling general paresis. In 1921 Witte [3] described a similar patient with an accumulation of metachromatic material in the pituitary, liver, kidney, and testes. The detailed account by Scholz in 1925 [4] of three children from one family with progressive leukodystrophy included histologic studies of celloidin and paraffin-embedded blocks that had been dehydrated in alcohol. Most lipids, including the sulfatides, would be removed by this procedure, and the metachromatic properties of the tissue were missed. Scholz thought that the stored material represented breakdown products of myelin and proposed that the primary abnormality might be a glial cell defect. Thirty years later von Hirsch and Peiffer [5] described an acetic acid–cresyl violet stain that changes to a brown color in tissues from patients with MLD. With this stain Peiffer found striking metachromasia in frozen sections of the original patient of Scholz [6]. Thus, the report of Scholz supplemented with the findings of Peiffer represents the first comprehensive description of the clinical and pathologic aspects of juvenile MLD. The disease entity which Scholz described became known as leukodystrophy, type Scholz. A third type of MLD that begins in the late infantile period was reported by Greenfield [7] in 1933. Feigin is credited with the first description of a congenital form [8].

A significant biochemical advance was made in 1958 when Jatzkewitz [9] and Austin [10] independently demonstrated a large excess of sulfatides in tissues from patients with MLD. The accumulation of this acidic lipid causes the metachromasia characteristic of this disease. Austin [11] in 1963 reported the deficiency of arylsulfatase A in MLD and the following year Mehl and Jatzkewitz [12] demonstrated a block in the metabolism of cerebroside sulfate (Fig. 44-1). Arylsulfatase A was subsequently identified as the heat-labile component of cerebroside sulfate sulfatase [13]. Mehl and Jatzkewitz [14] also described a heat stable factor that activates cerebroside sulfate sulfatase activity severalfold. In a rare patient with MLD [15], it is this factor rather than arylsulfatase A that is deficient. Another variant with associated signs of a mucopolysaccharidosis has been reported several times since 1965 [16]. In this disorder, known as *multiple sulfatase deficiency*, or *mucosulfatidosis*, at least nine different sulfatases are deficient [17].

SULFOLIPIDS

Structure and Biosynthesis

The term *sulfolipid* is applied to all sulfur-containing lipids. These consist of lipids containing sulfur in the sulfate form and proteolipids containing amino acids that include sulfur in a different oxidation state. The non-amino acid lipid sulfur exists in three major classes of compounds (Fig. 44-2):

1. The sulfated sphingolipids, galactosyl sulfatide and lactosyl sulfatide, are the major sulfate-containing lipids in the nervous system (Fig. 44-2A and B).

2. Sulfate is present in certain galactose-containing glycerolipids that are found in small concentrations in the nervous system and in the testes after puberty (Fig. 44-2C).

3. Steroid sulfates are of particular importance in the adrenal, testis, and placenta, and are also normally present in plasma, red blood cells, and the brain (Fig. 44-2D).

In MLD, the catabolism of sulfatides and sulfogalactoglycerolipids is impaired; in the rare variant of MLD associated with multiple sulfatase deficiency, the metabolism of steroid sulfates is, in addition, also affected.

Sulfatides

STRUCTURE   Thudichum [18, 19] first recognized the existence of a sulfur-containing lipid and named it sulfatide. Blix, in 1933 [20], reported the isolation of this substance and showed it to contain equimolar amounts of cerebronic acid, sphingosine, galactose, and sulfate. It was eventually proven to be a sulfate ester of cerebroside with the sulfate joined by an ester linkage to the C-3 hydroxyl of galactose [21, 22]. As is true for cerebrosides, the sphingosine base of sulfatides consists predominantly of C-18 sphingosine [23]. The structural formula of galactosyl sulfatide appears in Fig. 44-2A.

Both sulfatides and cerebrosides contain a high proportion of long-chain fatty acids and of fatty acids that contain a 2-hydroxy group. In fact, nearly all of the 2-hydroxy fatty acids found in brain lipids are constituents of these two glycolipids. In adult brain, 20 to 25 percent of sulfatide fatty acids contain the 2-hydroxy group with cerebronic (C24h:0), oxynervonic (C24h:1), and the 22 and 23 carbon saturated fatty acids predominating. In fetal and immature brain, the proportion of hydroxy fatty acids is smaller. The major non-hydroxy fatty acids in sulfatide of adult brain are nervonic acid (C24n:1) and lignoceric acid (C24n:0), whereas in fetal and immature brain medium-chain fatty acids (C16n:0, C18n:0, and C18n:1) predominate. The development of the pattern characteristic of adult brain coincides with myelination.

The fatty acid pattern of kidney sulfatides differs from that in the brain. The kidney sulfatides contain more than 10 times as much behenic acid (C22n:0) as those in brain. Kidney sulfatides also contain a higher proportion of lignoceric acid than nervonic acid; in brain the reverse holds true [24, 25].

In 1963 Martensson demonstrated a dihexoside ceramide sulfuric acid ester fraction in human kidney [26]. The structural sequence of this compound was shown to be identical with lactosylceramide [25] and to contain in addition a sulfate ester linkage involving C-3 of the galactose [27]. Figure 44-2B shows the structure of lactosyl sulfatide. As in galactosyl sulfatide, the predominant sphingosine base is C-18 sphingosine. The fatty acid composition of kidney lactosyl sulfatide resembles that of kidney galactosyl sulfatide; nearly one-half of the fatty acids contain a 2-hydroxy group [25].

BIOSYNTHESIS   The major synthetic pathway for the formation of cerebroside sulfate is probably through sulfation of galactocerebroside [28] by reaction with 3'-phosphoadenosine-5'-phosphosulfate (PAPS) as follows:

$$\text{PAPS + cerebroside} \longrightarrow \text{cerebroside-3-sulfate + PAP}$$

The reaction is catalyzed by a microsomal sulfotransferase that has been demonstrated in a variety of mammalian tissues [29–32]. A precursor–product relationship between cerebroside and sulfatide is supported by the close compositional relationship that exists between these two glycosphingolipids in the brain and in the kidney. The same enzyme will also transfer the sulfate moiety of PAPS to lactosylceramide to form lactosyl sulfatide [31–33]. A second sulfotransferase has also been described that will sulfate galactosylsphingosine and lactosylsphingosine [31–34]. The significance of this pathway is unclear since neither of these compounds have been described as natural constituents of brain.

Sulfatide synthesis is maximal during the period of myelination and proceeds more slowly in the adult. It is stimulated by cortisol [35] and reduced in neonatal hypothyroidism [36]. Both neurons and oligodendroglial cells have sulfatide-synthesizing capability but sulfotransferase activity is much more active in cells of glial origin [37, 38]. Established cell lines from renal tubule epithelium have also been shown to synthesize sulfatide [39].

Sulfogalactoglycerolipid   Diacyl and alkylacyl glycerol forms of sulfogalactoglycerolipid have been characterized. Together these two lipids account for 2.1 to 7.2 percent of the total sulfolipids in rat brain [40]. The structure of the alkylacyl form is 1-0-alkyl-2-0-acyl-3 (β-3'-sulfogalactosyl) glycerol (Fig. 44-2 C). Its common name, seminolipid, reflects the fact that it is the major sulfolipid of mammalian testes and sperm [41]. A sulfotransferase step is involved in the synthesis of each lipid, but it is not certain whether the same or different sulfotransferases are responsible [42, 43].

Steroid Sulfates   Steroid sulfates found in human tissues include conjugates of cholesterol, dehydroepiandrosterone, estrogen, androgen, and corticosteroid. Their synthesis is catalyzed by one or more steroid sulfotransferases with PAPS serving as the sulfate donor [for review see Ref. 44].

Sulfolipid Degradation

Desulfation is the first step in the enzymatic hydrolysis of the sulfolipids. Each of these sulfate esters with the exception of the steroid sulfates is a substrate for arylsulfatase A. This lysosomal enzyme was so designated because of its ability to desulfate such unphysiologic aromatic sulfate esters as p-nitrocatechol sulfate and 4-methylumbelliferyl sulfate (Fig. 44-3). The hydrolysis of these synthetic compounds leads to a chromogenic or fluorigenic product that simplifies the quantitative analysis of this enzyme. These substrates are also hydrolyzed by arylsulfatase B, another lysosomal enzyme involved in mucopolysaccharide metabolism, and by arylsulfatase C, a microsomal enzyme active in steroid sulfate catabolism (see Table 44-1). In the pathogenesis of MLD arylsulfatase A is significant because its deficiency in classical cases of this disease leads to the accumulation of its major physiologic sub-

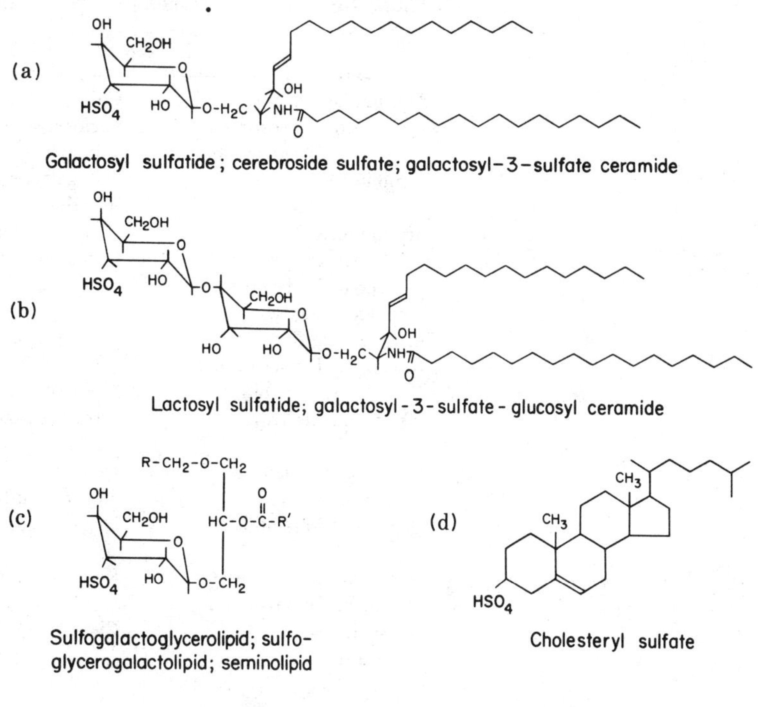

(a) Galactosyl sulfatide; cerebroside sulfate; galactosyl-3-sulfate ceramide

(b) Lactosyl sulfatide; galactosyl-3-sulfate-glucosyl ceramide

(c) Sulfogalactoglycerolipid; sulfo-glycerogalactolipid; seminolipid

(d) Cholesteryl sulfate

Figure 44-2   The structure of some sulfolipids. Note that a variety of fatty acyl groups and of sphingosine long-chain bases are found in naturally occurring sulfatides.

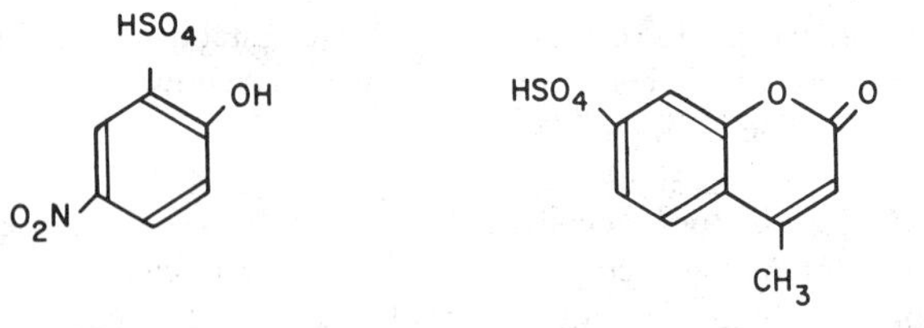

p-Nitrocatechol sulfate   4-Methylumbelliferyl sulfate

Figure 44-3 Synthetic substrates of arylsulfatase.

strate, cerebroside sulfate. In multiple sulfatase deficiency, all three arylsulfatases as well as other sulfate ester hydrolases listed in Table 44-1 are deficient.

Arylsulfatase A

STRUCTURAL AND PHYSICAL PROPERTIES   The arylsulfatases are found in all body tissues and fluids. Arylsulfatase A has been purified from a variety of sources including human liver [45–47], placenta [48, 49], and urine [50, 51]. It is an acidic glycoprotein with a low isoelectric point due to a high content of aspartic and glutamic acids. It also contains large amounts of proline. Ox liver [52] and sheep brain [53] arylsulfatase A contain respectively 10 and 25 percent carbohydrate. The enzyme binds tightly to conconavalin A [48, 50] and is modified by neuraminidase [52] and gentle periodate treatment [54] as would be anticipated of a glycoprotein. A high uptake sugar linked phosphorylated form and a low uptake non-phosphorylated form have been shown for sheep brain arylsulfatase A [54].

Arylsulfatase A undergoes a pH-dependent polymerization forming a tetramer below pH 5.5. Above pH 6.5, the enzyme exists as a monomer with a molecular weight of approximately 100,000. In human urine, the enzyme consists of two subunits of identical size of 50,000 daltons each [50]. Arylsulfatase A purified from human liver also consists of two subunits but of slightly different sizes [46, 47]. Multiple molecular forms of

arylsulfatase A have been demonstrated in enzyme preparations from human urine [51], leukocytes [55, 56], cultured fibroblasts [57, 58] and liver [57–59]. Treatment with neuraminidase eliminates the more acidic bands in certain enzyme preparations [57, 58]. In one study of liver arylsulfatase A [59], two forms with slightly differing properties were separated by polyacrylamide gel electrophoresis, an α-form that had a pH optimum of 4.6 and acted at low ionic strength, and a β-form that had a pH optimum of 5.15 and acted in a high ionic strength environment. Only the α-form had cerebroside sulfate-cleaving activity. Other studies of multiple components in arylsulfatase A preparations have not demonstrated any substrate differences among them.

CATALYTIC SITE   The active site of arylsulfatase A contains an essential histidine residue [60] and two or more arginine residues [61]. Many anions are inhibitors of the enzyme at concentrations in the millimolar range or lower. These include SO_4^{2-}, PO_4^{3-}, SO_3^{2-} and F^-. The reaction is also inhibited by Ag^+, Cu^{2+} and by carbonyl reagents in the presence of Cu^{2+}. Antibodies to arylsulfatase A have been shown in one study to increase enzyme activity [62] and in another to slightly decrease enzyme activity [63].

KINETICS   A time-dependent inactivation of arylsulfatase A occurs during its reaction with *p*-nitrocatechol sulfate (Fig. 44-4). Partial reactivation results on exposure to SO_4^{2-} or certain other anions. It has been proposed that the reaction between enzyme and substrate substantially modifies the enzyme with loss of secondary structure [65]. An enzyme-antibody complex also shows anomalous kinetics but the enzyme inactivation is significantly lower than for the native enzyme; presumably, this is because the antibody retards the process of structural rearrangement or covalent modification of the enzyme [63]. A similar inactivation of arylsulfatase A occurs during its hydrolysis of cerebroside sulfate, but no reactivation results on addition of SO_4^{2-} [66]. The anomalous kinetics of arylsulfatase A render it impossible to determine

Table 44-1 Human arylsulfatases and glycosaminoglycan sulfatases

Enzyme	Natural substrates	Deficiency states
Arylsulfatase A (EC 3.1.6.1, lysosomal) (EC 3.1.6.8, cerebroside sulfatase)	Galactosyl sulfatide Lactosyl sulfatide Sulfogalactosylsphingosine Sulfogalactoglycerolipid Ascorbic acid-2-sulfate	Metachromatic leukodystrophy Multiple sulfatase deficiency
Arylsulfatase B (EC 3.1.6.1, lysosomal N-acetylgalactosamine-4-sulfate sulfatase)	UDP-N-acetylgalactosamine-4-sulfate Dermatan sulfate Chondroitin-4-sulfate	Maroteaux-Lamy disease Multiple sulfatase deficiency
Arylsulfatase C (EC 3.1.6.1, microsomal) (EC 3.1.6.2, sterol sulfate, sulfohydrolase)	Dehydroepiandrosterone sulfate Pregnenolone sulfate Androstenediol-3-sulfate Estrone sulfate Cholesteryl sulfate	X-Linked ichthyosis Multiple sulfatase deficiency
Iduronide-2-sulfate sulfatase	Dermatan sulfate Heparan sulfate	Hunter disease Multiple sulfatase deficiency
Heparan-N-sulfamidase	Heparan sulfate	Sanfilippo disease type A Multiple sulfatase deficiency
N-acetylgalactosamine-6-sulfate sulfatase	Keratan sulfate	Morquio disease, type A Multiple sulfatase deficiency
N-acetylglucosamine-6-sulfate sulfatase	Chondroitin-6-sulfate	Mucopolysaccharidosis VIII Multiple sulfatase deficiency

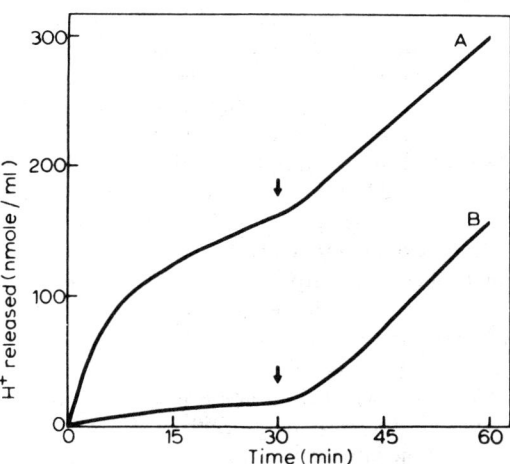

Figure 44-4 Time curves of "native" and "modified" ox liver arylsulfatase A. Modified arylsulfatase A was obtained by gel filtration and dialysis of a conventional assay mixture. Both native (*a*) and modified (*b*) enzymes were then incubated with *p*-nitrocatechol sulfate under standard conditions in a pH-stat, and the rate of cleavage was determined. At 30 min (*arrow*) SO_4^{2-} was added to both assays. Note the diminished activity of modified enzyme compared with native, prior to addition of SO_4^{2-}. *(From Nicholls and Roy [64].)*

initial reaction rates. This property may have little if any physiological significance since it occurs only with the monomeric form of the enzyme, whereas in its natural state in the lysosome the enzyme is probably in the dimeric form [67].

Substrate Specificity The cleavage of both *p*-nitrocatechol sulfate and cerebroside sulfate is catalyzed by the same enzyme. This conclusion is based on the copurification of both activities as well as on their common deficiency in MLD. For optimal in vitro activity of cerebroside sulfatase at ionic concentrations in the physiological range, a bile salt such as sodium cholate or taurodeoxycholate and Mn^{2+} are needed. The metal ion facilitates the formation of mixed micelles of detergent and cerebroside sulfate [68]. A heat-stable activator protein substitutes for the bile salt in vivo. This complementary factor is a nonenzymatic lysosomal glycoprotein with a molecular weight of 21,500 and isoelectric point of 4.3 [69, 70]. On a weight basis it is more effective than taurocholate. It forms a one-to-one complex with sulfatide that serves as the actual substrate of the enzyme [71]. In a system of very low ionic strength, purified arylsulfatase A can also hydrolyze cerebroside sulfate without the activator present.

Other galactosyl-3-sulfates can also be hydrolyzed by arylsulfatase A. These include lactosyl sulfatide [72], seminolipid [73, 74], and psychosine sulfate [74, 75]. The rates of hydrolysis for several natural and artificial substrates of arylsulfatase A are shown in Table 44-2. The activator of cerebroside sulfate sulfatase activity also stimulates the hydrolysis of seminolipid and the deacylated derivatives, lysoseminolipid and psychosine sulfate [74]. Ascorbic acid-2-sulfate is also a substrate for the enzyme [77]. The latter compound occurs throughout the body, but it apparently does not accumulate in MLD [78].

Arylsulfatase A does not hydrolyze chondroitin sulfate, cerebroside-6-sulfate or galactose-6-sulfate. It only feebly attacks tyrosine-O-sulfate, is inactive toward 5-hydroxytryptamine-O-sulfate, and has no phosphatase activity. Arylsulfatase B is discussed in Chap. 36, and arylsulfatase C in Chap. 49 of this text.

Physiologic Role

Sulfolipids share with other membrane lipids the dual capability of hydrophilic and hydrophobic interactions. In addition, their anionic charge allows combination with inorganic cations or organic amines to maintain the electrical neutrality of the membrane. Cerebroside sulfate (sulfatide), a major component of the myelin sheath [79], is located on the surface of this membrane [80] and is linked to basic proteins by ionic interactions [81]. It is believed to be involved in active sodium transport, serving as a cofactor for $[Na^+, K^+]$-dependent ATPase. The principal evidence in support of this hypothesis is the close correlation in many tissues of sulfatide concentrations with $[Na^+, K^+]$-ATPase activity [82], but there is at least as much evidence against this proposition. Within the kidney tubule cell, sulfatide and $[Na^+, K^+]$ ATPase have different topological locations [83]. Furthermore, neither antisulfatide antibodies nor treatment with cerebroside sulfatase appear to affect the activity of $[Na^+, K^+]$-dependent ATPase [83].

There is also evidence implicating sulfatide in the opiate binding site. It fulfills most of the structural requirements for an opiate receptor and the affinity with which it binds various opiates correlates well with their pharmacological potency [84, 85]. Antibodies to sulfatide antagonize the effect of morphine and β-endorphin on the periaquaductal gray region, which contains a high concentration of opiate and endorphin receptors [86]. Decreasing available sulfatide sites by treatment with azure A, a dye with high affinity for sulfolipids, also decreases the analgesic response to morphine [87]. In aqueous solutions of sulfatide, human β-endorphin adopts a partial helical conformation, possibly facilitating the electrostatic interaction between the protonated nitrogen of the opiates and the anionic groups at the binding site [88]. The sulfatide in myelin is probably not accessible for opiate binding because it is bound internally to basic protein [81].

A sulfolipid also appears to serve as a component of the (GABA) recognition site [89]. Preincubation of synaptic membrane suspensions with arylsulfatase A inhibits their ability to bind [³H]GABA. This effect can be blocked by known inhibitors of arylsulfatase A. Furthermore the degree of inhibition correlates directly with the *p*-nitrocatechol sulfate cleaving activity of the enzyme.

The sulfogalactoglycerolipids, because they are a myelin component and turn over rapidly during myelination, may have an important role in brain maturation [40]. They are also a major glycolipid of testes and spermatozoa and are thus important in spermatogenesis [41]. Steroid sulfates participate in detoxification reactions but may fulfill other membrane functions as well.

Table 44-2 Rate of hydrolysis of various sulfate esters by arylsulfatase A

Substrate	*μmol/min per milligram protein*
p-Nitrocatechol sulfate	160.0
4-Methylumbelliferyl sulfate	40.0
Ascorbic acid-2-sulfate	85.0
Cerebroside-3-sulfate	6.6
Seminolipid	5.0
Psychosine sulfate	3.0

SOURCE: Farooqui and Mandel [76].

CLINICAL MANIFESTATIONS

The six disorders that comprise the MLD group of diseases are summarized in Table 44-3. They are classified according to age of onset and biochemical defect. The most common forms are associated with deficiency of arylsulfatase A and are divided into late infantile, juvenile, and adult types.

Data on the age of onset for 55 cases published since 1977 and 15 cases from our own experience of the last 5 years are presented in Table 44-4. Most patients with the late infantile type develop clinical signs between ages 18 months and 2 years. Thereafter, the tempo of their disease is relatively rapid, with death occurring 1 to 7 years later.

The age of onset and duration of illness are far less stereotyped in the juvenile and adult variants. Many juvenile onset patients develop symptoms at about age 5 years, but a scattering of cases beginning in adolescence also suggests the possibility of two subgroups of juvenile MLD: an early-onset and a later-onset form. A similar subdivision occurs among the adult-onset cases. At least one-third become symptomatic at age 18 while the others develop the disease in the third, fourth, or a later decade. Those MLD patients whose symptoms begin around age 18 follow a clinical course that more closely resembles that of adult MLD than of juvenile MLD. This justifies their inclusion in the adult category of MLD [97] and suggests that the limit defining adult MLD be lowered below the age 21 milestone suggested by Austin [112] and adopted in previous editions of this text. A more appropriate age to demarcate the onset of adult-type cases of MLD might be 16 years. This is because there have been occasional reports of the disease first appearing at age 16 or 17 in the sib of a patient whose symptoms did not begin until after age 18 [91, 106]. Clearly, the same disease was evident in both so that age criteria should be established that will encompass both sibs under the same designation.

Late infantile and juvenile cases of MLD tend to have a shorter course than the adult cases, but the age of onset is not an entirely dependable indicator of disease duration. For example, very slow progression beyond a single decade has been observed in late infantile MLD [113], and in a juvenile case we have studied more than 20 years have passed since symptoms first appeared at age 5. In adult MLD, instances have been recorded of survival for 36 [112] and 42 years [107, 114] after the onset of clinical signs. For convenience, therefore, we retain the customary grouping of cases into late infantile, juvenile, and adult variants but acknowledge the heterogeneity that exists within each group with regard to age of onset and duration of illness.

There may be some regional variation in the relative frequency of the various forms of MLD (Table 44-5). In a report from Sweden [115] the late infantile form was found in 13 of 15 patients (87 percent) and in an English report [116] 13 of 17 (76 percent) were thus affected. A recent Finnish report [99] describes only two of nine patients with an onset before age 3. The authors of this report regard all of these patients as juvenile variants because they survived the age of 9 years. Using the age-of-onset concept to define the MLD variants separates two cases into the late-infantile class. The pre-1964 literature survey of Hollander [117] disclosed 67 percent of 60 cases with an onset of MLD typical of the late infantile variant. Our review of cases published since 1977 (Table 44-4) shows nearly equal numbers of cases of the late infantile and juvenile variants. Also, our own recent patient experience as well as that of Farrell [118] both suggest that approximately equal numbers of patients with these two variants are now being diagnosed. The adult variant occurred in 15 percent of Hollander's series [117]. In our own case experience and review of cases published during the last 5 years, the adult-onset variant accounted for 20 and 24 percent, respectively, of all cases. These somewhat higher frequencies are due in part to our use of 16 as the lower age limit for the onset of clinical signs in the adult-type

Table 44-3   Characteristics of MLD variants

Type	Age at onset, years	Main clinical manifestations	Spinal fluid protein	Nerve conduction velocity	Urinary sulfatide excretion	Arylsulfatase A activity	Other
Congenital	Birth	Apnea, cyanosis, seizures generalized weakness	Unknown	Unknown	Unknown	Unknown	
Late infantile	1–2	Developmental delay, ataxia, weakness, loss of speech, optic atrophy, progressive spastic quadriparesis	Elevated	Slowed	Elevated	Deficient	
Juvenile	4–6	Mental confusion, ataxia, clumsiness, postural abnormalities, optic atrophy, progressive spastic quadriparesis	Elevated	Slowed	Elevated	Deficient	
Adult	>16	Dementia, psychotic thinking, incontinence, ataxia, progressive spastic quadriparesis	Normal or elevated	Normal or slowed	Elevated	Deficient	
Multiple sulfatase deficiency	<1	Signs of late infantile MLD plus coarse facial features, deafness, ichthyosis, hepatosplenomegaly, skeletal anomalies	Elevated	Slowed	Elevated	Deficient	Excess urine mucopolysaccharide, Alder-Reilly granules in white blood cells, multiple sulfatases deficient
Cerebroside sulfate sulfatase activator deficiency	4–6	Signs of juvenile MLD	Elevated	Slowed	Elevated	Normal or mildly reduced	Deficiency of cerebroside sulfate sulfatase activator factor

Table 44-4 MLD case experience: Clinical subtypes classified by age of onset

Type	Subclass	Age of onset, year	Numbers of cases		References
			Authors' experience	Published reports, 1977–1981	
Late infantile		1–3	6	24	[90–101]
Juvenile	Early-onset	3–7	6	6	[93, 99, 102, 103]
	Later-onset	8–15	0	12	[93, 97–99, 102, 104, 105]
Adult	Early-onset	16–20	1	7	[91, 97, 99, 106]
	Later-onset	>20	2	6	[107–111]

case. Better techniques of diagnosis including more widespread use of enzyme analyses are also contributing to greater recognition of and therefore a greater relative frequency of the juvenile and adult-onset variants of MLD. Thus, one-fifth to one-quarter of all patients with MLD are probably of the adult-onset variety, and a very small percentage represent rare variants such as the congenital form, multiple sulfatase deficiency, and the sulfatase activator deficiency disorder. The majority of cases that remain are equally divided between the late infantile and juvenile forms.

Congenital MLD

The evidence for a separate congenital form of MLD has been based on histologic studies of two cases [8, 119]. Direct biochemical proof of either tissue storage of sulfatide or an enzyme deficiency are lacking.

Feigin [8] described deposits of granular metachromatic material in severely degenerated cystic white matter of a male infant born 6 weeks prematurely. From birth, he had periodic spells of apnea, cyanosis, and tonic-clonic movements. He died 6 weeks after birth. The other case was a newborn female who developed cyanosis, dyspnea, and generalized weakness and died 20 hours after birth [119]. Metachromatic material was scattered throughout white matter. In addition, ballooned nerve cells were found, and there was marked gliosis in the cerebral cortex and centrum semiovale. No metachromatic material was demonstrated in these enlarged neurons or in the kidney, liver, or lymph nodes, where large vacuolated cells were found.

It is conceivable that these cases represent an early stage in the clinical progression of late infantile MLD. Until both the pathology and pathological chemistry of further congenital cases can be documented, the existence of a genetically distinct congenital variant must remain conjectural.

Late Infantile MLD

The late infantile form of MLD begins insidiously between the first and second year. In some patients development is delayed, with poor speech acquisition and slowness in learning to walk. Staggering with frequent falling is a common presenting sign. Occasionally, ataxia and weakness may occur precipitously in association with an intercurrent infection, then subside in a few weeks, only to recur and progress 1 or 2 months later. In a few cases the disease is ushered in by the appearance of a peripheral neuropathy [120].

Hagberg has subdivided the clinical course of late infantile MLD into four stages based primarily on the degree of motor handicap [121].

Clinical Stage I Initially, most patients have flaccid weakness and hypotonia of both legs or of all four limbs. The deep tendon reflexes may be diminished or absent. Genu recurvatum is often present. A child who has already learned to walk becomes unsteady and requires support to stand or walk (Fig. 44-5). This stage lasts from a few months to 1 year or more.

Clinical Stage II In this stage the patient can sit up but can no longer stand. Mental regression is obvious. Speech deteriorates as a result of dysarthria and aphasia. Optic atrophy and a grayish discoloration of the macula are observed [98, 122]. Nystagmus is present. Muscle tone is increased in the legs, but the arms may remain hypotonic. Ataxia and truncal titubation become obvious. Intermittent pain occurs in the arms and legs, probably as a manifestation of peripheral nerve or root involvement. The progress of the disease is now rapid so that this stage lasts only a few months.

Clinical Stage III At this stage the child is bedridden and quadriplegic. Muscle tone is variable. There may be decorticate, decerebrate, or dystonic postures upon which hypertonic fits may be superimposed. Bulbar and pseudobulbar palsies occur causing difficulty in feeding and in maintaining the airway. The mental deficit is much more severe and speech is no longer distinct, but these children may still be able to smile and respond to their parents.

Clinical Stage IV In this final stage, patients appear to have lost all meaningful contact with their surroundings. They are blind, without speech, and without volitional movement. Usually they must be fed through a nasogastric or gastrostomy tube. In late infantile MLD, this final stage lasts for a few months to several years.

Juvenile MLD

Juvenile MLD designates those cases with an age onset

Table 44-5 Types of MLD by geographical location

Geographical location	Number of cases			Reference
	Late infantile	Juvenile	Adult	
Sweden	13	2		[115]
England	13	4		[116]
Finland	2	7		[99]
1964 Survey	40	11	9	[117]
Washington State	6	4		[118]
New England	6	6	3	Authors' experience

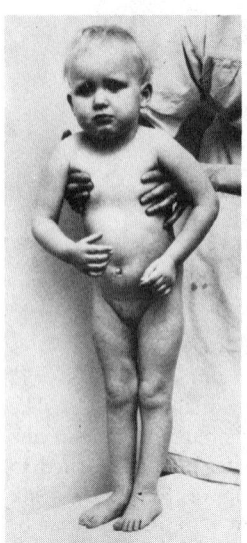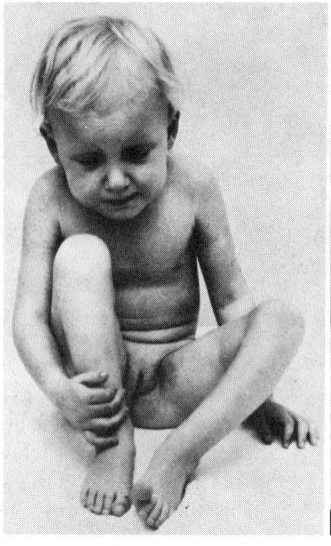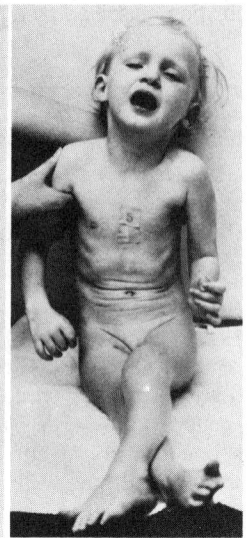

Figure 44-5 Metachromatic leukodystrophy in late infancy. *Left.* The child needs to be supported when standing. *Center.* She can no longer stand, even with support. *Right.* In the late stage of the disease of the patient is no longer able to sit; note the plantar-flexion of the foot and the general debility. *(From Hagberg [121].)*

between 3 and 16 years. The majority present during their first or second year of formal schooling with a fall-off in performance, confusion in following directions, day-dreaming, and abnormal sometimes bizarre behavior [103] (Fig. 44-6). Incontinence and gait clumsiness also occur early in the disease. Speech becomes slurred and signs of extrapyramidal dysfunction appear including postural abnormalities, increased muscle tone, and tremor. Within a year the child is no longer able to walk. The child then rapidly moves into stage III of the disease with pseudobulbar palsy, rigidly flexed arms, leg scissoring, and tonic spasms. In juvenile MLD beginning later in childhood or early adolescence, grand mal seizures are common [99]. Some cases have had a very slow course lasting longer than 20 years [102, 104, 113, 123], but the majority of juvenile MLD patients do not live beyond their teens.

Adult MLD

Adult MLD may begin at almost any age beyond puberty. The first appearance of the disease has been recorded in cases as young as 16 years [106] and as old as 62 years [108]. A 5- to 10-year survival is common, but in a few patients the course is much more rapid [108, 109] and in others the illness may progress slowly over several decades [104, 107, 112, 114]. The diagnosis is not often suspected during life so that until recently most cases were brought to light by a postmortem examination. Of the 13 cases reported since 1977 [91, 94, 99, 106–109, 111, 124] and 3 others that we have diagnosed, all but 2 [107, 109] were identified during life. The earlier recognition of this condition results in part from the increased use of lysosomal enzyme assays in the study of degenerative nervous system diseases.

A change in personality and poor school or job performance herald the onset of the disease. The individual becomes anxious, bewildered, apathetic, and emotionally labile. Defective visual-spatial discrimination, poor memory, disorganized thinking, and decreased mental alertness are found. Psychiatric attention is frequently sought because of symptoms of depression, schizophrenic-like psychosis, or chronic alcoholism. The patient may express feelings of depersonalization or paronoia and display an inappropriate affect. Actual loss of contact by the patient with the surroundings does not occur until late in the course of the disease. Combined with these intellectual and emotional changes are a general slowness and clumsiness of movement and urinary and sometimes fecal incontinence.

Rarely, the disease may first appear as a peripheral neuropathy [108, 124], but not all patients with adult MLD develop a peripheral neuropathy. Even in the presence of a neuropathy, deep tendon reflexes are hyperactive and muscle tone is increased indicating that the involvement of pyramidal and extrapyramidal systems is more significant in the pathophysiology of the disease. Dystonic movements and pareses occur which may involve one side of the body more than the other. In a more advanced stage of the disease, spastic tetraparesis, decorticate posturing, and pathological reflexes are present. Optic atrophy and horizontal nystagmus develop and occasionally there are generalized seizures. During the final stages of the disease, the patient is in a severely deteriorated state and is mute, blind, bedridden, and unresponsive.

Multiple Sulfatase Deficiency

This rare condition is of considerable theoretical interest since it apparently results from a single mutant gene affecting the expression of nine distinct enzymes [17]. A total of 14 cases have been described [125–129]. Onset of symptoms is during the first or second year of life. The clinical manifestations represent the summation of two diseases, late infantile MLD and a mucopolysaccharidosis (Fig. 44-7). The mucopolysaccharidosis-like features include coarse facial features, deafness, hepatosplenomegaly, and skeletal anomalies such as lumbar kyphosis and abnormalities of the sternum. In addition, ichthyosis is present. Corneal opacities do not occur. In general, the early "presymptomatic" development of children with multiple sulfatase deficiency is less advanced than that in late infantile MLD. Most children with multiple sulfatase deficiency never achieve normal gait or speech.

The laboratory findings also reflect the concurrence of two separate disease processes. The usual clinical pathological features of late infantile MLD are present along with findings that are typical of many mucopolysaccharidoses. Among these are Alder-Reilly granules in bone marrow and peripheral blood leukocytes, bone x-ray changes such as a J-shaped sella turcica and broad phalanges, and an increased urinary content of dermatan sulfate and heparan sulfate. Besides the arylsulfatase A deficiency, there is loss of activity of arylsulfatases B, C, two steroid sulfatases, and four other sulfatases that help to degrade mucopolysaccharides [17].

MLD without Arylsulfatase A Deficiency

Three patients have been reported who have a form of juvenile MLD without arylsulfatase A deficiency [130, 131]. Two are sibs whose parents were first cousins [130]. Their early development was normal. In one, a girl, behavioral abnormalities first appeared at age 4½ years. She also presented with an abnormal gait, a decrease in fine motor ability, and hyporeflexia. By age 6 years, she was functioning below a 6-month level and demonstrated a marked increase in tone and hyperreflexia. Her nerve conduction times were slowed. Light and electron microscopic studies of a sural nerve biopsy demonstrated the histopathologic features of MLD, and the sulfatide content of her urinary sediment was markedly elevated.

Her brother began to deteriorate at age 6 years and had a similar but more slowly progressive course. At age 19, he was incontinent, nonambulatory, and uncommunicative with extreme spasticity and hyperreflexia.

Enzyme studies of these two patients have demonstrated a

dissociation between the ability of their cultured skin fibroblasts to degrade cerebroside sulfate in vitro and in situ. The activity of arylsulfatase A and cerebroside sulfatase in their fibroblast homogenates was in the range typical of heterozygotes for MLD, but with intact growing fibroblasts loaded with [^{35}S]sulfatide a defect in sulfatide cleavage comparable to that in MLD patients was observed [130]. This defect was normalized by the addition of exogenous purified cerebroside sulfate sulfatase activator factor [15].

A third patient reported with this syndrome was also born to consanguine parents [131]. She is 21 years old and has a history of developmental delay, clumsiness, ataxia, muscle weakness, and progressive psychomotor deterioration. Her motor nerve conduction velocities were markedly slowed, and her sensory action potentials were unrecordable. Sural nerve biopsy and urinary excretion of sulfatide are typical of patients with classical MLD. Nevertheless, the arylsulfatase A activity in urine and leukocytes is normal. Presumably, she too lacks the activator protein needed for the in vivo hydrolysis of sulfatide; however, tissue culture correction experiments with added activator have not been reported in this case.

Arylsulfatase A Deficiency without MLD

Deficiency of arylsulfatase A may occur in the absence of any other laboratory evidence of MLD. Most cases of this type have been found in otherwise normal older relatives of patients

Figure 44-6 Juvenile MLD. *Left.* At age 5½ years, 1 year before onset of symptoms, the child is entirely normal. *Center.* At age 6 11/12 years the child has increasing gait difficulty and is unable to stand without support. *Right.* At age 8 10/12 years the patient is bedridden, has increasing difficulty in swallowing, and requires tube feeding. He is no longer able to speak, but recognizes his family and displays pleasure when people pay attention to him.

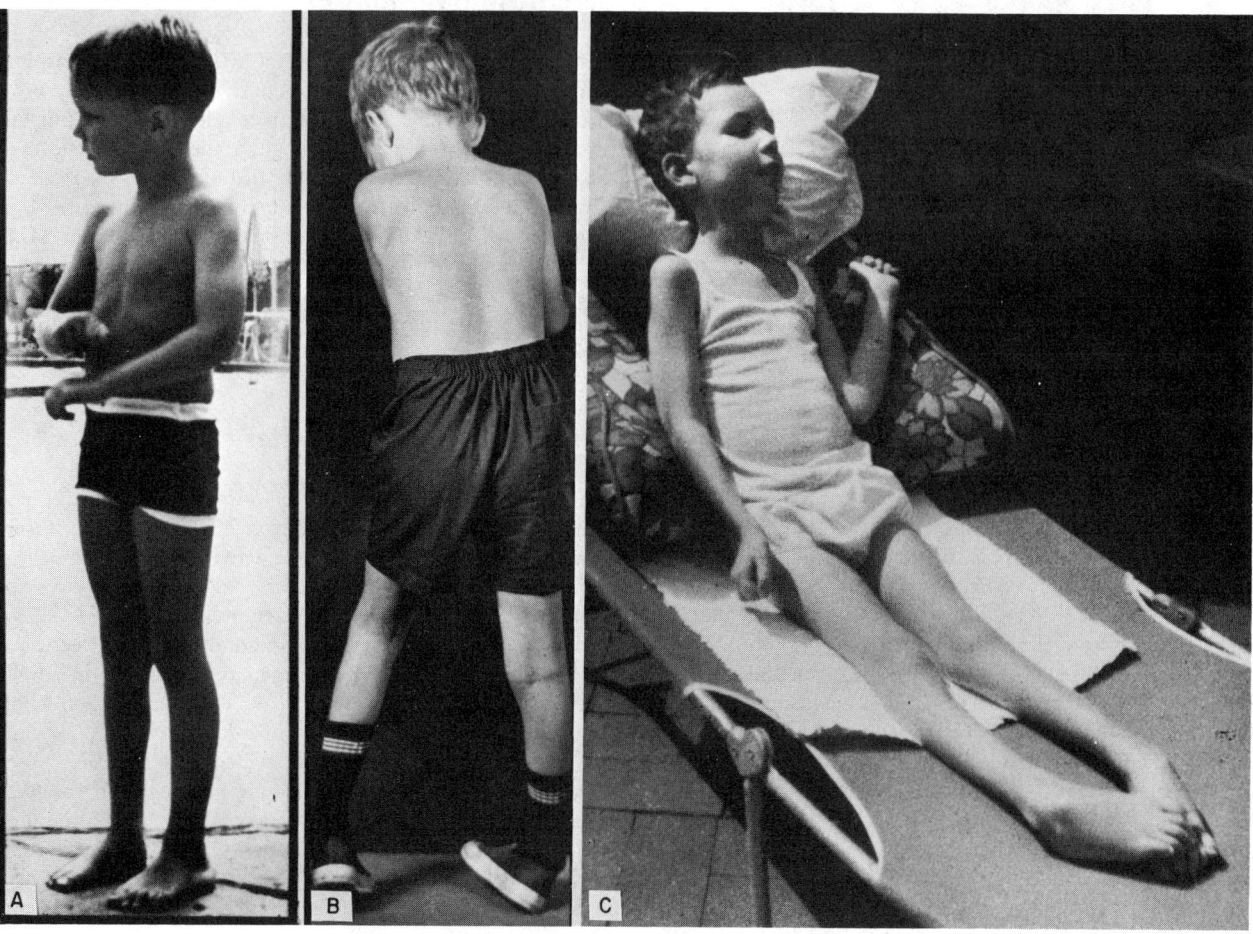

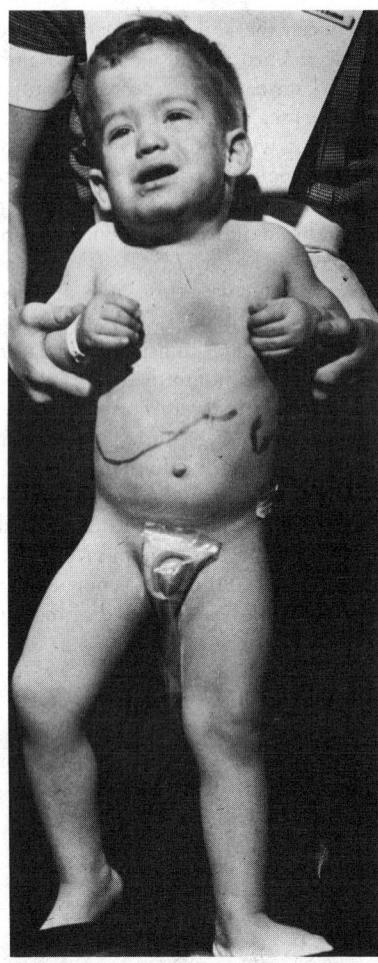

Figure 44-7 MLD variant with multiple sulfatase deficiencies in a child 26 months of age. Note enlarged head circumference, depressed bridge of nose, enlarged liver and spleen, pectus excavatum and incurved little finger. (From Murphy et al. [125].)

with MLD [123, 132–136]. These individuals do not have metachromatic deposits in peripheral nerve tissues and their urine content of sulfatide is normal [123, 137]. Thus, they themselves do not have MLD nor are they in a preclinical stage of MLD. This phenomenon has sometimes been described as *pseudo-arylsulfatase A deficiency* [136].

Rarely, an arylsulfatase A deficient relative of a patient with MLD actually may have neurological signs and symptoms suggestive of a leukodystrophy but of a type different from MLD [138]. In these persons it manifests as a progressive spastic paraparesis.

Arylsulfatase A deficiency has also been found in a few patients without any family history of MLD [139–141]. In nearly all such cases neurological disabilities were present that suggested disease of the central nervous system white matter. In these cases also the clinical signs differed from those of the classical forms of MLD, and ancillary studies failed to disclose in them any evidence of MLD. A major distinguishing feature is their retention of some sulfatidase activity in leukocytes. In contrast, patients with MLD are totally deficient in leukocyte sulfatidase activity [140]. It is possible that some cases previously described as unusual variants of MLD [142] may actually represent examples of this association of arylsulfatase A deficiency with a non-MLD type of neurological disease.

Available data do not make clear the relationship between the neurological disease and the enzyme deficiency. In two families without MLD that the authors have studied, the younger member of a pair of sibs with arylsulfatase A deficiency also had neurological disease. The healthy older sib was detected only in the course of a family study of the enzyme abnormality. The lack of complete congruence between the biochemical defect and clinical state even in the same family casts some doubt on a cause-and-effect relationship. There is the possibility that in some unspecified way this type of arylsulfatase A deficiency predisposes to demyelinating disease.

The gene for this low enzyme variant appears to be allelic with the MLD gene locus [143, 144] and its frequency is common. This would account for its frequent occurrence in MLD obligate heterozygotes, resulting in an apparent arylsulfatase A deficiency in such individuals. It is not possible to differentiate the MLD gene from this other allele since both are expressed in the heterozygote state by a reduction in enzyme activity to approximately 50 percent of normal. In the prenatal diagnosis of MLD it is important to determine whether either parent at risk for an MLD offspring also carries this additional mutation. The presence of this gene in the fetus together with a single dose of the MLD gene could lead to a false-positive diagnosis of MLD. Assays of sulfatide-cleaving activity in the cultured amniotic fluid cells can be used to circumvent this difficulty [136].

CLINICAL LABORATORY FINDINGS

Cerebrospinal Fluid Protein

In the early stages of late infantile MLD, the cerebrospinal fluid protein may be normal, but as the disease progresses through stage II the spinal fluid protein level may continue to rise. Eventually, in the chronic stages of the disease, the level of total protein may reach or exceed 100 mg/dl. A similar elevation in spinal fluid protein occurs in the cases of juvenile MLD that begin before age 7. The later onset cases of juvenile MLD may or may not exhibit any increase in spinal fluid protein. In most adult onset cases of MLD, cerebrospinal fluid protein is normal, but raised levels have been recorded in a few patients [107, 108].

Neurophysiological Studies

The electroencephalogram may be normal early in the course of the disease. As the disease advances, it becomes diffusely slow, exhibiting mainly 4- to 7-Hz activity but also some 2- to 4-Hz activity. In a few cases, occasional bursts of spikes or of asymmetric slow wave activity have been recorded [145].

In most cases motor nerve conduction velocity is decreased and sensory nerve action potentials are diminished in amplitude with prolonged latency to peak. These nerve conduction abnormalities may be present prior to the appearance of clinical symptoms and thus provide evidence of MLD in a presymptomatic stage [105, 146]. Some patients with the later onset form of juvenile MLD and with adult MLD may not exhibit any slowing of nerve conduction or any other electrophysiological evidence of a peripheral neuropathy, even in a clinically advanced stage of their disease.

Brainstem auditory evoked responses (BAER) represent a relatively new diagnostic tool for investigating leukodystrophies that has not yet been extensively tested in various forms of MLD. In one case of late infantile MLD tested by this technique at age 3 in a clinically advanced stage of this disease, an increase in latency of wave I was found and waves II to VII were totally absent [147].

Computerized Brain Tomography

With computed tomography (CT) scans of the brain it is possible to differentiate the white matter involvement of MLD from other cases of leukodystrophy [94] (Fig. 44-8). There is diffuse symmetrical loss of white matter density involving the entire centrum semiovale. The lateral perimeter appears scalloped and generally no contrast enhancement occurs. Ventricular dilitation is minimal in early onset cases of MLD, but older patients may show moderate enlargement of the ventricles. In CT scans of patients with adult MLD, the lateral ventricles can appear very large and cortical atrophy is prominent. All reported cases of MLD have been abnormal on CT scan [94] except for one case that was presymptomatic [148].

With a modification of the CT scan technique, it is possible to calculate the effective atomic number (Z^*) of the white matter [149]. In a chronic case of MLD, the Z^* was increased, a finding that is consistent with the sulfatide accumulation that is known to occur in this disease. In another case that had become symptomatic only 3 months earlier, the Z^* value suggested brain edema [149].

Gallbladder Imaging

Extensive deposition of sulfatide may occur on the mucosal surface of the gallbladder and interferes with its normal func-

Figure 44-8 Brain CT scans in MLD. *A*. A $5\frac{1}{2}$ year old boy with a 3-month history of blunted mentation, weakness, and ataxia. GE model 8800 scanner. Note bilateral symmetrical zones of decreased white matter density. In the frontal regions the white matter lesion extends to the surface of the anterior projection of the lateral ventricles. The ventricular system is normal. *(Courtesy Department of Radiology, Children's Hospital Medical Center, Boston.)* *B*. A 32-year-old woman with a 14-year history of progressive dementia, optic atrophy, and spastic tetraparesis. EMI scanner. Note cortical atrophy and nearly loss of white matter from the centrum semiovale. Gaping cortical sulci extend almost to the surface of the massively enlarged lateral ventricles. *(Courtesy Department of Radiology, Sidney Farber Cancer Institute, Boston.)*

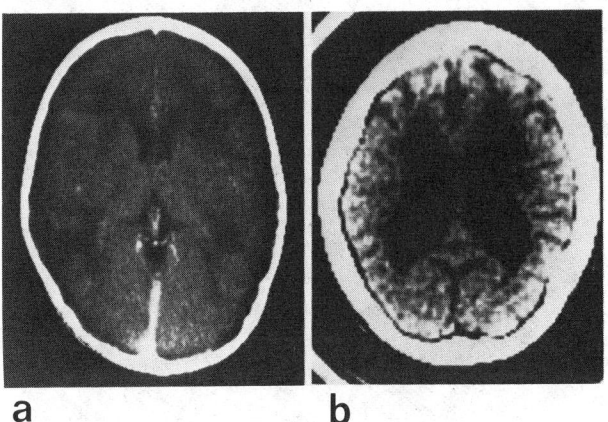

a   b

tioning. Serial examination of the gallbladder with oral cholecystography [150] or radionuclide scanning may show progressive loss of function. A completely nonfunctioning gallbladder has been demonstrated in patients as young as 2 years of age [95]. Polypoid filling defects have also been seen on oral cholecystography [151]. In one patient with adult MLD, symptoms dramatically worsened after gallbladder surgery [152].

HISTOPATHOLOGY

Metachromatic Deposits

The pathology of MLD consists primarily of demyelination and deposits of metachromatic granules in the central and peripheral nervous system. The metachromatic deposits are spherical masses 15 to 20 μm in diameter that stain brown in frozen tissue sections when treated with a 1% solution of acidified cresyl violet [5]. These masses have been observed not only in the nervous system but also in the kidney, urine, gallbladder, liver, pancreas, pituitary gland, adrenal cortex, retina, and testes.

The specificity of the cresyl violet staining reaction can be enhanced by viewing in polarized light with the polarizer and analyzer 90° out of phase [153]. Pseudoisocyanin [154], acriflavine [155], and trypaflavine-phosphotungstic acid [155] have also been used to demonstrate metachromatic granules in MLD. The material in the granules can also be stained with alcian blue in the presence of 0.8 *M* magnesium chloride [156], Sudan black and the periodic acid Schiff reaction. Preextraction of the tissue with lipid solvents such as alcohol, pyridine, petroleum ether, and chloroform-methanol abolishes the reaction with these stains. These staining characteristics suggest that the stored material is acidic glycolipid of the sulfatide type. Actual chemical analysis of metachromatic granules isolated from the white matter of an MLD brain has revealed a sulfatide content amounting to 39 percent of their total lipid content. The other lipid components were cholesterol and phosphatides [157]. Energy dispersive x-ray microanalysis of the membrane bound granules in dermal nerves has demonstrated a pronounced sulfur peak, further strengthening the concept that the specific storage materials in the metachromatic granules are sulfatides [96].

High resolution analysis of the storage granules by electron microscopy suggests that they are composed of several different types of inclusions. Prismatic and Tuffstone inclusions are especially characteristic. The lipid leaflets of prismatic inclusions appear in the form of little disks stacked in parallel prisms with a periodicity of approximately 5.8 nm. The orientation of the disks in adjacent leaflets may be oblique to one another creating a herringbone pattern (Fig. 44-9). A cross section of this type of inclusion assumes a hexagonal honeycomb pattern [159]. This type of inclusion has also been observed in cultured fibroblasts from MLD cases grown in the presence of sulfatides [158].

Tuffstone bodies consist of concentrically or radially arranged lamellae with a 5.8-nm spacing in a granular matrix and several vacuoles of varying sizes contained within a membrane bound lysosomal-like body (Fig. 44-10) [160]. The term *Tuffstone* derives from the fact that these inclusions resemble volcanic limestone. Inclusions common to other types of lipid

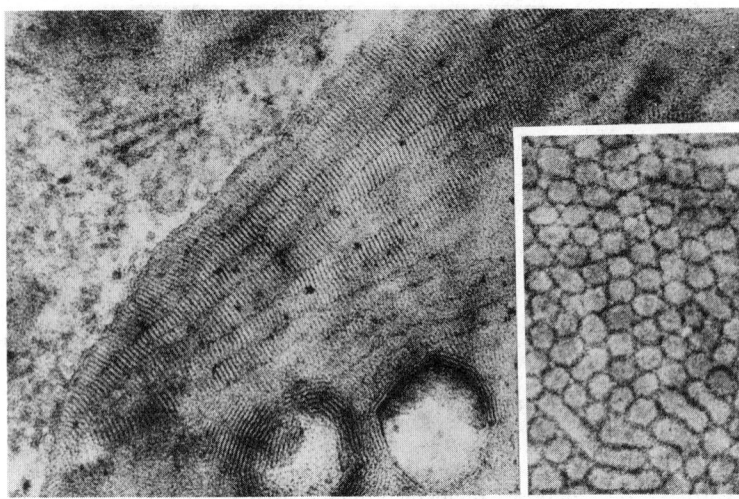

Figure 44-9 Inclusions found at autopsy in the brain of a patient with infantile MLD. The preparation was stained with a combination of uranyl acetate and lead acetate. Note the lamellar lipid leaflets with a herringbone pattern, and (inset) the honeycomb aspect of the same type of structure seen in a section approximately parallel to the lamellas. ×200,000 (From Rutsaert et al. [158].)

storage disease may also be observed in MLD. These include membranous cytoplasmic bodies, striated zebra bodies, granular bodies with weak osmophilia, and myelin figures [102].

Central Nervous System

The central white matter is reduced in amount and is firmer than normal, has a gray or sometimes brown discoloration, and in severely affected regions may show cavitation or spongy degeneration. Usually there is sparing of the U fibers, the subcortial association fibers between adjacent convolutions, and of myelin sheaths within the central gray nuclei and optic radiation. There is a moderate to severe loss of myelin sheaths, a diminished number of interfascicular oligodendrocytes [7], and a striking accumulation of metachromatic granules. These deposits are present in macrophages that are prominent in perivascular spaces and also may appear as free-lying bodies within the tissues. They also are found within oligodendrocytes even in areas where the myelin sheaths are relatively spared, and have been observed within the neurons of certain nuclei such as the dentate nucleus of the cerebellum, some nuclei of the brainstem, and the gray matter of the spinal ganglia [6, 101, 161]. The nerve cells of the cerebral cortex are usually spared. A reactive gliosis is found in the areas of demyelination, and there may be partial or complete loss of axis cylinders. An immunochemical study of MLD white matter has described intense staining of the myelin remnants with antiserum to basic protein, but severely affected white matter remained unstained by antiserum to myelin-associated glycoprotein [162].

The cerebellum is atrophic, with severe demyelination, prominent gliosis, and storage granules. There is a marked reduction in Purkinje cells and granule cells, and the axons of some of the surviving Purkinje cells show torpedolike swellings in the granular layer. The axon terminals of climbing fibers and mossy fibers in the cerebellar granular layer and molecular layer also are missing [100].

The retinal ganglion cells also accumulate metachromatic granules that appear under the electron microscope as laminated bodies with increased acid phosphatase activity similar to the lysosomal bodies of Tay-Sachs disease [110, 122]. Accumulations of metachromatic material also have been observed in retinal glial cells. The prismatic and Tuffstone inclusions

characteristic of MLD have not been described in the retina but have been found in optic nerve [163].

Peripheral Nervous System

A segmental demyelination occurs in the peripheral nervous system [164] with metachromatic granules present singly or in clusters in Schwann cells, in endoneural macrophages, and to a lesser degree in the Remak cells associated with unmyelinated nerve fibers. They are also seen as free-lying bodies between nerve fibers. Some observers report that the number of myelinated fibers is reduced [99, 152], but only in late infantile MLD has an actual count been made disclosing a myelinated fiber density that is below normal [102]. In the later onset cases, repeated axonal degeneration and regeneration causes hypertrophic changes that are reflected in palpably enlarged nerves. The microscopic appearance is of dense collagen deposits surrounding clusters of myelinated and unmyelinated axons in small onion-bulb formations [91, 99, 102].

Particular attention has been focused on the sural nerve, a sensory nerve in the leg that is frequently biopsied for diagnostic purposes. The inclusions present in this nerve are varied and

Figure 44-10 Tuffstone inclusion in the Schwann cell of a myelinated axon from a cutaneous nerve ×23,000. The inclusion at a higher magnification (inset) ×120,000. Note the granular matrix containing a mosaic of slender lamellae surrounding electron lucent vacuoles of varying sizes. (From Gebhart et al. [96].)

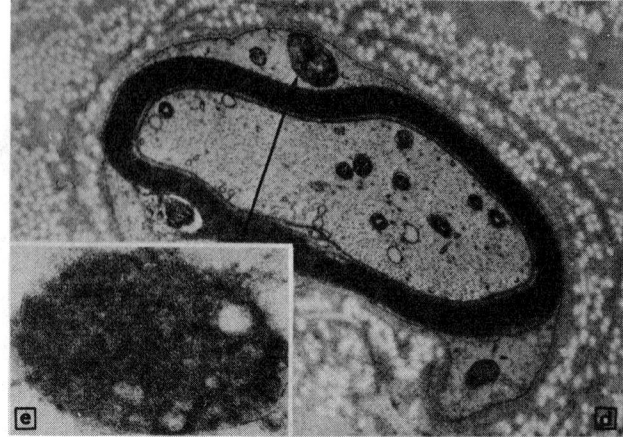

have the same ultrastructural appearance as those described above. Nerve specimens from the different clinical variants of MLD do not show any striking differences in the types of inclusions present. Observations similar to those in sural nerve have been made on cutaneous nerves [96] and intramuscular nerve fibers [108, 110].

Visceral Organs

Involvement of visceral organs has been observed in all patients whose tissues have been carefully examined [165]. Tissues with an excretory function are particularly affected. In the kidney, metachromatic material is present in the cells of the distal convoluted tubules (especially on the luminal side), the thin limb of the loop of Henle, and the collecting tubules, as well as in the tubule lumen and urine. The inclusions consist mainly of large lamellae, but some prismatic inclusions have been observed. The glomerulus and proximal convoluted tubule are normal [152, 166, 167]. A proximal renal tubular acidosis has been described in one patient with the late infantile form of MLD [95].

The gallbladder is small and fibrotic, and the mucosal cells and villi are distended with macrophages containing metachromatic material. In some cases multiple large polypoid masses or papillomatous fronds have been noted projecting from the mucosa into the lumen of the gallbladder [151]. Liver parenchymal cells, particularly at the periphery of the lobules, and the epithelial cells of the intrahepatic bile ducts contain abundant metachromatic material. There is similar but less striking involvement of the Kupffer cells and portal histiocytes [150, 166, 168]. Deposits of metachromatic lipids have been demonstrated in the islets of Langerhans [150, 169], the anterior pituitary [3, 165], and the adrenal cortex [3, 165]. Accumulation of metachromatic material in the testes has been reported only in adult patients [3, 165]. It is possible that this material was not sulfatide but seminolipid whose metabolism is also impaired in MLD. This sulfolipid normally is not formed in the testes until after puberty and therefore would not accumulate in patients with MLD who die before then. The reticuloendothelial system generally is not involved.

CHEMICAL PATHOLOGY

Central Nervous System

In late infantile MLD, white matter sulfatide levels are increased three- to tenfold (see Table 44-6). The levels of other myelin lipids, such as cholesterol and sphingomyelin, may be decreased by 30 to 50 percent, presumably secondary to the loss of myelin. Cerebroside levels are diminished out of proportion to those of other myelin lipids. They vary from less than 10 percent up to 50 percent of normal. Consequently, the cerebroside/sulfatide ratio, which in normal white matter is approximately 4, may be reduced in late infantile MLD to 0.5. The excess of sulfatide also has been noted in isolated myelin [157] including a preparation from a fetus with MLD [170]. Its chemical structure in late infantile MLD is the same as the sulfatide of normal white matter. Chemical analyses of a few cases of adult MLD have disclosed differences from late infan-

tile MLD. In adult MLD, the white matter sulfatide level is only moderately increased and contains more short-chain and saturated fatty acid and less unsaturated fatty acid than the sulfatide from normal white matter [171]. Also, there is more gray matter sulfatide accumulation in adult MLD than in late infantile MLD. In both types of MLD, a significant alteration also occurs in the fatty acid composition of white matter sphingomyelin and cerebrosides. The proportion of long-chain fatty acids is diminished, probably reflecting the loss of myelin with a return to the fatty acid pattern of immature white matter [24]. Cerebrosides in the peripheral nerve do not show this deficit in long-chain fatty acids [172].

Extraneural Tissues

Sulfatide concentrations are increased in the liver, gallbladder, kidney, and urine of MLD patients. The level in the liver is at least 10 times normal [173], 10 to 75 times normal in the kidney [24, 174], and 10 to 100 times normal in the urine [175, 176]. Both cerebroside sulfate and lactosylceramide sulfate are found. The ratio of these two sulfatides in the liver approaches 1 [177], in the gallbladder it is 5.8 [177], in the kidney it is 4 [176], and in the urine it is 20 to 30 [176]. The chemical structure of the sulfatides is typical of sulfatides present in normal kidney and differs from brain sulfatide. The close resemblance of the fatty acid pattern in urine sulfatides of MLD patients to normal kidney sulfatides supports the notion that the urine sulfatides reflect the chemical pathology of the kidney.

Multiple Sulfatase Deficiency

As in late infantile MLD, tissues from patients with multiple sulfatase deficiency contain the expected sulfatide excess. In addition, an increase of mucopolysaccharide levels has been demonstrated in the brain, liver, kidney, urine, and cultured skin fibroblasts. Both dermatan sulfate and heparan sulfate have been detected. Accumulation of cholesteryl sulfate has also been reported in the liver, kidney, plasma, and urine. An abnormality in the gray matter ganglioside pattern resembling that seen in Hurler's syndrome has also been detected [125–127, 173, 178].

ENZYME DEFECTS

Late Infantile, Juvenile, and Adult MLD

Arylsulfatase A Deficiency Deficiency in the activity of arylsulfatase A, the heat-labile component of cerebroside sulfatase, has been established as the primary enzymatic abnormality in the late infantile, juvenile, and adult variants of MLD. This deficiency was first demonstrated by Austin in the urine [179] and tissues [16] of patients with MLD. At the same time, Mehl and Jatzkewitz reported that MLD kidney was deficient in cerebroside sulfatase activity [12] and later that both enzyme activities were absent from the kidney, liver, and brain tissues of seven patients with MLD [13] (Fig. 44-11). Many other tissues and fluids from MLD patients have since been examined and also have been found deficient in arylsulfatase A

Table 44-6 Composition of cerebral white matter and kidney in metachromatic leukodystrophy, percent of dry weight

	Cerebral white matter				Kidney		
		Metachromatic leukodystrophy				Metachromatic leukodystrophy infantile	
		Infantile					
Components	Normal, 6 subjects, age range, 4–5 yr	Age, $3\frac{1}{4}$ yr	Age, $4\frac{1}{2}$ yr	Adult, age 29 yr	Normal, 3 subjects, all age 2 mo	Age, $3\frac{1}{4}$ yr	Age, $4\frac{1}{2}$ yr
Total lipids	55.6–61.9	39.9	40.9	50.1	9.4–10.5	10.8	12.5
Cholesterol	12.2–15.7	8.1	7.8	13.5	1.3–1.7	1.7	1.6
Phospholipids	28.0–30.6	17.1	14.1	22.4	7.4–8.5	6.8	5.6
Cephalins	14.4–16.5	8.1	5.1	9.0	3.3–4.0	2.0	1.6
Lecithins	8.5–9.9	6.9	7.9	8.7	2.6–3.4	3.6	3.0
Sphingomyelin	4.1–5.2	2.5	2.2	4.7	1.0–1.22	1.1	1.0
Cerebrosides	10.3–13.8	2.8	3.2	7.8	0.41–0.45	1.21	0.71
Sulfatides	1.7–4.1	12.8	15.8	6.5	0.09–0.17	1.26	4.60
Lipid hexosamine	0.05	0.08	0.09	0.03			
Nonlipid hexosamine	0.23	0.7	0.65				

activity. Those most frequently studied have been urine [179–181], peripheral leukocytes [182–184], and cultured skin fibroblasts [185] (Fig. 44-12), but the enzyme defect has also been demonstrated in serum [92, 188], tears [98, 189], saliva [190], cultured lymphocytes [191], and cultured bone marrow cells [192]. The loss of cerebroside sulfate sulfatase activity in MLD has also been repeatedly confirmed, particularly in peripheral leukocytes [140, 193, 194] and cultured skin fibroblasts [93, 193, 195]. In addition, there is defective catabolism of other natural substrates of arylsulfatase A. These include lactosylceramide sulfatide [72], sulfogalactosylsphingosine [75], seminolipid [196], and ascorbate-2-sulfate [78].

Purified arylsulfatase B has also been shown to hydrolyze cerebroside sulfate, although at a much slower rate than arylsulfatase A [197]. Consequently, the level of activity of this enzyme in MLD has been of some interest. Some reports have described reduced arylsulfatase B activity in kidney and brain white matter [13], leukocytes [184, 198], cultured bone marrow fibroblasts [192], and tears [98], but most studies have not shown any consistent abnormality of this enzyme in patients with MLD. Other lysosomal enzyme activities have been normal [199]. The presence of normal concentrations of the heat-stable activator of arylsulfatase A has also been documented in the common variants of MLD [200].

Properties of the Mutant Enzyme The most frequently used method for the determination of arylsulfatase A activity was developed for use with human urine and employs the chromogenic substance p-nitrocatechol sulfate [201]. Under a different set of reaction conditions, this artificial substrate will also measure arylsulfatase B activity. The assay conditions established for the assay of arylsulfatase A activity are supposed to minimize any contribution from the arylsulfatase B present. With this method, specimens from patients with MLD invariably demonstrate the presence of a small amount of residual enzyme activity. Several groups of investigators [202–204] have examined this activity by immunological methods to determine whether it represents true arylsulfatase A activity or a spillover of arylsulfatase B activity. Monospecific antibodies were prepared to purified arylsulfatase A and used to examine the antigenicity of the residual enzyme in Ochterlony double-diffusion plates. In each instance precipitin lines formed between the antibody and the MLD enzyme and indicated the presence of cross-reacting material (Fig. 44-13). The precipitin line of the normal enzyme-antibody complex exhibited arylsulfatase A activity, but no enzyme activity was observed in the precipitin line from the MLD samples. Based upon these findings and additional experiments with anti-arylsulfatase B antibody, Shapira and Nadler attributed all of the residual arylsul-

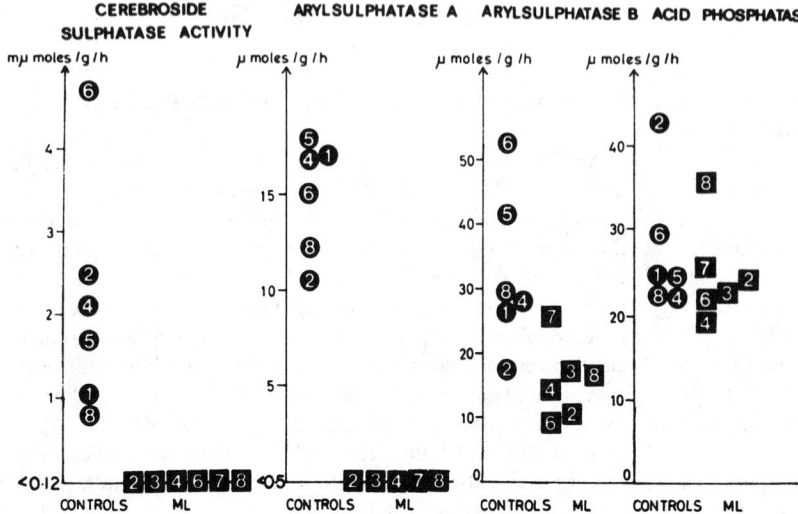

Figure 44-11 Deficiency of cerebroside sulfatase activity and arylsulfatase A activity in the renal cortex of patients with late infantile MLD. Circles represent the enzyme activities in control subjects, and the squares those in patients with late infantile MLD. (From Jatzkewitz and Mehl [13].)

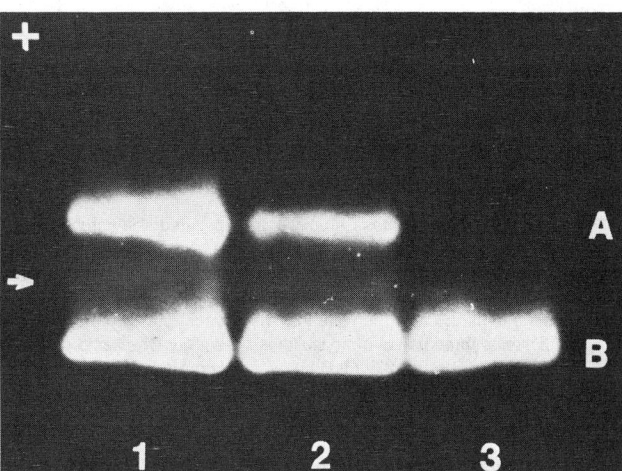

Figure 44-12 Fluorescent bands of arylsulfatase activity after electrophoresis of skin fibroblast extracts on cellulose acetate gel strips. Extracts were prepared from skin fibroblasts of normal individual (A), an individual heterozygous for MLD (B), and a patient with MLD (C). After application at the point indicated by the arrow, and subsequent electrophoresis and incubation of the strip in the presence of 4-methylumbelliferyl sulfate, bands of arylsulfatase A and B activity appeared under ultraviolet light, as indicated. *(From Rattazzi et al. [186], originally published in [187].)*

fatase A-like activity to normal arylsulfatase B activity [203]. In keeping with their conclusion is the observation that quantifiable cerebroside sulfate sulfatase activity is almost totally absent from MLD specimens when in vitro assays are employed to measure this activity.

There is also contrary evidence suggesting that some enzymatically active arylsulfatase A activity does persist in MLD. This has been directly measured after separation of arylsulfatase components in MLD tissues by isoelectric focusing [58, 197] (Fig. 44-14). Three main bands of arylsulfatase A activity appear when extracts of cultured skin fibroblasts are subjected to isoelectric focussing on cellulose acetate membranes [58]. A similar banding pattern occurs when the residual arylsulfatase A activity in cultured fibroblasts of patients with the late infantile form of MLD is examined by this technique. In contrast, the juvenile form of MLD exhibits only one band of enzyme activity corresponding to the major acidic band of activity in controls. Farrell et al. [58] have concluded that the mutant gene product in late infantile MLD is deficient in enzyme activity but is able to undergo the postribosomal modification that results in the three-band pattern. These investigators believe that the mutation in juvenile MLD not only reduces enzyme activity but blocks the ability of the gene product to undergo further postribosomal modification so that only one band of activity results. In a study of the properties of the mutant urine arylsulfatase A activity, Luijten et al. [204] also found greater similarities with the normal enzyme in a late infantile case than in the juvenile or adult cases that they studied. Other researchers also have described quantitative and qualitative differences in the residual arylsulfatase A activity of urine [205, 206] and liver [207, 208] from patients with different forms of MLD.

Biochemical Basis for Varying Ages of Onset in MLD

The difference in ages of onset between the late infantile, juvenile, and adult forms of MLD cannot be explained on the basis of quantitative differences in the level of mutant enzyme in cell-free homogenates. Most studies that have examined this question show no differences between clinical subtypes in their activity in vitro of residual arylsulfatase A [13, 193, 209, 210].

This result would be expected if the residual arylsulfatase A activity were unstable or otherwise lost its catalytic activity upon disruption of its intracellular milieu. The findings of in situ tissue culture experiments suggest that this might be happening [91, 209, 211].

Cultured skin fibroblasts from patients with MLD incorporate sulfatide that has been added to the growth media, accumulating it in sufficient amounts to stain metachromatically [211]. Normal cells also incorporate sulfatide but degrade it and do not develop metachromasia. Using [^{35}S]sulfatide, Porter et al. [209] found that the amount of this lipid that accumulated intracellularly was largest in cells derived from a patient with late infantile MLD and least in cells from a patient with adult MLD. Cells from patients with juvenile MLD stored an intermediate amount of sulfatide (Fig. 44-15). Also, the amount of hydrolysis, determined by the release of [^{35}S]sulfatide into the media, directly correlated with the latency of onset of symptoms.

Ultrastructural differences are also readily observable between cultured skin fibroblasts from late infantile and adult forms of MLD after exposure of the cells to sulfatide (91). The adult onset MLD cultures grown in media containing 20 μg/ml of sulfatide could not be distinguished from similarly treated control cells, whereas cultures of infantile MLD cells grown in the same media contained numerous lipid-laden lysosomes. In a medium containing 200 μg/ml both the adult onset and infantile MLD cell lines contained large numbers of dense lysosomes. Only occasional cells in the control cultures exposed to this environment were abnormal, containing vacuoles and few dense lysosomes. Thus, intact cells in culture are able to express subtle variations in their ability to cleave sulfatide that do not appear in cell-free homogenates.

Multiple Sulfatase Deficiency

In this disease sulfate-containing glycolipids, mucopolysaccharides, and steroids accumulate because of a deficiency of sev-

Figure 44-13 *Left.* Immunododiffusion of arylsulfatase A from normal human liver (N) and from liver of patients with MLD (ML) against monospecific absorbed antibody (Ab) to normal arylsulfatase A. The well at top right contained a preparation from liver of a patient with late infantile MLD; that at the bottom, a specimen from a patient with the juvenile form; and that at top left, from a patient with multiple sulfatase deficiency. The arrow indicates the single precipitin line of identity formed after diffusion for 24 h, showing protein in the three types of MLD which is antigenically equivalent to the arylsulfatase A in normal individuals. *Right.* Enzyme activity in the precipitin lines formed after diffusion of normal arylsulfatase A against its antibody. The same slide shown on the left was incubated in the presence of p-nitrocatechol sulfate; after development of color (due to formation of p-nitrocatechol) by exposure of alkali, the plate was photographed. The reverse negative, in which enzyme activity appears as white areas, is shown here. (Dashed lines show areas of maximal red color on original slide.) It will be noted that only the precipitin lines that formed in relation to normal arylsulfatase A (N) contained detectable enzymatic activity, not those lines formed in relation to MLD enzyme. *(From Stumpf et al. [202].)*

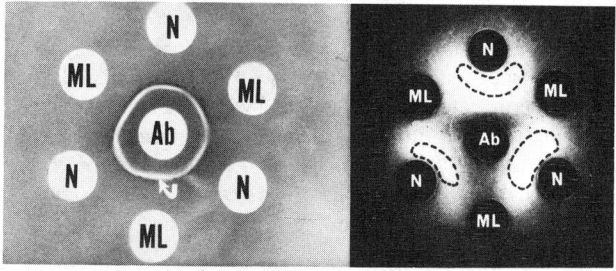

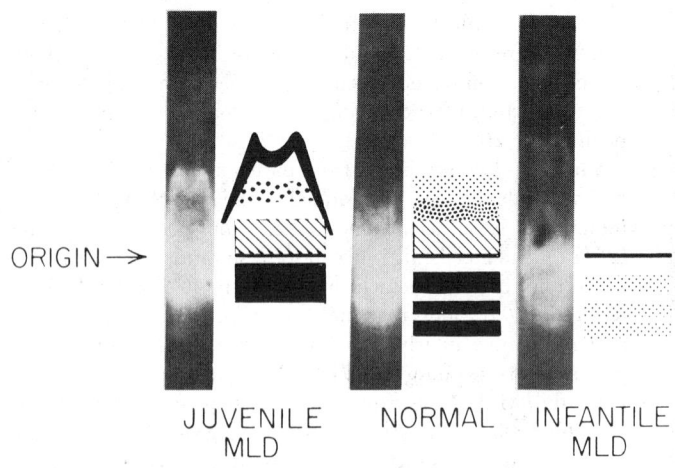

ORIGIN →

JUVENILE MLD   NORMAL   INFANTILE MLD

Figure 44-14 Arylsulfatase A activity from cultured skin fibroblasts separated by isoelectric focusing on cellulose acetate strips in a pH 4 to 6 ampholine mixture. Enzyme activity was located by incubating the strips in the presence of 4-methylumbelliferyl sulfate and then exposing them to ultraviolet light. Note that the extract from a normal cell line contains three bands of arylsulfatase A activity. The same pattern is observed in late infantile MLD but was only obvious after twentyfold concentration of the enzyme preparation. In juvenile MLD only one band of residual arylsulfatase A activity is visualized. The intense band at the origin probably represents acid-precipitated arylsulfatase B activity. *(From Farrell et al. [58].)*

eral different sulfatases [125–127, 173, 178]. Cultured skin fibroblasts from patients are deficient in arylsulfatases A, B, and C, cholesteryl sulfatase, dehydroepiandrosterone sulfatase, iduronide-2-sulfate sulfatase, heparan-N-sulfamidase, N-acetylgalactosamine-6-sulfate sulfatase, N-acetylgalactosamine-4-sulfate sulfatase (arylsulfatase B), and N-acetylglucosamine-6-sulfate sulfatase [17, 178]. Less complete studies of tissue sulfatases have disclosed deficits of arylsulfatases A, B, and C in kidney (Fig. 44-16C and D) and brain and of arylsulfatases A and C in the liver [125, 127, 213]. The activity of arylsulfatase B is reduced but not totally absent in liver [125] and fibroblasts [178]. Tissue levels of steroid sulfatase activities also are reduced to the limit of detection.

The activity of acid β-galactosidase is partially deficient in tissues [127] but is normal in fibroblasts [17], which suggests that the reduction in tissues is secondary to their storage of mucopolysaccharides. The activities of acid phosphatase, α-mannosidase, and α-fucosidase are normal or increased [125]. PAPS-sulfatase activity is also normal [127]. Tissue culture cocultivation experiments with Hurler's disease and type B Sanfilippo disease cell lines indicate that the activities of α-iduronidase and of α-N-acetylglucosaminidase are also normal [178].

The arylsulfatase A gene in multiple sulfatase deficiency is intact and can be expressed under suitable environmental conditions. In cultured skin fibroblasts grown in media containing an MEM-CO$_2$ buffer (pH<7.0), arylsulfatase A activity is less than one-tenth of normal. With the use of an MEM-HEPES buffer (pH 7.4) in the media, arylsulfatase A activity is expressed at levels 30 to 100 percent of normal [214]. Other sulfatases deficient in this disease do not appear to manifest these pH-dependent differences in activity. The addition of sodium thiosulfate to the culture medium results over a period of 1 to 2 months in higher intracellular levels of all deficient sulfatases with the possible exception of heparan-N-sulfamidase [215]. This effect is most pronounced for arylsulfatase A but does not completely restore its activity to normal. It is not observed in normal cells and is not present simply upon addition of this sulfate to cell homogenates.

The arylsulfatases A and B show the same properties including pH optima, isoelectric points (see Fig. 44-16D), and heat stability as the normal enzymes [178, 197, 216]. They also precipitate with antibodies specific for the normal arylsulfatases [17, 216, 217] (see Fig. 44-13). The amount of cross-reacting material (CRM) is less than normal but the activity/CRM ratio is normal. Consequently, it appears that these enzymes are qualitatively normal but reduced in activity because of decreased synthesis or increased degradation.

MLD without Arylsulfatase A Deficiency

Three living cases of this disorder have been investigated. In one case [130], leukocyte and fibroblast arylsulfatase A activity was reduced to one-half of that present in normal controls. In another unrelated case [131], the arylsulfatase A activity in leukocytes, fibroblasts, and urine was above the control range. The properties of the fibroblast enzyme from both cases were identical to the properties of normal fibroblast arylsulfatase A [15, 131].

In spite of apparently adequate arylsulfatase A activity, the hydrolysis of cerebroside sulfate by the cultured skin fibroblasts from these patients is markedly attenuated (Fig. 44-17). Supplementation of the fibroblasts from one case [131] with cerebroside sulfate sulfatase activator factor corrected the defect in cerebroside sulfate hydrolysis. The molecular basis for this variant is therefore considered to be a deficiency of the physiological activator protein required for in vivo sulfatide catabolism.

PATHOGENESIS OF MLD

The accepted biochemical defect in all forms of MLD is a deficiency in the enzymatic hydrolysis of sulfatide. This leads to a progressive accumulation of sulfatides, mainly within lysosomes. The storage process is not uniform in all tissues and organs and functional loss is not directly proportional to the amount of sulfatide that is deposited. On this basis, four categories of tissues may be defined:

1. Tissues that show little or no sulfatide accumulation and no tissue damage. These tissues include the heart, lung, spleen, skin, bones, and intestinal tract.

2. Tissues in which there is accumulation of sulfatide but no demonstrable impairment of functions. These tissues include the liver and the kidney.

3. Tissues in which there are sulfatide accumulation and evidence of impaired function, but which do not appear to contribute to the fatal outcome of the disease. This applies to

the gallbladder, which as already noted shows sulfatide accumulation and progressive functional impairment [151].

4. White matter of the nervous system.

The accumulation of sulfatide probably occurs independently in each organ. It is unlikely, for example, that sulfatide from the central nervous system is deposited within the kidney. The fatty acid composition of brain and kidney sulfatide are different [24], the sulfatide concentration in MLD serum is normal [218], and massive subcutaneous injections of sulfatide fail to produce kidney deposits in infant rats [219]. It is more probable that the increase in sulfatide observed in extraneural tissues reflects an in situ failure in the turnover of sulfatide that is normally present in plasma membranes of these tissues and serves other purposes than as a structural component of myelin. The tolerance of the kidney, gallbladder and other extraneural tissues for sulfatides may relate to the fact that the cells most involved in the storage process fulfill an excretory function and therefore can discharge the accumulating lipid from the cell into the urine, bile, or other fluid.

The demyelination that occurs in MLD appears to be secondary to sulfatide-induced changes within the cells responsible for myelin maintenance, namely the Schwann cells in the peripheral nervous system and the oligodendrocytes in the central nervous system. Changes in the subcellular organelles of these cells have been observed before any morphologic abnormalities in the myelin sheaths associated with them were detected. In a fetus with MLD aborted in the fifth month of gestation [220], an increase in lysosomes, some containing lamellar structured material, had been found in the cerebrum and cerebellum even though these tissues did not stain metachromatically and myelination had not yet begun. This increase in lysosomal bodies was even more marked in the oligodendroglial cells of the spinal cord. Although accumulations of metachromatic material were observed in the spinal cord oligodendrocytes, the morphologic appearance of the spinal cord myelin at this stage was normal. An increase in the number of lysosomes thus appears to be the earliest pathologic change resulting from the failure of sulfatide catabolism.

Neuropathologic study of two other MLD fetuses aborted in the fifth month of gestation have also demonstrated cellular abnormalities at a stage when myelin had either not yet developed or had appeared morphologically normal [170, 221]. Also, in nerve biopsies from patients with MLD, a normal myelin sheath is often observed together with abundant storage material in the Schwann cell belonging to the same internodal segment of the myelin sheath [222–224]. Therefore, it is the abnormal accumulation of sulfatide within the lysosomes of oligodendroglial and Schwann cells and the metabolic failure of these cells that precede and trigger the events that cause demyelination.

It has been suggested that myelin breakdown in MLD results from defective resorption of sulfatide from the innermost part of the myelin sheath. Catabolism of this layer of myelin is necessary for the axon to increase its cross-diameter during growth [225]. Even after maturity is reached, enzymatic failure in the resorption of myelin would prevent normal restructuring of the myelin sheath. Experiments with isotopic sulfate have confirmed the presence of two myelin compartments in adult rat myelin, one with a slow turnover rate and the other with a fast turnover rate [226]. Thus, both during growth and after the active growth phase is completed, sulfatase activity is needed to maintain the normal integrity of myelin.

Alternative pathogenetic mechanisms have also been suggested, but there is less evidence to support them. One is that the myelin formed in MLD has an abnormal composition and is therefore unstable. While it is true that the chemical composition of the myelin present in MLD white matter is abnormal [157, 227, 228], the quantity of metachromatic lipid that accumulates in an area of demyelination is considerably more than would be expected based upon the amount of sudanophilic lipid that is normally present. Another proposed mechanism is that sulfogalactosylsphingosine, a compound closely related to galactosylsphingosine, which is known to be highly cytotoxic, might accumulate and cause myelin breakdown because of the deficiency of sulfogalactosylsphingosine sulfatase in MLD [75].

GENETICS

The four forms of MLD—late infantile, juvenile, adult, and multiple sulfatase deficiency—appear to be genetically distinct. This is evident clinically in families that have more than one affected member. In such cases, the chronology of symp-

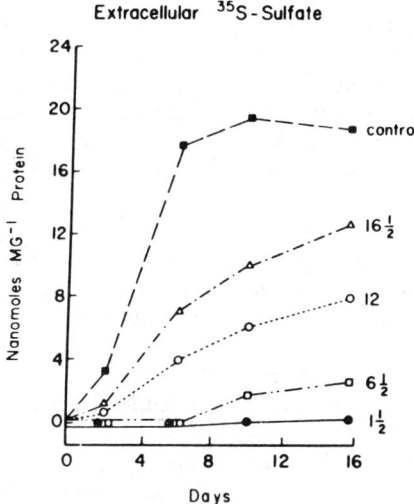

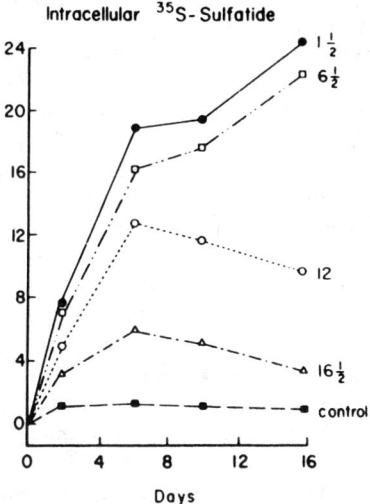

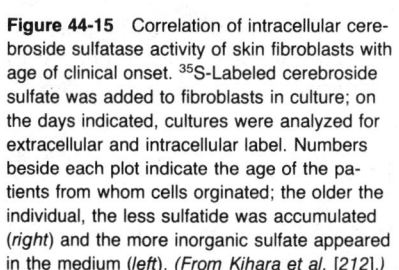

Figure 44-15 Correlation of intracellular cerebroside sulfatase activity of skin fibroblasts with age of clinical onset. ^{35}S-Labeled cerebroside sulfate was added to fibroblasts in culture; on the days indicated, cultures were analyzed for extracellular and intracellular label. Numbers beside each plot indicate the age of the patients from whom cells orginated; the older the individual, the less sulfatide was accumulated (right) and the more inorganic sulfate appeared in the medium (left). (From Kihara et al. [212].)

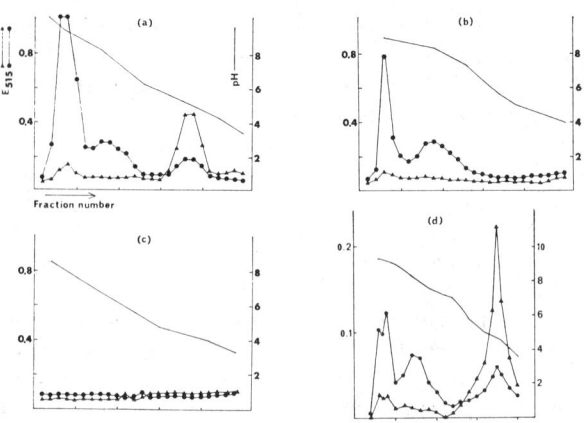

Figure 44-16 Arylsulfatase A and B patterns obtained by isoelectric focusing of kidney extracts from (a) a control, (b) an MLD patient, and (c) and (d) patients with multiple sulfatase deficiency. The sloping solid line indicates the pH of each fraction, ●——● combined arylsulfatase activity, and ▲——▲ arylsulfatase A activity. Incubation time for (a to c) was 1 hour, for (d) 6 hours. Note the absence of arylsulfatase A activity in MLD and the presence in multiple sulfatase deficiency of both enzyme activities only after a prolonged incubation. *(From Harzer, et al. [197].)*

tomatology and progression of the disease is the same. For at least one form, the multiple sulfatase deficiency syndrome, the difference in clinical subtypes of MLD is also expressed on the molecular level. Intergenic complementation experiments demonstrate that the gene for multiple sulfatase deficiency and those for other types of MLD are nonallelic. In somatic cell hybrids produced by fusing cultured fibroblasts from patients with these two conditions, arylsulfatase A activity is restored [215, 229]. Conversely, hybridizing cell lines from patients with late infantile and adult MLD does not restore arylsulfatase A activity, suggesting that the loci for these two variants are situated on the gene map too close to one another for intergenic complementation to occur and thus are allelic [230].

All varieties of MLD are transmitted through an autosomal recessive pattern of inheritance. This is deduced from the appearance of approximately equal numbers of affected individuals of each sex, the frequent occurrence of more than one affected individual in a sibship, the occasional association of parental consanguinity, and the presence of approximately one-half the normal level of arylsulfatase A in the parents of patients. In a few parents or siblings, the level of enzyme activity is reduced to 20 percent or less without any of the signs or symptoms of MLD present. These individuals appear to have two recessive traits, one for MLD and another for low enzyme activity without MLD [143, 144]. Assays for cerebroside sulfate sulfatase activity differentiate between these individuals and patients with true MLD. Such assays, however, do not distinguish carriers of an MLD gene apart from those carrying this other silent or null allele.

The overall incidence of MLD and the frequency of the trait for MLD are unknown. A decade ago in northern Sweden, the incidence of late infantile MLD was estimated to be 1:40,000 [115]. This probably represents a somewhat higher figure than can be expected elsewhere due to a clustering of 6 of the 13 cases surveyed in a single restricted geographic isolate. In the Habbanite Jewish community in Israel, 12 cases of late infantile MLD have been noted among 750 to 850 live births between 1950 and 1978 [231]. The very high incidence of MLD in this community (1.3 percent) is due to a 17 percent

carrier frequency and a marked tendency to consanguine marriages. Our own case experience would suggest an aggregate incidence figure for all forms of MLD of approximately 1 per 100,000 births.

The gene for the low enzyme allele not associated with MLD is probably quite common since it is often found in the parents of patients with MLD. By virtue of their status as obligate heterozygotes, these individuals already carry one allele for reduced enzyme activity. Thus the presence of another allele that also reduces their ability to produce active enzyme becomes readily apparent. In the general population this allele would not be separately discernible because it reduces enzyme activity to the same extent as the MLD gene and therefore cannot be differentiated from it.

The locus determining the expression of arylsulfatase A activity has been mapped with human-rodent somatic cell hybrids to chromosome 22 [232–234]. Arylsulfatase B activity was similarly examined and found to be concordant with β-hexosaminidase B activity, thus establishing its locus on chromosome 5 [233]. The chromosome assignment of a gene that might regulate the production of sulfatases and could be involved in the multiple sulfatase deficiency disorder has not yet been accomplished.

DIAGNOSIS

Clinical Evaluation

The initial signs of MLD may appear at any age from birth to the seventh decade. Therefore, this diagnosis should be considered whenever progressive white matter disease is encountered, regardless of the patient's age. The most common ages for the disease to begin are $1\frac{1}{2}$ to 2 years for the late infantile variant, 4 to 6 years for the juvenile variant, and 16 to 26 years for the adult variant. Intellectual loss, weakness, and incoordination are early signs that might suggest the diagnosis. Further involvement of the long tracts leads eventually to spastic tetraparesis and incontinence. Specific signs that help at this stage to confirm the diagnosis are the presence of optic atrophy and peripheral neuropathy.

The clinician with a high index of suspician for MLD will pursue this diagnostic possibility with certain clinical laboratory tests. The most useful are a cerebrospinal fluid examination for elevated protein, measurements of nerve conduction velocity, and a CT scan of the brain. In adult patients without peripheral neuropathy, nerve conduction and the level of cerebrospinal fluid protein may be normal, but all patients with a significant amount of symptomatology show changes on the CT scan that are characteristic of brain white matter disease [94]. The clinical investigation of the dysmorphic child with a possible diagnosis of multiple sulfatase deficiency should, in addition, include a skeletal x-ray series, examination of the peripheral smear for Alder-Reilly granules, and a urine spot test to rule out mucopolysacchariduria.

Biochemical Confirmation

Until recently, the diagnosis of MLD was most often confirmed by histologic examination of a sural nerve biopsy. Less invasive

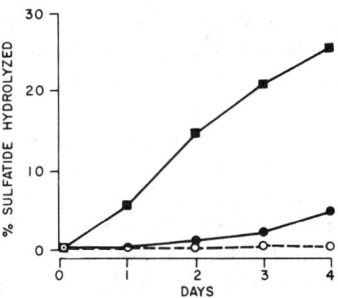

Figure 44-17 Hydrolysis of ³⁵S-sulfatide by intact growing fibroblasts from an MLD patient without arylsulfatase A deficiency ●——● a patient with classical late infantile MLD ○——○, and a normal control cell line ■——■. The free [³⁵S]sulfate present in the media on 4 consecutive days was analyzed and expressed as a percent of the labeled lipid added to the media at the beginning of the experiment. Note that the MLD variant cells cannot degrade sulfatide in vivo in spite of the substantial amounts of aryl-sulfatase A activity present in these cells. *(From Shapiro et al. [130].)*

attempts to identify accumulations of metachromatic material have employed biopsies of conjuctiva [98], skin [96], or cells of the urinary sediment [235]. As the molecular defects of the MLD group of diseases have become better understood, there has been increasing reliance on biochemical determinations so that tissue biopsies for histological study are now only being done in exceptional circumstances.

The most common biochemical parameter studied is the activity of arylsulfatase A. This enzyme can be reliably assayed using peripheral leukocytes and cultured skin fibroblasts. Aryl-sulfatase A activity is also present in urine but this is not a reliable source for diagnostic assays because the enzyme normally has a low specific activity in this fluid [179–181]. There-fore, the assay of urine arylsulfatase A is generally regarded as a screening procedure, and low levels of activity are followed up by analysis of leukocyte or fibroblast enzyme activity. Var-ious modifications [50, 99, 182] of the *p*-nitrocatechol sulfate method of Baum et al. [201] are used for the analysis. Each takes advantage of the fact that the contribution from arylsul-fatase B to the total enzyme activity can be minimized by inhi-bition of this enzyme with a high NaCl content in the reaction mixture. An alternative method has been developed that uti-lizes the fluorogenic substrate 4-methylumbelliferyl sulfate and Ag⁺ ions to inhibit arylsulfatase A activity specifically [236]. Measurements of enzyme activity are made in the presence and absence of Ag⁺. The difference between the two activities rep-resents the contribution for arylsulfatase A.

In order to improve the accuracy of the arylsulfatase A assay, several procedures have been developed to separate aryl-sulfatase A and B physically prior to their quantification. These have employed various forms of ion exchange chromatogra-phy [237, 238], electrophoresis [187, 239], and isoelectric focusing [58, 93]. With several of these techniques it is possible to visualize directly individual bands of enzyme activity. This provides the clinical chemist with an extra measure of confi-dence, particularly when assessing the significance of a defi-ciency in vitro in enzyme activity.

Several procedures have been described for labeling cerebro-side sulfate for use as an enzyme substrate [66, 140, 194, 240]. The advantage of the cerebroside sulfate sulfatase assay is that it can distinguish between the few normal individuals who have unusually low arylsulfatase A activity and patients with MLD (Fig. 44-18). Those with true MLD are totally deficient in activity toward this natural substrate, whereas the normal individuals with low arylsulfatase A activity will hydrolyze a

small amount of cerebroside sulfate [140]. The labeled sub-strate is also useful in tissue culture loading experiments for diagnosing the variant with cerebroside sulfate sulfatase acti-vator deficiency [15].

Urine sulfatide determinations are a useful adjunct to the enzyme analyses in the diagnosis of MLD [175, 176]. All cases of MLD, including multiple sulfatase deficiency and those due to the deficiency of the cerebroside sulfate sulfatase activator protein, excrete large amounts of sulfatide in the urine. Fresh urine is filtered and the cellular debris trapped on the filter is then extracted with organic solvents and its lipid content ana-lyzed. A less rigorous screening procedure for urine sulfatide has also been described [241]. Two types of clinical situations specifically require an assessment of the urinary sulfatide excretion: the patient with clinical signs of MLD but normal arylsulfatase A activity, and the patient with arylsulfatase A deficiency without other signs of MLD. In the first of these two classes of patients, an increase in urine sulfatide will suggest the diagnosis of cerebroside sulfate sulfatase activator protein deficiency. In the case of the second type of patient, the increased excretion of sulfatide will alert the clinician to a pre-symptomatic case of MLD, whereas a finding of normal urine sulfatide will exclude the MLD genotype.

Heterozygote Identification

Leukocyte and fibroblast assays for arylsulfatase A and cere-broside sulfatase can also be used to determine whether an individual is a carrier of the trait for MLD. This is most fre-quently done for the sibs and other family members of a patient with MLD and for their spouses. This information per-

Figure 44-18 Leukocyte sulfatidase activity in normal controls, patients with MLD, and obligate heterozygotes. A dialyzed leukocyte sonicate was incubated for 2 hours with [³H]sulfatide labeled in the sphingosine portion of the molecule. The mean for each group is indicated by arrows. Note that the enzyme activity in some heterozygotes was quite low but that only in the MLD cases was it totally absent. *(Adapted from Raghavan et al. [140].)*

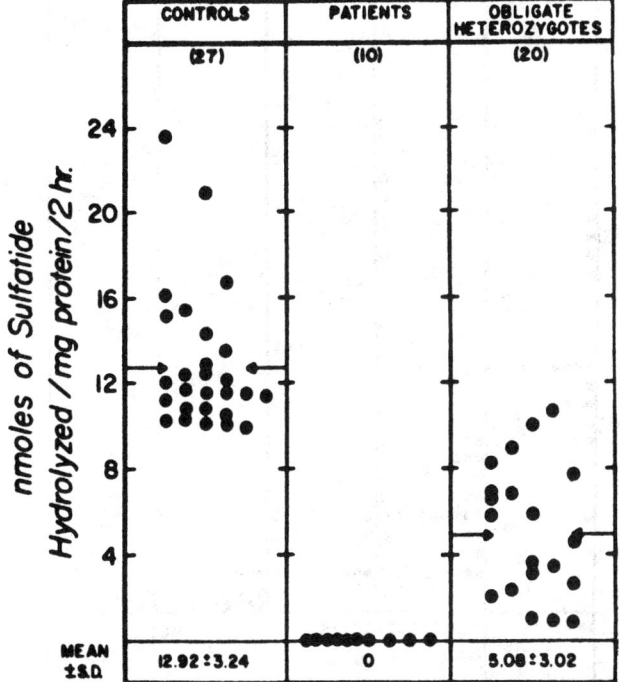

mits an estimate of their risk for having children with MLD [231]. There is some overlap in enzyme values at both ends of the heterozygote range, between those for normal individuals and carriers, and between those for affected homozygotes and carriers [183] (Fig. 44-19). This spread in activity is due partly to the protein polymorphism that characterizes any diverse population and partly to the relatively frequent occurrence of a non-MLD low activity allele in the normal population. If this low activity allele is present in an MLD heterozygote, the amount of leukocyte arylsulfatase A activity present may be so low as to suggest the disease state. When this occurs further enzyme testing using the natural substrate, cerebroside sulfate, is desirable. Heterozygote levels of enzyme activity vary less within a given family than among unrelated persons. Therefore, it is helpful in doing carrier ascertainment to test as many members of the same family as possible and compare their results with those obtained for the obligate heterozygotes in that family.

Prenatal Diagnosis

Prenatal diagnosis has been repeatedly and successfully accomplished for the late infantile and juvenile forms of MLD [161, 209, 210, 228] and is theoretically possible for other variants. The usual procedure is to determine the activity of arylsulfatase A in cultured amniotic fluid cells. Activity is normally low during the log phase of cell growth. Only after the cultured cell monolayer has reached confluency does a significant amount of enzyme activity appear. Therefore, careful attention must be paid to cell culture conditions and time of harvesting. In fam-

Figure 44-19 Arylsulfatase A (●) and B (○) levels in leukocytes from patients with late infantile (LI) MLD and juvenile (J) MLD, heterozygote parents, and healthy adults. Note the overlap in arylsulfatase A activity between patients and heterozygotes and between heterozygotes and controls. Also note that arylsulfatase B activity tends to be lower in patients and their parents than in controls. *(Adapted from Dubois et al. [184].)*

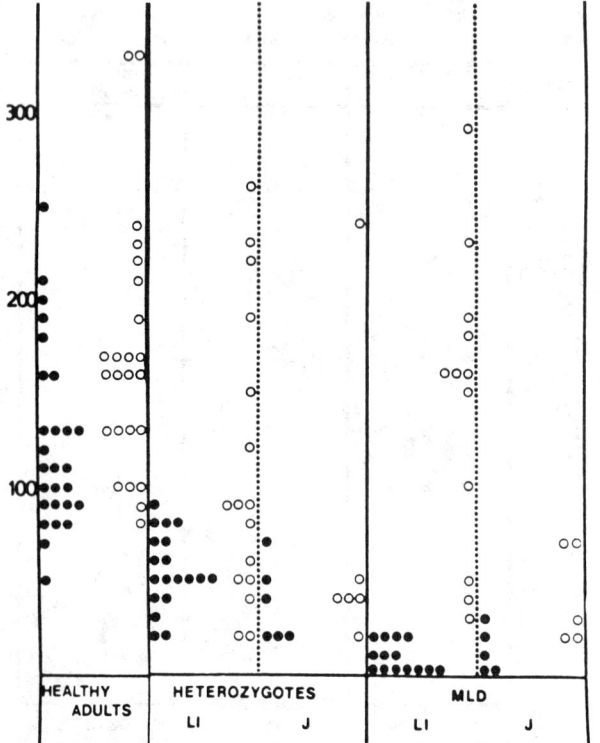

ilies that carry both the MLD allele and the unrelated low activity allele, additional tests are indicated beyond the arylsulfatase A assay usually performed in cell-free homogenates. A successful prenatal diagnosis in this circumstance has been performed by applying the cerebroside sulfate loading test to the growing amniotic fluid cells [136]. An in vitro assay of cerebroside sulfatase activity should also help to differentiate the affected fetus from one with the low arylsulfatase A activity variant without MLD. Direct assays of arylsulfatase A activity in amniotic fluid have also been used for the prenatal diagnosis of MLD [90, 242] but most authorities feel that this procedure is less reliable than enzyme methods utilizing cultured amniotic fluid cells. In a single case of multiple sulfatase deficiency, a low estriol level was found in maternal urine during gestation [129]. If confirmed in additional cases, this measurement might be of considerable value in the prenatal diagnosis of this variant.

TREATMENT

Currently, there exists no specific treatment that will halt the progression of MLD nor reverse its fatal outcome. The objectives in managment of a child or adult with this disease are to maintain useful function and meaningful interaction for as long as possible. The educational program of the juvenile MLD patient in kindergarden or first grade is adjusted to lowered expectations so that the child's participation in the school environment can continue. Patients with the adult onset variant can frequently continue for several years to enjoy the company of their family and perform useful chores in the familiarity of their own home. Eventually all mobility is lost and total supportive care becomes necessary. A permanent gastrostomy tube may be needed to assist in feeding and to maintain adequate nutrition. Passive physical therapy is utilized to prevent contractures that would otherwise cause nursing problems in the bedridden patient.

Attempts have been made to reduce sulfatide synthesis by the use of a diet low in vitamin A [243–245] or low in sulfur [246]. The rationale is that both vitamin A and sulfur are required for sulfatide synthesis. Unfortunately, neither approach has had favorable long-lasting effects.

Replacement therapy with normal enzyme is theoretically possible but has never been successfully applied to this or any other lysosomal storage disease that is almost exclusively due to brain dysfunction. Tissue culture experiments have shown that arylsulfatase A supplied to the nutrient media can enter cells deficient in arylsulfatase A degrading [^{35}S]sulfatide previously stored within them. This has been accomplished with MLD skin fibroblasts [195, 247], and with explants and dissociated cells from the brain of a fetus with MLD [170]. The targeting of enzyme into an oligodendroglial cell in vivo is a much more difficult task. Purified enzyme has twice been injected into children with MLD. In one instance, a pyrogenic reaction occurred [248]; in the second, high levels of enzyme activity were present transiently in the liver but no activity could be detected in a brain biopsy 8 hours after an intrathecal injection of the enzyme [249]. For enzyme replacement therapy to be successful in the future, several major problems must be circumvented. The enzyme will have to be targeted so that it can cross the blood-brain barrier and specifically enter those cells and subcellular sites where it is most needed. It must be stable, and it must somehow avoid the immunological surveillance system. These are formidable problems for which solutions are now actively being sought.

An alternative to the replacement of the missing enzyme with normal enzyme is the use of drugs that would activate or stabilize the mutant arylsulfatase A protein. The ability of an arylsulfatase A antibody to combine with the normal enzyme both to activate and stabilize it has prompted the suggestion that various drugs might be able to achieve the same result with the mutant enzyme protein that is present in the patient's cells [202]. For example, long-term thiosulfate treatment of skin fibroblasts cultured from a patient with multiple sulfatase deficiency substantially improved the capacity of these cells to catabolize sulfatide. Consequently, thiosulfate has been proposed as a treatment for this particular disease [215]. Acetosalicylate, another drug thought likely to increase residual arylsulfatase activity, has been administered to a patient with adult MLD [109]. After the medication trial leukocyte arylsulfatase A activity nearly doubled but was still less than 10 percent of the mean for the control group. The ultimate success of this type of approach requires that much more be learned about the physical and chemical properties of the mutant enzyme.

REFERENCES

1. DULANEY JT, MOSER HW: Sulfatide lipidosis: metachromatic leukodystrophy, in Stanbury JB, Wyngaarden JB, Fredrickson DS (eds): *The Metabolic Basis of Inherited Disease*, 4th ed. New York, McGraw-Hill, 1978, p 770n
2. ALZHEIMER, A: Beitrage zur Kenntnis der pathologischen Neurologia und ihrer Beziehung zu den Abbauvorgangen im Nervengewebe. *Nissl-Alzheimer's Histol Histopathol Arb*, 3:493, 1910
3. WITTE, F: Über pathologische Abbauvorgange im Zentralnervensystem. *Munch Med Wochenschr* 68:69, 1921
4. SCHOLZ W: Klinische, pathologisch-anatomische und erbbiologische Untersuchungen bei familiärer, diffuser Hirnsklerose im Kindesalter. *Z Gesamte Neurol Psychiat* 99:42, 1925
5. VON HIRSCH T, PEIFFER J: Über histologische Methoden in der Differentialdiagnose von Leukodystrophien und Lipoidosen. *Arch Psychiat Nervenkr* 194:88, 1955
6. PEIFFER J: Über die metachromatischen Leukodystrophien (Typ Scholz). *Arch Psychiatr Nervenkr* 199:386, 1959
7. GREENFIELD JG: A form of progressive cerebral sclerosis in infants associated with primary degeneration of the interfascicular glia. *J Neurol Psychopath* 13:289, 1933
8. FEIGIN I: Diffuse cerebral sclerosis (metachromatic leuko-encephalopathy). *Amer J Path* 30:715, 1954
9. JATZKEWITZ H: Zwei Typen von Cerebrosid-schwefelsaureestern als Sog. "Pralipoide" und Speichersubstanzen bei der Leukodystrophie, Typ Scholz (metachromatische Form der diffusen Sklerose). *Z Physiol Chem* 311:279, 1958
10. AUSTIN J: Metachromatic sulfatides in cerebral white matter and kidney. *Proc Soc Exp Biol Med* 100:361, 1959
11. AUSTIN JH, BALASUBRAMANIAN AS, PATTABIRAMAN TN, SARASWATHI S, BASU DK, BACHHAWAT BK: A controlled study of enzymatic activities in three human disorders of glycolipid metabolism. *J Neurochem* 10:805, 1963
12. MEHL E, JATZKEWITZ H: Evidence for the genetic block in metachromatic leukodystrophy (ML). *Biochem Biophys Res Commun* 19:407, 1965
13. JATZKEWITZ H, MEHL E: Cerebroside-sulfatase and arylsulfatase A deficiency in metachromatic leukodystrophy (ML). *J Neurochem* 16:19, 1969
14. MEHLE, JATZKEWITZ H: Eine Cerebrosidsulfatase aus Schweineniere. *Hoppe-Seylers Z Physiol Chem* 339:260, 1964
15. STEVENS RL, FLUHARTY AL, KIHARA H, KABACK MM, SHAPIRO LJ, MARSH B, SANDHOFF K, FISCHER G: Cerebroside sulfatase activator deficiency induced metachromatic leukodystrophy. *Am J Hum Genet*, in press
16. AUSTIN JH, ARMSTRONG D, SHEARER L: Metachromatic form of diffuse cerebral sclerosis. V. The nature and significance of low sulfatase activity: A controlled study of brain, liver and kidney in four patients with metachromatic leukodystrophy (MLD). *Arch Neurol* 13:593, 1965
17. BASNER R, VON FIGURA K, GLÖSSL J, KLEIN U, KRESSE H, MLEKUSCH W: Multiple deficiency of mucopolysaccharide sulfatases in mucosulfatidosis. *Pediat Res* 13:1316, 1979
18. THUDICHUM JLW: *A Treatise on the Chemical Constitution of Brain.* London, Baliere, 1884
19. THUDICHUM JLW: Die chemische Konstitution des Gehirns des Menschen und der Tiere. Tübingen, Franz Pietzeker, 1901
20. BLIX G: Zur Kenntnis der schwefelhaltigen Lipid Stoffe des Gehirns: Über cerbron Schwefelsaüre. *Z Physiol Chem* 219:82, 1933
21. YAMAKAWA T, KISO N, HANDA S, MAKITA A, YOKOYAMA S: On the structure of brain cerebroside sulfuric ester and ceramide dihexoside of erythrocytes. *J Biochem (Tokyo)* 52:226, 1962
22. STOFFYN P, STOFFYN A: Structure of sulfatides. *Biochim Biophys Acta* 70:218, 1963
23. STOFFYN PJ: The structure and chemistry of sulfatides. *J Am Oil Chem Soc* 43:69, 1966
24. MALONE MJ, STOFFYN P: A comparative study of brain and kidney glycolipids in metachromatic leukodystrophy. *J Neurochem* 13:1037, 1966
25. MARTENSSON E: Sulfatides of human kidney: Isolation, identification, and fatty acid composition. *Biochim Biophys Acta* 116:521, 1966
26. MARTENSSON E: On the sulfate containing lipids of human kidney. *Acta Chem Scand* 17:1174, 1963
27. STOFFYN A, STOFFYN P, MARTENSSON E: Structure of kidney ceramide dihexoside sulfate. *Biochim Biophys Acta* 152:353, 1968
28. HAUSER G: Labeling of cerebrosides and sulfatides in rat brain. *Biochim Biophys Acta* 84:212, 1964
29. BALASUBRAMANIAN AS, BACHHAWAT BK: Formation of cerebroside sulphate from 3′-phosphoadenosine 5′-phosphosulphate in sheep brain. *Biochim Biophys Acta* 106:218, 1965
30. MCKHANN GM, HO W: The *in vivo* and *in vitro* synthesis of sulphatides during development. *J Neurochem* 14:717, 1967
31. CUMAR FA, BARRA HS, MACCIONI HJ, CAPUTTO R: Sulfation of glycosphingolipids and related carbohydrates by brain preparations from young rats. *J Biol Chem* 243:3807, 1968
32. FARRELL DF, MCKHANN GM: Characterization of cerebroside sulfotransferase from rat brain. *J Biol Chem* 246:4694, 1971
33. FARRELL DF: Enzymatic sulphation of some galactose-containing sphingolipids in developing rat brain. *J Neurochem* 23:219, 1974
34. NUSSBAUM JL, MANDEL P: Enzymic synthesis of psychosine sulphate. *J Neurochem* 19:1789, 1972
35. DAWSON G, KERNES SM: Induction of sulfogalactosylceramide (sulfatide) synthesis by hydrocortisone (cortisol) in mouse G-26 oligodendroglioma cell strains. *J Neurochem* 31:1091, 1978
36. HARRIS RA, LOH HH: Brain sulfatide and non-lipid sulfate metabolism in hypothyroid rats. *Res Commun Chem Path Pharm* 24:169, 1979
37. BENJAMINS JA, GUANIERI M, MILLER K, SONNEBORN CM, MCKHANN GM: Sulfatide synthesis in isolated oligodendroglial and neuronal cells. *J Neurochem* 23:751, 1974
38. SARLIEVE, LL, NISKOVIC NM, FREYSZ L, MANDEL P, REBEL G: Ceramide galactosyltransferase and cerebroside sulphotransferase in chicken brain cellular fractions and glial and neuronal cells in culture. *Life Sci* 18:251, 1976
39. ISHIZUKA I, TADANO K, NAGATA N, NHMURA Y, NAGAI Y: Hormone-specific responses and biosynthesis of sulfolipids in cell lines derived from mammalian kidney. *Biochim Biophys Acta* 541:467, 1978
40. ISHIZUKA I, INOMATA M, UENO K, YAMAKAWA T: Sulphated glyceroglycolipid in rat brain. Structure, sulphation *in vivo* and accumulation in whole brain during development. *J Biol Chem* 253:898, 1978
41. KORNBLATT MJ, KNAPP A, LEVINE M, SCHACHTER H, MURRAY RK: Studies on the structure and formation during spermatogenesis of sulphoglycerogalactolipid of rat testis. *Can J Biochem* 52:689, 1974
42. SUBBA RAO G, NARCIA LN, PIERINGER J, PIERINGER RA: The biosynthesis of sulphogalactosyldiacylglycerol of rat brain *in vitro*. *Biochim J* 166:429, 1977
43. HANDA S, YAMATO K, ISHIZUKA I, SUZUKI A, YAMAKAWA T: Biosynthesis of seminolipid. *J Biochem (Tokyo)* 75:77, 1974
44. ROBERTS KD, LIEBERMAN S: The biochemistry of the 3β-hydroxy-Δ⁵-steroid sulfates, in Bernstein S, Solomon S (eds): *Chemical and Biological Aspects of Steroid Conjugation.* New York, Springer-Verlag, 1970, p 219
45. SHAPIRA E, NADLER HL: Purification and some properties of soluble human liver arylsulfatases. *Arch Biochem Biophys* 170:179, 1975
46. DRAPER RK, FISKUM GM, EDMOND J: Purification, molecular weight, amino acid, and subunit composition of arylsulfatase A from human liver. *Arch Biochem Biophys* 177:525, 1976
47. JAMES GT, AUSTIN JH: Studies in metachromatic leukodystrophy. XIV. Purification and subunit structure of human liver arylsulfatase A. *Clin Chim Acta* 98:103, 1979
48. FAROOQUI AA: Purification and properties of arylsulfatase A from human placenta. *Archs Int Physiol Biochim* 84:479, 1976
49. GNIOT-SZULZYCKA, J: Some properties of highly purified arylsulfatase A from human placenta. *Acta Biochim Pol* 21:247, 1974

50. STEVENS RL, FLUHARTY AL, SKOKUT MH, KIHARA H: Purification and properties of arylsulfatase A from human urine. *J Biol Chem* 250:2495, 1975

51. LUIJTEN JAFM, VAN DER HEIJDEN MCM, RIJKSEN G, STAAL GEJ: Purification and characterization of arylsulfatase A from human urine. *J Mol Med* 3:213, 1978

52. GRAHAM ERB, RAY AB: Sulfatase A as glycoprotein. *Biochim Biophys Acta* 329:88, 1973

53. BALASUBRAMANIAN KA, BACHHAWAT BK: Purification properties and glycoprotein nature of arylsulfatase A from sheep brain. *Biochim Biophys Acta* 403:113, 1975

54. DAS PK, BISHAYEE S: Differential localisation of phosphorylated and nonphosphorylated forms of arylsulfatase A in lysosomes. *FEBS Lett* 111:43, 1980

55. MANOWITZ P, GOLDSTEIN L, BELLOMO F: An improved method for arylsulfatase A detection of polyacrylamide slab gels. *Anal Biochem* 89:423, 1978

56. DUBOIS G, TURPIN JC, BAUMANN N: Arylsulfatases isoenzymes in metachromatic leukodystrophy/Detection of a new variant by electrophoresis. Improvement of quantitative assay. *Biomedicine* 23:116, 1975

57. STEVENS RL, FLUHARTY AL, KILLGROVE AR, KIHARA H: Microheterogeneity of arylsulfatase A from human tissues. *Biochim Biophys Acta* 445:661, 1976

58. FARRELL DF, MacMARTIN MP, CLARK AF: Multiple molecular forms of arylsulfatase A in different forms of metachromatic leukodystrophy (MLD). *Neurology* 29:16, 1979

59. DUBOIS G, BAUMANN N: *Identification of 2 Forms of Arylsulfatase A. Relations with Cerebroside in Liver and Brain.* Abstr. Seventh Meeting International Society for Neurochemistry, Jerusalem, 1979, p 306

60. LEE GD, VAN ETTEN RL: Evidence for an essential histidine residue in rabbit liver arylsulfatase A. *Arch Biochem Biophys* 171:424, 1975

61. JAMES GT: Essential arginine residues in human liver arylsulfatase A. *Arch Biochem Biophys* 197:57, 1979

62. NEUWELT E, STUMPF D, AUSTIN J, KOHLER P: A monospecific antibody to human sulfatase A: Preparation, characterization and significance. *Biochim Biophys Acta* 236:333, 1971

63. RYBARSKA-STYLINSKA J, VAN ETTEN RL: Antigen-antibody interactions and the anomalous kinetics of arylsulfatase A. *Biochim Biophys Acta* 570:107, 1979

64. NICHOLLS RG, ROY AB: The sulphatase of ox liver. XV. Changes in the properties of sulphatase A in the presence of substrate. *Biochim Biophys Acta* 242:141, 1971

65. WAHEED A, VAN ETTEN RL: The structural basis of the anomalous kinetics of rabbit liver arylsulfatase A. *Arch Biochem Biophys* 203:11, 1980

66. STINSHOFF K, JATZKEWITZ H: Comparison of the cerebroside sulphatase and the arylsulphatase activity of human sulphatase A in the absence of activators. *Biochim Biophys Acta* 377:126, 1975

67. WAHEED A, VAN ETTEN RL: The monomer-dimer association of rabbit liver arylsulfatase A and its relationship to the anomalous kinetics. *Biochim Biophys Acta* 194:215, 1979

68. JERFY A, ROY AB: Comparison of the arylsulfatase and cerebroside sulfatase activities of sulphatase A. *Biochim Biophys Acta* 293:128, 1973

69. FISCHER G, JATZKEWITZ H: The activator of cerebroside sulphatase. Purification from human liver and identification as a protein. *Hoppe-Seylers Z Physiol Chem* 356:605, 1975

70. MRAZ W, FISCHER G, JATZKEWITZ H: The activator of cerebroside sulphatase. Lysosomal localization. *Hoppe-Seyler's Z Physiol Chem* 357:1181, 1976

71. FISHER G, JATZKEWITZ H: The activator of cerebroside sulphatase. Binding studies with enzyme and substrate demonstrating the detergent function of the activator protein. *Biochim Biophys Acta* 481:561, 1977

72. HARZER K, BENZ HU: Deficiency of lactosyl sulfatide sulfatase in metachromatic leukodystrophy (sulfatidosis). *Hoppe-Seyler's Z Physiol Chem* 355:744, 1974

73. FLUHARTY AL, STEVENS RL, MILLER RT, KIHARA H: Sulfoglycerogalactolipid from rat testis: A substrate for pure human arylsulfatase A. *Biochem Biophys Res Commun* 61:348, 1974

74. FISHER G, REITER S, JATZKEWITZ H: Enzymic hydrolysis of sulphosphingolipids and sulphoglycerolipids by sulphatase A in the presence and absence of activator protein. *Hoppe-Seyler's Z Physiol Chem* 359:863, 1978

75. ETO Y, WIESMANN U, HERSCHKOWITZ NN: Sulfogalactosylsphingosine sulfatase: Characteristics of the enzyme and its deficiency in metachromatic leukodystrophy in human cultured skin fibroblasts. *J Biol Chem* 249:4955, 1974

76. FAROOQUI AA, MANDEL P: Recent developments in the biochemistry of globoid and metachromatic leucodystrophies. *Biomedicine* 26:232, 1977

77. FLUHARTY AL, STEVENS RL, MILLER RT, SHAPIRO SS, KIHARA H: Ascorbic acid-2-sulfate sulfohydrolase activity in human arylsulfatase A. *Biochim Biophys Acta* 429:508, 1976

78. MANOWITZ P, SHAPIRO SS, GOLDSTEIN L: Ascorbate-2-sulfate levels in metachromatic leukodystrophy patients. *Biochem Med* 18:274, 1977

79. NORTON WT, PODUSLO SE: Myelination in rat brain: Changes in myelin composition during brain maturation. *J Neurochem* 21:759, 1973

80. DUPOUEY P, ZALC B, LEFROIT-JOLY M, GOMES D: Localization of galactosylceramide and sulfatide at the surface of the myelin sheath: an immunofluorescence study in liquid medium. *Cell Mol Biol* 25:269, 1979

81. LONDON Y, VOSSENBERG FGA: Specific interaction of central nervous system myelin basic protein with lipid. *Biochim Biophys Acta* 478:478, 1973

82. HANSSON CG, KARLSSON KA, SAMUELSSON BE: The identification of sulphatides in human erythrocyte membrane and their relation to sodium-potassium dependent adenosine triphosphatase. *J Biochem* 83:813, 1978

83. ZALC B, HELWIG JJ, GHANDOUR MS, SARLIEVE L: Sulfatide in the kidney: how is this lipid involved in sodium chloride transport? *FEBS Lett* 92:92, 1978

84. LOH HH, CHO TM, WU YC, HARRIS RA, WAY EL: Opiate binding to cerebroside sulfate: A model system for opiate-receptor interaction. *Life Sci* 16:1811, 1975

85. LOH HH, LAW PY, OSTWALD T, CHO TM, WAY EL: Possible involvement of cerebroside sulfate in opiate receptor binding. *Fed Proc* 37:147, 1978

86. CRAVES FB, ZALC B, LEYBIN L, BAUMANN N, LOH HH: Antibodies to cerebroside sulfate inhibit the effects of morphine and β-endorphin. *Science* 207:75, 1980

87. LAW PY, HARRIS RA, LOH HH, WAY EL: Evidence for involvement of cerebroside sulfate in opiate receptor binding: Studies with azure A and Jimpy mutant mice. *J Pharmacol Exp Ther* 207:458, 1978

88. WU C. SC, LEE NM, LOH HH, YANG JT, LI CH: β-endorphin: Formation of α-helix in lipid solutions. *Proc Natl Acad Sci USA* 76:3656, 1979

89. EBADI M, CHWEH A: Inhibition by arylsulfatase A of Na-independent [^{3}H]-GABA and [^{3}H]-muscinol binding to bovine cerebellar synaptic membranes. *Neuropharmacology* 19:1105, 1980

90. RATTAZZI MC, DAVIDSON RG: Prenatal diagnosis of metachromatic leukodystrophy by electrophoretic and immunologic techniques. *Pediat Res* 11:1030, 1977

91. PERCY AK, KABACK MM, HERNDON RM: Metachromatic leukodystrophy: Comparison of early and late-onset forms. *Neurology* 27:933, 1977

92. HASHIMOTO T, MINATO H, KURODA Y, TOSHIMA K, OHARA K, MIYAO M: Monozygotic twins with presumed metachromatic leukodystrophy: Activity of arylsulfatase A in serum of patients and family. *Arch Neurol* 35:689, 1978

93. CHRISTOMANOU H, SANDHOFF K: Variation of arylsulfatase A: Comparative studies of arylsulfatase A with synthetic and natural substrates in three families with metachromatic leukodystrophy. *Neuropadiatrie* 9:385, 1978

94. BUONNANO FS, BALL MR, LASTER DW, MOODY DM, McLEAN WT: Computed tomography in late-infantile metachromatic leukodystrophy. *Ann Neurol* 4:43, 1978

95. RODRIGUEZ-SORIANO J, RIVERA JM, VALLO A, PRATS-VIÑAS JM, CASTILLO G: Proximal renal tubular acidosis in metachromatic leukodystrophy. *Helv Paediat Acta* 33:45, 1978

96. GEBHART W, LASSMANN H, NIEBAUER G: Demonstration of specific storage material within cutaneous nerves in metachromatic leukodystrophy. *J Cutaneous Path* 5:5, 1978

97. LUIJTEN JAFM, STAAL GEJ, WILLEMSE J: Metachromatic leukodystrophy and age: A comparative study of clinical, enzymological and ultrastructural findings. *Clin Neurol Neurosurg* 81:221, 1979

98. LIBERT J, VANHOFF F, TOUSSAINT D, ROOZITALAB H, KENYON KR, GREEN WR: Ocular findings in metachromatic leukodystrophy: An electron microscopic and enzyme study in different clinical and genetic variants. *Arch Ophthal* 97:1495, 1979

99. HALTIA T, PALO J, HALTIA M, ICÉN A: Juvenile metachromatic leukodystrophy: Clinical, biochemical and neuropathologic studies in nine cases. *Arch Neurol* 37:42, 1980

100. YAMANO T, OHTA S, SHIMADA M, OKADA S, YOTAKA T, SUGITA T, YABUCCHI H: Neuronal depletion of cerebellum in late infantile metachromatic leukodystrophy. *Brain Dev* 2:359, 1980

101. NASCIMENTO OJ, FREITAS MR, ALENCAR AA, COUTO BH: Metachromatic leukodystrophy: Report of a case. *Arq Neuropsiquiatr* 38:287, 1980

102. THOMAS PK, KING RHM, KOCEN RS, BRETT EM: Comparative ultrastructural observations on peripheral nerve abnormalities in the late infantile, juvenile and late onset forms of metachromatic leukodystrophy. *Acta Neuropath (Berl)* 39:237, 1977

103. GORDON N: The insidious presentation of the juvenile form of metachromatic leukodystrophy. *Postgrad Med J* 54:335, 1978

104. TAGLIAVINI F, PIETRINI V, PILLERI G, TRABATTONI G, LECHI A: Case report. Adult metachromatic leukodystrophy: Clinicopathological report of two familial cases with slow course. *Neuropath Applied Neurobiol* 5:233, 1979

105. CLARK JR, MILLER RG, VIDGOFF JM: Juvenile-onset metachromatic leu-

kodystrophy: Biochemical and electrophysiologic studies. *Neurology* 29:346, 1979

106. MANOWITZ P, KLING A, KOHN H: Clinical course of adult metachromatic leukodystrophy presenting as schizophrenia. *J Nerv Ment Dis* 166:500, 1978

107. MARKIEWICZ D, ADAMCZEWSKA-GONCERZEWICZ Z, ZELMAN IB, DYNECKI J, BIENIASZ J: A case of metachromatic leukodystrophy with a chronic course (clinical-morphological-biochemical study). *Neuropat Pol* 16:233, 1978

108. BOSCH EP, HART MN: Late adult-onset metachromatic leukodystrophy: Dementia and polyneuropathy in a 63 year old man. *Arch Neurol* 35:475, 1978

109. HOES MJAJM, LAMERS KJ, HOMMES OR, TER HAAR B: Adult metachromatic leukodystrophy: Arylsulfatase-A values in four generations of one family and some reflections about the genetics. *Clin Neurol Neurosurg* 80:174, 1978

110. GOEBEL HH, SHIMOKAWA K, ARGYRAKIS A, PILZ H: The ultrastructure of the retina in adult metachromatic leukodystrophy. *Am J Ophthal* 85:841, 1978

111. BESSON JAO: A diagnostic pointer to adult metachromatic leukodystrophy. *Brit J Psychiat* 137:186, 1980

112. AUSTIN J, ARMSTRONG D, FOUCH S, MITCHELL C, STUMPF D, SHEARER L, BRINER O: Metachromatic leukodystrophy (MLD). VIII. MLD in adults: Diagnosis and pathogenesis. *Arch Neurol* 18:225, 1968

113. KIHARA H: Metachromatic leukodystrophy, an unusual case with a subtle cerebroside sulfatase defect, in Buchwald N, Brazier MAB (eds): *Brain Mechanisms in Mental Retardation*. New York, Academic, 1975, p 501

114. ROIZIN L, SCHEINESSON G, EROS G: Comparative histological and histochemical studies of infantile and adult metachromatic leukodystrophy. *Pathol Eur* 3:286, 1968

115. GUSTAVSON K-H, HAGBERG B: The incidence and genetics of metachromatic leucodystrophy in northern Sweden. *Acta Pediatr Scand* 60:585, 1971

116. SCHUTTA HS, PRATT RTC, METZ H, EVANS KA, CARTER CO: A family study of the late infantile and juvenile forms of metachromatic leukodystrophy. *J Med Genet* 3:86, 1966

117. HOLLANDER H: Über metachromatische Leukodystrophie. II. Relation zwischen Erkrankungsalter und Verlaufsdauer. *Arch Psychiatr Z Neurol* 205:300, 1964

118. FARRELL D: Personal communication

119. BUBIS JJ, ADLESBERG L: Congenital metachromatic leukodystrophy. Report of a case. *Acta Neuropathol* 6:298, 1966

120. DESILVA KL, PEARCE J: Neuropathy of metachromatic leukodystrophy. *J Neurol Neurosurg Psychiatr* 36:30, 1973

121. HAGBERG B: Clinical symptoms, signs and tests in metachromatic leukodystrophy, in Folch-Pi J, Bauer H (eds): *Brain Lipids and Lipoproteins and the Leukodystrophies*. Amsterdam, Elsevier, 1963, pp 134–146

122. COGAN DG, KUWABARA T, MOSER H: Metachromatic leukodystrophy. *Ophthalmology* 160:2, 1970

123. KOLODNY EH, RAGHAVAN S, SPIELVOGEL C, GAJEWSKI A, LASCON AC, JUNGALWALA FB, LOTT IT, DULANEY JT, HOEFNAGEL D: Genetic heterogeneity in arylsulfatase A deficiency. *Neurology* 29:576, 1979

124. PILZ H, DVENSING I, HEIPERTZ R, SEIDEL D, LOWITZSCH K, HOPF HC, GOEBEL HH: Adult metachromatic leukodystrophy. I. Clinical manifestation in a female aged 44 years, previously diagnosed in the preclinical state. *Eur Neurol* 15:301, 1977

125. MURPHY JW, WOLFE HJ, BALASZ EA, MOSER HW: A patient with deficiency of arylsulfatase A, B, C and steroid sulfatase, associated with storage of sulfatide, cholesterol sulfate and glycosaminoglycans, in Bernsohn J, Grossman HJ (eds): *Lipid Storage Diseases: Enzymatic Defects and Clinical Implications*. New York, Academic, 1971, p 67

126. RAMPINI S, ISLER W, BAERLOCHER K, BISCHOFF A, ULRICH J, PLUSS H: Die Kombination von metachromatischer Leukodystrophie und Mucopolysaccharidose als selbstandiges Krankheitsbild (Mukosulfatidose). *Helv Paediatr Acta* 25:436, 1970

127. AUSTIN J: Studies in metachromatic leukodystrophy. XII. Multiple sulfatase deficiency. *Arch Neurol* 28:258, 1973

128. COUCHOT J, PLUOT M, SCHMAUCH M-A, PENNAFORTE F, FANDRE M: La mucosulfatidose: Étude de trois cas familiaux. *Arch Fr Pediatr* 31:775, 1974

129. STEINMANN B, MIETH D, GITZELMANN R: A newly recognized cause of low urinary estriol in pregnancy: Multiple sulfatase deficiency of the fetus. *Gynecol Obstet Invest* 12:107, 1981

130. SHAPIRO LJ, ALECK KA, KABACK MM, ITABASHI H, DESNICK RJ, BRAND N, STEVENS RL, FLUHARTY AL, KIHARA H: Metachromatic leukodystrophy without arylsulfatase A deficiency. *Ped Res* 13:1179, 1979

131. HAHN AF, GORDON BA, FELEKI V, HINTON GG, GILBERT JJ: A variant form of metachromatic leukodystrophy without arylsulfatase deficiency. *Ann Neurol*, in press

132. DUBOIS G, TURPIN JC, BAUMANN N: Absence of ASA activity in healthy father of a patient with metachromatic leukodystrophy. *N Engl J Med* 293:302, 1975

133. LOTT IT, DULANEY JT, MILUNSKY A, HOEFNAGEL D, MOSER HW: Apparent biochemical homozygosity in two obligatory heterozygotes for metachromatic leukodystrophy. *J Pediatr* 89:438, 1976

134. DUBOIS G, HARZER K, BAUMANN N: Very low arylsulfatase A and cerebroside sulfatase activities in leukocytes of healthy members of metachromatic leukodystrophy family. *Am J Hum Genet* 29:191, 1977

135. FLUHARTY AL, STEVENS RL, KIHARA H: Cerebroside sulfate hydolysis by fibroblasts from a metachromatic leukodystrophy parent with deficient arylsulfatase. *J Pediatr* 92:782, 1978

136. KIHARA H, HO C-K, FLUHARTY AL, TSAY KK, HARTLAGE PL: Prenatal diagnosis of metachromatic leukodystrophy in a family with pseudo arylsulfatase A deficiency by the cerebroside sulfate loading test. *Pediat Res* 14:224, 1980

137. LOTT IT, DULANEY JT: Sulfatide excretion in metachromatic leukodystrophy. *Am J Hum Genet* 29:228, 1977

138. KOLODNY EH, RAGHAVAN SS, LOTT IT, SERGAY SM: Low sulfatidase activity and demyelinating disease. *Neurology* 31(2):86, 1981

139. BUTTERWORTH J, BROADHEAD DM, KEAY AJ: Low arylsulfatase A activity in a family without metachromatic leukodystrophy. *Clin Genet* 14:213, 1978

140. RAGHAVAN SS, GAJEWSKI A, KOLODNY EH: Leukocyte sulfatidase for the reliable diagnosis of metachromatic leukodystrophy. *J Neurochem* 36:724, 1981

141. WEITER JJ, FEINGOLD M, KOLODNY EH, RAGHAVAN SS: Retinal pigment epithelial degeneration associated with leukocyte arylsulfatase A deficiency. *Am J Ophth* 90:768, 1980

142. NYBERG-HANSEN R: Metachromatic leukodystrophy: Two unusual cases of the late infantile form. *Z Neurol* 203:145, 1972

143. LANGENBECK U, DUNKER P, HEIPERTZ R, PILZ H: Inheritance of metachromatic leukodystrophy. *Am J Hum Genet* 29:639, 1977

144. ZLOTOGORA J, COHEN T, ELAIN E, BACH G: About the inheritance of the arylsulfatase A. *Pediatr Res* 14:963, 1980

145. BLOM S, HAGBERG B: EEG findings in late infantile metachromatic and globoid cell leucodystrophy. *Electroencephalogr Clin Neurophysiol* 22:253, 1967

146. PILZ H, HOPF HC: A preclinical case of late adult metachromatic leukodystrophy? *J Neurol Neurosurg Psych* 35:360, 1972

147. OCHS R, MARKAND ON, DEMYER WE: Brainstem auditory evoked responses in leukodystrophies. *Neurology* 29:1089, 1979

148. PROCOPIS PG: Computerised tomography in the leukodystrophies. *Clin Exp Neurol* 16:309, 1979

149. DUBAL L, WIGGLI U: Tomochemistry of the brain. *J Computer Assisted Tomography* 1:300, 1977

150. HAGBERG B, SOURANDER P, SVENNERHOLM L: Sulfatide lipidosis in childhood: Report of a case investigated during life and at autopsy. *Am J Dis Child* 104:644, 1962

151. KLEINMAN P, WINCHESTER P, VOLBERT F: Sulfatide cholecystosis. *Gastrointestinal Radiology* 1:99, 1976

152. JOOSTEN E, HOES M, GABREËLS-FESTEN A, HOMMES O, SCHUURMANS STEKHOVEN H, SLOOF JL: Electron microscopic investigation of inclusion material in a case of adult metachromatic leukodystrophy: Observations on kidney biopsy, peripheral nerve and cerebral white matter. *Acta Neuropath (Berl)* 33:165, 1975

153. DAYAN AD: Dichromism of cresyl violet-stained cerebroside sulfate ("sulfatide"). *J Histochem Cytochem* 15:421, 1967

154. BENZ HU, HARZER K: Metachromatic reaction of pseudoisocyanine with sulfatides in metachromatic leukodystrophy (MLD). I. Technique of histochemical staining. *Acta Neuropathol* 27:177, 1974

155. HOLLÄNDER H: A staining method for cerebroside-sulfuric esters in brain tissue. *J Histochem Cytochem* 11:118, 1963

156. LAMPERT IA, LEWIS PD: Staining of sulfatides in metachromatic leukodystrophy with Alcian blue at high salt concentrations. *Histochemistry* 43:269, 1975

157. SUZUKI K, SUZUKI K, CHEN GC: Isolation and chemical characterization of metachromatic granules from a brain with metachromatic leukodystrophy. *J Neuropathol Exp Neurol* 26:537, 1967

158. RUTSAERT J, MENU R, RESIBOIS A: Ultrastructure of sulfatide storage in normal and sulfatase-deficient fibroblasts in vitro. *Lab Invest* 29:527, 1973

159. GREGOIRE A, PERIER O, DUSTIN P: Metachromatic leukodystrophy, an electron microscopic study. *J Neuropathol Exp Neurol* 25:617, 1966

160. BISCHOFF A, ULRICH J: Amaurotische Idiotie in Verbindung mit Metachromatischer Leukodystrophie. *Acta Neuropath (Berl)* 8:292, 1967

161. MULLER D, PILZ H, MUELEN VT: Studies on adult metachromatic leukodystrophy. Part 1. Clinical, morphological and histochemical observations in two cases. *J Neurol Sci* 9:567, 1969

162. ITOYAMA Y, STERNBERGER N, QUARLES R, WEBSTER HDeF, RICHARDSON EP JR, COHEN S, MOSER HW: Successful immunocytochemical localization of myelin components in paraffin sections of human nervous tissue with preliminary observations on multiple sclerosis and metachromatic leukodystrophy lesions. *Trans Am Neurol Assoc* 103:216, 1978

163. GOEBEL HH, ARGYRAKIS A: Adult metachromatic leukodystrophy. *Am J Ophthal* 88:270, 1979

164. WEBSTER HDeF: Schwann cell alterations in metachromatic leukodystrophy: Preliminary phase and electron microscope observations. *J Neuropathol Expo Neurol* 21:534, 1962

165. WOLFE HJ, PIETRA GG: The visceral lesions of metachromatic leukodystrophy. *Am J Pathol* 44:921, 1964

166. RÉSIBOIS A: Electron microscopic studies of metachromatic leukodystrophy. IV. Liver and kidney alterations. *Path Europ* 6:278, 1971

167. TOGA M, BERARD-BADIER M, PINSARD N, GAMBARELLI D, HASSOUN J, TRIPIER MF: Etude clinique, histologique et ultrastructurale de quarte cas de leucodystrophie métachromatique infantile et juvénile. *Acta Neuropath (Berl)* 21:23, 1972

168. BARGETON E: The metachromatic form of leucodystrophy and its relationship to lipidosis and demyelination in other metabolic disorders, in Folch-Pi J, Bauer HJ (eds): *Brain Lipids and Lipoproteins, and the Leucodystrophies.* Amsterdam, Elsevier, 1963, p 90

169. DENNY-BROWN DE, RICHARDSON EP Jr, COHEN RB: Difficulty in walking and petit mal attacks in a child. *N Engl J Med* 267:1198, 1962

170. PODUSLO SE, TENNEKOON G, PRICE D, MILLER K, MCKHANN GM: Fetal metachromatic leukodystrophy: Pathology, biochemistry and a study of in vitro enzyme replacement in CNS tissue. *J Neuropathol Exp Neurol* 35:622, 1976

171. PILZ H, HEIPERTZ R: The fatty acid composition of cerebrosides and sulfatides in a case of adult metachromatic leukodystrophy. *Z Neurol* 206:203, 1974

172. MALONE MJ, STOFFYN P: Peripheral nerve glycolipids in metachromatic leukodystrophy. *Neurology* 17:1033, 1967

173. MOSER HW, SUGITA M, HARBISON MD, WILLIAMS M: Liver glycolipids, steroid sulfates and steroid sulfatases in a form of metachromatic leukodystrophy associated with multiple sulfatase deficiencies, in Volk BW, Aronson SM (eds): *Sphingolipids, Sphingolipidoses and Allied Disorders* (Adv Exp Med Biol, vol 19). New York, Plenum, 1972, p 429

174. MARTENSSON E, PERCY A, SVENNERHOLM L: Kidney glycolipids in late infantile metachromatic leukodystrophy. *Acta Paediatr Scand* 55:1, 1966

175. PHILIPPART M, SARLIEVE L, MEURANT C, MECHLER L: Human urinary sulfatides in patients with sulfatidosis (metachromatic leukodystrophy). *J Lipid Res* 12:434, 1971

176. PILZ H, MÜLLER D, LINKE I: Histochemical and biochemical studies of urinary lipids in metachromatic leukodystrophy and Fabry's disease. *J Lab Clin Med* 81:7, 1973

177. ABE T, ISHIBA S, FUKUYAMA Y: The lipid analysis and some characterization of sulfate-containing glycolipids of the mucous layer of the gall bladder from a patient with metachromatic leukodystrophy. *Japan J Exp Med* 47:129, 1977

178. ETO Y, WEISMANN UN, CARSON JH, HERSCHKOWITZ NN: Multiple sulfatase deficiencies in cultured skin fibroblasts: Occurrence in patients with a variant form of metachromatic leukodystrophy. *Arch Neurol* 30:153, 1974

179. AUSTIN J, MCAFEE D, SHEARER L: Metachromatic form of diffuse cerebral sclerosis. IV. Low sulfatase activity in the urine of nine living patients with metachromatic leukodystrophy (MLD). *Arch Neurol* 12:447, 1965

180. THOMAS GH, HOWELL RR: Arylsulfatase A activity in human urine: Quantitative studies on patients with lysosomal disorders including metachromatic leukodystrophy. *Clin Chim Acta* 36:99, 1972

181. HULTBERG B: Fluorometric assay of the arylsulphatases in human urine. *J Clin Chem Clin Biochem* 17:795, 1979

182. PERCY AK, BRADY RO: Metachromatic leukodystrophy: Diagnosis with samples of venous blood. *Science,* 161:594, 1968

183. KIHARA H, PORTER MT, FLUHARTY AL, SCOTT ML, DE LA FLOR SD, TRAMMELL JL, NAKAMURA RN: Metachromatic leukodystrophy: ambiguity of heterozygote identification. *Am J Mental Deficiency* 77:389, 1973

184. DUBOIS G, TURPIN JC, GEORGES MC, BAUMANN N: Arylsulfatases A and B in leukocytes: A comparative statistical study of late infantile and juvenile forms of metachromatic leukodystrophy and controls. *Biomedicine* 33:2, 1980

185. PORTER MT, FLUHARTY AL, KIHARA H: Metachromatic leukodystrophy: arylsulfatase-A deficiency in skin fibroblast cultures. *Proc Natl Acad Sci USA* 62:887, 1969

186. RATTAZZI MC, CARMODY PJ, DAVIDSON RG: Studies on human lysosomal β-D-N-acetyl hexosaminidase and arylsulfatase isoenzymes, in Markert CL (ed): *Isozymes. II. Physiological Function.* New York, Academic, 1974, p 439

187. RATTAZZI MC, MARKS JS, DAVIDSON RG: Electrophoresis of arylsulfatase from normal individuals and patients with metachromatic leukodystrophy. *Am J Hum Genet* 25:310, 1973

188. BERATIS NG, ARON AM, HIRSCHHORN K: Metachromatic leukodystrophy: Detection in serum. *J Peds* 83:824, 1973

189. JORDAN TW, CASEY B, WESTON HJ: Enzymic detection of metachromatic leukodystrophy patients and heterozygotes. *NZ Med J* 85:369, 1977

190. DENTANDT WR, JAEKEN J: Determination of lysosomal enzymes in saliva: Confirmation of the diagnosis of metachromatic leukodystrophy and fucosidosis by enzyme analysis. *Clin Chim Acta* 97:19, 1979

191. BERATIS NG, DANESINO C, HIRSCHHORN K: Detection of homozygotes and heterozygotes for metachromatic leukodystrophy in lymphoid cell lines and peripheral leukocytes. *Ann Hum Genet Lond* 38:485, 1975

192. BERATIS NG, FLEISHER LD, DANESINO C, HIRSCHHORN K: Arylsulfatase A deficiency in bone marrow fibroblasts of two different forms of metachromatic leukodystrophy. *J Lab Clin Med* 84:49, 1974

193. PERCY AK, KABACK MM: Infantile and adult-onset metachromatic leukodystrophy: Biochemical comparisons and predictive diagnosis. *N Engl J Med* 285:785, 1971

194. DUBOIS G, ZALC B, LESAUX F, BAUMANN N: Stearoyl [1-¹⁴C] sulfogalactosylsphingosine ([¹⁴C] sulfatide) as substrate for cerebroside sulfatase assay. *Anal Biochem* 102:313, 1980

195. PORTER MT, FLUHARTY AL, KIHARA H: Correction of abnormal cerebroside sulfate metabolism in cultured metachromatic leukodystrophy fibroblasts. *Science* 172:1263, 1971

196. YAMAGUCHI S, AOKI K, HANDA S, YAMAKAWA T: Deficiency of seminolipid sulphatase activity in brain tissue of metachromatic leucodystrophy. *J Neurochem* 24:1087, 1975

197. HARZER K, STINSHOFF K, MRAZ W, JATZKEWITZ H: The patterns of arylsulfatases A and B in human normal and metachromatic leucodystrophy tissues and their relationship to the cerebroside sulphatase activity. *J Neurochem* 20:279, 1973

198. HALTIA T, ICÉN A, PALO J: Arylsulphatase A and B in juvenile metachromatic leukodystrophy. *Clin Chim Acta* 95:255, 1979

199. HULTBERG B, ISAKSSON A, SJÖBLADS S, ÖCKERMAN PA: Acid hydrolases in serum from patients with lysosomal disorders. *Clin Chim Acta* 100:33, 1980

200. JATZKEWITZ H, STINSHOFF K: An activator of cerebroside sulphatase in human normal liver and in cases of congenital metachromatic leukodystrophy. *FEBS Lett* 32:129, 1973

201. BAUM H, DODGSON KS, SPENCER B: The assay of arylsulphatases A and B in human urine. *Clin Chim Acta* 4:453, 1950

202. STUMPF D, NEUWELT E, AUSTIN J, KOHLER P: Metachromatic leukodystrophy (MLD). X. Immunological studies of the abnormal sulfatase A. *Arch Neurol* 25:427, 1971

203. SHAPIRA E, NADLER HL: The nature of the residual arylsulfatase activity in metachromatic leukodystrophy. *J Pediatr* 86:881, 1975

204. LUIJTEN JAFM, VAN DER HEIJDEN, RIJKSEN G, WILLEMSE J, STAAL GEJ: Characterization of arylsulfatase A of three cases of metachromatic leukodystrophy: One of the late infantile, one of the juvenile and one of the adult variant. *J Mol Med* 3:227, 1978

205. STUMPF D, AUSTIN J: Metachromatic leukodystrophy (MLD). IX. Qualitative and quantitative differences in urinary arylsulfatase A in different forms of MLD. *Arch Neurol* 24:117, 1971

206. SUZUKI Y, MIZUNO Y: Juvenile metachromatic leukodystrophy: Deficiency of an arylsulfatase A component. *J Pediatr* 85:823, 1974

207. NEUWELT E, KOHLER PF, AUSTIN J: Methodology. Primary enzyme immunoassay (PEIA): Studies of the mutant enzyme in metachromatic leukodystrophy (primary enzyme immunoassay of arylsulfatase-A). *Immunochemistry* 10:767, 1973

208. SHAPIRA E, DEGREGORIO RR, NADLER HL: Immunologic studies of arylsulfatase A in normal and metachromatic leukodystrophy liver. *Pediat Res* 12:199, 1978

209. PORTER MT, FLUHARTY A, TRAMMELL J, KIHARA H: A correlation of intracellular cerebroside sulfatase activity in fibroblasts with latency in metachromatic leukodystrophy. *Biochem Biophys Res Commun* 44:660, 1971

210. PERCY AK, FARRELL DF, KABACK MM: Cerebroside sulphate (sulphatide) sulphohydrolase: An improved assay method. *J Neurochem* 19:233, 1972

211. PORTER MT, FLUHARTY AL, HARRIS SE, KIHARA H: The accumulation of cerebroside sulfates by fibroblasts in culture from patients with late infantile metachromatic leukodystrophy. *Arch Biochem Biophys* 138:646, 1970

212. KIHARA H, PORTER MT, FLUHARTY A: Enzyme replacement in cultured fibroblasts from metachromatic leukodystrophy, in Bergsma D, Desnick RJ, Bernlohr RW, Krivit W (eds): *Enzyme Therapy in Genetic Diseases* (Birth Defects: Original Article Series, vol IX, no 2). Baltimore, Williams & Wilkins, for the National Foundation—March of Dimes, 1973

213. ETO Y, RAMPINI A, WIESMANN U, HERSCHKOWITZ NN: Enzymic studies of sulphatases in tissues of the normal human and in metachromatic leukodystrophy with multiple sulphatase deficiencies: Arylsulfatases A, B, and C. Cerebroside sulphatase, psychosine sulphatase and steroid sulphatases. *J Neurochem* 23:1161, 1974

214. FLUHARTY AL, STEVENS RL, DE LA FLOR SD, SHAPIRO LJ, KIHARA H: Arylsulfatase A modulation with pH in multiple sulfatase deficiency disorder fibroblasts. *Am J Hum Genet* 31:574, 1979

215. KRESSE H, HOLTFRERICH D: Thiosulfate-mediated increase of arylsulfa-

tase activities in multiple sulfatase deficiency disorder fibroblasts. *Biochem Biophys Res Commun* 97:41, 1980

216. FLUHARTY AL, STEVENS RL, DAVIS LL, SHAPIRO LJ, KIHARA H: Presence of arylsulfatase A (ARS A) in multiple sulfatase deficiency disorder fibroblasts. *Am J Hum Genet* 30:249, 1978

217. FIDDLER MB, VINE D, SHAPRIA E, NADLER HL: Is multiple sulphatase deficiency due to defective regulation or sulphohydrolase expression? *Nature* 282:98, 1979

218. SVENNERHOLM E, SVENNERHOLM L: Isolation of blood serum glycolipids. *Acta Chem Scand* 16:1282, 1962

219. AUSTIN J: Recent studies in metachromatic and globoid forms of diffuse sclerosis, in Folch-Pi J, Bauer H (eds): *Brain Lipids and Lipoproteins and the Leukodystrophies.* Amsterdam, Elsevier, 1963, p 120

220. MEIER C, BISCHOFF A: Sequence of morphological alterations in the nervous system of metachromatic leukodystrophy: Light-and electronmicroscopic observations in the central and peripheral nervous system in a prenatally diagnosed foetus of 22-weeks. *Acta Neuropath (Berl)* 36:369, 1976

221. LEROY JG, VAN ELSEN A, MARTIN JJ, DUMON JE, HULET AE, OKADA S, NAVARRO C: Infantile metachromatic leukodystrophy: Confirmation of a prenatal diagnosis. *N Engl J Med* 288:1365, 1973

222. ARGYRAKIS A, PILZ H, GOEBEL HH, MULLER D: Ultrastructural findings of peripheral nerve in a preclinical case of adult metachromatic leukodystrophy. *J Neuropathol Exp Neurol* 36:693, 1977

223. AUREBECK G, OSTERBERG K, BLAW M, CHOU S, NELSON E: Electron microscopic observations on metachromatic leukodystrophy. *Arch Neurol* 11:273, 1964

224. GREGOIRE A, PERIER O, DUSTIN P: Metachromatic leukodystrophy, an electron microscopic study. *J Neuropathol Exp Neurol* 25:617, 1966

225. AUSTIN J: Metachromatic leukodystrophy (sulfatide lipidosis), in Hers HG, Van Hoof F, (eds): *Lysosomes and Lysosomal Storage Diseases.* edited by New York, Academic, 1973, p 411

226. DAVISON AN, GREGSON NA: Metabolism of cellular membrane sulpholipids in the rat brain. *Biochem J* 98:915, 1966

227. O'BRIEN JS, SAMPSON EL: Myelin membrane: A molecular abnormality. *Science* 150:1613, 1965

228. LEES MB, SAPIRSTEIN VS, REISS DS, KOLODNY EH: Carbonic anhydrase and 2'3' cyclic nucleotide 3'-phosphohydrolase activity in normal human brain and in demyelinating diseases. *Neurology* 30:719, 1980

229. HOROWITZ AL: Genetic complementation studies of multiple sulfatase deficiency. *Proc Natl Acad Sci USA*, 76:6496, 1979

230. KABACK MM, PERCY AK, KASSELBERG AG: *In vitro* studies in sulfatide lipidosis, in Volk BW, Aronson SM (eds): *Sphingolipids, Sphingolipidoses and Allied Disorders* (Adv Exp Med Biol, vol 19). New York, Plenum, 1972, p 451

231. ZLOTOGORA J, BACH G, BARAK V, ELIAN E: Metachromatic leukodystrophy in the Habbanite Jews: High frequency in a genetic isolate and screening for heterozygotes. *Am J Hum Genet* 32:663, 1980

232. BRUNS GAP, MINTZ BJ, LEARY AC, REGINZ VM, GERALD PS: Expression of human arylsulfatase-A in man-hamster somatic cell hybrids. *Cytogenet Cell Genet* 22:182, 1978

233. DELUCA C, BROWN JA, SHOWS TB: Lysosomal arylsulfatase deficiencies in humans: Chromosome assignments for arylsulfatase A and B. *Proc Natl Acad Sci USA*, 76:1957, 1979

234. HORS-CAYLA MC, HEUERTZ S, VAN CONG N, WEIL D, FRÉZAL J: Confirmation of the assignment of the gene for arylsulfatase A to chromosome 22 using somatic cell hybrids. *Hum Genet* 49:33, 1979

235. READ CR: Screening for metachromatic leukodystrophy. *J Clin Pathol* 20:301, 1967

236. CHRISTOMANOU H, SANDHOFF K: A sensitive fluorescence assay for the simultaneous and separate determination of arylsulphatases A and B. *Clin Chim Acta* 79:527, 1977

237. KOLODNY EH, MUMFORD RA: Arylsulfatases A and B in metachromatic leukodystrophy and Maroteaux-Lamy syndrome: Studies with 4-methylumbelliferyl sulfate, in Volk BW, Schneck L (eds): *Current Trends in Sphingolipidosis and Allied Disorders* (Adv Exp Med Biol, vol 68). New York, Plenum, 1976, p 239

238. HUMBEL R: Rapid method for measuring arylsulfatase A and B in leucocytes as a diagnosis for sulfatidosis, mucosulfatidosis and mucopolysaccharidosis VI. *Clin Chim Acta* 68:339, 1976

239. DUBOIS G, BAUMANN N: Arylsulfatase A and B of human leukocytes: Specific inhibitors and electrophoretic characterization. *Biochem Biophys Res Commun* 50:1129, 1973

240. FLUHARTY AL, DAVIS ML, KIHARA H: Simplified procedure for preparation of ^{35}S-labeled brain sulfatide. *Lipids* 9:865, 1974

241. AUSTIN JH: Metachromatic form of diffuse cerebral sclerosis. 2. Diagnosis during life by isolation of metachromatic lipids from urine. *Neurology* 7: 716, 1957

242. BØRRENSEN A-L, VAN DER HAGEN CB: Metachromatic leukodystrophy. II. Direct determination of arylsulphatase A activity in amniotic fluid. *Clin Genet* 4:442, 1973

243. MELCHIOR JC, CLAUSEN J: Metachromatic leukodystrophy in early childhood: Treatment with a diet deficient in vitamin A. *Acta Pediatr Scand* 57: 2, 1968

244. MOOSA A, DUBOWITZ V: Late infantile metachromatic leukodystrophy: Effect of low vitamin A diet. *Arch Dis Child* 46:381, 1971

245. WARNER JO: Juvenile onset metachromatic leucodystrophy: Failure of response on a low vitamin A diet. *Arch Dis Child* 50:735, 1975

246. MOSER HW, MOSER AB, MCKHANN GM: The dynamics of a lipidosis: Turnover of sulfatide, steroid sulfate, and polysaccharide sulfate in metachromatic leukodystrophy. *Arch Neurol* 17:494, 1967

247. WIESMANN UN, ROSSI EE, HERSCHKOWITZ NN: Treatment of metachromatic leukodystrophy in fibroblasts by enzyme replacement. *N Engl J Med* 284:672, 1971

248. AUSTIN JH: Studies in metachromatic leukodystrophy. XI. Therapeutic considerations, in Bergsma D, Desnick RJ, Bernlohr PW, Krivit W (eds): *Enzyme Therapy in Genetic Diseases* (Birth Defects: Original Article Series, vol IX, no 2). Baltimore, Williams & Wilkins, for the National Foundation—March of Dimes, 1973

249. GREENE HL, HUG G, SCHUBERT WK: Metachromatic leukodystrophy: Treatment with arylsulfatase A. *Arch Neurol* 20:147, 1969

45

FABRY'S DISEASE:
α-Galactosidase A Deficiency

ROBERT J. DESNICK

CHARLES C. SWEELEY

1. Fabry's disease *is an inborn error of glycosphingolipid catabolism resulting from the defective activity of the lysosomal hydrolase α-galactosidase A in tissues and fluids of affected hemizygous males. Most heterozygous female carriers of the gene have an intermediate level of enzymatic activity.*

2. *The enzymatic defect leads to the systemic deposition of glycosphingolipids with terminal α-galactosyl moieties, predominantly globotriaosylceramide (Gal-Gal-Glc-Cer) and, to a lesser extent, galabiosylceramide (Gal-Gal-Cer) and blood group B substances. These glycosphingolipid substrates are accumulated in body fluids and in the lysosomes of most visceral tissues, particularly of the vascular endothelium.*

3. *Hemizygous males have extensive deposition of glycosphingolipid in the endothelium, perithelium, and smooth muscle of blood vessels; in ganglion cells; in the heart, kidneys, and eyes; and in most other tissues. The clinical sequelae include onset of pain and paresthesias in the extremities and vessel ectasia (angiokeratoma) in skin and mucous membranes during childhood or adolescence. Corneal and lenticular opacities as well as hypohidrosis may be earlier findings. With increasing age, albuminuria, hyposthenuria, and lymphedema appear; severe renal impairment leads to hypertension and uremia. Death usually occurs from renal failure or from cardiac or cerebrovascular disease.*

4. *Heterozygous females may have an attenuated form of the disease; they can be asymptomatic, or rarely, as severely affected as hemizygous males. The most frequent clinical finding in females is the characteristic whorllike corneal epithelial dystrophy observed by slit-lamp examination.*

5. *The disorder is transmitted by an X-linked gene. Somatic cell hybridization studies have localized the structural gene locus for α-galactosidase A activity to a small region on the long arm of the X-chromosome, Xq22 → q24.*

6. *Confirmation of the clinical diagnosis in hemizygotes and heterozygotes requires the demonstration of deficient α-galactosidase A activity in plasma, leukocytes, or tears or increased levels of Gal-Gal-Glc-Cer in plasma or urinary sediment. Heterozygous females have intermediate levels of enzymatic activity and accumulated substrate.*

7. *Prenatal diagnosis can be accomplished by demonstration of deficient α-galactosidase A activity and an XY karyotype in cultured amniotic cells.*

8. *Low maintenance dosages of diphenylhydantoin or carbamazepine may provide relief of the excruciating pain and constant discomfort. Exploratory trials of direct enzyme replacement indicate the potential value of this therapeutic approach.*

Fabry's disease is an inborn error of glycosphingolipid metabolism resulting from deficient activity of the lysosomal enzyme α-galactosidase A. The enzymatic defect, transmitted by an X-linked gene, leads to the progressive deposition of neutral glycosphingolipids with terminal α-galactosyl moieties in most visceral tissues and fluids of the body. A trihexosylceramide, called globotriaosylceramide, or galactosyl-(α1 → 4)-galactosyl-(β1 → 4)-glucosyl-(β1 → 1')-ceramide (Gal-Gal-Glc-Cer), is the predominant glycosphingolipid accumulated in this disorder (Fig. 45-1). The birefringent deposits are primarily found in the lysosomes of endothelial, perithelial, and smooth-muscle cells of the cardiovascular-renal system. They accumulate to a lesser extent in reticuloendothelial, myocardial, and connective tissue cells of the cornea, kidney, and other tissues, and in ganglion and perineural cells of the autonomic nervous system.

Clinically, hemizygous males have a characteristic skin lesion which led to the descriptive name of *angiokeratoma corporis diffusum universale*. They also have acroparesthesias, episodic crises of excruciating pain, corneal and lenticular opacities, hypohidrosis, and cardiac and renal dysfunction. Death usually occurs in adult life from renal, cardiac, or cerebral complications of their vascular disease. Heterozygous females, who may exhibit the disease in an attenuated form, are most likely to show the corneal opacities. Over 350 affected males have been reported, most of them since 1960.

HISTORY

In 1898, two dermatologists, Anderson [1] in England and Fabry [2] in Germany, independently described the first patients with angiokeratoma corporis diffusum. Anderson designated his case as one of angiokeratoma. His original patient was a 39-year-old male who had proteinuria, finger deformities, varicose veins, and lymphedema. Because of the proteinuria, Anderson suspected that the disease was a generalized disorder and astutely suggested that abnormal vessels might be present in kidneys as well as in skin. Fabry originally made the diagnosis of purpura nodularis in a 13-year-old male whom he followed over the next 30 years [2–4]. He documented the presence of albuminuria [3], further described the cutaneous lesions, noting the presence of small vessel aneurysms [5], and subsequently classified his case to be one of angiokeratoma corporis diffusum, a designation that has persisted.

Several others made early contributions to the clinical description of the disease. Steiner and Voerner [6] and Gunther [7] described a male with anhidrosis and intermittent acroparesthesias that were aggravated by hot or cold weather. Examination of a skin biopsy showed atrophy of the sweat glands and aneurysmal dilatation of the capillaries. Weicksel [8] first described the characteristic corneal opacities and the vascular abnormalities in the retina and conjunctiva. In 1947, Pompen and coworkers [9, 10] reported the postmortem findings in two brothers who had the disease and died from renal failure. The most significant observation was the presence of abnormal vacuoles in blood vessels throughout their bodies.

Similar vacuoles were found about the nuclei of hypertrophied myocardial fibers. Although special stains were negative for fat and glycogen in their paraffin-embedded material, they suggested that the disease was a generalized storage disorder. Subsequently, Scriba [11] definitely established the lipid nature of the storage material. He observed birefringent lipid crystals in frozen sections of blood vessels, glomerular and tubular epithelium, spleen, adrenal glands, lymph nodes, and ganglion cells of the brain and peripheral nervous system. On the basis of these morphological findings, he concluded that the pattern of lipid storage was unlike that of glucosylceramide in Gaucher disease. Hornbostel and Scriba were the first to confirm the diagnosis histologically in a living patient by demonstrating a refractile lipid in vessels of a skin biopsy specimen [12]. Fessas et al. [13] demonstrated birefringent globules in the urinary sediment and found vacuolated macrophages in the bone marrow of an affected male.

The first description of pathologic involvement in heterozygous females was reported in 1958 by Wallace [14] and Colley et al. [15], who demonstrated vacuolated glomerular epithelial cells in autopsy material from a woman whose son died from this disorder. Subsequently, Burda and Winder [16] documented the occurrence and clinical features of the more limited manifestations in heterozygous females. Wise et al. [17] described the characteristic corneal opacities in females who were otherwise asymptomatic. Stiles and Opitz [18] and Opitz et al. [19] studied a large kindred and documented the X-linked inheritance of the disorder by pedigree analysis.

Chemical analyses have confirmed the lipid nature of the storage material. Early and incomplete studies indicated that a phospholipid might be involved [11, 20, 21], but in 1963, Sweeley and Klionsky [22] isolated and characterized two neutral glycosphingolipids—globotriaosylceramide (Gal-Gal-Glc-Cer) and galabiosylceramide (Gal-Gal-Cer)—from the kidney of a Fabry hemizygote obtained at autopsy [23, 24]. On the basis of these findings, they classified Fabry's disease as a sphingolipidosis. Subsequent chemical analyses of various Fabry tissues, including brain [25], plasma [26], urinary sediment [27–31], cultured skin fibroblasts [32], and most internal tissues [22, 25, 33–36] have demonstrated increased levels of Gal-Gal-Glc-Cer. Gal-Gal-Cer has been found increased in the kidney [22, 25, 34, 36], urinary sediment [27–31], pancreas [34], right heart structures, and lung [37]. In addition, the pancreatic accumulation of blood group B substances, glycosphingolipids with terminal α-galactosyl moieties, has been reported [38].

In 1967 Brady et al. [39] demonstrated that the enzymatic defect in this inborn error was the defective activity of ceramide trihexosidase, a lysosomal galactosylhydrolase required for the catabolism of Gal-Gal-Glc-Cer. Kint [40], using synthetic substrates, characterized the defective enzymatic activity as an α-galactosylhydrolase. Shortly thereafter, several laboratories independently demonstrated that the accumulated glycosphingolipid substrates, including blood group B substances, all had α-linked terminal galactosyl residues [41–46].

The elucidation of the specific enzymatic defect provided the ability to diagnose affected hemizygous males enzymatically, identify heterozygous carrier females [47–49], and diagnose hemizygous fetuses [50, 51]. In addition, pilot trials of α-galactosidase A replacement for the experimental treatment of patients with this lysosomal storage disease have been reported [52–54].

Various designations have been used to identify the disorder,

Figure 45-1 Globotriaosylceramide (galactosylgalactosylglucosylceramide).

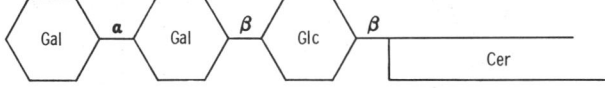

including Fabry's disease, Fabry-Anderson syndrome, angiokeratoma corporis diffusum universale, cardiovasorenal syndrome of Reuter-Pompen, hereditary dystopic lipidosis, glycosphingolipidosis, and tri- and dihexosylceramide lipidosis. In keeping with the terminology applied to other lipidoses and for the benefit of information retrieval, it would seem advisable to retain the commonly used eponym and to append the specific enzymatic defect. Thus, an appropriate designation is Fabry's disease: α-galactosidase A deficiency. Comprehensive reviews of the clinical, pathologic, chemical, and therapeutic studies are available [55–61].

CLINICAL FEATURES

The Hemizygote

Clinical manifestations of Fabry's disease are the sequelae of the anatomic and physiologic alterations produced by the progressive deposition of specific neutral glycosphingolipids in the tissues. Onset of the disease usually occurs during childhood or adolescence. Early manifestations include periodic crises of severe pain in the extremities (acroparesthesias), the appearance of vascular cutaneous lesions (angiokeratoma) as well as hypohidrosis and the characteristic corneal and lenticular opacities.

Pain The single most debilitating symptom of Fabry's disease is the pain. Two types of pain have been described: episodic crises and constant discomfort [17, 62]. The painful crises most often begin in childhood or in early adolescence and signal clinical onset of the disease [18]. Lasting from minutes to several days, these "Fabry crises" consist of agonizing, burning pain initially in the palms and soles. Often the pain will radiate to the proximal extremities and other parts of the body. The painful crises may be triggered by exercise, fatigue, emotional stress, or rapid climatic changes in temperature and humidity. With increasing age, the periodic crises usually decrease in frequency and severity. In some patients, they may occur more frequently and the pain can be so severe that the patient may contemplate suicide [16, 33]. Because the pain usually is associated with a low-grade fever and an elevated erythrocyte sedimentation rate, these symptoms frequently have led to the misdiagnosis of rheumatic fever, neurosis, or erythromelalgia [33, 62–64]. Attacks of abdominal or flank pain may simulate appendicitis or renal colic [65]. In addition

to these intermittent crises, most patients complain of nagging, constant discomfort in their hands and feet characterized by burning or tingling paresthesias [62]. The acroparesthesias may occur daily, usually during late afternoon, and may represent an attenuated form of the episodic excruciating crises. Although pain is a hallmark of the disease, it should be noted that about 10 to 20 percent of older patients deny a history of Fabry crises or acroparesthesias.

Skin Lesion Angiectases may be one of the earliest manifestations and may lead to diagnosis in childhood [18, 63]. There is a progressive increase in the number and size of these cutaneous vascular lesions with age. Classically, the angiokeratomas develop slowly as clusters of individual punctate, dark-red to blue-black angiectases in the superficial layers of the skin (Fig. 45-2). The lesions may be flat or slightly raised and do not blanch with pressure; there is a slight hyperkeratosis in larger lesions. The clusters of lesions are densest between the umbilicus and the knees and have a tendency toward bilateral symmetry. The hips, back, thighs, buttocks, penis, and scrotum are most commonly involved, but there is a wide variation both in the pattern of distribution and in the density of the lesions. Involvement of the oral mucosa and conjunctiva is common, and other mucosal areas may also be involved. Variants without the characteristic skin lesions have been reported [36, 66–78]. Although the angiectases may not be detected readily in some patients, careful examination of the skin, especially the scrotum and umbilicus, may reveal the presence of isolated lesions. In addition to these vascular lesions, anhidrosis, or more commonly, hypohidrosis is an almost constant finding.

Cardiac-Cerebral-Renal Manifestations With increasing age, the major morbid symptoms of the disease result from progressive infiltration of glycosphingolipid into the cardiovascular-renal system. Cardiac disease occurs in most hemizygous males; common clinical manifestations include anginal chest pain, myocardial ischemia and infarction, congestive heart failure, and cardiac enlargement [79–82]. These findings may be accentuated by systemic hypertension related to vascular involvement of renal parenchymal vessels. Mitral insufficiency and aortic stenosis are the most frequent valvular lesions [37, 83]. Involvement of the myocardium and possibly the conduction system results in electrocardiographic abnormalities which may show left ventricular hypertrophy, ST segment changes, and T wave inversion. Other abnormalities including arrhythmias and an abbreviated PR interval have

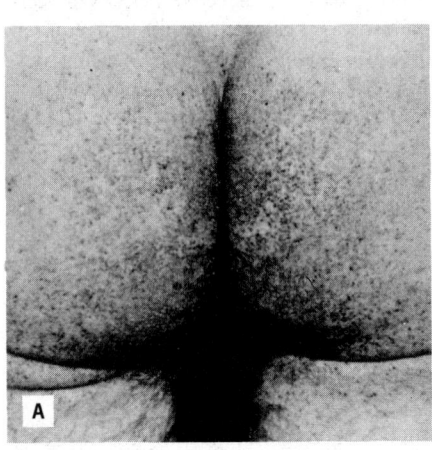

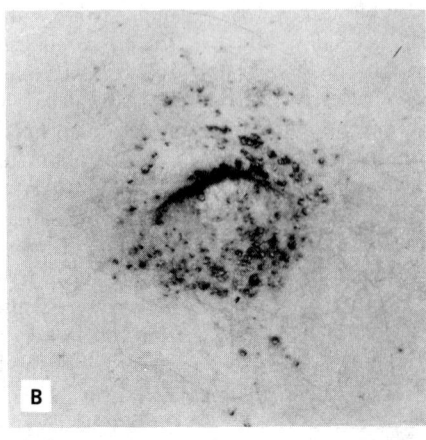

Figure 45-2 Clusters of dark-red to blue angiokeratomas (telangiectases) on the buttocks (A) and in the umbilical area (B) of a hemizygote with Fabry's disease.

been reported [84–88]. In two patients followed over 10 years, the PR interval decreased, indicating an accelerated atrioventricular conduction with progressive lipid deposition in the bundle of His [87]. Electrocardiographic patterns consistent with myocardial infarction have been seen rarely. One reported case with electrocardiographic changes indicating infarction had no evidence of myocardial necrosis at postmortem examination [81]. Echocardiographic studies reveal increased thickness of the interventricular septum and left ventricular posterior wall, particularly in adult males [89].

Cerebrovascular manifestations result primarily from multifocal small vessel involvement and may include thromboses [90], basilar artery ischemia [91] and aneurysm [92], seizures [93], hemiplegia [74, 91, 94], hemianesthesia [95], aphasia [14, 17], labyrinthine disorders [96], or frank cerebral hemorrhage [17]. Personality changes and psychotic behavior may appear with increasing age [97–99]. A transient state of disorientation and confusion may occur in association with electrolyte imbalance secondary to renal disease. Severe neurologic signs may be present without evidence of major thrombosis or hypertension [100–102] and are due presumably to multifocal small vessel occlusive disease. Death may result from vascular disease of the heart or brain.

Progressive glycosphingolipid deposition in the kidney results in proteinuria and other signs of renal impairment, with gradual deterioration of renal function and development of azotemia in middle age. During childhood and adolescence, protein, casts, red cells, and desquamated kidney and urinary tract cells may appear in the urine. Birefringent lipid globules with characteristic "Maltese crosses" can be observed free in the urine and within desquamated urinary sediment cells by polarization microscopy. With age, progressive renal impairment is evidenced by significant proteinuria, isosthenuria (specific gravities of 1.008 to 1.012), and alterations of other renal tubular functions including tubular reabsorption, secretion, and excretion [103]. Polyuria and a syndrome similar to vasopressin-resistant diabetes insipidus occasionally develop [104]. Gradual deterioration of renal function and azotemia usually occur in the third to fourth decades of life, although renal failure has been reported in the second decade [105]. Death most often results from uremia, unless chronic hemodialysis or renal transplantation is undertaken. The mean age at death of 94 males who were not treated for uremia was 41 years [106], but occasionally an affected individual has survived into his sixties [63, 107].

Ocular Features Although ocular lesions in Fabry's disease are present in all elements of the eye, involvement is most prominent in the cornea, lens, conjunctiva, and retina [108–121]. A characteristic corneal opacity, observed only by slit-lamp microscopic examination, is found in males with the disease and in most heterozygous females (Fig. 45-3). The opacities have been observed in a 6-month-old hemizygote [115]. The earliest lesion is a diffuse haziness in the subepithelial layer. Typically, the whorllike opacities are inferior and cream-colored, but they range from white to golden brown and may be very faint. In more advanced cases the opacities appear as whorled streaks extending from a central vortex to the periphery of the cornea [17, 80, 108]. An identical familial corneal dystrophy, termed cornea verticillata, was described by Gruber in 1946 [116]. Subsequent investigation of these patients revealed that they were hemizygotes and heterozygotes for Fabry's disease [67, 68, 117, 118]. An indistinguishable, drug-

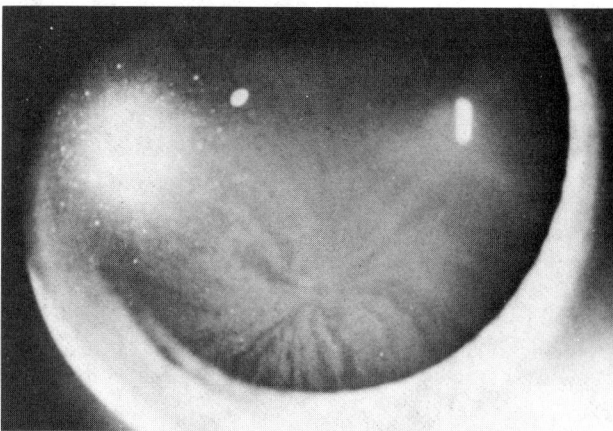

Figure 45-3 Corneal opacity in a heterozygote observed by slit-lamp microscopy. The corneal involvement results from subepithelial glycosphingolipid deposition. (*From Sher et al. [108]. Used by permission.*)

induced phenocopy of the Fabry corneal dystrophy occurs in patients on long-term chloroquine or amiodarone therapy [121, 122] (see "Genetics" section).

Two specific types of lenticular changes have been described (Fig. 45-4). A granular anterior capsular or subcapsular deposit has been observed in about one-third of a large series of hemizygous males, but not in heterozygous females. Typically, these lenticular opacities are bilateral and are inferior in position. They frequently appear in a "propellerlike" distribution, i.e., wedge-shaped with their bases near the lenticular equator and aligned radially with the apexes toward the center of the anterior capsule. A second, and possibly unique, lenticular opacity has been observed in both hemizygous and heterozygous individuals [108, 115]. It may be the first ocular manifestation to appear. The opacity is posterior, linear, and appears as a whitish, almost translucent, spokelike deposit of fine granular material on or near the posterior lens capsule. These lines usually radiate from the central part of the posterior cortex. This unusual opacity has been termed the *Fabry cataract* [108] and is best seen by retroillumination.

Conjunctival and retinal vascular lesions are common and represent part of the diffuse systemic involvement of vessels. These vascular lesions occur early in life in normotensive individuals and are characterized by mild to marked tortuosity of the conjunctival and retinal vessels (Fig. 45-5). There is an aneurysmal dilatation of thin-walled venules as well as angulation and segmental, sausagelike dilatation of veins typically seen on the inferior bulbar conjunctiva. As the disease progresses, retinal changes associated with the development of hypertension and uremia may be superimposed. Vision is not impaired by the vascular lesions in the conjunctiva and retina or by the dystrophy of the corneal epithelium. However, acute visual loss has occurred in hemizygotes as a result of unilateral total central retinal artery occlusion [108, 109].

Other ocular findings have included lid edema in the absence and presence of renal insufficiency [108, 110, 115], myelinated nerve fibers radiating from optic disc [108], mild optic atrophy [108–110], papilledema [110, 111, 121], peripapillary edema [112], nystagmus [110, 121], and internuclear ophthalmoplegia [113, 114].

Other Clinical Features Because of the widespread distribution of the lipid deposits, signs and symptoms of this disorder arise in many other organs and systems. Several patients

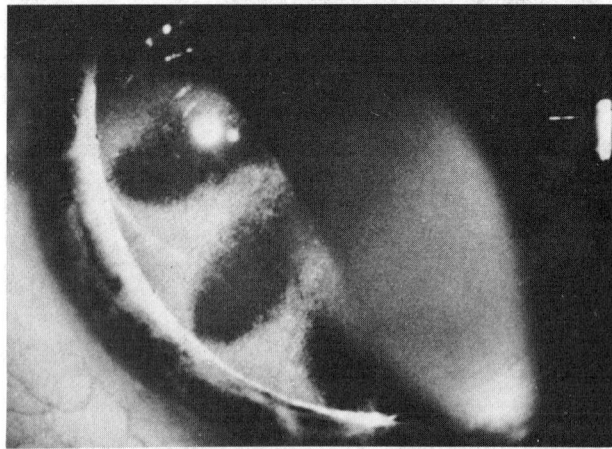

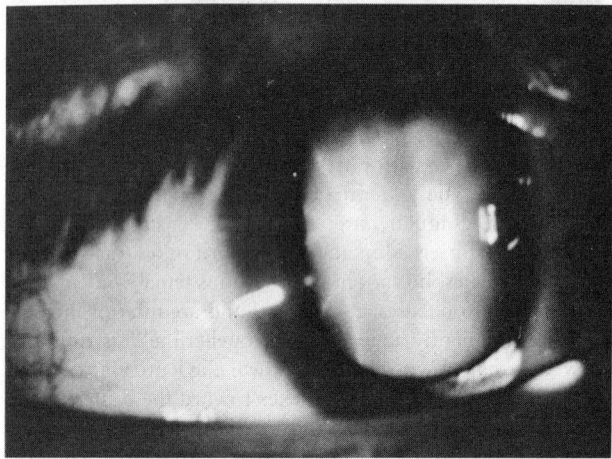

Figure 45-4 Lenticular changes include the anterior capsular opacity shown with a "propellerlike" distribution *(above)* and the posterior opacity or "Fabry cataract" *(below)*, which is best seen by retroillumination and may be unique to Fabry hemizygotes and heterozygotes. *(From Sher et al. [108]. Used by permission.)*

have had chronic bronchitis, wheezing respiration [17, 123], or dyspnea with alveolar capillary block [104]. Pulmonary function studies in older hemizygotes may show significant airflow obstruction, reduced diffusing capacity and a reduction in the $V_{max_{25}}$ values [124]. Roentgenographic studies may reveal hyperinflation or bullous disease. Smokers have greater airflow obstruction than expected from smoking alone [124]. In general, hemizygotes do not manifest significant clinical or functional pulmonary involvement on a primary basis [125]. Presumably the reported findings of pneumothorax, pleural effusions, and pulmonary edema were secondary to primary cardiac, vascular, or renal insufficiency. Primary pulmonary involvement has been reported in the absence of cardiac or renal disease [126]. In contrast to previous statements [24, 55], pulmonary involvement is not a frequent cause of death [125].

Lymphedema of the legs may be present in adulthood without hypoproteinemia, varices, or any clinically evident vascular disease [114]. This symptom presumably reflects the progressive glycosphingolipid deposition in the lymphatic vessels and lymph nodes. Many patients have varicose leg veins and hemorrhoids. Lipid deposits have been observed in the saphenous veins of a patient who underwent vein stripping for varices [127]. Priapism also has been reported [128, 129].

Episodic diarrhea and, to a lesser extent, nausea, vomiting, and flank pain are the most common gastrointestinal com-

plaints [130–132]. These symptoms may be related to deposition of glycosphingolipid in intestinal small vessels and in the autonomic ganglia of the bowel. Perforation of the small bowel has been described [132]. Although intestinal malabsorption has been reported [133], it is not a recognized feature of the disease. Radiologic studies reveal thickened, edematous folds and mild dilation of the small bowel, a granular appearing ileum, and the loss of haustral markings throughout the colon [130–132], particularly in the distal segments.

Anemia is probably due to decreased red blood cell survival [33, 134]. A decreased serum iron concentration [135], normal red blood cell fragility [135], and an elevated reticulocyte count [82] have been reported. Lipid-laden, foamy-appearing macrophages are present in the bone marrow [13]. The spleen is not enlarged.

Many patients have evidence of involvement of the musculoskeletal system. A characteristic permanent deformity arises from changes in the distal interphalangeal joint of the fingers

Figure 45-5 Retinal *(above)* and conjunctival *(below)* vascular lesions. Note the marked tortuosity of the retinal vasculature, especially veins, and the aneurysmal, angular, and segmental sausagelike dilatation of the conjunctival veins. *(From Sher et al. [108]. Used by permission.)*

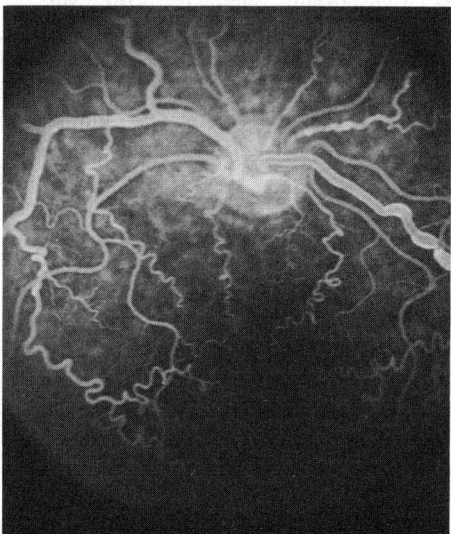

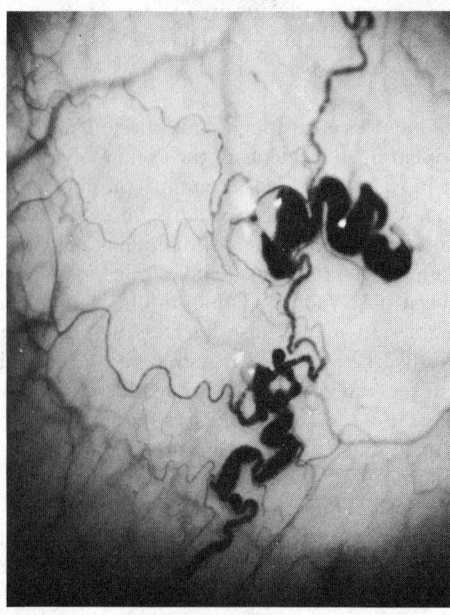

[17, 65, 136, 137], causing limited extension of the terminal joint [17]. Avascular necrosis of the head of the femur [138] or talus [66], multiple small infarctlike opacities in the femoral heads [139], and involvement of the metacarpals, metatarsals, and temporal mandibular joints [115] have been reported. Local severe osteoporosis in a dorsal vertebrae is recorded [90].

Many hemizygous males appear to have retarded growth or delayed puberty [127, 140] and sparse, fine facial [141] and body hair. In some kindreds, an acromegaliclike appearance has been reported [65, 66, 115, 141, 142]. Affected individuals may complain of fatigue and weakness and may be incapacitated for prolonged periods of time [10, 143].

The Heterozygote   Although biochemically documented heterozygotes may be completely asymptomatic throughout a normal life span, most have some symptoms of the disease [14–17, 65, 71, 145–151]. The clinical manifestations are usually limited and variable, but a few heterozygotes have been reported in whom the expression was comparable to that observed in severely affected hemizygous males [18, 79, 144]. In contrast, obligate heterozygotes (daughters of affected hemizygous males) without clinical or biochemical evidence of the disease have also been described [145]. Of more than 150 heterozygotes reported in the literature, corneal involvement is the most frequent and often the singular manifestation [17, 67, 68, 71, 106, 108, 146, 147]. Frequently the corneal dystrophy is more prominent than in affected males in the same family. Corneal lesions have been detected in a heterozygote as early as 3 years of age [106]. Biochemically documented or obligate heterozygous females without corneal opacities have been described [115, 119, 121, 145].

The skin lesions are much less prominent in affected females than in males, and often they are not clinically manifested [15, 67, 69, 71, 106]. The lesions may occur in the characteristic distribution. Isolated lesions may occasionally be seen on the breasts, lips, and trunk. The lesions have been detected in a heterozygote as early as 6 years of age [152].

Other manifestations include intermittent pain in the extremities [16, 71, 106, 141, 147, 153]; sensitivity to changes in environmental temperature [74, 141]; edema, particularly of the ankles [16, 17, 71, 74, 106]; vascular lesions in the conjunctiva and retina [68, 71, 74, 106, 141, 147]; and cardiovascular changes such as hypertension, electrocardiographic abnormalities, and left ventricular hypertrophy [15–17, 74, 106]. Basilar artery aneurysms have been reported [92]. Urologic symptoms in the heterozygotes include hyposthenuria [16, 74, 106, 141]; the occurrence of erythrocytes, leukocytes, and granular and hyaline casts in the urinary sediment [15, 16, 74, 106, 141]; proteinuria; and other signs of renal impairment [15–17, 71, 106, 141]. Mucosal lesions [16, 141], hypohidrosis [65, 106, 141], and diarrhea [99, 153] have been recorded less frequently. Heterozygotes may develop a distal interphalangeal arthritis.

Colley et al. [15] were the first to demonstrate lipid deposition histologically in the kidney of a 47-year-old heterozygote obtained at autopsy. Renal biopsy material from two affected male relatives appeared to be histologically identical to that of the heterozygote. Subsequently, Rahman et al. [65] found a birefringent substance in the cytoplasm of epithelial cells from the glomerular tufts of a 17-year-old heterozygote. Renal biopsy of a 3-year-old heterozygote demonstrated the characteristic glomerular lesion by electron microscopy [154], and skin biopsies from two heterozygotes (8 and 35 years old) contained deposits of lipid in the vascular endothelial and muscularis cells of clinically unaffected skin [141].

The clinical course and prognosis of heterozygotes and hemizygotes differs significantly. Heterozygotes experience little difficulty in adult life, when hemizygous males already have severe renal or cardiac involvement [16]. Although the life expectancy is much longer in heterozygous women, most become more symptomatic as they reach the seventh and eight decades of life. Death usually results from renal or cardiac insufficiency or both [16], although heterozygotes have expired from central nervous system complications [15, 155].

PATHOLOGY

Fabry's disease is characterized by widespread tissue deposits of crystalline glycosphingolipid which shows birefringence with typical Maltese crosses under polarizing miscroscopy. The glycosphingolipid is deposited in all areas of the body, occurring predominantly in the lysosomes of endothelial, perithelial, and smooth-muscle cells of blood vessels (Fig. 45-6), and to a lesser degree, in histiocytic and reticular cells of connective tissue. Lipid deposits are also prominent in epithelial cells of the cornea and glomeruli and tubules of the kidney, in muscle fibers of the heart, and in ganglion cells of the autonomic nervous system. Information is available from more than 30 publications in which the findings of one or more autopsies of hemizygous males were reported [9–11, 24, 34, 35, 63, 75, 79, 82, 156–166]. Autopsy findings of heterozygous females also have been described [14, 16, 153, 154].

Skin

The skin lesions (Fig. 45-7) are telangiectases or small superficial angiomas. After a silent period, cumulative vascular damage leads eventually to clinically apparent and progressive

Figure 45-6   Photomicrograph of a prostatic arteriole showing the hypertrophied, lipid-laden endothelial cells encroaching on the vascular lumen. Hematoxylin and eosin; magnification, ×600.

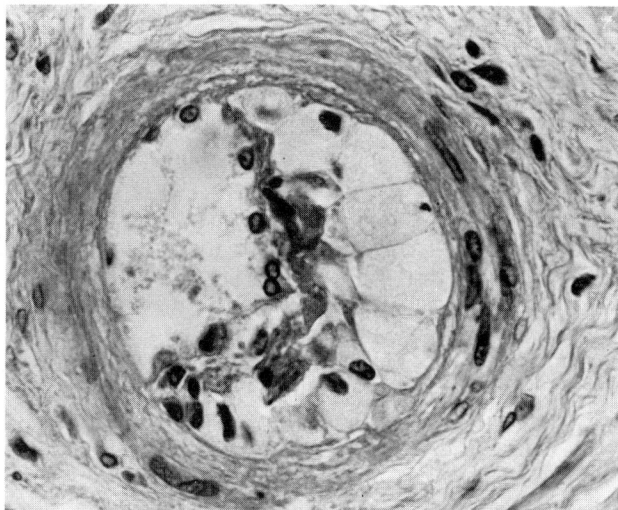

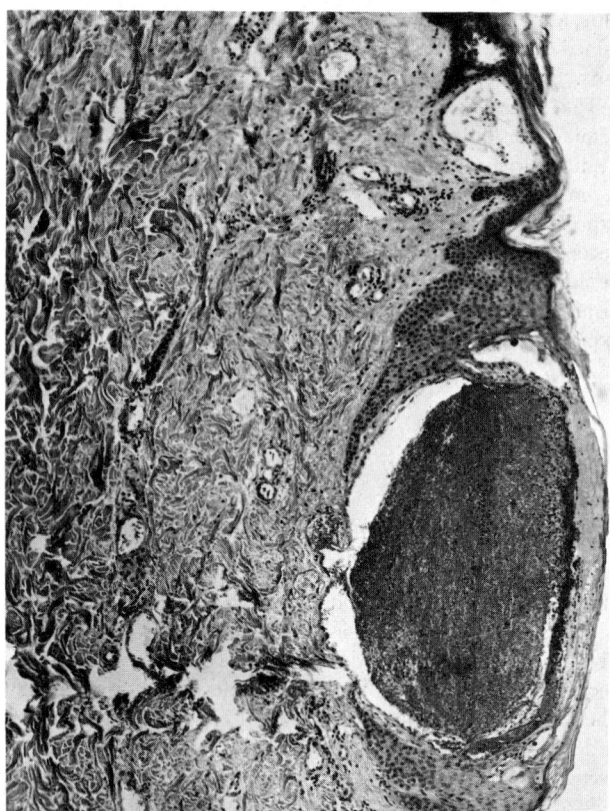

Figure 45-7 Photomicrograph of the skin lesion reveals dilated vascular channels of varying size in the upper dermis. The vessels may contain thrombi, and the overlaying epithelium may be thinned, ulcerated, and/or keratotic. Hematoxylin and eosin; magnification, ×65.

angiectases. This sequence is suggested by the biopsy finding of lipid deposits in areas of clinically normal skin [167, 168] or in patients with no skin lesions [169], and by recognition of patients who have visceral lesions but whose skin lesions either were of minimal consequence [36, 69, 170] or were delayed [171]. The earliest pathologic involvement was observed in the vascular endothelium and perithelium of clinically normal skin from a 1-year-old hemizygote [168].

Capillaries, venules, and arterioles contain pathologic lipid storage in the endothelium, perithelium, and smooth muscle [127, 160, 167, 172]. There is marked dilatation of the capillaries of the dermal papillae just below the dermis. Deeper vessels show less dilatation and aneurysm formation. Lipid stores have been noted in arrectores pilorum muscles [13, 127, 136, 147, 160, 167, 173], sweat gland epithelium [136, 173], and perineural cells [136, 160, 173–176]. Similar findings have been observed in gingival tissues [177, 178]. Atrophic [104] or scarce sweat and sebaceous glands have been reported.

The fully developed classic lesions are usually located in the upper dermis, where they may produce elevation, flattening, or hypertrophy of the epithelium. The larger lesions may have a slight to moderate keratosis, hence the term angiokeratoma. As in all forms of angiokeratomas, the hypertrophy and hyperkeratosis may be secondary to pressure on the epithelium by the underlying dilated vessel.

Angiokeratomas reportedly similar to or indistinguishable from the clinical appearance and distribution of the cutaneous lesions in Fabry's disease have been described in patients with other lysosomal storage diseases, including fucosidosis [179], adult-type neuraminidase deficiency [180, 181], and a recently

reported lysosomal disorder which presents with mental retardation and some features of the mucopolysaccharidoses [182]. Ultrastructural examination of these lesions reveals a distinct difference in the fine structure of the storage material [179, 180]. Clinical and pathologic details of the differential diagnosis of the skin lesions are available in reviews [167, 183–185].

Kidney

Accumulation of glycosphingolipids in the kidney is a progressive process, the earliest documentation of which was found in a 3-year-old heterozygote [154]. The earliest lesions [186, 187] are due to the accumulation of the glycosphingolipid in endothelial and epithelial cells of the glomerulus and of Bowman's space (Fig. 45-8) and in the epithelium of the loops of Henle and of distal tubules (Fig. 45-9). In later stages and, to a lesser degree, proximal tubules [14, 188], interstitial histiocytes, and fibrocytes [189] may show lipid accumulation. Lipid-laden distal tubular epithelial cells desquamate (Fig. 45-9) and may be detected in the urinary sediment [27].

Concurrently, renal blood vessels are also involved progressively and often extensively. An early finding is the presence of arterial fibrinoid deposits which may result from the necrosis of severely involved muscular cells [10, 99, 136, 170, 186]. Other histologic changes in the kidney are the sequelae of nonspecific, end-stage renal disease with evidence of severe arteriolar sclerosis, glomerular atrophy and fibrosis, pseudotubular

Figure 45-8 Photomicrograph of a glomerulus from a 35-year-old hemizygote. The epithelial cells of the parietal and visceral layers of Bowman's capsule show multiple vacuoles from which the stored glycosphingolipids were extracted. Zenker's fixation, paraffin embedding, hematoxylin and eosin; magnification, ×225.

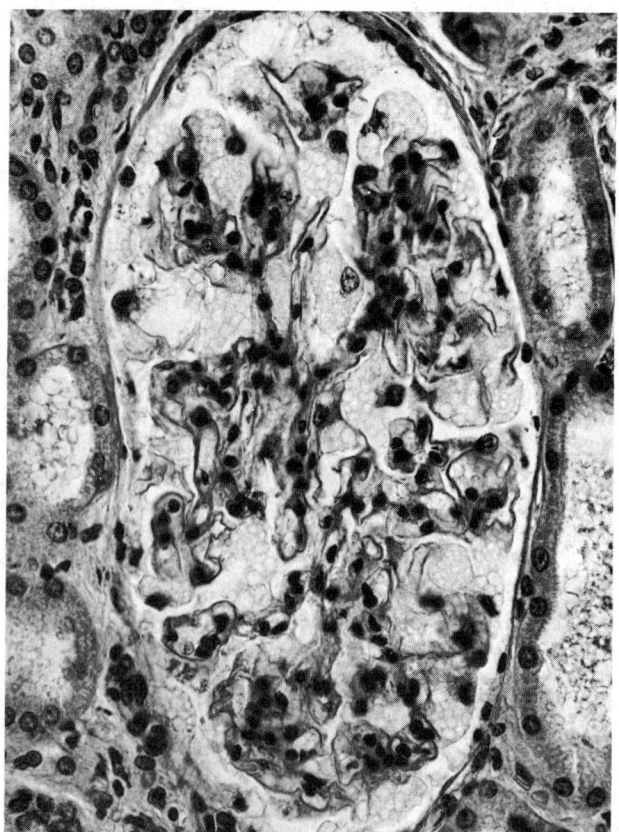

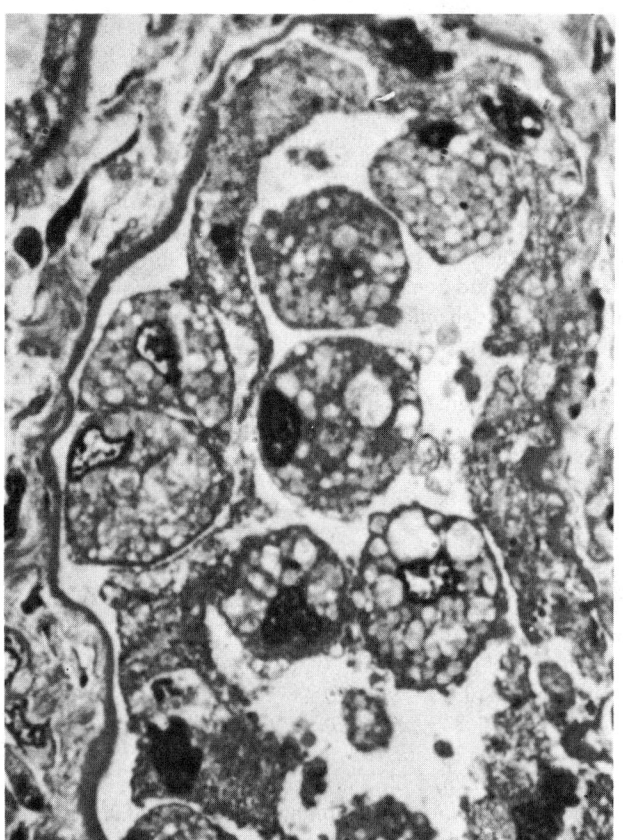

Figure 45-9 Photomicrograph of the lipid-laden cells in the lining and in the lumen of a renal tubule. Formalin fixation, postfixation in osmium tetroxide, and embedding in Vestopal; 1-mm thick section; magnification, ×1000.

proliferation of residual glomerular epithelium, tubular atrophy, and diffuse interstitial fibrosis. Renal size increases during the third decade of life, followed by a decrease in the fourth and fifth decades [190]. The renal involvement has been the subject of comprehensive reviews [103, 170, 188, 191–195].

Nervous System

Vascular involvement is prominent in the nervous system, as it is elsewhere in the body [24, 36, 164, 196–205]. The vascular involvement of the central and peripheral nervous system presumably accounts for the observation of minor EEG and EMG abnormalities in these patients [207]. In addition, vascular ischemia and lipid deposition in the perineurium may cause the peripheral nerve conduction abnormalities of slowed conduction velocities and distal latency, respectively [208]. In both heterozygotes and hemizygotes, glycosphingolipid deposition in nervous tissue appears to be limited to perineural sheath cells of peripheral nerves [24, 136, 164, 167, 173–175, 197–204], neurons of the peripheral and central autonomic nervous system [11, 36, 99, 164, 197–206], and certain primary neurons of somatic afferent pathways [99]. Lipid deposition was observed in Schwann cells by some [24, 206], but not by other investigators [200–203]. Qualitative [197–201] and quantitative [199, 206] studies of peripheral sensory neurons in sural nerves and spinal ganglia have shown preferential loss of small myelinated and unmyelinated fibers as well as small cell bodies of spinal ganglia [199, 200].

Brainstem centers that are involved include the nuclei graci-

lis and cuneatus, the dorsal automatic vagal nuclei, salivary nuclei, nucleus ambiguus, thalamus, reticular substance, mesencephalic nucleus of the fifth nerve, and the substantia nigra [199, 201, 205]. Hemisphere involvement has been noted in the amygdaloid, hypothalamic, and hippocampal nuclei [99, 196]. Recent studies have revealed abnormal lipid deposits in the fifth and sixth cortical layers of the inferior temporal gyrus, the Edinger-Westphal nucleus, the parasympathetic cell column, and the midline nucleus [200, 201]. Lipid storage in neuronal cells of the anterior and posterior lobes of the pituitary has been described [173]. Detailed reviews of the neurologic findings are available [136, 164, 201].

Eye

Histologically, abnormal glycosphingolipid deposits are found in endothelial, perivascular, and smooth-muscle cells of all ocular and orbital vessels [146, 173, 209–216], in smooth muscle of iris and ciliary body [211], in perineural cells, and in connective tissue of the lens and cornea [146, 173, 211, 212]. Inclusions have been localized in the epithelium of the conjunctiva, cornea, and lens [146, 173, 211–215], and by electron microscopy in the basal layer of conjunctival epithelial cells [146, 209] as well as in the surface epithelium. There may be hyperplasia and edema of corneal epithelial cells. Bowman's membrane appears normal, and no deposits have been observed in the stroma or endothelium by light or electron microscopy [146]. It has been suggested that the whorllike corneal dystrophic pattern may result from the formation of a series of subepithelial ridges or from the reduplication of the basement membrane [146, 212–214, 216].

Heart

The progressive deposition of glycosphingolipid in myocardial cells and valvular fibroblasts appears to be a primary cause of cardiac disease in hemizygotes and some heterozygotes [37, 79–81]. Gross cardiomegaly involving all chambers has been observed [37]. Most commonly, the left atrium and ventricle are enlarged and the ventricular walls and septum are markedly thickened. Right atrial and ventricular dilation and enlargement are variable findings. Within the myocardial cells, there is extensive glycosphingolipid deposition around the nucleus and between myofibrils. The vessels show marked hypertrophy of the endothelial cells and smooth-muscle cells secondary to lipid deposition.

Mitral and tricuspid valves have numerous lipid-laden cells embedded in fibrous tissue [37]. The most common valvular defect is thickening and interchordal hooding of the leaflets of the mitral valve, with normal chordae tendineae and either normal or thickened and shortened papillary muscles. The tricuspid valve may be similarly involved, while the aortic and pulmonary valves are usually normal. Clinical and pathologic features of cardiac involvement in both hemizygotes and heterozygotes have been reviewed [37, 79–81].

Other Tissues

Many other organs, including the liver, pancreas, testis, thyroid, prostate, urinary bladder, adrenal glands, and gastrointestinal tract, show involvement of the blood vessels, smooth muscle, ganglia, and nerves. In addition, vacuoles or lipid stores have been demonstrated in epithelial cells [10, 24], mucous glands [173], synovial membrane [64], smooth muscle of the bronchus [79], alveolar ciliated epithelial cells and goblet cells [124], and alveolar epithelial pneumocytes of type II [33]. No inclusions have been found in alveolar macrophages [124]. Involvement of reticuloendothelial cells has been noted in the bone marrow [13, 24, 74, 102, 143, 147, 148, 162, 183] and in the liver, spleen, and lymph nodes [11, 13, 68, 70, 82, 100, 154, 159, 161, 217]. Foam cells containing birefringent lipid droplets are nearly always present in the urinary sediment (Fig. 45-10). Involvement of the interstitial cells of the testis has been noted [173]. Hyalinization and loss of cross striations in skeletal muscle have been observed, as have alterations in the electromyogram [207, 218]. Only by electron microscopy have morphological changes in striated muscle been documented. Lamellar bodies were observed between the myofibrils and underneath the plasma membrane [202].

Histochemistry

Scriba [11] demonstrated that the accumulated lipid is birefringent and shows a Maltese cross configuration in polarized light, that it can be stained in frozen sections with lipid-soluble dyes, and that it may be removed from the tissues by the process of dehydration and embedding in paraffin. In most organs of the body, inclusions containing the lipid-staining material have been found. If lipid-solubilizing procedures are used, empty vacuoles are observed by light microscopy.

Studies with free-floating frozen sections and with blocks of formalin-fixed tissues demonstrate that most of the lipid crystals are retained through alcohol dehydration but are lost on exposure to xylene [24] or pyridine [172]. Exposure of formalin-fixed tissue to 3% potassium chromate for 1 week helps to preserve the lipid [172]. Improved fixation of the lipid deposits can be achieved with 1% calcium formol [127, 209, 219]. Diastase digestion of formalin-fixed frozen sections does not alter the subsequent intense staining of the lipids by the PAS (periodic acid Schiff) procedure. A comparison of various fixation and embedding techniques to preserve the storage material has been reported [220].

The presence of a phosphotungstic acid–positive matrix in electron micrographs [154] raises the question of mucopoly-

saccharide storage in the lesions, but other studies have indicated that the PAS-positive lipid [192] does not contain acid mucopolysaccharide [11, 24, 79, 209, 219], glycogen, phospholipid, sulfatide, or ganglioside [221, 222]. A modified PAS stain, specific for neutral glycosphingolipids [221], and a positive test for sphingosine [222] have served to confirm the chemical identification of the accumulated lipid. In addition, the normal and deficient activities of α-galactosidase A are localized largely in lysosomallike organelles in frozen tissues from normal and hemizygous individuals, respectively, by an enzymatic histochemical assay using 1-naphthyl-α-D-galacto-pyranoside as substrate and hexazonium pararosanilin as the diazo-coupling reagent [223]. Peroxidase-labeled *Bandeiraea simplicifolia* lectin, which is specific for α-D-galactosyl residues, also has been used to stain selectively the glycosphingo-lipid substrates [220].

Ultrastructure

The ultrastructural characteristics of the lesions and of the lipid inclusions in various tissues from hemizygous males have been described in more than 60 published reports. These have dealt with skin [33, 75, 99, 140, 167, 171, 174–176, 183, 185, 186, 189, 209, 222, 224–234], oral mucosa [231], gingiva [178], kidney [69, 136, 142, 143, 148, 154, 188, 189, 192–195, 220, 224, 225, 232–235], bone marrow [209, 237], gastrointestinal tract [33, 209], lymph node [162, 165], liver [154, 224, 235], spleen [154, 220, 235], heart [37, 79–81], skeletal muscle [202, 203, 206, 209, 223], lungs [33], cornea [212, 216], conjunctiva [146, 209, 210], pituitary gland [220], peripheral nerve [174, 197, 201–204, 206], synovial membrane [236], urinary sediment [237], cultured skin fibroblasts [238, 239], and isolated globotriaosylceramide [240]. The ultrastructural findings in the heart, kidney, lymph nodes, arterial blood vessels, and pancreas of a 73-year-old heterozygote have been described [241].

The size and location of the lipid-dense bodies suggest that enzyme-deficient lysosomes fail to hydrolyze Gal-Gal-Glc-Cer, which accumulates progressively and remains enclosed in membrane-lined secondary lysosomes and residual bodies, or following lysosomal rupture, as free intracytoplasmic bodies. Lipid-dense subparticles, ranging from 0.1 to 0.5 μm in diameter [154, 209, 226], aggregate and fuse into larger masses, which may measure up to 10 μm in diameter. These are often

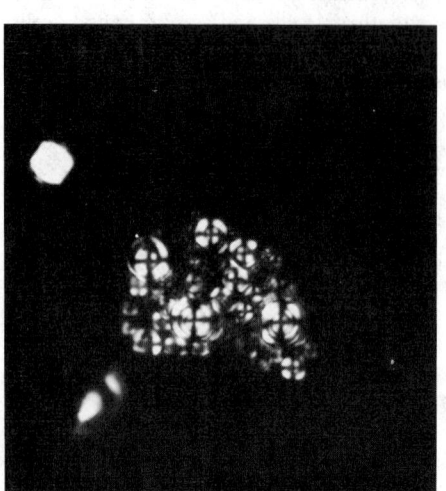
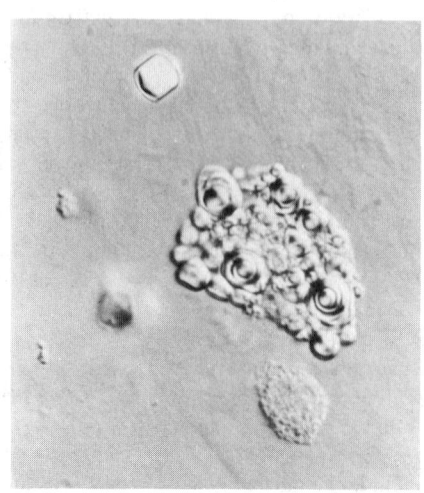

Figure 45-10 Photomicrographs of the urinary sediment from a heterozygote showing lipid accumulation (Maltese crosses) by polarization light microscopy *(left)* and interference contrast microscopy *(right)*. Magnification, ×1000.

limited by a single-unit membrane [*79, 140, 154, 169, 171, 189*], but when present in larger quantities, they may be free in the cytoplasm. Localization to the lysosomal apparatus is suggested by the prominence of pinocytic activity and multivesicular bodies [*171, 175*], by the demonstration of acid phosphatase within the inclusion-bearing bodies [*169–171*], and by analogy with the similar localization of other sphingolipid hydrolases [*242*].

Material examined at high resolution reveals a typical pattern of concentric or lamellar inclusions with alternating light- and dark-staining bands (Fig. 45-11). The periodicity of these bands has been reported variably as 4 to 5 μm [*77, 99, 162, 165, 169, 209, 231, 237*], 5 to 6 μm [*33, 140, 167, 174, 176, 204*], 6 to 6.5 μm [*154, 175, 226*], or as great as 9.8 μm [*189*]. The electron-dense component is 2 to 3 μm in thickness. These inclusions have coarser periods of 15 to 20 μm [*167, 176*]. The periodicity of the crystalline deposits observed in synovial membrane by electron microscopy has been estimated by the Fourier optical transform technique [*243*]. The tubular arrangement, which is observed with purified glucosylceramide and globotriaosylceramide [*240*], and in tissue deposits of lipids in Gaucher disease [*240, 244*], is rarely found in the tissues in Fabry's disease [*174, 209, 237*].

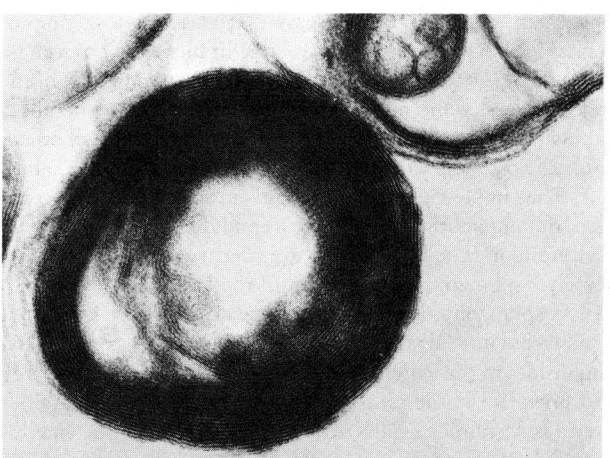

Figure 45-11 Electron photomicrograph of a portion of a cell in the urinary sediment of a hemizygote. The lamellar arrangement has the periodicity of 5 to 6 nm. Magnification, ×100,000.

BIOCHEMISTRY OF NEUTRAL GLYCOSPHINGOLIPIDS

Structure

The deficiency of α-galactosidase A activity in patients with Fabry's disease leads to the progressive accumulation of glycolipids with terminal α-galactosyl residues in most nonneural tissues and fluids of the body. These substances are structurally and metabolically members of a family of glycosphingolipids that is widely distributed in mammalian tissues as normal constituents of plasma membranes and possibly of subcellular membranes as well. The lipoidal moiety of glycosphingolipids is a hydrophobic biantennary structure called *ceramide*, which consists of a mixture of 4-sphingenine (sphingosine) and related long-chain aliphatic amines joined in amide linkages with various fatty acids. Carbohydrate groups are attached by a glycosidic linkage between the reducing end of the carbohydrate and the terminal hydroxyl group of the ceramide.

$$\text{Carbohydrate} \ldots \text{O} \text{---} \underset{\underset{\underset{CO(CH_2)_{22}CH_3}{|}}{\underset{NH}{|}}}{CH_2}\overset{\overset{HO}{|}}{C}H\overset{\overset{H}{|}}{C}HC=\overset{\overset{H}{|}}{C}(CH_2)_{12}CH_3$$

Ceramide

The glycosphingolipids involved in Fabry's disease are of the type called neutral glycosphingolipids, as contrasted with the gangliosides, which contain one or more acidic sialic acid groups, and the sulfo-glycosphingolipids (sulfatides), which contain a sulfate monoester group on the carbohydrate moiety.

In an aqueous environment, "water-soluble" glycosphingolipids such as gangliosides and blood group–active substances are, in reality, large molecular aggregates in which the carbohydrate groups extend out into the aqueous region, while the ceramide groups arrange themselves in a hydrophobic region resembling a bilayer lipid membrane. Less polar glycosphingolipids are insoluble in water but can be dispersed by incorporating them along with phospholipids and cholesterol or with various synthetic detergents into similar structures called mixed micelles or liposomes, which in tissues may have a characteristic multilamellar form. In living organisms, the glycosphingolipids are localized in the membranes of cells and in transport complexes such as lipoproteins. During their synthesis, and when exchanged from one membrane to another, they may be attached to cytosolic exchange proteins [*245*]. Glycosphingolipids of the plasma membrane are believed to be associated primarily with the outer half of the bilayer in such a way that the carbohydrate residues extend from the surface of the cell into the extracellular environment [*246*].

Ceramide Component The most common sphingolipid base in the neutral glycosphingolipids of human origin is 4-sphingenine (sphingosine), the chemistry of which is discussed in detail in several reviews [*247–249*]. It is generally accompanied by small amounts of sphinganine (dihydrosphingosine), chain-length analogues (C_{16} and C_{20}), and 4-hydroxysphinganine (phytosphingosine). In some instances these other forms are predominant, such as in brain gangliosides (rich in eicosasphing-4-enine) and some of the kidney and intestinal glycosphingolipids (rich in 4-hydroxysphinganine) especially those that contain 2-hydroxy fatty acids as well [*248, 250*].

The fatty acids of neutral glycosphingolipids are primarily saturated and monounsaturated compounds with chain lengths from C_{16} to C_{26}. The virtual absence of polyunsaturated fatty acids, such as linoleate and arachidonate, in these lipids distinguish them from phospholipids, triacyl-*sn*-glycerols and cholesteryl esters. Some tissues contain glycosphingolipids with high proportions of 2-hydroxy fatty acids. Examples are brain cerebroside [*251*], kidney cerebroside, and galabiosylceramide [*252*], and some of the neutral glycosphingolipids of erythrocyte membrane [*253*]. Comparisons of the fatty acid composition of various neutral glycosphingolipids are given in the previous edition of this text [*55*] and in several reviews [*254, 255*].

Carbohydrate Component The neutral glycosphingolipids contain a carbohydrate moiety that varies from a simple monosaccharide (cerebrosides) to large-branched oligosaccharides with 20 or more sugar residues. An attempt has been made to classify the neutral glycosphingolipids into families that bear structural or biosynthetic relationships to each other [256, 257]. These classifications are summarized in Table 45-1. The simplest glycosphingolipids in most tissues (except brain) of human origin are glucosylceramide (Glc-Cer) and lactosylceramide (Lac-Cer), which are precursors of more complex glycosphingolipids of several of the families.

Glycosphingolipids of the *globo* type are most predominant in many but not all of the nonneural tissues, in contrast to gangliosides of the *ganglio, lacto,* and *neolacto* type, which are most prevalent in the central nervous system. Globoside (globotetraosylceramide, GalNAc-Gal-Gal-Glc-Cer) is the major neutral glycosphingolipid in normal kidney [258], heart [259], and erythrocytes [260, 261], whereas Lac-Cer is the major component of the glycosphingolipids in leukocytes [262–264], platelets [265–270], liver [267, 268], spleen [269, 270], skeletal muscle [271], and most other nonneural tissues. In plasma, Glc-Cer is the principal component, but lipids of the globo type up to globotetraosylceramide are present [261]. In plasma these glycosphingolipids are distributed in the lipoproteins (Table 45-2), the highest proportion being in the low density

lipoprotein (LDL) fraction [272–278]. Glycosphingolipid antigens of the human erythrocyte P blood group system are also of the globo type. The P^k and P blood group activities were shown by immunochemical techniques to be globotriaosylceramide and globotetraosylceramide, respectively [279–281]. Table 45-3 gives the concentrations of neutral glycosphingolipids of the globo type in various normal human tissues and fluids.

Glycosphingolipids of the *gala* type are derived from galactosylceramide (Gal-Cer) instead of glucosylceramide. In the central nervous system Gal-Cer is the major neutral glycosphingolipid [282, 283]. It is associated primarily with myelin but has also been found in microsomes [284–286], isolated axonal fragments [287], and preparations of neurons [288]. It also occurs along with the sulfate derivative (sulfatide) in kidney [252, 289] and urinary sediment [27, 28] and is a minor constituent of human neutrophils [263]. The cerebroside fraction of human plasma contains a small proportion of Gal-Cer [290]. Galabiosylceramide (Gal-Gal-Cer) is a normal constituent of kidney [252] and is present in other tissues as well but in much lower quantities. More complex glycolipids of the gala type have not been reported.

The structures of glycosphingolipids with ABH and I blood group and Lewis antigen activities are summarized in Table

Table 45-1 Neutral glycosphingolipids of human origin*

Family	Chemical structure	Trivial name	Approved nomenclature	Suggested abbreviation
Globo	Glcβ1→1'Cer	Glucocerebroside	Glucosylceramide	GlcCer
	Galβ1→4Glcβ1→1'Cer	Lactosyl Ceramide	Lactosylceramide	LacCer
	Galα1→4GalB1→ 4Glcβ1→1'Cer	Ceramide trihexoside, trihexosyl ceramide	Globotriaosylceramide	GbOse₃Cer
	GalNAcβ1→3Galα1→ 4GalB1→4GlcB1→1'Cer	Globoside, cytolipin K	Globotetraosylceramide	GbOse₄Cer
Gala	Galβ1→1'Cer	Galactocerebroside	Galactosylceramide	GalCer
	Galα1→4Galβ1→1'Cer	Digalactosylceramide	Galabiosylceramide	GaOse₂Cer
Ganglio	GalNAcβ1→4Galβ1→ 4Glcβ1→1'Cer	Asialo G$_{M2}$	Gangliotriaosylceramide	GgOse₃Cer
	Galβ1→3GalNAcβ1→ 4Galβ1→4Glcβ1→1'Cer	Asialo G$_{M1}$	Gangliotetraosylceramide	GgOse₄Cer
Lacto	Galβ1→3GlcNAc(4←1αFuc)β1→ 3Galβ1→4Glcβ1→1'Cer	Leᵃ glycolipid	III⁴-α-Fucosyl-lactotetraosylceramide	III⁴-α-Fuc-LcOse₄Cer
	Galα1→3Gal(2←1αFuc)β1→ 3GlcNAcβ1→3Galβ1→4Glcβ1→1'Cer	Blood group B glycolipid	IV²-α-Fucosyl-IV³-α-galactosyl-lactotetraosylceramide	IV²-α-Fuc-IV³-α-Gal-LcOse₄Cer
Neolacto	Galβ1→4GlcNAcβ1→3Galβ1→ 4Glcβ1→1'Cer	Paragloboside	Neolactotetraosylceramide	LcnOse₄Cer
	Galβ1→3Galβ1→4GlcNAcβ1→ 3Galβ1→4Glcβ1→1'Cer		IV³-β-Galactosyl-neolactotetraosylceramide	IV³-β-Gal-LcnOse₄Cer
	Galβ1→4GlcNAc(3←1αFuc)β1→ 3Galβ1→4Glcβ1→1'Cer	X Hapten	III³-α-Fucosyl-neolactotetraosylceramide	III³-α-Fuc-LcnOse₄Cer
	Fucα1→2Galβ1→4GlcNAcβ1→ 3Galβ1→4Glcβ1→1'Cer	Blood group H-1 glycolipid	IV²-α-Fucosyl-neolactotetraosylceramide	IV²-α-Fuc-LcnOse₄Cer
	Galα1→3Gal(2←1αFuc)β1→ 4GlcNAβ1→3Galβ1→4Glcβ1→1'Cer	Blood group B-1 glycolipid	IV²-α-Fucosyl-IV³-α-galactosyl-neolactotetraosylceramide	IV²-α-Fuc-IV³-α-Gal-LcnOse₄Cer
	GalNAcα1→3Gal(2←1αFuc)β1→ 4GlcNAcβ1→3Galβ1→4Glcβ1→ 1'Cer	Blood group Aᵃ glycolipid	IV²-α-Fucosyl-IV³-α-N-acetylgalactosaminyl-neolactotetraosylceramide	IV²-α-Fuc-IV³-α-GalNAc-LcnOse₄Cer
	Fucα1→2Galβ1→4GlcNAcβ1→ 3Gal(6←1βGlcNAc4← 1βGal12← 1αFuc)β1→ 4GlcNAcβ1→3Galβ1→ 4Glcβ1→1'Cer	Blood group I glycolipid	IV⁶-β-Fucosyl-α1, 2galactosyl-β1, 4-N-acetylglucosaminyl-neolactohexaosylceramide	IV⁶-β-Fuc-α1, 2Galβ1, 4GlcNAc-LcnOse₆Cer

* For more complete information on glycosphingolipid structures, see Ref. 257.

Table 45-2 Distribution of neutral glycosphingolipids in lipoprotein fractions of normal human serum

| | *Mean percentage of total glycosphingolipid recovered†* | | | | | | | | | | | |
| | VLDL | | | | LDL | | | | HDL | | | |
Glycosphingolipid*	*(1)*	*(2)*	*(3)*	*(4)*	*(1)*	*(2)*	*(3)*	*(4)*	*(1)*	*(2)*	*(3)*	*(4)*
Glucosylceramide (Glc-Cer)	15	6	7	13	61	68	43	59	12	20	31	28
Galactosylceramide (Gal-Cer)	—	6	—	—	82	—	—	—	—	11	—	—
Lactosylceramide (Gal-Glc-Cer)	—	9	6	14	—	68	51	60	—	20	36	26
Globotriaosylceramide (Gal-Gal-Glc-Cer)	15	9	—	12	32	61	61	62	32	23	37	25
Globotetraosylceramide (GalNAc-Gal-Gal-Glc-Cer)	14	7	—	12	32	67	59	64	32	24	39	24

* Complete structural elucidations of these glycosphingolipids were not made; they were assumed to be of the globo type.
† These data were taken from the results of (1) van den Bergh and Tager [275]; (2) Clarke, Stoltz, and Mulcahey [273]; (3) Desnick, Zavoral, and Krivit [274]; and (4) Dawson, Kruski, and Scanu [272]. Data from these sources for percentage of glycosphingolipid recovered in the very high density lipoprotein or residue fraction not shown.

45-1. These substances are fucose-containing neutral glycosphingolipids of the *lacto* or *neolacto* type. Lactotriaosylceramide, GlcNAcβ1 → 3Ga1β1 → 4G1cβ1 → 1′Cer, is a minor component of human erythrocytes [291, 292] and human neutrophils [263]. It is the lowest molecular weight member of the lacto and neolacto families with a structural difference from the globo and ganglio families, and is a metabolic precursor of the A-, B- and H-active glycosphingolipids. The next higher molecular weight member of the neolacto type is paragloboside, neolactotetraosylceramide, which is a trace compound of erythrocyte membrane [292, 293], leukocytes [294], spleen [270, 289], muscle, and peripheral nerve [295]. It is the common structural core of the blood group H-active fucoglycosphingolipids of human erythrocytes [296–298], Le^a antigen of human adenocarcinoma [299], and blood group A- and B-active fuco-glycosphingolipids of human erythrocyte [38, 297] and pancreas [300]. In general, glandular epithelial tissues such as stomach, pancreas, and intestine are a rich source of these fucolipids, whereas parenchymatous organs and erythrocytes contain relatively much lower quantities.

Sulfatide, I³-sulfo-galactosylceramide, was first isolated from brain [301], where it is a major component of the acidic glycosphingolipid fraction [254, 282]. Kidney medulla contains an unusually high concentration of this glycosphingolipid [252, 254], as compared with other visceral organs. A more complex sulfo-glycolipid, II³-sulfo-lactosylceramide, was first isolated from human kidney by Martensson [252]. It accounts for about 30 percent of the total sulfo-glycosphingolipid fraction in the organ and for smaller proportions in small intestine [302] and gastric mucosa [303]. Structural studies of the material from human kidney suggest that it may contain some II³-sulfo-galabiosylceramide as well.

The chemistry and normal occurrence of the neutral glycosphingolipids and sulfo-glycosphingolipids have been reviewed in detail [256, 257].

Isolation and Quantitative Analysis

The neutral and acidic glycosphingolipids can be extracted from homogenates of tissues and from formed elements of blood, blood plasma, or serum; cultured cells; and urine or urinary sediment with a mixture of chloroform and methanol, as originally described by Folch et al. [304]. Although these solvents are generally mixed in a proportion of 2:1, other ratios (1:1 and 1:2) are preferred when good recoveries of highly polar constituents such as the blood group substances are of importance. Differential extraction of the glycosphingolipids after initial acetone or ethanol-ether treatment of tissues is especially useful with large-scale isolations [258, 305–308]. When the total lipids of chloroform-methanol extracts are partitioned into an upper aqueous methanol phase and a lower phase consisting of chloroform and small amounts of water and methanol, the neutral glycosphingolipids of molecular weights up to perhaps 1500 (pentaglycosylceramides) are distributed almost quantitatively into the lower phase with the phosphoglycerolipids, cholesterol, cholesterol esters, and triacyl-*sn*-glycerols, whereas more polar neutral glycosphingolipids and simple gangliosides are distributed between the two phases, and complex gangliosides nearly completely into the upper phase. Polar phosphoglycerolipids are generally removed from the crude neutral glycosphingolipid fraction by alkali-catalyzed methanolysis or chromatography on silicic acid [35, 252, 305, 309–311], Iatrobeads [312], or Florisil [34, 35, 252, 309, 313–315]. Chromatography on DEAE-cellulose can be used to remove acidic glycosphingolipids [252, 270, 305, 310, 311, 316–318]. On a modest scale, thin-layer chromatography is useful as a final purification step before characterization of the glycosphingolipid.

High performance liquid chromatography has been used for the separation and quantitative analysis of glycosphingolipids from a variety of tissues such as erythrocytes [318], myelin [319], brain [320–322], plasma [323], and liver [323]. Excellent separations have been obtained from perbenzoylated [324, 325] and O-acetyl-N-*p*-nitrobenzoyl derivatives [326], taking advantage of the ultraviolet absorption of these compounds for detection. Microparticulate silicas and reversed-phase columns containing covalently bonded hydrophobic alkyl groups have been utilized. Methods of isolation have been described more fully elsewhere [327–329].

Fatty acids and long-chain base constituents of the glycosphingolipids can be analyzed by gas-liquid chromatography

Table 45-3   Concentrations of neutral glycosphingolipids in various normal human tissues, mg/g wet weight

Source	Glucosylceramide (Glc-Cer)	Lactosyl- and Galabiosylceramide (Gal-Glc-Cer), (Gal-Gal-Cer)	Globotriaosylceramide (Gal-Gal-Glc-Cer)	Globotetraosylceramide (GalNAc-Gal-Gal-Glc-Cer)	Total	Reference
Kidney	0.10	0.16	0.37	0.64	1.27	[252]
	0.18	0.14	0.36	0.35	0.93	[270]
	—	—	—	—	1.0	[457]
Spleen	0.098	0.16	0.072	0.107	0.44	[270]
	—	—	—	—	0.8	[457]
Liver	0.041	0.10	0.045	0.035	0.20	[270]
	—	—	—	—	0.4	[457]
Placenta	0.022	0.044	0.056	0.11	0.23	[289]
Erythrocytes	0.004	0.014	0.015	0.09	0.124	[261]
Heart (ventricle)	0.06	0.014	0.018	0.034	0.126	[37]
Lung	0.19	0.15	0.06	0.05	0.45	[37]
Prostate	—	—	—	—	0.6	[457]

of the products after acid-catalyzed methanolysis [330]. The carbohydrate composition can be established by gas-liquid chromatography of trimethylsilylated methyl glycosides [261, 331] or acetylated alditols [331]. The arrangement of the sugars in the carbohydrate portion can be deduced by Smith degradation; methylation analysis, involving permethylation [332] and analysis of partially O-methylated hexitol acetates by gas-liquid chromatography and mass spectrometry [333]; mass spectroscopy of the intact permethylated glycosphingolipids [334]; proton [335, 336] and carbon 13 [337–339] nuclear magnetic resonance spectrometry; and sequential enzymatic degradation with specific exoglycosidases [340], which also establishes the anomeric configuration of each of the glycosidic linkages.

Function

The glycosphingolipids can be classified into three groups according to their role in cell surface phenomena [341]. The annular glycosphingolipids form a complex with a particular membrane protein and are not free to diffuse laterally in the membrane [342]. An example of this type is the proposed association of I^3-sulfo-galactosylceramide (sulfatide) with NA$^+$-K$^+$-ATPase as a K-selective cofactor [343].

The second class involves glycosphingolipids that function as cell surface receptors and antigenic markers. Examples are the cholera toxin [344], Sendai virus [345], and tetanus toxin receptors [346] and glycosphingolipids with blood group activity. The third type of glycosphingolipid is involved as a structural component of the membrane [347]. Examples of this type are the organization of Gal-Cer in myelin and perhaps the relationship of G_{M3} ganglioside (sialyl-lactosylceramide) with process formation in fibroblasts and other cell types.

Biosynthesis

Neutral glycosphingolipids are synthesized by sequential enzymatic reactions, involving the stepwise addition of monosaccharide units to acceptors which are the appropriate precursors for each enzyme. This process, in which sugar nucleotides serve as donors of the carbohydrate residues, requires the con-

certed action of a group of glycosyltransferases that may be closely associated in a subcellular membrane as a multienzyme complex. The synthesis of asparagine-linked glycoproteins involves the assembly of an oligosaccharide on a polyisoprenoid lipid (dolichol phosphate) [348] and transfer *en bloc* of the oligosaccharide to asparagine residues of newly synthesized protein in the lumen of the endoplasmic reticulum [349]. In contrast, the glycosyltransferases of glycosphingolipid synthesis catalyze the direct transfer of a sugar residue from the nucleotide derivative to an acceptor substrate, as illustrated below by a galactosyltransferase for the conversion of glucosylceramide to lactosylceramide.

$$\text{Glc-Cer} + \text{UDP-Gal} \xrightarrow[\text{Galactosyltransferase}]{} \text{Gal-Glc-Cer} + \text{UDP}$$

The further conversion of lactosylceramide to neutral glycosphingolipids of the globo, lacto, and neolacto types and conversion of ceramide to galabiosylceramide and sulfo-glycosphingolipids are summarized in Fig. 45-12.

The concept of membrane-bound multiglycosyltransferase systems for the synthesis of gangliosides was proposed in 1970 by Roseman [350]. Studies have shown that the glycosyltransferase activities are enriched in the synaptosomal fraction of embryonic chicken brain [351, 352], in the plasma membrane of mouse neuroblastoma cells [353], and in the endoplasmic reticulum and Golgi apparatus of rat liver [354–356] and bovine thyroid gland [357]. Similar complexes are assumed to be involved in the synthesis of the neutral glycosphingolipids. Recent results with hamster NIL cells suggest that the β- and α-N-acetylgalactosaminyltransferases required for conversion of globotriaosylceramide (Galα1 → 4Galβ1 → 4GlcCer of Fig. 45-12) to Forssman antigen (globo type pentaglycosylceramide, GalNAcα1 → 3GalNAcβ1 → 3Galα1 → 4Galβ1 → 4GlcCer of Fig. 45-12) exist in a complex [358]. The intermediate formed *in situ* from the β-N-acetylgalactosaminyltransferase, globotetraosylceramide (GalNAcβ1 → 3Galα1 → 4Galβ1 → 4GlcCer), was more readily converted to Forssman antigen than exogenously added globotetraosylceramide, indicating that these two glycosyltransferases may be tightly coupled in the membrane.

The mechanism of metabolic control within such multiglycosyltransferase systems is not well understood. The occurrence of the intermediates as well as end products in the pathway to globotetraosylceramide in kidney and erythrocytes, for example, raises the possibility of incomplete glycosylation under some circumstances or, alternatively, of the existence of separate multiglycosyltransferase systems for each glycosphingolipid found as a component of the cell. Studies of glycosphingolipid composition and pulse labeling of these lipids in normal and tranformed cells indicate that contact inhibition in confluent cultures [359], cell cycle [360], and the transforming genes are involved in the regulation of glycosphingolipid metabolism, but the mechanisms are not clear. It has been postulated that a cyclic AMP–dependent protein kinase may regulate the activity of a plasma membrane N-acetylgalactosaminyltransferase in neuroblastoma cells by covalent phosphorylation of the enzyme [361]. This is potentially of great importance, since some of the transforming genes of viruses, such as the *src* gene of various sarcoma viruses, yield products which are tyrosine phosphokinases [362–364]. The possibility that specific glycosyltransferases may be activated and others inactivated by phosphorylation is an attractive, though presently unsupported, mechanism for the regulation of glycosphingolipid metabolism.

Much of the evidence in support of the pathways shown in Fig. 45-12 has been obtained from in vitro studies with particulate enzyme preparations. The early work in this area was presented in a previous edition of this text [56] and has been summarized in several reviews [344, 350, 365–368]. The conversion of ceramide to Glc-Cer to Lac-Cer has been demonstrated in brain [369], spleen [370], intestine [371], and kidney subcellular particulate fractions [372]. Enzymatic activities for the two galactosyltransferase steps in the conversion of Glc-Cer to Lac-Cer (β-galactosyltransferase) and globotriaosylcer-

amide (α-galactosyltransferase) were shown to be different by heat inactivation and substrate inhibition studies [373]. The further conversion of globotriaosylceramide to globotetraosylceramide [374] and Forssman antigen [375, 376] involves β- and α-N-acetylgalactosaminyltransferase steps which are also assumed to be different enzymes [377]. Human peripheral lymphocytes contain I and i antigens [378], which have neolacto-type structures [379], and neutral glycosphingolipids of the globo type as well [380]. These cells incorporate [U-14C]galactose into Glc-Cer, Lac-Cer, globotriaosylceramide, and globoside, with the greatest amount of label recovered in Lac-Cer [381]. Phytohemagglutinin activation of the lymphocytes led to severalfold elevations of the radiolabel in these globo-type glycosphingolipids. In contrast, human blood neutrophils contain Lac-Cer and neolactotetraosylceramide as the major neutral glycosphingolipids, but no globotriaosylceramide or globoside [263]. This indicates that significant differences will be found in the glycosyltransferase activities of the two leukocyte cell types.

Steps in the pathway leading from lactosylceramide to blood group B–active glycosphingolipids have also been studied with cell-free particulate fractions. The synthesis of the blood group glycolipid precursor, GlcNAcβ1 → 3Galβ1 → 4GlcCer, from lactosylceramide was reported by Kijimoto et al. [375]. The biosynthesis of B–active glycosphingolipids involves two galactosyltransferases and an α-fucosyltransferase, which were shown to be present in rabbit bone marrow [382], bovine spleen [383], and a human neuroblastoma cell line, IMR-32 [384]. It has been shown that neolactotetraosylceramide and neolactopentaosylceramide are both substrates for α-fucosyltransferase, giving H_1 and B_1 blood group glycosphingolipids, respectively, and that these conversions are probably catalyzed by the same enzyme [384].

Figure 45-12 Steps in the biosynthesis of neutral glycosphingolipids from ceramide, involving sugar nucleotides and glycosyltransferases. See text for details.

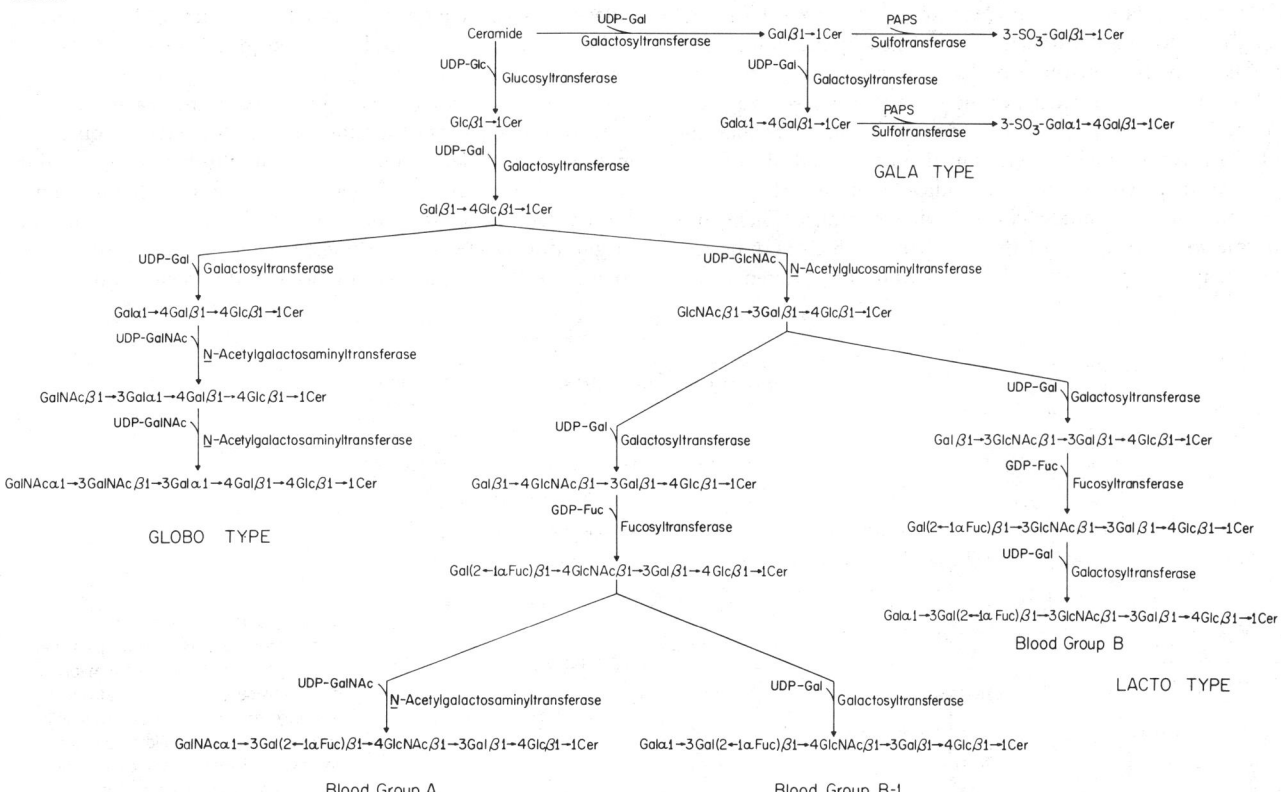

In plasma, the neutral glycosphingolipids are distributed among the lipoproteins, where they occur primarily in the low density (LDL) and high density (HDL) lipoprotein fractions [272–277]. These plasma pools of neutral glycosphingolipids appear to be synthesized in part in the liver, probably during the assembly of the lipoproteins [385], and the kinetics of their turnover in plasma after incorporation in vivo of [^{14}C]glucose [386, 387] or [6,6-^{2}H$_2$]glucose [388] are comparable to those observed with triacyl-sn-glycerols and phospholipids after pulse labeling with fatty acids or inorganic phosphate [389]. It was recently reported that HDL$_3$ stimulates glycosphingolipid synthesis in human leukocytes and fibroblasts [390]. Increased levels of particular glycosphingolipids were observed in the cells as well as the HDL$_3$ fraction—lactosylceramide in the case of leukocytes and globotriaosylceramide in the fibroblasts—requiring a mechanism of exchange of cellular glycosphingolipids with the HDL$_3$ in the medium. This is an interesting and possibly important finding, as it contrasts with previous analytic [261, 272] and metabolic studies [386] showing that the exchange of complex glycosphingolipids between erythrocytes and lipoproteins is minimal. The cholesterol components of LDL are utilized by various cells following uptake by a mechanism involving receptor-mediated endocytosis [391]. The endocytic vesicles fuse with lysosomes, in which the glycosphingolipids are assumed to be completely degraded. Studies with LDL-containing labeled ceramide indicate that this is the case [392].

Metabolism

Glycosphingolipids are degraded in a stepwise fashion by a family of specific exoglycosidases, as illustrated by the pathways shown in Fig. 45-13 for the metabolism of globotetraosylceramide, galabiosylceramide, and a blood group B–active hexaglycosylceramide. Reactions catalyzed by individual glycosidases involved in these pathways have been extensively studied in cell-free extracts. Some of the enzymes have been obtained in relatively pure form and their kinetic properties and substrate specificities determined. Virtually all of the glycosidases are glycoproteins with acidic pH optima. They occur predominantly but not exclusively in lysosomes. There are multiple forms of many of these enzymes, which may be related in part to their subcellular distribution, differences in

their substrate specificities, and chemical heterogeneity due to structurally different carbohydrate moieties or subunit proteins or both. The lysosomal glycosidases involved in glycosphingolipid metabolism have been the subject of several reviews [393–396].

Detergents are required to disperse glycosphingolipid substrates for in vitro assays of glycosidase activity. Catabolism of glycosphingolipids in vivo may involve protein complexes of the substrate glycolipids, since specific proteins have been shown to activate glycosphingolipid hydrolysis in vitro and they substitute for detergents in these assays [397–400]. Synthetic artificial substrates are often hydrolyzed at rates equal to or greater than those measured in vitro with glycosphingolipids. Substances such as the p-nitrophenyl and 4-methylumbelliferyl derivatives of hexoses and N-acetylhexosamines have been exploited in diagnostic assays of some of the glycosphingolipidoses, including Fabry's disease. These substances are generally used in assays to monitor activity during the purification of various lysosomal glycosidases.

Metabolism of the globotriaosylceramide from Fabry kidney in a cell-free system was first described in 1967 by Brady et al. [401]. Using a radiolabeled form of the glycosphingolipid, glycosidase activity was observed in particulate fractions from rat small intestine, spleen, kidney, brain, and liver. Information about the substrate specificity of this lysosomal glycosidase resulted from an observation by Kint in 1970 that leukocytes from hemizygous males with Fabry's disease were deficient in a thermally labile α-galactosidase activity measured with either p-nitrophenyl-α-galactoside or 4-methylumbelliferyl-α-galactoside [40]. It was subsequently shown by spectroscopic and enzymatic studies that the globotriaosylceramide from Fabry kidney has an α1 → 4 linkage in the terminal galactosyl moiety [41–45].

Using the artificial substrate assay, two forms of α-galactosidase activity have been observed in extracts of human liver, kidney, brain, spleen, and leukocytes [47, 402] and in plasma, urine, and tears [47, 48]. The thermally labile form, called α-galactosidase A, is the predominant type in most normal tissues. Multiple forms of α-galactosidase A have been observed in preparations from human liver or fibroblasts by staining starch gels with the fluorogenic substrate 4-methylumbelliferyl-α-galactoside [402–408], by assaying fractions of hepatic origin after isoelectric focusing [402, 409], and by isoelectric focusing of highly purified fractions of the splenic and placen-

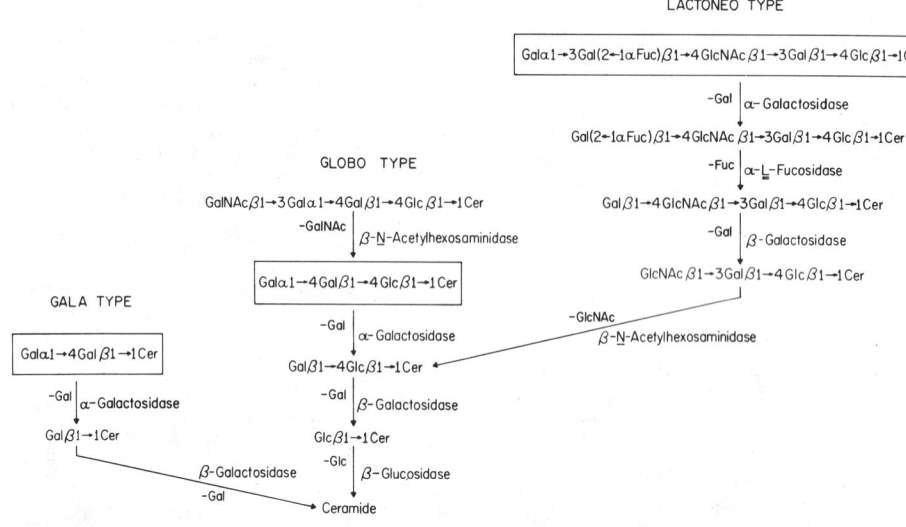

Figure 45-13 Pathway for the catabolism of neutral glycosphingolipids (neolacto, globo, and gala types) involving the stepwise hydrolysis of individual sugar residues by specific glycosyl hydrolases. The accumulated substrates in Fabry's disease—galabiosylceramide, globotriaosylceramide, and the blood group B glycosphingolipids—are indicated.

tal enzyme on slab gels [410]. The more thermally stable α-galactosidase B represents 20 percent or less of the total α-galactosidase activity in most tissues except brain, where it is the major form [411]. Both enzymes have been purified from various human tissues such as spleen, placenta, liver, kidney, plasma, and urine. The most recent procedures for liver [412], spleen [410], placenta [410, 413], and plasma [410, 414] have yielded α-galactosidases A and B of high purity. Other sources of α-galactosidase activity include coffee beans [415, 416], red lentil [417], soybean [418], yeast [419, 420], a protozoan [421], an *Escherichia coli* plasmid [422], and slime mold [423].

α-Galactosidase A

The A form of α-galactosidase is a relatively heat labile glycoprotein that catalyzes the hydrolysis of substrates possessing α-galactosidic residues, including various synthetic water-soluble substrates and naturally occurring glycosphingolipids and glycoproteins. Maximal activity of α-galactosidase A is obtained at about pH 4.5 with 4-methylumbelliferyl-α-galactoside. The Michaelis constant (K_m) of the reaction with this substrate is 2.6 ± 0.7 mM [47, 48, 55, 59, 410, 412, 424–427]. The highest specific activities obtained to date were reported with human liver [412], spleen, and placenta [410]. Variability in the specific activity of apparently homogeneous enzyme may reflect the degree to which the protein is denatured during the rather lengthy isolation procedure used by most investigators. This possibility is strengthened by the observation that the best yields (30 percent) and highest specific activities (45 ± 15 μmol 4-methylumbelliferone formed per milligram protein per minute) were obtained by a rapid isolation procedure employing lectin (Con A) and α-galactosylamine affinity chromatography steps [410]. The half-life of α-galactosidase A activity in vitro at 50 ± 5°C and pH 4.8 is 10 min [427]. Enzyme activity is inhibited by *myo*-inositol [47, 410, 424, 428–430], D-galactose [48], melibiose [410, 431], raffinose [410], and a ligand used in affinity chromatography, N-6-aminohexanoyl-α-D-galactosylamine [410].

The molecular weight of native α-galactosidase A from human tissues is approximately 101,000 [410, 412, 414, 427, 431]. Polyacrylamide gel electrophoresis in the presence of sodium dodecylsulfate (SDS) has consistently shown a diffuse band of subunits with an M_r of about 47,000 to 49,000 and higher molecular weight material with an M_r of about 65,000 [410, 413, 414, 431]. It has been reported that SDS gel electrophoresis of splenic α-galactosidase A of the highest specific activity gave only a single band at 49,800, which indicated that the enzyme probably has a homodimeric structure [410]. Studies of the molecular weight are complicated because the enzyme is a glycoprotein. The carbohydrate chains perturb chromatographic mobility and provide heterogeneity to the structure. It seems certain that α-galactosidase A contains one or more asparagine-linked complex oligosaccharide chains. The plasma form of the enzyme is the most anodic [isoelectric point (pI), 4.2] of the human α-galactosidase isoenzymes [410]. Multiple forms are observed upon horizontal slab isoelectric focusing of placental and splenic α-galactosidase A preparations [410, 427], as illustrated in Fig. 45-14. The pI of the tissue forms of α-galactosidase A range from 4.4 to as high as 5.1 [410].

The plasma and tissue forms of the enzyme are converted by

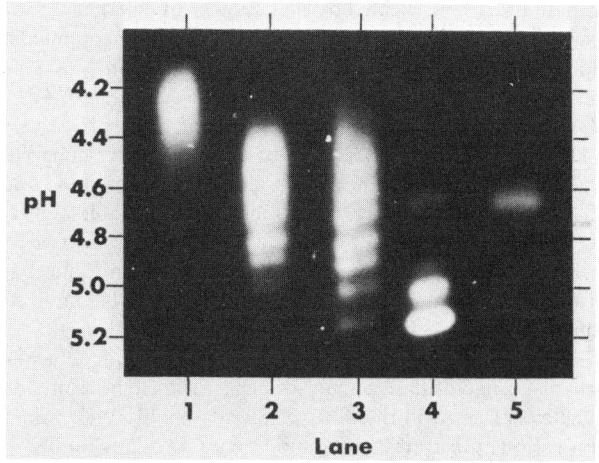

Figure 45-14 Isoelectric focusing of purified α-galactosidase A. *Lane 1*, plasma form; *lanes 2* and *3*, splenic forms (different preparations); *lane 4*, placental form; *lane 5*, placental α-galactosidase B. (*From* [65a]. *Used by permission. For details see* [410].)

neuraminidase to a single form with a sharp isoelectric focusing band of higher pI. Thus the heterogeneity is the result of variations in the amount of sialic acid on the carbohydrate chain. It has been suggested that the plasma form may contain 10 to 12 sialic acid residues, whereas the placental form of α-galactosidase A has only 1 or 2 residues [410]. This property is of considerable importance in connection with the circulatory half-life of enzyme infused into patients with Fabry's disease [54] and may also be a factor determining which organs acquire enzyme activity after infusion.

Lysosomal enzymes are synthesized in the endoplasmic reticulum, where nascent polypeptide chains are glycosylated by a process involving the *en bloc* transfer of a high mannose oligosaccharide to asparagine residues from a lipid-linked (dolichol phosphate) intermediate [349]. Subsequent posttranslational processing reactions in the endoplasmic reticulum and Golgi apparatus are required to remove some of the mannose residues and to introduce other sugars, including sialic acid, by a series of glycosyltransferase steps [432]. During the course of these reactions glycoproteins that are destined to become lysosomal enzymes are converted to a phosphodiester form by an unusual N-acetylglucosamine-1-phosphate transferase [433] and later to a monoester form with exposed mannose phosphate groups [434]. The presence of these mannose phosphate residues may be a signal in the glycoprotein processing pathway [435] and may also provide a ligand that is recognized by receptors on the inner aspect of lysosomal membranes [435, 436].

Assays of globotriaosylceramide hydrolysis by α-galactosidase A in vitro require the presence of detergent for optimal activity [49, 401, 425, 426, 428, 437]. Mixed micelles of the glycosphingolipid with sodium cholate [49, 401, 425], sodium taurocholate [428, 437, 438], and mixtures of sodium taurocholate and Triton X-100 [426] have been used. Alternatively, the hydrolysis of globotriaosylceramide can be stimulated by the addition of a heat-stable activator isolated from liver [439]. The activator is a glycoprotein that can replace the detergent in the determination of activity in vitro. Similar proteins have been isolated that stimulate the hydrolysis of G_{M1} and G_{M2} gangliosides [397–400] and glucosylceramide [440]. Whether these activators have a physiologic role is uncertain.

The kinetics of globotriaosylceramide hydrolysis by α-galactosidase A are complicated by the presence of detergent in the assay mixtures. Using mixed micelles of glycosphingolipid and cholate, taurocholate, or taurocholate plus Triton X-100, apparent K_m values have been reported [410, 412, 414, 425–428, 431, 437]. Assays carried out according to the procedures of Desnick et al. [47] or Dean and Sweeley [61] give apparent K_m values of about 0.2 mM with globotriaosylceramide and 0.3 mM with galabiosylceramide. Lineweaver-Burk plots [441] give nonlinear (sigmoidal) curves, as predicted by Gatt et al. [442] for enzymes with hydrophobic substrates in a micellar form. More accurate values of K_m and V_{max} may be obtained from Hill plots [443] or Eadie-Hofstee plots [444].

Normal leukocytes are reported to contain a unique acidic form of α-galactosidase activity, which appears to be related to α-galactosidase A on the basis of thermal lability, K_m values with various substrates, and inhibition by *myo*-inositol [445]. This activity was shown to have a much lower pI than that of tissue α-galactosidase A. This property permits the two forms to be completely separated from each other and from α-galactosidase B by isoelectric focusing [428, 445]. Whether this form of α-galactosidase A is the same as the most acidic forms in spleen, placenta, and liver is uncertain, though Salvayre et al. [445] were unable to demonstrate it in liver and kidney extracts.

α-Galactosidase B

The more heat stable form of α-galactosidase activity in human tissues, called α-galactosidase B, has been purified to apparent homogeneity from human liver [56, 427, 446] and human placenta [431]. The purified enzyme catalyzes the hydrolysis of several water-soluble synthetic substrates with terminal α-galactose or α-N-acetylgalactosamine residues and glycosphingolipids with these terminal sugars, such as globotriaosylceramide, which represents the type with terminal α-galactosyl residues, and Forssman antigen, which is of the type with terminal α-N-acetylgalactosamine residues. The molecular weight of the native enzyme is about 100,000 [427, 431] and that of apparently identical subunits is about 48,000 [431]. Although its pI (4.4) is similar to that of splenic α-galactosidase A, ion exchange chromatography allows separation of the two forms [410, 424]. The enzyme has a half-life in vitro of 120 min at 50°C and pH 4.8 [427]. It is not inhibited by *myo*-inositol but is strongly inhibited by N-acetylgalactosamine [427, 431].

Kinetic studies of α-galactosidase B indicate that it probably functions in vivo as an α-N-acetylgalactosaminidase rather than as an α-galactosidase. This conclusion was reached in 1977 by Dean et al. [447] and by Schram et al. [448] and confirmed in 1978 by Kusiak et al. [431]. While it was originally believed that α-galactosidase B might be a biosynthetic precursor of the A form [409, 449, 450], this possibility can be excluded on the basis of their different substrate specificities as well as the fact that antibodies raised against each of the purified enzymes do not cross-react with the other form [413, 424, 451, 452]. It has been concluded, therefore, that α-galactosidase B is probably identical to the α-N-acetylgalactosaminidases isolated independently from various sources by monitoring activity with *p*-nitrophenyl-α-N-acetylgalactosaminide [453]. It should be noted that a preparation of α-N-acetylgalactosaminidase from *Clostridium perfringens* does not share this property of hydrolyzing α-galactosides [454].

Conversion of α-galactosidase B to an "α-galactosidase A-like" form during purification and storage has been reported [451, 452]. The α-galactosidase A-like form has a lower K_m than α-galactosidase B, and its chromatographic behavior on DEAE-cellulose is similar to that of α-galactosidase A. It does not cross-react with anti-α-galactosidase A but is precipitated by anti-α-galactosidase B [451, 452].

BIOCHEMICAL ABNORMALITIES IN FABRY'S DISEASE

The Nature of Accumulated Glycosphingolipids

Globotriaosylceramide   The enzymatic defect in Fabry's disease leads to the widespread accumulation of globotriaosylceramide, Gal(α1 → 4)Gal(β1 → 4)Glc(β1 → 1')Cer, in endothelial and epithelial cells of many organs and in the cardiovascular system. Chemical analyses have shown that the accumulated glycosphingolipid isolated from kidney [22, 25, 35], heart [25], and lymph nodes of patients with Fabry's disease is identical with that of normal kidney [252, 258], spleen [308], and serum [311]. The positions of glycosidic linkages were assigned from the results of permethylation analysis, periodate oxidation products, and partial acid hydrolysis to lactosylceramide [22, 24, 455]. The anomeric configurations of these linkages were established by sequential hydrolysis with specific exoglycosidases and by proton nuclear magnetic resonance spectrometry [6, 41–45]. The fatty acid compositions of globotriaosylceramide from normal and Fabry tissue were given in a previous edition of this text [55]. The complete structure of this glycosphingolipid, shown in Fig. 45-15, has been chemically synthesized [456].

Galabiosylceramide   Galabiosylceramide, Gal(α1 → 4) Gal(β1 → 1')Cer, occurs in abnormally high concentrations in the kidneys [22–25], pancreas [34], and urinary sediment [27–31] of patients with Fabry's disease. Some of this glycosphingolipid may also occur abnormally in other tissues as well, such as lung and the right-sided heart structures [37]. The chemical structure of the carbohydrate moiety of the material obtained from Fabry kidney was established by permethylation studies [24, 35], nuclear magnetic resonance spectrometry [44], and sequential enzymatic hydrolysis by fig α-galactosidase and jackbean β-galactosidase [45]. The complete structure is shown in Fig. 45-15.

Blood Group B Glycosphingolipids   Formalin-fixed pancreas from a patient with Fabry's disease who had blood group B activity contained abnormal quantities of IV^2-α-fucosyl-IV^3-α-galactosyl-lactotetraosylceramide and IV^2-α-fucosyl-IV^3-α-galactosyl-neolactotetraosylceramide, two neutral glycosphingolipids that inhibit blood group B–specific hemagglutination [38]. These substances have been shown to occur in human erythrocytes [38, 297]. The structures of the glycosphingolipids from the Fabry pancreas were established by permethylation studies and cleavage of the terminal galactose unit by an α-galactosidase from ficin to yield products with the same chromatographic behavior and immunologic properties as H$_1$ and H$_2$ glycosphingolipids of human erythrocytes [38]. The complete structures of these blood group B–active glycosphingolipids are shown in Fig. 45-15.

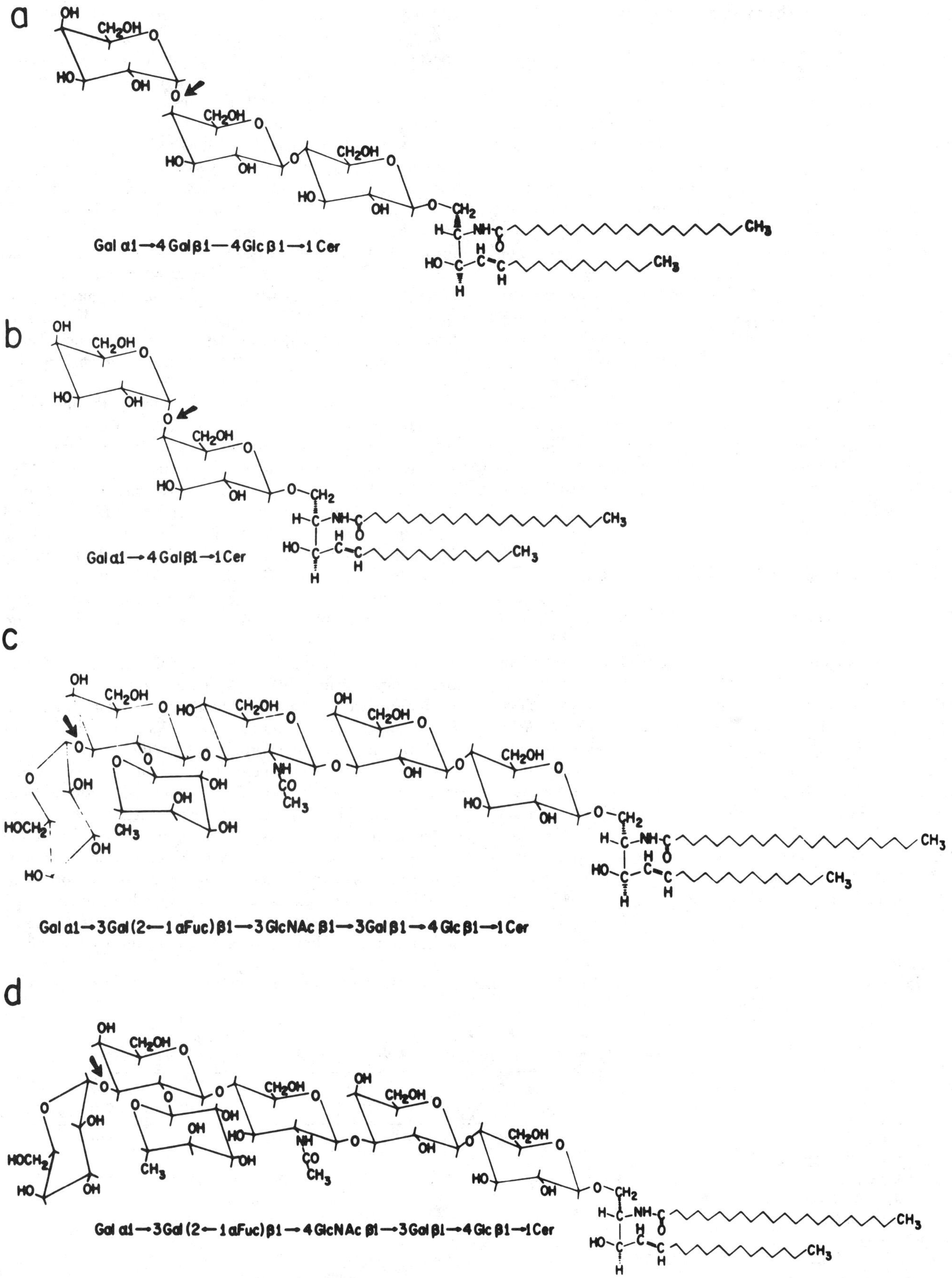

Gal α1→4 Gal β1→4 Glc β1→1 Cer

Gal α1→4 Gal β1→1 Cer

Gal α1→3 Gal (2←1 αFuc) β1→3 GlcNAc β1→3 Gal β1→4 Glc β1→1 Cer

Gal α1→3 Gal (2←1 αFuc) β1→4 GlcNAc β1→3 Gal β1→4 Glc β1→1 Cer

Figure 45-15 Complete chemical structures of the neutral glycosphingolipids that accumulate in Fabry's disease. *A.* Globotriaosylceramide, Gal-Gal-Glc-Cer, the major accumulated substrate. *B.* Galabiosylceramide, Gal-Gal-Cer. *C* and *D.* The blood group B antigenic glycosphingolipids which accumulate in blood group B and AB patients. The arrows indicate the α-galactosyl bonds which are normally cleaved by α-galactosidase A.

Abnormal Distribution in Tissues

The distribution of glycosphingolipids in the organs and tissues of patients with Fabry's disease has been investigated in several laboratories [25, 34, 35]. Increased concentrations of globotriaosylceramide were found in all sources analyzed [25, 27–32, 34–38, 200, 201, 267, 457, 458] except erythrocytes, which indicates that most tissues are involved in the catabolism of glycosphingolipids of the globo type. In one patient the magnitude of glycosphingolipid accumulation was 30- to 300-fold higher than normal levels [34]. The greatest levels of accumulation were observed in kidney, lymph nodes, vessels, prostate, and autonomic ganglia [24, 25, 35].

Accumulation of galabiosylceramide has been reported to occur only in the kidney [22, 24, 25, 34, 35], pancreas [34], heart [37], lungs [37], and urinary sediment [27]. The two blood group B–active neutral glycosphingolipids have only been found in one Fabry patient who had type B blood group specificity [38] but can be expected to occur abnormally in all patients with this blood type. Table 45-4 contains a summary of the average levels of the globo-type neutral glycosphingolipids and galabiosylceramide in plasma, urinary sediment, and cultured skin fibroblasts from hemizygotes, heterozygotes, and normal subjects.

The Primary Defect in Fabry's Disease

The primary biochemical defect in Fabry's disease is deficient activity of the lysosomal enzyme α-galactosidase A [39, 40] in the tissues and fluids of affected individuals. The deficient activity in hemizygotes and heterozygotes has been demonstrated with radiolabeled globotriaosylceramide [39] and chromogenic or fluorogenic substrates [40, 47, 48, 265, 402–405, 408, 409, 425, 438, 452]. Studies with chromogenic or fluorogenic substrates have revealed that affected hemizygotes have residual α-galactosidase activity which is approximately 10 to 25 percent of that observed in material from normal subjects [47, 48, 402, 403, 409, 424, 425, 437, 459]. The residual activity was determined to be due to the presence of α-N-acetylgalactosaminidase (α-galactosidase B) on the basis of differential thermostability [47, 48, 403, 404, 407–409, 424, 426, 428, 438]; substrate and inhibitor specificities [47, 48, 408, 424–426, 428, 430]; and kinetic [47, 48, 402, 406,

424–426, 428, 438], isoelectric or electrophoretic [406, 424, 426, 450], and immunologic properties [406, 424, 452]. Leukocytes from Fabry hemizygotes are deficient in α-galactosidase A as well as the related form that was reported to be uniquely present in normal leukocytes [445].

Immunologic techniques have been employed to determine the presence or absence of nonfunctional α-galactosidase A protein in hemizygotes with Fabry's disease. Using rabbit anti-human α-galactosidase A antibodies, Beutler and Kuhl [424, 460], Rietra et al. [452], and Hamers et al. [461] were unable to detect cross-reacting immunologic material (CRIM) in fibroblasts, leukocytes, urine or renal tissue from eight hemizygotes from seven unrelated Fabry families. Based on these findings, they independently concluded that the mutation(s) in these families were CRIM-negative. Thus, the inability to detect any residual α-galactosidase A activity in these Fabry sources was consistent with the absence of the enzyme protein.

Subsequently, Romeo et al. [462] reported the finding of residual α-galactosidase A activity in fibroblasts from five unrelated hemizygotes, including one patient previously reported to have about 20 percent residual activity [76, 463]. The residual α-galactosidase A activity was isolated and characterized using rabbit anti-human liver α-galactosidase A and B antibodies (which were absorbed with the other enzyme since they initially showed cross-reactivity) and DEAE-cellulose chromatography [462]. With the exception of the fifth hemizygote, who had about 20 percent of normal α-galactosidase A acterized using rabbit anti-human liver α-galactosidase A and B antibodies (which were absorbed with the other enzyme since they initially showed cross-reactivity) and DEAE-cellulose chromatography [462]. With the exception of the fifth hemizygote, who had about 20 percent of normal α-galactosidase A activity (see "Genetic Variants" section), the level of residual A activity in the fibroblasts from the four other hemizygotes was only about 3 percent of normal. This activity had an apparent K_m similar to that of normal α-galactosidase A but was thermostable and eluted more electronegatively on anion exchange chromatography. Rietra et al. suggested that the finding of residual α-galactosidase A activity in these four hemizygotes was artifactual due to the fact that a portion of the thermostable α-galactosidase B is rapidly converted, particularly during storage, to an "A-like" form which has some of the physical and kinetic properties of α-galactosidase A (i.e.,

Table 45-4   Mean concentrations of neutral glycosphingolipids in selected sources from normal subjects, heterozygotes, and hemizygotes with Fabry's disease

Glycosphingolipid	Plasma [26], nmol/ml			Urinary sediment [27], nmol/24 h urine			Cultured skin fibroblasts [556], nmol/g dry weight		
	Normal	Hetero-zygote	Hemi-zygote	Normal	Hetero-zygote	Hemi-zygote	Normal	Hetero-zygote	Hemi-zygote
Glycosylceramide (Glc-Cer)	9.8	7.7	7.8	40	148	64	440	420	620
Lactosylceramide (Gal-Glc-Cer)	5.5	5.8	4.7	58	151	204	200	200	600
Galabiosylceramide (Gal-Gal-Cer)	nd*	nd	nd	tr*	183	247	nd	nd	nd
Globotriaosylceramide (Gal-Gal-Glc-Cer)	2.1	4.5	7.6	26	405	1570	660	2260	2430
Globotetraosylceramide (GalNAc-Gal-Gal-Glc-Cer)	2.8	2.1	3.1	21	94	176	320	270	340

* nd = not detectable; tr = trace.

K_m toward artificial substrates, behavior on anion exchange chromatography), but retains the thermostability and immunologic properties of α-galactosidase B [451]. Their finding of an A-like form of α-galactosidase B in human and Fabry liver also has been confirmed in human placenta and lung during purification of α-galactosidase B by affinity chromatography [464].

Efforts in our laboratory also have been directed to evaluate the α-galactosidase A CRIM status in hemizygotes with Fabry's disease. Using a monospecific rabbit antibody to homogeneous placental α-galactosidase A (which does not cross-react with α-galactosidase B), the presence of CRIM has been evaluated by rocket immunoelectrophoresis in tissues from six unrelated Fabry hemizygotes who had no detectable α-galactosidase A by activity assay of the immunoprecipitated protein. To date, renal or splenic tissues from four hemizygotes were CRIM-negative, but CRIM corresponding to about 1 to 5 percent of normal enzyme protein levels was detected in the tissues of two other hemizygotes [465]. These findings support the presence of heterogeneity in the structural gene mutation in this disease (see "Genetics" section).

Thus, it can be reasonably concluded that the defective activity of α-galactosidase A is the primary biochemical defect in Fabry's disease. The inability to detect α-galactosidase A activity in affected hemizygotes is consistent with the accumulation of glycosphingolipid substrates with terminal α-galactosyl moieties. Furthermore, the intermediate levels of α-galactosidase activity in most heterozygous females (Fig. 45-16) is associated with a less severe accumulation of globotriaosylceramide and galabiosylceramide in plasma, urinary sediment, and cultured skin fibroblasts, as shown in Table 45-4. Finally, the observed transmission of the defective α-galactosidase A activity in families with Fabry's disease is consistent with the inheritance of a mutant gene for this catalytic gene product on the X chromosome.

PATHOPHYSIOLOGY

The pattern of glycosphingolipid deposition in Fabry's disease, particularly its predilection for vascular endothelial and smooth-muscle cells, is uniquely different from that seen in other glycosphingolipidoses [466]. The origin of the accumulated glycosphingolipid substrates has not been fully clarified. Certainly there is a significant contribution from the endogenous synthesis and subsequent lysosomal accumulation of terminal α-galactosyl–containing glycosphingolipids following autophagy of cellular membranous material containing these lipid substrates. Defective endogenous metabolism presumably is the major source of substrate accumulation in avascular sites, such as the cornea and in neural cells, which presumably are protected from the increased circulating levels of Gal-Gal-Glc-Cer by the blood-brain barrier. In addition, the turnover of Gal-Gal-Glc-Cer and particularly its precursor, globotetraosylceramide (globoside), which are present in higher concentrations in normal renal tissue than in any other tissue, is presumably responsible for the endogenous renal deposition of the Fabry substrate.

The unique cellular and tissue distribution of accumulated Gal-Gal-Glc-Cer, particularly in the vascular endothelium (Fig. 45-17) and smooth muscle, suggests that a significant

intracellular contribution may be derived by the endocytosis or diffusion of Gal-Gal-Glc-Cer from the circulation where the concentration is three- to tenfold higher than that of normal individuals. In Fabry hemizygotes and normal individuals, the circulating Gal-Gal-Glc-Cer is primarily transported in the LDL and HDL fractions (Table 45-2) [272–275]. In plasma from hemizygotes, the accumulated Gal-Gal-Glc-Cer is distributed in the LDL and HDL fractions in proportions similar to those in normal plasma, approximately 60 and 30 percent of recovered globotriaosylceramide, respectively [273, 274]. The finding that little, if any, substrate deposition occurs in Fabry hepatocytes (in contrast to the marked accumulation in Kupffer cells [154, 220, 224, 230]) supports the contention that Gal-Gal-Glc-Cer synthesized by the hepatocyte is associated with lipoprotein and secreted as a complex [467, 468]. In support of this concept is the fact that patients with hypercholesterolemia have proportional plasma elevations of both LDL and neutral glycosphingolipids including Gal-Gal-Glc-Cer [272, 468]. The circulating Gal-Gal-Glc-Cer then presumably gains access to vascular endothelial and smooth-muscle cells throughout the body by the high-affinity lipoprotein receptor-mediated uptake pathway [469–472]. Deposits in other tissues also may be derived to a lesser extent from receptor-independent diffusion or by nonadsorptive endocytosis [473, 474] of globoside- or Gal-Gal-Glc-Cer-lipoprotein complexes from the plasma. Since lysosomes in all cells are deficient in the α-galactosidase A activity needed to degrade glycosphingolipids of the globo type, the intermediate Gal-Gal-Glc-Cer accumulates within extended multivesicular bodies or, in more advanced stages, as free intracytoplasmic masses which may lead to cellular dysfunction or degeneration.

In addition to hepatocyte biosynthesis, glycosphingolipids are synthesized in the bone marrow, where they become incorporated into the membranes of the formed blood elements [26, 386, 387]. It has been postulated that erythrocyte globoside (GalNAc-Gal-Gal-Glc-Cer), the predominant glycosphingolipid of erythrocytes and the catabolic precursor of Gal-Gal-Glc-Cer (Fig. 45-13), may be another major metabolic source of the circulating pathogenic lipid. Globoside is presumably released into the circulation from senescent erythrocytes [22, 386] and is subsequently catabolized (presumably in the spleen) to Gal-Gal-Glc-Cer. In Fabry's disease, the Gal-Gal-Glc-Cer cannot be metabolized and may be partly released into the circulation, where it can be incorporated into both HDL and LDL fractions [467], or rapidly cleared by the liver as has been shown for intravenously administered neutral glycosphingolipids [475]. Thus, the turnover of erythrocyte and other membrane glycosphingolipids may contribute significantly to the substrate load in Fabry's disease. The dynamics and importance of the erythrocyte turnover in the glycosphingolipid accumulation process has been considered in depth by van den Bergh [476]. In addition, a minor amount of Gal-Gal-Glc-Cer may be "excreted" into the circulation from the secondary lysosomes of various cell types throughout the body. Since the glycosphingolipid cannot be catabolized in the circulation, it would slowly accumulate at a rate reflecting the turnover of various cells, the contribution from exocytosis, lipoprotein uptake, and diffusion.

The metabolism of at least two other compounds is also abnormal, as demonstrated by the accumulation of galabiosylceramide, Gal-Gal-Cer [24, 25, 27, 34–37], and the blood group B antigenic substances [38, 58]. Hemizygous and heterozygous individuals who are blood group type B or AB

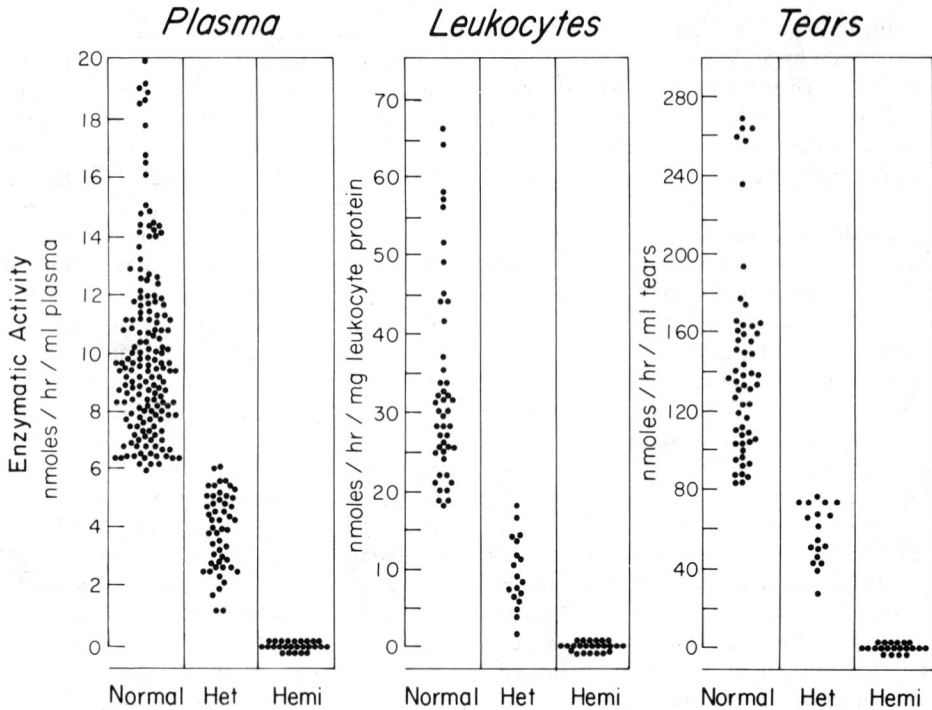

Figure 45-16 Levels of α-galactosidase A activity in plasma (or serum) [47], isolated leukocytes [47], and tears [48] from normal individuals and heterozygotes (Het) and hemizygotes (Hemi) with Fabry's disease. For methods of collection and enzyme assay using artificial substrates, see above references.

appear to be more severely affected, presumably due to the additional accumulation of B-specific glycosphingolipids [58, 477, 478]. Thus, the total amount of glycosphingolipids stored in a given tissue depends on time, the rate of accumulation from intracellular and circulatory sources, the possibilities for excretion, the individual's ABO blood type, and the presence or absence of residual α-galactosidase A activity.

That glycosphingolipid deposition is partly a function of time is illustrated by events after corneal biopsy. The regenerating corneal epithelium is initially clear but develops a golden haze within 3 months [479]. The rate of accumulation of lipid is probably determined by a number of factors. Perhaps the most important variable is the possible occurrence of residual activity of the mutant enzyme. Assuming that globoside from the erythrocyte membrane is a major precursor of accumulated Gal-Gal-Glc-Cer, factors affecting red blood cell survival and red blood cell mass may also be involved. Excretion of glycosphingolipids from the kidney and urogenital tract may be in the range of 0.1 to 6.0 mg/day [27]. There is little likelihood of appreciable excretion from other sites, although losses must occur into the bile and by desquamation of intestinal, corneal, or bronchial epithelium.

The pattern of glycosphingolipid accumulation, predominantly in the cardiovascular-renal system, best correlates pathophysiologically with the major clinical manifestations of the disease as selectively described below.

Vasculature Narrowing, dilatation, motor unresponsiveness, and instability of blood vessels are major features of the altered physiology of Fabry's disease. The swollen endothelial cells, often accompanied by endothelial proliferation [34], encroach upon the lumen (Figs. 45-6 and 45-17), causing a focal increase of intraluminal pressure, dilatation, and angiectases as well as peripheral ischemia or frank infarction. Such changes are frequently the precursors of thromboses and infarcts of the brain and other tissues. Muscle and peripheral nerve ischemia may contribute to the pain or fatigue [202, 207, 480].

There may be progressive aneurysmal dilatation of the weakened vascular wall. This process is apparent in the progressive dilatation and microaneurysm formation of the retinal and conjunctival vessels (Fig. 45-5) [36] and in the transition from normality to telangiectasia and frank angiokeratoma in the skin. The observation of angiokeratoma in patients with defective α-L-fucosidase [179] and α-neuraminidase [180, 181] activities suggests a common pathologic mechanism responsible for the occurrence of the cutaneous lesion in patients with different lysosomal hydrolase deficiencies.

Observed alterations of vasomotor control may reflect either the vascular lesions themselves or the extensive glycosphingolipid deposits in autonomic ganglia and perineural sheath cells. The alteration of vasomotor response has been compared to that seen in patients with cold injury [63]. Both hemizygotes and heterozygotes with Fabry's disease demonstrate an impaired ability for vasoconstriction, and the more severely involved hemizygotes show, in addition, an inability of vasodilatation. Such a combined vascular and neural lesion may also explain the clinically observed temperature intolerance.

Nervous System The involvement of peripheral and central autonomic nerve cells may be responsible for the paresthesias, pain, hypohidrosis, gastrointestinal symptoms such as nausea and diarrhea, and a variety of vague neurologic signs and symptoms. Fukuhara et al. [480] found marked degeneration of the secretory cells and myoepithelial cells of sweat glands by electron microscopy and proposed that the hypohidrosis was due to local lipid deposition rather than autonomic nervous system involvement. The episodic fevers may be related to lesions of the hypothalamus [164]. The observations of a selective decrease in the number of unmyelinated and small myelinated fibers in peripheral nerves [197, 200–203, 206] have led to the suggestion that the selective damage to these fibers may account for the hypohidrosis and pain production in this disorder. Studies of autonomic function revealed sympathetic and parasympathetic dysfunction, particularly in distal cutaneous responses [481]. Alternatively, it has been suggested that the lipid deposition in the vasa nervorum may lead to the acroparethesias rather than involvement of the autonomic nervous system [209, 480].

Kidney The observed disorders in renal function have their basis in lesions of the nephron and of the renal vasculature, and possibly in disorders of the posterior pituitary and hypothalamus. Early glycosphingolipid deposits antedate clinical signs and symptoms. During this early period, the lesions of the renal vasculature are less prominent than those of the nephron, and renal architecture is maintained [36]. The observed mild proteinuria may be explained by alteration of the glomerular epithelial cells and their foot processes [186, 188] or by increased desquamation of lipid-laden tubular epithelial cells.

Loss of renal concentrating ability, with polyuria [15, 192] and polydipsia [14, 147, 192], may occur well in advance of a significant decrease in glomerular filtration or evidence of renal failure [103]. The defect in concentrating ability may be due to decreased water permeability of the distal tubules and collecting ducts secondary to lipid deposition [186, 195]. The diabetes insipidus-like syndrome, which is not related to faulty electrolyte transfer in distal tubules [192], may result from tubular insensitivity to antidiuretic hormone [192] or to combined dysfunction of the renal tubular cells and lesions of the glycosphingolipid-laden supraoptic nucleus, an antidiuretic

center of the hypothalamus [141]. The later and more severe renal changes are the result of vascular lesions and of hypertension.

Heart The progressive deposition of glycosphingolipids in the myocardial cells, the valvular fibroblasts, and the coronary vessels is the primary cause of cardiac disease in hemizygotes and some heterozygotes [37, 79–81]. The frequent findings of left ventricular hypertrophy and mitral insufficiency are presumably related to the fact that the left ventricular myocardium and the mitral valve are the sites of the most marked lipid deposition in the heart [37]. The abnormally short PR interval and the finding of cardiomyopathy on ECG may be related to lipid deposition in the myocardium or conducting system or both [9, 85]. The marked deposition of Gal-Gal-Glc-Cer in the coronary arteries leads to myocardial ischemia and frank infarction [37, 79–81].

Other Involvement Pulmonary symptoms have been attributed to involvement of lung vasculature or bronchial and mucous gland epithelium [125]. The airflow obstruction may be due to the loss of the elastic recoil secondary to lipid deposition in the lung parenchyma [124]. The lymphedema presumably results from lymphatic obstruction or venous insufficiency secondary to lipid-laden endothelial cells.

Reports of growth retardation, delayed puberty [71, 140], abnormal beard [141], or impaired fertility [19, 482] associated with a decrease of gonadotropins [123], may correlate with observations of testicular atrophy [483] or with glycosphingolipid storage in anterior and posterior lobes of the pitu-

Figure 45-17 Electron micrograph of a section of an arteriole from a hemizygote, showing the marked accumulation of concentric lamellar inclusions in the lysosomes of the vascular endothelium. The progressive lysosomal deposition of the glycosphingolipid substrate leads to the narrowing and eventual occlusion of the vascular lumen. Magnification, ×25,000. *(Courtesy of Dr. J. G. White, University of Minnesota.)*

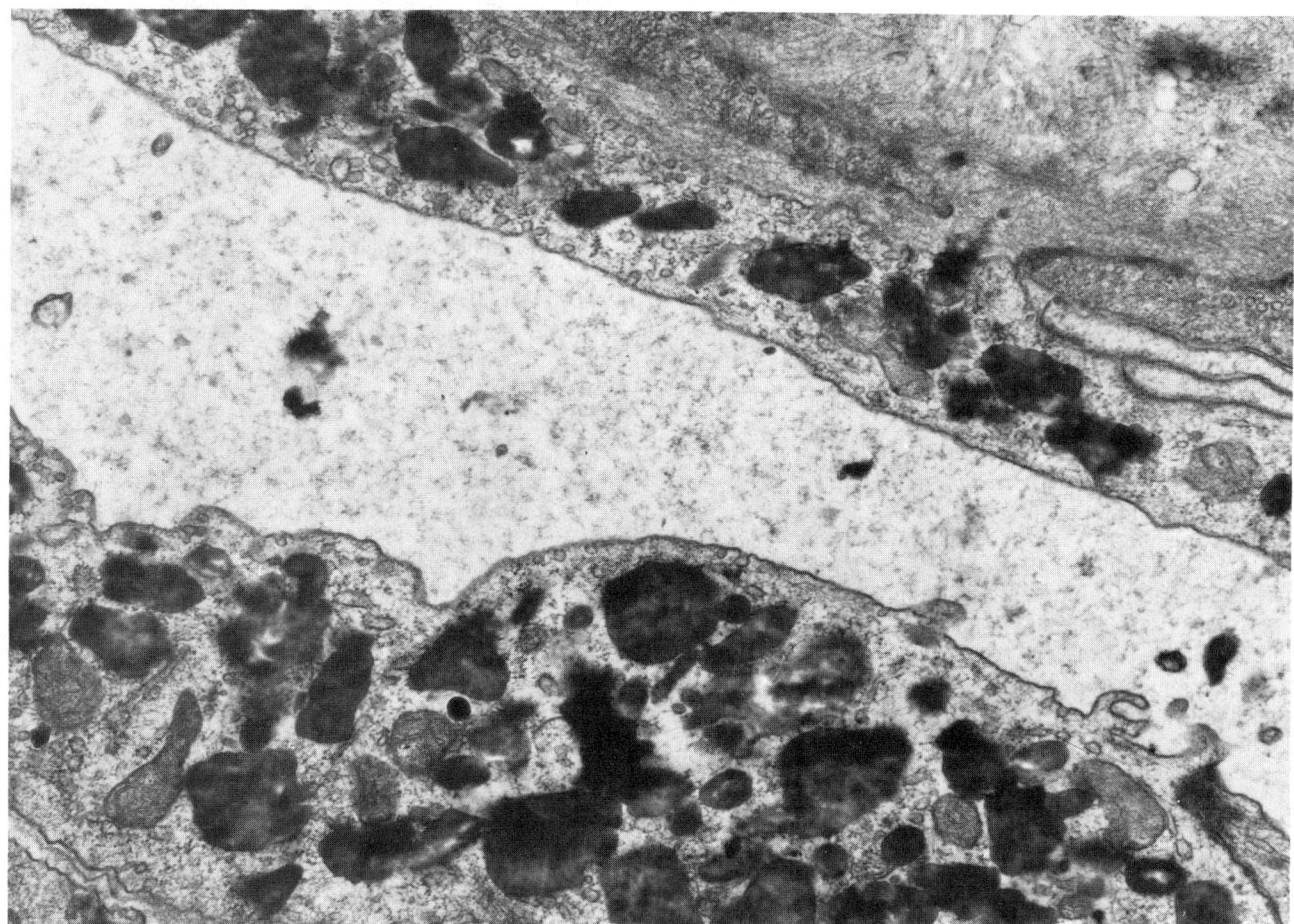

itary gland [*173, 220*] or in the interstitial cells of the testis [*99, 173*]. No explanations have been offered for the frequently observed acromegalylike appearance [*65, 66, 115, 141, 142*].

GENETICS

Mode of Inheritance

The genetics of Fabry's disease has been the subject of several reports [*19, 65, 71, 482, 484–486*]. The disease is transmitted by an X-linked structural gene which is presumably responsible for the gene product, α-galactosidase A [*39, 49*]. Of the sphingolipidoses, only in Fabry's disease is the gene encoding the mutant hydrolytic enzyme on the X chromosome [*487*]. The evidence for the X-linked inheritance of this disease has been reviewed in detail in the previous edition of this text [*55*].

The frequency of Fabry's disease has not been determined. The disease is rare, and we estimate that the incidence is about 1:40,000. Of the over 350 described cases of hemizygous males, most are Caucasian, but black [*77, 78, 105*], Latin American [*135, 145, 488, 489*], Egyptian [*490*], and Oriental [*158, 159, 200, 252, 491–493*] cases have been observed. Chromosome studies of affected males demonstrated only normal karyotypes [*36, 69, 71, 74, 193, 194*] with the exception of one hemizygote who was 47,XYY [*495*].

Regional Gene Assignment

As reviewed in the previous edition of this text [*55*], the locus of the Fabry gene was originally linked by recombination analysis to the well-established X-linked locus for the blood group antigen Xg^a [*19, 71, 193, 485*]. Although the linkage data for Xg^a and Fabry's disease were not strong [*55*], the most likely recombination fraction was 0.23 with wide 95 percent probability limits of 0.16 to 0.35. The Lod score was slightly less than 2.0, the value required for a formal level of significance. These data suggested that the Fabry gene was located on the short arm of the X chromosome [*55*]. More recent data obtained from somatic cell hybridization studies of human-hamster hybrid fibroblasts localized the α-galactosidase A structural gene to a small region on the long arm of the X chromosome, $Xq22 \rightarrow q24$ [*496–502*]. Since the Xg^a locus has been assigned to the region $Xp22 \rightarrow pter$ on the short arm [*503*], the original linkage relationship recently was reevaluated [*504*]. Analysis of additional data revealed that the sum of the Lods for the Xg^a-Fabry linkage were not consistent with linkage. The gene for human α-galactosidase B (α-N-acetylgalactosaminidase) has been assigned to chromosome 22 by somatic cell hybridization techniques [*504*], further distinguishing α-galactosidases A and B at the genic level.

In addition, the somatic cell hybridization studies suggested that both the human and hamster α-galactosidases were homodimers since an enzyme with an intermediate electrophoretic mobility was observed in hybrid cells containing X-chromosomes from both species [*496, 497, 499, 505*]. Using species-specific anti-α-galactosidase A antibodies, the hybrid enzyme was shown to contain immunologic determinants of both species [*506*]. Hybrid clones (derived from Fabry and Chinese hamster fibroblasts) which contained an active X

chromosome from each species did not express human α-galactosidase A or the hybrid enzyme. This suggests that the α-galactosidase A deficiency in Fabry's disease resulted from a structural gene mutation rendering the protein either immunologically undetectable or markedly unstable, as well as functionally inactive [*506*].

Penetrance and Variable Expressivity

The Fabry gene is highly penetrant in the hemizygote; no clinically normal sons of proven heterozygotes have had affected sons or carrier daughters. Clinical onset is variable, occurring usually during childhood [*507*], but may be delayed until the second or third decade [*34, 71, 73, 74, 104, 171, 508–510*]. Both intrafamilial and interfamilial variations in the clinical expression have been reported, the intrafamilial being less than the interfamilial variation [*36, 65, 482, 495, 511*]. It has been suggested [*65*] that modifying genes and environmental factors may be responsible for intrafamilial variations [*511*].

In heterozygous females penetrance is not complete, although the presence of the mutant gene may be demonstrated biochemically [*26, 29, 31, 47, 48, 67, 512*]. Expressivity in the heterozygote is variable, as exemplified by the range of clinical findings observed in eight daughters of an affected male [*513*]. Approximately 20 percent of the heterozygotes have some skin lesions, a smaller percentage have the characteristic intermittent pain in the extremities, and about 80 percent have the whorllike corneal dystrophy. Proven heterozygotes may be completely asymptomatic throughout a normal life span [*19*]. Franceschetti et al. [*67*] have identified clinically asymptomatic heterozygotes by their increased urinary Gal-Gal-Glc-Cer excretion. Obligate heterozygotes without any clinical manifestations and with normal levels of leukocyte α-galactosidase [*145, 512*] and urinary sediment glycosphingolipids have been reported [*145*]. In contrast, complete clinical [*79, 486, 514*] and biochemical [*486, 512, 514*] expression of the disease, as severe as in affected hemizygotes, has been documented in several heterozygotes.

The markedly variable expression of the Fabry gene in heterozygous females is anticipated for X-linked enzymatic deficiencies, although it is somewhat difficult to explain the high frequency of clinical involvement in these heterozygous individuals by the random X-inactivation hypothesis [*513, 515, 516*]. At the cellular level, this hypothesis predicts that heterozygotes for X-linked enzymatic defects will have two populations of cells, one clone with mutant and the other with normal enzymatic activity. Two such populations have been cloned from individual cultured skin fibroblasts from obligate heterozygotes, one with normal and the other with defective α-galactosidase A activities [*517*]. Ultrastructural examination of renal tissue from heterozygotes also demonstrated two populations of glomerular, interstitial, and vascular cells; one normal, the other in which glycosphingolipid deposition was observed [*186*]. Laboratory studies have not demonstrated metabolic cooperation between the two cell clones derived from these heterozygotes [*518*]. Preferential X inactivation has also been proposed to explain the clinical expression in Fabry heterozygotes [*513*]. It is of interest to speculate that some clinical manifestations may result in these women if more than 50 percent of normal α-galactosidase A activity is required to maintain its substrates at nonpathologic concentrations in certain cells or tissues. Biochemical studies of most heterozygotes reveal intermediate levels of α-galactosidase A activity (Fig.

45-16) and intermediate levels of Gal-Gal-Glc-Cer accumulation (Table 45-4). Further clinical and biochemical studies are required to elucidate the mechanism of clinical expression in the heterozygous state.

Phenocopies

A phenocopy is a phenotypic mimic or simulation of a specific genetic trait. Since a phenocopy is usually the result of environmental factors, it is not inherited. There are two such phenocopies for Fabry's disease, one which mimics the characteristic corneal opacity and another which causes renal functional and ultrastructural changes resembling those in hemizygotes. Since the diagnosis of Fabry's disease is often suspected from an eye examination or renal evaluation for proteinuria, these phenocopies have significant diagnostic import.

The whorllike keratopathy of Fabry's disease is readily distinguishable from the corneal opacities of other lysosomal storage diseases [110, 519] but is clinically [68, 110, 519, 520] and ultrastructurally [521] identical to the corneal dystrophy associated with long-term chloroquine or amidarone therapy [121, 122]. This observation suggested that chloroquine, a lysosomotropic agent [522], might induce a true biochemical, as well as morphological, phenocopy of the Fabry keratopathy [523]. This hypothesis was supported by determining the activities of selected lysosomal and cytoplasmic enzymes in cultured human cornea incubated with increasing concentrations of chloroquine diphosphate for 48 h [523]. As shown in Fig. 45-18, the α-galactosidase A activity decreased with increasing chloroquine concentrations, whereas the levels of other lysosomal enzymes were less markedly reduced or unchanged.

Chloroquine has been shown to concentrate rapidly in lysosomes [524–526], increase the intralysosomal pH [525–527], cause the formation of lysosomal inclusions [522, 525, 528], alter the rate of proteolysis, and decrease the activity of specific lysosomal hydrolases [524–528]. Based on these findings, it was proposed that the chloroquine-induced keratopathy resulted from the marked pH inactivation of lysosomal α-galactosidase A and the subsequent accumulation of Gal-Gal-Glc-Cer [523]. In support of this concept is the finding that corneal α-galactosidase A is more sensitive to increasing pH in vitro than other lysosomal hydrolases including α-galactosidase B, β-hexosaminidases A and B, β-galactosidase, and β-glucuronidase [529]. These findings demonstrate the likely

mechanism responsible for the phenocopy and represent the first biochemical elucidation of a human phenocopy.

Another tissue-specific phenocopy of Fabry's disease occurs in individuals who are environmentally exposed to silica dust. The pulmonary complications of silicolipoproteinosis are well described [530], but the renal manifestations of proteinuria and lipiduria have received little attention [531]. Ultrastructural examination of renal tissue from these individuals has revealed the typical electron-dense lamellar inclusions in the lysosomes of glomerular epithelial and endothelial cells and proximal and distal tubular cells observed in Fabry's disease [532, 533] (Fig. 45-19). The levels of α-galactosidase A and urinary sediment glycosphingolipids were normal in one such patient [533]. Although the mechanism responsible for the silica-induced phenocopy is unknown, the finding of such lesions in biopsied renal tissue should include silicosis as well as Fabry's disease in the differential diagnosis.

Genetic Variants

In 1971, Clarke et al. [76] described a 38-year-old Italian male who presented with proteinuria and hypercholesterolemia; biopsied renal tissue revealed histologic and ultrastructural abnormalities consistent with the diagnosis of Fabry's disease. There was no history of acroparesthesias, and no angiokeratoma or corneal opacities were observed. Urinary sediment glycosphingolipid analyses demonstrated levels of Gal-Gal-Glc-Cer in the heterozygote range and low levels of Gal-Gal-Cer [76]. Subsequently, he died at age 49 years after a second myocardial infarction [534]. His total α-galactosidase activity (A and B) in leukocytes was about 30 percent of normal. Crude extracts of cultured skin fibroblasts from this hemizygote were shown to have about 30 percent of normal total α-galactosidase activity which contained both thermolabile and thermostable components, had a lower apparent K_m (6 mM) toward the artificial substrate [compared to the normal value for α-galactosidase A (2 mM) or that of α-galactosidase B (20 mM) found in typical hemizygotes], and had about one-tenth of normal activity toward the radiolabeled natural substrate, Gal-Gal-Glc-Cer [463]. Subsequently, the residual α-galactosidase A in cultured fibroblasts was partially purified by anion exchange and immunologic techniques and shown to have kinetic and thermostability properties similar to normal α-galactosidase A. About 20 percent of normal α-galactosidase A

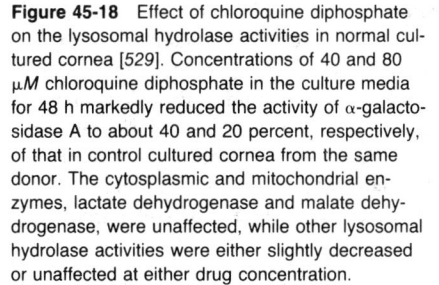

Figure 45-18 Effect of chloroquine diphosphate on the lysosomal hydrolase activities in normal cultured cornea [529]. Concentrations of 40 and 80 μM chloroquine diphosphate in the culture media for 48 h markedly reduced the activity of α-galactosidase A to about 40 and 20 percent, respectively, of that in control cultured cornea from the same donor. The cytosplasmic and mitochondrial enzymes, lactate dehydrogenase and malate dehydrogenase, were unaffected, while other lysosomal hydrolase activities were either slightly decreased or unaffected at either drug concentration.

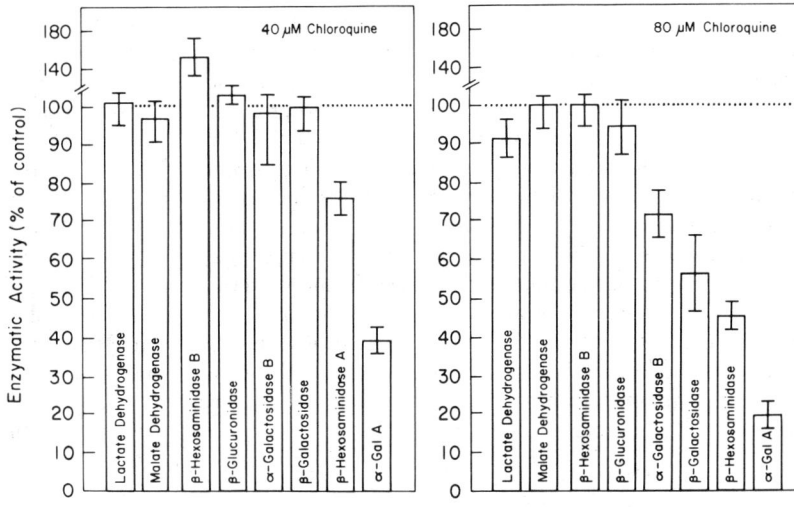

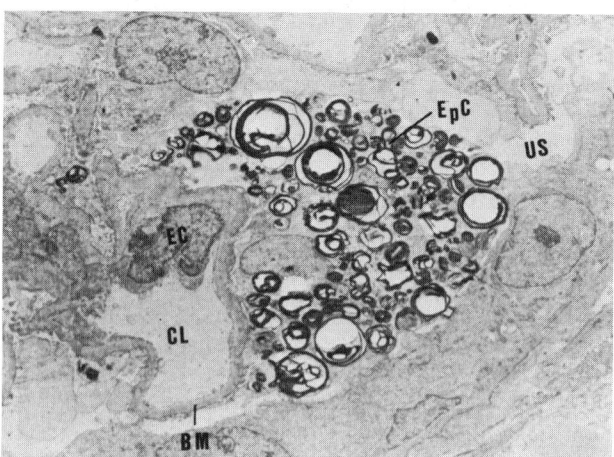

Figure 45-19 Electron photomicrograph showing the concentric lamellar inclusions in the glomerular epithelial cell (EpC) of a patient with silicosis. These lesions resemble the ultrastructural findings observed in Fabry's disease. EC, endothelial cell; CL, capillary lumen; US, urinary space; BM, basement membrane. Magnification, ×3750 (reproduced at 51 percent original size).

activity was detected in fibroblasts, but the amount of CRIM was not measured [462].

Recently, we evaluated a 42-year-old male with severe rheumatoid arthritis and proteinuria, who was referred following renal biopsy which revealed ultrastructural findings consistent with Fabry's disease [535, 536]. He denied a history of acroparesthesias or hypohidrosis. No angiokeratoma, corneal or lenticular opacities, or cardiac manifestations were found. Creatinine clearance and concentrating ability were normal. The level of α-galactosidase A activity, which was about 5 percent of normal in plasma, confirmed the diagnosis. His sister and daughter had heterozygous levels of plasma α-galactosidase A activity. Specific immunoprecipitation with monospecific anti-α-galactosidase A antibodies demonstrated residual A activity in granulocytes (6 percent of normal), lymphocytes (6 percent), lymphoblasts (14 percent), liver (8 percent), and cultured fibroblasts (24 percent). The immunoprecipitated residual A activity from fibroblasts had the same K_m value as the immunoprecipitated enzyme (2 mM) from normal fibroblasts. Compared to normal, the residual lymphoblast α-galactosidase A was more thermolabile at pH 4.6, 50°C ($t_{1/2}$ = 250 vs. 150 min) and significantly more pH unstable (pH 7.4 and 37°C: $t_{1/2}$ = 49 vs. 11 min), consistent with the extremely low enzyme level in plasma and urine. Interestingly, the levels of Gal-Gal-Glc-Cer in plasma and urinary sediment were 2.1 nmol/ml and 155 nmol/24 h, respectively, levels in the low heterozygote range. Urinary sediment Gal-Gal-Cer was 63 nmol/24 h. No lysosomal inclusions were observed in hepatocytes or Kupffer cells in biopsied liver. Rocket immunoelectrophoresis studies demonstrated that the level of α-galactosidase A activity corresponded to the amount of enzyme protein. These findings are consistent with a stability mutation, resulting in an enzyme with normal kinetics. In this variant, it appears that 6 to 20 percent of normal intracellular activity is sufficient to prevent the majority of the clinical manifestations of the disease. In addition, the finding of only 5 percent of enzymatic activity in the plasma and low levels of plasma Gal-Gal-Glc-Cer suggests that circulating enzyme is not required to catabolize the plasma substrate.

Genetic Nature of the Enzymatic Defect

It is intriguing to speculate on the molecular nature of the enzymatic defect in Fabry's disease. Although the number of unrelated hemizygotes studied to date is small, several different mutations involving the α-galactosidase A structural gene have been presumptively identified by biochemical and immunologic techniques. These include atypical variants with residual α-galatosidase A activity, classic hemizygotes with no detectable activity and very low, but detectable levels of enzyme protein, and classic hemizygotes with no detectable α-galactosidase A activity or enzyme protein.

Two Fabry variants with less severe clinical expression and residual α-galactosidase A activity have been recognized [76, 462, 463, 535] (see "Genetic Variants" section). In one hemizygous variant [535], 6 to 20 percent of normal α-galactosidase A activity and a proportionate amount of CRIM were found in various tissues with the exception of plasma, which had only 5 percent of the respective normal α-galactosidase A activities. The residual fibroblast α-galactosidase A was shown to have the same K_m but was more thermolabile and pH sensitive (particularly at values >7.0) than the normal enzyme. These findings were consistent with a structural gene mutation which altered the stability but not the substrate-binding or catalytic sites of the enzyme protein [535].

In the other hemizygous variant, the residual α-galactosidase A activities in fibroblasts and leukocytes were about 20 percent of respective normal levels [76, 462, 463]. Although the amount of CRIM was not determined, the partially purified fibroblast enzyme was found to have the same K_m value and thermostability properties as the normal enzyme. The differences in levels of residual activity in this patient [76, 462, 463] suggest that the defective α-galactosidase A in these two hemizygous variants resulted from different structural gene mutations. The frequency of such mutations is difficult to estimate since these patients may be asymptomatic or minimally involved and, therefore, may escape detection.

The second category includes hemizygous males who have the typical clinical expression of the disease, undetectable α-galactosidase A activity in all sources, and 1 to 5 percent of normal levels of enzyme protein (CRIM). The presence of CRIM indicates that these families have structural gene mutations that presumably render the enzyme protein noncatalytic and markedly unstable [537].

The third category includes the majority of hemizygotes studied. Clinically, these individuals have the classic phenotype and biochemically are CRIM-negative, i.e., no detectable α-galactosidase A activity or CRIM [537]. Several possible explanations may be advanced to account for these CRIM-negative mutations. First, the mutation(s) in these families may have altered the enzyme conformation such that its antigenic sites are not recognized by the anti-α-galactosidase A antibodies. It is unlikely that a rabbit polyvalent antibody preparation [538, 539] would not recognize many, if not most, structurally altered proteins analogous to the experience with other enzyme deficiency disorders [540]. A more likely explanation would be a point mutation(s) resulting in a markedly unstable α-galactosidase A protein which is rapidly degraded. Further investigation of the molecular nature of the CRIM-negative mutations may require the use of recombinant DNA techniques to obtain appropriate DNA probes to evaluate the possibility that the genetic defect(s) in these CRIM-negative kindreds result from chain terminating defects, mRNA processing defects, or partial or complete gene deletions analogous to those recently identified in the α- and β-thalassemias [541–545].

Genetic Counseling

Genetic counseling should be made available to all families in which the diagnosis of Fabry's disease is made. Inheritance of the Fabry gene from hemizygotes and heterozygotes should be considered, since both genotypes transmit the gene. All sons of hemizygous males will be unaffected, but all daughters will be obligate carriers of the gene. On the average, half the sons of heterozygous females will have the disease and half the daughters will be carriers. All possible carriers among close female relatives should be examined clinically and biochemically for heterozygote identification. Fabry's disease has been detected antenatally from cultured fetal cells and amniotic fluid obtained by amniocentesis (see "Prenatal Diagnosis" section).

DIAGNOSIS

Clinical Evaluation

Both hemizygotes and heterozygotes with Fabry's disease are discovered by deliberate investigation of the families of patients with the disease. The clinical diagnosis in hemizygous males is most readily made from the history and by observation of the characteristic skin lesions and corneal dystrophy. Differential diagnosis of the cutaneous lesions must exclude the angiokeratoma of Fordyce [546], angiokeratoma of Mibelli [547], and angiokeratoma circumscriptum [548]. The diagnosis of Fabry's disease has been made in some males during infancy [18, 168]. The most common childhood symptom before the appearance of the cutaneous lesions is recurrent fever in association with pain of the hands and feet [18, 511]. The disorder has often been misdiagnosed as rheumatic fever [18, 549, 560], neurosis, erythromelalgia [551], or collagen vascular disease [495].

Presumptive diagnosis of hemizygotes can be made by a careful ophthalmologic examination, demonstration of the birefringent inclusions in the urinary sediment (Fig. 45-10) or by skin or bone marrow biopsy. The observation of dilated, tortuous retinal and conjunctival vessels and particularly the characteristic corneal dystrophy observed by slit-lamp examination should aid in the diagnosis. Biopsied skin will reveal the characteristic refractile lipid inclusions (Maltese crosses) in blood vessels [168]. Lipid-containing macrophages may also be observed in bone marrow aspirates [13].

Women suspected of being heterozygous carriers of the Fabry gene should be carefully examined for evidence of the characteristic corneal opacity by slit-lamp microscopy [63, 68, 147] and for isolated skin lesions, particularly on the breasts, back, trunk, and posterolateral thighs. Detection may also be accomplished by the histologic finding of lipid-laden cells in biopsied skin [63], tissues, or in the urinary sediment [115, 143].

Biochemical Confirmation

All suspect hemizygotes should be confirmed biochemically by the demonstration of deficient α-galactosidase A activities in plasma or serum [47], leukocytes [40, 47, 552, 553], tears [48] (Fig. 45-16), biopsied tissues, or cultured skin fibroblasts [47, 402, 403, 409]. Alternatively, multiprocedural glycosphingolipid analyses can be accomplished to demonstrate the increased levels of Gal-Gal-Glc-Cer in urinary sediment [26–31, 193, 553, 554], plasma [26], or cultured skin fibroblasts [32, 555, 556] (Table 45-4). Suspect patients with angiokeratoma or corneal opacities and normal α-galactosidase A should be evaluated for α-L-fucosidase [180] or α-neuraminidase deficiencies [180, 182].

Suspect heterozygotes should be biochemically identified by their intermediate levels of α-galactosidase A activity in the above sources [512]. If borderline normal values of α-galactosidase A activity are obtained, then the enzyme levels should be determined in a series of single hair roots, which are presumably derived from single cells and should express either normal or hemizygous levels of activity [91, 558–562]. The genotypic diagnosis also may be made by the demonstration of increased concentrations of Gal-Gal-Glc-Cer and Gal-Gal-Cer in urinary sediment [26–31, 512, 553, 554]. Further documentation of heterozygosity, if necessary, can be accomplished by cloning cultured skin fibroblasts followed by the demonstration of two cell populations, normal and deficient, for α-galactosidase A activity [517].

Prenatal Diagnosis

Prenatal diagnosis of Fabry's disease has been accomplished by amniocentesis at approximately 14 weeks of gestation and biochemical analysis of the amniotic fluid components [50, 51, 563–566]. The prenatal diagnosis of an affected hemizygous male fetus minimally requires the demonstration of deficient α-galactosidase A activity and an XY karyotype in cultured amniotic cells. An early "indication" of the prenatal diagnosis can be obtained by determining the fetal sex (sex chromatin and fluorescent Y-body studies) [567] of the uncultured amniocytes and the α-galactosidase A and B activities in the amniotic fluid. These initial studies must be confirmed subsequently by determining the enzyme levels in cultured amniotic cells. In addition, the demonstration of accumulated Gal-Gal-Glc-Cer in the cell-free amniotic fluid will provide further diagnostic confirmation [566]. Using these techniques we have monitored 10 at-risk pregnancies and were able to confirm the prenatal diagnosis of 1 affected hemizygous fetus and of 5 unaffected males and four females (1 heterozygous, 3 normal) after delivery [566]. A microtechnique for the rapid prenatal diagnosis of affected hemizygotes using a microchemical analysis for α-galactosidase activity in isolated groups of cultured amniotic cells (each with 100 to 250 cells) has been developed [568–570] and used successfully [568, 569].

Biochemical and ultrastructural studies of tissues from fetuses with Fabry's disease have been reported [50, 563, 564]. Consistent with the prenatal diagnosis, the α-galactosidase A activity was defective in all tissues studied; increased concentrations of globotriaosylceramide were found in all tissues analyzed, with the exception of neural tissues [563]. Histologic and light-microscopic examination of various tissues were unremarkable, but ultrastructural examination revealed electron-dense concentric lamellar inclusions in the lysosomes of vascular endothelium, renal tubules, and epithelial and endothelial cells of renal glomeruli [563, 564]. Although lipid deposition was evident at 18 weeks of fetal life, the degree of substrate accumulation in fetal Fabry's disease was markedly less than that observed in fetuses affected with G_{M2} gangliosidosis type 1 [571] or type 2 [563, 572], diseases in which the substrate deposition and deteriorating clinical course occur rapidly. Reviews of the techniques, safety, and accuracy of prenatal metabolic diagnosis are available [573–578].

TREATMENT

Medical Management

In Fabry's disease the chronicity of the clinical events causes severe debilitation and incapacity that extends over years. The single most debilitating and morbid aspect of Fabry's disease is the excruciating pain. The pathophysiologic events that cause the incapacitating episodes of pain or the chronic burning acroparesthesias have not been clarified. In one patient, a spinal block was effective in the relief of the pain. This suggested that the origin of the pain was at the level of the peripheral nerves or the dorsal spinal ganglia [200]. Numerous drugs have been tried for the relief of these agonizing pains [17, 55]. The α-adrenergic blocking agent phenoxybenzamine, which increases peripheral vascular flow [98], has been tried and provided relief in one hemizygote on several occasions, but priapism and epistasis were early complications in two other hemizygotes [98, 579]. With the exception of centrally acting narcotic analgesics, which have been only partially effective, conventional analgesic agents have not been successful. Prophylactic administration of low maintenance dosages of diphenylhydantoin has been found to provide relief from the periodic crises of excruciating pain and constant discomfort in hemizygotes and heterozygotes [62]. The results of a double-blind triple crossover study indicated that patients maintained on diphenylhydantoin had a striking remission of Fabry crises and discomfort and that exacerbation of these episodes occurred when either an analgesic or placebo was substituted [62]. Lenior et al. [580] noted that carbamazepine also provided pain relief. The combination of diphenylhydantoin and carbamazepine significantly reduced the pain in an affected hemizygote [581]. Subsequent reports have further documented the effectiveness of diphenylhydantoin or carbamazepine or both in the prevention and amelioration of these debilitating pains [64, 202, 582]. Maintenance corticosteroid administration (e.g., prednisone, 7.5 mg daily) also has been reported to provide symptomatic relief of the pain [583].

Care of patients with regard to cardiac, pulmonary, and central nervous system manifestations remains nonspecific and symptomatic. Obstructive lung disease has been documented in older hemizygotes and heterozygotes, with more severe impairment in smokers [124]. Patients should be discouraged from smoking. Since renal insufficiency is the most frequent late complication in patients with this disease, chronic hemodialysis and renal transplantation have become life-saving procedures. In addition to treatment of the renal failure, kidney transplantation has been undertaken to determine if the allograft could provide normal α-galactosidase A for substrate metabolism [144, 584]. Hypothetically, the normal kidney might metabolize the accumulated substrate by uptake and catabolism within the allograft or by the release of the active enzyme into the circulation for uptake and metabolism in other tissues such as the vascular endothelium. Although biochemical or clinical improvement or both have been reported in several recipients [144, 584–589], no biochemical effect could be demonstrated in other recipients [590–593]. Thus, the use of renal allografts to alter the rate of progressive substrate accumulation remains controversial and further studies are required to determine the long-term biochemical effects of this strategy. In view of these results, renal transplantation should be undertaken only in patients with clinically significant renal failure.

At present, the most practical and effective therapy is preventive. Screening of all suspect heterozygotes, genetic counseling, and prenatal diagnostic studies should be made available to all at-risk families (see "Genetics" section). Family and vocational counseling should be provided, especially to families with affected children. Often, parents, teachers, or physicians misinterpret the excruciating pain experienced during childhood as psychosomatic, especially in the absence of any objective physical or laboratory findings. Since physical exertion, emotional stresses and fatigue, as well as rapid changes in the environmental temperature and humidity, can trigger these painful episodes, appropriate arrangements must be made with physical education teachers and other individuals to minimize or eliminate stressful activities. In addition, young hemizygotes should be allowed to pursue selected activities and be permitted to stop these activities at their own discretion. Within this perspective, reasonable occupational and vocational objectives should be pursued. Vocational counseling should discourage occupations which require significant manual dexterity, physical exertion, emotional stress, or exposure to rapid changes in temperature or humidity.

Enzyme Replacement

Attempts to replace the defective α-galactosidase A activity with normal enzyme have been undertaken in vitro and in vivo. Studies using partially purified α-galactosidase A from fig [594] and human spleen [595] supplied in the media of cultured skin fibroblasts from Fabry hemizygotes demonstrated the ability of the exogenous enzyme to gain access to and catabolize the accumulated substrate, Gal-Gal-Glc-Cer. These in vitro studies indicated the feasibility of enzyme replacement and in particular, demonstrated that low levels (5 percent) of exogenous enzyme were capable of effecting normalization of substrate metabolism.

Since the major morbid manifestations of Fabry's disease are the result of progressive substrate deposition in the vascular endothelium, efforts to alter the course of the disease must focus on the depletion of the vascular endothelial glycosphingolipid deposits. Alternatively, if the amount of circulating glycosphingolipid could be decreased, less substrate would be available for uptake into the vessel walls by the LDL receptor-mediated pathway (see "Pathophysiology" section). Several studies support the concept that substrate in endothelial lysosomes can be depleted. Endothelial cells from hemizygotes with Fabry's disease were observed to lose slowly the accumulated substrate from intracellular inclusion bodies with time in culture [466]. More specifically, fibroblast globotriaosylcer-amide was exchanged into the HDL$_3$ fraction of the media under conditions in which there were no changes in the neutral lipid or phospholipid composition [390]. Finally, the vascular endothelial inclusions in a sural nerve biopsy from a Fabry hemizygote were apparently depleted following successful transplantation into the sciatic nerves of nude mice [596]. After 4 months, the human graft was identified by the presence of lamellar inclusions in the transplanted perineural cells and the smooth-muscle cells of an epineural artery. Significantly, the inclusions in the endothelium of epineural arteries and in the endothelial and perithelial cells of capillaries in the endo-, peri-, and epineurium, which were observed prior to transplantation, were no longer present. These studies suggest possible mechanisms for glycosphingolipid exchange by endothelial cells (or other cell types) and hydrophobic sites on the circulating lipoproteins. There may be transport systems for the distribution of glycosphingolipids into (LDL receptor) and out (HDL exchange) of various cell types. Alternatively, circulating enzyme may be taken up by cells, particularly endothelial cells, for *in situ* metabolism. The elucidation of these mechanisms will provide increased understanding of the dynamic interrelationships betwen globotriaosylceramide pools in the body as well as their vascular catabolism. This information will be crucial to the development of effective therapy for Fabry disease which might include (1) the direct targeting of active α-galactosidase A to the vascular endothelium, (2) enzyme delivery to the hepatocyte to decrease the availability of substrate which is presumably complexed with lipoproteins for secretion, or (3) the removal of the circulating substrate by mechanical procedures (e.g., plasmapheresis).

Several in vivo exploratory studies of enzyme replacement have been undertaken to determine its effectiveness and whether such endeavors can affect the circulating accumulated substrate concentration. Normal plasma containing active enzyme has been administered to hemizygotes with Fabry's disease [52]. Although active enzyme and decreased levels of Gal-Gal-Glc-Cer were demonstrated in the recipients' plasmas, the half-life in the circulation of the infused enzymatic activity was relatively short ($t_{1/2} \sim 95$ min). Subsequently, Brady and coworkers [53] partially purified a tissue form of α-galactosidase A from human placenta and administered single doses intravenously to two patients (6000 and 11,000 units, respectively). The exogenous activity was more rapidly cleared from the recipient's circulation with half-lives of 10 and 12 min, respectively. The plasma substrate was decreased about 50 percent at 45 min with a return to the preinfusion level by 48 h. In addition, the administered activity was detected in percutaneously biopsied liver at 1 h [53].

Recently, we reported the results of a clinical trial involving multiple injections of purified splenic and plasma forms of α-galactosidase A into two brothers with Fabry's disease [54]. These trials confirmed the previously observed differences in clearance rates of enzyme from the circulation and demonstrated for the first time the different kinetics of depletion and reaccumulation obtained with enzyme purified from tissue and from plasma sources [597]. The differential plasma clearance of the glycoprotein enzymes was presumably related to differences in their posttranslational modifications. The splenic form, which was rapidly cleared from the circulation ($t_{1/2} = 10$ min), contained few sialic acid residues. The plasma form was highly sialylated and was retained in the circulation ($t_{1/2} = 70$ min) [54]. These results are in accord with the Ashwell model

for the prolonged retention of sialylated glycoproteins in the circulation and the rapid clearance of desialylated glycoproteins [598].

A marked difference in the clearance of circulating substrate was observed after the administration of these isoenzymes [54, 597, 599]. The splenic enzyme effected a rapid decrease in the plasma concentration of accumulated substrate. The level of the circulating substrate decreased to approximately 50 percent of the preinfusion values at 15 min after injection, followed by a rapid return to preinfusion levels by 2 to 3 h. In contrast, the plasma enzyme resulted in a prolonged depletion of the circulating substrate. At 2 h after injection, the levels of Gal-Gal-Glc-Cer were decreased to 30 to 50 percent of the preinfusion values. Significantly, low levels were retained up to 12 to 24 h, and the substrate levels slowly returned to preinfusion levels after 36 to 72 h. When the total amount of substrate cleared with time was calculated by integrating the mean concentrations of Gal-Gal-Glc-Cer, the plasma enzyme appeared to have cleared about 25 times more substrate over time than the splenic form. For each administration, the total amount of circulating lipid cleared, based on the respective recipient's plasma volume, was less than the potential quantity of natural substrate that the administered enzymatic activity could hydrolyze in vitro. When two doses were administered on subsequent days, the plasma substrate level was reduced into the normal range [597]. In addition, these clinical trials demonstrated that multiple doses of either partially purified enzyme, administered over a 117-day period, did not elicit an immune response in the recipients.

Due to the limitations of human experimentation, it is difficult to determine the site(s) of hydrolysis of the circulating substrate following enzyme replacement. The fact that little, if any, substrate is hydrolyzed in the plasma [53, 414, 600] suggests that it is catabolized at other sites. Based on the differential plasma clearance kinetics of the plasma and splenic enzymes, their demonstrated partial uptake by the liver [599], and their differential effects on the depletion of circulating substrate, it is likely that the liver is a major site for substrate catabolism. This concept is supported by the demonstration of hepatic globotetraosylceramide degradation in cats with Sandhoff disease following intravenous administration of β-hexosaminidase A [601]. This hypothesis would require the circulating substrate to exchange between the hepatic and circulating pools. Alternatively or additionally the substrate may be exchanged between circulating and endothelial pools [390]. These and other potential mechanisms to account for the plasma substrate depletion in vivo have been considered [54, 597, 600]. Clearly, further studies are required not only to determine the site of substrate catabolism, but also the long-term biochemical and clinical effects of chronic enzyme replacement.

Recently, fetal liver has been transplanted in three hemizygotes with Fabry's disease in an attempt to replace the deficient enzyme [602–604]. The rise and subsequent fall in the levels of serum α-fetoprotein evidenced the initial survival and subsequent maturation of the fetal cells. Following transplantation, the α-galactosidase A levels in serum and leukocytes were unchanged, and the substrate levels in urine and serum were slightly decreased. The recipients noted subjective clinical improvement (e.g., increased sweating, no acroparesthesias, slightly decreased angiokeratoma). The effectiveness of fetal liver transplantation must await the long-term evaluation of these recipients to document its efficacy.

Another approach that has been employed to deplete the accumulated circulating substrate is chronic plasmapheresis [605, 606]. Three plasmaphereses performed at 2-day intervals resulted in a 70 percent reduction of the level of circulating Gal-Gal-Glc-Cer to a value within the normal range. A total of 23 mg of substrate was removed. The plasma substrate levels slowly returned to preplasmapheresis levels in 5 days. The major question to be resolved is whether intervention by chronic plasmapheresis will deplete enough substrate, compared to that newly synthesized, so that the net result is decreased substrate deposition in the important target site, the vascular endothelium. Thus, further evaluation is required to determine the value of this strategy in Fabry's disease.

Recent reviews of the various approaches for the treatment of enzyme deficiency diseases are available [396, 607].

This work was supported in part by a grant (1-578) from the March of Dimes Birth Defects Foundation, grants (AM 15174 and AM 12434) from the National Institutes of Health, and a grant (RR-71) from the Clinical Research Centers Program of the Division of Research Resources, National Institutes of Health. The authors are grateful to Ms. Linda Lugo for preparation of the manuscript.

REFERENCES

1. ANDERSON W: A case of angiokeratoma. *Brit J Dermatol* 10:113, 1898
2. FABRY J: Ein Beitrag zur Kenntnis der Purpura haemorrhagica nodularis (Purpura papulosa hemorrhagica Hebrae). *Arch Dermatol Syph* 43:187, 1898
3. FABRY J: Zur Klinik und Atiolgie des Angiokeratoma. *Arch Dermatatol u. Syph* 123:294, 1916
4. FABRY J: Uber einen Fall von Angiokeratoma circumscriptum Am. linken Oberschenkel. *Dermatatol Ztschr* 22:1, 1915
5. FABRY J: Weiterer Beitrag zur Klinik des Angiokeratoma naeviforme (Naevus angiokeratosus). *Dermatatol Wchnschr* 90:339, 1930
6. STEINER L, VOERNER H: Angiomatosis miliaris: Eine ideiopathische Gefasserkrankung. *Deutsch Arch Klin Med* 96:105, 1909
7. GUNTHER H: Anhidrosis und Diabetes insipidus. *Z Klin Med* 78:53, 1913
8. WEICKSEL J: Angiomatosis, bzw. Angiokeratosis universalis (eine sehr seltene Haut-und Gafasskrankheit). *Deutsch Med Wschr* 51:898, 1925
9. RUITER M, POMPEN AWM, WYERS JJG: Uber interne und pathologische-anatomische Befunde bei Angiokeratoma corporis diffusum (Fabry). *Dermatologica (Basel)* 94:1, 1947
10. POMPEN AWM, RUITER M, WYERS JJG: Angiokeratoma corporis diffusum (universale) Fabry, as a sign of an unknown internal disease: Two autopsy reports. *Acta Med Scand* 128:234, 1947
11. SCRIBA K: Zur Pathogenese des Angiokeratoma corporis diffusum Fabry mit cardio-vasorenalem Symptomenkomplex. *Verh Deutsch Ges Pathol* 34:221, 1950
12. HORNBOSTEL H, SCRIBA K: Zur Diagnostik des Angiokeratoma Fabry mit kardio-vasorenalem Symptomenkomplex als Phosphatidspeicherungskrank-heit durch Probeexcision der Haut. *Klin Wschr* 31:68, 1953
13. FESSAS P, WINTROBE MM, CARTWRIGHT GE: Angiokeratoma corporis diffusum universale (Fabry): First American report of a rare disorder. *Arch Intern Med* 95:469, 1955
14. WALLACE HJ: Angiokeratoma corporis diffusum. *Brit J Dermatol* 70:354, 1958
15. COLLEY JR, MILLER DL, HUTT MSR, WALLACE HJ, DE WARDENER HE: The renal lesion in angiokeratoma corporis diffusum. *Brit Med J* 7:1266, 1958
16. BURDA CD, WINDER PR: Angiokeratoma corporis diffusum universale (Fabry's disease) in female subjects. *Am J Med* 42:293, 1967
17. WISE D, WALLACE HJ, JELLINCK EH: Angiokeratoma corporis diffusum: A clinical study of eight affected families. *Quart J Med* 31:177, 1962
18. STILES FD, OPITZ JM: Diffuse angiokeratosis (Fabry's disease) in children (abstract). *Meeting of the Midwest Society for Pediatric Research*. Chicago, November, 1963
19. OPITZ JM, STILES FC, WISE D, VON GEMMINGEN G, RACE RR, SANDER R, CROSS EG, DE GROOT WP: The genetics of angiokeratoma corporis diffusum (Fabry's disease), and its linkage with Xg(a) locus. *Am J Hum Genet* 17:325, 1965
20. RUITER M: Angiokeratoma corporis diffusum Syndrom und seine Hauterscheinungen: Ubersicht und eignene Erfahrungen der letzten zehn Jarh. *Hautarzt* 9:15, 1958
21. RUITER M: Milestones in dermatology: Angiokeratoma corporis diffusum. *Excerpta Med* 8:61, 1959
22. SWEELEY CC, KLIONSKY B: Fabry's disease: Classification as a sphingolipidosis and partial characterization of a novel glycolipid. *J Biol Chem* 238:3148, 1963
23. SWEELEY CC, KLIONSKY B: Fabry's disease: The isolation and characterization of a ceramide-trihexoside from kidney. *Abstracts, Sixth International Congress of Biochemistry*. New York, 1964
24. SWEELEY CC, KLIONSKY B: Glycolipid lipidosis: Fabry's disease, in Stanbury JB, Wyngaarden JB, Fredrickson DS (eds): *The Metabolic Basis of Inherited Disease*, 2d ed. New York, McGraw-Hill, 1966, p 618
25. CHRISTENSON-LOU HO: A biochemical investigation of angiokeratoma corporis diffusum. *Acta Pathol Microbiol Scand* 68:332, 1966
26. VANCE DE, KRIVIT W, SWEELEY CC: Concentrations of glycosyl ceramides in plasma and red cells in Fabry's disease: A glycolipid lipidosis. *J Lipid Res* 10:188, 1969
27. DESNICK RJ, SWEELEY CC, KRIVIT W: A method for the quantitative determination of the neutral glycosphingolipids in urine sediment. *J Lipid Res* 11:31, 1970
28. DESNICK RJ, DAWSON G, DESNICK SJ, SWEELEY EC, KRIVIT W: Diagnosis of glycosphingolipidoses by urinary sediment analysis. *N Engl J Med* 284:739, 1971
29. DESNICK RJ, KRIVIT W: Fabry's disease: Early detection and heterozygote identification by urine sediment glycolipid analyses. *Proceedings of the American Society for Human Genetics*. Austin, Texas, October 10, 1968
30. KREMER GJ, DENK R: Angiokeratoma corporis diffusum (Fabry). Lipid-chemische Untersuchungen des Harnsediments. *Klin Wschr* 46:24, 1968
31. PHILIPPART M, SARLIEVE L, MANACORDA A: Urinary glycolipids in Fabry's disease: Their examination in the detection of atypical variants and the presymptomatic state. *Pediatrics* 43:201, 1969
32. MATALON R, DORFMAN A, DAWSON G, SWEELEY CC: Glycolipid and mucopolysaccharide abnormality in fibroblasts of Fabry's disease. *Science* 164:1522, 1969
33. BAGDALE JD, PARKER F, WAYS PO, MORGAN TE, LAGUNOFF D, EIDELMAN S: Fabry's disease: A correlative clinical, morphologic, and biochemical study. *Lab Invest* 18:681, 1968
34. SCHIBANOFF JM, KAMOSHITA S, O'BRIEN JS: Tissue distribution of glycosphingolipids in a case of Fabry's disease. *J Lipid Res* 10:515, 1969
35. MIYATAKE T: A study on glycolipid in Fabry's disease. *Jap J Exp Med* 39:35, 1969
36. JENSEN E: On the pathology of angiokeratoma corporis diffusum (Fabry). *Acta Pathol Microbiol Scand* 68:313, 1966
37. DESNICK RJ, BLEIDEN LD, SHARP HL, MOLLER JH: Cardiac valvular anomalies in Fabry's disease: Clinical, morphologic and biochemical studies. *Circulation* 54:818, 1976
38. WHERRET JR, HAKOMORI S: Characterization of a blood group B glycolipid, accumulating in the pancreas of a patient with Fabry's disease. *J Biol Chem* 218:3046, 1973
39. BRADY RO, GAL AE, BRADLEY RM, MARTENSSON E, WARSHAW AL, LASTER L: Enzymatic defect in Fabry's disease: Ceramide trihexosidase deficiency. *N Engl J Med* 276:1163, 1967
40. KINT JA: Fabry's disease, α-galactosidase deficiency. *Science* 167:1268, 1970
41. BENSAUDE I, CALLAHAN J, PHILIPPART M: Fabry's disease as an α-galactosidosis: Evidence for an α-configuration in trihexosyl ceramide. *Biochem Biophys Res Commun* 43:913, 1971
42. CLARKE JTR, WOLFE LS, PERLIN AS: Evidence for a terminal α-D-galactopyranosyl residue in galactosyl-galactosyl-glucosyl-ceramide from human kidney. *J Biol Chem* 246:5563, 1971
43. HAKOMORI SI, SIDDIQUI B, LI YT, LI SC, HELLERQVIST CB: Anomeric structures of globoside and ceramide trihexoside of human erythrocytes and hamster fibroblasts. *J Biol Chem* 246:2271, 1971
44. HANDA S, ARIGA T, MIYATAKE T, YAMAKAWA T: Presence of α-anomeric glycosidic configurations in the glycolipids accumulated in kidney with Fabry's disease. *J Biochem (Tokyo)* 69:625, 1971
45. LI YT, LI SC: Anomeric configuration of galactose residues in ceramide trihexosides. *J Biol Chem* 246:3769, 1971
46. SWEELEY CC, MAPES CA, KRIVIT W, DESNICK RJ: Chemistry and metabolism of glycosphingolipids in Fabry's disease. *Adv Exp Med Biol* 19:287, 1972
47. DESNICK RJ, ALLEN KY, DESNICK SJ, RAMAN MK, BERNLOHR RW, KRIVIT W: Enzymatic diagnosis of hemizygotes and heterozygotes. Fabry's disease. *J Lab Clin Med* 81:157, 1973
48. JOHNSON DL, DEL MONTE MA, COTLIER E, DESNICK RJ: Fabry disease: Diagnosis of hemizygotes and heterozygotes by α-galactosidase A activity in tears. *Clin Chim Acta* 63:81, 1975
49. MAPES CA, ANDERSON RL, SWEELEY CC: Trihexosyl ceramide: Galactosyl

hydrolase in normal human serum and plasma and its absence in patients with Fabry's disease. *Fed Abstr* 29:409, 1970

50. BRADY RO, UHLENDORF BW, JACOBSON CB: Fabry's disease: Antenatal diagnosis. *Science* 172:172, 1971

51. DESNICK RJ, SWEELEY CC: Prenatal detection of Fabry's disease, in Dorfman A (ed): *Antenatal Diagnosis*. Chicago, University of Chicago Press, 1971, p 185

52. MAPES CA, ANDERSON RL, SWEELEY CC, DESNICK RJ, KRIVIT W: Enzyme replacement in Fabry's disease, an inborn error of metabolism. *Science* 169:987, 1970

53. BRADY RO, TALLMAN JF, JOHNSON WG, GAL AE, LEAHY WR, QUIRK JM, DEKABAN AS: Replacement therapy for inherited enzyme deficiency: Use of purified ceramidetrihexosidase in Fabry's disease *N Engl J Med* 289:9, 1973

54. DESNICK RJ, DEAN KJ, GRABOWSKI GA, BISHOP DF, SWEELEY CC: Enzyme therapy XII: Enzyme therapy in Fabry's disease: Differential enzyme and substrate clearance kinetics of plasma and splenic α-galactosidase isozymes. *Proc Nat Acad Sci USA* 76:5326, 1979

55. SWEELEY CC, KLIONSKY B, KRIVIT W, DESNICK RJ: Fabry's disease, in Stanbury JB, Wyngaarden JB, Fredrickson DS (eds): *The Metabolic Basis of Inherited Disease*, 3d ed. New York, McGraw-Hill, 1972, p 663

56. DESNICK RJ, KLIONSKY B, SWEELEY C: Fabry's disease. Defective α-galactosidase A, in Stanbury JB, Wyngaarden JB, Fredrickson DS (eds): *The Metabolic Basis of Inherited Disease*, 4th ed. New York, McGraw-Hill, 1978, p 810

57. KAHLKE W: Angiokeratoma corporis diffusum (Fabry's disease), in Schettler G (ed): *Lipids and Lipidoses*. Berlin, Springer, 1967, p 332

58. KINT JA, CARTON D: Fabry's disease, in Hers HG, van Hoof F (eds): *Lysosomes and Storage Diseases*. New York, Academic, 1973, p 347

59. WALLACE HJ: Anderson-Fabry disease. *Brit J Dermatol* 88:1, 1973

60. DESNICK RJ, O'DEA RF, KRIVIT W: Fabry's disease—angiokeratoma corporis diffusum universale, in Schettler G, Greten H, Schierf G, Seidel D (eds): *Hanbuch Der Inneren Medizin*, Bland VII(4): Fettstoffwechsel. Heidelberg, Springer-Verlag, 1977, p 597

61. DEAN K, SWEELEY C: Fabry disease, in Glew RH, Peters SP (eds): *Practical Enzymology of the Sphingolipidoses*. New York, Alan R. Liss, 1977, p 173

62. LOCKMAN LA, HUNNINGHAKE DB, KRIVIT W, DESNICK RJ: Relief of pain of Fabry's disease by diphenylhydantoin. *Neurology* 23:871, 1973

63. JOHNSTON AW, WELLER SD, WARLAND BJ: Angiokeratoma corporis diffusum. Some clinical aspects. *Arch Dis Child* 43:73, 1968

64. SHETH KJ, BERNHARD GC: The arthropathy of Fabry disease. *Arthr Rheumat* 22:781, 1979

65. RAHMAN AN, SIMCONE FA, HACKEL DB, HALL PW III, HIRSCH EZ, HARRIS JW: Angiokeratoma corporis diffusum universale (hereditary dystopic lipidosis). *Trans Assoc Am Physicians* 74:366, 1961

66. FONE DJ, KING WE: Angiokeratoma corporis diffusum (Fabry's syndrome). *Aust Ann Med* 13:339, 1964

67. FRANCESCHETTI AT, PHILIPPART M, FRANCESCHETTI A: A study of Fabry's disease. I. Clinical examination of a family with cornea verticillata. *Dermatologica (Basel)* 138:209, 1969

68. FRANCOIS J, SNACKEN J, STOCKMANS L: Fabry's disease (glycolipid lipidosis). *Pathol Eu* 3:347, 1968

69. HAMBURGER J, DORMONT J, DE MONTERA H, HINGLAIS NO: Sur une singuliere malformation familiale de l'epithelium renal. *Schweiz Med Wschr* 94:871, 1964

70. JOHNSTON AW: Fabry's disease without skin lesions. *Lancet* 1:1277, 1967

71. JOHNSTON AW, WARLAND BJ, WELLER SDV: Genetic aspects of angiokeratoma corporis diffusum. *Ann Hum Genet* 30:25, 1966

72. KEMP GL: Fabry's disease involving the myocardium and coronary arteries. *Vasc Dis* 4:100, 1967

73. URBAIN G, PEREMANS J, PHILIPART M: Fabry's disease without skin lesions? *Lancet* 1:1111, 1967

74. WALLACE RD, COOPER WJ: Angiokeratoma corporis diffusum universale (Fabry). *Am J Med* 39:656, 1965

75. WYERS HJF, BRUGGE RJ, POMPE CA, PIJPERS PM: Histologische Aspecten bij Ziekte van Fabry (angiokeratoma corporis diffusum). *Nederl T Geneesk* 109:548, 1965

76. CLARKE JTR, KNAACK J, CRAWHALL JC, WOLFE LS: Ceramide trihexosidosis (Fabry's disease) without skin lesions. *N Engl J Med* 284:233, 1971

77. VOLK BW, SCHNECK L, CLEMMONS JE, NICASTRI AD: Fabry's disease in a black man without skin lesions. *Neurology* 24:991, 1971

78. AINSWORTH SK, SMITH RM: A case study of Fabry's disease occurring in Black kindred without peripheral neuropathy or skin lesions. *Lab Invest* 38:373, 1978

79. FERRANS VJ, HIBBS RB, BURDA CD: The heart in Fabry's disease: A histochemical and electron microscopic study. *Am J Cardiol* 24:95, 1969

80. MOSSARD JM, JOSSOT G, WOLFE LS, BATZENSCHLAGER A, STOEBNER P, METZGER H: The heart in Fabry's disease. *Arch Mal Coeur* 65:495, 1972

81. BECKER AE, SCHOORL R, BALK AG, VAN DER HEIDE RM: Cardiac manifestations of Fabry's disease. Report of a case with mitral insufficiency and electrocardiographic evidence of myocardial infarction. *Am J Cardiol* 36:829, 1975

82. FALCK I, WEICKSEL A: Angiokeratoma corporis diffusum Fabry mit vasorenalem Symptomenkomplex. *Samml Selt Klin Falle* 13:20, 1957

83. DUCAN C, McLEOD EM: Angiokeratoma corporis diffusum universale (Fabry's disease): A case with gross myocardial involvement. *Aust Ann Med* 1:58, 1970

84. ROUDEBUSH CP, FOERSTER VM, BING OHL: The abbreviated PR interval of Fabry's disease. *N Engl J Med* 289:357, 1973

85. MEHTA J, TUNA N, MOLLER JH, DESNICK RJ: Electrocardiographic and vectorcardiographic abnormalities in Fabry's disease. *Am Heart J* 93:699, 1977

86. MEHTA J, TUNA N, MOLLER JH, DESNICK RJ: Electrocardiographic and vectorcardiographic correlates in Fabry's disease. *Adv Cardiol* 21:220, 1977

87. ROWE JW, CARALIS DG: Accelerated atrioventricular conduction in Fabry's disease: A case report. *Angiology* 29:562, 1978

88. MEHTA J, TUNA N, MOLLER JA, DESNICK RJ: Electrocardiographic and vectorcardiographic observations in Fabry's disease. *Adv Cardiol* 21:220, 1978

89. BASS JL, SHRIVASTAVA S, GRABOWSKI GA, DESNICK RJ, MOLLER JH: The M-mode echocardiogram in Fabry's disease. *Am Heart J* 100:807, 1980

90. BETHUNE JE, LANDRIGAN PL, CHIPMAN CD: Angiokeratoma corporis diffusum (Fabry's disease in two brothers). *N Engl J Med* 264:1280, 1961

91. BEAUDET AL, CASKEY CT: Detection of Fabry's disease heterozygotes by hair root analysis. *Clin Genet* 13:251, 1978

92. MAISEY DN, COSH JA: Basilar artery aneurysm and Anderson-Fabry disease. *J Neurol Neurosurg Psych* 43:85, 1980

93. VAN ROEY A, WELLENS W: Angiokeratoma corporis diffusum van Fabry. *Arch Belg Dermatol Syph* 17:325, 1961

94. DUPERRAT B: L'Angiokeratome diffus de Fabry (angiokeratoma corporis diffusum). *Presse Med* 67:1814, 1959

95. CURRY HB, FLEISHER TL: Angiokeratoma corporis diffusum: A case report. *J Am Med Assoc* 175:864, 1961

96. STOUGHTON RB, CLENDENNING WE: Angiokeratoma corporis diffusum (Fabry). *Arch Dermatol (Chicago)* 79:601, 1959

97. GUIN GH, SAINI N, BURNS WA, JONES WP: Diffuse angiokeratoma (Fabry's disease): Case report. *Milit Med* 141:259, 1976

98. LISTON EH, LEVINE MD, PHILIPPART M: Psychosis in Fabry's disease and treatment with phenoxybenzamine. *Arch Gen Psychiat* 29:402, 1973

99. STEWARD VW, HITCHCOCK C: Fabry's disease (angiokeratoma corporis diffusum): A report of 5 cases with pain in the extremities as the chief symptom *Pathol Eur* 3:377, 1968

100. BROWN A, MILNE JA: Diffuse angiokeratoma: Report of two cases with diffuse skin changes, one with neurological symptoms and splenomegaly. *Glasgow J Med* 33:361, 1952

101. DUPERRAT B, PLUVINAGE G: Angiokeratose diffuse de Fabry avec hemiplegie. *Bull Soc Med Hop Paris* 72:748, 1956

102. HOFMAN A, HAUSER W: Angiokeratoma corporis diffusum (Fabry) with cerebral manifestations. *Deutsch Z Nervenheik* 183:351, 1962

103. PABICO RC, ATANACIO BC, McKENNA BA, PAMURCOGLU T, YODAIKEN R: Renal pathologic lesions and functional alterations in a man with Fabry's disease. *Am J Med* 55:415, 1973

104. PARKINSON JE, SUNSHINE A: Angiokeratoma corporis diffusum universale (Fabry) presenting as suspected myocardial infarction and pulmonary infarcts. *Am J Med* 31:951, 1961

105. SHETH KJ, TAN TT, GOOD TA: Fabry's disease in a black kindred. *Am J Dis Child* 133:1178, 1979

106. COLOMBI A, KOSTYAL A, BRACHER R, GLOOR F, MAZZI R, THOLEN H: Angiokeratoma corporis diffusum—Fabry's disease. *Helv Med Acta* 34:67, 1967

107. JACOB W, GAHLEN W, DIEKMANN H: Zur differential-diagnosides Angiokeratoma Fabry und der Periarteriitis nodosa. *Arz Wsch* 8:551, 1953

108. SHER NA, LETSON RD, DESNICK RJ: The ocular manifestations in Fabry's disease. *Arch Ophthalmol* 97:671, 1979

109. SHER NA, REIFF W, LETSON RD, DESNICK RJ: Central retinal artery occlusion complicating Fabry's disease. *Arch Ophthalmol* 96:815, 1978

110. FRANCESCHETTI ATh: Etude ophthalmologique, genetique et biochimique de la maladie de Fabry. Thesis, Geneva, 1973

111. BLOOMFIELD SE, DAVID DS, RUBIN AL: Eye findings in the diagnosis of Fabry's disease: Patients with renal failure. *J Am Med Assoc* 240:647, 1978

112. VISKOPER JR, MERIN S: Angiokeratoma corporis diffusum (Fabry's disease) with renal, ocular and possibly cardiac involvement. *Isr J Med Sci* 6:640, 1970

113. SCHMIDT D, ZIMMERMAN H: Internukleare ophthalmoplegie dei morbus Fabry-Anderson. *Klin Monatsbl Augenheilkd* 162:361, 1973

114. GEMIGNANI F, PIETRINI Y, TAGLIAVINI F, LECHI A, NERI TM, ASINARI A, SAVI M: Fabry's disease with familial lymphedema of the lower limbs. *Eur Neurol* 18:84, 1979

115. SPAETH GL, FROST P: Fabry's disease: Its ocular manifestations. *Arch Ophthalmol (Chicago)* 74:760, 1965

116. GRUBER H: Cornea verticillata. *Ophthalmologica* 111:120, 1946

117. FRANCESCHETTI ATH: La Cornea verticillata (Gruber) et ses relations avec la maladie de Fabry (angiokeratoma corporis diffusum). *Ophthalmologica* 156:232, 1968

118. FRANCESCHETTI A, FRANCESCHETTI ATH: Cornea verticillata et maladie de Fabry. II Symp. Lipidoses Cerebrales, Coimbra/Curia (1967). *Pathol Eur* 3:369, 1968

119. FRANCOIS J: Heterozygotes for sex-linked traits and Mary Lyon's inactivation theory. *Proc IIId Intl Cong Human Genetics.* Chicago, 1966, p 423

120. FRANCESCHETTI ATH: Etude ophthalmologique, genetique, et biochimique de la maladie de Fabry. *Chron Dermatol (Roma)* 4:370, 1974

121. FRANCESCHETTI ATH: Fabry disease. Ocular manifestations, in Bergsma D, Bron AJ, Cotlier E (eds): *The Eye and Inborn Errors of Metabolism. Birth Defects: Orig. Art. Ser. XII (3).* New York, Alan R Liss, 1976, p 195

122. PETROHELOS, MA: Chloroquine induced ocular toxicity. *Ann Ophthalmol* 6:615, 1974

123. PRICE JH: Angiokeratoma corporis diffusum. *Brit J Dermatol* 67:105, 1955

124. ROSENBERG DM, FERRANS VJ, FULMER JD, LINE BR, BARRANGER JA, BRADY RO, CRYSTAL RG: Chronic airflow obstruction in Fabry's disease. *Am J Med* 68:898, 1980

125. BARTIMMON EE JR, GUSAN M, MOSER KA: Pulmonary involvement in Fabry's disease: A reappraisal. Follow up of a San Diego kindred and review of the literature. *Am J Med* 53:755, 1972

126. KARIMAN K, SINGLETARY WV JR, SIEKER HO: Pulmonary involvement in Fabry's disease. *Am J Med* 64:911, 1978

127. PITTELKOW RB, KIERLAND RR, MONTGOMERY H: Polariscopic and histochemical studies in angiokeratoma corporis diffusum. *Arch Dermatol* 76:59, 1957

128. WILSON SK, KLIONSKY BL, RHAMY RK: A new etiology of priapism: Fabry's disease. *J Urol* 109:646, 1973

129. FUNDERBURK SJ, PHILIPPART M, DALE G, CEDERBAUM SD, VYDEN JK: Priapism after phenoxybenzamine in a patient with Fabry's disease. *N Engl J Med* 290:630, 1974

130. ROWE JW, GILLIAM JI, WARTHIN TA: Intestinal manifestations of Fabry's disease. *Ann Intern Med* 81:628, 1974

131. FLYNN D, LAKE B, BOTHBY CB, YOUNG EP: Gut lesions in Fabry's disease without a rash. *Arch Dis Child* 47:26, 1972

132. BYRAN A, KNAUFT RF, BURNS WA: Small bowel perforation in Fabry's disease. *Ann Intern Med* 86:315, 1977

133. HALSTED CH, ROWE JW: Occurrence of celiac sprue in a patient with Fabry's disease. *Ann Intern Med* 83:524, 1975

134. KRIVIT W, VANCE DE, DESNICK R, WHITECAR JP, SWEELEY CC: Red cell physiology in Fabry's disease. *J Lab Clin Med* 12:906, 1968

135. KARR WJ JR: Fabry's disease (angiokeratoma corporis diffusum universale): An unusual syndrome with multiple system involvement and unique skin manifestations. *Am J Med* 27:829, 1959

136. GARCIN R, HEWITT J, GODLEWSKI S, LAUDAT P, DE MONTERA H, EMILE J: Les Aspects neurologiques de l'angiokeratose de Fabry. A propos de deux cas. *Presse Med* 75:435, 1967

137. LILIS M, VULCAN P, PERESECENSCHI G: Notes on a case of angiokeratoma corporis diffusum (Fabry's disease). *Rum Med Rev* 20:29, 1966

138. PITTELKOW RB, KIERLAND RR, MONTGOMERY H: Angiokeratoma corporis diffusum. *Arch Dermatol* 72:556, 1955

139. LACTOUX R: Angiokeratome diffus (angiokeratoma corporis diffusum) de Fabry. *Bull Soc Franc Dermatol Syph* 67:474, 1960

140. RUITER M, VAN MULLEN PJ: Electron microscopy of angiokeratoma corporis diffusum. *Dermatologica (Basel)* 138:346, 1969

141. DE GROOT WP: Angiokeratoma corporis diffusum Fabry (thesaurismosis hereditaria Ruiter-Pompen-Wyers). *Dermatologica (Basel)* 128:321, 1964

142. DEMPSEY H, HARTLEY MW, CARROLL J, BALINT J, MILLER RE, FROMMEYER WB: Fabry's disease (angiokeratoma corporis diffusum): Case report on a rare disease. *Ann Intern Med* 63:1059, 1965

143. DUBACH UC, GLOOR F: Fabry-Krankheit (Angiokeratoma corporis diffusum universale). Phosphatid-speicherkrankheit bei zwei Familien. *Deutsch Med Wschr* 91:241, 1966

144. DESNICK RJ, ALLEN KY, SIMMONS RL, WOODS JE, ANDERSON CF, NAJARIAN JS, KRIVIT W: Correction of enzymatic deficiencies by renal transplantation: Fabry's disease. *Surgery* 72:203, 1972

145. AVILA JL, CONVIT J, VELAZQUEZ-AVILA G: Fabry's disease: Normal α-galactosidase activity and urinary-sediment glycosphingolipid levels in two obligate heterozygotes. *Brit J Dermatol* 89:149, 1973

146. WEINGEIST TA, BLODI FC: Fabry's disease: Ocular findings in a female carrier. A light and electron microscopic study. *Arch Ophthalmol* 85:169, 1973

147. VON GEMMINGEN G, KIERLAND RR, OPITZ JM: Antiokeratoma corporis diffusum (Fabry's disease). *Arch Dermatol (Chicago)* 91:206, 1965

148. JEFFRIES JL, BARRETT JC: Medical grand rounds from the University of Alabama Medical Center. *South Med J* 56:518, 1963

149. RAHMAN AN: The ocular manifestations of hereditary dystopic lipidosis (angiokeratoma corporis diffusum universale). *Arch Ophthalmol (Chicago)* 69:708, 1963

150. SIGUIER F, DUPERRAT B, BETOURNE C, HANAUT A: Angiokeratose de Fabry, expression cutanée d' une maladie generale, nouvellement individualisée. *Bull Soc Med Hop Paris* 72:291, 1956

151. WALLACE HJ, COLLEY C: Angiokeratoma corporis diffusum. *Bull Soc Franc Dermatol Syph* 4:348, 1958

152. LENG-LEVY J, LE COULANT C, DAVID-CHAUSEE M, MALEVILLE H, GENIAWX M: Angiokeratose familiale des membres inferieurs. *Bull Soc Franc Dermatol Syph* 71:740, 1964

153. CAMPBELL AMG, HALFORD MEH: Syndrome of diarrhea and peripheral nerve changes due to generalized vascular disease. *Brit Med J* 2:1509, 1964

154. TONDEUR M, RESIBOIS A: Fabry's disease in children: An electron microscopic study. *Virchow Arch (Zellpath)* 2:239, 1969

155. LEDER AA, BOSWORTH WC: Angiokeratoma corporis diffusum universale (Fabry's disease) with mitral stenosis. *Am J Med* 38:814, 1965

156. RUITER M, POMPEN AWM, WIJERS HJG: Angiokeratoma corporis diffusum (universale) als sympton van een onbekende en nog niet beschreven inwendige ziekte. *Nederl T Genesk* 90:1757, 1946

157. WITSCHEL H, MEYER W: Der Morbus Fabry als Beispiel einer erblichen Lipoidspeicherkrankheit. *Klin Wschr* 46:72, 1968

158. NAKAO K, MIZUNO Y, KANO S, SANTO H, YANO Y, MIZOGUCHI H, UONO M, SHIBATA S: A case of angiokeratoma corporis diffusum (Fabry's disease). *J Jap Soc Intern Med* 56:369, 1967

159. UNONO M: Fabry's disease—from the standpoint of neuronal lipidosis. *Jap J Clin Med* 25:1587, 1967

160. RUITER M: Histological investigation of the skin in angiokeratoma corporis diffusum in particular with regard to the associated disturbance of phosphatid metabolism. *Dermatological (Basel)* 109:273, 1954

161. HORNBOSTEL H: Das Angiokeratoma corporis diffusum universale mit kardio-vasorenalem Symptomenkomplex als neuartige Thesaurismoseform. *Helv Med Acta* 19:388, 1952

162. GERMAIN P, CAULET T, GIRARD P, ETIENNE JC, ADNET JJ, HOPFNER C: Angiokeratose de Fabry familiale avec retentissement vasculaire et polyvisceral. *Bull Soc Med Hosp* 118:299, 1967

163. FALCK I: Angiokeratoma corporis diffusum Fabry mit vasorenalem Symptomenkomplex. *Samml Selt Klin Falle* 9:20, 1955

164. RAHMAN AN, LINDENBERG R: The neuropathology of hereditary dystopic lipidosis. *Arch Neurol (Chicago)* 9:373, 1963

165. CAULET T, GERMAIN P, J-J, HOPFNER C, PLUOT M: Deux cas familiaux de maladie de Fabry: Etude structurale et ultrastructurale. *Ann Anat Pathol (Paris)* 12:49, 1967

166. RAINE DN: Biochemical classification of the sphingolipidoses, in Allan JD, Raine DN, (eds): *Some Inherited Disorders of Brain and Muscle.* Edinburgh, Livingston, 1969, p 89

167. SAGEBIEL RW, PARKER F: Cutaneous lesions of Fabry's disease: Glycolipid lipidosis—Light and electron microscopic findings. *J Invest Dermatol* 50:208, 1968

168. BREATHNACH SM, BLACK MM, WALLACE HJ: Anderson-Fabry disease: Characteristic ultrastructural features in cutaneous blood vessels in a 1 year old boy. *Brit J Dermatol* 103:81, 1980

169. TARNOWSKI WM, HASHIMOTO K: New light microscopic skin findings in Fabry's disease. *Acta Dermatol-Venereol* 49:386, 1969

170. MOREL-MAROGER L, GANTER P, ARDAILOU R, CATHELINEAU G, RICHET G: Des rapports avec l'angiokeratose de Fabry et la cytodystrophie remale familiale. *Bull Soc Med Hop Paris* 117:149, 1966

171. HASHIMOTO K, GROSS BG, LEVER WF: Angiokeratoma corporis diffusum (Fabry): Histochemical and electron microscopic studies of the skin. *J Invest Dermatol* 44:119, 1965

172. RUITER M: Some further observations on angiokeratoma corporis diffusum. *Brit J Dermatol* 69:137, 1957

173. WITSCHEL H, MEYER W: Fabry's disease: Clinical and pathologic studies of a clinical case. *Klin Wschr* 46:305, 1968

174. BISCHOFF A, FIERZ U, REGLI G, ULRICH J: Peripheral neurological disorders in Fabry's disease (angiokeratoma corporis diffusum universale): Clinical and electron microscopic findings in a case. *Klin Wschr* 46:666, 1968

175. PERRELET A, FORSSMAN WG, FRANCESCHETTI AT, ROUILLER CA: A study of Fabry's disease. II. Light and electron microscopy. *Dermatologica (Basel)* 138:222, 1969

176. SAGEBIEL R, PARKER F: Electron microscopic observations relating Fabry's disease to other sphingolipidoses. *Clin Res* 14:273, 1966

177. BRINDLEY HP, ARCHARD HO, ALLING CC, JURGENS PE, JURGENS EH: Angiokeratoma corporis duffusum (Fabry's disease). *J Oral Surg* 33:199, 1975

178. YOUNG WG, SAUK JJ JR, PHILSTROM B, FISH AJ: Histopathology and electron and immunofluorescence microscopy of gingivitis granulomatosa

associated with glossitis and cheilitis in a case of Anderson-Fabry disease. *Oral Surg* 46:540, 1978

179. EPINETTE WW, NORINS AL, DREW AL, ZEMAN W, PATEL V: Angiokeratoma corporis diffusum with α-L-fucosidase deficiency. *Arch Dermatol* 107:755, 1973

180. MIYATAKE T, ATSUMI T, OBAYASHI T, MIZUNO Y, ANDO S, ARIGA T, MATSUI-NAKAMURA K, YAMADA T: Adult type neuronal storage disease with neuraminidase deficiency. *Ann Neurol* 6:232, 1978

181. LOONEN MCB, VDLUGT L, FRANKE CL: Angiokeratoma corporis diffusum and lysosomal enzyme deficiency. *Lancet* 2:785, 1974

182. MCCALLUM DI, MACADAM RF, JOHNSTON AW: Angiokeratoma corporis diffusum with features of a mucopolysaccharidosis. *J Med Genet* 17:21, 1980

183. FROST P, SPAETH GL, TANAKA Y: Fabry's disease: Glycolipid lipidosis. Skin manifestations. *Arch Intern Med* 117:440, 1966

184. IMPERIAL R, HELIWIG EB: Angiokeratoma: A clinicopathological study. *Arch Dermatol (Chicago)* 95:166, 1967

185. VAN MULLEM PJ, RUITER M: Electron microscopic study of the skin in angiokeratoma corporis diffusum. *Arach Klin Exp Dermatol* 226:453, 1966

186. GUBLER MC, LENOIR G, GRUNFLED J-P, ULMANN A, DROZ D, HABIB R: Early renal changes in hemizygous and heterozygous patients with Fabry's disease *Kidney Intl* 13:223, 1978

187. ULMANN A, LENOIR G, BAUMANN N, GRUNFELD J-P: Diagnostic de la maladie de Fabry. *Nouv Presse Med* 5:2697, 1976

188. MCNARY W, LOWENSTEIN LM: A morphological study of the renal lesion in angiokeratoma corporis diffusum universale (Fabry's disease). *J Urol* 93:641, 1965

189. RAE AI, LEE JC, HOPPER J: Clinical and electron microscopic studies of a case of glycolipid lipidosis. *J Clin Pathol* 20:21, 1967

190. STIENNON M, GOLDBERG MF: Renal size in Fabry's disease. *Urol Radiol* 2:17, 1980

191. FUNCK-BRENTANO JL, DORMON J, MERY JP, DE MONTERA H, MOREIRA M: Les Lesions renales de l'angiokeratose de Fabry: A propos d'une observation. *J Urol Nephrol* 70:826, 1964

192. HENRY EW, RALLY CR: The renal lesion in angiokeratoma corporis diffusum (Fabry's disease). *Can Med Assoc J* 89:206, 1963

193. MALMQVIST E, IVEMARK BI, LINDSTEN J, MAUNSBACH AB, MARTENSSON E: Pathologic lysosomes and increased urinary glycosylceramide excretion in Fabry's disease. *Lab Invest* 25:1, 1971

194. MIYASKI K: Renal accumulation of glycosphingolipids. Report of a case and review of the literature. *Nephron* 14:456, 1975

195. BURKHOLDER PM, UPDIKE SJ, WARE RA, REESE OG: Clinopathologic, enzymatic and genetic features in a case of Fabry's disease. *Arch Pathol Lab Med* 104:17, 1980

196. GRUNNET ML, SPILSBURY PR: The central nervous system in Fabry's disease. *Arch Neurol* 28:231, 1973

197. KOCEN RS, THOMAS PK: Peripheral nerve involvement in Fabry's disease. *Arch Neurol* 22:81, 1970

198. KAHN P: Anderson-Fabry disease: A histopathological study of three cases with observations on the mechanism of production of pain. *J Neurol Neurosurg Psych* 36:1053, 1973

199. OHNISHI A, DYCK PJ: Loss of small peripheral sensory neurons in Fabry disease. Histologic and morphometric evaluation of cutaneous nerves, spinal ganglia, and posterior columns. *Arch Neurol* 31:120, 1974

200. TABIRA T, GOTO I, KUROIWA Y, KIKUCHI M: Neuropathological and biochemical studies in Fabry's disease. *Acta Neuropathol* 30:345, 1974

201. SUNG JH, MASTRI AR, DESNICK RJ: Neuropathology and neural glycosphingolipid deposition in Fabry's disease. *J Neuropathol Exp Neurol* in press

202. TOME FMS, FARDEAU M, LEOIR G: Ultrastructure of muscle and sensory nerve in Fabry disease. *Acta Neuropathol* 38:187, 1977

203. SUNG JH: Autonomic neurons affected by lipid storage in the spinal cord of Fabry's disease: Distribution of autonomic neurons in the sacral cord. *J Neuropathol Exp Neurol* 38:87, 1979

204. FIERZ V, BISCHOFF A: Angiokeratoma corporis diffusum. *Dermatologica (Basel)* 137:277, 1968

205. RAHMAN AN: The pathological basis of neurophysiological dysfunctions in hereditary dystopic lipidosis (angiokeratoma corporis diffusum universale). *Clin Res* 10:393, 1962

206. SIMA AAF, ROBERTSON DM: Involvement of peripheral nerve and muscle in Fabry's disease. *Arch Neurol* 35:291, 1978

207. VISSER SL, DE GROOT WP: Electroencephalographic and electromyographic changes in a case of angiokeratoma corporis diffusum (Fabry's disease). *Confin Neurol* 32:25, 1970

208. SETH KJ, SWICK HM: Peripheral nerve conduction in Fabry's disease. *Ann Neurol* 7:319, 1980

209. FROST P, TANAKA Y, SPAETH GL: Fabry's disease—Glycolipid lipidosis: Histochemical and electron microscopic studies of two cases. *Am J Med* 40:618, 1966

210. LIBERT J, TONDEUR M, VAN HOOF F: The use of conjunctival biopsy and enzyme analysis in tears for the diagnosis of homozygotes and heterozygotes with Fabry disease. *Birth Defects: Orig Art Ser* 12:221, 1976

211. WITSCHEL H, MATHYL J: Morphological elements of the specific ocular changes in Morbus Fabry. *Klin Mbl Augenheilk* 154:599, 1969

212. FRANCOIS J, HANSSENS M, TEUCHY H: Corneal ultrastructural changes in Fabry's disease. *Ophthalmologica* 176:313, 1978

213. TRIPATHI RC, ASHTON N: Application of electron microscopy to the study of ocular inborn errors of metabolism, in Bergsma D, Bron AJ, Cotlier E (eds): *The Eye and Inborn Errors of Metabolism. Birth Defects: Orig Art Ser* 12:69, 1976

214. FRIEDMAN AH, RIEGEL EM, POKORNY KS, SUHAN J, RITCH RH, DESNICK RJ: Ocular pathology in Fabry's disease. *Survey Ophthalmol* in press

215. DUFIER JL, GUBLER MC, DHERMY P, LENOIR G, PAUPE J, HAYE C: La maladie de Fabry et ses manifestations ophthalmologiques. *J Fr Ophthalmol* 3:625, 1980

216. FONT RL, FINE BS: Ocular pathology in Fabry's disease. Histochemical and electron microscopic observations. *Am J Ophthalmol* 73:419, 1972

217. KNAPE BM, POLMAN HA: Fabry's disease diagnosed in childhood. *Nederl T Geneesk* 113:1418, 1969

218. DENK R, SOLLBERG G: Skelet Muskelbefunde beim Angiokeratoma corporis diffusum. *Hautarzt* 17:248, 1966

219. ADAMS CWM: *Neurohistochemistry*. Amsterdam, Elsevier, 1965

220. FARRAGINA T, CHURG J, GRISHAM E, STRAUSS L, PRADO A, BISHOP DF, SCHUCHMAN E, DESNICK RJ: Light and electron microscopic histochemistry of Fabry disease. *Am J Pathol* 103:247, 1981

221. LEHNER T, ADAMS CWM: Lipid histochemistry of Fabry's disease. *J Pathol Bactiol* 95:411, 1968

222. VAN MULLEM PJ, RUITER M: Histochemical studies on lipid metabolism in so-called Fabry's disease (angiokeratoma corporis diffusum). *Arch Klin Exp Dermatol* 232:148, 1968

223. GOSSRAU R: Uber den histochemischen Nachweis der β-glucuronidase, α-mannosidase and α-galactosidase mit 1-Naphthylglykosiden. *Histochemie* 36:367, 1973

224. HARTLEY MW, MILLER RE: Renal and vascular changes in Fabry's disease, a dysphospholipidosis. *L Cell Biol* 1963

225. HARTLEY MW, MILLER RE, LUPTON CH JR: Dysphospholipidosis in Fabry's disease: A light and electron microscopic study. *Alabama J Med Sci* 1:361, 1964

226. VAN MULLEM PJ, RUITER M: Electron microscopical investigation of the skin in angiokeratoma corporis diffusum. *Dermatologica (Basel)* 136:281, 1968

227. VAN MULLEM PJ, RUITER M: Fine structure of the skin in angiokeratoma corporis diffusum (Fabry's disease). *J Pathol* 101:221, 1970

228. RUITER M, DE GROOT WP: Methods of demonstration of lipid deposits in angiokeratoma corporis diffusum. *Dermatologica (Basel)* 135:75, 1967

229. TARNOWSKI WM, HASHIMOTO K: Lysosomes in Fabry's disease. *Acta Dermatol-Venereol* 48:143, 1968

230. ARCHARD HO, BRINDLEY HP: Ultrastructural observations of the oral mucosa in Anderson-Fabry disease. *J Oral Pathol* 4:273, 1975

231. HASHIMOTO K, LIEBERMAN P, LAMKIN N JR: Angiokeratoma corporis diffusum (Fabry's disease). *Arch Dermatol* 112:1416, 1976

232. SAVI M, OLIVETTI G, NERI TM, CURTONI C: Clinical, histopathological, and biochemical findings in Fabry's disease. A case report and family study. *Arch Pathol Lab Med* 101:536, 1977

233. SCHATZKI PF, KIPREOS B, PAYNE J: Fabry disease: Primary diagnosis by electron microscopy. *Am J Surg Pathol* 3:211, 1979

234. NAKAMURA T, KANEKO H, NISHINO I: Angiokeratoma corporis diffusum (Fabry disease): Ultrastructural studies of the skin. *Acta Dermatovener* 61:37, 1981

235. LOEB H, JONNIAUX G, DAVIS P, GREGOIRE PE, WOLFF P: Etude clinique, biochimique et ultrastructurelle de la maladie de Fabry chez l'enfant. *Helv Paediatr Acta* 23:269, 1968

236. DELBARRE F, LAOUSSADI S, KAHAN A, MENKES C, AUBOUY G: Le Rhumatisme des thesaurismoses a lipides. Arthropathies au cours de la carence en α-galactosidase A (maladie de Fabry). Etude ultrastructurale de la membrane synoviale avec mise en evidence de microcristaux dans les mitochondires des synoviocytes. *CR Acad Sci Paris* 288:579, 1979

237. TANAKA Y, FROST P, SPAETH GL: Figures myeliniques dans les cellules spumeuses de la maladie de Fabry. *Nouv Rev Franc Hemat* 5:425, 1965

238. MCLEAN J, STEWART G: Fabry's disease: Specific inclusions found on electron microscopy of fibroblast cultures. *J Med Genet* 11:133, 1974

239. YUASA T, FUKUMA M, TAKASHIMA S, TAKAKI R: Cultured skin fibroblasts in lipidoses. *Arch Pathol Lab Med* 104:321, 1980

240. LEE RF, BALCERZAK SP, WESTERMAN MP: Gaucher's disease: A morphologic study and measurements of iron metabolism. *Am J Med* 42:891, 1967

241. ROTH J, ROTH H: Elektronenmikroskopische Befunde an inneren Organen bei Morbus Fabry. *Virchows Arch A Pathol Anat Histol* 378:75, 1978

242. WEINREB NJ, BRADY RO, TAPPEL AL: The lysosomal localization of sphingolipid hydrolases. *Biochim Biophys Acta* 159:141, 1968

243. DUPOISOT H, CONSTANS A, DAURY G, DELBARE F, LAOUSSADI S: Etude par transformation Fourier optique, des depots de glycolipides dans le cas de la maladie de Fabry. *CR Acad Sci Paris* 288:783, 1979

244. JORDAN SW: Electron microscopy of Gaucher cells. *Exp Molec Pathol* 3:76, 1964

245. CRAIN RC, ZILVERSMIT DB: Net transfer of phospholipid by the nonspecific phospholipid transfer proteins from bovine liver. *Biochim Biophys Acta* 620:37, 1980

246. STECK TL, DAWSON G: Topographical distribution of complex carbohydrates in the erythrocyte membrane. *J Biol Chem* 239:2135, 1974

247. WIEGANDT H: Glycosphingolipids, in Paoletti R, Kritchevsky D (eds): *Advances in Lipid Research*. New York, Academic, 1971, p 249

248. KARLSSON KA: On the chemistry and occurrence of sphingolipid long-chain bases, in Sweeley CC (ed): *Chemistry and Metabolism of Sphingolipids*. Amsterdam, North-Holland Publishing Company, 1970, p 6

249. PROSTENIK M: Organic chemistry of sphingolipids, in Burton RM, Guerra FC (eds): *Fundamentals of Lipid Chemistry*. St. Louis, BI-Science International, 1974, p 307

250. PURO K, KERANEN A: Fatty acids and sphingosines of bovine-kidney gangliosides. *Biochim Biophys Acta* 187:383, 1969

251. SVENNERHOLD L, STALLVERG-STENHAGEN S: Changes in the fatty acid composition of cerebrosides and sulfatides of human nervous tissue with age. *J Lipid Res* 9:215, 1968

252. MARTENSSON E: Neutral glycolipids of human kidney. Isolation, identification and fatty acid composition. *Biochim Biophys Acta* 116:296, 1966

253. COLES E, FOOTE JL: Fatty acids of glycosphingolipids from pig blood fractions. *J Lipid Res* 11:433, 1970

254. MARTENSSON E: Glycosphingolipids of animal tissue, in Holman RT (ed): *Progress in the Chemistry of Fats and Other Lipids*. Oxford, Pergamon, 1969, p 367

255. SWEELEY CC, DAWSON G: Lipids of the erythrocyte, in Jamieson GA, Greewalt TJ (eds): *Red Cell Membrane Structure and Function*. Philadelphia, Lippincott, 1970, p 172

256. SWEELEY CC, SIDDIQUI B: Chemistry of glycolipids, in Pigman W, Horowitz M (eds): *Biochemistry of Mammalian Glycoproteins and Glycolipids*. New York, Academic, in press

257. MACHER BA, SWEELEY CC: Glycosphingolipids: Structure, biological source and nomenclature. *Meth Enzymol* 50C, 1978, p 236

258. MAKITA A: biochemistry of organ glycolipids. II. Isolation of human kidney glycolipids. *J Biochem Tokyo* 55:269, 1964

259. LEVIS GM, KARLI JN, MOULOPOULOS SC: Isolation and partial characterization of the neutral glycosphingolipids and gangliosides of the human heart. *Lipids* 14:9, 1979

260. KLENK E, LAUENSTEIN K: Uber die zuckerhaltigen Lipoide der Formbestandtiele des menschlichen Blutes. *Ztchr Physiol Chem* 288:220, 1951

261. VANCE DE, SWEELEY CC: Quantitative determination of the neutral glycosyl ceramides in human blood. *J Lipid Res* 8:621, 1967

262. HILDEBRAND J, STRYCKMANS P, VANHOUCHE J: Gangliosides in leukemic and non-leukemic human leukocytes. *Biochim Biophys Acta* 260:272, 1972

263. MACHER BA, KLOCK JC: Isolation and characterization of neutral glycosphingolipids of human neutrophils. *J Biol Chem* 255:2092, 1980

264. NARASIMHAN R, MURRAY RK: Neutral glycosphingolipids and gangliosides of human lung and lung tumors. *Biochem J* 176:199, 1979

265. SNYDER PD Jr, DESNICK RJ, KRIVIT W: The glycosphingolipids and glycosyl hydrolases of human blood platelets. *Biochem Biophys Res Commun* 46:1857, 1972

266. WOND CT, SCHICK PK: The effect of thrombin on the organization of human platelet membrane glycosphingolipids. The sphingosine composition of platelet glycolipids and ceramides. *J Biol Chem* 256:752, 1981

267. TAO RVP, SWEELEY CC, JAMIESON GA: Sphingolipid composition of human platelets. *J Lipid Res* 14:16, 1973

268. KWITEROVICH RO, SLOAN HR, FREDRICKSON DS: Glycolipids and other lipid constituents of normal human liver. *J Lipid Res* 11:322, 1970

269. DAWSON G: Detection of glycosphingolipids in small samples of human tissue. *Ann Clin Lab Sci* 2:274, 1972

270. SNYDER PD Jr, KRIVIT W, WEELEY CC: Generalized accumulation of neutral glycosphingolipids with G_{M2} ganglioside accumulation in the brain. *J Lipid Res* 13:128, 1972

271. CHIEN JL, HOGAN EL: Glycosphingolipids of skeletal muscle, in Sweeley CC (ed): *Cell Surface Glycolipids*. ACS Symp. Ser., 128. Washington, DC, 1980, p 135

272. DAWSON G, KRUSKI AW, SCANU AM: Distribution of glycosphingolipids in the serum lipoproteins of normal human subjects and patients with hypo- and hyper-lipidemias. *J Lipid Res* 17:125, 1976

273. CLARKE JTR, STOLTZ JM, MULCAHY MR: Neutral glycosphingolipids of serum lipoproteins in Fabry's disease. *Biochim Biophys Acta* 431:317, 1976

274. DESNICK RJ, ZAVORAL J, KRIVIT W: Unpublished results

275. VAN DEN BERGH FAJTM, TAGER JM: Localization of neutral glycosphingolipids in human plasma. *Biochim Biophys Acta* 441:391, 1976

276. CLARKE JTR, STOLTZ JM, GARNER JB: Stability of plasma low density lipoprotein with abnormal glycolipid composition from patients with Fabry's disease. *Atherosclerosis* 35:155, 1980

277. CHATTERJEE S, KWITEROVICH PO: Glycosphingolipids of human plasma lipoproteins. *Lipids* 11:462, 1976

278. CHATTERJEE S, KWITEROVICH PO, SEKERKE CS: Alterations in cell surface glycosphingolipids and their metabolism in familial hypercholesterolemic fibroblasts, in Sweeley CC (ed): *Cell Surface Glycolipids*. ACS Symp. Ser., 128. Washington, DC, 1980, p 265

279. NAIKI M, MARCUS DM: Human erythrocyte P and P^k blood group antigens: Identification as glycosphingolipids. *Biochim Biophys Res Commun* 60:1105, 1974

280. KOSCIELAK J, MILLER-PODRAZA H, KRAUZE R, CEDERGREN B: Glycolipid composition of blood group P erythrocytes. *FEBS Lett* 66:250, 1976

281. MARCUS DM, NAIKI M, KUNDU SK: Abnormalities in the glycosphingolipid content of human P^k and P erythrocytes. *Proc Nat Acad Sci USA* 73:3263, 1976

282. ETO Y, SUZUKI K: Brain sphingoglycolipids in Krabbe's globoid cell leukodystrophy. *J Neurochem* 18:503, 1971

283. NORTON WT, PODUSLO SE, SUZUKI J: Subacute sclerosing leukoencephalitis. II. Chemical studies including abnormal myelin and an abnormal ganglioside pattern. *J Neuropathol Exp Neurol* 25:582, 1966

284. CUMINGS JN, THOMPSON EJ, GOODWIN H: Sphingolipids and phospholipids in microsomes and myelin from normal and pathological brains. *J Neurochem* 15:243, 1968

285. CUZNER ML, DAVIDSON AN: The lipid composition of rat brain myelin and subcellular fractions during development. *Biochem J* 106:29, 1968

286. KISHIMOTO Y, AGRANOFF BW, RADIN NS, BURTON RM: Comparison of the fatty acids of lipids of subcellular brain fractions. *J Neurochem* 16:397, 1969

287. DEVRIES GH, NORTON WT: Evidence for the absence of myelin and the presence of galactolipid in an axon-enriched fraction from bovine CNS. *Fed Proc* 30:1248, 1971

288. RAGHAVAN S, KANFER JN: Ceramide galactoside of enriched neuronal and glial fractions from rat brain. *J Biol Chem* 247:1055, 1972

289. SVENNERHOLM L: Gangliosides and other glycolipids of human placenta. *Acta Chem Scand* 19:1506, 1965

290. WELLS HW, JONES M: Galactosylceramides in human plasma. *Am J Clin Pathol* 60:890, 1973

291. YAMAKAWA T, IIDA T: Immunochemical study on the red blood cells. I. Globoside, as the agglutinogen of the ABO system on erythrocytes. *Jap J Exp Med* 23:327, 1953

292. ANDO S, KOU J, ISOBE M, NAGAI Y, YAMAKAWA T: Existence of glucosaminyl lactosyl ceramide (Amino CTH-I) in human erythrocyte membranes as a possible precursor of blood group-active glycolipids. *J Biochem (Tokyo)* 79:625, 1976

293. SIDDIQUI B, HAKOMORI S: A ceramide tetrasaccharide of human erythrocyte membrane reacting with anti-type. XIV. Pneumococcal polysaccharide antiserum. *Biochim Biophys Acta* 330:147, 1973

294. WHERRETT JR: Characterization of the major ganglioside in human red cells and of a related tetrahexosyl ceramide in white cells. *Biochim Biophys Acta* 326:63, 1973

295. SVENNERHOLM L, BRUCE A, MANSSON JE, RAYNMARK BM, VANIER MT: Sphingolipids in human skeletal muscle. *Biochim Biophys Acta* 280:626, 1972

296. STELLNER K, WATANABE K, HAKOMORI S: Isolation and characterization of glycosphingolipids with blood group H specificity from membranes of human erythrocytes. *Biochemistry* 12:656, 1973

297. KOSCIELAK J, PIASEK A, GORNIAK H, GARDAS A, GREGOR A: Structures of fucose-containing glycolipids with H and B blood group activity and of sialic acid and glucosamine-containing glycolipid of human-erythrocyte membrane. *Eur J Biochem* 37:214, 1973

298. WATANABE K, HAKOMORI S: Status of blood group carbohydrate chains in ontogenesis and in oncogenesis. *J Exp Med* 144:644, 1976

299. HAKOMORI S, JEANLOZ RW: Isolation of a glycolipid containing fucose, galactose, glucose and glucosamine from human cancerous tissue. *J Biol Chem* 239:PC3606, 1964

300. HAKOMORI S, ANDREWS HD: Sphingoglycolipid with Le^b activity, and the co-presence of Le^a- and Le^b-glycolipid in human tumor tissue. *Biochim Biophys Acta* 202:225, 1970

301. THUDICHUM JLW: *The Chemical Constitution of the Brain*. London, Balliere, Tindall and Cox, 1884

302. McKIBBIN JM: The composition of the glycolipids in dog intestine. *Biochemistry* 8:379, 1969

303. SLOMIANY BL, SLOMIANY A, HOROWITZ MI: Sulfatides of hog gastric mucosa. *Biochim Biophys Acta* 348:388, 1974

304. FOLCH M, LEES M, SLOANE-STANLEY GH: A simple method for the isolation and purification of total lipids from animal tissues. *J Biol Chem* 226:497, 1957

305. VANCE WR, SHOOK CP III, MCKIBBIN JM: The glycolipids of dog intestine. *Biochemistry* 5:435, 1966

306. CARTER HE, ROTHFUS JA, GIGG R: Biochemistry of the sphingolipids. XII. Conversion of cerebrosides to ceramides and sphingosine: Structure of Gaucher cerebroside. *J Lipid Res* 2:228, 1961

307. GRAY JM: The isolation and partial characterization of the glycolipids of BP8/C3H ascites-sarcoma cells. *Biochem J* 94:91, 1965

308. MAKITA A, YAMAKAWA T: Biochemistry of organ glycolipid. I. Ceramideoligohexosides of human, equine, and bovine spleens. *J Biochem (Tokyo)* 51:124, 1962

309. GALLAI-HATCHARD JJ, GRAY GM: The isolation and partial characterization of the glycolipids from pig lung. *Biochim Biophys Acta* 116:532, 1966

310. YAMAKAWA T, IRIE R, IWANAGA M: The chemistry of lipid of posthemolytic residue or stroma of erythrocytes. IX. Silicic acid chromatography of mammalian stroma glycolipids. *J Biochem (Tokyo)* 48:490, 1960

311. SVENNERHOLM E, SVENNERHOLM L: The separation of neutral blood-serum glycolipids by thin-layer chromatography. *Biochim Biophys Acta* 70:441, 1963

312. ANDO S, ISOBE M, NAGAI Y: High performance preparative column chromatography of lipids using a new porous silica, iatro-beads. *Biochim Biophys Acta* 424:98, 1976

313. RADIN NS: Florisil chromatography. *Meth Enzymol* 14:268, 1969

314. PHILIPPART M, ROSENSTEIN B, MENKES JH: Isolation and characterization of the main splenic glycolipids in the normal organ and in Gaucher's disease: Evidence for the site of metabolic block. *Biochim Biophys Res Commun* 15:551, 1964

315. MIRAS CJ, MANTZOS JD, LEVIS JM: The isolation and partial characterization of glycolipids of normal human leucocytes. *Biochem J* 98:782, 1966

316. ROUSER G, KRITCHEVSKY G, YAMAMOTO A: Column chromatographic and associated procedures for separation and determination of phosphatides and glycolipids, in Marinetti GV (ed): *Lipid Chromatographic Analysis.* New York, Marcel Dekker, 1967, p 99

317. IWAMORI M, NAGAI Y: A new chromatographic approach to the resolution of individual gangliosides. *Biochim Biophys Acta* 528:257, 1978

318. YAMAZAKI T, SUZUKI A, HANDA S, YAMAKAWA T: Consecutive analysis of sphingoglycolipids on the basis of sugar and ceramide moieties by high performance liquid chromatography. *J Biochem (Tokyo)* 86:803, 1979

319. YAHARA S, KISHIMOTO Y, PODSULO J: High performance liquid chromatography of membrane glycolipids. Assessment of cerebrosides on the surface of myelin, in Sweeley CC (ed): *Cell Surface Glycolipids.* ACS Symp. Ser., 128. Washington, DC, 1980, p 15

320. NONAKA G, KISHIMOTO Y: Simultaneous determination of picomole levels of glucosyl and galactosylcerebroside, monogalactosyl diglyceride, and sulfatide by high performance liquid chromatography. *Biochim Biophys Acta* 572:423, 1979

321. TJADEN UR, KROL JH, von HOEVEN RP, OOMEN-MEULEMANS EPM, EMMELOT P: High pressure liquid chromatography of glycosphingolipids (with special reference to gangliosides). *J Chromatogr* 136:233, 1977

322. YAHARA S, MOSER HW, KOLODNY EH, KISHIMOTO Y: Reverse phase high performance liquid chromatography of cerebrosides, sulfatides, and ceramides. Microanalysis of homolog composition without hydrolysis and application to cerebroside analysis in peripheral nerves of adrenoleukodystrophy patients. *J Neurochem* 34:694, 1980

323. MCCLUER RH, ULLMAN MD: Preparative and analytical high performance liquid chromatography of glycolipids, in Sweeley CC (ed): *Cell Surface Glycolipids.* ACS Symp. Ser., 128. Washington, DC, 1980, p 1

324. MCCLUER RH, EVANS JE: Preparation and analysis of benzoylated cerebrosides. *J Lipid Res* 14:611, 1973

325. ULLMAN MD, MCCLUER RH: Quantitative analysis of plasma neutral glycosphingolipids by high performance liquid chromatography of their perbenzoyl derivatives. *J Lipid Res* 18:371, 1977

326. SUZUKI A, HANDA S, YAMAKAWA T: Separation of molecular species of higher glycolipids by high performance liquid chromatography of their O-acetyl-N-p-nitrobenzoyl derivatives. *J Biochem (Tokyo)* 82:1185, 1977

327. ESSELMAN WJ, LAINE RA, SWEELEY CC: Isolation and characterization of glycosphingolipids. *Meth Enzymol* 28:140, 1972

328. SKIPSKI VP: Thin-layer chromatography of neutral glycosphingolipids. *Meth Enzymol* 35:396, 1975

329. HAKOMORI S, WATANABE K: Blood group glycolipids of human erythrocytes, in Witting LA (ed): *Glycolipid Methodology.* Champaign, Illinois, Amer. Oil. Chem. Soc., 1976, p 13

330. GAVER RC, SWEELEY CC: Methods for methanolysis of sphingolipids and direct determination of long-chain bases by gas chromatography. *J Am Oil Chem Soc* 42:294, 1965

331. CHAMBERS RE, CLAMP JL: An assessment of methanolysis and other factors used in the analysis of carbohydrate-containing materials. *Biochem J* 125:1009, 1971

332. LAINE RA, STELLNER K, HAKOMORI S: Isolation and characterization of

333. BJORNDAL H, HELLERQVIST CG, LINDBERG B, SVENSSON S: Gas-liquid chromatography and mass spectrometry, in *Methylation Analysis of Polysaccharides,* intern ed, Agnew. Chem., 9:610, 1970

334. BREIMER ME, HANSSON GC, KARLSSON K-A, LEFFLER H, PIMLOTT W, SAMUELSSON BE: Selected ion monitoring of glycosphingolipid mixtures. Identification of several blood group type glycolipids in the small intestine of an individual rabbit. *Biomed Mass Spectrum* 6:231, 1979

335. DABROWSKI J, HANFLAND P, EGGE H: Structural analysis of glycosphingolipids by high resolution 'H nuclear magnetic resonance spectroscopy. *Biochemistry* 19:5652, 1980

336. FALK K-E, KARLSSON K-A, SAMUELSSON BE: Proton nuclear magnetic resonance analysis of anomeric structure of glycosphingolipids. *Arch Biochem Biophys* 192:191, 1979

337. SWEELEY CC, MOSKAL JR, NUNEZ H, MATSUURA F: Structural analysis of glycoconjugates by mass spectrometry of permethylated derivatives and by ^{13}C NMR spectroscopy, in Varmavuori A (ed): *Proceedings of 27th International Congress of Pure and Applied Chemistry.* New York, Pergamon, 1980, p 233

338. KOERNER TAW, CARY LW, LI S-C, LI YT: Carbon 13 NMR spectroscopy of a cerebroside. *J Biol Chem* 254:2326, 1978

339. SILLERUD LO, PRESTEGARD JH, YU RK, SCHAFER DE, KONIGSBURG WH: Assignment of the ^{13}C nuclear magnetic resonance spectrum of aqueous ganglioside G_{M1} micelles. *Biochemistry* 17:2619, 1978

340. LI Y-T: Enzymatic methods for structural analysis of complex carbohydrates, in Gregory JD, Jeanloz RW (eds): *Glyconjugate Research.* New York, Academic, 1979, vol 1, p 3

341. YAMAKAWA T, NAGAI Y: Glycolipid at the cell surface and their biological functions. *Trends Biol Sci* 3:128, 1978

342. NAGAI Y, IWAMORI M: Brain and thymus gangliosides: Their molecular diversity and its biological implications and a dynamic annular model for their function in surface membranes. *Mol Cell Biochem* 29:81, 1980

343. KARLSSON K-A: in Abrahamsson S, Pascher I (eds): *Structures of Biological Membranes.* New York, Plenum, 1977, p 245

344. FISHMAN PH, BRADY RO: The biosynthesis and function of gangliosides. *Science* 194:906, 1976

345. SVENNERHOLM L, FREDMAN P, ELWING H, HOLMGREN J, STRANNEGARD O: Gangliosides as receptors for cholera toxin, tetanus toxin and sendai virus, in Sweeley CC (ed): *Cell Surface Glycolipids.* ACS Symp. Ser., 128. Washington, DC, 1980, p 373

346. HANSSON H-A, HOLMGREN J, SVENNERHOLM L: Ultrastructural localization of cell membrane G_{M1} ganglioside by cholera toxin. *Proc Nat Acad Sci USA* 74:3782, 1977

347. ABRAHAMSSON S, DAHLEN G, LOFGREN H, PASCHER I, SUNDELL S: in Abrahamsson S, Pascher I (eds): *Structures of Biological Membranes.* New York, Plenum, 1977, p 1

348. PARODI A, LELOIR L: The role of lipid intermediates in the glycosylation of proteins in the eucaryotic cell. *Biochim Biophys Acta* 559:1, 1979

349. HUBBARD SC, ROBBINS P: Synthesis and processing of protein-linked oligosaccharides *in vivo. J Biol Chem* 254:4568, 1979

350. ROSEMAN S: The synthesis of complex carbohydrates by multiglycosyltransferase systems and their potential function in intercellular adhesion. *Chem Phys Lipids* 5:270, 1970

351. DEN H, KAUFMAN B, ROSEMAN S: Properties of some glycosyltransferases in embryonic chicken brain. *J Biol Chem* 245:6607, 1970

352. DiCESARE JC, DAINE JA: The enzymic synthesis of ganglioside. IV. UDP-N-acetylgalactosamine: (N-acetylneuraminyl)-galactosylglucosyl ceramide N-acetylgalactosaminyl-transferase in rat brain. *Biochim Biophys Acta* 231:385, 1971

353. STOOLMILLER AC, BITTNER SL: Localization of sialyltransferase activity in the plasma membrane of cultured mouse neuroblastoma cells. *J Cell Biol* 55:251a, 1972

354. KEENAN TW, MORRE DJ, BASU S: Ganglioside biosynthesis. Concentration of glycosphingolipid glycosyltransferases in Golgi apparatus from rat liver. *J Biol Chem* 249:310, 1974

355. RICHARDSON CL, KEENAN TW, MOORE DJ: Ganglioside biosynthesis, characterization of CMP-N-acetylneuraminic acid: Lactosylceramide sialyltransferase in Golgi apparatus from rat liver. *Biochim Biophys Acta* 488:88, 1977

356. RICHARDSON CL, MERRITT WD, KEENAN TW, MOORE DJ: Enzymatic synthesis of trisialoganglioside by particulate fractions of rat liver. *Experientia* 34:571, 1978

357. PACUSZKA T, DUFFARD RO, NISHIMURA RN, BRADY RO, FISHMAN PH: Biosynthesis of bovine thyroid gangliosides. *J Biol Chem* 253:5839, 1978

358. KIJIMOTO-OCHIAI S, YOKOSAWA N, MAKITA A: Mechanism for the biosynthesis of Forssman glycolipid from trihexosylceramide. *J Biol Chem* 255:9037, 1980

359. HAKOMORI S: Structures and organization of cell surface glycolipids:

membrane glycosphingolipids, in Korn ED (ed): *Methods in Membrane Biology.* New York, Plenum, 1974, p 205

Dependency on cell growth and malignant transformation. *Biochim Biophys Acta* 417:55, 1975

360. CHATTERJEE S, SWEELEY CC, VELICER LF: Glycosphingolipids of human KB cells grown in monolayer, suspension, and synchronized cultures. *J Biol Chem* 250:61, 1975

361. DAWSON G, McLAWHON RW, SCHOON G, MILLER RJ: Modulation of ganglioside synthesis by eukephalins, opiates, and prostaglandins. Role of cyclic AMP in glycosylation, in Sweeley CC (ed): *Cell Surface Glycolipids*. ACS Symp. Ser., 128. Washington, DC, 1980, p 359

362. ERICKSON RL, PURCHIO AF, ERICKSON E, COLLETT MS, BRUGGE IS: Molecular events in cells transformed by Rous sarcoma virus. *J Cell Biol* 87:319, 1980

363. HUNTER T, SEFTON BM: Transforming gene product of Rous sarcoma virus phosphorylates tyrosine. *Proc Nat Acad Sci USA* 77:1311, 1980

364. LEVINSON AD, OPPERMANN H, VARMUS HE, BISHOP JM: The purified product of the transforming gene of avian sarcoma virus phosphorylates tyrosine. *J Biol Chem* 255:11973, 1980

365. FISHMAN PH: Normal and abnormal biosynthesis of gangliosides. *Chem Phys Lipids* 13:305, 1974

366. SWEELEY CC, FUNG Y-K, MACHER BA, MOSKAL JR, NUNEZ HA: Structure and metabolism of glycolipids, in Walborg EE Jr (ed): *Glycoproteins and Glycolipids in Disease Processes*. ACS Symp. Ser., 80. Washington, DC, 1978, p 47

367. HAKAMORI S: Cell growth control and antigenic expression through membrane glycosphingolipids, in Gregory JD, Jeanloz RW (eds): *Glycoconjugate Research*. New York, Academic, vol 2, p 965

368. DAWSON G: Glycolipid biosynthesis, in Horowitz MI, Pigman W (eds): *The Glycoconjugates*. New York, Academic, 1978, vol 2, p 256

369. BASU S, KAUFMAN B, ROSEMAN S: Enzymatic synthesis of ceramide-glucose glycosyltransferases from embryonic chicken brain. *J Biol Chem* 243:5802, 1968

370. HAUSER G: The enzymatic synthesis of ceramide lactoside from ceramide glucoside and UDP-galactose. *Biochem Biophys Res Commun* 28:502, 1967

371. BOUHOURS J-F, GLICKMAN RM: Rat intestinal glycolipids. II. Distribution and biosynthesis of glycolipids and ceramide in villus and crypt cells. *Biochim Biophys Acta* 441:123, 1976

372. STOFFYN A, STOFFYN P, HAUSER G: Structure of trihexosylceramide biosynthesized *in vitro* by rat kidney galactosyltransferase. *Biochim Biophys Acta* 360:174, 1974

373. HILDEBRAND J, HANSEN G: Biosynthesis of lactosylceramide and triglycosylceramide by galactosyltransferases from rat spleen. *J Biol Chem* 244:5170, 1969

374. CHIEN JL, WILLIAM TJ, BASU S: Biosynthesis of a globoside-type glycosphingolipid by a β-N-acetylgalactosaminyltransferase from embryonic chicken brain. *J Biol Chem* 248:1778, 1973

375. KIJIMOTO S, ISHIBASHI T, MAKITA A: Biosynthesis of Forssman hapten from globoside by α-N-acetylgalactosaminyltransferase of guinea pig tissues. *Biochem Biophys Res Commun* 56:177, 1974

376. ISHIBASHI T, KIJIMOTO S, MAKITA A: Biosynthesis of globoside and Forssman Hapten from trihexosylceramide and properties of β-N-acetylgalactosaminyltransferase of guinea pig kidney. *Biochim Biophys Acta* 337:92, 1974

377. ISHIBASHI T, ATSUTA T, MAKITA A: Effects of uridine nucleotides and nucleotide pyrophosphatase on glycolipid α- and β-N-acetylgalactosaminyltransferase activities in guinea pig microsomes. *Biochim Biophys Acta* 429:759, 1976

378. PRUZANSKI W, SHUMAK KH: Biological activity of cold-reacting autoantibodies. *N Engl J Med* 297:583, 1977

379. WATANABE K, HAKAMORI S, CHILDS RA, FEIZI T: Characterization of a blood group I-active ganglioside. *J Biol Chem* 254:3221, 1979

380. STEIN KE, MARCUS DM: Glycosphingolipid of purified human lymphocytes. *Biochemistry* 16:5285, 1977

381. VAKIRTZI-LEMONIAS C, EVANGELATOS GP, KAPOULAS VM, LEVIS GM: Studies on glycosphingolipid biosynthesis by lectin-stimulated human lymphocytes. *Eur J Biochem* 109:541, 1980

382. BASU S: Biosynthesis *in vitro* and the pattern of lectin binding receptors in monkey kidney cell surfaces. *Biochem Biophys Res Commun* 66:1380, 1975

383. BASU S, BASU M, CHIEN JL: Enzymatic synthesis of a blood group H-related glycosphingolipid by an α-fucosyltransferase from bovine spleen. *J Biol Chem* 250:2956, 1975

384. PRESPER KA, BASU M, BASU S: Biosynthesis *in vitro* of fucose-containing glycosphingolipids in human neuroblastoma IMR-32 cells. *Proc Nat Acad Sci USA* 75:289, 1978

385. BROWN MS, KOVANEN PT, GOLDSTEIN JL: Regulation of plasma cholesterol by lipoprotein receptors. *Science* 212:628, 1981

386. DAWSON G, SWEELEY CC: *In vivo* studies on glycosphingolipid metabolism in porcine blood. *J Biol Chem* 245:410, 1970

387. TAO RVP: Biochemistry and metabolism of mammalian blood glycosphingolipids. PhD Thesis, Michigan State University, 1973

388. VANCE DE, KRIVIT W, SWEELEY CC: Metabolism of neutral glycosphingolipids in plasma of a normal human and a patient with Fabry's disease. *J Biol Chem* 250:8119, 1975

389. ENTENMAN C, CHAIKOFF IL, ZILVERSMIT DB: Removal of plasma phospholipids as a function of the liver: The effect of exclusion of the liver on the turnover rate of plasma phospholipids as measured with radioactive phosphorus. *J Biol Chem* 166:15, 1946

390. KWOK BCP, DAWSON G, RITTER MC: Stimulation of glycolipid synthesis and exchange by human serum high density lipoprotein-3 in human fibroblasts and leukocytes. *J Biol Chem* 256:92, 1981

391. GOLDSTEIN JL, BROWN MS: The LDL receptor locus and the genetics of familial hypercholesterolemia. *Ann Rev Genet* 13:259, 1979

392. CHEN WW: Metabolism of oleylsphingosine containing low density lipoprotein in cultured human fibroblasts. 72d Annual Meeting of Amer. Soc. Biol. Chem. 40:1693, 1981

393. DAWSON G: Glycolipid catabolism, in Horowitz MI, Pigman W (eds): *The Glycoconjugates*. New York, Academic, 1978, vol 2, p 285

394. GLEW RH, PETERS SP: *Practical Enzymology of the Sphingolipidoses*. New York, Alan R Liss, 1977

395. KUSIAK JW, QUIRK JM, BRADY RO: Ceramide trihexoside from human placenta. *Meth Enzymol* 50:529, 1978

396. DESNICK RJ (ed): *Enzyme Therapy in Genetic Diseases: 2*. New York, Alan R Liss, 1980

397. LI S-C, YIRABAYASHI Y, LI Y-T: A protein activator for the enzymatic hydrolysis of G_{M2}-ganglioside. *J Biol Chem* in press

398. HECHTMAN P: Characterization of an activating factor required for hydrolysis of G_{M2}-ganglioside catalyzed by hexosaminidase A. *Can J Biochem* 55:315, 1977

399. CONZELMAN E, SANDHOFF K: AB variant of infantile G_{M2}-gangliosidosis: Deficiency of a factor necessary for stimulation of hexosaminidase A-catalyzed degradation of ganglioside G_{M2} and glycolipid G_{A2}. *Proc Nat Acad Sci USA* 75:3979, 1978

400. LI S-C, NAKAMURA T, OGAMA A, LI Y-T: Evidence for the presence of two separate protein activators for the enzymic hydrolysis of G_{M1} and G_{M2} gangliosides. *J Biol Chem* 254:10592, 1979

401. BRADY RO, GAL AE, BRADLEY RM, MARTENSSON E: The metabolism of ceramide trihexosides. I. Purification and properties of an enzyme that cleaves the terminal galactose molecule of galactosylgalactosylglucosylceramide. *J Biol Chem* 242:1021, 1967

402. BEUTLER E, KUHL W: Biochemical and electrophoretic studies of α-galactosidase in normal man, in patients with Fabry's disease, and in Equidae. *Am J Hum Genet* 24:237, 1972

403. WOOD S, NADLER HL: Fabry's disease: Absence of an α-galactosidase isozyme. *Am J Hum Genet* 24:250, 1972

404. SNYDER PD JR, WOLD F, BERNLOHR RW, DULLUM C, DESNICK RJ, KRIVIT W, CONDIE RM: Enzyme therapy II. Purified human α-galactosidase A. Stabilization to heat and protease degradation by complexing with antibody and by chemical modification. *Biochim Biophys Acta* 350:432, 1974

405. BEUTLER E, GUINTO E, KUHL W: Variability of α-galactosidase A and B in different tissues of man. *Am J Hum Genet* 25:42, 1973

406. BEUTLER E, KUHL W: Relationship between human α-galactosidase isozymes. *Nat New Biol* 239:207, 1972

407. ROMEO G, DiMATTEO G, D'URSO M, LI S-C, LI Y-T: Characterization of human α-galactosidase A and B before and after neuraminidase treatment. *Biochim Biophys Acta* 391:349, 1975

408. KANO I, YAMAKAWA T: The properties of α-galactosidase remaining in kidney and liver of patients with Fabry's disease. *Chem Phys Lipids* 13:283, 1974

409. HO MW, BEUTLER S, TENNANT L, O'BRIEN JS: Fabry's disease: Evidence for a physically altered α-galactosidase. *Am J Hum Genet* 24:256, 1972

410. BISHOP DF, DESNICK RJ: Affinity purification of α-galactosidase A from human spleen, placenta and plasma with elimination of pyrogen contamination. *J Biol Chem* 256:1307, 1981

411. KINT JA, HUYS A: Effect of bacterial neuraminidase on the isoenzymes of acid hydrolases of human brain and liver, in Zamlotti V, Tettamanti G, Arrigoni M (eds): *Glycolipids, Glycoproteins and Mucopolysaccharides of the Nervous System*. New York, Plenum, 1972, p 273

412. DEAN KJ, SWEELEY CC: Studies on human liver α-galactosidases. I. Purification of α-galactosidase A and its enzymatic properties with glycolipid and oligosaccharide substrates. *J Biol Chem* 254:9994, 1979

413. MAYES JS, BEUTLER E: α-Galactosidase A from human placenta. *Biochim Biophys Acta* 484:408, 1977

414. BISHOP DF, SWEELEY CC: Plasma α-galactosidase A. Properties and comparisons with tissue α-galactosidases. *Biochim Biophys Acta* 525:399, 1978

415. MALHOTRA OP, SINGH H: Effect of kinetic paramaters and inhibitors on α-galactosidase of coffee beans. *Indian J Biochem Biophys* 13:316, 1976

416. CARCHON H, DeBRYNE CK: Purification and properties of coffee bean α-galactosidase. *Carb Res* 41:175, 1975

417. DEY PM, WALLENFELS K: Isolation and characterization of α-galactosidase from *Lens esculanta*. *Eur J Biochem* 50:107, 1974

418. HARPAZ N, FLOWERS HM, SHARON N: α-D-Galactosidase from soybeans destroying blood group B antigens. *Eur J Biochem* 77:419, 1977

419. LAZO PS, OCHOA AG, GASCON S: α-Galactosidase from *S. cerlsbergensis*. *Eur J Biochem* 77:375, 1977

420. LAZO PS, OCHOA AG, GASCON S: α-Galactosidase from *S. cerlsbergensis*: Structural and kinetic properties. *Arch Biochem Biophys* 91:316, 1978

421. YATES AD, MORGAN WTJ, WATKINS WM: Linkage-specific α-galactosidases from *T. foetus*. Characterization of the blood group B destroying enzyme as α1,3-galactosidase and the blood group P₁-destroying enzyme as a α1,4-α-galactosidase. *FEBS Lett* 60:281, 1975

422. SCHMID K, SCHMITT R: Raffinose metabolism in *E. coli* K12. Purification and properties of a new α-galactosidase specified by a transmissible plasmid. *Eur J Biochem* 67:95, 1976

423. KILPATRICK DC, STIRLING JL: Properties and developmental regulation of an α-galactosidase from *D. discoidem*. *Biochem J* 158:409, 1976

424. BEUTLER E, KUHL W: Purification and properties of human α-galactosidases. *J Biol Chem* 247:195, 1972

425. JOHNSON WG, BRADY RO: Ceramide trihexoside from human placenta. *Meth Enzymol* 28:849, 1972

426. HO MW: Hydrolysis of ceramide trihexoside by a specific α-galactosidase from human liver. *Biochem J* 133:1, 1973

427. BISHOP DF, DEAN KJ, SWEELEY CC, DESNICK RJ: Purification and characterization of human α-galactosidase isozymes, in Desnick RJ (ed): *Enzyme Therapy in Genetic Diseases: 2*. New York, Alan R Liss, 1980, p 17

428. KANO I, YAMAKAWA T: Human kidney α-galactosidases. Multiplicity and enzyme activities for ceramide trihexoside and some aryl α-galactosides. *J Biochem (Tokyo)* 75:347, 1974

429. LUSIS AJ, PAIGEN K: Properties of mouse α-galactosidase. *Biochim Biophys Acta* 437:487, 1976

430. CRAWHALL JC, BANFALVI M: Fabry's disease: Differentiation between two forms of α-galactosidase by myoinositol. *Science* 177:527, 1972

431. KUSIAK JW, QUIRK JM, BRADY RO, MOOK GE: Purification and properties of the two major isozymes of α-galactosidase from human placenta. *J Biol Chem* 253:184, 1978

432. KORNFELD S, LI E, TABAS I: The synthesis of complex type oligosaccharides. *J Biol Chem* 253:7771, 1978

433. REITMAN ML, KORNFELD S: UDP-N-acetylglucosamine: Glycoprotein N-acetylglucosamine-I-phosphotransferase. *J Biol Chem* 256:4275, 1981

434. WAHEED A, POHLMANN A, HASILIK A, VON FIGURA K: Subcellular location of two enzymes involved in the synthesis of phosphorylated recognition markers in lysosomal enzymes. *J Biol Chem* 256:4150, 1978

435. KAPLAN A, ACHORD DT, SLY WS: Phosphohexosyl components of a lysosomal enzyme are recognized by pinocytosis receptors on human fibroblasts. *Proc Nat Acad Sci USA* 74:2026, 1977

436. FISCHER HD, GONZALEZ-NORIEGA A, SLY WS: β-Glucuronidase binding to human fibroblast membrane receptors. *J Biol Chem* 255:5069, 1980

437. DEAN K, SUNG S-SJ, SWEELEY CC: Purification and partial characterization of human liver α-galactosidase. Is α-galactosidase B an α-N-acetylgalactosaminidase? *Fed Proc* 36:731, 1977

438. RIETRA PJGM, TAGER JM, BORST P: Detection and properties of an acid α-galactosidase (ceramide trihexosidase) in normal human urine. *Biochim Biophys Acta* 279:436, 1972

439. LI S-C, WAN C-C, MAZZOTTA MY, LI Y-T: Requirement of an activator for the hydrolysis of sphingoglycolipids by glycosidases of human liver. *Carb Res* 34:189, 1974

440. PETERS SP, COYLE C, COFFEE CJ, GLEW R, KULENSCHMIDT MS, ROSENFELD L, LEE YC: Purification and properties of a heat-stable glucocerebrosidase activating factor from control and Gaucher spleen. *J Biol Chem* 252:563, 1977

441. WILKINSON GN: Statistical estimations in enzyme kinetics. *Biochem J* 80:324, 1969

442. GATT S, BARENHOLZ Y, BORKOVSKI-KUBILER I, LEIBOVITZ-BEN GERSHON Z: Interaction of enzymes with lipid substrates, in Volk BW, Aronson SM (eds): *Sphingolipids, Sphingolipidoses and Allied Disorders*. New York, Plenum, 1972, p 237

443. HILL AV: A new mathematical treatment of changes of ionic concentration in muscle and nerve under the action of electric currents, with a theory as to their mode of excitation. *J Physiol (London)* 40:190, 1910

444. DOWEL JE, RIGGS DS: A comparison of estimates of Michaelis-Menton kinetic constants from various linear transformations. *J Biol Chem* 240:863, 1965

445. SALVAYRE R, MARET A, NEGRE A, DOUSTE-BLAZY L: Properties of multiple molecular forms of α-galactosidase and α-N-acetylgalactosaminidase from normal and Fabry leukocytes. *Eur J Biochem* 100:377, 1979

446. DEAN K, SWEELEY CC: Studies on human liver α-galactosidases. II. Purification and enzymatic properties of α-galactosidase B (α-N-acetylgalactosaminidase). *J Biol Chem* 254:10001, 1979

447. DEAN KJ, SUNG S-SJ, SWEELEY CC: The identification of α-galactosidase B

448. from human liver as an α-N-acetylgalactosaminidase. *Biochem Biophys Res Commun* 77:1411, 1977

448. SCHRAM AW, HAMERS MN, TAGER JM: The identity of α-galactosidase B from human liver. *Biochim Biophys Acta* 482:138, 1977

449. MAPES CA, SWEELEY CC: Interconversion of the A and B forms of ceramide trihexosidase from human plasma. *Arch Biochem Biophys* 158:297, 1973

450. KINT JA: On the existence and the enzymic interconversion of the isozymes of α-galactosidase in human organs. *Arch Intern Physiol Biochem* 79:633, 1971

451. SCHRAM AW, HAMERS MC, BROUWER-KELDER B, DONKER-KOOPMAN WE, TAGER JM: Enzymological properties and immunological characterization of α-galactosidase isozymes from normal and Fabry human liver. *Biochim Biophys Acta* 482:125, 1977

452. RIETRA PJGM, MOLENAAR JL, HAMERS MN, TAGER JM, BORST P: Investigation of the α-galactosidase deficiency in Fabry's disease using antibodies against the purified enzyme. *Eur J Biochem* 46:89, 1974

453. SUNG S-SJ, SWEELEY CC: Purification and partial characterization of porcine liver α-N-acetylgalactosaminidase. *J Biol Chem* 255:6589, 1980

454. LEVY GN, AMINOFF D: Purification and properties of α-N-acetylgalactosaminidase from *Clostridium perfringens*. *J Biol Chem* 255:11737, 1980

455. SWEELEY CC, SNYDER PD, GRIFFEN CE: Chemistry of glycosphingolipids in Faby's disease. *Chem Phys Lipids* 4:393, 1970

456. SHAPIRO D, ACHER AJ: Total synthesis of ceramide trihexoside accumulating with Fabry's disease. *Chem Phys Lipids* 197:206, 1978

457. KLIONSKY B, SWEELEY CC: Unpublished results

458. PARODI AJ, BEHRENS NH, LELOIR LF, CARMINATTI H: The role of polyprenol-bound saccharides as intermediates in glycoprotein synthesis in liver. *Proc Nat Acad Sci USA* 69:3268, 1972

459. RIETRA PJGM, VAN DEN BERGH FAJTM, TAGER JM: Properties of the residual α-galactosidase activity in the tissues of a Fabry hemizygote. *Clin Chim Acta* 62:401, 1975

460. BEUTLER E, KUHL W: Absence of cross-reactive antigen in Fabry disease. *N Engl J Med* 289:694, 1973

461. HAMERS MN, WISE D, EJIOFOR A, STRIJLAND A, ROBINSON D, TAGER JM: Relationship between biochemical and clinical features in an English Anderson-Fabry family. *Acta Med Scand* 206:5, 1979

462. ROMEO G, URSO M, PISACANE A, BLUM E, DE FALCO A, RUFFILLI A: Residual activity of α-galactosidase A in Fabry's disease. *Biochem Genet* 13:615, 1975

463. ROMEO G, CHILDS B, MIGEON BR: Genetic heterogeneity of α-galactosidase in Fabry's disease. *FEBS Lett* 27:161, 1972

464. LEAVY J, BISHOP DF, DESNICK RJ: Unpublished results

465. BISHOP DF, KOVAC C, DESNICK RJ: Unpublished results

466. JOHNSON DL, DESNICK RJ: Molecular pathology of Fabry's disease: Physical and kinetic properties of α-galactosidase A in cultured human endothelial cells. *Biochim Biophys Acta* 538:195, 1978

467. CLARKE JTR, STOLTZ JM: Uptake of radiolabeled galactosyl-(α1→4)-galactosyl-(β1→4)-glucosylceramide by human lipoproteins *in vitro*. *Biochim Biophys Acta* 441:165, 1976

468. ATZPODIEN W, KREMER GJ SCHNELLBACHER E: Konzentration und Verteilung der Plasmaglycosphingolipide bei verschiedenen Hyperlipoproteinamien. *Klin Wschr* 54:585, 1976

469. STEIN O, STEIN Y: High density lipoproteins reduce the uptake of low density lipoproteins by human endothelial cells in culture. *Biochim Biophys Acta* 431:363, 1976

470. GOLDSTEIN JL, BROWN MS: The low density lipoprotein pathway and its relation to atherosclerosis. *Ann Rev Biochem* 46:897, 1977

471. BROWN MS, KOVANEN PT, GOLDSTEIN JL: Regulation of plasma cholesterol by lipoprotein receptors. *Science* 212:628, 1981

472. VLODAVSKY I, FIELDING PE, FIELDING CJ, GOSPODAROWICZ D: Role of contact inhibition in the regulation of receptor-mediated uptake of low density lipoprotein in cultured vascular endothelial cells. *Proc Nat Acad Sci USA* 75:356, 1979

473. SHEPHARD J, BICKER S, LORIMER AR, PACKARD CJ: Receptor-mediated low density lipoprotein catabolism in man. *J Lipid Res* 20:999, 1979

474. SHEPHARD J, PACKARD CJ, BICKER S, LAWRIE TDV, MORGAN HG: Cholestyramine promotes receptor-mediated low-density lipoprotein catabolism. *N Engl J Med* 302:1219, 1980

475. BARKAI A, DiCESARE JL: Influence of sialic acid groups on the retention of glycosphingolipids in blood plasma. *Biochim Biophys Acta* 398:287, 1975

476. VAN DEN BERGH FAJ-ThM: Biochemical studies on Fabry's disease. Pathogenesis of glycosphingolipid accumulation and problems in therapy. Thesis, University of Amsterdam, 1978, p 75

477. KINT JA, DACREMONT G: ABO blood groups and lysosomal diseases. *N Engl J Med* 285:121, 1971

478. DESNICK RJ: Unpublished results

479. DILORENZY PA, KLEINFELD J, TELLMAN W, NAY L: Angiokeratoma corporis diffusum (Fabry's disease). *Acta Dermatovener (Stockholm)* 49:319, 1969

480. FUKUHARA N, SUZUKI M, FUJITA N, TSUBAKI T: Fabry's disease on the mechanism of the peripheral nerve involvement. *Acta Neuropathol* 33:9, 1975

481. CABLE WJL, KOLODNY EH, ADAMS RD: Fabry disease: A clinical demonstration of impaired autonomic function. *Neurology* 30:352, 1980 (abstract)

482. WISE D: Diffuse angiokeratoma (J. Fabry), in *Jadassohn's Handbuch des Haut und Geschlechtskrankheiten*. Berlin, Springer, 1966, vol 7, sec 743

483. VOGELBERG KH, SOLBACH HG, GRIES FA: Lipoidchemische Untersuchungen beim Angiokeratoma corporis diffusum (Fabry-syndrome). *Klin Wschr* 47:916, 1969

484. DE GROOT WP: Genetic aspects of the thesaurismosis lipoidica hereditaria Ruiter-Pompen-Wyers (angiokeratoma corporis diffusum Fabry). *Dermatologica (Basel)* 129:281, 1964

485. JOHNSTON AW, FROST P, SPAETH GL, RENWICK JH: Linkage relationships of the angiokeratoma (Fabry) locus. *Ann Hum Genet (London)* 32:369, 1969

486. DESNICK RJ: Biochemical and genetic studies of Fabry's disease. PhD thesis, University of Minnesota, 1970

487. BRADY RO: Genetics and the sphingolipidoses. *Med Clin N Am* 53:327, 1969

488. GARZA TOBA M: Angioqueratoma corporis diffusum. Comunicación de un caso clínico. *Medicina (Mexico)* 37:525, 1957

489. RODRIGUEZ O: Angioqueratomas. Comunicación de un caso de angioqueratoma corporis diffusum. *Dermatológica (Mexico)* 1:309, 1957

490. MADDEN FC: Papilliform lesions (lymphangioma) of the scrotum. Associated with multiple petechial spots on the trunk and limbs. *Brit Med J* 2:302, 1912

491. KUANG-YUAN Y: Angiokeratoma corporis diffusum universale (Fabry): Report of a case with lipoiduria. *Chinese Med J* 74:478, 1956

492. YEOH SA, ASAN P: Fabry's disease with tubular acidosis. *Singapore Med J* 8:275, 1967

493. YOSHITOSHI Y, NAJATA N, NAKAMURA T, MAEDA T: A case of Fabry's disease with special references to changes in the skin, urinary albumin, anhydroses and kidney function. *Naika* 15:555, 1965

494. DENDEN A, EBERLE P: Chromosomenanalysen beim Fabry-Anderson syndrom. *Besicht Deutsch Ophthal Gesell* 70:462, 1970

495. PIERIDES AM, HOLTI G, CROMBIE AL, ROBERTS DF, GARDINER SE, COLLING A, ANDERSON J: Study on a family with Anderson-Fabry's disease and associated familial spastic paraplegia. *J Med Genet* 13:455, 1976

496. GRZESCHIK K, GRZESCHIK A, BANHOF S, ROMEO G, SINISCALCO M, VAN SOMEREN H, MEERA KHAN P, WESTERVELD A, BOOTSMA D: X-linkage of human α-galactosidase. *Nat N Biol* 240:48, 1972

497. REBOURCET R, WEIL D, VAN CONG N, FREZAL J: Localisation d'un locus de structure de l'α-galactosidase sur le chromosome X par la méthode d'hybridation cellulaire homme-hamster. *CR Acad Sci (Paris)* 278:3379, 1974

498. BROWN JA, GOSS S, KLINGER HP, MILLER OJ, OHNO S, SINISCALO M: Report of the committee on the genetic constitution of the X and Y chromosomes. *Birth Defects: Orig. Art. Ser.* 12:54, 1976

499. MILLER OJ, SANGER R, SINISCALO M: Report of the committee on the genetic constitution of the X and Y chromosomes. *Cytogenet Cell Genet* 22:124, 1978

500. SHOWS TB, BROWN JA, HALLEY LL, GOGGIN AP, EDDY RL, BYERS MG: Assignment of α-galactosidase (αGAL) gene to the q22 qter region of the X chromosome in man. *Cytogenet Cell Genet* 22:541, 1978

501. DE LA CHAPELLE A, MILLER OJ: Report of the committee on the genetic constitution of chromosomes 10, 11, 12, X and Y. *Cytogenet Cell Genet* 25:47, 1979

502. WEIL D, VAN CONG N, REBOURCET R, GROSS MS, FREZAL J: Regional mapping of enzyme loci on human chromosomes 2, 17, 5 and X by use of somatic cell hybridization. *Cytogenet Cell Genet* 25:215, 1979

503. JOHNSTON AW, SANGER R: Linkage relationship of the loci for Anderson-Fabry disease and the Xg blood groups. *Ann Hum Genet* 45:155, 1981

504. DE GROOT PG, WESTERVELD A, MERRA KHAN P, TAGER M: Localization of a gene for human α-galactosidase B (=N-acetyl-α-D-galactosaminidase) on chromosome 22. *Hum Genet* 44:305, 1978

505. KHAN M, WESTERVELD A, WURZER-FIGURELLI EM, BOOTSMAN D: Alpha-galactosidase in man-Chinese hamster somatic cell hybrids, in *Human Gene Mapping 2, Birth Defects: Orig. Art. Ser.*, 11:205, 1975

506. HAMERS MN, WESTERVELD A, KHAN M, TAGER JM: Characterization of α-galactosidase isozymes in normal and Fabry human-Chinese hamster somatic cell hybrids. *Hum Genet* 36:289, 1977

507. DE GROOT WP: Fabry's disease in children. *Brit J Derm* 82:329, 1970

508. CALMETTES L, DEODATI F, DUPRE A, BEC P: Manifestations oculaires du syndrome de Fabry. *Bull Soc Ophthal France* 72:513, 1959

509. RHODES EL: Angiokeratoma corporis diffusum. *Proc Roy Soc Med Lond* 57:43, 1964

510. ZAKON SJ: Angiokeratoma corporis diffusum (Mibelli). *Arch Derm Syph (Chicago)* 51:155, 1945

511. SPENSE MW, CLARKE JTR, D'ENTREMONT DM, SAPP GA, SMITH ER, GOLDBLOOM AL, DAVAR G: Angiokeratoma corporis diffusum (Anderson-Fabry disease) in a single large family in Nova Scotia. *J Med Genet* 15:428, 1978

512. RIETRA PJGM, BROUWER-KELDER EM, DE GROOT WP, TAGER JM: The use of biochemical parameters for the detection of carriers of Fabry's disease. *J Mol Med* 1:237, 1976

513. ROPERS H-H, WIENKER TF, GRIMM T, SCHROETTER K, BENDER K: Evidence for preferential X-chromosome inactivation in a family with Fabry disease. *Am J Hum Genet* 29:361, 1977

514. DE GROOT WP, TAGER JM: Personal communication, 1974

515. LYON M: Gene action in the X-chromosome of the mouse (*Mus musculus* L.). *Nature (London)* 190:372, 1961

516. LYON M: Sex chromatin and gene action in the X-chromosome of mammals, in Moore KL (ed): *The Sex Chromatin*. Philadelphia, Saunders, 1966, p 370

517. ROMEO G, MIGEON BR: Genetic inactivation of the α-galactosidase locus in carriers of Fabry's disease. *Science* 170:180, 1970

518. GALJAARD H: Personal communication, 1975

519. BRON AJ, TIPATHI RC: Corneal disorders, in Goldberg MR (ed): *Genetic and Metabolic Eye Disease*. Boston, Little, Brown, 1974, p 281

520. FRANCOIS J: Cornea verticillata. *Docum Ophthalmol* 27:235, 1969

521. YAMADA E, SHIKANO S: *Electron Microscopic Atlas in Ophthalmology*. Igaku Shoin Ltd., Tokyo, 1972

522. DE DUVE C, DE BARSY T, POOLE B, TROUET A, TULKINS P, VAN HOOF F: Lysosomotropic agents. *Biochem Pharm* 23:2495, 1974

523. DESNICK RJ, DOUGHMAN DJ, RILEY FC, WHITLEY CB: Fabry Keratopathy: Molecular pathology of the chloroquine-induced phenocopy. *Am J Hum Genet* 26:26a, 1974

524. WIBO M, POOLE B: Protein degradation in cultured cells. II. The uptake of chloroquine by rat fibroblasts and the inhibition of cellular protein degradation and cathepsin B_1. *J Cell Biol* 63:430, 1974

525. FEDORKO ME, HIRSCH JG, COHN Z: Autophagic vacuoles produced in vitro. II. Studies on the mechanism of formation of autophagic vacuoles produced by chloroquine. *Cell Biol* 38:392, 1968

526. REIJNGOUD DJ, TAGER JM: Chloroquine accumulation in isolated rat liver lysosomes. *FEBS Lett* 64:231, 1976

527. HOMEWOOD CA, WARHURST DC, PETERS W, BAGGALEY VC: Lysosomes, pH and the antimalarial action of chloroquine. *Nature* 235:50, 1972

528. LIE SO, SCHOFIELD B: Inactivation of lysosomal function in normal cultured human fibroblasts. *Biochem Pharm* 22:3109, 1973

529. WHITLEY CB: *Studies of Heritable and Induced Lysosomopathies*. PhD thesis. University of Minnesota, 1977

530. ZISKIND M, JONES RN, WEILL H: State of the art: Silicosis. *Am Rev Respir Dis* 113:643, 1976

531. COPEZZUTO A: La funzionalita renale nei silicoti. *Folia Med* 46:697, 1963

532. KOLEV K, DOITSCHINOV D, TODOROV D: Morphologic alternations in the kidneys by silicosis. *Med Lav* 61:205, 1970

533. BANKS DE, MILUTINOVIC J, DESNICK RJ, GRABOWSKI GA, LAPP NL, BOEHLECKE BA: Silicon nephropathy mimicking Fabry's disease. *N Engl J Med* in review

534. CRAWHALL JC: Personal communication, 1981

535. BISHOP DF, GRABOWSKI GA, DESNICK RJ: Unpublished results

536. GRABOWSKI GA, BISHOP DF, DESNICK RJ: Unpublished results

537. BISHOP DF, KOVAC C, DESNICK RJ: Unpublished results

538. SLAUGHTER CA, COSEO MC, ABRAMS C, CANCRO MR, HARRIS H: The use of hybridomas in enzyme genetics, in Kennett RH, McKearn TJ, Bechtel KB (eds): *Monoclonal Antibodies*. New York, Plenum, 1980, p 103

539. PRAGER EM, WILSON AC: The dependence of immunochemical cross-reactivity upon sequence resemblance among lysozymes. 1. Micro-complement fixation studies. *J Biol Chem* 246:5978, 1971

540. SUTTON HE, WAGNER RP: Mutation and enzyme function in humans. *Ann Rev Genet* 9:187, 1975

541. KAN YW, HOLLAND J, DOZY A, VARMUS H: Demonstration of non-functional β-globin mRNA in homozygous β-thalassemia. *Proc Nat Acad Sci USA* 72:5140, 1975

542. KAN YW, HOLLAND J, DOZY A, CHARACHE S, KAZAZIAN H: Deletion of the β-globin structure gene in hereditary persistence of foetal haemoglobin. *Nature* 258:162, 1975

543. WETHERALL DJ, CLEGG JB: Recent developments in the molecular genetics of human hemoglobin. *Cell* 16:467, 1979

544. KANTOR JA, TURNER PH, NIENHUIS AW: Beta thalassemia: Mutations which affect processing of the β-globin mRNA precursor. *Cell* 21:149, 1980

545. PROUDFOOT NJ, SHANDER MHM, MANLEY JL, GEFLER ML, MANIATIS T: Structure and *in vitro* transcription of human globin genes. *Science* 209:1329, 1980

546. IMPERIAL R, HELIWIG EB: Angiokeratoma of the scrotum (Fordyce type). *J Urol* 98:379, 1967

547. TRAUB EF, TOLMACH JA: Angiokeratoma. Comprehensive study of the literature and report of a case. *Arch Dermatol Syph* 24:39, 1931

548. DAMMERT K: Angiokeratosis naeviformis—A form of naevus telangiectatieus lateralis (naevus flammeus). *Dermatologica* 130:17, 1965

549. ENDE M, PEABODY C: Angiokeratoma corporis diffusum universale (Fabry). *Virginia Med Monthly* 85:192, 1958

550. VINEYARD WR, KAMIN EJ: Angiokeratoma corporis diffusum. *Arch Dermatol* 82:817, 1960

551. CROSS EG: The familial occurrence of erythromelalgia and nephritis. *Can Med Assoc J* 87:1, 1962

552. BEUTLER E, KUHL W, MATSUMOTO F, PANGALIS G: Acid hydrolases in leukocytes and platelets of normal subjects and in patients with Gaucher's and Fabry's disease. *J Exp Med* 143:975, 1976

553. GOTO I, TABIRA T, NAWA A, KUROKAWA T, KUROIWA Y: Biochemical and genetic studies in two families with Fabry disease. *Arch Neurol* 31:45, 1974

554. PILZ H, DENDEN A: Glycolipidausscheidung im Urin bei einer Sippe mit Fabryscher Krankheit (angiokeratoma corporis diffusum). *Dtsch Med Wschr* 97:120, 1972

555. MAYES JS, SCHEERER JB, SIFERS RN, DONALDSON ML: Differential assay for lysosomal α-galactosidases in human tissues and its application to Fabry's disease. *Clin Chim Acta* 112:247, 1981

556. DAWSON G, MATALON R, DORFMAN A: Glycosphingolipids in cultured human fibroblasts. II. Characterization and metabolism in fibroblasts from patients with inborn errors of glycosphingolipid and mucopolysaccharide metabolism. *J Biol Chem* 247:5951, 1972

557. GRIMM T, WIENKER TF, ROPERS H-H: Fabry's disease: Heterozygote detection by hair root analysis. *Hum Genet* 32:329, 1976

558. PELTIER A, HERBEUVAL E, BRONDEAU MT, BELLEVILLE F, NABET P: Pseudo-clinical Fabry's disease without α-galactosidase deficiency. *Biomedicine* 26:194, 1977

559. EJIOFOR A, ROBINSON D, WISE D, HAMERS MN, TAGER JM: Hair root analysis in heterozygotes for Fabry's disease, in Gatt S, Freysz L, Mandel P (eds): *Enzymes of Lipid Metabolism.* New York, Plenum, 1978, p 719

560. SPENSE MW, GOLDBLOOM AL, BURGESS JK, D'ENTREMONT D, RIPLEY BA, WELDON KL: Heterozygote detection in angiokeratoma corporis diffusum (Anderson-Fabry disease). *J Med Genet* 14:91, 1977

561. VERMORKEN AJM, WETERINGS PJJM, SPIERENBURG GTh, VAN BENNEKOM CA, WIRTZ P, DE BRUYN CHMM, OEI TL: Fabry's disease: Biochemical and histochemical studies on hair roots for carrier detection. *Brit J Dermatol* 98:191, 1978

562. VERMORKEN AJM, VAN BENNEKOM CA, DE BRUYN CHMM, OEI TL: Heterozygote detection in Fabry's disease using mailed hair roots. *Brit J Dermatol* 103:101, 1980

563. DESNICK RJ, RAMAN MK, BENDEL RP, KERSEY J, LEE JC, KRIVIT W: Prenatal diagnosis of glycosphingolipidoses: Sandhoff's and Fabry's diseases. *J Pediatr* 83:149, 1973

564. MALOUF M, KIRKMAN HN, BUCHANAN PD: Ultrastructural changes in antenatal Fabry's disease. *Am J Pathol* 82:132, 1976

565. SORENSEN SA, HAHNEMANN N, MOHR J: Praenatal diagnostik af enzymdefelter belyst ved et tilfaelde of undersogelse for angiokeratoma corporis diffusum (Fabry's sygdom). *Ugeskr Laeg* 136:1636, 1974

566. DESNICK RJ, RAMAN MK, BENDEL RP: Unpublished results

567. CERVENKA J, GORLIN RJ, BENDEL RP: Prenatal sex determination. Detection of "Y body." *Obstet Gynec* 37:912, 1971

568. GALJAARD H, NIERMEIJER MF, HAHNEMANN N, MOHR J, SORENSEN SA: An example of rapid prenatal diagnosis of Fabry's disease using microtechniques. *Clin Genet* 5:368, 1974

569. GALJAARD H, HOOGEVEEN A, KEIJZER W, DE WIT-VERBECK Z, VLEKNOOT C: The use of quantitative cytochemical analyses in rapid prenatal detection and somatic cell genetic studies of metabolic diseases. *Histochem J* 6:491, 1974

570. BLADON MT, MILUNSKY A: Use of microtechniques for the detection of lysosomal enzyme disorders: Tay-Sachs disease. G$_{M1}$-gangliosidosis and Fabry disease. *Clin Genet* 14:359, 1978

571. SCHNECK L, ADACHI M, VOLK BW: Chemical pathology of Tay-Sachs disease in the fetus, in Volk BW, Aronson SM (eds): *Sphingolipids, Sphingolipidoses, and Allied Disorders.* New York, Plenum, 1972, p 385

572. DESNICK RJ, SHARP HL, KRIVIT W: *In utero* diagnosis of Sandhoff's disease. *Biochem Biophys Res Commun* 51:20, 1973

573. MILUNSKY A: *Genetic Disorders and the Fetus. Diagnosis, Prevention and Treatment.* New York, Plenum, 1979

574. GALJAARD H: *Genetic Metabolic Diseases: Early Diagnosis and Prenatal Analysis.* Amsterdam, Elsevier/North-Holland Biomedical, 1980

575. GRABOWSKI GA, DESNICK RJ: Prenatal metabolic diagnosis: Principles, pitfalls and prospects, in Latt A, Darlington GL (ed): *Prenatal Diagnosis: Cell Biological Approaches.* New York, Academic, in press

576. NICHD NATIONAL REGISTRY FOR AMNIOCENTESIS STUDY GROUP: Midtrimester amniocentesis for prenatal diagnosis, safety and accuracy. *J Am Med Assoc* 236:1471, 1976

577. SIMPSON NE, DALLAIRE L, MILLER JR, SIMINOVICH L, HAMERTON JL, MILLER J, MCKEEN C: Prenatal diagnosis of genetic disease in Canada: Report of a collaborative study. *Can Med Assoc J* 23:739, 1976

578. MRC WORKING GROUP ON AMNIOCENTESIS: An assessment of the hazards of amniocentesis. *Brit J Obstet Gynaecol* 85(Suppl. 2) 1978, p 1

579. FUNDERBURK SJ, PHILIPPART M, DALE G, CEDERBAUM SD, VYDEN JK: Priapism after phenoxybenzamine in a patient with Fabry's disease. *N Engl J Med* 290:630, 1974

580. LENOIR G, RIVRON M, GUBLER M-C, DUFIER J-L, TOME FSM, GUIVARCH M: La maladie de Fabry. Traitement du syndrome acrodyniforme par la carbamazepine. *Arch Franc Ped* 34:704, 1977

581. ATZPODIEN W, KREMER GJ, SCHNELLBACHER E, DENK R, HAFERKAMP G, BIERBACH H: Angiokeratoma corporis diffusum (Morbus Fabry). Biochemische diagnostik im blutplasma. *Dtsch Med Wschr* 100:423, 1975

582. DUPPERRAT B, PUISSANT A, SAURAT J-H, DELANOE J, DOYARD P-A, GRUNFELD J-P: Maladie de Fabry. Angiokeratomes presents a la naissance. Action de la diphenylhydantoine sur les crises douloureuses. *Ann Dermatol Syphil* 102:392, 1975

583. WADSKOV S, ANDERSON V, KOBAYASI T, SONDERGAARD J, SORENSON SA: On the diagnosis of Fabry's disease. *Acta Dermatovenev* 55:363, 1975

584. PHILIPPART M, FRANKLIN SS, GORDON A: Reversal of an inborn sphingolipidosis (Fabry's disease) by kidney transplantation. *Ann Intern Med* 77:195, 1972

585. DESNICK RJ, ALLEN KY, SIMMONS RL, WOODS JE, ANDERSON CF, NAJARIAN JS, KRIVIT W: Fabry disease: Correction of the enzymatic deficiency by renal transplantation, in Desnick RJ, Bernlohr RW, Krivit W (eds): *Enzyme Therapy in Genetic Diseases.* Baltimore, Williams & Wilkins, 1973, p 88

586. PHILIPPART M, FRANKLIN SS, GORDON A, LEEBER D, HULL AR: Studies on the metabolic control of Fabry's disease through kidney transplantation, in Volk BW, Aronson SM (eds): *Sphingolipids, Sphingolipidoses and Allied Disorders.* New York, Plenum, 1972, p 641

587. PHILIPPART M: Fabry disease: Kidney transplantation as an enzyme replacement technique, in Desnick RJ, Bernlohr RW, Krivit W (eds): *Enzyme Therapy in Genetic Diseases.* Baltimore, Williams & Wilkins, 1973, p 81

588. JACKY E: Fabrysche Erkrankung (Angiokeratoma corporis diffusum universale): Gunstiger Verlauf nach Nierentransplantation. *Schweiz Med Wschr* 106:703, 1976

589. BUHLER FR, THIEL G, DUBACH VC, ENDERLIN F, GLOOR F, THOLEN H: Kidney transplantation in Fabry's disease. *Brit Med J* 3:28, 1973

590. CLARKE JTR, GUTTMANN RD, WOLFE LS, BEAUDOIN JG, MOREHOUSE DD: Enzyme replacement therapy by renal allotransplantation in Fabry's disease. *N Engl J Med* 287:1215, 1972

591. SPENSE MW, MACKINNON KE, BURGESS JK, D'ENTREMONT DM, BELITSKY P, LANNON SG, MACDONALD AS: Failure to correct the metabolic defect by renal allotransplantation in Fabry's disease. *Ann Intern Med* 84:13, 1976

592. GRUNFELD JP, LEPORRIER M, DROZ D, BENSAUDE I, HINGLAIS N, CROSNIER J: Le transplantation renale chez les sujets atteints de maladie de Fabry. *Nour Presse Med* 4:2081, 1975

593. VAN DEN BERGH FAJTM, RIETRA PJGM, KOLK-VEGTER AJ, BOSCH E, TAGER JM: Therapeutic implications of renal transplantation in a patient with Fabry's disease. *Acta Med Scand* 200:249, 1976

594. DAWSON G, MATALON R, LI Y-T: Correction of the enzymatic defect in cultured fibroblasts from patients with Fabry's disease: Treatment with purified α-galactosidase from Ficin. *Pediatr Res* 7:684, 1973

595. JOHNSON DL, DESNICK RJ: Unpublished results

596. OHNISHI A, TATEISHI J, MATSUMOTO T, SHIDA K, KUROIWA Y: Fabry disease: Cellular expression of enzyme deficiency in nerve xenografts. *Neurology* 29:899, 1979

597. DESNICK RJ, DEAN KJ, GRABOWSKI G, BISHOP DF, SWEELEY CC: Enzyme therapy XVII: Metabolic and immunologic evaluation of α-galactosidase A replacement in Fabry disease, in Desnick RJ (ed): *Enzyme Therapy in Genetic Diseases:2.* New York, Alan R Liss, 1980, p 393

598. ASHWELL G, MORELL AG: The role of surface carbohydrates in the hepatic recognition and transport of circulating glycoproteins. *Adv Enzymol* 41:99, 1974

599. BISHOP DF, KOVAC CR, DESNICK RJ: Enzyme therapy XX: Further evidence for the differential *in vivo* fate of human splenic and plasma forms of α-galactosidase A in Fabry disease. Recovery of exogenous activity from hepatic tissue. in Callahan JW, Lowden JA (eds): *Lysosomes and Lysosomal Storage Diseases.* New York, Raven, 1981, p 381

600. SCHRAM AW, HAMERS MN, OLDENBROEK-HAVERLAMP E, STRIJLAND A, DE JONGE A, VAN DEN BERG FAThM, TAGER JM: Properties of immobilized fig α-galactosidase and effect on ceramide-3 content of plasma from patients with Fabry's disease. *Biochim Biophys Acta* 527:456, 1978

601. RATTAZZI MC, APPEL AM, BAKER HJ: Enzyme replacement in feline G$_{M2}$-gangliosidosis: Catabolic effects of human β-hexosaminidase A. *Pediatr Res* 15:567, 1981

602. TOURAINE JL, MALIK MC, TRAEGER J, PERROT H, MARIE I: Attempt at enzyme replacement by fetal liver transplantation in Fabry's disease. *Lancet* 1:1094, 1979

603. TOURAINE JL, MALIK MC, PERROT H, MAIRE I, REVILLARD JP, GROSSHANS E, TRAEGER J: Maladie de Fabry: Deux maladies ameliores par la greffe de cellules de foie foetal. *Nouv Presse Med* 8:1499, 1979

604. TOURAINE JL, MALIK MC: Fetal liver transplantation in Fabry's disease. *Proc. EBMT Meeting,* Sils Maria, 1980

605. MOSER HW, BATSHAW ML, MURRAY C, BRAINE H, BRUSILOW SW: Management of heritable disorders of the urea cycle and of Refsum's and Fabry's disease, in Papadatos CJ, Bartsocas CS (eds): *The Management of Genetic Disorders.* New York, Alan R Liss, 1979, p 183

606. MOSER HW, BRAINE H, PYERITZ RE, ULLMAN D, MURRAY C, ASBURY AK: Therapeutic trail of plasmapheresis in Refsum disease and in Fabry disease, in Desnick RJ (ed): *Enzyme Therapy in Genetic Diseases:2.* New York, Alan R Liss, 1980, p 491

607. DESNICK RJ, GRABOWSKI GA: Advances in the treatment of inherited metabolic diseases. *Adv Hum Genet* 11:281, 1981

46

THE GANGLIOSIDOSES

JOHN S. O'BRIEN

1. *Defects of ganglioside degradation can be divided into two groups, the G_{M1} gangliosidoses and the G_{M2} gangliosidoses. Each ganglioside storage disease appears to be transmitted as an autosomal recessive trait. The G_{M1} gangliosidoses are due to a deficiency of acid β-galactosidase. The G_{M2} gangliosidoses are due to deficiencies of hexosaminidase A or B, or both, or a deficiency of a factor (activator factor) which stimulates hexosaminidase A to cleave ganglioside G_{M2}.*

2. *The G_{M1} gangliosidoses include patients with acute infantile onset, rapid neurologic decline, and severe bony abnormalities, at one end of the spectrum, and normal intelligence and survival to adulthood at the other. At least five different subtypes are presently recognized, including those with chronic adult neurologic disease. All patients have severe deficiencies of acid β-galactosidase activity.*

3. *Acid β-galactosidase exists in several forms, monomeric (A_1), dimeric (A_2), and multimeric (A_3). A single monomeric subunit of 65,000 daltons is obtained after treatment of each form. The monomeric polypeptide A_1 appears to be coded by a single autosomal locus, located on the short arm of chromosome 3. The simultaneous loss of activity in all forms in patients with G_{M1} gangliosidosis is explained by a mutation at this locus. β-Galactosidase A is heterocatalytic, cleaving β-D-galactose from ganglioside G_{M1}, galac-*

tose-containing oligosaccharides, and other galacto-conjugates. The pleotropic effects of a single mutation affecting the locus for β-galactosidase A can be explained by a one gene–one polypeptide–many substrates model. Phenotypic variability among β-galactosidase A mutants may result from better residual activity of the mutant enzyme for one substrate than another. For example, patients with significantly higher residual activity for ganglioside G_{M1} than for galactose-containing oligosaccharides or proteoglycans may have severe bony involvement with minimal nervous system abnormalities due to the specific localization of each substrate in brain and bones, respectively. Patients with this phenotype, called Morquio syndrome type B (MPS IV B), have recently been described.

4. *Thus far, all human mutants for G_{M1} β-galactosidase are structural mutants, synthesizing nearly normal quantities of mutant enzyme. Several patients are proven K_m mutants. The number of different mutations which lead to β-galactosidase deficiency is not known, but it is probably large. The wide phenotypic variability present in patients with β-galactosidase mutations makes precise classification into numerous subtypes impractical. A general classification such as infantile, juvenile, or adult G_{M1} gangliosidosis is useful for instruction, clinical diagnosis, management, prognostication, and counseling. It seems*

945

inappropriate to classify patients having bony abnormalities but without cerebral defect as having G_{M1} gangliosidosis, since the term implies progressive neurologic deterioration and suggests a pessimistic prognosis.

5. *The G_{M2} gangliosidoses can be classified into infantile-, juvenile-, and adult-onset disorders. Similar to the G_{M1} gangliosidoses large phenotypic variability exists in this group of disorders. The four most common disorders are Tay-Sachs disease, caused by a severe deficiency of hexosaminidase A; Sandhoff disease, caused by a severe deficiency of hexosaminidase A and B; and juvenile G_{M2} gangliosidosis and adult G_{M2} gangliosidosis, caused by a deficiency of hexosaminidase A.*

6. *Tay-Sachs disease (TSD) is the most common ganglioside storage disease known. The heterozygote frequency for TSD mutation among Ashkenazi Jewish persons is 1 in 27. Heterozygotes can be reliably determined by serum assay. Mass screening programs have been carried out in 73 cities in 13 different countries with over 312,000 individuals tested since 1970. These community-based voluntary screening programs have led to the identification of over 250 at-risk carrier couples who have no history of TSD in their families. In such couples, prenatal diagnosis has led to identification of TSD in utero. TSD is the first example of a genetic disease in which the birth of an affected child has been prevented by mass screening for heterozygotes in at-risk populations.*

7. *The molecular genetics of hexosaminidase A and hexosaminidase B have been clarified. Both enzymes have molecular weights of approximately 100,000 and cleave N-acetylhexosamine from a variety of substrates, including lipids (asialo G_{M2}, globoside) and oligosaccharides. Only hexosaminidase A cleaves ganglioside G_{M2}. Hexosaminidase A is composed of two nonidentical subunits: the α chain, coded by a locus on chromosome 15, and the β chain, coded by a locus on chromosome 5. Hexosaminidase B is a tetrameric homopolymer of 25,000-dalton β subunits ($\beta_2\beta_2$). The structure of hexosaminidase A is still under investigation, but recent work suggests it is a trimer ($\alpha\beta_2$) with a single 58,000-dalton α chain and a pair of β chains. A third protein, an activator protein (or proteins), stimulates hexosaminidase A (but not hexosaminidase B) to cleave ganglioside G_{M2}. It is deficient in patients with AB(+) G_{M2} gangliosidosis.*

8. *A three-locus model explains the molecular genetics of G_{M2} gangliosidosis. Mutations at the α locus located on chromosome 15 lead to hexosaminidase A deficiency (TSD or juvenile or adult G_{M2} gangliosidosis). Mutations at the β locus located on chromosome 5 lead to hexosaminidase A and B deficiency (infantile, juvenile, or adult Sandhoff disease). Mutations at the activator locus (not mapped as yet) lead to AB(+) G_{M2} gangliosidosis.*

9. *A large number of unusual hex A and B variants have been described, and a nomenclature based upon the three-locus model has been proposed to classify them.*

10. *No specific therapy for the ganglioside metabolic disorders is available. Enzyme replacement therapy is not available. Prenatal diagnosis of affected fetuses by amniocentesis and enzyme assay, although admittedly imperfect, is the only preventive solution available for these fatal inborn errors of ganglioside metabolism. Animal models for G_{M1} gangliosidosis in dogs and cats and for Sandhoff disease in cats are now available and will be valuable in therapeutic studies.*

In 1881 Warren Tay, a British ophthalmologist, was the first to describe an inborn error of ganglioside metabolism. The condition he described is now known as Tay-Sachs disease, or G_{M2} gangliosidosis [1]. A second disorder, G_{M1} gangliosidosis, was discovered 84 years later in 1965 [2, 3]. At present, several additional distinct subtypes of both G_{M2} gangliosidosis and G_{M1} gangliosidosis are known, including juvenile and adult disorders. Each is caused by a metabolic defect in ganglioside breakdown resulting from deficiencies of ganglioside glycohydrolases (Fig. 46-1).

GANGLIOSIDE STRUCTURE AND LOCATION

Gangliosides are glycosphingolipids which contain sialic acid in their oligosaccharide chain. They were discovered by Ernst Klenk, who named them for their high concentration in "ganglion" cells, or neurons. At least ten different gangliosides occur in human brain [4], four of which comprise over 90 percent of the total. The major brain monosialoganglioside, G_{M1}, has the following abbreviated structure: galactosyl-$(1 \rightarrow 3)$-N-acetylgalactosaminyl $(1 \rightarrow 4)$-$[(2 \rightarrow 3)$-N-acetylneuraminyl]-galactosyl-$(1 \rightarrow 4)$ glucosyl-$(1 \rightarrow 1)$-[2-N-acyl]-sphingosine. Modifications of the same oligosaccharide chain occur. The chain is incomplete in some forms (G_{M2}, G_{M3}) and contains more sialic acid residues in others (G_{D1a}, G_{D1b}, and G_T). The normal distribution of the six major gangliosides in human brain is given in Table 46-1. There are significant differences in ganglioside content and pattern between different portions of the brain [5] and during development [5, 6].

In brain, gangliosides are localized primarily in nerve-ending membranes, with a high content in synaptic membranes [7]. Neuronal perikaryon preparations, which contain few dendrites, have a low ganglioside content [7]. Some gangliosides in nerve endings appear to originate from the cell body and move to the end of the nerve by rapid axonal transport [8]. Axons, myelin, astroglia, and oligodendroglia have a smaller ganglioside content than neuronal endings. Although brain has the highest content, gangliosides are present in most cell types in the body as well as in cultured cells.

Biosynthesis

The ganglioside biosynthetic pathway [9] in the mammalian nervous system involves the stepwise addition of monosaccharide units. The first sugar, glucose, is added to the hydroxyl

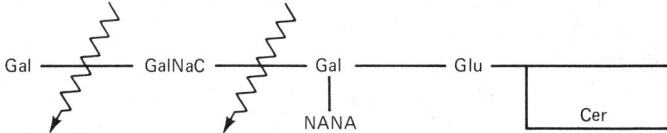

Figure 46-1 Structure of G_{M1} ganglioside, showing the sites of the enzymatic defects in the gangliosidoses.

group of ceramide. The remaining sugars are then added to the nonreducing end of the oligosaccharide chain. Specific glycosyltransferases catalyze the transfer of each monosaccharide unit, and the glycose units are donated by the corresponding sugar nucleotides (Fig. 46-2).

The pathway to G_{M1} involves the addition of five sugars in strict sequence by a multiglycosyltransferase system composed of five different glycosyltransferases [9]. A sixth step, possibly at a branch point, is catalyzed by a sialyltransferase apparently different from that which forms G_{D1a} (bottom of Fig. 46-2) and leads to the formation of G_{D1b}. This branch point may lead to the ultimate biosynthesis of more highly sialylated forms such a trisialogangliosides. The transferases appear to be specific with respect to the type of glycosidic bond and the stereospecific assignments of each linkage. The multiglycosyltransferase system has its highest activity in synaptosomal membranes. The fact indicates biosynthesis of ganglioside at the nerve end itself.

Although the pathway shown in Fig. 46-2 is the commonly accepted one, it may not be the only route of ganglioside biosynthesis [10]. Complete understanding will require purification and substrate specificity studies of each of the transferases.

GalNAc Transferase Deficiency (G_{M3} Gangliosidosis)

One patient with an apparent defect in ganglioside biosynthesis has been reported [11, 12]. He presented with rapidly progressive neurologic symptoms, including generalized hyporeflexia, motor weakness, dulled sensorium, and failure to thrive.

A relative increase in the concentration of G_{M3} and a deficiency of higher homologues such as G_{M1}, G_{D1a}, and G_{D1b} were found in the brain [11]. The activity of G_{M3} sialidase was normal in brain and liver, but the activity of G_{M3} UDP-N-acetylgalactosaminyltransferase was reduced to about 10 percent of normal [13].

A sib of this patient was born with the same disorder but had a normal brain ganglioside pattern. The common pathobi-

Table 46-1 Structure and distribution of brain gangliosides

| Structure | Nomenclature | Normal distribution of gangliosides | | | |
| | | Gray matter | | White matter | |
		Newborn	Adult	Newborn	Adult
Cer ⟵ 1 Glc 4 ←β— 1 Gal 3 ⟵ 2 NANA	GM₃	1.0	—	1.0	
Cer ⟵ 1 Glc 4 ←β— 1 Gal 4 ←β— 1 GalNac	GM₂	3.6	1.7	6.9	1.9
Cer ⟵ 1 Glc 4 ←β— 1 Gal 4 ←β— 1 GalNac 3 (2 NANA; ↑β 1 Gal)	GM₁	14.6	12.8	19.1	12.6
Cer ⟵ 1 Glc 4 ←β— 1 Gal 4 ←β— 1 GalNac 3 (2 NANA; ↑β 1 Gal 3; NANA 2)	GD₁ₐ	71.6	22.8	57.8	18.4
Cer ⟵ 1 Glc 4 ←β— 1 Gal 4 ←β— 1 GalNac 3 (2 NANA 8 ⟵ 2 NANA; ↑β 1 Gal)	GD₁ᵦ	1.8	23.5	2.1	30.4
Cer ⟵ 1 Glc 4 ←β— 1 Gal 4 ←β— GalNac 3 (2 NANA ⟵ 2 NANA; ↑β 1 Gal 3; NANA 2)	GT₁	7.3	31.2	3.4	27.9

NOTE: Cer, ceramide (acylsphingosine); Glc, glucose; Gal, galactose; galNac, N-acetylgalactosamine; NANA, N-acetylneuraminic acid.
SOURCE: Modified from Sloan and Fredrickson [10].

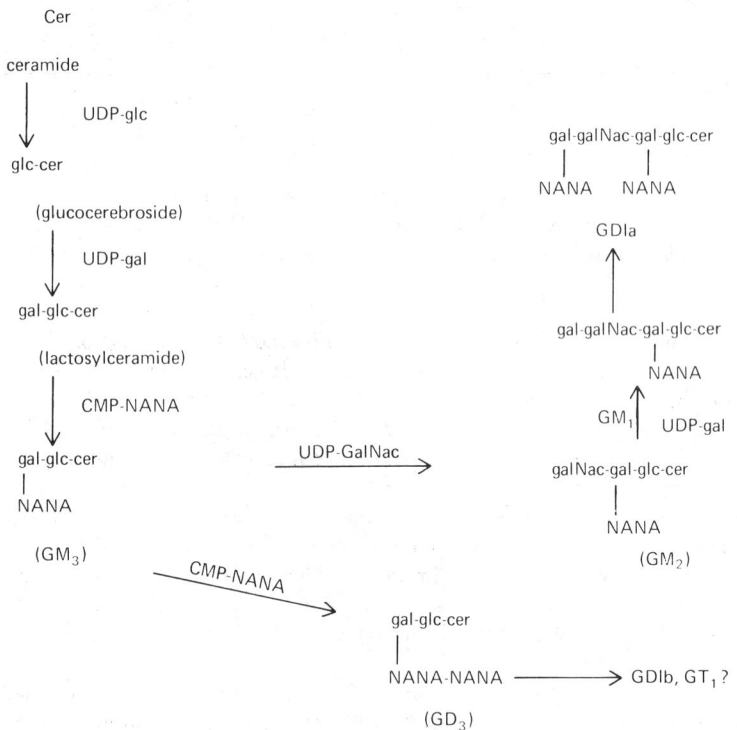

Figure 46-2 Roseman's proposed pathway of synthesis of G_{D1a}. (*From Roseman [9]. Used by permission.*)

ology that occurred in the two patients may be due to some entirely unrelated developmental anomaly [*14*]. A virus infection was suspected in the first patient [*14*]. At present, there is no evidence to include G_{M3} *gangliosidosis* (or *GalNAc transferase deficiency*) among the hereditary diseases of human beings.

GANGLIOSIDE CATABOLISM

Gangliosides are catabolized by the stepwise removal of sugar molecules at the nonreducing end of the oligosaccharide chain and catalyzed by exohydrolases [*15, 16*]. If a deficiency of one hydrolase exists, further breakdown is blocked, even though the remaining hydrolases in the pathway are present in normal amounts.

Although the sequence shown in Fig. 46-3 is the generally accepted scheme, precise kinetic rates for each of the steps in vivo have yet to be established. Minor pathways may exist, as indicated in Fig. 46-3. In the first reaction, the major trisialo-ganglioside, G_{T1b}, is converted to G_{D1b}, rather than G_{D1a}, and both are then converted to G_{M1}. The next catabolic step is the removal of the terminal galactose from G_{M1} to give ganglioside G_{M2}. G_{M2} is then hydrolyzed to G_{M3} by action of G_{M2} β-acetylgalactosaminidase. The sialic acid linked to the midchain galactose appears to be more resistant to removal than the other sialic acid residues. Nonreactivity appears to be due to steric hindrance imposed by *N*-acetylgalactosamine, which is bound to the C–4 hydroxyl of the same galactose as the sialic acid. G_{M3} sialidase next catalyzes the hydrolysis of neuraminic acid from G_{M3}, yielding lactosylceramide, which is itself hydrolyzed by a second β-galactosidase to give glucocerebroside. Glucocerebroside is hydrolyzed by glucocerebroside β-glucosidase to give ceramide, which is cleaved to sphingosine and fatty acids by ceramidase. Except for some sialidases which are extralysosomal [*15*], all the glycosidases responsible

for hydrolizing G_{M1} to ceramide appear to be located in lysosomes [*16*].

The steps in which sialic acid and *N*-acetylgalactosamine moieties are cleaved from G_{M2} are poorly understood. Both activities are extremely low and may be the rate-limiting ones in the sequence. Since the rates in vitro are so low, it is also probable that optimal assay conditions have yet to be worked out for each activity.

GANGLIOSIDE STORAGE DISEASES

Several G_{M1} and G_{M2} gangliosidosis variants are now known. For simplicity, the most common disorders are described first and unusual variants later. The reader should be aware that not all patients in each phenotypic grouping may have the same mutation. In fact, many patients probably are allelic compounds (heterozygous for two different mutations at the same locus) rather than homozygotes for a single mutation.

In general, the most common ganglioside storage disorders are characterized by (1) progressive mental and motor deterioration with onset in childhood and fatal outcome; (2) autosomal recessive inheritance; (3) neuronal lipidosis secondary to storage of ganglioside G_{M2} or ganglioside G_{M1}; (4) storage of structurally related glycolipids or oligosaccharides; and (5) absence or severe deficiency of specific lysosomal glycohydrolases. A nomenclature of the G_{M1} and the G_{M2} gangliosidoses based upon the clinical picture is given in Tables 46-2 and 46-3. The major clinical features of each disorder are given in Table 46-4.

Genetics

Each gangliosidosis appears to be genotypically distinct, and each phenotype breeds true. Multiple affected children in sibships have been phenotypically similar to probands. No reports have appeared in which more than one ganglioside storage disease has appeared in the same sibship.

For the following reasons, each ganglioside storage disease appears to be transmitted as an autosomal recessive trait. Parents of probands have been clinically normal. Sex ratios are nearly equal. Analysis of pedigrees, correcting for incomplete ascertainment, in TSD and in infantile G_{M1} gangliosidosis give ratios of affected to nonaffected children which are consistent with those expected for autosomal recessive inheritance [17, 18]. Most importantly, enzyme assays in families have demonstrated a segregation pattern consistent with autosomal recessive inheritance.

In the United States the frequency of TSD has been estimated by case ascertainment from mortality records [19–21]. These have given a heterozygote frequency of about 0.026 for Ashkenazi Jewish individuals (1 in 38) and about 0.0029 for non-Jewish individuals (1 in 344). It is estimated that 50 to 100 children with TSD were conceived in North America in 1970, 75 percent of whom were offspring of Jewish parents. Data on the heterozygote frequency for TSD have also come from mass screening by serum assays in Ashkenazi Jewish populations. The values found (Table 46-5) are higher than those obtained by case ascertainment. In California the heterozygote frequency is 0.034 (1 in 30), based on screening over 60,000 individuals [22]. The worldwide frequency ascertained by screening of 312,214 Jewish individuals in 14 countries is 0.041 (1 in 24) [22]. This figure is higher than actual since it is not corrected for inclusion of relatives of probands; the actual value is between 1 in 24 and 1 in 30. An unusually high heterozygote frequency (1 in 14) has been detected in Toronto, Canada. The frequency found on serum screening agreed with that calculated from case ascertainment [23]. The highest heterozygote frequency for TSD occurs in Ashkenazi Jewish individuals whose ancestors derive from the Balkan provinces of Grodno, Vilno, and Suwalki, Poland [10, 21], and it has been reported that a very high proportion of Toronto Jewish individuals trace their ancestry to this region [23].

Controversy exists concerning the reason for the high frequency of the TSD mutation in the Ashkenazi Jewish population. Selective advantage for the heterozygote [24] or the founder effect [25] have both been postulated as causative. The former has pointed to resistance to pulmonary tuberculosis

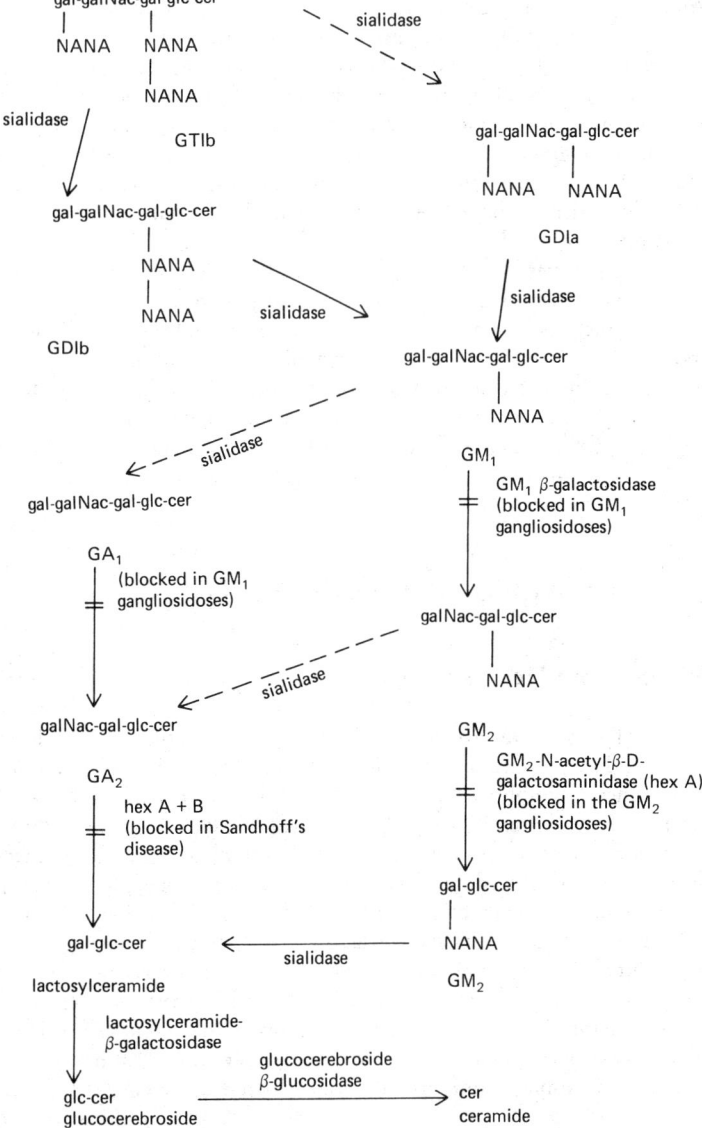

Figure 46-3 Pathways of G_{T1b} degradation to ceramide. Minor or questionable pathways are indicated by the dashed arrows. (*From Ledeen and Yu* [4]. *Used by permission.*)

Table 46-2 Nomenclature of G_{M1} gangliosidoses

Common name	Genetic classification	Year discovered	Number of patients known	Inheritance
Infantile G_{M1} gangliosidosis	βGal-2	1964	100	Autosomal recessive
Juvenile G_{M1} gangliosidosis	βGal-3	1968	20	Autosomal recessive
Adult G_{M1} gangliosidosis	βGal-4	1972	10	Autosomal recessive

among ancestors of TSD patients as a possible survival advantage [26]. The latter [25] proposes a disproportionate contribution from a founder originating from a Jewish community in Eastern Europe, with manifestation of the mutant gene later in history, and proposes that the present high incidence of affected individuals among Ashkenazi Jews is a transient phenomenon due to the chance encounter of recessive genes. The selective-advantage hypothesis might suggest a future increase in the frequency of TSD, whereas the founder-effect hypothesis predicts a decline.

The founder-effect hypothesis appears to best explain the high frequency of TSD reported among a group of French-Canadians living in Quebec [27] and among a group of non-Amish Pennsylvania Dutch [28]. In the Quebec study the frequency of the carrier status approximated that among Ashkenazi Jews (0.029), while in the Pennsylvania study it was somewhat lower (0.051). In each deme the population groups were clearly identifiable geographically and culturally and each had a common ancestral origin consistent with founder effect. Whether the mutation of hexosaminidase A in each deme is identical to that in "Ashkenazi Jewish TSD" is an open question.

The frequencies of the other ganglioside storage diseases are not known. Most cases have occurred in non-Jews from a variety of ethnic groups. Each of these disorders is much less common than TSD. An increased frequency of infantile G_{M1} gangliosidosis has been noted in Malta, perhaps as a result of inbreeding in a geographic isolate [29]. Data on the homozygote and heterozygote frequency of G_{M1} gangliosidosis in Malta have yet to be reported.

G_{M1} GANGLIOSIDOSIS

Phenotypic Descriptions

Infantile G_{M1} Gangliosidosis (Type 1)   In infantile G_{M1} gangliosidosis (generalized gangliosidosis, infantile with bony involvement) symptoms begin at birth or shortly thereafter. Edema of the extremities is often present. Appetite is poor, sucking is weak, and weight gain is subnormal. Ineffective swallowing may necessitate tube feeding. The patient may hold his head up but usually cannot crawl or sit unsupported. Sensorium is dull. Respirations are labored and irregular, and recurrent bronchopneumonia is frequent. Clonic-tonic convulsions often occur. If survival extends beyond the first year, the clinical picture is that of decerebrate rigidity with blindness, deafness, spastic quadriplegia, and unresponsiveness. Death due to bronchopneumonia usually occurs by age 2 years.

The appearance is that of a dull-looking, hypoactive, hypotonic infant. Facial abnormalities include frontal bossing, depressed nasal bridge, large low-set ears, and coarse features. Gingival hypertrophy and macroglossia are often present. The corneas are usually clear. Cherry-red spots, identical to those seen in Tay-Sachs disease, are present in about half the patients. Hepatosplenomegaly is usually evident within the first few months of life. Macrocephaly may develop but is not as frequent nor as massive as in TSD. Dorsolumbar kyphoscoliosis and hard, nontender enlargements of the epiphyseal joints, due to cartilaginous hypertrophy, may be prominent.

The radiologic changes are those of dysostosis multiplex. Deformities of the vertebral bodies and long bones consist of rarefaction, anterior beaking of vertebral bodies, periosteal cloaking of the long bones early in the course of the disease, spatulate ribs, shoe-shaped sella, and modeling deformities of pelvic, hand, and foot bones [30].

Pathologic changes include neuronal lipidosis, visceral histiocytosis, and cytoplasmic ballooning of renal glomerular epithelial cells. Neurons contain numerous cytoplasmic membranous bodies.

Visceral histiocytosis is prominent throughout the reticuloendothelial system. Foamy histiocytes are found in bone marrow, liver, spleen, lymph nodes, and most visceral organs. Renal glomerular epithelial cytoplasmic ballooning is prominent. The cells are filled with a material which is soluble in aqueous fixatives, leaving empty vacuoles after preparation for electron microscopy. Occasional lamellar lipid bodies are also seen in these cells. Similar clear vacuoles, found in epithelial cells in skin biopsies, facilitate the diagnosis (Fig. 46-4) [31].

Juvenile G_{M1} Gangliosidosis (Type 2)   The phenotype differs from that of the infantile disorder. Onset is later, the course is slower, and the bony abnormalities are milder. Mental and motor development is often normal during the first year. Appetite is good, weight gain is adequate, and developmental milestones are not delayed. Locomotor ataxia beginning at about 1 year of age is usually the initial symptom. Internal strabismus, loss of coordinated manipulative hand movements, loss of speech, and generalized moderate muscular weakness of both upper and lower extremities are early symptoms. Mental and motor deterioration often progress rapidly thereafter. Dulling of sensorium, lack of interest, and lethargy are present. Progressive spasticity of upper and lower extremities develops, and, with time, a state of decerebrate rigidity is reached. Seizures often occur after 16 months of age and may constitute a major problem in medical management. Recurrent infections, especially bronchopneumonia, are constant problems and usually lead to the patient's demise. The average life span has varied between 3 and 10 years [32, 33].

Coarsening of facial features is not evident. Internal strabismus and bilateral nystagmus may be present. Corneas are usually clear, and the retina and macula usually appear normal. Blindness may occur late in the coarse of the disease. Lymphocytes are vacuolated, and foamy histiocytes occur in the bone marrow. Hepatosplenomegaly is usually absent. Radiographic examination often reveals mild inferior beaking of one or more lumbar vertebral bodies, proximal beaking of metacarpal bones, especially the fifth, and modeling deformities of the pelvic bones. These radiologic changes are mild but can be of considerable diagnostic value. They have been noted as early as age 7 months, prior to neurologic symptoms [32].

Pathologic changes include neuronal lipidosis, which appears identical to but less prominent than that in the infantile type. Visceral histiocytosis is usually present but is not as florid as that seen in the infantile type. Renal glomerular cytoplasmic ballooning is similar to that in the infantile type.

Adult G_{M1} Gangliosidosis (Type 3)   Patients with this disorder have presented with progressive cerebellar dysarthria beginning in the juvenile period. In the best studied patients [34, 35], the picture has been that of progressive spasticity and ataxia. Intellectual impairment has been mild but with time loss of intellectual function is evident. Progression of symptoms is slow. Neurologic impairment may only be suspected 10 years after the initial symptoms. Seizures are uncommon and vision remains unimpaired. Thus far, no patients have expired.

Chemistry of Storage Substances

The sugar composition, fatty acid composition, sugar sequence, and glycosidic linkages of the stored compound are identical to those of normal ganglioside G_{M1} [18] (Fig. 46-1). G_{M1} storage is approximately 10 times normal in gray matter in both infantile and juvenile G_{M1} gangliosidosis, and 20 to 50 times normal in liver in the infantile type. In four patients studied with the juvenile type, visceral storage of G_{M1} was not found. The asialo-derivative of G_{M1} (G_{A1}) also accumulates in the brain to about 10 times normal levels.

Galactose-containing Oligosaccharides   Galactose-containing oligosaccharides accumulate in the viscera in G_{M1} gangliosidosis. The most abundant storage compound is an octasaccharide with the structure [36]:

Gal β1 ⟶ 4 GlcNac β1 ⟶ 2 Man α1 ⟶ 6
Gal β1 ⟶ 4 GlcNac β1 ⟶ 2 Man 61 ⟶ 3
Man β ⟶ 4 GlcNac

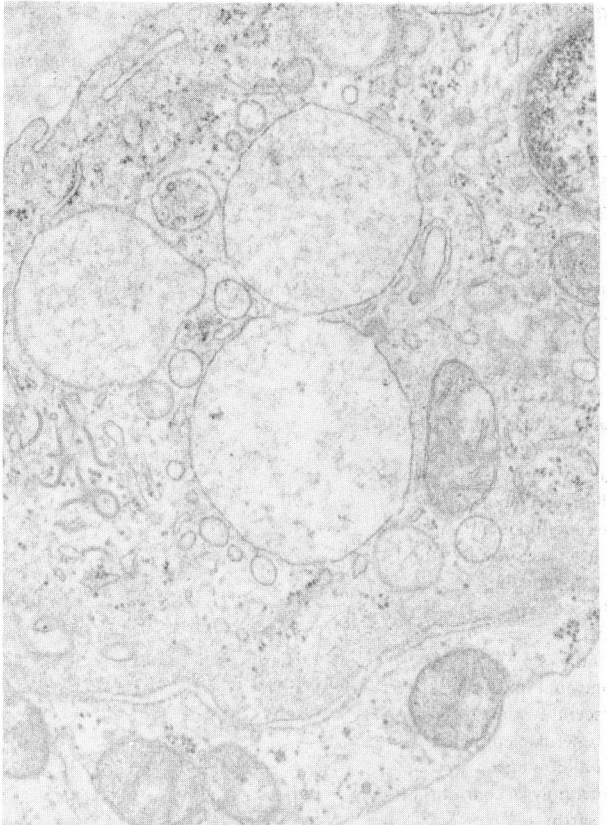

Figure 46-4 G_{M1} gangliosidosis, type 1. Electron microscopy of skin biopsy. Sweat gland secretory cell with four large membrane-bound clear vacuoles containing finely fibrillar material. Magnification, ×28,000.

When sialylated this compound is similar to the oligosaccharide side chain of a number of glycoproteins, such as erythrocyte stromal glycoprotein, transferrin, and immunoglobins. Its presence in the tissues (and in urine) in G_{M1} gangliosidosis can be explained by a block in glycoprotein catabolism at a step subsequent to cleavage of the oligosaccharide unit from the peptide chain by an endo-N-acetylglucosaminidase which hydrolyzes dichitobiose (N-acetylglucosaminyl-N-acetylglucosamine) linkages after action of neuraminidase, which hydrolyzes its sialic acid residues (Fig. 46-5). The gamut of oligosaccharides stored is truly amazing. Over 30 compounds have been detected and about 15 of them have been structurally defined [37]. The metabolic block (Fig. 46-5) provides the experiment of nature which allows the carbohydrate chemist

Table 46-3 Nomenclature of G_{M2} gangliosidoses

Common name	Genetic classification	Year discovered	Number of patients known	Inheritance
Tay-Sachs disease	Hex A-2, Hex B-1	1881	Thousands	Autosomal recessive
Sandhoff disease	Hex A-1, Hex B-2	1968	100	Autosomal recessive
Juvenile G_{M2} gangliosidosis	Hex A-3, Hex B-1	1968	50	Autosomal recessive
Adult G_{M2} gangliosidosis	Hex A-4, Hex B-1	1973	10	Autosomal recessive
AB(+) variant	Activator mutant	1968	5	Autosomal recessive

Table 46-4 Major clinical features of ganglioside storage diseases

	G_{M2} gangliosidoses				G_{M1} gangliosidoses		
	Tay-Sachs	Sandhoff disease	Juvenile	Adult	Infantile	Juvenile	Adult
Age at onset of symptom	3–6 mo.	3–6 mo.	2–6 yr.	Teens	Birth	6–20 mo.	Teens
Age at death	2–5 yr.	2–5 yr.	5–15 yr.	20+ yr.	$\frac{1}{2}$–2 yr.	3–10 yr.	20+ yr.
Mental-motor retardation	+	+	+	±	+	+	+
Facial appearance	Doll-like	Doll-like	Normal	Normal	Coarse	Normal	Normal
Edema	–	–	–	–	+	–	–
X-ray changes, long bones	–	–	–	–	+	Mild	Mild
X-ray changes, vertebrae	–	–	–	–	+	Mild	Mild
Vacuolated lymphocytes	–	–	–	–	+	+	±
Foam cells in marrow	–	–	–	–	+	+	±
Hepatomegaly	–	–	–	–	+	–	–
Splenomegaly	–	–	–	–	+	–	–
Cherry-red spot	90% +	+	–	–	50%	–	–
Retinitis pigmentosa	–	–	–*	±	–	–	–
Startle response to sound	+	+	+	–	+	+	–
Macrocephaly	+	+	–	–	Rarely	–	–
Macroglossia	–	–	–	–	+	–	–
Seizures	+	+	+	–	+	+	–
Blindness	Early	Early	Late	–	Early	Late	–
Neuronal lipidosis	+	+	+	+	+	+	+
Visceral histiocytosis	–	Mild	–	–	+	+	+
Glomerular epithelial ballooning	–	–†	–	–	+	+	?
Mucopolysacchariduria	–	–	–	–	±	±	?
Dysarthria	–	–	+	+	+	+	+
Spasticity-ataxia	–	–	+	+	–	+	+
Hypotonia	+	+	–	–	+	–	–

* Retinitis pigmentosa was noted late in the course of one patient, not in three others.
† Renal tubular epithelial cell vacuolization.

to determine the full gamut of β-D-galactose-terminal oligosaccharide residues in human glycoproteins [38]. An important task will be to determine which of these compounds (or others yet to be completely defined) [37] are responsible for such clinical symptoms as bony abnormalities, edema, seizures, and the like.

Enzyme Defect: Acid β-Galactosidase Deficiency

G_{M1} gangliosidosis is the first ganglioside storage disease shown to be caused by the absence of a degradative enzyme [39]. β-Galactosidase activity is strikingly deficient if ganglioside G_{M1} and galactose-containing glycoproteins [40] are used as substrates. The deficiency of β-galactosidase activity is not due to the presence of soluble endogenous inhibitors. Activities of other lysosomal enzymes, including acid phosphatase, β-glucosidase, and β-N-acetylglucosaminidase, are either normal or increased. Ganglioside G_{M1}–β-galactosidase activity is diminished to less than 0.1 percent of normal brain, liver [41], and cultured fibroblasts [18]. Brain β-galactosidase activities for galactocerebroside and ceramic lactoside (ceramic-glucose-galactose) are normal or increased when the appropriate assay is used [42]. The metabolic block involves the first step in G_{M1} breakdown (Fig. 46-3).

The diagnosis of G_{M1} gangliosidosis can be confirmed by β-galactosidase assays of leukocytes [43], urine [44], and cul-

tured fibroblasts [45, 18]. Heterozygotes are most easily detected by β-galactosidase assays of leukocytes. Levels between homozygotes and controls are found [43]. The enzyme is present in normal cultured amniotic cells obtained by amniocentesis in the second trimester of pregnancy, and β-galactosidase assay has been used for the prenatal diagnosis of at-risk fetuses [46–48].

Molecular Genetics of Acid β-Galactosidase Several different β-galactosidases, assayed using synthetic substrates, occur in human tissues [49]. Three of these, isoenzymes A_1 and A_2 (formerly called acid β-galactosidase A) and A_3 (formerly called acid β-galactosidase B) [50], are deficient in G_{M1} gangliosidosis. The activity of a fourth β-galactosidase, called *neutral β-galactosidase*, varies greatly in G_{M1} gangliosidosis, sometimes being elevated and sometimes diminished [18].

The following questions have arisen in considering the molecular genetics of the G_{M1} gangliosidosis [51]: Do all the A forms cleave galactose from all the stored compounds, or do they selectively cleave different substrates? Do they contain a common polypeptide which is coded by a single common autosomal locus? Is neutral β-galactosidase related to the A forms? What is the nature of the mutation in G_{M1} gangliosidosis—structural or regulatory? Are the mutations in infantile, juvenile, and adult types allelic or not? Can the storage of the different galactoconjugates be explained by a mutation at a single locus? Studies on purified acid β-galactosidase have provided answers to these questions.

Properties of Acid β-Galactosidases and Other β-Galactosidases

The major acid β-galactosidase isoenzymes β-galactosidase A_1 and A_2, have been purified to homogeneity from human liver and studied in detail [52, 53]. From A_1 is monomeric and spontaneously dimerizes to A_2 under appropriate conditions. Form A_3 is a multimer of A_1 [53].

β-Galactosidase A_1, A_2, and A_3 (Table 46-6) which possess pH optima (4.2 to 4.4) in the acid region are designated *acid β-galactosidases* [54]. Each is stimulated and stabilized by sodium chloride [55], is thermolabile, and cleaves aryl-β-D-galactoside linkages but not aryl-β-D-glucoside linkages. Each hydrolyzes β-linked galactose residues from G_{M1} [52, 56]. β-Galactosidase A_3 has a molecular weight (660,000) about 10 times higher than that of G_{A1} (65,000). Under appropriate conditions A_1 can be generated from A_3 [53]. A_3 is comprised solely of multimers of A_1 [57]. Monospecific antibodies prepared against homogeneous A_1 selectively precipitate A_2 and A_3 [52, 53]. Thus all the A forms possess a common polypeptide and appear to be coded by a common locus.

Neutral β-galactosidase (Table 46-6) possesses a more neutral pH optimum that the A forms and a lower molecular weight (57,000). It is inhibited by sodium chloride, is more heat stable than β-galactosidase A [55], and cleaves both aryl-β-D-galactoside and aryl-β-D-glucoside linkages, in contrast to the A forms. Neutral β-galactosidase does not cleave galactose from ganglioside G_{m1} or from asialofetuin [52, 56]. Neutral β-galactosidase from human liver does not absorb to conca-

navalin A–Sepharose columns and is readily separated from A_1 and A_3 by this means [56]. Monospecific anti-A antibodies do not precipitate neutral β-galactosidase [52]. Thus neutral β-galactosidase contains polypeptide different from the A forms and is coded by a separate genetic locus.

In normal human liver, using 4-methylumbelliferyl-β-galactoside (4MU-β-D-galactoside) or p-nitrophenyl-β-galactoside as substrates, approximately 85 percent of the activity assayed at pH 4.5 is due to A_1 (plus A_2), 10 percent to A_3, and 5 percent to neutral β-galactosidase. Variations from these values are obtained from individual to individual or when the chloride concentration or pH of the assay is varied. Neutral β-galactosidase has some β-galactosidase at the pH optimum of acid β-galactosidase, and if one equates 4-methylumbelliferyl-β-galactosidase activity with G_{M1} β-galactosidase activity, an error will result if neutral β-galactosidase is present. Neutral β-galactosidase must be removed prior to assay to avoid this error, or ganglioside G_{M1} must be used as the substrate.

Initially, patients with infantile G_{M1} gangliosidosis (type 1) appeared to have much lower activities of neutral β-galactosidase than those with juvenile G_{M1} gangliosidosis (type 2) [18]. This finding was not confirmed when larger numbers of patients were studied [59, 60]. It is now evident that the activity of neutral β-galactosidase in liver varies over a sevenfold range, both in patients with G_{M1} gangliosidosis and in normal controls, without apparent relationship to clinical status or subtype [61]. The reason for this large variability is not known. Unfortunately, since neutral β-galactosidase comigrates with β-galactosidase A_1 on gel electrophoresis, they can be con-

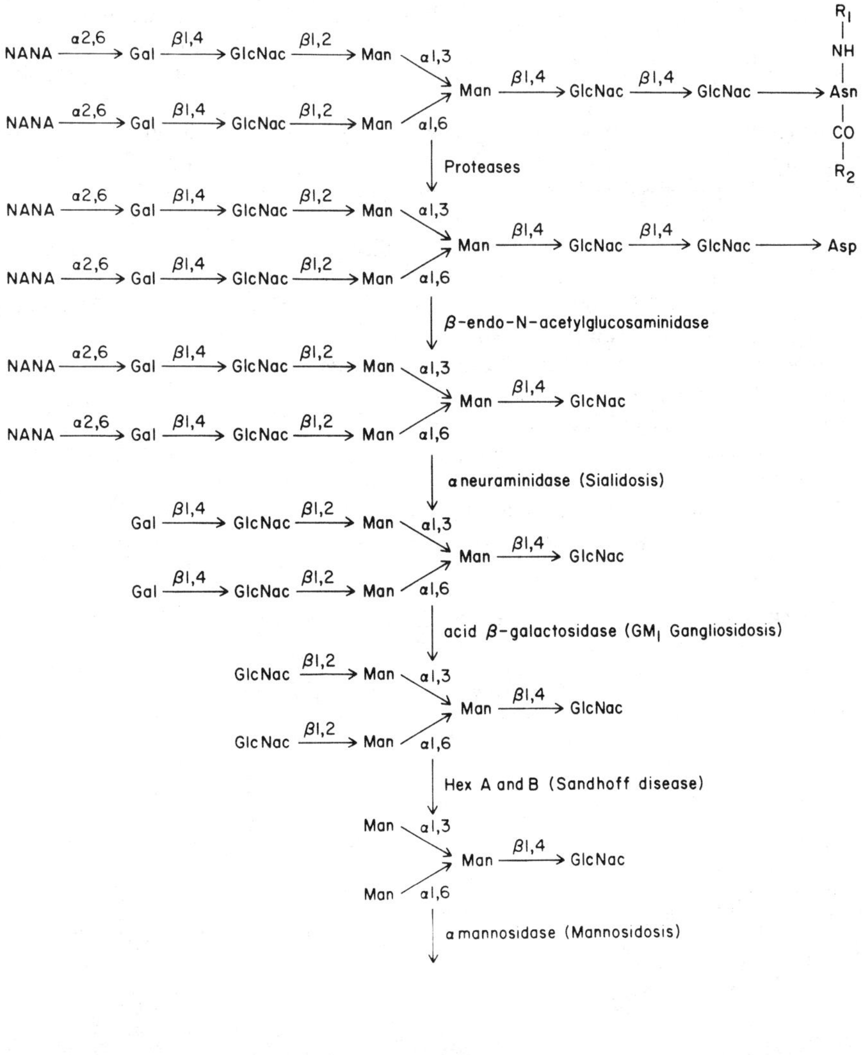

Figure 46-5 Scheme for degradation of asparaginyl-linked oligosaccharide in glycoproteins. Diseases resulting from block at each step are given.

Table 46-5 Heterozygote frequency of Tay-Sachs disease in Ashkenazi Jewish populations in some worldwide cities as shown by mass screening programs as of June 1980 [22]

City	Total tested	Total carriers	At-risk couples detected
Los Angeles	37,461	1,325	32
San Diego	9,674	281	10
San Francisco	14,570	571	12
Denver	1,753	115	1
Hartford-New Haven	5,534	170	0
Miami	6,045	234	14
Atlanta	3,345	156	6
Baltimore	16,769	817	10
Boston	11,119	479	9
Detroit	5,020	244	4
Minneapolis	4,289	159	3
Newark	7,385	293	8
New York (Bronx)	14,640	623	15
Brooklyn	46,289	1,539	17
Philadelphia	26,261	1,234	25
Houston	2,231	75	3
Richmond	3,600	83	0
USA total	259,121	10,111	212
Toronto	15,786	954	23
Montreal	14,407	750	4
Europe	1,436	80	2
Israel	15,530	527	18
South Africa	1,794	154	3
Worldwide	312,214	12,763	268

fused. The proposal that type 2 patients may be A(+) and type 1 patients A(−) [18] resulted from this overlap. It now appears that neutral β-galactosidase is not involved in the pathogenesis of G_{M1} gangliosidosis.

Neutral β-galactosidase has been strikingly deficient in liver tissue of subjects who expired from causes unrelated to β-galactosidase deficiency [62]. The benign deficiency of this enzyme suggests that it is not involved in storage disease.

Competitive inhibition studies indicate that the same catalytic site(s) on purified β-galactosidase A_1 cleaves G_{M1} and 4MU-β-D-galactoside [52]. Isoenzyme A_1 also cleaves lactose, N-acetyllactosamine, 4MU-α-L-arabinoside, and p-nitrophenyl-β-D-fucoside [52]. The latter two substrates are isomers of β-D-galactose, and the explanation for depressed hydrolysis of these substrates in G_{M1} gangliosidosis [63, 64] is apparent.

β-Galactosidase A_1 can cleave both β-D, 1–3 linkages, which occur in G_{M1}, and β-D, 1–4 linkages which appear in glycoproteins [52] (Fig. 46-5). Substrates cleaved poorly or not at all include galactosylhydroxylysine and galactosylhydroxylysine peptides from a proteolytic digestion of collagen, galactocerebroside, lactosylceramide, and monogalactosyldiglyceride [52].

If one measures the activities of galactocerebroside β-galactosidase, lactosylceramide β-galactosidase, and monogalactosyldiglyceride β-galactosidase during the purification of β-galactosidase A_1, these three activities do not copurify with A_1. Monospecific anti-A_1 antibodies do not precipitate galactocerebroside β-galactosidase, lactosylceramide β-galactosidase, or monogalactosyldiglyceride β-galactosidase from solution. Accordingly, these enzymatic activities are the properties of protein(s) different from β-galactosidase A_1 [52].

Thus the mutation in Krabbe's disease (Chap. 43), wherein there is a deficiency of galactocerebroside β-galactosidase [65] (and lactosylceramide β-galactosidase and monogalactosyldiglyceride β-galactosidase [42], is not allelic with the G_{M1} gangliosidosis mutation. Earlier findings that galactocerebroside β-galactosidase activities are not deficient in G_{M1} gangliosidosis [42] and that acid β-galactosidase activity is not deficient in Krabbe's disease [65] pointed to the same conclusion.

Two groups have reported partial or severe deficiencies of lactosylceramide β-galactosidase activity in G_{M1} gangliosidosis [66, 67]. The apparent explanation for these results is that the assay used, in which *crude* taurocholate is employed instead of *purified* taurocholate, stimulates acid β-galactosidase to cleave lactosylceramide [66]. With this assay, one finds a deficiency of lactosylceramide β-galactosidase in G_{M1} gangliosidosis. When purified taurocholate is the detergent, no deficiency is found.

The important conclusion is that the deficiency of lactosylceramide β-galactosidase activity in G_{M1} gangliosidosis appears to be due to methodologic peculiarities, not to production of the two enzymes by a common locus.

Human liver acid β-galactosidase appears to exist in vivo as a single monomeric polypeptide chain of 65,000 molecular weight or as multimers of A_1 [53]. Since acid β-galactosidase is monomeric, its polypeptide chain is apparently the product of a single autosomal locus.

Nature of the Mutation in G_{M1} Gangliosidosis

The genetic defect in G_{M1} gangliosidosis appears to be a mutation of the structural gene which codes for β-galactosidase A,

Table 46-6 Properties of β-galactosidases in human liver

Isoenzyme	Molecular weight	pH Optimum (4MUβGal)	Heat stability*	Effect of chloride	Cleaves 4MUβGal	Cleaves 4MUβGl	Cleaves G_{M1}	Cleaves asialofetuin
A_1	62,000	4.35	Labile	Stimulates	+	0	+	+
A_3	600,000–800,000	4.20	Labile	Stimulates	+	0	+	+
Neutral	57,000	5.80	Stable	Inhibits	+	+	0	0

* Heating at 37°C

† Values are approximate; assayed at pH 4.3 with 4MU-β-galactoside

NOTE: 4MUβGal = 4-methylumbelliferyl-β-galactoside; 4MUβGlc = 4-methylumbelliferyl-β-glucoside.

SOURCE: For references, see O'Brien [51].

located on the short arm (p12q21) of human chromosome 3 [68]. Liver samples from 11 patients with G_{M1} gangliosidosis (5 with infantile, 3 with juvenile, and 3 with "intermediate" phenotypes) contained normal or supranormal quantities of cross-reacting material to anti-β-galactosidase A_1 antibodies. This indicates that structurally altered β-galactosidase A was produced in all [51]. A similar result was obtained in the study of another patient [69]. Quantitative analyses of mutant β-galactosidase, determined immunologically, in infantile, juvenile, and adult G_{M1} gangliosidosis fibroblasts have given normal amounts of kinetically defective enzyme in each type and higher enzyme activity per units of immunoreactivity in the later onset patients [70].

One unusual patient (C. E.) with juvenile onset has an electrophoretic variant of β-galactosidase A_1 [61] with a more positive charge than normal. The enzyme from C. E. had a K_m that was five times normal with ganglioside G_{M1}. The mutant enzyme cross-reacted immunologically with normal β-galactosidase A antibodies but possessed only 1 percent of the normal catalytic activity per unit of antigenic activity. This is the first electrophoretic variant reported for a patient with lysosomal hydrolase deficiency disease.

Patient C. E. is a proven kinetic mutant, and many other patients are likely so. Since a single locus appears to code for the synthesis of β-galactosidase A_1 polypeptide, the mutations in all types of G_{M1} gangliosidosis studied thus far appear to be allelic. Structurally altered A protein is produced in nearly normal quantities in all cases. Somatic cell hybridization of cultured cells from patients with different types of G_{M1} gangliosidosis have failed to yield complementary β-galactosidase A in the mixed heterokaryons as a consequence of subunit rearrangements [71] as expected [51]. The finding of complementary activity in heterokaryons derived from fusions between type 2 cells and those from an unusual β-galactosidase-deficient patient, termed type 4 [71] has been explained. The type 4 patient has been shown to have sialidosis (α-neuraminidase deficiency) with secondary β-galactosidase deficiency [72] (see Chap. 38).

Explanation of the G_{M1} Gangliosidosis Phenotype

The phenotypic effects of a single gene mutation involving acid β-galactosidase may be explained by a one gene–one polypeptide–many substrates model [51] (Fig. 46-6). Acid β-galactosidase is *heterocatalytic*, cleaving β-D-linked galactose from several galactoconjugates [52]. Keratosulfatelike glycosaminoglycans (sulfated and sulfate, free), galactose-oligosaccharides,

glycoproteins with carbohydrate side chains similar to asialofetuin, G_{M1}, and asialo-G_{M1} are a few of the natural substrates known. Many others, yet to be defined, probably exist. A structural mutation giving rise to altered β-galactosidase A with impaired catalytic activity can simultaneously lead to the accumulation of multiple galactoconjugates affecting many organ systems, depending upon the nature, location, degree, and consequences of storage.

Multiple Phenotypes   One explanation for the multiplicity of G_{M1} gangliosidosis phenotypes is that different mutations exist which lead to different kinetic alterations of each mutant polypeptide. Two possibilities may be considered: (a) mutant A protein which possesses about the same residual activity for each natural substrate is synthesized; or (b) mutant A protein which possesses significantly different residual activities for different natural substrates is synthesized.

Possibility a may be the case in most infantile-onset patients in whom storage of gangliosides and galactoproteins is massive and residual activity for all substrates is less than 1 percent of normal. Many patients with juvenile onset also may belong to category a, since β-galactosidase activities for G_{M1} and galactoprotein (in this case asialofetuin) are deficient to about the same extent [61]. However, in most later onset patients, residual activity is 2 to 5 times higher in liver than in those with type 1 [61] and 5 to 30 times higher in cultured skin fibroblasts [73–74]. This difference in residual enzyme activity could account for the phenotypic differences, the rate of storage being slower in type 2 because of higher residual activity.

Mutations of type b, in which residual β-galactosidase activity is higher for one type of substrate than for another, might be expected from the differences in molecular size, ionic charge, solubility in water, nature of galactose linkage, and type of penultimate amino sugar in the natural substrates thus far known to be cleaved by acid β-galactosidase. Unusual phenotypes can be predicted. For example, if significant catalytic activity is retained for galactose-containing glycoconjugates, but not for G_{M1}, the phenotype will be that of rapid neurologic decline due to G_{M1} storage without significant bony deformities. Patients with this phenotype have been described [75]. Alternatively, if significant catalytic activity is retained for G_{M1} and not for galactose-containing glycoconjugates, the phenotype will be that of severe bony abnormalities due to storage of these compounds with minimal cerebral defect. Several patients with such a phenotype have recently been discovered.

MORQUIO SYNDROME, TYPE B (MPS, IV, B)   Four patients in four different sibships have presented with progressive severe skeletal dysplasia without neurologic impairment [76–78]. The first patient [76] had hip pain at age 8 due to progressive dysplastic changes of the pelvis and femoral heads. She also had vertebral platyspondyly and unusual modeling deformities of the vertebral bodies similar to those seen in the hereditary spondyloepiphysial dyplasias. On careful neurologic examination there was no impairment of mental or motor function. Both parents had half-normal levels of β-galactosidase activity in leukocytes, consistent with heterozygosity for primary mutation of β-galactosidase.

Three other patients with the same phenotype have been reported [77, 78] and an altered K_m of the mutant enzyme was evident in two [78]. This condition has been classified as mucopolysaccharidosis IV B. It appears inappropriate to designate

Activity in G_{M1} gangliosidosis	Binds to con A-Sepharose	Cross reacts with anti-A antibodies	% of Total activity†
Deficient	+	+	85
Deficient	+	+	10
Variable	0	0	5

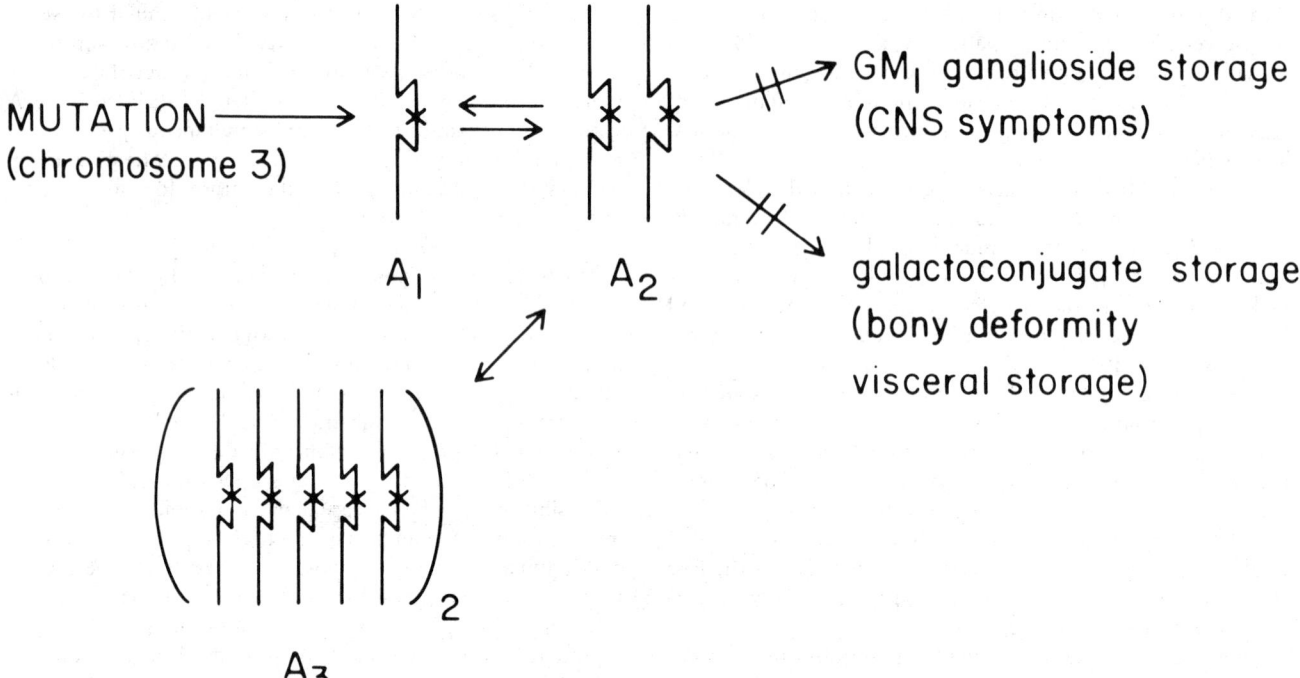

Figure 46-6 One gene—one polypeptide—many substrates model to explain the pleiotropic effect of a single mutation involving β-galactosidase A, which gives rise to the G_{M1} gangliosidosis phenotype. Although the model depicts a single amino acid substitution, other types of mutations could play a role. Isoenzyme A_3 is depicted as a decamer of A; the precise number of A subunits is unknown.

such patients as having G_{M1} gangliosidosis since this condition signifies a neurodegenerative disorder. The number of mutations which give rise to β-galactosidase deficiency and clinical disease is larger than previously thought, as expected with the model presented (Fig. 46-6).

A number of patients with β-galactosidase deficiency who were thought to be unusual G_{M1} gangliosidosis mutants [18] are now known to have sialidosis (α-neuraminidase deficiency [79, 80]. In such patients the β-galactosidase deficiency is secondary [79], but the underlying molecular basis for the low levels of activity are still poorly understood (see Chap. 38).

Classification

In the search for "new" mutants of acid β-galactosidase, clinicians should remain flexible in phenotypic classification. The "classical" phenotypes are useful trail markers in the search, but the searcher must be willing to ignore them as unknown territory is explored. It is likely that the number of different β-galactosidase mutations which lead to clinical disease is large, and compulsive overclassification of subtypes appears premature. A general classification such as "infantile," "juvenile," and "adult" G_{M1} gangliosidosis is useful for instruction, clinical diagnosis, management, prognostication, and counseling.

Animal Models

G_{M1} gangliosidosis has been reported in Siamese cats in the United States [81] and Japan [82], in a short-hair domestic cat in Cambridge [83], in Friesian cattle in Ireland [84], and in mixed breed beagles from Purdue University, Indiana [85]. Acid β-galactosidase has been documented as the primary defect in Siamese cats [86] and beagles [85, 87].

As in humans, hepatic oligosaccharides accumulate in affected cats, but their structures differ in that an extra N-acetylglucosamine residue is present [88]. Comparison of the mutant cat enzyme with the wild-type enzyme has been made [89]. The major differences include an altered K_m, increased thermolability, and altered molecular weight of the mutant enzyme [87]. The mutant and wild-type enzyme did not cross-react immunologically.

A similar comparison has been made between mutant and wild-type enzyme in G_{M1} beagles [90]. A striking deficiency of β-galactosidase (4 percent of normal) has been found in cultured fibroblasts and in tissues (brain and viscera) accompanied by oligosaccharide storage [91] and cerebral G_{M1} gangliosidosis [85]. Preliminary characterization of the mutant enzyme in frozen liver indicated identity to the wild-type enzyme but a deficiency of cross-reactive material [90].

More recent studies with fresher sources of tissue (fibroblasts) indicate normal quantities of immunoreactive mutant enzyme which is very thermolabile [91]. A preliminary study of the oligosaccharides stored in liver in the canine disorder has been made [91]. Examination by thin-layer chromatography (Fig. 46-7) reveals a difference between the mutant dog and human oligosaccharide patterns. The dog compounds are more polar and contain one extra N-acetylglucosamine residue at the reducing terminus than the human compounds. Structural analysis [91] reveals the major dog compound to be a nonasaccharide:

$$\text{Gal } \beta 1 \longrightarrow 4 \text{ GlcNac } \beta 1 \longrightarrow 2 \text{ Man } \alpha 1 \longrightarrow 6$$
$$\text{Gal } \beta 1 \longrightarrow 4 \text{ GlcNac } \beta 1 \longrightarrow 2 \text{ Man } \alpha 1 \longrightarrow 3$$
$$\text{Man } \beta 1 \longrightarrow 4 \text{ GlcNac } \beta 1 \longrightarrow 4 \text{ GlcNac}$$

It is important to characterize such animal mutants in detail since they can serve as experimental models for therapy. The beagle model is especially useful since breeding colonies have been established at Purdue University, Indiana, and at the University of California, San Diego. In the predicted era of gene therapy, such animals will be especially valuable in determining whether replacement of the cloned gene for β-galactosidase is an efficatious therapeutic approach.

G_{M2} GANGLIOSIDOSIS

Phenotypic Descriptions [18]

Tay-Sachs Disease Motor weakness usually begins between 3 and 6 months of age. The startle reaction, an extension response to sudden, sharp but not necessarily loud sounds, is a characteristic early symptom. After 6 months of age, motor weakness becomes obvious. The infant may crawl, sit unaided, and pull to a standing position but usually does not achieve the ability to walk. Mental and motor deterioration progress rapidly after 1 year of age. Feeding becomes a problem because of ineffective swallowing. Muscle tone is poor and generalized paralysis develops. After 18 months progressive deafness, blindness, convulsions, and spasticity appear and a state of decerebrate rigidity is reached. The patient usually dies from bronchopneumonia by 3 years of age. Many patients have a doll-like facial appearance with pale, transluscent skin, long eyelashes, fine hair, and delicate pink coloring. Cherry-red spots in the macular region are present in over 95 percent of the patients. This lesion may resemble a paint splotch in the first few days of life but gradually develops into a well-defined circular red spot within a white halo. Later the spot becomes darker and brownish in color as the macula degenerates, and opaque whitish streaks (lipid deposits?) along vessels may be observed. Progressively increasing head size (macrocephaly)

Figure 46-7 Thin-layer chromatogram of oligosaccharides from liver tissue. *A.* Normal dog extract; *B.* infantile G_{M1} gangliosidosis extract; *C.* dog G_{M1} gangliosidosis extract; and *D.* through *G.* purified oligosaccharides from dog G_{M1} gangliosidosis. Compounds 1 and 2 contain 6 sugars and compounds 3, 4, and 5 contain 9, 11, and 13 sugars, respectively. Note the slower migration of the dog compounds than the human compounds.

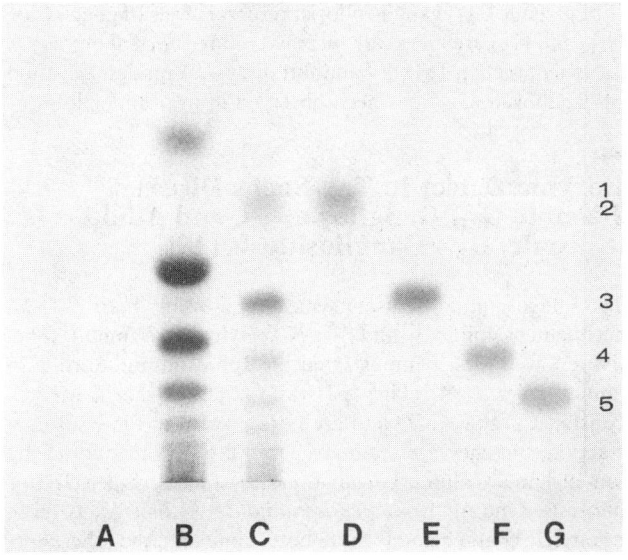

usually develops after 16 months of life and is due to cerebral gliosis rather than ventricular enlargement.

Pathologic changes include conspicuous neuronal lipidosis of cortical, autonomic, and rectal mucosal neurons. The cytoplasm of most neurons is ballooned and distended, and the nucleus is displaced to the periphery. Osmiophilic cytoplasmic membranous bodies accumulate within neurons. These are round structures comprised of tightly packed, circular membranes, each lamella having a cross-sectioned thickness of 5 nm (Fig. 46-8). The storage bodies are the site of intense acid phosphatase activity and, after isolation, have been shown to be comprised of large quantities of ganglioside G_{M2}.

Central demyelination occurs and appears to be secondary to axonal degeneration. Cortical gliosis is prominent. Pathologic changes are not evident in visceral organs, except for an occasional lipid inclusion body noted on ultrastructural examination.

Sandhoff Disease [18] The clinical and pathologic picture is similar to Tay-Sachs disease. Motor weakness begins within the first 6 months of life. The startle reaction to sound, early blindness, progressive mental and motor deterioration, doll-like faces, cherry-red spots, and macrocephaly are present. Occasional patients have had bony deformities similar to those noted in infantile G_{M1} gangliosidosis. Lymphocyte vacuolation is not prominent. Occasional foamy histiocytes are found in the bone marrow. Death due to bronchopneumonia usually occurs by 3 years of age.

Pathologic changes in the cortex are nearly identical to those seen in Tay-Sachs disease. Lipidosis of cortical, cerebellar, spinal, and autonomic neurons is prominent. Vacuolated histiocytes are present in lungs, spleen, lymph nodes, and bone marrow, but the degree of histiocytosis is less than that seen in Gaucher's or Niemann-Pick disease. Vacuolation of the tubular epithelial cells of the renal loops of Henle may be prominent, probably due to storage of *N*-acetylglucosamine-containing oligosaccharides. Ultrastructural studies reveal intracellular lamellar lipid inclusions and clear vacuolar material in these cells.

Juvenile G_{M2} Gangliosidosis with Hexosaminidase A Deficiency [18] Onset occurs between 2 and 6 years of age. Locomotor ataxia is the most prominent initial symptom. Loss of speech, progressive spasticity, athetoid posturing of hands and extremities, and minor motor seizures follow. All patients have deteriorated to a state of decerebrate rigidity. Blindness occurs late in the course of this disorder, in contrast to Tay-Sachs disease and Sandhoff disease, where early blindness is characteristic. Optic atrophy was present in two patients and retinitis pigmentosa was present in the terminal stages of a third, but a macular lesion has been reported only once. Death occurs between 5 and 15 years of age, often secondary to bronchopneumonia.

Hepatosplenomegaly, bony deformities, lymphocyte vacuolization, and foam cells in the bone marrow have not been described. Juvenile G_{M2} gangliosidosis is clinically similar to Batten-Spielmeyer-Vogt disease and has probably been misdiagnosed as such. Important differentiating features include prominent visual disturbances, macular degeneration, and retinitis pigmentosa early in the course of Batten-Spielmeyer-Vogt disease, and absence or late retinal involvement in juvenile G_{M2} gangliosidosis.

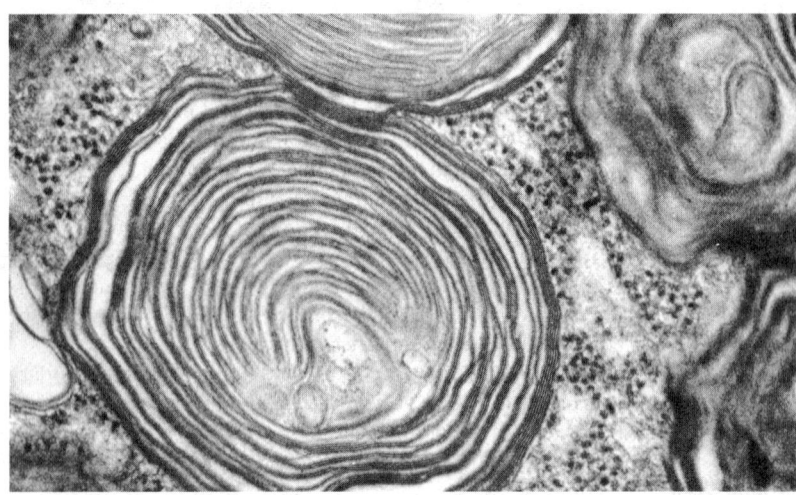

Figure 46-8 Cytoplasmic membranous body in neuron in Tay-Sachs disease. Original magnification, ×98,000.

Neuronal lipidosis is prominent. Neurons contain cytoplasmic inclusions of a mixed type. Cytoplasmic membranous bodies, similar to those seen in Tay-Sachs and Sandhoff disease, are present, but other bodies with a more random ordering, called pleomorphic lamellar bodies, are also present (Fig. 46-9). Visceral histiocytosis has not been described.

Adult (Chronic) G_{M2} Gangliosidosis with Hexosaminidase A Deficiency   The spectrum of the G_{M2} gangliosidoses has been broadened by the discovery of adults with this disorder [92]. The initial patients had a slowly progressive deterioration of gait and posture which began between 2 and 4 years of age. Atypical spinocerebellar degeneration was suggested since pes cavus, foot drop, spasticity, mild ataxia of limbs and trunk, dystonia, and dysarthria were present in addition to proximal muscle atrophy. Vision and optic fundi were normal, and verbal intelligence has been stable over two decades. An older sister expired at 16 years of age with the same disorder. Postmortem examination revealed diffuse neuronal storage predominating in subcortical areas and consisting of membranous cytoplasmic, zebra bodies and complex lamellar structures. An increased concentration of G_{M2} ganglioside was found in the brain. Hexosaminidase A activity was strikingly decreased in serum and leukocytes of the living patients, and in the parents it was in the range for carriers of TSD [92].

An additional patient has recently been detected at age 20 through a TSD screening program [93]. He was normal until age 16, when leg cramping began. By 18 years he had developed proximal muscle wasting, weakness, fasciculations, slight dysarthria, spasticity, and ataxia, but intelligence was normal. Diagnoses which were entertained included amyotrophic lateral sclerosis. Ophthalmologic examination, EEG, and nerve conduction velocity were normal. Rectal biopsy revealed lipidosis of myenteric plexus neurons containing "onion-skin" membranous cytoplasmic lysosomal inclusions by electron microscopy. Serum hexosaminidase A activity was totally deficient and assays of G_{M2} N-acetylgalactosaminidase activity gave no activity in cultured fibroblasts [93]. Assays of hexosaminidase A activity in both parents gave intermediate activities in serum and fibroblasts consistent with the heterozygote state. This patient differs from those described above since he had a symptom-free period to age 16 and had less severe cerebellar symptoms.

Chemistry

G_{M2}, G_{A2}, Globoside, and N-Acetylglucosamine-Oligosaccharide Storage   Cerebral levels of ganglioside G_{M2} are increased 100 to 300 times normal in Tay-Sachs and Sandhoff disease. The asialo-derivative of ganglioside G_{M2} (G_{A2}) accumulates to levels about 20 times normal. The ganglioside content of visceral organs is not significantly increased, but the ganglioside pattern is abnormal in that ganglioside G_{M2} comprises a higher proportion of total gangliosides than normal.

Much higher amounts of G_{A2} accumulate in the brain and viscera in Sandhoff disease than in Tay-Sachs disease. Globoside [Cer-Glc-Gal-Gal-Gal (NAc)] accumulates in large quantities in the viscera, especially the kidney and spleen, in Sandhoff disease. This probably accounts for the lipid inclusions found on ultrastructural examination. In addition, N-acetylglucosaminyl-oligosaccharides accumulate in the tissues and are excreted in urine in Sandhoff disease [37]. These appear to derive from degradation of glycoproteins (Fig. 46-5) and accumulate because of absence of both hexosaminidase A and B, each of which hydrolyzes them. Globoside and N-acetylglucosaminyl-oligosaccharides do not accumulate in TSD, since there is sufficient hexosaminidase B to degrade them.

In juvenile G_{M2} gangliosidosis, cerebral levels of ganglioside G_{M2} and G_{A2} are markedly increased above normal but not to the extent seen in TSD or Sandhoff disease. A modest elevation of ganglioside G_{M2} has been observed in liver and spleen.

Enzyme Defect in Tay-Sachs Disease, Juvenile G_{M2} Gangliosidosis, and Adult (Chronic) G_{M2} Gangliosidosis [18]

Two hexosaminidase isoenzymes (possessing both β-D-N-acetylglucosaminidase and β-D-N-acetylgalactosaminidase activities) were first demonstrated by Robinson and Stirling in human spleen [94]. They possess similar Michaelis-Menten constants (Table 46-7) and are both present in the lysosomal fraction, but they are readily separated from one another by ion-exchange column chromatography or starch-gel electrophoresis. One of these, *hexosaminidase A* (hex A), is more negatively charged and is more heat-labile than the other, *hex-*

osaminidase B (hex B). Both hex A and hex B have been found in all normal human tissues (except red cells), including leukocytes, serum, urine, tears, cultured skin fibroblasts, amniotic fluid, and cultured amniotic cells. A third enzyme, termed *hexosaminidase C*, is nonlysosomal and is not related to hex A or hex B [95].

In TSD, hex A activity is nearly absent [96, 97]. The deficiency was demonstrated using *p*-nitrophenyl, 4-methylumbelliferyl, and naphthyl-ASBI derivatives of both β-D-*N*-acetylglucosamine and β-D-*N*-acetylgalactosamine as substrates [96]. Brain activity of hex B in TSD is increased about 10 times normal and is probably due to lysosomal stimulation secondary to ganglioside storage, since the activities of other lysosomal hydrolases are also increased and hex B activity is not increased in tissues where ganglioside storage is minimal. The deficiency of hex A persists in cultured skin fibroblasts over many cellular generations [98].

A partial deficiency of hex A was found in the first several patients studied with juvenile G_{M2} gangliosidosis. As more patients have been analyzed using synthetic substrates, some have had a total deficiency of hex A and some have had hex A activities close to normal [18]. When G_{M2} ganglioside is used as substrate, activities have been nearly totally deficient [99]. In patients with only a slight deficiency of hex A, using synthetic substrates, prenatal diagnosis and carrier detection must be performed using ganglioside G_{M2} as substrate [99, 100].

In the two families with adult G_{M2} gangliosidosis described above, hex A activity was strikingly deficient, and parents had reduced activities consistent with autosomal recessive transmission of the trait. Since both families were of Ashkenazi Jewish ancestry, it is likely that the patients were heterozygous for two different mutations at the same locus (allelic compounds), one of these being the TSD allele and the second being a new mutant allele.

Diagnosis of Homozygotes and Carrier Detection   A serum assay, which exploits the different thermal stabilities of hex A and B, was developed in 1970 in the author's laboratory for the diagnosis of TSD and for carrier detection [101]. Patients with phenotypes similar to TSD, such as those with Niemann-Pick disease, infantile Gaucher's disease, and G_{M1} gangliosidosis, are not hex A deficient. Hex A is deficient in fetal TSD serum [102] and the assay can be used to diagnose TSD at birth using umbilical cord serum. The serum assay is especially valuable in unusual patients with TSD who do not have cherry-red spots in the macula [101].

Persons heterozygous for the TSD gene have intermediate reductions of hex A in serum, leukocytes, and cultured fibroblasts. The serum assay was initially designed to detect heterozygotes in families in which TSD had occurred [101]. The heat denaturation assay has subsequently been semiautomated and modified [103–105] for mass screening. The modifications include increasing substrate concentration for improved linearity, optimizing other conditions, and full automation. The automated assay has been the basis for mass screening for TSD carriers worldwide [103–105].

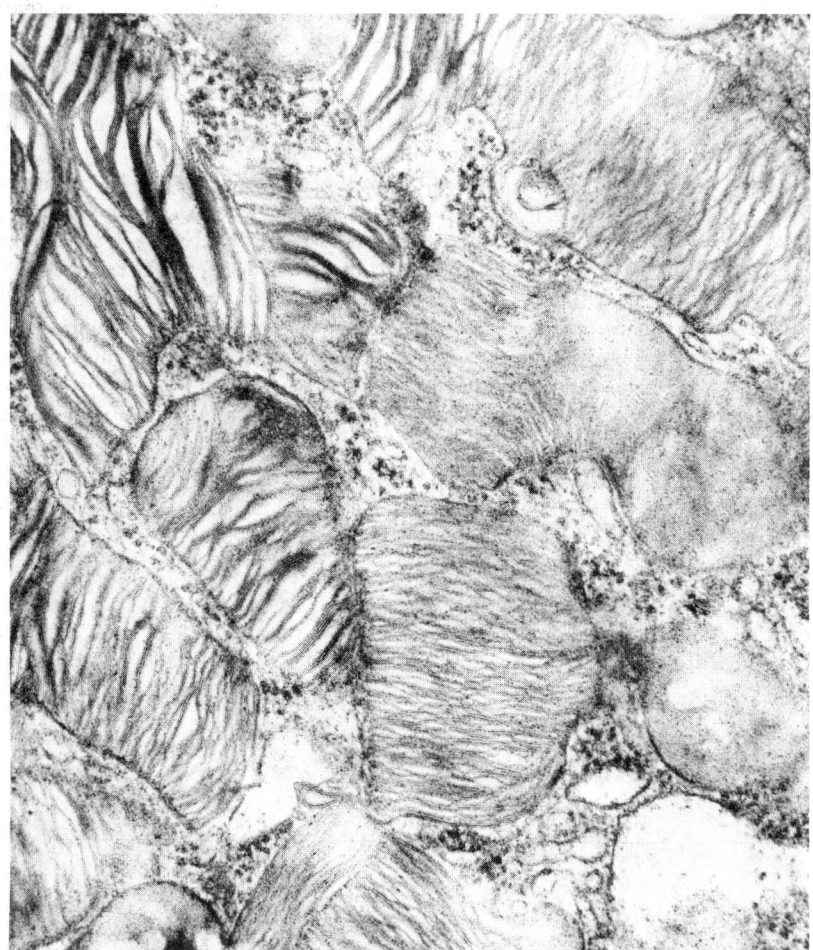

Figure 46-9   Pleomorphic inclusion bodies in the neuron in juvenile G_{M2} gangliosidosis. Original magnification, ×80,000.

Table 46-7   Some properties of human hexosaminidase A and B

	Hex A	Hex B
Isoelectric pH	5.4	7.9
Molecular weight	102,000	100,000
pH optimum	4.4	4.4
Amino-terminal amino acid	Blocked	Blocked
Carboxy-terminal amino acid	Serine	Aspartic or asparagine
Substrates cleaved	G_{M2}, G_{A2}, Globoside, hexosamine oligosaccharides	G_{A2}, globoside, hexosamine oligosaccharides
Subunit (mol. wt.)	α chain (58,000) β chain (25,000)	β chain (25,000)
Proposed structure	$\alpha\beta_2$	$\beta_2\beta_2$

NOTE: For references, see text.

The assay is accurate for genotype assignment in 96 percent of those tested. The remaining 4 percent fall into an inconclusive range arbitrarily defined to avoid false negative and false positive assignment (Fig. 46-10). When these inconclusive subjects are retested by the more accurate leukocyte assay, a confidence level greater than 99 percent in genotype designation is reached. The reliability of the automated serum assay was demonstrated by testing 256 relatives of patients with TSD [106, 107]. The heterozygote frequencies in each group of relatives were determined and a near-perfect correlation was found for the expected and observed carrier frequencies. Thus, the serum method neither overidentifies carriers (false positives) nor significantly misses them (false negatives).

A theoretical distribution curve for serum hex A levels in obligate carriers was plotted [106, 107] (Fig. 46-10). Individuals whose values fell within 1.7 standard deviations (SD) from the mean for known carriers were designated carriers and those whose values fell above 3 SD were designated noncarriers. The probability that the test would miss a TSD carrier has been calculated at less than 1 in 30,000 [106, 107].

In our earlier study [101] it was shown that reduced percentages of serum hex A in the carrier range (false positive) occurred in many patients with diabetes mellitus, with disorders involving tissue destruction such as myocardial infarction, hepatitis, and pancreatitis, and in normal pregnant women. In mass screening programs, such conditions are ascertained by a questionnaire at the time of testing, and the subjects are retested by leukocyte assay.

A high proportion of nonheterozygous women taking oral contraceptives have shown values in the inconclusive or heterozygous range [106, 107]. About 20 percent of women taking oral contraceptives have a false positive test. Fortunately, leukocyte activities of hex A remain unaltered, and this assay remains valid for genotype assignment. Tears can be used for the detection of heterozygotes, and the tear assay remains valid during pregnancy [108]. It is this group of subjects which comprises the largest proportion of "inconclusives" in mass screening programs.

In pregnant women the change in the serum hexosaminidase isoenzyme pattern after delivery is remarkably rapid. During pregnancy a gradual shift in serum hexosaminidase isoenzymes occurs, so that by 3 months of gestation all pregnant women tested have reduced proportions of heat-labile hexosaminidase, similar to TSD heterozygotes [109]. By 48 hours postpartem, the serum pattern returns to normal [109]. Increased activity of a heat-stable isoenzyme, called hexosaminidase P [110, 111], appears to cause the shift. This isoenzyme appears to be synthesized by liver, not placenta [112] and is apparently hormonally induced.

In screening programs [103–107] the problem of heterozygote detection in couples in which the wife is pregnant has been handled as follows. If the woman is more than 4.5 months pregnant, testing is not done since it is too late for pregnancy termination if the fetus has TSD. If the woman is less than 4.5 months pregnant, both are tested by serum hex A assay, the husband by serum assay, and the wife by leukocyte assay.

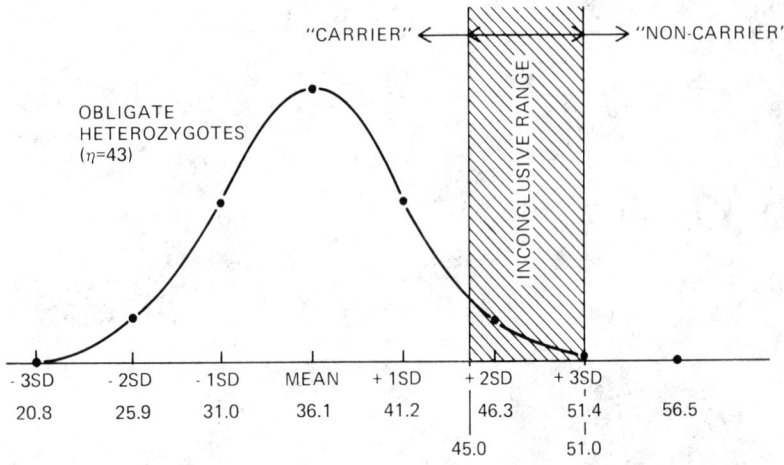

Figure 46-10   Serum hex A and carrier-noncarrier designation. A statistical basis for genotype assignment is derived from a normalized distribution curve of hex A levels in serum from obligate heterozygotes. An inconclusive area which is arbitrarily defined is indicated. Participants with serum hex A levels in this range require the follow-up leukocyte test before genotype is designated. (*From Kaback et al. [93]. Used by permission.*)

The studies [103–107] indicate that with appropriate precautions and with the methods used for serum assay, genotype assignment, and follow-up testing, a highly accurate determination can be made. In the first 10,000 individuals tested, no proven false positive serum carrier was identified [106, 107]. As discussed, the data suggest that false negative tests would be extremely rare.

The precise nature of those isoenzymes which have electrophoretic charges and thermal labilities intermediate between hex A and B [111] is not understood. As many as four to five bands of the p type and one to two bands of the I type have been found in human serum [113]. The electrophoretic mobility of the hexosaminidase isoenzymes in tissues differs from that in serum and some of the differences may be due to variations in the number of sialic acid residues in each isoenzyme [114, 115].

Implications of Mass Screening for TSD

Three criteria make the prospective prevention of TSD feasible: (1) the disorder occurs principally in a defined population group, Ashkenazi Jews; (2) a simple, accurate, and inexpensive carrier detection test is available, which can be automated for mass screening; and (3) the condition can be diagnosed in utero early enough to terminate pregnancies with TSD fetuses [116].

Mass screening for TSD heterozygotes has in general been carried out in community-based screening programs in which interested volunteers have participated in the organization and implementation of the screening effort. In Israel, screening of premarital Ashkenazi couples on a voluntary basis, referred through the Rabbinate, is operative [117]. Approximately 8000 couples marry each year in Israel.

The worldwide experience on screening for TSD heterozygotes through 1980 is summarized in Table 46-5. Screening has been carried out in 73 cities and 13 countries with 312,214 individuals tested since 1969. The program has identified 12,763 carriers and 268 at-risk couples with no family history of TSD. Among these couples, 252 pregnancies have occurred with 39 TSD fetuses identified prenatally; 212 unaffected offspring have been born.

Estimations of the effectiveness of the screening program in preventing the birth of a TSD baby can be made from a comparison of the anticipated versus actual incidence. In 1970 in North America, between 50 to 100 infants with TSD were born (80 percent were of Jewish ancestry) [18]. In 1980, 13 newly diagnosed patients with TSD were reported among the Ashkenazi Jewish population [22]. Assuming the same birth rate, the same pattern of marital selection of Ashkenazi Jewish individuals and reliable ascertainment, a 65 to 85 percent reduction in the incidence of TSD has occurred in North America in a decade, apparently as a result of the screening program.

This is the first example of prospective prevention of a genetic disease by mass screening for heterozygotes in an at-risk population [116]. Although TSD is a rare disorder, in the future the program may be used as a prototype model for prevention of other genetic diseases which occur in high-risk population groups. Since 82 percent of the cases of TSD are first-affected children in the family [118], only 18 percent can be prenatally detected if the birth of a TSD child is the tip-off that both parents are carriers. Large-scale screening for heterozy-

gotes and prospective prevention is necessary to detect most cases. When program costs are compared with the medical care costs which ensue for those TSD patients who are born if the screening program is not carried out, the program costs are about one-third to one-fifth the care costs [119, 120].

The psychological and sociological aspects of TSD screening are currently under study [121–123]. Such factors as anxiety generated by mass screening programs, stigmatization of heterozygotes, effectiveness of genetic counseling in information transfer, and compliance rates in community screening programs are being evaluated [122, 123]. Although anxiety generated from knowledge of carrier status appears minimal [122], public knowledge of genetics is scanty [123].

Prenatal Diagnosis of TSD

TSD has been the inborn error of metabolism most frequently diagnosed in utero [124]. Hex A and B are usually assayed in amniotic fluid, uncultured amniotic cells, and cultured amniotic fluid cells obtained by amniocentesis. Our group previously stressed the importance of carrying out the assay on cultured amniotic cells to make the diagnosis [102].

An estimate of the accuracy of the prenatal diagnosis of TSD can be made from the collected cases [22]. To 1980, 814 pregnancies have been monitored for TSD in 77 worldwide centers; 252 were in pregnancies ascertained to be at risk by carrier screening and 562 were ascertained by birth of a previous child with TSD. In 175 instances TSD was diagnosed prenatally and 168 abortions were carried out. In 3 the diagnosis was made too late for termination and in 4 instances abortion was refused. All 7 infants had TSD. In 150, confirmation of the diagnosis was made, but in 18 instances confirmation was not possible since material was unusable or unavailable. One child was diagnosed as having TSD at 9 months, after having been misidentified by amniocentesis as unaffected. Two other prenatal misdiagnoses have been reported, one false positive [124] and the other false negative [126]. In both instances cultured cells were not analyzed. This gives an error of 3 in 791 or 0.38 percent. In one pregnancy a "spontaneous" abortion occurred 1 week after amniocentesis. The low rate of fetal loss after mid-trimester amniocentesis is consistent with the results obtained by a study organized by the National Institutes of Child Health and Human Development on the safety and accuracy of mid-trimester amniocentesis in the United States [127].

Pitfalls in Prenatal Diagnosis   In spite of the remarkable success in prenatal diagnosis of TSD, several major pitfalls must be dealt with to achieve an accurate prenatal diagnosis [128]. Proper diagnosis of the proband is essential. Confusion of Tay-Sachs disease and Sandhoff disease may be troublesome, and misdiagnosis of the proband can be disastrous. Enzyme diagnosis is essential. The presence of twins can be a major problem. Unusual hexosaminidase variants (discussed below) may be ascertained only by using ganglioside G_{M2} as substrate. Both hex A and hex B are labile enzymes and may be inactivated during shipment, handling, or assay, leading to a disastrous artifact. This is especially true in dilute solutions such as amniotic cell or fibroblast homogenates [128]. Addition of protein, such as albumin, helps prevent such losses, but in very dilute solutions these may still occur. Contamination of amniotic taps with maternal blood or of cell cultures with maternal leukocytes may invalidate the results. Bacterial contamination must be studiously avoided since common gram-positive diplococci, such as *Mima polymorpha*, contain a hexosaminidase which migrates very close to hex A on gel electrophoresis [128].

In order to avoid such pitfalls, considerable expertise must be available. As a minimum, the collaboration of obstetricians experienced in amniocentesis, diagnosticians experienced in ultrasound technique, genetic counselors to advise and counsel, technicians expert in culturing amniotic cells, and biochemists experienced in enzyme assays and electrophoresis of hex A and B are necessary. Appropriate normal amniotic fluid samples must be run as controls with each high-risk tap. Final diagnosis must await results on cultured amniotic cells, whenever possible. Proper organization, precise timing, and error-free technique are essential at all steps. Centers without such expertise should not attempt the prenatal diagnosis of TSD or other gangliosidoses.

The author's recommended procedure for the prenatal diagnosis of TSD is as follows:

1. Ascertain that the disorder at risk is TSD by enzyme assay of affected patients or parents.

2. Amniocentesis, after ultrasound examination, by an experienced obstetrician, using the transabdominal approach, at 15 to 17 weeks gestation.

3. Removal of 10 to 30 ml of amniotic fluid, preferably not bloody, with all subsequent handling by sterile technique.

4. After centrifugation, tissue culture of amniotic cells, saving the cell-free fluid for assay.

5. Assay of total hexosaminidase and hexosaminidase A (heat-labile hexosaminidase) by the heat denaturation method in amniotic fluid, running normal controls and a bonafide TSD sample simultaneously. Gel electrophoresis after tenfold concentration of amniotic fluid and repeat determination of hex A and B (Fig. 46-11).

6. After adequate amniotic cell growth (average 3 weeks), repeat of step 5 above. The result should agree with that in step 5 and is the most reliable of the three samples.

7. Confirmation of the diagnosis, if possible, using fetal tissue, or if negative, using a sample such as umbilical cord serum or a portion of the cord itself, obtained from the infant at delivery.

Enzyme Defect in Sandhoff Disease and Juvenile Sandhoff Disease

The activities of both hex A and B are deficient in Sandhoff disease [129]. The deficiency is present in all tissues and body fluids that have been examined, including cultured skin fibroblasts and amniotic cells from affected fetuses [130, 131]. The deficiency has been documented using synthetic N-acetylglucosaminides and N-acetylgalactosaminides as well as G_{M2}, G_{A2}, and globoside [129], steroid-glucosaminides [132], and a heptasaccharide containing N-acetylgalactosamine [133] as substrates. The diagnosis of homozygotes is conveniently made by the hexosaminidase assay of serum [129] or cultured fibroblasts [134]. Heterozygote detection using serum has been demonstrated. Low total hexosaminidase and a low percentage of hex B are used as criteria [135, 136]. The demonstration by Lowden that hex B in Sandhoff disease heterozygotes is more thermolabile than normal suggests the presence of a heteropolymer of hex B comprised of both wild-type and mutant β chains which renders the enzyme thermolabile [137]. Sandhoff disease has been correctly diagnosed prenatally in two affected fetuses; both pregnancies were terminated [130, 131].

A patient with a juvenile form of Sandhoff disease has been described. He was normal until age 5 when slurred speech, ataxia, and mental decline became apparent. At 10 years he had generalized hypertonia, hyperreflexia, ataxia, and normal optic fundi [138]. A deficiency of hex B with preservation of some residual hex A activity in fibroblasts was demonstrated [139].

Several unusual variants of Sandhoff disease have been described, one with considerable hex A and B activity in serum but a striking reduction in tissues [140], and another who appears to be a genetic compound of two different β-chain mutations [141].

Other Unusual Hexosaminidase Variants

Variant AB(+) (Activator Factor Mutants) Several patients have been described with the clinical picture of TSD and massive cerebral accumulation of G_{M2} but with normal

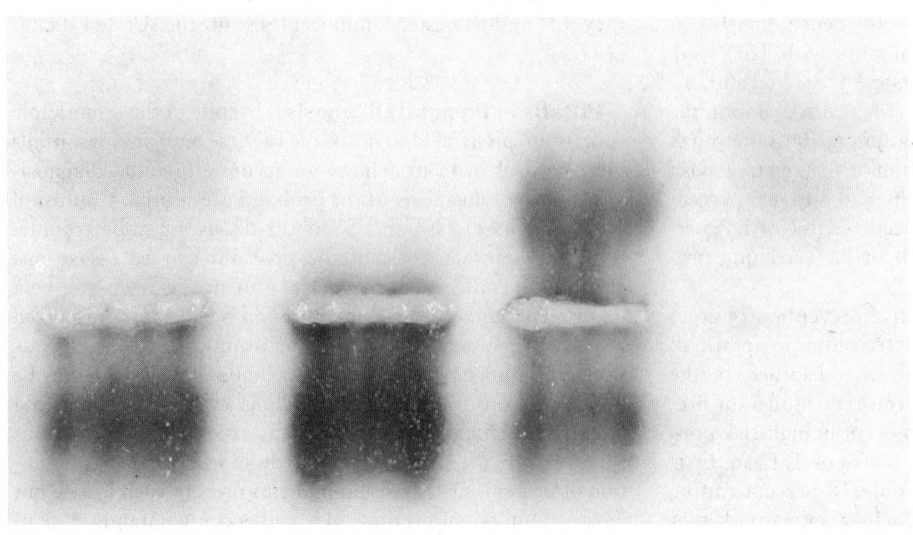

+

X

A

B

_

1   2   3   4

Figure 46-11 Starch-gel electrophoresis of hexosaminidases. *Lane 1*, Tay-Sachs disease liver homogenate contaminated with bacteria (*Mima polymorpha*); *lane 2*, Tay-Sachs disease homogenate uncontaminated; *lane 3*, normal liver homogenate; and *lane 4*, hexosaminidase from homogenate of *M. polymorpha* (X). Gels were stained with naphthol-ASBI-β-D-N-acetylglucosaminide. Note the close migration of the bacterial hexosaminidase (X) and normal human liver hex A (A).

activities of hex A and B when tested with synthetic substrates [92, 142–144]. When ganglioside G_{M2} was used as substrate, no activity was detected [144]. Conzelmann and Sandhoff [146] have shown that the defect is a severe deficiency of an activator protein, characterized from kidney, which is necessary for the in vivo interaction of ganglioside and enzyme. The activator appears to be comprised of two components, one with a molecular weight of 25,000, the other 60,000, and both are required for G_{M2} hydrolysis by hex A. The smaller component was found to be deficient in kidney from a patient with the AB(+) mutation (activator deficiency) [146].

An adult with G_{M2} gangliosidosis, but normal activity of hex A and B, has been described. He may be an adult variant of the AB(+) mutation [147]. Seizures began at age 18, followed by intellectual deterioration, nystagmus, facial paresis, uncoordination, hyperreflexia, and progressive motor weakness. Cortical biopsy revealed neuronal lipidosis and an eightfold increase in the concentration of ganglioside G_{M2}. Lipidosis of splenic sinusoidal cells, hepatocytes, and parenchymal cells of lymph nodes was evident.

The implications of the AB(+) mutation in the diagnosis of G_{M2} gangliosidosis are apparent. Assays of hex A and B using synthetic substrates or ganglioside G_{M2} cannot be used to make this diagnosis—a special assay is required. Especially intriguing is the possibility that a significant number of patients with adult-onset dementia include patients with G_{M2} or G_{M1} gangliosidosis, either due to a structural mutation of the enzyme or alteration of an activator. Although still unexplored, activator mutants leading to G_{M1} gangliosidosis could occur since a specific activator for G_{M1} hydrolysis exists [156].

Healthy Adults with Hex A Deficiency Three families have been described in which a striking deficiency of hex A (synthetic substrates) occurred in normal healthy adults [148–150]. In each family, women with the hex A deficiency had produced offspring with TSD. The hex A deficiency was nearly total in serum and leukocytes. Hex A deficiency was nearly complete in fibroblasts from affected members of two families [149, 150], but in the second family it was partial [148]. Using G_{M2} as substrate, reductions of activity to about one-half normal were found in leukocytes [151] and in fibroblasts [150, 152]. It has been proposed that these clinically normal hex A–deficient patients are allelic compounds consisting of the TSD allele and a second allele whose product lacks activity for synthetic substrates but retains activity for ganglioside G_{M2} [149, 150]. Heterozygotes for this second mutation have a reduction of hex A activity close to that seen in TSD heterozygotes.

This proposal has been strengthened by studies of a large Pennsylvania Dutch family in which TSD occurred [153]. A healthy adult female was assumed to represent the allelic compound since she had a remarkable deficiency of hex A in serum and leukocytes. Her activity of G_{M2} β-acetylgalactosaminidase is close to half normal, indicating TSD heterozygosity [18]. Levels of activity of hex A (synthetic substrate) in serum and leukocytes of those individuals presumed heterozygotes for the anomalous mutation are intermediate between those of controls and those from presumed heterozygotes for TSD. The enzyme activity studies, combined with the segregation pattern within this kindred, conform to the expectation of allelic segregation [153].

One normal adult male with no apparent hex A activity in serum or fibroblasts using synthetic substrates had half-normal

activity of G_{M2} N-acetylgalactosaminidase [150]. G_{M2} N-acetylgalactosaminidase activity could be immunoprecipitated using antibodies specific for the α-chain of hex A. This proved the presence of immunoreactive hex A which cleaved G_{M2} but not synthetic substrates [154].

Healthy Adult with Hex A and B Deficiency The absence of hex A and B activity (as shown with synthetic substrates) has been described in a normal adult male [155]. This individual was a clinically normal father of two children who died with the TSD phenotype. When G_{A2} was used as substrate, a value in the heterozygous range was found in his leukocytes. It was postulated that he was an allelic compound for the classic Sandhoff disease mutation and a second mutation which impaired activity against the artificial substrate but not for the natural substrate.

Properties of Hex A and B [18]

Hex A and hex B have molecular weights of approximately 100,000 (Table 46-7). Hex A has a lower isoelectric point than B. The amino terminals of hex A and B appear to be blocked, but the carboxyl-terminal amino acid of hex A appears to be serine and that of hex B aspartic acid (or asparagine). Antibodies raised against purified hex B cross-react with hex A. Conditions favoring subunit disassociation cause disaggregation of A and B to the smaller units.

Kinetic studies indicate that ganglioside G_{M2} is cleaved by hex A but not by hex B. Both enzymes cleave G_{A2} and globoside, as well as p-nitrophenyl and 4-methylumbelliferyl-β-acetylhexosaminidase. When these substrates are used, hex A and B have similar pH optima and kinetics (Table 46-7).

Fibroblast homogenates from patients with TSD and Sandhoff disease fail to hydrolyze N-acetylgalactosamine from a heptasaccharide derived from chondroitin-4-sulfate under conditions in which normal fibroblasts have activity. This suggests that hex A, but not B, cleaves N-acetylgalactosamine from this compound. Hex A and B apparently both cleave N-acetylglucosamine from steroid conjugates such as testosterone 17-β-N-acetylglucosaminide. Studies with a trisaccharide containing a terminal N-acetylglucosamine residue (isolated from hyaluronate) reveal that hex A cleaves the aminosugar at a rate 35 to 40 times that of hex B.

Hex A cleaves synthetic β-acetylhexosaminidase substrates at rates 100 to 6 million times higher than ganglioside G_{M2}, depending on the assay conditions and tissue source. A small-molecular-weight glycoprotein simulatory "factor," isolated from human liver [156] and kidney [146], simulates hex A to cleave G_{M2}. Geiger and Arnon [157] and Lee and Yoshida [158] purified hex A and B to homogeneity from human placenta and determined their properties. Hex A contained 1.65 residues of sialic acid per molecule and hex B contained none. Their molecular weights were 100,000 and 108,000, respectively. Both could be dissociated into 4 subunits of 25,000 molecular weight. Hex B contained only one type of polypeptide chain, the β chain, whereas hex A contained an equal proportion of β chains and α chains. The latter were more negatively charged than the former, with the charge difference apparently caused by a high proportion of acidic amino acids as well as sialic acid in the α chains.

Mahuran and Lowden [159] recently isolated hex A and B in homogeneous form from human placenta and studied their subunit compositions. They confirmed the previous finding that hex B is a tetramer of two pairs of β chains ($\beta_2\beta_2$) but found that hex A contains two β chains and one 50,000-molecular-weight α chain. They conclude that the α chain of hex A is either a 50,000-molecular-weight polypeptide or that two 25,000-molecular-weight chains are linked by nondisulfide cross-linkage (e.g., an isopeptide bond) with hex A having the structure ($\alpha\beta_2$).

Molecular Genetics of the G_{M2} Gangliosidoses

A three-locus model [160] coding for two separate polypeptide chains, α and β, of hex A and for activator protein appears to explain the molecular genetics of the G_{M2} gangliosidoses (Fig. 46-12). The α-chain locus, located on chromosome 15 [161, 162], is mutated in the hex A mutants (TSD, juvenile G_{M2} gangliosidosis with hex A deficiency, and adult G_{M2} gangliosidosis with hex A deficiency). The β-chain locus, located on chromosome 5, is mutated in the hex B mutants (Sandhoff disease and juvenile Sandhoff disease). The activator locus (or loci) is involved in the AB(+) mutants.

The model explains how the mutation in Sandhoff disease can lead to simultaneous loss of hex A and B activity [18] and

how restoration of hex A activity can occur in fusions of TSD and Sandhoff disease fibroblasts, the α subunit being derived from the Sandhoff disease fibroblasts and the β subunit from the TSD fibroblasts [18]. It explains why independent segregation of hex A and hex B occurs in somatic cell hybrids [161, 162]. The model provides the basis for the excellent results in heterozygote detection of TSD using the heat denaturation method [101]. Since both enzymes contain a common polypeptide chain, the β chain, they are closely related genetically and the ratio of one to the other obtained in the assay [101] is less variable than the ratio of hex A to other denominators such as volume and protein.

There are several important questions regarding the molecular genetics of the G_{M2} gangliosidoses which remain to be answered. The relationship of activator protein(s) to enzyme hydrolysis needs clarification. Assays for activators need to be devised. The genetic defect in TSD is still unclear: synthesis of altered α chains has been reported [163] but needs confirmation. The frequency of G_{M2} gangliosidosis among adults with dementia needs definition.

Figure 46-12 Three-locus model to explain the molecular genetics of G_{M2} gangliosidosis in humans. Hex A mutants include TSD, juvenile G_{M2} gangliosidosis, and adult Sandhoff disease. Activator mutants include infantile, juvenile, and adult AB mutants. More than one locus may be involved in generation of activator polypeptide.

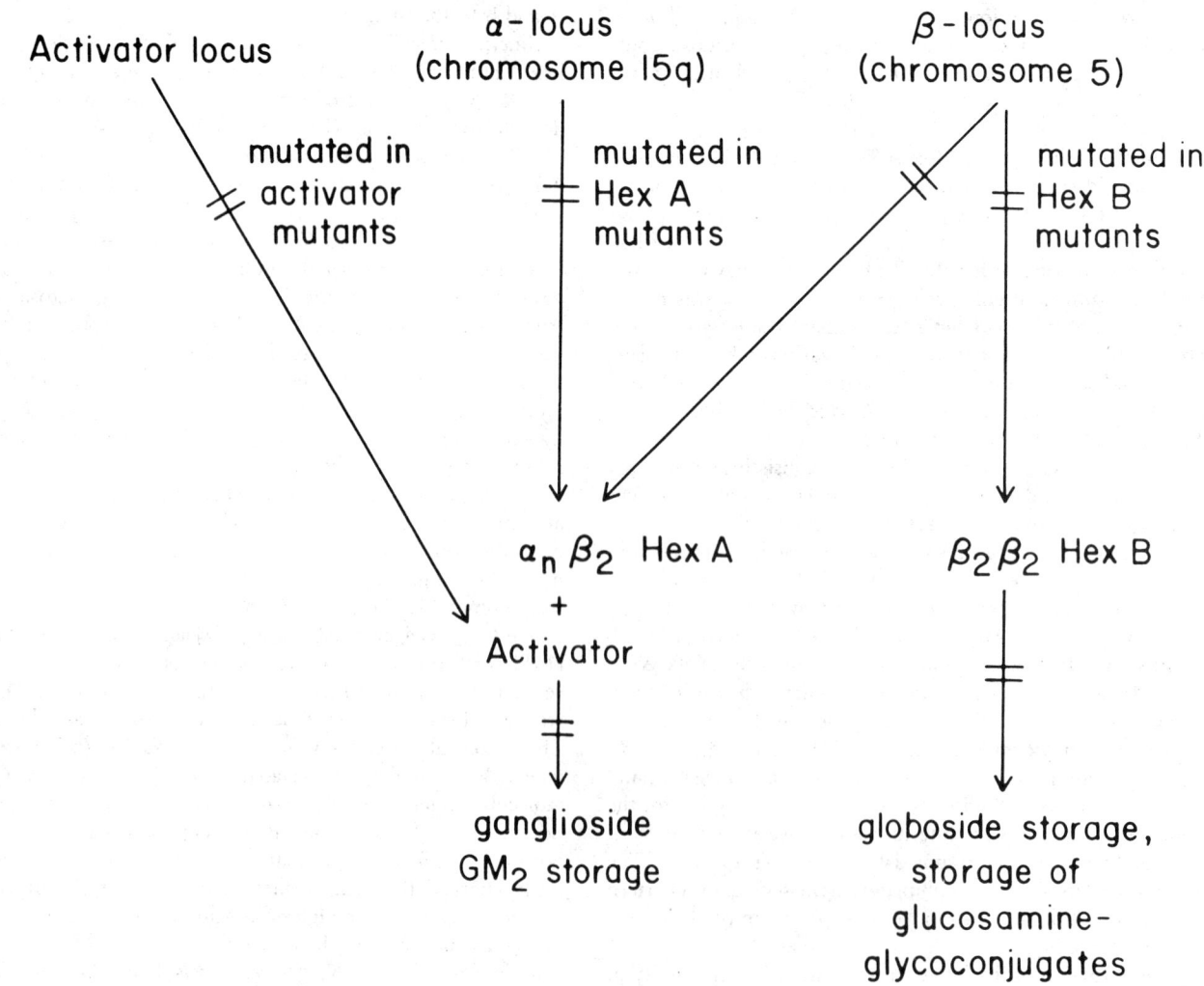

Nomenclature of the G_{M2} Gangliosidoses

As new mutations of hex A and hex B have been described, the literature has become confusing. This author has attempted to bring order out of chaos by proposing a nomenclature system based upon the assumed genetic defects in patients with G_{M2} gangliosidosis [164] (Table 46-8). The nomenclature is based upon the three-locus model (Fig. 46-12). With a few formal changes this nomenclature has been incorporated into the newly adopted *Guidelines for Human Gene Nomenclature* [165]. It has also been suggested that the designation "type 1," introduced previously by this author for TSD, be reserved for hex B variants, and that "type 3" be reserved for activator mutations [166].

Animal Models

G_{M2} gangliosidosis with deficiency of hex A and B (Sandhoff disease) has been reported in cats [167] and has been used by Rattazzi and coworkers [168, 169] to explore enzyme replacement therapy with human hex A. Hepatic uptake of human hex A was enhanced by administration of mannosans. Brain uptake was induced by cerebral oxygen embolism without neurologic damage. Enzyme levels of hex A, which were virtually zero in Sandhoff disease cats, were brought to 30 percent of normal in liver and 10 percent of normal in brain after enzyme administration. A marked reduction of G_{M2} and globoside storage in liver occurred, but there was no reduction of G_{M2} storage in brain cortex. These promising studies need to be carried further.

THERAPY

No specific therapy for the ganglioside storage diseases is available. Enzyme replacement has been attempted in two patients

Table 46-8 Nomenclature of G_{M2} gangliosidoses mutants

Described phenotype	Suggested phenotypic symbol	Suggested genotype	Phenotypic symbols and explanations
Normal	HEX A 1, HEX B 1	$HEX_\alpha{}^1 HEX_\alpha{}^1 HEX_\beta{}^1 HEX_\beta{}^1$	HEX A, HEX B
HEX A Mutants:			
Tay-Sachs disease	HEX A 2, HEX B 1	$HEX_\alpha{}^2 HEX_\alpha{}^2 HEX_\beta{}^1 HEX_\beta{}^1$	Absent HEX A
Juvenile G_{M2} gangliosidosis*	HEX A 3, HEX B1	$HEX_\alpha{}^3 HEX_\alpha{}^3 HEX_\beta{}^1 HEX_\beta{}^1$	Nearly complete deficiency of HEX A in some patients, intermediate HEX A deficiency in others.
Tay-Sachs disease with intermediate HEX A deficiency	HEX A 2-4, HEX B 1	$HEX_\alpha{}^2 HEX_\alpha{}^4 HEX_\beta{}^1 HEX_\beta{}^1$	Genetic compound of Tay-Sachs allele and anomalous HEX A allele, the latter with activity for synthetic but not natural substrates.
Normal subject with absent HEX A	HEX A 2-5, HEX B 1	$HEX_\alpha{}^2 HEX_\alpha{}^5 HEX_\beta{}^1 HEX_\beta{}^1$	Genetic compound of Tay-Sachs allele and anomalous HEX A allele, the latter with activity against natural but not synthetic substrates.
Normal subject with deficient HEX A	HEX A 2-6, HEX B 1	$HEX_\alpha{}^2 HEX_\alpha{}^6 HEX_\beta{}^1 HEX_\beta{}^1$	Genetic compound of Tay-Sachs allele and an anomalous HEX A allele which leads to reduction of HEX A synthesis.
Adult (chronic) G_{M2} gangliosidosis	HEX A 2-7, HEX B 1	$HEX_\alpha{}^2 HEX_\alpha{}^6 HEX_\beta{}^1 HEX_\beta{}^1$	Most patients are probably genetic compounds of Tay-Sachs allele and a new allelic mutation.
HEX B Mutants:			
Sandhoff disease	HEX A 1, HEX B 2	$HEX_\alpha{}^1 HEX_\alpha{}^1 HEX_\beta{}^2 HEX_\beta{}^2$	Variant O of Tay-Sachs disease.
Normal with deficient HEX A and HEX B	HEX A 1, HEX B 2-3	$HEX_\alpha{}^1 HEX_\alpha{}^1 HEX_\beta{}^2 HEX_\beta{}^3$	Genetic compound of Sandhoff's allele and an anomalous HEX B allele, the latter with activity for natural but not synthetic substrates.
Juvenile Sandhoff's disease	HEX A 1, HEX B 2-4	$HEX_\alpha{}^1 HEX_\alpha{}^1 HEX_\beta{}^2 HEX_\beta{}^4$	Most patients are probably genetic compounds of the Sandhoff's allele and a new allelic mutation.
Activator Mutants:			
Tay-Sachs disease with normal HEX A; (AB+) variant	HEX A 1, HEX B 1	$HEX_\alpha{}^1 HEX_\alpha{}^1 HEX_\beta{}^1 HEX_\beta{}^1$	Variant AB (+) of Tay-Sachs disease. Normal HEX A and B but deficiency of HEX A activator protein.
Adult AB+ mutation	HEX A 1, HEX B 1	$HEX_\alpha{}^1 HEX_\alpha{}^1 HEX_\beta{}^1 HEX_\beta{}^1$	Adult variant with activator protein deficiency.

* NOTE: Genetic compounds of HEX A 3 with HEX A 2 or HEX A 4 could give rise to juvenile or late infantile G_{M2} gangliosidosis with varying HEX A activities using artificial substrates. Variability of HEX A activity in juvenile G_{M2} gangliosidosis has been described.

with TSD, a 14-month-old child and a 7-week infant [170]. Treatment consisted of weekly intrathecal injections of pure hex A (1.0 to 1.5 mg), a dose equivalent to about 9 percent of the total brain hex A activity (this author's calculation), for 4 weeks in the older patient and 40 weeks in the younger one. Injection of the enzyme resulted in almost complete disappearance of G_{M2} from serum but no dissolution of G_{M2} membranous cystoplasmic bodies in the brain by electron microscopy. Both patients tolerated the injection without complications, but no clear-cut improvement was noted in either. Since the treatment was initiated in both an advanced and early stage and since very large doses of hex A were given, the authors conclude that hex A replacement therapy by this route is not beneficial in patients with TSD.

Proper recognition, early diagnosis, and immediate genetic counseling followed by contraception is the simplest, most effective means available for preventing the conception and birth of children with ganglioside storage diseases. Recognition of the phenotypes by primary physicians, pediatricians, neurologists, radiologists, pathologists, and geneticists is crucial. The diagnosis should be confirmed in all patients or in heterozygotes by enzyme assays wherever possible. Biopsies of liver, brain, or other tissues are no longer necessary for the diagnosis of most patients. Prenatal diagnosis of affected fetuses by amniocentesis and enzyme assay, although admittedly imperfect, is the only preventive solution available at present for these fatal inborn errors of ganglioside metabolism.

This work was supported by grants from the National Institutes of Health, Grant NS 08682; U.S. Public Health Service, Program Project Grant GM 17702; and the Gould Family Foundation Grant.

REFERENCES

1. TAY W: Symmetrical changes in the region of the yellow spot in each eye of an infant. *Trans Ophthalmol Soc UK* 1:155, 1881

2. O'BRIEN JS, STERN MB, LANDING BH, O'BRIEN JK, DONNELL GN: Generalized gangliosidosis. *Am J Dis Child* 109:338, 1965

3. GONATAS NK, GONATAS J: Ultrastructural and biochemical observations on a case of systemic late infantile lipidosis and its relationship to Tay-Sachs disease and gargoylism. *J Neuropathol Exp Neurol* 24:318, 1965

4. LEDEEN R, YU RK: Structure and enzymic degradation of sphingolipids, in Hers HG, van Hoof F (eds): *Lysosomes and Storage Diseases*. New York, Academic, 1973

5. SUZUKI K: The pattern of mammalian brain gangliosides. III. Regional and developmental differences. *J Neurochem* 12:169, 1965

6. VANIER MT, HOLM M, OHMAN R, SVENNERHOLM L: Developmental profiles of gangliosidosis in human and rat brain. *J. Neurochem* 18:581, 1971

7. NORTON WT, PODUSLO SE: Neuronal perikarya and astroglia of rat brain: Chemical composition during myelination. *J Lipid Res* 12:84, 1971

8. FORMAN DS, LEDEEN RW: Axonal transport of gangliosides in goldfish optic nerve. *Science* 177:630, 1972

9. ROSEMAN S: The synthesis of complex carbohydrates by multiglycosyltransferase systems and their potential function in intracellular adhesion. *Chem Phys Lipids* 5:270, 1970

10. SLOAN HR, FREDRICKSON DS: GM₂ Gangliosides: Tay-Sachs disease, in Stanbury JB, Wyngaarden JB, Fredrickson DS (eds): *Metabolic Basis of Inherited Disease*. 4th ed. New York, McGraw-Hill, 1972, p 615

11. MAX SR, MACLAREN NK, BRADY RO, BRADLEY RM, RENNELS MB, TANAKA J, GARCIA JH, CORNBLATH: GM₃ (Hematoside) sphingolipodystrophy. *N Engl J Med* 291:929, 1974

12. TANAKA J, GARCIA JH, MAX SR, VILORIA JE, KAMIJO Y, MACLAREN NK, CORNBLATH M, BRADY RO: Cerebral sponginess and GM₃ gangliosidosis: Ultrastructure and probable pathogenesis. *J Neuropathol Exp Neurol* 34:249, 1975

13. FISHMANN PH, MAX SR, TALLMAN JF, BRADY RO, MACLAREN NK, CORNBLATH M: Deficient ganglioside biosynthesis: A novel human sphingolipidosis. *Science* 187:68, 1975

14. BRADY RO: Inherited metabolic disease and the pathogenesis of mental retardation. *Ann Biol Clin* 36:113, 1978

15. OHMAN R, ROSENBERG A, SVENNERHOLM L: Human brain sialidase. *Biochemistry* 9:3774, 1970

16. VAES G: Digestive capacity of lysosomes, in Hers HG, van Hoof F (eds): *Lysosomes and Storage Diseases*. New York, Academic, 1973

17. KNUDSON AG: *Genetics and Disease*. New York, McGraw-Hill, 1965, p 13

18. For references see: O'BRIEN JS: GM₁ Gangliosidosis, in Stanbury, JS, Wyngaarden JB, Fredrickson DS (eds): *The Metabolic Basis of Inherited Disease*. 4th ed. New York, McGraw-Hill, 1978, p 841

19. ARONSON SM: Epidemiology, in Volk BW (ed): *Tay-Sachs Disease*. New York: Grune and Stratton, 1964, p 118

20. KOZINN PJ, WIENER H, COHEN P: Infantile familial amaurotic idiocy. *J Pediatr* 51:58, 1957

21. ARONSON SM, VOLK BW: Some epidemiologic and genetic aspects of Tay-Sachs disease, in Aronson SM, Volk BW (eds): *Cerebral Sphingolipidoses: a Symposium on Tay-Sachs Disease and Allied Disorders*. New York, Academic, 1962, p 375

22. KABACK M: *Summary of worldwide Tay-Sachs disease Screening and Detection*. Los Angeles, University of California, 1981

23. LOWDEN JA, LA RAMEE MA, LANG E, ZUKER S: Tay-Sachs heterozygote detection in mass-carrier screening in Toronto. *Clin Res* 20:930, 1972

24. MYRIANTHOPOULOS NC, ARONSON SM: Population dynamics of Tay-Sachs disease. I. Reproductive fitness and selection. *Am J Hum Genet* 18:313, 1966

25. CHASE GA, McKUSICK VA: Founder effect in Tay-Sachs disease. *Am J Hum Genet* 24:339, 1972

26. MYRIANTHOPOULOS NC, ARONSON SM: Population dynamics in Tay-Sachs disease. II. What confers the selective advantage upon the Jewish heterozygote?, in Volk BW, Aronson SM (eds): *Sphingolipids Sphingolipidoses and Allied Disorders*. New York, Plenum, 1972

27. ANDERMANN E, SCRIVER CR, WOLFE LS, DANSKY L, ANDERMANN F: Genetic Variants of Tay-Sachs Disease, in Kaback M (ed): *Tay-Sachs and Screening and Prevention*. New York, Alan R. Liss, 1977, p 161

28. KELLY TE, CHASE GA, KABACK MM, KUBOR K, McKUSICK VA: Tay-Sachs disease: High gene frequency in a non-Jewish population. *Am J Hum Genet* 27:287, 1975

29. STEPHENS R, PATRICK AD: Personal communication, 1975

30. SPRANGER JW, LANGER LO, WIEDEMANN HR: GM₁Gangliosidosis, in *Bone Dysplasias: An Atlas of Constitutional Disorders of Skeletal Development*. Philadelphia, W.B. Saunders, 1974, p 171

31. O'BRIEN JS, BERNETT J, VEATH ML, PAA D: Lysosomal storage disorders: Diagnosis by ultrastructural examination of skin biopsies. *Arch Neurol* 32:592, 1975

32. O'BRIEN JS: Ganglioside storage diseases, in Hirschhorn K, Harris H (eds): *Advances in Human Genetics*. New York, Plenum, vol 3, 1972, p 39

33. WOLFE LS, CALLAHAN J, FAWCETT JS, ANDERMANN P, SCRIVER C: GM₁ gangliosidosis without chondrodystrophy or visceromegaly: β-Galactosidase deficiency with gangliosidosis and the excessive excretion of a keratan sulfate. *Neurology* 20:23, 1970

34. WENGER DA, SATTLER M, MUELLER OT, MYERS GG, SCHNEIDER RS, NIXON GW: Adult GM₁ gangliosidosis: Clinical and biochemical studies on two patients and comparison to other patients called variant or adult GM₁ gangliosidosis. *Clin Genet* 17:323, 1980

35. STEVENSON RE, TAYLOR HA, PARKS SE: β-Galactosidase deficiency: Prolonged survival in three patients following early central nervous deterioration. *Clin Genet* 13:305, 1978

36. WOLFE LS, SENIOR RG, NG YING, KIN NMK: The structures of oligosaccharides accumulating in the liver of GM₁ gangliosidosis, type 1. *J Biol Chem* 249:1828, 1974

37. STRECKER G, MONTREUIL J: Glycoproteins et glycoproteinoses. *Biochemie* 61:1199, 1979

38. MONTREUIL J: Primary structure of glycoprotein glycans: Basis for the molecular biology of glycoproteins. *Adv Carbohyd Chem Biochem* 37:157, 1980

39. OKADA S, O'BRIEN JS: Generalized gangliosidoses: Beta-galactosidase deficiency. *Science* 160:1002, 1968

40. MACBRINN MC, OKADA S, HO MW, HU CC, O'BRIEN JS: Generalized gangliosidosis: Impaired cleave of galactose from a mucopolysaccharide and a glycoprotein. *Science* 163:946, 1969

41. NORDEN AGW, O'BRIEN JS: Ganglioside GM₁ β-galactosidase: Studies in human liver and brain. *Arch Biochem Biophys* 159:383, 1973

42. WENGER DA, SATTLER M, HIATT W: Globoid cell leucodystrophy: Deficiency of lactosyl ceramide beta-galactosidase. *Proc Nat Acad Sci USA* 71:854, 1974

43. SINGER HS, SCHAFER IA: White cell β-galactosidase activity. *N Engl J Med* 282:571, 1970

44. THOMAS GH: β-D-Galactosidase in human urine: Deficiency in generalized gangliosidosis. *J Lab Clin Med* 74:725, 1969

45. SLOAN HR, UHLENDORF BW, JACOBSON CB, FREDRICKSON DS: β-Galactosidase in tissue culture derived from human skin and bone marrow: Enzyme defect in GM₁ gangliosidosis. *Pediat Res* 3:532, 1969

46. LOWDEN JA, CUTZ E, CONEN PE, RUDD N, DORAN TE: Prenatal diagnosis of GM₁ gangliosidosis. *N Engl J Med* 288:255, 1973

47. KABACK MM, SLOAN HR, SONNEBORN M, HERNDON RM, PERCY AK: GM₁ gangliosidosis type I in utero: Detection and fetal manifestations. *J Pediatr* 82:1037, 1973

48. BOOTH CW, GERBIE AB, NADLER HL: Intrauterine diagnosis of GM₁ gangliosidosis, type 2. *Pediatrics* 52:521, 1973

49. ROBINSON D: Multiple forms of glycosidases in the normal and pathological states. *Enzyme* 18:114, 1974

50. CHEETHAM PS, DANCE NE, ROBINSON D: Isoenzymes of human liver β-galactosidase. *Biochem Soc Trans* 241, 1975

51. O'BRIEN JS: Molecular genetics of GM₁ β-galactosidase. *Clin Genet* 8:303, 1975

52. NORDEN AGW, TENNANT LL, O'BRIEN JS: GM₁ ganglioside β-galactosidase A: Purification and studies of the enzyme from human liver. *J Biol Chem* 249:7969, 1974

53. FROST RG, HOLMES EW, NORDEN AGW, O'BRIEN JS: Characterization of purified human liver acid β-galactosidases A₂ and A₃. *Biochem J* 175:181, 1978

54. HO MW, O'BRIEN JS: Stimulation of acid beta-galactosidase activity by chloride ions. *Clin Chim Acta* 30:531, 1970

55. HO MW, O'BRIEN JS: Differential effect of chloride ions on β-galactosidase isoenzymes: A method for separate assay. *Clin Chim Acta* 32:443, 1971

56. HO MW, CHEETHAM P, ROBINSON D: Hydrolysis of GM₁-ganglioside by human liver β-galactosidase isoenzymes. *Biochem J* 136:351, 1973

57. TENNANT LL, VEATH LM, O'BRIEN JS: Unpublished data, 1980

58. NORDEN AGW, O'BRIEN JS: Binding of human liver β-galactosidase to plant lectins insolubilized on agarose. *Biochem Biophys Res Commun* 56:193, 1974

59. SUZUKI Y, CROCKER A, SUZUKI K: GM₁ gangliosidosis: Correlation of clinical and biochemical data. *Arch Neurol* 24:48, 1971

60. VAN HOOF F: GM₁ Gangliosidosis, in Hers HG, van Hoof F (eds): *Lysosomes and Storage Diseases.* New York, Academic, 1973

61. NORDEN AGW, O'BRIEN JS: An electrophoretic variant of β-galactosidase with altered catalytic properties in a patient with GM₁ gangliosidosis. *Proc Nat Acad Sci USA,* 72:240, 1975

62. CHEETHAM PSJ, DANCE NE, ROBINSON DA: Benign deficiency of type B β-galactosidase in human liver. *Clin Chim Acta* 83:67, 1978

63. VAN HOOF F, HERS HG: The abnormalities of lysosomal enzymes in mucopolysaccharidoses. *Eur J Biochem* 7:34, 1968

64. HINDMAN J, COTLIER E: Glycosidases in normal human leucocytes and abnormalities in GM₁ gangliosidosis. *Clin Chem* 18:971, 1972

65. SUZUKI K, SUZUKI Y: Globoid cell leucodystrophy (Krabbe's disease). Deficiency of galactocerebroside β-galactosidase. *Proc Nat Acad Sci USA* 66:302, 1970

66. TANAKA H, SUZUKI K: Lactosylceramide β-galactosidase in human sphingolipidoses: Evidence for two genetically distinct enzymes. *J Biol Chem* 250:2324, 1975

67. LOWDEN JA, CALLAHAN JW, NORMAN MG, TAHIN M, PRICHARD JS: Juvenile GM₁ gangliosidosis; occurrence with absence of two β-galactosidase components. *Arch Neurol* 31:200, 1974

68. NAYLOR SL, LALLEY PA, ELLIOTT RW, BROWN JA, SHOWS TB: Evidence for homologous regions of human chromosome 3 and mouse chromosome 9 predicts location of human genes. *Am J Hum Genet* 32:159a, 1980

69. MEISLER M, RATTAZZI MC: Immunological studies of β-galactosidase in normal human liver and in GM₁ gangliosidosis. *Am J Hum Genet* 26:868, 1974

70. BEN-YOSEF Y, BURTON BK, NADLER HL: Quantification of the enzymatically deficient cross-reacting material in GM₁ gangliosidosis. *Am J Hum Genet* 29:575, 1977

71. KEIJZER W, DE WIT-VERBEEK HA, REUSER AJJ, HO MW, ROBINSON D: Genetic heterogeneity in GM₁ gangliosidosis demonstrated by somatic cell hybridization and enzyme assays in single heterokaryons. *Nature* 257:60, 1975

72. O'BRIEN JS: An explanation for complementation in GM₁ gangliosidosis. *Am J Hum Genet* 30:36A, 1978

73. O'BRIEN JS, NORDEN AGW: Nature of the mutation in adult β-galactosidase deficient patients. *Am J Hum Genet* 29:184, 1977

74. PINKSY L, MILLER J, SHANFIELD B, WALTERS G, WOLFE LS: GM₁ gangliosidosis in skin fibroblast cultures: Enzymatic differences between types 1 and 2 and observations on a third variant. *Am J Hum Genet* 26:563, 1974

75. FELDGES A, MUELLER HJ, BUEHLER E, STALDER G: GM₁ gangliosidosis. Part I: Clinical aspects and biochemistry. *Helv Paediatr Acta* 28:511, 1973

76. O'BRIEN JS, GUGLER E, GIEDION A, WIESSMANN U, HERSHKOWITZ N, MEIER C, LEROY J: Spondyloepiphyseal dysplasia, corneal clouding, normal intelligence and β-galactosidase deficiency. *Clin Genet* 9:495, 1976

77. ARBISSER AL, DONNELLY KA, SCOTT CI: Morquio-like syndrome with beta-galactosidase deficiency and normal hexosamine sulfatase activity: mucopolysaccharidosis IVB. *Am J Med Genet* 1:195, 1977

78. GROEBE H, KRINS M, SCHMIDBERGER H, VON FIGURA K, HARZER K, KRESSE E, PASCHKE E, SEWELL A, ULLRICH K: Morquio syndrome (mucopolysaccharidoses IVB) associated with β-galactosidase deficiency. Report of two cases. *Am J Hum Genet* 32:258, 1980

79. WENGER DA, TARBY TJ, WHARTON C: Macular cherry-red spots and myoclonus with dementia: Coexistent neuraminidase and β-galactosidase deficiencies. *Biochem Biophys Res Commun* 82:589, 1978

80. LOWDEN JA, O'BRIEN JS: Sialidosis: A review of human neuraminidase deficiency. *Am J Hum Genet* 31:1, 1979

81. BAKER HJ, LINDSEY JR: Feline GM₁ gangliosidosis. *Am J Pathol* 74:649, 1974

82. HANDA S, YAMAKAWA T: Biochemical studies in cat and human gangliosidosis. *J Neurochem* 18:1275, 1971

83. BLAKEMORE WF: GM₁ gangliosidosis in a cat. *J Comp Pathol* 82:179, 1972

84. DONNELLY WJC, SHEAHAN BJ, KELLY M: Beta-galactosidase deficiency in GM₁ gangliosidosis of Friesian calves. *Res Vet Sci* 15:139, 1973

85. READ DH, HARRINGTON DD, KEENAN TW, HINSMAN EJ: Neuronal visceral GM₁ gangliosidosis in a dog with β-galactosidase deficiency. *Science* 194:442, 1976

86. BAKER HJ, LINDSEY JR, MCKHANN GM, FARRELL DM: Neuronal GM₁ gangliosidosis in a Siamese cat with β-galactosidase deficiency. *Science* 174:838, 1971

87. HOLMES E, O'BRIEN JS: Feline GM₁ gangliosidosis: Characterization of the residual liver acid β-galactosidase. *Am J Hum Genet* 30:505, 1978

88. HOLMES EW, O'BRIEN JS: Hepatic storage of oligosaccha- and glycolipids in a cat affected with GM₁ gangliosidosis. *Biochem J* 175:945, 1978

89. HOLMES EW, O'BRIEN JS: Purification of acid β-galactosidase from feline liver. *Biochemistry* 18:952, 1979

90. RITTMANN LS, TENNANT LL, O'BRIEN JS: Dog GM₁ gangliosidosis: Characterization of the residual liver acid β-galactosidase. *Am J Hum Genet* 32:880, 1980

91. WARNER TG, O'BRIEN JS: Unpublished data, 1981

92. RAPIN I, SUZUKI K, SUZUKI K, VALSAMIS M: Adult (chronic) GM₂ gangliosidosis. Atypical spinocerebellar degeneration in a Jewish sibship. *Arch Neurol* 33:120, 1976

93. KABACK M, MILES J, YAFFE M, ITIBASHI H, MCINTYRE H, GOLDBERG M, MOHANDAS T: Hexosaminidase A (Hex A) deficiency in early adulthood: A new type of GM₂ gangliosidosis. *Am J Hum Genet* 30:31A, 1978

94. ROBINSON D, STIRLING JL: N-Acetyl-β-glucosaminidases in human spleen. *Biochem J* 107:321, 1968

95. BRAIDMAN I, CARROLL M, DANCE N, ROBINSON D, POENAM L, WEBER A, DREYFUS JC, OVERDIJK B, HOOGHWINKEL GJM: Characterization of human hexosaminidase C. *FEBS Lett* 41:181, 1974

96. OKADA S, O'BRIEN JS: Tay-Sachs disease: Generalized absence of a beta-D-N-actylhexosaminidase component. *Science* 165:698, 1969

97. SANDHOFF K: Variation of β-N-acetylhexosaminidase pattern in Tay-Sachs disease. *Eur Biochem Soc Lett* 4:351, 1969

98. OKADA S, VEATH ML, LEROY J, O'BRIEN JS: Ganglioside GM₂ storage diseases: Hexosaminidase deficiencies in cultured fibroblasts. *Am J Hum Genet* 23:55, 1971

99. O'BRIEN JS, NORDEN AGW, MILLER AL, FROST RG, KELLY TE: Ganglioside GM₂ N-acetyl-β-D-galactosaminidase and asialo GM₂(GA₂) N-acetyl-β-D-galactosaminidase: Studies in human skin fibroblasts. *Clin Genet* 11:171, 1977

100. O'BRIEN JS, TENNANT LL, VEATH ML, SCOTT CR, BUCKNALL WE: Characterization of unusual hexosaminidase A-deficient human mutants. *Am J Hum Genet* 30:602, 1978

101. O'BRIEN JS, OKADA S, CHEN A, FILLERUP DL: Tay-Sachs disease: Detection of heterozygotes and homozygotes by serum hexosaminidase assay. *N Engl J Med* 283:15, 1970

102. O'BRIEN JS, OKADA S, FILLERUP DL, VEATH ML, ADORNATO B, BRENNER PH, LEROY J: Tay-Sachs disease: Prenatal diagnosis. *Science* 172:61, 1971

103. KABACK MM, ZEIGER RS: Heterozygote detection in Tay-Sachs disease: a prototype community screening program for the prevention of genetic disorders, in Volk BW, Aronson SM (eds): *Sphingolipidoses and Allied Disorders.* New York, Plenum, 1972, p 613

104. KABACK MM: Thermal fractionation of serum hexosaminidase: Approaches to heterozygote detection and diagnosis of Tay-Sachs disease, in Ginsberg V, Neufeld E (eds): *Methods of Enzymology.* New York, Academic Press, 1973, p 862

105. LOWDEN JA, SKOMOROWSKI MA, HENDERSON F, KABACK MM: Automated assays of hexosaminidases in serum. *Clin Chem* 19:1345, 1973

106. KABACK MM, ZEIGER RS, REYNOLDS LW, SONNEBORN M: Tay-Sachs dis-

ease: A model for the control of recessive genetic disorders, in Motulsky AG, Lentz W (eds): *Proceedings of the 4th International Conference, Birth Defects.* Amsterdam, Exerpta Medica, 1973, p 248

107. KABACK MM, ZEIGER RS, REYNOLDS LW, SONNEBORN: Approaches to the control and prevention of Tay-Sachs disease, in Steinberg AG, Bearn AG (eds): *Progress in Medical Genetics.* New York, Grune and Stratton, vol 10, 1974, p 103

108. CARMODY PJ, RATTAZZI MC, DAVIDSON RG: Tay-Sachs disease. The use of tears for the detection of heterozygotes. *N Engl J Med* 289:1071, 1973

109. LOWDEN JA, LARAMEE M-A: Problems in prenatal diagnosis using sphingolipid hydrolase assays, in Volk BW, Aronson SM (eds): *Sphingolipids, Sphingolipidoses and Allied Disorders.* New York, Plenum, 1972, p 257

110. STIRLING JL: Separation and characterization of N-acetyl-β-glucosaminidases A and P from maternal serum. *Biochim Biophys Acta* 271:154, 1972

111. PRICE RG, DANCE N: The demonstration of multiple heat stable forms of N-acetyl-β-glucosaminidase in normal human serum. *Biochim Biophys Acta* 271:145, 1972

112. HUDDLESTON JF, CEFALO RC, LEE G, ROBINSON JC: An investigation of the gestational increase in serum hexosaminidase B. *Am J Obstet Gynecol* 111:804, 1971

113. HAYASE K, KRITCHEVSKY D: Separation and comparison of isoenzymes of N-acetyl-beta-D-hexosaminidase of pregnant serum by polyacrylamide gel electrofocusing. *Clin Chim Acta* 46:455, 1973

114. SWALLOW DM, STOKES DC, CORNEY G, HARRIS H: Differences between the N-acetylhexosaminidase isoenzymes in serum and tissues. *Ann Hum Genet (London)* 37:287, 1974

115. IKONNE JU, ELLIS RB: N-acetyl-β-D-hexosaminidase component A: Different forms in human tissues and fluids. *Biochem J* 135:457, 1973

116. KABACK MM, O'BRIEN JS: Tay-Sachs: Prototype for prevention of genetic disease. *Hosp Prac* 8:107, 1973

117. PADEH B, SHACHER S, BAT-MIRIAM KATZNELSON M, NAVON R, GOLDMAN M: Perspectives on screening and prevention of Tay-Sachs disease in Israel, in Kaback M, Rimoin D, O'Brien J (eds): *Tay-Sachs Disease: Screening and Prevention.* New York, Alan R Liss, 1977, p 47

118. SLOME D: The genetic basis of amaurotic family idiocy. *J Genet* 27:363, 1934

119. O'BRIEN JS: Tay-Sachs disease: From enzyme to prevention. *Fed Proc* 32:191, 1973

120. NELSON WB, SWINT JM, CASKEY CT: An economic evaluation of a genetic screening program for Tay-Sachs disease. *Am J Hum Genet* 30:160, 1978

121. KABACK MM, BECKER MH, RUTH MV: Sociologic studies in human genetics I: Compliance factors in a voluntary heterozygote screening program, in *Ethical, Social and Legal Dimensions of Screening for Human Genetic Disease.* Birth Defects Original Article Series, vol X, 1974, p 145

122. CHILDS B, GORDIS L, KABACK MM, KAZAZIAN HH: Tay-Sachs screening: Motives for participating and knowledge of genetics and probability. *Am J Hum Genet* 28:537, 1976

123. CHILDS B, GORDIS L, KABACK MM, KAZAZIAN HH: Tay-Sachs screening: Social and psychological impact. *Am J Hum Genet* 28:550, 1976

124. MILUNSKY A: *The Prenatal Diagnosis of Hereditary Disorders.* Springfield, Ill: Charles C Thomas, 1973, p 65

125. RATTAZZI MC, DAVIDSON RG: Prenatal detection of Tay-Sachs disease, in Dorfman A (ed): *Antenatal Diagnosis.* Chicago, University of Chicago Press, 1972, p 208

126. ELLIS RB, KONNE JU, PATRICK AD, STEPHENS R, WILLCOX P: Prenatal diagnosis of Tay-Sachs disease. *Lancet* 1:1144, 1973

127. LOWE CU, ALEXANDER D, BRYLA D, SIEGEL D: The safety and accuracy of mid-trimester amniocentesis. *D HEW Publ* 78:190, 1978

128. O'BRIEN JS: Pitfalls in the prenatal diagnosis of Tay-Sachs disease, in Kaback M, Rimoin D, O'Brien J (eds): *Tay-Sachs Disease: Screening and Prevention.* New York: Alan R. Liss, 1977, p 283

129. SANDHOFF K, HARZER K: Total hexosaminidase deficiency in Tay-Sachs disease (variant o), in Hers HG, van Hoof F (eds): *Lysosomes and Storage Diseases.* New York: Academic Press, 1973, p 345

130. DESNICK RJ, KRIVIT W, SHARP HR: In utero diagnosis of Sandhoff's disease. *Biochim Biophys Res Commun* 51:20, 1973

131. HARZER K, STENGEL-RUTKOWSKI S, GLEY EO, ALBERT A, MURKEN J-D, ZAHR V, HENKEL KP: Prenatale diagnose der G$_{M2}$ gangliosidose type 2 (Sandhoff-Jatzkowitz-Krankheit). *Dtsch Med Wschr* 100:106, 1975

132. TOMASI LG, FUKUSHIMA DK, KOLODNY EH: Steroid hexosaminidase activity in Tay-Sachs and Sandhoff-Jatzkewitz disease. *Neurology* 24:1158, 1974

133. THOMPSON JN, STOOLMILLER AG, MATALON R, DORFMAN A: N-Acetyl-β-hexosaminidase: Role in the degradation of glycosaminoglycans. *Science* 181:866, 1973

134. OKADA S, McCREA M, O'BRIEN JS: Sandhoff's disease (G$_{M2}$ gangliosidosis type 2): Clinical, chemical and enzyme studies in five patients. *Pediatr Res* 6:606, 1972

135. KOLODNY EH: Sandhoff's disease: Studies on the enzyme defect in homozygotes and detection of heterozygotes, in Volk BW, Aronson SM (eds): *Sphingolipidoses and Allied Disorders.* New York, Plenum, 1972, p 321

136. LOWDEN JA, IVES EJ, KEENE DL, BURTON AL, SKOMOROWSKI MA, HOWARD F: Carrier detection in Sandhoff's disease. *Am J Hum Genet* 30:38, 1978

137. LOWDEN JA: Evidence for a hybrid hexosaminidase isoenzyme in heterozygotes for Sandhoff disease. *Am J Hum Genet* 31:281, 1979

138. McLEOD PM, WOOD S, JAN JE, APPLEGARTH DA, DOLMAN CL: Progressive cerebellar ataxia, psychomotor retardation, and hexosaminidase deficiency in a 20 year old child: Juvenile Sandhoff disease. *Neurology* 27:571, 1977

139. WOOD S, MAC DOUGALL BG: Juvenile Sandhoff disease: Some properties of the residual hexosaminidase in cultured fibroblasts. *Am J Hum Genet* 28:489, 1976

140. SPENCE MW, RIPLEY BA, EMBIL JA, TIBBLES JA: A new variant of Sandhoff's disease. *Pediatr Res* 8:628, 1974

141. LANE AB, JENKINS T: Two variant hexosaminidase β-chain alleles segregating in a South African family. *Clin Chim Acta* 87:219, 1978

142. SANDHOFF K, HARZER K, WASSLE W, JATZKEWITZ H: Enzyme alteration and lipid storage in three variants of Tay-Sachs disease. *J Neurochem* 18:2469, 1971

143. KOLODNY EH, WALD I, MOSER HW, COGAN DG, KUBUWARA T: GM$_2$ Gangliosidosis without deficiency in the artificial substrate cleaving activity of hexosaminidase A and B *Neurology* 23:427, 1973

144. DE BAECQUE CM, SUZUKI K, RAPIN I, JOHNSON AB, WITHERS DL, SUZUKI K: GM$_2$ gangliosidosis, AB variant. *Acta Neuropathol* 33:207, 1975

145. SANDHOFF K, JATZKEWITZ H: The chemical pathology of Tay-Sachs disease, in Volk BW, Aronson SM (eds): *Sphingolipids, Sphingolipidosis and Allied Disorders.* New York, Plenum, 1972, p 305

146. CONZELMANN E, SANDHOFF K: AB Variant of infantile GM$_2$ gangliosidosis: Deficiency of a factor necessary for stimulation of hexosaminidase A–catalyzed degradation of ganglioside GM$_2$ and glycolipid GA$_2$. *Proc Nat Acad Sci* 75:3979, 1978

147. O'NEILL B, BUTLER AB, YOUNG E, FALK PM, BASS NH: Adult onset GM$_2$ gangliosidosis. *Neurology* 28:1117, 1978

148. VIDGOFF J, BUIST NRM, O'BRIEN JS: Absence of β-N-Acetyl-D-hexosaminidase A activity in a healthy woman. *Am J Hum Genet* 25:372, 1973

149. NAVON R, PADEH B, ADAM A: Apparent deficiency of hexosaminidase A in healthy members of a family with Tay-Sachs disease. *Am J Hum Genet* 25:287, 1973

150. O'BRIEN JS, TENNANT LL, VEATH ML, SCOTT CR, BUCKNALL WE: Characterization of unusual hexosaminidase A–deficient human mutants. *Am J Hum Genet* 30:602, 1978

151. TALLMAN JF, BRADY RO, NAVON R, PADEH B: Ganglioside catabolism in hexosaminidase A–deficient adults. *Nature* 252(5480):254, 1974

152. O'BRIEN JS, NORDEN AGW, MILLER AL, FROST RG, KELLY TE: Ganglioside GM$_2$ N-acetyl-β-D-galactosaminidase and asialo G$_{M2}$(G$_{A2}$) N-acetyl-β-D-galactosaminidase: Studies in human skin fibroblasts. *Clin Genet* 11:171, 1977

153. KELLY T, REYNOLDS LW, O'BRIEN JS: Segregation within a family of two mutant alleles for hexosaminidase A. *Clin Genet* 9:540, 1976

154. O'BRIEN JS, GEIGER B: Normal adult with absent HEX A: Immunoreactive HEX A is present. *Am J Hum Genet* 31:642, 1979

155. DREYFUS J-C, POENARU L, SVENNERHOLM L: Absence of hexosaminidase A and B in a normal adult. *N Engl J Med* 292:61, 1975

156. LI S-C, HIRABAYASHI Y, LI Y-T: A protein activator for the enzyme hydrolysis of G$_{M2}$ ganglioside. *J Biol Chem* 256:6234, 1981

157. GEIGER B, ARNON R: Chemical characterization and subunit structure of human N-acetylhexosaminidases A and B. *Biochemistry* 15:3484, 1976

158. LEE JES, YOSHIDA A: Purification and chemical characterization of human hexosaminidase A and B. *Biochem J* 159:535, 1976

159. MAHURAN D, LOWDEN JA: The subunit and polypeptide structure of hexosaminidases from human placenta. *Can J Biochem* 58:287, 1980

160. For review see BEUTLER E: The biochemical genetics of the hexosaminidase system in man. *Am J Hum Genet* 31:95, 1979

161. GILBERT F, KUCHERLAPATI R, CREAGAN RP, MURNANE MJ, DARLINGTON GI, RUDDLE FH: Tay-Sachs and Sandhoff's diseases: The assignment of genes for hexosaminidases A and B to individual human chromosomes. *Proc Nat Acad Sci USA* 72:263, 1975

162. LALLEY PA, RATTAZZI MC, SHOWS TB: Human β-D-N-acetyl-hexosaminidase A and B: Expression and linkage relationships in somatic cell hybrids. *Proc Nat Acad Sci USA* 71:1569, 1974

163. SRIVASTAVA SK, ANSARI NH: Altered α subunits in Tay-Sachs disease. *Nature* 273:245, 1978

164. O'BRIEN JS: Suggestions for a nomenclature for the G$_{M2}$ gangliosidoses making certain (possibly unwarrantable) assumptions. *Am J Hum Genet* 30:672, 1978

165. *Guidelines for Human Gene Nomenclature (1979).* Proceedings of the Fifth International Workshop on Human Gene Mapping, in press

166. Norby S: Nomenclature of GM$_2$ gangliosidosis. *Clin Genet* 17:320, 1980

167. Cork LC, Munnell JF, Lorenz MD, Murphy JN, Baker HJ, Rattazzi MC: GM$_2$ Ganglioside storage disease in cats with β-hexosaminidase deficiency. *Science* 196:1014, 1977

168. Rattazzi MC, Lanse SB, Mc Cullough RA, Nester JA, Jacobs EA: Towards enzyme replacement in GM$_2$ gangliosidosis: Organ disposition

and induced central nervous system uptake of human hexosaminidase in the cat. *Birth Defect Original Article Series* 16:179, 1980

169. Rattazzi MC, Appel AM, Baker HJ: Enzyme replacement in GM$_2$ gangliosidosis: reduction of glycolipid storage in visceral organs. *Am J Hum Genet* 32:51A, 1980

170. von Specht BU, Geiger B, Arnon R, Passell J, Keren G, Goldman B, Padeh B: Enzyme replacement in Tay-Sachs disease. *Neurology* 29:849, 1979

PART 6

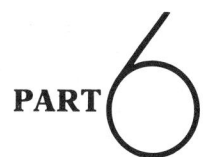

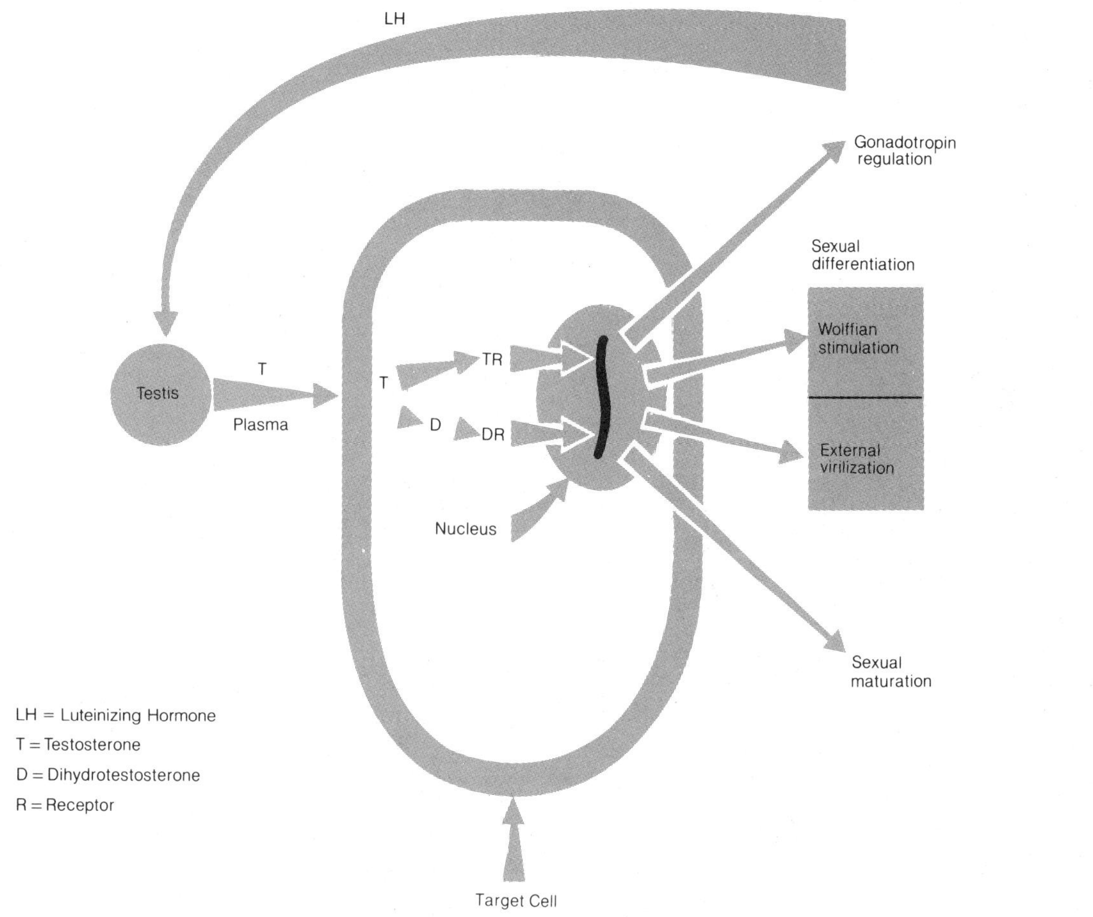

Testosterone metabolism

DISORDERS OF STEROID METABOLISM

47

CONGENITAL ADRENAL HYPERPLASIA AND RELATED CONDITIONS

MARIA I. NEW

BO DUPONT

KEVIN GRUMBACH

LENORE S. LEVINE

1. Congenital adrenal hyperplasia (CAH) is a family of disorders produced by enzymatic deficiencies of adrenal steroidogenesis. Oversecretion of ACTH secondary to impairment of cortisol synthesis leads to two abnormalities: (1) excessive synthesis of the steroid precursors proximal to the enzyme defect, and (2) accumulation of the products of those adrenal hormones whose synthesis is unimpaired by the enzyme deficiency.

2. The most frequent enzyme deficiency is that of 21 hydroxylation. Deficiencies of the enzymes 11β-hydroxylase, 3β-hydroxysteroid dehydrogenase (3β-HSD), 17α-hydroxylase, and cholesterol desmolase have also been reported. Ambiguous genitalia presenting at birth is the most prominent clinical feature of CAH due to 21-hydroxylase or 11β-hydroxylase deficiency in genetic females as a result of excessive prenatal secretion of adrenal androgens. In 3β-HSD, 17α-hydroxylase, and cholesterol desmolase deficiency, androgen synthesis is impaired and thus virilization of the genitalia in genetic males is incomplete. Salt wasting is associated with those forms of CAH with deficient mineralocorticoid production; in other forms hypertension may result from accumulation of steroid precursors with salt-retaining properties. Defects of 18-hydroxylase and 18-dehydrogenase cause a defect in aldosterone synthesis, while 17-hydroxysteroid reductase and 17,20-lyase deficiencies cause androgen deficiency without interrupting cortisol synthesis.

3. The adrenal zona fasciculata and zona glomerulosa appear to function as two separate glands; the fasciculata is primarily regulated by ACTH and the glomerulosa by the renin-angiotensin system. In CAH due to the 11β-hydroxylase deficiency, there is a defect in 11 and 18 hydroxylation in the fasciculata, while the activity of these enzymes in the glomerulosa is normal. The concept that the fasciculata and glomerulosa function as two separate glands has been applied to CAH due to 21-hydroxylase deficiency. A new hypothesis to explain the presence or absence of salt-wasting signs in 21-hydroxylase deficiency is as follows: (1) in both simple virilizers and salt wasters there is a fasciculata defect of 21-hydroxylation in both the 17-hydroxy and 17-deoxy pathways, and (2) in salt wasters there is a 21-hydroxylase defect in the glomerulosa as well, while in simple virilizers the glomerulosa is spared this defect. The ability of simple virilizers, but not salt wasters, to respond to renin-angiotensin stimulation with an increase in aldosterone secretion supports this hypothesis.

4. Each of the enzyme deficiencies causing CAH is inherited as an autosomal recessive trait. Close genetic linkage between the HLA complex and 21-hydroxylase deficiency has been demonstrated, and the 21-hydroxylase deficiency gene has been mapped in close proximity to the HLA-B genetic locus on chromosome 6. HLA genotyping, in addition to hormonal testing, is useful for the

detection of heterozygote carriers for 21-hydroxylase deficiency and prenatal diagnosis in families with an affected index case.

5. *Two nonclassical, HLA-linked forms of 21-hydroxylase deficiency are described: a late-onset form and an asymptomatic cryptic form. The degree of enzymatic deficiency ranges from severe in the classical form to milder in the late-onset and cryptic disorders, to a still milder deficiency detectable only with ACTH stimulation in heterozygotes for all three forms. It is proposed that there are allelic variants at the 21-hydroxylase genetic locus which produce different degrees of 21-hydroxylase deficiency, resulting in the phenotypic diversity of classical, late-onset, and cryptic 21-hydroxylase deficiency. It is also proposed that the cryptic disorder represents a genetic compound of the classical and mild 21-hydroxylase deficiency alleles. Studies of genetic linkage disequilibrium suggest that late-onset patients may also be genetic compounds, possessing both a mild and classical 21-hydroxylase deficiency allele.*

6. *A microfilter paper method for measuring 17-hydroxy-progesterone (17-OHP) for the neonatal diagnosis of 21-hydroxylase deficiency is described. The results of a pilot newborn screening program for CAH using the 17-OHP microfilter paper method has demonstrated that screening for this disorder is feasible. Further, 21-hydroxylase deficiency occurs with sufficient frequency to warrant screening. Measurement of 17-OHP and Δ^4-androstenedione in amniotic fluid make the prenatal diagnosis of 21-hydroxylase deficiency possible.*

7. *The fundamental aim of therapy in CAH is to provide replacement of the deficient hormones. Glucocorticoid administration both replaces the deficient cortisol and suppresses ACTH overproduction, resulting in a decrease in adrenal androgens which produce virilization and ultimate short stature. Mineralocorticoid supplements are required in the salt-wasting disorders. Mineralocorticoid administration is also recommended for patients with elevated plasma renin activity but no evident symptoms of salt wasting, in order to improve the control of androgen oversecretion. Recognition of this disorder is important in the sex assignment of newborns with ambiguous genitalia.*

Congenital adrenal hyperplasia (CAH) consists of a group of disorders involving adrenal steroidogenesis. Each disorder results from an inherited deficiency of one of the several enzymes necessary for normal steroid synthesis. The different enzyme deficiencies produce characteristic patterns of hormonal abnormalities; the clinical symptoms of the different forms of CAH depend on the particular hormones that are deficient or that are produced in excess.

The earliest documented description of CAH was by De Crecchio in 1865 [1]. This Neapolitan anatomist described a cadaver having a penis with first-degree hypospadias but no externally palpable gonads. Dissection revealed a vagina, uterus, fallopian tubes, ovaries, and markedly enlarged adrenals. It is interesting that the subject suffered a confusion of sex assignment, being declared a female at birth and a male 4 years

later. He conducted himself as a male sexually and socially. Since the original description of this remarkable case 100 years ago, investigators have unraveled the pathophysiology of the inborn errors of steroidogenesis.

STEROIDOGENESIS AND ENZYMATIC CONVERSIONS OF ADRENAL STEROID HORMONES

Steroidogenesis

The adrenal synthesizes three main classes of hormones: mineralocorticoids (17-deoxy pathway), glucocorticoids (17-hydroxy pathway), and sex steroids. A simplified scheme of adrenal steroidogenesis appears in Fig. 47-1. Each hydroxylation step is indicated and the newly added hydroxyl group is circled. ACTH acts on the adrenals to increase the conversion of cholesterol to pregnenolone. ACTH binds to receptors on the external membranes of adrenal cortical cells, stimulating increased synthesis of adenosine-3',5'-monophosphate (cyclic AMP). Cyclic AMP activates adrenal cellular phosphoprotein kinases which catalyze the side-chain cleavage, converting cholesterol to pregnenolone [2, 3].

A detailed discussion of the biochemistry of the defects in steroidogenesis in CAH is omitted here since a thorough discussion has been presented in other texts [4–6]. For the purposes of understanding the pathophysiology of CAH, the discussion below and reference to the simplified scheme in Fig. 47-1 will suffice.

Mineralocorticoids (17-deoxy Pathway)   Pregnenolone, a Δ^5-steroid, is converted to a biologically active Δ^4-steroid,

Figure 47-1 Simplified scheme for adrenal steroidogenesis. Each hydroxylation step is indicated and the newly added hydroxyl group is circled. *(From New and Levine [165]. Used by permission.)*

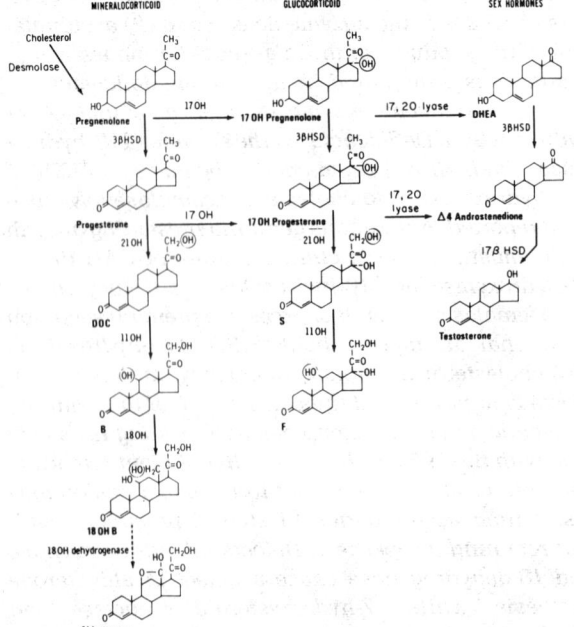

progesterone, by the enzymes 3β-hydroxysteroid dehydrogenase (3β-HSD) and isomerase. Progesterone is then hydroxylated at the C-21 position to form deoxycorticosterone (DOC), an active salt-retaining hormone. When DOC is hydroxylated at the C-11 position, corticosterone (B) is formed, which is a weak mineralocorticoid, but is the precursor of aldosterone, the most potent salt-retaining hormone [7]. Synthesis of aldosterone, a unique hormone because of the aldehyde group at C-18, is restricted to the outer zone of the adrenal cortex, the zona glomerulosa [8, 9]. Regulation of the zona glomerulosa differs from that of the other zones. The synthesis of aldosterone from corticosterone has not been entirely elucidated [9].

Glucocorticoids (17-Hydroxy Pathway) Glucocorticoid synthesis requires hydroxylation at the C-17 position. In studies of bovine adrenal cortex, negligible 17-hydroxylase activity has been found in the cells of the zona glomerulosa, in contrast to the active 17 hydroxylation occurring in the inner adrenal zona fasciculata [10]. A similar pattern of 17-hydroxylase activity is believed to exist in the human adrenal cortex and it is generally accepted that glucocorticoids and adrenal androgens, both of which depend on 17 hydroxylation for their synthesis, originate predominantly in the zona fasciculata. Pregnenolone and progesterone yield 17-hydroxypregnenolone and 17-hydroxyprogesterone (17-OHP), respectively, when hydroxylated at the C-17 position. The Δ^5-steroid 17-hydroxypregnenolone is converted to 17-OHP, a Δ^4-steroid, by enzymatic steps similar to those that convert pregnenolone to progesterone in the 17-deoxy pathway. When 17-OHP undergoes 21 hydroxylation, 11-deoxy-cortisol (S) is formed. 11-Deoxycortisol is further hydroxylated at C-11 to form cortisol (F), the most potent glucocorticoid in humans. Thus it can be seen from Fig. 47-1 that parallel hydroxylation steps at C-21 and C-11 of progesterone and 17-OHP result in the formation of corticosterone and cortisol, respectively. Although these steps are parallel, it has not been proved that the enzymes for 17-hydroxylated substrates are identical to those for 17-deoxy substrates.

Sex Hormones The main unconjugated C-19 steroid secreted by the adrenal cortex is dehydroepiandrosterone (DHEA). It results from the side-chain cleavage of the C-21 steroid, 17-hydroxypregnenolone, by the action of a desmolase enzyme. DHEA, a Δ^5-steroid with little androgenic activity, is converted to Δ^4-androstenedione, a moderately active androgen, by the 3β-HSD and isomerase enzymes. Δ^4-Androstenedione is reduced at the C-17 position to form testosterone. Testosterone is converted peripherally by the 5α-reductase enzyme to dihydrotestosterone. Both testosterone and dihydrotestosterone have androgenic activity, affecting different target tissues [11, 12].

Mechanism of Adrenal Steroid Regulation

The hypothalamic-pituitary-adrenal feedback is mediated through the circulating level of plasma cortisol. The central nervous system controls the secretion of ACTH, its diurnal variation, and its increase in stress via corticotrophin-releasing factor [13, 14]. Any condition that decreases cortisol secretion will result in increased ACTH secretion. In CAH, an enzyme

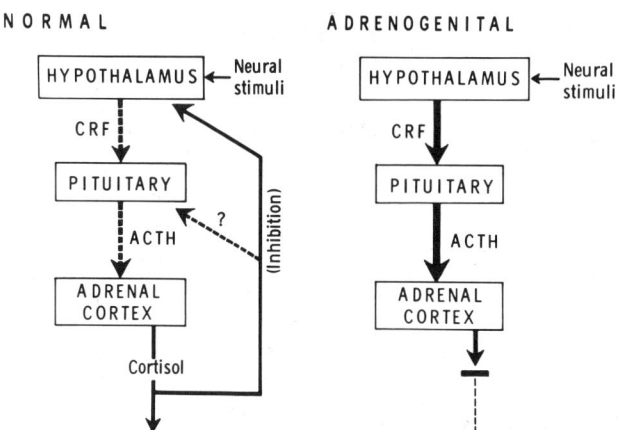

Figure 47-2 The regulation of cortisol secretion in normal subjects and in patients with congenital adrenal hyperplasia. *(From New and Levine [165]. Used by permission.)*

deficiency causes impaired cortisol synthesis, resulting in excessive ACTH secretion and hyperplasia of the adrenal cortex (Fig. 47-2).

Aldosterone secretion is regulated primarily by the renin-angiotensin system and is also stimulated directly by the serum K^+ concentration (Fig. 47-3). The juxtaglomerular apparatus of the kidney secretes the enzyme renin in response to the state of electrolyte balance and plasma volume. Renin cleaves renin substrate, an α_2-globulin produced by the liver, to release angiotensin I. Angiotensin I is then enzymatically converted to angiotensin II, a potent stimulator of aldosterone secretion. Although this scheme is generally accepted, there are many aspects of aldosterone regulation that remain unexplained [15, 16].

With respect to regulation and secretion, New and Seaman [17] have proposed that the zona glomerulosa and the zona fasciculata behave as two separate glands. According to this concept, steroidogenesis in the fasciculata is regulated by ACTH while that of the glomerulosa is regulated by the renin-angiotensin system such that (1) ACTH stimulates secretion of cortisol, corticosterone, and androgens by the zona fasciculata, and (2) angiotensin stimulates aldosterone secretion by the zona glomerulosa, with ACTH presumably exerting only a secondary influence on the secretion of aldosterone by the glomerulosa [13, 18, 19] (Fig. 47-4). Whereas the zona fasciculata lacks the enzyme necessary for the terminal step of aldosterone synthesis, the zona glomerulosa lacks the 17-hydroxylase activity required for the production of 17-hydroxy corticoids and androgens.

FETAL SEXUAL DEVELOPMENT

In order to understand the pathophysiology of CAH, it is necessary to discuss normal sexual differentiation. According to the hypothesis developed by Jost [20], normal differentiation of male genitalia is dependent on two functions of the fetal testis:

1. The testes secrete the fetal androgen, testosterone, which stimulates the Wolffian ducts to develop into the male internal genitalia (the epididymis, vas deferens, seminal vesicles, and

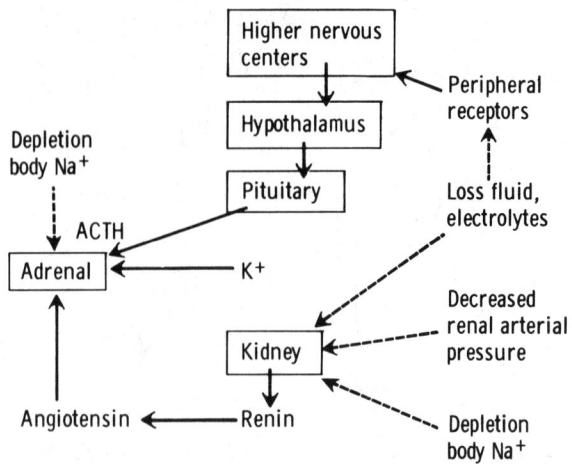

Figure 47-3 Regulation of aldosterone secretion. *(From New and Peterson, Pediatr Clin N Am 13:43, 1966. Used by permission.)*

ejaculatory ducts). Testosterone also induces differentiation of the male external genitalia when it is reduced in the target tissue to dihydrotestosterone, including elongation of the genital tubercle to form the glans penis and midline fusion of the labioscrotal folds and swellings to form the shaft of the penis and the scrotal sacs [11, 12]. In complete male differentiation the urethra opens at the tip of the penis. In the male, the normal source of androgen is the fetal testis, but androgen from any source can cause masculinization of the external genitalia.

2. The testes also secrete a nonsteroidal substance that inhibits development of the female internal genitalia (müllerian ducts). Thus the normal male is born without a uterus [21].

Since the fetal ovary secretes neither testosterone nor the factor necessary to inhibit the development of the müllerian structures, the normal female is born without male differentiation of the external genitalia (i.e., with female external genitalia) and without müllerian repression (i.e., with a uterus and fallopian tubes). This process is shown schematically in Fig. 47-5. Thus, the ovary does not play a determining role in sex differentiation.

Female fetuses exposed to high levels of androgen consequent to either CAH, an androgen-producing tumor in the mother, or maternal ingestion of androgens manifest virilization of the external genitalia but normal internal female genitalia [22, 23].

ENZYME DEFECTS IN CONGENITAL ADRENAL HYPERPLASIA

The following enzymatic deficiencies of steroidogenesis have been described:

21-hydroxylase: (i) simple virilizing, (ii) salt wasting*
11β-hydroxylase*
3β-hydroxysteroid dehydrogenase (3β-HSD)*
17α-hydroxylase*
    cholesterol desmolase*
18-hydroxylase (corticosterone methyl oxidase, type I)

*Indicates those disorders associated with cortisol deficiency.

18-dehydrogenase of 18-hydroxycorticosterone (corticosterone methyl oxidase, type II)
17β-hydroxysteroid dehydrogenase (17β-HSD)
17, 20-lyase

A summary of the clinical and biochemical features of these disorders appears in Table 47-1. It should be noted that sexual ambiguity is not a feature of the 18-hydroxylase (methyl oxidase, type I) and the 18-dehydrogenase of 18-hydroxycorticosterone (methyl oxidase, type II) deficiencies since in patients with these disorders sex hormone secretion is normal. The 17β-HSD defect may occur only in the gonad [24]; 17β-HSD activity is normally low in the adrenal gland, making exclusion of an adrenal defect difficult. It is included only for completeness. It is presumed that there is adrenal hyperplasia only in those defects associated with cortisol deficiency (entries marked with an asterisk in the preceding list).

21-Hydroxylase Deficiency

Simple Virilizing Adrenal Hyperplasia   Impairment of 21 hydroxylation is the most common enzymatic deficiency observed in CAH. Reference to Fig. 47-1 indicates that an enzymatic deficiency of 21-hydroxylase results in decreased cortisol synthesis. The decreased cortisol synthesis induces increased ACTH secretion, a phenomenon which has been demonstrated in the blood [13, 25, 26]. Consequent to the increased ACTH secretion, there is overproduction of cortisol precursors and sex steroids, the biosynthesis of which does not require 21-hydroxylase.

Early studies demonstrated that patients with 21-hydroxylase deficiency have excessive urinary pregnanetriol, the metabolite of 17-OHP [27, 28]. Urinary 17-ketosteroids, which result from the metabolism of DHEA, Δ^4-androstenedione, and testosterone, are also present in increased amounts. More recently, newly developed simple and reliable radioimmunoassays for circulating serum levels of adrenal steroids have provided a more accurate laboratory method for the diagnosis of CAH than can be provided by urinary steroid measurement alone. Criteria for the diagnosis of 21-hydroxylase

Figure 47-4 Regulation of adrenocortical steroidogenesis considering the fasciculata and glomerulosa as two separate glands. Dotted arrows indicate negative feedback. Symbols: P, progesterone; DOC, deoxycorticosterone; B, corticosterone; 17-OHP, 17-hydroxyprogesterone; S, 11-deoxycortisol; F, cortisol; Δ4, Δ4-androstenedione; DHEA, dehydroepiandrosterone; T, testosterone; 18OHDOC, 18-hydroxydeoxycorticosterone; 18OHB, 18-hydroxycorticosterone; ALDO, aldosterone.

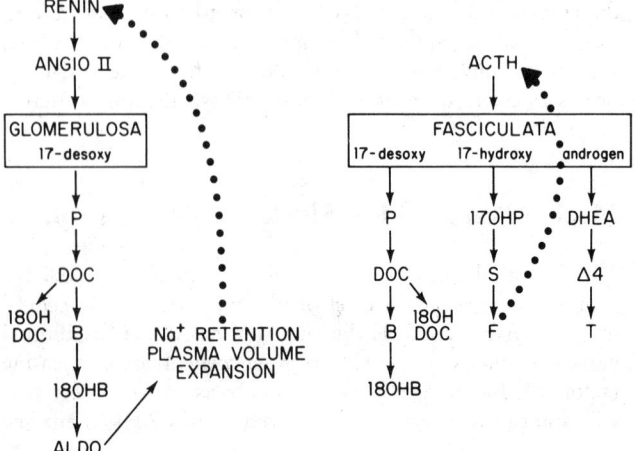

FETAL SEX DIFFERENTIATION

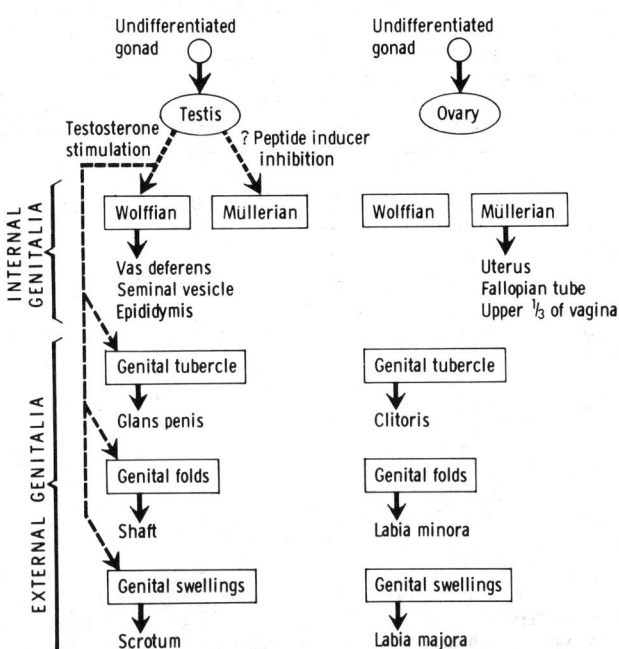

Figure 47-5 Fetal sex differentiation. *(From New and Levine [165]. Used by permission.)*

deficiency depend on the elevated levels of precursors and decreased levels of product [29, 30]. The excessive rise of serum 17-OHP with ACTH administration is at present the best indicator of a 21-hydroxylase deficiency. Concentrations of serum DOC and 11-deoxycortisol and of their urinary metabolites may fall within a normal or low-normal range, but their failure to rise appropriately in response to ACTH administration indicates deficient 21 hydroxylase.

The most prominent clinical feature of this form of CAH is virilization. Adrenocortical function begins at the end of the first trimester of gestation and, in cases of 21-hydroxylase deficiency, the developing fetus is exposed to the excessive adrenal androgens secreted by the hyperplastic adrenal cortex. From the previous discussion of normal and abnormal sexual differentiation, it is apparent that excessive androgens will cause virilization of the external genitalia, which depend on androgens for male differentiation. In the female fetus, the excessive fetal adrenal androgens masculinize the external genitalia and female pseudohermaphroditism results (Fig. 47-6). In rare cases the masculinization in females may be so profound that the urethra is penile [31]. Virilization of the genitalia in the genetic female is present only in the androgen-responsive external genitalia. Since the female fetus possesses ovaries and not testes, müllerian inhibiting factor is not produced and thus the female with 21-hydroxylase deficiency is born with a uterus and fallopian tubes. Although external genitalia in the genetic female may be ambiguous, the internal genitalia develop normally.

The specific character of the virilization in genetic females with 21-hydroxylase deficiency is somewhat puzzling. Affected females frequently present with labioscrotal fusion and a urogenital sinus, in addition to an enlarged clitoris. Although the clitoris is known to be sensitive to the masculinizing effects of androgens throughout fetal life and even postnatally, by the

twelfth week of gestation the vagina has fully separated from the urogenital sinus in females and these genital structures are no longer responsive to the virilizing influence of androgens. Studies have demonstrated that maternal ingestion of androgens after the twelfth fetal week, while stimulating clitoral enlargement, will not cause labioscrotal fusion or formation of a urogenital sinus [23]. Although the fetal adrenal gland is capable of synthesizing adrenal androgens by 11.5 weeks of gestation [32, 33], the main androgen resulting from incubation of fetal adrenal glands is Δ^4-androstenedione. It is therefore difficult to reconcile the variant timings of fetal adrenal steroidogenesis and labioscrotal differentiation with the profound virilization of the external genitalia often found in genetic females with 21-hydroxylase deficiency. It is possible that there is greater variability in the timing of these developmental events than is thought, such that in some individuals either the period of labioscrotal responsiveness to androgens is prolonged or the onset of fetal adrenal function occurs earlier, allowing labioscrotal fusion in some patients and clitoromegaly alone in others.

Another puzzling feature of the virilization is the status of the internal genital ducts in affected females. As expected, müllerian duct development is normal due to the absence of testes, which are required for secretion of müllerian inhibiting factor. It is suprising that Wolffian duct development is consistently absent in these virilized females, despite the elevated androgen levels. It has been suggested that higher local concentrations of testosterone are necessary for Wolffian stimulation than for virilization of external genitalia and that the local presence of a testis is required for the former [23]. Federman [22] has proposed that the adrenal androgens, which are oversecreted in the circulation in CAH, may not achieve sufficient concentrations in the Wolffian duct region. Wilson and Walsh [34] have pointed out that in animal experiments androgens administered into the maternal circulation can stimulate Wolffian development in female fetuses. They have also pointed out that the major androgen secreted in this disorder is Δ^4-androstenedione and that this androgen may not be sufficiently potent to induce Wolffian development. Thus the failure of Wolffian development and the variability in the virilization of the external genitalia is unexplained.

Clarification of the process of in utero virilization of females with CAH must await more detailed studies of fetal adrenal function and fetal sexual differentiation. Recently there has been a report of a female with 21-hydroxylase deficiency born with labioscrotal fusion but without clitoromegaly [35], an unexpected variation of the virilization in this disorder.

Males with 21-hydroxylase deficiency do not have genital abnormalities at birth. Postnatally, in untreated males as well as in untreated females, continued excessive androgen production results in rapid somatic growth, advanced epiphyseal maturation, progressive penile or clitoral enlargement, early appearance of facial, axillary, and pubic hair, and acne. Without treatment, early epiphyseal closure and short stature result.

Salt-wasting CAH   In the salt-wasting form of 21-hydroxylase deficiency, virilization occurs as in simple virilizing CAH, but in addition signs of adrenal insufficiency appear, including low serum sodium, high serum potassium, and vascular collapse. In the compensated or simple virilizing form, there is no deficiency of aldosterone secretion, while in the salt-wasting form aldosterone deficiency is present and may be profound. Life-threatening crises may occur within the first 2 weeks of life and therefore must be recognized soon after birth in order for treatment to be administered prior to a crisis.

11β-Hydroxylase Deficiency

A defect in 11β-hydroxylation results in the "hypertensive" form of CAH. As shown in Fig. 47-1, an enzymatic deficiency of 11β-hydroxylase results in decreased cortisol synthesis. As in simple virilizing CAH, the decreased cortisol synthesis induces increased ACTH secretion [36], with the resultant overproduction of cortisol precursors and androgens.

The most prominent clinical feature of 11β-hydroxylase deficiency is virilization. As in 21-hydroxylase deficiency, the external genitalia of the female fetus are masculinized by the excessive fetal adrenal androgen and female pseudohermaphroditism results. Internal female genitalia are normal. Postnatally, untreated males and females manifest progressive virilization and eventual short stature, as in 21-hydroxylase deficiency.

Hypertension is an additional finding in many but not all patients with this form of CAH. The hypertension is thought to result from the excessive production of DOC, an aldosterone precursor that acts as a mineralocorticoid. Although it has been reported that exogenous DOC administration can produce hypertension [37], it is not yet proven that the hyper-

Figure 47-6 Ambiguous genitalia in a newborn female with CAH due to 21-hydroxylase deficiency. Note the enlarged clitoris, single orifice on the perineum, and scrotalization of the labia majora.

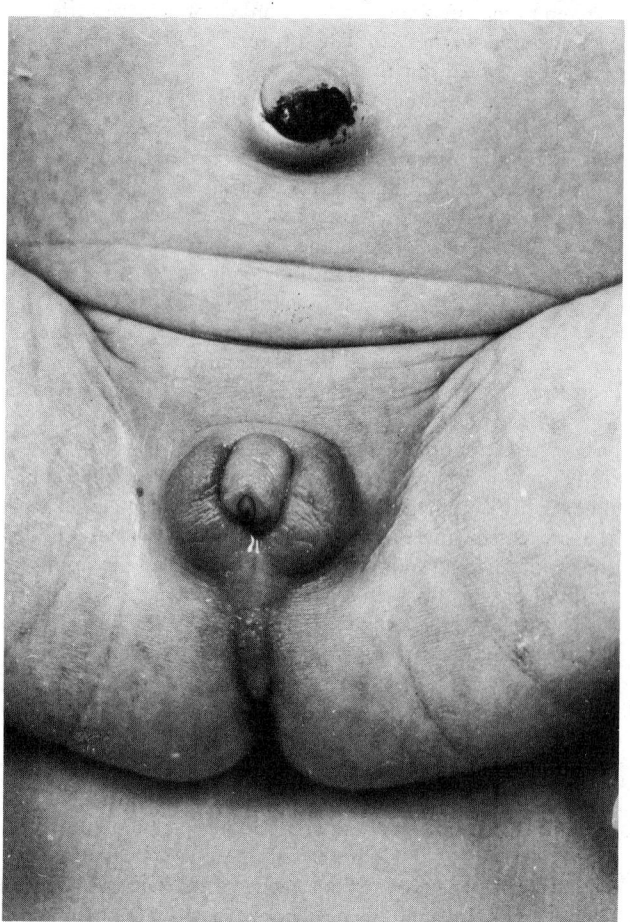

Table 47-1   Clinical and laboratory features of various forms of adrenal disorders of steroidogenesis

Clinical Features

| Newborn with sexual ambiguity | | Salt wasting | Hyper-tension | Postnatal virilization |
Female	Male			
+	0	0	0	+
+	0	+	0	+
+	0	0	+	+
+	+	+	0	0
0	+	0	+	0
0	+	+	0	0
0	0	+	0	0
0	0	+	0	0
?	+	−	−	+[e]

[a] Mostly THS.
[b] The values presented apply to the infant and very young child.
[c] Mostly Δ5,17-ketosteroids.
[d] Largely 18-hydroxy THA, which gives a Porter-Silber reaction.
[e] Only in males at puberty.
[f] This defect may occur only in the gonad.
NOTE: nl = normal. P'triol = pregnanetriol.

tension in 11β-hydroxylase deficiency is attributable to DOC.

DOC and 11-deoxycortisol (S) are the predominant precursors produced in 11β-hydroxylase deficiency. The concentrations of their urinary metabolites, including the 17-hydroxysteroids, are increased. Urinary pregnanetriol excretion is only modestly elevated in contrast to the marked elevation in 21-hydroxylase deficiency. There is overproduction of adrenal androgens and increased urinary excretion of 17-ketosteroids. Markedly increased serum levels and secretion rates of 11-deoxycortisol and DOC, which increase with ACTH administration, and suppressed plasma renin activity (PRA) distinguish the 11β-hydroxylase defect from 21-hydroxylase deficiency [17, 38–40].

3β-HSD Deficiency

An enzymatic deficiency of 3β-HSD, first described by Bongiovanni [41], results in decreased synthesis of all three classes of adrenal steroids. There is impaired secretion of aldosterone, cortisol, and testosterone, which leads to male pseudohermaphroditism and life-threatening salt wasting in infancy. An unexpected finding in female newborns with 3β-HSD deficiency has been slight clitoral enlargement, which may be attributable to the extremely high levels of DHEA, a weak androgen. Although secreted in very high amounts, DHEA is not a sufficiently potent androgen to masculinize the external genitalia in the male completely, although there are cases of males who have been almost completely masculinized [42]. Salt-wasting symptoms secondary to aldosterone deficiency are associated with 3β-HSD deficiency, although the salt wasting has varying degrees of severity.

Table 47-1 Clinical and laboratory features of various forms of adrenal disorders of steroidogenesis *(Continued)*

Enzyme deficiency	Laboratory Findings								
	Urinary excretion				Circulating hormones				
	17-KS	17-OH	P'triol	Aldo	17-OHP	Δ⁴	DHEA	Testosterone	Renin
21-Hydroxylase									
not salt wasting	↑↑	nl or ↓	↑↑	nl	↑↑	↑↑	nl or ↑ (DHEA/Δ⁴ ↓)	↑	nl or ↑
salt wasting	↑↑	↓	↑↑	↓	↑↑	↑↑	nl or ↑	↑	↑↑
11β-Hydroxylase	↑↑	↑↑ᵃ	↑	↓	↑	↑↑	↑	↑	↓↓
3β-HSDᵇ	↑ᶜ	↓↓	↑	↓	nl or ↑	nl or ↑	↑↑↑	↓ or nl	↑
17α-Hydroxylase	↓↓	↓↓	↓↓	↓	↓	↓	↓	↓	↓
Cholesterol desmolase	↓↓	↓↓	↓↓	↓↓	↓	↓	↓	↓	↑
18-Hydroxylase	nl	nl	nl	↓↓	nl	nl	nl	nl	↑
18-Dehydrogenase of 18 hydroxycortico-sterone (methyl oxidase, type II)	nl	↑ᵈ	nl	↓↓	nl	nl	nl		↑
17β-Hydroxysteroidᶠ dehydrogenase	nl ↑	nl	nl	nl	nl	↑↑	nl or ↑	nl or ↓ (Δ⁴/ T ↑↑)	nl

The urine of patients with 3β-HSD deficiency contains predominantly Δ⁵-steroids. Markedly elevated DHEA levels in plasma and excessive urinary excretion of the DHEA metabolite pregnenetriol are diagnostic of 3β-HSD deficiency [43]. Urinary pregnenetriol may also be elevated, and this is a potential source of confusion with a diagnosis of 21-hydroxylase deficiency if the overall pattern of urinary steroids is not carefully examined for the increased ratio of Δ⁵- to Δ⁴-steroids.

The 3β-HSD enzyme in the testes, adrenals, and liver may be under different genetic control. This could result in varying degrees of enzymatic deficiency in different organs and would explain the heterogeneity in the clinical presentation of the disorder. Thus the advent of male puberty, which has been described in some cases of 3β-HSD deficiency [42, 44], could occur when the testes are less affected than the adrenals.

17α-Hydroxylase Deficiency

A defect in 17α-hydroxylase results in diminished secretion of glucocorticoids and sex steroids and increased secretion of mineralocorticoids. Since the first description of a female with 17α-hydroxylase deficiency by Biglieri [45], additional cases in males and females have been reported [46–48]. In all cases there has been an overproduction of 17-deoxysteroids, especially corticosterone. The hypertension and hypokalemia have been attributed to the excessive DOC secretion. Untreated females with 17α-hydroxylase deficiency have had sexual infantilism. In males the androgen deficiency results in male pseudohermaphroditism. There is suppression of the müllerian ducts in males and the uterus and fallopian tubes are absent, indicating the normal production of müllerian inhibiting hormone.

Laboratory tests show decreased serum androgen levels and decreased urinary excretion of 17-ketosteroids and 17-hydroxycorticoids as expected as a consequence of the 17α-hydroxylase defect. Also reported in many cases are low aldosterone levels, a finding discussed in greater detail below in the section titled "Recent Advances in 21- and 11β-Hydroxylase Deficiencies."

Cholesterol Desmolase Deficiency

In 1955, Prader and Gurtner [49] described a male pseudohermaphrodite with severe salt wasting and impaired synthesis of all three classes of adrenal steroids: mineralocorticoids, glucocorticoids, and sex steroids. In this genetic male, female external genitalia with male internal genital ducts were found at autopsy. The enlarged adrenals were remarkable in that the cortical cells were filled with lipoid material consisting of cholesterol and cholesterol esters, which prompted the name *lipoid adrenal hyperplasia*.

Several patients with this biosynthetic defect have since been described [50, 51]. Most did not survive beyond infancy and died in adrenal crisis because of deficient mineralocorticoid and glucocorticoid production. The biosynthetic defect involves the side-chain cleavage converting cholesterol to pregnenolone. At least three enzymes are involved in this conversion: 20α-hydroxylase, 22R-hydroxylase and 20α, 22R-desmolase [52]. Degenhart [53] obtained biochemical evidence that the deficient enzyme in one patient was the cholesterol 20α-hydroxylase, but deficiency of any of these three enzymes would lead to profound adrenal insufficiency. The severe ambiguity of the external genitalia in the male suggests that the defect is also present in the testes. Affected females have normal genital development. Since the defect impairs aldosterone and DOC secretion as well, salt wasting is attributable to the lack of mineralocorticoid secretion. Few children have survived beyond early infancy [51]. As in Addison's disease of infancy, early recognition and proper treatment should permit survival of these infants. It is possible that patients with a mild form of this enzyme deficiency who do not have prominent salt wasting may have gone unrecognized, as may have occurred in some cases of 3β-HSD deficiency.

18-Hydroxylase Deficiency

Rare cases have been described of children with 18-hydroxylase deficiency, which results in a syndrome of profound salt wasting [54–56]. Dehydration, poor weight gain, and intermittent fever are early presenting symptoms, which become less marked with age. Initially, hyponatremia and hyperkalemia are present. One of the terminal steps in aldosterone synthesis, conversion of corticosterone to 18-hydroxycorticosterone, was shown to be defective. In this disorder there is no impairment of cortisol or sex steroid synthesis and genitalia are normal. Only aldosterone and its precursor 18-hydroxycorticosterone were shown to be deficient.

Deficiency of 18-Dehydrogenase of 18-Hydroxycorticosterone

This enzyme deficiency was first described by Ulick [57]; numerous other cases have been reported [9, 58]. A particularly high incidence of the disorder has been found in an inbred population of Iranian Jews [59]. The deficient aldosterone production and resultant salt-wasting symptoms found in these patients have been attributed to a defect in the enzymatic conversion of 18-hydroxycorticosterone (18-OHB) to aldosterone by the adrenal zona glomerulosa. The glucocorticoid and androgen pathways are thus spared in this enzyme deficiency and there is no excessive secretion of ACTH or genital abnormalities.

There is a broad range in the clinical severity of the disorder varying from cases of salt-wasting crises leading to infant death, to intermediate cases with short stature and postural hypotension, to asymptomatic adults whose deficiency was only detectable by biochemical screening. Correspondingly, variable levels of aldosterone secretion have been reported, indicating a variability in the severity of the enzyme defect. In some instances, normal or even elevated plasma aldosterone concentrations in salt-depleted patients lead to confusion in diagnosis. Although the aldosterone level may be normal, PRA is elevated and indicates a degree of sodium depletion.

A general rule in assessing enzyme activity in all of the errors of steroidogenesis described in this chapter is that the absolute level of hormone secretion may be less informative than the relation of a hormonal level to a given stimulus, such as a tropic hormone (ACTH or angiotensin). The best diagnostic measure for specifying the enzymatic defect is to examine the precursor-to-product ratio when the tropic hormone is increased. The diagnosis of 18-dehydrogenase deficiency can be made by comparing the secretion of aldosterone to the secretion of 18-OHB, as measured by their urinary metabolites. Thus the ratio of 18-OHB metabolite to aldosterone, normally less than 3.0, is often greater than 100 in untreated

patients. This suggests that the zona glomerulosa cannot effectively convert 18-OHB to aldosterone [59].

The term *corticosterone methyl oxidase, type II deficiency* has recently been adopted as a more accurate nomenclature for this enzyme disorder, and *corticosterone methyl oxidase, Type I deficiency* for 18-hydroxylase deficiency [9].

17β-HSD Deficiency

Deficiency of the 17β-HSD enzyme impairs only the synthesis of sex steroids and is another cause of male pseudohermaphroditism [24, 60–62]. With one exception [63], all previously reported genetic males were assigned to the female sex at birth because they were so incompletely masculinized. The conversion of Δ⁴-androstenedione to testosterone is impaired in the testes, although peripheral conversion of Δ⁴-androstenedione to testosterone is apparently still intact [24]. This suggests that the enzymes controlling 17β-HSD in the testes and the liver are under different genetic control. Elevated Δ⁴-androstenedione/testosterone ratios in peripheral and spermatic blood of older patients are diagnostic for 17β-HSD deficiency. In newborns and infants, hCG stimulation may be required to unmask the abnormal Δ⁴-androstenedione/testosterone ratio [64]. Conversion of estrone to estradiol is also impaired in 17β-HSD deficiency, but usually to a lesser degree. The defect is probably only expressed in the gonads and not in the adrenal gland and thus may not be detectable after castration.

17,20-Lyase Deficiency

The 17, 20-lyase enzyme deficiency results in male pseudohermaphroditism consequent to a defect in the conversion of 17-hydroxyprogesterone and 17-hydroxypregnenolone to C-19 steroids by testes and adrenals. Only sex steroid biosynthesis is affected in this form of male pseudohermaphroditism. Urinary pregnanetriolone, a metabolite of 17-hydroxyprogesterone, is increased and increases further after ACTH and hCG stimulation. Testosterone or DHEA excretion does not rise appreciably. Seven patients in a total of three different kindred with this disorder have been reported. All seven patients were genetic males [65–67].

The clinical and laboratory features of these various enzymatic disorders of adrenal steroidogenesis are summarized in Table 47-1.

RECENT ADVANCES IN 21- AND 11β-HYDROXYLASE DEFICIENCIES

The Fasciculata and Glomerulosa as Two Separate Glands

11β-Hydroxylase Deficiency In proposing that the adrenal zona fasciculata and zona glomerulosa function as two separate glands under different regulatory control, New and Seaman [17] suggested that an 11β-hydroxylase defect might occur only in the fasciculata, sparing the glomerulosa from an 11β-hydroxylase deficiency. The hypothesis attempted to account for the rise in aldosterone secretion observed in a patient with 11β-hydroxylase deficiency after excessive DOC levels were suppressed during treatment. According to the proposal, the fasciculata suffers from an 11β-hydroxylase defect and produces excessive DOC. Elevated circulating levels of DOC cause excessive renal tubular reabsorption of sodium, which suppresses renal renin production. Thus, the glomerulosa is deprived of the stimulation of the renin-angiotensin system required for aldosterone synthesis and low aldosterone secretion results (Fig. 47-7). When DOC secretion is suppressed by treatment, natriuresis occurs and renin-angiotensin levels consequently rise, stimulating the glomerulosa to synthesize aldosterone (Fig. 47-8). Because the glomerulosa, unlike the fasciculata, is spared the 11β-hydroxylase defect, it can respond to this stimulation with an appropriate increase in aldosterone secretion, and serum and urinary aldosterone levels rise.

This hypothesis was supported by subsequent reports [68–71] and has been confirmed by the recent extensive study of four patients with 11β-hydroxylase deficiency [40]. In this study, the fasciculata and glomerulosa were separately stimulated by ACTH and renin. Results in one patient are illustrated in Fig. 47-9. In the untreated state, when renin was suppressed consequent to excessive DOC secretion, ACTH stimulation resulted in a further increase of the markedly elevated levels of 11-deoxy steroids (DOC and its metabolite THDOC [tetrahydrodeoxycorticosterone]) while the levels of 11-hydroxylated steroids (aldosterone and 18-OHB) did not rise. This indicated impaired 11β hydroxylation in the ACTH-responsive zona fasciculata. In contrast, when ACTH was suppressed by dexamethasone and renin was stimulated by a low salt diet, the levels of the 11-hydroxylated steroids increased normally, demonstrating that the renin-responsive zona glomerulosa was not defective in 11β-hydroxylation.

The hormonal data reported in this study also corroborate the recent report of Ulick [72], who detected parallel deficiencies in both 11β and 18-hydroxylase function in patients with the hypertensive form of CAH. He proposed that 11β and 18 hydroxylation in the adrenal fasciculata are functionally related and may involve the same enzyme protein and catalytic site. As can be seen in Fig. 47-9, the failure of 18-hydroxydeoxycorticosterone (18-OHDOC) levels to rise in concert with DOC during ACTH stimulation suggests the presence of an 18-hydroxylase defect as well as an 11β-hydroxylase defect in the ACTH-stimulable zona fasciculata. The normal rise of 18-OHB levels with renin stimulation indicates that in the glomer-

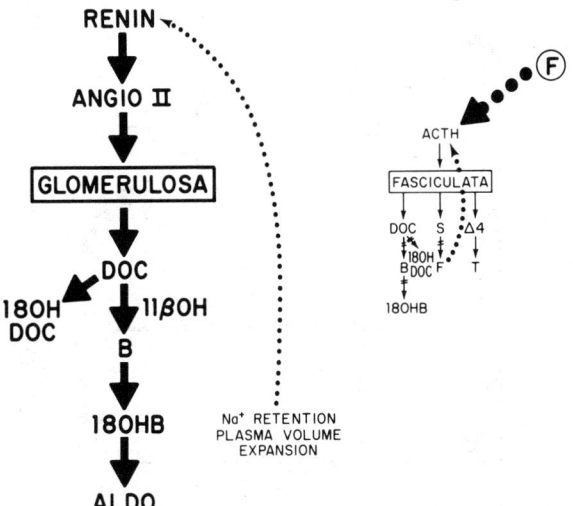

Figure 47-8 Regulation of adrenocortical steroidogenesis in treated 11β-hydroxylase deficiency. Dotted arrows indicate negative feedback. Elevated or diminished synthesis is indicated by relative size of print.   F represents glucocorticoid administered in therapy, suppressing fasciculata secretion of DOC and permitting renin-angiotensin stimulation of the glomerulosa which is not affected with an 11β-hydroxylase defect.

ulosa, 18-hydroxylase as well as 11β-hydroxylase activity remains unimpaired.

A number of studies have demonstrated inhibition of 11β- and 18-hydroxylase functions by androgens [73, 74]. It has been proposed that the elevated androgens observed in the hypertensive form of CAH are the major cause of the defective enzyme activity. Our data argue against this proposal. In the patients we studied, persistent 11β- and 18-hydroxylase deficiencies were demonstrated both when adrenal androgens were well suppressed and when increased with ACTH administration. In addition, in patients with simple virilizing CAH due to 21-hydroxylase deficiency aldosterone secretion, which requires 11β hydroxylation and 18 hydroxylation, is normal despite extremely high levels of androgens [17]. High androgen levels therefore do not inhibit the activity of the 11β-hydroxylase enzyme in 21-hydroxylase deficiency.

On the basis of this remarkable parallelism of 11β and 18 hydroxylation functions of the fasciculata zone, Ulick [72] proposed that both activities may reside in the same enzyme protein. Although it may seem surprising that one enzyme can catalyze hydroxylation at more than one position, Ulick pointed out the precedence for this in microbial steroid hydroxylases. In patients with a genetic defect in 11β hydroxylation, the presence of simultaneous defects in 11β and 18 hydroxylation in the fasciculata provides strong evidence for the parallelism of these two enzymatic functions in humans.

21-Hydroxylase Deficiency Additional evidence supporting the concept that the adrenal fasciculata and glomerulosa function as two separate glands has been gained from the recent study of patients with 21-hydroxylase deficiency. There has long been controversy over the biochemical basis for the differences between the simple virilizing and the salt-wasting forms of 21-hydroxylase deficiency. In both forms there is defective 21 hydroxylation of the 17-hydroxy steroids leading to elevation of 17-OHP and diminished production of cortisol [75]. The nature of the 21-hydroxylase defect in the 17-deoxy pathway remains less clear, although it is widely accepted that aldosterone is deficient in salt wasters and not in simple viril-

Figure 47-7 Regulation of adrenocortical steroidogenesis in untreated 11β-hydroxylase deficiency considering the fasciculata and glomerulosa as two separate glands. Dotted arrows indicate negative feedback. Elevated or diminished secretion levels are indicated by relative size of print. Note that the excessive secretion of DOC due to an 11β-hydroxylase defect impairing the conversion of DOC to B by the fasciculata results in suppression of the glomerulosa.

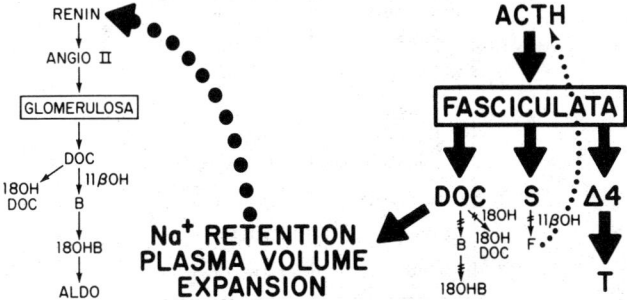

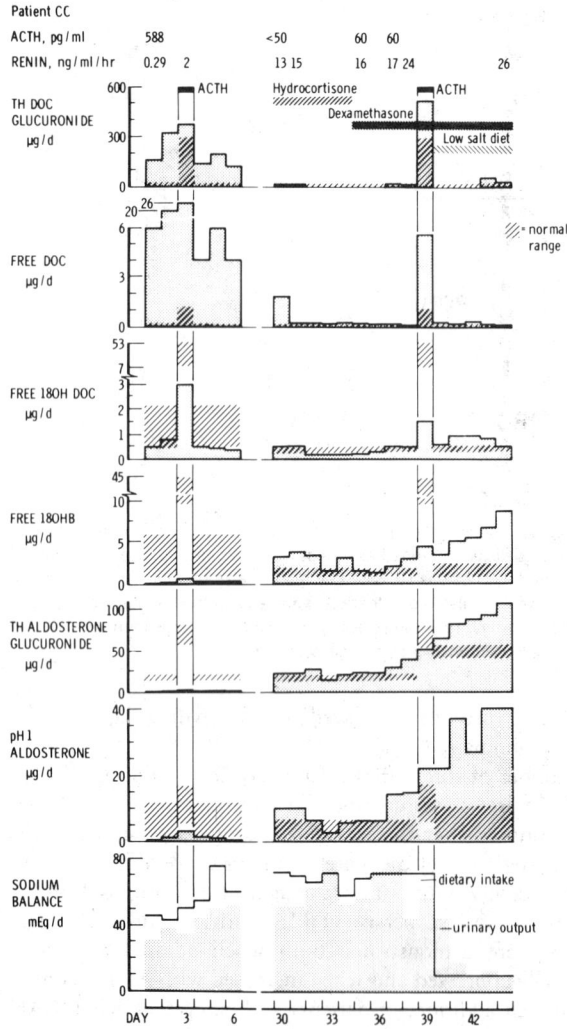

Figure 47-9 Metabolic balance and urinary hormone excretion in a prepubertal boy with 11β-hydroxylase deficiency during baseline, ACTH, dexamethasone, and dexamethasone and low salt periods. ▨, patient's response; ▨, normal control response.

izers. The hypotheses proposed to explain the different 21-hydroxylase syndromes are based either on a "one-enzyme" or a "two-enzyme" defect. Neither in vivo nor in vitro studies have been conclusive and results compatible with both theories have been reported [76].

The one-enzyme theory holds that one 21-hydroxylase enzyme is capable of 21 hydroxylation in both the 17-hydroxy and 17-deoxy pathways. The theory attributes the differences between salt-wasting and simple virilizing CAH to a different degree of enzymatic deficiency, the more severe deficiency leading to salt wasting [75, 77–79]. The two-enzyme theory postulates that two different enzymes regulate the different pathways. Thus the simple virilizers would have an enzymatic deficiency only in the 17-hydroxy pathway, whereas the salt wasters would have deficiencies in both the 17-hydroxy and 17-deoxy pathways of adrenal steroidogenesis. The two-enzyme theory is supported by reports of normal or even elevated aldosterone secretion in simple virilizers in contrast to the deficient aldosterone production in salt wasters [80–85].

Recent studies from our laboratory [86] have suggested a new hypothesis to explain the differences in salt-wasting and simple virilizing CAH. This hypothesis utilizes the two-gland model of the adrenal cortex and states: (1) in both simple vir-

ilizers and salt wasters, there is a fasciculata defect of 21 hydroxylation in both the 17-hydroxy and 17-deoxy pathways, and (2) in the salt waster there is a defect in 21 hydroxylation in the glomerulosa as well, while in the simple virilizer the glomerulosa is spared this defect. This hypothesis is schematically presented in Fig. 47-10. A sample of the data supporting this hypothesis is presented in Figs. 47-11 and 47-12.

In Fig. 47-11 the marked rise in progesterone together with the minimal response of DOC, corticosterone (B), and cortisol (F) to ACTH stimulation in both simple virilizers and salt wasters indicates a 21-hydroxylase defect for both the 17-hydroxy and 17-deoxy pathways in the ACTH-responsive zona fasciculata. The 21-hydroxylase deficiency in the zona fasciculata appears to be more severe in the salt wasters than in the simple virilizers since the response to ACTH demonstrates greater deficiency in the products of 21 hydroxylation in the salt wasters. When the fasciculata is then suppressed with dexamethasone and the glomerulosa is stimulated by renin during low sodium intake (Fig. 47-12), both normal subjects and simple virilizers have a rise in serum and urinary aldosterone and 18-OHB, which is indicative of normal glomerulosa 21-hydroxylase function. In contrast, the salt wasters show almost no increment in their aldosterone and 18-OHB levels in response to renin stimulation, as is consistent with a deficiency of 21 hydroxylation in the glomerulosa.

These data support the hypothesis that there is a 21-hydroxylase defect in the zona fasciculata of simple virilizers and salt wasters, whereas the zona glomerulosa is defective only in salt wasters and not in simple virilizers. The results show that in both normal subjects and in simple virilizers, the glomerulosa can increase aldosterone secretion in response to renin independently of precursor hormones of the fasciculata. In addition, the data indicate that there is one enzyme involved in the 21 hydroxylation of both 17-hydroxy and 17-deoxy pathways of adrenal steroidogenesis in the zona fasciculata.

Further evidence that the fasciculata and glomerulosa function as two glands has been provided by the study of 17α-

Figure 47-10 Pathway of adrenal steroidogenesis in the simple virilizing and salt-wasting forms of congenital adrenal hyperplasia due to 21-hydroxylase deficiency. *(From Kuhnle et al. [86]. Used by permission.)*

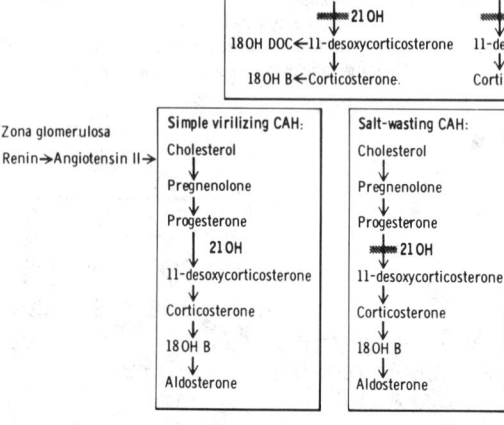

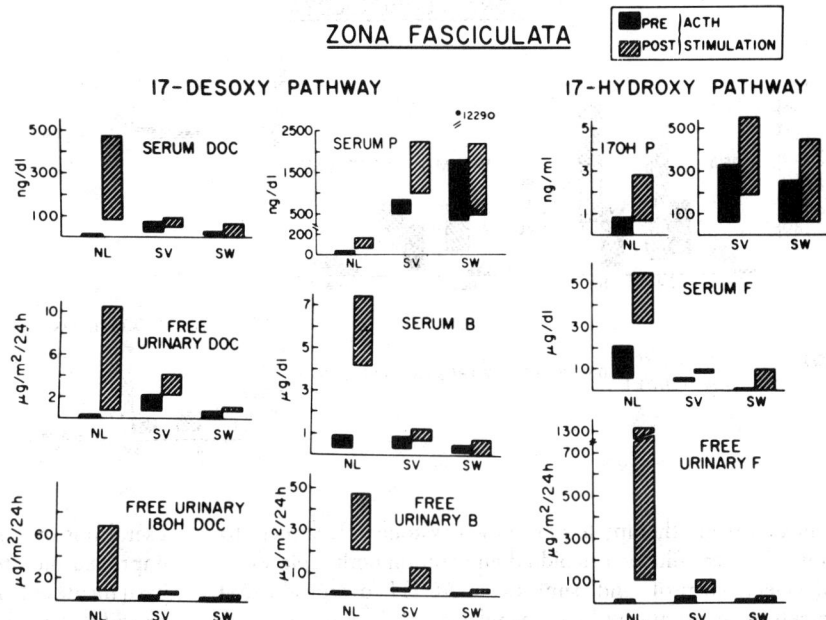

Figure 47-11 Hormonal response to ACTH stimulation of the zona fasciculata. NL, normal subject; SV, patient with the simple virilizing form of 21-hydroxylase deficiency; SW, patient with the salt-wasting form of 21-hydroxylase deficiency.

hydroxylase deficiency. Investigators found low aldosterone secretion in many of the reported cases of 17α-hydroxylase deficiency [45, 46, 87], despite the fact that a 17α-hydroxylase defect does not impair steroid synthesis in the 17-deoxy pathway. Biglieri [45] and Mantero [47] proposed that this hypoaldosteronism could be explained by the existence of an additional defect in 18-hydroxylase impairing aldosterone synthesis. Consideration of the fasciculata and glomerulosa as two separate glands obviates the need for proposing an additional enzyme deficiency [46]. According to the two-gland concept, the 17α-hydroxylase deficiency leads to overproduction of 17-deoxy steroids by the ACTH-responsive fasciculata. This results in excessive secretion of DOC and corticosterone by the fasciculata. The excessive DOC levels lead to suppressed renin secretion and a consequent failure of the renin-angiotensin stimulation of the glomerulosa necessary for aldosterone synthesis. When dexamethasone is administered, ACTH stimulation of the fasciculata is suppressed and DOC secretion diminishes, resulting in renin-angiotensin stimulation of the glomerulosa and a rise in aldosterone secretion. This result of dexamethasone treatment is similar to that observed in 11β-hydroxylase deficiency. The observed increase in aldosterone excretion with dexamethasone treatment makes it unnecessary to invoke a second enzyme defect of 18-hydroxylase to explain the hypoaldosteronism in the untreated state. Biglieri has recently reported his detailed examination of the dynamics of aldosterone secretion in treated and untreated 17α-hydroxylase deficiency [87] and proposes that both suppressed renin and an inhibitory influence of chronic ACTH stimulation are responsible for the low aldosterone secretion in the untreated state [88].

Thus in three genetic errors of steroidogenesis, 21-, 11β-, and 17α-hydroxylase deficiencies, there is evidence that the fasciculata and glomerulosa function separately and only the fasciculata may demonstrate the enzymatic defect [40, 46, 86].

The reports of elevated levels of DOC, corticosterone, and aldosterone in simple virilizing 21-hydroxylase deficiency remain perplexing. Proponents of the two-enzyme theory have contended that these findings demonstrate unimpaired 21

hydroxylation in the 17-deoxy pathway [85]. Others have attributed the elevated DOC to inhibition of 11 hydroxylation because of excessive androgens [89] or to an intraadrenal event caused by ACTH [90]. The reports of frequently elevated PRA in simple virilizers [84, 91] point to a different explanation. Consistent with the two-gland concept, it seems probable that these elevated renin levels are stimulating the unimpaired 17-deoxy pathway of the glomerulosa. The basis for this high renin activity in simple virilizers remains unclear since these patients appear capable of conserving sodium to the same degree as normal control subjects. It has been suggested that the oversecretion of aldosterone secondary to elevated renin is a compensatory response to natriuretic hormones secreted by the adrenals in patients with 21-hydroxylase deficiency [86, 92–95]. The existence of such hormones has not been proved, although a study by Kuhnle and colleagues [96] of patients with 21-hydroxylase deficiency provides new and additional evidence for the presence of an unknown mineralocorticoid antagonist in the enzyme disorder.

In summary, the findings presented herein provide further evidence that the zona fasciculata and zona glomerulosa can function as separate glands under different regulation [17]. These findings further suggest the possibility of separate genetic loci for the regulation of 21 and 11β hydroxylation in the fasciculata and the glomerulosa. The hormonal data indicate that within the fasciculata, only one genetic locus seems to regulate 21-hydroxylase enzyme activity in both the 17-hydroxy and 17-deoxy pathways.

TREATMENT

Endocrine Treatment

The fundamental aim of endocrine therapy in CAH is to provide replacement of the deficient hormones. Since 1949, when Wilkins et al. [97] and Bartter [98] discovered the efficacy of cortisone therapy for CAH due to 21-hydroxylase deficiency,

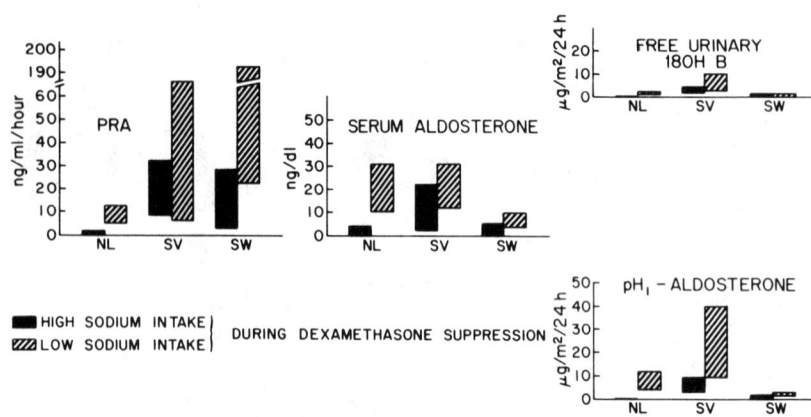

ZONA GLOMERULOSA

■ HIGH SODIUM INTAKE
▨ LOW SODIUM INTAKE } DURING DEXAMETHASONE SUPPRESSION

Figure 47-12 Hormonal response to sodium deprivation of the zona glomerulosa. See legend to Fig. 47-11 for explanation of abbreviations.

glucocorticoid therapy has been the keystone of treatment for this disorder. Glucocorticoid administration both replaces the deficient cortisol and suppresses ACTH overproduction, resulting in cessation of overstimulation of the adrenal cortex and amelioration of the noxious effects of oversecreted adrenal steroids. Proper replacement therapy in 21- and 11β-hydroxylase deficiency suppresses excessive adrenal androgen production, averting further virilization, slowing accelerated growth and bone age advancement to a more normal rate, and allowing a normal onset of puberty (Fig. 47-13). Glucocorticoid treatment also leads to remission of hypertension in 11β- and 17α-hydroxylase deficiency, presumably by suppressing oversecretion of DOC. Excessive glucocorticoid administration should be avoided since this produces Cushingoid facies, growth retardation, and inhibition of epiphyseal maturation. In the enzyme deficiencies impairing mineralocorticoid synthesis, the administration of salt-retaining steroid is required to maintain adequate sodium balance.

Increasing attention has been focused on the role of the renin-angiotensin system in the treatment of CAH. Although aldosterone levels are not deficient in the non-salt-wasting (simple virilizing) form of 21-hydroxylase deficiency, it has long been recognized that PRA is elevated in the non-salt-wasting as well as in the salt-wasting form [84, 91, 98–101.]. Despite the observation of elevated PRA, it has not been customary to supplement conventional glucocorticoid replacement therapy with the administration of salt-retaining steroids in cases of non-salt-wasting 21-hydroxylase deficiency. In a recent clinical study, Rösler and colleagues [79] demonstrated that the addition of salt-retaining hormone to glucocorticoid therapy in non-salt-wasting patients with elevated PRA does in fact improve the hormonal control of the disease.

Rösler showed that in patients with CAH due to 21-hydroxylase deficiency, the PRA was closely correlated to the ACTH level. Thus, when PRA was normalized by the added administration of 9α-fludrocortisone acetate, a steroid with salt-retaining activity, the ACTH level fell and excessive androgen stimulation by ACTH decreased (Fig. 47-14). The addition of salt-retaining steroids to the therapeutic regimen often made a decrease in the glucocorticoid dose possible. Normalization of PRA also resulted in improved statural growth in these patients, a finding which has been corroborated in subsequent reports [102, 103] (Fig. 47-15).

The newly developed steroid radioimmunoassays have been

useful not only for the initial diagnosis of CAH, but also for improved monitoring of hormonal control once therapy has been instituted. Serum 17-OHP and Δ⁴-androstenedione levels provide a sensitive index of biochemical control in 21-hydroxylase deficiency [104, 105]. In females and prepubertal males, but not in newborn and pubertal males, the serum testosterone level is also a useful index [104]. The combined determinations of PRA, 17-OHP, and serum androgens, as well as the clinical assessment of growth and pubertal status, must all be considered in adjusting the dose of glucocorticoid and salt-retaining steroid for optimal therapeutic control. Both in our clinic and in others, combinations of hydrocortisone and 9α-fludrocortisone acetate have proved to be highly effective treatment modalities [103].

Measurement of PRA can be used to monitor efficacy of treatment not only in 21-hydroxylase deficiency but also in other salt-losing forms of CAH (cholesterol desmolase and 3β-HSD deficiencies). It is also useful as a therapeutic index in those forms of CAH with mineralocorticoid excess and suppressed PRA (11β-hydroxylase and 17α-hydroxylase defi-

Figure 47-13 Habitus of pubertal girls with CAH due to 21-hydroxylase deficiency. Patient on the left was untreated until age 16 years; patient in the center was treated at age 9 years; patient on the right was treated at age 4 years. Note the progressively more feminine habitus with earlier treatment. *(From New and Levine [165]. Used by permission.)*

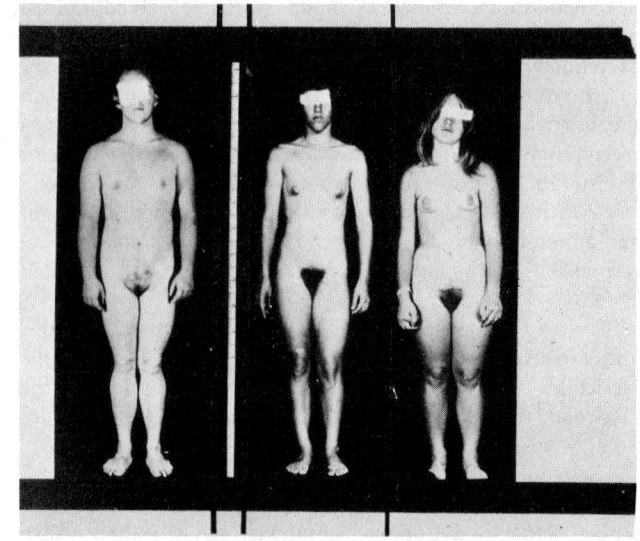

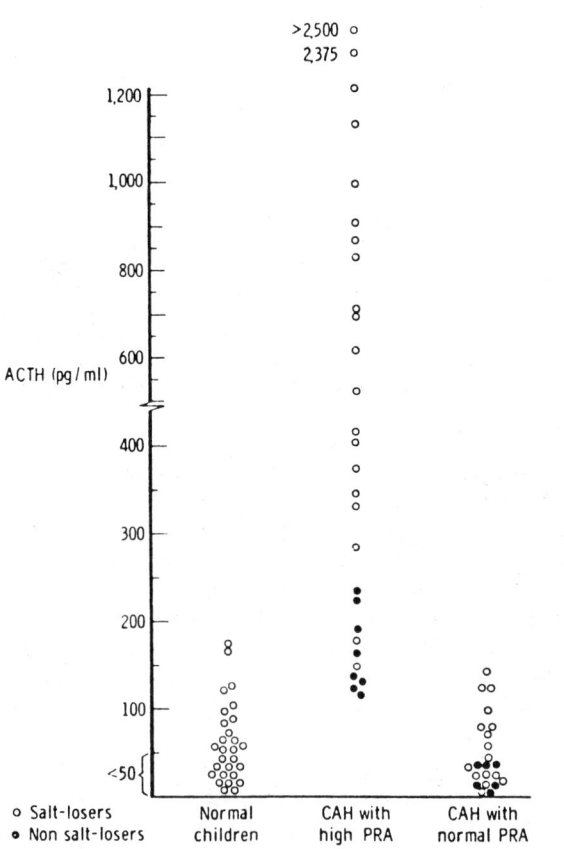

Figure 47-14 ACTH levels in normal children and in seven patients with CAH treated with constant replacement doses of glucocorticoids equivalent to 25 mg/(m²·day) of hydrocortisone. Samples were drawn between 0800 and 0900 h. Levels of PRA were high during the ad lib, normal, and low sodium diets. Normal PRA levels were achieved by sodium repletion with a high sodium diet and/or additional 9α-fludrocortisone acetate. *(From Rösler et al., [79]. Used by permission.)*

ciencies). In poor control, PRA is elevated in the salt-losing forms and suppressed in the mineralocorticoid excess forms (Fig. 47-16).

Sex Assignment

Sexual ambiguity at birth characteristic of male or female pseudohermaphroditism is a common presenting sign of CAH (see Table 47-1). In such cases, a rational and judicious choice of sex assignment is a critical aspect of treatment, since the decision of sex assignment has obvious lifelong implications. Determination of genetic sex by karyotype or buccal smear and the accurate diagnosis of the specific underlying enzymatic defect are essential in assessing a patient's potential for future sexual activity and fertility.

In cases of female pseudohermaphroditism to 21- or 11β-hydroxylase deficiency, a female sex assignment is appropriate. When medical treatment is begun early in life, the initially large and prominent clitoris shrinks slightly and, as the surrounding structures grow normally, it becomes much less prominent and surgical revision of the clitoris may not be required. When the clitoris is conspicuously enlarged or when the abnormal genitalia interfere with parent-child bonding, plastic surgery to correct the appearance of the clitoris should be carried out. Definitive vaginoplasty should, in general, be

performed in early childhood by an experienced gynecologic surgeon [106]. Because of the normal internal genitalia and gonads in these patients, normal puberty, fertility, and childbearing are possible when there is early therapeutic intervention. In view of this potential for normal female sexual development, it is unfortunate when, as a result of a hasty delivery room examination of the virilized external genitalia, affected females are improperly assigned and reared as males.

In cases of male pseudohermaphroditism due to enzyme deficiencies impairing androgen synthesis, a sex assignment consistent with the genetic sex—i.e., a male sex assignment—is not always optimal. Virilization of the genitalia in these children is frequently so extremely and irrevocably incomplete that the anatomy precludes normal male functioning. There are certain physiologic capacities which we consider integral to "normal" male sexual development: a capacity for intercourse, for urinating in a standing position, and for developing secondary sex characteristics adequate for the presentation of a male gender identity in society. Because these capacities are often severely compromised in genetic males with congenital disorders of sex steroid synthesis, a female sex assignment may be advisable. If the male pseudohermaphrodite is to be raised as a female, surgical correction of the genitalia and gonadectomy are required; with appropriate therapeutic measures, relatively normal, albeit infertile, female sexual activity and development are possible. In cases of impaired androgen synthesis, administration of sex steroids is usually required to induce development of appropriate sex characteristics at puberty—either

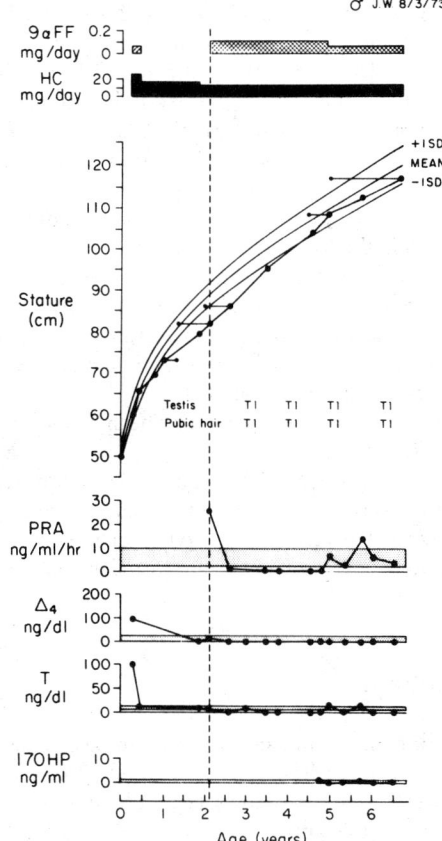

Figure 47-15 Growth curve of a patient with salt-wasting CAH before and after therapeutic control of PRA. Note that with renin suppression, hydrocortisone dose could be lowered, growth improved, and androgen suppression was maintained despite the decrease in hydrocortisone dose.

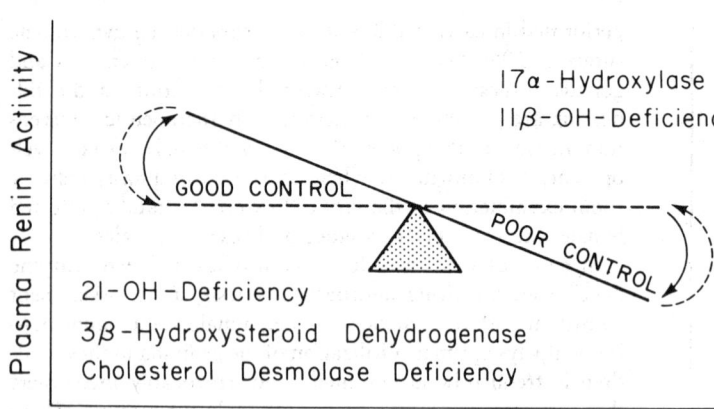

Figure 47-16 The pivotal role of monitoring PRA in various forms of CAH. In poor control, renin is elevated in 21-hydroxylase deficiency, 3β-hydroxysteroid deficiency, and cholesterol desmolase deficiency and decreases with proper mineralocorticoid treatment. In contrast, in 17α-hydroxylase deficiency and 11β-hydroxylase deficiency renin is suppressed in poor control and rises with proper treatment.

estrogens if the patient is to be reared as a female or androgens if reared as a male.

Society sees phenotype, not genotype. In assigning a sex of rearing to a male or female pseudohermaphrodite, the genetic sex is of less consideration than the physiologic and anatomic character of the genitalia and their potential for development and function. Because of the wide individual variability in the presentation of ambiguous genitalia in these patients, there can be no all-inclusive rules for sex assignment based solely on genetic sex or type of enzyme deficiency.

GENETICS

Population Studies

Several surveys have established that 21-hydroxylase deficiency is transmitted as an autosomal recessive trait [31, 107, 108]. Males and females are equally at risk [109]. With few exceptions [110], the clinical presentation—simple virilizing or salt wasting—is consistent within one family. In Europe and the USA recent estimates of the incidence of CAH due to 21-hydroxylase deficiency have been between 1:5000 and 1:15,000. In Alaska the incidence in Yupik Eskimos is unusually high, while the low incidence reported in Maryland may have been due to inadequate case ascertainment (Table 47-2). The gene frequency is estimated as approximately 1 in 100 and the carrier frequency as approximately 1 in 50 [111]. The salt-wasting variety occurs in about 50 to 80 percent of patients with 21-hydroxylase deficiency [112, 113]. A very high incidence of the salt-wasting variety has been found among the Yupiks [114].

The 11β-hydroxylase, 3β-HSD, and 17α-hydroxylase deficiencies are also transmitted as autosomal recessive traits but are much rarer than the 21-hydroxylase deficiency. The other enzyme defects are probably transmitted by an autosomal recessive gene as well.

HLA Linkage

The genes for HLA (human leukocyte antigens), cell surface antigens important in transplantation, are located on chromosome 6. The HLA complex consists of at least four genetic loci which code for the antigens HLA-A, HLA-B, HLA-C, and HLA-D/DR. Each of the loci is polymorphic and multiple

alleles have been demonstrated for each locus. In addition to the HLA loci several other loci have been mapped on chromosome 6 in close linkage with HLA [115, 116]. A detailed discussion of the HLA complex is given in Chapter 3.

Each individual inherits one chromosome 6 from his father and one from his mother. The HLA genes are codominantly expressed and the gene products of the HLA-A, -B, -C, and -D/DR loci from both parents are expressed on the surface of all nucleated cells. An example of an HLA genotype of an individual is written as follows:

$$\frac{\text{A3, Bw47(w4), Cw6, DR7}}{\text{A28, Bw35(w6), Cw4, DR5}}$$

in which one haplotype [the set of A3, Bw47(w4), Cw6, DR7] is inherited from one parent, while the other haplotype [A28, Bw35(w6), Cw4, DR5] is inherited from the other parent.

Close genetic linkage between HLA and CAH due to 21-hydroxylase deficiency was first described in 1977 [117]. In this study HLA genotyping of parents and children in six families with one or more child affected with CAH due to 21-hydroxylase deficiency was performed. In five of these families, all of the affected offspring were HLA identical and different from their unaffected sibs.

Subsequently, studies of 34 unrelated families with a total of

Table 47-2 Estimated incidence of CAH (21-hydroxylase deficiency)

Reference	Population	Patient/live births
Childs et al. [108]	Maryland, USA	1:67,000
Prader [49]	Zurich, Switzerland	1:5,041
Hubble†	Birmingham, England	1:7,255
Rosenbloom and Smith [110]	Wisconsin, USA	1:15,000
Hirschfeld and Fleshman [114]	Alaska, USA; Yupik Eskimo, USA	1:700* / 1:245
Qazi and Thompson‡	Toronto, Canada	1:13,000*
Mauthe et al.§	Munich, Germany	1:9,831
Muller et al. [111]	Tyrol, Austria	1:8,991
Werder et al. [160]	All of Switzerland	1:15,472

* Incidence was corrected for both variants of salt waster and non-salt waster.

† Hubble D: Congenital adrenal hyperplasia, in HALT KS, RAINE DM (eds): *Basic Concepts of Inborn Errors and Defects of Steroid Biosynthesis.* Edinburgh, London. Livingstone Press, 1966, pp 68–74.

‡ Quazi QH, Thompson MW: Incidence of salt-wasting form of congenital adrenal virilizing hyperplasia. *Arch Dis Child* 47:302, 1972.

§ Mauthe I, Laspe H, Knorr D: Zur Häufigkeit des kongenitalen adrenogenitalen Syndroms (AGS): Munchen:1963–1972. *Klin Padiat* 189:172, 1977.

48 patients were reported from New York and Zurich [118]. The findings of this study are illustrated in the two typical pedigrees shown in Fig. 47-17. As shown in Fig. 47-17A, the 3 affected sibs are HLA identical. In Figure 47-17B, the unaffected sibs are all HLA different from their affected sister.

Each parent is an obligate heterozygote carrier and has transmitted one HLA haplotype carrying the gene for 21-hydroxylase deficiency to the patient. Both HLA haplotypes of the patient are linked to the gene for 21-hydroxylase deficiency and therefore any member of the family who shares one HLA haplotype with the patient should also carry the gene for the enzyme defect. The brother and sister having only one haplotype linked to the gene for CAH are presumed heterozygotes. The sib sharing neither haplotype with the patient is presumed not to carry the gene for 21-hydroxylase deficiency. The HLA genotype is thus a marker for the CAH genotype.

Recent international studies reported at the Eighth International Histocompatibility Workshop have provided more detailed genetic mapping of the specific location of the 21-hydroxylase deficiency gene relative to the different loci that constitute the HLA complex. By examining cases of genetic recombination between HLA and the 21-hydroxylase defi-

ciency gene, these studies established that the 21-hydroxylase deficiency gene is located between the HLA-A locus and the centromere but is further away from the centromere than the glyoxylase I locus [119]. The studies of genetic recombination also suggest the possibility that there exists more than one HLA-linked genetic locus for 21-hydroxylase deficiency [76, 119].

Statistical methods of genetic analysis have established close genetic linkage between the 21-hydroxylase deficiency gene and HLA. The studies reported at the Eighth International Histocompatibility Workshop found a peak Lod score of 15.65 at a recombination frequency θ of 0.00 for linkage between HLA and 21-hydroxylase deficiency [119]. The Lod score is a statistical index of the certainty with which one can arrive at a conclusion of genetic linkage. A score of 15.65 means that the odds are $10^{15.65}$ to 1 that linkage exists. In humans, genetic linkage is considered established if the Lod score exceeds 3.00.

The loci mapped on chromosome 6 within the HLA linkage group are shown in Fig. 47-18. The 21-hydroxylase deficiency gene has been mapped within a range of 3 to 4 centimorgans.

Heterozygote Detection

Prior to the discovery that 21-hydroxylase deficiency is genetically linked to HLA, attempts were made to test for hormonal heterozygosity using the obligate heterozygote parents of children with CAH. A mild deficiency of 21-hydroxylase was demonstrated in parents by hormonal measurements by several investigators, although similar hormonal studies in the sibs of patients with CAH have been more difficult to interpret because of the inability to ascertain which sibs are carriers of the gene and which are genetically unaffected [120–131]. With the demonstration of linkage between the genes for HLA and 21-hydroxylase deficiency, HLA genotyping makes it possible to predict which sibs are carriers and which sibs are genetically unaffected. The method for utilizing HLA genotyping in the prediction is shown in Fig. 47-17B.

The prediction of heterozygosity by HLA genotyping has been validated by hormonal studies. We have found that family members predicted by HLA genotyping to be heterozygotes demonstrate a higher 17-OHP response to ACTH stimulation than do family members predicted to be genetically unaffected (Fig. 47-19) [132, 133]. Baseline 17-OHP concentrations in heterozygotes are indistinguishable from those in genetically unaffected subjects, and ACTH stimulation is required to unmask the presence of a mild 21-hydroxylase deficiency. Other investigators have corroborated the HLA genotyping prediction of heterozygosity by hormonal measurements [134–137]. Improved segregation of CAH heterozygotes from unaffected subjects in the adult female population has recently been obtained by pretreating these subjects with dexamethasone [135, 138, 139].

Nonclassical Variants of 21-Hydroxylase Deficiency

Virilization with menstrual disturbances presenting in later childhood or early adulthood associated with endocrinologic features consistent with 21-hydroxylase deficiency is a puz-

Figure 47-17 Pedigrees for two families with 21-hydroxylase deficiency. The HLA-haplotypes for the HLA-A, HLA-B, and HLA-C alleles are given in each family. The paternal haplotypes are labeled a and b, and the maternal haplotypes c and d. The parents are obligate heterozygous carriers for the 21-hydroxylase deficiency gene (denoted by the half-black symbols). The affected children are denoted by black symbols. In A, three affected sibs are HLA genotypically identical. In B, one affected child is HLA genotypically different from the three unaffected sibs. One sib who carries the parental a and d haplotypes is presumed to be a heterozygous carrier for 21-hydroxylase deficiency because he shares the haplotype with the patient. Another sib has the parental b and c haplotypes and shares the c haplotype with the patient, and should be a carrier of the 21-hydroxylase deficiency gene. The child with the b and d haplotypes should be normal for the gene. (From Levine et al. [118]. Used by permission.)

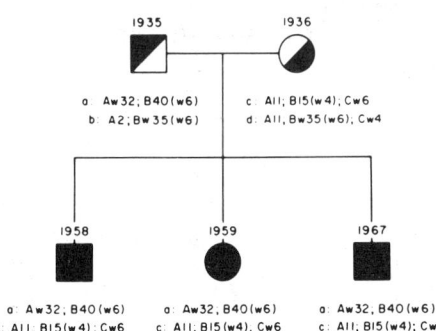

A.   FAMILY Zurich 7 (21-Hydroxylase Deficiency)

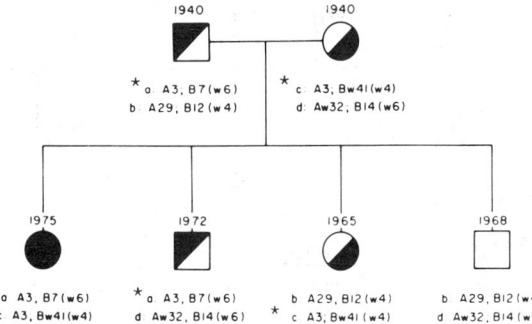

B.   FAMILY N.Y. 16 (21-Hydroxylase Deficiency)

HLA-LINKAGE GROUP

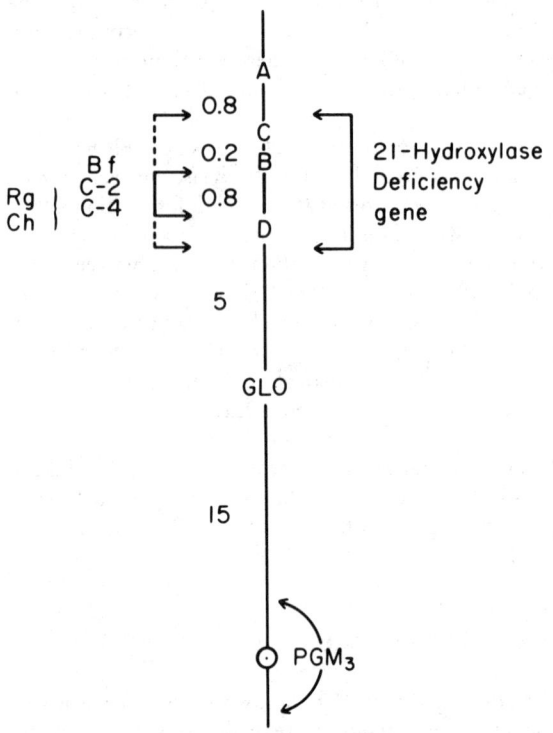

Figure 47-18 HLA linkage group on chromosome 6. The recombinant fractions for the known linkages between A:C, C:B, B:D, B:GLO, and GLO:PGM₃ are shown. The positions of the genes for factor B (Bf), complement C2 and complement C4 and Rodgers (Rg) and Chido (Ch) blood groups are also indicated. The 21-hydroxylase deficiency gene can be mapped between HLA-A and glyoxalase I (GLO). The most likely position of the 21-hydroxylase deficiency gene is very close to HLA-B. (*From Levine et al.* [118]. *Used by permission.*)

zling syndrome to which the term *late-onset* or "acquired" adrenal hyperplasia is applied [140–143]. Unlike patients with classic 21-hydroxylase deficiency, females with late-onset 21-hydroxylase deficiency show no evidence of in utero virilization and are born with normal vaginal and urethral orifices and no labial fusion. Both types of patients respond similarly to glucocorticoid treatment. The late presentation of a biochemical defect has raised the question as to whether this is the same inherited disorder as CAH with delayed presentation or is an "acquired" disorder distinct from CAH. Although initial studies suggested that the late-onset disorder was not HLA-linked [144, 145], more recent reports have provided evidence that this disorder is in fact also genetically linked to HLA [146–149], and it has been proposed that congenital and late-onset 21-hydroxylase deficiency are allelic variants [76, 148, 149].

Our HLA studies of families with classical 21-hydroxylase deficiency have also led us to uncover a new, cryptic form of 21-hydroxylase deficiency. In the course of HLA genotyping and hormonal testing, we encountered family members whose biochemical profiles were characteristic of 21-hydroxylase deficiency, although the clinical hallmarks commonly accompanying the disorder (eg., virilization, abnormal puberty and growth, infertility) were absent. The presence of hormonal abnormalities without clinical stigmata led us to designate this disorder as *cryptic* 21-hydroxylase deficiency. The hormonal

abnormalities which these cryptic family members demonstrated were similar to those observed in the late-onset form of 21-hydroxylase deficiency [150].

After further investigation we concluded that these asymptomatic family members were genetic compounds, having 21-hydroxylase deficiency as a result of inheriting two recessive genetic defects: (1) a severe 21-hydroxylase genetic defect shared with the index case with classical CAH (21-OH^{CAH}), and (2) a mild, cryptic variant of the 21-hydroxylase genetic defect (21-OH^{CRYPTIC}). The genotype 21-OH^{CAH}/21-OH^{CRYPTIC} was thus assigned to these family members with cryptic 21-hydroxylase deficiency.

Lod score analysis established close genetic linkage between HLA and the 21-OH^{CRYPTIC} gene [150]. The pedigrees of several families with members having the cryptic disorder are illustrated in Figs. 47-20 and 47-21 and the HLA genotypes denoted.

Zachmann and Prader [151, 152] also reported family members of patients with classical 21-hydroxylase deficiency whose hormonal responses are consistent with cryptic 21-hydroxylase deficiency. Zachmann and Prader proposed that these members were heterozygotes for the classical gene (21-OH^{CAH}/21-OH^{NORMAL}) with unusual manifestations, rather than genetic compounds as we have proposed. Our demonstration that family members predicted by HLA genotyping to be heterozygous for the cryptic gene (21-OH^{CRYPTIC}/21-OH^{NORMAL}) have a 17-OHP response to ACTH identical to that of family members predicted to be het-

Figure 47-19 Stimulated 17-OHP level and the stimulated 17-OHP/F ratio in prepubertal and early pubertal children, postpubertal males, and postmenarchal females. Gen. pop., general population (■ male; ● female; ▲ homozygous normal brother of a patient with CAH, based on HLA typing; △ homozygous normal sister, based on HLA typing). Het. pop., heterozygous population (■ father; ● mother; □ heterozygous brothers or heterozygous male family members, based on HLA typing; ○ heterozygous sisters or heterozygous female family members, based on HLA typing). The bar represents the range, the heavy horizontal line the mean. (*From Lorenzen et al.* [133]. *Used by permission.*)

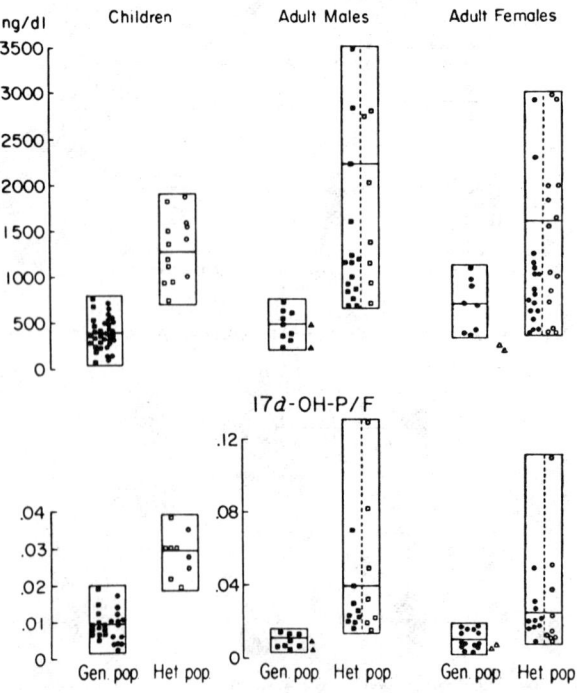

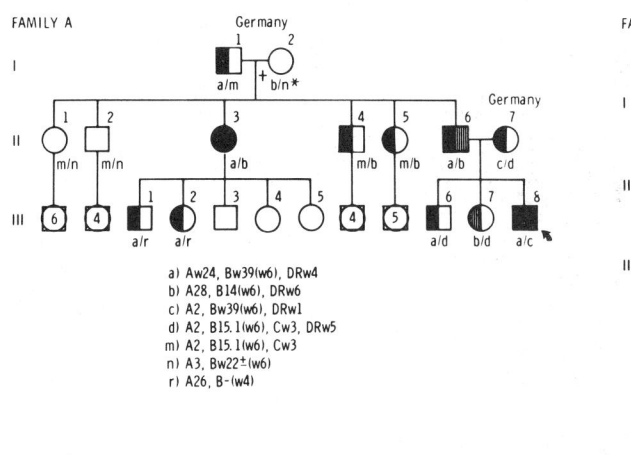

a) Aw24, Bw39(w6), DRw4
b) A28, B14(w6), DRw6
c) A2, Bw39(w6), DRw1
d) A2, B15.1(w6), Cw3, DRw5
m) A2, B15.1(w6), Cw3
n) A3, Bw22±(w6)
r) A26, B-(w4)

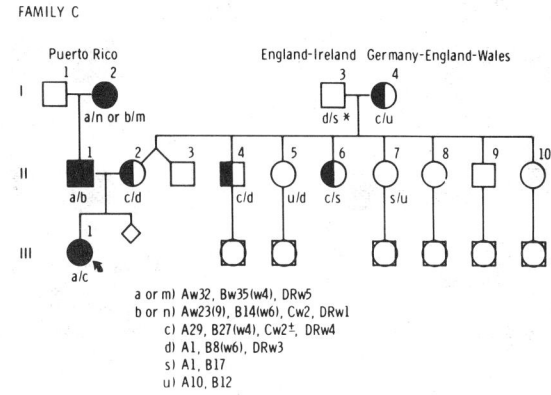

a or m) Aw32, Bw35(w4), DRw5
b or n) Aw23(9), B14(w6), Cw2, DRw1
c) A29, B27(w4), Cw2±, DRw4
d) A1, B8(w6), DRw3
s) A1, B17
u) A10, B12

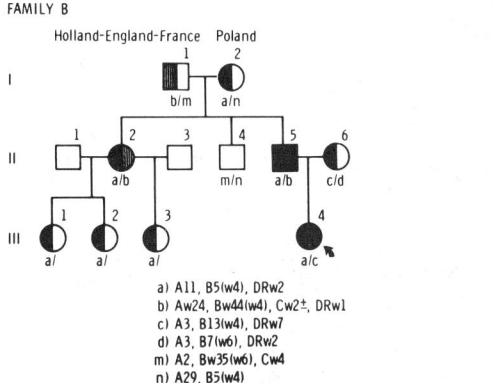

a) A11, B5(w4), DRw2
b) Aw24, Bw44(w4), Cw2±, DRw1
c) A3, B13(w4), DRw7
d) A3, B7(w6), DRw2
m) A2, Bw35(w6), Cw4
n) A29, B5(w4)

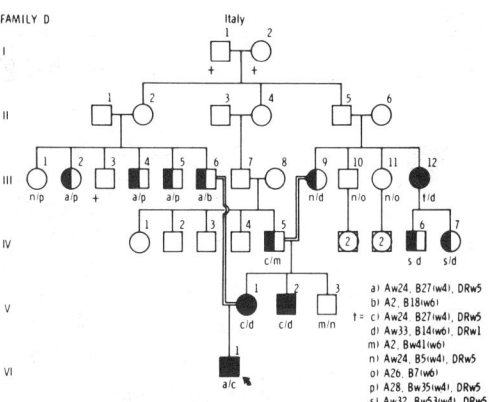

a) Aw24, B27(w4), DRw5
b) A2, B18(w6)
t = c) Aw24, B27(w4), DRw5
d) Aw33, B14(w6), DRw1
m) A2, Bw41(w6)
n) Aw24, B5(w4), DRw5
o) A26, B7(w6)
p) A28, Bw35(w4), DRw5
s) Aw32, Bw53(w4), DRw5

Figure 47-20 Pedigrees of families A to D. The HLA haplotypes for the HLA-A, HLA-B, HLA-C, and HLA-DR are indicated for each family member tested. The index case with CAH is assigned the haplotypes a/c. *Indicates haplotypes deduced from offspring. ◐ ◧ indicates heterozygous carriers of the severe deficiency gene for CAH. ● ◧ indicates family members with cryptic 21-hydroxylase deficiency, having both a severe and mild deficiency gene. ◐ ◧ indicates heterozygous carriers of the cryptic 21-hydroxylase deficiency gene. ⬡ indicates offspring, number if known.

erozygous for the classical gene (21-OH^{CAH}/21-OH^{NORMAL}) argues against the suggestion of Zachmann and Prader. In family H in Fig. 47-21, for example, members II-3, III-3, and III-4 all demonstrated hormonal responses characteristic of heterozygous carriers for a 21-hydroxylase deficiency gene. HLA genotyping revealed that they shared one HLA haplotype (b) with the cryptic family members (II-2, II-4) but no HLA haplotype with the index case with classical CAH (III-5). If, as proposed by Zachmann and Prader, the cryptic members II-2 and II-4 were simply unusual heterozygotes for the classical gene, members II-3, III-3, and III-4 would be predicted to be genetically unaffected (21-OH^{NORMAL}/21-OH^{NORMAL}). This prediction conflicts with the observed hormonal responses in these members, which clearly fall in the range for heterozygotes. Our proposal that these members have inherited a variant 21-OH^{CRYPTIC} gene from a family member with cryptic 21-hydroxylase deficiency is consistent with the hormonal findings.

An interesting biologic paradox which remains to be elucidated is the absence of clinical signs in patients with cryptic 21-hydroxylase deficiency, in contrast to the severe virilization noted in patients with late-onset 21-hydroxylase deficiency, despite the fact that both patient groups demonstrate similar biochemical abnormalities. Patients with the late-onset disorder are detected because of their clinical symptoms, whereas cryptic 21-hydroxylase deficiency has been detected only as a result of genetic and hormonal studies of classic CAH families.

Hormonal Standards for Genotyping 21-Hydroxylase Deficiency

We have developed a series of nomograms relating the baseline and ACTH-stimulated levels of 17-OHP, Δ^4-androstenedione (Δ^4), DHEA, the ration DHEA/Δ^4-androstenedione, and testosterone (T). These nomograms provide hormonal standards for assignment of the 21-hydroxylase deficiency genotype; i.e., patients whose hormonal values fall on the regression line within a defined group are assigned to that group [Figs. 47-22 to 47-27]. Clinical symptoms and signs must distinguish between the cryptic and late-onset forms of 21-hydroxylase deficiency, which are indistinguishable biochemically. Heterozygotes for classical and cryptic 21-hydroxylase deficiency demonstrate a similar hormonal response and are thus phenotypically indistinguishable. Our preliminary findings also indicate that heterozygotes for late-onset 21-hydroxylase deficiency are phenotypically indistinguishable from other heterozygotes for 21-hydroxylase deficiency.

The distribution of responses along a regression line suggests that there is a spectrum of enzymatic deficiency in these groups. Patients with classical CAH have the most severe deficiency, patients with cryptic or late-onset forms have a less severe deficiency, while heterozygotes for all three forms have

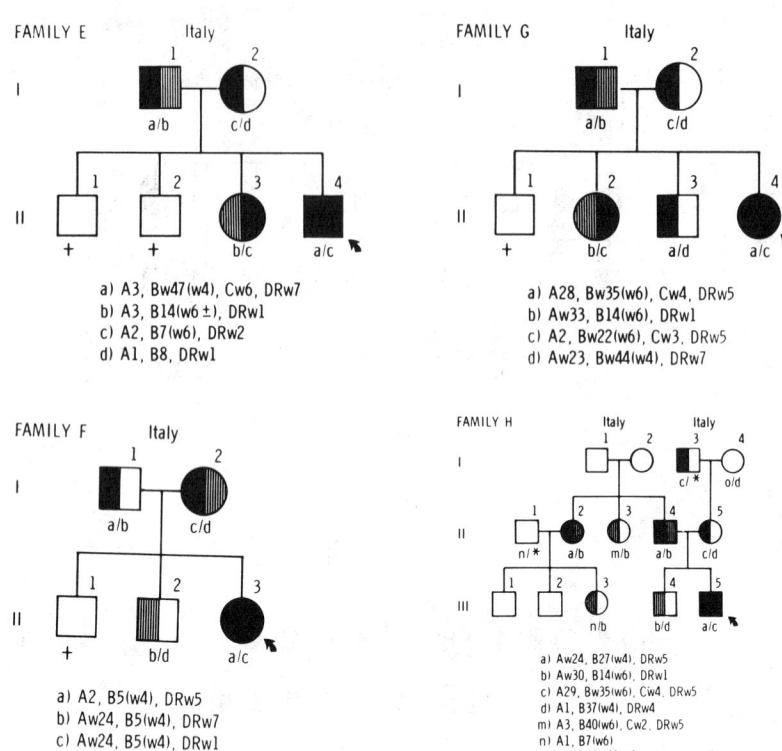

Figure 47-21   Pedigrees of families E to H. See Fig. 47-20 for symbols.

an even milder deficiency which is unmasked only upon ACTH stimulation. Hormonal values in family members predicted by HLA genotyping to be unaffected for 21-hydroxylase deficiency fall at the lowest point of the regression line and serve as the best control population for normal 21-hydroxylase activity. Those members of the general population whose responses are in the heterozygote range may actually be carriers of a gene for 21-hydroxylase deficiency.

Allelic Variants

In 1973, McKusick listed CAH due to 21-hydroxylase deficiency among the disorders in which the phenotypic diversity might be attributed to allelic series [153]. He noted that genetic compounds were an additional source of phenotypic diversity. Although the phenotypic variants of salt-wasting and simple virilizing CAH due to 21-hydroxylase deficiency have long been recognized, the new phenotypic variant of cryptic 21-hydroxylase deficiency has only recently been described [150].

We propose that there are allelic variants at the 21-hydroxylase locus which produce different degrees of 21-hydroxylase deficiency resulting in the phenotypic diversity of classical, cryptic, and late-onset 21-hydroxylase deficiency. According to the two-gland model in which the adrenal fasciculata and glomerulosa function separately (see above), we propose that the clinical spectrum of virilization is the result of allelism at the 21-hydroxylase locus in the fasciculata, while salt wasting is the result of a separate genetic defect. We further suggest that the cryptic form represents a genetic compound of the classical (or more severe) 21-hydroxylase deficiency allele and the less severe cryptic 21-hydroxylase deficiency allele. This postulate awaits proof by complementation studies. Ultimate proof may be obtained by sequencing the gene by recombinant DNA techniques and demonstrating the specific nature of the genetic mutation for each allelic variant.

One may anticipate that a similar degree of genetic heterogeneity is likely to be found in the other inherited enzyme defects of steroidogenesis. Thus the phenotypic variability already recognized in 11β-hydroxylase and 17β-HSD deficiency may be other examples of genetic heterogeneity.

Genetic Linkage Disequilibrium

Genetic linkage, which we have described for HLA and 21-hydroxylase deficiency, is distinguished from *genetic linkage disequilibrium,* which is the nonrandom association of particular alleles of different genetic loci (see Chap. 3). In patients with classical, late-onset, and cryptic 21-hydroxylase deficiency, certain HLA antigens appear with either a significantly increased or decreased frequency relative to their frequency in the general population. Thus not only are 21-hydroxylase deficiency and HLA genetically linked, but there is genetic linkage disequilibrium between the 21-hydroxylase deficiency alleles and certain HLA alleles.

The most significant association for classical 21-hydroxylase deficiency has been found for HLA-Bw47, where the combined relative risk is 15.4 [119]. Slight increases have also been reported for Bw51, Bw53, Bw60, and DR7. A review of the Bw47 positive haplotypes in patients with 21-hydroxylase deficiency reveals that this antigen frequently occurs on one particular haplotype: A3, Cw6, Bw47, DR7. Although the gene frequency for Bw47 in different Caucasian populations is always very low (<0.005), international studies have found that Bw47 appears with remarkable frequency among 21-hydroxylase CAH patients. In one particular region of England, the Bw47 frequency among CAH patients is nearly 50 percent. Several studies have also demonstrated that A1, B8, and DR3 are consistently decreased among 21-hydroxylase–deficient patients [118, 135, 154, 155].

Genetic linkage disequilibrium has also been reported for the variant forms of 21-hydroxylase deficiency [119, 146,

147]. Our latest study documents the significantly increased frequency of HLA-B14, DR1, and complement factor BfS in both late-onset and cryptic 21-hydroxylase deficiency [149]. The fact that these alleles tend to appear together on the same haplotype in patients with late-onset or cryptic 21-hydroxylase deficiency suggests that the HLA haplotype segment HLA-B14, DR1, BfS—rather than the individual HLA alleles—is highly associated with both these variant forms of 21-hydroxylase deficiency.

Our analysis of genetic linkage disequilibrium provides provocative evidence that some patients with late-onset 21-hydroxylase deficiency, similar to patients with cryptic 21-hydroxylase deficiency, may be genetic compounds possessing both a classical and variant 21-hydroxylase deficiency gene. In a few late-onset patients we have detected HLA-Bw47, an allele occurring with strikingly high frequency in association with the gene for classical 21-hydroxylase deficiency. In the family shown in Fig. 47-28, the appearance of Bw47 on haplotype c makes the presence of a classical deficiency gene highly likely. Because heterozygotes for the classical gene and heterozygotes for the late-onset gene are biochemically indistinguishable, hormonal tests provide no indication of whether the mother (I-2) carries a classical or late-onset gene on haplotype c. Conclusive proof for the presence of a classical 21-hydroxylase deficiency gene rests on the eventual appearance of a patient with classical 21-hydroxylase deficiency in the family pedigree. Indeed, in studying the family of a patient recently diagnosed as having congenital salt-wasting 21-hydroxylase deficiency, we found that the maternal grandmother has a hormonal response and medical history consistent with late-onset 21-hydroxylase deficiency. Particularly noteworthy is that the HLA haplotype which the grandmother shares with the patient with classical CAH (Fig. 47-29, haplotype a) contains Bw47, while the grandmother's other HLA haplotype contains B14, the HLA antigen most strongly associated with late-onset and cryptic 21-hydroxylase deficiency.

The finding that both the late-onset and cryptic 21-hydroxylase deficiency genes are associated with the same HLA haplotype segment (B14, DR1, BfS) suggests that these two variant genes are highly related. It is possible that individuals who have similar or identical nonclassical 21-hydroxylase deficiency alleles may express different clinical manifestations of their 21-hydroxylase defect, expressing either the late-onset or cryptic disorder. Similarly, the clinical distinction between the late-onset and cryptic disorders no longer appears as discrete as initially appreciated. We have found marked variability in the symptoms of the late-onset patients we have recently examined, ranging from precocious pubic hair growth without subsequent symptoms of virilization to more severe degrees of hirsutism, acne, menstrual disturbances, and stunted growth.

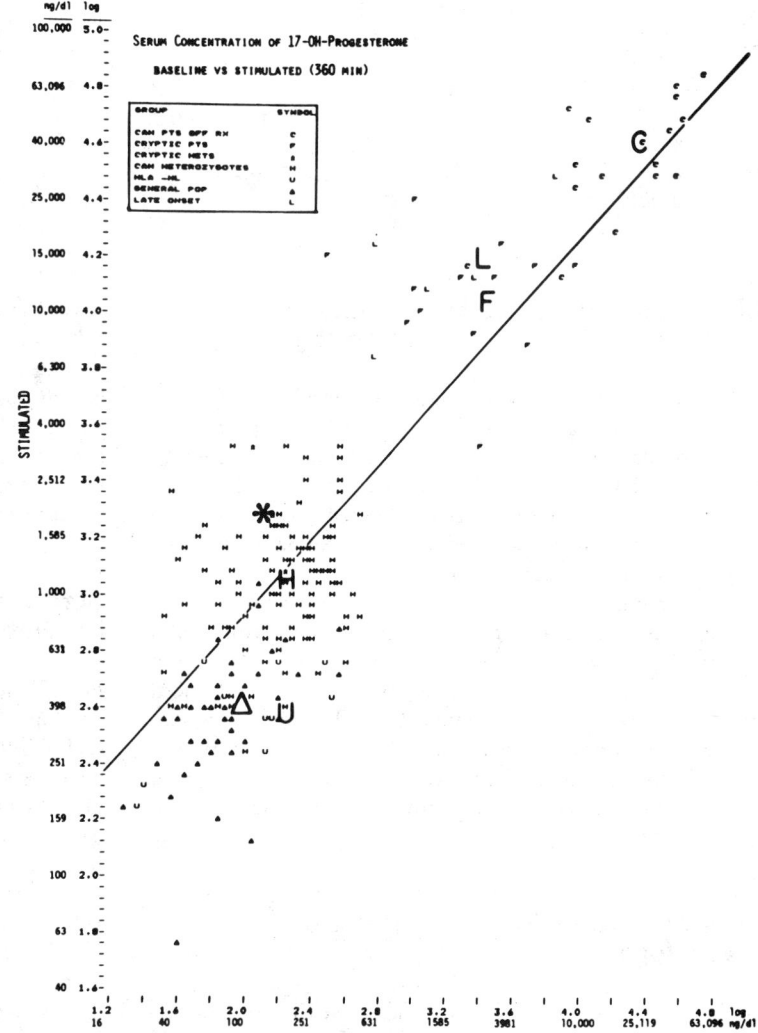

Figure 47-22 Nomogram relating baseline to ACTH stimulated serum 17-OHP concentration. Values for the log₁₀ and the antilog are indicated. The mean for each group is indicated by a large symbol. C = classic CAH patients off treatment; F = cryptic 21-hydroxylase deficiency patients; * = heterozygotes for cryptic 21-hydroxylase deficiency; H = heterozygotes for classic CAH; U = family members predicted by HLA genotyping to be genetically unaffected; Δ = general population; L = patients with late-onset 21-hydroxylase deficiency. The values for each group aggregate in descending order along the regression line. Note that the heterozygotes for the cryptic 21-hydroxylase defect are in the same range as the heterozygotes for the classical 21-hydroxylase defect.

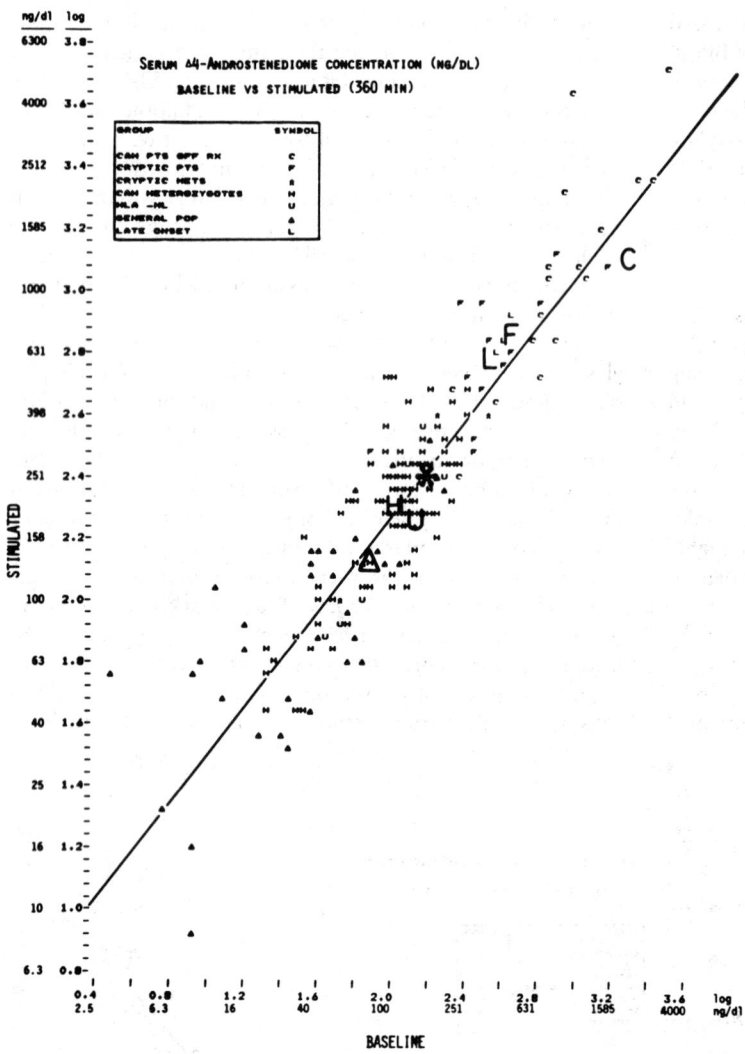

Figure 47-23 Nomogram relating baseline to the ACTH stimulated serum Δ⁴-androstenedione concentration. Values for the $\log_{10}$ and the antilog are indicated. The mean for each group is indicated by a large symbol. See legend to Fig. 47-22 for explanation of abbreviations. The values for each group aggregate in descending order along the regression line. Note that the values for the asymptomatic patients with cryptic 21-hydroxylase deficiency are in the same range as the symptomatic virilized females with late onset 21-hydroxylase deficiency.

Clinical Spectrum of 21-Hydroxylase Deficiency—Phenotypic Variability

It thus appears that 21-hydroxylase deficiency has a spectrum of clinical manifestations (Fig. 47-30), as well as a spectrum of enzymatic deficiencies, as reflected in the hormonal findings presented in Figs. 47-22 to 47-27. If 21-hydroxylase deficiency is similar to other autosomal recessive enzyme defects, we would predict that further studies will reveal patients whose clinical and biochemical abnormalities will be intermediate to those currently described. It may also be possible that the assignments by clinical criteria may change in the course of a lifetime. In one patient (Fig. 47-31), the symptoms of late-onset 21-hydroxylase deficiency, including pubic hair and advanced growth, were evident at 6 months of age. The symptoms subsequently disappeared but the biochemical abnormality persisted. Thus the clinical classification for this patient changed from late-onset to cryptic 21-hydroxylase deficiency within a span of 10 years.

HLA and Other Enzyme Defects of Steroidogenesis

Studies of families of patients with CAH due to 11β-hydroxylase deficiency [119] and 17α-hydroxylase deficiency [156]

have demonstrated that these enzyme defects are not genetically linked to HLA. In addition, hormonal studies have not provided a means for detecting heterozygote carriers for 11β-hydroxylase deficiency [157]. One study of corticosterone methyl oxidase, type II deficiency failed to demonstrate close genetic linkage with HLA, although a Lod score of 1.128 was reported and thus the possibility of genetic linkage could not be ruled out [158].

Screening for CAH and Future Population Studies

In 1977 neonatal screening for CAH became possible by the development of a microfilter paper method for measuring 17-OHP [159]. This method utilizes a heel stick blood specimen which is spotted onto filter paper and then analyzed for 17-OHP by radioimmunoassay. Results are shown in Fig. 47-32. The hormone is stable on filter paper and the filter paper specimens can be sent to an appropriate laboratory by surface mail.

Based on population surveys which indicate that the incidence of 21-hydroxylase deficiency is approximately 1:15,000 before screening (an incidence equal to that of phenylketonuria after screening), we and others have proposed that the newborn population also be screened for 21-hydroxylase deficiency [160]. Both classical and cryptic 21-hydroxylase deficiency have gone unrecognized in families in the general population [132, 150, 161].

The reliability and feasibility of the 17-OHP microfilter paper screening method has recently been proved by a pilot study screening all infants born in Alaska in a 19-month period [162]. A total of 11,177 consecutive newborns were screened on the third day of life. Of 644 newborn Yupik Eskimos screened, 2 were found to be affected with CAH and 1 of 7802 newborn Caucasians screened was affected (Table 47-3). All 3 affected patients had the salt-wasting form of CAH. Based on these data, a 95 percent confidence limit establishes a range for the incidence of salt-wasting CAH of between 1:892 to 1:2600 live births in Yupiks and 1:1400 to 1:31,000 live births in Caucasians (Table 47-3). The incidence of salt-wasting CAH in Yupiks agrees with the incidence previously predicted by case survey (1:292 to 1:896) in this population [114]. In Caucasians, the highest incidence of salt-wasting CAH allowed at the 95 percent confidence level based on screening data (1:1400) is far greater than the highest possible incidence predicted by case surveys (1:18,454 for salt-wasting CAH and 1:14,798 for salt-wasting and simple virilizing CAH combined) (Table 47-3). A larger screening sample size is needed to permit more definite conclusions about the frequency of the disorder. The false-positive and recall rates for the pilot screening program were 0.088 percent and 0.25 percent, respectively [162], figures that compare favorably with the rates in currently enacted screening programs for other disorders [163].

Figure 47-24 Nomogram relating baseline to ACTH stimulated serum testosterone concentration in females. Values for the log₁₀ and the antilog are indicated. The mean for each group is indicated by a large symbol. See legend to Fig. 47-22 for explanation of abbreviations. The values for each group aggregate in descending order along the regression line. Note that the values for the asymptomatic females with cryptic 21-hydroxylase deficiency are in the same range as the symptomatic virilized females with late-onset 21-hydroxylase deficiency.

PRENATAL DIAGNOSIS OF CAH

21-Hydroxylase Deficiency

Since the report by Jeffcoate et al. [164] of the prenatal diagnosis of CAH by elevated concentrations of 17-ketosteroids and pregnanetriol in the amniotic fluid of the affected fetus, several investigators have attempted the prenatal diagnosis by measurement of various hormones [165]. Most recently, elevated levels of 17-OHP [166–169] and Δ⁴-androstenedione [169] in the amniotic fluid of fetuses affected with CAH due to 21-hydroxylase deficiency have been reported.

HLA genotyping of amniotic cells has provided an additional method for prenatal diagnosis of 21-hydroxylase deficiency in a pregnancy at risk and has made possible the prediction of a heterozygous fetus [170]. When HLA genotyping of amniotic cells reveals that the fetus is HLA identical to the affected sib, the fetus is predicted to be affected. The HLA prediction of CAH genotype should always be corroborated by hormonal measurement of 17-OHP and Δ⁴-androstenedione in amniotic fluid. Caution must be exercised in interpreting results if multiple births are expected or if there is antigen sharing in the parents [170].

11β-Hydroxylase Deficiency

Recently, levels of 11-deoxycortisol and tetrahydrocortisol (THS) in amniotic fluid and THS in maternal urine have been found to be increased in pregnancies with fetuses affected with 11β-hydroxylase deficiency [171, 172]. This suggests that prenatal diagnosis of this disorder by hormonal measurement is feasible. Since this disorder is not genetically linked to HLA, HLA typing of amniotic cells is not helpful.

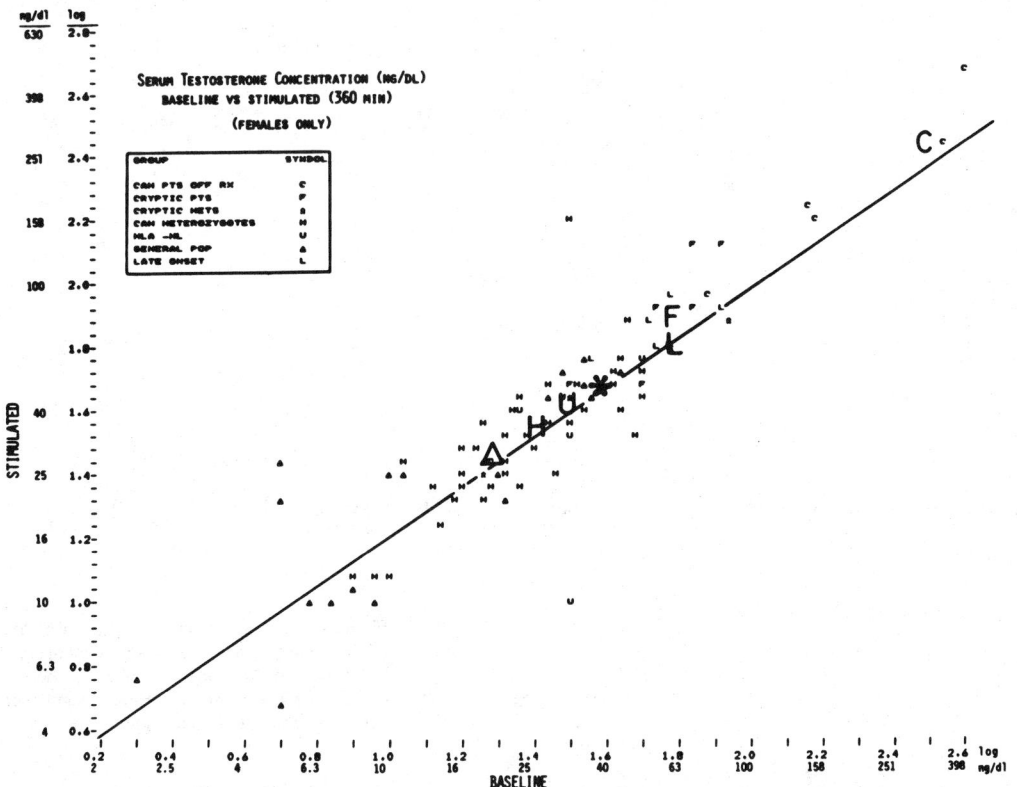

Table 47-3 Incidence of CAH

	Cases	Sample size	Estimated incidence	95th percentile confidence* limit of estimated rate	
				Lower	Upper
Yupik Eskimo (salt wasting)					
Alaska screening	2	644	1:322	1:89	−1:2661
Case survey[a]	14	6860	1:490	1:292	−1:896
Caucasian					
Alaska screening (salt waster only)	1	7802	1:7802	1:1400	−1:31,000
Case survey [b–f] (salt waster only)	106	2,343,895	1:22,112	1:18,454	−1:26,730
Case survey[b–d, f–i] (all 21-OH deficient)	215	3,619,891	1:16,836	1:14,798	−1:19,239

* Confidence level for extrapolation of a poisson variable.
[a] Hirschfeld and Fleshman [114]
[b] Muller et al. [111]
[c] Werder et al. [160]
[d] Rosenbloom AL, Smith DW: Congenital adrenal hyperplasia. *Lancet* 1:660, 1966.
[e] Qazi QH, Thompson MW: Incidence of salt-losing form of congenital adrenal virilizing hyperplasia. *Arch Dis Child* 47:302, 1972.
[f] Mauthe I, Laspe H, Knorr D: Zur Haufigkeit des kongenitalen adrenogenitalen Syndromes (AGS) München 1963–1972. *Klin Padiat* 189:172, 1980.
[g] Childs et al. [108]
[h] Prader A: Die Haufigkeit Des Kongenitalen Adrenogenitalen Syndroms. *Helv Paediat Acta* 13:426, 1958.
[i] Wilkins L: Adrenal disorders II. Congenital virilizing adrenal hyperplasia. *Arch Dis Child* 37:231, 1962.

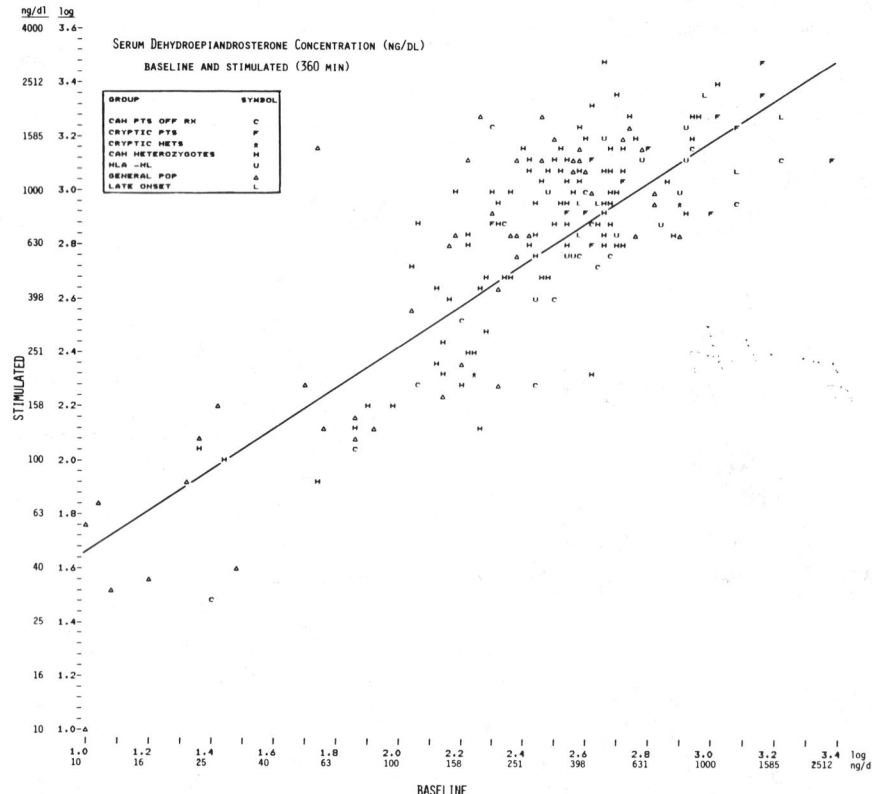

Figure 47-25 Nomogram relating baseline to ACTH stimulated serum DHEA concentration. Values for the log $_{10}$ and the antilog are indicated. Note that the serum DHEA concentration does not aggregate according to group.

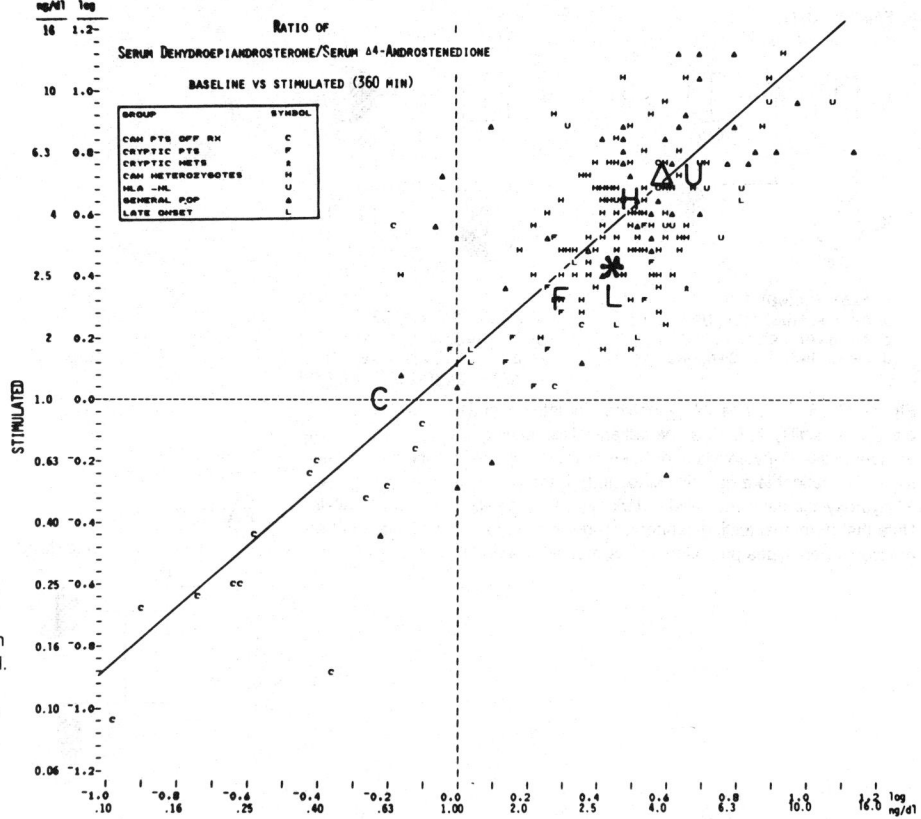

Figure 47-26 Nomogram relating baseline to ACTH stimulated ratio of serum DHEA/Δ⁴-androstenedione concentration. Values for log₁₀ and the antilog are indicated. The mean for each group is indicated by a large symbol. See legend to Fig. 47-22 for explanation of abbreviations. The values for each group aggregate in descending order along the regression line. Note that the ratio of DHEA/Δ4-androstenedione is lower in patients with CAH and that this group is easily distinguished from other groups by ratio.

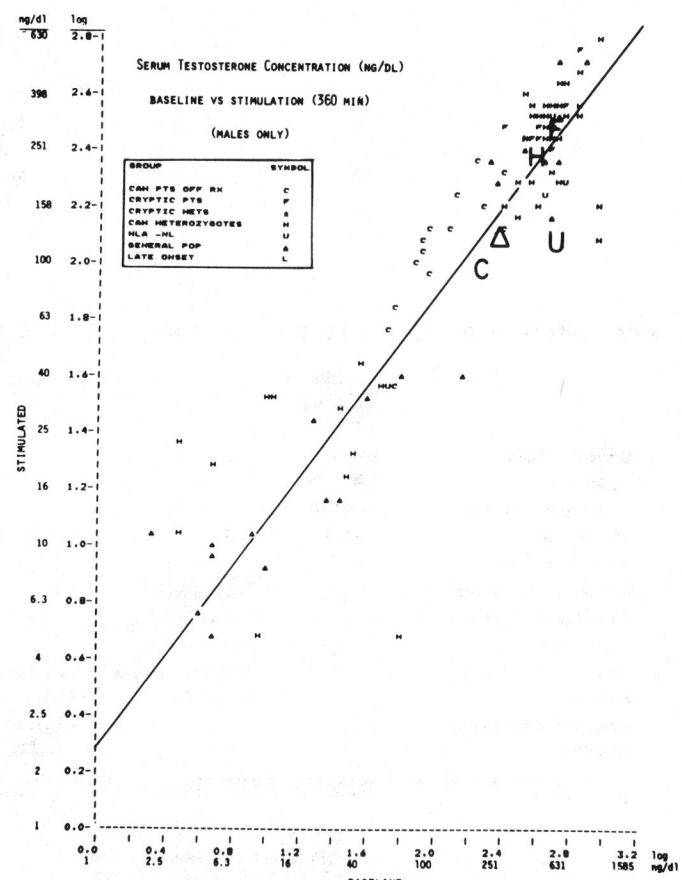

Figure 47-27 Nomogram relating baseline to the ACTH stimulated serum testosterone concentration in males. Values for the log₁₀ and the antilog are indicated. The mean for each group is indicated by a large symbol. See legend to Fig. 47-22 for explanation of abbreviations. Note that in males the serum testosterone does not distinguish the groups as it does in females.

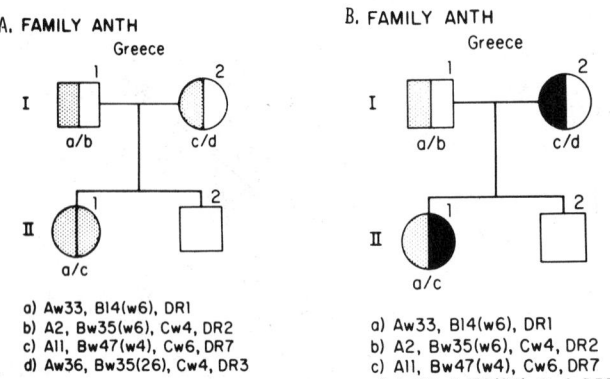

A. FAMILY ANTH
Greece

B. FAMILY ANTH
Greece

a) Aw33, B14(w6), DR1
b) A2, Bw35(w6), Cw4, DR2
c) A11, Bw47(w4), Cw6, DR7
d) Aw36, Bw35(26), Cw4, DR3

a) Aw33, B14(w6), DR1
b) A2, Bw35(w6), Cw4, DR2
c) A11, Bw47(w4), Cw6, DR7
d) Aw36, Bw35(26), Cw4, DR3

Figure 47-28   Two possible genotypes for late-onset 21-hydroxylase deficiency. Possibility A: Both of the patient's HLA haplotypes are linked to variant late-onset 21-hydroxylase deficiency alleles (spotted symbols). Possibility B: The patient is a genetic compound, possessing a Bw47-linked classic 21-hydroxylase deficiency allele (dark symbol) in addition to a variant allele. Note that hormonal testing cannot distinguish between the two different heterozygote genotypes proposed for the mother in A and B.

FAMILY DeW

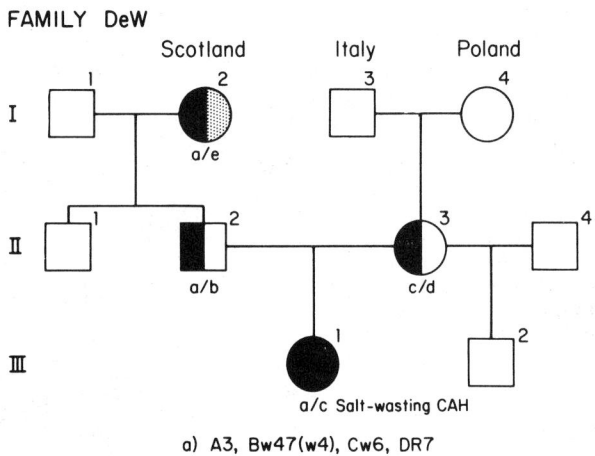

a) A3, Bw47(w4), Cw6, DR7
b) (A3), B7(w6)
c) A11, Bw35(w6), Cw4, DR5
d) A26, Bw22.1(w6), Cw3, DRw6.1
e) Aw24, B14(w6), DR1

Figure 47-29   Occurrence of classic and late-onset 21-hydroxylase deficiency in the same family. It is proposed that the grandmother (I-2) with late-onset 21-hydroxylase deficiency is a genetic compound, possessing both a Bw47-linked classic 21-hydroxylase deficiency allele and a B14-linked variant deficiency allele. See Fig. 47-28 for symbols.

CLINICAL SPECTRUM OF HLA-LINKED STEROID 21-HYDROXYLASE DEFICIENCY

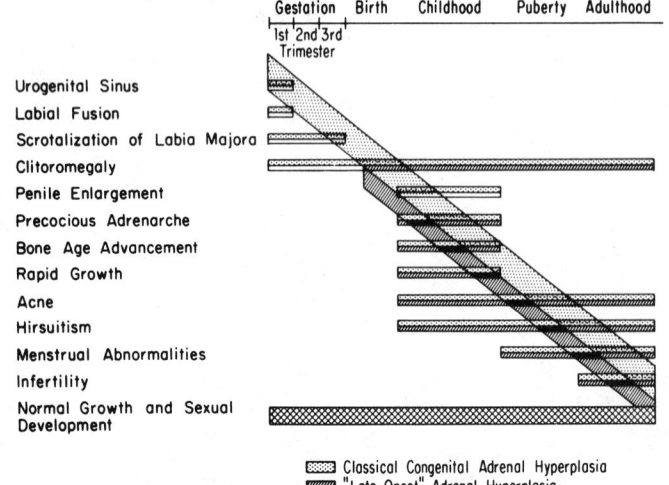

Classical Congenital Adrenal Hyperplasia
"Late-Onset" Adrenal Hyperplasia
Cryptic 21-Hydroxylase Deficiency

Figure 47-30   Clinical spectrum of 21-hydroxylase deficiency.

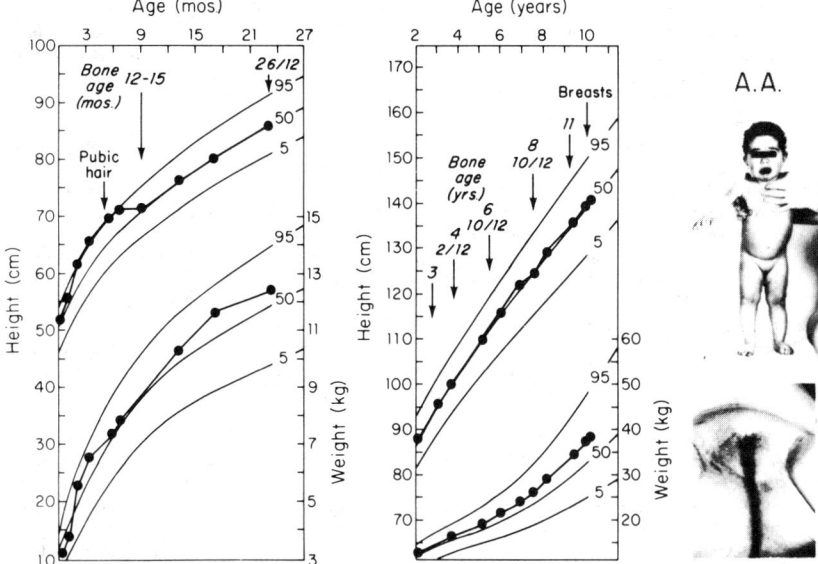

Figure 47-31 The changing clinical profile from late-onset to cryptic 21-hydroxylase deficiency. In this female, postnatal onset of virilization and growth acceleration was followed by a remittance of symptoms during childhood, despite persistence of hormonal abnormalities.

Figure 47-32 17α-OHP concentration in cord and capillary blood samples in infants with CAH. Ages of infants at diagnosis were as follows: ● = cord blood, △ = 2 days, □ = 4 days, ■ = 7 days, ▲ = 2 weeks, ○ = 4 weeks. Samples on treatment were taken from 5 days to 1 month after treatment was begun. The dashed line indicates upper limit of normal infants. The solid line indicates upper limit of pooled plasma in sick infants. Plasma samples were pipetted quantitatively and assayed. Cord blood samples were also quantitatively pipetted onto filter paper. Capillary samples were directly applied to filter paper without quantitation and a 3 mm disc punched out for analysis. (*From Pang et al. [159]. Used by permission.*)

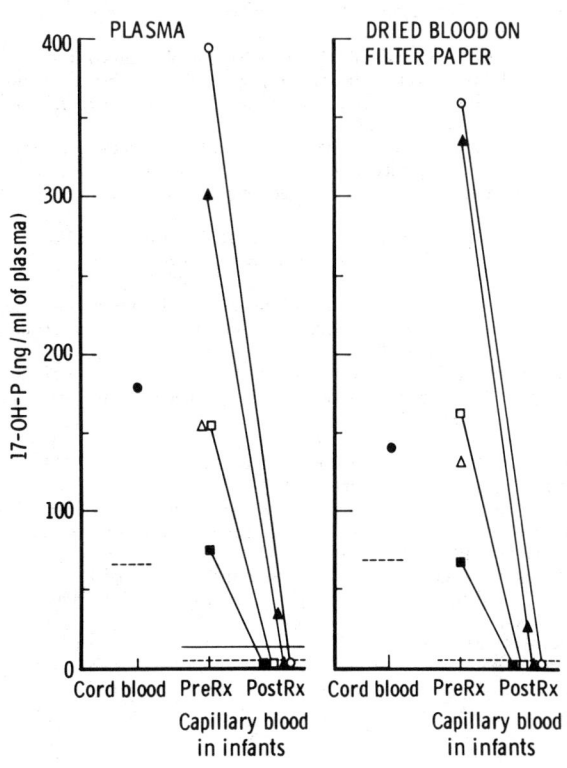

17-OH-PROGESTERONE CONCENTRATIONS OF CORD AND CAPILLARY BLOOD IN INFANTS

REFERENCES

1. DE CRECCHIO L: Sopra un caso di apparenze virile in una donna. *Morgagni* 7:1951, 1865
2. GARREN LD, GILL GN, MASUI H, WALTON GM: Mechanism of action of ACTH. *Rec Prog Horm Res* 27:433, 1971
3. HARDING BW: Synthesis of adrenal cortical steroids and mechanism of ACTH effects, in Degroot LJ, Cahill GF, Odell WD, Martini L, Potts JT, Jr. Nelson DH, Steinberger E, Winegrad AI (eds): *Endocrinology.* New York, Grune & Stratton, 1979, vol 2, p 1131
4. BONGIOVANNI AM, EBERLEIN WR, GOLDMAN AS, NEW MI: Disorders of adrenal steroid biogenesis. *Rec Prog Horm Res* 23:375, 1967
5. BONGIOVANNI AM: Congenital adrenal hyperplasia and related conditions, in Stanbury JB, Wyngaarden JB, Fredrickson DS (eds): *The Metabolic Basis of Inherited Disease.* 4th ed. New York, McGraw-Hill, 1978, p 868
6. FINKELSTEIN M, SHAEFER JM: Inborn errors of steroid biosynthesis. *Physiol Rev* 59:353, 1979
7. GAUNT R: Action of adrenal cortical steroids on electrolyte and water metabolism, in Christy NP (ed): *The Human Adrenal Cortex.* New York, Harper & Row, 1971, p 273
8. ULICK S, VETTER K: Simultaneous measurement of secretory rates of aldosterone and 18-hydroxycorticosterone. *J Clin Endocrinol Metab* 25:1015, 1965
9. ULICK S: Diagnosis and nomenclature of the disorders of the terminal portion of the aldosterone biosynthetic pathway. *J Clin Endocrinol Metab* 43:92, 1976
10. HARKINS JB, NELSON EB, MASTERS BSS, BRYAN GT: Preparation and properties of microsomal membranes from cells of beef adrenal cortex. *Endocrinology* 94:897, 1974
11. SIITERI PK, WILSON JD: Testosterone formation and metabolism during male sexual differentiation in the human embryo. *J Clin Endocrinol Metab* 38:113, 1974
12. PETERSON RE, IMPERATO-MCGINLEY J, GAUTIER T, STARLA E: Male pseudohermaphroditism due to steroid 5α-reductase deficiency. *Am J Med* 62:170, 1977
13. GANONG WF, ALPERT LC, LEE TC: ACTH and the regulation of adrenocortical secretion. *N Engl J Med* 290:1006, 1974
14. GANONG WF: Neurotransmitters and pituitary function: regulation of ACTH secretion. *Fed Proc* 39:2923, 1980
15. LARAGH JH, SEALEY JE: The renin-angiotensin-aldosterone hormonal system and regulation of sodium, potassium, and blood pressure homeostasis, in Orloff J, Berliner RW (eds): *Handbook of Physiology—Renal Physiology.* Baltimore, Maryland, Waverly Press, 1973, p 831
16. KOTCHEN TA, GUTHRIE GP: Renin-angiotensin-aldosterone and hypertension. *End Rev* 1:78, 1980

17. NEW MI, SEAMAN MP: Secretion rates of cortisol and aldosterone precursors in various forms of congenital adrenal hyperplasia. *J Clin Endocrinol Metab* 30:361, 1970

18. GANONG WF, BIGLIERI EG, MULROW PJ: Mechanisms regulating adrenocortical secretion of aldosterone and glucocorticoids. *Rec Prog Horm Res* 22:381, 1966

19. MASON PA, FRASER R, SEMPLE PF, MORTON JJ: The interaction of ACTH and angiotensin II in the control of corticosteroid plasma concentration in man. *J Steroid Biochem* 10:235, 1979

20. JOST A: Embryonic sexual differentiation, in Jones HW, Scott WW (eds): *Hermaphroditism, Genital Anomalies and Related Endocrine Disorders.* 2d ed. Baltimore, William & Wilkins, 1971, p 16

21. JOSSO N, PICARD JY, TRAN D: The antiMullerian hormone. *Rec Prog Horm Res* 33:117, 1977

22. FEDERMAN DD: *Abnormal Sexual Development.* Philadelphia, WB Saunders, 1968

23. GRUMBACH MM, VAN WYK JJ: Disorders of sex differentiation, in Williams RH (ed): *Textbook of Endocrinology.* 5th ed. Philadelphia, WB Saunders, 1974, p 423

24. VIRDIS R, SAENGER P, SENIOR B, NEW MI: Endocrine studies in a pubertal male pseudohermaphrodite with 17-ketosteroid reductase deficiency. *Acta Endocrinol* 87:212, 1978

25. SYDNOR KL, KELLEY VC, RAILE RB, ELY RS, SAYERS G: Blood adrenocorticotrophin in children with congenital adrenal hyperplasia. *Proc Soc Exp Biol Med* 82:695, 1953

26. BINOUX M, PHAM-HUU-TRUNC MT, GOURMELEN M, GIRARD F, CANLOBRE P: Plasma ACTH in adrenogenital syndrome. *Acta Pediatr Scand* 61:269, 1972

27. BONGIOVANNI AM, EBERLEIN WR, CARA J: Studies on metabolism of adrenal steroids in adrenogenital syndrome. *J Clin Endocrinol Metab* 14:409, 1954

28. BUTLER GC, MARRIAN GF: Isolation of pregnane-3,17,20-triol from urine of women showing adrenogenital syndrome. *J Biol Chem* 119:565, 1937

29. HUGHES IA, WINTER JSD: The application of a serum 17OH-progesterone radioimmunoassay to the diagnosis and management of congenital adrenal hyperplasia. *J Pediatr* 88:766, 1976

30. PANG S, LEVINE LS, CHOW D, FAIMAN C, NEW MI: Serum androgen concentrations in neonates and young infants with virilizing congenital adrenal hyperplasia (VCAH). *Clin Endocrinol* 11:575, 1979

31. WILKINS L: Adrenal disorders. II. Congenital virilizing adrenal hyperplasia. *Arch Dis Child* 37:231, 1962

32. BLOCH E: Fetal adrenal cortex: function and steroidogenesis, in McKerns KW (ed): *Functions of the Adrenal Cortex.* New York, Appleton-Century-Crofts, 1968, vol 2, p 721

33. VILLEE DB: Changes in fetal steroid metabolism with age. *Clin Pharmacol Ther* 14:705, 1973

34. WILSON JD, WALSH PC: Disorders of sexual differentiation, in Harrison JH, Gittes RF, Perlmutter AD, Stamey TA, Walsh PC (eds): *Campbell's Urology.* 4th ed. Philadelphia, WB Saunders, 1979, vol 2, 1979, p 1484

35. WOLFF PB, WILBOIS RP, WELDON VV, HAYMOND MW: Posterior fusion without clitoromegaly in a female with partial 21-hydroxylase deficiency. *J Pediatr* 91:951, 1977

36. BERSON SA, YALOW RS: Radioimmunoassay of ACTH in plasma. *J Clin Invest* 47:2725, 1968

37. PERERA GA, KNOWLTON AI, LOWELL A, LOEB RF: Effect of deoxycorticosterone acetate on the blood pressure of man. *J Am Med Assoc* 125:1030, 1944

38. BROWN RD, STROTT CA: Plasma deoxycorticosterone in man. *J Clin Endocrinol Metab* 32:744, 1971

39. EBERLEIN WR, BONGIOVANNI AM: Plasma and urinary corticosteroids in the hypertensive form of congenital adrenal hyperplasia. *J Biol Chem* 223:85, 1956

40. LEVINE LS, RAUH W, GOTTESDIENER K, CHOW D, GUNCZLER P, RAPAPORT R, PANG S, SCHNEIDER B, NEW MI: New studies of the 11 β-hydroxylase and 18-hydroxylase enzymes in the hypertensive form of congenital adrenal hyperplasia. *J Clin Endocrinol Metab* 50:258, 1980

41. BONGIOVANNI AM: The adrenogenital syndrome with deficiency of 3β-hydroxysteroid dehydrogenase. *J Clin Invest* 41:2086, 1962

42. PARKS GA, BERMUDEZ JA, ANAST CS, BONGIOVANNI AM, NEW MI: Pubertal boy with 3β-hydroxysteroid dehydrogenase defect. *J Clin Endocrinol Metab* 33:269, 1971

43. BONGIOVANNI AM: Urinary steroidal pattern of infants with congenital adrenal hyperplasia due to 3β-hydroxysteroid dehydrogenase deficiency. *J Steroid Biochem* 13:809, 1980

44. SCHNEIDER G, GENEL M, BONGIOVANNI AM, GOLDMAN AS, ROSENFELD RL: Persistent testicular Δ⁵-isomerase-3β-hydroxysteroid dehydrogenase (Δ⁵-3β-HSD) deficiency in the Δ⁵-3β-HSD form of congenital adrenal hyperplasia. *J Clin Invest* 55:681, 1975

45. BIGLIERI EG, HERRON MA, BRUST N: 17α-Hydroxylation deficiency in man. *J Clin Invest* 45:1946, 1966

46. NEW MI: Male pseudohermaphroditism due to 17α-hydroxylase deficiency. *J Clin Invest* 49:1930, 1970

47. MANTERO F, BUSNARDO B, RIONDEL A, VEYRAT R, AUSTONI M: Hypertension artérielle, alcalose hypokaliémique et pseudohermaphrodisme mâle par déficit en 17α-hydroxylase. *Schweiz Med Wochenschr* 101:38, 1971

48. MADAN K, SCHOEMAKER J: XY females with enzyme deficiencies of steroid metabolism: a brief review. *Hum Genet* 53:291, 1980

49. PRADER A, GURTNER HP: Das Syndrom des Pseudohermaphroditismus masculinus bei Kongenitaler Nebennierenrinden Hyperplasie ohne Androgen-Uberproduktion. *Helv Pediatr Acta* 10:397, 1955

50. CAMACHO AM, KOWARSKI A, MIGEON CJ, BROUGH AJ: Congenital adrenal hyperplasia due to a deficiency of one of the enzymes involved in the biosynthesis of pregnenolone. *J Clin Endocrinol Metab* 28:153, 1968

51. KIRKLAND RT, KIRKLAND JL, JOHNSON C, HORNING M, LIBRICK L, CLAYTON GW: Congenital lipoid adrenal hyperplasia in an eight-year-old phenotypic female. *J Clin Endocrinol Metab* 36:488, 1973

52. HOCHBERG RB, McDONALD PD, FELDMAN M, LIEBERMAN S: Studies on the biosynthetic conversion of cholesterol into pregnenolone. *J Biol Chem* 249:1277, 1974

53. DEGENHART HJ: A study of the cholesterol splitting enzyme system in normal adrenal and in adrenal lipoid hyperplasia. *Acta Paediatr Scand* 60:611, 1971

54. VISSER HKA, COST WS: A new hereditary defect in the biosynthesis of aldosterone: urinary C21-corticosteroid pattern in three related patients with a salt-losing syndrome, suggesting an 18-oxidation defect. *Acta Endocrinol* 47:589, 1964

55. DEGENHART HJ, FRANKENA L, VISSER HKA, COST WS, VAN SETERS AP: Further investigation of a new hereditary defect in the biosynthesis of aldosterone. Evidence for a defect in 18-hydroxylation of corticosterone. *Acta Physiol Pharmacol Neerl* 14:88, 1966

56. JEAN R, LEGRAND JC, MEYLAN F, RIEU D, ASTRUC J: Hypoaldosteronisme primaire par anomalie probable de la 18-hydroxylation. *Arch Franc Pediatr* 26:769, 1969

57. ULICK S, GAUTIER E, VETTER KK, MARKELLO JR, YAFFE S, LOWE CU: An aldosterone biosynthetic defect in a salt-losing disorder. *J Clin Endocrinol Metab* 24:669, 1964

58. VELDHUIS JD, KULIN HE, SANTEN RJ, WILSON TE, MELBY JC: Inborn error in the terminal step of aldosterone biosynthesis. *N Engl J Med* 303:117, 1980

59. ROSLER A, RABINOWITZ D, THEODOR R, RAMIREZ L, ULICK S: The nature of the defect in a salt-wasting disorder in Jews of Iran. *J Clin Endocrinol Metab* 44:279, 1977

60. SAEZ JM, DE PERETTI E, MORERA AM, DAVID M, BERTRAND J: Familial male pseudohermaphroditism with gynecomastia due to a testicular 17-ketosteroid reductase defect. I: studies in vivo. *J Clin Endocrinol Metab* 32:604, 1971

61. GOEBELSMANN U, HORTON R, MESTMAN JH, ARCE JJ, NAGATA Y, NAKAMURA RM, THORNEYCROFT IH, MISHELL DR: Male pseudohermaphroditism due to testicular 17β-hydroxysteroid dehydrogenase deficiency. *J Clin Endocrinol Metab* 36:867, 1973

62. GIVENS JR, WISER WL, SUMMITT RL, KERBER IJ, ANDERSEN RN, PITTAWAY DE, FISH SA: Familial male pseudohermaphroditism without gynecomastia due to deficient testicular 17-ketosteroid reductase activity. *N Engl J Med* 291:938, 1974

63. KNORR D, BIDLINGMAIER F, ENGELHARDT D: Reifenstein's syndrome, a 17β-hydroxysteroid-oxydoreductase deficiency? *Acta Endocrinol (Kbh),* suppl 173:37, 1973

64. LEVINE LS, LIEBER E, PANG S, NEW MI: Male pseudohermaphroditism due to 17-ketosteroid reductase deficiency diagnosed in the newborn period. *Pediatr Res* 14:480, 1980

65. ZACHMANN M, VOLLMIN JA, HAMILTON W, PRADER A: Steroid 17, 20-desmolase deficiency: a new cause of male pseudohermaphroditism. *Clin Endocrinol* 1:369, 1972

66. GOEBELSMANN U, ZACHMANN M, DAVAJAN V, ISRAEL R, MESTMAN JH, MISHELL DR: Male pseudohermaphroditism consistent with 17-20 desmolase deficiency. *Gynecol Invest* 7:138, 1976

67. FOREST MG, LECORNU M, DE PERETTI E: Familial male pseudohermaphroditism due to 17-20-desmolase deficiency, I. In vivo endocrine studies. *J Clin Endocrinol Metab* 50:826, 1980

68. GREGORY T, GARDNER LI: Hypertensive virilizing adrenal hyperplasia with minimal impairment of synthetic route to cortisol. *J Clin Endocrinol Metab* 43:769, 1976

69. ZACHMANN M, VOLLMIN JA, NEW MI, CURTIUS HCH, PRADER A: Congenital adrenal hyperplasia due to deficiency of 11β-hydroxylation of 17α-hydroxylated steroids. *J Clin Endocrinol Metab* 33:501, 1971

70. Sizonenko PC, Riondel AM, Kohlberg IJ, Paunier L: 11β-Hydroxylase deficiency: steroid response to sodium restriction and ACTH stimulation. *J Clin Endocrinol Metab* 35:281, 1972

71. Tan SY, Noth RH, Mulrow PJ: Deoxycorticosterone and 17-ketosteroids; elevated levels in adult hypertensive patients. *J Am Med Assoc* 240:123, 1978

72. Ulick S: Adrenocortical factors in hypertension, I. Significance of 18-hydroxy-11-deoxycorticosterone. *Am J Cardiol* 38:814, 1976

73. Molteni A, Skelton FR, Brownie AC: Effect of adrenalectomy on the development of androgen-induced hypertension. *Lab Invest* 23:429, 1970

74. McCall AL, Stern J, Dale SI, Melby JC: Adrenal steroidogenesis in methylandrostenediol-induced hypertension. *Endocrinology* 103:1, 1978

75. Bongiovanni AM, Eberlein WR: Adrenogenital syndrome: uncomplicated and hypertensive forms. *Pediatrics* 21:661, 1958

76. New MI, Dupont B, Pang S, Pollack M, Levine LS: An update of congenital adrenal hyperplasia. *Rec Prog Horm Res* 37:105, 1981

77. Blizzard RM, Liddle GW, Migeon CJ, Wilkins L: Aldosterone excretion in virilizing adrenal hyperplasia. *J Clin Invest* 38:1442, 1959

78. Kowarski A, Finklestein JW, Spaulding JS, Holman GH, Migeon CJ: Aldosterone secretion rate in congenital adrenal hyperplasia. A discussion of the theories on the pathogenesis of the salt losing form of the syndrome. *J Clin Invest* 44:1505, 1965

79. Rosler A, Levine LS, Schneider B, Novogroder M, New MI: The interrelationship of sodium balance, plasma renin activity and ACTH in congenital adrenal hyperplasia. *J Clin Endocrinol Metab* 45:500, 1977

80. Bryan GT, Kliman B, Bartter FC: Impaired aldosterone production in "salt-losing" congenital adrenal hyperplasia. *J Clin Invest* 44:957, 1965

81. Degenhart HG, Visser HKA, Wilmink R, Croughs W: Aldosterone and cortisol secretion rates in infants and children with congenital adrenal hyperplasia suggesting different 21-hydroxylation defects in "salt-losers" and "non-salt-losers." *Acta Endocrinol (Kbh)* 48:587, 1965

82. New MI, Miller B, Peterson RE: Aldosterone secretion in normal children and in children with adrenal hyperplasia. *J Clin Invest* 45:412, 1966

83. Bartter FC, Henkin RI, Bryan GT: Aldosterone hypersecretion in "non-salt-losing" congenital adrenal hyperplasia. *J Clin Invest* 47:1742, 1968

84. Simopoulos AP, Marshall JR, Delea CS, Bartter FC: Studies on the deficiency of 21-hydroxylation in patients with congenital adrenal hyperplasia. *J Clin Endocrinol Metab* 32:438, 1971

85. West CD, Atcheson JB, Stanchfield JB, Rallison ML, Chavre VJ, Tyler FH: Multiple or single 21-hydroxylases in congenital adrenal hyperplasia? *J Steroid Biochem* 11:1413, 1979

86. Kuhnle U, Chow D, Rapaport R, Pang S, Levine LS, New MI: The 21-hydroxylase activity in the glomerulosa and fasciculata of the adrenal cortex in congenital adrenal hyperplasia. *J Clin Endocrinol Metab* 52:534, 1981

87. Biglieri EG: Mechanisms establishing the mineralocorticoid hormone patterns in the 17α-hydroxylase deficiency syndrome. *J Steroid Biochem* 11:653, 1979

88. Biglieri EG, Chang B, Hirai J, Brust N, Rost CR, Schambelan M: Adrenocorticotropin inhibition of mineralocorticoid hormone production. *Clin Sci* 57:307, 1979

89. Sharma DC, Forchielli E, Dorfmann RJ: Inhibition of enzymatic steroid 11β-hydroxylation by androgens. *J Biol Chem* 238:572, 1963

90. Schambelan M, Rost GR, Sebastian A, Biglieri EG: Influence of the renin-angiotensin system (RAS), potassium (K) and ACTH on plasma levels of 18-hydroxycorticosterone (18-OHB) and aldosterone (A) in man. *Program and Abstracts, VI International Congress of Endocrinology*, Melbourne, 1980, p 241

91. Edwin C, Lanes R, Migeon CJ, Lee PA, Plotnick LP, Kowarski AA: Persistence of the enzymatic block in adolescent patients with salt-losing congenital adrenal hyperplasia. *J Pediatr* 95:534, 1979

92. Klein R: Evidence for and against the existence of a salt-losing hormone. *J Pediatr* 57:452, 1960

93. Prader A, Spahr A, Neher R: Erhoehte aldosteronausscheidung bein kongenitalen adrenogenitalen syndrom. *Schweiz Med Wochenschr* 85:45, 1955

94. Loras B, Haour F, Bertrand J: Exchangeable sodium and aldosterone secretion in children with congenital adrenal hyperplasia due to 21-hydroxylase deficiency. *Pediatr Res* 4:145, 1970

95. Schaison G, Couzinaet B, Gourmelen M, Elkik F, Bougneres P: Aggiotensin and adrenal steroidogenesis: Study of 21-hydroxylase-deficient congenital adrenal hyperplasia. *J Clin Endocrinol Metab* 51:1390, 1980

96. Kuhnle U, Land M, Marver D, New MI, Ulick S: Evidence for the secretion of a mineralocorticoid antagonist in congenital adrenal hyperplasia. *Program and Abstracts, Annual Meeting of the Endocrine Society*, Cincinnati, 1981

97. Wilkins L, Lewis, RA, Klein R, Rosemberg: The suppression of antigen secretion by cortisone in a case of congenital adrenal hyperplasia. *Bull. John Hopkins Hospital* 86:249–256

98. Bartter FC: Adrenogenital syndromes from physiology to chemistry (1950–1975), in Lee PA, Plotnick LP, Kowarski AA, Migeon CJ (eds): *Congenital Adrenal Hyperplasia*. Baltimore, University Park Press, 1977, p 9

99. Dillon MJ: Plasma renin activity and aldosterone concentrations in children: results in salt wasting states. *Arch Dis Child* 50:330, 1975

100. Godard C, Riondel AM, Veyrat R, Megevand A, Muller AF: Plasma renin activity and aldosterone in congenital adrenal hyperplasia. *Pediatrics* 41:883, 1968.

101. Strickland AL, Kotchen TA: A study of the renin-aldosterone system in congenital adrenal hyperplasia. *J Pediatr* 81:962, 1972

102. Kuhnle U, Pareira JA, Gunczler P, Rosler R, Levine LS, New MI: Effect of normalization of plasma renin activity on linear growth and pubertal development in various forms of aldosterone deficiency. *J Clin Endocrinol Metab* (Submitted for publication) 1982

103. Winter JSD: Current approaches to the treatment of congenital adrenal hyperplasia. *J Pediatr* 97:81, 1980

104. Korth-Schutz S, Virdis R, Saenger P, Chow DM, Levine LS, New MI: Serum androgens as a continuing index of adequacy of treatment of congenital adrenal hyperplasia. *J Clin Endocrinol Metab* 46:452, 1978

105. Golden MP, Lippe BM, Kaplan SA, Lavin N, Slavin J: Management of congenital adrenal hyperplasia using serum dehydroepiandrosterone sulfate and 17-hydroxyprogesterone concentrations. *Pediatrics* 61:67, 1978

106. Jones HW, Scott WW: *Hermaphroditism, genital anomalies and related endocrine disorders*. 2d ed. Baltimore, Williams & Wilkins, 1971

107. Prader A: Volkommen maenliche aussere Genitalentwicklung und Salzverlust-Syndrom bei Maedchen mit kongenitalen adrenogenitalem Syndrom. *Helv Paediatr Acta* 13:426, 1958

108. Childs B, Grumbach MM, Van Wyk JJ: Virilizing adrenal hyperplasia: a genetic and hormonal study. *J Clin Invest* 35:213, 1956

109. Baulieu EE, Peillon F, Migeon CJ: Adrenogenital syndrome, in Eisenstein AB (ed): *The Adrenal Cortex*. Boston, Little, Brown, 1967, p 553

110. Rosenbloom AL, Smith DW: Varying expression in salt losing in related patients with congenital adrenal hyperplasia. *Pediatrics* 38:215, 1966

111. Muller W, Prader A, Kofler J, Glatzl J, Geir W: Frequency of congenital adrenal hyperplasia. *Paediatr Paedol* 14:151, 1979

112. Cohen JM: Salt-losing congenital adrenal hyperplasia. *Pediatrics* 44:621, 1969

113. Rimoin DL, Schimke RN: *Genetic Disorders of the Endocrine Glands*. St. Louis, Mosby, 1971

114. Hirschfeld AG, Fleshman JK: An unusually high incidence of congenital adrenal hyperplasia in the Alaskan Eskimo. *J Pediatr* 75:492, 1969

115. Passarge E, Valentine-Thon E: Everything the pediatrician ever wanted to know about HLA but was afraid to ask. *Eur J Pediatr* 133:93, 1980

116. Farid NR, Bear JC: The human major histocompatibility complex and endocrine disease. *Endocrine Rev* 2:50, 1981

117. Dupont B, Oberfield SE, Smithwick EM, Lee TD, Levine LS: Close genetic linkage between HLA and congenital adrenal hyperplasia (21-hydroxylase deficiency). *Lancet* 2:1309, 1977

118. Levine LS, Zachmann M, New MI, Prader A, Pollack MS, O'Neill GJ, Yang SY, Oberfield SE, Dupont B: Genetic mapping of the 21-hydroxylase deficiency gene within the HLA linkage group. *N Engl J Med* 299:911, 1978

119. Dupont B, Pollack MS, Levine LS, O'Neill GJ, Hawkins B, New MI: Congenital adrenal hyperplasia and HLA: Joint report from the Eighth International Histocompatibility Workshop, in Terasaki, PI (ed): *Histocompatibility Testing 1980*. Los Angeles, UCLA Tissue Typing Laboratory, 1980, p 693

120. Cleveland WW, Nikezic M, Migeon CJ: Response to an 11β-hydroxylase inhibitor (SU-4885) in males with adrenal hyperplasia and in their parents. *J Clin Endocrinol Metab* 22:281, 1962

121. Hall R, Smith PA, Harkness RA, Smart GA: A study of the parents of patients with congenital adrenal hyperplasia: detection of the heterozygote. *Proc Roy Soc Med* 63:1040, 1970

122. Qazi QH, Hill JG, Thompson MW: Steroid studies in parents of patients with congenital virilizing adrenal hyperplasia. *J Clin Endocrinol Metab* 33:23, 1971

123. Lee PA, Gareis FJ: Evidence for partial 21-hydroxylase deficiency among heterozygote carriers for congenital adrenal hyperplasia. *J Clin Endocrinol Metab* 41:415, 1975

124. Gutai JP, Kowarski AA, Migeon CJ: The detection of the heterozygous carrier for congenital virilizing adrenal hyperplasia. *J Pediatr* 90:924, 1977

125. Krensky AM, Bongiovanni AM, Marino J, Parks J, Tenore A: Identification of heterozygote carriers of congenital adrenal hyperplasia by radioimmunoassay of serum 17-OH progesterone. *J Pediatr* 90:930, 1977

126. HOMOKI J, FAZEKAS ATA, TELLER WM: Urinary excretion of pregnane-triolone in parents of children with 21-hydroxylase deficiency: plasma 17α-hydroxyprogesterone in patients' relatives, in Lee PA, Plotnick LP, Kowarski AA, Migeon CJ (eds): *Congenital Adrenal Hyperplasia*. Baltimore, University Park Press, 1977, p 487

127. KNORR D, BIDLINGMAIER F, BUTENANDT O, SCHNAKENBURG KV, WAGNER W: Test for heterozygosity of congenital adrenal hyperplasia, in Lee PA, Plotnick LP, Kowarski AA, Migeon CJ (eds): *Congenital Adrenal Hyperplasia*, Baltimore, University Park Press, 1977, p 495

128. GUTAI JP, KOWARSKI A, MIGEON CJ: The detection of the heterozygous carrier for congenital virilizing adrenal hyperplasia. *J Pediatr* 90:924, 1977

129. GUTAI JP, LEE PA, JOHNSONBAUGH RE, GAREIS F, URBAN M, MIGEON CJ: Detection of the heterozygous state in siblings of patients with congenital adrenal hyperplasia due to 21-hydroxylase deficiency. *J Pediatr* 94:770, 1979

130. CHILD DF, BU'LOCK DE, ANDERSON DC: Adrenal steroidogenesis in heterozygotes for 21-hydroxylase deficiency. *Clin Endocrinol* 11:391, 1979

131. CASSORLA F, TENORE A, PARKS JS, MARINO J, BONGIOVANNI AM: Serum 21-deoxycortisol and 17-hydroxypregnenolone in parents of patients with congenital adrenal hyperplasia. *J Endocrinol Invest* 3:137, 1980

132. LORENZEN F, PANG S, NEW MI, DUPONT B, POLLACK MS, CHOW D, LEVINE LS: Hormonal phenotype and HLA-genotype in families of patients with congenital adrenal hyperplasia (21-hydroxylase deficiency). *Pediatr Res* 13:1356, 1979

133. LORENZEN F, PANG S, NEW MI, POLLACK MS, OBERFIELD S, DUPONT B, CHOW D, LEVINE LS: Studies of the C-21 and C-19 steroids and HLA genotyping in siblings and parents of patients with congenital adrenal hyperplasia due to 21-hydroxylase deficiency. *J Clin Endocrinol Metab* 50:572, 1980

134. GROSSE-WILDE HJ, WEIL J, SCHOLZ S, ALBERT E, BIDLINGMAIER F, KNORR D: Linkage studies between HLA-A, B, D alleles and congenital adrenal hyperplasia (CAH). *Pediatr Res* 12:1088, 1978

135. GROSSE-WILDE HJ, WEIL J, ALBERT E, SCHOLZ S, BIDLINGMAIER F, SIPPEL WG, KNORR D: Genetic linkage studies between congenital adrenal hyperplasia and the HLA blood group system. *Immunogenetics* 8:41, 1979

136. MAUSETH RS, HANSEN JA, SMITH EK, GIBLETT ER, KELLEY VC: Detection of heterozygotes for congenital adrenal hyperplasia: 21-hydroxylase deficiency—a comparison of HLA typing and 17-OH progesterone response to ACTH infusion. *J Pediatr* 97:749, 1980

137. SOBEL DO, GUTAI JP, JONES JC, WAGENER DK, SMITH W: Detection of heterozygote of 21-hydroxylase deficiency. *Lancet* 1:47, 1980

138. WEIL J, BIDLINGMAIER F, SIPPELL WG, BUTENANDT O, KNORR D: Comparison of two tests for heterozygosity in congenital adrenal hyperplasia (CAH). *Acta Endocrinol* 91:109, 1979

139. LEJEUNE-LENAIN C, CANTRAINE F, DUFRASNES M, PREVOLT F, WOLTER R, FRANCKSON JRM: An improved method for the detection of heterozygosity of congenital virilizing adrenal hyperplasia. *Clin Endocrinol* 42:575, 1980

140. NEWMARK S, DLUHY R, WILLIAMS G, POCHI P, ROSE L: Partial 11 and 21 hydroxylase deficiencies in hirsute women. *Am J Obstet Gynecol* 127:594, 1977

141. DECOURT MJ, JAYLE MF, BAULIEU E: Virilisme cliniquement tardif avec excrétion de prégnanetriol et insuffisance de la production du cortisol. *Ann Endocrinol* 18:416, 1957

142. BOUCHARD P, KUTTENN F, MOWSZOWICZ I, SCHAISON G, RAUX-EURIN M-C, MAUVAIS-JARVIS P: Congenital adrenal hyperplasia due to partial 21-hydroxylase deficiency. A study of five cases. *Acta Endocrinol* 96:107, 1981

143. ROSENWAKS Z, LEE PA, JONES GS, MIGEON CJ, WENTZ AC: An attenuated form of congenital virilizing adrenal hyperplasia. *J Clin Endocrinol Metab* 49:335, 1979

144. NEW MI, LORENZEN F, PANG S, GUNCZLER P, DUPONT B, POLLACK M, LEVINE LS: "Acquired" adrenal hyperplasia with 21-hydroxylase deficiency is not the same genetic disorder as congenital adrenal hyperplasia. *J Clin Endocrinol Metab* 48:52, 1979

145. MORILLO E, GARDNER LI: Genetics of acquired and congenital adrenal hyperplasia. *Lancet* 2:202, 1979

146. LARON Z, POLLACK MS, ZAMIR R, ROITMAN A, DICKERMAN Z, LEVINE LS, LORENZEN F, O'NEILL GJ, PANG S, NEW MI, DUPONT B: Late onset 21-hydroxylase deficiency and HLA in the Ashkenazi population: a new allele at the 21-hydroxylase locus. *Hum Immunol* 1:55, 1980

147. BLANKSTEIN J, FAIMAN C, REYES FI, SCHROEDER ML, WINTER JSD: Adult-onset familial adrenal 21-hydroxylase deficiency. *Am J Med* 68:441, 1980

148. MIGEON CJ, ROSENWAKS Z, LEE PA, URBAN MD, BIAS WB: The attenuated form of congenital adrenal hyperplasia as an allelic form of 21-hydroxylase deficiency. *J Clin Endocrinol Metab* 51:647, 1980

149. POLLACK MS, LEVINE LS, O'NEILL GJ, PANG S, LORENZEN F, KOHN B, RONDANINI GF, CHIUMELLO G, NEW MI, DUPONT B: HLA linkage and B14, DR1, BfS haplotype association with the genes for late onset and cryptic 21-hydroxylase deficiency. *Am J Hum Genet* 33:540, 1981

150. LEVINE LS, DUPONT B, LORENZEN F, PANG S, POLLACK M, OBERFIELD S, KOHN B, LERNER A, CACCIARI E, MANTERO F, CASSIO A, SCARONI C, CHIUMELLO G, RONDANINI GF, GARGANTINI L, GIOVANNELLI G, VIRDIS R, BARTOLOTTA E, MIGLIORI C, PINTOR C, TATO L, BARBONI F, NEW MI: Cryptic 21-hydroxylase deficiency in families of patients with classical congenital adrenal hyperplasia. *J Clin Endocrinol Metab* 51:1316, 1980

151. ZACHMANN M, PRADER A: Unusual heterozygotes of congenital adrenal hyperplasia due to 21-hydroxylase deficiency. *Acta Endocrinol* 87:557, 1978

152. ZACHMANN M, PRADER A: Unusual heterozygotes of congenital adrenal hyperplasia due to 21-hydroxylase deficiency confirmed by HLA tissue typing. *Acta Endocrinol* 95:542, 1979

153. MCKUSICK VA: Phenotypic diversity of human diseases resulting from allelic series. *Am J Hum Genet* 25:446, 1973

154. KLOUDA PT, HARRIS R, PRICE DA: HLA and congenital adrenal hyperplasia. *Lancet* 2:1046, 1978

155. POLLACK MS, LEVINE LS, ZACHMANN M, PRADER A, NEW MI, OBERFIELD S, DUPONT B: Possible genetic linkage disequilibrium between HLA and the 21-hydroxylase deficiency gene (congenital adrenal hyperplasia). *Transplant Proc* XI:1315, 1979

156. MANTERO F, SCARONI C, PASINI C, FAGIOLO U: No linkage between HLA and congenital adrenal hyperplasia due to 17-alpha-hydroxylase deficiency. *N Engl J Med* 303:530, 1980

157. PANG S, LEVINE LS, LORENZEN F, CHOW D, POLLACK M, DUPONT B, GENEL M, NEW MI: Hormonal studies with obligate heterozygotes and siblings of patients with 11β-hydroxylase deficiency congenital adrenal hyperplasia (CAH). *J Clin Endocrinol Metab* 50:586, 1980

158. BRAUTBAR C, THEODOR R, SACK J, LEVINE C, DUPONT B, LEVINE LS, SHARON R, SMALLER S, COHEN T, ROSLER A: HLA in a selective aldosterone biosynthetic defect due to type 2 corticosterone methyl-oxidase deficiency. *Tissue Antigens* 17:212, 1981

159. PANG S, HOTCHKISS J, DRASH AL, LEVINE LS, NEW MI: Microfilter paper method for 17-α-progesterone radioimmunoassay: its application for rapid screening for congenital adrenal hyperplasia. *J Clin Endocrinol Metab* 45:1003, 1977

160. WERDER EA, SIEBENMANN RE, KNORR-MURSET G, ZIMMERMANN A, SIZONENKO PC, THEINTZ P, GIRARD J, ZACHMANN M, PRADER A: The incidence of congenital adrenal hyperplasia in Switzerland: a survey of patients born in 1960 to 1974. *Helv Paediatr Acta* 35:5, 1980

161. PRICE DA, KLOUDA PT, HARRIS R: HLA and congenital adrenal hyperplasia linkage confirmed. *Lancet* 1:930, 1978

162. PANG S, MURPHEY W, LEVINE LS, SPENCE D, LEON A, LAFRANCHI S, SURVE A, NEW MI: A pilot newborn screening for congenital adrenal hyperplasia (CAH) at New York Hospital (NYH) and Alaska. *Pediatr Res* 15:512, 1981

163. LAFRANCHI SH, MURPHEY WH, FOLEY TP JR, LARSEN PR, BUIST NRM: Neonatal hypothyroidism detected by the northwest regional screening program. *Pediatrics* 63:180, 1979

164. JEFFCOATE TNA, FLIEGNERS JRH, RUSSELL SH, DAVIS JC, WADE AP: Diagnosis of the adrenogenital syndrome. *Lancet* 2:553, 1965

165. NEW MI, LEVINE LS: Congenital adrenal hyperplasia, in Harris H, Hirschhorn KK (eds): *Advances in Human Genetics*. London, Plenum Press, 1973, p 251

166. FRASIER SD, THORNEYCROFT IH, WEILL BA, HORTON R: Elevated amniotic fluid concentration of 17-hydroxyprogesterone in congenital adrenal hyperplasia. *J Pediatr* 86:310, 1975

167. NAGAMANI M, MCDONOUGH PG, ELLEGOOD JO, MAHESH VB: Maternal and amniotic fluid 17-hydroxyprogesterone levels during pregnancy: diagnosis of congenital adrenal hyperplasia in utero. *Am J Obstet Gynecol* 130:791, 1978

168. HUGHES IA, LAURENCE KM: Antenatal diagnosis of congenital adrenal hyperplasia. *Lancet* 2:7, 1979

169. PANG S, LEVINE LS, CEDERQVIST LL, FUENTES M, RICCARDI VM, HOLCOMBE JH, NITOWSKY HM, SACHS G, ANDERSON CE, DUCHON MA, OWENS R, MERKATZ I, NEW MI: Amniotic fluid concentrations of Δ5 and Δ4 steroids in fetuses with congenital adrenal hyperplasia due to 21-hydroxylase deficiency and in anencephalic fetuses. *J Clin Endocrinol Metab* 51:223, 1980

170. POLLACK MS, LEVINE LS, PANG S, OWENS RP, NITOWSKY HM, MAURER D, NEW MI, DUCHON M, MERKATZ IR, SACHS G, DUPONT B: Prenatal diagnosis of congenital adrenal hyperplasia (21-hydroxylase deficiency) by HLA typing. *Lancet* 1:1107, 1979

171. RÖSLER A, LEIBERMAN E, ROSENMANN A, BEN-UZILIO R, WEIDEMFELD J: Prenatal diagnosis of 11β-hydroxylase deficiency congenital adrenal hyperplasia. *J Clin Endocrinol Metab* 49:546, 1979

172. SCHUMERT Z, ROSENMANN A, LANDAU H, ROSLER A: 11-Deoxycortisol in amniotic fluid: prenatal diagnosis of congenital adrenal hyperplasia due to 11β-hydroxylase deficiency. *Clin Endocrinol* 12:257, 1980

48

THE ANDROGEN RESISTANCE SYNDROMES: 5α-Reductase Deficiency, Testicular Feminization, and Related Disorders

JEAN D. WILSON

JAMES E. GRIFFIN

MARK LESHIN

PAUL C. MACDONALD

1. The mechanism by which androgens act within target cells is similar to that of other steroid hormones: the hormone combines with a receptor protein in the cytosol of the cell and the receptor-hormone complex moves to the nucleus, attaches to chromatin, and promotes the formation of messenger RNA. However, androgen action differs from that of other steroids in two ways. First, testosterone, the major circulating androgen, must be converted to dihydrotestosterone before exerting certain of its actions. Second, androgens act during embryogenesis to convert the undifferentiated genital tract into the male phenotype. In this manner androgens promote differentiation of those tissues that serve as the major androgen target tissues in later life.

2. Hereditary defects that impede androgen action frequently cause resistance to the hormone both during later life and during embryogenesis, and hence frequently cause developmental defects of the male urogenital tract. Such defects in genetic men produce a phenotypic spectrum ranging from infertile but otherwise normal men to individuals with varying degrees of ambiguous genitalia to phenotypic women. In molecular terms, these disorders can be classified on the basis of the step in androgen action that is impeded by the individual mutations.

3. 5α-Reductase deficiency is an autosomal recessive enzyme defect that impairs the conversion of testosterone to dihydrotestosterone. As a consequence the internal male genital tract virilizes normally, but the external genitalia are predominantly female in character. The syndrome is the result of one of several mutations that impair the function of the 5α-reductase enzyme.

4. A variety of disorders influences the cytosolic androgen receptor that mediates the action of both testosterone and dihydrotestosterone. At least four phenotypic variants can be distinguished—complete testicular feminization, incomplete testicular feminization, the Reifenstein syndrome, and the infertile male syndrome, each of which is inherited as an X-linked trait. Absence of receptor function is found commonly in the phenotype of complete testicular feminization, but qualitative or quantitative defects in receptor function can be associated with all four variants.

5. A third type of disorder—termed receptor-positive resistance—also causes a spectrum of defects in male development and is associated with normal 5α-reductase activity and normal (or elevated) levels of androgen receptor. The underlying defect is presumed to lie at the intranuclear site or sites of action of the hormone-receptor complex.

6. Normal androgen action is essential for reproduction but not for the life of individuals. Because even slight abnormalities in androgen actions are usually mani-

fested by anatomic or functional abnormalities (and hence come to the attention of physicians frequently), the syndromes of androgen resistance provide a remarkable opportunity to utilize single-gene mutations for the simultaneous elucidation of the normal pathway of action of a hormone and of the pathogenesis of common abnormalities of human sexual development.

The fact that endocrine disease can result from resistance to hormonal action at the cellular level was first recognized by Albright and his colleagues, who deduced that pseudohypoparathyroidism is caused by peripheral resistance to the action of parathyroid hormone [1]. The second disorder that was shown to result from resistance to hormone action was the form of male pseudohermaphroditism known as testicular feminization, in which genetic males with testes differentiate as phenotypic women as the result of a single-gene defect [2]. In 1957 Wilkins observed that the administration of androgen to a patient with testicular feminization did not induce virilization [3], and a large body of subsequent information has documented that this disorder is due to resistance to the action of androgen during embryogenesis and postnatal life. Additional syndromes of androgen resistance have been delineated, ranging from other types of male pseudohermaphroditism to infertility in otherwise normal men [4].

Investigations along four lines have converged in recent years to provide insight into the underlying pathophysiology: (1) The essential role of androgen in the development of the male phenotype during embryogenesis has been established [5–8]. (2) Quantitative techniques have been developed to assess androgen and estrogen metabolism in intact subjects, and this information has provided insight into the pathogenesis of the various phenotypes that occur in different forms of androgen resistance [9, 10]. (3) Most disorders of androgen resistance are due to single-gene defects, and analysis of the patterns of inheritance has provided insight into the pathogenesis of the disorders and has been useful in defining distinct subgroups of subjects [11, 12]. (4) The molecular processes by which androgens act within cells have been identified [13–15], and techniques have been developed to assess these processes in biopsy material from affected subjects and in fibroblasts cultured from skin biopsies. As a consequence, we now have considerable insight into the functions of the various gene products required for normal androgen action.

The principal focus of this chapter is to describe the mechanisms by which androgens promote virilization of the normal male during embryogenesis as well as in postnatal life and to summarize the current concepts of the pathogenesis of the syndromes of androgen resistance.

DYNAMICS OF ANDROGEN AND ESTROGEN METABOLISM IN NORMAL MEN

The two principal androgens in male plasma are the testicular hormone testosterone and the adrenal steroid androstenedione. Testosterone is a potent hormone and also serves as the precursor (or prohormone) for two other active hormones—

estradiol and dihydrotestosterone (Fig. 48-1). [9, 10, 13]. Dihydrotestosterone is the intracellular mediator of certain androgen actions and also circulates in blood; the circulating hormone is derived primarily by conversion from testosterone in peripheral tissues and to a lesser extent by direct secretion into the circulation by the testes. The plasma level of dihydrotestosterone is on the average about one-tenth that of testosterone [13].

The exact function of estrogen in normal men remains to be established [16], although it has been suggested that the hormone serves a role in male sexual drive [17, 18]. Excess estrogen—either relative or absolute—causes profound feminization in men, particularly the induction of breast enlargement (gynecomastia) [19]. As a consequence, estrogen plays a major role in determining the final phenotype in several disorders of androgen action. For this reason it is imperative to understand the dynamics of estrogen and androgen production and metabolism in the normal man (Fig. 48-2). As measured by isotope-dilution techniques, the production rates of estradiol and estrone, respectively, average about 45 and 66 μg/day in normal men, and plasma production rates of testosterone and androstenedione, respectively, average about 5000 and 3000 μg/day [10]. Thus, the ratio of the production rate of testosterone to that of estradiol in normal men is about 100 to 1. All the estrone and about 85 percent of the estradiol is derived from peripheral conversion from androstenedione and testosterone. Thus, in normal men an average of only 6 to 10 μg estradiol is secreted directly into the circulation by the testes [9, 10]. Kelch et al. [20] and Weinstein et al. [21] reached a similar conclusion that estrogen in men is synthesized predominantly in peripheral tissues as the result of studies of differences in the concentration of estrogens in peripheral blood as compared to that in testicular venous blood of normal men. However, when large amounts of human chorionic gonadotropin (hCG) are administered to normal men (or when plasma luteinizing hormone (LH) activity is elevated in pathologic states), direct secretion of estrogen by the stimulated testes increases in proportion to the increase in the secretion of testosterone [21]. Thus, under normal conditions most estrogen in men is formed by peripheral aromatization of circulating androgens, but when gonadotropin concentrations are elevated the testis may secrete significant amounts of estrogen directly into the circulation. Feminization of men can result when the normal 100-fold excess of androgens to estrogens is disturbed either by an increase in estrogen production or by a decrease in testosterone formation (or action) under circumstances in which estrogen production remains appreciable [19].

MECHANISMS OF ANDROGEN ACTION

The current concepts of the mechanisms by which androgens exert their physiologic actions are summarized schematically in Fig. 48-3. Testosterone, the principal androgen secreted by the testis and the major androgen in plasma of men, circulates bound to two proteins, testosterone-binding globulin (TeBG, also termed sex-hormone-binding globulin or SHBG) and albumin [22, 23]. The protein-bound steroid is in dynamic equilibrium with unbound or free hormone, the latter comprising 1 to 3 percent of the total [22, 23]. Although the mech-

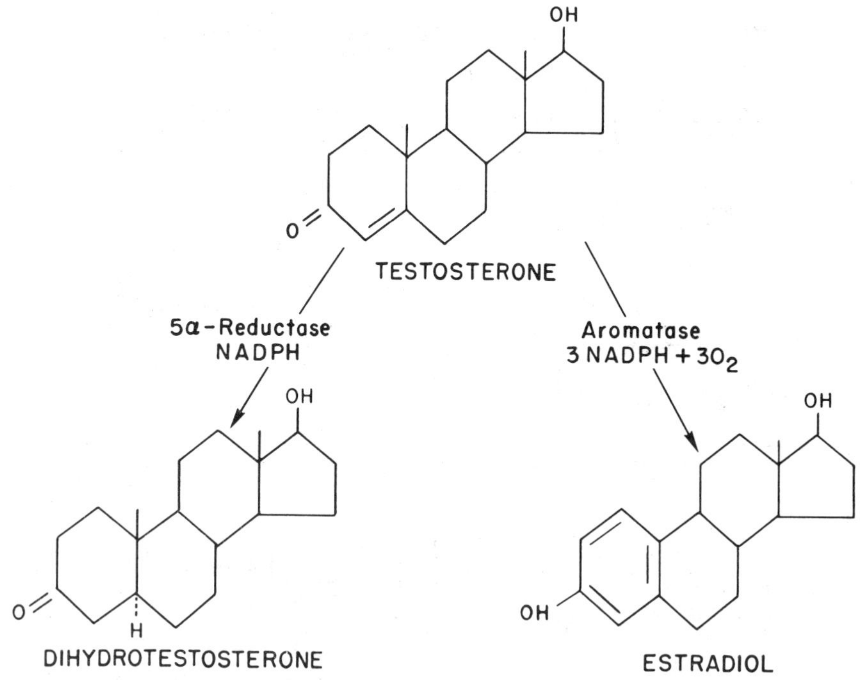

OH

O=

TESTOSTERONE

5α-Reductase
NADPH

Aromatase
3 NADPH + 3O₂

OH

O=

H

DIHYDROTESTOSTERONE

OH

OH

ESTRADIOL

Figure 48-1 The principal hormones formed from testosterone by the testes and in peripheral tissues.

anism of entry into cells may be more complex than simple passive diffusion through the plasma membrane, studies of androgen metabolism in the prostate suggest that the entry process is not energy dependent and that free steroid, rather than a steroid-protein complex, enters the prostate cell by a passive mechanism [24]. The fact that the concentration of testosterone in most androgen target tissues is lower than that of plasma is in keeping with this interpretation [25, 26].

Inside the cell testosterone undergoes one of two fates. It can be reduced to dihydrotestosterone by the 5α-reductase enzyme. This serves to keep the intracellular concentration of testosterone low and thus promotes the diffusion of testosterone into the cell down an activity gradient [24]. Either dihydrotestosterone or testosterone is bound to a high-affinity receptor protein in the cell cytoplasm. The androgen-receptor complexes (TR and DR) enter the nucleus, become attached to the chromatin of the cell, and in some way promote the transcription of messenger RNA (mRNA) [14, 15]. There is no uniform agreement on the size or properties of the androgen receptor or on the nature of the chemical transformations (if any) that the hormone-receptor complexes must undergo before becoming active, but it appears that the major native receptor in cytosol is large (8 S or greater) and that the form recoverable from the nuclear chromatin is smaller in size (4 S or less) [14, 15]. The mechanisms by which the androgen-receptor complexes affect the transcription of stored genetic information also is not known [14, 15].

Although dihydrotestosterone and testosterone bind to the same receptor protein, the biologic and genetic evidence is convincing that the two hormones perform different roles in androgen physiology. The testosterone-receptor complex is responsible for the regulation of the secretion of the gonadotropin LH by the hypothalamic-pituitary system, for the virilization of the Wolffian ducts during male phenotypic sex differentiation, and possibly for the promotion of spermatogenesis in the testis [13, 27]. The dihydrotestosterone-receptor complex, in contrast, is responsible for the formation of the male external genitalia and prostate during embryogenesis and

for most of the androgen-mediated events of sexual maturation at the time of male puberty (growth of facial and body hair, temporal hair recession, and maturation of external genitalia) [13, 27]. The reason that different species of one hormone perform different functions is unresolved, but since testosterone binds less avidly to the receptor than does dihydrotestosterone [28], it is possible that testosterone could effect all androgen functions if present in high enough concentrations.

In summary, the general processes by which all steroid hormones act are believed to be similar in that following passive entry of the hormone into a target tissue and binding to a receptor protein in the cell cytosol, the protein-hormone complex gains access to the nuclear chromatin and promotes the transcription (or effective translation) of mRNA. The action of androgens differs from that of other steroid hormones in at least two ways: (1) Many effects of testosterone, the major circulating androgen, are mediated by intracellular metabolites of the parent hormone, dihydrotestosterone and (possibly) estradiol. Thus, the sum of the physiologic effects of testosterone is comprised of the actions of testosterone itself and of its 5α-reduced and estrogenic metabolites. Since dihydrotestosterone cannot be converted to estrogen, its actions are purely androgenic. (2) During embryogenesis androgens actually promote the differentiation of those tissues that will be major sites of action for the hormone in postnatal life. In exerting this critical role in normal male sexual development, androgens exert their most fundamental action.

NORMAL MALE SEXUAL DEVELOPMENT

As formulated by Jost, normal sexual development in the mammalian embryo consists of three sequential, ordered, and interrelated processes [5–8]. The first of these involves the establishment of *chromosomal sex*. This is determined primar-

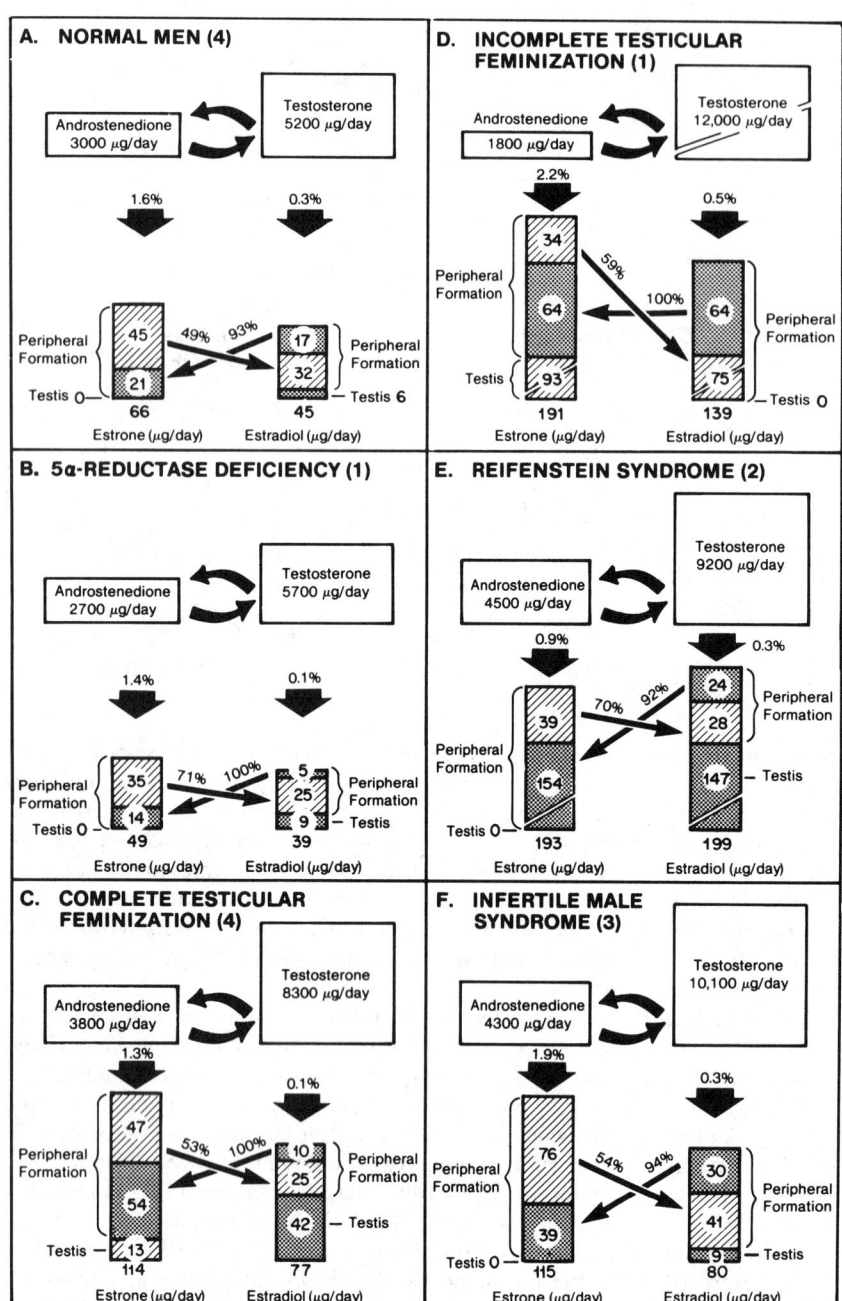

Figure 48-2 Dynamics of androgen and estrogen production in normal men and in 46,XY subjects with androgen resistance. *A.* Four normal men. *B.* One subject with 5α-reductase deficiency. *C.* Four subjects with complete testicular feminization. *D.* One woman with incomplete testicular feminization. *E.* Two men with Reifenstein syndrome. *F.* Three infertile men. The average production rates of androgen are indicated in the upper boxes, and the production rates of estrogen are shown at the bottom of each vertical bar. The extent of conversion of plasma testosterone and androstenedione to estradiol and estrone is indicated by the vertical arrows, and the interconversion of estrone and estradiol and of testosterone and androstenedione are indicated by the horizontal arrows. The sources of estradiol and estrone are indicated in the vertical bars. Thus, estradiol arises from plasma testosterone, from estrone, and from direct secretion by the testis, and estrone arises from plasma androstenedione, from estradiol, and in some instances from direct secretion by the testis. (*From Wilson et al.* [130], *Walsh et al.* [58], *Madden et al.* [124], *Aiman et al.* [137], *and MacDonald et al.* [10].)

ily by the sex chromosome constitution established at the time of fertilization. In the mammal the heterogametic sex (XY) is male, and the homogametic sex (XX) is female. In the second phase, chromosomal sex is translated into *gonadal sex.* The exact mechanisms by which the genetic information determines that an indifferent gonad differentiates into a testis in the male or an ovary in the female and secretes the hormones characteristic of the testis or ovary are not understood entirely, but the Y chromosome carries genetic determinants that induce the indifferent gonad to develop into a testis. These determinants are either identical to or closely linked to a differentiative antigen termed H-Y antigen [29, 30]. The final process, the translation of gonadal sex into *phenotypic sex,* is the direct consequence of the type of gonad formed and the resulting endocrine secretions of the fetal testis. In the formation of phenotypic sex, indifferent internal and external genital anlagen are con-

verted to a male or female form, and the sexual, behavioral, and functional characteristics are ultimately determined.

The embryologic processes involved in the development of phenotypic sex are summarized in Fig. 48-4. The internal genitalia arise from the Wolffian and müllerian ducts, both of which are present in early embryos of both sexes [31, 32]. The Wolffian ducts are the excretory ducts of the mesonephric kidney and are physically connected with the indifferent gonad. The müllerian duct forms secondarily from the Wolffian duct and is not contiguous with the gonad [33]. In the male the Wolffian ducts give rise to the epididymides, vasa deferentia, and seminal vesicles. In the female the müllerian ducts give rise to the fallopian tubes, uterus, and upper vagina. Thus, the internal genital tracts in males and females develop from different anlagen. In contrast, the external genitalia and urethra of both sexes develop from common anlagen, the urogenital

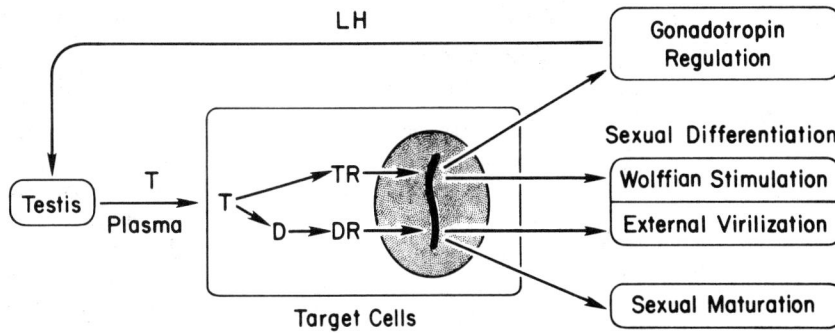

Figure 48-3 Schematic diagram of normal androgen physiology. LH, luteinizing hormone; T, testosterone; D, dihydrotestosterone; R, receptor.

sinus and the genital tubercle, folds, and swellings. In the male the urogenital sinus gives rise to the prostate and prostatic urethra and in the female to the lower two-thirds of the vagina and urethra. The genital tubercle is the anlage of the glans penis in the male and the clitoris in the female. The genital swellings become the labia majora or scrotum, and the genital folds develop into labia minora or the shaft of the penis [31, 32].

In the absence of the testes, as in the normal female or in male embryos castrated prior to the onset of phenotypic differentiation, the development of phenotypic sex proceeds along female lines [5–8]. Thus, masculinization of the fetus is the positive result of action by testicular secretions, whereas development of the female phenotype is passive in character, not requiring the action of a hormone from the fetal ovary. Under ordinary conditions development of the sexual phenotype conforms faithfully to the chromosomal or genetic sex, i.e., chromosomal sex determines gonadal sex, and gonadal sex in turn determines phenotypic sex.

Three hormones control the development of the male phenotype [27, 34, 35] (Table 48-1). Two of the hormones—müllerian inhibiting substance and testosterone—are secretory products of the fetal testes. Müllerian inhibiting substance is an incompletely characterized product of the embryonic testis, probably a macromolecule with a molecular weight greater than 15,000 that is secreted by the seminiferous tubules [36–39]. The substance causes regression of the müllerian ducts and consequently prevents development of the uterus and fallopian tubes in the male.

Testosterone is the principal androgen secreted both by the adult testis and by the fetal testis at the time of male phenotypic differentiation [40, 41]. The relation between the onset of testosterone formation by the human fetal testes and male phenotypic development is illustrated in Fig. 48-5. The onset of testosterone secretion corresponds closely to the onset of virilization of the embryo (at about 3 cm of development); the factors that regulate the initial secretion of testosterone at the

time of Leydig cell differentiation have not been defined. The present evidence suggests that the initiation and early maintenance of Leydig cell function is autonomous and that gonadotropin control of testosterone formation is acquired later during embryogenesis [42, 43].

On the basis of studies of androgen metabolism in embryos of several species including humans, it was deduced that testosterone promotes virilization of the urogenital tract in two different ways. Testosterone acts directly to stimulate the Wolffian ducts and induce development of the epididymides, vasa deferentia, and seminal vesicles. As illustrated in Fig. 48-5, differentiation of the Wolffian ducts into seminal vesicle and epididymis is completed in the human male embryo (≅ 9 cm of development) before the capacity to form dihydrotestosterone is acquired by these tissues [41]. In contrast, in the remaining tissues of the male urogenital tract (Fig. 48-5) testosterone acts as a prohormone for the third hormone of fetal virilization, namely dihydrotestosterone. Dihydrotestosterone, which does not appear to be synthesized in appreciable quantities by the fetal testes at the time of male phenotypic development [40, 41], is formed by enzymatic reduction of testosterone within the urogenital sinus and lower urogenital tract before male differentiation of these tissues takes place [41, 44–47]. Dihydrotestosterone acts in the urogenital sinus to induce formation of the male urethra and prostate and in the urogenital tubercle, swelling, and folds to cause the midline fusion, elongation, and enlargement that eventuate in the male external genitalia.

Because of technical difficulties inherent in the small amounts of embryonic tissues available for study, few studies have been conducted to characterize directly the receptor machinery for androgen action in embryonic tissues. As the result of studies of single-gene defects that impede androgen action it is now established that the schema shown in Fig. 48-3 is valid for the embryonic as well as for postnatal androgen action—namely a single high-affinity cytosolic receptor is

Table 48-1 Hormonal control of male phenotypic sex differentiation

		Phase of phenotypic differentiation		
Gonadal hormone	Intracellular hormone	Müllerian duct regression	Wolffian duct differentiation	Virilization of urogenital sinus and external genitalia
Müllerian inhibiting substance	?	+		
Testosterone	Testosterone and dihydrotestosterone		+	
				+

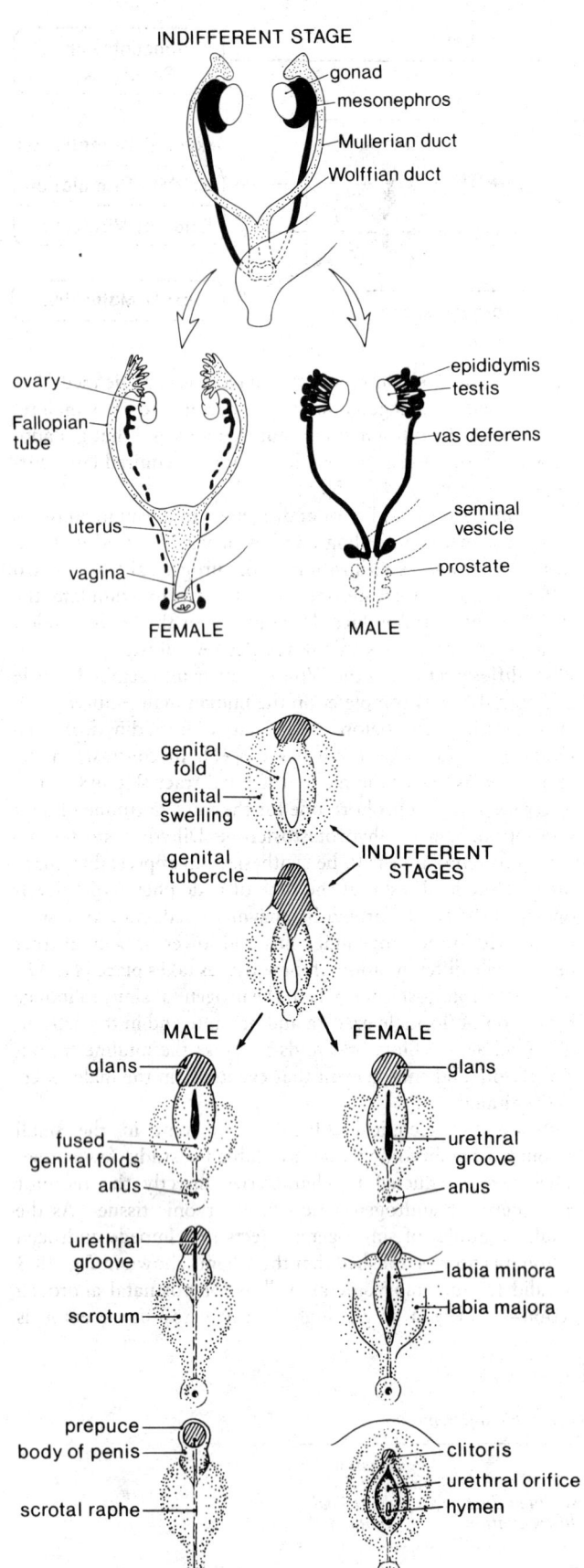

INDIFFERENT STAGE

gonad
mesonephros
Mullerian duct
Wolffian duct

ovary
Fallopian tube
uterus
vagina
FEMALE

epididymis
testis
vas deferens
seminal vesicle
prostate
MALE

genital fold
genital swelling
genital tubercle
INDIFFERENT STAGES

MALE
glans
fused genital folds
anus
urethral groove
scrotum
prepuce
body of penis
scrotal raphe

FEMALE
glans
urethral groove
anus
labia minora
labia majora
clitoris
urethral orifice
hymen

Figure 48-4 *A.* Phenotypic differentiation of the internal urogenital tract in male and female embryos. *B.* Phenotypic differentiation of the external genitalia in male and female embryos.

responsible for mediating the actions of both testosterone and dihydrotestosterone [4]. It is also established that the androgen-receptor mechanism is fundamentally the same in male and female embryos. Thus, when female embryos are exposed to androgens at the appropriate time in embryonic development, both the Wolffian ducts and external genitalia virilize in the characteristic male fashion [27, also see Chap. 47]. Thus, the differences in male and female phenotypic development are due solely to the action of hormones produced by the fetal gonads at the critical period of embryonic development and not to differences in the receptor machinery for the hormones.

DISORDERS OF SEXUAL DEVELOPMENT

A disturbance during embryogenesis at any step of sexual differentiation may give rise to a disorder of sexual development. On theoretical grounds, these disorders can be classified meaningfully in terms of the initial developmental stage influenced by the mutant gene, e.g., errors in chromosomal sex, errors in gonadal sex, or errors in phenotypic sex [11, 12, 48]. Such abnormalities may arise by several mechanisms, such as environmental insult (as ingestion of a virilizing drug during pregnancy), a nonfamilial aberration in the sex chromosomes (as in 45,X gonadal dysgenesis), a developmental birth defect of multifactorial etiology (as in most cases of hypospadias), or a hereditary disorder resulting from a single-gene mutation (as in the testicular feminization syndrome). In fact, at least 19 simply inherited disorders of sexual development are now recognized [11, 12].

Male pseudohermaphroditism is a disorder of phenotypic sex in which chromosomal and gonadal males do not develop as completely normal men, most commonly because of a single-gene mutation. Three general categories of such disorders have been delineated: the persistent müllerian duct syndrome, defects of testosterone formation, and the androgen resistance syndromes.

The persistent müllerian duct syndrome is a rare disorder characterized by normal male virilization but failure of müllerian regression, so that affected men have a uterus and fallopian tube(s) in addition to normal Wolffian structures [49]. This syndrome is believed to be caused by a deficiency of müllerian inhibiting substance or by resistance to its action.

Disorders of testosterone formation result either from poorly understood developmental abnormalities in the testis or from a deficiency in any of the five enzymes necessary for testosterone synthesis from cholesterol: 20,22-desmolase, 3β-hydroxysteroid dehydrogenase, 17α-hydroxylase, 17,20-desmolase, or 17β-hydroxysteroid dehydrogenase. The latter disorders result in a spectrum of defects in virilization of affected males and are discussed in detail in Chap. 47.

The third type of disorder and the focus of this chapter, androgen resistance, accounts for approximately three-fourths of cases of male pseudohermaphroditism [50–52]. Testosterone synthesis and müllerian duct regression are normal, but because of a defect in some aspect of androgen action, affected persons are resistant to the hormone during embryogenesis as

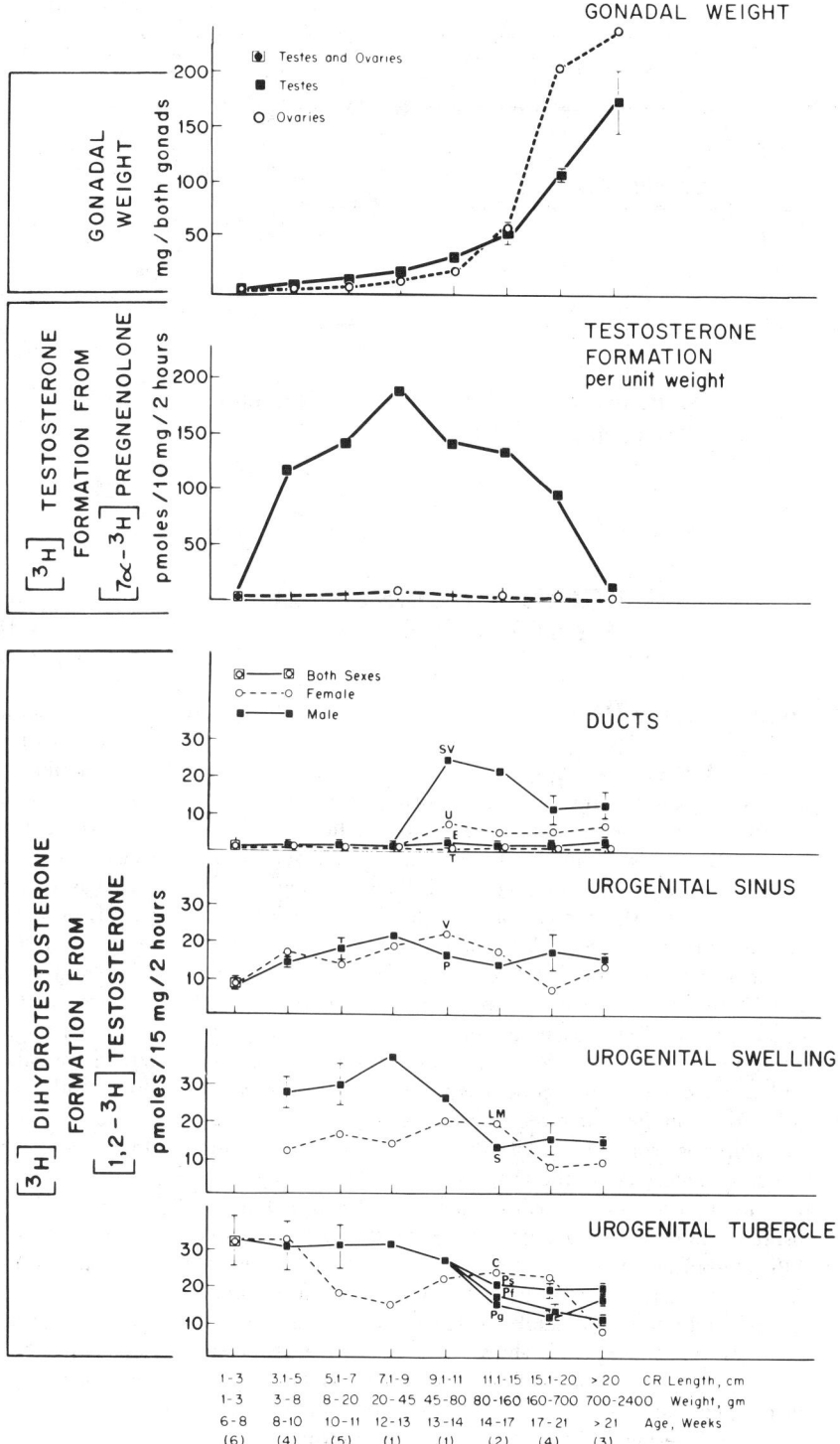

Figure 48-5 Testosterone formation and metabolism during phenotypic differentiation of the human male embryo. Gonadal weight (upper panel), testosterone formation by the gonads (second panel), and dihydrotestosterone formation by the urogenital tract (lower three panels) are charted as a function of age of the human embryo. Each value represents the mean for the number of measurements shown in parentheses at the bottom of the chart. (*From Siiteri and Wilson* [41].)

well as in the postnatal state. These abnormalities were originally delineated by studying patients with male pseudohermaphroditism in whom defects in virilization were associated with normal male (or high) production rates of testosterone. Subsequently, it has been recognized that incomplete defects in androgen action do not necessarily result in anatomic defects in male development but are manifested only as failure of sperm production in otherwise normal men. Thus, the spectrum of presentation of androgen resistance is broader than

envisioned originally. The molecular defects responsible for androgen resistance can occur at any one of the three major sites in the pathway of androgen action (Fig. 48-6): abnormalities in 5α-reductase, in the androgen receptor, or in the subsequent phases of androgen action. This last category has been termed receptor-positive resistance. There is considerable genetic heterogeneity in these disorders so that several mutations in the 5α-reductase enzyme and a variety of defects in the androgen receptor are now recognized.

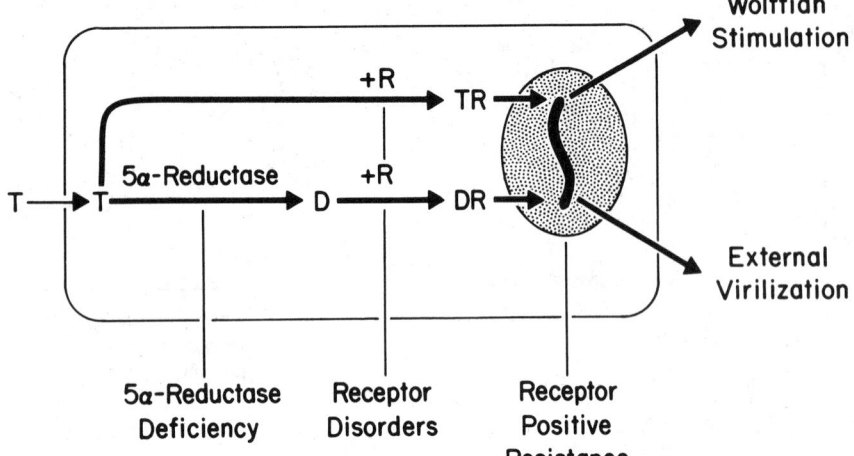

Figure 48-6 Classification of the androgen resistance syndromes based on the site of the defect in androgen action. T, testosterone; D, dihydrotestosterone; R, receptor protein.

THE ANDROGEN RESISTANCE SYNDROMES

5α-Reductase Deficiency

Clinical Features A specific form of hereditary male pseudohermaphroditism termed *pseudovaginal perineoscrotal hypospadias* was defined on clinical and genetic grounds in 1961 by Nowakowski and Lenz [53–55]. Subsequent patients were described by Simpson et al. [56] and by Opitz and coworkers [57]. Affected persons are 46,XY males who have an autosomal recessive disorder characterized by an external female phenotype at birth, bilateral testes, and normally virilized Wolffian structures that terminate or empty in the vagina. This entity (also termed familial incomplete male pseudohermaphroditism, type 2 [58]) constitutes a distinct disorder on genetic, phenotypic, and endocrine grounds and is now recognized to result from deficient conversion of testosterone to dihydrotestosterone. Thus, the disorder is now termed 5α-reductase deficiency. In the original description, normal male testosterone production was assumed to be a feature, but the disorder was described at a time when plasma testosterone was difficult to measure. In these early studies testosterone production was documented to be normal only in some affected individuals, and one of the families originally described with the syndrome was subsequently shown to have a hereditary defect in testosterone synthesis [59]. This problem emphasizes the overlapping nature of phenotypes in the various categories of male pseudohermaphroditism; this is the reason why it is mandatory to demonstrate a normal male level of testosterone (and of testosterone precursors) before a diagnosis of androgen resistance can be entertained.

The clinical features of 5α-reductase deficiency are summarized in Table 48-2 and include: (1) autosomal recessive inheritance; (2) severe perineoscrotal hypospadias with a dorsal, hooded prepuce and a ventral urethral groove that opens at the base of the phallus (illustrated in Fig. 48-7); (3) a blind vaginal pouch of variable size, opening either into a urogenital sinus or onto the perineum immediately behind the urethral orifice; (4) well-developed and histologically differentiated testes with normal epididymides, vasa deferentia, and seminal vesicles; (5) the absence of female internal genitalia; and (6) variable mas-

culinization and little or no breast enlargement at the time of expected puberty. Typically, affected individuals are raised as girls, despite the clitoromegaly that is usually present at birth.

Certain clinical features of the disorder deserve emphasis. The degree of masculinization at the time of expected puberty can be striking, with the habitus becoming masculine [56, 57, 60–62]; furthermore, in some [60–63] but not all [64], subjects who are untreated until later in life a reversal of gender role occurs at the time of expected puberty so that individuals raised as girls begin to function as men. The ejaculatory ducts usually terminate in the vagina. In some individuals no vaginal pouch is present, and the Wolffian duct derivatives terminate adjacent to the urethra on the perineum [58, 65]. No prostatic tissue is palpable, and no prostatic utricle can be demonstrated on cystoscopy. Thus, Wolffian derivatives are male in character, whereas the urogenital sinus and external genitalia are predominantly female [58, 61]. A radiogram of the lower Wolffian duct system from one such patient is illustrated in Fig. 48-8.

Endocrinology Simpson et al. characterized the basic endocrinologic features of 5α-reductase deficiency by demonstrating that normal male levels of testosterone in one affected individual rose even higher after administration of hCG and fell to the castrate range after removal of the testes [56]. They concluded that testosterone secretion is within the normal male range and is under normal feedback control. Subsequent studies have substantiated this interpretation.

Table 48-2 Clinical features of 5α-reductase deficiency

External phenotype: Female genitalia with some clitoromegaly at birth and variable virilization at expected time of puberty, normal male breast development
Internal phenotype: Testes; epididymides, vasa deferentia, and seminal vesicles empty into vagina; no müllerian duct derivatives
Karyotype: 46,XY
Inheritance: Autosomal recessive
Endocrinology
 Testosterone: Normal male plasma levels and production rates
 Estrogen: Normal male plasma levels and production rates
 Gonadotropin: Normal to slightly elevated plasma LH levels
Pathogenesis: Inability to form dihydrotestosterone

The endocrine characteristics of this syndrome appear to be quite consistent: (1) normal male to high levels of plasma testosterone and low levels of plasma dihydrotestosterone [58, 60, 61], (2) elevated ratios of plasma testosterone to dihydrotestosterone in adulthood and after stimulation with hCG in childhood [61, 62, 66], (3) elevated ratios of urinary 5β to 5α metabolities of androgen [61, 62, 67, 68], and (4) diminished conversion of testosterone to dihydrotestosterone in affected subjects [61, 62]. Levels of plasma LH are sometimes normal [58, 67] or more commonly slightly elevated (although not as elevated as in men with primary testicular failure or in patients with abnormalities of the androgen receptor [61, 62, 64, 69, 70]). Detailed studies of androgen and estrogen dynamics have been conducted in one patient (Fig. 48-2) [58]; plasma levels of androstenedione (1.1 ng/ml) and testosterone (6.9 ng/ml) and the plasma production rates of androstenedione (2.7 mg/day) and testosterone (5.2 mg/day) were in the range for normal young men. Estradiol production also was in the range for normal men in regard to the total production rate (45 μg/day), the amount secreted by the testis directly (9 μg/day), and the amount derived from the peripheral aromatization of plasma androgens (36 μg/day) [58]. These quantitative studies demonstrating normal male androgen and estrogen production provide a clearcut explanation for the failure of patients to undergo female breast development at the time of puberty and are in contrast to the situation in male pseudohermaphroditism due to disorders of the androgen receptor; in the latter disorders the variable feminization at puberty is associated with increased production of estrogen by the testes.

A major unresolved issue is why the external genitalia of patients with 5α-reductase deficiency virilize more at puberty than during embryogenesis. This problem is closely related to the unresolved question of why dihydrotestosterone formation is important in androgen physiology. The late virilization may be due to the presence of higher levels of plasma testosterone itself at puberty than during embryogenesis, to the accumulation of some dihydrotestosterone in plasma as a result of the action of the residual 5α-reductase demonstrable in all patients, or to some unidentified change in molecular or endocrine function with age.

Genetics Simpson et al. [56] and Opitz and coworkers [57] provided evidence that the disorder is due to the homozygous state of a rare autosomal recessive gene. Affected sibs are common, and consanguinity can be documented in approximately half of the cases. No evidence of heterozygous expression has been adduced in either men or women, and affected homozygous 46,XX sisters of affected males are phenotypically normal and have normal reproductive capacity [62]. Thus, the mutation appears to be silent in women. The prevalence of the disorder is uncertain, but it appears to be distributed widely and has been reported in individuals from Algeria [68], France [71], Mexico [64], Cyprus [67], Santo Domingo [60–63], Israel [70], Italy [69], and Pakistan [72], as well as from the United States [58, 65]. It is now established that more than one mutation of the enzyme causes functional impairment in enzyme activity [69, 73]. Such genetic heterogeneity is similar to that in other hereditary enzyme deficiencies and could be due to at least two causes. Distinct familial mutations may occur in the enzyme similar to those described for glucose-6-phosphate dehydrogenase [74]. Alternatively, there may be a smaller number of mutant alleles within the population, in which case either homozygosity for one mutation or heterozy-

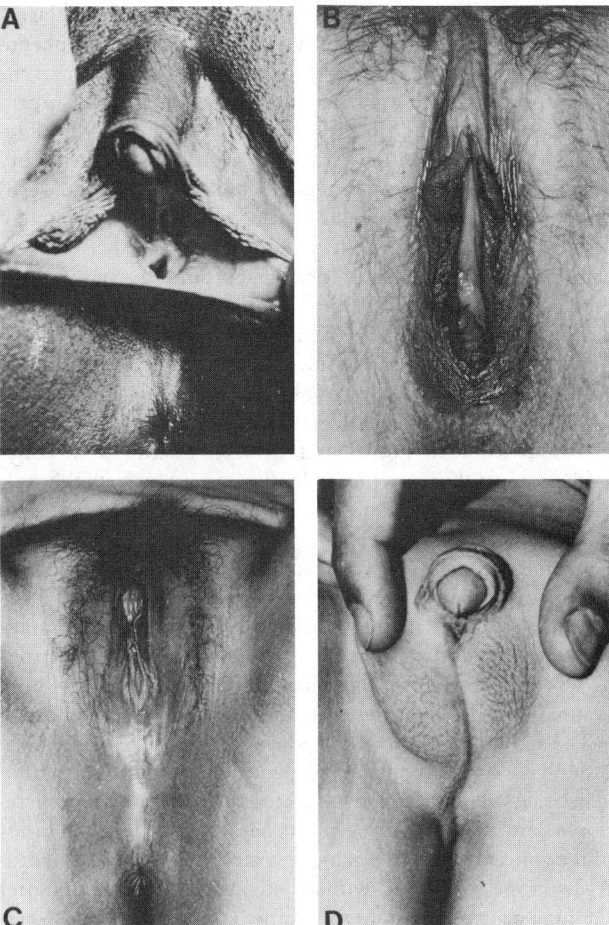

Figure 48-7 External genitalia of representative patients with defects of androgen action. *A.* 5α-reductase deficiency; the patient is the propositus from Walsh et al. [57]. *B.* Complete testicular feminization. *C.* Incomplete testicular feminization. (*From Madden et al. [120]*) *D.* Reifenstein syndrome. (*From Bowen et al. [126].*)

gosity for two different mutations of the same allele (i.e., a genetic compound) could result in clinical deficiency of the enzyme. The presence of consanguinity in a family enhances the likelihood that the defect in a given patient is the result of homozygosity for one mutant allele.

Pathogenesis The fact that dihydrotestosterone formation is essential for virilization of the external genitalia and male urethra, whereas testosterone itself causes male differentiation of the Wolffian ducts, was deduced from studies of androgen metabolism in embryos of several species [41, 44–47]. Consequently, it was predicted that impairment of dihydrotestosterone formation would result in male pseudohermaphroditism [75]. Specifically, it was expected that failure of dihydrotestosterone formation in a male embryo with normal testosterone synthesis would result in the phenotype observed in subjects with pseudovaginal perineoscrotal hypospadias, namely normal male Wolffian duct derivatives but defective masculinization of the urogenital sinus and external genitalia [75]. Substantiating evidence that this phenotype is the result of deficient production of dihydrotestosterone was obtained in 1974 by studies of two families with the disorder, one in Dallas [58] and the other in the Dominican Republic [60].

The initial studies in Dallas were performed in a 13-year-old 46,XY phenotypic girl who was ascertained because of primary amenorrhea. She had partial virilization and male plasma testosterone values. Because of the predominant female phenotype a decision was made to remove the testes and to repair the virilization of the external genitalia. Documentation at surgery of the presence of normal Wolffian duct structures—epididymides, vasa deferentia, seminal vesicles, and ejaculatory ducts—that terminated in a blind-ending vagina (Fig. 48-8) established the phenotype as that of pseudovaginal perineoscrotal hypospadias. Dihydrotestosterone formation was examined in tissue slices of foreskin, corpora cavernosa of the phallus, epididymis, and labia majora obtained from the subject at the time of surgery and compared with rates of formation in tissue slices from control patients and from subjects with other forms of male pseudohermaphroditism (Table 48-3). Dihydrotestosterone formation was virtually undetectable in tissues from the patient but clearly measurable in tissues from all control groups [58], a finding consistent with the view that deficiency in dihydrotestosterone formation is the cause of this distinctive phenotype.

A similar conclusion was reached by Imperato-McGinley et al. [60–63] from studies of an extensive pedigree of a family with the disorder in the Dominican Republic. The urinary excretion of androstanediol and androsterone (the end products of dihydrotestosterone metabolism) were low, as would be predicted if dihydrotestosterone formation were deficient.

The subsequent endocrine and enzymatic studies of this disorder have substantiated and expanded insight into the pathogenesis. As described above, decreased formation and excretion of 5α-reduced androgens is characteristic, and the ratios of the concentration of plasma testosterone to that of dihydrotestosterone (measured without stimulation in patients after the time of expected puberty or after stimulation of testosterone production by hCG in prepubertal years) can be used for diagnosis of the condition [60–63]. Alternatively, the ratios of the urinary etiocholanolone to androsterone can be measured [60–62]. It is of considerable interest that to date no patient has been described with total absence of plasma dihydrotestosterone, and it is not known the extent to which the partial virilization that occurs at puberty may be mediated by testosterone itself or by the small amounts of dihydrotestosterone that are present in the circulation.

The molecular features of the mutation have been characterized in fibroblasts cultured from the skin of patients with the disorder. 5α-Reductase activity is high on average in normal genital skin (foreskin, scrotum, labia majora) [76] and in fibroblasts cultured from normal genital skin [73, 77–80]. The

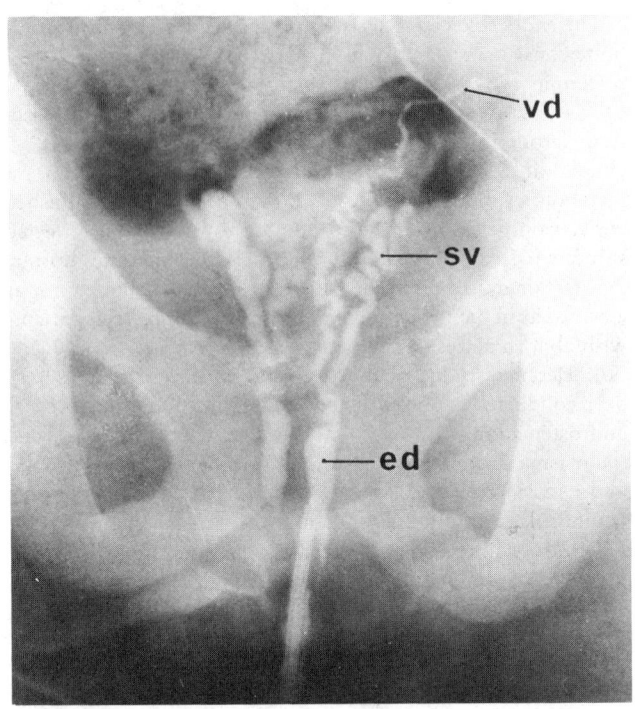

Figure 48-8 X-ray of the abdomen of a patient with 5α-reductase deficiency after the injection of diatrizoate sodium into the vasa deferentia at the time of abdominal exploration. vd, vas deferens; sv, seminal vesicles; ed, ejaculatory duct. The dye emptied into the vagina. (*From Walsh et al.* [58].)

enzyme catalyzes the 5α-reduction of many steroid hormones including cortisol [65]. The pH optimum of enzyme in homogenates of normal genital skin fibroblasts is 5.5 with a broad shoulder of activity extending over a more alkaline range [78]. Measurement of the activity in tissue homogenates at pH 5.5 has proved to be the most sensitive means to detect the enzyme deficiency. In homogenates prepared from cells grown from biopsies of genital skin from members of the original Dallas family, activity was virtually undetectable [78] (Fig. 48-9). Similar results (i.e., low rates of enzyme activity at all concentrations of substrate) were obtained in cells grown from skin biopsies from patients from eight other families that fulfill the endocrine, genetic, phenotypic, and enzymatic criteria for the diagnosis of 5α-reductase deficiency (Fig. 48-10). These ten families with deficient enzyme include the Dominican Republic family studied by Imperato-McGinley and coworkers [60–63]

Table 48-3 Dihydrotestosterone formation by tissue slices from normal subjects and from patients with various forms of androgen resistance

Group	Age range, yrs	Dihydrotestosterone formation [pmol/(h · 100 mg tissue) ± SEM]						
		Scrotum	Foreskin	Penis (corpora cavernosum)	Clitoris	Epididymis	Labia majora	Miscellaneous body skin
Miscellaneous control subjects	6–85	526 ± 60	211 ± 26	83 ± 17	210 ± 72	142 ± 32	183 ± 25	49 ± 6
5α-Reductase deficiency	13		8	0		3	0	
Complete testicular feminization	2–56					101 ± 15	72 ± 22	
Incomplete testicular feminization	26					71	319	19
Reifenstein syndrome	9	422	87					

Tissue slices (40 to 100 mg) were incubated with 0.5 μM [³H]testosterone, 10 mM glucose and Krebs-Ringer phosphate buffer, pH 7.4 in a total volume of 2.5 ml. After incubation for 1 h (genital tissue) or 2 h (miscellaneous body sites) the steroids were extracted and analyzed. Samples from 5 to 20 subjects were pooled for each of the control tissues analyzed, and 6 patients with complete testicular feminization were studied. The other groups represent 1 subject each.
SOURCES: Reproduced with permission from Walsh et al. [58] and Madden et al. [124].

and other families previously reported [67, 69] as well as seven previously undescribed families. In approximately half of these families consanguinity has been documented or is probable. Thus, deficiency of enzyme activity is the most common cause of the syndrome and results in a fairly uniform phenotype.

The picture became more complex when an affected family from Los Angeles was evaluated. The two affected members had characteristic endocrine findings of 5α-reductase deficiency, a clinical phenotype identical to that of previously characterized families, and profound deficiency of 5α-reductase in direct biopsy material [65]. However, activity of the enzyme in fibroblasts cultured from the genital skin of these subjects was within the normal range (labeled "unstable enzyme" in Fig. 48-10) [73]. Furthermore, in contrast to the situation in the previous cases, the enzyme from these patients had a normal pH optimum and a normal apparent K_m for testosterone. Affinity of the enzyme for reduced nicotinamide adenine dinucleotide phosphate, the cofactor for the reaction, was decreased and as a consequence the enzyme was unstable and exhibited a rapid turnover [73] (Fig. 48-11). Recently, enzyme activity in cells from another affected subject (labeled "unstable and deficient enzyme" in Fig. 48-10) was found to be intermediate in activity and to have an intermediate turnover rate as compared to that in fibroblasts from the Los Angeles family and normal controls [69]. We conclude that the qualitatively defective enzyme in these two families is probably synthesized at a normal rate but does not function normally within the cell and is degraded more rapidly than normal so that the steady state activity in intact cells is profoundly decreased.

Disorders of the Androgen Receptor

Disorders of the androgen receptor (Fig. 48-6) have been documented to result in several distinct phenotypes. Despite differences in clinical presentation and molecular pathology, these disorders are similar in regard to endocrinology, genetics, and basic pathophysiology.

Figure 48-9   5α-Reductase activity at pH 5.5 in homogenates of fibroblasts cultured from foreskin of a patient with 5α-reductase deficiency (○—○) and a normal control (●—●) as a function of testosterone concentration. (*From Moore, et al.* [78]).

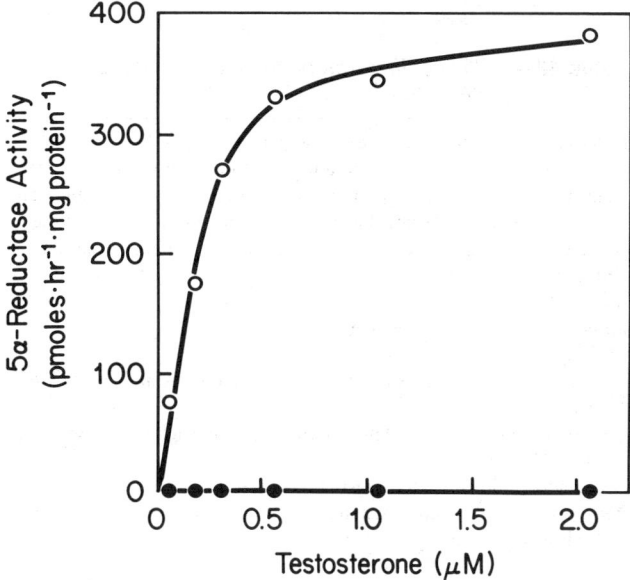

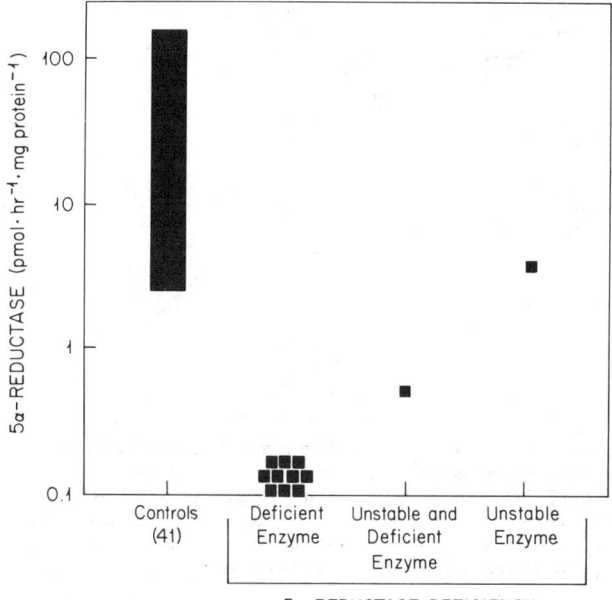

Figure 48-10   5α-Reductase activity in genital skin fibroblasts cultured from skin biopsies from 12 families with 5α-reductase deficiency. The range of pH 5.5 activity in 41 control subjects is illustrated in the black bar, and the activity in 12 patients from different families with 5α-reductase deficiency is shown in the individual points (■).

Clinical Features

COMPLETE TESTICULAR FEMINIZATION   The clinical features of complete testicular feminization are summarized in Table 48-4. The syndrome has been recognized for many years (reviewed in detail in [81]). A detailed clinical description was provided by de Quervain in 1923 [82], and extensive genetic studies of the disorder were reported by Dieffenbach in 1912 (cited in [81]) and by Perkins in 1933 [83]. Major insight into the pathogenesis of the disorder was afforded by two pioneering studies of the disease. In 1937 Pettersson and Bonnier deduced from pedigree and genetic analyses that affected individuals are genetic males, that the pattern of inheritance is consistent either with an X-linked recessive defect or a sex-limited autosomal mutation, and that the syndrome could best be explained by a failure of male induction in an embryo in which the fundamental trend is toward the female phenotype [84]. In 1953 Morris defined the disorder in greater detail [2]. In this paper, in which the term testicular feminization was first used, Morris reviewed 79 published cases that fulfilled the criteria for inclusion in the syndrome and added two new cases [2]. The disorder has been the subject of a number of subsequent reviews [81, 85–87]. The clinical findings are still those formulated by Morris and summarized in Table 48-4. The typical patient is seen by a physician either because of primary amenorrhea (postpubertally) or an inguinal hernia (prepubertally). Occasional patients are not diagnosed until later in life [88–89]. Breast development is that of a normal woman, and the general habitus and distribution of body fat are female in character (Fig. 48-12). Axillary and pubic hair are absent or scanty, but some vulvar hair is usually present. Facial and scalp hair are those of normal women. The external genitalia are unambiguously female, as illustrated in Fig. 48-7. The labia and clitoris are normal or somewhat underdeveloped. The vagina is blind-ending; although usually adequate for successful coitus,

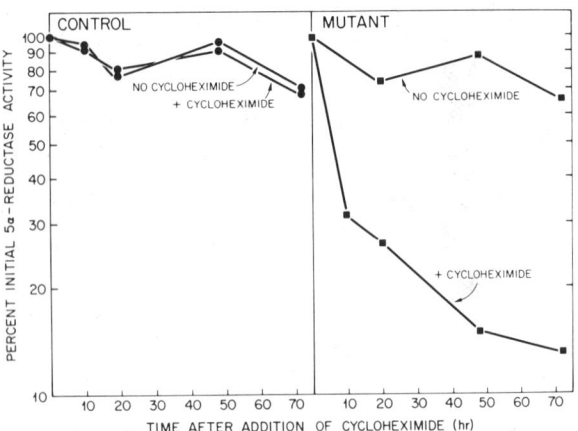

Figure 48-11 Stability of 5α-reductase in intact fibroblasts from a control subject and a patient with the unstable variant of 5α-reductase deficiency. On day 7 after plating 1 mM cycloheximide was added to half the samples of fibroblasts from a control and a mutant subject (the same subject labeled unstable enzyme in Fig. 48-10). 5α-Reductase was assayed in the whole cell at varying intervals. (*Redrawn from Leshin, et al. [73].*)

it may be absent or shallow. There is an absence of internal genitalia except for gonads that have the histologic features of undescended testes (normal or increased Leydig cells and seminiferous tubules without spermatogenesis). The testes may be located in the abdomen, along the course of the inguinal canal, or in the labia majora. Occasionally, remnants of müllerian or Wolffian origin can be identified in the paratesticular fascia or in fibrous bands extending from the testes. Morris [2] also noted the occurrence of tumors in the cryptorchid testes of affected subjects and concluded on the basis of bioassay data that the testes produce both androgens and estrogens, with the consequence that the disease could not be explained as the result of testicular inadequacy.

Subsequent studies in other laboratories have provided additional information about this disorder. The findings that nuclear chromatin is male in character [90, 91], that the chromosomal complement is 46,XY, and that the chromosomes are of normal structure [92–94] confirmed the deduction from pedigree analysis and gonadal histology that the affected individuals are genetic males. The presence of testes as well as the normal male expression of the H-Y antigen in cells of affected individuals indicate that the Y-linked genetic determinants for testicular differentiation function normally [95]. This interpretation is supported by the finding that the gonads in 47,XXY individuals with testicular feminization are testes [96]. It is of interest that affected subjects tend to be rather tall for women, averaging 171 cm in height in one series [81], that bone age corresponds to the chronologic age [81], and that tooth size is as large as in normal men (and larger than in normal women) [97]. The fact that height and tooth size are greater than those of normal women suggests that the effect of the Y chromosome on these parameters may not be mediated by androgens. Adrenal and thyroid function are normal, and there are no commonly associated clinical anomalies [81]. Intelligence is normal [98], and psychologic development is unmistakably feminine in regard to behavior, outlook, and maternal instincts [99].

Estimates of incidence vary from 1 in 20,000 to 1 in 64,000 male births [81, 100–102]. Through studies of buccal smears, it has been estimated that as many as 1 to 2 percent of girls with inguinal hernias may have the disorder [100–102]. In a nationwide survey in Japan, testicular feminization was the

most common form of primary resistance to hormone action, some 390 patients having been ascertained in a 10-year period [103]. This disorder is also the third most frequent cause of primary amenorrhea in women after gonadal dysgenesis and congenital absence of the vagina [104].

The most important insight into the nature of the disorder was the demonstration that these women have a profound resistance to the action of both exogenous and endogenous androgens. Wilkins [3] gave methyltestosterone in large doses to such a woman following castration and showed that there was no growth of sexual hair (despite documentation of the presence of pubic hair follicles by biopsy), no enlargement of the clitoris, no change in the voice, and no other obvious clinical effect. Subsequent work confirmed the lack of growth of pubic hair in response to androgen treatment [105, 106] and demonstrated as well a lack of response to exogenous androgens in regard to sebum production [106], failure of the expected decrease in thyroxine-binding globulin concentration in plasma [107, 108], diminished feedback on the secretion of LH by the pituitary [109], and no effect on phosphorus and nitrogen balance [110–112]. Thus, by every variable measured, resistance to the action of androgen appears to be virtually absolute in the complete form of testicular feminization.

The histologic characteristics of the testes are similar to those in cryptorchid testes due to other causes but differ in that spermatogenesis is virtually always absent (present in half of age-matched cryptorchid testes), germinal elements are detected only rarely, and adenoma formation of the Sertoli cells is frequent [113–115]. Although the number of Leydig cells per high-power field is increased [113], the total volume and number of Leydig cells is probably normal [116]. The Leydig cells vary considerably in size and degree of differentiation [117–118].

INCOMPLETE TESTICULAR FEMINIZATION   The term incomplete testicular feminization was introduced by Prader [119] and by Morris and Mahesh [120] to characterize subjects who resemble individuals with the complete disorder but who have some ambiguity of the external genitalia and who experience some virilization as well as feminization at puberty. The term was utilized subsequently in descriptions of various types of incomplete male pseudohermaphroditism, including individu-

Table 48-4 Clinical features of complete testicular feminization

External phenotype: Female external genitalia with underdevelopment of the labia and a blind-ending vagina, female habitus and breast development, paucity of axillary and pubic hair
Internal phenotype: Testes that may be intraabdominal, along the course of the inguinal canal, or in the labia; absent Wolffian and müllerian derivatives
Karyotype: 46,XY
Inheritance: X-linked recessive
Endocrinology:
   Testosterone: Normal or high male plasma levels and production rates
   Estrogen: Plasma levels and production rates higher than in normal men
   Gonadotropin: Elevated plasma LH levels
Pathogenesis: Complete resistance to all actions of testosterone and dihydrotestosterone

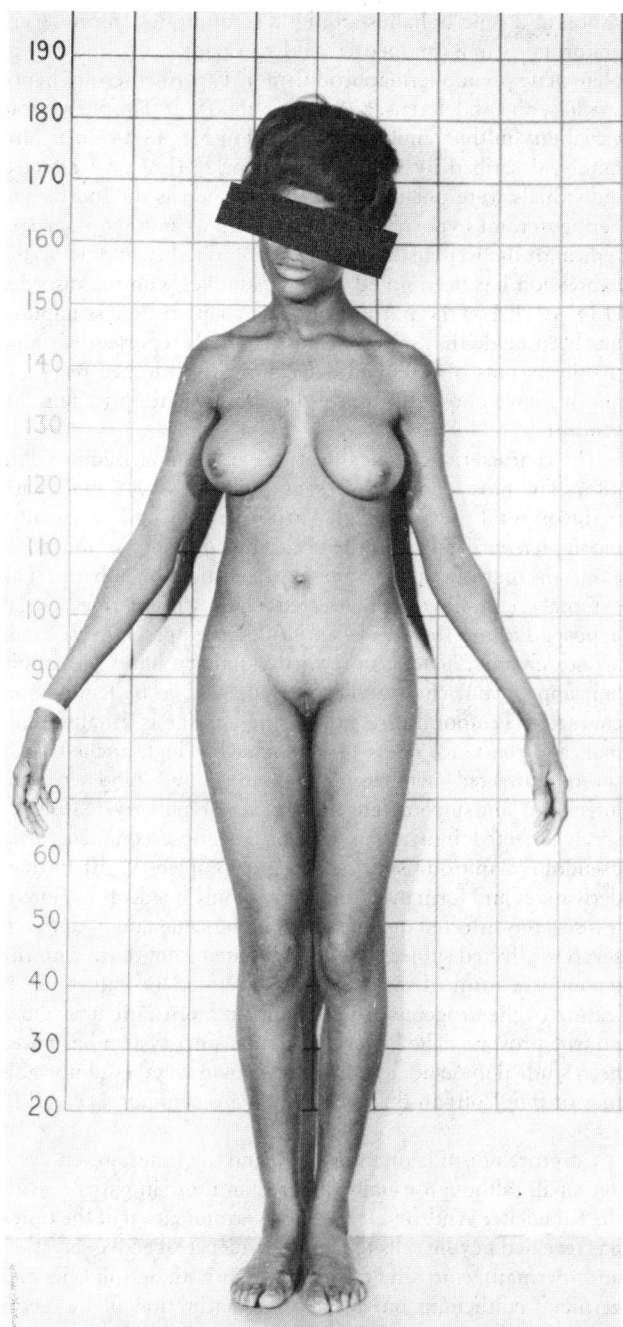

Figure 48-12 Photograph of patient with complete testicular feminization. (*From Wilson and Walsh [48].*)

in the abdomen or in the inguinal canals and are indistinguishable on histologic grounds from those in complete testicular feminization. The external genitalia are distinctive in that partial fusion of the labioscrotal folds and a variable degree of clitoromegaly are present (Fig. 48-8). The vagina, like that in complete testicular feminization, is short and ends blindly. At the expected time of puberty both variable feminization and partial virilization may take place. All müllerian duct derivatives are absent, but Wolffian duct structures are present; this latter feature, together with the partial virilization of the external genitalia, clearly separates the phenotype from that of testicular feminization. Not only are upper Wolffian duct structures present (epididymides and vasa deferentia), but in addition the terminal derivatives of the Wolffian ducts, including the ampullae of the vasa deferentia, the seminal vesicles, and the ejaculatory ducts are male in character (although probably underdeveloped in comparison with those of a normal man). The ejaculatory ducts empty into the vagina. Thus, the syndrome has certain features that resemble testicular feminization (female breast development), some that resemble 5α-reductase deficiency (presence of male Wolffian duct derivatives and ambiguous external genitalia), and some that resemble the Reifenstein syndrome (mixed virilization and feminization at the time of expected puberty).

The frequency of this disorder is uncertain, but in most series (including the personal experience of the authors) it is only about a tenth as frequent as the complete form of testicular feminization.

REIFENSTEIN SYNDROME   A number of families have been described in which individuals with hereditary male pseudohermaphroditism have a failure of virilization less complete than seen in patients with incomplete testicular feminization. In each family the disorder is inherited as an apparent X-linked recessive trait. Although the common phenotype is male, affected individuals within a given family may have a spectrum of abnormalities ranging from almost complete failure of virilization to nearly complete masculinization. The disorder has been described under a variety of terms, including Reifenstein syndrome [125, 126], Lubs syndrome [127], Gilbert-Dreyfus syndrome [128], Rosewater syndrome [129], and familial incomplete male pseudohermaphroditism, type 1 [130], but the most common appellation is that of the Reifenstein syn-

Table 48-5   Clinical features of incomplete testicular feminization

---

External phenotype: Clitoromegaly and partial fusion of the labioscrotal folds, female habitus and breast development, normal axillary and pubic hair
Internal phenotype: Testes that may or may not be cryptorchid, underdeveloped Wolffian duct derivatives that empty into the vagina, no müllerian duct derivatives
Karyotype: 46,XY
Inheritance: X-linked recessive
Endocrinology:
  Testosterone: Normal or high male plasma levels and production rates
  Estrogen: Plasma levels and production rates higher than in normal men
  Gonadotropin: Elevated plasma LH level
Pathogenesis: Partial resistance to the actions of testosterone and dihydrotestosterone

als with defects of testosterone synthesis, men with the Reifenstein syndrome, and many subjects for whom data are not available to determine the etiology of the underlying disorders. Nevertheless, certain of these patients constitute a distinct phenotype associated with resistance to androgen action; such patients have abnormalities of the androgen receptor and appear to be genetically distinct from other forms of androgen resistance [121–124].

The clinical features of this disorder are summarized in Table 48-5. Affected individuals have the habitus and general appearance of women (Fig. 48-13) and like women with the complete form of the disorder most commonly present because of primary amenorrhea. The karyotype is 46,XY; the testes are

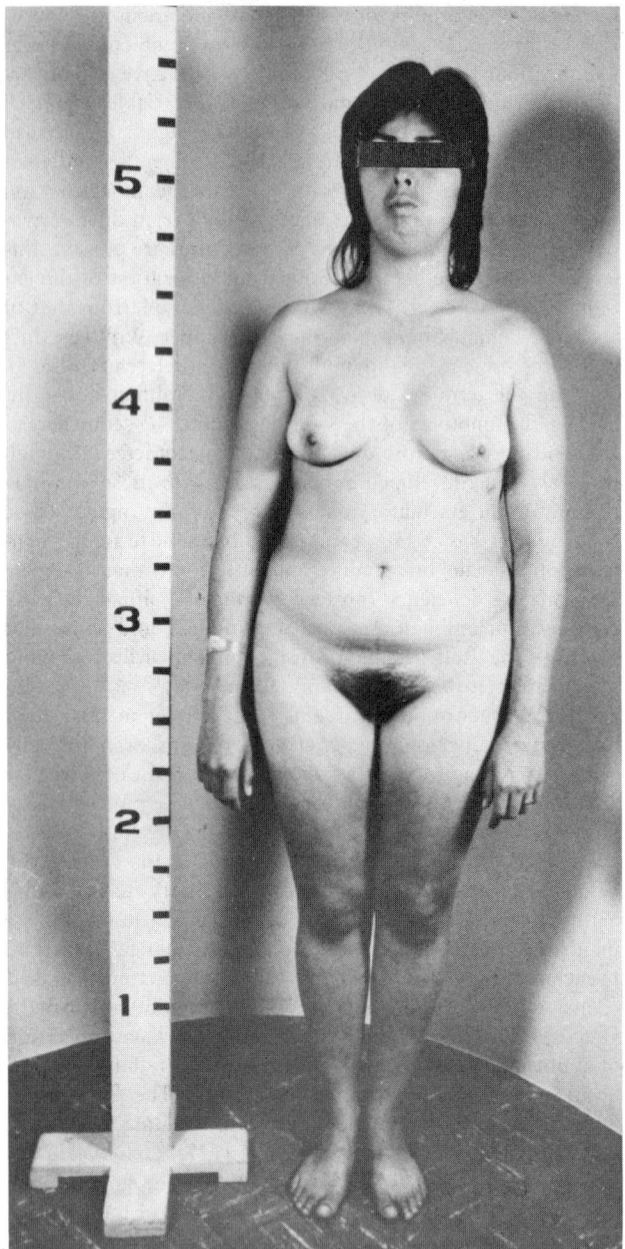

Figure 48-13 Photograph of patient with incomplete testicular feminization. *(From Madden et al. [124].)*

zation in 2 (microphallus and bifid scrotum) to a more severe abnormality in 8 (perineoscrotal hypospadias) to almost complete male pseudohermaphroditism in 1 (perineoscrotal hypospadias, no vas deferens, and a vaginal orifice). The phenotypic variability in this family is illustrated in Fig. 48-14. In a third family, described by Gardo and Papp [133], 3 of 4 affected individuals were phenotypic females, whereas the fourth had perineoscrotal hypospadias, bifid scrotum, and gynecomastia typical of the Reifenstein syndrome. Variability in phenotypic expression has been noted in other families with the disorder [134, 135]. For the purposes of this chapter, the assumption has been made that these various disorders represent variable manifestations of X-linked defects in the androgen receptor, and we have chosen to utilize the eponymic term Reifenstein syndrome.

The characteristic clinical features are summarized in Table 48-6. The most common presentation is a 46,XY male with perineoscrotal hypospadias, azoospermia and infertility, incomplete virilization at the usual time of puberty, and gynecomastia that develops at the expected time of puberty. The external genitalia of an affected child with perineoscrotal hypospadias are shown in Fig. 48-7. Development of secondary sex characteristics is noteworthy in that axillary and pubic hair appear, but chest and facial hair tend to be feminine in character. Temporal recession of the hairline is usually minimal, and the voice tends to be somewhat high-pitched. Less severely affected members may exhibit only a bifid scrotum, infertility, and incomplete virilization at puberty. More severely affected individuals can have almost complete male pseudohermaphroditism, including incomplete Wolffian duct derivatives and formation of a vagina; only by identification of less severely affected members within the same family can such severely affected subjects be differentiated from those with the incomplete form of testicular feminization. Incomplete virilization of the urogenital sinus results in a prostatic utricle but no true prostate. The lower ejaculatory duct system has never been studied in detail, and it is not known whether abnormalities of the Wolffian duct derivatives are common [126, 130, 132].

Cryptorchidism is often present, and the testes are on average small (although usually larger than those in patients with the Klinefelter syndrome). Histologic examination of the testes has revealed Leydig cells that show evidence of active secretion and spermatogenic tubules that contain both Sertoli cells and germinal epithelium but usually no maturation of the germ cells beyond the primary spermatocyte stage. Hyaline degeneration of the tubules is often found [126].

Certain features of the disorder are of particular interest. First, although affected individuals have been raised as women [132], most are raised as men. While the total number of reported subjects is small and no in-depth psychologic studies have been performed, gender identity in affected subjects raised as men appears to be unambiguously male in character, and some have had successful marriages. Second, infertility is the most consistent feature of the syndrome and appears to be the result of both defective spermatogenesis and of the anatomic abnormalities of the ejaculatory system.

INFERTILE MALE SYNDROME   In a family study of the Reifenstein syndrome, some affected men were identified who were infertile but otherwise phenotypically normal. They had the same apparent degree of androgen resistance, as assessed by endocrinologic criteria [130] and the same apparent degree

drome. Evidence that these disorders are in fact variable manifestations of a similar mutation was derived from pedigree analyses. Several large families have been described in which individual affected members exhibited phenotypes that vary from infertility in otherwise normal men to an extreme form of male pseudohermaphroditism in which the subjects have a vaginal orifice, no vas deferens, and severe hypospadias. The most extensive of these pedigrees is that reported originally by Ford [131] and subsequently by Walker et al. [132]. In this family the manifestations in 12 affected men ranged from moderate abnormalities (microphallus and gynecomastia) to intermediate defects of virilization (hypospadias) to defects of virilization (complete failure of scrotal fusion) so severe that 3 affected members were identified initially as females [132]. In the family reported originally by Bowen et al. [126] and subsequently by Wilson et al. [130], the phenotype in 11 affected family members also ranged from a moderate defect in virili-

Table 48-6 Clinical features of the Reifenstein syndrome

External phenotype: Usually a male with perineoscrotal hypospadias, normal axillary and pubic hair but scanty beard development and body hair; breast enlargement at time of expected puberty

Internal phenotype: Testes which are often cryptorchid, Wolffian duct structures vary in the degree of male development, no müllerian duct derivatives

Karyotype: 46,XY

Inheritance: X-linked recessive

Endocrinology:

Testosterone: Normal or high male plasma levels and production rates

Estrogen: Plasma levels and production rates higher than those in normal men

Gonadotropin: Elevated plasma LH levels

Pathogenesis: Variable resistance to the action of testosterone and dihydrotestosterone

of abnormality of the androgen receptor in cultured skin fibroblasts as did the more severely affected first-degree relatives [136]. Gynecomastia was variable and late in appearance. Thus, it was clear that individuals with the Reifenstein syndrome may have only mild phenotypic evidence of androgen receptor deficiency. Subsequently, it was established that some infertile men without a family history of the Reifenstein syndrome have endocrine evidence of androgen resistance, and the androgen resistance is associated with an abnormality of the androgen receptor similar to the defect demonstrated in individuals with familial Reifenstein syndrome [137]. The clinical features of these men are summarized in Table 48-7. Such individuals have normal male external genitalia, apparently normal Wolffian duct structures, and infertility due to absence or to an extreme deficiency in sperm production. The prevalence of this form of androgen resistance as a cause of male infertility is not established, but in one survey it appears to account for as much as a fifth to a third of infertility associated with idiopathic azoospermia or severe oligospermia [138]. Thus, the infertile male syndrome may be not only the most common form of abnormality of the androgen receptor but the most common form of primary resistance to the action of any hormone.

Endocrinology The endocrine pattern is similar in all forms of androgen-receptor disorders but has been best char-

acterized in complete testicular feminization. The early deductions by Morris [2] and by Wilkins [3] that androgen production in testicular feminization is normal have been confirmed and extended. For example, the conversion of radiolabeled precursors to testosterone by in vitro preparations of the testes of persons with complete testicular feminization is within normal limits [139–150]. Plasma levels of testosterone are either in the normal male range or somewhat higher than those of normal men [10, 141, 145, 147, 151–155], a phenomenon that is probably due to two factors: (1) the patients have elevated estrogen production rates (see below) that result in an increase in the level of plasma testosterone-binding globulin, and (2) blood production rates of testosterone tend to be somewhat higher than in normal men [10]. As in normal men the testes are responsible for the major portion of testosterone production [20, 144, 147, 156]. In one study of 6 affected subjects the daily production of testosterone averaged about 50 percent more than in normal men (8.3 versus 5.7 mg/day), but in individual subjects testosterone production was greater than that of the control men only in those with inguinal testes and not in those with intraabdominal testes [10] (Fig. 48-2).

The elevated testosterone production rate is presumably secondary to high levels of LH in plasma, which in turn is the consequence of defective feedback regulation because of resistance at the hypothalamic-pituitary level to the feedback effects of androgen on LH production [109, 153, 155, 157]. The elevated plasma LH level is the result of two interlocking phenomena—more frequent secretory episodes and greater amplitude of the secretory spikes as compared to normal [155]. The increase in plasma LH level after the administration of luteinizing hormone releasing hormone (LHRH) is within the normal range [155]. In virtually all studies, plasma levels of follicle stimulating hormone (FSH) have been normal [155]. Although there is failure of the negative feedback regulation of LH secretion by androgens in persons with testicular feminization, two types of evidence indicate that in the steady state LH secretion in these patients is regulated by estradiol. Namely, following castration plasma LH rises to even higher levels, and the administration of the antiestrogen compound clomiphene citrate to these individuals prior to castration results in a further increase in plasma LH [158].

The origin of estrogen in women with testicular feminization has been defined in detail and is illustrated in Fig. 48-2 [10]. In four women with complete testicular feminization the mean

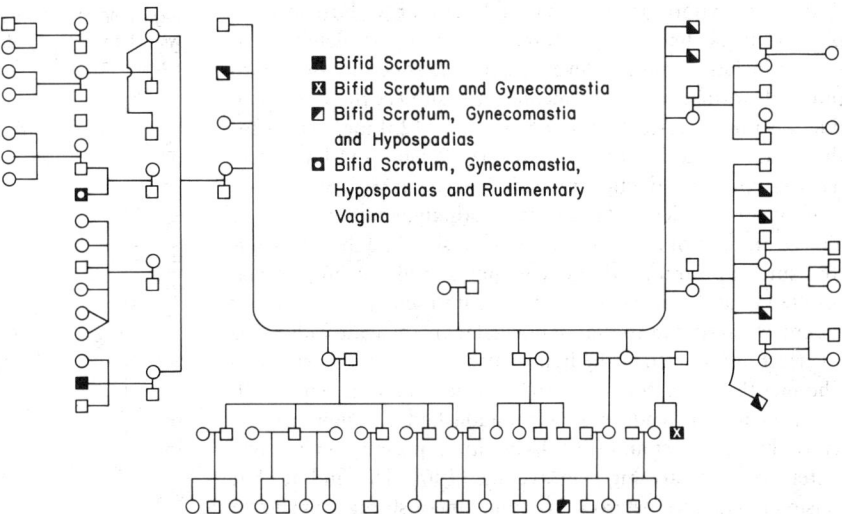

Figure 48-14 Pedigree of a family with Reifenstein syndrome. (*From Wilson et al.* [130].)

■ Bifid Scrotum
▨ Bifid Scrotum and Gynecomastia
▧ Bifid Scrotum, Gynecomastia and Hypospadias
▣ Bifid Scrotum, Gynecomastia, Hypospadias and Rudimentary Vagina

Table 48-7   Clinical features of the infertile male syndrome

External phenotype: Normal man with tendency to minimal male beard and body hair, occasional gynecomastia
Internal phenotype: Testes, infertility associated with azoospermia or extreme oligospermia, Wolffian duct structures of normal men, no müllerian duct derivatives
Karyotype: 46,XY
Inheritance: Probably X-linked recessive
Endocrinology:
  Testosterone: Plasma levels and production rates of normal men or slightly higher
  Estrogen: Production rates usually higher than in normal men
  Gonadotropin: Plasma LH levels usually elevated
Pathogenesis: Resistance to the action of androgen principally in the testes

production rates of estrone and estradiol, respectively, were 114 and 77 µg/day (as contrasted to 66 and 45 µg/day, respectively, in normal young men). The amount of estradiol production due to testicular secretion in these women averaged 42 µg/day (in contrast to a mean secretion rate of 6 µg/day by the testes of normal men). Thus, not only is the production rate of the potent estrogen estradiol increased, but in addition the major portion of this increased production is due to secretion by the testes. This is in keeping with the demonstration by Southren and coworkers [86, 143] that estrogen formation can be demonstrated in in vitro preparations of testes from subjects with testicular feminization and with the report by Kelch and coworkers [20] and by Laatikainen et al. [156] that spermatic vein estradiol concentrations are high in women with testicular feminization.

To summarize, resistance to the feedback regulation of LH production by circulating androgen results in elevated plasma LH levels, and this in turn results in the enhanced secretion of both testosterone and estradiol by the testes. The fact that gonadotropin levels rise even higher (and that symptoms of menopausal flushing develop) when the testes are removed is consistent with the view that gonadotropin secretion is under some type of regulatory control; presumably, in the steady state and in the absence of an effect of androgen, estrogen alone regulates LH secretion in subjects with testicular feminization. This feedback control is purchased at the expense of a higher plasma estrogen level than in normal men [109, 158].

Endocrine findings in incomplete testicular feminization and Reifenstein syndrome are remarkably similar to those in complete testicular feminization (Fig. 48-2). In incomplete testicular feminization plasma levels of testosterone are similar to those of normal men, and in one such subject the daily production rate of testosterone was greater (12.0 mg/day) [124] than the average in normal men [10]. Plasma LH levels and daily estrogen production rates and estrogen secretion by the testes were also elevated [124]. Interestingly, administration of a large amount of estradiol benzoate to simulate the preovulatory surge of estradiol that occurs in normally cycling women resulted in an LH surge in a subject with incomplete testicular feminization similar to that of normal women, again indicating an effect of estrogen at the hypothalamic-pituitary level [159]. The fact that gonadotropins are also elevated in persons with the Reifenstein syndrome was established through urinary assays by Bowen et al. [126]. In addition, plasma LH and testosterone levels are high on average [130]. The finding that plasma LH and testosterone are simultaneously high (as shown

in Fig. 48-15) again suggests that there is defective feedback control of LH secretion by testosterone at the hypothalamic-pituitary level. When LHRH is administered to subjects with Reifenstein syndrome, the surge in plasma LH is either normal or somewhat greater than normal [149, 155]. Furthermore, plasma LH does not decrease following administration of medroxyprogesterone acetate (Depo-Provera) [130], testosterone [161], or dihydrotestosterone [155]. These findings further substantiate the concept that the incomplete male differentiation during embryogenesis and the defective virilization at the expected time of puberty are the result of a defect in androgen action. Quantitative studies of the rates of androgen and estrogen formation have provided further insight into the phenotype in this disorder [130]. One such study is summarized in Fig. 48-2. The production rates for plasma testosterone (9.2 mg/day) and for the estradiol (199 µg/day) were high; three-fourths of the estradiol (147 µg), 10 times the normal amount, was secreted directly into the circulation, presumably from the testes [130].

The endocrine changes in men with infertility due to androgen resistance are similar to but less marked than those in subjects with other forms of androgen receptor defects (Fig. 48-2). Namely, plasma production rates of testosterone and plasma levels of LH are normal to high, and estradiol production rates are elevated [137].

It is possible to deduce from these findings the mechanism by which feminization occurs in individuals with defects of the androgen receptor. In each disorder androgen resistance usually results in a high mean level of plasma LH, elevated estradiol secretion by the testes, and the appearance of feminizing signs at puberty. There is, however, no direct relation between the absolute amount of estrogen secretion and the degree of feminization. Indeed, two phenotypic men with Reifenstein syndrome had estrogen secretion rates greater than any that have been found to date in any individual with either complete or incomplete testicular feminization [130]. We conclude that feminization in subjects with androgen resistance is dependent upon increased estradiol production after puberty, but that the degree of feminization is influenced by the severity of the androgen resistance. The effective ratio of estradiol to androgen at some cellular level must be the rate-limiting factor that determines the degree of feminization. It follows that the variable feminization that occurs in infertile men with androgen resistance is a function both of a less complete resistance to the

Figure 48-15 Serum testosterone in postpubescent men from one family with Reifenstein syndrome as a function of serum LH concentration. Same patients as in Fig. 48-14. (*From Wilson et al. [130].*)

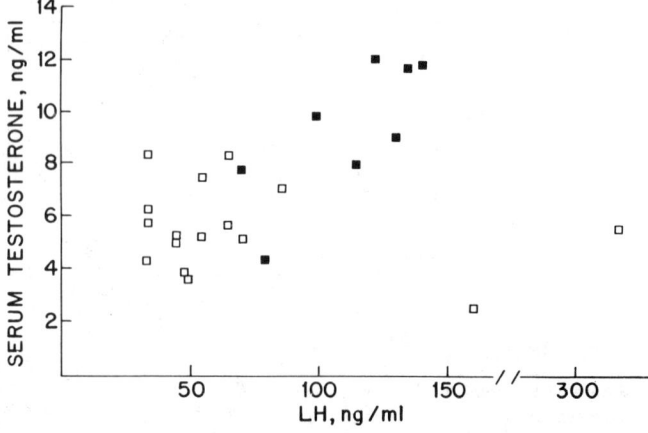

action of androgen at the cellular level and to the inconsistent increase in estradiol formation.

The metabolism of testosterone in the peripheral tissues of persons with the various receptor abnormalities, and in particular the conversion of testosterone to dihydrotestosterone, has been investigated in considerable detail. As shown in Table 48-3 dihydrotestosterone formation is low on average in skin slices from patients with complete testicular feminization [76, 121, 162], and in some patients the excretion of dihydrotestosterone metabolites in urine is also decreased [163, 164]. This decrease in 5α-reductase activity is believed to be secondary to the primary defect in androgen action that leads to a decrease in the mass of androgen target tissues (or organelles) that form dihydrotestosterone [165]. A defect in dihydrotestosterone formation is not manifested in fibroblasts cultured from skin biopsies from most such individuals [78]. Furthermore, in incomplete testicular feminization [124] and the Reifenstein syndrome [130] dihydrotestosterone formation in biopsied skin is normal (Table 48-3) as it is in fibroblasts cultured from skin [77–80]. Thus, on endocrine, genetic, and phenotypic grounds these individuals are clearly distinct from subjects with 5α-reductase deficiency.

Genetics The familial occurrence of complete testicular feminization was documented in 1912 [81], and by 1937 sufficient pedigree data were available for Pettersson and Bonnier [84] to conclude that the disorder could be explained either as an X-linked recessive trait or as an autosomal trait that is manifested only in genetic males. Since all affected individuals are infertile, these two possibilities could not be resolved by pedigree analysis. Furthermore, attempts to establish X linkage by studying the association between testicular feminization and other X-linked traits such as hemophilia and color blindness in specific pedigrees were uninformative [166–169]. So many crossovers occurred that it was possible to conclude only that if the trait is X-linked the genetic locus for the mutation is so far away from the loci for color blindness and hemophilia as to preclude mapping.

Two other types of evidence have accrued in favor of X-linkage. The disorder appears to be common in the animal kingdom, since similar mutations have been found in the dog [170], cow [171], rat [172], mouse [173], horse [174], and chimpanzee [175]. In the mouse the mutant gene was shown to be X-linked by mapping techniques [173]. Since there are no known instances in which X-linked genes in one species are autosomal in other species [176], documentation of X-linkage for the gene in the mouse has been interpreted as evidence for location of the mutation on the X chromosome in other species as well. In addition, Meyer et al. [177] found that a significant population of fibroblast clones cultured from an obligate heterozygote for complete testicular feminization had deficient androgen binding, whereas binding in the remaining clones approximated the normal range. This finding is compatible with random inactivation of one X-linked allele in each cell, as would be predicted by the Lyon hypothesis [178], and is indicative of the presence of the gene on the human X chromosome.

Although the ratio of genetic men to women in the affected sibships is 1:1, a preponderance of affected to normal men (4:1) has been observed repeatedly [179] since the original study of Pettersson and Bonnier [84]. Lenz has interpreted this apparent enrichment of affected to normal men as the result of a statistical artifact of selection, since the family with no or

only one affected member is less likely to be ascertained [180]. The fact that in the mouse the ratio of affected to normal males is 1:1 is in keeping with this view [173].

It would be of major importance for genetic counseling if a means were available for diagnosing the obligate heterozygote before pregnancy. Although Nowakowski and Lenz [53] reported that some carriers of the disorder have diminished body hair, no clearcut means of identifying the carrier has been established. The finding of Meyer et al. [177] that approximately half of fibroblast clones derived from the skin of heterozygous carriers have absent androgen binding makes it theoretically possible to diagnose such individuals in some families.

Although the familial occurrence of testicular feminization is the usual clinical finding, approximately a third of women with the typical phenotype and endocrine changes of complete testicular feminization have negative family histories. Since affected individuals cannot reproduce, the natural selection against persistence of the mutation is strong; it is believed that the majority of patients with negative family histories are the result of new mutations [81].

The family history in most cases of incomplete testicular feminization is uninformative. In at least one family the pattern of inheritance is compatible with X-linkage [182]. As originally pointed out by Morris and Mahesh [120], no convincing pedigree has been reported in which the complete and incomplete forms of testicular feminization coexist in the same family.

A number of pedigrees of the Reifenstein syndrome have been described in which the inheritance pattern, like that of testicular feminization, is compatible either with an X-linked recessive gene or with an autosomal mutation that is manifested only in genetic males [125, 126, 130–135, 161]. (One such pedigree is shown in Fig. 48-14 [130].) As in complete testicular feminization, linkage studies in three families have not resolved the question of whether an X-linked or an autosomal mutation is involved [126, 183, 184]. Nor has it been possible to utilize cloning studies of cultured human fibroblasts to resolve this issue as was done for complete testicular feminization.

The genetic basis for the infertile male syndrome is less clear. In most affected men described to date, the family history is uninformative [137]. In three instances multiple family members are affected, and the family pedigree in each is compatible with either X-linkage or autosomal inheritance manifested only in men (unpublished observations of the authors).

Indirect evidence suggests that each of these disorders is inherited as an X-linked trait. Each has been documented to involve the same gene product, namely the androgen receptor, and since X-linkage has been established in one of the disorders—complete testicular feminization—the implication is that X-linkage is common to all. The finding that all pedigree analyses in the various disorders (when informative) are compatible with X-linked inheritance and that X-linkage is known to be conservative among species [176] further support this interpretation. This is not to imply that a single mutation is common to the various disorders—only that a variety of mutations of the X chromosome in humans influence the amount and function of the androgen receptor.

Pathogenesis Androgen resistance in testicular feminization is due to abnormalities of the androgen receptor. The basic study that allowed this problem to be investigated was the observation by Keenan and coworkers that a specific dihydrotestosterone receptor protein is present in fibroblasts cultured from the skin of normal subjects [185, 186]. The receptor content is greater in fibroblasts cultured from genital skin sites (foreskin, scrotum, labia majora) than from nongenital sites [136]. The receptor has a dissociation constant of approximately 1 nM and is believed to be the same as the intracellular receptor protein in androgen target tissues (Fig. 48-3). Furthermore, Keenan et al. established that fibroblasts grown from some women with complete testicular feminization showed no detectable dihydrotestosterone binding [185], a finding that has been confirmed in other laboratories [136, 187]. The finding of absent binding in fibroblasts from some patients with testicular feminization is illustrated in Fig. 48-16 and provides an explanation for the profound resistance to all androgen actions in this disorder [Fig. 48-6]. Whether absent binding of dihydrotestosterone in such cases is due to true absence of the androgen receptor protein or whether the mutant protein is present but cannot bind the ligand is not known.

Recently, evidence has accrued indicating that other subjects with complete testicular feminization do have a qualitatively abnormal receptor protein (Fig. 48-16). Identification of such a phenomenon came first from studies of thermolability of binding [182] and subsequently from studies of stabilization of the receptor by sodium molybdate [188]. The initial studies involved fibroblasts from two sisters with complete testicular feminization who had about half the normal levels of binding under the usual assay conditions at 37°C and normal binding at 26°C. When the assay was performed at an elevated temperature (42°C) dihydrotestosterone binding decreased to less than a fifth that seen at 37°C (Fig. 48-16). The binding is rapidly restored on lowering the assay temperature to 37°C, suggesting that the alteration of the structure at elevated temperatures is reversible [182]. Similar receptor thermolability has been observed by Pinsky et al. [189]. Qualitative abnormalities of the receptor in subsequent experiments have also been iden-

tified by examining the ultracentrifugation characteristics of the cytosol receptor in the presence of molybdate, a compound that stabilizes the normal 8 S androgen receptor but not the receptor from many subjects with androgen resistance [188].

The characteristics of the androgen receptor in fibroblasts grown from biopsies of individuals from 35 families that fulfill the phenotypic and endocrine requirements to be designated androgen resistance, including 15 families with complete testicular feminization, are summarized in Fig. 48-17. Receptor has been designated as qualitatively abnormal when it is measurable in intact cells at 37°C and exhibits thermolability or inability to form an 8 S complex in the presence of molybdate, or both. In 9 such families binding was virtually undetectable in fibroblast monolayers at any temperature and was designated as absent. These families are representative of the receptor-negative category of testicular feminization identified in the early studies of the problem [136, 185–187].

The deduction that the deficiency of the receptor in fibroblasts grown from biopsies of these subjects reflects the in vivo situation has been substantiated by the demonstration that the androgen receptor was missing from the testis of a woman with complete testicular feminization [190]. These findings also indicate that the pathogenesis of androgen resistance in the human disorder is similar to that in the mouse with testicular feminization, since absence of the high-affinity cytosol androgen receptor protein in the mouse had been reported previously in several laboratories [191–196]. Such a defect could not be the explanation for the androgen resistance in the remaining families with complete testicular feminization. In five families with complete testicular feminization the receptor was measurable but was thermolabile in monolayers and/or unstable in fibroblast cytosol preparations, and in one family the receptor was normal in amount and stable (Fig. 48-17). Likewise, in the initial studies in fibroblasts grown from a subject with incomplete testicular feminization binding was about half normal. On the other hand, when binding in fibroblasts from affected individuals from seven families with incomplete testicular feminization was measured, a qualitative abnormality was demonstrated in four, a diminished amount of binding was present in one family, and no defect could be identified in the other two families (Fig. 48-17). Similarly, in the initial studies of the Reifenstein syndrome [136, 197–199] and the infertile male syndrome [137] the only defect identified was a diminished amount of binding. When this residual binding was reexamined and additional patients were studied, the androgen receptor was found to be qualitatively abnormal in two Reifenstein families and three infertile men and was diminished in amount in three Reifenstein families and four unrelated infertile men (Fig. 48-17) [188]. In affected subjects of four families (three with the phenotype of testicular feminization and one infertile male) no abnormality of the androgen receptor was demonstrable, in spite of endocrine evidence of profound androgen resistance (see "Receptor-Positive Resistance" below).

To summarize, absent binding appears to be associated with the syndrome of complete testicular feminization. Qualitatively abnormal receptors and decreased amounts of receptor are associated with a spectrum of phenotypes from female to male. We assume that those qualitative defects associated with complete testicular feminization are the result of mutations that impair the in vivo function of the receptor more severely than do those mutations that cause the infertile male syndrome. The category, designated "decreased amount of recep-

Figure 48-16 Androgen receptor assay in fibroblasts from a normal control and from patients with testicular feminization due to absent binding or abnormal receptor. Specific dihydrotestosterone binding in intact fibroblast monolayers as a function of dihydrotestosterone concentration was assessed at two temperatures (37°C and 42°C) in cells grown from a normal control subject (A), a patient with complete testicular feminization associated with absent binding (B), and two unrelated patients with complete testicular feminization associated with intermediate levels of dihydrotestosterone binding at 37°C (C and D). (From Griffin [182].)

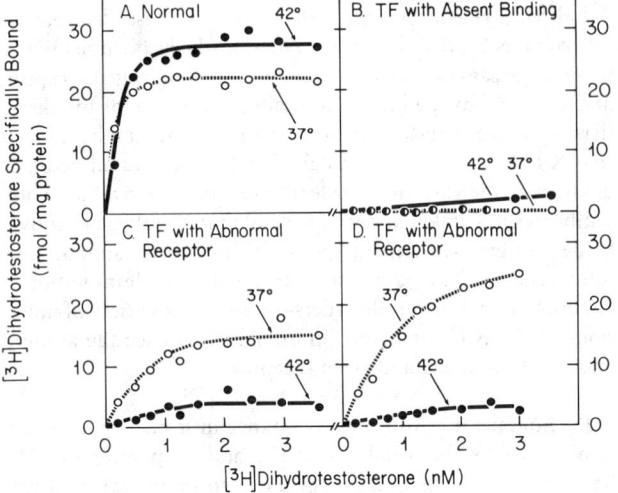

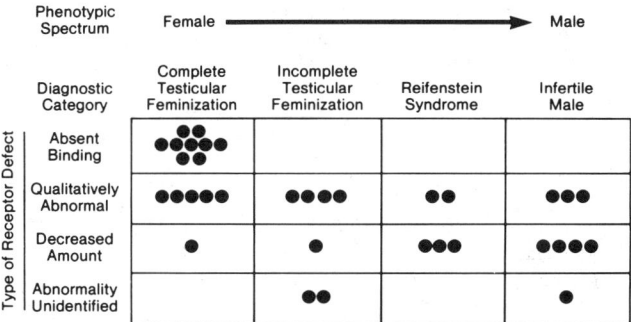

Figure 48-17 Androgen receptor assays in subjects from 35 families with androgen resistance and putative defects in the androgen receptor. The 35 families include 32 families with established defects of the androgen receptor and three with no abnormality identified (receptor-positive resistance). Absent binding is associated with the phenotype of complete testicular feminization, but the qualitative and quantitative defects in the receptor can be associated with a spectrum of phenotypes from complete testicular feminization to infertile men. (*Redrawn from Griffin and Durrant [188].*)

tor," is likewise a mixture of quantitative defects and qualitative abnormalities not yet identified. As more subtle tests of receptor function become available it will be possible to assess structure-function relationships more completely.

Receptor-Positive Resistance

A category of androgen resistance that does not appear to involve either the 5α-reductase or the androgen receptor was identified by Amrhein et al. [200] in three affected members of one family with the phenotype of testicular feminization and with normal 5α-reductase, normal amounts of androgen receptor, and normal nuclear localization of dihydrotestosterone. The subjects are 46,XY and have bilateral testes and normal or high levels of testosterone and LH in plasma. Subsequent subjects have been described with a variety of phenotypes ranging from incomplete testicular feminization to findings similar to those in the Reifenstein syndrome [201–204]. The site of the molecular abnormality in these patients is unclear (Fig. 48-6). It is possible that the receptor is qualitatively abnormal but that the defect is too subtle to be detected by present methods. In the four subjects we have assessed—labeled "abnormality unidentified" in Fig. 48-17—all parameters of receptor function studied to date are normal, including affinity of binding, turnover rate, nuclear localization of the hormone receptor complex [201], and stability of binding both to elevated temperature [182] and to ultracentrifugation [188]. Alternatively, the defect may reside at some step in androgen action distal to the receptor, such as the site of generation of specific RNA. Indeed, it is not established that a uniform defect is present; the disorder may be comprised of a heterogeneous group of molecular abnormalities.

Differential Diagnosis of the Androgen Resistance Syndromes

Suspicion of androgen resistance is based upon genital ambiguity at birth, abnormal sexual development, or unexplained infertility in a 46,XY man. The androgen resistance syndromes are clearly separable from male pseudohermaphroditism caused by defective müllerian duct regression. The uterus and fallopian tubes are absent in the former but present in the latter

[49]. Furthermore, they are separable from the androgen deficiency states by the presence of normal (or elevated) male levels of plasma testosterone and plasma LH following the time of expected puberty (Chap. 47). It is true that patients with abnormal testosterone formation because of defects in one of the several enzymes involved in testosterone biosynthesis may have partial enzyme deficiency, and as a consequence plasma testosterone levels in the steady state may approach those of a normal man, but such partial defects are accompanied by elevations in the plasma levels of androgen precursors. For example, in 17β-hydroxysteroid dehydrogenase deficiency, the most common enzyme defect in testosterone biosynthesis, the level of plasma androstenedione in adults is 5 to 20 times greater than in controls [59, 205–208], and in affected children plasma androstenedione after administration of hCG is 5 times normal [209–210]. Plasma testosterone levels can also be used to separate the androgen resistance syndromes from those disorders in which the testes are absent because of a variety of developmental defects, including pure gonadal dysgenesis and the testicular regression syndrome. Subjects with the latter condition may exhibit a broad spectrum of defects, varying from a phenotypically normal male to that of a female with absent müllerian duct derivatives [48, 211]. Children with androgen resistance can be separated from those with defective testosterone synthesis (due either to single enzyme defects or to developmental defects of the testis) by demonstrating that plasma testosterone increases (to levels greater than 3 ng/ml) after suitable treatment with hCG [212–214]. Likewise, subjects with mixed gonadal dysgenesis are separable from those with androgen resistance syndromes on the basis of the karyotype, the presence of testes bilaterally, or both [48].

Once the diagnosis of an androgen resistance syndrome is suspected, careful analysis of the family history, the phenotype, the endocrine profile, and androgen metabolism in cultured fibroblasts may be required before a specific diagnosis can be made. The criteria that are presently available for this purpose are summarized in Table 48-8. The diagnosis of the Reifenstein syndrome is usually suspected early in life since most subjects are phenotypic males with incomplete development of the external genitalia. The critical separation that must be made in a given patient is between complete testicular feminization on the one hand and 5α-reductase deficiency and incomplete testicular feminization on the other. A precise diagnosis is of utmost importance in the prepubertal years; if the correct diagnosis is either 5α-reductase deficiency or incomplete testicular feminization and the girl is allowed to enter puberty prior to castration, irreversible and disfiguring virilization may occur during pubescence, whereas if the diagnosis is complete testicular feminization, such girls can be allowed to complete puberty prior to removal of the testes. In most circumstances, this distinction can be reached in a straightforward manner on the basis of the family history, phenotype, and endocrine findings. Of particular importance is the fact that the ratio of plasma testosterone to dihydrotestosterone is greater than 20 in 5α-reductase deficiency and 20 or less in controls [61, 65]. Major problems can be encountered in establishing a diagnosis of 5α-reductase deficiency in young children. This is particularly true when the family history is uninformative or negative, and as a consequence it is not possible to determine whether the disorder is the result of a new mutation or an autosomal recessive state. In the prepubertal years assessment of ratios of plasma testosterone to dihydrotestosterone following stimulation of the testis with hCG may be useful in making the diagnosis [61]; in addition, in most instances of incomplete testicular feminization and 5α-reductase deficiency the external genitalia are slightly abnormal. In some patients the assessment of androgen metabolism and androgen binding in fibroblasts cultured from genital skin is helpful in establishing the diagnosis of androgen receptor abnormality or 5α-reductase deficiency [4]. The diagnosis of Reifenstein syndrome is usually based upon the family history, phenotype, and characteristic endocrine pattern; the diagnosis is less urgent since most of these subjects are assigned male gender at birth, and pubertal virilization is desired.

Treatment

Since no specific therapy is available to circumvent or reverse the abnormal development that takes place during embryogenesis, therapy is directed toward prevention of complications and adverse secondary effects of the mutations, appropriate hormone replacement or supplementation when necessary, and suitable psychological support.

The Psychological Problems   Subjects with the infertile male syndrome and complete testicular feminization, respectively, have unambiguous male and female phenotypes at birth and are raised in accordance. Individuals with 5α-reductase deficiency, incomplete testicular feminization, and the Reifenstein syndrome have varying degrees of abnormal external genitalia, and the correct diagnosis can be made in the newborn babies or quite early in life. Since gender identity is critical to psychological development and normal mental health, it is mandatory that gender assignment be made as early as possible, preferably at the time of birth in individuals with ambiguous external genitalia. A detailed discussion of the diagnostic procedures and of the various problems encountered in reaching a decision about gender assignment in infants with ambiguous genitalia is given elsewhere [48]. Once gender assignment is made the central obligation is to conduct any indicated surgery as early as feasible, to provide the appropriate hormonal environment at the time of expected puberty, and to assist affected individuals to adjust to their inevitable infertility. Vaginal agenesis can be corrected after the time of expected puberty by surgical or nonsurgical means [215].

At any age in life it is unwise to inform patients that their genetic sex and phenotypic sex do not coincide. When castration is indicated it should be explained that as a result of a hereditary defect the gonads are abnormal, that the resulting infertility is not treatable, and that because of the potential for tumor development the gonads should be removed at a suitable time. With appropriate counseling and reassurance, most persons with male pseudohermaphroditism that we have managed have made adequate adjustment, especially in the case of phenotypic women (complete and incomplete testicular feminization and 5α-reductase deficiency).

The Cryptorchid Testis   The most serious complication of the undescended testis in complete testicular feminization is the development of tumors [2, 81, 216, 217]. It is not known whether tumor incidence is more common in this disorder than in cryptorchidism of other causes. Approximately 1 in 64 undescended testes becomes malignant, and the frequency of tumor is about four times greater in abdominal than in inguinal testes [218]. The natural history of the tumors in subjects

Table 48-8   Current classification of the androgen resistance syndromes according to molecular, genetic, anatomic, and endocrine characteristics

Category	Nature of Defect		
5α-Reductase deficiency	Absent or unstable enzyme		
Receptor disorders	Absent binding	Qualitatively abnormal	Decreased amount
Complete testicular feminization	+	+	+
Incomplete testicular feminization		+	+
Reifenstein syndrome		+	+
Infertile male syndrome		+	+
Receptor-positive resistance	Uncertain		

with testicular feminization is not entirely clear, but some behave as true malignancies [217]. Therefore, it is generally accepted that the testes should be removed in women with complete testicular feminization. Since these patients undergo a normal pubertal growth spurt and feminize successfully at the time of expected puberty [2, 8], and since tumors rarely develop in cryptorchid testes until after this time, it is customary to delay castration until after secondary sexual maturation is completed. If, however, hernia repair is indicated in the prepubertal years or if the testes are in the inguinal region or the labia majora and cause discomfort, some physicians prefer to remove the testes at the time of herniorrhaphy. If the testes are removed prepubertally, estrogen therapy is required at the appropriate age to ensure normal growth and breast development. If castration is performed after pubescence, menopausal symptoms and other evidences of estrogen withdrawal supervene [2, 81], and suitable estrogen replacement is indicated.

The situation in regard to the development of tumors in intraabdominal testes in women with incomplete testicular feminization and 5α-reductase deficiency is uncertain, but presumably the same considerations would apply as in women with complete testicular feminization. To prevent disfiguring virilization that may take place, the testes should be removed in those with female gender assignment prior to the expected time of puberty if possible, and feminization should be induced with estrogens.

Cryptorchidism is also frequent in the Reifenstein syndrome [130] and should be corrected surgically. The case material is small, but in other forms of cryptorchidism development of tumors is rare following successful repair [218].

Gynecomastia in Men with Defects of the Androgen Receptor   In the instances in which gynecomastia has been studied histologically, it is indistinguishable from other forms of estrogen-induced gynecomastia [126]. In men with the Reifenstein syndrome [130] and in occasional infertile men [137], gynecomastia develops as the result of increased estrogen production and androgen resistance, as in both forms of testicular feminization [10, 124]. Since most Reifenstein subjects have

Table 48-8 Current classification of the androgen resistance syndromes according to molecular, genetic, anatomic, and endocrine characteristics *(Continued)*

	Phenotype						*Endocrine profile relative to normal men*		
Inheritance	*General*	*Wolffian ducts*	*Spermatogenesis*	*Urogenital sinus*	*External genitalia*	*Breast*	*Testosterone production*	*Estrogen production*	*Plasma LH*
Autosomal recessive	F	M	N or ↓	F	C	M	N	N	N or ↑
X-linked recessive	F	A	A	F	F	F	↑	↑	↑
X-linked recessive	F	M, V	A	F	C & PF	F	↑	↑	↑
X-linked recessive	M	V	A	V from M to F	IMD	F	↑	↑	↑
X-linked recessive	M	M	A or ↓	M	M	M to F	N or ↑	N or ↑	N or ↑
Uncertain	M or F	V	A	V	F to IMD	V	N or ↑	↑	↑

NOTE: M denotes male; F, female; N, normal; A, absent; V, variable; C, clitoromegaly; PF, posterior fusion; IMD, incomplete male development; ↓, decreased; and ↑, increased.

male gender assignment and male gender identity, the gynecomastia may be disfiguring as well as disturbing. The only form of therapy available is surgical removal. As in normal men who are castrated [19] gynecomastia can occasionally develop following castration of individuals with androgen resistance [219]. This is presumably due to the fact that estrogen formation from adrenal precursors continues unabated following removal of the testes [19]. Carcinoma of the breast has not been described in men with androgen resistance. Presumably the risk of cancer is small since it is an infrequent complication of other forms of gynecomastia [220].

Hormone Treatment Appropriate estrogen treatment is indicated in all phenotypic women following removal of the testes [2, 81, 87]. Supplemental androgen therapy has been used without success in men with Reifenstein syndrome [155, 161] and is not ordinarily needed in subjects with 5α-reductase deficiency who are raised as men. Whether treatment of men with 5α-reductase deficiency with supplemental dihydrotestosterone might promote more complete development of secondary sex characteristics is not known.

THE NATURE OF ANDROGEN RESISTANCE

Hormone resistance was originally defined as a lack of response to endogenous and exogenous hormone [221]. In the case of androgen resistance, it was assumed that the degree of resistance to the hormone is equal in all tissues at all times of life and that the phenotypic expression of such a disorder was inevitably male pseudohermaphroditism. As the complexity of androgen action has been further elucidated, the spectrum of the manifestations of androgen resistance has expanded beyond the original formulations. Not only do different androgen metabolites have different effects, but any one androgen may have different actions during different phases of life—

from embryogenesis to old age. Furthermore, at the clinical level androgen resistance can be documented in some but not all tissues of the same affected subject. Therefore, we have adopted a more complex classification of androgen resistance that is dependent on a combination of molecular, genetic, phenotypic, and endocrine characteristics (Table 48-8).

Subjects with 5α-reductase deficiency have a special type of androgen resistance—in these individuals certain target tissues that are resistant to the action of endogenous androgen (testosterone) presumably would have responded normally to the missing end product (dihydrotestosterone) if it had been administered at the appropriate time during embryogenesis. This condition is analogous to hereditary resistance to the action of vitamin D; in one form of this disorder, so-called vitamin D–dependent rickets, the subject is unable to synthesize the 1,25-dihydroxy vitamin D [222]. In contrast, persons with androgen receptor abnormalities and those with receptor-positive resistance appear to be equally unresponsive to all androgens.

Fibroblasts cultured from genital skin have proved to be useful in defining the defects that underlie these various disorders and in the classification of specific entities. In disorders such as 5α-reductase deficiency and testicular feminization, the cultured fibroblast symbolizes the whole body in that the molecular defect present in vivo in all androgen target tissues is also expressed in fibroblasts cultured from genital skin. The clinical manifestations of these disorders are consistent within families, and the molecular defects are uniform among tissues. The identification of qualitative abnormalities in the 5α-reductase and in the androgen receptor in fibroblasts cultured from some affected families provides additional support for the concept that the defect expressed in the fibroblast is, indeed, the primary genetic defect in the disorders.

For other conditions (e.g., the Reifenstein syndrome and infertility in some men) the reconstruction of the pathogenesis is less certain. Even within the same family the phenotypic expression of androgen resistance in these disorders varies from subject to subject and from tissue to tissue. Disorders of the androgen receptor are always associated with defective spermatogenesis and abnormal gonadotropin regulation, whereas the phenotypic abnormalities and degree of sexual maturation at puberty are variable (Table 48-8). This phenomenon is compatible with at least two possibilities. First, different factors may regulate the activity of the androgen receptor in different tissues in the intact organism. For example, phenotypic expression of the Reifenstein syndrome among individuals within the same family can vary from infertility to pseudovagina formation even though the same degree of receptor abnormality is demonstrable in vitro. This finding indicates that unidentified factors must modify hormone action in vivo. Second, different amounts of androgen receptor may be required for different in vivo actions of the hormone. Accordingly a partial defect (either qualitative or quantitative) in the production of the androgen receptor could cause more complete manifestations of androgen resistance in some tissues than in others. The fact that qualitative defects in the androgen receptor have been identified in some families with Reifenstein syndrome and male infertility indicates that the fundamental mutation in these disorders does primarily involve the androgen receptor. Thus, the receptor abnormality and the resulting androgen resistance probably cause the disorders, regardless of the mechanism of the incomplete expression of the hormone resistance among tissues and among individuals.

Androgen resistance associated with male pseudohermaphroditism is relatively common, and if androgen resistance is also a common cause of male infertility, it may prove to be more frequent than all other forms of primary hormone resistance combined [103, 221]. There are several possible reasons for this frequency. First, expression of androgen activity is required for reproduction but not for the life of the individual. As a consequence, those with even the most complete forms of androgen resistance have a normal life span. In contrast, severe mutations affecting the action of hormones essential for life (such as cortisol) probably result in fetal wastage [221]. Second, defects in androgen action result either in abnormal sexual development or in reproductive failure. As a consequence there is a high probability that even subtle defects in the cellular machinery required for normal androgen action eventually come to the attention of physicians. Third, since the gene that specifies the androgen receptor is X-linked, defects in the androgen receptor become clinically manifested in the hemizygous (XY) state. As a consequence, there is a high probability that a new mutation in the androgen receptor will be clinically evident. If the gene were autosomal, most mutations would probably be manifested only in the homozygous state.

As in other forms of hormone resistance, elucidation of the pathophysiology of the androgen resistance syndromes has been important in unraveling the normal pathway of androgen action. Each new type of androgen resistance that is recognized provides an opportunity for defining the nature of a specific reaction essential for the action of the hormone.

REFERENCES

1. ALBRIGHT F, BURNETT CH, SMITH PH, PARSON W: Pseudohypoparathyroidism—an example of "Seabright-Bantam syndrome." *Endocrinology* 30:922, 1942
2. MORRIS JM: The syndrome of testicular feminization in male pseudohermaphrodites. *Am J Obstet Gynecol* 65:1192, 1953
3. WILKINS L: Abnormal sex differentiation: hermaphroditism and gonadal dysgenesis, in *The Diagnosis and Treatment of Endocrine Disorders in Childhood and Adolescence*. 2d ed. Springfield, Ill, Charles C Thomas, 1957, p 258
4. GRIFFIN JE, WILSON JD: The syndromes of androgen resistance. *N Engl J Med* 302:198, 1980
5. JOST A: Recherches sur la différenciation sexuelle de l'embryon de lapin. *Arch Anat Microsc Morphol Exp* 36:271, 1946–47
6. JOST A: Problems of fetal endocrinology: The gonadal and hypophyseal hormones. *Recent Prog Horm Res* 8:379, 1953
7. JOST A: The role of fetal hormones in prenatal development. *Harvey Lect* 55:201, 1961
8. JOST A: Hormonal factors in the sex differentiation of the mammalian foetus. *Philos Trans R Soc Lond, Ser B*, 259:119, 1970
9. SIITERI PK, MACDONALD PC: Role of extraglandular estrogen in human endocrinology, in Greep RO, Astwood EB (eds): *Handbook of Physiology*. Sect 7: Endocrinology. Washington, American Physiological Society, vol II, 1973, p 615
10. MACDONALD PC, MADDEN JD, BRENNER PF, WILSON JD, SIITERI PK: Origin of estrogen in normal men and in women with testicular feminization. *J Clin Endocrinol Metab* 49:905, 1979
11. GOLDSTEIN JL, WILSON JD: Hereditary disorders of sexual development in man, in Motulsky AG, Lentz W (eds): *Birth Defects*. International Congress Series 310, Amsterdam, Excerpta Medica, 1974, p 165
12. WILSON JD, GOLDSTEIN JL: Classification of hereditary disorders of sexual development, in Bergsma D (ed): *Genetic Forms of Hypogonadism*. New York, Birth Defects: Original Article Series, vol 11, Stratton Corp, 1975, p 1
13. WILSON JD: Metabolism of testicular androgens, in Greep RO, Astwood EB (eds): *Handbook of Physiology*. Sect 7: Endocrinology, vol V, Male Reproductive System, Washington, American Physiological Society, 1975, p 491
14. WILLIAMS-ASHMAN HG: Metabolic effects of testicular androgens, in Greep RO, Astwood EB (eds): *Handbook of Physiology*. Sect 7: Endocrinology, vol V, Male Reproductive System, Washington, American Physiological Society, 1975, p 473
15. KATZENELLENBOGEN BS: Dynamics of steroid hormone receptor action. *Ann Rev Physiol* 42:17, 1980
16. MARCUS R, KORENMAN SG: Estrogens and the human male. *Ann Rev Med* 27:357, 1976
17. BAUM MJ, VREEBURG JTM: Copulation in castrated male rats following combined treatment with estradiol and dihydrotestosterone. *Science* 182:283, 1973
18. LARSSON K, SODERSTEN P, BEYER C: Induction of male sexual behavior by estradiol benzoate in combination with dihydrotestosterone. *J Endocrinol* 57:563, 1973
19. WILSON JD, AIMAN J, MACDONALD PC: The pathogenesis of gynecomastia. *Adv Int Med* 25:1, 1980
20. KELCH RP, JENNER MR, WEINSTEIN R, KAPLAN SL, GRUMBACH MM: Estradiol and testosterone secretion by human, simian, and canine testes, in males with hypogonadism and in male pseudohermaphrodites with the feminizing testes syndrome. *J Clin Invest* 51:824, 1972
21. WEINSTEIN RL, KELCH RP, JENNER MR, KAPLAN SL, GRUMBACH MM: Secretion of unconjugated androgens and estrogens by the normal and abnormal human testis before and after human chorionic gonadotropin. *J Clin Invest* 53:1, 1974
22. VIGERSKY RA, LORIAUX DL, HOWARDS SS, HODGEN GB, LIPSETT MB, CHRAMBACH A: Androgen binding proteins of testis, epididymis, and plasma in man and monkey. *J Clin Invest* 58:1061, 1976
23. ANDERSON DC: Sex-hormone-binding globulin. *Clin Endocrinol* 3:69, 1974
24. LASNITZKI I, FRANKLIN HR, WILSON JD: The mechanism of androgen uptake and concentration by rat ventral prostate in organ culture. *J Endocrinol* 60:81, 1974
25. SIITERI PK, WILSON JD: Dihydrotestosterone in prostatic hypertrophy. I. The formation and content of dihydrotestosterone in the hypertrophic prostate of man. *J Clin Invest* 49:1737, 1970
26. MOORE RJ, GAZAK JM, QUEBBEMAN JF, WILSON JD: Concentration of dihydrotestosterone and 3α-androstanediol in naturally occurring and androgen-induced prostatic hyperplasia in the dog. *J Clin Invest* 64:1003, 1979
27. WILSON JD: Sexual differentiation. *Ann Rev Physiol* 40:279, 1978
28. WILBERT DM, GRIFFIN JE, WILSON JD: Characterization of the cytosol androgen receptor of the human prostate. *Clin Res* 29:509A, 1981
29. WACHTEL SS: Immunogenetic aspects of abnormal sexual differentiation. *Cell* 16:691, 1979
30. OHNO S: The role of H-Y antigen in primary sex determination. *J Am Med Assoc* 239:217, 1978
31. PATTEN BM: *Human Embryology*. 2d ed. New York: McGraw-Hill, 1953, p 549
32. HAMILTON WJ, BOYD JD, MOSSMAN HW: *Human Embryology*. Baltimore: Williams and Wilkins, 1962, p 267
33. GRUENWALD P: The relation of the growing mullerian duct to the wolffian duct and its importance for the genesis of malformations. *Anat Rec* 81:1, 1941

34. GOLDSTEIN JL, WILSON JD: Genetic and hormonal control of male sexual differentiation. *J Cell Physiol* 85:365, 1975

35. GEORGE FW, WILSON JD: Sexual differentiation, in Beard RW, Nathanielsz PW (eds): *Fetal Physiology and Medicine*. In press

36. JOSSO N: Interspecific character of the mullerian-inhibiting substance: Action of the human fetal testis, ovary and adrenal on the fetal rat mullerian duct in organ culture. *J Clin Endocrinol Metab* 32:404, 1971

37. JOSSO N: Permeability of membranes to the mullerian-inhibiting substance synthesized by the human fetal testis *in vitro*: A clue to its biochemical nature. *J Clin Endocrinol Metab* 34:265, 1972

38. PICARD J-Y, TRAN D, JOSSO N: Biosynthesis of labelled anti-mullerian hormone by fetal testes: evidence for the glycoprotein nature of the hormone and for its disulfide-bonded structure. *Mol Cell Endocrinol* 12:17, 1978

39. DONAHUE PK, ITO, Y, PRICE JM, HERNDON WH III: Mullerian inhibiting substance activity in bovine fetal, newborn, and prepubertal testes. *Biol Reprod* 16:238, 1977

40. WILSON JD, SIITERI PK: Developmental pattern of testosterone synthesis in the fetal gonad of the rabbit. *Endocrinology* 92:1182, 1973

41. SIITERI PK, WILSON JD: Testosterone formation and metabolism during male sexual differentiation in the human embryo. *J Clin Endocrinol Metab* 38:113, 1974

42. CATT KJ, DUFAU ML, NEAVES WB, WALSH PC, WILSON JD: LH-hCG receptors and testosterone content during differentiation of the testis in the rabbit embryo. *Endocrinology* 97:1157, 1975

43. GEORGE FW, SIMPSON ER, MILEWICH L, WILSON JD: Studies on the regulation of the onset of steroid hormone biosynthesis in fetal rabbit gonads. *Endocrinology* 105:1100, 1979

44. WILSON JD, LASNITZKI I: Dihydrotestosterone formation in fetal tissues of the rabbit and rat. *Endocrinology* 89:659, 1971

45. WILSON JD: Testosterone uptake by the urogenital tract of the rabbit embryo. *Endocrinology* 92:1192, 1973

46. SULCOVA J, JIRASEK JE, STARKA L: Transformation of testosterone into dihydrotestosterone by the primordia of human genitalia and by the fetal suprascapular skin. *Steroids Lipids Res* 4:129, 1973

47. WILSON JD: Testosterone metabolism in skin. *Symp Dtsch Ges Endokrin.* 17:11, 1971

48. WILSON JD, WALSH PC: Disorders of sexual differentiation, in Harrison JH, Gittes RF, Perlmutter AD, Stamey TA, Walsh PC (eds): *Urology.* 4th ed, Philadelphia, WB Saunders, 1979, ch 42, vol 2, p 1484

49. SLOAN WR, WALSH PC: Familial persistent mullerian duct syndrome. *J Urol* 115:459, 1976

50. SAVAGE MO, CHAUSSAIN JL, EVAIN D, ROGER M, CANLORBE P, JOB JC: Endocrine studies in male pseudohermaphroditism in childhood and adolescence. *Clin Endocrinol* 8:219, 1978

51. CAMPO S, STIVEL M, NICOLAU G, MONTEAGUDO C, RIVAROLA M: Testicular function in postpubertal male pseudohermaphroditism. *Clin Endocrinol* 11:481, 1979

52. CAMPO S, MOTEAGUDO C, NICOLAU G, PELLIZZARI E, BELGOROSKY A, STIVEL M, RIVAROLA M: Testicular function in prepubertal male pseudohermaphroditism. *Clin Endocrinol* 14:11, 1981

53. NOWAKOWSKI H, LENZ W: Genetic aspects in male hypogonadism. *Recent Prog Horm Res* 17:53, 1961

54. LENZ W: Genetisch bedingte Storungen der weiblichen Fortpflanzungsfunktionen. *Med Welt* 1:16, 1962

55. LENZ W: Pseudohermaphroditismus masculinus externus mit Sckundarbehaarung und ohne Brustentwicklung (pseudovaginale, perineoskrotalehypospadie), in Becker PE (ed): *Humangenetik.* Stuttgart: Verlag, 1964, p 385

56. SIMPSON JL, NEW M, PETERSON RE, GERMAN J: Pseudovaginal perineoscrotal hypospadias (PPSH) in sibs, in Bergsma D (ed): *Birth Defects.* Original Article Series, Baltimore, Williams and Wilkins, vol 7, p 140

57. OPITZ JM, SIMPSON JL, SARTO GE, SUMMITT RL, NEW M, GERMAN J: Pseudovaginal perineoscrotal hypospadias. *Clin Genet* 3:1, 1972

58. WALSH PC, MADDEN JD, HARROD MJ, GOLDSTEIN JL, MACDONALD PC, WILSON JD: Familial incomplete male pseudohermaphroditism, type 2. Decreased dihydrotestosterone formation in pseudovaginal perineoscrotal hypospadias. *N Engl J Med* 291:944, 1974

59. GIVENS JR, WISER WL, SUMMITT RL, KERBER IJ, ANDERSEN RN, PITTAWAY DE, FISH SA: Familial male pseudohermaphroditism without gynecomastia due to deficient testicular 17-ketosteroid reductase activity. *N Engl J Med* 291:938, 1974

60. IMPERATO-MCGINLEY J, GUERRERO L, GAUTIER T, PETERSON RE: Steroid 5α-reductase deficiency in man: An inherited form of male pseudohermaphroditism. *Science* 186:1213, 1974

61. PETERSON RE, IMPERATO-MCGINLEY J, GAUTIER T, STURLA E: Male pseudohermaphroditism due to steroid 5α-reductase deficiency. *Am J Med* 62:170, 1977

62. IMPERATO-MCGINLEY J, PETERSON RE, GAUTIER T, STURLA E: Male pseudohermaphroditism secondary to 5α-reductase deficiency—a model for the role of androgens in both the development of the male phenotype and the evolution of a male gender identity. *J Steroid Biochem* 11:637, 1979

63. IMPERATO-MCGINLEY J, PETERSON RE, GAUTIER T, STURLA E: Androgens and the evolution of male-gender identity among male pseudohermaphrodites with 5α-reductase deficiency. *N Engl J Med* 300:1233, 1979

64. CANTÚ JM, CORONA-RIVERA E, DÍAZ M, MEDINA C, ESQUINCA E, CORTÉS-GALLEGOS V, VACA G, HERNÁNDEZ A: Post-pubertal female psychosexual orientation in incomplete male pseudohermaphroditism type 2 (5α-reductase deficiency). *Acta Endocrinol* 94:273, 1980

65. FISHER LK, KOGUT MD, MOORE RJ, GOEBELSMANN U, WEITZMAN JJ, ISAACS H JR, GRIFFIN JE, WILSON JD: Clinical, endocrinological, and enzymatic characterization of two patients with 5α-reductase deficiency: Evidence that a single enzyme is responsible for the 5α-reduction of cortisol and testosterone. *J Clin Endocrinol Metab* 47:653, 1978

66. SAENGER P, GOLDMAN AS, LEVINE LS, KORTHSCHUTZ S, MUECKE EC, KATSUMATA M, DOBERNE Y, NEW MI: Prepubertal diagnosis of steroid 5α-reductase deficiency. *J Clin Endocrinol Metab* 46:627, 1978

67. SAVAGE MO, PREECE MA, JEFFCOATE SL, RANSLEY PG, RUMSBY G, MANSFIELD MD, WILLIAMS DI: Familial male pseudohermaphroditism due to deficiency of 5α-reductase. *Clin Endocrinol* 12:397, 1980

68. KUTTENN F, MOWSZOWICZ I, WRIGHT F, BAUDOT N, JAFFIOL C, ROBIN M, MAUVAIS-JARVIS P: Male pseudohermaphroditism: A comparative study of one patient with 5α-reductase deficiency and three patients with the complete form of testicular feminization. *J Clin Endocrinol Metab* 49:861, 1979

69. IMPERATO-MCGINLEY J, PETERSON RE, LESHIN M, GRIFFIN JE, COOPER G, DRAGHI S, BERENYI M, WILSON JD: Steroid 5α-reductase deficiency in a 65 year old male pseudohermaphrodite: the natural history, ultrastructure of the testes and evidence for inherited enzyme heterogeneity. *J Clin Endocrinol Metab* 50:15, 1980

70. OKON E, LIVNI N, RÖSLER A, YORKONI S, SEGAL S, KOHN G, SCHENKER JG: Male pseudohermaphroditism due to 5α-reductase deficiency: ultrastructure of the gonads. *Arch Pathol Lab Med* 104:363, 1980

71. JAFFIOL C, ROBIN M, CORRATGE P, MIROUZE J: Société francaise d'endocrinologie. *Ann Endocrinol (Paris)* 39:47, 1978

72. GREENE SA, SYMES E, BROOK CGD: 5-α-reductase deficiency causing male pseudohermaphroditism. *Arch Dis Child* 53:751, 1978

73. LESHIN M, GRIFFIN JE, WILSON JD: Hereditary male pseudohermaphroditism associated with an unstable form of 5α-reductase. *J Clin Invest* 62:685, 1978

74. BEUTLER E, YOSHIDA A: Human glucose-6-phosphate dehydrogenase variants: a supplementary tabulation. *Ann Hum Genet* 37:151, 1973

75. WILSON JD: Recent studies on the mechanism of action of testosterone. *N Engl J Med* 287:1284, 1972

76. WILSON JD, WALKER JD: The conversion of testosterone to 5α-androstan-17β-ol-3-one (dihydrotestosterone) by skin slices of man. *J Clin Invest* 48:371, 1969

77. WILSON JD: Dihydrotestosterone formation in cultured human fibroblasts: comparison of cells from normal subjects and patients with familial incomplete male pseudohermaphroditism, type 2. *J Biol Chem* 250:3498, 1975

78. MOORE RJ, GRIFFIN JE, WILSON JD: Diminished 5α-reductase activity in extracts of fibroblasts cultured from patients with familial incomplete male pseudohermaphroditism, type 2. *J Biol Chem* 250:7168, 1975

79. MOORE RJ, WILSON JD: Steroid 5α-reductase in cultured human fibroblasts: biochemical and genetic evidence for two distinct enzyme activities. *J Biol Chem* 251:5895, 1976

80. PINSKY L, KAUFMAN M, STRAISFELD C, ZILAHI B, HALL C ST-G: 5α-reductase activity of genital and nongenital skin fibroblasts from patients with 5α-reductase deficiency, androgen insensitivity, or unknown forms of male pseudohermaphroditism. *Am J Med Genet* 1:407, 1978

81. HAUSER GA: Testicular feminization, in Overzier C (ed): *Intersexuality.* London, Academic, 1963, p 255

82. DE QUERVAIN F: Ein fall von pseudohermaphroditismus masculinus. *Schweiz Med Wochenschr* 53:563, 1923

83. PERKINS OC: Hereditary agenitalism. *Am J Surg* 21:104, 1933

84. PETTERSSON G, BONNIER G: Inherited sex-mosaic in man. *Hereditas* 23:49, 1937

85. HAUSER GA, KELLER M, KOLLER T, WENNER R, GLOOR F: Testikuläre feminisierung bei erwachsenen. *Schweiz Med Wochenschr* 87:1573, 1957

86. SOUTHREN AL: The syndrome of testicular feminization, in Levine R, Luft R (eds): *Advances in Metabolic Disorders.* New York, Academic, 1965, vol 2, p 227

87. SIMMER HH, PION RJ, DIGNAM WJ: In Selle WA (ed): *Testicular Feminization: Endocrine Function of Feminizing Testes, Comparison with Normal Testes.* Springfield, Ill, Charles C Thomas, 1965, pp 1–100

88. SCHINDLER A-M, CSANK-BRASSERT J: Late discovery of a case of testicular feminisation. *J Med Genet* 15:229, 1978

89. KHODR GS: An elderly patient with testicular feminization. *Fertil Steril* 32:708, 1979

90. STERN ON, VANDERVORT WJ: Testicular feminization in a male pseudo-hermaphrodite: Report of a case. *N Engl J Med* 254:787, 1956

91. GRUMBACH MM, BARR ML: Cytologic tests of chromosomal sex in relation to sexual anomalies in man. *Recent Prog Horm Res* 14:255, 1958

92. JACOBS PA, BAIKIE AG, COURT BROWN WM, FORREST H, ROY JR, STEWART JSS, LENNOX B: Chromosomal sex in the syndrome of testicular feminisation. *Lancet* 2:591, 1959

93. PUCK TT, ROBINSON A, TJIO JH: Familial primary amenorrhea due to testicular feminization: A human gene affecting sex differentiation. *Proc Soc Exp Biol Med* 103:192, 1960

94. CHU EHY, GRUMBACH MM, MORISHIMA A: Karyotypic analysis of a male pseudohermaphrodite with the syndrome of feminizing testes. *J Clin Endocrinol Metab* 20:1608, 1960

95. KOO GC, WACHTEL SS, SAENGER P, NEW MI, DOSIK H, AMAROSE AP, DORUS E, VENTRUTO V: H-Y antigen: expression in human subjects with the testicular feminization syndrome. *Science* 196:655, 1977

96. GERLI M, MIGLIORINI G, BOCCHINI V, VENTI G, FERRARESE R, DONTI E, ROSI G: A case of complete testicular feminisation and 47,XXY karyotype. *J Med Genet* 16:480, 1979

97. ALVESALO L, VARRELA J: Permanent tooth sizes in 46,XY females. *Am J Hum Genet* 32:736, 1980

98. MASICA DN, MONEY J, EHRHARDT AA, LEWIS VG: IQ, fetal sex hormones and cognitive patterns: studies in the testicular feminizing syndrome of androgen insensitivity. *Johns Hopkins Med J* 124:34, 1969

99. MONEY J, EHRHARDT AA, MASICA DN: Fetal feminization induced by androgen insensitivity in the testicular feminizing syndrome: effect on marriage and maternalism. *Johns Hopkins Med J* 123:105, 1968

100. JAGIELLO G, ATWELL JD: Prevalence of testicular feminisation. *Lancet* 1:329, 1962

101. GERMAN J, SIMPSON JL, MORILLO-CUCCI G, PASSARGE E, DEMAYO AP: Testicular feminisation and inguinal hernia. *Lancet* 1:891, 1973

102. PERGAMENT E, HEIMLER A, SHAH P: Testicular feminisation and inguinal hernia. *Lancet* 2:740, 1973

103. IMURA H, MATSUMOTO K, OGATA E, YOSHIDA S, IGARASHI Y, KONO T, MATSUKURA S: "Hormone receptor diseases" in Japan: A nation-wide survey for testicular feminization syndrome, pseudohypoparathyroidism, nephrogenic diabetes insipidus, Bartter's syndrome and congenital adrenocortical unresponsiveness to ACTH. *Folia Endocrinol Jap* 56:1031, 1980

104. ROSS GT, VANDE WIELE RL: The ovary, in Williams RH (ed): *Textbook of Endocrinology.* Philadelphia, WB Saunders, ch 7, 1974, p 368

105. SCHREINER WE: On a hereditary form of male pseudohermaphroditism ("testicular feminization"). *Geburtshilfe Frauenheilkd* 19:1110, 1959

106. GWINUP G, WIELAND RG, BESCH PK, HAMWI GJ: Studies on the mechanism of the production of the testicular feminization syndrome. *Am J Med* 41:448, 1966

107. VAGENAKIS AG, HAMILTON C, MALOOF F, BRAVERMAN LE, INGBAR SH: The concentration and binding of thyroxine in the serum of patients with the testicular feminization syndrome: Observations on the effects of ethinyl estradiol and norethandrolone. *J Clin Endocrinol Metab* 34:327, 1972

108. TREMBLAY RR, SCHLAEDER G, DUSSAULT JH: Effets de l'ethynil estradiol et des androgènes sur les parametres de la fonction thyroidienne dans le syndrome de pseudohermaphrodisme male avec feminisation testiculaire. *Union Med Can* 103:421, 1974

109. FAIMAN C, WINTER JSD: The control of gonadotropin secretion in complete testicular feminization. *J Clin Endocrinol Metab* 39:631, 1974

110. FRENCH FS, VAN WYK JJ, BAGGETT B, EASTERLING WE, TALBERT LM, JOHNSTON FR, FORCHIELLI E, DEY AC: Further evidence of a target organ defect in the syndrome of testicular feminization. *J Clin Endocrinol Metab* 26:493, 1966

111. VOLPE R, KNOWLTON TG, FOSTER AD, CONEN PE: Testicular feminization: A study of two cases, one with a seminoma. *Can Med Assoc J* 98:438, 1968

112. CASTANEDA E, PEREZ AE, GUILLEN MA, RAMIREZ-ROBLES S, GUAL C, PEREZ-PALACIOS G: Metabolic studies in a patient with testicular feminization syndrome. *Am J Obstet Gynecol* 110:1002, 1971

113. O'LEARY JA: Comparative studies of the gonad in testicular feminization and cryptorchidism. *Fertil Steril* 16:813, 1965

114. JIRASEK JE: Syndrom testikularni feminizace. *Cas Lek Cesk* 106:1083, 1967

115. JUSTRABO E, CABANNE F, MICHIELS R, BASTIEN H, DUSSERRE P, PANSIOT F, CAYOT F: A complete form of testicular feminisation syndrome; a light and electron microscopy study. *J Pathol* 126:165, 1978

116. FAULDS JS, LENNOX B: Leydig-cell hyperplasia in testicular feminization. *Lancet* 1:344, 1971

117. DAMJANOV I, DROBNJAK P, GRIZELJ V: Testicular feminization with immature Leydig cells—an ultrastructural demonstration. *Am J Obstet Gynecol* 110:594, 1971

118. MILLONIG G, MORANO E, BOLLERO E, VECCHIETTI G, ZANOIO L: Ultrastructural study of gonads in the complete and incomplete feminization syndrome. *Gynecol Obstet Invest* 9:16, 1978

119. PRADER A: Gonadendysgenesie und testikuläre feminisierung. *Schweiz Med Wochenschr* 87:278, 1957

120. MORRIS JM, MAHESH VB: Further observations on the syndrome, "testicular feminization." *Am J Obstet Gynecol* 87:731, 1963

121. ROSENFIELD RL, LAWRENCE AM, LIAO S, LANDAU RL: Androgens and androgen responsiveness in the feminizing testis syndrome: Comparison of complete and "incomplete" forms. *J Clin Endocrinol Metab* 32:625, 1971

122. CRAWFORD JD, ADAMS RD, KLIMAN B, FEDERMAN DD, ULFELDER HS, HOLMES LB: Syndromes of testicular feminization. *Clin Pediatr* 9:165, 1970

123. WINTERBORN MH, FRANCE NE, RAITI S: Incomplete testicular feminization. *Arch Dis Child* 45:811, 1970

124. MADDEN JD, WALSH PC, MACDONALD PC, WILSON JD: Clinical and endocrinological characterization of a patient with the syndrome of incomplete testicular feminization. *J Clin Endocrinol Metab* 40:751, 1975

125. REIFENSTEIN EC JR: Hereditary familial hypogonadism. *Clin Res* 3:86, 1947

126. BOWEN P, LEE CSN, MIGEON CJ, KAPLAN NM, WHALLEY PJ, McKUSICK VA, REIFENSTEIN EC JR: Hereditary male pseudohermaphroditism with hypogonadism, hypospadias, and gynecomastia (Reifenstein's syndrome). *Ann Intern Med* 62:252, 1965

127. LUBS HA JR, VILAR O, BERGENSTAL DM: Familial male pseudohermaphroditism with labial testes and partial feminization: Endocrine studies and genetic aspects. *J Clin Endocrinol Metab* 19:1110, 1959

128. GILBERT-DREYFUS S, SEBAOUN CA, BELAISCH J: Étude d'un cas familial d'androgynoïdisme avec hypospadias grave, gynécomastie et hyperoestrogénie. *Ann Endocrinol (Paris)* 18:93, 1957

129. ROSEWATER S, GWINUP G, HAMWI GJ: Familial gynecomastia. *Ann Intern Med* 63:377, 1965

130. WILSON JD, HARROD MG, GOLDSTEIN JL, HEMSELL DL, MACDONALD PC: Familial incomplete male pseudohermaphroditism, Type 1. Evidence for androgen resistance and variable clinical manifestations in a family with the Reifenstein syndrome. *N Engl J Med* 290:1097, 1974

131. FORD E: Congenital abnormalities of the genitalia in related Bathurst Island natives. *Med J Aust* 1:450, 1941

132. WALKER AC, STACK EM, HORSFALL WA: Familial male pseudohermaphroditism. *Med J Aust* 1:156, 1970

133. GARDO S, PAPP Z: Clinical variations of testicular intersexuality in a family. *J Med Genet* 11:267, 1974

134. PEREZ-PALACIOS G, ORTIZ S, LÓPEZ-AMOR E, MORATO T, FEBRES F, LISKER R, SCAGLIA H: Familial incomplete virilization due to partial end organ insensitivity to androgens. *J Clin Endocrinol Metab* 41:946, 1975

135. PITTAWAY DE, STAGE AH: Familial male pseudohermaphroditism with incomplete virilization. *Obstet Gynecol* 51:82s, 1978

136. GRIFFIN JE, PUNYASHTHITI K, WILSON JD: Dihydrotestosterone binding by cultured human fibroblasts: Comparison of cells from control subjects and from patients with hereditary male pseudohermaphroditism due to androgen resistance. *J Clin Invest* 57:1342, 1976

137. AIMAN J, GRIFFIN JE, GAZAK JM, WILSON JD, MACDONALD PC: Androgen insensitivity as a cause of infertility in otherwise normal men. *N Engl J Med* 300:223, 1979

138. AIMAN J, GRIFFIN JE: The frequency of androgen receptor deficiency in infertile men. *J Clin Endocrinol Metab*, 1982. In press

139. KASE N, MORRIS JM: Steroid synthesis in the cryptorchid testes of three cases of the "testicular feminization" syndrome. *Am J Obstet Gynecol* 91:102, 1965

140. DAVID RR, WIENER M, ROSS L, LANDAU RL: Steroid metabolism in the syndrome of testicular feminization. *J Clin Endocrinol Metab* 25:1393, 1965

141. PION RJ, DIGMAN WJ, LAMB EJ, MOORE JG, FRANKLAND MV, SIMMER HH: Testicular feminization. *Am J Obstet Gynecol* 93:1067, 1965

142. NEHER R, KAHNT FW, ROVERSI GD, BOMPIANI A: Steroid transformations in vitro by testicular tissue from two cases of testicular feminisation. *Acta Endocrinol* 49:177, 1965

143. SHARMA DC, DORFMAN RI, SOUTHREN AL: Steroid biosynthesis *in vitro* by feminizing testes. *Endocrinology* 76:966, 1965

144. FRENCH FS, BAGGETT B, VAN WYK JJ, TALBERT LM, HUBBARD WR, JOHNSTON FR, WEAVER RP: Testicular feminization: Clinical, morphological and biochemical studies. *J Clin Endocrinol Metab* 25:661, 1965

145. SOUTHREN AL, ROSS H, SHARMA DC, GORDON G, WEINGOLD AB, DORFMAN RI: Plasma concentration and biosynthesis of testosterone in the syndrome of feminizing testes. *J Clin Endocrinol Metab* 25:518, 1965

146. GRIFFITHS K, GRANT JK, WHYTE WG: Steroid biosynthesis *in vitro* by cryptorchid testes from a case of testicular feminization. *J Clin Endocrinol Metab* 23:1044, 1963

147. JEFFCOATE SL, BROOKS RV, PRUNTY FTG: Secretion of androgens and oestrogens in testicular feminization: Studies *in vivo* and *in vitro* in two cases. *Br Med J* 1:208, 1968

148. CARDIFF C, UDEN V, KILLINGER DW: Steroid biosynthesis in gonadal tissue from patients with testicular feminization. *Can J Biochem* 50:849, 1972

149. LOCKWOOD E, GHOSH PC, PENNINGTON GW, TIPTON R: Steroid excretion and metabolism by gonadal tissue from a subject with testicular feminization syndrome. *J Clin Pathol* 27:135, 1974

150. PEREZ-PALACIOS G, LAMONT KG, PEREZ AE, JAFFE RB: *De novo* formation and metabolism of steroid hormones in feminizing testes: Biochemical and ultrastructural studies. *J Clin Endocrinol Metab* 29:786, 1969

151. DESHPANDE N, WANG DY, BULBROOK RD, MCMILLAN M: Hormone studies in cases of testicular feminization. *Steroids* 6:437, 1965

152. TREMBLAY RR, FOLEY TP JR, CORVOL P, PARK IJ, KOWARSKI A, BLIZZARD RM, JONES HW JR, MIGEON CJ: Plasma concentration of testosterone, dihydrotestosterone, testosterone-oestradiol binding globulin, and pituitary gonadotrophins in the syndrome of male pseudohermaphroditism with testicular feminization. *Acta Endocrinol* 70:331, 1972

153. TREMBLAY RR, KOWARSKI A, PARK IJ, MIGEON CJ: Blood production rate of dihydrotestosterone in the syndrome of male pseudohermaphroditism with testicular feminization. *J Clin Endocrinol Metab* 35:101, 1972

154. JUDD HL, HAMILTON CR, BARLOW JJ, YEN SSC, KLIMAN B: Androgen and gonadotropin dynamics in testicular feminization syndrome. *J Clin Endocrinol Metab* 34:229, 1972

155. BOYAR RM, MOORE RJ, ROSNER W, AIMAN J, CHIPMAN J, MADDEN JD, MARKS JF, GRIFFIN JE: Studies of gonadotropin-gonadal dynamics in patients with androgen insensitivity. *J Clin Endocrinol Metab* 47:1116, 1978

156. LAATIKAINEN T, APTER D, WAHLSTRÖM T: Steroids in spermatic and peripheral vein blood in testicular feminization. *Fertil Steril* 34:461, 1980

157. ZARATE A, CANALES ES, SORIA J, CARBALLO O: Studies on the luteinizing hormone- and follicle-stimulating hormone-releasing mechanism in the testicular feminization syndrome. *Am J Obstet Gynecol* 119:971, 1974

158. MEDINA M, ULLOA-AGUIRRE A, FERNÁNDEZ MA, PÉREZ-PALACIOS G: The role of oestrogens on gonadotrophin secretion in the testicular feminization syndrome. *Acta Endocrinol* 95:314, 1980

159. HOCHMAN J, GANGULY M, WEISS G: Induction of an LH surge with estradiol benzoate in a patient with incomplete testicular feminization syndrome. *Obstet Gynecol* 49:17s, 1977

160. FLATAU E, JOSEFSBERG Z, PRAGER-LEWIN R, MARKMAN-HALABE E, KAUFMAN H, LARON Z: Response to LH-RH and HCG in two brothers with the Reifenstein syndrome. *Helv Paediat Acta* 30:377, 1975

161. LEONARD JM, BREMNER WJ, CAPELL PT, PAULSEN CA: Male hypogonadism: Klinefelter and Reifenstein syndromes, in Bergama D (ed): *Genetic Forms of Hypogonadism. Birth Defects: Original Article Series, New York, Stratton Corp, vol XI, no 4, 1975, p 17*

162. NORTHCUTT RC, ISLAND DP, LIDDLE GW: An explanation for the target organ unresponsiveness to testosterone in the testicular feminization syndrome. *J Clin Endocrinol Metab* 29:422, 1969

163. MAUVAIS-JARVIS P, FLOCH HH, BERCOVICI J-P: Studies on testosterone metabolism in human subjects with normal and pathological sexual differentiation. *J Clin Endocrinol Metab* 28:460, 1968

164. MAUVAIS-JARVIS P, BERCOVICI JP, CREPY O, GAUTHIER F: Studies on testosterone metabolism in subjects with testicular feminization syndrome. *J Clin Invest* 49:31, 1970

165. IMPERATO-MCGINLEY J, PETERSON RE, GAUTIER T, COOPER G, DANNER R, ARTHUR A, MORRIS PL, SWEENEY WJ, SHACKLETON C: Hormonal evaluation of a large kindred with complete androgen insensitivity: Evidence for secondary 5α-reductase deficiency. *J Clin Endocrinol Metab*, in press

166. STEWART JSS: Testicular feminisation and colour-blindness. *Lancet* 2:592, 1959

167. NILSSON IM, BERGMAN S, REITALU J. WALDENSTRÖM J: Haemophilia A in a "girl" with male sex-chromatin pattern. *Lancet* 2:264, 1959

168. SANGER R, TIPPETT P, GAVIN J, GOOCH A, RACE RR: Inheritance of testicular feminization syndrome: Some negative linkage findings. *J Med Genet* 6:26, 1969

169. HOLMBERG L: Genetic studies in a family with testicular feminization, haemophilia A and colour blindness. *Clin Genet* 3:253, 1972

170. SCHULTZ MG: Male pseudohermaphroditism diagnosed with aid of sex chromatin technique. *J Am Vet Med Assoc* 140:241, 1962

171. NES N: Testikulaer feminisering hos storfe. *Nord Vet Med* 18:19, 1966

172. BARDIN CW, BULLOCK L, SCHNEIDER G, ALLISON JE, STANLEY AJ: Pseudohermaphrodite rat: end organ insensitivity to testosterone. *Science* 167:1136, 1970

173. LYON MF, HAWKES SG: X-linked gene for testicular feminization in the mouse. *Nature (London)* 227:1217, 1970

174. KIEFFER NM, BURNS SJ, JUDGE NG: Male pseudohermaphroditism of the testicular feminizing type in a horse. *Equine Vet J* 8:38, 1976

175. EIL C, MERRIAM GR, BOWEN J, EBERT J, TABOR E, WHITE B, DOUGLASS EC, LORIAUX DL: Testicular feminization in the chimpanzee. *Clin Res* 28:624A, 1980

176. OHNO S: *Major Sex-Determining Genes*. New York, Springer-Verlag, 1979

177. MEYER WJ III, MIGEON BR, MIGEON CJ: Locus on human X chromosome for dihydrotestosterone receptor and androgen insensitivity. *Proc Nat Acad Sci USA* 72:1469, 1975

178. LYON MF: X-chromosome inactivation and developmental patterns in mammals. *Biol Rev* 47:1, 1972

179. TAILLARD W, PRADER A: Étude génétique du syndrome de feminisation testiculaire totale et partielle. *J Genet Hum* 6:13, 1957

180. LENZ W: Quelques remarques au sujet du travail de W Taillard et A Prader: Étude génétique du syndrome de feminisation testiculaire totale et partielle. *J Genet Hum* 8:199, 1959

181. HALDANE JBS: The rate of spontaneous mutation of a single gene. *J Genet* 31:317, 1935

182. GRIFFIN JE: Testicular feminization associated with a thermolabile androgen receptor in cultured human fibroblasts. *J Clin Invest* 64:1624, 1979

183. BREMNER WJ, OTT J, MOORE DJ, PAULSEN CA: Reifenstein's syndrome: Investigation of linkage to X-chromosomal loci. *Clin Genet* 6:216, 1974

184. OTT J, GOLDSTEIN JL, HARROD MJ: Linkage investigation of a large family with Reifenstein's syndrome. *Clin Genet* 7:342, 1975

185. KEENAN BS, MEYER WJ III, HADJIAN AJ, JONES HW, MIGEON CJ: Syndrome of androgen insensitivity in man: Absence of 5α-dihydrotestosterone binding protein in skin fibroblasts. *J Clin Endocrinol Metab* 38:1143, 1974

186. KEENAN BS, MEYER WJ III, HADJIAN AJ, MIGEON CJ: Androgen receptor in human skin fibroblasts: Characterization of a specific 17β-hydroxy-5α-androstan-3-one-protein complex in cell sonicates and nuclei. *Steroids* 25:535, 1975

187. KAUFMAN M, STRAISFELD C, PINSKY L: Male pseudohermaphroditism presumably due to target organ unresponsiveness to androgens: deficient 5α-dihydrotestosterone binding in cultured skin fibroblasts. *J Clin Invest* 58:345, 1976

188. GRIFFIN JE, DURRANT JL: The frequency of qualitative receptor defects in 32 families with androgen resistance. *Clin Res* 29:505A, 1981

189. PINSKY L, KAUFMAN M, SUMMITT RL: Congenital androgen insensitivity due to a qualitatively abnormal androgen receptor. *Am J Med Genet*, 10:91, 1981

190. TAMAYA T, NIOKA S, FURUTA N, BOKU S, MOTOYAMA T, OHONO Y, OKADA H: Preliminary studies on steroid-binding proteins in human testes of testicular feminization syndrome. *Fertil Steril* 30:170, 1978

191. BULLOCK LP, BARDIN CW, OHNO S: The androgen insensitive mouse: Absence of intranuclear androgen retention in the kidney. *Biochem Biophys Res Commun* 44:1537, 1971

192. GEHRING U, TOMKINS GM, OHNO S: Effect of the androgen-insensitivity mutation on a cytoplasmic receptor for dihydrotestosterone. *Nature [New Biol]* 232:106, 1971

193. BULLOCK LP, BARDIN CW: Androgen receptors in mouse kidney: A study of male, female and androgen-insensitive (tfm/y) mice. *Endocrinology* 94:746, 1974

194. ATTARDI B, OHNO S: Cytosol androgen receptor from kidney of normal and testicular feminized (Tfm) mice. *Cell* 2:205, 1974

195. GEHRING U, TOMKINS GM: Characterization of a hormone receptor defect in the androgen-insensitivity mutant. *Cell* 3:59, 1974

196. VERHOEVEN G, WILSON JD: Cytosol androgen receptor in submandibular gland and kidney of the normal mouse and the mouse with testicular feminization. *Endocrinology* 99:79, 1976

197. GRIFFIN JE, WILSON JD: Studies on the pathogenesis of the incomplete forms of androgen resistance in man. *J Clin Endocrinol Metab* 45:1137, 1977

198. AMREIN JA, KLINGENSMITH GJ, WALSH PC, MCKUSICK VA, MIGEON CJ: Partial androgen insensitivity. The Reifenstein syndrome revisited. *N Engl J Med* 297:350, 1977

199. THIES N, WARNE G, CONNELLY JF, MONTALTO J, FUNDER J, WALKER AC, WETTENHALL HNB: Familial incomplete male pseudohermaphroditism due to androgen insensitivity in an Australian aboriginal community. *Aust Pediatr J* 15:209, 1979

200. AMREIN JA, MEYER WJ III, JONES HW JR, MIGEON CJ: Androgen insensitivity in man: evidence for genetic heterogeneity. *Proc Nat Acad Sci USA* 73:891, 1976

201. COLLIER ME, GRIFFIN JE, WILSON JD: Intranuclear binding of [³H]dihydrotestosterone by cultured human fibroblasts. *Endocrinology* 103:1499, 1978

202. KEENAN BS, KIRKLAND JL, KIRKLAND RT, CLAYTON GW: Male pseudohermaphroditism with partial androgen insensitivity. *Pediatrics* 59:224, 1977

203. MAES M, LEE PA, JEFFS RD, SULTAN C, MIGEON CJ: Phenotypic variation in a family with partial androgen insensitivity syndrome. *Am J Dis Child* 134:470, 1980

204. KAUFMAN M, PINSKY L, BAIRD PA, MCGILLIVRAY BC: Complete androgen insensitivity with a normal amount of 5α-dihydrotestosterone-binding activity in labium majus skin fibroblasts. *Am J Med Genet* 4:401, 1979

205. SCHAISON G, SITRUK LR: Male pseudohermaphroditism due to testicular 17-ketosteroid reductase deficiency. *Horm Metab Res* 8:307, 1976

206. Akesode FA, Meyer WJ III, Migeon CJ: Male pseudohermaphroditism with gynaecomastia due to testicular 17-ketosteroid reductase deficiency. *Clin Endocrinol* 7:443, 1977

207. Virdis R, Saenger P, Senior B, New MI: Endocrine studies in a pubertal male pseudohermaphrodite with 17-ketosteroid reductase deficiency. *Acta Endocrinol* 87:212, 1978

208. Imperato-McGinley J, Peterson RE, Stoller R, Goodwin WE: Male pseudohermaphroditism secondary to 17β-hydroxysteroid dehydrogenase deficiency: gender role change with puberty. *J Clin Endocrinol Metab* 49:391, 1979

209. Harkness RA, Thistlethwaite D, Darling JAB, Skakkeback NE, Corker CS: 17 β-Hydroxysteroid oxidoreductase deficiency causing male pseudohermaphroditism in a child. *J Endocrinol* 67:16P, 1975

210. Levine LS, Lieber E, Pang S, New MI: Male pseudohermaphroditism due to 17-ketosteroid reductase deficiency diagnosed in the newborn period. *Pediatr Res* 14:480, 1980

211. Edman CD, Winters AJ, Porter JC, Wilson D, MacDonald PC: Embryonic testicular regression. A clinical spectrum of XY agonadal individuals. *Obstet Gynecol* 49:208, 1977

212. Scholler R, Roger M, Leymarie P, Castanier P, Toublanc JE, Canlorbe P, Job JC: Evaluation of Leydig-cell function in normal prepubertal and pubertal boys. *J Steroid Biochem* 6:95, 1975

213. Walsh PC, Curry N, Mills RC, Siiteri PK: Plasma androgen response to hCG stimulation in prepubertal boys with hypospadias and cryptorchidism. *J Clin Endocrinol Metab* 42:52, 1976

214. Forest MG: Pattern of the response of testosterone and its precursors to human chorionic gonadotropin stimulation in relation to age in infants and children. *J Clin Endocrinol Metab* 49:132, 1979

215. Wabrek AJ, Millard PR, Wilson WB Jr, Pion RJ: Creation of a neovagina by the Frank nonoperative method. *Obstet Gynecol* 37:408, 1971

216. Dewhurst CJ, Ferreira HP, Gillett PG: Gonadal malignancy in XY females. *J Obstet Gynaecol Br Commonw* 78:1077, 1971

217. O'Connell MJ, Ramsey HE, Whang-Peng J, Wiernik PH: Testicular feminization syndrome in three sibs: Emphasis on gonadal neoplasia. *Am J Med Sci* 265:321, 1973

218. MacNab GH: Maldescent of the testicle. *J R Coll Surg Edinb* 1:126, 1955

219. Andler W, Zachmann M: Spontaneous breast development in an adolescent girl with testicular feminization after castration in early childhood. *J Pediatr* 94:304, 1979

220. Hall PF: *Gynaecomastia.* Monographs of Federal Council of British Medical Association in Australia No. 2. Glebe, New South Wales: Australasian Medical Publishing Co, 1959

221. Verhoeven GFM, Wilson JD: The syndromes of primary hormone resistance. *Metabolism* 28:253, 1979

222. Brooks MH, Bell NH, Love L, Stern PH, Orfei E, Queener SF, Hamstra AJ, DeLuca HF: Vitamin-D-dependent rickets type II: resistance of target organs to 1,25-dihydroxyvitamin D. *N Engl J Med* 298:996, 1978

49

STEROID SULFATASE DEFICIENCY AND X-LINKED ICHTHYOSIS

LARRY J. SHAPIRO

1. Steroid sulfatase deficiency *(also called X-linked ich-thyosis) is an inborn error of metabolism inherited as an X-linked recessive trait. The disorder affects 1 in 6000 males. The enzymatic defect leads to several bio-chemical alterations in steroid metabolism, including diminished estrogen production from dehydroepiandrosterone sulfate during fetal life and accumulation of cholesterol sulfate in blood, skin, and other tissues postnatally. The effects of the enzymatic defect on androgen metabolism and upon androgen and estrogen hormone action have not been completely assessed, but gross disturbances are not clinically apparent.*
2. *The major clinical consequences of steroid sulfate deficiency involve ichthyosis and corneal opacities. The ichthyosis becomes apparent soon after birth in all completely deficient males. Heterozygous mothers may experience difficulties with parturition when pregnant with steroid sulfatase–deficient male fetuses, owing to diminished estrogen production by the placenta.*
3. *The mechanism by which steroid sulfatase deficiency causes ichthyosis is not completely clear, but may be related to the accumulation of cholesterol sulfate in the skin.*
4. *The diagnosis of X-linked ichthyosis due to steroid sulfatase deficiency can be made by measurement of the blood level of cholesterol sulfate (fifteen- to thirty-fold*
above normal in affected males). There is no effective therapy for X-linked ichthyosis.*
5. *The genetic locus coding for steroid sulfatase is located on the short arm of the X chromosome. It is one of the few X-linked loci that is not subject to X chromosome inactivation.*

In the past few years, a series of fortuitous observations with important implications for several areas of biomedical investigation have led to the delineation of steroid sulfatase deficiency as a human inborn error of metabolism. These developments have resulted from an amalgamation of clinical observations dating back more than a century with biochemical and genetic studies of more recent vintage. The pathogenesis of this disorder is not yet understood, but ongoing studies should be a rich source of new information in the areas of steroid metabolism, the mechanism of initiation of parturition, the physiology of normal and pathologic skin, and the organization and regulation of gene expression on the X chromosome.

SULFATED STEROIDS

Occurrence and Distribution

Sulfated steroids are relatively abundant compounds with

1027

unique chemical and physiologic properties conferred by their relative water solubility and retention of the capability for lipophilic interactions by virtue of the cyclopentanophenanthrene backbone. Early steroid chemists appreciated that prior acid hydrolytic treatment of urine considerably increased the yield of steroids extractable into organic solvents. The reason for this phenomenon was not understood until the 1930s, when several acid-labile steroid conjugates (glucuronides and sulfates) were first identified. Estrone sulfate was isolated from pregnant mare's urine in 1938 [1], and androsterone sulfate was found in 1942 [2]. Munson et al. reported the isolation of dehydroepiandrosterone sulfate (DHEAS) from human urine in 1944 [3]. Subsequent to these discoveries relatively little work was done on the steroid sulfates for some period of time. This can be ascribed to the difficulty of separating intact sulfoconjugates of steroids from one another by methods then available. Furthermore, early investigations had suggested that steroid conjugates were not biologically active. The general view which evolved was that steroid sulfates were merely water-soluble forms of the physiologically more interesting neutral steroids that were conjugated to prepare them for excretion in either the urine or the bile. In the late 1950s and early 1960s, this view of sulfated steroids was changed by the development of suitable analytic techniques (chiefly chromatographic) and the introduction of isotopically labeled steroid conjugates for use in physiologic studies. Since that time much interest has been focused on the production and metabolism of these steroids, if for no other reason than the sheer quantity of conjugates present in normal physiologic fluids. With the exception of cholesterol, DHEAS (60 to 500 μg/dl) and cholesterol sulfate (100 to 350 μg/dl) represent the most abundant sterols found circulating in plasma. A large number of steroid glucuronides and steroid sulfates have been identified in various physiologic fluids and tissues. A comprehensive consideration of the chemistry, distribution, physiology, and metabolism of all of the steroid sulfates is beyond the scope of the current discussion.

Several reviews have been written [4].

This chapter will focus specifically upon the 3β-hydroxy steroid sulfates and their metabolism in steroid sulfatase deficiency.

Sulfate esters of 3β-hydroxy steroids may be formed in a number of tissues. Essentially all biologic conjugation is catalyzed by sulfotransferases. Uniformly, the sulfate donor is 3'-phosphoadenosine-5'-phosphosulfate (PAPS). Formation of the high-energy PAPS is presumably mediated by an ATP-sulfurylase and APS-phosphokinase sulfate activating system. PAPS then becomes the donor of the sulfuryl group to a recipient steroid in a reaction catalyzed by the steroid sulfotransferase. The absolute number, distribution, and substrate specificities of steroid sulfotransferases are not yet entirely clear, but PAPS-mediated sulfation reactions have been demonstrated in adrenal glands, liver, skin, testes, ovary, jejunal mucosa, and placenta [5].

Roberts et al. elegantly demonstrated that sulfated steroids may be biosynthetically interconverted along pathways analogous to those followed by the parent unconjugated compounds [6]. These reactions may proceed without prior desulfation of the substrate (Fig. 49-1). This point was established by infusing a patient who had an adrenal tumor with cholesterol sulfate (CS) which was labeled with ^{3}H in the sterol nucleus and ^{35}S in the sulfate moiety. These workers were able to isolate DHEAS which had a ^{35}S/^{3}H ratio almost identical to that of the CS originally infused. Similar substrate functions have been dem-

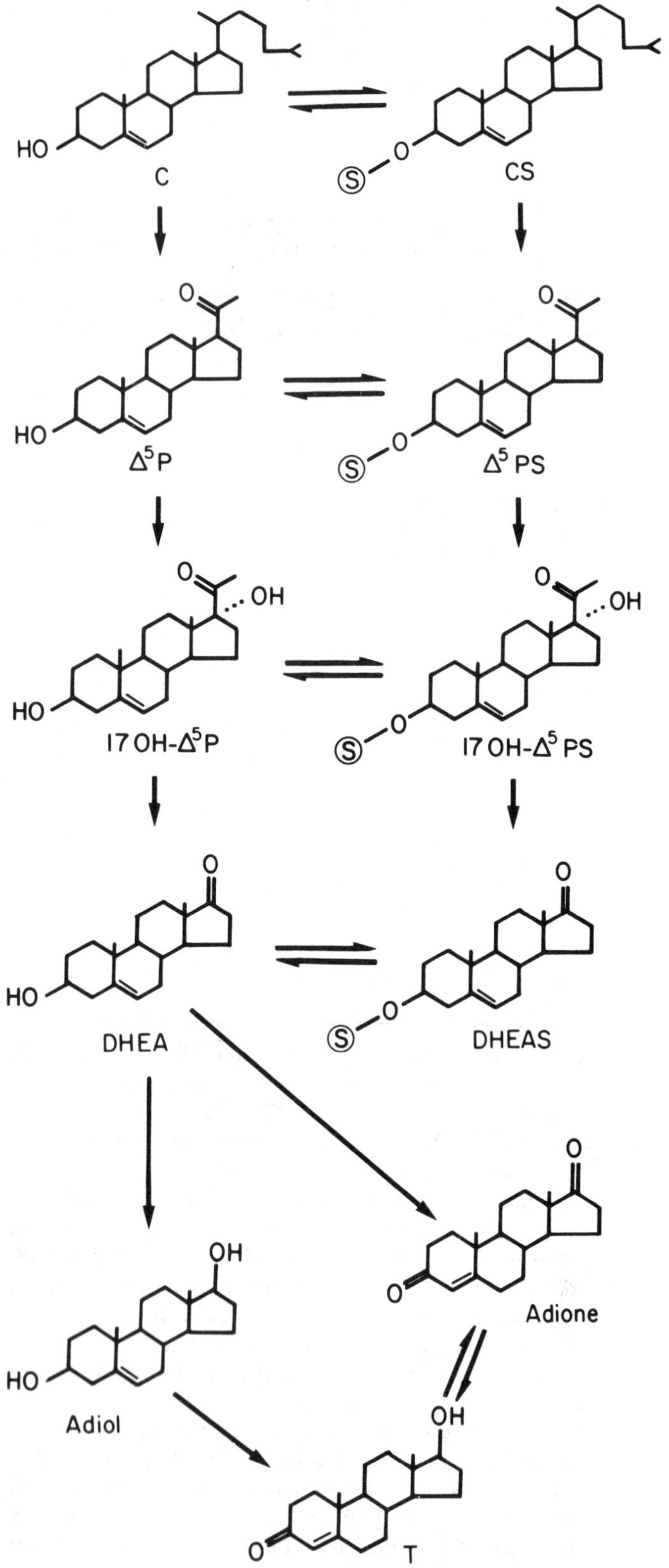

Figure 49-1 Metabolic pathways of free and sulfated 3β-hydroxy steroids. Known metabolic relationships of cholesterol (C), cholesterol sulfate (CS), pregnenolone (Δ^{5}P), pregnenolone sulfate (Δ^{5}PS), 17-hydroxy-pregnenolone (17OH-Δ^{5}P), 17-hydroxy-pregnenolone sulfate (17OH-Δ^{5}PS), dehydroepiandrosterone (DHEA), dehydroepiandrosterone sulfate (DHEAS), androstenediol (Adiol), androstenedione (Adione), and testosterone (T) are shown. The four sulfates shown can be converted to the corresponding free steroids by the action of steroid sulfatase, and the conjugates can be resynthesized by sulfotransferase(s) in the presence of PAPS. The quantitative importance of the various possible pathways is not always known and may vary developmentally, and from tissue to tissue. It is clear that under some conditions CS may be converted to DHEAS without desulfation.

onstrated for pregnenolone sulfate and DHEAS [7, 8, 9]. Although the existence of these pathways is well established, the physiologic role of sulfated steroids themselves and their quantitative importance as precursors of steroid hormones, is less clear.

Sterol Sulfates in Biologic Membranes

Cholesterol sulfate is present in a variety of tissues, including the adrenal gland, brain, liver, kidney, plasma, urine, feces, bile, aortic plaques, gallstones, red blood cell membranes, and seminal fluid [10, 12]. Physiologic function of this steroid, which is present at normal levels of 150 to 300 μg/dl of plasma, is unknown. There is a high concentration of CS in red blood cell membranes, and this compound when added exogenously to red blood cells or given in large doses to dogs can promote osmotic stability both in vivo and in vitro [13, 13a, 14]. This has led Bleau and coworkers to postulate a role in membrane stabilization for this amphipathic molecule. Recent observations in steroid sulfatase–deficient patients suggest that substantial increases in the amount of CS contained within red cell membranes can be well tolerated without apparent harmful effects upon red cell life span or function [15, 16]. Also of note is the identification of CS as a major constituent of the superficial stratum corneum layer of the epidermis. Cholesterol sulfate is greatly increased in this tissue in patients with steroid sulfatase deficiency, with probable significant pathologic effects [17]. Of further interest is the observation that CS is an integral component of sperm membranes and might theoretically be acted upon by the potent steroid sulfatase of the female genital tract [18, 18a, 19]. Lalumière et al. have postulated that the process of sperm capacitation might be mediated by steroid sulfatase, which could reduce the content of the membrane-associated CS, thereby preparing the sperm for fertilization. At the present time it may be presumed that sulfated sterols are important components of many cell membranes.

Sulfated Steroids as Metabolic Precursors of Biologically Active Hormones

For a number of years workers have attempted to explain the paradox of the large quantity of circulating steroid sulfates in the face of their relative biologic inactivity. Although CS may have surface-active or membrane properties which make it important in the metabolic economy of some cell types, obvious functions for other sulfates are not clear. Pregnenolone sulfate is not active per se. DHEAS fails to cause changes in activity of several enzymes modulated by free DHEA, and large doses of DHEAS given to human subjects seem to have little metabolic effect. Similarly, the large amounts of circulating estrogen sulfates appear incapable of interacting with estrogen receptors or exerting a biologic effect without prior hydrolysis [20, 21]. All of these findings led to the suggestion that steroid sulfates must be inactive end products of metabolism prepared for elimination or excretion in a water-soluble form.

Given that sulfated steroids are truly inactive as hormones themselves, an alternative model for their function would be as a reservoir or source of precursors for the production of more active hormones. Several pieces of evidence support this notion. First, the circulating half-life of most plasma steroid sulfates is longer than the corresponding free steroid, so that the sulfates are in fact more slowly metabolized or excreted [4].

Second, sulfated steroids may be acted upon by steroid sulfatase to yield active estrogens or other hormones in situ in target tissues. This has been demonstrated for estrogen sulfates in breast cancer cells [21] and in fetal sheep hypothalamus [22]. Third, steroid sulfates are substrates for a large number of steroid interconverting enzymes and, under appropriate circumstances, may be metabolized to a large number of active molecules. Much work over the past 15 years has been designed to investigate the *quantitative* importance of these reactions in normal hormone economy.

As mentioned previously, Roberts et al. showed the direct conversion of CS to DHEAS [6]. The fact that these experiments were accomplished in a patient with an adrenal carcinoma may account for some of the results. Other studies on normal subjects or fetuses failed to demonstrate efficient conversion of CS to adrenal steroids or other active metabolites [23–25]. Pregnenolone sulfate has been shown to be a precursor of placental progesterone biosynthesis during pregnancy [26, 27]. As will be described later, the large amounts of steroid sulfatase found in placenta probably render fetal-placental steroidogenesis somewhat unique in the quantitative utilization of sulfated steroids as substrates for hormone synthesis.

DHEAS and Androgen Production   DHEAS is present in considerable amounts in physiologic fluids. Its metabolism has been well studied. It is present at appreciable levels in cord blood but rapidly diminishes in concentration during the first months of life. Levels remain low until 5 to 7 years of age, when they begin a gradual rise to adult values [28–30]. On average this rise begins 1 or 2 years earlier in females than in males. This increased circulating DHEAS is presumably of adrenal origin and is the hallmark of the phase of pubertal development commonly referred to as adrenarche. Most of the DHEAS circulating in blood probably arises from adrenal secretion. Production rates for adults are on the order of 6 to 10 mg/day [4]. The normal human testis is probably not responsible for very much secretion of DHEAS, although small gradients between peripheral blood concentrations and spermatic vein concentrations have been identified [31].

A considerable controversy has surrounded the possible role of DHEAS and other sulfated 3β-hydroxy steroids as precursors or intermediates for testosterone production. A number of nongonadal tissues are capable of desulfating DHEAS to free DHEA in vitro and subsequently converting this steroid to androstenedione and then to testosterone (Fig. 49-1). Several workers have attempted to quantify the contribution of adrenally produced DHEAS to total body testosterone production. MacDonald et al. [32] and Chapdelaine et al. [33] found that between 3 and 12 percent of DHEAS may be converted to testosterone. This suggests that circulating DHEAS might be a significant precursor for testosterone production.

The methodology used by these workers involved the determination of the specific activity of urinary testosterone glucuronide following the administration of tritiated DHEAS. With this technique there is no assurance that the labeled testosterone formed from the labeled DHEAS ever entered the circulation intact to exert a metabolic effect. It is possible that the reaction sequence DHEAS → DHEA → androstenedione → testosterone → testosterone glucuronide could all have occurred in the liver and that no free testosterone was ever released.

Horton and Tait attempted to clarify this problem by determining the amount of free labeled testosterone formed in plasma during the continuous infusion of [³H]-DHEA [34]. They did not use the sulfated steroid but determined that the transfer constant of DHEA to testosterone was only 0.7 percent. This would mean that DHEA would serve as the precursor of about 15 percent of the circulating testosterone produced by an adult female, but only 1 percent or less of the testosterone produced by an adult male. DHEAS would presumably have given rise to even less testosterone. Thus, *circulating* DHEAS is probably not a quantitatively important precursor of blood-borne testosterone.

The role of intracellular DHEAS in testosterone production remains uncertain. Several authors have proposed a role for testicular steroid sulfatase in the regulation of testosterone production in response to human chorionic gonadotropin (hCG) [31, 35, 35a, 36, 38]. Administration of hCG to a variety of animals results in an increase in testicular steroid sulfatase activity. An analogous increase in adrenal steroid sulfatase activity is observed following ACTH administration. Furthermore, testicular homogenates contain substantial amounts of sulfated steroids. These are usually present in amounts considerably greater than the parent unconjugated steroids. Furthermore, testicular homogenates are capable of utilizing sulfated steroids as precursors for testosterone production. Thus it is possible, even if DHEAS and other sulfated 3β-hydroxy steroids are not quantitatively important as circulating precursors of testosterone, that locally formed sulfoconjugates may be important in testosterone biogenesis. Studies of testosterone production in steroid sulfatase–deficient patients should help to clarify this point since these patients should be unable to desulfate sulfoconjugate precursors and utilize them for testosterone synthesis. In this regard several measurements have been made which indicate normal circulating levels of testosterone associated with normal gonadotropin stimulation (Table 49-1) [16].

Steroid Sulfates as Precursors for Estrogens   Another important precursor function for DHEAS is in estrogen production during pregnancy. Several lines of evidence came together in the early 1960s to suggest that DHEAS was a major precursor of the large amounts of estrogens produced during normal pregnancy (Fig. 49-2). Several investigators observed that mothers who were carrying anencephalic fetuses had markedly diminished urinary estrogen excretion when compared to mothers pregnant with normal fetuses [39, 40]. Since anencephalic fetuses often have hypoplastic adrenal glands, it was suggested that the fetal adrenals might be the source of important precursors for estrogen production. DHEAS in the plasma of fetuses is present in appreciable concentrations [41,

42]. While the fetal adrenal glands are probably the major source of DHEAS used as a precursor for estrogen production, maternally secreted DHEAS may contribute as well. When pregnant women are given ACTH, enhanced estrogen production can be demonstrated, and when the maternal adrenals are suppressed with dexamethasone, estrogen production falls [43]. Pulkkinen, Warren, and Timberlake demonstrated that the placenta was a rich source of steroid sulfatase which could cleave DHEAS in perfusion experiments [44–46]. This desulfation could be achieved whether the placenta was perfused with DHEAS from either the maternal or from the fetal side. It had already been established that the placenta contained the necessary enzymatic activities to transform C_{19} steroids into estrogens once they had been desulfated [47]. This was validated for intact pregnant women in studies in which radioactively labeled DHEAS was administered and the conversion to labeled estradiol was determined [48]. At term 28 to 45 percent of the injected DHEAS was converted to 17β-estradiol. In subsequent experiments it was demonstrated that the conversion of DHEAS to estrogens was much more efficient when the DHEAS was injected via the umbilical vein. Further evidence to support an important role for sulfated steroids as precursors of estrogens was obtained by studying pregnancies affected with placental steroid sulfatase deficiency, as will be discussed below.

Steroid Sulfatase

A number of enzymes having the ability to hydrolyze sulfate ester bonds have been isolated from a variety of sources. Specifically, a group of arylsulfatases (arylsulfate sulfohydrolases), which catalyze the hydrolysis of a variety of arylsulfates, have been identified. These enzymes were originally grouped into type I and type II arylsulfatases [5]. The type I arylsulfatases are relatively nonspecific with regard to the sulfated substrate and are relatively insensitive to inhibition by sulfate and phosphate ions. Type II enzymes by contrast are inhibited by sulfate and phosphate and often are activated by chloride ions. They also show somewhat greater apparent specificity toward their substrates. Over the past several decades a number of type II arylsulfatases of animal origin have been isolated and carefully studied. They have generally been found to reside within the lysosomal compartment and to function at an acidic pH optimum. Arylsulfatase A and arylsulfatase B have been extensively studied and their respective natural substrates have been identified as cerebroside sulfate and dermatan sulfate. Deficiency of each of these enzymes has been identified in groups of

Table 49-1   Circulating metabolite and hormone levels in four adult patients with steroid sulfatase deficiency

	Subject 1	Subject 2	Subject 3	Subject 4	Normal range
Cholesterol sulfate (μg/dl)	3300	2800	4000	3400	100–300
Cholesterol (mg/dl)	213	159	204	112	140–280
DHEAS (μg/dl)	295	420	586	28	130–550
DHEA (ng/dl)	340	250	330	30	150–700
Androstenedione (ng/dl)	263	85	68	60	50–180
Testosterone (ng/dl)	644	965	521	397	>300
FSH (mIU/ml)	7.4	8.4	<2	11	<15
LH (mIU/ml)	14.3	17	10	18	<15
Estradiol (pg/ml)	42	85	43	61	10–50

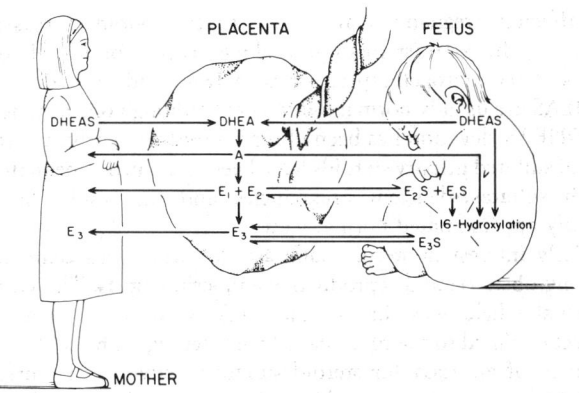

Figure 49-2 Schematic outline of fetal-maternal-placental estrogen biosynthesis. Total estrogen production increases several hundredfold during the course of a normal pregnancy. The primary substrate for this biosynthetic activity are C_{19} steroids, particularly DHEA, 16-hydroxy-DHEA, and their sulfates. Earlier in pregnancy, DHEAS supplied by the maternal adrenals is important, but later in gestation fetally derived DHEAS and 16-hydroxy-DHEAS are most significant. These precursors are supplied to the placenta where they are hydrolyzed by steroid sulfatase and metabolized by 3-β-hydroxy steroid dehydrogenase Δ5-isomerase and aromatization enzyme systems to give rise to estrogens. The estrogen present in largest quantities in normal pregnancies is estriol. E_1 = estrone, E_2 = estradiol, E_3 = estriol.

patients with inborn errors of metabolism leading to the various forms of metachromatic leukodystrophy (arylsulfatase A deficiency) and Maroteaux-Lamy syndrome (arylsulfatase B deficiency) [49, 50]. Both of these clinical disorders are discussed elsewhere in this volume (see Chaps. 36 and 44).

The type I arylsulfatase from animal tissues has been much less well studied. This arylsulfatase is also referred to as arylsulfatase C and is charcterized by a neutral pH optimum and a strong association with the microsomal fraction of tissue extracts. Until recently no procedures suitable for solubilization and purification have been reported. This has hampered the understanding of this enzyme or group of enzymes. In the early sixties Pulkkinen reported that the human placenta contains a great deal of an enzymatic activity capable of hydrolyzing estrone sulfate [44]. Warren and Timberlake reported the ability of placentas to hydrolyze DHEAS [45, 46]. Other microsomal steroid sulfatases with neutral pH optima have been identified which have activity against pregnenolone sulfate, DHEAS, and CS as well. These hydrolytic activities have been identified in a variety of tissues including liver, adrenal gland, testis, brain, and skin. The full extent of substrates for steroid sulfatase has not been firmly established. A variety of other structural analogs of these sulfate esters, such as vitamin D sulfate, are known to occur and might be acted upon by steroid sulfatase.

Considerable attention has been given to the number of steroid sulfatase enzyme molecules which might exist and whether any or all of them might be identical in activity to arylsulfatase C. Most of these considerations were hampered by the inability to solubilize and purify steroid sulfatase. Most early hypotheses were based on kinetic data which demonstrated slightly different pH optima for hydrolysis of the various substrates [51]. Furthermore, inhibition studies were taken as evidence for the presence of a multiplicity of steroid sulfatases [52–55]. It should be pointed out that the insoluble steroid sulfatase preparations generally do not follow classical Michaelis-Menton kinetics, and therefore determination of competitive versus noncompetitive inhibition is difficult. Numerous steroid inhibitors for this enzyme have been reported

[35–56]. At present it remains speculative whether these inhibitors function at the active site of the enzyme molecule and compete for substrate binding or whether they bind to some additional allosteric effector site.

Two successful attempts at solubilization and purification of steroid sulfatase activities have been published [54, 55]. One study involved human placenta as the starting material and one group studied the rat liver steroid sulfatase. All of these investigations have involved the use of the detergent miranol H2M, a zwitterionic surface-active agent which has been found empirically to release substantial amounts of activity in a nonsedimentable form. If this detergent is incorporated into the various buffer systems employed, classical purification techniques involving gel filtration, ion exchange, and electrophoresis can be employed. Steroid sulfatase activities purified by these groups as well as the characterizations of crude steroid sulfatase reported by others have resulted in molecular weights which have varied from 23,000 to over 1,000,000 [53, 57]. Some of the differences may be attributable to incomplete solubilization of the enzyme and the presence of either membrane fragments or multimeric aggregates of the enzyme.

In the studies of steroid sulfatase purification, kinetic data also might suggest the presence of several different steroid sulfatase enzymes. Furthermore, one of the groups reported differential enrichment of estrone sulfatase, DHEAS sulfatase, and cholesterol sulfatase activities [55], but no physical separation of any of these sulfatases has been achieved, even in highly purified enzyme preparations. The one possible exception is the finding of Hameister et al., who claim to have electrophoretically differentiated neutral 4-methylumbelliferyl sulfatase activity from DHEAS sulfatase activity [58]. This observation remains unconfirmed.

It is noteworthy that in steroid sulfatase deficiency produced by a single-gene inherited metabolic defect, activity against all of these sulfated substrates is lost. It is possible that the different pH optima for the various substrates could be accounted for by modulation of a single enzyme molecule. The problems in interpreting kinetic data have been mentioned. Therefore, until definitive physical separation of these various steroid sulfatase activities can be achieved, the simplest interpretation of the available data is that there is a single, or at most a very small number, of steroid sulfatases. This steroid sulfatase is probably encompassed within the activity usually referred to as microsomal arylsulfatase C. This term might also apply to a number of neutral sulfatases capable of hydrolyzing artificial sulfate esters.

PLACENTAL SULFATASE DEFICIENCY

In 1969, France and Liggins described two pregnancies of a New Zealand woman in which strikingly low estrogen excretion was noted [59]. Fetal growth and development appeared normal. At term, the patient was delivered by cesarean section of normal-appearing male infants without obvious defects. One placenta studied had a virtual absence of 3β-hydroxy steroid sulfatase activity, with preservation of other enzymes involved in estrogen biogenesis. These authors were able to study a subsequent pregnancy in another subject with similar findings. Studies both in vivo and in vitro demonstrated an inability to metabolize DHEAS to estrogens but normal function in converting DHEA to estrogens.

During the ensuing years, a substantial number of similar cases have been reported from around the world. This is in part due to the large-scale application of urinary estriol monitoring to assess fetal-maternal well being in pregnancy. To date, over 40 cases of *placental* steroid sulfatase deficiency have been reported [60–74]. Recognition has most often been the result of urinary estriol determinations performed because of some prior obstetric difficulty. In a smaller number of cases, the affected patients were identified without any ascertainment bias through large-scale estriol screening programs for detecting obstetric difficulties. The total 24-h excretion of urinary estrogen in women carrying affected progeny has been strikingly low. All values reported have been less than 3 mg/24 h even at term. Similarly, in those situations in which plasma estriol levels have been determined, striking diminution has been found. In most of these pregnancies confirmation of the biochemical diagnosis has been obtained through a variety of placental incubation studies with radioactively labeled steroid substrates.

In the well-documented cases an isolated defect in steroid sulfatase has been identified with preservation of the subsequent steps in estrogen biosynthesis, namely the 3β-hydroxy steroid dehydrogenase-isomerase step and the aromatase reaction. A variety of in vivo loading studies performed by administering DHEAS either into the maternal or fetal compartment in these pregnancies has failed to produce the expected augmentation of estrogen production. In contrast, when the product of the sulfatase reaction, free DHEA, is administered, a normal rise in estrogen is observed. Plasma levels of progesterone and of placental lactogen and hCG have been normal in affected pregnancies [66, 67]. In spite of the strikingly low estrogen production, affected pregnancies seem to progress normally, at least until the completion of 40 weeks gestation.

In the initial reports of the clinical features of steroid sulfatase deficiency, a relative refractoriness to the onset of labor, particularly in primigravidas, was noted [60]. Prolongation of pregnancy beyond 40 weeks was seen in a number of cases. Failure of cervical dilatation and effacement in spite of a normal uterine response to oxytocin was observed [63, 64, 72]. Therefore, quite a few of these pregnancies were terminated by cesarean section. In subsequent series, a substantial number of patients have been identified who were capable of being delivered by the normal vaginal route [16, 67, 72–74].

This phenomenon is reminiscent of that seen in other estrogen-deficient states such as hypoplasia of the fetal adrenal glands and pregnancies associated with anencephalic fetuses. In both of these clinical situations, maternal-fetal estrogen production is reduced, although not to the extreme levels seen in placental sulfatase deficiency. Furthermore, postterm gestations are not infrequent in these other clinical settings. After delivery the male infants resulting from pregnancies affected with steroid sulfatase deficiency are clinically normal and their placentas are without anatomic defects.

The prenatal metabolic consequences of steroid sulfatase deficiency have received considerable attention. In addition to the very low maternal urinary and plasma levels of estrogens already noted, the maternal urinary excretion of a variety of sulfated steroids is abnormal [75]. Most notably, the mean 24-h urinary 16-hydroxy DHEAS is elevated almost twentyfold above normal. Likewise, DHEAS levels in amniotic fluid

of affected pregnancies are seven- to twentyfold increased [66, 67]. In contrast to these findings, cord blood levels of the sulfated estrogenic precursors DHEAS and 16-hydroxy-DHEAS are usually normal [63, 65, 75] although one instance of DHEAS elevation has been observed [66]. Similarly, a variety of sulfated urinary steroids have been examined in neonates from sulfatase-deficient pregnancies and the results have closely approximated normal values.

Early interest in steroid sulfatase deficiency was centered among obstetric and reproductive endocrinologists. The view originally held was that steroid sulfatase deficiency was a defect confined to the placenta. More recently, with the development of an assay for steroid sulfatase activity in cultured fibroblasts, it has been possible to demonstrate the generalized nature of the enzyme defect [70]. The availability of the fibroblast assay facilitated widespread case finding and the performance of family studies which would otherwise not have been possible. Deficiency of steroid sulfatase activity in affected males has been documented in placenta, cultured fibroblasts, white blood cells, hair follicles, cultured epidermal cells, stratum corneum (scales and calluses), whole skin, and even fingernail clippings [59, 70, 76–79].

Three patients said to have a partial deficiency of steroid sulfatase activity in placenta and skin fibroblasts have been described [58]. They were recognized through diminished estrogen production during pregnancy and had 19 to 36 percent of normal steroid sulfatase activity.

STEROID SULFATASE DEFICIENCY AND X-LINKED ICHTHYOSIS

The availability of cell culture assays for steroid sulfatase activity has permitted family studies. Many authors had speculated on the X-linked nature of the enzyme defect based on initial observations that this disorder exclusively involved male fetuses. Pedigree studies using fibroblast assays were able to confirm the X-linked nature of inheritance, and this was validated by somatic cell genetic studies as described below [80]. Until recently, the opinion of a number of investigators working in the area was that children resulting from pregnancies affected by steroid sulfatase deficiency were phenotypically normal after the time of birth. Two groups independently observed that individuals with steroid sulfatase deficiency suffered from a unique dermatologic condition, ichthyosis [80, 81]. Furthermore, in several of the families under investigation, ichthyosis segregated as an X-linked trait, and there was complete concordance between steroid sulfatase deficiency and phenotypic ichthyosis [80]. These findings raised several questions about the relationship of steroid sulfatase deficiency and X-linked ichthyosis.

The genetic ichthyoses comprise a group of heritable disorders of the epidermis characterized by hyperkeratosis, or increased thickness of the stratum corneum [82, 82a]. A large number of syndromes associated with ichthyosis have been reported and there are many acquired forms of ichthyosis as well [83]. Three major genetically and clinically separable disorders in which ichthyosis is the primary feature have been described. These include a relatively severe autosomal recessively inherited condition known as lamellar ichthyosis, the somewhat milder disorders of autosomal dominant ichthyosis vulgaris, and X-linked ichthyosis [84]. It has been known for over a hundred years that ichthyosis can segregate in some families as an X-linked trait [85]. The work of Wells, Kerr, and Jennings in the early and middle 1960s provided clearcut genetic and clinical delineation of these various forms of ichthyosis [86–90]. These workers were able to demonstrate that autosomal dominant and X-linked ichthyosis were relatively common disorders, with the latter condition being present in approximately 1 in 6000 males studied in their population. They had reason to believe that they had complete ascertainment within the geographic area under consideration. They were able to show that X-linked ichthyosis differed from autosomal dominant ichthyosis vulgaris in age of onset, relative distribution of disease, severity, and a variety of histopathologic features (Tables 49-2 and 49-3).

Aside from the obvious differences in inheritance patterns, X-linked ichthyosis is characterized by onset between birth and 4 months of age, and involvement of the upper and lower limbs and trunk (Fig. 49-3). There is frequent involvement of the scalp and neck but sparing of the palms and soles. The nails and hair are normal. The scales are dark, large, and prominent. Histologically there is hyperkeratosis, with a normal or increased granular layer (Fig. 49-4) [89]. Finally, characteristic corneal opacities may be observed on slit-lamp examination [91]. These opacities have no effect on visual acuity and are said to be present occasionally in heterozygous females, although it is not clear whether the abnormalities in these women are much more frequent than in the normal population [91]. Although complaints of "dry skin" are often elicited from women who are obligate heterozygotes, objectively detectable ichthyosis is not seen. This is interesting in view of the unusual behavior of the steroid sulfatase locus with regard to X chromosome inactivation to be discussed below.

In the late 1960s X-linked ichthyosis became the subject of a number of genetic investigations in several parts of the world [92–97]. It was found to be an interesting genetic trait to which linkage analysis could be applied because of the relative frequency of the disorder, its known chromosomal location, and the apparent minimal effects on genetic fitness of the mutant allele which resulted in large pedigrees with several

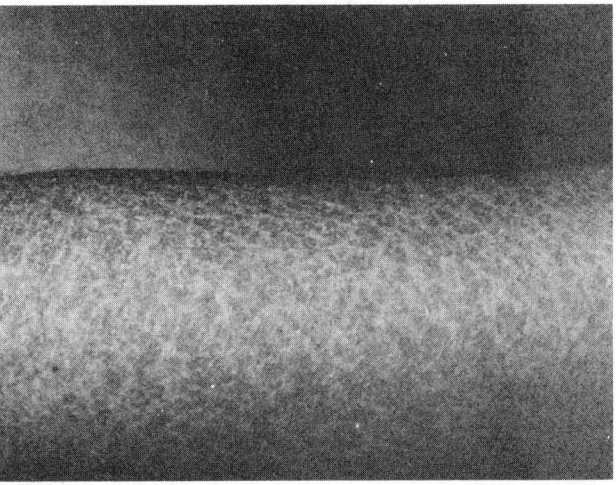

Figure 49-3 Photograph of forearm of 6-year-old boy with X-linked ichthyosis due to steroid sulfatase deficiency. The scales present were first noted at about 3 months of age and have become progressively larger, thicker, and darker. They are present on the extremities, trunk (particularly the flanks), neck, and scalp. The face is less severely affected. Symptoms are often milder during warmer weather and topical moisturizers are of limited benefit.

affected generations. Tests were made for linkage with other known X chromosome markers by family-study methods. Linkage with the glucose-6-phosphate dehydrogenase locus was clearly excluded but studies established definite and close linkage with the Xg blood group antigen locus.

Following the observation that patients with steroid sulfatase deficiency had a skin disorder clinically and genetically indistinguishable from X-linked ichthyosis, it seemed reasonable to ask whether some abnormality in sulfated steroid metabolism might be responsible for the extensively studied, common X-linked ichthyosis. Studies were performed involving patients from many parts of the world who were ascertained by virtue of their ichthyosis and without regard to obstetric or endocrinologic history. It was established that all patients who had pedigree documentation of X-linked ichthyosis and had no other associated defects had steroid sulfatase deficiency [78, 81, 98–100]. Patients with various other kinds of epidermal disorders were studied and found to have normal steroid sulfatase activity. It thus appeared that steroid sulfatase deficiency is a feature of most if not all cases of uncomplicated X-linked ichthyosis. It is of note that the obstetric histories obtained from the mothers of patients with X-linked ichthyosis rarely reflect any difficulties with parturition. The best synthesis of available clinical details at present would suggest that: (1) decreased estriol production during pregnancy and postnatal ichthyosis are consistently associated with steroid sulfatase deficiency, and (2) delayed onset of parturition and prolongation of labor are seen in only some and perhaps even a minority of patients.

A causal relationship between steroid sulfatase deficiency and X-linked ichthyosis is supported by observations on the relatively rare genetic disorder, multiple sulfatase deficiency [102–104]. This condition is inherited as an autosomal recessive single-gene disorder and results in deficiency of a variety of sulfatases in many tissues. Absent or reduced activity of lysosomal arylsulfatases A and B, iduronate sulfatase, heparan sulfatase, and several other nonlysosomal sulfatases, including steroid sulfatase, have been reported. The involved sulfatases are normally found in the lysosomal compartment or in the

Table 49-2 Clinical features of steroid sulfatase deficiency

In fetal life	In postnatal life
Low maternal urinary and serum estriol	Ichthyosis with onset from birth to 4 months
Male fetus	Corneal opacities
Delayed onset of labor (a variable feature)	Pedigree evidence of X-linked defect
Relative refractoriness of cervical dilatation during parturition (particularly primigravidas)	Increased cholesterol sulfate in plasma, red blood cells, and skin with rapidly migrating LDL
Apparent clinical normality in newborn period	Diminished steroid sulfatase activity with a variety of substances in numerous tissues
Elevated DHEAS and 16-hydroxy-DHEAS in maternal urine and amniotic fluid	
Absent placental 3β-hydroxy steroid sulfatase activity with normal dehydrogenase-isomerase and aromatase	

Table 49-3 Some genetic ichthyoses

	Inheritance	Biochemical defect	Associated abnormalities	Distinguishing histologic features
X-linked ichthyosis	X-linked	Steroid sulfatase	↓ Fetal estriol production	Hyperkeratosis with normal to ↑ granular layer
Lamellar ichthyosis	AR	—	None	Collodian membrane at birth, hyperkeratosis, parakeratosis, ↑ granular layer and prominent rete ridges
Ichthyosis vulgaris	AD	—	None	Mild hyperkeratosis ↓ or absent granular layer
Congenital ichthyosiform erythroderma	AR	—	Ectropion eclabion	
Bullous ichthyosiform erythroderma	AD	—	Blisters, verrucous scales	Marked hyperkeratosis, coarse keratohyalin granules, vacuolization of cells
Refsum's syndrome	AR	Phytanic acid α-hydroxylase	Retinitis pigmentosa polyneuritis, ataxia, deafness, anosmia	—
Sjogren-Larson	AR	—	Spasticity, mental retardation, short stature, brittle hair, hypoplasia of teeth, metaphysical dysplasia	—
Conradi's disease	AD & AR forms	—	Short limbed, short stature, stippled epiphyses, cataracts, joint contractures	—
Netherton's syndrome	AR	—	Trichorrhexis invaginata	—

NOTE: AR, autosomal recessive; AD, autosomal dominant

microsomal fraction of cell extracts. The enzymes involved in multiple sulfatase deficiency do not share common subunits and are encoded on different autosomes, as well as the X chromosome. No common posttranslational processing stops have been found. Patients who have steroid sulfatase deficiency from this unique mutation also have diminished estriol production during fetal life [105] and ichthyosis or other skin abnormalities postnatally [104]. This observation discounts the hypothesis that there is a close genetic linkage between steroid sulfatase deficiency and X-linked ichthyosis but no true cause-and-effect relationship.

Metabolic Studies in Steroid Sulfatase Deficiency

Initial ascertainment of steroid sulfatase–deficient subjects was the result of fetal maternal metabolic abnormalities. Decreased estriol production because of an inability of the placenta to metabolize sulfated precursors was the initial hallmark of this disorder. There is an impaired ability in vivo to convert DHEAS to estrogens, whether the precursors are supplied to the maternal or fetal compartment. Associated with these dynamic observations are increased steady state levels of DHEAS or 16-hydroxy-DHEAS in amniotic fluid and maternal urine [66, 67, 106]. Surprisingly, cord blood levels of these metabolites have been normal except in one investigation, and levels of DHEAS, pregnenolone sulfate, and androstenediol sulfate measured in adult subjects with X-linked ichthyosis have been investigated and found to be twenty to thirtyfold increased in plasma and red blood cell membranes of affected subjects postnatally [15]. Furthermore, electrophoretic mobil-

ity of low density lipoproteins (LDL) is increased in these subjects, presumably because of increased electronegativity resulting from incorporation of the charged sulfate ester [108]. Increased cholesterol content of stratum corneum from X-linked ichthyosis patients has also been described. This suggests a primary etiologic role for accumulation of this sterol in the pathogenesis of the skin lesions [17].

A number of forms of ichthyosis have been associated with abnormalities of lipid metabolism. Patients taking triparanol (MER-29) or nicotinic acid to lower serum cholesterol levels may develop ichthyosis [109, 110]. Essential fatty acid deficiency in experimental animals produces epidermal changes which include ichthyosis [111]. Vitamin A deficiency leads to scaling of the skin [112], and synthetic retinoids have proved to be useful therapeutically in several of the ichthyoses, but not in X-linked ichthyosis [113]. Some patients on retinoic acid therapy have developed hypertriglyceridemia [114, 114a]. Individuals with Refsum's disease frequently have ichthyosis and this is associated with epidermal accumulation of phytanic acid glycerides or esters of cholesterol [115–117]. Finally, at least one infant with the very severe "harlequin" ichthyosis has been found to have increased epidermal cholesterol ester content [118]. While it is difficult to reconcile all of these observations, the role of lipids in epidermal differentiation seems clear and suggests possibilities for further investigation regarding the relationship of CS accumulation to the development of X-linked ichthyosis.

While the plasma levels of DHEAS and CS in normal subjects are similar, there is a striking disparity in the metabolism of these compounds in steroid sulfatase–deficient individuals, and this remains to be completely explained [15] (Table 49-1). The source and quantitative kinetics of circulating CS have been examined. At least half of the CS produced daily is desulfated to free cholesterol or cholesterol esters [23]. Biliary-fecal excretion may account for the remainder [119]. In contrast, only a small percentage of DHEAS is normally desulfated [32, 33, 34, 120]. The metabolic fate of all of the daily production of DHEAS is not clear. DHEAS is more water soluble than CS and has a higher renal clearance rate [4]. The lack of increase in circulating DHEAS levels in steroid sulfatase–deficient patients thus confirms the relatively small contribution of desulfation to DHEAS disposal. Interestingly, free DHEA levels in these patients are normal. Free DHEA normally circulates in concentrations a thousandfold less than the corresponding sulfate. Therefore, even slow desulfation of DHEAS → DHEA may be important in maintaining levels of the unconjugated steroid. Normal levels of free DHEA in steroid sulfatase–deficient patients suggest that enzymatic desulfation of DHEAS may in fact not be important in the production of circulating DHEA.

Preliminary studies of pituitary-gonadal function have been performed in adult steroid sulfatase–deficient males [16] (Table 49-1). Affected individuals have normal plasma levels of testosterone and estradiol without requiring the stimulation of excessive gonadotropins. Fertility is, of course, well documented by virtue of the ability of affected individuals to transmit the mutant gene. As discussed in a previous section, the finding of large amounts of sulfated precursors in testicular homogenates and the demonstration of the ability of various preparations to use sulfated steroids as precursors for testosterone production have suggested a role for steroid sulfatase activity in the regulation of gonadal androgen biosynthesis. Although further studies are needed and the direct demonstration of enzyme deficiency in testicular tissue has not been achieved, the normal gonadal function of these patients suggests that pathways involving sulfated intermediates are not quantitatively important.

Steroid Sulfatase Deficiency and X Chromosome Inactivation

Considerable evidence has been assembled to suggest that a locus important in the expression of steroid sulfatase activity is

Figure 49-4 Histologic features in X-linked ichthyosis. A routine punch biopsy was performed from the forearm of the maternal grandfather of the boy shown in Fig. 49-3. This individual had documented steroid sulfatase deficiency and ichthyosis. No inflammatory changes are seen. There is marked thickening and delamination of the stratum corneum with a normal or slightly thickened granular layer.

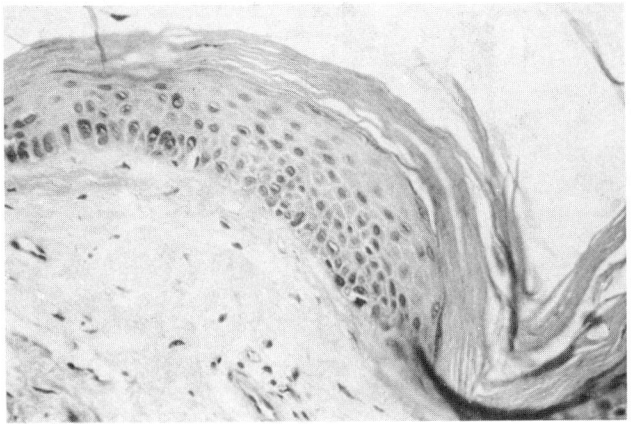

on the X chromosome. Recent investigations into the mechanism of control of expression of this locus have yielded unexpected dividends in knowledge about X chromosome inactivation. The phenomenon of X chromosome inactivation is observed in virtually all mammals [121, 122] and is discussed in Chap. 1.

Several problems in accepting the notion of complete inactivation of one of the X chromosomes in normal females and other individuals have been appreciated. Based on evolutionary considerations, Lyon suggested that X inactivation might not involve the entire X chromosome [123]. Clinicians have suspected this for some time. This is because individuals with X aneuploid states such as the Turner syndrome and Kleinfelter syndrome have clearly observable abnormalities [124]. If one of the two X's in a normal female somatic cell was completely inactivated, then one would anticipate no genetic difference between XY males with one copy of X chromosomal material, XO Turner individuals with one copy of X chromosomal material, and normal XX females who have two copies of X chromosomal material with one set of X-encoded genes inactivated. Likewise, if the second X in Kleinfelter males were completely functionally inactivated, one would not anticipate the clinical abnormalities so often observed. A variety of cytogenetic and clinical correlations have been drawn which permit proposal of a model in which some X chromosomal genes remain non-inactivated.

Until recently, the only specific locus for which there is any biochemical evidence supporting a non-inactivated region of the X involves the Xg^a blood group antigen system. The Xg^a antigen is a highly polymorphic marker in human populations. Race and Sanger were able to demonstrate the X-linked nature of antigen positivity by pedigree studies [125]. It is not possible, however, to separate two populations of red blood cells [Xg(a+) and Xg(a−)] in obligate heterozygotes, as one might expect. This is in spite of the fact that artificial mixtures of hemizygous Xg(a+) and Xg(a−) cells can be separated by immunologic techniques [126].

Other studies supporting the non-inactivation of Xg involved a chimeric twin pair, each of whom had blood group O and AB cells. The cells could easily be separated on the basis of their ABO blood group markers. The O cells were found to be Xg(a+) positive and the AB cells were Xg(a−) negative [127]. This demonstration of two populations of cells in one blood circulation indicated that the reason for failure of identification of clonal populations in other experiments was not due to the fact that the Xg^a antigen was synthesized in extra erythrocytic cells and secondarily taken up by the red cells. Furthermore, in females doubly heterozygous for X-linked sideroblastic anemia and Xg positivity, two populations of red cells may be separated by virtue of their size. These women fail to show mosaicism for the Xg^a expression patterns [128].

Perhaps the best evidence in support of non-inactivation of the Xg system comes from the work of Fialkow et al., who studied three women doubly heterozygous for hypoxanthine guanine phosphoribosyltransferase (HGPRT) deficiency (they were mothers of Lesch-Nyhan patients) and for Xg^a antigen positivity. By examination of the pedigrees and knowledge of the distribution of HGPRT-positive red cells in their peripheral blood, it was possible to provide strong evidence for non-inactivation of the Xg locus [129]. In spite of these findings, some doubt about the status of Xg inactivation has persisted [130, 131]. This is because it appears that the Xg locus may in fact be inactivated when it is positioned on a structurally abnormal X chromosome [132]. The partial inactivation question could not be resolved to a completely satisfactory degree because of the inability to study Xg in a somatic cell genetic system, as Xg^a is expressed only on the surface of erythroid cells.

As already discussed, a strong linkage exists between the locus for X-linked ichthyosis–steroid sulfatase deficiency and the Xg blood group locus. The advantage of studying steroid sulfatase deficiency is that it can be easily detected in cultured somatic cells and this locus can be subjected to analysis by somatic cell hybridization and related genetic techniques. When fibroblasts from obligate heterozygotes for steroid sulfatase deficiency were cloned, only a single population of cells with normal levels of steroid sulfatase was identified [133]. Additional work with hair follicles likewise substantiated a unimodal distribution of enzyme activities in women who should have had two populations of follicles if the region of the X encoding the steroid sulfatase locus were inactivated [77a]. Even when the women who were chosen as subjects were doubly heterozygous for steroid sulfatase deficiency and G-6-PD deficiency, no inactivation of the steroid sulfatase locus was observed [133]. These studies had an important built-in control in that the G-6-PD locus is known to undergo X inactivation. Therefore, it was possible to test the clones that were isolated from these women and to show that they derived from two populations of cells with regard to G-6-PD phenotypes. Thus, some clones were obtained in which the paternal X was active and other clones in which the maternal X was active. In spite of this, the single normal steroid sulfatase allele which these cells possessed was apparently never inactivated. Further studies utilizing somatic cell hybrids which retain only the inactive human X chromosome have likewise demonstrated that steroid sulfatase appears to be expressed by an otherwise inactivated X chromosome [134]. These somatic cell hybrids were produced by fusion of mouse fibroblast cells which lacked steroid sulfatase and human fibroblast cell lines derived from patients with X-autosome translocations. In such human subjects it is possible to distinguish the active from the inactive X morphologically. In the hybrids isolated with the "inactive" X chromosome, there was no expression of a number of known human X-linked markers including HGPRT, G-6-PD, and PGK (phosphoglycerate kinase) in spite of the presence of a cytologically identifiable X chromosome. Nonetheless, steroid sulfatase, which was electrophoretically and immunologically indistinguishable from normal human fibroblast steroid sulfatase, was produced by these hybrids.

Studies with steroid sulfatase–deficient patients and others with aberrations of X chromosome structure can likewise be used for purposes of delineating the region of the X chromosome that contains this interesting locus. Somatic cell hybrids have been produced between a variety of human cell lines containing translocations and mouse parental lines. By analysis of the segregation of the various fragments of the X chromosome and the concordance of these cytologic markers with the expression of human steroid sulfatase, it has been possible to assign the steroid sulfatase locus to the very distal tip of the short arm of the X chromosome [135, 136]. Recently this assignment was confirmed by a deletion mapping technique. Several informative patients have been identified in whom XY translocations involving the short arm of the X chromosome have occurred [137–139]. In those translocations which result in the deletion of the very distal tip of the X chromosome, steroid sulfatase deficiency and ichthyosis may be observed. The correlation of these findings is of considerable interest. All

of the X-linked genes which are known to undergo X chromosome inactivation and have received a regional assignment on the X chromosome have been shown to reside on the long arm of the X. Only steroid sulfatase and perhaps Xg have been mapped to the short arm of this chromosome. Thus, there is apparent functional and "anatomic" correlation. The short arm of the X chromosome pairs end to end with the Y chromosome during male meiosis, and it is deletion of the short arm of the X chromosome which produces many of the features of the Turner syndrome. It is therefore interesting to speculate that a group of genes located within this portion of the genome must be present in two dosages to produce normal female differentiation (Fig. 49-5).

Several interesting genetic issues remain to be clarified in regard to the steroid sulfatase locus. One question is whether

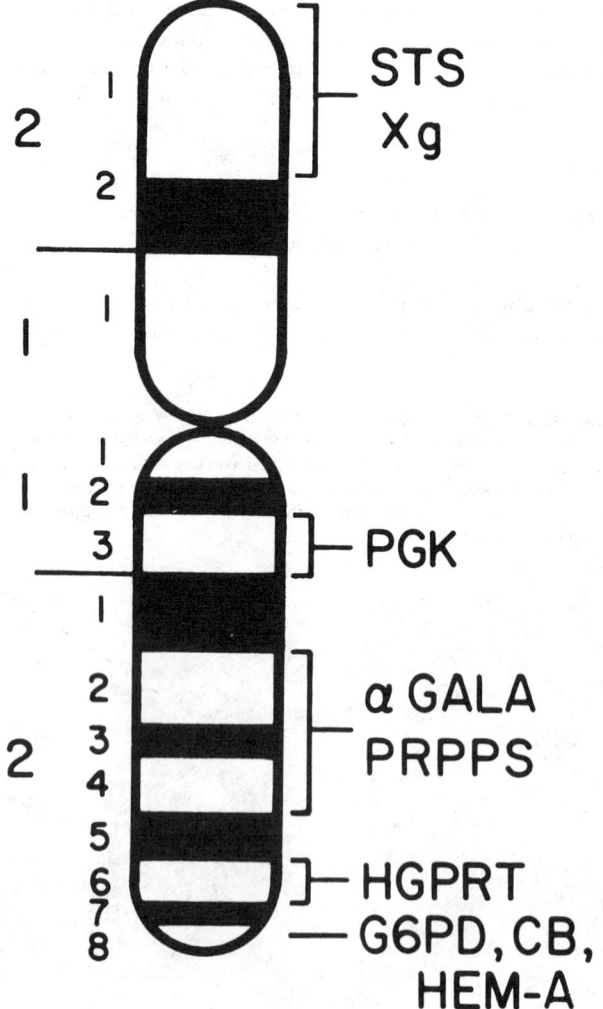

Figure 49-5 Schematic genetic map of the human X chromosome. The banding pattern shown conforms to the Paris Conference standards. At present at least 114 loci have been assigned to the X chromosome, primarily through pedigree analysis. A number of loci have now been regionally mapped largely as a result of somatic cell hybridization techniques employing X autosome translocation cell lines. Some assignments have been made by classical linkage analysis with known markers and at least one by radiation-induced chromosome fragmentation and somatic cell genetic analysis. Steroid sulfatase has been assigned to the region Xp22 → Xpter by using suitable translocations and by deletion mapping. STS = steroid sulfatase, Xg = blood group antigen, PGK = phosphoglycerate kinase, α-GALA = α-galactosidase A, PRPPS = phosphoribosyl pyrophosphate synthetase, HGPRT = hypoxanthine guanine phosphoribosyltransferase, G-6-PD = glucose-6-phosphate dehydrogenase, CB = color blindness, HEM-A = hemophilia A.

or not the steroid sulfatase locus escapes X inactivation when it is situated on a structurally abnormal X chromosome, as appears to be the case with Xg. A second question relates to the extent of genetic heterogeneity in steroid sulfatase deficiency. This disorder is one of the most common inborn errors of metabolism and appears in many populations around the world. To date, complementation studies and immunologic investigations have failed to disclose any differences between patients ascertained from diverse geographic areas [140]. A third question relates to gene dosage compensation at the steroid sulfatase locus. If this region truly escapes inactivation, one might anticipate that increasing enzyme activity would be found with increasing numbers of X's. One group has found a sex difference in enzyme levels in cultured fibroblasts [141], and another study observed similar differences in placentas from male and female fetuses [142]. Two other groups using leukocytes and hair follicles have not observed a gene dosage effect [76, 77a]. These differences will need to be reconciled.

CLINICAL MANAGEMENT

The diagnosis of X-linked ichthyosis can now be readily made both prenatally and postnatally. Typical clinical findings coupled with a characteristic family history are virtually diagnostic, but this impression can be confirmed by assay of steroid sulfatase activity in fibroblasts, epidermal derivatives including hair roots, and white blood cells. Elevated blood cholesterol sulfate (fifteen- to thirtyfold) is present as early as age 3 months and persists in affected patients at least to 74 years and can be used as a clinical marker. Prenatally, diminished estrogen production assessed in maternal urine or serum should be a good indicator in the third trimester. As far as the author is aware, no pregnancies that have been monitored prospectively in families ascertained solely through ichthyosis have demonstrated abnormal estrogen metabolism.

Mid-trimester prenatal diagnosis may be achieved through enzyme assay of cultured amniotic fluid cells and careful serum estriol determinations by a laboratory with extensive experience with estriols done at 18 to 20 weeks gestation. We have studied a single pregnancy that was correctly diagnosed in this fashion [16]. The indications for prenatal diagnosis must be carefully considered in advance. Improved management of pregnancy at term is one justification for such studies. Many ethical questions are raised by consideration of pregnancy termination for this *relatively* mild cosmetic defect.

Since the steroid sulfatase locus escapes inactivation, carrier detection in this disorder is apparently more feasible in steroid sulfatase deficiency than for many other X-linked disorders in which the extent of deviation from the expected 50:50 distribution can cause numerous difficulties [143]. Although experience is limited, it would seem that fibroblasts or white blood cells can be used for such determinations [76, 144]. Reliability still needs to be established.

No effective therapy for steroid sulfatase deficiency exists. The prenatal consequences of the enzyme defect can be handled expectantly and cesarean section used when indicated. The ichthyosis is relatively refractory to most topical agents. Oral synthetic retinoids which are useful in many of the other ichthyoses do not seem to benefit steroid sulfatase–deficient patients. Perhaps from our improved understanding of the biochemical basis of this disorder will come further information about pathogenesis and rational therapy.

REFERENCES

1. SCHACHTER B, MARRIAN GF: The isolation of estrone sulfate from the urine of pregnant mares. *J Biol Chem* 126:663, 1938
2. VENNING EH, HOFFMAN MM, BROWNE JSL: Isolation of androsterone sulfate. *J Biol Chem* 146:369, 1942
3. MUNSON PL, GALLAGHER, TF, KOCK FC: Isolation of dehydroisoandrosterone sulfate from normal male urine. *J Biol Chem* 152:67, 1944
4. ROBERTS DR, LIEBERMAN S: The biochemistry of the 3β-hydroxy-Δ⁵-steroid sulfates, in Bernstein S, Solomon S (eds): *Chemical and Biological Aspects of Steroid Conjugation.* New York, Springer-Verlag, 1970, p 219
5. ROY AB: Enzymological aspects of steroid conjugation, in Bernstein S, Solomon S (eds): *Chemical and Biological Aspects of Steroid Conjugation.* New York, Springer-Verlag, 1970, p 74
6. ROBERTS KD, BANDI L, CALVIN HI, DRUCKER WD, LIEBERMAN S: Evidence that steroid sulfates serve as biosynthetic intermediates. IV. Conversion of cholesterol sulfate *in vivo* to urinary C_{19} and C_{21} steroidal sulfates. *Biochem* 3:1983, 1964
7. ROBERTS KD, VAN DE WIELE RL, AND LIEBERMAN S: The conversion in vivo of dehydroisoandrosterone sulfate to androsterone and etiocholanolone glucuronides. *J Biol Chem* 236:2213, 1961
8. KELLIE AE: The metabolism of steroid conjugates: Androstenolone sulphate and glucuronoside. *J Endocrinol* 22:i–ii, 1961
9. CALVIN HI, VAN DE WIELE RL, LIEBERMAN S: Evidence that steroid sulfates serve as biosynthetic intermediates: In vivo conversion of pregnenolone-sulfate-S³⁵ to dehydroisoandrosterone sulfate–S³⁵. *Biochem* 2:648, 1963
10. DRAYER NM, LIEBERMAN S: Isolation of cholesterol sulfate from human blood and gallstones. *Biochem Biophys Res Commun* 18:126, 1965
11. DRAYER NM, LIEBERMAN S: Isolation of cholesterol sulfate from human aortas and adrenal tumors. *J Clin Endocrinol Metab* 27:136, 1967
12. MOSER HW, MOSER AB, ORR JC: Preliminary observations on the occurrence of cholesterol sulfate in man. *Arch Biochem Biophys* 116:146, 1966
13. BLEAU G, BODLEY FH, LONGPRÉ J, CHAPDELAINE A, ROBERTS KD: Cholesterol sulfate I. Occurrence and possible biological function as an amphipathic lipid in the membrane of the human erythrocyte. *Biochim Biophys Acta* 352:1, 1974
13a. LALUMIÈRE G, LONGPRÉ J, TRUDEL J, CHAPDELAINE A, ROBERTS KD: Cholesterol sulfate II. Studies on its metabolism and possible function in canine blood. *Biochim Biophys Acta* 394:120, 1975
14. BLEAU G, LALUMIÈRE G, CHAPDELAINE A, ROBERTS KD: Red cell surface structure. Stabilization by cholesterol sulfate as evidenced by scanning electron microscopy. *Biochim Biophys Acta* 375:220, 1975
15. BERGNER EA, SHAPIRO LJ: Increased cholesterol sulfate in plasma and red blood cell membranes of steroid sulfatase deficient patients. *J Clin Endocrinol Metab* 53:221, 1981
16. SHAPIRO LJ, unpublished observations
17. WILLIAMS ML, ELIAS PM: X-linked ichthyosis: Elevated cholesterol sulfate in pathologic stratum corneum. *Clin Res* 29:26 (abstract), 1981
18. BLEAU G, VANDENHEUVEL WJA: Desmosteryl sulfate and desmosterol in hamster epididymal spermatozoa. *Steroids* 24:549, 1974
18a. LALUMIÈRE G, BLEAU G, CHAPDELAINE A, ROBERTS KD: Cholesteryl sulfate and sterol sulfatase in the human reproductive tract. *Steroids* 27:247, 1976
19. LEGAULT Y, BLEAU G, CHAPDELAINE A, AND ROBERTS KD: The binding of sterol sulfates to hamster spermatozoa. *Steroids* 34:89, 1979
20. PAYNE AH, LAWRENCE CC, FOSTER DL, JAFFE RB: Intranuclear binding of 17-β estradiol and estrone in female ovine pituitaries following incubation with estrone sulfate. *J Biol Chem* 248:1598, 1973
21. VIGNON F, TERQUI M, WESTLEY B, DEROCQ D, ROCHEFORT H: Effects of plasma estrogen sulfates in mammary cancer cells. *Endocrinol* 106:1079, 1980
22. JENKIN G, HEAP RB: Formation of oestradiol-17β from oestrone sulphate by sheep foetal pituitary in vitro. *Nature* 259:330, 1976
23. GURPIDE E, ROBERTS KD, WELCH MT, BANDI L, LIEBERMAN S: Studies on the metabolism of blood-borne cholesterol sulfate. *Biochem* 5:3352, 1966
24. ROBERTS KD, BANDI L, LIEBERMAN S: The conversion of cholesterol-³H-sulfate-³⁵S into pregnenolone-³H-sulfate-³⁵S by sonicated bovine adrenal mitochondria. *Biochem Biophys Res Commun* 29:741, 1967
25. SOLOMON S: Formation and metabolism of neutral steroids in the human placenta and fetus. *J Clin Endocrinol Metab* 26:762, 1966
26. PION R, CONRAD SH, WOLF BJ: Pregnenolone sulfate—an efficient precourser for the placental production of progesterone. *J Clin Endocrinol Metab* 26:255, 1966
27. MATHUR RS, ARCHER DF, WIQVIST N, DICZFALUSY E: Quantitative assessment of the de novo sterol and steroid synthesis in the human foetoplacental unit. I. Synthesis and secretion of cholesterol and cholesterol sulphate. *Acta Endocrinol* 65:663, 1970
28. KORTH-SCHUTZ S, LEVINE LS, NEW MI: Dehydroepiandrosterone sulfate

(DS) levels, a rapid test for abnormal adrenal androgen secretion. *J Clin Endocrinol Metab* 42:1005, 1976

29. REITER EO, FAULDAUER VG, ROOT AW: Secretion of the adrenal androgen, dehydroepiandrosterone sulfate during normal infancy, childhood, and adolescence, in sick infants, and in children with endocrinologic abnormalities. *J Pediatr* 90:766, 1977

30. DE PERETTI E, FOREST MG: Patterns of plasma dehydroepiandrosterone sulfate levels in humans from birth to adulthood and evidence for testicular production. *J Clin Endocrinol Metab* 47:572, 1978

31. VIHKO R, RUOKONEN A: Regulation of steroidogenesis in testis. *J Steroid Biochem* 5:843, 1974

32. MACDONALD PC, CHAPDELAINE A, GONZALEZ O, GURPIDE E, VAN DE WIELE RL, LIEBERMAN S: Studies on the secretion and interconversion of the androgens. III. Results obtained after the injection of several radioactive C$_{19}$ steroids, singly or as mixtures. *J Clin Endocrinol* 25:1557, 1965

33. CHAPDELAINE A, MACDONALD PC, GONZALEZ O, GURPIDE E, VAN DE WIELE RL, LIEBERMAN S: Studies on the secretion and interconversion of the androgens. IV. Quantitative results in a normal man whose gonadal and adrenal function were altered experimentally. *J Clin Endocrinol* 25:1569, 1965

34. HORTON R, TAIT JF: *In vivo* conversion of dehydroisoandrosterone to plasma androstenedione and testosterone in man. *J Clin Endocrinol* 27:79, 1967

35. NOTATION AD, UNGAR F: Rat testis steroid sulfatase: 2. Kinetic study. *Steroids* 14:151, 1969

35a. NOTATION AD: Regulatory interactions for the control of steroid sulfate metabolism. *J Steroid Biochem* 6:311, 1975

36. DOMINGUEZ OV, VALENCIA SA, LOZA AC: On the role of steroid sulfates in hormone biosynthesis. *J Steroid Biochem* 6:301, 1975

37. VIHKO R, RUOKONEN A: Steroid sulphates in human adult testicular steroid synthesis. *J Steroid Biochem* 6:353, 1975

38. PAYNE AH: Testicular steroid sulfotransferases: Comparison to liver and adrenal steroid sulfotransferases of the mature rat. *Endocrinol* 106:1365, 1980

39. FRANDSEN VA, STAKEMANN G: The site of production of oestrogenic hormones in human pregnancy. *Acta Endocrinol* 38:383, 1961

40. FRANDSEN VA, STAKEMANN G: The site of production of oestrogenic hormones in human pregnancy II. *Acta Endocrinol* 43:184, 1963

41. MIGEON CJ, FELLER AR, HOLMSTROM EG: Dehydroepiandrosterone, androsterone, and 17 hydroxycorticosteroid levels in maternal and cord plasma in cases of vaginal delivery. *Johns Hopkins Hosp. Bull.* 97:415, 1955

42. SIMMER HH, EASTERLING WE, PION RJ, DIGNAM WJ; Neutral C$_{19}$-steroids and steroid sulfates in human pregnancy. I. Identification of dehydroepiandrosterone sulfate in fetal blood and quantification of this hormone in cord material, cord venous, and maternal peripheral blood in normal pregnancy at term. *Steroids* 4:125, 1964

43. SIITERI PK, MACDONALD PC: Placental estrogen biosynthesis during human pregnancy. *J Clin Endocrinol Metab* 26:751, 1966

44. PULKKINEN MO: Arylsulphatase and the hydrolysis of some steroid sulphates in developing organisms and placenta. *Acta Physiol Scand* 52 suppl 18:9, 1961

45. WARREN JC, TIMBERLAKE CE: Steroid sulfatase in the human placenta. *J Clin Endocrinol Metab* 22:1148, 1962

46. WARREN JC, TIMBERLAKE CE: Biosynthesis of estrogens in pregnancy: Precursor role of plasma dehydroisoandrosterone. *Obstet and Gynecol* 23:689, 1964

47. RYAN KJ: Biological aromatization of steroids. *J Biol Chem* 234:268, 1959

48. SIITERI PK, MACDONALD PC: The utilization of circulating dehydroisoandrosterone sulfate for estrogen synthesis during human pregnancy. *Steroids* 2:713, 1963

49. KOLODNY E, MOSER HW: Sulfatide lipidosis: Metachromatic leukodystrophy, in Stanbury JB, Wyngaarden JB, Fredrickson DS, et al (eds): *Metabolic Basis of Inherited Disease,* 5th ed. New York, McGraw-Hill 1982, p 751

50. MCKUSICK VA, NEUFELD E: The mucopolysaccharide storage diseases, in Stanbury JB, Wyngaarden JB, Fredrickson DS, et al (eds): *Metabolic Basis of Inherited Disease,* 5th ed. New York, McGraw-Hill 1982, pp

51. ZUCKERMAN NA, HAGERMAN DD: The hydrolysis of estrone sulfate by rat kidney microsomal sulfatase. *Arch Biochem Biophys* 135:410, 1966

52. FRENCH AP, WARREN JC; Properties of steroid sulphatase and arylsulphatase activities of human placenta. *Biochem J* 105:233, 1967

53. BLEAU G, CHAPDELAINE A, ROBERTS KD: Studies on mammalian and molluscan steroid sulfatase. Solubilization and properties. *Canad J Biochem* 49:234, 1971

54. IWAMORI M, MOSER HW, KISHIMOTO Y: Solubilization and partial purification of steroid sulfatase from rat liver: Characterization of estrone sulfatase. *Arch Biochem Biophys* 174:199, 1976

55. GAUTHIER R, VIGNEAULT N, BLEAU G, CHAPDELAINE A, ROBERTS KD: Solubilization and partial purification of steroid sulfatase of human placenta. *Steroids* 31:783, 1978

56. TOWNSLEY JD, SCHEEL, DA, RUBIN EJ: Inhibition of steroid 3-sulfatase by endogenous steroids. A possible mechanism controlling placental estrogen synthesis from conjugated precursors. *J Clin Endocrinol* 31:670, 1970

57. MCNAUGHT RW, FRANCE, JT: Studies of the biochemical basis of steroid sulphatase deficiency: Preliminary evidence suggesting a defect in membrane-enzyme structure, *J Steroid Biochem* 13:363, 1980

58. HAMEISTER H, WOLFF G, LAURITZEN CH, LEHMANN WO, HAUSER A, ROPERS HH: Clinical and biochemical investigations on patients with partial deficiency of placental steroid sulfatase. *Hum Genet* 46:199, 1979

59. FRANCE JT, LIGGINS GC: Placental sulfatase deficiency. *J Clin Endocrinol Metab* 29:138, 1969

60. FRANCE JT: Steroid sulphatase deficiency. *J Steroid Biochem* 11:647, 1979

61. CEDARD L, TCHOBROUSKY C, GUGLIELMINA R, MAILHAC M: Insuffisance oestrogenique paradoxale au cours d'une grossesse normale per défaut de sulfatase placentaire. *Bull Fed Soc Gynaecol Obstet Jan Fr* 23:16, 1971

62. FLIEGNER JRH, SCHINDLER I, BROWN JB: Low urinary oestriol excretion during pregnancy associated with placental sulphatase deficiency or congenital adrenal hypoplasia. *J Obstet Gynaecol Br Commonw* 79:810, 1971

63. FRANCE JT, SEDDON RJ, LIGGINS GC: A study of a pregnancy with low estrogen production due to placental sulphatase deficiency. *J Clin Endocrinol Metab* 36:1, 1973

64. OAKEY RE, CAWOOD MT, MACDONALD PR: Biochemical and clinical observations in a pregnancy with placental sulphatase and other enzyme deficiencies. *Clin Endocrinol* 3:131, 1974

65. TABEI T, HEINRICHS WL: Diagnosis of placental sulfatase deficiency. *Am J Obstet Gynecol* 124:409, 1976

66. OSATHANONDH R, CARICK J, RYAN KJ, TULCHINSKY D: Placental sulfatase deficiency: A case study. *J Clin Endocr Metab* 43:208, 1976

67. BRAUNSTEIN GD, ZIEL FH, ALLEN A, VAN DE VELDE R, WADE M: Prenatal diagnosis of placental steroid sulfatase deficiency. *Am J Obstet Gynecol* 126:716, 1976

68. BEDIN M, CONQUY P, ALSAT E, CEDARD L: Deficit en sulfatase placentaire. Etude clinique et biochimique de trois observations. *Nour Presse Med* 5:1889, 1976

69. CHADWICK JM, MURNAIN JR: Placental sulphatase deficiency causing low urinary oestriol excretion in pregnancy complicated by toxaemia. *Aust NZ J Obstet Gynecol* 16:119, 1976

70. SHAPIRO LJ, COUSINS L, FLUHARTY AL, STEVENS RL, KIHARA H: Steroid sulfatase deficiency. *Pediatr Res* 11:894, 1976

71. FRANCE JT, DOWNEY JA, MCNAUGHT RW, SEDDON RJ, LIGGINS GC: Placental sulphatase deficiency, in James VHT (ed): *Proceedings of the V International Congress of Endocrinology.* Hamburg, July 18–24, 1976. Amsterdam, Excerpta Medica, 2:319, 1977

72. LEHMAN WD, WOLF AS, LAURITZEN CH: Klinische und biochemische Untersuchungen bei drei graviden Patientinnen mit placentarem Sulfatasemangel. *Arch Gynak* 225:43, 1978

73. OAKEY RE: Placental sulphatase deficiency: Antepartum differential diagnosis from foetal adrenal hypoplasia. *Clin Endocrinol* 9:81, 1978

74. BEDIN M, ALSAT E, TANGUY G, CEDARD L: Deficit en sulfatase placentaire, in *Prenatal Endocrinology and Parturition.* Paris, Inserm, 1979 (in press)

75. TAYLOR NG, SHACKLETON CHL; Gas chromatographic steroid analysis for diagnosis placental sulfatase deficiency: A study of nine patients. *J Clin Endocrinol Metab* 49:78, 1979

76. EPSTEIN EH JR, LEVENTHAL ME: Steroid sulfatase of human leukocytes and epidermis and the diagnosis of recessive X-linked ichthyosis. *J Clin Invest* (in press)

77. MEYER JCh, GUNDMANN H-P, SCHNYDER UW: Determination of arylsulfatase C in hair follicles. *Arch Dermatol Res* 266:95, 1979

77a. DANCIS J, JANSEN V, HUTZLER J: Gene dose compensation in X-linked ichthyosis. *Pediatr Res* 14:521, 1980

78. KUBILUS J, TARCIO AJ, BADEN HP: Steroid-sulfatase deficiency in sex-linked ichthyosis. *Am J Hum Genet* 31:50, 1979

79. BADEN HP, HOOKER PA, KUBILUS J, TARASCIO A: Sulfatase activity of keratinizing tissues in X-linked ichthyosis. *Pediatr Res* 14:1347, 1980

80. SHAPIRO LJ, WEISS R, WEBSTER D, FRANCE JT: X-linked ichthyosis due to steroid-sulfatase deficiency. *Lancet* 70, 1978

81. KOPPE JG, MARINKOVIC-ILSEN A, RIJKEN Y, DE GROOT WP, JOBSIS AC: X-linked ichthyosis. A sulphatase deficiency. *Arch Dis Childhood* 53:803, 1978

82. HARPER PS: Genetic heterogeneity in the ichthyoses, in Marks R, Dykes PJ (eds): *The Ichthyoses.* New York, SP Medical & Scientific Books, Spectrum Publications, 1978, p 127

82a. GIANOTTI F: Inherited ichthyosiform dermatoses in infants and children, in Marks R, Dykes PJ (eds): *The Ichthyoses.* New York, SP Medical & Scientific Books, Spectrum Publications, 1978, p 137

83. GOLDSMITH LA: The ichthyoses. *Prog Med Genet* 1:185, 1976

84. WELLS RS, KERR CB: Genetic classification of ichthyosis. *Arch Dermat* 92:1, 1965

85. SEDGWICK W: On the influence of sex in heredity disease. *Br Foreign Med-Chiurg Rev* 31:445, 1863

86. KERR CB, WELLS RS: Sex-linked ichthyosis. *Ann Hum Genet,* 29:33, 1965

87. WELLS RS, KERR CB: Clinical features of autosomal dominant and sex-linked ichthyosis in an English population. *Br Med J* 1:947, 1966

88. WELLS RS, KERR CB: The histology of ichthyosis. *J Invest Dermat* 46:530, 1966

89. MERRETT JD, WELLS RS, KERR CB, BARR A: Discriminant function analysis of phenotype variates in ichthyosis. *Am J Hum Genet* 19:575, 1967

90. WELLS RS, JENNINGS MC: X-linked ichthyosis and ichthyosis vulgaris. *J Am Med Assoc* 202:485, 1967

91. SEVER RJ, FROST P, WEINSTEIN G: Eye changes in ichthyosis. *J Am Med Assoc* 206:2283, 1968

92. KERR CB, WELLS RS, SANGER R: X-linked ichthyosis and the Xg groups. *Lancet* ii:1369, 1964

93. ADAM A, ZIPRKOWSKI L, FEINSTEIN A, SANGER R, RACE RR: Ichthyosis Xg blood-groups, and protan. *Lancet* 1:877, 1966

94. WELLS RS, JENNINGS MC, SANGER R, RACE RR:Xg bloodgroups and ichthyosis. *Lancet* ii:493, 1966

95. FILIPPI G, MEERA KHAN P: Linkage studies on X-linked ichthyosis in Sardinia. *Am J Hum Genet* 20:564, 1968

96. ADAM A, ZIPRKOWSKI L, FEINSTEIN A, SANGER R, TIPPETT P, GAVIN J, RACE RR: Linkage relations of X-borne ichthyosis to the Xg blood groups and to other markers of the X in Israelis. *Am J Hum Genet, Long.* 32:323, 1969

97. WENT LN, DE GROOT WP, SANGER R, TIPPETT P, GAVIN J: X-linked ichthyosis: Linkage relationship with the Xg blood groups and other studies in a large Dutch kindred. *Ann Hum Genet (London)* 32:333, 1969

98. SHAPIRO LJ, BUXMAN MM, WEISS R, VIDGOFF J, DIMOND RL, ROLLER JA, WELLS RS: Enzymatic basis of typical X-linked ichthyosis. *Lancet* ii:756, 1978

99. SHAPIRO LJ: X-linked ichthyosis. *Int J Dermatol* 20:26, 1981

100. DE GROOT WP, JOBSIS AC, MARINKOVIC-ILSEN A, KOPPE JG, DE BRUIJN HWA: Sex-linked ichthyosis and placental sulphatase C deficiency. *Br J Dermatol* 103:73, 1980

101. JOBIS AC, DE GROOT WP, TIGGES AJ, DE BRUIJN HWA, RIJKEN Y, MEIJER AEFH, MARINKOVIC-ILSEN A: X-linked ichthyosis and X-linked placental sulfatase deficiency: A disease entity. *Am J Pathol* 99:279, 1980

102. AUSTIN J: Studies in metachromatic leukodystrophy XII. Multiple sulfatase deficiency. *Arch Neurol* 15:13, 1966

103. MURPHY JV, WOLFE HJ, BALAZS, MOSER HW: A patient with deficiency of arylsulfatases A, B, C, and steroid sulfatase associated with deficiency of sulfatide, cholesterol sulfate, and glycosaminoglycans, in Bernsohn J, Grossman HJ (eds): *Lipid Storage Diseases: Enzymatic Defects and Clinical Implications.* New York, Academic, 1971, p 67

104. DALANEY JT, MOSER HW: Sulfatide lipidosis: Metachromatic leukodystrophy, in Stanbury JB, Wyngaarden JB, Frederickson DS (eds): *Metabolic Basis of Inherited Disease.* 4th ed. New York, McGraw-Hill 1978, p 770

105. STEINMANN B, MIETH D, GITZELMANN R: A newly recognized cause of low urinary estriol in pregnancy: Multiple sulfatase deficiency of the fetus. *Gynecol Obstet Invest* 12:107, 1981

106. TAYLOR NG, SHACKLETON CHL: Gas chromatographic steroid analysis for diagnosis placental sulfatase deficiency: A study of nine patients. *J Clin Endocr Metab* 49:78, 1979

107. RUOKONEN A, OIKARINEN A, PALATSI R, HUHTANIEMI I: Serum steroid sulphates in ichthyosis. *Br J Dermatol* 102:245, 1980

108. EPSTEIN EH, KRAUSS RM, SHACKLETON CHL: X-linked ichthyosis: Increased blood cholesterol sulfate and electrophoretic mobility of low-density lipoprotein. *Science* 214:659, 1981

109. WINKELMANN RK, PERRY HO, ACHOR RU: Cutaneous syndromes produced as side effects of triparanol therapy. *Arch Dermatol* 87:372, 1963

110. FLESCH P: Inhibition of keratinizing structures by systemic drugs. *Pharmacol Rev* 15:653, 1963

111. LOWE NJ, STOUGHTON RB: Essential fatty acid deficient hairless mouse: a model of chronic epidermal hyperproliferation. *Br J Dermatol* 96:155, 1977

112. VAN SCOTT EJ, YU RJ: Metabolic basis for disturbed keratinization in ichthyosis and other diseases, in Marks R, Dykes PJ (eds): *The Ichthyoses.* New York, SP Medical & Scientific Books, Spectrum Publications, 1978, p 3

113. PECK GL, YODER FW: Treatment of disorders of keratinization with an oral stereoisomer of retinoic acid, in Marks R, Dykes PJ (eds): *The Ichthyoses.* New York, SP Medical & Scientific Books, Spectrum Publications, 1978, p 193

114. DICKEN CH, CONNOLLY SM: Eruptive xanthomas associated with isotretinon (13-cis-retinoic acid). *Arch Dermatol* 116:951, 1980

114a.KATZ RA, JORGENSEN H, NIGRA TP: Elevation of serum triglyceride levels from oral isotretinoin in disorders of keratinization. *Arch Dermatol* 116:1369, 1980

115. REFSUM S: Heredopathia atactica polyneuritiformis. *Acta Psychiatr Scand* (suppl) 38:9, 1946

116. ANTON-LAMPRECHT I: Zur ultrastructur hereditarer verhornungsstorungen: U ichthyosis beim Refsumsyndrome. *Arch Dermatol Forsch* 250:185, 1974

117. STEINBERG D: Phytanic acid storage disease (Refsum's Disease), in Stanbury JB, Wyngaarden JB, Fredrickson DS (eds): *Metabolic Basis of Inherited Disease,* 5th ed. New York, McGraw-Hill, 1982, p 731

118. BUXMAN MM, GOODKIN PE, FAHRENBACH WH, DIMOND RL: Harlequin ichthyosis with epidermal lipid abnormality. *Arch Dermatol* 115:189, 1979

119. ENEROTH P, NYSTROM E: Quantification of cholestryl sulfate and neutral sterol derivatives in human feces after purification on lipophilic sephadex gels. *Steroids* 11:187, 1968

120. ROSENFELD RS, HELLMAN L, GALLAGHER TF: Metabolism and interconversion of dehydroisoandrosterone and dehydroisoandrosterone sulfate. *J Clin Endocrinol Metab* 35:187, 1972

121. GARTLER SM, ANDINA RJ: Mammalian X-chromosome inactivation. *Adv Hum Genet* 7:99, 1976

122. LYON MF: Gene action on the X-chromosome of the mouse (Mus musculus). *Nature* 190:372, 1961

123. LYON MF: Evolution of X-chromosome inactivation in mammals. *Nature* 250:651, 1974

124. SIMPSON JL: *Disorders of Sexual Differentiation.* New York, Academic Press, 1976

125. RACE RR, SANGER R: *Blood Groups in Man,* 6th ed. Oxford, Blackwell, 1975

126. GORMAN JG, DIRE J, TREACY AM, CAHAN A: The application of $-Xg^a$ antiserum to the question of red cell mosaicism in female heterozygotes. *J Lab Clin Med* 61:642, 1963

127. DUCOS J, MARTY Y, SANGER R, RACE RR: Xg and X chromosome inactivation. *Lancet* ii:219, 1971

128. WEATHERALL DJ, PEMBREY ME, HALL EG, SANGER R, TIPPETT P, GAVIN J: Familial sideroblastic anaemia: Problem of Xg and X chromosome inactivation. *Lancet* ii:744, 1970

129. FIALKOW PJ: X-chromosome inactivation and the Xg locus. *Am J Hum Genet* 22:460, 1970

130. LAWLER SD, SANGER R: Xg blood-groups and clonal-origin theory of chronic myeloid leukaemia. *Lancet* i:584, 1970

131. FIALKOW PJ, LISKER R, GILBLETT ER, ZAVALA C: Xg locus: Failure to detect inactivation in females with chronic myelocytic leukaemia. *Nature* 226:367, 1970

132. POLANI PE, ANGELL R, GIANNELLI F, DE LA CHAPELLE A, RACE RR, SANGER R: Evidence that the Xg locus is inactivated in structurally abnormal X chromosomes. *Nature* 227:613, 1970

133. SHAPIRO LJ, MOHANDAS T, WEISS R, ROMEO G: Non-inactivation of an X-chromosome locus in man. *Science* 204:1224, 1979

134. MOHANDAS T, SPARKES RS, HELLKUHL B, GRZESCHIK KH, SHAPIRO LJ: Expression of an X-linked gene from an inactive human X chromosome in mouse-human hybrid cells: Further evidence for the noninactivation of the steroid sulfatase locus in man. *Proc Nat Acad Sci USA* 77:6759, 1980

135. MOHANDAS T, SHAPIRO LJ, SPARKES RS, SPARKES MC: Regional assignment of the steroid sulfatase–X-linked ichthyosis locus: Implications for a non-inactivated region on the short arm of human X chromosome. *Proc Nat Acad Sci USA* 76:5779, 1979

136. MULLER CR, WESTERVELD A, MIGL B, FRANKE W, ROPERS HH: Regional assignment of the gene locus for steroid sulfatase. *Hum Genet* 54:201, 1980

137. TIEPOLO L, ZUFFARDI O, FRACCARO M, DI NATALE D, GARGANTINI L, MULLER CR, ROPERS HH: Assignment by deletion mapping of the steroid sulfatase X-linked ichthyosis locus to Xp223. *Hum Genet* 54:205, 1980

138. AKESSON HO, HAGBERG B, WAHLSTROM J: Y-to-X chromosome translocation observed in two generations. *Hum Genet* 55:39, 1980

139. FERGUSON-SMITH MA, personal communication

140. SHAPIRO LJ, AND MOHANDAS T: Molecular genetics of X-linked ichthyosis. *Pediatr Res* 14:527, 1980

141. MULLER CR, MIGL B, TRAUPE H, AND ROPERS HH: X-linked steroid sulfatase: evidence for different gene-dosage in males and females. *Hum Genet* 54:197, 1980

142. LYKKESFELDT G, BACH JE, LYKKESFELDT AE: Sex specific difference in placental steroid sulfatase activity. *Lancet* 2:255, 1981

143. SHAPIRO LJ: Current status and future direction for carrier detection in lysosomal storage diseases, in Callahan JW, Lowden JA (eds): *Lysosomes and Lysosomal Storage Diseases.* New York, Raven Press, 1981, p 343

144. Muller CR, Migl B, Ropers HH, Happle R: Heterozygote detection in steroid sulphatase deficiency. *Lancet* 1:546, 1980

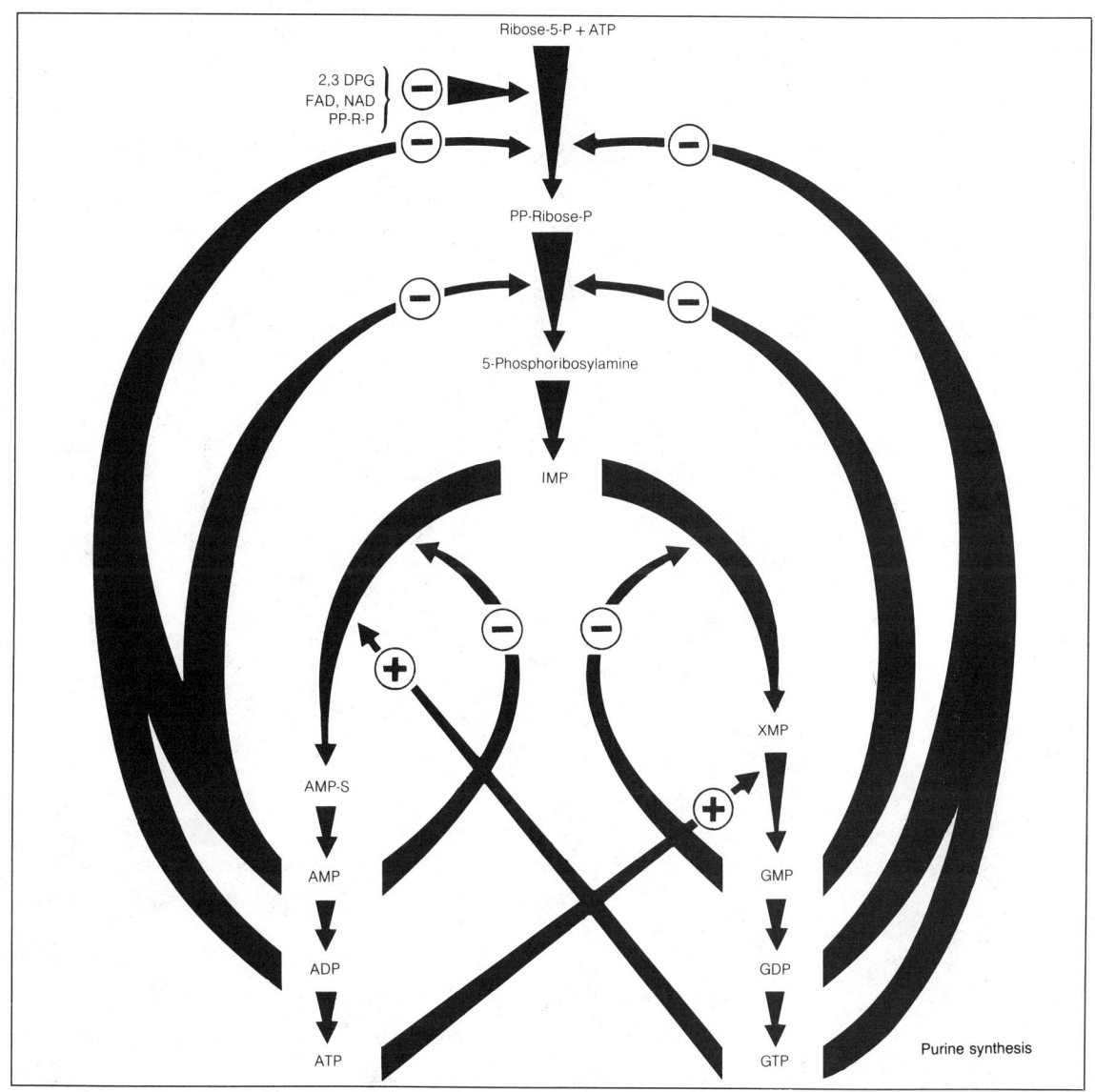

PART 7

Purine synthesis

DISORDERS OF PURINE AND PYRIMIDINE METABOLISM

50

GOUT

JAMES B. WYNGAARDEN

WILLIAM N. KELLEY

1. Gout is a clinical disorder manifested by hyperuricemia, recurrent attacks of acute arthritis ordinarily responsive to colchicine, and, in some instances, by tophaceous deposits of monosodium urate. The arthritis may become chronic and disabling. Rarely it is grotesquely deforming. Nephropathy is frequent in gout and sometimes a complication of gout, but more often it is due to other concurrent conditions. Nephrolithiasis is also common and often antedates articular gout.

2. Primary gout is a form of the disease that is attributable to an inborn error of metabolism. The category is biochemically and genetically heterogeneous. The largest subgroup consists of patients in whom the biochemical defect is as yet undefined. Many patients in this group can be shown to produce uric acid excessively, when studied by techniques for assessment of turnover of uric acid or of rate of incorporation of labeled precursors into uric acid. In many subjects there is a reduction in fractional renal urate clearance. In addition to genetic factors, dietary excesses of caloric and alcohol ingestion often appear to be important.

3. Three distinct genetically determined enzymatic defects have been defined that lead to marked hyperuricemia at an early age. These are glucose-6-phosphatase deficiency (von Gierke's glycogen storage disease), hypoxanthine-guanine phosphoribosyltransferase deficiency (complete and partial), and phosphoribosylpyrophosphate synthetase variants with increased catalytic activity. In the last two of these, markedly excessive production of purines appears to result from elevated intracellular levels of 5-phosphoribosyl-l-pyrophosphate (PP-ribose-P), a key substrate of the initial reaction of the purine pathway.

4. Overproduction of uric acid in patients with types of primary gout that have not yet been defined metabolically has been discussed in terms of availability of L-glutamine and PP-ribose-P, the substrates of the initial reaction, and in terms of possible excessive nucleotide catabolism in response to hexose ingestion.

5. Reduction of fractional renal urate clearance is most readily demonstrable in gouty patients when serum urate concentration values are artificially raised. The defect is most prominent in those patients with normal 24-h urinary uric acid excretion values. Some patients appear to exhibit this defect as the major or even the sole basis of hyperuricemia. This defect is present in many overproducers of uric acid, although not in patients with HGPRT deficiency, or with overactive variants of PP-ribose-P synthetase.

6. Solutions of the electrolyte composition of extracellular fluid are saturated with monosodium urate at a concentration of about 6.4 mg/dl. Perhaps an addi-

tional 5 percent (i.e., 0.3 to 0.4 mg/dl) is normally bound to nondiffusible elements of plasma. The most logical definition of hyperuricemia is one based not upon the statistical distribution of serum urate values in a population, but rather upon the limits of solubility of monosodium urate in body fluids.

7. *The prevalences of articular gout and of nephrolithiasis are strongly correlated with the height of the serum urate concentration value. In one population study the prevalences were 90 and 40 percent, respectively, in males with serum urate values 9 mg/dl or greater at mean age 58 years. An important factor favoring stone formation in gouty subjects is a tendency toward excretion of persistently acid urine.*

8. *There is significant variability of mean plasma urate values among certain racial groups, especially in the Pacific islands. For example, among adult male Maori, mean serum urate values are over 7 mg/dl, and the prevalence of tophaceous gout is 10 percent. In most populations, serum urate values are positively correlated with surface area and body weight.*

9. *The acute gouty attack is triggered by crystals of monosodium urate, which activate an inflammatory reaction. Colchicine is thought to interrupt the attack by suppressing the production of a low molecular weight chemotactic factor elaborated by the leukocyte following crystal ingestion.*

10. *In population studies hyperuricemia appears to be multifactorial and attributable to a combination of genetic and nongenetic factors. Genetic factors may include both cumulative gene action and single-gene effects. In studies of families or isolates the latter sometimes suggest autosomal dominant factors, sometimes sex-linked factors. Known enzymatic abnormalities associated with hyperuricemia are of several genetic types. HPRT deficiency and PP-ribose-P synthetase superactivity are X-linked. Glucose-6-phosphatase deficiency is an autosomal recessive trait.*

Gout is a term representing a heterogeneous group of diseases, which in their full development are manifest by (1) an increase in the serum urate concentration; (2) recurrent attacks of a characteristic type of acute arthritis, in which crystals of monosodium urate monohydrate are demonstrable in leukocytes of synovial fluid (Fig. 50-1); (3) aggregated deposits of monosodium urate monohydrate (tophi) occurring chiefly in and around the joints of the extremities and sometimes leading to severe crippling and deformity; and (4) uric acid urolithiasis. These manifestations occur in different combinations. Renal disease involving interstitial tissue, glomeruli, tubules, and blood vessels is common in gout, but the best current evidence is that nephropathy in gout is usually secondary to associated conditions such as hypertension, vascular disease, obstruction, infection, or glomerulonephritis rather than to urate crystals. We no longer include renal disease within a stringent definition of gout.

The biochemical hallmark and prerequisite of the disease is hyperuricemia, which can arise on the basis of several mechanisms operating singly or in combination. Documented mechanisms in different forms of gout include increased uric acid production and diminished uric acid clearance by the kidney. Four additional theoretical possibilities—an increase in purine absorption, an increase in binding of urate to nondiffusible elements of plasma, a decrease in extrarenal disposal of urate, and a decrease in urate catabolism (uricolysis)—have not been shown to play a role in the pathophysiology of the hyperuricemia of gout.

The pathologic mechanisms resulting in hyperuricemia are heterogeneous and complex. Some are genetically determined, others acquired. Hyperuricemia is common, and in the majority of its hosts, quite innocuous. We think a distinction should be drawn between a chemical abnormality that is usually innocent and a disease, which by definition produces symptoms, a dis-ease. Thus, asymptomatic hyperuricemia alone is not a disease. Hyperuricemia with renal stone is a disease but should not be called gout. We reserve the term *gout* to signify a disease with the characteristic articular manifestations or tophaceous involvements mentioned above.

Gout is classified as *primary* when it appears to be innate and is neither a consequence of an acquired disorder nor a late and subordinate manifestation of an inborn error that leads initially to a clinical disorder unlike gout. There are several distinct subtypes of primary gout. Probably all instances of primary gout have a hereditary basis, although the precise metabolic lesion and its genetic pattern have been identified in only a small percentage of cases in this category. Gout is classified as *secondary* when it develops as a consequence of another disorder or of its therapy, or as a late manifestation of an inborn error that initially presents quite unlike gout. There are many varieties and causes of secondary gout. The term *idiopathic gout* is used when assignment to either primary or secondary categories is uncertain. A classification of hyperuricemia and gout is presented in Table 50-1.

This chapter deals chiefly with varieties of gout that are genetically determined. A large portion of the inquiry is di-

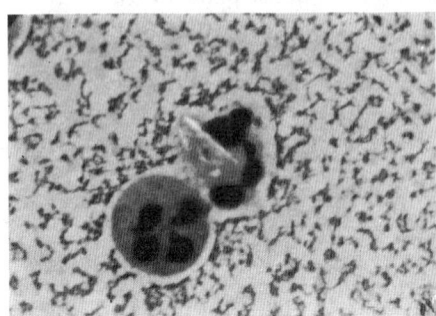
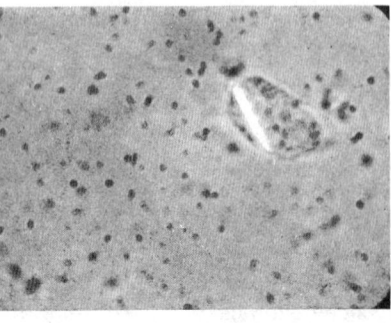

Figure 50-1 Crystals of sodium urate monohydrate in leukocytes of synovial fluid in acute gouty arthritis, as seen under polarized light.

Table 50-1 Classification of hyperuricemia and gout

Type	Metabolic disturbance	Inheritance
Primary		
Molecular defects undefined		
Normal excretion (85–90% of primary gout)	Overproduction of uric acid or underexcretion of uric acid or both (specific defects undefined; some reported to have reduced levels of an $\alpha_1 - \alpha_2$ urate-binding globulin in plasma)	Polygenic
Overexcretion (10–15% of primary gout)	Overproduction of uric acid (specific defects undefined)	Polygenic
Associated with specific enzyme defects		
PP-ribose-P synthetase variants; increased activity	Overproduction of PP-ribose-P and of uric acid	X-linked
Hypoxanthine-guanine phosphoribosyltransferase deficiency, partial	Overproduction of uric acid; increased purine biosynthesis *de novo* driven by surplus PP-ribose-P	X-linked
Secondary		
Associated with increased purine biosynthesis *de novo*		
Glucose-6-phosphatase deficiency or absence	Overproduction plus reduced renal clearance of uric acid; glycogen storage disease, type I (von Gierke)	Autosomal recessive
Hypoxanthine-guanine phosphoribosyltransferase deficiency "virtually complete"	Overproduction of uric acid; Lesch-Nyhan syndrome	X-linked
Associated with increased nucleic acid turnover	Overproduction of uric acid (chronic hemolysis, polycythemia, leukemia, lymphoma)	
Associated with decreased renal excretion of uric acid	Reduced renal functional mass	
	Inhibited tubular secretion of uric acid or enhanced tubular reabsorption of uric acid, or both	
Idiopathic	Normal or reduced renal clearance of uric acid	Unknown

rected toward the pathophysiology of hyperuricemia. For a more complete discussion of gout and hyperuricemia, including secondary gout, the reader is referred to the book by Wyngaarden and Kelley [1].

HISTORY

The clinical descriptions of gout can be traced to ancient medical literature [2].[1] Early Greek and Roman physicians possessed an intimate knowledge of its varied features. In the fifth century B.C., Hippocrates described gout as podagra, cheiagra, or gonagra, depending on whether the big toe, wrist, or knee was involved. Tophi were first described by Galen (A.D. 131 to 200). The term *gout,* introduced in the thirteenth century, is derived from the Latin *gutta,* a drop, and reflects an early belief that the disease was caused by a *noxa,* a poison, falling drop by drop into the joint.

Colchicine was known to Byzantine physicians as early as the fifth century A.D. under the name of *hermodactyl* (finger of

Hermes). A drug probably identical with colchicine was described in the Ebers papyrus (1500 B.C.). *Colchicum autumnale* (or meadow saffron) was introduced into Europe in 1763 by Baron Anton von Storch, physician to Empress Maria Theresa, and subsequently into this country by Benjamin Franklin. The term *colchicum* probably originates from a district in Asia Minor called Colchis.

The modern clinical history of gout began with Thomas Sydenham, whose unsurpassed description of the disease, drawn from 34 years of personal affliction, first clearly differentiated gout from other articular disorders [3]. The chemical history of gout began a century after Sydenham, when in 1776 Scheel discovered uric acid as a constituent of a kidney stone. Shortly thereafter Wollaston (1797) and Pearson (1798) demonstrated urate in the tophi of patients with gout. Another 50 years later, Garrod performed his historic experiments in which he demonstrated first by the murexide test [4] and later by his famous "thread" test (1854) [5] an increased amount of uric acid in the blood of gouty subjects.

At this time the structure of uric acid was unknown. With the establishment by Fischer in 1898 that uric acid was a purine compound, its potential relationship to the nucleic acid constituents adenine and guanine was appreciated, and a key role of purine metabolism in the pathophysiology of gout was recognized. The introduction of a reliable method for the

---

[1] Many of the historic references have been omitted. The interested reader is referred to the fourth edition of this text for early references [2].

determination of uric acid in the blood by Folin and Denis in 1913 greatly facilitated clinical and metabolic studies of gout. The pathways of enzymatic synthesis of purine compounds were elucidated by Buchanan, Greenberg, and others during the 1950s. The first specific enzymatic defect responsible for one subtype of adult primary gout, hypoxanthine guanine phosphoribosyltransferase deficiency, was discovered by Seegmiller and associates in 1967. The second, phosphoribosylpyrophosphate synthetase overactivity, was discovered by Sperling and colleagues in 1973.

Through the centuries, gout has enjoyed a royal patronage, and victims of gout have been favored subjects of caricatures, novels, and biographies. Many writers have compiled rosters of distinguished personages in history who have allegedly had gout. The list includes the Medici, Isaac Newton, Charles Darwin, Martin Luther, John Calvin, Benjamin Franklin, Ben Jonson, William Pitt, Samuel Johnson, Cotton Mather, and George IV of England. Illuminating articles on the history of gout those by Copeman [6], Hartung, Rodnan and Benedek, and Bywaters.

CLINICAL FEATURES OF GOUT

Asymptomatic Hyperuricemia

Asymptomatic hyperuricemia is that stage in which the serum urate level is raised but arthritic symptoms, tophi, or uric acid stones, have not yet appeared. This stage begins at puberty in the male at risk from the common form of gout but is usually delayed until the menopause in the female [7]. In patients with hyperuricemia secondary to a specific enzyme deficiency, this trait is present from birth. Renal calculi composed partially or wholly of uric acid may occur at any stage of gout; their significance in the prearticular stage is often overlooked. Rarely, tophi may antedate the development of articular gout.

Acute Gouty Arthritis

It is difficult to improve on Sydenham's [8] description of the acute attack:

> The victim goes to bed and sleeps in good health. About two o'clock in the morning he is awakened by a severe pain in the great toe; more rarely in the heel, ankle or instep. This pain is like that of a dislocation, and yet the parts feel as if cold water were poured over them. Then follow chills and shivers, and a little fever. The pain, which was at first moderate, becomes more intense. With its intensity the chills and shivers increase. After a time this comes to its height, accommodating itself to the bones and ligaments of the tarsus and metatarsus. Now it is a violent stretching and tearing of the ligaments—now it is a gnawing pain and now a pressure and tightening. So exquisite and lively meanwhile is the feeling of the part affected, that it cannot bear the weight of the bedclothes nor the jar of a person walking in the room. The night is passed in torture, sleeplessness, turning of the part affected, and perpetual change of posture; the tossing about of the body being as incessant as the pain of the tortured joint, and being worse as the fit comes on. Hence the vain effort, by change of posture, both in the body and the limb affected, to obtain an abatement of the pain.

The attack usually subsides spontaneously in a few days to a few weeks, and recovery following the initial episode is gener-

ally complete. About 50 percent of initial attacks involve the great toe (podagra). In 10 to 15 percent of patients the initial attack is bilateral or polyarticular [9]. Ninety percent of gouty patients experience attacks in the great toe at some time during the course of their disease. Next in order of frequency as sites of initial involvement are the instep, ankle, heel, knee, and wrist. Any joint in the body may be involved. The more distal the site of involvement, the more typical is the character of the attack.

Prevalence and Incidence   The prevalence of gout varies widely in different parts of the world [2]. A figure of 0.3 percent in Europe was recorded by Lawrence [10] in 1960, and of 0.26 percent in Great Britain by Currie [10a] in 1979. In the Heart Disease Epidemiology Study conducted in Framingham, Massachusetts, a prevalence of gouty arthritis of 0.2 percent was found in a population of 5127 subjects (2283 men and 2844 women) aged 30 to 59 years (mean age, 44). Fourteen years later the prevalence had increased to 1.5 percent of this population (mean age, 58), 2.8 percent in men, 0.4 percent in women [11]. Prevalence appears to be even higher among Filipino males in Northwestern North America, and very much higher among the Chamorros and the Carolinians in the Mariana Islands and in the Maori of New Zealand. In the last group the prevalence of gout is 10.3 percent in men and 4.3 percent in women [11]. Relationship of prevalence to the serum urate level is shown in Table 50-2, which summarizes the situation in the Framingham population admitted at mean age 44 and followed for 14 years.

During World Wars I and II acute gouty arthritis was uncommon in Europe. When protein again became plentiful, the prevalence returned to prewar levels. In Japan, where protein intake per capita has doubled since World War II, gout is now common. These and other observations underscore the importance of dietary and environmental influences in determining whether the genetic factor or factors are expressed in subjects at risk. Gout has long been considered a disease of middle and upper social classes. A study in Manchester, England, documented this belief, and a similar correlation noted in Pittsburgh led to the studies cited below on the distribution of serum urate values among members of various social and educational classes. Nevertheless, the disease is widely distributed and involves all nationalities and all social classes. It is said to be rare in African nationals, but it is common in American blacks.

Acute gout is preeminently a disease of the adult male. Since the time of Hippocrates it has been known that gout is uncommon in women. In large series, only 3 to 7 percent of the cases of primary gout are found in women, and these are chiefly in the postmenopausal group. In limited series, higher percentages of women are occasionally noted. These series may include cases of secondary gout complicating lead ingestion, hypertension, renal disease, or the use of diuretics.

Gout in women may be more severe and more destructive than in men. When gout is inherited from the mother, its onset may be at an earlier age, and it may be more severe than usual. A special form of familial gout and renal failure in young women has recently been described [12]. Gout is very rare in prepubertal children and, when it occurs, it may represent a form of gout associated with a specific enzymatic deficiency leading to the overproduction of urate [13, 14].

The usual form of primary gout is uncommon before the third decade, and its peak incidence in various series is in the

Table 50-2 Prevalence of gouty arthritis by maximum urate level in a population of mean age 58

Serum urate concentration, mg/100 ml	Men		Women	
	Fraction with gout	Percent with gout	Fraction with gout	Percent with gout
<6	8/1281	0.6	2/2665	0.08
6.0–6.9	15/790	1.9	5/151	3.3
7.0–7.9	27/162	16.7	4/23	17.4
8.0–8.9	10/40	25.0	0/4	0
9+	9/10	90.0	0/1	0
Total	69/2283	3.0	11/2844	0.4

SOURCE: From Hall et al. [11].

thirties, forties, or fifties. In general, the higher the serum urate level, the earlier the onset of gouty arthritis. In the population study in Framingham, Massachusetts, the cumulative incidence of gouty arthritis in men appeared to be approaching a plateau at mean age 58 years. This occurred in spite of the fact that only one-third of the men with urate levels of 8 mg/dl or more had experienced an attack of gout [11]. The age factor may explain the low fraction of 21 patients with gout among 5400 cases of arthritis (0.4 percent) in one United States Army Arthritis Center during World War II, compared with the usual frequency of 4 or 5 percent of gouty patients among all arthritic patients of civilian clinic populations in this country.

Plasma and Urinary Uric Acid No characteristic changes of plasma urate levels precede, accompany, or follow an acute attack of gouty arthritis [2]. There may be an elevation of urinary uric acid excretion values during the acute attack, perhaps mediated by the uricosuric action of corticosteroids secreted during the stress of gouty inflammation. Such a uricosuric effect would normally be anticipated to reduce the serum urate level, and perhaps this mechanism explains some of the normal values observed during acute attacks. In general, however, the values do not fall, and an increased production of uric acid, a consequence of leukocytosis, enhanced leukocyte turnover, and increased nucleic acid production, has been postulated as offsetting the effects of uricosuria. Intravenously administered deoxyribonuclease increases uric acid excretion in symptomatic gouty subjects (as well as in nongouty subjects with inflammatory disease) but not in gouty subjects in the asymptomatic phase, and these observations support the concept described above.

Mechanism of the Acute Attack Garrod [15] proposed in 1859 that the acute gouty paroxysm was triggered by precipitation of sodium urate crystals in the joint or neighboring tissues. In 1899, Freudweiler [16] reproduced acute gouty attacks by the injection of microcrystals of sodium urate, and also of other crystals such as those of hypoxanthine, or xanthine [17]. The subcutaneous injection of urate crystals was followed by the evolution of a histologically characteristic tophus [18].

For many years these observations were overlooked and when the measurement of serum and urinary uric acid revealed no characteristic changes during the acute attack and infusions of urate solutions or injections of them near, or into, the joints of gouty subjects evoked no inflammatory response, the concept of a direct role of urate in the pathogenesis of the acute attack fell into disfavor. Theories of primary vascular distur-

bance, metabolic abnormalities, endocrine imbalance, or allergy to food or bacterial products were then proposed [2].

In 1961 McCarty and Hollander [19] rediscovered crystals of sodium urate in gouty effusions, and recognized the diagnostic value of negatively birefrigent crystals within synovial fluid leukocytes during the acute attack. With polarized light [20] (Fig. 50-1) and a first-order red compensator, the urate crystal is yellow when oriented in parallel with the axis of the compensator and blue when perpendicular to it. Intracellular urate crystals are virtually constant in acute gouty arthritis and constitute the most reliable diagnostic criterion of the disease.

Following the recognition of crystals in gouty effusions (a confirmation of the *gutta-noxa* theory!) Faires and McCarty [21] and Seegmiller et al. [22] rediscovered the capacity of microcrystals of sodium urate to evoke an inflammatory response in the skin, subcutaneous tissues, and joints of animals and human beings. In humans, both normouricemic and gouty, the inflammatory response strikingly resembles the acute gouty attack. It may be successfully treated with or prevented by colchicine [23]. A similar response may also be evoked by crystals of calcium oxalate, calcium pyrophosphate dihydrate, sodium orotate, and certain steroids, but not by diamond dust [23].

SYNOVIAL MEMBRANE TOPHI IN ACUTE GOUT Agudelo and Schumacher [24] have observed microtophi in the synovial membrane 2 days after the onset of the first attack of acute gout. Synovial membrane tophi have been found by many observers during the acute attack, but in most instances gout had been present intermittently for one or more years [2]. Synovial membrane crystals may also be present in synovial biopsy material obtained from an asymptomatic joint during the intercritical phase [25]. In addition, there are chronic as well as acute inflammatory cells in the synovitis reaction of acute gout [24]. These findings suggest that acute gout may be superimposed on a joint in which urate deposition and low-grade chronic inflammation may have developed silently at an earlier time.

MONOSODIUM URATE CRYSTALS IN ASYMPTOMATIC JOINTS Recently, Weinberger and associates [26] also found urate crystals in aspirates of first metatarsophalangeal joints not previously involved in acute gouty attacks in six of nine gouty patients. These crystals were rod or needle shaped and almost entirely extracellular. These findings have been confirmed in about 75 percent of such aspirates. Monosodium urate crystals are very rare in asymptomatic hyperuricemic subjects who have never had a gouty attack. Crystals from asymptomatic joints tend to be shorter, to have blunter tips, and to have different proteins adherent to the surface than those found in acutely inflamed joints. Crystals aspirated from inflamed joints have immunoglobulin G and albumin adherent to the surface, whereas the crystals in asymptomatic joints do not [27].

MECHANISMS OF CRYSTAL FORMATION   The factors leading to precipitation of monosodium urate crystals in tissue and the mechanisms by which these crystals induce inflammation are poorly understood. Supersaturation of serum or synovial fluid with monosodium urate is a necessary but not sufficient precondition. In subjects with gouty synovitis the concentration of urate in the synovial fluid is usually equal to its concentration in serum [2]. Thus, an important question is what makes monosodium urate crystals form in some subjects but not in others in spite of a similarity in serum urate concentrations.

ROLE OF PROTEOGLYCANS   In 1892, Roberts [28] incubated pig tarsal bones in a saturated solution of sodium urate, and after 3 days noted the encrustation of tophaceouslike material on the cartilaginous articulating surface. At that time little was known of the macromolecules of cartilage, but its electrolyte composition had been determined. He proposed that precipitation occurred because of relatively high sodium concentrations in connective tissues as compared with serum and parenchymal organs.

The connective tissue sites of urate deposition are rich in polysaccharides. These are covalently bound to protein and are called proteoglycans. Cartilage and synovial fluid contain a series of proteoglycans, composed of protein and chondroitin sulfate or keratin sulfate. The linear polysaccharides are attached to the protein core like bristles on a brush. Certain of these markedly enhance the solubility of urate in buffers having molarities and hydrogen ion concentrations similar to those of most body fluids [29]. The integrity of the proteoglycan molecule is essential: unbound chondroitin sulfate or proteoglycan digested by trypsin does not augment urate solubility. Proteoglycan aggregates inhibit crystallization of urate from a supersaturated solution, but the effect is transient. There is doubt that this is an important effect in vivo [29].

The work of Dingle [30], Schubert and Hamerman [31], and others indicates that there is a continuous turnover of proteoglycan molecules. Katz and Schubert [29] suggest that when proteoglycan is enzymatically destroyed as a result of normal or accelerated connective tissue turnover, its binding capacity for urate is reduced. Because the tissue is relatively avascular, degradation will result in a sudden local increase in the concentration of free sodium urate. Crystals may precipitate from the supersaturated tissue fluids, with silent deposition in cartilage, bone, or tendon, or with activation of an acute synovitis. Perhaps destruction of connective tissue also releases bound sodium, resulting in an even greater increase in sodium activity and an enhanced tendency toward crystal formation through common ion effects, as first proposed by Roberts [28]. This formulation postulates that connective tissue storage of bound urate precedes crystallization and the acute attack. This point has not been critically examined in the laboratory, although it is known that cartilage has an affinity for absorbing urate in vitro. This hypothesis does not readily account for the poor correlation of urate crystal formation with the serum or synovial fluid urate concentration. It assumes that the postulated increase in urate concentration is localized to the layer of synovial fluid in intimate contact with cartilage, since the concentration of urate as measured in synovial fluid samples is not greater than the serum concentration in gout. This notion is consistent with the behavior of "unstirred layers" in physiologic fluid. Thus, a possible contributory role of connective tissue proteoglycans to urate storage and crystal formation is an attractive hypothesis.

TEMPERATURE DIFFERENTIALS AND URATE SOLUBILITY   Loeb [32] has emphasized the possible role of temperature in the initial precipitation of urate. The maximal equilibrium concentration of urate in the presence of 140 mM Na^+ drops from 6.8 mg/dl at 37°C to 4.5 mg/dl at 30°C (Table 50-3). A gradient exists between central body temperature and intraarticular temperatures of extremity joints. Hollander and colleagues [33] have measured joint temperatures with a filamentous copper-constantin thermocouple inserted through the bore of an aspiration needle. The intraarticular temperature of the normal knee joint is approximately 32°C (range, 30.5 to 32.8°C); that of the normal ankle joint is approximately 29°C.

Acute gout often begins at night and may follow exercise. Perhaps cooling of extremity joints during rest is a contributing factor in acute gout. Loeb [32] suggests that the cooler peripheral extracellular fluids may be supersaturated with sodium urate even at plasma urate concentration values usually considered normal. The phenomenon would be even more striking in the patient with basal hyperuricemia. A temperature effect could explain the tendency of urate to crystallize in more distal parts of the body, such as joints of the foot or the cartilage of the ears. In addition, Loeb proposes that the heat associated with inflammation may help to limit the process by enhancing the solubility of the urate crystals. In the chronically gouty joint with moderately active inflammation, temperatures of 36.6°C have been recorded, while in the acutely inflamed gouty knee temperatures may rise to 37°C [33].

TRAUMA AND AGING   Trauma has been implicated as a factor in the predisposition of joints of the lower extremity to gout. Acute gout often begins after exposure out of doors, e.g., "pheasant hunter's toe." The most frequently affected site is the first metatarsophalangeal joint of the great toe, a site that is subjected during walking to the greatest stress, in kilograms of weight per square centimeter of area, of any joint in the body. Mechanical damage to connective tissue might be a factor in the mechanism proposed by Katz and Schubert [29]. Trauma might flake off urate crystals from an articular crust and serve to trigger an attack. Other factors favoring crystal formation may include age-related changes in connective tissue and in the microvascular circulation. Any reduction in blood flow would

Table 50-3   Solubility of urate ion (U^-) as a function of temperature in the presence of 140 mM Na^+

Temperature, °C	Maximal equilibrium concentration of U^- in the presence of 140 mM Na^+, mg/100 ml
37	6.8
35	6.0
30	4.5
25	3.3
20	2.5
15	1.8
10	1.2

SOURCE: From Loeb [32]. (Reproduced by permission of *Arthritis and Rheumatism*.)

affect the rate of dissipation of a local increase in tissue urate concentration and also contribute to temperature differentials.

Simkin [34] has integrated several of the factors discussed above into an interesting proposal, based upon a purported effusion into or around a stressed or traumatized joint. He proposes a more rapid rate of reabsorption of fluid than of urate, resulting in a transient local increase in sodium urate concentration to levels exceeding solubility limits, resulting in a shower of urate crystals.

THE ROLE OF pH   Although a decrease in pH, resulting from production of lactic acid during anaerobic glycolysis of leukocytes, has been postulated to play a role in the propagation of the acute attack of gout [22], there is little evidence to support this hypothesis. In fact, monosodium urate is more soluble at pH 6 or 6.5 than at pH 7.4. A decrease in pH should lead to precipitation of uric acid rather than monosodium urate. Since the crystals present are monosodium urate, pH change would seem to be unimportant. The maximal pH drop during an attack is only 0.5 unit, probably inconsequential in terms of urate solubility.

Mediation of the Inflammatory Response   Urate crystals can activate Hageman factor of synovial fluid, which in turn may initiate a series of reactions leading to permeability-enhancing activity, kallikrein, and kinins. The concentration of kininlike peptides in synovial fluid may rise fiftyfold during crystal-induced attacks in humans, as it does during spontaneous attacks of gout, but this response is not specific for gout and also occurs in other inflammatory states such as rheumatoid arthritis [36]. These factors can induce vasodilation, increased vascular permeability, and leukocyte margination and emigration through the vessel wall. However, an inflammatory response to urate can also occur in the absence of this system. Phelps et al. [37] found in dogs that arthritis induced with urate crystals was not prevented by carboxypeptidase injected directly into the joint space or into the arterial supply to the joint. Carboxypeptidase inactivates bradykinin, but not kallikrein. In addition, Spilberg [38] has shown that monosodium urate crystals can induce an acute inflammatory synovitis in the chicken stifle joint even though these birds lack Hageman factor and do not have detectable kinin activity in their synovial fluid. These studies suggest that the kallikrein-kinin system is not an obligatory mediator of the inflammatory response of acute gout.

The complement systems may be involved in the acute inflammatory response to urate crystals as a concomitant or alternative activator. Naff and Byers [39] found that incubation of urate crystals with serum led to marked reduction of activity of C-4, C-2, C-3, and C-5, but to only a slight decrease in C-1. The reaction does not appear to require properdin, Hageman factor, or immunoglobulin G [40]. C5a [39] and a C5b-9 complex [41] are generated during incubation. Monospecific antibody to human C5 completely abolishes the generation of chemotactic activity when serum is incubated with urate crystals [41]. However, the effect on complement is lost by heating the urate crystals to 200°C [39], whereas the phlogistic characteristics of crystals are not abolished by heat [42]. Furthermore, complement levels are normal in synovial fluid during an acute attack of gouty arthritis [43], and depletion of C-3 and C-5 in rabbits and dogs by injection of purified cobra venom factor does not diminish the leukocyte response to urate

crystals in synovial fluid [42]. Thus, complement-mediated neutrophil chemotaxis is not an obligatory component of the inflammatory response to urate crystals.

ROLE OF THE LEUKOCYTE   The inflammatory response to urate crystals depends on the presence of polymorphonuclear leukocytes. In dogs rendered leukopenic with vancomycin [44] or with antipolymorphonuclear leukocyte serum [45], urate crystals fail to induce an inflammatory response; responsiveness is restored by cross circulation with replacement of leukocytes [44] or when time for recovery is allowed [45]. The initial event is phagocytosis of the urate crystals [24]. Agudelo et al. [46] have found that within 30 min of injection, some urate crystals have been taken up by the synovial lining cells and other mononuclear cells free in the joint fluid of the dog. Vasodilation, edema, and polymorphonuclear margination first appeared at 30 min, and were followed at 45 min by rising intraarticular pressure, at 60 min by the first detectable chemotactic activity, and at 75 min by a rising polymorphonuclear leukocyte count in the synovial fluid with phagocytosis of urate crystals. By 3.5 h there was intense focal polymorphonuclear infiltration of the synovium and 40 percent of synovial fluid polys contained crystals. At 48 h only 3 percent of synovial fluid polys contained crystals. Plasma cell and lymphocyte infiltration of the synovium was beginning.

Phelps [47] has shown that leukocytes release a factor chemotactic for other leukocytes within 11 min after phagocytosis of urate crystals. This factor, purified by Spilberg and colleagues [48], is a glycoprotein of molecular weight 8400. Human neutrophils have a specific receptor to which it binds, but erythrocytes and lymphocytes do not [49]. When purified factor is injected into an animal joint, it is highly inflammatory and produces a response with a lag phase that is shorter than is required following injection of urate crystals. Colchicine will prevent the response to urate crystals injected into joints [23]. Production of chemotactic factor in response to urate crystals is also suppressed by colchicine at levels equivalent to therapeutic concentrations [49, 50]. However, colchicine will not prevent the inflammatory response that follows the injection of purified chemotactic factor [50]. Thus, this factor may be central to the pathogenesis of the acute gouty attack. However, it may not be specific for gout. Induction of a chemotactic factor with very similar properties follows phagocytosis of heat-aggregated human gamma globulin [51], of calcium pyrophosphate dihydrate crystals [23, 52], or of diamond dust [23] by polymorphonuclear leukocytes. The factor is located chiefly in the lysosomal fraction of the cell but is also found in the media of the cell-crystal incubations, suggesting that the material finds its way to the exterior of the cell following exocytosis or cell death. Its appearance is blocked by inhibition of protein synthesis or by cytochalasin B, an inhibitor of phagocytosis. The generation of a chemotactic factor may represent a uniform response of PMNs, to the phagocytosis of calcium pyrophosphate dihydrate (CPPD), monosodium urate, and perhaps other crystals [52].

ENDOTOXINS AND ACUTE GOUT   In gouty subjects, urate crystals may be present in the synovial fluid of joints that have never experienced an acute attack [26] as well as in the synovium of joints during the quiescent phase between acute attacks [25]. Clearly, more than the presence of crystals is involved in the pathogenesis of the gouty paroxysm.

Acute gout may be precipitated by infection. Sicuteri [53]

reported that five of six patients with gouty arthritis, in remission at the time, suffered an especially violent painful attack upon the intravenous injection of small doses of a bacterial pyrogen, insufficient to cause fever. Acting on these clues, Van Arman et al. [54] investigated the possible role of a model bacterial endotoxin obtained from *Escherichia coli* in the experimental arthritis induced by urate crystals injected into the joints of dogs. Endotoxins are large highly charged molecules easily adsorbed onto reactive surfaces such as those presented by the urate crystal. When endotoxin-exposed crystals were instilled, the resultant inflammatory response was considerably more florid and intense than when endotoxin-free crystals were employed. More significantly, when a small dose of clean crystals that by itself caused no pain was injected into joints and endotoxin was given orally, a painful arthritis resulted. It was suggested that circulating endotoxin might be adsorbed onto the crystal and thus initiate an intense inflammatory response, but localization of endotoxin on the crystal was not demonstrated. It is not likely that adsorbed complement is essential in the attack. As pointed out above, crystals heated to 200°C to destroy previously adsorbed complement proved as effective in producing an inflammatory reaction in the joint as those with complement adherent. These studies focus attention on a factor or factors other than the crystal itself that initiate or perpetuate an acute gouty inflammation.

CYTOLOGIC STUDIES OF CRYSTAL INGESTION   Destruction of ingested urate crystals is observed by light microscopy. This has been attributed to enzymatic digestion by leukoperoxidases of the leukocyte [2].

Electron-microscopic studies of urate crystals within synovial fluid leukocytes show some crystals within lysophagosomes, others within the cytoplasm. Schumacher and Phelps [55] found that at 3 min (Fig. 50-2) the urate crystals were surrounded by a closely applied phagosome membrane. By 8 min there was distension and dissolution of some phagosome membranes and beginnning degranulation. By 30 min some cells were necrotic, and by 2 h some crystals appeared to lie free in the cytoplasm of viable cells (Fig. 50-3). Other crystals were surrounded by incomplete phagosome membranes, and in these cells necrosis was more frequent.

The weakly acidic groups of the monosodium urate molecule interact by hydrogen bonding with phosphate esters of the phospholipid membrane of the phagolysosome. In studies in vitro crystals of sodium urate rupture lysosomes and liposomes in media that do not constrain hydrogen bonding [56]. Lipo-

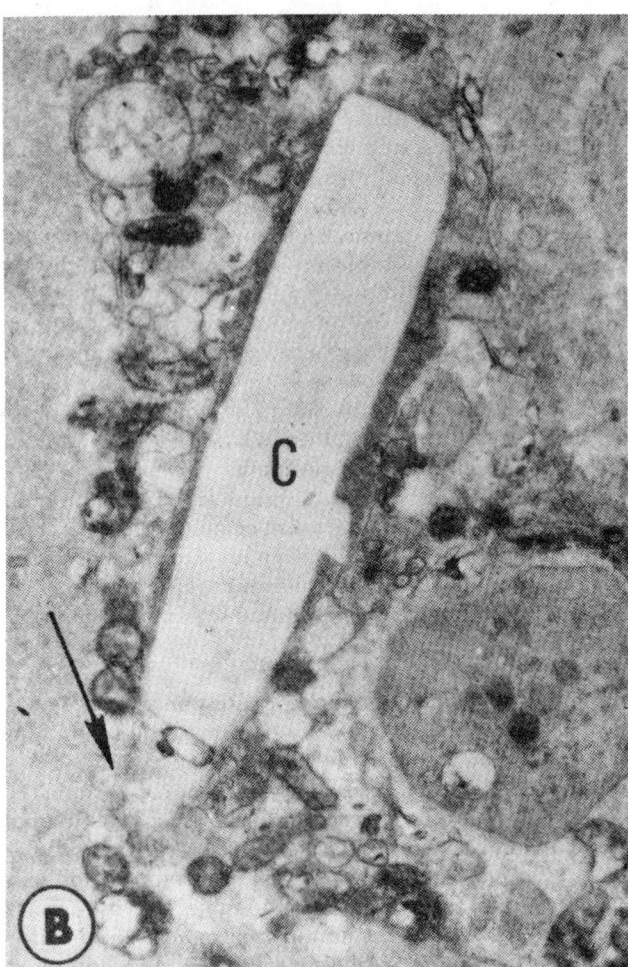

Figure 50-3   Dying polymorphonuclear leukocyte at 2 h. The crystal is surrounded by dense material and intact membrane at one end but is protruding from the dying PMN at the other (arrow). Note a loss of large portions of cell membrane and degeneration of organelles. A piece of viable cell at the lower right seems surrounded by the necrotic cell (×10,120). (*From Schumacher and Phelps* [55]; *reproduced by permission of* Arthritis and Rheumatism.)

somes are artificial lamellar arrays of phospholipids. These membranes are rendered susceptible to urate-induced lysis if they contain cholesterol and testosterone, but are refractory if they contain 17-β-estradiol. Weissmann and Rita [56] suggest that this effect of 17-β-estradiol may explain why men and chiefly postmenopausal women get gout.

On the basis of these studies the following series of events seems possible. Crystals of monosodium urate coated with IgG and albumin [27] are taken up within the phagosomes of the polymorphs. Phagosomes merge with primary lysosomes, and crystals come to lie within secondary lysosomes. A direct interaction of urate crystals with lysosomes takes place, perhaps by hydrogen bonding to cholesterol-rich, testosterone-containing membranes. The organelle perforates, injury results to the cell in general, and escape of leukocyte contents induces tissue injury and inflammation.

Disruption of the membrane around the crystals leads to a release into the cytoplasm of the crystal along with the lysosomal enzymes [57]. The crystals may then be available to be engulfed by other leukocytes, thus perhaps contributing to the perpetuation of the inflammatory response.

THE ROLE OF LYSOSOMAL ENZYMES   By whatever intermediary mechanisms are involved, it appears that lysosomal

Figure 50-2   Completely phagocytized crystal (C) at 3 min. Distinct phagosome membranes and crystal borders are seen (×20,025). (*From Schumacher and Phelps* [55]; *reproduced by permission of* Arthritis and Rheumatism.)

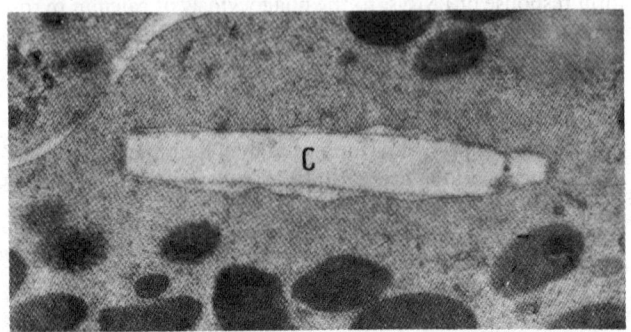

enzymes released in this process play a key role in both the acute inflammatory reaction and the destructive changes of gout, as in other forms of joint disease [57]. Lysosomes are viewed as components of a "common final pathway" of tissue damage [58]. In joints, lysosomes are found in synovial lining cells, cartilage cells, wandering and fixed macrophages, the pericytes of blood vessels, and the polymorphonuclear leukocytes which enter joint spaces from the blood. Leukocyte lysosomes contain a cationic protein that induces inflammation by disrupting mast cell granules, a protease which induces capillary permeability, and acid proteases capable of breaking down cartilage proteoglycans and of cleaving C-5 to C-5a. Perhaps further breakdown of proteoglycans in cartilage leads to further urate crystallization. Other factors such as the prostaglandins and cAMP may also play a role in the pathogenesis of the acute attack, but evidence is fragmentary at present.

Lysosomes of synovial cells contain a collagenase capable of attacking whole articular cartilage. The cleavage of collagen by synovial collagenase may be the rate-limiting step in cartilage degradation. Crystals of monosodium urate stimulate secretion of collagenase and PGE$_2$ by synovial fibroblasts in culture [59]. The collagenase is four times as active at 36°C as at 33°C [60] and may thus be activated by the "calor" of inflammation.

Why Are Acute Gouty Attacks Self-limited? The answer to this question is not known, but several contributing factors may be postulated: (1) In the later stages of an inflammatory response, although polymorphonuclear leukocytes and crystals are present, the latter are no longer intracellular. The arrest of phagocytosis, and of generation of chemotactic factor, may lead to a subsidence of inflammation [52]. (2) The increased heat of inflammation may increase urate solubility, diminishing the tendency toward new crystal formation, and favoring dissolution of existing crystals. (3) The increased blood flow may help to transport urate away from the joint and lessen the tendency toward formation of local regions of supersaturation. (4) Some of the ingested urate crystals may be destroyed by the myeloperoxidase of the leukocytes, thus diminishing the load of crystals released by ruptured cells and capable of perpetuating the inflammatory response. (5) Adrenocortical hormones secreted as a part of the alarm reaction of the acute attack may suppress the inflammatory process.

Interval Gout

Following the initial acute attack, the gouty subject enters an asymptomatic interval phase that may last from a few weeks to many years. In the experience of Gutman [61], 62 percent of new gouty patients suffered a second attack within a year and 78 percent within 2 years, whereas 7 percent had no recurrence for 10 years or more. In the natural history of the disease acute attacks recur with increasing frequency. Later attacks are often polyarticular, more severe, longer, and perhaps febrile. Roentgenographic changes may develop, and the attacks may abate more gradually than before, but the joints may nevertheless recover completely.

Chronic Gouty Arthritis

The time from the initial attack to the beginning of chronic symptoms or visible tophaceous involvement is highly vari-

able, ranging in one large series of untreated patients from 3 to 42 years, with an average of 11.6 years [62]. The development of tophi is correlated with the height of the serum urate concentration, the severity of renal involvement, and the duration of the disease, occurring primarily in subjects who have had gout for 6 to 10 years or more. Only 10 percent of patients will develop tophi with serum urate levels of 8 mg/dl or less, whereas 50 percent will do so when serum urate levels are above 9 mg/dl [63]. Acute attacks may be superimposed on the chronically affected joints, although late in the chronic phase they may disappear altogether.

The process of tophaceous deposition advances insidiously, and although the tophi themselves are relatively painless, there is often progressive stiffness and persistent aching of affected joints. Eventually extensive destruction of joints and large subcutaneous tophi may lead to grotesque deformities, particularly of hands and feet, and to progressive crippling (Fig. 50-4). The tense, shiny thin skin overlying the tophus may ulcerate and extrude white chalky or pasty material composed of myriads of fine needlelike crystals. Horace Walpole is said to have had more tophi than joints in his fingers, such that he could, when playing cards, "chalk a score with more ease and rapidity than any man in England" [64].

Prior to the advent of uricosuric agents, 50 to 70 percent of gouty patients developed visible tophi, permanent joint changes, or chronicity of symptoms [1, 2]. Since the introduction of prophylactic colchicine therapy and uricosuric drugs, the incidence of tophi has dropped substantially [65]. Pertinent data collected over a 25-year period in the clinic of Gutman and Yü are reproduced in Table 50-4. The further drop since 1968 probably reflects the introduction of allopurinol. With the increasing awareness of gout future incidence figures should be lower still. Unfortunately, when compliance is poor, the incidence of tophi still approaches the historic figures.

Pathology The pathognomonic lesion of gout is the *tophus*, a urate deposit surrounded by tissue exhibiting inflammatory and foreign body reactions. Because urate crystals are water-soluble, nonaqueous fixatives are necessary to preserve urate deposits in histologic sections. Urate crystals, if preserved in bulk, are brilliantly anisotropic when viewed with polarized light under the microscope. A useful though nonspecific staining technique is that of de Galantha, in which tissue is fixed in

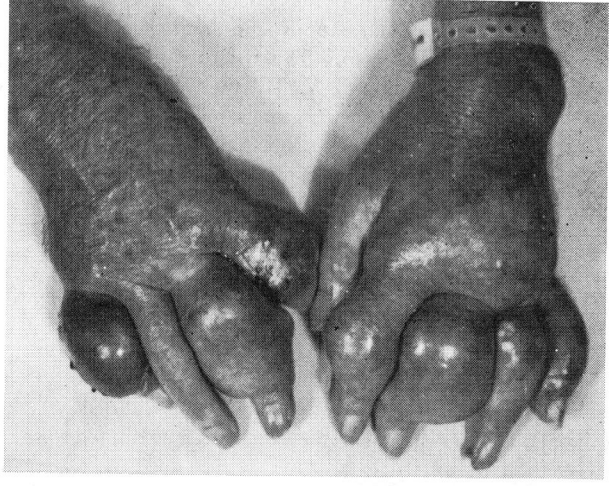

Figure 50-4 Chronic tophaceous gout of severe degree, with bulbous enlargements of several fingers. Note sparing of fourth finger of right hand. (*Courtesy of Dr. R. Wayne Rundles, Duke University Medical Center.*)

Table 50-4 Changing trend in the incidence of tophi and renal calculi in primary gout

Years	Patients (No.)	Tophi		Renal calculi	
		No.	%	No.	%
1948–1953	165	88	53	37	20
1954–1958	369	154	42	92	25
1959–1963	522	172	33	138	26
1964–1968	355	112	32	80	23
1969–1973	289	49	17	57	20
Total	1700	575		404	

SOURCE: Yü [65]. (Reproduced by permission of *The American Journal of Medicine.*)

absolute alcohol and stained with silver. Urate crystals are brown-black by this method. However, provided the initial fixation is with absolute alcohol, staining with hematoxylin and eosin is also usually successful, even though the bulk of the crystals may have been dissolved out.

Two general categories of mechanisms have been proposed for the deposition of urate in gout. Sokoloff [66] has grouped these as follows: (1) metastatic, implying that urate is deposited in tissues because excessive quantities are presented to them by circulating blood; and (2) dystrophic, implying that urate is deposited in tissues because the latter have undergone pathologic alteration rendering them susceptible to urate deposition. These two categories are not mutually exclusive. In gout, urate tends to deposit in cartilage, epiphyseal bone, periarticular structures, and kidneys. The deposits produce local necrosis and (unless the tissue is avascular) an ensuing foreign-body reaction with proliferation of fibrous tissue. The characteristic *tophaceous nodule* consists of multicentric deposits of urate crystals, an intercrystalline matrix, together with an inflammatory reaction and foreign-body granuloma. The crystals, proved by x-ray crystallography to be monosodium urate monohydrate [67], are acicular and arranged radially in small clusters. The internal structure of crystals of tophi suggests crystal formation about an electron-lucent nidal matrix [67a]. Granular and amorphous deposits have also been described. Calcific material deposited in the matrix may render the tophus radiopaque, and rarely this process may reach the proportions of heterotopic ossification. Protein, lipid, and polysaccharide components are found in the tophus. By immunohistologic techniques IgG, IgM, and small amounts of IgA are found in the intercrystalline matrix of gouty tophi [67b].

In the joint, cartilaginous degeneration, synovial proliferation, destruction of subchondral bone, proliferation of marginal bone, often synovial pannus, and sometimes fibrous or bony ankylosis may develop. The articular surface may be encrusted with urate (Fig. 50-5). The punched-out lesions of bones commonly seen in roentgenograms of gouty patients (Figs. 50-6 and 50-7) represent subchondral tophus deposits, which often communicate with the urate crust through erosions and defects in articular cartilage (Fig. 50-8).

Urate deposition in spinal joints is rare unless there is advanced tophaceous disease elsewhere in the skeleton [1, 2]. Urate may deposit in marrow spaces of vertebral bodies, as well as in the disk tissue itself (Figs. 50-9 and 50-10). Tophaceous softening of the odontoid process with subluxation of the first cervical vertebra has been reported, as well as cervical nerve root compression from a collapsed cervical disk which contained urate crystals. Paraplegia has been attributed to spi-

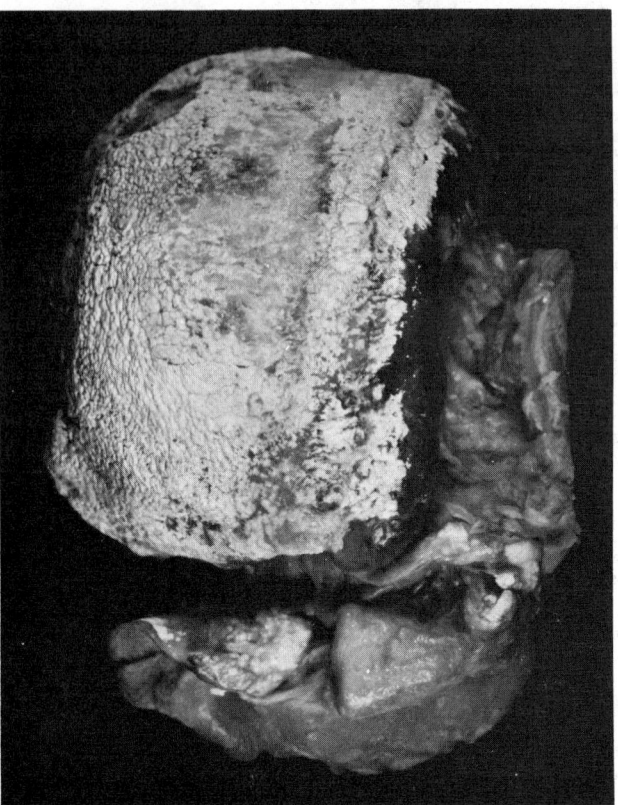

Figure 50-5 Extensive urate deposition on the articular cartilage of a femoral condyle of a patient with long-standing gout.

nal cord pressure from an extradural urate mass at the level of the tenth dorsal vertebra. Tophi may cause nerve compressions and the carpal tunnel and tarsal tunnel syndromes.

Tophaceous involvement of the sacroiliac joint may be found on x-ray examination. Aseptic necrosis of the hip is occasionally a manifestation of gout. The collapsed femoral head may contain urate crystals [1, 2].

Watts and associates [69] have demonstrated crystals of anhydrous uric acid, uric acid dihydrate, and monosodium urate monohydrate in the deltoid muscle of patients with untreated long-standing tophaceous gout.

Tophi are conspicuously absent from liver, spleen, and lungs. Also, tophi do not occur within the central nervous system even in advanced cases of gout. The concentration of uric acid is very low in spinal fluid [70], ranging in normal and gouty subjects from 0.25 to 1.0 mg/dl. The low concentration has been attributed to selective inpermeability of the blood-brain barrier to urates and to the absence of xanthine oxidase in the central nervous system.

Tophi commonly occur in the helix or antihelix of the ear (Fig. 50-11), the olecranon and patellar bursae, and tendons. Less commonly, they occur in the skin of fingertips, palms, or soles, the tarsal plates of the eyelids, the nasal cartilages, or the cornea or sclerotic coats of the eye. Rarely they occur in the corpus cavernosum and prepuce of the penis, tongue, epiglottis, vocal cords, and arytenoid cartilages.

Tophi have been described along the free margins of aortic, tricuspid, and mitral valves, appearing as small yellow-white plaques. They have also been identified as nodular deposits up to 1 cm in diameter within the mitral valve or its annulus, or within the myocardium. Diffuse deposits have been described in the interstitial connective tissue between the myofibrils.

Complete heart block has been attributed to a tophus in the conducting system [1, 2].

Renal Disease in Primary Gout

Renal disease is common in patients with primary gout. Ordinarily the process is only slowly progressive and does not materially reduce life expectancy. The incidence of proteinuria varies from 20 to 40 percent and shows a modest correlation with age. It may be intermittent or persistent; only rarely is the quantity heavy. Hypertension is approximately as common as albuminuria. Usually it is benign (see below).

The glomerular filtration rate is well preserved in many gouty subjects, but in others it gradually falls [71–73]. Decline in renal function appears to be correlated with aging, renal vascular disease and hypertension, renal calculi, pyelonephritis, or independently occurring nephropathy including that of lead nephropathy. Only rarely is it ascribable to gout alone. Hyperuricemia alone had no deleterious effect upon renal function during follow-up of 149 gouty subjects for periods ranging up to 22 years [72, 73].

Renal Hemodynamics

INULIN CLEARANCE   The majority of inulin clearance values in gouty subjects are within the normal range. In the study of Berger and Yü [72] of 524 male patients with gout, 23 percent had an inulin clearance of more than 130 ml/min, 51 percent had clearances between 90 and 130 ml/min, 22 percent below 90 ml/min, and 9 percent below 70 ml/min. The values showed a downward trend with age and at all intervals were about 30 ml/min lower in the 20 percent of patients with proteinuria than in those without. If hypertensive subjects are excluded, the age-related decline in glomerular filtration rate is not significantly greater in gouty than in control subjects [74].

C_{PAH} The mean value in 110 gouty subjects reported by Gutman and Yü [71] in 1957 was 414 ± 90 ml/(min · 1.73 m^2) (range, 208 to 722 ml). A comparison with the distribution of nongouty subjects of an equivalent age indicated a moderate but significant reduction in the effective renal plasma flow ($p <$

0.01 in all age groups) in patients with gout. The reduction in C_{PAH} was disproportionate to the minimal reduction of inulin clearances, especially in the older patients, and as a consequence the filtration fraction tended to rise with age from 0.19 to 0.25. Arterial hypertension was present in about half the subjects with a statistically significant increase in filtration fractions.

In a much larger study of 524 gouty patients reported from the same clinic in 1975 [72], C_{PAH} showed trends with age comparable to those in inulin clearance. In patients without proteinuria C_{PAH} values fell from 578 ± 95 ml/(min · 1.73 m^2) at ages 21 to 35 to 384 ± 73 ml/(min · 1.73 m^2) at ages 61 to 65 years. At all ages, C_{PAH} was lower in patients with proteinuria than in those without. The age-related changes in C_{PAH} (and also in C_{inulin}) in the gouty patients without proteinuria were no different from what would be expected in a similarly aging nongouty population [75].

The Kidney in Gout   The kidneys of patients with gout present a wide variety of changes whether the gout is primary or secondary [1, 2]. Of these changes, the only one distinctive of gout (but not diagnostic—see below) is the presence of urate crystals in the interstitium, medulla, or pyramids, and a surrounding giant-cell reaction. Crystals are also common within the collecting tubules of the medulla. Associated interstitial inflammatory and vascular changes are prominent, as are changes resulting from tubular obstruction, chronic infection, aging processes, or hypertension.

Upon gross examination the kidneys are equally affected and generally small. The subcapsular surface may show granularity with some coarser scars, and the cortex may be reduced in width. The medulla and pyramids may show small white specks and sometimes radiating white lines representing urate deposits. The pelvis may contain uric acid stones, and in these cases the pyramids may be reduced in size.

On microscopic examination [76, 77] the pathologic changes are found to be highly variable. Glomeruli may be normal in appearance or partially or completely hyalinized. The tubules may be normal, or may show atrophy, dilatation, or regeneration. The proximal tubules are likely to be spared. The interstitial tissue may show fibrosis and foci of lymphocytes, macrophages and plasma cells typical of chronic pyelo-

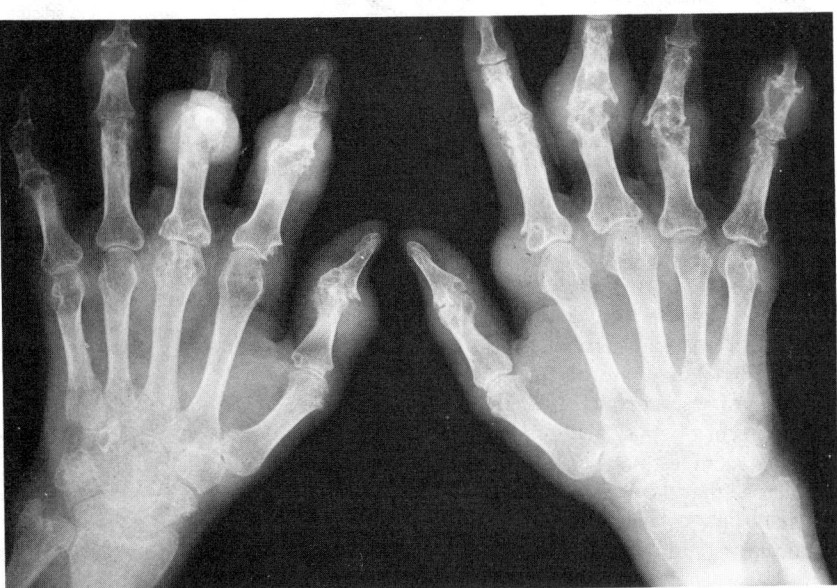

Figure 50-6 Chronic gouty arthritis of the hands. Note the extensive destruction of bone by urate deposits and the large soft-tissue tophi.

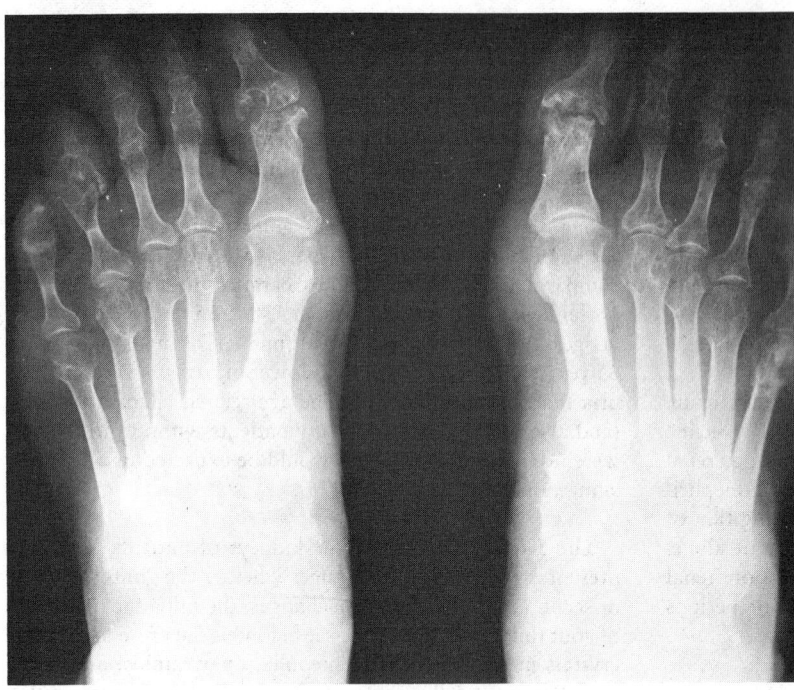

Figure 50-7 Chronic gouty arthritis of the feet of the patient shown in Fig. 50-6.

nephritis. The collecting tubules may be dilated and loaded with crystals, hyaline casts, and calcific concretions. The crystals may be elongated, rectangular, or so fragmented as to be amorphous. They are seen particularly well in alcohol-fixed material, but may be preserved in formalin-fixed tissue stained with hematoxylin-eosin, and then present a deep blue appearance [77]. The most characteristic locations of deposits of urate are the medullary interstitium, the pyramids, and the papillae (Figs. 50-12 and 50-13), where they may be surrounded by an accumulation of lymphocytes and foreign-body giant cells. In some cases there are collections of amyloidlike material in the medulla which do not give the specific staining reactions for amyloid. Arteries and arterioles show increased basophilia and degenerative changes which are sometimes out of proportion to the parenchymal damage. The vascular changes in the kidney may be associated with an increased incidence of large-vessel sclerosis elsewhere.

The traditional view [1, 2] has been that the renal lesions stem from deposits of urate formed in the convoluted tubules and flushed into the collecting tubules with resultant obstruction, dilation, and atrophy of the more proximal tubules and secondary necrosis and fibrosis. Crystals were detected in 93 percent of 191 patients with gout coming to autopsy, reviewed by Talbott and Terplan in 1960 [76]. In 25 percent the urate deposits had produced extensive structural alterations.

Percutaneous needle biopsy has permitted study of early changes of the kidney in gout. The information gained is limited, for only rarely is adequate medullary tissue obtained to disclose crystals in their commonest location. In addition, in some studies, specimens were fixed in aqueous formalin which readily dissolves urate crystals. Nevertheless, these studies have led to revised concepts of the sequence of events in the development of gouty nephropathy.

Greenbaum et al. [78] and Gonick and associates [79] emphasize that the earliest renal lesion is *interstitial* reaction. There is slight collagenous change and increase in cellularity of cortical interstitial tissue without an associated inflammatory infiltration. At this stage there may be no tubular abnormality. The increase in interstitial fibrosis is greater than expected for the age of the patient and may be present in subjects with normal blood pressure [78].

Gonick et al. [79] studied 28 biopsy and 42 autopsy specimens from patients with gout and concluded that the most characteristic early changes were uniform fibrillar thickening of glomerular capillary basement membranes, increased numbers of nuclei in capillary loops, and atrophy of Henle loops sometimes associated with brown pigment degeneration of epithelium and increased basophilia of arteries and arterioles. The interstitial changes were located in areas proximal to the changes in the Henle loops and spared the medullary and juxtamedullary cortex which is usually involved in infectious

Figure 50-8 Proximal phalanx of a finger. The surface of the articular cartilage is frayed and uneven. There is cartilaginous and bony overgrowth (lipping) at the articular margins. The two large circular defects (punched-out areas) in the articular cartilage and subchondral bone were lined with fibrous tissue infiltrated with large numbers of inflammatory cells and studded with masses of urate crystals. (*From Ludwig et al.* [68]; *reproduced by permission of* Annals of Internal Medicine.)

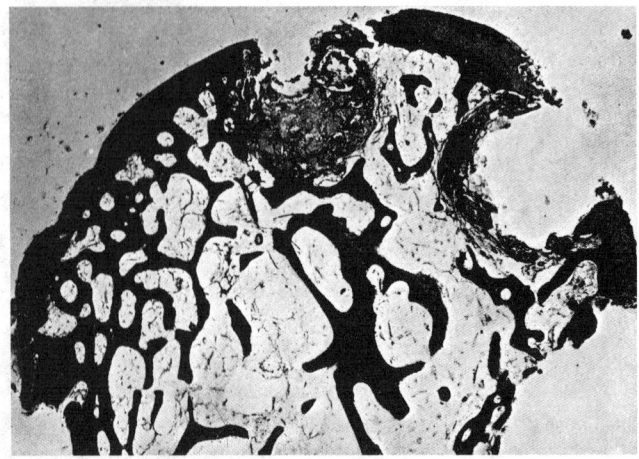

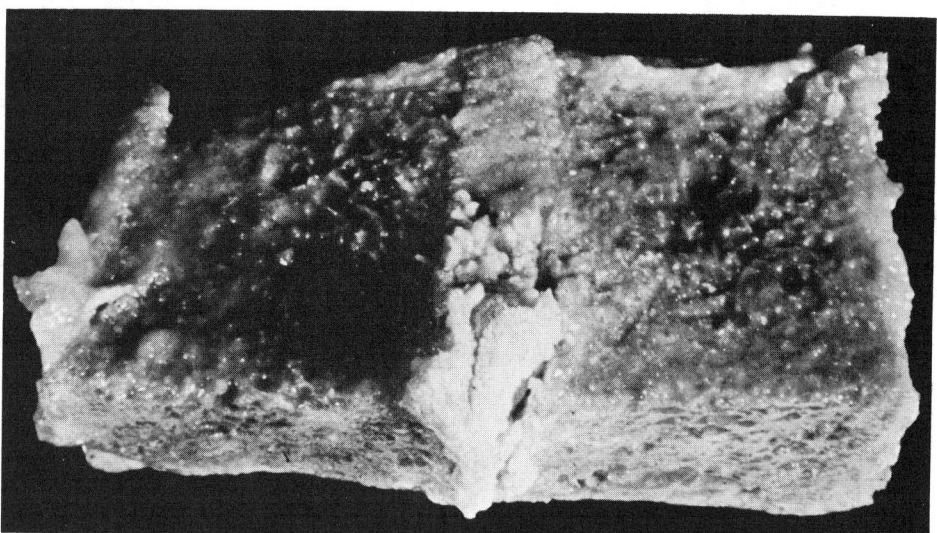

Figure 50-9 Ventral slice of a segment of vertebral column showing heavy urate deposits within the intervertebral disk and extending into the contiguous vertebral bodies.

pyelonephritis. Postmortem cultures were positive in only 4 percent of gouty kidneys. Thus, the interstitial changes in gout are probably not of infectious origin.

Gonick and associates observed tophaceous deposits in only 1 of 28 biopsy specimens and 4 of 42 necropsy kidneys. These frequencies are lower than in earlier studies in kidneys of patients with gout. The disparity is probably explained by the low yield of medullary tissue by needle biopsy [1, 2] and previous treatment of 35 percent of patients with uricosuric agents. According to Gonick et al. the glomerular changes of gout can be differentiated from those of nephrosclerosis or diabetic glomerulosclerosis, but Heptinstall [77] and Pardo et al. [80] do not agree that the lesion is distinctive.

In the human kidney the highest concentrations of urate are in the region of the Henle loops. This is a region also high in sodium concentration. These findings suggest that the initial damage to the tubular epithelium of Henle's loop may be a consequence of high local concentrations of sodium urate. The interstitial reaction may be a response to the deposition of microcrystalline sodium urate. Seegmiller and Frazier [81] showed by x-ray diffraction studies that crystals found in the renal interstitium of patients with chronic gout were monosodium urate monohydrate, not uric acid.

The renal medulla, pyramids, and interstitium are rich in acid mucopolysaccharide. Perhaps urate-binding proteoglycans such as those of Katz and Schubert [29] discussed above also play a role in the pathogenesis of renal tophi, in releasing high local concentrations of urate and of sodium, resulting in crystal formation within the renal parenchyma.

In advanced cases of gouty nephropathy, crystals are often found in the collecting ducts as well as in the interstitium. The formation of crystals in the collecting ducts should be related to the concentration of urate in tubular urine, the acidification process that converts monosodium urate to uric acid, and the very limited solubility of uric acid in acid urine. One would therefore predict that these crystals would be uric acid. Seegmiller and Frazier [81] have demonstrated by x-ray diffraction that the crystals found in the collecting ducts in patients with acute lymphoblastic leukemia are uric acid, not sodium urate. It is likely that kidneys with both interstitial and collecting duct crystals contain both urate and uric acid crystals, but this has not been proved.

Reports of several decades ago cited instances of "gout nephrosis" occurring without clinical evidence of gout. In four patients dying of renal insufficiency and purported to represent this syndrome [1, 2], the only tophaceous deposits were in the kidneys, and no uric acid analyses had been performed during life. Whether these cases represent hyperuricemic nephropathy occurring in the absence of or in advance of clinical gout, or whether they represent urate deposits laid down in end-stage kidney disease is difficult to decide in retrospect.

Verger et al. [82] examined the kidneys of 62 patients dying of renal insufficiency. In 17 they identified the tophi in the renal medulla. In alcohol-fixed section they found needlelike crystals having the characteristics of urate. The tophi were identical to those observed in primary gout. They attributed these tophi to the hyperuricemia of chronic renal insufficiency. Of the 17 patients, 4 had had attacks of articular gout considered to be secondary to renal insufficiency.

Linnane and colleagues [83] found urate deposits within medullary microtophi in 8 percent of unselected autopsies in Brisbane, Australia. In three-fourths of patients the microtophi were associated with a history of gouty arthritis or with primary renal disease, but in one-fourth of patients a retrospective

Figure 50-10 Urate crystals from the specimen shown in Fig. 50-9, viewed under polarized light.

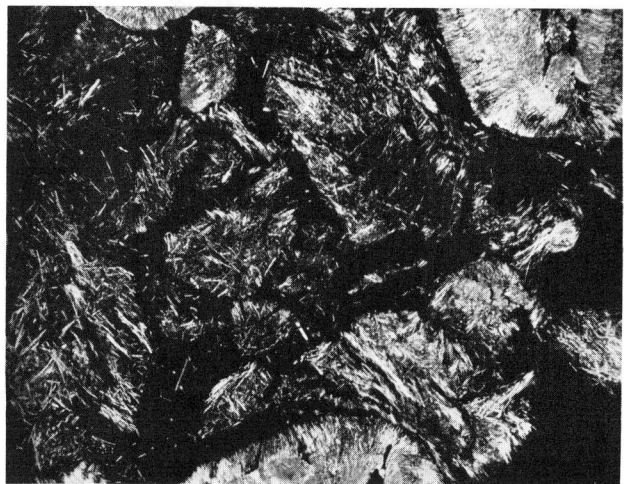

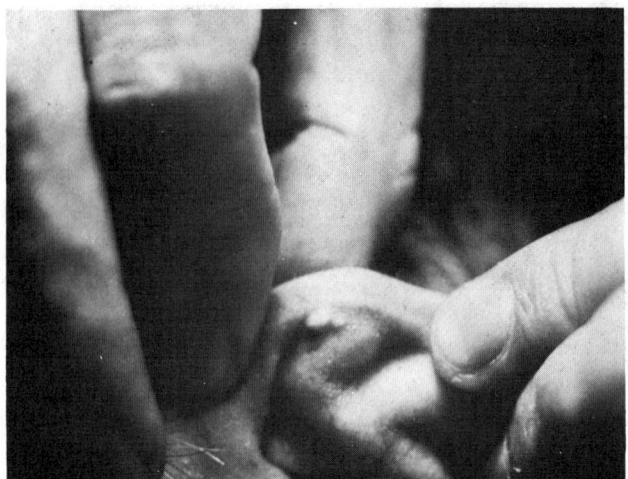

Figure 50-11 Tophus of the helix of the ear adjacent to the auricular tubercle.

survey of the medical record did not reveal any causative factor. These two studies indicate that a diagnosis of gout cannot be made post mortem solely on the basis of tophaceous deposits in the kidney.

Urolithiasis in Gout The incidence of renal calculi in various American or European series of gout is 5 to 33 percent [1, 2]. It is 75 percent in gouty subjects in Israel [84]. In the experience of Yü and Gutman [85], the incidence was 22 percent in 1258 patients with primary gout and 42 percent in 59 patients with gout secondary to hematologic disease. The incidence of urolithiasis is about 0.1 percent in the general population. In 40 percent of the cases of primary gout, lithiasis antedated acute arthritis, occasionally by more than 20 years. Uric acid nephrolithiasis is frequently associated with hyperuricemia without acute arthritis. About one-third of such patients give a family history of gout. In 84 percent of gouty subjects the stones are pure uric acid (not sodium urate); in 4 percent they are uric acid and calcium oxalate; in 12 percent, calcium oxalate or phosphate alone [85]. In Fessel's study the risk of urolithiasis was 1 stone in 852 patients per year in normouricemic controls, 1 in 295 patients per year in asymptomatic hyperuricemics, and 1 in 114 patients per year in patients with established gout [86].

Factors that predispose toward uric acid nephrolithiasis in gout include undue acidity of the urine, increased urinary excretion of uric acid, increased urinary concentration, and perhaps qualitative or quantitative abnormalities of urinary constituents that affect the solubility of uric acid [84].

Gouty patients have a tendency toward unusually acid urine, both in fasting morning specimens and throughout the day [1, 2, 85, 87], and a substandard rise of urinary pH in response to oral alkali. There is no correlation between urine pH and urinary uric acid excretion [85]. In the three-fourths of gouty subjects whose urinary uric acid values fall within the normal range, the high incidence of renal stones is probably in part related to low urinary pH. This, in turn, is a reflection of a low NH_4^+/titratable acidity ratio attributed by some to subnormal ammonium excretion at a given acid load or pH and by others to high values of titratable acidity [1, 2]. The deficit of ammonium excretion, when present, has been assigned to the effects of occult or measurable renal damage, aging, or high purine intake by some authors [1, 2] but is regarded as an intrinsic

defect in the production of ammonia, presumably from glutamine, by Gutman and Yü [88]. The pK_{a1} and pK_{a2} of uric acid are 5.75 and 10.3, respectively. Therefore at urinary pH values of 4.5 to 5 the predominant form is uric acid, not sodium urate. X-ray crystallographic studies have shown that the stones are uric acid [1, 2]. The solubility of uric acid is only one-seventeenth that of sodium urate in water at 37°C.

The prevalence of renal stones rises with increasing plasma urate levels in the general population (see Table 50-5) and approximates 50 percent when serum urate levels exceed 12 mg/dl in patients with gout [85]. The influence of hyperuricemia is probably chiefly significant as it affects urinary uric acid excretion. The prevalence of urolithiasis increases from 11 percent in patients with excretion values under 300 mg/day to 50 percent in patients with values over 1100 mg/day [85]. Patients with increased uric aciduria have an increased incidence of calcium oxalate stones [89, 90]. Urate (not uric acid) can participate in "heterogeneous nucleation" with calcium oxalate [91].

According to several authorities [1, 2] uric acid stones are formed only when supersaturation prevails and when there is a crystallation nucleus of organic matrix. Sperling and De Vries [92] conclude that urine is invariably supersaturated with uric acid if the pH is below 5.5 or 5.7. Uric acid stone formers have normal urinary uric acid solubility and a normal capacity to form supersaturated urine.

URIC ACID NEPHROLITHIASIS IN NONHYPERURICEMIC SUBJECTS   Only about 20 percent of patients without clinical gout who form uric acid stones are hyperuricemic [2]. In *idiopathic* uric acid nephrolithiasis, by definition occurring in patients with normal plasma and urinary uric acid values, a consistent finding, as in gouty and in otherwise asymptomatic hyperuricemic subjects, is a tendency toward a low urine pH. Several groups [1, 2] have reported reduced ammonium excretion and normal or increased titratable acidity in such patients, but Metcalfe-Gibson and associates [93] found normal ammonium excretion in relation to pH, except in patients with overt renal damage. Ammonium excretion per nephron was normal.

A familial form of uric acid lithiasis is found in Israel, in which patients are normouricemic and frequently hyperuricosuric, with unusually acid urines, in the absence of other abnormalities of renal function. Those patients have normal

Figure 50-12 Urate deposit in the medulla of kidney as seen in alcohol-fixed section, stained with hematoxylin and eosin (×250).

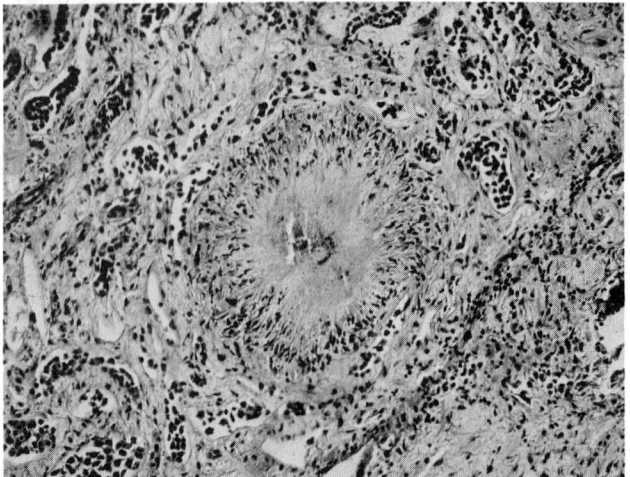

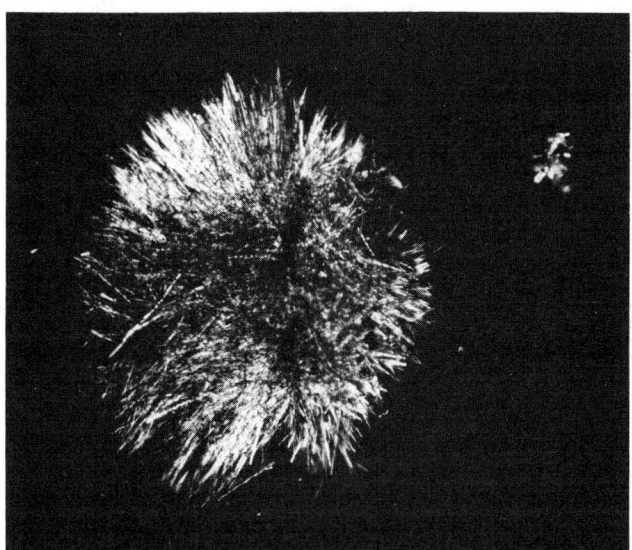

Figure 50-13 Section adjacent to that shown in Fig. 50-12, viewed under polarized light.

rates of ammonium excretion and elevated titratable acidity. The excretion of ammonium, with or without administration of an acid load is not lower than in control subjects of equivalent age. There is no apparent deficiency in urinary "solubilizers" of uric acid [94]. This disorder appears to be an inherited disease, distinct from gout, with an autosomal dominant mode of inheritance and high penetrance in both sexes [95].

The risk of uric acid stones is also increased in patients with ileostomies who exhibit increased renal conservation of sodium, a decreased urinary Na/K ratio, increased urinary acid excretion, and low urinary pH values [96].

Uric acid stones may at times be dissolved with protracted fluid and alkali therapy [84], but allopurinol is the treatment of choice (see below).

Association of Gout with Other Metabolic Disorders

Obesity The association of gout with obesity and overeating has been recognized for hundreds of years. In 6000 subjects in Tecumseh, Michigan, hyperuricemia was found in only 3.4 percent of those with a relative weight at or below the 20th percentile, in 5.7 percent of those between the 21st and 79th percentiles, and in 11.4 percent of those at or above the 80th percentile [97]. In a study of 460 people, Krizek [98] noted a highly significant correlation between serum urate and weight for both males and females. Gertler et al. [99] found a strong correlation between serum urate, weight, ponderal index, and somatotype. Other population studies also demonstrate a positive correlation between serum urate and weight or body surface area [1, 2, 100].

A large percentage of gouty patients show body weights above ideal values for age and height. Emmerson and Knowles [101] noted that subjects with primary gout were an average of 17.8 percent overweight (compared with patients with lead gout, who were an average of 1.3 percent overweight). Brochner-Mortensen [102] found that 78 percent of his gouty subjects were more than 10 percent overweight, and 57 percent were more than 30 percent overweight. Grahame and Scott [103] noted that 48 percent of 355 patients with gout were more

than 15 percent overweight. Fessel et al. [104] reported that their patients with asymptomatic hyperuricemia had significantly greater values for weight, triceps skin folds, subscapular skin folds, and a smaller value for ponderal index than the control group.

Weight reduction in obese people usually leads to a modest reduction of serum urate values. In one study of 67 hyperuricemic subjects, 49 exhibited a mean decrease in serum urate concentration of 1.6 mg/dl following a mean weight loss of 20 kg, but the other 18 showed a further elevation of their hyperuricemia [105].

Diabetes Mellitus Hyperuricemia has been reported in 2 to 50 percent of patients with diabetes, whereas gouty arthritis has been reported in from less than 0.1 percent to 9.0 percent of diabetic subjects [112]. Abnormal glucose tolerance tests have been noted in 7 to 74 percent of patients with gout, depending, in part, on the criteria used. When overt clinical diabetes is present in such patients, it tends to be mild. The common factor may well be obesity, which predisposes to both hyperuricemia and hyperglycemia. Engelhardt and Wagner [106] called attention to obesity as an integral part of a triad with gout and diabetes; others have also noted this association.

Despite the apparent high incidence of hyperuricemia in patients selected for diabetes, and of glucose intolerance in patients selected for gout, epidemiologic studies have not demonstrated any relation between gout and diabetes or between serum urate and blood glucose concentrations [97]. In such studies the mean serum urate concentration is actually lower in patients with overt diabetes. This has been attributed to the apparent uricosuric effect of high glucose blood levels [1, 2].

The recent observation that uric acid inhibits insulin secretion in the rat both in vitro and in vivo provides an interesting potential explanation for the putative relationship between hyperuricemia and glucose intolerance [107].

Hyperlipidemia Hypertriglyceridemia has been reported in 75 to 84 percent of patients with gout and hyperuricemia in up to 82 percent of patients with hypertriglyceridemia [1, 2]. Here, too, the common factor may be obesity. Gibson and Grahame [108] found that the mean serum triglyceride concentration of 50 male gouty subjects was elevated in comparison with that of a control group unmatched as to weight but was not significantly greater than that of an equally obese male control group without hyperuricemia. The gouty patients who drank alcohol excessively had a mean serum triglyceride level that was higher than that of their obesity-matched controls and that of nondrinking gouty patients. By contrast, serum triglyceride values were not elevated in lean gouty subjects in com-

Table 50-5 Prevalence of urinary calculi by maximum urate category in a population of mean age 58

Serum urate concentration, mg/100 ml	Men		Women	
	No.	Percent with stones	No.	Percent with stones
7.0+	212	12.7	28	7.1
8.0+	50	22.0	5	0
9.0+	10	40.0	1	0

SOURCE: From Hall et al. [11].

parison with matched controls. Further evidence against a direct relationship between hypertriglyceridemia and hyperuricemia is the observation that elevations of serum triglyceride concentration during Intralipid infusion have no effect upon the serum urate concentrations [109].

Although individual gouty subjects are frequently hypercholesterolemic, many studies have failed to show a correlation between serum urate and cholesterol values [1, 2]. Gibson and Grahame [108] reported that serum cholesterol values of their gouty patients did not differ significantly from either weight-matched or unmatched controls.

Hypertension Hypertension is present in one-fourth to one-half of patients with classic gout [1, 2]. For example, hypertension, with a diastolic blood pressure of 90 mmHg or more, was present in 52 percent of a group of 354 patients with gout reviewed by Grahame and Scott in 1970 [103]. In 9 percent it was severe, with a diastolic pressure of 130 mmHg or more. The incidence of both moderate and severe hypertension was unrelated to duration of gout, but that of moderate hypertension rose with increasing age of onset. The incidence of severe hypertension was greatest in the group with onset of gout in the second decade. Moderate hypertension was more common in obese than in nonobese subjects. The relative contributions of obesity, age, and coexistent renal disease to hypertension in gout have not been determined.

Hyperuricemia has been reported in 22 to 38 percent of untreated hypertensive persons. This is significantly greater than the prevalence of hyperuricemia expected in an unselected population. When therapy and renal disease are not excluded, the prevalence increases to 47 to 67 percent. The overall prevalence of gout in persons with hypertension has been variously reported as 2 to 12 percent [1, 2].

The prevalence of hyperuricemia in the general population rises with increases of diastolic *or* systolic blood pressure in both males and females. However, Grahame and Scott found no consistent pattern relating hyperuricemia to the interaction of diastolic *and* systolic blood pressures. Furthermore, when serum urate values were standardized for population variables of weight, age, and anthropometric measurements, there was only random variation of hyperuricemia and diastolic and systolic pressures in relation to one another [103]. Among Polynesian peoples also, hyperuricemia was associated with hypertension only when the group was also obese [110].

In an Israeli ischemic heart disease study of 10,000 male civil service workers age 40 or over published in 1972 [111], 9 of 90 variables studied were associated with the incidence of hypertension (systolic pressure of 160 mmHg *and* diastolic pressure of 95 mmHg, or over) to a degree that they would not be observed by chance alone more than one time in a hundred. Three of the nine variables represented different measurements of obesity. A fourth was the serum urate concentration, but the correlation between urate concentration and hypertension was not adjusted for age or relative body weight. In a different analysis of data collected in this study [112], the simple correlation coefficient between systolic blood pressure and serum urate concentration was 0.16. Of variables examined, only 1 percent of blood pressure variation could be accounted for by serum urate concentrations, compared with age, 8.9 percent; pulse, 6.0 percent; myocardial ischemia, 2.0 percent; weight/height ratio, 1.6 percent; and so on. In the population study of 6000 residents of Tecumseh, Michigan, in 1968 Myers et al. [97] found no correlation between serum urate concentrations

adjusted for age, sex, and relative body weight, and levels of blood pressure.

In contrast, Fessel [113] found that asymptomatic hyperuricemic subjects who developed hypertension (25 of 111 patients followed for a mean duration of 108 months) had body weight not statistically higher than the remainder.

The important study of Messerli and associates [114] suggests that unexplained hyperuricemia in patients with essential hypertension most likely reflects early renal vascular involvement, specifically nephrosclerosis. They measured glomerular filtration rate (GFR), renal and systemic hemodynamics, intravascular volume, and serum urate levels in normal subjects and in subjects with borderline or established hypertension. Serum urate levels correlated inversely with renal blood flow and directly with renal vascular and total peripheral vascular resistance. There was no correlation of serum urate levels with cardiac output, heart rate, intravascular volume, or GFR. Mild asymptomatic hyperuricemia was associated with reduced renal blood flow in the absence of changes in GFR. Other studies show a significant correlation between serum urate concentrations and plasma renin activity [115] as well as reduced renal clearance of uric acid following infusions of angiotensin or norepinephrine sufficient to raise diastolic blood pressure by 20 mmHg [116]. The common factor in all these situations may be reduced renal cortical blood flow [117]. Thus hyperuricemia may be an *expression* of vascular disease, rather than a risk factor *for* vascular disease and hypertension. Such a postulate would explain many of the associations discussed above, without supporting causal relationships between hyperuricemia and hypertension or arteriosclerosis.

Atherosclerosis and Coronary Heart Disease In 1951 Gertler and coworkers [99] noted a statistically significant excess of hyperuricemia in a group of young patients with coronary heart disease. Several other reports have noted the association of hyperuricemia with the manifestations of atherosclerosis [1, 2]. In Framingham [118], the incidence of coronary artery disease was twice as high in gouty subjects as in the male population with normal serum urate values but was not increased in hyperuricemic subjects who did not have clinically overt gout. In a study at Henry Ford Hospital of 280 gouty patients selected to exclude renal disease, hypertension, diabetes mellitus, or prior arterial thrombosis, there was an increased incidence of myocardial infarction during the fourth, fifth, and sixth decades [119]. On the other hand, a comparison of serum urate levels with extent of coronary artery disease in 1002 patients having coronary angiography disclosed no significant correlation [120]. In the Tecumseh study [97], there was no clear association between levels of blood pressure, blood sugar, or serum cholesterol and serum urate concentrations when adjustments were made for effects of age, sex, and relative weight. When these variables were taken into account, the figures showed that the serum urate levels of persons with coronary heart disease were not significantly different from the mean of the population. Myers et al. [97] concluded that an elevated serum urate concentration value could not be taken as an attribute associated with coronary heart disease. Emmerson [121], in a recent review, concludes that available data do not support a causal relationship between hyperuricemia and atherosclerosis.

The situation among the Polynesians is also complex but appears to confirm that hypertension, diabetes, and atherosclerosis are correlates of obesity rather than of hyperuricemia.

The Maori are hyperuricemic, obese, hypertensive, diabetic, and atherosclerotic. However, the Pukapukans, who are not westernized, are hyperuricemic but thin, nondiabetic, and non-atherosclerotic [110].

Hyperuricemia has been proposed as a risk factor for coronary heart disease [122]. Fessel [113] concludes that hyperuricemia predicts future cardiovascular disease independently of body weight. In 1356 men ages 60 to 69 with a serum urate value recorded in 1977, deaths from cardiovascular disease showed stepwise increases when deaths were arranged according to serum urate levels but not when arranged according to body weight. However, it was not stated that the 1356 men were free of renal disease, hypertension, diabetes or arteriosclerotic events in 1977. Thus hyperuricemia might have been a "marker for . . . vascular changes" [117] rather than a predictor of future disease.

Prognosis and Causes of Death

Available analyses of longevity in gout indicate a mortality rate closely approximating that of the general population. An example of observed and expected deaths in two groups of gouty patients (from Boston and Buffalo, respectively) is presented [123, 124] in Table 50-6.

Older textbooks often stated that one-half of gouty subjects died of renal failure, but we have been unable to locate data in support of this statement. Reports published in 1956 [125] and 1960 [176] documented renal failure as the cause of death in 22 to 25 percent of gouty patients. In 1972 Gutman [63] analyzed a 20-year experience with 1600 patients with primary gout. There were 38 deaths (18 percent of the cumulative mortality of 223 deaths) due to renal insufficiency, but 27 of these were related to such causes as malignant hypertension, chronic glomerulonephritis, or polycystic renal disease. Only 11 (6.9 percent of deaths) were attributed to gouty nephropathy. In a 30-year review of 2000 patients with primary gout from the same clinic in 1980 by Yü and Talbott [126], 7.7 percent of deaths from 1950 to 1967 and 6.6 percent of deaths from 1968 to 1979 were due to renal insufficiency unrelated to other primary diagnoses. Approximately 65 percent of deaths of gouty subjects were due to cardiovascular or cerebrovascular disease during 1950 to 1967. The majority of gouty males died of cardiac or cerebral vascular disease, or malignancies, in about the same proportions as in the general male population of the United States [126, 127]. Many authors have stressed increased severity of arteriosclerotic processes in primary gout, but the subject remains controversial, and the relationship of

these changes to hyperuricemia itself is not clear. In Framingham, Massachusetts, the incidence of coronary artery disease was not increased in hyperuricemic subjects without clinical gout [118]. In a series of 280 patients with primary gout followed for 5 to 10 years, myocardial infarction occurred in 22 instances, cerebral vascular occlusion in 20, and peripheral vascular occlusive disease in 9. Compared by decades with the Framingham and Tecumseh studies, there was a greater than anticipated incidence of myocardial infarction during the fourth, fifth, and sixth decades [119]. Although ischemic heart disease continues to be the most common cause of death in gout, the death rate from this cause has fallen in the last decade in gouty patients as in the general population [126].

The prognosis in the various forms of secondary gout is usually that of the underlying disorder.

URIC ACID IN BLOOD SERUM

Methods

The methods that are currently used to assay uric acid in blood and urine depend on chemical or enzymatic oxidation to allantoin [1, 2]. In the former, a chromogen is reduced concurrently with the oxidation to yield a chromophore which may be measured spectrophotometrically. In the latter, uricase (urate:oxygen oxidoreductase, EC 1.7.3.3) is used to catalyze the reaction, and the concentration of uric acid may be determined by direct spectrophotometry (following the change in absorbance at 292 nm during the reaction) or by measuring the amount of oxygen consumed or the amount of hydrogen peroxide produced. Alternatively, a chemical oxidizing agent may be employed, and colorimetric measurements made before and after treatment with uricase.

Colorimetric Methods The most widely used colorimetric methods depend on the reduction of sodium tungstate by uric acid. The difficulties inherent in these methods are four-fold: The tendency of uric acid to coprecipitate with the plasma proteins; the possible formation of turbidity in the final colored solutions; nonlinearity in relation to the color yield and amount of uric acid present over the range of uric acid concentrations commonly encountered; and interference by other reducing agents in plasma or urine. The potential interfering reducing agents include ascorbic acid, free thiols (e.g., thionene, cysteine, glutathione), salicylates and gentisic acid (a salicylate metabolite), homogentisic acid, caffeine, theophylline, theobromine, and their metabolites [260], L-dopa, very high concentrations of glucose, and certain chromogens retained in renal failure. The tendency of the phosphotungstic acid method to develop turbidity is obviated by the Archibald method, which substitutes polyanethol sodium sulfonate for the dangerous cyanide reagent [1, 2].

AUTOMATED COLORIMETRIC METHODS   Automated colorimetric methods of determining uric acid depend on the reduction of phosphotungstate or arsenotungstate or of a metal complex (e.g., cupric phenanthroline, neocuproine, or bathocuproine).

Most automated analyzer procedures work with dialysates and thus avoid the protein precipitation step. They appear to

Table 50-6   Observed and expected deaths in two groups of gouty patients

Source of patients	No. of patients	Total person-years*	Deaths	
			Occurred	Expected
Boston	54	948.5	23	24.5†
Buffalo VA Hospital	114	824	14	18.3‡

*From time of first observation until death or last observation.
† Expected on basis of age-specific death rates in 1947 for white males, United States.
‡ Expected on basis of age-specific death rates in 1952 for white males, United States.
SOURCE: From Talbott and Lilienfeld [124].

overestimate true urate by 0.4 to 1.0 mg/dl [128, 129]. The loose protein binding of urate may retard diffusion of urate and offset a tendency toward even higher readings based on nonspecificity of the colorimetric method.

The DuPont automatic clinical analyzer uses reduction of Cu(II)-2,2'-bicinchorinate chelate by uric acid. Falsely high values are noted in the presence of D,L-dopa, ampicillin, penicillin, methacillin, resorcinol, glutathione, and ascorbic acid [129].

Enzymatic Methods

URICASE DIFFERENTIAL SPECTROPHOTOMETRIC METHOD Uric acid has a characteristic ultraviolet absorption spectrum with a maximum at 292 nm and a molar absorption coefficient of 12,500 cm^2/mol at pH 9.4 [130]. In the presence of uricase, urate is converted to allantoin, which has no ultraviolet absorption at this wavelength. The resulting decrease in optical density at 292 nm provides a direct measure of the amount of uric acid present in the buffered assay mixture. This method, introduced by Kalckar and modified by Praetorius [131], is sensitive, accurate, and specific, and avoids errors inherent in colorimetric methods requiring precipitation of protein or involving some degree of nonspecificity in color development. The modification of Liddle et al. [132] avoids the need to plot graphically the fall in absorbance and introduces a biologic fluid blank to correct for changes in absorbance during the reaction due to substances other than uric acid. This modification facilitates the handling of numbers of samples with reasonable efficiency. It is the method of choice for research determinations.

MEASUREMENT OF HYDROGEN PEROXIDE FORMED The conversion of uric acid to allantoin, catalyzed by uricase, generates 1 mol of H_2O_2 for each mole of uric acid consumed. A number of modifications of the uricase method have been developed which are based on quantification of the H_2O_2 produced.

The underlying principle is that the reduction of hydrogen peroxide by either catalase (H_2O_2:H_2O_2 oxidoreductase, EC 1.11.1.6) or peroxidase (donor: H_2O_2 oxidoreductase, EC 1.11.1.7) is coupled to another oxidative reaction which yields a colored product. Thus, Kageyama [133] coupled catalase to the uricase reaction, oxidized methanol to formaldehyde, and measured colorimetrically the dihydrolutidine formed by condensation of formaldehyde with acetylacetone and ammonia:

$$Uric\ acid + 2H_2O + O_2 \xrightarrow{uricase} allantoin + CO_2 + H_2O_2$$

$$H_2O_2 + CH_3OH \xrightarrow{catalase} HCHO + 2H_2O$$

$$HCHO + acetylacetone + NH_3 \longrightarrow$$
$$3,5\text{-diacetyl-1,4-dihydrolutidine} + 3H_2O$$

A new method measures the formaldehyde yield in a centrifugal analyzer [134]. Sensitivity and precision were reported to be excellent. Several authors have coupled the uricase reaction with the hydrogen peroxide-peroxidase-catalyzed oxidation of a chromogen, such as O-dianisidine hydrochloride 3-methyl-2-benzothiazolinone hydrazone, and N,N-dimethylaniline, 2:4:6-tribromophenol and aminoantipyrine, 3,5-diacetyl-1,4-dihydrolutidine [2] or phenol and 4-aminophenazone [135]. Alternatively, the fluorescence of scopoletin may be abolished by oxidation with hydrogen peroxide in the presence of peroxidase [2]. Each of these modifications combines the specificity

of the uricase reaction with the simplicity of a colorimetric or fluorometric detection system.

Comparison of Methods

In a comparative survey of results of analysis of serum urate in clinical chemistry laboratories in the United Kingdom, Whitehead et al. [136] found that automated analyzer techniques gave more reproducible results than manual colorimetric methods, with the precision of manual uricase methods being intermediate.

Lum and Gambino [129] compared four methods for measuring uric acid over the range of 1 to 20 mg/100 ml. The DuPont automatic clinical analyzer, which measures uric acid by reduction of a copper chelate, gave values which averaged 13.06 mg/dl compared with an average value of 9.85 mg/dl by a manual uricase technique. An automated kinetic uricase method employing an enzyme from *Bacillus fastidiosus* gave an average result exactly the same as with the manual uricase method. The automated Archibald phosphotungstic acid method of Nishi [137] gave a mean value 0.79 mg/dl higher than the automated uricase procedure.

In a comparative study conducted at Duke Hospital serum samples were divided, one aliquot being analyzed by an automated method involving reduction of phosphotungstic acid and the other by a manual uricase-differential spectrophotometric method. The automated colorimetric method gave values that averaged 1 mg/dl higher than the uricase method at normal serum creatinine values. The range was 0 to 3.5 mg/dl higher, and the average difference increased slightly with rising serum creatinine values.

Normal Values

In plasma pH 7.4, about 98 percent of uric acid exists as the monoalkali salt. Human serum values vary with age and sex. In children, there is normally no sex difference in serum urate levels, which are lower than in adults, averaging about 3.6 mg/dl [138]. After puberty the levels rise in both sexes, but more in males. These differences have been attributed to higher renal clearances of urate in children than in adults and, among adults, in women than in men [2].

Sex- and age-specific mean serum urate values in nearly 6000 members of a healthy population in Tecumseh, Michigan [139], are shown in Fig. 50-14. Values in males reach a plateau in the early twenties and are essentially stable thereafter. Values in females are constant from age 20 to about age 40. With the menopause, the values rise further and approach [139, 140] or equal values in males.

The sex difference in urate levels in adults is found with all methods. The ratio of values in males to those in females averaged 1.19 in 11 published studies [2]. Figure 50-15 presents a good example of the distribution of serum urate values in the two sexes in a large healthy population. The values are distributed in bell-shaped curves with skewing towards higher levels. The curves are not bimodal, i.e., the curves for each sex do not separate the population into two distinct groups, one normal and one hyperuricemic. The serum urate concentration value is a continuous variable, much like height or blood pressure, and although the distribution is bell shaped, it is not gaussian [141]. Thus it is theoretically improper to define a normal

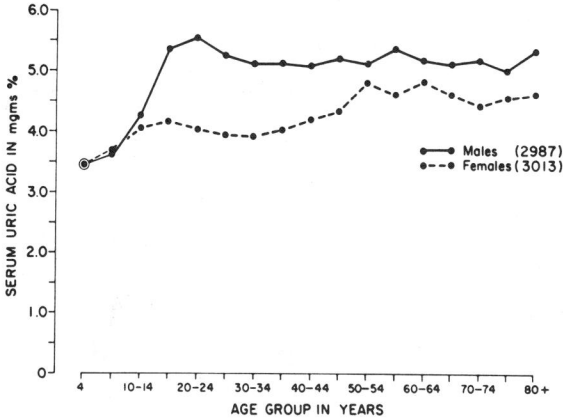

Figure 50-14 Sex- and age-specific mean serum urate values, determined with ultraviolet differential spectrophotometric (uricase) method, in the population of Tecumseh, Michigan, 1959 to 1960. (*From Mikkelsen et al. [139], with permission of* The American Journal of Medicine.)

range by statistical methods that assume parametric distribution. The upper limit of normal defined on the basis of the central 95 percent segment of the distribution (rather than the mean + 2 SD), is 7.3 mg/dl in postpubertal males and 5.9 mg/dl in postpubertal females [11] for a colorimetric method involving a protein precipitation step. With the enzymatic and spectrophotometric method, it ranges from 6.9 to 7.5 mg/dl in males and 5.7 to 6.6 in females in the United States and most of Europe (Table 50-7).

Ethnic Variations

The mean serum urate value is similar for American and European Caucasian men, North American Indians (Pima and Blackfeet of Arizona and the Haida of British Columbia), North American Negroes, Australians of European origin, full-blooded Hawaiians and national groups of Japanese, Chinese, Portuguese, and Caucasians living in Hawaii, and Filipinos living in the Philippines [2].

By contrast, other indigenous Pacific peoples have mean serum urate concentrations significantly higher than in Caucasian populations [2]. These include the Maoris of New Zealand and other Polynesians living in Rarotonga and Pukapuka in the Cook Islands and in American Samoa, two Micronesian groups in the Mariana and Western Caroline Islands (the Chamorros and Palauans), Micronesians on the Pacific island of Nauru [146], Japanese-Americans living in Hawaii [143], Filipinos living in Hawaii, Alaska, and other parts of the United States, Malaysians, and Chinese living in Malaysia but not those in Taiwan. In addition, mean serum urate values are higher in Australian aborigines and in Xavante Indians of Brazil than in Caucasians in the same regions.

No racial differences in serum urate values were observed between healthy Caucasians and Indians in India and Indonesia, but the mean values in both groups were lower than in most other studies.

Selected examples of ethnic variations in mean serum urate values are included in Table 50-7.

Association of Serum Urate Values with Other Variables

Anthropometric Factors Serum urate values show positive correlations with weight and with surface area in peoples of widely differing races and cultures throughout the world but exceptions exist among Hawaiians, Brazilian recruits, and a tribe of Australian aborigines, the Aurukun [2]. In epidemiologic studies body bulk (as estimated by body weight, surface area, or ponderal index) has proved to be one of the most important predictors of hyperuricemia [147].

Social Factors There is an association of serum urate values with "social class" or academic achievement (Table 50-7). Mean serum urate levels are higher in executives than in craftsmen [2]. They are also higher in Ph.D. scientists than in supervisors, and in supervisors than in craftsmen, at the Oak Ridge National Laboratory, and in medical than in high school students in Pittsburgh. Among university professors and Edinburgh business executives, urate levels showed a positive correlation with drive, achievement, range of activities, and leadership. Also, positive correlations exist between serum urate levels and Army aptitude test scores of inductees ($p = 0.03$), as well as between urate values and hemoglobin and serum protein values. The development of hyperuricemia in some Filipinos on moving to the United States has been ascribed to a change from a low purine, low protein diet to the typical American diet containing more meat.

Interaction of Hereditary and Environmental Factors Hyperuricemia is a continuously distributed variable and therefore unlikely to be determined by a simple Mendelian mechanism. The essentially unimodal curve suggests a characteristic of multiple and cumulative etiologies. As a biochemical trait, serum urate concentration would thus seem to fall in a category with cholesterol or glucose levels or even blood pressure, all biochemical traits which increasingly appear to have complex genetic backgrounds influenced in their manifestation

Figure 50-15 Distributions of serum urate values in the male and female populations of Tecumseh, Michigan, 1959 to 1960. Note skewness toward high values in both sexes. (*From Mikkelsen et al. [139], with permission of* The American Journal of Medicine.)

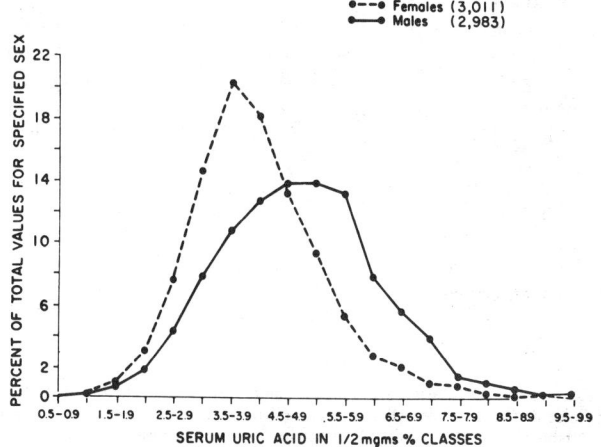

Table 50-7   Serum urate concentration values

Population, class, or group	Males			Females			Ref.*
	No.	Mean	SD	No.	Mean	SD	
Population							
Tecumseh, Mich.	2987	4.9	1.4	3013	4.2	1.2	
Framingham, Mass.†	2283	5.12	1.11	2844	4.00	0.94	
United States	22	5.32	0.93	18	4.32	0.81	
U.S. Army inductees	817	5.06	0.94				
U.S. prisoners (Caucasian)	90	5.01	1.11				
Denmark	150	5.10	1.19	150	4.00	0.94	
Finland	737	5.0	1.1	1048	4.0	1.0	
Wensleydale, England	436	4.46		475	3.70		
West Germany	265	4.86	1.32	119	4.05	1.29	
Australia (Caucasian)†	100	5.56	0.95	100	4.52	0.70	
France	23,923	5.88	1.19				
Thailand recruits (age 20)	710	4.96	0.90				
Thailand prisoners (ages 16–50)	300	4.74	0.97				
Florida, United States (ages ≧ 65)	634	6.35	1.41	1067	5.44	1.55	142
Quebec, Canada	558	5.80	1.32	633	4.74	1.10	144
England-Scotland	849	5.5	1.1	254	3.9	0.8	145
Social class							
Pittsburgh executives	339	5.73	1.21				
ORNL Ph.D. scientists	76	5.34	1.23				
U.S. craftsmen‡	532	4.77	1.13				
U.S. high school students	138	5.16					
University of Michigan professors	113	5.66	1.17				
Edinburgh executives	100	6.00	0.88				
Ethnic group							
American Negro	154	5.17					
North American Indians							
Pima	949§	4.89	1.19				
Blackfoot	1018§	4.22	1.19				
Haida	237	4.41	0.99				
Filipinos, in Seattle	118	6.29	1.29				
Subgroup I	92	5.80	0.89				
Subgroup II	26	8.07	0.89				
Filipinos in Hawaii	60	6.1	1.3				
Filipinos in Philippines	483	5.2	1.3				
Hawaiians (full bloods)	49	5.4	1.1				
Japanese-Americans in Hawaii	7971	5.99	1.51				143
Micronesians							
Chamorros							
California	164	6.4	1.4	151	4.9	1.3	
Guam	273	7.1	1.5	355	5.4	1.4	
Rota	122	7.2	1.4	149	5.4	1.2	
Palauans							
Koror	109	6.8	1.4	145	5.2	1.3	
Palelin	41	6.2	1.3	57	5.5	1.2	
Nger	69	6.7	1.3	89	4.9	1.4	
Polynesians							
Maori (New Zealand)	366	7.06	1.54	381	5.77	1.55	
Rarotongans	243	6.96	1.39	228	5.97	1.20	
Pukapukans	188	7.04	1.10	191	6.18	1.09	
Australian aborigines (Aurukan)	82	6.03	1.25	135	4.78	1.23	
Taiwan Chinese	247	4.99	0.91	120	3.87	0.78	
Malayan Chinese	298	6.11	1.29	106	4.52	0.98	
Malays	169	6.32	1.25	9	4.21	0.68	
Indians	141	3.60	0.70				

* Only references to new entries in this edition are given. Others may be found in Table 43-9 of the fourth edition of this text [2].
† Colorimetric methods. All other values determined by enzymatic spectrophotometric methods.
‡ Pittsburgh and ORNL (Oak Ridge National Laboratories).
§ Males and females about equally distributed in each group.

by multiple environmental factors. In commenting upon the associations of serum urate values with weight, surface area, obesity, intelligence, social status, achievement, hemoglobin, and serum proteins, Acheson and Chan [147] have expressed the situation well by stating, "The associates of a high uric acid are the associates of plenty."

Physical State of Urate in Plasma

The physiochemical state of urate in plasma has been a controversial subject for decades. Some early investigators claimed substantial binding of urate to nondiffusible elements of plasma, whereas others concluded that all urate was in true solution because it was readily ultrafiltrable and dialyzable [2].

In 1965 Alvsaker initiated a series of studies utilizing more sensitive techniques of gel filtration and immunoelectrophoresis which demonstrated reversible interactions between urate and four macromolecular components in human plasma. These components were albumin, low density β-lipoprotein, β_2-macroglobulins, and an α_1-α_2-globulin not identified with any known protein. Much of the binding was to albumin. The affinity of the α_1-α_2-globulin for urate was greater than that found with other proteins. It bound 33 times as much urate per milligram as albumin, but accounted for only about 0.4 mg/dl of urate in normal plasma [148]. The α_1-α_2 urate-binding globulin of plasma [149] is a glycoprotein of 67,000 M.W., with an isoelectric point of 4.6. It is the first human protein to be shown to contain ornithine [150].

The extent of urate binding to plasma proteins in vivo is uncertain. Widely varying percentages of bound urate have been described under different conditions of temperature, ionic strength, and buffer composition with native and delipidated protein [2]. Even with delipidated albumin, the association constant [151] is only 3.88×10^2 M^{-1} at 37°C, a value representing "binding" or "association" of little physiologic significance. Farrell et al. [152] found that workers who reported substantial binding had employed lithium urate, whereas those who reported low levels had used uric acid. In their own studies they found that 20 to 40 percent of added lithium urate was bound in 5 percent human serum albumin, and 35 to 55 percent in normal heparinized plasma at 37°C. By contrast the figures with uric acid were about 4 and 7 percent, respectively, under comparable conditions. In our laboratory a careful study of urate binding [153] discloses no more than 4 or 5 percent of urate bound to plasma protein, a figure agreeing with results of our earlier studies in vitro using equilibrium dialysis [2], as well as with more recent studies in vivo [154]. These studies confirm that the binding of uric acid to plasma proteins at 37°C is small and probably of little physiologic significance.

Alvsaker [148] described a reduced capacity of plasma from seven gouty patients to bind urate, which he attributed to a specific reduction in the plasma component which migrates as an α_1-α_2-globulin. This deficiency appeared to be inherited in an autosomal manner, and the patients exhibiting reduced levels were heterozygous for this defect [155]. Using equilibrium dialysis, Klinenberg and Kippen described reduced binding of urate in plasma proteins in 3 patients with severe tophaceous gout, although plasma from 17 other gouty subjects, including 3 with tophi, exhibited a normal urate-binding capacity. Bluestone and coworkers also reported that several drugs, including salicylates, phenylbutazone, sulfinpyrazone, and probene-

cid, reduce urate binding to plasma macromolecules in vitro. The relevance of these observations to the pathogenesis of gouty arthritis and the deposition of tophi remains to be established [2].

Definition and Significance of Hyperuricemia

Definitions of hyperuricemia based on distribution cutoffs encounter theoretical difficulties on several scores. These include (1) the asymmetry of the urate distributions, with skewness toward high values; (2) the bimodality of some frequency histograms, e.g., of Filipino males living in northwestern North America (Table 50-7); (3) the positive correlations of serum urate values with factors of plenty; and (4) possible racial differences.

A better definition of hyperuricemia is one based upon the limited solubility of sodium urate in extracellular body fluids. In extracellular fluid uric acid exists almost exclusively as monosodium urate. The solubility product of sodium urate in aqueous solution is 4.9×10^{-5}. On the basis of this value, aqueous solutions having the sodium content of serum, 0.13 M, are saturated with urate at 6.4 mg/dl at 37°C [156]. Allen et al. [157] and Loeb [32] have found that urate solubility in solutions of 140 meq/liter sodium content is 6.8 mg/dl. If one allows an additional 0.4 mg/dl for urate bound to the α_1-α_2-globulin, one may define the solubility limit of urate in plasma as about 7 mg/dl. Above this value, extracellular fluids are supersaturated with sodium urate, and the potentiality for precipitation of urate crystals exists. Supersaturated solutions of sodium urate are readily prepared in the laboratory. When plasma is subsequently incubated at 37°C, the concentration of uric acid falls as a result of the precipitation of crystals of monosodium urate monohydrate, and eventually plasma concentrations as low as 8.5 mg/dl are found.

The physiochemical definition of hyperuricemia is consistent with clinical experience. With the Folin method only 2 percent of 1190 determinations of serum urate values in 234 gouty patients in three laboratories were below 6 mg/dl [2]. Ninety-four percent of 177 serum analyses in 21 gouty patients exceeded 7 mg/dl. The prevalence of gout is high in ethnic groups whose mean serum uric acid values are above the American mean. The study of Seegmiller et al. [158] of the distribution of serum urate values of 940 nongouty males and 60 gouty males (Fig. 50-16), employing the enzymatic spectrophotometric method, shows an appreciable overlap of the distributions of values in nongouty and gouty subjects in the region of 6 to 7.5 mg/dl. Nine percent of gouty patients showed serum values below 7 mg/dl.

For purposes of population surveys, arbitrary normal limits of 7 mg/dl for males and 6 mg/dl for females have been suggested for the spectrophotometric method. In the Framingham study [11] 22 percent of the adult male population had serum urate levels of 6 mg/dl or more on a single determination, and 4.8 percent had levels of 7 mg/dl or more. If all determinations obtained over a 14-year period are considered, 9.3 percent had at least one value of 7 mg/dl or more. Diuretic therapy, renal disease, blood dyscrasia, or psoriasis accounted for no more than 3 percent of the hyperuricemic group. In the Tecumseh study [139] 6.42 percent of men had serum urate values greater than 7 mg/dl, and 6.27 percent of women had values greater than 6 mg/dl on a single determination.

The prevalence of hyperuricemia varies greatly among the

PER CENT

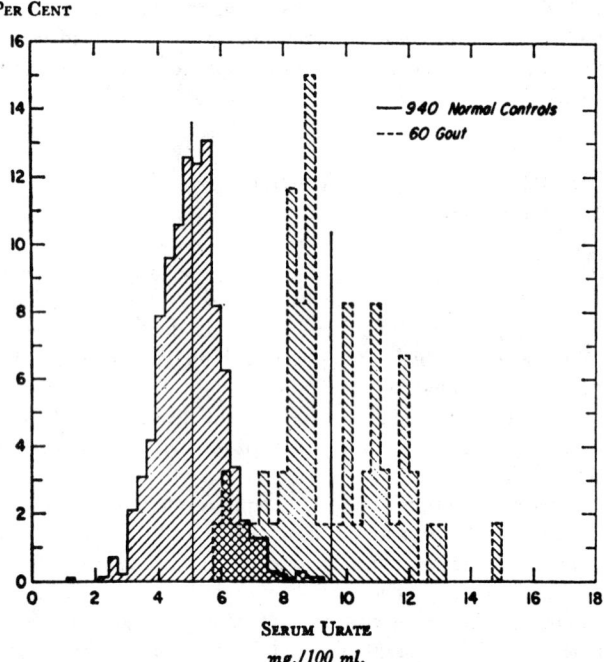

Figure 50-16 Distribution of serum urate values in a normal and gouty population. (*Reproduced from Seegmiller et al.* [*158*], *with permission of* The New England Journal of Medicine.)

peoples of the world. In Wensleydale, England, only 2.3 percent of serum urate values were 7 mg/dl or above in males or 6.0 mg/dl or above in females [159]. In a rural Finnish population, 5.2 percent of males and 1.2 percent of females had values of 7 mg/dl or above [160]. In France 17.6 percent of values in 23,923 men were 7 mg/dl or above [161]. By contrast, more than 40 percent of serum urate values of the New Zealand Maori, Rarotongans, and Pukapukans, three Polynesian groups, were 7 mg/dl or above in males and 6 mg/dl or above in females [110]. By these same definitions, more than 60 percent of men and women of the Micronesian island of Nauru are hyperuricemic [146].

In population studies the prevalences of gout, and of renal stones, are correlated with the height of the serum urate value in both males and females. Zalokar et al. [161], in a single-point survey of 4257 men of mean age 48.8 years in France, found prevalence rates for gout that increased from 4.7 percent in the group with serum urate values of 7 to 7.9 mg/dl, to 47.6 percent in the group with values over 10 mg/dl. The situation in the Framingham population admitted at mean age 44 and followed for 14 years is shown in Tables 50-2 and 50-5. In male subjects with serum urate values above 9 mg/dl at mean age 58, the prevalence of gout was 90 percent and of renal stones was 40 percent. The figures on the prevalence of stones at various serum urate levels in this population agree well with the prevalence values of stones in a large series of patients with gout in a referral practice [84].

Potential Pathophysiologic Mechanisms of Hyperuricemia

In theory, hyperuricemia could result from increased absorption of precursor purines or from increased plasma protein binding, increased production, decreased excretion, or decreased destruction of uric acid, or from some combination of these abnormalities.

A purine-free diet results in an average reduction of the serum urate level of 1 to 1.2 mg/dl in gouty subjects but, with rare exceptions, does not correct hyperuricemia [2]. Feeding of 4 g yeast RNA per day for 4 days results in comparable elevations of serum urate levels in nongouty [162] and gouty subjects [163]. Hyperuricemia has not been attributed to abnormal absorption of precursor purines.

There is considerable evidence that both increased production of uric acid and reduced renal clearance of uric acid play important roles in the pathogenesis of hyperuricemia in primary gout. This evidence will be considered in detail below.

Such uricolysis as occurs in humans [164] can be accounted for almost entirely by the action of intestinal flora upon uric acid entering the gastrointestinal tract in gastric, biliary, pancreatic, and intestinal secretions [165]. There is no evidence that extrarenal disposal of uric acid is diminished in gout; on the contrary, in gouty patients with reduced renal excretion of uric acid extrarenal disposal may constitute the chief route of disposal of urate. The topic of uricolysis will also be considered below, but first we will review the normal processes of synthesis and excretion of uric acid, and studies of these processes in patients with primary gout.

BIOCHEMISTRY OF PURINE COMPOUNDS

Biosynthesis of the Purine Ring

The origins of the individual atoms of the purine ring have been defined with labeled substrates in bacterial, avian, and mammalian systems [2]. Glycine contributes carbon atoms 4 and 5 and nitrogen atom 7. Carbon atoms 2 and 8 come from formate, carbon atom 6 comes from CO_2, nitrogen atoms 3 and 9 come from the amide-N of glutamine, and nitrogen atom 1 comes from aspartic acid (Fig. 50-17).

A key intermediate in the synthesis of purines is 5-phosphoribosyl-α-1-pyrophosphate (PP-ribose-P). This high-energy compound is involved in purine synthesis in two types of reactions: in one it is a substrate, together with L-glutamine, in the first specific reaction of purine synthesis *de novo* [166]; in the other it participates with purine bases in the direct synthesis of purine ribonucleotides by a condensation reaction with liberation of inorganic pyrophosphate [167]. PP-ribose-P is formed by transfer of the terminal pyrophosphate group of ATP to the carbon 1 of ribose-5-phosphate in a reaction catalyzed by PP-ribose-P synthetase [168].

$$\text{Ribose-5-phosphate} + \text{ATP} \xrightarrow{\text{Mg}^{2+}, \text{P}_i} \text{PP-ribose-P} + \text{AMP} \quad (1)$$

The first specific intermediate of purine synthesis *de novo* is 5-β-phosphoribosyl-1-amine [166]. In the reaction in which it is generated the α-pyrophosphate group of PP-ribose-P is displaced by the amide group of glutamine, and there is an inversion of the substituents to yield the β linkage characteristic of the glycosidic bond of all known ribonucleotides (Fig. 50-18).

$$\text{α-PP-ribose-P} + \text{glutamine} + \text{H}_2\text{O} \xrightarrow{\text{Mg}^{2+}} \text{β-phosphoribosylamine} + \text{glutamic acid} + \text{PP}_i \quad (2)$$

The reaction generating phosphoribosylamine is irreversible and is a potentially important reaction in the control of purine synthesis. The enzyme catalyzing this reaction, amidophospho-

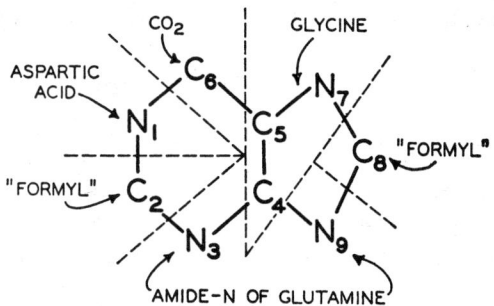

Figure 50-17 Origins of the atoms of the purine ring.

ribosyltransferase, will also function with ammonia in place of glutamine [169].

$$\alpha\text{-PP-ribose-P} + NH_3 \longrightarrow \beta\text{-phosphoribosylamine} + PP_i \quad (2a)$$

Mammalian mutant cells that lack amidophosphoribosyltransferase activity also lack aminophosphoribosyltransferase activity. Both reactions appear to be catalyzed by the same enzyme [170].

An alternative pathway for the synthesis of phosphoribosylamine by the direct reaction of ammonia with ribose-5-phosphate (R-5-P) was described in bacterial extracts by Nierlich and Magasanik [171].

$$Ribose\text{-5-P} + NH_3 + ATP \longrightarrow$$
$$\beta\text{-phosphoribosylamine} + PP_i + AMP \quad (2b)$$

There is also suggestive evidence for such a pathway in bacteria, in Ehrlich ascites cells, and in pigeon liver and white blood cell extracts [2]. Westby and Gots have described a *Sal-*

Figure 50-18 Biosynthesis of the purine ring. The encircled numbers in this figure and in Fig. 50-19 refer to numbered reactions in the text.

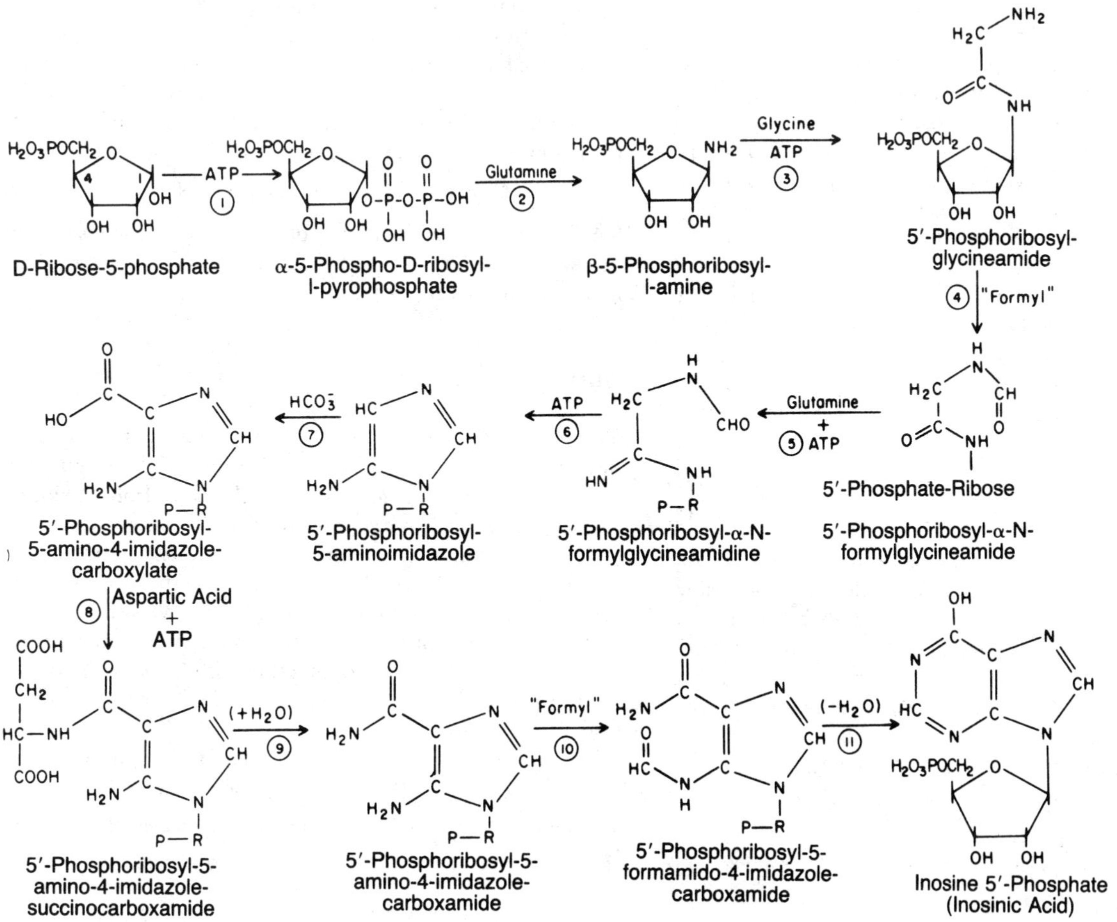

monella mutant that lacks any activity of amidophosphoribosyltransferase (pur F) and shows complete dependence upon exogenous purines for growth, even though activity of R-5-P aminotransferase is normal in lysates prepared from these mutants [172]. These results suggest that the R-5-P aminotransferase pathway does not operate in vivo.

The stepwise synthesis of the purine ring [2] is shown in Fig. 50-18. Phosphoribosylamine reacts with glycine to yield 5'-phosphoribosylglycineamide. ATP is involved as an energy source.

$$Phosphoribosylamine + glycine + ATP \xrightarrow{Mg^{2+}}$$
$$5'\text{-phosphoribosylglycineamide} + ADP + P_i \quad (3)$$

Thus at this early stage the fundamental components of the eventual polynucleotide structure of nucleic acids are already joined, and a combination of base, sugar, and phosphoric acid has been made.

Phosphoribosylglycineamide receives a one-carbon "formyl" unit from N^5,N^{10}-methenyl tetrahydrofolic acid.

$$Phosphoribosylglycineamide + N^5,N^{10}\text{-methenyl-THFA}$$
$$+ H_2O \longrightarrow 5'\text{-phosphoribosyl-}\alpha\text{-}N\text{-formylglycineamide}$$
$$+ THFA + H^+ \quad (4)$$

The formyl derivative then receives the amide group of glutamine to form the corresponding amidine compound, following which ring closure forms the five-membered imidazole ring. Each of these reactions requires ATP as an energy source and magnesium. Ring-closure requires potassium as well.

$$5'\text{-Phosphoribosylformylglycineamide} + glutamine + ATP +$$
$$H_2O \xrightarrow{Mg^{2+}} 5'\text{-phosphoribosyl-}\alpha\text{-}N\text{-formylglycineamidine} +$$
$$glutamic\ acid + ADP + P_i \quad (5)$$

5′-Phosphoribosyl-α-N-formylglycineamidine + ATP $\xrightarrow{Mg^{2+} K^+}$

$$\text{5′phosphoribosyl-5-aminoimidazole + ADP + P}_i \quad (6)$$

5′-Phosphoribosyl-5-aminoimidazole now receives a carboxyl group at C-4 by a reversible CO_2-fixation reaction which requires a high concentration of bicarbonate. The carboxyl serves as a point for the condensation of this intermediate with aspartic acid through an amide linkage involving another ATP as the source of energy. Hydrolysis of the intermediate yields a compound lacking only carbon atom 2 of a complete purine ribonucleotide.

5′-Phosphoribosylaminoimidazole + CO_2 $\rightleftharpoons$

$$\text{5′-phosphoribosyl-5-amino-4-imidazole carboxylate} \quad (7)$$

5′-Phosphoribosyl-5-amino-4-imidazole carboxylate +

aspartate + ATP $\xrightarrow{Mg^{2+}}$

5′-phosphoribosyl-5-amino-4-imidazolesuccinocarboxamide +

$$\text{ADP + P}_i \quad (8)$$

5′-Phosphoribosyl-5-amino-4-imidazolesuccinocarboxamide $\rightleftharpoons$

fumarate + 5′-phosphoribosyl-5-amino-4-imidazolecarboxamide (9)

5′-Phosphoribosyl-5-amino-4-imidazolecarboxamide receives a formyl group from a N^{10}-formyl-THFA, and ring closure completes the biosynthesis of the purine structure by forming inosine-5′-monophosphate (IMP).

5′-Phosphoribosyl-5-amino-4-imidazolecarboxamide +

N^{10}-formyl-THFA $\rightleftharpoons$

5′-phosphoribosyl-5-formamido-4-imidazolecarboxamide + THFA

$$(10)$$

5′-Phosphoribosyl-5-formamido-4-imidazolecarboxamide $\rightleftharpoons$

$$\text{IMP + H}_2O \quad (11)$$

Biosynthesis of AMP and GMP

IMP may be considered the parent purine compound. It is an intermediate in the formation of adenosine-5′-monophosphate (AMP) and guanosine-5′-monophosphate (GMP), the purine nucleotide components of nucleic acids (Fig. 50-19). The conversion of IMP to AMP occurs in two steps [2], involving an initial condensation of IMP with aspartic acid to form adenylosuccinic acid (AMP-S). Energy for this reaction is derived from guanosine triphosphate. Cleavage of AMP-S yields AMP and fumaric acid. This latter reaction is freely reversible. This reaction is analogous to the cleavage of SAICAR (reaction 9) and is probably catalyzed by the same enzyme, adenylosuccinase. Mutant strains of microorganisms and mammalian cells that lack the ability to catalyze one reaction cannot catalyze the other.

$$\text{IMP + L-aspartate + GTP} \xrightarrow{Mg^{2+}} \text{AMP-S + GDP + P}_i \quad (12)$$

$$\text{AMP-S} \rightleftharpoons \text{AMP + fumarate} \quad (13)$$

The conversion of IMP to GMP also occurs in two steps [2]: the first is the irreversible oxidation of IMP to xanthosine-5′-monophosphate (XMP), with nicotinamide adenine dinucleotide (NAD) as hydrogen acceptor; the second is the amination of XMP at the 2 position, and the specific amino donor of the reaction is the amide group of glutamine. The second step requires ATP as the source of energy. These reactions proceed according to the following overall schemes:

$$\text{IMP + NAD}^+ + \text{H}_2O \xrightarrow{K^+} \text{XMP + NADH + H}^+ \quad (14)$$

XMP + glutamine + ATP $\xrightarrow{Mg^{2+}}$

$$\text{GMP + glutamic acid + AMP + PP}_i \quad (15)$$

Nucleotide Interconversions and Catabolism

AMP may be deaminated to IMP by a specific AMP deaminase:

$$\text{AMP} \longrightarrow \text{IMP + NH}_3 \quad (20)$$

Mononucleotides may be split by 5′-nucleotidases, as well as by nonspecific phosphatases to yield nucleosides.

$$\text{Purine mononucleotide + H}_2O \longrightarrow \text{purine nucleoside + P}_i \quad (19)$$

Microsomal 5′-nucleotidase shows greater activity with AMP than with IMP or GMP [2]. Cytoplasmic 5′-nucleotidases are much more active against IMP and GMP than AMP [173, 174]. AMP catabolism appears to be by deamination to IMP rather than by cleavage to adenosine [175]. The chief source of adenosine is probably the cleavage of S-adenosylhomocysteine, a by-product of methylation reactions, to adenosine and homocysteine [176].

Adenosine is deaminated by adenosine deaminase to yield inosine:

$$\text{Adenosine + H}_2O \longrightarrow \text{inosine + NH}_3 \quad (21)$$

Adenosine may also be reconverted to AMP in a reaction catalyzed by adenosine kinase:

$$\text{Adenosine + ATP} \longrightarrow \text{AMP + ADP} \quad (18)$$

Purine nucleosides are split phosphorolytically to yield a free purine base plus ribose-1-phosphate:

$$\text{Purine nucleoside + P}_i \longrightarrow \text{purine base + ribose-1-P} \quad (17)$$

Erythrocyte purine nucleoside phosphorylase is active with inosine, guanosine, and to a lesser extent with xanthosine, but it does not cleave adenosine [177]. Hepatic purine nucleoside phosphorylase will cleave adenosine [178]. With inosine the equilibrium of this reaction lies far toward the nucleoside.

The free bases formed from these reactions are chiefly hypoxanthine and guanine. Small amounts of xanthine may be formed from XMP via xanthosine, but xanthine arises chiefly by action of guanase upon guanine:

$$\text{Guanase + H}_2O \longrightarrow \text{xanthine + NH}_3 \quad (22)$$

Small amounts of adenine may be formed from adenosine, but its chief precursor is 5′-methyl thioadenosine, an intermediate in spermidine synthesis [176].

Salvage Pathways

Two general mechanisms exist for the synthesis of ribonucleotides from purine bases or ribonucleosides which result from the catabolism of endogenous ribonucleotides, from the ingestion of purine-containing foods, or from the administration of purine compounds. These involve phosphoribosyltransferase reactions in which free bases condense with PP-ribose-P to form ribonucleotides in one step, or phosphorylase reactions in which free bases react with ribose-1-phosphate to form ribonucleosides, operating in conjunction with kinase reactions in which ribonucleosides are phosphorylated to form ribonucleotides.

The phosphoribosyltransferase reaction has the following general form:

$$\text{Base + PP-ribose-P} \rightleftharpoons \text{base-ribose-phosphate + PP}_i \quad (16)$$

This reaction is responsible for the conversion of purines,

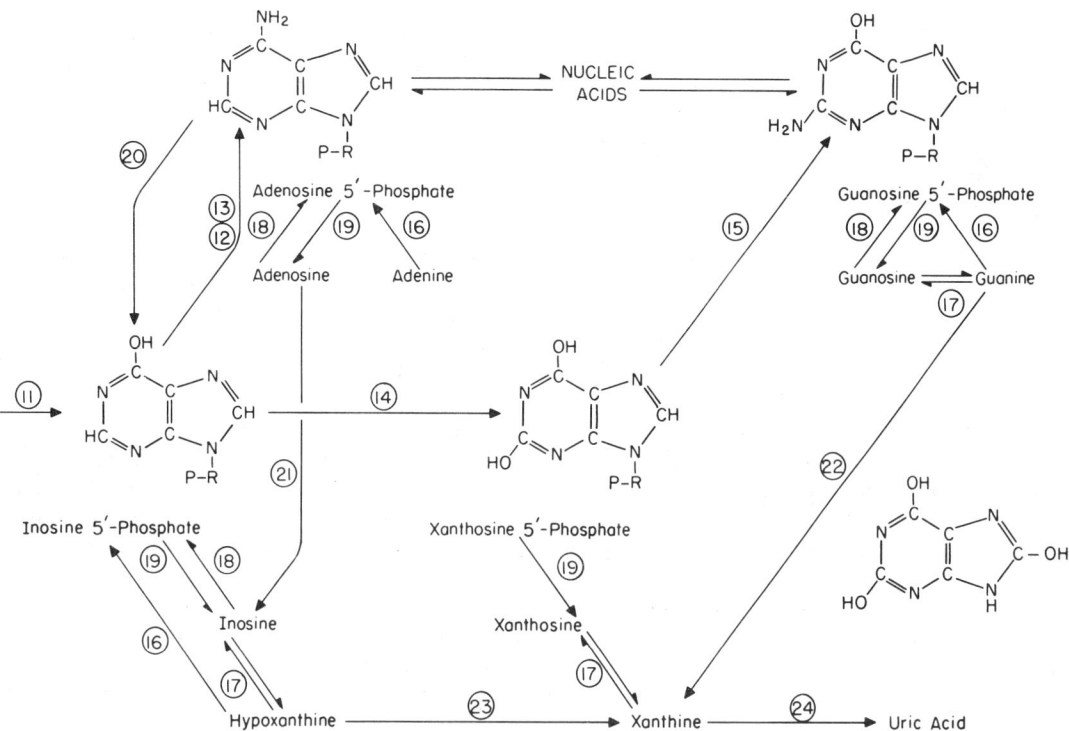

Figure 50-19 Biosynthesis of purine ribonucleotides, ribonucleosides, and bases.

pyrimidines, nicotinamide, and certain other nitrogenous bases to their respective ribonucleotides. Two different purine phosphoribosyltransferases have been identified. Adenine phosphoribosyltransferase (APRT) (EC 2.4.2.7) acts upon AIC and adenine [167] and will also accept adenine analogues such as 2,6-diaminopurine and 8-azadenine [2]. Hypoxanthine-guanine phosphoribosyltransferase (HPRT) (EC 2.4.2.8) acts upon hypoxanthine and guanine and upon xanthine but at only about 0.3 percent of the rate of the reaction with hypoxanthine or guanine [180]. HPRT will also catalyze the conversion of 6-thiopurine, 6-thioguanine, 8-azaguanine, allopurinol [181], and probably oxipurinol to their respective ribonucleotides. The K_{eq} of both phosphoribosyltransferases is far toward the ribonucleotide; a value of 290 has been estimated for APRT [182]. Deficiency states of both phosphoribosyltransferases have been described. APRT is discussed more fully in Chap. 52, HPRT in Chap. 51. Deficiency of purine nucleoside phosphorylase is discussed in Chap. 53.

The two-step pathway has the following form:

$$\text{Base} + \text{ribose-1-phosphate} \rightleftharpoons \text{base-ribose} + \text{P}_i \quad (17)$$

$$\text{Base-ribose} + \text{ATP} \longrightarrow \text{base-ribose-phosphate} + \text{ADP} \quad (18)$$

Studies in subjects who lack activity of HPRT, and of their cells in culture, indicate that the phosphoribosyltransferases are normally responsible for extensive recycling of purine bases into nucleotide pools. By contrast, recycling of hypoxanthine and guanine via the nucleoside phosphorylase-nucleoside kinase route is not very active. Kinases capable of phosphorylating inosine or guanosine have been described in animal tissues [183], and labeled inosine is incorporated into adenine and guanine nucleotides in liver of both normal and HPRT-deficient subjects [184]. These kinases appear to be absent in human fibroblasts [185]. Normally the action of purine nucleoside phosphorylase upon inosine or guanosine is probably largely degradative. The situation with adenosine is different.

Adenosine kinase is an active enzyme with an extensive distribution in mammalian tissues.

By either of these salvage pathways only one high energy bond, in the form of PP-ribose-P or ATP, is expended in the synthesis of a ribonucleotide, whereas synthesis of AMP or GMP *de novo* from glutamine and PP-ribose-P requires the expenditure of a minimum of six high energy bonds.

Formation of Uric Acid

Hypoxanthine is oxidized by xanthine oxidase to yield xanthine (reaction 23), which in turn is further oxidized by the same enzyme to yield uric acid (reaction 24) [186]. In humans, xanthine oxidase is found in high activity only in liver and small intestinal mucosa. Traces of activity are found in heart and skeletal muscle, kidney, and spleen, none in leukocytes, erythrocytes, stratum corneum, or fibroblasts in tissue culture. The enzyme is a flavoprotein containing iron and molybdenum, capable of oxidizing a wide variety of purines, aldehydes, and pteridines (see Chap. 55).

Because of the restricted distribution of xanthine oxidase and its great activity in liver, uric acid synthesis appears largely to be a hepatic process in humans. Presumably purine degradation products of other tissues are transported to the liver for further oxidation. Since human tissue does not contain uricase, uric acid is normally the end product of human purine metabolism. In bacterial systems free adenine is deaminated to form hypoxanthine, but mammalian tissues lack adenase activity. If adenine is not reconverted to its nucleoside or nucleotide, it may be excreted unchanged; normal human subjects excrete adenine in small quantities in urine [187]. When its concentration is raised, as in patients with adenine phosphoribosyltransferase deficiency (see Chap. 52), adenine is oxidized to 2,8-dioxyadenine by xanthine oxidase [188]. Hereditary deficiency of xanthine oxidase results in replacement of uric acid by xanthine (xanthinuria) and hypoxanthine as end products of purine metabolism. Xanthine oxidase and xanthinuria are discussed in Chap. 55.

Uric Acid Ribonucleoside Since the discovery of uric acid ribonucleoside in beef erythrocytes [189] and liver [190], the possibility has been entertained that this nucleoside is an intermediate of an alternative pathway of uric acid synthesis. Its existence in human erythrocytes has been claimed and denied [191]. Although Falconer and Gulland [190] originally concluded that the beef compound was a 9-N-ribosyl derivative, spectral studies [192] indicate that the ribosyl group is attached to the N3 position of uric acid [191]. This structure has been confirmed by synthesis. The ribonucleoside is cleaved to uric acid and ribose-1-phosphate by a phosphorylase found in several species. The ribonucleoside is formed from uric acid ribonucleotide [3-N-(5'-phosphoribosyl)uric acid], which is formed by a direct condensation of uric acid and PP-ribose-P [193] in a reaction catalyzed by orotate phosphoribosyltransferase (see Chap. 56). Therefore, the pathway does not result in net synthesis of uric acid. Small amounts of the ribonucleotide exist in beef erythrocytes. In addition, a phosphoribosyltransferase derived from *Lactobacillus plantarus* forms a 9-N-(5'-phosphoribosyl) uric acid [194]. 9-N-Ribosyluric acid has been identified in the urine of a patient deficient in purine nucleoside phosphorylase [195], and so presumably 9-N(5'-phosphoribosyl)uric acid is also formed in humans.

Economy of Purine Biosynthesis in the Mammal

Purine biosynthesis *de novo* is especially active in liver. All enzymes of purine biosynthesis, nucleotide interconversion, degradation, and base salvage are found in the soluble portion of the cell, except for uricase which, when present, is particulate and is found in lysosomes. Uricase is not present in birds, higher apes, and humans.

Nonhepatic tissues other than placenta appear capable of only limited synthesis of purines *de novo*. The mature erythrocyte actively synthesizes PP-ribose-P and purine ribonucleotides from free bases via phosphoribosyltransferase reactions, but it cannot synthesize phosphoribosylamine. Therefore, it is incapable of purine synthesis *de novo*. Reactions beyond 5'-phosphoribosyl-5-amino-4-imidazole-carboxamide are active in the erythrocyte, including those of nucleotide interconversion.

Data of Lajtha and Vane [196] suggest that nonhepatic tissues, e.g., bone marrow, are dependent upon an advanced purine precursor originating in liver as a source of nucleic acid purine bases. Mager and associates [197] assigned this function to ATP synthesized in liver and delivered to distant tissues by the erythrocyte.

Lerner and Lowy [198] examined this process in detail, by means of isotopic labeling of purine compounds of rat liver and subsequent perfusion of the liver with media or with rat or human red blood cells. The immediate hepatic product taken up by the erythrocyte appears to be adenosine. The red blood cell membrane contains adenosine kinase, and so the transported compounds are probably adenyl ribonucleotides. This process is reversed in peripheral tissues, adenosine being released from the erythrocytes to tissues capable of synthesis of ATP.

The critical role of phosphoribosyltransferase pathways in nonhepatic tissues is thus clear. In the presence of a limited capacity for purine synthesis *de novo*, and partial dependence upon purine imports, recovery of purine bases generated by catabolic reactions becomes a function of major importance to the cell. Because of the restricted distribution in humans of catabolic enzymes capable of acting upon free purines, those bases generated in nonhepatic or nonintestinal tissue are largely protected from catabolism and are available for recycling, unless lost from the cell and transported to the liver.

Catabolism of Ingested Nucleoproteins

Nucleic acids of dietary nucleoproteins are liberated in the intestinal canal by the action of proteolytic enzymes. Nucleic acids are degraded to nucleotides by nucleases and phosphodiesterases secreted by the pancreas. The nucleotides are chiefly hydrolyzed to nucleosides by various nucleotidases and phosphatases. The nucleosides may be absorbed intact, or they may be cleaved phosphorolytically to free bases. The small intestinal mucosa of humans is rich in nucleoside phosphorylase and xanthine oxidase, and ingested nucleoprotein purines may potentially be converted to uric acid in the gastrointestinal mucosa. The uric acid may be absorbed, or it may be further catabolized by intestinal bacteria. From experiments in which normal and gouty subjects ingested ^{15}N-labeled nucleic acid [199], it appeared that the purine moieties were converted to uric acid largely by direct routes without prior incorporation into body nucleic acids. However, small quantities of dietary nucleosides and even nucleotides may also be utilized directly for the synthesis of nucleic acids [200].

REGULATION OF PURINE BIOSYNTHESIS

Rate-determining Step

A number of arguments [2] collectively suggest that the first committed reaction, that in which L-glutamine and 5-phosphoribosyl-l-pyrophosphate form 5-phosphoribosyl-l-amine, is rate-determining for the entire sequence: (1) Phosphoribosylamine is the first specific purine precursor, and no branching of the succeeding pathway occurs prior to the synthesis of inosinic acid. (2) No intermediates of the *de novo* pathway accumulate unless a genetic or chemical block of a reaction is introduced, e.g., in bacteria or in tissue culture of surviving mammalian cells. (3) The activity of the first enzyme is regulated by purine ribonucleotides, but that of the second enzyme is not, and no functional inhibition is observed in the portion of the sequence from 5'-phosphoribosylglycineamide to inosine monophosphate (IMP) [201]. Although inhibition of the amidation of 5'-phosphoribosylformylglycineamide by AMP and GMP can be demonstrated with the isolated enzyme, the required concentrations of inhibitor ribonucleotides are unphysiologically high. (4) Bacterial purine auxotrophs grown on limiting concentrations of purines show derepression of synthesis of the first enzyme as well as of five others concerned with purine synthesis *de novo* [202]. (5) Measures which raise intracellular concentrations of PP-ribose-P accelerate purine biosynthesis; measures which lower PP-ribose-P concentrations reduce the rate of purine biosynthesis [203–205]. (6) The availability of glutamine can be rate-limiting for purine synthesis under certain circumstances [206].

As will be presented below, PP-ribose-P activates amidophosphoribosyltransferase, the enzyme that catalyzes the first reaction of purine biosynthesis, as well as serving as a substrate of that reaction. Thus its synthesis, and its concentration, secondarily control amidotransferase activity. The interrelationships of controls of PP-ribose-P synthetase and amidophosphoribosyltransferase will be examined in detail below. First we will discuss the individual enzymes, their substrates, and their regulators.

Phosphoribosylpyrophosphate Synthetase

PROPERTIES OF THE ENZYME   PP-ribose-P synthetase from all sources studied has an absolute requirement for inorganic phosphate, which acts as an allosteric activator. The apparent Michaelis constant of Ehrlich ascites cell enzyme for inorganic phosphate is 3.3 mM [207]. Removal of phosphate leads to immediate and complete loss of enzyme activity [208]. In Sperling's view, the rate of PP-ribose-P synthesis in liver is largely regulated by inorganic phosphate [209]. The enzyme also requires magnesium or manganese. With purified human PP-ribose-P synthetase the K_m value for ribose-5-phosphate is $3.3 \times 10^{-5}M$, and for magnesium ATP is $1.4 \times 10^{-5}M$ [208].

The smallest native form of enzyme from human erythrocytes [210] has a molecular weight of 60,000 and consists of two subunits of equal molecular weight. In the presence of saturating concentrations of ATP and magnesium chloride, the enzyme associates into two heavy forms with molecular weights of about 720,000 and 1.2 million. Ribose-5-phosphate does not alter the aggregation state of the enzyme. The associated enzyme appears to be the active form. Inhibition by ADP does not affect the state of molecular aggregation. Known intracellular concentrations of magnesium and ATP indicate that the enzyme probably exists in an aggregated state within the cell. In addition to the heterogeneity of molecular size, human PP-ribose-P synthetase exhibits striking electrophoretic heterogeneity. Electrophoretic variants of the erythrocyte enzyme were found in 2.5 percent of 200 subjects. In addition, human organs obtained at autopsy disclosed a unique electrophoretic mobility for nearly each organ of the same individual. These variants are postulated to represent posttranscriptional modifications of the enzyme [211].

The gene for PP-ribose-P synthetase is X-linked [212]. Several different mutations of PP-ribose-P synthetase have been described in gouty subjects, all resulting in increased rates of synthesis of PP-ribose-P. These are described below.

REGULATION OF ENZYME ACTIVITY   PP-ribose-P synthetase activity is dependent not only on concentrations of substrates and modifiers but also on concentrations of a number of end products of pathways for which PP-ribose-P is an essential substrate. From detailed analysis of enzymes from several sources, it is concluded that inhibitors interact at three different sites. Inhibition by ADP is competitive with respect to magnesium ATP. The K_i for ADP of 0.01 mM is well below its intracellular concentration in most mammalian tissues [208]. ADP changes the substrate-velocity plot from a hyperbolic to a sigmoidal function with increasing concentrations of inorganic phosphate [213].

PP-ribose-P and 2,3-diphosphoglycerate (2,3-DPG) both inhibit the enzyme competitively with respect to ribose 5-phosphate [208]. It seems unlikely that PP-ribose-P is an important inhibitor of its own synthesis under normal conditions since the K_i for PP-ribose-P, which is 0.05 mM, is approximately 10 times higher than its concentration in human cells [214]. However, the K_i of the enzyme for 2,3-DPG is approximately equal (5.3 mM) to its concentration in some tissues such as human erythrocytes. Therefore, 2,3-DPG may participate in the control of PP-ribose-P synthesis.

A large number of nucleotides, including AMP, ADP, GDP, GTP, IDP, ITP, TDP, NAD, NADPH, and FAD, inhibit PP-ribose-P synthetase by a third mechanism which is noncompetitive with respect to both magnesium ATP and ribose 5-phosphate [208, 215]. In general terms the di- and triphosphate derivatives are more potent inhibitors than the monophosphates. This group of inhibitors has a low affinity for the enzyme, presumably binds at a single site, and regulates by a mechanism called *heterogeneous metabolic pool inhibition.* This term means that the degree of inhibition depends on total nucleotide concentration and is largely independent of specific nucleotide composition. K_i values are high, and pairs of inhibitors do not act synergistically. Total inhibition of PP-ribose-P synthetase requires unphysiologically high concentrations of nucleotides. The relationships of these potential controls to those of the succeeding reaction are shown in Fig. 50-20.

Atkinson [216] postulates that the activity of a biosynthetic reaction is controlled by the "energy charge" of the cell, as well as by feedback inhibition:

$$\text{"Energy charge"} = \frac{\text{ATP} + \frac{1}{2}\,\text{ADP}}{\text{ATP} + \text{ADP} + \text{AMP}}$$

This concept predicts that the synthesis of PP-ribose-P will be inhibited by nucleoside diphosphates and monophosphates, irrespective of specific feedback effects.

α-PHOSPHORIBOSYL-1-PYROPHOSPHATE   Steady state levels of PP-ribose-P will be determined by the balance achieved between rates of production and of utilization. Data on intracellular concentrations of PP-ribose-P are fragmentary. Values in normal human erythrocytes range from 1.3 to 6.5 nmol/ml (approximately 0.002 to 0.007 mM) [204, 217, 218]. In normal human fibroblasts in culture they range up to 0.013 mM [219]. In mouse liver, Lalanne and Henderson [220] found basal fasting values of PP-ribose-P of about 50 nmol/g protein, equivalent to about 0.015 mM in liver water. In these studies liver was removed and then frozen. When liver is frozen *in situ* in anesthetized mice, hepatic PP-ribose-P concentrations of about 700 nmol/g protein are found, equivalent to 0.21 mM in cell water. These values are about equal to the K_m value of amidophosphoribosyltransferase for PP-ribose-P. These values increase 2.3 times 30 min following fructose infusion [221].

Figure 50-20   Feedback controls of sequential reactions of purine biosynthesis, catalyzed by PP-ribose-P synthetase and amidophosphoribosyltransferase. The first enzyme has at least three regulatory sites, the second at least two, as described in the text.

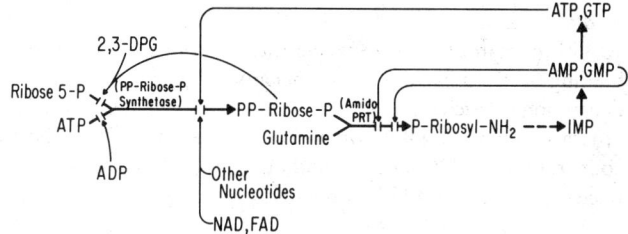

The mechanism is suggested to involve release of inhibition of PP-ribose-P synthetase, secondary to depletion of adenylnucleotides (including ADP, an inhibitor of PP-ribose-P synthetase) by fructose.

Lalanne and Henderson [220] found a twofold diurnal variation in hepatic PP-ribose-P levels in mouse liver, maximal values being reached at the seventh hour of a 14-h feeding period. Insulin, epinephrine, glucagon, tolbutamide, 2-deoxyglucose, and 2-ethylamino-1,3,4-thiadiazole (EA-TDA) all caused twofold or greater elevations of PP-ribose-P concentrations within 15 to 45 min. Greatest increases were caused by EA-TDA which in doses of 400 mg/kg led to a tenfold increase within 30 min to values of over 800 nmol/g protein.

Sperling et al. [222] have reported an increased availability of PP-ribose-P, which correlated with enhanced purine biosynthesis de novo, in immature leukemic granulocytes.

Methylene blue will raise the intracellular concentration of PP-ribose-P in Ehrlich ascites cells in vitro, in human fibroblasts in tissue culture, and in human erythrocytes in vitro [2], presumably by accelerating the regeneration of NADP in the oxidative pathway of glucose metabolism and thereby stimulating the rate of production of ribose-5-phosphate. Purine biosynthesis de novo is enhanced. In addition, ethanol has been shown to raise PP-ribose-P concentrations in isolated mouse hepatic cells [223].

PP-ribose-P concentration values are elevated in cells with deficient hypoxanthine-guanine phosphoribosyltransferase activity [224]. HPRT-deficient fibroblasts show accelerated rates of purine biosynthesis. Intracellular PP-ribose-P concentrations may be reduced by stimulating PP-ribose-P consumption with allopurinol, orotic acid, adenine, or 2,6-diaminopurine [2]. Such measures reduce the rate of purine biosynthesis de novo, except in HPRT-deficient cells which have a surfeit of PP-ribose-P.

Amidophosphoribosyltransferase

PROPERTIES OF THE ENZYME   This enzyme has been studied in bacteria, yeast, mammalian and avian liver [225], and in several human tissues [226–229]. PP-ribose-P is a specific substrate and cannot be replaced by α-D-ribofuranosyl-1,5-diphosphate, ribose-5-phosphate, or ribose-5-phosphate plus ATP [169]. In place of glutamine the enzyme will accept NH_3 and certain other amines [169].

The K_m for PP-ribose-P is 0.06 to 0.30 mM in pigeon liver [230, 231], 0.25 mM in human lymphoblasts [228], and 0.48 mM in human placenta [226]. The enzyme has an absolute requirement for a divalent cation, of which the most effective is magnesium. The K_m for glutamine ranges from 0.53 to 1.5 mM in rat liver [232]. The K_m of the human enzyme for glutamine is 1.0 to 4.5 mM [232]. The K_m for NH_3 is 2.0 to 3.8 mM with human lymphocytes [229] and placental enzymes [233]. With avian and placental enzyme, PP-ribose-P is bound first and produces a conformational change in the enzyme prior to binding of glutamine [225, 226]. The reaction is irreversible, and there is no evidence for an enzyme-bound intermediate [225].

With human placental enzyme there is cooperativity in the binding of PP-ribose-P. Hill coefficients range from 1.1 to 3.0, depending on the concentration of inorganic phosphate [232]. P_i is a competitive inhibitor of PP-ribose-P [226], it reduces cooperativity in PP-ribose-P binding [234], and it potentiates nucleotide inhibition [226] (see below). There is no coopera-

tivity of glutamine binding, but binding of NH_3 shows a Hill coefficient of 1.5 [233].

The glutamine site of human amidophosphoribosyltransferase is distinct from the NH_3 site, since glutamine utilization can be eliminated by covalent binding of the glutamine analogues azaserine and 6-diazo-5-oxo-L-norleucine (DON) without reduction in NH_3 utilization [233]. Although the sites are distinct, they apparently interact since binding of DON to the glutamine site eliminates the cooperativity in NH_3 binding.

The enzymes from Bacillus subtilis [235], Chinese hamster fibroblasts [236], murine erythroleukemia cells [232], and human placenta [237] are all extremely labile in vitro because of oxygen sensitivity. The enzyme from B. subtilis [235] is an iron-sulfur protein with a tetranuclear center (4Fe-4S) of the reduced high potential type [238]. Oxidation of the iron-sulfur center by oxygen is correlated with loss of catalytic activity [235]. Preliminary results suggest that human amidophosphoribosyltransferase has similar properties [232]. Ligands such as PP-ribose-P and purine nucleotides protect the enzyme from inactivation by oxygen.

REGULATION OF ENZYME ACTIVITY   Amidophosphoribosyltransferase is allosterically inhibited by purine ribonucleotide end products of the pathway. The first demonstration was that pigeon liver enzyme is inhibited by purine 5'-ribonucleotides but not by purine 2'- or 3'-ribonucleotides, 5'-deoxyribonucleotides, ribonucleosides, or free bases, nor by pyrimidine compounds [230]. The human enzyme shows similar sensitivities but is also inhibited by certain pyrimidine nucleotides at relatively high concentrations [226]. With enzyme from all sources effective ribonucleotides produce 100 percent inhibition at suitable concentrations. The inhibition is formally competitive with respect to PP-ribose-P; nevertheless, the enzyme may be totally desensitized to action of nucleotide inhibitors, while retaining catalytic activity [231, 239]. These results prove that inhibitors bind at regulatory sites that are distinct from binding sites of substrates.

Amidophosphoribosyltransferases from human placenta [226, 227], human lymphoblasts [228], pigeon liver [230], rat liver [231], and Aerobacter aerogenes [240] are inhibited equally well by adenyl and guanyl ribonucleotides. The enzyme from Schizosaccharomyces pombe [241] and the mouse spleen enzyme induced by Friend leukemia virus [242] are less sensitive to inhibition by AMP than by GMP. By contrast, enzyme from bakers' yeast [243] appears to be less sensitive to GMP than to AMP or ADP. Effectiveness of inhibitors of the human enzyme is in the order monophosphates > diphosphates > triphosphates [226].

With amidophosphoribosyltransferases from pigeon liver [231], A. aerogenes [240], S. pombe [241], human placenta [226], and L1210 cells [244] inhibitions by mixtures of ribonucleotides with the same substituent at position 6 are additive, whereas combinations of 6-amino- and 6-hydroxypurine ribonucleotides inhibit synergistically. Such pairs as AMP plus GMP or AMP plus IMP, which are unlike at position 6, produce inhibitions that significantly exceed predicted additive effects. The synergistic inhibition by mixtures of 6-amino- and 6-hydroxypurine ribonucleotides on the first step unique to their own biosynthesis should permit more effective curtailment of the pathway when both types of inhibitors are in surplus simultaneously but should result in a moderate control when an equivalent excess of only one kind of purine is present.

With enzyme pigeon liver [239] and human placenta [226], purine ribonucleotides change the PP-ribose-P substrate-velocity plot from hyperbolic to sigmoidal. This change is not produced when the variable substrate is glutamine. With increasing concentrations of AMP, and with PP-ribose-P as variable substrate, the Hill coefficient for human amidophosphoribosyltransferase increases from 1.1 to 2.7. Thus, interactions between the PP-ribose-P and nucleotide binding sites are cooperative. Synergistic inhibition by nucleotides can be completely overcome by high concentrations of PP-ribose-P.

Amidophosphoribosyltransferase from chicken and pigeon livers has a molecular weight of approximately 210,000 and contains 12 atoms of nonheme iron [231]. The pigeon liver enzyme [239] is composed of four electrophoretically identical subunits. The 200,000 M. W. form can be dissociated to 100,000 and 50,000 M. W. species. The largest form appears to be the active catalytic molecule and is stabilized by PP-ribose-P. In the presence of AMP the 100,000 M. W. form is favored and is inhibited [245].

Amidophosphoribosyltransferase from human placenta exists in two forms with molecular weights of 133,000 and 270,000 [227]. In the absence of added purine ribonucleotides or PP-ribose-P, the small and large forms of the enzyme are both demonstrable in the same tissue preparation. Purine ribonucleotides, alone or in combination, convert the small form of the enzyme to the large form. PP-ribose-P converts the large form of the enzyme to the small form. Enzyme activity correlates directly with amount of amidophosphoribosyltransferase present in small form (Fig. 50-21). Glutamine has no influence on these form interchanges. Conversion of the small to the large form in the presence of purine ribonucleotides is rapid (<2 min) at 4 or 37°C, whereas conversion of the large to the small form in the presence of PP-ribose-P is slow (>10 min) and takes place only at 25 to 37°C. The slow conversion of the large to the small form is associated with a lag phase before phosphoribosylamine synthesis reaches maximal velocity

Figure 50-21 Correlation of enzyme activity with the amount of the small form of human amidophosphoribosyltransferase. Activity is expressed in the cross-hatched area as percentage of maximal activity observed with 10 mM PP-ribose-P in the absence of AMP. The percentages of the enzyme present in the large and small forms were determined by separation in sucrose density gradients. Samples were assayed following preincubation in the presence of high concentrations of PP-ribose-P. (*From* Holmes et al. [227]; *reproduced by permission of* The Journal of Biological Chemistry.)

RELATIONSHIP OF HUMAN PRPP AMIDOTRANSFERASE ACTIVITY TO THE MOLECULAR FORM OF THE ENZYME

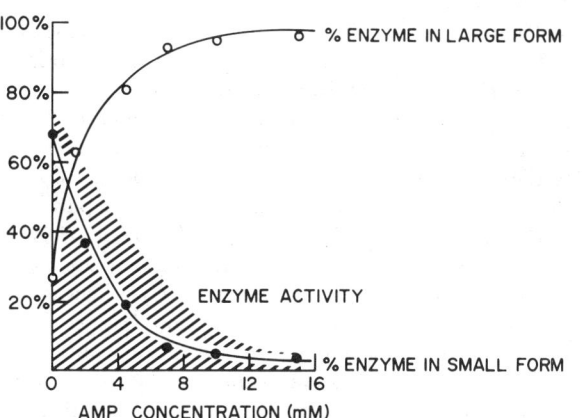

[246]. These findings suggest a model in which the 270,000 M. W. form is inactive and the 133,000 M. W. form is the catalytic species [227]. Conversion of the small form of amidophosphoribosyltransferase to the large form could represent polymerization of two molecules of active enzyme, or an association of one molecule of the small form with another protein of very similar molecular weight, shape, and charge (Fig. 50-22).

Rowe et al. [246a] find that the enzymes of the purine biosynthetic pathway can be copurified from pigeon liver by a method dependent upon the use of polyethylene glycol for enzyme stabilization and cofractionation. At PP-ribose-P concentrations below 0.3 mM the activity of amidophosphoribosyltransferase was rate limiting, and inhibition of this enzyme by AMP regulated the rate of purine ring synthesis. At higher concentrations of PP-ribose-P, aminoimidazole ribonucleotide synthetase, the fifth enzyme of the pathway, became rate limiting and was subject to inhibition by added AMP. Concentrations of about 0.5 mM PP-ribose-P were reported in mouse liver following fructose infusion by Itakura et al. [221].

REGULATION OF ENZYME AMOUNT   Relatively few studies have examined changes in rate of synthesis or degradation of amidophosphoribosyltransferase. Nierlich and Magasanik [247] demonstrated repression and derepression of six enzymes of purine biosynthesis in *A. aerogenes*, including three in the pathway leading to the synthesis of IMP. Activity of amidophosphoribosyltransferase varied coordinately with that of phosphoribosylformylglycineamidine synthetase, but noncoordinately with activity of the other enzymes, including that of phosphoribosylglycineamide synthetase, the second enzyme in the pathway.

McFall and Magasanik [248] have provided evidence that amidophosphoribosyltransferase may be repressed in an *L* strain of mouse fibroblasts cultured for several generations in adenine or guanosine. When offered to cells conditioned in this way, these agents produced a complete suppression of purine biosynthesis *de novo,* and all purines of soluble pools were then derived from exogenous supplements. By contrast, addition of adenine or guanosine to cells not previously exposed to purines produced only partial inhibition, and one-half of purines of soluble pools still arose by synthesis *de novo.*

Mouse spleen normally has no detectable amidophosphoribosyltransferase activity. However, following infection with Friend leukemia virus, activity of amidophosphoribosyltransferase appeared by the fourth day, increased rapidly to a peak of activity by the sixth to ninth day, and thereafter declined gradually over 2 to 4 weeks [242]. Enzyme activity was subject to purine ribonucleotide inhibition both in vivo and in vitro. Appearance of enzyme correlated with the extent of infiltration of spleen by tumor cells. Whether amidophosphoribosyltransferase was produced by derepression of host genome or by induction of viral genome is not known.

In the rat, a shift from a 5 to 50 percent casein diet results in a slight increase in activity of liver amidophosphoribosyltransferase in 1 week. Chicken liver amidophosphoribosyltransferase activity, which is normally about 10 times greater than that of rat liver [231, 249], triples on this regimen [249].

Total amidophosphoribosyltransferase activity, and presumably the amount of this enzyme, is increased in a number of malignant cell lines. This has been demonstrated by a comparison of hepatoma cell lines to normal liver, neoplastic to normal kidney, and leukemic to normal white blood cells

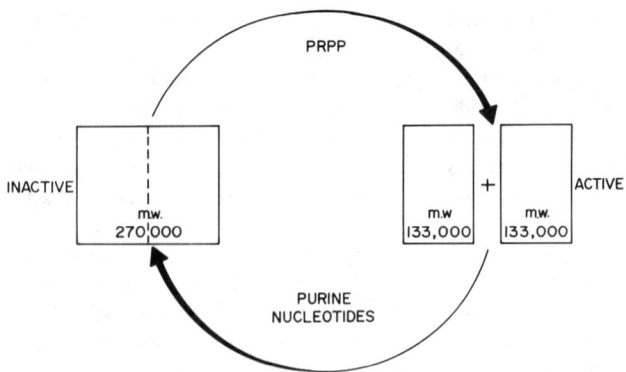

Figure 50-22 Model of interconversion of small (active) and large (inactive) forms of amidophosphoribosyltransferase. (*Courtesy of Dr. E. W. Holmes, Duke University Medical Center.*)

[232]. In rodent hepatomas, those lines with the fastest growth have the highest activities [250] and the largest amounts of amidophosphoribosyltransferase, as quantitated by antibody titration of amidophosphoribosyltransferase protein [251]. The gene for human amidophosphoribosyltransferase has been assigned to the pter → q21 region of chromosome 4 [252].

MUTANT FORMS OF AMIDOPHOSPHORIBOSYLTRANSFERASE A mutant form of amidophosphoribosyltransferase has been described in *S. pombe* [241], in which the enzyme is 10 times less sensitive to feedback inhibition by IMP and GMP than the enzyme from wild-type cells. An Ehrlich ascites cell line has been described in which exogenous guanine does not suppress purine biosynthesis to the same extent as in wild-type cells. It is presumed that amidophosphoribosyltransferase in these cells is less sensitive to feedback inhibition by purine ribonucleotides, since purine transport, nucleoside synthesis, and nucleotide catabolism are not altered in the mutant cell line [253]. A purine-requiring mutant of Chinese hamster ovary cells defective in both amidophosphoribosyltransferase and in phosphoribosylformylglycineamidine (FGAM) synthetase has been described [254] in which the low amidophosphoribosyltransferase activity is attributable to a "K_m mutation" at the glutamine site [255]. This is the first example of a mutant form of the enzyme from a mammalian source.

Coordination of Control of Early Steps of Purine Synthesis

There is debate in the literature whether PP-ribose-P synthetase or amidophosphoribosyltransferase is the more important enzyme in regulation of purine biosynthesis. The feedback controls operating on these two enzymes are summarized in Fig. 50-20. In some studies in tissue culture, e.g., those of Sperling and colleagues in fibroblasts [256] and in epithelial-like rat liver cells [257], the activation of PP-ribose-P synthetase by inorganic phosphate and the rate of PP-ribose-P synthesis appeared to be the limiting and controlling factors for purine ribonucleotide synthesis. In other studies, such as those of Hershfield and Seegmiller [258] in the WI-L2 line of diploid human lymphoblasts and of Allsop and Watts [259] in unstimulated and stimulated human lymphocytes, PP-ribose-P concentrations did not appear to play a central role, and end product feedback regulatory effects were thought to be more important for coordination of purine nucleotide synthesis.

Recent studies from Holmes's laboratory [221] provide data

indicating that the model illustrated in Fig. 50-20 is operational in vivo and that control of the two regulatory enzymes is coordinated. Adenyl nucleotide content of the liver of mice is decreased 35 percent by the intravenous infusion of fructose. Subsequently there is an increase of 2.3 times in PP-ribose-P concentration. This result most probably reflects the release of inhibition of PP-ribose-P synthetase resulting from the fall in concentration of one of its specific inhibitors, ADP. Before fructose infusion, only about 5 percent of amidophosphoribosyltransferase is in the small, active form; following fructose infusion, over 30 percent of amidophosphoribosyltransferase is present in the small form. Incorporation of ^{14}C-glycine into hepatic purines is increased threefold in conjunction with the shift of this amount of amidophosphoribosyltransferase from large to small form. These studies demonstrate that changes in the intracellular concentrations of adenyl ribonucleotides result in activation of PP-ribose-P synthetase, increased synthesis of PP-ribose-P, and activation of amidophosphoribosyltransferase (shift of large to small form) and that in association with these changes there is an increase in the rate of purine biosynthesis in the cell.

Regulation of Purine Ribonucleotide Interconversions

There are many short biosynthetic sequences by which one nucleotide is produced from another. Each of these reaction sequences is regulated by the end product which serves as an inhibitor of the first enzyme of the short pathway. The synthesis of AMP from IMP involves a two-step reaction sequence, the first of which is irreversible and requires GTP as a source of energy. This reaction is inhibited by AMP and GDP [260, 261]. The synthesis of GMP from IMP also involves two reaction steps. The first is irreversible and is inhibited by GMP [262]; the second requires ATP as an energy source. The combined influences of "forward" control, based on the availability of GTP and ATP, each of which is concerned with the synthesis of the other nucleotide, and of feedback inhibition, by which AMP and GMP each controls its own biosynthesis, may regulate the intracellular levels of adenyl and guanyl nucleotides.

In an *E. coli* mutant, transport of purine bases into the cell and conversion of IMP to AMP and GMP are inhibited during amino acid starvation. The effects can be explained by the accumulation of guanosine tetraphosphate [2] and the inhibitory effects of this substance on the membrane-localized purine phosphoribosyltransferases, on adenylosuccinate synthetase, and IMP dehydrogenase, the enzymes that catalyze these reactions.

AMP may be converted to IMP by adenylic deaminase and thus potentially serves as a source of guanyl ribonucleotides. The first enzyme of this pathway, adenylic deaminase, is stimulated by ATP and strongly inhibited by GTP and inorganic phosphate [263]. Under physiologic conditions the enzyme is 95 percent inhibited [264]. When the inhibition is released, uric acid is formed in large excess and biosynthesis of purines is increased. Hers and Van Den Berghe [265] have postulated that some cases of primary gout may be due to an abnormal AMP deaminase which is less sensitive to its physiologic inhibitors. This hypothesis will be discussed below. A genetic deficiency of myoadenylic deaminase is associated with a late-onset myopathy (Chap. 54). Adenosine may be converted to inosine by adenosine deaminase, and inosine may then be phosphorylated by ATP in the presence of inosine kinase [263].

Thus, this pathway may also serve as a source of guanyl nucleotides. The pathway adenosine → inosine → hypoxanthine → IMP → AMP-S → AMP → adenosine has been called the *adenosine cycle* [263]. A genetic deficiency of adenosine deaminase is associated with a severe combined immunodeficiency (Chap. 53). Cultured mammalian cells which are HGPRT- and adenosine kinase-deficient excrete considerably more purines into the medium than cells which are only HGPRT-deficient, because of reduced salvage of adenosine against the flow of this cycle. GMP may be converted to IMP and then serve as a source of adenyl nucleotides. The first enzyme of this pathway, GMP reductase, is strongly inhibited by ATP [262]. In addition, free guanine may be deaminated and reduced to hypoxanthine in mammalian tissue [266]. These last two reactions probably represent very minor pathways.

Ribonucleotide Cleavage In circumstances in which accelerated purine biosynthesis *de novo* results in production of a surfeit of IMP, there is a rapid conversion of the excess ribonucleotide to uric acid. The controls that lead to this result, rather than to continual expansion of pools of adenyl and guanyl nucleotides, may depend on tight regulation of nucleotide biosynthetic pathways plus improved competition of 5′-nucleotidase for IMP as its concentration is raised.

Zoref, de Vries, and Sperling [266a] have studied the comparative aspects of nucleotide metabolism in cultured fibroblasts obtained from normal subjects and from patients with HPRT deficiency or PP-ribose-P synthetase superactivity. The latter two defects result in both elevations of intracellular concentrations of PP-ribose-P and excessive purine biosynthesis *de novo*. In this study the rate of ^{14}C-formate incorporation into cellular purines and purines excreted into the medium was increased 6.5 times in cells with PP-ribose-P synthetase superactivity, 10 times in partial HPRT deficiency, and 13.5 times in complete HPRT deficiency. In normal cells 14 percent of newly formed labeled purines were excreted into the medium in 6 h. In HPRT deficiency this figure was 21 to 33 percent, in PP-ribose-P synthetase overactivity it was 50 percent. In all cases the extracellular purine was almost exclusively hypoxanthine. These studies confirm that synthesis of IMP in amounts greater than are needed for cellular metabolic needs results in prompt cleavage of IMP to inosine and hypoxanthine. Some information on control mechanisms may be obtained from review of nucleotidase activities in the cells.

5′-Nucleotidases have been isolated from a number of animal tissues. Two kinds have been purified from hepatic tissue. One is located in microsomes and plasma membranes [267]; the other has been found in the nonsedimentable fraction of liver homogenates [173, 174, 268].

Microsomal 5′-nucleotidases show greatest activity with 5′-AMP, 5′-CMP, and 5′-UMP, and less with 5′-IMP or 5′-GMP. K_m values for AMP are 10 to 40 μM, depending on the buffer employed and Mg^{2+} concentrations [2].

The cytoplasmic 5′-nucleotidases of chicken [173], rat, frog, and pig liver [174] all show highest activity with 5′-IMP and 5′-GMP, and are inhibited by inosine and guanosine. When dietary casein content is increased from 5 to 75 percent, the specific activities of cytosol 5′-nucleotidase and purine nucleoside phosphorylase of chicken liver and kidney increase by two- to threefold, whereas that of xanthine dehydrogenase of liver increases thirteenfold. The IMP-hydrolyzing activity is correlated with the serum uric acid concentration ($r = 0.84$, $p < 0.001$) [269].

Table 50-8 shows K_m values of several cytoplasmic 5′-nucleotidases, compared with K_m values of reactions of IMP leading to synthesis of AMP or GMP. Under resting and fed conditions, IMP concentration in mouse liver is 0.05 μmol per gram wet weight [221] or about 70 μM in liver cell water. This concentration is close to the K_m values of AMP-S synthetase and IMP dehydrogenase, but far below the K_m value of cytosolic 5′-nucleotidase. Thus AMP-S and XMP synthesis will be favored over cleavage of IMP. Following fructose infusion, there is rapid depletion of ATP and ADP, with increases of IMP concentrations to about 900 μM [221]. At this concentration of IMP both the synthetase and the dehydrogenase are probably saturated, whereas the nucleotidase will be functioning with a substrate concentration close to its K_m value. IMP cleavage to inosine should proceed actively.

Under steady state conditions adenyl nucleotides account for about 90 percent of the soluble nucleotides of the liver cell. Of these, about 10 percent is AMP, whose concentration is about 0.6 μmol per gram wet weight [221] or about 900 μM in liver cell water. AMP is protected from cleavage by the low activity of cytosolic nucleotidase with AMP [174] and the compartmentation of cytosolic AMP from microsomal enzymes [175, 270]. Its major catabolic pathway involves deamination to IMP. Under physiologic circumstances, AMP deaminase of liver is 95 percent inhibited [264]. The rate of allantoin production by isolated rat hepatocytes is accounted for by the residual 5 percent activity [265]. AMP deaminase may therefore be the limiting step in purine catabolism of intracellular nucleotides. This conclusion is further strengthened by studies of fructose-induced hyperuricemia.

Fructose-induced Hyperuricemia The rapid intravenous administration of fructose induces a prompt rise in serum and urinary uric acid levels in humans and in animals [271]. Animal experiments have shown that this effect is a consequence of the consumption of ATP in phosphorylation of fructose, and subsequent reactions that result in reduction of total adenyl nucleotides through conversion of AMP to IMP, cleavage of IMP, phosphorolysis of inosine, and oxidation of oxypurine bases [271]. Urinary inosine, hypoxanthine, xanthine, and uric acid all increase following fructose administration [272]. There is also a marked depletion of intracellular inorganic phosphate and of GTP in response to fructose infusion [271]. P_i and GTP are inhibitors of AMP deaminase. Even a limited release of inhibition will result in an increase in degradation of AMP to IMP and further catabolic products.

Fructose infusion also results in stimulation of purine biosynthesis *de novo*. ^{14}C-glycine incorporation into adenine nucleotides [273] and urinary uric acid [274, 275] is increased.

Table 50-8 Relative affinities of enzymes competing for inosine-5′-phosphate*

	K_m, μM IMP		
Source of tissue	Cytoplasmic 5′-nucleotidase	AMP-S synthetase	IMP dehydrogenase
Escherichia coli	800	30–77	14
Chicken liver	800		
Rat liver	400		
Rabbit heart		110	
Human placenta		37–70	14

* For references see [2].

This is probably a secondary consequence of a significant reduction in the hepatic content of ADP, a nucleotide that is thought to be a physiologically important inhibitor of PP-ribose-P synthetase. Intracellular PP-ribose-P concentrations rise within 30 min after fructose infusion and result in a sixfold increase in the amount of active amidophosphoribosyltransferase, the enzyme that catalyzes the first step of purine synthesis [221].

Equimolar infusions of sorbitol and xylitol have effects similar to those of fructose [276], whereas infusions of glucose and galactose do not [277]. However in glycogen storage disease type I the breakdown of glycogen also induces hyperuricemia. The absence of glucose-6-phosphatase allows the trapping of large quantities of hexose as glucose-6-phosphate and fructose-1,6-diphosphate with resulting ATP and P_i depletion and nucleotide catabolism [278], by mechanisms that appear to mimic those activated by fructose infusion.

Infusion of 15 g of ethanol in 5 min also results in increased production of uric acid by the liver, attributed to increased breakdown of preformed purine nucleotides. Ethanol reduces cellular content of inorganic phosphate and ATP in the liver and thus may also produce a fructoselike effect. In this study about 300 mg of uric acid was produced in response to ethanol infusion [278a].

Effects of Variations in Xanthine Oxidase Activity on Purine Biosynthesis

The rate at which free purine bases are removed will influence the rate of new synthesis of purine ribonucleotides. Inhibition of xanthine oxidase activity by allopurinol results in reduced rates of oxidation of hypoxanthine and xanthine, and enhanced reconversion of these bases to nucleotides. There is a concomitant reduction in the rate of synthesis of new purine ribonucleotides from low-molecular-weight precursors, presumably because of both enhanced competitive utilization of PP-ribose-P in the salvage reactions and heightened feedback inhibition of the amidophosphoribosyltransferase by reconstituted ribonucleotides. Within the limits of measurement, nucleotide levels remain constant in spite of very different rates of operation of the biosynthetic pathway [279].

Gouty subjects who are marked overexcretors of uric acid may show substantially increased levels of hepatic xanthine oxidase activity [280], possibly as an induced enzyme response triggered by other factors [281]. The increased xanthine oxidase activity, even if a secondary response, would be expected to lead to further enhancement of purine biosynthesis through reversal of the two mechanisms cited above, with maintenance of relative constancy of nucleotide levels.

A rather different situation exists in hepatoma cells, in which the enzymes concerned with regulation of purine nucleotide biosynthesis de novo are of very high activity, while the catalytic capacity of xanthine oxidase is unusually low. Weber and associates [282] have found raised activity values of enzymes of the oxidative limb of the pentose phosphate pathway, of PP-ribose-P synthetase, and of amidophosphoribosyltransferase in hepatoma cells, together with normal activity values of hypoxanthine-guanine phosphoribosyltransferase and depressed activity values of xanthine oxidase. There altered enzymatic relationships are found throughout the hepatoma cell series, beginning with the minimal deviation varieties and extending through the most highly malignant examples. This complex system appears to be poised to maximize purine nucleotide biosynthesis by both the de novo and salvage pathways to meet the demands of the hepatoma cell for accelerated nucleic acid production.

Inhibitors of Purine Biosynthesis *de novo*

Purine biosynthesis *de novo* can be inhibited by compounds which compete for PP-ribose-P in phosphoribosyltransferase reactions. Included in this group are orotic acid [219], allopurinol [283], adenine, and 2,6-diamino purine, all of which have been shown to reduce intracellular PP-ribose-P levels in erythrocytes in vivo or in cultured fibroblasts in vitro. The glutamine analogues, aza-L-serine and DON [2], inhibit the three steps of purine synthesis in which L-glutamine serves as substrate. The enzyme which catalyzes the conversion of 5'-phosphoribosylglycineamide to 5'-phosphoribosylformylglycineamide is 100 times more sensitive to azaserine than is amidophosphoribosyltransferase. Azaserine blocks the formation of a γ-glutamyl-enzyme complex through the formation of a stable compound with a sulfhydryl group on the enzyme surface. As a result 5'-phosphoribosylglycineamide accumulates in intact cells, or in tissue cultures treated with azaserine. In studies with such cells, the incorporation of labeled precursor into the accumulated 5'-phosphoribosylformylglycineamide provides an index of purine synthesis *de novo*. Both azaserine and DON have been shown to inhibit purine synthesis in humans, but they are too toxic for therapeutic use.

The purine analogues, 6-mercaptopurine, 6-thioguanine, 8-azaguanine, allopurinol, and 6-methylmercaptopurine ribonucleoside, inhibit the accumulation of 5'-phosphoribosylformylglycineamide in azaserine-treated tissues [284]. The inhibitions depend upon prior conversion of the base to ribonucleotide. Cultured fibroblasts deficient in HPRT activity are resistant to the lethal action of 6-mercaptopurine, 8-azaguanine, and 6-thioguanine, all of which require HPRT activity for conversion to their nucleotide form [284]. The ribonucleotide derivatives of these bases and of allopurinol act as pseudofeedback inhibitors of amidophosphoribosyltransferase [181].

5-Aminoimidazole-4-carboxamide (AIC) [285], adenine [286], 6-thiopurine [287], and azathioprine [288] inhibit purine synthesis *de novo* when administered in large doses in humans. The effects of azathioprine (6-imidazolylthiopurine) in inhibiting purine synthesis *de novo* are probably dependent upon its hydrolysis to 6-mercaptopurine and conversion of the latter substance to ribonucleotide form. Azathioprine does not inhibit purine synthesis in patients who are deficient in HPRT activity [288]. Adenine exhibits its effect even in HPRT-deficient fibroblasts in culture, which have very high levels of PP-ribose-P. Accordingly, the inhibition of purine synthesis *de novo* by AIC and adenine probably represents the activation of endogenous feedback control mechanisms by normal nucleotides derived from these bases, rather than competition for PP-ribose-P. AIC, adenine, 6-thiopurine, and azathioprine are themselves catabolized in part to uric acid, so that the net change in serum urate concentration is often quite small in spite of the fact that they inhibit purine synthesis [285, 286]. Hence, even if these drugs were nontoxic, their potential use as antihyperuricemic agents would be limited.

Methotrexate (4-amino-N^{10}-methylpteroylglutamic acid) inhibits the incorporation of single carbon fragments into positions 2 and 8 of the purine ring and thereby reduces purine synthesis in humans [289]. Hadacidine (N-formyl hydroxy-aminoacetic acid), an analogue of L-aspartate, inhibits the conversion of IMP to AMP-S [290], in concentrations that appear to have little effect upon the conversion of 5'-phosphoribosyl-5-amino-4-imidazole carboxylate to 5'-phosphoribosyl-5-amino-4-imidazolesuccinocarboxamide, a reaction in which aspartate also participates. Both methotrexate and hadacidine are too toxic for use as antihyperuricemic agents in humans.

Xanthine Oxidase Inhibitors Many inhibitors of xanthine oxidase are known [2] including 6-pteridylaldehyde and various purine analogues such as adenine, 2,6-diaminopurine, 6-thiopurine, 6-chloropurine, 4-diazoimidazole-5-carboxamide, symmetric triazines, allopurinol [4-hydroxypyrazolo-(3, 4-d) pyrimidine], and oxipurinol [2, 4-dihydroxypyrazolo-(3,4-d) pyrimidine].

Stimulation of Purine Biosynthesis *de novo*

2-Ethylamino-1,3,4-thiadiazole (EA-TDA) causes marked hyperuricemia and hyperuricaciduria. When administered to human subjects, it produced a severalfold increase in both the serum urate level and the urinary excretion of uric acid [291]. In animals [292] and in humans [293] a striking increase in the rate of purine biosynthesis *de novo* follows adminstration of the drug. In humans this is reflected in an increased incorporation of ^{14}C-glycine into uric acid, hypoxanthine, xanthine, adenine, guanine, and 7-methylguanine in the urine and an increased excretion rate of these compounds [293].

The mechanism responsible for this effect of EA-TDA appears to involve a marked increase in hepatic cell levels of PP-ribose-P [220], although just how this is brought about is unclear. EA-TDA also induces hepatic xanthine oxidase activity in humans [281]. The effect of the drug on purine metabolism in humans can be prevented by the simultaneous administration of nicotinamide at a dose four times greater than that of EA-TDA [293], and by nicotinic acid.

PRODUCTION OF URIC ACID IN GOUT

Chemical Balance

In theory, the rate of purine synthesis may be assessed from the difference between purine intake and excretion in the dynamic steady state. In practice this approach fails because the urinary excretion of uric acid represents a variable fraction of total purine turnover, and there are no convenient methods for the measurement of extrarenal disposal of urate. Purine intake may be reduced to levels of less than 3 mg purine-*N* per day by severe dietary purine restriction. The average urinary uric acid value then becomes a minimal estimate of purine production. Values in normal adults show a wide range (Table 50-9). Frequency histograms show skewness toward high values without evidence of bimodality. Normal urinary uric acid excretion values have been defined on a statistical basis as representing the range, mean ± 2 SD, of nongouty subjects studied under standard conditions of activity and dietary intake. With standard American diets from which purine-containing foods have been omitted, values in normal adult males range from 278 to 558 mg/day (mean 418 ± 70 mg) [71], or from 264 to 588 mg/day (mean 426 ± 81 mg) [294].

Table 50-9 Basal urinary uric acid excretion values, mg/day*

Diet	Males	Females
Purine-free formula diet	336 ± 39†	
Purine-free formula diet	361 ± 63	
Meat free–purine free	374	374
Low purine	401 ± 42	321 ± 34
Low purine	410	383
Low purine	416 ± 68	
Essentially free of purines	426 ± 81	

* For references see Table 43-11 in the fourth edition of this text [2].
† Mean ± SD.

Urinary uric acid values in males with primary gout extend from values of 150 mg/day or less to values of 2400 mg/day or more. Low values are found in patients with overt renal damage. In selected samples of gouty patients from 21 to 28 percent excreted quantities of urate exceeding the mean + 2 SD [71, 294], but the more general experience is that only 5 to 15 percent of patients with primary gout fall into this category. Such patients have arbitrarily been classified as *overexcretors* of uric acid. The theoretical possibility that an increased urinary excretion is secondary to a decreased extrarenal disposal of urate has been excluded by normal urinary recoveries of injected labeled uric acid in the majority of overexcretor patients [294]. Therefore, sustained overexcretion of uric acid is evidence for excessive synthesis of purines *de novo*. However, a normal urinary excretion of uric acid does not exclude overproduction of uric acid in gouty subjects, for in the hyperuricemic subject with reduced renal urate excretion, the disposal of urate by extrarenal processes may be much increased, occasionally accounting for over 80 percent of the urate turnover [294].

Since about 1950 the mechanisms and rates of uric acid production have been studied by means of two general types of biochemical techniques: (1) the turnover study, employing principles of isotope dilution; and (2) precursor administration, with evaluation of the rate and extent of conversion of the administered substance into uric acid. More recently, studies of purine metabolism in gout have been amplified by direct enzyme assays in human tissue and by the use of cell culture techniques.

The Miscible Pool of Uric Acid and Its Turnover

In the isotope dilution technique for measurement of the miscible pool of uric acid and the rate of its turnover [295] either [15]N- or ^{14}C-uric acid is injected intravenously, following which it mixes intimately with uric acid in the body. Urinary uric acid is isolated serially for several days, and the isotope concentration of each sample is determined. A first-order turnover process is assumed in which a constant fraction of the pool is replaced per unit time. This assumption leads to the expression

$$I_t = I_0 e^{-Kt} \tag{25}$$

the integrated form of which is

$$\log I_t = \log I_0 - Kt \tag{26}$$

where I_0 is the isotope concentration in body uric acid at $t = 0$, the moment of mixing; I_t is the isotope concentration at time t

thereafter; and K is the fraction of uric acid replaced per unit time. On semilogarithmic coordinates, a plot of log I_t versus t gives a straight line, where KI is the negative slope, and log I_0 is the intercept (Fig. 50-23). The miscible pool of uric acid is defined as the quantity of uric acid in the body of the recipient by which the injected uric acid is promptly diluted. The quantity of uric acid present in the miscible pool (A) may be calculated from knowledge of the amount of uric acid injected (a), of the concentration of isotope in it (I_i), and of the concentration of isotope in the uric acid of the body at the moment of mixing (I_0), by use of standard dilution equation:

$$(A + a) I_0 = aI_i \qquad (27)$$

By rearrangement,

$$A = a \frac{I_i}{I_0} - 1$$

The decline in the concentration of isotope in uric acid is a result of the continuous dilution of the labeled uric acid pool by new nonisotopic uric acid molecules. From knowledge of the fraction of the pool replaced per unit time (K) and the size of the miscible pool (A), the rate of addition of new labeled uric acid (KA) may be calculated [295].

Normal Values In subjects with normal serum urate concentrations straight lines are obtained in plots such as that of Fig. 50-24. This finding supports the assumptions made in the derivation of Eq. (26) and the validity of the calculations made from plots constructed from it. The majority of studies have employed the original technique of determining the isotope concentration of uric acid isolated from urine. Sorensen [165] has injected ^{14}C-uric acid intravenously and has calculated the specific activity of uric acid from the radioactivity value and uric acid content of a volume of serum, on the reasonable assumption that (in humans) all ^{14}C in serum is in the form of uric acid. This technique gives results that show a high correlation coefficient (0.96) with results obtained with uric acid isolated from urine [296].

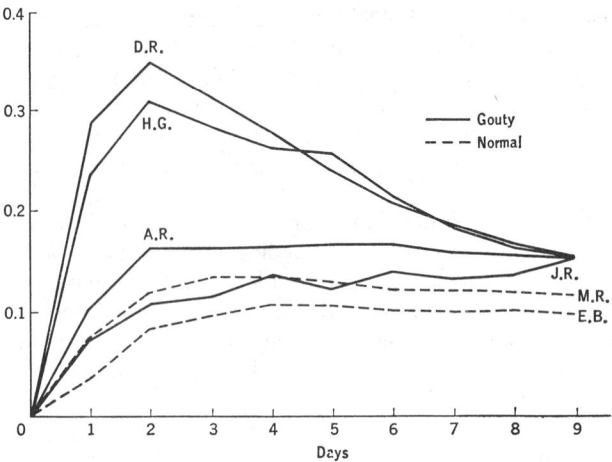

Figure 50-24 Concentration of ^{15}N in urinary uric acid following ingestion of glycine-^{15}N by normal and gouty subjects. (*From J. D. Benedict et al.* [302], *with permission of* The Journal of Clinical Investigation.)

POOL SIZE In about 30 normal male subjects [2], the rapidly miscible pool was an average of 1200 mg uric acid, with values ranging from 866 to 1650 mg. In five normal females, the pool ranged from 541 to 687 mg. When calculated on the basis of body weight, values averaged 16.3 mg/kg, with a range from 11.0 to 20.3 mg/kg [296].

TURNOVER RATE From the rate of decline in concentration of ^{15}N or ^{14}C in urinary uric acid, it was calculated that from 45 to 85 percent of the uric acid of the miscible pool was normally replaced each day by newly formed, nonisotopic molecules. The turnover of uric acid averaged 695 mg/day, with values ranging from 513 to 1108 mg/day. Rieselbach et al. [297] found a mean turnover of 743 mg in nine normal subjects, representing a production rate of 343 ± 36 mg/(m^2 · day). The quantity of uric acid entering the pool exceeds the amount recovered in urine by 100 to 365 mg/day [2, 164]. The significance of this surplus is discussed below (see "Uricolysis in Normal Humans" and "Uricolysis in Gout").

Values in Gouty Subjects

POOL SIZE In gouty subjects without tophi, the miscible pool is generally enlarged to 1600 to 4000 mg [2] (20.0 to 42.3 mg/kg in one series [296]). In patients with severe tophaceous disease it may reach 18,000 to 31,000 mg [298]. Even so, the value of the miscible pool may represent only a small fraction of the total urate in the body of gouty patients. In subjects with hyperuricemia, in particular those with tophi, plots of log I of urinary uric acid versus time may not be linear [296], indicating the presence of more than one exponential component. When such curvilinearity is ignored, and the plot is treated as though it was monoexponential, the best-fit estimate of the straight line underestimates the intercept and therefore overestimates pool size; hence it also overestimates turnover rate. Curvilinear plots can be analyzed in terms of a two-compartment model [296]. Such analyses may represent the soluble urate pool plus a variable portion of solid urate in slow exchange with that in solution. The turnover rate of the soluble pool plus the transfer rate between the first and second pools then more accurately represents the composite rate of synthesis of uric acid than calculations based on the single-compartment model. In one patient with tophaceous gout analyzed by Sorensen [299] according to the two-compartment model, the

Figure 50-23 Semilogarithmic plot of isotope concentration (^{15}N) in urinary uric acid versus time in days, following intravenous administration of (1,3)-^{15}N-uric acid to a normal subject. (*From Wyngaarden and Stetten* [164]; *Fig. 3B, replotted.*)

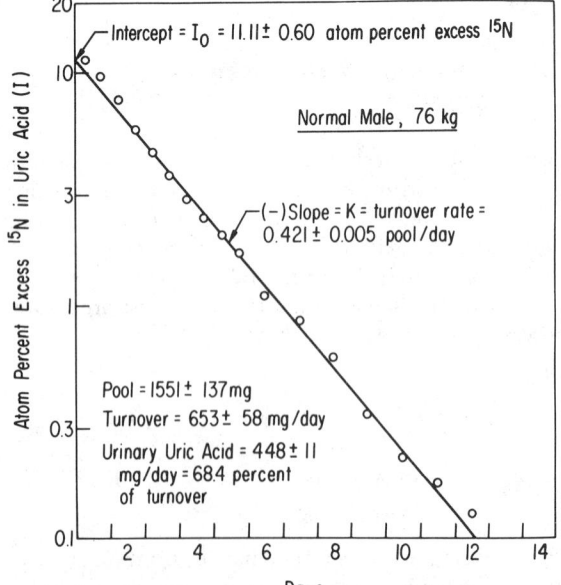

amount of uric acid in the tophaceous compartment in slow exchange with soluble uric acid was estimated to be 300 times larger than the rapidly miscible pool.

TURNOVER RATE The possibility of exchange of labeled urate of the miscible pool with unlabeled urate of the solid phase was recognized by Benedict et al. [295] in their initial presentation of the method. They cautioned that the turnover technique might not provide a dependable measure of the rate of synthesis of urate in subjects with tophaceous gout. By sequential extraction of a large tophus removed from a gouty subject who had been given ^{15}N-uric acid, they demonstrated that only the peripheral layers were readily exchangeable with urate in solution in body fluids [298].

In spite of this technical limitation, values for turnover of uric acid calculated on the basis of a one-compartment, single-exponential model agree very well with another calculation of rate of synthesis [294, 300], viz.,

$$\frac{\text{Basal urinary uric acid, mg/day}}{\substack{\text{Urinary recovery of injected isotopic uric acid,}\\ \text{fraction of administered dose}}}$$

The turnover rate is uniformly increased in gouty patients who overexcrete uric acid [2]. Values in excess of 2 g/day have been reported [2, 300]. In patients with normal uric acid excretion values, and without visible tophi, uric acid turnover values show extensive overlap with control values. For example, in eight such subjects, Scott et al. [296] found turnover values ranging from 616 to 1000 mg/24 h, compared with values of 552 to 838 in six nongouty controls. The mean values were 800 ± 130 mg/24 h and 693 ± 112 mg/24 h, respectively ($0.2 > p > 0.1$).

In those gouty patients whose miscible pool is within, or just above, the normal range, calculations may show that all urate measured in the miscible pool is in solution. In two patients meeting these criteria, Sorensen [299] found excessive turnover of uric acid. However, in five patients also meeting these criteria, Seegmiller et al. [294] found a normal turnover of uric acid, and these five patients also showed normal values of incorporation of isotopic glycine into uric acid (see below).

Incorporation of Labeled Precursors into Uric Acid

The rate of generation of uric acid has been studied in both normal and gouty subjects by observing the rate at which isotope appears in urinary uric acid when a labeled precursor is administered. Studies of this type have been performed with ^{15}N-glycine, 1-^{14}C-glycine, 2-^{14}C-glycine, U-^{14}C-glycine, ^{15}N-ammonium, ^{14}C-formate, 4-^{13}C- and 4-^{14}C-4-aminoimidazole-5-carboxamide, 8-^{14}C-hypoxanthine, and 8-^{14}C- and 8-^{13}C-adenine.

Incorporation of Labeled Glycine into Urinary Uric Acid Glycine serves as a specific precursor of carbon atoms 4 and 5 and nitrogen atom 7 of the purine ring. The rate of uric acid biosynthesis can be appraised by measurement of the incorporation of labeled glycine into urinary uric acid [301, 302]. The following discussion is based on studies of incorporation of 1-^{14}C-glycine, U-^{14}C-glycine, and ^{15}N-glycine under standardized experimental conditions.

After the subject has been prepared with a low purine diet for about 5 days, labeled glycine is fed with a light breakfast [301] or injected intravenously [303]. The labeled glycine will be diluted with glycine of dietary origin and with glycine of various extracellular and intracellular pools. Variations in the amount of diluting unlabeled glycine, and in size and turnover of hepatic glycine pools, could influence the specific activity of glycine incorporated into 5′-phosphoribosylglycineamide and into uric acid, quite apart from differences in rates of purine biosynthesis. However, measurements of enrichment of other products of glycine metabolism, such as hippurate [304] or creatinine [301], have not disclosed evidence of abnormal labeling or turnover kinetics of glycine in gout. Therefore, abnormalities of labeling of urinary uric acid in gouty subjects do not appear to derive from disturbances in glycine metabolism and may be attributed to differences in rates of purine biosynthesis or of dilutions within purine pools.

Each study must be interpreted in the light of appropriate controls. For example, one cannot compare results of studies of ^{15}N-glycine incorporation in gouty subjects with data of ^{14}C-glycine incorporation in controls. 1-^{14}C-Glycine is given in tracer doses of a few milligrams, whereas with ^{15}N-glycine doses of 0.1 g/kg are required. This quantity of ^{15}N-glycine is approximately equal to the free glycine pool in humans, which is 80 to 90 mg/kg [304]. Since glycine enters the purine biosynthetic sequence beyond the rate-limiting step of purine synthesis, one would anticipate that approximately one-half as much isotope would enter uric acid when such a glycine load is given as when a tracer dose is administered. Average incorporation values for ^{14}C and ^{15}N in control and gouty subjects, as well as a direct appraisal of this question in four control subjects given 1-^{14}C-glycine with and without carrier glycine [305], confirm this prediction.

When labeled glycine is administered to control subjects, urinary uric acid is isotopically labeled within the first few hours. Enrichment values reach a maximum by the second to fourth day and then gradually decline. Sometimes a secondary maximum is observed about the tenth to twelfth day. Urinary uric acid remains labeled at low levels for 6 months [286].

The immediate labeling of uric acid probably reflects the synthesis and prompt catabolism of purine ribonucleotides to purine bases and uric acid. The late secondary peak corresponds to the turnover of some of the more stable portions of RNA.

In the initial studies of Benedict et al. [301, 302] with ^{14}N-glycine, two gouty subjects who consistently excreted excessive quantities of uric acid in urine showed rapid rises of ^{15}N concentrations in urinary uric acid to values about three times normal (Fig. 50-24). Maximal values occurred earlier than in controls, and were followed by rapid declines in ^{15}N concentrations during succeeding days. These results reflected an exaggeration of the rate of incorporation of dietary glycine nitrogen into uric acid, and these findings were borne out by cumulative incorporation values of ^{15}N into uric acid three times greater than normal in these subjects. These authors postulated that the excess ^{15}N had appeared in urinary uric acid too rapidly to have traversed nucleic acids as intermediates. This is the origin of the concept of a "shunt pathway" by which intermediates bypass nucleic acids in their accelerated conversion to uric acid in primary gout. Subsequent evidence [306, 307] has suggested that this pathway may consist of the normal sequence: early precursors (including glycine) → inosinic acid → hypoxanthine → xanthine → uric acid, utilized in the overproducer gouty subject to excessive degree.

Benedict and associates [301, 302] also included in their initial studies three gouty subjects whose basal urinary uric acid excretion values were within the normal range. ^{15}N labeling of urinary uric acid fell within or only minimally above the normal range with respect to both enrichment and cumulative incorporation (Fig. 50-24). Although subsequent studies disclosed excessive incorporation of ^{15}N-glycine into urinary uric acid in some gouty patients with similar characteristics [296], in general the initial experience of Benedict and colleagues has been reproducible in other studies employing ^{15}N-glycine.

Because of concern that the large load of ^{15}N-glycine studies may have influenced the incorporation results, Wyngaarden [308, 309] repeated these studies employing tracer doses of 1-^{14}C-glycine and observed increased incorporation values in six of eight gouty subjects, including several without hyperuricaciduria. Subsequent studies in many laboratories throughout the world have confirmed and extended these observations.

For routine tracer studies designed to evaluate the rate of uric acid biosynthesis *de novo*, use of 1-^{14}C-glycine is preferable to use of ^{15}N-glycine, both because it is a more specific label and because its administration in a tracer dose obviates the kinetic and dilutional complications resulting from administration of gram quantities of glycine. The study is also technically easier and much cheaper.

Figure 50-25 summarizes the majority of 1-^{14}C-glycine incorporation values published through 1980. In gouty subjects with uric acid excretions of less than 590 mg/day, the cumulative incorporation of ^{14}C is excessive in one-half to two-thirds of patients. Mean incorporation values are 0.17 percent in 7 days in normal subjects, 0.28 percent in gouty subjects. In subjects with excretions of more than 590 mg/day, incorporation is invariably increased, often exceeding normal values by severalfold.

Figure 50-25 Summary of values of cumulative incorporation of ^{14}C into urinary uric acid in control and gouty subjects reported from 1957 through 1980.

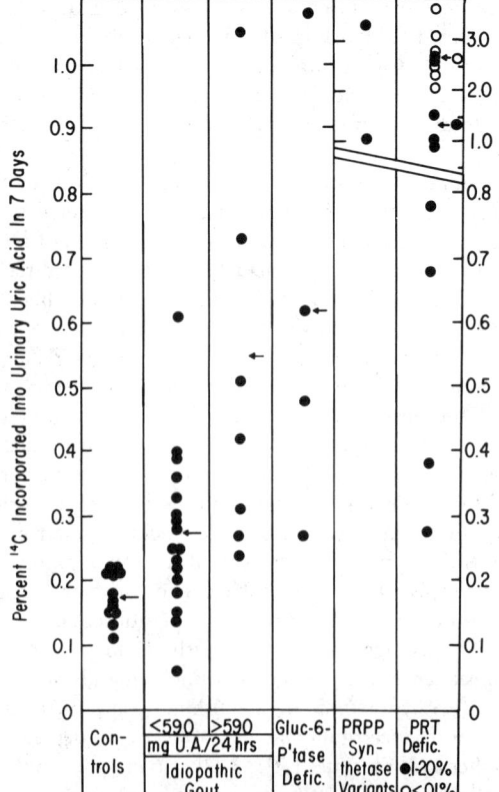

When studies of incorporation of ^{15}N-glycine into urinary uric acid have been repeated in the same individual a few months later, good agreement between paired values has been observed [302]. However, in one subject studied by Emmerson, controlled weight loss over a 2-year span, during which hyperuricemia and hyperuricaciduria reverted to normal, also led to reduction of a previously elevated 1-^{14}C-glycine incorporation value to normal [310]. Yü and Roboz [311] repeated ^{15}N-glycine incorporation studies in three gouty patients 13, 18, and 27 years after the first studies. All three were marked overexcretors of uric acid, but over the years the magnitude of the uric acid excretion had declined, entering the normal range in one of them. The magnitude of ^{15}N-glycine incorporation declined in each to about one-half of the earlier values, but each was still above the normal range. Each patient had lost some weight (18, 2, and 5 kg). Each patient had received allopurinol for years, but the drug had been discontinued for several months before the study. Thus, these two publications indicate that whatever metabolic abnormalities lead to uric acid overproduction and glycine overincorporation into uric acid, they are at least partially reversible in some subjects.

Incorporation of Labeled Glycine into Total Body Uric Acid   Newly synthesized isotopic urate will be diluted within an expanded uric acid pool in gouty subjects. In addition, as renal function deteriorates, the fraction of the urate turnover excreted in urine each day may decline, and that excreted into the gastrointestinal tract may increase. Several of the gouty subjects of Fig. 50-25 with apparently normal incorporation values had extensive tophaceous deposits and impaired renal function. These factors could mask overincorporation. Seegmiller and coworkers [294] have measured the fraction of intravenously injected uric acid (labeled with a different isotope) that was recovered in the urine during the experiment. If one assumes that the same fraction of uric acid synthesized *de novo* is recovered in urine during the same time, this procedure allows one to correct for the unrecovered component. In this study, two of five gouty subjects whose ^{14}C-glycine incorporation values were normal showed excessive incorporation values when appropriate corrections for extrarenal disposal were made. A number of additional examples have been published [300].

We consider glycine incorporation values to be indexes rather than definitive measurements of rates of purine production. There is no independent quantitative method for assessing purine production that is reliable under all circumstances. The 24-h urinary uric acid value generally represents about two-thirds of the turnover in normal persons, but in gouty subjects with renal damage it may be a much smaller fraction [294]. The turnover of uric acid, as determined by isotope dilution, may not be a measure of production in subjects in whom solid urate contributes to the dilution process. In gouty subjects with tophi, turnover measurements may overestimate uric acid production. Excretion measurements always underestimate production.

Incorporation of Glycine, 5-Aminoimidazole-4-carboxamide, Hypoxanthine, or Adenine into Urinary Purine Bases   In both nongouty and gouty subjects, 5-aminoimidazole-4-carboxamide (AIC) [285, 312] and adenine [286] are rapidly converted to uric acid, following initial conversion to ribonucleotide forms. In all of five gouty subjects studied [312], incorporation of AIC into uric acid was somewhat greater than normal, irrespective of urinary urate excretion.

The degree of abnormality was magnified when appropriate corrections were made for dilution factors within the urate pool and for uricolysis, on the basis of simultaneous studies with ^{14}C-uric acid.

In a similar study with 8-^{13}C-adenine [286] three gouty subjects who were known overproducers of uric acid incorporated twice as much ^{13}C into urate as two controls.

When AIC or adenine was administered together with ^{15}N-glycine, a marked and comparable suppression of incorporation of ^{15}N into urinary uric acid was observed in normal and gouty subjects [285, 286, 312]. This could be attributed to activation of feedback inhibition of purine synthesis by nucleotides derived from AIC and adenine, or to diversion of PP-ribose-P from purine synthesis *de novo* during conversion of AIC and adenine to ribonucleotides. Following the administration of 1-^{14}C-glycine, there is a prompt and striking labeling of urinary hypoxanthine, indicative of the normal operation of an IMP cleavage pathway. Early labeling of adenine and 7-methylguanine indicates that other nucleotides are also subject to cleavage shortly after formation. Labeled hypoxanthine administered intravenously is promptly converted to uric acid. Labeled adenine in tracer dose is only slowly and sparingly converted to uric acid [306], in contrast to larger doses, which are converted to uric acid more rapidly [286]. Labeled AIC gives rise to extensive labeling of all urinary purine bases, in particular hypoxanthine and xanthine [307]. These findings strengthen the concept that IMP cleavage contributes to the rapid synthesis of uric acid in normal and gouty persons.

OVERPRODUCTION OF
URIC ACID IN GOUT

All tracer studies discussed thus far involve the isolation of uric acid from urine and the determination of its isotopic enrichment, following the administration of labeled uric acid or some labeled precursor of uric acid. These studies have demonstrated the overproduction of uric acid in a substantial percentage of gouty subjects but have not disclosed the mechanism.

Present concepts of control of purine synthesis *de novo* suggest three general categories of abnormalities that may potentially lead to overproduction of uric acid. These are (1) metabolic defects that increase the *substrate levels* of L-glutamine or phosphoribosylpyrophosphate; (2) defects that increase the *amount* or intrinsic *activity* of the first enzyme of the pathway of purine synthesis; or (3) defects that reduce the concentrations of one or more *negative effectors* (nucleotide inhibitors) of the first enzyme.

Studies of mechanisms of hyperuricemia in primary gout of idiopathic varieties will be presented first. Information on hyperuricemia and gout occurring as a consequence of known specific enzyme defects will be presented thereafter.

Role of L-Glutamine in Primary Hyperuricemia and Gout

L-Glutamine is a cosubstrate for the putative rate-limiting step of purine biosynthesis *de novo*. In 1963 Gutman and Yü [88] proposed a defect in glutamine metabolism as the basis for excessive purine biosynthesis in primary gout. The initial elements of the hypothesis were (1) the reduced ability of many gouty subjects to form urinary ammonia in response to an acid load, and (2) disproportionate labeling of $N(3 + 9)$ of urinary uric acid in gouty subjects following an oral test dose of ^{15}N-glycine. Both N3 and N9 of the purine ring and a major portion of urinary ammonia are derived from the amide nitrogen of glutamine. Later observations provided additional arguments for the hypothesis: these were (3) reduced renal clearance of glutamine [313], and (4) elevated levels of glutamate in plasma [313, 314] in gout. These results first led to the hypothesis that renal glutaminase was deficient [88] and that such a deficiency would cause a deviation of glutamine from ammonia production into purine biosynthesis *de novo*. Later it was suggested that a glutamate dehydrogenase deficiency would divert glutamate toward glutamine and purine biosynthesis. However, there is no direct evidence that either glutaminase or glutamate dehydrogenase is deficient in subjects with gout.

Glutamine as a Regulatory Substance The concentration values of glutamine in human liver are not known. In fed rats mean values range from 2.3 to 7 mM in cell water [2]. These values are above the Michaelis constant (K_m) for glutamine of amidophosphoribosyltransferase of rat liver, though not saturating. The K_m for glutamine of human placental and lymphoblast amidophosphoribosyltransferase is 1.6 mM [226, 228], which is higher than the glutamine concentrations of plasma of 0.5 to 0.7 mM [2, 313, 315]. The rate of purine biosynthesis in cultured human fibroblasts is dependent on the concentration of glutamine in the medium, since these cells are unable to synthesize glutamine [206]. The rate of purine biosynthesis, assessed by means of ^{15}N-glycine incorporation into urinary uric acid, is increased on a high protein diet in both control and gouty humans [316]. This effect could operate by way of an increased supply of nitrogen and glutamine. In rats and mice the intraperitoneal injection of glutamine leads to a 1.7- to 2.5-fold increase in ^{14}C-glycine incorporation into purines of liver and kidney [317]. These results indicate that glutamine concentrations can be rate-limiting even in tissues that have high activities of glutamine synthetase.

Renal Ammonia Production in Gout Later in this chapter we review the data on reduced renal ammonia production in patients with primary gout, first proposed by Gutman and Yü [318] as an intrinsic component of the metabolic defect leading to overproduction of uric acid. They suggested that glutamine not utilized in renal ammonia production became a substrate stimulant of purine biosynthesis *de novo*. Others have viewed reduced ammonia production in gout as subtle manifestation of renal damage or of aging [2].

If the renal tubular synthesis of ammonia limits the amount of uric acid synthesized by the liver, one would anticipate an inverse relationship between urinary ammonia and uric acid production rates. Swales and coworkers [319] failed to find such an inverse relationship over a wide range of urinary ammonia levels in three subjects. Thus, uric acid excretion (and presumably production) appears to be independent of the renal utilization of glutamine to form ammonia. The significance of the deficit in the urinary excretion of ammonium therefore remains conjectural.

Glycine and Glutamine Turnover in Gout 1-^{14}C-Glycine serves as a specific label of C-4 of the purine ring. No detectable recycling of isotope from the degradation products of 1-^{14}C-glycine into other carbon atoms of uric acid occurs in normal [305, 320] or gouty subjects [305].

When $1\text{-}^{14}C,\alpha\text{-}^{15}N$-glycine was administered, the $^{15}N/^{14}C$ ratio in urinary uric acid was significantly above 1 in both nongouty and gouty subjects, indicating a greater incorporation of ^{15}N than could be attributed to the entry of the intact glycine molecule into the eventual purine structure [305, 320]. When the urate molecule was degraded into fractions representing N7 and N(1 + 3 + 9), the latter fraction was found to contain 23 to 34 percent of the total ^{15}N on day 1 in normal subjects, and from 34 to 50 percent on day 1 in six gouty subjects [320, 321]. These studies indicated that amino nitrogen derived from glycine was incorporated into the N1 of purines by way of aspartic acid and into N3 and N9 by way of the amide nitrogen of glutamine in both nongouty and gouty subjects.

Further dissection of the urate molecule by Gutman and Yü [88] disclosed that the increase in percentage of ^{15}N in the N(1 + 3 + 9) fraction in gouty subjects was entirely accounted for by an increase in the percentage of ^{15}N in N(3 + 9), relative to values in their control subjects. Representative values in three control subjects, three gouty normal excretors, and three gouty overexcretors are shown in Table 50-10.

In the original paper of Gutman and Yü [88], the preferential labeling of N(3 + 9) in the gouty subjects was provisionally attributed to "glutamine amide nitrogen containing an unduly high concentration of N^{15}." Sperling et al. [304] have reexamined this proposition in four gouty subjects, three of whom had specific metabolic defects in which the driving force of excessive purine biosynthesis was known to be surplus PP-ribose-P. One patient was a mild overproducer with "idiopathic gout"; one was a marked overproducer with high-grade but "partial" HPRT deficiency; two were extraordinary overproducers with superactive PP-ribose-P synthetases, though of different variant types. Following administration of ^{15}N-glycine, disproportionately high labeling of N(3 + 9) was observed in all the gouty subjects, most marked in the most flamboyant overproducers (Fig. 50-26). Thus, the original observation of Gutman and Yü was confirmed.

The precursor glycine pool was sampled by periodic administration of benzoic acid and isolation of urinary hippuric acid. Similarly, the precursor glutamine pool was sampled by means of periodic administration of phenylacetic acid and isolation of

Table 50-10   Intramolecular distribution of uric acid ^{15}N

	Atom percent excess			
Subjects	Uric acid-^{15}N	$^{15}N7$	$^{15}N1$	^{15}N (3 + 9)
Controls (3)	0.063 (100)*	0.172 (68)	0.067 (26)	0.009 (6)
Gout normal excretors (3)	0.099 (100)	0.247 (61)	0.090 (22)	0.034 (17)
Gout over-excretors (3)	0.308 (100)	0.699 (53)	0.286 (24)	0.141 (23)

* Numbers in parentheses below percentages are the percent of total.
SOURCE: Day 2 values from Gutman and Yü [88].

the amide nitrogen of urinary phenylacetylglutamine. The enrichments and turnover kinetics of hippurate and phenylacetylglutamine were normal in the gouty subjects [304]. Thus, the increased labeling of N7 and N(3 + 9) in gout could not be attributed to excessive enrichments of precursor pools, and instead appeared to represent the utilization of increased fractions of precursor glycine and glutamine pools for purine biosynthesis per unit of time.

A computer model simulating the kinetics of the relevant reactions was constructed [322], utilizing as input data the observed enrichments of hippurate and phenylacetylglutamine. The relationships of the enrichments of glutamine amide N to glycine N with time were such that accelerations in the rates of purine biosynthesis, based on increasing concentrations of PP-ribose-P, resulted in progressive increases in the theoretical ratio $^{15}N(3 + 9)/^{15}N(3 + 9 + 7)$ in uric acid during the first few hours following labeling of the glycine pool. Thus, the increased fractional labeling of N3 and N9 of uric acid in gouty overproducers fed ^{15}N-glycine appears to be related to accelerated kinetics of purine biosynthesis per se, and to be independent of the type of metabolic or molecular abnormality responsible for the process [304]. Therefore, the observations of Table 50-10 do not necessarily implicate a specific metabolic defect of glutamate or glutamine in gout.

Plasma and Urinary Amino Acids in Gout   Plasma glutamine values are normal in gout and range from 7 to 10 mg/dl or 0.5 to 0.7 mM in both normal and excessive excretors of uric acid [313, 315]. Concentration values of total amino acids in plasma, exclusive of proline and aspartic acid, are about 2.7 mM in both nongouty [313] and gouty subjects [313, 314]. One report of hyperaminoacidemia in gout (2.6 μmol/ml) is probably attributable to low values in the control group (2.02 μmol/ml), which included a large number of hospitalized subjects recovering from acute infectious illnesses [323]. Elevations of individual plasma amino acid values in gout largely disappear when protein intakes are standardized in the two groups [313]. An exception is glutamic acid, which remains higher than in controls [313, 314] even after casein loading of both groups [314].

Fasting plasma glutamate values average 68 to 72 μM in gouty subjects, compared with 45 to 51 μM in controls [313, 314]. Erythrocyte values average 214 to 243 μM in gouty subjects, compared with 216 μM in controls [314]. Following oral glutamate loading, plasma levels rise to maximal values at 2 h in both gouty and nongouty subjects, but the increment in concentrations resulting from a standard load was 200 μM in the gouty subjects and only 97 μM in the controls. In both groups

Figure 50-26   Intramolecular distribution of ^{15}N in uric acid, expressed as percentage of total ^{15}N found in N(3 + 9), following administration of ^{15}N-glycine to control and gouty subjects. The shaded area includes essentially all values in the three control subjects. (*From Sperling et al.* [304], *by permission of* The Journal of Clinical Investigation.)

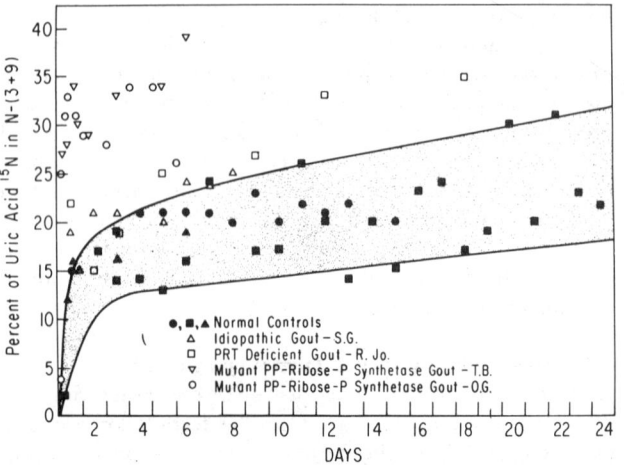

erythrocyte concentrations also rose substantially at 2 to 3 h, although the rise was slower and to higher peak values in the gouty subjects.

Elevations of plasma glutamate and urate concentrations develop at puberty in the asymptomatic hyperuricemic sons of gouty fathers. Plasma glycine values are distinctly lower in gouty subjects than in controls, and serine is slightly so [313].

The significance of the elevated plasma values of glutamate is difficult to assess. The turnover rates of free amino acid in plasma are very rapid, with half-lives ranging from 1 to 3 min. The half-life of glutamate is similar to that of other amino acids in dogs and humans. Free amino acids of erythrocytes are not in ready equilibrium with those of plasma. Their turnover is increased more than twentyfold during passage of erythrocytes through the capillary and sinusoid beds of liver and gut. These data suggest a direct transfer of amino acid between erythrocytes and tissue cells by a process that bypasses the plasma compartment. The transfer of amino acids by plasma and erythrocytes is frequently in opposite directions. At the time that liver is taking up amino acids from plasma, it is transferring amino acids to erythrocytes. Simultaneously, the fluxes in the gut and in skeletal muscle are in reverse directions [2].

The data on changes in concentrations of glutamate in plasma and erythrocytes of gouty subjects following glutamate or casein loads suggest a reduced rate of metabolism in the liver, and both a greater extent and more prolonged phase of transfer to erythrocytes in the liver. The latter may reflect the development of higher intrahepatic levels of glutamate and its slower metabolic disposition.

Role of Phosphoribosylpyrophosphate in Primary Hyperuricemia and Gout

In 1960 we postulated that an excess of PP-ribose-P was the cause of purine overproduction in some patients with primary gout [324]. This hypothesis was based on the excessive utilization of both glycine and a preformed purine analogue (aminoimidazolecarboxamide) for uric acid synthesis by certain gouty subjects, and the involvement of PP-ribose-P as a common substrate of both the *de novo* and salvage pathways.

The intracellular concentrations of PP-ribose-P are in the low ranges of the substrate-velocity curve of amidophosphoribosyltransferase (see above), and factors that raise their intracellular, perhaps chiefly intrahepatic, concentrations even slightly could have a significant influence on purine biosynthesis. The sigmoidal kinetics of the amidophosphoribosyltransferase reaction in the presence of nucleotide regulators is a reflection of a conformational change of the enzyme catalyzed by PP-ribose-P, resulting in enzyme activation. Thus synthesis of β-phosphoribosylamine is greatly increased by small increases in PP-ribose-P concentration within a critical range.

An excess of PP-ribose-P could result from overproduction of PP-ribose-P, or from its underutilization in some normally competing reaction. Each of the two rare examples of definitive enzymatic lesions in families with primary gout illustrates one of these mechanisms. The abnormally active PP-ribose-P synthetases result in PP-ribose-P overproduction; the HPRT deficiency states result in PP-ribose-P underutilization. These disorders are described below. They provide convincing demonstrations that excessive intracellular levels of PP-ribose-P result in remarkable accelerations of purine biosynthesis *de novo*. Whether these conditions are useful, if extreme, models of the mechanism of purine overproduction in patients with primary gout (in whom PP-ribose-P synthetase and HPRT activities are normal) is not currently known. Available data are summarized below.

Phosphoribosylpyrophosphate Turnover in Primary Gout The rate of turnover of PP-ribose-P has been assessed in control and gouty subjects by determination of the specific activity of the ribose moiety of PP-ribose-P following the administration of labeled glucose [325]. Net flux of carbon is from glucose-6-phosphate to ribose-5-phosphate via the oxidative limb of the hexose monophosphate shunt [326]. Normally, only a small fraction, perhaps one-sixth, of ribose-5-phosphate is converted to PP-ribose-P [326]. However, measures that increase the production of ribose-5-P may be reflected in an increased synthesis of PP-ribose-P and of purines (see above). An increase in turnover of PP-ribose-P from ribose-5-P should result in an increase in the specific activity of PP-ribose-P, provided that the pool of PP-ribose-P does not expand by a factor as large as the increase in PP-ribose-P production. The PP-ribose-P pool can be sampled periodically by administration of imidazoleacetic acid and isolation of its ribonucleoside derivative from the urine. The reactions occur in liver and are as follows:

Imidazoleacetic acid + ATP + PP-ribose-P ⟶
$$\text{IAA-ribose-P} + \text{ADP} + \text{PP}_i + \text{P}_i$$

$$\text{IAA-ribose-P} \longrightarrow \text{IAA-ribose} + \text{P}_i$$

A study was performed on seven control and nine gouty subjects, including three overexcretors of uric acid [325]. Specific activity values were determined in the ribose moiety of IAA-ribonucleoside isolated from the 0- to 10-h urine samples. Values in gouty subjects who excreted more than 600 mg uric acid per day were markedly increased, whereas those of subjects who excreted normal amounts were indistinguishable from controls. The results indicate an increase in turnover of PP-ribose-P in the three gouty overexcretors. The underlying metabolic defects in these patients are unknown, except that erythrocyte HPRT activity was normal in the one subject in whom it was assayed. The results in the gouty normal excretors do not exclude an increase in turnover of PP-ribose-P, for a raised rate of synthesis of PP-ribose-P could draw upon labeled glucose and unlabeled precursors equally, such that the specific activity of PP-ribose-P would remain unchanged, or, conversely, enhanced enrichment could be obscured by dilution within an enlarged PP-ribose-P pool.

Phosphoribosylpyrophosphate Concentrations in Gout Intracellular concentrations of PP-ribose-P are high in cultured fibroblasts of overproducer gouty subjects. These include patients with superactive variants of PP-ribose-P synthetase of three different subtypes [2], and patients with reduced HPRT activities due to enzyme deficiencies or kinetic abnormalities [2]. In addition Becker [327] has studied seven gouty overproducers of uric acid in whom PP-ribose-P synthetase and HPRT activities were normal but in whom fibroblast concentrations of PP-ribose-P were high. In two of this group intracellular concentrations of ribose-5-phosphate and rates of generation of PP-ribose-P were above normal. These results suggest a new subtype of primary gout resulting from an accelerated rate of generation of ribose-5-phosphate. This could result from a kinetic disturbance of either the oxidative or nonoxidative limb of the pentose phosphate pathway, because of an enzyme abnormality of the pathway itself or of another system which results in increased substrate flow through the pathway. The rate of purine biosynthesis *de novo*, as determined by measurement of accumulation of 5'-phosphoribosylformylglycine-amide in the presence of azaserine, was increased by 1.9 times to 6.3 over control values in all cell lines from overexcretors.

Concentrations of PP-ribose-P in erythrocytes of overproducer gouty subjects may or may not be elevated (Table 50-11). They are raised in patients with superactive PP-ribose-P synthetase variants and with high-grade HPRT deficiencies. Concentrations may be elevated in heterozygous carriers of HPRT deficiency whose erythrocyte enzyme activity values are in the intermediate range. However, erythrocyte PP-ribose-P concentrations may be normal in some heterozygotes for HPRT deficiency with evidence of abnormalities of purine production such as hyperuricemia, hyperuricaciduria, raised values of labeled glycine incorporation into uric acid, or increased turnover of the miscible uric acid pool [329]. Thus, normal erythrocyte values of PP-ribose-P do not exclude raised values in other tissues such as fibroblasts or, more importantly, liver. Normal values are found in erythrocytes of patients with glucose-6-phosphatase deficiency glycogen storage disease [204] where the enzyme defect is expressed in liver and kidney but not in the red cell.

Predicted hepatocellular concentrations and turnover of ribose-5-P and PP-ribose-P in specific genetic subtypes of gout are indicated in Table 50-12.

In most studies of other gouty subjects concentrations of PP-ribose-P are normal in erythrocytes and do not correlate with the height of the serum or urinary uric acid levels [2].

In one study of 43 young subjects (ages 10 to 23 years) with asymptomatic hyperuricemia, no individuals with raised values were found, and mean values were significantly *lower* than in the control group [328]. Interestingly, patients with active psoriasis are reported to have elevated PP-ribose-P concentrations in their erythrocytes [330].

The Japanese Sumo wrestlers maintain their massive size through gargantuan caloric intakes. They are enormously obese and show marked hypertriglyceridemia and hyperuricemia. They have recently been shown to have elevated erythrocyte concentrations of PP-ribose-P as well [331]. A significant positive correlation was found between plasma triglyceride and erythrocyte PP-ribose-P levels. There were no significant differences in erythrocyte PP-ribose-P synthetase, purine nucleoside phosphorylase, and HPRT activities between Sumo wrestlers and controls, but erythrocyte adenosine kinase, adenosine deaminase, and APRT activities and ATP concentrations were significantly raised in the Sumo wrestlers. Nishida et al. [331] postulate both increased turnover of adenine nucleotides and increased purine synthesis *de novo*. This study suggests analogies in metabolic interrelationships in Sumo wrestlers with those discussed immediately above, as well as with those discussed earlier in connection with fructose-induced hyperuricemia.

Phosphoribosylpyrophosphate Production Rates in Vitro In 1968, Hershko and coworkers [332] reported an increased rate of PP-ribose-P formation in erythrocytes from several gouty subjects. In 1971 Sperling and colleagues [333] extended these studies to 51 gouty subjects with urinary uric acid excretion values greater than 800 mg/day and normal HPRT activities, and found a mean increase of 35 percent ($p < 0.001$) in the incorporation values of adenine, hypoxanthine, and guanine into erythrocyte nucleotides during a 45-min incubation period. These results suggested an increase in the mean rate of generation of PP-ribose-P in this group of subjects. However, the spread of values was wide, and the majority of individual results fell within the normal range.

Further study of the patient with the most remarkable rates of purine base incorporation led to the discovery of the first example of gout resulting from a superactive mutant of PP-ribose-P synthetase [334]. All other patients with high values have now also been investigated for the possibility of an abnormality of PP-ribose-P synthetase activity, with negative results. Studies in the United States [214] have failed to show increased rates of production of PP-ribose-P in erythrocytes of patients with the common forms of primary gout.

Variations of Phosphoribosylpyrophosphate Concentration in Liver Purine biosynthesis *de novo* is ordinarily most active in liver. In the study of mechanisms of purine overproduction in primary gout, one would like to know the rates

Table 50-11 PP-Ribose-P concentration values in human erythrocytes, μM

Ref.	Controls	Primary hyperuricemia and gout, normal excretors	Lesch-Nyhan Hemizygote	Lesch-Nyhan Heterozygote	Partial HGPRT deficiency Hemizygote	Partial HGPRT deficiency Heterozygote	PP-Ribose-P synthetase variants	Glycogen storage disease type 1
	2.6 ± 0.7 [28]*	2.6 ± 0.7 [28]						
	4.4 ± 1.8 [12]		35.3 (21–50) [3]	4.2 (1.5–6.5) [3]				
	3.1 ± 0.5 [10]	2.7 ± 0.5 [14]	38.8 ± 4.0 [7]		4.6 ± 1.3 [3]			2.2, 2.4 [2]
	3.0 ± 0.3 [10]	2.8 ± 0.4 [17]†						
328‡	1.3 ± 0.4 [13]	0.9 ± 0.3 [43]						
	6.1 ± 3.1 [9]						13.1, 17.3 [2]	
	8.0 ± 1.0 [13♂]§							
	11.6 ± 2.8 [18♀]§			8.5 (6.0–10.1) [4]		17.7 (10.1–25.2) [6]		

* Numbers of subjects in brackets.
† Eleven of 17 patients studied while on allopurinol, which lowers PP-ribose-P concentrations.
‡ New entry. References to other studies can be found in Table 43-14 of the fourth edition of this text [2].
§ Assayed by a method that utilizes endogenous APRT, blocks new synthesis of PP-ribose-P by addition of 2,3-DPG, and avoids a heat and filtration step. Values by this method are higher than those obtained with earlier methods.

Table 50-12 Predicted intracellular concentrations and turnovers of ribose 5-phosphate and phosphoribosylpyrophosphate in specific genetic subtypes of gout

Ribose 5-P		PP-Ribose-P		
Concentration	Turnover	Concentration	Turnover	Subtype
↑	↑	↑	↑	Glucose 6-phosphatase ↓
				Pentose phosphate pathway ↓
N or ↓	↑	↑	↑	PP-ribose P synthetase ↑
N	N	↑	↑	HPRT ↓
N or ↓	↑	N or ↓	↑	Amidophosphoribosyl-transferase ↑ or feedback resistance

of production and steady state concentrations of phosphoribosylpyrophosphate in the liver and how these may be influenced by dietary factors, drugs, and hormones. Since studies of this type are unavailable in humans, attempts have been made to obtain relevant data in animals. Lalanne and Henderson [220] reported a twofold diurnal variation of phosphoribosylpyrophosphate concentrations in quick-frozen liver of mice. Animals were fed a chow diet between 1800 and 0800 h. Hepatic PP-ribose-P values reached a maximum at 0100 h, then declined and stayed at basal levels between 0800 and 1800 h. Intraperitoneal injections of insulin, epinephrine, glucagon, tolbutamide, or 2-deoxyglucose (all of which should elevate intrahepatic concentrations of glucose-6-phosphate) brought about prompt, transient increases of ten- or twelvefold in liver phosphoribosylpyrophosphate concentrations. These studies provide some insight into mechanisms by which environmental factors could influence the rates of uric acid production in gout, if, for example, patients with primary gout regulated the production of phsophoribosylpyrophosphate less effectively than normal when exposed to certain dietary, physiologic, or pharmacologic stimuli.

Krebs and Eggleston [335] have summarized the regulation of the pentose phosphate cycle in rat liver. The rate of the cycle is controlled at the glucose-6-phosphate dehydrogenase (G-6-PD) step. In response to a diet containing excess carbohydrate the capacity of G-6-PD and 6-phosphogluconate dehydrogenase may increase up to tenfold within 3 days. G-6-PD is inhibited by NADPH; when the ratio [NADPH]/[NADP⁺] is greater than 8, inhibition is almost complete. The calculated ratio in rat liver in vivo is 100. Thus, the enzyme must be almost completely inhibited in vivo, unless this ratio is changed. The main NADPH-consuming process is the synthesis of fatty acid from carbohydrate where two molecules of NADPH are used for each acetyl CoA added to a fatty acid chain. Fatty acid synthesis occurs when the diet contains excess carbohydrate, i.e., when more carbohydrate is ingested than can be broken down or deposited as glycogen. Thus, in the presence of carbohydrate excess and active lipogenesis, the inhibition of G-6-PD by NADPH will be released, and the flux through the pentose phosphate pathway will be increased. The additional pentose phosphate will be potentially available for synthesis of PP-ribose-P and purine ribonucleotides. Gumaa and McLean [336] have found a correlation in rats between the rate of lipogenesis and the rate of purine biosynthesis de novo following carbohydrate feeding. They attribute the relationship to the regeneration of NADP during lipogenesis and the control of the oxidative limb of the pentose phosphate pathway by the [NADPH]/[NADP] ratio. NADPH inhibition of G-6-PD will also be released by reaction of the cofactor with oxidized glu-

tathione (GSSG) in the reaction catalyzed by glutathione reductase (see below). The main source of GSSG is the glutathione peroxidase reaction which utilizes hydrogen peroxide, an important source of which is the oxidation of hypoxanthine and xanthine by xanthine oxidase. Thus, obesity, hypertriglyceridemia, purine nucleotide biosynthesis, and uric acid production may be linked by these metabolic relationships.

Role of Abnormal Properties of Amidophosphoribosyltransferase

When 5-amino-4-imidazolecarboxamide (AIC) [285], adenine [286], azathioprine [288], or allopurinol [337] is administered to normal subjects, there is inhibition of purine biosynthesis de novo. Comparable inhibition is found in normal excretor and overexcretor gouty subjects, except that patients who are HPRT-deficient do not respond to azathioprine or allopurinol with suppression in purine production [288, 300]. They do respond normally to adenine [286], which is converted to adenylic acid by APRT and (in tissue culture) to 6-methylmercaptopurine ribonucleoside [338], which is converted to its ribonucleotide by adenosine kinase and then behaves as an analogue of inosinic acid [284]. Thus, in gouty subjects, including those who are HPRT-deficient, both the 6-aminopurine ribonucleotide and 6-hydroxypurine ribonucleotide control sites of the amidophosphoribosyltransferase are intact. This has also been demonstrated directly in leukocyte extracts [339].

In 1968, Henderson and coworkers [338] found that fibroblasts cultured from two remarkable overproducer gouty subjects were relatively insensitive to the effects of adenine, hypoxanthine, and 6-methylmercaptopurine ribonucleoside on the early steps of purine biosynthesis. They postulated an alteration of one of the regulatory sites of amidophosphoribosyltransferase. However, both fibroblast lines had elevated levels of PP-ribose-P, a finding inconsistent with the proposed defect. Both these subjects have since been found to have increased PP-ribose-P synthetase activities [339]. The insensitivity to nucleotides was probably due to the increased concentration of PP-ribose-P. Thus, there are as yet no examples of gout attributable to overactive or improperly regulated amidophosphoribosyltransferase.

Increased Activity of Amidophosphoribosyltransferase
There is at present no evidence for or against this concept in hyperuricemic subjects, for current techniques do not permit the direct assay of amidophosphoribosyltransferase activity in accessible tissue in humans.

Role of Possible Deficiencies of Ribonucleotide Regulators in Primary Hyperuricemia and Gout

The modulations of activities of PP-ribose-P synthetase and amidophosphoribosyltransferase by purine ribonucleotides fail to reach total inhibition of purine biosynthesis *de novo* because of their continuous removal into other cofactors and nucleic acids, and catabolism to free bases and uric acid. The latter process is opposed by APRT and HPRT reactions, which reconvert purine bases to ribonucleotides. Continuous purine overproduction could result from any process that increases the rate of removal of purine ribonucleotides or decreases the rate of operation of salvage pathways, particularly in liver where the bulk of purine biosynthesis *de novo* takes place. The hyperuricemia induced by fructose infusion in normal subjects, or by hypoglycemia in patients with glucose-6-phosphatase deficiency, has been explained in terms of the first mechanism [271, 278].

In hyperuricemia secondary to increased nucleic acid turnover, e.g., in polycythemia vera or chronic hemolytic anemia, the continuous removal of ribonucleotides into nucleic acids is presumed to release the early enzymes of purine biosynthesis from inhibition, resulting in compensatory increases in rates of purine production *de novo*. Rapid degradation of nucleotides could have the same effect in specific hyperuricemic patients. In one overproducer gouty subject studied by Seegmiller et al. [286], the rate constant of turnover of labeled adenine was twice that found in two other gouty subjects and two controls. In addition, fibroblasts cultured from a gouty patient who had an abnormally rapid rate of breakdown of azathioprine to uric acid in vivo showed a twentyfold increase in the rate of deamination of adenylic acid to inosinic acid [338]. These two studies form part of the basis of a postulated increase in activity of AMP deaminase in primary gout, put forward by Hers and van den Berghe [265]. This hypothesis will be discussed below.

In patients with HPRT deficiency, the reduced conversion of hypoxanthine, guanine, and xanthine to ribonucleotides may result in reduced levels of regulatory nucleotides. However, analyses of nucleotide content in cultured fibroblasts [224] or lymphoblasts [340] of Lesch-Nyhan patients do not support this hypothesis. Subjects who are partially deficient in APRT activity do not show abnormalities of purine metabolism attributable to this defect [341].

In patients treated with allopurinol there is both a reduced formation of uric acid due to inhibition of xanthine oxidase [337] and a partial inhibition of purine biosynthesis *de novo*, manifested by a reduction in total purine excretion (uric acid + xanthine + hypoxanthine) [337, 342], and a lower rate of incorporation of isotopic glycine into urinary uric acid [343]. The reduction in rate of purine biosynthesis *de novo* presumably results from inhibition of xanthine oxidase activity, increased reconversions of hypoxanthine and xanthine to ribonucleotide stages, and the combined effects of raised concentrations of regulatory ribonucleotides and reduced concentration of PP-ribose-P because of its enhanced consumption in the phosphoribosyltransferase reaction. Predictably, this effect of allopurinol on total purine excretion does not occur in patients who are deficient in HPRT activity [300, 344].

The synergistic nature of feedback inhibition of the amido-phosphoribosyltransferase by adenyl and guanyl nucleotides suggests that relaxation of control could result from a nonoptimal ratio of 6-aminopurine ribonucleotides and 6-hydroxy-purine ribonucleotides. Weissmann and Gutman [345] proposed a nucleotide imbalance in explanation of the increased excretion of 7-methyl-8-hydroxyguanine and decreased excretion of 6-succinoaminopurine in acute gout. Patients with gout given 1-^{14}C-glycine show greater than normal labeling of urinary 7-methylguanine, but not of urinary adenine [306]. These observations are tantalizing, but no conclusions can be drawn at present.

Xanthine Oxidase Activity in Gout

Carcassi et al. [280] described a fourfold mean increase of hepatic xanthine oxidase activity in eight patients with gout and excessive excretion of uric acid. Jejunal xanthine oxidase activity was normal. Although such an alteration could theoretically be a primary cause of increased uric acid synthesis in some patients, several studies suggest that the raised activity of xanthine oxidase is secondary to increased purine ribonucleotide production resulting from other disturbances. The highest activity for xanthine oxidase was found in a patient with HPRT deficiency as the primary defect [281]. Xanthine oxidase is a readily induced enzyme whose activity in liver is increased by high protein feeding in rats [346], by injections of xanthine in protein-depleted mice [347], or by administration of inosine in chicks [348]. In humans, feeding of ribonucleic acid, hypoxanthine, or 2-ethylamino-1, 3-thiadiazole, or infusion of fructose, results in elevation of hepatic xanthine oxidase activity [281]. The increases following oral administration of RNA are equal in magnitude to those found in the gouty overexcretors. Nevertheless, an increase in hepatic xanthine oxidase activity, whether primary or secondary, should enhance the rate of conversion of hypoxanthine and xanthine to uric acid, reduce the amount of hypoxanthine available for reconversion to regulatory purine ribonucleotides, spare PP-ribose-P for purine biosynthesis *de novo*, and provide additional H_2O_2 for oxidation of NADPH, by way of GSSG, thus possibly increasing the rate of PP-ribose-P production. This state of affairs in the gouty subject is the reverse of the situation created by allopurinol and may help to explain the sensitivity of overproducer gouty subjects to the inhibitory effects of allopurinol. Hepatic xanthine oxidase may participate in regulating the rate of purine biosynthesis *de novo* in gout, whether its activity is increased by induction or inhibited by drugs.

Purine Biosynthesis *de novo* in Isolated Cells in Gout

^{14}C-glycine incorporation into adenine and guanine residues of DNA and "insoluble" RNA of leukocytes of subjects with primary gout was reported to be greater than in controls [349, 350], but it was also greater in leukocytes of patients with chronic renal failure and of normal females, but normal in males with asymptomatic hyperuricemia. Clearly, this method is too insensitive to be useful. Kamoun et al. [351] studied the incorporation of ^{14}C-formate into N-formyl glycinamide ribonucleotide (FGAR) by human leukocytes when the subsequent reaction was blocked with azaserine. The average synthesis of labeled FGAR was higher in gouty subjects without therapy than in controls, but the overlap of values was extensive. Incorporation values were not elevated in patients with hyperuricemia secondary to renal insufficiency. This method appears to give results that are similar to those obtained with ^{14}C-glycine in vivo, although a direct comparison of the two techniques has not been conducted in the same individuals.

EXCRETION OF URIC ACID IN GOUT

Renal Mechanisms of Uric Acid Excretion in Normal Humans

Studies of the renal handling of uric acid have generated models of two-, three-, and four-component systems. Initially it was thought that uric acid was processed in humans by glomerular filtration followed by extensive though incomplete tubular reabsorption [352]. Next, a three-component system was proposed on the basis of evidence for tubular secretion of uric acid in animals and humans [353]. More recently several investigators have proposed a four-component model: of glomerular filtration, early proximal tubular reabsorption, tubular secretion, and finally postsecretory tubular reabsorption (Fig. 50-27) [354–356].

Within the vertebrate phylum there is an impressive variety of patterns for the renal disposition of uric acid [2, 357]. In some animals, e.g., birds, reptiles, guinea pigs, Dalmatian coach hounds, and certain species of monkeys, net secretion of urate is the rule. In others net reabsorption is the rule, e.g., rats, non-Dalmatian dogs, cats, several species of New World monkeys, the great apes, and humans. The rabbit occupies an intermediate position, some specimens demonstrating net secretion, others net reabsorption. In many of these species there is evidence for bidirectional transport [2, 358]. The species most

nearly comparable to the human in the renal handling of urate is the chimpanzee, and next the *Cebus* monkey. The ratio C_{urate}/GFR is about 0.07 to 0.11 in these species [27], as in humans. Both species respond appropriately to substances that are uricosuric in humans [2]. The discussion that follows emphasizes studies performed in humans or in these lower primates.

Glomerular Filtration of Uric Acid   Glomerular ultrafiltration of uric acid was first conclusively demonstrated by micropuncture studies of Bowman's space in the snake and frog in which urate concentrations in the glomerular fluid were the same as in plasma. Studies in the rat also demonstrate nearly complete ultrafilterability of urate [359, 360]. It is reasonable to assume that ultrafiltration of uric acid also occurs in humans.

Whether all urate in plasma is freely filtrable at the glomerulus is uncertain. As reviewed above, some urate may be bound to plasma protein. This fraction is thought to be less than 5 percent. Thus, it may not be strictly valid to assume that the filtered load of urate can be estimated by the product of plasma urate concentration × glomerular filtration rate. There may be a small systematic error in the calculation of the fractional excretion of uric acid, i.e., the quantity of uric acid excreted/quantity of uric acid filtered, and also in the calculation of the quantity of uric acid reabsorbed.

An important variable not previously considered is a monophasic circadian fluctuation in fractional uric acid excretion (uric acid clearance/creatinine clearances) with afternoon values about 50 percent greater than those obtained during the night [361]. Variations in fractional uric acid clearance did not correspond with variations in creatinine clearance, which showed a biphasic rhythm with highest values in the morning and evening hours. Thus the fluctuations in fractional uric acid clearance probably reflect variations of tubular to a greater extent than glomerular processes.

Reabsorption of Uric Acid   Comparisons of renal clearances of uric acid with those of inulin or creatinine disclose a mean ratio of about 0.07 to 0.10 in normal human subjects. If complete glomerular ultrafiltration of plasma urate is assumed, such clearance ratios indicate tubular reabsorption of at least 90 to 93 percent of filtered urate.

Figure 50-27   Five possible models for urate transport in humans. The stippled arrows represent filtered urate, solid arrows represent urate reabsorption, and open arrows indicate either tubular secretion of urate or urate remaining in tubular fluid after reabsorption. Numerical values indicate hypothetical orders of magnitude of the transport processes. A. The traditional view, in which most filtered urate is reabsorbed and all secretion takes place subsequently. B. No presecretory reabsorption takes place; all reabsorption occurs distally to secretion. C and D. Varying amounts of pre- and postsecretory reabsorption take place. E. Secretion and reabsorption could occur simultaneously along a substantial length of the renal tubule. (*From Rieselbach and Steele [354], by permission of The American Journal of Medicine.*)

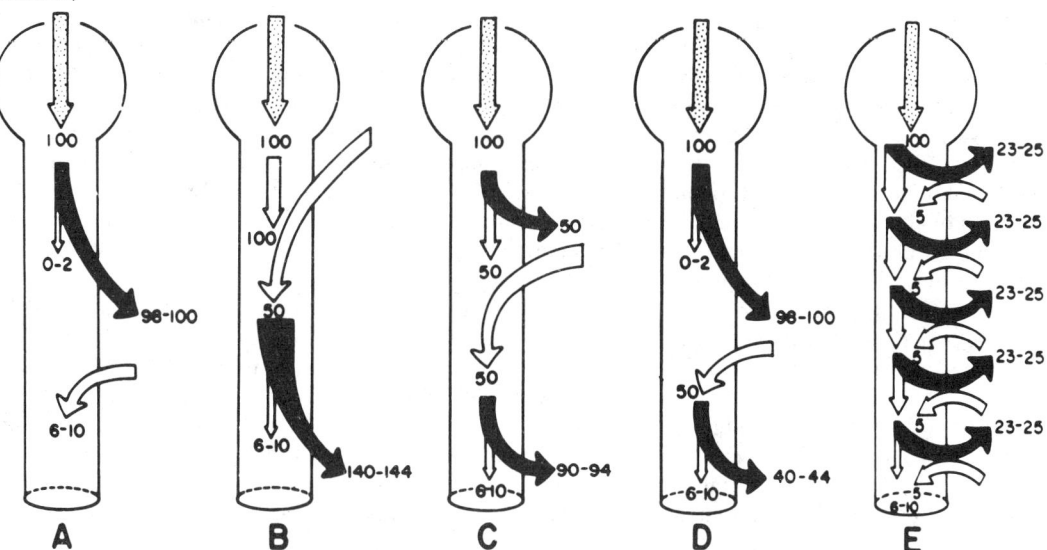

In 1950, Berliner et al. [352] infused lithium urate into volunteers, producing marked hyperuricemia. As the filtered load of urate was raised, the difference between filtered and excreted urate increased progressively. They concluded that the maximum rate of urate reabsorption (T_m) was about 15 mg/(min · 1.73 m^2) of surface area in normal humans, but pointed out that the capacity for urate reabsorption was so great that it almost certainly remained unsaturated under normal circumstances. They discussed urate excretion at filtered loads of less than T_m in terms of the affinity of the reabsorptive system for urate and the influence of flow rates. This excellent study did not consider urate secretion, which in 1950 was regarded as limited to birds and reptiles.

Almost all studies of uric acid reabsorption indicate that the process takes place in the proximal tubule. Most localizations have been made with the stop-flow technique. In animals exhibiting net reabsorption of urate under control conditions[2], mongrel dog, cat, Cebus monkey, and certain rabbits, a distinct reabsorptive concentration minimum is seen in samples corresponding to the proximal tubule. In some animals in which a secretory peak is seen under control conditions [2], the Dalmatian, guinea pig, and certain other rabbits, inhibition of secretion by probenecid allows demonstration of proximal reabsorption by the stop-flow technique.

In studies in the rat employing microperfusion and microinjection techniques and ^{14}C-urate, proximal tubular reabsorption has been observed in both early and late segments of the proximal tubule [2]. Free-flow micropuncture studies following the fate of intravenously injected ^{14}C-urate have also demonstrated reabsorption in the first part of the proximal tubule, and in agreement with other studies [360] disclosed secretion in the late proximal tubule [357]. The pattern is one of net proximal reabsorption with some secretion of urate in that segment [358].

Micropuncture and microperfusion experiments in the rat employing *chemical* determinations of urate [362, 363] support the concept of bidirectional transport of urate in the proximal tubule, but the data suggest that the secretory flux exceeds the reabsorptive. Since in the whole kidney net reabsorption is the rule, such results require a major reabsorptive site for urate beyond the proximal tubule in the rat. Henle's loop has been suggested [362]. However, since signs of so large a secretory flux do not appear in studies which employ ^{14}C-urate, it is possible that results with the chemical method are complicated by intrarenal synthesis of uric acid in the rat [364].

Results of free-flow micropuncture studies in *Cebus albifrons* are essentially in accord with results of stop-flow experiments in specifying that most urate reabsorption occurs in the proximal tubule [365]. However, distal tubular fluid contains a greater fraction of filtered urate than does final urine. This finding, confirmed in additional animals [358], may signify reabsorption of a small fraction of filtered or secreted urate in collecting ducts. Thus, although net urate reabsorption occurs largely in proximal tubules in all animals in which the process has been localized (with the exception of the rat, where it may take place in the loop of Henle), the possibility exists of reabsorption in more distal segments, at least in certain animals.

NATURE OF THE REABSORPTIVE MECHANISM   Available evidence suggests that urate reabsorption occurs by a mechanism of *active transport*. In lower animals ouabain and metabolic poisons inhibit urate reabsorption [2]. In nonhuman primates

and humans the concentration of uric acid in urine may approach one-tenth the concentration in plasma during diuresis and inhibition of urate secretion with pyrazinoate [366]. In free-flow micropuncture samples in the chimpanzee and monkey the concentrations of urate average 0.6 of the concentrations in plasma, and in individual samples may be as low as 0.2 [358]. Thus, urate reabsorption may occur against a concentration gradient. According to Weiner and Fanelli [358] the transepithelial potential difference in the proximal tubule is too small to account for this phenomenon by passive forces.

The response of proximal sodium reabsorption to changes in extracellular fluid volume or filtration fraction has been attributed to changes of hydrostatic and effective oncotic pressure ("physical factors") in the peritubular capillaries [367]. Tubular reabsorption of many solutes in addition to sodium is affected. Uric acid is among the solutes that respond to changes in "physical factors" [368].

The pH of the fluid in the proximal tubule is approximately the same as that of plasma [369]. Since the pK_{a_1} of uric acid is 5.75, over 98 percent of this compound will be in the form of the monovalent urate ion in the proximal tubule. Excretion of uric acid is largely independent of changes of pH of urine [370], but acidification is a distal tubular function, and would not be expected to affect proximal processes. In highly acidified distal tubular fluid, uric acid will be minimally ionized. One might anticipate that uric acid would then undergo reabsorption by nonionic diffusion. If so, the contribution to urate reabsorption is too small to be readily detected, for unlike other weak organic acids, the overall process of uric acid reabsorption does not follow principles of nonionic diffusion [358].

Secretion of Uric Acid   As indicated above, net secretion of urate occurs in birds, reptiles, guinea pigs, Dalmatian coach hounds, some individual rabbits, and certain species of monkeys. Also in virtually all animals that exhibit net tubular reabsorption of urate, there is evidence of bidirectional urate transport.

In mammals in which net urate secretion is normal stop-flow studies indicate that secretion is a function of the proximal tubule. Studies with isolated rabbit tubules localize secretion to the proximal straight tubule with little if any secretion in the proximal convoluted tubule or the cortical collecting tubule [371]. In contrast, net secretion of uric acid can be demonstrated in the proximal convoluted tubule of the pig during free-flow micropuncture [372]. Proximal tubular secretory flux of urate has also been demonstrated in mongrel dogs and *C. albifrons* [379], in which net reabsorption is normal. In addition, small secretory fluxes for urate in the distal nephron have been reported in the *Cebus* monkey as well as in the dog in some experiments, although not in others [2]. Thus, while evidence for proximal secretory flux seems convincing, that for an additional small distal secretory flux in mammals is inconclusive.

The first evidence for uric acid secretion in humans was published in 1950 when Praetorius and Kirk [373] reported the case of a young man with a plasma urate concentration of less than 0.6 mg/dl, and a urate/inulin clearance ratio of 1.46. Subsequently, Gutman and coworkers [374] achieved urate/inulin clearance ratios as high as 1.23 in normal subjects following urate loading, mannitol diuresis, and large doses of probenecid. Each of these studies indicated net tubular secretion of urate in humans under these special conditions. The biphasic effects of salicylate upon uric acid excretion are interpreted as representing inhibition of urate secretion at low salicylate doses, with urate retention, plus inhibition of urate reabsorption at higher salicylate doses, with urate diuresis [375].

The site within the human nephron where uric acid secretion ocurs is not definitely established. In a study of this process in humans, the proximal nephron transported uric acid from plasma to tubular fluid but the distal nephron was unable to do so [376].

NATURE OF THE SECRETORY PROCESS   In animals in which net secretion occurs, urate moves into the proximal lumen against a concentration gradient and against a small electrical potential difference. Thus, the process qualifies as an active transport mechanism. In animals in which net movement of urate is reabsorptive, secretory flux of urate normally proceeds in the direction of a favorable concentration gradient. However, the process can be inhibited by certain chemicals [2] and possesses specificity, and therefore cannot represent simple diffusion. Weiner and Fanelli [358] have evidence that the mechanism is capable of transport against a gradient and is therefore active. In the chimpanzee the mercurial diuretic mersalyl is sufficiently uricosuric to unmask net secretion of urate. These results suggest a model involving two oppositely oriented active transport systems in the proximal tubule. Recent studies utilizing isolated brush border membrane vesicles from rabbit kidney confirm that active nature of uric acid transport [377].

SECRETION OF OTHER ORGANIC ANIONS   Several authors have proposed that urate is secreted by the same mechanism responsible for the secretion of other organic anions, e.g., p-aminohippurate (PAH) [2]. Two types of observation support the concept that urate and PAH are secreted by different transport systems. In the reptile, transport of PAH and urate is not strictly coextensive along the nephron [378]. In chimpanzees [366, 379] and humans [380], pyrazinoate reduces urate excretion to very low levels at concentrations that do not influence clearance or T_m of PAH.

A number of organic acids will inhibit uric acid excretion in animals and humans. These include lactate [381], β-hydroxybutyrate [382], acetoacetate [382], branched chain keto acids [383], and salicylate [375]. These effects have been interpreted as representing inhibition of tubular secretion of urate [375, 384], for which there is evidence in micropuncture studies [385].

Postsecretory Reabsorption   A number of observations have proved difficult to accommodate within the model of filtration, early proximal reabsorption, and later proximal secretion. In patients with Wilson's disease [386] and Hodgkin's disease [387], and hypouricemia associated with raised renal urate clearance values, pyrazinamide suppresses the increased uricaciduria. Also, in both chimpanzees [388] and humans [353, 389] the uricosuric response to probenecid is virtually abolished by pretreatment with pyrazinamide or pyrazinoate. Finally, the uricosuric respones to intravenous chlorothiazide [353] or volume expansion with hypertonic sodium chloride [390] are substantially diminished by pretreatment with pyrazinamide. If these effects were to be interpreted within the three-component model, one would need to conclude that the

renal tubular dysfunctions of Wilson's and Hodgkin's diseases, and the administration of probenecid, chlorothiazide, and saline solution, resulted in enhanced tubular secretion of urate which was suppressible by pyrazinamide.

In 1973, Steele and Boner [389], Steele [391], and Diamond and Paolino [355] proposed a more tenable model to account for these observations, in which extensive postsecretory reabsorption of urate was postulated. In this model the effects of pyrazinamide are explained in terms of reduced secretory delivery to the late reabsorptive sites. The location of the postsecretory reabsorptive process could be coextensive with the secretory mechanism, or separate and distal to it, or both. The latter possibilities are supported in some animals by evidence for urate reabsorption beyond the proximal tubule, as cited above. Sorensen and Levinson [392] have described one patient who exhibited an exaggerated increase in the ratio of uric acid to creatinine clearance after RNA loading. A reduced uricosuric response of this patient to benzbromarone led them to suggest that this patient had a reduced postsecretory reabsorption of uric acid.

Quantitative Estimates of Reabsorption and Secretion   Bidirectional uric acid transport in humans is established by the evidence cited above. However, the relative contributions of tubular reabsorption and tubular secretion to uric acid excretion have been difficult to ascertain. In human beings mean urate/inulin (or creatinine) ratios of 1.23 to 1.46 have been observed in unusual situations [373, 374]. In the chimpanzee a ratio of 1.78 was observed following administration of mersalyl [358]. These figures provide minimal estimates of unidirectional urate secretion, for there is no evidence in any of these studies that urate reabsorption was reduced to zero or that secretion was unimpaired by the drugs or procedures employed. The data suggest that secretion may be of the same order of magnitude as filtration, and therefore that reabsorption may be very much greater than might be deduced from control clearance periods.

Attempts to quantitate secretion and reabsorption are further complicated by the recent demonstration that at least 7 percent of the uric acid excreted in the urine in the rat is synthesized in the kidney (nephrogenic uric acid) [364]. The first attempt to estimate transport constants gave an apparent K_m of 0.41 mM and V_{max} of 4.7 pmol/(min·mm) for net secretory flux in the rat proximal tubule [393].

THE PYRAZINAMIDE SUPPRESSION TEST   Following administration of pyrazinamide, urinary uric acid excretion is transiently reduced to very low levels without change of glomerular filtration rate [394, 395]. Studies in the dog [396] and rat [397] established that pyrazinamide was a potent inhibitor of tubular secretion of uric acid. The increased urinary uric acid excretion that followed oral administration of RNA or intravenous infusion of lithium urate [163] in humans was substantially suppressed by pyrazinamide. The pyrazinamide suppression test [391] rests on the assumptions that pyrazinamide blocks tubular secretion of urate completely and has no effect on tubular reabsorption of urate. It was introduced as a means for evaluating the relative contributions of incomplete tubular reabsorption of filtered urate and of secreted urate to the excretory process.

The test is performed by determining uric acid excretion before and immediately after the administration of pyrazinamide or its metabolite, pyrazinoic acid (PZA), in a dose sufficient to give maximal suppression of uric acid excretion. The decrement in uric acid excretion after PZA administration has been taken as a quantitative measure of uric acid secretion. In addition, the difference between filtered load of uric acid and uric acid excretion at the time of maximal PZA effect has been taken as a quantitative measure of uric acid reabsorption. On the basis of this test, reabsorption of filtered urate was judged to be 98 to 99 percent complete in normal humans. Tubular secretion was judged to account for 80 to 85 percent of excreted uric acid in normal persons [394, 398].

The model as initially constructed envisioned reabsorption occurring early and secretion late within the proximal tubule and made no allowance for postsecretory reabsorption. The likely existence of postsecretory reabsorption compromises the use of pyrazinamide in the dissection of renal processes of urate handling, for reduction in delivery of the secretory load to later reabsorptive sites could affect the percentage of urate reabsorbed at these sites. It is also not established that PZA blocks secretion completely, or that it is without effect upon reabsorption even in the relatively small doses used. Weiner and Tinker [399] have shown that very large doses of PZA cause a uricosuric response in the dog and chimpanzee. These results suggest that large doses of PZA inhibit uric acid reabsorption as well as secretion. Kramp et al. [400] have demonstrated directly by micropuncture that PZA inhibits uric acid reabsorption in the proximal nephron of the rat. In view of these limitations, results obtained with the pyrazinamide test in humans, even when its interpretation takes account of postsecretory reabsorption [354], must be regarded as tentative.

Some Effects on Renal Clearance of Uric Acid

ESTROGENS   The serum urate concentration is relatively low in children, increases in males and to a lesser extent also in females at puberty, and in females again at the menopause. Changes in renal urate clearance are at least partly responsible. The mean clearance of uric acid is 2.3 and 1.2 ml/min higher in females than in males [2]. Nicholls and associates [401] found that exogenous estrogens produced a significant increase in mean C_{urate} values from 6.3 to 9.1 ml/min in 22 transexual males.

REDUCED NEPHRON POPULATION   In the chronically diseased kidney, urate secretion is markedly reduced in association with a striking increase in the fractional excretion of filtered urate. When renal disease is severe, as much as 45 percent of filtered urate may escape reabsorption and be excreted. Thus although substrate-regulated tubular secretion is the principal homeostatic mechanism for urate excretion in normal and moderately diseased kidneys, glomerular filtration assumes this role in far advanced renal disease [402].

Renal Mechanisms of Uric Acid Excretion in Gout

Uric Acid Clearance and Excretion Rates   A careful comparison of uric acid clearances and excretion rates over wide but comparable ranges of filtered loads of urate indicates that most gouty subjects have a lower C_{urate}/C_{inulin} ratio than nongouty subjects (Table 50-13) [71, 162, 403]. This ratio

increases in gouty subjects as in normal controls when the plasma urate level is raised by feeding of RNA or by infusion of lithium urate, but higher plasma urate values are required in gouty subjects to achieve a given clearance ratio [404, 405]. When the data from these and other studies were plotted by Simkin [406] on semilogarithmic coordinates as rates of uric acid excretion at various serum urate levels, the excretion curve was shifted such that gouty subjects required serum urate values about 2 mg/dl higher than those of controls in order to achieve equivalent uric acid excretion rates (Fig. 50-28). The displacement of the curve in gouty subjects is not a consequence of sustained hyperuricemia, for in leukemic subjects the rates of uric acid excretion are generally normal or increased in relation to the titration curve in nongouty subjects. Most patients with idiopathic gout will exhibit the renal defect as defined by the abnormal substrate-velocity curve. In Simkin's analysis of six published studies the kidneys of overproducer gouty subjects (38 of the 73 gouty patients) were "no less handicapped" than those of other gouty subjects [406]. Patients with gout due to one of the specific enzymatic defects usually exhibit a normal uric acid/inulin (or creatinine) clearance ratio [162].

Theoretically, the shift in the substrate-velocity curve in gouty subjects could be due to (1) reduced filtration of uric acid, (2) enhanced reabsorption, or (3) decreased secretion. Attempts to localize the site of the defect of uric acid transport in the nephron have been thwarted by the limitations of available techniques. The only technique used to differentiate among these possibilities has been the pyrazinamide suppression test. The problems in the interpretation of the pyrazinamide suppression test results are such that specific conclusions based on this test alone are difficult to justify. At present there are no unequivocal data to establish any one of these three mechanisms.

Glomerular Filtration   About 5 percent of plasma urate may be bound in vivo, and not freely filterable at the glomerulus. Enhanced binding of urate to proteins in gouty subjects could result in precisely the abnormal substrate-velocity curve described above. At present, however, there is no evidence for such enhanced binding in gouty subjects studied in the United States or in Europe. In fact, reduced urate binding to proteins has been described in some gouty subjects [155].

Tubular Reabsorption   Increased reabsorption of uric acid as a cause of the altered substrate-velocity curve has not received serious consideration. On the basis of the pyrazinamide suppression test, reabsorption appeared to be 98 percent complete, with most of the uric acid appearing in the final urine arising from secretion. However, bidirectional transport of uric acid is underestimated by the pyrazinamide suppression test; secretion and reabsorption are more extensive than previously supposed. Since reabsorption of secreted urate occurs, the extent of reabsorption in the nephron may be in excess of 100 percent of the filtered urate. Thus, increased reabsorption could theoretically be a factor in the pathogenesis of hyperuricemia.

Tubular Secretion   Rieselbach and associates [297] have postulated diminished renal urate secretion *per nephron* as a basis for hyperuricemia in some patients with primary gout without demonstrable overproduction of uric acid. This postu-

Table 50-13 Uric acid clearance (ml/min) reported by six authors in gouty subjects and normal controls

Authors*	Date	Place	Gout No.	Gout Mean CUA¶	Control No.	Control Mean CUA¶
Gutman and Yü	1957	United States	150	7.5	61	8.7
Nugent and Tyler	1959	United States	6	6.2	7	8.5
Seegmiller et al.	1962	United States	5†	5.5		
			5‡	6.2	7	7.0
			6§	8.7		
Lathem and Rodnan	1962	United States	11	6.0	10	7.5
Houpt and Ogryzlo	1964	Canada	30	5.0	22	7.0
Snaith and Scott	1970	Great Britain	-46	3.6	46	5.8

* For references see Table 43-17 in the fourth edition of this text [2].
† Uric acid production in normal range.
‡ Moderate overproduction of uric acid.
§ Marked overproduction of uric acid.
¶ Clearance of uric acid, in ml/min.

late was based on the pyrazinamide suppression test, the reliability of which has been questioned. According to the current interpretation of the test by Steele [391], the data presented in support of decreased secretion in these patients could be reinterpreted as enhanced reabsorption distal to the urate secretory site. Nevertheless, decreased secretion could lead to the abnormal velocity substrate curve and should be considered further.

ORGANIC ACID EXCRETION   There are several mechanisms whereby an alteration in the transport of an organic acid could be related to a defect of urate secretion in gouty subjects. Certain organic acids may share a secretory site with uric acid. An increased secretion of an organic acid sharing such a transport system could competitively inhibit the tubular secretion of uric acid. Alternatively, the reduced secretion of an organic acid could reflect a defective secretory system, which might also be limited in uric acid transport.

A number of naturally occurring organic acids reduce the renal excretion of uric acid, presumably by inhibiting its tubular secretion. Elevated concentrations of lactate and β-hydroxybutyrate are important causes of secondary hyperuricemia. These observations led to the proposal that the renal defect in uric acid transport could be related to a subtle abnormality in organic acid metabolism in some patients with gout. Kramer et al. [407] found a normal excretion of total organic acids in the urine in 32 gouty subjects. However, analysis of Krebs cycle organic acids in 12 of these patients revealed a decreased excretion of citrate in all 12, an increased excretion of lactate in five, and an increased excretion of succinate-fumarate in three. Unfortunately, plasma concentrations could not be measured, so the renal handling of these compounds could not be estimated.

Other Renal Functional Abnormalities in Gout

Ammonia Excretion   Perhaps the best studied and still most controversial renal abnormality in subjects with gout relates to the production of ammonia. Gutman and Yü [318] reported that when ^{15}N-glycine is administered to gouty subjects, the first-day and cumulative ^{15}N-ammonium values are less than those found in control subjects. The average cumulative values in 7 days were 3.38 percent of administered ^{15}N in controls, 2.54 percent in gouty normal excretors, and 1.61 percent in gouty overexcretors. The enrichment values were the same in all groups: 2.61 to 2.72 atoms percent excess ^{15}N. Thus, the deficit in the gouty subjects was attributable to a decrease in the quantity of ammonia produced. Ammonium/creatinine ratios averaged 0.27 ± 0.09 in 77 gouty subjects, as compared with 0.41 ± 0.10 in 17 nongouty subjects with comparable urinary pH values. In 83 gouty subjects with a urinary pH of less than 5.7 the mean net deficit in the elimination of ammonia was 8 μeq/min when compared with 46 nongouty controls excreting urine of the same pH [318].

L-Glutamine of plasma is the immediate precursor of perhaps 80 percent of urinary ammonia.

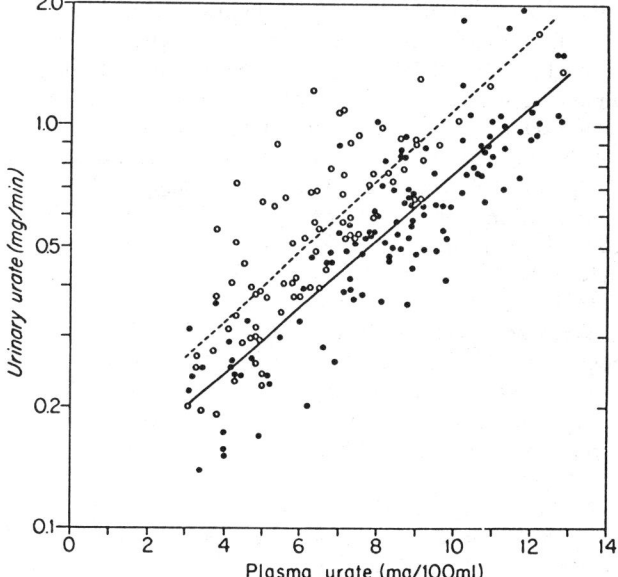

Figure 50-28 Urate excretion at varying concentrations of plasma urate. Urinary urate is expressed in mg/(min · 100 ml) of glomerular filtrate. The slopes of the normal (O———O) and gout (●———●) regressions are not significantly different from each other. The average gouty individual must have a serum urate 1.7 mg/dl higher than normal in order to equal the normal rate of urate excretion. (From P. A. Simkin, in Purine Metabolism in Man—II, edited by M. M. Müller, E. Kaiser, and J. E. Seegmiller, p. 41. Plenum, New York, 1977. Also, Ref. 406.)

L-Glutamine is often regarded as a storage form of ammonia-N:

$$\alpha\text{-Ketoglutarate} + NH_3 + NADH + H^+ \rightleftharpoons \text{L-glutamate} + H_2O + NAD^+$$

$$\text{L-Glutamate} + NH_3 + ATP \longrightarrow \text{L-glutamine} + H_2O + P_i + ADP$$

The reversible fixation of ammonia by α-ketoglutarate is catalyzed by glutamic acid dehydrogenase, an enzyme subject to complex regulation by purine ribonucleotides and certain steroids. The reaction of L-glutamate, NH_3, and ATP is catalyzed by glutamine synthetase, an enzyme found in high activity in liver, cerebral cortex, and rat kidney, but apparently absent from dog kidney [2].

Two glutaminases are present in the kidney and liver. One, designated as glutaminase I, is activated (or stabilized) by phosphate and splits off the amide nitrogen of glutamine to form glutamic acid and ammonia. Its pH optimum is 8; it is found in the mitochondria. The other, designated as glutaminase II, is in reality a glutamine-transaminase-ω-deamidase system and is activated by α-keto acids. α-Ketoglutaramide is the hypothetical direct precursor of ammonia. The pH optimum of this enzyme is about 9, and it is found in the soluble fraction of the cell.

The tendency of gouty subjects to excrete an inappropriately acid urine has been discussed above (see "Urolithiasis in Gout"). This has been confirmed by many workers and generally attributed to the preferential excretion of an acid load as an increase in titratable acidity rather than as an increase in urinary ammonia [2].

Plante and coworkers [409] noted that the apparent defect in ammonium excretion in gouty subjects was not present in patients on a low purine diet, but they did not reexamine the same patients during the ingestion of normal or high purine diets. Metcalfe-Gibson et al. [93] found no abnormally low values of ammonium excretion in hyperuricemic subjects with creatinine clearance values above 65 ml/min.

Falls [410] has carefully reinvestigated urinary acidification and ammonium excretion in 10 gouty and 10 control subjects with normal renal function. He found that gouty patients do not establish a greater pH gradient across the distal tubule than normal subjects but that gouty patients tend to handle an acid load by preferentially excreting titratable acid rather than ammonium. This modest defect in ammonia production was best elicited during dietary restriction of phosphate. He also pointed out that there was no restriction in the diffusion of ammonia, as might have been expected if the reduced ammonium excretion were due to occult renal disease.

Gibson et al. [411] have confirmed the more acid urine, and the preferential excretion of titratable acidity rather than ammonia, in gout. With prolonged ammonium chloride administration, ammonium excretion increased but urate production fell. On allopurinol, ammonium production fell, but titratable acid excretion was unchanged. They propose a metabolic association between ammonia and uric acid that cannot be explained by their common derivation from glutamine, and they suggest that the association may be explained by the purine nucleotide cycle which is a proven source of ammonia (from deamination of AMP [412]).

Amino Acid Excretion in Gout   The possibility that a defect in uric acid transport or metabolism may be related to an alteration of amino acid metabolism has attracted considerable attention. Although total amino acid concentrations in plasma are normal in gout [323, 413], those of glutamate average about 50 percent greater than normal in gouty subjects as well as in their asymptomatic hyperuricemic sons [323, 414]. Renal clearance of glutamate is normal in gouty subjects but clearances of serine and threonine and especially of glutamine are low even after protein restriction [413, 415].

Excretion of Purine Bases in Gout

Normal urine contains about 30 mg/day of purines other than uric acid. These include xanthine, hypoxanthine, 1-methylhypoxanthine, guanine, 1-methylguanine, 7-methylguanine, N^2-methylguanine, 7-methyl-8-hydroxyguanine, adenine, and 6-succinoaminopurine [187, 306, 345, 416]. Their normal excretion values are given in Table 50-14. The origins of adenine, guanine, hypoxanthine, xanthine, and of the methylated adenines and guanines have been discussed. Succinoadenine is the aglycone of adenylosuccinic acid, the intermediate in the conversion of IMP to AMP. 7-Methyl-8-hydroxyguanine arises from 7-methylguanine by action of human liver xanthine oxidase [417]; bovine milk xanthine oxidase will not catalyze this reaction [306].

The urinary excretions of trace purine and pyrimidine bases are not increased in patients with primary gout during the interval phase (Table 50-14). Some years ago it was claimed that excretion of 7-methyl-8-hydroxyguanine was slightly increased and that of 6-succinoaminopurine slightly decreased during acute attacks [345], but with additional data on the range of values in normal subjects the validity of these interpretations is now unclear. Also, mean excretion values of pseudouridine (5-ribosyluracil), a constituent of soluble and ribosomal RNA, have been reported to be slightly higher in gouty subjects than in controls, but here also further experience has indicated a wide range of values in normal subjects, and the validity of the interpretation is uncertain. There is no correlation between urinary uric acid and pseudouridine excretion values in gout. These patterns in gout are unlike those found in leukemic subjects, in whom excretion levels of many bases are often much increased. There is thus no substantial evidence to suggest that increased nucleic acid turnover is the basis of hyperuricemia in primary gout [2].

Extrarenal Disposal of Uric Acid in Gout

Uricolysis in Normal Humans   Urinary recoveries of injected uric acid are incomplete in normal subjects. The average of 14 studies with uric acid-^{15}N was 75.6 percent [2].

Studies of the turnover of uric acid in normal persons show that the quantity of uric acid synthesized per day is greater than the quantity appearing in urine. In studies with uric acid-^{15}N [303] or uric acid-^{14}C [165], the fraction of the turnover appearing in urine is essentially the same as the fraction of injected uric acid recovered in urine. Thus a significant quantity of uric acid is disposed of by routes other than the kidney.

In initial studies with uric acid-^{15}N, small but significant concentrations of ^{15}N were found in urinary urea and ammonia [295]. Subsequently, when a relatively large quantity of uric acid-1,3-^{15}N was administered intravenously to a normal subject [164], about 25 percent of the isotope was found in urinary allantoin, urea, and ammonia and fecal nitrogen. In

Table 50-14 Some purines and pyrimidines excreted in human urine, mg/day

	Normal range*	Primary gout*
Adenine	0.3–6.2	0.9–1.5
Guanine	0.2–1.3	0.1–0.4
Hypoxanthine	3.1–13.2	4.8–13.7
Xanthine	3.7–8.7	2.3–6.5
6-Succinoaminopurine	0.5–1.5	0.2–3.3
7-Methylguanine	2.2–7.8	3.9–8.4
7-Methyl-8-hydroxyguanine	0.6–2.2	1.2–3.4
N^2-Methylguanine	0.3–0.6	0.2–0.3
1-Methylhypoxanthine	0.2–0.7	0.2–0.8
4-Amino-5-imidazolecarboxamide	0.5–1.3	
Uracil	3.7–13.7	3.7–5.6
Pseudouridine	18–178	32–134

* In some instances dietary purines were not restricted.
SOURCE: For references see Table 43-12 in the fourth edition of this text [2].

studies with uric acid-2-^{14}C, a comparable percentage of administered isotope was recovered in respiratory CO_2, urinary urea, allantoin and allantoic acid, and feces [165]. In patients with biliary catheters given uric acid-^{15}N, labeled products were recovered in bile [418]. These results suggested that uricolysis occurred in the intestinal tract.

SITES OF URICOLYSIS   When labeled uric acid was administered orally to normal subjects, only 9 to 11 percent was excreted unchanged in urine [2]. With uric acid-^{15}N, 47 percent of the ^{15}N was recovered in urinary urea in 3 days. With uric acid-2-^{14}C, only 2.4 percent appeared in urea, but 55 percent of the ^{14}C was excreted as respiratory CO_2 [165]. An additional 16.3 percent was recovered in feces, 83 to 91 percent of this amount being found within the intestinal bacteria themselves.

To verify the role of the intestinal flora in uricolysis in humans, the degradation of intravenously administered uric acid was studied in a normal subject before and after an effective bacteriostasis was achieved with concomitant sulfonamide, streptomycin, and neomycin [165]. The quantity of ^{14}C recovered in various degradation products was reduced from 22.5 to 3.0 percent during drug treatment (Table 50-15). Many intestinal organisms destroy uric acid [164].

Sorenson [165] estimated that 100 mg uric acid or more enters the alimentary tract in saliva, gastric juice, and bile. An equal quantity may enter in pancreatic and intestinal juices. These quantities of uric acid are adequate to account for the degradation of one-third of the uric acid normally turned over each day.

A trivial amount of uricolysis may occur within the tissues of human beings. Two enzyme systems can destroy uric acid in vitro at physiologic pH. These are verdoperoxidase and cytochromecytochrome oxidase. Cells of the myeloid series contain verdoperoxidase. The peroxidative reaction yields allantoin and CO_2 as the initial products [419]. Ames et al. [420] propose that uric acid serves as an antioxidant and is destroyed in tissues by oxygen radicals in a similar reaction.

Uricolysis in Gout   Urinary recoveries of injected ^{14}N-uric acid [418] or ^{14}C-uric acid [165] have ranged from 35 to 54 percent in gouty subjects. All these values are lower, on the average, than those found in nongouty subjects. These results suggest an enhanced rather than reduced rate of extrarenal

disposal in gouty subjects. In addition, the fraction of the daily turnover of uric acid recovered in urine is smaller in gouty than in normal subjects. In hyperuricemic individuals larger than normal quantities of uric acid enter the intestinal tract. Pollycove et al. [421] have reported an increased yield of $^{14}CO_2$ from injected ^{14}C-uric acid in hyperuricemic subjects. Thus, no substantial evidence exists to implicate failure of tissue or intestinal uricolysis in the hyperuricemia of gout. On the contrary, enhanced enteral uricolysis is a compensatory factor in gout, tending to lessen hyperuricemia and constituting the major process of disposal of uric acid in certain patients with severe renal insufficiency [299].

GOUT ASSOCIATED WITH SPECIFIC ENZYMATIC DEFECTS

Glucose-6-Phosphatase Deficiency in Gout

Patients with glycogen storage disease type I (glucose-6-phosphatase deficiency) have hyperuricemia from infancy and may develop gouty arthritis by the end of the first decade of life, sometimes of disabling severity [2]. Chronic tophaceous gout and nephropathy may be the major cause of morbidity in these patients as they become adults. Over 40 cases of glycogen storage disease and gout have been recorded. In addition, in some cases of "primary juvenile gout," the clinical history and physical findings suggest underlying glycogen storage disease [2].

Hyperuricemia in glycogen storage disease type I is marked, often in the range of 10 to 16 mg/dl of plasma [422, 423]. Two distinct pathophysiologic mechanisms contribute to the hyperuricemia of this disorder. They are reduced renal clearance of uric acid because of the presence of marked hyperlactic acidemia and increased production of uric acid, possibly a consequence of enhanced nucleotide catabolism followed secondarily by an increased rate of purine biosynthesis *de novo*.

Patients with glucose-6-phosphatase deficiency are unable to produce free glucose from phosphorylated carbohydrates. Recurrent hypoglycemia acts as a stimulus both to glycogenolysis and gluconeogenesis. One consequence is hyperlactic acidemia [422]. Blood lactate levels may be 50 mg/dl or more (normal 5 to 18 mg/dl). Lactate suppresses tubular secretion of

Table 50-15 Recovery of intravenously administered uric acid-2-^{14}C in excretory products (5 to 10 days) before and after establishment of effective bacteriostasis of the intestinal tract

Excretory product	Recovery of ^{14}C, percent of dose	
	Before bacteriostasis	During bacteriostasis
Urinary uric acid	69.0 (10 days)	55.7 (5 days)
Urinary allantoin	2.1	1.8
Urinary allantoic acid	0.2	
Urinary urea	2.2	0.7
Expired carbon dioxide	10.9	0.5
Fecal products	7.1	0.0
Total recovery in degradation products	22.5	3.0

SOURCE: From L. B. Sorensen [165].

uric acid. Renal clearances of uric acid are low in type I glycogen storage disease [422].

The hyperuricemia of type I glycogen storage disease is also associated with an excessive uric acid production. Uric acid excretion values are high when expressed in terms of body weight [423]. The urinary uric acid/creatinine ratio may be >0.75 [424]. By tracer methods, both the turnover of the urate pool and 1-^{14}C-glycine incorporation into urinary urate may be excessive [423, 425] (Table 50-16).

There is now reason to question the postulate that overproduction of uric acid in this disorder is a consequence of overproduction of phosphoribosylpyrophosphate secondary to shunting of phosphorylated carbohydrate intermediates into the pentose phosphate pathway [423]. Roe and Kogut [426] found in 1977 that within 30 min after the injection of glucagon, patients with glycogen storage disease type I showed a significant increase in plasma urate levels and a two- to threefold increase in urinary uric acid excretion. Such a rapid increase in urate levels was thought probably to result from enhanced nucleotide catabolism rather than from a direct effect upon the rate of purine synthesis *de novo*. An increase in purine biosynthesis *de novo* follows an increase in nucleotide catabolism when fructose is infused into humans or animals, as discussed above. Greene and associates showed in 1978 that glucagon administration in glycogen storage disease type I [278] led to phosphorylase activation, hepatic glycogen breakdown, an increase in hepatic glucose-6-phosphate and fructose-1,6-diphosphate, and depletion of hepatic ATP and inorganic phosphate. The last two changes resemble those caused by fructose infusion, which have been shown to result in degradation of preformed AMP to uric acid, and release of feedback inhibition of early steps of purine biosynthesis [221]. Greene et al. [278] postulated that hypoglycemia in glycogen storage disease type I, which is known to stimulate glycogenolysis [422], initiates a similar chain of events leading to depletion of ATP and P_i in the liver, increased nucleotide catabolism, and uric acid formation followed by enhanced purine biosynthesis *de novo*.

If hypoglycemia does contribute to hyperuricemia by such mechanisms, its prevention should reduce hyperuricemia. Prevention of hypoglycemia by continuous nasogastric infusions of a high glucose diet for 24 h a day for 14 days [278] was associated first with an increased excretion of uric acid (which correlated with a decrease in blood lactate concentration) and then with a decreased excretion of uric acid to levels less than during pretreatment. This second phase was marked by a lowering of serum urate concentrations to normal. The second phase of serum and urinary uric acid changes suggests that uric acid production was decreased by treatment. These findings confirm and extend those of Burr et al. [427].

Since hyperuricemia in untreated glycogen storage disease type I is usually in a range where the probability of gout or gouty nephropathy is high, treatment is indicated even though the patient is young and asymptomatic with respect to gout. The hyperuricemia can be reduced with allopurinol but responds less well to uricosuric agents, perhaps because substances such as lactic acid interfere with the pharmacologic effects of probenecid in a manner analogous to that of salicylates, as suggested by Jakovcic and Sorensen [425]. In published cases, normal plasma urate values have rarely been achieved. Prevention of hypoglycemia is a superior approach and also reduces hyperlipidemia and promotes growth [426, 427].

Hyperuricemia has also been described in an undefined type of glycogen storage disease with normal hepatic glucose-6-phosphatase activity [428]. In this instance, renal retention of urate appeared to be related, at least in part, to hyperlactic acidemia.

Increased Phosphoribosylpyrophosphate Synthetase Activity and Gout

In 1972, Sperling and colleagues [429] demonstrated a markedly accelerated rate of PP-ribose-P synthesis in two gouty brothers with flamboyant overproduction of urate, and showed [334] that this was a consequence of altered kinetic properties of PP-ribose-P synthetase. Subsequently, five additional families have been discovered in which excessive rates of PP-ribose-P synthesis can be attributed to abnormalities of this enzyme. The first patient to be identified had had repeated episodes of renal colic since age 18, with a near-fatal episode of uric acid nephropathy at age 20. Attacks of acute gout occurred at ages 20 and 36. Basal serum urate concentration was 13.6 mg/dl, and the 24-h urinary uric acid excretion was 2400 mg. ^{15}N-Glycine incorporation into urinary uric acid was tenfold greater than in controls, and occurred 2 to 4 h following glycine feeding (Fig. 50-29). Cumulative ^{15}N incorporation was 3.32 percent in 7 days [304] (Table 50-17). Activities of hypoxanthine-guanine phosphoribosyltransferase (HPRT) were normal [332, 429]. These results suggested an increase in the rate of generation of PP-ribose-P, and this was convincingly demonstrated in erythrocytes during a 2-h incubation [332, 429].

Table 50-16 Turnover and synthesis of uric acid in glycogen storage disease, type I

Subject*	Sex	Age, yr	Serum urate, mg/100 ml	Pool size, mg	Turnover rate, pool/day	Turnover uric acid, mg/day	Excretion uric acid, mg/day
Normal control subjects	6 M 2 F	26 (19–38)	4.3 (2.9–5.5)	978 (541–1290)	0.62 (0.46–0.80)	590 (431–729)	429 (357–536)
Patients with type I glycogen storage disease	M	14	10.9	1380	0.85	1176	528
	M	17	16.4	2843	0.48	1365	569
	F	19	14.7	1917	0.61	1175	343
	M	34	15.0	1920	0.42	807	362
	M	18	17.0	2251	0.39	884	318

* For references see Table 43-19 in the fourth edition of this text [2].

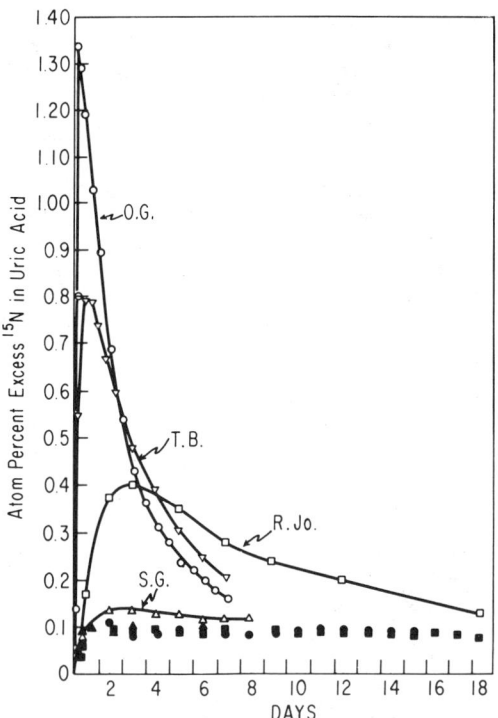

Figure 50-29 ^{15}N enrichment of urinary uric acid in two gouty patients with overactive PP-ribose-P synthetases (O.G. and T.B.), one gouty patient with partial HPRT deficiency (R.Jo.), one patient with idiopathic gout (S.G.), and three control subjects (solid symbols). (*From Sperling et al. [304], by permission of* The Journal of Clinical Investigation.)

Hemolysates of the index case contained excessive PP-ribose-P synthetase activity at inorganic phosphate concentrations of 0.48 to 0.88 mM, but normal activity at phosphate concentration above 2 mM [332, 334] (Fig. 50-30). Experiments employing hemolysates either from this subject or from a normal control, mixed with dialyzed hemolysate from the opposite subject, resulted in only additive enzyme activities. Thus, the enhanced rate of PP-ribose-P generation reflected an abnormality of the enzyme. This result could have been due either to increased sensitivity of PP-ribose-P synthetase to activation by inorganic phosphate or to reduced sensitivity to inhibition by regulatory compounds normally present in the erythrocyte, such as AMP, ADP, GDP, and 2,3-DPG. The activation of the partially purified enzyme by inorganic phosphate was normal. Its affinities for ribose-5-phosphate, ATP, and inorganic phosphate also were normal. However, its sensitivity to inhibition by nucleotides and 2,3-DPG was markedly reduced

[334]. The PP-ribose-P synthetase from these cells was inhibited by GDP, ADP, 2,3-DPG, and AMP, but an average of 45, 5, 2, and 1.5 times higher concentrations, respectively, were required to inhibit the mutant enzyme to the same extent as the normal enzyme. Thus the PP-ribose-P synthetase was structurally altered in some way which rendered it relatively resistant to control by nucleotides at their usual concentrations within cells, but did not reduce catalytic activity.

One brother, who also suffered from recurrent gout and uric acid lithiasis, showed similarly increased rates of PP-ribose-P synthesis, but a normal brother, three sons, both parents, and one maternal aunt were found to have normal synthetic rates of PP-ribose-P in hemolysates [429, 430].

Becker and coworkers [431, 432] subsequently discovered a second family (B. Family, Table 50-17) with a different variant of PP-ribose-P synthetase, also leading to sustained overproduction of PP-ribose-P, marked hyperuricemia and uricaciduria, and gout. The propositus, T.B, excreted 1200 to 1600 mg uric acid per day, had normal HPRT activity in erythrocytes [339], incorporated ^{15}N-glycine into urinary uric acid excessively [304] (Fig. 50-29), and had elevated concentrations of PP-ribose-P in cultured fibroblasts [338]. Erythrocytes and fibroblasts from the patient, one brother, and a daughter, all of whom overproduced uric acid, showed increases of PP-ribose-P synthetase activity of 2.5 to 3 times. Hemolysates and partially purified enzyme preparations showed greater enzyme activity at all concentrations of inorganic phosphate tested, up to at least 50 mM (Fig. 50-31). Normal affinities for substrates and normal sensitivities to purine nucleotide end products were demonstrated [339]. Immunologic studies involving antibody-inhibition titration showed an increased specific activity of the enzyme with a normal number of enzyme molecules per erythrocyte [431]. Thus, the PP-ribose-P synthetase abnormality in this family results in a two- to threefold increase in catalytic activity per molecule. The mutant enzyme exhibited an increase in thermal lability at 55°C [432]. This provides evidence for a structural alteration of the enzyme as the cause of the increased specific activity.

The patient with the third variant (B.P.) was selected for further study on the basis of gout, gross overproduction of purines [338], normal erythrocyte HPRT activity, reduced

Recovery of isotope in urinary uric acid in 7 days

Turnover excreted, %	Administered uric acid, %	Administered glycine	
		Uncorrected, %	Corrected, %
73	73	0.24	0.32
(65–82)	(63–82)	(0.16–0.29)	(0.27–0.37)
45	54	1.09	2.02
42	39	0.61	1.56
29	35	0.48	1.37
45	42	0.26	0.62
36	32	0.11	0.34

Figure 50-30 Effect of inorganic phosphate concentration on PP-ribose-P synthetase activity in hemolysates of normal subject (●———●) and of patient O.G. (○———○). (*From Sperling et al. [334], by permission of* Biochemical Medicine.)

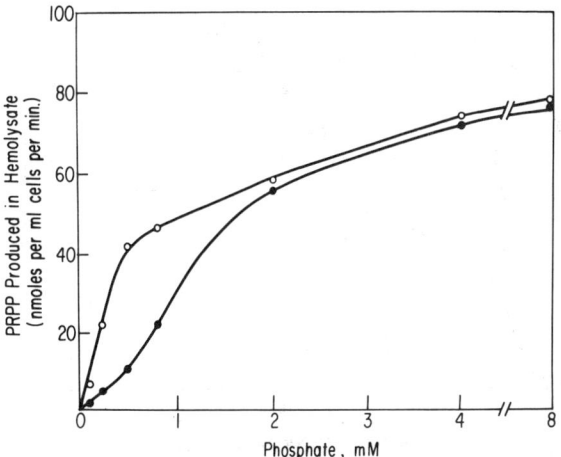

Table 50-17 Turnover and synthesis of uric acid in PP-ribose-P synthetase overactivity

Subject*	Sex	Relation to propositus	Age, yr	Serum urate, mg/100 ml	Pool size, mg	Turnover uric acid, mg/day	Excretion uric acid, mg/day	Excretion uric acid, mg/g C
Normal								
control	6 M		26	4.3	978	590	429	M472 ± 99
subjects	2 F		(19–38)	(2.9–5.5)	(541–1290)	(431–729)	(357–536)	F596 ± 110
G. Family								
O.G.	M	Propositus	35	13.5			2400	1410
H.G.	M	Brother		13.6			2250	1320
A.G.	M	Brother		6.0				
	M	Father		6.7			880	550
	F	Mother		5.3			1100	1000
B. Family								
T.B.	M	Propositus	53	10.4	2130	1490	1241–1600	830
H.B.	M	Brother	43	9.6			950–1100	650
J.B.	M	Brother	50					
B.B.	M	Son	15					
Y.B.	F	Wife	40					
C.B.	F	Daughter	16	6.2			890	550
P. Family								
B.P.	M	Propositus		9.7	3930	2370	1529	

* For references see Table 43-20 in the fourth edition of this text [2].

concentrations of ribose-5-phosphate, and elevated concentrations of PP-ribose-P in fibroblasts growing in vitro [338, 432]. The defect in the propositus of this family appears to be an increased affinity of PP-ribose-P synthetase for one of its substrates, ribose-5-phosphate [432]. Thus, at any concentration of ribose-5-phosphate below saturation, this mutant form of the enzyme will catalyze the synthesis of PP-ribose-P at a faster than normal rate.

A fourth variant studied by Becker and coworkers [433] represents a combination of the defects identified in the first and second families. In this patient, the elevated PP-ribose-P synthetase activity was due to both an abnormal resistance of the enzyme to feedback inhibition by purine nucleotides and a hyperbolic rather than sigmoidal activation curve with increasing phosphate concentrations. The total activity per immunoreactive enzyme molecule was twice normal.

Two additional variants have been reported by Lejeune et al. [434]. The PP-ribose-P synthetase from one of these patients exhibited an increased affinity for P_i, while that of the second appeared to be resistant to feedback inhibition by ADP. Finally, Muller and Frank [435] have reported a 53-year-old male with benign symmetric lipomatosis and purine overproduction, in whom activities of APRT and HPRT were within the normal ranges. His serum urate concentration was 8.9 mg/dl, his 24-h uric acid excretion was 850 mg, and his U-^{14}C-glycine incorporation into urinary uric acid was 0.54 percent in 7 days compared with control values of 0.13 and 0.24 percent. Erythrocyte PP-ribose-P synthetase activity was 52.1 nmol/h per milligram of protein, compared with values in eight controls of 24.0 ± 2 nmol/h per milligram of protein. It is not clear whether the defect in this patient is related to the lipomatosis, which had its onset a year or two after hyperuricemia was discovered at age 50. In favor of a primary enzyme defect are the family history of a brother with presumed primary gout and without lipomatosis, and the finding of normal PP-ribose-P synthetase activity in a second unrelated patient with benign symmetric lipomatosis.

The net result of all types of defects is an excessive rate of generation of PP-ribose-P. Increased PP-ribose-P synthetase activity represents a specific genetic subtype of gout. This class of defects is probably rare.

Other Studies Green and Martin [215] have reported a mutant form of PP-ribose-P synthetase from mutagenized hepatoma cells that overproduce purines, in which the properties of the synthetase are remarkably similar to those of the enzyme in subject O.G. (Table 50-17 and Ref. 304).

Figure 50-31 PP-ribose-P synthetase activity in dialyzed hemolysates from patient H.B. as a function of inorganic phosphate concentration.
●———●, mean values in hemolysates from 15 normal subjects;
○———○, hemolysate from patient H.B. (*From Becker, et al.* [431a], *by permission of* The American Journal of Medicine.)

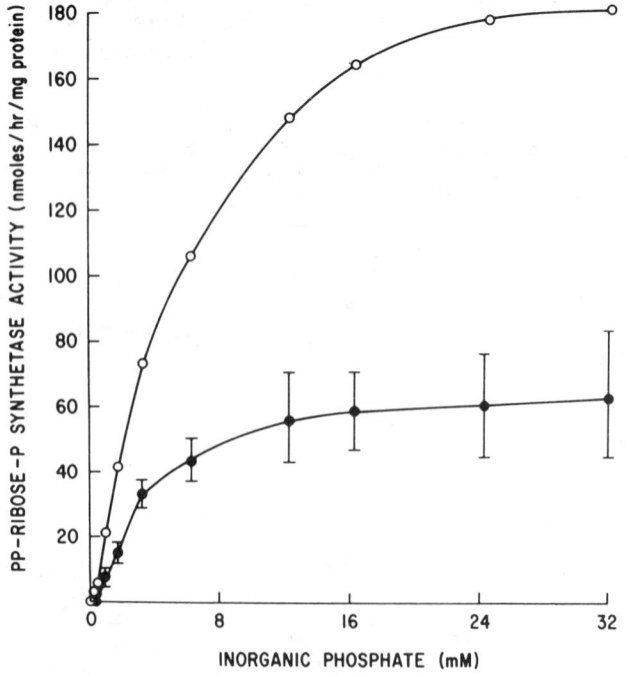

Turnover excreted, %	Administered uric acid, %	Recovery of isotope in urinary uric acid in 7 days	
		Administered glycine, %	
		Uncorrected	Corrected
73	73	0.24	0.32
(65–82)	63–82	0.16–0.29	(0.27–0.37)
		3.32	
72	61	1.11	1.44
67	72	1.24	1.85

Hypoxanthine-Guanine Phosphoribosyltransferase Deficiency in Gout

Virtually complete deficiency of this enzyme activity is associated with a syndrome of choreoathetoses, spasticity, mental retardation, and a bizarre compulsive self-mutilation, known as the Lesch-Nyhan syndrome [436]. There is prodigious overproduction and overexcretion of uric acid, and renal stones and secondary renal damage are common. In a few patients, a severe gouty arthritis has occurred. All the patients are males, and the disorder is X-linked. The Lesch-Nyhan syndrome is considered in Chap. 51.

Among adult gout patients with marked overproduction of uric acid, some have been found to have a high-grade, but partial, deficiency of HPRT activity [437]. The syndrome of partial HPRT deficiency is also considered in detail in Chap. 51, but a brief inclusion is warranted here. The incidence of this enzyme defect in the gouty population is low. A total of 18 patients were described in a general review of the topic written in 1968 [300]. Included were several who had been reported earlier as examples of juvenile gout associated with hyperexcretion of uric acid or with neurologic abnormalities. Sperling et al. [438] found only 1 subject with a partial deficiency of HPRT activity among 52 adult male gouty overproducers of urate. HPRT deficiency appears to be present in less than 2 percent of gouty subjects [439].

Presenting symptoms in partial HPRT deficiency may be typical acute gouty arthritis, renal stones, crystalluria, or neurologic dysfunction. Gouty arthritis usually presents in the second or third decade. Three-quarters of patients have formed renal stones; half of these occurred before age 10. In 20 percent of patients there have been neurologic manifestations, including mental retardation, mild spastic quadriplegia, dysarthria, cerebellar ataxia, and seizures. These suggest a relationship to the debilitating disease found in patients with complete HPRT deficiency.

Gouty subjects with HPRT deficiency tend to have rather high serum urate values. Most have been above 10 mg/dl. Urinary uric acid excretion is elevated unless renal failure is present, often being well above 1000 mg/day (Fig. 51-4). Patient T.S. of Fig. 51-4, whose uric acid excretion falls within the normal range, had a glomerular filtration rate of only 10 ml/min. Turnover studies in T.S. disclosed a urate production of 1693 mg/day, of which only 34 percent was disposed of in the urine.

Turnover studies with labeled uric acid have disclosed enlarged urate pools and increased urate turnovers [300]. $1\text{-}^{14}\text{C}$-glycine incorporation into urinary uric acid is excessive, particularly after correction for extrarenal disposal. In the initial five patients studied values ranged from 0.88 to 3.94 percent of administered glycine in 7 days. These values are somewhat less than may be found in patients with complete HPRT deficiency (4.3 to 6.1 percent) but very much greater than in normal subjects (0.1 to 0.3 percent). There is an overlap with values found in gouty overproducers with normal HPRT activity (0.4 to 1.9 percent). In patients with HPRT deficiency given $1\text{-}^{14}\text{C}$-glycine, the peak specific activity values in urinary uric acid occur earlier than in normal individuals. These results indicate that excessive purine production in these patients is the result of increased purine synthesis *de novo*.

HPRT Activity Patients with the partial enzyme defect exhibit levels of HPRT activity in erythrocytes ranging from 0.01 to nearly 30 percent of normal [300, 438, 439]. There are several striking exceptions to this generalization. In at least one patient with clinical features characteristic of the partial enzyme defect there was no detectable HPRT activity in circulating erythrocytes [440]. In two unrelated patients levels of activity in circulating erythrocytes or leukocytes were approximately normal [441–443]. In the first patient there is an alteration in kinetic constants (increased K_m for PP-ribose-P) such that the enzyme apparently does not function properly in vivo even though activity appears to be normal when assayed in vitro at saturating concentrations of substrates [441, 442]. This particular patient exemplifies the difficulty that may exist in making the proper diagnosis and underscores the importance of careful kinetic studies of the enzyme in patients suspected of having this disease on clinical grounds. In the second patient the mutant form of the enzyme exhibited normal kinetic constants but had an enhanced sensitivity to inhibition by purine nucleotides [443]. Thus, in this patient as well the function of the enzyme in vivo may be substantially less than would be apparent on the basis of assay in vitro.

The extent of the overlap of erythrocyte HPRT activity between patients with the Lesch-Nyhan syndrome and patients with the partial deficiency indicates that the clinical features cannot be reliably predicted on the basis of an assay of HPRT in erythrocytes alone. The level of HPRT activity in erythrocytes does not necessarily reflect the level of activity in other tissues. In addition, as illustrated above, function of the enzyme in vivo may not always be directly related to assayable activity in vitro.

While the level of HPRT activity in erythrocytes from patients with the partial enzyme defect often differs between families, it is usually the same within a family. In addition, in two members of one family, there is substantially more activity with hypoxanthine (10 percent of normal) than with guanine as substrate (0.5 percent of normal) [437]. These observations suggest that the mutations leading to a partial loss of enzyme activity may also be different among the families studied. Further evidence for this was obtained by study of thermal inactivation of the HPRT enzymes obtained from six patients in three families. The mutant enzyme obtained from two members of one family was very resistant to heat; that from three members of another family was very sensitive to heat; and that from one patient in a third family was slightly more sensitive to heat than the normal enzyme. A mixture of the dialyzed hemolysates from members of the first two families showed the expected intermediate sensitivity of the enzyme mixture to heat, demonstrating that no labilizing or stabilizing factors were present in the hemolysates. These findings suggest heterogeneity of mutations on the structural gene for HPRT. The pathogenesis of excessive uric acid production in partial HPRT deficiency is discussed in Chap. 51.

CURRENT HYPOTHESES

The Glutaminase Hypothesis

On the basis of the findings of reduced ammonia production in gout and of preferential labeling of N(3 + 9) following administration of ^{15}N-glycine to gouty subjects, a block of glutaminase I activity was proposed by Gutman and Yü [88]. This hypothesis, as a general mechanism in gout, has been disproved by the finding of normal activities of phosphate-activated glutaminase (glutaminase I), pyruvate-activated glutaminase (glutaminase II), and nonactivated glutaminase in renal biopsy tissue from four gouty subjects by Pollak and Mattenheimer [444]. In rebuttal, Yü and Gutman [318] have cited the need for a functional assay of glutaminase I in vivo, by measurement of transrenal glutamine differences at various urinary pH values in nongouty and gouty subjects.

The Glutamic Acid Dehydrogenase Hypothesis

The reaction catalyzed by glutamic acid dehydrogenase appears to operate chiefly in the direction of α-ketoglutaric acid. The observations that plasma levels of glutamic acid are elevated in gout, both in the fasting state and following casein or glutamate feeding, are viewed by Yü et al. [313] and by Pagliara and Goodman [314] as supporting a suggestion first made by Frieden [445] that faulty control or reduced activity of glutamic acid dehydrogenase could result in diversion of glutamic acid toward glutamine and purine biosynthesis.

Glutathione Reductase Variants and Gout

Long [445a] has reported a rank order association of hyperuricemia with increased enzymatic activity of a series of variant glutathione reductases. Of 28 black patients with gout, 23 were found to have a fast glutathione reductase variant. The fast variant is 28 percent more active than the normal enzyme and is associated with a mean serum urate level of 7.24 mg/dl and often with gout (Table 50-18) [445b]. Elevated activity of erythrocyte glutathione reductase has also been observed in a group of Caucasians with untreated primary gout [445c].

Table 50-18 Frequency of glutathione reductase phenotypes in general black population and in black males with gout or other medical illnesses

GSSG-R phenotype	General black population, percent	Black male patients	
		Gout	Other illnesses
S	75.16	5	150
FS	23.06	15	40
F	1.78	8	6

SOURCE: From W. K. Long [445b].

Glutathione reductase catalyzes the reduction of glutathione by NADPH + H$^+$ with generation of NADP, the cofactor of the first two reactions of the pentose phosphate pathway. Long has proposed that increased glutathione reductase activity results in excess synthesis of pentose phosphate compounds including PP-ribose-P and that this leads to excessive purine production, hyperuricemia, and gout [445a]. Wasserzug et al. [445d] failed to find increased glutathione reductase activity in hemolysates of 52 gouty patients in Israel, but none of the subjects was either black or an overexcretor of urate. Glutathione reductase activity was increased, and its electrophoretic mobility faster, in subjects with glucose-6-phosphate dehydrogenase deficiency, which was not the case in Long's patients [445b]. Activity of glutathione reductase is increased in certain other diseases and by certain vitamins, e.g., nicotinamide and riboflavin [445e], but rates of purine production or possible associations with hyperuricemia have not been reported.

Adenosine Monophosphate Deaminase Variants and Gout

Hers and Van Den Berghe [265] propose that primary hyperuricemia is caused by the presence of an abnormal AMP deaminase that is less sensitive than the normal enzyme to its physiologic inhibitors. Their studies suggest that the rate-limiting step in the degradation of adenyl nucleotides in the liver is the conversion of AMP to IMP by AMP deaminase and that this enzyme is normally 95 percent inhibited by inorganic phosphate and GTP. Fructose-induced hyperuricemia is explained by a decrease in intrahepatic concentrations of P_i and GTP during fructose metabolism and a resulting degradation of adenyl nucleotides to uric acid. By analogy, they suggest that an abnormal AMP deaminase, perhaps less sensitive to its inhibitors, mainly P_i and GTP, would permit a continuous increase in the rate of degradation of adenyl nucleotides to IMP, inosine, oxypurine bases, and uric acid, and result in hyperuricemia and gout. Direct enzymatic evidence in support of the hypothesis has been obtained in a postmortem sample of liver from one gouty patient. AMP deaminase in this liver was partially resistant to inhibition by GTP at concentrations that completely inhibited the normal enzyme [446].

Idiopathic Gout

Many authors have classified the large group of gouty patients with an undefined biochemical lesion into two discrete subgroups, termed metabolic (overproducer) and renal gout.

Although this may be a useful functional distinction on the basis of the more obvious pathologic mechanism underlying the hyperuricemia, in our view the evidence does not support such a categorical differentiation. In a large percentage of patients evidence for both processes can be found if appropriately detailed studies are performed.

1. Some patients with urinary uric acid values that fall within the normal range show an excessive turnover (production) of the uric acid pool [299].

2. Many patients with normal urinary uric acid values show excessive incorporation of ^{14}C-glycine into urinary uric acid [308]. Some patients with apparently normal incorporation values show excessive incorporation when corrections are made for an expanded uric acid pool or extrarenal disposal of uric acid [294].

3. Patients with apparently normal values of incorporation of ^{15}N-glycine into urinary uric acid may nevertheless show excessive incorporation of ^{15}N into N(3+9) of uric acid [88].

4. Reduced fractional renal urate clearances are not restricted to gouty subjects with normal urinary uric acid values. The kidneys of 38 overproducer subjects were "no less handicapped" with respect to uric acid clearance than those of 35 subjects with normal total urinary uric acid values [406].

5. Both overproduction and overexcretion of uric acid, and reduced renal clearance of uric acid, may be reversible with weight loss and disappearance of hypertension in the same subject [310].

There appears to be extensive coexistence of metabolic and renal factors in the pathogenesis of hyperuricemia in many patients with primary gout. Nevertheless, pure forms of metabolic and renal gout also exist. For example, patients with partial HPRT deficiency or PP-ribose-P superactivity do not appear to have reduced fractional clearance of uric acid [162]. Similarly some gouty families with reduced renal uric acid clearance show no evidence for overproduction of, or isotope overincorporation into, uric acid [325]. The proportion of such pure forms is uncertain. Those with pure metabolic gout (PP-ribose-P synthetase variants, HPRT deficiency) probably represent no more than 1 to 2 percent of the total. In a recent survey of the gouty population of Queensland, Australia, Emmerson estimated that no more than 7 percent could be considered to represent primary renal gout.

The relationship between excessive purine production and reduced renal urate clearance is not clear, but since both appear to be reversible derangements, they may have linked metabolic mechanisms. The hypothesis of Hers and van den Berghe [265] forms a basis for a more general speculation. Their hypothesis of a genetically altered AMP deaminase does not require obesity or alcoholism as an essential component and could apply to nonobese abstemious gouty subjects. Other gouty subjects might require the stimulus of caloric excess or alcohol to induce nucleotide breakdown, which could occur in persons with normal AMP deaminase as a fructoselike effect or in persons with AMP-deaminase variants with lesser dietary stress. The brief reports [448, 449] of excessive hyperuricemic and hyperuricosuric responses of gouty subjects to fructose loads become especially interesting from the point of view of the AMP-deaminase hypothesis. The prompt production of uric acid from adenyl nucleotides, and the secondary acceleration of purine biosynthesis *de novo* following fructose administration, have been discussed and explained above. Could

excessive deamination of AMP provide other products that might explain some of the other features of gout? For example, AMP deamination yields one mol of NH_3 for each mol of IMP. Does conversion of the excess NH_3 to glutamic acid explain the hyperglutamatemia of gout? Fructose infusions also result in excess lactate production. Do related intrarenal responses account for effects upon secretion in the gouty kidney?

The metabolic responses to caloric and alcohol excess may also rest upon a relationship between lipogenesis and purinogenesis, as presented earlier in this chapter. Feeding raises hepatic PP-ribose-P concentrations in mice [220]. Extreme obesity is associated with hyperuricemia and with raised levels of PP-ribose-P in erythrocytes in Sumo wrestlers [331]. Alcohol increases the production of PP-ribose-P in hepatocytes in vitro [223]. Glucose stimulates PP-ribose-P synthesis in Ehrlich ascites cells [203], and glucose, fructose and mannose increase uric acid production in *Cebus* monkeys [447]. Caloric and alcohol excess may also contribute to hyperuricemia by driving purine synthesis *de novo* through the primary production of excess amounts of PP-ribose-P.

HEREDITY

Familial Incidence of Gout

The familial nature of gout has been recognized since antiquity. Galen ascribed gout to "debauchery, intemperance and an hereditary trait." English observers have reported a familial incidence of gout of 38 to 81 percent in their cases [450]. In series reported from the United States the familial incidence has generally been from 6 to 18 percent [2], but the true familial incidence may be higher, as reflected in figures ranging up to 75 percent [451], obtained after persistent questioning. Among hyperuricemic relatives of gouty subjects, the incidence of gout averaged 20 percent in five series reviewed by Smyth [452] (Table 50-19).

Asymptomatic Hyperuricemia in Families of Gouty Patients

The first recorded observation of asymptomatic hyperuricemia in the family of a patient with gout was by Folin and Lyman in 1913 [453]. In 1937 Jacobson found hyperuricemia in a son of each of two men with gout, and a brother of a third [454]. The first extensive study was by Talbott [455], who reported in 1940 that 25 percent of 136 asymptomatic blood relatives of 27 gouty persons had hyperuricemia. Smyth et al. [7] in the

Table 50-19 Hyperuricemia in relatives of gouty patients

No. of gouty patients	No. of relatives	No. of gouty relatives	No. of hyperuricemic relatives	Percent hyperuricemic
27	136	3	34	25
19	87	3	21	24
44	136	0	16	11
3	29	11	21	72
32	261	16	71	27

SOURCE: From C. J. Smyth [452].

United States and Hauge and Harvald [140] in Denmark found similar prevalences (24 and 27 percent) in groups of 87 and 261 relatives, respectively. In other studies prevalences as high as 72 percent [456] have been recorded.

Hypothesis of an Autosomal Dominant Gene   The first studies of hyperuricemia in families of gouty subjects led to the conclusion that hyperuricemia was determined by an autosomal dominant gene whose penetrance was low, especially in women (Fig. 50-32). Smyth et al. [7] found that a frequency diagram of serum urate values among relatives of gouty patients was bimodal for both males and females, with nadirs of 6 and 5 mg/dl, respectively. Using these critical levels, they classified 10 of 48 male relatives and 11 of 39 females as hyperuricemic. The distribution of hyperuricemic individuals in 19 pedigrees conformed rather closely with expectation if such kindreds were segregated according to the presence or absence of a dominant autosomal gene for hyperuricemia. In this mode of inheritance, the ratio of hyperuricemic to normal offspring of matings in which only one parent is hyperuricemic should be 1:1. There were no hyperuricemic sons among 14 below the age of 16 years. However, when sons above age 16 years were considered, the ratio was six hyperuricemic to seven normal sons. Thus the data on male relatives were in agreement with the hypothesis of dominant autosomal inheritance if one assumes that the metabolic change resulting in hyperuricemia is not manifested in males until the age of puberty. Among daughters of the same matings, two of six below age 16 years and two of four above 16 years were hyperuricemic.

Stecher et al. [457] have published data which permit similar analyses. A frequency distribution of serum urate values of 137 relatives of gouty persons (excluding spouses) was shifted toward high values in comparison with a similar plot of 1024 determinations on individuals from the general hospital population. It was also suggestively bimodal, the nadir being 6.0 to

6.4 mg/dl, and 23 of 147 determinations on 137 relatives fell above this range. Among relatives, they observed hyperuricemia in 15 to 21 percent of mothers, brothers, sisters, and sons, but in none of 45 daughters of index cases. These workers also tentatively concluded that hyperuricemia was an autosomal dominant trait with low penetrance in both sexes, but lower in females than in males. When this conclusion was put to numerical test for male offspring only, a correction being applied for small family size, the expected number of hyperuricemic individuals was 31. Actually 26 were found among 51 men. These figures were regarded as showing satisfactory conformity with the expected 1:1 ratio. The data were then used to estimate penetrance. Since 26 hyperuricemic sons were observed where 31 were expected, the penetrance was estimated at about 84 percent in heterozygote males. And since there were only 8 hyperuricemic females compared with 54 hyperuricemic males, despite the nearly equal sex distribution of the 203 individuals of the study, the penetrance was estimated to be about one-seventh as high in women as in men, or about 14 percent. Since no daughters of gouty patients were hyperuricemic, among 45 tested, no critical analysis could be applied in the case of female offspring. Both groups excluded X-linked inheritance on the basis of male-to-male transmission. Also a recessive genetic transmission pattern was excluded by Stecher et al. [457] on the basis of a probability analysis. In neither of these studies was a rigorous statistical analysis performed to exclude a unimodal distribution with skewness toward high values.

Hypothesis of Multifactorial Inheritance   The hypothesis of an autosomal dominant genetic control of hyperuricemia was questioned by Hauge and Harvald [140] following their study of 261 sibs of 32 gouty subjects. These writers con-

Figure 50-32 Pedigree of family with primary gout, normal uric acid production, and low renal clearance of uric acid. Elliptocytosis is also present in the pedigree but discordant with respect to hyperuricemia.

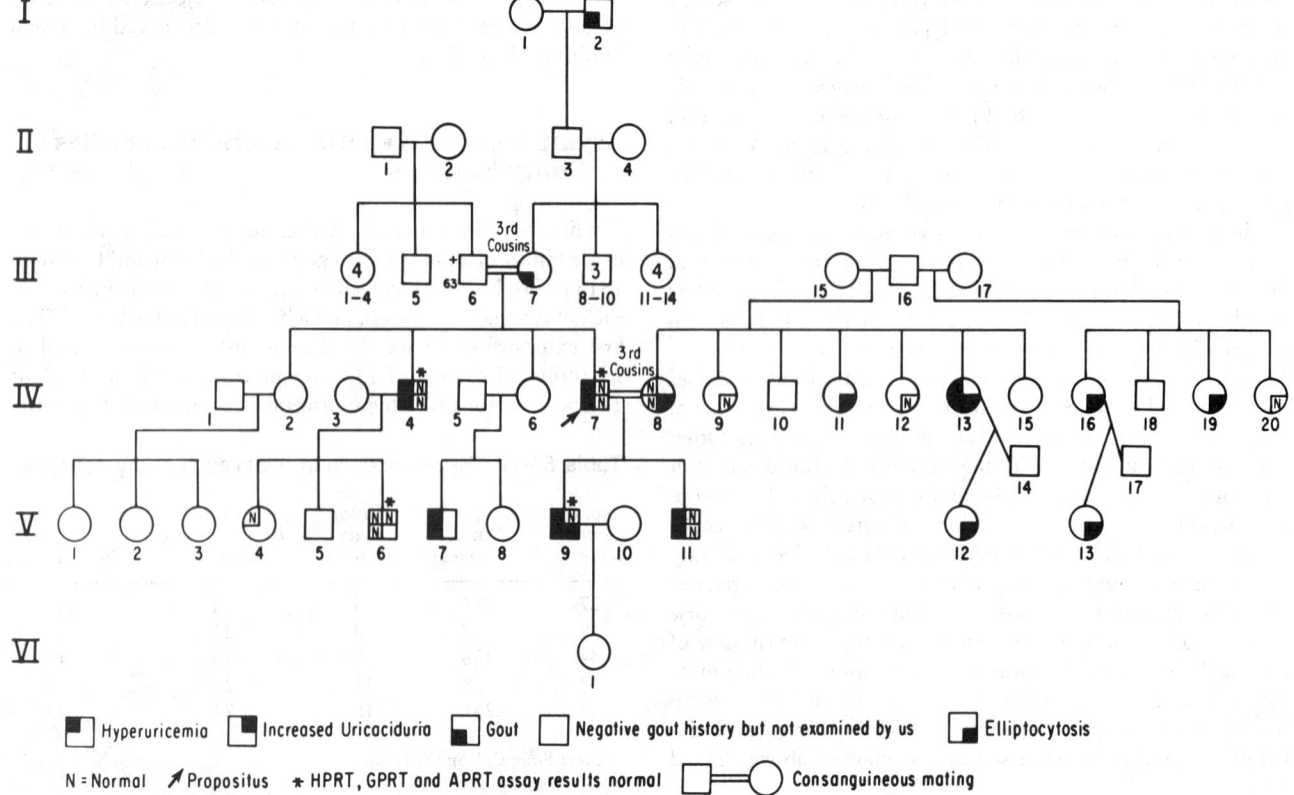

cluded that hyperuricemia was a polygenic trait. Plots of serum uric acid values in both controls and relatives fitted unimodal distributions. No clear separation could be made between normal and abnormal uric acid values, although the mean values for both male and female relatives of gouty patients were higher than the mean values of their respected control groups. The data on male sibs conformed satisfactorily to the sum of two normal distributions, but those on female relatives did not. The writers therefore excluded inheritance due to a single autosomal dominant gene and concluded that to the extent that the higher uric acid values observed in these sibs as compared with the control group were genetically determined, multifactorial inheritance was responsible.

In 1965, Neel and associates [458] restudied 271 members of 19 families first studied 18 years earlier by Smyth et al. [7] because of a gouty propositus. The new results showed a significant skewing to the right, and the evidence for bimodality was less convincing than earlier. The hypothesis of multifactorial inheritance was considered at least as tenable as the "one-gene hyperuricemia" hypothesis.

Hyperuricemia in Population Studies

A study of 2000 Blackfoot and Pima Indians showed an association of hyperuricemia with obesity and surface area, but in addition there were strong hereditary determinants of serum urate levels, which appeared to be polygenic. Transmission patterns suggested that some of the genes were autosomal dominants and others possibly X-linked dominants [459]. The studies of Mikkelsen et al. [139, 460] of 6000 residents of Tecumseh, Michigan, and of Hall et al. [11] of 5000 residents of Framingham, Massachusetts, also favored multifactorial inheritance. The frequency histograms showed skewness toward high values without evidence of bimodality.

In contrast, the population studies of Lawrence et al. [10] in England, of Cobb and associates of Pittsburgh executives and medical students, of Decker et al. of Filipino males living in northwestern North America, and of Burch et al. of the Chamorros and Carolinians of the Mariana Islands all showed bimodal distribution of serum uric acid values [2]. Accordingly, these studies appear to support the dominant-gene hypothesis.

When all available data are considered, they suggest a possible synthesis of views. In the species at large, the serum uric acid concentration is controlled by multiple genes. The probability of selecting out an apparently dominant genetic factor increases when the basis of selection is racial, when the group is an isolate, or when the study concerns several generations of families in which gout occurs, as in the studies of Smyth et al. [7] and Stecher et al. [457]. Evidence for polygenic control will be more prominent when the population is heterogeneous or when only sibs of gouty subjects are studied, as in the investigations of Hague and Harvald [140].

Further progress in understanding the heredity of hyperuricemia will require a definition of the precise biochemical mechanism of hyperuricemia in each isolate or family, and study of the transmission of that trait.

X-linked Hyperuricemia

HPRT Deficiency   As pointed out in Chap. 51, hypoxanthine-guanine phosphoribosyltransferase deficiency is an X-linked condition, clinically manifest in fully expressed form only in the hemizygous male. A representative pedigree of complete deficiency (Lesch-Nyhan syndrome) is shown in Fig. 51-9, and one of partial deficiency in Fig. 50-33. Examples of complete [436] or partial [300] deficiencies among half-brothers are known. In both instances the half-brothers were related through their mothers. No examples of male-to-male transmission of HPRT deficiency have been identified. The gene coding for HPRT is located on the long arm of the X chromosome between the genes coding for PP-ribose-P synthetase [461] and glucose-6-phosphate dehydrogenase [462].

Heterozygous subjects may be mildly hyperuricemic, may show greater than normal quantities of uric acid in their urine, may show abnormalities of kinetics of uric acid synthesis or turnover, and may show values of erythrocyte HPRT activity intermediate between normal values and values in deficient subjects [329, 380]. All these abnormalities are more prevalent among heterozygotes for the "partial" enzyme defect than for the complete deficiency. At least three heterozygotes have had attacks of monoarticular arthritis thought to be gout.

PP-Ribose-P Synthetase Variants   The gene for PP-ribose-P synthetase has been localized on the X chromosome on the basis of separation of two clones of cells expressing distinct phenotypes with respect to PP-ribose-P synthetase from heterozygous female members of two families with structurally altered forms of the enzyme [463, 464] and of cotransference of the enzyme with HPRT as well as additional X-linked enzymatic markers in human-hamster hybrid clones [212]. The gene has been assigned to a position on the long arm of the X, between the loci for α-galactosidase and HPRT [212].

Most of the subjects identified with variant PP-ribose-P synthetase activity and gout have been males. There are no recorded instances of male-to-male transmission. In the first family described with PP-ribose-P synthetase superactivity two brothers were affected. Both parents had normal serum urate levels, but the mother excreted 1100 mg uric acid a day, and her fibroblasts incorporated more than normal quantities of ^{14}C-formate into soluble purines [465]. In the second family (Fig. 50-34) two brothers and one daughter were affected.

The mother in the first family and the daughter in the second were the subjects later shown to have two populations of cells with respect to enzyme phenotype [463, 464]. Thus the pedigrees are consistent with X-linkage, although prior to the cloning studies an autosomal dominant pattern of inheritance was not excluded.

THERAPY

The objectives of therapy differ in acute gouty arthritis, interval gout, and chronic tophaceous gout. Current concepts and practices in the treatment of primary and secondary gout are presented in detail elsewhere [1]. This discussion will be limited to the *mechanisms of the actions* of drugs that have specific effects in gout or upon purine metabolism.

Acute Gout

The acute gouty attack may be treated with colchicine, phen-

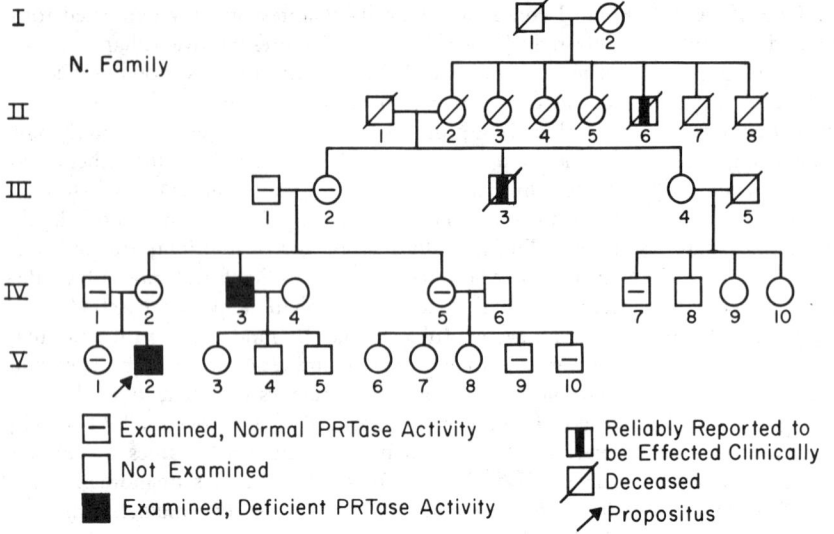

I   N. Family

☐— Examined, Normal PRTase Activity
☐ Not Examined
◼ Examined, Deficient PRTase Activity

▯▮ Reliably Reported to be Effected Clinically
◿ Deceased
↗ Propositus

Figure 50-33 Pedigree of a family with partial HPRT deficiency, gout, and spinocerebellar ataxia. (*Reproduced from Kelley et al.* [300], *with permission of* Annals of Internal Medicine.)

ylbutazone, oxyphenbutazone, indomethacin, naproxen, ibuprofen, and other nonsteroidal anti-inflammatory agents, ACTH, or corticoids. The possible mechanism of action of colchicine will be discussed below.

Colchicine The response of the inflammatory reaction of acute gouty arthritis to colchicine (Fig. 50-35) has long been considered specific, but this time-honored axiom has been questioned in reports of responses of acutely inflamed joints of serum sickness, experimental arthritis, sarcoid arthritis, rheumatoid arthritis, and the inflammation associated with hydroxyapatite calcific tendinitis [1, 2]. Some of the disagreement results from the varying criteria for an adequate colchicine response. Wallace et al. [466] noted a typical response to oral colchicine in 75 percent of 58 patients with gout (major subsidence of objective changes of joint inflammation within 48 h, and no recrudescence of inflammation within 7 days), and in only 4 of 37 patients with a variety of other articular disorders. Response to colchicine given intravenously may be more specific for gouty arthritis.

The nature of anti-inflammatory action of colchicine in gout has been one of the mysteries of medicine, but recent studies by Spilberg [50] showing that colchicine blocks the production of a leukocyte chemotactic factor in response to crystal ingestion (see "Mediation of the Inflammatory Response" above) may at long last offer a decisive clue to the mechanism of its action. Following its intravenous infusion, colchicine rapidly enters cells. It inhibits the movement of granules within the cell as well as the secretion of cellular components to the exterior. Specific examples [1, 2] of the effects of colchicine include (1) inhibition of insulin secretion from pancreatic beta cells, (2) inhibition of iodine and thyroxine secretion from the thyroid gland, (3) inhibition of TSH secretion by the pituitary gland, (4) inhibition of catecholamine secretion by adrenal medulla or axons, (5) stimulation of steroid secretion by adrenal tumor cells in culture, (6) decreased aggregation of melanin in frog skin, (7) decreased release of histamine from mast cells, (8) decreased release of lysosomal hydrolases to the cell exterior by phagocytes, (9) decreased amylase secretion by parotid tissue, (10) inhibition of collagen transport to the extracellular space, (11) stimulation of collagenase production in cultured mammalian cells, (12) impairment of the renal reponse to antidiuretic hormone, (13) inhibition of axonal transport, and (14)

production of denervationlike changes in mammalian skeletal muscle.

It seems likely that many of these effects of colchicine can be attributed to its interaction with a subunit protein of microtubules, with which colchicine forms a reversible covalent complex [467, 468]. Microtubules form a part of the internal cytoskeleton, which is critical to a number of cellular events, including formation of the mitotic spindle and movement of granules.

Colchicine inhibits a variety of leukocyte functions, including [1, 2] leukocyte adhesiveness, ameboid motility, mobilization, chemotaxis, random motility under the influence of urate, degranulation of lysosomes, and leukocyte metabolism during phagocytosis. In addition, colchicine blocks kinin release from plasma under the influence of leukocytes. However, the most potent inhibitory effects of colchicine are on chemotaxis and random motility of leukocytes under the influence of urate.

Colchicine does not alter serum concentration or renal excretion of uric acid, nor does it have any significant effect on

Figure 50-34 Pedigree of family with PP-ribose-P synthetase mutant of high specific activity. (*From Becker et al.* [431a], *by permission of* The American Journal of Medicine.)

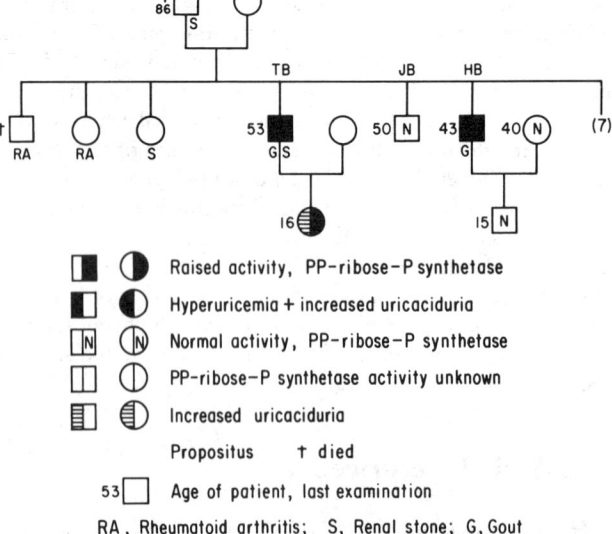

▮▮ ◖ Raised activity, PP-ribose-P synthetase
▮▮ ◖ Hyperuricemia + increased uricaciduria
▯N̄ Ⓝ Normal activity, PP-ribose-P synthetase
▯ ◖ PP-ribose-P synthetase activity unknown
▤ ◑ Increased uricaciduria

   Propositus   † died

53☐ Age of patient, last examination

RA , Rheumatoid arthritis;   S, Renal stone;   G, Gout

STRUCTURE OF COLCHICINE

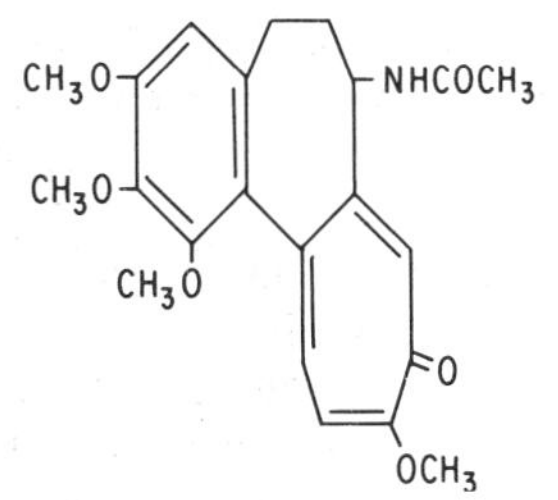

Figure 50-35 Structure of colchicine.

the miscible pool of uric acid or the rate of its turnover [298].

Regulation of Serum Urate Level

Four approaches have been employed in attempts to reduce serum urate levels in hyperuricemic subjects. These include (1) reduction of uric acid synthesis by dietary means—restriction of purine, protein, ethanol, or caloric intake; (2) promotion of increased uric acid excretion by the administration of uricosuric agents; (3) destruction of urate within the body by the administration of uricase; (4) inhibition of uric acid synthesis by the administration of agents which either inhibit xanthine oxidase or purine synthesis *de novo*, or both.

The efficacy of dietary measures has been touched upon elsewhere in this chapter. Influences upon rates of both production of purines and excretion of uric acid have been cited, but the full scope of these complex interrelationships is not yet known. In addition to the obvious effect of the restriction of purine intake upon the production of uric acid, protein restriction in and of itself reduces the rate of purine synthesis *de novo* in both normal and gouty humans [316]. Although caloric restriction in obese gouty subjects is recommended, and alcohol and purine restriction are also prudent, the advent of well-tolerated antihyperuricemic agents has rendered severe dietary measures unnecessary in most gouty patients.

This section will deal with the pharmacologic therapy of hyperuricemia or uricaciduria. Indications for therapy include recurrent attacks of acute gouty arthritis or of uric acid nephrolithiasis, or demonstrable accumulations of monosodium urate as visible or radiographically detectable tophi. Asymptomatic hyperuricemia is not an indication for therapy with drugs, unless serum urate levels are in a range where acute gouty attacks, early tophaceous gout, uric acid nephrolithiasis, or hyperuricemic nephropathy become statistically likely. From data presented elsewhere in this chapter, a critical value of 9 mg/dl or above is suggested. In other hyperuricemic subjects, one can afford to wait for an attack of acute gout or of uric acid stone before instituting therapy. Mild hyperuricemia by itself does not appear to be associated with a more rapid decline of renal function than occurs in nonhyperuricemic subjects of equivalent age [72, 86].

When administration of an antihyperuricemic drug is indicated, the objective of treatment is to reduce the serum urate level to 6 mg/dl or lower and to maintain it in this range indefinitely. No resolution of tophi occurs unless the serum level is brought below 7 mg/dl [469], but if lower levels are achieved, striking reductions in the size of visible tophi and some regeneration and recalcification of bone matrix may take place [469,

470]. The shift of the uric acid balance in tissues from positive to negative occurs as a consequence of the lowering of serum uric acid levels to values sufficiently undersaturated to permit the dissolution of tophi. In addition, the frequency of attacks of acute gout may eventually be considerably reduced in patients by the adequate control of hyperuricemia, although shortly after the institution of therapy acute attacks may continue.

Uricosuric Drugs This category of compounds includes [2] salicylates, cinchophen, probenecid, phenylbutazone and its derivatives, sulfinpyrazone and *p*-nitrophenylbutazone, zoxazolamine, dicoumarol, ethyl biscoumacetate, phenylindandione, acetoheximide, glycine, azauridine, orotic acid, ethyl *p*-chlorophenoxyisobutyric acid, benziodarone, benzbromaron, chlorprothixene, ticrynafen, indacrinone, and certain radiographic agents. At the present time probenecid and sulfinpyrazone are most widely employed in this country; benzbromarone, and zoxazolamine are used in Europe as well.

All these compounds increase the excretion of uric acid without causing a significant change in the glomerular filtration rate. Several have been shown to have a paradoxical effect upon uric acid excretion, consisting of an inhibition of excretion at low doses and an enhancement at high doses. The explanation of this biphasic response has been discussed above.

Striking reductions of the miscible pool of uric acid have been demonstrated after the administration of adequate doses of salicylates [298], probenecid [471], phenylbutazone [303, 472], and cortisone [473]. These are probably accounted for entirely by the increment in urate excretion [303].

The uricosuric actions of probenecid, sulfinpyrazone, and zoxazolamine are suppressed by salicylates in human beings, in part because they countermand the inhibition of tubular reabsorption of uric acid produced by uricosuric drugs. The mechanism is complex, however, and also involves effects upon the tubular secretion of uric acid by salicylates and competition between salicylates and sulfinpyrazone for binding sites on transporting plasma proteins and perhaps elsewhere [474]. Probenecid, phenylbutazone, and salicylates are reported to reduce urate binding to protein. Sulfinpyrazone may have a similar though less striking effect [475]. Such an action could at best account for only a fraction of their uricosuric effects.

EFFECT ON URIC ACID SECRETION The uricosuric effects of several drugs [2], including glycine [2], benziodarone, azapropazone, and the x-ray contrast agents, have been attributed to enhanced tubular secretion of urate. This hypothesis was based on the finding that prior administration of pyrazinamide (PZA) partially or completely blocked the uricosuric effects of these drugs. At the time these studies were done, urate secretion was thought to occur beyond all urate reabsorptive sites in the proximal renal tubules. However, the uricosuric action of these drugs could also be explained by an effect upon reabsorption of uric acid at a postsecretory site.

THERAPEUTIC EFFECTS Agents such as probenecid [469] and sulfinpyrazone [476] have been dramatically effective in the control of hyperuricemia and the prevention and resolution of tophi in a large segment of the gouty population. Nevertheless, in spite of careful management, a significant percentage of patients is not brought under ideal control. In one large clinic,

27 percent of the patients receiving probenecid failed to achieve serum urate levels of less than 7 mg/dl [469]. In another study with various agents, only half of 64 patients achieved levels of 6 mg/dl [477]. Leading causes of failure were drug intolerance, concomitant salicylate ingestion, and renal impairment. In the experience of de Seze et al. [478] and Kuzell et al. [476], about one-third of patients eventually became intolerant of probenecid. Tolerance for sulfinpyrazone is reported to be better than for probenecid. At times, combinations of uricosuric drugs prove superior to the use of one drug alone [479].

The use of uricosuric agents adds to the risk of urinary stone formation and does not result in the improvement of impaired renal function, though further progression of renal damage may be arrested [480].

Uricase Infusion of purified uricase results in a transient reduction in serum urate levels [481, 482]. An increased renal clearance of uric acid accounts for part of the observed effect [482]. Rapid development of antibodies results in diminished effectiveness of repeated injections [483] and occasionally anaphylaxis [484]. Recent development of a very active microbial urate oxidase has led to a renewed interest in this form of therapy [484, 485]. The microbial and animal enzymes are immunologically unrelated [485]. Urate oxidase from *Candida utilis* was covalently attached to polyethylene glycol with retention of 11 percent of activity [486]. In five subjects a single intravenous dose resulted in the rapid *disappearance* of serum urate for 32 h, without toxic effects. Urinary uric acid was largely replaced by allantoin. No long-term studies have yet been reported.

Allopurinol Allopurinol (4-hydroxypyrazolo [3,4-*d*] pyrimidine) is an analogue of hypoxanthine in which the positions of N7 and C8 are reversed [487] (Fig. 50-36). Allopurinol is metabolized to oxipurinol (the 4,6-dihydroxy analogue) by xanthine oxidase [488]. Oxipurinol is also an inhibitor of xanthine oxidase. The Michaelis constant of allopurinol is some fifteen- to twentyfold lower than that of xanthine, whereas that of oxipurinol is comparable to that of xanthine [488]. Allopurinol shows substrate-competitive kinetics. Both allopurinol and oxipurinol produce pseudoirreversible inactivation

of xanthine oxidase. Inactivation occurs when allopurinol and the enzyme are incubated in the absence of substrate, but enzyme activity can be restored by prolonged dialysis. Oxipurinol has no effect on the enzyme alone, but inactivates in the presence of xanthine when molecular oxygen is the hydrogen acceptor [489].

Allopurinol has a half-life in vivo of only 2 to 3 h [490]. Since allopurinol and oxipurinol both inhibit the oxidation of allopurinol, the half-life of allopurinol increases as the level of xanthine oxidase inhibition increases. Three to ten percent of an administered dose is excreted with a clearance rate approximately equal to the GRF [490]. Most of the allopurinol (45 to 65 percent) is rapidly oxidized to oxipurinol in vivo, with a portion being converted to 1-N(5'-ribosyl) allopurinol [491] and 1-N-(5'-phosphoribosyl) allopurinol [217]. Most of the oxipurinol formed is excreted unchanged by the kidney, with a half-life ranging from 13.5 to 28 h [490, 492]. Small portions are metabolized to 7-N-(5'ribosyl) oxipurinol [493] and also to the corresponding 5'-phosphoribosyl derivatives [493a] (Fig. 50-36). Factors which affect uric acid excretion generally alter oxipurinol excretion in a similar manner [493]. Because of its prolonged half-life oxipurinol may be primarily responsible for xanthine oxidase inhibition in vivo when allopurinol is administered [488]. Although allopurinol is the more effective of the two agents when the two are compared orally, this reflects the relatively poor absorption of oxipurinol in the gastrointestinal tract [494].

Allopurinol has a number of additional effects. Through its action upon xanthine oxidase it inhibits trytophan pyrrolase [495], probably by limiting the availability of H_2O_2 for use by the latter enzyme. In vitro, allopurinol also inhibits purine nucleoside phosphorylase [177, 491] and pyrimidine deoxyribosyltransferase [496]. It activates, and at higher concentration inhibits, urate oxidase [497]. In ribonucleotide linkage, allopurinol inhibits early enzymes of both purine and pyrimidine biosynthesis. Its inhibition of amidophosphoribosyltransferase was described above. The increased urinary excretion of orotic acid and orotidine in patients receiving allopurinol [498, 499] has been traced to the inhibition of orotidylic decarboxylase by allopurinol ribonucleotide. The action occurs also in HPRT-deficient subjects [500]. Furthermore, high concentrations of both allopurinol and oxipurinol inhibit purine biosyn-

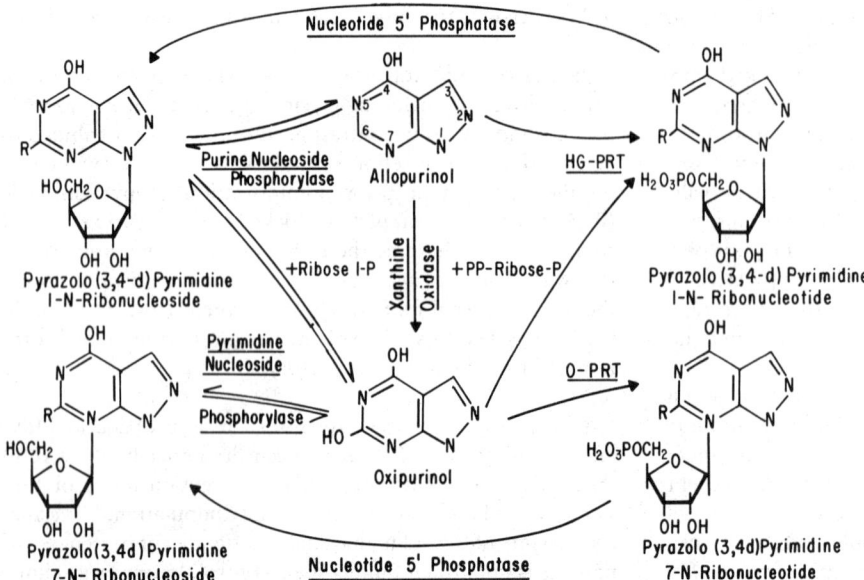

Figure 50-36 Reactions of allopurinol and its oxidation product oxipurinol. Enzymes are underlined. R = H-(allopurinol) or HO-(oxipurinol).

thesis *de novo* in azaserine-treated HPRT-deficient fibroblasts in culture [283]; they also inhibit the orotidylic decarboxylase of HPRT-deficient cells. These actions are also dependent upon the presence of PP-ribose-P and upon the activity of another enzyme, orotate phosphoribosyltransferase, which converts oxipurinol to 7-*N*-(5′-phosphoribosyl) oxipurinol, analogous to the 3-*N*-(5′phosphoribosyl) purines described above (Fig. 50-36).

Allopurinol therapy results in an eightfold increase in activity of both the orotate phosphoribosyltransferase and the orotidylic decarboxylase of erythrocytes [501], apparently through stabilization mechanism rather than as an effect upon enzyme synthesis or turnover [502].

Thiopurinol (mercapto pyrazolo-pyrimidine), although developed for use as a xanthine oxidase inhibitor, apparently reduces uric acid synthesis without a concomitant increase in oxypurine excretion [503]. This effect has also been postulated to reflect inhibition of purine biosynthesis *de novo*, although this remains to be documented.

The administration of allopurinol to subjects with normal renal function is followed by a prompt decrease in the serum and urinary uric acid values within 24 to 48 h. These reach minimal values in 4 days to 2 weeks and remain relatively constant over prolonged periods of time [504, 505]. Inhibition of urate production by allopurinol is accompanied by increased amounts of the precursors, hypoxanthine and xanthine, in the urine, usually within 4 to 6 h [490]. Only trivial changes occur in the excretion of other urinary purine bases [498]. The combined increase in hypoxanthine and xanthine, though striking, usually falls far short of balancing the decrement in uric acid (see below). Withdrawal of allopurinol results in a return to pretreatment serum urate levels within a few days. Occasional more prolonged effects are associated with delayed excretion of oxipurinol [506].

Normal serum urate values can be achieved in all but a few patients. The doses required to reduce the elevated levels to normal average 200 to 300 mg/day for patients with mild disease and 400 to 600 mg/day for those with moderately severe tophaceous disease; rarely, doses of 700 to 1000 mg/day have been required. The average dose required to maintain the serum urate level between 6.0 and 6.9 mg/dl is 300 mg/day. In most patients allopurinol need not be initiated at a low dose. In some patients with frequent episodes of gout, however, beginning with a low dose will lessen the probability of precipitating a series of incapacitating attacks. Because of the long biologic half-life of the active metabolite, oxipurinol, it is not necessary to divide the doses nor to space them throughout the day. A single 300-mg tablet has been shown to be as effective as three divided doses of 100 mg each [507].

By the selection of the appropriate dose of allopurinol it is possible to reduce the serum urate level to normal or, if desired, to hold it as low as 2 or 3 mg/dl indefinitely, unless renal function is markedly limited. Even then, appreciable reduction of serum urate values can be achieved with allopurinol.

When allopurinol is given, serum oxypurine levels rise only slightly, reaching 0.5 to 1.0 mg/dl [337, 508] or, rarely, 2 mg/dl [342] because of the high renal clearance of oxypurines. The oxypurine levels achieved are well below the solubility limits of hypoxanthine or xanthine in serum.

THERAPEUTIC EFFECTS   An extensive clinical experience attests to the usefulness of allopurinol as an antihyperuricemic

agent in gout. Resolution of tophi occurs gradually with the maintenance of normal serum urate levels and is frequently extensive by 6 to 12 months. Slower improvement can be anticipated in patients with renal insufficiency. Destructive arthritis improves. There is a corresponding improvement in functional status. The progression of nephropathy appears to halt in most patients [2, 505].

Formation of uric acid stones can be virtually abolished with allopurinol. The drug has found wide utility in the treatment of idiopathic uric acid nephrolithiasis, as it has in management of nephrolithiasis in otherwise asymptomatic hyperuricemia and in frankly gouty subjects. In addition, it has proved very useful in controlling the marked hyperuricemia and hyperuricaciduria and urinary crystalluria that may accompany aggressive therapy of lymphoma or leukemia. A variety of forms of secondary gout have been effectively treated with allopurinol [2].

COMBINED USE OF ALLOPURINOL AND A URICOSURIC AGENT
Uricosuric agents may be used concurrently with allopurinol to hasten mobilization of urate deposits [505, 509]. Combined therapy may be particularly effective in the patient with extensive tophaceous deposits (and good renal function) where substantial amounts of preformed urate must be eliminated. The administration of a uricosuric agent to a patient receiving allopurinol usually results in appreciable increases of urinary uric acid excretion and a further decline in serum urate level [505]. Allopurinol lengthens the biologic half-life of probenecid and thus potentiates its uricosuric effect [510]. On the other hand, uricosuric drugs increase the clearance of oxipurinol in humans [488, 493] and thus diminish the degree of xanthine oxidase inhibition. They cause either no change or a decrease in excretion of oxypurines in patients receiving allopurinol [493].

COMPLICATIONS OF ALLOPURINOL THERAPY   *Acute attacks of gout* The frequency of gouty attacks may remain unchanged or may increase on initiation of therapy. Typical attacks have occurred with serum urate levels as low as 2 mg/dl and comparably low urinary urate excretions. On the basis of these experiences, we recommend that daily colchicine be given during the first 6 to 12 months of therapy of gout with allopurinol. After excess urate has been mobilized, attacks will be rare, provided normal serum urate levels are maintained.

Xanthine renal stones   More than one-half the urinary oxypurine increase observed with allopurinol therapy consists of xanthine [498], a sparingly soluble compound in acid and neutral urine [508]. The levels attained with full doses of allopurinol equal those which in xanthinuric subjects (who lack xanthine oxidase activity as an inborn error of metabolism) have caused formation of urinary calculi composed of xanthine (see Chap. 55). Thus far, development of xanthine crystalluria or lithiasis as a complication of allopurinol therapy has not been observed in any patient given the drug for treatment of idiopathic gout or uric acid stones.

Rare instances of xanthine stone formation induced by allopurinol therapy have been reported in other circumstances. These have occurred in four children with the Lesch-Nyhan syndrome [511–514] and in one adult with partial HPRT deficiency [515]. In addition xanthine stones have been reported in an adult with lymphosarcoma given allopurinol [516]. Several of these patients excreted approximately 1500 mg uric acid a day prior to allopurinol therapy. One child, who received allopurinol 9 mg/kg, excreted as much as 800 mg xanthine a day while on therapy [511, 517]. Another case occurred in a 9-year-old American boy with Burkitt's lymphoma, who was given 600 mg allopurinol a day. He excreted 1976 mg of oxypurines, 240 to 950 mg orotic acid, and 640 to 1530 mg orotidine daily in the urine, and passed many crystals identified as xanthine [518]. Allopurinol should be given cautiously and in minimal doses to patients with extraordinarily great uric acid excretion values, particularly those with inability to reutilize hypoxanthine and xanthine because of HPRT deficiency.

Oxipurinol crystal deposition   Watts et al. have demonstrated microcrystalline deposits of oxipurinol as well as of hypoxanthine and xanthine in muscle biopsy specimens of patients receiving allopurinol for treatment of gout. There are no recognizable clinical consequences of this phenomenon. The concentration of hypoxanthine and xanthine in muscle is considerably less than observed in patients congenitally deficient in xanthine oxidase [519].

In addition, one instance of formation of oxipurinol sludge and stones in the urinary tract has been reported in an 8-year-old boy given both allopurinol and oxipurinol orally in doses of 15 and 37.5 mg/kg, respectively [520]. Surgical intervention was required because of urinary tract obstruction. Both sludge and stones showed infrared spectra virtually the same as those with authentic oxipurinol, and unlike the spectrums of allopurinol and uric acid. Oxipurinol nephrolithiasis has also been reported in a patient with regional enteritis given allopurinol for uric acid renal stones [521].

Toxicity of allopurinol   Serious toxicity of allopurinol therapy appears to be rare. A small percentage of patients (perhaps 5 percent) find it necessary to discontinue the drug [510]. Allopurinol may lead to the development of gastrointestinal intolerance, skin rashes, sometimes with fever, occasionally toxic epidermal necrolysis, alopecia, bone marrow suppression with leukopenia and thrombocytopenia, agranulocytosis, hepatitis, granulomatous liver disease, severe jaundice, fatal hepatic necrosis and vasculitis. The incidence of side effects of all kinds may be about 20 percent [510]. Toxic effects tend to occur more often in the presence of renal insufficiency.

Skin rashes are more frequent and serious in patients receiving allopurinol and ampicillin. In the Boston Collaborative Drug Surveillance Program [522], 2.1 percent of 283 patients receiving allopurinol without ampicillin, 7.5 percent of 1257 patients receiving only ampicillin, and 22.4 percent of 67 hospitalized patients receiving allopurinol and ampicillin experienced drug rashes. Although it could not be determined whether the threefold greater risk of drug rash in patients taking ampicillin plus allopurinol was associated with allopurinol or hyperuricemia, it would be prudent not to prescribe these two drugs together. Sometimes allopurinol can be successfully reinstituted for treatment of gout after a cutaneous reaction [523].

EFFECT OF ALLOPURINOL ON PURINE SYNTHESIS *DE NOVO*
In most patients the replacement of urinary uric acid by the oxypurines, hypoxanthine and xanthine, is less than stoichiometric [337, 342, 505, 508, 524]. The deficit ranges from 10 to 60 percent, and in patients with normal HPRT activity is roughly proportional to the pretreatment level of uric acid excretion (Fig. 50-37) [300, 342, 505, 508, 524]. The total

deficit may amount to several hundred milligrams of total purines (uric acid plus oxypurines) a day [337, 342, 505]. In addition, the reduction in total purine excretion is associated with a decreased incorporation of isotopic glycine into urinary uric acid [525]. This effect of allopurinol requires normal HPRT activity (Fig. 50-37) [300, 526] and could be due to a combination of factors, including (1) depletion of PP-ribose-P [217]; (2) reduction in purine biosynthesis *de novo* due to the inhibitory action of purine ribonucleotides derived from IMP on PP-ribose-P synthetase and amidophosphoribosyltransferase [231]; and (3) reduction of purine biosynthesis *de novo* by the inhibitory effect of allopurinol ribonucleotide on amidophosphoribosyltransferase [181]. Studies by Elion and Nelson [527] suggest that the last possibility is probably not biologically very important. Tissue levels of allopurinol ribonucleotide in human liver are probably less than 0.0001 mM, and concentrations of di- or triphosphates of allopurinol or oxipurinol are not present at the 10^{-9} M level, reflecting the absence in mammalian tissues of kinases for inosinic and xanthylic acids.

EFFECTS OF ALLOPURINOL IN PATIENTS DEFICIENT IN HYPOXANTHINE-GUANINE PHOSPHORIBOSYLTRANSFERASE ACTIVITY
Allopurinol exerts its predicted effect upon xanthine oxidase in HPRT-deficient subjects. Uric acid levels in blood and urine are reduced, and urinary oxypurines are increased. However, in contrast to results in other subjects, there is a stoichiometric replacement of urinary uric acid by hypoxanthine and xanthine in HPRT-deficient subjects [300, 519] (Fig. 50-37). Similarly, no reduction of total purine excretion occurs in response to azathioprine [288]. These anomalous responses are attributed to the HPRT deficiency itself, as inhibition of purine synthesis *de novo* requires prior conversion of these analogue bases to ribonucleotide form [181, 199, 284]. No reduction of intracellular PP-ribose-P content occurs on incubation of HPRT-deficient erythrocytes with allopurinol [217].

In spite of the HPRT deficiency, allopurinol does result in orotidinuria in children with the Lesch-Nyhan syndrome. Furthermore, in HPRT-deficient fibroblasts studied in vitro, high concentrations of both allopurinol and oxipurinol inhibit an early step of purine synthesis *de novo*, probably amidophosphoribosyltransferase [283]. These effects probably involve the formation of oxipurinol-7-N-ribonucleotide, which is an analogue of the purine-3-N-ribonucleotides, and whose formation is also catalyzed by orotate phosphoribosyltransferase [499] (Fig. 50-36).

OTHER EFFECTS OF ALLOPURINOL   Allopurinol inhibits growth of several *Leishmania* species in vitro [528, 529]. Allopurinol ribonucleoside is even more effective than free allopurinol [529, 530]. In these organisms allopurinol is sequentially converted to allopurinol mononucleotide and 4-aminopyrazolo[3,4-*d*]pyrimidine mono-, di-, and trinucleotides. The latter are incorporated into RNA [531]. The metabolism of allopurinol is the same in intracellular as in extracellular forms [531]. These studies offer promise of a new chemotherapeutic approach for the treatment of leishmaniasis.

Allopurinol antagonizes the growth-inhibitory activity of 5-fluorouracil in leukemic cell lines in culture [532] and reduces the mortality of 5-fluorouracil (5-FU) in mice and rats by almost twofold [533]. It is proposed that orotate accumulation within the cell consequent to inhibition of orotidine 5-monophosphate decarboxylase by oxipurinol ribonucleotide

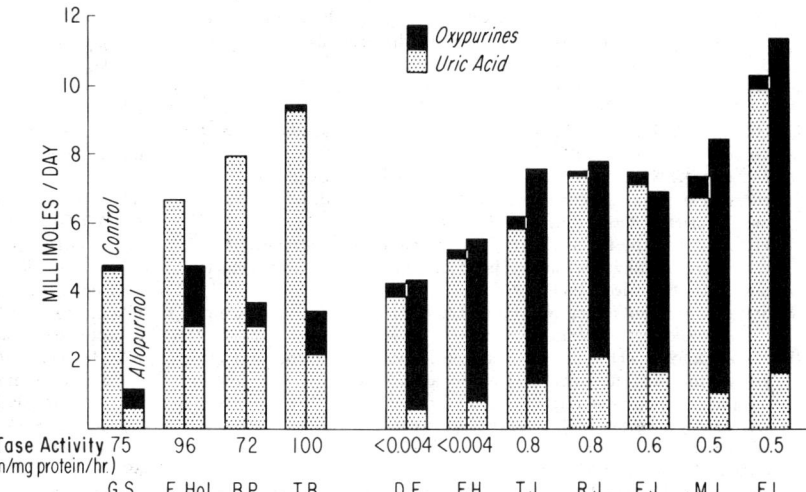

Figure 50-37 Effects of allopurinol on total purine excretion in patients who produce excessive quantities of uric acid. Comparison in patients with normal, virtually completely deficient, and partially deficient hypoxanthine-guanine phosphoribosyltransferase (HPRT) activity. The height of each bar represents total purine excretion, oxypurines plus uric acid. (*From Kelley et al.* [300], *with permission of* Annals of Internal Medicine.)

competes with the activation of 5-FU via orotate phosphoribosyltransferase [533].

Allopurinol increases bone marrow depression during treatment with cyclophosphamide [534]. Allopurinol does not significantly influence the serum half-life of unchanged cyclophosphamide but does cause an elevation of serum concentrations of drug metabolites [535].

Allopurinol apparently increases the toxicity of adenine arabinoside, perhaps because a metabolite, hypoxanthine arabinoside, is further metabolized to xanthine arabinoside by xanthine oxidase [536].

Long-term allopurinol administration (14 to 28 days) inhibits theophylline metabolism [537]. 1-Methylxanthine appears in urine, at the expense of 1-methyluric acid [538].

A controlled, double-blind study of allopurinol therapy in muscular dystrophy failed to confirm earlier claims of benefit [539].

REFERENCES

1. WYNGAARDEN JB, KELLEY WN: *Gout and Hyperuricemia.* New York, Grune & Stratton, 1976
2. WYNGAARDEN JB, KELLEY WN: Gout, in Stanbury JB, Wyngaarden JB, Fredrickson DS (eds): *Metabolic Basis of Inherited Disease*, 4th ed. New York, McGraw-Hill, 1978, p 916
3. SYDENHAM T: *Tractatus de podagra et hydrope.* London, G. Kettilby, 1683
4. GARROD AB: Observations on certain pathological conditions of the blood and urine in gout, rheumatism and Bright's disease. *Trans Med Chir Soc Edinburgh* 31:83, 1848
5. GARROD AB: On the blood and effused fluids in gout, rheumatism and Bright's disease. *Trans Med Chir Soc Edinburgh* 37:49, 1854
6. COPEMAN WSC: *A Short History of the Gout and the Rheumatic Diseases.* Berkeley, University of California Press, 1964
7. SMYTH CJ, COTTERMAN CW, FREYBERG RH: The genetics of gout and hyperuricemia: Analysis of nineteen families. *J Clin Invest* 27:749, 1948
8. SYDENHAM T: *The Works of Thomas Sydenham*, translated by RG Latham. London, Sydenham Society, 1850, vol II
9. HADLER NM, FRANCK WA, BRESS NM: Acute polyarticular gout. *Am J Med* 56:715, 1974
10. LAWRENCE JS: Heritable disorders of connective tissue. *Proc R Soc Med* 53:522, 1960
10a. CURRIE WJC: Prevalence and incidence of the diagnosis of gout in Great Britain. *Ann Rheum Dis* 38:101, 1979
11. HALL AP, BARRY PE, DAWBER TR, McNAMARA M: Epidemiology of gout and hyperuricemia: A long-term population study. *Am J Med* 42:27, 1967
11a. BRAUER GW, PRIOR IAM: Prospective study of gout in New Zealand Maoris. *Ann Rheum Dis* 37:466, 1978

12. SIMMONDS HA, WARREN DJ, CAMERON JS, POTTER CF, FAREBROTHER DA: Familial gout and renal failure in young women. *Clin Nephrol* 14:176, 1980
13. KOLB FO, DE LALLA OF, GOFMAN JW: The hyperlipemias in disorders of carbohydrate metabolism: Serial lipoprotein studies in diabetic acidosis with xanthomatosis and in glycogen storage disease. *Metabolism* 4:310, 1955
14. LESCH M, NYHAN WL: A familiar disorders of uric acid metabolism and central nervous system function. *Am J Med* 36:561, 1964
15. GARROD AB: *A Treatise on Gout and Rheumatic Gout (Rheumatoid Arthritis)*, 3d ed. London, Longman, 1876
16. FREUDWEILER M: Experimentelle untersuchungen uber das Wesen der Gichtknoten. *Dtsch Arch Klin Med* 63:266, 1899
17. FREUDWEILER M: Experimentelle untersuchungen über die Entstehung der Gichtknoten. *Dtsch Arch Klin Med* 69:155, 1901
18. HIS WJ: Schicksal und Wirkungen des säuren harnsäuren Natrons in Bauch und Gelenkhohle des Kaninchens. *Dtsch Arch Klin Med* 67:81, 1900
19. McCARTY DJ JR, HOLLANDER JL: Identification of urate crystals in gouty synovial fluid. *Ann Intern Med* 54:452, 1961
20. McCARTY DJ JR: Phagocytosis of urate crystals in gouty synovial fluid. *Am J Med Sci* 243:288, 1962
21. FAIRES JS, McCARTY DJ JR: Acute synovitis in normal joints of man and dog produced by injections of microcrystalline sodium urate, calcium oxalate and corticosteroid ester. *Arthritis Rheum* 5:295, 1962
22. SEEGMILLER JE, HOWELL RR, MALAWISTA SE: Inflammatory reaction to sodium urate: Its possible relationship to genesis of acute gouty arthritis. *JAMA* 180:469, 1962
23. TSE R, PHELPS P: Polymorphonuclear leukocyte motility in vitro: V. Release of chemotactic activity following phagocytosis of calcium pyrophosphate crystals, diamond dust and urate crystals. *J Lab Clin Med* 76:403, 1970
24. AGUDELO CA, SCHUMACHER HR: The synovitis of acute gouty arthritis: A light and electron microscopic study. *Hum Pathol* 4:265, 1973
25. SCHUMACHER HR, KULKA JP: Needle biopsy of the synovial membrane: Experience with the Parker-Pearson technique. *N Engl J Med* 286:416, 1972
26. WEINBERGER A, SCHUMACHER HR, AGUDELO CA: Urate crystals in asymptomatic metatarsophalangeal joints. *Ann Intern Med* 91:56, 1979
27. TILIAKOS N, WILSON CH JR: The proteinic coating of urate crystals from asymptomatic joints: A clue to their nonpathogenicity. *Arthritis Rheum* 24:S83, 1981 (abstract)
28. ROBERTS W: The Croonian lectures. On the chemistry and therapeutics of uric acid gravel and gout. *Br Med J* 2:61, 1892
29. KATZ WA, SCHUBERT M: The interaction of monosodium urate with connective tissue components. *J Clin Invest* 49:1783, 1970
29a. PERRICONE E, BRANDT KD: Enhancement of urate solution by connective tissue. I. Effect of proteoglycan aggregates and buffer action. *Arthritis Rheum* 21:453, 1978
30. DINGLE JT: Synthesis and degradation of connective tissue in organ cultures, in *Advanced Study Institute on Structure and Function of Connective and Skeletal Tissue.* London, Butterworth, 1965, p 431
31. SCHUBERT M, HAMERMAN D: *A Primer on Connective Tissue Biochemistry.* Philadelphia, Lea & Febiger, 1968
32. LOEB JN: The influence of temperature on the solubility of monosodium urate. *Arthritis Rheum* 15:189, 1972

33. HOLLANDER JL, STONER EK, BROWN EM JR, DE MOOR P: Joint temperature measurements in the evaluation of anti-arthritic agents. *J Clin Invest* 30:701, 1951

34. SIMKIN PA: The pathogenesis of podagra. *Ann Intern Med* 86:230, 1977

35. HOWELL DS: Preliminary observations on local pH in gouty tophi and synovial fluid. *Arthritis Rheum* 8:736, 1965

36. MELMON K, WEBSTER ME, GOLDFINGER SE, SEEGMILLER JE: The presence of a kinin in inflammatory synovial effusion from arthrides of varying etiologies. *Arthritis Rheum* 10:13, 1967

37. PHELPS P, PROKOP DJ, MCCARTY DD: Crystal induced inflammation in canine joints. III. Evidence against bradykinin as a mediator of inflammation. *J Lab Clin Med* 68:443, 1966

38. SPILBERG I: Urate crystal arthritis in animals lacking Hageman factor. *Arthritis Rheum* 17:143, 1974

39. NAFF GB, BYERS PH: Complement as a mediator of inflammation in acute gouty arthritis. I. Studies on the reaction between human serum complement and sodium urate crystals. *J Lab Clin Med* 81:747, 1973

40. GICLAS PC, GINSBERG MH, COOPER NR: Immunoglobulin G independent activation of the classical complement pathway by monosodium urate crystals. *J Clin Invest* 63:759, 1979

41. RUSSELL IJ, MAUSEN CF, KOLB LM, KOLB WP: Activation of the fifth component of human complement in human serum by urate crystals. *Arthritis Rheum* 24:S82, 1981 (abstract)

42. SPILBERG I, OSTERLAND CK: Anti-inflammatory effect of the trypsin-kallikrein inhibitor in acute arthritis induced by urate crystals in rabbits. *J Lab Clin Med* 76:472, 1970

43. FOSTIROPOULOUS K, AUSTEN KT, BLOCK KJ: Total hemolytic complement and second component of complement activity in serum and synovial fluid. *Arthritis Rheum* 8:219, 1965

44. PHELPS P, MCCARTY DJ JR: Crystal induced inflammation in canine joints. II. Importance of polymorphonuclear leukocytes. *J Exp Med* 124:115, 1966

45. CHANG Y-H, GRALLA EJ: Suppression of urate crystal-induced canine joint inflammaiton by heterologous anti-polymorphonuclear leukocyte serum. *Arthritis Rheum* 11:145, 1968

46. AGUDELO CA, SCHUMACHER HR, PHELPS P: Sequence of synovial changes in urate crystal-induced arthritis in the dog. *Arthritis Rheum* 15:100, 1972

47. PHELPS P: Appearance of chemotactic activity following intraarticular injection of monosodium urate crystals: Effect of colchicine. *J Lab Clin Med* 76:622, 1970

48. SPILBERG I, GALLAGHER A, MEHTA JM, MANDELL B: Urate crystal-induced chemotactic factor. Isolation and partial characterization. *J Clin Invest* 58:815, 1976

48a. SPILBERG I, MEHTA J: Demonstration of a specific neutrophil receptor for a cell-derived chemotactic factor. *J Clin Invest* 63:85, 1979

49. PHELPS P: Polymorphonuclear leukocyte motility in vitro. V. Colchicine inhibition of chemotactic activity formation after phagocytosis of urate crystals. *Arthritis Rheum* 13:1, 1970

50. SPILBERG I, MANDELL B, MEHTA J, SIMCHOWITZ L, ROSENBERG D: Mechanism of action of colchicine in acute urate-crystal induced arthritis. *J Clin Invest* 64:775, 1979

51. ZIGMOND SH, HIRSCH JG: Leukocyte locomotion and chemotaxis: New methods for evaluation and demonstration of a cell-derived chemotactic factor. *J Exp Med* 137:387, 1973

52. SPILBERG I, GALLAGHER A, MANDELL B: Calcium pyrophosphate dihydrate (CPPD) crystal-induced chemotactic factor: Subcellular localization, role of protein synthesis and phagocytosis. *J Lab Clin Med* 89:817, 1977

53. SICUTERI T: Sensitization of nociceptors by 5-hydroxytryptamine in man: Pharmacology of pain. *Proc 3d International Pharmacol Meeting* 9:70, 1968

54. VAN ARMAN CG, CARLSON RP, KLING PJ, ALLEN DJ, BONDI JV: Experimental gouty synovitis caused by bacterial endotoxin absorbed onto urate crystals. *Arthritis Rheum* 17:439, 1974

55. SCHUMACHER HR, PHELPS P: Sequential changes in human polymorphonuclear leukocytes after urate crystal phagocytosis. An electron microscopic study. *Arthritis Rheum* 14:513, 1971

56. WEISSMANN G, RITA GA: Molecular basis of gouty inflammation: Interaction of monosodium urate crystals with lysosomes and liposomes. *Nature (New Biol)* 240:167, 1972

57. WEISSMANN G: Crystals, lysosomes and gout. *Adv Intern Med* 19:239, 1974

58. ZWAIFLER N: A speculation on the pathogenesis of joint inflammation in rheumatoid arthritis. *Arthritis Rheum* 8:289, 1965

59. HASSELBACHER P, MCMILLAN RM, VATER CA, HAHN J, HARRIS ED JR: Monosodium urate monohydrate (MSUM) crystals stimulate secretion of collagenase and PGE$_2$ by synovial fibroblasts: A model of joint destruction in chronic gouty arthritis. *Arthritis Rheum* 24:S77, 1981 (abstract)

60. HARRIS ED JR, MCCROSKERY PA: The influence of temperature and fibril

61. stability on degradation of cartilage collagen by rheumatoid synovial collagenase. *N Engl J Med* 290:1, 1974

61. GUTMAN AB: Gout, in Beeson P, McDermott W (eds): *Textbook of Medicine*, 12th ed. Philadelphia, Saunders, 1958, p 595

62. HENCH PS: The diagnosis of gout and gouty arthritis. *J Lab Clin Med* 22:48, 1936

63. GUTMAN AB: Views on the pathogenesis and management of primary gout. *J Bone Joint Surg* 54A:357, 1972

64. TOYNBEE P: *The Letters of Horace Walpole*. Oxford, Clarendon, 1904

65. YÜ T-F: Milestones in the treatment of gout. *Am J Med* 56:676, 1974

66. SOKOLOFF L: The pathology of gout. *Metabolism* 6:230, 1957

67. HOWELL RR, EANES ED, SEEGMILLER JE: X-ray diffraction studies on the tophaceous deposits in gout. *Arthritis Rheum* 6:97, 1963

67a. PRITZKER KPH, ZAHN CE, NYBERG SC, LUK SC, HOUPT JB: Ultrastructure of urate crystals in gout. *J Rheumatol* 5:7, 1978

67b. HASSELBACHER P, SCHUMACHER HR: Immunoglobulin in tophi and on the surface of monosodium urate crystals. *Arthritis Rheum* 21:353, 1978

68. LUDWIG AP, BENNETT GA, BAUER W: Rare manifestation of gout: Widespread ankylosis simulating rheumatoid arthritis. *Ann Intern Med* 11:1248, 1938

69. WATTS RWE, SCOTT JT, CHALMERS RA: Microscopic studies on skeletal muscle in gouty patients treated with allopurinol. *Q J Med* 40:1, 1971

70. WYNGAARDEN JB: Uric acid, in Piersol GM (ed): *The Cyclopedia of Medicine, Surgery, Specialties*. Philadelphia, Davis, 1955, p 341

71. GUTMAN AB, YÜ T-F: Renal function in gout: With a commentary on the renal regulation of urate excretion and the role of the kidney in the pathogenesis of gout. *Am J Med* 23:600, 1957

72. BERGER L, YÜ T-F: Renal function in gout. IV. An analysis of 524 gouty subjects including long-term follow-up studies. *Am J Med* 59:605, 1975

73. YÜ T-F, BERGER L, DORPH DJ, SMITH H: Renal function in gout. V. Factors influencing the renal hemodynamics. *Am J Med* 67:766, 1979

74. GIBSON T, HIGHTON J, POTTER C, SIMMONDS HA: Renal impairment and gout. *Ann Rheum Dis* 39:417, 1980

75. DAVIES DF, SHOCK NW: Age changes in glomerular filtration rate, effective renal plasma flow and tubular excretory capacity in adult males. *J Clin Invest* 29:496, 1950

76. TALBOTT JH, TERPLAN KL: The kidney in gout. *Medicine* 39:405, 1960

77. HEPTINSTALL RH: *Pathology of the Kidney*. Boston, Little, Brown, 1966

78. GREENBAUM D, ROSS JH, STEINBERG VL: Renal biopsy in gout. *Br Med J* 1:1502, 1961

79. GONICK HC, RUBINI ME, GLEASON IO, SOMMERS SC: The renal lesion in gout. *Ann Intern Med* 62:667, 1965

80. PARDO V, PEREZ-STABLE E, FISHER ER: Ultrastructure studies in hypertension. III. Gouty nephropathy. *Lab Invest* 18:143, 1968

81. SEEGMILLER JE, FRAZIER PD: Biochemical considerations of the renal damage of gout. *Ann Rheum Dis* 25:668, 1966

82. VERGER D, LEROUX-ROBERT GP, RICHET G: Depots d'urate intrarenaux chez les insuffisants renaux chroniques hyperuricemiques. *Urol Nephrol* 73:314, 1967

83. LINNANE JW, BURRY AF, EMMERSON BT: Urate deposits in the renal medulla: Prevalence and associations. *Nephron* 1982, in press

84. ATSMON A, DE VRIES A, FRANK M: *Uric Acid Lithiasis*. Amsterdam, Elsevier, 1963

85. YÜ T-F, GUTMAN AB: Uric acid nephrolithiasis in gout. Predisposing factors. *Ann Intern Med* 67:1133, 1967

86. FESSEL WJ: Renal outcomes of gout and hyperuricemia. *Am J Med* 67:74, 1979

87. GIBSON T, SIMMONDS HA, RODGERS V, POTTER C: The abnormal excretion of acid in gout—a metabolic clue? *Rev Rheum Abst 15th Int Congr Rheumatology*. Paris, June 1981, no 0822

88. GUTMAN AB, YÜ T-F: An abnormality of glutamine metabolism in primary gout. *Am J Med* 35:820, 1963

89. COE FL: Hyperuricosuric calcium oxalate nephrolithiasis. *Kidney Int* 13:418, 1978

90. PAK CYC, BRITTON F, PETERSON R, WARD D, NORTHCUTT C, BRESLAN NA, MCGUIRE J, SAKHAEE K, BUSH S, NICAR M, MORMAN DA, PETERS P: Ambulatory evaluation of nephrolithiasis. Classification, clinical presentation and diagnostic criteria. *Am J Med* 69:19, 1980

91. PAK CYC, BARILLA DE, HOLT K, BRINKLEY L, TOLENTINSO R, ZERWEKH JE: Effect of oral purine load and allopurinol on the crystallization of calcium salts in urine of patients with hyperuricosuric calcium urolithiasis. *Am J Med* 65:593, 1978

92. SPERLING O, DE VRIES A: Studies on the etiology of uric acid lithiasis. p 2. Solubility of uric acid in urine specimens from normal subjects and patients with idiopathic uric acid lithiasis. *J Urol* 92:331, 1964

93. METCALFE-GIBSON A, MCCALLUM FM, MORRISON RBI, WRONG O: Urinary excretion of hydrogen ion in patients with uric acid calculi. *Clin Sci* 28:325, 1965

94. SPERLING O, DE VRIES A, KEDEM O: Studies on the etiology of uric acid lithiasis. IV. Urinary nondialyzable substance in idiopathic uric acid lithiasis. *J Urol* 94:286, 1965

95. DE VRIES A, FRANK M, ATSMON A: Inherited uric acid lithiasis. *Am J Med* 33:880, 1962

96. CLARKE AM, MCKENZIE RG: Ileostomy and the risk of urinary uric acid stones. *Lancet* 2:395, 1969

97. MYERS A, EPSTEIN FH, DODGE HJ, MIKKELSEN WM: The relationship of serum uric acid to risk factors in coronary heart disease. *Am J Med* 45:520, 1968

98. KRIZEK V: Serum uric acid in relation to body weight. *Ann Rheum Dis* 25:456, 1966

99. GERTLER MM, GARN SM, LEVINE SA: Serum uric acid in relation to age and physique in health and in coronary artery disease. *Ann Intern Med* 34:1421, 1951

100. BRENNAN PJ, SIMPSON JM, BLACKET RB, MCGILCHRIST CA: The effects of body weight on serum cholesterol, serum triglycerides, serum urate and systolic blood pressure. *Aust NZ J Med* 10:15, 1980

101. EMMERSON BT, KNOWLES BR: Triglyceride concentrations in primary gout and gout of chronic lead nephropathy. *Metabolism* 20:721, 1971

102. BROCHNER-MORTENSEN K: One hundred gouty patients. *Acta Med Scand* 106:81, 1941

103. GRAHAME R, SCOTT JT: Clinical survey of 354 patients with gout. *Ann Rheum Dis* 29:461, 1970

104. FESSEL JW, SIEGELAUB AB, JOHNSON ES: Correlates and consequences of asymptomatic hyperuricemia. *Arch Intern Med* 132:44, 1973

105. HEYDEN S: The working man's diet. II. Effect of weight reduction in obese patients with hypertension, diabetes, hyperuricemia, and hyperlipidemia. *Nutr Metab* 22:141, 1978

106. ENGELHARDT HT, WAGNER EL: Gout, diabetes mellitus and obesity, a poorly recognized syndrome. *South Med J* 43:51, 1950

107. SCOTT FW, TRICK KD, STAVRIC B, BRAATEN JT, SIDDIQUI Y: Uric acid-induced decrease in rat insulin secretion. *Proc Soc Exp Biol Med* 166:123, 1981

108. GIBSON T, GRAHAME R: Gout and hyperlipidaemia. *Ann Rheum Dis* 33:298, 1974

109. GIBSON T, KILBOURN K, HORNER I, SIMMONDS HA: Mechanism and treatment of hypertriglyceridaemia in gout. *Ann Rheum Dis* 38:31, 1979

110. PRIOR AIM, ROSE BS, HARVEY HPB, DAVIDSON F: Hyperuricaemia, gout, and diabetic abnormality in Polynesian people. *Lancet* 1:333, 1966

111. KAHN HA, MEDALIE JH, NEUFELD HN, RISS E, GOLDBOURT U: The incidence of hypertension and associated factors: The Israel ischemic heart disease study. *Am Heart J* 84:171, 1972

112. SIVE PH, MADALIE JH, KAHN HA, NEUFELD HN, RISS E: Distribution and multiple regression analysis of blood pressure in 10,000 Israeli men. *Am J Epidemiol* 93:317, 1971

113. FESSEL WJ: High uric acid as an indicator of cardiovascular disease. Independence from obesity. *Am J Med* 68:401, 1980

114. MESSERLI FH, FROHLICH ED, DRESLINSKI GR, SUAREZ DH, ARISTIMUNO GG: Serum uric acid in essential hypertension: An indicator of renal vascular involvement. *Ann Intern Med* 93:817, 1980

115. SAITO I, SARUTA T, KONDO K, NAKAMURA R, OGURO T, YAMAGAMI K, OZAWA Y, KATO E: Serum uric acid and the renin-angiotensin system in hypertension. *J Am Geriat Soc* 26:241, 1978

116. FERRIS TF, GORDEN P: Effect of angiotensin and norepinephrine upon urate clearance in man. *Am J Med* 44:359, 1968

117. Editorial. Hypertension and uric acid. *Lancet* 1:365, 1981

118. HALL AP: Correlation among hyperuricemia, hypercholesterolemia, coronary artery disease and hypertension. *Arthritis Rheum* 8:846, 1965

119. VIOZZI FJ, BLUHM GB, RIDDLE JM: Gout and arterial thrombosis. *Henry Ford Hosp Med J* 20:119, 1972

120. ALLARD C, GOULET C: Serum uric acid: Not a discriminator of coronary heart disease in men and women. *Can Med Assoc J* 109:986, 1973

121. EMMERSON BT: Atherosclerosis and urate metabolism. *Aust NZ J Med* 9:451, 1979

122. KOHN PM, PROZAN GB: Hyperuricemia: Relationship to hypercholesteremia and acute myocardial infarction. *JAMA* 170:1909, 1959

123. UNGERLEIDER HE: The internist and life insurance. *Ann Intern Med* 41:124, 1954

124. TALBOTT JH, LILIENFELD A: Longevity in gout. *Geriatrics* 14:409, 1959

125. MAYNE JG: Pathological study of the renal lesions found in 27 patients with gout. *Ann Rheum Dis* 15:61, 1956 (abstract)

126. YÜ T-F, TALBOTT JH: Changing trends in mortality in gout. *Semin Arthritis Rheum* 10:1, 1980

127. RAKIC MT, VALKENBURG HA, DAVIDSON RT, ENGELS JP, MIKKELSEN WM, NEEL NV, DUFF IF: Observations on the natural history of hyperuricemia and gout. I. An eighteen year follow-up of nineteen gouty families. *Am J Med* 37:862, 1964

128. CROWLEY LV, ALTON FI: Automated analysis of uric acid. *Am J Clin Pathol* 49:285, 1968

129. LUM G, GAMBINO SR: Comparison of four methods for measuring uric acid: Copper-chelate, phosphotungstate, manual uricase, and automated kinetic uricase. *Clin Chem* 19:1187, 1973

130. BERGMANN F, DIKSTEIN S: The relationship between spectral shifts and structural changes in uric acids and related compounds. *J Am Chem Soc* 77:691, 1955

131. PRAETORIUS E: An enzymatic method for determination of uric acid by ultraviolet spectrophotometry. *Scand J Clin Lab Invest* 1:222, 1949

132. LIDDLE L, SEEGMILLER JE, LASTER L: Enzymatic spectrophotometric method for determination of uric acid. *J Lab Clin Med* 54:903, 1959

133. KAGEYAMA N: A direct colorimetric determination of uric acid in serum and urine with uricase-catalase system. *Clin Chim Acta* 31:421, 1971

134. WHITE RM, CROSS RE, SAVORY J: Enzyme-coupled measurement of uric acid in serum with a centrifugal analyzer. *Clin Chem* 23:1538, 1977

135. KLOSE S, STOLTZ M, MUNZ E, PORTENHAUSER R: Determination of uric acid on continuous flow (AutoAnalyzer II and SMA) systems with a uricase/phenol/4-aminophenazone color test. *Clin Chem* 24:250, 1978

136. WHITEHEAD TP, BROWNING DM, GREGORY A: A comparative survey of the result of analysis of blood serum in clinical chemistry laboratories in the United Kingdom. *J Clin Pathol* 26:435, 1973

137. NISHI HH: Determination of uric acid: Adaptation of the Archibald method on the AutoAnalyzer. *Clin Chem* 13:12, 1967

138. HARKNESS RA, MICOL AD: Plasma uric acid levels in children. *Arch Dis Child* 44:773, 1969

39. MIKKELSEN WM, DODGE HJ, VALKENBURG H: The distribution of serum uric acid values in a population unselected as to gout or hyperuricemia. Tecumseh, Michigan, 1959–1960. *Am J Med* 39:242, 1965

140. HAUGE M, HARVALD B: Hereditary in gout and hyperuricemia. *Acta Med Scand* 152:247, 1955

141. ELVEBACK LR, GUILLIER CL, KEATING FR: Health, normality, and the ghost of Gauss. *JAMA* 211:69, 1970

142. STEWART RB, YOST RL, HALE WE, MARKS RG: Epidemiology of hyperuricemia in an ambulatory elderly population. *J Am Geriat Soc* 27:552, 1979

143. YANO K, RHOADS GG, KAGAN A: Epidemiology of serum uric acid among 8000 Japanese-American men in Hawaii. *J Chron Dis* 30:171, 1977

144. MUNAN L, KELLY A, PETIT-CLERC C: Population serum urate levels and their correlates: The Sherbrooke regional study. *Am J Epidemiol* 103:369, 1976

145. STURGE RA, SCOTT JT, KENNEDY AC, HART DP, BUCHANAN WW: Serum uric acid in England and Scotland. *Ann Rheum Dis* 36:420, 1977

146. ZIMMET PZ, WHITEHOUSE S, JACKSON I, THOMA K: High prevalence of hyperuricemia and gout in an urbanized Micronesian population. *Br Med J* 1:1237, 1978

147. ACHESON RM, CHAN YK: The prediction of serum uric acid on haemoglobin and other factors in the general population. *Lancet* 2:277, 1966

148. ALVSAKER JO: Uric acid in human plasma. V. Isolation and identification of plasma proteins interacting with urate. *Scand J Clin Lab Invest* 18:227, 1966

149. AAKESSON I, ALVSAKER JO: The urate-binding alpha$_{1-2}$globulin: Isolation and characterization of the protein from human plasma. *Eur J Clin Invest* 1:281, 1971

150. SLETTEN K, AAKESSON I, ALVSAKER JO: Presence of ornithine in the urate-binding a$_1$-a$_2$globulin. *Nature [New Biol]* 231:118, 1971

151. CAMPION DS, BLUESTONE R, KLINENBERG JR: Uric acid: Characterization of its interaction with human serum albumin. *J Clin Invest* 52:2283, 1973

152. FARRELL PC, POPOVICH RD, BABB AL: Binding levels of urate ions in human serum albumin and plasma. *Biochim Biophys Acta* 243:49, 1971

153. KOVARSKY J, HOLMES E, KELLEY WN: Absence of significant urate binding to human serum proteins. *J Lab Clin Med* 93:85, 1979

154. POSTLETHWAITE AE, GUTMAN RA, KELLEY WN: Salicylate-mediated increase in urate removal during hemodialysis: Evidence for urate binding to protein in vivo. *Metabolism* 23:771, 1974

155. ALVSAKER JO: Genetic studies in primary gout: Investigations on the plasma levels of the urate-binding α_1-α_2 globulin in individuals from two gouty kindreds. *J Clin Invest* 47:1254, 1968

156. PETERS JP, VAN SLYKE KK: *Quantitative Clinical Chemistry*, 2d ed. Baltimore, Williams & Wilkins, 1946

157. ALLEN DJ, MILOSOVICH G, MATTOCKS AM: Inhibition of monosodium urate crystal growth. *Arthritis Rheum* 8:1123, 1965

158. SEEGMILLER JE, LASTER L, HOWELL RR: Biochemistry of uric acid and its relation to gout. *N Engl J Med* 268:712, 1963

159. POPERT AJ, HEWITT JV: Gout and hyperuricemia in rural and urban populations. *Ann Rheum Dis* 20:154, 1962

160. ISOMAKI HA, TAKKUNEN H: Gout and hyperuricemia in a Finnish rural population. *Acta Rheumatol Scand* 15:112, 1969

161. ZALOKAR J, LELLAUCH J, CLAUDE JR, KUNTZ D: Serum uric acid in 23,923 men and gout in a subsample of 4,257 men in France. *J Chron Dis* 25:305, 1972

162. SEEGMILLER JE, GRAYZEL AI, HOWELL RR, PLATO C: The renal excretion of uric acid in gout. *J Clin Invest* 41:1094, 1962

163. YÜ T-F, BERGER L, GUTMAN AB: Renal function in gout. II. Effect of uric acid loading on renal excretion of uric acid. *Am J Med* 33:829, 1962

164. WYNGAARDEN JB, STETTEN D JR: Uricolysis in normal man. J Biol Chem 203:9, 1953

165. SORENSEN LB: The elimination of uric acid in man studied by means of C^{14}-labeled uric acid. Scand J Clin Lab Invest 12:1, 1960

166. HARTMAN SC, BUCHANAN JM: Biosynthesis of purines. XXI. 5-Phosphoribosylpyrophosphate amidotransferase. J Biol Chem 233:451, 1958

167. FLAKS JG, ERWIN MJ, BUCHANAN JM: Biosynthesis of the purines. VI. The synthesis of adenosine 5'-phosphate and 5'-amino-4-imidazole-carboxamide ribotide by a nucleotide pyrophosphorylase. J Biol Chem 228:201, 1957

168. KORNBERG A, LIEBERMAN I, SIMMS ES: Enzymatic synthesis and properties of 5-phosphoribosylpyrophosphate. J Biol Chem 215:389, 1955

169. HARTMAN SC: Phosphoribosyl pyrophosphate amidotransferase: Purification and general catalytic properties. J Biol Chem 238:3024, 1963

170. HOLMES EW, KING GL, LEYVA A, SINGER SC: A purine auxotroph deficient in phosphoribosylpyrophosphate amidotransferase and phosphoribosylpyrophosphate aminotransferase activities with normal activity of ribose-5-phosphate aminotransferase. Proc Natl Acad Sci USA 73:2458, 1976

171. NIERLICH DP, MAGASANIK B: Alternative first steps of purine biosynthesis. J Biol Chem 236:PC32, 1961

172. WESTBY CA, GOTS JS: Genetic blocks and unique features in the biosynthesis of 5'-phosphoribosyl-N-formylglycinamide in Salmonella typhimurium. J Biol Chem 244:2095, 1969

173. ITOH R, MITSUI A, TSUSHIMA K: 5'-Nucleotidase of chicken liver. Biochim Biophys Acta 146:151, 1967

174. ITOH R, MITSUI A, TSUCHIMA K: Properties of 5'-nucleotidase from hepatic tissue of higher animals. J Biochem 63:165, 1968

175. VAN DEN BERGHE G, VAN POTTELSBERGHE C, HERS H-G: A kinetic study of the soluble 5'-nucleotidase of rat liver. Biochem J 162:611, 1977

176. KREDICH NM, HERSHFIELD MS: Adenosine deaminase deficiency, in Stanbury JB, Wyngaarden JB, Fredrickson DS, Goldstein JL, Brown MS (eds): The Metabolic Basis of Inherited Disease, 5 ed. New York, McGraw-Hill, 1983, chap 53

177. KRENITSKY TA, ELION GB, HENDERSON AM, HITCHINGS GH: Inhibition of human purine nucleoside phosphorylase: Studies with intact erythrocytes and the purified enzyme. J Biol Chem 243:2876, 1968

178. ZIMMERMAN TP, GERSTEN N, MIECH RP: Adenine and adenosine metabolism in liver. Proc Am Assoc Cancer Res 11:87, 1970 (abstract)

179. FERRO AJ, BARRETT A, SHAPIRO SK: Kinetic properties and the effect of substrate analogues on 5'-methylthioadenosine nucleosidase from Escherichia coli. Biochim Biophys Acta 438:487, 1976

180. KELLEY WN, ROSENBLOOM FM, HENDERSON JF, SEEGMILLER JE: Xanthine phosphoribosyltransferase in man: Relationship to hypoxanthine-guanine phosphoribosyltransferase. Biochem Biophys Res Comm 28:340, 1967

181. MCCOLLISTER RJ, GILBERT WR JR, ASHTON DM, WYNGAARDEN JB: Pseudofeedback inhibition of purine synthesis by 6-mercaptopurine ribonucleotide and other purine analogues. J Biol Chem 239:1560, 1964

182. HORI M, HENDERSON JF: Kinetic studies with adenine phosphoribosyltransferase. J Biol Chem 241:3403, 1966

183. PIERRE RJ, LEPAGE GA: Formation of inosine-5'-monophosphate by a kinase in cell-free extracts of Ehrlich ascites cells in vitro. Proc Soc Exp Biol Med 127:432, 1968

184. WADA Y, ARAKAWA T, KOIZUMI K: Lesch-Nyhan syndrome: Autopsy findings and in vitro study of incorporation of C-8-inosine into uric acid, guanosine-monophosphate an adenosine-monophosphate in the liver. Tohoku J Exp Med 95:253, 1968

185. FRIEDMANN T, SEEGMILLER JE, SUBAK-SHARPE JH: Evidence against the existence of guanosine and inosine kinases in human fibroblasts in tissue culture. Exp Cell Res 56:425, 1969

186. BERGMANN F, DIKSTEIN S: Studies on uric acid and related compounds. III. Observations on the specificity of mammalian xanthine oxidase. J Biol Chem 223:765, 1956

187. WEISSMANN B, BROMBERG PA, GUTMAN GB: The purine bases of human urine. II. Semiquantitative estimation and isotope incorporation. J Biol Chem 224:423, 1957

188. WYNGAARDEN JB, DUNN JT: 8-Hydroxyadenine as the intermediate in the oxidation of adenine to 2,8-dihydroxyadenine by xanthine oxidase. Arch Biochem Biophys 70:150, 1957

189. DAVIS AR, NEWTON EB, BENEDICT SR: The combined uric acid in beef blood. J Biol Chem 54:595, 1922

190. FALCONER R, GULLAND JM: The constitution of purine nucleosides. Pt VIII. Uric acid riboside. J Chem Soc C p 1369, 1939

191. FORREST HS, HATFIELD D, LAGOWSKI JM: Uric acid riboside. Pt I. Isolation and reinvestigation of the structure. J Chem Soc C p 963, 1961

192. CARTER CE, POTTER JL: Distribution and properties of uric acid riboside. Fed Proc II:195, 1952

193. HATFIELD D, WYNGAARDEN JB: 3-Ribosylpurines. II. Studies on (3-ribosylxanthine)5'-phosphte and on ribonucleotide derivatives of certain uracil analogues. J Biol Chem 29:2587, 1964

194. HATFIELD D, GREENLAND RA, STEWART HL, WYNGAARDEN JB: Biosynthesis of a new uric acid ribonucleotide. Biochim Biophys Acta 91:163, 1964

195. COHEN A, DOYLE D, MARTIN DW JR, AMMANN AN: Abnormal purine metabolism and purine overproduction in a patient deficient in purine nucleoside phosphorylase. N Engl J Med 295:1449, 1976

196. LAJTHA LG, VANE JR: Dependence of bone marrow cells on the liver for purine supply. Nature (Lond) 182:191, 1958

197. MAGER J, HERSHKO A, ZEITLIN-BECK R, SHOSHAMI T, RAZIN A: Turnover of purine nucleotides in rabbit erythrocytes. I. Studies in vivo. Biochim Biophys Acta 149:50, 1967

198. LERNER MH, LOWY BA: The formation of adenosine in rabbit liver and its possible role as a direct precursor of erythrocyte adenine nucleotides. J Biol Chem 249:959 1974

199. WILSON D, BEYER A, BISHOP C, TALBOTT JH: Urinary uric acid excretion after the ingestion of isotopic yeast nucleic acid in the normal and gouty human. J Biol Chem 209:227, 1954

200. ROLL PM, BROWN GB, DE CARLO FJ, SCHULTZ AS: The metabolism of yeast nucleic acid in the rat. J Biol Chem 180:333, 1949

201. WYNGAARDEN JB, SILBERMAN HR, SADLER JH: Feedback mechanisms influencing purine ribotide synthesis. Ann NY Acad Sci 75:45, 1958

202. MOMOSE H, NISHIKAWA H, SHUS I: Regulation of purine nucleotide synthesis in Bacillus subtilis. J Biochem 59:325, 1966

203. HENDERSON JR, KHOO KY: Synthesis of 5-phosphoribosyl-1-pyrophosphate from glucose in Ehrlich ascites tumor cells in vitro. J Biol Chem 240:2349, 1965

204. GREENE ML, SEEGMILLER JE; Elevated erythrocyte phosphoribosylpyrophosphate in X-linked uric aciduria: Importance of PRPP concentration in the regulation of human purine biosynthesis. J Clin Invest 48:32a, 1969 (abstract)

205. KELLEY WN, FOX IH, WYNGAARDEN JB: Essential role of phosphoribosylpyrophosphate (PRPP) in regulation of purine biosynthesis in cultured human fibroblasts. Clin Res 18:457, 1970

206. RAIVIO KO, SEEGMILLER JE: Role of glutamine in purine synthesis and interconversions. Clin Res 19:161, 1971 (abstract)

207. WONG PCL, MURRAY AW: 5-Phosphoribosyl pyrophosphate synthetase from Ehrlich ascites tumor cells. Biochemistry 8:1508, 1969

208. FOX IH, KELLEY WN; Human phosphoribosyl-pyrophosphate synthetase: Kinetic mechanism and end-product inhibition. J Biol Chem 247:2126, 1972

209. SPERLING O: In Ciba Foundation Symposium on Purine and Pyrimidine Metabolism. Amsterdam, Elsevier 48:347, 1977

210. FOX IH, KELLEY WN: Human phosphoribosylpyrophosphate synthetase: Distribution, purification and properties. J Biol Chem 246:5739, 1971

211. LEBO RV, MARTIN DW JR: Electrophoretic heterogeneity of 5-phosphoribosyl-1-pyrophosphate synthetase within and among humans. Biochem Genet 16:905, 1978

212. BECKER MA, YEN RCK, ITKIN P: Regional localization of the gene for human phosphoribosylpyrophosphate synthetase on the X chromosome. Science 203:1016, 1979

213. ROTH DG, SHELTON E, DENEL TF: Purification and properties of phosphoribosylpyrophosphate synthetase from rat liver. J Biol Chem 249:291, 1974

214. FOX I, KELLEY WN: Phosphoribosylpyrophosphate (PRPP) in man: Biochemical and clinical significance. Ann Intern Med 74:424, 1971

215. GREEN CD, MARTIN DW JR: Characterization of a feedback resistant phosphoribosylpyrophosphate synthetase from cultured, mutagenized hepatoma cells that overproduce purines. Proc Natl Acad Sci USA 70:3698, 1973

216. ATKINSON DE: The energy charge of the adenylate pool as a regulatory parameter: Interaction with feedback modifiers. Biochemistry 7:4030, 1968

217. FOX IH, WYNGAARDEN JB, KELLEY WN: Depletion of erythrocyte phosphoribosylpyrophosphate in man, a newly observed effect of allopurinol. N Engl J Med 283:1177, 1970

218. VAN MARIS AGCCM, TAX WJM, OEI TL, DE BRUYN CHMM, KLEIN F, GEERTS SJ, VEERKAMP JH, VALKENBURG HA: Phosphoribosylpyrophosphate and enzymes of purine metabolism in erythrocytes from young hyperuricemic males. Biochem Med 23:263, 1980

219. KELLEY WN, FOX IH, WYNGAARDEN, JB: Regulation of purine biosynthesis in cultured human cells. I. Effects of orotic acid. Biochim Biophys Acta 215:512, 1970

220. LALANNE M, HENDERSON JF: Effects of hormones and drugs on phosphoribosylpyrophosphate concentrations in mouse liver. Can J Biochem 53:394, 1975

221. ITAKURA M, SABINA RL, HEALD PW, HOLMES EW: Basis for control of purine biosynthesis by purine ribonucleotides. J Clin Invest 67:994, 1981

222. SPERLING O, BROSH S, BOER P, KUPFER B, BENHAMIN D, WEINBERGER A, PINKHAS J: De novo synthesis of purine nucleotides and metabolic availability of phosphoribosylpyrophosphate in leukemic leukocytes. Biomedicine 31:20, 1979

223. NISHIDA Y, KAMATANI N, YANO E, AKAOKA I: Influences of ethanol on 5-phosphoribosyl-1-pyrophosphate concentration and purine metabolizing enzyme activities in the mouse liver. *Biochem Med* 21:86, 1979

224. ROSENBLOOM FM, HENDERSON JF, CALDWELL IC, KELLEY WN, SEEGMILLER JE: Biochemical bases of accelerated purine biosynthesis de novo in human fibroblasts lacking hypoxanthine-guanine phosphoribosyltransferase. *J Biol Chem* 243:1166, 1968

225. WYNGAARDEN JB: Glutamine phosphoribosylpyrophosphate amidotransferase, in Horecker B, Stadtman E (eds): *Current Topics in Cellular Regulation.* New York, Academic, 1972, vol 5, p 135

226. HOLMES EW, MCDONALD JA, MCCORD JM, WYNGAARDEN JB, KELLEY WN: Human glutamine phosphoribosylpyrophosphate amidotransferase: Kinetic and regulatory properties. *J Biol Chem* 248:144, 1973

227. HOLMES EW, WYNGAARDEN JB, KELLEY WN: Human glutamine phosphoribosylpyrophosphate amidotransferase: Two molecular forms interconvertible by purine ribonucleotides and phosphoribosylpyrophosphate. *J Biol Chem* 248:6035, 1973

228. WOOD AW, SEEGMILLER JE: Properties of 5-phosphoribosyl-1-pyrophosphate amidotransferase from human lymphoblasts. *J Biol Chem* 248:138, 1973

229. REEM GH: Enzymatic synthesis of phosphoribosylamine in human cells. *J Biol Chem* 249:1696, 1974

230. WYNGAARDEN JB, ASHTON DM: The regulation of activity of phosphoribosylpyrophosphate amidotransferase by purine ribonucleotides: A potential feedback control of purine biosynthesis. *J Biol Chem* 234:1492, 1959

231. CASKEY CT, ASHTON DM, WYNGAARDEN JB: The enzymology of feedback inhibition of glutamine phosphoribosylpyrophosphate amidotransferase by purine ribonucleotides. *J Biol Chem* 239:2570, 1964

232. HOLMES EW: Kinetic, physical, and regulatory properties of amidophosphoribosyltransferase. *Adv Enzyme Reg* 44:215, 1981

233. KING GL, BOUNOUS CG, HOLMES EW: Human placental amidophosphoribosyltransferase. Comparison of the kinetics of glutamine and ammonia utilization. *J Biol Chem* 253:3933, 1978

234. KOVARSKY J, EVANS MC, HOLMES EW: Regulation of human amidophosphoribosyltransferase: Interaction of orthophosphate, PP-ribose-P and purine ribonucleotides. *Can J Biochem* 56:334, 1978

235. WONG JY, MEYER E, SWITZER RL: Glutamine phosphoribosylpyrophosphate amidotransferase from *Bacillus subtilis*. A novel iron-sulfur protein. *J Biol Chem* 252:7424, 1977

236. ITAKURA M, MEADE J, HOLMES EW: Protection of amidophosphoribosyltransferase from O$_2$ inactivation in the cell: A potential mechanism for controlling purine biosynthesis. *Fed Proc* 38:671, 1979

237. ITAKURA M, HOLMES EW: Human amidophosphoribosyltransferase. An oxygen-sensitive iron-sulfur protein. *J Biol Chem* 254:333, 1979

238. AVERIL BA, DWIREDI A, DEBRUNNER P, VOLLMER SJ, WONG JY, SWITZER RL: Evidence for a tetra-nuclear iron-sulfur center in glutamine phosphoribosylpyrophosphate amidotransferase from *Bacillus subtilis*. *J Biol Chem* 255:6007, 1980

239. ROWE PB, COLEMAN MD, WYNGAARDEN JB: Glutamine phosphoribosylpyrophosphate amidotransferase: Catalytic and conformation heterogeneity of the pigeon liver enzyme. *Biochem* 9:1498, 1970

240. NIERLICH DP, MAGASANIK B: Regulation of purine ribonucleotide synthesis by end product inhibition. *J Biol Chem* 240:358, 1965

241. NAGY M: Regulation of the biosynthesis of purine nucleotides in *Schizosaccharomyces pombe*. I. Properties of the phosphoribosylpyrophosphate: Glutamine amidotransferase of the wild strain and of a mutant desensitized towards feedback modifiers. *Biochim Biophys Acta* 198:471, 1970

242. REEM GH, FRIEND C: Phosphoribosylamidotransferase: Regulation of activity in virus-induced murine leukemia by purine nucleotides. *Science* 157:1203, 1967

243. SATYANARAYANA T, KAPLAN JG: Regulation of the purine pathway in bakers' yeast. Activity and feedback inhibition of phosphoribosyl-pyrophosphate amidotransferase. *Arch Biochem Biophys* 142:40, 1971

244. GRINDEY GB, LOWE JK, DIVEKAR AY, JAKALA MT: Potentiation by guanine nucleosides on the growth-inhibitory effects of adenosine analogs on L1210 and sarcoma 180 cells in culture. *Cancer Res* 36:379, 1976

245. ITOH R, HOLMES EW, WYNGAARDEN JB: Pigeon liver amidophosphoribosyltransferase: Ligand-induced alterations in molecular and kinetic properties. *J Biol Chem* 251:2234, 1976

246. SINGER SC, HOLMES EW: Human glutamine phosphoribosylpyrophosphate amidotransferase: Hysteretic properties. *J Biol Chem* 252:7959, 1977

246a. ROWE PB, MCCAIRNS E, MADSEN G, SAUER D, ELLIOTT H: De novo purine synthesis in avian liver. *J Biol Chem* 253:7711, 1978

247. NIERLICH DP, MAGASANIK B: Control by repression of purine biosynthetic enzymes in aerogenes. *Fed Proc* 22:476, 1963 (abstract)

248. MCFALL E, MAGASANIK B: The control of purine biosynthesis in cultured mammalian cells. *J Biol Chem* 235:2103, 1960

249. KATUNUMA N, MATSUDA Y, KURODA Y: Phylogenic aspects of different regulatory mechanisms of glutamine metabolism. *Adv Enzyme Regul* 8:73, 1970

250. KATUNUMA N, WEBER G: Glutamine phosphoribosylpyrophosphate amidotransferase: Increased activity in hepatomas. *FEBS Lett* 49:53, 1974

251. TSUDA M, KATUMUMA K, MORRIS HP, WEBER G: Purification, properties and immunititration of hepatoma glutamine phosphoribosylpyrophosphate amidotransferases. *Cancer Res* 39:305, 1979

252. STANLEY W, CHU EHY: Assignment of the gene for phosphoribosylpyrophosphate amidotransferase to the pter → q21 region of human chromosome 4. *Cytogenet Cell Genet* 22:228, 1978

253. HENDERSON JF, CALDWELL IE, PATERSON ARP: Decreased feedback inhibition of a 6-methylmercaptopurine resistant tumor. *Cancer Res* 27:1773, 1967

254. OATES DC, VANNAIS D, PATTERSON D: A mutant of CHO-K1 cells deficient in two nonsequential steps of de novo purine biosynthesis. *Cell* 20:797, 1980

255. HOLMES EW: Unpublished data

256. ZOREF-SHANI E, SPERLING O: Dependence of the metabolic fate of IMP on the rate of total IMP synthesis. Studies in cultured fibroblasts from normal subjects and from purine-overproducing mutant patients. *Biochim Biophys Acta* 607:503, 1980

257. BASHKIN P, SPERLING O: Some regulatory properties of purine biosynthesis de novo in long-term cultures of epithelial-like rat liver cells. *Biochim Biophys Acta* 538:505, 1978

258. HERSHFIELD MS, SEEGMILLER JE: Regulation of *de novo* purine synthesis in human lymphoblasts: Similar rates of *de novo* synthesis during growth by normal cells and mutants deficient in hypoxanthine-guanine phosphoribosyltransferase activity. *J Biol Chem* 252:6002, 1977

259. ALLSOP W, WATTS RWE: The amidophosphoribosyltransferase (EC 2.4.2.14) and ribosephosphate pyrophosphokinase (EC 2.7.6.1) activities, and phosphoribosylpyrophosphate content of unstimulated and stimulated human lymphocytes. *J Molec Med* 3:105, 1978

260. WYNGAARDEN JB, GREENLAND RA: The inhibition of succinoadenylate kinosynthetase of *Escherichia coli* by adenosine and guanosine 5'-monophosphates. *J Biol Chem* 238:1054, 1963

261. VAN DER WEYDEN MB, KELLEY WN: Human adenylosuccinate synthetase: Partial purification, kinetic, and regulatory properties of the enzyme from placenta. *J Biol Chem* 249:7282, 1974

262. MAGER J, MAGASANIK B: Guanosine 5'-phosphate reductase and its role in the interconversion of purine nucleotides. *J Biol Chem* 235:1474, 1960

263. CHAN T-S, ISHII K, LONG C, GREEN H: Purine excretion by mammalian cells deficient in adenosine kinase. *J Cell Physiol* 81:315, 1973

264. HERS H-G: The mechanism of adenosine triphosphate depletion in the liver after a fructose load. A kinetic study of liver adenylate deaminase. *Biochem J* 162:601, 1977

265. HERS H-G, VAN DEN BERGHE G: Enzyme defect in primary gout. *Lancet* 1:585, 1979

266. BISWAS BB, ABRAMS R: Formation of hypoxanthine from guanine in rat liver extracts. *Arch Biochem Biophys* 92:507, 1961

266a. ZOREF E, DE VRIES A, SPERLING O: Kinetic aspects of purine metabolism in cultured fibroblasts. A comparative study of cells from patients overproducing purines due to HGPRT deficiency and PRPP synthetase superactivity. *Monogr Hum Genet* 10:96, 1978

267. SONG CS, NISSELBAUM JS, TANDLER B, BODANSKY O: Partial solubilization of protein and 5'-nucleotidase from microsomal membranes of rat liver by ultrasonic irradiation. *Biochim Biophys Acta* 150:303, 1968

268. ITOH R, TSUSHIMA K: Comparison of adaptations to diet of enzymes involved in uric acid production from IMP in chickens and rats. *J Biochem* 75:715, 1974

269. ITOH R, TSUSHIMA K: Changes in 5'-nucleotidase activity in chick liver during development and dietary treatment. *Biochim Biophys Acta* 273:229, 1972

270. TUCKER-PIAN C, BAKAY B, NYHAN WL: 5'-Nucleotidase: Solubilization, radiochemical analysis, and electrophoresis. *Biochem Genet* 17:995, 1979

271. VAN DEN BERGHE G: Metabolic effects of fructose in the liver. *Curr Top Cell Reg* 13:97, 1978

272. FOX IH, KELLEY WN: Studies on the mechanism of fructose-induced hyperuricemia in man. *Metabolism* 21:713, 1972

273. SCHWARZMEIER JD, MARKTL W, MOSER K, LUIF A: Fructose induced hyperuricemia. *Res Exp Med* 162:341, 1974

274. EMMERSON BT: Effect of oral fructose on urate production. *Ann Rheum Dis* 33:276, 1974

275. RAIVIO KO, BECKER MA, MEYER LJ, GREENE ML, MUKI G, SEEGMILLER JE: Stimulation of human purine synthesis de novo by fructose infusion. *Metab Clin Exp* 24:861, 1975

276. FORSTER H, MEYER E, ZIEGE M: Erhohung von serum-harnsaure und serumbilirubin nach hochdosierten infusionen von sorbit, xylit und fructose. *Klin Wochenschr* 48:878, 1970

277. NARINS RG, WEISBERG JS, MYERS AR: Effects of carbohydrates on uric acid metabolism. *Metabolism* 23:455, 1974

278. GREENE HL, WILSON FA, HEFFERAN O, TERRY AB, MORAN JR, SEONIN AE, CLAUS TH, BURR IM: ATP depletion, a possible role in the pathogen-

esis of hyperuricemia in glycogen storage disease Type I. *J Clin Invest* 62:321, 1978

278a. GRUNST J, DIETZE G, WICKLMAYR M: Effect of ethanol on uric acid production of human liver. *Nutri Metab* 21:138, 1977

279. ELION GB, NELSON DJ: Ribonucleotides of allopurinol and oxipurinol in rat tissues and their significance in purine metabolism, in Sperling O, de Vries A, Wyngaarden JB (eds): *Purine Metabolism in Man.* New York, Plenum, 1974, p 639

280. CARCASSI A, MARCOLONGO R JR, MARINELLO E, RIARIO-SFORZA G, BOGGIANO C: Liver xanthine oxidase in gouty patients. *Arthritis Rheum* 12:17, 1969

281. MARCOLONGO R, MARINELLO E, POMPUCCI G, PAGANI R: The role of xanthine oxidase in hyperuricemic states. *Arthritis Rheum* 17:430, 1974

282. WEBER G, PRAJDA N, JACKSON RC: Key enzymes of IMP metabolism: Transformation and proliferation-linked alterations in gene expression, in Weber G (ed): *Advances in Enzyme Regulation.* Oxford, Pergamon, 1976, vol 14, p 3

283. KELLEY WN, WYNGAARDEN JB: Effects of allopurinol and oxipurinol on purine synthesis in cultured human cells. *J Clin Invest* 49:602, 1970

284. BROCKMAN RW: Metabolism and mechanisms of action of purine analogues, in *Exploitable Molecular Mechanisms and Neoplasia.* Baltimore, Williams & Wilkins, 1969, p 435

285. SEEGMILLER JR, LASTER L, STETTEN D JR: Incorporation of 4-amino-5-imidazolecarboxamide-4-C^{13} into uric acid in the normal human. *J Biol Chem* 216:653, 1955

286. SEEGMILLER JE, KLINENBERG JR, MILLER J, WATTS RWE: Suppression of glycine-N^{15} incorporation into urinary uric acid by adenine-8-C^{13} in normal and gouty subjects. *J Clin Invest* 47:1193, 1968

287. SORENSEN LB: Mechanism of excessive purine biosynthesis in hypoxanthine guanine phosphoribosyltransferase deficiency. *J Clin Invest* 49:968, 1970

288. KELLEY WN, ROSENBLOOM FM, SEEGMILLER JE: The effect of azathioprine (Imuran) on purine synthesis in clinical disorders of purine metabolism. *J Clin Invest* 46:1518, 1967

289. KRAKOFF IH, BALIS ME, MAGILL JW, NARY D: Studies of purine metabolism in neoplastic diseases. *Med Clin North Am* 45:521, 1961

290. SHIGEURA HT, GORDON CN: The mechanism of action of hadacidin. *J Biol Chem* 237:1937, 1963

291. KRAKOFF IH, MAGILL GB: Effects of 2-ethylamino-1,3,4 thiadiazole HCl on uric acid production in man. *Proc Soc Exp Biol Med* 91:470, 1956

292. BAUMAN N, WYNGAARDEN JB: Regulation of purine biosynthesis in the mouse. *Fed Proc* 23:324, 1964

293. SEEGMILLER JE, GRAYZEL AI, LIDDLE L, WYNGAARDEN JB: The effect of 2-ethylamino-1,3,4-thiadiazole on the incorporation of glycine into urinary purines and uric acid in man. *Metabolism* 12:507, 1963

294. SEEGMILLER JE, GRAYZEL AI, LASTER L, LIDDLE L: Uric acid production in gout. *J Clin Invest* 40:1304, 1961

295. BENEDICT JD, FORSHAM PH, STETTEN D JR: The metabolism of uric acid in the normal and gouty human studied with the aid of isotopic uric acid. *J Biol Chem* 181:183, 1949

296. SCOTT JT, HOLLOWAY VP, GLASS HI, ARNOT RN: Studies of uric acid pool size and turnover rate. *Ann Rheum Dis* 28:366, 1969

297. RIESELBACH RE, SORENSEN LB, SHELP WD, STEELE TH: Diminished renal urate secretion per nephron as a basis for primary gout. *Ann Intern Med* 73:359, 1970

298. BENEDICT JD, FORSHAM PH, ROCHE M, SOLOWAY J, STETTEN D JR: The effect of salicylates and adrenocorticotropic hormone on the miscible pool of uric acid in gout. *J Clin Invest* 29:1104, 1950

299. SORENSEN LB: The pathogenesis of gout. *Arch Intern Med* 109:379, 1962

300. KELLEY WN, GREENE ML, ROSENBLOOM FM, HENDERSON JF, SEEGMILLER JE: Hypoxanthine-guanine phosphoribosyltransferase deficiency in gout. *Ann Intern Med* 70:155, 1969

301. BENEDICT JD, ROCHE M, YÜ T-F, BIEN EJ, GUTMAN AB, STETTEN D JR: Incorporation of glycine nitrogen into uric acid in normal and gouty man. *Metabolism* 1:3, 1952

302. BENEDICT JD, YÜ T-F, BIEN EJ, GUTMAN AB, STETTEN D JR: A further study of the utilization of dietary glycine nitrogen for uric acid synthesis in gout. *J Clin Invest* 32:775, 1953

303. WYNGAARDEN JB: The effect of phenylbutazone on uric acid metabolism in two normal subjects. *J Clin Invest* 34:256, 1955

304. SPERLING O, WYNGAARDEN JB, STARMER CF: The kinetics of intramolecular distribution of ^{15}N in uric acid after administration of [^{15}N] glycine: A reappraisal of the significance of preferential labeling of N−(3 + 9) of uric acid in primary gout. *J Clin Invest* 52:2468, 1973

305. GUTMAN AB, YÜ T-F, BLACK H, YALOW RS, BERSON SA: Incorporation of glycine 1-C^{14} glycine 2-C^{14} and glycine-N^{15} into uric acid in normal and gouty subjects. *Am J Med* 25:917, 1958

306. WYNGAARDEN JB, BLAIR AE, HILLEY L: On the mechanism of overproduction of uric acid in patients with primary gout. *J Clin Invest* 37:579, 1958

307. WYNGAARDEN JB, SEEGMILLER JE, LASTER L, BLAIR AE: The utilization of hypoxanthine, adenine and 4-amino-5-imidazolecarboxamide for uric acid synthesis in man. *Metabolism* 8:455, 1959

308. WYNGAARDEN JB: Overproduction of uric acid as the cause of hyperuricemia in primary gout. *J Clin Invest* 36:1508, 1957

309. WYNGAARDEN JB: Normal glycine-C^{14} incorporation into uric acid in primary gout. *Metabolism* 7:374, 1958

310. EMMERSON BT: The effect of weight reduction on urate metabolism, in Sperling O, De Vries A, Wyngaarden JB (eds): *Purine Metabolism in Man.* New York, Plenum, 1974, vol 41B, p 429

311. YÜ T-F, ROBOZ J: Long-term follow-up of incorporation of ^{15}N from glycine into uric acid in gout. *Am J Med* 70:797, 1981

312. SEEGMILLER JE, LASTER L, STETTEN D JR: Uric acid formation in patients with gout: The incorporation of 4-amino-5-imidazolecarboxamide-C^{13} into uric acid. *Ninth Int Congr Rheumatic Diseases,* Toronto, Canada, June 23–28, 1957, vol 2, p 207

313. YÜ T-F, ADLER M, BOBROW E, GUTMAN AB: Plasma and urinary amino acids in primary gout, with special reference to glutamine. *J Clin Invest* 48:885, 1969

314. PAGLIARA AS, GOODMAN AD: Elevation of plasma glutamate in gout, its possible role in the pathogenesis of hyperuricemia. *N Engl J Med* 281:767, 1969

315. SEGAL S, WYNGAARDEN JB: Plasma glutamine and oxypurine content in patients with gout. *Proc Soc Exp Biol Med* 88:342, 1955

316. BIEN EJ, YÜ T-F, BENEDICT JD, GUTMAN AB, STETTEN D JR: The relation of dietary nitrogen consumption to the rate of uric acid synthesis in normal and gouty man. *J Clin Invest* 32:778, 1953

317. FEIGELSON M, FEIGELSON P: Relationships between hepatic enzyme induction, glutamate formation, and purine nucleotide biosynthesis in glucocorticoid action. *J Biol Chem* 241:5819, 1966

318. GUTMAN AB, YÜ T-F: Urinary ammonium excretion in primary gout. *J Clin Invest* 44:1474, 1965

319. SWALES GD, KOPSTEIN J, WRONG OM: Renal excretion of ammonia and urate production: Examination of Gutman-Yü hypothesis. *Metabolism* 21:541, 1972

320. HOWELL RR, SPEAS M, WYNGAARDEN JB: A quantitative study of recycling of isotope from glycine-1-C^{14}, α-N^{15} into various subunits of the uric acid molecule in a normal subject. *J Clin Invest* 40:2976, 1961

321. GUTMAN AB, YÜ T-F, ADLER M, JAVITT NB: Intramolecular distribution of uric acid-N^{15} after administration of glycine-N^{15} and ammonium-N^{15} chloride to gouty and nongouty subjects. *J Clin Invest* 41:623, 1962

322. STARMER CF, SPERLING O, WYNGAARDEN JB: A kinetic model for the intramolecular distribution of ^{15}N in uric acid in patients with primary gout fed ^{15}N-glycine. *Math Biosci* 25:105, 1975

323. KAPLAN D, BÉRNSTEIN D, WALLACE SL, HALBERSTAM D: Serum and urinary amino acids in normouricemic and hyperuricemic subjects. *Ann Intern Med* 62:658, 1965

324. WYNGAARDEN JB: Gout, in Stanbury JB, Wyngaarden JB, Fredrickson DS (eds): *Metabolic Basis of Inherited Disease.* New York, McGraw-Hill, 1960, p 679

325. JONES OW JR, ASHTON DM, WYNGAARDEN JB: Accelerated turnover of phosphoribosylpyrophosphate, a purine nucleotide precursor, in certain gouty subjects. *J Clin Invest* 41:1805, 1962

326. KATZ J, ROGNSTAD R: The labeling of pentose phosphate from glucose-^{14}C and estimation of the rates of transaldolase, transketolase, the contribution of the pentose cycle, and ribosephosphate synthesis. *Biochemistry* 6:2227, 1967

327. BECKER MA: Gout with purine overproduction: Patterns of fibroblast phosphoribosylpyrophosphate and ribose-5-phosphate concentrations and generation. *Arthritis Rheum* 18:385, 1975 (abstract)

328. VAN MARIS AGCCM, TAX WJM, OEI TL, DE BRUYN CHMM, KLEIN F, GEERTS SJ, VEERKAMP JH, VALKENBURG HA: Phosphoribosylpyrophosphate and enzymes of purine metabolism in erythrocytes from young hyperuricemic males. *Biochem Med* 23:263, 1980

329. EMMERSON BT, WYNGAARDEN JB: Purine metabolism in heterozygous carriers of hypoxanthine-guanine phosphoribosyltransferase deficiency. *Science* 166:1533, 1969

330. BALO-BANGA JM, LEIBINGER J, MOLNAR L, KIRALY K: The effect of retinoic acid on the synthesis of phosphoribosylpyrophosphate in human erythrocytes in psoriasis. *Dermatologica* 157:45, 1978

331. NISHIDA Y, HAYASHI E, AKAOKA I, YOSHIMURA T: Hyperuricemia in Japanese Sumo wrestlers. *Revue du Rhumatisme. Abstracts 15th Int Congr Rheumatology.* Paris, June 1981, no 0823

332. HERSHKO A, HERSHKO C, MAGER J: Increased formation of 5′phosphoribosyl-1-pyrophosphate in red blood cells of some gouty patients. *Israel J Med Sci* 4:939, 1968

333. SPERLING O, OPHIR R, DE VRIES A: Purine base incorporation into erythrocyte nucleotides and erythrocyte phosphoribosyltransferase activity in primary gout. *Rev Eur Etud Clin Biol* 16:147, 1971

334. SPERLING O, PERSKY-BROSH S, BOER P, DE VRIES A: Human erythrocyte phosphoribosylpyrophosphate synthetase mutationally altered in regulatory properties. *Biochem Med* 7:389, 1973

335. KREBS HA, EGGLESTON LV: The regulation of the pentose phosphate cycle in rat liver, in Weber G (ed): *Advances in Enzyme Regulation.* Oxford, Pergamon, 1974, vol 12, p 421

336. GUMAA KA, McLEAN P: Factors controlling the flux of glucose through the pentose phosphate pathway. *Postgrad Med J* 47:403, 1971

337. RUNDLES RW, WYNGAARDEN JB, HITCHINGS GH, ELION GB, SILBERMAN HR: Effects of a xanthine oxidase inhibitor on thiopurine metabolism, hyperuricemia and gout. *Trans Assoc Am Physicians* 76:126, 1963

338. HENDERSON JF, ROSENBLOOM FM, KELLEY WN, SEEGMILLER JE: Variations in purine metabolism of cultured skin fibroblasts from patients with gout. *J Clin Invest* 47:1511, 1968

339. HOLMES EW, WYNGAARDEN JB, KELLEY WN: The regulation of PRPP amidotransferase in man. *Clin Res* 21:87, 1973 (abstract)

340. NUKI G, ASTRIN K, BRENTON D, CRUIKSHANK M, LEVER J, SEEGMILLER J: Purine and pyrimidine nucleotide pools in azaguanine resistant human lymphoblasts deficient in hypoxanthine-guanine phosphoribosyltransferase. *Proc Am Soc Hum Genet*, Atlanta, Oct. 24–27, 1973 (abstract)

341. KELLEY WN, LEVY RI, ROSENBLOOM FM, HENDERSON JF, SEEGMILLER JE: Adenine phosphoribosyltransferase deficiency: A previously underscribed genetic defect in man. *J Clin Invest* 47:2281, 1968

342. YÜ T-F, GUTMAN AB: Effects of allopurinol [4-hydroxypyrazolo(3,4-d) pyrimidine] on serum and urinary uric acid in primary and secondary gout. *Am J Med* 37:885, 1964

343. EMMERSON BT: Discussion, symposium on allopurinol. *Ann Rheum Dis* 25:622, 1966

344. KELLEY WN, ROSENBLOOM FM, MILLER J, SEEGMILLER JE: An enzymatic basis for variation in response to allopurinol. *N Engl J Med* 278:287, 1968

345. WEISSMANN B, GUTMAN AB: The identification of 6-succinoaminopurine and of 8-hydroxy-7-methylguanine as normal human urinary constituents. *J Biol Chem* 229:239, 1957

346. ROWE PB, WYNGAARDEN JB: The mechanism of dietary alterations in rat hepatic xanthine oxidase levels. *J Biol Chem* 241:5571, 1966

347. MANGONI A, PENNETTI V, SPADONI MA: Aumento adattivo di xantinossidasi in topini alimentati con diete a diverso contenuto proteico. *Boll Soc Ital Biol Sper* 31:1397, 1955

348. DELLA CORTE E, STIRPE F: Regulation of xanthine dehydrogenase in chick liver. *Biochem J* 102:520, 1967

349. DIAMOND HS, FRIEDLAND M, HALBERSTAM D, KAPLAN D: Glycine C^{14} incorporation into nucleic acid purine by leukocytes obtained from normal and gouty subjects. *Ann Rheum Dis* 28:275, 1969

350. CHANG GM, FAM A, LITTLE AM, MALKIN A: The uptake of glycine ^{14}C into the adenine and guanine of DNA and insoluble RNA of human leukocytes. *Adv Exp Med Biol* 41B:407, 1974

351. KAMOUN P, CHANARD J, BRAMI M, FUNCK-BRENTANO JL: Purine biosynthesis de novo by lymphocytes in gout. *Clin Sci Mol Med* 54:595, 1978

352. BERLINER RW, HILTON JG, YÜ T, KENNEDY TJ JR: The renal mechanism for urate excretion in man. *J Clin Invest* 29:396, 1950

353. GUTMAN AB, YÜ T-F: A three-component system for regulation of renal excretion of uric acid in man. *Trans Assoc Am Physicians* 74:353, 1961

354. RIESELBACH RE, STEELE TH: Influence of the kidney upon urate homeostasis in health and disease. *Am J Med* 56:665, 1974

355. DIAMOND HS, PAOLINO JS: Evidence for a post-secretory reabsorptive site for uric acid in man. *J Clin Invest* 52:1491, 1973

356. LEVINSON DJ, SORENSEN LB: Renal handling of uric acid in normal and gouty subjects: Evidence for a 4-component system. *Ann Rheum Dis* 39:173, 1980

357. ROCH-RAMEL F, PETERS G: Urinary excretion of uric acid in nonhuman mammalian species. *Handbook Exp Pharmacol* 51:211, 1978

358. WEINER IM, FANELLI GM JR: Renal urate excretion in animal models. *Nephron* 14:33, 1975

359. ROCH-RAMEL F, DIEZI-CHOMETY F, DE ROUGEMONT D, TELLIER M, WIDMER J, PETERS G: Renal excretion of uric acid in the rat: A micropuncture and microperfusion study. *Am J Physiol* 230:768, 1976

360. ROCH-RAMEL F: Renal excretion of uric acid in mammals. *Clin Nephrol* 12:1, 1979

361. LANG F, GREGER R, OBERLEITHNER H, GRISS E, LANG K, PASTNER D, DITTRICH P, DEETJEN P: Renal handling of urate in healthy man in hyperuricaemia and renal insufficiency: Circadian fluctuation, effect of water diuresis and of uricosuric agents. *Eur J Clin Invest* 10:285, 1980

362. GREGER R, LANG F, DEETJEN P: Handling of uric acid by the rat kidney. I. Microanalysis of uric acid in proximal tubular fluid. *Pfluegers Arch* 324:279, 1971

363. GREGER R, LANG F, DEETJEN P: Handling of uric acid by rat kidney. II. Microperfusion studies on bidirectional transport of uric acid in the proximal tubule. *Eur J Physiol* 335:257, 1972

364. CHIN TY, CACINI W, ZMUDA MJ, QUEBBEMANN AJ: Quantification of renal uric acid synthesis in the rat. *Am J Physiol* 238:F481, 1980

365. ROCH-RAMEL F, WEINER IM: Excretion of urate by the kidney of *Cebus* monkeys: A micropuncture study. *Am J Physiol* 224:1369, 1973

366. FANELLI GM JR, WEINER IM: Pyrazinoate excretion in the chimpanzee:

367. MARTINO JA, EARLEY LE: Demonstration of a role of physical factors as determinants of the nutriuretic response to volume expansion. *J Clin Invest* 46:1963, 1967

368. WEINMAN EJ, EKNOYAS G, SUKI WN: The influence of the extracellular fluid volume on the tubular reabsorption of uric acid. *J Clin Invest* 55:283, 1975

369. MALNIC G, AIRES MM, GIEBISCH GG: Micropuncture study of renal tubular hydrogen ion transport in the rat. *Am J Physiol* 222:147, 1972

370. WEINER IM, MUDGE GH: Renal tubular mechanisms for excretion of organic acids and bases. *Am J Med* 36:743, 1964

371. CHONKO AM: Urate secretion in isolated rabbit renal tubules. *Am J Physiol* F545, 1980

372. ROCH-RAMEL F, WHITE F, VOWLES L, SIMMONDS HA, CAMERON JS: Micropuncture study of tubular transport of urate and PAH in the pig kidney. *Am J Physiol* 239:F107, 1980

373. PRAETORIUS E, KIRK JE: Hypouricemia: With evidence for tubular elimination of uric acid. *J Lab Clin Med* 35:865, 1950

374. GUTMAN AB, YÜ T-F, BERGER L: Tubular secretion of urate in man. *J Clin Invest* 38:1778, 1959

375. YÜ T-F, GUTMAN AB: Study of the paradoxical effects of salicylate in low, intermediate and high dosage on the renal mechanisms for excretion of urate in man. *J Clin Invest* 38:1298, 1959

376. PODEVIN R, ARDAILLOU R, PAILLARD F, FONTANNELE J, RICHET G: Etude chez l'homme de la cinetique d'apparition dans purine de l'acide urique 2 ^{14}C. *Nephron* 5:134, 1968

377. BOUMENDIL-PODEVIN EF, PODEVIN RA, PRIOL C: Uric acid transport in brush border membrane vesicles isolated from rabbit kidney. *Am J Physiol* 236:F519, 1979

378. SHANNON JA: The excretion of uric acid by the chicken. *J Cell Comp Physiol* 11:135, 1938

379. MAY DG, WEINER IM: The renal mechanisms for the excretion of *m*-hydroxybenzoic acid in *Cebus* monkeys: Relationships to urate transport. *J Pharmacol Exp Ther* 176:407, 1971

380. BONER G, STEELE TH: Relationship of uric acid and PAH secretion in man. *Am J Physiol* 225:100, 1973

381. YÜ T-F, SIROTA JH, BERGER L, HALPERN M, GUTMAN AB: Effect of sodium lactate infusion on urate clearance in man. *Proc Soc Exp Biol Med* 96:809, 1957

382. GOLDFINGER S, KLINENBERG JR, SEEGMILLER JE: Renal retention of uric acid induced by infusion of beta-hydroxybutyrate and acetoacetate. *N Engl J Med* 272:351, 1965

383. SCHULMAN JD, LUSTBERG TJ, KENNEDY JL, MUSELES M, SEEGMILLER JE: A new variant of maple syrup urine disease (branched chain ketoaciduria): Clinical and biochemical evaluation. *Am J Med* 49:118, 1970

384. GUTMAN AB, YÜ T-F: Renal mechanisms for regulation of uric acid excretion, with special reference of normal and gouty man. *Semin Arthritis Rheum* 2:1, 1972

385. GERGER R, LANG F, DEETJEN P: Handling of uric acid by rat kidney. II. Microperfusion studies on bidirectional transport of uric acid in the proximal tubule. *Eur J Physiol* 335:257, 1972

386. WILSON DM, GOLDSTEIN NP: Renal urate excretion in patients with Wilson's disease. *Kidney Int* 4:331, 1973

387. BENNETT JS, GOTTLIEB AJ, BOND D, SINGER I, GOTTLIEB AJ: Hypouricemia in Hodgkin's disease. *Ann Intern Med* 76:751, 1972

388. FANELLI GM JR, BOHN DH, REILLY SS: Renal urate transport in the chimpanzee. *Am J Physiol* 220:613, 1971

389. STEELE TH, BONER G: Origins of the uricosuric response. *J Clin Invest* 52:1368, 1973

390. MANUEL MA, STEELE TH: Pyrazinamide suppression of the uricosuric response to sodium chloride infusion. *J Lab Clin Med* 83:417, 1974

391. STEELE TH: Urate secretion in man: The pyrazinamide suppression test. *Ann Intern Med* 79:734, 1973

392. SORENSEN LB, LEVINSON DJ: Isolated defect in post-secretory reabsorption of uric acid. *Ann Rheum Dis* 39:180, 1980

393. WEINMAN EJ, SANSOM SC, STEPLOCK DA, SHETH AU, KNIGHT TF, SENEKJIAN HO: Secretion of urate in the proximal convoluted tubule of the rat. *Am J Physiol* 239:F383, 1980

394. STEELE TH, RIESELBACH RE: The renal mechanism for urate homeostasis in normal man. *Am J Med* 43:868, 1967

395. YÜ T-F, BERGER L, STONE DJ, WOLF J, GUTMAN AB: Effects of pyrazinamide and pyrazinoic acid on urate clearance and other discrete renal functions. *Proc Soc Exp Biol Med* 96:264, 1957

396. YÜ T-F, BERGER L, GUTMAN AB: Suppression of the tubular secretion of urate by pyrazinamide in the dog. *Proc Soc Exp Biol Med* 107:905, 1961

397. DAVIS BB, FIELD JB, RODNAN GP, KEDES LH: Localization and pyrazinamide inhibition of distal transtubular movement of uric acid-2-^{14}C with a modified stop-flow technique. *J Clin Invest* 44:716, 1965

398. GUTMAN A, YÜ T-F, BERGER L: Renal function in gout. III. Estimation of

tubular secretion and reabsorption of uric acid by use of pyrazinamide (pyrazinoic acid). *Am J Med* 47:575, 1969

399. WEINER IM, TINKER JP: Pharmacology of pyrazinamide: Metabolic and renal function studies related to the mechanism of drug-induced urate retention. *J Pharmacol Exp Ther* 180:411, 1972

400. KRAMP RA, LASSITER WE, GOTTSCHALK CW: Urate-2-¹⁴C transport in the rat nephron. *J Clin Invest* 50:35, 1971

401. NICHOLLS A, SNAITH ML, SCOTT JT: Effect of estrogen therapy on plasma and urinary levels of uric acid. *Br Med J* 1:449, 1973

402. STEELE TH, RIESELBACH RE: The contribution of residual nephrons within the chronically diseased kidney to urate homeostasis in man. *Am J Med* 43:876, 1967

403. SNAITH ML, SCOTT JT: Uric acid clearance in patients with gout and normal subjects. *Ann Rheum Dis* 30:285, 1971

404. WYNGAARDEN JB: Gout. *Adv Metab Dis* 2:2, 1965

405. NUGENT CA, MacDIARMID WD, TYLER FH: Renal excretion of urate in patients with gout. *Arch Intern Med* 113:115, 1964

406. SIMKIN PA: Uric acid excretion in patients with gout. *Arthritis Rheum* 22:98, 1979

407. KRAMER HJ, LU E, GONICK HC: Organic acid excretion patterns in gout. *Ann Rheum Dis* 31:137, 1972

408. OWEN EE, ROBINSON RR: Amino acid extraction and ammonia metabolism by the human kidney during the prolonged administration of ammonium chloride. *J Clin Invest* 42:263, 1963

409. PLANTE GE, DURIVAGE J, LEMIEUX G: Renal excretion of hydrogen in primary gout. *Metabolism* 17:377, 1968

410. FALLS WF JR: Comparison of urinary acidification and ammonium excretion in normal and gouty subjects. *Metabolism* 21:433, 1972

411. GIBSON T, SIMMONDS HA, RODGERS V, POTTER C: The abnormal excretion of acid in gout—a metabolic clue? *Revue du Rhumatisme. Abstracts 15th Int Congr Rheumatology.* Paris, June 1981, no 0822

412. LOWENSTEIN JM: Ammonia production in muscle and other tissues. The purine nucleotide cycle. *Physiol Rev* 52:382, 1972

413. YÜ T-F, ADLER M, BORROW E, GUTMAN AB: Plasma and urinary amino acids in primary gout, with special reference to glutamine. *J Clin Invest* 48:885, 1969

414. GUTMAN AB, YÜ T-F: Hyperglutamatemia in primary gout. *Am J Med* 54:713, 1973

415. KAPLAN D, DIAMOND H, WALLACE SL, HALBERSTAM D: Amino acid excretion in primary hyperuricaemia. *Ann Rheum Dis* 28:180, 1969

416. WEISSMAN B, BROBERG PA, GUTMAN AB: The purine bases of human urine. I. Separation and identification. *J Biol Chem* 224:407, 1957

417. SKUPP S, AYVAZIAN JH: Oxidation of 7-methylguanine by human xanthine oxidase. *J Lab Clin Med* 73:909, 1969

418. BUZARD J, BISHOP C, TALBOTT JH: The fate of uric acid in the normal and gouty human being. *J Chron Dis* 2:42, 1955

419. HOWELL RR, WYNGAARDEN JB: On the mechanism of peroxidation of uric acids by hemoproteins. *J Biol Chem* 235:3544, 1960

420. AMES BN, CATHCART R, SCHWIERS E, HOCHSTEIN P: Uric acid provides an anti-oxidant defense in humans against oxidant- and radical-caused aging and cancer: A hypothesis. *Proc Natl Acad Sci USA* 78:6858, 1981

421. POLLYCOVE M, TOLBERT BM, LAWRENCE JH, HARMAN D: Uric acid metabolism: The oxidation of uric acid in normal subjects and patients with gout, polycythemia and leukemia. *Clin Res Proc* 5:38, 1957 (abstract)

422. HOWELL RR, ASHTON DM, WYNGAARDEN JB: Glucose-6-phosphatase deficiency glycogen storage disease: Studies on the interrelationships of carbohydrate, lipid, and purine abnormalities. *Pediatrics* 29:553, 1962

423. KELLEY WN, ROSENBLOOM FM, SEEGMILLER JE, HOWELL RR: Excessive production of uric acid in Type I glycogen storage disease. *J Pediatr* 72:488, 1968

424. KAUFMAN JM, GREENE ML, SEEGMILLER JE: Urine uric acid to creatinine ratio: A screening test for inherited disorders of purine metabolism. *J Pediatr* 73:583, 1968

425. JAKOVCIC S, SORENSEN LB: Studies of uric acid metabolism in glycogen storage disease associated with gouty arthritis. *Arthritis Rheum* 10:129, 1967

426. ROE TF, KOGUT MD: The pathogenesis of hyperuricemia in glycogen storage disease type I. *Pediatr Res* 11:664, 1977

427. BURR IM, O'NEILL JA, KARZON DT, HOWARD J, GREENE HL: Comparison of the effects of total parenteral nutrition, continuous intragastric feeding, and portacaval shunt on a patient with type I glycogen storage disease. *J Pediatr* 85:792, 1974

428. BRIGGS JM, HAWORTH JC: Liver glycogen disease (report of a case of hyperuricemia, renal calculi and no demonstrable enzyme defect). *Am J Med* 36:443, 1964

429. SPERLING O, EILAM G, PERSKY-BROSH S, DE VRIES A: Accelerated erythrocyte 5-phosphoribosyl-1-pyrophosphate synthesis: A familial abnormality associated with excessive uric acid production and gout. *Biochem Med* 6:310, 1972

430. DE VRIES A, SPERLING O: Familial gouty malignant uric acid lithiasis due to mutant phosphoribosylpyrophosphate synthetase. *Urologe A* 12:153, 1973

431. BECKER MA, KOSTEL PJ, MEYER LJ, SEEGMILLER JE: Human phosphoribosylpyrophosphate synthetase: Increased enzyme specific activity in a family with gout and excessive purine synthesis. *Proc Natl Acad Sci USA* 70:2749, 1973

431a.BECKER MA, MEYER LJ, SEEGMILLER JE: Gout with purine overproduction due to increased phosphoribosyl-pyrophosphate synthetase activity. *Am J Med* 55:232, 1973

432. BECKER MA, MEYER LJ, KOSTEL PJ, SEEGMILLER JE: Increased 5-phosphoribosyl-1-pyrophosphate (PRPP) synthetase activity and gout: Diversity of structural alterations of the enzyme. *J Clin Invest* 53:4a, 1974 (abstract)

433. BECKER MA, RAIVIO KO, BAKAY B, ADAMS WB, NYHAN WL: Variant human phosphoribosylpyrophosphate synthetase altered in regulatory and catalytic functions. *J Clin Invest* 65:109, 1980

434. LEJEUNE E, BOUVIER M, MOUSSON B, LLORCA G, BALTASSAT P: Anomalies de la phosphoribosylpyrophosphate synthetase dans deux cas de goutte a debut precose. *Rev Rhum* 46:457, 1979

435. MULLER MM, FRANK O: Lipid and purine metabolism in benign symmetric lipomatosis, in Sperling O, De Vries A, Wyngaarden JB (eds): *Purine Metabolism in Man.* New York, Plenum, 1974, p 509

436. SEEGMILLER JE, ROSENBLOOM FM, KELLEY WN: An enzyme defect associated with a sex-linked human neurological disorder and excessive purine synthesis. *Science* 155:1682, 1967

437. KELLEY WN, ROSENBLOOM FM, HENDERSON JF, SEEGMILLER JE: A specific enzyme defect in gout associated with overproduction of uric acid. *Proc Natl Acad Sci USA* 57:1735, 1967

438. SPERLING O, FRANK M, OPHIR R, LIBERMAN UA, ADAM A, DE VRIES A: Partial deficiency of hypoxanthine-guanine phosphoribosyltransferase associated with gout and uric acid lithiasis. *Rev Eur Etud Clin Biol* 15:942, 1970

439. YÜ T-F, BALIS ME, KRENITSKY TA, DANCIS J, SILVERS DN, ELION GP, GUTMAN AB: Rarity of X-linked partial hypoxanthine-guanine phosphoribosyltransferase deficiency in a large gouty population. *Ann Intern Med* 76:255, 1972

440. DE BRUYN CHMM, OEI TL, GEERDINK RA, LOMMEN EJP: An atypical case of hypoxanthine-guanine phosphoribosyltransferase deficiency (Lesch-Nyhan syndrome). *Clin Genet* 4:353, 1973

441. SORENSEN L, BENKE PJ: Biochemical evidence for a distinct type of primary gout. *Nature (Lond)* 213:1122, 1967

442. BENKE PJ, HERRICK N: Azaguanine-resistance as a manifestation of a new form of metabolic overproduction of uric acid. *Am J Med* 52:547, 1972

443. FOX IH, DWOSH IL, MARCHANT PJ: Hypoxanthine-guanine phosphoribosyltransferase characteristics of a mutation in a patient with gout. *J Clin Invest* 56:1239, 1975

444. POLLAK VE, MATTENHEIMER H: Glutaminase activity in the kidney in gout. *J Lab Clin Med* 66:564, 1965

445. FRIEDEN C: Glutamate dehydrogenase. V. The relation of enzyme structure to the catalytic function. *J Biol Chem* 238:3286, 1963

445a.LONG WK: Association between glutathione reductase variants and plasma uric acid concentration of a Negro population. Program abstracts, p. 14a. *American Society of Human Genetics,* Indianapolis, October 1970

445b.LONG WK: Glutathione reductase in red blood cells: Variant associated with gout. *Science* 155:712, 1967

445c.LONG WK: Red blood cell glutathione reductase in gout. *Science* 138:991, 1962

445d.WASSERZUG O, SZEINBERG A, SPERLING O: Erythrocyte glutathione reductase in gout and in glucose-6-phosphate dehydrogenase deficiency. *Monogr Hum Genet* 9:16, 1978

445e.BEUTLER E: Effect of flavin compounds on glutathione reductase activity: In vivo and in vitro studies. *J Clin Invest* 48:1957, 1969

446. VAN DEN BERGHE G, HERS H-G: Abnormal AMP deaminase in primary gout. *Lancet* 2:1090, 1980

447. SIMKIN PA: Hexose infusions in *Cebus* monkeys: Effects on uric acid metabolism. *Metabolism* 21:1029, 1972

448. STIRPE F, DELLA CORTE E, BONETTI E, ABBONDANZA A, ABBATI A, DE STAFANO F: Fructose-induced hyperuricemia. *Lancet* 2:1310, 1970

449. DIPAOLO N, MARCOLONGO R: Fructose-induced hyperuricemia. Abstract 33.11, *Seventh Eur Rheumatology Congr.* Brighton, England, 1971

450. COHEN J: Gout, in Copeman WSC (ed): *Textbook of the Rheumatic Diseases.* Edinburgh, Livingstone, 1955, p 361

451. TALBOTT JH: Gout. *J Chron Dis* 1:338, 1955

452. SMYTH CJ: Hereditary factors in gout: A review of recent literature. *Metabolism* 6:218, 1957

453. FOLIN O, LYMAN H: On the influence of phenylquinolin carbonic acid (Atophan) on uric acid elimination. *J Pharmacol Exp Ther* 4:539, 1913

454. JACOBSON BM: The uric acid in the serum of gouty and non-gouty individuals: Its detection by Folin's recent method and its significance in the diagnosis of gout. *Ann Intern Med* 11:1277, 1937

455. TALBOTT JH: Serum urate in relatives of gouty patients. *J Clin Invest* 27:749, 1940

456. WILSON D, COLLINS DH, MARSON RM: Gout: Discussion. *Proc R Soc Med* 44:285, 1951

457. STECHER RM, HERSH AH, SOLOMON WM: The hereditary of gout and its relationship to familial hyperuricemia. *Ann Intern Med* 31:595, 1949

458. NEEL JV, RAKIC MT, DAVIDSON RI, VALKENBURG HA, MIKKELSEN WM: Studies on hyperuricemia. II. A reconsideration of the distribution of serum uric acid values in the families of Smyth, Cotterman, and Freyberg. *Am J Hum Genet* 17:14, 1965

459. BURCH TA, O'BRIEN WM, REED R, KURLAND LT: Hyperuricemia and gout in Mariana Islands. *Ann Rheum Dis* 25:114, 1966

460. FRENCH JG, DODGE HJ, KJELSBERG MO, MIKKELSEN WM, SCHULL WJ: A study of familial aggregation of serum uric acid levels in the population of Tecumseh, Michigan. *Am J Epidemiol* 86:214, 1967

461. BECKER MA, YEN RCK, ITKIN P: Regional localization of the gene for human phosphoribosylpyrophosphate synthetase on the X-chromosome. *Science* 203:1016, 1979

462. GOSS SJ, HARRIS H: New method for mapping genes in human chromosomes. *Nature* 255(5511):680, 1975

463. ZOREF E, DE VRIES A, SPERLING O: Evidence for X-linkage of phosphoribosylpyrophosphate synthetase in man: Studies with cultured fibroblasts from a gouty family with mutant feedback resistant enzyme. *Hum Hered* 27:73, 1977

464. YEN RCK, ADAMS WB, LAZAR C, BECKER MA: Evidence for X-linkage of human phosphoribosylpyrophosphate synthetase. *Proc Natl Acad Sci USA* 75:482, 1978

465. ZOREF E, DE VRIES A, SPERLING O: Mutant feedback-resistant phosphoribosylpyrophosphate synthetase associated with purine overproduction and gout. *J Clin Invest* 56:1093, 1975

466. WALLACE SL, GERNSTEIN D, DIAMOND H: Diagnostic value of the colchicine therapeutic trial. *JAMA* 199:525, 1967

467. BORISY GG, TAYLOR EW: The mechanism of action of colchicine: Binding of colchicine-³H to cellular protein. *J Biol Chem* 34:525, 1967

468. WEISENBERG RC, BORISY GG, TAYLOR EW: The colchicine-binding protein of mammalian brain and its relation to microtubules. *Biochemistry* 7:4466, 1968

469. GUTMAN AB, YÜ T-F: Protracted uricosuric therapy in tophaceous gout. *Lancet* 2:1258, 1957

470. BARTELS EC: Treatment of gout. *Metabolism* 6:297, 1957

471. SIROTA JH, YÜ T-F, GUTMAN AB: Effect of Benemid [*p*-(di-*n*-propylsulfamyl)-benzoic acid] on urate clearance and other discrete renal functions in gouty subjects. *J Clin Invest* 31:692, 1952

472. YÜ T-F, SIROTA JH, GUTMAN AB: Effect of phenylbutazone (3,5-dioxo-1,2-diphenyl-4-*N*-butylpyrazolidine) on renal clearance of urate and other discrete renal functions in gouty subjects. *J Clin Invest* 32:1121, 1953

473. BISHOP C, GARNER W, TALBOTT JH: Pool size, turnover rate, and rapidity of equilibration of injected isotopic uric acid in normal and pathological subjects. *J Clin Invest* 30:879, 1951

474. YÜ T-F, DAYTON PG, GUTMAN AB: Mutual suppression of the uricosuric effects of sulfinpyrazone and salicylate: A study in interactions between drugs. *J Clin Invest* 42:1330, 1963

475. BLUESTONE R, KIPPEN I, KLENENBERG JR, WHITEHOUSE MW: Effect of some uricosuric and anti-inflammatory drugs on the binding of uric acid to human serum albumin in vitro. *J Lab Clin Med* 76:85, 1970

476. KUZELL W, GLOVER R, GIBBS J, BLAU R: Effect of anturane on serum uric acid and cholesterol in gout: A long term study. *Acta Rheumatol Scand Suppl* 8:31, 1964

477. THOMPSON GR, DUFF IF, ROBINSON WD, MIKKELSEN WM, FALINDEZ H: Long term uricosuric therapy in gout. *Arthritis Rheum* 5:384, 1962

478. DE SEZE S, RYCKEWAERT A, CARIOT M, KAHN MF, D'ANGLEJAN G: Le traitement uricosurique de la goutte. *Congrès Internatinal de la goutte ed de la lithiase urique*, Evian, Sept. 4–6, 1964, p 297

479. SEEGMILLER JE, GRAYZEL AI: Use of the newer uricosuric agents in the management of gout. *JAMA* 173:1076, 1960

480. ROBINSON WD: The present status of colchicine and uricosuric agents in management of primary gout. *Arthritis Rheum* 8:865, 1965

481. LONDON M, HUDSON PB: Uricolytic activity of purified uricase in two human beings. *Science* 125:937, 1957

482. ROYER R, VINDEL J, LAMARCHE M, KISSEL P: Modalities of purine excretion during enzyme treatment of gout and other hyperuricemic conditions with urate oxidase. *Presse Med* 76:2325, 1968

483. FITZGERALD O, FITZPATRICK DA, MCGEENEY KF: Urate oxidase treatment for hyperuricaemia. *Lancet* 1:525, 1975

484. ZITTOUN R, DAUCHY F, TEILLAUD C, BARTHELEMY M, BOUCHARD P: Le traitement des hyperuricemies en hematologie par l'urate-oxydase et l'allopurinol. *Ann Med Interne* 172:479, 1965

485. FITZPATRICK DA, FITZGERALD O, MCGEENEY KF: Immunological aspects of urate oxidase therapy in hyperuricaemia. *Irish J Med Sci* 146:155, 1977

486. DAVIS S, PARK YK, ABUCHOWSKI A, DAVIS FF: Hypouricaemic effect of polyethyleneglycol modified urate oxidase. *Lancet* 2:281, 1981

487. ROBINS RK: Potential purine antagonists. I. Synthesis of some 4,6-substituted pyrazolo 3,4-*d* pyrimidines. *J Am Chem Soc* 78:784, 1956

488. ELION GB: Enzymatic and metabolic studies with allopurinol. *Ann Rheum Dis* 25:608, 1966

489. MASSEY V, KOMAI H, PALMER G, ELION GB: On the mechanism of inactivation of xanthine oxidase by allopurinol and other pyrazolo (3,4-*d*) pyrimidines. *J Biol Chem* 245:2837, 1970

490. ELION GB, KOVENSKY A, HITCHINGS GH, METZ E, RUNDLES RW: Metabolic studies of allopurinol, an inhibitor of xanthine oxidase. *Biochem Pharmacol* 15:863, 1966

491. KRENITSKY TA, ELION GB, STRELITZ RA, HITCHINGS GH: Ribonucleoside of allopurinol and oxoallopurinol. *J Biol Chem* 242:2675, 1967

492. HANDE K, REED E, CHABNER B: Allopurinol kinetics. *Clin Pharmacol Ther* 23:598, 1978

493. ELION GB, YÜ T-F, GUTMAN AB, HITCHINGS GH: Renal clearance of oxipurinol, the chief metabolite of allopurinol. *Am J Med* 45:69, 1968

493a. NELSON DJ, BRIGGE CJL, KRASNY HC, ELION GB: Formation of nucleotides of [6-¹⁴C] allopurinol and [6-¹⁴C] oxipurinol in rat tissues and effects on uridine nucleotide pools. *Biochem Pharmacol* 22:2003, 1973

494. CHALMERS RA, KROMER H, SCOTT JT, WATTS RWE: A comparative study of the xanthine oxidase inhibitors, allopurinol and oxipurinol in man. *Clin Sci* 35:353, 1968

495. CHYTIL F: Activation of liver tryptophan oxygenase by adenosine 3'5'-phosphate and by other purine derivatives. *J Biol Chem* 243:893, 1968

496. GALLO RC, PERRY S, BREITMAN TR: Inhibition of human leukocyte pyrimidine deoxynucleoside synthesis by allopurinol and 6-mercaptopurine. *Biochem Pharmacol* 17:2185, 1968

497. TRUSEVE R, WILLIAMS V: The effect of allopurinol on urate oxidase acticity. *Biochem Pharmacol* 17:165, 1968

498. KELLEY WN, WYNGAARDEN JB: The effect of dietary purine restriction, allopurinol and oxipurinol on the urinary excretion of ultraviolet absorbing compounds. *Clin Chem* 16:707, 1970

499. KELLEY WN, BEARDMORE TD: Allopurinol: Alteration in pyrimidine metabolism in man. *Science* 169:388, 1970

500. BEARDMORE TD, FOX IH, KELLEY WN: Effect of allopurinol on pyrimidine metabolism in the Lesch-Nyham syndrome. *Lancet* 2:830, 1970

501. BEARDMORE TD, CASHMAN JS, KELLEY WN: Mechanism of allopurinol-mediated increase in enzyme activity in man. *J Clin Invest* 51:1823, 1972

502. GROBNER W, KELLEY WN: Effect of allopurinol and its metabolic derivatives on the configuration of human orotate phosphoribosyltransferases and orotidine 5'-phosphate decarboxylase. *Biochem Pharmacol* 24:379, 1975

503. DELBARRE F, AUSCHER C, DEGERY A, BROUILHET H, OLIVIER J-L: Le traitement de la dyspurine goutteuse par la mercaptopyrazolopyrimidine (MPP:thiopurinol). *Presse Med* 76:2329, 1968

504. WYNGAARDEN JB, RUNDLES RW, METZ EN: Allopurinol in the treatment of gout. *Ann Intern Med* 62:842, 1965

505. RUNDLES RW, METZ EN, SILBERMAN HR: Allopurinol in the treatment of gout. *Ann Intern Med* 64:229, 1966

506. RUNDLES RW, WYNGAARDEN JB, HITCHINGS GH, ELION GB: Drugs and uric acid. *Annu Rev Pharmacol* 9:345, 1969

507. RODNAN G, ROBIN JA, TOLCHIN SF: Efficacy of a single daily dose of allopurinol in gouty hyperuricemia, in Sperling O, de Vries A, Wyngaarden JB (eds): *Purine Metabolism in Man*. New York, Plenum, 1974, p 571

508. KLINENBERG JR, GOLDFINGER SE, SEEGMILLER JE: The effectiveness of the xanthine oxidase inhibitor allopurinol in the treatment of gout. *Ann Intern Med* 62:639, 1965

509. KUZELL WC, SEEACH LM, GLOVER RP, JACKMAN AE: Treatment of gout with allopurinol and sulphinpyrazone in combination and with allopurinol alone. *Ann Rheum Dis* 25:634, 1966

510. TJANDRAMAGA TB, GUTMAN AB: Observations on the disposition of probenecid in patients receiving allopurinol. *Pharmacology* 8:259, 1972

511. SORENSEN LB: Seminars on the Lesch-Nyhan syndrome: Management and treatment. Discussion. *Fed Proc* 27:1097, 1968

512. GREENE ML, FUJIMOTO WY, SEEGMILLER JE: Urinary xanthine stones—a rare complication of allopurinol therapy. *N Engl J Med* 280:426, 1969

513. MIZUNO T, SEGAWA M, KURUMADA T: Clinical and therapeutic aspects of the Lesch-Nyhan syndrome in Japanese children. *Neuropaediatrie* 2:38, 1970

514. MANZKE H: Xanthine stone formation subsequent to allopurinol therapy. *Dtsch Med Wochenschr* 99:918, 1974

515. SPERLING O, BROSH S, BOER P, LIBERMAN UA, DE VRIES A: Urinary xanthine stones in an allopurinol-treated gouty patient with partial deficiency of hypoxanthine-guanine phosphoribosyltransferase. *Israel J Med Sci* 14:288, 1978

516. BAND PR, SILVERBERG DS, HENDERSON JF, ULAN RA, WENSEL RH, BANERJEE TK, LITTLE AS: Xanthine nephropathy in a patient with lymphosarcoma treated with allopurinol. *N Engl J Med* 283:354, 1970

517. WYNGAARDEN JB: Allopurinol and xanthine nephropathy. *N Engl J Med* 283:371, 1970

518. ABLIN A, STEPHENS GG, HIRATA T, WILSON K, WILLIAMS HE: Nephropathy, xanthinuria, and orotic aciduria complicating Burkitt's lymphoma treated with chemotherapy and allopurinol. *Metabolism* 21:771, 1972

519. WATTS RWE, SNEEDEN W, PARKER RA: A quantitative study of skeletal-muscle purines and pyrazolo (3,4-*d*) pyrimidines. *Clin Sci* 41:153, 1971

520. LANDGREBE AR, NYHAN WL, COLEMAN M: Urinary tract stones resulting from the excretion of oxypurinol. *N Engl J Med* 292:626, 1975

521. STOTE RM, SMITH LH, DUBB JW, MOYER TP, ALEXANDER F, ROTH JLA: Oxypurinol nephrolithiasis in regional enteritis secondary to allopurinol therapy. *Ann Intern Med* 92:384, 1980

522. BOSTON COLLABORATIVE DRUG SURVEILLANCE PROGRAM: Excess of ampicillin rashes associated with allopurinol or hyperuricemia. *N Engl J Med* 286, 505, 1972

523. FAM AG, PATON TW, CHAITON A: Reinstitution of allopurinol therapy for gouty arthritis after cutaneous reactions. *Can Med Assoc J* 123:128, 1980

524. DELBARRE F, AMOR B, AUSCHER C, DEGERY A: Treatment of gout with allopurinol, a study of 106 cases. *Ann Rheum Dis* 25:627, 1966

525. EMMERSON BT: Discussion, symposium on allopurinol. *Ann Rheum Dis* 25:621, 1966

526. KELLEY WN, ROSENBLOOM FM, MILLER J, SEEGMILLER JE: An enzymatic basis for variation in response to allopurinol. *N Engl J Med* 278:287, 1968

527. ELION GB, NELSON DJ: Ribonucleotides of allopurinol and oxipurinol in rat tissues and their significance in purine metabolism, in Sperling O, De Vries A, Wyngaarden JB (eds): *Purine Metabolism in Man.* New York, Plenum, 1974, p 639

528. MARR JJ, BERENS RL: Antileishmanial effect of allopurinol. II. Relationship of adenine metabolism in *Leishmania* species to the action of allopurinol. *J Infect Dis* 136:724, 1977

529. BERENS RL, MARR JJ, MELSON DJ, LaFON SW: Antileishmanial effect of allopurinol and allopurinol ribonucleoside on intracellular forms of *Leishmania donovani. Biochem Pharmacol* 29:2397, 1980

530. NELSON DJ, LaFON SW, TUTTLE JV, MILLER WH, MILLER RL, KRENITSKY TA, ELION GB, BERENS RL, MARR JJ: Allopurinol ribonucleoside as an antileishmanial agent. Biological effects, metabolism, and enzymatic phosphorylation. *J Biol Chem* 254:11544, 1979

531. NELSON DJ, BUGGE CJL, ELION GB, BERENS RL, MARR JJ: Metabolism of pyrazolo(3,4-*d*) pyrimidines in *Leishmania braziliensis* and *Leishmania donovani.* Allopurinol, oxipurinol, and 4-amino-pyrazolo(3,4-*d*) pyrimidine. *J Biol Chem* 254:3959, 1979

532. SCHWARTZ PM, HANDSCHUMACHER RE: Selective antagonism of 5-fluorouracil cytotoxicity by 4-hydroxypyrazolopyrimidine (allopurinol) *in vitro. Cancer Res* 39:3095, 1979

533. SCHWARTZ PM, DUNIGAN JM, MARSH JC, HANDSCHUMACHER RE: Allopurinol modification of the toxicity and antitumor activity of 5-fluorouracil. *Cancer Res* 40:1885, 1980

534. BOSTON COLLABORATIVE DRUG SURVEILLANCE PROGRAM: Allopurinol in relation to bone marrow depression. *JAMA* 227:1036, 1974

535. WITTEN J, FREDERICKSON PL, MONRIDSEN HT: The pharmacokinetics of cyclophosphamide in man after treatment with allopurinol. *Acta Pharmacol Toxicol* 46:392, 1980

536. FRIEDMAN HN, GRASELA T: Adenine arabinoside and allopurinol—possible adverse drug interaction. *N Engl J Med* 304:423, 1981

537. MANFREDI RL, VESELL ES: Inhibition of theophylline metabolism by long-term allopurinol administration. *Clin Pharmacol Ther* 29:224, 1981

538. GRYGIEL JJ, WING LMH, FARKAS J, BIRKETT DJ: Effects of allopurinol on theophylline metabolism and clearance. *Clin Pharmacol Ther* 26:660, 1979

539. MENDELL JR, WIECHERS DO: Lack of benefit of allopurinol in Duchenne dystrophy. *Muscle Nerve* 2:53, 1979

51

CLINICAL SYNDROMES ASSOCIATED WITH HYPOXANTHINE-GUANINE PHOSPHORIBOSYLTRANSFERASE DEFICIENCY

WILLIAM N. KELLEY

JAMES B. WYNGAARDEN

1. The Lesch-Nyhan syndrome *is an inherited disorder associated with a virtually complete deficiency of an enzyme of purine metabolism, hypoxanthine-guanine phosphoribosyltransferase (HPRT). The disease is characterized by the excessive production of uric acid and certain characteristic neurologic features, including self-mutilation, choreoathetosis, spasticity, and mental retardation.*

    A partial deficiency of HPRT is also associated with an excessive production of uric acid, but these patients go on to develop a severe form of gout, often with uric acid nephrolithiasis, rather than the neurologic and behavioral abnormalities associated with the Lesch-Nyhan syndrome.

2. *The abnormalities of purine metabolism are present at birth in patients with both clinical syndromes and may lead to hyperuricemia, uric acid crystalluria, and stone formation early in life. Other direct complications of the purine overproduction and hyperuricemia, such as gouty arthritis, tophaceous deposits, and monosodium urate deposits within the kidney, may not develop for many years.*

3. *At birth the patients with the Lesch-Nyhan syndrome generally have no apparent central nervous system dysfunction. Developmental retardation usually begins at about 3 to 4 months of age, and by the age of 2 years other neurologic manifestations of the syndrome are*

usually present. No characteristic pathologic changes have been noted in the central nervous system at the time of autopsy.

4. *Deficiency of HPRT is generalized to all tissues in patients with these two syndromes. Studies of the mutant HPRT from these patients and their cells indicate that the mutation is on the structural gene and that there is considerable genetic heterogeneity among patients deficient in HPRT.*

5. *The deficiency of HPRT is associated with an increased intracellular concentration of 5-phosphoribosyl-1-pyrophosphate (PP-ribose-P). This is probably at least partly responsible for both the increased rate of purine biosynthesis de novo, and for the increased amounts of the enzyme adenine phosphoribosyltransferase found in erythrocytes from these patients.*

6. *The mechanism by which the deficiency of HPRT produces the central nervous system disorder characteristic of this disease remains unknown.*

7. *HPRT is coded by deoxyribonucleic acid (DNA) in the X chromosome in humans. Hemizygous males are affected with the disease, which is transmitted through heterozygous females. Heterozygotes may exhibit biochemical evidence of excessive purine synthesis and hyperuricemia, although generally they remain asymptomatic. Detection of the heterozygous state is most reliable in cultured fibroblasts; HPRT activity is usu-*

ally normal in erythrocytes obtained from heterozygotes for the Lesch-Nyhan syndrome although heterozygotes for the partial enzyme defect usually exhibit reduced activity in erythrocytes.

8. Patients lacking HPRT activity exhibit several distinctive pharmacogenetic features. They are resistant to the effects of allopurinol and certain other purine analogues on purine synthesis de novo, but they are slightly more sensitive to the inhibitory effects of allopurinol on xanthine oxidase.

9. Allopurinol should be used to prevent or reverse the consequences of the excessive uric acid synthesis. No therapy has been successful so far in treating the devastating central nervous system dysfunction characteristic of the Lesch-Nyhan syndrome.

A deficiency of the enzyme hypoxanthine-guanine phosphoribosyltransferase (HPRT) (Fig. 51-1) is associated with two clinical syndromes in humans [1, 2]. A *virtually complete deficiency* of the enzyme occurs in patients with the *Lesch-Nyhan syndrome,* which is manifested clinically by hyperuricemia, excessive production of uric acid, and certain characteristic neurologic features including self-mutilation, choreoathetosis, spasticity, and mental retardation [3]. Death usually occurs in the second or third decade from infection or renal failure. In contrast, patients with *a partial deficiency* of HPRT have a *severe form of gout* with hyperuricemia and excessive production of uric acid. Approximately 20 percent of the patients in this latter group have neurologic manifestations, including mental retardation, mild spastic quadriplegia, dysarthria, cerebellar ataxia, and seizures, but they do not develop self-mutilation. Patients with partial HPRT deficiency appear to have a normal life expectancy. HPRT is X-linked and thus both clinical syndromes occur only in males.

CLINICAL FEATURES

Central Nervous System Function

Patients with the Lesch-Nyhan syndrome generally appear normal at birth. Although hypotonia, recurrent vomiting, and difficulty with secretions occur in some patients during the first

3 months of life [3], the earliest consistent abnormality is a delay in motor development that appears by 3 to 4 months of age. Between 8 months and 1 year, extrapyramidal signs develop. These signs are characterized by fine athetoid movements of the hands and feet and by dystonia and chorea. The athetosis, which is similar to that associated with asphyxia, birth injury, and hyperbilirubinemia, accounts at least in part for the dysarthria that appears later in life [5]. At about 1 year, signs of pyramidal tract involvement, such as hyperreflexia, sustained ankle clonus, extensor plantar responses, and scissoring of the legs also develop. These findings preclude ambulation in the older patient.

The most striking neurologic feature of the Lesch-Nyhan syndrome is compulsive self-destructive behavior (Fig. 51-2). Between 2 and 16 years of age, affected children begin to bite their fingers, lips, and buccal mucosa. This compulsion for self-mutilation becomes so extreme that it may be necessary to keep the elbows in extension with splints, or to wrap the hands with gauze or restrain them in some other manner. In several patients mutilation of lips could only be controlled by extraction of teeth.

The compulsive urge to inflict painful wounds appears to grip the patient irresistibly. Often he will be content until one begins to remove an arm splint. At this point a communicative patient will plead that the restraints be left alone. If one continues in freeing the arm, the patient will become extremely agitated and upset. Finally, when completely unrestrained, he will begin to put the fingers into his mouth. An older patient will plead for help, and if one then takes hold of the arm that has previously been freed, the patient will show obvious relief. If help is not forthcoming, a painful and often severe injury may be inflicted. The apparent urge to bite fingers is often not symmetrical. In many patients it is possible to leave one arm unrestrained without concern, even though freeing the other would result in an immediate attempt at self-mutilation.

Retarded children with a variety of other disorders will also often exhibit finger biting as well as other types of self-destructive behavior, but mutilation leading to a loss of tissue seems to be unique to the Lesch-Nyhan syndrome. Severe self-biting also occurs in a number of neurologic disorders characterized by loss of pain sensation [6], but study of patients with the Lesch-Nyhan syndrome has failed to reveal any sensory abnormalities.

These patients also attempt to injure themselves in other ways, by hitting their heads against inanimate objects or by placing their extremities in dangerous places, such as in between the spokes of a wheelchair. If the hands are unrestrained, their mutilation becomes the patient's main concern, and effort to inflict injury in some other manner seems to be sublimated.

Patients with this syndrome also exhibit unusual aggressiveness toward others. They will strike at those around them, including children, nurses, physicians, relatives, and friends. A typical maneuver is a swing at the physician in an apparent attempt to knock glasses off. This is done in a peculiarly jovial but extremely aggressive manner and is usually followed by an apology. In addition, some patients will spit and use abusive language, often apologizing while doing so.

The degree to which self-mutilation and aggressiveness occur is quite variable. One patient exhibited no behavioral abnormality other than mental deficiency until the age of 16, when he first developed self-mutilation. Other patients have tended to improve as they became older. Behavior may also

Figure 51-1 The reaction catalyzed by hypoxanthine-guanine phosphoribosyltransferase with hypoxanthine as substrate.

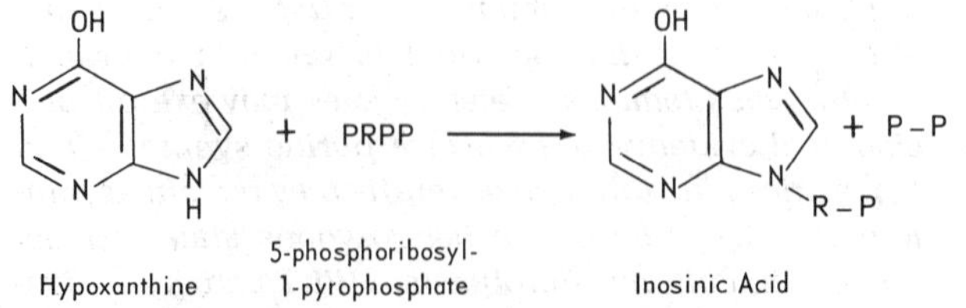

Hypoxanthine + PRPP (5-phosphoribosyl-1-pyrophosphate) → Inosinic Acid + P–P

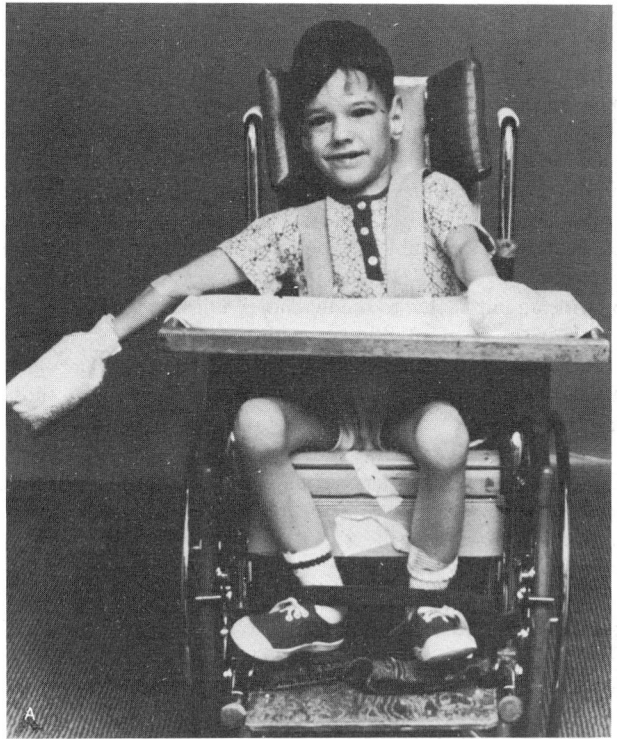

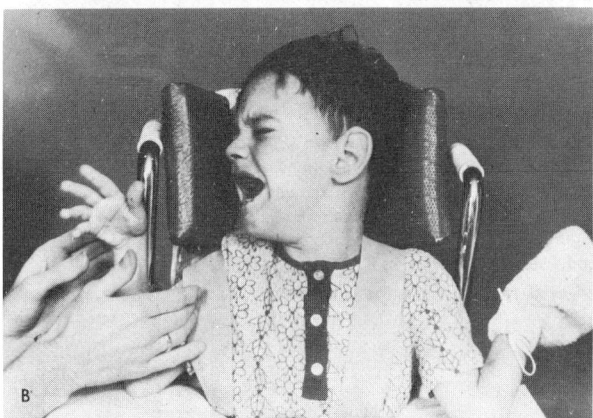

Figure 51-2 *A.* Patient H.D. *B.* Note agitated appearance and the attempt by the patient to bite his fingers after the wrapping is removed from his hands.

improve with prolonged hospitalization. The degree of mutilation and aggressiveness varies from day to day, depending at least in part on surrounding events.

These patients respond to stressful situations by increased agitation, episodes of opisthotonic posturing, and increasing attempts at self-mutilation. Munsat et al. [7] have compared the aggressiveness that they direct toward others upon being disturbed with "sham rage." In the older patient the internal struggle between the desire to inflict injury and the attempt to control this urge can be quite overt.

Most patients with the Lesch-Nyhan syndrome appear to be mentally deficient. IQ testing by routine methods usually gives values ranging from 39 to 65. Their poor performance on formal testing is in part related to dysarthria and choreoathetosis, which make communication difficult. One patient was found to have normal intelligence when testing was designed to minimize these factors [8].

Approximately 50 percent of patients reported in the literature have had seizures. In several instances these have been

attributed to some apparently unrelated event such as hypocalcemia [9] or hypoglycemia [10]. The seizures in some patients have been interpreted as decerebrate cerebellar fits [11].

Routine studies of cerebrospinal fluid are uniformly normal. Electromyograms and nerve conduction velocities are also normal [12]. Electroencephalograms may be normal or may show diffuse slowing.

Most patients with partial HPRT deficiency have a normal neurological examination. In one large series [4], six of eighteen patients had some evidence of neurologic dysfunction. Three patients had a spinocerebellar disorder and one had a history of seizures; three of these four patients were mentally retarded. The remaining two patients of the six appeared to have acquired neurologic disorders unrelated to partial HPRT deficiency. Three sibs with partial HPRT deficiency and no neurologic involvement are shown in Fig. 51-3.

Hyperuricemia and Overproduction of Uric Acid

All patients with the Lesch-Nyhan syndrome exhibit excessive production of uric acid. Although the daily excretion of uric acid may not be in excess of that seen in normal adults, the values are extremely high when one considers the small size of these patients. The excretion of uric acid ranges from 25 to 143 mg per kilogram of body weight per day [13, 14] compared with an upper limit in normal children of 18 mg per kilogram of body weight per day [13].

Figure 51-3 Three brothers in one family with "partial" hypoxanthine-guanine phosphoribosyltransferase deficiency.

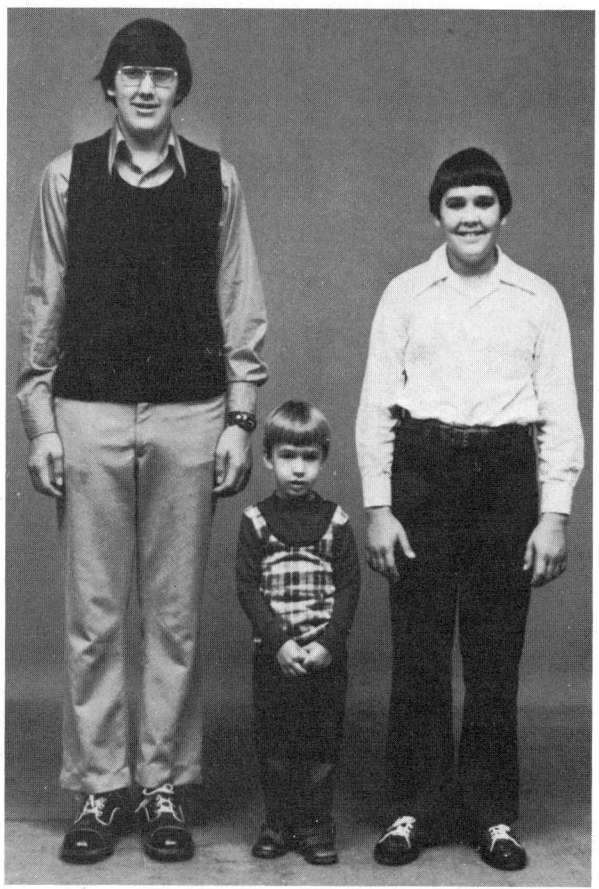

All patients with a partial deficiency of HPRT also produce excessive quantities of uric acid. The excretion of uric acid reflects this overproduction in most instances (Fig. 51-4A) especially when corrected for body weight (Fig. 51-4B). In some patients the level of uric acid excretion, even when adjusted for body weight, approaches that observed in patients with the Lesch-Nyhan syndrome (Fig. 51-4B).

The excretion of uric acid can also be expressed in relation to creatinine excretion, another index of body mass. As indicated in Fig. 51-5, the ratio of uric acid to creatinine concentration in urine samples obtained from patients with the Lesch-Nyhan syndrome and partial HPRT deficiency is uniformly higher than in age-matched controls. The consistency of this elevated ratio, the ease of collecting random urine samples, and the simplicity of the chemical determinations make the uric acid/creatinine ratio in urine an excellent, although non-specific, screening test for these disorders [15]. Although false negative results are unusual, several other disorders also associated with excessive uric acid production, such as type I glycogen storage disease and certain lymphoproliferative disorders, will cause an occasional false positive test result.

The increased quantity of uric acid excreted in the urine leads to uric acid crystalluria in patients with each syndrome at some time. The finding of orange crystals on a diaper during the first few weeks of life has occasionally been the first sign observed by the mother [16]. Unfortunately, this is rarely brought to the attention of the physician, and even when recognized these crystals are easily mistaken for some other urinary constituent such as cystine. Many patients progress to symptomatic uric acid nephrolithiasis, and this may lead to obstructive uropathy with severe and unrelenting azotemia. Such a course has been a common cause of death during the first decade of life in untreated patients with the Lesch-Nyhan

syndrome. At least 75 percent of patients with partial HPRT deficiency have a history of uric acid stones, and in 50 percent of the patients uric acid nephrolithiasis precedes the development of gout.

The excessive production of uric acid also leads to hyperuricemia in both clinical syndromes. The serum urate concentration usually ranges from 7 mg/dl to as high as 18 mg/dl in the absence of renal insufficiency, but in an occasional patient, particularly before puberty, a random value will fall within the normal range [12, 17, 18]. The serum urate concentration may provide an initial clue to the diagnosis, but because of its variability it is not an infallible screening test.

It is unusual for patients with the Lesch-Nyhan syndrome to develop gouty arthritis. In contrast, gout is common in those with partial HPRT deficiency occurring in all patients over the age of 13 years in one large series [4]. Onset as late as 65 years has been noted by others. Tophi will appear ultimately in patients with both syndromes if the hyperuricemia is not treated effectively.

Hematologic Abnormalities

At least 10 of the patients initially reported with the Lesch-Nyhan syndrome, or partial HPRT deficiency, were anemic prior to the occurrence of renal insufficiency [4, 14, 18–24]. Catel and Schmidt described the anemia in their patient as megaloblastic in character [21]. A number of investigators

Figure 51-4 Daily uric acid excretions in patients producing excessive quantities of uric acid. Comparison of patients with normal, partially deficient, and virtually completely deficient hypoxanthine-guanine phosphoribosyltransferase (HPRT) activity. A. Excretion values in milligrams per day (upper limit of normal is 590 mg/day). B. Excretion values in milligrams per kilogram of body weight per day (upper limit of normal is 7 mg per kilogram of body weight per day). (From Kelley et al. [4]).

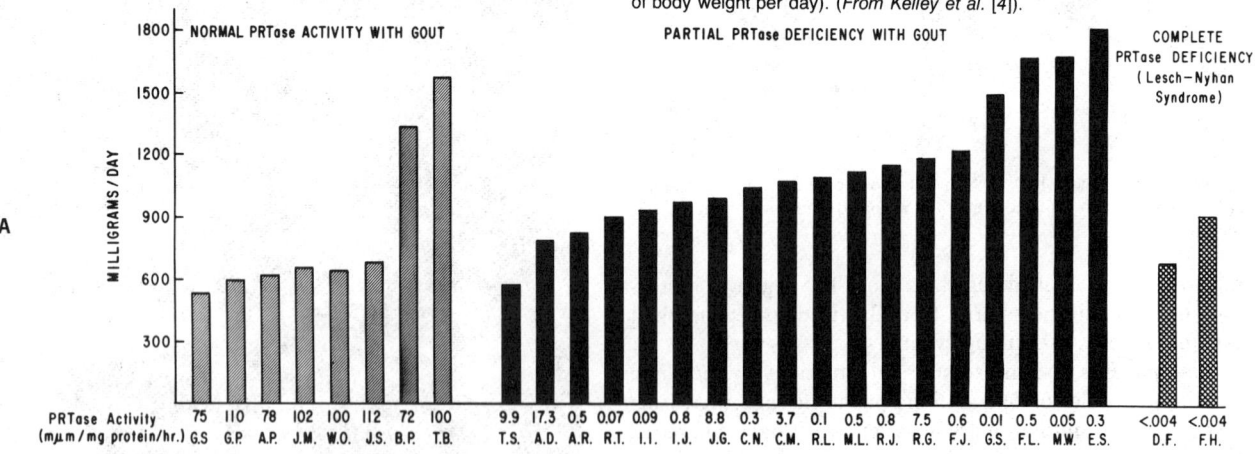

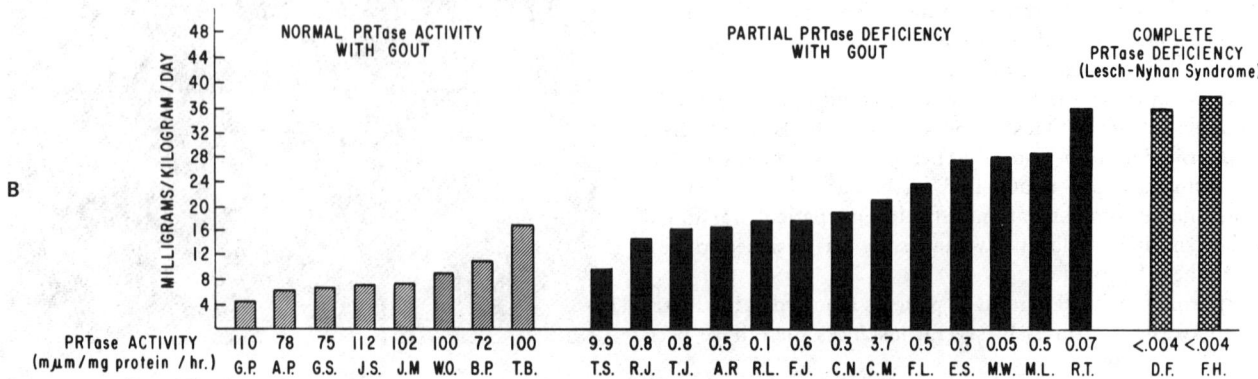

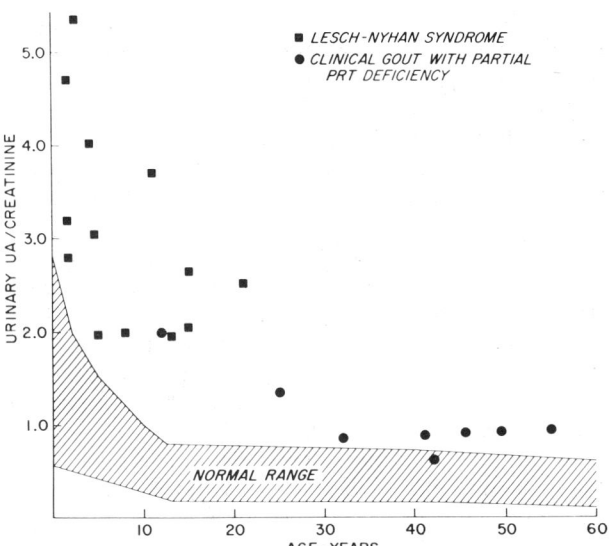

Figure 51-5 Ratio of uric acid to creatinine concentration in urine samples obtained from patients with the Lesch-Nyhan syndrome (complete HPRT deficiency) and those with gout and a partial deficiency of HPRT. The normal range represents the mean ± 2 SD in a total of 284 control subjects of various ages. (*From Kaufman et al.* [15].)

have confirmed the presence of macrocytic erythrocytes in the peripheral blood and megaloblastic changes in the bone marrow [4, 22–24]. These changes may be present even in the absence of overt anemia. Possible mechanisms for these morphologic changes and approaches to therapy will be considered later.

Infections

The development of bacterial infections in patients with the Lesch-Nyhan syndrome may be more common than previously recognized. The occurrence of furuncles and periungual infections has usually been attributed to the unusual frequency of contaminated self-inflicted wounds. Nonetheless, such infections may occur in areas where antecedent trauma does not seem to have occurred. Death in patients with the Lesch-Nyhan syndrome is often due to pneumonia or urinary tract infections with sepsis; infections of this type have usually been attributed to aspiration or underlying uric acid nephropathy, respectively. One study has suggested that patients with the Lesch-Nyhan syndrome may have some degree of B lymphocyte immunologic dysfunction, as reflected in B-cell lymphocytopenia, reduced levels of IgG in the serum, and low levels of isohemagglutinins [25]. In addition, there appears to be reduced blastogenesis in the presence of pokeweed mitogen. T-cell function seems to be normal. More recent studies, however, have not confirmed these observations in patients with the Lesch-Nyhan syndrome. There is no evidence of a consistent abnormality of immune dysfunction in patients with partial HPRT deficiency.

Associated Congenital Defects

Some of the congenital defects frequently observed in children with the Lesch-Nyhan syndrome, such as clubfeet and bilaterally dislocated hips, may be the result of the severe spasticity. Other congenital abnormalities have also been seen which are

not necessarily related to the basic disease process. These include Hirschsprung's disease [18], imperforate anus [26], and bilateral cryptorchism [10, 27].

Roentgenographic Findings

There are no specific x-ray findings in either syndrome. Most patients with the Lesch-Nyhan syndrome have bilaterally dislocated hips. Tophaceous deposits in older patients with partial HPRT deficiency may be apparent as lytic bone lesions on x-ray. An intravenous pyelogram may suggest radiolucent stones or, if renal disease is present, small kidneys with poor function. There is usually some delay in bone age in those with the complete enzyme deficiency, but it is not as marked as the retardation in height and weight [28]. Pneumoencephalography and computerized tomography (CT) scans usually show ventricular dilatation consistent with bilateral cortical atrophy in those with central nervous system disease [3, 7, 13, 14, 20, 29].

Pathology

There are no reports to date of pathological abnormalities or autopsies in patients with partial HPRT deficiency. At least nine patients dying with the Lesch-Nyhan syndrome have been autopsied [16, 18, 27, 29–33]. In addition to the evidence of growth retardation and self-mutilation, a consistent finding has been bilaterally shrunken kidneys with striking deposits of monosodium urate and uric acid.

There are no distinctive pathologic changes in the central nervous system. The findings described by Sass et al. [29], which include demyelinative and vascular lesions of the cerebral and cerebellar white matter, degeneration of the granules in Purkinje cells, multiple small chronic infarcts, and the presence of De Galantha staining material, can probably be attributed to the severe uremia preceding death. Partington and Hennen [18] noted occasional perivascular birefringent crystals that were not uric acid in the alcohol-fixed brain of one patient. One of the two original patients reported by Lesch and Nyhan was autopsied at the National Institutes of Health in 1966. Gross examination disclosed a brownish pigmentation over the cerebral cortex, but this could not be detected histologically in either formalin- or alcohol-fixed tissue [30]. The patient originally described by Riley [19] was found at autopsy to have thinning of the cerebellar cortex and loss of cells in the granular layer [27]. Autopsies on at least four additional cases, by routine histologic methods, have failed to reveal any significant changes in the central nervous system [16, 31–33]. Detailed studies by more powerful methods, including electron microscopy, are needed.

BIOCHEMICAL FEATURES

Regulation of Purine Metabolism

Purine synthesis, interconversion, and degradation and the regulation of these processes have been considered in detail in the previous chapter and will only be summarized here.

The purine nucleotides, guanylic acid (GMP) and adenylic

acid (AMP), can be synthesized by several mechanisms (Fig. 51-6). The free purine bases can be converted directly to their respective ribonucleotides by the appropriate purine phosphoribosyltransferase in the presence of PP-ribose-P [34, 35]. In addition, GMP and AMP can be synthesized *de novo* from smaller precursors including PP-ribose-P, glutamine, glycine, aspartate, formate, and bicarbonate through a common intermediate, inosinic acid (IMP) [36–38].

Data obtained in bacterial [39], avian [40, 41], and mammalian [42–45] systems indicate that AMP and GMP inhibit amidophosphoribosyltransferase, the initial and rate-limiting step of purine biosynthesis *de novo*, by interacting at separate sites on the enzyme termed the 6-amino and 6-hydroxy sites, respectively. Inhibition of the human enzyme by purine nucleotides is competitive with respect to PP-ribose-P, and the kinetics of the reaction shift from a hyperbolic to a sigmoidal function when PP-ribose-P is the variable substrate. AMP and GMP are also inhibitors of formylglycinamide ribonucleotide (FGAR) amidotransferase, although the importance of this feedback site to the control of the rate of purine synthesis *de novo* is not established [46].

A regulatory role of PP-ribose-P was suggested by several observations in human cell culture as well as in humans in vivo [47–51]. Under normal conditions, depletion of PP-ribose-P in vitro and in vivo decreases the rate of purine biosynthesis *de novo* [47–50]. Elevation of PP-ribose-P by several different mechanisms is associated with an increased rate of purine bio-

synthesis *de novo* [48, 52, 53]. In addition, when PP-ribose-P concentrations are initially elevated and then reduced to levels that are still supranormal, there is no inhibitory effect on purine biosynthesis *de novo* [47]. Finally, the normal intracellular concentration of PP-ribose-P is considerably less than the Michaelis constant established for amidophosphoribosyltransferase in lower organisms [39, 54–56] or in mammalian cells [43].

The mechanism by which PP-ribose-P and purine ribonucleotides interact to regulate the activity of amidophosphoribosyltransferase was provided by direct study of the enzyme from a human source. Two forms of human amidophosphoribosyltransferase are apparent following gel filtration; the small form has a molecular weight of about 133,000 and the large form a molecular weight of about 270,000 [45]. The larger species appears to be catalytically inactive, whereas the smaller species appears to be catalytically active. Purine ribonucleotides shift the active smaller species to the inactive larger molecular species; PP-ribose-P converts the large inactive species back to the small active species. The importance and nature of this regulatory mechanism is discussed further in Chap. 50.

The next branch point in the pathway leading to the synthesis *de novo* of AMP and GMP occurs with the synthesis of

Figure 51-6 Outline of purine metabolism. (*1*) Amidophoshoribosyltransferase; (*2*) hypoxanthine-guanine phosphoribosyltransferase; (*3*) PP-ribose-P synthetase; (*4*) adenine phosphoribosyltransferase; (*5*) adenosine deaminase; (*6*) purine nucleoside phosphorylase; (*7*) 5'-nucleotidase; (*8*) xanthine oxidase.

INBORN ERRORS OF PURINE METABOLISM IN MAN

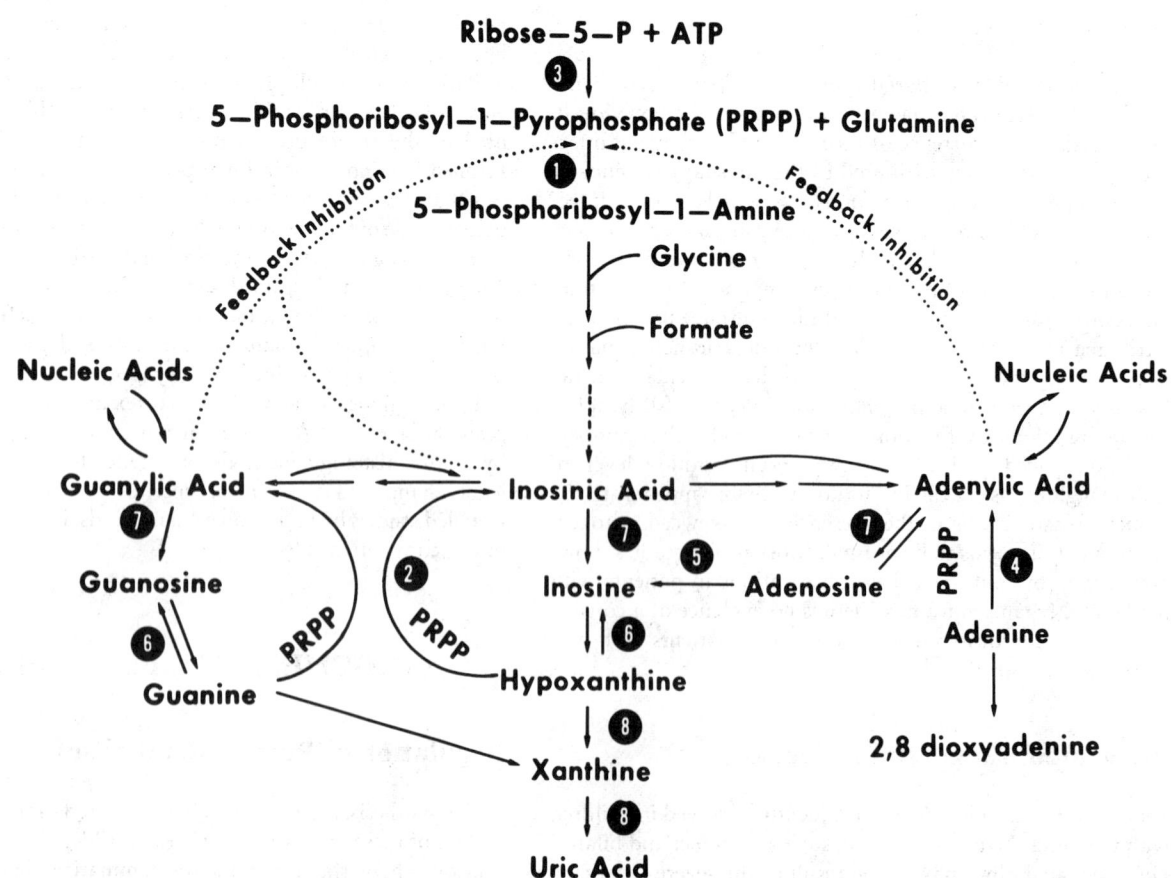

IMP. In bacterial systems each nucleotide appears to regulate its own formation *de novo* by inhibiting the appropriate nucleotide interconversion: GMP inhibits inosinic dehydrogenase that catalyzes the formation of xanthylic acid (XMP) from IMP [58, 59], and AMP inhibits the formation of adenylosuccinic acid (AMP-S) from IMP that is catalyzed by adenylosuccinate synthetase [60]. An analysis of the regulation of adenylosuccinate synthetase [61] and IMP dehydrogenase [62] from a human source suggests, however, that the utilization of IMP by each of the alternative pathways may be governed by the intracellular concentration of GTP, a substrate of AMP-S synthetase with a K_m ranging from 31 to 72 μmol [61]. On the other hand, guanosine triphosphate (GTP) is an inhibitor of IMP dehydrogenase [62]. As IMP is formed, it is utilized for the synthesis of XMP, GMP, guanosine diphosphate (GDP), and GTP. As GTP reaches a critical concentration in the cell, probably in the micromolar range, it will increase the activity of AMP-S synthetase, allowing IMP to be effectively utilized in the synthesis of AMP. As GTP reaches a higher level, not only can it promote the flux of IMP in the direction of AMP, but it can then function as a direct inhibitor of the conversion of IMP to XMP. Finally, AMP and GMP also inhibit their respective purine phosphoribosyltransferases, adenine phosphoribosyltransferase (APRT) and HPRT, and thereby regulate their synthesis from the free purine bases [63, 64].

Regulation of purine biosynthesis and purine interconversions by end-product repression of enzyme synthesis is important in bacterial systems [65, 66], but in humans this mechanism has not been shown conclusively to play a significant role in the regulation of purine synthesis or metabolism.

Enzyme Defect

In 1967 Seegmiller, Rosenbloom, and Kelley [1] described a virtually complete deficiency of an enzyme of purine metabolism, hypoxanthine-guanine phosphoribosyltransferase, in erythrocyte lysates from three patients and in cultured skin fibroblasts from a fourth patient with this disorder. In 1968 Kelley et al. [4] described a partial deficiency of the same enzyme in patients with a severe form of gout. The enzyme defect was subsequently confirmed in other tissues including liver, brain, and leukocytes as well as in cultured skin fibroblasts and erythrocytes from many similarly affected patients with both clinical syndromes [4, 67, 68] (Tables 51-1, 51-2, and 51-3).

Properties of the Normal Enzyme

Hypoxanthine-guanine phosphoribosyltransferase (HPRT) (EC 2.4.2.8) catalyzes the transfer of the phosphoribosyl moiety of 5-phosphoribosyl-1-pyrophosphate (PP-ribose-P) to the 9 position of hypoxanthine and guanine to form IMP or GMP, respectively (Fig. 51-1). The human enzyme has been studied extensively [64]. The enzyme binds 6-oxo or 6-thio purines, but not 6-amino compounds. An amino group in the 2 position of the purine ring enhances binding, whereas a hydroxyl group at the 2 position decreases binding. The imidazole ring also is important, but itself is not sufficient for binding. Although certain 1-methyl derivatives are bound to the enzyme, purines that are methylated at other nitrogens in the purine ring are not bound. Therefore, in addition to hypoxanthine and guanine,

Table 51-1 Specific activity of hypoxanthine-guanine phosphoribosyltransferase (HPRT) in erythrocyte hemolysates in hyperuricemic subjects

Subject*	HPRT activity, mμmol/h per milligram protein		
	Hypoxanthine	Guanine	Adenine
Normal (32), mean ± SD	103 ± 18	103 ± 21	31.1 ± 6.0
Hyperuricemia, mean ± SD	99 ± 13	106 ± 10	31.2 ± 5.3
Normal uric acid production (6)			
Excessive uric acid production, mean ± SD	103 ± 18	104 ± 22	30.4 ± 5.3
Normal enzyme (10)			
Complete deficiency (9) (Lesch-Nyhan syndrome)			
J.W.	<0.01	<0.004	58
J.S.	<0.01	<0.004	39
D.F.	<0.01	<0.004	53
B.M.	<0.01	<0.004	49
M.B.	<0.01	<0.004	56
S.M.	<0.01	<0.004	51
F.H.	<0.01	<0.004	94
M.W.	<0.01	<0.004	65
T.S.	<0.01	<0.004	71
Partial deficiency (18)			
J. Family			
F.J.	1.3	0.6	46
R.J.	1.5	0.8	43
T.J.	1.8	0.8	56
L. Family			
F.L.	11.8	0.5	74
M.L.	8.7	0.5	64
S₁. Family			
T.S.	9.9	9.5	39
D. Family			
A.D.	12.2	17.3	33
G. Family			
J.G.	9.4	8.8	32
R.G.	9.2	7.5	38
S₂. Family			
G.S.	0.03	0.009	58
I. Family			
T.I.	0.06	0.09	32
R. Family			
A.R.	0.9	0.5	48
M. Family			
C.M.	2.7	3.7	26
T. Family			
R.T.	0.06	0.07	36
M.W.	0.06	0.05	29
R.L.	0.09	0.10	44
N. Family			
C.N.	0.3	0.3	35
E.S.	0.4	0.3	39

* Number of subjects in parentheses.
SOURCE: Kelley et al. [4]. Reproduced by permission of *Annals of Internal Medicine*.

xanthine, allopurinol, 6-mercaptopurine, 8-azaguanine, and 6-thioguanine also serve as substrates for the human enzyme. The Michaelis constants for hypoxanthine and guanine with the human HPRT from erythrocytes are 1.7×10^{-5} M and 5.0×10^{-6} M, respectively [64, 69, 70]. Similar values are

Table 51-2 Specific activity of hypoxanthine-guanine phosphoribosyltransferase (HPRT) and guanase in human liver

Subject	Storage at −20° C, months	HPRT activity, mμmol/h per milligram protein			Guanase activity, nmol/h per milligram protein
		Hypoxanthine	Guanine	Adenine	
Controls					
B.G.	0	41	66	155	1439
B.G.	1		54	118	1497
F.H.	1	18	30	139	2372
H.C.	6.5	25	31	163	917
Mutant					
E.W.	6.5	<1.0	<1.0	264	1546

SOURCE: Kelley [68].

observed for the HPRT obtained from beef liver [71], rat brain [72], and adenocarcinoma 755 cells [73].

As in mammalian cells, HPRT exists as a single enzyme in *Saccharomyces* [74, 75]. These reactions, however, are catalyzed by two separate enzymes in bacterial cells. In *Salmonella typhimurium* [76, 77] and in *Escherichia coli* [78], one enzyme uses guanine and xanthine as substrate and has relatively low but significant activity with hypoxanthine as substrate, whereas a separate enzyme has a high affinity for hypoxanthine with relatively low activity with guanine and xanthine as substrate. In contrast, the protozoan, *Leishmania donovani*, has one enzyme which catalyzes the phosphoribosyl transfer to hypoxanthine and guanine and a second which catalyzes this reaction for xanthine [79].

The only compound known to serve as a donor of the phosphoribosyl moiety for HPRT from any source is PP-ribose-P. The K_m value for PP-ribose-P is approximately 2.5×10^{-4} M [70], 5.5×10^{-5} M [71], and 2×10^{-4} M [72] with the enzyme from human erythrocytes, beef liver, and rat brain, respectively. The K_m value for PP-ribose-P in adenocarcinoma 755 cells varies from 3.6×10^{-5} to 1.2×10^{-4} M, depending on the purine base that is present [73]. The enzyme has an absolute requirement for magnesium, and dimagnesium PP-ribose-P appears to be the preferred substrate [64]. The enzyme is most active at magnesium concentrations ranging from 5 to 20 mM. At higher concentrations marked inhibition of the enzyme occurs unless very high concentrations of PP-ribose-P are also present.

In most published studies, plots of activity versus substrate concentration show a hyperbolic curve with increasing concentrations of PP-ribose-P except at very low ratios of magnesium to PP-ribose-P [64]. At low magnesium concentrations, a sigmoidal curve is observed with an increasing concentration of PP-ribose-P [64]. In addition, Craft et al. [80] have reported that HPRT from human erythrocytes exhibits sigmoidal kinetics at a pH of 7.5 or less, whereas hyperbolic kinetics are observed at a more alkaline pH. These investigators reported that the enzyme exhibited sigmoidal kinetics with increasing PP-ribose-P concentrations irrespective of the concentration of magnesium.

The predominant enzyme mechanism appears to be dependent on the concentration of magnesium relative to that of PP-ribose-P [64, 81]. Under essentially all conditions, PP-ribose-P binds to the enzyme first, and the purine nucleotide product is released last [64, 69]; the order in which the purine base is bound and pyrophosphate is released appears to be related to the concentration of magnesium. At magnesium concentrations that are only moderately in excess of the PP-

ribose-P concentration, the enzyme (E) exhibits an ordered mechanism in which the binding of PP-ribose-P is followed by the binding of purine base with the formation of a ternary complex, E:PP-ribose-P:purine. Pyrophosphate release is then followed by the release of the nucleotide product. At magnesium concentrations that are in large excess of the PP-ribose-P concentration, the enzyme exhibits a ping-pong mechanism in which the binding of PP-ribose-P is followed by the release of pyrophosphate and the formation of an enzyme ribosylphosphate intermediate. The purine base then adds to the enzyme, and the nucleotide product is released. The enzyme from a number of sources has been reported to be inhibited by the products of the reaction, GMP and IMP, as well as other purine ribonucleotides [69, 72]. In general, the inhibition is competitive with respect to magnesium PP-ribose-P. HPRT can also be inhibited or inactivated by GMP dialdehyde [82] and by periodate oxidation [83]. Unfortunately, it is still not possible to utilize inhibitors such as these to develop an animal model of HPRT deficiency.

In most studies, HPRT has been found to exist free in the cytoplasm. Gutensohn and Guroff [72] have noted a small but significant portion of the enzyme in synaptosomes from rat brain. Studies of the tissue distribution of the enzyme from human [67], rhesus monkey [84], rat [72, 85], and mouse [85] tissue all indicate that enzyme activity is highest in the brain. In humans the highest activity within the brain appears to be in the basal ganglia [67], whereas in the rat [72, 86] distribution of the enzyme within the central nervous system is more homogeneous. Activity in gray matter is twice as high as in white matter [86]. Enzyme activity is also characteristically noted to be relatively high in leukocytes, fibroblasts, and gonadal tissue.

In general terms, HPRT activity is highest in rapidly dividing tissues. For example, in rat brain there is a threefold increase in HPRT activity during the first 15 to 20 days of life [72, 87]. In rabbit embryos during the first 3 days of development, there is also a rapid increase in HPRT activity [88]. In the postimplantation period of embryonic development, the increase in activity parallels the increase in the weight of the embryo [81]. The HPRT activity is significantly increased in leukocytes from patients with acute myelocytic leukemia in relapse as compared with leukocytes from normal subjects [89]. While HPRT activity increases for the first 48 h after phytohemagglutinin-induced transformation of lymphocytes, the increase in activity parallels the increase in total protein [90]. Finally, human lymphoblasts in long-term culture have the highest activity observed in any human cell.

There has been considerable controversy related to the subunit structure of the human HPRT [91–95]. Most agree that the subunit molecular weight of the protein is in the range of 24,000 to 26,000. The major question is whether the native enzyme exists normally as a dimer, trimer, or tetramer of this subunit. Several authors have concluded from a comparison of the apparent molecular weights of the subunit and native protein that the enzyme exists as a trimer in its native form [92, 94, 96], and others have suggested that the enzyme is normally present as a dimer [91] or a tetramer [95]. Several more direct lines of evidence have provided strong evidence now that the enzyme normally exists as a tetramer (or, more accurately, as a dimer of dimers). The first evidence was provided by covalent crosslinkage of the purified enzyme which revealed four protein bands indicating the presence of a tetramer which had a pattern most suggestive of a dimer of dimers [95]. In more recent studies, careful analysis of the active HPRT heteropolymer in human-mouse hybrids revealed that the protein was present both as a dimer and as a tetramer; the equilibrium was influenced by the ionic strength of the enzyme solvent [97]. The physical properties of the enzyme from Chinese hamster cells [98], mouse liver [96], rat brain [99], and rat liver [100] are similar in many ways to the human enzyme. Immunologic studies suggest some variability among mammalian species [101]. Antibody to normal human HPRT does not inhibit Chinese hamster or mouse HPRT activity [101, 102]. Antibody to rat HPRT does not inhibit rabbit or human HPRT [72].

A number of studies have demonstrated the presence of electrophoretic variants of normal human HPRT. Arnold and Kelley [91, 103], Davies and Dean [104], Muller and Stemberger [105], and Bakay and Nyhan [106] have reported multiple electrophoretic forms of the human erythrocyte enzyme demonstrated by isoelectric focusing. In addition, Rubin et al. [107] recovered two peaks of HPRT activity after diethylaminoethyl (DEAE)-cellulose chromatography of the human enzyme, and Bakay and Nyhan [106, 108] observed four different areas of apparent HPRT activity after electrophoresis of crude hemolysate or purified enzyme on polyacrylamide gels. Gutensohn and Guroff [72] have also reported three peaks of HPRT activity during DEAE-cellulose chromatography of a partially purified preparation of HPRT from rat brain. In contrast to erythrocytes and brain, HPRT exhibits only a single electrophoretic species in cultured lymphoblasts [109] and fibroblasts [110].

Several findings suggest that the electrophoretic heterogeneity is due to a nongenetic alteration of the protein [91, 103]. A single genetic event leads to a virtually complete deficiency of the enzyme in all tissues in humans. It, therefore, seems unlikely that there are multiple genes coding for the enzyme. The enzyme is known to be coded by DNA in the X chromosome. Since all the studies by Arnold and Kelley demonstrating electrophoretic heterogeneity by isoelectric focusing were done with erythrocytes from male subjects, multiple alleles cannot account for the observed electrophoretic heterogeneity [91]. In addition, if the electrophoretic variation were on a genetic basis, the relative amounts of each variant should be comparable among different subjects and the electrophoretic mobility characteristic of each variant should be stable, which is not the case. More recently, Nesbitt, et al. [111] have provided evidence to suggest that in the mouse chromosome 7 controls the electrophoretic mobility of HPRT in erythrocytes but not in other tissues.

The nature of the posttranscriptional alteration in the protein remains unclear. The native impure preparation, as well as each of the highly purified electrophoretic variants, exhibits a similar Stokes radius and molecular weight. In addition, the electrophoretic variants are immunologically identical and do not contain detectable amounts of sialic acid or ribosylphosphate [91, 109]. Possible explanations for the electrophoretic heterogeneity, which are consistent with available data, include differential amidation or phosphorylation of the molecule, but there is no direct evidence to support either of these possibilities. Although the mechanism remains unclear, the observation that the substrate specificity, product inhibition, and degree of substrate inhibition are the same for each of the electrophoretic variants suggests that the electrophoretic heterogeneity is not of major functional significance.

Mutant Forms of the Enzyme

Mutations affecting the activity of HPRT have been known for many years in bacteria and in several lines of cultured mammalian cells [112–114]. Indeed, some of the earliest studies [115, 116] of cell hybridization utilized cells lacking HPRT activity. As noted earlier, the first report of a deficiency of this enzyme in humans was published in 1967 by Seegmiller, Rosenbloom, and Kelley [1]. While the initial patients had the Lesch-Nyhan syndrome, shortly thereafter Kelley et al. [2] found that some adult patients with gout also had a deficiency of HPRT. These patients differed from the first subjects in that they did not have the devastating neurologic and behavioral features characteristic of the Lesch-Nyhan syndrome. In addition, they generally had a less striking deficiency of the enzyme in erythrocytes. The deficiency of HPRT is demonstrable in all tissues including cultured fibroblasts, lymphoblasts, and amniotic fluid cells.

Table 51-3 Specific activity of hypoxanthine-guanine phosphoribosyltransferase (HPRT) and guanase in human basal ganglia

| Subject | Storage at −20° C, months | HPRT activity, mμmol/h per milligram protein | | | Guanase activity, nmol/h per milligram protein |
		Hypoxanthine	Guanine	Adenine	
Controls					
B.G.	0	843	1137	43	3786
B.G.	1	685	715	37	5027
F.H.	1	315	413	27	2662
Mutant					
E.W.	6.5	<4	<4	71	6839

SOURCE: Kelley [68].

The initial studies of the activity of the mutant forms of HPRT in man suggested that two major classes existed: those with no detectable activity and those with significantly reduced but easily detectable activity in erythrocytes [4, 68]. Those in the former group were obtained from patients with the classic Lesch-Nyhan syndrome; those in the latter group were obtained from patients with gout. In the last several years, this distinction with respect to enzyme activity in erythrocytes has become somewhat less satisfactory. For example, it is now clear that a very low but measurable level of HPRT activity can be consistently detected in fibroblasts, leukocytes, and erythrocytes from some patients with the classic Lesch-Nyhan syndrome [70, 117–122]. Indeed, the level of activity observed in erythrocytes from several patients with the Lesch-Nyhan syndrome overlaps the activity present in erythrocytes from some patients with gout. Despite the overlap in erythrocytes, it may still be true that the higher the activity in tissues such as brain, the less severe the neurologic disease and the more likely that the patient will have only the gouty diathesis. Unfortunately, it is impossible to predict the level of activity present in other tissues, such as brain or liver, from an assessment of activity in circulating erythrocytes or cultured fibroblasts. To further complicate matters, attempts to compare HPRT activity in extracts and intact cells have frequently shown a poor correlation [123]. If functional activity could be determined reliably in these tissues in vivo, this might help resolve the question of whether factors other than the level of HPRT activity could modify the central nervous system disease. At any rate, it appears now that there is a virtually continuous spectrum of enzyme activity in mutant hemizygous subjects with HPRT deficiency ranging from undetectable to about 50 percent of normal.

The wide variability of HPRT activity between mutant hemizygotes from different families and the similarity of enzyme activity among affected individuals within the same family provided the initial clue for striking genetic heterogeneity at the HPRT locus in man. Although alterations in primary structure have not been defined for any mutant form of HPRT, differences in the physical properties of the unpurified enzyme from various families have provided further evidence for this hypothesis. Aberrations, in addition to reduced activity, include increased enzyme thermolability [2, 124, 125], enhanced thermostability [1], altered electrophoretic mobility [4, 125–128], increased sensitivity to inhibition by products [125], resistance to inhibition by-products [118], altered substrate specificity [2], altered Michaelis constants [70, 124, 129, 130], and altered stability in vivo [119]. Based on this type of information there appear to be at least 10 or 12 different mutant forms of the enzyme. Unfortunately, it may be misleading to propose alterations in primary structure based on study of the protein in an unpurified state since the milieu may have unpredictable effects on the results obtained.

Most patients studied to date with HPRT deficiency have exhibited a reduced level of cross reactive material which closely approximates the reduced enzyme activity [134–137]. In each patient in whom this is the case, the absolute specific activity of the enzyme is normal [136]. When the absolute specific activity is normal, it is assumed that the mutation involving HPRT is such that the enzyme protein intrinsically has normal catalytic activity but that it is synthesized at a reduced rate or degraded at an accelerated rate. Indeed, careful analysis of mutant HPRT in mutagenized mouse cells suggests that this is the case in this experimental condition [138]. To date, only

three patients have been found to have levels of CRM that are normal or greater than normal despite markedly reduced enzyme activity [128, 134–136, 139]. In two patients there is a striking alteration in kinetic constants [70, 139] while the third patient appears to be an example of a V_{max} mutation [136].

Wilson et al. [136] have recently purified erythrocyte HPRT to >94 percent purity from five unrelated patients with HPRT deficiency. Sufficient protein was available in four of the five patients for evaluation of subunit structure and charge under denaturing conditions. HPRT from one patient (L.P.) was more acidic than normal by denaturing isoelectric focusing; this mutant protein has been named $HPRT_{Toronto}$. In a second patient (G.S.), the mutation has resulted in a protein with a more rapid migration than normal during SDS gel electrophoresis. Since the charge and absolute specific activity of this protein are normal, the altered migration in SDS is more likely to be due to a structurally induced altered affinity of the mutant HPRT for SDS than to a reduced subunit molecular weight. This mutant protein has been named $HPRT_{London}$. The mutant protein from a third patient (E.S.) had a more basic isoelectric point than normal under denaturing conditions. This mutant protein termed $HPRT_{Kinston}$ was previously shown to have altered Michaelis constants [70]. A fourth patient (I.V.) had a mutant protein that also differed from normal in that its isoelectric point was more basic as in the alteration noted in $HPRT_{Kinston}$. The mutant protein could be differentiated from $HPRT_{Kinston}$ in that it had a markedly reduced V_{max}. Hence, this protein has been termed $HPRT_{Munich}$. Each of these mutant forms of human HPRT has been confirmed with the enzyme isolated from lymphoblastoid cells cultured from each patient [139a]. Furthermore, the use of lymphoblastoid cells has allowed the elucidation of an additional variant, $HPRT_{Ann Arbor}$. A summary of findings in the five mutants is provided in Table 51-4.

A large number of mutants selected for HPRT deficiency in cell culture have been carefully studied immunologically from mouse [140], Chinese hamster cell lines [141–144], and human lymphoblasts [145]. These studies clearly demonstrate a number of different mutations, at least some of which are on the structural gene for the enzyme.

Associated Biochemical Abnormalities

The activities of several erythrocyte enzymes are altered in patients with a deficiency of HPRT.

Adenine Phosphoribosyltransferase   Adenine phosphoribosyltransferase (APRT), which catalyzes the synthesis of adenylic acid from adenine and PP-ribose-P (Fig. 51-7), is increased in erythrocytes from patients with a "complete" deficiency of HPRT [1, 68] as well as in many patients with a "partial" deficiency [4]. Greene et al. [146] have demonstrated that PP-ribose-P stabilizes purified APRT in vitro. In addition, PP-ribose-P concentrations are increased in erythrocytes from patients lacking HPRT [49, 106]. Based on these observations, Greene et al. [146] suggested that stabilization of APRT in vivo by the increased PP-ribose-P levels may lead to a diminished rate of degradation of the enzyme and thus to an increased activity. Support for this hypothesis came with the findings that both APRT activity [146, 147] and enzyme protein [133] were more stable in circulating erythrocytes from patients with the Lesch-Nyhan syndrome than from normal subjects, and

Table 51-4 Comparison of lymphoblast and erythrocyte hypoxanthine-guanine phosphoribosyltransferase

Subject	Enzyme	Source	Absolute specific activity, milliunits/g CRM	Migration during native polyacrylamide gel electrophoresis (relative to normal)	Apparent subunit molecular weight, $\times 10^{-3}$	Isoelectric points
Normal	Normal	Lymphoblast	44 ± 3	—	26.0	6.00
		Hemolysate	38 ± 5		26.0	6.6, 6.2, 6.0
L.P.	HPRT$_{\text{Toronto}}$	Lymphoblast	28 ± 5	Anodal	26.0	5.75
		Hemolysate	42 ± 8		26.0	6.2, 6.0, 5.8
G.S.	HPRT$_{\text{London}}$	Lymphoblast	74 ± 13	No change	25.0	6.00
		Hemolysate	51 ± 7		25.0	6.6, 6.2, 6.0
I.V.	HPRT$_{\text{Munich}}$	Lymphoblast	1.4 ± 0.4	Cathodal	26.5	6.40
		Hemolysate	1.3 ± 0.1		26.5	6.9, 6.6, 6.2
E.S.	HPRT$_{\text{Kinston}}$	Lymphoblast	0.21	Cathodal	26.0	6.20
		Hemolysate			26.0	6.9, 6.6, 6.2
C. Family	HPRT$_{\text{Ann Arbor}}$	Lymphoblast	41 ± 9	No change	26.0	5.85
		Hemolysate	41 ± 11		26.0	

that there was a direct relationship between the intracellular content of PP-ribose-P and the activity of APRT in erythrocytes [148]. However, APRT activity is normal in cultured cells deficient in HPRT including human fibroblasts [149], mouse neuroblastoma cells [150], and human lymphoblasts [151, 152] in spite of increased concentrations of PP-ribose-P in each of these cell types. In addition, erythrocytes from patients with an elevation of PP-ribose-P synthetase activity have elevated levels of PP-ribose-P but normal APRT activity [153, 154]. Finally, in one family with HPRT deficiency, reduced APRT activity is reported [155]. Thus the mechanism and significance of the altered APRT activity remains to be defined in patients with HPRT deficiency.

Inosine 5′-Monophosphate Dehydrogenase The activity of IMP dehydrogenase, which catalyzes the conversion of IMP to XMP (Fig. 51-7), is elevated in erythrocytes [156] but not in leukocytes [156], fibroblasts [156, 157], or muscle [156] from patients with HPRT deficiency. Pehlke et al. [156] demonstrated that after prolonged dialysis of hemolysates from HPRT-normal (HPRT$^+$) and HPRT-deficient (HPRT$^-$) subjects, IMP dehydrogenase activity was the same in preparations from both sources. Lommen et al. [158] suggest that this increase in activity is due to the complete insensitivity of IMP dehydrogenase from patients with HPRT deficiency to 2,3-diphosphoglycerate, which is present in high concentrations in erythrocytes and is normally a strong inhibitor of the enzyme in this cell type. The mechanism responsible for and the significance of this apparent alteration of IMP dehydrogenase in HPRT$^-$ subjects remain undefined.

Purine Nucleotides Erythrocytes from patients with the Lesch-Nyhan syndrome have reduced concentrations of ATP, ADP, and AMP with a normal concentration of GTP [159]. The concentration of ATP is also reduced to one-third of normal in platelets from patients with the Lesch-Nyhan syndrome [160]. A relationship between the activity of IMP dehydrogenase and intracellular content of purine ribonucleotides has not been examined further.

Orotate Phosphoribosyltransferase and Orotidine 5′-Phosphate Decarboxylase Beardmore et al. [161] noted three- to tenfold increases in activities of orotate phosphoribosyltransferase (OPRT) and orotidine 5′-phosphate decarboxylase (ODC) in erythrocytes from patients with HPRT defi-

ciency. These enzymes catalyze the conversion of orotic acid to uridine 5′-phosphate (Fig. 51-7). These increases in enzyme activity also appear to be restricted to erythrocytes. In contrast to the previous examples, the increased activity of OPRT and ODC cannot be attributed to either enzyme stabilization or resistance of the enzyme to a dialyzable inhibitor. Treatment with allopurinol is also associated with an apparent increased activity of these two enzymes [162, 163]. The administration of this drug could not account for the observed increase in activity, since the drug had been discontinued in all patients for a sufficient time for activity to return to normal, and several patients had never received allopurinol prior to testing. The mechanism and the significance of the increased activity of OPRT and ODC in patients with HPRT deficiency also remain unclear.

Cells from four patients with the Lesch-Nyhan syndrome have also been found to show an increased incorporation of labeled aspartate and decreased incorporation of labeled orotate into the nucleus [164]. The latter observation seems to be inconsistent with the changes noted above.

Phosphoribosylpyrophosphate (PP-Ribose-P) Synthetase and PP-Ribose-P Martin et al. [165] and more recently Reem [166] have reported a two- to fourfold increase in the activity of PP-ribose-P synthetase in fibroblasts and lymphoblasts cultured from patients with either a partial or a complete deficiency of HPRT as well as in HPRT$^-$ rat hepatoma cells (Fig. 51-7). These differences in levels of PP-ribose-P synthetase activity in HPRT fibroblasts are more readily demonstrable at physiologic concentrations of inorganic phosphate from 1 to 10 mM than at 50 mM [167]. PP-ribose-P synthetase activity is normal in erythrocytes obtained from patients with HPRT deficiency [168].

An elevated intracellular concentration of PP-ribose-P has been demonstrated in erythrocytes [49, 146] and in cultured fibroblasts [169] from patients with the Lesch-Nyhan syndrome. The elevated concentration in fibroblasts appears to be due to decreased utilization of the compound rather than to increased synthesis [169]. The possible importance of this abnormality to the excessive rate of purine biosynthesis *de novo* is discussed later in this chapter.

Pyrimidine Nucleotides Nuki et al. [170] have shown that concentrations of uridine diphosphate (UDP), uridine triphosphate (UTP), and cytidine triphosphate (CTP) are

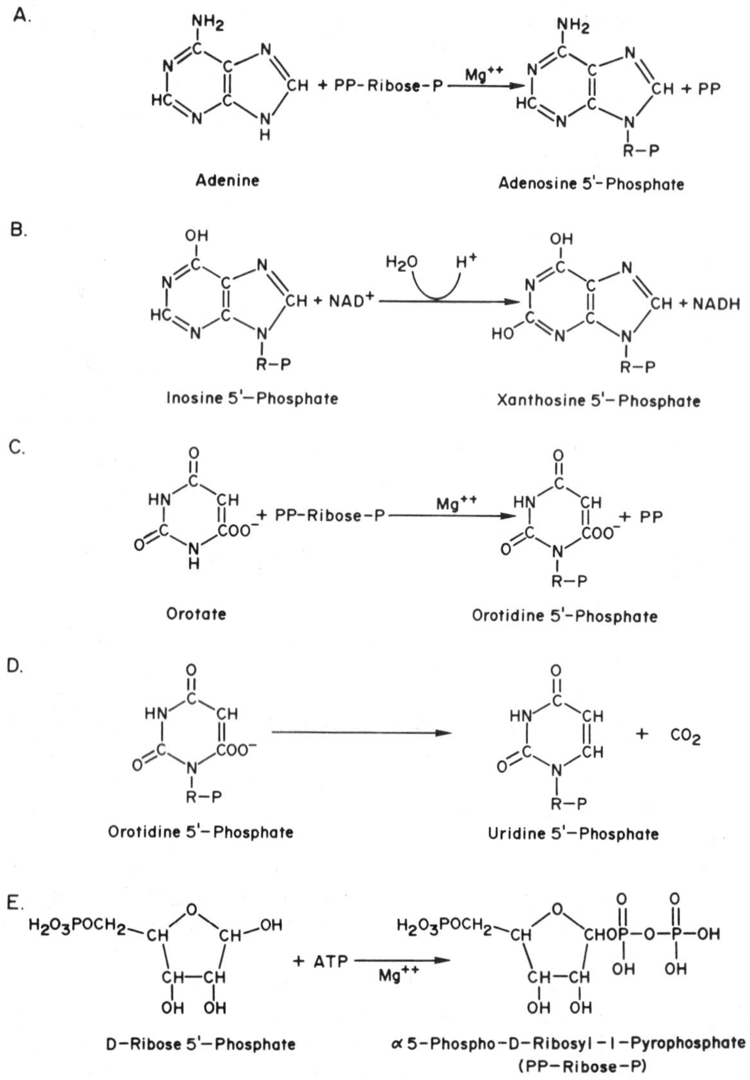

A.

Adenine   Adenosine 5'-Phosphate

B.

Inosine 5'-Phosphate   Xanthosine 5'-Phosphate

C.

Orotate   Orotidine 5'-Phosphate

D.

Orotidine 5'-Phosphate   Uridine 5'-Phosphate

E.

D-Ribose 5'-Phosphate   α 5-Phospho-D-Ribosyl-1-Pyrophosphate
(PP-Ribose-P)

Figure 51-7 Reactions catalyzed by enzymes which exhibit increased activity in patients deficient in HPRT. *A.* Adenine phosphoribosyltransferase. *B.* Inosine 5'-phosphate dehydrogenase. *C.* Orotate phosphoribosyltransferase. *D.* Orotidine 5'-phosphate decarboxylase. *E.* PP-ribose-P synthetase.

increased two- to sixfold in lymphoblasts cultured from one patient lacking HPRT, as well as in 15 clones of HPRT-deficient cells selected following mutagenesis. The increased levels of these pyrimidine nucleotides are presumably secondary to the increased availability of PP-ribose-P, which is both a potent activator of the glutamine-dependent carbamoyl phosphate synthetase that catalyzes the initial step of pyrimidine biosynthesis *de novo* [171], and an essential and possibly rate-limiting substrate for the step of the pathway catalyzed by OPRT [172]. The increase in activity of OPRT and ODC described above could also possibly contribute to the elevation in the concentration of pyrimidine nucleotides.

Cell Fusion

Hybridization of HPRT⁻ cells with cells containing normal HPRT activity promises to provide considerable information on the regulation of HPRT as well as further insight into the nature of the enzyme deficiency in humans. Watson et al. [173] developed mouse-human hybrids using A9 mouse fibroblasts (a line of L cells resistant to azaguanine and deficient in HPRT) and various human cells with normal HPRT activity, including a permanent lymphoblastoid cell line, a fibroblast line derived from human embryonic lung tissue, and phytohemagglutinin-

stimulated human peripheral blood lymphocytes. As expected, the hybrid cells, which were capable of growing in HAT medium (hypoxanthine, amethopterin, and thymidine), had substantial HPRT activity. In three of the five lines examined in detail, the HPRT activity was of murine rather than of human origin [173]. Bakay et al. [174, 175] reported essentially the same findings in chick-mouse hybrids in which the HPRT⁻ cell was the 1-R mouse cell line, another subline of the L strain of mouse fibroblasts. In the latter study [175], HPRT⁻ as well as HPRT⁺ human cells appeared to increase the level of rodent HPRT activity in HPRT⁻ mouse cells after cell fusion. Each of these studies was interpreted as providing evidence for derepression of the murine HPRT locus. Watson et al. [173] also pointed out that they could not exclude an increased reversion frequency from HPRT⁻ to HPRT⁺ as an explanation for their findings. Since the amount of CRM present in the hybrid cells is not reported in either study, the possibility that the increase in activity was due to the activation of the mutant enzyme also cannot be excluded. Sekiguchi and Sekiguchi [176] have also described the appearance of HPRT activity in hybrid cells derived from diploid clones of Chinese hamster cells deficient in HPRT activity. Again, it is not possible to determine whether enzyme activation or depression is the mechanism responsible for the increased activity observed in this study; both alternatives exist. Whatever the mechanism, each of these studies indicates that there are at least two cistrons that can affect HPRT activity in cultured cells.

Over the last 20 years, several investigators have reported that the addition of exogenous DNA resulted in the appearance of HPRT activity in cells lacking activity of this enzyme [177, 178]. McBride and Ozer [179] have used metaphase chromosomes from Chinese hamster fibroblasts, which are HPRT[+], to transform mouse A9 cells, which are HPRT[−]. Cells that survived in HAT selective media were found to have HPRT activity, and the enzyme present had the properties of the Chinese hamster cell enzyme. While the exact molecular basis for this intriguing observation remains to be defined, it has now been amply confirmed [180, 181], and this phenomenon has now been used as a method for gene mapping [181].

Metabolic Cooperation

The phenomenon of metabolic cooperation [182–191] appears to be unrelated to the control of HPRT activity or synthesis. Under normal conditions, cells lacking HPRT are unable to incorporate radioactive hypoxanthine into nucleic acids. However, when cells with normal HPRT activity come into contact with cells lacking activity, there is substantial incorporation of the labeled hypoxanthine into nucleic acids in the mutant cells. Although the mechanism responsible for metabolic cooperation is not totally explained, several studies suggest that normal cells synthesize the radioactive nucleotide IMP, which is then transferred to the mutant cells as nucleotide or as a product of the nucleotide [187, 188]. DeBruyn and Oei [192] have recently reported that membranes from either normal or HPRT[−] cells will, when added to a culture of fibroblasts deficient in HPRT, allow the incorporation of labeled exogenous IMP into the cells. On the basis of this observation, they suggest an IMP-transporting system in the membrane. Such a transport system could account for many of the observations relevant to metabolic cooperation. Ashkenazi and Gartler [193] have reported that crude extracts from HPRT[+] cells (lysed by sonication in saline and centrifuged at 10,000 × gravity for 20 min) apparently correct the defect in HPRT[−] cells. The corrective factor was destroyed by pronase, and the apparent HPRT activity was observed even in the presence of cycloheximide. Ashkenazi and Gartler suggest that the corrective factor is a protein. Their study differed from most others in that freshly trypsinized cells were used as recipients and the pattern of labeling was primarily cytoplasmic rather than nuclear or nucleolar, as ordinarily seen with metabolic cooperation. The transient nature of metabolic cooperation distinguishes it from the transfer of genetic material described in the previous section.

Ghost-mediated Transfer

Recently a method has been developed to introduce macromolecules into cells by means of fusing preloaded erythrocyte ghosts with mammalian cells using inactivated Sendai virus [194–196] or polyethylene glycol [197]. This technique has been successfully used to load human HPRT into HPRT[−] Chinese hamster ovary cells [197] and to load suppressor tRNA from other species into HPRT[−] Chinese hamster cells thus suppressing the mutation [198].

RELATIONSHIP OF THE BIOCHEMICAL ABNORMALITIES TO CLINICAL FINDINGS

Pathogenesis of the Excessive Uric Acid Production

The excessive production of uric acid characteristic of patients with HPRT deficiency results from an accelerated rate of purine biosynthesis de novo. [^{14}C]- or [^{15}N]Glycine is rapidly incorporated into uric acid, and the cumulative incorporation into urinary uric acid over a 7-day period may be as much as 20 times normal (Table 51-5) [3, 4, 26]. The strikingly increased turnover rate of the uric acid pool in these patients is a reflection of the increased rates of uric acid synthesis and excretion.

Hypoxanthine and xanthine, the immediate precursors of uric acid, are readily converted to uric acid by the ample quantities of xanthine oxidase in the liver, so that only a moderate increase in the total urinary excretion of these compounds is observed. In normal persons xanthine is usually excreted in excess of hypoxanthine because of reutilization of hypoxanthine into IMP. In patients with the Lesch-Nyhan syndrome, the absence of HPRT is associated with an inability to convert hypoxanthine into IMP and a substantial increase in the excretion of hypoxanthine relative to that of xanthine [199, 200].

Increased urinary excretion of another purine intermediate, 4-aminoimidazole-5-carboxamide, has also been reported in two patients with this syndrome [201, 202]. The significance of this finding is difficult to evaluate, since this compound is also elevated in the urine of patients depleted of folic acid [203], and patients with HPRT deficiency may be deficient in this vitamin [4]. In at least one patient the elevated excretion of 4-aminoimidazole-5-carboxamide was reduced by 50 percent with oral folic acid, 10 mg/day [193]. After stabilization for up to 27 days on this dose of folic acid, urinary levels of this compound were still about 5 times greater than normal.

There are at least three possible mechanisms by which a deficiency of HPRT could result in excessive purine synthesis. First, the deficiency could lead to enhanced purine synthesis by virtue of decreased concentrations of either IMP or GMP, since these nucleotides are potential inhibitors of purine biosynthesis de novo [43, 45]. Attempts to measure intracellular levels of IMP and GMP in these cells have been of only limited value, partly because of the very low intracellular concentration of these compounds under normal conditions. Where they have been measured, they appeared to be normal [151, 169, 204, 205]. Second, the increased concentration of PP-ribose-P characteristic of HPRT deficiency could increase purine biosynthesis de novo by providing more substrate for the enzyme which catalyzes the presumed limiting step of this pathway, amidophosphoribosyltransferase. Finally, the "drain" of hypoxanthine into uric acid in the absence of reutilization could have some effect unrelated to either IMP or PP-ribose-P [206]. In our view, the altered concentration of PP-ribose-P is the most important factor responsible for the accelerated rate of purine biosynthesis de novo occurring with HPRT deficiency. The critical role of PP-ribose-P in the regulation of purine biosynthesis de novo is discussed earlier in this chapter and more fully in the previous chapter.

The tissues responsible for excessive production of purines in HPRT deficiency are unknown. Although most studies on

Table 51-5   Incorporation of isotopically labeled uric acid and glycine into urinary uric acid in patients with HPRT deficiency

Subject	Reference	Serum urate, mg/dl	Urinary uric acid		Urate pool size		Turnover rate, pools/day	Turnover	
			mg/24 h	mg/kg per 24 h	mg	mg/kg		mg/day	mg/kg per day
Normal adults		<7.0	<600		866–1587		0.45–0.85	513–1108	
Normal children		3.6±1.2		<18					
Lesch-Nyhan syndrome									
D.F.	[59]	12.4	659	33.9	1130	58.3	1.02	1150	59.4
F.H.	[59]	10.0	828	38.7	1690	79.0	0.98	1650	77.1
M.W.	[3]	9.9	669	46.8	530	37.1	2.06	1090	76.2
E.W.	[3]	8.9	712	43.7	787	48.3	1.61	1270	77.9
S.M.	[116]	7.2	911		833		1.55	1294	
Partial HPRT deficiency								1592	24.6
F.J.	[4]	11.7	1237	18.4	2567	39.6	0.62	1645	21.1
R.J.	[4]	10.8	1159	14.9	2050	26.3	0.80	2424	34.6
F.L.	[4]	15.0	1674	23.9	3000	42.9	0.81	1945	49.9
M.L.	[4]	10.4	1132	29.0	2192	56.2	0.89	1693	29.2
T.S.	[4]	14.7	571	9.8	3078	53.1	0.55		

purine synthesis and its regulation have involved the liver, other tissues can also synthesize purines *de novo*. Circulating leukocytes [207, 208] as well as fibroblasts [169, 209] and lymphoblasts [152] cultured in vitro from patients deficient in HPRT activity appear to exhibit accelerated rates of purine synthesis *de novo* similar to the rates observed in vivo. An increase in the rate of the early steps of purine biosynthesis *de novo* has also been demonstrated in mouse neuroblastoma [150] and human lymphoblasts [151] selected for a deficiency of HPRT following mutagenesis. More recent studies have suggested that the maximal rates of purine biosynthesis in cultured HPRT⁻ and HPRT⁺ cells are the same during growth in purine-free media [204, 205, 210]; the difference between HPRT⁺ and HPRT⁻ cells noted in earlier studies is attributed to feedback inhibition of normal cells in the presence of hypoxanthine (and hence IMP) rather than to an abnormal increase of purine synthesis in HPRT⁻ cells. In the latter cell type hypoxanthine is unable to form IMP because of the absence of HPRT activity, and thus purine synthesis is not inhibited under these conditions as it is in normal cells. The inhibition of purine biosynthesis *de novo* in HPRT⁺ fibroblasts grown in fetal calf serum (containing purines) can be overcome at high media concentrations of inorganic phosphate, and maximal rates of purine biosynthesis are thus also the same in HPRT⁺ and HPRT⁻ cells [204]. These studies emphasize that the use of cultured cells with HPRT deficiency to study mechanisms of purine overproduction is critically dependent on media conditions, and that great caution must be exercised in extrapolating these results to patients with HPRT deficiency.

Unfortunately, clinical studies on the location and nature of the accelerated purine biosynthesis *de novo* in patients with HPRT deficiency are limited. The most relevant of these studies relate to the central nervous system (CNS). The capacity for purine synthesis *de novo* exists in the CNS [211], and indirect evidence suggests that excessive purine synthesis may occur in the brain in patients with the Lesch-Nyhan syndrome. The concentration of hypoxanthine and xanthine in cerebrospinal fluid (CSF) is 4 times higher than in normouricemic control patients [67, 212]. In addition, the concentration of these oxypurines in CSF is nearly 3 times higher than the simultaneous plasma concentration, whereas the normal CSF/plasma ratio is

0.33 [67] (Table 51-6). The elevated concentration of oxypurines in the CSF could be the result of transport from the plasma against a concentration gradient [213, 214], but more likely reflects an accelerated production of purines within the CNS. The CNS lacks xanthine oxidase activity, so that hypoxanthine and xanthine are not further oxidized to uric acid within this tissue. The concentration of uric acid in the CSF is consistently normal in patients with the Lesch-Nyhan syndrome [67].

Irrespective of the sources of accelerated purine biosynthesis in patients with HPRT deficiency, the actual overproduction of uric acid is probably restricted to the liver since for practical purposes the enzyme responsible for catalyzing the formation of uric acid is limited to the liver [215].

Pathogenesis of CNS Dysfunction

The mechanism by which a decrease in HPRT activity produces the neurologic dysfunction observed in the Lesch-Nyhan syndrome and in some patients with partial HPRT deficiency remains unclear. The most compelling arguments against a causal role of uric acid in the CNS dysfunction are the demonstration of normal concentrations of uric acid in the CSF of all patients examined [67, 212] and the failure of antihyperuricemic therapy to alter CNS function. Although an elevated concentration of oxypurines occurs in patients with the Lesch-Nyhan syndrome [67], the finding of a similar concentration of hypoxanthine and xanthine in the CSF from two patients with a partial deficiency of HPRT and who show no evidence of CNS dysfunction suggests that these compounds are not in themselves responsible for the CNS disease [4] (Table 51-6).

The first biochemical evidence of an abnormality of CNS function related to a pathway not directly associated with purine metabolism came with the observation by Rockson et al. [219] and later Lake et al. [220] who noted an alteration in the activity of dopamine β-hydroxylase (DBH) in plasma from patients with HPRT deficiency who also exhibited self-mutilation. In addition, both groups observed an absent pressor response to acute sympathetic stimulation [219, 220]. Sub-

7-Day recovery of isotope into urinary uric acid

Percent turnover excreted	Administration uric acid	Administered glycine	
		Uncorrected	Corrected
55–76	57–77	<0.22	<0.30
		<0.15	
58	61	2.49	4.29
50	54	3.16	6.08
61		2.37	3.89
56		2.05	3.66
70	71	3.67	5.19
75	81	0.99	1.22
70	66	0.69	1.03
70	73	2.74	3.81
58	75	2.62	3.94
34	32	0.29	0.88

sequently, HPRT⁻ cells have been shown to have a marked deficiency of monoamine oxidase activity [221–225]. The relevance of these observations to the pathogenesis of the CNS dysfunction remains unclear. Recent studies of brain tissue obtained from patients with the Lesch-Nyhan syndrome at the time of autopsy have shown normal activities of both dopamine β-hydroxylase and monamine oxidase [225a]. Nevertheless, several indexes of dopamine neuron function are markedly and significantly reduced, including concentrations of dopamine, homovanillic acid, and dihydroxyphenylacetic acid, and activities of dopa decarboxylase and tyrosine hydroxylase (Table 51-7).

It is possible that a toxic product may accumulate or that a compound necessary for normal CNS function may be deficient as a direct result of the enzyme defect. The observations in humans [67], rhesus monkey [79], and rat [211] that HPRT activity is normally higher in the CNS than in any other tissue, and that the activity of amidophosphoribosyltransferase, the probable rate-limiting step in the pathway *de novo*, is low in the CNS [211], suggest that the brain may be unusually dependent on the salvage pathway for the synthesis of IMP and GMP. The possibility exists, therefore, that in the absence of HPRT, the CNS may be unable to maintain intracellular concentrations of GMP, IMP, or perhaps the cyclic nucleotides, necessary for normal function. McKeran et al. [226] have

shown that cells heavily dependent on the salvage pathways for purine nucleotide synthesis grow poorly in culture. They suggest that the CNS disease characteristic of the Lesch-Nyhan syndrome may be due in part to impaired cellular proliferation. In support of this thesis, they note that mothers of affected hemizygotes have remarked on the feebleness of intrauterine contractions. In addition, they point out that postmortem brain weight was reduced in four of the six patients in whom data were available.

In the absence of HPRT activity, the purine nucleotide GMP must be synthesized entirely *de novo*. The increased activity of the pathway *de novo* could lead to depletion of certain cofactors, such as ATP or folic acid, and deficiencies of these critical substances could also impair normal development or limit normal function. There are no data available which would allow further consideration of these possibilities.

A number of animal studies have provided exciting clues to possible understanding of the behavioral abnormalities characteristic of the Lesch-Nyhan syndrome. Several examples may be cited. The administration of caffeine, a methylated xanthine, produces self-mutilation in rats [216, 217] (Fig. 51-8). Ungerstedt [218] produced unilateral destruction of a dopamine pathway in the nigrostriatal system with the dopamine analogue 6-hydroxydopamine, and under certain conditions he noted unilateral self-mutilation. Relationships between cGMP, GTP [227], AMP cyclase [228] and dopamine sensitivity are becoming more apparent. In addition, guanine is involved in the synthesis of biopterin which, in turn, is involved in catecholamine biosynthesis [229]. Finally, hypoxanthine is an inhibitor of the diazepam binding site in the central nervous system and thus hypoxanthine itself may have a neuromodulatory role [230].

Several studies have suggested an alteration in glycine levels, although the precise role if any of such a change remains uncertain. Cells deficient in HPRT have a twofold increase of free intracellular glycine [223]. In addition, HPRT deficient patients with the Lesch-Nyhan syndrome exhibit an elevated concentration of glycine in the CSF as well as an increased excretion of this compound in the urine [231].

Pathogenesis of Megaloblastic Anemia

Several patients with HPRT deficiency have had megaloblastic changes in the bone marrow, macrocytic erythrocytes, and a low serum folate concentration [4]. In addition, HPRT deficient fibroblasts exhibit an increased growth requirement for

Table 51-6 Oxypurine and uric acid concentration in plasma and cerebrospinal fluid (mg/dl)

Subject	Uric acid			Oxypurines†		
	CSF	Plasma	CSF/plasma	CSF	Plasma	CSF/plasma
Control (7)	0.29	4.3	0.07	0.13	0.18	0.72
Complete HPRT* deficiency (5)	0.32	8.2	0.04	0.55	0.20	2.75
Partial HPRT* deficiency (4)						
F.L.	1.25	14.1	0.09	0.32	0.12	2.56
M.L.	0.39	9.8	0.04	0.45	0.15	3.02
T.J.	0.72	7.5	0.10	0.44	0.19	2.32
C.M.	1.32	10.9	0.11	0.23		

* HPRT = hypoxanthine-guanine phosphoribosyltransferase.
† Hypoxanthine and xanthine.
SOURCE: Kelley et al. [4]. Reproduced by permission of *Annals of Internal Medicine*.

Table 51-7 Indexes of dopamine-neuron function in putamen from patients with the Lesch-Nyhan syndrome

Substance	Control	Lesch-Nyhan syndrome
	(7)	(3)
Dopamine (μg/g tissue)	5.0 ± 0.5	0.5 ± 0.2*
Homovanillic acid (μg/g tissue)	9.9 ± 1.5	1.8 ± 0.5*
Dihydroxyphenylacetic acid (μg/g tissue)	1.0 ± 0.3	0.3 ± 0.1
Dopa decarboxylase, nmol CO_2/mg protein per 2 h	5.3 ± 1.5	0.6 ± 0.2*
Tyrosine hydroxylase, mmol CO_2/100 mg protein per 2 h	8.1 ± 1.4	1.6 ± 0.4*

* $p < 0.01$ vs. controls
While data shown are from the putamen, similar results were noted in tissue from caudate nucleus, external pallidum, and nucleus accumbens. Values in the substantia nigra were not significantly different from normal.
SOURCE: K. G. Lloyd et al. [225a].

adenine which can be overcome by high concentrations of folic acid [232]. One interpretation of these findings is that the accelerated rate of purine synthesis *de novo* leads to an increased utilization of folate, an essential cofactor at two sites in the pathway *de novo*. Adenine is readily converted to AMP and then to IMP. These purine nucleotides inhibit amidophosphoribosyltransferase and thereby reduce the rate of *de novo* synthesis, and presumably the rate of folate utilization. It is not known whether the deficiency of folate observed in vivo is due to its increased utilization or is even related to anemia. The finding by Van Der Zee et al. [233] that the megaloblastic anemia in their patient failed to respond to exogenous folate but did respond to adenine indicates that additional factors may be important [233].

GENETICS

The familial nature of this syndrome was recognized in the original report by Lesch and Nyhan [3]. The patients have not had any unique ethnic background. Although most patients are Caucasian, the disease has been described in at least five Oriental and three Negro families.

Major clinical manifestations only occur in affected males, and transmission is through carrier females. In all large pedigrees the pattern of inheritance has been consistent with either an X-linked or sex-limited mode of transmission [234, 235] (Figs. 51-9 and 51-10). The absence of male-to-male transmission, a critical test of X-linked inheritance, cannot be evaluated in patients with the Lesch-Nyhan syndrome because they do not reproduce. The finding of patients with a partial deficiency of the same enzyme was particularly valuable in this regard, since they have a milder disease and do reproduce. No male-to-male transmission of the defect has been observed in this latter group [4] and this is consistent with the enzymes being coded by DNA on the X chromosome. X-linked inheritance would also account for the absence of parental consanguinity in spite of the rarity of the disease.

Using fibroblasts in culture it has been possible to demonstrate that obligate heterozygotes for the severe enzyme defect are mosaics in terms of HPRT activity. With a radioautographic technique, 60 percent of the cells from an obligate heterozygote appeared to have normal activity, whereas the remaining 40 percent had no detectable activity [236] (Figs. 51-11 and 51-12). The two cell populations have also been separated by cloning techniques and selective chemical treatment [237–239]. These findings provided substantial support for the X-linked mode of inheritance and are consistent with the Lyon hypothesis [240]. The ultimate evidence for the X-linked nature of HPRT came from an examination of the expression of human HPRT in human-rodent hybrids which

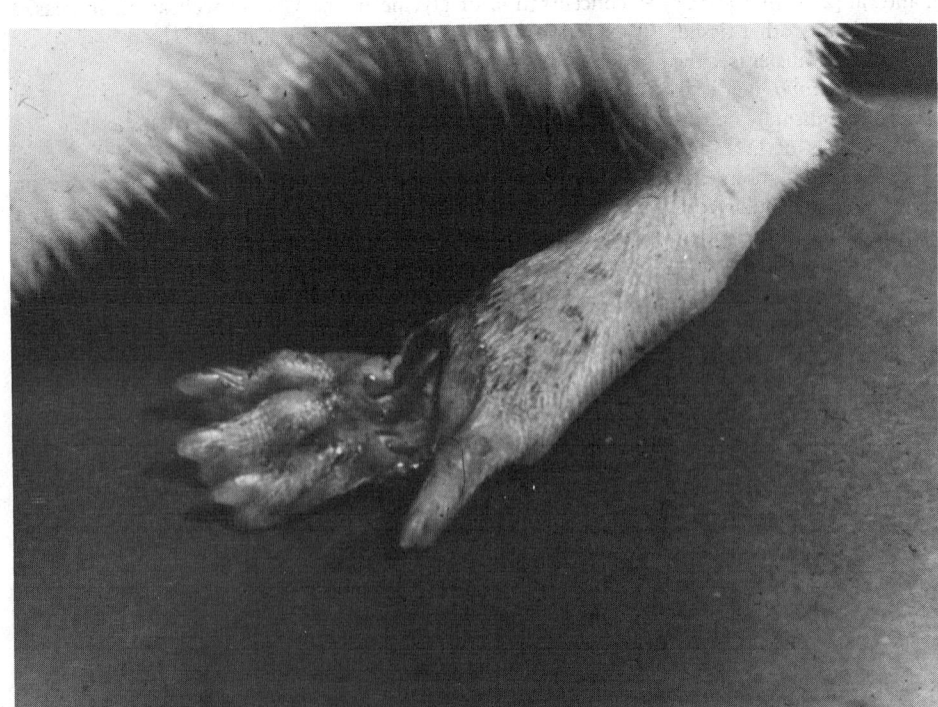

Figure 51-8 Mutilation produced in the rat by administration of caffeine. (*Courtesy of Dr. F. M. Rosenbloom.*)

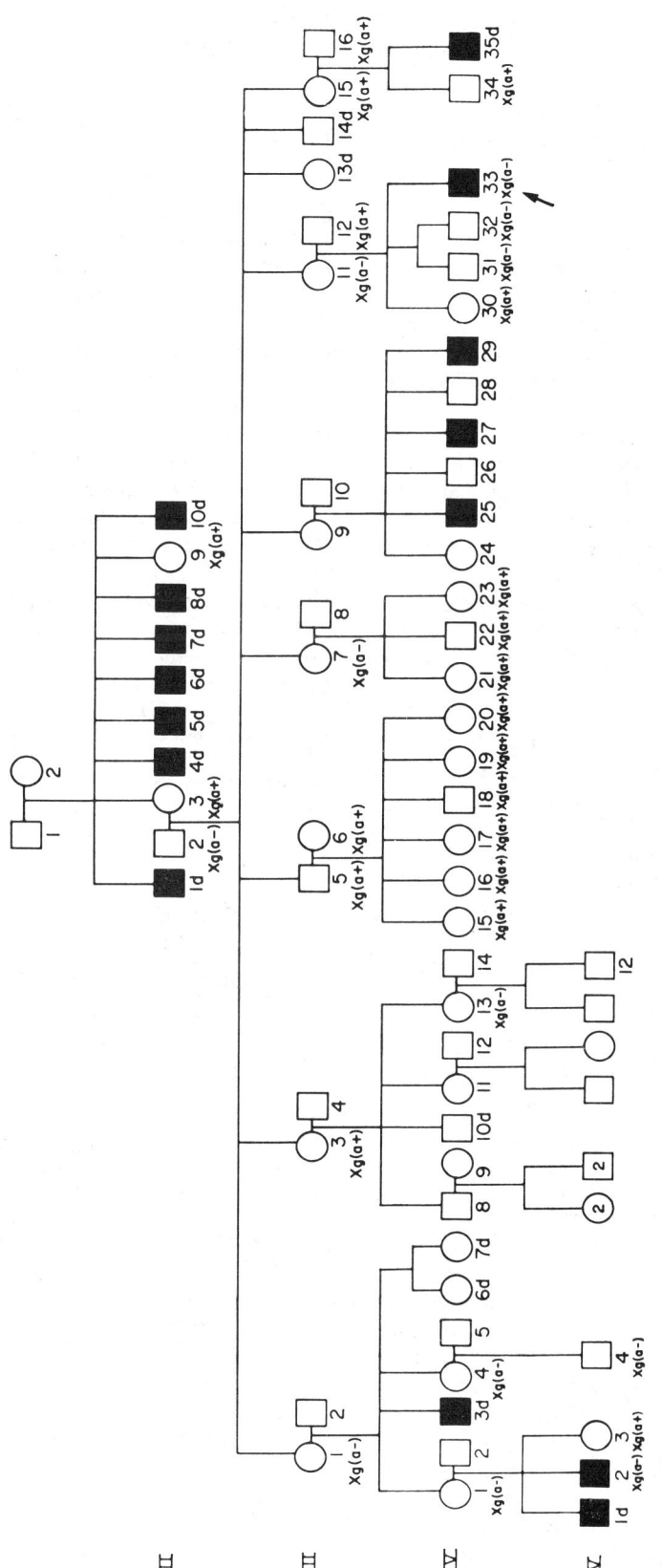

Figure 51-9 Pedigree of the family of patient D.B. (*From Nyhan, Fed. Proc., 27, 1091, 1968.*)

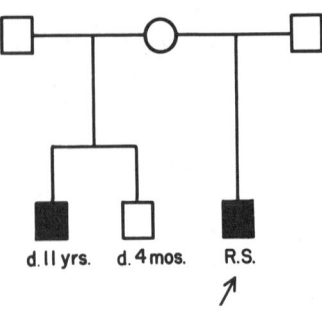

Figure 51-10 Pedigree of the family of patient R.S., suggesting X-linked inheritance. (*From Nyhan, Fed. Proc., 17, 1091, 1968.*)

retain the human X chromosome [181]. These studies demonstrated that the gene coding for HPRT is located on the long arm of the X chromosome, between the genes coding for PP-ribose-P synthetase [241] and glucose-6-phosphate dehydrogenase [181].

Several observations indicate that heterozygotes for a deficiency of HPRT exhibit subtle abnormalities of purine metabolism in vivo. Although they are generally asymptomatic clinically, an elevated serum urate concentration has been noted in a number of such subjects, and at least three have had recurrent monoarticular arthritis clinically thought to represent gout. In addition, several heterozygotes have excreted greater than normal quantitites of uric acid in their urine [4, 16, 242]. Finally, studies on the incorporation of [14C]glycine into urinary uric acid in heterozygous individuals have demonstrated a moderate increase in the rate of purine synthesis de novo [4, 242, 243] (Table 51-8). Based on the data cited above, some cases of gout in the female occurring after menopause may be related to heterozygosity for HPRT deficiency.

Emmerson and Wyngaarden [242] and Emmerson et al. [244] have demonstrated an intermediate level of HPRT activity in subjects heterozygous for the partial enzyme defect. Obligate heterozygotes for the complete enzyme defect, cannot be reliably detected by assay of the enzyme in erythrocyte lysates. Several studies have demonstrated both directly [245] and indirectly [246] that the mutant enzyme is not present in circulating erythrocytes from proven heterozygotes for the complete defect; in most cases total enzyme activity has also been within the normal range [68, 247]. The most likely explanation for this seeming paradox is that hematopoietic precursor cells with a marked reduction of HPRT activity are unable to proliferate in the presence of cells with normal HPRT activity. A low level of activity such as that found with the partial defect allows the cells to proliferate and mature. Support for this hypothesis is provided by McKeran et al. [226] who found that myeloid progenitor cells from bone marrow in patients with HPRT deficiency grew poorly in culture, whereas a similar sample obtained from a heterozygous carrier for the complete enzyme defect gave rise to colonies which were mostly (15 of 17 clones) positive with regard to HPRT activity.

Although initial attempts to detect mosaicism in circulating lymphocytes were unsuccessful [247], Albertini and DeMars [248] using cultured phytohemagglutinin-stimulated lymphocytes found that HPRT⁻ lymphocytes constituted 5 to 10 percent of the total population in three sisters ranging in age from 7 to 17 years. They failed to find a similar HPRT⁻ population in the mother, a proven heterozygote. These results led them to suggest that selection against HPRT⁻ cells may not be absolute and may be age related. The observation by DeBruyn and Oei [249] that transformation of lymphocytes by phytohemagglu-

tinin is associated with an apparent increase in HPRT activity in cells derived from patients with HPRT deficiency may account for the low percentage of HPRT⁻ cells noted by Albertini and DeMars. Although promising, the reliability of this technique for routine demonstration of heterozygosity at the HPRT locus has yet to be demonstrated.

Gartler et al. [250] were the first to use hair follicles for detection of heterozygosity at the HPRT locus. Cells of the scalp exhibit a degree of clonal growth. Since a single hair follicle starts from a small number of cells, the probability is great of finding a follicle in which only one of the X-linked alleles is expressed. Analysis of hair follicles for HPRT activity reveals three types of follicles [250]: one type with normal HPRT activity; a second type with no HPRT activity; and a third type composed of both HPRT⁺ and HPRT⁻ cells, that gives an intermediate activity value. The finding of HPRT⁻ follicles in a possible carrier would be taken as evidence, therefore, of heterozygosity at the HPRT locus. The value of this technique has been confirmed in most [251–255] but not all [252, 256] families studied. The technique is rapid and may be used in the initial evaluation of family members when there is some urgency in determining heterozygosity. The test is not infallible, and a result suggesting the absence of heterozygosity at the HPRT locus should be confirmed using cultured skin fibroblasts. We have found that hair follicle testing is tedious and generally not only less reliable but more difficult than tissue culture methods, particularly in the field, where a skin biopsy can be obtained and leisurely transported to the labo-

Figure 51-11 Radioautographs of fibroblasts from an affected child incubated with (*A*) [³H]hypoxanthine and (*B*) [³H]adenine. Black granules throughout the nucleus and cytoplasm show distribution of ³H-labeled purine base incorporated into trichloroacetic acid precipitable RNA. (*Courtesy of Dr. F. M. Rosenbloom.*)

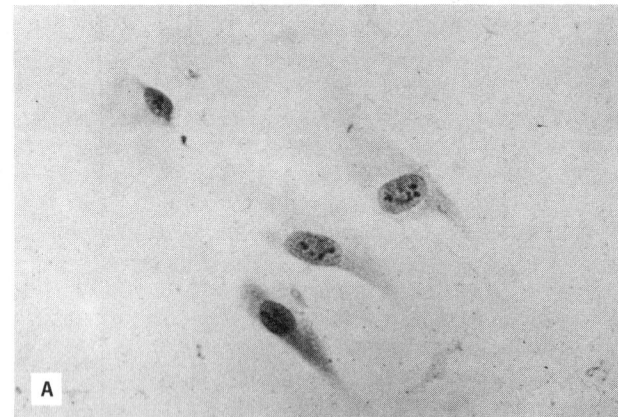

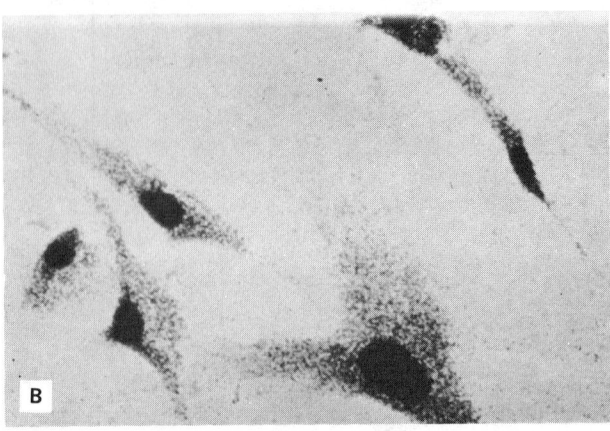

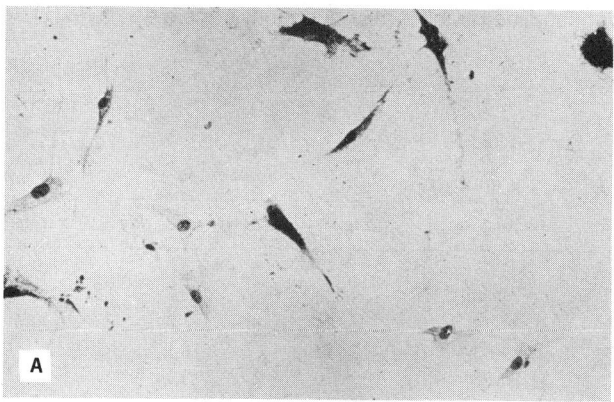

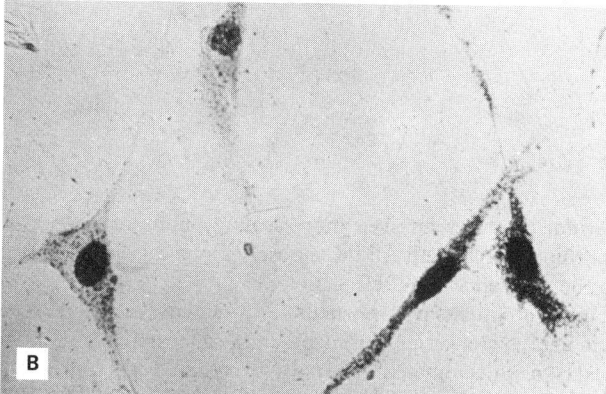

Figure 51-12 Radioautographs of fibroblasts from an obligate heterozygote incubated with [³H]hypoxanthine, demonstrating the presence of two cell populations. *A.* ×160. *B.* ×400. (*Courtesy of Dr. F. M. Rosenbloom.*)

ratory for explanting. If there is no urgency and a tissue culture facility is available, we recommend using one of the cell culture techniques involving growth of HPRT⁻ cells in selective media for the routine evaluation of families at risk [239, 257].

In an analysis of 176 female members of 47 independent kindreds of patients with the Lesch-Nyhan syndrome, only 4 propositi were found to have mothers who were homozygous normal [258]. According to Haldane's principle, if one assumes genetic equilibrium, one-third of all affected males per generation would represent new mutations. Possible explanations for the unexpectedly low number of homozygous normal mothers include a higher mutation rate in males [259] or perhaps somatic or half-chromatid mutations in an X-linked lethal disease [260]. The proportion of new mutants among heterozygotes was not significantly different from expected. In those cases in which the heterozygous mother of an affected individual was a new mutant the age of her parents was higher than the mean parental age in the population. This suggested a paternal age effect on X-linked mutations.

Culture of cells obtained from amniotic fluid has allowed the heterozygous [261] as well as the hemizygous [262] state to be diagnosed in utero. In at least three cases the diagnosis of HPRT deficiency has been made in utero and the pregnancy has been interrupted.

Pharmacogenetics

In addition to the naturally occurring substrates for HPRT, a number of purine analogues are converted to their nucleotide

derivatives by this enzyme. Several of these, including 6-mercaptopurine (and its nitroimidazole derivative, azathioprine), 3-azaguanine, and allopurinol, are used clinically. The deficiency of HPRT in humans is associated with an altered response to certain effects of these drugs both in vivo and in vitro.

The administration of azathioprine to patients with normal HPRT activity leads to a striking reduction in purine synthesis *de novo* that is often accompanied by a decrease in both serum and urinary uric acid values [265] (Fig. 51-13). This is presumably due to hydrolysis of azathioprine to 6-mercaptopurine, which is then converted to its ribonucleotide by HPRT. The ribonucleotide derivative of 6-mercaptopurine, but not the free base, is an inhibitor of human amidophosphoribosyltransferase [43]. In patients lacking HPRT activity, azathioprine has no effect on synthesis of purines *de novo* [4, 132, 265, 266] (Fig. 51-14). In addition, absence of this enzyme in lymphocytes obtained from these patients is associated with a loss of the ability of azathioprine to suppress phytohemagglutinin-induced transformation of lymphocytes as measured by incorporation of [³H]thymidine into DNA [267]. Resistance to the potential inhibitor effects of 6-mercaptopurine on purine synthesis *de novo* has also been demonstrated in cultured fibroblasts derived from these patients [1]. Resistance to azathioprine and 6-mercaptopurine could be of potential clinical significance in subjects either hemizygous or heterozygous for HPRT deficiency if circumstances were to occur such as a malignancy, a life-threatening connective tissue disease, or an organ transplantation in which one of these drugs was medically indicated.

Figure 51-13 The effect of azathioprine treatment on the serum urate and 24-h urinary uric acid excretion of a gouty patient who produces excessive quantities of uric acid. (*From Kelley et al. [265].*)

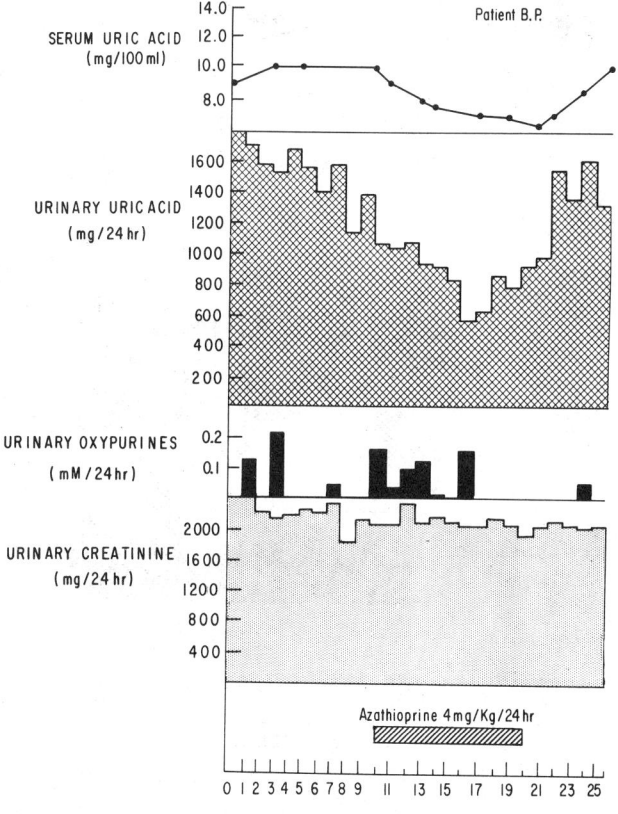

Table 51-8 Uric acid metabolism in females heterozygous for hypoxanthine-guanine phosphoribosyltransferase (HPRT) deficiency

Subject	Serum urate, mg/dl	Urinary uric acid		Urate pool size		Turnover rate, pools/day	Turnover		Percent turnover excreted
		mg/24 h	mg/kg per 24 h	mg	mg/kg		mg/day	mg/kg per day	
Normal adults	<7.0	<600	—	866–1587	—	0.45–085	513–1108	—	55–7–6
B.W.	4.4	367	9.2	535	13.4	0.85	455	11.4	81
R.W.	4.6	348	5.6	881	14.3	0.63	552	8.9	63
D.W.	9.1	499	9.2	1699	31.2	0.58	990	18.2	50
I.J.	7.5	773	11.1	1811	26.0	0.68	1232	17.7	63
R.L.	4.9	761	13.4	868	15.3	0.98	853	15.0	89
L.B.	5.1	400	7.0	834	14.6	0.64	535	9.4	75
C.B.	4.8	586	8.8	1026	15.4	0.74	763	11.4	—
V.B.	4.3	665	11.4	734	12.6	1.20	884	15.1	75
M.B.	4.4	631	11.1	—	—	—	—	—	—

* 6 Days.
SOURCE: Modified from Emmerson [243].

The effects of allopurinol in patients lacking HPRT activity differ in several distinctive ways from its effects in normal subjects: (1) Allopurinol does not have its usual inhibitory effect on purine biosynthesis *de novo* [268–270] (Fig. 51-15). (2) Allopurinol does not reduce erythrocyte PP-ribose-P concentration [271]. (3) A normally occurring ribonucleoside derivative of allopurinol does not appear in the urine [212]. (4) Allo-

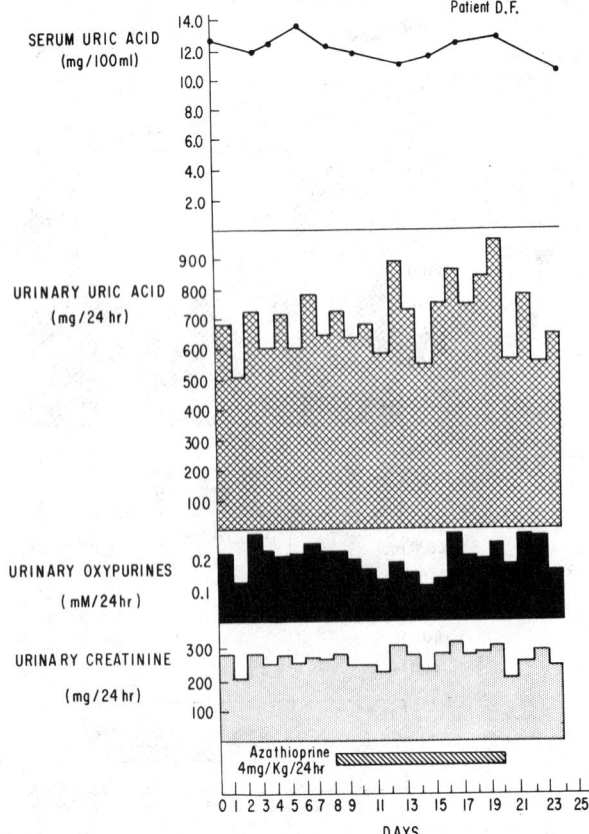

Figure 51-14 The effect of azathioprine treatment on the serum urate and 24-h urinary uric acid excretion of a patient with the Lesch-Nyhan syndrome. (*From Kelley et al.* [265].)

purinol produces an even more striking inhibitory effect on xanthine oxidase [4]. All these observations can be attributed to the deficiency of HPRT activity.

In most patients with normal HPRT activity, the decrease in uric acid excretion produced by allopurinol is not accompanied by a stoichiometric increase in excretion of the immediate precursors of uric acid, hypoxanthine and xanthine. This decrease in total purine excretion reflects a decrease in the rate of purine synthesis [272], an effect probably due to a combination of factors (Fig. 51-16) including (1) an increased conversion of hypoxanthine to IMP, (2) the conversion of allopurinol to its ribonucleotide, and (3) a depletion of intracellular PP-ribose-P as a result of either mechanism (1) or (2). Both IMP and allopurinol ribonucleotide are inhibitors of amidophosphoribosyltransferase, whereas the free bases are not; therefore, an increase in their formation could lead to a decrease in purine biosynthesis *de novo*. In addition, since PP-ribose-P is an essential and rate-limiting substrate for this reaction, a decrease in its concentration could also decrease purine synthesis. Both of these possible inhibitory mechanisms depend on the presence of HPRT.

The failure of allopurinol to reduce purine synthesis *de novo* in HPRT-deficient patients results in an increase in excretion of hypoxanthine and xanthine that roughly equals the decrease in uric acid excretion. Although hypoxanthine usually predominates in the urine under these conditions, the excretion of xanthine can be high enough to exceed solubility limits. Four of the seven patients who have developed xanthine stones while on allopurinol have been patients with the Lesch-Nyhan syndrome [273–276], and one was partially HPRT deficient [277].

Patients lacking HPRT appear to be somewhat more sensitive to the inhibitory effect of allopurinol on xanthine oxidase than the normal person [4] (Fig. 51-17). This may be due to the failure of allopurinol to be metabolized to its ribonucleotide derivative, leaving more of the free bases allopurinol and oxipurinol to inhibit xanthine oxidase. The serum urate concentration also tends to drop faster once xanthine oxidase is inhibited because of the rapid turnover of uric acid in these patients. The partial deficiency of HPRT does not protect the patient from a hypersensitivity reaction to the drug [278].

Table 51-8 Uric acid metabolism in females heterozygous for hypoxanthine-guanine phosphoribosyltransferase (HPRT) deficiency (*Continued*)

| Administered uric acid | *7-Day recovery of isotope into urinary uric acid* | | C urate, ml/(min · 1.73 m²) | C creatinine, ml/(min 1.73 m²) | Percent C urate/ creatinine × 100 |
| | Administered glycine | | | | |
	Uncorrected	Corrected			
55–77	<0.22	<0.30	—	—	—
75*	0.50*	0.67*	7.5	64	11.7
66	0.38	0.58	4.2	71	5.9
55	0.64	1.16	6.5	64	10.2
66	0.77	1.17	7.1	98	7.2
92	1.27	1.38	20.1	123	16.3
73	0.46	0.63	9.6	77	12.5
83	0.45	0.54	10.7	117	9.1
91	0.42	0.46	13.7	130	10.5
—	0.49	—	11.8	135	8.7

TREATMENT

The life-threatening aspects of HPRT deficiency toward which therapy should be primarily directed are (1) excessive uric acid synthesis and (2) the CNS dysfunction when present. For the former, therapy is well defined and effective; unfortunately, no therapy has yet proved beneficial for the latter.

Excessive Uric Acid Synthesis

Since allopurinol effectively lowers the uric acid content of both serum and urine in these patients, this drug can be used to prevent uric acid stone formation, uric acid and urate nephropathy, gouty arthritis, and the development of tophi. When these findings are already present, progression can be stopped, and some reversal may be achieved. For these reasons every patient with the Lesch-Nyhan syndrome or partial HPRT deficiency should be treated with allopurinol. Unless allopurinol is also administered, uricosuric drug therapy probably should not be used in this setting because of the extremely large load of uric acid already being presented to the kidney. In most patients without tophi, allopurinol alone will be adequate to maintain a normal serum urate concentration, and a uricosuric drug will not be needed. The possibility of xanthine stone formation during allopurinol treatment [273–277] can be minimized by increasing urine flow. This potential complication should not deter the use of allopurinol in this disease. Allopurinol has not been shown to affect the progression of CNS dysfunction in either a beneficial or detrimental manner, although only a few patients with this syndrome have been treated with allopurinol from birth.

Central Nervous System Dysfunction

Approaches toward prevention or correction of the CNS dysfunction remain experimental. Since these children have no apparent abnormalities in CNS function at birth and because no distinctive pathologic changes are noted on routine gross and histologic study of the brain postmortem, it seems possible that this aspect of the disease may be preventable or treatable. Several major problems continue to plague this area of investigation. First, the pathogenesis of the disease remains unclear. Second, there are few dependable and objective methods of

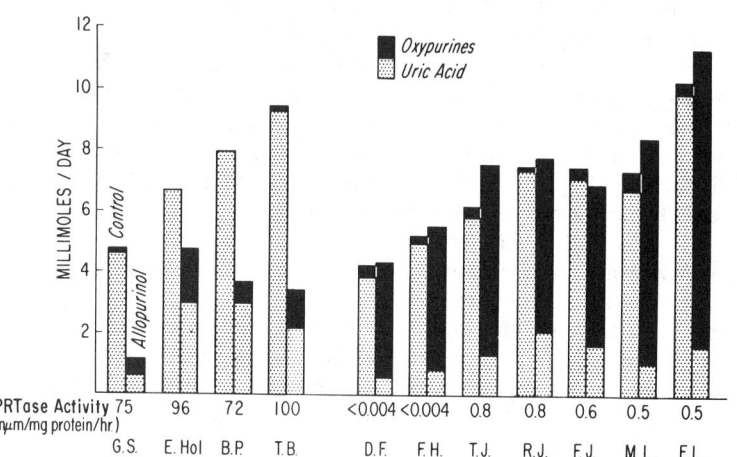

Figure 51-15 Effect of allopurinol on total purine excretion in subjects that produce excessive quantities of uric acid. "Partial" HPRT deficiency (T.J., R.J., F.J., M.L., and F.L.) and "complete" HPRT deficiency (D.F. and F.H.). (*From Kelley* [*68*]. *Reproduced by permission of Federation Proceedings.*)

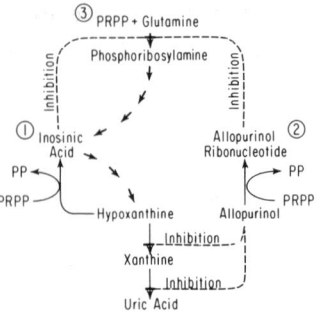

Figure 51-16 Possible mechanisms to account for the inhibitory effect of allopurinol on *de novo* purine synthesis. These include (*1*) an increased conversion of hypoxanthine to inosinic acid, (*2*) a direct conversion of allopurinol to its ribonucleotide, and (*3*) a depletion of intracellular P-ribose-PP.

evaluating subtle changes in neurologic function in these patients. Finally, the patients seem to improve generally when they receive the care and attention associated with hospitalization. This is particularly true when they are transferred from the environment of a large institution to a clinical research facility. Evaluation of results of therapy should consider these factors before conclusions are drawn.

A major experimental approach in treating the CNS dysfunction has been directed toward replacing the presumed but undocumented deficiency of either GMP or IMP. The administration of GMP or AMP has been tried without evidence of clinical improvement [14]. This might be anticipated, since these purine nucleotides cross cell membranes poorly if at all. Guanosine has been tried with the hope that it would be converted to GMP by guanosine kinase [4]. The patient did not improve clinically. In one patient, the daily oral administration of 20 to 40 mg inosine per kilogram of body weight produced no change in uric acid excretion [12] and no clinical improvement during the course of the study. The free bases hypoxanthine or guanine would not be effective, since they cannot be converted to their nucleotides in the absence of HPRT.

Adenine appeared to be a reasonable therapeutic agent for several reasons. Adenine is readily converted to AMP by APRT and might then increase IMP or GMP levels by way of purine interconversion pathways and by inhibiting microsomal 5'-nucleotidase. In addition, formation of AMP and consumption of PP-ribose-P should reduce the rate of purine synthesis *de novo*. Because of these theoretical considerations and the observations that (1) exogenous adenine is required for the normal growth of fibroblasts derived from patients deficient in HPRT, (2) erythrocyte levels of adenine nucleotides are reduced [159], and (3) the urinary excretion of adenine and adenosine is lower than normal in these patients [279], adenine seemed to be a good agent to try. Two patients have been treated from birth with adenine [277]. Both went on to develop the CNS abnormalities characteristic of the Lesch-Nyhan syndrome. Several older patients have also been treated with adenine without apparent success [159, 233, 281–283]. One 9-year-old patient was treated with 1500 mg adenine daily for nearly 2 months [233]; although this produced a striking improvement in his megaloblastic anemia, no changes in neurologic behavior were noted [283]. In two other studies adenine did seem to lead to some improvement in the neurologic disorder [284, 285]. In each case therapy had to be discontinued due to the nephrotoxicity of 2,8-dioxyadenine, the major metabolic product of adenine [286]. This occurred in spite of the concomitant use of allopurinol to inhibit xanthine oxidase,

which catalyzes the oxidation of adenine to 2,8-dioxyadenine.

2,6-Diaminopurine is also converted to its nucleotide by APRT and can then be converted to GMP [287]. This compound has been used in preliminary studies without apparent benefit [12].

Several patients had been depleted of folate, and the apparent adenine requirement of cultured fibroblasts can be replaced with high concentrations of folate. In one patient treated from birth with adenine plus folic acid, the CNS manifestations occurred at the expected time [288]. The use of folic acid in a number of older patients has uniformly been of no benefit to the neurologic disease [256].

In one instance, low plasma levels of glutamine were observed, and these were returned to normal on a regimen of glutamate supplementation which led to an improved appetite and increased protein intake. The suggestion was made that behavior improved on this regimen [289]. It seems likely that improvement may have been attributable to nutritional factors or to supportive measures, such as padding and restraining of hands and exemplary nursing care. The administration of glutamine to one 8-year-old patient produced no apparent benefit [290].

Magnesium is an essential cofactor for HPRT. Benke et al. [288] noted that the addition of magnesium at nontoxic concentrations up to 20 mM increased the rate of growth of fibroblasts derived from patients with HPRT deficiency and led to an apparent increase in HPRT activity in the mutant cells. Magnesium supplementation in one patient, however, was of no apparent value [291].

Based on the observation that aggressive behavior in rats induced by transection of olfactory bulbs could be alleviated by administration of L-5-hydroxytryptophan, Mizuno and Yugari [292] treated four patients with the Lesch-Nyhan syndrome, ages 19 months to 12 years, with this compound at daily doses ranging from 1 to 8 mg per kilogram of body weight for up to 36 weeks. They reported that a daily dose as small as 1.2 mg per kilogram of body weight administered

Figure 51-17 The effect of allopurinol administration on the concentration of urate in serum of hyperuricemic patients. Comparison of effects in patients with the Lesch-Nyhan syndrome and patients with normal hypoxanthine-guanine phosphoribosyltransferase activity. (*Adapted from Kelley et al.* [4].)

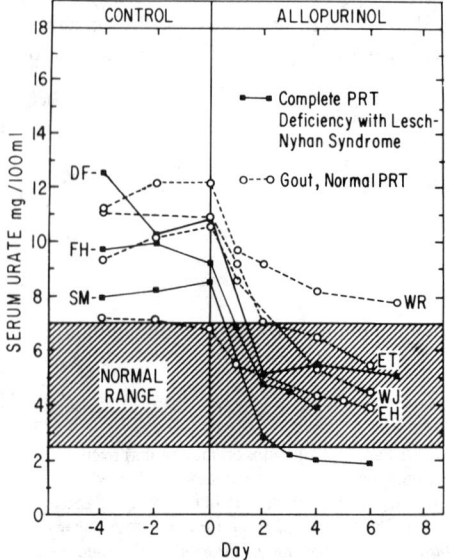

orally led to complete control of the self-mutilation in all four patients and that this manifestation reappeared in each patient within 15 h after discontinuation of treatment. Nyhan et al. [293] used the combination of 5-hydroxytryptophan and carbidopa, an inhibitor of peripheral decarboxylase, in seven patients with the Lesch-Nyhan syndrome. Although some patients seemed to improve, all relapsed in 1 to 3 months despite continuation of therapy. We have observed no improvement in four patients treated with L-5-hydroxytryptophan in daily doses up to 8 mg per kilogram of body weight for up to 4 weeks [294].

Several attempts have been made to activate or replace HPRT. Arnold and Kelley [295] noted that dietary purine restriction was associated with a severalfold increase in HPRT activity in circulating erythrocytes derived from patients with HPRT deficiency. On the other hand, restriction of purines in the diet for up to 6 months in one 9-year-old patient led to no apparent improvement in his behavior. The discovery of a patient with the Lesch-Nyhan syndrome with a mutant form of HPRT that exhibits normal activity at high concentrations of substrates, PP-ribose-P and hypoxanthine, suggested that attempts to elevate the intracellular levels of these compounds might be beneficial [70]. Unfortunately, administration of hypoxanthine, guanine, methylene blue, and ribose (the latter two compounds in an attempt to increase the synthesis of PP-ribose-P) to this patient for several days led to no apparent improvement [296]. Watts et al. [282] noted no improvement in motor function in a 4-year-old patient after exchange blood transfusion. There was a small, transient decrease in serum urate concentration, with no change in urinary uric acid excretion values. Surprisingly, erythrocyte HPRT activity did not fall below 10 percent of normal for more than 90 days. Similarly negative findings were reported by Edwards et al. [297], who found neither metabolic changes nor improvement in CNS function following blood transfusion.

Other agents found to be of no therapeutic benefit include orotic acid [298], L-tryptophan [292], tetrabenazine [282], thiopropazate [282], chlorpromazine [282], and α-methyldopa [256].

Behavioral methods of treatment recently have been reported to be beneficial. This includes the extinction of injurious behavior plus reinforcement of alternative behavior that is not self-injurious [299–302]. Such therapy has not been proven to be useful over the long term at home [302].

Future approaches to therapy using enzyme replacement with erythrocyte ghosts or liposome trapped enzyme hold promise [303] as do approaches using chromosome or DNA mediated transfer of the HPRT gene [304, 305].

Despite the absence of specific therapy for the CNS manifestations of complete HPRT deficiency, it is possible to make the patient more comfortable by supportive measures and drug treatment. Patients are apparently less agitated when restrained in such a manner that they cannot mutilate. For the fingers and hands this can be achieved satisfactorily with elbow splints, heavy wrappings about the hands, or restraints on the wheelchair. The patients appear more calm when sitting up during their hours awake so long as they are adequately restrained and their wheelchairs are heavily padded and cannot be easily overturned. For mutilation of the lips, nothing short of tooth extraction has proven to be of benefit in some patients. We recommend waiting until lip biting becomes apparent before extracting the teeth involved, since (1) this manifestation may be markedly delayed in onset, (2) it is dif-

ficult to predict which teeth will cause the most serious difficulty, and (3) extraction of teeth may lead to a reduction in caloric intake. Many patients eventually develop severe inanition. It is not clear whether this is a reflection of the basic genetic defect or is due to poor feeding. Only a rare patient can adequately feed himself. For this reason, part of the therapeutic program must include feeding by parents or institutional personnel.

Drugs that appear to be helpful with regard to the movement disorder include diazepam, haloperidol, and phenobarbital. Levodopa has also been reported to be of some value [292]. Evidence that the adrenergic nervous system may be abnormal in patients with the complete enzyme defect suggests that some of these drugs may interact in a specific way with the dopaminergic system.

Therapeutic Abortion

The preferred form of therapy for complete HPRT deficiency at the present time is prevention. As discussed earlier, HPRT deficiency can be diagnosed in utero, and in at least two cases the disease was prevented by abortion. Several problems exist which deserve comment.

Two distinct clinical syndromes are associated with a deficiency of HPRT; one leads to the devastating and untreatable neurologic and behavioral disorder, and the other leads to gout. It is extremely important to differentiate between these two clinical syndromes before recommending abortion; the Lesch-Nyhan syndrome should be prevented in this manner, whereas the partial HPRT deficiency syndrome does not warrant this approach. Unfortunately, one cannot always differentiate between the two syndromes by the activity of HPRT in circulating erythrocytes. At present, the best way to determine which clinical syndrome an HPRT-deficient fetus is destined to develop is by family history. The two syndromes have never been observed in the same family. Thus, if the Lesch-Nyhan syndrome has occurred previously in the family, it is virtually certain that an HPRT-deficient male fetus will develop the same disease, and abortion should be recommended. From a practical standpoint, the importance of differentiating between the carrier states of the two syndromes is not yet critical, because heterozygotes for these disorders are only sought for in families known to have an HPRT-deficient member, whose clinical status will already have been defined.

With the development of methods of screening for heterozygosity in the future, precise differentiation will become mandatory.

VARIANTS AND PHENOCOPIES

Nyhan et al. [306] have reported a 3-year-old boy who exhibited excessive purine synthesis and hyperuricemia in addition to mental retardation, dysplastic teeth, absence of tears on crying, absence of speech, and unusual autistic behavior. There was no self-mutilation or choreoathetosis. Erythrocyte HPRT activity was normal, but APRT activity was increased. If the kinetic constants for HPRT from this patient are normal, he may represent another inborn error of purine metabolism associated with abnormal behavior.

Hooft et al. [307] have studied a young girl with delayed psychomotor development, mutilation of fingers and buccal mucosa, choreoatheosis, episodes of opisthotonos, and generalized spasticity. Serum urate concentrations were 3.5 to 5.0 mg/dl, but excessive purine synthesis was manifest in the excretion of 35.0 to 45.0 mg uric acid per kilogram of body weight per day and the incorporation of 1.7 percent of an intravenously administered dose of [^{14}C]glycine into urinary uric acid in 7 days. Both parents were normal clinically. This patient has most of the classic features of the Lesch-Nyhan syndrome, except that by both clinical and chromosomal analysis she is female. Other differences include (1) parental consanguinity, (2) a relatively late peak in the incorporation of isotopic glycine into urinary uric acid, (3) persistent normouricemia in the absence of antihyperuricemic agents, and (4) marked improvement with allopurinol therapy to the point that she was able to walk. Additional biochemical information is awaited, including determination of HPRT activity.

Bazelon et al. [308] have described three females with hyperuricemia, mental retardation, and mutilation of the lips and hands. These subjects differ from patients with the Lesch-Nyhan syndrome in that urinary excretion of uric acid is normal, HPRT activity is normal, and there is no choreoathetosis, spasticity, or severe growth retardation.

It is not surprising that other patients are being described who exhibit some degree of neurologic disease and hyperuricemia [309], since the latter finding occurs with a relatively high frequency in the general population. An increased excretion of uric acid will no doubt prove to be a more significant finding than an elevated serum urate concentration when associated with one of the neurologic or behavioral disorders described here.

Preliminary studies suggesting a less stable HPRT with altered isoelectric points in patients with Gilles de la Tourette's syndrome [310] have not been confirmed by others.

REFERENCES

1. SEEGMILLER JE, ROSENBLOOM FM, KELLEY WN: An enzyme defect associated with a sex-linked human neurological disorder and excessive purine synthesis. Science 155:1682, 1967
2. KELLEY WN, ROSENBLOOM RM, HENDERSON JR, SEEGMILLER JE: A specific enzyme defect in gout associated with overproduction of uric acid. Proc Natl Acad Sci USA 57:1735, 1967
3. LESCH M, NYHAN WL: A familial disorder of uric acid metabolism and central nervous system function. Am J Med 36:561, 1964
4. KELLEY WN, GREENE ML, ROSENBLOOM FM, HENDERSON JF, SEEGMILLER JE: Hypoxanthine-guanine phosphoribosyltransferase in gout. Ann Intern Med 70:155, 1969
5. DREIFUSS FE, NEWCOMBE DS, SHAPIRO SL, SHEPPARD GL: X-linked primary hyperuricemia (hypoxanthine-guanine phosphoribosyltransferase deficiency encephalopathy). J Ment Defic Res 12:100, 1968
6. GILLESPIE JB, PERUCCA LG: Congenital generalized indifference to pain (congenital analgia). Am J Dis Child 100:124, 1960
7. MUNSAT TL, KLINENBERG J, CARREL RE, MENKES J: Defects in purine metabolism and neurologic disease. Bull Los Angeles Neurol Soc 33:101, 1968
8. SCHERZER AL, ILSON JB: Normal intelligence in the Lesch-Nyhan syndrome. Pediatrics 44:116, 1969
9. MARKS JF, BAUM J, KELLE DK, KAY JL, MACFARLEN A: Lesch-Nyhan syndrome treated from the early neonatal period. Pediatrics 42:357, 1968
10. SMITH MG, BLAND JH, KELLEY WN, SEEGMILLER JE: Unpublished observations
11. HOEFNAGEL D: Seminars on the Lesch-Nyhan syndrome: Discussion. Fed Proc 27:1045, 1967
12. BERMAN PH, BALIS ME, DANCIS J: Congenital hyperuricemia, an inborn error of purine metabolism associated with psychomotor retardation, athetosis, and self-mutilation. Arch Neurol 20:44, 1969
13. MICHENER WM: Hyperuricemia and mental retardation with athetosis and self-mutilation. Am J Dis Child 113:195, 1967
14. ROSENBERG D, MONNET P, MAMELLE JL, COLOMBEL M, SALLE B, BOVIER-LAPIERRE M: Encephalopathie avec troubles du metabolisme des purines. Presse Med 76:2333, 1968
15. KAUFMAN JM, GREENE ML, SEEGMILLER JE: Urine uric acid to creatinine ratio: Screening test for disorders of purine metabolism. J Pediatr 73:583, 1968
16. HOEFNAGEL D, ANDREW ED, MIREAULT NG, BERNDT WO: Hereditary choreoathetosis, self-mutilation, and hyperuricemia in young males. N Engl J Med 273:130, 1965
17. VANBOGAERT L, DAMME JV, VERSCHUEREN M: Sur un syndrome professif d'hypertonie extrapyramidale avec osteoarthropathies goutteuses chez deux freres. Rev Neurol 114:15, 1966
18. PARTINGTON MW, HENNEN BKE: The Lesch-Nyhan syndrome: Self-destructive biting, mental retardation, neurological disorder and hyperuricemia. Dev Med Child Neurol 9:563, 1967
19. RILEY JD: Gout and cerebral palsy in three-year-old boy. Arch Dis Child 35:293, 1960
20. LABRUNE B, CARTIER M, HAMET MM, BONNENFANT F, VELIN J, RIBIERRE M, MALLET R: Encephalopathie familiale avec hyperuricemie. Presse Med 76:2337, 1968
21. CATEL W, SCHMIDT J: Uber familiare gichtische Diathese in Verdundung mit zerebralen und renalen Symptomen bei einem Kleinkind. Dtsch Med Wochenschr 84:2145, 1959
22. MARIE J, ROYER P, RAPPAPORT R: Hyperuricemie congenitale avec troubles neurologiques, renaux et sanguinis. Arch Fr Pediatr 24:501, 1967
23. MANZKE H: Hyperuricamie mit cerebralparese Syndrom eines hereditaren Purenstoffwechselleidens. Helv Paediatr Acta 22:258, 1967
24. VAN DER ZEE SPM, MONNENS LAH, SCHRETLEN EDAM: Hereditary disorder of purine metabolism with cerebral affection and megaloblastic anemia. Ned Tijdschr Geneeskd 112:1475, 1968
25. ALLISON AC, WATTS RWE, HOVI T, WEBSTER ADB: Immunological observations on patients with Lesch-Nyhan syndrome, and on the role of de novo purine synthesis in lymphocyte transformation. Lancet Dec. 13, 1975, p 1179
26. NYHAN WL, OLIVER WJ, LESCH M: A familial disorder of uric acid metabolism and central nervous system function. II. J Pediatr 67:257, 1965
27. SEEGMILLER JE: Summary: Pathology and pathologic physiology. Fed Proc 27:1042, 1968
28. SKYLER JS, NEELON FA, ARNOLD WJ, KELLEY WN, LEBOVITZ HE: Growth retardation in the Lesch-Nyhan syndrome. Acta Endocrinol 75:3, 1974
29. SASS JK, ITABASHI HH, DEXTER RA: Juvenile gout with brain involvement. Arch Neurol 13:639, 1965
30. ROSENBLUM WI, ROSENBLOOM FM, SEEGMILLER JE: Unpublished results
31. RENUART AW: Personal communication
32. CRUSSI FG, ROBERTSON DM, HISCOX JL: The pathological condition of the Lesch-Nyhan syndrome. Am J Dis Child 118:501, 1969
33. BASSERMANN R, GUTENSOHN W, SPRINGMANN JS: Pathological and immunological observations in a case of Lesch-Nyhan syndrome. Eur J Pediatr 132:93, 1979
34. KORNBERG A, LIEBERMAN I, SIMS ES: Enzymatic synthesis of purine nucleotides. J Biol Chem 215:417, 1955
35. KORN ED, REMY CN, WASILEYKO HC, BUCHANAN JM: Biosynthesis of nucleotides from bases by partially purified enzymes. J Biol Chem 217:875, 1955
36. BUCHANAN JM, HARTMAN SC: Enzymatic reactions in synthesis of the purines. Adv Enzymol 21:199, 1959
37. BUCHANAN JM: The enzymatic synthesis of the purine nucleotides. Harvey Lect 54:104, 1960
38. GUTMAN AB, YU TF: Uric acid metabolism in normal man and in primary gout. N Engl J Med 273:252, 313–321, 1965
39. NIERLICH DP, MAGASANIK B: Regulation of purine ribonucleotide synthesis by end product inhibition: The effect of adenine and guanine ribonucleotides on the 5'-phosphoribosylpyrophosphate amidotransferase of Aerobacter aerogenes. J Biol Chem 240:358, 1965
40. WYNGAARDEN JB, ASHTON DM: The regulation of activity of phosphoribosylpyrophosphate amidotransferase by purine ribonucleotides: A potential feedback control of purine biosynthesis. J Biol Chem 234:1492, 1959
41. CASKEY CT, ASHTON DM, WYNGAARDEN JB: The enzymology of feedback inhibition of glutamine phosphoribosylpyrophosphate amidotransferase by purine ribonucleotides. J Biol Chem 239:270, 1964
42. HENDERSON JF: Feedback inhibition of purine biosynthesis in ascites tumor cells. J Biol Chem 237:2631, 1962
43. HOLMES EW, MCDONALD JA, MCCORD MM, WYNGAARDEN JB, KELLEY WN: Human glutamine phosphoribosylpyrophosphate amidotransferase: Kinetic and regulatory properties. J Biol Chem 248:144, 1973
44. WOOD AW, SEEGMILLER JE: Properties of 5-phosphoribosyl-l-pyrophosphate amidotransferase from human lymphoblasts. J Biol Chem 248:138, 1973

45. HOLMES EW, WYNGAARDEN JB, KELLEY WN: Human glutamine phosphoribosylpyrophosphate amidotransferase: Two molecular forms interconvertible by purine ribonucleotide and phosphoribosylpyrophosphate. *J Biol Chem* 248:6035, 1973

46. HOWARD WJ, APPEL SI: Control of purine biosynthesis: FGAR amidotransferase (abstract). *Clin Res* 16:344, 1968

47. KELLEY WN, FOX IH, WYNGAARDEN JB: Regulation of purine biosynthesis in cultured human cells. I. Effects of orotic acid. *Biochim Biophys Acta* 215:512, 1970

48. KELLEY WN, FOX IH, WYNGAARDEN JB: Essential role of phosphoribosylpyrophosphate (PRPP) in regulation of purine biosynthesis in cultured human fibroblasts. *Clin Res* 18:457, 1970

49. FOX, IH, KELLEY WN: Phosphoribosylpyrophosphate in man: Biochemical and clinical significance. *Ann Intern Med* 74:424, 1971

50. KELLEY WN, GREENE ML, FOX IH, ROSENBLOOM FM, LEVY RH, SEEGMILLER JE: Effects of orotic acid on purine and lipoprotein metabolism in man. *Metabolism* 19:1025, 1970

51. SPERLING O, BROSH S, BOER P, KUPFER B, BENJAMIN D, WEINBERGER A, PINKHAS J: De novo synthesis of purine nucleotides and metabolic availability of phosphoribosylpyrophosphate in leukemic leukocytes. *Biomedicine* 31:20, 1979

52. HENDERSON JF, KHOO MKY: Synthesis of 5-phosphoribosyl-l-pyrophosphate from glucose in Ehrlich ascites tumor cells in vitro. *J Biol Chem* 240:2349, 1965

53. LINDSAY RH, ASH AG, HILL JB: TSH stimulation of orotic acid conversion of pyrimidine nucleotides and RNA in bovine thyroid. *Endocrinology* 84:534, 1969

54. ROTTMAN F, GUARINO AJ: The inhibition of phosphoribosylpyrophosphate amidotransferase activity by cordecepin monophosphate. *Biochim Biophys Acta* 89:465, 1964

55. NAGY M: Regulation of the biosynthesis of purine nucleotides in Schizosaccharomyces pombe. I. Properties of the phosphoribosylpyrophosphate glutamine amidotransferase of the wild strain and of a mutant desensitized towards feedback modifiers. *Biochim Biophys Acta* 198:471, 1970

56. ROWE PB, COLEMAN MD, WYNGAARDEN JB: Glutamine phosphoribosylpyrophosphate amidotransferase: Catalytic and conformational heterogeneity of the pigeon liver enzyme. *Biochemistry* 9:1498, 1970

57. ITAKURA M, SABINA RL, HEALD PW, HOLMES EW: Basis for the control of purine biosynthesis by purine ribonucleotides. *J Clin Invest* 67:994, 1981

58. MAGASANIK B, KARIBIAN D: Purine nucleotide cycles and their metabolic role. *J Biol Chem* 235:2672, 1960

59. MAGER J, MAGASANIK B: Guanosine 5'-phosphate reductase and its role in the interconversion of purine nucleotides. *J Biol Chem* 235:1474, 1960

60. WYNGAARDEN JB, GREENLAND RA: The inhibition of succinoadenylate kinosynthetase of *Escherichia coli* by adenosine and guanosine 5'-monophosphates. *J Biol Chem* 238:1054, 1963

61. VAN DER WEYDEN MB, KELLEY WN: Human adenylosuccinate synthetase: Partial purification, kinetic and regulatory properties of the enzyme from placenta. *J Biol Chem* 249:7282, 1974

62. HOLMES EW, PEHLKE DM, KELLEY WN: The role of human inosinic acid dehydrogenase in the control of purine biosynthesis de novo. *Biochim Biophys Acta* 364:209, 1974

63. HENDERSON JF: Kinetic properties of hypoxanthine-guanine and adenine phosphoribosyltransferase. *Fed Proc* 27:1053, 1968

64. KRENITSKY TA, PAPAIOANNOU R, ELION GB: Human hypoxanthine phosphoribosyltransferase. I. Purification, properties and specificity. *J Biol Chem* 244:1263, 1969

65. NIERLICH DP, MAGASANIK B: Control by repression of purine biosynthetic enzymes in *Aerobacter aerogenes*. *Fed Proc* 22:476, 1963

66. MOMOSE H, NISHIKAWA H, KATSUYA N: Genetic and biochemical studies of 5'-nucleotide fermentation. II. Repression of enzyme formation in purine nucleotide biosynthesis in *Bacillus subtilis* and derivation of derepressed mutants. *J Gen Appl Microbiol* 11:211, 1965

67. ROSENBLOOM FM, KELLEY WN, MILLER J, HENDERSON JF, SEEGMILLER JE: Inherited disorder of purine metabolism: Correlation between central nervous system dysfunction and biochemical defects. *JAMA* 202:175, 1967

68. KELLEY WN: Hypoxanthine-guanine phosphoribosyltransferase deficiency in the Lesch-Nyhan syndrome and gout. *Fed Proc* 27:1047, 1968

69. HENDERSON JF, BROX LW, KELLEY WN, ROSENBLOOM FM, SEEGMILLER JE: Kinetic studies of hypoxanthine-guanine phosphoribosyltransferase. *J Biol Chem* 243:2514, 1969

70. MCDONALD JA, KELLEY WN: Lesch-Nyhan syndrome: Altered kinetic properties of mutant enzyme. *Science* 171:689, 1971

71. HAGEN C: Effect of purine analogues on IMP-pyrophosphorylase. *Biochim Biophys Acta* 293:105, 1973

72. GUTENSOHN W, GUROFF G: Hypoxanthine-guanine phosphoribosyltransferase from rat brain (purification kinetic properties, development and distribution). *J Neurochem* 19:2139, 1972

73. HILL DL: Hypoxanthine phosphoribosyltransferase and guanine metabolism of adenocarcinoma 755 cells. *Biochem Pharmacol* 19:545, 1970

74. DEGROODT A, WHITEHEAD EP, HESLOT H, PIORIER L: The substrate specificity of purine phosphoribosyltransferases in *Schizosaccharomyces pompe*. *Biochem J* 122:415, 1971

75. SCHMIDT R, WIEGAND H, REICHERT U: Purification and characterization of the hypoxanthine-guanine phosphoribosyltransferase from *Saccharomyces cerevisiae*. *Eur J Biochem* 93:355, 1979

76. GOTS JS, BENSON CE, SHUMAS SR: Genetic separation of hypoxanthine and guanine-xanthine phosphoribosyltransferase activities by deletion mutations in *Salmonella typhimurium*. *J Bacteriol* 112:910, 1972

77. CHOU JY, MARTIN RG: Purine phosphoribosyltransferases of *Salmonella typhimurium*. *J Bacteriol* 112:1010, 1972

78. MILLER RL, RAMSEY GA, KRENITSKY TA, ELION GB: Guanine phosphoribosyltransferase from *Escherichia coli*, specificity and properties. *Biochemistry* 11:4723, 1972

79. TUTTLE JV, KRENITSKY TA: Purine phosphoribosyltransferase from *Leishmania donovani*. *J Biol Chem* 255:909, 1980

80. CRAFT JA, DEAN BM, WATTS RWE, WESTWICK WJ: Studies on human erythrocyte IMP: pyrophosphate phosphoribosyltransferase. *Eur J Biochem* 15:367, 1970

81. SALERNO C, GIACOMELLO A: Human hypoxanthine guanine phosphoribosyltransferase. The role of magnesium ion in a phosphoribosylpyrophosphate-utilizing enzyme. *J Biol Chem* 256:3671, 1981

82. JOHNSON LA, GORDON RB, EMMERSON BT: Inactivation of hypoxanthine guanine phosphoribosyltransferase by guanosine dialdehyde: An active site directed inhibitor. *Biochem Med* 22:33, 1979

83. GUTENSOHN W, JAHN H: Irreversible inhibition of hypoxanthine phosphoribosyltransferase: Further studies on the specificity of periodate-oxidized GMP. *Hoppe-Seyler's Z Physiol Chem* 358:939, 1977

84. KRENITSKY TA: Tissue distribution of purine ribosyl- and phosphoribosyltransferases in the rhesus monkey. *Biochim Biophys Acta* 179:506, 1969

85. MURRAY AW: Purine-phosphoribosyltransferase activities in rat and mouse tissues and in Ehrlich ascites-tumor cells. *Biochem J* 100:664, 1966

86. ADAMS A, HARKNESS RA: Developmental changes in purine phosphoribosyltransferases in human and rat tissues. *Biochem J* 160:565, 1976

87. ALLSOP J, WATTS RWE: Activities of amidophosphoribosyltransferase (EC 2.4.2.14) and the purine phosphoribosyltransferases (EC 2.4.2.7 and 2.4.2.8), and the phoshoribosylpyrophosphate content of rat central nervous system at different stages of development. *J Neurol Sci* 46:221, 1980

88. EPSTEIN CJ: Phosphoribosyltransferase activity during early mammalian development. *J Biol Chem* 245:3289, 1970

89. SMITH JL, OMURA GA, KRAKOFF IH, BALIS ME: IMP and AMP: Pyrophosphate phosphoribosyltransferase in leukemic and normal human hematocytes. *Proc Soc Exp Biol Med* 136:1299, 1971

90. RAIVIO KO, HOVI T: Purine reutilization in phytohemagglutin in stimulated human T-lymphocytes. *Exper Cell Res* 116:75, 1978

91. ARNOLD WJ, KELLEY WN: Human hypoxanthine-guanine phosphoribosyltransferase: Purification and subunit structure. *J Biol Chem* 246:7398, 1971

92. OLSEN AS, MILMAN G: Subunit molecular weight of human hypoxanthine-guanine phosphoribosyltransferase. *J Biol Chem* 249:4038, 1974

93. STRAUSS M: Determination of the subunit molecular weight of hypoxanthine-guanine phosphoribosyltransferase from human erythrocytes by recovery of enzyme activity from sodium dodecyl sulphate gels. *Biochim Biophys Acta* 410:426, 1975

94. MUENSCH H, YOSHIDA A: Purification and characterization of human hypoxanthine/guanine phosphoribosyltransferase. *Eur J Biochem* 76:107, 1977

95. HOLDEN JA, KELLEY WN: Human hypoxanthine-guanine phosphoribosyltransferase: Evidence for tetrameric structure. *J Biol Chem* 253:4459, 1978

96. HUGHES SH, WAHL GM, CAPECCHI MR: Purification and characterization of mouse hypoxanthine-guanine phosphoribosyltransferase. *J Biol Chem* 250:120, 1975

97. JOHNSON GG, EISENBERG LR, MIGEON BR: Human and mouse hypoxanthine-guanine phosphoribosyltransferase: Dimers and tetramers. *Science* 203:174, 1979

98. OLSEN, AS, MILMAN G: Chinese hamster hypoxanthine-guanine phosphoribosyltransferase. *J Biol Chem* 249:4030, 1974

99. GUTENSOHN W, HUBER M, JAHN H: Facilitated purification of hypoxanthine phosphoribosyltransferase. *Hoppe-Seyler's Z Physiol Chem* 357:1379, 1976

100. NATSUMEDA Y, YOSHINO M, TSUSHIMA K: Hypoxanthine-guanine phosphoribosyltransferase from rat liver: Effects of magnesium 5-phosphoribosyl-1-pyrophosphate on the chemical modification and stability of the enzyme. *Biochim Biophys Acta* 483:63, 1977

101. HELD KR, KAHAN B, DEMARS R: Adenine phosphoribosyltransferase and hypoxanthine-guanine phosphoribosyltransferase immunoprecipitation reactions in human-mouse and human-hamster cell hybrids. *Humangenetik* 30:23, 1975

102. ARNOLD WJ, CASKEY CT, KELLEY WN: Unpublished observation
103. KELLEY WN, ARNOLD WJ: Human hypoxanthine-guanine phosphoribo-syltransferase: Studies on the normal and mutant forms of the enzyme. *Fed Proc* 32:1656, 1973
104. DAVIES MR, DEAN BM: The heterogeneity of erythrocyte IMP: Pyrophosphate phosphoribosyltransferase and purine nucleoside phosphorylase by isoelectric focusing. *FEBS Lett* 18:283, 1971
105. MULLER MM, STEMBERGER H: Immunological studies of hypoxanthine-guanine phosphoribosyltransferase in Lesch-Nyhan syndrome, in Sperling O, DeVries A, Wyngaarden JB (eds): *Purine Metabolism in Man.* New York, Plenum, 1974 p 187
106. BAKAY B, NYHAN WL: Heterogeneity of hypoxanthine guanine phospho-ribosyltransferase from human erythrocytes. *Arch Biochem Biophys* 168:26, 1975
107. RUBIN CS, DANCIS J, YIP LC, NOWINSKI RC, BALIS ME: Purification of IMP: Pyrophosphate phosphoribosyltransferases, catalytically incompe-tent enzymes in Lesch-Nyhan disease. *Proc Natl Acad Sci USA* 68:1461, 1971
108. BAKAY B, NYHAN WL: The separation of adenine and hypoxanthine-guanine phosphoribosyl transferases isoenzymes by disc gel. *Biochem Genet* 5:81, 1971
109. WILSON JM, KELLEY WN: Unpublished observation
110. ZANNIS VI, GUDAS LJ, MARTIN DW JR: Characterization of the subunit composition of HGPRTase from human erythrocytes and cultured fibro-blasts. *Biochem Genet* 18:1, 1980
111. NESBITT MN, BAKAY B, BOHDAN, GARDNER MB, DAY C: Isoenzyme pattern of HPRT in murine erythrocytes: Control by an autosomal locus. *Biochem Genet* 17:957, 1979
112. DAVIDSON JD, BRADLEY TR, ROOSA RA, LAW LW: Purine nucleotide pyrophosphorylases in 8-azaguanine-sensitive and resistant P 388 leuke-mias. *Natl Cancer Inst Monogr* 29:789, 1962
113. LITTLEFIELD JW: The inosinic acid pyrophosphorylase activity of mouse fibroblasts partially resistant to 8-azaguanine. *Proc Natl Acad Sci USA* 50:568, 1963
114. BROCKMAN RW, DEBOVADI CS, STUTTS P, HUTCHINSON DJ: Purine ribo-nucleotide pyrophosphorylase and resistance to purine analogues in *Strep-tococcus faecalis. J Biol Chem* 236:1471, 1961
115. SZYBALSKA W, SZYBALSKI EH: Drug sensitivity as a genetic marker for human cell lines. *Univ Mich Med Bull* 28:277, 1962
116. LITTLEFIELD JW: Selection of hybrids from matings of fibroblasts in vitro and their presumed recombinants. *Science* 145:709, 1964
117. FUJIMOTO WY, SEEGMILLER JE: Hypoxanthine-guanine phosphoribosyl-transferase deficiency: Activity in normal, mutant and heterozygote cul-tured human skin fibroblasts. *Proc Natl Acad Sci USA* 65:577, 1970
118. KELLEY WN, MEADE JC: Studies on hypoxanthine-guanine phosphoribo-syltransferase in fibroblasts from patients with the Lesch-Nyhan syn-drome: Evidence for genetic heterogeneity. *J Biol Chem* 246:2953, 1971
119. ARNOLD WJ, MEADE JC, KELLEY WN: Hypoxanthine-guanine phospho-ribosyltransferase: Characteristics of the mutant enzyme in erythrocytes from patients with the Lesch-Nyhan syndrome. *J Clin Invest* 51:1805, 1972
120. MIZUNO T, SEGAWA M, KURUMADA T, MARUYAMA H, ONISAWA J: Clin-ical and therapeutic aspects of the Lesch-Nyhan syndrome in Japanese children. *Neuropaediatrie* 2:38, 1970
121. SORENSEN LB: Mechanism of excessive purine biosynthesis in hypoxan-thine-guanine phosphoribosyltransferase deficiency. *J Clin Invest* 49:968, 1970
122. DANCIS J, YIP LC, COX RP, PIOMELLI S, BALIS ME: Disparate enzyme activity in erythrocytes and hematocytes: A variant of hypoxanthine phos-phoribosyltransferase deficiency with an unstable enzyme. *J Clin Invest* 52:2068, 1973
123. UITENDAAL MP, DEBRUYN CHMM, OEI TL, HOSLI P: Molecular and tissue-specific heterogeneity in HPRT deficiency. *Biochem Genet* 16:1187, 1978
124. SPERLING O, BOER P, EILAM G, DEVRIES A: Altered kinetic properties of erythrocyte phoshoribosylpyrophosphate synthetase in excessive purine production. *Eur J Clin Biol Res* 17:703, 1972
125. BALIS ME, YIP LC, YU TF, GUTMAN AB, COX R, DANCIS J: Unstable HPRTase in subjects with abnormal urinary oxypurine excretion, in Sperl-ing O, DeVries A, Wyngaarden JB (eds): *Purine Metabolism in Man.* New York, Plenum, 1974, p 195
126. BAKAY B, NYHAN WL: Activation of variants of hypoxanthine-guanine phosphoribosyl transferase by the normal enzyme. *Proc Natl Acad Sci USA* 69:2523, 1972
127. BAKAY B, NYHAN WL: Electrophoretic properties of hypoxanthine-guanine phosphoribosyltransferase in erythrocytes of subjects with Lesch-Nyhan syndrome. *Biochem Genet* 6:139, 1972
128. GUTENSOHN W, JAHN H: Partial deficiency of hypoxanthine-phosphoribo-syltransferase: Evidence for a structural mutation in a patient with gout. *Eur J Clin Invest* 9:43, 1979
129. BENKE PM, HERRICK N: Azaguanine-resistance as a manifestation of a new form of metabolic overproduction of uric acid. *Am J Med* 52:547, 1972
130. SWEETMAN L, BORDEN M, LESH P, BAKAY B, BECKER MA: Diminished affinity for purine substrates as a basis for gout with mild deficiency of hypoxanthine-guanine phosphoribosyltransferase, in Muller MM, Kaiser E, Seegmiller JE (eds): *Purine Metabolism in Man II: Regulation of Path-ways and Enzyme Defects.* New York, Plenum, 1977, p 319
131. KAISER WP, STERMBERGER H, MULLER MM: Der Nachweis von enzym-portein der hypoxanthin-guanin-phosphoribosyltransferase bei Lesch-Nyhan syndrome. *Klin Wochenschr* 51:88, 1973
132. MULLER MM, STERMBERGER H: Biochemische und immulogische unter-suchungen der hypoxanthin-guanin-phosphoribosyltransferase in den erythrozyten von Lesch-Nyhan-patienten. *Wein Klin Wochenschr* 86:127, 1974
133. YIP LC, DANCIS J, METHIESON B, BALIS ME: Age induced changes in adenosine monophosphate: Pyrophosphate phosphoribosyltransferase and inosine monophosphate: Pyrophosphate phosphoribosyltransferase from normal and Lesch-Nyhan erythrocytes. *Biochemistry* 13:2558, 1974
134. UPCHURCH KS, LEYVA A, ARNOLD WJ, HOLMES EW, KELLEY WN: Hypo-xanthine-guanine phosphoribosyltransferase deficiency: Association of reduced catalytic activity with reduced levels of immunologically detect-able enzyme protein. *Proc Natl Acad Sci USA* 72:4142, 1975
135. GHANGAS GS, MILMAN G: Radioimmune determination of hypoxanthine phosphoribosyltransferase cross-reacting material in erythrocytes of Lesch-Nyhan patients. *Proc Natl Acad Sci USA* 72:4147, 1975
136. WILSON JM, BAUGHER BW, LANDA L, KELLEY WN: Human hypoxan-thine-guanine phosphoribosyltransferase: Purification and characteriza-tion of mutant forms of the enzyme. *J Biol Chem* 256:10306, 1981
137. BAKAY B, GRAF M, CAREY S, NYHAN WL: Study of immunoreactive mate-rial in patients with deficient HPRT activity, in Muller MM, Kaiser E, Seegmiller JE (eds): *Purine Metabolism in Man II: Regulation of Pathways and Enzyme Defects.* New York, Plenum, 1977, p 361
138. CAPECCHI MR, CAPECCHI NE, HUGHES SH, WAHL G: Selective degrada-tion of abnormal protein in mammalian tissue culture cells. *Proc Natl Acad Sci USA* 71:4732, 1974
139. RIJKSEN G, STAAL GEJ, VANDERVLIST MJM, BEEMER FA, TPOOST J, GUTENSOHN W, VAN LAARHOVEN JPRM, DEBRUYN CHMM: Partial hypoxanthine-guanine phosphoribosyl transferase deficiency with full expression of the Lesch-Nyhan syndrome. *Hum Genet* 57:39, 1981
139a. WILSON JM, BAUGHER BW, MATTES PM, DADDONA PE, KELLEY WN: Human hypoxanthine-guanine phosphoribosyltransferase: Demonstration of structural variants in lymphoblastoid cells derived from patients with a deficiency of the enzyme. *J Clin Invest* (in press)
140. WAHL GM, HUGHES SH, CAPECCHI MR: Immunological characterization of hypoxanthine-guanine phosphoribosyl transferase mutants of mouse L cells: Evidence for mutations at different loci in the HGPRT gene. *J Cell Physiol* 85:307, 1974
141. BEAUDET AL, ROUFA DJ, CASKEY CT: Mutations affecting the structure of hypoxanthine: Guanine phosphoribosyltransferase in cultured Chinese hamster cells. *Proc Natl Acad Sci USA* 70:320, 1973
142. FENWICK RG JR, CASKEY CT: Mutant Chinese hamster cells with a ther-mosensitive hypoxanthine-guanine phosphoribosyltransferase. *Cell* 5:115, 1975
143. KRUH GD, FENWICK RG, CASKEY CT: Structural analysis of mutant and revertant forms of Chinese hamster hypoxanthine-guanine phosphoribo-syltransferase. *J Biol Chem* 256:2878, 1981
144. FENWICK RG, SAWYER TH, KRUH GD, ASTRIN KH, CASKEY CT: Forward and reverse mutations affecting the kinetics and apparent molecular weight of mammalian HGPRT. *Cell* 12:383, 1977
145. EPSTEIN J, LEYVA A, KELLEY WN, LITTLEFIELD JW: Mutagen-induced dip-loid human lymphoblast variants containing altered hypoxanthine guanine phosphoribosyltransferase. *Somatic Cell Genet* 3:135, 1977
146. GREENE ML, BOYLE JA, SEEGMILLER JE: Substrate stabilization: Geneti-cally controlled reciprocal relationship of 2 human enzymes. *Science* 167:337, 1970
147. RUBIN CS, BALIS ME, PIOMELLI S, BERMAN PH, DANCIS J: Elevated AMP pyrophosphorylase activity in congenital IMP pyrophosphorylase defi-ciency (Lesch-Nyhan disease). *J Lab Clin Med* 74:732, 1969
148. GORDON RB, THOMPSON L, EMMERSON BT: Erythrocyte phosphoribosyl-pyrophosphate concentrations in heterozygotes for hypoxanthine-guanine phosphoribosyltransferase deficiency. *Metabolism* 23:921, 1974
149. KELLEY WN: Studies on the adenine phosphoribosyltransferase enzyme in human fibroblasts lacking hypoxanthine-guanine phosphoribosyltransfer-ase. *J Lab Clin Med* 77:33, 1971
150. WOOD AW, BECKER MA, MINNA JD, SEEGMILLER JE: Purine metabolism in normal and thioguanine-resistant neuroblastoma. *Proc Natl Acad Sci USA* 70:3880, 1973
151. NUKI G, LEVER J, SEEGMILLER JE: Biochemical characteristics of 8-aza-guanine resistant human lymphoblast mutants selected in vitro, in Sperling O, DeVries A, Wyngaarden JB (eds): *Purine Metabolism in Man.* New York, Plenum, 1974, p 255
152. WOOD AW, BECKER MA, SEEGMILLER JE: Purine nucleotide synthesis in lymphoblasts cultured from normal subjects and a patient with Lesch-Nyhan syndrome. *Biochem Genet* 9:261, 1973

153. SPERLING O, EILAM G, BROSH SP, DEVRIES A: Accelerated erythrocyte synthesis: A familial abnormality associated with excessive uric acid production and gout. *Biochem Med* 6:310, 1972

154. BECKER MA, MEYER LJ, SEEGMILLER JE: Gout with purine overproduction due to increased phosphoribosylpyrophosphate synthetase activity. *Am J Med* 55:232, 1973

155. ITIABA K, MELANCON SB, DALLAIRE L, CRAWHALL JC: Adenine phosphoribosyl transferase deficiency in association with subnormal hypoxanthine phosphoribosyl transferase in families of Lesch-Nyhan patients. *Biochem Med* 19:252, 1978

156. PEHLKE DM, MCDONALD JA, HOLMES EW, KELLEY WN: Inosinic acid dehydrogenase activity in the Lesch-Nyhan syndrome. *J Clin Invest* 51:1398, 1972

157. SWEETMAN L, NYHAN WL: Further studies of the enzyme composition of mutant cells in X-linked uric aciduria. *Arch Intern Med* 130:214, 1974

158. LOMMEN EJP, DEABREU RA, TRIJBELS JMF, SCHRETLEN EDAM: The IMP dehydrogenase catalysed reaction in erythrocytes of normal individuals and patients with hypoxanthine-guanine phosphoribosyltransferase deficiency. *Acta Paediatr Scand* 63:140, 1974

159. LOMMEN EJP, VOGELS GD, VAN DER ZEE SPM, TRIJBELS JMF, SCHRETLEN EDAM: Concentrations of purine nucleotides in erythrocytes of patients with the Lesch-Nyhan syndrome before and during oral administration of adenine. *Acta Paediatr Scand* 60:642, 1971

160. RIVARD GE, IZADI P, LAZERGON J, MCLAREN JD, PARKER C, FISH CH: Functional and metabolic studies of platelets from patients with Lesch-Nyhan syndrome. *Br J Haematol* 31:245, 1975

161. BEARDMORE TD, MEADE JC, KELLEY WN: Increased activity of two enzymes of pyrimidine biosynthesis de novo in erythrocytes from patients with the Lesch-Nyhan syndrome. *J Lab Clin Med* 81:43, 1973

162. FOX RM, ROYSE-SMITH D, O'SULLIVAN WJ: Orotidinuria induced by allopurinol. *Science* 168:861, 1970

163. BEARDMORE TD, CASHMAN JS, KELLEY WN: Mechanism of allopurinol mediated increase in enzyme activity in man. *J Clin Invest* 51:1823, 1972

164. MARTINEZ-RAMON A, GRISOLIA S: Increased incorporation of aspartate and decreased incorporation of orotate in fibroblasts from Lesch-Nyhan patients as revealed by autoradiography. *Biochem Biophys Res Comm* 96:1011, 1980

165. MARTIN DW, GRAF LH, MCROBERTS JA, HARRISON TM: Evidence that the gene for hypoxanthine-guanine phosphoribosyltransferase controls the concentration of the enzyme, phosphoribosylpyrophosphate synthetase, abstracted. *Clin Res* 23:263A, 1975

166. REEM GH: Purine metabolism in murine virus-induced erythroleukemic cells during differentiation in vitro. *Proc Natl Acad Sci USA* 72:1630, 1975

167. TORRELIO BM, PAZ MA: Increased phosphoribosylpyrophosphate synthetase activity in fibroblasts of hypoxanthine-guanine phosphoribosyl transferase deficient patients. *Biochem Biophys Res Comm* 87:380, 1979

168. LEYVA A, HOLMES, EW, KELLEY WN: Unpublished observations

169. ROSENBLOOM FM, HENDERSON JF, CALDWELL IC, KELLEY WN, SEEGMILLER JE: Biochemical basis of accelerated purine biosynthesis de novo in human fibroblasts lacking hypoxanthine-guanine phosphoribosyltransferase. *J Biol Chem* 243:1166, 1968

170. NUKI G, ASTRIN K, BRENTON D, CRUIKSHANK M, LEVER J, SEEGMILLER JE: Purine and pyrimidine nucleotide pools in azaguanine resistant human lymphoblasts deficient in HGPRT, abstracted. *Am J Hum Genet* 25:56A, 1973

171. TATIBANA M, KATSUYA S: Control of pyrimidine biosynthesis in mammalian tissues. V. Regulation of glutamine-dependent carbamyl phosphate synthetse: Activation by 5-phosphoribosyl-1-pyrophosphate and inhibition by uridine triphosphate. *J Biochem (Tokyo)* 72:549, 1972

172. SHOAF WT, JONES E: Uridylic acid synthesis in Ehrlich ascites carcinoma: Properties, subcellular distribution, and nature of enzyme complexes of the six biosynthetic enzymes. *Biochemistry* 12:4039, 1973

173. WATSON B, GORMLEY IP, GARDINER SE, EVANS HJ, HARRIS H: Reappearance of murine hypoxanthine-guanine phosphoribosyltransferase activity in mouse A9 cells after attempted hybridization with human cell lines. *Exp Cell Res* 75:401, 1972

174. BAKAY B, CROCE CM, KOPROWSKI H, NYHAN WL: Restoration of hypoxanthine phosphoribosyltransferase activity in mouse IR cells after fusion with chick embryo fibroblasts. *Proc Natl Acad Sci USA* 70:1998, 1973

175. BAKAY B, NYHAN WL, CROCE CM, KOPROWSKI H: Reversion in expression of hypoxanthine-guanine phosphoribosyltransferase following cell hybridization. *J Cell Sci* 17:567, 1975

176. SEKIGUGHI T, SEKIGUCHI R: Interallelic complementation in hybrid cells derived from Chinese hamster diploid clones deficient in hypoxanthine-guanine phosphoribosyltransferase activity. *Exp Cell Res* 77:391, 1973

177. SZYBALSKI EH, SZYBALSKA W: Genetics of human cell lives. IV. DNA-mediated heritable transformation of a biochemical trait. *Proc Natl Acad Sci USA* 48:2026, 1962

178. FRIEDMAN T, SUBAK-SHARPE JH, FUJIMOTO W, SEEGMILLER JE: The possible DNA-mediated abortive transformation of human fibroblasts in tissue culture, abstracted. *Am J Hum Genet* p 525, 1969

179. MCBRIDE OW, OZER HL: Transfer of genetic information by purified metaphase chromosomes. *Proc Natl Acad Sci USA* 70:1258, 1973

180. WULLEMS GJ, VAN DER HORST K, BOTTSMA D: Incorporation of isolated chromosomes and induction of hypoxanthine phosphoribosyltransferase in Chinese hamster cells. *Somatic Cell Genet* 1:137, 1975

181. GOSS SJ, HARRIS H: New method for mapping genes in human chromosomes. *Nature* 255(5511):680, 1975

182. SUBAK-SHARPE H, BURK RR, PITTS JD: Metabolic cooperation by cell to cell transfer between genetically different mammalian cells in tissue culture. *Heredity* 21:342, 1966

183. FRIEDMAN T, SEEGMILLER JE, SUBAK-SHARPE JH: Metabolic cooperation between genetically marked human fibroblasts in tissue culture. *Nature* 220:272, 1968

184. SUBAK-SHARPE JH, BURK RR, PITTS JD: Metabolic cooperation between biochemically marked mammalian cells in tissue culture. *J Cell Sci* 4:353, 1969

185. DANCIS J, COX RP, BERMAN PH, JANSEN V, BALIS ME: Cell population density and phenotypic expression of tissue culture fibroblasts from heterozygotes of Lesch-Nyhan disease (inosinate pyrophosphorylase deficiency). *Biochem Genet* 3:609, 1969

186. COX RP, KRAUSS MR, BALIS ME, DANCIS J: Evidence for transfer of enzyme production as the basis of metabolic cooperation between tissue culture fibroblasts of Lesch-Nyhan disease and normal cells. *Proc Natl Acad Sci USA* 67:1573, 1970

187. PITTS JD: Molecular exchange and growth control in tissue culture, in Wolstenholme GEW, Knight J (eds): *Ciba Foundation on Growth Control in Cell Cultures.* London, Churchill and Livingstone, 1971, p 89

188. COX RP, KRAUSS MR, BALIS ME, DANCIS J: Communication between normal and enzyme deficient cells in tissue culture. *Exp Cell Res* 74:251, 1972

189. VANZEELAND AA, VANDIGGELEN MCE, SIMONS JWIM: Effect of calf serum on toxicity of 8-azaguanine. *Mutat Res* 14:355, 1972

190. COX RP, KRAUSS MR, BALIS ME, DANCIS J: Metabolic cooperation in cell culture: Studies of the mechanisms of cell interaction. *J Cell Physiol* 84:237, 1974

191. BOLS NC, KANE AB, RINGERTZ NR: Restoration of metabolic cooperation in heterokaryons between HGPRT-deficient mouse A9 fibroblasts and chick embryo erythrocytes. *Somatic Cell Genet* 5:1045, 1979

192. OEI TL, DEBRUYN CHMM: Studies on metabolic cooperation using different types of normal and hypoxanthine-guanine, phosphoribosyltransferase (HGPRT) deficient cells, in Sperling O, DeVries A, Wyngaarden JB (eds): *Purine Metabolism in Man.* New York, Plenum, 1974, p 237

193. ASHKENZAI YE, GARTLER SM: A study of metabolic cooperation utilizing human mutant fibroblasts. *Exp Cell Res* 64:9, 1971

194. FURUSAWA M, NISHIMURA T, YAMAIZUMI M, OKADA Y: Injection of foreign substances into single cells by cell fusion. *Nature* 249:449, 1974

195. LOYTER A, ZAKAI N, KULKA RG: "Ultramicroinjection" of macromolecular or small particles into animal cells: A new technique based on virus-induced cell fusion. *J Cell Biol* 66:292, 1975

196. SCHLEGEL RA, RECHSTEINER MC: Microinjection of thymidine kinase and mammalian cells by fusion with red blood cells. *Cell* 5:371, 1975

197. KALTOFT K, CELIS JE: Ghost mediated transfer of human hypoxanthine-guanine phosphoribosyltransferase into deficient chinese hamster ovary cells by means of polyethylene glycol-induced fusion. *Exper Cell Res* 115:423, 1978.

198. CAPECCHI MR, VON DER HAAR RA, CAPECCHI NE, SVEDA MM: The isolation of a suppressible nonsense mutant in mammalian cells. *Cell* 12:371, 1977

199. BALIS ME, KRAKOFF IH, BERMAN PH, DANCIS J: Urinary metabolites in congenital hyperuricosuria. *Science* 156:1122, 1967

200. BALIS ME: Aspects of purine metabolism. *Fed Proc* 27:1067, 1968

201. NEWCOMBE DS, LAPES M, THOMSON C, WRIGHT EY: Urinary excretion of 4-amino-5-imidazolecarboxamide in X-linked primary hyperuricemia. *Clin Res* 15:45, 1967

202. PIGNERO A, GILIBERTI P, TANCREDI F: Effect of the treatment with folic acid on urinary excretion pattern of aminoimidazolecarboxamide in the Lesch-Nyhan syndrome, in *Perspectives in Inherited Metabolic Diseases,* vol 1, 1978

203. HERBERT V, STREIFF RR, SULLIVAN LW, MCGEER PL: Deranged purine metabolism manifested by aminoimidazolecarboxamide excretion in megaloblastic anemias, hemolytic anemia, and liver disease. *Lancet* 2:45, 1964

204. HERSHFIELD MS, SEEGMILLER JE: Regulation of de novo purine synthesis in human lymphoblast. *J Biol Chem* 252:6002, 1977

205. SNYDER FF, CRUIKSHANK MK, SEEGMILLER JE: A comparison of purine metabolism and nucleotide pools in normal and hypoxanthine-guanine phosphoribosyltransferase-deficient neuroblastoma cells. *Biochim Biophys Acta* 543:556, 1978

206. EDWARDS NL, RECKER D, FOX IH: Overproduction of uric acid in hypo-

xanthine-guanine phosphoribosyltransferase contribution by impaired purine salvage. *J Clin Invest* 63:922, 1979

207. SPERLING O, BROSH S, DE VRIES A: Synthesis of purine nucleotides in leukocytes from normal and hypoxanthine-guanine phosphoribosyltransferase-deficient subjects. *Isr J Med Sci* 11:1221, 1975

208. POMPUCCI RM, MICHELI V: Evidence for purine biosynthesis in human leukocytes. *Experientia* 31:1137, 1975

209. ROSENBLOOM FM, HENDERSON JF, KELLEY WN, SEEGMILLER JE: Accelerated purine biosynthesis de novo in skin fibroblasts deficient in hypoxanthine-guanine phosphoribosyltransferase activity. *Biochim Biophys Acta* 166:258, 1968

210. TAYLOR MW, TOKITO M, GUPTA KC: Lack of enhanced purine biosynthesis in HGPRT and Lesch-Nyhan cells. *Hum Hered* 29:187, 1979

210a. ZOREF SHANI E, SPERLING O: Characterization of purine nucleotide metabolism in cultured fibroblasts with deficiency of hypoxanthine-guanine phosphoribosyl transferase and with super activity of phosphoribosylpyrophosphate synthetase. *Enzyme* 25:413, 1980

211. HOWARD WJ, KERSON LA, APPEL SH: Synthesis de novo of purines in slices of rat brain and liver. *J Neurochem* 17:121, 1970

212. SWEETMAN L: Urinary and cerebrospinal fluid oxypurine levels and allopurinol metabolism in the Lesch-Nyhan syndrome. *Fed Proc* 27:1055, 1967

213. LASSEN UV: Hypoxanthine transport in human erythrocytes. *Biochim Biophys Acta* 135:146, 1967

214. BERLIN RD: Purine: Active transport by isolated choroid plexus. *Science* 163:1194, 1969

215. WYNGAARDEN JB: Hereditary xanthinuria, in Stanbury JB, Wyngaarden JB, Fredrickson DS (eds): *The Metabolic Basis of Inherited Diseases*, 4th ed. New York, McGraw-Hill, 1978

216. BOYD EM, DOLMAN M, KNIGHT LM, SHEPPARD EP: The chronic oral toxicity of caffeine. *Can J Physiol Pharmacol* 43:995, 1965

217. ROSENBLOOM FM, KELLEY WN, SEEGMILLER JE: Unpublished results

218. UNGERSTEDT V: Postsynaptic supersensitivity after 6-hydroxydopamine induced degeneration of the nigrostriatal dopamine system. *Acta Physiol Scand* 367:69, 1971

219. ROCKSON S, STONE R, VAN DER WEYDEN M, KELLEY WN: Lesch-Nyhan syndrome: Evidence for abnormal adrenergic function. *Science* 186:934, 1974

220. LAKE CR, ZIEGLER MG: Lesch-Nyhan syndrome: Low dopamine-β-hydroxylase activity and diminished sympathetic response to stress and posture. *Science* 196:905, 1977

221. BREAKEFIELD XO, CASTIGLIONE CM, EDELSTEIN SB: Monoamine oxidase activity decreased in cells lacking hypoxanthine phosphoribosyltransferase activity. *Science* 192:1018, 1976

222. ROTH JA, BREAKEFIELD XO, CASTIGLIONE CM: Monamine oxidase and catechol-o-methyltransferase in cultured human skin fibroblasts. *Life Sciences* 19:1705, 1976

223. SKAPER SD, SEEGMILLER JE: Hypoxanthine-guanine phosphoribosyltransferase mutant glioma cells: Diminished monoamine oxidase activity. *Science* 194:1171, 1976

224. EDELSTEIN SB, CASTIGLIONE CM, BREAKEFIELD XO: Monoamine oxidase activity in normal and Lesch-Nyhan fibroblasts. *J Neurochem* 31:1247, 1978

225. SINGH S, WILLER I, KLUSS EM, GOEDDE HW: Monoamine oxidase and catechol-o-methyltransferase activity in cultured fibroblasts from patients with maple syrup urine disease, Lesch-Nyhan syndrome and healthy controls. *Clin Genet* 15:153, 1979

225a. LLOYD KG, HORNYKIEWICZ O, DAVIDSON L, SHANNAK K, FARLEY I, GOLDSTEIN M, SHIBUYA M, KELLEY WN, FOX IH: Biochemical evidence of dysfunction of brain neurotransmitters in the Lesch-Nyhan syndrome. *N Engl J Med* 305:1106, 1981

226. MCKERAN RO, HOWELL A, ANDREWS TM, WATTS RWE, ARLETT CF: Observations on the growth in vitro of myeloid progenitor cells and fibroblasts from hemizygotes and heterozygotes for "complete" and "partial" HGPRT deficiency, and their relevance to the pathogenesis of brain damage in the Lesch-Nyhan syndrome. *J Neurol Sci* 22:183, 1974

227. ROUFOGALIS BD, THORNTON M, WADE DN: Nucleotide requirement of dopamine sensitive adenylate cyclase in synaptosomal membranes from the striatum of rat brain. *J Neurochem* 27:1533, 1976

228. NIEOULLON A, CHERAMY A, GLOWINSKI J: Nigral and striatal dopamine release under sensory stimuli. *Nature* 269:340, 1977

229. BUFF K, DAIRMAN W: Biosynthesis of biopterin by two clones of mouse neuroblastoma. *Mol Pharm* 11:87, 1975

230. SKOLNICK P, MARANGOS PJ, GOODWIN FK, EDWARDS M, PAUL S: Identification of inosine and hypoxanthine as endogenous inhibitors of [³H] diazepam binding in the entral nervous system. *Life Sciences* 23:1473, 1978

231. SWEETMAN L, BORDEN M, KULOVICH S, KAUFMAN I, NYHAN WL: Altered excretion of 5-hydroxyindoleacetic acid and glycine in patients with the Lesch-Nyhan disease, in Muller MM, Kaiser E, Seegmiller JE (eds): *Purine Metabolism in Man II: Regulation of Pathways and Enzyme Defects*. New York, Plenum, 1977, p 398

232. FELIX JS, DEMARS R: Purine requirement of cells cultured from humans affected with Lesch-Nyhan syndrome (hypoxanthine-guanine phosphoribosyltransferase deficiency). *Proc Natl Acad Sci USA* 62:536, 1969

233. VAN DER ZEE SPM, SCHRETLEN EDAM, MONNENS LAH: Megaloblastic anemia in the Lesch-Nyhan syndrome. *Lancet* 1:1427, 1968

234. SHAPIRO SL, SHEPPARD GL, DREIFUSS FE, NEWCOMBE DS: X-linked recessive inheritance of a syndrome of mental retardation with hyperuricemia. *Proc Soc Exp Biol Med* 122:609, 1966

235. NYHAN WL, PESEK J, SWEETMAN L, CARPENTER DG, CARTER CH: Genetics of an X-linked disorder of uric acid metabolism and cerebral function. *Pediatr Res* 1:5, 1967

236. ROSENBLOOM FM, KELLEY WN, HENDERSON JF, SEEGMILLER JE: Lyon hypothesis and X-linked disease. *Lancet* 2:305, 1967

237. MIGEON BR, DER KALOUSTIAN VM, NYHAN WL, YOUNG WJ, CHILDS B: X-linked hypoxanthine-guanine phosphoribosyltransferase deficiency: Heterozygote has two clonal populations. *Science* 160:425, 1968

238. SALZMANN J, DEMARS R, BENKE P: Single allele expression at an X-linked hyperuricemia locus in heterozygous human cells. *Proc Natl Acad Sci USA* 60:545, 1968

239. MIGEON BR: X-linked hypoxanthine-guanine phosphoribosyltransferase deficiency: Detection of heterozygotes by selective medium. *Biochem Genet* 4:377, 1970

240. LYON MF: Gene action in the X-chromosome of the mouse (Musmusculus L). *Nature (London)* 190:372, 1961

241. BECKER MA, YEN RCK, ITKIN P: Regional localization of the gene for human phosphoribosylpyrophosphate synthetase on the X-chromosome. *Science* 203:1016, 1979

242. EMMERSON BT, WYNGAARDEN JB: Purine metabolism in heterozygous carriers of hypoxanthine-guanine phosphoribosyltransferase deficiency. *Science* 166:1535, 1969

243. EMMERSON BT: Urate metabolism in heterozygotes of HGPRTase deficiency, in Sperling O, De Vries A, Wyngaarden JB (eds): *Purine Metabolism in Man*. New York, Plenum, 1974, p 237

244. EMMERSON BT, THOMPSON CJ, WALLACE DC: Partial deficiency of hypoxanthine-guanine phosphoribosyltransferase: Intermediate enzyme deficiency in heterozygote red cells. *Ann Intern Med* 76:285, 1972

245. MCDONALD JA, KELLEY WN: Lesch-Nyhan syndrome: Absence of the mutant enzyme in erythrocytes of a heterozygote for both normal and mutant hypoxanthine-guanine phosphoribosyltransferase. *Biochem Genet* 6:21, 1972

246. NYHAN WL, BACKAY B, CONNOR JD, MARKS JF, KEELE DK: Hemizygous expression of glucose-6-phosphate dehydrogenase in erythrocytes of heterozygotes for the Lesch-Nyhan syndrome. *Proc Natl Acad Sci USA* 65:214, 1970

247. DANCIS J, BERMAN PH, JANSEN V, BALIS ME: Absence of mosaicism in the lymphocyte in X-linked congenital hyperuricosuria. *Life Sci* 7:587, 1968

248. ALBERTINI RJ, DEMARS R: Mosaicism of peripheral blood lymphocyte-populations in females heterozygous for the Lesch-Nyhan mutation. *Biochem Genet* 11:397, 1974

249. DEBRUYN CH, OEI TL: Incorporation of ³H-hypoxanthine in phytohemagglutinin-stimulated HGPRT deficient lymphocytes, in Sperling O, De Vries A, Wyngaarden JB (eds): *Purine Metabolism in Man*. New York, Plenum, 1974, p 229

250. GARTLER SM, SCOTT RC, GOLDSTEIN JL, CAMPBELL B: Lesch-Nyhan syndrome: Rapid detection of heterozygotes by the use of hair follicles. *Science* 172:572, 1971

251. GOLDSTEIN JL, MARKS JF, GARTLER SM: Expression of two X-linked genes in human hair follicles of double heterozygotes. *Proc Natl Acad Sci USA* 68:1425, 1971

252. SILVERS DN, COX P, BALIS ME, DANCIS J: Detection of heterozygotes in Lesch-Nyhan disease by hair-root analysis. *N Engl J Med* 286:390, 1972

253. FRANCKE U, BAKAY B, NYHAN WL: Detection of heterozygous carriers of the Lesch-Nyhan syndrome by electrophoresis of hair root lysates. *J Pediatr* 82:472, 1973

254. MCKERAN RO, ANDREWS TM, HOWELL A, GIBBS DA, WATTS RWE: Biochemical studies on the carrier state in the Lesch-Nyhan syndrome, abstracted. *Clin Sci Mol Med* 45:17p, 1973

255. DEBRUYN CHM, OEI TL, TER HAAR BGA: Studies on hair roots for carrier detection in HGPRT deficiency. *Clin Genet* 5:449, 1974

256. KELLEY WN: Unpublished observation

257. FELIX JS, DEMARS R: Detection of females heterozygous for the Lesch-Nyhan mutation by 8-azaguanine-resistant growth of cultured fibroblasts. *J Lab Clin Med* 77:596, 1971

258. FRANCKE U, FELSENSTEIN J, GARTLER SM, MIGEON BR, DANCIS J, SEEGMILLER JE, BAKAY B, NYHAN WL: The occurrence of new mutants in the X-linked recessive Lesch-Nyhan disease. *Am J Hum Genet* 28:123, 1976

259. HALDANE KBS: The mutation rate of the gene for hemophilia and its segregation ratios in males and females. *Ann Eugen* 13:262, 1947

260. GARTLER SM, FRANCKE U: Half-chromatid mutations: Transmission in humans? *Am J Hum Genet* 27:218, 1975

261. FUJIMOTO WY, SEEGMILLER JE, UHLENDORF BW, JACOBSON CB: Biochemical diagnosis of an X-linked disease in utero. *Lancet* 2:511, 1968

262. DEMARS R, SARTO G, FELIX JS, BENKE P: Lesch-Nyhan mutation: Prenatal detection with amniotic fluid cells. *Science* 164:1303, 1969

263. BOYLE JA, RAIVIO KO: Lesch-Nyhan syndrome: Preventive control by prenatal diagnosis. *Science* 169:688, 1970

264. BAKAY B, FRANCKE U, NYHAN WL, SEEGMILLER JE: Experience with detection of heterozygous carriers and prenatal diagnosis of Lesch-Nyhan disease, in Muller MM, Kaiser E, Seegmiller JE (eds): *Purine Metabolism in Man II: Regulation of Pathways and Enzyme Defects.* New York, Plenum, 1977, p 351

265. KELLEY WN, ROSENBLOOM FM, SEEGMILLER JE: The effects of azathioprine (Imuran) on purine synthesis in clinical disorders of purine metabolism. *J Clin Invest* 46:1518, 1967

266. NYHAN WL, SWEETMAN L, CARPENTER DG, CARTER CH, HOEFNAGEL D: Effects of azathioprine in a disorder of uric acid metabolism and cerebral function. *J Pediatr* 72:111, 1968

267. BROWN RS, KELLEY WN, SEEGMILLER JE, CARBONE PP: The action of thiopurines in lymphocytes lacking hypoxanthine-guanine phosphoribosyltransferase, abstracted. *J Clin Invest* 47:12a, 1968

268. NEWCOMBE DS, SHAPIRO SL, SHEPPARD GL, DREIFUSS FE: Treatment of X-linked primary hyperuricemia with allopurinol. *JAMA* 198:315, 1966

269. SWEETMAN L, NYHAN WL: Excretion of hypoxanthine and xanthine in genetic disease of purine metabolism. *Nature (London)* 215:859, 1967

270. KELLEY WN, ROSENBLOOM FM, MILLER J, SEEGMILLER JE: An enzymatic basis for variation in response to allopurinol. *N Engl J Med* 278:287, 1968

271. FOX IH, WYNGAARDEN JB, KELLEY WN: Depletion of erythrocyte phosphoribosylpyrophosphate in man: A newly observed effect of allopurinol. *N Engl J Med* 283:1177, 1970

272. EMMERSON BT: Discussion. Session I. Biochemistry and metabolism. Symposium on allopurinol. *Ann Rheum Dis* 25:(Suppl. 6):621, 1966

273. SORENSEN LB: Seminars on the Lesch-Nyhan syndrome: Management and treatment: Discussion. *Fed Proc* 27:1097, 1968

274. GREENE ML, FUJIMOTO WY, SEEGMILLER JE: Urinary xanthine stones: A rare complication of allopurinol therapy. *N Engl J Med* 280:426, 1969

275. MANZKE H: Xanthine stone formation subsequent to allopurinol therapy. *Dtsch Med Wochenschr* 99:918, 1974

276. MIZUNO T, SEGAWA M, KURUMADA T: Clinical and therapeutic aspects of the Lesch-Nyhan syndrome in Japanese children. *Neuropaediatrie* 2:38, 1970

277. SPERLING O, BROSH S, BOER P, LIBERMAN UA, DE VRIES A: Urinary xanthine stones in an allopurinol-treated gouty patient with partial deficiency of hypoxanthine-guanine phosphoribosyltransferase. *Is J Med Sci* 14:288, 1978

278. WEISS EB, FORMAN P, ROSENTHAL IM: Allopurinol-induced arteritis in partial HGPRTase deficiency: Atypical seizure manifestation. *Arch Int Med* 138:1743, 1978

279. SWEETMAN L, NYHAN WL: Detailed comparison of the urinary excretion of purines in a patient with Lesch-Nyhan syndrome and a control subject. *Biochem Med* 4:121, 1970

280. BENKE PJ, ANDERSON J: Use of folic acid, adenine, and bicarbonate in newborn twins with the Lesch-Nyhan syndrome. *Pediatr Res* 3:356, 1969 (abs)

281. NYHAN WL: The Lesch-Nyhan syndrome. *Ann Rev Med* 24:41, 1973

282. WATTS RWE, MCKERAN RO, BROWN E, ANDREWS TM, GRIFFITHS MI: Clinical and biochemical studies on treatment of Lesch-Nyhan syndrome. *Arch Dis Child* 49:693, 1974

283. VAN DER ZEE SPM, LOMMEN EJP, TRIJBELS JMF, SCHRETLEN EDAM: The influence of adenine on the clinical features and purine metabolism in the Lesch-Nyhan syndrome. *Acta Paediatr Scand* 59:259, 1970

284. DEMUS A, KAISER W, SCHAUB J: The Lesch-Nyhan syndrome. Metabolic studies during administration of adenine. *Z Kinderheilkd* 114:119, 1973

285. NISSIM S, CIOPI ML, BARZAN L, PASERO G: Behavioral changes during adenine therapy in Lesch-Nyhan syndrome, in Sperling O, De Vries A, Wyngaarden JB (eds): *Purine Metabolism in Man.* New York, Plenum, 1974, p 677

286. PHILIPS FS, THIERSCH JB, BENDICH A: Adenine intoxication in relation to in vivo formation and deposition of 2,8-dioxyadenine in renal tubules. *J Pharmacol Exp Ther* 104:20, 1952

287. HAMILTON L: Utilization of purines for nucleic acid synthesis in man. *Nature (London)* 172:457, 1953

288. BENKE PJ, HERRICK N, SMITEN L, ARADINE C, LAESSIG R, WOLCOTT GJ: Adenine and folic acid in the Lesch-Nyhan syndrome. *Pediatr Res* 7:729, 1973

289. GHADIMI H, BHALLA CK, KIRSCHENBAUM DM: The significance of the deficiency state in Lesch-Nyhan disease. *Acta Paediatr Scand* 59:233, 1970

290. WOOD MH, FOX RM, VINCENT L, REYE C, O'SULLIVAN WJ: The Lesch-Nyhan syndrome: Report of three cases. *Aust NZ J Med* 2:57, 1972

291. BENKE PJ, HERBERT A, HERRICK N: In vitro effects of magnesium ions on mutant cells from patients with the Lesch-Nyhan syndrome. *N Engl J Med* 289:446, 1973

292. MIZUNO TI, YUGARI Y: Self-mutilation in Lesch-Nyhan syndrome. *Lancet* 1:761, 1974 (letter to the editor)

293. NYHAN WL, JOHNSON HG, KAUFMAN IA, JONES KL: Serotonergic approaches to the modification of behavior in the Lesch-Nyhan syndrome. *Appl Res Mental Retard* 1:25, 1980

294. VAN DER WEYDEN MB, KELLEY WN: Unpublished observations

295. ARNOLD WJ, KELLEY WN: Dietary induced variations of hypoxanthine-guanine phosphoribosyltransferase activity in patients with the Lesch-Nyhan syndrome. *J Clin Invest* 52:970, 1973

296. FOX IH, KELLEY WN: Unpublished observations

297. EDWARDS NL, JERYC W, LIEBERMAN C, FOX IH: Enzyme replacement therapy in the Lesch-Nyhan syndrome. *Clin Res* 28:129A, 1980

298. SEEGMILLER JE: Unpublished observations

299. DUKER P: Behaviour control of self-biting in a Lesch-Nyhan patient. *J Mental Deficiency Res* 19:11, 1975

300. ANDERSON L, DANCIS J, ALPERT M, HERMAN L: Punishment learning and self-mutilation in Lesch-Nyhan disease. *Nature* 265:461, 1977

301. BULL M, LAVECCHIO F: Behaviour therapy for a child with Lesch-Nyhan syndrome. *Develop Med Child Neurol* 20:368, 1978

302. GILBERT S, SPELLACY E, WATTS RWE: Problems in the behavioural treatment of self-injury in the Lesch-Nyhan syndrome. *Develop Med Child Neurol* 21:795, 1979

303. DESNICK RJ, FIDDLER MB, DOUGLAS SD, HUDSON LDS: Enzyme therapy II: Immunologic considerations for replacement therapy with unentrapped, erythrocyte- and liposome-entrapped enzymes, in Gatt S, Freysz L, Mandel P (eds): *Enzymes of Lipid Metabolism.* New York, Plenum, 1978, p 753

304. PETERSON JL, MCBRIDE OW: Cotransfer of linked eukaryotic genes and efficient transfer of hypoxanthine phosphoribosyltransferase by DNA-mediated gene transfer. *Proc Natl Acad Sci USA* 77:1583, 1980

305. LESTER SC, LEVAN SK, STEGLICH C, DEMARS R: Expression of human genes for adenine phosphoribosyltransferase and hypoxanthine-guanine phosphoribosyltransferase after genetic transformation of mouse cells with purified human DNA. *Somatic Cell Genet* 6:241, 1980

306. NYHAN WL, JAMES JA, TEBERG AJ, SWEETMAN L, NELSON LG: A new disorder of purine metabolism with behavioral manifestations. *J Pediatr* 74:20, 1969

307. HOOFT C, VAN NEVEL C, DE SCHAEPDRYVER AF: Hyperuricosuric encephalopathy without hyperuricemia. *Arch Dis Child* 43:734, 1968

308. BAZELON M, STEVENS H, DAVIS M, SEEGMILLER JE, GREEN M: Mental retardation, self-mutilation and hyperuricemia in females. *Trans Am Neurol Assoc* 93:187, 1968

309. ROSENBERG AL, BARTHOLOMEW BA: Hyperuricemia and neurologic deficits: A family study, abstracted. *Arthritis Rheum* 17:837, 1968

310. VANWOERT MH, YIP LC, BALIS ME: Purine phosphoribosyltransferase in Gilles de la Torette syndrome. *New Engl J Med* 296:210, 1977

52

ADENINE PHOSPHORIBOSYLTRANSFERASE DEFICIENCY:
2,8-Dihydroxyadenine Lithiasis

H. ANNE SIMMONDS

KAREL J. VAN ACKER

1. Adenine phosphoribosyltransferase (APRT) deficiency is a supposedly rare inherited disorder of purine metabolism. The enzyme defect results in an inability to salvage the purine base adenine which (in the absence of any other significant pathway of metabolism in humans) is oxidized via the 8-hydroxy intermediate by xanthine oxidase to 2,8-dihydroxyadenine (2,8-DHA). It is associated with the excretion of excessive amounts of this insoluble purine and the possible formation of kidney stones.

2. Clinical symptoms—colic, hematuria, urinary tract infection, and dysuria—are due to 2,8-DHA stone or gravel formation and may be present from birth. Two of the eighteen homozygotes have been completely symptomless. Six others presented in acute renal failure, three of whom have suffered permanent and severe renal damage, indicating a wide spectrum of clinical expression of the defect.

3. Except for the excretion of adenine and its metabolites no other biochemical abnormalities have so far been recorded. Purine production and excretion is considered normal, indicating that APRT is not vital for the overall control of purine metabolism in humans. Neither homozygotes nor heterozygotes show any evidence of immunodeficiency.

4. Normally, adenine metabolites account for 20 to 30 percent of the total purine excretion even on a low purine intake. The source of this endogenous adenine is probably the polyamine pathway, of which adenine is a metabolic by-product. However, adenine in the diet may be a precipitating factor in the expression of the more severe clinical manifestations of the defect.

5. Exogenous adenine is itself toxic in different systems in vitro and may produce 2,8-DHA nephrotoxicity in a variety of animal models, and in humans with normal APRT activity, through adenine overload. Adenine and 2,8-DHA are secreted by the human kidney, and 2,8-DHA is protein-bound. Both factors tend to minimize toxicity in tissues other than the kidney in vivo.

6. APRT is a dimer of molecular weight approximately 38,000. Normal kinetics, electrophoretic mobility, and heat stability have been demonstrated for the enzyme from heterozygotes. These data, together with the presence of cross-reacting material in homozygotes and the considerable heterogeneity in clinical expression, suggest the defect is due to a mutation on a structural gene coding for the enzyme.

7. The gene coding for human APRT is located on the long arm of chromosome 16. The defect is inherited in an autosomal recessive manner. Heterozygotes generally have no clinical or biochemical abnormality; in the majority of instances heterozygote activity in red cell lysates is approximately 25 percent of normal

activity and variable in white cells, fibroblasts, and rectal mucosa. Intact red cells from heterozygotes show normal conversion of adenine at physiologic concentrations of substrate and P_i. APRT-deficient cells are resistant to the deleterious effects of 2,6-diaminopurine and other analogues.

8. *A relatively high frequency of heterozygosity has been noted in several population studies (0.4 to 1.0 per hundred). This suggests that homozygosity for the defect may be more frequent than currently recognized, presumably due to the wide range of clinical expression coupled with the problems of diagnosis.*

9. *Diagnosis of the defect has presented problems in the past. 2,8-DHA stones were erroneously confused with uric acid because of the structural similarity of these purines, which leads to identical chemical reactivity. Homozygotes may be identified by the adenine as well as the 2,8-DHA excreted in the urine; from the 2,8-DHA in the stones by UV, IR, mass spectrometry, or x-ray crystallography; and by the absence of APRT activity in lysed erythrocytes, but correct diagnosis will be impossible if transfusion has formed an essential part of the treatment.*

10. *Treatment includes dietary purine restriction and high fluid intake. Allopurinol [10 mg/kg per day, or 5 mg/kg per day if renal function is poor] has prevented further 2,8-DHA excretion and stone formation. It is suggested that the use of alkali be avoided.*

Deficiency of the purine salvage enzyme adenine phosphoribosyltransferase (APRT; EC 2.4.2.7) is inherited as an autosomal recessive trait. The chief clinical manifestation directly related to the metabolic defect is urolithiasis. This is not an invariable finding, but when present can lead to serious complications. The stones were previously mistaken for uric acid stones [1–3]. Eighteen homozygotes, thirteen males and five females, have been identified to date [4–15]. Initially the defect was reported only in children [1–13], but recently five adults have been described [14, 14a, 14b, 14e, 15], all but one [14a] in the Japanese literature.

CLINICAL FEATURES

Clinical symptoms in APRT deficiency occur only when 2,8-dihydroxyadenine (2,8-DHA) stones are formed in consequence of the enzyme defect (Fig. 52-1) and may vary from benign to life-threatening [1–15]. 2,8-DHA crystalluria can occur without clinical symptoms [5], and the abnormality is then detected only during family investigation [5, 11]. Brief case histories from three patients representing the most extreme forms of expression (Table 52-1) are as follows:

PATIENT 1   This boy, born in January 1973, had passed gravel since birth and small stones and crystals from 9 months, accompanied by abdominal colic, dysuria, and pain in the urethra [5]. Clinical investigation was normal except for laxity of joints. Laboratory data, including uric acid levels in serum and urine, were not contributory. Crystals in the urine were interpreted as "uric acid" and examination of the stones by con-

ventional techniques revealed "pure uric acid." The patient was treated with allopurinol (200 mg/day) and bicarbonate (0.3 g/day) with little diminution in stone formation. During a further investigation at 2 years, 7 months the clinical and biochemical picture was the same, but examination of the urine by specialized techniques showed appreciable amounts of adenine and its oxidation products. Reexamination of the stones by UV, IR, and mass spectrometry showed the principal constituent to be not uric acid but 2,8-DHA [2, 3]. Subsequent determination of APRT activity in erythrocyte lysates revealed almost undetectable levels (Table 52-1). Mixing with normal erythrocytes gave intermediate values, excluding enzyme inhibition. Treatment with low purine diet and allopurinol (10 mg/kg per day) without bicarbonate led to an almost immediate disappearance of the stones and crystals from the urine. On annual reinvestigation the patient's condition has remained excellent for more than 6 years.

PATIENT 2   This healthy male sib of patient 1, born in March 1969, was found to have increased amounts of adenine and its metabolites in the urine during the family study [5, 16]. APRT activity in erythrocyte lysates was also negligible (Table 52-1). The past history was negative. No clinical abnormalities were found except for marked laxity of the joints. There was no stone formation, but the same round crystals were present in the urinary sediment. Other laboratory investigations were within normal limits. No treatment was given, except a low purine diet, and no change in the clinical situation has occurred over 6 years.

PATIENT 3   This girl, born October 1974 [8, 9], was the second child of unrelated Caucasian parents living on macrobiotic vegetarian diets. The child was well until the age of 2 when she complained of frequent abdominal pains, had a poor appetite, and lacked energy. At age 3 she had an episode of hematuria. In February 1979, she was admitted to hospital with abdominal pains, vomiting, diarrhea, increasing drowsiness, had been anuric for 16 h and was deeply comatose. Different investigations pointed to renal insufficiency which appeared to be caused by renal calculi as shown by ultrasound echography and retrograde pyelography. After peritoneal dialysis for 10 days the clinical situation and renal function improved. Bilateral pyelolithotomy was performed and many soft, gray, crumbly stones removed. They were found to consist of 2,8-DHA. The erythrocyte APRT levels were falsely raised because of a recent blood transfusion, but later measurements confirmed a complete APRT deficiency (Table 52-1). Renal biopsy at the time of pyelolithotomy showed interstitial fibrosis and chronic inflammation (Fig. 52-2). A number of crystals were seen within the tubular lumens but mainly in the interstitial tissue where some had initiated a giant-cell reaction. Treatment was started with allopurinol (5 mg/kg per day) and a low purine diet. Renal function 3 years later is still markedly impaired.

PATTERN OF EXPRESSION OF APRT DEFICIENCY

These patients are typical of the variable pattern of expression summarized in Table 52-1. In those children with 2,8-DHA urolithiasis, the whole scale of symptoms associated with stone

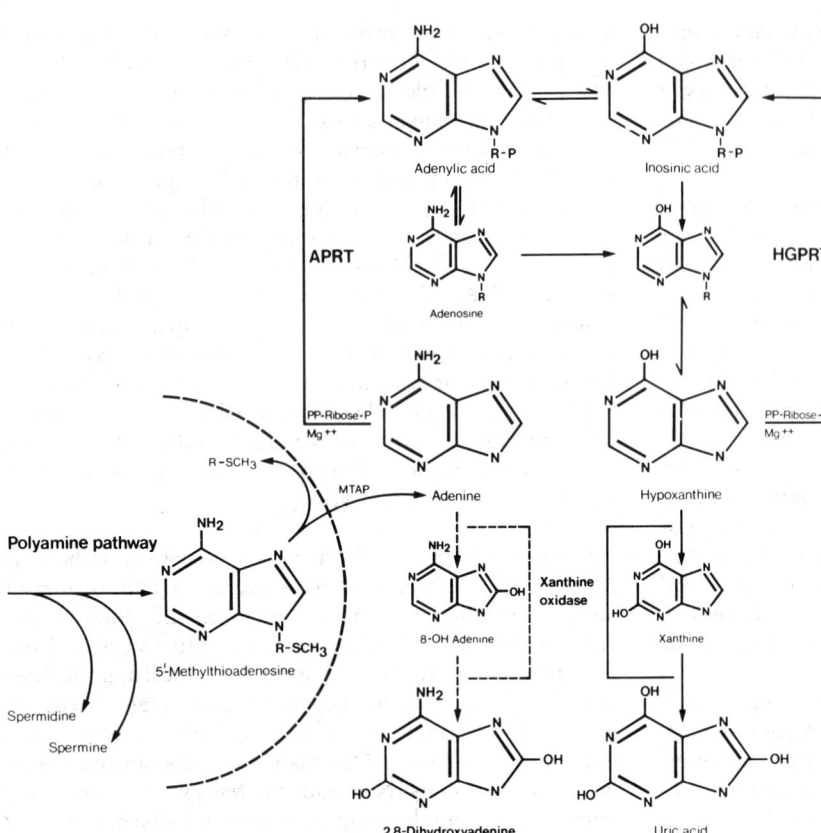

Figure 52-1 Metabolic pathways for the formation and disposal of adenine in humans. Adenine is normally converted by APRT to adenylic acid. In the absence of this enzyme it is oxidized by xanthine oxidase via the 8-hydroxy intermediate to 2,8-dihydroxyadenine. Significant amounts of adenine are not formed from adenosine by intact cells in vitro. Formation of adenine from 5'-methylthioadenosine has been demonstrated, indicating that the polyamine pathway, and not purine metabolism, is the likely source of adenine formation in vivo. APRT, adenine phosphoribosyltransferase; HGPRT, hypoxanthine-guanine phosphoribosyltransferase; MTAP, 5'-methylthioadenosine phosphorylase; R-SCH$_3$, 5'-methylthioribose-1-phosphate.

formation was observed within the first 2 years: fever from urinary tract infection, macroscopic hematuria, dysuria, urinary retention, and abdominal colic. In two cases acute anuric renal failure drew attention to the underlying lithiasis [8, 9, 12]. Once the diagnosis of urolithiasis had been made it generally took considerable time before the exact nature of the stone was recognized and appropriate treatment given. Most stones were considered to be uric acid stones, either on the ground of chemical analysis [1, 2, 6, 8, 12] or because of their radiolucency together with "uric acid" crystals in the urine [13]. Only in recent cases [7, 8, 10, 11, 13, 14, 14a, 14f], undoubtedly due to the use of more appropriate techniques and better knowledge of the disease, was the correct diagnosis made shortly after recognition of the urolithiasis. Laxity of the joints observed in two sibs has been shown to be inherited independently of APRT deficiency [5]. The spectrum of clinical manifestations in adults is also broad (Table 52-1). Case 11 first presented with urolithiasis at age 42, confirming that homozygotes may remain asymptomatic for many years [14a].

Heterozygotes have not previously had any specific clinical symptoms, but the fathers of cases 2, 3, and 4 passed stones [5, 7], one of them identified as calcium oxalate [7]. Lithiasis was also reported in the grandparents of case 1 [4]. The formation of stones by case 10, an apparent heterozygote, is therefore of considerable interest. The possibility that this case may also have had factitiously raised erythrocyte APRT levels because of other factors such as a blood transfusion, as in case 5, has been excluded [15a].

BIOCHEMICAL FEATURES OF APRT DEFICIENCY

Subjects with complete APRT deficiency generally have normal levels of uric acid in plasma and urine, although slightly raised levels have been noted initially [1–5, 8, 9, 12]. Total purine end product (uric acid + precursor oxypurines and adenine derivatives) has also been normal [0.05 to 0.1 mmol/(kg · 24 h)], with adenine metabolites making up to 20 to 30 percent of this total [7, 8, 11, 16, 17]. Three different adenine derivatives are excreted in the defect: adenine, 8-hydroxyadenine (8-HA), and 2,8-dihydroxyadenine (2,8-DHA) in the proportion of approximately 1:0.03:1.5, as shown by several different reports [5, 7, 11, 16, 17]. The excretion of 8-HA in APRT deficiency confirms earlier studies in vitro [18] that adenine, unlike uric acid, is oxidized by xanthine oxidase via the 8-, not the 2-hydroxy intermediate.

No other abnormal purines or pyrimidines have been detected in plasma and urine, and heterozygotes do not excrete detectable amounts of adenine or its metabolites [5, 7, 11, 16]. Consequently further details of three patients recently reported in the Japanese literature with urolithiasis and "heterozygote levels" of APRT are awaited with interest [14, 14d, 15]. Erythrocytes from both homozygotes and heterozygotes for APRT deficiency have normal ATP and 5-phosphoribosylpyrophosphate (PP-ribose-P) levels [19, 20]. The former observation indicates that the erythrocyte must maintain its adenine nucleotide pool predominantly through the action of adenosine kinase [21]. The latter, together with the normal PP-ribose-P synthetase activity [19] and purine production [16, 17] suggests that APRT, unlike its companion salvage enzyme hypoxanthine-guanine phosphoribosyltransferase (HPRT) [22], is not critical for cellular economy, and that adenine salvage is not vital for the overall regulation of purine metabolism in humans [9, 23].

Apart from the abnormal adenine metabolites excreted, all other biochemical and hematologic factors studied have been normal in homozygotes [1–13, 14a].

Immunology. Lymphocyte function has been investigated in homozygotes from two families and heterozygotes in their immediate kindred [7, 24]. T- and B-cell function were within normal limits as judged from lymphocyte transformation studies after stimulation with phytohemagglutinin, pokeweed mitogen, and concanavalin A, E-rosette formation, lymphocyte membrane immunoglobulins, cutaneous sensitivity tests, and serum immunoglobulins. C3, C4, and total hemolytic complement were also normal [7, 24]. From these studies it can be concluded that APRT is not vital for normal immune function. Also from the clinical standpoint, and unlike two other enzyme defects in purine metabolism [25], APRT deficiency is not characterized by an increased susceptibility to recurrent infection [4–13].

KINETIC PROPERTIES OF NORMAL HUMAN APRT

APRT catalyzes the synthesis of adenylic acid (AMP) from adenine and PP-ribose-P (Fig. 52-1). The reaction is inhibited by its product AMP, and also by IMP, GMP, and all three di- and triphosphates, with guanylates the most effective [26, 27]. Low concentrations of the last stimulate APRT activity; pH-dependent stimulation by ATP also occurs [28]. The relatively nonspecific nucleotide inhibition contrasts with HPRT, for which AMP is not an inhibitor [29, 30]. Metal ions and sulf-

hydryl binding agents may also inhibit APRT activity [31]. The enzyme binds 6-amino purines (adenine, 2- and 8-azaadenine, 2-fluoroadenine, 2,6-diaminopurine), 6-mercaptopurine (6-MP) and also 4-amino-5-imidazolecarboxamide (AICA) [32].

The enzyme is active over a broad pH range [33]. The Michaelis constant (K_m) for the reaction of adenine with adenine phosphoribosyltransferase from human erythrocytes is 1.4 to 2.7×10^{-6} M [34]. The K_m for PP-ribose-P is approximately 6×10^{-6} M [31, 34]. Adenine and PP-ribose-P may not be present on the enzyme simultaneously, Mg PP-ribose-P possibly binding first, followed by adenine [31]. As with HPRT the enzyme appears dependent on both magnesium and PP-ribose-P, with an absolute requirement for divalent cations [31]. The enzyme is widely distributed in body tissues [35], with the highest specific activity in nucleated cells [32]. It is considered to exist free in the cytoplasm [32].

Human APRT has been assayed by several different techniques [32, 36, 37]. Different laboratories report the mean specific activity of APRT in erythrocyte hemolysates (dialyzed or undialyzed) at being between 20 to 30 nmol/h per milligram of protein (or hemoglobin) [36–42]. Most give a value around 24 ± 5 nmol/h per milligram of hemoglobin. Heterozygotes for APRT deficiency generally have less than 50 percent of normal activity, the majority showing levels 25 to 30 percent of the normal mean [20, 37–42].

Studies of APRT activity in different human tissues have generally been undertaken as an adjunct to investigation of HPRT activity [35, 38, 43]. APRT activity is lower than HPRT activity in erythrocytes, but both activities are higher and of the same order in leukocytes, platelets, and fibroblasts [20, 41, 44–46]. The highest activity is found in liver where it exceeds HPRT activity threefold [35]. It is also in similar excess over HPRT in muscle, but here the specific activity of both is extremely low [35]. Although APRT activity is relatively high in brain, it is still tenfold less than that of HPRT [35]. The properties of the normal enzyme in other mammalian species and bacterial systems are discussed in two excellent reviews [47, 48].

Role of PP-Ribose-P in APRT Activity

A direct correlation is considered to exist between intracellular PP-ribose-P and APRT activity in erythrocytes [49]. Intact red cells from heterozygotes for APRT deficiency show normal substrate conversion at high levels of adenine and P_i (PP-ribose-P–generating conditions). This indicates enzyme activation by PP-ribose-P [19]. PP-ribose-P apparently stabilizes APRT in vitro [50]. It has been suggested that the increased erythrocyte APRT levels in HPRT-deficient subjects [51, 52, 53] (also found in liver and brain [35]) could result from diminished degradation through stabilization by the raised levels of PP-ribose-P in vivo [50, 54, 55]. Despite raised PP-ribose-P levels APRT activity is, however, normal in HPRT-deficient cells in culture [56–59]. By contrast both PP-ribose-P levels and purine synthesis were normal in APRT-deficient lymphocyte cell lines [60]. Erythrocyte lysate APRT activity is also increased in hereditary orotic aciduria (OPRT:ODC deficiency) but PP-ribose-P levels are normal in this defect [61, 62]. Erythrocyte APRT activity is also increased in purine nucleoside phosphorylase (PNP) deficiency [63] as are PP-ribose-P levels [63, 64] but the latter are normal in PNP-

Figure 52-2 Renal biopsy taken at pyelolithotomy in case 5 (Table 52-1), showing rosette-shaped crystals of 2,8-DHA in the tubular lumen, and crystalline debris within the interstitium (arrows), dilated tubules, interstitial edema, and infiltrate. These findings are identical with earlier animal models of adenine, xanthine, or uric acid nephropathy [109].

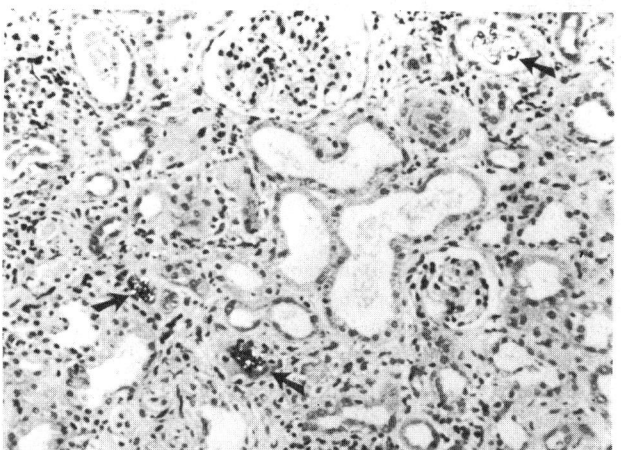

Table 52-1 Clinical features in 10 patients with 2,8-DHA lithiasis, and 2 asymptomatic sibs with almost complete APRT deficiency

| Case | Year of birth | Onset of symptoms | | Diagnosis | |
		Age, yr (sex)	Type	Original	Age at correct diagnosis, yr
1	1970	$2\frac{6}{12}$ (M)	Repeated emission small stones with dysuria	"Uric acid" stones removed at surgery	$3\frac{9}{12}$
2	1973	Birth (M)	Repeated passage small stones, dysuria and colics	Spontaneous emission of "uric acid" stones	$2\frac{7}{12}$
3	1969	(M)	Never ill	Asymptomatic sib of Case 2	$6\frac{5}{12}$
4	1975	1 (F)	Repeated attacks abdominal pain, urinary tract infection	Radiolucent calculi by IVU	$1\frac{7}{12}$
5	1974	2 (F)	Abdominal pain, lack of energy, poor appetite, eventual acute anuric renal insufficiency	Acute renal failure due to bilateral renal calculi	$4\frac{6}{12}$
6	1975	2 (M)	Recurrent urinary tract infection, later emission of calculi	Calculi at surgery diagnosed as "calcium oxalate"	$2\frac{5}{12}$
7	1965	(F)	Never ill	Asymptomatic sib of Case 6	14
8	1967	$1\frac{5}{12}$ (M)	Anorexia, fatigue, acute anuric renal failure	Bilateral hydronephrosis "uric acid" stones requiring series of operations at $1\frac{5}{12}$	11
9	1974	6 (M)	Abdominal pain and hematuria	Radiolucent stone by IVU, "uric acid" crystals in urine	$6\frac{1}{2}$
10	1940	25 (M)	Flank pain	Radiolucent stone in left ureter	38
11	1938	42 (F)	Hematuria, right renal colic	"Uric acid" calculi at surgery	43
12	1948	8 (M)	Repeated passage small stones, dysuria, fever, and flank pain	Uremia 1972, Staghorn calculus (100 g: "Struvite plus an unidentified purine compound")	¶

* Creatinine clearance or GFR   § 6 months later
† Uncorrected   ¶ No further data available
‡ Falsely raised due to transfusion   NOTE: LPD = low purine diet; GFR = glomerular filtration rate.

deficient fibroblasts [64]. These apparent contradictions suggest that other explanations should be sought for the raised APRT levels in HPRT and OPRT:ODC deficiency. A recent report of Lesch-Nyhan kindreds partially deficient in both APRT and HPRT, but with normal PP-ribose-P levels, is likewise contradictory [65]. By contrast, HPRT activity was normal in homozygotes and heterozygotes for APRT deficiency in most reports [1–5, 7, 8, 11, 12, 17, 20, 37–39, 66].

Role of APRT in Adenine Transport

Adenine apparently penetrates rapidly into mammalian cells but the mode of transport is poorly understood. Suggestions involving phosphoribosyltransferases in the membrane [67, 68] have been questioned [69, 70]. A saturable process [69] involving simple diffusion with subsequent cytoplasmic phos-

phoribosylation, dependent on APRT and PP-ribose-P availability, has recently been proposed [70]. In accordance with this hypothesis it has been demonstrated that adenine is not accumulated against a concentration gradient in APRT-deficient Chinese hamster fibroblast clones [71].

Physical Properties of the Purified Normal Enzyme

Considerable variation in the molecular weight of APRT from different sources was originally reported [48]. Recent reports utilizing more efficient purification methods concur that mammalian APRT is a dimer of molecular weight approximately 38,200 [72] consisting of two identical subunits of molecular weight 18,000 [72] and 20,000 [73] for the human erythrocyte [72] and rodent enzymes [73], respectively. Since antibody

Table 52-1 Clinical features in 10 patients with 2,8-DHA lithiasis, and 2 asymptomatic sibs with almost complete APRT deficiency (Continued)

| Correct diagnosis based on: | Length of follow-up, yr | GFR ml/(min·1.73 m²)* | | Treatment | APRT activity nmol/(h·mgHb) | Ref. |
		Diagnosis	Present			
Investigation of hyperuricemia: APRT in RBCs	None	56	Lost to follow-up	Water (1.5l), bicarbonate 2 g/24 h	0.002	[1, 4]
Adenine in urine, 2,8-DHA in stones	6	105	90	LPD, allopurinol 10 mg/kg per day. High fluids	<0.3	[2, 3, 5]
Adenine in urine during family study	6	106	102	LPD and high fluids only	<0.25	[5]
2,8-DHA in stones removed by surgery	5	83	90	Allopurinol 10 mg/kg per day, LPD, high fluids	0.61	[6, 7]
2,8-DHA in stones at surgery	3	8.5	14	LPD, allopurinol 5 mg/kg per day	11.0‡ <0.01§	[8, 9]
2,8-DHA in stones	3	100	"Normal"¶	Allopurinol 7, later 14 mg/kg per day	<0.005	[10, 11]
APRT in RBCs during family study	3	Not given	¶	Allopurinol 14 mg/kg per day	<0.004	[11]
2,8-DHA in urine, APRT in RBC's (stones no longer available)	2 5/12	Blood urea 200 mg/dl	22 (10 yr), 3.9 (12 yr) Chronic dialysis (12 yr)	Allopurinol 100 mg/day	<0.02% of normal	[12]
2,8-DHA in stone after surgery	2	Normal¶	¶	Allopurinol 100 mg/day	<0.006	[13]
2,8-DHA in stones	3	Blood urea 19 mg/dl	Not given	Allopurinol 300 mg/day	3.4	[14]
2,8-DHA in stone	<1	85†	85†	Allopurinol 300 mg/day	<0.5	[14a]
2,8-DHA in stone re-examined in 1979	Lost to follow-up in 1973	Hemodialysis 1973¶	¶	¶	Not done	[14b]

from the latter cross-reacts with the human enzyme, a common evolutionary past is suggested [73]. APRT exists predominantly as a single electrophoretic species when examined on polyacrylamide gels [74] or starch gels [75], but two differently charged species, a major and relatively minor peak, have been noted by isoelectric focusing [41].

THE MUTANT ENZYME

Detailed studies have now been reported in the English literature in ten individuals homozygous for the defect [1–13, 14a]. An additional eight have been identified recently [14, 14b, 14f, 15], seven of them in Japan [14, 14b–14e, 15]. More details of these subjects are necessary. In general APRT activity in eryth-

rocyte lysates has varied from essentially undetectable in some [4, 9, 11–13] to extremely low, though measureable, in others [5, 7]. This has led to the suggestion that the latter represent "partial" deficiencies [12], presumably by comparison with HPRT deficiency. Studies in intact erythrocytes from the homozygotes of these families failed to detect nucleotide formation under any conditions [19], confirming homozygosity for the defect and suggesting that intact cells may be a better guide to enzyme competence in inborn errors of metabolism. Interestingly, in intact red cells at physiologic levels of adenine and P_i, obligate heterozygotes showed APRT activity indistinguishable from healthy controls [19], despite APRT activity much less than 50 percent in their lysed cells [5, 7]. The majority of heterozygotes have levels 25 to 30 percent of the normal mean [37–43].

The finding of levels of this order in three Japanese patients with 2,8-DHA lithiasis [14, 14d, 15] is unusual and warrants further study. Certainly the results in case 5 indicate the potential pitfalls attached to the diagnosis of inborn errors of metabolism exclusively from a single estimation of erythrocyte lysate activity [76].

Lymphocytes and fibroblasts from homozygotes also lack APRT activity [11, 17]. Obligate heterozygotes have intermediate levels, but both normal and abnormal levels have been reported in leukocytes, fibroblasts, and rectal mucosa from families in which only heterozygotes were found [20, 41].

Properties of the Mutant Enzyme

Detailed studies of the catabolic, immunochemical, and electrophoretic properties of APRT from six unrelated families have been published recently [77]. In four homozygotes both immunoreactive protein and APRT were less than 1 percent of control levels. APRT activity in 26 heterozygotes was approximately 25 percent of normal, while immunoreactive protein ranged from 22 to 112 percent [77]. These studies provide the first clear evidence for a variety of mutations in the structural gene for APRT [77], in agreement with earlier suggestions [41].

As mentioned above the specific activity in lysed erythrocytes from the majority of heterozygotes is generally 25 percent rather than the more usual 50 percent of normal activity [37–43]. This finding, together with the recent confirmation that the human enzyme is a dimer of identical subunits [72], supports the contention that protein-protein interaction of two normal subunits is essential for the expression of APRT activity [37, 43].

Studies of the mutant enzyme in heterozygotes have shown normal heat stability and kinetic parameters [47, 55], end-

product inhibition, substrate affinity, and generally a normal half-life in circulating erythrocytes [41]. Reports of an abnormally short half-life [41] may be due to abnormal degradation of APRT in the erythrocyte aging process [55]. Elevated erythrocyte APRT levels have been noted in newborns [78] and patients with megaloblastic anemia and reticulocytoses [79], confirming the general pattern of increased enzyme activity in immature erythrocytes.

GENETICS

The gene that codes for APRT synthesis in humans is apparently located on the long arm of chromosome 16 [80], as shown by hybridization studies [81], while in the mouse this gene has been assigned to chromosome 8 [82]. HPRT-deficient A9 mouse fibroblasts used for mouse-human hybrids are also APRT-deficient [83]. In human cells with trisomy 16X increased APRT activity has been found [84]. The majority of subjects homozygous for APRT deficiency have been Caucasian, including an Arab family [7], but the defect has been identified in Japanese kindreds [14, 14b–14e, 15], excluding any specific ethnic origin. Extensive studies in one large kindred (Fig. 52-3) have confirmed that APRT deficiency is inherited in an autosomal recessive manner with high penetrance

Figure 52-3 Pedigree of patient B.Dh (case 2, Table 52-1) and his asymptomatic sib (case 3) showing the high penetrance also noted in the kindred of other homozygotes, and the absence of any other heterozygote in the father's kindred, suggesting a spontaneous mutation. The numbers refer to the level of APRT activity in lysed erythrocytes for the heterozygotes. The high proportion of enzyme levels, approximately 25 percent of the control mean (24.5 ± 4.8 nmol/h per milligram of hemoglobin) was also a feature in other kindreds.

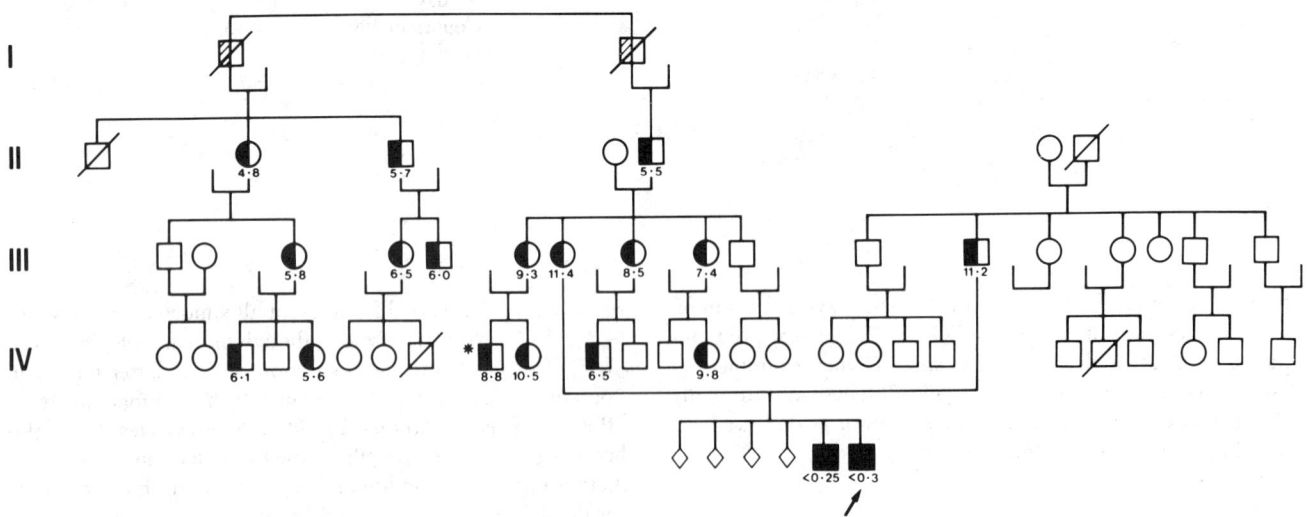

□ ○ Normal

◪ Dead, not studied

◪ Dead, presumed heterozygote

◧ ◐ Partial APRT deficiency

■ Complete APRT deficiency

◇ Spontaneous abortion

✳ Hyperuricaemia

／ Propositus

[85], as suggested from limited studies in the immediate family members of other homozygotes [1, 7, 11, 12, 13] and earlier studies in heterozygotes [20, 37, 39, 40, 66].

Consanguinity has been demonstrated in the kindred of two homozygous individuals [7, 14].

Heterozygosity for APRT Deficiency

Heterozygosity for APRT deficiency was originally described by Kelley et al. [37], long before identification of homozygotes for the defect. This was an incidental finding during the screening for HPRT deficiency [37]. Five such families were originally investigated in detail [20, 22, 37, 39, 66]. Initial observations suggesting links between abnormal lipid metabolism [37], hyperuricemia and gout [20], and partial deficiency [37, 39] were not substantiated [40, 41, 42]. These variables were found with equal frequency in family members with normal enzyme activity [40] or in the normal population [39–41].

In humans four different population studies have put the prevalence of heterozygosity for APRT deficiency at between 0.41 and 1.1 percent [37, 38, 40, 41]. This is a relatively high frequency and accords with the abnormally high rate of mutation at the APRT locus reported in different cell lines (10^{-3} to 10^{-7}) [86–89]. Reversion of mutation has also been observed in culture in both Chinese hamster and mouse cells selected in azaserine medium [89].

The relatively high level of heterozygosity for the APRT-deficient gene in humans suggests homozygosity of the order of 1/100,000 or more. The possibility that death in utero may occur is supported by the four spontaneous abortions in family 2 [5, 85]. In addition, the potentially lethal nature of the defect, when unrecognized or misdiagnosed as in two homozygotes [9, 12], the asymptomatic status in some homozygotes [5, 11], and the difficulties of diagnosis [6, 9, 17], may have contributed to lack of adequate recognition in the past. Future awareness should allow determination of the real prevalence of homozygosity and establish whether the defect is more frequent than its recent description suggests.

TOXICITY AND STONE FORMATION

The nephrotoxicity of 2,8-DHA is due to its insolubility at any pH. Solubility in water at pH 6.5 is 1.53 ± 0.04 mg/liter (approximately 9×10^{-6} M) [90]. Unlike uric acid, significant increase in solubility does not occur within the physiologic pH range for human urine [1]. Human urine at 37°C appears to exhibit enhanced capacity for solubilizing 2,8-DHA. Solubility in vitro is 2.68 ± 0.84 mg/liter at pH 5.0 and 4.97 ± 1.49 mg/liter at pH 7.8 [90]. 2,8-DHA may remain supersaturated in urine in vitro at levels of 40.38 ± 3.33 mg/liter for 16 h, while levels as high as 96 mg/liter have been noted in vivo in patients receiving oral adenine [90]. Levels up to 0.5 mmol/liter (~80 mg/liter) have been noted in a growing asymptomatic homozygote [16], confirming supersaturation in vivo of 2,8-DHA in APRT deficiency. Varying ability to supersaturate the urine may thus explain the existence of affected and asymptomatic sibs in two families [5, 11]. The apparent lack of 2,8-DHA toxicity to other tissues in vivo may be related to the high

degree of protein binding [91] coupled with active secretion of 2,8-DHA by the human kidney [92]; 92 percent of a high dose of [^{14}C]2,8-DHA was recovered in the urine of rats 24 h after IV injection. High retention with very high specific activity was found only in the kidney [93], confirming this hypothesis.

The nephrotoxicity of 2,8-DHA was first noted, as early as 1898, during the feeding of adenine to animals [94]. Since then, 2,8-DHA nephrotoxicity has been demonstrated in most mammalian species, the severity varying with the route and length of time of adenine administration and the species [95, 96]. The threshold varies, the pig tolerating the highest doses [95]. In all species little 2,8-DHA was formed at doses below 10 mg/kg [95–98]. With increasing dosage insoluble yellowish spheres of 2,8-DHA appeared in the urine with crystals in tubular lumens [94, 98]. Higher doses and longer periods produced extensive deposits not only within tubules, but also within the interstitium, with progressive renal failure and death [98]. Renal pathology in these animal studies corresponded closely with the findings in case 5 (Fig. 52-2) and confirmed acute intratubular crystal deposition as the primary event [8, 9] in this nephropathy.

Adenine and Red Cell Preservation

Much of the recent work in this field has been related to the investigation of the potential toxicity of blood to which adenine has been added to prolong its shelf life from 3 to 6 weeks [99, 100], a practice common in Sweden and the western U.S.A. [99, 100]. Adenine levels equivalent to 10 to 15 mg/kg apparently do not produce 2,8-DHA crystals in normal humans [99–104]. A fatal instance occurred in a patient receiving a massive dose (equivalent to 95 mg/kg) who developed impaired renal function [101]. Intratubular birefringent rosette-shaped crystals were found at autopsy [101]. Although 10 to 15 mg/kg is considered nontoxic [99, 100], the possibility that toxicity could occur in heterozygotes for APRT deficiency should be considered, particularly in view of the possible frequency of the defect in the population.

In Vitro Toxicity of Adenine Compounds

Under the influence of APRT the purine analogues 2,6-diaminopurine (2,6-DAP), 2- and 8-azaadenine (2-AA, 8-AA), 2-fluoroadenine (2-FA) and 6-mercaptopurine (6-MP) are converted to ribonucleotides which are toxic to the cell [48, 80, 86–89]. Fibroblasts with normal APRT are therefore killed in media containing these analogues, as opposed to APRT-deficient fibroblasts which grow normally, with heterozygote cells showing variable values [105]. Drug resistance has also been used to select spontaneous mutations at the APRT locus [86–89].

Adenine itself, in the absence of APRT, is toxic to human lymphoblasts [106] and other cell lines in vitro [107]. Adenine may be inhibitory to lymphocyte-mediated cytolysis through elevation of S-adenosyl-l-homocysteine levels [108]. The normal clinical and immunologic status of two homozygous sibs [5, 24], despite 6 years of allopurinol therapy [135] in the younger brother (in whom adenine accumulation could occur) must argue against significant adenine toxicity in vivo. Presumably rapid excretion by an active kidney secretory mechanism [92] ensures that circulating adenine levels are low.

Long-term follow-up studies will be vital, particularly in homozygotes in whom renal function is defective [109].

ADENINE METABOLISM IN HUMANS

Adenine Metabolism and the Regulation of Purine Production in Humans

Studies with [^{14}C]adenine have contributed to our understanding of adenine metabolism in animals and humans [91, 93, 99, 103]. In one study in the rabbit [110] less than 10 percent of the label was incorporated into nucleic acids, but extensive incorporation into the soluble nucleotides occurred, predominantly in the kidney and small intestine, with little in the brain or skeletal muscle. Large amounts of free adenine and hypoxanthine were excreted within 24 h in the urine, the former with the same specific activity. Thus the body pools of adenine must normally be very small. A slow subsequent rate of isotope elimination reflected the incorporation and turnover of body mononucleotide pools. Similar results have been found in humans [99, 103].

Earlier isotope studies have shown an identical pattern and also demonstrated inhibition of *de novo* purine synthesis by adenine in normal [41] and gouty humans [112]. This reduced purine synthesis did not result in diminished uric acid excretion. This was explained in part by a prompt conversion of adenine to uric acid [111]. The clinical use of adenine in the Lesch-Nyhan syndrome has been based on the assumption, derived from such experiments, that adenine causes feedback inhibition of purine synthesis [112].

Adenine therapy has proved generally ineffective in the Lesch-Nyhan syndrome [113, 114, 115] and has actually precipitated 2,8-DHA nephropathy in spite of allopurinol therapy [116, 117]. Other studies have demonstrated that adenine-induced reduction in synthesis *de novo* to be a transitory phenomenon, due to diminution in the pool of available PP-ribose-P [118], which accords with other data and the general ineffectiveness of therapy [114]. Furthermore, a loading test for the diagnosis of latent hyperuricemia in patients who form oxalate stones, based on the rapid catabolism of approximately 1 g of adenine and guanine to uric acid, is further proof that adenine will increase uric acid levels rather than correct them [119]. This practice is equally dangerous, with its real risk of nephrotoxicity.

Origin of the Adenine in APRT Deficiency

Homozygotes for APRT deficiency eliminate up to 100 mg (750 μmol) of adenine and its oxidation products per 24 h [5, 7, 11]. The ubiquitous distribution of the APRT enzyme in human tissue had long been puzzling in view of extremely low adenine levels in blood (1.13 ± 0.41 μmol/liter; 0.64 ± 0.15 μmol/liter; 0.07 μmol/liter [120, 121, 102]) and almost undetectable levels [25], or less than 1.5 mg (11 μmol)/24 h in the urine of normal humans [120, 122]. Furthermore, unlike hypoxanthine and guanine, no significant pathway for the formation of adenine from adenosine (or vice versa) via PNP has been demonstrated in mammalian cells [19, 123, 124], as distinct from bacterial and other cells [125]. The high activity of APRT in normal cells had made it difficult to study this point. Studies in intact cells from APRT-deficient homozygotes

(forming an effective adenine trap) have thus been extremely useful and have confirmed the insignificance of this pathway in either direction in humans [19]. Some activity of adenosine phosphorylase has been demonstrated in one study in APRT-deficient erythrocyte lysates [11]. It required high and unphysiologic substrate levels and is unlikely to be of significance in vivo [11, 123].

The original description of adenine (and traces of 2,8-DHA) excretion in adenosine deaminase (ADA) deficiency [121], suggested significance for this pathway in vivo. The adenine was subsequently shown in reality to be deoxyadenosine degraded in the cationic systems used [25]. Studies with ADA-deficient intact erythrocytes have also failed to demonstrate any significant PNP activity with adenine or adenosine as substrate [126].

Dietary Sources of Adenine The source of the adenine compounds excreted in APRT deficiency has thus been the subject of considerable interest. Detailed studies of the effect of dietary purine restriction on urinary excretion levels demonstrated only a slight reduction in total urinary adenine metabolites [16, 127]. This suggested an endogenous origin for most of the adenine compounds excreted. Nevertheless, diet can be an important precipitating factor in the most severe clinical expression of the defect, as indicated by the acute renal failure and permanent renal damage in the child [8, 76, 109] fed a diet rich in adenine-containing compounds [128].

Polyamine Pathway and Endogenous Adenine

The polyamine pathway [129], of which adenine is a metabolic by-product (Fig. 52-1), now appears to be the most likely source of endogenous adenine in humans [76]. Recent studies have demonstrated the production in vitro of adenine from 5'-methylthioadenosine through the action of 5'-methylthioadenosine phosphorylase (MTAP). The enzyme, which has an absolute requirement for phosphate [130], catalyzes the last step of this pathway and has been found in different mammalian tissues [131], including lymphocytes [132]. The erythrocyte enzyme has a specific activity in the range (6 to 14 nmol/h per milligram of hemoglobin) [133]. Production of adenine via this route in vivo thus seems most likely. The extent remains to be established.

The polyamine pathway is active in dividing or regenerating tissue [129]. The level of adenine metabolites excreted by homozygotes would be consistent with the normal activity of this pathway [134]. Detailed studies over 6 years in two homozygotes have shown a remarkable constancy in the daily excretion of adenine metabolites as a percentage of the total daily purine excretion (20 to 30 percent). Both tend to parallel the increase in body weight, which would support the polyamine pathway as the endogenous source of cellular adenine [135].

DIAGNOSIS OF 2,8-DHA LITHIASIS

2,8-DHA is an analogue of uric acid indistinguishable from it in routine chemical testing [1, 2, 6, 76]. It reacts mole for mole as uric acid in colorimetric analysis (phosphomolybdate and murexide tests). The two compounds may also be mistaken if only the alkaline UV spectrum is examined [1], or when stone material is analyzed by thermogravimetric analysis [6]. Both stones are radiolucent [4, 5]. These factors have been responsible for the earlier and frequent misdiagnosis of the stones as "uric acid" stones [6, 76, 136, 137] (Table 52-1).

Simple guidelines for correct stone identification include the macroscopic appearance of the stones. 2,8-DHA stones are whitish to pale gray, rough, and friable [1, 2], in contrast to uric acid stones which are generally yellowish, smooth, hard, and crush with difficulty [6] [76]. 2,8-DHA is resistant to the action of uricase [135] and will also be separated in the acid, but not the alkaline fraction by a technique employing wet chemistry [6]. Final confirmation may be obtained from the UV spectrum in both acid and alkali, infrared, mass spectrometry, and x-ray crystallography [1, 2, 10, 12, 13, 138]. The diagnosis of uric acid stones should always be suspect, especially in children who are otherwise normal. The stones are generally 90 to 98 percent 2,8-DHA, the remainder being predominantly uric acid [1, 2].

Diagnosis of Asymptomatic Subjects

Homozygotes for the defect, particularly asymptomatic subjects, can also be identified by the adenine compounds excreted in the urine [2, 16]. A new technique, isotachophoresis [6, 25], is superior to HPLC [12] in this regard. Coelution problems with methylated xanthine derivatives may lead to a false adenine peak when using HPLC in subjects not on caffeine-free diets [76, 135]. The estimation of APRT activity in erythrocyte lysates will identify both homozygotes and heterozygotes for APRT deficiency. The latter cannot be detected by any other means. It should again be stressed that false and near-normal results may be obtained if (as in case 5) the clinical condition on admission has necessitated blood transfusion [8, 9].

TREATMENT AND PROGNOSIS

Diet In all homozygotes, particularly those with urolithiasis, a low purine diet is recommended [5] since dietary adenine can contribute to the severity of the clinical manifestation. The child [8] presenting in acute renal failure was from a commune consuming diets rich in lentils and other grain and vegetable extracts, all foods with a reputedly high adenine content [128].

Therapy 2,8-DHA formation may be controlled by allopurinol but some 8-HA is still excreted [5]. Allopurinol therapy has not reduced the total level of adenine compounds excreted by homozygotes (still 20 to 30 percent of total purine excretion) [135], but has rearranged the proportion so that adenine becomes the major urinary component [5, 7, 11, 16]. One study also showed that allopurinol was ineffective in reducing the absorption of dietary purine in homozygotes, in contrast to its apparently beneficial effect in this regard in controls [16, 127]. This indicates that dietary purine restriction will always be necessary in APRT deficiency. The apparent lack of effect of allopurinol on total oxypurine excretion (xanthine plus hypoxanthine plus uric acid), on either a low or a high purine diet [16, 127], was questioned in another report [11], but urinary xanthine and hypoxanthine were unfortunately not measured [11].

A high fluid intake is encouraged, and the use of allopurinol *without* alkali is advised [4, 5, 6, 7, 13, 136]. The solubility of 2,8-DHA is not altered within the physiologic pH range [4, 11]. Indeed, three different observations have suggested that use of alkali may even be contraindicated [5, 7, 13]. Allopurinol at 10 mg/kg per day has eliminated 2,8-DHA from the urine in most cases. It has been reduced to 5 mg/kg per day in a child with permanent renal damage [8] because of the well-documented retention of oxipurinol (the active metabolite of allopurinol) in renal failure [139], with its risk of bone marrow depression [140]. When possible, plasma oxipurinol levels should be monitored and dosage adjusted accordingly. A careful watch should be kept on all hematologic factors.

Prognosis The ultimate prognosis clearly depends on the renal function at the time of diagnosis [135]. The importance of early diagnosis and treatment should be stressed. The long-term effect of xanthine oxidase inhibition, with its attendant potential for increasing circulating adenine levels, particularly where renal function is impaired, remains to be established.

REFERENCES

1. CARTIER P, HAMET M: Une nouvelle maladie métabolique: le deficit complet en adénine-phosphoribosyltransférase avec lithiase de 2,8-dihydroxyadénine. *C R Acad Sci (Paris)* 279:883, 1974
2. SIMMONDS HA, VAN ACKER KJ, CAMERON JS, SNEDDEN W: The identification of 2,8-dihydroxyadenine, a new component of urinary stones. *Biochem J* 157:485, 1976
3. SIMMONDS HA, VAN ACKER KJ, CAMERON JS, SNEDDEN W: A new cause of urinary calculi: 2,8-dihydroxyadenine stones in supposed "uric acid" crystalluria, in Fleisch H, Robertson WG, Smith LH, Vahlensieck W (eds): *Urolithiasis Research.* New York, Plenum Press, 1976, p. 517
4. DEBRAY H, CARTIER P, TEMSTET A, CENDRON J: Child's urinary lithiasis revealing a complete deficit in adenine phosphoribosyltransferase. *Pediatr Res* 10:762, 1976
5. VAN ACKER KJ, SIMMONDS HA, POTTER CF, CAMERON JS: Complete deficiency of adenine phosphoribosyltransferase: Report of a family. *N Engl J Med* 297:127, 1977
6. SIMMONDS HA, POTTER CF, SAHOTA A, CAMERON JS, ROSE GA, BARRATT TM, WILLIAMS DI, ARKELL DG, VAN ACKER KJ: Adenine phosphoribosyltransferase deficiency presenting with supposed uric acid stones; pitfalls of diagnosis. *J R Soc Med* 71:791, 1978
7. BARRATT TM, SIMMONDS HA, CAMERON JS, POTTER CF, ROSE GA, ARKELL DG, WILLIAMS DI: Complete deficiency of adenine phosphoribosyltransferase. A third case presenting as renal stones in a young child. *Arch Dis Child* 54:25, 1979
8. GREENWOOD MC, DILLON MJ, SIMMONDS HA, BARRATT TM, PINCOTT JRL, METREWELLI C: Renal failure due to 2,8-dihydroxyadenine urolithiasis. *Eur J Pediatr,* 1982, in press
9. SIMMONDS HA, BARRATT TM, WEBSTER DR, SAHOTA A, VAN ACKER KJ, CAMERON JS, DILLON MJ: Spectrum of 2,8-dihydroxyadenine urolithiasis in complete APRT deficiency, in Rapado A, Watts RWE, De Bruyn CHMM (eds): *Purine Metabolism in Man III, 122A.* New York, Plenum Press, 1980, p 337
10. REVEILLAUD RJ, DAUDON M, PROTAT MF, VINCENS A, GRAVELEAU D: Lithiase 2,8-dihydroxyadéninique: un nouveau cas dépisté par analyse infra-rouge. *Nouv Presse Med* 8:2965, 1979
11. CARTIER P, HAMET M, VINCENS A, PERIGNON JL: Complete adenine phosphoribosyltransferase (APRT) deficiency in two siblings: Report of a new case, in Rapado A, Watts RWE, De Bruyn CHMM (eds): *Purine Metabolism in Man III, 122A.* New York, Plenum Press, 1980, p 343
12. SCHABEL F, DOPPLER W, HIRSCH-KAUFFMANN M, GLATZL J, SCHWEIGER M, BERGER H, HEINZ-ERIAN P: Hereditary deficiency of adenine phosphoribosyltransferase. *Paediatr Paedol* 15:233, 1980
13. JOOST J, DOPPLER W: The 2,8-dihydroxyadenine stone in childhood. *Urology,* 1982, in press
14. KURODA M, MIKI T, KIYOHARA H, USAMI M, NAKAMURA T, KOTAKE T, TAKEMOTO M, SONODA T: Urolithiasis composed of 2,8-dihydroxyadenine due to partial deficiency of adenine phosphoribosyltransferase. *Jpn J Urol* 71:283, 1980
14a. GAULT MH, SIMMONDS HA, SNEDDEN W, DOW D, CHURCHILL DN, PENNEY H. Urolithiasis due to 2,8-dihydroxyadenine in an adult. *N Engl J Med* 305:1570, 1981
14b. TAKEMOTO M, NAGANO S: Urolithiasis containing 2,8-dihydroxyadenine: Report of a case. *Acta Urol (Jpn)* 25:265, 1979
14c. NORO T, NOBUHARA R, OGIWARA M, TSUYUKI K, MIYAJIMA T, MATSU-

OKA T: A case of 2,8-dihydroxyadenine lithiasis in a child who had repeated symptoms of renal insufficiency. *Clin Urol (Jpn)* 34:271, 1980

14d. TAKEUCHI H, UCHIDA M, NAKAMURA T: An interesting case of a urinary trace stone in a child (2,8-dihydroxyadenine). *Uric Acid Research (Jpn)* 4:113, 1980

14e. OSADA T, INCUE T, HIRANO A, TANAKA K, OGITA Z-, ISOBE M, HAYASHI S-: A case of 2,8-dihydroxyadenine lithiasis revealing a complete deficit in adenine phosphoribosyltransferase. *Clin Urol (Jpn)* 34:981, 1980

14f. MORGON JW, NICKERSON JF: Personal communication, 1981

15. YAMAMOTO H. Two cases of 2,8-dihydroxyadenine stone. Personal communication, 1981

15a. KOTAKE T. Personal communication, 1981

16. SIMMONDS HA, VAN ACKER KJ, CAMERON JS, McBURNEY A: Purine excretion in complete adenine phosphoribosyltransferase deficiency, in Müller MM, Kaiser E, Seegmiller JE (eds): *Purine Metabolism in Man II*, 76B, New York, Plenum Press, 1977, p. 304

17. CARTIER P, HAMET M, PERIGNON JL: Lithiase urinaire de l'enfant. Possibilité d'un déficit héréditaire en adénine phosphoribosyltransférase. *Nouv Presse Med* 9:1767, 1980

18. WYNGAARDEN JB, DUNN JT: 8-Hydroxyadenine as the metabolic intermediate in the oxidation of adenine to 2,8-dihydroxyadenine by xanthine oxidase. *Arch Biochem Biophys* 70:150, 1957

19. DEAN BM, PERRETT D, SIMMONDS HA, SAHOTA A, VAN ACKER KJ: Adenine and adenosine metabolism in intact erythrocytes deficient in adenosine monophosphate—pyrophosphate phosphoribosyltransferase: A study of two families. *Clin Sci Mol Med* 55:407, 1978

20. FOX IH, MEADE JC, KELLEY WN: Adenine phosphoribosyltransferase deficiency in man. Report of a second family. *Am J Med* 55:614, 1973

21. DEAN BM, PERRETT D: Studies on adenine and adenosine metabolism by intact human erythrocytes using high-performance liquid chromatography. *Biochim Biophys Acta* 437:1, 1976

22. CARTIER P: Les déficits enzymatiques du métabolisme des purines. Symposium Interdisciplinaire sur l'hyperuricémie, Paris, 1975, p 160

23. SEEGMILLER JE: Genetic defects in human purine metabolism leading to urolithiasis, in Fleisch H, Robertson WG, Smith LH, Vahliensieck W (eds): *Urolithiasis Research*. New York, Plenum Press, 1976, p 147

24. STEVENS WJ, PEETERMANS ME, VAN ACKER KJ: Immunological investigation in adenine phosphoribosyltransferase (APRT) deficiency. *Clin Exp Immunol* 36:364, 1979

25. SIMMONDS HA, SAHOTA A, POTTER CF, CAMERON JS: Purine metabolism and immunodeficiency: Urinary purine excretion as a diagnostic screening test in adenosine deaminase and purine nucleoside phosphorylase deficiency. *Clin Sci Mol Med* 54:579, 1978

26. HENDERSON JF, GADD REA, PALSER HM, HORI M: Mechanisms of inhibition of adenine phosphoribosyltransferase by adenine nucleosides and nucleotides. *Can J Biochem* 48:573, 1969

27. HENDERSON JF, HORI M, PALSER HM, GADD REA: Kinetic studies of inhibition of adenine phosphoribosyltransferase by guanylate. *Biochim Biophys Acta* 268:70, 1972

28. MURRAY AW, WONG PCL: Stimulation of adenine phosphoribosyltransferase by adenosine triphosphate and other nucleoside triphosphates. *Biochem J* 104:669, 1967

29. KRENITSKY TA, PAPAIOANNOU R, ELION GB: Human hypoxanthine phosphoribosyltransferase. 1. Purification, properties and specificity. *J Biol Chem* 244:1263, 1969

30. KRENITSKY TA, NEIL SM, ELION GB, HITCHINGS GH: Adenine phosphoribosyltransferase from monkey liver. *J Biol Chem* 244:4779, 1969

31. SRIVASTAVA SK, BEUTLER E: Purification and kinetic studies of adenine phosphoribosyltransferase from human erythrocytes. *Arch Biochem Biophys* 142:426, 1971

32. ARNOLD WJ, KELLEY WN: Adenine phosphoribosyltransferase, in Hoffee PA, Jones ME (eds): *Methods in Enzymology, 51*. New York, Academic Press, 1978, p 568

33. THOMAS CB, ARNOLD WJ, KELLEY WN: Human adenine phosphoribosyltransferase. *J Biol Chem* 248:2529, 1973.

34. DEAN BM, WATTS RWE, WESTWICK WJ: Human erythrocyte AMP pyrophosphate phosphoribosyltransferase (EC 2.4.2.7) *FEBS Lett* 1:179, 1968

35. ROSENBLOOM FM, KELLEY WN, MILLER J, HENDERSON JF, SEEGMILLER JE: Inherited disorder of purine metabolism. Correlation between central nervous system dysfunction and biochemical defects. *J Am Med Assoc* 202:103, 1967

36. CARTIER P, HAMET M: Les activités purine-phosphoribosyltransfériques des globules rouges humains. Technique de dosage. *Clin Chim Acta* 20:205, 1968

37. KELLEY WN, LEVY RI, ROSENBLOOM FM, HENDERSON JF, SEEGMILLER JE: Adenine phosphoribosyltransferase deficiency—A previously undescribed genetic defect in man. *J Clin Invest* 47:2281, 1968

38. SRIVASTAVA SK, VILLACORTE D, BEUTLER E: Correlation between adenylate metabolising enzymes and adenine nucleotide levels of erythrocytes during blood storage in various media. *Transfusion* 12:190, 1972

39. DELBARRE F, AUSCHER C, AMOR B, deGERY A, CARTIER P, HAMET M: Gout with adenine phosphoribosyltransferase deficiency. *Biomedicine* 21:82, 1974

40. JOHNSON LA, GORDON RB, EMMERSON BT: Adenine phosphoribosyltransferase: A simple spectrophotometric assay and the incidence of mutation in the normal population. *Biochem Genet* 15:256, 1977

41. FOX IH, LA CROIX S, PLANET G, MOORE M: Partial deficiency of adenine phosphoribosyltransferase in man. *Medicine* 56:515, 1977

42. VAN ACKER KJ, SIMMONDS HA, CAMERON JS: Complete deficiency of adenine phosphoribosyltransferase: Report of a family, in Müller MM, Kaiser E, Seegmiller JE (eds): *Purine Metabolism in Man II, 76A*. New York, Plenum Press, 1977, p 295

43. WYNGAARDEN JB: Phosphoribosyltransferase (PRT) and adenine PRT (APRT) deficiency states in man—new inborn errors of purine metabolism. *Ann Intern Med* 70:229, 1969 (editorial)

44. SMITH JL, OMURA GA, KRAKOFF JH, BALIS EM: IMP and AMP: pyrophosphate phosphoribosyltransferase in leukemic and normal human leucocytes. *Proc Soc Exp Biol Med* 136:1299, 1971

45. JERUSHALMY Z, SPERLING O, PINKHAS J, KRYNSKA M, DE VRIES A: Enzymes of purine metabolism in platelets: Phosphoribosylpyrophosphate synthetase and purine phosphoribosyltransferases. *Adv Exp Med Biol* 41:159, 1973

46. RIVARD G, IZADI P, LAZERSON J, McLAREN JD, PARKER C, FISH CH: Functional and metabolic studies of platelets from patients with Lesch-Nyhan syndrome. *Br J Haematol* 31:245, 1975

47. RAIVIO KO, SEEGMILLER JE: The role of phosphoribosyltransferases in purine metabolism, in Horecker BL, Stadman ER (eds): *Current Topics in Cellular Regulation*. London, Academic Press, 1970, p 201

48. ARNOLD WJ: Purine salvage enzymes, in Kelley WN, Weiner IM (eds): *Uric Acid*. Berlin, Springer-Verlag, 1978, p 61

49. GORDON RB, THOMPSON L, EMMERSON BT: Erythrocyte phosphoribosylpyrophosphate concentrations in heterozygotes for hypoxanthine-guanine phosphoribosyltransferase deficiency. *Metabolism* 23:921, 1974

50. GREENE ML, BOYLE JA, SEEGMILLER JE: Substrate stabilization: Genetically controlled reciprocal relationship of two human enzymes. *Science* 167:887, 1970

51. KELLEY WN, GREENE ML, ROSENBLOOM FM, HENDERSON JF, SEEGMILLER JE: Hypoxanthine-guanine phosphoribosyltransferase deficiency in gout. *Ann Intern Med* 70:155, 1969

52. SEEGMILLER JE, ROSENBLOOM FM, KELLEY WN: An enzyme defect associated with a sex-linked human neurological disorder and excessive purine synthesis. *Science* 155:1682, 1967

53. KELLEY WN: Hypoxanthine-guanine phosphoribosyltransferase deficiency in the Lesch-Nyhan syndrome and gout. *Fed Proc* 27:1047, 1968

54. RUBIN CS, BALIS ME, PIOMELLI S, BERMAN PH, DANCIS J: Elevated AMP pyrophosphorylase activity in congenital IMP pyrophosphorylase deficiency (Lesch-Nyhan disease). *J Lab Clin Med* 74:732, 1969

55. YIP LC, DANCIS J, MATHIESON B, BALIS NE: Age-induced changes in adenosine monophosphate pyrophosphate phosphoribosyltransferase and inosine monophosphate pyrophosphate phosphoribosyltransferase from normal and Lesch-Nyhan erythrocytes. *Biochemistry* 13:2558, 1974

56. KELLEY WN: Studies on the adenine phosphoribosyltransferase enzyme in human fibroblasts lacking hypoxanthineguanine phosphoribosyltransferase. *J Lab Clin Med* 77:33, 1971

57. WOOD AW, BECKER MA, MINNA JD, SEEGMILLER JE: Purine metabolism in normal and thioguanine-resistant neuroblastoma. *Proc Natl Acad Sci USA* 70:3880, 1973

58. NUKI G, LEVER J, SEEGMILLER JE: Biochemical characteristics of 8-azaguanine resistant human lymphoblast mutants selected in vitro, in Sperling O, De Vries A, Wyngaarden JB (eds): *Purine Metabolism in Man, 41B*. New York, Plenum Press, 1974, p 255

59. WOOD AW, BECKER MA, SEEGMILLER JE: Purine nucleotide synthesis in lymphoblasts cultured from normal subjects and a patient with Lesch-Nyhan syndrome. *Biochem Genet* 9:261, 1973

60. SPECTOR EB, HERSHFIELD MS, SEEGMILLER JE: Purine reutilization and synthesis de novo in long term human lymphocyte cell lines deficient in adenine phosphoribosyltransferase activity. *Somat Cell Genet* 4:253, 1978

61. SIMMONDS HA, WEBSTER DR, BECROFT DHO, POTTER CF: Purine and pyrimidine metabolism in hereditary orotic aciduria: Some unexpected effects of allopurinol. *Eur J Clin Invest* 10:33, 1980

62. FOX IH, KELLEY WN: Observations of altered intracellular phosphoribosylpyrophosphate (PP-ribose-P) in human diseases, in Sperling O, De Vries A, Wyngaarden JB (eds): *Purine Metabolism in Man, 41B*. New York, Plenum Press, 1974, p 471

63. SAHOTA A, SIMMONDS HA: Unpublished observations, 1980

64. COHEN A, DOYLE D, MARTIN DW Jr, AMMANN AJ: Abnormal purine metabolism and purine overproduction in a patient deficient in purine nucleoside phosphorylase. *N Engl J Med* 295:1449, 1976

65. ITIABA K, MELANCON SB, DALLAIRE L, CRAWHALL JC: Adenine phosphoribosyltransferase deficiency in association with subnormal hypoxanthine

phosphoribosyltransferase in families of Lesch-Nyhan patients. *Biochem Med* 19:252, 1978

66. EMMERSON BT, GORDON RB, THOMPSON L: Adenine phosphoribosyltransferase deficiency: Its inheritance and occurrence in a female with gout and renal disease. *Aust NZ J Med* 5:440, 1975

67. HOCHSTADT-OZER J, STADTMAN ER: The regulation of purine utilization in bacteria. *J Biol Chem* 246:5312, 1971

68. DE BRUYN CHMM, OEI TL: Incorporation of purine bases by intact red blood cells, in Müller MM, Kaiser E, Seegmiller JE (eds): *Purine Metabolism in Man II, 76B*. New York, Plenum Press, 1977, p 139

69. ZYLKA JM, PLAGEMANN PGW: Purine and pyrimidine transport by cultured Novikoff cells. Specificities and mechanism of transport and relationship to phosphoribosylation. *J Biol Chem* 250:5756, 1975

70. CARTIER PH: Adenine uptake by isolated rat thymocytes. *J Biol Chem* 255:4574, 1980

71. WITNEY FR, TAYLOR MW: Role of adenine phosphoribosyltransferase in adenine uptake in wild-type and APRT mutants of CHO. *Biochem Genet* 16:917, 1978

72. HOLDEN JA, MEREDITH GS, KELLEY WN: Human adenine phosphoribosyltransferase: Affinity purification, subunit structure, amino acid composition and peptide mapping. *J Biol Chem* 254:6951, 1979

73. TAYLOR MW, HERSHEY HV: Purification and characterisation of mammalian adenine phosphoribosyltransferases, in Rapado A, Watts RWE, De Bruyn CHMM (eds): *Purine Metabolism in Man III, 122B*. New York, Plenum Press, 1980, p 130

74. BAKAY B, TELFER MA, NYHAN WL: Assay of hypoxanthineguanine and adenine phosphoribosyltransferases. A simple screening test for the Lesch-Nyhan syndrome and related disorders of purine metabolism. *Biochem Med* 3:230, 1969

75. MOWBRAY S, WATSON B, HARRIS H: A search for electrophoretic variants of human adenine phosphoribosyltransferase. *Ann Hum Genet* 36:153, 1972

76. SIMMONDS HA: 2,8-dihydroxyadeninuria, or when is a uric acid stone not a uric acid stone? *Clin Nephrol* 12:195, 1979

77. WILSON JM, DADDONA PE, SIMMONDS HA, VAN ACKER KJ, KELLEY WN: Human adenine phosphoribosyltransferase: Immunochemical quantitation and protein blot analysis of mutant forms of the enzyme. *J Biol Chem*, 1982, in press

78. BORDEN M, NYHAN WL, BAKAY B: Increased activity of adenine phosphoribosyltransferase in erythrocytes of normal newborn infants. *Pediatr Res* 8:31, 1974

79. FOX IH, DOTTEN DA, MARCHANT PJ, LA CROIX S: Acquired increases of human erythrocyte purine enzymes. *Metabolism* 25:571, 1976

80. TISCHFIELD JA, RUDDLE FH: Assignment of the gene for adenine phosphoribosyltransferase to human chromosome 16 by mouse-human somatic cell hybridization. *Proc Natl Acad Sci USA* 71:45, 1974

81. KUSANO T, LONG C, GREEN H: A new reduced human-mouse somatic cell hybrid containing the human gene for adenine phosphoribosyltransferase. *Proc Natl Acad Sci USA* 68:82, 1971

82. KOZAK C, NICHOLS E, RUDDLE FH: Gene linkage analysis in the mouse by somatic cell hybridisation: Assignment of adenine phosphoribosyltransferase to chromosome 8 and α-galactosidase to the X chromosome. *Somat Cell Genet* 1:371, 1975

83. COX RP, KRAUSS MR, BALIS ME, DANCIS J: Mouse fibroblasts A9 are deficient in HGPRT and APRT. *Am J Hum Genet* 26:272, 1974

84. MARIMO B, GIANNELLI F: Gene dosage effect in human trisomy 16. *Nature* 256:204, 1975

85. VAN ACKER KJ, SIMMONDS HA, POTTER CF, SAHOTA A: Inheritance of adenine phosphoribosyltransferase (APRT) deficiency, in Rapado A, Watts RWE, De Bruyn CHMM (eds): *Purine Metabolism in Man, III, 122A*. New York, Plenum Press, 1980, p 349

86. JONES GE, SARGENT PA: Mutants of cultured Chinese hamster cells deficient in adenine phosphoribosyltransferase. *Cell* 2:43, 1974

87. TAYLOR MW, PIPKORN JH, TOKITO MK, POZZATTI RD JR: Purine mutants of mammalian cell lines: III control of purine biosynthesis in adenine phosphoribosyltransferase mutants of CHO cells. *Somat Cell Genet* 3:195, 1977

88. REUSER AJJ, MINTZ B: Mouse teratocarcinoma mutant clones deficient in adenine phosphoribosyltransferase and developmentally pluripotent. *Somat Cell Genet* 5:781, 1979

89. TISCHFIELD JA, TRILL JJ, LEE YK, COY K, TAYLOR MW: Genetic instability at the adenine phosphoribosyltransferase locus in mouse L-cells. *Proc Natl Acad Sci USA*, 1982, in press

90. PECK CC, BAILEY FJ, MOORE GL: Enhanced solubility of 2,8-dihydroxyadenine (DOA) in human urine. *Transfusion* 17:383, 1977

91. STERN IJ, COSMAS F, GARVIN PJ: The occurrence and binding of 2,8-dioxyadenine in plasma. *Transfusion* 13:382, 1972

92. ERICSON A, GROTH T, NIKLASSON F, DE VERDIER C-H: Plasma concentration and renal excretion of adenine and 2,8-dihydroxyadenine after administration of adenine in man. *Scand J Clin Lab Invest* 40:1, 1980

93. DEVENUTO F, WILSON SM, BILLINGS TA, SHIELDS CE: In vivo distribution

of injected ^{14}C-dioxyadenine in tissues and organs of normal rats. *Transfusion* 16:24, 1976

94. MINKOWSKI O: Untersuchungen zur Physiologie und Pathologie der Harnsaure bei saugetieren. *Arch Exp Pathol Pharmakol* 41:375, 1898

95. CAMERON JS, SIMMONDS HA, CADENHEAD A, FAREBROTHER D: Metabolism of intravenous adenine in the pig, in Miller MM, Kaiser E, Seegmiller JE (eds): *Purine Metabolism in Man II, 76A*. New York, Plenum Press, 1977, p 496

96. SHIELDS CE, LOPAS H, BIRNDORF NI: Investigation of nephrotoxic effects of adenine and its metabolic product 2,8-dioxyadenine, on primates *(Macaca Irus)*. *J Clin Pharmacol* 10:316, 1970

97. KLAIN GJ, MEIKLE AW, SULLIVAN FJ, ROGERS GB: Metabolic effects of dietary adenine on kidney of rats. *Fed Proc* 29:366, 1970 (abstract)

98. LINDBLAD G, JANSSON G, FALK J: Adenine toxicity: A three-week intravenous study in dogs. *Acta Pharmacol Toxicol* 32:246, 1973

99. BARTLETT GR: Metabolism by man of intravenously administered adenine. *Transfusion* 17:367, 1977

100. WESTMAN BJM: Serum creatinine and creatinine clearance after transfusion with ACD-adenine blood and ACD blood. *Transfusion* 12:371, 1972

101. FALK JS, LINDBLAD GTO, WESTMAN BJM: Histopathological studies on kidneys from patients treated with large amounts of blood preserved with ACD-adenine. *Transfusion* 12:376, 1972

102. DE VERDIER CH, ERICSON A, NIKLASSON F, WESTMAN M: Adenine metabolism in man. 1. After intravenous and peroral administration. *Scand J Clin Lab Invest* 37:567, 1977

103. BARTLETT GR: Formation of oxyadenine metabolites in the rabbit after intravenous administration of adenine. *Transfusion* 17:351, 1972

104. ROTH GJ, MOORE CL, KLINE WE, POSKITT TR: The renal effect of intravenous adenine in humans. *Transfusion* 15:116, 1975

105. VAN DE VIJVER AM: Ein selectieve groeitechniek voor het aantonen van het mutante gen van adenine phosphoribosyltransferase in diploide huidfibroblasten van de mens. Thesis, Antwerpen, 1977

106. HERSHFIELD MS, SNYDER FF, SEEGMILLER JE: Adenine and adenosine are toxic to human lymphoblast mutants defective in purine salvage enzymes. *Science* 197:1284, 1977

107. HENDERSON JF, SCOTT FW: Inhibition of animal and invertbrate cell growth by naturally occurring purine bases and ribonucleosides. *Pharmacol Ther* 8:539, 1980

108. ZIMMERMAN TP, WOLBERT G, DUNCAN GS, ELION GB: Adenosine analogues as substrates and inhibitors of S-adenosylhomocysteine hydrolase in intact lymphocytes. *Biochemistry* 19:2252, 1980

109. FAREBROTHER DA, PINCOTT JR, SIMMONDS HA, WARREN DJ, DILLON MJ, CAMERON JS: Uric acid crystal induced nephropathy: Evidence for a specific renal lesion in a gouty kindred. *J Pathol* 135:159, 1981

110. BARTLETT GR: Metabolism of intravenously administered adenine and inosine in the rabbit, in Chaplin H Jr, Jaffé ER, Lenford C, Valeri CR (eds): *Preservation and Red Blood Cells*. Washington, DC, Natl Acad Sci, 1973, p 215

111. WYNGAARDEN JB, SEEGMILLER JE, LASTER L, BLAIR AE: Utilization of hypoxanthine, adenine and 4-amino-5-imidazolecarboximide for uric acid synthesis in man. *Metabolism* 8:455, 1959

112. SEEGMILLER JE, KLINENBERG JR, MILLER J, WATTS RWE: Suppression of glycine-^{15}N incorporation into urinary uric acid by adenine-8-^{13}C in normal and gouty subjects. *J Clin Invest* 47:1193, 1968

113. VAN DER ZEE SPM, LOMMEN EJP, TRIJBELS JMF, SCHRETLEN EDAM: The influence of adenine on the clinical features and purine metabolism in the Lesch-Nyhan syndrome. *Acta Paediatr Scand* 59:259, 1970

114. WATTS RWE, MCKERAN RO, BROWN E, ANDREWS TM, GRIFFITHS MI: Clinical and biochemical studies on treatment of Lesch-Nyhan syndrome. *Arch Dis Child* 49:693, 1974

115. BEYER P, BIETH D, LUTZ D, GEISERT J, BOILLETOT A: Une nouvelle observation du syndrome de Lesch-Nyhan: essai de traitement par l'adénine. *Arch Fr Pediatr* 32:293, 1975

116. DEMUS A, KAISER W, SCHAUB J: The Lesch-Nyhan syndrome. Metabolic studies during administration of adenine. *Eur J Pediatr* 114:119, 1973

117. CECCARELLI M, CIOMPI ML, PASERO G: Acute renal failure during adenine therapy in Lesch-Nyhan syndrome, in Sperling O, De Vries A, Wyngaarden JB (eds): *Purine Metabolism in Man, 41B*. New York, Plenum Press, 1974, p 671

118. MARKO P, GERLACH E, ZIMMER HG, PECHÁN I, CREMER T, TRENDELENBURG C: Interrelationship between salvage pathway and synthesis de novo of adenine nucleotides in kidney slices. *Hoppe-Seyler's Z Physiol Chem* 350: 1669, 1969

119. SCHNEEBURGER W, BACH D, HESSE A, VAHLENSIECK W: Circadian excretion of uric acid on a standard diet and purine load in Ca-oxalate stone formers and healthy controls, in Smith LH, Robertson WG, Finlayson B (eds): *Urolithiasis: Clinical and Basic Research*. New York, Plenum Press, 1981, p 51

120. HAMET M: Le microdosage de l'adénine par une méthode de cinétique enzymatique-dilution isotopique. *Ann Biol Clin* 33:131, 1975

121. MILLS CG, SCHMALSTIEG FC, TRIMMER KB, GOLDMAN AS, GOLDBLUM RM: Purine Metabolism in adenosine deaminase deficiency. *Proc Natl Acad Sci USA* 73:2867, 1976

122. KELLEY WN, WYNGAARDEN JB: Effect of dietary purine restriction, allopurinol, and oxipurinol on urinary excretion of ultraviolet absorbing compounds. *Clin Chem* 16:707, 1970

123. ZIMMERMAN TP, GERSTEN NB, ROSS AF, MIECH RP: Adenine as a substrate for purine nucleoside phosphorylase. *Can J Biochem* 49:1050, 1971

124. SNYDER FF, HENDERSON JF: Alternative pathways of deoxyadenosine and adenosine metabolism. *J Biol Chem* 248:5899, 1973

125. HAMET M, BONISSOL C, CARTIER P: Activities of enzymes of purine and pyrimidine metabolism in nine mycoplasma species, in Rapado A, Watts RWE, De Bruyn CHMM (eds): *Purine Metabolism in Man III, 122B*. New York, Plenum Press, 1980, p 231

126. SAHOTA A, SIMMONDS HA, POTTER CF, WATSON JG, HUGH-JONES K, PERRETT D: Adenosine and deoxyadenosine metabolism in the erythrocytes of a patient with adenosine deaminase deficiency, in Rapado A, Watts RWE, De Bruyn CHMM (eds): *Purine Metabolism in Man III, 122A*. New York, Plenum Press, 1980, p 397

127. SIMMONDS HA, VAN ACKER KJ, POTTER CF, WEBSTER DR, KASIDAS GP, ROSE GA: Influence of purine content of diet and allopurinol on uric acid and oxalate excretion levels, in Smith LH, Robertson WG, Finlayson B (eds): *Urolithiasis: Clinical and Basic Research*. New York, Plenum Press, 1981

128. CLIFFORD AJ, STORY DL: Levels of purines in foods and their metabolic effects in rats. *J Nutr* 106:435, 1975

129. JÄNNE J, POSO H, RAINA A: Polyamines in rapid growth and cancer. *Biochim Biophys Acta* 473:241, 1978

130. PEGG AE, WILLIAMS-ASHMAN HG: Phosphate-stimulated breakdown of 5'-methylthioadenosine by rat ventral prostate. *Biochem J* 115:241, 1969

131. FERRO AJ, WROBEC NC, NICOLETTE JA: 5'-methylthioribose-1-phosphate: A product of partially purified rat liver 5'-methylthioadenosine phosphorylase activity. *Biochim Biophys Acta* 570:65, 1979

132. FERRO AJ, VANDENBARK AA, MARCHITTO K: The role of 5'-methylthioadenosine phosphorylase in 5'-methylthioadenosine-mediated inhibition of lymphocyte transformation. *Biochim Biophys Acta* 588:294, 1979

133. SAHOTA A, SIMMONDS HA: Unpublished observations, 1980

134. KREDICH NM: Personal communication, 1980

135. SIMMONDS HA, CAMERON JS, DILLON MJ, BARRATT TM, VAN ACKER KJ: 'Uric acid' stones in children—problems of diagnosis and treatment in a new defect—adenine phosphoribosyltransferase deficiency, in *Proceedings of Workshop on Uric Acid Lithiasis*, Tel Aviv, 1981, in press

136. VAN ACKER KJ, SIMMONDS HA: Erfelijke Adenine fosforibosyltransferase (APRT) deficiëntie. *Tidschr Geneeskunde* 36:497, 1980

137. SIMMONDS HA: Harnsteine bei Kindern. *MMW* 121:1654, 1979

138. REVEILLAUD RJ, DAUDON M, PROTAT MF, AYROLE G, VINTHERHARDER V: Purine metabolism and urolithiasis. *Kidney Int* 3:452, 1979 (abstract)

139. ELION GB, BENEZRA FM, BEARDMORE TD, KELLEY WN: Studies with allopurinol in patients with impaired renal function, in Rapado A, Watts RWE, De Bruyn CHMM (eds): *Purine Metabolism in Man III, 122A*. New York, Plenum Press, 1980, p 263

140. SHAPIRO S: Allopurinol and bone-marrow depression. *Lancet* 2:412, 1974 (letter)

53

IMMUNODEFICIENCY DISEASES CAUSED BY ADENOSINE DEAMINASE DEFICIENCY AND PURINE NUCLEOSIDE PHOSPHORYLASE DEFICIENCY

NICHOLAS M. KREDICH

MICHAEL S. HERSHFIELD

1. Heritable deficiency of either adenosine deaminase (ADA) or purine nucleoside phosphorylase (PNP) causes abnormalities in purine nucleoside metabolism that are selectively toxic to lymphocytes and result in immune deficiency disease. Most patients with ADA deficiency lack both cell-mediated (T-cell) and humoral (B-cell) immunity and have severe combined immunodeficiency disease (SCID). PNP-deficient children have a severe defect in cell-mediated immunity but retain relatively normal humoral immunity.

2. Both conditions are inherited in an autosomal recessive manner and result from mutations in the structural gene for either ADA or PNP. Approximately 40 to 50 cases of ADA-deficient SCID and 9 cases of PNP deficiency have been reported. The diagnosis is made by finding an absence of one or the other enzyme in a hemolysate of the patient's erythrocytes. Heterozygotes for both conditions have normal immune function and in most cases approximately one-half normal erythrocyte enzyme levels.

3. Studies of immune function in ADA deficiency reveal a relative lack of T and B cells with marked, absolute lymphopenia, absence of specific antibodies and isohemagglutinins, negative skin test reactions to infectious and chemical agents, and failure of peripheral lymphocytes to respond to stimulation by lectins and allogenic cells. Findings in PNP deficiency are similar except for the presence of B cells and antibodies.

4. Levels of the ADA substrates adenosine and deoxyadenosine are elevated in the plasma or urine of ADA-deficient children, and dATP accumulates in their erythrocytes and peripheral blood mononuclear cells. PNP-deficient children are usually hypouricemic and hypouricosuric but excrete abnormally large amounts of total purines as the PNP substrates inosine, guanosine, deoxyinosine, and deoxyguanosine; plasma inosine and guanosine are abnormally high as well.

5. Erythrocyte S-adenosylhomocysteine hydrolase activity is markedly diminished in ADA deficiency, owing to its irreversible "suicidelike" inactivation by deoxyadenosine. A lesser deficiency of erythrocyte S-adenosylhomocysteine hydrolase activity also occurs in PNP deficiency as a result of the slow inactivation of this enzyme by inosine.

6. Of the several mechanisms proposed for the pathogenesis of the immune defect in ADA deficiency, two are currently favored: dATP accumulation and S-adenosylhomocysteine toxicity. dATP is believed to accumulate preferentially in ADA-deficient T lymphocytes and inhibits ribonucleotide reductase; a resultant decrease in dCTP and possibly other deoxyribonucleotides would then lead to inhibition of DNA replication and cell division. S-Adenosylhomocysteine may accumulate as a result of increased adenosine levels or inactivation of S-adenosylhomocysteine hydrolase by deoxyadenosine; S-adenosylhomocysteine would in turn

inhibit S-adenosylmethionine–mediated transmethylation reactions vital to lymphocyte division and function.

7. *Accumulation of dGTP in T lymphocytes with resultant inhibition of ribonucleotide reductase and DNA replication has been proposed as an explanation for the T-cell defect in PNP deficiency.*

8. *Unless special measures are taken, ADA-deficient children usually die before age 2 from overwhelming infection. Bone marrow transplantation from an HLA-A and HLA-B identical donor is the preferred treatment and has resulted in virtually complete immune reconstitution in several patients. Enzyme replacement therapy in the form of repeated transfusions with irradiated packed erythrocytes from normal donors has improved immune function in some ADA-deficient children.*

   Transplantation and packed erythrocyte transfusion therapy have been used in PNP deficiency with only limited success.

Immunodeficiency states are frequently classified according to whether they involve cellular immunity, humoral immunity, or both [1]. Cellular immunity requires the participation of several different cell types, of which the thymus-dependent lymphocyte, or *T cell*, is the most characteristic. Immunoglobulin is the predominant element in humoral immunity, and its production is dependent upon a class of lymphocytes termed *B cells*. Although a significant degree of interdependence makes it impossible to dissect these two divisions of the immune system from each other completely, it is clear that primary immune defects do occur that dramatically affect one form of immunity while leaving the other relatively intact. Severe combined immunodeficiency disease (SCID) is a term used to describe a syndrome in which both cellular and humoral immunity are severely impaired.

Although several different types of heritable, or primary, immunodeficiency disease had been recognized and categorized on the basis of clinical and pathologic criteria, until 1972 none had ever been associated with a specific, known molecular defect. In that year Eloise Giblett and her collaborators [2] described two patients with SCID and virtually complete absence of erythrocyte adenosine deaminase (ADA). As Dr. Giblett relates the story [3], she was engaged in testing genetic marker systems in blood as part of a project evaluating patients receiving human transplants. Among the polymorphic enzymes analyzed in her laboratory was ADA, an activity she found to be absent in a specimen from a 2-year-old child with SCID, who was being considered for a bone marrow transplant. Shortly thereafter, she obtained a blood sample from a second SCID patient, unrelated to the first, and it too was found to lack ADA. Within a year four additional ADA-deficient SCID patients were described [4–6], making it quite clear that these two conditions are closely related.

Dr. Giblett and her colleagues then established a screening program in which other enzymes of purine and pyrimidine metabolism were assayed in patients with various immune disorders. In 1975 these efforts were rewarded with the discovery of the first case of purine nucleoside phosphorylase (PNP) deficiency, found in a 5-year-old girl with a defect in cellular immunity but with apparently normal humoral immunity [7]. Additional cases were soon reported by others [8–12].

CLINICAL ASPECTS

As the historical account suggests, the most conspicuous clinical consequence of heritable ADA or PNP deficiency is immunodeficiency, manifested as a predisposition to recurrent and persistent infections. Almost all ADA-deficient patients have SCID, whereas a T-cell defect predominates in PNP-deficient individuals, who have impaired cellular immunity and normal or even hyperactive B-cell function.

ADA Deficiency

Severe Combined Immunodeficiency   Heritable SCID is a rare disorder that is caused by at least several, and probably many different, primary genetic defects [1]. The condition is X-linked in approximately one-third of cases and has an autosomal recessive mode of inheritance in the others. Of the latter a reasonable estimate is that a third are due to ADA deficiency [13].

In most cases the immune defect is present in partial or complete form at birth, or at least at 1 to 2 months of age, which may be the earliest that a clinical picture of recurrent infection prompts an evaluation of immune function. Initially, infection involves those areas with greatest exposure to organisms, i.e., skin and gastrointestinal and respiratory systems. A variety of infectious agents are encountered, including various bacteria, fungi, viruses, and protozoa, both ordinary and opportunistic pathogens. Candidiasis is almost invariably present, usually first as just "diaper rash," then as a more extensive infection involving skin, oral mucosa, and vagina. Diarrhea, which is believed to be secondary to abnormal intestinal flora, is a common feature and may seriously compromise nutrition. Physical growth and development are delayed in most SCID patients. Unless special measures are taken, these children usually die from overwhelming infection and sepsis before 2 years of age.

Approximately 85 to 90 percent of ADA-deficient patients initially present with a form of SCID that, on the basis of clinical appearances, cannot be distinguished with confidence from the disease found in patients with normal ADA [14]. Most often a history of multiple infections during the first few months of life first prompts medical attention, or in some instances the defect is ascertained at birth because of an older sib, often deceased, with suspected or proven immunodeficiency. For the most part, physical findings are unremarkable except for evidence of infection and the absence of lymph nodes and pharyngeal lymphoid tissue.

Prominence of the costochondral junctions, a so-called rachitic rosary, may also be noted in ADA deficiency [14]. Three patients have been described with various neurologic abnormalities including spasticity, head lag, movement disorders, nystagmus, and inability to focus [15, 16]. Although the relationship of these disturbances to ADA deficiency is unclear, their improvement with enzyme replacement therapy suggests that loss of ADA leads to an accumulation of toxic metabolites that can disturb neurologic function [16]. Fine, sparse hair, anatomic malformations of the urinary tract, and transient renal tubular acidosis have also been reported [14], but so rarely that their association with ADA deficiency may be only coincidental.

In contrast to those ADA-deficient patients who present

with classical SCID, the remaining 10 to 15 percent have a milder disease characterized by later age of onset and relative sparing of humoral immunity. In several cases immune function was found to deteriorate over the course of months or years until typical SCID prevailed, implying a cumulative effect of ADA deficiency on the immune system [17–19].

Radiographic Features X-ray studies show, as in other forms of SCID, absence of a thymic shadow and suggest diminution or lack of adenoids. Of special note is the finding in about two-thirds of ADA patients of a characteristic cupping and flaring of the anterior rib ends, which is responsible for the rachitic rosary [20]. This abnormality is also seen in rickets and a number of other conditions, but its presence in the clinical setting of suspected immunodeficiency should alert one to the possibility of ADA deficiency. Other x-ray abnormalities include pelvic dysplasia, shortening of the vertebral transverse processes with flattening or convexity of their ends, platyspondyly, and unusually thick growth arrest lines [20]. None of these x-ray changes is specific for ADA deficiency and in our present state of knowledge may be construed as nonspecific reactions to metabolic insult [21].

Laboratory Findings Laboratory studies show lymphopenia ranging from severe to moderate, with absolute lymphocyte counts generally less than 500 per cubic millimeter. Eosinophilia has been reported in some patients, but other blood elements are normal in number. Abnormal platelet function in vitro has been described [22, 23]. Lymphocytes, when present, usually bear none of the surface markers by which B cells and T cells are routinely identified. Skin tests for delayed hypersensitivity to Candida, streptokinase, streptodornase, dinitrochlorobenzene, and other agents are negative, and, when attempted, skin grafts are not rejected. In vitro lymphocyte responses to lectins such as phytohemagglutinin and concanavalin A, to specific antigens, and to allogenic cells are attenuated or absent. Total immunoglobulin levels may be only slightly depressed at birth because of the maternal contribution of IgG, but IgM and IgA, which ordinarily do not pass the placental barrier, are often absent. IgG levels decline as maternal antibodies are cleared, and by 1 or 2 months of age pronounced hypogammaglobulinemia signals the patient's lack of humoral immunity. Antibody responses to specific antigens such as tetanus toxoid usually cannot be elicited, and blood group isoagglutinins are absent in patients with SCID.

The prerequisite finding for the diagnosis of ADA-deficient SCID is, of course, the demonstration of very low or immeasurable levels of ADA. Because of its ready availability, an erythrocyte hemolysate is routinely used as an enzyme source, but in many instances peripheral lymphocytes and other tissues have been assayed as well and found to lack ADA activity. One can also find elevated levels of the ADA substrates adenosine and 2'-deoxyadenosine in the plasma and urine of many patients (Table 53-1).

Pathology The cartilaginous growth plates of ADA-deficient children lack proliferative cells and column formation in the hypertrophic zone and show interrupted areas of calcified cartilage with poor trabecular formation. These changes correspond to the x-ray abnormalities already described and are unlike those seen in other metaphyseal chondrodysplasias [24].

Early studies on thymic histopathology suggested a significant difference between ADA-deficient patients and SCID patients with normal ADA [25]. In the latter group the thymus was described as embryonal, with small nests of undifferentiated epithelial cells and an absence of Hassall's bodies, a picture presumed to represent a defect in the early stages of thymic differentiation. In contrast, the thymus in several ADA-deficient children showed areas of differentiated epithelium and Hassall's bodies, which suggested some degree of normal thymic development and subsequent involution. A later study, however, failed to find consistent differences between these two groups of SCID patients [21].

Other ADA Abnormalities Shortly after the first description of ADA deficiency in SCID, a report appeared of a 10-year-old !Kung tribesman in South-West Africa, who lacked erythrocyte ADA while retaining normal immune function [26]. Subsequent studies showed that this individual, who appears to be homozygous for a mutant ADA allele common among the !Kung (gene frequency of about 0.11) [27], has ADA activities in his erythrocytes, leukocytes, and cultured fibroblasts that are 2 to 3 percent, 10 to 12 percent, and 26 percent, respectively, of normal [28]. Immune function was still normal when reevaluated at age 18 [29].

An additional interesting case of ADA deficiency in an immunocompetent individual was discovered as the result of a newborn screening program in New York State. As in the !Kung tribesman, this child's erythrocytes were found to contain virtually no ADA, but his peripheral mononuclear cells had ADA activity that was 24 percent of a control value and very heat labile [30]. In both cases, it is believed that the reduced levels of ADA activity found in tissues other than erythrocytes are adequate to preserve immune function and that the near absence of erythrocyte ADA is caused by the time-dependent inactivation of a relatively unstable mutant enzyme in cells that cannot synthesize new protein.

Erythrocyte ADA levels that are 40 to 70 times normal have been described in individuals from two unrelated families [31, 32]. This condition is associated with a 50 percent reduction in erythrocyte ATP and a mild to fully compensated, Coombs' negative, nonspherocytic hemolytic anemia. Lymphocyte ADA levels and immune function appear to be normal. In one family a pedigree analysis showed an autosomal dominant form of inheritance, and biochemical studies suggested that the elevated levels of ADA are due to increased quantities of a normal enzyme [31].

PNP Deficiency

The clinical feature common to all nine PNP-deficient patients thus far described is a defect in cellular immunity in conjunction with relatively normal humoral immunity [7–12, 33]. Children have presented between 4 months and 9 years of age with infections involving skin, lung, middle ear and mastoids, and urinary tract. In keeping with current concepts regarding the role of cellular immunity, infections with nonbacterial agents such as Candida albicans, varicella, vaccinia, and cytomegalovirus have been the most common and troublesome in these patients. Although several children have received live virus immunization without complication, two others developed generalized vaccinia, which for one proved fatal [10]. The neurologic abnormalities described in two patients [8, 12] may

Table 53-1 Purine compounds in plasma, serum, and urine of ADA- and PNP-deficient patients

A. Plasma or serum, ADA and PNP deficiency*

Compound	Controls, μM	ADA deficiency, μM	PNP deficiency, μM	References
Adenosine	<0.5	0.7–6.7		[155, 160, 245, 284]
Deoxyadenosine	<0.1	0.15–1.8		[245, 284]
Inosine	Undetectable		14–115	[7, 8, 12, 35, 82, 256, 285]
Guanosine	Undetectable		6–29	[8, 82, 285]
Urate	220 ± 60		100–150	[7, 12, 35, 256, 285]

B. Urine, ADA deficiency*

	Adenosine	Deoxyadenosine	References
Control, μmol/24 h	<2	Undetectable	
ADA deficiency,	<2–5.6	60–124	[163, 286]
Control, μmol/g uric acid	<4.2	<0.6	[287]
ADA deficiency, μmol/g uric acid	15.7	193	
Control, μM	<0.3, 5.4 ± 4.5	<2, <0.01	[190, 288]
ADA deficiency, μM	1.38, 5.6	300, 68	
ADA deficiency, mmol/mol creatinine	4.5 ± 1.2	50 ± 16	[289]

C. Urine, PNP deficiency*

Compound	Controls, mmol/24 h (mmol/g creatinine)	PNP deficiency, mmol/24 h (mmol/g creatinine)	References
Inosine	undetectable	1.3–4.3 (4.5–16)	[7, 12, 35, 163, 256, 259, 285]
Deoxyinosine	undetectable	1.7, 0.4 (4.7)	[35, 163, 259]
Guanosine	undetectable	0.61–2.3 (1.4–7.7)	[7, 12, 35, 163, 256, 259, 285]
Deoxyguanosine	undetectable	0.82, 0.53 (2.3)	[35, 163, 259]
Uric acid	(2.8–5.2)†	0.01–1.19 (0.16–3.13)	[7, 12, 35, 163, 256, 259, 285]
Uric acid equivalents (mg/mg creatinine)	0.48–0.88†	1.9–5.1	[7, 12, 35, 163, 256, 259, 285]

*Data have, where possible, been recalculated for purposes of comparison of values in common units.
†Data for children from Balis ME, Krakoff IH, Berman PH, Dancis J: *Science* 156:1122, 1967.

represent complications of viral infection rather than direct consequences of PNP deficiency per se.

X-rays may show absence of a thymic shadow, but none of the bone abnormalities characteristic of ADA deficiency has been noted in PNP-deficient patients. Anemia has occurred in several children, and at one point was the most conspicuous feature in the first PNP-deficient patient described, whose hypoplastic bone marrow had earlier suggested a diagnosis of Diamond-Blackfan syndrome [7]. Autoimmune hemolytic anemia has been observed in two patients [11, 12].

Studies of immune function in PNP deficiency show lymphopenia, a paucity of peripheral T cells as determined by E-rosetting with sheep erythrocytes, diminished or absent lymphocyte responses to phytohemagglutinin and allogenic cells, and negative delayed hypersensitivity skin tests. One patient, diagnosed retrospectively, suffered a fatal graft-versus-host reaction following transfusion with unirradiated whole blood [8, 34]. Tests of humoral immunity typically show normal levels of immunoglobulins, isohemagglutinins, and specific antibodies. The finding of autoimmune hemolytic anemia in two patients and in a third of rheumatoid factor, a positive LE preparation, antinuclear antibody, and a positive Coombs' test [33] has led to speculation that impairment of T-suppressor cell activity in PNP deficiency can actually lead to a hyperactive state of humoral immunity (see discussion in [33]).

Assays of erythrocyte lysates and other tissues show only trace to immeasurable levels of PNP activity. Most patients have marked hypouricemia and hypouricosuria, but actually excrete excessive amounts of total purine, which are found in the urine as inosine, guanosine, 2'-deoxyinosine, 2'-deoxyguanosine, and uric acid 9-N-ribonucleoside [35]. High levels of inosine and guanosine are found in patients' sera as well (Table 53-1).

GENETIC ASPECTS

ADA Deficiency

Genetics and Chemistry of the Normal Enzyme ADA catalyzes the irreversible deamination of adenosine and 2'-deoxyadenosine to inosine and 2'-deoxyinosine, respectively (Fig. 53-1). The enzyme exists in many different physical forms, which can be accounted for by a combination of genetic polymorphism and a system of isoenzymes generated by post-translational modifications and binding to a noncatalytic glycoprotein.

The use of specific histochemical stains for enzyme activity has allowed characterization of ADA isoenzymes by their mobility during starch-gel electrophoresis [36]. The pattern given by erythrocyte lysates is relatively simple, consisting of one major and two minor bands, and has been used extensively to study ADA genetic polymorphism. In the phenotype designated ADA 2 each of the three erythrocyte isoenzymes has a slightly slower anodal mobility than that of its counterpart in the predominant ADA 1 phenotype. A combination of the two patterns is seen in the ADA 2,1 phenotype and indicates codominant expression of two alleles, designated ADA^1 and ADA^2, at an autosomal locus. This conclusion has been confirmed by pedigree analyses [36]. Thus, ADA 1, ADA 2, ADA 2,1 are the phenotypes corresponding to the genotypes ADA^1/ADA^1, ADA^2/ADA^2, and ADA^2/ADA^1, respectively. ADA^2 is much less common than ADA^1 and has a gene frequency of 0.03 to 0.11 in populations described as "Negro," "English," and "Asian Indian" [36].

Examination of tissues other than erythrocytes shows more complicated isoenzyme patterns, which in large part are tissue-specific [37]. Most if not all of these "tissue isoenzymes" are of higher molecular weight than the erythrocyte enzymes [37, 38] and arise from interaction of the ADA catalytic moiety with a protein termed *binding protein* or *complexing protein* [39]. Variations in the carbohydrate content of binding protein may account for the different tissue isoenzymes noted on electrophoresis [40, 41]. The erythrocyte isoenzymes contain no binding protein and presumably reflect posttranslational modifications of the catalytic subunit itself [42, 43].

The catalytic moiety of ADA from several human tissues has been purified to homogeneity and is a single polypeptide chain with a molecular weight of 36,000 to 38,000 [42, 43]. The locus coding for this protein has been assigned to the long arm of human chromosome 20 [44], more specifically 20q13.2→qter [45]. The binding protein also has been exten-

sively purified [41, 46] and is a dimer with a native molecular weight of about 190,000. One native molecule of binding protein has been found to bind two molecules of catalytic ADA [41]. No catalytic activity or physiologic role for binding protein has yet been described. Genes on chromosomes 2 and 6 are both required for the expression of binding protein in cultured cells [47, 48].

The Primary Genetic Defect Studies using patient tissues have not only delineated the nature of the genetic defect in ADA deficiency but have also aided our understanding of the relatedness of ADA isoenzymes. The finding that ADA-deficient children lack both erythrocyte and tissue isoenzymes indicates that there is a component common to all forms of ADA that is missing or defective in this condition [49]. Binding protein is normal in ADA deficiency as determined from direct assays [50] and from the fact that addition of tissue extracts from an ADA-deficient child to normal erythrocyte enzyme results in the formation of tissue isoenzymes [51].

At the time of the first description of ADA deficiency it was suggested that the actual genetic lesion in these children might be a deletion extending from the ADA locus into a nearby gene that was in some way required for immune function [2]. Thus it was speculated that the loss of ADA in these children might only be accidental and not responsible per se for SCID. This possibility now seems most unlikely in view of the demonstration of mutant enzymes possessing residual activity but differing from normal with respect to kinetic properties, electrophoretic mobility, and heat stability [50, 52–55]. The reactivity of these enzymes with antibody to normal ADA [50, 54, 55] leaves little doubt that they are products of a mutant ADA locus. Since large deletions are unlikely to give proteins with such recognizable properties, it appears that a mutation in the ADA locus itself is sufficient to cause both ADA deficiency and SCID. Considerable heterogeneity has been demonstrated among mutant proteins, which is probably responsible in part for the variability in expression of SCID in ADA deficiency.

Prevalence, Inheritance, and Diagnosis Approximately 40 to 50 families with ADA-deficient SCID have been identified. The actual prevalence of this condition has not been determined, but prospective screening of 1,000,000 newborns in New York State detected only one case of partial ADA deficiency with normal immune function and no children with ADA-deficient SCID [13].

Consistent with our knowledge of the molecular genetics of ADA, family studies have shown an autosomal recessive mode of inheritance for ADA-deficient SCID, with most obligate heterozygotes having approximately half-normal levels of erythrocyte ADA. Because of an overlap between normal individuals and some obligate heterozygotes, erythrocyte ADA levels are reliable for the identification of only 90 percent of carriers [56]. ADA levels in cultured skin fibroblasts and amniotic cells are too variable to be useful in heterozygote detection [52].

Occasionally ADA polymorphism can be exploited to identify carriers of a mutant or "null" gene, as was demonstrated in a family in which three sibs with ADA 1 phenotypes were born to ADA 1 and ADA 2 parents [57]. One would have expected ADA 2,1 offspring in this situation; therefore the ADA 2 parent (in this case the mother) must have contributed a null gene. Similar cases have been reported in families of ADA-deficient children [58, 59].

Although unsuitable for the detection of carriers, assay of

Figure 53-1 Reactions catalyzed by ADA and PNP.

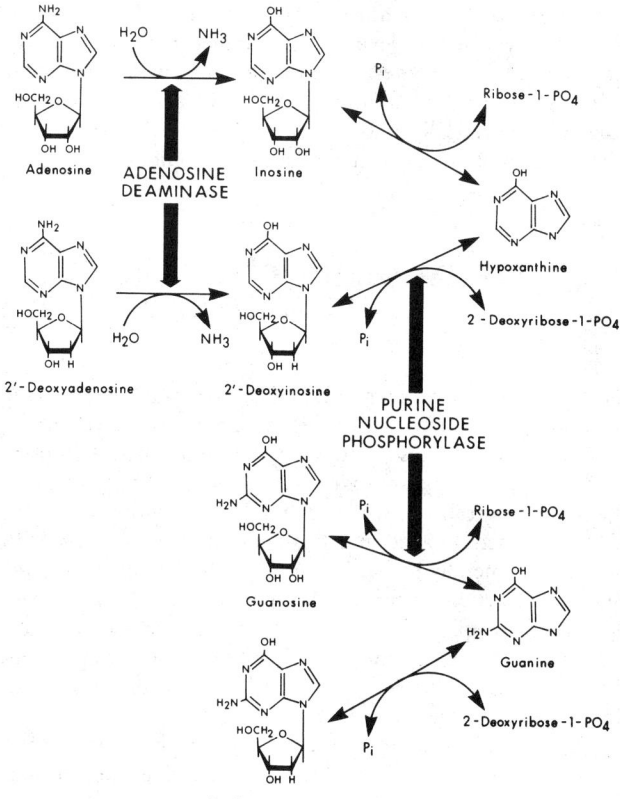

ADA in cultured amniotic cells has been used successfully in the prenatal diagnosis of ADA deficiency [60, 61]. By means of a sensitive microradioassay, ADA can be measured in as few as 1000 cells within 14 days after amniocentesis [62]. Other assays are suitable for newborn screening [63, 64].

PNP Deficiency

Genetics and Chemistry of the Normal Enzyme   PNP catalyzes the reversible phosphorolysis of inosine, guanosine, and their 2'-deoxy derivatives to give either hypoxanthine or guanine and the appropriate pentose-1-phosphate (Fig. 53-1). K_m values of 44 to 60 μM have been reported for these nucleosides with the human erythrocyte enzyme [65, 66]. Although the equilibrium constant in the direction of nucleoside formation is rather high (K_{eq} is 54 for inosine [67] and 2'-deoxyinosine [68] formation), intracellular phosphorolysis occurs readily, probably as a result of inorganic phosphate concentrations that are higher than those of ribose-1-phosphate or 2-deoxyribose-1-phosphate. The mammalian enzyme has no significant activity with adenosine as a substrate [69]. Hence, both ADA and PNP are required in the sequential degradation of adenosine and 2'-deoxyadenosine to hypoxanthine.

Human PNP has been extensively purified from several different tissues including erythrocytes [66, 70–72], placenta [73], granulocytes [74] and cultured fibroblasts [75]. In each case the native enzyme has been found to be a trimer composed of subunits with identical molecular weights. The erythrocyte enzyme has a native molecular weight of 87,000 to 94,000 with a subunit molecular weight of 30,000 to 32,000 [71, 72, 76]. Similar values have been reported for the enzymes isolated from other tissues.

As in the case of ADA, electrophoretic separations of native PNP show an extensive system of isoenzymes, which arise from a common gene product and vary from one tissue to another [77]. There is no evidence for a noncatalytic, PNP-binding protein. The most complicated pattern is found in erythrocytes where at least seven isoenzymes can be demonstrated. Isoenzymes with a slower anodal mobility predominate in young erythrocytes, and older cells have greater amounts of the more rapidly migrating species [78]. The patterns in placenta, granulocytes, and cultured fibroblasts are much simpler, consisting of only two or three isoenzymes which correspond to the slowest erythrocyte bands. From these findings it has been suggested that the slowest migrating band is the primary gene product, or at least most closely related to such, and that other bands arise from time-dependent, posttranslational modifications [78] which are likely to be more extensive in erythrocytes than in tissues with a significant rate of protein turnover.

The separation of erythrocyte PNP subunits by isoelectric focusing has shown four major and two minor forms with the same molecular weights but with different pIs [71]. Given a trimeric structure and the estimated charge differences between the four major components, one would predict the generation of twelve electrophoretically distinguishable native isoenzymes if all combinations of subunits were permitted. The fact that only seven are usually noted may be due to technical difficulties in obtaining sufficient resolution and sensitivity.

The locus for human PNP is on the long arm of chromosome 14 [79]. Although variant alleles of PNP have been described, they are very rare, and the locus is not polymorphic in the populations tested [77]. Studies of isoenzyme patterns in individuals heterozygous for such rare alleles provided some of the earliest evidence for the trimeric structure of the native enzyme [77].

The Primary Genetic Defect   Considerable evidence indicates that the genetic defect in PNP-deficient patients lies in the PNP gene locus itself. Patients from two unrelated families have been found to have residual erythrocyte PNP activities that differ from each other and from normal with respect to kinetic parameters, isoelectric point, and sensitivity to sulfhydryl reagents [80, 81]. Two patients from one of these families have PNP with an altered electrophoretic mobility, 0.5 percent of normal enzyme activity, and about 50 percent of normal reactivity with specific antibody [80, 82]. Studies of obligate heterozygotes have shown varying amounts of immunologically reacting protein with little or no enzyme activity, indicating the presence of catalytically inactive PNP protein [82]. In one family, a mutant protein could not be demonstrated in the patient but was present in both consanguine parents [3, 82, 83]. Two-dimensional protein gels and peptide maps of the PNP purified from the parents have shown what is believed to be two forms of mutant subunit with molecular weights that are 300 to 500 greater than normal [83, 84].

The molecular heterogeneity found in these different cases of PNP deficiency indicates that different mutations at the same locus can lead to similar biochemical and clinical results, a finding common to many inborn errors of metabolism.

Prevalence, Inheritance, and Diagnosis   In spite of a heightened awareness of PNP deficiency among immunologists and other clinicians, a total of only nine patients in six families has been described, making this a very rare condition. Both males and females are affected, and based on the molecular genetics of PNP as well as on family studies, PNP deficiency must be considered an autosomal recessive condition. In most cases erythrocyte PNP levels have been reported as half-normal in obligate heterozygotes. The presence of a low serum urate in a child with recurrent infections should suggest PNP deficiency. Theoretically it should be possible to diagnose PNP deficiency in utero by assaying cultured amniotic cells.

METABOLISM OF PURINE NUCLEOSIDES

Several observations suggest that ADA serves a "detoxifying" function particularly essential to lymphoid tissue. (1) Inhibition of ADA enhances the toxicity of its substrates. Adenosine and deoxyadenosine are toxic to ADA-deficient cells at micromolar concentrations, while millimolar concentrations of the ADA products inosine and deoxyinosine are not. (2) ADA activity is generally higher in lymphoid than nonlymphoid tissues. ADA activity increases in lymph draining from antigen-stimulated lymph nodes in sheep [85] and increases in and is excreted by mitogen-stimulated peripheral blood lymphocytes [86]. (3) ADA deficiency causes selective lymphopenia and immunodeficiency.

There is now general agreement that lymphopenia in ADA deficiency results from toxic effects of adenosine and deoxyadenosine and also that T-cell dysfunction in PNP deficiency may result from toxicity of one of its substrates, deoxyguanosine. These nucleosides are toxic to nonlymphoid as well as to lymphoid cells in tissue culture, so that understanding the basis for selective lymphotoxicity in vivo requires information at three levels, regarding: (1) the factors that govern the production and disposal of purine nucleosides, both at the cellular level and in intact individuals; (2) the biochemical actions of purine nucleosides that can contribute to their toxicity; and (3) the basis for selective toxicity of nucleosides to lymphoid cells.

We will briefly review the normal metabolism of purine nucleosides as a framework for considering the mechanisms of their toxicity to cultured cells, and their metabolism in ADA- and PNP-deficient patients.

Sources of Purine Nucleosides

The concentration of urate in plasma, approximately 200 to 450 μM, and the amount excreted daily in the urine, approximately 2 to 4 mmol, far exceed those values for any other extracellular purine. Adenosine concentration in plasma has been reported in the range of 0.05 to 0.5 μM (Table 53-1). Concentrations of other purine ribo- and deoxyribonucleosides are even lower, being usually reported as "undetectable," probably less than 0.05 μM. Intracellular purines exist almost exclusively as 5'-phosphorylated nucleoside derivatives (nucleotides and nucleic acids), or in other forms in which the hydroxyl group on the 5' carbon of the pentose moiety of the nucleoside is replaced by amino acids (S-adenosylmethionine and its derivative, S-adenosylhomocysteine). Free nucleosides are formed in the degradation of these compounds.

Some adenosine must be formed in all living cells from the hydrolysis of S-adenosylhomocysteine derived from S-adenosylmethionine–dependent methyl transfer reactions. Metabolic balance studies in which the intake and excretion of methylated compounds were determined in normal adults suggest that 14 to 23 mmol of adenosine is generated from S-adenosylhomocysteine daily [87]. Methylation of guanidinoacetic acid to form creatine alone accounts for about 85 percent of the total S-adenosylhomocysteine formed. This reaction occurs in the liver. In other tissues a variety of transmethylation reactions involving nucleic acids, proteins, phospholipids, biogenic amines, and other methyl acceptors account for the remainder of the adenosine derived from this route.

The potential sources of nucleotides and nucleic acids that may undergo degradation to nucleosides include (1) diet, (2) senescent cells, (3) living cells in their normal metabolic state, and (4) ischemic cells, or cells treated with inhibitors of energy metabolism (largely a laboratory phenomenon).

Labeled nucleic acids fed to mice were rapidly broken down, but most of the nucleosides formed were further catabolized in liver and intestine and excreted without gaining access to the systemic circulation [88]. This appears to be the case in humans [89]. Absorption of nucleosides derived from dietary nucleotides would be expected to increase in ADA- or PNP-deficient patients, a possibility which has not yet been studied.

Dissolution of cells derived from senescent bone marrow may be the major source of nucleotides and nucleic acids that are degraded to nucleosides. A variety of extracellular, membrane-bound, lysosomal, and cytoplasmic nucleases, nucleo-

tidases, and phosphatases exist that might participate in this process, but in general physiologic roles have not yet been firmly established for specific enzymes. One enzyme that has received considerable attention is the "ecto" 5'-nucleotidase (EC 3.1.3.5) present on the external surface of the plasma membrane [90, 91]. The preferred substrate for the ectoenzyme from guinea pig polymorphonuclear leukocytes is AMP with a K_m of 10.6 μM [91]. This enzyme has been shown to catalyze the "vectorial" dephosphorylation of extracellular AMP, facilitating its entry as adenosine into lymphocytes [92] and cardiac muscle [93]. Involvement of ecto-5'-nucleotidase in the degradation of intracellular nucleotides has been questioned, both because of its extracellular location and because it is strongly inhibited by purine and pyrimidine nucleoside triphosphates. Direct evidence against such involvement has been obtained in studies with rat polymorphonuclear leukocytes [94].

AMP is generated within living cells from ATP-requiring processes and from turnover of RNA, particularly of the 3'-terminal polyadenylate region of messenger RNA. It is unclear to what extent adenosine is produced from intracellular AMP. Under normal metabolic conditions reconversion of AMP to ATP is highly efficient. In contracting skeletal muscle this involves the intermediate steps of deamination of AMP to IMP, followed by resynthesis of AMP, catalyzed by adenylosuccinate synthetase and lyase (the "purine nucleotide cycle" discussed in Chap. 54). In other tissues AMP is directly rephosphorylated. An intracellular "adenosine cycle" has been proposed to operate in living cells under physiologic conditions [95], which involves the sequence, AMP → adenosine → inosine → hypoxanthine → IMP → AMP. Direct attempts have been made to quantitate adenosine produced in the first step in the postulated cycle. Under culture conditions that would support normal cellular respiration very little evidence of adenosine production occurred in Ehrlich ascites cells [96], rat liver [97], rat leukocytes [94], or in normal or adenosine kinase–deficient WI-L2 human lymphoblasts [98–100], in studies where deamination or both deamination and rephosphorylation of adenosine were prevented. There is little evidence to support the physiologic operation within cells of the so-called adenosine cycle. Some release of adenosine by adipose tissue [101] and well-oxygenated liver has been observed [102, 103].

Although dephosphorylation of intracellular AMP is probably not a physiologic source of adenosine in most tissues, some adenosine is produced by conditions that cause the net degradation of adenine nucleotides, such as myocardial anoxia [104] or treatment of cells with metabolic poisons. An attempt has been made to determine the relative extents to which degradation of intracellular AMP under these circumstances proceeds by the route AMP → adenosine → inosine, or by direct deamination to IMP followed by dephosphorylation to inosine. In Ehrlich ascites cells treated with 2-deoxyglucose more than 80 percent of the adenylate broken down was directly deaminated to IMP, and less than 20 percent was dephosphorylated [105]. Fructose-induced adenine nucleotide catabolism in rat liver also proceeded via the AMP → IMP pathway [97]; formation of adenosine was only observed when AMP deaminase was inhibited by high concentrations of coformycin. Adenosine formation was not observed in studies of KCN-treated rat leukocytes [94]; neither inhibitors of ADA nor antiserum to ecto-5'-nucleotidase altered the production of inosine from intracellular ATP, findings also consistent with degradation via the AMP → IMP, rather than the AMP → adenosine route. In studies of human WI-L2 lymphoblasts starved for glucose and oxygen or treated with inhibitors of oxidative phosphorylation, adenosine formation was observed only when the adenylate energy charge (ATP + $\frac{1}{2}$ ADP/ATP + ADP + AMP) fell to less than 0.6 from its value of 0.9 under physiologic conditions [100].

Production of inosine and guanosine has not been as extensively studied as that of adenosine, either with regard to the enzymes involved (except for ADA) or the magnitude of production by cultured cells. It is likely that little guanosine is produced within living cells from GMP, except when energy metabolism is severely compromised, but is derived mainly from catabolism of nucleotides of dead cells. Inosine is derived from dephosphorylation of IMP, as well as from deamination of adenosine. IMP may be the primary source of inosine in vivo, since ADA deficiency does not decrease the excretion of uric acid, an appreciable fraction of which is derived from inosine.

It is unlikely that appreciable purine deoxyribonucleosides are generated in living cells. Deoxyribonucleoside triphosphate pools are usually 1 percent or less than those of the corresponding ribonucleotides, and they are primarily committed to DNA polymerization. "Turnover" of DNA as such does not occur, except for some excision of nucleotides as part of repair or recombinational processes. Deoxyadenosine and deoxyguanosine are probably derived mainly from degradation of DNA from dead cells or diet. Release of deoxyadenosine from DNA of nucleated erythrocyte precursors by the action of phagocytizing mouse macrophages has been demonstrated [106].

Metabolic Fate of Purine Nucleosides

Entry of exogenous purine and pyrimidine nucleosides into cells is efficient and involves facilitated diffusion mediated by elements that recognize the presence of the pentose sugar rather than the nature of the base. Drugs that are potent inhibitors of adenosine transport, such as nitrobenzylthioinosine, nitrobenzylthioguanosine, or dipyridamole, inhibit transport of both purine and pyrimidine ribo-and deoxyribonucleosides [107–109]. An adenosine-resistant mutant of S49 mouse lymphoma cells was incapable of transporting not only adenosine but a number of other purine and pyrimidine nucleosides, confirming the concept of a single nucleoside transport system [110].

In normal cells adenosine undergoes essentially two reactions: phosphorylation to AMP, catalyzed by adenosine kinase, and deamination to inosine, catalyzed by ADA. The K_m values for adenosine of human adenosine kinase from placenta [111], red cells [112], and WI-L2 lymphoblasts [113] range from 0.4 to 3 μM, considerably less than values reported for human ADA, 25 to 74 μM, [38, 43, 114, 115]. In most tissue and cell extracts that have been studied, the total activity of ADA exceeds that of adenosine kinase. A few careful studies of alternative rates of adenosine utilization in intact cells have shown that phosphorylation exceeds deamination only at low concentrations of adenosine. As the concentration of adenosine increases, adenosine kinase becomes saturated and is also subject to both substrate and product inhibition [111, 116]. In mitogen-stimulated human peripheral blood lymphocytes [86] and in the WI-L2 line of human B lymphoblastoid cells [99]

deamination far exceeded phosphorylation above 5 μM external adenosine (Fig. 53-2). In unstimulated peripheral blood lymphocytes deamination exceeded phosphorylation by tenfold at all adenosine concentrations above 0.5 μM [86]. An adenosine phosphorylase activity has been reported to exist in rat liver and in some rodent tumor lines [117]. In rat liver cleavage of adenosine to adenine occurred only at approximately 0.25 percent of the rates of deamination or phosphorylation.

Deoxyadenosine is below present limits of accurate measurement in plasma (~0.1 μM). The K_m of ADA for deoxyadenosine is in the range of 7 to 40 μM, comparable to that for adenosine, and the maximal rate of its deamination by ADA is about 30 percent that of adenosine [38, 115, 118]. Deamination was by far the major route of deoxyadenosine metabolism in studies of several mouse tissues and human erythrocytes [119]. By using the appropriate maximal velocities and Michaelis constants determined in extracts of rat thymocytes, it was calculated that the ratio of deamination:phosphorylation would be greater than 2000:1 at 0.1 μM deoxyadenosine, and greater than 200:1 even at 1 mM; analogous ratios for adenosine were 3:1 and 80:1 [118]. Phosphorylation only plays a significant role in deoxyadenosine metabolism in ADA deficiency, as discussed below.

Taken together, the results of available studies suggest that in normal individuals deoxyadenosine is almost exclusively deaminated, while phosphorylation is a significant route, and in some tissues with low ADA activity the major route, of adenosine metabolism. Dephosphorylation of IMP must be an important source of inosine since uric acid excretion is not affected by ADA deficiency. This implies that production of its precursors inosine and guanosine is undiminished.

Metabolism of PNP substrates by routes other than phosphorolysis is minimal, although not as well studied as the metabolism of ADA substrates. There has been no corroborated evidence for the operation of enzymes that phosphorylate inosine, deoxyinosine, or guanosine in intact mammalian cells, although some enzymes do show limited activity with these nucleosides. Phosphorylation of deoxyguanosine in PNP deficiency will be discussed below.

Figure 53-2 Ratio of the rates of [^{14}C]adenosine phosphorylation and deamination by intact human WI-L2 lymphoblasts, as a function of the concentration of [^{14}C]adenosine. (*From Snyder et al. [99]. Used by permission.*)

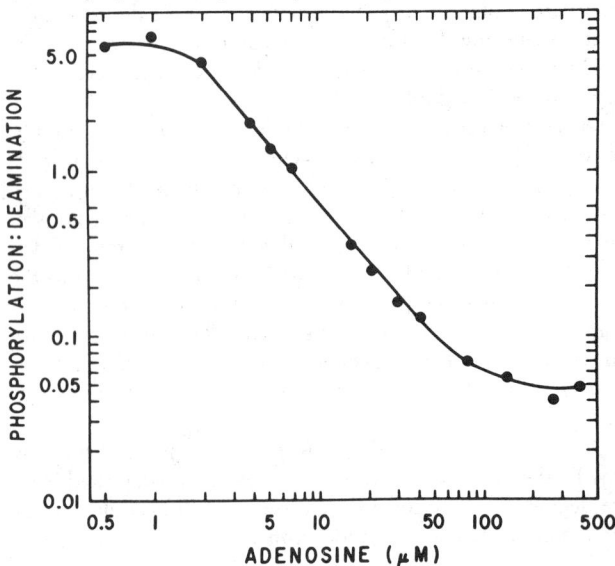

PATHOGENESIS

Cultured Cell Models of ADA Deficiency

Toxic effects of some naturally occurring purines in the 10^{-4} to 10^{-3} M range were first recognized in attempts to characterize the growth requirements of cultured cells, and in conjunction with studies of cytotoxic purine analogues (see reviews [120–122]). The tumor cells and fibroblasts used in these studies possessed the normal complement of nucleoside catabolizing enzymes. In more recent studies lymphoid cells lacking ADA activity have been employed as a more appropriate model for identifying toxic effects of adenosine and deoxyadenosine that might cause lymphopenia in the 0.5 to 10 μM range found in the plasma of ADA-deficient children.

The severe lymphopenia, small size, and poor health of children with ADA deficiency has limited biochemical and functional studies of their lymphoid cells. In one study, peripheral lymphocytes with 8 percent of normal ADA activity were obtained from a child with incomplete enzyme deficiency who had a severe defect in T-cell function but normal immunoglobulin levels [123]. Fifty μM adenosine caused a 50 percent inhibition of the response of these cells to phytohemagglutinin, compared with 500 μM adenosine required to inhibit normal lymphocytes to the same extent. Epstein-Barr virus–transformed B lymphoblastoid cell lines from patients with partial ADA deficiency and some degree of humoral immune function have also been established in culture and shown to be more sensitive to ADA substrates than normal B-cell lines [124]. It has been more convenient for most investigators studying the basis for toxicity of ADA substrates to use lymphoid cells derived from normal individuals which are then cultured with ADA inhibitors. Potent inhibitors with a high degree of specificity for ADA were originally developed to slow the degradation of adenosine analogues with chemotherapeutic potential. Of these agents, coformycin, EHNA [erythro-9-(2-hydroxy-3-nonyl)adenine], and 2'-deoxycoformycin (Pentostatin), with inhibitory constants of 1×10^{-11}, 1.6×10^{-9}, and 2.5×10^{-12} M, respectively [125], have been widely used to achieve tissue culture models of severe (≥98 percent) ADA deficiency.

A consistent observation in all these models in vitro is that ADA inhibition is not particularly toxic to lymphoid cells cultured in the absence of exogenous ADA substrates per se. This presumably reflects the limited production of deoxyadenosine in living cells, and the capacity of adenosine kinase to metabolize nontoxically the adenosine that is generated from S-adenosylhomocysteine cleavage. On the other hand, ADA inhibition greatly enhances the toxicity of exogenous adenosine and deoxyadenosine. For example, in the absence of ADA inhibitors 50 μM adenosine did not block the response of human peripheral blood lymphocytes to phytohemagglutinin, even when cultured in horse serum that lacked ADA activity. The same concentration of adenosine inhibited blastogenesis by 95 percent and caused significant cell death in the presence of a nontoxic concentration of coformycin sufficient to inhibit ADA by 95 percent [86]. Similar enhancement of adenosine and deoxyadenosine toxicity by nontoxic concentrations of ADA inhibitors has been reported in numerous studies of both human and rodent lymphoid and nonlymphoid cells. Adenosine toxicity to ADA-inhibited cells is usually manifested in the range of 5 to 50 μM, and deoxyadenosine at 0.2 to 50 μM.

Variation in sensitivity is related in part to differences among cell types and species in the way nucleosides are metabolized or exert their effects and partly to differences in experimental design. ADA inhibitors themselves do cause toxicity at concentrations much higher than required to inhibit ADA, presumably related to their weaker interaction with other enzymes, such as AMP deaminase [126–128].

Specific Mechanisms of Adenosine and Deoxyadenosine Toxicity

The major toxic effects of adenosine, deoxyadenosine, and their metabolites that have been considered as potential causes of the immune dysfunction in ADA deficiency are summarized in Fig. 53-3. Prior to 1977 most attention was focused upon two mechanisms involving adenosine, the first mediated through its effects on cyclic AMP levels, and the second, pyrimidine starvation, mediated by excessive conversion of adenosine to other adenine nucleotides. Since 1977, interest has shifted to effects of dATP accumulation from deoxyadenosine and to effects of both adenosine and deoxyadenosine that impair the catabolism of S-adenosylhomocysteine.

Cyclic AMP as a Mediator of Adenosine Toxicity

Adenosine has effects on several biologic processes that are thought to be physiologic and mediated by changes in the intracellular concentration of cyclic AMP (cAMP). The literature dealing with these effects is too extensive to be reviewed here, but the effects include its actions as a vasodilator, as an inhibitor of platelet aggregation and lipolysis, as a stimulator of steroidogenesis, and as both an inhibitor and stimulator of histamine release. Increases or decreases in cAMP levels observed in some adenosine-treated cells appear to result from direct interaction of adenosine with outer cell membrane–associated adenylate cyclase, first suggested by studies with guinea pig brain slices [129]. Membrane-binding sites for adenosine, distinct from the adenosine transport system, have been identified by direct binding studies of fat cells [130] and by indirect methods on human peripheral blood lymphocytes [131, 132].

Initial consideration that adenosine toxicity to ADA-inhibited lymphoid cells might also be mediated by cAMP arose from the finding that the ability of adenosine to inhibit the capacity of mouse peritoneal lymphocytes to kill ascites tumor cells was greatly enhanced by EHNA, and that inhibition of killing was associated with a transient two- to fourfold increase in lymphocyte cAMP concentration [133]. Transient increases in cAMP also occur in adenosine-treated mouse lymphocytes [134] and in human peripheral blood lymphocytes [131, 132]. For example, 10-min incubation of human peripheral lymphocytes with 10 μM adenosine produced a maximal increase in cAMP of about fivefold which persisted for 40 min [131]. Toxicity was not evaluated in these studies. Among other elevated adenine nucleotide pools, two- to threefold elevation in cAMP was found in the peripheral blood lymphocytes of one ADA-deficient patient [135].

Studies predating discovery of ADA deficiency had shown that at millimolar concentrations exogenous cAMP blocked the mitogenic response of human peripheral blood lymphocytes [136]. Later studies with HeLa cells [137, 138] and human WI-L2 lymphoblasts [139] showed that the toxicity of exogenous cAMP was due to its slow conversion to adenosine.

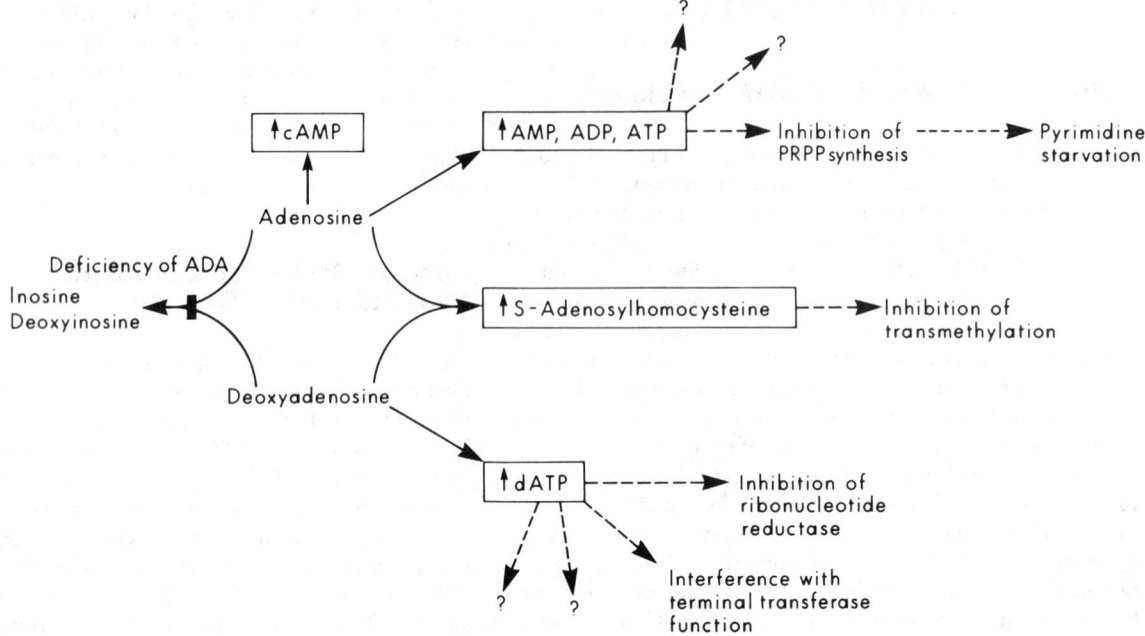

Figure 53-3 Effects of adenosine and deoxyadenosine that have been considered as potential causes of immune dysfunction in ADA deficiency.

At concentrations sufficient to inhibit growth, adenosine failed to increase intracellular cAMP in HeLa cells [138], phytohemagglutinin-stimulated human lymphocytes [140], or in ADA-inhibited WI-L2 lymphoblasts [141]. Furthermore, although inhibitors of adenosine transport such as dipyridamole and nitrobenzylthioinosine enhance the effects of adenosine on cAMP accumulation [130, 131], a mutant of mouse S49 lymphoma cells incapable of transporting adenosine was almost completely resistant to its growth inhibitory effects [110]. The converse was also demonstrated: unimpaired toxicity of adenosine to S49 mutants that lack either adenylate cyclase, cAMP-dependent protein kinase, or other functions necessary for expression of the actions of cAMP [142]. Thus, there does not appear to be compelling evidence that cAMP is the major metabolite responsible for the growth inhibitory effects of adenosine to ADA-inhibited lymphoid cells.

Inhibition of Pyrimidine Synthesis by Adenosine
Depletion of UTP pools was first observed as a cause of growth inhibition by adenosine in HeLa cells [137] and in mouse fibroblasts [143]. Shortly after the appearance of reports of ADA deficiency, these studies were extended to mouse and human lymphoblasts [144]. Depletion of pyrimidine nucleotides was accompanied by a decrease in intracellular phosphoribosylpyrophosphate (PRPP), accumulation of orotic acid, and diminished incorporation of radiolabeled aspartate into pyrimidine nucleotides [138, 139, 141, 143, 144]. These findings indicated a block in pyrimidine biosynthesis de novo at the level of the PRPP-dependent conversion of orotate to orotidylic acid (see Chap. 56). Growth inhibition by adenosine could be partially prevented by exogenous uridine, a PRPP-independent source of pyrimidine nucleotides. The fact that adenosine did not deplete pyrimidines in a mutant mouse fibroblast line that lacked adenosine kinase indicated a requirement for conversion of adenosine to adenine nucleotides [143]. This mutant and an adenosine kinase–deficient Chinese hamster cell line [145] were 70 and 300 times more resistant to adenosine than their parent lines. Additional studies of the effects of 5 to 100

μM adenosine on ADA-inhibited S49 mouse lymphoma cells [146], L1210 murine leukemia cells [147], GMA32 Chinese hamster ovary cells [148], and human fibroblasts [149], have confirmed to one degree or another the associated biochemical findings of ATP pool expansion of up to twofold, depletion of PRPP concentration, and impaired utilization of orotate for pyrimidine biosynthesis. The depletion in PRPP concentration caused by adenosine presumably results from inhibition of PRPP synthesis caused by excessive synthesis of adenine nucleotides. This may result from direct inhibition of PRPP synthetase by nucleotides [150] or from depletion of intracellular inorganic phosphate [151] (see Chap. 50 in which regulation of this enzyme is presented in detail). Diminished synthesis of ribose-5-PO$_4$ resulting from inhibition of the oxidative branch of the pentose phosphate pathway by adenosine has also been proposed as a cause of decreased PRPP synthesis [141].

Exposure of phytohemagglutinin-stimulated human peripheral lymphocytes for 24 h to $10^{-5}M$ adenosine and $10^{-5}M$ coformycin increased ATP content fourfold and decreased UTP and GTP content by 40 percent and 70 percent, respectively [147]. Uridine did not prevent inhibition of the mitogenic response in this study, or in another in which the mitogen used was concanavalin A, and EHNA the ADA inhibitor [152]. Unequivocal evidence that adenosine toxicity does not result from pyrimidine starvation alone was obtained in studies of adenosine kinase–deficient mutants of the WI-L2 human B lymphoblastoid cell line [153]. Adenosine was found to be as toxic to the ADA-inhibited mutant as to its parent, and uridine, which only partially prevented toxicity to the parent, had no effect with the mutant. These studies indicated that a form of adenosine toxicity existed that did not require its conversion to nucleotides. Nucleotide-independent, uridine-resistant adenosine toxicity was subsequently shown to result from S-adenosylhomocysteine accumulation (see below).

The possibility that pyrimidine starvation caused by unrestricted phosphorylation of adenosine might be the basis for the immune defect in ADA deficiency [144] initially received considerable attention because of the potential for reversal of this metabolic block with exogenous uridine, and because of reports of expanded ATP pools in blood cells of some ADA-deficient patients [15, 135]. As will be discussed below, there is now some doubt about the degree to which ATP pool expansion generally occurs in ADA deficiency. Nevertheless, in one study in which a four- to eightfold increase in ATP and ADP concentrations was found in the peripheral lymphocytes of an ADA-deficient child, UTP and CTP pools in these cells were not diminished [135]. Uridine did not enhance the capacity of peripheral lymphocytes from ADA-deficient children to respond to mitogens in vitro [135, 154]. In addition, no evidence of abnormal orotic acid excretion was found in the urine of an affected patient [155, 156].

dATP Toxicity Tattersall et al. [157] reported in 1975 that $10^{-3}M$ deoxyadenosine expanded dATP pools and inhibited mitogenesis in phytohemagglutinin-stimulated human peripheral blood lymphocytes. The first reports of the enhancement of deoxyadenosine toxicity by ADA inhibitors [158] and examination of the effects of deoxyadenosine on deoxyribonucleotide pools in ADA-inhibited murine lymphocytic leukemia cells [159] appeared in 1977. The observations that drew the most attention to the possible role of deoxyadenosine toxicity mediated by dATP pool expansion in causing immunodeficiency were the discoveries of dATP accumulation in the erythrocytes [160, 161] and deoxyadenosine in the urine [162, 163] of ADA-deficient patients.

In the first patients studied by Coleman et al. [161] dATP and dADP were definitively identified by high-pressure liquid chromatography, gas chromatography–mass spectrometry, and by showing that the abnormal triphosphate substituted for authentic dATP as a substrate for DNA polymerase. The concentration of dATP found was 157 nmol per 10^9 erythrocytes, compared with less than 0.1 nmol in normal erythrocytes. dATP concentrations of 340 to 1100 nmol per milliliter packed red cells were found in three immunodeficient, ADA-deficient children studied by Cohen et al. [160]. Less than 20 nmol dATP per milliliter packed cells was found in a fourth enzyme-deficient but immunocompetent child, and less than 8 nmol/ml in control erythrocytes. In both of the above studies ATP concentrations were about the same in the red cells of patients and controls.

Earlier reports that had indicated ATP pool expansion in erythrocytes and lymphocytes of ADA-deficient children had not mentioned dATP accumulation. Some reasons for the failure to identify dATP include (1) the use of enzymatic assays that do not distinguish between ATP and dATP, (2) use of high-pressure liquid chromatographic columns that do not adequately resolve ribo- and deoxyribonucleotides, and (3) the degradation of deoxyadenosine and its nucleotide derivatives to give adenine during acid extraction of cells, or during slow conventional ion-exchange chromatography under acidic conditions. This lability accounts for the finding of high concentrations of adenine in the urine of one ADA-deficient patient [155]. Another factor that may have prevented recognition of dATP is the decline in its concentration (half-life ~2.5 days [160]) that occurs after transfusion of ADA-deficient patients with irradiated red cells from normal donors (Fig. 53-4).

When the proper analytic techniques are used, expansion of the dATP pool is easily established, particularly in nondividing cells such as mature erythrocytes and peripheral lymphocytes in which the dATP pool is normally very small. The concentration of ATP in these cells is about a hundredfold higher, so

that a much larger accumulation of ATP than dATP must occur to permit recognition of ATP pool expansion. Thus ATP pool size is not a sensitive index of excessive phosphorylation of adenosine. Efficient reutilization of adenosine probably does occur in ADA deficiency, since: (1) the concentration of adenosine in plasma of normal individuals is below the K_m values of about 1 μM for adenosine kinase [111–113] and S-adenosylhomocysteine hydrolase [164], and is elevated ten- to fiftyfold to the 2 to 7 μM range in ADA deficiency; and (2) the urinary excretion of deoxyadenosine, present in the 0.5 to 2 μM range in ADA-deficient plasma, is much greater than that of adenosine (Table 53-1), and deoxyadenosine is also less efficiently "recaptured" as nucleotide by ADA-deficient cells than is adenosine (see below).

DIFFERENTIAL ACCUMULATION OF dATP AND SENSITIVITY TO DEOXYADENOSINE   The strongest evidence for an important role of dATP in mediating deoxyadenosine toxicity comes from studies of ADA-inhibited mutant lymphoid cell lines. Nucleoside transport–deficient mutants of mouse S49 lymphoma cells were twentyfold less sensitive than their parent line to deoxyadenosine toxicity, as were mutants with normal transport capacity but with an incapacity to phosphorylate the nucleoside [165]. Similarly, phosphorylation-defective mutants of human WI-L2 lymphocytes were five- to tenfold more resistant than parental cells to deoxyadenosine [113, 166]. Dipyridamole, an inhibitor of nucleoside transport, prevented both growth inhibition and dATP accumulation in ADA-inhibited human T lymphoblastoid cells exposed to 50 μM deoxyadenosine [167].

Both mouse [168, 169] and human [124, 167, 170–172] T

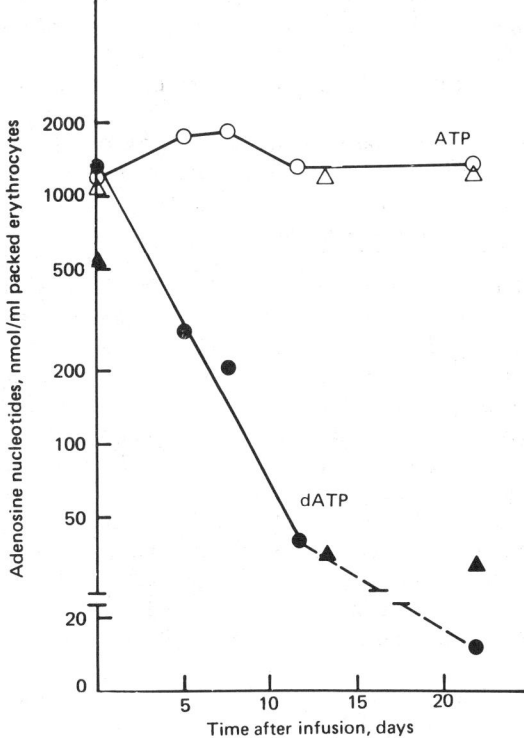

Figure 53-4 Disappearance of dATP from the erythrocytes of two ADA-deficient patients after transfusion with normal erythrocytes. Concentrations of ATP (O,△) and dATP (●,▲) were determined in samples drawn from patient A (O,●) and from patient B (△,▲) at the indicated times after erythrocyte transfusion. The half-life of dATP after transfusion in patient A is approximately 2.5 days. (From Cohen et al. [160]. Used by permission.)

lymphoblastoid cell lines are more sensitive to the toxic effects of deoxyribonucleosides than are B-cell lines, and this correlates with enhanced capacity of T cells to accumulate deoxynucleotides. For example, dATP increased from 31 to 172 pmol per 10^6 cells in an ADA-inhibited human T-cell line after 1 h exposure to 50 μM deoxyadenosine but no detectable increase occurred in a B-cell line [167]. Growth of the T-cell line was inhibited 50 percent by 5 μM deoxyadenosine, but 50 μM deoxyadenosine inhibited growth of the B-cell line by only 15 percent. In another study the concentration of deoxyadenosine required to inhibit growth by 50 percent (EC_{50}) was 2.3 μM for three different human T-cell lines, compared with 53 μM for three B-cell lines [170]. In the T-cell lines dATP increased from 50 to 600 pmol per 10^6 cells on exposure to 20 μM deoxyadenosine for 4 h, while no detectable increase occurred in the B-cell lines. In contrast, ADA-inhibited B- and T-cell lines are about equally sensitive to adenosine toxicity [124], which, as discussed below, is largely mediated by a nucleotide-independent mechanism. The greater capacity of T lymphoid cells than B cells to accumulate dATP may be significant since approximately 15 percent of patients with ADA deficiency have shown some evidence of B-cell function, but absent T cells and severely impaired cell-mediated immunity [141].

ENZYMES CAPABLE OF PHOSPHORYLATING DEOXYADENOSINE   Accumulation of dATP in ADA-deficient cell lines exposed to deoxyadenosine depends upon the relative rates of the kinases involved in the successive phosphorylation of deoxyadenosine to dAMP, dADP, and dATP; the rate of utilization of the triphosphate in DNA synthesis; and the rates of degradation of the nucleotides. Of these, greatest attention has been focused upon the initial phosphorylation of deoxyadenosine to dAMP and upon the analogous formation of dGMP from deoxyguanosine. Both adenosine kinase and deoxycytidine kinase are capable of phosphorylating deoxyadenosine, but with much less efficiency than the substrates for which they are named. Adenosine kinase purified from rabbit liver [173] used deoxyadenosine as substrate about 10^{-4} as efficiently as adenosine [174], and the enzyme from human placenta [175] 1 percent or 16 percent as well, depending upon the conditions of assay [111]. The K_m for adenosine of adenosine kinase from WI-L2 human lymphoblasts is 3 μM, compared with 540 μM for deoxyadenosine [113]. For various preparations of deoxycytidine kinase, K_m values for deoxycytidine have ranged from 2 to 16 μM [176–178], compared with 0.12 to 0.73 mM for deoxyadenosine [113, 177, 178]. Deoxyguanosine is also a substrate for deoxycytidine kinase, with K_m values reported in the range of 0.3 to 3 mM [177–179]. The V_{max} values of calf thymus deoxycytidine kinase for deoxyadenosine and deoxyguanosine phosphorylation were fourteen- and sixfold greater than for deoxycytidine [178]. Phosphorylation of both purine deoxynucleosides by deoxycytidine kinase is strongly inhibited by dCTP [177]. A mitochondrial enzyme with a K_m of 6 μM for deoxyguanosine, but without activity towards deoxycytidine, has been isolated from calf thymus [179]. A cytoplasmic deoxyadenosine-deoxyguanosine kinase that may be distinct from deoxycytidine kinase has also been isolated from calf thymus [180, 181]. It is also inhibited by dCTP and has K_m values for deoxyadenosine and deoxyguanosine of 0.7 mM and 1.1 mM, respectively.

Deoxycytidine kinase is largely confined to lymphoid tissues in the rat and mouse, with highest activity in thymus [182]. A

similar distribution of "deoxyadenosine kinase" was found in extracts of autopsy tissues obtained from human infants [183, 184]. Kinase activities for deoxyadenosine and deoxyguanosine cochromatographed with deoxycytidine kinase in human thymic extracts but were resolved from adenosine kinase, which showed no preferential distribution in lymphoid tissues. Based on these results and the implicit assumption that adenosine kinase does not utilize deoxyadenosine as a substrate, the suggestion was made that deoxycytidine kinase is the physiologic deoxyadenosine kinase, and that accumulation of dATP in ADA deficiency should be confined to lymphoid tissue [183]. However, erythrocytes, which contain adenosine kinase but virtually no deoxycytidine kinase, do accumulate large amounts of dATP in ADA-deficient patients. Other nonlymphoid tissues from these patients have not been examined for evidence of dATP accumulation.

DEOXYADENOSINE PHOSPHORYLATION IN KINASE-DEFICIENT LYMPHOID CELL LINES   Given large differences between T and B lymphoid cell lines in their sensitivity to deoxyadenosine, and in their capacity to accumulate dATP, the question of the relative contributions of adenosine kinase and deoxycytidine kinase to deoxyadenosine phosphorylation in various tissues assumes some importance. Direct answers to this question have been obtained in studies of dATP accumulation by mutant lymphoid cell lines that lack adenosine or deoxycytidine kinase or both.

In S49 cells (a mouse T-lymphoma line) about 70 percent of total deoxyadenosine phosphorylating activity in extracts is inhibitable by adenosine and 30 percent by deoxycytidine [165], a result which is also characteristic of mouse tissues in general [184]. A deoxycytidine kinase–deficient mutant of S49 was as sensitive as its parent to deoxyadenosine ($EC_{50} \cong 4$ μM), while adenosine kinase–deficient mutants were three- to fivefold less sensitive [165]. Both the wild type and deoxycytidine kinase–deficient lines increased dATP from below 20 to about 200 μM after 4 h exposure to 50 μM deoxyadenosine, while no increase in dATP was detected in the adenosine kinase–deficient mutant. Adenosine kinase thus appears to be entirely responsible for dATP accumulation in S49 cells.

A survey of extracts of human lymphoid tissues indicated that deoxycytidine was a better inhibitor than adenosine of deoxyadenosine phosphorylation [184]. The K_m values for deoxyadenosine of partially purified deoxycytidine kinase (120 μM) and adenosine kinase (540 μM) from the WI-L2 human B-cell line [113] would also suggest that deoxycytidine kinase might be the more efficient deoxyadenosine kinase. Extracts of an adenosine kinase–deficient mutant of the WI-L2 B-cell line possessed 85 to 90 percent of parental deoxyadenosine kinase activity [113, 185], and a deoxycytidine kinase–deficient mutant retained less than 10 percent [166]. However, the deoxycytidine kinase–deficient mutant and wild type cells were equally sensitive to deoxyadenosine ($EC_{50} \cong 50$ μM), while the adenosine kinase–deficient mutant was three- to sixfold less sensitive [113, 166]. When wild type and adenosine kinase–deficient cells were exposed to 0.1 to 1 mM deoxyadenosine for 4 and 24 h, total deoxyadenosine nucleotides increased from 8 to 11, to a maximum of 145 nmol per 10^9 cells in the parent, but to only 19 to 22 nmol per 10^9 cells in the adenosine kinase mutant [113]. Accumulation of dATP from deoxyadenosine was unimpaired by loss of deoxycytidine kinase [166]. Thus, adenosine kinase acts as the physiologic deoxyadenosine kinase in this human B-cell line. In contrast, in the CEM human T lymphoblastoid cell line both deoxycytidine kinase and adenosine kinase are active in phosphorylating deoxyadenosine, with deoxycytidine kinase predominating at low concentrations of deoxyadenosine, and adenosine kinase at higher, consistent with their relative K_m values for deoxyadenosine [184, 186, 187].

DEOXYNUCLEOTIDE DEGRADATION IN T AND B LYMPHOBLASTS   It is clear that the difference in capacity of various cell lines to accumulate dATP must be regulated by factors in addition to the relative kinetic constants of adenosine kinase and deoxycytidine kinase for deoxyadenosine. Thus, the rates of dATP accumulation by human T- and B-cell lines differ by ten- to a hundredfold, but the deoxyadenosine phosphorylating activities in extracts of these cells differ by less than threefold [184, 187]. One hypothesis that has attracted interest is that differences in rates of nucleotide catabolism may account for the different capacities of T and B lymphoid cells to accumulate toxic nucleotides.

Ecto-5'-nucleotidase activity was found to be much higher in B than T lymphoblastoid cell lines, and was proposed as a factor that might limit deoxynucleotide accumulation in B cells [172, 188]. As discussed earlier, there is considerable doubt that this ectoenzyme is involved in the catabolism of intracellular nucleotides. Furthermore, human null lymphoblastoid lines possess high ecto-5'-nucleotidase activity, but are as sensitive to deoxynucleoside toxicity as are T cells [189]. Human B-cell lines with very low levels of ecto-5'-nucleotidase activity, established from peripheral lymphocytes of an ADA-deficient patient, showed no increase in sensitivity to deoxyadenosine [190]. B cells, but not T cells or null cells, also possess an ecto-ATPase which is distinct from ecto-5'-nucleotidase [191], but there is no evidence that this enzyme acts on intracellular nucleotides.

There has been a recent report of a cytoplasmic deoxynucleotidase activity in human lymphoid cell extracts [192]. The enzyme partially purified from WI-L2 cells had highest activity with dIMP, but also degrades dAMP, dGMP, and dTMP, with K_m values in the 300 to 600 μM range, about 1000 times higher than the intracellular concentrations of these deoxynucleotides. The activity of this enzyme varied widely among several human lymphoblastoid cell lines, with no more than a threefold difference in extracts of T and B lines, comparable to the difference in their deoxyadenosine kinase activities [170].

Until thorough studies of the rates and regulation of deoxynucleotide catabolism by intact T and B cells are conducted, and the putative enzyme (or enzymes) involved in this process have been better characterized, it would seem premature to conclude that nucleotide catabolism accounts for the difference in capacity of B and T cells to accumulate dATP. Other possibilities exist that have not been fully pursued. For example, dCTP is a powerful inhibitor ($K_i \sim 0.16 \mu M$) of deoxyadenosine kinases from calf thymus [177, 180, 181]. Differences in regulation of dCTP pool size in T and B cells might explain the finding that deoxycytidine kinase, although assayable in extracts of both T and B cells, does not function effectively as a deoxyadenosine kinase in B cells [113, 166].

INHIBITION OF RIBONUCLEOTIDE REDUCTASE   Deoxyribonucleotide synthesis de novo, via the reduction, catalyzed by ribonucleotide reductase (EC 1.17.4.1), of ADP, GDP, CDP, and UDP to their corresponding 2'-deoxy derivatives, is a stringently regulated process that maintains steady state con-

centrations of deoxynucleoside triphosphates (dNTP) at a level sufficient to support only a few minutes of DNA polymerization [193–195]. A balanced production of dATP, dGTP, dCTP, and dTTP appears to be achieved by complex allosteric effects of these compounds and ATP on ribonucleotide reductase. According to a recent review [196] ATP is a general activator, and dATP a general inhibitor, of the reduction of all four substrates. dGTP and dTTP act to inhibit CDP reduction and dGTP also inhibits UDP reduction. Reduction of ADP and GDP are stimulated by dGTP and dTTP, respectively. K_i values for dATP as an inhibitor of the reduction of CDP, UDP, GDP, and ADP were, respectively, 40, 55, 1500, and 4 μM for the enzyme purified from the Molt-4 human T-cell line [197]. K_i values for dGTP as an inhibitor of CDP and UDP reduction by this enzyme were 25 to 47 μM, and 1.5 to 4.3 μM.

Inhibition of DNA synthesis by deoxyadenosine was first demonstrated in 1959 in Ehrlich ascites cells [198] and was later attributed to inhibition of ribonucleotide reductase by dATP [199–201]. Exogenous deoxyguanosine and thymidine also inhibit DNA synthesis in many cells, and this effect is the basis for the "thymidine block" technique for synchronizing populations of cultured cells. Several observations made in nonlymphoid cells between 1959 and 1976 indicated that accumulation of dATP, dGTP, and dTTP derived from their respective deoxynucleosides is lethal to dividing cells, primarily because of inhibition of the CDP reductase activity associated with ribonucleotide reductase, and that lethality could be prevented by deoxycytidine [122, 202–205]. Deoxyadenosine-resistant mutants of the 3T6 mouse fibroblast line were shown to contain increased ribonucleotide reductase activity that was resistant to inhibition by dATP [206, 207]. These mutants also had increased pools of dCTP. Since 1977 these observations have all been confirmed by laboratories studying lymphoid cell lines as follows:

1. As discussed above, deoxynucleoside toxicity is diminished in lymphoid cells incapable or inefficient at converting them to deoxynucleotides.

2. Depletion of appropriate dNTP pools occurs in lymphoid cells treated with toxic deoxynucleosides. For example, exposure of S49 cells to 50 μM deoxyadenosine + 10 μM EHNA for 4 h depleted dCTP, dGTP, and dTTP pools 99 percent, 80 percent, and 67 percent, respectively [165], and exposure to 100 μM deoxyguanosine for 2 to 7 h depleted dCTP by 88 to 99 percent [208]. Decrease in dCTP to undetectable levels occurred in the human T-cell line Molt-4 after a 1-h incubation with 50 μM deoxyadenosine or deoxyguanosine [209].

3. Deoxyguanosine-resistant mutants of mouse S49 lymphoma cells were about fivefold less sensitive to deoxyadenosine, and ten- to twentyfold less sensitive to deoxyguanosine and thymidine than parental cells [210]. Basal levels of the four dNTPs were 2 to 5 times higher in the mutant, and equivalent expansion of dCTP, dGTP, or dTTP pools by incubation with the corresponding deoxynucleoside caused much less depletion of dCTP in the mutant than in its parent. Ribonucleotide reductase in this mutant was also less sensitive to dATP inhibition. A dGTP-insensitive reductase was found in another deoxyguanosine-resistant S49 mutant [211].

4. Deoxycytidine has been reported in numerous studies to protect partially various lymphoid cell lines from the toxic effects of deoxyadenosine and deoxyguanosine [122]. This protection probably results in many cases from inhibition of phosphorylation of the purine nucleosides by deoxycytidine

kinase, as discussed above, rather than to bypass of ribonucleotide reductase inhibition by repletion of the dCTP pool, or to the ability of deoxycytidine to reverse dTTP pool depletion owing to synthesis of thymidylate via deamination of dCMP [169]. On the other hand, protection by deoxycytidine from thymidine toxicity to human CEM T cells has been convincingly shown to be related to repletion of dCTP pools, since dTTP accumulation via thymidine kinase was unaffected by deoxycytidine [212].

Some observations regarding deoxyadenosine toxicity to cultured lymphoid cells are clearly not consistent with the ribonucleotide reductase hypothesis. For example, deoxycytidine did not prevent deoxyadenosine toxicity to ADA-inhibited mouse L5178Y lymphoma cells, even though it completely prevented dCTP pool depletion [159]. Nor did various combinations of deoxycytidine, thymidine, and deoxyguanosine restore growth to ADA-inhibited WI-L2 lymphoblasts treated with deoxyadenosine [113]. Ribonucleotide reductase activity is related to cell cycle events; its activity is very low in nondividing or resting cells and rises dramatically at the onset of S phase [193]. In unstimulated peripheral blood lymphocytes, a population of largely nondividing cells, ribonucleotide reductase is barely detectable and does not appreciably increase during the first 23 h after phytohemagglutinin stimulation. Between 23 and 31 h its activity increases rapidly and reaches a peak at 50 to 54 h, which is 150 to 200 times higher than initially present [213, 214]. Pools of all four dNTPs also remain at very low levels prior to 23 h and then rise sharply to peak values by 50 h, coincident with the time course for DNA synthesis. Despite absence of DNA synthetic activity and very low levels of ribonucleotide reductase during the first 24 h after exposure to mitogen, 50 μM deoxyadenosine + 1 μM deoxycoformycin inhibited leucine uptake during this prereplicative period [215]. Addition of deoxyadenosine to lymphocytes 72 h after mitogen, when DNA synthesis was active, did produce decreases in dNTP pools consistent with ribonucleotide reductase inhibition [157], but the proliferative response was most effectively inhibited when deoxyadenosine was added during the first 24 h, and inhibition was markedly reduced when addition of deoxyadenosine was delayed beyond 24 h [215]. All of these results suggest the existence of mechanisms of deoxyadenosine toxicity that do not involve ribonucleotide reductase.

EFFECTS OF dATP ACCUMULATION ON TERMINAL TRANSFERASE   Terminal deoxynucleotidyl transferase (terminal transferase, EC 2.7.7.31) is a unique type of DNA polymerase that is capable of adding deoxynucleotide residues to the 3'-hydroxyl ends of DNA primers in the absence of a template strand. It occurs only in thymic lymphocytes and in bone marrow lymphocytes thought to be T-cell precursors. While its function is unknown there have been suggestions that, by virtue of its capacity to introduce new DNA sequences at gaps in DNA, terminal transferase might be involved in generating immunologic diversity [216–221]. Because the composition of sequences generated by terminal transferase is partly a function of the relative abundances of its dNTP substrates, it has been suggested that a marked increase in dATP pool size could modify the terminal transferase product and possibly interfere with some function essential to lymphocyte function or replication in ADA deficiency [161]. In the presence of manganese ions dATP, but not other dNTPs, is also a potent inhibitor of

terminal transferase [222]. At present there are no studies to support any role for terminal transferase in contributing to deoxyadenosine toxicity to cultured lymphoid cells that contain this enzyme, and other mechanisms must account for its toxicity to lymphoid cells that lack terminal transferase.

S-Adenosylhomocysteine Toxicity   S-Adenosylmethionine–mediated transmethylation reactions contribute to the metabolism of many different classes of biologic molecules [223]. Postsynthetic methylation is involved in the processing or functioning of DNA, mRNA, rRNA, tRNA, small nuclear RNA, and numerous proteins, and in the synthesis or further metabolism of various small molecules, including creatine, neurogenic amines, and certain phospholipids. Furthermore, a growing body of evidence suggests that certain methylation reactions play a role in specialized cellular phenomena such as leukocyte chemotaxis [224, 225], initiation of the mitogenic response of lymphocytes [226], neurosecretion [227], mast cell degranulation [228], β-adrenergic receptor activity [229, 230], and membrane function in general [230–232]. Methylation of eukaryote DNA may be involved in cell differention [233–235]. Inhibition of transmethylation has been shown to interfere with these processes in various experimental systems, and in the context of ADA deficiency to contribute to the toxic effects of adenosine and deoxyadenosine on lymphoid cells.

All transmethylation reactions give S-adenosylhomocysteine as a product (Fig. 53-5), which through its further metabolism, catalyzed by S-adenosylhomocysteine hydrolase (EC 3.3.1.1) [236], accounts for the production of 14 to 23 mmol of adenosine and an equivalent amount of homocysteine per day in a normal adult [87]. S-Adenosylhomocysteine is a potent inhibitor, competitive with S-adenosylmethionine, of virtually all transmethylation reactions examined (K_i values of 10^{-7} to $10^{-5}M$ for different methyltransferases [237]), and therefore must be kept at low levels to ensure normal operation of methylation-dependent processes. Since hydrolysis of S-adenosylhomocysteine is a reversible and thermodynamically unfavorable reaction (K_{eq} of $1.4 \times 10^{-6}M$), maintenance of low steady state concentrations of this potentially toxic metabolite requires efficient metabolism of adenosine and homocysteine. In fact, deamination and phosphorylation of adenosine and removal of homocysteine via transsulfuration and remethylation (Chap. 25) are efficient, permitting S-adenosylhomocysteine to be kept at one-tenth or less than the concentration of its precursor, S-adenosylmethionine.

Recognition of these metabolic factors influencing S-adenosylhomocysteine catabolism has led to speculation that the elevated levels of adenosine found in ADA-deficient children might increase cellular S-adenosylhomocysteine and cause some degree of inhibition of critical transmethylation reactions. Studies in model systems indicate that this is indeed a major mechanism of adenosine toxicity to ADA-inhibited S49 mouse [238] and WI-L2 human lymphoid cell lines [239], and to mitogen-stimulated human peripheral blood lymphocytes [240]. Adenosine concentrations of 10 to 50 μM, which inhibit cell growth in these systems, give three- to twentyfold increases in S-adenosylhomocysteine to levels that approximate those of S-adenosylmethionine (Fig. 53-6). Because inhibition of transmethylation reactions by S-adenosylhomocysteine is competitive with S-adenosylmethionine, the ratio S-adenosylmethionine/S-adenosylhomocysteine, sometimes called the *methylation index*, should theoretically be a better indicator of the capacity of a cell to transmethylate than is the concentration of

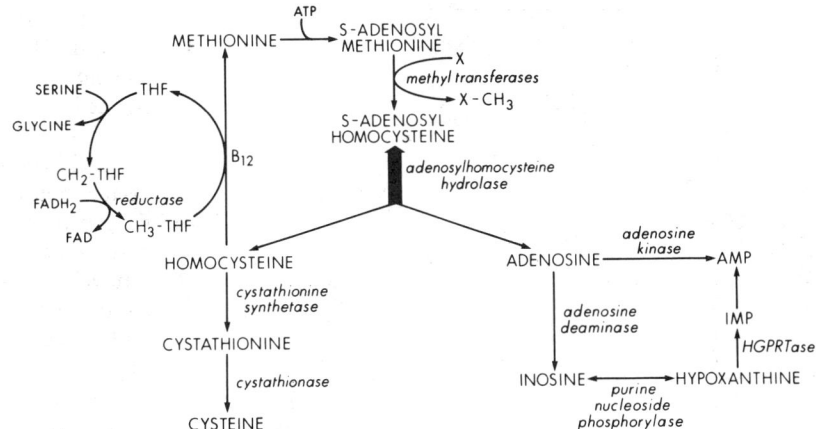

Figure 53-5 The transmethylation pathway, showing the relationships between methionine, homocysteine, and adenosine metabolism. Because of the reversibility of the *S*-adenosylhomocysteine hydrolase reaction, an increase in adenosine concentration, as would occur from a lack of ADA, is accompanied by a higher steady state level of *S*-adenosylhomocysteine, a potent inhibitor of methyl transfer reactions.

either compound alone. The methylation index fell from control values of 10 or greater in the cells studied to values of 3 or less at toxic concentrations of adenosine, and as predicted inhibition of both DNA (Fig. 53-7) and RNA methylation accompanied these changes in methylation index. Homocysteine enhanced the toxicity of adenosine by greatly accentuating *S*-adenosylhomocysteine accumulation.

These same biochemical events were shown to account for the finding that adenosine remained toxic to an adenosine kinase–deficient mutant of the WI-L2 lymphoblast line, even in the presence of uridine [153, 239]. In addition, homocysteine was found to be selectively toxic to the ADA-inhibited adenosine kinase–deficient mutant in the absence of any exogenous adenosine. This toxicity was also associated with *S*-adenosylhomocysteine accumulation, and presumably involved condensation of homocysteine with endogenously synthesized adenosine that accumulated in the mutant. These experiments demonstrate that toxicity results from *S*-adenosyl-

homocysteine accumulation per se, and not from potential effects of exogenous adenosine, i.e., mediated by its phosphorylation or by its interaction with the cell surface adenylate cyclase system.

A second mechanism by which ADA deficiency might increase intracellular *S*-adenosylhomocysteine has been proposed as a result of the discovery that *S*-adenosylhomocysteine hydrolase is capable of forming a stable complex with adenosine and is in fact the principal high-affinity "adenosine-binding protein" present in the cytoplasm of mammalian cells [164, 241]. Deoxyadenosine, among other analogues of adenosine, including the antiviral agent adenine arabinoside, was found to bind to this enzyme and cause its irreversible inactivation by a process akin to "suicide inactivation" [242] (Fig. 53-8). The inactivation constant for deoxyadenosine, K_i, was 66 μM, and its $V_{\max}$ was approximately 0.12 per minute. Inactivation by deoxyadenosine and adenine arabinoside involves the irreversible reduction of the tightly bound NAD cofactor that is essential for catalytic activity [243, 244].

Since hydrolysis constitutes the major route of *S*-adenosylhomocysteine catabolism in eukaryotes, inactivation in vivo of *S*-adenosylhomocysteine hydrolase to below a critical level should cause *S*-adenosylhomocysteine accumulation independent of any effects of adenosine. Inactivation of this enzyme intracellularly by deoxyadenosine has been shown to cause *S*-adenosylhomocysteine accumulation in ADA-inhibited WI-L2 lymphoblasts [113]. Of significance with respect to the pathogenesis of SCID in ADA deficiency is that the erythrocytes of three ADA-deficient children were found to possess less than 2 percent of control *S*-adenosylhomocysteine hydrolase activity [245]. This is a unique example of suicide inactivation as a mechanism for the production of a secondary enzyme deficiency in an inborn error of metabolism (Fig. 53-9). The extent to which *S*-adenosylhomocysteine hydrolase inactivation occurs in vivo in lymphoid cells of ADA-deficient children remains to be established.

A Pharmacologic Model of ADA Deficiency in Vivo
Studies of the effects of adenosine and deoxyadenosine on ADA-inhibited cultured cells have provided the primary experimental basis for hypotheses regarding the pathogenesis of SCID in ADA deficiency. Phenomena related to two of the mechanisms discussed above have thus far been shown to occur in vivo: dATP pool expansion and inactivation of *S*-adenosylhomocysteine hydrolase by deoxyadenosine, but no direct information has been obtained to shed light on the nature of the biochemical events that precede the development

Figure 53-6 Effects of adenosine on growth and intracellular *S*-adenosyl-homocysteine (AdoHcy) in an adenosine kinase–deficient derivative of the human lymphoblast line WI-L2. This strain is resistant to adenosine-induced pyrimidine starvation, but its growth is still inhibited by adenosine. Cells were cultured with 5 μM of the ADA inhibitor EHNA and adenosine as indicated. *S*-Adenosylmethionine was approximately 100 nmol per 10⁹ cells. *S*-Adenosylhomocysteine was measured at 4 h and growth after 72 h. (*From Kredich, Hershfield, and Johnston* [290]. *Used by permission.*)

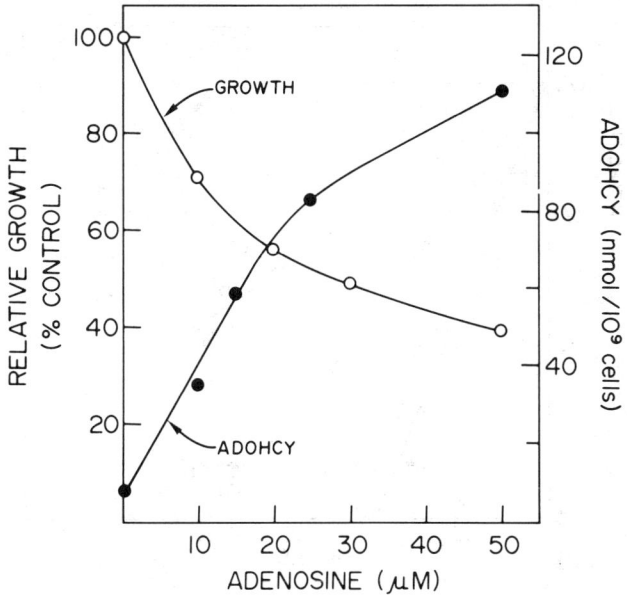

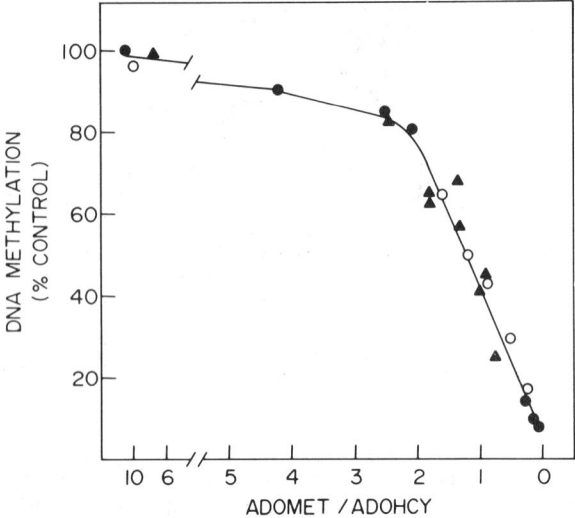

Figure 53-7 Relationship of DNA methylation to the ratio S-adenosylme-thionine/S-adenosylhomocysteine (AdoMet/AdoHcy, the methylation index) in the human lymphoblastoid cell line WI-L2 (O), an adenosine kinase–deficient derivative of WI-L2 (●), and in phytohemagglutinin-stimulated human peripheral lymphocytes (▲). Cells were treated with the ADA inhibitor EHNA and with varying concentrations of adenosine ± homocysteine to achieve low values of AdoMet/AdoHcy. (*From Kredich, Hershfield, and Johnston* [290]. *Used by permission.*)

of lymphopenia. Circulating mononuclear cells from patients have been examined in some cases, but these cells generally lack lymphoid surface markers, do not respond to mitogens in vitro, and may not be representative of a more sensitive population of cells that had been depleted by the metabolic defect.

Deoxycoformycin, a very tightly bound inhibitor of ADA that produces long-lasting ADA deficiency in vivo, has recently been used experimentally in the treatment of various malignancies. The drug appears to be effective against some lymphatic leukemias, particularly those of T-cell origin [246–250], and has also produced marked and selective depletion of nonmalignant lymphocytes in patients with nonlymphoid tumors [247]. Although only limited reports of its use in the latter have been published, detailed studies of the biochemical changes that occur between the time of induction of ADA deficiency and the lysis of malignant lymphoblasts that occurs 1 to several days later have been made in several patients with T-cell leukemia. These studies have provided a unique pharmacologic model of heritable ADA deficiency in vivo.

The most striking effects of treatment with deoxycoformycin, when given in doses sufficient to maintain virtually complete inhibition of ADA in erythrocytes and malignant lymphoblasts for 3 to 5 days, are (1) rise in plasma deoxyadenosine with concomitant urinary excretion of large amounts of deoxyadenosine. Plasma deoxyadenosine is highest during the period of active cell lysis, and in patients with impaired renal function may reach levels as high as 100 μM. Levels in the 0.5 to 2 μM range, typical of the genetic disease, occur in patients with normal renal function who do not undergo massive cytolysis, either because their tumor is unresponsive or because they are treated in remission. Elevated levels of adenosine also occur, but with greater variability than with deoxyadenosine and less adenosine is excreted in the urine. (2) Accumulation of dATP in both erythrocytes and lymphoblasts occurs gradually, reaching levels observed in the

genetic disease over a period of days (Fig. 53-10). In erythrocytes, dATP accumulation is accompanied by a fall in ATP content. This may proceed to nearly complete replacement of red cell ATP by dATP, which is accompanied by a fall in hematocrit without marked bilirubinemia, suggesting extravascular hemolysis [249]. The cause of ATP depletion has not been established. This phenomenon has not been observed in the genetic disease, possibly reflecting lower steady state levels of deoxyadenosine. In two patients who died during deoxycoformycin treatment, elevated dATP levels were found in both kidney and liver, and exceeded levels in spleen [250]. Thus dATP accumulation is not a unique property of lymphoid tissues. (3) Within hours of onset of ADA inhibition there is an abrupt fall in S-adenosylhomocysteine hydrolase activity in erythrocytes to nearly undetectable levels (Fig. 53-10), even before a measurable increase in plasma deoxyadenosine or in erythrocyte dATP can be appreciated [246, 251]. S-Adenosylhomocysteine hydrolase activity declines more slowly in malignant lymphoblasts, reflecting their capacity for new protein synthesis. In one patient with T-cell leukemia studied by us [251], detailed serial measurements were made of lymphoblast S-adenosylhomocysteine and S-adenosylmethionine levels during several courses of deoxycoformycin treatment. In each case a reproducible fall in the ratio S-adenosylmethionine/S-adenosylhomocysteine (methylation index) from more than 20:1 to less than 5:1 was observed within hours of the onset of treatment (Fig. 53-11). This was accompanied by a fall in plasma homocysteine levels and occurred while lymphoblasts still possessed significant S-adenosylhomocysteine hydrolase activity. Although no rise in plasma adenosine was detected, it seems likely that this rapid increase in S-adenosylhomocysteine concentration resulted from reversal of the physiologic direction of the hydrolase reaction, with sequestration of adenosine (and homocysteine) as S-adenosylhomocysteine in cells. Elevated S-adenosylhomocysteine levels were maintained in the malignant cells during the period of maximal hydrolase inactivation (80

Figure 53-8 Kinetics of inactivation of human lymphoblast S-adenosylhomocysteine hydrolase by deoxyadenosine. The rate of loss of enzyme activity is first-order and saturates at high concentrations of deoxyadenosine, indicating that inactivation proceeds from an enzyme-deoxyadenosine complex. Other studies established that deoxyadenosine binds to the enzyme active site and that inactivation is irreversible, consistent with a suicidelike process. (*From Hershfield* [242]. *Used by permission.*)

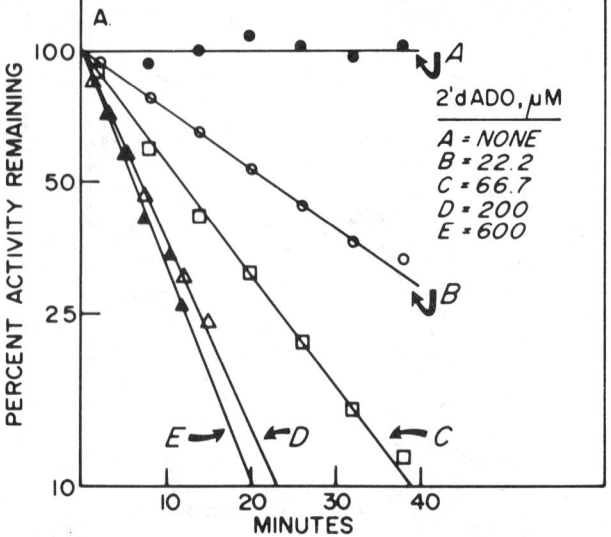

ONE MUTATION , TWO ENZYME DEFICIENCIES

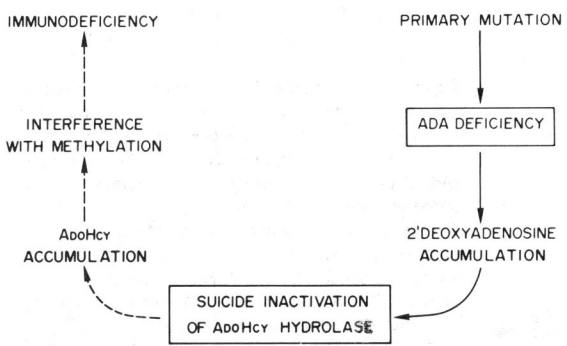

Figure 53-9 A single mutation causing primary deficiency of ADA also results in a secondary deficiency of erythrocyte *S*-adenosylhomocysteine hydrolase owing to the accumulation of its suicide substrate deoxyadenosine. The dashed line suggests a mechanism, inhibition of transmethylation by *S*-adenosylhomocysteine, by which deficiency of *S*-adenosylhomocysteine hydrolase in lymphoid cells might contribute to the clinical consequences of the primary inborn error. (*From Hershfield and Kredich* [291]. *Used by permission.*)

to 95 percent), causing a maximal decrease in methylation index to about 3:1. Some evidence of impaired methylation of newly synthesized lymphoblast RNA was observed, the degree of inhibition corresponding to the decrease in methylation index (Fig. 53-11).

Failure of lymphoid leukemia to respond to deoxycoformycin appears in some cases to correlate with failure to sustain elevated plasma deoxyadenosine levels [252]. In at least one patient treated over a period of 5 months, a cell population eventually emerged with diminished capacity to accumulate dATP, despite marked elevation in plasma deoxyadenosine levels [251]. ADA inhibition and *S*-adenosylhomocysteine hydrolase inactivation in these cells indicated continued capacity to transport both deoxycoformycin and deoxyadenosine. Reduction of the lymphoblast methylation index to below 5:1 was associated with marked cytolysis, although the overall response to treatment was more short-lived than during the early stages of treatment when marked dATP accumulation occurred. These results suggest that accumulation of both dATP and *S*-adenosylhomocysteine contribute to the lymphopenia associated with pharmacologic ADA deficiency.

Significant toxicity to nonlymphoid organs has occurred in a substantial proportion of patients treated with deoxycoformycin and may be related to the high levels of deoxyadenosine or to effects of deoxycoformycin unrelated to its role as an ADA inhibitor.

Pathogenetic Mechanisms in PNP Deficiency

Deoxyguanosine Toxicity Of the four nucleosides that accumulate in the plasma or urine of PNP-deficient patients (Table 53-1), guanosine and deoxyguanosine have been found to be more toxic to a variety of cultured cell lines with normal PNP activity than are inosine and deoxyinosine [122, 204–206, 208]. Deoxyguanosine, like deoxyadenosine and thymidine, has also been shown to be selectively toxic to T compared with B cells [124, 167, 171, 189, 253]. Interpretation of such results is complicated both because of phosphorolysis of these nucleosides and because guanine itself is toxic. The T lymphopenia of PNP-deficient patients and the current absence of

potent PNP inhibitors have prevented studies with PNP-deficient human T cells, perhaps the most appropriate cell model for examining the pathogenesis of the immune defect in this disease. Studies of a B-cell line established from peripheral blood lymphocytes of a PNP-deficient patient [124], and of a PNP-deficient mutant selected from the S49 mouse T lymphoma cell line [211], have permitted direct studies of the toxic effects of PNP substrates.

Since both of these PNP-deficient lymphoid cell lines grew normally in the absence of PNP substrates, the enzyme deficiency per se is not toxic. Guanosine, 0.5 mM, did not inhibit growth of the B-cell line [124], and had an EC$_{50}$ of greater than 1 mM with the T-cell mutant [211]. This probably reflected the inability of mammalian cells to phosphorylate guanosine [121]. Deoxyguanosine produced 50 percent growth inhibition of both PNP-deficient [211] and wild type S49 cells [208, 254] at 10 to 25 μM, but had no effect on growth of the PNP-deficient human B-cell line at 0.5 mM [124]. This enhanced toxicity to T cells correlates with their greater ability to accumulate dGTP. Deoxyguanosine toxicity to PNP-deficient S49 cells requires both an intact nucleoside transport system and deoxycytidine kinase [211].

Figure 53-10 Correlation of plasma deoxyadenosine concentration (*A*) with lymphoblast dATP levels (*B*), *S*-adenosylhomocysteine hydrolase activity (*C*), and white blood cell count (*D*) in a 13-year-old male with refractory T-cell leukemia during treatment with the ADA inhibitor deoxycoformycin. Complete inhibition of lymphoblast ADA was achieved on day 5. The peak concentration of deoxyadenosine was 104 μM (day 7). In contrast the highest concentration of plasma adenosine achieved was 2.1 μM on day 4 (not shown). Arrows in the figure indicate days on which leukapheresis was performed to lower the white cell count, prior to the onset of cell lysis on day 6. (*From Mitchell, Koller, and Heyn* [246]. *Used by permission.*)

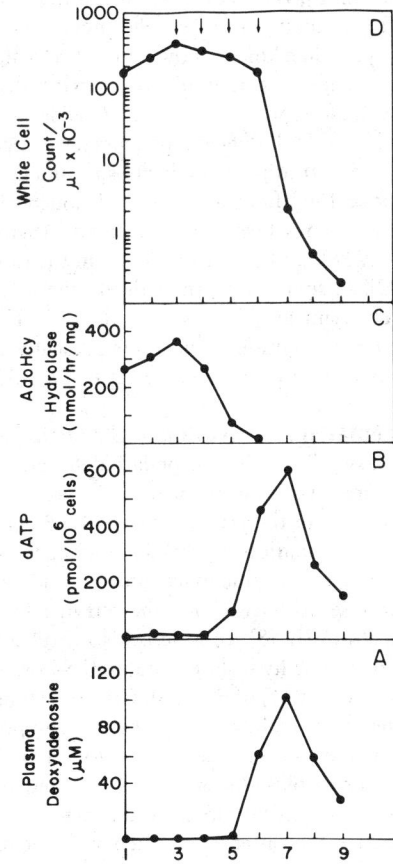

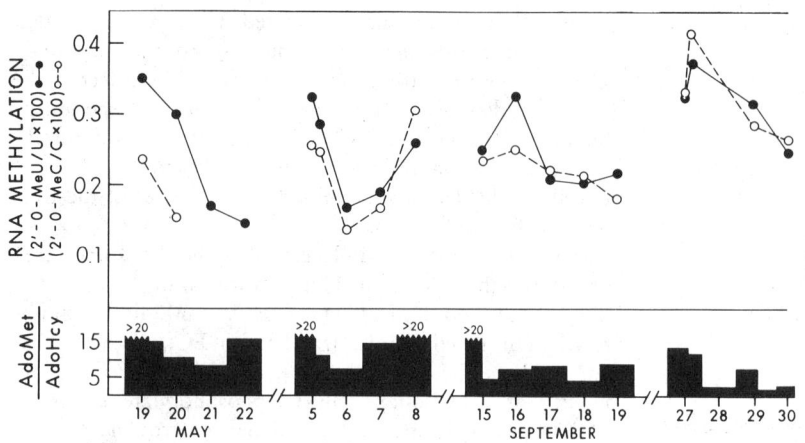

Figure 53-11 Effects of 2′-deoxycoformycin treatment on lymphoblast methylation index and RNA methylation in a patient with T-cell acute leukemia. Four courses of treatment are depicted in which the methylation index (AdoMet/AdoHcy) and extent of RNA methylation (measured as 2′-O-methyluridine and 2′-O-methylcytidine) were measured in peripheral lymphoblasts. The first point in each sequence represents a *zero-time* control value obtained just before administration of 2′-deoxycoformycin. The abbreviations are: 2′-O-MeU/U, ratio of 2′-O-methyluridine to uridine in RNA; 2′-O-MeC/C, ratio of 2′-O-methylcytidine to cytidine in RNA. (*From unpublished data of the authors and [251].*)

Toxicity of deoxyguanosine to a variety of cultured cells, including human peripheral blood lymphocytes and T-cell lines is associated with dGTP accumulation and with depletion of dCTP and inhibition of DNA synthesis. This suggests inhibition by dGTP of the CDP reductase activity of ribonucleotide reductase [205–207, 210, 211]. Partial protection by deoxycytidine, shown in many of these studies, is consistent with this mechanism. Inhibition of phosphorylation of deoxyguanosine by deoxycytidine kinase could also explain those findings. Isolation of a deoxyguanosine-resistant, PNP-deficient S49 mutant with an altered ribonucleotide reductase [210, 211] is more specific evidence for the ribonucleotide reductase hypothesis.

Normally undetectable in red cells, dGTP accumulation has been found to be 2 to 8 nmol per milliliter of erythrocytes in PNP deficiency [255], values that are far less than the accumulation of dATP occurring in ADA deficiency. This reflects the very low deoxycytidine kinase activity in red cells and the ability of red cell adenosine kinase to phosphorylate deoxyadenosine (see above). No reports of elevated dGTP levels in peripheral lymphocytes of PNP-deficient patients have appeared, nor have plasma concentrations of deoxyinosine and deoxyguanosine been reported in affected patients, although plasma inosine concentration has been reported in the 18 to 115 μM range [35, 82, 256], and guanosine levels in the range of 6 to 29 μM [8, 82]. In some cases, these determinations may also include the deoxynucleosides. Nevertheless, dGTP-mediated inhibition of ribonucleotide reductase is presently considered the most likely cause of the T-cell defect in PNP deficiency.

Inosine-mediated Inactivation of *S*-Adenosylhomocysteine Hydrolase Recently a secondary deficiency of *S*-adenosylhomocysteine hydrolase to below 15 percent of control levels was reported in the erythrocytes of PNP-deficient children [257]. An explanation for this finding appears to be that inosine is a weak, irreversible inactivator of *S*-adenosylhomocysteine hydrolase with a K_I for the enzyme from human placenta of 5.9 mM [258]. Inosine is also a substrate for *S*-adenosylhomocysteine hydrolase–catalyzed *S*-inosylhomocysteine synthesis, with a K_m of 9.3 mM. Given the long life span of erythrocytes, their inability to synthesize new protein, and the high plasma inosine concentration found in PNP deficiency, a rate of hydrolase inactivation only a few percent per day in excess of the normal rate in erythrocytes would be sufficient to produce the observed deficiency. It seems unlikely that significant hydrolase depletion would occur in cells capable of enzyme turnover, so that *S*-adenosylhomocysteine accu-

mulation via this mechanism is not likely to contribute to the clinical consequences of PNP deficiency. As discussed above, inosine is not toxic to PNP-deficient lymphoblasts, even at millimolar concentrations [211], and at such concentrations produced only partial and transient decreases in *S*-adenosylhomocysteine hydrolase activity in WI-L2 lymphoblasts [258].

Purine Overexcretion The hypouricemia and hypouricosuria that occur in PNP deficiency are easily explained by the block in synthesis of the uric acid precursors, guanine and hypoxanthine. These purine bases are also substrates for hypoxanthine-guanine phosphoribosyltransferase, so that the major salvage pathway for purine nucleotide synthesis is also eliminated by complete PNP deficiency. As in the case of primary deficiency of hypoxanthine-guanine phosphoribosyltransferase (Chap. 51), the metabolic consequence of impaired purine salvage in PNP deficiency is also overproduction of purines *de novo*. This overproduction results in, and was discovered as, an overexcretion of the end products of purine catabolism, the nucleoside substrates for PNP [35]. For example, a 10-kg PNP-deficient child excreted in 24 h 0.08 mmol of uric acid, and 1.78, 0.71, 0.40, and 0.53 mmol each of inosine, guanosine, deoxyinosine, and deoxyguanosine, with total purine excretion of 3.59 mmol. A 12.8-kg control child excreted 0.92 mmol total purines, 95 percent as uric acid [259]. Thus far no clinical consequences of this purine overexcretion have been noted. This largely reflects the greater solubility of these nucleosides compared with uric acid.

In hypoxanthine-guanine phosphoribosyltransferase deficiency two mechanisms may cause purine overproduction: diminished synthesis of feedback inhibitory nucleotides that regulate the rate of the early enzymes in the purine biosynthetic pathway *de novo*, and increased intracellular concentration of PRPP, a rate-limiting substrate for the first step in the pathway *de novo*, as well as for the missing phosphoribosyltransferase (Chap. 51). In contrast to the finding of markedly elevated PRPP concentrations in the cultured fibroblasts of hypoxanthine-guanine phosphoribosyltransferase–deficient patients, fibroblasts from a PNP-deficient patient had normal levels of PRPP [35]. Based upon studies of the regulation of purine synthesis *de novo* in which generation of PRPP from inosine was demonstrated in hypoxanthine-guanine phosphoribosyltransferase–deficient cultured human lymphoblasts, a model has been proposed that could account for the differences with respect to fibroblast PRPP content in these two genetic diseases of purine salvage, and for the tendency common to both to overproduce purines *de novo* [98]. In hypoxanthine-guanine phosphoribosyltransferase deficiency, reutilization of the purine bases derived from phosphorolysis of purine nucleosides by PNP is deficient, but salvage of ribose-1-PO₄, after isomerization to ribose-5-PO₄, can still occur, resulting in an increase in steady state concentration of PRPP. In PNP deficiency there is an equal block in salvage of both the purine base and ribosyl moieties of the PNP substrates, so that this source of excess PRPP is eliminated. In both diseases there is a block in salvage synthesis of feedback inhibitory purine nucleotides, and this could account for the increased activity of the *de novo* pathway in each case (Fig. 53-12).

Figure 53-12 Schema depicting factors that may affect the cellular content of phosphoribosylpyrophosphate (PRPP), purine nucleotide synthesis, and the urinary excretion of purines in normal individuals (I), and in patients with genetic deficiencies of hypoxanthine-guanine phosphoribosyltransferase (HGPRT)(II) and purine nucleoside phosphorylase (PNP)(III). In normal individuals there is a "balanced" reutilization, via HGPRT-catalyzed IMP synthesis, of the ribose and purine base moieties generated by PNP-catalyzed phosphorolysis of inosine and guanosine, with a fraction of the hypoxanthine and guanine being converted to uric acid. In HGPRT deficiency virtually all of the hypoxanthine and guanine are converted to uric acid, while the ribose-1-PO₄ generated by the PNP reaction continues to be reutilized by cells, contributing to an increased steady state concentration of PRPP. Both increased PRPP concentration and diminished salvage synthesis of feedback-inhibitory nucleotides result in enhanced synthesis of purine nucleotides via the *de novo* pathway. In PNP deficiency inosine and guanosine, rather than uric acid, are the end products of purine catabolism. There is an equivalent block in formation, and hence reutilization, of both the ribose and purine bases ordinarily generated by the PNP reaction. Therefore, there is no increase in steady state concentration of PRPP in cells capable of purine synthesis *de novo*, and the diminished salvage synthesis of feedback-inhibitory nucleotides alone accounts for enhanced synthesis *de novo* of purine nucleotides. (*Modified from Hershfield and Seegmiller [98]. Used by permission.*)

I. NORMAL

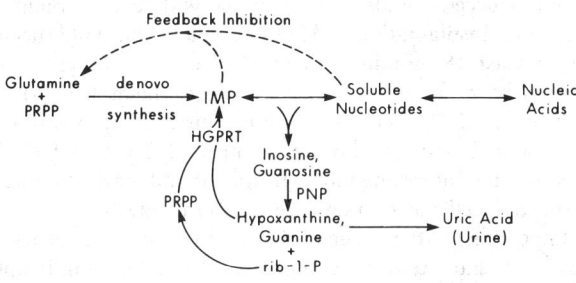

II. HGPRT DEFICIENCY

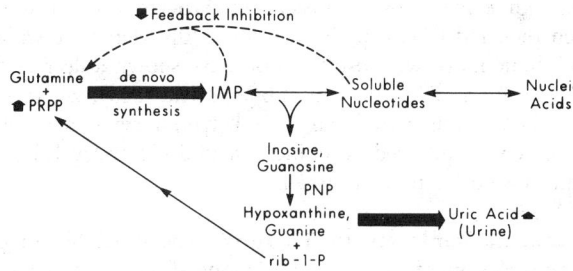

III. PNP DEFICIENCY

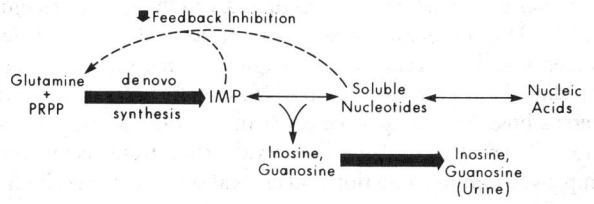

Basis for Selective Immune Dysfunction in ADA and PNP Deficiencies

Attempts have been made to account for the "purinogenic" immune deficiency diseases by a common mechanism, and the most obvious candidate thus far considered is the "ribonucleotide reductase" hypothesis (Fig. 53-13). Although it is not yet known to what extent nonlymphoid cells, other than erythrocytes, accumulate dATP or dGTP in affected patients, the facility with which T lymphocytes trap deoxyadenosine and deoxyguanosine as these nucleotides in vitro is striking. Both nucleosides are substrates for deoxycytidine kinase, a lymphospecific enzyme with greater functional activity in T than in B cells (though adenosine kinase also functions as a deoxycytidine kinase in intact cells), and both are much more toxic to T than to B cells. Both dATP and dGTP inhibit ribonucleotide reductase. For these reasons inhibition of DNA synthesis by this mechanism has been proposed as a single cause of the clinical consequences of both ADA and PNP deficiency. This mechanism seems most acceptable when considering the isolated defect in cellular immunity in PNP deficiency, and the absence of T cells in ADA deficiency, but it fails to explain the occurrence of a profound deficit in B-cell function in ADA but not in PNP deficiency. Nor can inhibition of ribonucleotide reductase account for the disappearance of nondividing peripheral blood lymphocytes in deoxycoformycin-treated patients, nor for the probably related ability of deoxyadenosine to inhibit prereplicative protein synthesis in ADA-inhibited, mitogen-stimulated, peripheral lymphocytes in vitro.

Thus far no direct evidence has been obtained that peripheral lymphocytes are especially predisposed to S-adenosylhomocysteine accumulation, or to its deleterious effects, but there are theoretical reasons for considering both possibilities. The low metabolic activity in circulating lymphocytes would lead to a greater extent of S-adenosylhomocysteine hydrolase inactivation by deoxyadenosine than would occur in cells capable of more rapid protein turnover. In addition, human resting peripheral blood lymphocytes have low levels of S-adenosylmethionine (compared to lectin-stimulated cells and cultured lymphoblasts [238–240]), which would be expected to accentuate the toxic effects of any increase in S-adenosylhomocysteine by giving a lower value for the methylation index.

Low S-adenosylmethionine levels may account for peculiarities in rRNA metabolism that have been noted in human resting peripheral blood lymphocytes in which, in contrast to lectin-stimulated lymphocytes and other cultured cells, approximately 50 percent of the 45S precursor rRNA transcribed in the nucleus is degraded and never reaches the cytoplasm as mature 18S rRNA [260]. Processing of 45S rRNA into mature 18S and 28S rRNA is believed to require extensive methylation and can be inhibited in HeLa cells by methionine deprivation [261] or by the methionine analogue ethionine [262]. A phenomenon similar to the 18S rRNA "wastage" found in resting lymphocytes has also been induced in cultured human myeloma cells by adenosine [263], which can inhibit transmethylation through its ability to increase S-adenosylhomocysteine levels. These observations suggest that resting peripheral blood lymphocytes, in which S-adenosylmethionine levels are low, are already marginal in their ability to methylate. Therefore, small increases in S-adenosylhomocysteine, due either to impaired adenosine metabolism or to inactivation of S-adenosylhomocysteine hydrolase, could further compromise methyl-

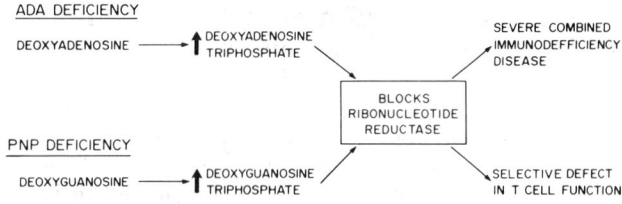

Figure 53-13 The "ribonucleotide reductase" hypothesis. It has been proposed that the immune defects in both ADA and PNP deficiency result from inhibition of ribonucleotide reductase, owing to the selective accumulation of dATP or dGTP by lymphoid cells, causing inhibition of DNA synthesis.

ation capacity, causing ribosome depletion and preventing the burst of prereplicative protein synthesis that occurs after lectin stimulation. The absence of 18S rRNA wastage in phytohemagglutinin-treated peripheral blood lymphocytes [260] may be a reflection of the five- to tenfold increase in S-adenosylmethionine levels found within 24 h after lectin stimulation [240].

ADA levels are higher in lymphocytes than in most other tissues [264]. Thus, lymphocytes may rely on deamination of adenosine to a greater extent than other cells to pull the S-adenosylhomocysteine hydrolase reaction in the hydrolytic direction. If this is true, loss of ADA could lead to greater accumulation of S-adenosylhomocysteine in lymphocytes than in cells that are more dependent upon adenosine phosphorylation or homocysteine metabolism to permit efficient catabolism of S-adenosylhomocysteine. Conversely, high levels of ADA in lymphocytes would provide these cells with increased tolerance to high levels of homocysteine and could account for the fact that patients with homocystinuria are not immunodeficient.

The fact that the effects of adenosine and deoxyadenosine on S-adenosylhomocysteine hydrolysis may operate in ADA deficiency, but not in PNP deficiency, could explain the more severe impairment in both T- and B-cell function that occurs in the former. With regard to a role for impaired methylation in causing B-cell dysfunction, it is intriguing that agammaglobulinemia was found in a patient with heritable deficiency of transcobalamin II, a major plasma cobalamin binding protein (Chap. 23), and that this deficit in humoral immunity was corrected by pharmacologic doses of vitamin B₁₂ [265]. Remethylation of homocysteine by methyl tetrahydrofolate is one of only two or three known cobalamin-dependent reactions in humans (Chap. 23), and in individuals on a normal diet is required to generate sufficient labile methyl groups for methylation purposes [87]. It is possible, therefore, that impaired methylation explains the B-cell defect in this patient with transcobalamin II deficiency.

ATP and GTP subserve functions not only as precursors of RNA and as phosphate donors, but also as sources of energy for specific cellular processes and as effectors that modify the function of proteins in all cellular compartments. In contrast, dATP and dGTP serve much more limited functions, which may all be related to DNA replication in the nucleus. In ADA and PNP deficiencies these deoxynucleotides are found at abnormally high concentrations, and in addition may occur in abnormal cellular locations. They may act essentially as substrate analogue inhibitors of reactions that have evolved with specificity for purine ribonucleotides, and not inconceivably as suicide substrates for some, based upon the example of S-adenosylhomocysteine hydrolase. If the remarkable diversity of toxic effects attributable at present to deficiencies of ADA

and PNP are any indication, one may predict that others will be discovered before the next version of this chapter is written.

TREATMENT

In both ADA and PNP deficiency, as in all immunodeficiency states, supportive care consisting of varying degrees of isolation and antisepsis combined with vigorous antibiotic therapy for specific infections comprise an essential aspect of patient care. It is particularly important to avoid exposure to common childhood viral illnesses such as varicella, and immunization with live virus is contraindicated. Forms of specific therapy are discussed below.

ADA Deficiency

Transplantation   The current treatment of choice for SCID is bone marrow transplantation from a histocompatible donor. A successful outcome with minimal graft-versus-host reaction depends on donor-host identity at the HLA-A and HLA-B loci as well as nonreactivity in mixed lymphocyte culture [266]. Experience thus far indicates that patients lacking ADA are as likely to respond with engraftment and restoration of immune function as those who have normal ADA [267], and at least three ADA-deficient children have achieved long-term immune reconstitution (18 to 43 months) from such treatment [268, 269].

Some success has also been achieved with fetal liver and thymic cell transplantation in ADA deficiency. One child survived for at least 18 months with restored immune function [17]. Others have shown only partial improvement from similar treatment [270, 271]. In another instance transfusion of peripheral blood lymphocytes from an HLA-A and HLA-B identical parent resulted in engraftment and marked improvement in T-cell function and clinical status [272].

Engraftment after tissue transplantation for ADA deficiency has been characterized by chimerism for circulating lymphocytes, most or all of which are of donor origin and contain ADA. Erythrocytes generally are of host origin and lack ADA, although evidence for transient erythrocyte chimerism has been reported in two patients [269, 270]. Metabolic studies after bone marrow transplantation have shown a decrease in erythrocyte dATP to normal in one patient [269], whereas in the child given peripheral blood lymphocytes an initial decrease was followed by an increase in dATP to levels higher than those prior to engraftment [272].

Enzyme Replacement Therapy   The feasibility of enzyme replacement therapy for ADA deficiency was first suggested by experiments in vitro showing that the responsiveness of a patient's peripheral blood lymphocytes to lectin stimulation was enhanced by addition of ADA to the culture medium [154]. This observation led to treatment of ADA-deficient patients with exogenous enzyme given in the form of frozen, irradiated (to eliminate lymphocytes that might cause graft-versus-host disease), packed erythrocytes from normal donors [15]. Given at 2- to 4-week intervals, such transfusions have improved immune function and clinical status in some children

[15, 16, 273, 274] but not others [275, 276]. A review of ten such patients showed that of the five whose response was judged good, all had residual T-cell and B-cell function prior to treatment, while the four who did not respond had no such residual function [277]. A fair response was obtained in one patient with some T-cell but no B-cell function prior to treatment. Thus, the benefits of erythrocyte transfusion appear to depend in large part on the amount of remaining immune function that can be "rescued" by enzyme replacement.

Although thymosine alone is of no apparent benefit in ADA deficiency, in one child an increase in lymphocyte count and improved responsiveness to lectin stimulation in vitro were obtained only with a combination of this thymus-derived factor and erythrocyte transfusion [274]. Many children have received plasma in conjunction with erythrocyte transfusions, but there have been no studies showing any advantage of this combination over packed erythrocytes alone.

Erythrocyte ADA can be increased to near-normal levels by repeated transfusions and decays with a half-life of 3 to 4 weeks [277]. Lymphocyte ADA is not affected by such therapy [15]. Erythrocyte transfusions have decreased plasma levels of adenosine [160] and deoxyadenosine [16, 274, 285] and urinary excretion of deoxyadenosine [16]. Reductions in erythrocyte dATP of 90 percent or more are observed [16, 160, 273] and reflect not only the metabolic state of transfused cells, but probably a loss of dATP from remaining ADA-deficient erythrocytes as well. In one study lymphocyte dATP decreased from three times normal after 10 weeks of transfusion therapy to a normal level after 40 weeks [278]. Lymphocyte dCTP and dTTP levels were normal or elevated during this entire time. Unfortunately the effects of enzyme replacement therapy on lymphocyte deoxyribonucleotide metabolism could not be fully assessed in this patient because pretreatment samples were not available.

Metabolite Replacement The only reported attempt to correct a putative dCTP deficiency by oral administration of deoxycytidine was unsuccessful [277]. It has been suggested that deamination of this nucleoside by intestinal cytidine deaminase may prevent its absorption intact, and that parenteral administration might be required to insure delivery to lymphocytes, but there are no published reports of such therapy.

PNP Deficiency

The small total number of PNP-deficient patients and a tendency for several of these to do reasonably well without specific therapy have made it difficult to evaluate different forms of treatment. From experience obtained in the treatment of other heritable immunodeficiencies, one might expect that immune reconstitution could be achieved by bone marrow or other tissue transplantation, but this approach has been used in only one known PNP-deficient patient. This child, who was discovered to have been PNP-deficient only several years after her death, received a series of fetal thymus transplants for what was recognized at the time as a severe defect in cellular immunity complicated by generalized vaccinia and candidiasis [34]. Significant but transient improvements in clinical status and laboratory measurements of cellular immunity were noted after the first two transplants, but the child died of lymphosarcoma shortly after the third.

Irradiated erythrocyte transfusions have been given to four patients in the hope that enzyme replacement therapy might achieve results similar to those reported for some ADA-deficient patients. In two children no improvement was noted [279, 280], while in the others some increases in T-cell rosetting and responsiveness to phytohemagglutinin were observed [281, 282]. In the latter two children measurements of purine metabolites during transfusion therapy showed a marked decrease in urinary excretion of inosine, guanosine, deoxyinosine, deoxyguanosine, and total purines; increased plasma and urinary urate; and significant reductions in erythrocyte dGTP. In one patient mononuclear-cell dGTP was normal during transfusion therapy [282]. The significance of this finding is unknown because pretreatment levels were not determined.

Administration of thymosin to one patient for 9 months resulted in substantially improved T-cell function in vitro, but development of an allergic reaction to the drug finally required its discontinuation [283]. Studies on mechanisms of nucleoside toxicity in model systems have prompted the use of several different metabolites in the treatment of PNP deficiency. Some improvements in T-cell rosetting and responsiveness to phytohemagglutin in vitro were noted in two patients receiving oral uridine, but not in a third [33, 283]. Oral deoxycytidine had no effect in the one child who received it [281]. Parenteral use of this compound has not been reported.

REFERENCES

1. ROSEN FS: Immune deficiencies: An overview, in Gelfand EW, Dosch H-M (eds): *Biological Basis of Immunodeficiency.* New York, Raven Press, 1980, p 1
2. GIBLETT ER, ANDERSON JE, COHEN F, POLLARA B, MEUWISSEN HJ: Adenosine deaminase deficiency in two patients with severely impaired cellular immunity. *Lancet* 2:1067, 1972
3. GIBLETT ER: Adenosine deaminase and purine nucleoside phosphorylase deficiency: How they were discovered and what they may mean, in Elliot K, Whelan J (eds): *Enzyme Defects and Immune Dysfunction, Ciba Foundation Symposium 68.* New York, Excerpta Medica, 1979, p 3
4. DISSING J, KNUDSEN JB: Adenosine deaminase deficiency and combined immunodeficiency syndrome. *Lancet* 2:1316, 1972
5. OCHS HD, YOUNT JE, GIBLETT ER, CHEN SH, SCOTT CR, WEDGEWOOD RJ: Adenosine-deaminase deficiency and severe combined immunodeficiency syndrome. *Lancet* 1:1393, 1973
6. POLLARA B, PICKERING RJ, MEUWISSEN HJ: Combined immunodeficiency disease and adenosine deaminase deficiency, an inborn error of metabolism. *Pediatr Res* 7:362, 1973
7. GIBLETT ER, AMMANN AJ, WARA DW, SANDMAN R, DIAMOND LK: Nucleoside-phosphorylase deficiency in a child with severely defective T-cell immunity and normal B-cell immunity. *Lancet* 1:1010, 1975
8. STOOP JW, ZEGERS BJM, HENDRICKX GFM, SIEGENBEEK VAN HEUKELOM LH, STAAL GEJ, DE BREE PK, WADMAN SK, BALLIEUX RE: Purine nucleoside phosphorylase deficiency associated with selective cellular immunodeficiency. *N Engl J Med* 296:651, 1977
9. BIGGAR WD, GIBLETT ER, OZERE RL, GROVER BD: A new form of nucleoside phosphorylase deficiency in two brothers with defective T-cell function. *J Pediatr* 92:354, 1978
10. VIRELIZIER JL, HAMET M, BALLET JJ, REINERT P, GRISCELLI C: Impaired defense against vaccinia in a child with T-lymphocyte deficiency associated with inosine phosphorylase defect. *J Pediatr* 92:358, 1978
11. CARAPELLA-DE LUCA E, AIUTI F, LUCARELLI P, BRUNI L, BARONI CD, IMPERATO C, ROOS D, ASTALDI A: A patient with nucleoside phosphorylase deficiency, selective T-cell deficiency, and autoimmune hemolytic anemia. *J Pediatr* 93:1000, 1978
12. RICH KC, ARNOLD WJ, PALELLA T, FOX IH: Cellular immune deficiency with autoimmune hemolytic anemia in purine nucleoside phosphorylase deficiency. *Am J Med* 67:172, 1979
13. HIRSCHHORN R: Incidence and prenatal detection of adenosine deaminase deficiency and purine nucleoside phosphorylase deficiency, in Pollara B, Pickering RJ, Meuwissen HJ, Porter IH (eds): *Inborn Errors of Specific Immunity.* New York, Academic Press, 1979, p 5
14. HIRSCHHORN R: Clinical delineation of adenosine deaminase deficiency, in Elliot K, Whelan J (eds): *Enzyme Defects and Immune Dysfunction, Ciba Foundation Symposium 68.* New York, Exerpta Medica, 1979, p 35

15. POLMAR SH, STERN RC, SCHWARTZ AL, WETZLER EM, CHASE PA, HIRSCHHORN R: Enzyme replacement therapy for adenosine deaminase deficiency and severe combined immunodeficiency. *N Engl J Med* 295:1337, 1976

16. HIRSCHHORN R, PAPAGEORGIOU PS, KESARWALA HH, TAFT LT: Amelioration of neurologic abnormalities after "enzyme replacement" in adenosine deaminase deficiency. *N Engl J Med* 303:377, 1980

17. ACKERET C, PLUSS HJ, HITZIG WH: Hereditary severe combined immunodeficiency. *Pediatr Res* 10:67, 1976

18. HIRSCHHORN R: Defects of purine metabolism in immunodeficiency diseases, in Schwartz RS (ed): *Progress in Clinical Immunology*. New York, Grune and Stratton, 1977, vol 3, p 67

19. COHEN F, CEJKA J, CHANG C-H, BROUGH AJ, ROWE BJ, GAINES PJ: Adenosine deaminase deficiency and immunodeficiency, in Pollara B, Pickering RJ, Meuwissen HJ, Porter IH (eds): *Inborn Errors of Specific Immunity*. New York, Academic Press, 1979, p 401

20. WOLFSON JJ, CROSS VF: The radiographic findings in 49 patients with combined immunodeficiency, in Meuwissen HJ, Pickering RJ, Pollara B, Porter IH (eds): *Combined Immunodeficiency Disease and Adenosine Deaminase Deficiency: A Molecular Defect*. New York, Academic Press, 1975, p 255

21. HIRSCHHORN R, VAWTER GF, KIRKPATRICK JA JR, ROSEN FS: Adenosine deaminase deficiency: Frequency and comparative pathology in autosomally recessive severe combined immunodeficiency. *Clin Immunol Immunopathol* 14:107, 1979

22. SCHWARTZ AL, POLMAR SH, STERN RC, COWAN DH: Abnormal platelet aggregation in severe combined immunodeficiency disease with adenosine deaminase deficiency. *Br J Haematol* 39:189, 1978

23. LEE CH, EVANS SP, ROZENBERG MC, BAGNARA AS, ZIEGLER JB, VAN DER WEYDEN MB: In vitro platelet abnormality in adenosine deaminase deficiency and severe combined immunodeficiency. *Blood* 53:465, 1979

24. CEDERBAUM SD, KAITILA I, RIMOIN DL, STIEHM ER: The chondro-osseous dysplasia of adenosine deaminase deficiency with severe combined immunodeficiency. *J Pediatr* 89:737, 1976

25. HUBER J, KERSEY J: Pathologic features, in Meuwissen HJ, Pickering RJ, Pollara B, Porter IH (eds): *Combined Immunodeficiency Disease and Adenosine Deaminase Deficiency: A Molecular Defect*. New York, Academic Press, 1975, p 279

26. JENKINS T: Red-blood-cell adenosine deaminase deficiency in a "healthy" !Kung individual. *Lancet* 2:736, 1973

27. JENKINS T, LANE AB, NURSE GT, HOPKINSON DA: Red cell adenosine deaminase (ADA) polymorphism in Southern Africa, with special reference to ADA deficiency among the !Kung. *Ann Hum Genet* 42:425, 1979

28. JENKINS T, RABSON AR, NURSE GT, LANE AB: Deficiency of adenosine deaminase not associated with severe combined immunodeficiency. *J Pediatr* 89:732, 1976

29. JENKINS T, LANE AB: The red cell adenosine deaminase polymorphism in Southern African populations with particular reference to the !Kung of Tsumkwe, Southwest Africa/Namibia, in Pollara B, Pickering RJ, Meuwissen HJ, Porter IH (eds): *Inborn Errors of Specific Immunity*. New York, Academic Press, 1979, p 73

30. HIRSCHHORN R, ROEGNER V, JENKINS T, SEAMAN C, PIOMELLI S, BORKOWSKY W: Erythrocyte adenosine deaminase deficiency without immunodeficiency. Evidence for an unstable mutant enzyme. *J Clin Invest* 64:1130, 1979

31. VALENTINE WN, PAGLIA DE, TARTAGLIA AP, GILSANZ F: Hereditary hemolytic anemia with increased red cell adenosine deaminase (45- to 70-fold) and decreased adenosine triphosphate. *Science* 195:783, 1977

32. MIWA S, FUJII H, MATSUMOTO N, NAKATSUJI T, ODA S, ASANO H, ASANO S: A case of red-cell adenosine deaminase overproduction associated with hereditary hemolytic anemia found in Japan. *Am J Hematol* 5:107, 1978

33. AMMAN AJ: Immunologic aberrations in purine nucleoside phosphorylase deficiencies, in Elliot K, Whelan J (eds): *Enzyme Defects and Immune Dysfunction, Ciba Foundation Symposium 68*. New York, Exerpta Medica, 1979, p 55

34. STOOP JW, EIJSVOOGEL VP, ZEGERS BJM, BLOK-SCHUT B, VAN BEKKUM DW, BALLIEUX RE: Selective severe cellular immunodeficiency: Effect of thymus transplantation and transfer factor administration. *Clin Immunol Immunopathol* 6:289, 1976

35. COHEN A, DOYLE D, MARTIN DW JR, AMMANN AJ: Abnormal purine metabolism and purine overproduction in a patient deficient in purine nucleoside phosphorylase. *N Engl J Med* 295:1449, 1976

36. SPENCER N, HOPKINSON DA, HARRIS H: Adenosine deaminase polymorphism in man. *Ann Hum Genet* 32:9, 1968

37. EDWARDS YH, HOPKINSON DA, HARRIS H: Adenosine deaminase in human tissues. *Ann Hum Genet* 35:207, 1971

38. AKEDO H, NISHIHARA H, SHINKAI K, KOMATSU K, ISHIKAWA S: Multiple forms of human adenosine deaminase. I. Purification and characterization of two molecular species. *Biochim Biophys Acta* 276:257, 1972

39. NISHIHARA H, ISHIKAWA S, SHINKAI K, AKEDO H: Multiple forms of human adenosine deaminase. II Isolation and properties of a conversion factor from human lung. *Biochim Biophys Acta* 302:429, 1973

40. SWALLOW DM, EVANS L, HOPKINSON DA: Several of the adenosine deaminase isozymes are glycoproteins. *Nature* 269:261, 1977

41. DADDONA PE, KELLEY WN: Human adenosine deaminase binding protein. Assay, purification, and properties. *J Biol Chem* 253:4617, 1978

42. SCHRADER WP, STACY AR, POLLARA B: Purification of human erythrocyte adenosine deaminase by affinity column chromatography. *J Biol Chem* 251:4026, 1976

43. DADDONA PE, KELLEY WN: Human adenosine deaminase: Purification and subunit structure. *J Biol Chem* 252:110, 1977

44. TISCHFIELD JA, CREAGAN RP, NICHOLS EA, RUDDLE FH: Assignment of a gene for adenosine deaminase to human chromosome 20. *Hum Hered* 24:1, 1974

45. PHILLIP T, LENOIR G, ROLLAND MO, PHILLIP I, HAMET M, LAURAS B, FRAISSE J: Regional assignment of the ADA locus on 20q13.2 → qter by gene dosage studies. *Cytogenet Cell Genet* 27:187, 1980

46. SCHRADER WP, STACY AR: Purification and subunit structure of adenosine deaminase from human kidney. *J Biol Chem* 252:6409, 1977

47. KOCH G, SHOWS TB: A gene on human chromosome 6 functions in assembly of tissue-specific adenosine deaminase isozymes. *Proc Natl Acad Sci USA* 75:3876, 1978

48. KOCH G, SHOWS TB: Somatic cell genetics of adenosine deaminase expression and severe combined immunodeficiency disease in humans. *Proc Natl Acad Sci USA* 77:4211, 1980

49. HIRSCHHORN R, LEVYTAKA V, POLLARA B, MEUWISSEN HJ: Evidence for control of several different tissue-specific isozymes of adenosine deaminase by a single genetic locus. *Nature, New Biol* 246:200, 1973

50. DADDONA PE, FROHMAN MA, KELLEY WN: Human adenosine deaminase and its binding protein in normal and adenosine deaminase-deficient fibroblast cell strains. *J Biol Chem* 255:5681, 1980

51. HIRSCHHORN R: Conversion of human erythrocyte-adenosine deaminase activity to different tissue specific isozymes. Evidence for a common catalytic unit. *J Clin Invest* 55:661, 1975

52. CHEN SH, SCOTT CR, SWEDBERG DR: Heterogeneity for adenosine deaminase deficiency: Expression of the enzyme in cultured skin fibroblasts and amniotic fluid cells. *Am J Hum Genet* 27:46, 1975

53. HIRSCHHORN R, BERATIS N, ROSEN FS: Characterization of residual enzyme activity in fibroblasts from patients with adenosine deaminase deficiency and combined immunodeficiency: Evidence for a mutant enzyme. *Proc Natl Acad Sci USA* 73:213, 1976

54. CARSON DA, GOLDBLUM R, SEEGMILLER JE: Quantitative immunoassay of adenosine deaminase in combined immunodeficiency disease. *J Immunol* 118:270, 1977

55. DADDONA PE, FROHMAN MA, KELLEY WN: Radioimmunochemical quantitation of human adenosine deaminase. *J Clin Invest* 64:798, 1979

56. SCOTT CR, CHEN SH, GIBLETT ER: Detection of the carrier state in combined immunodeficiency disease associated with adenosine deaminase deficiency. *J Clin Invest* 53:1194, 1974

57. BRINKMANN B, BRINKMAN M, MARTIN H: A new allele in red cell adenosine deaminase polymorphism: ADA°. *Hum Hered* 23:603, 1973

58. CHEN SH, SCOTT CR, GIBLETT ER: Adenosine deaminase: Demonstration of a "silent" gene associated with combined immunodeficiency disease. *Am J Hum Genet* 26:103, 1974

59. CHEN SH, SCOTT CR, GIBLETT ER, LEVIN AS: Adenosine deaminase deficiency: Another family with a "silent" ADA allele and normal ADA activity in two heterozygotes. *Am J Hum Genet* 29:642, 1977

60. HIRSCHHORN R, BERATIS N, ROSEN FS, PARKMAN R, STERN R, POLMAR S: Adenosine-deaminase deficiency in a child diagnosed prenatally. *Lancet* 1:73, 1975

61. HIRSCHHORN R: Prenatal diagnosis and heterozygote detection in adenosine deaminase deficiency, in Güttler F, Seakins JWT, Harkness RA (eds): *Inborn Errors of Immunity and Phagocytosis*, Lancaster, MTP Press, 1979, p 121

62. AITKEN DA, KLEIJER WJ, NIERMEIJER MF, HERBSCHLEB-VOOGT E, GALJAARD, H: Prenatal detection of a probable heterozygote for ADA deficiency and severe combined immunodeficiency disease using a microradioassay. *Clin Genet* 17:293, 1980

63. NAYLOR EW, ORFANOS AP, GUTHRIE R: An improved screening test for adenosine deaminase deficiency. *J Pediatr* 93:473, 1978

64. ITO K, SAKURA N, USUI T, UCHINO H: Screening for primary immunodeficiencies associated with purine nucleoside phosphorylase deficiency of adenosine deaminase deficiency. *J Lab Clin Med* 90:844, 1977

65. LEWIS AS, LOWY BA: Human erythrocyte purine nucleoside phosphorylase: Molecular weight and physical properties. A Theorell-Chance catalytic mechanism. *J Biol Chem* 254:9927, 1979

66. KIM BK, CHA S, PARKS RE JR: Purine nucleoside phosphorylase from human erythrocytes. I. Purification and properties. *J Biol Chem* 243:1763, 1968

67. KALCKAR HM: The enzymatic synthesis of purine ribosides. *J Biol Chem* 167:477, 1947

68. Friedkin M: Desoxyribose-1-phosphate. II The isolation of crystalline desoxyribose-1-phosphate. *J Biol Chem* 184:449, 1950

69. Zimmerman TP, Gersten NB, Ross RF, Miech RP: Adenine as substrate for purine nucleoside phosphorylase. *Can J Biochem* 49:1050, 1971

70. Agarwal RP, Parks RE Jr: Purine nucleoside phosphorylase from human erythrocytes. IV. Crystallization and some properties. *J Biol Chem* 244:644, 1969

71. Zannis V, Doyle D, Martin DW Jr: Purification and characterization of human erythrocyte purine nucleoside phosphorylase and its subunits. *J Biol Chem* 253:504, 1978

72. Osborne WR: Human red cell purine nucleoside phosphorylase. Purification by biospecific affinity chromatography and physical properties. *J Biol Chem* 255:7089, 1980

73. Ghangas G, Reem GH: Characterization of the subunit structure of human placental nucleoside phosphorylase by immunochemistry. *J Biol Chem* 254:4233, 1979

74. Wiginton DA, Coleman MS, Hutton JJ: Characterization of purine nucleoside phosphorylase from human granulocytes and its metabolism of deoxyribonucleosides. *J Biol Chem* 255:6663, 1980

75. Zannis VI, Gudas LJ, Martin DW Jr: Characterization of the subunits of purine nucleoside phosphorylase from cultured normal human fibroblasts. *Biochem Genet* 17:621, 1979

76. Stoeckler JE, Agarwal RP, Agarwal KC, Schmid K, Parks RE Jr: Purine nucleoside phosphorylase from human erythrocytes: Physiochemical properties of the crystalline enzyme. *Biochemistry* 17:278, 1978

77. Edwards YH, Hopkinson DA, Harris H: Inherited variants of human nucleoside phosphorylase. *Ann Hum Genet* 34:395, 1971

78. Turner BM, Fisher RA, Harris H: An association between the kinetic and electrophoretic properties of human purine-nucleoside-phosphorylase isozymes. *Eur J Biochem* 24:288, 1971

79. Creagan RP, Tan YH, Chen S, Tischfield JA, Ruddle FJ: Mouse/human somatic cell hybrids utilizing human parental cells containing a (14:22) translocation: Assignment of the gene for nucleoside phosphorylase to chromosome 14, in Bergsma D (ed): *Human Gene Mapping*. New York, The National Foundation, 1973

80. Fox IH, Andres CM, Gelfand EW, Biggar D: Purine nucleoside phosphorylase deficiency: altered kinetic properties of a mutant enzyme. *Science* 197:1084, 1977

81. Wortmann RL, Andres CM, Kaminska J, Gelfand EW, Arnold W, Rich K, Fox IH: Biochemical heterogeneity in purine nucleoside phosphorylase deficiency. *Arthritis Rheum* 21:603, 1978

82. Osborne WR, Chen SH, Giblett ER, Biggar WD, Ammann AA, Scott CR: Purine nucleoside phosphorylase deficiency. Evidence for molecular heterogeneity in two families with enzyme-deficient members. *J Clin Invest* 60:741, 1977

83. Gudas LJ, Zannis VI, Clift SM, Amman AJ, Staal GE, Martin DW Jr: Characterization of mutant subunits of human purine nucleoside phosphorylase. *J Biol Chem* 253:8916, 1978

84. McRoberts JA, Martin DW Jr: Submolecular characterization of a mutant purine-nucleoside phosphorylase. *J Biol Chem* 255:5605, 1980

85. Hall JG: Adenosine deaminase activity in lymphoid cells during antibody production. *Aust J Exp Biol Med Sci* 41:93, 1963

86. Snyder FF, Mendelsohn J, Seegmiller JE: Adenosine metabolism in phytohemagglutinin-stimulated human lymphocytes. *J Clin Invest* 58:654, 1976

87. Mudd HS, Poole JR: Labile methyl balances for normal humans on various dietary regimens. *Metabolism* 24:721, 1975

88. Sonoda T, Tatibana M: Metabolic fate of pyrimidines and purines in dietary nucleic acids ingested by mice. *Biochim Biophys Acta* 521:55, 1978

89. Wilson D, Beyer A, Bishop C, Talbott JH: Urinary uric acid excretion after ingestion of isotopic yeast nucleic acid in the normal and gouty human. *J Biol Chem* 209:227, 1954

90. De Pierre JW, Karnovsky ML: Ecto-enzymes of the guinea pig polymorphonuclear leukocyte. *J Biol Chem* 249:7111, 1974

91. De Pierre JW, Karnovsky ML: Ecto-enzymes of the guinea pig polymorphonuclear leukocyte II. Properties and suitability as markers for the plasma membrane. *J Biol Chem* 249:7121, 1974

92. Fleit H, Conklyn M, Stebbins RD, Silber R: Function of 5'-nucleotidase in the uptake of adenosine from AMP by human lymphocytes. *J Biol Chem* 250:8889, 1975

93. Frick GP, Lowenstein JM: Vectorial production of adenosine by 5'-nucleotidase in the perfused rat heart. *J Biol Chem* 253:1240, 1978

94. Newby AC: Role of adenosine deaminase, ecto-(5'-nucleotidase) and ecto-(non-specific phosphatase) in cyanide-induced adenosine monophosphate catabolism in rat polymorphonuclear leucocytes. *Biochem J* 186:907, 1980

95. Chan T-S, Ishii K, Long C, Green H: Purine excretion by mammalian cells deficient in adenosine kinase. *J Cell Physiol* 81:315, 1973

96. Brox LW, Henderson JF: The "adenosine cycle" is not a significant route of purine metabolism in mammalian cells. *Can J Biochem* 54:200, 1976

97. Van Den Berghe G, Van Pottelsberghe C, Hers H-G: A kinetic study of the soluble 5'-nucleotidase of rat liver. *Biochem J* 162:611, 1977

98. Hershfield MS, Seegmiller JE: Regulation of de novo purine synthesis in human lymphoblasts. Similar rates of de novo synthesis during growth by normal cells and mutants deficient in hypoxanthine-guanine phosphoribosyltransferase activity. *J Biol Chem* 252:6002, 1977

99. Snyder FF, Trafzer RJ, Hershfield MS, Seegmiller JE: Elucidation of aberrant purine metabolism. Application of hypoxanthine-guanine phosphoribosyltransferase—and adenosine kinase-deficient mutants, and IMP dehydrogenase—and adenosine deaminase-inhibited human lymphoblasts. *Biochim Biophys Acta* 609:492, 1980

100. Matsumoto SS, Raivio KO, Seegmiller JE: Adenine nucleotide degradation during energy depletion in human lymphoblasts. Adenosine accumulation and adenylate energy charge correlation. *J Biol Chem* 254:8865, 1979

101. Schwabe U, Ebert R, Erbler HC: Adenosine release from isolated fat cells and its significance for the effects of hormones on cyclic 3',5'-AMP levels and lipolysis. *Naunyn-Schmiedbergs Arch Pharmacol* 276:133, 1973

102. Lerner MH, Lowy BA: Formation of adenosine in rabbit liver and its role as a direct precursor of erythrocyte nucleotides. *J Biol Chem* 249:259, 1974

103. Pritchard JB, O'Connor N, Oliver JM, Berlin RD: Uptake and supply of purine compounds by the liver. *Am J Physiol* 229:967, 1975

104. Rubio R, Berne RM, Katori M: Release of adenosine in reactive hyperemia of the dog heart. *Am J Physiol* 216:56, 1969

105. Lomax CA, Henderson JF: Adenosine formation and metabolism during adenosine triphosphate catabolism in Ehrlich ascites tumor cells. *Cancer Res* 33:2825, 1973.

106. Chan TS: Purine excretion by mouse peritoneal macrophages lacking adenosine deaminase activity. *Proc Natl Acad Sci USA* 76:925, 1979

107. Plagemann PGW, Richey DP: Transport of nucleosides, nucleic acid bases, choline and glucose by animal cells in culture. *Biochim Biophys Acta* 344:263, 1974

108. Berlin RD, Oliver JM: Membrane transport of purine and pyrimidine bases and nucleosides in animal cells. *Int Rev Cytol* 42:287, 1975

109. Paterson ARP, Babb LR, Paran JH, Cass CE: Inhibition by nitrobenzylthioinosine of adenosine uptake by asynchronous HeLa cells. *Mol Pharmacol* 13:1147, 1977

110. Cohen A, Ullman B, Martin DW Jr: Characterization of a mutant mouse lymphoma cell with deficient transport of purine and pyrimidine nucleosides. *J Biol Chem* 254:112, 1979

111. Palella TD, Andres CM, Fox IH: Human placental adenosine kinase: Kinetic mechanism and inhibition. *J Biol Chem* 255:5264, 1980

112. Meyskens FL, Williams HE: Adenosine metabolism in human erythrocytes. *Biochim Biophys Acta* 240:170, 1971

113. Hershfield MS, Kredich NM: Resistance of an adenosine kinase–deficient human lymphoblastoid cell line to effects of deoxyadenosine on growth, S-adenosylhomocysteine hydrolase inactivation, and dATP accumulation. *Proc Natl Acad Sci USA* 77:4292, 1980

114. Osborne WRA, Spencer N: Partial purification and properties of the common inherited forms of adenosine deaminase from human erythrocytes. *Biochem J* 133:117, 1973

115. Agarwal RP, Sagar SM, Parks RE Jr: Adenosine deaminase from human erythrocytes: Purification and effects of adenosine analogs. *Biochem Pharmacol* 24:693, 1975

116. Henderson JF, Mikoshiba A, Chu SY, Caldwell IC: Kinetic studies of adenosine kinase from Ehrlich ascites tumor cells. *J Biol Chem* 247:1972, 1972

117. Divekar AY: Adenosine phosphorylase activity as distinct from inosine-guanosine phosphorylase activity in sarcoma 180 cells and rat liver. *Biochim Biophys Acta* 422:15, 1976

118. Snyder FF, Lukey T: Purine ribonucleoside and deoxyribonucleoside metabolism in thymocytes. *Adv Exp Med Biol* 122B:259, 1980

119. Snyder FF, Henderson JF: Alternative pathways of deoxyadenosine and adenosine metabolism. *J Biol Chem* 248:5899, 1973

120. Fox IH, Kelley WN: The role of adenosine and 2'-deoxyadenosine in mammalian cells. *Ann Rev Biochem* 47:655, 1978

121. Henderson JF, Scott FW: Inhibition of animal and invertebrate cell growth by naturally occurring purine bases and ribonucleosides. *Pharmacol Ther* 8:539, 1980

122. Henderson JF, Scott FW, Lowe JK: Toxicity of naturally occurring purine deoxyribonucleosides. *Pharmacol Ther* 8:573, 1980

123. Uberti J, Lightbody JJ, Wolf JW, Anderson JA, Reid RH, Johnson RM: The effect of adenosine on mitogenesis of ADA-deficient lymphocytes. *Clin Immunol Immunopathol* 10:446, 1978

124. Ochs UH, Chen S-H, Ochs HD, Osborne WRA, Scott CR: Deoxyribonucleoside toxicity on adenosine deaminase and purine nucleoside phosphorylase positive and negative cultured lymphoblastoid cells, in Pollara B, Pickering RJ, Meuwissen HJ, Porter IH (eds): *Inborn Errors of Specific Immunity*. New York, Academic Press, 1979, p 191

125. AGARWAL RP, SPECTOR T, PARKS RE JR: Tight-binding inhibitors-IV. Inhibition of adenosine deaminases by various inhibitors. *Biochem Pharmacol* 26:359, 1977

126. DEBATISSE M, BUTTIN G: The control of cell proliferation by performed purines: A genetic study. II. Pleiotropic manifestations and mechanisms of a control exerted by adenylic purines on PRPP synthesis. *Somatic Cell Genet* 3:513, 1977

127. AGARWAL RP, PARKS RE JR: Potent inhibition of muscle 5'-AMP deaminase by the nucleoside antibiotics coformycin and deoxycoformycin. *Biochem Pharmacol* 26:663, 1977

128. HENDERSON JF, BROX L, ZOMBOR G, HUNTING D, LOMAX CA: Specificity of adenosine deaminase inhibitors. *Biochem Pharmacol* 26:1967, 1977

129. SATTIN A, RALL TW: The effect of adenosine and adenine nucleotides on the cyclic adenosine 3',5'-phosphate content of guinea pig cerebral cortex slices. *Mol Pharmacol* 6:13, 1970

130. MALBON CC, HERT RC, FAIN JN: Characterization of [³H]adenosine binding to fat cell membranes. *J Biol Chem* 253:3114, 1978

131. MARONE G, PLAUT M, LICHTENSTEIN LM: Characterization of a specific adenosine receptor on human lymphocytes. *J Immunol* 11:2153, 1978

132. SCHWARTZ AL, STERN RC, POLMAR SH: Demonstration of an adenosine receptor on human lymphocytes in vitro and its possible role in the adenosine deaminase-deficient form of severe combined immunodeficiency. *Clin Immunol Immunopathol* 9:499, 1978

133. WOLBERG G, ZIMMERMAN TP, HIEMSTRA K, WINSTON M, CHU LC: Adenosine inhibition of lymphocyte-mediated cytolysis: Possible role of cyclic adenosine monophosphate. *Science* 187:957, 1975

134. ZENSER TV: Formation of adenosine 3',5'-monophosphate from adenosine in mouse thymocytes. *Biochim Biophys Acta* 404:202, 1975

135. SCHMALSTIEG FC, NELSON JA, MILLS GC, MONAHAN TM, GOLDMAN AS, GOLDBLUM RM: Increased purine nucleotides in adenosine deaminase-deficient lymphocytes. *J Pediatr* 91:48, 1977

136. HIRSCHHORN RJ, GROSSMAN J, WEISSMANN G: Effect of cyclic 3',5'-adenosine monophosphate and theophylline on lymphocyte transformation. *Proc Soc Exp Biol Med* 133:1361, 1970

137. KAUKEL E, FURHMANN U, HILZ H: Divergent action of cAMP and dibutyryl cAMP on macromolecular synthesis in Hela S3 cultures. *Biochem Biophys Res Commun* 48:1516, 1972

138. HILZ H, KAUKEL E: Divergent action mechanism of cAMP and dibutyryl cAMP on cell proliferation and macromolecular synthesis in HeLA S3 cultures. *Mol Cell Biochem* 1:229, 1973

139. SNYDER FF, SEEGMILLER JE: The adenosine-like effect of exogenous cyclic AMP upon nucleotide and PP-ribose-P concentrations of cultured human lymphoblasts. *FEBS Lett* 66:102, 1976

140. SMITH JW, STEINER AI, PARKER CW: Human lymphocyte metabolism. Effects of cyclic and noncyclic nucleotides on stimulation by phytohemagglutinin. *J Clin Invest* 50:442, 1971

141. SNYDER FF, HERSHFIELD MS, SEEGMILLER JE: Cytotoxic and metabolic effects of adenosine and adenine on human lymphoblasts. *Cancer Res* 38:2357, 1978

142. ULLMAN B, COHEN A, MARTIN DW JR: Characterization of a cell culture model for the study of adenosine deaminase and purine nucleoside phosphorylase-deficient immunologic disease. *Cell* 9:205, 1976

143. ISHII K, GREEN H: Lethality of adenosine for cultured mammalian cells by interference with pyrimidine biosynthesis. *J Cell Sci* 13:429, 1973

144. GREEN H, CHAN T-S: Pyrimidine starvation induced by adenosine in fibroblasts and lymphoid cells: Role of adenosine deaminase. *Science* 182:836, 1973

145. MCBURNEY MW, WHITMORE GF: Mutants of Chinese hamster cells resistant to adenosine. *J Cell Physiol* 85:87, 1975

146. GUDAS LJ, COHEN A, ULLMAN B, MARTIN DW JR: Analysis of adenosine-mediated pyrimidine starvation using cultured wild-type and mutant mouse T-lymphoma cells. *Somatic Cell Genet* 4:201, 1978

147. HARRAP KR, PAINE RM: Adenosine metabolism in cultured lymphoid cells. *Adv Enzyme Regul* 15:169, 1977

148. DEBATISSE M, BUTTIN G: The control of cell proliferation by performed purines: A genetic study. I. Isolation and preliminary characterization of Chinese hamster lines with single or multiple defects in purine "salvage pathways." *Somatic Cell Genet* 3:497, 1977

149. FOX IH, BURK L, PLANET A, GOREN M, KAMINSKA J: Pyrimidine nucleotide biosynthesis; A study of normal and purine enzyme-deficient cells. *J Biol Chem* 253:6794, 1978

150. BAGNARA AS, LETTER AA, HENDERSON JF: Multiple mechanisms of regulation of purine biosynthesis de novo in intact tumor cells. *Biochim Biophys Acta* 374:259, 1974

151. PLANET G, FOX IH: Inhibition of phosphoribosylpyrophosphate synthesis by purine nucleosides in human erythrocytes. *J Biol Chem* 251:5839, 1976

152. CARSON DA, SEEGMILLER JE: Effect of adenosine deaminase inhibition upon human lymphocyte blastogenesis. *J Clin Invest* 57:274, 1976

153. HERSHFIELD MS, SNYDER FF, SEEGMILLER JE: Adenine and adenosine are toxic to human lymphoblast mutants defective in purine salvage enzymes. *Science* 197:1284, 1977

154. POLMAR SH, WETZLER EM, STERN RC, HIRSCHHORN R: Restoration of in vitro lymphocyte responses with exogenous ADA in a patient with severe combined immunodeficiency. *Lancet* 2:743, 1975

155. MILLS GC, SCHMALSTIEG FC, TRIMMER KB, GOLDMAN AS, GOLDBLUM RM: Purine metabolism in adenosine deaminase deficiency. *Proc Natl Acad Sci USA* 73:2867, 1976

156. MILLS GC, SCHMALSTIEG FC, NEWKIRK KE, GOLDBLUM RM: Cytosine and orotic acid in urine of immunodeficient children. *Clin Chem* 25:419, 1979

157. TATTERSALL MHN, GANESHAGURU K, HOFFBRAND AV: The effect of external deoxyribonucleosides on deoxyribonucleoside triphosphate concentrations in human lymphocytes. *Biochem Pharmacol* 24:1495, 1975

158. LAPI L, COHEN SS: Toxicities of adenosine and 2'-deoxyadenosine in L cells treated with inhibitors of adenosine deaminase. *Biochem Pharmacol* 26:71, 1977

159. LOWE JK, GOWANS B, BROX L: Deoxyadenosine metabolism and toxicity in cultured L5178Y cells. *Cancer Res* 37:3013, 1977

160. COHEN A, HIRSCHHORN R, HOROWITZ SD, RUBINSTEIN A, POLMAR SH, HONG R, MARTIN DW: Deoxyadenosine triphosphate as a potentially toxic metabolite in adenosine deaminase deficiency. *Proc Natl Acad Sci USA* 75:472, 1978

161. COLEMAN MS, DONOFRIO J, HUTTON JJ, HAHN L, DAOUD A, LAMPKIN B, DYMINSKI J: Identification and quantitation of adenine deoxynucleotides in erythrocytes of a patient with adenosine deaminase deficiency and severe combined immunodeficiency. *J Biol Chem* 253:1619, 1978

162. SIMMONDS HA, PANAYI GS, CORRIGALL V: A role for purine metabolism in the immune response: Adenosine-deaminase activity and deoxyadenosine catabolism. *Lancet* 1:60, 1978

163. SIMMONDS HA, WATSON JG, HUGH-JONES K, PERRETT D, SAHOTA A, POTTER CF: Deoxynucleoside excretion in adenosine deaminase deficiency and purine nucleoside phosphorylase deficiency, in Pollara B, Pickering RJ, Meuwissen HJ, Porter IH (eds): *Inborn Errors of Specific Immunity*. New York, Academic Press, 1979, p 377

164. HERSHFIELD MS, KREDICH NM: S-Adenosylhomocysteine hydrolase is an adenosine-binding protein: A target for adenosine toxicity. *Science* 202:757, 1978

165. ULLMAN B, GUDAS LJ, COHEN A, MARTIN DW JR: Deoxyadenosine metabolism and cytotoxicity in cultured mouse T lymphoma cells: A model for immunodeficiency disease. *Cell* 14:365, 1978

166. ULLMAN B, LEVINSON BB, HERSHFIELD MS, MARTIN DW JR: A biochemical genetic study of the role of specific nucleoside kinases in deoxyadenosine phosphorylation by cultured human cells. *J Biol Chem* 256:848, 1981

167. MITCHELL BS, MEJIAS E, DADDONA PE, KELLEY WN: Purinogenic immunodeficiency diseases: Selective toxicity of deoxyribonucleosides for T cells. *Proc Natl Acad Sci USA* 75:5011, 1978

168. HORIBATA K, HARRIS AW: Mouse myelomas and lymphomas in culture. *Exp Cell Res* 60:61, 1970

169. REYNOLDS EC, HARRIS AW, FINCH LR: Deoxyribonucleoside triphosphate pools and differential thymidine sensitivities of cultured mouse lymphoma and myeloma cells. *Biochim Biophys Acta* 561:110, 1979

170. CARSON DA, KAYE J, SEEGMILLER JE: Differential sensitivity of human leukemic T cell lines and B cell lines to growth inhibition by deoxyadenosine. *J Immunol* 121:1726, 1978

171. GELFAND EW, LEE JJ, DOSCH HM: Selective toxicity of purine deoxynucleosides for human lymphocyte growth and function. *Proc Natl Acad Sci USA* 76:1998, 1979

172. CARSON DA, KAYE J, MATSUMOTO S, SEEGMILLER JE, THOMPSON L: Biochemical basis for the enhanced toxicity of deoxyribonucleosides toward malignant human T cell lines. *Proc Natl Acad Sci USA* 76:2430, 1979

173. MILLER RL, ADAMCZYK DL, MILLER WH: Adenosine kinase from rabbit liver: Purification by affinity chromatography and properties. *J Biol Chem* 254:2339, 1979

174. MILLER RL, ADAMCZYK DL, MILLER WH, KOSZALKA GW, RIDEOUT JL, BEACHMAN LM, CHAO EY, HAGGERTY JJ, KRENITSKY TA, ELION GB: Adenosine kinase from rabbit liver: II. Substrate and inhibitor specificity. *J Biol Chem* 254:2346, 1979

175. ANDRES CM, FOX IH: Purification and properties of human placental adenosine kinase. *J Biol Chem* 254:11388, 1979

176. MOMPARLER RL, FISCHER GA: Mammalian deoxynucleoside kinases I. Deoxycytidine kinase: Purification, properties and kinetic studies with cytosine arabinoside. *J Biol Chem* 243:2498, 1968

177. IVES DH, DURHAM JP: Deoxycytidine kinase: Kinetics and allosteric regulation of the calf thymus enzyme. *J Biol Chem* 245:2285, 1970

178. KRENITSKY TA, TUTTLE JV, KOSZALKA GW, CHEN IS, BEACHMAN LM, RIDEOUT JL, ELION GB: Deoxycytidine kinase from calf thymus: Substrate and inhibitor specificity. *J Biol Chem* 251:4055, 1976

179. GOWER WR, CARR MC, IVES DH: Deoxyguanosine kinase: Distinct molecular forms in mitochondria and cytosol. *J Biol Chem* 254:2180, 1979

180. KRYGIER V, MOMPARLER RL: Mammalian deoxynucleoside kinases II.

Deoxyadenosine Kinase: Purification and properties. *J Biol Chem* 246:2745, 1971

181. KRYGIER V, MOMPARLER RL: Mammalian deoxynucleoside kinases. III Deoxyadenosine kinase: Inhibition by nucleotides and kinetic studies. *J Biol Chem* 246:2752, 1971

182. DURHAM JP, IVES DH: Deoxycytidine kinase I. Distribution in normal and neoplastic tissues and interrelationships of deoxycytidine and 1β-D-arabinofuranosylcytidine phosphorylation. *Mol Pharmacol* 5:358, 1969

183. CARSON DA, KAYE J, SEEGMILLER JE: Lymphospecific toxicity in adenosine deaminase deficiency and purine nucleoside phosphorylase deficiency: Possible role of nucleoside kinase(s). *Proc Natl Acad Sci USA* 74:5677, 1977

184. CARSON DA, KAYE J, WASSON DB: Differences in deoxyadenosine metabolism in human and mouse lymphocytes. *J Immunol* 124:8, 1980

185. WILLIS RC, CARSON DA, SEEGMILLER JE: Adenosine kinase initiates the major route of ribavirin activation in a cultured human cell line. *Proc Natl Acad Sci USA* 75:3042, 1978

186. HERSHFIELD MS, KREDICH NM: Effects of adenosine deaminase inhibition on transmethylation, in Tattersall MNH, Fox RM (eds): *Nucleosides in Cancer Treatment.* New York, Academic Press, 1981, p 161

187. HERSHFIELD MS, FETTER JE, SMALL WC, BAGNAR AS, WILLIAMS SR, ULLMAN B, MARTIN DW JR, WASSON DB, CARSON DA: Effects of mutational loss of adenosine kinase and deoxycytidine kinase on deoxyATP accumulation and deoxyadenosine toxicity in cultured CEM human T-lymphoblastoid cells. *J Biol Chem*, in press, 1982

188. WORTMANN RL, MITCHELL BS, EDWARDS NL, FOX IH: Biochemical basis for differential deoxyadenosine toxicity to T and B lymphoblasts: Role for 5'-nucleotidase. *Proc Natl Acad Sci USA* 76:2434, 1979

189. FOX RM, TRIPP EH, PIDDINGTON SK, TATTERSALL MHN: Sensitivity of leukemic human null lymphocytes to deoxynucleosides. *Cancer Res* 40:3383, 1980

190. THOMPSON LF, SEEGMILLER JE: Adenosine deaminase deficiency and severe combined immunodeficiency disease. *Adv Enzymol* 51:167, 1980

191. FOX RM, PIDDINGTON SK, TRIPP EH, TATTERSALL MHN: Ecto-ATPase deficiency in cultured human T and null leukemic lymphocytes: A biochemical basis for thymidine sensitivity. *J Clin Invest* 68:544, 1981

192. CARSON DA, KAYE J, WASSON DB: The potential importance of soluble deoxynucleotidase activity in mediating deoxyadenosine toxicity in human lymphoblasts. *J Immunol* 126:348, 1981

193. NORDENSKJÖLD BA, SKOOG L, BROWN NC, REICHARD P: Deoxyribonucleotide pools and deoxyribonucleic acid synthesis in cultured mouse embryo cells. *J Biol Chem* 245:5360, 1970

194. REICHARD P: Control of deoxyribonucleotide synthesis *in vitro* and *in vivo. Adv Enzyme Regul* 10:3, 1972

195. WALTERS RA, TOBEY RA, RATLIFF RL: Cell-cycle dependent variations of deoxyribonucleoside triphosphate pools in Chinese hamster cells. *Biochim Biophys Acta* 319:336, 1973

196. THELANDER L, REICHARD P: Reduction of ribonucleosides. *Ann Rev Biochem* 48:133, 1979

197. CHANG C-H, CHEN Y-C: Effects of nucleoside triphosphates on human ribonucleotide reductase from molt-4F cells. *Cancer Res* 39:5087, 1979

198. KLENOW H: On the effect of some adenine derivatives on the incorporation *in vitro* of isotopically labelled compounds into the nucleic acids of Ehrlich ascites tumor cells. *Biochim Biophys Acta* 35:412, 1959

199. MUNCH-PETERSEN A: Formation *in vitro* of deoxyadenosine triphosphate from deoxyadenosine in Ehrlich ascites cells. *Biochim Biophys Res Comm* 3:392, 1960

200. KLENOW H: Further studies on the effect of deoxyadenosine on the accumulation of deoxyadenosine triphosphate and inhibition of deoxyribonucleic acid synthesis in Ehrlich ascites tumor cells *in vitro. Biochim Biophys Acta* 61:885, 1962

201. MOORE EC, HURLBERT RB: Regulation of mammalian deoxyribonucleotide biosynthesis by nucleotides as activators and inhibitors. *J Biol Chem* 241:4802, 1966

202. MORRIS NR, FISCHER GA: Studies concerning the inhibition of cellular reproduction by deoxyribonucleosides I. Inhibition of the synthesis of deoxycytidine by a phosphorylated derivative of thymidine. *Biochim Biophys Acta* 68:84, 1963

203. BJURSELL G, RIECHARD P: Effects of thymidine on deoxyribonucleoside triphosphate pools and deoxyribonucleic acid synthesis in Chinese hamster ovary cells. *J Biol Chem* 248:3904, 1973

204. SCHACHTSCHABEL DO, CUNZE P: Inhibition of cell division and induction of chromosome aberrations in cultured Ehrlich ascites tumor cells by deoxyguanosine. *Humangenetik* 10:127, 1971

205. THEISS JC, MORRIS NR, FISCHER GA: Pyrimidine nucleotide metabolism in L5178Y murine leukemia cells: Deoxycytidine protection from deoxyguanosine toxicity. *Cancer Biochem Biophys* 1:211, 1976

206. MEUTH M, GREEN H: Alterations leading to increased ribonucleotide reductase in cells selected for resistance to deoxynucleosides. *Cell* 3:367, 1974

207. MEUTH A, AUFREITER E, REICHARD P: Deoxyribonucleotide pools in

mouse-fibroblast cell lines with altered ribonucleotide reductase. *Eur J Biochem* 71:39, 1976

208. CHAN T-S: Deoxyguanosine toxicity on lymphoid cells as a cause for immunosuppression in purine nucleoside phosphorylase deficiency. *Cell* 14:523, 1978

209. WILSON JM, MITCHELL BS, DADDONA PE, KELLEY WN: Purinogenic immuno-deficiency diseases: Differential effects of deoxyadenosine and deoxyguanosine on DNA synthesis in human T lymphoblasts. *J Clin Invest* 64:1475, 1979

210. ULLMAN B, CLIFT SM, GUDAS LJ, LEVINSON BB, WORMSTED MA, MARTIN DE JR: Alterations in deoxyribonucleotide metabolism in cultured cells with ribonucleotide reductase activities refractory to feedback inhibition by 2'-deoxyadenosine triphosphate. *J Biol Chem* 255:8308, 1980

211. ULLMAN B, GUDAS LJ, CLIFT SM, MARTIN DW JR: Isolation and characterization of purine-nucleoside phosphorylase-deficient T-lymphoma cells and secondary mutants with altered ribonucleotide reductase: Genetic model for immunodeficiency disease. *Proc Natl Acad Sci USA* 76:1074, 1979

212. FOX RM, TRIPP EH, TATTERSALL MHN: Mechanism of deoxycytidine rescue of thymidine toxicity in human T-leukemic lymphocytes. *Cancer Res* 40:1718, 1980

213. MUNCH-PETERSEN B, TYRSTED G, DUPONT B: The deoxyribonucleoside 5'-triphosphate (dATP and dTTP) pools in phytohemagglutinin-stimulated and non-stimulated human lymphocytes. *Exp Cell Res* 79:249, 1973

214. TYRSTED G, GAMULIN V: Cytidine 5'-diphosphate reductase activity in phytohemagglutinin stimulated human lymphocytes. *Nucleic Acids Res* 6:305, 1979

215. UBERTI J, LIGHTBODY JJ, JOHNSON RM: The effect of nucleosides and deoxycoformycin on adenosine and deoxyadenosine inhibition of human lymphocyte activation. *J Immunol* 123:189, 1979

216. BOLLUM FJ: Terminal deoxynucleotidyl transferase: Biological studies. *Adv Enzymol* 47:347, 1978

217. CHANG LMS: Development of terminal deoxynucleotidyl transferase activity in embryonic calf thymus gland. *Biochem Biophys Res Commun* 44:124, 1971

218. KUNG PC, SILVERSTONE AE, MCCAFFREY RP, BALTIMORE D: Murine terminal deoxynucleotidyl transferase: Cellular distribution and response to cortisone. *J Exp Med* 141:855, 1975

219. GREGOIRE KE, GOLDSCHNEIDER I, BARTON RW, BOLLUM FJ: Intracellular distribution of terminal deoxynucleotidyl transferase in rat bone marrow and thymus. *Proc Natl Acad Sci USA* 74:3993, 1977

220. BALTIMORE D: Is terminal deoxynucleotidyl transferase a somatic mutagen in lymphocytes? *Nature* 248:409, 1974

221. BOLLUM FJ: Terminal deoxynucleotidyl transferase: Source of immunological diversity? in Zahn R (ed): *Karl-August-Forster Lectures.* Wiesbaden, W. Germany, Franz Steiner Verlag Gmbh, 1975, vol 14, p 1

222. MODAK MJ: Biochemistry of terminal deoxynucleotidyl transferase. Mechanism of manganese-dependent inhibition by deoxyadenosine 5'-triphosphate and biological implications. *Biochemistry* 12:2679, 1979

223. SALVATORE F, BOREK E, ZAPPIA V, WILLIAMS-ASHMAN HG, SCHLENK F: *The Biochemistry of S-Adenosylmethionine.* New York, Columbia University Press, 1977

224. O'DEA RF, VIVEROS OH, AXELROD J, ASWANIKUMAR S, SCHIFFMAN E, CORCORAN BA: Rapid stimulation of protein carboxymethylation in leukocytes by a chemotactic peptide. *Nature* 272:462, 1978

225. PIKE MC, KREDICH NM, SNYDERMAN R: Requirement of S-adenosyl-L-methionine-mediated methylation for human monocyte chemotaxis. *Proc Natl Acad Sci USA* 75:3928, 1978

226. HIRATA F, TOYOSHIMA S, AXELROD J, WAXDAL MJ: Phospholipid methylation: A biochemical signal modulating lymphocyte mitogenesis. *Proc Natl Acad Sci USA* 77:862, 1980

227. DILIBERTO EJ JR, VIVEROS OH, AXELROD J: Subcellular distribution of protein carboxymethylase and its endogenous substrates in the adrenal medulla: Possible role in excitation-secretion coupling. *Proc Natl Acad Sci USA* 73:4050, 1976

228. ISHIZAKA T, HIRATA F, ISHIZAKA K, AXELROD J: Stimulation of phospholipid methylation, Ca²⁺ influx, and histamine release by bridging of IgE receptors on mast cells. *Proc Natl Acad Sci USA* 77:1903, 1980

229. STRITTMATTER WJ, HIRATA F, AXELROD J: Phospholipid methylation unmasks cryptic β-adrenergic receptors in rat reticulocytes. *Science* 204:1205, 1979

230. HIRATA F, STRITTMATTER WJ, AXELROD J: β-Adrenergic receptor agonists increase phospholipid methylation, membrane fluidity, and β-adrenergic-adenylate cyclase coupling. *Proc Natl Acad Sci USA* 76:368, 1979

231. HIRATA F, AXELROD J: Enzymatic synthesis and rapid translocation of phosphatidylcholine by two methyltransferases in erythrocyte membranes. *Proc Natl Acad Sci USA* 75:2348, 1978

232. HIRATA F, AXELROD J: Enzymatic methylation of phosphatidylethanolamine increases erythrocyte membrane fluidity. *Nature* 275:219, 1978

233. HOLLIDAY R, PUGH JE: DNA modification mechanisms and gene activity during development. *Science* 187:226, 1975

234. RAZIN A, RIGGS AD: DNA methylation and gene function. *Science* 210:604, 1980

235. JONES PA, TAYLOR SM: Cellular differentiation, cytidine analogs and DNA methylation. *Cell* 20:85, 1980

236. DE LA HABA G, CANTONI GL: The enzymatic synthesis of S-adenosyl-L-homocysteine from adenosine and homocysteine. *J Biol Chem* 234:603, 1959

237. BORCHARDT RT: Synthesis and biological activity of analogues of adenosylhomocysteine as inhibitors of methyltransferases, in Salvatore F, Borek E, Zappia V, Williams-Ashman HG, Schlenk F (eds): *The Biochemistry of Adenosylmethionine*. New York, Columbia University Press, 1977, p 151

238. KREDICH NM, MARTIN DW JR: Role of S-adenosylhomocysteine in adenosine-mediated toxicity in cultured mouse T-lymphoma cells. *Cell* 12:931, 1977

239. KREDICH NM, HERSHFIELD MS: S-Adenosylhomocysteine toxicity in normal and adenosine kinase-deficient lymphoblasts of human origin. *Proc Natl Acad Sci USA* 76:2450, 1979

240. JOHNSTON JM, KREDICH NM: Inhibition of methylation by adenosine in adenosine deaminase-inhibited, phytohemagglutinin-stimulated human lymphocytes. *J Immunol* 123:97, 1979

241. SAEBO J, UELAND PM: An adenosine 3':5'-monophosphate adenosine-binding protein from mouse liver. Association with S-adenosylhomocysteinase activity. *FEBS Lett* 96:125, 1978

242. HERSHFIELD MS: Apparent suicide inactivation of human lymphoblast S-adenosylhomocysteine hydrolase by 2'-deoxyadenosine and adenine arabinoside. A basis for direct toxic effects of analogs of adenosine. *J Biol Chem* 254:22, 1979

243. HERSHFIELD MS: Alternate reactions of S-adenosylhomocysteine hydrolase. *Fed Proc* 39:1858, 1980

244. ABELES RH, TASHJIAN AH, FISH S: The mechanism of inactivation of S-adenosylhomocysteinase by 2'-deoxyadenosine. *Biochem Biophys Res Commun* 95:612, 1980

245. HERSHFIELD MS, KREDICH NM, OWNBY DR, OWNBY H, BUCKLEY R: In vivo inactivation of erythrocyte S-adenosylhomocysteine hydrolase by 2'-deoxyadenosine in adenosine deaminase-deficient patients. *J Clin Invest* 63:807, 1979

246. MITCHELL BS, KOLLER CA, HEYN R: Inhibition of adenosine deaminase results in cytotoxicity to T lymphoblasts in vivo. *Blood* 56:556, 1980

247. SMYTH JF, PAINE RM, JACKMAN AL, HARRAP KR, CHASSIN MM, ADAMSON RH, JOHNS DG: The clinical pharmacology of the adenosine deaminase inhibitor 2'-deoxycoformycin. *Cancer Chemother Pharmacol* 5:93, 1980

248. PRENTICE HG, GANESHAGURU K, BRADSTOCK KF, GOLDSTONE AH, SMYTH JF, WONKE B, JANOSSY G, HOFFBRAND AV: Remission induction with the adenosine deaminase inhibitor 2'-deoxycoformycin in thy-lymphoblastic leukemia. *Lancet* 2:170, 1980

249. SIAW MFE, MITCHELL BS, KOLLER CA, COLEMAN MS, HUTTON JJ: ATP depletion as a consequence of adenosine deaminase inhibition in man. *Proc Natl Acad Sci USA* 77:6157, 1980

250. GREVER MR, SIAW MFE, JACOB WF, NEIDHART JA, MISER JS, COLEMAN MS, HUTTON JJ, BALCERZAK SP: The biochemical and clinical consequences of 2'-deoxycoformycin in refractory lymphoproliferative malignancy. *Blood* 57:406, 1981

251. HERSHFIELD M, KREDICH N, FALLETTA J, KINNEY T, MITCHELL B, KOLLER C: An in vivo model of adenosine deaminase (ADA) deficiency. *Clin Res* 29:513, 1981

252. KOLLER CA, MITCHELL BS, GREVER MR, MEJIAS E, MALSPEIS L, METZ EN: Treatment of acute lymphoblastic leukemia with 2'-deoxycoformycin: Clinical and biochemical consequences of adenosine deaminase inhibition. *Cancer Treat Rep* 63:1949, 1979

253. OCHS UH, CHEN S-H, OCHS HD, OSBORNE WRA, SCOTT CR: Purine nucleoside phosphorylase deficiency: A molecular model for selective loss of T cell function. *J Immunol* 122:2424, 1979

254. GUDAS LJ, ULLMAN B, COHEN A, MARTIN DW JR: Deoxyguanosine toxicity in a mouse T lymphoma: Relationship to purine nucleoside phosphorylase-associated immune dysfunction. *Cell* 14:531, 1978

255. COHEN A, GUDAS LJ, AMMANN AJ, STAAL GEJ, MARTIN DW JR: Deoxyguanosine triphosphate as a possible toxic metabolite in the immunodeficiency associated with purine nucleoside phosphorylase deficiency. *J Clin Invest* 61:1405, 1978

256. EDWARDS NL, GELFAND EW, BIGGAR D, FOX IH: Partial deficiency of purine nucleoside phosphorylase: Studies of purine and pyrimidine metabolism. *J Lab Clin Med* 91:736, 1978

257. KAMINSKA JE, FOX IH: Decreased S-adenosylhomocysteine hydrolase in inborn errors of purine metabolism. *J Lab Clin Med* 96:141, 1980

258. HERSHFIELD MS: Proposed explanation for S-adenosylhomocysteine hydrolase deficiency in purine nucleoside phosphorylase and hypoxanthine guanine phosphoribosyltransferase-deficient patients. *J Clin Invest* 67:696, 1981

259. SIMMONDS HA, SAHOTA A, POTTER CF, CAMERON JS, WADMAN SK: Purine metabolism and immunodeficiency: Urinary purine excretion as a diagnostic screening test in adenosine deaminase and purine nucleoside phosphorylase deficiency. *Clin Sci Mol Med* 54:579, 1978

260. COOPER HL: Ribosomal nucleic acid production and growth regulation in human lymphocytes. *J Biol Chem* 244:1946, 1969

261. VAUGHAN MH JR, SOEIRO R, WARNER JR, DARNELL JE JR: The effects of methionine deprivation on ribosome synthesis in HeLa cells. *Proc Natl Acad Sci USA* 58:1527, 1967

262. WOLF SF, SCHLESSINGER D: Nuclear metabolism of ribosomal RNA in growing, methionine-limited, and ethionine-treated HeLa cells. *Biochemistry* 16:2783, 1977

263. BYNUM JW, VOLKIN E: Wasting of 18S ribosomal RNA by human myeloma cells cultured in adenosine. *J Cell Physiol* 88:197, 1976

264. ADAMS A, HARKNESS RA: Adenosine deaminase activity in thymus and other human tissues. *Clin Exp Immunol* 26:647, 1976

265. HITZIG WH, DOHMANN U, PLUSS HJ, VISCHER D: Hereditary transcobalamin II deficiency: Clinical findings in a new family. *J Pediatr* 85:622, 1974

266. O'REILLY RJ, PAHWA R, DUPONT B, GOOD RA: Severe combined immunodeficiency: Transplantation approaches for patients lacking an HLA genotypically identical sibling. *Transplant Proc* 10:187, 1978

267. KENNY AB, HITZIG WH: Bone marrow transplantation for severe combined immunodeficiency disease. *Eur J Pediatr* 131:155, 1979

268. PARKMAN R, GELFAND EW, ROSEN FS, SANDERSON A, HIRSCHHORN R: Severe combined immunodeficiency and adenosine deaminase deficiency. *N Engl J Med* 292:714, 1975

269. CHEN SH, OCHS HD, SCOTT CR, GIBLETT ER, TINGLE AJ: Adenosine deaminase deficiency: Disappearance of adenine deoxynucleotides from a patient's erythrocytes after successful marrow transplantation. *J Clin Invest* 62:1386, 1978

270. KEIGHTLEY RG, LAWTON AR, COOPER MD, YUNIS EJ: Successful fetal liver transplantation in a child with severe combined immunodeficiency. *Lancet* 2:850, 1975

271. HONG R, SCHULTE-WISSERMANN H, HOROWITZ S, BORZY M, FINLAY J: Cultured thymic epithelium in severe combined immunodeficiency. *Transplant Proc* 10:201, 1978

272. RICH KC, RICHMAN CM, MEJIAS E, DADDONA P: Immunoreconstitution by peripheral blood leukocytes in adenosine deaminase-deficient severe combined immunodeficiency. *J Clin Invest* 66:389, 1980

273. DYMINSKI JW, DAOUD A, LAMPKIN BC, LIMOUZE S, DONOFRIO J, COLEMAN MS, HUTTON JJ: Immunological and biochemical profiles in response to transfusion therapy in an adenosine deaminase-deficient patient with severe combined immunodeficiency disease. *Clin Immunol Immunopathol* 14:307, 1979

274. RUBINSTEIN A, HIRSCHHORN R, SICKLICK M, MURPHY RA: In vivo and in vitro effects of thymosin and adenosine deaminase on adenosine-deaminase-deficient lymphocytes. *N Engl J Med* 300:387, 1979

275. SCHMALSTIEG FC, MILLS GC, NELSON JA, MAY LT, GOLDMAN AS, GOLDBLUM RM: Limited effect of erythrocyte and plasma infusions in adenosine deaminase deficiency. *J Pediatr* 93:597, 1978

276. TSUCHIYA S, ARAI N, KUDO M, KONNO T, TADA K, YOKOYAMA S: Effect of adenosine deaminase replacement therapy on a child with adenosine deaminase deficiency with severe combined immunodeficiency disease. *Tohoku J Exp Med* 128:251, 1979

277. POLMAR SH: Enzyme replacement and other biochemical approaches to the therapy of adenosine deaminase deficiency, in Elliot K, Whelan J (eds): *Enzyme Defects and Immune Dysfunction, Ciba Foundation Symposium 68*. New York, Exerpta Medica, 1979, p 213

278. HUTTON JJ, WIGINTON DA, COLEMAN MS, FULLER SA, LIMOUZE S, LAMPKIN BC: Biochemical and functional abnormalities in lymphocytes from an adenosine deaminase-deficient patient during enzyme replacement therapy. *J Clin Invest* 68:413, 1981

279. SANDMAN R, AMMANN AJ, GROSE C, WARA DW: Cellular immunodeficiency associated with nucleoside phosphorylase deficiency. *Clin Immunol Immunopathol* 8:247, 1977

280. GELFAND EW, DOSCH H-M, BIGGAR WD, FOX IH: Partial purine nucleoside phosphorylase deficiency: Studies of lymphocyte function. *J Clin Invest* 61:1071, 1978

281. ZEGERS BJM, STOOP JW, STAAL GEJ, WADMAN SK: An approach to the restoration of T cell function in a purine nucleoside phosphorylase deficient patient, in Elliot K, Whelan J (eds): *Enzyme Defects and Immune Dysfunction, Ciba Foundation Symposium 68*. New York, Exerpta Medica, 1979, p 231

282. RICH KC, MEJIAS E, FOX IH: Purine nucleoside phosphorylase deficiency: Improved metabolic and immunologic function with erythrocyte transfusions. *N Engl J Med* 303:973, 1980

283. AMMAN AJ, WARA DW, ALLEN T: Immunotherapy and immunopathologic studies in a patient with nucleoside phosphorylase deficiency. *Clin Immunol Immunopathol* 10:262, 1978

284. HIRSCHHORN R, ROEGNER V, RUBINSTEIN A, PAPAGEORGIOU P: Plasma deoxyadenosine, adenosine, and erythrocyte deoxyATP are elevated at birth in an adenosine deaminase-deficient child. *J Clin Invest* 65:768, 1980

285. Siegenbeek Van Heukelom LH, Akermann JWN, Staal JEJ, De Bruyn CHMM, Stoop JW, Zegers BJM, De Bree PK, Wadman SK: A patient with purine nucleoside phosphorylase deficiency: Enzymological and metabolic aspects. *Clin Chim Acta* 74:271, 1977
286. Donofrio J, Coleman MS, Hutton JJ, Daoud A, Lampkin B, Dyminski J: Overproduction of adenine deoxynucleosides and deoxynucleotides in adenosine deaminase deficiency with severe combined immunodeficiency disease. *J Clin Invest* 62:884, 1978
287. Hirschhorn R, Papageorgiou P, Rubinstein A, Rosen FS: Transfusion vs. bone marrow transplantation in combined immunodeficiency. *Clin Res* 27:507A, 1979
288. Kuttesch JF, Schmalstieg FC, Nelson JA: Analysis of adenosine and other adenine compounds in patients with immunodeficiency diseases. *J Liquid Chromatogr* 1:97, 1978
289. Mills GC, Goldblum RM, Newkirk KE, Schmalstieg FC: Urinary excretion of purines, purine nucleosides, and pseudouridine in adenosine deaminase deficiency. *Biochem Med* 20:180, 1978
290. Kredich NM, Hershfield MS, Johnston JM: Role of methylation in adenosine toxicity in adenosine deaminase inhibited cells, in Pollara B, Pickering RJ, Meuwissen HJ, Porter IH (eds): *Inborn Errors of Specific Immunity*. New York, Academic Press, 1979, p 261
291. Hershfield MS, Kredich NM: Suicide-like inactivation of intracellular adenosylhomocysteine hydrolase by 2'-deoxyadenosine: A mechanism which may contribute to the immune dysfunction in adenosine deaminase deficiency, in Pollara B, Pickering RJ, Meuwissen HJ, Porter IH (eds): *Inborn Errors of Specific Immunity*. New York, Academic Press, 1979, p 269

54

MYOADENYLATE DEAMINASE DEFICIENCY

JUDITH L. SWAIN

RICHARD L. SABINA

EDWARD W. HOLMES

1. Muscle AMP deaminase (EC 3.5.4.6) deficiency *is a relatively benign disorder characterized clinically by muscle fatigue following exercise. It has been reported in 26 patients and has also been demonstrated in approximately 2 percent of 770 muscle biopsy specimens submitted for pathologic examination for a wide array of indications.*

2. *The enzyme deficiency appears to be inherited as an autosomal recessive trait with equal sex distribution.*

3. *Of the reported patients, 77 percent have had easy fatigability, cramps, or myalgias following exercise; 67 percent first experienced their postexercise-related symptoms in childhood or as a teenager. Patients exhibit muscle dysfunction only and AMP deaminase activity is normal in other tissues.*

4. *Exercise does not lead to NH_3 and IMP production in skeletal muscle as in normal subjects, and muscle ATP and total purine content fall with exercise to a greater extent than in controls. ATP concentration may remain depressed for hours.*

5. *The myopathy in patients with AMP deaminase deficiency indicates that this enzyme and the purine nucleotide cycle of which it is one component play an important role in skeletal muscle metabolism during exercise.*

The purine nucleotide cycle (Fig. 54-1), of which the AMP deaminase reaction is one component, is thought to play an important role in skeletal muscle function for several reasons. The activities of all three enzymes in the purine nucleotide cycle are severalfold greater in skeletal muscle than any other organ, and the activity of AMP deaminase is approximately 100 times greater than that of the other two enzymes [1–3]. During exercise NH_3 production and IMP content of skeletal muscle increase in proportion to the work performed by the muscle [1–7], indicating increased AMP deaminase activity under these conditions. Activation of myoadenylate deaminase and increased flux through the purine nucleotide cycle during exercise lead to an increase in energy production through the generation of intermediates for the citric acid cycle from amino acids and through stimulation of glycolysis [1–3, 5–7]. Thus, one might anticipate that a high-grade deficiency of myoadenylate deaminase activity and disruption of the purine nucleotide cycle could lead to skeletal muscle dysfunction.

In 1978 Fishbein et al. described five patients with a history of skeletal muscle dysfunction following mild to moderate exercise [8]. In these patients myoadenylate deaminase activity was virtually absent. Twenty-one additional patients with myoadenylate deaminase deficiency have been described; 67 percent of these patients have had postexercise-related muscle dysfunction, cramping, or myalgias [8–15]. Data from three

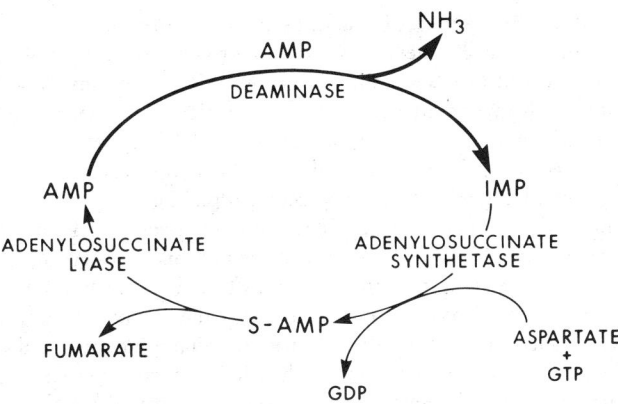

Figure 54-1 Purine nucleotide cycle.

different institutions suggest that this myopathy may be relatively common, since approximately 2 percent of 770 muscle biopsies submitted for pathologic evaluation have been found to be deficient in AMP deaminase activity [8, 10, 15].

CLINICAL FEATURES

The clinical features and laboratory abnormalities reported in the first 26 patients with myoadenylate deaminase deficiency are summarized in Table 54-1. Males account for 54 percent; 77 percent of patients developed fatigue, cramps, or myalgias following moderate to vigorous exercise. Weakness was found in only 27 percent of patients, and muscle wasting has not been reported. Myoglobinuria followed strenuous exercise in only 1 patient. The median age at the time of diagnosis of myoadenylate deaminase deficiency is 22 years, with a range of 1.5 to 70 years. Of patients noted, 39 percent had onset of symptoms in childhood and 28 percent as teenagers.

Increased serum creatine kinase activity has been found in 56 percent of patients. In a number of cases serum creatine kinase activity was normal at rest and only increased into the abnormal range following exercise. EMG may be normal, but minor abnormalities were described in 58 percent of patients undergoing this test. Results of muscle biopsy, examined by routine histochemical stains and electron microscopy, have varied from no pathologic findings to mild abnormalities in distribution of fiber type, with or without minimal changes in fiber size. Histochemical stain for AMP deaminase activity has been negative in all 25 patients tested, and myoadenylate deaminase activity has been virtually absent (0–6.2 percent of control) in all patients. No NH_3 is produced following ischemic forearm exercise in patients with myoadenylate deaminase deficiency, and this test has been used to screen patients for this enzyme deficiency. This test is not specific for myoadenylate deaminase deficiency, but it does appear to be a sensitive screening procedure since all 7 patients with this enzyme deficiency failed to produce NH_3 during ischemic forearm exercise, whereas lactate production was normal.

Illustrative Cases

Case 1 The patient studied by Di Mauro et al. [12], a 37-

Table 54-1

I. Clinical features of AMP deaminase deficiency

Sex: 14/26 male

Age at time of diagnosis
  Mean: 31 years
  Median: 22 years
  Range: 1.5 to 70 years

Age at time of onset of symptoms
  Infancy (<2 years): 1 out of 18 (6%)
  Childhood (2–12): 7 out of 18 (39%)
  Teenage (13–19): 5 out of 18 (28%)
  Young adult (20–40): 1 out of 18 (6%)
  Older adult (>40): 4 out of 18 (22%)

Postexercise symptoms
  Easy fatigue, cramps, myalgia: 20 out of 26 (77%)

Weakness without exercise
  7 out of 26 (27%)

Hypotonia
  2 out of 26 (8%)

Other clinical diagnoses
  1—Hypokalemic periodic paralysis—age 22
  1—Amyotrophic lateral sclerosis—age 68
  1—Kugelberg-Welander syndrome—age 56
  2—Influenza-like illness preceded onset of symptoms—ages 68 and 70

II. Laboratory abnormalities in patients with AMP deaminase deficiency

Elevated serum CPK
  10 out of 18 (56%)

Myopathic EMG
  5 out of 12 (42%)

Failure to produce NH_3 on ischemic testing
  7 out of 7 (100%)

Abnormal muscle biopsy
  10 out of 19 (53%)   AML and K.W.—denervation (2)
               Post-flu—necrosis, fiber degeneration (2)
               Mild abnormalities— ↓ type I (1)
               Mild abnormalities— ↑ type I (1)
               Mild abnormalities— ↑ type 2 (1)
               Mild abnormalities— ↓ type 2 (1)
               Mild abnormalities—Change in fiber size (2)

Negative histochemical stain for AMP deaminase
  25 out of 25 (100%)

AMP deaminase activity on direct assay
  0–6% of normal; no crossreactive antigen in 10 patients

year-old male, reported symptoms of cramping pain in the calves and aching in the hand, forearm, and shoulder muscles after moderately strenuous exercise since adolescence. After age 30, his symptoms increased in severity, forcing him to abandon jobs as a machinist, garbage collector, and laundry worker. Muscle bulk and strength were normal. There was no family history of consanguinity or neuromuscular disease. Serum creatine kinase activity varied from 513 to 1100 U/liter (normal <225), with the highest activity occurring on the morning after a day of intense physical activity. EMG was normal except for an increased number of polyphasic potentials (>12 percent). Following ischemic exercise there was a normal rise in plasma lactate, but no increase in plasma NH_3. AMP deaminase activity was not detectable in muscle by histochemical stain or by enzymatic assay. Routine light and electron microscopic examinations of the muscle biopsy were normal. This patient also had gouty arthritis. It is questionable whether there is a relationship between the two diseases, since none of the other myoadenylate deaminase–deficient patients are reported to have gout.

Case 2 Sabina et al. [14] described a 36-year-old female who noted easy fatigability and exercise-induced muscle aches since childhood. She first experienced significant impairment of her daily activities at age 21. Over the next 15 years there was gradual progression of symptoms to the point that activities such as dressing, walking from one room to another, and climbing one flight of stairs led to fatigue and myalgias. This patient found that a rest period of several hours was required following even mild activity before her strength returned to baseline. To complete simple house chores she alternated periods of activity with periods of rest. Physical examination revealed normal muscle mass and no weakness. Serum creatine kinase activity was normal at rest, and routine EMG studies were normal. Following ischemic forearm exercise plasma lactate concentration increased 2.5 times, while plasma NH_3 concentration did not increase. Routine microscopic examination of the muscle biopsy was normal except for the presence of scattered small, angular fibers. No AMP deaminase activity was detectable by histochemical stain, and AMP deaminase activity was less than 0.3 percent of controls on direct assay.

Comment

These two case reports illustrate the typical clinical findings in patients with myoadenylate deaminase deficiency. Not all patients with an absence of AMP deaminase activity on muscle biopsy fit this picture (Table 54-1). For example, two patients had clinical findings consistent with a primary neuronal disorder—amyotrophic lateral sclerosis and Kugelberg-Welander syndrome. The first patient reported with myoadenylate deaminase deficiency was diagnosed as having primary hypokalemic periodic paralysis. Two patients with myoadenylate deaminase deficiency first sought medical attention for muscle symptoms at approximately 70 years of age following an influenzalike illness. Another patient presented at 1.5 years of age with delayed motor and speech development, as well as prominent hypotonia. It is not clear what relationship, if any, the deficiency of myoadenylate deaminase activity bears to the neuromuscular disorders exhibited by these patients. As will be discussed in subsequent sections of this chapter, the postexercise symptoms experienced by the great majority (77 percent) of patients may be explained by the deficiency of myoadenylate deaminase and disruption of the purine nucleotide cycle. The deficiency of myoadenylate deaminase activity found in patients with the clinical diagnosis of other neuromuscular diseases may represent the coincidental finding of a relatively common enzyme deficiency in patients in whom muscle biopsy is performed as a routine part of their diagnostic evaluation.

The severity and age of onset of postexercise symptoms are variable in patients with myoadenylate deaminase activity. The reactions catalyzed by AMP deaminase and the other enzymes in the purine nucleotide cycle (Fig. 54-1) play an important role in the metabolism of the fast-twitch glycolytic fiber following vigorous exercise (see "Purine Nucleotide Cycle"). In contrast, this series of reactions does not appear to play a major role in the metabolism of slow-twitch oxidative fibers. Thus some of the variability in postexercise symptoms associated with myoadenylate deaminase deficiency may be related to individual differences in the proportion of fast-twitch glycolytic versus slow-twitch oxidative fibers in a given muscle group. Changes in fiber type occur with aging and conditioning, and are additional variables that may affect the severity as well as age of onset of postexercise symptoms. The severity of postexercise symptoms may also be affected by the amount of work required of a given muscle. Since the purine nucleotide cycle is used to its capacity only after the anaerobic threshold is exceeded, patients who modify their habits to avoid strenuous activity may experience minimal symptoms from AMP deaminase deficiency.

PURINE NUCLEOTIDE CYCLE

Three enzymes participate in the purine nucleotide cycle (Fig. 54-1): AMP deaminase (AMP aminohydrolase; EC 3.5.4.6), adenylosuccinate synthetase (EC 6.3.4.4), and adenylosuccinate lyase (EC 4.3.2.2). At first glance this series of reactions might appear to be a futile cycle, i.e., AMP → IMP → AMP. However, each turn of the cycle results in the utilization of 1 molecule of aspartate and GTP and the production of 1 molecule of fumarate and NH_3.

Before discussing the potential role(s) that this cycle plays in muscle function, it may be helpful to review the data which establish the fact that during exercise flux through the cycle increases in skeletal muscle. Extracts of muscle cytosol produce AMP from IMP and aspartate in the presence of GTP. When 2-deoxyglucose is added to provide an energy drain (i.e., to induce catabolism of ATP to AMP), adenine nucleotides disappear and IMP and NH_3 accumulate [16]. These experiments show that the cycle of IMP → AMP → IMP is operative in muscle extract and demonstrate that while deamination of AMP is the immediate source of NH_3 production, the amino group of aspartate is the ultimate source of this nitrogen.

Several laboratories have shown that the purine nucleotide cycle is operative in vivo [2–7, 17]. Biopsies obtained from the hind limbs of rodents following nerve stimulation or treadmill running demonstrate the following sequence of biochemical changes: (1) In fast-twitch glycolytic muscle the ATP concentration falls when the capacity for energy production by substrate oxidation is exceeded. (2) The resultant increase in AMP and ADP production coupled with the decreases in ATP concentration leads to an increase in AMP deaminase activity (see section on control of AMP deaminase below). (3) IMP accumulates in an amount that is almost stoichiometric with the decrease in adenine nucleotides. (4) NH_3 content of the muscle increases stoichiometrically with IMP, and spillover of additional NH_3 into the blood leads to an increase in plasma NH_3 concentration. (5) Aspartate concentration in the muscle falls while fumarate, malate, and citrate concentrations increase. This sequence of events demonstrates that following vigorous exercise AMP deaminase activity increases in muscle, and activation of this enzyme in turn leads to increased flux through the purine nucleotide cycle. These experiments establish a central role for AMP deaminase in the control of flux through this cycle.

It is difficult to quantify the flux through the purine nucleotide cycle, and consequently it has been difficult to estimate the extent to which flux is increased during exercise. Several studies indicate that flux through the cycle is increased substantially during exercise. Meyer, Dudley, and Terjung [5] have shown that blood NH_3 concentration increases 5.5 times in the rat following vigorous exercise. This magnitude of increase in blood NH_3 cannot be accounted for by the stoichiometric conversion of ATP to IMP and suggests that a substantial proportion of the NH_3 released into the blood is derived from aspartate through the purine nucleotide cycle. Aragon and Lowenstein [3] have demonstrated that citrate, isocitrate, and succinate concentrations in muscle increase following exercise, and that at least 72 percent of this expansion of the pool of citric acid cycle intermediates is derived from aspartate via the purine nucleotide cycle. These studies demonstrate that the IMP which accumulates during exercise in skeletal muscle is continuously recycled to AMP and back to IMP.

During the rest period following vigorous muscle contraction, IMP is converted first to adenylosuccinate and then to AMP [3, 5–7]. Since the capacity for ATP synthesis is greater than the rate of ATP utilization in resting muscle, any AMP formed from IMP rapidly accumulates in the muscle as ATP. Thus, the IMP which accumulates during exercise is used to restore the ATP pool during rest. In most studies the ATP pool is fully repleted after 15 to 30 min of rest [3, 5–7].

Sequential muscle biopsies have also been obtained in human subjects at rest, following exercise, and during the period of recovery [18]. Changes in IMP and adenine nucleotide content of human skeletal muscle are similar to those reported in animal experiments [3, 5–7]. Blood NH_3 concentration increases following vigorous exercise, and the increase in NH_3 concentration is proportional to the work load [19]. Ischemic forearm exercise also leads to NH_3 production by human skeletal muscle [8, 12, 14]. These results indicate that AMP deaminase activity and flux through the purine nucleotide cycle are increased in human skeletal muscle, much as in rodent skeletal muscle, following exercise.

In rodents different types of muscle fibers utilize the purine nucleotide cycle to varying degrees. In fast-twitch glycolytic fibers (type IIb) the capacity for substrate oxidation and ATP synthesis is exceeded at relatively low work loads, and consequently ATP catabolism leads to increased flux through the purine nucleotide cycle. In contrast, in slow-twitch oxidative fibers (type I) the capacity for ADP phosphorylation and ATP synthesis is not exceeded even during vigorous exercise, and little to no increase in flux through the purine nucleotide cycle occurs even after vigorous contraction [5–7]. Although slow-twitch fibers contain all the enzymes of the purine nucleotide cycle, albeit in lower activity than in fast-twitch muscle [20], AMP deaminase activity and flux through the cycle are not increased in this fiber type because ATP concentrations do not fall significantly with muscle contraction [5, 7]. Fast-twitch oxidative fibers (type IIa) are intermediate between type IIb and I fibers in their ability to maintain ATP pools following muscle contraction. Flux through the purine nucleotide cycle can be increased in this fiber type following exercise, but the work load required to decrease ATP content in type IIa fibers and to initiate the increase in flux through the cycle is considerably greater than that required in type IIb fibers [5–7].

As mentioned earlier these differences in metabolism between types I, IIa, and IIb fibers may account for some of the variability in symptoms exhibited by patients with myoadenylate deaminase deficiency. Since the reactions of the purine nucleotide cycle appear to be used sparingly in all types of muscle fibers at rest, disruption of the cycle by myoadenylate deaminase deficiency would not be expected to produce muscle dysfunction at rest. The extent to which AMP deaminase activity and flux through the purine nucleotide cycle increase during exercise is largely dependent upon the amount of ATP depletion produced. Since type IIb fibers are depleted of ATP at the lowest work loads, one would expect that disruption of the purine nucleotide cycle by myoadenylate deaminase deficiency would have the greatest effect on the function of fast-twitch glycolytic fibers. Type IIa fibers would be less severely affected, and type I fibers should be essentially unaffected by myoadenylate deaminase deficiency.

Several mechanisms have been proposed to explain the role of the purine nucleotide cycle in muscle function. One hypothesis is that the increase in flux through the purine nucleotide cycle during exercise serves to maintain the adenylate energy charge of the myocyte under these conditions [2, 21, 22]. The adenylate energy charge would be maintained through the following mechanism: The increase in AMP deaminase activity that occurs during exercise would prevent AMP accumulation following ATP catabolism, and this in turn would displace the adenylate kinase reaction toward ATP formation. A second hypothesis is that the local production of NH_3 would act in conjunction with the decrease in ATP to stimulate the activity of phosphofructokinase and enhance the rate of glycolysis [22]. It has also been suggested that the increase in IMP concentration may contribute to activation of glycogen phosphorylase and further enhance glycolysis [23]. Still another hypothesis is that the generation of fumarate, malate, and citrate from aspartate would provide a mechanism by which intermediates of the citric acid cycle could be replenished during a time of increased demand for ATP production [3]. Finally, the accumulation of IMP may provide a mechanism for preserving the pool of purine nucleotides during exercise, and this reservoir of IMP may be used to replete the ATP pool rapidly during recovery [14]. These proposed mechanisms are not mutually exclusive and more than one, or all, may have validity. Studies in patients with myoadenylate deaminase deficiency are beginning to provide insight into the relative importance of these proposed mechanisms for the role of the purine nucleotide cycle in muscle function.

AMP Deaminase

There are several isoenzymes of AMP deaminase. Different tissues contain varying proportions of these isoenzymes, and the properties of these isoenzymes are quite distinct [24–26]. At least three isoenzymes of AMP deaminase have been identified on the basis of kinetic, physical, and immunologic properties. Isoenzyme A is found only in skeletal muscle and diaphragm; isoenzyme B is the predominant form in liver, kidney, and testes; isoenzyme C is the only form in heart muscle; and hybrids of isoenzymes B and C are found in brain, lung, and spleen [24–26]. Studies in patients with myoadenylate deaminase deficiency suggest that some, if not all, of these isoenzymes are products of different genes, since skeletal muscle is the only tissue deficient in AMP deaminase activity in patients with this disorder [8, 12, 27].

During the course of development the total amount of AMP deaminase activity in a given tissue may vary, as well as the relative distribution among isoenzyme species [28]. In rat skeletal muscle, total AMP deaminase activity increases as much as eightfold from birth to adulthood [29]. Fast-twitch white type (IIb) fibers contain two- to threefold more AMP deaminase activity than slow-twitch red (type I) fibers [20]. Although some studies have suggested that red and white skeletal muscle contain different isoenzymes of AMP deaminase [30], others have found little difference in the kinetic properties of AMP deaminase from red and white muscle [26]. In some species there appears to be a change in the kinetic properties, and possible isoenzyme type, during development [28, 31]. A shift in isoenzyme type has also been observed when myocytes are grown in culture [28], and this may explain the finding of AMP deaminase activity in cells grown from a muscle biopsy specimen of a patient with well-documented myoadenylate deaminase deficiency [12].

Myoadenylate deaminase (isoenzyme A) has been purified to homogeneity from many mammalian sources, including humans [32–34]. The native molecular weight of the enzyme from rat skeletal muscle is 238,000, and following treatment with denaturing agents such as guanidine hydrochloride or sodium dodecylsulfate the enzyme dissociates into a single polypeptide with a molecular weight of approximately 60,000 [33]. The enzyme from rabbit skeletal muscle has a native molecular weight of approximately 270,000 and is composed of a single subunit of approximately 69,000 [34]. All data are consistent with the conclusion that AMP deaminase from skeletal muscle is composed of four polypeptide chains, and tryptic maps suggest that these subunits are identical. The amino acid composition of this protein is not unusual and it does not appear to contain substantial amounts of carbohydrate.

AMP deaminase is closely associated with contractile proteins in the myocyte. Histochemical studies have demonstrated that AMP deaminase is bound to the myofibril in the region of the A band [35] and that 2 mol of native enzyme are bound to 1 mol of myosin [36]. AMP deaminase binds to a specific region of myosin, i.e., heavy meromyosin or subfragment 2, and the association between AMP deaminase and myosin may play a role in controlling the activity of this enzyme (see below).

AMP deaminase from skeletal muscle is a complex allosteric enzyme, the activity of which is influenced by many ligands. Human myoadenylate deaminase exhibits a high degree of specificity for 5'-AMP [32, 37]. The velocity with 5'-dAMP is only 4 percent of that with 5'-AMP, and essentially no deaminase activity is observed with ATP, ADP, 3'-AMP, 2'-AMP, or adenosine. Other isoenzymes of AMP deaminase exhibit varying degrees of activity with these potential substrates [37].

Studies in vitro and in vivo suggest that myoadenylate deaminase exhibits a striking increase in activity in muscle during exercise (see section on purine nucleotide cycle above). Experiments that attempt to mimic conditions found in resting muscle in vitro suggest that AMP deaminase is inhibited by as much as 80 to 90 percent under these conditions [38]. Many factors have been identified that affect myoadenylate deaminase activity in vitro: adenylate energy charge; ratio of purine nucleoside triphosphates to diphosphates to monophosphates; concentration of K^+, H^+, Pi, and creatine phosphate; and binding to myosin [26, 33, 35, 45]. Changes in one or more of these variables are thought to lead to the release of inhibition of AMP deaminase and the increase in activity of this enzyme during exercise. It is not established how each of the above factors influences AMP deaminase activity, but the data obtained by Ashby and Frieden [41] from kinetic and binding studies have led these investigators to propose a model that explains many of the regulatory properties of this enzyme. These investigators suggest that the enzyme has three distinct types of purine nucleotide binding sites: a catalytic site that binds AMP, an inhibitory site that binds purine nucleoside triphosphates, and a stimulatory site that binds all types of purine nucleotides, but binds diphosphates in preference to monophosphates, and monophosphates in preference to triphosphates. K^+ ions affect the activity of the enzyme through cooperative effects on the catalytic site. Nucleoside triphosphates (ATP and GTP) bind avidly to the inhibitory site and produce indirect effects on cooperativity at the catalytic site. Nucleoside diphosphates and monophosphates (ADP, GDP, AMP, and GMP) bind avidly to the stimulatory site and indirectly decrease the affinity of the inhibitory site for nucleoside triphosphates. IMP, a product of the reaction, also binds to the stimulatory site and may under some conditions lead to enzyme activation. In resting muscle, purine nucleoside triphosphates are present in considerable excess relative to diphosphates and monophosphates. Following vigorous work, nucleoside triphosphate content decreases, producing a lower concentration of ligands for binding at the inhibitory site. Nucleoside diphosphate and monophosphate content increases, leading to higher ligand concentrations for binding at the stimulatory site and secondarily decreasing the affinity of the inhibitory site for nucleoside triphosphates. AMP content increases, providing more substrate and probably enhanced enzyme activity by binding of this monophosphate at the stimulatory site. This model accommodates a close correlation between the increase in AMP deaminase activity and the drop in adenylate energy charge that occurs with exercise [18, 46]. The drop in myocyte pH that follows exercise may also contribute to the increase in AMP deaminase activity, since the pH optimum for this enzyme is 6.5 [40]. Changes in creatine phosphate concentration probably do not play a role in controlling the activity of this enzyme [42]. The effect of AMP deaminase binding to myosin on the control of enzyme activity has not been thoroughly evaluated, but may prove to be important since the myosin components participating in this reaction bind to the nucleoside triphosphate, or inhibitory site, of AMP deaminase [36].

A number of potent inhibitors of AMP deaminase have been identified and may prove useful in defining the role of this enzyme in muscle function. Coformycin and 2'-deoxycoformycin, potent inhibitors of adenosine deaminase, are less potent inhibitors of AMP deaminase (K_i of 2×10^{-8} and 4×10^{-7}, respectively) [47]. The nucleotide derivatives, coformycin-5'-phosphate and 2'-deoxycoformycin-5'-phosphate, are considerably more potent inhibitors of AMP deaminase (K_i of 6×10^{-11} and 1×10^{-9}, respectively) [48].

METABOLIC DEFECTS IN PATIENTS

Animal studies suggest that the isoenzyme of AMP deaminase found in skeletal muscle is different from that found in other tissues on the basis of physical, kinetic, and immunologic properties. Thus, it is not surprising that AMP deaminase activity is normal in erythrocytes, leukocytes, and fibroblasts from patients with a deficiency of this enzyme in skeletal muscle [8, 12, 27]. These results provide strong support for the conclusion that myoadenylate deaminase is the product of a gene that is distinct from genes for other isoenzymes of AMP deaminase.

AMP deaminase is apparently the only enzymatic activity affected in the muscle of these patients, since assays for creatine kinase, adenosine deaminase, phosphorylase, and phosphofructokinase are normal [8, 9, 12, 14]. The deficiency of AMP deaminase activity can be detected with a nonquantitative histochemical stain or by direct enzymatic assay, in which case the activity varies from 0 to less than 6 percent of that found in biopsy specimens from patients with other types of myopathies (Table 54-1). Mixing experiments have ruled out a diffusible inhibitor of the enzyme [8, 12]. In 10 of the patients for whom analyses are reported, the deficiency of AMP deaminase activity is associated with the absence of protein antigenically related to myoadenylate deaminase [11, 27, 49]. The rabbit antibody used to perform these studies is specific for the myoadenylate isoenzyme and readily detects AMP deaminase protein in crude homogenates from a variety of human muscles. Based on results of immunologic studies, a portion or all of the residual AMP deaminase activity detected in biopsy specimens may be accounted for by contamination with erythrocytes or other blood components [27, 49]. These observations suggest that AMP deaminase deficiency is the consequence of an absence of myoadenylate deaminase protein, or if the protein is present, that it is structurally altered such that it is no longer recognized by antibody to the native enzyme.

One would anticipate that several metabolic abnormalities might be observed in patients with myoadenylate deaminase deficiency. If flux through the purine nucleotide cycle, and AMP deaminase activity in particular, is required for NH_3 production during exercise, then patients with myoadenylate deaminase deficiency should not increase venous NH_3 concentration following exercise. As shown in Table 54-2, normal subjects produce both NH_3 and lactate following ischemic forearm exercise. Fishbein et al. [8] have demonstrated a positive correlation between the amounts of NH_3 and lactate produced under these exercise conditions. In contrast the patient with myoadenylate deaminase deficiency exhibits little if any rise in venous NH_3 concentration following ischemic exercise, while lactate production is normal (Table 54-2).

In normal subjects vigorous exercise is associated with a 20 to 40 percent drop in ATP content of the muscle [18, 46], and in association with the decrease in adenine nucleotides there is a stoichiometric increase in IMP (Table 54-3). Within 15 to 30 min of rest the IMP concentration has returned to control levels and the ATP pool has been repleted. In the patient with myoadenylate deaminase deficiency a less strenuous exercise protocol is associated with a greater drop in the adenine nucle-

otide content of muscle (Table 54-3). In the myoadenylate deaminase–deficient patient there is no detectable increase in the IMP content of muscle following exercise. There is a greater increase in content of adenosine, inosine, and hypoxanthine in muscle of the AMP deaminase–deficient patient following exercise, but the purine nucleosides and bases that accumulate account for less than 50 percent of the purine lost from the adenine nucleotide pool [14]. Thus, during exercise the total purine content of skeletal muscle falls in the myoadenylate deaminase–deficient patient, while in the normal subject the total purine nucleotide content (ATP + ADP + AMP + IMP) changes very little. As a consequence of this loss of purine, the ATP pool of skeletal muscle from the myoadenylate deaminase–deficient patient is repleted more slowly during the rest period that follows exercise (Table 54-3).

A model illustrating the proposed differences in purine nucleotide metabolism in skeletal muscle of the normal individual compared with the patient with myoadenylate deaminase deficiency is shown in Fig. 54-2. Since ATP is the only source of energy for muscle contraction [50], the drop in ATP and prolonged time required for ATP repletion following exercise may account for the postexercise symptoms observed in the patient with myoadenylate deaminase deficiency.

As discussed earlier, several mechanisms have been proposed to explain the role of the purine nucleotide cycle in muscle function. The studies of myoadenylate deaminase–deficient patients reviewed here permit one to begin to assess the relative importance of these putative mechanisms. It has been proposed that the increased production of NH_3 [22] or IMP [23] or both during exercise may be the signals that stimulate the rate of glycolysis in the muscle. Since patients with myoadenylate deaminase deficiency produce neither NH_3 nor IMP upon exercise, yet lactate production is normal, these two compounds cannot be the only signals responsible for the enhanced rate of glycolysis observed following exercise. Another hypothesis is that AMP deaminase activity is required to maintain the adenylate energy charge in muscle during exercise [2, 21, 22, 43]. Apparently, other reactions are also capable of removing AMP since the adenylate energy charge falls to a comparable degree in myoadenylate deaminase–deficient and normal muscle during exercise [14]. Considerable evidence reviewed earlier indicates that activation of AMP deaminase and increased flux through the purine nucleotide cycle during exercise lead to the production of potential substrates from aspartate and other amino acids for use in the citric acid cycle. The disproportionate drop in ATP content of muscle relative to work load in the myoadenylate deaminase–deficient patient is consistent with the hypothesis that increased flux through the purine

Table 54-2 Results of ischemic exercise testing in normal and AMP deaminase–deficient subjects

Ischemic exercise testing	NH_3 production, μmol/liter		Lactate production, meq/liter	
	Patient	Controls*	Patient	Controls*
Baseline	20	30 ± 12	1.7	1.5 ± 0.5
0 min	30	111 ± 68	4.2	5.4 ± 2.5
2 min	32	117 ± 50	3.4	5.1 ± 1.5
6 min	28	98 ± 49	2.7	4.0 ± 1.5
10 min	32	70 ± 35	2.6	3.3 ± 1.6

* $n = 20$ normal volunteers
NOTE: Results are presented as the mean ± 1 SD

Table 54-3   Change in nucleotide content of normal and AMP deaminase–deficient skeletal muscle with exercise

	Rest		Exercise		30–45 min recovery		145 min recovery
	Control	Patient	Control	Patient	Control	Patient	Patient
ATP	4.86	4.35	3.92	3.05	4.65	3.37	4.12
TAN*	5.51	5.03	4.73	3.99	5.34	3.96	4.73
ΔTAN*	—	—	−0.78	−1.04	−0.17	−1.07	−0.30
IMP	N.D.†	0.01	0.74	N.D.†	0.22	0.03	0.01

* TAN = total adenine nucleotides (ATP + ADP + AMP)

NOTE: For comparison all data are expressed in micromoles of nucleotide per gram of wet weight. Results for control subjects were obtained from Sahlin et al. [18] and for the AMP deaminase–deficient patient from Sabina et al. [14]. The data of Sahlin et al. were converted from micromoles per gram of dry weight to wet weight by assuming that 80 percent of muscle weight is water. The data of Sabina et al. were recalculated from that originally published [14] based on the recent demonstration that results normalized by wet weight alone may give spurious values [53]. Biopsies were obtained from the vastus lateralis in both groups of patients. The five control subjects were biopsied at the point of exhaustion following bicycle exercise at 80 percent or greater of their maximum work load. The AMP deaminase–deficient patient was biopsied after 15 min of step-up exercise on a 12-in platform at 17–19 steps per minute.

† N.D. = not determined

nucleotide cycle during exercise makes a significant contribution to energy production in the myocyte. The hypothesis that IMP accumulation provides a reservoir of purine nucleotide to be used for repletion of the ATP pool during recovery from exercise may also have some validity, since the time required for restoration of the ATP concentration found in resting muscle is prolonged in the patient with myoadenylate deaminase deficiency.

GENETICS

The mode of inheritance of myoadenylate deaminase deficiency has not been well characterized. Metabolic and enzy-

Figure 54-2   Comparison of purine metabolism in muscle from normal subject and patient with myoadenylate deaminase deficiency.

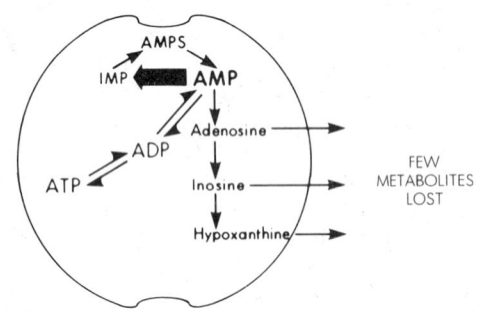

A.   NORMAL MUSCLE CELL

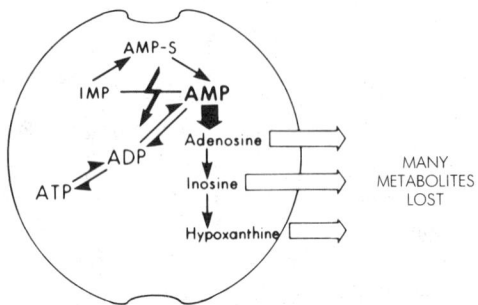

B.   MYOADENYLATE DEAMINASE DEFICIENT MUSCLE CELL

matic studies of patients and families with this disorder have been slow because these experiments require biopsy of skeletal muscle, the only tissue that expresses the deficiency of AMP deaminase. Consequently, large numbers of family members have not been evaluated. Two kindreds have been studied. Mothers of two children with essentially complete deficiency of myoadenylate deaminase have each exhibited approximately 50 percent of control AMP deaminase activity [12, 15]. These data suggest that the complete deficiency of AMP deaminase requires two abnormal alleles at the AMP deaminase locus. The finding of approximately equal numbers of males and females with AMP deaminase deficiency is consistent with an autosomal recessive mode of inheritance.

TREATMENT

Because of the relatively recent recognition of myoadenylate deaminase deficiency there has not been sufficient time to evaluate treatment regimens in these patients. From limited biochemical data from muscle biopsies, one might expect that therapeutic programs aimed at enhancing the rate of repletion of the ATP pool might be beneficial. One approach that has been successful in increasing the rate of ATP synthesis in myocardium of the rat is the administration of ribose [51]. Ribose increases the rate of synthesis of PP-ribose-P through increasing the availability of ribose-5-phosphate. The increase in PP-ribose-P content of the cell could enhance salvage and *de novo* synthesis of purine nucleotides. If this regimen were combined with allopurinol administration to increase the availability of salvageable purines such as hypoxanthine, it might be possible to restore the ATP pool more rapidly following exercise in these patients.

Another potential approach to therapy is a graduated exercise program aimed at increasing the relative proportion of type IIa and type I muscle fibers. As discussed previously, the greater oxidative capacity of type IIa and type I fibers, compared to type IIb fibers, makes these muscle fibers less dependent upon AMP deaminase and the purine nucleotide cycle. Studies in human volunteers indicate that conditioning programs can produce skeletal muscle that contains a greater proportion of type IIa and type I fibers [52]. Thus, an exercise program designed to increase the proportion of these fiber types might improve exercise tolerance. However, patients with myoadenylate deaminase deficiency should be cautioned against unsupervised strenuous exercise as this could lead to undesirable sequellae such as rhabdomyolysis and myoglobinuria.

REFERENCES

1. LOWENSTEIN JM: Ammonia production in muscle and other tissues: The purine nucleotide cycle. *Physiol Rev* 52:382, 1972
2. LOWENSTEIN JM, GOODMAN MN: The purine nucleotide cycle in skeletal muscle. *Fed Proc* 37:2308, 1978
3. ARAGON JJ, LOWENSTEIN JM: The purine-nucleotide cycle: Comparison of the levels of citric acid cycle intermediates with the operation of the purine nucleotide cycle in rat skeletal muscle during exercise and recovery from exercise. *Eur J Biochem* 110:371, 1980
4. GOODMAN MN, LOWENSTEIN JM: The purine nucleotide cycle: Studies of ammonia production by skeletal muscle in situ and in perfused preparations. *J Biol Chem* 252:5054, 1977
5. MEYER RA, DUDLEY GA, TERJUNG RL: Ammonia and IMP in different skeletal muscle fibers after exercise in rats. *J Appl Physiol* 49:1037, 1980
6. MEYER RA, TERJUNG RL: AMP deamination and IMP reamination in working skeletal muscle. *Am J Physiol* 239:C32, 1980
7. MEYER RA, TERJUNG RL: Differences in ammonia and adenylate metabolism in contracting fast and slow muscle. *Am J Physiol* 237:C111, 1979
8. FISHBEIN WN, ARMBRUSTMACHER VW, GRIFFIN JL: Myoadenylate deaminase deficiency: A new disease of muscle. *Science* 200:545, 1978
9. ENGEL AG, POTTER CS, ROSEVEAR JW: Nucleotides and adenosine monophosphate deaminase activity of muscle in primary hypokalaemic periodic paralysis. *Nature* 202:670, 1964
10. SCHUMATE JB, KATNIK R, RUIZ M, KAISER K, FRIEDEN C, BROOKE MH, CARROLL JE: Myoadenylate deaminase deficiency. *Muscle and Nerve* 2:213, 1979
11. FISHBEIN WN, GRIFFIN JL, MAGARAJAN K, WINKERT JW, ARMBRUSTMACHER VW: Myoadenylate deaminase deficiency: Association with collagen disease. *Clin Res* 27:37A, 1979
12. DIMAURO S, MIRANDA AF, HAYS AP, FRANCK WA, HOFFMAN GS, SCHOENFELDT RS, SINGH N: Myoadenylate deaminase deficiency: Muscle biopsy and muscle culture in a patient with gout. *J Neurol Sci* 47:191, 1980
13. SCHUMATE JB, KAISER KK, CARROLL JE, BROOKE MH: Adenylate deaminase deficiency in a hypotonic infant. *J Pediatr* 96:885, 1980
14. SABINA RL, SWAIN JL, PATTEN BM, ASHIZAWA T, O'BRIEN WE, HOLMES EW: Disruption of the purine nucleotide cycle: A potential explanation for muscle dysfunction in myoadenylate deaminase deficiency. *J Clin Invest* 66:1419, 1980
15. KELEMEN J, RICE DR, BRADLEY WG, MUNSAT TL, DIMAURO S, HOGAN EL: Familial aches, cramps and pains syndrome. Manuscript in preparation
16. TORNHEIM K, LOWENSTEIN JM: The purine nucleotide cycle: The production of ammonia from aspartate by extracts of rat skeletal muscle. *J Biol Chem* 247:162, 1972
17. HETTLEMAN BD, SABINA RL, HOLMES EW, SWAIN JL: The biochemical basis of skeletal muscle dysfunction in hypophosphatemia. *Circulation* 64:IV-64, 1981
18. SAHLIN K, PALMSKOG G, HULTMAN E: Adenine nucleotide and IMP content of the quadriceps muscle in man after exercise. *Pfleug Arch Eur J Physiol* 374:193, 1978
19. WILKERSON JE, BATTERSON DL, HORVATH SM: Exercise-induced changes in blood ammonia levels in humans. *Eur J Appl Physiol* 37:255, 1977
20. WINDER WW, TERJUNG RL, BALDWIN KM, HOLLOSZY JO: Effect of exercise on AMP deaminase and adenylosuccinase in rat skeletal muscle. *Am J Physiol* 227:1411, 1974
21. TORNHEIM K, LOWENSTEIN JM: The purine nucleotide cycle: Interactions with oscillations of the glycolytic pathway in muscle extracts. *J Biol Chem* 249:3241, 1974
22. TORNHEIM K, LOWENSTEIN JM: The purine nucleotide cycle: Control of phosphofructokinase and glycolytic oscillations in muscle extracts. *J Biol Chem* 250:6304, 1975
23. ARAGON JJ, TORNHEIM K, LOWENSTEIN JM: On a possible role of IMP in the regulation of phosphorylase activity in skeletal muscle. *FEBS Lett* 117:suppl K56, 1980

24. OGASAWARA N, GOTO H, YASUKAZU Y, WATANABE T: Distribution of AMP-deaminase isozymes in rat tissue. *Eur J Biochem* 87:297, 1978
25. OGASAWARA N, GOTO H, WATANABE T: Isozymes of rat AMP deaminase. *Biochim Biophys Acta* 403:530, 1975
26. SOLANO C, COFFEE CJ: Differential response of AMP deaminase isoenzymes to changes in the adenylate energy charge. *Biochem Biophys Res Commun* 85:564, 1978
27. FISHBEIN WN, DAVIS JI, NAGARAJAN K, WINKERT JW, FOELLMER JW: Immunologic distinction of human muscle adenylate deaminase from the isozyme in human peripheral blood cells: Implications for myoadenylate deaminase deficiency. *Arch Biochem Biophys* 205:360, 1980
28. SAMMONS DW, CHILSON OP: AMP deaminase: Stage-specific isoenzymes in differentiating chick muscle. *Arch Biochem Biophys* 191:561, 1978
29. KALETHA K: Changes of the heat sensibility of AMP-deaminase from rat skeletal muscle in the course of postnatal development. *Int J Biochem* 6:471, 1975
30. RAGGI A, BERGAMINI C, RONCA G: Isozymes of AMP deaminase in red and white skeletal muscles. *FEBS Lett* 58:19, 1975
31. KALETHA K, ZYDAWO M: Differences in thermal susceptibility of the kinetics of AMP-aminohydrolase from foetal and postnatal chick muscle. *Int J Biochem* 2:20, 1971
32. MAKAREWICZ W, STANKIEWICZ A: Purification of AMP-deaminase from human skeletal muscle on 5'-AMP sepharose 4B. *Int J Biochem* 7:245, 1976
33. COFFEE CJ: AMP deaminase from rat skeletal muscle. *Methods Enzymol* 51:490, 1978
34. BOOSMAN A, CHILSON OP: Subunit structure of AMP-deaminase from chicken and rabbit skeletal muscle. *J Biol Chem* 251:1847, 1976
35. ASHBY B, FRIEDEN C, BISCHOFF R: Immunofluorescent and histochemical localization of AMP deaminase in skeletal muscle. *J Cell Biol* 81:361, 1979
36. ASHBY B, FRIEDEN C: Interaction of AMP aminohydrolase with myosin and its subfragments. *J Biol Chem* 252:1869, 1977
37. STANKIEWICZ A, SPYCHALA J, MAKAREWICZ W: Comparative studies on muscle AMP-deaminase—III. Substrate specificity of the enzymes from man, rabbit, rat, hen, frog and pikeperch. *Comp Biochem Physiol* 66B:529, 1980
38. COFFEE CJ, SOLANO C: Rat muscle 5'-adenylic acid aminohydrolase. *J Biol Chem* 252:1606, 1977
39. RAHIM ZHA, LUTAYA G, GRIFFITHS JR: Activation of AMP aminohydrolase during skeletal-muscle contraction. *Biochem J* 184:173, 1979
40. SOLANO C, COFFEE CJ: Comparison of AMP deaminase from skeletal muscle of acidotic and normal rats. *Biochim Biophys Acta* 582:369, 1979
41. ASHBY B, FRIEDEN C: Adenylate deaminase. Kinetic and binding studies on the rabbit muscle enzyme. *J Biol Chem* 253:8728, 1978
42. WHEELER TJ, LOWENSTEIN JM: Creatine phosphate inhibition of adenylate deaminase is mainly due to pyrophosphate. *J Biol Chem* 254:1484, 1979
43. CHAPMAN AG, ATKINSON DE: Stabilization of adenylate energy charge by the adenylate deaminase reaction. *J Biol Chem* 248:8309, 1973
44. RAGGI A, RANIERI-RAGGI M: Negative homotropic cooperativity in rat muscle AMP deaminase. *Biochim Biophys Acta* 566:353, 1979
45. WHEELER TJ, LOWENSTEIN JM: Adenylate deaminase from rat muscle: Regulation by purine nucleotides and orthophosphate in the presence of 150 mM KCl. *J Biol Chem* 254:8994, 1979
46. SUTTON JR, TOEWS CJ, WARD GR, FOX IH: Purine metabolism during strenuous muscle exercise in man. *Metabolism* 29:254, 1980
47. AGARWAL RP, PARKS RE JR: Potent inhibition of muscle 5'-AMP deaminase by the nucleoside antibiotics coformycin and deoxycoformycin. *Biochem Pharmacol* 26:663, 1977
48. FRIEDEN C, GILBERT HR, MILLER RL: Adenylate deaminase: Potent inhibition by 2'-deoxycoformycin 5'-phosphate. *Biochem Biophys Res Commun* 91:278, 1979
49. FISHBEIN WN, ARMBRUSTMACHER VM, GRIFFIN JL: Myoadenylate deaminase deficiency: Verification on repeat biopsy, fresh or frozen, and origin of the residual enzyme. *IRCS Med Sci Biochem* 9:103, 1981
50. MOMMAERTS, WFHM: *Muscular Contraction: A Topic in Molecular Physiology.* New York, Interscience Publishers, 1950
51. ZIMMER HG, GERLACH E: Stimulation of myocardial adenine nucleotide biosynthesis by pentoses and pentitols. *Pfluegers Arch* 376:223, 1978
52. SALTIN B, HENRIKSSON J, NYGAARD E, ANDERSEN P: Fiber types and metabolic potentials of skeletal muscles in sedentary man and endurance runners. *Ann NY Acad Sci* 301:3, 1977
53. SABINA RL, HOLMES EW, SWAIN JL: Re-evaluation of methods for normalizing nucleotide data in percutaneous biopsies of skeletal muscle. Manuscript in preparation.

55

HEREDITARY XANTHINURIA

EDWARD W. HOLMES

JAMES B. WYNGAARDEN

1. Xanthinuria *is a rare disorder characterized by the replacement of uric acid by xanthine and hypoxanthine in urine. When dietary purines are restricted, there is a virtual absence of uric acid in serum and urine. The disorder of purine metabolism can be subdivided into two types. Classical xanthinuria, or isolated deficiency of xanthine oxidase, has been reported in 45 well-documented cases, 28 of them in males. In 58 percent of these cases, the patients were asymptomatic, and the metabolic defect was an incidental finding. In 33 percent of the subjects, xanthine calculi of the urinary tract developed. In 4 of the 45 a myopathy was present, associated in 3 with crystalline deposits of hypoxanthine and xanthine in muscle. Recurrent polyarthritis was noted in 3 patients but crystals have not been demonstrated in synovial fluid or tissue. A new subtype of xanthinuria has been described in which the deficiency of xanthine oxidase is associated with a deficiency of another molybdenum-containing enzyme, sulfite oxidase. Two patients have been reported to have a combined deficiency of these two enzymes as a result of defects in molybdenum metabolism. In these individuals the neurologic symptoms attributable to sulfite oxidase deficiency overshadow the symptoms of xanthine oxidase deficiency.*

2. *There is a gross deficiency of xanthine oxidase activity in xanthinuria. Jejunal, hepatic, and renal tissue, as well as colostrum, show absent or extremely low enzyme activity toward hypoxanthine, xanthine, and xanthopterin with either oxygen or NAD as the electron acceptor.*

3. *Several additional patients have formed xanthine stones in childhood and may have xanthinuria. Many of the adults who have formed xanthine stones have clearly not had a defect in xanthine oxidase activity, for in several instances normal or elevated serum uric acid levels were found. Circumstantial evidence, such as the finding of xanthine deposits in the renal parenchyma in one case, suggests that xanthine excretion may have been excessive in a few, but this is unproved.*

4. *All available data on genetic factors are consistent with an autosomal recessive pattern of inheritance. In two families some of the presumed obligate heterozygotes showed moderate increases in urinary oxypurine excretion, although they had normal levels of uric acid in serum and in urine.*

Hereditary xanthinuria is a rare disorder characterized by a gross deficiency of xanthine oxidase activity in the tissues, by the excretion of xanthine and hypoxanthine as the chief end products of purine metabolism, and by low concentrations of uric acid in serum and urine. There are well-documented reports of more than 45 patients with this disorder [1–36]. Although the true prevalence of xanthinuria is not known, discovery of 3 cases in a random survey of 137,194 serum urate analyses suggests a prevalence of 1:45,000 [32].

About 40 cases of xanthine stones have been recorded since they were first identified by Marcet in 1817 [37]. In some patients, chiefly adults, serum or urinary uric acid values were normal, and xanthine was only a minor component of the calculus. At least seven xanthine stones occurred in subjects under age 15 who may have had hereditary xanthinuria, but since xanthine excretion studies were not performed, the relationship is uncertain [38–49].

CLINICAL FEATURES

Xanthinuria can be subdivided into two types. Classical xanthinuria, or isolated deficiency of xanthine oxidase, has been recognized since 1954. There have been 45 patients with well-documented xanthinuria of the classical form described in the literature, and the clinical features and biochemical findings in these patients are summarized in Table 55-1. In 1978 Duran et al. [33] described a new subtype of xanthinuria in which the deficiency of xanthine oxidase was associated with a deficiency of sulfite oxidase. The clinical presentation of patients with the combined deficiencies of xanthine oxidase and sulfite oxidase encompasses the clinical and biochemical features of classical xanthinuria and those of isolated sulfite oxidase deficiency. Table 55-1 also summarizes the clinical features and biochemical findings for patients with combined deficiencies of xanthine oxidase and sulfite oxidase.

In classical xanthinuria only 42 percent of the patients describe symptoms referable to the deficiency of xanthine oxidase. Thus, the majority of the patients are asymptomatic and are usually discovered by the finding of a very low serum urate concentration during investigation of presumably unrelated medical problems or during screening tests in a population health survey. In 15 of 45 subjects, xanthine calculi of the urinary tract developed; in 1 it led to mild calyceal clubbing, and in another to hydronephrosis and eventual nephrectomy. In 4 patients a myopathy was present, associated in 3 with crystalline deposits of xanthine and hypoxanthine. Recurrent polyarthritis was noted in 3 patients. It has been suggested that this symptom may represent crystal-induced synovitis [50], but neither hypoxanthine nor xanthine crystals have been demonstrated in synovial fluid or tissue.

In patients with combined deficiencies of xanthine oxidase and sulfite oxidase the clinical features of sulfite oxidase deficiency [51–53] overshadow those of xanthine oxidase deficiency. These patients have severe neurologic abnormalities which include mental retardation, major motor seizures, and cerebral atrophy. In addition they have ocular lens dislocation.

Illustrative Cases

Case 1 In 1954 Dent and Philpot [1] described a 4½-year-old girl with hematuria who passed a smooth oval calculus weighing 0.9 g. It was nonopaque to x-rays, contained only traces of calcium and mag-

Table 55-1 Clinical features and biochemical data on reported cases of classical xanthinuria (isolated deficiency of xanthine oxidase) and cases of combined xanthine oxidase and sulfite oxidase deficiencies.

I. Classical xanthinuria (isolated xanthine oxidase deficiency)*

	Mean	Range
Age, yrs	29.7	1.5–80
Sex	62% Male	
Serum urate concentration, mg/dl	0.55	0–1.44
Urinary uric acid excretion, mg/24 h	22.9	0–81.2
Serum oxypurine concentration, mg/dl	0.56	0.1–0.96
Urinary oxypurine excretion, mg/24 h	316.9	55–557
Percent urinary oxypurine that is xanthine	79%	42–95
Renal calculi	33%	
Myopathy	8.9%	
Arthropathy	6.7%	
Xanthine oxidase activity		
Liver	0–10% of control (6 pts)	
Jejunum	0–5.7% of control (11 pts)	
Rectum	25% of control (1 pt)	
Kidney	10% of control (1 pt)	
Colostrum	0% of control (1 pt)	

II. Combined deficiencies of xanthine oxidase and sulfite oxidase†

	Congenital form	Acquired form
Age	3 wks	20 yrs
Sex	Female	Male
Serum urate concentration, mg/dl	0.67	1.0
Urinary uric acid excretion, mg/g of creatinine	11.8	100‡
Serum oxypurine concentration, mg/dl	Not reported	Not reported
Urinary oxypurine excretion, mg/g of creatinine	961	Not reported
Percent urinary oxypurine that is xanthine	85%	Not reported
Renal calculi	+	–
Neurologic symptoms	+	+
Lens dislocation	+	–
Xanthine oxidase activity		
Liver	6% of control	Not reported
Jejunum	0% of control	Not reported

* Data compiled for 45 patients [1–32]
† Data compiled for 2 patients [33–36]
‡ Milligrams of uric acid excreted per 24 hours

nesium, and was almost ash-free. In the murexide test it gave a reddish-brown color quite unlike that of uric acid. By paper chromatography, extracts of the stone matched xanthine exactly. Xanthine excretion was 176 mg/day, or 607 mg/g creatinine. Uric acid excretion was 30 mg/day, and plasma urate was 0.5 mg/dl.

This patient was restudied at age 9 by Dickinson and Smellie [2]. She had no further calculi but had developed clubbing of the calyces of the left kidney. As measured by specific enzymatic methods, plasma oxypurines were 0.75 mg/dl, and plasma uric acid was 0.2 mg/dl. The renal clearance of oxypurines was 94 ml/min per 1.73 m² body surface area, a value equivalent to 82 percent of the simultaneous endogenous creatinine clearance (normal is 10 to 20 percent). When the patient was given a low purine diet, uric acid was not detectable in fresh urine and plasma. Urinary hypoxanthine was equivalent to 10 to 20 percent of xanthine.

At age 14 a pyelogram showed some persistent clubbing of the left renal calyces, with reduction of size of the left kidney (10.5 cm) compared with the right (14 cm). At age 19 she was normotensive and in good health [50].

Case 2   In 1964 Engleman and colleagues [3, 4] described a 23-year-old black woman suffering from pheochromocytoma and heart failure who was found to have a very low serum urate value. In addition, she was mentally retarded, with an IQ of 53, had congenital skeletal abnormalities, and on a later admission, exhibited a glucose-6-phosphate dehydrogenase deficiency [50]. There was no clinical or radiologic evidence of urinary calculi. Further study disclosed diminished amounts of uric acid and increased quantities of oxypurines in both serum and urine. The renal clearance of oxypurines was 87 percent of the endogenous creatinine clearance. The increased excretion of uric acid which normally follows the ingestion of 5-amino-4-imidazole carboxamide was replaced by an approximately equivalent increase in the urinary excretion of xanthine [4]. With three different assays, xanthine oxidase activities of the patient's jejunal mucosa and liver corresponded to no more than 0.1 percent of activities found in specimens from control subjects. No evidence was found for an inhibitor of xanthine oxidase in intestinal mucosa or blood [3, 4]. By age 27 she had developed muscle cramps in her legs following walking or strenuous exercise. A muscle biopsy specimen contained numerous crystals which were identified as xanthine and hypoxanthine [10, 54].

Case 3   Bradford et al. [8] described a 62-year-old Puerto Rican woman, with a 30-year history of mild psoriasis, who entered Bellevue Hospital because of acute monoarticular arthritis. This became migratory and polyarticular, affecting ankles, knees, elbows, wrists, and hands over a 6-week period, with fever to 104°F (40°C). The etiology of the arthritis was not established, but the finding of a serum uric acid of 0.8 to 1.1 mg/dl prompted study of xanthinuria. On a low purine diet, urinary uric acid ranged from 0 to 38.5 mg/day; urinary xanthine, from 125 to 325 mg/day; and urinary hypoxanthine, from 27 to 76 mg/day.

Case 4   In 1969, Chalmers et al. [9] reported a 31-year-old black male from Guyana who had been an active athlete until 3 years earlier, when he developed "tight sensations" at the back of both thighs and calves. Examination disclosed no vascular abnormalities, and the neurologic findings were normal except for universally sluggish reflexes and absent ankle jerks. Muscle strength was normal, no muscle tenderness was found at rest or following exertion, and there was no myotonia, but the calves felt firmer than normal. The finding of a very low serum urate value led to further investigation in the hospital, where the mean of four determinations was 0.78 mg/dl. Plasma oxypurines, calculated as xanthine, were 0.29 mg/dl. Urinary excretion values were uric acid, 12 to 52 mg; xanthine, 245 mg; and hypoxanthine, 19 mg/24 h. No xanthine oxidase activity was demonstrated by histochemical techniques in a jejunal biopsy specimen. Electromyographic studies were in keeping with a diffuse myopathic process. Four muscle biopsies were performed over a period of 12 months. A striking feature was the unusually high average diameter of muscle fibers, which also showed increased numbers of centrally placed muscle nuclei. A few of the fibers contained intensely staining rodlike inclusions, which on electron microscopy consisted of aggregations of electron-dense material, much of which was crystalline in appearance. By polarized light, phase contrast, and interference microscopy, the optical properties of the crystals were compatible with their being hypoxanthine and xanthine [10, 54]. Identification of crystals from this patient and from the patient of case 2 was subsequently accomplished by high-resolution mass spectrometry [55].

Case 5   In 1978, Duran et al. [33, 34] described a 3-week-old female who had all of the biochemical features of xanthinuria, i.e.,

hypouricemia (0.2 to 1.1 mg/dl), hypouricosuria (11.8 mg of uric acid excreted per gram of creatinine), increased excretion of oxypurines (817 mg xanthine and 144 mg of hypoxanthine per gram of creatinine), and virtual absence of xanthine oxidase activity (not detectable in jejunum, 6 percent of control in liver). This patient was different from the classical patient with xanthinuria in that she had severe neurologic abnormalities. The patient was admitted to the hospital because of feeding difficulties since birth. Examination at that time demonstrated typical tonic-clonic seizures, nystagmus, enophthalmus, bilateral ocular lens dislocation, and a ring of Brushfield spots. The skull was asymmetric with frontal bossing. Electroencephalogram showed diffuse irregularities, and the pneumoencephalogram demonstrated widened ventricles and periventricular atrophy [35]. Liver biopsy demonstrated a deficiency of sulfite oxidase activity as well as of xanthine oxidase activity. In addition, the urine of this patient contained excessive quantities of sulfite, S-sulfocysteine, taurine, and thiosulfate. Sulfate, the product of the sulfite oxidase reaction, was diminished in the urine of this patient. These neurologic findings and abnormalities of sulfur metabolism are typical of those described in patients with an isolated deficiency of sulfite oxidase [51–53]. Subsequent studies have provided an explanation for the combined deficiency of xanthine oxidase and sulfite oxidase in this patient [35]. Both of these enzymes require a molybdenum cofactor for catalytic activity (see below), and this cofactor was not found in the liver of this patient even though the serum concentration of molybdenum was normal. Follow-up studies in this patient have revealed no improvement in clinical symptoms in spite of numerous manipulations of sulfur content of the diet. At age 14 months small brownish concretions were noticed on her diaper and the calculi were proved to be xanthine stones [33]. It is not clear at this time whether this congenital disorder is a genetic disease. If it is inherited, it is likely to be autosomal recessive since neither parent nor an older brother has any of the biochemical features of xanthine oxidase deficiency or sulfite oxidase deficiency.

Case 6   In 1979 Abumrad et al. [36] described a 20-year-old male with the short bowel syndrome maintained for 18 months on total parenteral nutrition who developed hypouricemia (1 mg/dl) and hypouricosuria (100 mg uric acid excreted per day). Following infusion of commercially available amino acid solutions he experienced headaches, night blindness, irritability, lethargy, and became comatose. Urinary excretion of sulfite and thiosulfate were increased while excretion of sulfate was decreased. Treatment with ammonium molybdate reversed the biochemical abnormalities in purine and sulfur metabolism, and relieved the neurologic symptoms. It was suggested from these results that acquired deficiency of molybdenum led to a decrease in the activity of both xanthine oxidase and sulfite oxidase. This conclusion is supported by studies with rats made molybdenum-deficient by feeding tungsten [56, 57]. These animals develop simultaneous deficiencies of xanthine oxidase and sulfite oxidase activities.

Comment   The association of xanthinuria and pheochromocytoma in case 2 is probably fortuitous. Plasma from eight other patients with pheochromocytoma studied by Engleman et al. [4] contained normal amounts of uric acid, and urine from the xanthinuric patient of Dent and Philpot contained normal amounts of catecholamines and their metabolites [1]. In the patient of Frezal et al. [7] urinary excretion of vanillylmandelic acid was normal.

The association of xanthinuria and hemochromatosis in one patient is also probably coincidental [5]. In 4 of 11 patients with proved hemochromatosis in whom serum uric acid values were available, the values were normal [5]. The patient with xanthinuria described by Engleman and associates [4] developed iron deficiency anemia and hypoferremia that responded promptly to oral iron administration. Seegmiller and associates [58] later found a normal absorption of ^{59}Fe and a normal incorporation of absorbed iron into erythrocytes of this patient.

As will be discussed below, the association of xanthine oxidase and sulfite oxidase deficiencies is not fortuitous. Since both of these enzymes require a molybdenum cofactor for catalytic activity and since studies with experimental animals have demonstrated that molybdenum deficiency leads to the simultaneous loss of both activities [56, 57], there is a sound biochemical explanation for the associated loss of xanthine oxidase and sulfite oxidase activities in patients with molybdenum deficiency or a defect in the synthesis of molybdenum cofactor (see below).

XANTHINE OXIDASE

Oxidation of hypoxanthine to xanthine and xanthine to uric acid (Fig. 55-1) may be catalyzed by either *xanthine oxidase* (EC 1.2.3.2), in which case oxygen is the terminal electron acceptor, or *xanthine dehydrogenase* (EC 1.2.1.37), in which case NAD functions as the electron acceptor. Although xanthine oxidase and xanthine dehydrogenase have been given separate numbers by the Enzyme Commission, it is not clear that these two activities are distinct proteins. Xanthine dehydrogenase from a number of mammalian sources can be converted to xanthine oxidase by treatments such as incubation at 37°C for several hours or limited proteolysis with trypsin [59–64a]. Apparently, oxidation of reduced sulfhydryls to disulfides is one mechanism by which the dehydrogenase can be converted to an oxidase, since the dehydrogenase activity can be restored by incubation of the oxidase with reductants such as dithiothreitol or dithioerythritol [60–64]. Conversion of the dehydrogenase to an oxidase by trypsin treatment is associated with the loss of a peptide of approximately 20,000 daltons which is rich in reduced sulfhydryl content and is essential for dehydrogenase activity [63]. Purification procedures in the past which did not protect the enzyme from oxidation or proteolysis may account for the failure of earlier reports to recognize that the great majority of the enzyme activity was present in the form of a dehydrogenase rather than an oxidase.

Other studies also suggest that xanthine oxidase activity is derived in vitro from xanthine dehydrogenase. When both activities have been purified from rat liver the enzymes are indistinguishable in their absorption spectra, cofactor composition, and electrophoretic behavior on 5 percent polyacrylamide gels [59]. These observations, combined with the reports that both xanthine oxidase and xanthine dehydrogenase activities are reduced or absent in tissues from xanthinuric subjects, suggest that both activities are the product of one gene. However, it may be premature to conclude that all of the xanthine oxidase activity detected in tissue extracts is derived from an in vitro transformation of the xanthine dehydrogenase. A recent study has reported that as much as 20 percent of the xanthine oxidase activity found in the intestine of mice is immunologically and catalytically different from the xanthine oxidase produced in vitro from xanthine dehydrogenase [64].

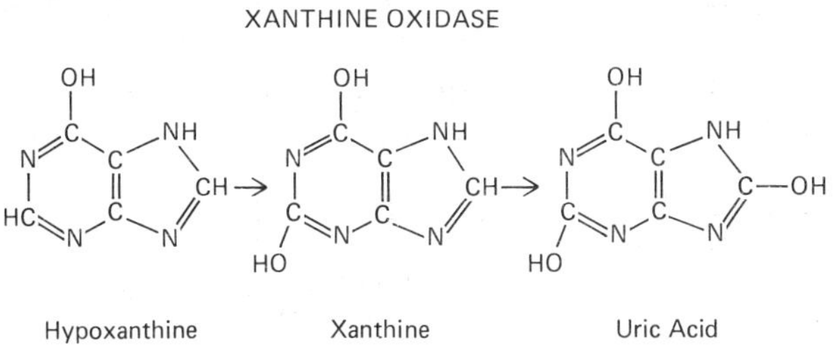

This study raises the possibility that some of the xanthine oxidase activity detected in extracts may be distinct from xanthine dehydrogenase. Possibly this non-xanthine dehydrogenase–related xanthine oxidase activity accounts for some of the residual activity found in tissue extracts from xanthinuric subjects.

Data from several laboratories indicate that oxidation of hypoxanthine and xanthine in most mammalian tissues is catalyzed in vivo by the xanthine dehydrogenase activity [50, 59–64]. In extracts from human liver the dehydrogenase activity is substantially greater than the oxidase activity. This suggests that NAD rather than oxygen is the primary electron acceptor in vivo in humans [50, 62]. Consequently, it would be more correct to state that xanthinuria results from a deficiency of xanthine dehydrogenase activity, but inasmuch as the bulk of the literature on the subject refers to the enzyme as "xanthine oxidase," and since assays of its activity in tissues of xanthinuric subjects have almost exclusively examined its oxidase function, we will retain the more common name in this discussion. In the limited cases where both activities have been determined in the tissues of xanthinuric subjects, both the xanthine oxidase and dehydrogenase activities have been markedly reduced or absent.

Substrate Specificity

Xanthine oxidase is not a highly discriminating enzyme. It attacks a variety of substrates, including aldehydes, pteridines, and purines other than hypoxanthine and xanthine. 6-Mercaptopurine [64a] is oxidized to 6-thiouric acid. Allopurinol is oxidized to oxipurinol (alloxanthine) [65–67]. Aldehyde oxidase (EC 1.2.3.1), a closely related molybdenum enzyme, may also catalyze the oxidation of allopurinol to oxipurinol [68]. Xanthine oxidase does not attack methylxanthines other than the 1-methyl compound [69]. The human liver enzyme oxidizes 7-methylguanine to 7-methyl-8-hydroxyguanine [70].

Molecular Weight and Cofactors

The molecular weight of the enzyme from milk is 275,000 [71, 72] to 300,000 [73]; from pig liver, 288,000 [74]; and from chicken liver, 300,000 [75]. The bovine milk enzyme can be dissociated into subunits of 150,000 daltons in guanidine hydrochloride or acid [73]. Amino acid analyses of the purified milk enzyme disclose no unusual percentage composition [76]

Bovine milk xanthine oxidase contains 2 g-atom molybdenum, 2 FAD residues, 8 g-atom nonheme iron, and 8 mol labile sulfide per molecular weight of 300,000 [77]. Different Mo/FAD/Fe ratios have been reported for the enzyme obtained from mammalian intestine and liver and from avian liver [78], but these differences may reflect inadvertent removal of cofactors during purification.

As pointed out earlier molybdenum is an essential cofactor for xanthine oxidase activity [56, 57, 79], and deficiency of the molybdenum cofactor can result in the clinical picture of xanthinuria [33–36]. Recent studies have identified the molybdenum cofactor from xanthine oxidase as a novel pterin with an unknown substitution at the 6 position [80]. Activity of the cofactor requires that the pterin moiety be present in a reduced form. This cofactor is stored in the outer membrane of the

Figure 55-1 Conversion of hypoxanthine to xanthine and of xanthine to uric acid by xanthine oxidase. Structures are shown in their lactim forms.

XANTHINE OXIDASE

Hypoxanthine   Xanthine   Uric Acid

mitochondria [81]. In one xanthinuric patient who has been carefully studied no molybdenum cofactor could be detected in hepatic tissue [35]. Liver extract from this patient had no detectable xanthine oxidase activity even though the apoprotein was readily observable on immunodiffusion plates. The xanthine oxidase apoprotein could not be activated by incubation in vitro with molybdenum cofactor. Since the molybdenum cofactor required for xanthine oxidase activity is identical with that required for sulfite oxidase activity [80], it is not surprising that patients with dietary deficiency of molybdenum or congenital absence of molybdenum cofactor exhibit the simultaneous loss of xanthine oxidase and sulfite oxidase activities [33–36].

Flavin-free enzyme is devoid of xanthine oxygen reductase activity and can be reconstituted by a short incubation with FAD [82]

Mechanism of Action

The complexity of xanthine oxidase approaches that of enzyme systems with multiple intermediates, such as the respiratory chain. Electron flow during purine oxidation is first to molybdenum, which is reduced from valence of $+6$ to $+5$ or $+4$, from molybdenum to iron sulfide to FAD, and terminally from $FAD \cdot H_2$ to oxygen or, anaerobically, to methylene blue, cytochrome c, NAD, or other acceptor [79, 82, 83]. Under anaerobic conditions lower valence states of molybdenum are detected [77]. The inhibitory action of allopurinol and oxipurinol apparently involves complex formation with enzyme-bound molybdenum in the Mo^{4+} state and is dependent upon prior reduction of the enzyme by substrate [67]. Binding studies with [^{14}C]oxipurinol suggest that 1 mol purine is bound per mol of molybdenum, and therefore that there are two active sites per molecule of enzyme [67]. This accords with the observation that the enzyme can be dissociated into halves [73].

Distribution and Synthesis

The distribution of xanthine oxidase in mammalian and avian tissues varies from species to species [62, 84]. In most mammals, liver and small-intestinal mucosa are rich sources. In human beings these are the only tissues that normally show abundant xanthine oxidase activity, although significant traces of activity exist in kidney, spleen, and skeletal and heart muscle [85]. Activity has been detected inconstantly in marrow of leukemic children [86], but not in circulating normal leukocytes [85]. Although activity is undetectable in serum of normal persons, individuals with acute infectious hepatitis and jaundice may have striking levels of activity in serum [87, 88]. Xanthine oxidase has also been detected in the urine from patients with urinary tract infections, but not in sterile urine [89]. Xanthine oxidase is regularly present in human milk.

Hepatic xanthine oxidase activity falls sharply with induced dietary deficiencies of iron or molybdenum in experimental animals [91]. Hepatic xanthine oxidase levels can be altered tenfold by changes of dietary protein intake in the rat [92]. Restoration of normal values following a shift from a low to a normal protein diet involves accelerated synthesis of new enzyme protein. In human beings [93] hepatic xanthine oxidase activity is increased two- to fourfold following feeding of RNA, hypoxanthine, or 2-ethylamino-1,3,4-thiadiazole, or by the infusion of fructose.

Regulation of hepatic synthesis and degradation of xanthine oxidase has been studied in a number of animal models. Results of studies in an avian model suggest that synthesis is proportional to levels of messenger RNA, and formation of the active enzyme follows synthesis of an inactive precursor [94]. Degradation is preceded by the formation of a second inactive enzyme species [94]. The following agents or conditions have been demonstrated to affect xanthine oxidase synthesis or degradation or both in chicken liver: dietary protein, dietary amino acids, starvation, insulin, carbamyl reagents which are vitamin B_6 antagonists such as hydrazine and amino-oxy-acetate, 6-aminonicotinamide, reserpine, monoamine oxidase inhibitors, and melatonin (reviewed in [94]). In mammalian systems the following agents or conditions have been shown to alter hepatic xanthine oxidase activity: increase in dietary protein intake [92], vitamin E deficiency [95], malignant transformation [96], and androgen/estrogen balance [97].

METABOLIC DEFECTS IN XANTHINURIA

Xanthine Oxidase Activity

The findings of Dent and Philpot [1] that xanthine had replaced uric acid as the chief end product of purine metabolism in their patients, and of Dickinson and Smellie [2] that the plasma level of oxypurines was elevated, pointed toward a deficiency of xanthine oxidase activity in xanthinuria. Watts, Engleman, and associates [3] subsequently demonstrated less than 0.1 percent of normal activity in jejunal mucosa and liver biopsy material from their patient. Activity was deficient using xanthine, hypoxanthine, or xanthopterin as substrate and was not restored by addition of FAD, molybdenum, or ferric iron. Xanthine dehydrogenase activity measured with addition of methylene blue as electron acceptor was also missing. Residual activity was abolished by heating the homogenate to 100°C for several minutes and by the inhibitors allopurinol and pteridyl-aldehyde.

Deficiency of hepatic, intestinal, renal, or milk xanthine oxidase activity has been reported in 16 additional patients. Assay values have ranged from "no detectable activity" to more than 10 percent of control values (25 percent of control values in rectal mucosa). In a postpartum patient with xanthinuria, enzyme activity was missing in colostrum [98]. The report of missing activity in leukocytes in a Spanish family [16] is difficult to evaluate, since Watts et al. [85] were unable to detect any xanthine oxidase activity in intact or sonicated leukocytes from normal subjects. Assay methods differed in the various laboratories, and limits of accuracy and sensitivity were not given. Accordingly, it is not yet known whether the apparent variations in levels of residual activity represent methodological limitations, heterogeneity of the genetic and molecular defect, or assay of a xanthine oxidase–like activity which is unrelated to xanthine dehydrogenase.

Muscle Hypoxanthine and Xanthine Content

Concentrations of hypoxanthine and xanthine in skeletal muscle of two patients have been determined by Parker, Snedden, and Watts [55, 99] using quantitative high-resolution mass spectrometry. The results are given in Table 55-2. In another patient oxypurine content of muscle was also found increased (25).

Plasma Purine Concentration Values

Normal plasma contains from 0.1 to 0.3 mg oxypurines per deciliter [100, 101], of which hypoxanthine appears to be the major component. Plasma oxypurine concentrations have been recorded in 26 xanthinuric patients and have ranged from 0.1 to 0.96 mg/dl, with a mean of 0.56 mg/dl (Table 55-1). In one patient in whom the plasma oxypurines were analyzed separately, 90 percent was xanthine [17]; while in another patient only 35 percent was xanthine [28].

Serum uric acid concentrations ranged from 0 to 1.44 mg/dl with a mean of 0.55 mg/dl (Table 55-1). On a purine-restricted diet virtually all values were less than 1.0 mg and were often less than 0.5 mg/dl. An exception is the patient of Terhorst [11], commented on below.

Purine Excretion

Urinary excretion of xanthine normally ranges from 4.1 to 8.6 mg/day (average 6.1) and of hypoxanthine from 5.9 to 13.2 mg/day (average 9.7) [102]. Auscher et al. [21] report an increased quantity of 7-methylguanine (10 mg) and no detectable 7-methyl-8-hydroxyguanine in the urine of their xanthinuric subject. Castro-Mendoza et al. [16] report a sixfold increase in urinary adenine in one of their subjects. Adenine and guanine excretions have been normal whenever measured in other xanthinuric subjects [16, 21, 22].

In reported cases of xanthinuria the excretion of hypoxanthine plus xanthine ranged from 55 to 557 mg/day with a mean of 317 mg/day (Table 55-1). Uric acid excretion ranged from 0 to 81 mg/day with a mean of 23 mg/day. The urinary uric acid is at least in part of endogenous origin, for in the patient of Engleman et al. [^{14}C]xanthine given intravenously was converted to [^{14}C]uric acid found in serum and urine. It was calculated that the low level of xanthine oxidase activity detected in liver and intestinal mucosa was sufficient to account for the small amounts of uric acid excreted, 2 to 12 mg/day [4].

An exceptional case was reported by Terhorst [11] of a man with a serum urate concentration of 3.15 mg/dl who excreted 670 mg xanthine per day, but also 269 mg uric acid per day. Xanthine oxidase activity was not measured. Presumably his degree or type of deficiency of xanthine oxidase differs from most other reported patients.

In all patients the urinary excretion of xanthine has greatly exceeded that of hypoxanthine (average 79 percent xanthine,

range 42 to 95 percent) (Table 55-1). The ratio of xanthine to hypoxanthine is reduced in some xanthinuric subjects given allopurinol [4, 22] but not in others [21]. The predominance of xanthine may be attributable to a low level of residual activity of xanthine oxidase in some subjects.

An additional and perhaps more important explanation for the preponderance of urinary xanthine has emerged from isotope dilution studies of the dynamics of the miscible pools of hypoxanthine and xanthine in two xanthinuric patients. Engleman et al. [4] calculated an immediate xanthine pool of 144 mg, with a turnover of 264 mg/day. Their patient excreted 126 mg xanthine and only 52 mg hypoxanthine. In a second patient (Table 55-3), Bradford et al. [8] showed that the initial pool of xanthine was 73 mg and of hypoxanthine, 118 mg. Daily turnovers of these pools were calculated to be 276 and 960 mg, respectively. Of these quantities 79 percent of the xanthine turnover (219 mg) was excreted in urine, compared with only 5.7 percent of the hypoxanthine turnover (54 mg). Qualitatively similar results were obtained by Ayvazian and Skupp [103], who found utilization of administered purines greatest with adenine, intermediate with hypoxanthine, and least with xanthine.

These data disclose a considerable reutilization, or "salvage," of hypoxanthine, but little reutilization of xanthine in the tissues of human beings. Although the same phosphoribosyltransferase, which efficiently catalyzes the conversion of hypoxanthine and guanine to their respective ribonucleotides, also catalyzes the reutilization of xanthine, it does so at less than 1 percent of the rate of the reaction with hypoxanthine [104]. Accordingly, a much larger percentage of xanthine produced each day is permanently lost from the purine nucleotide pool, and in the absence (or severe deficiency) of xanthine oxidase activity is excreted unchanged.

Renal Handling of Xanthine

Studies showing a renal clearance of oxypurines approaching that of the glomerular filtration rate in the original patient of Dent and Philpot suggested to Dickinson and Smellie [2] that there were two metabolic defects, one of xanthine oxidase deficiency and another of renal tubular reabsorption of xanthine. A high renal clearance of oxypurines was also found in the patient of Engleman and associates [4]. However, when serum oxypurine levels were raised in normal subjects to those found in xanthinuria, either by administration of a xanthine oxidase inhibitor [105] or by infusion of xanthine [4], the clearance of oxypurines rose from normal values of 0.1 to 0.2 of the filtered load to 0.7 to 1.9 times the endogenous creatinine clearance. The high clearances found in xanthinuria may therefore be regarded as a normal response to the elevated serum levels of oxypurines. It is not necessary to postulate a separate tubular defect in handling of xanthine.

IDENTIFICATION OF XANTHINE STONES

Xanthine stones are rare. Hsieh and Hsu [49] found 1 pure xanthine calculus in 760 cases of urinary calculi. Herring [106] found 4 stones containing xanthine among 10,000 urinary calculi. Of these, 1 was pure xanthine (possibly the one obtained

Table 55-2 Concentration of hypoxanthine and xanthine in skeletal muscle from xanthinuric and control subjects

Subject	Hypoxanthine, ng/mg dry wt	Xanthine, ng/mg dry wt
Patient	350 ± 40	315 ± 30
Control	22 ± 3	<50
Patient	240 ± 30	450 ± 40
Control	29 ± 3	<50

SOURCE: Parker, Snedden, and Watts [55]

Table 55-3 Dimensions and turnover of purine pools in a xanthinuric patient

Purine	Miscible pool, mg	Turnover mg/day	Urinary excretions, mg/day	Turnover excreted/day, %
Hypoxanthine	118	960	54.5	5.7
Xanthine	72.5	276	219	79
Uric acid	19	11	6.5	61

SOURCE: Bradford et al. [8]

from Hsieh and Hsu), and 3 contained 5 to 19 percent xanthine.

The majority of xanthine stones have been described as brownish or brown-yellow, smooth, round or oval, friable, easily cut with a razor, and white and laminated inside. A few have been irregular in shape. They have ranged in size from a few millimeters in diameter to the size of a hen's egg [38] and in weight from "a few grains" to 3 g [18] or more [45]. Xanthine stones are nonopaque to x-rays unless calcium is trapped within the stone.

A variety of methods have been used for identification of xanthine in the stone. Most of these leave much to be desired, and identification should be based upon the highly sensitive and specific methods now available, including differential spectrophotometry, paper and column chromatography, and x-ray crystallography [49]. Methods for detection of xanthine in stones are given elsewhere [107]. A detailed description of the two types of crystal structure found in xanthine stones is given by Hsieh and Hsu [49].

Other Cases of Xanthine Stones

Xanthine stones have been found in patients ranging from 2 to 72 years of age [38–49]. Three-quarters of the subjects have been males. Two-thirds of the xanthine stones have been "pure" and one-third, "mixed." The mixed stones have frequently contained uric acid, calcium oxalate, or phosphate in addition to xanthine.

Except in the patients described in Table 55-1, urinary excretion of xanthine has not been measured, nor has hypouricemia been reported in any other patient with xanthine stones. The level of blood or serum urate has been normal [39, 45, 48] or even somewhat high [44] in the few patients studied, all of them adults. In two Duke Hospital patients who had passed mixed xanthine–uric acid stones, excretions of xanthine and of other urinary purines [108] were normal, and serum uric acid levels were not low. A third subject, a woman who had passed stones since early childhood, had pure xanthine stones at age 28. No uric acid analyses were performed, and she has since been lost to follow-up.

It is clear that not all patients who form xanthine stones have a deficiency of xanthine oxidase activity. Among the patients with xanthine stones are several about whom a strong suspicion exists that xanthine excretion may have been elevated.

Taylor and Taylor [45] reported a 60-year-old male who has xanthine stones weighing 12 g. If xanthine excretion were normal in this subject (6 mg/day), these stones would represent quantitative precipitation and retention of the cumulative urinary xanthine excretion of 6 years. In addition, seven cases of xanthine stone formation have involved children under age 15,

an age group in which the suspicion of an underlying metabolic defect is high. For example, the 2-year-old Taiwanese girl from whom surgeons removed a pure xanthine stone weighing 0.2 g [49] may very well have xanthinuria. Unfortunately the critical studies required to establish the presence or absence of xanthinuria have not been performed in these subjects.

Ichikawa [47] reported a 44-year-old male who had a left nephrectomy after a lengthy history of hematuria and negative study for urinary calculi. The kidney was grossly normal but on palpation was studded with numerous small nodules. The cut surface disclosed many small holes with brownish, granular concretions, which were round or oval, smooth, and friable. Chemical tests showed these to be xanthine, and some tubules contained xanthine casts.

GENETICS

Of the 45 known patients with xanthinuria, 17 have been females and 28 males. Only 3 have been blacks. The xanthinuric subject examined by Dent and Philpot [1] had 13 relatives who showed no abnormal excretion values of xanthine and had normal urinary values of uric acid. These included an only sister, both parents, and three surviving grandparents. None gave a history of renal stone, and the parents were not related. The paternal aunts and the three children of the patient of Ayvazian [5] had ample uric acid in urine; urinary oxypurines were not measured. The mother of the patient of Engleman and associates had normal uric acid and oxypurine levels in plasma and urine and normal xanthine oxidase activity in jejunal mucosa [4]. The patient has no sibs, and the father was not available for study. All 3 sibs of the patient of Sperling et al. [13] had normal plasma urate values.

The family reported by Cifuentes Delatte and Castro-Mendoza [6] included two brothers with near total replacement of urinary uric acid by xanthine and a sister who excreted 60 to 83 mg oxpurines per day in addition to 371 to 421 mg uric acid per day. In a second Spanish family described by Castro-Mendoza et al. [16], oxypurine excretion was normal in all sibs and offspring of xanthinuric subjects. In the study of a large xanthinuric kindred by Wilson and Tapia [20], 3 of 21 possible heterozygotes tested (Fig. 55-2) showed elevated urinary excretion values of oxypurines: 73, 38, and 116 mg/day on a low purine diet. All had normal plasma and urinary uric acid values.

Temperville et al. [29] studied a kindred with three xanthinuric subjects and found no relationship between the deficiency of xanthine oxidase and HLA type or the blood groups ABO, Rh, Pi, and Gm.

All known data are consistent with the interpretation that xanthinuria is an autosomal recessive disorder. No abnormalities have been detected in most of the presumed obligate heterozygotes, but in two families some possible heterozygotes showed elevated urinary oxypurine excretion values. These findings, taken together with the variable range of residual enzyme activity values, indicate probable heterogeneity of the genetic and molecular defect.

A deficiency of xanthine oxidase activity, probably genetic, has been discovered in a dachshund that produced xanthine urinary stones [109].

TREATMENT

Prevention of xanthine stone formation in predisposed individuals depends upon recognition of the low solubility of xanthine in acid solutions. The pK_{a1} of xanthine is 7.7, and the pK_{a2} is 10.6 [110]. Dent and Philpot [1] found that 100 ml normal urine at 26°C dissolved 6.7, 6.5, and 16.5 mg xanthine at a pH of 5.8, 7.0, and 8.1, respectively.

A high fluid intake and maintenance of a large urinary volume would appear to be indicated, as in all instances of stone formation. Oral alkali may be useful in specific instances, but the hazards of continuous alkali therapy must be borne in mind. Furthermore, alkalinization produces only a modest increase in the solubility of xanthine compared with its effect upon uric acid (Table 55-4) [50, 111]. Although xanthine excretion is independent of diet in normal subjects [108], dietary purines would no doubt add to the burden of xanthine excretion and should be limited. Allopurinol therapy in high doses reversed the xanthine/hypoxanthine ratio in two patients [4, 22] and might be useful in xanthinuric people with xanthine stones and residual xanthine oxidase activity. The potential advantage of substitution of the more soluble hypoxanthine for a portion of xanthine is clear from Table 55-4. Methylxanthines, such as caffeine and theophylline, are very much more soluble than xanthine and are not metabolized by xanthine oxidase. It is unnecessary to prohibit their use in xanthinuric subjects.

In managing patients with a combined deficiency of xanthine oxidase and sulfite oxidase, the neurologic symptoms resulting from sulfite oxidase deficiency are more devastating clinically than those resulting from xanthine oxidase deficiency. Consequently, most attention has been focused on the treatment of the neurologic symptoms and correction of the sulfite oxidase deficiency. In the patient reported by Abumrad et al. [36] treatment with 300 to 500 µg of ammonium molybdate per day replaced the dietary deficiency of molybdenum, corrected the disorders of both purine and sulfur metabolism, and markedly ameliorated the neurologic symptoms attributed to sulfite oxidase deficiency. The patient with no detectable

molybdenum cofactor in the liver was treated with oral ammonium molybdate (200 µg/day) without significant improvement in biochemical parameters or neurologic symptoms [35]. Allopurinol therapy with $NaHCO_3$ supplements was also tried in this patient because of xanthine calculi, but there was no reduction in the incidence of xanthine calculi or change in the ratio of xanthine to hypoxanthine in the urine. Restriction of methionine and cysteine reduced urinary output of abnormal sulfur metabolites but had no demonstrable effect on clinical symptoms during a short therapeutic trial.

Table 55-4 Solubility of purines in body fluids

Fluid	pH	Uric acid, mg/100 ml	Xanthine, mg/100 ml	Hypoxanthine, mg/100 ml
Serum	7.4	7	10	115
Urine	5	15	5	140
Urine	7	200	13	150

SOURCE: Klinenberg et al. [111]

REFERENCES

1. DENT CE, PHILPOT GR: Xanthinuria, an inborn error (or deviation) of metabolism. *Lancet* 1:182, 1954
2. DICKINSON CJ, SMELLIE JM: Xanthinuria. *Br Med J* 2:1217, 1959
3. WATTS RWE, ENGLEMAN K, KLINENBERG JR, SEEGMILLER JE, SJOERDSMA A: The enzyme defect in a case of xanthinuria. *Biochem J* 90:4P, 1964
4. ENGLEMAN K, WATTS RWE, LINENBERG JR, SJOERDSMA A, SEEGMILLER JE: Clinical, physiological, and biochemical studies of a patient with xanthinuria and pheochromocytoma. *Am J Med* 37:839, 1964
5. AYVAZIAN JH: Xanthinuria and hemochromatosis. *N Engl J Med* 270:18, 1964
6. CIFUENTES-DELATTE L, CASTRO-MENDOZA HJ: Xanthinuria familiar. *Rev Clin Esp* 107:244, 1967
7. FREZAL J, MALASSENET R, CARTIER P, FESSARD C, ROY C, REY J, LAMY M: Sur un cas de xanthinurie. *Arch Fr Pediatr* 24:129, 1967
8. BRADFORD MJ, KRAKOFF IH, LEEPER R, BALIS ME: Study of purine metabolism in a xanthinuric female. *J Clin Invest* 47:1325, 1968
9. CHALMERS RA, JOHNSON M, PALLIS C, WATTS RWE: Xanthinuria with myopathy (with some observations on the renal handling of oxypurines in the disease). *Q J Med* 38:493, 1969
10. CHALMERS RA, WATTS RWE, BITENSKY L, CHAYEN J: Microscopic studies on crystals in skeletal muscle from two cases of xanthinuria. *J Pathol* 99:45, 1969
11. TERHORST B: Xanthinsteine und Xanthinurie: Ein kasuisticher Beitrag. *Z Urol Nephrol* 62:37, 1969

Figure 55-2 Kindred of a family with hereditary xanthinuria in which heterozygote expression was found. *(From Wilson and Tapia [20]. Used by permission.)*

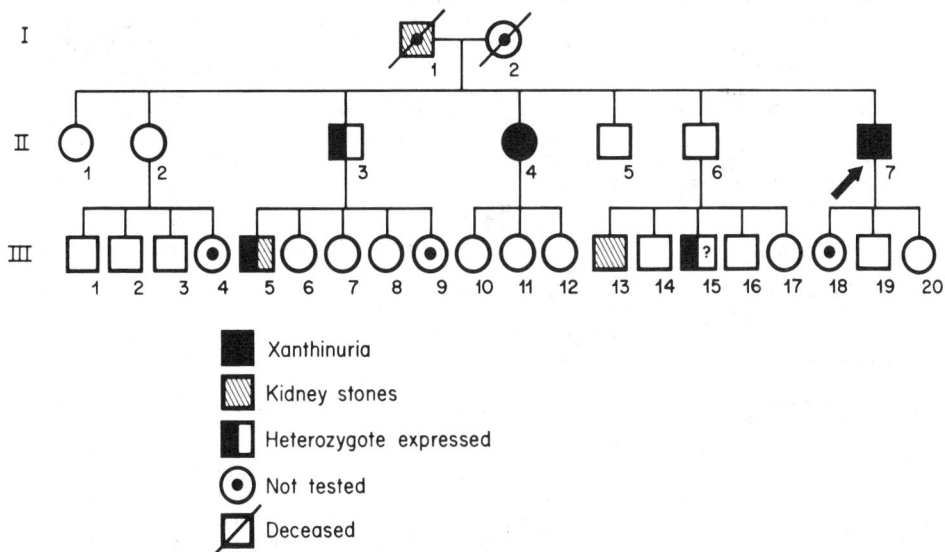

Xanthinuria

Kidney stones

Heterozygote expressed

Not tested

Deceased

12. KUTTER D, HUMBEL R, BISDORFF J: Biochemische Untersuchungen bei einem typischen Fall von Xanthinurie. *Dtsch Med Wochenschr* 95:1269, 1970

13. SPERLING O, LIBERMAN UA, FRANK M, DeVRIES A: Xanthinuria: An additional case with demonstration of xanthine oxidase deficiency. *Am J Clin Pathol* 55:351, 1971

14. CURNOW DH, MASAREL JR, CULLEN KM, McCALL MG: Xanthinuria discovered in population screening. *Br Med J* 1:403, 1971

15. CLERC M, BARBIER M: Lecalcul renal d'un sujet deficitaire en xanthine-oxydase. *Bull Soc Pathol Expt* 64:527, 1971

16. CASTRO-MENDOZA HJ, CIFUENTES-DELATTE LC, RAPADO YAR: Una neuva observacion de xanthinuria familiar. *Rev Clin Exp* 124:341, 1972

17. SORENSEN LB, TESAR JT, ELLMAN MH, COLWELL N: A new case of xanthinuria. *Am J Med* 53:690, 1972

18. FRAYHA RA, SALTI IS, HAICLAR GIA, AL-KHALIDI U, HEMADY K: Hereditary xanthinuria and xanthine urolithiasis: An additional 3 cases. *J Urol* 109:871, 1973

19. DE VOOGHT HJ, VON DE KAMP JJP, VAN GERDEREN HH, BERNINI LF, BOOGAART AM: Een xanthinesteen by een kind met xanthinurie: Enkele beschouwingen over een Zeldaure "inborn error of metabolism." *Ned Tijdschr Geneeskd* 117:976, 1973

20. WILSON DM, TAPIA HK: Xanthinuria in a large kindred, in Sperling D, DeVries A, Wyngaarden JB (eds): *Purine Metabolism in Man*. Plenum, New York, 1974, p 343

21. AUSCHER C, PASQUIER C, MERCIER N, DELBARRE F: Urinary excretion of 6 hydroxylated metabolite and oxypurines in a xanthinuric man given allopurinol or thiopurinol, in Sperling D, DeVries A, Wyngaarden JB (eds): *Purine Metabolism in Man*. New York, Plenum, 1974, p 663

22. HOLMES EW, MASON DH, GOLDSTEIN LI, BLOUNT RE, KELLEY WN: Xanthine oxidase deficiency: Studies in a previously unreported case. *Clin Chem* 20:1076, 1974

23. SIMMONDS HA, LEVIN B, CAMERON JS: Variations in allopurinol metabolism by xanthinuric subjects. *Clin Sci Mol Med* 47:173, 1974

24. RAPADO A, CASTRO-MENDOZA HJ, CASTRILLO JM, FRUTOS M, CIFUENTES-DELATTE L: Xanthinuria as a cause of hypouricemia in liver disease. *Br Med J* II:560, 1975

25. ISAACS H, HEFFRON JJA, BERMAN L, BADENHORST M, PICKERING A: Xanthine, hypoxanthine, and muscle pain. Histochemical and biochemical observations. *S Afr Med J* 49:1035, 1975

26. KITAMURA T, KAWAMURA J, KITAGAWA R, OGAWA A: Xanthine stone and xanthinuria associated with retrocaval ureter: Report of a case and a review of the literature. *Jpn J Urol* 67:670, 1976

27. AUSCHER C, PASQUIER C, DE GERY A, WEISSENBACH R, DELBARRE, D: Xanthinuria: Study of a large kindred with familial urolithiasis and gout. *Biomed Exp* 27:57, 1977

28. CARTIER P, PERIGNON JL: Xanthinuria. *Nov Presse Med* 7:1381, 1978

29. TEMPERVILLE B, GODIN M, DUBOIS D, FILLASTRE JP: A propos de trois observations de xanthinurie familiale: Revue de la litterature. *Sem Hop Paris* 55:1899, 1979

30. MITNICK PD, BECK LH: Hypouricemia and malignant neoplasms. *Arch Intern Med* 139:1186, 1979

31. CURIEL P, BANDINELLI R: Pregnancy in a woman with xanthinuria: Study of amniotic fluid uric acid. *Am J Obstet Gynecol* 134:721, 1979

32. MORIMI PL, BANDINELLI R, CURIEL P: Hypouricemia and xanthinuria. Observation of 3 cases. *Minerva Med* 70:873, 1979

33. DURAN M, BEEMER FA, HEIDEN CVD, KORTELAND J, DE BREC PK, BRINK M, WADMAN SK: Combined deficiency of xanthine oxidase and sulfite oxidase: A defect of molybdenum metabolism or transport. *J Inher Metab Dis* 1:175, 1978

34. HEIDEN CVD, BEEMER FA, BRINK W, WADMAN SK, DURAN M: Simultaneous occurrence of xanthine oxidase and sulfite oxidase deficiency. A molybdenum dependent inborn error of metabolism. *Clin Biochem* 12:206, 1979

35. JOHNSON JL, WAUD WR, RAJAGOPALAN KV, DURAN M, BEEMER FA, WADMAN SK: Inborn errors of molybdenum metabolism: Combined deficiencies of sulfite oxidase and xanthine dehydrogenase in a patient lacking the molybdenum cofactor. *Proc Natl Acad Sci* 77:3715, 1980

36. ABUMRAD NN, SCHNEIDER AJ, STEEL DR, ROGERS LS: Acquired molybdenum deficiency *Clin Res* 27:774A, 1979

37. MARCET A: *An Essay on the Chemical History and Medical Treatment of Calculous Disorders*. 2d ed., rev. and enlarged. London, Strahan and Spottiswoode for Longman, 1819

38. KRETSCHMER HL: Xanthine calculi: Report of a case and a review of the literature. *J Urol* 38:183, 1937

39. RATNER M, STRASBERG A: A case of xanthine calculosis. *Can Med Assoc J* 40:563, 1939

40. HYMAN A, LEITER HE: A case of xanthine calculi. *J Mount Sinai Hosp* 8:84, 1941

41. BUTT AJ, HOLLIMAN HE, JR: Xanthine calculus: A case report. *J Urol* 52:89, 1944

42. GERSH IJ, MELTZER HL: Xanthine urinary calculi: Two cases. *J Urol* 55:169, 1946

43. BERMAN LS: Twenty-second case of xanthine urinary calculus. *J Urol* 60:420, 1948

44. PEARLMAN CK: Xanthine urinary calculus *J Urol* 64:799, 1950

45. TAYLOR WN, TAYLOR JN: Xanthine calculus: Case report. *J Urol* 68:659, 1952

46. MACKEY JF, JR: Xanthine calculus. *Mo Med* 50:617, 1953

47. ICHIKAWA T: Xanthine calculi of kidney. *J Urol* 72:770, 1954

48. JORDON H: Multiple Xanthinsteinbildung: Bericht uber einen Fall. *Dtsch Z Verdau Stoffwechselkr* 15:143, 1955

49. HSIEH HF, HSU TC: Xanthine calculus: A case report. *J Formosan Med Assoc* 62:83, 1963

50. SEEGMILLER JE: Hereditary xanthinuria, in Bondy PK, Rosenberg LE (eds): *Duncan's Diseases of Metabolism*. Philadaelphia, Saunders, 1974, p 739

51. MUDD SH, IRREVERRE F, LASTER L: Sulfite oxidase deficiency in man: Demonstration of the enzymatic defect. *Science* 156:1599, 1967

52. IRREVERRE F, MUDD SH, KEIZER WD, LASTER L: Sulfite oxidase deficiency: Studies of a patient with mental retardation, dislocated lenses, and abnormal urinary excretion of S-sulfo-L-cysteine, sulfite, and thiosulfate. *Biochem Med* 1:187, 1967

53. SHIH VE, ABROMS IF, JOHNSON JL, CARNEY M, MANDELL R, ROBB RM, CLOHERTY JP, RAJAGOPALAN KV: Sulfite oxidase deficiency: Biochemical and clinical investigations of a hereditary metabolic disorder in sulfur metabolism. *N Engl J Med* 297:1022, 1977

54. CHALMERS RA, WATTS RWE, PALLIS C, BITENSKY L, CHAYEN J: Crystalline deposits in striped muscle in xanthinuria. *Nature* 221:170, 1969

55. PARKER R, SNEDDEN W, WATTS RWE: The mass-spectrometric identification of hypoxanthine and xanthine ("oxypurines") in skeletal muscle from two patients with congenital xanthine oxidase deficiency (xanthinuria). *Biochem J* 115:103, 1969

56. JOHNSON JL, RAJAGOPALAN KV, COHEN HJ: Molecular basis of the biological function of molybdenum. Effect of tungsten on xanthine oxidase and sulfite oxidase in the rat. *J Biol Chem* 249:859, 1974

57. COHEN HJ, JOHNSON JL, RAJAGOPALAN KV: Molecular basis of the biological function of molybdenum. Developmental patterns of sulfite oxidase and xanthine oxidase in the rat. *Arch Biochem Biophys* 164:440, 1974

58. SEEGMILLER JE, ENGLEMAN K, KLINENBERG JR, WATTS RWE, SJOERDSMA A: Xanthine oxidase and iron. *N Engl J Med* 270:534, 1964

59. STIRPE E, DELLA CORTE, E: The regulation of rat liver xanthine oxidase: Conversion in vitro of the enzyme activity from dehydrognease (type D) to oxidase (type O). *J Biol Chem* 244:3855, 1969

60. DELLA CORTE E, STIRPE F: The regulation of rat liver xanthine oxidase: Involvement of thiol groups in the conversion of the enzyme activity from dehydrogenase (type D) into oxidase (type O) and purification of the enzyme. *Biochem J* 126:739, 1972

61. BATELLI MG, LORENZONI E, STIRPE F: Milk xanthine oxidase type D (dehydrogenase) and type O (oxidase). *Biochem J* 131:191, 1973

62. KRENITSKY TA, TUTTLE JV, CATTAU EL JR, WONG P: A comparison of the distribution and electron acceptor specificities of xanthine oxidase and aldehyde oxidase. *Comp Biochem Physiol* 49B:687, 1974

63. WAUD WR, RAJAGOPALAN KV: The mechanism of conversion of rat liver xanthine dehydrogenase from an NAD^+-dependent form (type D) to an O_2-dependent form (type O). *Arch Biochem Biophys* 172:365, 1976

64. KRENITSKY TA, TUTTLE JV: Xanthine oxidase activities: Evidence for two catalytically different types. *Arch Biochem Biophys* 185:370, 1978

64a. SILBERMAN HR, WYNGAARDEN JB: 6-Mercaptopurine as substrate and inhibitor of xanthine oxidase. *Biochim Biophys Acta* 47:178, 1961

65. FEIGELSON P, DAVIDSON JD, ROBINS RK: Pyrazolopyrimidines as inhibitors and substrates of xanthine oxidase. *J Biol Chem* 226:993, 1957

66. ELION GB: Enzymatic and metabolic studies with allopurinol. *Ann Rheum Dis* 25:608, 1966

67. MASSEY V, KOMAI H, PALMER G, ELION G: On the mechanism of inactivation of xanthine oxidase by allopurinol and other pyrazolo [3,4-d] pyrimidines. *J Biol Chem* 245:2837, 1970

68. HUH K, YAMAMOTO I, GOHDA E, IWATA H: Tissue distribution and characteristics of xanthine oxidase and allopurinol oxidizing enzymes. *Jpn J Pharmacol* 26:719, 1976

69. DE RENZO, EC: Chemistry and biochemistry of xanthine oxidase. *Adv Enzymol* 17:293, 1956

70. SKUPP S, AYVAZIAN JH: Oxidation of 7-methylguanine by human xanthine oxidase. *J Lab Clin Med* 73:909, 1969

71. ANDREWS P, BRAY RC, EDWARDS, P, SHOOTER KV: The chemistry of xanthine oxidase. II. Ultracentrifuge and gel-filtration studies on the milk enzyme. *Biochem J* 93:627, 1964

72. HART LI, McGARTOLL MA, CHAPMAN HR, BRAY RC: The composition of milk xanthine oxidase. *Biochem J* 116:851, 1970

73. NELSON CA, HANDLER P: Preparation of bovine xanthine oxidase and the subunit structures of some iron flavoproteins. *J Biol Chem* 243:5368, 1968

74. BRUMBY PE: Ph.D. thesis. University of Sheffield, 1963

75. RAJAGOPALAN KV, HANDLER P: Purification and properties of chicken liver xanthine dehydrogenase. *J Biol Chem* 242:409, 1967

76. BRAY RC, MALMSTROM BG: The chemistry of xanthine oxidase. 12. The amino acid composition. *Biochem J* 93:633, 1964

77. MASSEY V, BRUMBY PE, KOMAI H, PALMER G: Studies on milk xanthine oxidase: Some spectral and kinetic properties. *J Biol Chem* 244:1682, 1969

78. MEHLER AH: *Introduction to Enzymology.* New York, Academic, 1957, p 178

79. BRAY RC, CHISHOLM J, HART LI, MERIWETHER LS, WATTS DC: Studies on the composition and mechanism of action of milk xanthine, in Slater EC (ed): *Flavines and Flavoproteins.* Amsterdam, Elsevier, 1966, p 117

80. JOHNSON JL, HAINLINE BE, RAJAGOPALAN KV: Characterization of the molybdenum cofactor of sulfite oxidase, xanthine oxidase, and nitrate reductase. *J Biol Chem* 255:1783, 1980

81. JOHNSON JL, JONES HP, RAJAGOPALAN KV: In vitro reconstitution of demolybdosulfite oxidase by a molybdenum cofactor from rat liver and other sources. *J Biol Chem* 252:4994, 1977

82. KOMAI H, MASSEY V, PALMER G: The preparation and properties of deflavo xanthine oxidase. *J Biol Chem* 244:1692, 1969

83. OLSON JS, BALLOU DP, PALMER G, MASSEY V: The mechanism of action of xanthine oxidase. *J Biol Chem* 249:4363, 1974

84. AL-KHALIDI, UAS, CHAGLASSIAN TH: The species distribution of xanthine oxidase. *Biochem J* 97:318, 1965

85. WATTS RWE, WATTS JEM, SEEGMILLER LE: Xanthine oxidase activity in human tissues and its inhibition by allopurinol (4-hydroxypyrazolo [3,4-d] pyrimidine). *J Lab Clin Med* 66:688, 1965

86. DUNN JT, WYNGAARDEN JB: Unpublished data

87. SHAMMA'A MH, NASRALLAH S, CHAGLASSIAN T, KACHADURIAN AK, AL-KHALIDI UAS: Serum xanthine oxidase: a sensitive test of acute liver injury. *Gastroenterology* 48:226, 1965

88. GILER S, SPERLING O, BROSCH S, URCA I, DEVRIES A: Serum xanthine oxidase in jaundice. *Clin Chim Acta* 63:37, 1975

89. GILER S, HENIG EF, URCA I, SPERLING O, DEVRIES A: Urine xanthine oxidase activity in urinary tract infection. *J Clin Pathol* 31:444, 1978

90. MORGAN EJ: The distribution of xanthine oxidase. *Biochem J* 20:1282, 1926

91. BRAY RC: Xanthine oxidase, in Boyer P, Lardy H, Myrbach K (eds): *The Enzymes,* 2d ed. New York, Academic Press, 1963, vol. VII, p 533

92. ROWE PB, WYNGAARDEN JB: The mechanism of dietary alterations in rat hepatic xanthine oxidase levels. *J Biol Chem* 241:5571, 1966

93. MARCOLONGO R, MARINELLO E, POMPUCCI G, PAGANI R: The role of xanthine oxidase in hyperuricemic states. *Arthritis Rheum* 17:430, 1974

94. THOMPSON JM, NICKELS JS, FISHER JR: Synthesis and degradation of xanthine dehydrogenase in chick liver: In vivo and in vitro studies. *Biochim Biophys Acta* 568:157, 1979

95. CATIGNANI GL, CHYTIL F, DARBY WJ: Vitamin E deficiency: Immunochemical evidence for increased accumulation of liver xanthine oxidase. *Proc Natl Acad Sci* 71:1966, 1974

96. PRAJDA N, MORRIS HP, WEBER G: Imbalance of purine metabolism in hepatomas of different growth rates as expressed in behavior of xanthine oxidase. *Cancer Res* 36:4639, 1976

97. LEVINSON DJ, CHALKER D: Rat hepatic xanthine oxidase activity. Age and sex specific differences. *Arthritis Rheum* 23:77, 1980

98. OLIVER I, SPERLING O, LIBERMAN UA, FRAN M, DEVRIES A: Deficiency of xanthine oxidase activity in colustrum of xanthinuric female. *Biochem Med* 5:279, 1971

99. PARKER R, SNEDDEN W, WATTS RWE: The quantitative determination of hypoxanthine and xanthine ("oxypurines") in skeletal muscle from two patients with congenital xanthine oxidase deficiency (xanthinuria). *Biochem J* 116:317, 1970

100. SEGAL S, WYNGAARDEN JB: Plasma glutamine and oxypurine content in patients with gout. *Proc Soc Exp Biol Med* 88:342, 1955

101. JORGENSEN S: Hypoxanthine and xanthine accumulated in stored human blood: Determination of relative amounts by spectrophotometry. *Acta Pharmacol Toxicol* 11:265, 1955

102. WEISSMANN B, BROMBERG PA, GUTMAN AB: The purine bases of human urine. II. Semiquantitative estimation and isotope incorporation. *J Biol Chem* 224:423, 1957

103. AYVAZIAN JH, SKUPP S: The study of purine utilization and excretion in a xanthinuric man. *J Clin Invest* 44:1248, 1965

104. KELLEY WN, ROSENBLOOM FM, HENDERSON JF SEEGMILLER JE: Xanthine phosphoribosyltransferase in man: Relationship to hypoxanthine-guanine phosphoribosyltransferase. *Biochem Biophys Res Commun* 28:340, 1967

105. KLINENBERG JR, GOLDFINGER S, MILLER J, SEEGMILLER JE: The effectiveness of a xanthine oxidase inhibitor in the treatment of gout. *Arthritis Rheum* 6:779, 1963

106. HERRING LC: Observations on the analysis of ten thousand urinary calculi. *J Urol* 88:545, 1962

107. WYNGAARDEN JB: Xanthinuria, in Stanbury JB, Wyngaarden JB, Fredrickson DS (eds): *The Metabolic Basis of Inherited Disease,* 1st ed. New York, McGraw-Hill, 1960, p 761

108. WEISSMANN B, BROMBERG PA, GUTMAN AB: The purine bases of human urine. I. Separation and identification. *J Biol Chem* 224:407, 1957

109. DELBARRE F, HOLTZER A, AUSCHER C: Xanthine urinary lithiasis in a dachshund: Deficiency, probably genetic, of the xanthine oxidase system. *C R Acad Sci [D] (Paris)* 269:1449, 1969

110. BERGMANN F, DIKSTEIN S: The relationship between spectral shifts and structural changes in uric acids and related compounds. *J Am Chem Soc* 77:691, 1955

111. KLINENBERG JR, GOLDFINGER SF, SEEGMILLER JD: The effectiveness of a xanthine oxidase inhibitor allopurinol in the treatment of gout. *Ann Intern Med* 62:639, 1965

56

HEREDITARY OROTIC ACIDURIA

WILLIAM N. KELLEY

1. *Hereditary orotic aciduria type I is a rare genetic disorder usually characterized by failure of normal growth and development, hypochromic anemia associated with a megaloblastic marrow resistant to the usual hematinic agents, and excessive urinary excretion of orotic acid. A second form of the disease (type II) has been described, which is indistinguishable clinically but which exhibits a different enzymatic defect.*
2. *The excessive excretion of orotic acid in the homozygous type I patient is secondary to a block in its further metabolism because of deficient activities of orotate phosphoribosyltransferase and orotidine-5'-phosphate decarboxylase. There is also overproduction of orotic acid, perhaps due to the accumulation of PP-ribose-P. In hereditary orotic aciduria type II, orotidine-5'-phosphate decarboxylase is deficient, but orotate phosphoribosyltransferase is increased in activity.*
3. *The patient with hereditary orotic aciduria is a "pyrimidine auxotroph," requiring pyrimidine replacement therapy for survival. Uridine alone results in a hematologic remission, marked improvement in growth and development, and a decrease in urinary orotic acid. Glucocorticoid therapy is partially effective, but the mechanism of this response is obscure.*
4. *Hereditary orotic aciduria is transmitted as an autoso-*
mal trait. Heterozygotes have partial enzyme deficiencies of orotate phosphoribosyltransferase and orotidine-5'-phosphate decarboxylase and excrete increased amounts of orotic acid in the urine but are asymptomatic.*
5. *The loss of two adjacent enzyme activities in hereditary orotic aciduria type I is consistent with a defect in a genetic control mechanism. The most likely explanation for this observation is that orotate phosphoribosyltransferase and orotidine-5'-phosphate decarboxylase activities relate to a single multifunctional protein or that the two enzymes are closely related in a complex requiring the integrity of both proteins for maintenance of normal activity.*

Hereditary orotic aciduria is a rare genetic disorder of pyrimidine metabolism usually characterized by retarded growth and development, hypochromic anemia associated with a megaloblastic marrow unresponsive to usual hematinic therapy, and excessive urinary excretion of orotic acid [1–4]. Replacement with uridine leads to a clinical and hematologic remission and to a reduction in the excretion of orotic acid. Studies of hemic cells, liver homogenates, and fibroblasts grown in tissue culture have demonstrated reduced activities of both orotate

1202

phosphoribosyltransferase (OPRT) and orotidine-5'-phosphate decarboxylase (ODC), sequential enzymes which catalyze the conversion of orotic acid to uridine-5'-phosphate (Fig. 56-1) [5–7]. More recently a single patient with an isolated deficiency of ODC activity has been discovered, indistinguishable clinically from the prototype disorder [2]. In this discussion hereditary orotic aciduria will be used as a general description, with the specific disorders designated as type I (double enzyme defect) and type II (isolated deficiency of ODC).

Hereditary orotic aciduria is the prototype of disordered pyrimidine metabolism and has several features which lend added importance to its investigation [8]: (1) It represents the only specific disorder of pyrimidine nucleotide synthesis so far elucidated in humans. (2) The phenotype can be partially simulated by the use of a pharmacologic agent. (3) Pyrimidine auxotrophism in humans is perhaps the clearest example of a human auxotrophism. (4) The "pyrimidine starvation" of hereditary orotic aciduria illustrates the importance of intracellular metabolic control mechanisms.

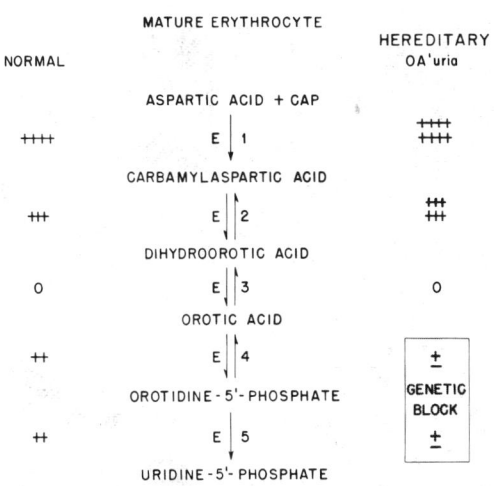

Figure 56-1 Site of the double enzyme block in hereditary orotic aciduria, as measured in the mature erythrocyte. Increased activities of aspartate transcarbamylase and dihydro-orotase represent release of end-product repression. Dihydro-orotic dehydrogenase activity is absent in the mature erythrocyte. E1, aspartate transcarbamylase; E2, dihydro-orotase; E3, dihydro-orotic dehydrogenase; E4, orotate phosphoribosyltransferase; E 5, orotidine-5'-monophosphate decarboxylase.

CLINICAL FEATURES

Only nine patients with hereditary orotic aciduria are known to the author. Seven are related to an enzymatic deficiency of OPRT or ODC or both. Two are atypical and appear to represent different disorders. Case reports of two will be summarized.[1]

Patient J.R. [1]. This white male infant, the product of a normal delivery at full term, weighed 8 lb, 9 oz at birth and appeared to be in good health until the age of 3 months. He was then observed to be pale, lethargic, and somnolent and had repeated respiratory infections and chronic diarrhea, with large, pale, foul-smelling stools. His hemoglobin was 6 g/dl. This anemia failed to respond to iron, ascorbic acid, folic acid, cobalamin, or crude liver concentrate.

When first studied at age 9 months, the patient was pale and weak but well developed and well nourished. The scleras appeared blue, and the edge of the liver and tip of the spleen were palpable. There was no atrophy of his tongue. There was outward torsion of the left tibia but no other skeletal abnormalities. No neurologic abnormalities were found. Laboratory studies revealed a severe hypochromic anemia (hemoglobin, 6.7 g; erythrocytes, 2.8 million/mm^3), with striking anisocytosis and poikilocytosis (Fig. 56-2). There was leukopenia (leukocytes, 2050/mm^3) with monocytosis, but a normal platelet count. The bone marrow was hypercellular, and there were striking abnormalities of the megaloblastic type in cells of both the granulocytic and erythrocytic series. Urinalysis was normal, except for a moderate number of crystals which were later proved to be orotic acid.

The clinical course of patient J.R. has been presented in detail elsewhere [1]. Appropriate diagnostic studies, including failure of therapeutic response, excluded deficiency of cobalamin, folic acid, pyridoxine, or iron as contributing to the anemia. Studies of hemoglobin abnormalities, thalassemia, and erythremic myelosis (di Guglielmo's syndrome) were also negative. There was a partial hematologic remission during glucocorticoid therapy without reversal of the bone marrow abnormalities. Throughout his course, large numbers of crystals precipitated from the urine on standing or,

occasionally, within the urinary tract. On several occasions urethral obstruction, and on one occasion right ureteral obstruction, occurred. These crystals were identified as orotic acid by a series of tests described elsewhere [1]. Orotic acid excretion was variable but usually was in the range of 800 to 1400 mg/24 h. When the child was treated with a yeast extract containing a mixture of pyrimidine nucleotides, there was a prompt reticulocytosis, rise of hemoglobin to normal, disappearance of marrow megaloblasts, and striking reduction in urinary orotic acid (Fig. 56-3). The prompt improvement in his general health was equally marked. He gained weight for the first time in 18 months and recovered from an apparent retardation in walking, talking, and general activity. After approximately 3 months, nucleotide therapy was discontinued because it was poorly tolerated. It was planned to reinstitute treatment with other preparations, but there was a prompt relapse. Death occurred shortly thereafter, secondary to varicella (Fig. 56-3). Autopsy showed only generalized varicella.

The patient's three sibs and his parents exhibited no clinical or hematologic abnormalities. Studies on the R family are presented in the section on "Genetics."

Patient D.G. [9, 10, 11]. This male infant, a quarter-caste Maori from New Zealand, weighed 9 lb, 2 oz at birth and seemed to grow and develop normally for the first 2 to 3 months. Beginning at about age 3 months he appeared pale and apathetic and was retarded in motor development. At age 13 months, at which time he could not sit unsupported, he received a short course of treatment with chloramphenicol for bronchopneumonia. He was discovered to be severely anemic (hemoglobin, 4.6 g/dl) and leukopenic (leukocytes, 2400/mm^3). Further investigation revealed a megaloblastic marrow and a low serum iron (11 μg/dl), but there was no hematologic response to iron, folic acid, cobalamin, pyridoxine, or thyroxine. Additional studies seemed to exclude blood loss, malabsorption, hepatic disease, or renal disease as contributing causes of his illness.

When examined at age 17 months at the Auckland Hospital, he was a pale, lethargic child with an alternating strabismus, weighing 21½ lb (< 3d percentile). Although there were no specific neurologic abnormalities, his general physical and mental development appeared to be retarded. He was unable to sit up alone but could maintain a sitting position. There was sparse growth of short, fine hair; and his fingernails failed to grow over a period of several months. The spleen tip was palpable. There was no glossitis. The

---

[1] Detailed case reports of other patients with this disorder may be found in the corresponding chapter of the previous edition of this book.

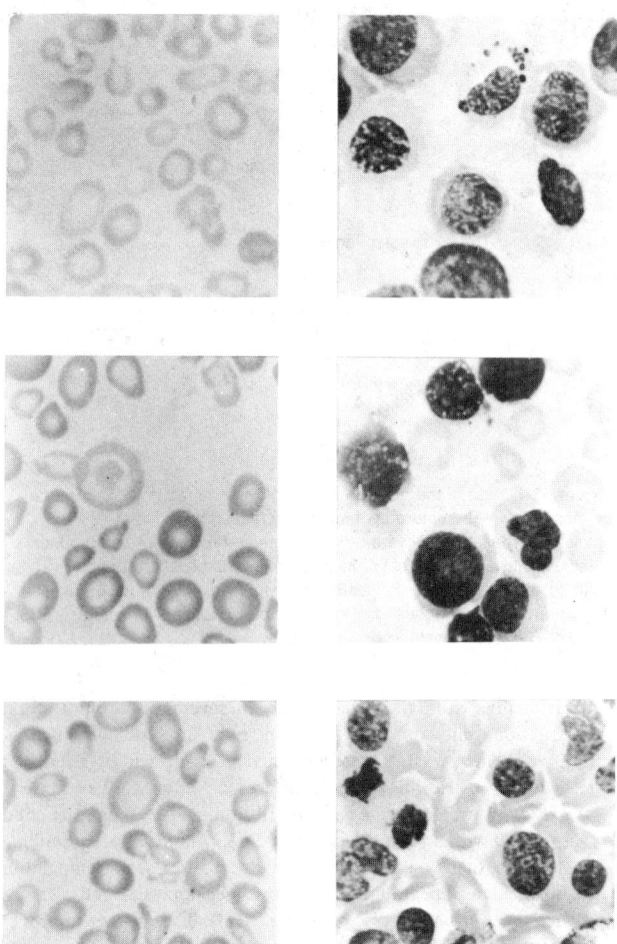

Figure 56-2 Peripheral blood *(left)* and bone marrow preparations *(right)* from three patients with untreated hereditary orotic aciduria. *A.* Patient J.R.; *B.* patient D.G.; *C.* patient J.P. (of Table 56-1.)

initial hemoglobin was 8.0 g/dl, and the smear showed hypochromic cells with marked anisocytosis and poikilocytosis (Fig. 56-2). The presence of megaloblastic changes in the bone marrow was confirmed. There was histamine-fast achlorhydria. Serum levels of cobalamin and folic acid were normal. On standing a urine specimen developed a heavy, flocculent precipitate of fine, needle-shaped crystals (Fig. 56-4) with the ultraviolet absorption spectrum of orotic acid. The excretion of orotic acid averaged 1.15 g daily. Absence of OPRT and ODC activities was demonstrated in frozen erythrocytes. A brief trial of cytidylic acid therapy was given, following which the patient was treated with oral uridine (Fig. 56-5). There was a rapid hematologic response to uridine, most marked when the initial dose of 0.75 g was increased to 1.5 g daily (see Fig. 56-6). One month after the beginning of uridine therapy, the hemoglobin was 13.7 g/dl, the hematocrit was 44 percent, and the bone marrow was normoblastic. Orotic acid excretion decreased to approximately 0.2 and 0.3 g/24 h. There was an accompanying improvement in general health, with weight gain, increased strength and activity, and renewed growth of hair and nails. Relapse occurred on uracil therapy (1.5 g/day). Treatment was continued at a dose of approximately 150 mg uridine per kilogram body weight in divided doses. Although there was initial rapid improvement in intellectual skills on uridine, his IQ (Wechsler scale) at age 7 was in the range of 73 to 81. Slight alternating convergent strabismus continues, and there are small areas of scleral pigmentation. On uridine feeding, his hemoglobin, platelets, and leukocytes have remained normal; orotic acid excretion has stabilized in the range of 0.4 to 0.6 g/day; and serum urate and immunoglobulins have been normal [10]. More recent studies conducted while receiving uridine revealed

an elevated excretion rate of uric acid [722 to 1092 mg/24 h or 13.4 to 20.2 mg/(kg · day)] with an increased uric acid clearance (30 ml/min) [11]. No renal complications have resulted from this level of excretion of orotic acid or uric acid in spite of crystalluria.

Extensive family studies have not as yet been carried out. The father, of Irish descent, has reduced levels of OPRT and ODC in his erythrocytes. A hydrocephalic sib died of a subdural hematoma. No orotic acid was found in his urine. At the time of writing, no studies have been carried out on the patient's mother, who is three-fourths Maori, or on an older male sib, who is reported to be in good health.

Some of the clinical and laboratory findings in the reported patients with hereditary orotic aciduria have been summarized in Table 56-1. Seven have been male and two female. With the exception of C.P., the patients appeared to be normal at birth. Typically, poor growth and development were evident during the first few months of life, with lassitude, pallor, and nonspecific "failure to thrive." No characteristic neurologic picture was found, although three patients (D.G., J.P., T.H.) had strabismus. Splenomegaly was noted in two. Other abnormalities seen in single patients were kyphoscoliosis, hernias, abnormalities of the hair and nails, outward torsion of the left tibia, a notched eyelid margin, optic atrophy, retinal degeneration, dilated lateral ventricles, and atrophy of the frontal cortex. Patient D.B. deviated most radically from the above pattern in that growth and development were normal. She presented with fatigue and symptoms related to crystalluria at age 7½. Although the clinical description is abbreviated, the atypical Spanish patient, J.G., also seemed to have normal somatic development when studied at age 10. Patients D.G., T.H., J.P., and J.G. have impaired intellectual development (IQs about 80), whereas patient D.B. is superior in mental capacity (IQ 133).

The most specific early finding was severe hypochromic anemia, with marked anisocytosis and poikilocytosis associated with erythroid hyperplasia and atypical megaloblastic changes in the bone marrow. An equally consistent finding was leukopenia (except in J.G.), but thrombocytopenia was not observed (Table 56-1). In each patient the hematologic abnormalities failed to respond to an array of hematinic agents. In patients J.R. and J.P., glucocorticoid therapy improved the anemia significantly without reversing the megaloblastic changes in the marrow. This form of treatment was not tried on the other seven patients. In each patient except S.Y., the degree of orotic aciduria was sufficient to result in spontaneous crystallization in urine specimens (Fig. 56-4); in three patients (J.R., J.P., and D.B.), partial obstruction of the urinary tract occurred. The response to uridine replacement therapy was prompt, including reticulocytosis; rise of hemoglobin; reversal of megaloblastosis; and improvement in general health, growth, and development (except in patient D.B., in whom no blunting of growth and development had occurred). Leukopenia also was reversed, but one patient required larger doses of uridine for effective therapy. A partial hematologic remission was obtained with folic or folinic acid in patient J.G. When measured quantitatively, the urinary excretion of orotic acid was found to decrease but not to disappear (Figs. 56-3 and 56-5). In only one family (J.G.) has the clinical disorder appeared more than once. The atypical disease in these sibs is probably different from hereditary orotic aciduria. The inheritance of hereditary orotic aciduria will be considered in detail in the section on "Genetics." Consanguinity was documented only in the M. family.

Table 56-1 Clinical findings in patients with hereditary orotic aciduria

Patient; sex	Onset of symptoms	Age at diagnosis	Clinical features	Physical examination	Urine and urinary tract	Hb	WBC	Platelets	Response to treatment
J. R.; M 1	3 mo	1 yr	Weakness, lethargy, diarrhea, repeated infections; mental and motor development apparently normal	Pallor, splenomegaly, outward torsion of left tibia	Gross crystalluria; ureteral and urethral obstruction	6.7	2050	260,400	Partial response to glucocorticoids; early response to pyrimidines; death from varicella off treatment
D. G.; M 9, 10	3 mo	1½ yr	Failure to thrive, retarded motor development, alternating strabismus	Splenomegaly, strabismus, weakness, fine short hair	Heavy crystalluria	4.6	2400	220,000	Good response to uridine, 1500 mg/day orally
J. P.; M 11	7 mo	1½ yr	Failure to thrive, strabismus, slow motor development; at age 1½ yr, tested at 9-mo level (Gesell)	Pallor and strabismus	Crystalluria with partial ureteral obstruction	4.8	1500	213,000	Partial response to glucocorticoids; good response to uridine, 1500 mg/day orally
T. H.; F 6	2 mo	10 mo	Weakness, bilateral strabismus, normal size	Heart murmur of interventricular septal defect; strabismus	Crystalluria	7.8	3300	570,000	Good response to uridine, 1500 mg/day orally
D. B.; F 14	6½ yr	7½ yr	Fatigue, back and flank pain; normal mental and physical development	Small notch at margin of right upper eyelid; soft systolic murmur over pulmonic area	Crystalluria and hematuria; symptoms probably related to crystalluria	7.4	3200	300,000	Response to uridine, 150 mg/(kg · day); leukopenia response last
C. P.; M 2	Birth	4 mo	Failure to thrive, generalized hypertonicity	Kyphoscoliosis, hernias, scaphoid skull	Crystalluria	6.3	2600	364,000	Early response to uridine, 150 mg/(kg · day); death from meningitis and pneumonia
P. M.; M 2, 3	5½ mo	6-7 mo	Failure to thrive with retarded motor development	Seborrheic dermatitis and fine dry hair	Crystalluria	7.4	?	?	Response to uridine, 15 mg/(kg · day)
J. G.; M. 15, 16	3 mo	5 yr	Anemia, normal growth and development	Not described	Crystalluria	8.5	10,000	270,000	Partial response to folic and folinic acids; no apparent response to uridine
S. Y.; M 17	3 mo	9 mo	Mental retardation; megaloblastic anemia	Motor retardation		8.2	5250		Not recorded

BIOCHEMISTRY OF PYRIMIDINES

Biosynthesis

The sequence of events leading to the synthesis of pyrimidine nucleotides, as in the purine pathway, was initially elucidated in nonmammalian organisms. Subsequently, the validity of this pathway has been largely confirmed in mammalian cells including those from human beings. The pyrimidine nucleotides can be synthesized *de novo* or by the reutilization of preformed pyrimidine bases or ribonucleosides.

Pathway *de Novo* The synthesis of uridine-5′-phosphate (UMP) *de novo* is summarized in Fig. 56-7 and several excellent reviews are available [19–21]. The initial step unique to pyrimidine biosynthesis *de novo* in mammalian species is the formation of carbamyl phosphate (CAP). CAP is an unstable, high-energy intermediate which serves as the donor of the car-

bamyl moiety in the synthesis of citrulline as part of the urea cycle and of carbamylaspartate, an intermediate in the formation of pyrimidines. In aqueous solution at physiologic pH, CAP is in equilibrium with phosphate and cyanate. Its enzymatically governed carbamylation reactions with amino groups are analogous to chemical reactions of cyanate to yield the same products.

In prokaryotes the synthesis of CAP required for the synthesis of pyrimidines and the urea cycle is catalyzed by one enzyme [22]. In eukaryotes the synthesis of CAP is catalyzed by two different enzymes [23]. Carbamyl-phosphate synthetase I (CPS I) catalyzes the synthesis of CAP to be utilized largely in the urea cycle (designated CAParg).

$$2 \text{ ATP} + \text{NH}_4^+ + \text{HCO}_3^- \xrightarrow[\text{Mg}^{2+}]{\text{acetylglutamate}} \text{CAParg} + 2 \text{ AMP} + P_i$$

This enzyme is located in the inner membrane of the mitochondrion of the liver and, to a lesser extent, the kidney and the small intestine [24]. It utilizes ammonia as a nitrogen donor and is activated by *N*-acetylglutamate or one of its analogues

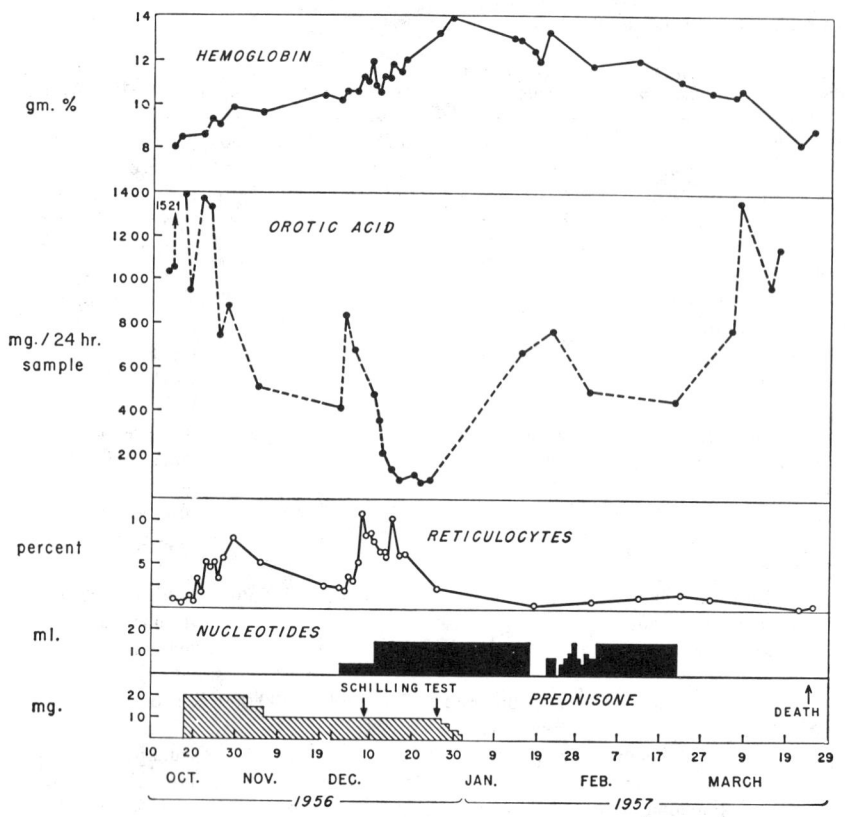

Figure 56-3 Changes in hemoglobin, reticulocytes, and urinary orotic acid in patient J.R. during treatment with prednisone and a mixture of nucleotides (uridylic acid, 115 mg/ml; cytidylic acid, 269 mg/ml).

[25]. This enzyme appears at the stage of metamorphosis during which the ammonotelic tadpole becomes a ureotelic frog [26].

Carbamyl-phosphate synthetase II (CPS II) catalyzes the synthesis of CAP to be utilized primarily for the formation of pyrimidine nucleotides *de novo* (designated CAPpyr). This carbamyl-phosphate synthetase, originally described in mushrooms [27], has now been demonstrated in microorganisms [28], yeasts [29], plants [30], and animal tissues [31–33]. It is found in most fetal [34] and adult tissues, although its activity is highest in the GI tract, spleen, thymus, and testis [35]. CPS II has the greatest affinity for glutamine as a nitrogen donor, although NH_4^+ may also serve as an effective substrate [36].

$$2 \text{ ATP} + \text{glutamine} + HCO_3^- + H_2O \xrightarrow[Mg^{2+}]{K^+}$$
$$CAPpyr + 2 \text{ ADP} + P_i + \text{glutamate}$$

The K_m of the enzyme in mouse spleen is 5×10^{-5} M for glutamine, 1×10^{-2} M for HCO_3^-, and 3 to 5×10^{-3} M for Mg ATP [37, 38].

In mammalian tissues CPS II is cytoplasmic and is found in a complex with the second and third enzymes of pyrimidine biosynthesis *de novo*, aspartate transcarbamylase and dihydroorotase [39–51]. One gene appears to code for a single multienzyme polypeptide; this multienzyme protein has been referred to as complex A, CAD or, more recently, pyr 1–3 [21]. The subunit molecular weight of this multifunctional protein is 200,000 to 220,000, with a native structure that appears to reflect multiples of three subunits, i.e., a trimer, hexamer, nonomer, etc. Aspartate transcarbamylase (20,000 daltons) is located on one end of the molecule and the integrity of this segment seems to be required for aggregation of the 200,000- to 220,000-dalton monomer described above [47].

Presumably the very low activity of CPS II and the low intracellular concentration of CAPpyr are compensated and explained by existence of the multifunctional protein with aspartate transcarbamylase and dihydro-orotase activity in addition to CPS II activity. For example, the concentration of pyrimidine-specific CAP in *Neurospora* is less than the molar concentration of the enzyme complex [52].

The channeling of CAP into either the pyrimidine pathway or the urea cycle, depending on how and where it is synthesized, is not complete under all circumstances. In rat liver slices, some mitochondrial CAP may escape into the cytoplasm [53, 54]. A genetically induced block in the utilization of CAPpyr for pyrimidine biosynthesis in *Neurospora* may lead to its utilization in the synthesis of arginine; similarly a block in the utilization of CAParg for arginine biosynthesis in this organism may lead to the availability of this compound for pyrimidine synthesis [55]. Finally, absence of CPS II activity in yeast does not lead to a requirement for pyrimidines [29]. This sug-

Figure 56-4 Sediment of crystalline orotic acid in the urine of patient D.G.

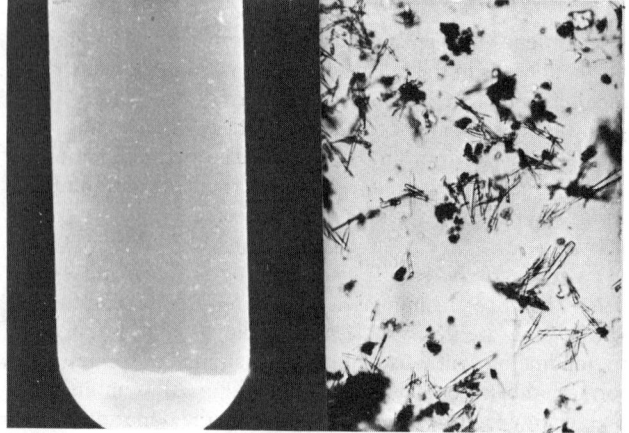

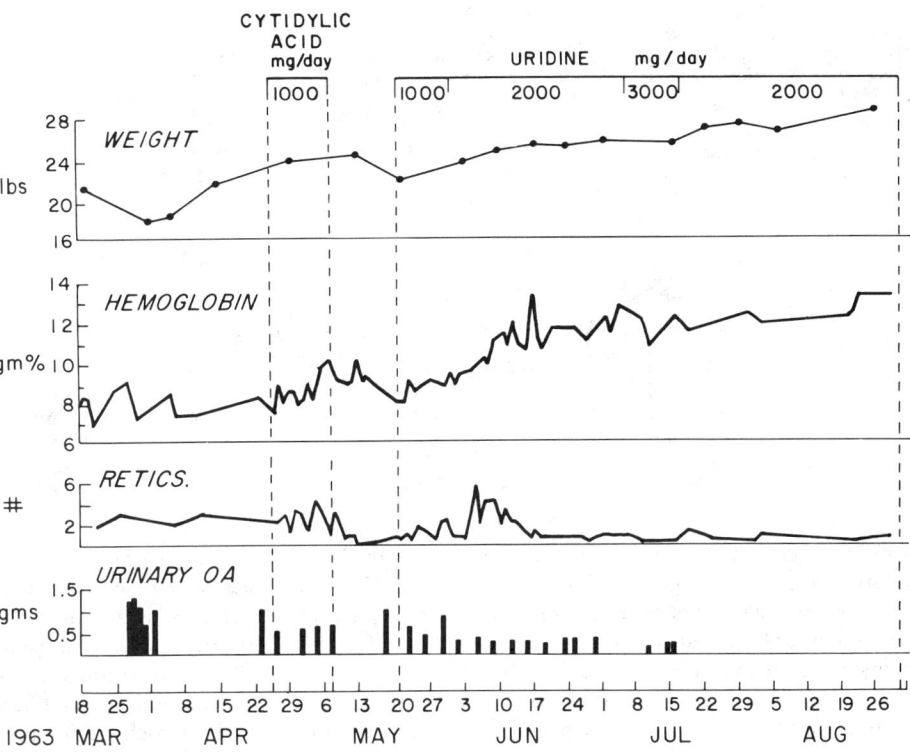

Figure 56-5 Changes in weight, hemoglobin, reticulocytes, and urinary orotic acid in patient D.G. during treatment with cytidylic acid and with uridine.

D.G. 19 Mos. Hereditary Orotic Aciduria

gests that CAP synthesized by CPS I can be utilized for pyrimidine biosynthesis under these conditions. There is evidence based on clinical observations to be described later that CAParg in human cells can also be utilized for the synthesis of pyrimidines in certain circumstances.

CAP can also be formed by the phosphorolytic cleavage of citrulline [56]. Carbamate kinase catalyzes the interconversion of carbamate and CAP in microorganisms, but this reaction does not appear to be an important source of CAP [57, 58].

$$NH_2COO^- + ATP \longrightarrow CAP + ADP$$

The possibility that "carbamyl carriers" may exist, such as citrulline, or, by analogy with bacterial studies, creatine, allantoin, and urea [59], has not been confirmed.

Aspartate transcarbamylase (EC 2.1.3.2., ATCase) catalyzes the irreversible carbamylation of L-aspartate by CAP to form carbamylaspartate.

$$CAP + L\text{-aspartate} \longrightarrow carbamylaspartate (CAA)$$

This enzyme is widely distributed in mammalian tissues. Highest activities are found in the testis, spleen, intestine, bone marrow, and liver [60]. The crystalline enzyme from *Escherichia coli* has been extensively studied in several laboratories as a model system for allosteric interactions [61–64]. It is available in gram quantities and can be dissociated readily into separable catalytic and regulatory subunits. Activity is reduced by sulfhydryl-reactive agents and also is inhibited by certain inorganic anions [65]. Aspartate transcarbamylase has been studied in bacteria, fungi, higher plants [66], birds, Ehrlich ascites cells [67], rat, and human beings [68].

The mammalian enzyme differs significantly from the enzyme from *E. coli*. The K_m for CAP ranges from $2 \times 10^{-6} M$ to $3 \times 10^{-5} M$ and for aspartate from 2 to $8 \times 10^{-3} M$ for the enzyme from rat liver [69], mouse spleen [70], and Ehrlich ascites tumor cells [39]. The kinetic mechanism [70, 71] which

is ordered and sequential with CAP binding first, aspartate binding second, carbamylaspartate dissociating first, and phosphate dissociating second, is the same as in *E. coli*.

The major fate of carbamylaspartate is ring closure to form dihydro-orotic acid, a reaction catalyzed by dihydro-orotase (EC 3.5.2.3).

Carbamylaspartate ⟶ dihydro-orotic acid

This reaction, described originally in bacteria [72–74], has been confirmed in a variety of other cells including human hemic cells [68, 75–77], intestinal mucosa [78], and cultured fibroblasts [7]. In human beings, the enzyme can be conveniently assayed in circulating erythrocytes and leukocytes [68]. In human tissue, activity appears to be particularly high in fat [79].

The reaction catalyzed by dihydro-orotase is reversible with

Figure 56-6 Hemoglobin and reticulocyte response in patient T.H. following uridine administration. Lack of response to treatment with iron, vitamin D, cobalamin, and folic acid is demonstrated. *(From Rogers et al. [6]. Used by permission.)*

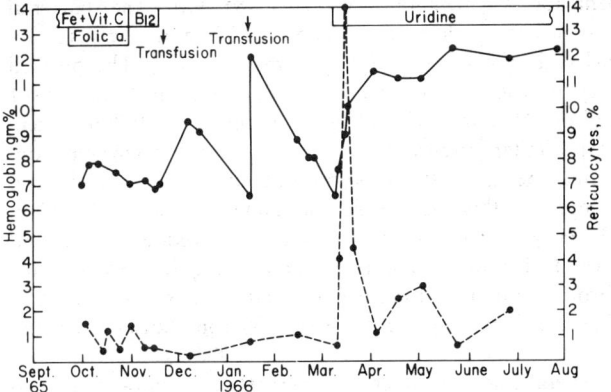

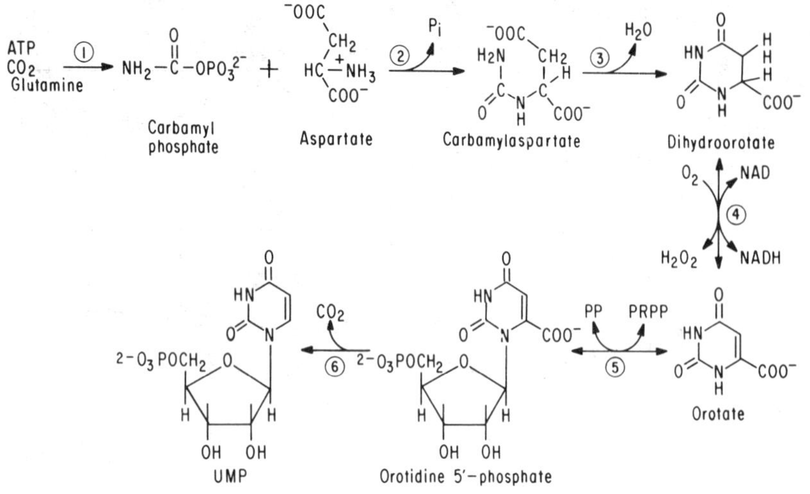

Figure 56-7 Pyrimidine biosynthesis *de novo. 1.* Carbamyl-phosphate synthetase, *2.* aspartate transcarbamylase, *3.* dihydro-orotase, *4.* dihydro-orotic acid dehydrogenase, *5.* orotate phosphoribosyltransferase, and *6.* orotidine-5'-monophosphate decarboxylase.

a pH-independent equilibrium constant ($K_{eq} = $ [L-DHO]/[L-CAsp^{2-}][H$_3$O$^+$]) of $1.51 \pm 0.02 \times 10^6$ liters/mol at 37° [80]. The Michaelis constants are highly pH dependent [80], but at physiologic pH they range from 1.2 to 2.8×10^{-4} M for carbamylaspartate [81] and 0.4 to 2.5×10^{-4} M for L-dihydro-orotate [81]. The hydrolysis of dihydro-orotate to carbamylaspartate resembles the cleavage of a peptide bond, and hence the mechanism may be similar to that catalyzed by carboxypeptidase A [82], a zinc-containing enzyme. Indeed, pure dihydro-orotase from *Clostridium oroticum* contains zinc [83], which is necessary for catalytic activity [84]. No requirement for divalent metals has been noted for the enzyme from any other source. In its action the enzyme is also comparable with hydropyrimidine hydrase, an enzyme which catalyzes the hydrolysis of dihydrouracil and dihydrothymine to their respective carbamyl compounds [85].

5-Carboxymethylhydantoinase catalyzes the reversible ring closure of carbamylaspartate to form the corresponding hydantoin.

Carbamylaspartate ⟶ 5-carboxymethylhydantoin

It was described first in *Zymobacterium oroticum* [72]. It has limited distribution in bacteria and is absent in rat liver and human leukocytes and erythrocytes [68]. There is no evidence to support its participation in mammalian pyrimidine metabolism.

Dihydro-orotic acid is reversibly oxidized to orotic acid to form the pyrimidine ring in a reaction catalyzed by dihydro-orotic acid dehydrogenase (EC 1.3.3.1) [86]. Dihydro-orotic dehydrogenase has been crystallized from *Z. oroticum* and studied extensively in several laboratories as a model for the behavior of metalloflavoproteins [85–92]. The bacterial enzyme has a molecular weight of 120,000 and contains 2 mol FMN, 2 mol FAD, and 4 g-atoms iron [88]. The purified enzyme from *Neurospora* is a lipoprotein which contains 1 mol of FMN and 1.2 mol of ferric iron per 120,000 protein [93]. Similar studies are not available on the enzyme from human beings. Little is known about the natural electron acceptor of this enzyme from a mammalian source [39, 94]. The enzyme from rat liver produces superoxide radicals, and several electron acceptors including ubiquinone and cytochrome b provide entry into the electron transport chain [95]. The iron may play a role in the electron transport process [93].

Several lines of evidence suggest that dihydro-orotic acid

dehydrogenase is separate from both the first three enzyme activities of pyrimidine biosynthesis *de novo,* which exist as pyr 1–3, as well as the last two, pyr 5,6. It is associated with the outer surface of the inner membrane of the mitochondrion [96, 97] in contrast to the cytosolic location of the other five enzyme activities of the pathway. This location of the enzyme in the mitochondrion presumably allows the product of pyr 1–3 in the cytosol, dihydro-orotate, to pass freely through the outer mitochondrial membrane to reach dihydro-orotic acid dehydrogenase, and the orotic acid produced by the reaction is readily able to diffuse back into the cytosol to serve as a substrate for the next reaction. Presumably, if this reaction catalyzed by dihydro-orotic acid dehydrogenase occurred in the cytosol, any accumulation of dihydro-orotate would tend to reverse the previous reaction catalyzed by dihydro-orotase, thus forcing the enzyme to catalyze an inefficient accumulation of carbamylaspartate. In addition to the unique intracellular location of this enzyme as compared to the others of pyrimidine biosynthesis *de novo,* mutants at the locus coding for dihydro-orotic acid dehydrogenase in Chinese hamster cells have a selective deficiency of the enzyme with no alteration in the activities of either pyr 1–3 or pyr 5,6 [98].

Dihydro-orotic acid dehydrogenase activity is found in all tissues of the rat. It is highest in liver, heart, kidney, and brain [99]. While the activity in human tissue is also high in heart, kidney, and liver [79], it is found also in human leukocytes [68], intestinal mucosa [78], and cultured fibroblasts [100]. The absence of dihydro-orotic acid dehydrogenase activity in the mature human erythrocyte and its presence in reticulocytes [68, 101] suggest that the enzyme is lost during cell maturation, with a resulting block in pyrimidine synthesis *de novo* at the stage of orotic acid formation [101]. Dihydro-5-azaorotic acid is a specific inhibitor of the enzyme [102]. The K_m in mammalian tissue for dihydro-orotate ranges from 1 to 2×10^{-4} M [39, 99].

Orotate phosphoribosyltransferase (EC 2.4.2.10, OPRT) catalyzes the formation of orotidine-5'-phosphate from orotic acid and 5-phosphoribosyl-1-pyrophosphate (PP-ribose-P) in the presence of Mg^{2+}.

Orotate + PP-ribose-P $\xrightarrow{Mg^{2+}}$ orotidine-5'-phosphate + PP$_i$

This reaction, which is specific for 2,6-diketopyrimidines, is similar to that which is involved in the conversion of free purine bases to purine ribonucleotides. The enzyme is widely distributed in rodent [103] and human [104] tissues and appears to be located entirely in the cytoplasm.

Considerable evidence now supports the concept that OPRT activity is closely related to the catalytic activity of the next enzyme in the pathway, orotidine-5'-phosphate decarboxylase (EC 4.1.1.23, ODC). The first evidence for this was provided by the description of the deficiency of both OPRT and ODC in orotic aciduria [5]. Subsequently, mutant cells produced in the laboratory have also shown a parallel increase [105, 106] or decrease [105–107] in the activity of both OPRT and orotidine-5'-phosphate. In each case, the activities associated with pyr 1–3 and dihydro-orotic acid dehydrogenase have been unaffected by the mutation. The two enzyme activities may reside in a single multifunctional protein similar to pyr 1–3, or the two enzymes may exist as a complex whose aggregation is dependent on the integrity of both enzymes. This multienzyme protein or complex has been termed complex U or pyr 5,6 [21].

Recent studies of this putative multienzyme protein or complex have failed to define clearly its molecular nature. Working with mouse Ehrlich ascites cells, Trout and Jones [51] noted four different aggregation states of pyr 5,6 with apparent molecular weights of 45,400, 78,000, 92,800, and 118,000. They have interpreted the 45,400-dalton and 92,800-dalton species as the monomer and dimer, respectively, with the 78,000-dalton and 118,000-dalton species postulated to represent the aggregation of the monomer and dimer with an as yet unidentified molecule with a molecular weight of 29,000. These studies led the authors to suggest that OPRT and ODC activities exist as part of the same multifunctional protein.

Multiple molecular species of OPRT and ODC have also been noted in human tissues [108, 109]. Brown and O'Sullivan [109] have provided evidence that human OPRT and ODC exist as an enzyme complex rather than as a multifunctional protein. They have purified both enzyme activities from human liver [110]. Further studies of the activities from erythrocytes have led the authors to suggest that OPRT exists as a polypeptide with a subunit molecular weight of 13,000, while ODC is a separate peptide with a subunit molecular weight of 20,000. Each enzyme appears to exist as a dimer, and a putative dimer of ODC with one subunit of OPRT is also described. The native enzyme complex is proposed to be a dimer of both OPRT and ODC with a molecular weight of 62,000. Further studies will be necessary to resolve these apparent differences between the OPRT and ODC in mouse and human tissues.

The K_m values of orotic acid have ranged from 2×10^{-6} M to 5×10^{-5} M [39, 111–120] while the K_m for PP-ribose-P ranges from 2×10^{-5} M to 1×10^{-4} M [39, 111–113, 121]. Although orotate appears to be the best substrate for the mammalian enzyme, it also functions with a number of other compounds including uracil, xanthine, and uric acid [122]. The enzyme-catalyzed reaction in yeast proceeds through the use of a bi bi ping pong kinetic mechanism under conditions of optimal Mg^{2+} concentrations [123, 124]. Reproducible, but very low, activity of this enzyme has been found in mature human erythrocytes. Although activities of the enzyme in leukocytes have been low and variable in sonicated cell preparations, more reproducible results are obtained when cells are lysed by freeze-thawing. This reaction is the only known pathway for orotidine-5'-phosphate synthesis, a small amount of which is irreversibly dephosphorylated to orotidine.

ODC catalyzes the irreversible decarboxylation of orotidine-5'-phosphate (OMP) to uridine-5'-phosphate (UMP).

$$OMP \longrightarrow UMP + CO_2$$

As noted above, in most studies this enzyme has been found in the cytosol as a complex or multifunctional protein with the enzyme catalyzing the preceding step, OPRT. Monophasic, biphasic, and triphasic kinetics have been reported. Two Michaelis constants were noted for OMP using the enzyme from yeast [125] and human beings [126]; the low K_m was 4.5 $\times 10^{-7}$ M, whereas the high K_m was 2.4×10^{-6} M. More recently, Brown et al. [127] reported triphasic kinetic constants which were related to the molecular size of the protein; i.e.; 2.5×10^{-5} M for monomer, $3 \times 10^{\times 6}$ M for dimer, and 6×10^{-7} M for tetramer in human erythrocytes. Tax and Veerkamp [128] also report triphasic kinetics of human erythrocyte ODC with values of 8.2×10^{-8} M, 1.7×10^{-6} M, and 3.3×10^{-5} M using conditions where concentrations of OMP were $< 3 \times 10^{-6}$ M, although no attempt was made to correlate these with molecular size. In contrast, only a single K_m (3×10^{-7} M) was noted for OMP in the four different molecular species of pyr 5,6 from Ehrlich ascites cells [129]. A single K_m of 9×10^{-6} M also has been noted for preparations of the enzyme from cow brain [130].

The reactions leading to the synthesis of UMP are summarized in Fig. 56-7.

Alternative Synthetic Pathways *de Novo* Uracil undergoes a series of degradative reactions in mammalian systems to form β-alanine, carbon dioxide, and ammonia. In theory, by reversal of these steps, uracil might be formed *de novo* from simple precursors by a pathway not involving orotic acid. Evidence is reviewed elsewhere that this pathway does not normally operate in mammalian tissues [131]. In a preliminary report, a high rate of incorporation of carbamyl-β-alanine ribonucleotide and dihydrouridylic acid into ribonucleic acid of avian liver was found [116]. This possible alternate pathway remains to be confirmed.

Reutilization Pathway This term refers to the utilization of preformed pyrimidine bases available from nucleotide turnover or from dietary sources. The formation of UMP from uracil and uridine represents a potentially important reutilization process (Fig. 56-8). Uracil may be converted directly to UMP in the presence of PP-ribose-P by the reaction catalyzed by OPRT [117–119].

$$Uracil + PP\text{-}ribose\text{-}P \xrightarrow{Mg^{2+}} UMP + PP_i$$

In mammalian tissue the more important pathway involves the prior formation of uridine. The conversion of uracil to uridine is catalyzed by uridine phosphorylase (EC 2.4.2.3).

$$Uracil + ribose\text{-}1\text{-}phosphate \longrightarrow uridine + P_i$$

This enzyme is widely distributed in mammalian tissues [120,

Figure 56-8 Pyrimidine nucleotide interconversions. *7.* CMP kinase, *8.* nucleoside diphosphate kinase, *9.* CTP synthetase, *10.* uridine phosphorylase, and *11.* uridine kinase.

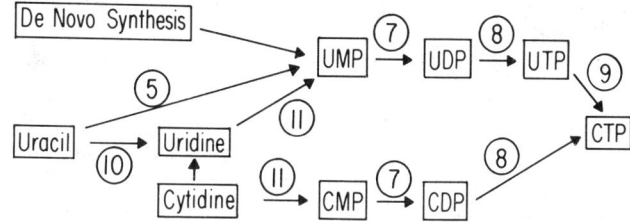

132]. It is also active for the 5-halogenated derivatives and 5-methyluracil but is not active for cytosine, orotic acid, thymine, or the purine bases [117, 133, 134]. A separate enzyme, deoxythymidine phosphorylase, catalyzes the conversion of uracil or thymine to the deoxyribonucleoside derivative in the presence of deoxyribose-1-phosphate [135–137].

$$\text{Thymine + deoxyribose-1-phosphate} \longrightarrow \text{deoxythymidine} + P_i$$

A second reaction involves the conversion of thymine to deoxythymidine in the presence of deoxyuridine and deoxythymidine synthetase.

$$\text{Thymine + deoxyuridine} \longrightarrow \text{deoxythymidine + uracil}$$

Uridine is converted to UMP in a reaction catalyzed by uridine kinase (EC 2.7.1.48).

$$\text{Uridine + Mg ATP} \longrightarrow \text{UMP + Mg ADP}$$

This enzyme, which has been extensively studied in Ehrlich ascites tumor cells [138], can also use cytidine, 5-fluorouridine, 5-fluorocytidine, and 6-azauridine, but not 5-methyluridine, deoxyuridine, deoxythymidine, or purine nucleosides. An alteration in this enzyme appears to account, at least in some cases, for resistance to 5-fluorouracil [139, 140] and possibly 6-azauridine [141].

Thymidine may be converted to thymidine-5'-phosphate in the reaction catalyzed by thymidine kinase (EC 2.7.1.75).

$$\text{Deoxythymidine + Mg ATP} \longrightarrow \text{dTMP + Mg ADP}$$

The enzyme is also widely distributed in human tissues. Both uridine kinase [142] and thymidine kinase [143, 144] are present in fetal and adult liver in different forms. Deoxycytidine is converted to its deoxyribonucleotide derivative by an enzyme which is separate from thymidine kinase [145]. Deoxycytidine or cytidine also can be deaminated to the respective uridine derivatives by a pyrimidine nucleoside deaminase which is present in a variety of animal tissues but apparently is particularly high in human liver [146–148]. Most of the halogenated derivatives are also substrates for the enzyme.

Interconversion

The pyrimidine ribonucleoside monophosphates (as well as the deoxyribonucleoside derivatives) can be phosphorylated to the di- and triphosphates (Fig. 56-8). Pyrimidine deoxynucleoside monophosphates, as well as the nucleoside monophosphates, are converted to the diphosphate derivatives by at least two enzymes in mammalian tissue [149]. The substrate specificity for one enzyme is CMP, UMP, and dCMP and for the other, dTMP and dUMP. Adenosine-5'-triphosphate or dATP can function as the phosphate donor; dUMP is converted to dTMP in a reaction catalyzed by thymidylate synthetase and requiring tetrahydrofolate and magnesium.

$$\text{dUMP + 5,10-methylene-5,6,7,8-tetrahydrofolate} \xrightarrow{Mg^{2+}}$$
$$\text{dTMP + 7,8-dihydrofolate}$$

This enzyme is not regulated in mammalian cells by the level of dTTP within the cell but appears to be controlled by the availability of folic acid derivatives [150]. Amethopterin blocks this step as a result of inhibition of dihydrofolate reductase necessary for the formation of the tetrahydrofolate derivative. The deamination of dCMP to form dUMP occurs in a reaction catalyzed by deoxycytidylate deaminase. The diphosphate derivatives are converted to the triphosphates in a reaction requiring

another nucleoside triphosphate and nucleoside diphosphokinase. This enzyme has been well studied from several different mammalian sources [151, 152]. Mammalian nucleoside diphosphate kinase can act equally on purine and pyrimidine ribonucleotide and deoxyribonucleotide diphosphates. The high activity of this enzyme in most tissues, coupled with its relative nonspecificity, makes the enzyme an unlikely site for control of nucleotide synthesis [152].

The reduction of nucleoside diphosphates to their deoxy forms appears to be a crucial and probably the exclusive biosynthetic pathway for the synthesis of deoxyribonucleotides from ribonucleotides in mammalian cells. This reduction appears to be similar in bacterial and mammalian cells in its requirement for reduced lipoate or thioredoxin and thioredoxin reductase [153–157]:

$$\text{Thioredoxin—S}_2 + \text{NADPH} + H^+ \longrightarrow$$
$$\text{thioredoxin (SH)}_2 + \text{NADP}^+ \quad (1)$$

$$\text{Nucleoside diphosphate + thioredoxin (SH)}_2 + \text{ATP} \xrightarrow{Mg^{2+}}$$
$$\text{deoxynucleoside diphosphate + thioredoxin—S}_2 \quad (2)$$

UTP can be aminated in the presence of glutamine or NH_3, ATP, Mg^{2+}, and CTP synthetase to yield CTP. In animal tissues, including Novikoff hepatoma cells, glutamine appears to be a more important substrate for this enzyme than ammonia [158–160]. The pathways involved in the synthesis of UTP and CTP are summarized in Fig. 56-8.

Degradation

The degradation of pyrimidines proceeds largely through the formation of uracil or thymine [161]. The pyrimidine nucleotides are catabolized to the ribonucleosides in reactions catalyzed by 5'-nucleotidase. In addition to the ubiquitous 5'-nucleotidases (EC 3.1.3.5), which react with a broad spectrum of nucleotides as substrate [162–167], a 5'-nucleotidase is present in human erythrocytes which is highly specific for pyrimidine nucleotides [168, 169]. In descending order of effectiveness, substrates for this enzyme are UMP, dUMP, CMP, dCMP, and TMP; OMP was apparently not studied. An impure preparation of the enzyme was strongly inhibited by adenosine, adenine, guanine, guanosine, and inosine, with a number of other purines and pyrimidines exhibiting less effect. Cytidine is deaminated to uridine in the reaction catalyzed by cytidine aminohydrolase (EC 3.5.4.5). The ribonucleosides, uridine and thymidine, are broken down to the free bases by pyrimidine nucleoside phosphorylase. Uracil is converted to dihydrouracil in a reaction catalyzed by dihydrouracil dehydrogenase (EC 1.3.1.2) [170]

$$\text{Uracil + NADP}^+ \longrightarrow \text{dihydrouracil + NADPH}$$

(Thymine is degraded in a similar reaction.) Dihydrouracil and dihydrothymine are then hydrolyzed to their respective carbamyl-β-amino acids in a reaction catalyzed by dihydropyrimidinase (EC 3.5.2.2).

$$\text{Dihydrouracil} \longrightarrow \text{ureidopropionate}$$

The products of this reaction are then degraded to the corresponding amino acid, CO_2, and ammonia in a reaction catalyzed by β-ureidopropionase (EC 3.5.1.6).

A potential degradative pathway also exists for orotic acid. By a reversal of reactions described in Fig. 56-7, orotic acid may be reduced to dihydro-orotic acid and subsequently hydrolyzed to carbamylaspartate. The carbamylaspartate may be irreversibly converted to aspartate, carbon dioxide, and ammonia by ureidosuccinase (carbamylaspartase), a reaction which has been studied only in bacteria [171]. Carbamylaspartate may also undergo decarboxylation to form carbamyl-β-alanine [172], which in turn is irreversibly decarbamylated [173]. Through the operation of this degradative pathway, orotic acid is converted to an amino acid (aspartate or β-alanine), carbon dioxide, and ammonia. Evidence reviewed elsewhere suggests that this degradative pathway is not quantitatively important [174, 175].

Regulation of Pyrimidine Biosynthesis *de Novo*

Control of Enzyme Activity   Several enzymes involved in the biosynthesis *de novo* of pyrimidine nucleotides may play a role in the regulation of the pathway. The reaction catalyzed by carbamyl-phosphate synthetase II (CPS II) is the first which is unique to the synthesis of pyrimidines *de novo* in mammals and thus is a potential site of regulation for the pathway. There is now considerable evidence to support this thesis. Based on the available Michaelis constants of the enzyme from mammalian tissue [37], it is probably saturated with respect to HCO_3^- and glutamine but not ATP. Enzyme preparations from human liver [36], mouse Ehrlich ascites tumor cells [39], mouse spleen [31, 32], and other species show sigmoidal kinetics at the sub-saturating concentrations of ATP which are likely to exist in vivo. An end product of pyrimidine biosynthesis, UTP, inhibits the enzyme from a variety of mammalian tissues in a manner which is competitive with respect to ATP [31, 32, 37, 38, 43, 176]. This inhibition by UTP is associated with a shift in the configuration of the multienzyme protein partially purified from rat liver [45]. PP-ribose-P, an essential substrate for both purine and pyrimidine nucleotide synthesis, activates the enzyme by decreasing the $S_{0.5}$ for ATP but has no effect on V_{max} [38]. Thus an increase in the activity of CPS II could theoretically result from an increase in the concentration of PP-ribose-P or ATP as well as a reduction of UTP. CPS I, which appears to be involved predominantly in the synthesis of urea, is not inhibited by UTP nor is it activated by PP-ribose-P. In addition, aspartate transcarbamylase from mammalian sources, unlike the bacterial enzyme, is not inhibited by end products of pyrimidine biosynthesis [42, 177–180]. The existence of these two enzymes as part of a multifunctional protein probably allows for the rapid and efficient conversion of CAP-pyr to carbamylaspartate. Thus, although CAP is an inhibitor of glutamine synthetase [181], it seems unlikely that it plays a role in regulation of the pathway by a mechanism such as the control of glutamine levels. The final enzyme in the multifunctional protein, dihydro-orotase, is also not inhibited by pyrimidine ribonucleotides, although it is inhibited by orotic acid [67, 182]. D-Galactosamine-mediated depletion of uridine nucleotides in the intact rat liver leads to a marked (twenty-fold) increase in the incorporation of [14C]bicarbonate into pyrimidine nucleotides [81]. These considerations, in addition to estimation of pool sizes and labeling of intermediates in the pathway [183], have led to the suggestion that, at least under some conditions, CPS II is the limiting step in the pathway.

In Ehrlich ascites tumor cells [39], the V_{max} of OPRT is the lowest of the six enzymes involved in the biosynthesis *de novo* of pyrimidine nucleotides. This has led to the suggestion that

this enzyme may be rate-limiting for the pathway in some circumstances. Since PP-ribose-P is an activator of CPS II and a substrate for OPRT, the effect of PP-ribose-P must be taken into account when comparing the two enzymes. In so doing, Shoaf and Jones [39] note that OPRT should be limiting at all concentrations of PP-ribose-P. For example, at a PP-ribose-P concentration of 0.1 m*M*, which is nearly physiologic in Ehrlich ascites tumor cells (0.28 to 0.66 m*M*) [184], CPS II is activated to levels 10 times normal (assuming that the enzyme is not saturated with ATP), whereas OPRT would be at half maximal activity [39]. The K_m of OPRT for PP-ribose-P is approximately 10 times higher than the intracellular concentration of PP-ribose-P in human cells. Thus the rate of this reaction, and perhaps the entire pathway, appears to be regulated by the level of PP-ribose-P. Indeed, the synthesis of RNA in rat liver appears to be limited by the availability of PP-ribose-P [69]. The toxicity of adenosine in cell culture, which is associated with an accumulation of orotate and is reversible with uridine [185], may be due to a decreased level of PP-ribose-P. More recent studies utilizing permeabilized cells [186], manipulation of mutant cells [187], and examination of the effects of added nucleosides [188] provide further evidence of the limiting nature of OPRT under certain conditions. Although OPRT is subject to product inhibition of both OMP and pyrophosphate, it is not likely that the level of OMP, due to its rapid metabolism, has any regulatory importance within the cell.

Orotidine-5'-phosphate decarboxylase (ODC) is sensitive to inhibition by pyrimidine and purine ribonucleotides [128, 189–193]. This provides another potential site of regulation of pyrimidine biosynthesis *de novo*, although it is not thought to be important under physiologic conditions.

Currently, it appears that CPS II predominates as the major control point, unless the cellular ATP levels rise at a time when both PP-ribose-P and uridine nucleotide pools are low; at which time OPRT becomes the rate-limiting step and thus the point of control.

Chen and Jones [194] have shown in Ehrlich ascites tumor cells that conditions associated with inhibition of ODC and an accumulation of orotic acid will lead to the accumulation of CAP, dihydro-orotic acid, and orotidine due to the inhibition of dihydro-orotic acid dehydrogenase, dihydro-orotase, and ODC, respectively, by the orotic acid. These observations demonstrate that under certain abnormal conditions, other reactions may become limiting and that under these conditions, a measure of the conversion of NaH [14C]orotic acid will underestimate the rate of pyrimidine biosynthesis *de novo*. This "ripple effect" may also have relevance to the accumulation of pyrimidine intermediates in patients with orotic aciduria [21].

Control of Enzyme Levels   The existence of CPS II, aspartate transcarbamylase, and dihydro-orotase in a multifunctional protein allows the coordinate regulation of the first three enzymes to be greatly simplified. There are now numerous examples where changes in the activity of CPS II are associated with coordinate changes in the activities of aspartate transcarbamylase and dihydro-orotase [47–49, 130, 195–198]. One group has recently shown that cells selected for resistance to *N*-(phosphoracetyl)-L-aspartate (PALA) have elevated levels of pyr 1–3 as a result of an increased amount of a mRNA that is approximately 8000 nucleotides in length, which is 2000 nucleotides larger than the minimal size required to code for a protein of $M_r = 200,000$ [48, 199]. The coordinate increase in activity of CPS II, aspartate transcarbamylase, and dihydro-orotase associated with resistance to PALA is due therefore to gene amplification of the multifunctional protein capable of catalyzing all three reactions. It is not known if a similar mechanism is responsible for the increased activity of pyr 1–3 observed in rapidly growing tissue [32, 200], in neoplastic tissue [201], in fetal liver [202], in neonatal cerebellum [203], in mouse submaxillary gland after ingestion of isoproterenol [195], or in phytohemagglutinin-mediated blast transformation of human lymphocytes [196, 203]. There is some evidence to suggest that PP-ribose-P may increase pyr 1–3 levels by acting at the gene level as well as by the activation of CPS II described above [204].

The levels of OPRT and ODC activity also usually vary in parallel. The activities of both enzymes increase in cultured human cells following the addition of azauridine [205], barbituric acid [206], and perhaps oxipurinol [207]. In addition, cultured cells selected for resistance to azauridine [105, 106], pyrazofurin [105] or 5-fluorouracil [106] exhibit increased activity of both enzyme activities. An increase in the activity of both OPRT and ODC is noted in neonatal erythrocytes [208] and in erythrocytes from patients with prednisone-responsive congenital hypoplastic anemia [209] and a coordinate decrease in the activities of both is noted in erythrocytes of patients with folate or B_{12} deficiency [210]. Finally, treatment of patients with allopurinol or oxipurinol increases the activity of both enzymes eightfold in circulating erythrocytes and of ODC by 70 percent in circulating leukocytes [211, 14]. In rat hepatoma, the addition of uridine leads to a 70 percent decrease in the synthesis de novo of pyrimidine nucleotides and to a 70 percent decrease in the levels of both OPRT and ODC [212]. The return of OPRT and ODC activity to control levels following removal of uridine can be blocked with inhibitors of RNA and protein synthesis [212]. Depletion of UTP with N-galactosamine leads to an increase in OPRT and ODC activity in liver, which correlates with an increased synthesis of UMP.

Although changes in the levels of activity of OPRT and ODC suggest that regulation of enzyme synthesis and degradation may be important in the control of pyrimidine metabolism, several limitations should be discussed. In no case in mammalian cells has the actual level of OPRT or ODC protein been shown to change with the conditions described above. Extreme lability has been a characteristic of both enzyme activities when attempts have been made to extract or purify them in vitro. Thus, the level of activity observed in vitro is not only a reflection of synthesis and degradation of the enzyme in situ but also possibly a result of the loss (or gain) of activity with extraction as the enzyme(s) is dissociated from membranes or other partners in the complex. If a substantial loss of activity occurs with extraction, then agents appearing to increase enzyme activity may do so predominantly, if not entirely, by stabilizing the particular enzyme to the extraction procedure. This mechanism may well account for the increase in OPRT and ODC activity observed in circulating erythrocytes obtained from patients receiving allopurinol. The ribonucleotide derivatives of allopurinol and its major metabolic product, oxipurinol, are potent inhibitors of ODC. In addition, they shift the conformation of the enzyme complex to a larger, more stable species [108] and thereby stabilize the two enzymes [108]. In at least one study [14], there was no change in the half-life of the enzyme observed in erythrocytes from patients being treated with allopurinol. Thus, stabilization did not appear to occur in vivo. In addition, an apparent absolute increase in activity could be shown by incubation of mature erythrocytes with either drug in vitro. This effect could not be attributed to enzyme induction, since mature erythrocytes are unable to synthesize proteins. The apparent increase in activity could not be attributed to stabilization of the enzyme to degradation, since activity actually increased. A similar apparent increase in ODC activity not dependent on new protein synthesis is noted following the addition of oxipurinol to cultured lymphoblasts [213]. Each of these observations would be best explained if the drug in question were stabilizing OPRT and ODC during the extraction procedure. The observation that the increase in OPRT and ODC activity observed in vivo is not accompanied by a detectable increase in the conversion of orotic acid to pyrimidine nucleotides is also consistent with this thesis [14]. Thus, elucidation of the role of enzyme synthesis and degradation in the control of OPRT and ODC activity must await more definitive studies of the level of each enzyme protein.

Whatever mechanisms of control predominate, it is clear that they favor the ultimate synthesis of the triphosphates. Fields and Brox [214] have noted in human lymphocytes and cultured lymphoblasts that the intracellular concentration of UTP is over 6 times higher than the concentration of UDP and at least 40 times higher than UMP. Likewise the concentration of CTP is at least five times higher than CMP.

Interaction of Purines and Pyrimidines

The important interrelationship between purines and pyrimidines implicit in the preceding discussion deserves further comment. As noted earlier, PP-ribose-P plays a potential regulatory role at two different steps in the synthesis of pyrimidines de novo. It is an activator of the enzyme CPS II, which catalyzes the initial step unique to pyrimidine biosynthesis de novo. In addition, it may serve an essential role in the apparent induction of pyr 1–3. Finally, it is an essential and probable rate-limiting substrate for OPRT, which catalyzes the conversion of orotic acid to orotidine-5′-phosphate. PP-ribose-P is also an essential and rate-limiting substrate for three reactions involved in the synthesis of purine nucleotides, amidophosphoribosyltransferase, hypoxanthine-guanine phosphoribosyltransferase, and adenine phosphoribosyltransferase. Thus an increase in the intracellular concentration of PP-ribose-P may increase the rate of both pyrimidine and purine biosynthesis, whereas a decrease in the concentration may have the opposite effect. This may provide the cell with one mechanism for coordinating the synthesis of purine and pyrimidine nucleotides to be used in the synthesis of nucleic acids. It also follows that a metabolic block in one pathway may alter the other. For example, a deficiency of hypoxanthine-guanine phosphoribosyltransferase leads to reduced consumption of PP-ribose-P and accumulation of this compound in the cell. This increase in the intracellular concentration of PP-ribose-P, as predicted from the above, is associated with a two- to sixfold increase in the intracellular concentration of UDP, UTP, and CTP [215]. It remains to be determined if this increase in pyrimidine nucleotides is due to an increase in the rate of pyrimidine biosynthesis de novo.

A reduction in the intracellular content of PP-ribose-P due to a deficiency of PP-ribose-P synthetase is associated with orotic aciduria and hypouricemia [18]. This suggests that the synthesis de novo of both purine and pyrimidine nucleotides may be reduced in this setting. This will be discussed in more detail later. The possibility that purine metabolism may be deranged in certain disorders of pyrimidine metabolism (to be discussed later) has not been carefully evaluated.

Adenosine-5'-triphosphate is also an activator of the enzyme CPS II, which catalyzes the initial step of pyrimidine biosynthesis *de novo*. Based on the K_m of the enzyme from mammalian sources and the intracellular concentration of ATP, this potential regulatory function of ATP may be important in vivo. Thus an increase in the levels of purine nucleotides, specifically ATP, may lead to an increase in the synthesis of pyrimidine nucleotides and vice versa. There is no experimental verification of this important interrelationship.

Adenosine is toxic to cultured mammalian cells [185, 216]. The inhibition of cell growth produced by adenosine in mouse fibroblasts [217, 185] and human lymphoblastoid cells [212] is associated with an increase in the pools of ATP, ADP, and GTP; a decrease in the pools of UDP, UTP, and CTP; and a decrease in the incorporation of [14C]aspartate into uridine nucleotides, together with an accumulation of [14C]orotic acid. The toxicity is prevented by exogenous uridine. These observations suggest that adenosine in some manner inhibits the conversion of orotic acid to OMP. The toxicity of adenosine is reduced by the presence of adenosine deaminase [218], which catalyzes the conversion of adenosine to inosine, or the absence of adenosine kinase, which catalyzes the conversion of adenosine to AMP. This suggests that the conversion of adenosine to AMP may play a role in the toxicity of adenosine. Although adenosine-mediated inhibition of PP-ribose-P synthesis [219] would be a satisfactory explanation for these observations, there are no further data available relevant to this thesis. A single mutation in a variant mouse cell line (A9, which is deficient in hypoxanthine-guanine phosphoribosyltransferase and adenine phosphoribosyltransferase) leads to resistance to both adenosine and 6-azauridine [220]; the mechanism remains to be established.

Several purine bases and nucleosides, including adenine, adenosine, guanine, and guanosine, are capable of preventing the apparent induction of pyr 1–3 associated with blast transformation [204] and of inhibiting the pyrimidine-specific 5'-nucleotidase in human erythrocytes [168]. The general applicability and relevance of these observations to the control of pyrimidine metabolism remains to be established.

Economy of Pyrimidine Metabolism in Human Beings

Absorption   The normal dietary content of orotic acid is not known. Orotic acid was first discovered in milk 60 years ago [221]. More recent measurements confirm its presence in cow's milk (50 to 100 mg/liter) [222], and especially in food milk powders, where the level is about 130 mg/100 g. Tax et al. [223], however, noted only 16 mg orotic acid per 100 g of milk powder. If the former values are correct, a powdered milk diet could reach 0.125 percent orotic acid [224, 225]. While human milk has a high content of the pyrimidines, cytidine monophosphate, and uridine monophosphate, only trace amounts of orotic acid are present [225]. While the content of orotic acid in other dietary constituents is not known, it may be very low. For example, very low levels of orotic acid are present in animal tissue; even in diets containing 1 percent orotic acid by weight, the free compound cannot be demonstrated in rat liver [174].

As a highly insoluble pyrimidine, orotic acid is not readily absorbed. In rats, from 2 to 59 percent of the radioactivity recovered after the oral administration of [14C]orotate was found in the feces [174]. While no data are available on the absorption of orotic acid in human beings, some is absorbed, as indicated by the partial efficacy of large oral doses of orotic acid in the treatment of pernicious anemia [226]. Urinary orotic acid excretion is no different in infants who were breast-fed as compared to those who received milk powder (and an estimated 10 mg orotic acid per day) [223]. Active transport of other pyrimidine bases occurs in the small intestine, with considerable structural specificity required [227]. There is no evidence that dietary orotic acid is a quantitatively important source of pyrimidines.

Excretion   Urinary orotic acid excretion appears to be highest in the newborn (median 12.1 with a range from 6 to 29 μmol per gram creatinine). Children up to the age of 12 months excrete somewhat less orotic acid (median 5.4 with a range from 1.7 to 34 μmol per gram creatinine) than the newborn but considerably more than older children, whether hospitalized (median 2.2 with a range from 0.7 to 3.9 μmol per gram creatine) or not (median trace with a range from trace to 1.7 μmol per gram creatinine) [228]. The normal adult excretes approximately 1.4 mg orotic acid in the urine per 24 h.

Orotic acid is actively secreted by the avian renal tubule, and this secretory mechanism is inhibited by probenecid [229]. In the rat, orotic acid is actively secreted from plasma to bile, from hepatic cells in vivo and from liver slices in vitro [230]; biliary secretion is inhibited by probenecid and p-aminohippurate. Considerable species variability appears to exist [231].

In human beings, several observations suggest that orotic acid is cleared by the kidney by both glomerular filtration and tubular secretion. During infusion of ring-labeled [14C]orotic acid in human beings, the clearance of radioactivity approached that of creatinine clearance [232]. During drug-induced orotic aciduria (see below) the clearance of orotic acid exceeds glomerular filtration. In addition, infused orotic acid increases the clearance of uric acid, presumably by competing for a common renal transport mechanism [233]. Renal clearance studies have not been possible in human beings in the absence of induced orotic aciduria, since no orotic acid is detectable in plasma by using either a sensitive isotope-dilution technique [68] or an enzymatic spectrophotometric method [234]. Orotic acid in bile and gastrointestinal secretions has not been studied.

The thousand-fold increase in the excretion of orotic acid in hereditary orotic aciduria is presumably due to an increased plasma concentration, although this has not been carefully examined. A primary renal tubular defect in the reabsorption of orotic acid seems unlikely in hereditary orotic aciduria in view of the enzyme defects to be described.

In normal humans there is usually no detectable dihydroorotate [235] in the urine, whereas the urinary excretion of carbamylaspartate ranges from 5.5 to 24.1 μmol/24 h [235].

Pharmacology of Orotic Acid

The effect of pharmacologic doses of orotic acid has been assessed on several occasions. Rundles and Brewer [226] reported a partial and transient remission of pernicious anemia in 9 of 11 patients who were treated with 3 to 6 g orotic acid per day orally. The mechanism of this response is unknown. A diet high in orotic acid leads to severe fatty liver in the rat, associated with a block in the synthesis and release of β-lipoproteins [236–238]. There is an accompanying increase in the hepatic content of uridine nucleotides (two- to fourfold increase), associated with a decrease in adenine nucleotides [174, 239]. In addition, apoproteins isolated from orotic acid–induced fatty liver are deficient in N-acetylglucosamine, galactose, and N-acylneuraminic acid [240]. Adenine [174], allopurinol [241, 242], 5,5′-diphenyl-2-thiohydantoin [241], D-thyroxin [241], and clofibrate [243] prevent or reverse fat accumulation in the liver induced by orotic acid. The administration of orotic acid does not appear to produce a fatty liver in mouse, chick, monkey, or human beings [244, 249]. In humans, the short-term administration of orotic acid leads to a modest, though statistically significant, decrease in plasma pre-β-lipoprotein, β-lipoprotein, and triglyceride concentrations [245]. Orotic acid also increases the clearance of uric acid [233, 245, 246] and reduces the synthesis of purine nucleotides de novo [245]. The latter effect appears to be due to the depletion of PP-ribose-P [245, 247]. Several authors [248, 249] have noted a decrease in the plasma bilirubin concentration in human infants with neonatal jaundice treated with 200 to 300 mg orotic acid per day; this effect has not been confirmed by others [250, 251]. Orotic acid has been reported to increase myocardial contractility during cardiac hypertrophy in the rat [252] and the rabbit [253]. A trial of orotic acid in human beings following acute myocardial infarction is said to have reduced the incidence of congestive heart failure and the mortality rate [254]. Orotic acid has also been reported to counteract galactose-induced cataract formation [224], to nullify the diabetogenic action of alloxan [224], and to protect the liver against the hepatotoxicity of a low-dose mixture of hepatotoxic substances (carbon tetrachloride, chlorophenothane, and 9,10-dimethyl-1,2-benzanthracene) [255] or D-galactosamine [256]. This latter effect of orotic acid has been attributed to correction of uridine monophosphate depletion following the conversion of D-galactosamine to UDP-galactosamine [256].

PATHOGENESIS OF OROTIC ACIDURIA

Hereditary Orotic Aciduria

Enzyme Defect The excessive excretion of orotic acid characteristic of patients with orotic aciduria could derive from an increased absorption from the diet, an increased clearance by the kidney, an increased rate of biosynthesis, or a decreased rate of metabolism. Evidence reviewed above indicates that excessive intestinal absorption could not account for the level of orotic acid excretion. The low plasma level of orotic acid (undetectable by current techniques) makes it unlikely that a renal tubular defect contributes to its excessive urinary excretion.

In the initial clinical studies of the first patient with orotic aciduria, the administration of a mixture of pyrimidine nucleotides led to a complete hematologic remission, a remarkable improvement in general well-being, and a prompt reduction in orotic acid excretion. This indicated a block in the pathway of pyrimidine biosynthesis at the conversion of orotic acid to UMP (Fig. 56-7). Further evidence was provided from the observation that both parents and two of the three sibs of this initial patient had reduced activity of OPRT and ODC in erythrocytes [5]. The deficiency of both enzymes was demonstrated directly in the second patient [257], and this double enzyme defect has subsequently been confirmed in six of the seven patients with markedly elevated urinary orotic acid levels reported since that time. The defect has also been demonstrable in leukocytes, liver homogenates, and cultured skin fibroblasts.

OPRT and ODC activities have been undetectable in erythrocytes or leukocytes from all patients with type I hereditary orotic aciduria. In addition, levels of OPRT and ODC activity have ranged from less than 2 percent of normal to 5 percent of normal under control conditions in cultured skin fibroblasts from four of the patients described. The patient described by Rogers et al. [6] exhibited a complete absence of OPRT and ODC in erythrocytes, approximately 5 percent of normal activity for both enzymes in fibroblasts, and levels of OPRT and ODC activity in liver which were 1 percent and 25 percent, respectively, of the activity observed in normal liver. It has been difficult to be certain that these low levels of apparent OPRT and ODC activity in patients with type I hereditary orotic aciduria do, in fact, represent residual activity of these two enzymes in mutant cells. An increase in the excretion of orotic acid in two patients after the administration of allopurinol, a drug which results in the inhibition of ODC [14], suggests, however, that a low level of activity may be present in vivo in some patients. This is further supported by the increased orotidine excretion observed in several patients [14]. Possibly such residual activity is the factor which allows the marginal survival of the occasional homozygous patient with type I hereditary orotic aciduria.

In one patient OPRT was normal in erythrocytes, whereas ODC was markedly deficient [2, 3]. This patient, lacking only ODC activity, was termed as having type II hereditary orotic aciduria in order to separate him from patients deficient in both enzymes. In this patient over a 3-year period of follow-up, OPRT activity in erythrocytes was found to decrease from a high normal value to a level of approximately 2 percent of normal [3]. While the explanation for this change is unclear, it was associated with the institution of therapy with uridine. Repeated assessment of OPRT and ODC activity in patients with type I hereditary orotic aciduria has disclosed no change in the activity of either enzyme.

Nature of the Genetic Defect Hereditary orotic aciduria is the only genetic disease so far detected in humans in which two sequential enzymes are involved. This has led to interesting speculation concerning the nature of the defect. A single mutation could lead to a double enzyme defect if both reactions were catalyzed by the same protein. The evidence for and against this possibility has been reviewed earlier in this chapter. A second possibility is that separate proteins may catalyze these sequential reactions, but they are intimately associated in a complex which is essential for the maintenance of activity. A mutation affecting the structure of one of the two enzymes could lead to a deficiency of the other if this structural change interfered with the integrity of the complex and disruption of the complex led to a loss of activity of the other enzyme. Thus, a mutation in the gene coding for ODC could possibly lead to a deficiency of both enzymes.

The development by Krooth and his colleagues of cell strains from patients with orotic aciduria provided an important tool for the study of the mechanism of the double enzyme defect in hereditary orotic aciduria and the control of pyrimidine biosynthesis in human diploid cells. Growth of the mutant homozygous cells in the presence of certain inhibitors of pyrimidine biosynthesis, 6-azauridine, 5-azaorotic acid, and barbituric acid (which inhibit, respectively, the activities of ODC, OPRT and dihydro-orotic dehydrogenase), leads to an increase in the activities of both OPRT and ODC [205, 206]. Enzyme levels have been produced in mutant cells which are comparable with those found in normal cell strains. While, as discussed earlier, the mechanism responsible for this increase in activity remains to be defined, the ability to increase the levels of OPRT and ODC activity to normal in mutant cells allowed a further examination of the properties of these two enzymes. Worthy et al. [126] found that the ODC–OPRT in fibroblasts derived from patient T.H. with orotic aciduria exhibited a different net charge and a different heat stability when compared with the two enzymes from normal human fibroblasts grown under identical conditions. These observations do not allow, however, a clear resolution of the question of whether the two enzymes exist in a complex or whether they represent two activities of a multifunctional protein. Clearly, additional studies, including peptide maps of the OPRT and ODC isolated from mutant cells, will be necessary to define further this possibility.

A double enzyme defect could be the result of a deletion involving two contiguous genes. If the structural genes coding for OPRT and ODC are adjacent on the human chromosome, a single deletion might overlap both genes. The presence of the double enzyme defect in all but one subject so far studied makes such a fortuitously situated defect unlikely. In addition, a deletion would usually be expected to lead to a reduction of the activity of an involved enzyme to zero. The rise of OPRT and ODC activities to normal levels in tissue culture during growth in 6-azauridine has been noted in cell strains from at least four unrelated patients. This indicates that a deletion is not likely. A deficiency of both enzymes could also be due to a mutation in a gene affecting a regulatory mechanism controlling the synthesis or degradation of these two sequential enzymes in pyrimidine biosynthesis. While the increase in the activities of both enzymes in fibroblasts grown in the presence of certain inhibitors of pyrimidine biosynthesis is consistent with a regulatory defect, the presence of altered enzyme structure, for which evidence was provided in patient T.H., is not. Evidence has been obtained in yeast [259] and in diploid cell strains from patients with homozygous orotic aciduria type I [206]. This suggests that levels of enzymes in pyrimidine biosynthesis may be sequentially induced by certain intermediates, especially dihydro-orotic acid. Krooth [260] has suggested that the primary defect in hereditary orotic aciduria may be an inappropriate excretion of (or inability to concentrate) orotic acid or other precursors by cells, with resultant failure of induction or stabilization of the subsequent two enzymes. This interesting hypothesis is open to experimental verification.

Consequences of the Enzyme Defect   The patients studied with type I hereditary orotic aciduria have excreted 600 to 1500 mg orotic acid per day. If normal values obtained in adults (Fig. 56-9) [261] are applicable in relationship to surface area in childhood, this is an increase of 3000- to 5000-fold in urinary orotic acid. Carbamylaspartic acid excretion in the urine was elevated to levels of at least twice normal in patients J.P. [41.5 μmol/(24 h $\cdot$ 1.73 m^2)] and D.G. [71.4 μmol/(24 h $\cdot$

1.73 m^2)] during therapy with uridine [235]. Dihydro-orotic acid was not detectable in urine from normal subjects or from two patients with hereditary orotic aciduria [235]. In patients J.P. and D.G., urinary orotidine excretion was 15.8 mg and 18.4 mg/24 h, respectively; in patients T.H. and D.B., urinary orotidine excretion was 34.8 mg and 21.0 mg per gram creatinine, respectively. This represents an increase of twenty- to fortyfold. The relatively small degree of orotidinuria, in spite of the rise of precursor orotic acid, suggests a marked but not complete deficiency of OPRT. Patient P.M. excreted 286 mg orotic acid per 24 h and 48 mg orotidine per 24 h in the urine prior to the initiation of therapy. This level of urinary orotidine excretion may be higher than that observed in other patients and presumably reflects the substantial residual OPRT activity in this patient.

Studies of the incorporation of ring-labeled orotic acid into urinary pseudouridine (5-ribosyluracil) have suggested that the synthesis *de novo* of pyrimidine bases is approximately 0.6 g/24 h in adults [232]. This value is similar to that of purine turnover, as estimated from the rate of uric acid synthesis [262]. Thus the excretion of orotic acid at levels up to 8 g/(24 h $\cdot$ 1.73 m^2) in patients with hereditary orotic aciduria suggests a marked increase in the rate of orotic acid synthesis. In all patients studied there was a reduction in the rate of orotic acid excretion (from 0.7 to 1.5 g to 0.1 to 0.2 g/24 h) during the clinical and hematologic remission produced by oral pyrimidine replacement therapy. In patient P.M., uridine therapy was associated with a marked decrease in the urinary excretion of both orotic acid and orotidine. Since the enzyme defects remain unchanged, this appears to represent a reduced rate of orotic acid synthesis. This putative reduction in orotic acid synthesis and excretion could be attributable to the operation of one of two types of metabolic regulatory mechanisms discussed above: end-product repression of enzyme synthesis and feedback inhibition in which the pyrimidine nucleotides suppress or inhibit the activity of one or more enzymes acting early in pyrimidine synthesis, especially carbamyl-phosphate synthetase.

The conversion of 1 mol orotic acid to OMP consumes 1 mol PP-ribose-P. Thus the deficiency of OPRT may lead to an accumulation of PP-ribose-P analogous to the accumulation of this substrate in patients deficient in hypoxanthine-guanine phosphoribosyltransferase [263]. The effect of PP-ribose-P as an activator of the initial step unique to the synthesis of orotic acid has been described. Thus if PP-ribose-P accumulates in patients with orotic aciduria, this may account for the increased rate of orotic acid synthesis observed in these patients. While PP-ribose-P levels were normal in erythrocytes obtained from one homozygous and two heterozygous OPRT-deficient subjects [264], there has been no attempt to assess the concentration or availability of PP-ribose-P in liver or other nucleated cells.

In an attempt to determine if enzymatic activities prior to the site of the block were increased, as a possible reflection of enzyme control, studies were carried out on aspartate transcarbamylase and dihydro-orotase in erythrocytes. With a possible single exception, erythrocyte activities of these enzymes were normal in all subjects presumed to be heterozygous for hereditary orotic aciduria (Fig. 56-10). This would be anticipated in subjects without clinical or laboratory evidence of pyrimidine deficiency, although presumed heterozygotes did excrete a small excess of orotic acid in the urine (Fig. 56-9). On the other hand, in the homozygous deficient subject, D.G., both enzymes were greatly increased in activity in circulating eryth-

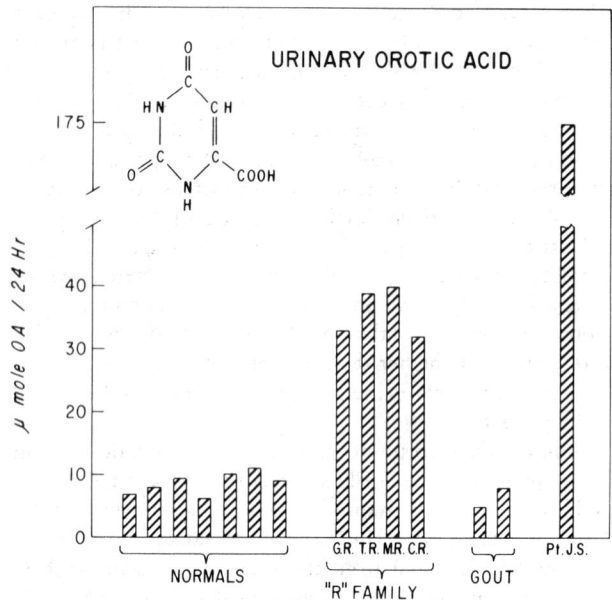

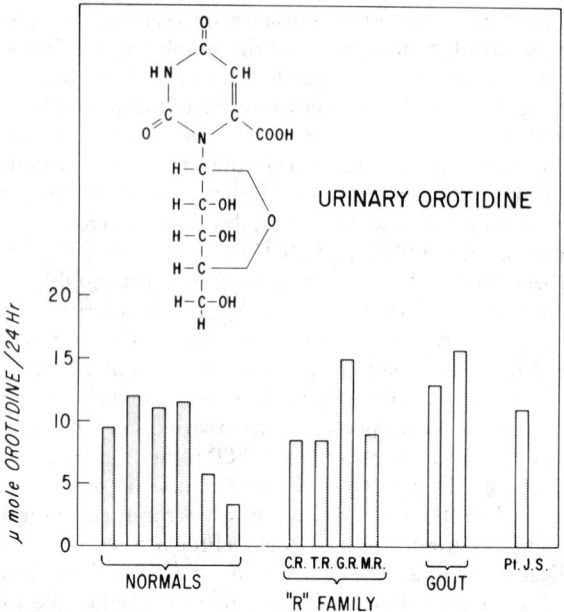

Figure 56-9 Urinary excretion of orotic acid and orotidine in normal subjects, in presumed heterozygotes of hereditary orotic aciduria, and in two patients with gout. *(From Lotz et al. [261]. Used by permission.)*

rocytes (Fig. 56-10) and returned to normal on treatment with uridine. Dihydro-orotase was similarly elevated in erythrocytes from patient D.B. [15]. Prior to treatment with uridine, OPRT activity was normal in erythrocytes from patient P.M., who had a selective deficiency of ODC [2]. OPRT activity in this patient dropped to 2 percent of normal during uridine therapy [3]. Similar studies have not yet been carried out in diploid cell strains from patients with hereditary orotic aciduria under conditions of pyrimidine starvation in vitro. The mechanism responsible for these changes in apparent levels of enzyme activity remains unclear.

Relationship to Clinical Manifestations The metabolic derangement in hereditary orotic aciduria is primarily that of pyrimidine nucleotide deficiency. The clinical manifestations of the disease presumably result from a deficiency of compounds necessary for the synthesis of nucleic acids and certain critical cofactors. There is no evidence in human beings that accumulation of orotic acid per se is deleterious, except that it may occasionally obstruct urine flow with crystalline deposits. The toxic properties of administered orotic acid are presumably related to its further metabolism and resulting nucleotide imbalance or a PP-ribose-P depletion [245, 265, 266]. The enzymatic block in the conversion of orotic acid to uridine-5'-phosphate should be protective against this mode of toxicity in hereditary orotic aciduria.

The most striking clinical feature has been megaloblastosis, which is associated with hypochromia of the erythrocytes. A critical discussion of megaloblastosis is beyond the scope of this chapter. It has been suggested that megaloblastosis results from a selective defect in DNA synthesis which interferes with mitosis [267]. It is a provocative finding, therefore, that hereditary orotic aciduria is associated with megaloblastosis, since the genetic block occurs at a position in the pyrimidine biosynthetic sequence which should result equally in deficient formation of both RNA and DNA. Possibly limited amounts of pyrimidine nucleotides are more efficiently used for RNA than for DNA synthesis. The megaloblasts in hereditary orotic aciduria are not as large as those found in pernicious anemia or folic acid deficiency, and the cellular abnormalities are considerably more striking in the more mature red blood cell precur-

sors. The degree of microcytosis and hypochromia in circulating erythrocytes (Fig. 56-2) also differs from that usually found in other megaloblastic anemias. These differing structural abnormalities may reflect the coexistence of deficient RNA production and therefore reduced protein synthesis in these patients, with a block in the common pathway of pyrimidine nucleotide synthesis. This speculation is not yet supported by experimental evidence. There is no specific information on the cause of the mental retardation, although presumably this too reflects a relative nucleotide deficiency at some crucial period of development of the central nervous system.

Orotic Aciduria from Other Causes

Orotic aciduria occurs when the rate of synthesis of orotic acid exceeds the rate at which OPRT is able to catalyze the synthe-

Figure 56-10 Activities of aspartate transcarbamylase and dihydro-orotase in erythrocyte preparations from control subjects; from presumed heterozygotes from the R., and S., and G. families; and from patient D.G. The elevated activities in D.G. returned to normal levels during uridine treatment (see Fig. 56-5).

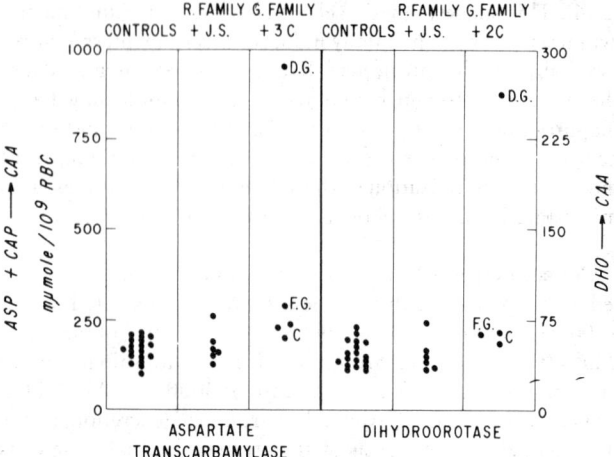

sis of OMP. In hereditary orotic aciduria, the capacity of the cell to handle this transformation is reduced due to a deficiency of OPRT. Wada et al. [18] described an infant with orotic aciduria, hypouricemia, severe mental retardation, and megaloblastic changes in the bone marrow. Orotic acid excretion was 35 mg/day. Further investigation of the patient revealed a low rate of urinary uric acid excretion (42 to 74 mg/day), an erythrocyte content of PP-ribose-P that was 65 percent of normal, and an apparent deficiency of PP-ribose-P synthetase activity. Presumably the orotic aciduria and perhaps the megaloblastic anemia and mental retardation are due to a reduced conversion of orotic acid to OMP as a result of the lowered concentration of PP-ribose-P. OPRT and ODC activity has not yet been assayed in this patient.

Several drugs produce orotic aciduria as a result of the inhibition of OPRT or ODC or both. A disorder of pyrimidine metabolism somewhat analogous to genetically induced orotic aciduria is produced in human beings by the administration of the antineoplastic agent 6-azauridine [233, 268]. Following its enzymatic conversion to 6-azauridine-5'-phosphate, this substance is a specific competitive inhibitor of the decarboxylation of orotidine-5'-phosphate to form uridine-5'-phosphate (Fig. 56-7) [269]. When it is used in therapeutic doses, there is a prompt urinary excretion of both orotic acid (up to 12 g/24 h) and orotidine (up to 10 g/24 h) (Fig. 56-11). 6-Azauridine therapy decreases orotic acid decarboxylation in the intact subject [175] or in leukocytes isolated from the patient under treatment [270]. The increased urinary excretion of orotidine is presumably due to the accumulation and concomitant dephosphorylation of orotidine-5'-phosphate to orotidine as a result of the inhibition of ODC. The increased urinary excretion of orotic acid may be due to inhibition of OPRT by the increased concentration of OMP [22] or possibly by 6-azauridine-5'-phosphate itself. There is no evidence that orotidine can be further metabolized to orotic acid. Although administration of 6-azauridine simulates many of the features of the genetic disease, a major point of dissimilarity lies in the absence of marked orotidinuria in type I hereditary orotic aciduria. This is probably due to the more marked reduction of OPRT in patients with a genetically determined deficiency of this enzyme. Prolonged administration of 6-azauridine to patients without hematologic disease has produced a mild anemia and often, but not invariably, a megaloblastic bone marrow. This anemia has not simulated closely the hypochromic, megaloblastic anemia of hereditary orotic aciduria, perhaps because severe anemia has not been produced. The antibiotic pyrazofurin also inhibits ODC and as a result leads to orotic aciduria and orotidinuria [271–273].

The administration of allopurinol and oxipurinol in human beings is also accompanied by a striking increase in the excretion of orotidine (up to 300 mg/day) and of orotic acid (up to 300 mg/day) [211, 274]. Studies in vivo and in cell culture demonstrate that the orotidinuria results from inhibition of ODC. It seems likely that the inhibition of ODC is due largely to the formation of 1-N-ribosyloxipurinol-5'-phosphate, 7-N-ribosyloxipurinol-5'-phosphate, and possibly allopurinol ribo-

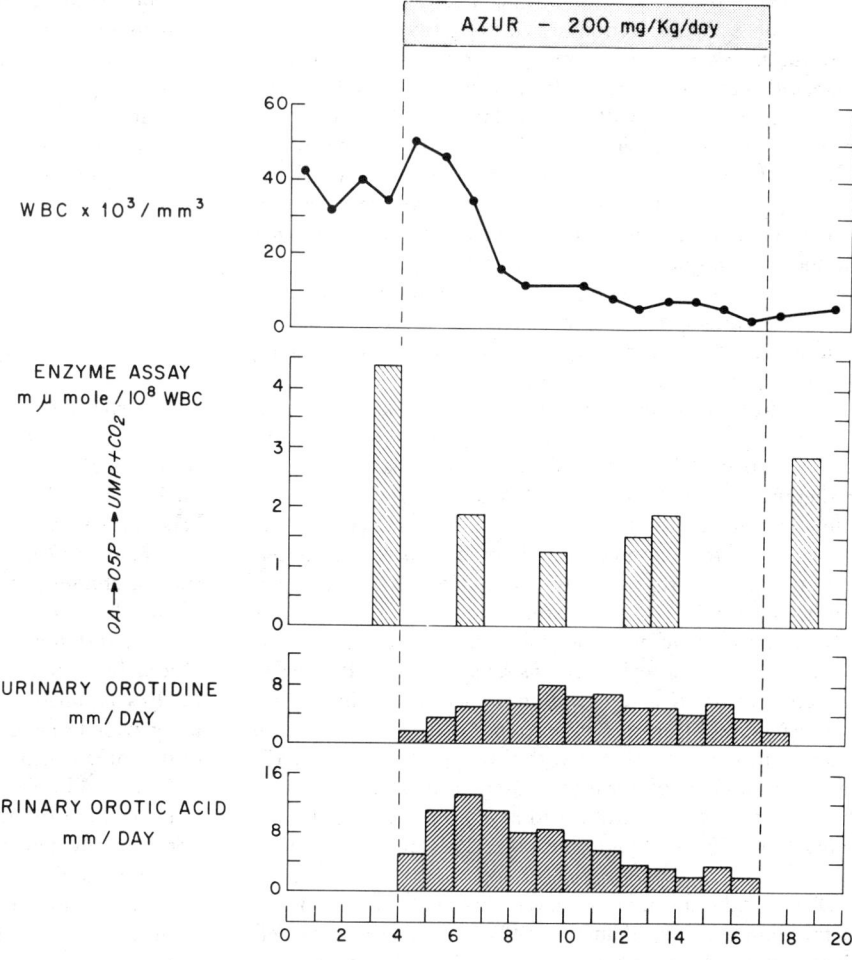

Figure 56-11 Effect of 6-azauridine treatment on a patient with chronic myelocytic leukemia. There was a prompt, coincident orotic aciduria and orotidinuria and a block in the metabolism of orotic acid by isolated leukocytes. *(From Fallon et al. [270]. Used by permission.)*

nucleotide, all of which are nucleotide derivatives of oxipurinol or allopurinol and are potent inhibitors of the enzyme [211, 274–277]. The orotic aciduria may be due, as described above, to an inhibition of OPRT by the increased concentration of OMP or of one or more of the metabolites of allopurinol or oxipurinol described above. In addition, the activity of OPRT may be reduced after allopurinol administration by a reduction in the intracellular content of PP-ribose-P. The administration of allopurinol produces a substantial reduction of erythrocyte PP-ribose-P content, which occurs 3 to 5 h after administration of the drug [278]. The administration of allopurinol to rats is associated with a transient decrease in UMP and UDP pools in the liver, whereas UTP levels are actually elevated; no change is observed in the level of uridine nucleotides in the kidney [279]. These studies suggest that, at least in the rat, any reduction of intracellular pyrimidine nucleotides due to the inhibition of pyrimidine biosynthesis de novo is rapidly corrected, presumably by an enhanced conversion of uridine to UMP. There is no evidence that the long-term administration of allopurinol in human beings is associated with any of the clinical manifestations of hereditary orotic aciduria other than an increased excretion of orotic acid. As discussed earlier, the administration of allopurinol or oxipurinol leads to an apparent eightfold increase in the activity of OPRT and ODC. There is no concomitant reduction in the excretion of orotic acid or orotidine associated with the apparent increase in activity. Although several additional drugs in clinical use, such as sodium aurothiomalate [280, 281] and chlorpromazine [282], have been reported to inhibit OPRT or ODC, it is not known if they produce orotic aciduria.

There are several situations in which orotic aciduria appears to occur as a result of an increased production of orotic acid. Increased excretion of orotic acid, uracil, and uridine has been noted in most children with hyperammonemia due to ornithine transcarbamylase deficiency [283–297]; for exception, see Ref. 288. In one patient urinary orotic acid was 240 mg/dl on a normal protein diet, falling to undetectable levels on a very low protein diet. In several patients the excretion of orotic acid paralleled the blood ammonia concentration [287, 289]. It was postulated that carbamyl phosphate might accumulate in this disorder secondary to the partial block in citrulline synthesis, resulting in a secondary increase in pyrimidine synthesis by way of aspartate transcarbamylase [283].

An increased excretion of orotic acid also occurs in other disorders of the urea cycle, including argininosuccinicaciduria [287, 290], citrullinemia [270, 287], and lysinuric protein intolerance [287]. Presumably, CAParg accumulates in the mitochondrion as a result of the block in the urea cycle, which allows it to diffuse into the cytoplasm. The increased concentration of CAP in the cytoplasm raises the rate of orotic acid synthesis, since CAP is beyond the major site of feedback control prior to orotic acid formation in mammalian systems. While this remains to be demonstrated directly, the marked reduction in orotic acid excretion on a low-protein diet and the correlation of orotic acid excretion with blood ammonia concentration are consistent with this hypothesis [283, 287]. An abnormality of ornithine transcarbamylase and an increased excretion of orotic acid have been observed in some patients with Reye's syndrome [291, 292] but not in others [287].

Orotic aciduria can be produced experimentally in animals by the administration of ammonia [290, 293], by arginine deficiency [294–296], and by amino acids [297]. The administration of ammonia presumably increases the formation of CAP,

while arginine deficiency leads to a decreased utilization of CAP as a result of the decreased synthesis of ornithine. An increased excretion of orotic acid has also been noted in infants on total parenteral nutrition during periods of hyperammonemia [224]. While the hyperammonemia in this setting is corrected by the infusion of arginine [298], the effect of arginine on orotic acid excretion in these infants has not been studied. These findings provide further evidence that an increased intramitochondrial concentration of CAP is capable of increasing pyrimidine synthesis. These studies further suggest that this may occur even in the presence of normal urea cycle enzymes.

In one patient described by Neimann et al. [16, 17], orotic aciduria was found, but the nature of the defect has remained unclear. There was a severe macrocytic anemia with a megaloblastic marrow but no leukopenia in both the proband J.G. and his sister. Three other sibs were normal. While the enzyme defect was not defined, it probably did not represent a block in uridine synthesis because there was no response to uridine, thymine, thymidine, or cytosine. There was a partial response to folic and folinic acid.

Patients with the Lesch-Nyhan syndrome due to a virtually complete deficiency of hypoxanthine-guanine phosphoribosyltransferase (HPRT) have elevated intracellular levels of pyrimidine nucleotides [215], but orotic aciduria is not present [275]. This may be due to an increased rate of conversion of orotic acid to OMP as a result of the increased levels of PP-ribose-P or the increased activity of OPRT and ODC observed in patients with HPRT deficiency [299].

Cohen et al. [300] reported an increased excretion of orotic acid in two patients with purine nucleoside phosphorylase (PNP) deficiency. Essentially normal levels of orotic acid excretion have been subsequently reported in a number of other patients with PNP deficiency [301–303]. In addition, a study of cultured cells from patients with PNP deficiency also showed no abnormalities of pyrimidine biosynthesis de novo [304].

GENETICS

The existence of a partial enzyme defect in presumed heterozygotes with hereditary orotic aciduria type I has allowed a convenient means to determine its mode of inheritance (Figs. 56-12 and 56-13). A survey was made of the available members of the R. family using the activity of ODC in erythrocytes as a marker [305, 306]. The range and mean values of the enzyme studies performed on a normal control group and on 63 members of the affected family are summarized in Fig. 56-14. The 18 family members with low enzyme levels were provisionally considered heterozygous for hereditary orotic aciduria. It is assumed that the proband was homozygous, although his enzyme levels were not determined. Both parents and two of the three sibs of this original patient had reduced activities of OPRT and ODC, and were presumably heterozygotes. The transmission of the defect was apparent through four generations, as shown in the pedigree (Figs. 56-15). The minor degree of consanguinity of the parents appeared to be irrelevant. No increased incidence of abortions, neonatal death, or anemia could be established in the family. Two other pedigrees have been subsequently published with similar patterns of transmission of the trait [6]. Family studies carried out on hereditary

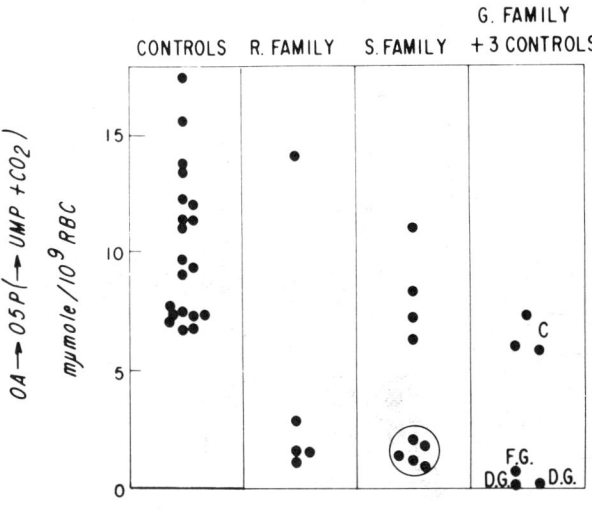

Figure 56-12 Activity of orotate phosphoribosyltransferase in erythrocyte preparations from control subjects and members of the R., S., and G families. The circle encloses five determinations over a period of 1 year in a presumed heterozygote in the S. family. C, controls obtained in New Zealand; D.G., two determinations on patient D.G.; F.G., father of D.G.

orotic aciduria type II similarly suggest autosomal recessive transmission [3]. In the family described by Worthy et al. [126], the nature of the defect in cultured fibroblasts appeared to be different with cells from each of the two heterozygotes (parents) studied. This suggests that the mutation in each parent was different. The absence of parental consanguinity is consistent with this finding.

From these studies it can be concluded that orotic aciduria is transmitted as an autosomal recessive disease. Heterozygotes exhibit decreased activities of OPRT and ODC and excrete a slightly increased amount of orotic acid in the urine. They do not appear to be deficient in pyrimidine nucleotide production, as is indicated by absence of symptoms, of anemia, and of the pattern of "pyrimidine starvation" in their pyrimidine biosynthetic pathway.

The frequency of the heterozygous trait of hereditary orotic aciduria in the general population has not been established. In the initial study of the enzyme defect, subject J.S. was discov-

ered in a series of about 40 controls. Whether he represents a heterozygote or a homozygote of a milder variant is unclear. In a subsequent study of approximately 200 specimens from donors at a blood bank, no heterozygotes were discovered by the erythrocyte-ODC assay [307]. More recently, Rogers et al. [308] found two unrelated heterozygotes in a survey of 1358 mentally retarded subjects. In studies of the family of T.H., a new heterozygote was discovered in an unrelated in-law [6]. Three other presumed heterozygotes were then found in this "I family." Several authors [3, 309] have noted a skewed frequency distribution of OPRT and ODC activity in hemolysates from apparently normal individuals. While the basis of the non-Gaussian distribution of enzyme activity remains unexplained, this type of distribution complicates the use of an arithmetic mean as a basis for comparison of heterozygote activity levels as well as for the detection of heterozygotes. Fox et al. [3] have emphasized the importance of demonstrating both reduced OPRT and ODC activity and an elevated excretion of orotic acid before accepting identification of the heterozygote as definitive. The latter requirement has been simplified by the introduction of a screening test for an elevated excretion of orotic acid and orotidine [310]. Unfortunately, these two criteria are further complicated by the finding that an increased excretion of orotic acid can be observed after the administration of several different drugs as well as in a number of conditions other than hereditary orotic aciduria. For these reasons we would also emphasize the importance of appropriate pedigree analysis in the assignment of heterozygosity at this locus. To summarize, heterozygote detection should include determination of OPRT and ODC activity in circulating erythrocytes, and estimation of urinary orotic acid excretion after discontinuation of all drugs if possible, followed by interpretation of the pedigree based on the inclusion of similar data collected from other family members.

Although some patients have undoubtedly escaped detection, homozygous hereditary orotic aciduria must be very rare, in that resistant megaloblastic anemia of infancy is rare. The rarity of this disease suggests that a homozygous defect in the

Figure 56-14 Activities of orotidine-5′-monophosphate decarboxylase in erythrocytes from control subjects and from members of the R. family. *(From Fallon et al. [270]. Used by permission).*

Figure 56-13 Activity of orotidine-5′-monophosphate decarboxylase in erythrocyte preparations from control subjects; from members of the R., S., and G. families; and from patient J.P. Abbreviations are as in Fig. 56-12.

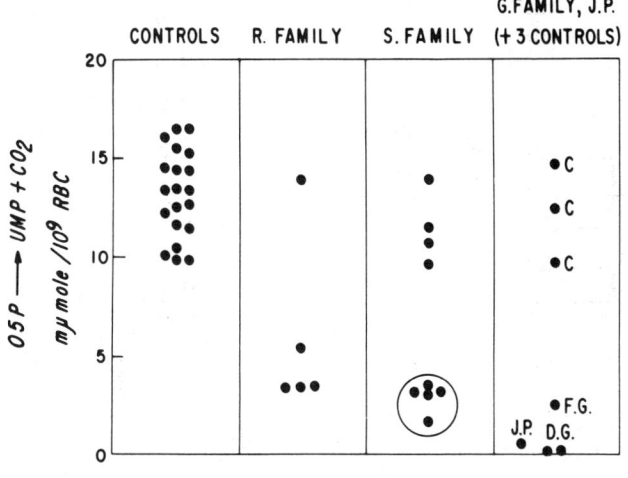

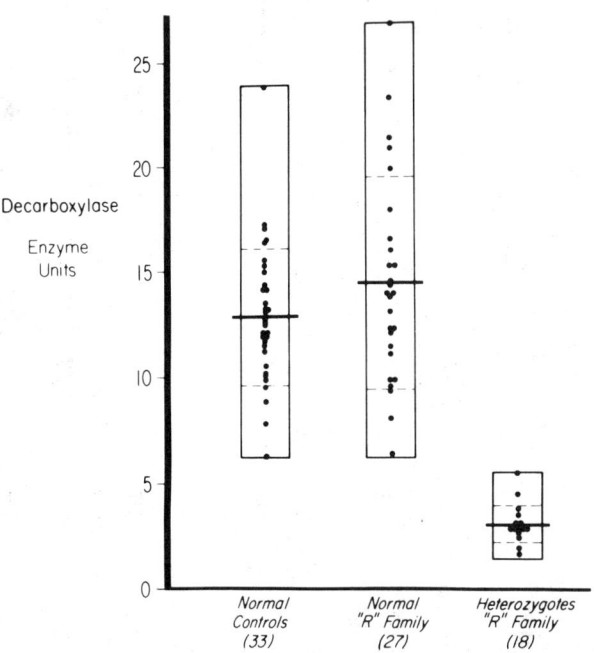

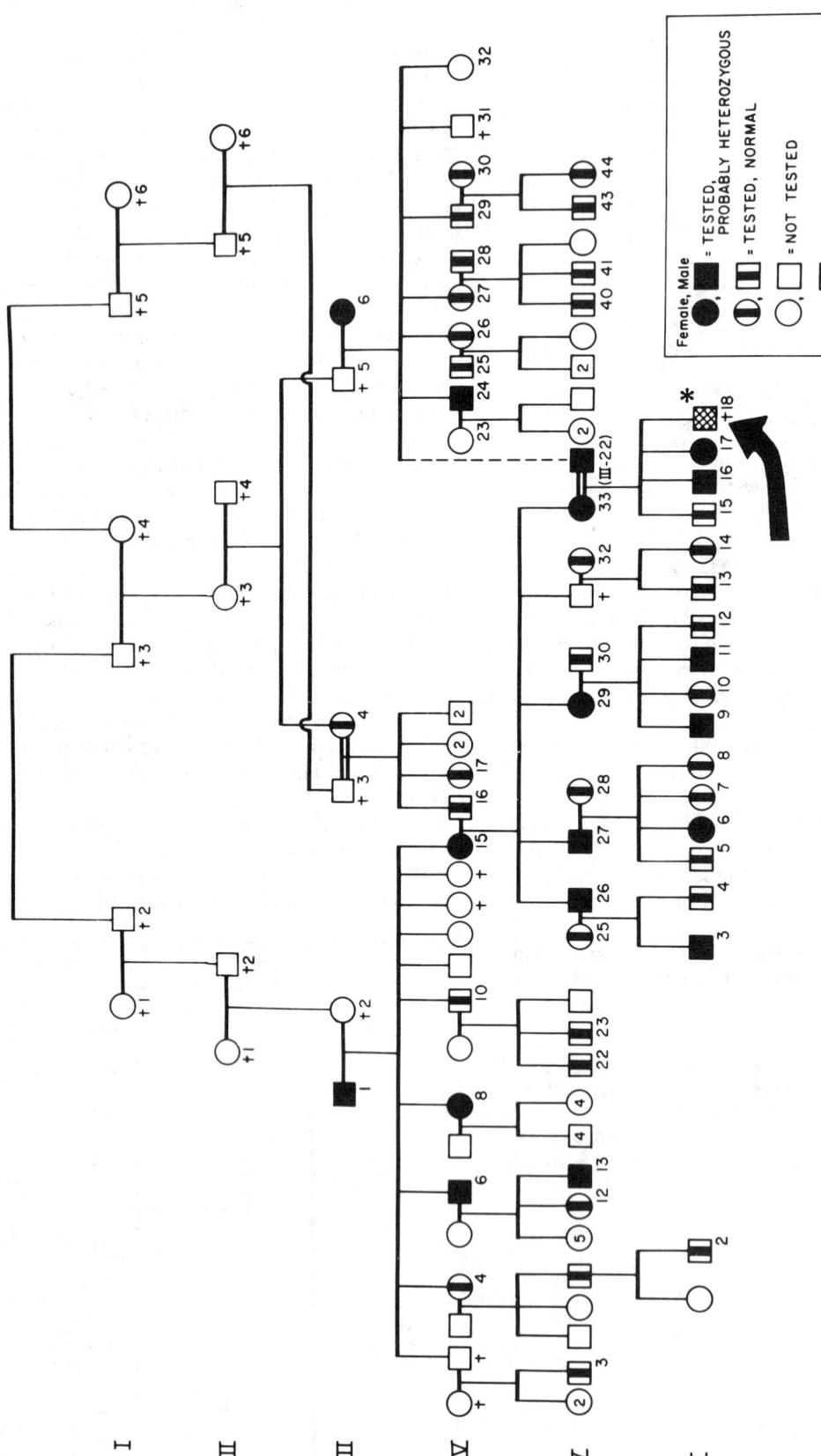

Figure 56-15 Pedigree of the R. family. The proband, patient J.R., is marked by an arrow. Presumed heterozygotes were identified in members of all four surviving generations. (*From Fallon et al.* [270]. *Used by permission.*)

pathway of pyrimidine biosynthesis *de novo* may usually be lethal. By analogy, mutants of *E. coli* are known which have "hereditary orotic aciduria" in that they exhibit a block at OPRT or ODC and accumulate orotic acid in the medium [*311, 312*]. These organisms fail to grow in the absence of an exogenous source of pyrimidines. As noted above, OPRT and ODC activities are not absent in diploid cell strains from patients with orotic aciduria [*7, 15*] but rather have approximately 0.4 to 5.0 percent of the activity of control cell lines. It is possible that this residual activity allows the marginal survival of an occasional homozygous case of hereditary orotic aciduria. The role of salvage synthesis of pyrimidine nucleotides from pyrimidine bases or nucleosides in the diet or released during catabolism has not been investigated in these patients but may also be important.

TREATMENT

Disability in hereditary orotic aciduria appears to be related to pyrimidine nucleotide deficiency and, to a much lesser degree, to toxicity of accumulated precursors. Glucocorticoid therapy led to a partial hematologic remission in two of the patients (J.R. and J.P.) without reversal of the megaloblastic marrow. The mechanism of this response is not clear. Oral replacement therapy with a mixture of yeast nucleotides in patient J.R. led to a rapid improvement in the general clinical state, a hematologic remission, and a decrease in urinary orotic acid (Fig. 56-3) [*1*]. This preparation caused gastrointestinal symptoms. All the surviving patients are now being treated with oral uridine in divided doses approximating 100 to 150 mg/(kg · day). The details of therapy and response have been summarized in the case reports earlier in the chapter and are summarized for patient D.G. in Fig. 56-5 and for patient T.H. in Fig. 56-6. Attempts at maintenance therapy with uracil were unsuccessful in two patients [*1, 10*]. A trial of allopurinol therapy in an attempt to increase OPRT and ODC activity was unsuccessful in two patients [*14*]. In general, hematologic abnormalities have responded promptly and completely to full doses of uridine, as have growth and development. In spite of normal growth, two of the patients still have mental deficiency (D.G. and J.P.). Patient D.B. was reported to have an IQ of 133. The severe illness which may occur (patient C.P.) and the residual impairment of mental function indicate the importance of early diagnosis and treatment.

Prenatal diagnosis might be attempted in order to allow pyrimidine therapy from birth or possibly termination of the pregnancy [*4, 313*]. It is possible that uridine treatment of the mother might prevent or reduce the occurrence of congenital abnormalities (such as those noted in Table 56-1), although the ability of uridine to cross the placental barrier has not been established.

Dr. L. H. Smith was the coauthor of this chapter in the previous edition of this book. His contribution is gratefully acknowledged.

REFERENCES

1. HUGULEY CM JR, BAIN JA, RIVERS S, SCOGGINS R: Refractory megaloblastic anemia associated with excretion of orotic acid. *Blood* 14:615, 1959

2. Fox RM, O'SULLIVAN WJ, FIRKIN BG: Orotic aciduria: Differing enzyme patterns. *Am J Med* 47:332, 1969

3. Fox RM, WOOD MJ, ROYSE-SMITH D, O'SULLIVAN WJ: Hereditary orotic aciduria: Types I and II. *Am J Med* 55:791, 1973

4. SEEGMILLER JE: Hereditary orotic aciduria, in Bondy PK (ed): *Duncan's Diseases of Metabolism.* Philadelphia, Saunders, 1969, p 570

5. SMITH LH JR, SULLIVAN M, HUGULEY CM JR: Pyrimidine metabolism in man. IV. The enzymatic defect of orotic aciduria. *J Clin Invest* 40:656, 1961

6. ROGERS LE, WARFORD LR, PATTERSON RB, PORTER FS: Hereditary orotic aciduria. I. A new case with family studies. *Pediatrics* 42:415, 1968

7. HOWELL RR, KLINENBERG JR, KROOTH RS: Enzyme studies on diploid cell strains developed from patients with hereditary orotic aciduria. *John Hopkins Med J* 120:81, 1967

8. SMITH LH JR: Hereditary orotic aciduria: Pyrimidine auxotrophism in man. *Am J Med* 38:1, 1965

9. BECROFT DMO, PHILLIPS LI: Hereditary orotic aciduria and megaloblastic anaemia: A second case, with response to uridine. *Brit Med J* 1:547, 1965

10. BECROFT DMO, PHILLIPS LI, SIMMONDS A: Hereditary orotic aciduria: Long-term therapy with uridine and trial of urcail. *J Pediatr* 75:885, 1969

11. WEBSTER DR, SIMMONDS HA, POTTER CF, BECROFT DMO: Purine and pyrimidine metabolism in hereditary orotic aciduria during a 15 year follow-up study. *Adv Exp Med Biol* 122B:203, 1979

12. HAGGARD ME, LOCKHART LH: Megaloblastic anemia with orotic aciduria. *Am J Dis Child* 113:733, 1967

13. HAGGARD ME: Personal communication

14. BEARDMORE TD, CASHMAN JS, KELLY WN: Mechanism of allopurinol mediated increase in enzyme activity in man. *J Clin Invest* 51:1823, 1972

15. TUBERGEN DG, KROOTH RS, HEYN RM: Hereditary orotic aciduria with normal growth and development. *Am J Dis Child* 118:864, 1969

16. NEIMANN N, NAJEAN Y, SCIALOM C, BOULARD M, PIERSON M, BERNARD J: Etude d'un cas d'anemie megaloblastique de l'enfant avec excretion anormale d'acide orotique. *Nouv Rev Fr Hematol* 5:445, 1963

17. NAJEAN AY: Personal communication

18. WADA Y, NISHIMURA Y, TANABU M, YOSHIMURA Y, IINUMA K, YOSHIDA T, ARAKAWA T: Hypouricemic, mentally retarded infant with a defect of 5-phosphoribosyl-1-pyrophosphate synthetase of erythrocytes. *Tohoku J Exp Med* 113:149, 1974

19. SHAMBAUGH GE III: Pyrimidine biosynthesis. *Am J Clin Nutr* 32:1290, 1979

20. MAKOFF AJ, RADFORD A: Genetics and biochemistry of carbamoyl phosphate biosynthesis and its utilization in the pyrimidine biosynthetic pathway. *Microbiol Rev* 42:307, 1978

21. JONES ME: Pyrimidine nucleotide biosynthesis in animals: Genes, enzymes, and regulation of UMP biosynthesis. *Ann Rev Biochem* 49:253, 1980

22. O'DONOVAN GA, NEUHARD J: Pyrimidine metabolism in microorganisms. *Bacteriol Rev* 34:278, 1970

23. COHEN PP: Biochemical aspects of metamorphosis: Transition from ammonotelism to ureotelism. *Harvey Lect* 60:119, 1966

24. JONES ME, ANDERSON AD, ANDERSON C, HODES S: Citrulline synthesis in rat tissues. *Arch Biochem* 95:499, 1961

25. SCHOOLER JM, FAHIEN LA, COHEN PP: 2-Acetoxyglutarate as an activator of carbamyl phosphate synthetase. *J Biol Chem* 238:1909, 1963

26. METZENBERG RL, MARSHALL M, PAIK WK, COHEN PP: The synthesis of carbamyl phosphate synthetase in thyroxin-treated tadpoles. *J Biol Chem* 236:162, 1961

27. LEVENBERG B: Role of L-glutamine as donor of carbamyl nitrogen for the enzymatic synthesis of citrulline in *Agaricus bisporus. J Biol Chem* 237:2590, 1962

28. PIERARD A, WIAME JM: Regulation and mutation affecting a glutamine dependent formation of carbamyl phosphate in *Escherichia coli. Biochem Biophys Res Commun* 15:76, 1964

29. LACROUTE F, PIERARD A, GRENSON M, WIAME JM: The biosynthesis of carbamoyl phosphate in *Saccharomyces cerevisiae. J Gen Microbiol* 40:127, 1965

30. O'NEAL D, NAYLOR AW: Purine and pyrimidine nucleotide inhibition of carbamyl phosphate synthetase from pea seedlings. *Biochem Biophys Res Comun* 31:322, 1968

31. TATIBANA M, ITO K: Carbamylphosphate synthetase of the hematopoietic mouse spleen and the control of pyrimidine biosynthesis. *Biochem Biophys Res Comun* 26:221, 1967

32. TATIBANA M, ITO K: Control of pyrimidine biosynthesis in mammalian tissues. I. Partial purification and characterization of glutamine-utilizing carbamyl phosphate synthesis of mouse spleen and its tissue distribution. *J Biol Chem* 244:5403, 1969

33. HAGER SE, JONES ME: Initial steps in pyrimidine synthesis in Ehrlich ascites carcinoma in vitro. II. The synthesis of carbamyl phosphate by a soluble, glutamine-dependent carbamyl phosphate synthetase. *J Biol Chem* 242:5667, 1967

34. SHAMBAUGH GE, MITZGER BE, FREINKEL N: Glutamine-dependent carbamyl phosphate synthetase in placenta and fetal structures of the rat. *Biochem Biophys Res Commun* 42:155, 1971

35. TATIBANA M, SHIGESADA K: Two carbamyl phosphate synthetase of mammals: Specific roles in control of pyrimidine and urea biosynthesis. *Adv Enzyme Regul* 10:249, 1972

36. GRILLOW MA, PINNA GG, CASOLO L: Carbamylphosphate synthetases in human liver. *Int J Biochem* 23:447, 1973

37. LEVINE RL, HOOGENRAAD NJ, KRETCHMER N: Regulation of activity of carbamoyl phosphate synthetase from mouse spleen. *Biochemistry* 10:3694, 1971

38. TATIBANA M, SHIGESADA K: Control of pyrimidine biosynthesis in mammalian tissues. V. Regulation of glutamine-dependent carbamyl phosphate synthetase: Activation by 5-phosphoribosyl 1-pyrophosphate and inhibition by uridine triphosphate. *J Biochem (Tokyo)* 72:549, 1972

39. SHOAF WT, JONES ME: Uridylic acid synthesis in Ehrlich ascites carcinoma: Properties, subcellular distribution, and nature of enzyme complexes of the six biosynthetic enzymes. *Biochemistry* 12:4039, 1973

40. SHOAF WT, JONES MF: Initial steps in pyrimidine synthesis in Ehrlich ascites carcinoma. *Biochem Biophys Res Commun* 45:796, 1971

41. SHOAF WT, JONES MF: Enzyme complexes of the pyrimidine pathway in Ehrlich ascites tumor cells. *Fed Proc* 31:473, 1972

42. HOOGENRAAD NJ, LEVINE RL, KRETCHMER N: Copurification of carbamoyl phosphate synthetase and aspartate transcarbamoylase from mouse spleen. *Biochem Biophys Res Commun* 44:981, 1971

43. ITO K, UCHINO H: Control of pyrimidine biosynthesis in human lymphocytes: Simultaneous increase in activities of glutamine-utilizing carbamyl phosphate synthetase and aspartate transcarbamylase in phytohemagglutinin-enzyme co-purification. *J Biol Chem* 248:389, 1973

44. MORI M, TATIBANA M: Dissociation by elastase digestion of enzyme complex catalyzing the initial steps of pyrimidine biosynthesis in rat liver. *Biochem Biophys Res Commun* 54:1525, 1973

45. MORI M, ISHIDA H, TATIBANA M: Aggregation states and catalytic properties of the multienzyme complex catalyzing the initial steps of pyrimidine biosynthesis in rat liver. *Biochemistry* 14:2622, 1975

46. MORI M, TATIBANA M: Purification of homogeneous glutamine-dependent carbamyl phosphate synthetase from ascites heptoma cells as a complex with aspartate transcarbamylase and dihydroorotase. *J Biochem (Tokyo)* 78:239, 1975

47. DAVIDSON JN, PATTERSON D: Alteration in structure of multifunctional protein from Chinese hamster ovary cells defective in pyrimidine biosynthesis. *Proc Natl Acad Sci USA* 76:1731, 1979

48. WAHL GM, PADGETT RA, STARK GR: Gene amplification causes overproduction of the first three enzymes of UMP synthesis in N-(phosphonacetyl)-L-aspartate-resistant hamster cells. *J Biol Chem* 254:8679, 1979

49. PATTERSON D, CARNRIGHT DV: Biochemical genetic analysis of pyrimidine biosynthesis in mammalian cells. I. Isolation of a mutant defective in the early steps of de novo pyrimidine synthesis. *Som Cell Genet* 3:483, 1977

50. COLEMAN PF, SUTTLE DP, STARK GR: Purification from hamster cells of the multifunctional protein that initiates de novo synthesis of pyrimidine nucleotides. *J Biol Chem* 252:6379, 1977

51. TRAUT TW, JONES ME: Interconversion of different molecular weight forms of the orotate phosphoribosyltransferase orotidine-5'-phosphate decarboxylase enzyme complex from mouse Ehrlich ascites cells *J Biol Chem* 254:1143, 1979

52. WILLIAMS LG, BERNHARDT SA, DAVIS RH: Evidence for two discrete carbamyl phosphate pools in Neurospora. *J Biol Chem* 246:973, 1971

53. NATALE PJ, TREMBLAY GC: On the availability of intramitochondrial carbamoyl phosphate for the extra mitochondrial biosynthesis of pyrimidines. *Biochem Biophys Res Commun* 37:512, 1969

54. BOURGET PA, NATALE PJ, TREMBLAY GC: Pyrimidine biosynthesis in rat liver: Studies on the source of carbamoyl phosphate. *Biochem Biophys Res Commun* 45:1109, 1971

55. DAVIS RH: Metabolite distribution in cells. Two carbamyl phosphate gradients and their sources can be discerned in Neurospora. *Science* 178:835, 1972

56. SMITH LH JR, REICHARD P: Enzymic synthesis of carbamylaspartate from citrulline in extracts from rat liver mitochondria. *Acta Chem Scand* 10:1024, 1956

57. PIERARD A, GLANSDORFF N, MERGEAY M, WIAME JM: Control of the biosynthesis of carbamoyl phosphate in *Escherichia coli*. *J Mol Biol* 14:23, 1965

58. MARSHALL M, COHEN PP: A kinetic study of the mechanism of crystalline carbamate kinase. *J Biol Chem* 241:4197, 1966

59. JONES ME: Carbamyl phosphate. *Science* 140:1373, 1963

60. YOUNG JE, PROGER MD, ATKINS IC: Comparative activities of aspartate transcarbamylase in various tissues of the rat. *Proc Soc Exp Biol Med* 125:860, 1967

61. YATES RA, PARDEE AB: Control of pyrimidine biosynthesis in *Escherichia coli* by a feed-back mechanism. *J Biol Chem* 221:757, 1956

62. CHANGEUX JP, GERHART JC, SCHACHMAN HK: Allosteric interactions in aspartate transcarbamylase. I. Binding of specific ligands to the native enzyme and its isolated subunits. *Biochemistry* 7:531, 1968

63. HERVE GL, STARK GR: Aspartate transcarbamylase: Amino terminal analyses and peptide maps of the subunits. *Biochemistry* 6:3743, 1967

64. WEBER K: New structural model of *E. coli* aspartate transcarbamylase and the amino acid sequence of the regulatory polypeptide chain. *Nature (London)* 218:1116, 1968

65. KLEPPE K: Aspartate transcarbamylase from *Escherichia coli*. I. Inhibition by inorganic anions. *Biochim Biophys Acta* 122:450, 1966

66. STEIN LI, COHEN PP: Correlation of growth and aspartate transcarbamylase activity in higher plants. *Arch Biochem* 109:429, 1965

67. BRESNICK E, HITCHINGS GH: Feedback control in Ehrlich ascites cells. *Cancer Res* 21:105, 1961

68. SMITH LH JR, BAKER FA: Pyrimidine metabolism in man. I. The biosynthesis of orotic acid. *J Clin Invest* 38:798, 1959

69. FAUSTO N: The control of RNA synthesis during liver regeneration. OMP pyrophosphorylase and decarboxylase activities in normal and regenerating liver. *Biochim Biophys Acta* 182:66, 1969

70. HOOGENRAAD NJ: Reaction mechanism of aspartate transcarbamylase from mouse spleen. *Arch Biochem Biophys* 161:76, 1974

71. PORTER RW, MODEBE MO, STARK GR: Aspartate transcarbamylase: Kinetic studies of the catalytic subunit. *J Biol Chem* 244:1846, 1969

72. LIEBERMAN I, KORNBERG A: Enzymatic synthesis and breakdown of a pyrimidine, orotic acid. II. Dihydroorotic acid, ureidosuccinic acid, and 5-carboxymethylhydantoin. *J Biol Chem* 207:911, 1954

73. YATES RA, PARDEE AB: Pyrimidine biosynthesis in *Escherichia coli*. *J Biol Chem* 221:743, 1956

74. SANDER EG, HEEB MJ: Purification and properties of dihydroortase from *Escherichia coli* B. *Biochim Biophys Acta* 227:442, 1971

75. SMITH LH JR, BAKER FA: Pyrimidine metabolism in man. III. Studies on leukocytes and erythrocytes in pernicious anemia. *J Clin Invest* 39:15, 1960

76. SMITH LH JR, SULLIVAN M: Feedback inhibition by fluorinated pyrimidines. *Biochim Biophys Acta* 39:554, 1960

77. SMITH LH JR, SULLIVAN M, BAKER FA, FREDRICK E: Inhibition of dihydroorotase in pyrimidine biosynthesis. *Cancer Res* 20:1059, 1960

78. SHAFRITZ DA, SENIOR JR: Synthesis of pyrimidine nucleotide precursors in human and rat small intestinal mucosa. *Biochim Biophys Acta* 141:32, 1967

79. KROOTH RS: Studies on the regulation of uridine 5-monophosphate synthesis in human diploid cells. *Symp Intern Soc Cell Biol* 9:43, 1970

80. CHRISTOPHERSON RI, JONES ME: Interconversion of carbamyl-1-aspartate and L-dihydroorotate by dihydroorotase from mouse Ehrlich ascites carcinoma. *J Biol Chem* 254:12506, 1979

81. KENNEDY J: Dihydroorotase from rat liver: Purification, properties and regulatory role in pyrimidine biosynthesis. *Arch Biochem Biophys* 160:358, 1974

82. MAKINEN MW, KUO LC, DYMOWSKI JJ, JAFFER S: Catalytic role of the metal ion of carboxypeptidase A in ester hydrolysis. *J Biol Chem* 254:356, 1979

83. TAYLOR WH, TAYLOR ML, BALCH WE, GILCHRIST PS: Purification and properties of dihydroorotase, a zinc-containing metalloenzyme in *Clostridium oroticum*. *J Bacteriol* 127:863, 1976

84. SANDER EG, WRIGHT LD, MCCORMICK DB: Evidence for function of a metal ion in the activity of dihydroorotase from *Zymobacterium oroticum*. *J Biol Chem* 240:3628, 1965

85. WALLACH DP, GRISOLIA S: The purification and properties of hydropyrimidine hydrase. *J Biol Chem* 26:277, 1957

86. LIEBERMAN I, KORNBERG A: Enzymatic synthesis and breakdown of a pyrimidine, orotic acid. I. Dihydro-orotic dehydrogenase. *Biochim Biophys Acta* 12:223, 1953

87. FRIEDMAN HD, VENNESLAND B: Crystalline dihydroorotic dehydrogenase. *J Biol Chem* 235:1526, 1960

88. ALEMAN V, HANDLER P: Dihydroorotate dehydrogenase. I. General properties. *J Biol Chem* 242:4087, 1967

89. ALEMAN V, HANDLER P, PALMER G, BEINERT H: Studies on dihydroorotate dehydrogenase by electron paramagnetic resonance spectroscopy. II. Electron paramagnetic resonance and optical spectra and titrations. *J Biol Chem* 243:2560, 1968

90. ALEMAN V, HANDLER P, PALMER G, BEINERT H: Studies on dihydroorotate dehydrogenase by electron paramagnetic resonance spectroscopy. III. Kinetic studies by rapid freezing. *J Biol Chem* 243:2569, 1968

91. MILLER RW, KERR CT: Dihydroorotate dehydrogenase. III. Interactions with substrates, inhibitors, artificial electron acceptors, and cytochrome c. *J Biol Chem* 241:5597, 1966

92. EAKIN RT, MITCHELL HK: A mitochondrial dihydroorotate oxidase system in *Neurospora crassa*. *Arch Biochem Biophys* 134:160, 1969

93. MILLER RW: Dihydroorotate dehydrogenase (neurospora). *Methods Enzymol* 51:63, 1978

94. MILLER RW, KERR CT, CURRY JR: Mammalian dihydro-orotate-ubiquinone reductase complex. *Can J Biochem* 46:1099, 1968

95. FORMAN HJ, KENNEDY J: Superoxide production and electron transport in oxidation of dihydro-orotic acid. *J Biol Chem* 250:4322, 1975

96. KARIBIAN D: Dihydro-orotate dehydrogenase of *Escherichia coli* K12: Effects of Triton X-100 and phospholipids. *Biochim Biophys Acta* 302:205, 1973

97. CHEN J-J, JONES ME: The cellular location of dihydroorotate dihydrogenase: Relation to de novo biosynthesis of pyrimidines. *Arch Biochem Biophys* 176:82, 1976

98. STAMATO TD, PATTERSON D: Biochemical genetic analysis of pyrimidine biosynthesis in mammalian cells. II. Isolation and characterization of a mutant of chinese hamster ovary cells with defective dihydroorotate dehydrogenase (E.C. 1.3.3.1) activity. *J Cell Physiol* 98:459, 1979

99. KENNEDY J: Distribution, subcellular localization, and product inhibition of dihydroorotate oxidation in the rat. *Arch Biochem Biophys* 157:369, 1973

100. WUU K-D, KROOTH RS: Dihydroorotic acid dehydrogenase activity of human diploid cell strains. *Science* 160:539, 1968

101. LOTZ M, SMITH LH JR: The effect of reticulocytosis in the rabbit on the activities of enzymes in pyrimidine biosynthesis. *Blood* 19:593, 1962

102. SANTILLI V, SKODA J, GUT J, SORM F: Dihydro-5-azaorotic acid: The first specific inhibitor of dihydro-orotate dehydrogenase. *Biochim Biophys Acta* 155:623, 1968

103. PAUSCH J, KEPPLER D, DECKER K: Activity and distribution of the enzymes of uridylate synthesis from orotate in animal tissues. *Biochim Biophys Acta* 258:395, 1972

104. GROBNER W, KELLEY WN: Unpublished results

105. SUTTLE DP, STARK GR: Coordinate overproduction of orotate phosphoribosyltransferase and orotidine-5'-phosphate decarboxylase in hamster cells resistant to pyrazofurin and 6-azauridine. *J Biol Chem* 254:4602, 1979

106. LEVINSON BB, ULLMAN B, MARTIN DW JR: Pyrimidine pathway variants of cultured mouse lymphoma cells with altered levels of both orotate phosphoribosyltransferase and orotidylate decarboxylase. *J Biol Chem* 254:4396, 1979

107. PATTERSON D: Isolation and characterization of 5-fluorouracil-resistant mutants of chinese hamster ovary cells deficient in the activities of orotate phosphoribosyltransferase and orotidine 5'-monophosphate decarboxylase. *Som Cell Genet* 6:101, 1980

108. GROBNER W, KELLEY WN: Effect of allopurinol and its metabolic derivatives on the configuration of human orotate phosphoribosyltransferase and orotidine 5'-phosphate decarboxylase. *Biochem Pharmacol* 24:379, 1975

109. BROWN GK, O'SULLIVAN WJ: Subunit structure of the orotate phosphoribosyltransferase–orotidylate decarboxylase complex from human erythrocytes. *Biochemistry* 16:3235, 1977

110. CAMPBELL MT, GALLAGHER ND, O'SULLIVAN WJ: Multiple molecular forms of orotidylate decarboxylase from human liver, *Biochem Med* 17:128, 1977

111. LIEBERMAN I, KORNBERG A, SIMMS ES: Enzymatic synthesis of pyrimidine nucleotides: Orotidine-5'-phosphate and uridine-5'-phosphate. *J Biol Chem* 215:403, 1955

112. HOLMES WL: Studies on the mode of action of analogues of orotic acid: 6-Uracilsulfonic acid, 6-uracilsulfonamide, and 6-uracil methylsulfone. *J Biol Chem* 223:677, 1956

113. KASBEKAR DK, NAGABHUSHANAM A, GREENBERG DM: Purification and properties of orotic acid-decarboxylating enzymes from calf thymus. *J Biol Chem* 239:4245, 1964

114. HOFFMAN DH, SWEENEY MJ: Orotate phosphorybosyltransferase and orotidylic acid decarboxylase activities in liver and Morris hepatomas. *Cancer Res* 13:1109, 1973

115. KESSEL D, DEACON J, COFFEY B, BAKAMJIAN A: Some properties of a pyrimidine phosphoribosyltransferase from murine leukemia cells. *Mol Pharmacol* 8:731, 1972

116. MOKRASCH LC, GRISOLIA S: Incorporation of hydropyrimidine derivatives in ribonucleic acid with liver preparations. *Biochim Biophys Acta* 27:226, 1958

117. CANELLAKIS ES: Pyrimidine metabolism. II. Enzymatic pathways of uracil anabolism. *J Biol Chem* 227:329, 1957

118. GOLDBERG AR, MACHLEDT JH, PARDEE AB: On the action of fluorouracil on leukemia cells. *Cancer Res* 26:1611, 1966

119. REYES P: The synthesis of 5-fluorouridine 5'-phosphate by a pyrimidine phosphoribosyltransferase of mammalian origin. I. Some properties of the enzyme from P1534J mouse leukemia cells. *Biochemistry* 8:2057, 1969

120. BROCKMAN RW, ANDERSON EP: Pyrimidine analogues, in Hochster RM, Quastel JH (eds): *Metabolic Inhibitors*. New York, Academic, 1963, vol I, p 239

121. BERNHARDT SA, DAVIS RH: Carbamoyl phosphate compartmentation in Neurospora: Histochemical localization of aspartate and ornithine transcarbamoylases. *Proc Natl Acad Sci USA* 69:1868, 1972

122. HATFIELD D, WYNGAARDEN JB: 3-Ribosylpurines. I. Synthesis of (3-ribosyluric acid) 5'-phosphate and (3-ribosylxanthine) 5'-phosphate by a pyrimidine ribonucleotide pyrophosphorylase of beef erythrocytes. *J Biol Chem* 239:2580, 1964

123. VICTOR J, GREENBERG LB, SLOAN DL: Studies of the kinetic mechanism of orotate phosphoribosyltransferase from yeast. *J Biol Chem* 254:2647, 1979

124. VICTOR J, LEO-MENSAH A, SLOAN DL: Divalent metal ion activation of the yeast orotate phosphoribosyltransferase catalyzed reaction. *Biochemistry* 18:3597, 1979

125. FYFE JA, MILLER RL, KRENITSKY TA: Kinetic properties and inhibition of orotidine 5'-phosphate decarboxylase. *J Biol Chem* 248:3801, 1973

126. WORTHY TE, GROBNER W, KELLEY WN: Hereditary orotic aciduria: Evidence for a structural gene mutation. *Proc Natl Acad Sci USA* 71:3031, 1974

127. BROWN GK, FOX RM, O'SULLIVAN WJ: Interconversion of different molecular weight forms of human erythrocyte orotidylate decarboxylase. *J Biol Chem* 250:7352, 1975

128. TAX WJM, VEERKAMP JH: Inhibition of orotate phosphoribosyltransferase and orotidine-5'-phosphate decarboxylase of human erythrocytes by purine and pyrimidine nucleotides. *Biochem Pharmacol* 28:829, 1979

129. JONES MD, KAVIPURAPU PR, TRAUT TW: Orotate phosphoribosyltransferase orotidylate decarboxylase (Ehrlich ascites cell). *Methods Enzymol* 51:55, 1978

130. APPEL SH: Purification and kinetic properties of brain orotidine 5'-phosphate decarboxylase. *J Biol Chem* 243:3924, 1968

131. REICHARD P: The enzymatic synthesis of pyrimidines. *Adv Enzymol* 21:263, 1959

132. KIT S: Nucleotides and nucleic acids, in Greenberg DM (ed): *Metabolic Pathways*, 3d ed. New York, Academic, 1970, vol IV, p 69

133. PAEGE LM, SCHLENK F: Bacterial uracil riboside phosphorylase. *Arch Biochem Biophys* 40:42, 1952

134. KRENITSKY TA, BARCLAY M, JACQUEZ JA: Specificity of mouse uridine phosphorylase: Chromatography, purification, and properties, *J Biol Chem* 239:805, 1964

135. FRIEDKIN M, ROBERTS D: The enzymatic synthesis of nucleosides. I. Thymidine phosphorylase in mammalian tissue. *J Biol Chem* 207:245, 1954

136. ZIMMERMAN M, SEIDENBERG J: Deoxyribosyl transfer. I. Thymidine phosphorylase and nucleoside deoxyribosyltransferase in normal and malignant tissues. *J Biol Chem* 239:2618, 1964

137. ZIMMERMAN M: Deoxyribosyl transfer. II. Nucleoside: Pyrimidine deoxyribosyltransferase activity of three partially purified thymidine phosphorylases. *J Biol Chem* 239:2622, 1964

138. SKOLD O: Uridine kinase from Ehrlich ascites tumor: Purification and properties. *J Biol Chem* 235:3273, 1960

139. REICHARD P, SKOLD O, KLEIN G: Possible enzymatic mechanism for the development of resistance against fluorouracil in ascites tumours. *Nature (London)* 183:939, 1959

140. SKOLD O: Studies on resistance against 5-fluorouracil. IV. Evidence for an altered uridine kinase in resistant cells. *Biochim Biophys Acta* 76:160, 1963

141. KORBECKI M, PLAGEMANN PGW: Competitive inhibition of uridine incorporation by 6-azauridine in uninfected and mengovirus-infected Novikoff hepatoma cells (34266). *Proc Soc Exp Biol Med* 132:587, 1969

142. KRYSTAL G, WEBB TE: Multiple forms of uridine kinase in normal and neoplastic rat liver. *Biochem J* 124:1943, 1971

143. BRESNICK E, THOMPSON VB, MORRIS HP, LIEBELT AG: Inhibition of thymidine kinase activity in liver and hepatomas by TTP and d-CTP. *Biochem Biophys Res Commun* 16:278, 1964

144. KLEMPERER HC, HAYNES GR: Thymidine kinase in rat liver during development. *Biochem J* 103:541, 1968

145. KIT S, DUBBS DR, PIEKARSKI LJ, HSU TC: Deletion of thymidine kinase activity from L cells resistant to bromodeoxyuridine. *Exp Cell Res* 31:297, 1963

146. ZICHA B, BURIC L: Deoxycytidine and radiation response: Exceedingly high deoxycytidine aminohydrolase activity in human liver. *Science* 163:191, 1969

147. CREASEY WA: Studies on the metabolism of 5-iodo-2'-deoxycytidine in vitro: Purification of nucleoside deaminase from mouse kidney. *J Biol Chem* 238:1772, 1963

148. TOMCHICK R, SASLAW LD, WARAVDEKAR VS: Mouse kidney cytidine deaminase: Purification and properties. *J Biol Chem* 243:2534, 1968

149. SUGINO Y, TERAOKA H, SHIMONO H: Metabolism of deoxyribonucleotides. I. Purification and properties of deoxycytidine monophosphokinase of calf thymus. *J Biol Chem* 241:961, 1966

150. FREARSON PM, KIT S, DUBBS DR: Deoxythymidylate synthetase and deoxythymidine kinase activities of virus-infected animal cells. *Cancer Res* 25:737, 1965

151. NAKAMURA H, SUGINO Y: Metabolism of deoxyribonucleotides. III. Purification and some properties of nucleoside dephosphokinase of calf thymus. *J Biol Chem* 241:4917, 1966a

152. MOURAD N, PARKS RE JR: Erythrocytic nucleoside dephosphokinase. II. Isolation and kinetics. *J Biol Chem* 241:271, 1966

153. MOORE EC, REICHARD P: Enzymatic synthesis of deoxyribonucleotides. VI. The cytidine dephosphate reductase system from Novikoff hepatoma. *J Biol Chem* 239:3453, 1964

154. LARSSON A, REICHARD P: Enzymatic synthesis of deoxyribonucleotides. IX. Allosteric effects in the reduction of pyrimidine ribonucleotides by the ribonucleoside diphosphate reductase system of Escherichia coli. *J Biol Chem* 241:2533, 1966

155. MOORE EC, HURLBERT RB: Regulation of mammalian deoxyribonucleotide biosynthesis by nucleotides as activators and inhibitors. *J Biol Chem* 241:4802, 1966

156. LARSSON A: Enzymatic synthesis of deoxyribonucleotides. III. Reduction of purine ribonucleotides with an enzyme system from *Escherichia coli* B. *J Biol Chem* 238:3414, 1963

157. MOORE EC: A thioredoxin-thioredoxin reductase system from rat tumor. *Biochem Biophys Res Commun* 29:264, 1967

158. HURLBERT RB, KAMMEN HO: Formation of cytidine nucleotides from uridine nucleotides by soluble mammalian enzymes: Requirements for glutamine and guanosine nucleotides. *J Biol Chem* 235:443, 1960

159. SALZMAN NP, EAGLE H, SEBRING ED: The utilization of glutamine, glutamic acid, and ammonia for the biosynthesis of nucleic acid bases in mammalian cell cultures. *J Biol Chem* 230:1001, 1958

160. EIDINOFF ML, KNOLL JE, MARANO B, CHEONG L: Purine studies. I. Effect of DON (6-diazo-5-oxo-L-norleucine) on incorporation of precursors into nucleic acid pyrimidines. *Cancer Res* 18:105, 1958

161. CANELLAKIS ES: Pyrimidine metabolism. I. Enzymatic pathways of uracil and thymine degradation. *J Biol Chem* 221:315, 1956

162. LEVENE PA, DILLON RT: Intestinal nucleotidase. *J Biol Chem* 88:753, 1930

163. HEPPEL LA, HILMOE RJ: 5′-Nucleotidases. *Methods Enzymol* 2:546, 1955

164. SONG CS, BODANSKY O: Purification of 5′-nucleotidase from human liver. *Biochem J* 101:5c, 1966

165. LEVIN SJ, BODANSKY O: The double pH optimum of 5′-nucleotidase of bull seminal plasma. *J Biol Chem* 241:51, 1966

166. WIDNELL CC, UNKELESS JC: Partial purification of a lipoprotein with 5′-nucleotidase activity from membranes of rat liver cells. *Proc Natl Acad Sci USA* 61:1050, 1968

167. DRUMMOND GI, YAMAMOTO M: Nucleotide phosphomonoesterases, in Boyer PD (ed): *The Enzymes.* New York, Academic, 1960, vol IV, pp 337–354

168. PAGLIA DE, VALENTINE WN: Characteristics of a pyrimidine specific 5′ nucleotidase in human erythrocytes. *J Biol Chem* 250:7973, 1975

169. HARLEY EH, HEATON A, WICOMB W: Pyrimidine metabolism in hereditary erythrocyte pyrimidine 5′ nucleotidase deficiency. *Metabolism* 27:1743, 1978

170. GRISOLIA S, CARDOSO SS: The purification and properties of hydropyrimidine dehydrogenase. *Biochim Biophys Acta* 25:430, 1957

171. LIEBERMAN I, KORNBERG A: Enzymatic synthesis and breakdown of a pyrimidine orotic acid. III. Ureidosuccinase. *J Biol Chem* 212:909, 1955

172. GRISOLIA S, CARAVACA J, CARDOSO S, WALLACH DP: Metabolism of dihydropyrimidines and related compounds. *Fed Proc* 16:189, 1957

173. CARAVACA J, GRISOLIA S: Enzymatic decarbamylation of carbamyl β-alanine and carbamyl β-aminoisobutyric acid. *J Biol Chem* 231:357, 1958

174. VON EULER LH, RUBIN RJ, HANDSCHUMACHER RE: Fatty livers induced by orotic acid. II. Changes in nucleotide metabolism. *J Biol Chem* 238:2464, 1963

175. RABKIN MT, FREDERICK EW, LOTZ M, SMITH LH JR: Pyrimidine metabolism in man. V. The measurement in vivo of the biochemical effect of antineoplastic agents in animal and human subjects. *J Clin Invest* 41:871, 1962

176. ITO K, NAKANISHI S, TERADA M, TATIBANA M: Control of pyrimidine biosynthesis in mammalian tissues. II. Glutamine utilizing carbamoyl phosphate synthetase of various experimental tumors: Distribution, purification, and characterization. *Biochim Biophys Acta* 220:477, 1970

177. CURCI MR, CONACHIE WD: An attempt to find pyrimidine inhibitors of a mammalian aspartate carbamoyltransferase. *Biochim Biophys Acta* 85:338, 1964

178. BRESNICK E, MOSSE H: Aspartate carbamoyltransferase from rat liver. *Biochem J* 101:63, 1966

179. KOSKIMIES O, OLIVER I, HURWITZ R, KRETCHMER N: Aspartate transcarbamoylase: Distribution in various tissues and identification of three molecular forms. *Biochem Biophys Res Commun* 42:1162, 1971

180. PRAGER MD, YOUNG JE, ATKINS IC: A study of the possible role of feedback inhibition of aspartate transcarbamylase in regulation of pyrimidine synthesis in human leukocytes. *J Lab Clin Med* 70:768, 1967

181. TATE SS, MEISTER A: Regulation of rat liver glutamine synthetase: Activation by α-ketoglutarate and inhibition by glycine, alanine, and carbamyl phosphate. *Proc Natl Acad Sci USA* 68:781, 1971

182. HAGER SE, JONES ME: Initial steps in pyrimidine synthesis in Ehrlich ascites carcinoma in vitro. I. Factors affecting the incorporation of ^{14}C-bicarbonate into carbon 2 of the uracil ring of the acid soluble nucleotides. *J Biol Chem* 240:4556, 1965

183. HISATA T, TATIBANA M: Control of de novo pyrimidine biosynthesis in mammalian tissues: Levels and turnover of early intermediates in mouse spleen in vivo. *Eur J Biochem* 105:155, 1980

184. ELLIOT WH: Glutamine synthesis. *Methods Enzymol* 2:337, 1955

185. ISHII K, GREEN H: Lethality of adenosine for cultured mammalian cells by interference with pyrimidine biosynthesis. *J Cell Sci* 13:429, 1973

186. CHEN J-J, JONES ME: Effect of 5-phosphoribosyl-pyrophosphate on de novo pyrimidine biosynthesis in cultured Ehrlich ascites cells made permeable with dextran sulfate 500. *J Biol Chem* 254:2697, 1979

187. GUDAS LJ, COHEN A, ULLMAN B, MARTIN DW JR: Analysis of adenosine deaminase medicated pyrimidine starvation using cultured wild type and mutant mouse T-lymphoma cells. *Som Cell Genet* 4:201, 1978

188. CRANDALL DE, LOVATT CJ, TREMBLAY GC: Regulation of pyrimidine biosynthesis by purine and pyrimidine nucleosides in slices of rat tissues. *Arch Biochem Biophys* 188:194, 1978

189. APPEL SH, PETTIS P: Regulation of brain orotidylic decarboxylase activity. *Fed Proc* 26:292, 1967

190. BLAIR DGR, POTTER VR: Inhibition of orotidylic acid decarboxylase by uridine 5′-phosphate. *J Biol Chem* 263:2503, 1961

191. BLAIR DGR, STONE JE, POTTER VR: Formation of orotidine 5′-phosphate by enzymes from rat liver. *J Biol Chem* 235:2379, 1960

192. CREASEY WA, HANDSCHUMACHER RE: Purification and properties of orotidylate decarboxylases from yeast and rat liver. *J Biol Chem* 236:2058, 1961

193. TRAUT TW, JONES ME: Inhibitors of orotate phosphoribosyltransferase and orotidine-5′-phosphate decarboxylase from mouse Ehrlich ascites cells: A procedure for analyzing the inhibition of a multi-enzyme complex. *Biochem Pharmacol* 26:2291, 1977

194. CHEN J-J, JONES ME: Effect of 6-azauridine on de novo pyrimidine biosynthesis in cultured Ehrlich ascites cells: Orotate inhibition of dihydroorotase and dihydroorotate dehydrogenase. *J Biol Chem* 254:4908, 1979

195. ROUX JM, HOOGENRAAD NJ, KRETCHMER N: Biosynthesis of pyrimidine nucleotides in mouse salivary glands stimulated with isoproterenol. *J Biol Chem* 248:1196, 1973

196. ITO K, UCHINO H: Control of pyrimidine biosynthesis in human lymphocytes: Induction of glutamine-utilizing carbamyl phosphate synthetase and operation of orotic acid pathway during blastogenesis. *J Biol Chem* 246:4060, 1971

197. ALLEN CM, JONES ME: Decomposition of carbamylphosphate in aqueous solutions. *Biochemistry* 3:1238, 1964

198. DAVIDSON JN, CARNRIGHT DV, PATTERSON D: Biochemical genetic analysis of pyrimidine biosynthesis in mammalian cells. III. Association of carbamyl phosphate synthetase, aspartate transcarbamylase, and dihydroorotase in mutants of cultured chinese hamster cells. *Som Cell Genet* 5:175, 1979

199. PADGETT RA, WAHL GM, COLEMAN PF, STARK GR: N-(Phosphonacetyl)-L-aspartate–resistant hamster cells overaccumulate a single mRNA coding for the multifunctional protein that catalyzes the first steps of UMP synthesis. *J Biol Chem* 254:974, 1979

200. REYES P, INTRESS C: Coordinate behavior of orotate phosphoribosyltransferase and orotidylate decarboxylase in developing mouse liver and brain. *Life Sci* 22:577, 1978

201. YIP MCM, KNOX WE: Glutamine-dependent carbamyl phosphate synthetase: Properties and distribution in normal and neoplastic rat tissues. *J Biol Chem* 245:2199, 1970

202. HAGER SE, JONES ME: A glutamine-dependent enzyme for the synthesis of carbamyl phosphate for pyrimidine biosynthesis in fetal rat liver. *J Biol Chem* 242:5674, 1967

203. WEICHSEL ME, HOOGENRAAD NJ, LEVINE RL, KRETCHMER N: Pyrimidine biosynthesis during development of rat cerebellum. *Pediatr Res* 6:682, 1972

204. ITO K, UCHINO H: Control of pyrimidine biosynthesis in human lymphocytes: Inhibitory effect of guanine and guanosine on induction of enzymes for pyrimidine biosynthesis de novo in phytohemogglutin-stimulated lymphocytes. *J Biol Chem* 251:1427, 1976

205. PINSKY L, KROOTH RS: Studies on the control of pyrimidine biosynthesis in human diploid cell strains. I. Effect of 6-azauridine on cellular phenotype. *Proc Natl Acad Sci USA* 57:925, 1967

206. PINSKY L, KROOTH RS: Studies on the control of pyrimidine biosynthesis in human diploid cell strains. II. Effects of 5-azaorotic acid, barbituric acid, and pyrimidine precursors on cellular phenotype. *Proc Natl Acad Sci USA* 57:1267, 1967

207. KROOTH RS, LAM GFM, CHEN KIANG SY: Oxipurinol and orotic aciduria: Effect on the orotidine-5′-monophosphate decarboxylase activity of cultured human fibroblasts. *Cell* 3:55, 1974

208. TAX WJM, VEERKAMP JH, SCHRETLEN EDAM: Pyrimidine metabolism in erythrocytes of the newborn. *Biol Neonate* 35:121, 1979

209. ZIELKE HR, OZAND PT, LUDDY RE, ZINKHAM WH, SCHWARTZ AD, SEVDALIAN DA: Elevation of pyrimidine enzyme activities in the RBC of patients with congenital hypoplastic anaemia and their parents. *Br J Haematol* 42:381, 1979

210. VANDER WEYDEN MB, COOPER M, FIRKIN BG: Altered erythrocyte pyrimidine activity in vitamine B₁₂ or folate deficiency. *Br J Haematol* 42:85, 1979

211. FOX RM, ROYSE-SMITH D, O'SULIVAN WJ: Orotidinuria induced by allopurinol. *Science* 168:861, 1970

212. HOOGENRAAD NJ, LEE DC: Effect of uridine on de novo pyrimidine biosynthesis in rat hepatoma cells in culture. *J Biol Chem* 249:2763, 1974

213. BECKER ME, ARGUBRIGHT KF, FOX RM, SEEGMILLER JE: Oxipurinol-associated inhibition of pyrimidine synthesis in human lymphoblasts. *Mol Pharmacol* 10:657, 1974

214. FIELDS T, BROX L: Purine and pyrimidine pool sizes and purine base utilization in human lymphocytes and cultured lymphoblasts. *Can J Biochem* 52:441, 1974

215. NUKI G, ASTRIN K, BRENTON D, CRUISHANK M, LEVER J, SEEGMILLER J: Purine and pyrimidine nucleotide pools in azaguanine resistant human lymphoblasts deficient in HGPRT. *Am J Hum Genet* 25:56a, 1973 (abstract)

216. KROOTH RS: Properties of diploid cell strains developed from patients with an inherited abnormality of uridine biosynthesis. *Cold Spring Harbor Symp Quant Biol* 29:189, 1964

217. GREEN H, CHAN T-S: Pyrimidine starvation induced by adenosine in fibroblasts and lymphoid cells: Role of adenosine deaminase. *Science* 182:836, 1973

218. MCBURNEY MW, WHITMORE GF: Mutants of chinese hamster cells resistant to adenosine. *J Cell Physiol* 85:87, 1975

219. FOX IH: The inhibition of phosphoribosylpyrophosphate synthesis by purine nucleosides in human erythrocytes. *J Biol Chem* 251:5839, 1976

220. HASHMI S, MAY SR, KROOTH RS, MILLER OJ: Concurrent development of resistance to 6-azauridine and adenosine in a mouse cell line. *J Cell Physiol* 86:191, 1975

221. BISCARO G, BELLONI E: Uber die Orotsaure. *Ann Soc Chim Milano* 11:1, 1905, *Chem Zentralbl* 2:64, 1905

222. KOBATA A, SUZUOKI J, KIDA M: Acid-soluble nucleotides of milk. I. Quantitative and qualitative differences of nucleotide constituents in human and cow milk. *J Biochem (Tokyo)* 51:277, 1962

223. TAX WJM, VEERKAMP JH, SCHRETLEN EDAM: The urinary excretion of orotic acid and orotidine, measured by an isotope dilution assay. *Clin Chim Acta* 90:217, 1978

224. LEVINE RL, HOOGENRAAD NJ, KRETCHMER N: A review: Biological and clinical aspects of pyrimidine metabolism. *Pediatr Res* 8:724, 1974

225. OKONKOYO PO, KINSELLA JE: Orotic acid in food milk powders. *Am J Clin Nutr* 22:532, 1969

226. RUNDLES RW, BREWER SS JR: Hematologic responses in pernicious anemia to orotic acid. *Blood* 13:99, 1958

227. SCHANKER LS, JEFFREY JJ: Structural specificity of the pyrimidine transport process of the small intestin. *Biochem Pharmacol* 11:961, 1962

228. BACHMANN C, COLOMBO JP: Determination of orotic acid in children's urine. *J Clin Chem Clin Biochem* 18:293, 1980

229. VOLLE Rl, GREEN RE, PETERS L, HANDSCHUMACHER RE, WELCH AD: Renal tubular excretion studies with pyrimidine derivatives and analogues. *J Pharmacol Exp Ther* 136:353, 1962

230. HANSCHUMAHER RE, COLERIDGE J: Hepatic and biliary transport of orotate and its metabolic consequences. *Biochem Pharmacol* 28:1977, 1978

231. DURSCHLAG RP, ROBINSON JL: Species specificity in the metabolic consequences of orotic acid consumption. *J Nutr* 110:822, 1980

232. WEISSMANN SM, EISEN AZ, FALLON H, LEWIS M, KARON M: The metabolism of ring-labeled orotic acid in man. *J Clin Invest* 41:1546, 1962

233. FALLON HJ, FREI E III, BLOCK J, SEEGMILLER JE: The uricosuria and orotic aciduria induced by 6-azauridine. *J Clin Invest* 40:1906, 1961

234. ROSENBLOOM FM, SEEGMILLER JE: An enzymatic spectrophotometric method for determination of orotic acid. *J Lab Clin Med* 63:492, 1964

235. SMITH LH JR, GILMOUR L: Determination of urinary carbamylaspartate and dihydro-orotate in normal subjects and in patients with hereditary orotic aciduria. *J Lab Clin Med* 86:1047, 1975

236. STANDERFER SB, HANDLER P: Fatty liver induced by orotic acid feeding. *Proc Soc Exp Biol Med* 90:270, 1955

237. CREASEY WA, HANKIN L, HANDSCHUMACHER RE: Fatty livers induced by orotic acid. I. Accumulation and metabolism of lipids. *J Biol Chem* 236:2064, 1961

238. WINDMUELLER HG, LEVY RI: Total inhibition of hepatic betalipoprotein production in the rat by orotic acid. *J Biol Chem* 242:2246, 1967

239. MARCHETTI M, PUDDU P, CALDARERA CM: Liver acid soluble nucleotides in orotic acid-fed rats. *Biochim Biophys Acta* 61:826, 1962

240. POTTENGER LA, FRAZIER LE, DuBIEN LH, GETZ GS, WISSTER RW: CHO composition of lipoprotein apoproteins isolated from rat plasma and from

241. the livers of rats fed orotic acid. *Biochem Biophys Res Commun* 54:770, 1973

241. ELWOOD JC, RICHERT DA, WESTERFELD WW: A comparison of hypolipidemic drugs in the prevention of an orotic acid fatty liver. *Biochem Pharmacol* 21:1127, 1972

242. WINDMUELLER HG, VON EULER LH: Prevention of orotic acid–induced fatty liver with allopurinol. *Proc Soc Exp Biol Med* 136:98, 1971

243. NOVIKOFF PM, ROHEIM PS, NOVIKOFF AB, EDELSTEIN D: Production and prevention of fatty liver in rats fed clofibrate and orotic acid diets containing sucrose. *Lab Invest* 30:732, 1974

244. VALLI EA, SARNA DAR, SARMA PS: Species specificity in orotic acid induced fatty liver. *Indian J Biochem* 5:120, 1968

245. KELLEY WN, GREENE ML, FOX IH, ROSENBLOOM FM, LEVY RI, SEEGMILLER JE: Effects of orotic acid on purine and lipoprotein metabolism in man. *Metabolism* 19:1025, 1970

246. DELBARRE F, AUSCHER C: Traitment de la goutte par l'acide uracil-6-carboxylique et ses derives. *Presse Med* 71:1765, 1963

247. KELLEY WN, FOX IH, WYNGAARDEN JB: Regulation of purine biosynthesis in cultured human cells. I. Effects of orotic acid. *Biochim Biophys Acta* 215:512, 1970

248. MATSUDA L, SHIRAHATA T: Effects of aspartic acid and orotic acid upon serum bilirubin levels in new born infants. *Tohoku J Exp Med* 90:133, 1966

249. KINTZEL HW, HINKEL GK, SCHWARZE R: The decrease in the serum bilirubin levels by orotic acid. *Acta Paediatr Scand* 60:1, 1971

250. CUTILLO S, MELONI T, DORE A: Effect of orotic acid upon serum bilirubin in newborn infants with erythrocyte G-6-PD deficiency. *Acta Paediatr Scand* 63:143, 1974

251. GRAY DWG, MOWAT AP: Effects of aspartic acid, orotic acid and glucose on serum bilirubin concentrations in infants born before term. *Arch Dis Child* 46:123, 1971

252. KOLOS G, WILLIAMS JF, HICKIE JB: Biochemical studies in myocardial hypertrophy and metabolic support of the acutely stressed myocardium. *Adv Cardiol* 12:106, 1974

253. MEERSON FZ: The myocardium in hyperfunction, hypertrophy and heart failure. *Circ Res* 24/25:1, 1969

254. LUKOMSKII PE, et al.: Kardiologiia 1, 1(in Russian), 1967. Quoted by Meerson FZ, in The myocardium in hyperfunction, hypertrophy and heart failure. *Circ Res* 25(suppl II):153, 1969

255. PATES MM, TSEITINA AY, POMERANTSEVA II, TUNITSKAYA TA, KURKMA VS, TURETSKAYA IM: Protective action of orotic acid on the liver following exposure to low doses of toxic substances. *Chem Abstr* 70:56116e, 1969

256. DECKER K, KEPPLER D, RUDIGIER J, DONISCHKE W: Cell damage by trapping of biosynthetic intermediates: The role of uracil nucleotides in experimental hepatitis. *Hoppe Seyler's Z Physiol Chem* 352:412, 1971

257. SMITH LH, HUGULEY CM, BAIN JA: Hereditary orotic aciduria, in Stanbury JB, Wyngaarden JB, Fredrickson DS (eds): *The Metabolic Basis of Inherited Disease.* New York, McGraw-Hill, 1966, p 739

258. BAIN JA, HUGULEY CM JR: Unpublished observations

259. LACROUTE F: Regulation of pyrimidine biosynthesis in *Saccharomyces cerevisiae. J Bacteriol* 95:824, 1968

260. KROOTH RS: Studies on the regulation of UMP synthesis in human diploid cells, in Padykula H (ed): *Control Mechanisms in Expression of Cellular Phenotype.* New York, Academic, 1970

261. LOTZ M, FALLON HJ, SMITH LH JR: Excretion of orotic acid and orotidine in heterozygotes of congenital orotic aciduria. *Nature (London)* 1997:194, 1963

262. SEEGMILLER JE, GRAYZEL AI, LASTER L, LIDDLE L: Uric acid production in gout. *J Clin Invest* 40:1304, 1961

263. ROSENBLOOM FM, HENDERSON JF, CALDWELL IC, KELLEY WN, SEEGMILLER JE: Biochemical bases of accelerated purine biosynthesis de novo in human fibroblasts lacking hypoxanthine-guanine phosphoribosyltransferase. *J Biol Chem* 243:1166, 1968

264. FOX IH, KELLEY WN: Phosphoribosylpyrophosphate in man. Biochemical and clinical significance. *Ann Intern Med* 74:424, 1971

265. RAJALAKSHMI S, HANDSCHUMACHER RE: Control of purine biosynthesis de novo by orotic acid in vivo and in vitro. *Biochim Biophys Acta* 155:317, 1968

266. BLOOMFIELD RA, LETTER AA, WILSON RP: Effect of orotic acid on the lipid and acid-soluble nucleotide concentrations in avian liver. *Biochim Biophys Acta* 187:266, 1969

267. THORELL B: Studies on the formation of cellular substances during blood cell production. *Acta Med Scand* (Suppl) 200:1, 1947

268. CARDOSO SS, CALABRESI P, HANDSCHUMACHER RE: Alterations in human pyrimidine metabolism as a result of therapy with 6-azauridine. *Cancer Res* 21:1551, 1961

269. HANDSCHUMACHER RE: Orotidylic acid decarboxylase: Inhibition studies with azauridine 5'phosphate. *J Biol Chem* 235:2917, 1960

270. FALLON HJ, LOTZ M, SMITH LH JR: Congenital orotic aciduria: Demon-

stration of an enzyme defect in leukocytes and comparison with drug-induced orotic aciduria. *Blood* 20:700, 1962

271. OHNUMA T, ROBBOZ J, SHAPIRO ML, HOLLAND JF: Pharmacological and biochemical effects of pyrazofurin in humans. *Cancer Res* 37:2043, 1977

272. CADMAN EC, DIX DE, HANDSCHUMACHER RE: Clinical, biological and biochemical effects of pyrazofurin. *Cancer Res* 38:682, 1978

273. MOYER JD, HANDSCHUMACHER RE: Selective inhibition of pyrimidine synthesis and depletion of nucleotide pools by N-(phosphonacetyl)-L-aspartate. *Cancer Res* 39:3089, 1979

274. KELLEY WN, BEARDMORE TD: Allopurinol: Alteration in pyrimidine metabolism in man. *Science* 169:388, 1970

275. BEARDMORE TD, FOX IH, KELLEY WN: Effect of allopurinol on pyrimidine metabolism in the Lesch-Nyhan syndrome. *Lancet* 2:830, 1970

276. HATFIELD D, WYNGAARDEN JB: 3-Ribosylpurines. II. Studies on (3-ribosylxanthine) 5'-phosphate and on ribonucleotide derivatives of certain uracil analogues. *J Biol Chem* 239:2587, 1964

277. BEARDMORE TD, KELLEY WN: Mechanism of allopurinol mediated inhibition of pyrimidine biosynthesis. *J Lab Clin Med* 78:696, 1971

278. FOX IH, WYNGAARDEN JB, KELLEY WN: Depletion of erythrocyte phosphoribosylpyrophosphate in man, a newly observed effect of allopurinol. *N Engl J Med* 283:1177, 1970

279. NELSON DJ, BUGGE CJL, KRASNY HC, ELION GB: Formation of nucleotides of [6-^{14}C]oxipurinol in rat tissues and effects on uridine nucleotide pools. *Biochem Pharmacol* 22:2003, 1973

280. WESTWICK WJ, ALLSOP J, GUMPEL JM, WATTS RWE: Studies on pyrimidine biosynthesis in the granulocytes of patients receiving gold therapy for rheumatoid arthritis. *Q J Med New Series* 43:170, 231, 1974

281. WESTWICK WJ, ALLSOP J, WATTS RWE: The effect of gold salts on the biosynthesis of uridine nucleotides in human granulocytes. *Biochem Pharmacol* 23:153, 1974

282. KLUBES P, FAY PJ, CERNA I: Effects of chlorpromazine on cell wall biosynthesis and incorporation of orotic acid into nucleic acids in *Bacillus megaterium*. *Pharmacol* 20:265, 1971

283. LEVIN B, ABRAHAM JM, OBERHOLZER VG, BURGESS EA: Hyperammonaemia: A deficiency of liver ornithine transcarbamylase: Occurrence in mother and child. *Arch Dis Child* 44:152, 1969

284. CORBEEL LM, COLOMBO JB, VAN SANDE M, WEBER A: Periodic attacks of lethargy in a baby with ammonia intoxication due to a congenital defect in ureogenesis. *Arch Dis Child* 44:681, 1969

285. SUNSHINE P, LINDENBAUM JD, LEVY HL, FREEMAN JM: Hyperammonemia due to a defect in hepatic ornithine transcarbamylase. *Pediatrics* 50:100, 1972.

286. MACLEOD P, MACKENZIE S, SCRIVER CR: Partial ornithine carbamyl transferase deficiency: An inborn error of the urea cycle presenting as orotic aciduria in a male infant. *Can Med Assoc J* 107:405, 1972

287. VAN GENNIP AH, VAN BREE-BLOM EJ, GRIFT J, DEBREE PK, WADMAN SK: Urinary purines and pyrimidines in patients with hyperammonemia of various origins. *Clin Chim Acta* 104:227, 1980

288. KANG ES, SNODGRASS PJ, GERALD PS: Ornithine transcarbamylase deficiency in the newborn infant. *J Pediatr* 82:642, 1973

289. GOLDSTEIN AS, HOOGENRAAD NJ, JOHNSON JD, FUKANAGA K, SWIEREZEWSKI E, CANN HM, SUNSHINE P: Metabolic and genetic studies of a family with ornithine transcarbamylase deficiency. *Pediatr Res* 8:5, 1974

290. STATTER M, RUSSEL A, ABZERG-HOROWITZ S, PUISON A: Abnormal orotic acid metabolism associated with acute hyperammonaemia in the rat. *Biochem Med* 9:1, 1974

291. THALER MM, HOOGENRAAD NJ, BOSWELL M: Reye's syndrome due to a novel protein variant of ornithine transcarbamylase deficiency. *Lancet* 2:438, 1974

292. THALER MM: Role of ornithine transcarbamylase in Reye's syndrome. *N Engl J Med* 291:797, 1974 (letter)

293. BELLINGER JF, BUIST NRH: Rapid column-chromatographic measurement of orotic acid. *Clin Chem* 17:1132, 1971

294. MILNER JA, VISEK WJ: Orotic aciduria and arginine deficiency. *Nature (London)* 245:211, 1973

295. HASSAN AS, MILNER JA: Orotic acid biosynthesis in arginine-deficient rats. *Arch Biochem Biophys* 194:24, 1979

296. COSTELLO MJ, MORRIS JG, ROGERS QR: Effect of dietary arginine level on urinary orotate and citrate excretion in growing kittens. *J Nutr* 110:1204, 1980

297. HATCHWELL LC, MILNER JA: Amino acid induced orotic aciduria. *J Nutr* 108:578, 1978

298. HEIRD WC, NICHOLSON JF, DRISCOLL JM, SCHULLINGER JN, WINTERS RW: Hyperammonemia resulting from intravenous alimentation using a mixture of synthetic L-amino acids. A preliminary report. *J Pediatr* 81:162, 1972

299. BEARDMORE TD, MEADE JC, KELLEY WN: Increased activity of two enzymes of pyrimidine biosynthesis de novo in erythrocytes from patients with the Lesch-Nyhan syndrome. *J Lab Clin Med* 81:43, 1973

300. COHEN A, STAAL GEJ, AMMANN AJ, MARTIN DW JR: Orotic aciduria in two unrelated patients with inherited deficiencies of purine nucleoside phosphorylase. *J Clin Invest* 60:491, 1977

301. EDWARDS L, GELFAND EW, BIGGAR D, FOX IH: Partial deficiency of purine nucleoside phosphorylase: Studies of purine and pyrimidine metabolism. *J Lab Clin Med* 91:736, 1978

302. SIMMOND HA, POTTER CF, SAHOTA A, CAMERON JS, WEBSTER DR, BECROFT DMO: Absence of oroticaciduria in adenosine deaminase deficiency and purine nucleoside phosphorylase deficiency. *Clin Exp Immunol* 34:42, 1978

303. VAN GENNIP AH, GRIFT J, DEBREE PK, ZEGERS BJM, STOOP JW, WADMAN SK: Urinary excretion of orotic acid, orotidine and other pyrimidines in a patient with purine nucleoside phosphorylase deficiency. *Clin Chim Acta* 93:419, 1979

304. FOX IH, BURK L, PLANET G, GOREN M, KAMINSKA J: Pyrimidine nucleotide biosynthesis. A study of normal and purine enzyme-deficiency cells. *J Biol Chem* 253:6794, 1978

305. FALLON HJ, SMITH LH JR, LOTZ M, GRAHAM JB, BURNETT CH: Hereditary orotic aciduria. *Trans Assoc Am Phys* 76:214, 1963

306. FALLON HJ, SMITH LH JR, GRAHAM JB, BURNETT CH: A genetic study of hereditary orotic aciduria. *N Engl J Med* 270:878, 1964

307. HOWARD B, SMITH LH JR: Unpublished observations

308. ROGERS LE, NICOLAISON AK, HOLT JG: Hereditary orotic aciduria: Results of a screening survey. *J Lab Clin Med* 85:287, 1975

309. GROBNER W, KELLEY WN: Unpublished observations

310. ROGERS LE, PORTER FS: Hereditary orotic aciduria. II. A urinary screening test. *Pediatrics* 42:423, 1968

311. SMITH LH JR, LOTZ M: Studies on congenital orotic aciduria: Comparison of orotic acid metabolism in microorganisms. *J Lab Clin Med* 61:211, 1963

312. BECKWITH JR, PARDEE AB, AUSTRIAN R, JACOB F: Coordination of the synthesis of the enzymes in the pyrimidine pathways of *E. coli*. *J Mol Biol* 5:618, 1962

313. NADLER HL: Prenatal detection of genetic defects. *J Pediatr* 74:132, 1969

57

XERODERMA PIGMENTOSUM

JAMES E. CLEAVER

1. Xeroderma pigmentosum (XP) is a disease in which patients show a high incidence of sunlight-induced skin cancers. It is inherited as an autosomal recessive disease. Two major clinical forms are seen. One involves predominantly the skin, while the other includes a variety of neurologic disorders. Together, these diseases occur at a frequency of about 1 in 250,000 in North America.
2. Within these two clinical classes of XP, complementation analysis has allowed a further classification into at least eight groups. The nonneurologic forms of XP are groups C, E, F, and "variant"; the neurologic forms consist of groups A, B, D, and G. Cultured cells from patients in each group restore DNA repair mechanisms when fused with cells from any of the other groups, suggesting that at least eight different gene products are defective.
3. Cells from all groups of XP show varying degrees of hypersensitivity to killing and mutagenesis by UV light and chemical carcinogens.
4. Patients with XP groups A through G are deficient in gene products that are required for the initial step of excision of damaged DNA.
5. Patients with the XP variant are deficient in a gene product that in normal cells permits accurate semiconservative replication past damaged sites in DNA.
6. Patients with all forms of XP show high levels of UV light–induced mutagenesis. This implies a mutational mechanism in the development of sunlight-induced skin cancers.

Several kinds of skin disease are caused by alterations in the normal resistance of the skin to sunlight. These occur either because of (1) a loss in the shielding afforded by melanin, exemplified by albinism [1]; (2) the deposition of sensitizing compounds in the skin, exemplified by porphyria [2]; or (3) a decrease in the capacity of cells to repair or replicate damage induced by sunlight, exemplified by xeroderma pigmentosum (XP) [3, 4]. In albinism and the porphyrias the amount of damage caused by sunlight to the genetic material (DNA) is increased; in XP the amount of damage is unchanged, but repair and replication are diminished or altered [3, 4] (Fig. 57-1). The major clinical feature that results from this loss is a high incidence of sunlight-induced skin cancers [3–8] (Fig. 57-2).

An important distinction should be made between the concepts of hypersensitivity to DNA-damaging agents and of defects in repair of damaged DNA [3]. A large variety of diseases are known in which cells or tissues exhibit abnormal responses to one or more kinds of DNA-damaging agents, i.e., they are hypersensitive [3]. Only in a few of these diseases, especially the various forms of XP, is the hypersensitivity

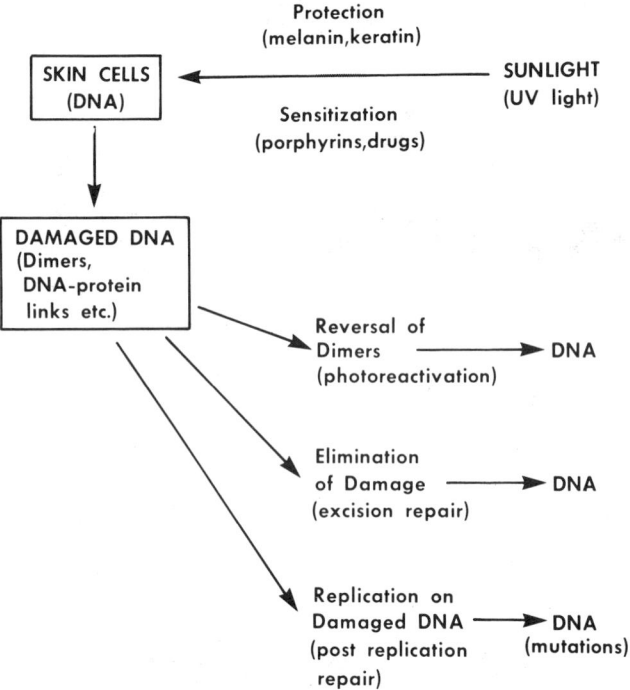

Figure 57-1 Schematic diagram of processes leading to damaged DNA in skin cells and three processes that repair damaged DNA. Damage to DNA of skin cells is caused by absorption of UV light; increased damage results if protection afforded by melanin is lost (e.g., albinism) or if photosensitizers are present in the skin (e.g., porphyrias). Damage is repaired by direct reversal (photoreactivation) or by excision and replacement (excision repair). Semiconservative replication of damaged templates may introduce errors (mutations) by a variety of mechanisms.

caused by a defect in the repair of damaged DNA [5, 6]. In other hypersensitivity diseases there may be more complex abnormalities, such as alterations in both semiconservative replication [9] and repair [10, 11] as seen in ataxia telangiectasia after x-irradiation, and alteration in the recovery of DNA replication as seen in Cockayne's syndrome after irradiation by ultraviolet (UV) light [12]. These are discussed in more detail below.

DNA REPAIR PATHWAYS

At least three different biochemical repair systems operate in damaged cells to safeguard DNA from permanent damage [3, 4]. These systems, photoreactivation, excision repair, and postreplication repair (Fig. 57-1), exist in most cells of most tissues. They are especially important in the skin where they mend damage to DNA caused by the UV rays (~ 300 nm) present in sunlight. In addition, some of the repair systems can mend damage to DNA caused by chemical carcinogens [13]. These systems protect internal tissues against the carcinogenic and mutagenic consequences of exposure to chemicals that damage DNA.

Photoreactivation simply reverts the damaged DNA to the normal chemical state without removing or exchanging any material from DNA. The photoreactivation system is specific for one form of damage induced by UV light, the cyclobutane pyrimidine dimer. Photoreactivation cleaves these dimers, but the system has no versatility in modifying other damaged sites.

The existence and importance of this system in human tissue is not generally agreed upon. Its demonstration in cell culture [14–18] is difficult, although it has been demonstrated directly in human skin [19].

Excision repair, in contrast, is extremely versatile and can mend a large variety of UV-light, x-ray, and chemically induced forms of damage to DNA [13]. This system excises damaged single strands of DNA and replaces them with a new sequence of bases according to the requirements of Watson-Crick base pairing imposed by the intact strand of DNA opposite the original damaged site. Excision repair is of central importance in the recovery of cells from radiation damage. It employs a wide variety of enzymes with different specificities and mechanisms for removal of damage.

The third system is exceedingly complex and is less easily defined as a specific system for handling damage in DNA. It involves multiple mechanisms by which semiconservative DNA replication can take place despite the presence of damage or incomplete excision repair in one strand of DNA [3, 4, 20]. Part of this set of mechanisms is known as post replication repair, which may be nothing more than an operational term for a particular type of DNA replication by which intact new strands of DNA can be synthesized despite the presence of unexcised damage on the parental template strands [20].

Figure 57-2 Xeroderma pigmentosum (group C) patient, 24 years of age, with moderately severe symptoms including large lentigines on the face that were not found on this patient's XP sibs. (Lynch et al. [36]. Used by permission.)

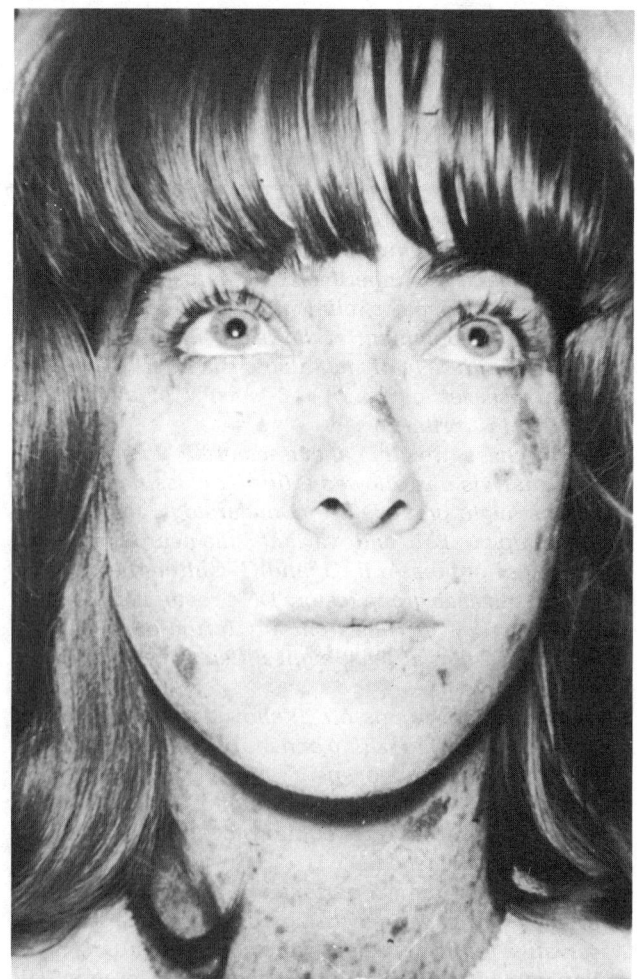

At one time XP was thought to be a disease involving a single defect in one of the repair systems [5], but it now appears that the three main repair systems may be interrelated or may have enzymes in common [3, 6], and several may be altered in patients with XP. Consequently, a full understanding of the biochemistry of XP and the relationship between the biochemistry and the clinical symptoms may be much more complicated than was first realized. Because the outstanding clinical characteristic of XP is marked predisposition for patients to develop skin cancers after exposure to sunlight, the disease comprises a unique conjunction of environmental, genetic, and biochemical factors in the etiology of cancer [8, 21]. The elucidation of its biochemical basis should thus provide clues to understanding the genetic changes involved in carcinogenesis by many physical and chemical agents.

CLINICAL FEATURES OF XP

XP is an autosomal recessive skin disease in which homozygotes show a marked tendency to develop skin cancers from exposure to sunlight [8, 21–24]. Heterozygotes are generally asymptomatic [25, 26]. There is no known linkage to other inherited diseases, HLA antigens [27], or to chromosomal abnormalities. Many patients are children of consanguine marriages, particularly in areas of the world in which such marriages are common, including parts of North Africa, especially Egypt [28–31], Israel [32], and Japan [33]. The disease is found among all racial groups at a frequency of about 1 in 250,000 in the general population, but it is about 10 times more frequent in Egypt, for unexplained reasons.

The disease was first described by Hebra and Kaposi [23], who considered the possible roles of both inheritance and sunlight in the disease and also noted the occurrence of an internal peritoneal tumor in one patient.

The nature and severity of cutaneous, ocular, and neurologic symptoms vary widely with genetic makeup and amount of sun exposure [8, 21]. The disease typically begins in the first years of life with an abnormal erythemal response. There may be a prolonged latent period, atypical stain morphology, edema, and blistering on minimal sun exposure. The minimal erythemal dose is lower than normal, and the erythemal response can be used in early diagnosis before other skin changes develop [34]. After several years of life, other skin changes, including excessive freckling, keratoses, and cancers, develop to varying degrees in different patients (Fig. 57-2). Pigmentary changes involving disturbances in melanocyte structure and function [35] and frequent recurrences of cancers in sun-exposed regions of the skin are the characteristic features on which diagnosis is based. These cancers involve all cell types that receive sun exposure: squamous and basal cell carcinomas, malignant melanomas, keratoacanthomas, angiomas, and sarcomas [8, 21, 36] (Table 57-1). Ocular involvement includes at least mild conjunctivitis and photophobia (Table 57-2). A few patients who exhibit a wide spectrum of characteristic cutaneous and ocular findings have been unambiguously diagnosed as having XP even though the erythemal response is normal [34]. This may be a distinctive feature of the form of XP known as the XP variant or pigmented xerodermoid [34, 37, 41], but this form can only be diagnosed fully by biochemical tests [41, 42].

Table 57-1   Cutaneous manifestations of XP

Erythema and bullae (acute sun sensitivity in infancy)
Freckles
Xerosis (dryness) and scaling
Hypopigmentation
Telangiectasia
Atrophy
Tumors
Actinic keratoses
Basal and squamous cell carcinomas
Malignant melanomas
Others (keratoacanthomas, angiomas, fibromas, sarcomas)

SOURCE: Robbins et al. [21].

The neurologic disorders associated with XP were first described by deSanctis and Cacchione [43] under the term *xerodermic idiocy.* This designation includes a wide range of neurologic symptoms: microcephaly with progressive mental deficiency, retarded skeletal development, sensorineural deafness, chorioathetosis, ataxia, and eventual quadriparesis [43–46] (Table 57-3). Few of the XP patients with neurologic disorders exhibit the full range of symptoms described as "the deSanctis-Cacchione syndrome," but common neurologic findings include microcephaly, mental deficiency, and areflexia [21, 46]. Postmortem studies of the brain fail to show distinctive morphological or cellular abnormalities other than nonspecific neuronal loss [21, 45]. This loss may be due to atrophy or to arrested development associated with the microcephaly.

The frequency of cancers other than on the skin in XP patients is uncertain, partly because of the early death of some patients from generalized consequences of their skin disease and partly because of inadequate reporting. A number of occurrences have been reported of leukemia, bronchial carcinoma, peritoneal cancer, glioblastoma, and squamous carcinoma of the tongue (Table 57-4). Whether the frequency will be found higher than in age-matched controls is an important question yet to be resolved.

Management of XP patients involves a combination of genetic counseling of the affected family [36], the prevention of actinic damage by minimizing sunlight exposure, and prompt surgical removal or chemotherapy of lesions when they become apparent. Genetic counseling is directed toward acquainting the patients and their parents with the inherited aspects of the disease and its rarity, the probability of familial relationship between the two parents, the 25 percent probability of the disease appearing among subsequent offspring, and the improbability of the patient's having affected children [36]. Prevention of actinic damage is achieved by avoiding UV light and sunlight as far as practicable, wearing protective clothing and glasses, and growing long hair. Sunscreens based on titanium dioxide compounds [47] or on para-aminobenzoic acid [48, 49] and thick makeup can all be effective. Keratoses or tumors can be removed by any standard dermatologic procedure including biopsy, dermabrasion, electrodesiccation, curettage, surgery, or cryosurgery [50–53]. Topical treatments with 5-fluorouracil can also be effective, although there is a tendency for tumors to become refractory [45–54]. More drastic systemic chemotherapy is necessitated in advanced cases of metastatic cancers, but these are frequently terminal, and death ensues either from the metastases or from bacteremia or pneumonia consequent to general debilitation. X-ray therapy

Table 57-2 Ocular abnormalities associated with XP

Lids
  Blepharitis
  Erythema, pigmentation, keratoses
  Atrophy leading to entropion, ectropion, loss of cilia, and loss of
    lower lid
  Neoplasms
    Papillomas
    Epitheliomas of free border of lid
    Basal and squamous cell carcinomas
Conjunctiva
  Conjunctivitis with photophobia, lacrimation, edema
  Pigmentation, telangiectasia
  Dryness
  Symblepharon
  Inflammatory nodules
  Neoplasms
    Intraepithelial epitheliomas
    Squamous cell carcinomas
Cornea
  Exposure keratitis with edema, cellular invasion, vascularization
  Dryness
  Opacification
  Ulceration and scarring
  Neoplasms
Iris
  Iritis
  Synechiae
  Atrophy
  Neoplasms

SOURCE: Robbins et al. [21].

may be ill-advised because of the general degeneration of the skin and the possibility of a hypersensitivity response.

PRODUCTION OF CELLULAR DAMAGE BY SUNLIGHT

Sunlight is the major environmental agent that precipitates the clinical symptoms of XP by damaging cutaneous cells. An understanding of the biochemical defects in XP requires knowledge of the way the damaging wavelengths in sunlight are absorbed by macromolecules and the nature of the damage that is produced.

The wavelengths of sunlight extend into the near UV region, the shortest detectable being about 300 nm. This lower limit slightly overlaps the upper region of the absorption spectra of nucleic acids and proteins. Energy in this region of overlap is absorbed by macromolecules in the skin producing harmful effects that include erythema, burns, and actinic carcinogenesis [55–57]. Comparisons between direct sunlight and shortwave UV light (254 nm) indicate that sunlight in the midwestern U.S. is equivalent in germicidal activity to about 0.1 to 0.2 J per square meter of surface per minute [J/(m²·min)] of 254 nm UV light [58, 59]. Since normal human cells in culture have a D_{37}[1]

---

[1] The D_{37} is the dose required to reduce survival to 0.37 from the initial value of 1.0, and in target theory [60] corresponds to the dose required to produce an average of one lethal hit on the sensitive target of an irradiated organism when the survival curve is exponential.

of only about 3 to 5 J/m² of radiation at 254 nm, the direct exposure of human proliferating cells to sunlight can result in significant amounts of cell killing.

Light at the UV end of the sun's spectrum produces its biologic effects through absorption of quanta in molecules that have unsaturated chemical bonds, such as aromatic amino acids in proteins and purine and pyrimidine components of DNA and RNA. The action spectra for production of DNA damage (pyrimidine dimers) [61], cell killing [62, 63], production of chromosomal aberrations [67], and induction of unscheduled DNA synthesis (i.e., DNA synthesis not associated with the normal cell cycle) [65] are all similar, exhibiting maximum efficiency from 260- to 280-nm wavelengths. Although there is negligible energy in this region of the sun's spectrum there is sufficient overlap of the shortest end of the sun's spectrum with the longer wavelength side of the absorption spectrum for DNA for significant photochemical reaction to occur.

One of the best characterized photoproducts formed in DNA by absorption of UV light is the cyclobutane pyrimidine dimer (Fig. 57-3). This is formed between adjacent pyrimidines in the same strand of DNA by the formation of new bonds between the 5 positions and between the 6 positions on the pyrimidine rings. At least four possible isomers (forms I to IV) [66] can be formed by irradiating frozen solutions of pyrimidines; the form I (meso) dimer corresponds to the one formed in DNA and can be isolated from sunlight and UV-irradiated cells and skin [59, 67, 69]. Numerous biologic effects, such as cell killing, production of chromosomal aberrations, mutagenesis, and carcinogenesis, can be attributed to this photoproduct in DNA [61–70]. Other photoproducts have biologic effects in some circumstances. These include the unstable cytosine hydrate and, at relatively high doses, locally denatured regions, DNA-protein crosslinks, and single strand breaks [70].

In addition to damaging DNA directly, sunlight can also produce chemical carcinogens by photochemical alteration of low molecular weight compounds [71]. Such chemical carcinogens can damage DNA. Repair of this chemically induced damage is accomplished by systems similar to those that repair UV-induced damage [13, 72], which are discussed above.

Table 57-3 Neurologic abnormalities associated with XP

Microcephaly
Higher cortical dysfunction
  Progressive mental deterioration
  Low intelligence
  Emotional lability
  Abnormal electroencephalogram
Basal ganglia and cerebellar involvement
  Choreoathetosis
  Ataxia
Extrapyramidal and pyramidal involvement
  Spasticity
  Extensor plantar responses
  Achilles tendon shortening
Cranial nerve involvement
  Sensorineural deafness
Lower motor neuron involvement
  Hyporeflexia or areflexia
  Neuropathic electromyogram and muscle biopsy

SOURCE: Robbins et al. [21].

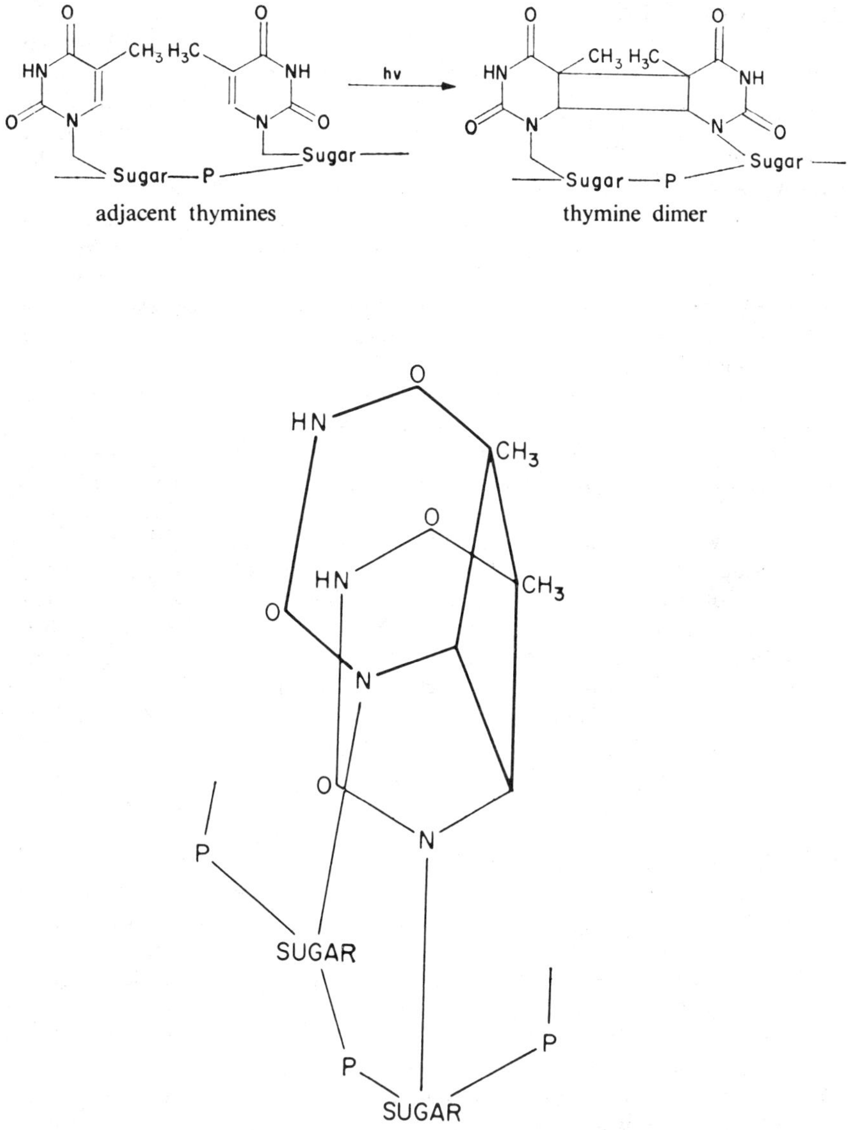

Figure 57-3 Cyclobutane pyrimidine dimer (type I, meso) formed by UV light in DNA. *Top,* adjacent thymines on same strand of DNA absorb a quantum of UV light (hv) and form 5-5 and 6-6 bonds to produce the cyclobutane dimer. *Bottom,* perspective view showing approximate structure of dimer in DNA with pyrimidine rings stacked one above the other.

CELLULAR CHARACTERISTICS OF XP

Most studies that have contributed to delineation of the cellular and biochemical aspects of XP have been based on fibroblast cultures from the skin. For an inherited disease such as XP, the results obtained are assumed to be typical of most somatic cells.

Fibroblast cultures can be obtained from XP patients by punch biopsy or by surgical removal of small pieces of skin. Cells are established in culture by routine procedures[2] [75]. XP cultures have no special nutritional requirements and have lifetimes and growth rates in vitro similar to those from normal

[2] Representative cultures are available from cell banks in both the American Type Culture Collection, 12301 Parkway Drive, Rockville, Maryland, and the Mammalian Genetic Mutant Cell Repository, Institute for Medical Research, Copewood Street, Camden, New Jersey. In comparative studies, the nomenclature adopted to identify XP cell lines is the following form: "XP number letter designation of laboratory or city of origin." Thus, cell lines from Rotterdam are XP1RO, XP2RO, etc.; those from San Francisco are XP1SF, XP2SF, etc.; those from Bethesda are XP1BE, XP2BE, etc. Other letters are chosen as appropriate. Heterozygotes are correspondingly identified as XPH1SF, XPH2SF, etc.

individuals [26]. Occasionally, cultures grow slowly in the initial period after biopsy. This refractoriness to culture may be a result of the atrophied state of the biopsied skin rather than a feature of XP itself.

Table 57-4   Frequency of case reports of nonskin tumors in XP patients

Tumor type	No. of cases*
Leukemia, acute lymphatic	1
Leukemia, myelogenous	1
Tongue	10
Mouth	1
Sarcoma testis	1
Brain (medulloblastoma, glioblastoma)	2
Thyroid	1
Breast carcinoma	1
Bronchial carcinoma	2
Peritoneal carcinoma	1

* See Refs. [26, 169].

Chromosomal Features

Cultured cells from most XP patients have a normal karyotype (Fig. 57-4). Distinctive karyotypic changes characteristic for some diseases with a high cancer incidence, such as Down's syndrome, Klinefelter's syndrome, and Bloom's syndrome [22] are not seen in XP, although karyotypic changes have occasionally been reported in XP cells. For example, two sisters with the deSanctis-Cacchione syndrome had different karyotypes, one normal and the other with an extra chromosome, but these karyotypic changes seemed unrelated to the disease [74]. In another patient characteristic reciprocal exchanges were identified in a small percentage of the cells [75], but this may have been related to the treatment the patient had been undergoing or may merely have been an idiosyncrasy. In one instance a sibling of an affected patient appeared to have a small proportion of normal cells and milder clinical symptoms [76].

Spontaneous and induced sister chromatid exchange (SCE) can be visualized in human fibroblasts by a combination of growth in bromodeoxyuridine and staining with a photochemical reaction plus Giemsa [77, 78] (Fig. 57-4). XP cells show a normal frequency of spontaneous SCEs [79], but a greater than normal frequency after exposure to UV light and most chemical carcinogens (Fig. 57-5) [80, 81]. Similarly, XP cells show more chromosome aberrations than normal cells after exposure to UV light and chemical carcinogens [82, 83].

Sensitivity of Colony Formation to DNA Damage

The number of cells in culture that can grow after UV irradiation can be used as an in vitro measurement of sensitivity and can be correlated with the sensitivity of patients to sunlight and their neurologic disorders.

The first demonstration of the high sensitivity of XP cells to UV light was based on a determination of total protein per culture 10 days after irradiation [84], but this important clue

to the cellular basis of XP was generally ignored. Several years later it was found that the colony-forming ability of cells from subjects with most forms of XP is much more sensitive than that of normal cells to UV light; the sensitivity increase corresponds to a dose-modifying factor between 3 and 10 [85–89]. Fibroblast cultures from patients that exhibit neurologic abnormalities are generally the most sensitive (Figs. 57-6 and 57-7) [89]. XP cells are also more sensitive to 4-nitroquinoline-1-oxide, benz[a]anthracene, and a variety of aromatic amides, but are normal in response to N-methyl-N'-nitro-N-nitroso-guanidine [87, 88, 90, 91].

Fibroblasts from some XP patients who are clinically typical but are without neurologic complications do not exhibit a great increase in UV sensitivity [37, 38, 89, 90] (e.g., XP7TA and XP30RO in Fig. 57-6). These are classified as XP variant or pigmented xerodermoid cases. If caffeine is added to the medium after irradiation, however, the amount of cell killing is greatly increased in these fibroblasts, whereas those from normal individuals and from most XP patients are unaffected (Fig. 57-6). Caffeine at high concentrations alters the regulation of semiconservative DNA replication [93], which then acts synergistically with the biochemical defect in these XP cells. This empirical characteristic, together with others to be described later, provides diagnostic tests for classifying this distinct form of XP—the XP variant.

Host Cell Reactivation

The ability of UV-damaged viruses to survive in infected cells is dependent on the genetic constitution of the cells. This is because most viruses depend on cellular enzymes for their reproduction. The degree of dependence is greater for the smaller viruses [e.g., simian virus 40 (SV40)] than for the larger ones (e.g., herpes simplex, cytomegalovirus) [76]. Irradiation of a virus suspension before infecting the host cells damages the viral DNA and inactivates a certain fraction of the viruses. The fraction inactivated depends on the host cell's ability to repair the damaged DNA in the infecting viruses. The extent of

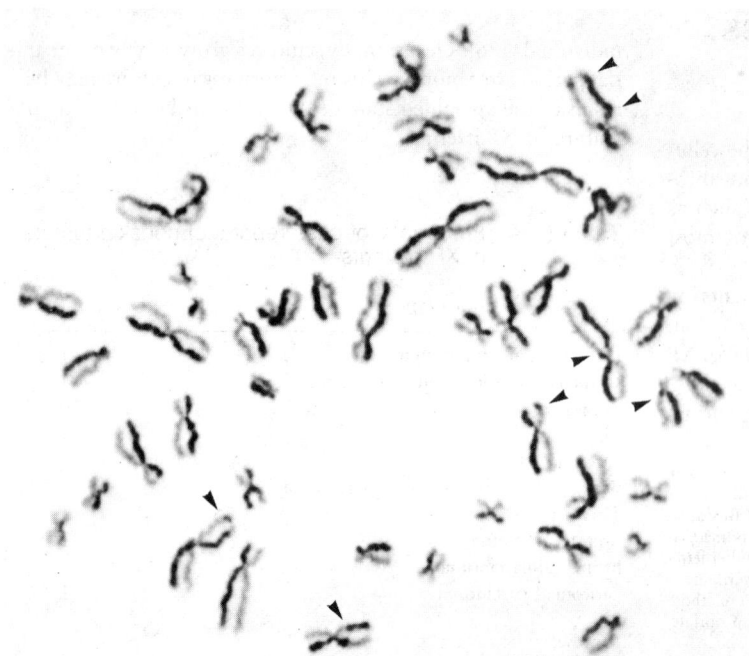

Figure 57-4 Karyotype of XP25RO, a deSanctis-Cacchione syndrome patient, stained by the fluorescent dye–Giemsa method to discriminate between sister chromatids [77–81]. Seven sister chromatid exchanges (arrows) can be seen in this particular cell. The karyotype is indistinguishable from that of a normal individual. (Wolff et al. [79]. Used by permission.)

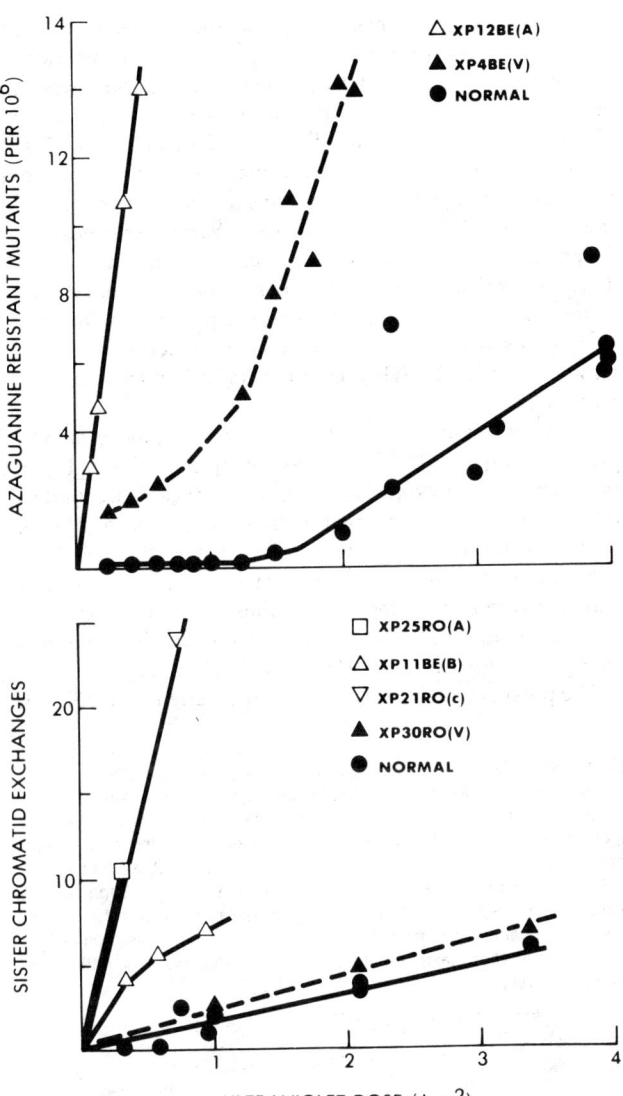

Figure 57-5 Relative frequencies of UV-induced mutations to 8-azaguanine (20μm) resistance or of sister chromatid exchanges in normal (●), excision-defective XP (▽, △, □) and XP variant (▲) cells as a function of ultraviolet dose. *Top,* mutation frequencies. *(Redrawn from Maher et al. [102, 103].)* Bottom, SCE frequencies. *(Redrawn from deWeerd-Kastelein et al. [81].)*

this host cell reactivation by various cell types often parallels the cells' ability to survive radiation damage. The survival of various UV-damaged viruses, including vaccinia [94, 95], herpes simplex virus [95, 96], adenovirus [97, 98], and SV40 [99], is therefore less in XP cells than in normal cells (Fig. 57-8). All of these are DNA viruses that replicate in the cell nucleus. There are, in addition, reports suggesting that UV-damaged RNA viruses, which replicate in the cytoplasm, also show reduced survival in XP cells. This is true for the free RNA but not the intact virion from encephalomyocarditis virus [94].

The D_{37} of irradiated viruses grown in XP cells is about 20 times less than in normal cell strains for adenovirus [97, 98] and about 3 times less for herpes virus [95, 96]. The D_{37} for adenovirus in XP cells corresponds to the production of about one pyrimidine dimer per viral genome. As would be expected from cell-killing results, irradiated adenoviruses grown in XP variant cells show reductions in survival of a factor of only about 2 compared to those grown in normal cells [100].

These observations imply that the enzymes responsible for

the survival of radiation-damaged cells and viruses in culture function reasonably well in patients with the variant form of XP, but are severely deranged in patients with more typical forms of XP. Nevertheless, patients with both forms of XP show similar skin symptoms. Thus, both types of genetic defects may predispose equally to carcinogenesis in vivo.

Induction of Mutations by UV Light

A small proportion of the cells that recover from irradiation carry mutations in the form of base-pair changes or deletions in the DNA. These are thought to arise from faulty replication of DNA that contains damaged bases. Some mutations can be detected by growing cells in drugs that are lethal analogues of normal metabolites (e.g., 8-azaguanine or 6-thioguanine as analogues of purines) and observing the growth of mutant cells that have acquired resistance. In human cells in culture only a few gene loci are amenable to quantitative study of mutagenesis. One that has been studied extensively is involved in the defective pathway of the Lesch-Nyhan syndrome [101] (see Chap. 51). The key step in this pathway consists of an enzyme, hypoxanthine-guanine phosphoribosyltransferase (HGPRT), that attaches a phosphoribosyl group to 8-azaguanine so that it can be incorporated into DNA. Resistant mutants produced by irradiation can survive high concentrations of 8-azaguanine because HGPRT activity has been lost. Other gene loci amenable to study are those that regulate binding of toxic chemicals to membrane proteins such as the ouabain resistance locus or the diphtheria toxin resistance locus.

The frequency with which cells resistant to 6-thioguanine, ouabain, diphtheria toxin, etc., are produced by irradiation with UV light or exposure to chemical carcinogens is greater in all XP cells, including XP variants, than in normal cells [102–104] (Fig. 57-5). This implies that the genetic defects in all XP cells confer increased mutability. The similar responses of all the XP cells in this mutagenesis assay contrast with the variability in their responses in the UV light toxicity assay (Figs. 57-6 and 57-7). This observation implies that the hypersensitive XP cells (later to be defined as the excision-defective groups A through G) have lost a system that normally repairs UV-induced damage in such a way as to avoid the errors that lead to mutations. In the XP variant, the damage is repaired in such a way as to allow cell survival. However, the repair system has lost fidelity and so produces a high frequency of mutations.

BIOCHEMICAL CHARACTERISTICS OF XP

Excision Repair Pathways

The first studies of cultured fibroblasts from patients with the common and the neurologic forms of XP [5, 105] showed that both classes of patients are defective to varying degrees in their ability to perform excision repair of damaged DNA (Figs. 57-9 and 57-10). This normally is accomplished by several different repair enzyme systems with different mechanisms and efficiencies for removing various kinds of damaged DNA bases [3, 4, 106]. The sites of damage and rates of repair are influenced by

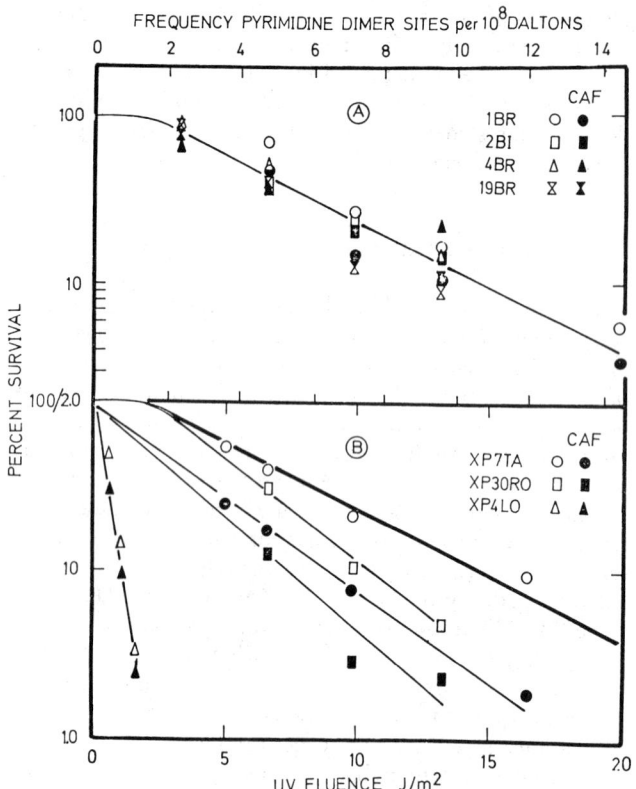

Figure 57-6 UV inactivation curves for normal and XP fibroblasts irradiated and grown in medium with or without 1 μm caffeine. The dose is expressed in both J/m² and the estimated number of pyrimidine dimers per 10^8 daltons DNA. *A.* Normal human fibroblasts, strains 1BR, 2BI, 4BR, 19BR, grown without (○, □, △, ⊠, respectively) or with 1 μm caffeine (●, ■, ▲, ⊠, respectively). *B.* XP fibroblasts, strains XP7TA and XP30RO (XP variants) and XP4LO (a deSanctis-Cacchione syndrome patient). Cells grown without (○, □, △, respectively) or with (●, ■, ▲, respectively) 1 μm caffeine. *(From Arlett et al. [92]. Used by permission.)*

endonucleases, has blurred the distinction between the nucleotide and base excision repair pathways. One of the features thought to distinguish nucleotide from base excision was that nucleotide excision involved an initial cleavage of the 3′,5′-phosphodiester bond on the 5′ side of the dimer (Fig. 57-10), whereas base excision involved cleavage of the glycosylic bond releasing a damaged base and leaving an apurinic-apyrimidinic site. However, UV endonucleases from *Micrococcus luteus* and T4 phage–infected *Escherichia coli* are now known to catalyze a glycosylic cleavage of the thymine deoxyribose bond on the 5′-thymine of the dimer [115]. This mechanism may not occur in *E. coli* itself, however, where a true endonucleolytic cleavage may operate [116]. Whether it occurs in human cells is currently unknown.

The polymerization step of excision repair may be catalyzed predominantly by DNA polymerase β[117], although some involvement of polymerase α cannot be excluded completely [118]. The final step of repair is the sealing of the 5′,3′ gap, a reaction catalyzed by polynucleotide ligase.

Excision repair requires a temporary relaxation of nucleosomal structure so that repaired regions are more accessible to exogenous nucleases (Fig. 57-9) [107–110]. This temporary change may involve poly(ADP-ribose)$_n$ [119, 120].

The process by which new bases are inserted into DNA dur-

the organization of DNA in the nucleus, which consists of histone particles around which 200 base pairs of DNA are wrapped to form each structural unit (nucleosome) [107, 110].

Two major pathways of excision repair, the nucleotide and base excision repair pathways, operate on different kinds of damage in DNA [3, 4, 106]. The nucleotide pathway removes pyrimidine dimers and large chemical adducts to DNA (e.g., benzo[*a*]anthracene adducts, methoxypsoralen monoadducts, acetoxyacetylaminofluorene adducts) and replaces the damaged site with a relatively long newly synthesized polynucleotide strand whose length seems to be related to the length of the DNA associated with one nucleosome [109]. The base excision pathway removes DNA bases that have undergone relatively small degrees of modification, such as alkylation or deamination, and replaces them with a relatively small patch of DNA. This is accomplished either by excision and resynthesis of a short region or by direct insertion of free bases [111]. A further type of excision repair has recently been found in human cells which is induced by growth in low concentrations of alkylating agents. This is the adaptation pathway [112]. It is efficient when there are low levels of damage and may operate by direct removal of the alkyl group itself [112–114].

Detailed analysis of the enzymes responsible for the first step in removal of pyrimidine dimers in some bacteria, the UV

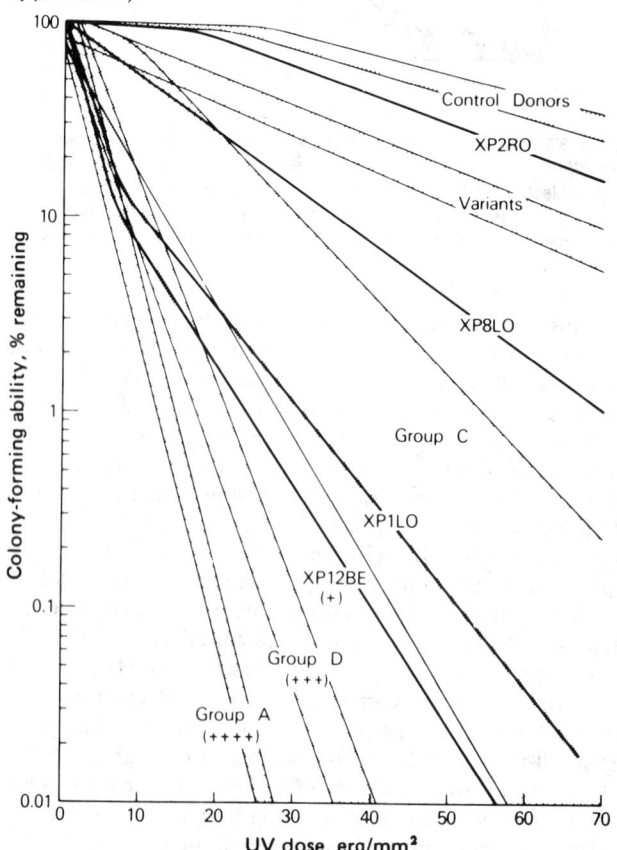

Figure 57-7 UV (254 nm) inactivation curve for fibroblasts from normal and various XP patients. Each complementation group (A-E, variant) is represented either by a range encompassing data from several patients in that group or as single line for data from a single patient (i.e., the exceptional group A patients with little neurologic involvement: XP1LO, XP8LO, XP12BE, and group E, XP2RO). The severity of neurologic abnormalities is indicated by: ++++, numerous clinical manifestations by age 7; +++, numerous clinical manifestations between ages 7 and 12; + areflexia and abnormal electroencephalogram at age 10. *(From Andrews et al. [89]. Used by permission.)*

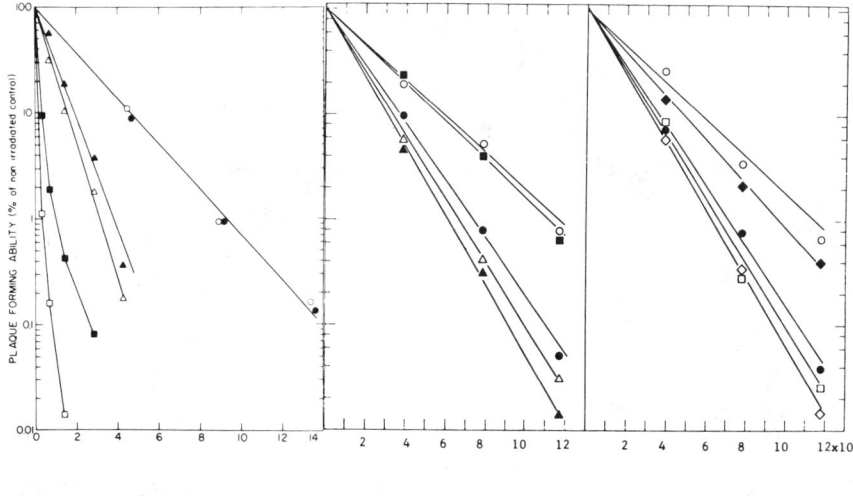

Figure 57-8 UV inactivation curve of adenovirus 2 irradiated in suspension and grown in various normal, XP, and XP variant cells. *Left,* ○, ● normal fibroblasts; ▲, △, ■, □, XP homozygote fibroblasts. *(From Day [98]. Used by permission.) Center and right,* ○, ■, ◆, normal cell lines; ○, ▲, △, ◇, □, XP variant fibroblasts *(From Day [100]. Used by permission.)*

ing repair has been given various names according to the methods used for study (for a full description of methods see [4, 121]). Autoradiographic methods (Fig. 57-18) of detection gave rise to the term *unscheduled synthesis* [122]. Cesium chloride isopycnic gradient methods led to the term *repair replication* [123], which is also used in the bromouracil photolysis method [124]. The term *radiation-stimulated* [³H]*thymidine incorporation* [37] describes an increase in total radioactivity incorporated into DNA by excision repair in cells in which normal DNA synthesis is naturally low (e.g., lymphocytes, plateau-phase tissue cultures), or is depressed by inhibitors of semiconservative DNA synthesis. These various terms all describe the same biochemical process and are essentially equivalent. The different methods are chosen according to the cells or tissues under study. A conclusion derived from the use of each of the methods is that the patches that replace excised dimers are large, up to 100 bases long [4, 5, 124, 125], and contain both purines and pyrimidines [13]. These long patches are probably formed through continuous exonucleolytic degradation of DNA strands beyond the site of the dimer initially excised.

The continuous excision of dimers (Fig. 57-11) and insertion of the bases (Figs. 57-12, 57-13) occurs with a very low frequency of strand breaks [4, 126–133]. This suggests that during excision repair a dynamic balance is established between strand breakage and rejoining. The actual number of sites involved in excision repair at any instant is small, no more than about 1 in 2×10^8 daltons of DNA. Only about 1 percent of the dimers produced in DNA by a dose of 10 J/m² is involved in excision at any instant. The excision rate must therefore be dictated by the enzymes involved in the early steps of repair, which presumably move from site to site repairing different sites in sequence.

DEFECTIVE REPAIR IN XP

Cells from patients with XP excise pyrimidine dimers and carry out repair replication at rates that are between 0 and 90 percent of normal [134, 136] (Figs. 57-11–57-13). Cells from affected sibs usually carry out these processes at similar rates. Those XP cell lines that do not excise a detectable number of dimers also have low levels of repair replication, and those that

excise at only a slightly reduced level also show only slightly reduced rates of repair replication. The reductions are similar in all tissues thus far investigated, including skin in vivo [136], peripheral lymphocytes [37], fibroblasts [5], and liver cell cultures [137]. Patients with the XP variant exhibit normal levels of both dimer excision and repair replication [37, 38, 41, 42].

Photoreactivation in XP

Photoreactivation is a DNA repair system that is absolutely specific for pyrimidine dimers and is therefore important only in repair of UV damage, unlike the more versatile excision repair system. It involves a single enzyme that binds to dimers and, on subsequent exposure to light between 300 and 600 nm, cleaves them [14–17, 137–139]. The monomerized thymines remain in DNA and no material is excised from DNA by this process. The cellular effect of photoreactivation is observed as the mitigation by visible light of many UV-induced effects caused by dimers in DNA, such as cell killing, mutagenesis, and production of chromosome aberrations [4, 138]. For a decade or more it was generally assumed that in spite of the widespread distribution of photoreactivation in prokaryotes and eukaryotes [138, 139], it was completely absent from all placental mammals [4, 14, 138–140] and was therefore of no interest in the biochemistry of XP. A reevaluation became necessary when an enzyme was isolated from human cells that had properties in vitro resembling those of photoreactivating enzymes from nonmammalian species [15–17]. This enzyme is different from those found in other organisms because it has optimum activity at lower ionic strength (about 0.02M) and an action spectrum extending further into the visible region than the prokaryotic enzyme [15–17]. The prokaryotic photoreactivating enzyme is inactive at yellow and longer wavelengths, but the human enzyme is active at yellow wavelengths and inactive at red and longer wavelengths. Because of these differences the human enzyme may play a different role in the cell.

To this day, demonstration of efficient photoreactivation is almost the sole prerogative of one research group [15–17, 19], and attempts to confirm the existence of this repair system by several other groups have been unsuccessful or ambiguous [18, 140–142]. The role of this system in the resistance to UV-induced skin changes in humans thus remains controversial.

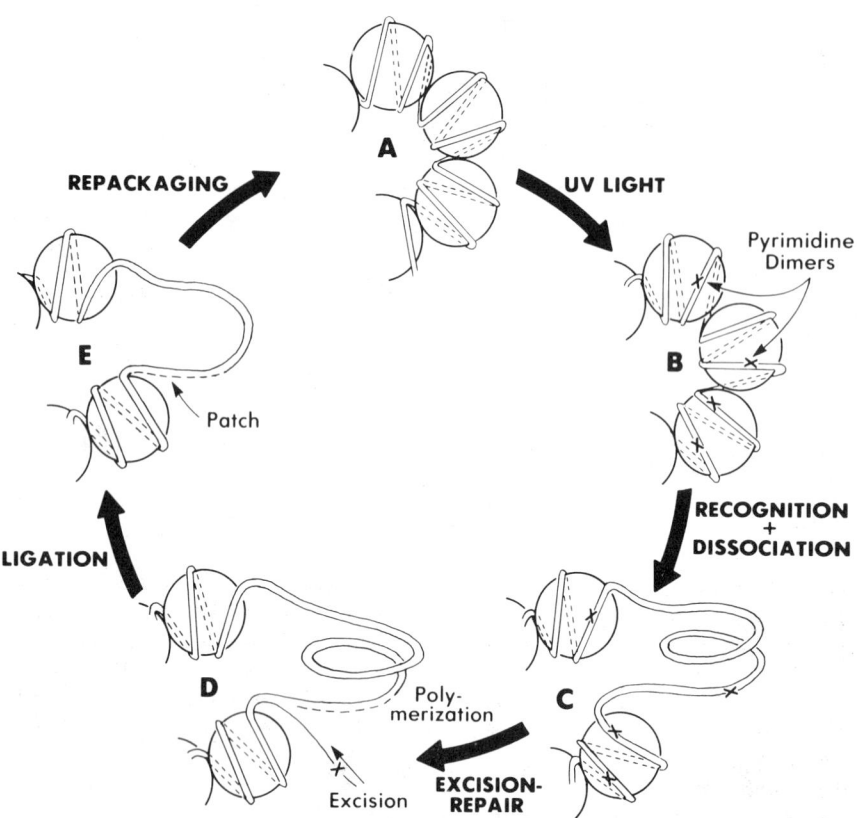

REPACKAGING

UV LIGHT

Pyrimidine Dimers

RECOGNITION + DISSOCIATION

Patch

LIGATION

Polymerization

Excision

EXCISION-REPAIR

Figure 57-9 Heuristic scheme for excision repair of damaged sites on DNA in mammalian chromatin. The first step involves mechanisms that recognize damage and dissociate nucleoproteins to make the DNA accessible to repair enzymes. This is followed by sequential incision by a UV endonuclease, excision by an exonuclease, repair replication by a DNA polymerase, sealing of the patch by a polynucleotide ligase, and final reassembly and repackaging of nucleoprotein. (*Reproduced by permission of J.E. Cleaver, in D. Scott, B.A. Bridges, F.H. Sobels (eds.): Progress in Genetic Toxicology Elsevier/North Holland Biomedical Press 1977, pp. 29–42.*)

Repair of Damage from Chemical Mutagens and Carcinogens in XP

Most chemical mutagens and carcinogens cause damage to many cellular components, but the damage they cause to DNA is probably paramount. In response to damage from some mutagens and carcinogens, XP cells perform the same amounts of excision repair and have the same sensitivity to killing as do normal cells [13, 88, 143, 144], while in response to damage from other carcinogens, XP cells perform less excision repair and have greater sensitivity than normal cells [13, 87, 88, 90, 91, 144–146]. Since XP cells also respond normally to x-ray-induced damage, but not to UV-induced damage, the chemicals to which XP cells respond normally can be considered "x-ray-like" and those to which XP cells are sensitive "UV-like" [13] (Table 57-5). In normal cells x-ray-like chemicals appear to cause damage that is repaired by much smaller excision repair patches (1 to 3 bases) than the damage caused by the UV-like chemicals (up to 100 bases) [4, 147, 148].

The response of XP cells to various carcinogens and mutagens appears to depend on the type of damage to DNA and the extent to which repair of the damage requires enzymes that are deficient in XP cells. Damage is caused by the reaction between cellular components and electrophilic carcinogens or mutagens ("ultimate carcinogens") [149]. Some carcinogenic and mutagenic chemicals are electrophilic in their native state (e.g., alkylating agents such as methyl methanesulfonate, propane sulfone, methyl nitrosourea), whereas others require metabolic conversion by cellular enzymes before becoming electrophilic (e.g., 4-nitroquinoline-1-oxide, acetylaminofluorene, benz[a]-anthracene). Reactions between chemical carcinogens and DNA produce alkylated bases and phosphate groups, covalent

adducts between bases and carcinogens, and strand breaks. The relative proportions of these various classes of damage depend on the carcinogen in question. Many chemical carcinogens induce several kinds of DNA damage, each of which might be repaired by different types of excision repair. Thus, ethylnitrosourea produces a variety of alkylated bases in DNA, including N-7 and N-3 ethyladenine, which are repaired by an N-glycosylase (base excision pathway); phosphotriesters that are not repaired at all; and 0,6-ethylguanine that is repaired by a combination of the nucleotide and base excision pathways and the adaptation pathway [112, 150]. Thus, the classification of agents with respect to repair refers to the predominant response to the quantitatively most frequent repairable lesions.

Damage that does not involve a strand break requires different recognition and endonucleolytic action for initiating excision than does strand break damage, which may not even require a specific endonuclease. Breaks may be produced directly as a part of the damage (as in x-ray-induced damage) or may appear as a result of enzymatic action on damaged (alkylated) bases in which a base is removed by an N-glycosylase reaction, as for example on N-7 and N-3 ethyladenine [151]. Other damage, which does not involve breaks or alkylated bases, tends to involve several bases (e.g., pyrimidine dimers) or adducts between bases and relatively large chemical groups (e.g., 4-nitroquinoline-1-oxide adducts to purines). The classification of carcinogens therefore implies that excision repair of damage induced by UV-like carcinogens involves the enzyme(s) of UV repair that are defective in XP cells. Excision repair of x-ray-like damage or damage from alkylating agents bypasses those defects. The precise biologic significance of the classification into x-ray-like and UV-like carcinogens for carcinogenesis is unclear at present although the categories correspond approximately to nucleotide and base repair or large patch versus small patch repair [13, 147]. Both categories include strong and weak carcinogens. The categories do not appear to correlate in any simple manner with the mutagenic and carcinogenic potential of a chemical.

GENETICS

Genetic Heterogeneity in XP

Genetic heterogeneity in XP patients whose cells are defective in excision repair is suggested by the different residual activities of repair replication and by the different clinical patterns. Underlying these quantitative differences are genetic differences between patients that can be analyzed by somatic cell hybridization. Cells from different XP patients can be hybridized in culture under the influence of inactivated Sendai virus or polyethylene glycol (Fig. 57-14), to produce multinucleated cells with nuclei from each XP patient (heterokaryons). Heterokaryons from some combinations of XP patients exhibit complementation and increased repair, whereas other combinations remain repair-deficient [6, 21, 152–157]. If complementation occurs, it is an indication that the cell types contain defects in different genes. Numerous studies in which cells from many patients were hybridized in pairs have demonstrated at least seven complementation groups among patients who are deficient in excision repair [6, 21, 152–157] (Table 57-6). This implies that the initial step of pyrimidine dimer excision, which appears to be the action of a single UV endonuclease, actually requires the normal function of at least 7 distinct genes.

Table 57-5 Classification of carcinogens and mutagens on the basis of the total amount of DNA repair in XP cells*

Agents causing damage that is repaired defectively in XP cells	Agents causing damage that is repaired normally in XP cells
UV light	X-rays
Methoxypsoralen adduct	Bromouracil photoproducts
4-Nitroquinoline-1-oxide	Dimethyl sulfate
Bromobenz [a] anthracene	Methyl methanesulfonate
Benz [a] anthracene epoxide	N-methyl-N'-nitro-N-nitrosoguanine
1-Nitropyridine-1-oxide	
Acetylaminofluorene	Methyl nitrosourea
Aromatic amides	ICR 170

* The measurements of repair are biased toward those lesions in DNA that predominate and that are repaired more rapidly with larger patches. Therefore, quantitatively minor lesions, such as those from x-rays that are defectively repaired or from 4NQO that are normally repaired, will not be resolved in measurements of the total amount of repair.
SOURCE: Refs. 4, 13, 87, 88, 90, 91, 143–147, 205.

Distribution of Complementation Groups and the Gene Structure in XP

The existence of seven distinct complementation groups in XP patients probably indicates intergenic, rather than intragenic, complementation. The affected genes may play a role as both structural and regulatory genes in the formation of one or more enzymes mediating the early steps of excision repair. One hypothesis consistent with the observed kinetics of excision and strand breakage is that the excision, replication, and ligation enzymes act in a coordinated way by means of an enzyme complex, as first suggested by Haynes [158]. This complex might contain seven different peptides. A defect in any one of the peptides might interfere with the action of the complex. Recent isolation of repair enzyme activity [159] and estimates

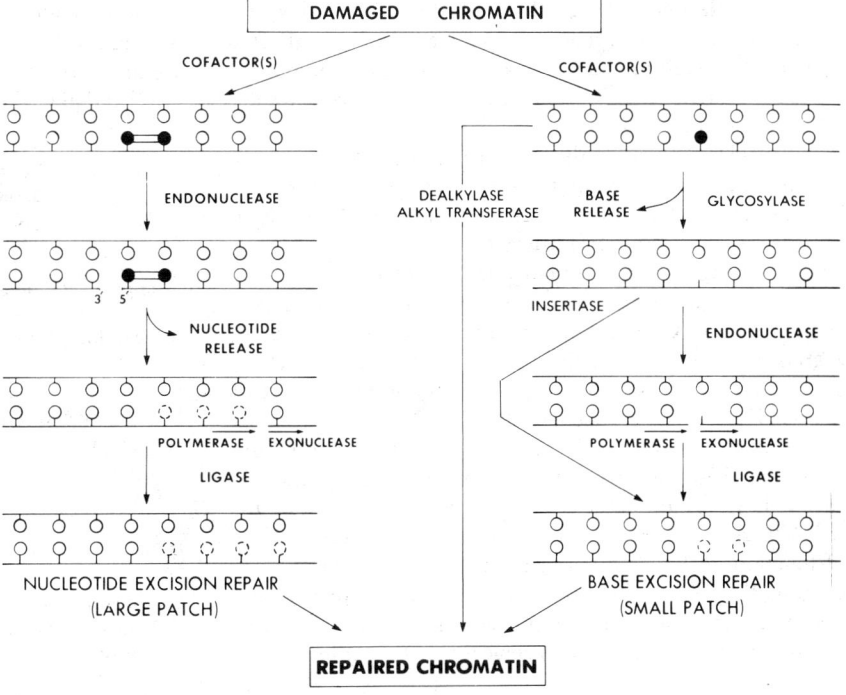

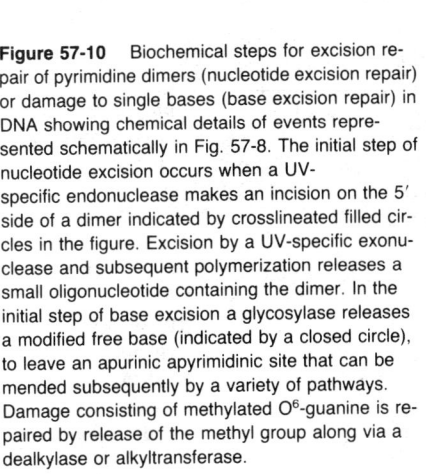

Figure 57-10 Biochemical steps for excision repair of pyrimidine dimers (nucleotide excision repair) or damage to single bases (base excision repair) in DNA showing chemical details of events represented schematically in Fig. 57-8. The initial step of nucleotide excision occurs when a UV-specific endonuclease makes an incision on the 5' side of a dimer indicated by crosslineated filled circles in the figure. Excision by a UV-specific exonuclease and subsequent polymerization releases a small oligonucleotide containing the dimer. In the initial step of base excision a glycosylase releases a modified free base (indicated by a closed circle), to leave an apurinic apyrimidinic site that can be mended subsequently by a variety of pathways. Damage consisting of methylated O⁶-guanine is repaired by release of the methyl group along via a dealkylase or alkyltransferase.

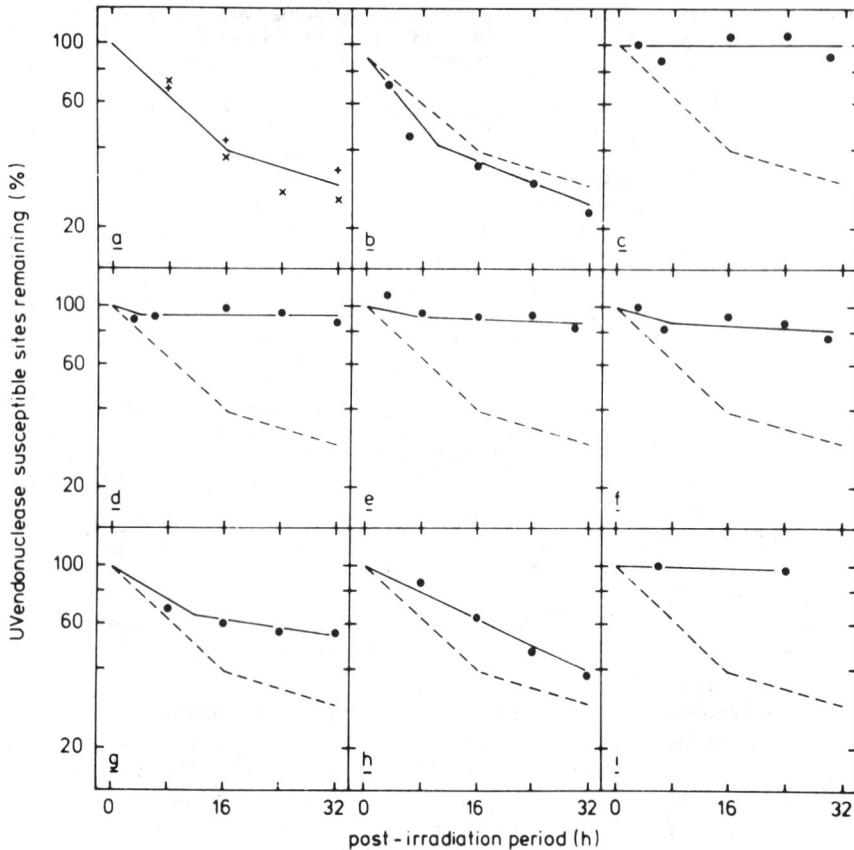

Figure 57-11 Time course of disappearance of UV endonuclease susceptible sites (pyrimidine dimers) from the DNA of normal human cells and cells from each complementation group of XP after radiation at 254 nm. After specified periods of post-UV incubation, cell samples were assayed to determine the number of dimers remaining in the extracted DNA. The percentages shown for the incubated samples are relative to those found for the parallel nonincubated ones, and normalized to 100 percent for the number of dimers present immediately after irradiation. *Panel a*, two normal cell lines. The other panels give data for one patient from each XP group: *b*, XP variant; *c*, group A; *d*, group B; *e*, group C; *f*, group D; *g*, group E; *h*, group F; *i*, group G. The dashed lines indicate the mean response of normal cells.

of its apparent molecular weight in excess of 10⁶ [160, 161] support the idea of an enzyme complex.

The number of patients from each complementation group observed so far in four countries is shown in Table 57-7. There are two major groups, A and C. The next most frequent are group D and variant, with the remaining groups B, E, F, and G thus far represented by only one or two families. A low frequency of group C cases among Japanese [33] was predicted in a study by Neel et al. [162]. Based on the relatively low frequency of consanguine marriages among parents of affected individuals, Neel and coworkers suggested that the number of genetic loci involved in XP was fewer in Japanese than in Caucasian populations.

A consideration from these various population studies is whether the complementation groups thus far discovered represent different alleles or genes and whether complementation involves intercistronic or intracistronic events. Most of the complementation groups contain one or more patients who are known to come from consanguine marriages. Accordingly, cells within one complementation group are probably homozygous at a particular locus, and the relative frequencies of each group can be used for a hypothesis about the structure of the repair enzymes and the gene loci.

The high frequency of occurrence of groups A and C suggests that these patients may have mutations in genes that encode large proteins involved in an early step of incision for which there are many potentially mutable sites resulting in loss of function [28]. The infrequent occurrence of other groups suggests that these may represent small proteins or polypeptides with few potential mutational sites at risk, or proteins whose function comes under stringent selection criteria.

Characteristics of Complementation Groups

Group A This group (Fig. 57-15) usually corresponds to the most severe clinical form of XP in which there are both skin symptoms and central nervous system disorders. Most patients exhibit disorders from birth and correspond to the clinical category of the deSanctis-Cacchione syndrome and xerodermic idiocy [43, 46]. Excision repair is very low in these cells, which are about tenfold more sensitive than normal to killing by UV light and many carcinogens (Figs. 57-6, 57-7). They are also about fourfold more sensitive to methyl methanesulfonate [163] and have slightly reduced levels of apurinic endonuclease

Table 57-6 Levels of unscheduled DNA synthesis and clinical symptoms in the complementation groups of XP

Complementation groups	Percent of normal repair	Representative cell lines
A:Neurologic form	2–5	XPPKSF, XP25RO, XP1LO, XP17SF, XP12BE
B:Neurologic form (and symptoms of Cockayne's syndrome)	3–7	XP11BE
C:Common form	10–20	XP4RO, XP12SF
	5–15	XP1BE
D:Neurologic form	25–50	XP5BE, XP6BE, XP2NE, XP3NE
E:Common form	40–50	XP2RO, XP3RO
F:Common form	18	
G:Neurologic form	<2	XP3BR, XP2BI

[164]. They may also exhibit hypersensitivity to sister chromatid exchange induction by alkylating agents [80].

There are exceptions to these general characteristics of group A cells. One British case, XP8LO, exhibited about 30 percent of normal excision repair and higher survival after UV than other group A cells. This patient is without CNS disorders [165].

One Egyptian case (a 35-year-old male, XP13CA), had a low level of unscheduled synthesis typical of most group A cells, but the patient was neurologically normal, had normal stature, and was fertile [26] (Fig. 57-16). Two other group A patients, XP12BE and XP1LO, also show minimal neurologic abnormalities, and the cells have higher survival after UV irradiation than the majority in group A [21, 89]. In one Italian family group A sibs exhibited different clinical symptoms, only one having disorders of the CNS [76]. In cell cultures it appeared that the sib without CNS disorder had higher repair on average due to a subpopulation of cells with normal repair mixed with typical group A cells.

Therefore, although group A patients usually have the associated neurologic abnormalities of the deSanctis-Cacchione syndrome several are known who are neurologically normal, implying that the skin and central nervous system abnormalities can segregate independently.

Figure 57-12 Autoradiographs of normal and XP cells irradiated with 30 J/m² of UV light and labeled for 3 h with [³H]thymidine (10 μCi/ml, 21.9 Ci/mmol). A. Normal (JEC) cells, nonirradiated; B. normal (JEC) cells, irradiated; C. repair-deficient XP23SF cells, irradiated; D. partially repair deficient XP20SF cells, irradiated; E. XP variant cells, irradiated. (From J. E. Cleaver, unpublished data, 1975.)

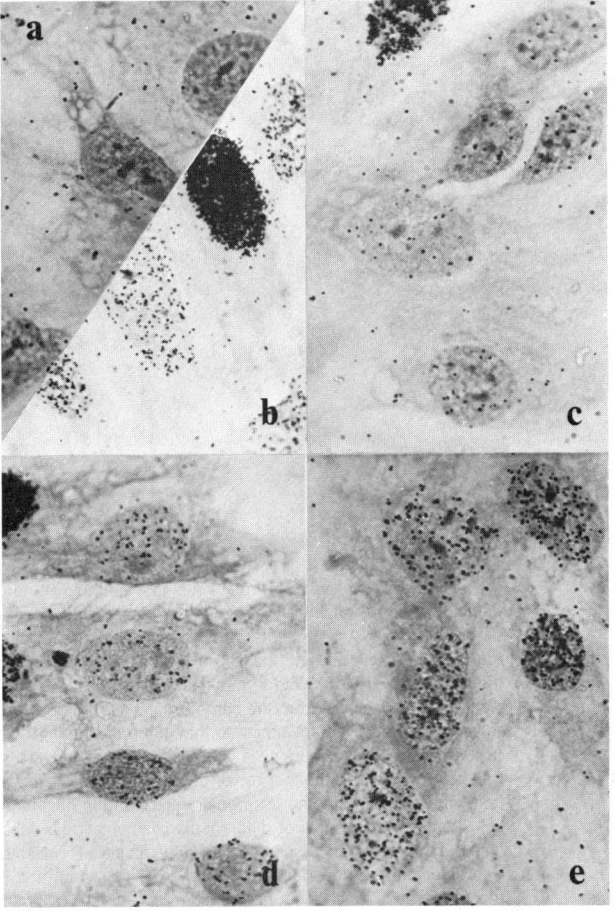

Table 57-7 Relative frequencies of various XP complementation groups among different populations [26, 28]

Population	A	B	C	D	E	F	G	Variant
North America	3	1	5	5	0	0	0	2
Europe and Britain	10	0	14	8	2	0	2	5
Japan	21	0	1	1	0	1	0	9
Egypt	7	0	12	0	0	0	0	5

Complementation group (no. of patients)

Group B There is only one reported patient (Fig. 57-17) in this group (XP1BE). The patient died of acute hypertension at age 33 and remains perplexing because of symptoms both of XP and of Cockayne's syndrome [21]. She had reduced stature, deafness and mental retardation, immature sexual development, premature senility, absence of subcutaneous fat, and optic nerve and retinal pigment degeneration characteristic of Cockayne's syndrome. Acute sun sensitivity, ocular changes, and cutaneous malignancy at age 18 were typical of XP. The conjunction of two extremely rare disorders in one patient is statistically unlikely, so that this constellation of symptoms may be regarded as characteristic of this group unless or until other cases are identified. Cells from this patient have low levels of excision repair and are very sensitive to killing by UV light.

Group C This is one of the largest groups (Fig. 57-2). Patients are found worldwide, although infrequently in Japan compared to elsewhere [21, 28, 33]. It is often referred to as the common or classic form of XP. The patients show only skin disorders. These vary considerably in severity depending on the climate. Tumors of the tongue have been observed in several patients [26, 166]. Cells have low but heterogeneous levels of excision repair (10 to 20 percent of normal) and are less sensitive to killing by UV light and chemical carcinogens than in groups A and D [21, 89].

One exceptional patient (XP1MI), exhibited symptoms of XP, systemic lupus erythematosus, and a marginal degree of mental retardation [167]. Cells from this patient had typical DNA repair levels but were the most UV sensitive of any in group C [89]. The only two reported instances of central nervous system tumors in XP patients, XP106LO [168], and a Hawaiian patient [169], are in this group.

Group D Patients in group D resemble those in group A in exhibiting both skin and CNS disorders, although the latter may occasionally develop later in life than in group A [46, 168]. Representatives of this group are slightly more common in Britain than elsewhere, but their distribution is not as restricted as groups B, F, G. Excision repair is low (10 to 20 percent), as in group C cells, but functionally poorer. Some evidence suggests that the amount of unscheduled DNA synthesis is higher than expected from the low amount of dimer excision observed in these cells [135]. Cells are almost as sensitive to cell killing as are group A cells [89]. Cells in this group are claimed to have reduced levels of apurinic endonuclease [164, 170], but this was not confirmed in another study [174].

Group E Patients in this rare group exhibit mild degrees of

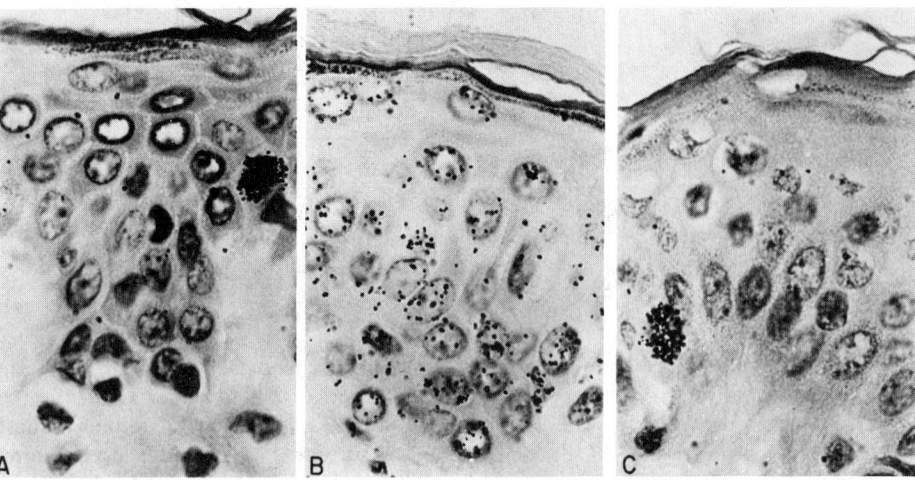

Figure 57-13 Autoradiograph of human skin that was irradiated *in situ* from above with 13.6 × 10³ J/m² of UV light, injected locally with [³H]thymidine, and biopsied 1 h later. *A.* Normal nonirradiated skin showing an occasional cell undergoing semiconservative replication labeled in the basal layer. *B.* Normal irradiated skin showing cells labeled throughout the epithelium by excision repair. *C.* XP skin, irradiated but showing labeling only from semiconservative replication in the basal layer and no excision repair. *(From Epstein et al. [136]. Used by permission.)*

skin symptoms and are neurologically normal [21]. The level of excision repair is high (greater than 50 percent of normal) and the cells are only slightly more sensitive than normal to UV damage.

Group F The only two representatives of this group have been described in Japan (XP230S and XP2YO) [156]. The skin symptoms were relatively mild and the patients had no neurologic abnormalities. Although excision repair was low (10 per-

cent of normal unscheduled synthesis), the cells showed an intermediate degree of sensitivity to killing by UV light and a high degree of excision of pyrimidine dimers.

Group G Two representatives of this group have been described in England, XP3BR, XP2BI [157, 172]. Both had mental retardation, microcephaly, and sun sensitivity, but tumors were not observed in either XP3BR at age 6 or XP2BI at age 17. The cells showed extremely low levels of dimer exci-

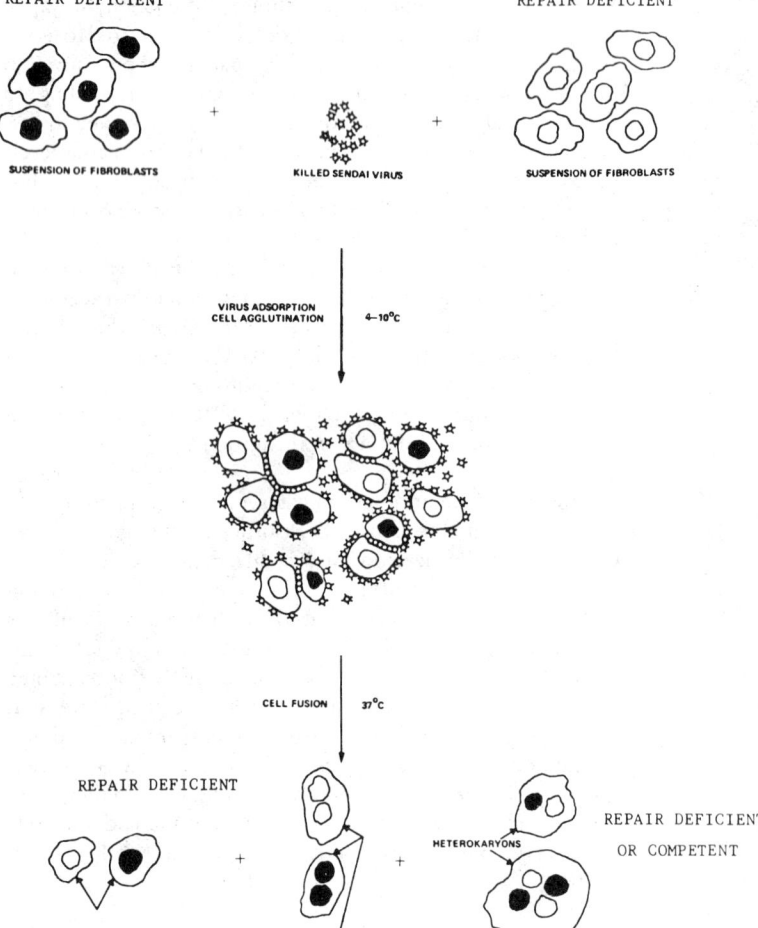

Figure 57-14 Schematic representation of cell fusion under the influence of inactivated Sendai virus as it is employed to detect complementation between different genetic defects. Fibroblasts from two XP patients who are both repair-deficient (denoted by dark and light nuclei) are allowed to agglutinate in the cold and fuse at 37°C to form multinucleate cells. Multinucleate cells with nuclei from the same cell line (homokaryons) will exhibit a repair defect similar to that of the original mononuclear cells. Multinucleate cells with nuclei from each cell line (heterokaryons) will be either repair-deficient or repair-competent, depending on whether the repair defects in the original cell lines are in the same or different complementation groups. One complementation group will usually comprise XP patients with defects in a single gene that codes for an enzyme, and enzyme subunit, or a single polypeptide.

sion and unscheduled synthesis and were as sensitive as groups A and D to killing by UV light.

Unusual for XP cell lines was the slightly increased sensitivity of XP3BR to lethal effects of x-rays. This is not generally observed in other XPs or even XP2BI. XP3BR has a D_o of 72 rads as compared to 102 rads for XP2BI and a range of 97 to 180 rads for normal cells [172, 173].

XP Variant Patients in this group (Fig. 57-18) have mild to severe skin symptoms and normal CNS. It is found worldwide and is a frequent and distinct group from all the other XP groups, even though it is not often clinically identifiable without cell culture studies. Originally defined as a clinically recognized XP without any biochemical defect in excision repair [37, 38], it was actually recognized earlier under the clinical designation pigmented xerodermoid [39, 40, 41]. With careful clinical investigation these patients may be recognized by relatively mild symptoms and the absence of an enhanced erythemal response, but this is insufficient for unambiguous diagnosis.

Slight alterations in late stages of excision repair have been reported [41, 131–133], but these are of unknown importance. The high level of mutagenesis [102, 174] with near-normal levels of cell survival after UV irradiation [89] could be interpreted as indicating that an inherited disorder in excision repair has made this system error-prone. The outstanding feature of this form of XP is that after UV irradiation replication forks appear to stop or to be interrupted during semiconservative replication at every site of DNA damage. This radiation effect on replication is exaggerated by growth in 1 mM caffeine [41, 42], which stimulates many new replication forks [93], and survival is concomitantly diminished [92]. These observations can be explained if it is assumed that normal cells and cells from XP groups A through G have gene product(s) that normally facilitate replication without interruption at damaged sites, and that XP variant cells have lost one or more of these gene product(s) [41]. This is correlated with a reduced rate of recovery of DNA replication after UV irradiation [175].

Whether the variant group is homogeneous or will have multiple subgroups is not known, but the clinical heterogeneity is suggestive. The pigmented xerodermoid family of Jung et al. [39, 40], although biochemically identical to other XP variants, is unusual because no clinical symptoms were evident until after the age of 40, and patients lived into their eighties. This mildness of symptoms contrasts with other variant families from comparable environments in whom the disease is quite severe [41, 168].

XP Heterozygotes

Clinical and laboratory investigations of XP heterozygotes have failed to uncover consistent clinical or cellular abnormalities [25, 26, 28, 176]. In a study of XP cases in the United States [25] the majority of XP heterozygotes were asymptomatic, although a few families in one geographical location had nonmelanoma skin cancers. In Egypt no skin abnormalities were seen in nearly 100 heterozygotes, despite the severe skin abnormalities seen in homozygotes and the intense sunlight [26, 28].

Studies of DNA repair in cell cultures from heterozygotes

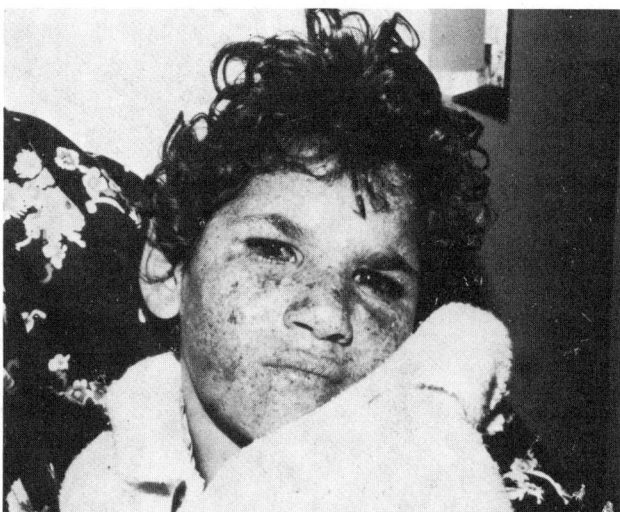

Figure 57-15 XP patient (complementation group A) exhibiting full spectrum of neurologic abnormalities first described by deSanctis and Cacchione [43], including microcephaly, mental retardation, and stunted growth. *(Photograph kindly supplied by Dr. J. German, N.Y. Blood Center.)*

also fail to detect any consistent DNA repair defect, although slight reductions in repair have been reported in occasional studies at high UV doses [176, 177, 178]. In one study fusion of heterozygote with homozygote cells produced multinucleated cells, each of which contained many repair-deficient nuclei and one heterozygous XP nucleus. Slight reductions in repair were then evident in comparison with normal cells [177]. Also, a slightly slower rate of dimer excision from DNA of heterozygote as compared to normal cells has been observed at high UV doses [178].

Measurements of host cell reactivation of irradiated adenovirus [97] or herpes virus [179] did not show any differences between normal and XP heterozygotes. However, measurements of the rate of production of viral antigen from irradiated adenovirus did show lower rates in heterozygotes [180].

The XP gene therefore only appears to have a significant effect on clinical symptoms and DNA repair when present in the homozygous state.

ISOLATION OF EXCISION REPAIR ENZYMES

Enzymes for the first step of repair would be expected to have unique properties related to their action on UV photoproducts. The enzymes for the later stages of excision repair (polymerases and a ligase) probably do not have unique properties because they operate on molecules in which specific damage has been excised. The later stages of repair may be performed by some of the polymerases [181] and the ligases [182] already identified and characterized in animal tissues. The situation may resemble that in *E. coli*, where several different polymerases can play a role in excision repair depending on the genetic and physiologic state of the cell, although the preferred mode involves polymerase I [183].

Identification of a UV-specific endonuclease involved in an early step of repair in human cells has been much more difficult

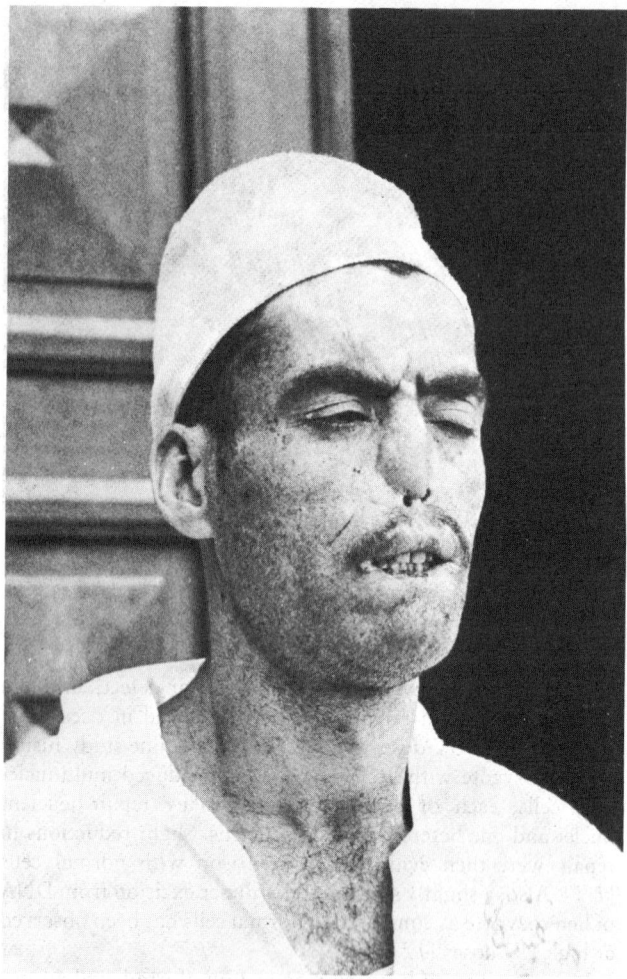

Figure 57-16 Exceptional XP patient (XP13CA) from complementation group A exhibiting skin abnormalities, including the consequence of invasive carcinoma of the nose, but with normal neurologic status, unlike most group A patients (compare Fig. 57-15). *(Photograph kindly supplied by Dr. J. German, N.Y. Blood Center.)*

than anticipated, mainly because of uncertainty in defining precisely the activity of the enzyme to be measured in any assay in crude or partially purified extracts. The most obvious function, and one that proved successful in isolating bacterial enzymes, is the ability of a UV-specific endonuclease to make nicks in UV-irradiated supercoiled DNA [183, 184]. Experiments based on this kind of substrate have identified enzyme activity that nicks UV-irradiated DNA in human (HeLa) cells [185, 186], embryonic lung [184], adult skin fibroblasts [184, 186], rat liver [187], numerous XP fibroblast cell lines [184, 186], and calf thymus [188]. This nicking activity does not appear to be involved in the repair of pyrimidine dimers because it nicks only about 1 percent of the dimers present in the UV-irradiated substrates [184, 185, 188], and because specific monomerization of dimers by photoreactivation in vitro does not alter the nicking activity of these extracts on the substrate [184]. Thus this enzyme activity does not have one of the properties required of a UV-specific endonuclease—that of nicking specifically close to dimers in DNA. It is therefore either an enzyme involved in repair of other kinds of lesions than dimers or is a less specific endonuclease. Examples of enzymes that will make nicks at a low frequency in UV-irradiated DNA in a manner similar to that seen with animal cell

extracts include the S1 nuclease from *Aspergillus oryzae* [189] and a nuclease from *Neurospora crassa* [190].

Because nicking activity has not proved to be a satisfactory assay system, a more specific one has been devised that is closely related to the enzyme's function in vivo—the ability of a cell extract to excise pyrimidine dimers in vitro [191, 192]. This assay measures the function of several enzymes together (at least a UV endonuclease and a UV exonuclease) and is therefore not an assay for UV endonuclease alone. Extracts from normal human cells have the capacity to excise dimers from DNA in vitro, but this activity is easily destroyed by freezing and thawing or excessive sonication during preparation of the extracts [192, 193].

Unfrozen extracts from both normal and XP cells (complementation groups A and C) can excise dimers from UV-irradiated *E. coli* DNA [192]. On this basis, even XP cells that cannot perform excision repair in vivo still perform normal repair in vitro [192]. This suggests either that the defect is more complex than first envisaged and is not simply a missing UV-specific endonuclease [105, 126] or that the excision observed in vitro is mediated by other enzymes that do not serve this function in the cell. When cell extracts were compared for their ability to excise dimers from both exogenous purified DNA and their own DNA still associated with nucleoprotein, extracts from XP cells (complementation groups A and C)

Figure 57-17 XP patient (XP1BE) from complementation group B exhibiting skin and neurologic characteristics that have been ascribed to both XP and Cockayne's syndrome. *(From Robbins et al. [121]. Used by permission.)*

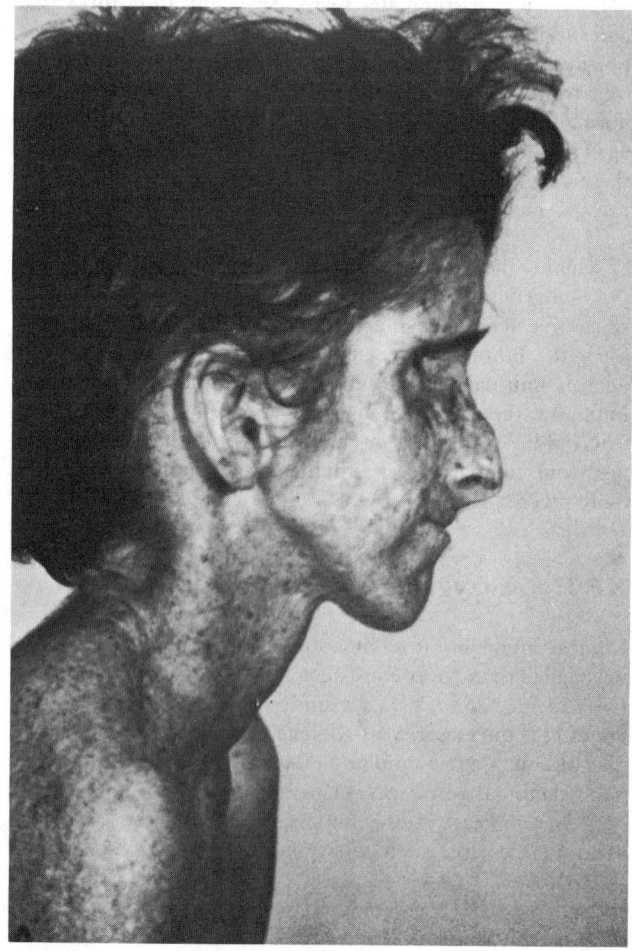

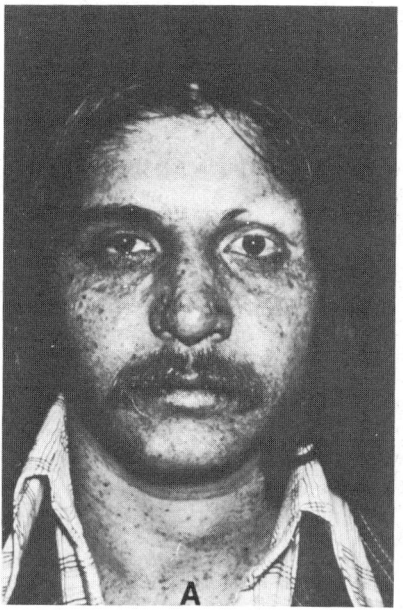 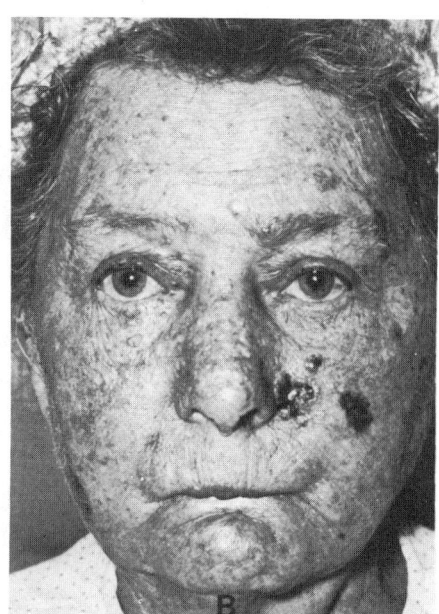

Figure 57-18 XP variants (A:XP115LO; B:XP5MA) exhibiting skin symptoms characteristic of XP and normal neurologic status. *(Photographs kindly provided by Drs. H. Hofmann and E. G. Jung (A) and F. Gianelli (B).)*

excised dimers only from exogenous DNA and not from DNA in chromatin. Thus the defect in these XP cells may lie in some factor that governs the accessibility of dimers in the DNA.

PRENATAL DIAGNOSIS OF XP

Once the main biochemical features of XP were delineated, the assays were adapted for use in prenatal diagnosis. Cell suspensions can be obtained from amniotic fluid by transabdominal puncture during the second half of the first trimester of pregnancy and used to grow fibroblasts in tissue culture representative of the fetus. Fibroblasts from normal fetuses have normal capacities for excision repair [85, 124], whereas those from XP fetuses are expected to be defective.

It is only possible to identify a family at risk for the XP genotype when one homozygous child has already appeared in the family. Prenatal diagnosis was first achieved in such a family by Ramsay et al. [194].

Speed is paramount in tests for DNA repair in amniocentesis specimens. One of the main purposes is to provide a family with reliable information on which to base a decision whether to interrupt pregnancy within the time period allowed by law. Autoradiographic analysis of DNA repair and many other assays for excision repair deficiency or postreplication repair deficiency can be completed in a few days. The longest delay is due to the time required for fibroblast cultures to develop from amniocentesis cell suspensions (about 1 week or longer). Autoradiographic analysis can be done on smaller cultures and is technically easier than most other assays. In the first successful prenatal diagnosis of XP [194], fibroblast cultures were ready to assay for unscheduled synthesis 6 days after amniocentesis, and autoradiography was completed in 3 days.

One potential problem in all amniocentetic tests is that of an error in diagnosis because of contamination of a sample with unrepresentative cells (e.g., nonviable or maternal cells). Usually the presence of nonviable cells can be excluded because they will be lost from cultures during the first days of growth. The probability of contamination with maternal cells is low (of

the order of 0.5 percent or less) and can be excluded for male fetuses by observing sex chromatin in interphase or karyotypic analysis. The risk of false diagnosis should be less than 1 in 500.

Prenatal diagnosis and the possibility of subsequent abortion raises numerous ethical questions in XP as in many other hereditary disorders. These questions may be difficult in the common form of XP because the patient is usually physically and mentally normal, except for the progressive skin disease which can be minimized with treatment.

OTHER HYPERSENSITIVITY DISEASES

XP is only one of a large number of human disorders in which cells (fibroblasts, lymphocytes, etc.) are more sensitive than normal (i.e., hypersensitive) to DNA damaging agents (Table 57-8). Only for XP, however, is there a clear correlation between the hypersensitivity to UV light, the biochemical defect in DNA repair, and the etiology of the disease. In several of the hypersensitive diseases abnormalities have been found in DNA replication rather than repair. Other diseases in which there is only about twofold more sensitivity than normal appear more difficult to attribute to specific defects in repair or replication of DNA; secondary or more subtle defects may be involved.

Ataxia telangiectasia (AT) is a lymphoreticular disorder that culminates in lymphatic malignancy [10, 195]. This disorder involves a complex spectrum of defects in repair of lesions in DNA caused by ionizing radiation [10, 195] or chemical agents [196, 197]. In addition, DNA replication is resistant to inhibition by x-rays [9, 198]. There also appears to be a reduced amount of poly(ADP-ribose) synthesis after x-irradiation.

Cockayne's syndrome is a premature aging syndrome that includes sensitivity to UV light and some chemicals [199–201]. Repair of UV damage is normal [202], but DNA replication is inhibited by UV and fails to recover [12].

Fanconi's anemia is a disease involving a deficiency in bone

Table 57-8 Hypersensitive diseases

Disease	Agent	D_o ratios*	References
Xeroderma pigmentosum (A, C, D)	UV (Chem. Carc.)	5–10	[89, 92]
XP variant	UV	1.6	[89, 92]
Ataxia telangiectasia	X-rays	2.9–3.5	[10, 195]
AT heterozygotes	X-rays	0.9–1.2	[195]
Fanconi's anemia	Mitomycin-C	4–15	[203]
	X-rays	1–2	[215, 216]
Cockayne's syndrome	UV	4.6	[199–201]
Cockayne's heterozygotes	UV	1.8	[199, 200]
Chediak-Higashi syndrome	UV	2.2	[217]
Retinoblastoma (hereditary)	X-rays	1.2–1.5	[215, 218]
Huntington's chorea	X-rays	1.25–2.0	[214]
Partial trisomy 13	X-rays	1.6–2.0	[215]
Progeria	X-rays	1.1–1.6	[215, 216]
Werner's syndrome	X-rays	1.1–1.6	[216]
Gardner's syndrome (hereditary polyposis coli)	X-rays	1 ~ 2	[219]

* This is the ratio of the losses required to reduce the survival of normal and affected cell lines by 63 percent as estimated from the exponential portion of survival curves.

development and bone marrow function. Although cells are markedly hypersensitive to DNA-DNA crosslinking agents [203] the biochemical defect is poorly understood and results have thus far been quite variable [203–206].

Patients with Bloom's syndrome have high spontaneous frequencies of lymphatic and other malignancies [75], baseline sister chromatid exchanges [207], and somatic cell mutation [208]. No consistent hypersensitivity, other than that involving SCEs [209], nor any defect in DNA repair has been demonstrated in Bloom's syndrome [202, 210]

DNA REPAIR AND CARCINOGENESIS IN XP

One theory of carcinogenesis [211] invokes an accumulation of genetic damage as part of the underlying mechanism. Environmental mutagens are postulated to damage some critical region(s) of the genome of somatic cells [212]. If the damage is not repaired before DNA replication occurs, then that region becomes the site of a somatic mutation. If the somatic mutation occurs in genes involved in growth control, then such a mutation might be an early event in carcinogenesis. Incomplete, inefficient, or inaccurate repair in some hereditary diseases should therefore be correlated with increased carcinogenesis. Carcinogenesis induced by radiation or chemicals in normal individuals would then be due to the normal amount of inaccuracy present in repair, or perhaps to inhibition of repair by the damaging agents themselves, or replication of a damaged region before repair was complete. XP would be an example of increased damage remaining in DNA during replication, with a resultant accumulation of mutations. AT might be an example of premature replication, despite DNA damage, with a similar accumulation of mutations.

Carcinogenesis often appears to proceed by a two-step process, the first being the initiation event and the second, which often occurs much later, the promotional event. One theory of carcinogenesis would correlate initiation with the induction of somatic mutations, and promotion with an alteration in the expression of the mutations (e.g., by induction of aneuploidy, which produces haploid cells which can express recessive mutations generated by the initiating carcinogenic event). The effects of the tumor promoter, phorbol ester, appear to be at the later stage involving cell-cell communication and mutation expression [213].

Substantial evidence from microorganisms and mammalian cells supports a theory in which initiating events in carcinogenesis are akin to mutagenic events caused by damage to DNA. Generally there is a high correlation between the mutagenic activity of a chemical and its carcinogenic activity [212]. In XP there is a correlation between high levels of carcinogenesis and susceptibility to UV-induced mutagenesis [3, 8, 21, 102–104] in all forms of the disease, both excision repair defective and variant, although UV-induced rearrangements of DNA in the form of SCEs are only elevated in excision defective XPs. In other diseases, however, the correlations are weaker. In AT cells mutagenesis from x-rays appears normal in spite of the hypersensitivity to x-rays [214].

These kinds of results suggest that the various cellular factors studied experimentally, such as DNA damage, repair, mutation, and transformation, are but a few of the complex mechanisms involved in carcinogenesis. Further elucidation of details of the biochemical, cellular, and clinical characteristics of XP should provide a better understanding of one kind of carcinogenesis, but might have implications for carcinogenesis in general.

This work was supported by the U.S. Department of Energy.

REFERENCES

1. FITZPATRICK TB, QUEVEDO WC JR: Albinism in Stanbury JB, Wyngaarden JB, Fredrickson DS (eds): *The Metabolic Basis of Inherited Disease*, 4th ed. New York, McGraw-Hill, 1977
2. MEYER US, SCHMID R: The porphyrias, in Stanbury JB, Wyngaarden JB, Fredrickson DS (eds): *The Metabolic Basis of Inherited Disease*, 4th ed. New York, McGraw-Hill, 1977
3. CLEAVER JE: DNA damage, repair systems and human hypersensitive diseases. *J Environ Pathol Toxicol* 3:53, 1980
4. CLEAVER JE: Repair processes for photochemical damage in mammalian cells, in Lett JT, Adler H, Zelle M (eds): *Advances in Radiation Biology*. New York, Academic, 1974, vol 4, p 1

5. CLEAVER JE: Defective repair replication of DNA in xeroderma pigmentosum. *Nature (London)* 218:652, 1968

6. CLEAVER JE, BOOTSMA D: Xeroderma pigmentosum: Biochemical and genetic characteristics. *Ann Rev Genet* 9:19, 1975

7. CLEAVER JE: DNA damage and repair in light-sensitive human skin disease. *J Invest Dermatol* 54:181, 1970

8. ROOK A, WILKINSON DS, EBLING FJG (eds): *Textbook of Dermatology.* Oxford, Blackwell, 1968, vol 1

9. PAINTER RB, YOUNG B: Radiosensitivity in ataxia telangiectasia: A new explanation. *Proc Natl Acad Sci,* 77:7315, 1980

10. PATERSON MC, SMITH BP, LOHMAN PHM, ANDERSON AK, FISHMAN L: Defective excision repair of γ-ray-damaged DNA in human (ataxia telangiectasia) fibroblasts. *Nature* 260:444, 1976

11. TAYLOR AMR, HARNDEN DG, ARLETT CF, HARCOURT SA, LEHMANN AR, STEVENS S, BRIDGES BA: Ataxia telangiectasia: A human mutation with abnormal radiation sensitivity. *Nature* 258:427, 1975

12. LEHMANN AR, KIRK-BELL S, MAYNE L: Abnormal kinetics of DNA synthesis in ultraviolet light irradiated cells from patients with Cockayne's syndrome. *Cancer Res* 39:4237, 1979

13. CLEAVER JE: DNA repair with purines and pyrimidines in radiation- and carcinogen-damaged normal and xeroderma pigmentosum human cells. *Cancer Res* 33:362, 1973

14. CLEAVER JE: Photoreactivation: A radiation repair mechanism absent from mammalian cells. *Biochem Biophys Res Comm* 24:569, 1966

15. SUTHERLAND BM: Photoreactivating enzyme from human leukocytes. *Nature (London)* 248:109, 1974

16. SUTHERLAND BM, RICE M, WAGNER EK: Xeroderma pigmentosum cells contain low levels of photoreactivating enzyme. *Proc Natl Acad Sci* 72:103, 1975

17. SUTHERLAND JC, SUTHERLAND BM: Human photoreactivating enzyme. Action spectrum and safelight conditions. *Biophys J* 15:435, 1975

18. MORTELMANS K, CLEAVER JE, FRIEDBERG EC, PATERSON MC, SMITH BP, THOMAS GH: Photoreactivation of thymine dimers in UV-irradiated human cells: Unique dependence on culture conditions. *Mutat Res* 44:433, 1977

19. SUTHERLAND BM, HARBER LC, KOCHEVAR IE: Pyrimidine dimer formation and repair in human skin. *Cancer Res* 40:3181, 1980

20. PARK SD, CLEAVER JE: Postreplication repair: Questions of its definition and possible alteration in xeroderma pigmentosum cell strains. *Proc Natl Acad Sci* 76:3927, 1979

21. ROBBINS JH, KRAEMER KH, LUTZNER MA, FESTOFF BW, COON HG: Xeroderma pigmentosum. An inherited disease with sun sensitivity, multiple cutaneous neoplasms, and abnormal DNA repair. *Ann Intern Med* 80:221, 1974

22. MCKUSICK VA: *Mendellian Inheritance in Man. Catalogs of Autosomal Dominant, Autosomal Recessive, and X-Linked Phenotypes,* 3d ed. John Hopkins Press, Baltimore, 1971, p 294

23. HEBRA F, KAPOSI M: *On Diseases of the Skin, Including the Exanthemata.* Tay W (trans). London, New Sydenham Society, 1874, vol 3, p 252

24. COCKAYNE EA: *Inherited Abnormalities of the Skin and Its Appendages,* London, Oxford University Press, 1933, p 93

25. SWIFT M, CHASE C: Cancer in families with xeroderma pigmentosum. *J Nat Cancer Inst* 62:1415, 1979

26. CLEAVER JE, ZELLE B, HASHEM N, EL-HEFNAWI MH, GERMAN J: Xeroderma pigmentosum in patients from Egypt. II. Preliminary correlations of epidemiology, clinical symptoms and molecular biology. *J Invest Derm,* 77:96, 1981

27. HODGE SE, BERKEL AI, GATTI RA, BODEI E, SPENCE MA: Ataxia telangiectasia and xeroderma pigmentosum: No evidence of linkage to HLA. *Tissue Antigens* 15:313, 1980

28. HASHEM N, BOOTSMA D, KEIJZER W, GREENE AE, CORIELL L, THOMAS GH, CLEAVER JE: Clinical characteristics, DNA repair, and complementation groups in xeroderma pigmentosum patients from Egypt. *Cancer Res* 40:13, 1980

29. MARSHALL J: *Skin Diseases in Africa.* Capetown, Maskew Miller, 1964, p 91

30. EL-HEFNAWI H, RASHEED A: Xeroderma pigmentosum. A comprehensive study of a further 34 cases in the United Arab Republic. *Gaz Egypt Soc Dermatol Venereol* 1:189, 1966

31. EL-HEFNAWI H: Xeroderma pigmentosum in Demis D, Crounse R, Dobson R (eds): *Clinical Dermatology.* New York, Harper & Row, 1972, unit 19-7, vol 4, p 1

32. BERLIN C, TAGER A: Dermatitis solaris in children. A herald manifestation of xeroderma pigmentosum. *Arch Dermatol* 85:41, 1962

33. TAKEBE H, MIKI Y, KOZUKA T, FURUYAMA J, TANAKA K, SASAKI MS, FUJIWARA Y, AKIBA H: DNA repair characteristics and skin cancers of xeroderma pigmentosum patients in Japan. *Cancer Res* 37:490, 1977

34. RAMSAY CA, GIANNELLI F: The erythemal action spectrum and deoxyribonucleic acid repair synthesis in xeroderma pigmentosum. *Brit J Dermatol* 92:49, 1975

35. GUERRIER CJ, LUTZNER MA, DEVICO V, PRUNIERAS M: An electronmicroscopial study of the skin in 18 cases of xeroderma pigmentosum. *Dermatologica* 146:211, 1973

36. LYNCH HT, ANDERSON DE, SMITH JL, HOWELL JB, KRUSH AJ: Xeroderma pigmentosum, malignant melanoma, and congenital ichthyosis. *Arch Dermatol* 96:625, 1967

37. BURK PG, LUTZNER MA, CLARKE DD, ROBBINS JH: Ultraviolet-stimulated thymidine incorporation in xeroderma pigmentosum lymphocytes. *J Lab Clin Med* 77:759, 1971

38. CLEAVER JE: Xeroderma pigmentosum: Variants with normal DNA repair and normal sensitivity to ultraviolet light. *J Invest Dermatol* 58:124, 1972

39. JUNG EG: New form of molecular defect in xeroderma pigmentosum. *Nature (London)* 228:361, 1970

40. HOFMANN H, JUNG EG, SCHNYDER UW: Pigmented xerodermoid: First report of a family. *Bull Cancer* 65:347, 1978

41. CLEAVER JE, ARUTYUNYAN RM, SARKISIAN T, KAUFMANN WK, GREENE AE, CORIELL L: Similar defects in DNA repair and replication in the pigmented xerodermoid and the xeroderma pigmentosum variants. *Carcinogenesis* 1:647, 1980

42. LEHMANN AR, KIRK-BELL S, ARLETT CF, PATERSON MC, LOHMAN PHM, DE WEERD-KASTELEIN EA, BOOTSMA D: Xeroderma pigmentosum cells with normal levels of excision repair have a defect in DNA synthesis after UV-irradiation. *Proc Natl Acad Sci* 72:219, 1975

43. DESANCTIS C, CACCHIONE A: L'idiozia xerodermica. *Riv Sper Freniatr* 56:269, 1932

44. REED WB, MAY SB, NICKEL WR: Xeroderma pigmentosum with neurological complications. The deSanctis Cacchione syndrome. *Arch Dermatol* 91:224, 1965

45. REED WB, LANDING B, SUGARMAN G, CLEAVER JE, MELNYK J: Xeroderma pigmentosum. Clinical and laboratory investigation of its basic defect. *J Am Med Assoc* 207:2073, 1969

46. THRUSH DC, HOLTI G, BRADLEY WG, CAMPBELL MI, WALTON JN: Neurological manifestations of xeroderma pigmentosum in two siblings. *J Neurol Sci* 22:91, 1974

47. SMITHERS DW, WOOD JH: Xeroderma pigmentosum. An attempt at cancer prophylaxis. *Lancet* 1:945, 1952

48. PATHAK MA, FITZPATRICK TB, FRENK E: Evaluation of topical agents that prevent sunburn—Superiority of paraaminobenzoic acid and its ester in ethyl alcohol. *N Engl J Med* 280:1459, 1969

49. WILLIS I, KLIGMAN AM: Aminobenzoic acid and its esters. The quest for more effective sunscreens. *Arch Dermatol* 102:405, 1970

50. BROCKINGTON WS, POSTLETHWAIT RW: Xeroderma pigmentosum. *Am Surg* 18:50, 1952

51. MOORE C, IVERSON PC: Xeroderma pigmentosum. Showing common skin cancers plus melanocarcinoma controlled by surgery. *Cancer* 7:377, 1954

52. GLEASON MC: Xeroderma pigmentosum—Five-year arrest after total resurfacing of the face. *Plast Reconstr Surg* 46:577, 1970

53. EPSTEIN EH, BURK PG, COHEN IK, DECKERS P: Dermatome shaving in the treatment of xeroderma pigmentosum. *Arch Dermatol* 105:589, 1972

54. CARTER VH, SMITH KW, NOOJIN RO: Xeroderma pigmentosum. Treatment with topically applied flourouracil. *Arch Dermatol* 98:526, 1968

55. SETLOW RB: The wavelengths in sunlight effective in producing skin cancer: A theoretical analysis. *Proc Natl Acad Sci* 71:3363, 1974

56. EPSTEIN JH: Ultraviolet carcinogenesis. *Photophysiology* 5:235, 1970

57. BLUM HF: *Carcinogenesis by Ultraviolet Light.* Princeton, NJ, Princeton University Press, 1959

58. HARM W: Use of an *E. coli uvr⁻ rec⁻ mutant* for monitoring the germicidal activity of sunlight. *Radiat Res* 39:517, 1969 (abstr)

59. TROSKO JE, KRAUSE D, ISOUN M: Sunlight-induced pyrimidine dimers in human cells *in vitro. Nature (London)* 228:358, 1970

60. ZIMMER KG: *Studies on Quantitative Radiation Biology* Griffith HD (trans). New York, Hafner, 1961

61. ROTHMAN RH, SETLOW RB: An action spectrum for cell killing and pyrimidine dimer formation in Chinese hamster V-79 cells. *Photochem Photobiol* 29:57, 1979

62. TODD P, COOHILL TP, MAHONEY JA: Responses of cultured Chinese hamster cells to ultraviolet light of different wavelengths. *Radiat Res* 35:390, 1968

63. KANTOR GJ, SUTHERLAND JC, SETLOW RB: Action spectra for killing nondividing normal human and xeroderma pigmentosum cells. *Photochem Photobiol* 31:459, 1980

64. CHU EHY: Effects of ultraviolet radiation on mammalian cells. I. Induction of chromosome aberrations. *Mutat Res* 2:75, 1965

65. ICHIHASHI M, RAMSAY CA: The action spectrum and dose response studies of unscheduled DNA synthesis in normal human fibroblasts. *Photochem Photobiol* 23:103, 1975

66. SMITH KC: An isomer of the cyclobutane-type thymine dimer produced in the presense of adenine. *Biochem Biophys Res Commun* 25:426, 1966

67. PATHAK MA, KRAMER DM, GUNGERICH U: Formation of thymine dimers in mammalian skin by ultraviolet radiation *in vivo. Photochem Photobiol* 15:177, 1972

68. SETLOW RB: Molecular changes responsible for ultraviolet inactivation of the biological activity of DNA, in Pavan C, Chagas C, Frota-Pessoa O, Caldas LR (eds): *Mammalian Cytogenetics and Related Problems in Radiobiology.* New York, Macmillan, 1964, p 291

69. SETLOW RB: Cyclobutane-type pyrimidine dimers in polynucleotides. *Science* 153:379, 1966

70. SMITH KC, HANAWALT PC: *Molecular Photobiology: Inactivation and Recovery.* New York, Academic, 1969

71. BLACK HS, LO WB: Formation of a carcinogen in human skin irradiated with ultraviolet light. *Nature (London)* 234:306, 1971

72. BROWN AJ, FICKEL TH, CLEAVER JE, LOHMAN PHM, WADE MH, WATERS R: Overlapping pathways for repair of damage from ultraviolet light and chemical carcinogens in human fibroblasts. *Cancer Res* 39:2522, 1979

73. HARRIS M: *Cell Culture and Somatic Variation.* New York, Holt, 1964

74. WALTIMO O, IIVANAINEN M, HOKKANEN E: Xeroderma pigmentosum with neurological manifestations. Family studies of two affected sisters, one of them with a chromosome abnormality, and report of one separate case. *Acta Neurol Scand* 43(suppl 31):66, 1967

75. GERMAN J: Genes which increase chromosomal instability in somatic cells and predispose to cancer. *Prog Med Genet* 8:61, 1972

76. STEFANINI M, KLEIJER W, DALPRA L, ELLI R, PORRO MN, NICOLETTI B, NUZZO F: Differences in the levels of UV repair and in clinical symptoms in two sibs affected by xeroderma pigmentosum. *Hum Genet* 634:1, 1980

77. KATO H: Spontaneous sister chromatid exchanges detected by a BUdR-labeling method. *Nature (London)* 251:70, 1974

78. PERRY P, WOLFF S: New Giemsa method for the differential staining of sister chromatids. *Nature (London)* 251:156, 1974

79. WOLFF S, BODYCOTE J, THOMAS GH, CLEAVER JE: Sister chromatid exchange in xeroderma pigmentosum cells that are defective in DNA excision repair or post-replication repair. *Genetics* 81:349, 1975

80. WOLFF S, RODIN B, CLEAVER JE: Sister chromatid exchanges induced by mutagenic carcinogens in normal and xeroderma pigmentosum cells. *Nature* 265:347, 1977

81. DE WEERD-KASTELEIN EA, KEIJZER W, RAINALDI G, BOOTSMA D: Induction of sister chromatid exchanges in xeroderma pigmentosum cells after exposure to ultraviolet light. *Mutat Res* 45:253, 1977

82. PARRINGTON JM, DELHANTY JDA, BADEN HP: Unscheduled DNA synthesis, UV-induced chromosome aberrations and SV40 transformation in cultured cells from xeroderma pigmentosum. *Ann Hum Genet* 35:149, 1971

83. SASAKI MS: DNA repair capacity and susceptibility to chromosome breakage in xeroderma pigmentosum cells. *Mutat Res* 20:41, 1973

84. GARTLER SM: Inborn errors of metabolism at the cell culture level, in Fishbein M (ed): *Second International Congress on Congenital Malformations.* New York, International Medical Congress, 1964, p 94

85. CLEAVER JE: DNA repair and radiation sensitivity in human (xeroderma pigmentosum) cells. *Int J Radiat Biol* 18:557, 1970

86. GOLDSTEIN S: The role of DNA repair in aging of cultured fibroblasts from xeroderma pigmentosum and normals. *Proc Soc Exp Biol Med* 137:730, 1971

87. TAKEBE H, FURUYAMA JI, MIKI Y, KONDO S: High sensitivity of xeroderma pigmentosum cells to the carcinogen 4-nitroquinoline-1-oxide. *Mutat Res* 15:98, 1972

88. STICH HF, SAN RHC, KAWAZOE Y: Increased sensitivity of xeroderma pigmentosum cells to some chemical carcinogens and mutagens. *Mutat Res* 17:127, 1973

89. ANDREWS AD, BARRETT SF, ROBBINS JH: Xeroderma pigmentosum neurological abnormalities correlate with colony-forming ability after ultraviolet radiation. *Proc Natl Acad Sci* 75:1984, 1978

90. STICH HF, SAN RHC: DNA repair synthesis and survival of repair deficient human cells exposed to the K-region epoxide of benz(a)anthracene. *Proc Soc Exp Biol Med* 142:155, 1973

91. MAHER WM, BIRCH N, OTTO JR, McCORMICK JJ: Cytotoxicity of carcinogenic aromatic amides in normal and xeroderma pigmentosum fibroblasts with different DNA repair capabilities. *J Nat Cancer Inst* 54:1287, 1975

92. ARLETT CF, HARCOURT SA, BROUGHTON BC: The influence of caffeine on cell survival in excision proficient and excision deficient xeroderma pigmentosum and normal human cell strains following ultraviolet light irradiation. *Mutat Res* 33:341, 1975

93. PAINTER RB: Effect of caffeine on DNA synthesis in irradiated and unirradiated mammalian cells. *J Mol Biol* 143:289, 1980

94. ZAVADOVA Z: Host-cell repair of vaccinia virus and of double stranded RNA of encephalomyocarditis virus. *Nature New Biol* 233:123, 1971

95. LYTLE CD, AARONSON SA, HARVEY E: Host-cell reactivation in mammalian cells. II. Survival by herpes simplex virus and vaccinia virus in normal human and xeroderma pigmentosum cells. *Int J Radiat Biol* 22:159, 1972

96. RABSON AS, TYRRELL SA, LEGALLAIS FY: Growth of ultraviolet-damaged herpes virus in xeroderma pigmentosum cells. *Proc Soc Exp Biol Med* 132:802, 1969

97. DAY RS III: Studies on repair of adenovirus 2 by human fibroblasts using normal, xeroderma pigmentosum, and xeroderma pigmentosum heterozygous strains. *Cancer Res* 34:1965, 1974

98. DAY RS III: Cellular reactivation of ultraviolet-irradiated human adenovirus 2 in normal and xeroderma pigmentosum fibroblasts. *Photochem Photobiol* 19:9, 1974

99. AARONSON SA, LYTLE CD: Decreased host-cell reactivation of irradiated SV40 virus in xeroderma pigmentosum. *Nature (London)* 228:359, 1970

100. DAY RS III: Xeroderma pigmentosum variants have decreased repair of UV-damaged DNA. *Nature (London)* 253:748, 1975

101. KELLEY WN, WYNGAARDEN JB: The Lesch-Nyhan syndrome, in Stanbury JB, Wyngaarden JB, Fredrickson DS (eds): *The Metabolic Basis of Inherited Disease*, 4th ed. New York, McGraw-Hill, 1977

102. MAHER VM, OUELETTE LM, CURREN RD, McCORMICK JJ: Frequency of ultraviolet light-induced mutations is higher in xeroderma pigmentosum variant cells. *Nature* 261:593, 1976

103. MAHER VM, DORNEY DJ, MENDRALA AL, KONZE-THOMAS B, McCORMICK JJ: DNA excision-repair processes in human cells can eliminate the cytotoxic and mutagenic consequences of ultraviolet irradiation. *Mutat Res* 62:311, 1979

104. GLOVER TW, CHANG CC, TROSKO JE, LI SS: Ultraviolet light induction of diphtheria toxin-resistant mutants of normal and xeroderma pigmentosum human fibroblasts. *Proc Natl Acad Sci* 76:3982, 1979

105. CLEAVER JE: Xeroderma pigmentosum: A human disease in which an initial stage of DNA repair is defective. *Proc Natl Acad Sci* 63:428, 1969

106. CLEAVER JE: DNA repair and its coupling to DNA replication in eukaryotic cells. *Biochim Biophys Acta* 516:489, 1978

107. McGHEE JD, FELSENFELD G: Nucleosome structure. *Ann Res Biochem* 49:115, 1980

108. BODELL WJ: Nonuniform distribution of DNA repair in chromatin after treatment with methylmethane sulfonate. *Nucleic Acids Res* 4:2619, 1977

109. CLEAVER JE: Nucleosome structure controls rates of excision repair in DNA of human cells. *Nature* 270:451, 1977

110. SMERDON MJ, TLSTY TD, LIEBERMAN MW: Distribution of ultraviolet-induced DNA repair synthesis in nuclease sensitive and resistant regions of human chromatin. *Biochemistry* 17:2377, 1978

111. DEUTSCH WA, LINN S: DNA binding activity that is from cultured human fibroblasts that is specific for partially depurinated DNA and that inserts purines into apurinic sites. *Proc Natl Acad Sci* 76:141, 1979

112. SAMSON L, SCHWARTZ JL: Evidence for an adaptive DNA repair pathway in CHO and human skin fibroblast cell lines. *Nature* 287:861, 1980

113. KARRAN P, LINDAHL T, GRIFFIN B: Adaptive response to alkylating agents involves alteration *in situ* of O^{-6}-methylguanine residues in DNA. *Nature* 280:76, 1979

114. PEGG A: Enzymatic removal of O^{-6}-methylguanine from DNA by mammalian cell extracts. *Biochem Biophys Res Commun* 84:166, 1978

115. HASELTINE WA, GORDON LK, LINDAN CP, GRAFSTROM RH, SHAPER NL, GROSSMAN L: Cleavage of pyrimidine dimers in specific DNA sequences by a pyrimidine dimer DNA glycosylase of *M. luteus. Nature* 285:634, 1980

116. DEMPLE B, LINN S: DNA N-glycosylases and UV repair. *Nature* 287:203, 1980

117. HUBSCHER U, KUENZLE CC, SPADARI S: Functional roles of DNA polymerases β and α. *Proc Natl Acad Sci* 76:2316, 1979

118. CIARROCCHI G, JOSE JG, LINN S: Further characterization of a cell-free system for measuring replicative and repair DNA synthesis with cultured human fibroblasts and evidence for the involvement of DNA polymerase α in DNA repair. *Nucleic Acids Res* 7:1205, 1979

119. DURKACZ BW, OMIDIJI O, GRAY DA, SHALL S: (ADP-ribose)n participates in DNA excision repair. *Nature* 283:593, 1980

120. BERGER NA, SIKORSKI GW, PETZOLD SJ, KUROHARA KK: Defective poly(adenosine diphosphoribose)n synthesis in xeroderma pigmentosum. *Biochemistry* 19:289, 1980

121. CLEAVER JE: Methods for studying repair of DNA damaged by physical and chemical carcinogens. In Busch H (ed): *Methods in Cancer Research.* New York, Academic, 1975, vol II, p 123

122. DJORDJEVIC B, TOLMACH LJ: Responses of synchronous population of HeLa cells to ultraviolet irradiation at selected stages of the generation cycle. *Radiat Res* 32:327, 1967

123. PETTIJOHN D, HANAWALT PC: Evidence for repair-replication of ultraviolet damaged DNA in bacteria. *J Mol Biol* 9:395, 1964

124. REGAN JD, SETLOW RB, LEY RD: Normal and defective repair of damaged DNA in human cells: A sensitive assay utilizing the photolysis of bromodeoxyuridine. *Proc Natl Acad Sci* 68:708, 1971

125. EDENBERG H, HANAWALT PC: Size of repair patches in the DNA of ultraviolet-irradiated HeLa cells. *Biochim Biophys Acta* 272:361, 1972

126. SETLOW RB, REGAN JD, GERMAN J, CARRIER WL: Evidence that xeroderma pigmentosum cells do not perform the first step in the repair of ultraviolet damage to their DNA. *Proc Natl Acad Sci* 64:1035, 1969

127. CLEAVER JE: Sedimentation of DNA from human fibroblasts irradiated with ultraviolet light: Possible detection of excision breaks in normal and repair-deficient xeroderma pigmentosum cells. *Radiat Res* 57:207, 1974

128. CLEAVER JE, THOMAS GH, TROSKO JE, LETT JT: Excision repair (dimer excision, strand breakage and repair replication) in primary cultures of eukaryotic (bovine) cells. *Exp Cell Res* 74:67, 1972

129. KLEIJER WJ, HOEKSEMA JL, SLUYTER ML, BOOTSMA D: Effects of inhibitors on repair of DNA in normal human and xeroderma pigmentosum cells after exposure to X-rays and ultraviolet irradiation. *Mutat Res* 17:385, 1973

130. BEN-HUR E, BEN-ISHAI R: DNA repair in ultraviolet light irradiated HeLa cells and its reversible inhibition by hydroxyurea. *Photochem Photobiol* 13:337, 1971

131. FORNACE AJ JR, KOHN FW, KANN HE JR: DNA single-strand breaks during repair of UV damage in human fibroblasts and abnormalities of repair in xeroderma pigmentosum. *Proc Natl Acad Sci* 73:39, 1976

132. DINGMAN CW, KAKUNAGA T: DNA strand breaking and rejoining in response to ultraviolet light in normal human and xeroderma pigmentosum cells. *Int J Radiat Biol* 30:55, 1976

133. DUNN WC, REGAN JD: Inhibition of DNA excision repair in human cells by arabinofuranosyl cytosine: Effects on normal and xeroderma pigmentosum cells. *Mol Pharmacol* 15:367, 1976

134. BOOTSMA D, MULDER MP, POT F, COHEN JA: Different inherited levels of DNA repair replication in xeroderma pigmentosum cell strains after exposure to ultraviolet irradiation. *Mutat Res* 9:507, 1970

135. ZELLE B, LOHMAN PHM: Repair of UV-endonuclease-susceptible sites in the 7 complementation groups of xeroderma pigmentosum A through G. *Mutat Res* 62:363, 1979

136. EPSTEIN JH, FUKUYAMA K, REED WB, EPSTEIN WI: Defect in DNA synthesis in skin of patients with xeroderma pigmentosum demonstrated *in vivo*. *Science* 168:1477, 1970

137. DUPUY JM, LAFFORET D, RACHMAN F: Xeroderma pigmentosum with liver involvement. *Helv Paediatr Acta* 29:213, 1975

138. HARM W, RUPERT CS, HARM H: Photoenzymatic repair of DNA. I. Investigation of the reaction by flash illumination, in Beers RF Jr, Herriott RM, Tilghman RC (eds): *Molecular and Cellular Repair Processes*. Baltimore, Johns Hopkins University Press, 1972, p 53

139. COOK JS: Photoenzymatic repair in animal cells, in Beers RF Jr, Herriott RM, Tilghman RC (eds): *Molecular and Cellular Repair Processes*. Baltimore, Johns Hopkins University Press, 1972, p 79

140. COOK JS, McGRATH JR: Photoreactivating-enzyme activity in Metazoa. *Proc Natl Acad Sci* 58:1359, 1967

141. LYTLE CD, BENANE SG, STAFFORD JE: Host cell reactivation in mammalian cells. V. Photoreactivation studies with herpes virus in marsupial and human cells. *Photochem Photobiol* 23:331, 1975

142. HARM H: Damage and repair in mammalian cells after exposure to nonionizing radiations. III. Ultraviolet and visible light irradiation of cells of placental mammals, including humans, and determination of photorepairable damage *in vitro*. *Mutat Res* 69:167, 1980

143. CLEAVER JE: Repair of alkylation damage in ultraviolet-sensitive (xeroderma pigmentosum) human cells. *Mutat Res* 12:453, 1971

144. KLEIJER WJ, LOHMAN PHM, MULDER MP, BOOTSMA D: Repair of X-ray damage in DNA of cultivated cells from patients having xeroderma pigmentosum. *Mutat Res* 9:517, 1970

145. Setlow RB, Regan JD: Defective repair of N-acetoxy-2-acetylaminofluorene—induced lesions in the DNA of xeroderma pigmentosum cells. *Biochem Biophys Res Commun* 16:1019, 1972

146. STICH HF, SAN RHC, MILLER JA, MILLER EC: Various levels of DNA repair synthesis in xeroderma pigmentosum cells exposed to the carcinogens N-hydroxy- and N-acetoxy-2-acetylaminofluorene. *Nature New Biol* 238:9, 1972

147. REGAN JD, SETLOW RB: Two forms of repair in the DNA of human cells damaged by chemical carcinogens and mutagens. *Cancer Res* 34:3318, 1974

148. PAINTER RB, YOUNG BR: Repair replication in mammalian cells after X-irradiation. *Mutat Res* 14:225, 1972

149. MILLER EC, MILLER JA: Biochemical mechanisms of chemical carcinogenesis, in Busch H (ed): *The Molecular Biology of Cancer*. New York, Academic, 1974, p 377

150. BODELL WJ, SINGER B, THOMAS GH, CLEAVER JE: Evidence for removal at different rates of O-ethylphosphotriesters in two human fibroblast cell lines. *Nucleic Acids Res* 6:2819, 1979

151. SINGER B, BRENT TP: Human lymphoblasts contain glycosylase activity excising N-3 and N-7 methyl and ethyl purines but not O-6-alkylguanine or l-alkylguanine. *Proc Natl Acad Sci* 78:856, 1981

152. DE WEERD-KASTELEIN EA, KEIJZER W, BOOTSMA D: Genetic heterogeneity of xeroderma pigmentosum demonstrated by somatic cell hybridization. *Nature New Biol* 238:80, 1972

153. KRAEMER KH, COON HG, PETTIGA RA, BARRETT SF, RAHE AE, ROBBINS JH: Genetic heterogeneity in xeroderma pigmentosum. Complementation groups and their relationship to DNA repair rates. *Proc Natl Acad Sci* 72:59, 1975

154. DE WEERD-KASTELEIN EA, KEIJZER W, BOOTSMA D: A third complementation group in xeroderma pigmentosum. *Mutat Res* 22:87, 1974

155. KRAEMER KH, DE WEERD-KASTELEIN EA, ROBBINS JH, KEIJZER W, BARRETT SF, PETINGA RA, BOOTSMA D: Five complementation groups in xeroderma pigmentosum. *Mutat Res* 33:327, 1975

156. ARASE S, KOZUKA T, TANAKA K, IKENAGA M, TAKEBE H: A sixth complementation group in xeroderma pigmentosum. *Mutat Res* 59:143, 1979

157. KEIJZER W, JASPERS NGJ, ABRAHAMS PJ, TAYLOR AMR, ARLETT CF, ZELLE B, TAKEBE H, KANMONT PDS, BOOTSMA D: A seventh complementation group in excision deficient xeroderma pigmentosum. *Mutat Res* 62:183, 1979

158. HAYNES RH: General discussion. *Radiat Res Suppl* 6:232, 1966

159. WALDSTEIN EA, PELLER S, SETLOW RB: UV-Endonuclease from calf thymus with specificity toward pyrimidine dimers in DNA. *Proc Natl Acad Sci* 76:3746, 1978

160. GRUENERT DC, CLEAVER JE: Repair of ultraviolet damage in human cells also exposed to agents that cause strand breaks, crosslinks, monoadducts and alkylations. *Chem Biol Interact* 33:163, 1981

161. PARK SD, CHOI KH, HONG SW, CLEAVER JE: Inhibition of excision repair of ultraviolet damage in human cells by exposure to methylmethane sulfonate. *Mutat Res* 82:365, 1981

162. NEEL JV, KODANI M, BREWER R, ANDERSON RC: The incidence of consanguineous matings in Japan, with remarks on the estimation of comparative gene frequencies and the expected rate of appearance of induced recessive mutations. *Am J Hum Genet* 1:156, 1949

163. THIELMANN HW, WITTE I: Correlation of the colony-forming abilities of xeroderma pigmentosum fibroblasts with repair-specific DNA incision reactions catalyzed by cell-free extracts. *Arch Toxicol* 44:197, 1980

164. KUHNLEIN U, PENHOET EE, LINN S: An altered apurinic endonuclease activity in group A and group D xeroderma pigmentosum fibroblasts. *Proc Natl Acad Sci* 73:1169, 1976

165. DE WEERD-KASTELEIN EA, KEIJZER W, SABOUR M, PARRINGTON JM, BOOTSMA D: A xeroderma pigmentosum patient having a high residual activity of unscheduled DNA synthesis after UV is assigned to complementation Group A. *Mutat Res* 37:307, 1976

166. KRAEMER KH: Xeroderma pigmentosum, in Demis DJ, Dobson RL, McGuire J (eds): *Clinical Dermatology*. 4:unit 19-7, 1, 1980

167. HANANIAN J, CLEAVER JE: Xeroderma pigmentosum exhibiting neurological disorders and systemic lupus erythematosus. *Clin Genet* 17:39, 1980

168. PAWSEY SA, MAGNUS IA, RAMSAY CA, BENSON PF, GIANELLI F: Clinical, genetic and DNA repair studies on a consecutive series of patients with xeroderma pigmentosum. *Quart J Med* 48:179, 1979

169. GOLDSTEIN N, HAY-ROE V: Prevention of skin cancer with a PABA in alcohol sunscreen in xeroderma pigmentosum. *Cutis (Jan)* 61, 1975

170. KUHNLEIN U, LEE B, PENHOET E E, LINN S: Xeroderma pigmentosum fibroblasts of the group D lack an apurinic DNA endonuclease species with a low apparent K_m. *Nucleic Acids Res* 5:951, 1978

171. MOSES RE, BEAUDET AL: Apurinic endonuclease activities in repair-deficient human cell lines. *Nucleic Acids Res* 5:463, 1978

172. ARLETT CF, HARCOURT SA, LEHMANN AR, STEVENS S, FERGUSON-SMITH MA, MOSLEY WN: Studies on a new case of xeroderma pigmentosum (XP3BR) from complementation group G with cellular sensitivity to ionizing radiation. *Carcinogenesis* 1:745, 1980

173. COX R, MASSON WK: Radiosensitivity in cultured human fibroblasts. *Int J Rad Biol* 38:575, 1980

174. MYHR BC, TURNBULL D, DIPAOLO JA: Ultraviolet mutagenesis of normal and xeroderma pigmentosum variant fibroblasts. *Mutat Res* 62:341, 1979

175. CLEAVER JE, THOMAS GH, PARK SD: Xeroderma pigmentosum variants have a slow recovery of DNA synthesis after irradiation with ultraviolet light. *Biochim Biophys Acta* 564:122, 1979

176. CLEAVER JE, CARTER DM: Xeroderma pigmentosum variants: Influence of temperature on DNA repair. *J Invest Derm* 60:29, 1973

177. GIANELLI F, PAWSEY SA: DNA repair synthesis in human heterokaryons. II. A test for heterozygosity in xeroderma pigmentosum and some insight into the structure of the defective enzyme. *J Cell Sci* 15:163, 1974

178. RITTER MA: Reduced DNA repair in xeroderma pigmentosum (XP) heterozygotes in *Sixth International Congress of Radiation Research*. Tokyo, Japan, Toppan Printing Co., 1979, p 264

179. SELSKY CA, GREER S: Host-cell reactivation of ultraviolet irradiated and chemically treated herpes simplex virus 1 by xeroderma pigmentosum, xeroderma pigmentosum heterozygotes and normal skin fibroblasts. *Mutat Res* 50:395, 1978

180. RAINBOW AJ: Reduced capacity to repair irradiated adenovirus in fibroblasts from xeroderma pigmentosum heterozygotes. *Cancer Res* 40:3945, 1980

181. WEISSBACH A: DNA polymerases. *Cell* 5:101, 1975

182. LINDAHL T, EDELMAN GM: Polynucleotide ligase from myeloid and lymphoid tissues. *Proc Natl Acad Sci* 61:680, 1968

183. GROSSMAN L: Enzymes involved in the repair of DNA in Lett JT, Adler H,

Zelle M (eds): *Advances in Radiation Biology*. New York, Academic, 1974, vol 4, p 77

184. BACCHETTI S, VAN DER PLAS A, VELDHUISEN G: A UV-specific endonucleolytic activity present in human cell extracts. *Biochem Biophys Res Commun* 48:662, 1972

185. BRENT TP: Repair enzyme suggested by mammalian endonuclease activity specific for ultraviolet-irradiated DNA. *Nature New Biol* 239:172, 1972

186. DUKER NJ, TEEBOR GW: Different ultraviolet DNA endonuclease activity in human cells. *Nature (London)* 255:82, 1975

187. VAN LANCKER JL, TOMURA T: Purification and some properties of a mammalian repair endonuclease. *Biochim Biophys Acta* 353:99, 1974

188. BACCHETTI S, BENNE R: Purification and characterization of an endonuclease from calf thymus acting on irradiated DNA. *Biochim Biophys Acta* 390:285, 1975

189. SHISHIDO K, ANDO T: Cleavage of ultraviolet light-irradiated DNA by single strand-specific S1 endonuclease. *Biochem Biophys Res Commun* 59:1380, 1974

190. KATO AC, FRASER MJ: Action of single-strand specific *Neurospora crassa* endonuclease on ultraviolet light-irradiated native DNA. *Biochim Biophys Acta* 312:645, 1973

191. COOK K, FRIEDBERG EC, SLOR H, CLEAVER JE: Excision of thymine dimers from specifically incised DNA by extracts of xeroderma pigmentosum cells. *Nature* 256:235, 1975

192. MORTELMANS K, FRIEDBERG EC, SLOR H, THOMAS G, CLEAVER JE: Defective thymine dimer excision by cell-free extracts of xeroderma pigmentosum cells. *Proc Natl Acad Sci* 73:2757, 1976

193. SLOR H, LEV-SOBE T, FREIDBERG EC: Evidence for inactivation of DNA repair in frozen and thawed mammalian cells. *Mutat Res* 45:137, 1947

194. RAMSAY CA, COLTART TM, BLUMT S, PAWSEY SA, GIANELLI F: Prenatal diagnosis of xeroderma pigmentosum. Report of the first successful case. *Lancet* 2:1109, 1974

195. PATERSON MC, ANDERSON AK, SMITH BP, SMITH PJ: Enhanced radiosensitivity of cultured fibroblasts from ataxia telangiectasia heterozygotes manifested by defective colony-forming ability and reduced DNA repair replication after hypoxic γ-irradiation. *Cancer Res* 39:3725, 1979

196. SCUDIERO DA: Decreased DNA repair synthesized defective colony forming ability of ataxia telangiectasia fibroblast cell strains treated with N-methyl-N′-nitro-N-nitrosoguanidine. *Cancer Res* 40:984, 1980

197. SMITH PJ, PATERSON MC: Defective DNA repair and increased lethality in ataxia telangiectasia cells exposed to 4-nitroguinoline-1-oxide. *Nature* 287:747, 1980

198. EDWARDS MJ, TAYLOR AMR: Unusual levels of (ADP-ribose)$_n$ and DNA synthesis in ataxia telangiectasia cells following γ-ray irradiation. *Nature* 287:745, 1980

199. SCHMICKEL RD, CHU EHY, TROSKO JE, CHANG CC: Cockayne syndrome: A cellular sensitivity to ultraviolet light. *Pediatrics* 60:135, 1977

200. WADE MH, CHU EHY: Effects of DNA damaging agents on cultured fibroblasts derived from patients with Cockayne syndrome. *Mutat Res* 59:49, 1979

201. CHANG WS, TARONE RE, ANDREWS AD, WHANG-PENG JS, ROBBINS JH: Ultraviolet light-induced sister chromatid exchanges in xeroderma pigmentosum and in Cockayne syndrome lymphocyte cell lines. *Cancer Res* 38:1601, 1978

202. AHMED FE, SETLOW RB: Excision repair in ataxia telangiectasia, Fanconi's anemia, Cockayne syndrome, and Bloom's syndrome after treatment with ultraviolet radiation and N-acetoxy-2-acetylaminofluorene. *Biochim Biophys Acta* 521:805, 1978

203. FUJIWARA Y, TATSUMI M, SASAKI MS: Cross-link repair in human cells and is possible defect in Fanconi's anemia cells. *J Mol Biol* 113:635, 1977

204. FORNACE AJ, LITTLE JB, WEICHSELBAUM, RR: DNA repair in a Fanconi's anemia fibroblast cell strain. *Biochim Biophys Acta* 561:99, 1979

205. KAYE J, SMITH CA, HANAWALT PC: DNA repair in human cells containing photoadducts of 8-methoxypsoralen or angelicin. *Cancer Res* 40:696, 1980

206. POON PK, O'BRIEN RL, PARKER JW: Defective DNA repair in Fanconi's anemia. *Nature (London)* 250:223, 1974

207. CHAGANTI RSK, SCHONBERG S, GERMAN J: A manyfold increase in sister chromatid exchanges in Bloom's syndrome lymphocytes. *Proc Nat Acad Sci* 71:4508, 1974

208. WARREN ST, SCHULTZ RA, CHANG CC, TROSKO JE: Elevated spontaneous mutation rate in Bloom's syndrome fibroblasts. Proceedings of the 31st Meeting of the American Society of Human Genetics, New York, 1980, p 161A

209. KREPINSKY AB, RAINBOW AJ, HEDDLE JA: Studies on the ultraviolet light sensitivity of Bloom's syndrome fibroblasts. *Mutat Res* 69:357, 1980

210. REMSEN JF: Repair of damage by N-acetoxy-2-acetylaminofluorene in Bloom's syndrome. *Mutat Res* 72:151, 1980

211. BURNET M: Cancer—A biological approach. I. The processes of control. *Brit Med J*, April 6, 779, 1957

212. AMES BN: The detection of chemical mutagens with enteric bacteria, in *Chemical Mutagens, Principles and Methods for Their Detection*. Plenum, New York, 1971, vol 1, p 267

213. CHANG CC, TROSKO JE, WARREN ST: *In vitro* assay for tumor promoters and antipromoters. *J Environ Pathol Toxicol* 2:43, 1978

214. ARLETT CF: Survival and mutation in gamma-irradiated human cell strains from normal or cancer-prone individuals, in Okada S, Imamura M, Terashima T, Yamaguchi H (eds): *Radiation Research*. Publ Japanese Association for Radiation Research, Japan, 1980, p 596

215. WEICHSELBAUM RR, NOVE J, LITTLE JB: X-ray sensitivity of fifty-three human diploid fibroblast cell strains from patients with characterized genetic disorders. *Cancer Res* 40:920, 1980

216. ARLETT CF, HARCOURT SA: Survey of radiosensitivity in a variety of cell strains. *Cancer Res* 40:926, 1980

217. TANAKA H, ORII T: High sensitivity but normal DNA-repair activity after UV irradiation in Epstein-Barr virus-transformed lymphoblastoid cell lines from Chediak-Higashi syndrome. *Mutat Res* 72:143, 1980

218. WEICHSELBAUM RR, NOVE J, LITTLE JB: X-ray sensitivity of diploid fibroblasts from patients with hereditary or sporadic retinoblastoma. *Proc Natl Acad Sci* 75:3962, 1978

219. LITTLE JB, NOVE J, WEICHSELBAUM RR: Abnormal sensitivity of diploid skin fibroblasts from a family with Gardner's syndrome to the lethal effects of X-irradiation, ultraviolet light and mitomycin-C. *Mutat Res* 70:241, 1980

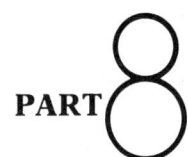

PART 8

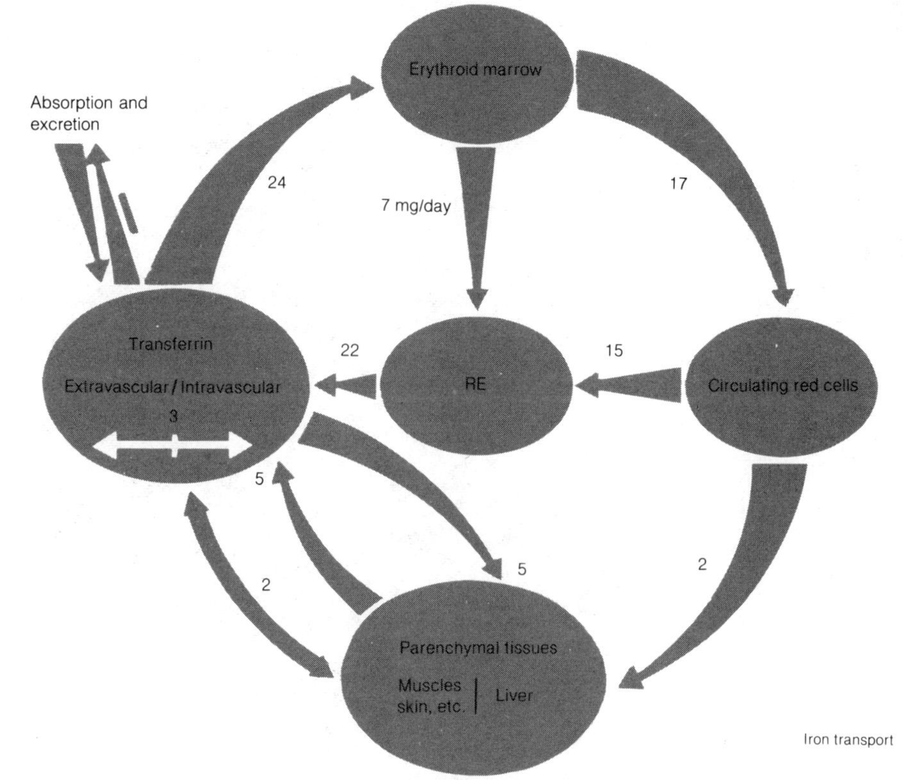

Erythroid marrow
Absorption and
excretion
24
7 mg/day
17
Transferrin
Extravascular / Intravascular
3
22
RE
15
Circulating red cells
5
5
2
2
Parenchymal tissues
Muscles
skin, etc.
Liver
Iron transport

DISORDERS OF METAL METABOLISM

58

HEREDITARY DISORDERS OF COPPER METABOLISM IN WILSON'S DISEASE AND MENKES' DISEASE

DAVID M. DANKS

1. *The importance of copper enzymes determines that copper is essential for human health. It is also a very toxic ion. Consequently a complex series of copper transport processes must exist to deliver copper to the sites of enzyme synthesis. The details of these processes are not known.*

2. *Copper homeostasis depends on a balance between intestinal copper absorption and biliary excretion of copper in an unabsorbable form. Separate processes may be involved in the liver for storage and biliary excretion of copper and for production of the copper binding protein, ceruloplasmin. It is not certain whether ceruloplasmin has a function in copper transport or whether it is merely a copper enzyme present in serum serving ferroxidase, and other, functions.*

3. *In Wilson's disease biliary excretion of copper and incorporation into ceruloplasmin are both severely impaired. The basic lesion underlying these two disturbances is not yet known. Defective biliary excretion leads to accumulation of copper in the liver with progressive liver damage and subsequent overflow to the brain causing involuntary movements and loss of coordination. Deposition in the cornea produces Kayser-Fleischer rings, and accumulation in other sites may cause renal tubular damage, osteoporosis, and arthropathy.*

4. *Symptoms of liver disease may occur in children over*

8 *years or in young adults, but acute onset is surprisingly frequent, and hemolysis is often pronounced. Neurologic effects are more frequent in adults up to middle age. It is important to remember this treatable disease in all patients with chronic liver disease and in all adults with neurologic symptoms referable to the basal ganglia.*

5. *The classic diagnostic features of Kayser-Fleischer rings, low plasma ceruloplasmin concentration, increased plasma nonceruloplasmin copper, and increased urinary copper excretion are found in all patients with neurologic manifestations, but in only 70 to 90 percent of those with clinical liver involvement. Increased liver copper concentration (>300 μg per gram dry weight) is a reliable finding, and lack of incorporation of ^{64}Cu or ^{67}Cu into ceruloplasmin over 48 h is the most definitive test available.*

6. *Inheritance is autosomal recessive. The prevalence is of the order of 1 in 100,000 live births. Sibs must be carefully investigated. Heterozygote detection by isotope studies is only 80 to 90 percent reliable.*

7. *Treatment with penicillamine is effective. Long-term results are excellent, but the 3- to 6-month lag before improvement occurs may be too long in patients with acute liver failure. Side effects are less frequent than generally thought, and dangers in the use of penicillamine in pregnancy do not appear great.*

8. *In Menkes' disease defective intestinal absorption*

leads to copper deficiency. The same defect which prevents copper absorption and causes copper to accumulate in mucosal cells is present in most other body cells, including cultured fibroblasts. Thus, copper given parenterally does not fully correct the deficient synthesis of copper enzymes. The molecular defect producing these effects is not yet identified.

9. *Defective synthesis of copper enzymes explains many features of the disease. These include abnormal and depigmented (steely) hair, a characteristic facies, hypothermia, arterial degeneration due to defective elastin synthesis, neuronal degeneration especially in the cerebellum, osteoporosis, and metaphyseal fractures. Death usually occurs before 2 years. Treatment has not yet been found to alter the course of the disease significantly.*

10. *Inheritance is X-chromosomal. Mottled mutants of a strain of mice appear to be homologous. Their study is contributing greatly to progress in understanding the disease. Prenatal diagnosis is well established in a few laboratories, using the altered copper metabolism observed in cultured cells. Heterozygote detection is made difficult by mosaic X-chromosome inactivation but can usually be achieved by taking multiple skin biopsies or by cloning cells.*

11. *Further genetic defects of copper metabolism may be expected and may be sought among patients with liver diseases, those with defects of connective tissue or keratin formation, and in neurologic diseases. Several forms of liver disease show severe copper accumulation (primary biliary cirrhosis and Indian childhood cirrhosis). This may be primary or secondary.*

NORMAL COPPER METABOLISM AND HOMEOSTASIS

Two genetic defects of copper transport have been known for 40 and 10 years, respectively. It is frustrating that neither can yet be described in precise molecular terms. One of these, Wilson's disease, shows autosomal recessive inheritance and appears to involve a defect in hepatic copper metabolism. The other, Menkes' disease, is X-linked in inheritance. Its basic defect is more widespread in the body, affecting cellular transport of copper. Since normal copper metabolism undoubtedly involves more than two active processes, further genetic defects of copper metabolism may be anticipated. Some forms of liver diseases showing marked copper retention may be candidates.

Certain aspects of normal copper metabolism are reviewed as a background to discussion of these diseases. Much original work dealt with in major reviews of copper metabolism [1–5] is not referred to directly in this chapter. The same approach is adopted with the two diseases, especially with Wilson's disease which has been reviewed frequently and exhaustively.

Copper is an essential micronutrient for humans and animals. It is an integral component of a number of important enzymes [1] (Table 58-1). Copper has been described in other enzymes,

Table 58-1 Copper enzymes in human beings

Common name	Functional role	Known or expected consequence of deficiency
Cytochrome oxidase	Electron transport chain	Uncertain
Superoxide dismutase	Free radical detoxification	Uncertain
Tyrosinase	Melanin production	Failure of pigmentation
Dopamine β-hydroxylase	Catecholamine production	Neurologic effects, type uncertain
Lysyl oxidase	Cross-linking of collagen and elastin	Vascular rupture
Ceruloplasmin	Ferroxidase;? other roles	Anemia
Enzyme not known	Cross-linking of keratin (disulphide bonds)	Pili torti

but further evidence is required before accepting them as true copper enzymes. Copper is also a very toxic ion. Consequently efficient methods must exist for transporting copper to the sites where it is required without allowing toxic accumulation of the free ions. Harmful effects of both deficiency and excess are well documented in humans and in animals [1–3, 5].

Copper Homeostasis

The normal adult human body contains 70 to 100 mg of copper. Homeostasis depends upon a balance between intestinal absorption and biliary excretion, other means of intake and loss being insignificant (Table 58-2). Absorption and excretion are normally in the range of 1 to 5 mg daily. Copper can be absorbed through the skin if applied in solution, and small amounts are even absorbed from metallic copper during prolonged contact with the skin and from copper-containing intrauterine contraceptive devices. Little copper is excreted in the urine. Some is lost in the sweat.

Intestinal Absorption [6]   Direct evidence regarding the site and mechanism of absorption is lacking in humans. Absorption from the upper small intestine has been demonstrated in chickens and in rats. Both species show two processes, a rapid transport system of low capacity which is inhibited by anoxia or by dinitrophenol, and a slower process which is less readily inhibited and has a greater capacity. In the rat and mouse the absorptive process of neonatal animals differs from that observed in adult animals, probably because of the transient existence of pinocytosis—this is probably peculiar to rodents, but human neonates have not been studied. The malabsorption of copper in babies with Menkes' disease indicates that absorption is an active process in humans. The similarity of the disturbance of absorption in Menkes' disease and in mottled mice suggests similarity in the normal processes of humans and mice.

The role of metallothionein in the intestinal absorption of copper is not clear [6]. In rats, zinc diminishes copper absorption by inducing increased production of metallothionein in mucosal cells, which then bind copper preferentially [7]. Most of the bound copper is lost when cells are shed from the villi. Since excessive zinc administration has been shown to induce copper deficiency in humans [8], similar absorptive mechanisms may operate. Evidence that metallothionein changes with the copper content of the diet is not impressive [6].

The overall rate of absorption of copper has been observed in many humans to whom ^{64}Cu or ^{67}Cu has been administered. Absorption of 40 to 70 percent of an oral dose was found by three different methods in four normal subjects [9]. Others have reported similar results. Copper isotopes become detectable in the blood quickly after oral administration. The peak level of radioactivity occurs by 90 to 150 min. This suggests a site of absorption high in the intestine.

Copper in the Plasma   Most of the copper absorbed from the intestine is found to be attached to albumin in the early hours after administration. A small amount is attached to amino acids or small peptides. Copper given as ^{64}Cu or ^{67}Cu is cleared from the plasma rapidly, reaching 10 percent of the initial level after intravenous administration in 20 to 25 min [10, 11]. External counting shows preferential uptake by the liver [9], but some uptake by all tissues. Difficulty in allowing for the blood present in each tissue complicates these assessments.

Albumin binds copper at a specific amino-terminal tripeptide site (Asp-Ala-His in humans), with the histidine residue having special significance [12]. Bovine, rat, and human albumins differ in residues 1 and 2, yet they bind copper well. Dog albumin has tyrosine at position 3 and binds copper poorly. The susceptibility of dogs to copper poisoning has been attributed to this, but pig albumin has a similar deficiency in copper binding. However, pigs are tolerant of copper excess. No comments have been made on the status of copper metabolism in the various reports of human analbuminemia. More copper can be dialyzed from dog plasma than from that of other species. This suggests that amino acids take over the copper transport role in this species. Prealbumin has six additional amino acids on its amino-terminal end [12] and does not bind copper. This may prevent copper from leaving the liver as albumin is exported.

The mechanism of uptake of copper by the liver is not well defined. An intermediary role for a copper histidine combination with transient formation of albumin-copper-histidine complexes has been suggested.

Over 90 percent of the copper in human plasma is present in ceruloplasmin, a blue α_2-globulin glycoprotein whose function is still poorly defined, even after 30 years of intense interest [13]. Radioactive copper starts to appear in ceruloplasmin within a few hours of intravenous administration and rises in a linear fashion over at least 7 days, reaching 5 to 6 percent of the dose administered by that time [11]. Computer analysis suggests a rapid phase and a slower phase involving hepatic storage. Both processes are defective in Wilson's disease, whereas only the rapid phase is reduced in primary biliary cirrhosis [11].

Ceruloplasmin, and therefore serum copper, levels are increased by a variety of factors, including pregnancy, oral contraceptives, and diseases which cause "acute-phase" reactions (Table 58-3). Genetic factors also influence the levels seen in different normal individuals [14], and a dominantly inherited symptomless condition of hypoceruloplasminemia has been described [15]. For all these reasons a single measurement of serum copper concentration is not a good indicator of copper nutrition [16]. Nevertheless, severe copper deficiency leads to a reduction in serum copper, and two measurements separated by a few days during which copper replacement therapy is given may be useful in diagnosing copper deficiency of less severe degree [17].

The noceruloplasmin component of serum copper is not easily measured but can be estimated by calculation and appears to vary little in healthy persons or in most diseases. This component is increased in Wilson's disease, but not in Menkes' disease or in copper deficiency, and persists even when no ceruloplasmin can be detected. A massive increase is seen in acute copper poisoning and in acute hemolytic crises in Wilson's disease.

It is generally assumed that copper in the liver is a store available to other tissues in circumstances of copper deficiency. This role has been claimed particularly in sheep and in young babies who are born with very high liver copper levels and can survive long periods on artificial milk feeding with very low copper content without developing features of copper deficiency [18]. The method by which copper is transferred from the liver to other tissues is not known. Some have assumed that ceruloplasmin plays a role in transport just because there is so much present [13]. Opinions remain sharply divided [5]. The little concrete evidence that does exist suggests a preferential role of ceruloplasmin in delivery of copper to cytochrome C oxidase [19]. Studies of the exchange of copper with ceruloplasmin suggest that the protein may need to be degraded in order to release copper. Albumin is another candidate for this transport role.

The Role of the Liver   The liver plays a central role in copper homeostasis, being the principal recipient of recently absorbed copper, the organ with the highest (and most variable) copper content and the principal organ of excretion. Some major species differences are apparent, especially between sheep and other species.

Kinetic analyses using computer curve fitting models have been used in rats [20], in sheep [18], and in humans [11, 21, 22]. In the rat the simplest model involves three interconnected functional compartments in the liver related to storage, biliary excretion, and ceruloplasmin production [20]. Some have argued that the disturbance of both ceruloplasmin production and biliary excretion in Wilson's disease implies a common mode of access to these two compartments. It is interesting that these same two processes are greatly reduced in efficiency in the sheep, in which a simpler model suffices to explain the findings [18].

In rats, and probably in humans, biliary excretion varies in response to liver copper load [3, 5] and therefore indirectly in response to copper intake. This tends to prevent chronic copper accumulation. In sheep, biliary excretion is much less responsive to intake and is hardly affected by liver copper lev-

Table 58-2   Copper homeostasis in humans—normal and abnormal. Approximate figures based on assumed normal dietary copper intake of 4 mg daily.

	Normal	Wilson's disease	Menkes' disease
Intestinal absorption	2 mg	2 mg	0.1–0.2 mg
Biliary excretion	2 mg	0.2–0.4 mg	Not known
Urinary excretion	0.04 mg	1 mg	Increased
Net balance	Zero	Positive	Negative

Table 58-3   Change in ceruloplasmin levels (mg/liter) with age and status—range of levels

Cord blood	20–130
6 months	200–400
2 years	300–500
Adult males	200–400
Adult females	200–400
Effect of	
Acute infection	+ 50%
Oral contraceptive	+ 100%
Pregnancy (3d trimester)	+ 100%

els. This allows accumulation of high levels if intake is excessive [18]. This permits sheep to cope with "feast and famine" circumstances of copper supply, but leaves them susceptible to copper poisoning when pasture deficiencies are replaced too enthusiastically. Symptomless accumulation of copper may occur for long periods followed by abrupt hemolytic crises, a sequence similar to that seen in Wilson's disease [1, 23]. Humans and rats are both quite resistant to chronic copper toxicity [1].

Most of the copper found in bile is in a form (or forms) which cannot be reabsorbed. There is no effective enterohepatic circulation of copper [5]. No consensus has yet been reached concerning the molecular form (forms) or copper complexes in bile. A small amount of copper which enters the bile rapidly after oral administration may be reabsorbed. Reabsorption also occurs by pinocytosis in young rodents and has been suggested in young babies on very low copper intakes [5].

The form in which copper is stored in the liver has also been investigated extensively but without complete resolution [5]. Much of the copper occurs in the supernatant fraction attached to metallothionein. Copper bound to a polymerized form of metallothionein is found attached to heavy lysosomes. In differential centrifugation experiments these particles were initially confused with mitochondria, which led to terms like mitochondriocuprein. It seems unlikely that the bonding of copper to metallothionein is reversible. Release might involve degradation of the protein, which has a half-life of only 17 h [6].

Other Tissues   The role of the kidney in copper homeostasis is usually discussed with a brief statement about the small amount of copper excreted in the urine. However, it seems likely that copper bound to amino acids is filtered through the glomerulus and reabsorbed in the tubules along with these amino acids. Intravenous loading with histidine leads to a considerable increase in urinary copper excretion in humans (and to massive excretion of zinc) [24]. In Menkes' disease and mottled mice renal copper levels are much increased, and urinary losses are high considering the low levels of copper in the serum.

Most other tissues act merely as recipients of the copper required to form their copper enzymes. Several of these are ubiquitous (Table 58-1).

The distribution of copper in the normal brain corresponds approximately to the distribution of catecholamine neurons, as might be expected considering that dopamine β-hydroxylase is a copper enzyme. Presumably all parts of the brain contain copper in cytochrome C oxidase and superoxide dismutase.

The Copper Enzymes   The copper enzymes listed in Table 58-1 all require incorporation of copper during their synthesis. Copper is required for apoenzyme synthesis, but excess copper does not superinduce enzyme production [17]. The detailed mechanisms by which copper is made available to the sites of enzyme synthesis are unknown, but they appear to differ from one enzyme to another, and from one tissue to another, at least in the rat. For example, copper deficiency reduces superoxide dismutase levels more than cytochrome C oxidase in liver, but the reverse pattern occurs in heart and muscle [25].

CERULOPLASMIN   This is the best known but least understood copper protein. Indeed only recently has there been conclusive evidence that this 132,000-molecular-weight glycoprotein has just one polypeptide chain [13]. Previous claims of multiple subunits have been resolved by showing several sites which are very susceptible to proteolytic cleavage. The protein contains six atoms of copper per molecule. It can oxidize Fe(II) to Fe(III), thereby allowing release of iron from ferritin and attachment to transferrin. However, patients with Wilson's disease or Menkes' disease who have no detectable ceruloplasmin do not often develop anemia [26, 28]. Ceruloplasmin can oxidize a number of biogenic amines in vitro but is not proved to play this role in vivo. It also inhibits lipid peroxidation. It responds as an acute phase reactant, but no function in inflammation has been found. Its role in copper transport is debated [5]. The fact that failure of other copper enzymes is not seen in patients with Wilson's disease indicates that any role in copper transport is not indispensable.

The other copper enzymes listed in Table 58-1 are less reduced in copper deficiency, but effects due to their inadequate function make up the syndrome of copper deficiency [28].

METALLOTHIONEIN   This is the other major enigma among the copper proteins [3, 6, 29]. The principal doubts relate to whether one, two, or many metallothioneins exist. This small protein(s) is very difficult to handle because the numerous cysteine residues are easily oxidized during extraction and purification, especially when copper is attached to the protein. Biochemists who have worked extensively on this subject recently drew up a list of facts which they regarded as established, including amino acid sequences of human MT-1 and MT-2 and the MT's of several other species. The proceedings of this symposium [29] include many papers on the properties of these curious metal binding proteins. They are further discussed by Bremner [6].

It seems probable that metallothioneins are important in binding excess metal ions in most cells of the body and that they exercise some control over intestinal and renal absorption. Intestinal metallothionein is sensitive to induction by certain metals (especially zinc and cadmium) but not very sensitive to induction by copper [6]. The metallothioneins probably play important roles in metal excretion and storage, but a role in transport is not yet defined.

Copper Deficiency

The effects of nutritional copper deficiency have been reviewed recently [28, 30] and are mostly what might be predicted from the known functions of copper enzymes (Tables 58-1 and 58-4). Interesting differences in the effects are seen in different species. For instance, sheep are very resistant to the vascular effects but sensitive to neurologic consequences, whereas vascular lesions predominate in pigs and poultry. Anemia, neutropenia, and osteoporosis have been the main features observed in human nutritional copper deficiency, but in Menkes' disease damage to brain and arteries is most pronounced, with no anemia or neutropenia. The former may just reflect severe and prolonged deficiency, but the absence of hematologic effects is difficult to explain.

Human copper deficiency has been described as part of a general nutritional deficiency in Peruvian children; in young babies; in adults receiving parenteral alimentation with copper-deficient solutions, especially when these are used after extensive gut resection; and in adults treated with large doses of zinc for defective wound healing or for sickle cell disease [8]. Chronic low-grade deficiency may become a problem in western countries because removal of copper is important in achieving long shelf life for prepared foods [28].

Copper Poisoning

Acute copper poisoning is seen frequently in India where it is a popular method of suicide [2]. Accidental poisoning is occasionally seen in young children in western cities [31]. Acute irritation and damage to the intestine cause vomiting and diarrhea with bleeding. Circulatory collapse may occur early. Over the next 2 or 3 days acute liver failure, acute renal failure, and severe hemolysis may occur. Nonceruloplasmin copper levels are greatly increased. Chronic copper poisoning is very rare in patients without preexisting liver disease but has been described in some industrial situations [2]. The normal human liver has a great excretory capacity. Moderately excessive intake may be important in patients with chronic liver disease. Recirculating copper-lined water systems may produce water with a remarkably high copper content if the water is soft.

Table 58-4 Effects seen in nutritional copper deficiency in human beings, sheep, rats, pigs, and in Menkes' disease

Effect	Human beings	Sheep	Rats	Pigs	Menkes' disease
Anemia	+	+	+	+	−
Neutropenia	+	+	+	+	−
Abnormal hair structure	±	++	+	+	++
Depigmentation	±	+	+	+	+
Arterial rupture	?	−	+	++	++
Myocardial fibrosis	?	−	+	+	−
Osteoporosis	+	+	+	++	+
Emphysema	?	−	+	−	+
Cerebellar ataxia	−	+*	+*	+*	+
Other brain damage	−	+*	+*	+	++

* Seen only after fetal copper deficiency.

Animal Models (Tables 58-5 and 58-6)

Discovery and study of animals with defects identical to those in human genetic diseases allow studies which are impossible in patients. Mottled mice appear to have a mutation homologous to that in Menkes' disease [32, 33]. Conservation of the genetic content of the mammalian X chromosome throughout evolution makes homology of the mutations very probable. Many Bedlington terriers have a hepatic copper storage disease which may prove to be similar to Wilson's disease [20, 34]. Normal sheep have some characteristics in common with Wilson's disease (see above).

Discovery of further animal mutants affecting copper transport would be a powerful method of identifying the various components of the normal copper transport process. Crinkled mice show reduced pigmentation, sparse fur, and a high mortality in the first week or two after birth. They have been claimed to suffer from a copper deficiency disorder [35], but others have refuted this claim [5]. Copper supplements have been claimed to ameliorate the quaking [35], in a myelin-deficient mutant mouse, but this has not yet been confirmed by other groups.

WILSON'S DISEASE (HEPATOLENTICULAR DEGENERATION)

Readers are referred to the fourth edition of this text [4] for reference to early publications. Only those critical to statements made here are cited, and even then only one or two most recent papers are given.

Described as a clinical entity by Kinnear-Wilson in 1912, this rare autosomal recessively inherited disease was related to copper accumulation in liver and brain in the 1940s. It is frustrating to realize how little progress has been made in understanding the defect in copper transport in over 30 years. Despite ignorance about the basic defect, effective treatment has been available since 1956, when Walshe introduced penicillamine.

Basic Defect and Pathogenesis

Although the basic defect in Wilson's disease is still not known, a certain amount is understood about the pathogenesis, enough to give some logical basis to diagnosis and treatment. But first a statement made in many genetics and medical texts must be refuted: Wilson's disease is *not* caused by a molecular defect in ceruloplasmin. A number of workers have studied the ceruloplasmin present in patients with Wilson's disease without showing any structural abnormality. A small number of patients have quite normal levels of ceruloplasmin. Heterozygotes do not show the consistent reduction in ceruloplasmin which would be expected if this were the primary defect.

The two fundamental disturbances of copper metabolism in Wilson's disease are (1) a gross reduction in the rate of incorporation of copper into ceruloplasmin, and (2) a considerable reduction in biliary excretion of copper. The models of hepatic copper metabolism in the rat propose separate functional pools of copper for ceruloplasmin production and for biliary excretion [20]. Interference with both processes by a single mutation suggests the existence of some preceding common pathway of entry to both these pools.

Decreased biliary excretion has been demonstrated by several workers [21, 36]. Indirect methods gave figures between 20 and 40 percent of normal [21]. Direct measurement in two patients showed an even greater reduction [36]. Since intestinal absorption is normal in Wilson's disease, the consequence is a substantial positive net copper balance (Table 58-2). Increased renal losses do little to redress this situation.

The immediate effect is accumulation of copper in the liver, a progressive process which may continue for many years with only minor effects upon the liver cells in some patients. In others the accumulation of copper leads to severe liver damage, which may cause death from liver failure by the age of 8 to 10 years. The level of nonceruloplasmin copper rises in the plasma, leading to increased renal excretion of copper and to deposition of copper in various extrahepatic tissues—cornea (Kayser-Fleischer rings), brain, especially basal ganglia (lenticular degeneration), kidney (renal tubular damage), muscles, bones, and joints. This seems the most probable sequence of events, but it has not been proved. Deposition in all tissues from the beginning is also possible, though less likely. Kayser-Fleischer rings are frequently absent in asymptomatic homozygotes, sometimes lacking in childhood cases with hepatic symptoms, but almost always found in adults with brain symptoms. Development of corneal deposits during a period of observation of an asymptomatic sib aged 32 has been described [37]. These facts and the rarity of neurologic presentation before 10 to 12 years are all in keeping with the sequence of events suggested. Development of neurologic symptoms due to lenticular copper deposition in a 5-year-old girl who accumulated massive amounts of copper secondary to the recessively inherited cholestatic syndrome of Åagenes also provides further circumstantial support for the idea of overflow from the liver [38], as does the development of Kayser-Fleischer rings in patients with copper overload in other types of liver disease [39, 40].

Much effort has gone into study of the distribution and form of copper within liver cells in Wilson's disease and in other situations involving hepatic copper accumulation in order to understand the mechanism of liver cell damage [5, 41–45]. Young patients with Wilson's disease tend to show copper spread diffusely in the cytoplasm, whereas the increased copper in the liver of normal neonates and in primary biliary cirrhosis tends to be in lysosomes. Chemically, cytoplasmic copper tends to be attached to monomeric metallothionein and lysosomal copper to polymeric complexes of metallothionein. In older patients with Wilson's disease and well compensated liver disease, the copper is mainly lysosomal.

Why should liver damage develop rapidly in some patients and not in others? Allelic differences in the mutant gene might be responsible. While there is a tendency toward similar presenting features in sibs, there are many reports of childhood hepatic symptoms in one sib and an adult neurologic presentation in another. Variability within a large inbred Japanese kindred also shows that allelic heterogeneity is not the whole explanation [46] (see "Genetics" section). Variation in dietary copper intake may be important. The ages of onset of both hepatic and neurologic findings are earlier in Japanese reports than in western countries [46]. Perhaps high intake from copper from cooking vessels is important, but this is not true in

Taiwan [47]. Finally, intercurrent hepatic viral infections may be important. The number of patients presenting with acute onset of hepatic symptoms or with multiple acute episodes is too high to ignore. In an unpublished study of 52 cases of childhood cirrhosis in London in 1961 the author found only 3 children with an impressive history suggesting posthepatitic cirrhosis—all 3 had Wilson's disease. In childhood liver disease one commonly finds multiple causative factors in those patients who develop cirrhosis. A number of viruses are probably capable of damaging a liver already suffering from chemical injury.

The disturbance of ceruloplasmin production in Wilson's disease has been studied by many groups, but little has been added to the original observations of the early 1950s. Use of ^{67}Cu has allowed measurements to continue for as long as 7 days, and even at this stage no definite incorporation of labeled isotope (administered intravenously) into ceruloplasmin could be detected [11]. Others have observed low levels of incorporation [22]. It is hard to interpret these findings in view of the existence of affected homozygotes who have low normal levels of ceruloplasmin. None of these particular patients appears to have been studied with ^{67}Cu. Some authors have blamed dilution of isotope in a large intrahepatic pool, but hepatic storage of a similar degree in primary biliary cirrhosis and other liver diseases causes only a mild reduction (or no change) in isotope incorporation. It seems that the ceruloplasmin present in these cases of Wilson's disease must be drawing copper from a pool into which the administered isotope is not entering [11, 22].

Many theories have been proposed to explain cell damage in copper accumulation [42, 45], including oxidation of lipids in membranes, binding to proteins and to nucleic acids, free radical generation, and many others. Certainly cell necrosis seems to be the final result in each of the affected organs.

The hemolytic crises seen in some patients are accompanied by very high levels of nonceruloplasmin copper comparable to those seen in acute copper poisoning. Indeed, the symptoms of hemolysis, acute tubular damage, and acute hepatic necrosis are similar. Sudden massive release of copper from the liver seems likely. In some cases this is caused by infarction of a large regenerative nodule in a cirrhotic liver. Acute viral infection with widespread liver cell damage and release of copper may be involved in other patients. Similarly in sheep acute hemolytic crises occur in chronic copper overdosage after large amounts of copper have accumulated in the liver [1, 23].

The most important and most surprising result of research in recent years is the observation of increased levels of copper in cultured fibroblasts from patients with Wilson's disease—an observation made independently in three different laboratories, each experienced with copper studies in cell culture through work on Menkes' disease [48–50]. This result is surprising because the defect in copper transport seemed likely to be confined to the liver with its specialized mechanism for copper excretion and therefore not likely to be manifested in cultured fibroblasts. This is important because the basic defect should now be more accessible to study.

Another important new finding is the defect in hepatic copper metabolism which occurs as a common autosomal recessive trait in Bedlington terriers [20, 34] (Table 58-5). There are obvious differences from Wilson's disease in the lack of involvement of organs other than the liver and in the course of the liver disease, which resembles more closely the events seen in sheep given excessive amounts of copper. Nonetheless study

Table 58-5 Comparison of Wilson's disease with copper storage in Bedlington terriers and in sheep

	Wilson's disease	Bedlington terriers	Normal sheep	Copper-loaded sheep
Hepatic copper accumulation (μg/g dry weight)	++ (200–3000)	+++ (2000–12000)	+ (300–600)	+++ (2000–8000)
Reduced biliary excretion of copper	++	+	+	+
Reduced ^{67}Cu incorporation into ceruloplasmin	+++	++	+	+
Liability to hemolytic crisis	+	++	–	++
Chronic liver cell damage	++	+/–	–	+/–
Overflow to other tissues	++	+/–	–	+/–

of these dogs may throw new light on Wilson's disease. It is surprising how little use has been made of sheep as a model of Wilson's disease.

Clinical Features

Patients with Wilson's disease most often appear with liver disease or with neurologic symptoms. A substantial number have symptoms of both types. Series from general hospitals show about equal numbers in each of these three categories [46, 47, 51–53]. Children with Wilson's disease may die with acute liver failure without a correct diagnosis in centers not keenly interested in the disease [54–57]. The large classical published series almost certainly underestimate the frequency with which liver disease is the presenting problem. These patients quite often lack some of the classic signs and laboratory findings [56], and some are slow to accept them as true cases of Wilson's disease.

Other presenting symptoms include acute hemolytic crises, joint symptoms, renal stones, and renal tubular acidosis. Wilson's disease is *not* a cause of mental retardation, despite its presence in lists of biochemical causes of retardation in some texts and reviews.

Although liver disease may cause symptoms at any age beyond about 6 years, this form of presentation is most frequent between 8 and 16 years. Females are a little more likely to present in this way; males more often appear first with neurologic features [51]. Neurologic symptoms are unusual before the age of 12 years, if one excludes hepatic coma.

Almost any symptom of liver disease may occur. Jaundice, vomiting, and malaise are frequent. Acute episodes may recur. All young patients with chronic or recurrent liver disease should be investigated for Wilson's disease (see below). Acute hemolysis occurs frequently in acute hepatic episodes and may appear without obvious features of liver disease [58]. Investigation reveals the underlying liver abnormalities.

Dysarthria and deterioration of coordination of voluntary movements are the most frequent neurologic symptoms. These are often accompanied by involuntary movements and by disorders of posture and tone. Pseudobulbar palsy may develop early in the illness in some patients and is the mode of death in many untreated cases. Deterioration in intellectual function

and disturbances of behavior are infrequent in the early stages, but usual later. It is unwise either to make or to dismiss the diagnosis on clinical signs alone. All patients in whom any of the neurologic features develop between the ages of 8 and 60 years should be investigated for Wilson's disease.

Evidence of bone and joint disorders can be found in many patients with Wilson's disease. These were found in 24 of 32 patients in one series [53, 59, 60]. The most frequent findings are osteoporosis, osteomalacia, reduction in the joint spaces of limbs and spine, osteophytes around large joints, and ligamentous laxity. Most of these changes are asymptomatic. Back or joint pain or stiffness occurs in less than 20 percent of older patients. Penicillamine therapy seems not to prevent (or to cause) these effects. Acute arthritis may occur as a complication of penicillamine therapy [59].

Renal stones have been described in 7 of 45 patients with Wilson's disease [61] and were present at the time of diagnosis in 4. Inadequate acidification of urine because of renal tubular malfunction has been blamed, along with hypercalciuria. Most patients with Wilson's disease show some elements of tubular malfunction, and some have the full picture of the Fanconi syndrome, including aminoaciduria, glycosuria, alkaline urine, and rickets. Poor growth and acidosis due to the renal lesion may be the presenting features.

The Kayser-Fleischer ring is the most important sign of Wilson's disease. It is a yellow-brown (dull copper colored) granular deposit on Descemet's membrane at the limbus of the cornea, usually seen earliest and most densely at the upper and lower poles [37]. When fully developed the rings are easily seen with the naked eye or ophthalmoscope, but at early stages a slit-lamp is required, especially when the irides are green-brown. The rings are present in 100 percent of patients with neurologic presentation and about 95 percent of all patients. Our experience in a pediatric hospital shows that absence of Kayser-Fleischer rings is considerably more frequent (over 30 percent) among children presenting with relatively acute liver disease. Certainly absence of the rings does not exclude Wilson's disease as a cause of hepatic symptoms. The rings are often (usually) absent in asymptomatically affected sibs of clinical cases [37]. Sunflower cataracts occur in a smaller proportion of cases (15 to 20 percent) [37]. Both these ocular signs improve with effective penicillamine chelation.

Table 58-6 Comparison of Menkes' disease with mouse mutants suggested as models

	Menkes' disease	Brindled (Mo^br/y) mice	Blotchy (Mo^blo/y) mice	Crinkled (cr/cr) mice
Inheritance	XL	XL	XL	AR
Hair deformity	+ +	+	+	−
Hair follicle reduction	−	−	−	+
Hair keratin disulphide deficiency	+	+	+	−
Arterial elastin abnormality	+ +	+/−	+	−
Lysyl oxidase deficiency (skin)	+	+	+	−
Life expectancy	1–2 years	13–15 days	6–18 months	70% die by 20 days
Liver copper reduced	+	+	+	Debated [35]
Kidney and intestinal copper increased	+	+	+	−

Kayser-Fleischer rings have been described in a small number of patients with massive hepatic copper accumulation in primary biliary cirrhosis [39, 40] and other liver diseases [40, 62].

Laboratory Findings

Typically serum ceruloplasmin is greatly reduced and the nonceruloplasmin copper is increased, giving a net reduction in serum copper. Urinary copper excretion is increased, and this increase is greatly augmented by penicillamine administration. Liver copper is greatly increased. Typical figures are quoted in Table 58-7.

Each of these test results may give misleading information. First of all, it is essential to be certain that the serum copper and ceruloplasmin results are compatible with one another. Multiplying the ceruloplasmin result in milligrams per liter by 3.0 gives its contribution to serum copper in micrograms per liter (division by 63.6 gives micromoles per liter). In normal subjects this figure is 90 to 95 percent of total serum copper. If it is double the serum copper reported, then the laboratory has made an error in one or another measurement. In Wilson's disease nonceruloplasmin copper may be as high as 200 to 300 μg/liter (3 to 5 μmol/liter). Higher levels are seen only in episodes of acute liver failure or acute hemolysis (also in acute copper poisoning). Copper-contaminated tubes or bottles may be responsible for overestimation of serum or urine copper.

Apart from these technical problems the ceruloplasmin concentration may fall in acute liver failure in patients who do not have Wilson's disease or rise to normal at such times in patients who do [63]. Considerable numbers of cases with normal ceruloplasmin levels have been reported, especially in younger patients with liver disease.

Urine copper is very variable in normal persons. Some authors have suggested measuring urine excretion after penicillamine. Various regimens of dosage and collection periods have been used, but none has been standardized enough to be reliable.

Liver biopsy with assay of copper content by graphite furnace atomic absorption spectrometry (or neutron activation) is by far the most reliable test [57]. The technique of collection of the biopsy and of assay must be meticulous in order to avoid contamination. Uneven distribution of copper in the liver may give spurious results in either direction if too small a sample is assayed. Samples above 5 mg (5 to 10 mm of needle biopsy core) should give reliable results, provided the tissue is parenchymal and not just fibrous tissue from a cirrhotic liver. Histochemical assessment is not reliable [43, 45].

The ultimate test for Wilson's disease is demonstration of negligible incorporation of radioactive copper into ceruloplasmin [64]. Indeed this is the best current method of defining the disease. This is usually studied by simply counting total plasma radioactivity for 48 h after giving the radiocopper. Intravenous administration is recommended in order to avoid the compounding influence of variable rates of absorption. ^{67}Cu would be ideal for this test but is not yet generally available. A dose of 500 μCi of ^{64}Cu is required in an adult. Blood should be drawn at 5 to 10 min, 1h, 2h, 4h, 24 h, and 48 h. The first 4 samples should be counted soon after the 4-h sample is taken and the other 2 samples soon after taking. This is because the 12-h half-life of ^{64}Cu can cause very low count rates in the 4-, 24-, and 48-h samples if they are held for counting when all samples have been taken (Fig. 58-1). Normal subjects show a steady secondary rise in corrected counts in the plasma from 4 h through to 48 h as the ^{64}Cu appears in newly synthesized ceruloplasmin. In Wilson's disease corrected counts fall progressively and the 48-h level is less than half the 4-h result. Intermediate results (i.e., smaller secondary rise) are seen in some heterozygotes and in patients with copper retention in other forms of liver disease.

Other tests show the effects of damage to various organs. Liver function test abnormalities have no specific pattern. Aminoaciduria, glycosuria, and defective urinary acidification occur in many diseases affecting renal tubules. Anemia (normochromic) is not frequent, except when there is hemolysis, but thrombocytopenia (50 percent of cases) and neutropenia (30 percent of cases) are more frequent [26].

Some have claimed that marked glycogen accumulation in hepatocyte nuclei is a specific histologic feature, but most now agree that the hepatic changes are variable and nondiagnostic [42, 65]. Indeed the liver changes can mimic other diseases usually diagnosed with some confidence by experienced liver pathologists, e.g., chronic active hepatitis [66]. Much has been written about histochemical identification of copper in liver sections [42, 43]. The differences in staining of copper attached to different ligands are interesting. These methods show nicely the uneven distribution of copper in Wilson's disease. No

Table 58-7 Typical copper measurements in Wilson's disease.

	Wilson's disease	Normal (adults)
Serum ceruloplasmin		
OD units/ml	0–0.25	0.25–0.49
mg/liter	0–200	200–400
Serum copper (μmol/liter)	3–10	11–24
Urinary copper (μg/24 h)		
Untreated	100–1000	<40
On penicillamine,		
250 mg every 6 h	1500–3000	100–600
Liver copper (μg/g dry weight)	200–3000	20–50

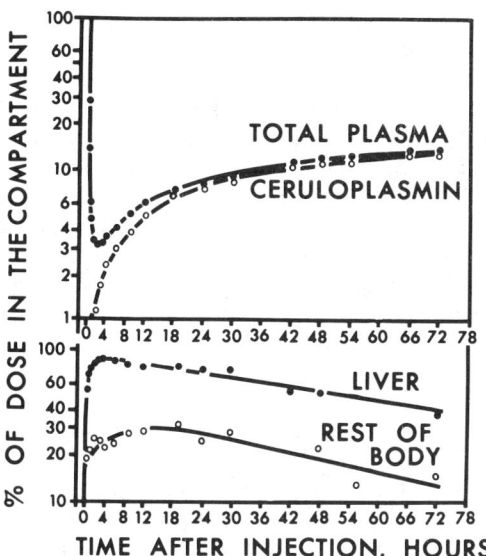

Figure 58-1 Changes in radioactivity in plasma and ceruloplasmin and in liver and other body tissues after intravenous administration of ^{64}Cu. *(Courtesy of Dr. A. Sass Kortsak).*

method is sufficiently reliable to replace copper assay in diagnosis.

EEG changes are rarely helpful in the diagnosis of the neurologic disorder [67], but CT scan may reveal radiolucency of the basal ganglia [68].

The accumulation of copper in cultured fibroblast cells is not yet sufficiently established as a constant finding for use in diagnosis but may become the most sensitive marker of the Wilson's genotype [49, 50].

Diagnosis

The essential first step toward diagnosis of Wilson's disease is to exclude it formally in patients with chronic liver disease and in all patients over 12 years of age with relevant neurologic symptoms and signs. Liver disease in children or young adults is Wilson's disease until proved otherwise, but one may bend a little in conditions like alcoholic cirrhosis in adults. It is probably the most frequent cause of chronic liver disease in childhood and certainly the most frequent treatable cause. Even in adults one must remember that summation of multiple causes is common in chronic liver disease and that Wilson's disease can present with liver symptoms even in late middle age [69].

In children and young adults one should seriously consider Wilson's disease in acute hepatitis if the course is unusual in any way—e.g., severe, prolonged, or recurrent, or associated with hemolysis.

Many authorities have emphasized the need to keep Wilson's disease in mind [65, 70], but most physicians have ignored the most reliable method for ensuring that the diagnosis is not missed. This is to measure the copper content of the initial liver biopsy in every patient with chronic liver disease [56, 57].

One may go through the standard procedures of slit-lamp examination of the eyes and measurements of serum copper, ceruloplasmin, and urine copper, but if one is already doing a liver biopsy to confirm chronic liver disease and to classify it histologically, then measurement of copper will provide defi-

nite information. It is in childhood liver disease that these classical tests are most likely to prove misleadingly normal [56]. Any patient with chronic liver disease deserves absolute exclusion of Wilson's disease.

This approach may introduce some confusion, since not all patients with high levels of liver copper (over 300 μg per gram dry weight) have Wilson's disease. Some have copper accumulation secondary to other liver diseases. One then uses ^{64}Cu administration to resolve this point. As a bonus one makes a diagnosis of copper retention in these other liver diseases, which may warrant chelation treatment (see below).

In patients with neurologic manifestations one may have no other reason to do a liver biopsy. Here the classical signs and tests are much more reliable. Slit-lamp examination and measurement of serum copper, ceruloplasmin, and urine copper comprise sufficient investigation. Further tests should be entertained only if negative results conflict with particularly characteristic clinical features. Liver biopsy may sometimes be needed to assess the condition of the liver after Wilson's disease has been diagnosed; the opportunity to measure the copper content should be taken.

A diagnosis of Wilson's disease should always lead to examination and investigation of sibs (see below).

Treatment and Prognosis

The management of Wilson's disease was revolutionized by Walshe's introduction of penicillamine in 1956. In the early years a mixture of D- and L-isomers was used, and toxic reactions, especially a nephrotic syndrome and pyridoxine deficiency, were frequent. This caused concern about penicillamine which as persisted inappropriately into the era of pure D-penicillamine usage. Experience has also proved that low copper diets and administration of sulphides to block copper absorption are not necessary.

Therapy now consists of the oral administration of D-penicillamine, generally 1 g daily divided into two doses. Some patients require up to 3 g daily. This can be given safely in adults. The dose in children is not well defined, but initially 500 mg daily is probably reasonable for those under 10 years, and 1 g afterward. In all patients 24-h urinary copper excretion should be monitored, with adjustment of dose to achieve losses of over 2 mg/day in the early stages of treatment. After a year or two the amount of copper available decreases and excretion of over 1 mg/day is satisfactory.

Beneficial clinical effects take some time—weeks for neurologic improvement and months for improvement in liver function. Consequently it is difficult to save patients who are diagnosed only in advanced stages of liver failure or in an acute fulminant hepatic episode [52, 65, 71]. One must somehow keep the patient alive for 3 to 6 months until improvement occurs. The levels of nonceruloplasmin plasma copper may be extraordinarily high during acute episodes (up to 100 μmol/liter). These levels undoubtedly set up a vicious circle of cell damage and copper release. Some method for rapid removal of large amounts of copper is needed. Albumin infusion (to increase copper binding capacity) and peritoneal dialysis (adding albumin to the dialysate) are moderately effective, as is exchange transfusion. Hemodialysis was followed by a rise in serum copper and rapid death in two patients [71]. Further study of the role and safety of hemodialysis is needed. Plasmapheresis proved the most powerful method of removing copper in a recent case under the author's care. All too often these measures fail. The solution is early diagnosis before fulminant episodes occur.

L-Dopa may be useful in the control of neurological symptoms which are not reversed by penicillamine or while awaiting a response.

The outcome with modern treatment is mainly determined by the amount of damage which has occurred before treatment is started. A normal life span with normal health seems likely for patients diagnosed before cirrhosis or neurologic effects appear. Treatment stops active liver damage, and the degree of fibrosis may diminish quite remarkably. Even patients with ascites and other features of chronic hepatic decompensation may return to good health. Many of the neurologic effects may also be reversible. It is difficult to predict how much improvement will occur in an individual patient.

Liver transplantation has been used in a few patients with far advanced liver disease [72]. The correction of all features of the disease favors the "liver overflow" hypothesis of pathogenesis. Exchange of the prognosis of treated Wilson's disease for that of liver transplantation is clearly a bad bargain, except when liver disease has proved irreversible or when death is imminent.

Side-effects occasionally occur with D-penicillamine. Skin rashes and thrombocytopenia are most frequent; nephrotic syndrome and acute arthritis may develop [59]. Cessation of therapy and slow reintroduction usually suffice, and a short course of corticosteroids may help prevent these hypersensitivity effects. Bone marrow aplasia or persistent nephrotic syndrome may prevent continuation of penicillamine. Triethylenetetramine hydrochloride is the best alternative chelator in this situation [73].

Two other approaches to therapy have been proposed: oral administration of zinc to reduce copper absorption [74], and sauna baths to promote copper loss in sweat [75]. Neither seems likely to supplant penicillamine as the main method of treatment.

Over 50 pregnancies have been reported in patients in good clinical health on penicillamine treatment, without serious symptoms during pregnancy and with normal babies [76, 77]. Two reports have described babies with unusual connective tissue changes born to women on penicillamine therapy for cystinuria and rheumatoid arthritis [78, 79]. Interference with collagen cross-linking by penicillamine was blamed. Other reports suggest that these occurrences are rare [76, 77, 80]. For the present it seems reasonable to continue penicillamine during pregnancy if the disease has been treated for a relatively short time. In long-treated patients no clinical effects are seen during rests from therapy for 6 or 9 months, and cessation during pregnancy might be preferable.

Genetics

Autosomal recessive inheritance is well supported in studies in the United States [81], Japan [46], Taiwan [47], Israel [82], and Canada [83] by the frequency of the disease in sibs and by parental consanguinity. The prevalence of the disease is not known accurately. Experience in Melbourne suggests a figure in the range of 1 in 50,000 to 1 in 100,000 live births.

Heterogeneity (allelic and nonallelic) is the rule in genetic diseases and must be anticipated in Wilson's disease. The variability of disease effects and of age of onset is in keeping with such heterogeneity, but environmental variables such as cop-

per intake and virus infections may also be important. One large kindred described from an isolated Japanese island with a population of only 300 contained patients presenting at ages ranging from 6 years to 25 years, some with hepatic and some with neurologic symptoms [46], yet all the patients must have been homozygous for the same allele. Caution is necessary in attempting to define genetic heterogeneity by using crude clinical criteria. This kindred and many smaller families show that hepatic and neurologic cases may occur in sibs. The mild neurologic symptoms described in New York in middle-aged Jewish immigrants from eastern Europe may indicate one genetic variant [81]. Differences between Jewish and Arab patients in Israel seem rather striking [82].

Heterozygotes do not have clinical manifestations. Approximately 20 percent have lowered levels of ceruloplasmin (and serum copper) [84]. A reduced secondary rise in plasma radioactivity after ^{64}Cu or ^{67}Cu is seen in heterozygotes as a group but cannot identify all heterozygotes. Another approach, measuring urinary excretion of copper and copper isotope after intravenous administration of isotope, has been described [85].

Genetic Counseling

Sibs of a patient with Wilson's disease have a 1 in 4 risk of developing the disease. These sibs should be examined for liver or neurologic disease, for Kayser-Fleischer rings, and by measuring serum copper, serum ceruloplasmin, and urinary copper. Patients older than the index case may be assumed to be unaffected if no abnormalities are detected. Younger sibs should be investigated more fully using liver biopsy or ^{64}Cu studies if initial test results are normal. The risk of affected children is very low.

Investigation of potential heterozygotes has little value, because available tests are not better than 80 to 90 percent reliable and cannot therefore be interpreted when applied to individuals with low *a priori* risks of being heterozygotes (e.g., spouses of relatives who may be heterozygotes).

Prenatal Diagnosis/Presymptomatic Diagnosis

Prenatal diagnosis has not been possible, but the recent findings in cultured cells raise this possibility. Many would doubt the place of prenatal diagnosis in a disease of late onset for which effective treatment is available.

Mass screening of newborn babies has been suggested, and simple methods of measuring serum ceruloplasmin exist. The very low levels seen in normal newborn babies (Table 58-3) make recognition at this age uncertain. Early symptomatic diagnosis of cases through constant awareness should be sufficient.

Copper Retention in Other Forms of Liver Disease

Copper retention occurs in forms of liver disease other than Wilson's disease; some of these patients may prove to have genetic defects of copper metabolism and may gain places of their own in future editions of this volume (Table 58-8). Their study may throw light on the pathogenesis of Wilson's disease. Some may cause diagnostic confusion, and copper chelation may be beneficial.

Copper retention may be expected in any form of chronic liver disease which interferes with biliary excretion. Prolonged mechanical obstruction of the bile ducts, as in extrahepatic biliary atresia, causes a progressive rise in liver copper, but the variation is considerable [86]. In other forms of liver disease copper accumulation is even more variable, and sometimes severe [39, 62, 86–88]. A few forms of liver disease are more consistently associated with copper retention.

Primary Biliary Cirrhosis   This disease shows a consistent and gross hepatic copper retention [42]. Promising responses to penicillamine therapy have been described [89]. Isotope studies indicate a disturbance of the initial rapid phase of incorporation of freshly injected copper into ceruloplasmin [11]. This may be a specific secondary effect in this disease, which is not usually familial and may have an autoimmune basis. The possibility of a primary defect in copper metabolism cannot be dismissed.

Copper retention has been described in other patients with neonatal cholestatic liver disease [62, 88].

Indian Childhood Cirrhosis   This is a familial and probably genetically determined disease. An extreme degree of hepatic copper accumulation has recently been found [42, 45, 90] and may prove to be primary. The effects of penicillamine therapy have not been reported. Abnormal copper metabolism has been investigated in cultured fibroblasts from four patients with negative results (J. Camakaris, unpublished results).

Åagenes Syndrome   This syndrome (lymphedema and cholestasis from birth) [91] was accompanied by progressive and rapid copper accumulation in one patient, who developed lenticular degeneration terminally at the age of 5 years and copper deposition in the brain [38]. Other patients with this recessive disorder should be studied.

The Arterioductular Hypoplasia Syndrome [92]   This syndrome is frequently associated with copper retention which may be secondary to abnormalities of the small bile ducts in this autosomal dominant condition.

Table 58-8   Liver copper in various liver diseases associated with copper retention

	Liver copper (μg/g dry weight)	Ref
Normal	20–50	
Wilson's disease	200–3000	
Primary biliary cirrhosis	100–2000	
Indian childhood cirrhosis	1000–5000	[45, 90]
Extrahepatic biliary atresia	30–500	[86, 87]
Åagenes syndrome (1 case)	1195	[38]
Arterioductular hypoplasia (7 cases)	71, 243, 288, 327, 1440, 1545, 2119*	

* From AL Smith, J Deutsch, and DM Danks: unpublished data. Other figures not referenced are composite data from numerous articles.

MENKES' (STEELY-HAIR) DISEASE

In this section citations of references are restricted to those essential to establish facts and to the most recent articles. General reviews [33] are not so numerous as for Wilson's disease.

The clinical features, neuropathology, and X-linked inheritance were clearly described by Menkes in 1962 [93]. A small number of case reports added to the range of features and confirmed the pattern of inheritance over the next decade. Discovery of a defect in copper metabolism in 1972 [27, 94] explained the pleiotropic features and triggered a new burst of interest in the disease. The combination of brain changes, like those of copper-deficient sheep, with arterial abnormalities, like those seen in copper-deficient pigs, had suggested copper deficiency. Hunt's discovery [32] of similar disturbances of copper metabolism in the X-linked mottled mutants in mice provided an animal model which appears to be homologous. The suggestion of homology rests on the close similarity of all aspects of copper metabolism in the murine and human mutants and on the remarkable conservation of X-chromosomal gene content in mammals [33].

At first a simple defect in intestinal absorption seemed possible, but disturbances of copper transport in many tissues became apparent, to the great frustration of those endeavoring to treat the disease with parenteral copper therapy.

A number of terms have been used for this disease. *Menkes' steely-hair disease* acknowledges the role of the discoverer and the similarity of the hair changes to the abnormalities of wool seen in copper-deficient sheep (known as steely-wool for many years) and describes the hair quite accurately. The hair is not "kinky" like the hair of negroid races or the wool of normal sheep. Trichopoliodystrophy, X-linked copper malabsorption and X-linked copper deficiency are terms which have also been used.

Basic Defect and Pathogenesis

In spite of many papers on copper metabolism in patients, in cultured cells, and in mottled mice the basic genetic defect is not fully defined. The presence of phenotypic effects in cultured cells and the availability of an animal model provide opportunities for further progress in understanding the disease and learning more about normal copper metabolism.

A graded series of mottled mutant mice has been studied since the mid-1950s, principally because the visible coat color mosaicism (Fig. 58-2) of the heterozygous females was of value in defining the single active X chromosome hypothesis. Mottled males (Mo/y) die in utero, brindled males ($Mo^{br/y}$) die at 14 days, and blotchy males ($Mo^{bo/y}$) live to adult life [32]. There are other mutants of intermediate severity. Allelism has been assumed but cannot be stringently proved by breeding experiments, because of X chromosome inactivation. Cell culture studies using fusion of cells from males with two different mutations will be required. These methods may also prove homology of the human and murine mutants.

In the following paragraphs mouse and human studies are described. Homology is assumed [33]. The data from cell cultures are mostly from human cell lines (but confirmed in the mice), whereas studies of tissue distribution of copper in vivo rest particularly on experiments in mice (with enough human evidence to believe that they apply to both species) [33].

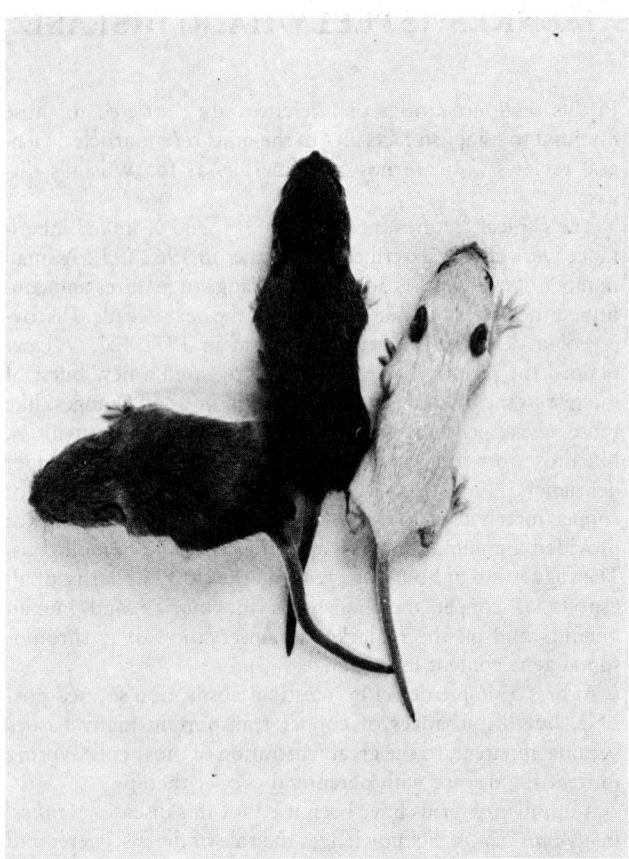

Figure 58-2 Brindled mutant mice—affected male (Mo^br/y)—showing depigmentation and growth failure; heterozygote (Mo^br/+) littermate is of normal size but shows the brindled coat.

Fibroblast cells from patients or affected mice (brindled or blotchy) accumulate abnormal amounts of copper (five times normal) [48, 95–97] and yet show reduced levels of lysyl oxidase, a copper enzyme [98]. Thus the basic cellular defect seems to cause copper to accumulate to abnormal levels in a form or location which renders it inaccessible for the synthesis of copper enzymes [33]. Less complete data show a similar situation for superoxide dismutase and cytochrome oxidase (M. Phillips, unpublished results). In untreated patients and the mutant mice copper levels are reduced in plasma (very low ceruloplasmin levels) [27, 94] and in all tissues excepting gut mucosa and kidney [27, 32, 94, 99–103], where levels are greatly increased (Table 58-9). Parenteral administration of copper quickly restores ceruloplasmin and plasma copper to normal [94], thus hepatic copper metabolism appears to be relatively normal, a suggestion borne out by most of the experimental results available [33, 104]. Radiocopper given intravenously accumulates to an abnormal extent in most tissues of affected mice other than the liver [105]. Observations on tissue copper levels in treated patients are not available.

The findings in the average patient diagnosed at 3 or 4 months of age are confusing, because the tendency of tissues other than liver to accumulate excessive amounts of copper is partly masked by overall copper deficiency secondary to malabsorption of copper [33, 94]. One finds high copper levels in tissues that have sufficient access to copper for accumulation—intestinal mucosa and kidney. All other tissues show low levels. Prenatally, copper supply is less constrained (not totally unconstrained because placental transfer is diminished

[106] and there is an increased level of copper in tissues other than liver, where the partial constraint on supply shows up as reduced copper storage [107, 108] (Table 58-9).

In most tissues (other than liver) the copper enzymes are relatively deprived of copper, even when plenty of copper is available in the plasma and even when cellular copper levels are elevated. The mottled fur of the heterozygous female mice immediately tells one that this is so. These animals do not show overall copper deficiency, yet tyrosinase does not have access to copper in the affected patches, where the pigment cells have presumably inactivated X chromosomes bearing the normal allele.

The clinical manifestations of Menkes' disease are mostly explicable in terms of failure of copper enzymes. The structural changes in the hair are due to defective disulphide bonding in keratin [27, 94], as seen in copper-deficient sheep. Depigmentation is presumably due to tyrosinase deficiency [109]. The arterial disease is principally the result of defective elastin formation secondary to lysyl oxidase deficiency [98]. The roles of catecholamine deficiency secondary to dopamine β-hydroxylase (DBH) malfunction, of cytochrome oxidase deficiency, and of superoxide dismutase deficiency in the neurologic and circulatory disturbances are hard to disentangle [110, 111]. Suggestions of an important role for DBH deficiency in the brain lesions seem reasonable. Brindled mice show reduced brain catecholamines and brain symptoms; blotchy mice have normal catecholamine levels and no neurologic symptoms [110].

The Cellular Phenotype The cellular phenotype of Menkes' disease and of the mottled mutations should be stated in more detail [33, 48, 95, 97] (Table 58-10). It comprises: (1) increased copper content; (2) normal initial uptake of copper; (3) excessive retention of radiocopper after 24-h exposure; (4) diminished release of the isotope during further incubation in isotope-free medium; (5) inability to grow in low copper medium, and (6) increased susceptibility to toxic effects of added copper. Any proposed basic defect must explain these findings.

It is obvious that an alteration of metallothionein could be involved. Several investigators have proposed different alterations of this (these) enigmatic protein(s) [112, 113]. Most of the excess copper in the cells is bound to low molecular weight proteins. Some have proposed that these are metallothioneins with reduced ability to bind copper, while others that they are normal metallothioneins superinduced by copper accumulating because of a defect in some other part of the copper transport system of the cell. Still others have claimed that these proteins have an amino acid content quite different from that of metallothionein [111]. These workers did not take the precautions necessary to protect copper metallothionein from oxidation during purification [5, 111].

The question remains open at present. Possible basic defects include: (1) a mutant metallothionein or other copper transport molecule which binds copper too avidly or is resistant to normal turnover; (2) lack of an enzyme needed to release copper from the protein concerned; (3) deficiency of some copper extrusion process with secondary superinduction of metallothionein to bind the accumulated copper; (4) constitutive production of normal metallothionein.

The location of the copper in the cells is not known for certain. A recent article suggests that the copper is not really in the cells but is sequestered on the surface of cultured cells or in

Table 58-9 Copper levels in serum and tissues in Menkes' disease and in brindled mice

	Normal baby (6–12 months)	Typical Menkes' disease	Normal fetus (20 weeks)[107]	Menkes' disease fetus (20 weeks)[107]	Normal mice (11 days)[100]	Mo^br/y mice (11 days)[100]	Mo^br/y mice (11 days)[100]
Serum, μmol/liter	11–24	2–6	NK	NK	76	24	58
Liver, μg/g dry weight	50–120	10–20	36*	12*	169	13	25
Brain, μg/g dry weight	20–30	1–7	0.4*	1.0*	12	3	8
Kidney, μg/g dry weight	10–20	240	0.8*	17.0*	16	50	112
Duodenal mucosa, μg/g dry weight	7–29	50–90	NK	NK	16	41	44

NOTE: Results for typical Menkes' disease represent a range of personal experience and published cases. Figures for mice are presented as mean only—more detailed figures are in the original report [100].
* μg/g wet weight.

the brush border of enterocytes [114]. It is difficult to reconcile these results with the findings of copper bound to low molecular weight proteins, a finding reported by many separate investigators.

Clinical Features

The key components of the clinical syndrome are abnormal hair, progressive cerebral degeneration, hypopigmentation, bone changes, arterial rupture and thrombosis, and hypothermia [27, 33, 115].

Premature delivery is frequent, as are neonatal hypothermia and hyperbilirubinemia. Hypothermia may also occur in older babies. In the neonatal period the child's appearance is usually normal with fine normal hair, but some have trichorrhexis nodosa and monilethrix and the unusual facies may be apparent. Neonatal symptoms may resolve, and the baby may seem normal during the next 2 or 3 months, although growth may be slow. Other babies may show continued symptoms. By about 3 months of age the more flagrant symptoms of developmental delay, loss of early development skills, and convulsions appear. Cerebral degeneration then dominates the clinical picture along with various vascular complications, particularly subdural hematoma.

The hair becomes tangled, lusterless, and grayish or ivory colored, with a stubble of broken hairs palpable over the occiput and temporal regions where the hair rubs on the sheets. Pili torti is found microscopically (Fig. 58-3). The facies is quite characteristic, with pudgy cheeks and abnormal eyebrows (Fig. 58-4A), and is recognizable even in babies who have no hair (Fig. 58-4B). Skeletal x-rays show osteoporosis and widening of the flared metaphyses with spiky protrusions at the edges. These may fracture [27, 116, 117]. Rib fractures are common. Wormian bones are usually seen in the skull. The combination of these bony changes with a subdural hematoma may lead to the erroneous diagnosis of child abuse [118]. CT scan or air studies may show macroscopic patches of brain destruction. Arteriograms show elongation, tortuosity, and variable caliber of major arteries throughout the brain, viscera, and limbs, with areas of localized dilatation and other areas of marked narrowing [27, 116, 119] (Fig. 58-5). Emphysema, bladder diverticula

[119], retinal degeneration, and iris cysts [120] have been described.

Survival varies between 3 months and 3 years, but is most often about 12 months. One patient lived in a decerebrate state until 12 years (R.R. Howell, personal communication).

Variants and Related Conditions One mildly affected patient has been described who presented at the age of 2 years with mild mental retardation and marked cerebellar ataxia [121]. Pili torti was present, bone changes were mild, and arteriography showed generalized elongation and uniform dilatation of the arteries. CT scan was normal.

Recently, apparent, X-linked inheritance of a disease comprising mental retardation, dystonia, and chorea with malabsorption of copper and low serum copper has been described [121a]. No other clinical features of copper deficiency were present, although arteriography was not performed. Liver copper was low in one boy and high in the other. No cell culture studies were reported. The nature of this disorder is not clear.

An X-linked form of cutis laxa has been described as showing reduced levels of lysyl oxidase in skin biopsies and in fibroblast cultures [121b]. The patients had low levels of serum copper. This combination has been observed in other families (D. W. Hollister, personal communication).

Table 58-10 Findings of Menkes' disease in cultured fibroblastic cells in our laboratory [95]

	Normal cells	Menkes' cells
Copper content (μg/10^6 cells)		
In normal medium	0.023 ± 0.013†	0.282 ± 0.091
With added copper (6 μg/ml)	0.113 ± 0.074†	0.770 ± 0.156
^{64}Cu content after 24 h* (μg ^{64}Cu/10^6 cells)	0.004 ± 0.001†	0.060 ± 0.019†
^{64}Cu efflux over subsequent 24 h in culture (percentage of content at 24 h)	70–90%	0–5%

* Calculated from corrected counts using the initial specific activity [95].
† Standard deviation.

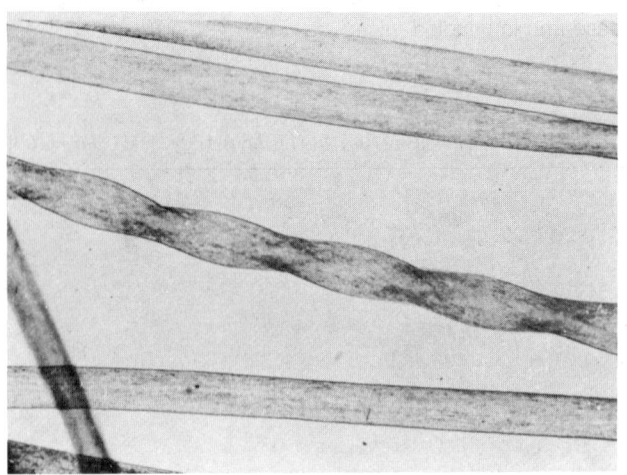

Figure 58-3 Pili torti.

Laboratory and Cell Culture Findings

Serum copper and ceruloplasmin levels are very low. Interpretation is difficult in the first 2 or 3 weeks of life, when the ceruloplasmin and serum copper levels are low in normal babies (Table 58-3). Cord blood levels in affected babies fall within the normal range [115]. During the next 2 weeks the levels fall even lower, whereas those in normal babies rise quite quickly. Diagnosis can be made with confidence by 2 weeks [115]. This creates a practical problem in assessing new sons in affected families or when neonatal hypothermia raises the possibility of Menkes' disease.

The liver content of copper is grossly reduced, and duodenal or jejunal biopsy specimens show greatly increased copper content [99] (Table 58-11). Oral ^{64}Cu is poorly absorbed, and when given intravenously is cleared from plasma and incorporated into ceruloplasmin quite normally [27, 122, 123]. Typical copper measurements are shown in Table 58-11.

The disturbances of copper handling in cultured cells described above (Table 58-10) comprise the most definitive test for the disease [95–97, 103]. Fibroblastic, amniotic, or lymphoid cells all show these changes, although the exact figures differ slightly in the three cell types. The influence of the phase of cell growth at the time of testing is troublesome with fibroblastic and amniotic cells. Use of confluent cultures which have been held in a nondividing state by reducing the fetal calf serum in the medium gives the most reproducible results in our experience [95]. Special care is needed in prenatal diagnosis using amniotic cells.

Reduced levels of various copper enzyme activities have been demonstrated but are of little diagnostic assistance. Noradrenaline is decreased and dopamine is increased in cerebrospinal fluid, as expected in dopamine β-hydroxylase deficiency (W.D. Grover, personal communication). Hair keratin analysis shows defective disulphide bonding [94].

Pathology

Gross and microscopic pathology is abundant in this disease. Arteries show precocious degenerative changes with elongation, aneurysmal dilatations, rupture, stenoses, and areas of intimal proliferation and of thrombosis. Microscopically, the fragmentation, disruption, and reduplication of the internal elastic lamina is quite extreme, especially in large arteries [27]

Figure 58-4 Typical facies of Menkes' disease in two unrelated cases, *A.* with and *B.* without visible hair.

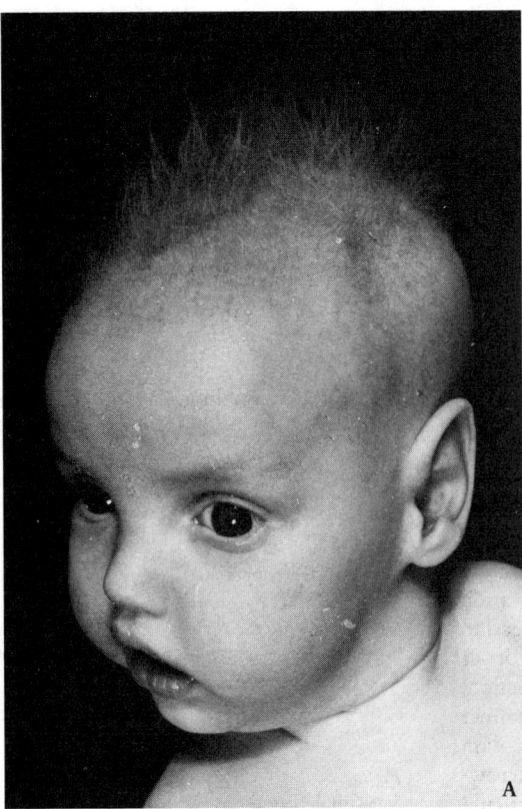

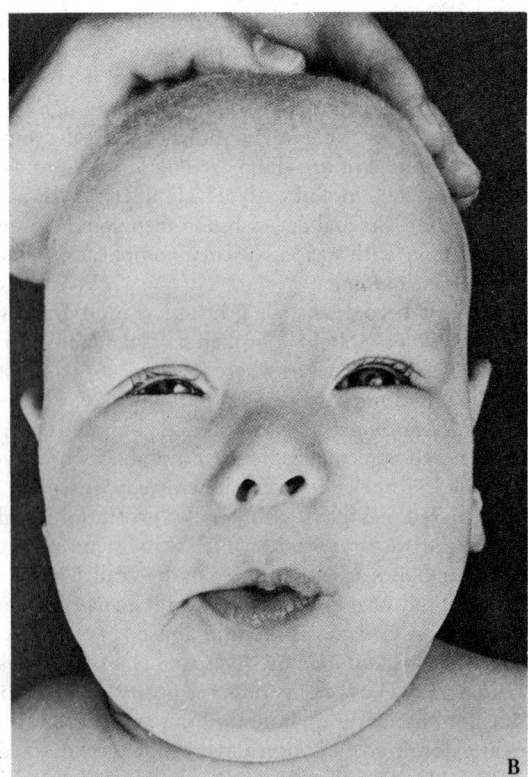

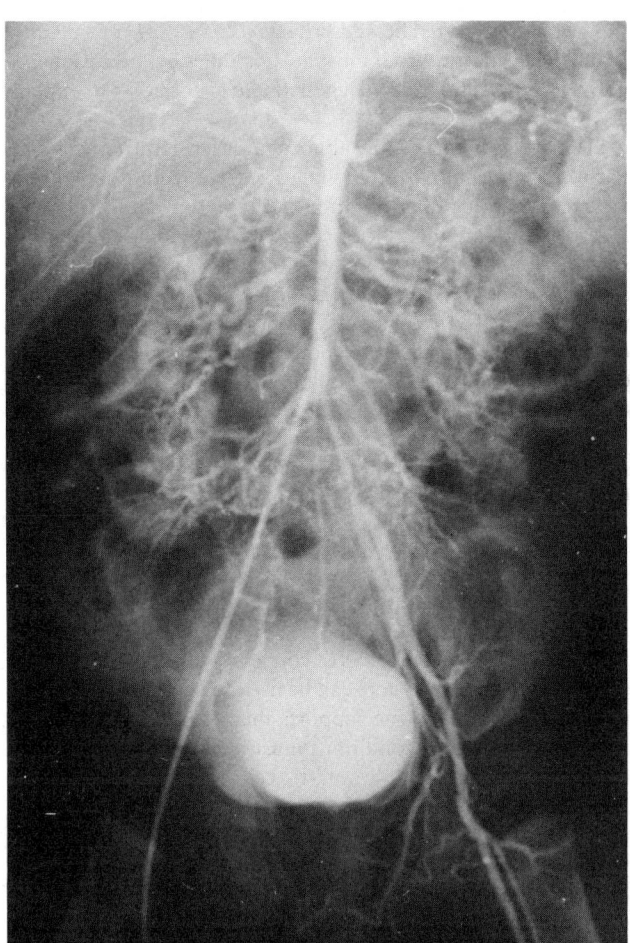

Figure 58-5 Aortogram showing tortuosity, elongation, patchy dilatation, and areas of stenosis of many arteries.

(Fig. 58-6). The intima may be thickened and subintimal plaques may include elastic fibril fragments (Fig. 58-6). Ultrastructural changes suggest defective formation of elastin rather than disruption of elastic fibers [124]. Elastin fibers in the skin show abnormal microfibrillary components and deficient formation of mature elastin, although collagen fibrils appear normal [124]. In cartilage, irregularity and abnormal variability of size of collagen fibrils have been described [119].

Neuronal destruction is widespread in the cerebral cortex and in the cerebellum, and there is associated gliosis [93, 125–127]. The changes in the cerebellum are particularly severe, with neuronal loss in the internal granule cell layer and molecular layer. Many Purkinje cells are lost, and the remaining cells show an unusual elaboration of dendritic sprouts from the cell body and grotesque proliferation of the dendritic tree which has been considered unique to this disease [125–127]. The pronounced involvement of the cerebellum fits in well with the marked cerebellar ataxia seen in the mildly affected boy described above [121].

Myelin is deficient in such a damaged brain but could be secondary to neuronal loss. Chemical markers of myelin destruction are found. In the late stages of the disease brain infarction and hemorrhage secondary to arterial disease are seen.

Changes in skeletal muscle (glycogen accumulation, mitochondrial disorganization) [125], in the iris (microcysts in pigment epithelian), and retina (marked in ganglion cells) [120] have been described.

Diagnosis

The diagnosis can be made with confidence from the clinical and radiologic features once one or two cases have been seen. Microscopic examination of the hair is helpful, even in a mild case. Low levels of serum copper and ceruloplasmin will usually clinch the diagnosis. If doubt persists, assay of copper in gut mucosal or liver biopsy specimens may be used, or studies of cell cultures. The latter comprise the ultimate test, showing marked abnormality even in the mild case [121] in whom the reductions of ceruloplasmin and serum copper are too slight to be interpreted (Table 58-11).

Treatment

No form of treatment has yet proved to be truly effective. Copper has been administered parenterally in a number of different forms—copper sulphate, copper chloride, copper EDTA, copper glycinate, copper histidinate, and copper albumin complex. Copper nitriloacetate is the only form of copper that has proved to be absorbed from the intestine in these patients [128]. All these forms of treatment have corrected the hepatic copper deficiency and have restored normal levels of serum copper. Some improvement has resulted, but in most cases there has been continuing cerebral degeneration and a fatal outcome. Restoration of normal brain copper levels has not been described [115, 128]. One patient is making encouraging progress at age $4\frac{1}{2}$ years. His motor development is quite good. Speech is delayed. There is no ataxia. Joint laxity and skin laxity are pronounced. Treatment with copper histidinate (600 μg copper per day) began in the second month, before symptoms developed, and has continued (A. Sass Kortsak, personal communication).

It is probable that many of the effects of the disease are already established in utero and that postnatal treatment cannot be fully effective. Nevertheless, the search should continue for some chemical form of copper which can bypass the disturbance in copper transport and deliver the copper to the copper enzymes that require it, especially in the brain. The sensitivity of affected cells in culture to toxic effects of excess copper may indicate that delivery of too much copper may also prove injurious.

Since some of the more serious effects of the disease may be the result of defective catecholamine synthesis, trials of mono-

Table 58-11 Typical copper measurements in Menkes' disease at usual age of diagnosis

	Menkes' disease (3–12 months)	Mild Menkes' disease [121] (2 years)	Normal (3–12 months)
Serum ceruloplasmin			
OD units/ml	<0.08	0.20	>0.25
mg/liter	<50	160	>200
Serum copper, μmol/liter	<6	9.5	>12
Liver copper, μg/g dry weight	10–20	18	140–70*
Duodenal copper, μg/g dry weight	50–80	98	7–29

* Higher levels observed in younger babies.

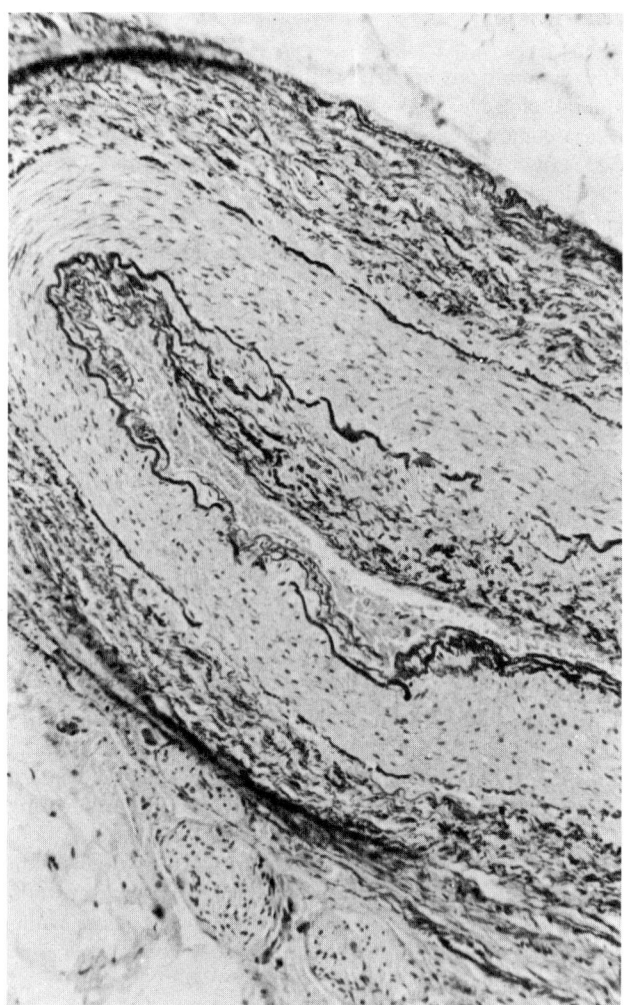

Figure 58-6 Section of large artery showing fragmentation and reduplication of the internal elastic lamina and intimal thickening.

amine oxidase inhibitors seemed warranted. We have used trancyclypramine sulphate in two children without benefit.

Treatment of the brindled mice has proved surprisingly simple and effective. A single dose of 50 μg copper as Cu^+ given on day 7 restores normal growth and allows survival to at least 1 year (middle aged for mice) [105]. The relative immaturity of mice at birth may be important, the seventh postnatal day being equivalent to mid third trimester for humans.

Genetics and Genetic Heterogeneity

Numerous pedigrees show X-linked recessive inheritance. This is supported by the mosaic skin depigmentation seen in a Negro heterozygous female [129], and the pili torti seen in some heterozygotes [27]. We have seen patchy sun tanning in one heterozygote. Full manifestations of the disease have been described in one Japanese girl, the sister of a severely affected male [130].

Experience in Melbourne in 1966 to 1971 suggested an incidence of 1 in 35,500 live births [27]. Extension of the period of collection of cases to 1980 has modified this figure to 1 in 90,000. The true figure is presumably in the range 1 in 50,000 to 1 in 100,000. The earlier period must have included a chance cluster of cases—so often a problem with initial observations on a genetic disease.

The mildly affected boy described recently [121] presumably is an allelic variant. Proof must await studies by cell fusion (see above). Others have also suggested allelic variation to explain less striking differences [115].

Heterozygotes may show abnormalities in cultured cells similar to those seen in affected males, but X chromosome inactivation confounds interpretation. Only about half of obligate heterozygotes are identified by studies on a single skin biopsy specimen [95, 131]. Use of two or three biopsies from separate sites improves the diagnostic accuracy, as does cloning of the fibroblastic cells grown from a biopsy specimen [132]. Development of a test using hair roots seems desirable. At present one can say that presence of pili torti, of mosaic skin pigmentation, or of abnormal cell culture results suggests heterozygosity in a female relative. Measurement of placental copper levels seems to be a good method of diagnosing heterozygotes when females are born into affected families [108].

Prenatal Diagnosis

Any or all of the disturbances of copper metabolism in cultured cells that are described here can be used for prenatal diagnosis. Experience in Melbourne supports the use of all four characteristics. Cell culture conditions must be standardized. Ideally the test should include fibroblastic cells from an affected relative, normal amniotic cells, and amniotic cells from an affected male. ^{64}Cu retention after 24 h alone has been used successfully in 42 pregnancies [108], but the test has proved vulnerable to changes in the phase of cell culture and the copper content of the medium. Release of ^{64}Cu during a subsequent 24 h of growth in media without isotope is least affected by culture variables and therefore the most reliable single test. Nevertheless, I prefer to use multiple tests.

Prenatal diagnosis should probably be concentrated in a few laboratories heavily involved with research in cellular copper metabolism until more experience has accumulated. The high level of copper found in the placenta allows confirmation of the diagnosis in terminated pregnancies and is useful in diagnosis of heterozygotes [108].

REFERENCES

1. UNDERWOOD EJ: *Trace Elements in Human and Animal Nutrition*, 4th ed. New York, Academic, 1977
2. MASON KE: A conspectus of research on copper metabolism and requirements in man. *J Nutr* 109:1979, 1979
3. EVANS GW: Copper homeostasis in the mammalian system. *Physiol Rev* 53:535, 1973
4. SASS-KORTSAK A, BEARN AG: Hereditary disorders of copper metabolism—Wilson's disease (hepatolenticular degeneration) and Menkes' disease (kinky-hair or steely-hair syndrome), in Stanbury JB, Wyngaarden JB, Fredrickson DS (eds): *The Metabolic Basis of Inherited Disease*, 4th ed., New York, McGraw-Hill, 1978
5. CIBA FOUNDATION SYMPOSIUM 79: *Biological Roles for Copper.* Amsterdam, Excerpta Medica, 1980
6. BREMNER I: Absorption, transport and distribution of copper, in CIBA Foundation Symposium 79: *Biological Roles for Copper.* Amsterdam, Excerpta Medica, 1980, p 23
7. HALL AC, YOUNG BW, BREMNER I: Intestinal metallothionein and the mutual antagonism between copper and zinc in the rat. *J Inorg Biochem* 11:57, 1979
8. PRASAD AG, BREWER GJ, SCHOOMAKER EB, RABBONI P: Hypocupremia induced by zinc therapy in adults. *J Am Med Assoc* 240:2166, 1978
9. STRICKLAND GT, BECKNER WM, LEU M-L: Absorption of copper in homozygotes and heterozygotes for Wilson's disease and controls: Isotope tracer studies with ^{67}Cu and ^{64}Cu. *Clin Sci* 43:617, 1972

10. SMALLWOOD RA, McILVEEN B, ROSENOER VM, SHERLOCK S: Copper kinetics in liver disease. *Gut* 12:139, 1971

11. VIERLING JM, SHRAGER MA, RUMBLE WF, AAMODT R, BERMAN MD, JONES EA: Incorporation of radiocopper into ceruloplasmin in normal subjects and in patients with primary biliary cirrhosis and Wilson's disease. *Gastroenterology* 74:652, 1978

12. PETERS T JR: Serum albumin: Recent progress in the understanding of its structure and biosynthesis. *Clin Chem* 23:5, 1977

13. FIREDEN E: Ceruloplasmin: A multi-functional metalloprotein of vertebrate plasma, in CIBA Foundation Symposium 79: *Biological Roles of Copper*. Amsterdam, Excerpta Medica, 1980, p 93

14. COX DW: Factors influencing serum ceruloplasmin levels in normal individuals. *J Lab Clin Med* 68:893, 1966

15. EDWARDS CQ, WILLIAMS DM, CARTWRIGHT GE: Hereditary hypoceruloplasminemia. *Clin Genet* 15:311, 1979

16. SOLOMONS NW: On the assessment of zinc and copper nutriture in man. *Am J Clin Nutr* 32:856, 1979

17. DANKS DM: Diagnosis of trace metal deficiency—With emphasis on copper and zinc. *Am J Clin Nutr* 34:278, 1981

18. WEBER KM, BOSTON RC, LEAVER DD: A kinetic model of copper metabolism in sheep. *Aust J Agric Res* 31:773, 1980

19. LINDER MC, MOOR JR JR: Plasma ceruloplasmin: Evidence for its presence in and uptake by heart and other organs of the rat. *Biochim Biophys Acta* 499:329, 1977

20. OWEN CA JR: Copper and hepatic function, in CIBA Foundation Symposium 79: *Biological Roles of Copper*. Amsterdam, Excerpta Medica, 1980, p 267

21. STRICKLAND GT, BECKNER WM, LEU M-L, O'REILLY S: Turnover studies of copper in homozygotes and heterozygotes for Wilson's disease and controls: Isotope tracer studies with ^{67}Cu. *Clin Sci* 43:605, 1972

22. GIBBS K, WALSHE JM: Studies with radioactive copper (^{64}Cu and ^{67}Cu); The incorporation of radioactive copper into ceruloplasmin in Wilson's disease and in primary biliary cirrhosis. *Clin Sci* 41:189, 1971

23. HOWELL JMcC: The pathology of chronic copper poisoning in sheep, in Kirchgessner M (ed): *Proceedings of 3d International Symposium on Trace Element Metabolism in Man and Animals*. Friesing-Weihenstephan, Arbeitskreis fur Tierernahrungs forschung, 1978, p 536

24. HENKIN RI: Metal-albumin-amino acid interactions: Chemical and physiological interrelationships, in Friedman M (ed): *Protein-Metal Interactions*. New York, Plenum, 1974, p 15

25. PAYNTER DI, MOIR RJ, UNDERWOOD EJ: Changes in activity of the Cu-Zn superoxide dismutase enzyme in tissues of the rat with changes in dietary copper. *J Nutr* 109:1570, 1979

26. HOAGLAND HC, GOLDSTEIN NP: Hematologic (cytopenic) manifestations of Wilson's disease (hepatolenticular degeneration). *Mayo Clin Proc* 53:498, 1978

27. DANKS DM, CAMPBELL PE, STEVENS BJ, MAYNE V, CARTWRIGHT E: Menkes' kinky hair syndrome: An inherited defect in copper absorption with widespread effects. *Pediatrics* 50:188, 1972

28. DANKS DM: Copper deficiency in humans, in CIBA Foundation Symposium 79: *Biological Roles of Copper*. Amsterdam, Excerpta Medica, 1980, p 209

29. KAGI JHR, NORDBERG M (eds): *Metallothionein*, Basel, Birkauser, 1979

30. HAMBIDGE KM: Trace elements in pediatric nutrition. *Adv Pediatr* 24:191, 1978

31. WALSH FM, CROSSON FJ, BAYLEY M, McREYNOLDS J, PEARSON BJ: Acute copper intoxication: Pathophysiology and therapy with a case report. *Am J Dis Child* 131:149, 1977

32. HUNT DM: Primary defect in copper transport underlies mottled mutants in the mouse. *Nature* 249:852, 1974

33. DANKS DM: Copper transport and utilisation in Menkes' syndrome and in mottled mice. *Inorg Perspect Biol Med* 1:73, 1977

34. TWEDT DC, STERNLIEB I, GILBERTSON SR: Clinical morphologic and chemical studies on copper toxicosis of Bedlington terriers. *J Am Vet Assoc* 175:269, 1979

35. HURLEY LS, KEEN CL, LONNERDAL B: Copper in fetal and neonatal development, in CIBA Foundation Symposium 79: *Biological Roles of Copper*. Amsterdam, Excerpta Medica, 1980, p 227

36. GIBBS K, WALSHE JM: Biliary excretion of copper in Wilson's disease. *Lancet* 2:538, 1980

37. WIEBERS DO, HOLLENHORST RW, GOLDSTEIN NP: The ophthalmologic manifestation of Wilson's disease. *Mayo Clin Proc* 52:409, 1977

38. SMITH AL, DANKS DM: Secondary copper accumulation with neurological damage in children with chronic liver disease. *Brit Med J* 2:1400, 1978

39. FLEMING CR, DICKSON ER, WAHNER HW, HOLLENHORST RW, McCALL JT: Pigmented corneal rings in non-Wilsonian liver disease. *Ann Intern Med* 86:285, 1977

40. FROMMER D, MORRIS J, SHERLOCK S, ABRAMS J, NEWMAN S: Kayser-Fleischer-like rings in patients without Wilson's disease. *Gastroenterology* 72:1331, 1977

41. GOLDFISCHER S, POPPER H, STERNLIEB I: The significance of variations in the distribution of copper in liver disease. *Am J Pathol* 99:715, 1980

42. STERNLIEB I: Copper and the liver. *Gastroenterology* 78:1615, 1980

43. JAIN S, SCHEUER PJ, ARCHER B, NEWMAN SP, SHERLOCK S: Histological demonstration of copper and copper-associated protein in chronic liver diseases. *J Clin Pathol* 31:784, 1978

44. OWEN CA, DICKSON ER, GOLDSTEIN NP, BAGGENSTOSS AH, McCALL JT: Hepatic subcellular distribution of copper in primary biliary cirrhosis: Comparison with other hyperhepatocupric states and review of the literature. *Mayo Clin Proc* 52:73, 1977

45. POPPER H, GOLDFISCHER S, STERNLIEB I, NAYAK NC, MADHAVAN, TV: Cytoplasmic copper and its toxic effects: Studies in Indian childhood cirrhosis. *Lancet* 1:1205, 1979

46. ARIMA M, SANO I: Genetic studies of Wilson's disease in Japan. *Birth Defects Orig Art Ser* 4(2):54, 1968

47. STRICKLAND GT, FROMMER D, LEU M-L, POLLARD R, SHERLOCK S, CUMMINGS JN: Wilson's disease in the United Kingdom and Taiwan. *Quart J Med* 42:619, 1973

48. GOKA TJ, STEVENSON RE, HEFFERAN PM, HOWELL RR: Menkes' disease a biochemical abnormality in cultured human fibroblasts. *Proc Natl Acad Sci USA* 73:604, 1976

49. CHAN WY, CUSHING W, COFEMAN MA, RENNERT OM: Genetic expression of Wilson's disease in cell culture: A diagnostic marker. *Science* 208:299, 1980

50. CAMAKARIS J, ACKLAND L, DANKS DM: Phenotype expression of Wilson's disease in cultured fibroblasts. *J Inher Metab Dis* 3:155, 1980

51. STRICKLAND GT, LEU M-L: Wilson's disease: Clinical and laboratory manifestations in 40 patients. *Medicine* 54:113, 1975

52. WALSHE JM: The physiology of copper in man and its relation to Wilson's disease. *Brain* 90:149, 1967

53. DOBYNS WB, GOLDSTEIN NP, GORDON H: Clinical spectrum of Wilson's disease (hepatolenticular degeneration). *Mayo Clin Proc* 54:35, 1979

54. SASS-KORTSAK A: A Wilson's disease: A treatable cause of liver disease in children. *Pediatr Clin N Am* 22:963, 1975

55. ODIEVRE M, VEDRENNE J, LANDRIEU P, ALAGILLE D: Les formes hepatiques "pures" de la maladie de Wilson chez l'enfant: a propos de dix observations. *Arch Franc Pediat* 31:215, 1974

56. DANKS DM, STEVENS BJ: Diagnosis of Wilson's disease in children with liver disease: A report of two families. *Lancet* 1:22, 1969

57. PERMAN JA, WERLIN SL, GRAND RJ, WATKINS JB: Laboratory measures of copper metabolism in the differentiation of chronic active hepatitis and Wilson's disease in children. *J Pediatr* 94:564, 1979

58. ISER JH, STEVENS BJ, STENING GF, HURLEY TH, SMALLWOOD RA: Hemolytic anemia of Wilson's disease. *Gastroenterology* 67:290, 1974

59. GOLDING DN, WALSHE JM: Arthropathy of Wilson's disease: Study of clinical and radiological features in 32 cases. *Ann Rheumat Dis* 36:99, 1977

60. CANELAS HM, CARVALHO N, SCAFF M, VITULE A, BARBOSA ER, AZEVEDO EM: Osteoarthropathy of hepatolenticular degeneration. *Acta Neurol Scand* 57:481, 1978

61. WIEBERS DO, WILSON DM, McLEOD RA, GOLDSTEIN NP: Renal stones in Wilson's disease. *Am J Med* 67:249, 1979

62. KAPLINSKY C, STERNLIEB I, JAVITT N, ROTEM Y: Familial cholestatic cirrhosis associated with Kayser-Fleischer rings. *Pediatrics* 65:782, 1980

63. WALSHE JM, BRIGGS J: Ceruloplasmin in liver disease: A diagnostic pitfall. *Lancet* 2:263, 1962

64. STERNLIEB I, SCHIENBERG IH: The role of radiocopper in the diagnosis of Wilson's disease. *Gastroenterology* 77:138, 1979.

65. STERNLIEB I: Diagnosis of Wilson's disease. *Gastroenterology* 74:787, 1978

66. SCOTT J, GOLLAN JL, SAMOURIAN S, SHERLOCK S: Wilson's disease, presenting as chronic active hepatitis. *Gastroenterology* 74:645, 1978

67. WESTMORELAND BF, GOLDSTEIN NP, KLASS DW: Wilson's disease: Electroencephalographic and evoked potential studies. *Mayo Clin Proc* 49:401, 1974

68. NELSON RF, GUZMAN DA, GRAHOVAC Z, HOWSE DCN: Computerized cranial tomography in Wilson's disease. *Neurology* 29:866, 1979

69. FITZGERALD MA, GROSS JB, GOLDSTEIN NP, WAHNER HW, McCALL JT: Wilson's disease (hepatolenticular degeneration) of late adult onset. *Mayo Clin Proc* 50:438, 1975

70. CARTWRIGHT GE: Diagnosis of treatable Wilson's disease. *N Engl J Med* 298:1347, 1978

71. HAMLYN AN, GOLLAN JL, DOUGLAS AP, SHERLOCK S: Fulminant Wilson's disease with hemolysis and renal failure: Copper studies and assessment of dialysis regimes. *Brit Med J* 2:660, 1977

72. DU BOIS RS, RODGERSON DO, MARTINEAU G, SHROTER G, GILES G, LILLY J, HALGRIMSON CG, STARZL TE: Orthotopic liver transplantation for Wilson's disease. *Lancet* 1:505, 1971

73. WALSHE JM: Copper chelation in patients with Wilson's disease. *Quart J Med* 42:441, 1973

74. HOOGENRAAD TU, VAN DEN HAMER CJA, KOEVOET R, DE RUYTER KORVER EGWM: Oral zinc in Wilson's disease. *Lancet* 2:1262, 1978

75. SUNDERMAN PW, HOHNADEL PC, EVENSON MA, WANNAMAKER BB, DAHL

BS: Excretion of copper in sweat of patients with Wilson's disease during sauna bathing. *Ann Clin Lab Sci* 74:407, 1974

76. WALSHE JM: Pregnancy in Wilson's disease. *Quart J Med* 46:73, 1977
77. SCHEINBERG IH, STERNLIEB I: Pregnancy in penicillamine-treated patients with Wilson's disease. *N Engl J Med* 293:1300, 1975
78. MJØLNEROD OK, RASMUSSEN K, DOMMERUD SA, GJERULDSEN ST: Congenital connective-tissue defect probably due to D-penicillamine treatment in pregnancy. *Lancet* 1:673, 1971
79. LINARES A, ZARRANZ JJ, RODRIGUEZ-ALARCON J, DIAZ-PEREZ JL: Reversible cutis laxa due to maternal D-penicillamine treatment. *Lancet* 2:43, 1979
80. LYLE WH: Penicillamine in pregnancy. *Lancet* 1:606, 1978
81. BEARN AG: Genetic analysis of Wilson's disease. *Ann Hum Genet* 24:33, 1960
82. PASSWELL J, ADAM A, GARFINKEL D, STREIFFLER M, COHEN BE: Heterogeneity of Wilson's disease in Israel. *Isr J Med Sci* 13:15, 1977
83. COX DW, FRASER FC, SASS-KORTSAK A: A genetic study of Wilson's disease: Evidence for heterogeneity. *Am J Hum Genet* 24:646, 1972
84. GIBBS K, WALSHE JM: A study of the ceruloplasmin concentrations found in 75 patients with Wilson's disease, their kinships and various control groups. *Quart J Med* 48:1, 1979
85. GIBBS K, HANKA R, WALSHE JM: The urinary excretion of radiocopper in presymptomatic and symptomatic Wilson's disease, heterozygotes and controls: Its significance in diagnosis and management. *Quart J Med* 47:349, 1978
86. REED GB, BUTT EM, LANDING BH: Copper in childhood liver disease: A histologic, histochemical and chemical survey. *Arch Pathol* 93:249, 1972
87. SMALLWOOD RA, WILLIAMS HA, ROSENOER VM, SHERLOCK S: Liver copper levels in liver disease: Studies using neutron activation analysis. *Lancet* 2:1310, 1968
88. EVANS J, NEWMAN S, SHERLOCK S: Liver copper levels in intrahepatic cholestasis of childhood. *Gastroenterology* 75:875, 1978
89. DEERING TB, DICKSON ER, FLEMING CR, GEALL MG, McCALL JT, BAGGENSTOSS AH: Effects of D-penicillamine on copper retention in patients with primary biliary cirrhosis. *Gastroenterology* 72:1208, 1977
90. TANNER MS, PORTMANN B, MOWAT AP, WILLIAMS R, PANDIT AN, MILLS CF: Increased hepatic copper concentration in Indian childhood cirrhosis. *Lancet* 2:4524, 1979
91. ÅAGENAES O: Hereditary recurrent cholestasis with lymphoedema: Two new families. *Acta Paediatr Scand* 63:465, 1974
92. ALAGILLE D, ODIEVRE M, GAUTIER M, DOMMERGUES JP: Hepatic ductular hypoplasia associated with characteristic facies, vertebral malformations, retarded physical, mental and sexual development, and cardiac murmur. *J Pediatr* 86:63, 1975
93. MENKES JH, ALTER M, STEIGLEDER GK, WEAKLEY DR, SUNG JH: A sex-linked recessive disorder with retardation of growth, peculiar hair and focal cerebral and cerebellar degeneration. *Pediatrics* 29:764, 1962
94. DANKS DM, STEVENS BJ, CAMPBELL PE, GILLESPIE JM, WALKER-SMITH J, BLOMFIELD J, TURNER B: Menkes' kinky-hair syndrome. *Lancet* 1:110, 1972
95. CAMAKARIS J, DANKS DM, ACKLAND L, CARTWRIGHT E, BORGER P, COTTON RGH: Altered copper metabolism in cultured cells from human Menkes' syndrome and mottled mouse mutants. *Biochem Genet* 18:117, 1980
96. CHAN W-Y, GARNICA AD, RENNERT OM: Cell culture studies of Menkes kinky hair syndrome. *Clin Chim Acta* 88:495, 1978
97. BERATIS NG, PRICE P, LA BADIE G, HIRSCHHORN K: ^{64}Cu metabolism in Menkes' and normal cultured skin fibroblasts. *Pediatr Res* 12:699, 1978
98. ROYCE PM, CAMAKARIS J, DANKS DM: Reduced lysyl oxidase activity in skin fibroblasts from patients with Menkes' syndrome. *Biochem J* 192:579, 1980
99. DANKS DM, CARTWRIGHT E, STEVENS BJ, TOWNLEY RRW: Menkes' kinky hair disease: Further definition of the defect in copper transport. *Science* 179:1140, 1973
100. CAMAKARIS J, MANN JR, DANKS DM: Copper metabolism in mottled mouse mutants: Copper concentrations in tissues during development. *Biochem J* 180:597, 1979
101. HUNT DM, PORT AE: Trace element binding in the copper deficient mottled mutants in the mouse. *Life Sci* 24:1453, 1979
102. EVANS GW, REIS BL: Impaired copper homeostasis in neonatal male and adult female brindled (Mo^{br}) mice. *J Nutr* 108:554, 1978
103. PRINS HW, VAN DEN HAMER CJA: Primary biochemical defect in copper metabolism in mice with a recessive X-linked mutation analogous to Menkes' disease in man. *Inorg Biochem* 10:19, 1979
104. MANN JR, CAMAKARIS J, DANKS DM, WALLICZEK EG: Copper metabolism in mottled mouse mutants: Copper therapy of brindled (Mo^{br}) mice. *Biochem J* 180:605, 1979
105. MANN JR, CAMAKARIS J, DANKS DM: Copper metabolism in mottled

mouse mutants: Distribution of ^{64}Cu in brindled (Mo^{br}) mice. *Biochem J* 180:613, 1979
106. MANN JR, CAMAKARIS J, DANKS DM: Copper metabolism in mottled mouse mutants: Defective placental transfer of ^{64}Cu to foetal brindled (Mo^{br}) mice. *Biochem J* 186:629, 1980
107. HEYDORN K, DAMSGAARD E, HORN N, MIKKELSEN M, TYGSTRUP I, VESTERMARK S, WEBER J: Extra-hepatic storage of copper. A male foetus suspected of Menkes' disease. *Humangenetik* 29:171, 1975
108. HORN N: Menkes' X-linked disease: Prenatal diagnosis of hemizygous males and heterozygous female. *Prenat Diag* 1:107, 1981
109. HOLSTEIN TJ, FUNG RQ, QUEVEDO WC, BIENIEKI TC: Effect of altered copper metabolism induced by mottled alleles and diet on mouse tyrosinase. *Pro Soc Exp Biol Med* 162:264, 1979
110. HUNT DM: Catecholamine biosynthesis and the activity of a number of copper-dependent enzymes in the copper-deficient mottled mouse mutants. *Comp Biochem Physiol* 57:79, 1977
111. HUNT DM: Copper and neurological function, in CIBA Foundation Symposium 79: *Biological Roles of Copper*. Amsterdam, Excerpta Medica, 1980
112. PRINS HW, VAN DEN HAMER CJA: Abnormal copper-thionein synthesis and impaired copper utilization in mutated brindled mice: Model for Menkes' disease. *J Nutr* 110:151, 1980
121a. HAAS RH, ROBINSON A, EVANS K, LASCELLES PT, DUBOWITZ V: An X-linked disease of the nervous system with disordered copper metabolism and features differing from Menkes' disease. *Neurology (NY)*, 31:852, 1981
121b. BYERS PH, SIEGEL RC, HOLBROOK KA, NARAYANAN AS, BORNSTEIN P, HALL JG: An X-linked cutis laxa: Defective cross-link formation in collagen due to decreased lysyl oxidase activity. *N Engl J Med*, 303:61, 1980
113. CHAN W-Y, GARNICA AD, RENNERT OM: Inducibility of metallothionein biosynthesis in cultured normal and Menkes' kinky hair disease fibroblasts: Effects of copper and cadmium. *Pediatr Res* 13:197, 1979
114. HORN N, JENSEN OA: Menkes syndrome: Subcellular distribution of copper determined by an ultrastructural histochemical technique. *Ultrastruct Pathol* 1:237, 1980
115. GROVER WD, JOHNSON WC, HENKIN RI: Clinical and biochemical aspects of trichopoliodystrophy. *Ann Neurol* 5:65, 1979
116. WESENBERG RL, GWINN JL, BARNES GR: Radiological findings in the kinky-hair syndrome. *Radiology* 92:500, 1969
117. KOZLOWSKI K, McCROSSIN R: Early osseous abnormalities in Menkes' kinky-hair syndrome. *Pediatr Radiol* 8:191, 1979
118. ADAMS PC, STRAND RD, BRESNAN MJ, LUCKY AW: Kinky hair syndrome: Serial study of radiological findings with emphasis on similarity to the battered child syndrome. *Radiology* 112:401, 1974
119. HARA K, OOHIRA A, NOGAMI, H, WATANABE K, MIYAZAKI S: Kinky hair disease: Biochemical, histochemical, and ultrastructural studies. *Pediatr Res* 13:1222, 1979
120. SEELENFREUND MH, GARTNER S, VINGER PF: The ocular pathology of Menkes' disease. *Arch Ophthalmol* 80:718, 1968
121. PROCOPIS P, CAMAKARIS J, DANKS DM: A mild form of Menkes' syndrome. *J Pediatr*, 1981 (in press)
122. LUCKY AW, HSIA YE: Distribution of ingested and injected radiocopper in two patients with Menkes' kinky-hair disease. *Pediatr Res* 13:1280, 1980
123. DEKABAN AS, AAMODT R, RUMBLE WF, JOHNSTON GS, O'REILLY S: Kinky hair disease. Study of copper metabolism with use of ^{64}Cu. *Arch Neurol* 32:672, 1975
124. OAKES BW, DANKS DM, CAMPBELL PE: Human copper deficiency: Ultrastructural studies of the aorta and skin in a child with Menkes' syndrome. *Exp Mol Pathol* 25:82, 1976
125. GHATAK NR, HIRANO A, POON TP, FRENCH JH: Trichopoliodystrophy. II. Pathological changes in skeletal muscle and nervous system. *Arch Neurol* 26:60, 1972
126. HIRANO A, LLENA JF, FRENCH JH, GHATAK NR: Fine structure of the cerebellar cortex in Menkes' kinky-hair disease. X-chromosome-linked copper malabsorption. *Arch Neurol* 34:52, 1977
127. VUIA O, HEYE D: Neuropathologic aspects in Menkes' kinky hair disease (trichopoliodystrophy). *Neuropadiatrie* 5:329, 1974
128. GROVER WD, SCRUTTON MC: Copper therapy in trichopoliodystrophy. *J Pediatr* 86:216, 1975
129. VOLPINTESTA EJ: Menkes' kinky hair syndrome in a black infant. *Am J Dis Child* 128:244, 1974
130. IWAKAWA Y, NIWA T, TOMITA M: Menkes' kinky hair syndrome: Report on an autopsy case and his female sibling with similar clinical manifestations. *Brain Devel (Tokyo)* 11:260, 1979
131. HORN N: Menkes' X-linked disease: Heterozygous phenotypic uncloned fibroblast cultures. *J Med Genet* 17:257, 1980
132. HORN N, MOOY P, McGUIRE VM: Menkes X-linked disease: Two clonal cell populations in heterozygotes. *J Med Genet* 17:262, 1980

59

IDIOPATHIC HEMOCHROMATOSIS

THOMAS H. BOTHWELL

ROBERT W. CHARLTON

ARNO G. MOTULSKY

1. Hemochromatosis *is the term applied when organ structure and function are impaired by the presence of excessive quantities of iron in the parenchymal cells. The iron is stored predominantly as hemosiderin, and at least 15 g is found at the time of clinical presentation. The liver, heart, pancreas, endocrines, skin, and joints are principally affected, and cirrhosis, cardiomyopathy, diabetes mellitus, hypogonadism, pigmentation, and arthritis are the usual manifestations.*

2. *The iron enters the body either via the gastrointestinal tract, as a consequence of a failure of the mechanism limiting the absorption of dietary iron, or in the hemoglobin of transfused blood. Idiopathic hemochromatosis is the result of an inborn error of metabolism which leads to enhanced absorption. In thalassemia major and other refractory anemias characterized by a hyperplastic marrow with a large degree of ineffective erythropoiesis, intestinal absorption is also enhanced, and the iron overload is usually compounded by multiple transfusions.*

3. *The metabolic defect responsible for the excessive absorption of iron in idiopathic hemochromatosis has not been elucidated. The reticuloendothelial cells, as well as the upper intestinal mucosal cells, release more iron to the plasma than is needed. As a result they contain very little of the superfluous iron, and the binding capacity of the iron transport protein in plasma, trans-ferrin, is saturated. The reason why iron absorption is enhanced in those hyperplastic anemias, both genetic and acquired in which erythropoiesis is largely ineffective, is also not known.*

4. *Idiopathic hemochromatosis is an autosomal recessive disease. The gene for the disease is situated close to the HLA-A locus on the short arm of chromosome 6. The gene is present in the heterozygous state in 8 to 10 percent of some Caucasian populations, with approximately 3 in 1,000 of the population being homozygous. Phenotypic expression in homozygotes is dependent on the presence of sufficient quantities of absorbable iron in the diet. The average American diet permits a maximal positive daily iron balance of 2 to 4 mg in males, and the age of overt clinical presentation is thus usually 40 years or older.*

The clinical spectrum of homozygous idiopathic hemochromatosis has markedly altered with the discovery of many patients with early manifestations of the disease. The classical clinical pattern is only found in a small fraction of homozygotes carrying the iron-loading gene. In women, menstruation and the smaller dietary intake diminish the positive balance so that full phenotypic expression occurs at a later age and 10 times less often than in men. In countries such as India where the bioavailable iron content of the average diet is low, clinically manifest hemochromatosis has not

*been reported, and in Australia the large meat con-
sumption contributes to the high prevalence there.
Alcohol plays a part in many patients, contributing to
the organ damage and the iron loading.*

5. *The diagnosis of fully developed idiopathic hemochromatosis is made by establishing the presence of massive iron overload with a parenchymal distribution and
normal erythropoiesis. The finding of an elevated
plasma iron concentration with saturation of the iron-
binding capacity and a markedly raised plasma ferritin
concentration should lead to needle biopsy of the liver,
which provides a specimen for both chemical analysis
and histologic examination.*

6. *Once clinical manifestations have appeared, iron overload is eventually fatal unless the iron is eliminated.
The common causes of death are cardiac failure,
arrhythmia, hepatic failure, hepatoma or other malignancy, or the complications of diabetes. Elimination of
the iron is most conveniently achieved in idiopathic
hemochromatosis by weekly venesections of 5 to 6 dl
blood. These must be continued for up to 3 years
depending on the amount of iron in the body. Thereafter a venesection every 3 to 4 months is sufficient to
prevent reaccumulation of the iron. Removal of the iron
prolongs survival, cures the cardiomyopathy and the
skin pigmentation, and arrests the liver damage. Diabetes may improve, but hypogonadism and arthropathy do not, and hepatoma may develop even years
later.*

7. *The incomplete reversal of the effects of iron overload
by removal of the iron, and in particular the high incidence of hepatoma and other malignancies, oblige the
physician who discovers a patient with idiopathic
hemochromatosis to identify all homozygotes among
sibs. HLA typing followed by investigation of plasma
iron and ferritin and total iron-binding capacity can
establish the diagnosis of homozygous idiopathic
hemochromatosis in the absence of signs and symptoms. If venesections can be instituted before organ
damage has occurred, the consequences of phenotypic
expression of the disease can be avoided. Adult male
sibs who are at 25 percent genetic risk have the highest
probability of developing clinical manifestations.*

    *Heterozygotes in families with a clinically identified
patient will be detected by HLA typing. They may show
minor deviation in iron metabolism and with the passage of time some male heterozygotes can acquire a
minor iron load. Clinical manifestations of idiopathic
hemochromatosis have not yet been reported in such
carriers. No test for the detection of heterozygotes in the
population at large exists.*

8. *Hemochromatosis secondary to refractory anemia
must be treated with iron chelators. The best of these is
the iron-specific deferoxamine, but it must be given
parenterally.*

Although iron is the second most abundant metal in the earth's
crust, it exists almost exclusively in the ferric (Fe^{3+}) state,
which greatly reduces its accessibility. As a result, humans have
difficulty in acquiring enough from the environment for their
needs, and iron deficiency is a worldwide problem. In contrast,

iron overload is extremely uncommon and arises only in very
special circumstances. The occasional association of cirrhosis
with heavy hepatic deposits of the iron-containing compound
hemosiderin was first recognized toward the end of the last
century and the name *hemochromatosis* was given to the condition [1]. Idiopathic hemochromatosis is now known to be the
result of an inherited metabolic defect or defects, in which
excessive quantities of iron are absorbed from the diet. At the
same time it has become apparent that iron overload can arise
in other ways and that it may give rise to similar metabolic,
pathologic, and clinical consequences. Iron absorption inappropriate to body needs occurs in a number of refractory anemias caused by genetic defects, such as thalassemia major. An
additional factor in such subjects is the repeated transfusion of
blood, the hemoglobin iron thus bypassing the mechanism
which controls iron absorption. Multiple transfusions may
also give rise to iron overload in refractory anemias in which
absorption is not enhanced, such as aplastic anemia. Finally,
iron overload occurs in many South African blacks who have
no genetic defect but who absorb more iron than they require
from alcoholic beverages brewed in iron drums. In order to
understand iron overload and its metabolic consequence it is
essential to have a background knowledge of the normal content and distribution of iron in the body and of the processes
involved in the maintenance of iron balance.

The body of a healthy adult male contains between 3 and 4 g
iron [2]. The major portion is in the iron porphyrin complexes,
hemoglobin, myoglobin, and a variety of heme-containing
enzymes (Table 59-1). There are also many nonheme enzymes
which either contain iron or which require it as a cofactor. The
remaining iron in the body is stored as ferritin and hemosiderin, in which forms it is relatively nonreactive. The size of this
reserve of iron depends on the previous iron nutrition of the
individual and normally varies between 0 and 1000 mg. The
subsequent discussion will be confined to the storage complexes, since in iron overload the superfluous iron is present in
these forms. In addition, consideration will be given to the
iron-transport protein transferrin, which plays a key role in the
distribution of iron within the body.

THE METABOLISM OF IRON

Storage Iron

The diffuse, soluble, mobile fraction of storage iron is called
ferritin, and the insoluble, aggregated deposits are known as
hemosiderin [3]. Most of the storage iron in the body is normally in the form of ferritin, but with increasing degrees of iron
overload the proportion of hemosiderin rises progressively.
Ferritin consists of a protein shell surrounding an iron core.
Hemosiderin is a degraded form of ferritin in which the iron
cores are no longer associated with intact protein shells, the
result perhaps of the action of oxidizing agents [5] or partial
digestion following autophagocytosis [6, 7]. The ferritin core
has a maximum diameter of about 6 nm and can contain up to
4500 iron atoms [12] in the form of hydrous ferric oxide–
phosphate micelles (Fig. 59-1) [13, 14]. Horse spleen ferritin
protein is made up of 24 subunits, which on x-ray crystallography appear to be identical. Recent sequencing studies indicate that each subunit is made up of 174 amino acids and has a

Table 59-1   Iron-containing compounds in human beings.

		Milligrams in a 75-kg male (approximate)	Milligrams per kilogram (approximate)
Functional compounds	Hemoglobin	2300	31
	Myoglobin	320	4
	Heme enzymes	80	1
	Nonheme enzymes	100	1
		2800	37
Storage complexes	Ferritin	700	9
	Hemosiderin	300	4
		1000	13
Total		3800	50

molecular weight of 19,760 [16]. This means that the molecular weight of the apoferritin monomer is 473,000. The inner cavity of the ferritin molecule communicates with the exterior via six channels which decrease in diameter from 1.7 nm at the inner surface to 0.9 to 1.3 nm at the outer surface [17]. It is through these channels that iron enters and leaves the molecule.

Although ferritins are closely similar in all species [18], preparations of ferritin from various tissues exhibit a good deal of heterogeneity even within the same subject. These differences are well illustrated by electrofocusing. The isoelectric points (pI) for human liver and spleen ferritins range between 5.3 and 5.8, while heart contains ferritins with pI values between 4.8 and 5.2; the values for kidney ferritins are intermediate [19]. A plausible explanation for the presence of so many isoferritins in tissue has been propounded by Drysdale [20], namely that the variants consist of differing proportions of two subunits, the one (H) with a molecular weight of 21,000 and the other (L) with a molecular weight of 19,000. The H subunit is postulated to predominate in the more acidic ferritins present in the heart, and the L subunit in the more basic ferritins of liver and spleen. The proposal has not gone unchallenged. It has been claimed that the bands obtained on isoelectric focusing are artifacts caused by the pH gradient and that there is actually a continuous distribution of ferritin molecules of varying pI but the same subunit structure [21]. According to this view the differences in net charge on individual ferritin molecules, and the differences in size and antigenicity, represent posttranslational surface changes.

Whether the existence of isoferritins has physiologic significance is not known. While they all appear to be able to store iron reversibly, there is some evidence of differences in the rate of iron uptake in vitro [21]. More basic ferritins are synthesized in states of iron overload and more acidic ones by tumors, but these findings are by no means uniform [22].

Uptake and Release of Iron by Ferritin   When iron enters tissues, their ferritin content rises. This is due not only to the incorporation of iron into preexisting apoferritin but also to the specific stimulation of apoferritin synthesis. Accelerated apoferritin synthesis is detectable within 10 min of the entry of iron and is maximal within 5 h [23]. This may be due to an increase in ferritin messenger RNA [24], or in the proportion of subunits converted into apoferritin [25]. While apoferritin synthesis occurs preferentially on free polyribosomes, as much as 20 percent may be made on membrane-bound polyribosomes [26, 27].

Observations in vitro suggest that iron deposition in ferritin involves the oxidation of Fe^{2+}, which is catalyzed by the apo-ferritin with molecular oxygen as electron acceptor [28]. This is followed by hydrolysis and deposition of the ferric oxyhydroxide in the interior of the protein shell. Iron stored as ferritin is readily available for deployment in functional compounds when required. Rat liver ferritin has a half-life of about 50 to 70 h [23].

There is morphological evidence that lysosomes are involved in its breakdown [29]; the iron so released may be converted to hemosiderin, solubilized and stored again in fresh ferritin molecules, or incorporated into functional compounds. Iron can also be mobilized from ferritin without disruption of the molecule. This has been achieved in vitro using either Fe^{3+} chelators [30] or reducing agents such as cysteine, glutathione, and ascorbic acid [31]. However, the rates at which iron is mobilized by such means is slower than occurs physiologically. Of the biologic reductants that have been tested, by far the most rapid are the reduced riboflavins [32]. It has been proposed that NADH is responsible for reducing the riboflavins in the reaction (Fig. 59-2)[33].

Although ascorbic acid does not appear to be of crucial importance for the normal release of iron from ferritin, there is evidence that it does play some role in the mobilization of storage iron. When ascorbic acid deficiency is present there is a partial block in the release of iron from reticuloendothelial cells, which is rapidly corrected when ascorbic acid is administered [34, 35]. It is possible that ascorbic acid is required for the retrieval of hemosiderin iron, since another feature of

Figure 59-1   Diagrammatic representation of ferritin molecules. On the left is a partially filled ferritin molecule with a hydrous Fe(III) oxide microcrystal growing from a nucleation center inside the apoferritin shell: the arrows indicate addition and release of iron (or phosphate) at the microcrystal surface. For the single perfect microcrystal shown, addition and release would be expected to follow a "last-in–first-out" principle. On the right is a nearly full ferritin molecule containing three microcrystals not perfectly aligned: added ions (such as phosphate), represented by black circles, might be expected to bind both at crystalline surfaces and within the "imperfections." Ions bound within these faults would be released after those at surface positions. (*From Harrison [14]. Used by permission.*).

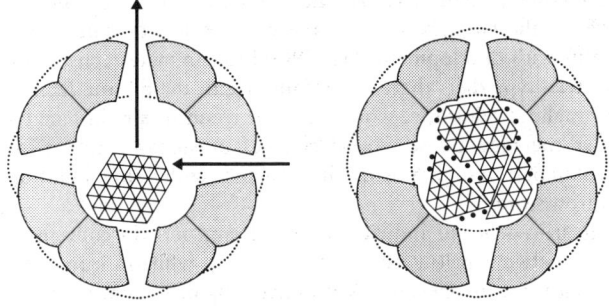

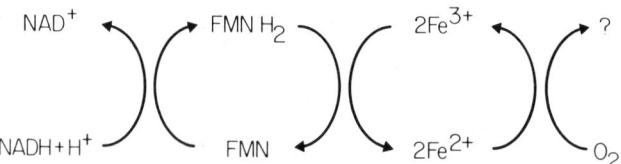

Figure 59-2 A proposed mechanism for the mobilization of iron from ferritin [33]. Reduced nicotinamide adenine dinucleotide (NADH) reduces flavin mononucleotide (FMN), which then reduces the Fe^{3+} of ferritin to Fe^{2+}, which then exits from the ferritin core. Ferrous iron is deposited in ferritin by oxidation with molecular oxygen.

experimental ascorbic acid deficiency is an increased hemosiderin/ferritin ratio in the storage depots, which rapidly returns to normal when the ascorbic acid deficiency is corrected [34].

Sites of Iron Storage   In normal subjects most of the body's iron reserve is present in roughly equal proportions in the liver, bone marrow, and skeletal muscles [2]. In the liver 95 percent of the ferritin is in hepatocytes [36], while most of the hemosiderin, which becomes visible with concentrations of iron greater than 0.25 mg/g, is present in Kupffer cells [37]. This may be due to the fact that there is less space available for storage in Kupffer cells, as they are less than one-tenth the size of hepatocytes [38]. Storage iron in the bone marrow and spleen is confined to reticuloendothelial cells, and there is some evidence that the iron in skeletal muscle is also located in reticuloendothelial cells lying between the muscle fibers rather than in the muscles themselves [39]. The iron stored in hepatocytes is derived from plasma transferrin [40] and to a lesser extent from hemoglobin-haptoglobin and heme-hemopexin complexes [41]. Reticuloendothelial cells derive their iron from broken-down red cells.

Plasma Ferritin as a Measure of Storage Iron   Minute amounts of ferritin normally circulate in the plasma [42]. This ferritin has a low iron content [43, 44] and probably has the same molecular weight as spleen ferritin [43]. While its origin is speculative, there is some evidence that it arises from reticuloendothelial cells [45]. The fact that a large proportion of the protein is glycosylated is in keeping with the concept that it is a secretory protein, perhaps arising in membrane-bound polyribosomes [3, 46]. Ferritin has a half-life in the plasma of only about 10 min [47–49] and is almost completely taken up by hepatocytes [50, 51].

In normal subjects there is a close correlation between the plasma ferritin concentration and the size of the body iron stores, with each microgram per liter of ferritin being equivalent to about 8 mg storage iron [52]. The geometric mean value of plasma ferritin for normal adult males has been found to be approximately 100 µg/liter and for premenopausal females about one-third of this [53]. The marked variations at different ages in the two sexes reflect the changes in iron nutritional status with development (Fig. 59-3) [47]. In males consuming western-type diets there is a steady rise in the plasma ferritin throughout adult life, while a similar trend occurs in females after the menopause. These changes presumably reflect, at least in part, a slight positive iron balance with a slow build-up in iron stores.

In iron-deficient individuals the plasma ferritin concentration is always below 12 µg/liter [53–55], while in iron overload it is greatly elevated. With increasing degrees of overload the relationship between the plasma ferritin concentration and

the size of the body iron stores becomes less precise. There are three possible reasons. First, the tissue damage associated with severe iron overload may lead to the release of ferritin from necrosed cells, especially hepatocytes [46, 56]. Second, there is some evidence that the secretion of glycosylated ferritin from reticuloendothelial cells eventually reaches a plateau, perhaps reflecting a maximum rate of synthesis [46]. Third, in guinea pigs ascorbic acid deficiency has been shown to produce falsely low plasma ferritin concentrations [57], and iron overload predisposes to ascorbic acid deficiency (see later section of this chapter). A simple relationship between the plasma ferritin concentration and the size of the iron stores should therefore not be assumed with ferritin values above 4000 µg/liter, or in patients who have received more than 100 units of transfused blood [46].

There are several situations in which the plasma ferritin concentrations may be inappropriately high for the size of the body iron stores. The first, *hepatic damage,* has already been mentioned. It can occur in both acute and chronic conditions, and particularly high values have been noted with viral and drug-induced liver disease [55, 56, 58]. The source of the ferritin in such circumstances is damaged hepatocytes. Raised ferritin concentrations are also a feature of *inflammation,* and in one study a mean value of 350 µg/liter (range 10 to 1650 µg/liter) was found in 39 patients with various infections [55]. While some of the elevation could be ascribed to the partial block in reticuloendothelial iron release, with the consequential increase in reticuloendothelial iron stores that is a feature of infection, this explanation did not appear to be the only factor. Other types of inflammatory reaction, such as those produced by endotoxin, surgical procedures [59] and rheumatoid arthritis [60] have also been associated with high plasma ferritin concentrations, as have a number of *neoplasms* [3, 61], including hepatoma [62, 63], breast cancer [43, 64], and acute leukemia [3, 65, 66]. It is not clear whether the raised concentrations in neoplastic diseases are due to the production of specific carcinofetal ferritins, to liver damage, or to disturbances in iron metabolism induced by the tumor [3].

Transferrin

Proteins specialized for the transport of iron (transferrins) have evolved in parallel with dependence on hemoglobin for oxygen

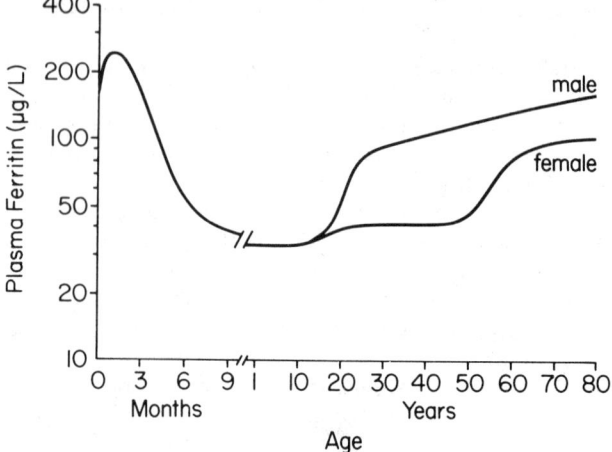

Figure 59-3 The mean plasma ferritin concentrations in American males and females at different ages. (*From Siimes, Addiego, and Dallman* [47]. *Used by permission.*)

transport and appear to be essential for the efficient distribution of iron [2]. Transferrin in the plasma picks up iron from donor cells, binds it very tightly, and delivers it to specific receptors on recipient cells. Only with such a system can the iron requirements of the erythroid marrow and the placenta, which are as much as a hundredfold greater than those of other tissues, be met. As much as 50 to 60 percent of the total amount of plasma transferrin is present in extracellular fluids, including lymph, cerebrospinal fluid, and edema fluid [67]. There is increasing evidence that transferrins are involved in intracellular as well as extracellular iron transport, e.g., in the transfer of iron across the intestinal mucous membrane during absorption [68, 69].

Transferrin is a single-chain polypeptide with two iron-binding sites, each residing in its own domain comprising about half the molecule [70]. The molecular weight is 76,000 [71], and it has a prolate ellipsoid shape with an axial ratio of 1:3, decreasing to 2:5 when iron is bound [72]. Two identical doubly branched carbohydrate chains terminating in sialic acid are attached to asparaginyl residues [73, 74]. Some 21 genetic variants have been identified by electrophoresis [75, 76]. They probably represent single amino acid substitutions, since no differences in molecular weight, carbohydrate content, or iron distribution have been established. Although a number of tissues can synthesize transferrin, the origin of most of the plasma transferrin is the liver [77]. Transferrin half-life in the plasma is about 8 days. In normal subjects it is present in amounts capable of binding about 330 µg iron per deciliter of plasma. The concentration rises in iron deficiency and falls in iron overload; there is thus an inverse relationship with the plasma ferritin concentration [55]. Factors which lower the plasma transferrin concentration other than an increase in the body iron stores are the nephrotic syndrome and protein-losing enteropathies, protein malnutrition, hemolysis, and inflammation of various origins including infections, rheumatoid arthritis, myocardial infarction, and malignant neoplasms [2]. An increased transferrin concentration is found not only when the body iron reserve is diminished but also in pregnancy, even when there is no iron deficiency, and in women taking estrogen-containing contraceptives [2]. The iron-binding capacity of transferrin is normally only about one-third saturated, so that the plasma iron concentration is of the order of 120 µg/dl. There is a considerable circadian variation, with a morning peak and an evening trough, due principally to variation in the donation of iron to transferrin by the cells of the reticuloendothelial system [78, 79]. In addition to the circadian fluctuation there are sizable day-to-day variations. Variation in the quantity of iron stored in the body has little effect until the iron reserve has been exhausted, when the concentration falls. In iron deficiency anemia the transferrin saturation is diminished by the reduced plasma iron concentration and the increased transferrin concentration [80]. The plasma iron concentration may be temporarily reduced by a transient imbalance between supply and demand, for example on starting treatment of pernicious anemia with vitamin B_{12}. The concentration is also lowered by the defective release of reticuloendothelial iron induced by inflammation, whether of infective, traumatic, neoplastic, or other origin. This has been shown to be secondary to increased ferritin synthesis within reticuloendothelial cells [81]. The concomitant fall in transferrin concentration means that the transferrin saturation is not as low as it is in iron deficiency.

The Binding and Release of Transferrin Iron Transferrin binds iron in the ferric (Fe^{3+}) form together with car-

bonate, or perhaps bicarbonate [82]. During the binding there is a transformational change and a characteristic salmon-pink color develops with an absorption maximum at 465 nm. The phenolic hydroxide groups of two tyrosine residues [84], at least one nitrogen ligand [85], two histidyl residues [86] [which may contribute the nitrogen ligand(s)], and possibly a water molecule [87], are required for binding at each site. The binding is markedly pH-dependent, being maximal (association rate of about $1024M-1$) above pH 7; dissociation commences at pH 6.5 and is virtually complete by pH 4.5. The binding constants at the two sites appear not to be identical [88], and differential loading can be achieved by substituting anions such as nitrilotriacetate or citrate for the physiologic carbonate, or other metals for iron [84, 89]. Differential release also occurs when the pH is lowered and with certain chelators [83]. Such observations have lent support to the view that iron is preferentially removed from one or other of the binding sites by different tissues [90]. While experiments apparently demonstrating this phenomenon have been reported, the methodological problems are formidable and the validity of the conclusions has been questioned [83, 91–93]. Such objections do not appear to apply to a recent study in which rabbit reticulocytes were incubated with diferric rabbit transferrin, and the proportions of diferric, N-terminal monoferric, C-terminal monoferric, and apotransferrin were determined at intervals [94]. The C-terminal monoferric species appeared initially about twice as fast as apotransferrin, indicating that iron was being removed preferentially from the N-terminal site of the diferric transferrin. Later the rate of appearance of apotransferrin was similar to the rate of disappearance of diferric transferrin, and eventually the concentration of both monoferric species declined. Both sites could therefore donate iron to the reticulocytes. Nevertheless, there is no in vivo evidence that the distribution of transferrin iron among the different tissues is affected by binding to one or the other site. It is generally agreed that the amount of transferrin iron taken up by erythroid precursors and other tissues is dependent on the degree of saturation of the transferrin [95–98], the rate of iron delivery being considerably greater from diferric transferrin than from monoferric transferrin [92, 99].

During the delivery of iron to red cell precursors the transferrin is initially adsorbed to the red cell membrane. This is a very rapid and nonspecific process, probably dependent on electrostatic forces [100], and is a function of the transferrin concentration[101]. A stronger attachment to specific receptors develops during the fixation phase, and this requires metabolic energy [102]. These receptors have been isolated from immature erythroid cell membranes and partially characterized [103–105], as have transferrin receptors on placenta [106, 107] and other tissues. The evidence indicates that the transferrin iron–receptor complex is transported into the interior of the cell by endocytosis before the iron is released by an energy-dependent process [108]. In vitro evidence suggests that the release of the iron is preceded by a reaction with H^+, possibly liberating the carbonate [109]. The apotransferrin is then returned to the plasma.

Internal Iron Exchange

Over the last several years general agreement has been obtained on quantitative aspects of internal iron exchange in health and disease [96, 110]. These concepts have largely been developed from studies in which the transferrin has been labeled with radioiron. Two approaches have been used. In one, the exchange of iron between plasma transferrin and individual tissues has been studied in vivo and in vitro. In the other, attempts have been made to characterize all internal iron exchange, in particular the behavior of the erythroid marrow, by detailed analysis of the patterns of disappearance of transferrin-bound radioiron from the circulation and its subsequent reappearance in erythrocytes.

Plasma iron follows three main pathways (Fig. 59-4). By far the largest fraction goes to the erythron, with virtually all this iron being incorporated into hemoglobin. Radioiron appears within circulating erythrocytes after an interval during which cell maturation takes place within the marrow. There is some "wastage" as a result of intramedullary death of some red cells. These cells are either phagocytosed in the reticuloendothelial system, or the hemoglobin released from them is bound to haptoglobin and transported to hepatocytes [41]. The second pathway of internal iron exchange is from plasma transferrin to parenchymal cells, particularly those of the liver. The flow of iron along this pathway is normally small, but if there is a decrease in erythroid marrow uptake, virtually all the plasma iron can be deposited in the liver parenchyma [40]. The third pathway is one in which iron leaves the circulation and passes into the extravascular tissues.

Most of the iron entering the plasma for distribution by transferrin is contributed by the cells of the reticuloendothelial system. This iron is derived mainly from hemoglobin catabolism, but there is also a contribution from storage compounds. A much smaller fraction is donated by other tissues, particularly those containing significant portions of the body iron reserve, such as hepatocytes. About 3 percent of the plasma iron turnover is normally iron absorbed from the diet by the mucosal cells of the upper small intestine. Unless the body iron stores are exhausted, the supply of iron to the plasma pool is capable of adjustment within wide limits to match changing demands. The requirement for transferrin iron is determined by the state of activity of the major recipient, the erythroid marrow. Thus in chronic hemolytic states, the quantity of iron passing through the plasma can increase six- to eightfold, while it diminishes to one-third on descending from high altitudes when erythropoiesis comes to a virtual standstill [40]. The regulation of reticuloendothelial iron release proceeds rapidly so that there are only transient changes in the plasma iron con-

centration. Little is known of how this homeostasis is achieved. Apart from the placenta in pregnancy, the number of parenchymal cell receptors for transferrin is not known to vary in a manner similar to the number of erythroid precursors. Parenchymal uptake of transferrin iron does vary, however, the determinant being the amount of transferrin iron in the plasma [96]. Parenchymal iron loading therefore occurs to an increasing degree as the transferrin iron saturation rises above the normal one-third.

External Iron Exchange

For adequate iron nutrition a positive iron balance is necessary during childhood and adolescence. In this way the growing demand of the body for functional iron is satisfied and storage depots are gradually built up. Thereafter the amounts absorbed from the diet must at least match the average daily losses from the body. Additional amounts must be absorbed to meet the requirements of pregnancy and to replace any abnormal losses through blood donation or hemorrhage.

Iron Excretion   Iron is lost from the body physiologically by desquamation of surface cells from the skin, gastrointestinal and urinary tracts, and from the minimal gastrointestinal blood loss which occurs even in healthy individuals. There are also very low concentrations of extracellular iron in the sweat, bile, and urine. In women the losses incurred through menstruation and pregnancy must be added. Using a variety of chemical and radioisotopic techniques it has been possible to define these losses in moderately precise terms. Total daily iron losses in adult males amount to between 0.9 and 1 mg [12 to 14 $\mu g/(kg \cdot day)$] [111]. Most of this is from the gastrointestinal tract, with 0.45 mg due to blood loss and 0.15 mg from bile and desquamated cells [111]. A further 0.2 to 0.3 mg is shed from the skin, while daily urinary iron losses amount to 0.1 mg.

Skin losses are not increased significantly by the excessive sweating that occurs in hot, humid climates. Basal iron losses are affected only to a limited degree by the iron content of the body. They are reduced to about half in iron deficiency [112] and may be increased up to twice normal in states of iron overload [111].

Because of their smaller surface areas, basal daily losses in women would be expected to be correspondingly less than in men, about 0.7 to 0.8 mg. The mean normal menstrual losses when expressed in terms of daily iron balance are approximately 0.5 mg, but there is considerable variation, and it has been calculated that in 5 percent of normal women the figure is greater than 1.4 mg [113]. During pregnancy the requirement is even greater, since an expanding maternal red cell mass and a growing fetus and placenta must be supplied. When these various requirements are added to the basal losses, it has been calculated that about 1 g iron is needed for each pregnancy [2]. This is equivalent to an average daily requirement of between 5 and 6 mg throughout the last two trimesters. Not all this iron is lost to the body, since that present in the expanded maternal red cell mass is returned to stores at the end of pregnancy.

Iron Absorption   The amount of iron absorbed from the diet at any one time is dependent on three factors—the quantity of iron, the composition of the diet, and the behavior of the mucosa of the upper small bowel.

Figure 59-4   The approximate amounts of iron, in milligrams per day, exchanging between different body compartments in a 70-kg subject. These data are largely based on ferrokinetic analyses. (*From Bothwell, et al. [2]. Used by permission.*)

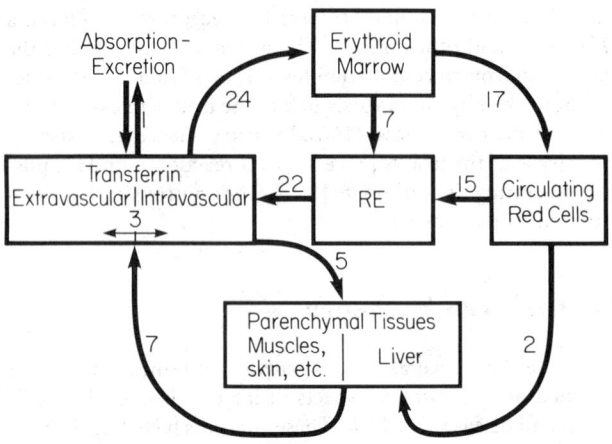

DIETARY IRON CONTENT   Typical western diets usually contain about 6 mg iron per 1000 kcal, with surprisingly little variation from meal to meal [114]. In certain circumstances the iron content is appreciably increased by extrinsic iron, either in the form of dirt or from the surface of containers or cooking vessels. The former is usually of very low bioavailability [115, 116], but iron derived from pans or skillets can add significantly to the absorbable iron intake, especially when the pH of the food being prepared in them is low [117]. This is strikingly illustrated by the traditional alcoholic beverages brewed in iron containers by South African blacks, whose daily iron intake may be increased from about 15 mg to as much as 100 mg as a result [118].

BIOAVAILABILITY OF IRON   Variations in the bioavailability of food iron are of greater importance for iron nutrition than is the amount of iron in the diet. Of prime importance is the difference between the bioavailability of heme iron, which is easily absorbed whatever the dietary composition, and nonheme iron, which is usually of low bioavailability and markedly affected by other ingredients in the meal [2]. When three major grain staples were fed as single foodstuffs, absorption of the iron contained within them was uniformly low (1 to 7 percent). In contrast, the absorption of fish and meat iron varied between 12 and 22 percent [119, 120]. Heme iron is well absorbed because it is taken up by mucosal cells as such, and the iron within it is therefore not exposed to the effects of the many ligands in the diet that inhibit iron absorption [121]. There is another reason why meat has an important effect on iron nutrition: it promotes the absorption of the various forms of nonheme iron present in a mixed diet [122]. The reason for this is not known, but it may relate to the release of amino acids during digestion which form complexes with iron that remain soluble in spite of the rise in pH during transit through the upper small intestine [123]. The other important promoter of the absorption of nonheme iron is ascorbic acid [124, 125], which not only is a powerful reductant, but also binds iron in equimolar amounts. Its action is dose-dependent and it is effective in a number of dietary settings [124–126]. It plays a particularly critical role when little or no meat is present, and it is therefore essential to know the ascorbic acid content of a diet when considering its iron nutritive value [127].

A number of inhibitors of iron absorption have been recognized [128]. On the basis of in vitro studies it has been suggested that carbonates, oxalates, phosphates, and phytates form large polymeric complexes with iron which are poorly absorbed [129], but their role in vivo remains uncertain. The only dietary constituents that have been unequivocally shown to inhibit the absorption of nonheme food iron are bran [130], the tannates in Indian tea [131], and the phosphoprotein in egg yolk [132]. A negative correlation between iron absorption and fecal bulk has suggested that factors in vegetable fibers may have an inhibiting effect [133]. Further studies indicate that pectin may be one such factor, but that cellulose has no effect on nonheme iron absorption [134].

The effects of the secretions of the upper intestinal tract on nonheme iron absorption must be added to those of exogenous dietary ligands. During peptic digestion a part of the nonheme iron in food is rendered ionizable [135]. In addition, heme is split from its globin bond [136]. Gastric hydrochloric acid plays a key role and has been shown to be necessary for the adequate absorption of ferric iron salts [137, 138] and of nonheme food iron [139]. This is presumably because polymeric

iron complexes are less likely to form at low pH. While other components of the gastric juices must obviously be relevant to iron absorption in that they promote digestion with release of iron from food, they do not contain a specific carrier [139]. There is also no evidence that pancreatic, biliary, and intestinal secretions have any direct effect on iron absorption [2].

MUCOSAL BEHAVIOR   The most active site of iron absorption is the duodenum and upper jejunum [140, 141]. There are two components to the absorptive mechanism, *uptake* from the lumen of the gut into the intestinal epithelial cells, and *transfer* into the body. In animal studies it has been shown that the uptake of iron is linear over a wide range (0.1 to 5.0 mM), but the slope of the line varies depending on the body's iron requirement [142]. A proportion of the iron entering the mucosal cell is transferred to the portal circulation within minutes. Transfer continues at a much slower rate for 12 to 24 h, but some of the iron is stored as ferritin and is eventually discarded when the mucosal cell exfoliates [143, 144]. The relative proportions of iron that follow these alternative pathways depend on the requirement for iron, transfer being enhanced when iron deficiency is present and ferritin formation being maximal when the body is replete with iron [145]. The carrier transporting iron through mucosal cells has been identified as a protein similar to but not identical with plasma transferrin [68, 69].

There is now abundant evidence that the amount of iron absorbed at any one time is markedly influenced by the body iron content (Fig. 59-5). If the body iron content is diminished a high proportion of the available iron is absorbed, and as the body iron content rises the percentage of absorption falls [146–148]. Absorption is therefore inversely related to the plasma ferritin concentration, which reflects the body iron reserve [53, 148–151]. In early animal experiments a direct relationship was also noted between iron absorption and the rate of erythropoiesis [152], but in humans the situation is more complicated. Absorption is not enhanced in chronic hemolytic states such as hereditary spherocytosis [153], but there are exceptions. The most notable is thalassemia major, in which progressive iron overload occurs, partly because of the

Figure 59-5   The inverse relationship between the percentage absorption of a 3-mg dose of ferrous iron and the nonheme marrow iron concentration in a group of 50 subjects. (*From Bezwoda et al.* [148]. *Used by permission.*)

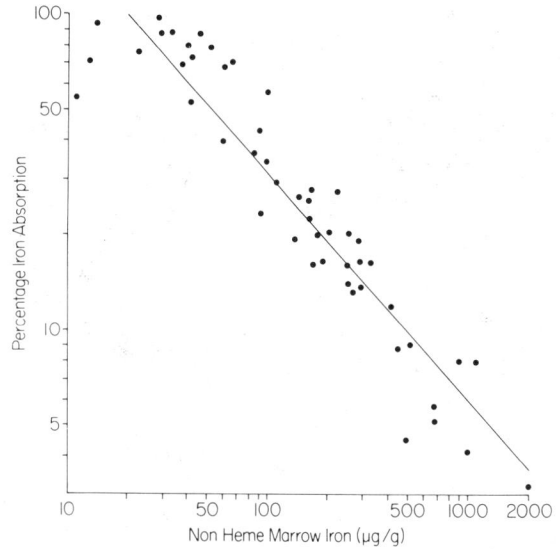

regular blood transfusions but also because iron absorption is inappropriately high [154–156]. The iron-loading anemias are those characterized by markedly ineffective erythropoiesis [2]. In these conditions the rate of iron absorption is greatest in subjects with the lowest hemoglobin concentrations [155, 156].

While the rate of absorption varies under certain circumstances, the control mechanisms have not been elucidated. It has been suggested that the regulation is a local one, perhaps mediated by changes in the luminal secretions, the brush border receptors for iron, the intracellular transport protein, or ability of the cells to sequester ferritin [157–160], but no definitive evidence favors any of these possibilities [2]. Attempts to demonstrate that the plasma iron-transport system regulates iron absorption have been equally unsuccessful [161, 162], as have those involving a search for some humoral controlling mechanism [163]. Perhaps the most plausible of current hypotheses is that the iron content of individual tissues is itself a regulating factor [164]. A labile pool of iron available to transferrin is assumed to be present in all body tissues, the size of the pool in each tissue being proportional to the iron stores in that tissue. Iron uptake from transferrin is determined by the requirements of the erythroid marrow, and each tissue supplies iron to transferrin in proportion to its iron pool (Fig. 59-6) [165]. Thus a decrease in tissue iron content results in an increased entrance of iron from the gut, while a rise in plasma iron turnover due to enhanced erythropoietic activity also results in increased iron absorption. Recent experimental evidence supporting the hypothesis has been obtained in rats [163]. When the requirement for transferrin iron was increased by the exchange transfusion of blood containing many reticulocytes, there was a doubling in the rate of tissue iron donation within minutes, with no detectable change in the plasma iron concentration. It was concluded that iron turnover through the plasma is primarily determined by the number of tissue receptors for transferrin iron, and that the amount of iron supplied by each donor tissue, including the intestinal mucosa, is dependent on the output from other donor tissues.

Figure 59-6 The regulation of internal iron exchange. The plasma iron turnover is visualized as a conveyer belt driven by the uptake of transferrin iron by erythroid precursors. The amount of iron released at any one time from donor sites onto transferrin is dependent on the amounts of iron being removed by the erythroid precursors [165].

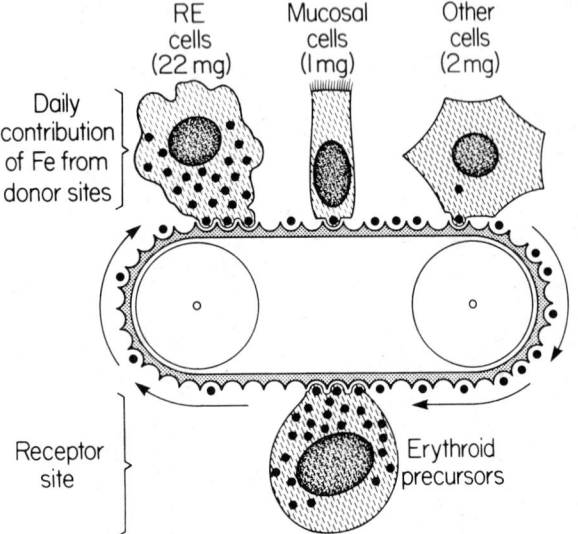

The mechanism by which donor tissue output of iron is regulated to match changing requirements still eludes explanation.

Quantitative Aspects of Iron Absorption Although the daily intake of dietary iron normally varies between 10 and 20 mg, the amount absorbed is much less than this. In the iron-replete adult male consuming a mixed western diet the amount of iron absorbed each day matches the obligatory basal losses of about 1.0 mg. In the female absorption is somewhat greater during her reproductive years, since menstruation increases physiologic losses to about 1.4 mg daily [113]. The absorptive behavior of the intestinal mucosa changes in an attempt to maintain the body iron content at optimal levels, but the amount of dietary iron that can be absorbed is limited because of its restricted bioavailability. Absorption rises to only 3 to 4 mg daily when the body is depleted of iron and falls to less than 0.5 mg daily when iron overload is present (Fig. 59-7). These figures underline the small amount of daily external iron exchange in relation to the total body iron content.

One final point merits comment. The figures for iron absorption given in the previous paragraph relate to people consuming western-type diets. In countries such as India, in which the population subsists on cereal diets containing little meat or ascorbic acid, the iron is even less bioavailable, and the ability of the body to step up absorption is therefore even more restricted.

IDIOPATHIC HEMOCHROMATOSIS

An inherited metabolic abnormality, the nature of which has still to be established, idiopathic hemochromatosis, leads to the absorption of more iron than is required, and in a proportion of affected individuals massive quantities may eventually be present in the body [2]. The process extends over many years. When the diagnosis is made *clinically*, cirrhosis and skin pigmentation are almost always present, often accompanied by diabetes mellitus, hypogonadism, arthritis, and cardiac failure. Even in the early stages the plasma iron concentration is high and the plasma transferrin is saturated with iron. Deposits of hemosiderin in the liver and other organs become more and more prominent as the years pass. Organ damage occurs only after markedly increased concentrations of stored iron have accumulated. It is important to stress the quantitative aspect of the iron overload. Cirrhosis with mild or even moderate hemosiderosis is relatively common and must be differentiated from idiopathic hemochromatosis. Failure to distinguish between the two conditions has in the past led to confusion. In order to avoid this pitfall one of the quantitative approaches discussed in a later section should be adopted.

Genetics of Idiopathic Hemochromatosis

Mode of Inheritance For a review of the genetic principles underlying the following discussion see Chap. 1. Idiopathic hemochromatosis is an inherited disease, since abnormalities in iron metabolism can consistently be demonstrated among relatives of affected patients [166]. This is not the case

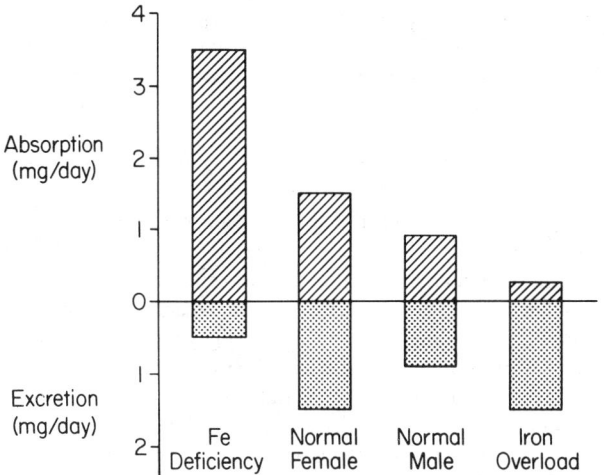

Figure 59-7 A diagrammatic representation of the average amounts of iron absorbed and excreted daily by normal, iron-deficient and iron-loaded subjects consuming a western-type diet.

in families of cirrhotic patients with increased liver iron [167]. For many years the finding of detectable abnormalities in iron metabolism among children or parents of patients suggested autosomal dominant inheritance of the disease. More detailed studies of many families, however, has established that the vertical transmission of overt and full-blown clinical hemochromatosis is relatively rare, although it is usual to find minor abnormalities in iron metabolism among children and parents as well as sibs. Full-blown clinical hemochromatosis is most frequently seen in adult males [166]. Genetic analysis of such data led to the hypothesis that idiopathic hemochromatosis is an autosomal recessive condition with expression of the full clinical disease largely limited to adult males, while the minor abnormalities in iron metabolism apparent in other family members were manifestations of the heterozygous carrier state [168, 169]. The problems of delayed clinical expression and the low manifestation rate in females made interpretation difficult, and no consensus regarding the mode of inheritance existed until recently.

HLA STUDIES CLARIFY AUTOSOMAL RECESSIVE TRANSMISSION A fortuitous observation that HLA-A3 was frequently found among patients with hemochromatosis [170] was confirmed in many series of patients of European origin [171–179] and has clarified the mode of inheritance [180]. While HLA-A3 occurs in no more than 30 percent of persons of European origin, it was present in 73 percent of 384 hemochromatotic patients in a collective series [166]. HLA-B14 was also more frequently found than among controls [166]. In contrast, the frequencies of HLA-A3 and HLA-B14 in patients with cirrhosis and increased liver iron did not differ from those in controls [181]. Many different diseases have been observed to be associated with one or several HLA alleles (see Chap. 3). While the pathogenetic explanation of such "associations" often remains poorly understood [182], the possibility of genetic linkage (i.e., the physical proximity of the HLA locus to a disease-producing gene) must always be considered, particularly when HLA association occurs with a monogenic disease such as idiopathic hemochromatosis [183]. Family investigations indicated that a gene for idiopathic hemochromatosis is located in close proximity to the supergene for HLA (including

loci for HLA-A, B, C, D, and others) on the short arm of chromosome 6, since such a gene is usually transmitted together with the adjoining HLA haplotype [184, 185]. Sibs with overt hemochromatosis in a given family usually share both their HLA haplotypes, i.e., have identical HLA alleles on both maternal and paternal chromosomes. Thus, a chromosomal segment comprising a gene for idiopathic hemochromatosis and a linked group of HLA genes is contributed by *both* father and mother to each affected offspring (Fig. 59-8) [186]. These data establish homozygosity and autosomal recessive inheritance for the disease. The genetic locus for hemochromatosis is clearly distinct from any of the HLA loci, since different HLA-A alleles—not only HLA-A3—may be found in various hemochromatotic kindreds. HLA-A3—B14 is the most common haplotype. Among all homozygous hemochromatotic patients who are HLA-A3 positive, about 70 percent carry a single dose of the A3 allele, while the remainder are homozygous for HLA-A3 [166]. Recombination between the HLA-A and HLA-B loci has been observed in hemochromatosis [187], but the distance between the idiopathic hemochromatosis gene and HLA-A is very small, and recombinants between these loci are very rare [185]. A recombination fraction of 1 percent has been calculated [183]. The gene for idiopathic hemochromatosis therefore appears to be located closer to the HLA-A locus than to the other HLA loci. Whether it is distal to the HLA-A locus or between the HLA-A and HLA-B loci remains unknown.

PREVALENCE AND GENETIC FREQUENCIES Fully developed idiopathic hemochromatosis is uncommon but not excessively rare. By 1935, 350 well-documented cases had been reported [189], and during the next 20 years there were another 800 [4]. Since 1955 many further reports have appeared [2]. Phenotypic expression of the HLA-linked iron-loading gene obviously depends not only on the gene frequency in the population but also on the amount of iron which can be absorbed from the average diet. Because this is limited, as has already been discussed, iron overload of any cause occurs infrequently in most communities. In a study in which the storage iron concentrations in almost 4000 liver specimens from 18 different countries were measured, only 3 were found to be more than 5 times normal concentration and none of these was anywhere near the hemochromatotic range of 20 to 50 times normal [189]. In

Figure 59-8 Hypothetical distribution of iron-loading alleles, each designated by an HLA haplotype, among family members of a patient (1) with fully developed idiopathic hemochromatosis. The topographic relationships between the gene (■) and the HLA loci (o) are diagrammatic approximations. The mother of the patient has two number 6 chromosomes, designated a and b, of which chromosome a carries the mutant allele of the hemochromatosis locus. In the father the mutant allele occurs on the sixth chromosome that is designated c. The patient inherited both mutant genes and is a homozygote.

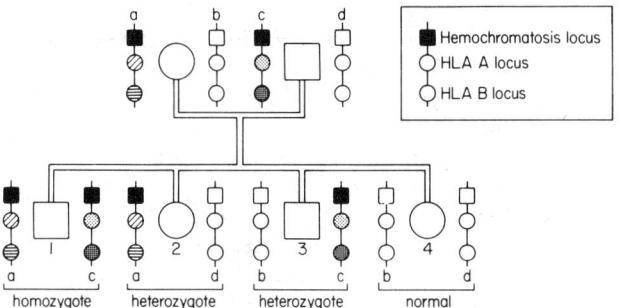

addition, none of more than 3000 apparently normal individuals in the Seattle, Washington, area had a plasma ferritin concentration approaching that found in idiopathic hemochromatosis [190]. In one comprehensive review the prevalence of clinically or pathologically identifiable idiopathic hemochromatosis was estimated to be 1 in 20,000 hospital admissions and 1 in 7000 deaths [4]. The prevalence in Olmstead County, Minnesota, was calculated to be 4 per 100,000 [1], but in Glasgow, Scotland, it was as high as 1 in 556 male necropsies [191].

More recent data from Utah (USA) and Brittanny (France) indicate that the HLA-linked genetic defect does indeed occur a good deal more commonly than its clinical expression suggests [186, 192]. In these studies the heterozygote carriers of the iron-loading gene were identified in families of affected homozygotes by HLA typing. As many as 8.4 percent and 10.5 percent, respectively, of the two populations were considered to be heterozygote carriers, yielding calculated homozygote frequencies of 1 in 319 (Utah) and 1 in 400 (Brittany). While biased ascertainment may have affected these figures, they suggest that the HLA-linked iron-loading gene is one of the most common abnormal genes, at least in some populations. The similar frequencies among two different populations of European origin is striking.

With relatively rare autosomal recessive diseases one expects to find a higher frequency of consanguinity among parents of affected patients, but this would be less likely with more common genes such as this one. The increased frequency of consanguinity in one of the early French studies is therefore hard to interpret [169, 193]. One would need to hypothesize that there is a series of rare hemochromatosis alleles (h^1, h^2, h^3, . . .) which in the homozygous state (i.e., h^1h^1, h^2h^2, h^3h^3, etc.), but *not* in the compound heterozygous state (i.e., h^1h^2, h^2h^3, h^1h^3, . . .) are capable of producing the clinical picture of idiopathic hemochromatosis. Genetic heterogeneity for idiopathic hemochromatosis remains a possibility, and the existence of other genes in addition to the hemachromatosis locus linked to the HLA complex cannot be excluded. The hypothesis of two different discrete genes on chromosome 6 as the cause of hemochromatosis is unlikely [166].

If the HLA-linked iron-loading gene is common, matings between homozygous individuals and heterozygote carriers would not be infrequent. Even with a homozygote frequency of 1/10,000 (q^2), 2 percent of the population would be heterozygote carriers (2pq), and therefore 2 percent of all matings by homozygotes would be with a carrier. If the data from France and Utah are representative, then the frequency is even higher. Since 50 percent of the children of homozygote × heterozygote matings would be homozygotes, the explanation for the observed "vertical" pedigree pattern mimicking autosomal dominant inheritance (i.e., pseudodominance) is apparent.

ORIGIN OF THE GENE The reason for the high frequency of the HLA-linked iron-loading gene is unknown. It is possible that in the past heterozygotes had a selective advantage if they absorbed more dietary iron and were therefore relatively protected against developing iron deficiency with its deleterious effects [180]. It is conceivable that the accumulation of larger body iron reserves improved survival during infancy, childhood, and pregnancy or conferred a higher fertility in comparison with the rest of the population. As a result, there would have been a gradual increase in the frequency of the gene. Selection against subjects homozygous for idiopathic hemo-

chromatosis is minimal, since the disease exerts its harmful effects only after the reproductive period is over, at a time when such patients have transmitted their abnormal genes to their offspring. Alternatively, it is possible that the gene reached a high frequency because of "hitchhiking" with the closely linked HLA complex. According to this hypothesis, positive selection of an unknown nature would have resulted from possession not of the iron-loading gene, but of some other gene or genes in the HLA cluster.

The high frequency of HLA-A3 in affected individuals could mean that all iron-loading genes that are tagged with that HLA marker had a common origin. A mutation leading to increased iron absorption might have arisen on a chromosome carrying the HLA-A3 allele. Because of tight linkage, recombination would not have separated these genes over the generations, so that all current HLA-A3 alleles in idiopathic hemochromatosis might be derived from a common ancestor in whom the mutation first occurred. Current data show an excess of HLA-A3 genes in patients from Germany, France, Belgium, England, Scotland, and Ireland, as well as from Australia and the United States. A Celtic origin, with spread of the gene by migration, has been postulated to account for these findings [166]. Alternatively, multiple mutations may have occurred and selective factors of an unknown nature may have preserved the linkage over many generations. This hypothesis would require a special selective advantage for the HLA-A gene (or a closely linked gene) over other HLA-A alleles. In this connection, examination of HLA types in affected populations other than those of European origin will be of interest. Were the HLA-A3 linkage with the iron-loading gene to be found in non-European patients also, then a common origin would be unlikely and some selective advantage would seem a more probable explanation.

Nature of the Metabolic Abnormality

The nature of the metabolic abnormality responsible for the accumulation of iron in subjects homozygous for the HLA-linked iron-loading gene awaits definition. From a theoretical standpoint it could be due to a defect or defects at a number of sites. These include the lumen of the gut, the mucosal cells of the upper small intestine, plasma transferrin, the liver, and the reticuloendothelial system.

Initial claims that gastric secretions contain a glycoprotein ("gastroferrin") which normally inhibits iron absorption and that this protein is absent in idiopathic hemochromatosis [194] have not been confirmed in subsequent studies [195, 196]. Of more interest has been the observation that there is less ferritin than would be expected in the mucosal cells of the upper gut [157] although this too was not confirmed in a subsequent study [197]. It has also been shown that a larger proportion than normal of the iron taken up by mucosal cells is transferred into the body [145, 198, 199]. Further evidence implicating an abnormality in mucosal behavior has recently been obtained in in vitro studies in which increased uptake of iron by the mucosal cells of the duodenum from patients has been demonstrated [200]. The nature of this defect has not been defined. The possibility that the increased absorption of iron might be secondary to an abnormality in the transferrin of plasma has been investigated, but with negative results. Transferrin from subjects with idiopathic hemochromatosis takes up and releases iron normally [201, 202]. Furthermore, studies in families whose members exhibit transferrin variants have shown that there is no suggestion of genetic linkage between the structural gene for transferrin and the HLA locus [203]. A claim based on kinetic studies that the liver has an abnormal affinity for iron in the condition [204] does not seem tenable, since iron stored in the hemochromatotic liver is readily mobilized in response to venesection [2]. The increased hepatic uptake of radioiron after both oral and intravenous administration can be ascribed to the saturation of the iron-binding capacity of the transferrin [1205]. The suggestion that a deficiency of xanthine oxidase might be responsible for the condition [206] is no longer acceptable, since it is now known that the enzyme is not involved in the mobilization of iron from ferritin and thus does not affect iron transport [67, 207]. Recently interest in the liver was rekindled by the demonstration of an abnormal hepatic isoferritin pattern in patients with fully developed idiopathic hemochromatosis [208], but similar changes were later found in other varieties of iron overload [44, 209], and the pattern reverts to normal after the removal of the excess iron [210].

Further insight into the possible sites or site of the metabolic defect in subjects homozygous for the HLA-linked iron-loading gene is provided by the distribution of the excess iron in those individuals who have developed the clinical disease. In every other variety of iron overload large amounts are present in the reticuloendothelial cells, particularly of the spleen, bone marrow, and liver, with variable involvement of the parenchymal cells of the liver and other organs [2]. In idiopathic hemochromatosis the parenchymal cells contain virtually all the hemosiderin deposits, and the reticuloendothelial system very little [211]. On the basis of these findings it has been suggested that intestinal and reticuloendothelial cells have a common defect in that they do not store iron normally, so that increased amounts of iron are delivered via the plasma to hepatocytes and other parenchymal cells [2]. Some support for this contention has been obtained in kinetic studies involving reticuloendothelial function in idiopathic hemochromatosis [79]. A defect in storing iron which is common to intestinal and reticuloendothelial cells is certainly compatible with a number of observations in the condition. Such a defect would explain the paucity of iron present in both of these cell types, the increased iron absorption, and the saturation of circulating transferrin with iron, both of which are noted long before the accumulation of large amounts of iron. The deposition of iron in hepatocytes and other parenchymal tissues would then be expected to occur only as a passive consequence of the saturated transferrin [212].

Environmental Factors

While there is no longer any room for doubt that idiopathic hemochromatosis is an inherited metabolic disorder, environmental factors play an important part in its phenotypic expression. It is obvious that surplus iron cannot be accumulated unless the diet provides more available iron than is required to replace obligatory losses and to allow for growth, pregnancy, and lactation. Even if the iron-loading genes are inherited, therefore, iron overload sufficient to produce organ damage and clinical manifestations can develop only very rarely in a country like India, where the bioavailability of the dietary iron is poor, iron deficiency is rife, and storage iron concentrations in the liver are low. Indeed, the disease does not appear to have been reported in this country. On the other hand, the heavy per capita consumption of meat, which contains bioavailable iron in the form of heme and promotes the absorption of the non-heme iron in the meal, must contribute to the high prevalence and relatively early age of presentation of fully developed hemochromatosis in Australia [145, 213].

Individuals who increase their iron intake by using iron cooking utensils or consuming iron-containing medicinal preparations accelerate the appearance of the clinical phase of the disease. On the negative side of the iron balance equation, hookworm infestation could cause the elimination through intestinal blood loss of any superfluous iron absorbed, and regular blood donation would have a similar effect.

Alcohol and Iron Overload The place of alcohol deserves special mention. In most published series a high proportion of patients with fully developed idiopathic hemochromatosis have been more than moderate users of alcohol [2]. This was largely responsible for the view that idiopathic hemochromatosis is not a metabolic disorder, but merely alcoholic or nutritional cirrhosis in subjects whose dietary intake of iron has been high [215]. Certainly, the association of alcoholic cirrhosis with increased quantities of hepatic hemosiderin has been frequently observed. In Southern African blacks the severity of the unique variety of iron overload still commonly encountered there is closely related to the quantity of home-brewed alcohol consumed by the affected individual. There appear to be several reasons for these associations [216].

The most obvious reason is the iron present in some varieties of alcoholic beverage. The beers indigenous to Southern Africa are based on millet and maize and are often brewed in pots or drums made of iron. During fermentation the iron content rises as the pH falls: the final mean concentration in one study was 40 mg/liter [217]. The alcohol content is low and large quantities are regularly consumed by many adult males, so that an additional 50 to 100 mg iron in a highly bioavailable form is ingested each day. This is several times more than the normal total dietary iron intake. The high bioavailability of the iron, equivalent to that of an inorganic ferric salt [217], must be ascribed to the fermentation process, since equivalent amounts of iron added to porridge prepared from the ingredients before fermentation are very poorly absorbed [218]. This phenomenon has been investigated, and it appears that several factors are involved. These are the removal (by filtration through cloth) of most of the grits, which inhibit iron absorption; perhaps the alcohol itself, by potentiating the absorption of ferric iron; and probably certain small-molecule fermentation products which serve as solubilizing ligands [218]. Alcoholic beverages in other parts of the world, notably certain red wines, have also been found to contain significant amounts of iron. While concentrations of up to 90 mg/liter have been reported [219], values greater than 15 mg/liter are uncommon [215, 220]. The average for Italian wines was found to be only 6 mg/liter for the red and about half this for the white wine [221]. The bioavailability of this iron cannot be assumed because of the inhibitory effect of tannins, which are present particularly in red wine. Only a mean of 6.8 percent of the 10.9 mg iron per liter of Swiss red wine was absorbed by fasting normal subjects [222].

While the use of alcohol can increase iron intake, most varieties of alcoholic beverage do not contain significant quantities. Distilled spirits in particular contain virtually none. Additional reasons must therefore be sought for the association between alcohol and iron overload. The enhancement of the absorption of ferric iron by alcohol mentioned above was demonstrated with a solution of ferric chloride in the fasting state and appears to be ascribable to the stimulation of HCl secretion [223]. Scotch whisky inhibits iron absorption under comparable circumstances [222], and ethanol had no effect on the absorption of nonheme iron from a standard meal [222]. Moreover, alcohol abuse can produce atrophic gastritis and hypochlorhydria, which would retard iron absorption. Another possibility is that absorption is enhanced by an indirect mechanism, such as the ineffective erythropoiesis and increased plasma iron turnover resulting from the disordered folate metabolism which alcohol induces [216, 224]. Alternatively, organ damage produced by alcohol may lead to increased iron absorption. The pancreas has been implicated [225], but later work has not substantiated this [226–228]. The evidence indicating that liver disease might be responsible is weightier, since a number of workers observed enhanced iron absorption in some patients with cirrhosis [229–233]. Portacaval anastomosis seems to lead to an increase in the density of hemosiderin deposition in the liver cells [234], but whether the body's store of iron is really increased or merely redistributed is less certain [2]. Absorption was not found increased on direct measurement [235].

The situation is thus far from clear. Alcohol abuse is certainly not always associated with an increase in the body iron content. In two carefully documented Swedish studies the iron stores were found to be within the normal range [236, 237] and in a group of distilled-liquor drinkers were actually lower than normal. Only 7 percent of 157 alcoholics with liver disease studied in London had significant histologic siderosis, and the degree of siderosis correlated *inversely* with the daily alcohol intake [238]. Slight increases in the amount of hemosiderin on histologic examination of the liver or in the hepatic nonheme iron concentration could be due to a decreased liver mass, or redistribution of the iron from other storage sites, or from hemoglobin if anemia is present. On the other hand, there can be no doubting the validity of the association in idiopathic hemochromatosis. Alcohol must contribute to the organ damage associated with the iron overload, and therefore accelerate the onset of the clinical phase of the condition. This cannot be the only reason, however, since the iron load of those subjects with idiopathic hemochromatosis who have an alcoholic history has been found to be 50 percent higher than that of abstemious individuals [239]. In addition iron overload does occur in alcoholics who are not homozygous for the HLA-linked iron-loading gene, although instances where the severity reaches the hemochromatotic range are rare outside Southern Africa.

A final syndrome in which iron overload and alcohol are associated deserves brief consideration, namely *porphyria cutanea tarda* (see Chap. 60). In this condition hepatic heme synthesis is disordered due to a deficiency of the enzyme uroporphyrinogen decarboxylase [240, 241]. It appears that there is a genetic predisposition in most patients [242], but that exogenous factors, including alcohol and iron overload, play an important part in the phenotypic expression. The urinary excretion of uroporphyrin, and usually also of coproporphyrin, is increased, and during clinical exacerbations there is vesication, ulceration, hypertrichosis, pigmentation, and thickening of the skin [243, 244]. The majority of patients give a history of prolonged consumption of excessive quantities of alcohol, and liver biopsy specimens usually show some degree of siderosis, although it is usually only mild to moderate [242].

The condition is commonly encountered in siderotic South African blacks [2] and has also been reported in association with iron overload of other types [1]. Support for the suggestion that siderosis plays a part in the production of the clinical manifestations is provided by reports that a marked decrease in porphyrin excretion has followed the treatment of the iron overload by repeated venesections [245–248]. Some experimental observations may be relevant. Rats fed hexachlorobenzene become porphyric much more readily if they have been given large doses of iron dextran intraperitoneally, and the rate of uroporphyrin synthesis in vitro is significantly increased by the addition of ferritin and cysteine [249]. Moreover, ferrous iron inhibits the deficient enzyme uroporphyrinogen decarboxylase, and stimulates porphyrin synthesis [240, 241]. Iron overload is certainly not invariably present, and in siderotic individuals clinical and biochemical improvement may occur before significant amounts of iron have been removed by phlebotomy [246]. The association with alcoholism may be a direct one or may merely reflect the association between iron overload and the consumption of alcohol. It nevertheless seems clear that both the hereditary enzyme deficiency and an acquired factor must be present, and that the latter is frequently iron overload, with or without alcohol. In this context, it is of interest that the relative importance of different exogenous factors may be changing, and that estrogen-containing oral contraceptives now represent a significant exacerbating factor [250].

Factors Influencing the Distribution of Iron in Iron Overload

As was mentioned in the previous section, the pattern of iron distribution in fully developed idiopathic hemochromatosis is a unique one, since most of the iron is confined to parenchymal cells throughout the body. Factors that appear to influence the distribution of iron in other forms of iron overload include the route of entry of the iron, the rate of red cell production and the degree of ineffective erythropoiesis, the duration of the disease, the ascorbic acid nutrition, and the transferrin saturation.

In aplastic anemias erythropoiesis is obviously inhibited, and the superfluous iron enters in the form of the hemoglobin in the transfused blood. As the cells reach the end of their life span they are engulfed by reticuloendothelial cells and the iron is deposited there. With time, some distribution to parenchymal tissues occurs, and indeed in pure red cell aplasia of childhood marked parenchymal involvement may eventually develop [251]. On the other hand, in those anemias where much of the erythropoiesis in the hypercellular marrow is ineffective, the location of the iron is mostly parenchymal [151]. There appear to be several reasons for this. The plasma iron turnover is increased to several times normal and the transferrin saturation is raised, both of which accelerate parenchymal uptake of iron [212]. In some of these conditions, notably β thalassemia major, the transferrin is fully saturated, and iron that is not bound by transferrin is present in the plasma [252, 253]. Such iron is deposited in parenchymal tissues [2]. Dietary iron absorption is enhanced [154] in addition to the iron loading via transfusion, and iron entering the portal venous system is removed by hepatocytes if the binding capacity of transferrin is exceeded [254]. The extra hemoglobin released into the plasma by the disintegration of the faulty erythrocytes which are produced in great numbers by the marrow is also taken up by the hepatocytes [41].

It might perhaps be anticipated that the distribution of the iron when the overload is due only to the entry of increased amounts from the intestine would be predominantly parenchymal, but except for idiopathic hemochromatosis this is not so. If experimental animals are given large amounts of oral iron, the deposits are almost entirely reticuloendothelial [2]. As mentioned above, in Southern African blacks iron overload develops as a consequence of the long-term ingestion of large amounts of beer containing highly bioavailable iron [118]. Iron overload of hemochromatotic proportions results in many subjects, mainly adult males with 20 or so years of regular beer drinking [255]. Reticuloendothelial siderosis is always very marked, particularly in the spleen, the bone marrow, and the Kupffer cells, but the hepatocytes contain equally heavy deposits of hemosiderin. Other parenchymal cells are not involved. The condition can therefore be distinguished from idiopathic hemochromatosis by histologic examination of the liver [256].

Since the excess iron in Southern African blacks enters the portal system from the intestine, hepatocyte involvement is hardly surprising, but the reason for the reticuloendothelial localization of the remainder of the iron is not quite so obvious. In many of these subjects ascorbic acid deficiency probably contributes to the retention of the iron by the reticuloendothelial cells. (The reason why iron overload predisposes to ascorbic acid deficiency is discussed in the following section.) With the superimposition of the inadequate dietary intake of ascorbic acid which is common among urban black South Africans, the deficiency is frequently severe and frank clinical scurvy is even seen. In scorbutic guinea pigs disordered release of iron to the plasma by the reticuloendothelial cells has been demonstrated, and these cells accumulate hemosiderin as a result [34]. In iron-overloaded South African blacks the injection of ascorbic acid produces an immediate rise in the plasma iron concentration, suggesting that reticuloendothelial iron release may be defective in them also. The predominantly reticuloendothelial localization of the iron in experimental oral iron overload is seen even when species not susceptible to scurvy are used, and this indicates that ascorbic acid deficiency cannot be solely responsible. The main reason may simply be that since much of the absorbed iron becomes incorporated into hemoglobin in the marrow, the reticuloendothelial release of the iron from catabolized hemoglobin is reduced in proportion [258]. The same argument could obviously be applied to idiopathic hemochromatosis, and the need to postulate a factor that prevents reticuloendothelial loading in the genetic disease is therefore apparent.

It is worth noting that the micronodular cirrhosis in black Southern Africans with iron overload is associated with an increased deposition of hemosiderin in parenchymal cells, particularly in the heart, pituitary, thyroid, and adrenal glands, and pancreas [259]. Although micronodular cirrhosis is found much more commonly in alcoholic subjects with severe iron overload than in those with little or no iron [259, 260], the parenchymal cell deposits in the cirrhotic individuals cannot be ascribed simply to the large quantity of iron in the body, since they are not seen in noncirrhotic subjects with equally heavy iron overload. The reason probably lies in the transferrin saturation, which is higher in the cirrhotic group [2]. This leads to increased uptake of plasma iron by parenchymal cells. Why cirrhosis should be associated with a rise in the transferrin sat-

uration is not known. Whatever the explanation, cirrhosis cannot be invoked as the reason for the parenchymal distribution of the iron in idiopathic hemochromatosis, since very severe parenchymal loading with cardiac failure and hypogonadism has been observed in the absence of cirrhosis [261] and even in the absence of hepatic fibrosis [239].

Relation between Iron Overload and Tissue Damage

While the chronic toxicity of iron was disputed at one stage [215], the similarity of the findings in fully developed idiopathic hemochromatosis and in the other varieties of iron overload, such as that found in Southern African blacks and that occurring in association with various anemias, is difficult to explain on any other basis. The common denominator to tissue damage is the presence of high concentrations of iron in parenchymal tissues over long periods of time. Although massive deposits of iron in reticuloendothelial cells may be associated with fibrosis, particularly in the spleen, the deleterious effects are certainly minimal in comparison to those produced by parenchymal deposits.

In all varieties of iron overload *hepatic portal fibrosis* is found. Its severity has been shown to be related to the quantity of iron in the liver in Southern African blacks [255, 262] and in subjects with chronic refractory anemias [263]. Liver biopsies performed on affected relatives of subjects with idiopathic hemochromatosis indicate that the portal cirrhosis, which is virtually always present in the fully developed disease [4, 188], is preceded by the accumulation of excessive iron [264, 265]. Liver damage is arrested and even reversed by iron chelation therapy in thalassemia major [266], and by phlebotomy therapy in idiopathic hemochromatosis [214, 267, 268]. *Cardiopathy* is the commonest cause of death in untreated idiopathic hemochromatosis, especially in young subjects [269], and in thalassemia major [270, 271]. Once cardiac failure develops, death soon follows unless the iron is removed [2], when complete recovery is the rule [272–277]. *Hypogonadism* is almost invariable in patients with idiopathic hemochromatosis and in those children with thalassemia major who survive until the age of puberty [155, 278, 279]. In both types of patients the hypogonadism is secondary to pituitary dysfunction [280]. If the build-up of iron can be retarded while keeping the hemoglobin concentration up, prepubertal growth improves and secondary sex characteristics may develop. Once hypogonadism is established in idiopathic hemochromatosis, removal of iron does not lead to improvement. *Diabetes* is a feature not only of fully developed idiopathic hemochromatosis but also of the iron overload found in Southern African blacks and in patients with chronic anemias; abnormal glucose tolerance has been reported in 50 percent of β thalassemia homozygotes [281].

Mechanisms of Chronic Iron Toxicity

There is evidence suggesting that iron produces cell damage by weakening lysosomal membranes so that acid hydrolases are released into the cytoplasm. The action on the membranes may be via the catalysis of the formation of free radicals that produce lipid peroxidation [282–284]. The concentration of the antioxidant vitamin E has been reported to be diminished

[285–287]. In animal experiments iron accumulates in hepatocyte lysosomes on iron loading, and in fully developed idiopathic hemochromatosis the histologic appearance may be consistent with such localization [265, 288]. The lysosomes from the livers of subjects with various types of iron overload are more fragile than normal in vitro, and there is increased lysosomal enzyme activity [282, 283]. Lysosomal fragility increases in proportion to the hemosiderin content [289]. These abnormalities return to normal on removing the iron [290]. Freely proliferating Chang liver cells grown in a culture containing large concentrations of iron (ferric nitrilotriacetate) accumulate up to 50 times their normal iron content and can survive for over 26 weeks without showing evidence of lysosomal damage [291]. On the other hand, slowly proliferating cultures die within 4 to 5 weeks.

Fibrosis is a feature of most organs containing excessive amounts of storage iron, even when there is little or no evidence of parenchymal cell damage. There is some evidence to suggest that iron stimulates collagen synthesis [292], and also that iron chelators inhibit it [293, 294].

Another consequence of iron overload is ascorbic acid depletion. This was first documented in Southern African blacks, in whom the observed clinical association between frank scurvy and iron overload [295] led to the discovery that in such subjects a proportion of the available dietary ascorbic acid is irreversibly oxidized. Administration of large amounts of ascorbic acid to normal subjects soon leads to the excretion of most of the dose unchanged in the urine, but if iron overload is present there is an increase in the excretion of the oxidation product, oxalic acid [296]. With physiologic amounts of ascorbic acid the major oxidation product is carbon dioxide [297]. Since ferric iron catalyzes the first step in the oxidation sequence in vitro, the accumulation of ferric iron in the tissues is presumably responsible. The severity of the resultant ascorbic acid deficiency is determined by the dietary intake of ascorbic acid. Clinical scurvy is seen in siderotic Johannesburg blacks mainly in late winter and early spring, when the dietary ascorbic acid content is at its lowest. Even in well-nourished subjects with iron overload, mild to moderate ascorbic acid deficiency is frequently demonstrable, for example by measurement of the leukocyte ascorbic acid concentration. This deficiency is seen frequently in idiopathic hemochromatosis and iron-loading anemias as well as in dietary iron overload [257, 298–300].

Chronic low-grade ascorbic acid deficiency may have metabolic consequences even if it does not reach scorbutic proportions. Tryptophan metabolism has been reported to be adversely affected [301]. Of possibly greater significance is the circumstantial evidence that chronic ascorbic acid deficiency can lead to osteoporosis. Osteoporosis of the spine [295, 296] and the femoral head [302] is frequently present in middle-aged South African black males with iron overload, although in other populations osteoporosis in middle-aged males is extremely uncommon. The usual variety of osteoporosis in other populations, that occurring in elderly women, is not common in black South African women. The relationship of the osteoporosis in black males to iron overload was established by a necropsy study in which the mineral density of iliac crest bone was shown to be inversely correlated with the concentration of storage iron in the liver [303]. The ascorbic acid nutrition of these subjects is also inversely related to the severity of the iron overload [303]. In experimental animals and in children scurvy causes osteoporosis [2], presumably because ascorbic acid is needed for osteogenesis, for the synthesis of bone collagen, the formation of osteoid, and for osteoblast maturation. The expected reduction in bone formation surface was found when semiquantitative microradiography was applied to the osteoporotic bones of guinea pigs deficient in ascorbic acid, but there was also an increase in bone resorption surface [304]. In iron-overloaded blacks with osteoporosis the bone resorption surface was also increased [304]. Experiments with radiocalcium suggested that these subjects have both reduced bone formation and enhanced bone resorption. When ascorbic acid was administered the urinary calcium excretion fell [305]. It has been postulated that the iron overload leads to chronic ascorbic acid deficiency and that this in turn produces osteoporosis. Support for the hypothesis was provided by an experiment with guinea pigs [304]. On a diet that kept the control animals healthy, the group overloaded with iron by repeated injections of iron dextran had very low hepatic ascorbic acid concentrations and diminished bone mineral density after several months. These changes were prevented by administering large parenteral ascorbic acid supplements to a third group.

Osteoporosis has been described in fully developed idiopathic hemochromatosis [306, 307]. The prevalence has not been established, but will probably be influenced by the amount of ascorbic acid in the habitual diet.

Pathogenesis of Symptomatic Hemochromatosis

The clinical manifestations of idiopathic hemochromatosis appear in those subjects homozygous for the HLA-linked iron-loading gene whose diets have permitted the accumulation of toxic quantities of iron. In such individuals the body iron content is between 15 and 40 g, 5 to 10 times the normal quantity [5]. All of the additional iron is in storage compounds that are increased 20 to 50 times [2, 4, 188, 214, 226]. Unless additional amounts of bioavailable iron are regularly ingested, not more than 3 to 5 mg/day can be absorbed from the average western-type diet [196, 308, 309]. The obligatory daily iron losses in adult males are about 0.9 mg, increasing to perhaps 2 to 3 mg as the body iron content rises.

It is obvious that the net accumulation of 20 to 40 g surplus iron takes many years. Most subjects are therefore 40 to 60 years of age at the time of diagnosis, although a number of younger patients have been described, including some in early adulthood [261] and even children [310]. The clinical manifestations of the disease are encountered approximately 10 times as frequently in males as in females. This is due, at least in part, to the more gradual accumulation of iron by females resulting from losses through menstruation, pregnancy, and lactation, and amounting to a lifetime total of between 5 and 15 g [2]. The quantities of absorbable iron in the diet are rarely sufficient to permit a significant positive balance in the face of these losses, even though the absorptive mechanism is set to do so. It is therefore not surprising that the age of onset of clinical manifestations tends to be younger in males than in females [4] and also that many affected females give a history of scanty menstruation for several years preceding the onset of symptoms [4].

At the time of diagnosis of hemochromatosis the absorption of iron may be found to be raised [311], but it is usually within the normal range [1, 2]. Since the body's requirement for iron normally determines the absorption rate, it is apparent that a normal absorption rate in the presence of the grossly enlarged iron stores is actually inappropriately high. Iron absorption in such subjects is greater than would be anticipated from the plasma ferritin concentration, which reflects the body store of iron [52, 312]. During phlebotomy therapy absorption rises to high levels, and it may remain above normal for years after phlebotomies have been discontinued [916, 235, 313, 314]. These observations suggest that in subjects who are homozygous for the HLA-linked iron-loading gene, iron absorption is subject to the usual influences, but that the setting of the control mechanism is higher than normal.

Pathologic Findings in the Full-Blown Disease

The storage iron concentration is highest in the liver and pancreas, reaching 50 to 100 times the normal figures, whereas in the thyroid it is usually about 25 times normal, and in the heart and adrenal gland between 10 and 15 times normal. In organs such as the skin, spleen, kidney, and stomach it is only about 5 times normal. The surplus iron is predominantly in the form of hemosiderin and is visible on histologic examination, particularly after staining with potassium ferrocyanide. Another pigment, "hemofuscin," has also been observed, but it is not specific to hemochromatosis. It is probably a lipofuscin and is also found in old age and in cachectic states. In addition to iron, levels of various trace metals may be increased in hemochromatosis [2]. The observed relationship between the concentrations of manganese and iron in the livers of subjects with the disease is compatible with experimental evidence suggesting that the two metals are absorbed by a similar mechanism [315].

Skin The characteristic pigmentation is due to melanin in the deeper layers of the epidermis, associated with increased amounts of hemosiderin in only about half of the cases. When present the hemosiderin is most obvious in the sweat glands, but deposits can also be seen in vascular endothelium and in the connective tissue of the corium. Atrophy of the epidermis and dermis has also been noted [316].

Liver The liver is usually considerably enlarged, the average weight being 2400 g, and is rusty red in color. A fine monolobular cirrhosis is almost invariably present, the lobules being typically separated by the wide bands of the fibrous tissue. A characteristic pattern of fibrosis and lobular disruption has been recognized in nonalcoholic subjects [317]. In young subjects lesser degrees of fibrosis may occur [261], and it may rarely be absent despite massive iron overload and damage to other tissues [239]. The striking feature in every case is the heavy deposition of hemosiderin granules in the hepatocytes. These deposits are scattered throughout the lobules, but a centripetal predominance can be discerned. The degree of hemosiderosis may vary from zone to zone and from lobule to lobule, tending to be less in areas of regeneration [2]. The bile duct epithelium also invariably contains heavy deposits of hemosiderin, but the amounts in Kupffer cells and in the fibrous connective tissue are far less than in some other forms of iron overload. The hepatocytes are mostly normal in size and staining quality but may be larger at the edge of the lobules, with more prominent nucleoli and chromatin [318], especially in subjects with a history of excessive alcohol intake in whom

fatty change may also be present. As the cells degenerate their nuclei become pyknotic and they release their iron to fibroblasts at the lobular periphery and in the portal spaces. Hepatoma complicates a proportion of the cases [4] and cholangiomas have also been reported [2].

Some insight has been gained into the pathologic findings in the liver during the long period prior to clinical manifestations. This information comes from examination of liver biopsies that have been performed on relatives of known patients because their plasma iron concentrations and transferrin saturations were high, they excreted excessive amounts of iron in the urine after the injection of an iron chelator, or, more recently, because their plasma ferritin concentrations were raised [187, 210, 264, 319, 320]. A complete spectrum from normality to the fully developed disease has been observed. In the early stages discrete granules of hemosiderin can be seen in the hepatocytes, either finely dispersed throughout the liver lobules or in focal scattered areas, especially peripherally. When greater quantities are present the hemosiderin is aggregated into coarser masses and is more uniformly distributed. Marked hemosiderosis is associated with a slight to moderate increase in portal tract fibrosis, while true monolobular cirrhosis is the rule in the fully developed clinical disease.

Pancreas In the established case the pancreas is firm and rusty in color. Fibrosis is almost invariably present and the gland structure is disorganized. There is degeneration of acinar epithelium, and the islets of Langerhans are usually decreased in number [188]. Hemosiderin deposits are more marked in the exocrine than in the endocrine cells.

Endocrine Tissues Although fibrosis is not a feature, hemosiderin deposits are prominent in the epithelial cells of the thyroid, the parathyroid, and the anterior pituitary glands. In the adrenal glands they are usually confined to the zona glomerulosa of the cortex. Testicular atrophy, particularly of the germinal epithelium, is present in about a quarter of patients, but hemosiderin deposits are usually scanty.

Heart The heart is typically enlarged, the weight often being two or three times normal. The ventricular walls are thickened and iron pigment is visible in the myocardial fibers, especially in the perinuclear region. Deposits tend to be less heavy in the atrial myocardium, and in conducting, as opposed to contracting, tissue. Degeneration, fragmentation, and necrosis of myocardial cells with fibrosis and interstitial edema have been described [2, 321].

Joints Synovial lining cells are heavily laden with hemosiderin, the type B cells more than the type A, in contrast to rheumatoid arthritis. Some fibrous thickening of the synovium has been described in certain cases [322–325]. Associated degenerative changes include separation of the superficial cartilage and clumping of the chondrocytes, as well as calcification of the fibrocartilage and hyaline cartilage [325].

Other Organs Hemosiderin is usually found in the mucosal cells of the stomach, and gastric biopsy has been suggested as a diagnostic procedure [2]. In contrast, there is virtually none in the upper small bowel, a striking point of difference from dietary iron overload. Only small amounts of iron are present in the renal tubules [188], in striated muscle, and in the choroid plexus, but the deposits in the salivary and lacrimal glands and in the submucous glands of the respiratory tract are usually heavy. Lymph nodes, especially those draining markedly siderotic organs, may also contain hemosiderin.

The average weight of the spleen is about 400 g, somewhat above normal. Congestive changes secondary to portal hypertension are often present [188]. Hemosiderin deposits are not prominent and are usually confined to the capsule, blood vessel walls, and trabeculae. The iron concentrations in the spleen are low in comparison to other varieties of iron overload [261]. The histologic examination of bone marrow smears is a convenient means of assessing the storage iron status under all other circumstances, but it is unreliable in idiopathic hemochromatosis [2]. Chemical analysis of bone marrow trephine samples from subjects with idiopathic hemochromatosis confirms that the concentrations are not significantly raised [211]. This emphasizes how minimal is the reticuloendothelial involvement in the disease.

Clinical Features in the Full-Blown Disease (Fig. 59-9)

Skin Pigmentation is virtually always present, although it may have developed so insidiously as not to have attracted the patient's notice. It is particularly prominent in exposed areas and old scars. It involves the conjunctiva and lid margin in about 30 percent of patients and the oral mucosa in 10 to 15 percent [316, 326]. The skin has a bronze color except in those individuals in whom iron deposits are present in addition to the melanin, when the color is slate gray. The skin is typically fine and soft with scanty facial, pubic, and axillary hair. Xerosis ranging in severity up to generalized ichthyosis has been reported in almost half the patients in a recent series [316].

Liver The liver is almost always firm and enlarged, and splenomegaly is found in about 50 percent of subjects. Severe portal hypertension is much less common than with Laennec's cirrhosis, and esophageal varices are seen less frequently. Clinical evidence of ascites is also not common and in a recent series was associated with cardiac failure [239]. Palmar erythema and spider angiomas may be present, but gynecomastia is unusual.

Hepatic function is typically not seriously deranged provided the individual does not drink alcohol excessively [4,

239]. The serum albumin concentration is frequently within the normal range [239], and in half or more of the patients the plasma glutamic oxalacetic transaminase, alkaline phosphatase, and bilirubin concentrations are not elevated, and the prothrombin time is not prolonged. Minor changes in protein patterns have been recorded but are usually nonspecific and merely reflect impaired liver function or diabetes. The liver disease in idiopathic hemochromatosis usually runs a prolonged and benign course, but episodes of acute hepatic failure may occur, often provoked by blood loss or surgical procedures, and 25 percent of subjects eventually die of complications such as coma or gastrointestinal hemorrhage.

Hepatoma is an important late complication, and cholangiomas have also been reported [2]. Malignant change is suggested by the onset of unexplained weight loss, fever, nodular enlargement of the liver, ascites, jaundice, abdominal pain, anemia, or insulin insensitivity [4]. In a number of series the incidence of hepatoma has been about 14 percent. Once cirrhosis has developed the risk appears not to be diminished by the successful removal of the iron [277], and with the resultant reduction in deaths due to cardiac and hepatic failure the figure may be expected to rise. No fewer than 29 percent of the treated patients in a recent study died of hepatoma [277].

Abdominal Pain Abdominal pain occurs quite frequently and is often the presenting symptom. An aching sensation in the epigastrium or right hypochondrium which may persist for long periods is the most frequently encountered type. It has been shown to have a variety of causes, including peptic ulceration, hepatoma, variceal bleeding, ascites, cholecystitis, and nephrolithiasis [239]. More puzzling are the descriptions of the acute onset of severe pain, often associated with shock [327]. A suggestion that the release of ferritin into the circulation could be responsible does not seem to be tenable [328, 329]. It seems more likely that such episodes are due to gram-negative septicemia [330]. *Escherichia coli* or *Pasteurella pseudotuberculosis* have been cultured from the blood or the peritoneum of several patients [327, 331]. The saturated transferrin found in subjects with idiopathic hemochromatosis has been thought to increase their susceptibility to such episodes. The patients are thought to be deprived of the bacteriostatic effect of unsaturated transferrin that has been ascribed to its sequestration of the iron needed by microorganisms for multiplication. In experimental animals the injection of iron enhances bacterial virulence [2], but there is little clinical evidence that individuals with saturated transferrin are more susceptible to infection. Furthermore, infection causes the transferrin saturation to fall.

Diabetes Symptoms ascribed to the onset of diabetes, including weight loss, lassitude, and weakness, are frequently present at the time of diagnosis, and diminished glucose tolerance can be demonstrated in most subjects. In the past it was assumed that the diabetes of hemochromatosis is due to damage to the islets of Langerhans. Low levels of circulating insulin have indeed been demonstrated in some patients [332, 332a], but it is now apparent that factors unassociated with hemochromatosis are also involved. The prevalence of diabetes among first-degree relatives of diabetic patients with idiopathic hemochromatosis is much higher than among the first-degree relatives of nondiabetic hemochromatotics [332]. The diabetes in such relatives is associated with the high levels of circulating insulin [333, 334]. In addition to the familial pre-

Figure 59-9 The frequency with which various symptoms and signs occur in fully developed idiopathic hemochromatosis. (*From Bothwell et al. [2]. Used by permission.*)

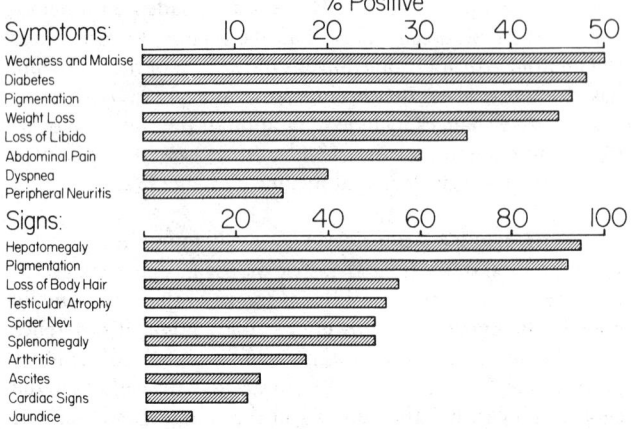

disposition to develop diabetes, the hepatic damage of hemochromatosis may play a part, since cirrhosis is associated with both insulin resistance [335] and hyperglucagonemia [336]. In summary, the diabetes that occurs in idiopathic hemochromatosis is not simply the result of damage to the pancreas by iron but appears to involve the expression of clinical diabetes in genetically predisposed persons with iron-induced pancreatic injury and cirrhosis.

Although it has been stated that the vascular complications of diabetes occur uncommonly in idiopathic hemochromatosis [188], nephropathy, neuropathy, retinopathy, and peripheral vascular disease, either singly or together, have been reported in a significant percentage of patients [2, 332]. The prevalence of retinopathy among subjects who have been diabetic for 10 or more years appears to be similar to that in nonhemochromatotic diabetics [337], although it may not be as severe [338]. It seems probable, therefore, that the complications of diabetes will be seen more commonly with improved survival [339].

Hypogonadism   Diminished sexual function is a relatively frequent finding in idiopathic hemochromatosis and is almost invariable in young subjects. Loss of libido, testicular atrophy, impotence, amenorrhea, and sparse body hair are common. The body hair may be scanty for many years before other manifestations of the disease appear. These are typical features of cirrhosis, but in hemochromatosis may be present before liver function is significantly impaired. Moreover, the gynecomastia which is characteristic of other varieties of cirrhosis is uncommon in idiopathic hemochromatosis. There is clear evidence of pituitary insufficiency in a proportion of these subjects [2, 340]. In a comparison between two groups with testicular atrophy, the majority of those with idiopathic hemochromatosis had low concentrations of luteinizing hormone, while in those with other types of cirrhosis the concentrations were in the normal range [341]. Low basal gonadotropin concentrations or low responses to gonadotropin-releasing hormone have been demonstrated in a high proportion of hemochromatotic subjects with low plasma testosterone concentrations and clinical hypogonadism [342]. A decrease in prolactin reserve has also been described in some patients [343]. In contrast, the secretion of other trophic pituitary hormones is not impaired, although mild hypothyroidism or hypoadrenalism has been reported in a small proportion of patients [2, 344].

Heart   Cardiac manifestations are the presenting feature in only 15 percent of cases, but arrhythmias or cardiac failure eventually develop in more than one-third, the average age of onset being 56 years [239]. Ischemic heart disease may play a part in some of these individuals.

The onset may be acute, cardiac failure developing within a few days, and the pulmonary congestion and peripheral edema may be very severe. Clinically the picture is usually that of a congestive cardiomyopathy with bilateral ventricular dilatation. On radiographic investigation the cardiac profile has a globular appearance with decrease in the amplitude of the cardiac pulsations. Restrictive features have also been described [2, 345].

Arrhythmias indicate a poor prognosis. Ventricular ectopic beats are the commonest manifestations, but supraventricular and ventricular tachycardias, ventricular fibrillation, and varying degrees of heart block may also occur [2]. Other rather nonspecific ECG changes such as low voltage, left-axis deviation, and flattening or inversion of T waves may be noted.

With better control of diabetes and infection, cardiac complications are probably the commonest cause of death [4]. In young subjects cardiac complications are more frequently the presenting features, and almost always the cause of death, which follows within a year of diagnosis unless the excess iron is removed [2]. The cardiac symptoms and signs may initially be aggravated by venesection to remove the iron and caution should be exercised [346] (see "Treatment" section).

Joints   Although the arthropathy of hemochromatosis was recognized only relatively recently [347], it has been reported in from 25 percent to 75 percent of patients [1, 323, 324, 348] and may be the presenting feature [349, 350]. While it has been thought to be a complication of idiopathic hemochromatosis only [324], there is a description of the development of arthropathy in a subject with transfusional siderosis [351]. The pathogenesis has not been elucidated. The typical initial complaint is of pain and stiffness in the metacarpophalangeal joints, particularly the second and third ones, with subsequent swelling and deformity. The ulnar deviation of rheumatoid arthritis is not a feature. Involvement of the larger joints follows, especially the knees, shoulders, hips, and lower back. The condition is usually not seriously disabling, although it can be. In some subjects attacks of acute inflammatory synovitis are superimposed on the chronic degenerative arthropathy. This pseudogout is associated with the precipitation of calcium pyrophosphate crystals, and it has been suggested that the iron inhibits pyrophosphatase, the enzyme that hydrolyzes pyrophosphate to the more soluble orthophosphate.

The characteristic radiologic features are those of chondrocalcinosis, with small cysts, irregularity of the articular surface, and sclerosis and loss of joint space affecting typically the second and third metacarpophalangeal joints. Similar changes are present in the carpal bones and in the inferior radioulnar joints. Venesection treatment does not improve the arthropathy [323], and in some cases the deposits of hemosiderin in the synovium and articular cartilage persist [322]. Indeed, the arthritis may develop only after the venesections have been completed.

Hematology   Changes in the blood are not remarkable in subjects with idiopathic hemochromatosis, and this clearly distinguishes them from individuals whose iron overload is secondary to anemia. In idiopathic hemochromatosis the rates of red cell production and destruction are normal, and erythropoiesis is effective [40]. Mild macrocytosis consistent with the liver disease may occur [4], and also mild leukopenia and thrombocytopenia, presumably the result of hypersplenism. In about half the subjects iron-containing macrophages can be demonstrated in buffy-coat preparations of venous blood [352]. A rise in the leukocyte count, if not ascribable to infection, uncontrolled diabetes, or cardiac failure, should suggest the emergence of a hepatoma [2]. Blood coagulation studies are usually normal except for the hypoprothrombinemia that may accompany the liver disease.

Diagnosis

The diagnosis of full-blown idiopathic hemochromatosis should be suspected from the history and the characteristic physical findings and confirmed by demonstrating the presence of grossly increased iron stores through laboratory investigations. Recognition of the classic triad of cirrhosis, diabetes, and hyperpigmentation is relatively easy, but cases will be missed unless hemochromatosis is thought of whenever these findings are encountered individually, and also as a possible cause of cardiopathy, arthritis, impotence or sterility, abdominal pain, or asymptomatic hepatomegaly, alone or in combination. In reaching a diagnosis the presence and extent of associated organ damage should be established, but a detailed discussion of the special tests used for the assessment of hepatic, cardiac, endocrine, or pancreatic function is beyond the scope of this chapter.

In order to document the iron overload the *plasma iron concentration*, the *percentage saturation of transferrin*, and the *plasma ferritin concentration* should first be estimated. Results suggesting iron overload should lead to *needle biopsy of the liver*. The plasma iron concentration is typically over 200 μg/dl. The unsaturated iron-binding capacity appears to be up to 30 to 40 μg/dl, but this is due to methodologic deficiencies as the transferrin is actually fully saturated [353]. The only exceptions are due to intercurrent infection or hepatoma. The total iron-binding capacity is usually diminished, since the liver synthesizes less transferrin in response to the iron overload. An extremely high plasma iron concentration has occasionally been reported. Under these circumstances the iron is probably mainly in the form of ferritin released from damaged hepatocytes, but it has also been observed in one subject during a phlebotomy program at a time when he appeared to be well [2].

A high plasma iron concentration with saturation or near saturation of the transferrin is thus an almost invariable finding in subjects homozygous for the HLA-linked iron-loading gene, but it does not necessarily indicate that clinically significant iron overload is present, since it is found even before the body iron content is significantly increased [187, 320, 354]. Moreover, a high plasma iron concentration is also a feature of anemias characterized by ineffective erythropoiesis, which indeed are frequently associated with secondary iron overload. On both counts, therefore, further investigation is imperative.

The plasma ferritin concentration has proved to be a most useful diagnostic tool in subjects with idiopathic hemochromatosis [55, 56, 355, 356] and other forms of iron overload [357–359]. In untreated fully developed idiopathic hemochromatosis the values are typically several thousand micrograms per liter, and although the quantity of iron in the body cannot be calculated with absolute precision (see earlier section), the progress of venesection therapy can be monitored by following the decrease in the ferritin concentration [239]. Valuable though this test has proved to be, it is not infallible, and both false-positive and false-negative results occur. Causes of an elevated plasma ferritin concentration other than enlarged iron stores have been considered in a previous section. Falsely low concentrations are found only very rarely, but three families have been described in which the asymptomatic relatives of patients with full-blown idiopathic hemochromatosis had normal plasma ferritin concentrations in spite of considerably increased iron stores [360, 361]. We have not yet observed this anomaly, although it has been reported to occur in as many as 5 percent of the relatives [362]. Whether it represents a different variety of hemochromatosis, an impairment in the production of plasma ferritin, or an antigenic variation resulting in a falsely low estimate is not yet clear.

A noninvasive means of distinguishing between high plasma

ferritin concentrations reflecting iron overload and those caused by acute liver injury, inflammation, or neoplasm is the measurement of the *chelator-induced urinary iron excretion*. The quantity of iron excreted correlates with the amount of mobilizable storage iron in the body [363, 364]. The iron-specific chelator deferoxamine is usually used [362, 365–368], but the nonspecific diethylenetriamine pentaacetic acid (DPTA) [369] and a number of other agents have also been tried. While experimental evidence suggests that iron is chelated by deferoxamine from both reticuloendothelial cells and hepatic parenchymal cells [50], clinical studies indicate a closer relationship between the amount excreted and the quantity of storage iron in parenchymal tissues [239, 370]. A convenient method is to inject 10 mg deferoxamine per kilogram of body weight intramuscularly and measure the iron content of the urine passed during the following 24 h [237]. Various elaborations have been described [365], but they are unnecessary for the diagnosis of iron overload [2, 370].

The total amount of storage iron in the body can also be estimated by performing *weekly phlebotomies*. Iron is mobilized from the tissue deposits to replace that in the blood removed by venesection, and the hemoglobin concentration is maintained until the stored iron is exhausted. In normal subjects this occurs between the third and fourth weeks, after the removal of about 1 g iron as hemoglobin, but in full-blown idiopathic hemochromatosis the phlebotomies can be continued for many months. The quantity of iron removed obviously reflects the amount of storage iron originally present, and it can be calculated from the volume of blood removed and its hemoglobin concentration [4].

Needle biopsy of the liver provides a specimen which can be examined both histologically and chemically. On histologic examination the association of portal cirrhosis with hepatic iron deposition can be documented, and the predominantly parenchymal localization of the hemosiderin helps to distinguish idiopathic hemochromatosis from other forms of iron overload [256]. The diagnosis should be confirmed by measuring the concentration of iron present in the biopsy specimen, using either simple chemical estimations [371] or atomic absorption spectrophotometry [72].

Radioiron absorption studies have no place in the diagnosis of fully developed hemochromatosis since values within the normal range are found in most cases [1]. On the other hand, the measurement of radioiron absorption may be helpful in uncovering affected relatives if the storage iron status of the individual is taken into account [312], and a test relating the plasma ferritin concentration to the postprandial plasma iron concentration has been described [314].

Other methods of diagnosis have been used in the past but have fallen into disfavor because they are not quantitative and are unreliable. They include the demonstration of hemosiderin in the urine, in the skin, in the stomach mucosa, and in the reticuloendothelial cells of the bone marrow [2]. Claims that ferrokinetic measurements can be used to distinguish between cirrhosis with hyperferremia and idiopathic hemochromatosis are no longer accepted, the earlier finding of greater nonerythroid iron turnover possibly being ascribable to incomplete transferrin binding of the injected radioiron [40].

Differential Diagnosis

The differential diagnosis of fully developed idiopathic hemochromatosis poses only two real problems. The first disappears if the degree of iron overload is established quantitatively, since this enables cirrhosis of alcoholic or nutritional origin to be distinguished from hemochromatosis even if a fair amount of hemosiderin is visible on histologic examination. Once it is clear that iron overload of hemochromatotic severity is present, it remains only to determine whether the hemochromatosis is the result of the inheritance of the HLA-linked iron-loading genes or not. The presence of thalassemia or one of other chronic anemias which may lead to iron loading can usually be easily recognized, although in thalassemia intermedia and refractory sideroblastic anemia a hemoglobin concentration closer to the normal can lead to diagnostic error. It is only the rare patient (outside southern Africa) who has consumed large amounts of absorbable iron for prolonged periods of time, usually together with alcohol, who poses a real problem. At least some of the subjects who develop significant iron overload under such circumstances may be idiopathic hemochromatosis heterozygotes. The cellular distribution of the iron would be expected on the basis of the findings in black South Africans (see previous section) to provide the distinguishing feature, namely a much greater involvement of the reticuloendothelial system in those individuals whose iron overload is not ascribable even partially to genetic predisposition, and histologic examination of the liver may therefore be helpful. Finally, investigation of the relatives, especially if it includes HLA typing, should reveal the genetic factor.

Treatment

Diabetes and hepatic and cardiac failure should be managed along conventional lines. Loss of libido and secondary sexual characteristics often benefit by the administration of androgens [2]. In addition to this supportive treatment, it is essential to undertake definitive therapy in the form of the *removal of the excess iron*. The method of choice is repeated venesection [2]. The quantity of iron removed with each pint of blood naturally depends on the hemoglobin concentration, but it is about 200 to 250 mg. The erythroid marrow responds to the induced anemia by stepping up the rate of erythropoiesis, and iron to replace that which has been removed is mobilized from the tissues. Most patients tolerate the removal of a pint of blood every week for prolonged periods, and even more frequent venesections may be possible [272]. Before initiating the venesection program it is important to assess the degree of cardiac involvement, clinically and by special investigations including radiography, electrocardiography, and echocardiography [372]. Since myocardial irritability, with attendant arrhythmias, may be aggravated by the mobilization of free iron, continuous infusions of deferoxamine (see later section) should be administered while the initial venesections are cautiously performed. Beta-adrenergic blocking agents have proved to be valuable for controlling supraventricular tachycardias.

The hemoglobin concentration initially falls somewhat, but the hematocrit soon returns to within 10 percent of its initial level (Fig. 59-10). It should be measured before each weekly phlebotomy, and the plasma iron and ferritin concentrations should be estimated each month, so that progress with the elimination of the excess iron can be monitored. Two to three years of venesection therapy is usually required to remove the iron, but in some patients less is present and the treatment

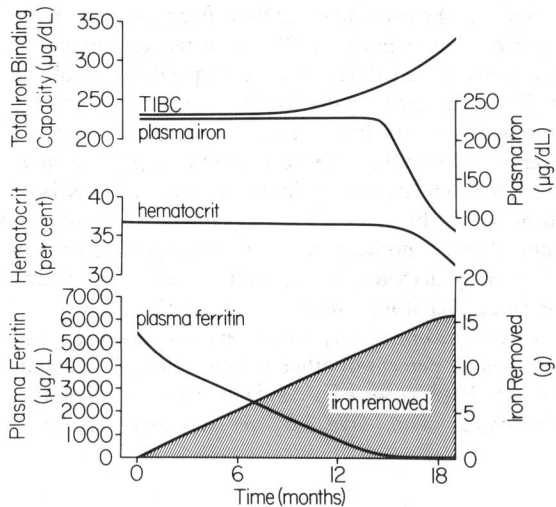

Figure 59-10 Serial changes in the hematocrit, plasma iron concentration, total iron-binding capacity, and plasma ferritin concentration in a subject with idiopathic hemochromatosis on repeated venesection therapy. (*From Bothwell et al. [2]. Used by permission.*)

correspondingly shorter [274]. After the excess has been eliminated reaccumulation can be prevented by venesecting every 2 to 3 months. Typically the plasma iron concentration remains high until tissue iron stores are almost exhausted, but occasionally a pseudo iron-deficient state may occur while abundant iron is still present in the tissues. This may be due to the development of a hepatoma, or else to ascorbic acid deficiency, which inhibits the mobilization of storage iron [34]. If the venesection rate is reduced for a period a satisfactory response usually returns. Ascorbic acid supplements can be administered, but this should be done cautiously since there is some evidence that the repair of the ascorbic acid deficiency may result in parenchymal cell damage, notably to the myocardium [373], perhaps by facilitating lipid peroxidation [374]. The ascorbic acid deficiency, which is a consequence of iron overload (see previous section), may thus actually be protective.

The plasma albumin concentration is usually well maintained during the venesection program, although it is reasonable to prescribe a moderately high protein diet. In alcoholic subjects the liver damage may lead to hypoproteinemia, and plasma may have to be replaced. If the restrictive form of cardiomyopathy is present it may be necessary to infuse plasma while the venesection is being performed in order to prevent hypovolemic shock [2]. It is not worth attempting to restrict the dietary intake of iron, since the amount absorbed is small in relation to the quantities being removed.

Chelating agents, of which the iron-specific deferoxamine is the best, can be used to remove excess iron from the body. Indeed, chelation is the only treatment available for the iron overload secondary to refractory anemias, but the rate of removal of iron is slower than with venesection unless continuous daily infusion techniques are used [358, 375, 376]. Deferoxamine is expensive and the parenteral route of administration inconvenient. The search for orally effective agents continues [377].

Prognosis

If the iron is not removed, the 5-year survival rate after diagnosis is 18 percent, and the 10-year survival rate 6 percent

[277]. Removing the iron improves these figures to 66 percent and 32 percent, respectively [277]. Death before removal of the iron can be completed occurs more frequently in alcoholic subjects [239]. The cardiopathy usually regresses [2], and the pigmentation disappears. Improvement in hepatic function has been observed in about half the treated subjects [277]. Apparent reduction in the degree of fibrosis in the liver has been reported by some observers [214, 268], but portal hypertension is not affected, nor are the other consequences of iron overload, namely diabetes, hypogonadism, and arthropathy. The incidence of hepatoma and other tumors remains high. Of treated subjects in one study, 29 percent eventually died of hepatoma, and 22 percent of other malignancies [277]. Hepatoma has not been reported in individuals with idiopathic hemochromatosis who have not yet developed cirrhosis [378].

The Widening Clinical Spectrum of Idiopathic Hemochromatosis

The availability of the HLA system as a linked marker for the iron-loading gene has made it possible to define the distinction between homozygotes and heterozygotes among the relatives of patients with fully developed idiopathic hemochromatosis. The ability to detect a genetic disease prior to the development of clinical signs and symptoms usually changes our understanding of its symptomatology, and it becomes apparent that the pattern of clinical manifestations among many "affected" persons is often considerably less severe than was suggested earlier [379]. This has proved to be the case with idiopathic hemochromatosis. It is now known that many homozygous individuals are asymptomatic [192] and that the classic triad of hepatomegaly, skin pigmentation, and diabetes mellitus is uncommon [187]. In fact, some homozygotes have none of these features. In a study of 35 homozygotes, 14 of whom were probands, only half the subjects had hepatomegaly, cirrhosis, and skin pigmentation, while diabetes was present in fewer than 10 percent and cardiac failure in none [127]. The plasma ferritin concentration was actually found to be normal in a small proportion of male homozygotes, although the hepatic iron concentration was always raised (Fig. 59-11) [187]. Complete saturation of the transferrin and increased liver iron was the rule only after the age of 20 years, and clinical manifestations were seen only in adults [187, 192]. With advancing age

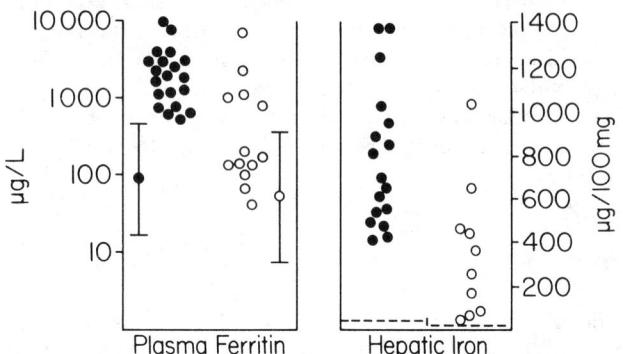

Figure 59-11 Serum ferritin and hepatic iron concentrations in male (closed circles) and female (open circles) subjects homozygous for the HLA-linked iron-loading gene. The normal mean value (±SD) for serum ferritin is shown, as is the upper limit of normal (broken lines) for hepatic iron concentration. *(From Edwards et al. [187]. Used by permission.)*

iron loading increased, reaching a peak in the fifth decade (Fig. 59-12) [192], and it is obvious that the risk of developing the clinical disease increased in parallel. The "textbook" description of clinical and pathologic idiopathic hemochromatosis therefore represents only the most severe end of the spectrum, and a recent study in Sweden suggests that adults, and especially males, with unexplained elevation of the serum transaminases ("transaminitis") should be investigated for iron overload [379a]. These studies have confirmed that female homozygotes are much less frequently affected clinically, the main reason being, as already discussed, that they lose a significant amount of iron with each menstrual period.

Heterozygotes   Carriers (2pq) are naturally always much more numerous than affected homozygotes (q^2). If the frequency of homozygosity for the HLA-linked iron-loading gene is 1/10,000 there would be 200 times as many carriers as homozygotes, and even with the high homozygote frequencies found in Utah and in Brittany there would be 40 to 50 times as many carriers as homozygotes.

At present heterozygotes can be identified only by HLA typing among the relatives of iron-loaded homozygous individuals. There is no test that will detect heterozygote carriers in the general population. The mean values for the various laboratory tests of iron metabolism (plasma iron concentration, transferrin saturation, plasma ferritin concentration, liver iron concentration) have been found somewhat higher in such heterozygotes than in normal subjects, but in general they were closer to the normal values than to those found in abnormal homozygotes (Table 59-2) [186, 192, 192a]. The liver iron concentration did gradually increase with age, with the result that by middle age 20 to 30 percent of heterozygotes had accumulated sufficient iron to qualify as a minor iron load (defined as more than 50 percent transferrin saturation or a hepatic iron load of more than 30 μg/100 mg in men and more than 20 μg/100 mg in women) (Fig. 59-12) [186, 192]. No heterozygotes had any *clinical* manifestation of iron overload. No further changes were observed after 45 years of age. It is conceivable that factors such as alcoholism, excess iron intake, porphyria cutanea tarda, or accelerated erythropoiesis might lead to the occasional clinical expression of overt iron-storage disease among heterozygotes. However, it should be noted that the prevalence of the HLA-A3 and HLA-B14 antigens, which occur with increased frequency in subjects with idiopathic hemochromatosis, is not increased in subjects with iron overload accompanying alcoholic liver disease [181]. This suggests they are not heterozygous for the HLA-linked iron-loading gene. It would nevertheless be of interest to have details on the drinking habits of those heterozygotes who have been found to have accumulated a minor iron load [192]. Idiopathic refractory sideroblastic anemia may sometimes be associated with a single allele for idiopathic hemochromatosis, since there is a higher frequency of HLA-A$_3$ in such patients [380]. Similarly, iron overload–associated myopathy may develop in some patients on maintenance hemodialysis because they carry a single HLA-linked iron-loading gene [381]. Heterozygosity for this gene may therefore be the reason why only certain patients develop iron overload under a variety of circumstances.

It has been suggested that the level of iron fortification of flour in the USA should be increased [382]. While there is little doubt that the resulting increase in the amount of absorbable iron in the average diet would cause clinical manifestations to occur more frequently and at a younger age in affected homo-

Table 59-2 Iron status of male subjects (normal subjects, heterozygotes, and homozygotes for the HLA-linked iron-loading gene) in Utah*

	Normal subjects			Heterozygotes			Homozygotes†		
	No.	Mean	95% limit	No.	Mean	95% limit	No.	Mean	95% limit
Age, years	44	33	0–77	67	33	0–75	13	48	25–70
Serum iron, µg/dl	44	106	50–162	67	135	62–208	13	244	173–307
Transferrin saturation, %	44	32	14–50	67	44	19–69	13	95	80–100
Serum ferritin,‡ µg/liter	41	93	16–542	64	96	15–617	12	2099	565–11560
Urinary iron,§ mg/24 h	19	1.3	0.4–2.2	38	1.6	0.2–3.0	12	11.2	4.4–26.5
Parenchymal stainable cell iron, grade	22	0.2	0–1	22	1.1	0–3	12	3.9	3.4
Hepatic iron, µg/100 mg	22	12	0–29	22	96	0–282	10	877	486–1417

* Data rearranged from Cartwright and coworkers [192].
† Majority identified because of signs and symptoms of fully developed idiopathic hemochromatosis.
‡ Geometric mean.
§ After deferoxamine 15 µg per kilogram of body weight intramuscularly.

zygotes, it remains conjectural as to whether it would have any deleterious effects on the great majority of heterozygotes [383]. From what is commonly known of iron balance it would be expected that there would be an increase in the iron stores in such individuals, but not to levels that would be potentially harmful. In fact, Sweden has had a program of iron fortification similar to that proposed for the United States in operation for a number of years, and there is as yet no evidence that heterozygotes have been adversely affected [384]. At the same time it is mandatory that the situation in Sweden be carefully and repeatedly monitored.

Detection of Affected Family Members Since idiopathic hemochromatosis is a treatable genetic disease, every effort must be made to detect subjects homozygous for the iron-loading gene. The combination of HLA typing and studies of iron status allows the identification of such subjects among the relatives of patients with the clinically manifested disease long before clinical manifestations have occurred. Once a diagnosis of idiopathic hemochromatosis is made in any patient, all male sibs past the age of 10 years should be tested for HLA type and iron status. The latter studies should include the plasma iron concentration, the transferrin saturation, and the

plasma ferritin concentration. If a sib's HLA haplotypes are found to be identical to those of the patient, it is highly likely that such a person is homozygous for the disease, and if the measures of iron status suggest significant iron loading, a liver biopsy for assay of the liver iron concentration should be performed and periodic venesections should be instituted in those with raised iron stores. If this is done it is probable that the clinical damage of iron overload, including liver tumors, can be prevented. Haplotype-identical sibs who do not show evidence of a significant iron load should be restudied every 2 to 3 years in order to detect the earliest manifestations of iron accumulation. The initial investigation of female sibs can perhaps be deferred until after the age of 20 years, since the rate of iron loading is less rapid in them and clinical manifestations occur in consequence much less frequently and at a later age.

Identification of affected individuals in the latent phase of the disorder should make it possible to study the cellular dynamics of iron metabolism in heterozygotes and homozygotes in much more detail. If it is possible to identify the basic defect in idiopathic hemochromatosis, then it is hoped that tests can be developed to detect carriers and homozygotes in the population at large and not just in the affected families of individuals who have already accumulated significant amounts of iron.

Figure 59-12 Hepatic iron concentrations as a function of age in males homozygous (●) and heterozygous (○) for the HLA-linked iron-loading gene. The normal range is indicated by the cross-hatched area. (*From Cartwright et al.* [192]. *Used by permission.*)

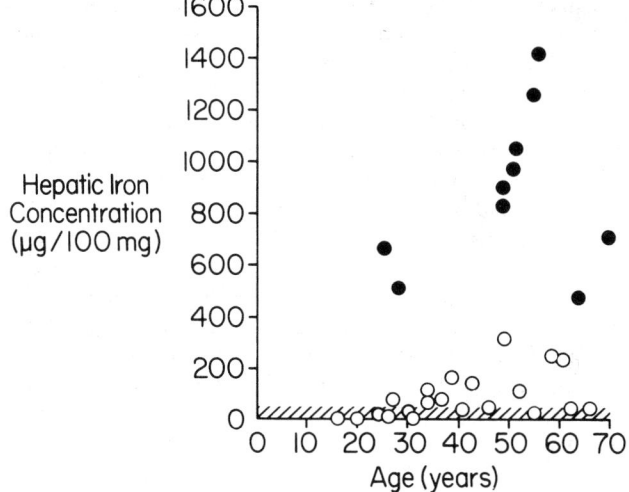

HEMOCHROMATOSIS IN HEREDITARY ANEMIAS

Clinical and pathologic features similar to those found in idiopathic hemochromatosis have been reported in a number of patients suffering from a variety of chronic anemias [2]. These fall into distinct groups on the basis of the degree of erythropoietic activity in the bone marrow. The first includes patients with hypoplastic anemia who are maintained on repeated blood transfusions over many years. Since each pint of blood contains 250 mg iron, tissue concentrations of storage iron in the range found in idiopathic hemochromatosis are often reached and may even be exceeded, but the overt pathologic and metabolic consequences tend to be milder because of the initial predominantly reticuloendothelial localization of the iron (see previous section). When reports of 20 such individuals were analyzed, only 1 had developed cirrhosis of the liver, although 4 had impaired glucose tolerance and 5 overt diabetes [269]. In a recent study disturbed glucose tolerance and endocrine function were noted in several multiply transfused subjects with hypoplastic anemias. This indicated that enough redistribution of iron occurs from reticuloendothelial into parenchymal tissues for disorders of cellular function to occur [385]. In the chronic anemias in which the bone marrow is hyperplastic but in which erythropoiesis is largely ineffective in terms of delivery of viable red cells into the circulation, there is heavy hepatocyte loading and parenchymal deposits in other tissues, and the full hemochromatosis syndrome is typically seen [2]. The reasons for the difference in iron distribution have been considered in a previous section. This group comprises thalassemia major and sometimes thalassemia intermedia, hereditary and acquired sideroblastic anemias, pyridoxine-responsive anemias, and a variety of other anemias associated with blocks in the incorporation of iron into hemoglobin [2].

By far the commonest of these conditions are the thalassemic syndromes (see Chap. 77). Their prevalence varies in different parts of the world [271, 386, 387]. Subjects heterozygous for any of the thalassemic genes do not accumulate excessive amounts of iron [156, 271, 278]. On the other hand, iron overload often is a feature of patients carrying two different abnormal genes (e.g., β thalassemia–hemoglobin E disease). In general, the most severe degrees of iron overload are encountered in patients with β thalassemia major. It is due not only to the repeated blood transfusions. Severe iron overload noted in subjects who have received little or no donor blood indicates that absorption of iron from the diet is increased [269]. This abnormality in iron absorption has been confirmed by radioisotope studies [154, 388]. Whether the tendency to absorb inappropriate amounts of iron is secondary to the exuberant but ineffective erythropoietic activity is not certain. The reduction in absorption that occurs when erythropoiesis is inhibited by keeping the hemoglobin concentration near the normal range via transfusion [278] is consistent with this interpretation. On the other hand, it is theoretically possible that some subjects with thalassemia major carry a genetic defect which is responsible for increased iron absorption [389]. In this connection it is of interest that certain individuals with idiopathic sideroblastic anemia associated with iron overload have been shown to be heterozygous for the HLA-linked iron-loading gene [379]. Clinically manifested hemochromatosis may therefore develop in such subjects when the sideroblastic factor is also present.

Pathologic and Clinical Features

The iron load in frequently transfused patients with thalassemia major is about 20 g by the age of 10 years [278]. This figure is equivalent to the average amount found at the time clinical manifestations occur in idiopathic hemochromatosis. In individuals who survive for 20 years the figure is a good deal higher, usually between 80 and 100 g. The hemochromatosis of thalassemia is similar to that seen in young and very severely affected patients with idiopathic hemochromatosis. *Cardiac manifestations* are the most serious for survival; they become particularly prominent in the second decade of life and are essentially those of a cardiomyopathy [155, 156, 278]. In one study of 41 patients with refractory anemia, 39 of whom had

thalassemia major, 26 had developed congestive cardiac failure and 19 pericarditis [270]. The heart was dilated and hypertrophied and on microscopy large amounts of iron were present in muscle cells and histiocytes, with extensive fibrosis and focal degeneration. In another analysis of 305 patients, the majority of the 52 deaths had occurred at an early age because of anemia or infection [156]. The age at death in the 21 who succumbed to iron overload ranged between 11 and 23 years, with the terminal event in every case being cardiac failure. If the teens are reached, *endocrine failure* becomes prominent [266, 390]. Failure or severe retardation of puberty is the most common manifestation and is associated with absence or retardation of the adolescent growth spurt. While maintaining the hemoglobin concentration at higher levels does improve the early growth rate, severe growth retardation nevertheless becomes obvious between 9 and 11 years [155, 156, 278, 391, 392]. Its exact cause is not known; but it is not due to growth hormone deficiency [271, 393]. Overt *diabetes mellitus* is frequently found among older patients, and even when it is not present laboratory evidence of abnormal pancreatic endocrine function can be demonstrated in the majority of patients [393, 394]. *Liver disease* is a constant feature. In the first decade hepatomegaly with cirrhosis is usually well established and is uniformly found in heavily transfused patients [156]. In a series of 32 liver biopsies a good correlation between the severity of the fibrosis and both the age of the patient and the liver iron concentration was found [263]. At iron concentrations of less than 0.6 g/100 g progression was relatively slow, but thereafter it accelerated. At all stages the iron is located in both reticuloendothelial cells and hepatocytes, with increasing parenchymal deposition occurring when the liver iron concentration is greater than 0.75 g/100 g [263]. Splenectomy has been reported to promote parenchymal loading in the liver and to accelerate the development of cirrhosis [395–397]. This can be ascribed to the rise in the mean transferrin saturation from between 62 and 74 percent to 90 percent which occurs after splenectomy [387]. A last factor aggravating liver damage in thalassemia major is serum hepatitis [279].

Management

The management of thalassemia major changed in 1964 following the demonstration that children transfused frequently in order to maintain a higher hemoglobin concentration were a good deal healthier and lived just as long as undertransfused patients [398]. Although the iron loading is accelerated by the additional units of blood, absorption of dietary iron is diminished at higher hemoglobin concentrations with the result that the total accumulation may not be much greater [278]. On such therapy growth is normal until about 9 years of age, but then the complications resulting from the iron overload appear. It is obviously desirable to remove as much iron as possible, and in recent years deferoxamine has been increasingly used for this purpose. There is evidence that worthwhile results have been achieved [399, 400]. While it does not appear to be possible to prevent the accumulation of iron during the first few years of life with daily intramuscular injections of 0.5 to 1 g deferoxamine, an equilibrium can be reached at tissue iron concentrations significantly lower than in untreated patients [266, 298]. Hepatic fibrosis may be arrested, and preliminary results suggest that cardiotoxicity may be diminished and survival prolonged. It is not clear whether this is due to the removal of iron only, since deferoxamine has been shown to inhibit collagen synthesis in fibroblast culture [293].

A number of workers have tried to increase the amount of iron eliminated by finding more effective ways of administering the deferoxamine. Continuous intravenous infusion mobilizes more iron than intramuscular injections, but this is obviously not feasible for long-term daily treatment. Continuous subcutaneous infusion has been shown to be almost as effective, and the development of small infusion pumps has made the method a practical one for home use (Fig. 59-13) [358, 376, 401]. It is now usually given only overnight since urinary iron losses are almost as great as when it is continued for 24 h [358, 375, 376, 402–404]. A dose of 20 mg/(kg·day) is usual, although larger amounts have also been tried [358, 376]. While the long-term effects of such therapy are not yet known, initial results are promising in that it is now possible to induce a negative balance in patients on high transfusion regimens [358, 373, 376, 403, 404]. Since different chelators have different modes of action, combinations have been used. Thus, diethylenetriamine pentaacetate (DTPA) in a dosage of 1 to 3 g may be added to the transfused blood, although it is too toxic for continuous administration.

The use of ascorbic acid in therapy is more controversial. As was mentioned in a previous section, subclinical ascorbic acid deficiency is commonly associated with various forms of iron overload, and this is true also of thalassemia major [405, 406]. Deferoxamine mobilizes iron less efficiently when ascorbic acid deficiency is present, and correction of the deficiency causes a mean twofold increase in urinary iron excretion. As a result, ascorbic acid has been widely used as an adjunct to chelator therapy [155, 156]. The wisdom of this approach has been questioned [373]. The ascorbic acid deficiency resulting from iron overload causes a partial block in the release of iron from reticuloendothelial cells [34]. It is therefore theoretically possible that its administration in a disease such as thalassemia major may lead to a relocation of iron from the reticuloendothelial system, where it is relatively innocuous, to the vulnerable parenchymal tissues. It has also been suggested that ascorbic acid facilitates the lipid peroxidation which is the presumptive mechanism of cellular iron toxicity [374]. Support for the view that the administration of ascorbic acid is hazardous has been provided by the demonstration of objective deterioration in cardiac function in 8 of 11 thalassemic subjects [373]. Function improved in 5 of them when the ascorbic acid was stopped. While other workers have not found evidence that ascorbic acid has deleterious effects [407], it should probably not be given to iron-loaded patients who are not receiving regular chelation therapy, or to massively iron-loaded patients just starting on deferoxamine therapy [156]. The dose should not exceed 200 mg daily and should be the smallest one necessary to achieve augmented iron excretion [373]. In addition, cardiac function should be monitored regularly. The results of several studies indicate that this can be effectively achieved in thalassemia major by echocardiography [372, 373, 408].

Another approach that is currently being explored in the treatment of thalassemia major is the transfusion of young red cells (neocytes) [409]. While this allows the interval between transfusions to be lengthened significantly so that the iron loading is slowed down, the approach is technically difficult and must still be regarded as experimental. Finally, the enhanced absorption of dietary iron, which adds significantly to the iron loading, can be diminished by the simple measure of drinking tea with meals [410] because the tannins in tea are potent inhibitors of iron absorption [131].

While current therapeutic approaches using iron chelators are promising, it must be pointed out that they are expensive and complicated and are therefore unsuitable for application in many areas where thalassemia major is common. It is hoped that in the future there will be combinations of chelators with differing and complementary modes of action which can be given in depot form or preferably orally [377, 411, 412].

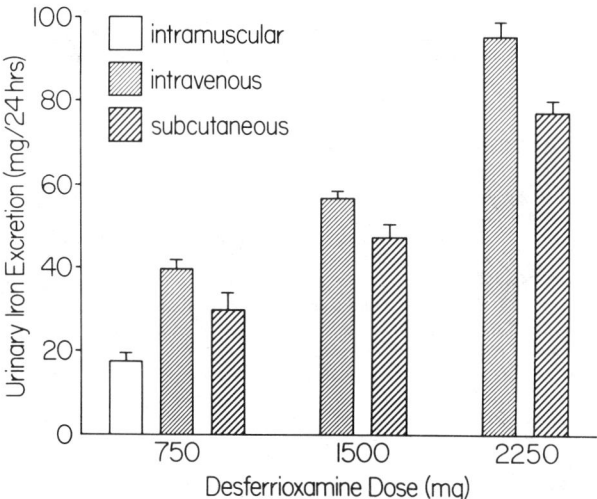

Figure 59-13 A comparison of the effects on urinary iron excretion of intermittent intramuscular injections of deferoxamine with those of continuous subcutaneous and continuous intravenous administration. Mean values (±SE) are given at three different dosage levels in patients with iron overload secondary to multiple transfusions. (*After Propper et al.* [358]. *Used by permission.*)

REFERENCES

1. FAIRBANKS VF, FAHEY JL, BEUTLER E: In *Clinical Disorders of Iron Metabolism.* New York, Grune & Stratton, 1971
2. BOTHWELL TH, CHARLTON RW, COOK JD, FINCH CA: *Iron Metabolism in Man.* Oxford, Blackwell, 1979
3. WORWOOD M: Serum Ferritin. *Crit Rev Clin Lab Sci* 10:171, 1979
4. FINCH SC, FINCH CA: Idiopathic hemochromatosis, an iron storage disease. *Medicine* 34:381, 1955
5. LYNCH SR, LIPSCHITZ DA, BOTHWELL TH, CHARLTON RW: Iron and the reticuloendothelial system, in Jacobs A, Worwood M (eds): *Iron in Biochemistry and Medicine.* New York, Academic, 1974, p 563
6. TRUMP BF, VALIGORSKY JM, ARSTILA AU, MERGNER WJ, KINNEY TD: The relationship of intracellular pathways of iron metabolism to cellular iron overload and the iron storage diseases. *Am J Path* 72:295, 1973
7. TRUMP BF, ARSTILA AU, VALIGORSKY JM, BARRETT LA: Subcellular aspects of ferritin metabolism, in Chrichton RR (ed): *Proteins of Iron Storage and Transport in Biochemistry and Medicine.* Amsterdam, North-Holland, 1975, p 343
8. CHRICHTON RR, COLLET-CASSARD D, PONCE-ORTIZ Y, WAUTERS M, ROMAN F, PAQUES E: Ferritin comparative structural studies, iron deposition and mobilization, in Brown EB, Aisen P, Fielding J, Chrichton RR (eds): *Proteins of Iron Metabolism.* New York, Grune & Stratton, 1977, p 13
9. CHRICHTON RR, PONCE-ORTIZ Y, KOCH MHJ, PARFAIT R, STUHRMANN HB: Isolation and characterization of phytoferritin from pea (*Pisum sativum*) and lentil (*Lens esculenta*). *Biochem J* 171:349, 1978
10. LAUFBERGER MV: Sur la cristallisation de la ferritine. *Bull Soc Chim Biol* 19:1575, 1937
11. GRANICK S: Structure and physiological functions of ferritin. *Physiol Rev* 31:489, 1951
12. CHRICHTON RR: The biochemistry of ferritin. *Br J Haemat* 24:677, 1973

13. HARRISON PM: Ferritin: an iron-storage molecule. *Seminars in Hemat* 14:55, 1977
14. HARRISON PM: The structure and function of ferritin, in *Iron Metabolism. Ciba Foundation Symposium 51* (new series). Amsterdam, Elsevier, 1977, p 19
15. HOARE RJ, HARRISON PM, HOY TG: The molecular structure and metal-ion binding sites of horse-spleen apoferritin, in Chrichton RR (ed): *Proteins of Iron Storage and Transport in Biochemistry and Medicine.* Amsterdam, North-Holland, 1975, p 231
16. CHRICHTON RR: Personal communication
17. HARRISON PM, BANYARD SH, HOARE RJ, RUSSELL SM, TREFFRY A: The structure and function of ferritin, in *Iron Metabolism. Ciba Foundation Symposium 51* (new series). Amsterdam, Elsevier, 1977, p 19
18. CHRICHTON RR, HUEBERS H, HUEBERS E, COLLET-CASSARD D, PONCE Y: Comparative studies on ferritin, in Chrichton RR (ed): *Proteins of Iron storage and transport in Biochemistry and Medicine.* Amsterdam, North-Holland, 1975, p 193
19. POWELL LW, MCKEERING L, HALLIDAY JW: Microheterogeneity of tissue ferritins in iron storage disease, in Chrichton RR (ed): *Proteins of Iron Storage and Transport in Biochemistry and Medicine.* Amsterdam, North-Holland, 1975, p 367
20. DRYSDALE JW: Ferritin phenotypes: structure and metabolism, in *Iron Metabolism. Ciba Foundation Symposium 51* (new series). Amsterdam, Elsevier, 1977, p 41
21. RUSSELL SM, HARRISON PM: Heterogeneity in horse ferritins. A comparative study of surface change, iron content and kinetics of iron uptake. *Biochem J* 175:91, 1978
22. WAGSTAFF M, WORWOOD M, JACOBS A: Properties of human tissue iso-ferritins. *Br J Haematol* 173:969, 1978
23. DRYSDALE JW, MUNRO HN: Regulation of synthesis and turnover of ferritin in rat liver. *J Biol Chem* 241:3630, 1966
24. ZAHRINGER J, KONIJN AM, BAGLIGA BS, MUNRO HN: Mechanism of iron induction of ferritin synthesis. *Biochem Biophys Res Comm* 65:583, 1975
25. DRYSDALE JW, SHAFRITZ DA: Induction of ferritin by iron, in Chrichton RR (ed): *Proteins of Iron Storage and Transport in Biochemistry and Medicine.* Amsterdam, North-Holland, 1975, p 319
26. REDMAN CM: Biosynthesis of serum proteins and ferritin by free and attached ribosomes of rat liver. *J Biol Chem* 244:4308, 1969
27. KONIJN AM, BAGLIGA BS, MUNRO HN: Synthesis of liver ferritin on free and membrane-bound polyribosomes of different sizes. *FEBS Lett* 37:249, 1973
28. CHRICHTON RR: Interactions between iron metabolism and oxygen activation, in *Oxygen Free Radicals and Tissue Damage, Ciba Foundation Series No. 65* (new series). Amsterdam, Elsevier/North-Holland 1979, p 57
29. LINDER MC, MUNRO HN: Metabolic and chemical features of ferritins, a series of iron inducible tissue proteins. *Am J Pathol* 72:263, 1973
30. PAPE L, MULTANI JS, STITT C, SALTMAN P: The mobilization of iron from ferritin by chelating agents. *Biochem* 7:613, 1968
31. BIELIG HJ, BAYER E: Synthetisches Ferritin, ein Eisen (III) Komplex des Apoferritins. *Naturwissenschaften* 42:125, 1955
32. SIRIVECH S, FRIEDEN E, OSAKI S: The release of iron from horse spleen ferritin by reduced flavins. *Biochem J* 143:311, 1974
33. OSAKI S, SIRIVECH S: Identification and partial purification of a ferritin reducing enzyme in liver. *Fed Proc* 30:1292 (abstract), 1971
34. LIPSCHITZ DA, BOTHWELL TH, SEFTEL HC, WAPNICK AA, CHARLTON RW: The role of ascorbic acid in the metabolism of storage iron. *Br J Haematol* 20:155, 1971
35. HILTON JW, CHO CY, SLINGER SJ: Effect of graded levels of supplemental ascorbic acid in practical diets fed to Rainbow Trout (*Salmo gairdneri*) *J Fish Res Can* 35:431, 1978
36. COOK JD, HERSHKO C, FINCH CA: Storage iron kinetics. I. Measurements of the cellular distribution of ^{59}Fe in rat liver. *J Lab Clin Med* 80:613, 1972
37. CHARLTON RW, BOTHWELL TH: Hemochromatosis: dietary and genetic aspects, in Brown EB, Moore CV (eds): *Progress in Hematology.* New York, Grune & Stratton, 1966, vol 5, p 298
38. WEIBEL ER, STAUBLI W, GNAGI HR, HESS FA: Correlated morphometric and biochemical studies on the liver cell. 1. Morphometric model, stereologic methods, and normal morphometric data for rat liver. *J Cell Biol* 42:68, 1969
39. TORRANCE JD, CHARLTON RW, SCHMAMAN A, LYNCH SR, BOTHWELL TH: Storage iron in 'muscle.' *J Clin Pathol* 21:495, 1968
40. FINCH CA, DEUBELBEISS K, COOK JD, ESCHBACH JW, HARKER LA, FUNK DD, MARSAGLIA G, HILLMAN RS, SLICHTER S, ADAMSON JW, GANZONI A, GIBLETT ER: Ferrokinetics in man. *Medicine* 49:17, 1970
41. HERSHKO C, COOK JD, FINCH CA: Storage iron kinetics. II. The uptake of hemoglobin iron by hepatic parenchymal cells. *J Lab Clin Med* 80:624, 1972
42. ADDISON GM, BEAMISH MR, HALES CN, HODGKINS M, JACOBS A, LLEWELLIN P: An immunoradiometric assay for ferritin in the serum of normal

43. WORWOOD M, DAWKINS S, WAGSTAFF M, JACOBS A: Purification and properties of ferritin from human serum. *Biochem J* 157:97, 1976
44. AROSIO P, YOKOTA M, DRYSDALE JW: Characterization of serum ferritin in iron overload: Possible identity to natural apoferritin. *Br J Haematol* 36:199, 1977
45. SIIMES MA, DALLMAN PR: New kinetic role for serum ferritin in iron metabolism. *Br J Haematol* 28:1, 1974
46. WORWOOD M, CRAGG SJ, JACOBS A, MCLAREN C, RICKETTS C, ECONOMIDOU J: Binding of serum ferritin to concanavalin A: Patients with homozygous B thalassemia and transfusional iron overload. *Br J Haematol* 46:409, 1980
47. SIIMES MA, ADDIEGO JE, DALLMAN PR: Ferritin in serum: Diagnosis of iron deficiency and iron overload in infants and children. *Blood* 43:581, 1974
48. POLLOCK AS, LIPSCHITZ DA, COOK JD: The kinetics of serum ferritin. *Proc Soc Exp Biol Med* 157:481, 1978
49. HALLIDAY JW, MACK U, POWELL LW: The kinetics of serum and tissue ferritins: relation to carbohydrate content. *Br J Haematol* 42:535, 1979
50. LIPSCHITZ DA, DUGARD J, SIMON MO, BOTHWELL TH, CHARLTON RW: The site of action of desferrioxamine. *Br J Haematol* 20:395, 1971
51. HERSHKO C, COOK JD, FINCH CA: Storage iron kinetics. III. Study of desferrioxamine action by selective radioiron labels of RE and parenchymal cells. *J Lab Clin Med* 81:876, 1973
52. WALTERS GO, MILLER FM, WORWOOD M: Serum ferritin concentration and iron stores in normal subjects. *J Clin Path* 26:770, 1973
53. COOK JD, LIPSCHITZ DA, MILES LEM, FINCH CA: Serum ferritin as a measure of iron stores in normal subjects. *Am J Clin Nutr* 27:681, 1974
54. JACOBS A, MILLER E, WORWOOD M, BEAMISH MR, WARDROP CA: Ferritin in the serum of normal subjects and patients with iron deficiency and iron overload. *Br Med J* 4:206, 1972
55. LIPSCHITZ DA, COOK JD, FINCH DA: A clinical evaluation of serum ferritin. *N Engl J Med* 290:1213, 1974
56. PRIETO J, BARRY M, SHERLOCK S: Serum ferritin in patients with iron overload and with acute and chronic liver disease. *Gastroenterology* 68:525, 1975
57. ROESER HP, HALLIDAY JW, SIZEMORE DJ, NIKLES A, WILLGOSS D: Serum ferritin in ascorbic acid deficiency. *Br J Haematol* 45:457, 1980
58. ZUYDERHOUDT FMJ, JOMING GGA, DE HAAN JG, SAMSON G, VAN GOOL J: Rat liver storage iron and plasma ferritin during D-galactosamine-HCl–induced hepatitis. *Clin Sci* 58:321, 1980
59. ELIN RJ, WOLFF SM, FINCH CA: Effect of induced fever on serum iron and ferritin concentrations in man. *Blood* 49:147, 1977
60. SMITH RJ, DAVIS P, THOMSON AB, WADSWORTH LD, FACKRE P: Serum ferritin levels in anemia of rheumatoid arthritis. *J Rheumatol* 4:389, 1977
61. SIIMES MA, WANG WC, DALLMAN PR: Elevated serum ferritin in children with malignancies. *Scandinav J Haematol* 19:153, 1977
62. HAZARD JT, YOKOTA M, AROSIO P, DRYSDALE JW: Immunologic differences in human isoferritins: Implications for immunologic quantitation of serum ferritin. *Blood* 49:139, 1977
63. KEW MC, TORRANCE JD, DERMAN D, SIMON M, MACNAB GM, CHARLTON RW, BOTHWELL TH: Serum and tumour ferritin in primary liver cancer. *Gut* 19:294, 1978
64. MARCUS DM, ZINBERG N: Measurement of serum ferritin by radioimmunoassay: Results in normal individuals and patients with breast cancer. *J Nat Canc Inst* 55:791, 1975
65. WORWOOD M, SUMMERS M, MILLER F, JACOBS A, WHITTAKER JA: Ferritin in blood cells from normal subjects and patients with leukaemia. *Br J Haematol* 28:27, 1974
66. PARRY DH, WORWOOD M, JACOBS A: Serum ferritin in acute leukaemia at presentation and during remission. *Br Med J* 1:245, 1975
67. AWAI M, BROWN EB: Examination of the role of xanthine oxidase in iron absorption by the rat. *J Lab Clin Med* 73:366, 1969
68. POLLACK S, LASKY FD: A new iron-binding protein isolated from intestinal mucosa. *J Lab Clin Med* 87:670, 1976
69. HUEBERS H, HUEBERS E, RUMMEL W, CRICHTON RR: Isolation and characterization of iron-binding proteins from rat intestinal mucosa. *Eur J Biochem* 66:447, 1976
70. EVANS RW, WILLIAMS J: Studies on the binding of different iron donors to human serum transferrin and isolation of iron-binding fragments from the N- and C-terminal regions of the protein. *Biochem J* 173:543, 1978
71. ROBERTS RC, MAKEY DG, SEAL US: Human transferrin. *J Biol Chem* 241:4907, 1966
72. BEZKOROVAINY A, ZSCHOCKE RH: Structure and function of transferrins I. Physical, chemical and iron-binding properties. *Arzeim-Forsh (Drug Res)* 24:476 1974
73. JAMIESON GA, JETT M, DE BARNARDO SL: The carbohydrate sequence of the glyco-peptide chains of the human transferrin. *J Biol Chem* 246:3686, 1971

subjects and patients with iron deficiency and iron overload. *J Clin Pathol* 25:236, 1972

74. Spik G, Bayard B, Fournet B, Strecker G, Bouquelet S, Montreuil J: Studies on glycoconjugates. LXIV. Complete structure of two carbohydrate units of human serotransferrin. *FEBS Lett* 50:296, 1975

75. Giblett ERJ: Transferrin. In: *Physiological Pharmacology*. New York: Academic, 1974 vol V, p 555

76. Putman FW: Transferrin, in Putman FW (ed): *The Plasma Proteins*. 2nd ed. New York, Academic, 1975, vol 1, p 266

77. Lane RS: Transferrin, in Allison AL (ed): *Structure and Function of Plasma Proteins*. New York, Plenum, 1976, vol 2, p 53

78. Lynch SR, Simon M, Bothwell TH, Charlton RW: Circadian variation in plasma iron concentration and reticuloendothelial iron release in the rat. *Clin Sci Molec Med* 45:331, 1973

79. Fillet G, Marsaglia G: Idiopathic hemochromatosis (IH). Abnormality in RBC transport of iron by the reticuloendothelial system (RES). *Proceedings of the XVIIIth Meeting of the American Society for Hematology*, 1975, p 53

80. Bainton DF, Finch CA: The diagnosis of iron deficiency anemia. *Am J Med* 37:62, 1964

81. Konijn AM, Hershko C: Ferritin synthesis in inflammation I. Pathogenesis of impaired iron release *Br J Haematol* 37:7, 1977

82. Bates GW, Schlabach MR: The reaction of ferric salts with transferrin. *J Biol Chem* 248:3228, 1973

83. Harris DC: Functional equivalence of iron bound to human transferrin at low pH or high pH. *Biochim Biophys Acta* 496:563, 1977

84. Luk CK: Study of the nature of the metal-binding sites and estimate of the distance between the metal-binding sites in transferrin using trivalent lanthanide ions as fluorescent probes. *Biochemistry* 10:2838, 1971

85. Aasa R, Aisen P: An electron paramagnetic resonance study of the iron and copper complexes of transferrin. *J Biol Chem* 243:2399, 1968

86. Aisen P, Liebman A: The role of the anion-binding site of transferrin and its interaction with the reticulocyte. *Biochim Biophys Acta* 304:797, 1973

87. Koenig SH, Schillinger WE: Nuclear magnetic relaxation dispersion in protein solutions. II. Transferrin. *J Biol Chem* 244:6520, 1969

88. Aisen P, Liebman A, Zweier J: Stoichiometric and site characteristics of the binding of iron to human transferrin. *J Biol Chem* 253:1930, 1978

89. Donovan JW, Beardslee RA, Ross KD: Formation of monoferric ovotransferrins in the presence of chelates. *Biochem J* 153:631, 1976

90. Fletcher J, Huehns ER: Function of transferrin. *Nature* 218:1211, 1968

91. Pootrakul P, Christensen A, Josephson B, Finch CA: The role of transferrin in determining internal iron distribution. *Blood* 49:957 1977

92. Huebers H, Huebers E, Csiba E, Finch CA: Iron uptake from diferric and monoferric transferrin species by rat reticulocytes. *J Clin Invest* 62:944, 1978

93. Van Der Heul C, Kroos MJ, Van Noort WL, Van Eijk HG: No functional difference of the two iron-binding sites of human transferrin in vitro. *Clin Sci* 60:185, 1981

94. Van Baarlen J, Brouwer JT, Leibman A, Aisen P: Evidence for the functional heterogeneity of the two sites of transferrin in vitro. *Br J Haematol* 46:417, 1980

95. Morgan EH, Laurell CB: Studies on the exchange of iron between transferrin and reticulocytes. *Br J Haematol* 9:471, 1963

96. Cook JD, Marsaglia G, Eschbach JW, Funk DD, Finch CA: Ferrokinetics: a biologic model for plasma iron exchange in man. *J Clin Invest* 49:197, 1970

97. Fletcher J: The plasma clearance and liver uptake of iron from transferrin of low and high iron saturation. *Clin Sci* 41:395, 1971

98. Brown EB: Evidence supporting the concept of heterogeneity of iron atoms bound to transferrin in the rat, in Crichton RR (ed): *Proteins of Iron Storage and Transport in Biochemistry and Medicine*. New York, American Elsevier, 1975, p 97

99. Skarberg K, Eng K, Huebers H, Marsaglia G & Finch C: Plasma iron kinetics in man. An explanation for the effect of plasma iron concentration. *Proc Nat Acad Sci (US)* 75:1559, 1978

100. Morgan EH: Transferrin and transferrin iron, in Jacobs A, Worwood M (eds): *Iron in Biochemistry and Medicine*. London and New York, Academic, 1974, p 29

101. Baker E, Morgan EH: The kinetics of the interaction between rabbit transferrin and reticulocytes. *Biochemistry* 8:1133, 1969

102. Morgan EH, Baker E: The effect of metabolic inhibitors on transferrin and iron uptake and transferrin release from reticulocytes. *Biochim Biophys Acta* 184:442, 1969

103. Witt DP, Woodworth RC: Identification of transferrin receptor of rabbit reticulocyte. *Biochem Am Chem Soc* 17:3913, 1978

104. Vanbockxmeer FM, Morgan EH: Transferrin receptors during rabbit reticulocyte maturation. *Biochim Biophys Acta* 584:76, 1979

105. Steiner M: Identification of the binding-site for transferrin in human reticulocytes. *Biochim Biophys Res Commun* 94:861, 1980

106. Seligman PA, Schleicher RB, Allen RH: Isolation and characterization of the transferrin receptor from human-placenta. *J Biol Chem* 254:9943, 1979

107. Loh TT, Higuchi DA, Van Bockxmeer FM, Smith CH, Brown EB: Transferrin receptors in the human placental microvillous membrane. *J Clin Invest* 65:1182 1980

108. Kaylis SG, Morgan EH: Iron uptake by immature erythroid cells.'Mechanism of dependence on metabolic energy. *Biochim Biophys Acta* 464:389, 1977

109. Morgan EH: Studies on the mechanism of iron release from transferrin. *Biochim Biophys Acta* 580:312, 1979

110. Ricketts C, Jacobs A, Cavill I: Ferrokinetics and erythropoiesis in man: the measurement of effective erythropoiesis, ineffective erythropoiesis and red cell life span using ^{59}Fe. *Br J Haematol* 31:65, 1975

111. Green R, Charlton RW, Seftel H, Bothwell T, Mayet F, Adams B, Finch C, Layrisse M: Body iron excretion in man. A collaborative study. *Am J Med* 45:336, 1968

112. Dubach R, Moore CV, Callender S: Studies in iron transportation and metabolism. IX. The excretion of iron as measured by the isotope technique. *J Lab Clin Med* 45:599, 1955

113. Hallberg L, Hogdahl A-M, Nilsson L, Rybo G: Menstrual blood loss—a population study. Variation at different ages and attempts to define normality. *Acta Obstet Gynec Scand* 45:320, 1966

114. United States Department of Health, Education and Welfare, Publication No. 722, Ten states nutrition survey, 1972

115. Derman D, Sayers M, Lynch SR, Charlton RW, Bothwell TH, Mayet F: Iron absorption from a cereal diet containing cane sugar fortified with ascorbic acid. *Br J Nutr* 38:261, 1977

116. Hallberg L, Bjorn-Rasmussen E, Garby L, Pleehachinda R, Suwanik R: Iron absorption from South-East Asian diets and the effect of iron fortification. *Am J Clin Nutr* 31:1403, 1978

117. Moore CV: Iron nutrition and requirement. *Scand J Haemat Series Haematologica* 6:1, 1965

118. Charlton RW, Bothwell TH, Seftel HC: Dietary iron overload, in Callender ST (ed): *Clinics in Haematology*. London, W.B. Saunders, 1973, vol 2, p 383

119. Layrisse M, Cook JD, Martinez C, Roche M, Kuhn IN, Walker RB, Finch CA: Food iron absorption: A comparison of vegetable and animal foods. *Blood* 33:430, 1969

120. Martinez-Torres C, Layrisse M: Nutritional factors in iron deficiency: food iron absorption, in Callender ST (ed): *Clinics in Haematology*. London, W.B. Saunders, 1973, vol 2, p 339

121. Raffin SB, Woo CH, Roost KT, Price DC, Schmid R: Intestinal absorption of hemoglobin iron: Cleavage by mucosal heme oxygenase. *J Clin Invest* 54:1344, 1974

122. Layrisse M, Martinez-Torres C, Cook JD, Walker R, Finch CA: Iron fortification of food: Its measurement by the extrinsic tag method. *Blood* 41:333, 1973

123. Hallberg L, Bjorn-Rasmussen E, Howard L, Rossander L: Dietary heme iron absorption. *Scand J Gastroenterol* 14:769, 1979

124. Sayers MH, Lynch SR, Jacobs P, Charlton RW, Bothwell TH, Walker RB, Mayet F: The effects of ascorbic acid supplementation on the absorption of iron in maize, wheat and soya. *Br J Haematol* 24:209, 1973

125. Bjorn-Rasmussen E, Hallberg L: Iron absorption from maize. Effect of ascorbic acid on iron absorption from maize supplemented with ferrous sulphate. *Nutr Metabol* 16:94, 1974

126. Derman DP, Bothwell TH, MacPhail AP, Torrance JD, Bezwoda WR, Charlton RW, Mayet FGH: Importance of ascorbic acid in the absorption of iron from infant foods. *Scand J Haematol* 25:193, 1980

127. Monsen ER, Hallberg L, Layrisse M, Hegsted DM, Cook JD, Mertz W, Finch CA: Estimation of available dietary iron. *Am J Clin Nutr* 31:134, 1978

128. Forth W, Rummel W: Iron absorption. *Physiol Rev* 53:724, 1973

129. Conrad ME: Factors affecting iron absorption, in Hallberg L, Harwerth HG, Vannotti A (eds): *Iron Deficiency, Pathogenesis, Clinical Aspects, Therapy*. London & New York, Academic, 1970

130. Bjorn-Rasmussen E: Iron absorption from wheat bread: Influence of various amounts of bran. *Nutr Metabol* 16:101 1974

131. Disler PB, Lynch SR, Charlton RW, Torrance JD, Bothwell TH: The effect of tea on iron absorption. *Gut* 16:193, 1975

132. Halkett JAE, Peters T, Ross JF: Studies on the deposition and nature of egg yolk iron. *J Biol Chem* 231:187, 1958

133. Olsson H, Isaksson B, Norrby A, Solvell L: Food iron absorption in iron deficiency. *Am J Clin Nutr* 31:106, 1978

134. Monnier L, Colette C, Aguirre L, Mirouze J: Evidence and mechanism for pectin-reduced intestinal inorganic iron absorption in idiopathic hemochromatosis. *Am J Clin Nutr* 33:1125, 1980

135. Jacobs A, Greenman DA: Availability of food iron. *Br Med J* 1:673, 1969

136. Conrad ME, Benjamin BI, Williams HL, Foy AL: Human absorption of hemoglobin iron. *Gastroenterology* 53:5, 1967

137. Jacobs P, Bothwell TH, Charlton RW: Role of hydrochloric acid in iron absorption. *J Appl Physiol* 19:187, 1964

138. Cook JD, Brown GM, Valberg LS: The effect of achylia gastrica on iron absorption. *J Clin Invest* 43:1185, 1964
139. Bezwoda W, Charlton R, Bothwell T, Torrance J, Mayet F: Gastric hydrochloric acid and iron absorption. *J Lab Clin Med* 92:108, 1978
140. Chirasiri L, Isak G: The effect of acute haemorrhage and acute haemolysis on intestinal iron absorption in the rat. *Br J Haematol* 12:611, 1966
141. Wheby MS: Site of iron absorption in man. *Scandinav J Haematol* 7:56, 1970
142. Thomson ABR, Valberg LS: Kinetics of intestinal iron absorption in the rat: effect of cobalt. *Am J Physiol* 220:1080, 1971
143. Conrad ME Jr, Crosby WH: Intestinal mucosal mechanisms controlling iron absorption. *Blood* 22:406, 1963
144. Charlton RW, Jacobs P, Torrance JD, Bothwell TH: The role of ferritin in iron absorption. *Lancet* 2:762, 1963
145. Powell LW, Campbell CB, Wilson E: Intestinal mucosal uptake of iron and iron retention in idiopathic haemochromatosis as evidence for a mucosal abnormality. *Gut* 11:727, 1970
146. Kuhn IN, Layrisse M, Roche M, Martinez C, Walker RB: Observations on the mechanism of iron absorption. *Am J Clin Nutr* 21:1184, 1968
147. Kuhn IN, Monsen ER, Cook JD, Finch CA: Iron absorption in man. *J Lab Clin Med* 71:715, 1968
148. Bezwoda WR, Bothwell TH, Torrance JD, Macphail AP, Charlton RW, Kay G, Levin J: The relationship between marrow iron stores, plasma ferritin concentrations and iron absorption. *Scand J Haematol* 22:113, 1979
149. Walters GO, Jacobs A, Worwood M, Trevett D: Iron absorption in normal subjects and patients with idiopathic hemochromatosis: Relationship with serum ferritin concentration. *Gut* 16:188, 1975
150. Charlton RW, Derman D, Skikne B, Lynch SR, Sayers MH, Torrance JD, Bothwell TH: Iron stores, serum ferritin and iron absorption, in Brown EB, Aisen P, Fielding J, Crichton RR (eds): *Proteins of Iron Metabolism*. New York, Grune & Stratton, 1977, p 387
151. Heinrich HC, Bender-Gotze C, Gabbe EE, Bartels H, Oppitz KH: Absorption of inorganic iron ($^{59}Fe^{2+}$) in relation to iron stores in pancreatic exocrine insufficiency due to cystic fibrosis. *Klin Wschr* 55:587, 1977
152. Bothwell TH, Pribilla WF, Mebust W, Finch CA: Iron metabolism in the pregnant rabbit. Iron transport across the placenta. *Am J Physiol* 193:615, 1958
153. Bender-Gotze C, Heinrich HC, Gabbe EE, Oppitz KH, Schafer KH, Schroter W, Whang DH: Intestinal iron absorption under the influence of available storage iron and erythroblastic hyperplasia. *Z Kinderheilk* 118:283, 1975
154. Heinrich HC, Gabbe EE, Oppitz KH, Whang DH, Gotze Ch B, Schafer KH, Schroter W, Pfau AA: Absorption of inorganic and food iron in children with heterozygous and homozygous beta thalassemia. *A Kinderheik* 115:1, 1973
155. Modell CB: Total management of thalassaemia major. *Arch Dis Child* 52:489, 1977
156. Modell CB: Advances in the use of iron-chelating agents for the treatment of iron overload, in Brown EB (ed): *Progress in Hematology*. New York, Grune & Stratton, 1979, vol XI, p 267
157. Crosby WH: Editorial review. The control of iron balance by the intestinal mucosa. *Blood*, 22:44, 1963
158. Charlton RW, Jacobs P, Torrance JD, Bothwell TH: The role of the intestinal mucosa in iron absorption. *J Clin Invest* 44:543, 1965
159. Huebers H, Huebers E, Crichton RR: Isolation and characterisation of rat mucosal ferritin. *FEBS Lett* 44:302, 1974
160. Huebers H, Huebers E, Forth W, Rummel W: Iron absorption and iron-binding proteins in intestinal mucosa of mice with sex-linked anaemia. *Hoppe-Seylers Z Physiol Chem* 355:1159, 1974
161. Schade SG, Felsher BF, Conrad ME: An effect of intestinal motility on iron absorption. *Proc Soc Exp Biol Med* 130:757, 1969
162. Levine PH, Levine AJ, Weintraub L: The role of transferrin in the control of iron absorption: Studies on a cellular level. *J Lab Clin Med* 80:333, 1972
163. Rosenmund A, Gerber S, Huebers H, Finch C: Regulation of iron absorption and storage iron turnover. *Blood*, 56:30, 1980
164. Cavill I, Worwood M, Jacobs A: Internal regulation of iron absorption. *Nature* 256:328, 1975
165. Hershko C: Storage iron regulation, in Brown EB (ed): *Progress in Hematology*. New York, Grune & Stratton, 1977, p 105
166. Simon M, Alexandre J-L, Rauchet R, Genetet B, Bourel M: The genetics of hemochromatosis. *Prog Med Genet* 4:135, 1980
167. Powell LW: Iron storage in relatives of patients with haemochromatosis and in relatives of patients with alcoholic cirrhosis and haemosiderosis. A comparative study of 27 families. *Quart J Med* 34:427, 1965
168. Scheinberg IH: The genetics of hemochromatosis. *Arch Int Med* 132:126, 1973

169. Saddi R, Feingold J: Idiopathic haemochromatosis: An autosomal recessive disease. *Clin Genet* 5:234, 1974
170. Simon M, Pawlotsky Y, Bourel M, Fauchet R, Genetet B:Hemochromatose idiopathique: maladie associee a l'antigene tissulaire HL-A3? *Nouv Presse Med* 4:1432, 1975
171. Walters JM, Watt PW, Steven FM, et al:HLA antigens in haemochromatosis. *Br Med J* 4:520, 1975
172. Shewan WG, Mouat SA, Allan TM: HLA antigens in haemochromatosis. *Br Med J* 1:281, 1976
173. Bomford A, Eddleston ALWF, Kennedy LA, Batchelor LH, Williams R: Histo-compatibility antigens as marker of abnormal iron metabolism in patients with idiopathic haemochromatosis and their relatives. *Lancet* 1:327, 1977
174. Morris PJ, Vaughan H, Tait BD, Mackay R: Histo-compatibility antigens (HLA): Association with immunopathic diseases and with response to microbial antigens. *Aust NZ J Med* 7:616, 1977
175. Henke J, Ungar W: HLA-antigens in idiopathic haemochromatosis (I.H.) preliminary report. *Z Immunitaetsforsch Immunobiol* 154:41, 1978
176. Laukens P, Versieck J, De Potter E, Barbier F: Association of HLA antigens with idiopathic hemochromatosis. *Gastroenterology* 75:1351, 1978
177. Simon M, Bourel M, Genetet B, Fauchet R, Edan G, Brissot P: Association of HLA antigens with idiopathic hemochromatosis. *Gastroenterology* 75:3151, 1978
178. Lipinski M, Hors J, Salaeun JP, Saddi R, Passa P, Lafaurie S, Feingold N, Dausset J: Idiopathic hemochromatosis: Linkage with HLA. *Tissue Antigens* 11:471, 1978
179. Dyrszka H, Eberhardt G, Eckert G: HLA-phenotype and hemochromatosis in Germany. *Gastroenterology* 75:555, 1978
180. Motulsky AG: Genetics of hemochromatosis. *N Engl J Med* 301:1291, 1979
181. Simon M, Bourel M, Genetet B, Fauchet R, Edan G, Brissot P: Idiopathic hemochromatosis and iron overload in alcoholic liver disease: differentiation by HLA phenotypes. *Gastroenterology* 73:655, 1977
182. Motulsky AG: The HLA complex and disease. Some interpretations and new data in cardiomyopathy. *N Engl J Med* 300:918, 1979
183. Kidd KK: Genetic linkage and haemochromatosis. *N Engl J Med* 301:209, 1979
184. Simon M, Bourel M, Genetet B, Fauchet R: Idiopathic hemochromatosis. Demonstration of recessive transmission and early detection by family HLA typing. *N Engl J Med* 297:1017, 1977
185. Kravitz K, Skolnick M, Cannings C, Carmelli D, Baty B, Amos B, Johnson A, Mendel N, Edwards C, Cartwright G: Genetic linkage between hereditary hemochromatosis and HLA *Am J Hum Genet* 31:601, 1979
186. Beaumont CM, Simon M, Fauchet R, Hespel JP, Brissot P, Benetet B, Bourel M: Serum ferritin as a possible marker of the hemochromatosis allele. *N Engl J Med* 301:169, 1979
187. Edwards CO, Cartwright GE, Skolnick MH, Amos DB: Homozygosity for hemochromatosis: clinical manifestations. *Ann Int Med* 93:519, 1980
188. Sheldon JH: *Haemochromatosis*. London, Oxford University Press, 1935
189. Charlton RW, Hawkins DM, Mavor MO, Bothwell TH: Hepatic storage iron concentrations in different population groups: *Am J Clin Nutr* 23:358, 1970
190. Cook JD, Finch CA, Smith N: Evaluation of the iron status of a population. *Blood* 48:449, 1976
191. MacSween RNM, Scott AR: Hepatic cirrhosis: a clinicopathological review of 520 cases. *J Clin Path* 26:936, 1973
192. Cartwright GE, Edwards CQ, Kravitz K, Skolnick M, Amos DB, Johnson A, Buskjaer L: Hereditary hemochromatosis. Phenotypic expression of the disease. *N Engl J Med* 301:175, 1979
192a.Bassett ML, Halliday JW, Powell LW: HLA typing in idiopathetic hemochromatosis: Distinction between homozygotes and heterozygotes with biochemical expression. *Hepatology* 1:120, 1981
193. Debre R, Dreyfus J-C, Frezal J, Labie D, Lamy M, Maroteaux P, Schapira F, Schapira G: Genetics of haemochromatosis. *Ann Hum Genet* 23:16, 1958
194. Luke CG, Davis PS, Deller DJ: Gastric iron binding in haemochromatosis, secondary iron overload, cirrhosis and diabetes. *Lancet* 2:844, 1968
195. Wynter CVA, Williams R: Iron-binding properties of gastric juice in idiopathic haemochromatosis. *Lancet* 2:534, 1968
196. Bezwoda WR, Disler PB, Lynch SR, Charlton RW, Torrance JD, Derman D, Bothwell TH, Walker RB, Mayet F: Patterns of food iron absorption in iron-deficient white and Indian subjects and in venesected haemochromatotic patients. *Br J Haematol* 33:265, 1976
197. Halliday JW, Mack U, Powell LW: Duodenal ferritin content and structure. *Arch Intern Med* 138:1109, 1978

198. BOENDER CA, VERLOOP MC: Iron absorption, iron loss and iron retention in man: studies after oral administration of a tracer dose of ^{59}FeSO4 and ^{131}BaSO$_4$. Br J Haematol 17:45, 1969

199. MARX JJM: Mucosal uptake, mucosal transfer and retention of iron, measured by whole body counting. Scand J Haematol 23:293, 1979

200. COX TM, PETERS TJ: In vitro studies of duodenal iron uptake in patients with primary and secondary iron storage disease. Quart J Med 49:249, 1980

201. BOTHWELL TH, JACOBS P, TORRANCE JD: Studies on the behaviour of transferrin in idiopathic haemochromatosis. S Afr J Med Sci 27:35, 1962

202. WHEBY MS, BALCERZAK SP, ANDERSON P, CROSBY WH: Brief report: clearance of iron from hemochromatotic and normal transferrin in vivo. Blood 24:765, 1964

203. JENKINS T, BOTHWELL TH: Unpublished observations

204. POLLYCOVE M: Hemochromatosis, in Stanbury JB, Wyngaarden JB, Fredrickson DS (eds): The Metabolic Basis of Inherited Diseases. 4th ed. New York, McGraw-Hill, 1978, p 1128

205. BATEY RG, PETTIT JE, NICHOLAS AW, SHERLOCK S, HOFFBRAND AV: Hepatic iron clearance from serum in treated hemochromatosis. Arch Dermatol 113:161, 1977

206. MAZUR A, SACKLER M: Haemochromatosis and hepatic xanthine oxidase. Lancet, 1:254, 1967

207. GREEN R, LEVIN NW, SAMASSA D, CHARLTON RW, BOTHWELL TH: The effect of allopurinol on iron metabolism. S Afr Med J 42:776, 1968

208. POWELL LW, ALPERT E, ISSELBACHER KJ, DRYSDALE JW: Abnormality in tissue isoferritin distribution in idiopathic haemochromatosis. Nature 250:333, 1974

209. POWELL LW, HALLIDAY JW, McKEERING LV, TWEEDALE R: Alterations in serum and tissue isoferritins in disease states. II. Hemochromatosis and malignant disease, in Brown EB, Aisen P, Fielding J (eds): Proteins of Iron Metabolism. New York, Grune & Stratton, 1977, p 61

210. HALLIDAY JW, McKEERING LV, TWEEDALE R, POWELL LW: Serum ferritin in haemochromatosis: Changes in the isoferritin composition during venesection therapy. Br J Haematol 36:395, 1977

211. BRINK B, DISLER P, LYNCH S, JACOBS P, CHARLTON R, BOTHWELL T: Patterns of iron storage in dietary iron overload and idiopathic hemochromatosis. J Lab Clin Med 88:725, 1977

212. COOK JD, BARRY WE, HERSHKO C, FILLET G, FINCH CA: Iron kinetics with emphasis on iron overload. Am J Path 72:337, 1973

213. SAINT EG: Haemochromatosis. Med J Austral 50:137, 1963

214. GRACE ND, POWELL LW: Iron storage disorders of the liver. Gastroenterology 64:1257, 1974

215. MACDONALD RA: In Hemochromatosis and Hemosiderosis. Springfield, Charles C Thomas, 1964

216. CONRAD ME, BARTON JC: Anemia and iron kinetics in alcoholism. Semin Hematol 17:149, 1980

217. BOTHWELL TH, SEFTEL H, JACOBS P, TORRANCE JD, BAUMSLAG N: Iron overload in Bantu subjects. Studies on the availability of iron in Bantu beer. Am J Clin Nutr 14:47, 1964

218. DERMAN DP, BOTHWELL TH, TORRANCE JD, BEZWODA WR, MACPHAIL AP, KEW MC, SAYERS MH, DISLER PB, CHARLTON RW: Iron absorption from maize (Zea mays) and sorghum (Sorghum vulgare) beer. Br J Nutr 43:271, 1980

219. PERMAN G: Hemochromatosis and red wine. Acta Med Scand 182:281, 1967

220. BARRY M: Iron overload: Clinical aspects, evaluation and treatment, in Callender S (ed): Clinics in Haematology. London, W.B. Saunders, 1973, vol 2, p 405

221. ANGUISSOLA AB: The nutritional value of wine as regards its iron content, in Harwerth HG, Vannotti A (eds): Iron Deficiency, Pathogenesis, Clinical Aspects Therapy. New York, Academic, 1970, p 71

222. CELADA A, RUDOLF H, DONATH A: Effect of a single ingestion of alcohol on iron absorption. Am J Hematol 5:225, 1978

223. CHARLTON RW, JACOBS P, SEFTEL H, BOTHWELL TH: Effect of alcohol on iron absorption. Br Med J 2:1427, 1964

224. CELADA A, RUDOLF H, DONATH A: Effect of experimental chronic alcohol ingestion and folic acid deficiency on iron absorption. Blood 54:906, 1979

225. DAVIS AE, BADENOCH J: Iron absorption in pancreatic disease. Lancet 2:6, 1962

226. MURRAY MJ, STEIN N: Does the pancreas influence iron absorption? A critical review of information to date. Gastroenterology 51:694, 1966

227. BALCERZAK SP, PETERNEL WW, HEINLE EW: Iron absorption in chronic pancreatitis. Gastroenterology 53:257, 1967

228. KAVIN H, CHARLTON RW, JACOBS P, BOTHWELL TH: Effect of the exocrine pancreatic secretions on iron absorption. Gut 8:556, 1967

229. CALLENDER ST, MALPAS JS: Absorption of iron in cirrhosis of liver. Br Med J 2:1516, 1964

230. GREENBERG MS, STROHMEYER G, HINE GJ, KEENE WR, CURTIS G, CHALMERS TC: Studies in iron absorption. III. Body radioactivity measurements of patients with liver disease. Gastroenterology 46:651, 1964

231. FRIEDMAN BI, SCHAEFER JW, SCHIFF L: Increased iron-59 absorption in patients with hepatic cirrhosis. J Nucl Med 7:594, 1966

232. BOTHWELL TH: Total iron loss and relative importance of different sources, in Hallberg L, Harwerth HG, Vannotti A (eds): Iron Deficiency. Pathogenesis, Clinical Aspects, Therapy. London, New York, Academic, 1970, p 151

233. AUZEPY P, VALETTE H, ALBESSARD F, DEPARIS M: Cardiomyopathie alcoholique avec hyperdideremie par absorption digestive exageree du fer. Ann Med Interne 125:923, 1974

234. CONN HO: Portacaval anastomosis and hepatic haemosiderin deposition: a prospective, controlled investigation. Gastroenterology 62:61, 1972

235. WILLIAMS R, WIlliams HS, SCHEUER PJ, PITCHER CS, LOIZEAN E, SHERLOCK S: Iron absorption and siderosis in chronic liver disease. Quart J Med 36:151, 1967

236. LUNDVALL O, WEINFELD A, LUNDIN P: Iron stores in alcohol abusers. I. Liver iron. Acta Med Scand 185:259, 1969

237. LUNDVALL O, WEINFELD A: Iron stores in alcohol abusers. II. As measured with the desferrioxamine test. Acta Med Scand 185:271, 1969

238. JAKOBOVITS AW, MORGAN MY, SHERLOCK S: Hepatic siderosis in alcoholics. Am J Digest Dis 24:305, 1979

239. MILDER MS, COOK JD, STRAY S, FINCH C: Idiopathic hemochromatosis, an interim report. Medicine 59:34, 1980

240. KUSHNER JP, STEINMULLER DP, LEE GR: The role of iron in the pathogenesis of porphyria cutanea tarda. II. Inhibition of uroporphyrinogen decarboxylase. J Clin Invest 56:661, 1975

241. KUSHNER JP, BARBUTO AJ, LEE GR: An inherited enzymatic defect in porphyria cutanea tarda. Decreased uroporphyrinogen decarboxylase activity. J Clin Invest 58:1089, 1976

242. HINES JD: Effects of alcohol on inborn errors of metabolism: porphyria cutanea tarda and hemochromatosis. Seminars Hemat 17:113, 1980

243. LUNDVALL O, WEINFELD A, LUNDIN P: Iron storage in porphyria cutanea tarda. Acta Med Scand 188:37, 1970

244. RAMSAY CA, MAGNUS IA, TURNBULL A, BAKER H: The treatment of porphyria cutanea tarda by venesection. Quart J Med 43:1, 1974

245. EPSTEIN JH, REDEKER AG: Porphyria cutanea tarda: A study of the effect of phlebotomy. N Engl J Med 279:1301, 1968

246. KALIVAS JT, PATHAK MA, FITZPATRICK TB: Phlebotomy and iron overload in porphyria cutanea tarda. Lancet 1:1184, 1969

247. SAUER GF, FUND DD: Iron overload in cutaneous pophyria. Arch Intern Med 124:190, 1969

248. TURNBULL A, BAKER H, VERNON-ROBERTS B, MAGNUS IA: Iron metabolism in porphyria cutanea tarda and in erythropoietic protoporphyria. Quart J Med 42:341, 1973

249. KUSHNER JP, LEE GR, NACHT S: The role of iron in the pathogenesis of porphyria cutanea tarda. J Clin Invest 51:3044, 1972

250. GROSSMAN MF, BICKERS DR, POH-FITZPATRICK MB, DELEO VA, HARBER LC: Porphyria cutanea tarda. Clinical features and laboratory findings in 40 patients. Am J Med 67:277, 1979

251. DIAMOND LK, ALLEN DM, MAGILL FB: Congenital (erythroid) hypoplastic anemia. A 25 year study. Am J Dis Child 102:403, 1961

252. HERSHKO C, GRAHAM G, BATES GW, RACHMILEWITZ EA: Non-specific serum iron in thalassemia—abnormal serum iron fraction of potential toxicity. Br J Haematol 40:255, 1978

253. GRAHAM G, BATES GW, RACHMILEWITZ EZ, HERSHKO C: Non-specific serum iron in thalassemia: quantitation and chemical reactivity. Am J Hemat 6:207, 1979

254. WHEBY MS, UMPIERRE G: Effect of transferrin saturation on iron absorption in man. N Engl J Med 271:1391, 1964

255. MACPHAIL AP, SIMON MO, TORRANCE JD, CHARLTON RW, BOTHWELL TH, ISAACSON C: Changing patterns of dietary iron overload in black South Africans. Am J Clin Nutr 32:1272, 1979

256. BOTHWELL TH, ABRAHAMS C, BRADLOW BA, CHARLTON RW: Idiopathic and Bantu hemochromatosis. Comparative histological study. Arch Pathol 79:163, 1965

257. WAPNICK AA, LYNCH SR, KRAWITZ P, SEFTEL HC, CHARLTON RW, BOTHWELL TH: Effects of iron overload on ascorbic acid metabolism. Br Med J 3:704, 1968

258. BOTHWELL TH, BRADLOW BA: Siderosis in the Bantu. A combined histopathological and chemical study. Arch Pathol 70:279, 1960

259. ISAACSON C, SEFTEL H, KEELEY KJ, BOTHWELL TH: Siderosis in the Bantu. The relationship between iron overload and cirrhosis. J Lab Clin Med 58:845, 1961

260. BRADLOW B, DUNN J, HIGGISON J: The effect of cirrhosis on iron storage. Am J Pathol 39:221, 1961

261. CHARLTON RW, ABRAHAMS C, BOTHWELL TH: Idiopathic hemochromatosis in young subjects. Clinical, pathological and chemical findings in four patients. Arch Pathol 83:132, 1967

262. BOTHWELL TH, ISAACSON C: Siderosis in the Bantu. A comparison of the incidence in males and females. Br Med J 1:522, 1962

263. RISDON RA, BARRY M, FLYNN DM: Transfusional iron overload: the relationship between tissue iron concentration and hepatic fibrosis in thalassemia. J Pathol 116:83, 1975

264. BOTHWELL TH, COHEN I, ABRAHAMS OL, PEROLD SM: A familial study in idiopathic hemochromatosis. *Am J Med* 27:730, 1959

265. SCHEUER PJ, WILLIAMS R, MUIR AR: Hepatic pathology in relatives of patients with haemochromatosis. *J Pathol* 84:53, 1962

266. BARRY M, FLYNN DM, LETSKY EA, RISDON RA: Long term chelation therapy in thalassaemia major: Effect on liver iron concentration, liver histology and clinical progress. *Br Med J* ii:16, 1974

267. KNAUER CM, GAMBLE CN, MONROE LS: The reversal of hemochromatic cirrhosis by multiple phlebotomies: Report of a case. *Gastroenterology* 49:667, 1965

268. WEINTRAUB LR, CONRAD ME, CROSBY WH: The treatment of hemochromatosis by phlebotomy. *Med Clin N Am* 50:1579, 1966

269. BOTHWELL TH, FINCH CA: *Iron Metabolism.* Boston, Little, Brown, 1962

270. ENGLE ME, ERLANDSON IG, SMITH CH: Late cardiac complications of chronic, severe, refractory anemia with hemochromatosis. *Circulation* 30:698, 1964

271. MODELL CB, MATTHEWS R: Thalassemia in Britain and Australia, in Bergsma D, Cerami A, Peterson CM, Graziano JH (eds): *Iron Metabolism and Thalassemia.* New York, Alan R Liss, 1976, p 13

272. CROSBY WH: Treatment of haemochromatosis by energetic phlebotomy. One patient's response to the letting of 55 liters of blood in 11 months. *Br J Haematol* 4:82, 1958

273. ACAR J, SLAMA R, LEBORGNE P, HERREMAN F, DELZANT JF, PAN-LAUBRE C: Coeur et hemochromatose: Aspects particuliers. *Coeur Med Intern* 6:17, 1967

274. WILLIAMS R, SMITH PM, SPICER EJF, BARRY M, SHERLOCK S: Venesection therapy in idiopathic haemochromatosis: An analysis of 40 treated and 18 untreated patients. *Quart J Med* 38:1, 1969

275. SKINNER C, KENMORE ACF: Haemochromatosis presenting as congestive cardiomyopathy and responding to venesection. *Br Heart J* 35:466, 1973

276. JACHUCK SK, RAI GS, FOSSARD C: Cardiac involvement in idiopathic haemochromatosis and the effect of venesection. *Postgrad Med J* 50:276, 1974

277. BOMFORD A, WILLIAMS R: Long term results of venesection therapy in idiopathic haemochromatosis. *Quart J Med* (new series) 45:611, 1976

278. MODELL CB: Transfusional haemochromatosis, in Kief H (ed): *Iron Metabolism and its Disorders.* Amsterdam, Exerpta Medica, 1975, p 230

279. O'BRIEN RT: Iron overload: clinical and pathologic aspects in pediatrics. *Sem Hematol* 14:115, 1977

280. LANDAU H, SPITZ IM, CIVIDALLI G, RACHMILEWITZ EA: Gonadotrophin, thyrotrophin and prolactin reserve in thalassemia. *Clin Endocrinol* 9:163, 1978

281. SAUDEK CA, PETERS TJ: Organelle pathology in primary and secondary haemochromatosis with special reference to lysosomal changes. *Br J Haematol* 40:239, 1978

282. PETERS TJ, SEYMOUR CA: Acid hydrolase activities and lysosomal integrity in liver biopsies from patients with iron overload. *Clin Sci Molec Med* 50:75, 1976

283. PETERS TJ, SELDEN C, SEYMOUR CA: Lysosomal disruption in the pathogenesis of hepatic damage in primary and secondary haemochromatosis, in Jacobs A (ed): *Iron Metabolism, Ciba Foundation Symposium 51* (new series). Amsterdam, Elsevier/North-Holland, 1977, p 317

284. JACOBS A: Iron overload—clinical and pathologic aspects. *Sem Hematol* 14:89, 1977

285. GOLBERG L, SMITH JP, MARTIN LE: The effects of intensive and prolonged administration of iron parenterally in animals. *Br J Exper Path* 38:297, 1957

286. HYMAN CB, LANDING B, ALFIN-SLATER R, KOZAK L, WEITZMAN J, ORTEGA JA: DL-Alpha-Tocopherol, iron and lipofuscin in thalassemia. *NY Acad Sci* 232:211, 1974

287. RACHMILEWITZ EA, LUBIA BH, SHOHET SB: Lipid membrane peroxidation in -thalassemia major. *Blood* 47:496, 1976

288. RICHTER GW: The iron-loaded cell—the cytopathology of iron storage. *Am Assoc Path Bact* 91:363, 1978

289. SELDEN C, OWEN M, HOPKINS JMP, PETERS TJ: Studies on the concentration and intracellular localization of iron proteins in liver biopsy specimens from patients with iron overload with special reference to their role in lysosomal disruption. *Br J Haematol* 44:593, 1980

290. SEYMOUR CA, PETERS TJ: Organelle pathology in primary and secondary haemochromatosis with special reference to lysosomal changes. *Br J Haematol* 40:239, 1978

291. HOY TG, JACOBS A: Iron overload and toxicity in cell cultures. *Br J Haematol* 46:329, 1980

292. IANCU TL, NEUSTEIN HB, LANDING BH: The liver in thalassemia major: ultrastructural observations, in *Iron Metabolism, Ciba Foundation Symposium 51* (new series). Amsterdam. Elsevier/North-Holland, 1977, p 293

293. HUNT J, RICHARDS RJ, HARWOOD RJ, JACOBS A: The effect of desferrioxamine on fibroblasts and collagen formation in cell cultures. *Br J Haematol* 41:69, 1979

294. ROJKING M, DUNN MA: Hepatic fibrosis. *Gastroenterology* 76:849, 1979

295. SEFTEL HC, MALKIN C, SCHAMAN A, ABRAHAMS C, LYNCH SR, CHARLTON RW, BOTHWELL TH: Osteoporosis, scurvy and siderosis in Johannesburg Bantu. *Br Med J* 1:642, 1966

296. LYNCH SR, SEFTEL HC, TORRANCE JD, CHARLTON RW, BOTHWELL TH: Accelerated oxidative catabolism of ascorbic acid in siderotic Bantu. *Am J Clin Nutr* 20:641, 1967

297. HANKES LV, JANSEN CR, SCHMAELER M: Ascorbic acid catabolism in Bantu with hemosiderosis (scurvy). *Biochem Med* 9:244, 1974

298. MODELL CB, BECK J: Long-term desferrioxamine therapy in thalassemia. *Ann NY Acad Sci* 232:201, 1974

299. O'BRIEN RT: Ascorbic acid enhancement of desferrioxamine-induced urinary iron excretion in thalassemia major. *Ann NY Acad Sci* 232:221, 1974

300. BRISSOT P, DEUGNIER Y, LETREUT A, REGNOUARD F, SIMON M, BOUREL M: Ascorbic acid status in idiopathic hemochromatosis. *Digestion* 17:479, 1978

301. HANKES LV: Influence of iron and ascorbic acid on tryptophan metabolism in man. *Acta Vitamin Enzymol (Milan).* 29:174, 1975

302. SOLOMON L, BEIGHTON P: Rheumatic disorders in the South African negro. Part III. Idiopathic necrosis of the femoral head. *S Afr Med J* 49:1825, 1975

303. LYNCH SR, BERELOWITZ I, SEFTEL HC, MILLER GB, KRAWITZ P, CHARLTON RW, BOTHWELL TH: Osteoporosis in Johannesburg Bantu males. Its relationship to siderosis and ascorbic acid deficiency. *J Clin Nutr* 20:799, 1967

304. WAPNICK AA, LYNCH SR, SEFTEL HC, CHARLTON RW, BOTHWELL TH, JOWSEY J: The effect of siderosis and ascorbic acid depletion on bone metabolism, with special reference to osteoporosis in the Bantu. *Br J Nutr* 25:367, 1971

305. LYNCH SR, SEFTEL HC, WAPNICK AA, CHARLTON RW, BOTHWELL TH: Some aspects of calcium metabolism in normal and osteoporotic Bantu subjects with special reference to the effects of iron overload and ascorbic acid depletion. *S Afr J Med* 35:45, 1970

306. DELBARRE F: L'osteoporose des hémochromatoses. *Sem de Hop* 36:3279, 1960

307. DU LAC T, DELOUX G, DENIL R: Arthropathies et chondrocalcinoses au cours des hémochromatoses. *Rev Rheum* 34:758, 1967

308. BOTHWELL TH, CHARLTON RW: Absorption of iron, in De Graff AC (ed): *Annual Review of Medicine.* Palo Alto, Annual Reviews, vol 21, 1970, p 145

309. BJÖRN-RASMUSSEN E, HALLBERG L, ISAKSSON B, ARVIDSSON B: Food iron absorption in man. Applications of the two-pool extrinsic tag method to measure heme and non-heme iron absorption from the whole diet. *J Clin Invest* 53:247, 1974

310. PERKINS KW, McINNES IWS, BLACKBURN CRB, BEAL RW: Idiopathic haemochromatosis in children. Report of a family. *Am J Med* 39:118, 1965

311. LOSOWSKY MS, WILSON AR: Whole-body counting of the absorption and distribution of iron in haemochromatosis. *Clin Sci* 32:151, 1967

312. VALBERG LS, GHENT CN, LLOYD DA, FREI JV, CHAMBERLAIN MJ: Iron absorption in idiopathic hemochromatosis: Relationship to serum ferritin concentration in asymptomatic relatives. *Clin Invest Med* 2:17, 1979

313. SARGENT T, SAITO H, WINCHELL HS: Iron absorption in hemochromatosis before and after phlebotomy therapy. *J Nucl Med* 12:660, 1971

314. MILDER MS, COOK JD, FINCH CA: The influence of food iron absorption on the plasma iron level in idiopathic hemochromatosis. *Acta Haematologica,* 60:65, 1978

315. DIEZ-EWALK M, WEINTRAUB LR, CROSBY WH: Interrelationship of iron and manganese metabolism. *Proc Sec Exp Biol Med* 129:448, 1968

316. CHEVRANT-BRETON J, SIMON M, BOUREL M, FERRAND B: Cutaneous manifestations of idiopathic hemochromatosis. *Arch Dermatol* 113:161, 1977

317. POWELL LW, KERR JFR: The pathology of the liver in hemochromatosis, in Ioachim HL (ed): *Pathobiology Annual.* New York, Appleton-Century-Crofts, 1975, p 317

318. BLOCK M, MOORE G, WASI P, HAIBY G: Histogenesis of the hepatic lesion in primary hemochromatosis, with consideration of the pseudo-iron deficient state produced by phlebotomies. *Am J Pathol* 47:89, 1965

319. BRICK IB: Liver histology in six asymptomatic siblings in a family with hemochromatosis: genetic implications. *Gastroenterology,* 40:210, 1961

320. EDWARDS CO, CARROLL M, BRAY P, CARTWRIGHT GE: Hereditary hemochromatosis: Diagnosis in siblings and children. *N Engl J Med* 297:7, 1977

321. BUJA LM, ROBERTS WC: Iron in the heart. Etiology and clinical significance. *Am J Med* 51:209, 1971

322. KRA SJ, HOLLINGSWORTH JW, FINCH SC: Arthritis with synovial iron deposition in a patient with hemochromatosis. *N Engl J Med* 272:1268, 1965

323. HAMILTON E, WILLIAMS R, BARLOW KA, SMITH PM: The arthropathy of idiopathic haemochromatosis. *Quart J Med* 37:171, 1968

324. DORFMANN H, SOLNICA J, MENZA CD, DE SEZE S: Les arthropathies des hemochromatoses. *Sem Hop* 45:516, 1969

325. ATKINS CJ, MCIVOR J, SMITH PM, HAMILTON E, WILLIAMS R: Chondrocalcinosis and arthropathy: Studies in haemochromatosis and in idiopathic chondrocalcinosis. *Quart J Med* 39:71, 1970

326. DAVIES G, DYMOCK I, HARRY J, WILLIAMS R: Deposition of melanin and iron in ocular structures in hemochromatosis. *Br J Ophthalmol* 56:338, 1972

327. MACSWEEN RNM: Acute abdominal crises, circulatory collapse and sudden death in haemochromatosis. *Quart J Med* 35:589, 1966

328. REISSMANN KR, DIETRICH MR: On the presence of ferritin in the peripheral blood of patients with hepatocellular disease. *J Clin Invest* 35:588, 1956

329. AUNGST CW: Ferritin in body fluids. *J Lab Clin Med* 71:517, 1968

330. JONES NL: Irreversible shock in haemochromatosis. *Lancet* 1:569, 1962

331. YAMASHIRO KM: Pasteurella pseudotuberculosis. Acute sepsis with survival. *Arch Intern Med* 128:605, 1971

332. DYMOCK IW, CASSAR J, PYKE DA, OAKLEY WG, WILLIAMS R: Observations on the pathogenesis, complications and treatment of diabetes in 115 cases of haemochromatosis. *Am J Med* 52:203, 1972

332a. SADDI R, FEINGOLD J: Idiopathic haemochromatosis and diabetes mellitus. *Clin Gen* 5:272, 1974

333. BALCERZAK SP, MINTZ DH, WESTERMAN MP: Diabetes mellitus and idiopathic hemochromatosis. *Am J Med Sci* 255:53, 1968

334. POZZA G, GHIDONI A: Studies on the diabetic syndrome of idiopathic haemochromatosis. *Diabetologia* 4:83, 1968

335. MEGYESI C, SAMOLS E, MARKS V: Glucose tolerance and diabetes in chronic liver disease. *Lancet* 2:1051, 1967

336. SHERWIN R, JOSHI P, HENDLER R, FELIG P, CONN HO: Hyperglucagonemia in Laennec's cirrhosis. *N Engl J Med* 290:239, 1974

337. GRIFFITHS JD, DYMOCK IW, DAVIES EWG, HILL DW, WILLIAMS R: Occurrence and prevalence of diabetic retinopathy in hemochromatosis. *Diabetes* 20:766, 1971

338. PASSA P, ROUSSELIE F, GAUVILLE C, CANIVET J: Retinopathy and plasma growth hormone levels in idiopathic hemochromatosis with diabetes. *Diabetes* 26:113, 1977

339. SIMON M, VONGSAVANTHONG S, JEHAN J-P, RONSSEY M, BOUREL M: Diabete et hemochromatose. II; Diabete de l'hemochromatose idiopathique et diabete commun. *Sem Hop Paris* 49:2133, 1973

340. STOCKS AE, MARTIN FIR: Pituitary function in hemochromatosis. *Am J Med* 45:839, 1968

341. STOCKS AE, POWELL LW: Pituitary function in idiopathic haemochromatosis and cirrhosis of the liver. *Lancet* 2:298, 1972

342. BEZWODA WR, BOTHWELL TH, VAN DER WALT LA, KRONHEIN S, PIMSTONE BL: An investigation into gonadal dysfunction in patients with idiopathic hemochromatosis. *Clin Endocrin* 6:377, 1977

343. LEVY CL, CARLSON HE: Decreased prolactin reserve in hemochromatosis. *J Clin Endocrinol Metab* 47:444, 1978

344. Case records of the Massachusetts General Hospital, Case 17-1979: *N Engl J Med* 300:969, 1979

345. CUTLER DJ, ISNER JM, BRACEY AW, HUFNAGEL CA, CONRAD PW, ROBERTS WC, KERWIN DM, WEINTRAUB AM: Hemochromatosis heart disease: An unemphasized cause of potentially reversible restrictive cardiomyopathy. *Am J Med* 69:923, 1980

346. JAQUET P, CODACCIONE JC, FABRE M: Accident mortel apres deux saignees au cours du traitement d'une hemochromatose. *Diabete,* 15:70, 1967

347. SCHUMACHER HR JR: Hemochromatosis and arthritis. *Arthr Rheum* 7:41, 1964

348. FRANCON F, EPINEY J, BLAUCHARD H, JOLY L, VISNIKS E, DIAZ R: Contribution a l'etude des arthropathies de l'hemochromatose. *Press Med* 76:1809, 1968

349. GORDON DA, CLARKE PV, OGRYZLO MA: The chondrocalcific arthropathy of iron overload. *Arch Intern Med* 134:21, 1974

350. M'SEFFAR A, FORNASIER VL, FOX IH: Arthropathy as the major clinical indicator of occult iron storage disease. *J Am Med Assoc* 238:1825, 1977

351. ABBOTT DF, GRESHAM GA: Arthropathy in transfusional siderosis. *Br Med J* 1:418, 1972

352. YAM LT, FINKEL HE, WEINTRAUB LR, CROSBY WH: Circulating iron-containing macrophages in hemochromatosis. *N Engl J Med* 279:512, 1968

353. COOK JD: Methods to determine plasma iron and total iron-binding capacity, in Halberg L, Harwerth HG, Vannotti A (eds): *Iron Deficiency, Pathogenesis, Clinical Aspects, Therapy.* London and New York, Academic 1969, p 397

354. BASSETT ML, HALLIDAY JW, POWELL LW: Early detection of idiopathic haemochromatosis: Relative value of serum ferritin and HLA typing. *Lancet* 2:4, 1979

355. BEAMISH MR, WALKER R, MILLER F, WORWOOD M, JACOBS A, WILLIAMS R, CORRIGALL A: Transferrin iron, chelatable iron and ferritin in idiopathic haemochromatosis. *Br J Haematol* 27:219, 1974

356. POWELL LW, HALLIDAY JW, COWLISHAW JL: Relationship between serum ferritin and total body iron stores in idiopathic haemochromatosis. *Gut* 19:538, 1978

357. LETSKY EA: A controlled trial of long-term chelation therapy in homozygous β-thalassaemia, in Bergsma D, Cerami A, Peterson CM, Graziano JH (eds): *Iron Metabolism and Thalassaemia.* New York, Alan R. Liss, 1976, p 31

358. PROPPER RD, COOPER B, RAFO RR, NIENHUIS AW, ANDERSON WF, BUNN HF, ROSENTHAL A, NATHAN DG: Continuous subcutaneous administration of deferoxamine in patients with iron overload. *N Engl J Med* 297:418, 1977

359. HUSSAIN MA, DAVIS LA, LAULICHT M, HOFFBRAND AV: Value of serum ferritin estimation in sickle cell anaemia. *Arch Dis Child* 53:319, 1978

360. WANDS JR, ROWE JA, MEZEY SE, WATERBURY LA, WRIGHT JR, HALLIDAY JW, ISSELBACHER KJ, POWELL LW: Normal serum ferritin concentrations in precirrhotic hemochromatosis. *N Engl J Med* 294:302, 1976

361. ROWE JW, WANDS JR, MEZEY E, WATERBURY LA, WRIGHT JR, TOBIN J, ANDRES R: Familial hemochromatosis: Characteristics of the precirrhotic stage in a large kindred. *Medicine* 56:197, 1977

362. HALLIDAY JW, RUSSO AM, COWLISHAN JL, POWELL LW: Serum ferritin in diagnosis of haemochromatosis. *Lancet* 2:621, 1977

363. SMITH PM, MILLER JPG, PITCHER CS, LESTAS AN, DYMOCK IW, WILLIAMS R: The differential ferrioxamine test in the management of idiopathic haemochromatosis. *Lancet* 2:402, 1969

364. WALKER RJ, MILLER JPG, DYMOCK IW, SHILKIN KB, WILLIAMS R: Relationship of hepatic iron concentration to histochemical grading and to total chelatable body iron in conditions associated with iron overload. *Gut* 12:1011, 1971

365. FIELDING J: Desferrioxamine chelatable body iron. *J Clin Pathol* 20:668, 1967

366. BALCERZAK SP, WESTERMAN MP, HEINLE EW, TAYLOR FH: Measurement of iron stores using deferoxamine. *Ann Intern Med* 68:518, 1968

367. HEDENBERG L: Studies on iron metabolism with desferrioxamine in man—experimental and clinical studies. *Scandinav J Haematol* (suppl 6):5, 1969

368. CUMMING RLD, MILLAR JA, SMITH JA, GOLDBERG A: Clinical and laboratory studies on the action of desferrioxamine. *Br J Haematol* 17:257, 1969

369. POWELL LW, THOMAS MJ: Use of diethylenetriamine penta-acetic acid (DTPA) in the clinical assessment of total body iron stores. *J Clin Path* 20:896, 1967

370. HARKER L, FUNK DD, FINCH CA: Evaluation of storage iron by chelates. *Am J Med* 45:105, 1968

371. BARRY M, SHERLOCK S: Measurement of liver-iron concentration in needle biopsy specimens. *Lancet* 1:100, 1971

372. HENRY WL, NIENHUIS AW, WIENER M, MILLER DR, CANALE VC, PIOMELLI S: Echo-cardiographic abnormalities in patients with transfusion-dependent anemia and secondary myocardial iron deposition. *Am J Med* 64:547, 1978

373. NIENHUIS AW, BENZ EJ, PROPPER R, CORASH L, ANDERSON F, BORER J: Thalassemia major: Molecular and clinical aspects. *Ann Intern Med* 91:883, 1979

374. GRAZIANO JH: Potential usefulness of fine radical scavengers in iron overload, in Bergsma D, Cerami A, Peterson CM, Graziano JH (eds): *Iron Metabolism and Thalassemia.* New York, Alan R. Liss, 1976, p 135

375. HUSSAIN MAM, FLYNN DM, GREEN N, HOFFBRAND AV: Effect of dose, time and ascorbate on iron excretion after subcutaneous desferrioxamine. *Lancet* 1:977, 1977

376. PIPPARD MJ, CALLENDER ST, WEATHERALL DJ: Intensive iron-chelation therapy with desferrioxamine in iron-loading anaemias. *Clin Sci Mol Med* 54:99, 1978

377. CERAMI A, GRADY RW, PETERSON CM, BHARGAVA KK: The status of new iron chelators. *NY Acad Sci* 425, 1980

378. POWELL LW, BASSETT ML, HALLIDAY JW: Hemochromatosis: 1980 update. *Gastroenterology* 78:374, 1980

379. MOTULSKY AG: Biased ascertainment and the natural history of disease. *N Engl J Med* 298:1197, 1978

379a. OLSSON KS: Personal communication

380. CARTWRIGHT GE, EDWARDS CO, SKOLNICK EMH, FLMOS DB: Association of HLA-linked hemochromatosis with idiopathic refractory sideroblastic anemia. *J Clin Invest* 65:989, 1980

381. BREGMAN H, GELFAND MC, WINCHESTER JF, MANZ HJ, KNEPSHIELD JK, SCHRINER GE: Iron-overload-associated myopathy in patients on maintenance haemodialysis: A histocompatibility-linked disorder. *Lancet* 2:882, 1980

382. WADDELL J, SASSOON HG, FISHER JD, CARR CJ: A review of the significance of dietary iron on iron storage phenomena. Life Sciences Research Office, Federation of American Societies for Experimental Biology, Maryland, 1972

383. BOTHWELL TH, DERMAN D, BEZWODA WR, TORRANCE JD, CHARLTON RW: Can iron fortification of flour cause damage to genetic susceptibles (idiopathic haemochromatosis and β-thalassaemia major)? Hum Genet, suppl 1, 1978, p 131

384. HALLBERG L, BENGTSSON C, GARBY L, LENNARTSSON J, ROSSANDER L, TIBBLIN E: An analysis of factors leading to a reduction in iron deficiency in Swedish women. Bull World Health Org 57:947, 1979

385. SCHAFER AI, CHERON RG, DLUHY R, COOPER B, GLEASON RE, SOELDNER JS, BUNN HF: Clinical consequences of acquired transfusional iron overload in adults. N Engl J Med 304:319, 1981

386. LOUKOPOULOS D: Present status of treatment of thalassemia in Greece, in Bergsma D, Cerami A, Petersen CM, Graziano JH (eds): Iron Metabolism in Thalassemia. New York, Alan R Liss, 1976, p 1

387. WASI P, POOTRAKUL P: Personal communication

388. PIPPARD MJ, CALLENDER ST, WARNER GT, WEATHERALL DJ: Iron absorption and loading in β-thalassemia intermedia. Lancet 2:819, 1979

389. CROSBY WH: Hemochromatosis and hemolytic disease. Arch Intern Med 140:894, 1980

390. MCINTOSH N: Endocrinopathy in thalassemia major. Arch Dis Child 51:195, 1976

391. JOHNSON FE, KROGMAN WM: Patterns of growth in children with thalassemia major. Ann NY Acad Sci 232:667, 1974

392. NECHELES TF, CHUNG S, SABBAH R, WHITTEN D: Intensive transfusion therapy in thalassemia major: An eight-year follow-up. Ann NY Acad Sci 232:179, 1974

393. LASSMAN MN, O'BRIEN RT, PEARSON HA, WISE JK, DONABEDIAN RK, FELIG P, GENEL M: Endocrine evaluation in thalassemia major. Ann NY Acad Sci 232:226, 1974

394. LASSMAN MN, GENEL M, WISE JK, HENDLER R, FELIG P: Carbohydrate homeostasis and pancreatic islet cell function in thalassemia. Ann Intern Med 80:65, 1974

395. WITZLEBEN CL, WYATT JP: The effect of long survival on the pathology of thalassemia major. J Pathol Bact 82:1, 1961

396. BERRY CL, MARSHALL WC: Iron distribution in the liver of patients with thalassemia major. Lancet 1:103, 1967

397. OKON E, LEVU IS, RACHMILEWITZ EA: Splenectomy, iron overload and liver cirrhosis in β-thalassemia major. Acta Haematol 56:142, 1976

398. WOLMAN IJ: Transfusion therapy in Cooley's anemia: Growth and health as related to long-range hemoglobin levels, a progress report. Ann NY Acad Sci 119:736, 1964

399. CONSTANTOULAKIS M, ECONOMIDOU J, KARAGIORGA M, KATSANTONI A, GYFTAKE E: Combined long-term treatment of hemosiderosis with desferrioxamine and DTPA in homozygous β-thalassaemia. Ann NY Acad Sci 232:193, 1974

400. SESHADRI R, COLEBATCH JH, GORDON P, EKERT H: Long-term administration of desferrioxamine in thalassaemia major. Arch Dis Child 49:631, 1974

401. GRAZIANO JH, MARKENSON A, MILLER DR, CHANG H, BESTAK M, MEYERS P, PISCIOTTO P, RIFKIND A: Chelation therapy in beta thalassaemia major. I. Intravenous and subcutaneous deferoxamine. J Pediatr Surg 13:25, 1978

402. COOPER B, BUNN HF, PROPPER RD, NATHAN DG, ROSENTHAL DS, MOLONEY WC: Treatment of iron overload in adults with continuous parenteral deferrioxamine. Am J Med 63:958, 1977

403. COHEN A, SCHWARTZ E: Decreasing iron stores during intensive chelation therapy. NY Acad Sci 405, 1980

404. PIOMELLI S, GRAZIANO J, KARPATKIN M, DUDELL GG, HART D, HILGARTNER M, KUSUM K, VALDES-CRUZ M, VORA S: Chelation therapy, transfusion requirement, and iron balance in young thalassemic patients. NY Acad Sci 409, 1980

405. CHARLTON RW, BOTHWELL TH: Iron, ascorbic acid and thalassemia, in Bergsma D, Cerami A, Peterson CM, Graziano JH (eds): Iron Metabolism in Thalassemia. New York, Alan R Liss, 1976, p 63

406. NIENHUIS AW, DELEA C, AAMODT R, BARTTER F, ANDERSON WF: Evaluation of desferrioxamine and ascorbic acid for the treatment of chronic iron overload, in Bergsma D, Cerami A, Peterson CM, Graziano JH, (eds): Iron Metabolism and Thalassemia. New York, Alan R Liss, 1976, p 177

407. HOFFBRAND AV, GORMAN A, LAULICHT M, GARIDI M, ECONOMIDOU J, GEORGIPOULOU P, HUSSAIN MAM, FLYNN DM: Improvement in iron status and liver function in patients with transfusional iron overload with long-term subcutaneous desferrioxamine. Lancet 1:947, 1979

408. LEON MB, BORER JS, BACHARACH SL, GREEN MV, BENZ EJ, GRIFFITH P, NIENHAUS AW: Detection of early cardiac dysfunction in patients with severe beta-thalassemia and chronic iron overload. N Engl J Med 301:1143, 1979

409. PROPPER RD, BUTTON LN, NATHAN DG: New approaches to the transfusion management of thalassemia. Blood, 55:55, 1980

410. DE ALARCON PA, DONOVAN M-E, FORBES GB, LANDAW SA, STOCKONAN JA: Iron absorption in the thalassemia syndromes and its inhibition by tea. N Engl J Med 300:5, 1979

411. GRADY RW: The development of new drugs for use in iron chelation therapy, in Bergsma D, Cerami A, Peterson CM, Graziano JH (eds): Iron Metabolism in Thalassemia. New York, Alan R Liss, 1976, p 161

412. PITT CG, GUPTA G, ESTES WE, ROSENKRANTZ H, METTERVILLE AL, CRUMBLISS AL, PALMER RA, NORDQUEST KW, SPRINKEL-HARDY KA, WHITCOMB DR, BYERS BR, ARCENEUX JEL, GAINES CG, SCIORTINO CV: The selection and evaluation of new chelating agents for the treatment of iron overload. J Pharmacol Exp Ther 208:12, 1979

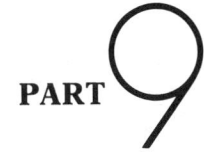

PART 9

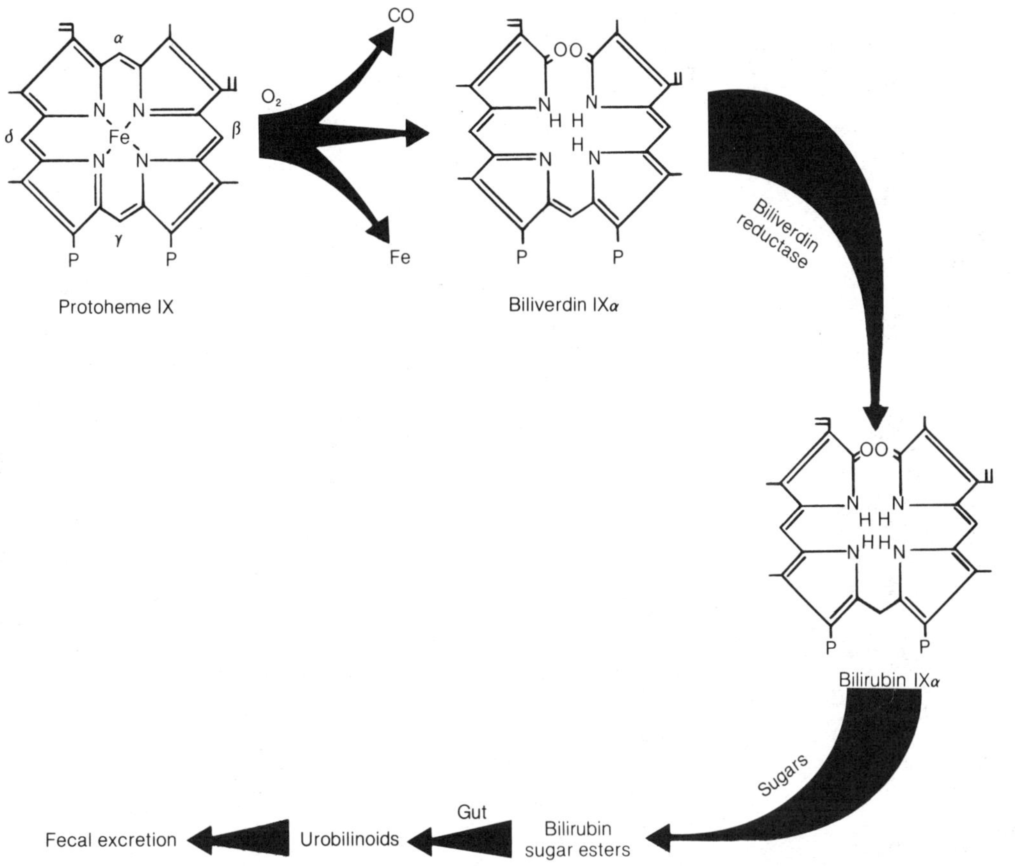

α
δ
β
γ
Fe
N
P
Protoheme IX
O_2
CO
Fe
Biliverdin IXα
Biliverdin reductase
Bilirubin IXα
Sugars
Bilirubin sugar esters
Gut
Urobilinoids
Fecal excretion

Heme metabolism

DISORDERS OF PORPHYRIN AND HEME METABOLISM

60

THE PORPHYRIAS

ATTALLAH KAPPAS

SHIGERU SASSA

KARL E. ANDERSON

The porphyrias are inherited and acquired disorders in which there are partial defects in enzymes of the heme biosynthetic pathway. These diseases are classified as either hepatic or erythroid in origin depending on the principal site of expression of the gene defect in each disorder. In all of the inherited forms of human porphyria, environmental factors (including nonheritable metabolic factors) play a vital role in determining clinical expression of the gene abnormality. In this respect the porphyrias represent a paradigm of the manner in which environmental and genetic factors may interact in the pathogenesis of human disease.

1. Congenital erythropoietic porphyria (CEP) *is the most striking of the porphyrias in terms of the marked severity of cutaneous photosensitivity and scarring which it may produce. Patients with CEP usually have hemolysis which may be severe and may serve as a further stimulus for increased porphyrin production in the bone marrow. Neurological disturbances do not occur. This autosomal recessive disorder is extremely rare. Porphyrins which are overproduced are primarily of the type I series, and the genetic defect in this disorder is probably a deficiency of uroporphyrinogen III cosynthase. Avoidance of sunlight and treatment of secondary infections of the skin are very important in the management of this disease. Hemolysis may improve after splenectomy.*

2. Erythropoietic protoporphyria (EPP) *is an autosomal dominant disorder due to a deficiency of ferrochelatase, the last enzyme of the heme biosynthetic pathway. The disease is characterized by mild to moderate photosensitivity, but unlike CEP there is little or no hemolysis. Excess protoporphyrin is found in erythroid cells, plasma, bile, and feces. Progressive hepatic damage associated with marked protoporphyrin deposition in the liver is a severe and often fatal complication that occurs in a minority of EPP patients. Gene expression at the clinical level is highly variable, such that some carriers of the genetic defect for this disorder have normal red cell porphyrin levels and no photosensitivity. Avoidance of sunlight is important in the prevention of cutaneous symptoms, and oral β-carotene is often helpful in reducing photosensitivity.*

3. Acute intermittent porphyria (AIP). *This hepatic porphyria is inherited in an autosomal dominant fashion and is characterized by a deficiency of porphobilinogen (PBG) deaminase activity. PBG deaminase activity is approximately 50 percent of normal in all tissues examined (i.e., red blood cells, skin, cultured fibroblasts, mitogen-stimulated lymphocytes, amniotic cells, and liver). Porphyrin overproduction is relatively minor, and therefore there is no photosensitivity. AIP is latent before puberty. The degree of clinical expression of AIP after puberty is highly variable, despite the fact that PBG deaminase deficiency is the same in clini-*

cally latent and clinically expressed AIP. The clinical syndrome is more frequent in females than in males. Hormonal, drug, and nutritional factors predispose to full expression of the disease probably by inducing hepatic δ-aminolevulinic acid (ALA) synthase, the rate-limiting enzyme for heme biosynthesis in the liver. The majority (~90 percent) of individuals who inherit the gene defect for AIP (i.e., PBG deaminase deficiency) remain clinically latent throughout adult life. Subtle endocrine abnormalities, including a demonstrated deficiency of hepatic steroid 5α-reductase activity in clinically expressed AIP, may underlie the increased susceptibility of the small number (~10 percent) of AIP gene carriers who develop clinical symptoms. The steroid 5α-reductase deficiency is absent in AIP gene carriers in whom the disease has never become clinically manifest. The symptoms of AIP are largely neurovisceral in character, and may be due to pharmacologic effects of porphyrin precursors on nervous tissue, although this is not fully established. Clinical management includes symptomatic therapy during acute attacks, a high carbohydrate intake, intravenous glucose or hematin, prevention of exposure to harmful drugs, and screening of family members to detect gene carriers of AIP who may be at potential risk by exposure to various chemicals.

4. *Hereditary coproporphyria (HCP) is generally a milder disorder than AIP, but it can cause similar neurovisceral symptoms; it is associated with overproduction of coproporphyrin III as well as excretion of the porphyrin precursors ALA and PBG during acute exacerbations of the disease. The underlying genetic defect of HCP is reflected in a 50 percent deficiency of coproporphyrinogen III oxidase. This defect is inherited as an autosomal dominant trait. One case of HCP, homozygous for the gene defect, has been described. Clinical expression of HCP is dependent upon the same metabolic, chemical, and environmental factors that seem to affect clinical expression of the gene defect in AIP, and clinical management of HCP is also similar to that for AIP. In HCP coproporphyrinogen III accumulates in the liver. The oxidized porphyrin is also found in plasma and skin, and it accounts for the photosensitivity observed in some patients.*

5. *Variegate porphyria (VP) has been recognized in many populations but is most common in South African whites. Inheritance is autosomal dominant in nature. The underlying genetic defect involves a deficiency in the activity of either protoporphyrinogen oxidase or ferrochelatase. Hormones, drugs, and metabolic factors influence clinical expression of the gene defect in VP, as has been observed in AIP and in HCP. Clinically expressed VP is characterized by the same neurovisceral symptoms as in AIP. Photosensitivity due to the accumulation of porphyrins in plasma and skin is more common than in HCP. Clinical management is similar to that for AIP and HCP.*

6. *Porphyria cutanea tarda (PCT) is the most common form of porphyria and usually begins in middle or late adult life. Males are affected more frequently than females. Patients with PCT have mild to severe photosensitivity and frequently have evidence of liver disease. Alcohol, estrogens, and hepatic siderosis are common predisposing factors. PCT patients have an increased risk for the development of hepatocellular carcinoma, especially when the disease is of long duration. A deficiency of hepatic uroporphyrinogen decarboxylase activity appears to characterize all cases of PCT. In PCT patients with an apparently uncommon genetic form of this disease, the enzyme deficiency can also be demonstrated in erythrocytes, lymphocytes, and cultured skin fibroblasts. This familial form of PCT is autosomal dominant; homozygotes have also been described. In most cases of PCT there is no family history of the disease. Although some investigators have suggested that there is an inherited uroporphyrinogen decarboxylase defect expressed in red cells as well as hepatic cells in virtually all PCT patients, others have reported that patients with sporadic PCT have an abnormal activity of this enzyme only in the liver. Therefore it is still not established that a genetic defect in uroporphyrinogen decarboxylase is present in all cases of PCT. Hexachlorobenzene and other chlorinated hydrocarbons can inhibit uroporphyrinogen decarboxylase in the liver and produce a syndrome that closely resembles PCT without affecting the activity of the red cell enzyme. The deficiency of hepatic uroporphyrinogen decarboxylase in PCT results in a complex pattern of porphyrin excretion, which includes excess production of the isocoproporphyrin series, a distinctive feature of this disease. PCT can be successfully treated by phlebotomy, which reduces iron stores in the liver. Avoidance of alcohol and estrogens is important in the therapy of this disease.*

The hepatic and erythropoietic porphyrias of humans are inherited and acquired disorders characterized by defects in specific enzymes of the heme biosynthetic pathway, increased accumulation and excretion of chemical intermediates in heme synthesis, and a variety of clinical manifestations among which neurological abnormalities and cutaneous photosensitivity dominate. Disorders of porphyrin-heme metabolism are not limited to humans. There are certain naturally occurring animal porphyrias of genetic origin as well as porphyrias that can be induced experimentally by a variety of chemicals in normal animals and in certain tissue preparations, such as cultured liver cells. These animal and experimental models of the porphyrias have provided important insights into the regulatory mechanisms by which cellular porphyrin and heme metabolism is controlled. Indeed, in few other categories of metabolic and genetic disorders has there been such a close parallel between the human condition and the model disorders that can be produced in the laboratory, nor so direct a relevance of information obtained in studies of experimental systems to the pathogenesis and therapy of the human disease.

There has been an eruption of new knowledge within recent years concerning (1) the biochemistry of heme, (2) the characteristics of the enzymes in the biosynthetic pathway, (3) the manner in which these enzymes are regulated, and (4) the biological implications of the perturbations of heme metabolism that are of genetic origin, as in the human porphyrias, or which are produced by chemicals such as steroids, drugs, carcinogens, and other environmental agents. Perhaps the strongest impetus for the intensification of research in heme biology has derived from the recent recognition that heme, as the prosthetic group of cytochrome P_{450}, plays a crucial role in the oxidative transformation of an extraordinary variety of chemicals of endogenous and exogenous origin. For this reason the clinical porphyrias have become of increasing interest not only to physicians but also to biochemists, pharmacologists, and other basic scientists whose research focuses on chemical biotransformations and problems of host-environment interaction. In the latter respect the human porphyrias are exemplary disorders for study. In every major form of these diseases, a clear environmental or chemical factor—whether it be sunlight in the erythropoietic porphyrias or drugs and hormones in the hepatic porphyrias—influences the clinical expression of the disorder in the genetically susceptible individual.

A reasonably extensive knowledge of heme biochemistry is essential to an understanding of the biochemical characteristics and genetic and metabolic aberrations that distinguish each of the human porphyrias. The initial section of this chapter therefore defines in considerable detail the enzymology and regulatory mechanisms for heme metabolism in the liver and in erythroid cells. Clinical descriptions of the individual porphyric disorders follow and include the biochemical characteristics of these diseases and the nature of the gene defects that have been defined.

NOMENCLATURE, STRUCTURE, AND FUNCTION OF PORPHYRINS

The biosynthesis of heme requires 8 mol of glycine and 8 mol of succinyl CoA. The first intermediate of this biosynthetic pathway is δ-aminolevulinic acid (ALA), a 5-carbon amino ketone, which is formed by the condensation of glycine activated by pyridoxal 5'-phosphate, and "active succinate" (i.e., succinyl CoA) [1]. Two molecules of ALA are converted to porphobilinogen (PBG), which is a monopyrrole, and PBGs are in turn condensed to form porphyrins (consuming four PBG molecules per one molecule of porphyrin), which are cyclic tetrapyrroles. Porphyrins are the immediate precursors of the various hemes, chlorophylls, and cobalamins. There are a number of excellent reviews on the developmental history of porphyrin and heme biosynthesis and readers are referred to these for detailed coverage of topics in this field [2–7].

Nomenclature and Structures

Porphyrins are metal-free cyclic tetrapyrroles. Porphyrin nomenclature was developed by Hans Fischer and his school at Munich and the terminology employed by this group has hitherto been used widely. The system of nomenclature of tetrapyrroles, however, is currently in a state of flux [7, 8], and the International Union of Pure and Applied Chemistry (IUPAC) and the International Union of Biochemistry (IUB) recently issued new recommendations concerning the nomenclature of tetrapyrroles [9]. These recommendations were thought necessary because the Fischer nomenclature is not systematic, utilizes a large number of trivial names, and therefore is difficult to learn readily. In this review it has seemed preferable to utilize the traditional (Fischer) system because it still remains the one used by the principal workers in this field, and most

nomenclature appearing in the literature of the past is based primarily on the Fischer system. The IUPAC-IUB nomenclature is referred to wherever it seems appropriate.

According to Fischer's system of nomenclature [10] the basic ring structure of porphyrins is represented by the compound he termed "porphin," shown in Fig. 60-1. Rings are designated from the upper left as ring A, B, C, and D and these are joined by the four methene bridges, α, β, γ, and δ. Hydrogens at the β position of the pyrrole ring (positions as 2, 4, 6, and 8 in the Fischer model or 3, 8, 13, and 18 in the IUPAC system) in porphyrins are substituted by alkyl groups, conferring a complex diversity on porphyrins. For example, each pyrrole ring in etioporphyrin I (2,4,6,8-tetraethyl-1,3,5,7-tetramethylporphin, according to Fischer) contains one methyl and one ethyl substituent. There are four possible isomers of etioporphyrin, i.e., types I, II, III, and IV as shown in Table 60-1. Naturally occurring porphyrins are all etio-type porphyrins. Each porphyrin isomer is defined in a way that corresponds to the appropriate etioporphyrin.

The new nomenclature recommended by the IUPAC-IUB is summarized in a 30-page document. [9]. There are two important aspects of this new proposal. First, the fundamental macrocycle is designated as a *porphyrin* instead of a *porphin* as in the older system (Fig. 60-1). Second, all carbon and nitrogen atoms of the porphyrin macrocycle are numbered 1 to 24, whereas in the Fischer system only the outer carbon atoms of the pyrrole ring are numbered (Fig. 60-1). The carbon atoms at the methene bridges (the *meso*-carbons) formerly designated by the Greek letters α, β, γ, and δ are now numbered 5, 10, 15, and 20 (Fig. 60-1). The IUPAC system retains eleven well-established trivial names as well as the designation of the positional isomers in the coproporphyrin, uroporphyrin, and etioporphyrin series (Table 60-1). Thus virtually all trivial names for the common porphyrins found in normal subjects and in porphyria patients are retained in the recent IUPAC nomenclature.

Porphyrins display a distinctive absorption spectrum allowing them to be readily identified in biological fluids or tissues. The absorption spectrum of porphyrins consists of the *Soret band*, a major absorption band in the 400-nm region, and four smaller absorption bands at longer wavelengths between 500 nm and 630 nm, with decreasing intensity in absorbance toward the red (Fig. 60-2a). The Soret band generally has a 10 to 15 times greater absorption (molar extinction coefficient of ~2 to 5×10^5) than the next major band (band IV), which

Figure 60-1 Structure and nomenclature of the porphyrin macrocycle. *Porphin* (Fischer nomenclature) or *porphyrin* (IUPAC nomenclature) is the basic structure of biologically occurring ring tetrapyrroles. The systems differ in the numeration of the carbon and nitrogen atoms of the macrocycle.

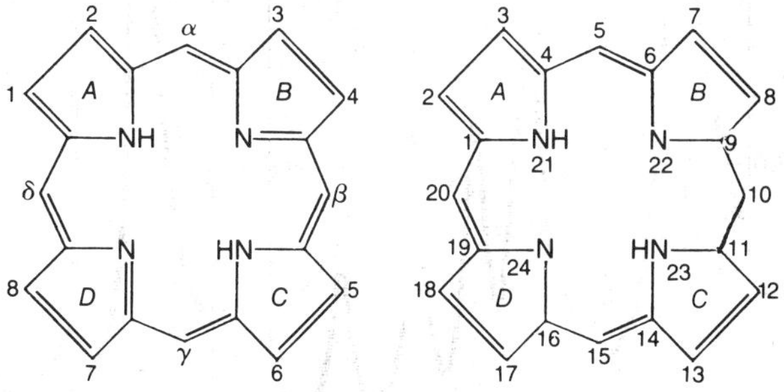

Porphin
(Fischer Numeration)

Porphyrin
(IUPAC-"1-24" Numeration)

occurs at around 500 nm. With the formation of a porphyrin dication in aqueous HCl, or the formation of the metal complex of a porphyrin [11, 12], the four bands in the longer wavelength region are replaced by two, the so-called α and β bands (Fig. 60-2b).

Metal-free porphyrins emit an intense red fluorescence upon excitation by long wavelength ultraviolet light (~400 nm). In acidic solution two strong emission bands corresponding to those of the two longest wavelength absorption bands are produced (Fig. 60-2b). Spectrofluorometric methods provide a far more sensitive means of detection of porphyrins in biological systems than does visible light absorption spectrophotometry [13]. Porphyrin chelates with those metals having no unpaired electrons (e.g., Mg, Zn, Sn) also display strong fluorescence upon illumination with long wavelength ultraviolet light. Thus while all free porphyrins and the porphyrin chelates with diamagnetic metals fluoresce, porphyrin chelates with paramagnetic metals do not fluoresce. For example, the magnesium-porphyrin chelate chlorophyll fluoresces, whereas iron-protoporphyrin IX (i.e., heme) does not.

The water solubility of porphyrins becomes greater with increases in the number of carboxylic acid side chains. Thus, uroporphyrin (8-carboxylate porphyrin) is most water-soluble, followed by coproporphyrin (4-carboxylate porphyrin) and protoporphyrin (2-carboxylate porphyrin) in decreasing order. Protoporphyrin is so hydrophobic that it is excreted only into bile, while uro- and coproporphyrin can be excreted in urine.

Actions

Although free porphyrins occur in nature in small quantities, no known function has been assigned to them. In contrast, heme, chlorophyll, and corrin, which are Fe-, Mg-, and Co-chelates of porphyrins or of porphyrin derivatives respectively, carry out crucial biological functions. For example, heme (ferroprotoporphyrin IX) is the prosthetic group for a number of hemoproteins. These include myoglobin and hemoglobin, which carry out oxygen binding or transport; mitochondrial cytochromes aa_3, b, c, and c_3, which are important in trans-

ferring electrons; microsomal cytochrome P_{450}, which catalyzes mixed function oxidations; catalase, which decomposes H_2O_2; peroxidase, which activates H_2O_2; and tryptophan pyrrolase, which catalyzes the oxidation of tryptophan. Recently, heme has also been shown to be the prosthetic group of prostaglandin endoperoxide synthetase and indoleamine dioxygenase [14, 15].

In most hemoproteins heme is associated with its apoprotein noncovalently through coordination of the iron atom with a nitrogen atom of an amino acid side chain. Therefore it is possible by proper chemical methods to separate heme and apoprotein quantitatively. There is also evidence that certain frac-

Table 60-1 Structures and trivial names of porphyrins

Name	2 / 1	3 / 2	7 / 3	8 / 4	12 / 5	13 / 6	17 / 7	18 / 8
Etioporphyrin I	M	E	M	E	M	E	M	E
Etioporphyrin II	M	E	E	M	M	E	E	M
Etioporphyrin III	M	E	M	E	M	E	E	M
Etioporphyrin IV	M	E	E	M	E	M	M	E
Uroporphyrin I	A	P	A	P	A	P	A	P
Uroporphyrin III	A	P	A	P	A	P	P	A
Heptacarboxylate porphyrin III	M	P	A	P	A	P	P	A
Hexacarboxylate porphyrin III	M	P	M	P	A	P	P	A
Pentacarboxylate porphyrin III	M	P	M	P	A	P	P	M
Dehydroisocoproporphyrin III	M	V	M	P	A	P	P	M
Coproporphyrin I	M	P	M	P	M	P	M	P
Coproporphyrin III	M	P	M	P	M	P	P	M
Protoporphyrin IX	M	V	M	V	M	P	P	M
Mesoporphyrin IX	M	E	M	E	M	P	P	M
Hematoporphyrin IX	M	HE	M	HE	M	P	P	M
Deuteroporphyrin IX	M	H	M	H	M	P	P	M

The header above the data reads:
Substituent* with *IUPAC† numeration:* (2, 3, 7, 8, 12, 13, 17, 18) and *Fischer numeration:* (1, 2, 3, 4, 5, 6, 7, 8).

* Substituent abbreviations: M, —CH$_3$; E, —C$_2$H$_5$; A, —CH$_2$COOH; P, —CH$_2$CH$_2$COOH; V, —CH=CH$_2$; HE, —CHOHCH$_3$.
† The International Union of Pure and Applied Chemistry.

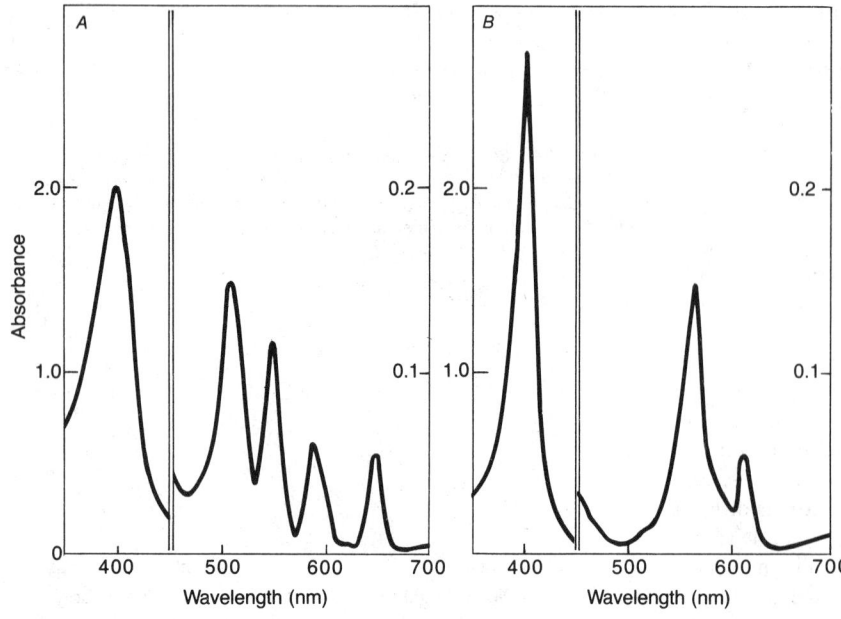

Figure 60-2 Absorption spectra of protoporphyrin IX. *A*. Protoporphyrin IX dimethylester in CHCl$_3$. *B*. Protoporphyrin IX in 1 *N* HCl. The typical absorption spectrum of protoporphyrin IX in an organic solvent is shown in *A* and consists of an intense Soret band and four smaller absorption peaks in the longer wavelength region of the spectrum. Formation of the porphyrin dication in HCl leads to the spectral changes shown in *B*.

tions of heme in the endoplasmic reticulum are not bound in cytochromes. For example, some of the heme in cytochrome b₅ exists in a freely exchangeable form [16–19]. Exogenously administered heme can also associate with certain apocytochromes [20–22] to form hemeproteins as it does with apohemoglobin [23]. In contrast, heme c in cytochrome c is covalently bound to the protein moiety by two thioether bonds between the two vinyl groups of the heme and two cysteinyl residues of the apocytochrome. Cytochrome P_{450} is a unique CO-binding hemeprotein with anomalous spectral behavior. For example the CO complex of reduced P_{450} has an intense absorption band only at 450 nm. With ethyl isocyanide as an exogenous ligand, on the other hand, cytochrome P_{450} displays a spectral change in which two bands in the Soret region appear. These unusual spectral properties disappear when the cytochrome is converted by various treatments in vitro to a nonfunctional form called P_{420}.

Fluorescence of porphyrins is related to their properties as photodynamic sensitizers. Upon illumination at ultraviolet wavelengths and in the presence of molecular oxygen, metal-free and diamagnetic metalloporphyrins cause photodynamic effects on multicellular organisms, cells, subcellular structures, and biomacromolecules [24]. Porphyrin-sensitized injury of cells appears to be the result of photodynamic damage to plasma and lysosomal membranes; injury to cells can also result from activation of the complement system [24, 25]. Animals and humans treated with porphyrins show characteristic photosensitization symptoms. These symptoms include intense itching, erythema, edema, pigmentation, ulceration and scarring of the skin, and in severe photosensitization reactions cardiocirculatory effects such as hypotension and collapse [26]. Porphyrins can sensitize the photooxidation of small organic molecules and of certain amino acids via singlet oxygen generation [27, 28]. For example, illumination of mice pretreated with hematoporphyrin by light at ultraviolet wavelengths leads to hypertrophy of the epithelium followed by tumor formation [29], while hematoporphyrin taken up by glioma cells can photodynamically destroy the tumor [30]. These photodynamic effects are not observed with porphyrins chelated with paramagnetic metal atoms such as Fe, Co, Cr, or Mn. Uroporphyrin has recently been shown to stimulate collagen synthesis in cultured human skin fibroblasts [30a]. This effect appears to be an interesting example of "dark effect" of a porphyrin.

ENZYMES AND CHEMICAL INTERMEDIATES OF THE HEME BIOSYNTHETIC PATHWAY

The biochemical pathway for the formation of heme is illustrated in Fig. 60-3. Shemin and Rittenberg [31, 32] in elegant studies, demonstrated the arrangement in the porphyrin macrocycle of the carbon and nitrogen atoms originating from the eight glycine and succinic acid molecules that are the precursors of porphyrins. Subsequently it was shown that the α carbon atom of glycine is utilized to label both the pyrrolic ring carbons and the methene bridge carbons [33, 34]. Shemin and Russell proposed that the 5-carbon amino ketone ALA is the product of the condensation of glycine and succinate. Cookson and Rimington [35] identified the structure of PBG, a substance known to occur in the urine of patients with

acute intermittent porphyria [36]. Both ALA and PBG were shown to be precursors in the formation of porphyrins and heme [37–40]. There are eight enzymes involved in the synthesis of heme. The first and the last three of these enzymes are localized in the mitochondria; the intermediate enzymes are localized in the cytosol. Normal values for activities of enzymes in the heme biosynthetic pathway in several human tissues are summarized in Table 60-2, and the alterations of these enzymic activities in the various human porphyrias are summarized in Table 60-3.

δ-Aminolevulinic Acid Synthase (ALA Synthase) [Succinyl CoA:Glycine C-Succinyl Transferase (Decarboxylating), (EC 2.3.1.37)]

The first reaction in the heme biosynthetic pathway is catalyzed by a mitochondrial enzyme, ALA synthase, which condenses glycine and succinyl CoA to form ALA. This enzymatic reaction was first identified in the photosynthetic bacterium *Rhodopseudomonas spheroides* [41, 42]. Subsequently the enzymatic activity has been demonstrated in a variety of species and tissues including microorganisms [43]; yeast [44], avian [45] and mammalian liver cells [46–48]; mammalian erythroid cells [49]; mouse Harderian gland [50]; rat kidney [51], heart [52], and brain [53]; and insects [54], as well as in the liver of normal human subjects and in patients with hepatic porphyrias (see Table 60-3).

Purification of ALA Synthase The purification of ALA synthase has proven to be quite difficult, probably because the enzyme is present in minute quantities and is very unstable. The reported molecular weight of ALA synthase has varied greatly depending on the source and method of preparation. The enzyme may also form aggregates with other proteins [55, 56]. Nevertheless several laboratory groups have been able to purify the enzyme to homogeneity by taking proper precautions to avoid aggregation. Whiting and Granick [57] purified liver mitochondrial ALA synthase to homogeneity from chick embryos that had been treated with chemical inducers of the enzyme, namely 2-allyl-2-isopropylacetamide (AIA) and 1,4-dihydro-3,5-dicarbethoxycollidine (DDC). Under nondenaturing conditions the purified enzyme was shown by polyacrylamide gel electrophoresis to have a molecular weight of 87,000. By sodium dodecyl sulfate (SDS)-polyacrylamide gel electrophoresis, the molecular weight was 49,000, which suggested that the enzyme exists as a dimer consisting of two identical subunits. A molecular weight of 120,000 [58] has been reported for rat liver mitochondrial ALA synthase. A smaller molecular weight of 77,000 was reported [55] when precautions were taken to avoid aggregation.

Properties of Mitochondrial ALA Synthase Mitochondrial ALA synthase partially purified from rabbit, rat, and guinea pig liver has K_m values for glycine, succinyl CoA, and pyridoxal 5'-phosphate in the range of 5 to 19 mM, 60 to 200 μM, and 1 to 10 μM, respectively [55, 56, 59–61]. The relatively high K_m (i.e., low affinity) of the enzyme for glycine, raises the possibility that the enzyme activity may be regulated by the physiological concentration of glycine in liver [62]. Indeed, the administration of p-aminobenzoic acid or sodium benzoate, which increases glycine metabolism via other path-

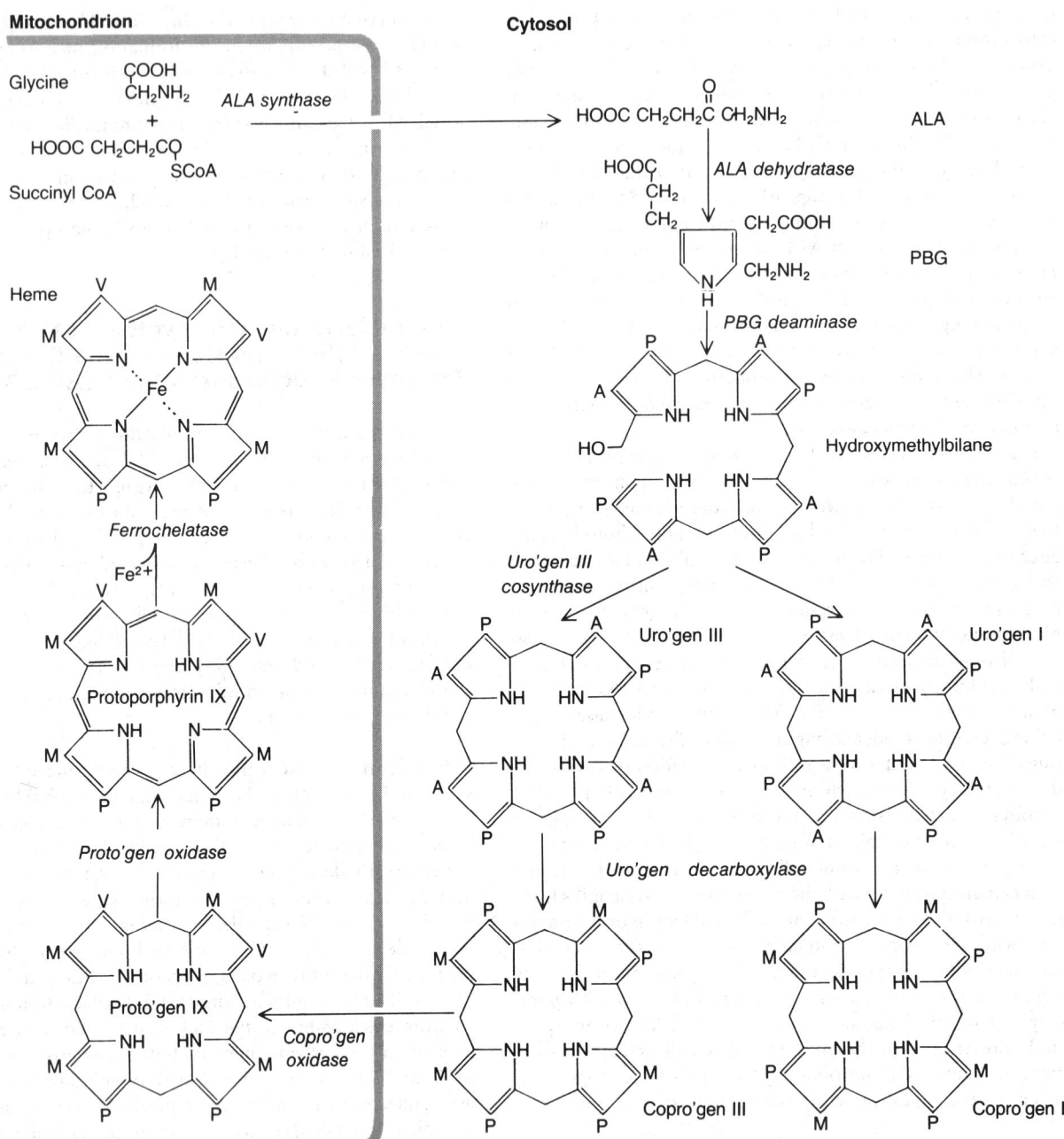

Figure 60-3   The heme biosynthetic pathway. Subcellular distribution of enzymes and intermediates in the synthesis of heme is shown. A, —CH₂·COOH; M. —CH₃; P, —CH₂·CH₂·COOH; V, —CH=CH₂

ways, is known to suppress the increase in activity of hepatic ALA synthase caused by DDC [63, 64].

The V_{max} of the purified rat liver mitochondrial ALA synthase is 2000 nmol/h per milligram of protein [58], while it is over 20,000 nmol/h per milligram of protein for the chick embryo liver enzyme [57].

Cytosolic ALA Synthase   Normally, ALA synthase activity is found only in mitochondria. By providing a succinyl CoA generating system to the enzyme assay mixture, a substantial increase of the enzyme activity can also be detected in rat liver cytosol after animals are treated with AIA, a potent inducer of ALA synthase [55, 65, 66]. An increase in cytosolic ALA synthase has also been reported in rat kidney [67] and in mouse [68] and chicken liver [69]. Cytosolic ALA synthase is believed to be a newly synthesized form of the enzyme that is in transit from cytoplasmic ribosomes to mitochondria [55, 66].

Cytosolic ALA synthase from rat liver can be purified to apparent homogeneity and has a molecular weight of 250,000, either by polyacrylamide gel electrophoresis under nondenaturing conditions or by gel filtration [70–72]. It appears to be an enzyme complex which is considerably larger than mitochondrial ALA synthase [73]. When this enzyme was analyzed by SDS-polyacrylamide gel electrophoresis, three protein bands having molecular weights of 120,000, 79,000, and 51,000 were observed [72]. This finding suggests that the apparent single form of the enzyme with a molecular weight of 250,000 is in reality an enzyme complex that can be split into three different components under denaturing conditions. When the 250,000-dalton form of the enzyme was fractionated by sucrose density gradient centrifugation, the active enzyme was recovered as a single protein species with a molecular weight of 110,000 and this fraction yielded a single protein with a molecular weight of 51,000 by SDS-polyacrylamide gel electrophoresis [72]. The catalytically active species of cytosolic ALA synthase freed from inactive subunits can also be obtained by treating the 250,000-dalton form with papain and by further purification through sucrose density gradient centrifugation [74]. The purified preparation from the papain-treated enzyme had molecular weights of 110,000 and 51,000 in sucrose density gradient centrifugation and in SDS-poly-acrylamide gel electrophoresis respectively. These findings suggest that cytosolic ALA synthase of the rat liver consists of a dimer of two identical subunits having a molecular weight of 51,000 and two catalytically inactive subunits having molecular weights of 79,000 and 120,000. The purified active ALA synthase from rat liver cytosol after AIA induction has a specific activity of 73,000 nmol/h per milligram of protein at 37°C; and isoelectric point of 8.2; and a pH optimum for the reaction of 7.6 [74]. The K_m value for succinyl CoA is 11 μM for both the papain-treated and untreated enzyme, whereas the K_m for glycine is 7.5 μM and 2.5 μM for the papain-treated enzyme and the untreated enzyme respectively [74].

When a specific antibody against the catalytically active subunit (51,000 daltons) of cytosolic ALA synthase was used, it was found that the antibody recognized cytosolic and mitochondrial ALA synthase equally [74]. This finding provides strong support for the view that cytosolic ALA synthase is immunochemically identical to the enzyme in the mitochondria and is a precursor protein in transit into the mitochondria. Incorporation of purified cytosolic ALA synthase of rat liver into mitochondria in vitro has also been demonstrated [75].

Turnover of ALA Synthase in the Liver   The half-life of

mitochondrial ALA synthase is short (e.g., only 34 min in fetal rat liver [76], 70 min in adult rat liver [47, 66, 77], and 180 min in cultured chick embryo liver cells [78]). The half-life of cytosolic ALA synthase in rat liver is only 20 min, which is even shorter than that of the mitochondrial enzyme [48, 66, 77], and presumably represents a composite of enzyme degradation in the cytosol and transport of the enzyme into mitochondria. ALA synthase appears to have one of the most rapid turnover rates of the proteins in mitochondria and its half-life is far shorter than the average half-life of mitochondrial proteins in general (approximately 5 days) [17]. Only ornithine decarboxylase is known to have a shorter half-life ($t_{\frac{1}{2}} = 11$ min) [79]. The short half-life of ALA synthase is a suitable property for its regulatory role in heme formation. Control of the rate of synthesis of the enzyme in liver is believed to be the major mode of regulation of heme biosynthesis. In bone marrow mitochondria, a mitochondrial protease that is specific for ALA synthase has been found [80] and purified to homogeneity [81]. It is attractive to postulate that, in bone marrow and perhaps in other tissues, the level of mitochondrial ALA synthase may be regulated in part by this specific protease.

The Reaction Mechanism   The following mechanism has been elucidated for the reaction catalyzed by ALA synthase purified from *R. spheroides* [82–84] (Fig. 60-4). (1) Glycine forms a Schiff base with pyridoxal 5'-phosphate which is bound to the enzyme yielding a stable carbanion. (2) A proton (R-configuration) is removed from the methylene carbon atom of glycine. (3) Succinyl CoA condenses to the carbanion to form α-amino-β-ketoadipic acid with the loss of CoA. (4) α-Amino-β-ketoadipic acid is decarboxylated to yield ALA. The proton on the methylene carbon atom of glycine that is lost at

Table 60-2 Normal values* of heme pathway enzymes† in human tissues

Enzyme	Liver	Erythroid cells	Fibroblasts	Lymphocytes
ALA synthase, nmol/h of ALA per gram	24 [736]	49.2[b,d][259]	5.34[a] [257]	116[a,i] [175]
ALA dehydratase, nmol/h of PBG per gram	1080, 1340 [800]	2513[e] [136]	115‡[a]	290[a,i] [175]
PBG deaminase, nmol/h of Uro I per gram	2.75 [166]	35.7[e] [169]	6.14[a,h] [174]	6.05[a,i] [175] 10.3[a,j] [175]
Uroporphyrinogen III cosynthase, nmol/h of Uro III per gram	—	6636[c,e,f] [153]	8775[a,f] [153]	—
Uroporphyrinogen decarboxylase, nmol/h of Copro per gram	174[a] [190]	717[a] [191]	313[a] [198]	480[a,k] [907a]
Coproporphyrinogen oxidase, nmol/h of Proto per gram	224[a] [232]	—	87[a] [433]	73[a,k] [233]
Protoporphyrinogen oxidase, nmol/h of Proto per gram	—	—	300[a] [262]	658[a,k] [819a]
Ferrochelatase, nmol/h of Heme per gram	352 [257]	18.4[b,d] [259]	3.74[a,g] [257] 6.2[g] [241]	313[a,k] [819a]
Protoporphyrin formation from added ALA, nmol/h of Proto per gram	—	—	4.10[a,l] [174] 2.02[a,m] [174]	7.92[a,i,l] [538] 2.02[a,i,m] [538]

* Only mean values are cited in this table.

† In order to make comparisons of enzymatic activities, certain assumptions were made to recalculate reported data so that they can be expressed per g tissue per h of incubation:

[a] assuming 150 mg of protein per gram of tissue	[d] bone marrow	[h] at 60°C	[l] with EDTA
[b] assuming 2 × 10⁸ erythroblasts per gram of bone marrow	[e] erythrocytes	[i] mitogen-stimulated lymphocytes	[m] without EDTA
[c] assuming 300 mg hemoglobin per gram of erythrocytes	[f] at 31°C	[j] EB-virus transformed lymphocytes	[n] asuming that uroporphyrinogen III is used as substrate (~5 times faster than 5-carboxylate porphyrinogen I)
	[g] protoporphyrin as substrate	[k] non-stimulated lymphocytes	

‡ Sassa et al., unpublished.

Table 60-3 Activities of heme pathway enzymes in human porphyrias

Enzyme	Disease displaying abnormal activity	Liver	Bone marrow	Erythrocytes	Fibroblasts	Lymphocytes
ALA synthase, nmol/h of ALA per gram	AIP	171 [736] ↑ 160 [737] ↑ 264–455 [166] ↑	—	—	Normal [172, 257]	Normal [175]
	HCP	234 [802] ↑	—	—	—	—
	VP	505 [738] ↑	—	—	—	—
PBG deaminase, nmol/h of Uro I per gram	AIP	≤1.1 [166] ↓	—	18.0 [169] ↓	1.86 [174] ↓	2.61 [175] ↓
Uroporphyrinogen III cosynthase, nmol/h of Uro III, per gram	CEP	—	—	966 [153] ↓	2647 [153] ↓	—
Uroporphyrinogen decarboxylase, nmol/h of Copro I per gram	PCT (sporadic)	81 [190] ↓	—	Normal [191, 198]	Normal [198]	Normal [907a]
	PCT (familial)					
	Patients	—	—	77 [191] ↓	—	262 [907a] ↓
	Carriers	—	—	80 [191] ↓	—	—
Coproporphyrinogen oxidase, nmol/h of Proto per gram	HCP					
	Homozygote	—	—	—	4.2 [433]* ↓↓	1.2 ↓↓
	Heterozygote	—	—	—	31–57 [433] ↓	20~32 [233] ↓
Protoporphyrinogen oxidase, nmol/h of Proto per gram	VP (?)	—	—	—	135 [262] ↓	361 [819a] ↓
Ferrochelatase, nmol/h of Heme per gram	EPP	44.2 [257] ↓	4.4 [259] ↓	—	0.54 [257] ↓	75 [819a] ↓
	VP (?)	—	—	—	3.6 [241] ↓	—
Protoporphyrin formation from added ALA, nmol/h of Proto per gram	AIP	—	—	—	1.44 [174] ↓ (control 4.10)	3.75 [175] ↓ (control 7.92)
	EPP	—	—	—	—	4.79 [175] ↑ (control 2.02)

* ↓ ↓ Especially marked

step (1) is specifically that of the R-configuration while the one having the S-configuration is incorporated into ALA [82]. Succinyl CoA is not required for the proton removal reaction [85]. Heme, an allosteric effector of the enzyme activity, has, however, no effect on the loss of the proton from glycine [85]. Decarboxylation of α-amino-β-ketoadipic acid to ALA occurs on the enzyme and then ALA is released into the medium from the pyridoxal-enzyme complex [84].

The Effect of Heme on ALA Synthase   There is a substantial body of evidence indicating that the level of ALA synthase in the liver is regulated by the end product of the biosynthetic pathway, heme. Three possible mechanisms have been proposed for the feedback regulatory effect of heme on ALA synthase and all may be important to some degree. (1) The activity of purified ALA synthase is inhibited (~50 percent) in vitro by hemin[1] at concentrations of ~10 to 50 μM [55–57, 59]. The enzyme activity in crude homogenates is not inhibited by hemin [86]. (2) The transport of cytosolic ALA synthase into mitochondria is inhibited by hemin [87]. In rats treated

with AIA and hemin, a considerable increase of cytosolic ALA synthase is observed with a concomitant decrease of mitochondrial ALA synthase activity in comparison with rats treated with AIA alone [87]. These findings indicate that hemin inhibits the transfer of cytosolic ALA synthase into mitochondria. (3) Hemin represses the synthesis of ALA synthase. Hemin repression of the enzyme synthesis occurs at a concentration of 0.1×10^{-6} M [88], which is considerably less than the concentration required for inhibition of the enzyme activity (10 to 50×10^{-6} M) [55–57, 59]. The action of hemin in the regulation of ALA synthase is discussed further in a later section.

ALA Formation via a Pathway Not Involving Glycine and Succinyl CoA   With only a few exceptions, ALA synthase activity, which utilizes succinate and glycine, has not been found in plant cells. Greening etiolated leaves and cotyledons incorporate [14C]glutamate or α-ketoglutarate but not [14C]succinyl CoA or glycine [89] into ALA. Thus the pathway for ALA formation in most plants does not involve glycine or succinyl CoA. In this reaction, C-1 of glutamate becomes C-5 of ALA via the formation of an intermediate, γ,δ-dioxovalerate (DOVA) [90] (Fig. 60-5). Transamination of DOVA to ALA then occurs as has been shown in extracts of *Chlorella* [91], bean leaves [92], and *R. spheroides* [93]. Whether or not chlorophyll formation is exclusively associated with the DOVA pathway is uncertain [94]. For example, in green algae

[1] *Heme* is ferroprotoporphyrin IX, i.e., the iron (Fe^{2+}) chelate of protoporphyrin IX. Heme is readily autooxidized in vitro to the ferric (Fe^{3+}) form, called ferriprotoporphyrin IX, or *hemin*. In this form, there is one residual positive charge, and the chelate is usually isolated as a halide (e.g., hemin chloride). In alkaline solution, the halide is replaced by the hydroxyl ion, forming *hematin*.

both the classical ALA synthase reaction involving glycine and succinyl CoA as well as the DOVA pathway have been demonstrated [95].

A reaction similar to that catalyzed by DOVA transaminase has been found in mammalian cells. Varticovski et al. [96] purified DOVA transaminase from bovine liver mitochondria. The enzyme had a molecular weight of 240,000. The K_m for DOVA was 2.4×10^{-4} M. Pyridoxal 5'-phosphate was required as a cofactor. Total DOVA transaminase activity was found to be considerably greater than that of ALA synthase in bovine liver, suggesting that this enzyme may play a significant role in ALA formation in mammalian cells as well. It is not known whether the level of this enzyme activity is increased when more heme synthesis is necessary or whether it, like ALA synthase, is inhibited by heme. Recently it has been reported that DOVA transaminase in mammalian liver and kidney is associated with another enzymic activity, i.e., alanine:glyoxylate transaminase [96a]. The activity of the latter is much greater than that of the former, and the reaction favors glycine formation. The role of DOVA transaminase in the regulation of heme formation in animal tissues thus remains to be elucidated.

The Assay of ALA Synthase Activity   ALA synthase activity is generally determined in tissue homogenates or in isolated mitochondrial fractions by the use of a colorimetric method [46, 47, 66, 97]. Cellular homogenates or mitochondria are incubated with glycine and pyridoxal 5'-phosphate in buffer. The ALA formed in the reaction mixture is converted to a pyrrole (2-methyl-3-acetyl-4-[3-propionic acid] pyrrole) by condensation with 2,4-pentanedione, which then combines with Ehrlich's aldehyde reagent to form a chromogen with a maximal absorption at 553 nm [98]. In this assay, succinyl CoA is generated from citrate by intact mitochondria. The assay therefore requires freshly prepared homogenates or mitochondria. Ethylenediaminetetraacetic acid (EDTA) [47, 97] or levulinic acid [62] is included in the assay mixture to prevent the loss of ALA by the ALA dehydratase reaction. Succinylacetone also may be useful to inhibit ALA utilization [99]. Fluoride is sometimes included in the assay and is known to increase ALA synthase activity, probably by inhibiting rapid breakdown of ATP which is required for succinyl CoA formation [100, 101]. It is important to isolate ALA pyrrole before the Ehrlich color salt formation. Aminoacetone is formed by aminoacetone synthase during the reaction and aminoacetone pyrrole also reacts with the reagent. Separation of ALA pyrrole and aminoacetone pyrrole can be carried out by DOWEX ion exchange column chromatography [98, 102] or alternatively by solvent extraction [45, 97]. Solvent extraction employing methylene chloride removes more than 90 percent of the aminoacetone pyrrole without loss of ALA pyrrole [97]. It is important to note that there are two general types of Ehrlich's reagent described in the literature. The modified Ehrlich's reagent described by Mauzerall and Granick [98] (2% w/v p-dimethylaminobenzaldehyde and 0.32% w/v HgCl$_2$ in a mixture of 1.87 N perchloric acid and 14.6 N acetic acid) gives rise to color that is twice as intense as that produced by the standard Ehrlich's reagent (2% w/v p-dimethylaminobenzaldehyde in 6 N HCl).

A simple and sensitive method to determine ALA synthase activity in cultured chick embryo liver cells has been developed by Sinclair and Granick [62]. Liver cells are incubated with an assay mixture for ALA synthase, and under these conditions,

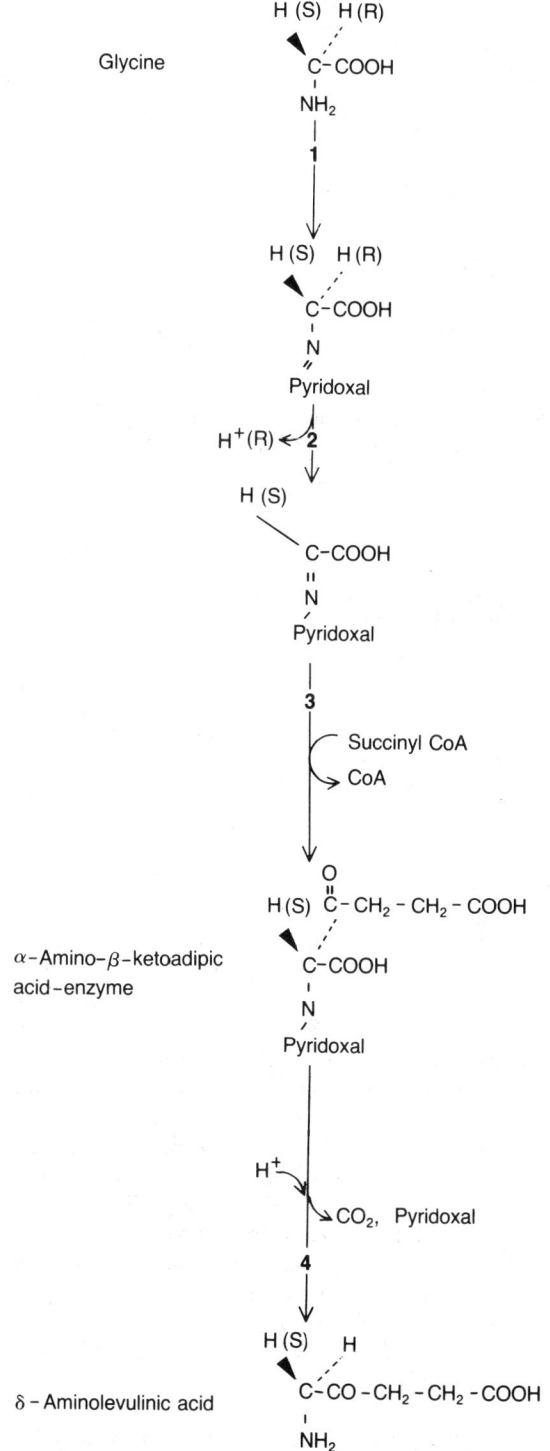

Figure 60-4   The reaction catalyzed by ALA synthase. 1. Glycine forms a Schiff base with pyridoxal 5'-phosphate-enzyme complex. 2. A proton (R-configuration) is removed from the methylene carbon atom of glycine. 3. The succinyl group is transferred from succinyl CoA to form α-amino-β-ketoadipic acid. 4. After decarboxylation of the intermediate, a proton is stereospecifically inserted and free ALA is released [82–84].

much of the ALA formed is excreted into the medium at a linear rate for at least 5 h [103] and can be quantitated colorimetrically. When a 10-cm light-path cuvette is utilized, the method requires as little as 0.5 mg protein for an assay and the lowest detection level for ALA is approximately 300 pmol/ml medium [62].

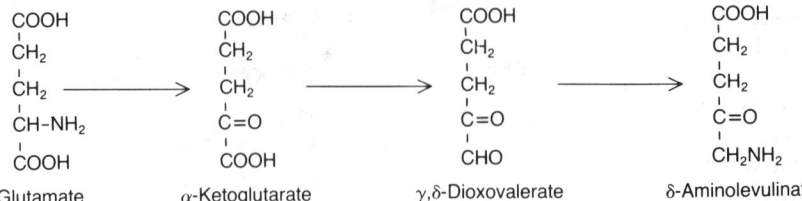

Figure 60-5 Formation of ALA in plant cells. The formation of ALA does not involve glycine or succinyl CoA. Instead C-1 of an α-ketoglutarate or glutamate is incorporated into C-5 of ALA via γ,δ-dioxovalerate [90]. An enzyme which catalyzes the transamination of γ,δ-dioxovalerate to ALA has also been demonstrated in bovine liver [96].

A more sensitive assay for ALA synthase is based on the incorporation of [14C]succinate into ALA. A variety of methods have been described to isolate [14C]ALA from the assay mixture, most of which depend on ion-exchange chromatography using DOWEX 50 resin [52, 101, 104–107]. Such radiochemical methods have been adapted for tissues containing low ALA synthase activity, such as the adrenal [108], heart [67, 109, 110], kidney [67], brain [67], testes [111], normal bone marrow cells [112], and cultured mouse Friend-virus transformed cells [107].

δ-Aminolevulinic Acid Dehydratase (ALA Dehydratase) [δ-Aminolevulinate Hydrolase (EC 4.2.1.24)]

ALA dehydratase is a cytosolic enzyme that has been characterized in animals [113], plants [114], and bacteria [115]. The enzyme catalyzes the condensation of two molecules of ALA with a loss of two molecules of water to form the monopyrrole PBG (Fig. 60-6).

The Reaction Mechanism The enzymatic mechanism of ALA dehydratase can be summarized as follows (Fig. 60-6): one molecule of ALA forms a covalent bond to the enzyme through the formation of a Schiff's base between the ε-amino group of a lysine residue and the keto group of ALA (Fig. 60-6a). This stabilized carbanion then participates in an aldol condensation with a second ALA molecule with the removal of one water molecule (Fig. 60-6b) [116]. The first ALA molecule bound to the enzyme ultimately forms the acetic acid side chain in PBG by this mechanism. The ALA molecule initially bound to ALA dehydratase is the one that becomes the propionic acid substituent of PBG [117]. The purified enzyme obtained from bovine liver and human erythrocytes is pale yellowish in color and spectral analysis and kinetic studies suggest that pyridoxal 5'-phosphate may be bound to the enzyme [118]. Pyridoxal 5'-phosphate competitively inhibits human erythrocyte ALA dehydratase [118]. Its precise role in the enzyme reaction is not known.

Properties ALA dehydratase purified from mammalian erythrocytes [119, 120] and liver [121, 122] displays maximal activity in the presence of Zn and sulfhydryl compounds such as β-mercaptoethanol, cysteine, reduced glutathione, and dithiothreitol. Enzyme activity is quickly lost when oxidation of its sulfhydryl groups takes place upon exposure to air or by inhibition of sulfhydryl groups by sulfhydryl inhibitors or by removal of Zn by a chelator such as EDTA [122].

Purified bovine liver ALA dehydratase contains two cysteine residues, two histidine residues, and one Zn. The histidine residues appear to be involved in Zn binding at the catalytic site of the enzyme [122]. If Zn is removed in the absence of oxygen and the apoenzyme is kept under anaerobic conditions, the enzyme remains fully active [122]. These findings suggest that

Zn protects the essential SH groups of the enzyme from oxidation, presumably by coordination with them [123], but that the metal itself is not required for catalytic activity if the essential SH groups are protected by other means. Interestingly, Cd can also protect the enzyme activity [123].

ALA dehydratase is an enzyme consisting of multiple subunits of identical molecular weight. The molecular weight of the purified enzyme from a variety of sources is 250,000 to 280,000. There is controversy concerning the number of subunits, with estimates ranging from 6 to 14 per enzyme molecule [121, 124–126]. Recent evidence suggests that ALA dehydratase from bovine liver [127] and from human erythrocytes [118] consists of 8 identical subunits. Electron-microscopic analysis of the bovine enzyme was also compatible with a structure consisting of 8 subunits [127]. ALA dehydratases purified from different mammalian tissues are remarkably similar [128]; the molecular weights are approximately 280,000; K_m values for ALA are ~1 to 4×10^{-4} M; and V_{max} values are ~20 to 24 μmol/h per milligram of protein, 37°C.

Inhibitors Lead is a potent inhibitor of erythrocyte ALA dehydratase [129], and presumably displaces Zn from the enzyme [122]. Lead-inhibited ALA dehydratase can be reactivated by the addition of Zn or dithiothreitol, both of which reduce the binding of lead to the enzyme. Levulinic acid, an analogue of ALA, inhibits the enzyme activity by competing with ALA for binding to the catalytic site [130]. Hemin has been reported to be a competitive inhibitor of mouse liver ALA dehydratase [124] but is a noncompetitive inhibitor of the enzyme from guinea pig liver and red cells [131]. 3,4,5-Aminotriazole inhibits the enzyme but only at relatively high concentrations and its mechanism of inhibition is not clearly established. The most potent inhibitor of the enzyme is probably succinylacetone (4,6-dioxoheptanoic acid), which is found in urine and blood of patients with hereditary tyrosinemia [132]. As shown in Fig. 60-7, succinylacetone is a structural analogue of ALA; it is a strong competitive inhibitor of purified ALA dehydratase from bovine liver or human red cells. The K_i of succinylacetone for the bovine enzyme is 5×10^{-8} M, which is about 1/10,000 of the K_m of the enzyme for ALA [99].

Inheritance ALA dehydratase in liver, kidney, spleen [124, 133], and red cells [134] shows a three- to fourfold range of interindividual variability of activity in animals and humans. Such differences in enzyme activity in mice are due to differences in the rate of synthesis of ALA dehydratase, and this is determined by at least two codominant alleles at the Lv locus. The Lv locus is known to occur in very close vicinity to brown b, in linkage group VIII [135]. Mouse strains homozygous for the Lv^a allele have approximately 3 times higher ALA dehydratase activity than strains homozygous for Lv^b alleles. The heterozygotes (Lv^a/Lv^b) show an intermediate level of the enzyme activity [133]. Erythrocyte ALA dehydratase in the human population also shows a three- to fourfold range of enzyme activity. Identical twins have very similar values of the

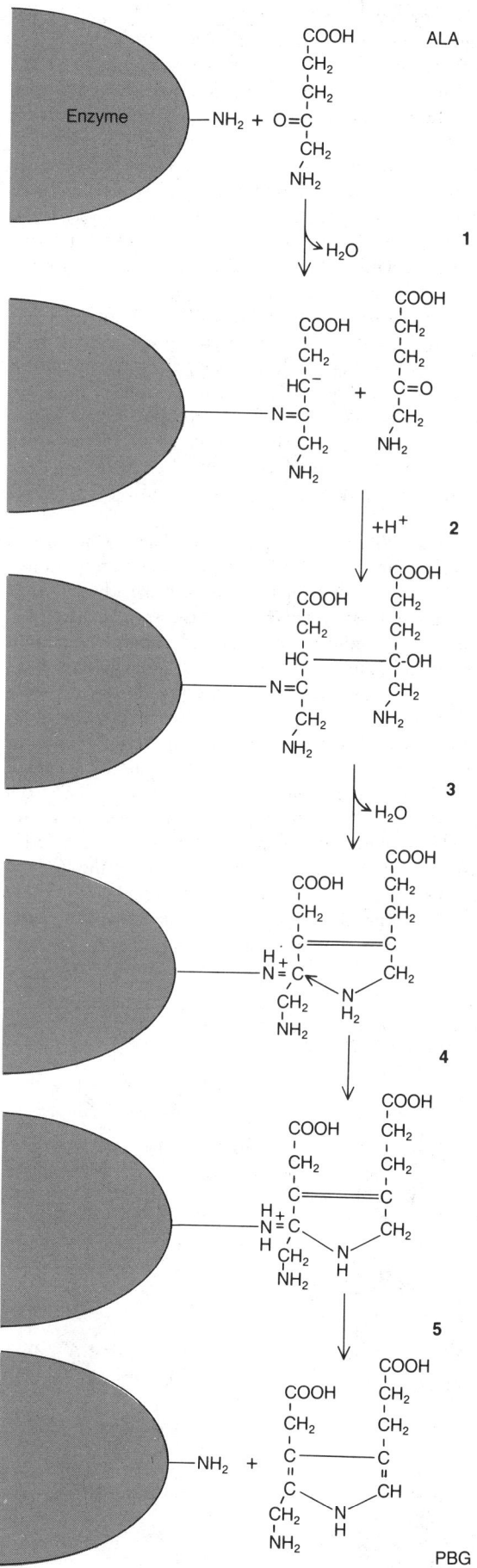

enzyme activity, and sibs have a much closer distribution of the enzyme activity than do nonsibs [136]. This strongly suggests genetic control of the enzyme synthesis in humans.

Developmental Changes ALA dehydratase activity of erythroid cells changes during erythroid maturation. Experiments using cultured erythroid precursor cells indicate that ALA dehydratase activity increases early and sharply during erythroid differentiation. For example, ALA dehydratase activity is greatly increased in mouse Friend erythroleukemia cells when erythroid differentiation is induced by dimethylsulfoxide [107] or hexamethylene bisacetamide [86] or in K562 human erythroleukemia cells treated with hemin [137]. ALA dehydratase activity increases early during erythroid differentiation and precedes the appearance of hemoglobin [86, 107, 137].

With the maturation of reticulocytes into mature erythrocytes, the enzyme activity falls. ALA dehydratase activity in mouse reticulocytes is approximately 15 times higher than in mature erythrocytes [134]. A similar decline of the enzyme activity with red cell age is also observed in human red cells [138]. An almost linear correlation between the level of erythrocyte ALA dehydratase activity and the reticulocyte count has also been found in rats [139]. High levels of ALA dehydratase activity (severalfold greater than that in adult liver) are also present in fetal rodent liver [124, 131, 140]. High levels of ALA dehydratase activity in fetal mouse and guinea pig livers fall quickly during the prenatal period (3 to 5 days prior to birth), and enzyme activity is lowest at or soon after birth. The enzyme activity then gradually rises to adult levels (which average one-third the fetal level) during the first month. In the mouse, the rapid fall of liver ALA dehydratase activity prior to birth occurs when erythroid precursor cells disappear from this organ [124].

A genetic deficiency of ALA dehydratase has been reported in three families. In one family the inherited ALA dehydratase deficiency was ~50 percent of normal and all subjects remained clinically unaffected [141]. In the two other families, the enzyme activity was below 1 percent of normal values in two subjects who were characterized by repeated intermittent acute manifestations of neurological symptoms similar to those of acute intermittent porphyria (AIP) and about 50 percent of normal in some first-degree relatives [142, 143].

Assay ALA dehydratase is assayed by incubating homogenates of tissues with ALA and then determining colorimetrically the amount of PBG generated enzymatically, after reacting the latter with modified Ehrlich's reagent [98]. It is necessary to maintain an optimum pH for the reaction (pH 6.3 to 6.7), to include sulfhydryl compounds such as DTT or GSH, and to maintain the zinc cation at the catalytic site in the enzyme.

Figure 60-6 The reaction catalyzed by ALA dehydratase. 1. The first molecule of ALA is bound covalently to the enzyme through a Schiff base between the ε-amino group of a lysine residue and the keto group of ALA. 2. This stabilized carbanion then participates in an aldol condensation with a second ALA molecule, with the removal (3) of one water molecule. 4. A proton is then transferred from the amino group of the second ALA molecule to the ε-amino group of lysine. 5. The enzyme is released, and after intramolecular rearrangement a PBG molecule is formed [116].

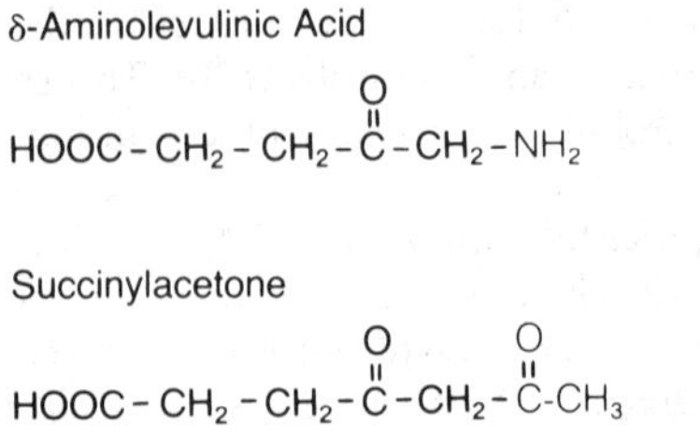

δ-Aminolevulinic Acid

$$HOOC-CH_2-CH_2-\overset{\overset{\displaystyle O}{\|}}{C}-CH_2-NH_2$$

Succinylacetone

$$HOOC-CH_2-CH_2-\overset{\overset{\displaystyle O}{\|}}{C}-CH_2-\overset{\overset{\displaystyle O}{\|}}{C}-CH_3$$

Figure 60-7 Structures of ALA and succinylacetone. The 4-oxopentanoic acid structure shown in bold letters is common to both ALA and succinylacetone, making the latter a potent competitive inhibitor in the ALA dehydratase reaction.

Porphobilinogen (PBG) Deaminase [Porphobilinogen Ammonia-Lyase (Polymerizing) (EC 4.3.1.8)] (Uroporphyrinogen I Synthase) and Uroporphyrinogen III Cosynthase

The step subsequent to PBG formation is the synthesis of the first macrocyclic intermediate of the heme pathway, uroporphyrinogen. Chemical condensation of four molecules of PBG can yield four possible uroporphyrinogen isomers [35, 144] (Fig. 60-8), but enzyme-catalyzed reactions yield only the type I and III isomers of uroporphyrinogen (Fig. 60-8). In the presence of PBG deaminase, only uroporphyrinogen I is formed from PBG, whereas when both PBG deaminase and uroporphyrinogen III cosynthase are present uroporphyrinogen III is formed. In the type III isomer one of the PBG molecules (ring D) is reversed (Fig. 60-8). PBG deaminase has frequently been referred to as uroporphyrinogen I synthase. However, according to the most recent evidence [145, 146], the enzyme does not directly produce uroporphyrinogen as a product but forms a straight chain tetrapyrrole, hydroxymethylbilane, which can then cyclize spontaneously to yield the macrocyclic tetrapyrrole, uroporphyrinogen I. Thus, in a strict sense the enzyme should be called methylbilane synthase or PBG deaminase. The latter term has also been used in the past and will be used in this chapter.

Reaction Mechanism   The way in which the two enzymes (PBG deaminase and uroporphyrinogen III cosynthase) interact in the assembly of PBG molecules to form uroporphyrinogens has been one of the most puzzling problems in the biochemistry of this field. Considerable progress has been made recently. Using ^{13}C nuclear magnetic resonance spectroscopy and specifically labeled [13C]PBG, Battersby et al. [147] have demonstrated that PBG deaminase catalyzes the joining of four PBG molecules in head-to-tail fashion to generate a linear tetrapyrrole or unrearranged bilane (Fig. 60-9) In this process the amino group of ring A is displaced, presumably by a nucleophilic group on PBG deaminase. In the absence of uroporphyrinogen III cosynthase, this product is released from the enzyme as hydroxymethylbilane, which then cyclizes gradually to form uroporphyrinogen I (Fig. 60-9). In the presence of the cosynthase as well as the deaminase the hydroxymethylbilane is rapidly transformed into uroporphyrinogen III [148] and no traces of hydroxymethylbilane remain [145]. There is also evidence suggesting an association or complex of the deaminase and cosynthase molecules, which would account for the rapid enzymatic formation of uroporphyrinogen III [149–151]. The assembly of the four pyrrole rings of the unrearranged bilane has been shown to start with ring A, followed by the stepwise

additions of rings B, C, and D in a clockwise fashion [146]. The rearrangement of ring D to form the asymmetrical uroporphyrinogen III occurs after formation of the linear tetrapyrrole and just prior to closure of the macrocycle ring (Fig. 60-9).

Normal human erythrocytes [152] and mouse spleen [148] contain excess cosynthase relative to deaminase activity, which favors the predominant synthesis of type III uroporphyrinogen in these tissues. Even in tissues with cosynthase activity that is lower than in red cells and spleen such as brain, muscle, testis, heart, kidney, liver, and lung in mice (i.e., ~1.6 to 5.5 units per milligram of cosynthase activity) deaminase activity is much lower [148]. PBG deaminase activity is quite low in most normal tissues and corresponds almost to the level of ALA synthase activity. In contrast, in erythrocytes from human patients or cattle with congenital erythropoietic porphyria, cosynthase activity is greatly reduced (~40 percent of normal) [153, 154] and this disease is accompanied by overproduction and excretion of uroporphyrinogen I. The fox squirrel is a species which naturally has a low cosynthase activity and excretes large amounts of uroporphyrinogen I in urine [155].

Properties   PBG deaminase purified from spinach leaves has a specific activity of ~1000 units per milligram of protein (1 unit = 1 nmol of uroporphyrinogen formed per hour) [150], while deaminase from R. spheroides has a specific activity of ~30,000 units per milligram of protein. Recently PBG deaminase has also been purified to homogeneity from human erythrocytes (activity ~2300 units per milligram of protein) [156]. The pH optimum of the deaminase from human erythrocytes is 8.2, and the K_m is 6 μM [156]. Molecular weights of deaminases from human and other sources are in the range of 36,000 to 40,000 [156, 158, 159]. Deaminase purified from human erythrocytes can be separated into five forms on DEAE cellulose chromatography or SDS-polyacrylamide gel electrophoresis [156]. The least charged form of the five isomers is considered to be the native enzyme, while the other forms have been proposed to be enzyme-substrate complexes in which intermediates (mono-, di-, tri-, and tetrapyrrole) are

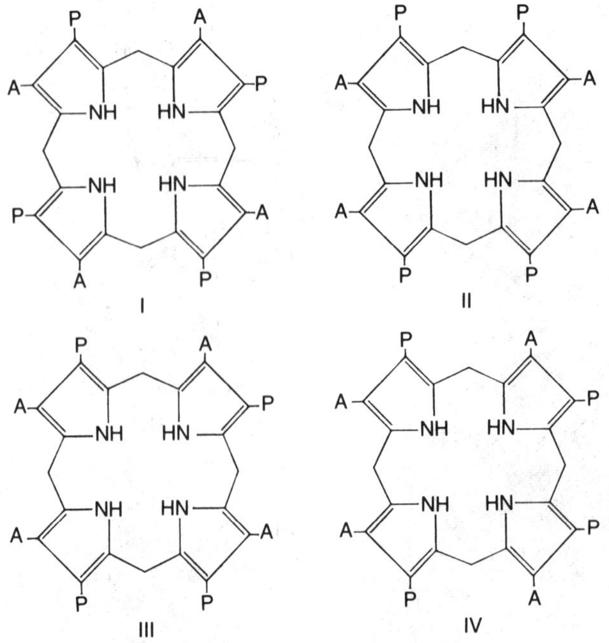

Figure 60-8 The four isomers of uroporphyrinogen. The only isomers found in nature are types I and III; and only isomer III can proceed to the formation of heme. A, —CH₂·COOH; P, —CH₂·CH₂·COOH

bound [156]. These enzyme intermediates are apparently highly stable and exhibit all the properties compatible with covalently bound substrates [160]. Although the hypothesis that the five forms of deaminase represent enzyme-substrate intermediates is attractive, Miyagi et al. [159] have reported a sixth form of deaminase which can be separated by SDS-poly-acrylamide gel electrophoresis; discrepancies in the data from these groups have not been elucidated.

Lead has also been reported to inhibit the activity of eryth-rocyte PBG deaminase in vitro [161], although concentrations required are higher than those found in lead poisoning and there is no inhibition of the enzyme activity in erythrocytes from patients with plumbism. A dialyzable factor that has a protective effect on the lead-inhibited deaminase has been purified from rat liver and has been determined to be a pter-oylpolyglutamate derivative [162]. Folic acid, which may serve as a precursor for pteroylglutamate, has also been reported to produce both clinical and biochemical improvement in some patients with AIP [163].

Inheritance Recently the gene locus encoding human PBG deaminase has been assigned to chromosome 11 by using human/mouse somatic cell hybrids [164]. This is the first instance in which a successful gene assignment has been made for an enzyme in the heme biosynthetic pathway in man.

PBG deaminase activity is decreased to about one-half of the normal value in tissues such as liver [165–167], erythrocytes [168–171], cultured fibroblasts [172–174], lymphocytes [175], and amniotic cells [174, 176] of patients with AIP. This enzymatic deficiency reflects the primary genetic defect of this disease and characterizes both clinically manifest patients as well as latent gene carriers of the disorder.

Assay for PBG Deaminase PBG deaminase activity is measured by the formation of uroporphyrinogen from PBG. Uroporphyrinogen, after oxidation to uroporphyrin, can be determined spectrophotometrically [158, 177] or fluorometri-cally [168, 169]. PBG consumption and tetrapyrrole formation are stoichiometric using a homogeneously purified deaminase from *Chlorella* [178], but loss of PBG can result in falsely higher values of the enzyme activity when crude tissues or par-tially purified enzyme preparations are used [179]. The dis-crepancy between PBG consumption and uroporphyrinogen formation can also be due in part to another enzyme that metabolizes PBG (i.e., PBG oxygenase). PBG oxygenase has been found in rat liver and brain, wheat germ, spinach chloro-plasts [180, 181], and in human erythrocytes [182] and is inducible by phenobarbital as well as the steroids progesterone and pregnenolone in rat liver [181].

Assay for Uroporphyrinogen III Cosynthase The enzyme catalyzes the formation of uroporphyrinogen III from PBG only in the presence of PBG deaminase [39, 183]. Since the rate of PBG consumption is principally determined by PBG deaminase, PBG loss in the reaction cannot be used as a mea-

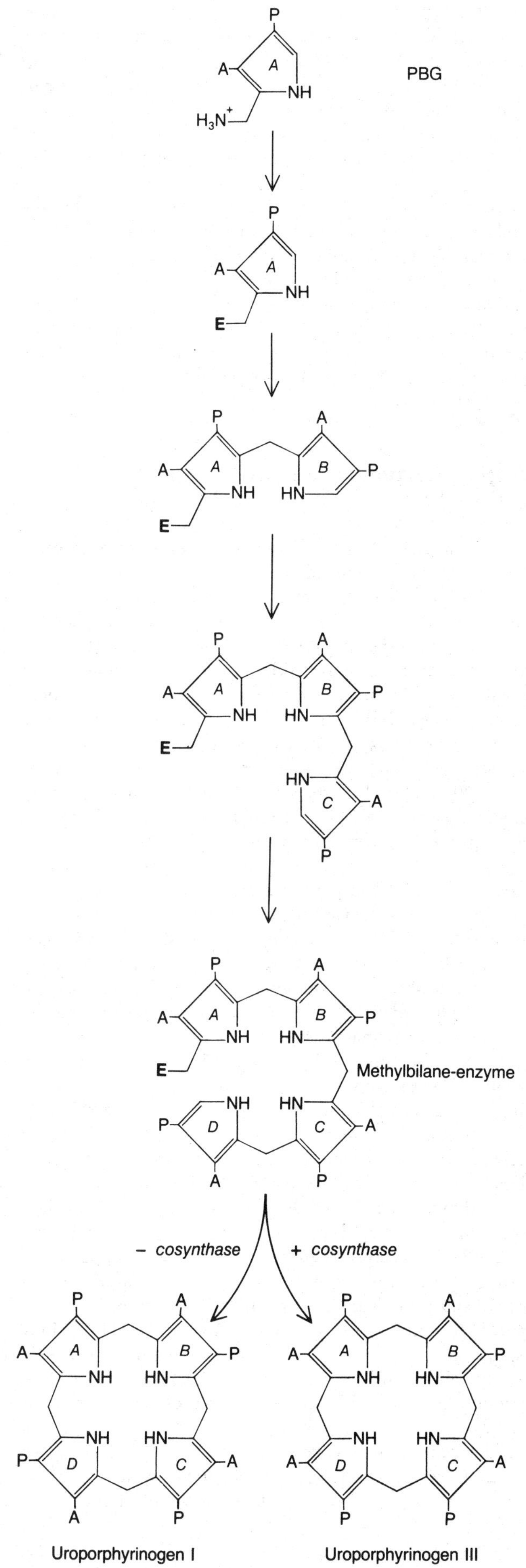

PBG

Methylbilane-enzyme

− cosynthase   + cosynthase

Uroporphyrinogen I   Uroporphyrinogen III

Figure 60-9 Formation of uroporphyrinogen I and III from PBG. PBG de-aminase catalyzes the condensation of four PBG molecules in a head-to-tail fashion to yield a linear unrearranged bilane. This is released from the en-zyme as hydroxymethylbilane which cyclizes nonenzymatically to form uro-porphyrinogen I. Thus the product of the PBG deaminase catalyzed reaction is not a porphyrinogen, therefore the enzyme should no longer be referred to as uroporphyrinogen I synthase. In the presence of uroporphyrinogen III cosynthase, hydroxymethylbilane is converted to uroporphyrinogen III [147, 148]. E, PBG deaminase; A, —CH₂·COOH; P, —CH₂·CH₂·COOH.

sure of cosynthase activity. Levin [148] determined uroporphyrinogen III cosynthase activity in the presence of a partially purified deaminase by measuring the rates of disappearance of PBG and the percent uroporphyrinogen found as the type III isomer. Using this method, he and his associates described a deficiency of cosynthase activity in hemolysates [148] and in fibroblasts from bovine [184] and human subjects with CEP [185].

Recent evidence by Battersby et al. [145] indicates that the product of the PBG deaminase reaction is hydroxymethylbilane and that this compound is rapidly converted to uroporphyrinogen III by the addition of uroporphyrinogen III cosynthase as noted above. It is therefore possible to determine cosynthase activity directly by the use of hydroxymethylbilane as substrate [186] in the absence of PBG deaminase, and this may prove to be the most precise method for quantitation of cosynthase activity.

Uroporphyrinogen Decarboxylase (EC 4.1.1.37)

A cytosolic enzyme, uroporphyrinogen decarboxylase catalyzes the sequential removal of the four carboxyl groups of the acetic acid side chains in uroporphyrinogen to yield coproporphyrinogen [187]. The enzyme decarboxylates all four isomers of uroporphyrinogen, but the naturally most abundant type III isomer appears to be decarboxylated most rapidly, followed by type IV, II, and I isomers in decreasing order [187–189]. There is no evidence that there is more than one enzyme for the four successive decarboxylation steps from the eight carboxylate uroporphyrinogen to the four carboxylate coproporphyrinogen [190, 191]. In fact, the reaction catalyzed by uroporphyrinogen decarboxylase yields from uroporphyrinogen, hepta-, hexa-, penta-, and tetracarboxylate porphyrinogens.

Properties Uroporphyrinogen decarboxylase is active only on porphyrinogen substrates and not on the corresponding porphyrins [192]. Partially purified uroporphyrinogen decarboxylase from mouse spleen has a K_m of approximately 1 $\times$ 10^{-6} M for uroporphyrinogens I and III [193]. The enzyme from R. spheroides [194] seems to require a cofactor, but the enzyme from mammalian sources, including human erythrocytes [188], does not. With uroporphyrinogen III as substrate the order of decarboxylation of acetate groups on each pyrrolic ring proceeds in a clockwise fashion starting from ring D (Fig. 60-10) [195]. The affinity of the enzyme for the substrate decreases with each decline in the number of carboxylic groups in the substrate, from the K_m value of 0.5 $\times$ 10^{-6} M for uroporphyrinogen to 8 $\times$ 10^{-6} M in the case of pentacarboxylate porphyrinogen [189]. Type I and III porphyrinogens with the same number of carboxyl groups appear to be decarboxylated at the same active center, whereas decarboxylation of porphyrinogen substrates with different numbers of carboxylic groups appears to occur at four different active centers [196]. In a mixture of [14C]uroporphyrinogens, series III isomers are decarboxylated much faster than series I isomers, the discrimination occurring mainly in the first step of decarboxylation [197].

The enzyme activity is decreased in the liver [190, 198] as well as in erythrocytes [199–201] of patients with PCT and is reduced in livers of rats fed with hexachlorobenzene [202–204]. The enzyme has an apparently long half-life, and does not show decay for at least 10 h after treatment with cycloheximide [197]. Iron removal by venesection is known to be highly beneficial in the treatment of PCT [206–212]. An experimental porphyria inducible with 2,3,7,8-tetrachlorodibenzo-p-dioxin (TCDD or dioxin) in normal mice does not occur in animals made iron deficient by phlebotomy [213]. Rats with genetic [214] or acquired [215, 216] siderosis are more susceptible to hexachlorobenzene porphyria than nonsiderotic rats. The effect of iron on the enzyme activity in vitro, however, remains controversial [205, 216a].

The Assay and Genetic Deficiency The principle of the assay is to determine the rate of conversion of uroporphyrinogen to coproporphyrinogen [217]. One method uses as substrate ^{3}H-labeled uroporphyrinogen, which is prepared enzymatically from [^{3}H]PBG [193, 199, 200, 205]. Other methods utilize porphyrinogens prepared by reduction of the corresponding porphyrins with sodium amalgam [190, 196]. Since a single enzyme appears to catalyze all four decarboxylation steps from uro- to coproporphyrinogen, 5-carboxylate porphyrinogen can be used as substrate and provides an assay from which it is easier to interpret the data since there is only a single product of the reaction (coproporphyrinogen) in vitro. Curiously, investigators using an enzymatic method to prepare substrate for the reaction by preincubating PBG with PBG deaminase have reported diminished uroporphyrinogen decarboxylase activity in erythrocytes from most patients with PCT [199–201], while those who have used chemical reduction of 5-carboxylate porphyrin or uroporphyrin to prepare the enzyme substrate have found such a decrease in the liver [190] but not in erythrocytes of patients with sporadic PCT. The latter workers however, did find decreased uroporphyrinogen decarboxylase in erythrocytes from patients with familial PCT (see discussion of PCT). The demonstration of a 50 percent decrease of uroporphyrinogen decarboxylase in hemolysates from subjects with familial PCT using 8-, 7-, 6-, or 5-carboxylate porphyrinogen as substrate [191] supports the existence of a single decarboxylase for these successive decarboxylation reactions.

Coproporphyrinogen Oxidase (EC 1.3.3.3)

Coproporphyrinogen oxidase is a mitochondrial enzyme that removes the carboxyl group and the two hydrogens from the propionic acid groups of pyrrole rings A and B of coproporphyrinogen to form vinyl groups at these positions (Fig. 60-11). The reaction thus yields a divinyl compound, protoporphyrinogen IX [187]. This mitochondrial enzyme can be readily solubilized without use of detergents [218–220] and evidently is not membrane-bound. Elder and Evans [221] using a technique for preferentially rupturing the outer mitochondrial membrane [222] demonstrated that coproporphyrinogen oxidase is situated in the intermembrane space of rat liver mitochondria. The oxidase activity was not released as completely as adenylate kinase or sulfite oxidase, which typify intermembrane space enzymes. Thus Elder and Evans [221] suggested that coproporphyrinogen oxidase may be loosely bound to one of the membrane surfaces surrounding the intermembrane space. These findings are consistent with the observations of Grandchamp et al. [223] that coproporphyrinogen

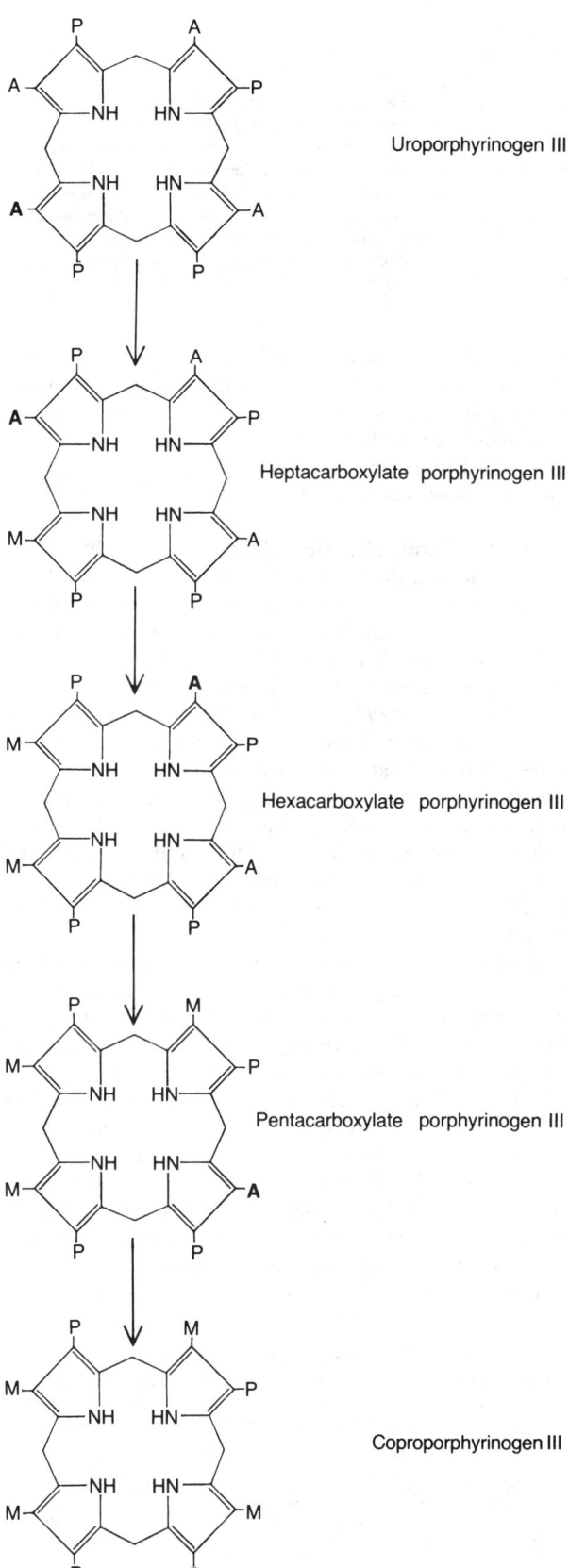

Uroporphyrinogen III

Heptacarboxylate porphyrinogen III

Hexacarboxylate porphyrinogen III

Pentacarboxylate porphyrinogen III

Coproporphyrinogen III

Figure 60-10 Formation of coproporphyrinogen from uroporphyrinogen. The decarboxylation of the four acetic acid groups in uroporphyrinogen III proceeds clockwise around the macrocycle starting from ring D to yield the four methyl groups in coproporphyrinogen III [195]. The sequence of decarboxylations is indicated by bold letters. A, —CH₂·COOH; M, —CH₃; P, —CH₂·CH₂·COOH

oxidase is present in the intermembrane space, with a fraction loosely bound to the inner mitochondrial membrane. The intermembrane localization of coproporphyrinogen oxidase implies that either protoporphyrinogen IX or protoporphyrin IX must cross the inner membrane since heme is formed within the inner membrane.

Properties and Reaction Mechanism   The reaction catalyzed by coproporphyrinogen oxidase requires the presence of molecular oxygen. The enzyme can act on the type III and IV isomers of coproporphyrinogen, but not on types I or II [218, 219, 224]. The purified enzyme from bovine liver has a molecular weight of 74,000 as measured by gel filtration and 71,000 as measured by SDS-polyacrylamide gel electrophoresis, and it probably is a monomeric protein [225]. The purified bovine liver enzyme has a specific activity of 6920 nmol/h protoporphyrinogen formed per milligram of protein and a K_m of 4.8×10^{-5} M. No known cofactor for this enzyme activity has been identified. This oxidase is unusual in that it does not contain any metals and that its activity is unaffected by treatment with metal chelators [225].

The mechanism of the coproporphyrinogen oxidase dependent reaction accounts for the following characteristics of this oxidative decarboxylation: the decarboxylation proceeds only at the β-carbon atom of the propionate side chains, with a stereospecific loss of one of the hydrogen atoms [226, 227]. It appears that aerobic and anaerobic organisms utilize different oxidants for the decarboxylation. In aerobic organisms, molecular oxygen is the oxidant. The reaction involves removal of a hydride ion with simultaneous decarboxylation, probably yielding β-hydroxypropionate as an intermediate [228]. In contrast, removal of the hydride ion from the β-carbon atom in anaerobic organisms appear to be facilitated by S-adenosylmethionine [227]. Studies using a chemically modified coproporphyrinogen oxidase or synthetic porphyrin substrates have led Yoshinaga and Sano [230] to suggest that one tyrosine residue is involved in the active site of the enzyme and that formation of a vinyl group from a β-hydroxypropionate side chain is much faster at position 2 than at position 4. An intermediate 3-carboxylate porphyrinogen in the decarboxylation of hydroxypropionic porphyrin to protoporphyrin IX was also isolated by high performance liquid chromatography and was characterized by field desorption mass spectrometry to be harderoporphyrinogen. The corresponding porphyrin was originally isolated from the Harderian gland of rodents [231].

Assay and Inheritance   A sensitive radiochemical method for the determination of coproporphyrinogen oxidase activity has been described by Elder and Evans [221]. The method measures the rate of production of $^{14}CO_2$ from the radiolabeled substrate [^{14}C]coproporphyrinogen III. The enzymatic activity is reported to be decreased by approximately 50 percent in the majority of patients with hereditary coprophyria (HCP) [232, 233]. This disorder is inherited as an autosomal dominant trait. In a case of HCP with severe clinical symptoms, a nearly complete deficiency of coproporphyrinogen oxidase activity was reported [234], with a 50 percent deficiency of the enzyme activity found in both parents of the proband. This case represents a homozygous coproporphyrinogen oxidase deficiency and is a proven example of the homozygous state for a gene defect among the dominantly inherited porphyrias in man.

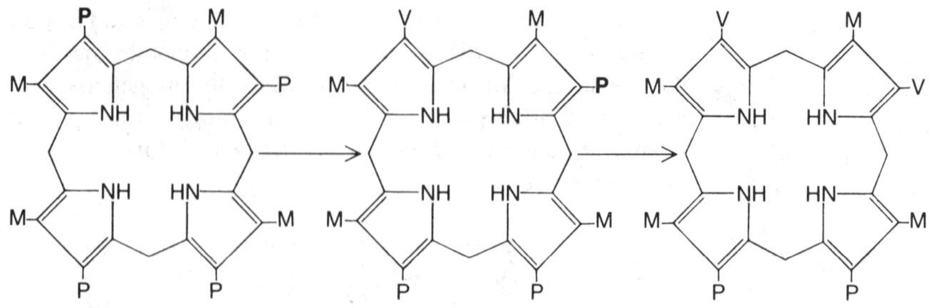

Figure 60-11 Formation of protoporphyrinogen IX from coproporphyrinogen III. The propionic acid group in ring A is first decarboxylated to a vinyl group yielding harderoporphyrinogen (a 3-carboxylate porphyrinogen); then another decarboxylation takes place on ring B of harderoporphyrinogen to yield protoporphyrinogen IX. The sequence of decarboxylations is indicated by bold letters. M, —CH₃; P, —CH₂·CH₂·COOH; V, —CH=CH₂

Protoporphyrinogen Oxidase

Protoporphyrinogen IX can be readily oxidized to protoporphyrin IX in vitro under aerobic conditions at physiologic temperature and pH (Fig. 60-12). An enzyme that catalyzes this oxidation step has also been identified in yeast [235], *Escherichia coli* [236, 237], rat liver, human fibroblasts, human erythrocytes, human leukocytes [238], and beef liver [218]. Protoporphyrinogen oxidase has been purified from rat liver mitochondria and has been shown to have a molecular weight of 35,000, a K_m of 11 μM, a V_{max} of 8.7 nmol/min per milligram of protein, and an absolute requirement for oxygen for activity. The same enzyme purified from yeast has a molecular weight of 180,000 and a K_m of 4.8 μM [235]. The enzyme acts specifically on protoporphyrinogen IX and does not catalyze the oxidation of coproporphyrinogen I, coproporphyrinogen III, or uroporphyrinogen I. Sulfhydryl reducing agents such as reduced glutathione or cysteine at low concentrations can stimulate the enzyme activity [238]. In *E. coli*, fumarate [237] and nitrate [239] serve as alternative electron acceptors to replace oxygen in the oxidation of protoporphyrinogen IX under anaerobic conditions, but the nature of the primary electron acceptor in eukaryotic systems has not been elucidated. Since the enzymic conversion of protoporphyrinogen IX to protoporphyrin IX is not inhibited by cyanide, 2,4-dinitrophenol, or azide, disulfide bonds are not essential for activity [235]. Hemin (50 μM) inhibits the enzyme activity by approximately 50 percent, and the inhibition is apparently noncompetitive and irreversible [235].   Human skin fibroblasts have protoporphyrinogen oxidase activity of 2 to 3 nmol/h of protoporphyrin formed per milligram of protein [238, 240], and rat liver mitochondria are known to contain ~10 to 12 nmol/h of protoporphyrin per milligram of protein [240]. Fibroblasts from patients with variegate porphyria (VP), but not erythropoietic protoporphyria (EPP), were reported to have decreased levels of protoporphyrinogen oxidase activity [240]. The primary gene defect of VP remains controversial, since Viljoen et al. [241] have reported a ferrochelatase deficiency in VP.

Ferrochelatase (Protoheme-Ferrolyase, EC 4.99.1.1)

The final step of heme biosynthesis is the insertion of iron into protoporphyrin IX (Fig. 60-13). This reaction can take place in the absence of an enzyme [242, 243], and the rate and quantitative incorporation of iron into protoporphyrin IX under these conditions can be significant at least in vitro. An enzyme that catalyzes the insertion of iron into protoporphyrin IX clearly exists in nature and has been variously termed *protoheme-ferrolyase, heme synthetase, iron incorporating*

enzyme, and *ferrochelatase*. This enzymatic activity has been demonstrated in a variety of tissues and species both in prokaryotic and eukaryotic cells. In rat liver cells, the enzyme is firmly associated with the inner mitochondrial membrane [244–246]. The enzyme activity is also found in plant chloroplasts and chromatophores of photosynthetic bacteria [3].

Properties and Reaction Mechanism Unlike other enzymatic steps in the heme biosynthetic pathway which utilize porphyrinogens (hexahydroporphyrins), ferrochelatase utilizes protoporphyrin IX as substrate. In addition to protoporphyrin IX, other 2-carboxylate porphyrins, e.g., deutero- and mesoporphyrin (Table 60-1), serve as good substrates for this enzyme in vitro [244, 247, 248]. Only the reduced form of iron (Fe^{2+}) is incorporated into protoporphyrin IX by the enzyme [249]. Co^{2+} and Zn^{2+} are more efficient enzyme substrates than Fe^{2+} [247]. Therefore various rates of ferrochelatase activity are obtained depending on which metal and porphyrin substrates are used [247]. There is also experimental evidence that suggests more than one ferrochelatase in pig liver [248, 249], but conclusive proof of this finding has not been obtained.

Ferrochelatase has been purified to apparent homogeneity from rat liver mitochondria [250, 250a]. The molecular weight of the purified enzyme was reported to be either 63,000 [250] or 42,000 [250a] as determined by SDS-polyacrylamide gel electrophoresis. The enzyme is enriched in lysine (11 percent) and hydrophobic amino acid residues (48 percent) [250a]. The purified enzyme has a specific activity of 3500 nmol protoheme formed per 30 min per milligram of protein; an optimum pH of 7.8; and a K_m of 28.5 μM. These properties were determined using iron and protoporphyrin IX as substrates [250a]. The enzyme activity is markedly stimulated by the addition of fatty acids, while it is inhibited by metals such as Co, Zn, Pb, Cu, or Mn [250a].

Figure 60-12 Formation of protoporphyrin IX from protoporphyrinogen IX. In this conversion, a hydrogen atom is removed from each of the four methene bridge carbons, and two hydrogens are removed from pyrrolic nitrogens, as indicated. M, —CH₃; P, —CH₂·CH₂·COOH; V, —CH=CH₂

Protoporphyrinogen IX   Protoporphyrin IX

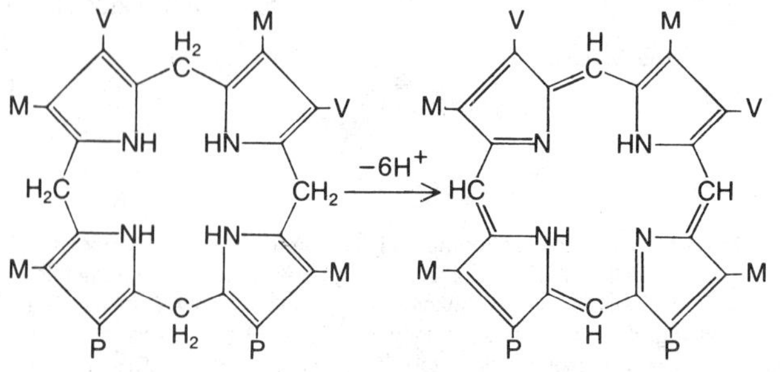

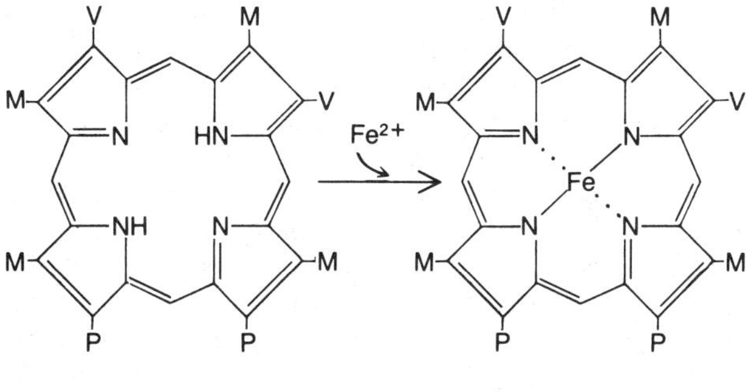

Protoporphyrin IX   Heme

Figure 60-13 Formation of heme from protoporphyrin IX and iron. M, —CH$_3$; P, —CH$_2$·CH$_2$·COOH; V, —CH=CH$_2$

Inhibitors Treatment of rodents [251, 252] and chick embryos with DDC [253, 254] produces a marked inhibition of ferrochelatase activity although it has no effect when added in vitro to the enzyme preparation [255]. A substance inhibitory for ferrochelatase has been isolated from livers of mice and rats treated with DDC and was shown to be an N-methylprotoporphyrin [255a] derived from liver heme [255, 256]. Treatment with cyclohexamide, an inhibitor of protein synthesis, decreased induction of ALA synthase caused by DDC [252], but did not affect the formation of the inhibitor of ferrochelatase [255].

Genetics Ferrochelatase deficiency has been reported in tissues from patients with EPP [257–259] and from cattle with the same disorder [260]. The cattle disease is inherited as an autosomal recessive trait while the human disease is inherited as an autosomal dominant trait. The enzyme activity was reported to be normal in patients with VP [261, 262], but there are also reports of decreased ferrochelatase activity in tissues from patients with this disorder [241, 263].

Assay The measurement of ferrochelatase activity requires the addition of sulfhydryl reducing agents and phospholipids for maximal activity. Reduced glutathione (GSH), cysteine, or mercaptoethanol are commonly used reducing agents that help to prevent the oxidation of the metal substrate under the anaerobic incubation condition. Exposure of the reaction mixture to air after incubation appears to be sufficient to terminate the reaction. Negatively charged phospholipid micelles markedly stimulate the activity of a partially purified ferrochelatase from avian erythrocytes [264, 265]. Crude enzymatic preparations do not require the addition of phospholipids for activity, possibly because there are sufficient endogenous lipids in such preparations. It appears that lipids may facilitate the solubilization of the otherwise poorly soluble porphyrin substrate or provide a proper environment to induce a conformational change in the enzyme so that it can interact with its substrates in a suitable manner.

Ferrochelatase activity has been measured by three different methods. (1) ^{59}Fe is used as a metal substrate, and the radioactivity in the purified heme fraction is determined after the reaction. This method is the most sensitive [247], but it is tedious and great care must be taken to ascertain the purity and the complete recovery of the radioactive heme product [266]. (2) Formation of heme is determined by the pyridine hemochromogen assay [249, 253]. This method gives the most unequivocal result, but it has a low sensitivity. Greater sensitivity has been reported using mesoporphyrin (Table 60-1)

rather than protoporphyrin as substrate [267]. The alkaline pyridine mesohemochromogen has an absorption peak distinct from that of the background protohemochromogen derived from preexisting tissue heme. The enzyme activity determined with one type of porphyrin or metal substrate may differ from that determined with another substrate [268]. For example, using protoporphyrin IX as the porphyrin substrate, it has been shown that DDC inhibits ferrochelatase activity [269] but does not inhibit cobalt chelatase activity [251]. When Co^{2+} and mesoporphyrin are used as substrates, DDC inhibits cobalt mesoheme formation [252]. (3) Disappearance of the porphyrin substrate during incubation is determined as a measure of ferrochelatase activity. Loss of porphyrin substrate may occur by reactions other than ferrochelatase, such as photocatalyzed oxidation reactions. Moreover, sufficient substrate concentrations must be provided to maintain a linear rate of product formation throughout the incubation, and ideally for the product formation greater than 90 percent of the substrate should remain at the end of incubation. This would make the porphyrin disappearance assay insensitive.

REGULATION OF HEME BIOSYNTHESIS

Biosynthesis of heme in the liver is controlled largely by the rate of production of ALA synthase [45, 270]. This mitochondrial enzyme catalyzes the first step of heme biosynthesis. The activity of this enzyme is at a rate-limiting level, and it is feedback-regulated by the intracellular concentration of heme.

In organs such as liver, where little cell multiplication or division occurs, it is logical to have a negative feedback control by the end product at the level of the rate-limiting step. In untreated liver cells in vivo or in culture, ALA synthase activity is very low, but its activity is increased in response to a variety of xenobiotics and natural steroids [45, 46, 271–273]. The induction of ALA synthase is suppressed by treatment with hemin [45, 103, 274–276] at concentrations as low as 10^{-7} M.

In erythroid cells the regulation of heme synthesis may not be controlled by ALA synthase alone. Although ALA synthase may be rate-limiting for hemoglobin formation in avian embryonic erythroid cells [277], it appears not to be rate-limiting for heme formation in mammalian erythroid cells [23, 86, 137]. Whether this discrepancy reflects species differences or the difference between embryonic and adult hemopoietic cells is not known. It should be noted that in contrast to the liver, the erythron responds to a stimulus to heme synthesis mainly by increasing its cell number. It is perhaps appropriate therefore for regulatory influences on hemoglobin synthesis in the erythron to act primarily on the process of cell differentiation to meet changing requirements for heme in this tissue.

Heme Synthesis in the Liver

Of the ALA produced in rat liver, as much as 65 percent is utilized for the formation of microsomal cytochrome P$_{450}$, about 15 percent for the synthesis of catalase in the peroxisomes, 6 percent for the formation of mitochondrial cytochromes, and 8 percent for the formation of cytochrome b$_5$

[277a]. Total bilirubin production in normal humans has been estimated to be about 5 to 8 μmol bilirubin daily per kilogram of body weight [278]. Liver cells normally make about 15 percent of the heme that is synthesized in the body [270]. It requires approximately 54 mg of ALA per day for this amount of hepatic heme synthesis. The remainder of heme formation takes place in the bone marrow for the synthesis of hemoglobin which requires approximately 304 mg of ALA per day. In AIP the liver may form as much ALA as the normal bone marrow does. This suggests that the rate of ALA synthesis is an important controlling step for heme formation in liver.

ALA Synthase and Its Rate-limiting Nature in the Liver   There is much evidence for the rate-limiting nature of ALA synthase in the liver [45, 46]. (1) The activity of ALA synthase in normal liver is very low (30 to 100 nmol/h of ALA per gram of mouse liver [279]). As noted above, another enzyme that is present at a similarly low level is PBG deaminase (35 to 60 nmol/h of PBG used per gram of mouse liver [279]). Thus under conditions of increased ALA production, ALA and PBG can accumulate and be excreted in excess amounts. The third enzyme of the heme pathway which has a relatively low activity is ferrochelatase (0.4 nmol/min of heme formed per milligram of mitochondrial protein in rat liver, or about 1200 nmol/h of heme per gram of liver [244]), but its activity is normally higher than that of ALA synthase and PBG deaminase. (2) ALA synthase activity can be markedly increased by treatment of animals with a variety of chemicals which results in the accumulation of porphyrins in the liver. The increase of enzyme activity is the result of increased synthesis *de novo* of the enzyme which can be abolished by inhibitors of RNA or protein synthesis. (3) The uninduced level of ALA synthase is sufficient to make the amount of heme that is necessary for daily maintenance of liver hemoproteins.

The enzyme level appears to increase in many instances when more heme needs to be made, for example, for increased cytochrome P_{450} synthesis. (4) In contrast to the very low level of ALA synthase, other enzymatic activities of the heme biosynthetic pathway are usually present in excess. For example, administration of ALA to rats and mice results in the induction of heme oxygenase [280], in an increase in bilirubin production [281], and in repression of ALA synthase [282, 283]. These findings suggest that ALA is readily converted to heme. Hepatic heme can also be labeled with radioactive ALA and, in cultured rat hepatocytes, ALA treatment has been reported in one study to increase the level of cytochrome P_{450} [282]. These data suggest that ALA administration enhances the rate of heme synthesis in the liver, although increases in hepatic hemoprotein concentration may not always be detectable or consistent [281]. (5) The rate of turnover of ALA synthase is very rapid, a property appropriate for an enzyme catalyzing a rate-limiting reaction. The half-life of ALA synthase in rat liver is approximately 70 min [77]; it is 3 h in mouse liver [284] and in cultured chick embryo liver cells [78]. The half-life of mitochondrial ALA synthase is in fact close to the shortest among all mitochondrial proteins, which generally turn over with a half-life of approximately 5 days.

Control by Glycine   ALA synthase has an unusually high K_m (i.e., a low affinity) for glycine. K_m's of ~5 to 19 mM for mammalian mitochondrial ALA synthase have, for example,

been reported. The concentration of glycine in the chick embryo liver is about 1 mM [285]. The hepatic concentration of glycine (which is tenfold greater than that in human plasma) suggests an active transport mechanism for glycine; but this concentration of the amino acid is only one-fifth to one-twentieth of the K_m for ALA synthase. The seemingly insufficient concentration of glycine for ALA synthase may in part be due to the high activity of glycine acyltransferase or the glycine cleavage system [286] in liver mitochondria [287, 288]. This raises the possibility that the activity of hepatic ALA synthase in vivo may also be regulated by the glycine concentration. On the supposition that ALA synthase activity follows Michaelis-Menten kinetics, an increase in the substrate concentration from the K_m value by a factor of 2 would result in a 33 percent increase in the rate of product formation, while an increase of the substrate concentration from 0.1 of the K_m, as in the case of glycine in liver, to 0.2, would yield 83 percent more product [289]. In chick embryo liver, the glycine concentration rose from 1 to 3 mM when protein synthesis was inhibited by cycloheximide, and this treatment was shown to be accompanied by a 60 percent increase in ALA synthase activity as determined without added glycine [285]. The glycine cleavage system would function in the direction of glycine synthesis in the presence of thiol compounds [286] and this system potentially may thus be important in the regulation of ALA synthase activity. Treatment of rats with *p*-aminobenzoic acid or sodium benzoate reverses the experimental porphyria induced by DDC [63]. Both benzoic acid derivatives yield glycine conjugates which can be readily excreted by the kidney, thereby decreasing the hepatic glycine concentration. Consistent with this hypothesis, Piper et al. [63] demonstrated that the administration of glycine prevents the reversal by *p*-aminobenzoic acid or sodium benzoate of the porphyria elicited by DDC.

Control by Heme   Hepatic ALA synthase formation can be controlled by intracellular heme or hemin administered exogenously. The intracellular heme concentration can be affected by a number of factors. Direct inhibition of ALA synthase by hemin ($K_i \sim 2 \times 10^{-5}$ M) [59], does not appear to be a physiologically important process, but in contrast the formation of ALA synthase is suppressed at much lower heme concentrations. For example, repression of ALA synthase formation in cultured chick embryo liver cells maintained in a serum-free medium takes place at a hemin concentration of 10^{-7} M [88, 276] (Fig. 60-14). Kr (i.e., the concentration of hemin which reduces the rate of synthesis of ALA synthase by half) is dependent in part on the presence of serum proteins in the medium. In the presence of 10 percent fetal bovine serum, an unusually high Kr of 2×10^{-6} M was reported [45], while in the presence of human serum albumin, the Kr was found to be as low as ~1 to 2×10^{-8} M [290, 291] (Fig. 60-14). Human serum albumin is known to bind hemin with a dissociation constant of 2×10^{-8} M in tris buffer [292] and this complex may be more readily taken up by hepatocytes. These data suggest that heme-mediated control of ALA synthase is principally at the level of enzyme synthesis rather than by enzyme inhibition. End product inhibition of ALA synthase activity cannot be ruled out completely because heme is synthesized within the mitochondria, where ALA synthase is also localized. A study by Wolfson et al. [293] indicated that heme generated in mitochondria was not sufficient to inhibit ALA synthase activity.

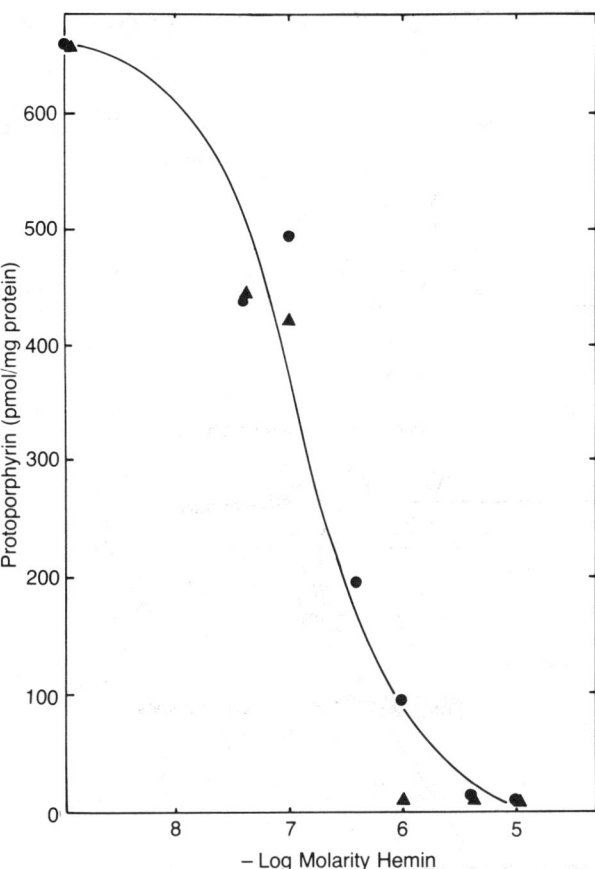

Figure 60-14 Inhibitory effect of hemin on protoporphyrin formation induced by the 5β-steroid metabolite, etiocholanolone, in cultured chick embryo liver cells. Similar inhibition by hemin is exerted against the inducing action of the barbiturate analogue AIA. (*From Sassa, Bradlow, and Kappas [276]. By permission of the Journal of Biological Chemistry.*)

In cultured liver cells, hemin repression of ALA synthase formation takes place immediately after its addition to medium [78]. This suggests that exogenously added hemin can rapidly enter a repressor "free" heme pool. Several heme binding proteins exist in the cytosol of liver [294] and intestinal cells [295] which facilitate the uptake of heme. Conversely, efflux of heme from mitochondria may also be facilitated by heme-binding proteins. Efflux is also inversely related to mitochondrial energy levels [296]. In liver cell cultures treated with hemin, ALA synthase decays with a half-life of approximately 3 h which is similar to the half-life determined by the use of an inhibitor of protein synthesis [78]. Findings in cultured avian embryonic liver cells suggest that hemin either shortened the lifetime of the mRNA for ALA synthase or interfered specifically with the synthesis of ALA synthase at the posttranscriptional level [78, 275] (Fig. 60-15). More recent evidence suggests that hemin may also repress the synthesis of the mRNA for ALA synthase [297] (Fig. 60-15).

Hemin administration to rats pretreated with ALA interferes with the transport of the cytosolic form of ALA synthase into the mitochondria [66]. This results in a decrease in mitochondrial ALA synthase and an accumulation in the cytosol of ALA synthase (Fig. 60-15). This mechanism involving enzyme transport intracellularly therefore could also control the level of ALA synthase present in the mitochondria. Whether such a mechanism applies to the induction of ALA synthase in general

is not yet established, since when rats [298] or mice [284] were treated with DDC, hemin administration did not result in an accumulation of ALA synthase in the cytosol. The transfer of purified ALA synthase into mitochondria has been demonstrated in vitro [75]. The effect of hemin on this process in vitro has not been reported.

Many chemicals induce synthesis of ALA synthase and cause overproduction of ALA, PBG, and porphyrins in the liver. Induction of ALA synthase by 5α- and 5β-epimeric pairs of natural C-19 and C-21 steroids is shown in Fig. 60-16. 5α- and 5β-metabolites of steroid hormones endogenous to humans stimulate ALA synthase formation in chick embryo hepatocytes. Among these compounds many 5β-steroids were found to be more potent inducers than their corresponding 5α-epimers in this action [276]. Induction of ALA synthase appears to be largely the result of transcriptional induction of the mRNA for ALA synthase because the induction can be prevented by inhibitors of RNA synthesis (Fig. 60-15).

Although it is attractive to speculate that the induction of ALA synthase is always due to derepression of enzyme synthesis by heme depletion [291, 299]. Under some circumstances heme depletion may occur without induction of ALA synthase. For example, inhibition of heme synthesis alone by desferrioxamine mesylate [103, 300] in the absence of a chemical inducer does not cause marked induction of ALA synthase. It has been postulated that DDC induces ALA synthase by inhibiting ferrochelatase, thereby causing heme depletion. This explanation is not entirely adequate since a DDC analogue was found to induce ALA synthase without inhibiting ferrochelatase activity [301]. DDC inhibits ferrochelatase nearly completely at doses far lower than those that induce ALA synthase, and the ferrochelatase inhibition is sustained long after ALA synthase levels return to normal [253]. Administration of cobaltous chloride [302–305] or cobalt protoporphyrin [306] to rats leads to a marked decrease in microsomal heme and a rapid decline, rather than an induction, in ALA synthase. Mn, a potent inhibitor of ferrochelatase, causes a marked reduction in the concentration of cytochrome P_{450} and catalase [307], but without affecting ALA synthase [308]. These findings suggest that heme depletion alone is not sufficient to account for the induction of ALA synthase and that certain chemicals may cause induction of ALA synthase independent of changes in heme concentration.

There is much evidence to suggest that the induction response of hepatic ALA synthase to certain chemicals can be enhanced by concurrent heme depletion or inhibition of heme synthesis [103, 253, 254, 300], although heme depletion alone may not lead to induction of ALA synthase. There are three general experimental conditions under which cellular heme balance can be affected (Fig. 60-15). (1) Certain chemicals such as AIA [271, 309, 310] and many related unsaturated compounds [311–317] destroy cytochrome P_{450} heme, leading to an accumulation of abnormal "green" pigments in the liver. These green pigments show all the properties of N-alkylated porphyrin species and can be considered as products of heme degradation by allyl-containing compounds [318]. A clear correlation exists between the fall of cytochrome P_{450} and hepatic heme content caused by AIA [271, 319], but the apoprotein of cytochrome P_{450} is not apparently damaged by AIA, since decreased levels of cytochrome P_{450} and its associated hydroxylase activities can be restored by exogenous hemin [21, 22, 320]. (2) Compounds like DDC or griseofulvin cause a rapid

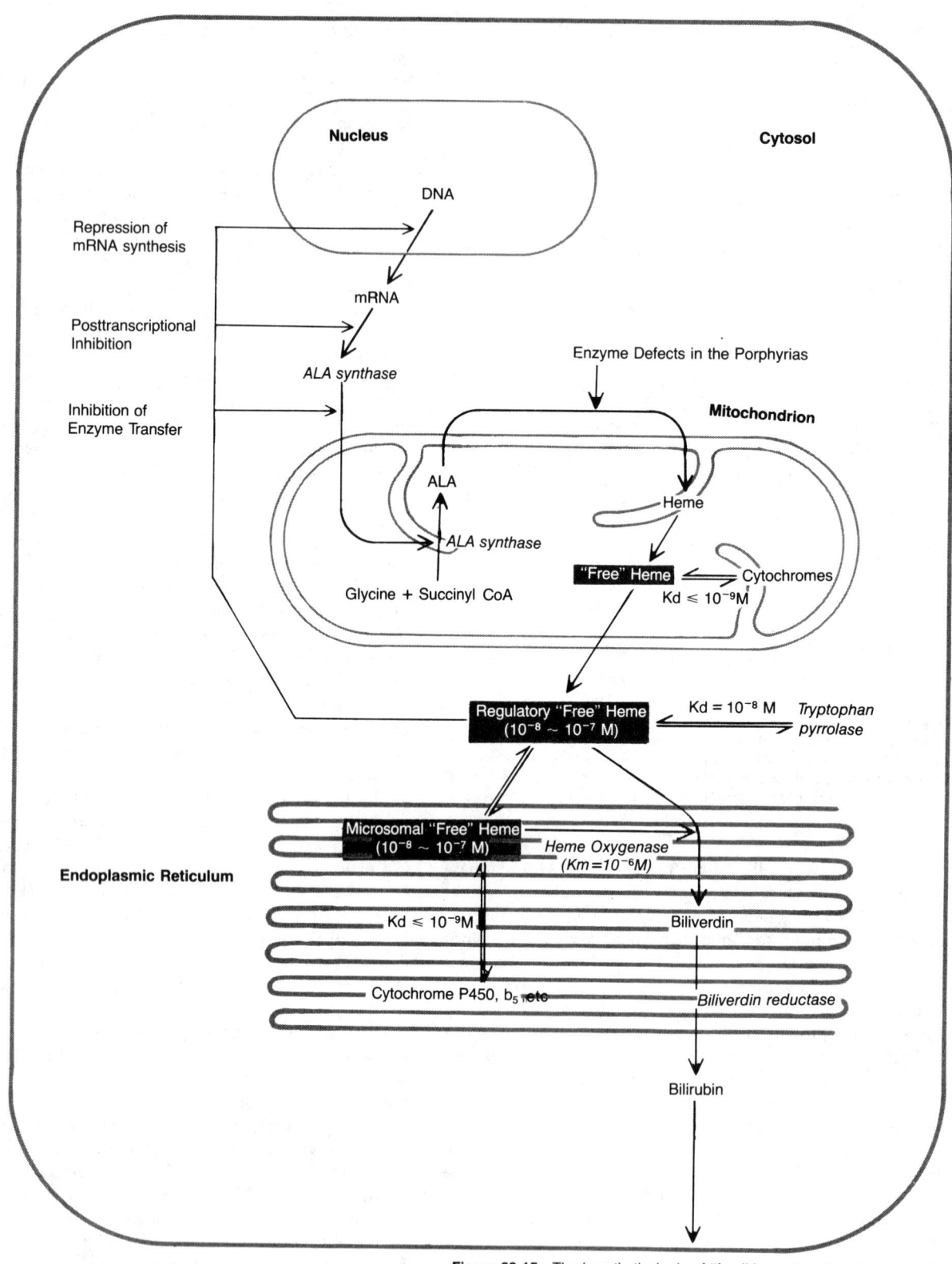

Figure 60-15 The hypothetical role of "free" heme in cellular heme metabolism.

inhibition of ferrochelatase [252–254], thus leading to a decrease in heme formation. Animals treated with DDC [321] or griseofulvin [256] accumulate green porphyrins in the liver that are distinct from those observed after AIA treatment and such compounds display a profound inhibitory activity toward ferrochelatase. (3) Phenobarbital and related compounds, on the other hand, probably reduce the concentration of regula-

tory "free" heme (which is in the range of $\sim 10^{-8}$ to 10^{-7} M) by increased synthesis of apocytochrome P_{450} [322, 323]. It has been shown for example that the apoprotein for cytochrome P_{450} is increased in rat liver after treatment with phenobarbital and lead [20].

The regulatory role of heme with respect to its own biosynthesis and catabolism can be best explained by assuming the existence of one or more free heme pools, as outlined in the hypothetical scheme shown in Fig. 60-15. *Free heme* can be considered as heme that is either synthesized very recently and not yet bound as the prosthetic group of specific hemeproteins, or possibly heme that has just been released from hemeproteins. Free heme pools probably exist, at least, in mitochondria, cytosol, and endoplasmic reticulum. All free heme pools are presumed to be very small and probably turn over very rapidly. Although the existence of free heme pools remains hypothetical, there is good evidence that such pools must in fact exist as functional entities in the liver cell. For example, a certain fraction of heme can be quickly labeled 1 to 2 h after a brief pulse of [^{14}C]glycine in the rat [324]. The appearance of this labeled heme is so immediate that it cannot be derived from hemeproteins [270]. This implies the existence of a rapidly synthesized heme fraction that can be considered to be a free heme pool. In cultured adult rat hepatocytes, 20 percent of newly formed heme is directly converted to bile pigment without being incorporated into hepatic hemeproteins [324a].

As illustrated in Fig. 60-15, free heme pools may affect heme biosynthesis and catabolism in a number of ways. (1) Free heme in mitochondria may regulate the rate of synthesis of subunits of cytochrome oxidase that are synthesized in the mitochondrial ribosomes. (2) Cytosolic free heme may repress the rate of synthesis of ALA synthase, or induce heme oxygenase, the enzyme that degrades heme to bile pigment. This fraction plays a critically important role in the biosynthesis and catabolism of heme, and thus can be considered as "regulatory" heme. (3) Microsomal free heme may regulate the activity of heme oxygenase in addition to serving as substrate for the enzyme. These free heme fractions probably reach equilibrium with each other very rapidly in part because of their rapid turnover. Thus an increase in mitochondrial or microsomal free heme can exert a repressor activity on ALA synthase formation via cytosolic free heme. Some fraction of the heme of cytochrome b_5 and cytochrome P_{450} is known to exist as an exchangeable heme pool which may be considered as a microsomal free heme pool. No information is yet available for assessing mitochondrial free heme even by indirect means. Thus in the liver free heme is presumed to control the rate of heme formation in a negative feedback fashion primarily by affecting the level of ALA synthase, while at higher concentra-

tions it may be considered to control positively the rate of heme catabolism by inducing heme oxygenase.

The cytosol free heme concentration in the liver is known to affect the saturation of tryptophan pyrrolase. This rate-limiting enzyme of tryptophan metabolism exists in two forms, heme-free apoenzyme and heme-containing holoenzyme. Hormones such as glucocorticoids induce apoenzyme synthesis and tryptophan inhibits enzyme degradation, both of which lead to an enhanced level of the enzyme. In animals treated with phenobarbital and phenylbutazone, an increase of tryptophan pyrrolase has been shown to occur, presumably reflecting the increased heme synthesis induced by drug treatment [325]. Inhibition of heme synthesis and increased destruction or utilization of heme all decrease the saturation of tryptophan pyrrolase [326]. Based on the decrease of heme saturation in the pyrrolase by DDC plus phenylbutazone, Badawy [326] calculated that the largest amount of heme that could be removed from tryptophan pyrrolase was 0.093 μmol. This exchangeable heme in the pyrrolase is probably in equilibrium with free heme and its concentration is very close to that which inhibits the synthesis of ALA synthase (i.e., Kr = 0.1 μM [88]).

Compounds that destroy free heme or inhibit heme formation are usually strong inducers of ALA synthase. In particular the most marked induction of ALA synthase occurs when animals are treated with two compounds (such as DDC and phenobarbital [252, 327] or DDC and AIA [57]) that affect heme biosynthesis by different mechanisms. Potentiation of ALA synthase induction by AIA can also be produced by simultaneous treatment with desferrioxamine [300] or Ca Mg EDTA [103] or a small dose of DDC [253, 254]. Both desferrioxamine and Ca Mg EDTA chelate iron, and DDC inhibits ferrochelatase activity. Thus Ca Mg EDTA or a low dose of DDC (which can inhibit ferrochelatase without inducing ALA synthase) leads to a potentiation of ALA synthase formation caused by other inducing chemicals such as phenobarbital.

This situation is analogous to that in the human hepatic porphyrias in which a deficiency of an enzyme activity of the heme biosynthetic pathway (e.g., a 50 percent deficiency of PBG deaminase in AIP) reflects the primary gene defect. One-half of the normal level of enzymatic activity appears to be sufficient to maintain normal hepatic heme synthesis in porphyric subjects during remission or in clinically latent gene carriers who

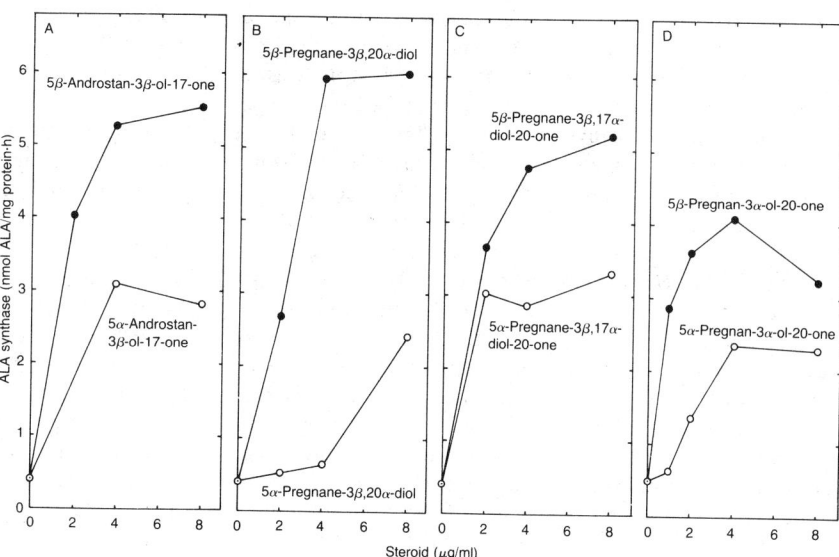

Figure 60-16 Effects of natural steroids on the induction of ALA synthase in cultured chick embryo liver cells. ALA synthase activity was determined after incubation of cells with steroids for 20 h. (*From Sassa, Bradlow, and Kappas [276]. By permission of the Journal of Biological Chemistry.*)

also carry the same enzymatic deficiency as in the clinically manifest porphyric subjects. When the liver has to increase its heme formation significantly in response to chemical treatment or exposure to drugs, environmental agents, etc., particularly in circumstances in which hepatic cytochrome P_{450} formation is induced, the primary enzyme deficiency then can become rate-limiting for heme formation, resulting in a decrease in the regulatory free heme concentration. The regulatory mechanism for synthesis of ALA synthase is then freed from heme repression and the susceptibility of ALA synthase to induction would then become increased.

This hypothesis suggests that an endogenously or exogenously derived inducer of ALA synthase could contribute to activation of ATP and related disorders. A circulating inducer(s) of ALA synthase has in fact been demonstrated in sera of patients with AIP in relapse, but not in remission [328, 329]. A circulating inducer may also be present in normal sera but in an inactive conjugated form, since inducer activity can be also demonstrated in normal sera following treatment with β-glucuronidase [330]. In those individuals with clinical expression of AIP, it also is possible that free heme concentrations are reduced but perhaps this is not the case in carriers whose disorder has remained clinically latent. This idea is supported by the fact that barbiturates and related compounds precipitate acute clinical attacks in patients with AIP, while they are not porphyrogenic in normal human subjects or normal animals (although they can become porphyrogenic when heme synthesis is inhibited by certain agents in experimental animals) [252, 254].

Certain drugs and chemicals are implicated in the exacerbation of the hepatic porphyrias in humans and in the induction of experimental porphyria in animals. Only a few chemicals (e.g., AIA and DDC) are able both to induce hepatic ALA synthase and produce a porphyric condition in animals. These chemicals usually carry special groupings (such as an allyl group in AIA), or they specifically inhibit heme synthesis (such as DDC or griseofulvin) [311]. In contrast, a large number of chemicals of diverse structure characterized principally by their relatively high lipid solubility [311] have been implicated in the clinical exacerbation of the hereditary hepatic porphyrias of humans [331, 332]. Chemicals in the latter group appear to induce hepatic ALA synthase and cause acute porphyria in gene carriers of the hepatic porphyrias. There are in these disorders preexisting deficiencies of enzymes in the heme biosynthetic pathway which "sensitize" ALA synthase to the induction stimulus. It remains uncertain whether or not all latent gene carriers of the hereditary hepatic porphyrias can be exacerbated by the ingestion of such chemicals, since clinical experience indicates that many gene carriers are apparently not affected by drugs that are usually highly provocative in other individuals carrying the same gene defect. Moreover, an explanation for the very high rate of complete clinical latency (about 90 percent) of PBG deaminase deficient individuals is not apparent since it seems highly unlikely that all such individuals have escaped exposure to the multitude of drugs, environmental agents, and other chemicals which are known to provoke the AIP clinical syndrome in a small number of these subjects. Thus important aspects of the relation between chemical exposure and the regulation of heme metabolism in clinically active as compared with clinically latent gene carriers for the hereditary hepatic porphyrias remain undefined.

Consistent with the idea that heme formation in the liver becomes limited during chemically induced acute attacks of the hepatic porphyrias, infusion of hematin has been shown to be, in some patients, an effective therapy in acute exacerbations of AIP [333–336]. In experimental animals or in cultured liver cells, hematin is known to block the induction of ALA synthase caused by foreign chemicals and natural steroids [45, 78, 103, 276, 337]. The original trial of hematin infusion in a patient with clinically manifest AIP resulted in a dramatic reduction of serum ALA and PBG and suggested that hematin infusion produced a decrease in the level of hepatic ALA synthase activity [338]. Subsequently, a number of acutely ill AIP patients have received this mode of treatment. Watson et al. [335, 336] summarized their experience with hematin therapy in 22 patients with acute porphyria and observed prompt recovery on 25 occasions in 31 acute attacks in 20 patients.

Among other possibilities relating to heme regulation in the porphyrias, heme destruction by hepatic heme oxygenase activity has been little studied in human subjects. Induction of heme oxygenase in isolated chick embryo liver cell suspensions takes place when the hemin concentration exceeds $5 \times 10^{-7}\,M$ [299]. The same liver cells, grown as a monolayer culture, required $8 \times 10^{-6}\,M$ hemin for induction of heme oxygenase [339]. Marked induction of this enzymatic activity occurs in rats after treatment with heme, certain organic chemicals including organometals, and a wide variety of inorganic metals [302, 303, 306, 340–342]. Heme oxygenase induction by these agents is usually accompanied by substantial cellular depletion of cytochrome P_{450} and hepatic heme. Thus, a mechanism operating at the level of heme degradation, as well as one operating at the level of heme synthesis could potentially serve to control the level of regulatory free heme, resulting in an alteration of ALA synthase formation. For example, agents (such as divalent metals [302, 303, 340, 341, 343], endotoxin [282], or organic chemicals [311, 342]) that stimulate the synthesis de novo of heme oxygenase might be able to deplete the regulatory free heme pool. Divalent metals cause an early (within 1 to 2 h) suppression of hepatic ALA synthase which is then followed by a rebound increase of the enzyme (12 to 16 h) [303, 305] which has been shown to represent synthesis de novo of enzyme protein. Adrenalectomy [344] and starvation also cause increased heme oxygenase activity and result in enhanced induction of ALA synthase. Starvation is also known to precipitate acute porphyric symptoms in some patients with hereditary hepatic porphyria [345, 346] and these clinical attacks can be prevented by the feeding of a high carbohydrate diet [347]. Interestingly, in late pregnancy in rats ALA synthase is quite refractory to induction by AIA [344, 348]. If a similar phenomenon occurred in humans, it might account for the fact that most patients with hereditary hepatic porphyria tolerate pregnancy well, despite the great increase in steroid production that accompanies gestation.

Heme Synthesis in Erythroid Cells

It has generally been believed that heme biosynthesis in non-hepatic tissues is regulated by a mechanism similar to that in the liver, i.e., a negative feedback control on the synthesis of ALA synthase. Early findings were compatible with this hypothesis [277, 349]. Recent studies utilizing more extensive and detailed analyses in a number of model systems suggest that there are distinct regulatory features of heme biosynthesis in erythroid cells [107, 137, 350–353].

In their original pioneering work, Levere and Granick [277, 349] demonstrated that in developing chick blastoderms incubated in vitro, hemoglobin appeared 48 h after the initiation of incubation. If ALA was added to the culture medium, hemoglobin appeared about 12 h earlier [277, 349, 354–356]. Addition of inhibitors of protein synthesis, but not of RNA synthesis, prevented the development of hemoglobin formation, whereas neither prevented formation of heme. It has been suggested that globin mRNA is already present in the early blastoderm cells but not ALA synthase, and that heme stimulates the translation of globin mRNA. Induction of heme and hemoglobin synthesis [354], as well as the formation of ALA synthase [357], occurs after treatment of cultured blastoderms with a number of naturally occurring steroids, and actinomycin D, an inhibitor of RNA synthesis, can block this action of steroids [354]. Such steroids are also capable of inducing erythroid colonies in human bone marrow cells in culture [358] and of inducing ALA synthase and porphyrins in cultured chick embryo liver in vitro [272, 273, 276, 359], in chick embryo liver in ovo [276, 360], and in isolated rat liver cell suspension [361]. Other potent inducers of hepatic ALA synthase of exogenous origin (such as AIA or DDC) do not affect the levels of ALA synthase in erythroid preparations [362].

More recent studies using murine erythroleukemia cells, human erythroleukemia cells in culture, and normal bone marrow colonies in vitro suggest that the regulation of heme biosynthesis in erythroid cells is not exerted through a feedback control by heme on ALA synthase formation. Mouse Friend-virus transformed erythroleukemia cells normally continue to divide and multiply in culture without showing erythroid features such as hemoglobin formation [363]. When these cells are treated with dimethylsulfoxide (DMSO) or a variety of other compounds, the cells undergo erythroid differentiation and display many characteristics of normal erythroid cells, including hemoglobin [363, 364]. It has been found that a clone of Friend cells (T3-C1-2) increases ALA synthase, and globin mRNA at around 24 h [365], ALA dehydratase at 36 h, PBG deaminase at 48 h, and hemoglobin at 96 h after DMSO treatment [107]. This sequential induction of heme pathway enzymes has been shown to occur in other clones of Friend cells [86, 353] or with other inducing chemicals [86], and the sequence of induction of enzymes is in the same order of the enzymes in the heme biosynthetic pathway [86, 107, 353]. The activities of heme pathway enzymes including ALA synthase in untreated Friend cells are sufficient to synthesize enough heme for hemoglobin formation during erythroid differentiation [107, 353]. Nonetheless, heme pathway enzymes increase in these cells after DMSO treatment. These findings suggest that the rate at which the enzymatic reactions are catalyzed is much smaller than the V_{max} determined in vitro and that the rate of heme formation also depends on the availability of substrates for these enzymatic steps.

A similar earlier induction of ALA synthase than of hemoglobin is observed also with treatment of cultured chick blastoderms with the 5β-steroid etiocholanolone [357]. In normal human bone marrow cultures PBG deaminase increases on the fourth day, while hemoglobin increases on the seventh day in response to erythropoietin treatment [350].

The fact that not only ALA synthase but also other enzymes in the heme biosynthetic pathway are increased during erythroid differentiation indicates that ALA synthase is not the rate-limiting enzyme for heme formation in erythroid cells. For example, the addition of ALA to Friend cells in which ALA synthase, ALA dehydratase, and PBG deaminase have already been increased by treatment with DMSO does not accelerate heme formation [107, 365]. A clone of Friend cells has also been isolated in which the induction of ALA synthase in response to inducers occurs normally, but the cells lack the ability to form heme for hemoglobin formation [351, 352]. Clearly there is not always a correlation between ALA synthase activity and heme content in erythroid cells.

These studies also point to the importance of ferrochelatase, the final enzyme of heme biosynthesis in controlling the rate of heme formation in erythroid cells. Evidence which substantiates the rate-limiting role of ferrochelatase in erythroid cells is as follows: (1) Hemoglobin formation does not occur until ferrochelatase activity increases in Friend cells treated with DMSO, despite the fact that other enzymatic activities of the heme pathway have increased considerably earlier than the increase in ferrochelatase activity [107, 353]. (2) Hemin, but not ALA, PBG, or protoporphyrin, can increase hemoglobin in undifferentiated Friend cells [23, 366, 367]. (3) In a mutant clone of Friend cells which have the normal induction responses of ALA synthase, ALA dehydratase, and PBG deaminase, but are not able to make hemoglobin after DMSO treatment (presumably due to an enzyme block after PBG deaminase), DMSO plus hemin can correct for the defect of hemoglobin formation [351, 352]. (4) Treatment of a wild-type clone of Friend cells with hemin can cause not only increased synthesis of hemoglobin but also increased levels of ALA synthase, ALA dehydratase, PBG deaminase, and ^{59}Fe incorporation into heme. Increases in ALA synthase activity by hemin treatment in erythroid cells are in striking contrast to the effect of hemin in the liver, where it suppresses the synthesis of ALA synthase. A similar finding of hemin-mediated induction of heme pathway enzymes, including that of ALA synthase, has been reported in human erythroleukemia cells [137]. Hemin, but not ALA, stimulates hemoglobin formation in normal mouse bone marrow cultures [368]. (5) The ferrochelatase deficiency in EPP appears to be expressed in terms of protoporphyrin accumulation mainly in erythroid tissue, although ferrochelatase is presumably deficient in all tissues. This suggests that deficient ferrochelatase may become rate-limiting in erythroid cells but not in nonerythroid tissues.

Concerning the effect of hemin on heme formation in erythroid cells, two lines of contrasting evidence exist. An early observation by Karibian and London [369] that the incorporation of radiolabeled glycine, but not ALA into heme, was decreased by hemin treatment suggested that hemin may directly inhibit ALA synthase activity in reticulocytes. This does not establish hemin inhibition of ALA synthase activity conclusively however, since by direct measurement the activity of ALA synthase is not affected in vitro by hemin even at a concentration as high as 10^{-4} M [86], and incorporation of ^{59}Fe into heme (i.e., the ferrochelatase reaction) is also strongly inhibited by hemin treatment [23]. Neuwirt and Ponka [370] also reported that the principal role of hemin in heme synthesis in erythroid cells is to regulate the transport of iron into reticulocytes to serve as the substrate for ferrochelatase. As discussed earlier, treatment of mouse Friend cells or human K562 erythroleukemia cells with hemin brings about an increase, rather than a decrease in ALA synthase activity, followed by increases in enzymes in the heme pathway and in hemoglobin concentration [23, 137]. It should also be noted that in the fetal rodent liver, which is highly erythropoietic, ALA synthase activity is constitutively high [371, 372] and cannot be suppressed by hemin treatment [76]. Likewise, fetal ALA synthase is suppressed by aminotriazole treatment rather than increased as is the case with adult rat liver ALA synthase, and a reversal of the aminotriazole suppression of the fetal enzyme can be brought about by treatment with hemin [76]. Recently it has been reported that ALA synthase from the fetal liver is similar to that of the adult erythropoietic form, but different from the adult liver form of the enzyme using an affinity column composed of AMP (6-amino) and CoA (sulfhydryl) carboxyhexyl-Sepharose [373]. This finding raises the interesting possibility that ALA synthase in erythroid and liver cells may be distinct isozymes.

The sequential induction of enzymes in the heme biosynthetic pathway, as well as hemin-mediated stimulation of heme biosynthesis in erythroid cells stands in considerable contrast to the situation which is observed in the liver. In some bacteria [374] the structural genes for the enzymes of the heme biosynthetic pathway are linked in a sequential manner, but this is not so in other bacteria [375]. A cocistronic transcription of structural genes in a sequential manner is also not likely in the case of heme pathway enzymes in erythroid cells, because such a mechanism would produce almost simultaneous induction of enzymes, while the observed time differences in enzyme induction and hemoglobin formation during erythroid differentiation ranges over a 3-day period [86, 107]. It appears more likely that the sequential induction of enzymes in the heme biosynthetic pathway may be due to activation of a set of temporal genes [376] that programs the output of structural genes for these enzymes during cellular differentiation and thereby acts as a biological clock. In certain variant clones of mouse Friend cells, early events in the biosynthesis of heme (i.e., ALA synthase, ALA dehydratase, and PBG deaminase) can be induced independently of the late processes of heme formation including ferrochelatase, but not vice versa. This suggests that the biological clock in these cells is defective [86, 351]. Clearly induction of the complete sequence, including both the early and the late steps of heme biosynthesis, is necessary for erythroid differentiation to be completed.

Heme Synthesis in Other Cell Types   Control of heme biosynthesis in cell types other than liver and erythroid cells has been little studied. It appears that the regulation of heme biosynthesis in nonhepatic tissues is not similar to that in the liver. For example, potent inducers of hepatic ALA synthase do not increase ALA synthase activity in the Harderian gland of mice [50]; heart [109], adrenal gland [108], testis [111], brain [53], and spleen [362] in the rat; or in cultured human amniotic cells [176]. On the other hand, specific hormones increase the level of ALA synthase activity in nonhepatic target tissues. For example, adrenocorticotropic hormone increases ALA synthase activity in the adrenal gland [108], human chorionic gonadotropin increases the enzyme activity in the testis [111], and erythropoietin increases ALA synthase in the spleen [362].

The effect of hemin on ALA synthase activity in nonhepatic tissues is also quite different from liver. Hemin does not suppress ALA synthase in mouse Harderian gland [50] and heart

[109], adrenal gland [108], and testis in the rat [111]. As described earlier, ALA synthase in the fetal liver, which is largely erythroid, is also refractory to treatment with hemin [61]. Changes in ALA synthase activity in fetal guinea pig liver are correlated with the change in the erythropoietic activity in this organ [373]. Thus the enzymatic activity of fetal liver reflects by and large that of erythroid cells.

The effects of nutritional factors and other treatments may also vary depending on the tissue. Starvation causes increases of ALA synthase in the liver and in the adrenal gland [108] but decreases the enzyme activity in the heart [108, 377] and has no effect on the brain enzyme [53]. Treatment of rats with cobaltous chloride causes a transient decrease of ALA synthase activity followed by a rebound increase of the enzyme activity in the liver at 16 h after treatment [341], while cardiac ALA synthase remains suppressed at this time [377].

Nonhepatic tissues obtained from patients with acute hepatic porphyrias fully express the deficiency of the heme pathway enzyme relevant to their disease in cell culture, e.g., skin fibroblasts or lymphocytes, and the enzyme deficiency in these cells is almost certainly similar to that found in the liver. Cultured skin fibroblasts [172, 173] or mitogen-stimulated lymphocytes [175] from patients with AIP do not show elevated ALA synthase activity in spite of a major deficiency of PBG deaminase. These findings suggest either that heme deficiency does not occur in isolated cultured cells to the same extent as in the livers of patients with active AIP, or that ALA synthase in cells derived from nonhepatic tissues in culture is not controlled by the intracellular free heme concentration. It is likely that latent gene carriers of AIP must have normal ALA synthase activity in liver since they seldom excrete excessive quantities of ALA or PBG in urine. Thus, the findings in these subjects are biochemically analogous to those in cultured skin fibroblasts and lymphocytes, i.e., they display a PBG deaminase deficiency but normal ALA synthase activity.

Patients with acute porphyric attacks suffer from various neurological disturbances, particularly those involving the autonomic nervous system. Watson [378] postulated that a heme deficiency involving cytochrome P_{450} may develop in central nervous system tissues, leading to a decrease in the activity of the cytochrome P_{450} associated mixed function oxidases. Whether a deficiency of cytochrome P_{450} occurs in the nervous system is not known, but there is evidence that central nervous system cells contain cytochrome P_{450} [379] and that they can form porphyrins from ALA [280] and might be capable of forming heme from appropriate precursors. For example, cultured dorsal root ganglion cells from chick embryo [380] and mouse [381] can form protoporphyrin from ALA. Thus the heme pathway enzymes, at least from ALA dehydratase to ferrochelatase, are present in these cultured cells. This enzymatic capacity is predominant in Schwann cells rather than in neuronal cells [380], and is subject to inhibition by environmental chemicals such as lead [382]. These findings provide a potential explanation for demyelination of nerve fibers in vivo and for deterioration of neuronal functions that may be dependent on normally functioning Schwann cells [383]. Hemin treatment of dorsal root ganglion cultures can limit the extent of the demyelination produced by lead [383]. It is possible therefore that neuronal cells may depend to some extent on the supply of heme or of heme precursors which may be provided by surrounding nonneuronal elements such as Schwann or other supporting cells. A similar cellular symbiotic relationship with respect to heme is also known to occur in protozoan-bacterium symbiosis [384].

CLASSIFICATION OF THE HUMAN PORPHYRIAS

The human porphyrias are a group of related but nonetheless distinct diseases. They are all clearly inborn errors of metabolism, with the exception of *porphyria cutanea tarda*, in which the prevalence of a genetic determinant of the disease still remains unclear. All are characterized by an autosomal dominant mode of inheritance except for *congenital erythropoietic porphyria,* which is an autosomal recessive disorder. Specific enzymatic defects have now been defined in the majority of the porphyrias and it is likely that all forms of these diseases will be characterized by distinct biochemical lesions in the near future.

The major porphyrias are classified as either erythropoietic or hepatic in type [385, 386] depending on whether the overproduction of porphyrins or porphyrin precursors takes place primarily in the erythron or the liver (Table 60-4). Clinical features, modes of inheritance, patterns of excretion of porphyrins, and their precursors and assays for specific enzymic deficiencies are important in diagnosing the various types of porphyria. Symptomatically the two most important clinical features in these diseases are (1) neurological manifestations in AIP, HCP, and VP, in which there is also, during clinical exacerbations, excess accumulation and excretion of the porphyrin precursors ALA and PBG; and (2) cutaneous photosensitivity (except in AIP). Porphyrias that are accompanied by neuropathic changes are sometimes referred to as *acute porphyrias,* and those characterized by photosensitivity have been termed *cutaneous porphyrias.* Although such terms are of descriptive value, they do not clearly differentiate the different types of porphyria, and the use of more precise diagnostic terminology should be encouraged. "Latent" cases can probably be found in all types of human porphyria [386]. The term *latent* is also imprecise because a porphyric disorder may be biochemically fully manifest (in terms of an enzyme deficiency or excess porphyrin or porphyrin precursor production) despite a complete lack of clinical expression of the disease.

Although enzyme defects are found in many tissues in certain of the porphyric disorders, such defects may not be of equal consequence in all tissues. In the erythropoietic porphyrias, for example, there are increased levels of porphyrins in the bone marrow and circulating erythrocytes, whereas porphyrin accumulation in liver is much less prominent or even absent. In the hepatic porphyrias, pathway intermediates are overproduced primarily in the liver and the levels of red cell porphyrins show little or no increase. Nevertheless certain clinical features are found in both the erythropoietic porphyrias and certain of the hepatic porphyrias—a prominent example being cutaneous photosensitivity. Thus excess porphyrins can enter the plasma and the skin from either erythroid tissue or the liver and produce skin photosensitivity.

Finally, as will be evident from the descriptions which follow of the specific forms of porphyria, three types of hereditary hepatic porphyria (AIP, HCP, and VP) show a number of common features in their clinical presentations. Striking among these is the highly variable penetrance of the disorders. The reason why the gene defects of these porphyrias often do not produce overt disease is not known. A central question concerning the pathogenesis of these disorders will be resolved when the basis for this phenomenon is defined.

CONGENITAL ERYTHROPOIETIC PORPHYRIA

Definition

Congenital erythropoietic porphyria (CEP) is an extremely rare disease that has been variously termed congenital porphyria, erythropoietic porphyria, or Günther's disease. It is inherited in an autosomal recessive pattern. The affected homozygote is characterized by marked increases in porphyrins in the bone marrow (Fig. 60-17), red cells, urine, and feces. Excreted porphyrins are predominantly type I rather than III. Studies in vitro of cells from patients indicate impaired formation of the type III isomers relative to type I isomers, and suggest a deficiency of uroporphyrinogen III cosynthase activity, but the precise enzyme defect is not yet firmly established. CEP is usually a severe disorder with marked skin photosensitivity beginning soon after birth and considerably shortened life expectancy. The disease is associated with hemolysis and increased uptake of porphyrin-laden red cells in an enlarged spleen. The degree of hemolysis is variable and is a varying stimulus to the bone marrow, which can further accentuate the production of excess porphyrins.

Prevalence

This is perhaps the rarest of the human inherited porphyrias. A total of only 60 cases was gathered from the literature up to 1972 by Marver and Schmid [387]. In earlier years some patients described as having this disorder may in fact have had PCT [386, 388]. With modern diagnostic methods this confusion should no longer occur. The prevalence of the disease is the same in males and females, and there is no clear racial predominance.

Clinical Manifestations

The earliest sign of CEP may be reddish-colored urine beginning at birth. Pink staining of diapers by urine and meconium have been observed [389]. Skin photosensitivity generally begins before 5 years of age, is usually severe, and is manifested by blistering of the epidermis, with formation of bullae and vesicles containing serous fluid. These often rupture and can become infected. The fluid in these vesicles may contain red cells and leukocytes, and may also be fluorescent due to the presence of porphyrins. These cutaneous features in CEP have

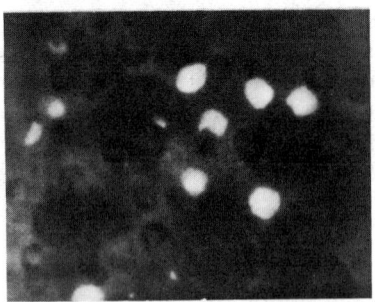

Figure 60-17 Fluorescence photomicrograph of a bone marrow smear from a patient with CEP showing considerable variation in porphyrin red fluorescence (shown in white) among the cells. (*Courtesy of I. Bossenmaier, Watson Laboratory, University of Minnesota School of Medicine, Minneapolis, Minn.*)

been termed *hydroa aestivale* because of their increased severity during the summer, when there is greater exposure to sunlight. Lesions occur on the face and hands or on other sun-exposed areas of the skin. Skin friability is also increased in these areas. Hypertrichosis is prominent, and fine hair growth may cover much of the face and extremities. Hypo- and hyperpigmentation also occur.

Particularly distressing is the cutaneous scarring and deformities that develop gradually in many patients due to the recurrent formation of vesicles and bullae. Secondary infection can also contribute to this process. The eyelids, nose, and ears are particularly susceptible to scarring and mutilation (Fig. 60-18). Corneal scarring can occur and can cause blindness if bilateral [390–392]. Nails and fingers may be deformed and partially lost. Porphyrins are deposited in the teeth such that they show reddish fluorescence with ultraviolet illumination. The teeth characteristically are reddish-brown in color even in normal light—an appearance which is termed *erythrodontia*. This process of porphyrin deposition, which can involve both the deciduous and permanent teeth and the skeleton as well, may be due to an affinity of calcium phosphate for porphyrins [5, 393].

Patients may have symptoms and signs of anemia, which usually is due to hemolysis. Some cases have presented with hemolytic anemia even before developing skin lesions.

In five reported cases of CEP, symptoms began in adult life [391, 394–396]. Erythrodontia is likely to be absent with late onset of the disease because porphyrins are deposited in the dentine during development of the teeth [391]. Surprisingly, one case has been reported with only mildly increased red cell porphyrin levels despite other typical features of CEP, including bone marrow fluorescence [395].

Neuropathic symptoms and sensitivity to drugs, hormones, or diet, which are characteristic of AIP and several other porphyrias, are not found in CEP. Sunlight, or other sources of ultraviolet radiation, and skin trauma are therefore the major environmental factors that play a role in clinical expression of this hereditary porphyria. Endogenous factors that can alter severity of the disease are poorly understood, but clearly the degree of associated hemolysis is an important influence.

Hematologic and Pathologic Features

Hemolysis is found in most if not all cases, although there may be adequate compensation by the bone marrow such that anemia is absent. Splenomegaly is present in almost all cases.

Abnormalities in peripheral red cells include anisocytosis, poikilocytosis, polychromasia, basophilic stippling, and increased reticulocytes and nucleated red cells. Absent serum haptoglobin, increased plasma iron turnover, decreased red cell survival, and increases in serum unconjugated bilirubin and in fecal urobilinogen are also indications of a hemolytic process. Unexplained exacerbations and remissions of hemolysis occur [397, 398].

An intrinsic erythrocytic abnormality appears to account in large part for hemolysis in CEP. Autohemolysis tests may indeed be mildly abnormal and suggest an intrinsic abnormality of some type [399–401]. Excess porphyrins in erythrocytes may predispose to hemolysis. Hausmann [402] noted that hematoporphyrin added to red cells in vitro caused them to lyse on exposure to light. Although osmotic resistance is reportedly normal in CEP [389], Watson et al. [403, 404] suggested that in both human and bovine CEP the red cells that are rich in uroporphyrin are osmotically more fragile. Reduced activities of some glycolytic and other enzymes have been noted in red cells in bovine CEP [405], but the evidence in the human disease is conflicting [406, 407]. Zail et al. [398] and Haining et al. [401] could find no clear evidence for a metabolic defect outside the heme pathway in CEP red cells. Therefore it seems unlikely that abnormal porphyrin metabolism in CEP may produce alterations in other metabolic pathways in erythrocytes to account in part for an increased rate of cell destruction. There is little evidence for an extrinsic red cell abnormality causing hemolysis. The direct Coombs' test result is positive occasionally [399, 401, 408] and has been attributed to transferrin carried by reticulocytes [392]. Moreover, normal red cells survived normally when transfused into a CEP patient [399], whereas survival times of cells from CEP patients were subnormal when given to subjects without porphyria [399, 401]. Interestingly, normal red cells in which porphyrin (mostly coproporphyrin III) content was raised by incubation of the cells with ALA in vitro survived normally when reinfused, suggesting that high red cell porphyrin content does not prejudice survival of red cells in the circulation [409]. However, this study did not duplicate the porphyrin pattern characteristic of CEP red cells.

The spleen is the major site for removal of abnormal red cells in CEP [401], and splenomegaly probably develops in response to the increased uptake of such cells from the circulation. Intravascular hemolysis may also occur and result in excretion of large amounts of iron in the urine [391]. Considerable hematinemia may be detectable.

An enlarged spleen can itself increase the random uptake and destruction of erythrocytes in CEP, as in hypersplenism associated with other disorders. Thrombocytopenia and leukopenia can occur in association with splenomegaly in CEP, and the former may be accompanied by symptoms of bleeding, such as purpura and epistaxis [389, 391, 394, 395, 410]. Splenectomy is considered in CEP patients when anemia or thrombocytopenia is pronounced.

Severe anemia is unusual in CEP, but anemia contributed to the death of two patients [411, 412]. In another case marked anemia requiring many transfusions was due in part to folic acid deficiency [400]. Petry, the well known CEP patient studied by Hans Fischer and coworkers (Fig. 60-18), was thought to have died with pernicious anemia and splenomegaly, but the published autopsy findings are more suggestive of a hemolytic anemia [410]. Erythroid hypoplasia can occur in CEP during acute infections [401] and perhaps other intercurrent illnesses, and if prolonged this could contribute to anemia.

Early studies suggested that there may be two populations of erythroid cells in the marrow and blood of CEP patients [386, 388]. This suggestion was based on fluorescent microscopic examination of marrow smears which showed fluorescence in only about half of the erythroid cells in the late normoblast and early reticulocyte stages of development (Fig. 60-17). Circulating erythrocytes also show variable fluorescence. Red cell survival appears to be nonuniform in CEP. Approximately one-half of the red cells have a half-life of 20 days or less, and the rest show intermediate or normal survival, at least as indicated by study of cells after labeling with [^{15}N]glycine [413–415]. Moreover, variations in such measurements with time have been found in the same patient [397, 416], and London et al. [417] found red cell survival to be normal in one CEP patient they studied by the same method. Such discrepant observations are perhaps not surprising since the severity of hemolysis can vary so greatly in this disorder. Since porphyrin content is not evenly distributed in CEP erythrocytes, uniform survival rates for the entire population of circulating cells might not be expected. Watson et al. have reported [403, 404] that in both human and bovine CEP the uroporphyrin-rich cells are more osmotically fragile, and that when bovine CEP cells are transfused into a normal animal, erythrocyte uroporphyrin declines more rapidly than protoporphyrin, suggesting more rapid destruction of the cells containing uroporphyrin.

The concept of separate "porphyroblast" and normal erythroid cell populations in CEP is difficult to explain on a genetic basis unless mosaicism is assumed. Also it has been shown that the percentage of fluorescent normoblasts in the bone marrow of human [418] and bovine CEP can be altered if anemia is induced by phlebotomy. And although protoporphyrin predominates in erythrocytes of cattle with CEP, bleeding results in marked increases of uroporphyrin and coproporphyrin in red cells [404, 419]. Therefore it seems more likely that all developing erythroid cells carry the mutant alleles for CEP [418], and that porphyrin fluorescence is more detectable microscopically in some normoblasts than in others for reasons related to cell maturation and perhaps other influences on the bone marrow that are incompletely understood [399].

Although hemolysis is the predominant cause of anemia in CEP there may also be a substantial degree of erythroid cell destruction and heme breakdown before these cells are released from the bone marrow. Such ineffective erythropoiesis is suggested by studies showing an increased incorporation of [^{15}N]glycine into "early-labeled" bile pigment in CEP [414, 417], and heavy deposits of iron in the marrow in some cases [391]. This phenomenon might be accounted for in part by extrusion of heme-containing (hemosiderin-staining) nuclei from maturing normoblasts in the marrow even without cell destruction. Also, red cell phagocytosis has been noted microscopically in marrow preparations from some CEP patients [397]. Incorporation of [^{15}N]ALA into fecal urobilins was normal in one child with CEP studied by Nicholson et al. [420]. This indicated that in contrast to heme in the erythron the turnover of hepatic heme and its conversion to bile pigment is not increased. Hepatic ALA synthase was reported to be normal in this disease [421].

Calculations show that the porphyrin content of circulating red cells, although markedly increased, cannot account for the daily output of porphyrin in urine and feces in CEP, and the erythroid cells in the marrow would appear to account for most of this markedly excessive porphyrin production [386, 401, 422]. The bone marrow characteristically shows erythroid hyperplasia. Morphological studies of the bone marrow indicate that there is no substantial block in the erythroid maturation process, and there is no evidence that hemoglobin synthesis is impaired [401, 423]. Therefore hyperplasia of the marrow can be regarded primarily as a response to hemolysis, but in addition there are morphologic abnormalities in marrow erythroid cells. There are many fluorescent erythroblasts, and this porphyrin fluorescence is principally in the nuclei of these cells [388, 389, 400, 407, 422, 424]. Porphyrin fluorescence is not found in all stages of erythroid maturation but is confined mostly to late normoblasts and early reticulocytes [388, 418]. Other changes may include vacuolated nuclei and cytoplasmic inclusions and granules; such abnormalities may have some specificity for CEP [388, 407], although they apparently are not observed in all cases [401]. These morphological abnormalities are probably related in some manner to the accumulation and eventual extrusion of massive amounts of excess porphyrins from bone marrow erythroid cells. Benzidine staining indicates that heme is also increased in erythroblast nuclei [388], and as previously mentioned the loss of these nuclei containing excess heme may contribute much of the so-called early-labeled component of bile pigment in these patients [425]. Thus the presence of erythroid hyperplasia, erythroid cells containing porphyrin fluorescence, and associated abnormalities in erythroid cell morphology are consistent with an overproduction of porphyrins in the marrow and an erythropoietic response to hemolysis.

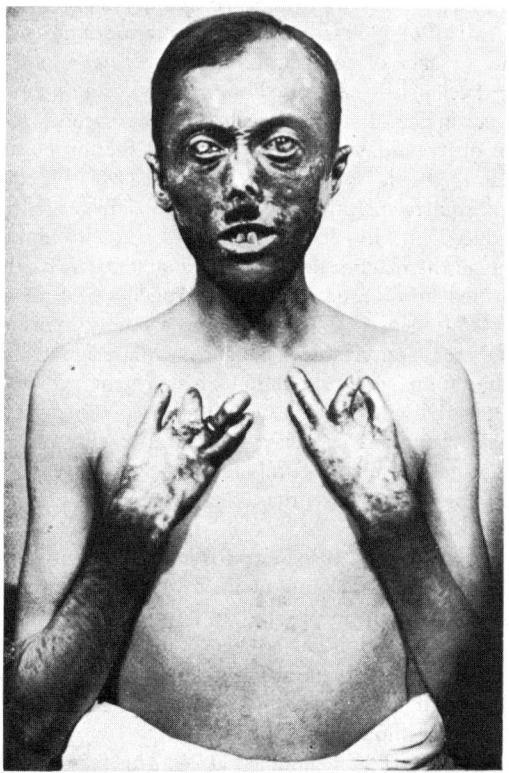

Figure 60-18 Destructive cutaneous manifestations of CEP in an adult who survived to age 34. This is the famous patient, Petry, who provided specimens to Hans Fischer for early studies in porphyrin chemistry. (*From Günther [390]. By permission of Springer-Verlag.*)

Porphyrin content in the spleen is frequently but variably increased, and perhaps bears a relationship to the rate of red cell destruction in this organ [385, 395, 422]. Liver porphyrin content is usually not greatly increased, but large amounts of porphyrin can be present in the liver in some CEP patients without evidence of liver damage [399]. Excess porphyrin may also be found in Kupffer cells [403]. Cirrhosis develops in some patients with CEP [5, 388, 426]. It is uncertain how often liver damage results from the disease itself or from treatments such as blood transfusions.

Biochemical Findings

Urine porphyrin excretion in CEP is greater than in other types of human porphyria and can be in the range of 50 to 100 mg daily (normal urine porphyrin excretion ranges up to about 0.3 mg daily). In CEP this is mostly uroporphyrin and coproporphyrin and there is a great predominance of the type I isomers (Table 60-4). Uroporphyrin III and coproporphyrin III excretion is also somewhat increased [5, 401, 410, 427], and excretion of 5-, 6-, and 7-carboxylated porphyrins is also excessive. Porphyrins are generally excreted in the free form and not complexed with zinc, and usually not as porphyrinogens [386]. Fecal porphyrin excretion is also increased, and consists mostly of coproporphyrin (predominantly type I); fecal uroporphyrin and protoporphyrin may also be increased, but this is variable. Urine porphyrin excretion can fluctuate with disease activity, and urine color may vary from pink to dark red depending upon the porphyrin content. Despite marked porphyrinuria, the excretion of the porphyrin precursors ALA and PBG is not increased in CEP.

In most reported cases the circulating erythrocytes contain large amounts of uroporphyrin I and lesser though still excessive amounts of coproporphyrin I. Red cell protoporphyrin may be normal or somewhat increased. In some atypical cases of CEP, protoporphyrin may be considerably increased and be the major excess porphyrin in red cells, as described in more detail below. Plasma uroporphyrin and coproporphyrin concentrations are also increased. Excess plasma porphyrins, which can enter the skin and produce photosensitivity, are probably derived from the increased porphyrin content in red cells and bone marrow erythroblasts [386, 399, 410, 422, 424]. The bone marrow porphyrin content greatly exceeds that of circulating erythrocytes or other tissues [388, 428]. Marrow porphyrins in CEP consist mostly of uroporphyrin and to a lesser extent, coproporphyrin [428].

Excess porphyrins (mostly uroporphyrin and coproporphyrin) are also found in the spleen and, less frequently, in the liver in CEP. Protoporphyrin may also be increased and be greater in the liver than in the spleen [399]. The intermediate 7-, 6-, and 5-carboxylate porphyrins may also be greater in the liver than in other tissues in CEP [399, 426]. Although porphyrins are excreted in the oxidized state, there are indications that porphyrinogens may accumulate to some degree in tissues such as the spleen [386, 399] and at times perhaps be excreted in the urine as well [399].

Activity of PBG deaminase is greater than normal in circulating red cells, and the significance of this is discussed below. Small amounts of ALA synthase may also escape from normoblasts in the marrow and blood of CEP patients and be increased in plasma [429].

Genetic Defect

Available genetic data indicate an autosomal recessive mode of inheritance for CEP. Estimates of affected subjects in reported sibships and a high estimated rate of consanguinity (minimum of 13 percent) are consistent with recessive inheritance [5]. Moreover parents or children of CEP patients have never been reported to have the disease. The prevalence is about equal in males and females and there is no significant birth order effect [5].

Biochemical evidence for autosomal recessive inheritance of a partial metabolic defect can be identified in some presumed heterozygotes. Heilmeyer et al. [165, 424, 430] observed slightly increased erythrocyte uroporphyrin in the parents and some sibs of two CEP patients. Darocha [431] found increased erythrocyte uroporphyrin and coproporphyrin in the parents and one sib of a CEP patient. Pain et al. [394] made similar observations, but in non-first degree relatives of a CEP patient. Studies by Levin and coworkers [185, 432] suggest a partial uroporphyrinogen III cosynthase deficiency in heterozygotes for CEP, as discussed below.

Uroporphyrinogen III cosynthase activity in CEP patients has not been assayed using the specific enzyme substrate. It has only recently been clearly established that the substrate for this enzyme is actually a hydroxymethylbilane, the synthesis of which is catalyzed by PBG deaminase [186] (see earlier discussion). Nonetheless, studies by Romeo and Levin [153], in which CEP red cell lysates were incubated with PBG in the presence of excess added PBG deaminase (partially purified from mouse spleen), and the ratio of uroporphyrin III to uroporphyrin I formed then determined at the end of the incubation, do provide evidence for a partial cosynthase deficiency in this disease (Fig. 60-19). Their findings [153] suggested that uroporphyrinogen III cosynthase activity was decreased by about two-thirds in erythrocytes from five CEP patients. Similar findings in four patients were recently reported by Deybach et al. [396]. No evidence for an inhibitor of the enzyme or for the presence of competing enzyme activity was found in CEP red cells [153]. As noted above, there is an intermediate deficiency in parents and some sibs of CEP patients [185, 396]. Similar observations have been made in CEP fibroblasts [184, 433], and red cells from animals with CEP [185, 432] (in cattle and fox squirrels). Although cosynthase activity is considerably reduced in CEP, it is not absent, and variation among patients in the magnitude of the residual activity, particularly in cultured fibroblasts, indicate heterogeneity of the genetic defect [184]. Since CEP is probably a recessive disorder in which there is appreciable residual cosynthase activity, a structural mutation with production of a protein with impaired enzyme activity seems plausible. Increased resistance of the residual enzyme activity to heat denaturation may also indicate an abnormal enzyme protein [432], but the precise nature and mechanism of the cosynthase defect remains to be established.

It has been noted also that cosynthase activity normally decreases in vitro, probably by inactivation of the enzyme, as the formation of uroporphyrinogen I by added PBG deaminase proceeds [153, 154]. It has not been demonstrated that inactivation of cosynthase can occur in this manner in vivo. Uroporphyrinogen III cosynthase is widely distributed in tissues and, at least in the mouse, tissue levels of the cosynthase greatly exceed those for PBG deaminase [154]. This may explain why

Table 60-4 Classification of the major human porphyrias

Classification	Deficient enzyme	Inheritance	Major presenting symptoms		Increased erythrocyte porphyrins*	Excess excretion of ALA, PBG, porphyrins*	
			Photosensitivity	Neurovisceral		Urine	Stool
Erythropoietic							
Congenital erythropoietic porphyria	Uroporphyrinogen III cosynthase	Autosomal Recessive	Present (severe)	Absent	Uro‡ Copro‡	Uro‡ Copro‡	Copro‡
Erythropoietic protoporphyria	Ferrochelatase	Autosomal Dominant	Present	Absent	*Proto*	Absent	Proto
Hepatic							
Acute intermittent porphyria	PBG deaminase	Autosomal Dominant	Absent	Present	Absent	ALA, *PBG*	—
Hereditary coproporphyria	Coproporphyrinogen oxidase	Autosomal Dominant	Present	Present	Absent	ALA, PBG Copro	Copro
Variegate porphyria	Protoporphyrinogen oxidase or ferrochelatase	Autosomal Dominant	Present	Present	Absent	ALA, PBG Copro	Copro Proto
Porphyria cutanea tarda	Uroporphyrinogen decarboxylase	†	Present	Absent	Absent	Uro, 7-carboxylate porphyrin	Isocopro

* Findings of major diagnostic importance are in italics.
† Autosomal dominant inheritance has been documented in some families but not others.
‡ Type I isomers.
NOTES: ALA, δ-aminolevulinic acid; PBG, porphobilinogen; Uro, uroporphyrin; Copro, coproporphyrin; Proto, protoporphyrin; Isocopro, isocoproporphyrin.

porphyria does not develop in individuals who are heterozygous for a deficiency of this enzyme.

Watson et al. [423, 434] and Heilmeyer [430], on the other hand, have favored the idea that the primary genetic abnormality in CEP may be overproduction and increased activity of either PBG deaminase or ALA synthase. A constitutive regulator mutation [423, 434] or perhaps a structural gene mutation that results in an increased activity in one or both of these enzymes [434] could be responsible for such an increase. Such a mutation could conceivably lead to production of hydroxymethylbilane in amounts exceeding the activity of available uroporphyrinogen III cosynthase in erythroid cells, such that the nonenzymatic formation of uroporphyrinogen I would be increased and an excess of uroporphyrin I and coproporphyrin I would be produced. ALA synthase overproduction seems less likely, because ALA and PBG do not accumulate in CEP [434]. Published data are compatible with either a partial deficiency of the cosynthase or a primary increase in PBG deaminase in CEP [153, 404, 434]. However, a primary overproduction of PBG deaminase would have to be very considerable to exceed the normal activity of the cosynthase. More specific assays for the cosynthase should settle this question in the future.

The only evidence for PBG deaminase overproduction in CEP is increased activity of this enzyme in peripheral red cells [404, 434, 435, 436]. This finding could, however, reflect hemolysis and a compensatory increased erythropoiesis and reticulocytosis in these patients [185], rather than a primary overproduction of this enzyme. In nonporphyric disorders associated with hemolysis and reticulocytosis, such as sickle-cell anemia, PBG deaminase is substantially increased (up to 10 times normal) [138]. A similar phenomenon is observed in mutant mice with hemolytic anemias [134]. In CEP patients increases (1.5 to 2 times) in ALA synthase [435], ALA dehydratase [435, 437], PBG deaminase [437], ferrochelatase

[435], and glucose-6-phosphate dehydrogenase (G-6-PD) [398] have also been noted in bone marrow or erythrocytes. These changes may also be a reflection of increased hematopoiesis. Such an interpretation is supported by the finding in two CEP families that in heterozygotes the cosynthase was reduced by about 50 percent while the deaminase was normal; deaminase was increased only in homozygotes who had even lower levels of cosynthase activity and also some evidence of hemolysis [396]. To our knowledge PBG deaminase has not been measured in nonerythroid tissues or cultured fibroblasts of CEP patients, which would be relevant to examining the question of an inherited increase in this enzyme.

If a defect in uroporphyrinogen III cosynthase is the primary inherited defect in CEP (Fig. 60-19), it does not result in a complete absence of uroporphyrin III formation [438]. Production and excretion of the type III isomers are in fact increased in this disorder [185], although not to the same degree as of the type I isomers. Certain findings in CEP, such as hematinemia and increased stercobilin excretion, suggest that the rate of formation of heme is also greater than normal [334, 423], as expected in a hemolytic state. Porphyrin formation from added ALA in cultured fibroblasts of CEP patients is also not impaired, even though these cells are markedly deficient in apparent cosynthase activity [433]. Since nonenzymatic uroporphyrinogen III formation seems unlikely as a source of adequate amounts of this intermediate for heme formation, it is likely that some cosynthase, perhaps as a protein with impaired enzymatic activity, is produced in CEP, such that residual cosynthase activity is indeed present in the tissues of these patients. In erythroid cells of CEP patients uroporphyrinogen III formation could nonetheless be inefficient, and could occur only at the expense of increased production of uroporphyrinogen I (Fig. 60-19). This would be consistent with the idea that the pathophysiology of CEP results more from accu-

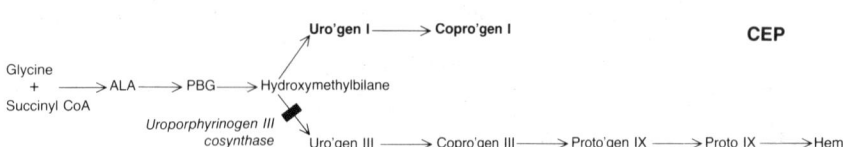

Figure 60-19 The enzymatic defect in the heme pathway in CEP is a partial deficiency of uroporphyrinogen III cosynthase activity. The deficiency in enzyme activity is sufficiently severe in homozygotes to make inefficient the formation of uroporphyrinogen III, such that normal or increased heme synthesis in the bone marrow occurs only with marked overproduction of the type I isomers of uroporphyrinogen and coproporphyrinogen, as shown in bold letters. ALA, δ-aminolevulinic acid; PBG, porphobilinogen; Uro'gen, uroporphyrinogen; Copro'gen, coproporphyrinogen; Proto'gen, protoporphyrinogen; Proto, protoporphyrin.

mulation of series I porphyrins than from a deficiency of uroporphyrinogen III and heme formation. Residual cosynthase and the ability of the bone marrow to increase the synthesis of this enzyme to some degree suggest that it is responsive to normal control mechanisms in CEP patients, such that hemolysis can stimulate erythropoiesis and increase the production of both types I and III porphyrins.

As mentioned above, red cell PBG deaminase activity is greatly increased in the presence of an increased proportion of young circulating erythrocytes, as in patients as well as mice with various hemolytic states [134, 138]. Moreover studies by Sassa [86, 107, 351] in murine erythroleukemia cells stimulated to differentiate and make hemoglobin in culture indicate that erythropoiesis results in the sequential induction of representative heme pathway enzymes, namely ALA synthase, ALA dehydratase, PBG deaminase, and ferrochelatase. It is not known whether uroporphyrinogen III cosynthase takes part in this sequential induction process when erythropoiesis is stimulated. Cosynthase activity is considerably greater in younger red cells than in older cells [185]. Zail et al. [398] found that red cells obtained from a CEP patient during hemolytic phases and incubated in vitro with ALA generated mostly type I porphyrins, whereas during a nonhemolytic phase cells generated predominatly porphyrins of the type III series. Heilmeyer et al. [424] also noted a shift in porphyrin synthesis from type I to type III isomers after splenectomy and remission of hemolysis in a CEP patient. Investigations by Watson et al. [404] in bovine CEP suggest that in younger circulating red cells there is a greater excess of the deaminase relative to the cosynthase as compared with older cells. A greater enzyme imbalance in younger cells may help explain the fact that excess porphyrin production is greatly accentuated in CEP when erythropoiesis is stimulated [398, 404]. The cosynthase moreover is thought to interact with PBG deaminase, perhaps as a multienzyme complex, and such an enzyme interaction may be important in the normal and efficient formation of uroporphyrinogen III [149, 151]. Therefore relative activities and enzyme interactions between the deaminase and the cosynthase during differentiation of erythroid cells in CEP merit further study.

The finding of increased erythrocyte protoporphyrin in some patients with CEP, and regularly in bovine CEP, also does not preclude a cosynthase deficiency. During some stages of normal erythroid development, ferrochelatase is rate-limiting for heme formation [86, 107]. Moreover this enzyme may also be influenced by a variety of endogenous factors, including age-related changes prior to the reticulocyte stage of erythrocyte maturation [428, 439], and individual and species variations. It has been suggested, for example, that the activity of ferrochelatase in mature normoblasts and reticulocytes may decrease more rapidly than the activity of ALA synthase [428, 439, 440]. There is also evidence that X chromosomal loci may regulate heme pathway enzymes such as ALA synthase and

ferrochelatase [441]. Thus genetic and developmental factors unrelated to the presumed cosynthase defect can influence heme pathway enzymes and erythrocyte porphyrin patterns. This, in addition to possible genetic heterogeneity at the level of cosynthase activity, could provide considerable potential for phenotypic variation in this disease.

Diagnosis

CEP should be suspected in a patient with severe photosensitivity beginning in childhood. Very rarely, skin lesions do not develop until adult life. Diagnosis must be based on proper laboratory evaluation to exclude other types of porphyria associated with photosensitivity, namely EPP, PCT, HCP, and VP. It is necessary to demonstrate that erythrocyte *and* urine porphyrins are increased, as CEP is the only major type of human porphyria in which marked increases in both are found. Full evaluation of porphyrin metabolism including quantitation of type I and III isomers is recommended to provide a proper diagnosis and better understanding of this rare disease and its possible variants.

Heterozygotes can be detected by studying uroporphyrinogen III cosynthase activity in cultured fibroblasts [185]. CEP can be detected in utero in a mother without manifest porphyria by examination of amniotic fluid. If the fetus has inherited the disease, the amniotic fluid has a red-brown discoloration due to the presence of porphyrins. It is important to distinguish this from fetal death, wherein amniotic fluid may be similar in color but will not fluoresce on exposure to ultraviolet light [442]. Detection of CEP in the fetus by testing amniotic fluid cells grown in culture should be possible but has not yet been accomplished [443]. Normal cosynthase activity in such cells from one pregnant patient with CEP was recently described and the infant was later confirmed not to have inherited the disease [444]. Occasionally patients with CEP become pregnant; excess porphyrins from the mother may cross the placenta and accumulate in the fetus, but then disappear from the infant within a few days after birth [426]. Recently a normal level of amniotic fluid coproporphyrin was found in a CEP patient carrying a normal fetus [444].

Unusual Types of CEP and CEP-like Porphyrias

Patients with CEP and atypical features are of interest because they indicate that this disease may be genetically heterogeneous. On the other hand, atypical cases may be phenotypic variations of a single genetic defect or of closely related defects due to influences that are not well defined at present.

Patients in whom the disease begins in adult life are examples [391, 394]. It has also been suggested that late-onset cases may be heterozygotes for CEP [391]. However, recent biochemical studies in two adult-onset cases of CEP, which included measurements of uroporphyrinogen III cosynthase and family studies, indicated a homozygous state with marked reduction of erythrocyte cosynthase activity in both [396].

A case reported by Haining et al. [401, 418] was typical for CEP, except that protoporphyrin was the major erythrocyte porphyrin. When this patient was treated by hypertransfusion, erythrocyte porphyrins decreased as expected (see Treatment), and red cell protoporphyrin declined more slowly than uroporphyrin. When anemia was produced by phlebotomy, the red cell uroporphyrin concentration rose more rapidly than protoporphyrin, and for a period of time the concentration of uroporphyrin exceeded that for protoporphyrin in the red cells [418]. This patient was one of five CEP patients reported to have deficient erythrocyte uroporphyrinogen III cosynthase by Romeo and Levin [153]. In another report, uroporphyrin predominated in red cells on some occasions and protoporphyrin at others in a CEP patient [399]. There are also a number of reported cases in which erythocyte protoporphyrin content was considerably increased and exceeded levels of uroporphyrin [391, 396, 399, 401, 431, 436, 455, 456], and in two cases cosynthase deficiency has been noted [396]. Two further cases studied by Moore et al. [436] had evidence of a cosynthase defect in erythrocytes. Bovine CEP is also characterized by reduced cosynthase activity [148] and large amounts of protoporphyrin in circulating red cells. Thus although a predominance of protoporphyrin in red cells is unusual in CEP, it is not inconsistent with the diagnosis or with a cosynthase defect.

These observations indicate that the pattern of red cell porphyrins in CEP, although largely determined by an inherited enzyme abnormality, can be influenced also by other factors related to red cell maturation in the bone marrow. In the bone marrow uroporphyrin fluorescence is associated primarily with cells (late normoblasts, early reticulocytes) that are released into the circulation more rapidly when erythropoiesis is stimulated [418]. Protoporphyrin fluorescence of fresh blood and marrow smears is quite labile [418], and its changes with bone marrow erythroid maturation have not been defined as well as have those of uroporphyrin in CEP. Ferrochelatase may become limiting under certain conditions of bone marrow stimulation and result in protoporphyrin accumulation.

A Norwegian boy had clinical and biochemical findings which were in general typical for CEP [445, 448], but unlike more classical cases of CEP, the urine porphyrins consisted mostly of uroporphyrin and 7-carboxylate porphyrins, and smaller amounts of the 6-, 5-, and 4-carboxylate porphyrins. Also, protoporphyrin predominated in erythrocytes rather than uroporphyrin and coproporphyrin as in more typical cases. The uroporphyrin and coproporphyrin in urine were mostly type I, whereas the intermediate porphyrins, including large amounts of 7-carboxylate porphyrin, were mostly isomer III. Small amounts of isocoproporphyrin and an apparent porphyrin peptide conjugate were also present [445, 448]. Large amounts of uroporphyrin and 7-carboxylate porphyrin were demonstrated in bone marrow. This patient excreted substantial amounts of porphyrinogens in urine which could be oxidized to porphyrins in vitro, and the proportion of porphyrinogens excreted was greater during periods when he was shielded from light [446]. Similar features have been described in bovine CEP during the winter when there is less light exposure. Eriksen et al. [446] suggested that light exposure could

increase the oxidation of excess porphyrinogens to porphyrins in their patient and thereby increase porphyrin-related photodamage to erythrocytes and skin cells. The bulk of the excess porphyrins appeared to originate in the marrow, based on the finding of large amounts of uroporphyrin and 7-carboxylate porphyrin in that tissue [447]. In view of the large amounts of certain type III porphyrins, it was also suggested that a uroporphyrinogen III cosynthase defect was unlikely, and that the excess excretion of isocoproporphyrin suggested inhibition of the decarboxylation of 5-carboxylate porphyrinogen III to coproporphyrinogen III [447]. This patient did, however, excrete very large amounts of uroporphyrin I and coproporphyrin I, and the presence of isocoproporphyrin could suggest a hepatic component to the excess porphyrin production [448].

Two somewhat similar cases were described in Spain by Piñol-Aguadé et al. [449–451]. In the first case uroporphyrin exceeded coproporphyrin in urine, and protoporphyrin predominated in red cells [449]. Hemolysis was mild. Porphyrins in the second case were studied in greater detail. There was a predominance in urine of 5-carboxylate porphyrin, and substantial amounts also of uroporphyrin, 6-carboxylate porphyrin, coproporphyrin, 7-carboxylate porphyrin, and isocoproporphyrin. Stool contained mostly protoporphyrin, and some isocoproporphyrin and intermediate porphyrins [451]. These cases have been termed *hepatoerythrocytic* because the mixture of porphyrins, including isocoproporphyrin, suggested an hepatic component; the first case also had early cirrhosis and considerable porphyrin fluorescence in the liver. Two sibs with a similar form of porphyria were described by Simon et al. [452]. Urine porphyrins were mostly 8-, 7-, and 5-carboxylate porphyrins, erythrocytes contained protoporphyrin, and there were small increases in fecal coproporphyrin levels. Liver tissue and bone marrow showed porphyrin fluorescence. Deletion of the short arm of chromosome 18 and 18-trisomy were also noted in these patients [453].

Elder et al. [454] has suggested recently that a total of seven atypical cases of erythropoietic porphyria, including those of Eriksen [445–447], Pinõl-Aguadé [449–451], and Simon [452–453] should be termed *hepatoerythropoietic porphyria*. Moreover they described profound decreases to levels of 7 to 8 percent of normal in uroporphyrinogen decarboxylase activity in red cells and cultured fibroblasts from three cases available for study. Their findings indicate that these patients are in fact homozygous for the enzyme defect found in familial PCT. Thus in atypical cases of erythropoietic porphyria, particularly when there is excess excretion of isocoproporphyrins, homozygous familial PCT should be considered.

Treatment

Therapy of CEP is generally only partially successful. Patients should be shielded from sunlight as much as possible, and trauma to the skin avoided. Sunscreen lotions and quinine ointments may be of some benefit [426]. Secondary bacterial infections of the skin should be treated promptly to avoid scarring. Cellulitis and other severe infections sometimes develop and require hospitalization and treatment with systemic antibiotics.

Splenectomy may benefit patients with CEP by reducing the degree of hemolysis and with it the stimulation of red cell production in the bone marrow. Although improvement following this procedure has been reported in some cases [389, 399,

410], it has not occurred in others [392, 400]. In an individual case of CEP it is difficult to determine the contribution of an enlarged spleen per se to the hemolytic process [401]. Splenectomy is likely to be most beneficial when there is reduced red cell survival and the spleen can be demonstrated to be removing the bulk of the red cells that disappear from the circulation. Increased hemolysis some months after splenectomy, to a degree approaching that seen preoperatively, may be explained by the gradual development of phagocytic activity in other organs after splenectomy, such as the liver [399]. It has also been pointed out that improvement with splenectomy in some reported cases may have been partly due to the transfusions which were given at the time of surgery [438]. Bleeding symptoms due to thrombocytopenia may also respond to splenectomy [394], but in at least one case thrombocytopenia did not improve [400].

Transfusion and the induction of polycythemia can also reduce porphyrin formation in CEP [418]. After transfusion to hematocrit levels between 50 and 60 percent, porphyrin excretion was reduced by only about one-half in one case studied in detail by Haining et al. [418]. Bone marrow erythropoiesis, erythropoietin production, plasma iron turnover, and iron uptake by the bone marrow also decreased with transfusion in this patient [418]. Transfusion has been employed chronically in some CEP patients to suppress porphyrin production, but hazards such as iron overload and hepatitis greatly reduce its usefulness [438].

Intravenous hematin therapy was studied in one patient by Watson et al. [438]. After 3 days of treatment decreases in plasma, erythrocyte, and urine porphyrins were observed. These responses were somewhat delayed when compared with improvements that have been documented in porphyrin precursor excretion in some of the hepatic porphyrias, suggesting that in CEP hematin may act on the bone marrow and not in the liver to reduce porphyrin production [438]. From this interesting case study it was suggested that hematin may exert a negative feedback action on the heme biosynthetic pathway, and in particular ALA synthase, in developing normoblasts and perhaps in reticulocytes. On the other hand there was also some evidence that hematin might have suppressed erythropoiesis in this patient in that the number of circulating normoblasts was reduced transiently. This is of some concern because CEP can be complicated by periods of bone marrow hypoplasia and an associated worsening of anemia. Therefore further study is needed to define whether hematin acts on porphyrin synthesis directly or indirectly via an alteration in erythroid maturation in CEP. Also heme can inhibit release of iron from transferrin in erythroid cells in experimental systems [457, 458]. Hematin may benefit patients with sideroblastic anemias [459] when the disease is associated with impaired porphyrin-heme synthesis and increased erythroid cell uptake of iron, but the consequence of any altered iron uptake in CEP erythroid cells as a result of hematin treatment is at present difficult to predict.

Oral β-carotene is an effective treatment in EPP (see below) which is a much milder disease than CEP. There are several reports that it may improve light tolerance at least to a degree in CEP as well [460, 461], and further evaluation is warranted.

Alkalinization of the urine can increase the output of coproporphyrin but not uroporphyrin [462–464]. Short-term alkalinization, while increasing urine coproporphyrin output somewhat in two CEP patients, did not produce clinical improvement [465]. Prednisolone may improve the anemia and thrombocytopenia in some patients [391, 394, 408], but not others [391, 392], and other signs improve less frequently. Treatment with pyridoxine, adenosine monophosphate, and inosine have also been tried with little or no success [400, 401, 466]. Chloroquine has been given to some patients but has not been clearly shown to be beneficial [389, 392, 436].

CEP in Animals

A rare autosomal recessive form of this disorder has been described in cattle, particularly of the Holstein and shorthorn breeds. The clinical and biochemical findings are very similar to CEP in humans. Thus there is markedly increased excretion of uroporphyrin I and coproporphyrin I in urine and lesser increases in isomer III porphyrin excretion. Total porphyrins are mostly uroporphyrin, coproporphyrin, and 5-carboxylate porphyrin, with very little 7-carboxylate porphyrin. There is no excretion of isocoproporphyrin [448]. As in the human disease, studies of red cells from affected animals suggest a deficiency of uroporphyrinogen III cosynthase (with no evidence of an enzyme inhibitor) [148] and increased PBG deaminase [467]. Labeled iron and erythrocyte kinetic studies indicate destruction of developing erythroid cells in the bone marrow and decreased survival of circulating erythrocytes, presumably due to an intracorpuscular defect [468].

A difference from most cases of human CEP is a marked increase in red cell protoporphyrin concentration in the bovine disease. Moreover, although bone marrow uroporphyrin and coproporphyrin content greatly exceeds red cell concentrations of these porphyrins, as in human CEP, the disease in cattle is characterized by red cell protoporphyrin concentrations that exceed bone marrow protoporphyrin content [428]. Erythrocyte protoporphyrin can also exceed bone marrow protoporphyrin content in nonporphyric animals in which erythropoiesis is increased experimentally by phenylhydrazine-induced hemolysis, prior bleeding, or hypoxia [428, 469]. Protoporphyrin in red cells of these porphyric cattle is free and not complexed with Zn [428]. Red cell protoporphyrin in bovine CEP has a half-life comparable to that of hemoglobin, as shown by studies in porphyric calves in which these compounds were labeled by injecting radiolabeled precursors (glycine and ALA) [428]. Red cell–free protoporphyrin in CEP (at least when labeled by ALA injection) has a half-life of several months, which is much longer than, for example, in human EPP (see below) and may explain at least in part the prominence of erythrocyte protoporphyrin in bovine CEP [428]. Red cell survival in normal cattle has been estimated at about 160 days [468]. Increased plasma porphyrins and skin photosensitivity probably originate mostly from bone marrow uroporphyrin and coproporphyrin production, rather than from porphyrins in circulating red cells, as is believed to be the case also in human CEP.

CEP has also been described in cats, swine, and the fox squirrel. This disease is an autosomal dominant disease in swine, and photosensitivity is not prominent [470–472]. In domestic short-haired cats [473, 474] the disease is also autosomal dominant. In a family of Siamese cats the clinical features included severe anemia, hepatosplenomegaly, and renal disease, and the mode of inheritance was uncertain [475]. In fox squirrels all individuals of the species have porphyria and appear to suffer little or no disability [476]. CEP in these species has been less studied than in cattle, but a deficiency of uroporphyrinogen III cosynthase has been found in the fox squirrel [155, 477].

ERYTHROPOIETIC PROTOPORPHYRIA

Definition

Erythropoietic protoporphyria (EPP) is an autosomal dominant disorder first clearly described by Magnus et al. [478] in 1961 and characterized by mild to moderate photosensitivity and excess protoporphyrin in red cells and feces. It is probably due to a genetic defect in ferrochelatase, the last enzyme in the heme biosynthetic pathway. Excess protoporphyrin in red cells is present as the free porphyrin rather than as zinc-protoporphyrin. There is considerable variability in severity of the disease, and some obligate heterozygotes may have normal erythrocyte porphyrin levels and no photosensitivity. The reason why some gene carriers manifest EPP while others do not is poorly understood. Other terms used for this disease include protoporphyria [439] and erythrohepatic protoporphyria [479].

Prevalence

EPP is the most common of the erythropoietic porphyrias. It was not recognized until recently because it generally produces only mild skin lesions and is not associated with porphyrinuria. Its prevalence has not been precisely estimated, but De Leo et al. [480] found over 300 published case reports up to 1976. The disorder appears more common in Caucasians, but occurs in patients from diverse racial backgrounds, including Negroes [481].

Clinical Features

The most characteristic clinical findings in a recent series of 32 cases are summarized in Table 60-5. Photosensitivity, which is generally much less severe than in CEP, usually begins in childhood and occurs on sun-exposed areas such as the face and dorsal aspects of the hands (Fig. 60-20). Photosensitivity is usually worse in spring and summer. Distinctive cutaneous fea-

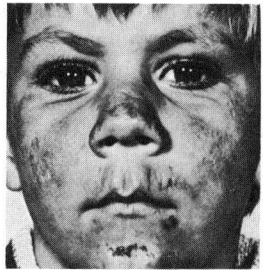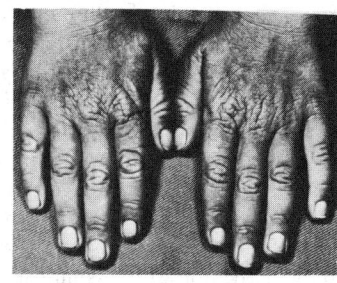

Figure 60-20 EPP in a 6-year-old boy, showing ulcerations and scarring on the face, labial grooving, coarse, thickened skin on the hands, and loss of lanulae of the fingernails. (*From Schmidt, Smither, Thomsen, and Lintrup* [483]. *By permission of Archives of Dermatology.*)

tures include itching and painful erythema and swelling of light-exposed areas of the skin; these can all develop within a few minutes of sun exposure. Diffuse edema of the skin may resemble angioneurotic edema. Vesicles and bullae may occur but are usually sparse [482]. Petechiae and purpuric lesions are also described. Occasionally patients may present with burning and itching without objective signs of skin damage. Lichenification of the skin, leathery pseudovesicles, and nail changes are occasionally pronounced [483–485]. There may be some residual scarring from vesicles or from occasional severe skin swelling with necrosis, but severe scarring of the skin and resulting marked deformities of the face and digits do not occur. Labial grooving is sometimes noted. Skin pigment changes are unusual. Increased friability of the skin with minor trauma and hirsutism (as in CEP, VP, and PCT) are not characteristic of EPP. Fluorescence of the teeth is not found. The nervous system is not affected, and there is no known sensitivity to drugs as in the hepatic porphyrias. There is no change in the color of the urine, as porphyrin excretion is increased only in the bile and feces.

The mechanism whereby protoporphyrin produces skin damage is not fully understood. The skin is maximally sensitive to light in the 400-nm range in EPP patients, which corresponds closely to the Soret band (i.e., the characteristic discrete maximal absorption range) for porphyrins [478]. The fact that cutaneous reactions to 400-nm light can be prevented by short-term occlusion of arterial flow to the forearm in a porphyria patient suggests that O_2 is a requirement, as in many photochemical reactions in vitro [482]. The light absorption spectrum of protoporphyrin is also identical to the action spectrum for photohemolysis of EPP erythrocytes in vitro, a phenomenon also requiring O_2 [486]. Skin fibroblasts in culture [487] and liver subcellular fractions [488] have also been used to study mechanisms of photooxidative cell damage. Protoporphyrin injection in guinea pigs also produces skin photosensitivity. It is believed that absorbed light induces an excited energy state of the porphyrin molecule, and that this can be released as fluorescence or can produce chemical reactions leading to the formation of free radicals and singlet oxygen and ultimately to cell damage [24, 486, 489, 490]. Available evidence favors singlet oxygen as the most important reactive oxygen species in porphyrin-mediated cytotoxicity [489]. Peroxidation of lipids [486] or oxidation of amino acids and cross-linking of proteins in cell membranes [491, 492] can accompany this process. In erythrocytes the cross-linking of proteins such as spectrin may reduce cell deformability [493], and in reticulocytes in vitro photoactivated protoporphyrin can inhibit globin synthesis and induce cross-linking of hemoglobin molecules [494]. The hydrophobic portion of the pro-

Table 60-5 Common clinical features of EPP from a series of 32 cases [480]

Symptoms and signs	Percent incidence
Burning	97
Edema	94
Itching	88
Erythema	69
Scarring	19
Vesicles	3
Anemia	27
Cholelithiasis	12
Abnormal liver study results	4

toporphyrin molecule allows it to penetrate lipoid monolayers in vitro and the porphyrin can under some conditions interact with amino groups on proteins [495]. Protoporphyrin is more readily taken up by mitochondria and can impair mitochondrial respiration and other functions to a greater degree than more water soluble porphyrins such as uroporphyrin [488, 489]. Mitochondrial damage may therefore be more important than lysosomal damage in the photosensitivity of EPP [487, 488]. Studies in vitro by Gigli et al. [25, 496, 497] suggest that photoactivation of the complement system may occur in EPP and be a factor in skin damage. Other possible mediators include histamine and kinins [482].

The microcirculation in the upper dermis is particularly affected in EPP. Amorphous material is deposited around cutaneous blood vessels in this disorder; this contains plasma proteins including immunoglobulins and complement components [496, 498] in addition to a predominance of neutral glycoprotein and lesser amounts of acid glycosaminoglycans and lipids [499–501]. Skin histopathology resembles that found in PCT, despite differences in the gross appearance of the skin in these two disorders [502]. This histological picture can be reproduced by irradiation with long-wavelength UV light of mice treated with griseofulvin, which produces a hepatic type of protoporphyria [503]. Fine structural alterations of the skin in EPP include multilayered and fragmented basement membranes and fine fibrillar material in and around the walls of small blood vessels, corresponding to the amorphous changes seen by light microscopy [504].

There is little evidence that EPP is associated with impaired erythropoiesis or abnormal iron metabolism [259, 478, 505–507]. Nevertheless mild anemia, hypochromia, and microcytosis have been noted in some cases in the apparent absence of other causes [259, 480] and may be more common than previously recognized [508]. Suurmond [563] described four children with EPP and associated mild anemia and reticulocytosis (red cell survival was normal in the one case studied) in whom there was a poor response to oral iron treatment. Hemolysis is not commonly observed or is very mild in EPP, unless due to complications or intercurrent illnesses. In cases complicated by liver disease (see below) hemolysis may be more pronounced and be associated with splenomegaly [509]. Studies of iron metabolism and the observation that with phlebotomy iron deficiency anemia develops rapidly suggest that depletion of iron stores may be relatively common in EPP even in the absence of iron deficiency anemia [507].

Fluorescence due to protoporphyrin accumulation in the bone marrow is detectable in maturing bone marrow erythroid cells, and this appears to become maximal soon after the loss of the nucleus. Thus nucleated erythroid cells display little or no fluorescence and bone marrow fluorescence is almost entirely found in reticulocytes [259, 440, 510]. Protoporphyrin content in peripheral red cells declines with age, and fluorescence is nonuniform when peripheral blood smears are examined by fluorescence microscopy [440]

Liver function is usually normal in EPP. There are few data on liver protoporphyrin content in EPP, but histological observations suggest that some increase in protoporphyrin is not uncommon in the liver. This is visible as a dark brown pigment which is birefringent under polarizing microscopy and crystalline by electron microscopy [511]. Protoporphyrin content sometimes appears greatly increased in the absence of evidence of liver damage. Chronic liver disease can be a significant complication in a minority of EPP patients [485, 512]. Advanced

liver disease can even on occasion be the presenting manifestation of EPP [513]. In 1979 Bloomer reviewed 15 case reports in the literature of patients with EPP who died as a result of cirrhosis and liver failure [512]. The patients consisted of nine males and six females between the ages of 11 and 60 years. In such cases there was marked deposition of protoporphyrin in hepatocytes, Kupffer cells, portal histiocytes, and bile canaliculi. Iron overload was not a feature. Early stages of this complication appear to be heralded by increasing levels of red cell and plasma protoporphyrin, sometimes increased photosensitivity, and abnormalities in liver function tests. Urine coproporphyrin may also increase in EPP patients with liver disease [514, 515].

The pathogenesis of liver damage in such individuals is poorly understood. Few have had evidence of other causes of liver damage which might decrease hepatobiliary function and predispose to the retention of protoporphyrin in the liver. Liver damage may therefore result from protoporphyrin accumulation itself, perhaps because this porphyrin is insoluble in water and tends to form crystalline structures in liver cells when it accumulates in excess [512, 516]. Excess protoporphyrin may particularly impair mitochondrial function in liver cells [515] and decrease hepatic bile formation [517]. An enterohepatic circulation of protoporphyrin may also predispose to its retention in the liver [518]. On at least three occasions, serious hepatic lesions have developed in two members of the same family [485, 514, 519, 520]. Although severe hepatic complications may develop only in a minority of patients with EPP, factors that may increase the production and delivery of protoporphyrin to the liver, or impair its biliary excretion should be avoided in EPP patients. Such factors may include iron deficiency, fasting, and oral contraceptive agents [512, 521].

Gallstones have also been reported in a substantial number of EPP patients [522]. These stones are fluorescent [6], are composed at least in part of protoporphyrin, and some have appeared to produce symptoms at an unusually young age. The factors which determine protoporphyrin solubility in bile and the mechanism by which stones form in EPP patients are poorly understood.

Biochemical Findings

Protoporphyrin is the only heme pathway intermediate that accumulates to a substantial degree in EPP. Because of its poor solubility in water it can only be excreted in bile regardless of its tissue of origin. Protoporphyrin concentrations are increased in erythrocytes, plasma, bile, and feces (Table 60-4). Urine porphyrins and porphyrin precursors, on the other hand, are normal. Protoporphyrin in blister fluid of EPP patients is likely to originate from plasma, although other possibilities have been discussed [523].

PBG deaminase can be somewhat increased in circulating erythrocytes of EPP patients [524], suggesting perhaps a slight degree of hemolysis and increased release of younger erythroid cells from the marrow. PBG deaminase has been shown to decrease with red cell age in EPP patients [525] as in CEP (see earlier discussion), normal persons, and patients with other erythroid disorders [138]. Increased red cell uroporphyrinogen decarboxylase in EPP has been reported by one laboratory [526] but not another [200]; such an increase might reflect a mild reticulocytosis [526].

Plasma levels of hemopexin may be somewhat subnormal in

EPP and PCT but not in AIP. This could reflect slight hemolysis or increased plasma porphyrin levels, since this protein binds porphyrins in addition to heme. Hemopexin is synthesized normally but catabolized at an increased rate in EPP [527, 528].

The origin of the excessive amounts of protoporphyrin excreted in EPP has been extensively studied. Red cells in the circulation would appear to be an insufficient source, unless the erythrocytic protoporphyrin pool were to turn over daily [479, 529]. In EPP patients protoporphyrin begins to accumulate in bone marrow normoblasts just before the nucleus is lost, and this continues through the reticulocyte stage until mitochondria are lost from the cell [440, 510]. Protoporphyrin formation by EPP bone marrow preparations incubated with porphyrin precursors (glycine and α-ketoglutarate) in vitro is markedly increased [530]. Bone marrow reticulocytes are therefore a likely major source of protoporphyrin in EPP. In circulating erythrocytes protoporphyrin content then declines markedly with red cell aging, a phenomenon not observed or at least much less marked in other states in which red cell protoporphyrin is increased, such as iron deficiency anemia and lead poisoning [440, 510]. Thus all of the excess red cell protoporphyrin does not remain in the cell for its full life span in EPP, but is able to diffuse quite rapidly into the plasma [510]. This occurs because red cell protoporphyrin is free, and not chelated with Zn as in lead poisoning and iron deficiency. In the latter disorders, which are not associated with photosensitivity, Zn-protoporphyrin is bound to hemoglobin, probably in the heme binding site, and remains in the cell for as long as it circulates. Free protoporphyrin, on the other hand, is bound less readily than Zn-protoporphyrin to hemoglobin within the red cell and diffuses more easily into plasma [510, 531].

Free protoporphyrin does, nevertheless, bind much more strongly to hemoglobin than to proteins that transport this porphyrin in plasma, namely albumin and hemopexin. Therefore the flux of free protoporphyrin in EPP from erythroid cells to plasma and bile appears to be greatly dependent upon the ability of the liver to take up protoporphyrin efficiently and excrete it in bile [532]. The binding site of free protoporphyrin to the hemoglobin molecule is controversial [531–533].

It is likely that more protoporphyrin diffuses into plasma from bone marrow reticulocytes than from cells in the circulation, and that this accounts for the bulk of protoporphyrin excreted daily in bile and feces [439, 510]. Earlier isotopic studies gave indirect evidence that the liver is also a source of excess porphyrin formation in EPP [420, 479, 505], although it was not possible to quantitate the relative contributions that were postulated for hepatic and erythroid tissues [420]. Moreover some short-term periods of calorie restriction in an EPP patient produced transient abrupt increases in fecal protoporphyrin excretion; a response mediated by the "glucose effect" on hepatic ALA synthase was suggested [534]. Unsupervised dieting and intermittent starvation may have exacerbated EPP and resulted in fatal hepatic disease in a case reported by Scott et al. [521], but the more recent realization that erythroid-free protoporphyrin can diffuse and turn over so rapidly in EPP has diminished the apparent potential of the liver as an important contributor of excess protoporphyrin in this disease [510]. Nevertheless liver ALA synthase may be increased in some EPP patients [520, 529, 535] even though normal cytochrome P$_{450}$ levels do not suggest impaired heme formation [520].

The occurrence of protoporphyrin deposition in liver and clinically significant liver disease in some EPP patients might support a hepatic component of protoporphyrin production in EPP. However, impaired hepatobiliary function could result from increased protoporphyrin presented to the liver from the erythron or other tissue sources, as is suggested by studies in which protoporphyrin has been shown to reduce bile flow in the isolated perfused rat liver [517]. The development of liver dysfunction from whatever cause might further predispose to hepatic protoporphyrin accumulation.

If protoporphyrin does accumulate in the liver, there is evidence from griseofulvin-treated mice [532, 536] that it can also diffuse back into plasma and be taken up by red cells in the circulation. In griseofulvin-treated mice excess protoporphyrin originates from liver production, and the process of transfer to erythrocytes is such that protoporphyrin content increases with red cell age, which is opposite to what is observed in human EPP [532]. Uptake across the red cell membrane appears to determine the rate of this process, and subsequent binding of the porphyrin to hemoglobin in erythrocytes takes place more readily than uptake into the cell [532]. This phenomenon can occur at liver protoporphyrin concentrations considerably below those found in patients with EPP-associated cirrhosis [519]. Lamon et al. [525] described a complex EPP patient with a history of hepatic involvement treated previously by splenectomy and cholestyramine, who at the time of study had erythrocyte protoporphyrin concentrations that increased with red cell age. This interesting observation appears similar to the phenomenon in griseofulvin-treated mice described above. Evidence against a hepatic component of protoporphyrin production was obtained in the same patient, however, in that hematin therapy failed to reduce protoporphyrin in plasma, feces, or red cells [525]. A 6-year-old child reported by Porter and Lowe [509], in whom EPP was complicated by liver disease, portal hypertension, splenomegaly, and hemolytic anemia, also suggests that protoporphyrin from erythroid cells can be deposited in the liver and produce liver damage. In this patient splenectomy relieved the hemolytic process and the associated bone marrow stimulation, and there was considerable improvement in liver function, disappearance of protoporphyrin from the liver, and no further photosensitivity even though erythrocyte protoporphyrin actually increased. The bone marrow clearly appeared to be the predominant source of excess liver protoporphyrin in this patient [509].

Genetic Defect

Assays of ferrochelatase activity in bone marrow or bone marrow reticulocytes [259, 515], liver, cultured fibroblasts [257], and blood or buffy coat lysates [259, 524, 537] strongly suggest that this enzyme is deficient in EPP (Fig. 60-21). A partial deficiency of ferrochelatase has also been demonstrated functionally in cultured skin fibroblasts [258] and mitogen-stimulated lymphocytes of EPP patients [548] by incubating these cells with ALA and measuring protoporphyrin accumulation [548]. The technique of measuring protoporphyrin formation after incubating cells with ALA is similar to that used in earlier studies of ALA conversion to protoporphyrin in cultured cells from AIP patients [174, 175]. In cells from EPP patients, protoporphyrin accumulation from ALA was substantially greater than in normal cells, and the responses to added iron [258, 538] or Ca-Mg-EDTA (an iron chelator) [548] were smaller than in normal cells, as might be expected for cells partially

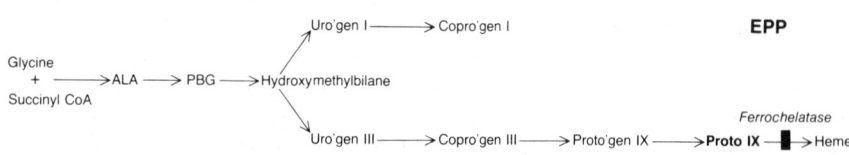

Figure 60-21 The enzymatic defect in the heme pathway in EPP is a partial deficiency of ferrochelatase activity. The enzyme defect results in protoporphyrin accumulation (bold letters) primarily in erythroid cells in some heterozygotes, even though hemoglobin synthesis is not impaired. ALA, δ-aminolevulinic acid; PBG, porphobilinogen; Uro'gen, uroporphyrinogen; Copro'gen, coproporphyrinogen; Proto'gen, protoporphyrinogen; Proto, protoporphyrin.

deficient in ferrochelatase activity [548]. Therefore, it would appear that in EPP, ferrochelatase activity is deficient in all body tissues. The many observations in vivo in patients described above would indicate, nevertheless, that the deficient enzyme becomes rate-limiting for protoporphyrin metabolism to heme primarily in the erythron and especially in bone marrow reticulocytes.

This porphyria is inherited in an autosomal dominant pattern [539–541]. Chromosomal abnormalities have not been described, except in a case with deletion of the long arm of chromosome 18 in whom the presence of EPP may have been coincidental [542] and in another case who had EPP with Klinefelter's syndrome [543]. There is much individual variability in severity of clinical expression and in the degree of altered porphyrin metabolism in EPP. Some obligate carriers have no increases in erythrocyte porphyrin content. Plasma and fecal protoporphyrin content may be more sensitive indicators of the genetic defect in some individuals than in others. Functional assessment of ferrochelatase activity in mitogen-stimulated lymphocytes and study of the effects of various amounts of added ALA, Fe, and Ca-Mg-EDTA in this system indicate that ferrochelatase activity is approximately one-half of normal [548]. All individuals who have inherited this disease are heterozygous. EPP may therefore be determined by a mutant allele that results in little or no enzymatically active ferrochelatase, and the one-half of normal enzyme activity is probably due to the normal allele in these individuals.

The activity of ferrochelatase in various tissue lysates of EPP patients has been reported to be only 10 to 25 percent of normal [257, 259, 263, 524, 537], which is considerably lower than might be expected for an autosomal dominant enzyme deficiency [258, 548]. Given the technical difficulty of directly measuring this mitochondrial enzyme in tissues with very low enzyme activity, it appears that indirect assessment by studying the conversion of ALA to protoporphyrin and the degree of protoporphyrin accumulation may more accurately reflect the functional activity of ferrochelatase, at least in cultured cells [544, 548]. A reduction of the enzyme to levels of 10 to 25 percent of normal would suggest more complex genetic mechanisms for the enzyme deficiency [263], as would kinetic data from studies of ferrochelatase in cultured fibroblasts, which indicate the presence of an enzyme inhibitor or a reduced apparent K_m for a porphyrin substrate [545]. A multimeric enzyme might conceivably be markedly reduced in activity in heterozygotes with a structural gene defect, but a recent report of the isolation and purification of rat liver ferrochelatase does not describe the enzyme as a multimer [250]. A mutant allele in EPP may alter membrane lipids or other aspects of the mitochondrial environment for ferrochelatase. Phospholipids are known to support ferrochelatase activity. However, mitochondrial structure is normal in EPP, and other aspects of mitochondrial function that have been examined are also normal [258, 545]. Kramer and Viljoen [546] reported altered heat

stability of ferrochelatase in intact or lysed marrow cell suspensions from EPP patients. This and an inability of EPP fibroblasts to incorporate Zn into protoporphyrin, an activity possibly mediated by ferrochelatase in normal cells, suggested that EPP is associated with a structurally variant form of ferrochelatase [546]. Zn chelation by protoporphyrin can occur nonenzymatically, or may be catalyzed by an enzyme other than ferrochelatase [547].

The interindividual variability among heterozygotes in erythrocyte protoporphyrin concentrations and degree of sensitivity to light is poorly explained. Few obligate heterozygotes with normal or nearly normal levels of protoporphyrin in red cells have in fact been studied. Our investigations of protoporphyrin formation from ALA in mitogen-stimulated lymphocytes in one family suggest that ferrochelatase activity may be lower in subjects with manifest EPP than in those with clinically latent disease [548]. Influences on ferrochelatase in addition to the primary genetic defect may therefore determine the degree of clinical expression of this disease. The nature of such additional influences remains to be defined. It seems plausible that these might influence the synthesis or activity of the product of the normal allele in EPP heterozygotes, since as noted above the gene product of the mutant allele may result in little or no ferrochelatase activity. There is some evidence in mice [441] suggesting other genetic influences on ferrochelatase activity during erythroid maturation and hemoglobin formation, and there may be genetic or acquired defects in this enzyme in some forms of sideroblastic anemia [549, 550]. Such genetic influences on ferrochelatase or on growth rates of hemopoietic cells [551] have so far been associated particularly with the X chromosome. There has been some suggestion that clinical expression of human EPP is more marked in males [541] and EPP does appear to be somewhat more commonly reported in males than in females [48, 541, 552]. Moreover EPP may occasionally be accompanied by features of a sideroblastic anemia [521]. In chickens a translocation involving a sex chromosome (Z) and chromosome 1 profoundly alters ferrochelatase activity in at least one tissue (uterus), and Schwartz and coworkers [553] suggested that a structural or regulatory gene for this enzyme might be located on one of these chromosomes. The observation that in EPP patients the levels of protoporphyrin in blood and stools are poorly correlated [529] may also indicate considerable individual variability in the rate of diffusion of protoporphyrin out of erythroid cells or in other steps in the transfer of protoporphyrin from the erythron to bile.

ALA synthase activity may be increased in the bone marrow [259, 435, 554] in some but not all cases and is also increased in the liver [529, 535] and in buffy coat preparations from whole blood [524]. As discussed by Bottomley et al. [259], the normal erythrocyte protoporphyrin content of approximately 10^{-6} M is below the optimal concentration (10^{-5} M) for maximal heme formation in vitro, such that the protoporphyrin concentration could have a rate-limiting role for heme synthesis even if ferrochelatase is partially deficient. ALA synthase is not increased in EPP fibroblasts, perhaps because the requirements for heme synthesis in these cells can be met by a partially deficient level of ferrochelatase. ALA synthase formation would not then be derepressed [257, 258].

Treatment

Mathews-Roth reported in 1970 [555] that oral administration of β-carotene improved the skin symptoms in three EPP patients. Previously she and Sistrom had shown that carotenoid pigments protected bacteria from photooxidative damage [556] and mice from porphyrin photosensitivity [557]. β-Carotene also protects fibroblasts in culture from porphyrin photodamage [558]. The clinical benefit of β-carotene has subsequently been substantiated in much larger series of patients with EPP [559–561]. Tolerance to sunlight is improved in most patients, sometimes very greatly, and this is usually maximal 1 to 3 months after beginning treatment. A dose of 120 to 180 mg daily in adults is usually required to maintain serum carotene levels in the recommended range of 600 to 800 µg/dl [480]. Discoloration of the skin from carotenemia is usually mild and not troublesome to most patients. No other side effects have been described from treatment with pure preparations of β-carotene [480, 560]. Porphyrin levels are not significantly altered by the drug. The mechanism of action of β-carotene is not fully established. Excitation of protoporphyrin by ultraviolet light can result in formation of singlet oxygen or free radicals and there is evidence that these can be quenched by β-carotene [560]. This drug appears to be less effective in CEP and PCT, and for nonporphyric disorders associated with skin photosensitivity [560]. It may provide some protection from photosensitivity after injection of hematoporphyrin in humans [562].

Other treatments have been tried in EPP patients with little or no success. These include antihistamines, sunscreen preparations, aminoquinoline antimalarials, adenosine monophosphate, inosine, vitamin E [480, 563], and zinc [547]. Topical dihydroxyacetone and lawsone (naphthoquinone), which act on keratin to darken the skin, may be useful in some patients [480, 564].

Cholestyramine has been reported to reduce liver protoporphyrin content and photosensitivity in a few patients with EPP [512, 565, 566]. This anion exchange resin may interrupt the enterohepatic circulation of protoporphyrin and increase its removal from the body. Although these initial observations are promising for treating EPP patients with hepatic involvement, further studies are needed. Use of other porphyrin adsorbants have also been considered [485]. Splenectomy has been carried out in a few patients [509, 525] and may be of substantial benefit when EPP is complicated by hemolysis and splenomegaly [509].

Other measures which may be important in the management of EPP include the avoidance of iron deficiency, calorie restriction, and drugs or hormones that may impair hepatic excretory function [512, 521, 567].

Bovine EPP

This disease represents the only genetic porphyria other than CEP known to occur in animals. Unlike the human disease, bovine EPP is an autosomal recessive disorder [260]. Homozygous animals have photosensitivity and marked elevation in circulating red cell protoporphyrin content. The maximal level of protoporphyrin is about seven times that found in erythrocytes in human EPP. There is little or no increase in urine porphyrins, and stool protoporphyrin excretion is considerably increased. As in the human disease, erythrocyte protoporphyrin is not chelated with zinc. Ferrochelatase activity was shown to be only 10 percent of normal in liver, kidney, heart, spleen, and lung of homozygous animals [260]. A functional deficiency of the enzyme could also be shown in cultured skin fibroblasts, and an intermediate defect demonstrated in heterozygous cattle [544].

ACUTE INTERMITTENT PORPHYRIA

Definition

Acute intermittent porphyria (AIP) is an autosomal dominant disorder in which the basic genetic defect is a deficiency of PBG deaminase. Expression of this mutant gene at the level of PBG deaminase appears to be relatively constant, in that this enzyme activity is near 50 percent of normal in all tissues that have been examined and in all subjects who are heterozygotes for AIP. The active clinical syndrome is not determined by a deficiency in PBG deaminase alone. Clinical expression is highly variable and is determined in part by other factors such as steroid hormones, certain of their metabolites, drugs, and nutrition, which are thought to influence the disorder by altering ALA synthase and porphyrin-heme synthetic rates in the liver. Symptoms usually occur as intermittent attacks after puberty, are more common in women than in men, and may occur in relation to hormonal fluctuations with the menstrual cycle. As in HCP, VP, acute porphyria with ALA dehydratase deficiency, plumbism, and perhaps certain patients with hereditary tyrosinemia as well, the symptoms are due to little-understood effects of the disease on the nervous system. Visceral autonomic neuropathy with abdominal pain, ileus, and peripheral neuropathy that can progress to total paralysis are especially prominent manifestations.

The majority (about 90 percent) of subjects who inherit PBG deaminase deficiency remain clinically latent and may never have excess excretion of ALA and PBG. They are presumed to be at risk if exposed to harmful drugs and other factors known to exacerbate AIP, although this presumption is precautionary in nature and not established with certainty in the majority of clinically latent individuals. Increased excretion of ALA and PBG in urine is not found in most heterozygotes who have never had symptoms, but is almost always found even between attacks in individuals in whom the disease has become clinically expressed. Other terms for this disease have included intermittent acute porphyria, pyrroloporphyria, and Swedish porphyria.

Prevalence

In most countries AIP appears to be more common than other genetic porphyrias. It produces neurological symptoms similar to those of HCP and VP. The disease occurs in many races but is probably most common in Scandinavia, Britain, and Ireland. For the population of Sweden, the prevalence was estimated to be 1.5 in 100,000 based on a survey using urine ALA and PBG determinations [568]. Allowing for a high frequency of latent carriers with normal urine ALA and PBG excretion, Wetterberg [569] estimated that the prevalence would be about 7.7 in 100,000 in Sweden. The highest known prevalence (100 in 100,000) is in Lapland. This estimate was based on urine PBG determinations, and all AIP subjects there appear to be related to a single family. The prevalence of AIP is greatly influenced by genetic drift [570].

Surveys using PBG deaminase measurements in the general population have not been carried out, partly because in erythrocytes of AIP patients, which are the cells most conveniently assayed, the range of PBG deaminase activity overlaps the normal range to some degree (see below). Erythrocyte PBG deaminase measurement is most useful in detecting gene carriers in families of known AIP patients. Extensive screening of AIP families can be expected to increase greatly the recognized prevalence of AIP heterozygotes.

Clinical Features

This disease remains clinically latent in most (about 90 percent) individuals. In the minority of PBG deaminase deficient subjects who become ill, the symptoms are usually nonspecific and therefore may not suggest the proper diagnosis unless there is a high index of suspicion. Abdominal pain and a variety of neurovisceral and circulatory disturbances probably all originate from effects of the disease on the nervous system. Photosensitivity rarely if ever occurs [6]. Symptoms have been reported before puberty [571–573] but this is exceptional.

The most common symptoms and signs in AIP, summarized from three large series of patients [574–576] are shown in Table 60-6. Especially noteworthy are abdominal pain and other gastrointestinal complaints, symptoms referrable to the peripheral and central nervous systems, and signs of sympathetic overactivity such as tachycardia and hypertension. Symptoms are characteristically intermittent, although long-term follow-up has revealed a high incidence (~40 percent) of chronic hypertension [577]. Attacks may develop very rapidly and then resolve after a period of days or sometimes weeks in an unpredictable fashion—determined in part by factors that may have exacerbated the disease. Advanced paralysis and death are unlikely to occur unless the diagnosis is made late and the patient is in the meantime treated inadvertently with harmful drugs [578]. Chronic symptoms such as continuing pain, depression, anxiety, and other emotional complaints are difficult to evaluate in AIP patients. Other causes (including drug dependence) should be considered, but it is likely that symptoms in patients with excess excretion of ALA or PBG are due to low-grade continuing activity of the disease itself [6, 579].

Acute attacks usually begin with abdominal pain, although there may be premonitory symptoms such as restlessness, irritability, or discomfort in the chest or back. Constipation or, less frequently, diarrhea may precede and accompany an abdominal crisis. Nausea and vomiting often follow the onset of abdominal pain. Distension due to ileus is common. Bladder dysfunction may result in urinary retention, dysuria, urgency, or incontinence. Pain in the extremities is also common, is often described as muscle pain, and is a manifestation of early peripheral neuropathy. Objective motor weakness does not occur during many attacks even though abdominal pain and ileus may be severe. Motor paresis is an indication that an attack may be more prolonged and debilitating.

The neuropathy in AIP is primarily motor. Weakness often begins in the proximal muscles, and more commonly in the arms than in the legs. Tendon reflexes are usually decreased or absent when neuropathy is advanced, but reflexes may be little affected especially in early stages [580]. Motor innervation to proximal muscles may have a particular sensitivity to metabolic disturbances in porphyria, perhaps related to the stress entailed in their weight-bearing function [580]. Symmetrical or asymmetrical paresis in the extremities may occur and can also be strikingly focal [578, 580]. Cranial nerve involvement can occur, and most commonly the tenth and seventh cranial nerves are affected. Rarely, blindness may result from involvement of optic nerves or the occipital lobes [576, 581, 582]. Sensory symptoms including paresthesias, dysesthesias, and

Table 60-6   Incidence of symptoms and signs in acute intermittent porphyria

Symptoms and signs	Percent incidence		
	Waldenström, 1957 [574], 321 cases	Goldberg, 1959 [575], 50 cases	Stein and Tschudy, 1970 [576], 46 cases
Abdominal pain	85	94	95
Vomiting	59	88	43
Constipation	48	84	48
Diarrhea	9	12	5
Limb, head, neck, or chest pain	—	52	50
Muscle weakness	42	68	60
Sensory loss	9	38	26
Convulsions	10	16	20
Respiratory paralysis	14	10	9
Mental symptoms	55	58	40
Hypertension	40	54	36
Tachycardia	28	64	80
Fever	37	14	9

numbness, with areas of loss of touch and pain sensation may also occur. Muscle weakness may progress and eventuate in respiratory and bulbar paralysis and death. Even advanced stages of porphyric neuropathy are potentially reversible.

Mental disturbances, which include insomnia, anxiety, depression, disorientation, hallucinations, and paranoia, may be severe during acute attacks. Patients may be violent and difficult to control. If porphyria has not been recognized, patients may be treated with drugs that further worsen the disease. Some patients with acute symptoms have been regarded as hysterical [578]. Chronic mental symptoms can also occur, and depression is the most common of these. Insomnia, restlessness, and anxiety may also occur chronically. Abnormal electroencephalograms may be found even in the absence of seizures and suggest an organic brain syndrome.

Few surveys for AIP in psychiatric patients have been reported. In one study 2500 consecutive patients were screened using a qualitative test for PBG in urine (Watson-Schwartz test) and 35 positive results were obtained [583]. Using qualitative and quantitative assays for PBG deaminase four AIP cases were detected in 917 patients at another psychiatric hospital [584]. Ideally, such surveys should be carried out using quantitative assays for urine PBG and erythrocyte PBG deaminase for reasons discussed below.

Seizures are not uncommon during severe exacerbations. Seizures in a patient with AIP are a problem in differential diagnosis and treatment, because they may be a neurological manifestation of AIP, sometimes are due to hyponatremia, or may be due to causes unrelated to porphyria. Treatment is difficult because all antiseizure drugs, with the exception of bromides, have the potential for adversely affecting this disease (see below) [585–587]. Hyponatremia is sometimes due to inappropriate ADH secretion [588], which can reflect damage to the supraoptic nuclei of the hypothalamus, as has been suggested from autopsy findings in some patients [579, 589]. Hyponatremia during acute attacks is not pathognomonic of inappropriate antidiuretic hormone (ADH) secretion, however, and may result simply from vomiting, diarrhea, and poor intake. Some AIP patients have unexplained reductions in total blood and red cell volumes [590], and when this occurs with hyponatremia and evidence of increased ADH secretion the latter can be considered an appropriate response [591]. One such patient who succumbed to the disease had large numbers of vacuoles in the supraoptic and paraventricular nuclei. These findings can reflect a strong stimulus to ADH secretion and do not always represent porphyric degeneration of neurosecretory cells [591]. Patients with hyponatremia and reduced blood volume clearly should not be treated by fluid restriction, as would be proper therapy for inappropriate ADH secretion [590]. Eales et al. [592] in a study of 45 acute porphyric attacks (mostly in patients with VP) concluded that inappropriate ADH secretion is an uncommon cause of hyponatremia and that salt depletion from gastrointestinal loss and poor intake or from excess renal sodium loss is much more frequent. Mild idiopathic impairment of renal function is not infrequent in patients with AIP or VP who have frequent attacks, and it has been suggested but not proven that ALA is nephrotoxic [592, 593]. Less well defined electrolyte abnormalities including hypomagnesemia may also develop in AIP [579]. Hypercalcemia from prolonged immobilization due to paralysis has been reported [594].

Tachycardia and hypertension are very common during attacks of acute porphyria. This may reflect an overactivity of the sympathetic nervous system, and be accompanied by restlessness, coarse or fine tremors, and excess sweating. Catecholamine excretion is often markedly increased during porphyria attacks. Sudden death may occur in such patients, perhaps as a result of cardiac arrhythmias [580, 591].

Abdominal pain in AIP is usually steady and severe although there may be a colicky component due to areas of spasm and distension of the gut. The pain may simulate other abdominal illnesses, especially appendicitis. Porphyria is accompanied usually by little or no fever, and leukocytosis is generally mild or absent. Examination seldom shows abdominal tenderness or signs of peritoneal irritation despite severe pain and often markedly reduced bowel motility. Abdominal pain in porphyria is thought to result from an autonomic neuropathy and not from an inflammatory process.

At the end of an attack, abdominal pain may clear in a matter of hours. Muscle paresis may disappear within a few days. After a severe and prolonged attack there may be residual muscle weakness, but complete or partial improvement in muscle function can follow over a period of months. Recovery from paresis may be incomplete [595]. Goldberg [575] noted that complete recovery of motor function and mental health may sometimes take several years. With proper management and support and avoidance of harmful drugs (see below), the long-term prognosis in AIP is "far from gloomy" [577].

Neurological Dysfunction Pathological changes in the nervous system have been reported from autopsied cases and in a few cases in which nerve biopsies have been taken [580, 596, 597]. The fact that some patients who die during acute attacks show little neuropathological change suggests that a metabolic disturbance is the initial insult, and the histological changes occur only with longer and more severe attacks [580, 598]. Vacuolization and chromatolysis of neurons have been described in anterior horn cells, dorsal root ganglia, splanchnic motor cells, cranial nerve nuclei, and the hypothalamus [580, 596]. The last changes may relate to increased ADH secretion [579]. Demyelinization has been described in peripheral and autonomic nerves and to a lesser degree in the cerebral cortex and cerebellum. Porphyric neuropathy is probably a "dying back" process wherein neuron damage and axonal degeneration precede demyelinization [580, 599, 600]. The hypothesis has also been put forward that a disturbance in myelin metabolism is an essential step in the neuropathy [575] but most evidence appears to point to neuronal degeneration as the primary process [580, 599].

Electrophysiological studies also suggest that an acute axonal neuropathy occurs in AIP [601–603]. In early stages this may be reversible, and is followed by a dying back type of axonal degeneration only in more prolonged attacks [601]. Electromyography shows fibrillation and other evidence of muscle denervation, whereas motor conduction velocity, which reflects the status of the myelin sheath, is less commonly affected. A single report [604] that motor and sensory conduction are frequently slow even in latent AIP and VP is exceptional, but it is difficult to compare these results with other studies because a special method (antidromal blocking) was used to measure conduction in slowly conducting motor fibers. This was reduced in the latent AIP group, whereas maximum motor conduction velocity as in other studies was not affected [603, 604]. Sensory neurons are less affected. Electrophysiological data also suggest that neuropathy in AIP may be accompanied by impaired release of acetylcholine from nerve endings

[601]. Blockade of cholinergic neurotransmission with overactivity of adrenergic nervous functions is consistent with what is observed during acute attacks of AIP, and with the results in vitro of Feldman et al. [605] and Hubbard and Quastel [606].

The mechanism of damage to nervous tissue in AIP is poorly understood [596]. Since PBG deaminase is deficient in all tissues of AIP patients so far examined (see below), this enzyme defect is probably found in the nervous system as well. One hypothesis is that PBG deaminase deficiency limits the formation of heme and important hemeproteins in neurons or supporting cells [607]. The heme content of nervous tissue is relatively small, but cytochromes including cytochrome P_{450} have been identified in brain tissue [379] and obviously support vital cell functions as in other tissues. ALA synthase is present in rat brain and displays developmental changes [53] and regional distribution [608], but whether this enzyme plays a rate-limiting function, as in the liver, has not been demonstrated. Moreover in brain the enzyme is not affected by a number of factors known to induce liver ALA synthase and to exacerbate symptoms in AIP patients [53]. Studies of 9000 g supernatant fractions from rabbit brain indicate that, unlike the liver, free pools of apocytochrome P_{450} may exist in nervous tissue and be capable of complexing with added heme to form functional holocytochrome [609]. Goldberg [575] suggested that an unknown substance produced by the heme pathway in the liver might be essential for nervous system function and that production of this "substance X" might be blocked in AIP. Heme itself could in fact be transported to neurons from other cells such as hepatocytes or glial cells [378, 380–382]. However, there is as yet no direct evidence for this, and De Matteis et al. [609a] have reported that intravenously administered [^{14}C]heme does not enter the brain. Present knowledge of heme metabolism and regulation in neural tissue is therefore insufficient to assess the consequences of a presumed PBG deaminase deficiency in the nervous system.

Alternatively, it has been postulated that ALA or PBG might in some manner be toxic to the nervous system. This idea is favored by increases in production of these precursors in AIP patients during acute attacks [596]. Although increased ALA and PBG excretion is found in some clinically latent heterozygotes for AIP, symptoms of AIP never occur when porphyrin precursor excretion is normal [596]. If excess amounts of these materials do alter neural function in AIP, it is likely that they would originate from nonnervous tissues, particularly the liver, because ALA synthase appears to be noninducible in brain [53]. ALA appears to be taken up by tissues more readily than PBG, whereas the opposite seems the case with respect to passage across the blood-brain barrier [338]. The ability of ALA to cross the blood-brain barrier is quite limited [610], but in rats and mice this can nonetheless occur at plasma concentrations close to those observed in porphyria patients [611–613] and brain ALA can remain elevated after blood levels have returned to normal [613]. Moreover rabbit brain slices can concentrate ALA in vitro [596, 614]. ALA and PBG are found in spinal fluid of patients during acute porphyric attacks [338, 600, 615]. Phenobarbital does not increase ALA uptake into brain or alter the amount of exogenous ALA excreted in urine [614, 616]. Uptake of labeled ALA is greater in the hypothalamus than in other areas of the brain in the rat, a finding that may relate to the development of inappropriate ADH secretion in acute porphyria [610].

Early studies indicated that ALA and PBG have no pharmacological effects in animals [617–621], and porphobilin (an oxidation product of PBG) has no effect on behavior, blood pressure, or pulse when injected as a bolus into rats [622]. Studies of rats with AIA-induced porphyria, however, provided some evidence for neurotoxic effects possibly due to porphyrin precursors: these animals excreted excess ALA and PBG, were somnolent [623], had weakness and ataxia of the hind legs [624], and increased susceptibility to convulsions induced by isonicotinic acid hydrazide or 4-methoxymethylpyridoxal [625]. Recent work has shown that ALA administration to rodents causes behavioral effects [611, 626], and that ALA has transitory behavioral effects when directly administered into the central nervous system [610, 627]. Both ALA and PBG have been shown to induce convulsions when injected into the lateral ventricle of the rat [610, 628]. ALA appears to enter cells more readily than PBG and can then be converted to porphyrins in substantial amounts, but the toxic potential of porphyrins derived in this manner from excess ALA has been little studied [280, 620, 629].

Effects of porphyrin precursors on nerve-muscle function have been more convincingly demonstrated in vitro. ALA, PBG, and also porphobilin, inhibit transmitter (acetylcholine) release in the rat hemidiaphragm [605, 630, 631]. ALA is structurally similar to γ-aminobutyric acid (GABA) and may activate GABA receptors in motor and sensory neurons [632–634]. Barbiturates facilitate the synaptic actions of GABA, and could therefore also potentiate the GABAergic effects of ALA [633]. ALA can also inhibit [Na^+, K^+]ATPase [635], impair Na^+ and water transport across frog skin [636, 637], depolarize muscle fibers [638], inhibit frog skeletal muscle response to electrical or nerve stimulation [639], depress ventral and dorsal root potentials in the frog spinal cord [640], and inhibit contractile activity of the rabbit duodenum [641]. These effects occur mostly at concentrations (10^{-4} to 10^{-3} M) greater than those found in spinal fluid of AIP patients [615, 631], although plasma levels may sometimes be in this range [641]. ALA can, however, inhibit potassium depolarization-induced GABA release from preloaded synaptosomes in vitro at much lower concentrations (10^{-5} M) [634, 642]. Moreover the uptake system for ALA into brain tissue could limit egress of ALA from brain to spinal fluid and result in brain ALA concentrations that are about one-half those of plasma [612, 626, 633]. ALA may therefore act as an agonist at presynaptic GABA receptors in the nervous system.

Increased excretion of pyrrolic material other than PBG, noted as an Ehrlich-positive spot on chromatograms of human urine, has been reported in some patients with AIP or schizophrenia. This "mauve factor" has been very difficult to characterize. It was initially thought to be kryptopyrrole (2,4-dimethyl-3-ethyl-pyrrole) [644] but has recently been identified as an oxidized form of hemopyrrole, hydroxyhemopyrrolene-5-one [645, 646]. The origin of this compound is unknown, but it and related pyrroles may have biological effects including influences on the heme pathway [647]. But as methods for its measurement have improved, its role in porphyria and schizophrenia appears to have become less certain [648]. Brown-colored pigments identified as dipyrrylmethenes also occur in the urine of AIP patients and are more likely to have been formed from PBG than by catabolism of porphyrins [649].

Hypertension and tachycardia correlate with the amount of excess catecholamine excretion in attacks of AIP [650, 651]. The cause of the increased catecholamines is unclear. Studies employing intact platelets as a model system for norepinephrine uptake indicate that uptake is blocked by ALA or PBG in cells from AIP patients but not in normal cells. Thus reuptake of norepinephrine by adrenergic neurons may in some manner be impaired in AIP patients [651]. Autonomic neuropathy and denervation of baroreceptors may be other mechanisms contributing to elevated catecholamines [651, 652].

Precipitating Factors Most heterozygotes for PBG deaminase deficiency remain asymptomatic through all or most of their lives. Certain precipitating factors cause the disease to become clinically expressed. The majority of these factors appear to act by inducing ALA synthase, the rate-limiting enzyme for hepatic heme synthesis. Under some circumstances it is possible also that activity of the deficient PBG deaminase may be further reduced in the liver, but this has not been directly shown. In a given patient a number of predisposing factors may exist and each may contribute to the exacerbation of AIP.

Endogenous hormones are probably the most important additional factors that result in clinical expression of the PBG deaminase defect in heterozygotes for AIP. This is indicated by: (1) the rarity of symptoms or of excess PBG excretion before puberty, (2) more common clinical expression of AIP in women than in men, (3) fluctuation of severity in relation to the menstrual cycle and pregnancy in some women, (4) reports that oral contraceptive steroids can exacerbate AIP or in other instances suppress activity of the disease by reducing the endogenous production of hormones, and (5) the demonstration in patients who have been ill with AIP of alterations in steroid hormone metabolism that predispose to the excess production of steroid hormone metabolites that experimentally are inducers of ALA synthase in liver.

The increased susceptibility to develop attacks after puberty and the greater incidence of symptoms in women points to an important role of sex hormones in this disease. In AIP it is not established which endogenous hormones are primarily responsible for clinical expression of the disease. Androgens are suspect because large amounts are produced by the adrenals and gonads in both men and women, and their metabolites, especially those with the 5β structural configuration, are potent inducers of hepatic ALA synthase. Female sex hormones may play an important role as well, and in rat liver ALA synthase has been shown to fluctuate with the normal female estrus cycle [653]. Many so-called estrogenic effects have been noted in AIP patients, such as hyperlipidemia, impaired BSP metabolism, and increased thyroid hormone binding globulin (see below). Estrogens are relatively weak inducers of ALA synthase when compared with androgen metabolites, progesterone, or progesterone metabolites in animal systems. Progesterone can also increase heme breakdown in vivo in women, although the site of this action is not established [654, 655]. Greater changes in progesterone production occur during the menstrual cycle than for estrogens, and cyclical attacks are most common in the luteal (premenstrual) phase when progesterone levels are highest. There are no gross abnormalities in progesterone metabolism in AIP [657], but patients are likely to have an abnormal sensitivity to this hormone, as they do to barbiturates, etc. Progesterone administration has been reported to cause attacks of AIP [658]. Welland et al. [659] noted that ethynylestradiol administration (0.3 to 0.45 mg daily) produced increased ALA and PBG excretion in seven AIP patients maintained on a constant diet but only one had

symptoms suggesting an exacerbation. Increased ALA and PBG excretion also occurred when an elderly man with latent porphyria (probably VP or HCP) was given stilbestrol 5 mg per os daily by Watson et al. [660]. Many synthetic steroids including estrogens and progestins have a 17α-ethynyl substituent on the steroid molecule, and it has been recently shown that when large doses of such synthetic steroids are given to animals they can interact with cytochrome P_{450} to destroy the heme moiety of cytochrome P_{450} and form "green pigments" in the liver [314–317]. A similar destruction of cytochrome P_{450} heme occurs with the porphyrogenic agent AIA [311]. Thus some synthetic steroids may have particular inducing effects on ALA synthase that relate to their capacity to increase heme breakdown and differ from those of natural steroids. For this and other reasons (see Treatment) the results of studies in which AIP patients have been treated with synthetic sex steroids are difficult to interpret.

Because so many subjects with PBG deaminase deficiency remain clinically latent despite normal hormonal and reproductive function, more subtle differences in steroid hormone metabolism in clinically latent and clinically expressed AIP have been investigated. In these studies defective 5α-reduction of steroid hormones in patients with AIP and a history of clinical expression of the disease has been described in the majority of patients examined (Figs. 60-22 and 60-23) [662–665]. This alteration in hormone biotransformation, which results in an activity of 5α-reductase in liver which averages about one-half of normal (Fig. 60-23), is not found in clinically latent gene carriers [665] and therefore represents a clear hormone metabolic difference between this group of PBG deaminase deficient subjects and those in whom AIP has become clinically expressed. The defect is confined to the liver, which metabolizes the bulk of endogenous steroid hormones, and does not appear to affect steroid 5α-reductase activity in skin [666]. Impaired steroid 5α-reduction is important in AIP as it favors compensatory formation of 5β-steroid metabolites, and many of the latter steroids are known to be more potent inducers of ALA synthase than are their corresponding 5α-epimers [272, 273, 276]. Interestingly, Paxton et al. [667] found increased urinary outputs of 5β-steroids in urine and higher than normal concentrations of such steroids in the blood of patients with AIP during acute attacks. Observations in a single parent-patient set [169] indicated that while the propositus showed both the PBG deaminase deficiency and the 5α-reductase defect, her father (who also carried the AIP gene defect) had entirely normal steroid metabolism, while her mother had normal PBG deaminase activity but a greater defect in 5α-reduction than the propositus [169]. This family lineage, in which a genetic determinant could account in part for the 5α-reductase deficiency, must be rare since hereditary aberrations of 5α-reductase are extremely uncommon, and study of several other parent-propositus sets have demonstrated the 5α-reductase deficiency only in the propositus [665]. Therefore, even though patterns of steroid hormone metabolism in animals and humans can be substantially influenced by genetic factors [668–670], and although there is a well-documented description in humans of a genetic defect in at least one steroid 5α-reductase [671], it appears likely that impaired steroid 5α-reduction in clinically expressed AIP is primarily an acquired abnormality. Genetic influences other than PBG deaminase deficiency may be nonetheless important in clinical expression of AIP. Susceptibility to development of impaired steroid 5α-reduction may, for example, be subject to genetic control and

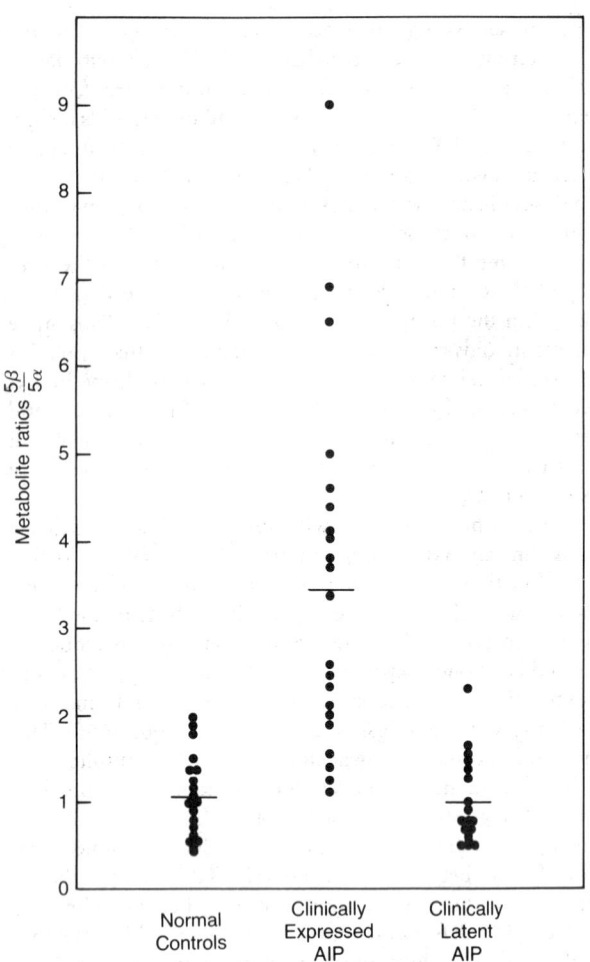

Figure 60-22 Disproportionate generation of 5β- as compared with 5α-steroid metabolites from radiolabeled testosterone in patients with AIP and a history of prior clinical expression of the disease, in contrast to normal testosterone metabolism in subjects carrying the gene defect of AIP but in whom the disease has never been expressed clinically. This abnormality of steroid metabolism can also be demonstrated with other C_{19} steroids such as dehydroisoandrosterone. (*From Anderson, Bradlow, Sassa, and Kappas* [665]. *By permission of the American Journal of Medicine.*)

that certain drugs may precipitate AIP attacks in part by acting through the endocrine system, or that endogenous humoral agents in such patients may have biological properties that lead to a defect in steroid 5α-reduction and also provoke the disease. Endogenous substances that induce ALA synthase in cultured cells have been identified in sera of patients with clinically expressed AIP [328, 329]. Regardless of its mechanism, the occurrence of the defect in 5α-reduction of steroid hormones in clinically expressed AIP patients and its absence in clinically latent individuals who inherit AIP indicates that subtle endocrine abnormalities are implicated in clinical expression of the disease.

Exacerbations of AIP can occur during pregnancy [574]. Worsening of symptoms during pregnancy has been associated with the use of barbiturates and perhaps reduced caloric intake, but most studies indicate that patients generally do well during pregnancy [677, 678]. This is surprising because progesterone levels are markedly increased during pregnancy and this hormone and its metabolites are potent inducers of liver ALA synthase [276, 674]. As reviewed elsewhere [679], the hepatic metabolism of progesterone is not fully defined, and only about one-half of a radiolabeled tracer dose of the hormone is accounted for by urinary excretion of progesterone metabolites. A significant portion of the remainder is excreted in bile and feces. The major metabolite in urine is 5β-pregnane-3α,20α-diol glucuronide. This compound and 5-pregnane-3β,20α-diol disulfate are the predominant biliary metabolites, but there is biliary excretion of 5α-pregnane metabolites as well. During late pregnancy progesterone appears to be largely reduced to 5α-pregnane compounds [680], and such metabolites are weaker inducers of ALA synthase as compared with 5β-compounds [276]. There is also evidence that progesterone can increase the 5α-reduction of testosterone and other C_{19} steroids [681] and could thereby reduce the formation of porphyrinogenic 5β-metabolites of androgens. Also, in the pregnant rat hepatic ALA synthase becomes highly refractory to induction by the porphyrogenic agent AIA [348, 682], and it is possible that the human liver enzyme may also become refractory to induction during gestation. Humoral agents have also been found in human serum during late pregnancy and the early postpartum period that can markedly inhibit the porphyrinogenesis elicited in cultured liver cells by a wide variety of chemicals [329]. Thus, there are a number of beneficial metabolic changes during pregnancy that can account in part for the absence of acute attacks in most AIP patients, despite an apparently adverse hormonal environment from the great increases in steroid hormone production that take place during gestation.

Drugs are frequently the direct cause of AIP attacks, and many patients do well after the proper diagnosis is made and harmful drugs are avoided. Nevertheless some patients continue to have exacerbations of AIP even though drugs are not ingested. Drugs are rarely reported to cause acute symptoms of porphyria in children with PBG deaminase deficiency [571, 586]. For example, in our clinic we have followed one prepubertal female with PBG deaminase deficiency (detected as part of a large family study) who was treated with phenobarbital and diphenylhydantoin for epilepsy by her neurologist for several years prior to the diagnosis of latent AIP and for some time thereafter; this patient has never displayed elevated PBG in urine or symptoms of porphyria. She is now postpubertal. Drug use is no longer necessary since the epilepsy has subsided, and she continues to have normal excretion of porphyrin pre-

this susceptibility may be greater in PBG deaminase-deficient individuals who develop active AIP as compared with those in whom AIP remains clinically latent. With regard to additional heritable influences, genetic control of δ-aminolevulinate synthase induction has been demonstrated in animals [672], and there is evidence in man for genetic control of tissue responsiveness to steroid hormones [673].

How a major defect in steroid 5α-reduction may be acquired in some AIP patients is not clear. The defect is not due to abnormal porphyrin metabolism per se, since it is not found in patients with PCT [662, 663]. Moreover it probably is not a dietary effect because a high carbohydrate intake, as is encouraged in AIP patients, enhances rather than inhibits steroid 5α-reduction in vivo in normal subjects [674]. Neonatal imprinting, which can influence adult patterns of hormone metabolism, is a possibly important influence on the steroid 5α- and 5β-reductases in humans [675] and deserves further study. Such a process could predispose to a detrimental pattern of hormone metabolism in some PBG deaminase-deficient subjects. Also, phenobarbital can impair steroid 5α-reduction, at the same time enhancing cytochrome P_{450} mediated oxidation of drugs [676]. This finding raises the interesting possibility

cursors. Thus drugs alone may not necessarily exacerbate AIP, unless the hormonal milieu or other factors—perhaps unique to only a small population of PBG deaminase-deficient individuals—favor the induction of ALA synthase. This view is supported by a recent large retrospective study of risk from anesthetic use in AIP and VP in which it was concluded that barbiturates or other inducing drugs quite frequently are detrimental to patients who already have acute symptoms of porphyria but seldom exacerbate latent disease [683]. Nonetheless drugs known to be potentially harmful should be avoided in AIP patients and in all relatives found to have PBG deaminase deficiency, including children, since it remains at present unpredictable which individuals with the enzyme deficiency will prove sensitive to provocation of their disease by such substances.

Barbiturates are most notorious for producing exacerbations of AIP. Their introduction in 1903 produced a great increase in the number of severe AIP cases and led to more widespread recognition of the disease. Goldberg in 1959 [575] noted that paralysis occurred much more commonly when a patient had taken a barbiturate than when an acute attack developed without barbiturate intake. Unrecognized cases can be expected to fare better now that these agents are less used as minor tranquilizers and sedatives than in the past. Short-acting intravenous barbiturates are still widely employed for induction of anesthesia, and their use can elicit severe and sometimes

Figure 60-23 Deficient 5α-reduction of the adrenal steroid 11-hydroxyandrostenedione in patients with clinically expressed AIP, and normal 5α-reduction of this steroid in clinically latent AIP. Metabolism of this adrenal steroid provides a specific assessment of hepatic steroid 5α-reductase activity for this hormonal substrate because this compound is normally metabolized almost exclusively by 5α-reduction. (*From Anderson, Bradlow, Sassa, and Kappas [665]. By permission of the American Journal of Medicine.*)

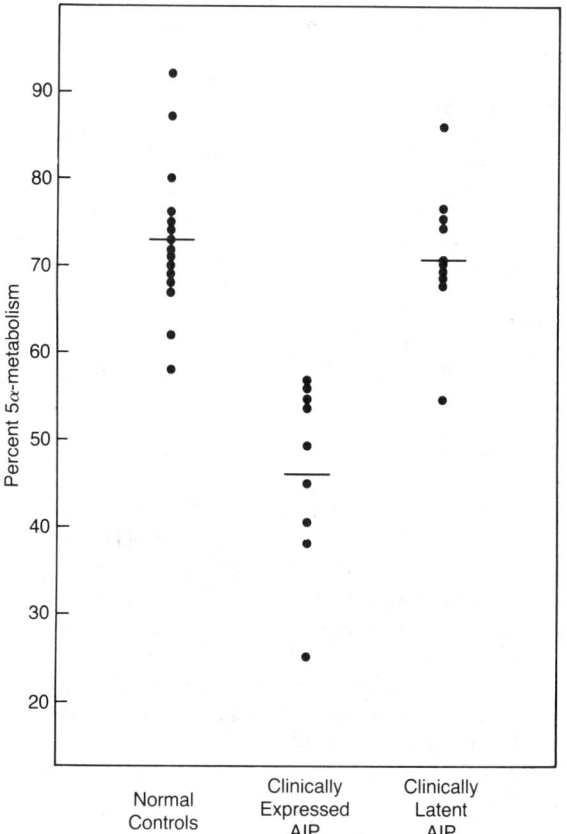

lethal exacerbations of AIP in previously unrecognized carriers of this genetic disease.

Most harmful drugs have the capacity to alter heme metabolism in the liver and to induce ALA synthase. The latter may result from induction of cytochrome P_{450}, which increases the demand for newly synthesized heme in the liver, and therefore causes an increased formation of the rate-limiting enzyme for heme formation, ALA synthase. Induction of ALA synthase also may occur by other mechanisms. Therefore all drugs that can induce ALA synthase or cytochrome P_{450} or lead to increased hepatic heme destruction in humans, experimental animals, or cultured liver cells should be avoided in AIP. Inducing effects of drugs are dose-related, and doses that cause induction in experimental systems may on a body-weight basis greatly exceed doses employed clinically. On the other hand, some drugs are harmful to porphyria patients but have never been shown to induce ALA synthase or cytochrome P_{450}; the sulfonamide antibiotics are an important example of this. Sulfonamides appear to act by inhibiting liver PBG deaminase and thereby accentuating the deficiency of this enzyme in the liver of AIP patients [685].

As shown in Table 60-7, a number of drugs (designated category I) have been implicated on many occasions as causing attacks of AIP, HCP, or VP in susceptible individuals and should be particularly avoided. A few drugs in this group are not known themselves to induce attacks but are closely related chemically to known harmful drugs. Almost all compounds in category I also induce ALA synthase or otherwise perturb liver heme biosynthesis in animals or cultured liver cells. Additional drugs can induce heme synthesis in experimental systems (category II). Although seldom or never reported as harmful in porphyria patients, these should be used with caution and only when an alternative medication known to be safe is not suitable. Drugs in category III are with some exceptions not porphyrinogenic in experimental systems; the few that are porphyrinogenic are weakly so and have appeared safe when given to patients. Drugs in this category are also preferably avoided because experience in patients with porphyria is limited. Drugs in category IV are regarded as safe based on extensive clinical experience and the absense of porphyrinogenic effects in model systems. Other reviews and lists relating to drug use in the acute porphyrias have also been published [6, 332, 685–687]. Choice of anesthetic agents has been recently studied in animal models and reviewed [683, 688–690].

Few drugs are definitely known to induce ALA synthase in human liver. Anticonvulsants (phenobarbital or diphenylhydantoin) are the only drugs other than alcohol [691] demonstrated in tissue obtained by liver biopsy in humans to be associated with increased ALA synthase activity [692] to our knowledge. A number of other drugs in categories I and II (Table 60-7) may increase cytochrome P_{450} content or function in humans and are therefore suspected to increase liver heme synthesis. But for many other drugs no information is available as to their safety for use in porphyric subjects. There is therefore a need to screen drugs for their capacity to induce ALA synthase and cytochrome P_{450} in order that such data may provide guidance in the treatment of AIP patients. The most convenient and sensitive test systems include the chick embryo liver in ovo (particularly after treatment with a ferrochelatase inhibitor to enhance porphyrin accumulation) [254] and cultured chick embryo liver cells [45, 273]. A number of other test systems have also been proposed [326, 693, 694].

Nutrition is another important influence on the clinical

Table 60-7 Categories of safe and unsafe drugs for AIP, HCP, and VP*

I. *Unsafe*
Barbiturates [574, 576, 686, 805]
Sulfonamide antibiotics [576, 686, 805]
Sulfonmethane (Sulfonal) [1006]
Sulfonethylmethane (Trional) [1006]
Meprobamate [331, 686, 1007]
Isopropylmeprobamate [1007]
Glutethimide [331, 686, 1008]
Aminoglutethimide [1008]
Methyprylon [331, 686, 1008]
Ethchlorvynol [685]
Carbromal [1009]
Ethinamate [1009]
Diphenylhydantoin [331, 576, 585, 587, 686, 1010]
Mephenytoin [686, 1008]
Succinimides [1007, 1008]
Pyrazolone preparations [686]
Griseofulvin [45, 346]
Ergot preparations [331, 686]
Danazol [773, 774]
Synthetic estrogens, progestins [331, 686, 772]
Carbamazepine [686, 1010]
Valproic acid [587, 686, 1011]
Primadone [686]
Trimethadione [686, 1008]
Diclophenac [686, 1012]
Novobiocin [686]
N-Butylscopolammonium bromide [686]
Tolbutamide [45, 331, 1008]
Tolazamide [1009]
Chlorpropamide [331, 1008, 1009]

II. *Potentially unsafe*
2-Allyloxy-3-methylbenzamide [1013]
Alfaxolone [688, 1014]
Alfadolone acetate [688, 1014]
Hydralazine [254]
Clonidine [254]
Phenoxybenzamine [254]
o,p¹-DDD [1008]
Tolazamide [346]
Methyldopa [331]
Alkylating agents [685]
Tranylcypromine [1008]
Theophylline [685]
Spironolactone [254]
Rifampicin [1015]
Pargyline [254, 1008]

Bemegride [685]
Nikethamide [685, 1008, 1009]
Pentylenetetrazole [685, 1008]
Metyrapone [1008]
Food additives [678, 685]
Pyrazinamide [685, 687]
Pentazocine [331]
Chloroquine [331]
Heavy metals [331, 685, 1016]
Fluroxene [1017]
Etomidate [688]
Ketamine [690]

III. *Probably safe*
Diazepam [686, 1008]
Chlordiazepoxide [686, 1008]
Dicumarol [6]
Digoxin [686]
Imipramine [685]
Chloramphenicol [686, 1008]
Nitrofurantoin [6]
Mandelamine [6]
Rauwolfia alkaloids [6]
Diphenhydramine [1008]
Vitamin B group [6]
Vitamin C [6]
Neostigmine [6]
Prostigmin [6]
Propoxyphene [6]
Propanidid [6]
Nitrous oxide [6]
Methylphenidate [1008]
Guanethidine [6]

IV. *Safe*
Narcotic analgesics [254, 686]
Chloral hydrate [254, 575]
Phenothiazines [254, 686]
Penicillin and derivatives [6]
Aspirin [686]
Acetaminophen [686]
Streptomycin [6]
Tetracycline [6]
Glucocorticoids [6]
Propranolol [6]
Bromides [585, 587, 678]
Insulin [685]
Atropine [685]
Amitryptyline [686]

* Drugs are not listed alphabetically; barbiturates and sulfonamide antibiotics are at the top of the list of unsafe drugs on the basis of extensive reports in the literature.

expression of AIP [345, 348, 695]. A low calorie intake, usually instituted in an effort to lose excess weight, is a common contributing cause of attacks. Welland et al. [345] demonstrated that a 60 to 80 percent reduction in optimal calorie intake in AIP patients was associated with a significant rise in the urinary excretion of both ALA and PBG. The isocaloric partial substitution of fat for protein, or for both protein and carbohydrate, also increased porphyrin precursor excretion. These changes were reversible on return to an optimal dietary intake. Excretion of PBG was decreased if added carbohydrate was given to a patient already on an adequate diet [345] or if

carbohydrate intake was increased from 150 g to 300 g daily (substituting carbohydrate for fat) [695]. Glycerol may be useful as a substitute for glucose [695]. Felsher and Redeker [348] have noted also the potential of caloric or carbohydrate restriction to precipitate acute symptoms as well as to increase porphyrin precursor excretion in AIP. Even brief periods of starvation during weight reduction, during postoperative periods, or with intercurrent illnesses should be avoided in patients with this disease [348].

Starvation enhances and glucose or protein can repress the inducing effect of AIA on ALA synthase and PBG excretion in animals [347, 624, 696]. An adequate explanation for this "glucose effect" on ALA synthase remains elusive [697]. A number of possible mechanisms, including catabolite repression and mediation by cyclic AMP are unlikely [347, 697, 698]. Repression of ALA synthase is probably mediated by glucose itself or perhaps G-6-P. Efficient precursors of hepatic glucose, such as fructose and glycerol also repress the enzyme [698]. The effect of glucose is not prevented by impaired glucose utilization in animals. In patients the benefit of glucose is apparently not enhanced by simultaneous administration of insulin [695]. Other mechanisms that have been suggested include increased glucuronidation of porphyrinogenic endogenous steroids [273, 360] and increased levels of NADPH, ATP, or glycogen [697]. Tschudy [697] concluded that none of the proposed mechanisms fully explains all the experimental and clinical data on the glucose effect on ALA synthase in the liver.

Infections, other intercurrent illnesses, and major surgery may precipitate acute attacks of AIP. The mechanisms involved are not established, but reduced food intake is probably important. Under situations of metabolic stress the production of steroid hormones as well as their ALA synthase-inducing metabolites can also increase and contribute to activation of AIP [579, 667].

Other Organ Systems   The liver in AIP contains excess PBG and sometimes porphyrin, but is usually otherwise normal. AIP can be described as a disorder affecting hepatic heme biosynthesis but generally not impairing overall hepatic function. Mild unexplained abnormalities in liver function, especially minimally increased serum transaminases, and nonspecific morphological changes are not uncommon. The latter are less severe than in PCT [699]. Alterations in cortisol metabolism in AIP also suggest liver damage [700]. Impaired excretion of BSP is not uncommon in clinically expressed AIP and is often seen in the absence of other abnormalities in liver function. Patients with abnormal BSP retention studied by Stein et al. [701], for example, had normal clearances of indocyanine green and radiolabeled bilirubin. The second component of the biexponential decay of BSP in plasma was delayed in some AIP patients, and this suggests either normal uptake of the dye by the liver but impaired biliary excretion with enhanced reflux into the circulation [701] or a defect in glutathione conjugation. Hepatic glutathione content is reduced in experimental porphyria due to AIA [702, 703]. Cirrhosis and hemosiderosis can occasionally be found in AIP [591]. Several AIP patients also had Gilbert's syndrome [576, 701, 704].

AIP can be associated with reduced red cell and total blood volumes [590]. Blood hemoglobin content is generally normal and these reductions probably reflect abnormalities in regulation of salt and water metabolism. There appears to be no impairment of hemoglobin synthesis in this disease. Patients are usually not anemic, and have normal rates of total bilirubin production, which is mostly of erythroid origin, and normal hepatic bilirubin production as determined by studies using radiolabeled glycine and ALA [590, 705].

It is estimated that approximately 40 percent of AIP patients have hypercholesterolemia [579, 706], and this is due to an increase in low density or β-lipoprotein concentration [707]. Glycerides on the other hand are normal. Whether there is a specific metabolic or genetic relationship between hypercholesterolemia and AIP has not been established. It is possible that hypercholesterolemia may be induced by a high carbohydrate intake in some patients. Hyperlipidemia has been noted in animals with chemically induced porphyria [706, 708, 709] and in humans exposed to the potent porphyrogenic chemical TCDD [710].

A number of endocrine abnormalities apart from inappropriate ADH secretion and deficient steroid 5α-reductase activity have been noted in AIP patients. Mild impairment of glucose tolerance, sometimes with an exaggerated but delayed insulin response, is not uncommon [712], but frankly diabetic responses are seldom observed [695]. Inappropriate release of growth hormone after a glucose load was reported in several AIP patients [713] but was not a feature in a later study [695]. The development of late-onset diabetes has not been associated with a worsening in the clinical course of an AIP patient followed in our clinic [674].

Patients with AIP sometimes have increased thyroxine and thyroxine-binding globulin levels in serum in spite of euthyroidism [714, 715]. In some patients this may be a manifestation of mild liver dysfunction [714]. Hyperthyroidism can occur in AIP patients [716, 717], and it has been suggested that porphyria can itself be a "neurogenic" cause of that disorder [717].

Haust and Haegy [711] have demonstrated perchlorate-induced radiolabeled iodide loss from the thyroid gland in patients with hereditary hepatic porphyrias or lead poisoning. This may suggest an alteration of thyroid peroxidase leading to impaired iodide organification in such disorders of porphyrin metabolism. Thyroid peroxidase is a hemeprotein that, as with tryptophan pyrrolase in the liver, may not be fully saturated with its heme prosthetic group and thus can be subject to regulation by the availability of heme [711].

Endocrine derangements that suggest hypothalamic involvement have been reported in AIP. Other than inappropriate ADH secretion, these include diabetes insipidus, galactorrhea [579], and an isolated deficiency of ACTH secretion [718].

One patient with AIP had primary aldosteronism [719]. Attacks of porphyria continued after removal of the aldosteronoma.

AIP has been reported in association with a number of other uncommon diseases, including systemic lupus erythematosus [720], relapsing pancreatitis [704], and transient hyperamylasemia or macroamylasemia [6, 721] and also with Gilbert's syndrome [704]. It is unclear whether these are chance associations or if there are pathogenetic links between AIP and these disorders.

Biochemical Findings

During acute attacks, patients with AIP excrete markedly excessive quantities of ALA and PBG in urine (Table 60-4). PBG excretion is generally in the range of 50 to 200 mg/day in ill AIP patients, and ALA excretion (mg/day) is about one-half that for PBG [619]. In individuals in whom the disease has become clinically expressed, the excretion of ALA and PBG usually remains increased between attacks as well. Further increases during exacerbations can often be demonstrated [722]. Concentrations of uroporphyrin and other porphyrins may be increased in AIP patients with high ALA and PBG levels, and probably result partly from nonenzymatic formation of uroporphyrin from PBG. Since increased porphyrins in the urine of AIP patients are predominantly of the isomer III series, it has been suggested that they may originate from metabolism of porphyrin precursors in nonhepatic tissues [723]. Extensive metabolism of ALA to porphyrins can indeed occur in nonhepatic tissues of animals after ALA loading [280]. PBG is itself a colorless compound, and reddish urine in AIP is due to increased porphyrins and also to the formation of porphobilin, a spontaneous degradation product of PBG. Nonenzymatic formation of both uroporphyrin and porphobilin is favored by acid, heat, or exposure to light. Urine may also contain brown dipyrrylmethenes [649, 724]. Stool porphyrins are normal or only mildly increased in AIP [725].

PBG is most readily detected by the formation of a reddish-purple chromogen with Ehrlich's aldehyde (p-dimethylamino-benzaldehyde). The preferred method for measuring urine PBG is that developed by Mauzerall and Granick [98] and includes the separation of PBG from interfering substances in urine by a simple and rapid anion exchange column technique, followed by addition of Ehrlich's reagent and quantitation by spectrophotometry. Positive urines are obvious also by visual inspection at this stage. This method is sensitive and very few false-positive results have been reported, although patients treated with phenothiazines sometimes show an atypical green-blue chromogen by this method [726]. Quantitative measurement of daily PBG output is useful for providing an index of disease activity over time in an AIP patient. Prepacked plastic columns for this method are commercially available. An additional "piggy-back" cation exchange column can be used for the separation and quantitation of ALA [98].

The Watson-Schwartz test [727, 728] is more widely used to detect excess PBG in urine, even though it is only slightly more rapid than the column method, is less sensitive, does not quantitate PBG, more commonly gives false-positive results, and is more subject to misinterpretation. In this method Ehrlich's reagent is added directly to an equal volume of urine. Compounds other than PBG, including urobilinogen, indole, and others that are poorly characterized, can also react with the aldehyde to form chromogens. For differentiation, extractions with chloroform and butanol are carried out; with these solvents and at the proper pH the PBG chromogen remains in the aqueous phase. Positive results in surveys using the Watson-Schwartz test have been highly variable, ranging from 0 in 1000 to 47 in 91 in eight studies, and this is undoubtedly due to problems of interpretation of color that may remain in the aqueous phase after extraction [6, 569]. If the Watson-Schwartz test is used, positive results should always be confirmed on the same sample by the column method. The Hoesch test, wherein a few drops of urine are added to a larger volume of Ehrlich's reagent, has also been advocated for bedside screening [729, 730]. The basis of this test is that PBG chromogen forms and is visible in strongly acid solution such as Ehrlich's reagent, whereas urobilinogen produces no color under these conditions. This test is similar in sensitivity to the Watson-Schwartz test but is less sensitive and specific than the Mauzerall-Granick method [730, 731].

Normal serum contains little or no ALA and PBG (10 μg/dl or less), whereas in acute exacerbations of AIP levels of PBG may increase to 20 to 300 μg/dl (0.8 to 12×10^{-6} M). ALA levels are usually less than one-half of the serum PBG levels (when expressed as μg/dl) in such patients, whereas the reverse is the case in lead poisoning [167]. Excess PBG has been found at autopsy in the liver and kidney, and the liver may also con-

tain some uroporphyrin [386, 575]. Marked increases in liver ALA and PBG with normal porphyrin content have also been noted at autopsy [600].

Genetic Defect

AIP is one of the few autosomal dominant disorders in which a specific enzyme deficiency has been clearly established. Decreased activity of PBG deaminase has been demonstrated in the liver [166, 167], erythrocytes [136, 168, 171, 732], cultured skin fibroblasts [172–174, 732], cultured amniotic cells [174, 732], and mitogen-stimulated lymphocytes [175] of AIP patients. Thus this enzyme deficiency has been shown in all tissues so far examined. PBG deaminase activity is about 50 percent of normal in tissues of AIP subjects. Considerably greater reductions in the enzyme have been noted in the liver in some cases, particularly at autopsy, but this may partly reflect postmortem alterations [167].

PBG deaminase is most readily measured in erythrocytes (Fig. 60-24). Although the mean enzyme activity is about 50 percent of the mean for normal subjects, a wide range of values is obtained and some overlap occurs between the normal and AIP groups [169]. There is little intraindividual variation in normal or AIP subjects tested repeatedly. The deficient enzyme activity does not vary with disease activity in AIP. Little or no overlap occurs when the enzyme is measured in cultured fibroblasts (Fig. 60-25) or mitogen-stimulated lymphocytes (Fig. 60-26) [174, 175, 732]. Red cell PBG deaminase, which is known to vary strikingly with red cell age [134, 138], also shows considerable interindividual variation (about threefold). Studies in twins indicate that this interindividual variation in the general population is in large part genetically determined [136].

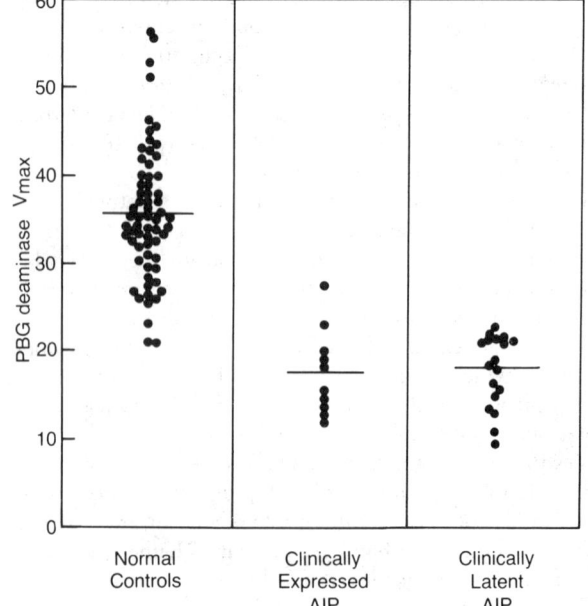

Figure 60-24 Erythrocyte PBG deaminase activities in normal subjects, patients with clinically expressed AIP, and individuals with clinically latent AIP. Activity of this enzyme is approximately 50 percent deficient in clinically expressed or latent AIP subjects and does not vary with disease activity. There is some overlap between the AIP and normal ranges of this enzyme activity in red cells.

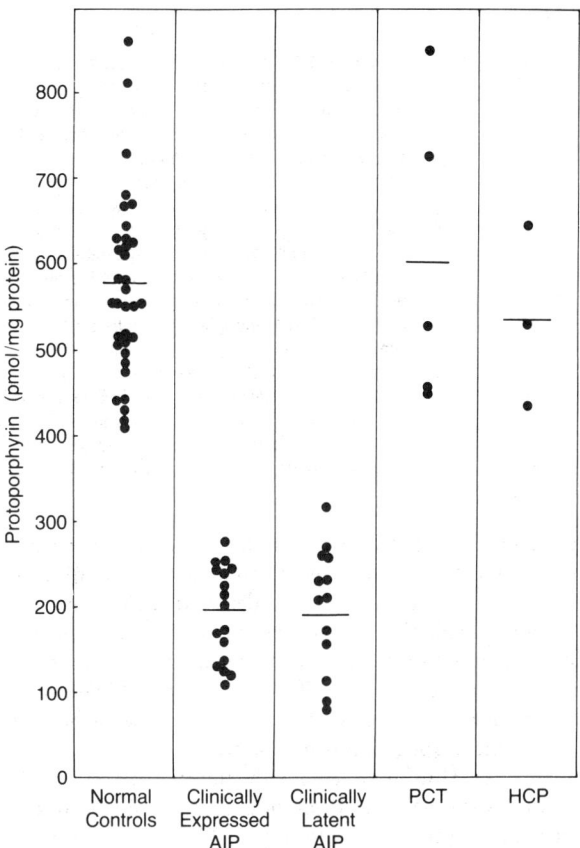

Figure 60-25 Metabolism of added ALA to protoporphyrin in cultured skin fibroblasts of normal subjects and patients with AIP, HCP, and PCT. PBG deaminase is rate-limiting for ALA metabolism to protoporphyrin in these cells; thus the PBG deaminase defect in AIP is reflected by a ~50 percent reduction in protoporphyrin formation. Coproporphyrinogen oxidase deficiency in HCP, and uroporphyrinogen decarboxylase deficiency in PCT do not limit ALA metabolism to protoporphyrin in these cells.

It is generally agreed that an approximately 50 percent deficiency of PBG deaminase is the basic inherited enzyme defect in AIP, but the precise nature of the enzyme deficiency remains obscure. Kinetic studies on crude lysates from erythrocytes or cultured lymphocytes indicate that the enzyme V_{max} is reduced, but the K_m, heat stability, and electrophoretic mobility are not appreciably different from the enzyme in normal red cell lysates [136, 170, 175]. A number of explanations for this are possible [175, 733]. The mutant allele could result in little or no enzyme activity because of deletion of all or part of the structural gene for PBG deaminase, or it might produce a structurally abnormal mRNA or enzyme protein that is rapidly degraded. The half-normal enzyme activity would then represent the gene product of the normal allele in heterozygotes for AIP. Alternatively, a regulatory gene or portion of DNA other than the structural DNA sequence for PBG deaminase may control synthesis of this enzyme, and a heterozygous mutation involving a regulatory gene or DNA sequence could result in reduced production of normal enzyme protein by structural genes for PBG deaminase [175]. Recent immunological studies of PBG deaminase in AIP families by Anderson et al. [733] using anti-human PBG deaminase, revealed evidence of a structural gene mutation (in the form of excess immunoreactive material relative to enzyme activity) in 1 of 22 unrelated AIP families. Excess immunoreactive material was found in all five AIP gene carriers studied in this family. Thus there is

clearly a potential for genetic heterogeneity among families with AIP [733]. Further studies are needed, but at present it appears that a structural gene mutation producing an abnormal and stable enzyme protein with subnormal or absent PBG deaminase activity is the exception rather than the rule in AIP, and that in other families unstable gene products, gene deletions, or regulatory genetic defects may eventually be demonstrated.

The structural gene for PBG deaminase has been localized on chromosome 11 in humans [164]. Studies in AIP families have shown absence of linkage between the PBG deaminase defect and known gene markers on chromosomes 1, 2, 6, and 9 [6, 734, 735]. Family studies have not been carried out using known markers on chromosome 11 to our knowledge.

Increased liver ALA synthase activity was described in AIP patients [600, 736–738] before the inherited deficiency in PBG deaminase was recognized. It was in fact initially postulated [736] that induction of ALA synthase might represent the primary enzyme abnormality in this disease. When the primacy of the PBG deaminase defect was recognized, it was suggested that this enzyme deficiency might result in heme deficiency in the liver and derepression of ALA synthase [168, 171], but there is no direct evidence that the PBG deaminase defect of itself results in a heme deficiency in tissues of AIP patients. ALA synthase induction during acute attacks is therefore an important phenomenon in the pathogenesis of the clinical syndrome of AIP and probably results in large part from exposure to drugs, hormones, or nutritional factors that are known to induce this enzyme (Fig. 60-27 and Table 60-8).

In individuals who inherit PBG deaminase deficiency, reduced hepatic heme synthesis is not a necessary consequence. PBG deaminase activity normally exceeds ALA synthase activity somewhat (Table 60-2), such that a 50 percent decrease in its activity would not be expected to cause a significant impairment of heme formation. Studies in vivo of labeled glycine and ALA metabolism in AIP patients also indicate that liver heme formation is not impaired [590, 705, 739]. In clinically latent heterozygotes for AIP, there is usually normal excretion of ALA and PBG in urine despite the PBG deaminase deficiency. This suggests that there is little or no induction of ALA syn-

Figure 60-26 Demonstration of the PBG deaminase deficiency of AIP in mitogen-stimulated lymphocytes. The enzyme activity increases markedly in normal cells when cultured in vitro for 4 days. However PBG deaminase activity in cells from AIP patients reaches levels only about one-half of those in cells from normal individuals. (*From Sassa, Zalar, and Kappas [175]. By permission of the Journal of Clinical Investigation.*)

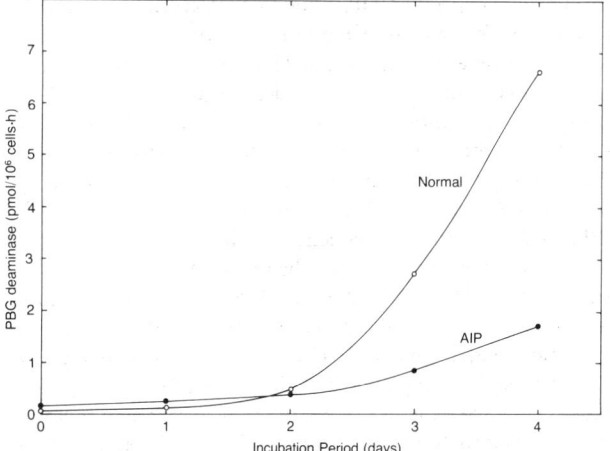

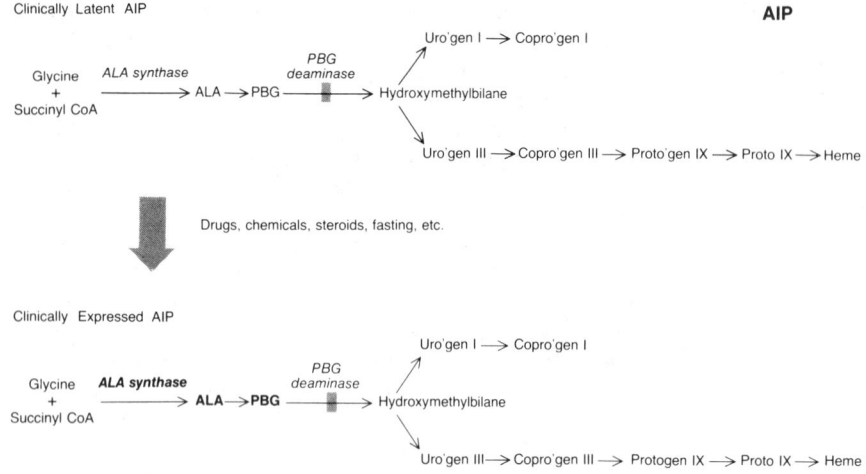

Figure 60-27 The enzymatic defect in AIP is a partial (~50 percent) deficiency of PBG deaminase activity. The extent of the enzyme deficiency is the same in clinically latent (*top*) and clinically expressed AIP (*bottom*) subjects. Full clinical expression of the AIP gene defect occurs with exposure to factors such as hormones, drugs, etc. which appear to activate the disease primarily by inducing ALA synthase (*bold letters*) in the liver. Activation of the disease is associated with excess production and excretion of ALA and PBG (*bold letters*). A similar transition from clinically latent to clinically expressed disease characterizes HCP and VP. ALA, δ-aminolevulinic acid; PBG, porphobilinogen; Uro'gen, uroporphyrinogen; Copro'gen, coproporphyrinogen; Proto'gen, protoporphyrinogen; Proto, protoporphyrin.

thase in the liver (Table 60-8) and therefore no significant lack of heme production; cytochrome P_{450}-mediated drug metabolism is normal in these individuals [740]. Moreover in AIP skin fibroblasts in culture there is no evidence of heme deficiency or ALA synthase induction [173, 174, 741].

Although the PBG deaminase defect in AIP is of itself unlikely to impair heme formation in the absence of heme pathway stimulation, the enzyme defect may become rate-limiting when greater hepatic heme formation is necessary in response to drugs, hormones, or other factors that induce cytochrome P_{450}. Under such circumstances a greater induction of ALA synthase might be required to provide sufficient PBG substrate for the deficient deaminase and to maintain a nearly adequate rate of heme formation for cytochrome P_{450}, other cellular hemeproteins, and for the regulatory "free" heme pool. If increased hepatic heme synthesis is suboptimal in a clinically expressed AIP patient with increased hepatic heme requirements, a reduction in the free heme content in the liver would occur and thereby derepress ALA synthase production. Induction of ALA synthase might then increase heme synthesis and provide much of the increased heme requirement for hemeprotein synthesis despite the PBG deaminase deficiency; in this process there is a loss of ALA and PBG from the pathway. Thus the PBG deaminase defect in AIP may accentuate the ALA synthase induction response to drugs and hormones, although it may not be sufficient of itself to elicit increased formation of ALA synthase and clearly cannot alone account for the clinical syndrome of AIP.

In clinically expressed AIP, wherein ALA synthase is induced and there is presumably a reduced pool of free heme in the liver, cytochrome P_{450} (as assessed indirectly by drug metabolism rates) is reduced in some patients but not others [740, 742] despite the known presence of inducing factors in the circulation in this disease [328, 329]. This suggests a deficient induction response for hemeprotein synthesis in the presence of the partial defect in PBG deaminase in such individuals [740]. In this regard, experimental studies utilizing the chick embryo liver in ovo treated with chemicals (desferrioxamine or a small dose of DDC) that partially block ferrochelatase support the idea that a partial block in a heme pathway enzyme can impair cytochrome P_{450} induction while enhancing the ALA synthase-inducing effects of chemicals in the liver [254]. Decreased cytochrome P_{450} may sometimes be related to additional factors such as high carbohydrate intake, which is known to reduce the rates of oxidative drug metabolism by the liver in normal subjects [743].

These considerations imply that the regulatory free heme pool in hepatocytes is quite sensitive to minor degrees of heme deficiency and can be substantially depleted with little alteration in heme availability for hemeprotein synthesis. This is a reasonable assumption because the free heme pool is very small and turns over rapidly and therefore should be highly sensitive to small changes in liver heme content, and because the binding affinity of heme to apocytochromes is estimated to be very high ($K_d \sim 10^{-9}$ M). Thus in patients with clinically expressed AIP in whom ALA synthase has been induced and the PBG deaminase defect has become rate-limiting for PBG metabolism, the regulatory or free heme pool in the liver may become depleted. The sequence in which these several events occur can probably vary, e.g., the regulatory heme pool may initially be depleted by some mechanism; an increased requirement for cytochrome P-450 production may develop; the heme moiety of this cytochrome may be degraded at an excessive rate by a variety of factors. Any of these processes would lead to derepression of ALA synthase formation. The concentration of PBG in normal liver is very low ($<10^{-6}$ M) and is probably less than the K_m for PBG deaminase ($\sim 10^{-6}$ M), so that a decrease in this enzyme activity might be compensated by an increase in sub-

Table 60-8 Classification of individuals who have inherited the PBG deaminase defect of AIP, based on clinical and biochemical features*

	Adults		Children
Biochemical and clinical features	Clinically expressed	Clinically latent	Clinically latent
Deficient PBG deaminase	Present	Present	Present
Increased hepatic ALA synthase	Present	(?)	(?)
Increased urinary ALA and PBG	Present	Absent†	Absent
Impaired hepatic steroid 5α-reductase	Present†	Absent	(?)
Inducer(s) of ALA synthase in serum	Present†	(?)	(?)
Clinical syndrome	Present	Absent	Absent

* PBG deaminase is equally deficient in all gene carriers and does not vary with disease activity. Children and most adults who are AIP gene carriers remain clinically latent; only a minority of adults develop clinical expression of the disease. Thus in adults there are two populations of AIP gene carriers who may differ in their susceptibility to clinical expression of the gene defect of AIP. The metabolic differences between these two populations of PBG deaminase-deficient individuals have not been fully defined. They include a deficiency of hepatic steroid 5α-reductase activity in most gene carriers who have clinical AIP but not in those classified as clinically latent. It is unlikely that hepatic ALA synthase activity is elevated in children or in most clinically latent adults, but this question has not been examined.
† Characteristic of most subjects in these categories.

strate (i.e., PBG) concentration [166, 168]. ALA synthase also has a high K_m for substrate (glycine) and it is possible that under some circumstances an increase in production of ALA and PBG can occur even without induction of ALA synthase [62]. Nevertheless it seems unnecessary to invoke this explanation for increased ALA and PBG production by the liver in AIP because hepatic ALA synthase is increased when this disease has become clinically expressed. Because of ALA synthase induction and an increased supply of PBG to the deficient deaminase, overall cellular heme synthesis and content may not be reduced substantially in clinically expressed AIP. This concept of a "compensated block" [5] can explain a maintenance of nearly normal rates of hepatic heme synthesis and the excess production and excretion of ALA and PBG in patients with clinically expressed AIP. However, there is no clear evidence that a compensated block with ALA synthase induction is present in subjects with clinically latent AIP, the majority of whom excrete normal amounts of ALA and PBG.

The ALA synthase induction response to a given inducing agent may not be the same for all individuals carrying the PBG deaminase defect of AIP. Studies in inbred strains of mice suggest that the degree of ALA synthase induction to a porphyrogenic drug (i.e., DDC) is controlled by genetic factors [672]. Such strain differences also occur in rats [214]. It is likely that similar genetic regulation of induction of this enzyme will eventually be demonstrated in humans.

Recently, an activator of PBG deaminase has been identified and purified from rat liver. The compound is probably a pteroylpolyglutamate derivative which may serve as a cofactor for the enzyme reaction [162, 744]. Whether altered availability of such a cofactor may play a role in activation of AIP deserves study.

Diagnosis

Measurements of PBG deaminase in red cells and PBG in urine are the primary means of recognizing patients with this disorder. Proper use of these and other diagnostic measurements is important because AIP is much more likely to produce severe and sometimes fatal neuropathy if the diagnosis is delayed. Most symptoms of AIP are nonspecific and the diagnosis in a symptomatic patient may not be obvious by history and physical examination until harmful drugs have been administered and motor neuropathy ensues. A variety of incorrect diagnoses can be made, most of which as noted by Waldenström [578] "seem to be rather well founded when one does not know anything about the acute porphyria of the patient." Delay in correct diagnosis can be avoided (1) by maintaining a high index of suspicion when evaluating patients with suggestive symptoms and (2) by screening relatives of known AIP patients to detect clinically latent heterozygotes before symptoms develop so that harmful drugs and other factors can be avoided. AIP is rare compared to other diseases that may produce similar symptoms, and if cases are to be detected at an early stage physicians and clinical laboratories should be prepared to test a large number of patients even though very few will be found to have porphyria. Unfortunately no single laboratory test is sufficient to exclude AIP completely, and if AIP is suspected, evidence for the related disorders HCP and VP should also be sought.

A quantitative test for urine PBG (see Biochemical Findings) should be performed in patients suspected of having AIP. Qualitative tests such as the Watson-Schwartz test can be used if their lower sensitivity is kept in mind and if positive results can be confirmed by a more specific and quantitative method [98] on the same urine specimen. A normal PBG level on a later urine sample does not completely exclude the possibility that PBG was increased when an initial urine sample was obtained, although transient elevation of urine PBG is less common in AIP than in HCP and VP. Acute symptoms occurring when urine PBG excretion is normal are probably not due to AIP.

Erythrocyte PBG deaminase should be measured in patients suspected of having AIP, although the immediate need for this test in an acutely ill patient is less than is the measurement of urine PBG. Urine and stool porphyrins should be assessed also because VP and HCP can produce identical symptoms. PBG deaminase is not reduced in these disorders and PBG may be only transiently increased. A simple quantitative assay for total urine porphyrins, such as that described by Schwartz et al. [745], and a qualitative stool porphyrin test [746] and measurement of urine PBG generally suffice in screening for VP and HCP.

There is a wide range for PBG deaminase activity in red cells in normal and AIP subjects. A few normal individuals have red cell enzyme values in or near the AIP range, some AIP patients have normal values, and there is an equivocal range in which results are nondiagnostic (Fig. 60-24). Activity may be increased in hemolytic disorders [138] and in patients with hepatic disease [747]; activity may be decreased in uremia [748]. In these situations diagnostic accuracy is increased by measuring urine PBG, carrying out a family pedigree study to detect other AIP gene carriers, or by measuring PBG deaminase in cultured fibroblasts [174] or mitogen-stimulated lymphocytes [175]. A qualitative spot test for erythrocyte PBG deaminase has been described [584], but it is unlikely to be useful because, even with a quantitative assay, results are not always definitive.

In following patients with AIP, it is useful to measure ALA and PBG output because these usually decrease with improvement in clinical status. Decreases in plasma ALA and PBG may occur even more promptly, particularly with hematin treatment. Measurement of PBG in plasma is probably more reliable than ALA because plasma ALA may be considerably overestimated when colorimetric methods are used [749]. A gas-liquid chromatographic method may be preferable for measuring plasma ALA [750], but there is as yet little experience with this method in porphyria patients.

The measurement of erythrocyte PBG deaminase is the mainstay for detecting clinically latent gene carriers in families of AIP patients (Fig. 60-28) [168–170, 751]. Since most heterozygotes for AIP do not have increased PBG excretion, many more gene carriers will be detected by the enzyme assay than by urine PBG measurements. Since some individuals in a family may have equivocal levels of this enzyme in red cells, family evaluations are facilitated if pedigree analysis (which will often suggest obligate carriers and normals) and urine PBG measurements are also carried out [169, 751, 752]. Erythrocyte PBG deaminase may be physiologically increased in normal infants during the first few months of life [753]. Values obtained during this period should be interpreted with caution and probably repeated at a later time. The red cell assay has so greatly increased our ability to detect clinically latent AIP (Fig. 60-28) that measures to provoke an increase in ALA and PBG excretion by giving phenobarbital, estrogen [660], or a glycine load [754] should rarely if ever be used. Provocative tests particularly with phenobarbital are likely to be hazardous [660], and an absence of response does not fully exclude AIP.

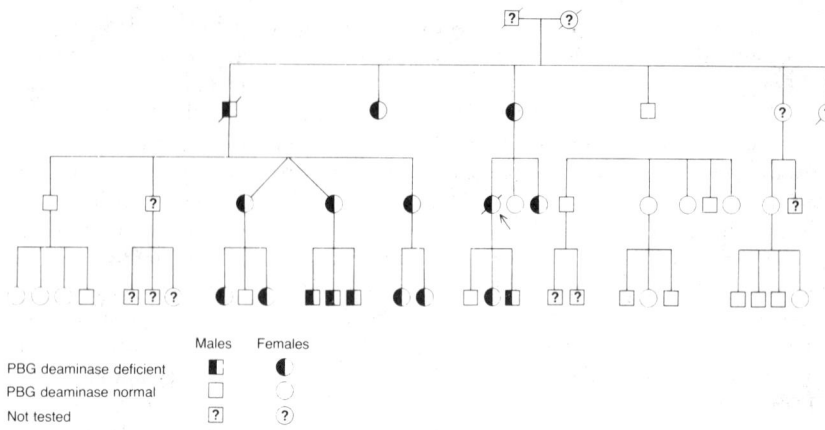

Figure 60-28 Lineage of a patient with AIP. As shown by studies of erythrocyte PBG deaminase, the AIP gene defect was inherited from the patient's mother and transmitted to two of her three children. Sixteen clinically latent gene carriers of AIP were also detected in this lineage. Only two adult gene carriers had increased urinary excretion of PBG, and in the 10 years since this AIP lineage was identified only the propositus, indicated by an arrow, developed the clinical syndrome of AIP.

PBG deaminase deficient
PBG deaminase normal
Not tested

Males   Females

Treatment

Patients with acute porphyric attacks generally require narcotic analgesics for relief of pain and usually are unable to maintain an adequate food intake. Hospitalization is recommended for relief of symptoms, administration of intravenous fluids including glucose, and for reinstitution of oral feedings when tolerated. The clinical course may be difficult to predict, and careful observation as to the precipitating cause of the attack and observation for neurological complications are best carried out in hospital. Even in a known AIP patient, other diseases including appendicitis should be considered as possible causes of abdominal pain.

Precipitating factors such as infections should be treated appropriately. Drugs known to be harmful in porphyria or those for which knowledge as to their safety is lacking should be discontinued (Table 60-7). Carbohydrate should be administered orally or intravenously (usually as 10 percent dextrose) in amounts of at least 300 to 500 g daily. Hyponatremia may result either from inappropriate ADH secretion (which requires fluid restriction) or from excess gastrointestinal or renal salt loss (which necessitates salt and fluid repletion). Especially when inappropriate ADH secretion is suspected, serum electrolytes should be monitored during intravenous glucose treatment because this generally entails administration of considerable volumes of fluid.

Pain should be treated with a narcotic analgesic such as morphine, meperidine, or codeine. Other less potent pain medications are usually of little use. Since porphyric attacks often remit rapidly there is little addiction potential, although drug addiction can become a problem in some patients with frequent attacks or chronic symptoms. Anxiety and other emotional symptoms and nausea or vomiting are usually best treated with chlorpromazine or another phenothiazine. These drugs also are helpful in controlling pain. AIP patients may not require, and often find unpleasant, large doses of phenothiazines. Chloral hydrate may be given for insomnia, and diazepam in low doses is probably safe to use as a minor tranquilizer.

The response to a high carbohydrate intake may range from dramatic to imperceptible. Patients who do not respond to 300 g carbohydrate daily may improve when the intake is increased to 450 to 500 g daily [579]. The rationale for this treatment is that carbohydrate can prevent the induction of ALA synthase by porphyrinogenic influences [347]. Carbohydrate can be given orally in any form such as sucrose, glucose polymers, or as foods rich in carbohydrate. Intravenous fructose (levulose) is also effective [755]. Glycerol can lower porphyrin precursor excretion in AIP and may also benefit these patients [695].

Intravenous infusion of hematin has been effective in reducing levels of ALA and PBG in serum and urine of patients with AIP [333, 336, 338, 756–760] and is more dramatic and dependable than glucose treatment. It has been the clinical impression that when patients were treated during acute attacks, symptoms and neurological signs resolved more quickly with hematin treatment than would have otherwise been expected, but controlled studies have not been reported and would be valuable in view of the unpredictable course of acute attacks and the consequent difficulty in judging responses to treatment. Chronic symptoms or acute neurological deficits that have already progressed to severe neuronal damage are unlikely to respond to this treatment [336, 756, 759]. Lamon et al. [758] found that monthly premenstrual attacks could be prevented in a 33-year-old woman with AIP by weekly hematin infusions. The patient served as her own control during nontreatment periods. Similar benefit has been noted in another patient to whom hematin was given twice monthly and timed carefully to cover the luteal phase of the menstrual cycle [674].

Hematin for intravenous infusion is prepared from outdated human blood by standard methods and given to patients only after being shown to be sterile and pyrogen-free. It is not effective by mouth [759]. For intravenous infusion, doses of 100 to 400 mg (maximum recommended dose 4 mg per kilogram of body weight) have been given over periods of about 15 min to several hours. Hematin clearance from plasma in patients is biexponential, with the rapid component having a half-life of 4.5 to 15.5 h and the slower a half-life of 16 to 53.3 h [759, 761]. Plasma hemopexin falls rapidly after hematin infusion and its catabolism is markedly accelerated [528]. The two components of the hematin clearance curve may be explained by initial saturation of hemopexin by hematin and rapid uptake into liver, followed by binding to albumin and more gradual transfer from albumin to hemopexin as the latter is resynthesized and becomes available for heme binding [761–763]. A response to hematin may not be observed for up to 48 h after hematin administration [757] as might be expected for recovery of neuronal function. Heme repression of ALA synthase has been amply documented in the liver of experimental animals (see earlier discussion) and in buffy coat preparations after hematin administration to an AIP patient [764]. The decrease in ALA in urine and plasma is often greater than that for PBG [759]. Hematin is detectable in plasma for up to 5 days after infusion [761]. Therefore, its effect may be prolonged significantly beyond the time of infusion [338].

When administered in amounts or at a rate exceeding the capacity for hepatocellular uptake and plasma binding hematin may appear in bile [765] and in urine. One AIP patient given 1000 mg of hematin in 15 min, an excessive dose, developed gross hematinuria followed by transient acute renal failure presumably due to acute tubular necrosis [766]. Renal impairment has not occurred with more conventional doses. Phlebitis is a common side effect. Hematin may be taken up by erythroblasts in addition to the liver, which would explain the responses to this treatment that have been reported in patients with CEP [334], EPP [525], and lead poisoning [767]. Responses in the latter disorders were less apparent than in AIP.

Of potential concern in patients who are treated repeatedly with hematin is the ability of this compound to induce heme oxygenase. In patients and mice with severe chronic hemolytic anemias there is no repression in heme biosynthesis or cytochrome P_{450} in the liver despite increased uptake of endogenous heme into hepatocytes [97, 768]. This is probably because of an adaptive increase in heme oxygenase activity [97]. Repeated hematin infusions might similarly increase heme oxygenase activity and reduce its therapeutic effectiveness in AIP.

Treatment with exogenous steroids to suppress ovulation has been reported to prevent acute attacks in some women with AIP when the attacks are associated with the menstrual cycle [6, 769, 770]. Benefit may be derived from synthetic estrogens, progestins, or androgens when each is given alone, as well as from oral contraceptive steroid combinations. Thus suppression of ovulation and lowering of endogenous sex hormone production may be the effective mechanism [769]. Oophorectomy [6, 770] and in our experience natural menopause do not produce prompt or dependable remission of AIP. Oral contraceptive steroids can also worsen symptoms in AIP [771], and in particular many progestins are capable of inducing ALA synthase [772]. This paradox is difficult to explain. Perhaps doses of these steroids are important, and it is possible that if contraceptive steroids are not started early enough in the menstrual cycle to suppress ovulation their effects will be additive to the actions of endogenously secreted steroid hormones, and their use would then be deleterious. As noted earlier, synthetic steroids with an ethynyl substituent can cause increased breakdown of cytochrome P_{450} heme, and such compounds should probably be avoided in AIP patients. Danazol is an example of such compounds [773, 774].

Evidence of sympathetic overactivity in acute porphyria has led to a variety of treatments including splanchnicectomy, reserpine, guanethidine, phenoxybenzamine, and propranolol [650, 775]. Such treatments have been uncontrolled, and their clinical value is not established. Most attention has been given to treatment with the β-adrenergic blocking drug propranolol [775, 776]. This drug can reduce tachycardia and hypertension in acute porphyric attacks. In some patients abdominal pain is also alleviated [775, 776]. Observations, also uncontrolled, suggest that the drug may reduce porphyrin precursor excretion in some patients with AIP or VP [777, 778]. Even in low doses, propranolol may pose a significant hazard in AIP patients with hypovolemia and incipient cardiac failure in whom catecholamine secretion is an important compensatory mechanism [779]. In female rats and in cultures of chick embryo liver cells the induction of ALA synthase by AIA or DDC is reduced by propranolol [780, 781]. This is probably due to nonspecific membrane effects rather than β-adrenergic blockade since both the D- and L-isomers of the drug can have this action [781]. These and some other membrane-active drugs also may inhibit amino acid uptake into liver cells [782]. Therefore propranolol may not have a specific biochemical effect in acute porphyric attacks and should probably only be used when necessary to control tachycardia, hypertension, or other signs of sympathetic overactivity. The drug has been used in a similar fashion in thyrotoxicosis and in psychiatric disorders [783].

Studies on treatment of patients with 3,5,3′-triiodothyronine have shown a partial correction in the 5α-reductase defect in AIP. The improvement in steroid hormone metabolism was modest compared to that seen in myxedema patients and did not appear to alter the clinical course of AIP. Since the AIP patients studied were euthyroid, this treatment was sometimes associated with mild symptoms of hyperthyroidism [662, 784]. A therapeutic trial with thyroid analogues that act primarily on the liver may be warranted in the future.

Other treatments for which there is little evidence for benefit in AIP include dexamethasone or other glucocorticoids to suppress endogenous adrenal androgen production [667], administration of zinc salts [785, 786], chelating agents, pyridoxine [678, 785, 787], adenosine monophosphate [788], vitamin E [789], and hemodialysis [790]. Recent evidence that folic acid is a cofactor for PBG deaminase may warrant study of folate metabolism and folic acid treatment in patients with AIP. Preliminary uncontrolled observations in three patients suggest that it may be useful [163].

HEREDITARY COPROPORPHYRIA

Definition

Hereditary coproporphyria (HCP) is another form of hereditary hepatic porphyria. Clinical manifestations closely resemble those for AIP, although it is usually a milder disorder. Photosensitivity can also occur. The fundamental biochemical abnormality is a partial (approximately 50 percent) deficiency of coproporphyrinogen oxidase, which is inherited as an autosomal dominant trait. Clinical expression is highly variable and is determined by the same additional factors that determine clinical expression in AIP and VP. A single well-documented case of homozygous HCP with a much more severe deficiency of coproporphyrinogren oxidase and with marked symptoms has been described.

Prevalence

HCP appears to be much less common than AIP. Most cases have been reported in Britain, Europe, and North America [791], but the prevalence has not been carefully estimated and there is no obvious racial predominance.

Clinical Findings

HCP generally presents with neurovisceral symptoms that are virtually identical to those in AIP. Photosensitivity due to accumulation of coproporphyrin occurs in a minority of patients. In a review of 111 reported cases including 28 of their own, Brodie et al. [792] noted that the most common symptomatic manifestations in patients were abdominal pain (80 percent), vomiting (34 percent), cutaneous photosensitivity (29 percent), neurological involvement (23 percent), psychiatric symptoms (23 percent), and constipation (20 percent). The disease is generally less severe than AIP, and only a few patients dying of respiratory paralysis have been reported [793, 794]. Clinically latent cases with increased coproporphyrin excretion in stool and sometimes in urine are very common in families of HCP patients, and most of these individuals never become clinically manifest. There is usually little or no abnormality of hepatic function in HCP.

This disease can be exacerbated by the same drugs that are dangerous to patients with AIP. The review by Brodie et al. [792] revealed that drugs, and usually phenobarbital, were responsible for initiating HCP attacks in 54 percent of patients. As in AIP there is a female predominance in subjects who become ill with the disease, and attacks may occur in association with menstrual cycle, pregnancy, or treatment with oral contraceptive steroids [792, 795, 796]. The disease is generally latent before puberty. Haeger-Aronsen et al. [791] reported a 13-year-old prepubertal patient who developed severe symptoms when treated for seizures with phenobarbital, but they pointed out that increased production of sex hormones could have already occurred at this age. Studies by Paxton et al. [795] indicate that as in AIP increased production of 17-oxysteroids and reduced metabolism of androgens via the 5α-reductase pathway in liver occurs in HCP patients who are prone to clinical exacerbations of the disease, although this steroid metabolic deficiency has not yet been demonstrated by more specific radiolabeled tracer techniques [663, 664]. Thus, as in AIP there is an important role for endogenous sex hormones in the clinical expression of this disease. Decreased hepatic function from hepatitis or other causes may cause increased porphyrin retention and worsening of cutaneous photosensitivity [232, 797].

A case of homozygous HCP in a 22-year-old woman whose parents were first cousins was reported by Grandchamp et al. [234]. The patient had hypertrichosis and increased skin pigmentation at 4 years of age and an acute porphyric attack at age 10 and again at age 20 when pregnant. Homozygous HCP was also suspected in a patient reported earlier by Berger and Goldberg [797].

Biochemical Findings

This disease is characterized by increased excretion of coproporphyrin, mostly type III, in the urine and stool (Table 60-4). Increased coproporphyrin excretion, particularly in stool, is found in many asymptomatic individuals with inherited coproporphyrinogen oxidase deficiency. Fecal porphyrins in HCP generally show a great predominance of coproporphyrin with little increase in protoporphyrin, whereas in VP the amounts of these porphyrins are often approximately equal. Fecal coproporphyrin may be partially in the form of copper coproporphyrin [798]. During acute attacks, increased urinary excretion of ALA, PBG, and uroporphyrin occurs, although these more often revert to normal than is the case in AIP. As described below, coproporphyrinogen oxidase activity is reduced by approximately 50 percent in all heterozygotes for HCP, whereas increased ALA and PBG excretion and increased hepatic ALA synthase activity occur in association with clinical exacerbations. In the single documented case of homozygous disease, the oxidase activity was markedly reduced (to about 2 percent of control values) in lymphocytes, and the excretion of ALA, PBG, uroporphyrin, and coproporphyrin was considerably increased [234].

Genetic Defect

Approximately one-half of normal activity of coproporphyrinogen oxidase has been found in cultured fibroblasts [232], circulating lymphocytes [233, 799], and buffy coat preparations [792] of HCP patients, and also in some of their first-degree relatives in a pattern consistent with autosomal dominant inheritance. Coproporphyrinogen oxidase cannot be assayed in erythrocytes, which do not contain mitochondria. The exact nature of the defect in this enzyme has not been determined. The K_m of the enzyme is the same in cultured fibroblasts derived from patients and normal subjects, and mixing experiments show no evidence of an inhibitor. Since enzyme activity is about one-half of normal in HCP cells, it is likely that the mutant gene product has little or no enzyme activity [232]. This is indicated also by the finding of markedly reduced activity of the oxidase (only 2 percent of normal) in lymphocytes of a homozygous case of HCP [234]. PBG deaminase is normal in HCP.

Coproporphyrinogen oxidase is normally present in considerable excess in the liver, and has been estimated to be 30 times greater than PBG deaminase activity [232]. It is not immediately evident that a reduction in coproporphyrinogen oxidase of only 50 percent could limit the further biotransformation of coproporphyrinogen and why acute attacks are associated also with excess excretion of ALA and PBG. Elder et al. [232] have suggested that the concentration of coproporphyrinogen III in human liver is probably below the K_m for coproporphyrinogen oxidase, so that the reaction rate is determined by substrate concentration. When the heme pathway is stimulated, an increased coproporphyrinogen III concentration may occur at the expense of greater loss of this intermediate from the liver cell, as loss of this porphyrinogen appears to occur more readily than, for example, uroporphyrinogen [232]. This increased loss of coproporphyrinogen under conditions in which there is a stimulus to heme synthesis could accentuate the metabolic significance of a partial defect in coproporphyrinogen oxidase. Increased ALA and PBG excretion during acute attacks (Fig. 60-29) is explainable by induction of ALA synthase and the normally low level of PBG deaminase in liver [232]. Measurements of liver ALA synthase in a limited number of patients indicates that this enzyme is increased during acute attacks when urinary ALA and PBG excretion rises but not during periods of remission when porphyrin precursor output is normal [801, 802]. Porphyrins do not accumulate in liver [791]. Coproporphyrinogen and coproporphyrin appear to be efficiently transported into bile or plasma from hepatocytes.

Increased ALA synthase activity probably occurs only in the presence of drug, hormonal, or nutritional factors that are known to induce this enzyme, although the coproporphyrinogen oxidase defect may limit the capacity for increased hepatic heme formation to a sufficient degree that there is increased

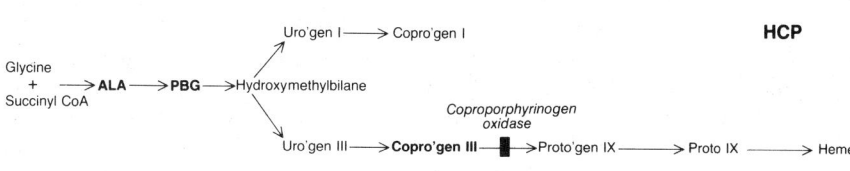

Figure 60-29 The enzyme defect in HCP is a deficiency of coproporphyrinogen oxidase activity. This enzyme defect favors the accumulation of coproporphyrinogen III (*bold letters*). As in AIP, full clinical expression of the disease occurs in the presence of factors that induce ALA synthase; this and the near rate-limiting activity of normal PBG deaminase causes ALA and PBG (*bold letters*) to accumulate during exacerbations of the disease. ALA, δ-aminolevulinic acid; PBG, porphobilinogen; Uro'gen, uroporphyrinogen; Copro'gen, coproporphyrinogen; Proto'gen, protoporphyrinogen; Proto, protoporphyrin.

sensitivity to such inducing factors. The oxidase is normally present in substantial excess. For example, PBG deaminase is the rate-limiting enzyme for conversion of ALA to protoporphyrin in cultured skin fibroblasts from both normal and HCP subjects [174, 433]. Fasting in pigs can decrease coproporphyrinogen oxidase activity [803]. If true in humans, this could accentuate the deficiency of this enzyme in HCP.

Diagnosis

Patients with HCP generally present with the same neurovisceral attacks found in AIP and VP. HCP should be suspected in those patients with acute porphyric attacks having normal PBG deaminase in red cells, cultured lymphocytes, or fibroblasts (see discussion of AIP). Urinary findings in HCP and VP are generally identical, with coproporphyrin as the predominant porphyrin and excess ALA, PBG, and perhaps uroporphyrin occurring especially during acute attacks. Stool porphyrins in HCP show a distinctive and marked excess of coproporphyrin, as demonstrated by thin layer or high-performance liquid chromatographic methods.

It is also desirable to confirm a deficiency of coproporphyrinogen oxidase by direct measurement, but assays for this enzyme are not widely available. Families of HCP patients should be screened for excess stool porphyrins, because in the absence of an assay for the oxidase, this remains the most sensitive method for detecting clinically latent gene carriers. Children who are heterozygotes for coproporphyrinogen oxidase deficiency may not excrete excess coproporphyrin until about 10 years of age [233].

Treatment

Acute attacks of HCP are treated in the same manner as AIP. Photosensitivity associated wth liver dysfunction may be responsive to cholestyramine, although the value of this drug has not been fully established [796].

VARIEGATE PORPHYRIA

Definition

Variegate porphyria (VP) is so termed because it can present with neurovisceral symptoms, cutaneous photosensitivity, or both. Like AIP and HCP it displays autosomal dominant inher-

itance but is clearly distinct etiologically from these other forms of hereditary hepatic porphyria. The basic genetic defect in VP is believed to be either a deficiency of protoporphyrinogen oxidase, or a type of defect in ferrochelatase that is different from that found in EPP. VP is also known as *porphyria variegata, protocoproporphyria* or *South African genetic porphyria.* "Mixed porphyria" may refer to either VP or HCP and is a term that should no longer be used. "Porphyria cutanea tarda hereditaria" was the term used in the past before VP and PCT were clearly distinguished.

Prevalence

VP is particularly common among South African whites, and it is estimated that 3 of every 1000 whites in that country have inherited the disease [804, 805]. Detailed investigations by Dean [804, 805] indicate that most cases in South Africa can be traced back to a man or his wife who were married in 1688 shortly after each had emigrated from Holland to South Africa. This is an example of genetic drift or the so-called founder effect. VP has since been recognized in many other races, including orientals, and is generally less common than AIP. The estimated prevalence of VP in Finland is 1.3 per 100,000 [806].

MacAlpine et al. [807] have suggested that some members of British royalty have suffered from VP, and this disease has therefore been called the "Royal Malady." This conclusion is based largely on retrospective analysis of symptoms—which are characteristically nonspecific in VP as in other hereditary hepatic porphyrias—and there is very little published laboratory data from living descendants to confirm the validity of the diagnosis in this royal lineage [805].

Clinical Features

VP usually presents with signs and symptoms of acute porphyria and like HCP is often clinically indistinguishable from AIP. Cutaneous photosensitivity occurs in at least one-third of patients but usually is more chronic and occurs apart from acute neurological symptoms [808]. In a survey of 300 patients, Eales and coworkers [593] noted that the most common complaints or signs were abdominal pain (occurring in 100 percent of patients), tachycardia (83 percent), vomiting (78 percent), constipation (64 percent), hypertension (63 percent), neuropathy (~60 percent), back pain (23 percent), confusion (~36 percent), bulbar paralysis (27 percent), and other mental problems (23 percent). Skin manifestations were present in 85 percent of patients in this series. Solar sensitivity is thus much more common than in HCP. Other common features include fever (38 percent), urinary frequency (30 percent), and dysuria (28 percent) [808].

The clinical features of abdominal pain and neuropathy are identical to those described for AIP. Skin manifestations are similar to those described for PCT. For example, increased fragility of sun-exposed areas of the skin is quite common. Vesicles, bullae, increased pigmentation, and hypertrichosis also occur. Cutaneous lesions are less common in patients residing in northern latitudes than in South Africa [809].

Hyponatremia with evidence of sodium depletion is common in South African patients with VP. This is often associated with renal dysfunction which suggests a toxic effect of the disease on the kidney, perhaps mediated by ALA [593]. Inappropriate ADH secretion seems a less common cause of hyponatremia, at least in South African patients [593]. As in AIP and HCP there is usually little or no hepatic dysfunction in VP.

The same factors that exacerbate AIP and HCP are detrimental to patients with VP. With use of oral contraceptives, women with VP seem especially prone to develop increased photosensitivity. The disease is clinically latent before puberty, and endogenous hormones clearly play a role in clinical expression of this disorder. Steroid 5α-reduction is commonly impaired in VP patients when the disease has become clinically expressed [674], although this was not observed in the single earlier patient studied [810]. Advice as to use of drugs in VP also corresponds to that for AIP. Perlroth et al. [811] found that in two patients with VP, caloric restriction was detrimental to the disease, particularly near the time of menses, whereas increased carbohydrate or protein intake was beneficial.

Biochemical Findings

The most characteristic finding is an increase in stool protoporphyrin content. Stool coproporphyrin (mostly isomer III) is also increased, usually to a lesser degree than protoporphyrin, but can equal or sometimes exceed protoporphyrin in VP. The stool coproporphyrin fraction in VP includes meso- and deuteroporphyrins which are derived in the gut from protoporphyrin. In HCP the increase in stool coproporphyrin is marked and protoporphyrin shows little or no increase. Stool porphyrins can be normal until near the age of puberty in subjects who inherit VP [806, 809, 812, 813]. The fecal *X-porphyrin fraction* (defined as ether-acetic acid–insoluble porphyrins extracted with urea-Triton) is increased in VP to a greater degree than in other porphyrias. In VP this fraction is predominantly *X-porphyrin*, a term referring to a heterogeneous group of porphyrin-peptide conjugates. In PCT this fraction consists mostly of uroporphyrin and 7-carboxylate porphyrin [814, 815].

Previously it was thought that fecal porphyrins characteristically decrease and urine porphyrins increase reciprocally during exacerbations of VP [816], but it is now recognized that both usually increase, particularly when there are neurovisceral symptoms [806]. This may vary with the factor that precipitates an exacerbation and whether the symptoms are predominantly cutaneous or neurological. "Reciprocity" in routes of porphyrin excretion may be important when exacerbating factors act to increase photosensitivity by reducing biliary excretion of porphyrin [816], as do estrogens, rather than by increasing liver ALA synthase, as do barbiturates.

Large amounts of ALA and PBG are excreted in urine during acute attacks. Coproporphyrin (mostly type III) is often increased as well, and excess uroporphyrin may form nonenzymatically from excess PBG. Between attacks, urine ALA and PBG commonly are normal or only slightly increased. A characteristic porphyrin complex, termed *Pu* [817], is found in plasma of many patients with VP and also HCP. It is a complex between coproporphyrin and a nonpeptide molecule (perhaps a lipid) [593, 817], and its significance is currently unknown. Studies of serum hemopexin in VP have given conflicting results [806].

Increased ALA synthase activity has been reported in the liver in VP patients [166, 435, 738], and this enzyme activity presumably increases substantially during acute attacks. Thus excess urinary ALA and PBG probably originate from the liver in this disease as in AIP. Hepatic porphyrin levels are not increased in VP; porphyrinogens have not been specifically measured [818]. Day et al. [818] have suggested that excess fecal and urine porphyrins in VP originate from the intestine and the renal tubules respectively, although the evidence for this is indirect.

Genetic Defect

Accumulation of protoporphyrin suggested that ferrochelatase might be deficient in this disease (Fig. 60-30). Pimstone et al. [819] were unable to show a difference in muscle ferrochelatase activity between normal and VP subjects. Nonetheless others reported that this enzyme is approximately 50 percent deficient in normoblast preparations [263] and cultured fibroblasts [241] of VP patients. Normal results were also reported using buffy coat preparations [820].

Protoporphyrinogen oxidase is the most recently described enzyme in the heme biosynthetic pathway [238, 821, 822], and its discovery led to the suspicion that it might be deficient in VP (Fig. 60-30) [822]. Recent studies by Brenner and Bloomer [262] with cultured skin fibroblasts suggest that protoporphyrinogen oxidase deficiency is indeed the primary genetic defect, whereas they found ferrochelatase to be normal. Protoporphyrinogen oxidase was found to be about 43 percent of normal in sonicates of fibroblasts from VP patients, as might be expected for an autosomal dominant trait, and this finding suggests that the product of the mutant gene has little or no enzyme activity. The enzyme activity has also been shown to be decreased in lymphocytes of VP patients [819a].

When ALA is added to VP fibroblasts, protoporphyrinogen does not accumulate, and protoporphyrin levels increase to the same degree as in normal cells, whereas in EPP protoporphyrin accumulation in fibroblasts [262] or mitogen-stimulated lymphocytes with ALA incubation is about twice normal [538]. Therefore ferrochelatase is clearly limiting for ALA metabolism to heme in such cells from normal, VP, or EPP subjects, and a one-half of normal activity of protoporphyrinogen oxidase does not appear to limit ALA metabolism to protoporphyrin in cultured fibroblasts. This is similar to what has been observed with cultured cells from HCP patients with one-half of normal activity of coproporphyrinogen oxidase (see above), and suggests that, as in HCP, factors that induce ALA synthase in the liver but not in other cells such as fibroblasts are important in full expression of disordered porphyrin metabolism in VP. Hepatic cytochrome P_{450} content is not reduced in this disorder [823]. This indicates that the enzyme deficiency does not impair heme formation sufficiently to reduce formation of this hemeprotein. Under the influence of factors which increase

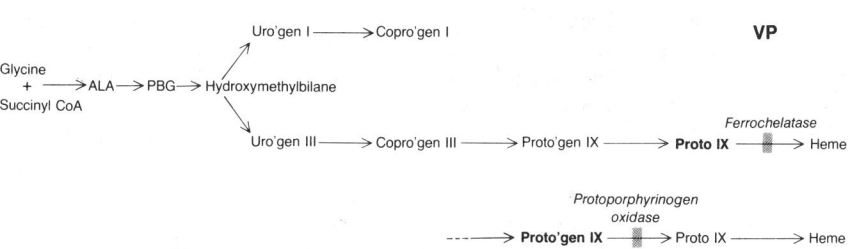

Figure 60-30 The enzyme defect in VP is a deficiency either of ferrochelatase or protoporphyrinogen oxidase activity, probably the latter. Either would favor the accumulation of protoporphyrinogen or protoporphyrin (*bold letters*) in this disorder. As in AIP, the disease becomes fully expressed in the presence of additional factors that appear to act primarily by inducing ALA synthase. During exacerbations of the disease induction of ALA synthase coupled with the normally low levels of PBG deaminase results in accumulation of ALA and PBG (*bold letters*). ALA, δ-aminolevulinic acid; PBG, porphobilinogen; Uro'gen,uroporphyrinogen; Copro'gen, coproporphyrinogen; Proto'gen, protoporphyrinogen; Proto, protoporphyrin.

demand for heme formation the deficient enzyme may sufficiently limit heme formation to reduce the size of the regulatory heme pool in liver cells and result in the induction of ALA synthase.

Watson et al. [824, 825] have described in part an interesting kindred in which the propositus had clear-cut VP with neurological complications, four relatives had clinically latent VP, and two others had chemical features of PCT which included excretion of large amounts of isocoproporphyrin in the feces. VP and the inherited form of PCT (see below) are believed to be genetically distinct diseases. Therefore perhaps two separate genetic diseases were coincidentally present in this family, or two individuals may have had an acquired form of PCT. Eales and coworkers [593] have also alluded to porphyrin excretion patterns with features of PCT in approximately 10 percent of their patients with known VP.

Diagnosis

VP should be considered in any patient with signs and symptoms suggesting acute porphyria. In VP the activity of PBG deaminase is normal, which differentiates this disorder from AIP, and the stool porphyrin pattern, as described above, distinguishes it from HCP. On occasion, examination of the composition of the X-porphyrin fraction may help differentiate VP from PCT [815]. This is seldom necessary, however, because in PCT the pattern of excess urinary 8- and 7-carboxylate porphyrin and fecal isocoproporphyrin as determined chromatographically is characteristic.

Normal levels of ALA and PBG in urine cannot be relied upon to exclude VP, because these may revert to normal quickly after an acute episode of neurological symptoms. As in AIP the precise causal relationship between the porphyrin precursors and neurological symptoms is still unclear, and it may be more difficult to correlate clinical symptoms with levels of ALA and PBG in this disease than in AIP.

Stool porphyrin screening of family members of VP patients is strongly recommended. The advantages of detecting clinically asymptomatic subjects are great, as in AIP and HCP. Increased stool porphyrins may be less common in VP heterozygotes if they are tested before puberty [804, 812, 813]. Fecal porphyrins may also be lower in elderly heterozygotes [804]. Nonetheless screening of fecal porphyrins is useful in family members of any age [826]. Examination of protoporphyrinogen oxidase in cultured fibroblasts [241] or in lymphocytes [819a] should prove to be even more useful in the detection of VP carriers.

Treatment

Acute exacerbations are treated as in AIP. Glucose [593, 811] and hematin [335, 756] have been reported to be effective. Propranolol is reportedly beneficial [593, 775, 777], but as with AIP controlled studies have not been carried out. Although effective in PCT, in which there is considerable porphyrin deposition in the liver, chloroquine treatment seems of little value [827]. Administration of D-penicillamine was associated with subjective improvement and decreased fecal and urine porphyrin concentrations in one Chinese patient with VP [812]. A number of other treatments, including hemodialysis, phlebotomy, alkalinization of urine, and β-carotene, have not proved successful [790, 828]. A broad-brimmed hat, gloves, and clothes that at least partially prevent exposure of the arms and legs to sunlight may be helpful in protecting against photosensitivity [804, 805]. Some patients with this disease have had difficulty obtaining life insurance. This is unfortunate because, as in AIP and HCP, the risk of dying from VP is remote once it is recognized [804, 805]. Abortion should not be advised simply because of the risk that a child may have VP; the disorder remains clinically latent in most individuals who inherit it [804, 805]. Similar considerations apply to the other autosomal dominant porphyrias, AIP and HCP.

A marked decline in acute attacks and mortality has occurred in South Africa in recent years [593]. This is due to better treatment of acute attacks, particularly the use of glucose and, when necessary, respiratory support, screening for latent cases in families of known VP patients, and avoidance of harmful drugs [593].

PORPHYRIA CUTANEA TARDA

Definition

Porphyria cutanea tarda (PCT) is generally a disease of adults and is usually sporadic. A family history of PCT is unusual. Nonetheless families with more than one affected member and kindreds suggesting autosomal dominant inheritance have been described. Porphyrins accumulate in the liver, pass into the blood, and are excreted in stool and urine. Urine contains mostly uroporphyrin and 7-carboxylate porphyrin, and the stool may contain considerable amounts of porphyrins including the isocoproporphyrin series. Cutaneous photosensitivity is the major symptom, and the disease does not produce neurological dysfunction. Uroporphyrinogen decarboxylase is decreased in the liver in all cases and, at least in familial PCT, in other tissues as well. The complex and distinctive pattern of porphyrin excretion is explainable by a deficiency of this enzyme in the liver. Liver damage from alcohol or other causes, increased hepatic iron, and estrogens are important contributing factors in the pathogenesis of PCT. A disorder similar to PCT occurs when humans or laboratory animals are exposed to hexachlorobenzene or related chlorinated hydrocarbons. This disease is also known as symptomatic porphyria, porphyria cutanea symptomatica, or idiosyncratic porphyria.

Prevalance

PCT is the most common of the porphyrias, but its prevalence has not been accurately estimated in most localities. It appears more common in countries in which alcohol consumption is high, such as in many Western countries and among the Bantu population in South Africa [804, 805, 829]. Almost 700 cases were known in 1974 in Prague alone [829]. PCT has been more common in men, perhaps due to greater alcohol intake. More recently the relative frequency of female patients has been increasing due in part to oral contraceptive use, postmenopausal estrogen treatment, and alcohol ingestion [831, 832]. The disease usually occurs in late adult life but onset at younger ages is now more common than in the past [832]. PCT rarely occurs in children, and if it does it is more likely to be familial [191, 833, 834]. Other than its relation to liver disease, PCT occurs also in association with diabetes mellitus [832, 835], systemic or discoid lupus erythematosus [836–839], other immunological disorders [837, 840, 841], and in uremic patients undergoing hemodialysis [842, 843] more frequently than would be expected by chance.

Clinical Features

Cutaneous lesions develop on sun-exposed areas such as the face, dorsa of the hands, forearms, and in women on the legs and feet. Skin lesions may be more frequent during the summer than winter but unlike EPP they may not occur immediately after sunlight exposure. Small white plaques, termed *milia*, are common and may precede or follow the formation of fluid-filled vesicles and bullae (Fig. 60-31). Increased friability of the skin over sun-exposed areas is also very common, and minor

Figure 60-31 Large bullae on the dorsum of the hand of a patient with PCT. *(From L. C. Harber [1018] by permission of Harper & Row.)*

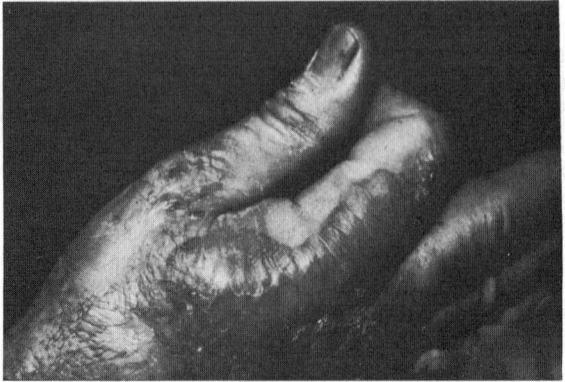

trauma may lead to the formation of bullae or denuded areas. Eroded areas and bullae may crust over and heal slowly; they are then replaced by thin or atrophic skin which may gradually return to normal over a period of months if, with treatment, the disease goes into remission. Facial hypertrichosis is also frequent and occasionally is the presenting complaint even in the absence of bullae or vesicles. A violaceous or erythematous hue to the face is also notable in some patients. Scarring, altered pigmentation, and thickening of the skin may occur. On occasion, thickening, scarring, and calcification of the skin may be striking and progressive and lead to an appearance of the face, scalp, and hands closely resembling systemic sclerosis or scleroderma. This *pseudoscleroderma* is usually confined to sun-exposed areas, and there is no involvement of internal organs as in systemic sclerosis.

Skin biopsies may reveal subepidermal bullae with deposition of periodic acid-Schiff staining material in and around the walls of cutaneous blood vessels. Fine fibrillar material may be deposited at the dermal-epidermal junction as in VP and may relate to excessive fragility of the skin [482, 502]. Deposition of immunoglobulins, especially IgG, and complement is seen by immunofluorescent methods around dermal vessels and at the epidermal junction. Sclerodermatous lesions are not distinguishable histologically from those in systemic scleroderma [844]. As noted earlier, uroporphyrin has been shown to stimulate collagen synthesis in cultured human skin fibroblasts, a finding which suggests a specific role for this porphyrin in producing the sclerodermatous skin changes in PCT [30a].

There is a history of heavy or moderately heavy alcoholic intake in most PCT patients, but many are not frank alcoholics in that alcohol has not impaired their normal functions or caused other symptoms of ill health, and patients often stop drinking with little difficulty. Liver function tests or biopsies usually reveal at least a degree of liver cell damage. Red fluorescence can be demonstrated in all cases on unfixed sections of liver [845, 846] or in paraffin embedded sections if properly processed [847]. Porphyrins are mostly in the cytoplasm rather than nuclei if sections are prepared without contact with water, which can cause an artifactual redistribution of porphyrin fluorescence [845]. Liver histopathology commonly consists of increased iron in hepatocytes and Kupffer cells, inflammation, necrosis, fatty change, and needlelike inclusions which are fluorescent and birefringent [699, 823, 846, 848]. Florid alcoholic hepatitis and fatty changes are unusual [846]. Cirrhosis may occur in as many as a third of cases, but is much less common in many series [832, 846, 848]. Distorted lobular architecture is more common in older PCT patients [846] and cirrhosis considerably more common at autopsy [849]. Electron microscopy shows needlelike lucent areas probably in lysosomes, and rather nonspecific changes including paracrystalline inclusions in mitochondria [848, 850]. Liver function tests that are most commonly abnormal include serum transaminase, γ-glutamyltranspeptidase, and BSP clearance [851]. Histological abnormalities in PCT are often not diagnostic of alcoholic liver damage, and other causes of liver cell damage may be important in some patients. A few patients may have evidence of persistent hepatitis B [852]. It has also been suggested that liver damage may relate in some manner to an underlying metabolic defect in PCT [846].

Associated factors are of considerable importance in PCT, although how they contribute to the pathogenesis of the disease is not fully understood. Liver cell damage, iron overload, and estrogens appear to be the most important of these contributing factors. Hepatic siderosis is very common but by liver biopsy is usually mild or moderate and not so severe as in untreated hemochromatosis. Nonetheless in PCT the serum iron and ferritin concentrations are generally increased. There is often an unexplained mild or moderate erythrocytosis in untreated PCT and its relationship to iron overload, if any, is unclear. Ferrokinetic and iron absorption studies have shown iron stores and absorption to be normal or increased, with a wide range of variation [211, 853–857]. Alcohol and liver disease are known to increase iron absorption, and this may contribute to siderosis in some patients. High levels of dietary iron may be important in some populations, as in the Bantu. Hemochromatosis is not commonly associated with porphyria [858]. Thus PCT clearly cannot be explained by iron overload alone. Rats with hepatic siderosis excrete a greater proportion of urinary porphyrins as uroporphyrin, but do not develop porphyria even when ethanol is also administered [859]. In addition most individuals who consume alcohol in large amounts or have liver damage from other causes do not develop PCT.

Men who are treated with estrogens for prostatic cancer [832, 860–862] and women given estrogens alone or as oral contraceptive combinations [831, 832, 863, 864] may develop PCT. The fact that the disease is associated with liver disease, alcohol abuse, and rarely Klinefelter's syndrome [865, 866], which in males are conditions often associated with gynecomastia and other signs of feminization, suggests that altered endogenous hormone metabolism may contribute to the development of PCT. As reviewed elsewhere [679] the feminizing effects of liver dysfunction in alcoholics may relate more to an increase in the ratio of endogenous estrogens to testosterone rather than to relatively small increases in plasma estrogen levels alone. Thus alterations in endogenous hormones that favor increased estrogenic effects may contribute to the development of PCT in some individuals. Estrogens alone, however, have never been shown to produce a condition resembling PCT in animals, and all human subjects exposed to estrogens do not develop PCT. Thus, these steroid hormones appear to influence the expression of underlying metabolic defect in individuals who are already susceptible to the development of PCT.

Exposure of animals to hexachlorobenzene or a number of other chlorinated cyclic hydrocarbons can produce a porphyria that mimics PCT very closely [203, 204, 866, 867, 869, 870]. This was shown after a massive outbreak of a PCT-like syndrome occurred in 1956 in eastern Turkey when seed wheat to which hexachlorobenzene had been added as a fungicide was used for food by a large impoverished population [871–874]. Photosensitivity with bullae, scarring, hyperpigmentation, and marked hypertrichosis was common. Porphyria in this population was more common in children than in adults, and because of increased hair growth and pigmentation many were described as having "monkey disease." The incidence was slightly greater in males than in females. An average interval of about 6 months was calculated between exposure and the development of symptoms. Early periods of illness were often accompanied by irritability, colic, anorexia, weakness, and red or brown urine. Painless arthritis was especially common in children. Many breast-fed infants in some villages died of a condition known locally as "pink sore" which was characterized by weakness, convulsions, and cutaneous annular erythema, and this illness may have resulted from hexachlorobenzene in breast milk [874, 875]. Older children and adults who developed porphyria and complained of irritability and weakness may have had the neurological involvement that has

been observed in hexachlorobenzene-treated animals [867, 868]. Moreover in these animals it is unclear whether weakness results from the induced porphyria or from a direct toxic effect of hexachlorobenzene on the nervous system. Cripps and coworkers [874] reexamined 32 patients with "porphyria turcica" 20 years after the initial illness, and found that although many had sequelae (scarring, increased pigment, hypertrichosis, pinched facies with perioral scarring, short stature, and contracted hands and fingers), porphyrin excretion had returned to normal or nearly normal levels without treatment. This disease originally developed in old Turkish settlers as well as immigrant Turks and Kurds. This is evidence against, but does not exclude a genetic predisposition [872, 874].

Smaller outbreaks and isolated cases of PCT from exposure to other cyclic chlorinated hydrocarbons, including di- and trichlorophenols and 2,3,7,8-tetrachlorodibenzo-p-dioxin (TCDD, or dioxin), have also been reported [710, 876–878]. In subjects exposed to TCDD, porphyrin fluorescence in the liver is quite prevalent, even with little or no increase in urine porphyrins [710]. Improved industrial hygiene can substantially reduce the prevalence of PCT and excess uroporphyrinuria [879]. Abnormalities in porphyrin metabolism in laboratory animals or cultured liver cells similar to those in hexachlorobenzene porphyria can be produced also by polychlorinated biphenyls (PCB), TCDD, and polybrominated biphenyls (PBB) [880–883]. The possibility is worth considering that inapparent exposure to such industrial and environmental chemicals may predispose to the development of some cases of sporadic PCT.

A number of cases of PCT have occurred in patients undergoing hemodialysis for chronic renal failure [842, 843, 884–886]. Photosensitivity in dialysis patients can also occur in the absence of porphyria, for reasons which are obscure. Alcohol intake and iron therapy may have contributed to the development of PCT in some of these. A role for unknown chemicals perhaps leached from the dialysis tubing was also suggested. One patient clearly had familial PCT, with decreased uroporphyrinogen decarboxylase in his red cells and in those of his mother and sister [885]. Familial PCT was said to be present in another case also, but evidence was not presented [886]. Even though uroporphyrin I binds poorly to plasma proteins and is soluble in water, hemodialysis is surprisingly ineffective in removing porphyrins from plasma in these patients [843], although better recovery of porphyrins in the dialysate was reported with use of a high-permeability membrane [885].

The risk of hepatocellular carcinoma is clearly increased in patients with PCT, and in several recent series the incidence has ranged from 4 to 47 percent [846, 849]. The highest incidence was found in an autopsy series [849]. These tumors rarely contain porphyrins in large amounts [846]. Chronic liver damage in general may predispose to such tumors, and iron deposition could also be a factor. Porphyrins themselves may bind to DNA and play a role in carcinogenesis [887]. Moreover many of the chemicals that can produce PCT-like syndromes in animals are carcinogenic, which suggests that inapparent chemical exposures may produce PCT and also predispose to hepatic malignancy.

As mentioned earlier, there is an apparent association between PCT and systemic lupus erythematosus and other autoimmune disorders [836–839]. Twenty cases in which lupus erythematosus (usually systemic) and PCT coexisted were described up to 1975 [888]. It is of interest that one patient (reported twice) with Klinefelter's syndrome and PCT also had systemic lupus erythematosus [865, 866], and there is a known association between Klinefelter's syndrome and systemic lupus [866]. Nonetheless the majority of patients with PCT do not have serological evidence of autoimmunity [889], and the deposition of immunoglobulins and complement in the skin of these patients may not represent an immune response [502]. Recent work indicates that complement activation and chemotactic activity is generated in human serum by ultraviolet light when uroporphyrin is present at concentrations similar to those found in PCT [497]. Thus there may be a link between endogenous porphyrin accumulation and activation of the immune system. PCT also occurs rarely in patients with hemolytic anemias [890].

Biochemical Findings

A complex pattern of porphyrin excretion is characteristic of PCT. Porphyrins are increased in the liver, plasma, urine, and stool (Table 60-4). Porphyrin precursor excretion is normal except for a slight increase in ALA in some patients. The urine contains mostly uroporphyrin and 7-carboxylate porphyrin, with lesser amounts of coproporphyrin, 5-, and 6-carboxylate porphyrins [891] (Fig. 60-32). Normal urinary porphyrin composition is 70 percent coproporphyrin (70 percent of which is isomer III), 15 percent uroporphyrin (90 percent isomer I), 3 percent 7-carboxylate porphyrin, 1 to 2 percent 6-carboxylate porphyrin, and 5 percent 5-carboxylate porphyrin (5-7-carboxylate porphyrins being mostly isomer III) [892]. Excess uroporphyrin in PCT urine is predominantly isomer I, whereas 7- and 6-carboxylate porphyrins are mostly type III, and 5-carboxylate porphyrin and coproporphyrin are approximately equal mixtures of isomers I and III [455, 893–895, 898]. Isomer composition of urine porphyrins is similar in PCT due to hexachlorobenzene as in sporadic cases but with somewhat

more uroporphyrin III [455]. Substantial excretion of unoxidized uroporphyrinogen is uncommon [895].

Dehydroisocoproporphyrin is prominent in bile in PCT and in rats with hexachlorobenzene porphyria [896]. The major porphyrins in stool are often isocoproporphyrins (Fig. 60-32), and smaller amounts of these may also appear in urine [896, 897]. Coproporphyrin, 7-carboxylate porphyrin and uroporphyrin may also be increased in stool [898]. The X-porphyrin fraction is usually increased but as was noted earlier contains principally uroporphyrin and 7-carboxylate porphyrin rather than porphyrin-peptide conjugates [815]. Total porphyrins in stool are in general increased to a lesser degree than in VP or HCP, whereas urine porphyrins usually exceed levels in the latter two disorders. Nevertheless, it is estimated that in PCT more total porphyrins are excreted daily in feces than in urine [891]. In the feces of Turkish patients with hexachlorobenzene porphyria there was a predominance of "coproporphyrin" as separated by solvent extraction [860]; this presumably included excess isocoproporphyrins.

Plasma porphyrins are increased [899, 900], and the porphyrin distribution pattern is similar to the urine, with small amounts of isocoproporphyrin sometimes being present [817, 834]. Levels of porphyrin in the skin are also increased, and more so in areas not exposed to light. This suggests that light destroys porphyrins which reach the skin [901, 902]. Increased liver porphyrins in PCT are composed mostly of uroporphyrin and 7-carboxylate porphyrin. The isomer patterns in the fecal and liver porphyrins have been very similar to those of urine porphyrins in the few PCT patients that have been so examined [455, 891, 894].

Not only does fecal porphyrin exceed urine porphyrin excretion in PCT, but total excretion of the type III isomers predominates over excretion of the type I isomers. This includes isocoproporphyrins which are derived from the type III series as described below [891]. Thus the most hydrophobic porphyrins appear to be excreted readily in PCT, whereas the hydrophilic 8- and 7-carboxylate porphyrins are preferentially stored in the liver. As Elder [891] has noted, total porphyrin excretion is about 6 μmol/day in PCT, and if porphyrin accumulates in the liver at an equal rate it would still take months to reach levels observed in patients' livers, which often are in the range of 0.22 to 2.0 μmol per gram wet weight. Immediate red fluorescence upon ultraviolet illumination suggests that these accumulate as the oxidized porphyrins rather than as porphyrinogens. In hexachlorobenzene porphyria in rats, liver porphyrins rise and eventually level off, suggesting saturation of binding or storage sites in liver cells [891]. In the presymptomatic phase of PCT, a smaller proportion of 8- and 7-carboxylate porphyrins may be excreted [898], and this suggests that these porphyrins are preferentially stored in the liver during this time [891].

Estimates by Elder [891] of daily rates of series I and III porphyrin excretion in PCT and normal rates of liver heme formation as calculated from hepatic bilirubin production for a 70-kg subject by Berk et al. [903] are shown in Table 60-9. Since formation of uroporphyrinogen III is required for heme synthesis, the total daily formation of uroporphyrinogen III greatly exceeds daily uroporphyrinogen I formation even in PCT. Nevertheless series I porphyrins are clearly produced in excess, since in normal subjects less than 1 percent of the uroporphyrinogen formed is the type I isomer and a much greater fraction is produced as the type I isomer in PCT (Table 60-9) [891].

Figure 60-32 Thin layer chromatogram visualized under ultraviolet light of stool and urine porphyrins (as their methyl ester derivatives) in a patient with PCT. Three columns of porphyrin methyl ester standards are also shown. Large amounts of isocoproporphyrin in the stool and uroporphyrin and 7-carboxylate porphyrin in urine are characteristic of this disease. The band labeled as isocoproporphyrin in the fecal porphyrin chromatogram may also contain deethylisocoproporphyrin. The method is previously described [1019].

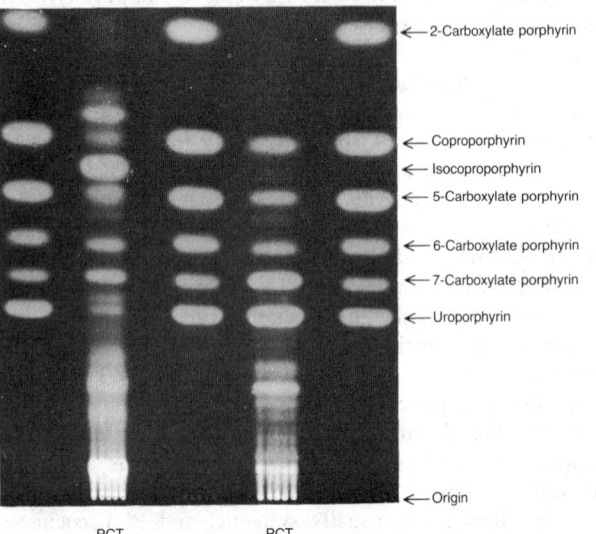

← 2-Carboxylate porphyrin

← Coproporphyrin
← Isocoproporphyrin
← 5-Carboxylate porphyrin

← 6-Carboxylate porphyrin

← 7-Carboxylate porphyrin

← Uroporphyrin

← Origin

PCT   PCT
(Stool)   (Urine)

Table 60-9   Formation of porphyrinogen intermediates by uroporphyrinogen decarboxylase and coproporphyrinogen oxidase in the liver in PCT*

Porphyrinogen (III series)	Substituents and their locations							
	1	2	3	4	5	6	7	8
Uroporphyrinogen	A↓	P	A↓	P	A	P	P	A↓
5-Carboxylate porphyrinogen	M	P	M	P	A↓	P	P	M
Coproporphyrinogen	M	P	M	P	M	P	P	M
Dehydroisocoproporphyrinogen	M	V	M	P	A↓	P	P	M
Harderoporphyrinogen	M	V	M	P	M	P	P	M
Protoporphyrinogen IX	M	V	M	V	M	P	P	M

* The metabolism of the acetate to methyl substituents by the decarboxylase is impaired (↓, A to M reactions) and there is accumulation of substrates for this enzyme in their oxidized forms (i.e., uroporphyrin, 7-, 6-, and 5-carboxylate porphyrins). Formation of dehydroisocoproporphyrinogen via a normally minor pathway by coproporphyrinogen oxidase (the P → V reaction indicated by the curved arrow) is accentuated in PCT with accumulation of dehydroisocoproporphyrinogen and porphyrins derived from it by oxidation and bacterial metabolism in the gut. Because of the decarboxylase deficiency, further metabolism of dehydroisocoproporphyrinogen to harderoporphyrinogen via the minor pathway is also impaired. The numbering system for locations of carbon atoms and substituents is according to Fischer [10].

M, —CH₃; A, —CH₂COOH; P, —CH₂CH₂COOH; V, —CH=CH₂.

Violin (or "phyriaviolin") is an uncharacterized pigment which may be excreted in amounts of 1 to 5 mg daily in the urine of PCT patients [904]. Its significance is unknown although it may be derived from bile pigments. Plasma hemopexin and albumin levels may both be reduced in this disease [527].

Genetic Defect

At present it is useful to divide PCT into three types: (1) sporadic cases in which there is no evidence of the disease in other family members, (2) familial cases in which there is evidence of autosomal dominant inheritance, and (3) cases due to exposure to halogenated aromatic hydrocarbons. In practice, all cases cannot be classified on these grounds alone because relatives cannot always be adequately studied to determine a pattern of inheritance, and chemical exposures can be inapparent and also occur in families rather than solely in individuals. Moreover there often are no distinctive clinical features by which to classify individual cases. Thus in familial PCT the same associated factors as in sporadic cases may often be required to bring out full clinical and biochemical expression of the disease [891, 905]. There are indications that in childhood cases of familial PCT evidence of liver dysfunction is often absent and serum iron levels frequently are normal [191, 834, 906, 907]. In most series the screening of available relatives suggests that familial PCT is much less common than the sporadic disease [834, 891, 905]. However, de Verneuil and Nordmann [907a] reported 14 cases of familial-type PCT (with decreased erythrocyte uroporphyrinogen decarboxylase) among 78 cases of the disease.

There is general agreement that in familial PCT there is an approximately 50 percent deficiency of uroporphyrinogen decarboxylase in liver, erythrocytes [191, 907], and presumably other tissues, and that this enzyme defect is inherited as an autosomal dominant biochemical trait (Fig. 60-33). In familial PCT this enzyme is also approximately one-half of normal in cultured skin fibroblasts. In such families onset of the disease in presumed heterozygotes during childhood and the occurrence of photosensitivity in more than one family member are common, although many clinically latent carriers have normal urine and fecal porphyrin levels. Erythrocyte uroporphyrinogen decarboxylase is equally reduced in clinically latent and affected family members who inherit this disorder [191]. Since familial PCT has been described only recently as a distinct entity and is quite uncommon in most series, many of its clinical and biochemical features remain to be defined better. Experience does suggest, however, that exogenous factors including alcohol, iron, and estrogens can contribute to activation of familial PCT, and that phlebotomy is often useful [907]. As discussed earlier the finding that in familial PCT uroporphyrinogen decarboxylase activity is about one-half of normal when 8-, 7-, 6-, or 5-carboxylate porphyrinogens (type I isomers) are used as substrate is of interest in terms of the mechanism of the decarboxylase reaction, and suggests that all four decarboxylations are carried out by the same enzyme [191]. There is evidence for this also from studies of the enzyme in avian erythrocytes [908]. Moreover decarboxylase activities for uroporphyrinogen and 5-carboxylate porphyrinogen have been copurified from human red cells [190].

Recently Elder et al. [454] have presented evidence that people with *hepatoerythropoietic porphyria* (HEP) are in fact homozygous for the decarboxylase defect found in familial PCT. In studies of three of the seven reported cases of HEP they found uroporphyrinogen decarboxylase activity to be 7 to 8 percent of normal in both erythrocytes and cultured fibroblasts of the patients, and about one-half of normal in a single parent available for study. Thus, familial PCT appears to be the second genetic porphyria in humans that can present both in the heterozygous and homozygous state. Increased red cell protoporphyrin in these cases who are homozygous for familial PCT was explained [454] as being due to accumulation of 8- to 5-carboxylate porphyrinogen intermediates in marrow erythroid cells during hemoglobin synthesis, followed by their transfor-

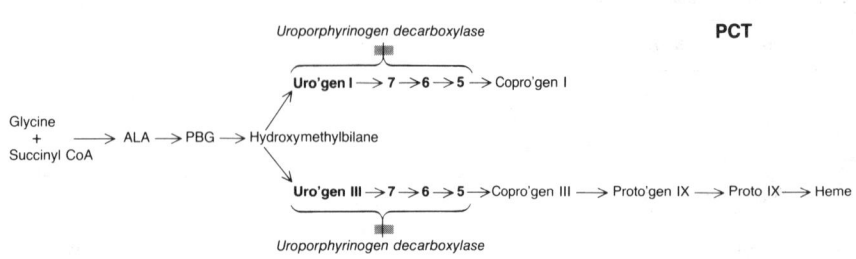

Figure 60-33 PCT is associated with a deficiency of uroporphyrinogen decarboxylase activity in liver which can result in the accumulation of porphyrins corresponding to the porphyrinogen (*bold letters*) substrates for this enzyme. In familial PCT the enzyme deficiency is also found in erythrocytes, lymphocytes, and fibroblasts. As a result of the enzyme deficiency in liver 7-, 6-, and 5-carboxylate porphyrinogens as well as uroporphyrinogen itself accumulate since all serve as substrates for the enzyme. ALA, δ-aminolevulinic acid; PBG, porphobilinogen; Uro'gen, uroporphyrinogen; Copro'gen, coproporphyrinogen; Proto'gen, protoporphyrinogen; Proto, protoporphyrin.

mation to protoporphyrin after hemoglobin synthesis was complete.

A genetic predisposition has long been suspected in the majority of cases of PCT, because alcohol, liver disease, mild iron overload, and estrogens alone or in combination have seemed insufficient explanations for even the sporadic disease [574, 860]. Recent descriptions of an association between PCT and certain histocompatibility antigens at the HLA locus strengthens this suspicion [909, 910], but it is still not established that an underlying inherited defect of uroporphyrinogen decarboxylase is present in so-called sporadic cases. The liver enzyme is clearly deficient in all cases of PCT (Fig. 60-33) [198, 199, 911]. Liver coproporphyrinogen oxidase is normal, and the reduced ratio of uroporphyrinogen decarboxylase to coproporphyrinogen oxidase explains the characteristic increase in excretion of isocoproporphyrin (Fig. 60-34) [198]. Several laboratories have reported [191, 198, 823] that uroporphyrinogen decarboxylase is not deficient in red cells of patients with the sporadic disease. Elder et al. [198] also found normal activity of this enzyme in cultured skin fibroblasts. Sporadic PCT would thus be similar to hexachlorobenzene porphyria in rats, in which uroporphyrinogen decarboxylase is decreased in the liver (shown in uroporphyrinogen, 7-, or 5-carboxylate porphyrinogen as substrate) [870, 912] but not in other tissues including red cells [912]. In contrast, others have reported a deficiency of the red cell enzyme in all PCT patients and that this deficiency is inherited as an autosomal dominant trait; they would argue that virtually all cases of PCT are probably familial [199–201]. Doss et al. [911] found the red cell enzyme to be deficient in about 40 percent of their sporadic cases.

This controversy may result in part from geographic differences in patient populations, but differences in methodology are probably more important. In studies showing decreased enzyme activity in red cells of sporadic PCT patients, the uroporphyrinogen decarboxylase assay employed tritiated uroporphyrinogen I generated from labeled PBG by preincubation with excess PBG deaminase; after incubation the total amount of products (7-, 6-, 5-, and 4-carboxylate porphyrinogens) formed were measured [199, 200]. This assay essentially measures the rate of decarboxylation of uroporphyrinogen I to 7-carboxylate porphyrinogen I [200]. Felsher et al. [200] recalculated their data and found that the "composite" rate of decarboxylation of uroporphyrinogen III to coproporphyrinogen was not different in normal and PCT red cells. Some investigators finding normal enzyme activity in sporadic patients' red cells employed uroporphyrinogen III [198, 526] or 5-carboxylate porphyrinogen III [198] as substrate and measured coproporphyrinogen formation, while others used uroporphyrinogen I [191] or uroporphyrinogen III [526] as

substrate and measured the sum of 7-, 6-, 5-, and 4-carboxylate porphyrinogen formation [191]. Blekkenhorst et al. [823] employed the same assay as Kushner et al. [199] and reported normal uroporphyrinogen decarboxylase in PCT red cells. Del C. Rios de Molina et al. [526] also found normal red cell enzyme activity in PCT using uroporphyrinogen III as substrate and measuring formation of 7-, 6-, 5-, and 4-carboxylate porphyrinogens or coproporphyrinogen alone. Decarboxylation of 5-carboxylate porphyrinogen was also normal in fibroblasts in the sporadic disorder [198]. Felsher et al. [200] suggested that the initial decarboxylation of uroporphyrinogen III but not the final 5-decarboxylation might be reduced in PCT red cells. However, uroporphyrinogen and 5-carboxylate porphyrinogen appear to undergo decarboxylation by the same enzyme in human erythrocytes [190]. Thus present evidence weighs mostly against the idea that there is a mutation in sporadic PCT which selectively alters one of the stepwise decarboxylations of uroporphyrinogen in erythrocytes while impairing all decarboxylation steps in the liver.

It is conceivable that the liver and red cell enzymes are in some manner under separate genetic control, and that the decarboxylase deficiency in liver in some sporadic PCT cases is inherited [198]. Familial and sporadic cases may not be comparable because liver dysfunction can be less common in familial PCT [526]. Brodie et al. [913] found that erythrocyte uroporphyrinogen decarboxylase was not decreased in their sporadic PCT patients, whereas PBG deaminase was increased. Other reports [914, 915] also suggest that PBG deaminase, which is a highly sensitive index for an increased proportion of young erythrocytes [138], was increased in some PCT patients. Moreover uroporphyrinogen decarboxylase activity was higher in one group of controls who were alcoholics than in another group with nonalcoholic liver diseases [913]. These results suggest that metabolic influences on red cell uroporphyrinogen decarboxylase in PCT patients may be complex. Genetic controls and other potential influences, such as red cell aging, on the erythrocyte enzyme merit further study and might clarify some questions concerning activity of the enzyme in circulating red cells of PCT patients.

Thus it is at present uncertain whether there is a genetic defect involving uroporphyrinogen decarboxylase in the majority of PCT patients. If an inherited defect of this enzyme is present in sporadic cases, it must differ from the defect that has been established in patients with familial PCT.

The relationship of iron, alcohol, and estrogens to liver uroporphyrinogen decarboxylase deficiency in PCT is still incompletely understood. It is reported that the enzyme activity in mammalian liver is inhibited by addition of ferrous iron in vitro [205], whereas others report an opposite effect [823].

Iron overload in rats is not required for inhibition of uropor-phyrinogen decarboxylase by hexachlorobenzene [870], although earlier observations implied such a requirement [204]. Hexachlorobenzene treatment does not itself increase liver iron content. Nonetheless, hexachlorobenzene porphyria and the associated decrease in decarboxylase activity in rats occurs more quickly and is greatly enhanced by iron [203, 215]. Uroporphyrinogen decarboxylase inhibition by TCDD is prevented by an iron deficiency state [212]. Hence, normal or greater levels of tissue iron may be required for decarboxylase inhibition by chlorinated hydrocarbons. Iron could act in part by changing the redox state of the liver cell cytoplasm and promoting the oxidation of uroporphyrinogen and other porphyrinogen substrates to porphyrins and thereby increasing their escape from the pathway. The finding that iron overload in hexachlorobenzene-treated rats increases in the liver the free or unbound NAD/NADH ratio (as determined indirectly by the lactate/pyruvate ratio) supports this idea [204]

The time course of liver changes induced by hexachloroben-zene or TCDD is complex and poorly explained. Induction of cytochrome P_{450} occurs early, and precedes the development of porphyria, decarboxylase inhibition, and increased ALA synthase activity [204, 916, 917]. Metabolism of hexachloro-benzene to products that bind covalently to cellular macromol-ecules appears to be necessary before inhibition of the decar-boxylase and porphyria occurs. This applies also to certain other halogenated hydrocarbons that can produce a porphyria resembling PCT [918–920]. The onset of hexachlorobenzene porphyria can be hastened by siderosis in rats [204]. Moreover naturally occurring levels of liver nonheme iron appeared to correlate with rapidity of induction of porphyria by this chem-ical in two strains of rats [214]. Hexachlorobenzene porphyria in iron-overloaded rats is associated with decreased levels of incorporation of [^{14}C]succinate into the heme moiety of cyto-chrome P_{450} [204]. Although iron overload alone can also reduce microsomal heme content and [^{14}C]ALA incorporation into heme [921], there is evidence that the delayed develop-ment of porphyria from TCDD treatment in mice without iron overload is also associated with reduced cytochrome P_{450} lev-els [917]. This differs from human PCT, in which cytochrome P_{450} is not reduced, as noted below.

Porphyria from hexachlorobenzene is also enhanced by estradiol administration in rats, whereas androgens, proges-tins, and alcohol had little or no such effect [922]. Chronic alcohol feeding in rats has been reported to decrease uropor-phyrinogen decarboxylase somewhat in the liver and also in the spleen [923]. These findings indicate that additional factors contributing to the development of PCT, such as alcohol, iron, and estrogens, act on the heme pathway primarily at or near

the level of uroporphyrinogen decarboxylase rather than by induction of ALA synthase. Increase in the latter enzyme in animals treated with chlorinated hydrocarbons occurs only when there is a progressive decrease in the decarboxylase and therefore appears to be a secondary event.

Available evidence in PCT patients indicates that iron, alco-hol, and estrogens do not alter decarboxylase activity in human liver or erythrocytes in vivo. Thus Elder et al. [198] found no correlation between iron content and uroporphyrin-ogen decarboxylase activity in liver tissue from patients with PCT or alcoholic liver disease, and the enzyme was not decreased in alcoholic liver disease in the absence of porphyria. Alcohol intake and iron status also did not appear to affect red cell uroporphyrinogen decarboxylase activity in studies by Felsher et al. [200]. Thus the red cell enzyme was not signifi-cantly different in a group of untreated PCT patients and in a postphlebotomy group (studied when hemoglobin and reticu-locyte alterations after phlebotomy had returned to normal) and was not influenced by a history of heavy alcohol intake [200]. There is conflicting evidence as to whether there is a sex difference in the activity of the human red cell enzyme (lower in females) [199] or whether exogenous estrogens can decrease the red cell enzyme activity [198–200].

There is little to suggest that iron, alcohol, or estrogens con-tribute to PCT by inducing ALA synthase. None of these agents is a potent inducer of this enzyme in human or animal livers. Iron itself does not induce hepatic ALA synthase in ani-mals, although it may accentuate the effects of other inducers of this enzyme [859, 924]. Alcohol intake may increase ALA synthase slightly in PCT patients [691] and in rats [859]. PCT patients are not sensitive to more potent inducers of ALA syn-thase such as phenobarbital. In animals treated with chlori-nated hydrocarbons, a delayed increase in ALA synthase occurs only when a decrease in uroporphyrinogen decarboxyl-ase develops. This suggests that the increase in ALA is a sec-ondary event that results from the marked reduction of decar-boxylase activity.

Recent studies of genetically controlled responsiveness to TCDD and hexachlorobenzene in rodents indicate that inher-ited factors can influence the development of PCT other than by simply decreasing the levels of decarboxylase activity in liver and other tissues. Jones and Sweeney [917, 925] showed in backcrossing experiments that susceptibility to the porphyrogenic effect of TCDD segregates with the Ah locus in two inbred strains of mice. This locus determines responsive-ness of aryl hydrocarbon hydroxylase and a number of other pathways of xenobiotic metabolism to induction by TCDD. Genes (Ah, ah) at this locus (or perhaps closely linked genes) did not affect control levels of uroporphyrin in urine or liver

Figure 60-34 Origin of isocoproporphyrins in PCT. 5-Carboxylate porphyrinogen III (5-C'gen III) accumulates (*bold letters*) due to the defi-ciency of uroporphyrinogen decarboxylase, and can undergo metabolism by coproporphyrinogen oxidase to form dehydroisocoproporphyrinogen (dehydroisocopro'gen). This compound also ac-cumulates (*bold letters*) because its further metabolism to harderoporphyrinogen is impaired by the decarboxylase deficiency. Isocoproporphy-rins are derived from dehydrocoproporphyrino-gen. ALA, δ-aminolevulinic acid; PBG, porphobi-linogen; Uro'gen, uroporphyrinogen; Copro'gen, coproporphyrinogen; Proto'gen, protoporphyrino-gen; Proto, protoporphyrin.

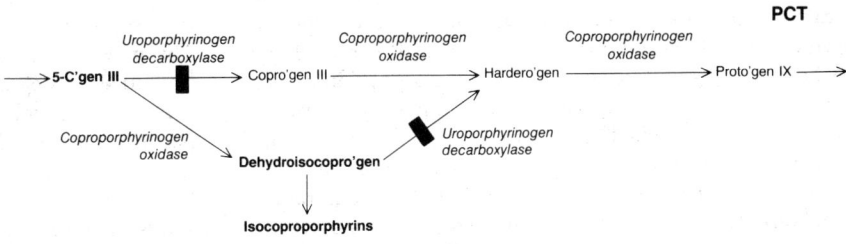

decarboxylase, but only the degree of response to TCDD treatment. The mechanism of this intriguing relationship remains to be determined [917]. Smith et al. [214] studied two strains of rats with markedly different susceptibility to hexachlorobenzene porphyria, and as noted above found that nonheme iron content correlated with this susceptibility. The inbred Agus strain had higher nonheme iron content and developed porphyria more rapidly than the randomly bred Porton strain (Wistar derived). Agus rats also showed greater inhibition of liver uroporphyrinogen decarboxylase and stimulation of ALA synthase. These strain differences did not correlate with differences in hexachlorobenzene content in liver. In contrast, the Agus strain was less susceptible to 3,5-diethoxycarbonyl-1,4-dihydrocollidine, a porphyrogenic chemical that acts by a different mechanism [214]. Genetic factors that determine liver iron content and influence the severity of PCT could exist in humans as well.

Reduced hepatic uroporphyrinogen decarboxylase activity and associated or compensatory changes in other heme pathway enzymes can provide a reasonable explanation for the complex pattern or porphyrin overproduction in PCT (Fig. 60-33). Decreased uroporphyrinogen decarboxylase activity would cause accumulation of uroporphyrinogen III, which is then oxidized to uroporphyrin III. To maintain a normal rate of heme formation there may be a compensatory increase in formation of uroporphyrinogen III and the other porphyrinogen intermediates between uroporphyrinogen III and coproporphyrinogen III. The 7-, 6-, and 5-carboxylate porphyrinogens may accumulate, and then undergo oxidation to corresponding porphyrins, because they are all intermediate substrates for the deficient decarboxylase. Moreover less carboxylated intermediate substrates may competitively inhibit decarboxylation of substrates with more carboxylate groups [196]. As noted earlier, the decarboxylase is probably a single enzyme, although it may have more than one active site [196, 908]. There is no strong or direct evidence for a selective mutation that reduces only one decarboxylation or impairs only one active site of the enzyme.

Elder [891, 926] demonstrated that in rat liver 5-carboxylate porphyrinogen III can be metabolized to dehydroisocoproporphyrinogen (Fig. 60-34). This occurs, as indicated in Table 60-9, by dehydrogenation-decarboxylation of the propionic acid substituent at the 2 position by coproporphyrinogen oxidase. The propionic acid group at the 4 position is not altered. The formation of dehydroisocoproporphyrinogen is favored not only by excess 5-carboxylate porphyrinogen III formation but also by decreased formation of coproporphyrinogen III, both of which result from a deficiency in uroporphyrinogen decarboxylase activity (Fig. 60-34). 5-Carboxylate porphyrinogen III has less affinity than coproporphyrinogen III for coproporphyrinogen oxidase (K_m = 25 to 30 μM and 1 to 2 μM, respectively) and reduced availability of the preferred substrate therefore favors the formation of isocoproporphyrinogen from 5-carboxylate porphyrinogen III. Dehydroisocoproporphyrinogen can itself be metabolized in the liver by decarboxylation of the remaining acetate substituent at the 5 position by uroporphyrinogen decarboxylase, to harderoporphyrinogen (3-carboxylate mono-vinyl porphyrinogen) (Fig. 60-34) and thence to heme. Whether dehydroisocoproporphyrinogen is formed in normal liver is uncertain, but if so it is rapidly metabolized in this manner to harderoporphyrinogen and heme, whereas it may accumulate in PCT because decarboxyl-

ation is impaired [927]. Therefore in PCT the hepatic uroporphyrinogen decarboxylase deficiency results in the accumulation of dehydroisocoproporphyrinogen both by favoring its formation and by impairing its further decarboxylation to harderoporphyrinogen. Elder [891] has also suggested that excess hepatic dehydroisocoproporphyrinogen in PCT may competitively inhibit coproporphyrinogen oxidase. A compensatory increase in coproporphyrinogen III formation to maintain heme synthesis followed by its partial loss from hepatocytes and subsequent oxidation would then explain increased coproporphyrin III excretion.

Excess dehydroisocoproporphyrin is excreted in bile of PCT patients and rats with hexachlorobenzene porphyria [896]. In the intestine bacterial enzymes probably act on the vinyl group (at the 2 position) to give isocoproporphyrin and de-ethylisocoproporphyrin, which are the major fecal porphyrins of this series in PCT and rat hexachlorobenzene porphyria. Fecal mesoporphyrins and deuteroporphyrins are derived from protoporphyrin in the same manner [896].

Increased excretion of series I porphyrins in PCT suggests that another enzyme deficiency, namely decreased hepatic uroporphyrinogen III cosynthase, is present in PCT [723, 891, 928]. Kushner et al. [929] found that ferrous iron can inhibit this enzyme in vitro. Therefore excess iron may explain the excess of series I porphyrins in PCT. Some patients have normal non-heme iron concentrations in the liver. Levin [930] suggested that the cosynthase may also be inhibited by porphyrins and porphyrinogens that accumulate in the liver, in view of studies showing that these compounds can impair the enzyme from mouse spleen.

Since uroporphyrinogen III exceeds uroporphyrinogen I formation in PCT, while excretion of the type I isomer of uroporphyrin exceeds that of the type III isomer, there appears to be preferential decarboxylation of type III uroporphyrinogen isomer [891]. Unexpectedly, no differences between the K_m and V_{max} for the I and III isomers of uroporphyrinogen have been found for the mammalian enzyme by some investigators [193, 929, 931]. Others found that uroporphyrinogen III was metabolized more readily than uroporphyrinogen I by the rat liver [197, 932] or human erythrocyte enzyme [196]. A preferential utilization of uroporphyrinogen III seems likely and would partly explain why excretion of the type III isomers of 7-, 6-, 5-, and 4-carboxylate porphyrins equals or exceeds excretion of the corresponding type I isomers in PCT [891]. Purified rat liver decarboxylase can metabolize uroporphyrinogen I to coproporphyrinogen I without accumulation of the intermediate porphyrinogens; similar characteristics of the human enzyme, namely more rapid decarboxylation of 7-carboxylate porphyrinogen I than III [196, 931], could account in part for the large proportion of the type III isomers of 7-, 6-, and 5-carboxylate porphyrins excreted in PCT [526, 932]. Coproporphyrin I is more readily excreted in bile than coproporphyrin III, and diminished hepatic function and biliary excretion can increase the proportion of coproporphyrin I excreted in urine [933]. This may alter the ratio of coproporphyrin I and III in urine at least to some degree in some PCT patients.

Increased porphyrin excretion, detected mostly by solvent partition methods, has suggested the presence of latent PCT in relatives in at least 10 to 15 percent of PCT patients [824, 825, 891, 906, 934–937]. Moreover increased liver porphyrin stores in some family members may be more common than excess porphyrin excretion [906]. Doss et al. [723, 894, 938] have studied porphyrin excretion by thin layer chromatography techniques and have identified various patterns, termed *chronic hepatic porphyria types A, B, C,* and *D,* which may represent early sequential stages of PCT. Progression from type A to type D has not yet been observed in the same patient. Nonetheless it seems likely that in chronic liver disease and in families of PCT patients such biochemical abnormalities may be more common than the full clinical syndrome of PCT [891].

Liver ALA synthase in this disease may be slightly to moderately increased [738, 939–941] or normal [166, 800, 819]. Conflicting reports on ALA synthase activity in PCT may result from differences in patient selection and methods of measuring the enzyme. More specific assays for ALA synthase have provided values closer to normal [891]. ALA synthase can be shown to be increased in cirrhosis [942] especially if an exogenous system for generation of succinyl CoA is included in the enzyme assay [691]. This matter is complicated by observations [692] that ALA synthase in human liver may be underestimated unless such an exogenous system for succinyl CoA generation is included, and this has not been done in assays in PCT patients. It has been suggested [692] that defective bile acid synthesis in liver disease could lead to accumulation of intermediates in bile acid synthesis, some of which (e.g., di- and trihydroxycoprostanes) are potent inducers of hepatic ALA synthase [943].

Heme is probably synthesized at a normal rate in the liver of PCT patients. Little or no increase in ALA synthase activity occurs in PCT because only small increases in ALA and porphyrinogen synthesis are required to account for the excess porphyrins excreted. Normal liver ALA synthase activity and rates of heme formation have been estimated to be considerably greater than the rate of porphyrin excretion in PCT (Table 60-10) [692, 736, 800]. In hexachlorobenzene-treated rats the activity of uroporphyrinogen decarboxylase remains well above that required for the normal rate of heme formation in rat liver [870]. Studies with [^{14}C]ALA also suggest that heme synthesis is normal in PCT [739]. Moreover there is no impairment of oxidative drug metabolism in PCT, and in fact cytochrome P$_{450}$ levels have been reported to be increased [823, 944]. Studies by Blekkenhorst et al. [823, 945] suggest that in PCT and in hexachlorobenzene porphyria in the rat there may be an increase in cytochrome P$_{448}$.

Graef et al. [946] reported that steroid 5α-reductase activity in rats is reduced by hexachlorobenzene feeding and suggested that a consequent overproduction of 5β-metabolites may contribute to the development of this porphyria. Impaired 5α-reductase activity is probably a significant factor in determining the clinical expression of AIP and perhaps HCP and VP. In PCT, on the other hand, the 5α-reduction of androgens in vivo is not impaired [663]. Whether steroid hormone metabolism is altered in humans with porphyria from exposure to hexachlorobenzene or related chemicals is not known.

Diagnosis

Clinical findings in PCT are quite characteristic but are not diagnostic in themselves because similar skin lesions occur in certain other porphyric and nonporphyric disorders associated with cutaneous photosensitivity. Skin manifestations of VP are especially similar to those in PCT. The diagnosis of PCT therefore requires reliable laboratory confirmation. PCT can usually be differentiated from other types of porphyria if both urine and stool are examined by the traditional solvent partition methods to separate "uroporphyrin" and "coproporphyrin" fractions in urine and "coproporphyrin" and "protoporphyrin" in stool. These methods do not permit individual measurement of 7-, 6-, and 5-carboxylate porphyrins or the isocoproporphyrin series. The uroporphyrin fraction includes 8- and 7-carboxylate porphyrins, and coproporphyrin includes 4- and 5-carboxylate porphyrins as well as isocoproporphyrins. In PCT uroporphyrin exceeds coproporphyrin in urine, and the coproporphyrin fraction predominates in feces. Fecal porphyrin levels are usually not increased as much as in patients with photosensitivity due to EPP, VP, or HCP.

To recognize the characteristic patterns of porphyrin excretion in PCT it is advantageous to separate and measure the different porphyrin species by thin-layer or high performance liquid chromatography [891]. A chromatographic pattern showing a predominance in the urine of 8- and 7-carboxylate porphyrins and an increase in isocoproporphyrin in stool is virtually diagnostic of PCT (Fig. 60-32). For quantitation it is useful to calculate the ratio of isocoproporphyrin to coproporphyrin in feces (ratio > 0.1 in PCT), since some isocoproporphyrin may be excreted by normal subjects (ratio < 0.01 in normals and patients with VP) [891, 947]. Isocoproporphyrin may be increased also in urine. Porphyrin isomer analysis is not required for diagnosis of PCT.

Plasma porphyrin content is always increased in PCT patients with skin lesions as well as in other photocutaneous porphyrias [817, 899, 948, 949]. Thus a normal plasma porphyrin level can rapidly exclude these diagnoses. This requires a sensitive fluorometer and special handling of plasma samples, because with light exposure porphyrins in plasma can be destroyed rapidly. Plasma and fecal porphyrin analysis is particularly important in the differential diagnosis of photosensitivity in hemodialysis patients with little or no urine output.

Treatment

Patients should be advised to cease exposure to alcohol or other agents judged to have contributed to the development of PCT. Some patients improve dramatically when use of alcohol is discontinued [934], but the result is quite unpredictable, and it is generally advisable to begin phlebotomy as well.

Treatment by phlebotomy was introduced by Ippen in 1961 [209, 210]. It is still the standard treatment for PCT and can induce remissions in the great majority of patients [934]. The original aim was to decrease to normal the mild or moderately

Table 60-10 Daily porphyrin excretion in PCT patients compared with the rate of hepatic heme synthesis in normal subjects.

	μ*mol/day*	*Reference*
Excretion of series I porphyrins (PCT)	4–5	[891]
Excretion of series III porphyrins (PCT)	8–9	[891]
Liver heme formation (normal subjects)	90–100	[903]

The data demonstrate that the marked porphyrinuria in PCT still represents only a small fraction of the normal daily production of porphyrins-heme. Thus the porphyrinuria in PCT does not require the induction of ALA synthase.

elevated blood hemoglobin levels that characterize PCT and perhaps to channel excess heme pathway intermediates to hemoglobin production in the bone marrow [210]. A more accepted rationale for this treatment is that reduction of excess iron in the liver has a beneficial effect on porphyrin metabolism in PCT, perhaps by removing the proposed inhibitory effects of iron on uroporphyrinogen III cosynthase and uroporphyrinogen decarboxylase [205, 929]. The disease can be reactivated after phlebotomy by iron replenishment [950]. The aim is therefore to reduce gradually body iron stores and thereby promote the removal of iron from the liver. Initially about 500 ml of blood can be removed at 1- to 2- week intervals. Later the intervals between phlebotomies can be lengthened, especially after there is evidence that an iron deficiency state is developing. Blood hemoglobin should generally not fall below 10 to 11 g/dl and perhaps should be maintained at a higher level in elderly patients. Serum iron levels should be brought down to the range of 50 to 60 µg/dl [844]. Serum ferritin levels may provide an even better index of iron status in PCT patients undergoing phlebotomy [212]. In a recent series a mean of 5.4 phlebotomies and a period of 6.2 months (range 2 to 16 months) was required to bring about a clinical remission [832]. Ippen treated 351 patients between 1959 and 1976 and found that about one-third had remissions lasting 6 to 16 years (sometimes after two or three relapses had occurred), an approximately equal number had no relapses for 2 to 4 years, and in the remainder treatment or follow-up was incomplete [210]. He suggests that phlebotomy be continued until urine porphyrin output falls below 0.5 mg/liter [210]. Absence of new skin lesions is the first clinical sign of improvement, but eventually even cutaneous scarring and pseudoscleroderma can disappear [934]. Sclerodermoid changes showed little or no improvement in one series [844]. Generally, clinical remission is preceded by biochemical improvement [832]. New skin lesions are unlikely when porphyrin excretion falls below 100 nmol/day [891] or when plasma porphyrin content is below 1 µg/dl [900]. Abnormal patterns of porphyrin excretion may eventually become normal [951]. Liver function abnormalities also improve with phlebotomy [952]. Hepatic fluorescence, needlelike inclusions, and siderosis can also be expected to decrease or disappear with this treatment, but other liver histological abnormalities may not [846, 953]. There are also suggestions that desferrioxamine may be effective in some patients [853].

An adverse effect of chloroquine in PCT was first described by Linden et al. [954]. Moreover, PCT has been unmasked by chloroquine treatment in some patients who were given this drug for systemic lupus erythematosus [955–957] or when given for malaria prophylaxis [958]. When chloroquine is given to PCT patients, there is a marked increase in uroporphyrin and 7-carboxylate porphyrin excretion, and this is accompanied by fever, malaise, nausea, and increase in serum transaminase and ferritin levels. These effects, which may be accompanied by increased cutaneous lesions, are transient and are followed in a few days by a prolonged period of remission [212, 959–961]. Chloroquine produces a decrease in liver uroporphyrin content but does not reduce hepatic siderosis, at least acutely [960]. An increase in iron excretion in urine may occur in some patients [962, 963]. Remission can occur in spite of continued treatment with estrogen for prostatic carcinoma [960]. Chloroquine is markedly concentrated in liver, particularly in lysosomes and mitochondria and is known also to form molecular complexes with porphyrins [964, 965]. In rats made

porphyric with DDC, the drug produces increased porphyrinuria without serum transaminase elevation or further induction of ALA synthase. Thus the action of chloroquine to increase porphyrin excretion does not result from hepatic toxicity per se or from induction of ALA synthase and stimulation of the heme biosynthetic pathway but largely from removal of porphyrin from the liver as a molecular complex with the drug. Increased iron excretion may also contribute [962, 966] and is reportedly a more likely mechanism in studies of response to chloroquine in siderotic hexachlorobenzene-treated rats [962]. A transient increase in porphyrin excretion may not occur in rats with hexachlorobenzene porphyria when they are treated with chloroquine [962, 967].

The hepatotoxicity observed in PCT patients has nonetheless discouraged the use of chloroquine for treating this disorder. Moreover the response to chloroquine may be incomplete and phlebotomy still may be required for a full remission [212]. Nevertheless, in general, good results have been obtained in treating patients with small doses of chloroquine (e.g., 125 mg twice weekly) or hydroxychloroquine until the urine uroporphyrin excretion diminishes. Further studies with low-dose regimens seem warranted, particularly when repeated venesection is contraindicated [961–963, 968–971]. Some patients initially given a low dose of one of these drugs have eventually required higher doses to induce a remission, and since treatment is prolonged the risk of other adverse effects of chloroquine, especially retinopathy, must be considered [963]. Hemosiderin deposition in the liver is decreased in some patients after low dose chloroquine treatment, but liver histopathology is otherwise unchanged [972].

The excretion of coproporphyrin but not uroporphyrin in urine can be increased by alkalinization [464]. Sodium bicarbonate orally has been employed for treating PCT patients with some apparent benefit [462, 463]. Whether improvement resulted only from this treatment is uncertain since many patients also decreased their intake of alcohol [463]. Other treatments tried in PCT patients have included p-aminobenzoic acid [973], cholestyramine, vitamin E, pyridoxal phosphate, and adenosine monophosphate [789, 844].

OTHER DISORDERS OF PORPHYRIN METABOLISM

Porphyria with Hepatic Tumors

The risk of primary hepatocellular carcinoma is considerably increased in PCT patients. These tumors are viewed as complications of PCT and are not responsible for the disease. PCT patients may also develop more common cancers in other organs, such as the colon, lung, or prostate, and these sometimes metastasize to the liver. Very rarely porphyria is associated with hepatic tumors that themselves contain and presumably produce excess porphyrins. Such cases may resemble PCT, but the clinical and biochemical picture is quite variable since all such tumors may not share a single biochemical defect in porphyrin metabolism.

The best-known case was an 80-year-old woman with recent onset of photosensitivity who was found to have a large 11 × 10.5-cm liver cell adenoma [974]. Excess porphyrins were found in the tumor, urine, and feces. By solvent partition methods the uroporphyrin fraction exceeded coproporphyrin in the urine, but in contrast to PCT, protoporphyrin was the predominant porphyrin in the feces. The adenoma contained uroporphyrin and lesser amounts of protoporphyrin, coproporphyrin, and 3-carboxylate porphyrin by paper chromatography. There was no evidence of porphyria in relatives. The patient improved after the adenoma was removed and died from another cause 2 years later. At autopsy no tumor was found and no porphyrins were detectable in the liver.

Berman et al. [975] reported 11 cases of PCT with cirrhosis and hepatocellular carcinoma. In one there was red fluorescence in the tumor under ultraviolet light. Two other cases of nonresectable malignant liver cell tumors containing porphyrins have been reported [976, 977]. One had predominantly uroporphyrin in the urine and fecal porphyrins were also increased [976], whereas in the second urine porphyrins were normal and fecal porphyrins were moderately increased (mostly consisting of protoporphyrin). In one case the tumor contained additional unusual 2- and 3-carboxylate porphyrins [978].

Thus histological features and patterns of porphyrin excretion in porphyrin-producing hepatic tumors are variable. They are nevertheless of considerable interest and merit detailed study because they may represent defects in enzymes of the heme pathway associated, albeit rarely, with neoplastic transformation of liver cells.

Erythropoietic Coproporphyria

A 22-year-old woman with symptoms suggesting EPP but with a markedly increased erythrocyte coproporphyrin content has been described by Heilmeyer and coworkers [430, 979]. Red cell uroporphyrin and protoporphyrin, urine ALA, and fecal protoporphyrin were only slightly increased. Similar symptoms occurred in a paternal cousin. This may represent a distinct form of genetic porphyria which resembles EPP clinically but is characterized by accumulation of coproporphyrin rather than protoporphyrin in erythrocytes. Further cases have not been described and the enzymatic defect remains to be defined.

Lead Poisoning

Plumbism can present with symptoms that are strikingly similar to those in AIP, such that a number of patients have been misdiagnosed initially as having porphyria [980–982]. If proper biochemical testing is available, these diseases can be readily differentiated.

Lead concentrates particularly in erythroid cells where it can inhibit at least two enzymes of heme biosynthesis, ALA dehydratase and ferrochelatase. Other heme pathway enzymes are inhibited by higher concentrations of the heavy metal. Excess intermediates accumulate in these cells or are excreted in urine. Much less inhibition of heme biosynthesis occurs in the liver of animals and patients with lead intoxication. Studies with radiolabeled ALA in subjects with lead intoxication and marked inhibition of ALA dehydratase in erythrocytes revealed no evidence of inhibition of heme synthesis in the liver [983]. Moreover there is little or no decrease in the content of cytochrome P_{450}, the major hemoprotein in terms of heme utilization for its synthesis, in the liver of subjects or animals with

lead intoxication [984]. Because lead poisoning affects primarily the erythron rather than the liver, it can be viewed as an acquired form of erythropoietic porphyria. As in the hepatic porphyrias, many of the major symptoms are due to neuropathic changes.

Inhibition of ALA dehydratase by lead results in excess urinary excretion of ALA with little or no increase in PBG. The active site of this enzyme contains sulfhydryl groups, which bind lead avidly. The active site is normally protected by zinc, which can be displaced by lead. Reversal of lead inhibition by DTT or zinc of ALA dehydratase can be shown in vitro in red cell lysates and is a sensitive index of excess lead exposure [129, 732, 985].

Ferrochelatase inhibition by excess lead results in accumulation of protoporphyrin in erythroid cells. Porphyrin accumulation occurs at a relatively earlier stage in the development of clinical lead poisoning and precedes inhibition of hemoglobin synthesis and anemia. The detection of excess protoporphyrin is a sensitive indicator of excess lead but somewhat less so than the assay for ALA dehydratase inhibition. Excess protoporphyrin in red cells of patients with plumbism is complexed with zinc. Therefore it should not be referred to as "free erythrocyte protoporphyrin." Zn-protoporphyrin remains in red cells for the duration of their life span in the circulation, and therefore does not fall quickly after treatment.

Urinary coproporphyrin excretion is also increased in lead poisoning. This suggests inhibition of coproporphyrinogen oxidase. However, this enzyme is not inhibited by lead in vitro [225]. Excess coproporphyrin excretion is a less sensitive indicator of lead poisoning than are the other effects of lead on the heme pathway noted above.

Lead can produce metabolic abnormalities unrelated to the heme pathway. Plumbism is associated, for example, with an acquired deficiency of pyrimidine-specific 5'-nucleotidase in red cells [986]. A hereditary form of this enzyme deficiency occurs and is accompanied, as in lead intoxication, by hemolysis and basophilic stippling of erythrocytes. In both disorders the enzyme deficiency appears to impair dephosphorylation of pyrimidine 5'-nucleoside monophosphates to soluble products that can diffuse out of erythroid cells. Pyrimidine nucleotides then accumulate and impair RNA breakdown, thereby giving rise to basophilic stippling [986]. The biochemical basis for many other manifestations of lead poisoning remain unexplained.

Hereditary Tyrosinemia (see also Chap. 13)

Urine from patients with this inborn error of amino acid metabolism has recently been found to contain succinylacetone (4,6-dioxoheptanoic acid), which is a by-product of the pathway for tyrosine degradation. Because of its structural similarity to ALA (Fig. 60-7) succinylacetone is a potent inhibitor of ALA dehydratase [99, 132]. Serum also contains succinylacetone. This provides an explanation for the marked inhibition of this enzyme in erythrocytes and liver of these patients and for symptoms resembling acute porphyria that occur during relapse of this disease, including abdominal pain, hypertension, tachycardia, and increased catecholamine excretion [132, 987]. The accumulation of succinylacetone and succinylacetoacetate points to decreased activity of fumarylacetoacetase as the primary genetic defect in tyrosinemia [132]. Low activity of 4-hydroxyphenylpyruvate dioxygenase also occurs in this disease, and this does not appear to be due to a circulating inhibitor. Children with tyrosinemia also develop renal tubular defects, chronic liver disease, and hepatocellular carcinoma. It is not known whether excess accumulation of tyrosine metabolites or ALA contributes directly to any of these complications.

Acute Porphyria with ALA Dehydratase Deficiency

Doss et al. [142, 143] recently described two unrelated males who in their teens developed symptoms, including severe neuropathy, suggesting AIP. Each had marked increases in urinary ALA excretion and markedly reduced erythrocyte ALA dehydratase. Activity of this enzyme was less than 1 percent of normal, and in contrast to lead poisoning there was little restoration of ALA dehydratase activity after in vitro treatment with 1,4-dithiothreitol. The urine also contained excess porphyrin, at least 95 percent of which was coproporphyrin III. Erythrocyte protoporphyrin was mildly increased, whereas fecal porphyrins were normal. The authors [142] noted that the excess excretion of coproporphyrin III was similar to that seen after ALA loading in normal subjects. This suggests that ALA may be metabolized to coproporphyrin in tissues other than the liver [723]. Family studies showed intermediate reductions of ALA dehydratase activity in some first-degree relatives, and this is consistent with autosomal recessive inheritance. The mode of inheritance needs to be more firmly established.

These patients appear to have a new form of hereditary hepatic porphyria with clinical features very similar to those in AIP. The nature of the ALA dehydratase defect in unclear. In contrast to lead poisoning, in which the enzyme activity can be restored to normal in vitro by addition of sulfhydryl reagents, in this hereditary condition there is little increase in enzyme activity with addition of 1,4-dithiothreitol [142]. Whether this disease is activiated by hormones, drugs and nutritional factors is as yet unknown; the onset of symptoms in both patients at age 15 suggests that hormonal changes associated with puberty may be important in its pathogenesis.

Another family with an approximately 50 percent deficiency of ALA dehydratase in erythrocytes was reported by Bird et al. [141]. This deficiency was not associated with symptoms or disordered porphyrin precursor metabolism. Members of this family were perhaps heterozygous for a defect similar to that in the two families reported by Doss and coworkers [142]. ALA dehydratase is normally present in considerable excess, such that only a marked deficiency would be expected to be associated with disease.

Hereditary Sideroblastic Anemia with Pyridoxine Responsiveness

A form of hereditary sideroblastic anemia is accompanied by decreased ALA synthase activity in erythroblasts and responds to treatment of the patient with large doses of pyridoxal phosphate. Aoki et al. [988] found in two patients that affinity of the apoenzyme for pyridoxal phosphate was not decreased in this disease, but the apoenzyme was highly sensitive to a mitochondrial protease that degrades ALA synthase and certain other pyridoxal enzymes in bone marrow erythroid and granulocytic cells. Activity of the protease itself was normal.

Hypercatabolism of a structurally abnormal ALA synthase therefore may be responsible for this genetic disorder, although other mechanisms could also explain increased enzyme degradation by the protease. It was considered likely but not proven that pyridoxine in large doses in some manner stabilizes the enzyme and slows its rate of catabolism [988].

This is an interesting and presently unique instance of an abnormality in a heme pathway enzyme resulting in enhanced enzyme degradation. Whether this was acquired or inherited in the two cases studied by Aoki et al. [988] is unclear. Others have described inherited cases of sideroblastic anemia responsive to pyridoxine, and in these cases decreased erythroid ALA synthase has been demonstrated [550, 989]. Inheritance in some cases is X-linked recessive. Other forms of the disease may exist. In primary sideroblastic anemia inheritance is less evident, and although ALA synthase in bone marrow is decreased there is no response to pyridoxine. In patients with primary sideroblastic anemia studied by Aoki [990], there were multiple enzymatic defects in erythroblast mitochondria, but the sensitivity of ALA synthase to the mitochondrial protease in these cases was normal.

Porphyrinuria

Excess urinary excretion of porphyrins can complicate other illnesses, particularly those associated with hepatic dysfunction or increased erythropoiesis. Porphyrinuria in patients with liver disease or anemia is generally confined to excess coproporphyrin excretion [991, 993]. Excess coproporphyrinuria in chronic hemolytic disorders may sometimes relate in part to iron overload and the resulting liver dysfunction [994]. Such "secondary" porphyrinurias are seldom in themselves associated with clinical manifestations [6].

Increased porphyrin excretion can be due to a number of factors in patients with liver disease. These include (1) impaired activity of uroporphyrinogen decarboxylase in patients who may be regarded as having a subclinical stage of PCT, (2) increased ALA synthase activity or decreased efficiency of utilization of porphyrinogen intermediates [349, 692], and (3) decreased biliary excretion of porphyrin which leads to a compensatory increase in urinary excretion. The latter primarily affects coproporphyrin excretion because uroporphyrin is not excreted in bile to a significant extent and little or no protoporphyrin is excreted in urine under any circumstance. As mentioned in the discussion of HCP, coproporphyrinogen is also postulated to leak out of hepatocytes more readily than other porphyrinogen intermediates [232], which may explain why coproporphyrin, its autooxidation product, is normally the predominant porphyrin in urine.

Coproporphyrin in normal urine is approximately 70 percent isomer III and 30 percent isomer I [892, 995, 996]. Coproporphyrin is excreted primarily in bile, and this occurs by a carrier-mediated mechanism that favors the transport of the symmetrical type I isomer [933]. Therefore when hepatic excretory function is impaired, as by ethynylestradiol administration in the rat, there is a proportional decrease in the excretion of both isomers and thus an increase in the ratio of coproporphyrin I to coproporphyrin III in urine. Measurement of this ratio is likely to be a sensitive index of impaired liver function in a variety of hepatic diseases [933]. In particular, in the Dubin-Johnson syndrome, in which a defect in bile canicular transport of organic anions is inherited as an autosomal recessive trait, the coproporphyrin I/coproporphyrin III isomer ratio is markedly increased. In other liver diseases, or in response to alcohol intake, total urinary coproporphyrin excretion is increased, largely due to increased coproporphyrin III production probably in the liver [991, 992]. The Dubin-Johnson syndrome in contrast is accompanied by decreased excretion of coproporphyrin III. Intermediate increases in the I/III ratio are noted in heterozygotes, and this represents the only dependable means of detecting such individuals [997, 1000]. The possibility that this altered ratio could be due to decreased uroporphyrinogen III cosynthase activity has been excluded by direct measurement of this enzyme in liver and red cells of patients with this syndrome [1001]. When endogenous (particularly hepatic) formation of coproporphyrinogen III is enhanced in normal subjects by ALA loading, an increase in formation and biliary excretion of protoporphyrin can result, in addition to increased urinary excretion of coproporphyrin III, and serum bilirubin also increases [723, 1002, 1003]. There is much less of an increase in coproporphyrin I excretion in bile or urine than of coproporphyrin III after ALA loading, suggesting that even large amounts of exogenous ALA cannot produce a significant increase in the formation of coproporphyrin I.

In the Dubin-Johnson syndrome ALA loading results in enhanced biliary excretion of protoporphyrin and little increase in urinary coproporphyrin III excretion [1003]. This may indicate impaired transport of coproporphyrinogen III from hepatocytes to blood, and a carrier-mediated mechanism at the liver cell plasma membrane was suggested to be defective in this disease [1003]. Such a defect would be analogous to the defective transport mechanism at the bile canaliculus. To our knowledge the mechanism by which coproporphyrinogen III from hepatocytes finally appears as coproporphyrin III in urine has not been established, and could involve biliary secretion as well as an enterohepatic circulation. Koskelo and Mustajoki [1004] suggest that in this disease coproporphyrin I excretion is shifted from bile to urine, but they found isomer III excretion to be decreased via both routes. Coproporphyrin III or perhaps a derivative may accumulate in liver lysosomes and itself account both for the characteristic hepatocellular pigment that is one of the hallmarks of the disorder as well as for decreased coproporphyrin III excretion [1004]. Direct evidence for this idea is lacking. A developmental hepatic excretory defect similar to that in the Dubin-Johnson syndrome may be present in the normal fetus and infant [1005].

REFERENCES

1. SHEMIN D, RUSSELL CS: Delta-aminolevulinic acid, its role in the biosynthesis of porphyrins and purines. *J Am Chem Soc* 75:4873, 1953
2. RIMINGTON C: Biosynthesis of haemoglobin. *Br Med Bull* 15:19, 1959
3. LASCELLES J: *Tetrapyrrole Biosynthesis and its Regulation.* New York, Amsterdam, Benjamin, 1964
4. MARKS GS: *Heme and Chlorophyll.* Princeton, NJ, Van Nostrand, 1969, p 208
5. MEYER UA, SCHMID R: The porphyrias, in Stanbury JB, Wyngaarden JB, Fredrickson DS (eds): *The Metabolic Basis of Inherited Disease,* 4th ed. New York, McGraw-Hill, 1978, p 1166
6. TSCHUDY DP, LAMON JM: Porphyrin metabolism and the porphyrias, in Bondy PK, Rosenberg LE (eds): *Duncan's Diseases of Metabolism,* 8th ed. Philadelphia, Saunders, 1980, p 939
7. EALES L: Clinical chemistry of the porphyrins, in Dolphin D (ed): *The Porphyrins,* vol VI. New York, Academic Press, 1979, p 663
8. KARLSON P: The nomenclature of tetrapyrroles. A report. *Hoppe-Seyler's Z Physiol Chem* 362:7, 1981
9. IUPAC-IUB JOINT COMMISSION ON BIOCHEMICAL NOMENCLATURE (JCBN): Nomenclature of tetrapyrroles: Recommendations 1978. *Eur J Biochem* 108:1, 1980
10. FISCHER H, ORTH H: *Die Chemie des Pyrrols,* vols I, II, III. New York, Johnson Reprint Co (Akademische Verlag Gueleschaft m.b.h., Leibzig, 1934), 1968
11. FALK JE: *Porphyrins and Metalloporphyrins,* vol 2. New York, Elsevier, 1964
12. WILLIAMS RJP: The properties of metalloporphyrins. *J Chem Soc Commun,* 1956, p 299
13. FUHRHOP JH, SMITH KM: Laboratory methods, in *Porphyrin and Metalloporphyrin Research.* Amsterdam, Elsevier, 1975, p 1
14. HEMLER M, LANDS WEM, SMITH WL: Purification of the cyclo-oxygenase that forms prostaglandins: Demonstration of two forms of iron in the holoenzyme. *J Biol Chem* 251:5575, 1976
15. VAN DER OUDERAA FJ, BUYTENHEK M, SLIKKERVEER LJ, VAN DORP DA: On the haemoprotein character of prostaglandin endoperoxide synthetase. *Biochim Biophys Acta* 572:29, 1979
16. BOCK KW, SIEKEVITZ P: Turnover of heme and protein moieties of rat liver microsomal cytochrome b$_5$. *Biochem Biophys Res Commun* 41:374, 1970
17. DRUYAN R, DEBERNARD B, RABINOWITZ M: Turnover of cytochromes labeled with δ-aminolevulinic acid-^{3}H in rat liver. *J Biol Chem* 244:5874, 1969
18. NEGISHI M, OMURA T: Presence of apo-cytochrome b$_5$ in microsomes from rat liver. *J Biochem* 67:745, 1970
19. HARA T, MINAKAMI S: Presence of apo-cytochrome b$_5$ in microsomes. Incorporation of radioactive heme to the cytochrome in vitro. *J Biochem (Tokyo)* 67:741, 1970
20. CORREIA MA, MEYER UA: Apocytochrome P-450: Reconstitution of functional cytochrome with hemin in vitro. *Proc Natl Acad Sci USA* 72:400, 1975
21. CORREIA MA, FARRELL GC, SCHMID R, ORTIZ DE MONTELLANO PR, YOST GS, MICO BA: Incorporation of exogenous heme into hepatic cytochrome P-450, *in vivo. J Biol Chem* 254:15, 1979
22. FARRELL GC, CORREIA MA: Structural and functional reconstitution of hepatic cytochrome P-450 *in vivo:* Reversal of allylisopropylacetamide-mediated destruction of the hemoprotein by endogenous heme. *J Biol Chem* 255:10128, 1980
23. GRANICK JL, SASSA S: Hemin control of heme biosynthesis in mouse Friend-virus transformed erythroleukemia cells in culture. *J Biol Chem* 253:5402, 1978
24. SPIKES JD: Porphyrins and related compounds as photodynamic sensitizers. *Ann NY Acad Sci* 244:496, 1975
25. LIM HW, PEREZ HD, GOLDSTEIN IM, GIGLI I: Complement-derived chemotactic activity is generated in human serum containing uroporphyrin after irradiation with 405 nm light. *J Clin Invest* 67:1072, 1981
26. BLUM HF: *Photodynamic Action and Diseases Caused by Light.* New York, Reinhold, 1941
27. JONI G, GALIAZZO G, SCOFFONE E: Photodynamic action of porphyrins on aminoacids and proteins. I. Selective photooxidation of methionine in aqueous solution. *Biochemistry* 8:2868, 1969
28. SPIKES JD, MACKNIGHT ML: Dye-sensitized photooxidation of proteins. *Ann NY Acad Sci* 171:149, 1970
29. BUNGELER W: Über den Einfluss photosensibilisierender Substanzen auf die Entstehung von Hautgeschwülsten. *Z Krebsforsch* 46:130, 1937
30. DIAMOND I, McDONAGH AF, WILSON CB, GRANELLI SG, NIELSEN S, JAENICKE R: Photodynamic therapy of malignant tumors. *Lancet* ii:1175, 1972
30a. VARIGOS G, SCHILTZ JR, BICKERS D: Uroporphyrin I stimulation of collagen biosynthesis in human skin fibroblasts. A unique dark effect of porphyrin. *J Clin Invest* 69:129, 1982
31. SHEMIN D, RITTENBERG D: The biological utilization of glycine for the synthesis of the protoporphyrin of hemoglobin. *J Biol Chem* 166:621, 1946
32. SHEMIN D, RITTENBERG D: The life-span of the human red blood cell. *J Biol Chem* 166:627, 1946
33. RADIN NS, RITTENBERG D, SHEMIN D: The role of glycine in the biosynthesis of heme. *J Biol Chem* 184:745, 1950
34. GRINSTEIN M, KAMEN MD, MOORE CV: Observation on the utilization of glycine in the biosynthesis of hemoglobin. *J Biol Chem* 174:767, 1948
35. COOKSON GH, RIMINGTON C: Porphobilinogen. *Biochem J* 57:476, 1954
36. WESTALL RG: Isolation of porphobilinogen from the urine of a patient with acute porphyria. *Nature* 170:614, 1952
37. SHEMIN D: The succinate-glycine cycle. The role of δ-aminolevulinic acid in porphyrin synthesis, in Wolstenholme GWE, Miller ECP (eds): *Ciba Foundation Symposium on Porphyrin Biosynthesis and Metabolism,* London, Churchill, 1955, p 4
38. BOGORAD L: Intermediates in the biosynthesis of porphyrins from porphobilinogen. *Science* 121:878, 1955

39. BOGORAD L: The enzymatic synthesis of porphyrin from porphobilinogen. I. Uroporphyrin I. *J Biol Chem* 233:501, 1958

40. MAUZERALL D, GRANICK S: Porphyrin biosynthesis in erythrocytes. III. Uroporphyrinogen and its decarboxylase. *J Biol Chem* 232:1141, 1958

41. KIKUCHI G, KUMAR A, TALMAGE P, SHEMIN D: The enzymatic synthesis of δ-aminolevulinic acid. *J Biol Chem* 233:1214, 1958

42. GIBSON KD, LAVER WG, NEUBERGER A: Initial stages in the biosynthesis of porphyrins. 2. The formation of δ-aminolaevulinic acid from glycine and succinyl-coenzyme A by particles from chicken erythrocytes. *Biochem J* 70:71, 1958

43. TAIT GH: Coproporphyrinogenase activities in extracts of *Rhodopseudomonas spheroides* and *Chromatium* strain D. *Biochem J* 128:1159, 1972

44. PORRA RJ, BARNES R, JONES OTG: The level and sub-cellular distribution of δ-aminolaevulinate synthase activity in semianaerobic and aerobic yeast. *Hoppe-Seyler's Z Physiol Chem* 353:1365, 1972

45. GRANICK S: The induction *in vitro* of the synthesis of δ-amino-levulinic acid synthetase in chemical porphyria: A response to certain drugs, sex hormones, and foreign chemicals. *J Biol Chem* 241:1359, 1966

46. GRANICK S, URATA G: Increase in activity of δ-aminolevulinic acid synthetase in liver mitochondria induced by feeding of 3,5-dicarbethoxy-1,4-dihydrocollidine. *J Biol Chem* 238:821, 1963

47. MARVER HS, TSCHUDY DP, PERLROTH MG, COLLINS A: δ-Aminolevulinic acid synthetase. I. Studies in liver homogenates. *J Biol Chem* 241:2803, 1966

48. MARVER HS, COLLINS A, TSCHUDY DP, RECHCIGL M, JR: δ-Aminolevulinic acid synthetase. II. Induction in rat liver. *J Biol Chem* 241:4323, 1966

49. TAKAKU F, WADA O, SASSA S, NAKAO K: Heme synthesis in normal and leukemic leukocytes. *Cancer Res* 28:1250, 1968

50. MARGOLIS FL: Regulation of porphyrin biosynthesis in the Harderian gland of inbred mouse strains. *Arch Biochem Biophys* 145:373, 1971

51. SARDESAI VM, LENAGHAN R, ROSENBERG JC: Tissue delta-aminolevulinic acid synthetase activity in hemorrhagic shock. *Biochem Med* 6:366, 1972

52. CONDIE LW, TEPHLY TR: δ-Aminolevulinic acid synthetase. Sensitive methods in liver for hemoprotein biosynthesis, in Fleischer S, Packer L (eds): *Methods in Enzymology*, vol 52 (Biomembranes), part C. New York, Academic, 1978, p 350

53. PATERNITI JR, SIMONE JJ, BEATTIE DS: Detection and regulation of δ-aminolevulinic acid synthetase activity in the rat brain. *Arch Biochem Biophys* 189:86, 1978

54. BRATTSTEN LB, WILKINSON CF: Properties of 5-aminolaevulinate synthetase and its relationship to microsomal mixed-function oxidation in the Southern Armyworm (*Spodoptera eridania*). *Biochem J* 150:97, 1975

55. WHITING MJ, ELLIOTT WH: Purification and properties of solubilized mitochondrial δ-aminolevulinic acid synthetase and comparison with the cytosol enzyme. *J Biol Chem* 247:6818, 1972

56. KAPLAN BH: δ-Aminolevulinic acid synthetase from the particulate fraction of liver of porphyric rats. *Biochim Biophys Acta* 235:381, 1971

57. WHITING MJ, GRANICK S: δ-Aminolevulinic acid synthase from chick embryo liver mitochondria. I. Purification and some properties. *J Biol Chem* 251:1340, 1976

58. PATERNITI JR, BEATTIE DS: δ-Aminolevulinic acid synthetase from rat liver mitochondria: Purification and properties. *J Biol Chem* 254:6112, 1979

59. AOKI Y, WADA O, URATA G, TAKAKU F, NAKAO K: Purification and some properties of δ-aminolevulinate (ALA) synthetase in rabbit reticulocytes. *Biochem Biophys Res Commun* 42:568, 1971

60. SCHOLNICK PL, HAMMAKER LE, MARVER HS: Soluble δ-aminolevulinic acid synthetase of rat liver. I. Some properties of the partially purified enzyme. *J Biol Chem* 247:4126, 1972

61. WOODS JS, MURTHY VV: δ-Aminolevulinic acid synthetase from fetal rat liver: Studies on the partially purified enzyme. *Mol Pharmacol* 11:70, 1975

62. SINCLAIR P, GRANICK S: Two methods for determining the activity of δ-aminolevulinate synthetase within intact liver cells in culture. *Anal Biochem* 79:380, 1977

63. PIPER WN, CONDIE LW, TEPHLY TR: The role of substrates for glycine acyl transferase in the reversal of chemically induced porphyria in the rat. *Arch Biochem Biophys* 159:671, 1973

64. TEPHLY TR, CONDIE LW, PIPER WN: The role of substrates for glycine acyl transferase and the role of sulfanylamide and acetate in the reversal of chemically-induced porphyria in the rat. *Enzyme* 16:187, 1973

65. PATTON GM, BEATTIE DS: Studies on hepatic δ-aminolevulinic acid synthetase. *J Biol Chem* 248:4467, 1973

66. HAYASHI N, YODA B, KIKUCHI G: Mechanism of allylisopropylacetamide-induced increase of δ-aminolevulinate synthetase in liver mitochondria. IV. Accumulation of the enzyme in the soluble fraction of rat liver. *Arch Biochem Biophys* 131:83, 1969

67. BARNES R, JONES MS, JONES OTG, PORRA RJ: Ferrochelatase and δ-aminolevulinate synthetase in brain, heart, kidney, and liver of normal and porphyric rats. *Biochem J* 124:633, 1971

68. IGARASHI J, HAYASHI N, KIKUCHI G: δ-Aminolevulinate synthetases in the liver cytosol fraction and mitochondria of mice treated with allylisopropylacetamide and 3,5-dicarbethoxy-1,4-dihydrocollidine. *J Biochem* 80: 1091, 1976

69. OHASHI A, KIKUCHI G: Mechanism of allylisopropylacetamide-induced increase of δ-aminolevulinate synthetase in liver mitochondria. VI. Multiple molecular forms of δ-aminolevulinate synthetase in the cytosol and mitochondria of induced cock liver. *Arch Biochem Biophys* 153:34, 1972

70. KIKUCHI G, OHASHI A, HAYASHI N: Studies on the conversion of the cytosol δ-aminolevulinate synthetase to the mitochondrial enzyme. *Ann Clin Res* 8(Suppl 17):74, 1976

71. OHAHSI A, KIKUCHI G: Studies on the mechanism of the conversion of cytosol δ-aminolevulinic acid synthase to the mitochondrial enzyme in the liver of the allylisopropylacetamide-treated rat. *Arch Biochem Biophys* 178:607, 1977

72. OHASHI A, KIKUCHI G: Purification and some properties of two forms of δ-aminolevulinic synthase from rat liver cytosol. *J Biochem (Tokyo)* 85:239, 1979

73. HAYASHI N, YODA B, KIKUCHI G: Differences in molecular sizes of δ-aminolevulinate synthetases in the soluble and mitochondrial fractions of rat liver. *J Biochem (Tokyo)* 67:859, 1970

74. NAKAKUKI M, YAMAUCHI K, HAYASHI N, KIKUCHI G: Purification and some properties of δ-aminolevulinate synthase from the rat liver cytosol fraction and immunochemical identity of the cytosolic enzyme and the mitochondrial enzyme. *J Biol Chem* 255:1738, 1980

75. OHASHI A, SINOHARA H: Incorporation of cytosol δ-aminolevulinate synthase of rat liver into the mitochondria in vitro. *Biochem Biophys Res Commun* 84:76, 1978

76. WOODS JS: Studies on the role of heme in the regulation of δ-aminolevulinic acid synthetase during fetal hepatic development. *Mol Pharmacol* 10:389, 1974

77. TSCHUDY DP, MARVER HS, COLLINS A: A model for calculating messenger RNA half-life: Short-lived messenger RNA in the induction of mammalian δ-aminolevulinic acid synthetase. *Biochem Biophys Res Commun* 21:480, 1965

78. SASSA S, GRANICK S: Induction of δ-aminolevulinic acid synthetase in chick embyro liver cells in culture. *Proc Natl Acad Sci USA* 67:517, 1970

79. RUSSELL DH, SNYDER SH: Amine synthesis in regenerating rat liver: Extremely rapid turnover of ornithine decarboxylase. *Mol Pharmacol* 5:253, 1969

80. AOKI Y, URATA G, TAKAKU F, KATSUNUMA N: A new protease inactivating δ-aminolevulinic acid synthetase in mitochondria of human bone marrow. *Biochem Biophys Res Commun* 65:567, 1975.

81. AOKI Y: Crystallization and characterization of a new protease in mitochondria of bone marrow cells. *J Biol Chem* 253:2026, 1978

82. ZAMAN Z, JORDAN PM, AKHTAR M: Mechanism and stereochemistry of the 5-aminolaevulinate synthetase reaction. *Biochem J* 135:257, 1973

83. AKHTAR M, ABBOUD MM, BARNARD G, JORDAN P, ZAMAN Z: Mechanism and stereochemistry of enzymic reactions involved in porphyrin biosynthesis. *Philos Trans R Soc Lond (Biol)* B273:117, 1976

84. ABBOUD MM, JORDAN PM, AKHTAR M: Biosynthesis of 5-aminolevulinic acid. Involvement of a retention-inversion mechanism. *J Chem Soc Chem Commun*, 1974, p 643

85. LAGHAI A, JORDAN PM: A partial reaction of δ-aminolevulinic acid synthetase from *Rhodopseudomonas spheroides*. *Biochem Soc Trans* 4:52, 1976

86. SASSA S: Control of heme biosynthesis in erythroid cells, in Rossi GB (ed): *Erythropoiesis and Differentiation in Friend Leukemia Cells*, EMBO Workshop on CNR. Amsterdam, Elsevier North-Holland Biochem Press, 1980, p 219

87. HAYASHI N, KURASHIMA Y, KIKUCHI G: Mechanism of allylisopropylacetamide-induced increase of δ-aminolevulinate synthetase in liver mitochondria. V. Mechanism of regulation by hemin of the level of δ-aminolevulinate synthetase in rat liver mitochondria. *Arch Biochem Biophys* 148:10, 1972

88. GRANICK S, SINCLAIR P, SASSA S, GRIENINGER G: Effects by heme, insulin, and serum albumin on heme and protein synthesis in chick embryo liver cells cultured in a chemically defined medium, and a spectrofluorometric assay for porphyrin composition. *J Biol Chem* 250:9215, 1975

89. BEALE SI, CASTELFRANCO PA: The biosynthesis of δ-aminolevulinic acid in higher plants. II. Formation of ^{14}C-δ-aminolevulinic acid from labeled precursors in greening plant tissues. *Plant Physiol* 53:297, 1974

90. BEALE SI, GOUGH SP, GRANICK S: Biosynthesis of δ-aminolevulinic acid from the intact carbon skeleton of glutamic acid in greening barley. *Proc Natl Acad Sci USA* 72:2719, 1975

91. GASSMAN M, PLUSCEC J, BOGORAD L: δ-Aminolevulinic acid transaminase in *Chlorella vulgaris*. *Plant Physiol* 43:1411, 1968

92. GASSMAN M, PLUSCEC J, BOGORAD L: δ-Aminolevulinic acid transaminase from *Chlorella* and *Phaseolus*. *Plant Physiol* 41(Suppl):xiv, 1966

93. NEUBERGER A, TURNER JM: γ-δ-Dioxovalerate aminotranferase activity in *Rhodopseudomonas spheroides*. *Biochim Biophys Acta* 67:342, 1963

94. PORRA RJ, GRIMME LH: Tetrapyrrole biosynthesis in algae and higher plants: A discussion of the importance of the 5-amino-laevulinate synthase and the dioxovalerate transaminase pathways in the biosynthesis of chlorophyll. *Int J Biochem* 9:883, 1978

95. KLEIN O, DÖRNEMANN D, SENGER H: Two biosynthetic pathways to 5-aminolevulinic acid in algae. *Int J Biochem* 12:725, 1980

96. VARTICOVSKI L, KUSHNER JP, BURNHAM BF: Biosynthesis of porphyrin precursors: Purification and characterization of mammalian L-alanine γ-δ-dioxovaleric acid aminotransferase. *J Biol Chem* 355:3742, 1980

96a. NOGUCHI T, MORI R: Biosynthesis of porphyrin precursors in mammals. Identity of alanine: γ,δ-Dioxovalerate aminotransferase with alanine: glyoxylate aminotransferase. *J Biol Chem* 256:10335, 1981

97. SASSA S, KAPPAS A, BERNSTEIN SE, ALVARES AP: Heme biosynthesis and drug metabolism in mice with hereditary hemolytic anemia: Heme oxygenase induction as an adaptive response for maintaining cytochrome P-450 in chronic hemolysis. *J Biol Chem* 254:729, 1979

98. MAUZERALL D, GRANICK S: The occurrence and determination of δ-aminolevulinic acid and porphobilinogen in urine. *J Biol Chem* 219:435, 1956

99. SASSA S, YOSHINAGA T, STONER E, LEVINE LS, NEW MI, KAPPAS A: Succinylacetone: A potent inhibitor of heme synthesis produced in tyrosinemia. *Clin Res* 29:569A, 1981

100. YODA B, SCHACTER BA, ISRAELS LG: δ-Aminolevulinic acid synthetase assay in chicken liver homogenates and particulate fractions. *Anal Biochem* 66:221, 1975

101. BONKOWSKY HL, POMEROY JS: Assay of δ-aminolevulinic acid synthetase in homogenates of mouse, rat, and human liver: Species differences in requirement for an exogenous succinyl CoA-generating system. *Anal Biochem* 91:82, 1978

102. MARVER HS, TSCHUDY DP, PERLROTH MG, COLLINS A, HUNTER G JR: The determination of aminoketones in biological fluids. *Anal Biochem* 14:53, 1966

103. SASSA S, KAPPAS A: Induction of δ-aminolevulinate synthase and porphyrins in cultured liver cells maintained in chemically defined medium: Permissive effects of hormones on the induction process. *J Biol Chem* 252:2428, 1977

104. EBERT PS, TSCHUDY DP, CHOUDHRY JN, CHIRIGOS MA: A simple micro method for the direct determination of δ-amino[^{14}C]levulinic acid production in murine spleen and liver homogenates. *Biochim Biophys Acta* 208:236, 1970

105. IRVING EA, ELLIOTT WH: A sensitive radiochemical assay method for δ-aminolevulinic acid synthetase. *J Biol Chem* 244:60, 1969

106. STRAND LJ, SWANSON AL, MANNING J, BRANCH S, MARVER HS: Radiochemical micro-assay for δ-aminolevulinic acid synthetase in hepatic and erythroid tissues. *Anal Biochem* 47:457, 1972

107. SASSA S: Sequential induction of heme pathway enzymes during erythroid differentiation of mouse Friend leukemia virus-infected cells. *J Exp Med* 143:305, 1976

108. CONDIE LW, BARON J, TEPHLY TR: Studies on adrenal δ-aminolevulinic acid synthetase. *Arch Biochem Biophys* 172:123, 1976

109. BRIGGS DW, CONDIE LW, SEDMAN RM, TEPHLY TR: δ-Aminolevulinic acid synthetase in the heart. *J Biol Chem* 251:4996, 1976

110. ISRAELS LG, SCHACTER BA, YODA B, GOLDENBERG GJ: δ-Aminolevulinic acid transport, porphyrin synthesis and heme catabolism in chick embryo liver and heart cells. *Biochim Biophys Acta* 372:32, 1974

111. TOFILON PJ, PIPER WN: Measurement and regulation of rat testicular δ-aminolevulinic acid synthetase activity. *Arch Biochem Biophys* 201:104, 1980

112. TANAKA M, BOTTOMLEY SS: Bone marrow Δ-aminolevulinic acid synthetase activity in experimental sideroblastic anemia. *J Lab Clin Med* 84:92, 1974

113. GIBSON KD, NEUBERGER A, SCOTT JJ: The purification and properties of δ-aminolevulinic acid dehydrase. *Biochem J* 61:618, 1955

114. GRANICK S: Enzymatic conversion of delta-aminolevulinic acid to porphobilinogen. *Science* 120:1105, 1954

115. BURNHAM BF, LASCELLES J: Control of porphyrin biosynthesis through a negative-feedback mechanism: Studies with preparations of delta-aminolaevulate synthetase and delta-aminolaevulic dehydratase from *Rhodopseudomonas spheroides*. *Biochem J* 87:462, 1963

116. NANDI DL, SHEMIN D: δ-Aminolevulinic acid dehydratase of *Rhodopseudomonas spheroides*. III. Mechanism of porphobilinogen synthesis. *J Biol Chem* 243:1236, 1968

117. JORDAN PM, SEEHRA JS: Mechanism of action of 5-aminolevulinic acid dehydratase: Stepwise order of addition of the two molecules of 5-aminolevulinic acid in the enzymatic synthesis of porphobilinogen. *J Chem Soc Chem Commun*, 1980, p 240

118. ANDERSON PM, DESNICK RJ: Purification and properties of δ-aminolevulinic acid dehydratase from human erythrocytes. *J Biol Chem* 254:6924, 1979

119. FINELLI VN, MURTHY L, PEIRANO WB, PETERING HG: δ-Aminolevulinate dehydratase, a zinc dependent enzyme. *Biochem Biophys Res Commun* 60:1418, 1974

120. FINELLI VN, KLAUDER DS, KARAFFA MA, PETERING HG: Interaction of zinc and lead on δ-aminolevulinate dehydratase. *Biochem Biophys Res Commun* 65:303, 1975

121. CHEH A, NEILANDS JB: Zinc, an essential metal ion for beef liver δ-aminolevulinate dehydratase. *Biochem Biophys Res Commun* 55:1060, 1973

122. TSUKAMOTO I, YOSHINAGA T, SANO S: The role of zinc with special reference to the essential thiol groups in δ-aminolevulinic acid dehydratase of bovine liver. *Biochim Biophys Acta* 570:167, 1979

123. BEVAN DR, BODLAENDER P, SHEMIN D: Mechanism of porphobilinogen synthase: Requirement of Zn^{2+} for enzyme activity. *J Biol Chem* 255:2030, 1980

124. DOYLE D, SCHIMKE RT: The genetic and developmental regulation of hepatic δ-aminolevulinate dehydratase in mice. *J Biol Chem* 244:5449, 1969

125. GURBA PE, SENNETT RE, KOBES RD: Studies on the mechanism of action of δ-aminolevulinate dehydratase from bovine and rat liver. *Arch Biochem Biophys* 150:130, 1972

126. WILSON EL, BURGER PE, DOWDLE EB: Beef-liver 5-aminolevulinic acid dehydratase: Purification and properties. *Eur J Biochem* 29:563, 1972

127. WU WH, SHEMIN D, RICHARDS KE, WILLIAMS RC: The quarternary structure of δ-aminolevulinic acid dehydratase from bovine liver. *Proc Natl Acad Sci USA* 71:1767, 1974

128. SHEMIN D: δ-Aminolevulinic acid dehydratase, in Boyer PD (ed): *The Enzymes*, 3d ed, vol VII. New York, Academic, 1972, p 323

129. GRANICK JL, SASSA S, GRANICK S, LEVERE RD, KAPPAS A: Studies in lead poisoning. II. Correlations between the ratio of activated and inactivated δ-aminolevulinic acid dehydratase of whole blood and the blood lead level. *Biochem Med* 8:149, 1973

130. BEALE SI: The biosynthesis of δ-aminolevulinic acid in *Chlorella*. *Plant Physiol* 45:505, 1970

131. WEISSBERG JB, VOYTEK PE: Liver and red cell porphobilinogen synthase in the adult and fetal guinea pig. *Biochim Biophys Acta* 364:304, 1974

132. LINDBLAD B, LINDSTEDT S, STEEN G: On the enzymic defects in hereditary tyrosinemia. *Proc Natl Acad Sci USA* 74:4641, 1977

133. COLEMAN DL: Purification and properties of δ-aminolevulinate dehydratase from tissues of two strains of mice. *J Biol Chem* 241:5511, 1966

134. SASSA S, BERNSTEIN SE: Levels of δ-aminolevulinate dehydratase, uroporphyrinogen-I synthase, and protoporphyrin IX in erythrocytes from anemic mutant mice. *Proc Natl Acad Sci USA* 74:1181, 1977

135. HUTTON JJ, COLEMAN D: Linkage analyses using biochemical variants in mice. II. Levulinate dehydratase and autosomal glucose 6-phosphate dehydrogenase. *Biochem Genet* 3:517, 1969

136. SASSA S, GRANICK S, BICKERS DR, LEVERE RD, KAPPAS A: Studies on the inheritance of human erythrocyte δ-aminolevulinate dehydratase and uroporphyrinogen synthetase. *Enzyme* 16:326, 1973

137. HOFFMAN R, IBRAHIM N, MURNANE MJ, DIAMOND A, FORGET BG, LEVERE RD: Hemin control of heme biosynthesis and catabolism in a human leukemia cell line. *Blood* 56:567, 1980

138. ANDERSON KE, SASSA S, PETERSON CM, KAPPAS A: Increased erythrocyte uroporphyrinogen-I-synthetase, δ-aminolevulinic acid dehydratase and protoporphyrin in hemolytic anemias. *Am J Med* 63:359, 1977

139. DAVIS JR, AVRAM MJ: Developmental changes in delta-aminolevulinic acid dehydratase (ALAD) activity and blood reticulocyte percent in the developing rat: A brief note. *Mech Ageing Dev* 7:123, 1978

140. FRESHNEY RI, PAUL J: The activities of three enzymes of heme synthesis during hepatic erythropoiesis in the mouse embryo. *J Embryol Exp Morphol* 26:313, 1971

141. BIRD TD, HAMERNYIK P, NUTTER JY, LABBE RF: Inherited deficiency of delta-aminolevulinic acid dehydratase. *Am J Hum Genet* 31:662, 1979

142. DOSS M, VON TIEPERMANN R, SCHNEIDER J, SCHMID H: New type of hepatic porphyria with porphobilinogen synthase defect and intermittent acute clinical manifestation. *Klin Wochensch* 57:1123, 1977

143. DOSS M, VON TIEPERMANN R, SCHNEIDER J: Acute hepatic porphyria syndrome with porphobilinogen synthase defect. *Int J Biochem* 12:823, 1980

144. MAUZERALL D: The thermostability of porphyrinogens. *J Am Chem Soc* 82:2601, 1960

145. BATTERSBY AR, FOOKES CJR, MATCHAM GWJ, MCDONALD E, GUSTAFSON-POTTER KE: Biosynthesis of the natural porphyrins: Experiments on the ring closure steps and with the hydroxy-analogue of porphobilinogen. *J Chem Soc Chem Commun* 539, 1979

146. BATTERSBY AR, FOOKES CJR, MATCHAM GWJ, MCDONALD E: Order of

assembly of the four pyrrole rings during biosynthesis of the natural porphyrins. *J Chem Soc Chem Commun* 539, 1979

147. BATTERSBY AR, HODGSON GL, HUNT E, McDONALD E, SAUNDERS J: Biosynthesis of porphyrins and related macrocycles. VI. Nature of the rearrangement process leading to the natural type III porphyrins. *J Chem Soc [Perkin I]*, 1976, p 273

148. LEVIN EY: Uroporphyrinogen III cosynthetase in bovine erythropoietic porphyria. *Science* 161:907, 1968

149. FRYDMAN, RB, FEINSTEIN G: Studies on porphobilinogen deaminase and uroporphyrinogen III cosynthetase from human erythrocytes. *Biochim Biophys Acta* 350:358, 1974

150. HIGUCHI M, BOGORAD L: The purification and properties of uroporphyrinogen I synthases and uroporphyrinogen III cosynthase. Interactions between the enzymes. *Ann NY Acad Sci* 244:401, 1975

151. ROSSETTI MV, JUKNAT DE GERALNIK AA, KOTLER M, FUMAGALLI S, BATTLE DEL C AM: Occurrence of multiple molecular forms of porphobilinogenase in diverse organisms: The minimum quaternary structure of porphobilinogenase is a promoter of one deaminase and one isomerase domain. *Int J Biochem* 12:761, 1980

152. STEVENS E, FRYDMAN RB, FRYDMAN B: Separation of porphobilinogen deaminase and uroporphyrinogen III cosynthetase from human erythrocytes. *Biochim Biophys Acta* 158:496, 1968

153. ROMEO G, LEVIN EY: Uroporphyrinogen III cosynthetase in human congenital erythropoietic porphyria. *Proc Natl Acad Sci USA* 63:856, 1969

154. LEVIN EY: Uroporphyrinogen III cosynthetase from mouse spleen. *Biochemistry* 7:3781, 1968

155. LEVIN EY, FLYGER V: Erythropoietic porphyria of the fox squirrel *Sciurus niger*. *J Clin Invest* 52:96, 1973

156. ANDERSON PM, DESNICK RJ: Purification and properties of uroporphyrinogen I synthase from human erythrocytes. Identification of stable enzyme-substrate intermediates. *J Biol Chem* 255:1993, 1980

157. LLAMBIAS EBC, BATTLE DEL C AM: Porphyrin biosynthesis VIII: Avian erythrocyte porphobilinogen deaminase-uroporphyrinogen III cosynthetase, its purification, properties, and the separation of its components. *Biochim Biophys Acta* 227:180, 1971

158. JORDAN PM, SHEMIN D: Purification and properties of uroporphyrinogen I synthetase from *Rhodopseudomonas spheroides*. *J Biol Chem* 248:1019, 1973

159. MIYAGI K, KANESHIMA M, KAWAKAMI J, NAKADA F, PETRYKA ZJ, WATSON CJ: Uroporphyrinogen I synthase from human erythrocytes: Separation, purification, and properties of isoenzymes. *Proc Natl Acad Sci USA* 76:6172, 1979

160. JORDAN PM, BERRY A: Mechanism of action of porphobilinogen deaminase: The participation of stable enzyme substrate covalent intermediates between porphobilinogen and the porphobilinogen deaminase from *Rhodopseudomonas spheroides*. *Biochem J* 195:177, 1981

161. PIPER WN, TEPHLY TR: Differential inhibition of erythrocyte and hepatic uroporphyrinogen I synthetase activity by lead. *Life Sci* 14:873, 1974

162. PIPER WN, VAN LIER RBL: Pteridine regulation of inhibition of hepatic uroporphyrinogen I synthetase activity by lead chloride. *Mol Pharmacol* 13:1126, 1977

163. WIDER DE XIFRA EA, BATTLE DEL C AM, STELLA AM, MALAMUD S: Acute intermittent porphyria: Another approach to therapy. *Int J Biochem* 12:819, 1980

164. MEISLER M, WANNER L, EDDY RE, SHOWS TB: The UPS locus encoding uroporphyrinogen I synthase is located on human chromosome 11. *Biochem Biophys Res Commun* 95:170, 1980

165. HEILMEYER L, CLOTTEN R, HEILMEYER L JR: *Disturbances in Heme Synthesis* (translated by M Steiner). Springfield, Ill, Charles C Thomas, 1966

166. STRAND LJ, FELSHER BF, REDEKER AG, MARVER HS: Enzymatic abnormality in heme biosynthesis in acute intermittent porphyria: Decreased hepatic conversion of porphobilinogen to porphyrins and increased delta-aminolevulinic acid synthetase activity. *Proc Natl Acad Sci USA* 67:1315, 1970

167. MIYAGI K, CARDINAL RA, BOSSENMAIER I, WATSON CJ: The serum porphobilinogen and hepatic porphobilinogen deaminase in normal and porphyric individuals. *J Lab Clin Med* 78:683, 1971

168. STRAND LJ, MEYER UA, FELSHER BF, REDEKER AG, MARVER HS: Decreased red cell uroporphyrinogen I synthetase activity in intermittent acute porphyria. *J Clin Invest* 51:2530, 1972

169. SASSA S, GRANICK S, BICKERS DR, BRADLOW HL, KAPPAS A: A microassay for uroporphyrinogen I synthase, one of three abnormal enzyme activities in acute intermittent porphyria, and its application to the study of the genetics of this disease. *Proc Natl Acad Sci USA* 71:732, 1974

170. MAGNUSSEN CR, LEVINE JB, DOHERTY JM, CHEESMAN JO, TSCHUDY DP: A red cell enzyme method for the diagnosis of acute intermittent porphyria. *Blood* 44:857, 1974

171. MEYER UA, STRAND LJ, DOSS M, REES AC, MARVER HS: Intermittent acute porphyria: Demonstration of a genetic defect in porphobilinogen metabolism. *N Engl J Med* 286:1277, 1972

172. MEYER UA: Intermittent acute porphyria: Clinical and biochemical studies of disordered heme biosynthesis. *Enzyme* 16:334, 1973

173. BONKOWSKY HL, TSCHUDY DP, WEINBACH EC, EBERT PS, DOHERTY JM: Porphyrin synthesis and mitochondrial respiration in acute intermittent porphyria: Studies using cultured human fibroblasts. *J Lab Clin Med* 85:93, 1975

174. SASSA S, SOLISH G, LEVERE RD, KAPPAS A: Studies in porphyria IV. Expression of the gene defect of acute intermittent porphyria in cultured human skin fibroblasts and amniotic cells: Prenatal diagnosis of the porphyric trait. *J Exp Med* 142:722, 1975

175. SASSA S, ZALAR GL, KAPPAS A: Studies in porphyria VII: Induction of uroporphyrinogen-I synthase and expression of the gene defect of acute intermittent porphyria in mitogen-stimulated human lymphocytes. *J Clin Invest* 61:499, 1978

176. SASSA S, LEVERE RD, SOLISH G, KAPPAS A: Studies on the porphyrin-heme biosynthetic pathway in cultured human amniotic cells. *J Clin Invest* 53:70a, 1974

177. GRANDCHAMP B, PHUNG N, GRELIER M, NORDMANN Y: The spectrophotometric determination of uroporphyrinogen I synthetase activity. *Clin Chim Acta* 70:113, 1976

178. SHIOI Y, NAGAMINE M, KUROKI M, SASA T: Purification by affinity chromatography and properties of uroporphyrinogen I synthetase from *Chlorella regularis*. *Biochim Biophys Acta* 616:300, 1980

179. YUAN M, RUSSELL CS: Porphobilinogen derivatives as substrates for porphobilinogenase. *FEBS Lett* 46:34, 1974

180. FRYDMAN RB, TOMARO ML, WANSCHELBAUM A, ANDERSEN EM, AWRUCH J, FRYDMAN B: Porphobilinogen oxygenase from wheat germ: Isolation, properties and products formed. *Biochemistry* 12:5253, 1973

181. TOMARO ML, FRYDMAN RB, FRYDMAN B: Porphobilinogen oxygenase from rat liver: Induction, isolation and properties. *Biochemistry* 12:5263, 1973

182. FRYDMAN RB, TOMARO ML, FRYDMAN B: Porphobilinogen oxygenase from human erythrocytes. *Clin Chim Acta* 97:269, 1979

183. BOGORAD L: The enzymatic synthesis of porphyrins from porphobilinogen. II. Uroporphyrin III. *J Biol Chem* 233:510, 1958

184. ROMEO G, KABACK MM, LEVIN EY: Uroporphyrinogen III cosynthetase activity in fibroblasts from patients with congenital erythropoietic porphyria. *Biochem Genet* 4:659, 1970

185. ROMEO G, GLENN BL, LEVIN EY: Uroporphyrinogen III cosynthetase in asymptomatic carriers of congenital erythropoietic porphyria. *Biochem Genet* 4:719, 1970

186. BATTERSBY AR, FOOKES CJR, MATCHAM GWJ, McDONALD E: Biosynthesis of the pigments of life: Formation of the macrocycle. *Nature* 285:17, 1980

187. GRANICK S, MAUZERALL D: Enzymes of porphyrin synthesis in red blood cells. *Ann NY Acad Sci* 75:115, 1958

188. CORNFORD P: Transformation of porphobilinogen into porphyrins by preparations from human erythrocytes. *Biochem J* 91:64, 1964

189. SMITH AG, FRANCIS JE: Decarboxylation of porphyrinogens by rat liver uroporphyrinogen decarboxylase. *Biochem J* 183:455, 1979

190. ELDER GH, TOVEY JA: Uroporphyrinogen decarboxylase activity of human tissues. *Biochem Soc Trans* 5:1470, 1977

191. DE VERNEUIL H, AITKEN G, NORDMANN Y: Familial and sporadic porphyria cutanea: Two different diseases. *Hum Genet* 44:145, 1978

192. BATTLE DEL C AM, GRINSTEIN M: Porphyrin biosynthesis. II. Phyriaporphyrinogen III. A normal intermediate in the biosynthesis of protoporphyrin IX. *Biochim Biophys Acta* 82:13, 1962

193. ROMEO G. LEVIN EY: Uroporphyrinogen decarboxylase from mouse spleen. *Biochim Biophys Acta* 230:330, 1971

194. HOARE DS, HEATH H: Intermediates in the biosynthesis of porphyrins from porphobilinogen by *Rhodopseudomonas spheroides*. *Nature* 181:1592, 1958

195. JACKSON AH, SANCOVICH HA, FERRAMOLA AM, EVANS N, GAMES DE, MATLIN SA, ELDER GH, SMITH SG: Macrocyclic intermediates in the biosynthesis of porphyrins. *Philos Trans R Soc Lond [Biol]* 273:119, 1975

196. DE VERNEUIL H, GRANDCHAMP B, NORDMANN Y: Some kinetic properties of human red cell uroporphyrinogen decarboxylase. *Biochim Biophys Acta* 611:174, 1980

197. SMITH AG, FRANCIS JE: Investigations of rat liver uroporphyrinogen decarboxylase: Comparisons of porphyrinogens I and III as substrates and the inhibition by porphyrins. *Biochem J* 195:241, 1981

198. ELDER GH, LEE GB, TOVEY JA: Decreased activity of hepatic uroporphyrinogen decarboxylase in sporadic porphyria cutanea tarda. *N Engl J Med* 299:274, 1978

199. KUSHNER JP, BARBUTO AJ, LEE GR: An inherited enzymatic defect in porphyria cutanea tarda: Decreased uroporphyrinogen decarboxylase activity. *J Clin Invest* 58:1089

200. FELSHER BF, NORRIS ME, SHIH JC: Red-cell uroporphyrinogen decarboxylase activity in porphyria cutanea tarda and in other forms of porphyria. *N Engl J Med* 299:1095, 1978

201. TIEPERMANN VON R, DOSS M: Uroporphyrinogen-Decarboxylase in Erythrocyten: Untersuchungen zum primären genetischer Enzymdefekt bei chronische hepatischer Porphyrie. *J Clin Chem Clin Biochem* 16:513, 1978

202. TALJAARD JJF, SHANLEY BC, DEPPE WM, JOUBERT SM: Decreased uroporphyrinogen decarboxylase activity in "experimental symptomatic porphyria." *Life Sci* 10(pt 2):887, 1971

203. TALJAARD JJF, SHANLEY BC, DEPPE WM, JOUBERT SM: Porphyrin metabolism in experimental hepatic siderosis in the rat. II. Combined effect of iron overload and hexachlorobenzene. *Br J Haematol* 23:513, 1972

204. TALJAARD JJF, SHANLEY BC, DEPPE WM, JOUBERT SM: Porphyrin metabolism in experimental hepatic siderosis in the rat. III. Effect of iron overload and hexachlorobenzene on liver haem biosynthesis. *Br J Haematol* 23:587, 1972

205. KUSHNER JP, STEINMULLER DP, LEE GR: The role of iron in the pathogenesis of porphyria cutanea tarda. II. Inhibition of uroporphyrinogen decarboxylase. *J Clin Invest* 56:661, 1975

206. DANBY CWE, KOVAL A, WYLLIE J: Acquired porphyria cutanea tarda: Two cases treated by repeated phlebotomies. *Can Med Assoc J* 94:1358, 1966

207. EPSTEIN JH, REDEKER AG: Porphyria cutanea tarda symptomatica (PCT-S): A study of the effect of phlebotomy therapy. *Arch Dermatol* 92:286, 1965

208. HICKMAN R, SAUNDERS SJ, EALES L: Treatment of symptomatic porphyria by venesection. *S Afr Med J* 41:456, 1967

209. IPPEN H: Allgemeine Symptome. Der spaten Hautporphyrie (Porphyria cutanea tarda) als Hinweise für deren Behandlung. *Dtsch Med Wschr* 86:127, 1961

210. IPPEN H: Treatment of porphyria cutanea tarda by phlebotomy. *Semin Hematol* 14:253, 1977

211. SAUNDERS SJ: Iron metabolism in symptomatic porphyria. *S Afr J Lab Clin Med* 9:277, 1963

212. SWEENEY GD, JONES KG: Porphyria cutanea tarda: Clinical and laboratory features. *Can Med Assoc J* 120:803, 1979

213. SWEENEY GD, JONES KG, COLE FM, BASFORD D, KRETYNSKI F: Iron deficiency prevents liver toxicity of 2,3,7,8-tetrachlorodibenzo-p-dioxin. *Science* 204:332, 1979

214. SMITH AG, CABRAL JRP, DE MATTEIS F:: A difference between two strains of rats in their liver non-haem iron content and in their response to the porphyrogenic effect of hexachlorobenzene. *Chem Biol Interact* 27:353, 1979

215. LOUW M, NEETHLING AC, PERCY VA, CARSTENS M, SHANLEY BC: Effects of hexachlorobenzene feeding and iron overload on enzymes of haem biosynthesis and cytochrome P-450 in rat liver. *Clin Sci Mol Med* 53:111, 1977

216. BLEKKENHORST GH, DAY RS, EALES L: The effect of bleeding and iron administration on the development of hexachlorobenzene-induced rat porphyria. *Int J Biochem* 12:1013, 1980

216a. WOODS JS, KARDISH R, FOWLER BA: Studies on the action of porphyrinogenic trace metals on the activity of hepatic uroporphyrinogen decarboxylase. *Biochem Biophys Res Comm* 103:264, 1981

217. BOGORAD L: Porphyrin synthesis III. Uroporphyrinogen decarboxylase, in Colowick SP, Kaplan NO (eds): *Methods in Enzymology*, vol V. New York, Academic Press, 1962, p 893

218. SANO S, GRANICK S: Mitochondrial coproporphyrinogen oxidase and protoporphyrin formation. *J Biol Chem* 236:1173, 1961

219. BATTLE DEL C AM, BENSON A, RIMINGTON C: Purification and properties of coproporphyrinogenase. *Biochem J* 97:731, 1965

220. POULSON R, POLGLASE WJ: Aerobic and anaerobic coproporphyrinogenase activities in extracts from *Saccharomyces cerevisiae*. Purification and characterization. *J Biol Chem* 249:6367, 1974

221. ELDER GH, EVANS JO: Evidence that the coproporphyrinogen oxidase activity of rat liver is situated in the intermembrane space of mitochondria. *Biochem J* 172:345, 1978

222. GREENAWALT JW: The isolation of outer and inner mitochondrial membranes. *Methods Enzymol* 31:310, 1974

223. GRANDCHAMP B, PHUNG N, NORDMANN Y: The mitochondrial localization of coproporphyrinogen III oxidase. *Biochem J* 176:97, 1978

224. PORRA RJ, FALK JE: The enzymic conversion of coproporphyrinogen III into protoporphyrin IX. *Biochem J* 90:69, 1964

225. YOSHINAGA T, SANO S: Coproporphyrinogen oxidase. I. Purification, properties and activation by phospholipids. *J Biol Chem* 255:4722, 1980

226. ZAMAN Z, ABBOUD MM, AKHTAR M: Mechanism and stereochemistry of vinyl group formation in heme biosynthesis. *J Chem Soc Chem Commun* 1263, 1972

227. BATTERSBY AR, BALDAS J, COLLINS J, GRAYSON DH, JAMES KJ, McDONALD E: Mechanism of biosynthesis of the vinyl groups of protoporphyrin IX. *J Chem Soc Chem Commun* 1265, 1972

228. SANO S: 2,4-Bis(β-hydroxypropionic acid)deuteroporphyrinogen IX, a possible intermediate between coproporphyrinogen III and protoporphyrin IX. *J Biol Chem* 241:5276, 1966

229. TAIT GH: 5-Aminolaevulinate synthetase of *Micrococcus denitrificans*. *Biochem J* 128:32P, 1972

230. YOSHINAGA T, SANO S: Coproporphyrinogen oxidase. II. Reaction mechanism and role of tyrosine residues on the activity. *J Biol Chem* 255:4727, 1980

231. JACKSON AH, JONES DM, PHILIP G, LASH TD, BATTLE DEL C AM, SMITH SG: Synthetic and biosynthetic studies of porphyrins. IV. Further studies of the conversion of coproporphyrinogen-III to protoporphyrin-IX: Mass spectrometric investigations of the incubation of specifically deuterated coproporphyrinogen-III with chicken red cell haemolysates. *Int J Biochem* 12:681, 1980

232. ELDER GH, EVANS JO, THOMAS N, COX R, BRODIE MJ, MOORE MR, GOLDBERG A, NICHOLSON DC: The primary enzyme defect in hereditary coproporphyria. *Lancet* ii:1217, 1976

233. GRANDCHAMP B, NORDMANN Y: Decreased lymphocyte coproporphyrinogen III oxidase activity in hereditary coproporphyria. *Biochem Biophys Res Commun* 74:1089, 1977

234. GRANDCHAMP B, PHUNG N, NORDMANN Y: Homozygous case of hereditary coproporphyria. *Lancet* ii:1348, 1977

235. POULSON R, POLGLASE WJ: The enzymic conversion of protoporphyrinogen IX to protoporphyrin IX: Protoporphyrinogen oxidase activity in mitochondrial extracts of *Saccharomyces cerevisiae*. *J Biol Chem* 250:1269, 1975

236. POLGLASE WJ, WHITLOW KJ, POULSON R: Regulation of porphyrin biosynthesis in *E. coli*. *Fed Proc* 34:692, 1975

237. JACOBS NJ, JACOBS JM: Fumarate as alternate electron acceptor for the late steps of anaerobic heme synthesis in *Escherichia coli*. *Biochem Biophys Res Commun* 65:435, 1975

238. POULSON R: The enzymic conversion of protoporphyrinogen IX to protoporphyrin IX in mammalian mitochondria. *J Biol Chem* 251:3730, 1976

239. JACOBS NJ, JACOBS JM: Nitrate, fumarate, and oxygen as electron acceptors for a late step in microbial heme synthesis. *Biochim Biophys Acta* 449:1, 1976

240. BRENNER DA, BLOOMER JR: A fluorometric assay for measurement of protoporphyrinogen oxidase activity in mammalian tissue. *Clin Chim Acta* 100:259, 1980

241. VILJOEN DJ, CAYANIS E, BECKER DM, KRAMER S, DAWSON B, BERNSTEIN R: Reduced ferrochelatase activity in fibroblasts from patients with porphyria variegata. *Am J Hematol* 6:185, 1979

242. KASSNER RJ, WALCHAK H: Heme formation from Fe(II) and porphyrin in the absence of ferrochelatase activity. *Biochim Biophys Acta* 304:294, 1973

243. TOKUNAGA R, SANO S: Comparative studies on nonenzymic and enzymic protoheme formation. *Biochim Biophys Acta* 264:263, 1972

244. JONES MS, JONES OTG: The structural organization of heme synthesis in rat liver mitochondria. *Biochem J* 113:507, 1969

245. McKAY, R, DRUYAN R, GETZ GS, RABINOWITZ M: Intramitochondrial localization of δ-aminolevulate synthetase and ferrochelatase in rat liver. *Biochem J* 114:455, 1969

246. BUGANY H, FLOTHE L, WESER U: Kinetics of metal chelatase of rat liver mitochondria. *FEBS Lett* 13:92, 1971

247. JOHNSON A, JONES OTG: Enzymic formation of hemes and other metalloporphyrins. *Biochim Biophys Acta* 93:171, 1964

248. PORRA RJ, JONES OTG: Studies on ferrochelatase. 2. An investigation of the role of ferrochelatase in the biosynthesis of various haem prosthetic groups. *Biochem J* 87:186, 1963

249. PORRA RJ, JONES OTG: Studies on ferrochelatase. 1. Assay and properties of ferrochelatase from a pig liver mitochondrial extract. *Biochemistry* 87:181, 1963

250. MAILER K, POULSON R, DOLPHIN D, HAMILTON AD: Ferrochelatase: Isolation and purification via affinity chromatography. *Biochem Biophys Res Commun* 96:777, 1980

250a. TAKETANI S, TOKUNAGA, R: Rat liver ferrochelatase. Purification, properties and stimulation by fatty acids. *J Biol Chem* 256:12748, 1981

251. TEPHLY TR, HASEGAWA E, BARON J: Effect of drugs on heme synthesis in the liver. *Metabolism* 20:200, 1971

252. DE MATTEIS F, ABBRITTI G, GIBBS AH: Decreased liver activity of porphyrin-metal chelatase in hepatic porphyria caused by 3,5-diethoxycarbonyl-1,4-dihydrocollidine. *Biochem J* 134:717, 1973

253. RIFKIND AB: Maintainance of microsomal hemoprotein concentrations following inhibition of ferrochelatase activity by 3,5-diethoxycarbonyl-1,4-dihydrocollidine in chick embryo liver. *J Biol Chem* 254:4636, 1979

254. ANDERSON KE: Effects of antihypertensive drugs on hepatic heme biosynthesis, and evaluation of ferrochelatase inhibitors to simplify testing of drugs for heme pathway induction. *Biochim Biophys Acta* 543:313, 1978

255. TEPHLY TR, GIBBS AH, INGALL G, DE MATTEIS F: Studies on the mech-

anism of experimental porphyria and ferrochelatase inhibition produced by 3,5-diethoxycarbonyl-1,4-dihydrocollidine. *Int J Biochem* 12:993, 1980

255a. ORTIZ DE MONTELLANO PR, BEILAN HS, KUNZE KL: N-Methylprotoporphyrin IX: Chemical synthesis and identification as the green pigment produced by 3,5-diethoxycarbonyl-1,4-dihydrocollidine treatment. *Proc Natl Acad Sci USA* 78:1490, 1981

256. DE MATTEIS F, GIBBS AH: Drug-induced conversion of liver haem into modified porphyrins: Evidence for two classes of products. *Biochem J* 187:285, 1980

257. BONKOWSKY HL, BLOOMER JR, EBERT PS, MAHONEY MJ: Heme synthetase deficiency in human protoporphyria: Demonstration of the defect in liver and cultured skin fibroblasts. *J Clin Invest* 56:1139, 1975

258. BLOOMER JR, BRENNER DA, MAHONEY MJ: Study of factors causing excess protoporphyrin accumulation in cultured skin fibroblasts from patients with protoporphyria. *J Clin Invest* 60:1354, 1977

259. BOTTOMLEY SS, TANAKA M, EVERETT MA: Diminished erythroid ferrochelatase activity in protoporphyria. *J Lab Clin Med* 86:126, 1975

260. RUTH GR, SCHWARTZ S, STEPHENSON B: Bovine protoporphyria: The first nonhuman model of this hereditary photosensitizing disease. *Science* 198:199, 1977

261. LANGELAAN DE, LOSOWSKY MS, TOOTHILL C: Heme synthetase activity in human blood cells. *Clin Chim Acta* 27:453, 1970

262. BRENNER DA, BLOOMER JR: The enzymatic defect in variegate porphyria. Studies with human cultured skin fibroblasts *N Engl J Med* 302:765, 1980

263. BECKER DM, VILJOEN JD, KATZ J, KRAMER S: Reduced ferrochelatase activity: A defect common to porphyria variegata and protoporphyria. *Br J Haematol* 36:171, 1977

264. YONEYAMA Y, SAWADA H, TAKESHITA M, SUGITA Y: The role of lipids in heme synthesis. *Lipids* 4:1, 1969

265. SAWADA H, TAKESHITA M, SUGITA Y, YONEYAMA Y: Effect of lipid on protoheme ferro-lyase. *Biochim Biophys Acta* 178:145, 1969

266. PORRA RJ, VITOLS KS, LABBE RF, NEWTON NA: Studies on ferrochelatase: The effects of thiols and other factors on the determination of activity. *Biochem J* 104:321, 1967

267. PORRA RJ: A rapid spectrophotometric assay for ferrochelatase (E.C.4.99.1.1) in preparations containing high concentrations of haemoglobin, in Doss M (ed): *Porphyrins in Human Diseases*. Basel, S Karger, 1976, p 123

268. TEPHLY TR: Inhibition of liver hemoprotein synthesis, in De Matteis F, Aldridge WM (eds): *Heme and Hemoproteins—Handbook of Experimental Pharmacology*, vol 44. Berlin, Springer-Verlag, 1978, p 81

269. ONISAWA J, LABBE RF: Effects of diethyl-1,4-dihydro-2,4,6-trimethylpyridine-3,5-dicarboxylate on the metabolism of porphyrins and iron. *J Biol Chem* 238:724, 1963

270. GRANICK S, SASSA S: δ-Aminolevulinic acid synthetase and the control of heme and chlorophyll synthesis, in Vogel HJ (ed): *Metabolic Regulation*, vol 5. New York, Academic 1971, p 77

271. DE MATTEIS F: Loss of heme in rat liver caused by the porphyrogenic agent 2-allyl-2-isopropylacetamide. *Biochem J* 124:767, 1971

272. GRANICK S, KAPPAS A: Steroid induction of porphyrin synthesis in liver cell culture. I. Structural basis and possible physiological role in the control of heme formation. *J Biol Chem* 242:4587, 1967

273. KAPPAS A, GRANICK S: Steroid induction of porphyrin synthesis in liver cell culture II: The effects of heme, uridine diphosphate glucuronic acid and inhibitors of nucleic acid and protein synthesis on the induction process. *J Biol Chem* 243:346, 1968

274. TOMITA Y, OHASHI A, KIKUCHI G: Induction of δ-aminolevulinate synthetase in organ culture of chick embryo liver by allylisopropylacetamide and 3,5-dicarbethoxy-1,4-dihydrocollidine. *J Biochem* 75:1007, 1974

275. TYRELL DLG, MARKS GS: Drug-induced porphyrin biosynthesis. V. Effect of protohemin on the transcriptional and post-transcriptional phases of δ-aminolevulinic acid synthetase induction. *Biochem Pharmacol* 21:2077, 1972

276. SASSA S, BRADLOW HL, KAPPAS A: Steroid induction of δ-aminolevulinic acid synthase and porphyrins in liver: Structure-activity studies on the permissive effects of hormones on the induction process. *J Biol Chem* 254:10011, 1979

277. LEVERE RD, GRANICK S: Control of hemoglobin synthesis in the cultured chick blastoderm by δ-aminolevulinic acid synthetase: Increase in the rate of hemoglobin formation with δ-aminolevulinic acid. *Proc Natl Acad Sci USA* 54:134, 1965

277a. SASSA S, KAPPAS A: Genetic, metabolic, and biochemical aspects of the porphyrias, in Harris H, Hirschhorn (eds): *Adv Hum Genet*. New York, Plenum Press, 1981, vol 11, p 121

278. BERK PD, RODKEY FL, BLASCHKE TF, COLLISON HA, WAGGONER JG: Comparison of plasma bilirubin turnover and carbon monoxide production in man. *J Lab Clin Med* 83:29, 1974

279. HUTTON JJ, GROSS SR: Chemical induction of hepatic porphyria in inbred strains of mice. *Arch Biochem Biophys* 141:284, 1970

280. ANDERSON KE, DRUMMOND GS, FREDDARA U, SARDANA MK, SASSA S, KAPPAS A: Porphyrogenic effects of and induction of heme oxygenase *in vivo* by δ-aminolevulinic acid. *Biochim Biophys Acta*, 676:289, 1981

281. SONG CS, MOSES HL, ROSENTHAL AS, GELB NA, KAPPAS A: The influence of postnatal development on drug-induced hepatic porphyria and the synthesis of cytochrome P-450. *J Exp Med* 134:1349, 1971

282. BISSELL DM, HAMMAKER LE: Cytochrome P-450 heme and the regulation of hepatic heme oxygenase activity. *Arch Biochem Biophys* 176:91, 1976

283. BISSELL DM, HAMMAKER LE: Cytochrome P-450 heme and the regulation of δ-aminolevulinic acid synthetase in the liver. *Arch Biochem Biophys* 176:103, 1976

284. GAYATHRI AK, RAO MRS, PADMANABAN G: Studies on the induction of δ-aminolevulinic acid synthetase in mouse liver. *Arch Biochem Biophys* 155:299, 1973

285. COWTAN ER, YODA B, ISRAELS LG: Cycloheximide enhanced porphyrin synthesis in chick embryo liver: Association with an increase in the hepatic glycine pool. *Arch Biochem Biophys* 155:194, 1973

286. KIKUCHI G: The glycine cleavage system: Composition reaction mechanism, and physiological significance. *Mol Cell Biochem* 1:169, 1973

287. KIELLEY RK, SCHNEIDER WC: Synthesis of p-aminohippuric acid by mitochondria of mouse liver homogenates. *J Biol Chem* 187:869, 1950

288. SCHACHTER D, TAGGART JV: Glycine N-acylase: Purification and properties. *J Biol Chem* 208:263, 1954

289. GRANICK S, BEALE SI: Hemes, chlorophylls, and related compounds: Biosynthesis and metabolic regulation, in Meister A (ed): *Advanced Enzymology and Related Areas of Molecular Biology*. New York, Wiley, 1978, p 33

290. SINCLAIR PR, GRANICK S: The transport of hemin and protoporphyrin across the plasma membrane of chick embryo liver cells in culture. *Ann Clin Res* 8(Suppl 17):250, 1976

291. SRIVASTAVA G, BROOKER JD, MAY BK, ELLIOTT WH: Haem control in experimental porphyria. The effect of haemin on the induction of δ-aminolaevulinate synthase in isolated chick-embryo liver cells. *Biochem J* 188:781, 1980

292. BEAVAN GH, HUA CHEN S, D'ALBIS A, GRATZER WB: A spectroscopic study of the haemin-human-serum-albumin system. *Eur J Biochem* 41:539, 1974

293. WOLFSON SJ, BARTCZAK A, BLOOMER JR: Effect of endogenous heme generation on δ-aminolevulinic acid synthase activity in rat liver mitochondria. *J Biol Chem* 254:3543, 1979

294. KETTERER B, SRAI KS, CHRISTODOULIDES L: Haem-binding proteins of the rat liver cytosol. *Biochim Biophys Acta* 428:683, 1976

295. TENHUNEN R, GRÄSBECK R, KOUVONEN I, LUNDBERG M: An intestinal receptor for heme: Its partial characterization. *Int J Biochem* 12:713, 1980

296. ROMSLO I, HUSBY P: Iron, porphyrin and heme transport in mitochondria. *Int J Biochem* 12:709, 1980

297. WHITING MJ: Synthesis of δ-aminolaevulinate synthase by isolated liver polyribosomes. *Biochem J* 158:391, 1976

298. HAYASHI N: Regulation of the amount of hepatic mitochondrial δ-aminolevulinic acid synthase. *Seikagaku* 51:420, 1979

299. SRIVASTAVA G, BROOKER JD, MAY BK, ELLIOTT WH: Induction of hepatic δ-aminolevulinate synthase by heme depletion and its possible significance in the control of drug metabolism. *Biochem Int* 1:64, 1980

300. SINCLAIR P, GRANICK S: Heme control on the synthesis of delta-aminolevulinic acid synthetase in cultured chick embryo liver cells. *Ann NY Acad Sci* 244:509, 1975

301. COLE SPC, MARKS GS: Structural requirements in dihydropyridines for ferrochelatase inhibition and δ-aminolevulinic acid synthetase induction. *Int J Biochem* 12:989, 1980

302. MAINES MD, KAPPAS A: Cobalt induction of hepatic heme oxygenase with evidence that cytochrome P-450 is not essential for this enzymatic activity. *Proc Natl Acad Sci USA* 71:4293, 1974

303. MAINES MD, KAPPAS A: Cobalt stimulation of heme degradation in the liver: Dissociation of microsomal oxidation of heme from cytochrome P-450. *J Biol Chem* 250:4171, 1975

304. NAKAMURA M, YASUKOCHI Y, MINAKAMI S: Effect of cobalt on heme biosynthesis in rat liver and spleen. *J Biochem* 78:373, 1975

305. DE MATTEIS F, GIBBS AH: The effect of cobaltous chloride on liver haem metabolism in the rat. Evidence for inhibition of haem synthesis and for increased heam degradation. *Ann Clin Res* 8:13, 1976

306. DRUMMOND GS, KAPPAS A: Profound and long-sustained depression of cytochrome P-450 levels *in vivo* by cobalt-heme administration: Implications for studies in chemical biology. Fifth International Symposium on Microsomes and Drug Oxidations, Tokyo, Japan, 1981, in press

307. WAGNER GS, DINAMARCA ML, TEPHLY TR: Studies on ferrochelatase activity: Role in regulation of hepatic heme biosynthesis, in Doss M (ed): *Porphyrins in Human Diseases*, Basel, S Karger, 1976, p 111

308. DRUMMOND GS, KAPPAS A: Manganese and zinc blockade of enzyme

induction: Studies with microsomal heme oxygenase. *Proc Natl Acad Sci USA* 76:5331, 1979

309. DE MATTEIS F: Rapid loss of cytochrome P-450 and heme caused in the liver microsomes by the porphyrogenic agent 2-allyl-2-isopropyl-acetamide. *FEBS Lett* 6:343, 1970

310. DE MATTEIS F: Loss of microsomal components in drug induced liver damage in cholestasis and after administration of chemicals which stimulate heme catabolism. *Pharmacol Ther* 2:693, 1978

311. DE MATTEIS F: Hepatic porphyrias caused by 2-allyl-2-isopropyl-acetamide, 3,5-diethoxycarbonyl-1,4-dihydrocollidine, griseofulvin and related compounds, in DeMatteis F, Aldridge WN (eds): *Heme and Hemoproteins, Handbook of Experimental Pharmacology*, vol 44. New York, Springer-Verlag, 1978, p 129

312. LEVIN W, SERNATINGER E, JACOBSON M, KUNTZMAN R: Destruction of cytochrome P-450 by secobarbital and other barbiturates containing allyl groups. *Science* 176:1341, 1972

313. IOANNIDES C, PARKE DV: The effect of allyl compounds on hepatic microsomal mixed function oxidation and porphyrogenesis. *Chem Biol Interact* 14:241, 1976

314. ORTIZ DE MONTELLANO PR, MICO BA: Destruction of cytochrome P-450 by ethylene and other compounds. *Mol Pharmacol* 18:128, 1980

315. ORTIZ DE MONTELLANO PR, KUNZE KL: Self-catalyzed inactivation of hepatic cytochrome P-450 by ethynyl substrates. *J Biol Chem* 255:5578, 1980

316. WHITE INH, MULLER-EBERHARD U: Decreased liver cytochrome P-450 in rats caused by norethindrone or ethynyloestradiol. *Biochem J* 166:57, 1977

317. WHITE INH: Metabolic activation of acetylene substituents to derivatives in the rat causing the loss of hepatic cytochrome P-450 and haem. *Biochem J* 174:853, 1978

318. DE MATTEIS F, CANTONI L: Alteration of the porphyrin nucleus of cytochrome P-450 caused in the liver by treatment with allyl-containing drugs: Is the modified porphyrin N-substituted? *Biochem J* 183:99, 1979

319. BRADSHAW JJ, ZIMAN MR, IVANETICH KM: The degradation of different forms of cytochrome P-450 *in vivo* by fluroxene and allyl-iso-propylacetamide. *Biochem Biophys Res Commun* 85:859, 1978

320. FARRELL GC, SCHMID R, KUNZE KL, ORTIZ DE MONTELLANO PR: Exogenous heme restores *in vivo* functional capacity of hepatic cytochrome P-450 destroyed by allylisopropylacetamide. *Biochem Biophys Res Commun* 89:456, 1979

321. DE MATTEIS F, GIBBS AH, TEPHLY TR: Inhibition of protohaem ferrolyase in experimental porphyria: Isolation and partial characterization of a modified porphyrin inhibitor. *Biochem J* 188:145, 1980

322. BARON J, TEPHLY TR: Further studies on the relationship of the stimulatory effects of phenobarbital and 3,4-benzpyrene on hepatic heme synthesis to their effects in hepatic microsomal drug oxidations. *Arch Biochem Biophys* 139:410, 1970

323. RAJAMANICKAM C, SATYANARAYANA RAO R, PADMANABAN G: On the sequence of reactions leading to cytochrome P-450 synthesis: Effect of drugs. *J Biol Chem* 250:2305, 1975

324. YANNONI CA, ROBINSON SH: Early-labelled haem in erythoid and hepatic cells. *Nature* 258:330, 1975

324a. GRANDCHAMP B, BISSELL DM, LICKO V, SCHMID R: Formation and disposition of newly synthesized heme in adult rat hepatocytes in primary culture. *J. Biol Chem* 256:11287, 1981

325. BADAWY AAB, EVANS M: The effects of chemical porphyrogens and drugs on the activity of rat liver tryptophan pyrrolase. *Biochem J* 136:885, 1973

326. BADAWY AAB: Tryptophan pyrrolase, the regulatory free haem and hepatic porphyrias: Early depletion of haem by clinical and experimental exacerbations of porphyria. *Biochem J* 172:487, 1978

327. DE MATTEIS F, GIBBS AH: Stimulation of liver 5-aminolevulinate synthetase by drugs and its relevance to drug-induced accumulation of cytochrome P-450. *Biochem J* 126:1149, 1972

328. KAPPAS A, SONG CS, SASSA S, LEVERE RD, GRANICK S: The occurrence of substances in human plasma capable of inducing the enzyme δ-aminovulinate synthetase in liver cells. *Proc Natl Acad Sci USA* 64:557, 1969

329. RIFKIND AB, SASSA S, MERKATZ IR, WINCHESTER R, HARBER L, KAPPAS A: Stimulators and inhibitors of hepatic porphyrin formation in human sera. *J Clin Invest* 53:1167, 1974

330. STRAND LJ, MARVER H: Determination of δ-aminolevulinic acid synthetase (ALA-S) in cell culture: Naturally occurring inducers in normal human plasma. *Clin Res* 18:345, 1970

331. WETTERBERG L: Internationell enkät om farliga och ofarliga läkemedel vid akut intermittent porfyri. *Kakartidningen* 73:4090, 1976

332. MOORE MR: International review of drugs in acute porphyria—1980. *Int J Biochem* 12:1089, 1980

333. WATSON CJ, JEELANI DHAR G, BOSSENMAIER I, CARDINAL R, PETRYKA ZJ: Effect of hematin in acute porphyric relapse. *Ann Intern Med* 79:80, 1973

334. WATSON CJ, BOSSENMAIER I, CARDINAL R, PETRYKA ZJ: Repression by hematin of porphyrin biosynthesis in erythrocyte precursors in congenital erythropoietic porphyria. *Proc Natl Acad Sci USA* 71:278, 1974

335. WATSON CJ, PIERACH CA, BOSSENMAIER I, CARDINAL R: Postulated deficiency of hepatic heme and repair by hematin infusions in the "inducible" hepatic porphyrias. *Proc Natl Acad Sci USA* 74:2118, 1977

336. WATSON CJ, PIERACH CA, BOSSENMAIER I, CARDINAL R: Use of hematin in the acute attack of the "inducible" hepatic porphyrias. *Adv Intern Med* 23:265, 1978

337. WAXMAN AD, COLLINS A, TSCHUDY DP: Oscillations of hepatic δ-aminolevulinic acid synthetase produced *in vivo* by heme. *Biochem Biophys Res Commun* 24:675, 1966

338. BONKOWSKY HL, TSCHUDY DP, COLLINS A, DOHERTY J, BOSSENMAIER I, CARDINAL R, WATSON CJ: Repression of the overproduction of porphyrin precursors in acute intermittent porphyria by intravenous infusions of hematin. *Proc Natl Acad Sci USA* 68:2725, 1971

339. MAINES MD, SINCLAIR P: Cobalt regulation of heme synthesis and degradation in avian embryo liver cell culture. *J Biol Chem* 252:219, 1977

340. MAINES MD, KAPPAS A: Studies on the mechanism of induction of haem oxygenase by cobalt and other metal ions. *Biochem J* 154:125, 1976

341. MAINES MD, KAPPAS A: Metals as regulators of heme catabolism. *Science* 198:1215, 1977

342. ROSENBERG D, DRUMMOND GS, CORNISH HC, KAPPAS A: Prolonged induction of hepatic haem oxygenase and decreases in cytochrome P-450 content by organotin compounds. *Biochem J* 190:465, 1980

343. DRUMMOND GS, KAPPAS A: Metal ion interactions in the control of haem oxygenase induction in liver and kidney. *Biochem J* 192:637, 1980

344. SARDANA MK, SASSA S, KAPPAS A: Adrenalectomy enhances the induction of heme oxygenase and the degradation of cytochrome P-450 in liver. *J Biol Chem* 255:11320, 1980

345. WELLAND FH, HELLMAN ES, GADDIS EM, COLLINS A, HUNTER GW JR, TSCHUDY DP: Factors affecting the excretion of porphyrin precursors by patients with acute intermittent porphyria. I. The effects of diet. *Metabolism* 13:232, 1964

346. FELSHER BF, REDEKER AG: Acute intermittent porphyria: Effect of diet and griseofulvin. *Medicine* 46:217, 1967

347. TSCHUDY DP, WELLAND FH, COLLINS A, HUNTER G JR: The effect of carbohydrate feeding on the induction of δ-aminolevulinic acid synthetase. *Metabolism* 13:396, 1964

348. PAUL S, BICKERS DR, LEVERE RD, KAPPAS A: Inhibited induction of hepatic δ-aminolevulinate synthetase in pregnancy. *FEBS Lett* 41:192, 1974

349. LEVERE RD, GRANICK S: Control of hemoglobin synthesis in the cultured chick blastoderm. *J Biol Chem* 242:1903, 1967

350. SASSA S, URABE A: Uroporphyrinogen I synthase induction in normal human bone marrow cultures: An early and quantitative response of erythroid differentiation. *Proc Natl Acad Sci USA* 76:5321, 1979

351. SASSA S, GRANICK JL, EISEN H, OSTERTAG W: Regulation of heme biosynthesis in mouse Friend virus-transformed cells in culture, in Murphy MJ (ed): *In Vitro Aspects of Erythropoiesis*. New York, Springer-Verlag, 1978, p 135

352. EISEN H, KEPPEL-BALLIVET F, GEORGOPOULOS CP, SASSA S, GRANICK J, PRAGNELL I, OSTERTAG W: Biochemical and genetic analysis of erythroid differentiation in Friend-virus-transformed murine erythroleukemia cells, in Clarkson B, Marks PA, Till JE (eds): *Differentiation of Normal and Neoplastic Hematopoietic Cells*, vol 5. Cold Spring Harbor Lab, Cold Spring Harbor Conference on Cell Proliferation, 1978, p 277

353. RUTHERFORD T, THOMPSON GG, MOORE MR: Heme biosynthesis in Friend erythroleukemia cells: Control by ferrochelatase. *Proc Natl Acad Sci USA* 76:833, 1979

354. LEVERE RD, KAPPAS A, GRANICK S: Stimulation of hemoglobin synthesis in chick blastoderms by certain 5β-androstane and 5β-pregnane steroids. *Proc Natl Acad Sci USA* 58:985, 1967

355. WAINWRIGHT SD, WAINWRIGHT LK: Regulation of the initiation of hemoglobin synthesis in the blood island cells of chick embryos. I. Qualitative studies on the effects of actinomycin D and δ-aminolevulinic acid. *Can J Biochem* 44:1543, 1966

356. WAINWRIGHT SD, WAINWRIGHT LK: Regulation of the initiation of hemoglobin synthesis in the blood island cells of chick embryos. II. Early onset and stimulation of hemoglobin formation induced by exogenous δ-aminolevulinic acid. *Can J Biochem* 45:344, 1967

357. IRVING RA, MAINWARING WIP, SPOONER PM: The regulation of haemoglobin synthesis in cultured chick blastoderms by steroid related to 5β-androstane. *Biochem J* 154:81, 1976

358. URABE A, SASSA S, KAPPAS A: The influence of steroid hormone metabolites on the *in vitro* development of erythroid colonies derived from human bone marrow. *J Exp Med* 149:1314, 1979

359. STEPHENS JK, FISCHER PWF, MARKS GS: Porphyrin induction: Equivalent effects of 5αH and 5βH steroids in chick embryo liver cells. *Science* 197:659, 1977

360. KAPPAS A, SONG CS, LEVERE RD, SACHSON RA, GRANICK S: The induction of δ-aminolevulinic acid synthetase *in vivo* in chick embryo liver by natural steroids. *Proc Natl Acad Sci USA* 61:509, 1968

361. EDWARDS AM, ELLIOTT WH: Induction of δ-aminolevulinic acid synthetase in isolated rat liver cells by steroids. *J Biol Chem* 250:2750, 1975

362. WADA O, SASSA S, TAKAKU F, YANO Y, URATA G, NAKAO K: Different responses of the hepatic and erythropoietic δ-aminolevulinic acid synthetase of mice. *Biochim Biophys Acta* 148:585, 1967

363. FRIEND C, SCHER W, HOLLAND JG, SATO T: Hemoglobin synthesis in murine virus-induced leukemic cells *in vitro*: Stimulation of erythroid differentiation by dimethylsulfoxide. *Proc Natl Acad Sci USA* 68:378, 1971

364. MARKS PA, RIFKIND RA: Erythroleukemic differentiation. *Ann Rev Biochem* 47:419, 1978

365. ROSS J, IKAWA Y, LEDER P: Globin messenger RNA induction during erythroid differentiation of cultured leukemia cells. *Proc Natl Acad Sci USA* 69:3620, 1972

366. ROSS J, SAUTNER D: Induction of globin mRNA accumulation by hemin in cultured erythroleukemic cells. *Cell* 8:513, 1976

367. DABNEY BJ, BEAUDET AL: Increase in globin chains and globin mRNA in erythroleukemia cells in response to hemin. *Arch Biochem Biophys* 179:106, 1977

368. PORTER PN, MEINTS RH, MESNER K: Enhancement of erythroid colony growth in culture by hemin. *Exp Hematol* 7:11, 1979

369. KARIBIAN D, LONDON IM: Control of heme synthesis by feedback inhibition. *Biochem Biophys Res Commun* 18:243, 1965

370. NEUWIRT DJ, PONKA P: *Regulation of Haemoglobin Synthesis.* The Hague, Netherlands, Martinus Nijhoff Medical Division, 1977

371. WOODS JS, DIXON RL: Perinatal differences in delta-aminolevulinic acid synthetase activity. *Life Sci* 9(Pt II):711, 1970

372. WOODS JS, DIXON RL: Studies on the perinatal differences in the activity of hepatic δ-aminolevulinic acid synthetase. *Biochem Pharmacol* 21:1735, 1972

373. BISHOP DF, KITCHEN H, WOOD WA: Evidence for erythroid and nonerythroid forms of δ-aminolevulinate synthetase. *Arch Biochem Biophys* 206:380, 1981

374. TIEN W, WHITE DC: Linear sequential arrangement of genes for the biosynthetic pathway of protoheme in *Staphylococcus aureus. Proc Natl Acad Sci USA* 61:1392, 1968

375. POWELL KA, COX R, MCCONVILLE M, CHARLES HP: Mutations affecting porphyrin biosynthesis in *Escherichia coli. Enzyme* 16:65, 1973

376. PAIGEN K: Temporal genes and developmental programs, in Armendares S, Lisker R (eds), Ebling FJG, Henderson IW (co-eds): *Human Genetics.* Amsterdam, Excerpta Med, 1977, p 33

377. SEDMAN RM, TEPHLY TR: Cardiac δ-aminolevulinic acid synthetase activity: Effects of fasting, cobaltous chloride and hemin. *Biochem Pharmacol* 29:795, 1980

378. WATSON CJ: Hematin and porphyria (editorial). *N Engl J Med* 293:605, 1975

379. COHN J, ALVARES AP, KAPPAS A: On the occurrence of cytochrome P-450 and aryl hydrocarbon hydroxylase activity in rat brain. *J Exp Med* 145:1607, 1977

380. WHETSELL WO JR, SASSA S, BICKERS D, KAPPAS A: Studies on porphyrin-heme biosynthesis in organotypic cultures of chick dorsal root ganglion. I. Observations on neuronal and non-neuronal elements. *J Neuropathol Exp Neurol* 37:497, 1978

381. WHETSELL WO JR, SASSA S, KAPPAS A: Studies on effects of chronic lead exposure upon porphyrin biosynthesis and myelin in cultures of mouse dorsal root ganglia (DRG). *J Neuropathol Exp Neurol* 38:348, 1979

382. SASSA S, WHETSELL WO JR, KAPPAS A: Studies on porphyrin-heme biosynthesis in organotypic cultures of chick dorsal root ganglion. II. The effect of lead. *Environ Res* 19:415, 1979

383. WHETSELL WO JR, KAPPAS A: Protective effect of exogenous heme against lead toxicity in organotypic cultures of mouse dorsal root ganglia (DRG): Electron microscopic observations. *J Neuropathol Exp Neurol* 40:334, 1981

384. CHANG K-P, CHANG C, SASSA S: Heme biosynthesis in bacterium-protozoan symbiosis: Enzymic defects in host hemoflagellates and complemental role of their intracellular symbiotes. *Proc Natl Acad Sci USA* 72:2479, 1975

385. WATSON CJ, LOWRY PT, SCHMID R, HAWKINSON VE, SCHWARTZ S: The manifestations of the different forms of porphyria in relation to chemical findings. *Trans Assoc Am Physicians* 64:345, 1951

386. SCHMID R, SCHWARTZ S, WATSON CJ: Porphyrin content of bone marrow and liver in the various forms of porphyria. *Arch Intern Med* 93:167, 1954

387. MARVER HS, SCHMID R: The porphyrias, in Stanbury JB, Wyngaarden JB, Fredrickson DS (eds): *The Metabolic Basis of Inherited Disease,* 3d ed. New York, McGraw-Hill, 1972, p 1087

388. SCHMID R, SCHWARTZ S, SUNDBERG RD: Erythropoietic (congenital) porphyria: A rare abnormality of the normoblasts. *Blood* 10:416, 1955

389. VARADI S: Haematological aspects in a case of erythropoietic porphyria. *Br J Haematol* 4:270, 1958

390. GÜNTHER H: In Schittenhelm A (ed): *Handbuch der Krankheiten des Blutes und der blutbildenden Organe,* vol 2. Berlin, Springer-Verlag, 1925

391. KRAMER S, VILJOEN E, MEYER AM, METZ J: The anemia of erythropoietic porphyria with the first description of the disease in an elderly patient. *Br J Haematol* 11:666, 1965

392. KAUFMAN BM, VICKERS HR, RAYNE J, RYAN TJ: Congenital erythropoietic porphyria: Report of a case. *Br J Dermatol* 79:210, 1967

393. SVEINSSON SL, RIMINGTON C, BARNES HD: Complete porphyrin analysis of pathological urines. *Scand J Clin Lab Invest* 1:2, 1949

394. PAIN RW, WELCH FW, WOODROFFE AJ, HANDLEY DA, LOCKWOOD WH: Erythropoietic uroporphyria of Günther first presenting at 58 years with positive family studies. *Br Med J* 3:621, 1975

395. WESTON MJ, NICHOLSON DC, LIM CK, CLARK KG, MACDONALD A, HENDERSON MA, WILLIAMS R: Congenital erythropoietic uroporphyria (Günther's disease) presenting in a middle aged man. *Int J Biochem* 9:921, 1978

396. DEYBACH JC, DE VERNEUIL H, PHUNG N, NORDMANN Y, PUISSANT A, BOFFETY B: Congenital erythropoietic porphyria (Günther's disease): Enzymatic studies on two cases of late onset. *J Lab Clin Med* 97:551, 1981

397. GRAY CH, MUIR IMH, NEUBERGER A: Studies in congenital porphyria. 3. The incorporation of ^{15}N into the haem and glycine of haemoglobin. *Biochem J* 47:542, 1950

398. ZAIL SS, KRAWITZ P, VILJOEN E, KRAMER S: The anaemia of erythropoietic porphyria. II. Studies of some red cell intermediates. *Br J Haematol* 13:60, 1967

399. ROSENTHAL IM, LIPTON EL, ASROW G: Effect of splenectomy on porphyria erythropoietica. *Pediatrics* 15:663, 1955

400. GROSS S: Hematologic studies on erythropoietic porphyria: A new case with severe hemolysis, chronic thrombocytopenia, and folic acid deficiency. *Blood* 23:762, 1964

401. HAINING RG, COWGER ML, SHURTLEFF DB, LABBE RF: Congenital erythropoietic porphyria. I. Case report, special studies and therapy. *Am J Med* 45:624, 1968

402. HAUSMANN W: Die Sensibilisierende Wirkung des Hämatoporphyrins. *Biochem Z* 30:276, 1911

403. WATSON CJ, PERMAN V, SPURRELL FA, HOYT HH, SCHWARTZ S: Some studies of the comparative biology of human and bovine erythropoietic porphyria. *Arch Intern Med* 103:436, 1959

404. WATSON CJ, BOSSENMAIER I, CARDINAL R: Formation of porphyrin isomers from porphobilinogen by various hemolysates of red cells from bovine and human subjects with erythropoietic (Uro-) porphyria. *J Clin Chem Clin Biochem* 7:119, 1969

405. ZINKL J, KANEKO JJ: Erythrocytic enzymes and glycolytic intermediates in the normal bovine and in bovine erythropoietic porphyria. *Comp Biochem Physiol* 45 (A):463, 1973

406. CARUSO P, CONTI F: Bioenzymology of porphyric erythrocyte. *Panminerva Med* 5:321, 1963

407. LARIZZA P: The problem of erythropoietic porphyria in the light of the latest advances of biochemistry and morphology. *Panminerva Med* 4:315, 1962

408. CHATTERJEA JB: Correspondence: Erythropoietic porphyria. *Blood* 24:806, 1964

409. KRAMER S, SIVE J, BECKER D, VILJOEN D, METZ J: Intracellular porphyrin concentration and erythrocyte life-span. *Scan J Haematol* 9:114, 1972

410. ALDRICH RA, HAWKINSON V, GRINSTEIN M, WATSON CJ: Photosensitive or congenital porphyria with hemolytic anemia. I. Clinical and fundamental studies before and after splenectomy. *Blood* 6:685, 1951

411. SIMARD H, BARRY A, VILLENEUVE B, PETITCLERC C, GARNEAU R, DELÂGE J-M: Porphyrie érythropoïétique congénitale. *Can Med Assoc J* 106:1002, 1972

412. SATO A, TAKAHASI N: A new form of congenital hematoporphyria: Oligochromemia, porphyrinuria (megalosplenica congenita). *Am J Dis Child* 32:325, 1926

413. GRAY CH, NEUBERGER A: Studies in congenital porphyria. I. Incorporation of ^{15}N into coproporphyrin, uroporphyrin and hippuric acid. *Biochem J* 47:81, 1950

414. GRAY CH, NEUBERGER A, SNEATH PHA: Studies in congenital porphyria. II. Incorporation of ^{15}N in the stercobilin in the normal and in the porphyric. *Biochem J* 47:87, 1950

415. GRAY CH: Isotope studies in porphyria. *Br Med Bull* 8:229, 1952

416. GRINSTEIN M, ALDRICH RA, HAWKINSON V, LOWRY P, WATSON CJ: Photosensitive or congenital porphyria with hemolytic anemia. II. Isotopic studies of porphyrin and hemoglobin metabolism. *Blood* 6:699, 1951

417. LONDON IM, WEST R, SHEMIN D, RITTENBERG D: Porphyrin formation and hemoglobin metabolism in congenital porphyria. *J Biol Chem* 184:365, 1950

418. HAINING RG, COWGER ML, LABBE RF, FINCH CA: Congenital erythropoietic porphyria. II. The effects of induced polycythemia. *Blood* 36:297, 1970

419. RUNGE W, WATSON CJ: The effect of bleeding on the proportion of red fluorescing forms among the total normoblasts of bovine porphyric bone marrow. *Blood* 33:119, 1969

420. NICHOLSON DC, COWGER ML, KALIVAS J, THOMPSON RPH, GRAY CH: Isotopic studies of the erythropoietic and hepatic components of congenital porphyria and "erythropoietic" protoporphyria. *Clin Sci* 44:135, 1973

421. NAKAO K: Biochemical aspects of porphyria. *Jpn J Med* 7:103, 1968

422. WATSON CJ, PERMAN V, SPURRELL FA, HOYT HH, SCHWARTZ S: Some studies of the comparative biology of human and bovine porphyria erythropoietica. *Trans Assoc Am Physicians* 71:196, 1958

423. WATSON CJ, RUNGE W, TADDEINI L, BOSSENMAIER I, CARDINAL R: A suggested control gene mechanism for the excessive production of types I and III porphyrins in congenital erythropoietic porphyria. *Proc Natl Acad Sci USA* 52:478, 1964

424. HEILMEYER VL, CLOTTEN R, KERP L, MERKER H, PARRA CA, WETZEL HP: Porphyria erythropoietica congenita Günther. *Dtsch Med Wochenschr* 51:2449, 1963

425. WATSON CJ: Some recent advances in the problem of erythropoietic porphyria. *Acta Med Scand* 179 (Suppl):25, 1966

426. KENCH JE, LANGLEY FA, WILKINSON JF: Biochemical and pathological studies of congenital porphyria. *Q J Med* 22:285, 1953

427. TADDEINI L, WATSON CJ: The clinical porphyrias. *Semin Hematol* 5:335, 1968

428. SCHWARTZ S, O'CONNOR N, STEPHENSON BD, ANDERSON AS, JOHNSON LW, JOHNSON J: Turnover of erythrocyte protoporphyrin, with special reference to bovine porphyria and iron deficiency anemia. *Ann Clin Res* 8 (Suppl):203, 1976

429. MIYAGI K, WATSON CJ: δ-Aminolevulinic acid synthetase activity in human plasma: Relation to erythropoiesis and evidence of induction in erythropoietic porphyria. *Blood* 39:13, 1972

430. HEILMEYER L: The erythropoietic porphyrias. *Acta Haematol (Basel)* 31:137, 1964

431. DAROCHA T: Family study in congenital erythropoietic porphyria. *S Afr J Lab Clin Med* 17 (special issue):231, 1971

432. LEVIN EY: Comparative aspects of porphyria in man and animals. *Ann NY Acad Sci* 241:347, 1974

433. GRANDCHAMP B, DEYBACH JC, GRELIER M, DE VERNEUIL H, NORDMANN Y: Studies of porphyrin synthesis in fibroblasts of patients with congenital erythropoietic porphyria and one patient with homozygous coproporphyria. *Biochim Biophys Acta* 629:577, 1980

434. MIYAGI K, PETRYKA ZJ, BOSSENMAIER I, CARDINAL R, WATSON CJ: The activities of uroporphyrinogen synthetase and cosynthetase in congenital erythropoietic porphyria (CEP). *Am J Hematol* 1:3, 1976

435. MASUYA T: Pathophysiological observations on porphyrias. *Acta Hematol Jpn* 32:465, 1969

436. MOORE MR, THOMPSON GG, GOLDBERG A: The biosynthesis of haem in congenital (erythropoietic) porphyria. *Int J Biochem* 9:933, 1978

437. HEILMEYER L, CLOTTEN R: Die Störung der Porphyrinsynthese bei der Güntherschen Porphyria congenita. *Acta Hematol* 34:65, 1965

438. ROMEO G: Analytical review, enzymatic defects of hereditary porphyrias: An explanation of dominance at the molecular level. *Hum Genet* 39:261, 1977

439. SCHWARTZ S, JOHNSON JA, STEPHENSON BD, ANDERSON AS, EDMONDSON PR, FUSARO RM: Erythropoietic defects in protoporphyria: A study of factors involved in labelling of porphyrins and bile pigments from ALA-³H and glycine-¹⁴C. *J Lab Clin Med* 78:411, 1971

440. CLARK KGA, NICHOLSON DC: Erythrocyte protoporphyrin and iron uptake in erythropoietic protoporphyria. *Clin Sci* 41:363, 1971

441. BENOFF S, BRUCE SA, SKOULTCHI AI: X-Linked control of globin mRNA and hemoglobin production in erythroleukemia-lymphoma cell hybrids. *Somatic Cell Genet* 6:15, 1980

442. KAISER IH: Brown amniotic fluid in congenital erythropoietic porphyria. *Obstet Gynecol* 56:383, 1980

443. NITOWSKY HM, SASSA S, NAKAGAWA A, JAGANI N: Prenatal diagnosis of congenital erythropoietic porphyria. *Pediatr Res* 12:455, 1978

444. DEYBACH JC, GRANDCHAMP B, GRELIER M, NORDMANN Y, BOUÉ J, DE BERRANGER P: Prenatal exclusion of congenital erythropoietic porphyria (Günther's disease) in a fetus at risk. *Hum Genet* 53:217, 1980

445. HOFSTAD F, SEIP M, ERIKSEN L: Congenital erythropoietic porphyria with a hitherto undescribed porphyrin pattern. *Acta Paediatr Scand* 62:380, 1973

446. ERIKSEN L, HOFSTAD F, SEIP M: Congenital erythropoietic porphyria. The effect of light shielding. *Acta Paediatr Scand* 62:385, 1973

447. ERIKSEN L, ERIKSEN N: Porphyrin distribution and porphyrin excretion in human congenital erythropoietic porphyria. *Scand J Clin Lab Invest* 33:323, 1974

448. RIMINGTON C, WITH TK: Porphyrin studies in congenital erythropoietic porphyria. *Dan Med Bull* 20:5, 1973

449. PIÑOL AGUADÉ J, CASTELLS A, INDACOCHEA A, RODÉS J: A case of biochemically unclassifiable hepatic porphyria. *Br J Dermatol* 81:270, 1969

450. PIÑOL AGUADÉ J, HERRERO C, ALMEIDA J, CASTELLS MAS A, FERRANDO J, DE ASPRER J, PALOU A, GIMÉNEZ A: Porphyrie hépato-érythrocytaire: Une nouvelle forme de porphyrie. *Ann Dermatol Venereol* 102:129, 1975

451. PIÑOL AGUADÉ J, HERRERO C, ALMEIDA J, SMITH SG, BELCHER RV: Thin layer chromatography and counter-current analysis in porphyrias. *Br J Dermatol* 93:277, 1975

452. SIMON N, BERKÓ GY, SCHNEIDER I: Hepato-erythropoietic porphyria presenting as scleroderma and acrosclerosis in a sibling pair. *Br J Dermatol* 96:663, 1977

453. SIMON N, HUNYADI J, SZÖRÉNYI A, SZEMERE G: Deletion des kurzen Armes des chromosoms nr. 18 und 18er Trisomie bei einem Geschwisterpaar mit Porphyrie ungewöhnlicher Erscheinungsform. *Hautarzt* 24:185, 1973

454. ELDER GH, SMITH SG, HERRERO C, MASCARO JM, LECHA M, MUNIESA AM, CZARNECKI DB, BRENAN J, POULOS V, DE SALAMANCA RE: Hepatoerythropoietic porphyria: A new uroporphyrinogen decarboxylase defect on homozygous porphyria cutanea tarda? *Lancet* i: 916, 1981

455. CHU TC, CHU EJ: Porphyrin patterns in different types of porphyria. *Clin Chem* 13:371, 1967

456. POULOS V, LOCKWOOD WH: Unclassified porphyrias. *Int J Biochem* 12:959, 1980

457. POŇKA P, NEUWIRT J: (Annotation) Haem synthesis and iron uptake by reticulocytes. *Br J Haematol* 28:1, 1974

458. POŇKA P, NEUWIRT J, BOROVÁ J: The role of heme in the release of iron from transferrin in reticulocytes. *Enzyme* 17:91, 1973

459. HINES J, HARRIS J, BONKOWSKY H, GRASSO J, GOODMAN A: Intravenous hematin in refractory sideroblastic anemia. *Clin Res* 28:769a, 1980

460. SEIP M, THUNE PO, ERIKSEN L: Treatment of photosensitivity in congenital erythropoietic porphyria (CEP) with beta-carotene. *Acta Derm Venereol (Stockh)* 54:239, 1974

461. MATHEWS-ROTH MM: Beta carotene in congenital porphyria (letter). *Arch Dermatol* 115:641, 1979

462. WIEGAND SE, COPEMAN PWM, PERRY HO: Metabolic alkalinization in porphyria cutanea tarda. *Arch Dermatol* 100:544, 1969

463. PERRY HO, MULLANAX MG, WIEGAND SE: Metabolic alkalinization therapy in porphyria cutanea tarda. *Arch Dermatol* 102:359, 1979

464. BOURKE E, COPEMAN PWM, MILNE MD, STOKES GS: Effect of urinary pH on excretion of porphyrins. *Lancet* i:1394, 1966

465. STRETCHER GS: Erythropoietic porphyria: Two cases and the results of metabolic alkalinization. *Arch Dermatol* 113:1553, 1977

466. GAJDOS A, GAJDOS-TÖRÖK M: The therapeutic effect of adenosine-5-monophosphoric acid in porphyria. *Lancet* ii:175, 1961

467. BATTLE DEL C AM, WIDER DE, XIFRA EA, STELLA AM, BUSTOS N, WITH TK: Studies on porphyrin biosynthesis and the enzymes involved in bovine congenital erythropoietic porphyria. *Clin Sci* 57:63, 1979

468. KANEKO JJ: Erythrokinetics and iron metabolism in bovine porphyria erythropoietica. *Ann NY Acad Sci* 104:689, 1963

469. SCHMID R, SCHWARTZ S, WATSON CJ: Porphyrins in the bone marrow and circulating erythrocytes in experimental anemia. *Proc Soc Exp Biol Med* 75:705, 1950

470. CLOUE NT, STEPHENS EH: Congenital porphyria in pigs. *Nature* 153:252, 1944

471. JØRGENSEN SK, WITH TK: Congenital porphyria in swine and cattle in Denmark. *Nature* 176:156, 1955

472. JØRGENSEN SK, WITH TK: Porphyria in domestic animals: Danish observations in pigs and cattle and comparison with human porphyria. *Ann NY Acad Sci* 104:701, 1963

473. TOBIAS G: Congenital porphyria in a cat. *J Am Vet Med Assoc* 145:462, 1964

474. GLENN BL, GLENN HG, OMTVEDT IT: Congenital porphyria in the domestic cat (Felis catus): Preliminary investigation on inheritance pattern. *Am J Vet Res* 29:1653, 1968

475. GIDDENS WE Jr, LABBE RF, SWANGO LJ, PADGETT GA: Feline congenital erythropoietic porphyria associated with severe anemia and renal disease. Clinical, morphological, and biochemical studies. *Am J Pathol* 80:367, 1975

476. TURNER WJ: Studies on porphyria. I. Observations on the fox squirrel (Sciurus niger). *J Biol Chem* 118:519, 1937

477. FLYGER V, LEVIN EY: Congenital erythropoietic porphyria. *Am J Pathol* 87:269, 1977

478. MAGNUS IA, JARRETT A, PRANKERT TAJ, RIMINGTON C: Erythropoietic protoporphyria: A new porphyria syndrome with solar urticaria due to protoporphyrinaemia. *Lancet* ii:448, 1961

479. SCHOLNICK P, MARVER HS, SCHMID R: Erythropoietic protoporphyria: Evidence for multiple sites of excess protoporphyrin formation. *J Clin Invest* 50:203, 1971

480. DE LEO VA, POH-FITZPATRICK M, MATHEWS-ROTH M, HARBER LC:

Erythropoietic protoporphyria: 10 years experience. *Am J Med* 60:8, 1976

481. Poh-Fitzpatrick MB: Erythropoietic porphyrias: Current mechanistic, diagnostic, and therapeutic considerations. *Semin Hematol* 14:211, 1977

482. Magnus IA: The cutaneous porphyrias. *Semin Hematol* 5:380, 1968

483. Schmidt HG, Snitker G, Thomsen K, Lintrup J: Erythropoietic protoporphyria: A clinical study based on 29 cases in 14 families. *Arch Dermatol* 110:58, 1974

484. Bopp C, Bakos L, da Graca Busko M: Erythropoietic protoporphyria. *Int J Biochem* 12:909, 1980

485. Eales L: Liver involvement in erythropoietic protoporphyria (EPP). *Int J Biochem* 12:915, 1980

486. Goldstein BD, Harber LC: Erythropoietic protoporphyria: Lipid peroxidation and red cell membrane damage associated with photohemolysis. *J Clin Invest* 51:892, 1972

487. Wakulchik SD, Schiltz JR, Bickers DR: Photolysis of protoporphyrin-treated human fibroblasts *in vitro*: Studies on the mechanism. *J Lab Clin Med* 96:158, 1980

488. Sandberg S: Protoporphyrin-induced photodamage to mitochondria and lysosomes from rat liver. *Clin Chim Acta* 111:55, 1981

489. Sandberg S, Romslo I: Porphyrin-induced photodamage at the cellular and the subcellular level as related to the solubility of the porphyrin. *Clin Chim Acta* 109:193, 1981

490. Bodaness RS, Chan PC: Singlet oxygen as a mediator in the hematoporphyrin-catalyzed photooxidation of NADPH to NADP$^+$ in deuterium oxide. *J Biol Chem* 252:8554, 1977

491. De Goeij AFPM, Van Steveninck J: Photodynamic effects of protoporphyrin on cholesterol and unsaturated fatty acids in erythrocyte membranes in protoporphyria and in normal red blood cells. *Clin Chim Acta* 68:115, 1976

492. Schothorst AA, Van Steveninck J, Went LN, Suurmond D: Photodynamic damage of the erythrocyte membrane caused by protoporphyrin in protoporphyria and in normal red blood cells. *Clin Chim Acta* 39:161, 1972

493. Dubbelman TMAR, De Bruijne AW, Van Steveninck J: Photodynamic effects of protoporphyrin on red blood cell deformability. *Biochem Biophys Res Commun* 77:811, 1977

494. Malik Z, Breitbart H: Cross-linking of hemoglobin and inhibition of globin synthesis in reticulocytes induced by photoactivated protoporphyrin. *Acta Haematol (Basel)* 64:304, 1980

495. Stenhagen E, Rideal EK: The interaction between porphyrins and lipoid and protein monolayers. *Biochem J* 33:1591, 1939

496. Gigli I, Schothorst AA, Soter NA, Pathak MA: Erythropoietic protoporphyria: Photoactivation of the complement system. *J Clin Invest* 66:517, 1980

497. Lim HW, Gigli I: Role of complement in porphyrin-induced photosensitivity. *J Invest Dermatol* 76:4, 1981

498. Baart De La Faille-Kuyper EH, Cormane RH: The occurrence of certain serum factors in the dermal-epidermal junction and vessel walls of the skin in lupus erythematosus and other (skin) diseases. *Acta Derm Venereol (Stockh)* 48:578, 1968

499. Peterka ES, Fusaro RM, Goltz RW: Erythropoietic protoporphyria. II. Histological and histochemical studies of cutaneous lesions. *Arch Dermatol* 92:357, 1965

500. Sasai Y: Erythropoietic protoporphyria. Histochemical study of hyaline material. *Acta Derm Venereol (Stockh)* 53:179, 1973

501. Ryan EA: Histochemistry of the skin in erythropoietic protoporphyria. *Br J Dermatol* 78:501, 1966

502. Epstein JH, Tuffanelli DL, Epstein WL: Cutaneous changes in the porphyrias (a microscopic study). *Arch Dermatol* 107:689, 1973

503. Hönigsmann H, Gschnait F, Konrad K, Stingl G, Wolff K: Mouse model for protoporphyria. III. Experimental production for chronic erythropoietic protoporphyria-like skin lesions. *J Invest Dermatol* 66:188, 1976

504. Ryan EA, Madill GT: Electron microscopy of the skin in erythropoietic protoporphyria. *Br J Dermatol* 80:561, 1968

505. Gray CH, Kulczycka A, Nicholson DC, Magnus IA, Rimington C: Isotope studies on a case of erythropoietic protoporphyria. *Clin Sci* 26:7, 1964

506. Holti G, Magnus IA, Rimington C: Erythropoietic protoporphyria in sisters. *Br J Dermatol* 75:225, 1963

507. Turnbull A, Baker H, Vernon-Roberts B, Magnus IA: Iron metabolism in porphyria cutanea tarda and in erythropoietic protoporphyria. *Q J Med* 42:341, 1973

508. Mathews-Roth MM: Anemia in erythropoietic protoporphyria. *JAMA* 230:824, 1974

509. Porter FS, Lowe BA: Congenital erythropoietic protoporphyria. I. Case reports, clinical studies and porphyrin analyses in two brothers. *Blood* 22:521, 1963

510. Piomelli S, Lamola AA, Poh-Fitzpatrick MB, Seaman C, Harber LC: Erythropoietic protoporphyria and Pb intoxication: The molecular basis for difference in cutaneous photosensitivity. I. Different rates of disappearance of protoporphyrin from the erythrocytes, both *in vivo* and *in vitro*. *J Clin Invest* 56:1519, 1975

511. Klatskin G, Bloomer JR: Birefringence of hepatic pigment deposits in erythropoietic protoporphyria. *Gastroenterology* 67:294, 1974

512. Bloomer JR: Pathogenesis and therapy of liver disease in protoporphyria. *Yale J Biol Med* 52:39, 1979

513. Singer JA, Plaut AG, Kaplan MM: Hepatic failure and death from erythropoietic protoporphyria. *Gastroenterology* 74:588, 1978

514. Thompson RPH, Molland EA, Nicholson DC, Gray CH: 'Erythropoietic' protoporphyria and cirrhosis in sisters. *Gut* 14:934, 1973

515. Romslo I, Hovding G, Hamre E, Laerum OD: Porphyrin production and liver involvement in a patient with erythropoietic protoporphyria. *Scand J Clin Lab Invest* 38:529, 1978

516. Wolff K, Wolff-Schreiner E, Gschnait F: Liver inclusions in erythropoietic protoporphyria. *Eur J Clin Invest* 5:21, 1975

517. Avner DL, Lee RG, Berenson MM: Protoporphyrin-induced cholestasis in the isolated *in situ* perfused rat liver. *J Clin Invest* 67:385, 1981

518. Ibrahim GW, Watson CJ: Enterohepatic circulation and conversion of protoporphyrin to bile pigment in man. *Proc Soc Exp Bio Med* 127:890, 1968

519. Bloomer JR, Phillips MJ, Davidson DL, Klatskin G: Hepatic disease in erythropoietic protoporphyria. *Am J Med* 58:869, 1975

520. Pimstone NR, Webber BL, Blekkenhorst GH, Eales L: The hepatic lesion in protoporphyria: Preliminary studies of haem metabolism, liver structure and ultrastructure. *Ann Clin Res* 8 (Suppl 17):122, 1976

521. Scott AJ, Ansford AJ, Webster BH, Stringer HCW: Erythropoietic protoporphyria with features of a sideroblastic anemia terminating in liver failure. *Am J Med* 54:251, 1973

522. Cripps DJ, Scheuer PJ: Hepatobiliary changes in erythropoietic protoporphyria. *Arch Pathol Lab Med* 80:500, 1965

523. Gog, Wiersema-Van H, De Wilde-Verburg MW, Suurmond D: Determination of protoporphyrin in plasma and suction-blister fluid from light-irradiated and non-irradiated skin in protoporphyria patients. *Dermatologica* 151:9, 1975

524. Brodie MJ, Moore MR, Thompson GG, Goldberg A, Holti G: Haem biosynthesis in peripheral blood in erythropoietic protoporphyria. *Clin Exp Dermatol* 2:381, 1978

525. Lamon JM, Poh-Fitzpatrick MB, Lamola AA: Hepatic protoporphyrin production in human protoporphyria: Effects of intravenous hematin and analysis of erythrocyte protoporphyrin distribution. *Gastroenterology* 79:115, 1980

526. Del C Rios De Molina M, De Calmanovici W, Grinstein M, San Martin De Viale: Erythrocyte porphyrinogen carboxy-lyase activity in porphyria cutanea tarda and certain other human porphyrias. *Clin Chim Acta* 108:447, 1980

527. Muller-Eberhard U, Liem HH, Mathews-Roth M, Epstein JH: Plasma levels of hemopexin and albumin in disorders of porphyrin metabolism. *Proc Soc Exp Biol Med* 146:694, 1974

528. Wochner RD, Spilberg I, Iio A, Liem HH, Muller-Eberhard U: Hemopexin metabolism in sickle-cell disease, porphyrias, and control subjects: Effects of heme injection. *N Engl J Med* 290:822, 1974

529. Cripps DJ, MacEachern WN: Hepatic and erythropoietic protoporphyria: δ-Aminolevulinic acid synthetase, fluorescence, and microfluorospectrophotometric study. *Arch Pathol* 91:497, 1971

530. Porter S: Congenital erythropoietic porphyria. II. An experimental study. *Blood* 22:532, 1963

531. Lamola AA, Piomelli S, Poh-Fitzpatrick MB, Yamane T, Harber LC: Erythropoietic protoporphyria and lead intoxication: The molecular basis for difference in cutaneous photosensitivity. II. Different binding of erythrocyte protoporphyrin to hemoglobin. *J Clin Invest* 56:1528, 1975

532. Poh-Fitzpatrick MB, Lamola AA: Comparative study of protoporphyrins in erythropoietic protoporphyria and griseofulvin-induced murine protoporphyria. *J Clin Invest* 60:380, 1977

533. Van Steveninck J, Dubbelman TMAR, De Goeij AFPM, Went LN.: Binding of protoporphyrin to hemoglobin in red blood cells of patients with erythropoietic protoporphyria. *Hemoglobin* 1:679, 1977

534. Redeker AG, Sterling RE: The "glucose-effect" in erythropoietic protoporphyria. *Arch Inten Med* 121:446, 1968

535. Miyagi K: The liver ALA-synthetase activity in erythropoietic protoporphyria by means of the new micromethod. *J Kyushu Hematol Soc* 17:397, 1967

536. Nakao K, Wada O, Takaku F, Sassa S, Yano Y, Urata G: The origin of the increased protoporphyrin in erythrocytes of mice with experimentally induced porphyria. *J Lab Clin Med* 70:923, 1967

537. De Goeij AFPM, Christianse K, Van Steveninck J: Decreased haem synthetase activity in blood cells of patients with erythropoietic protoporphyria. *Eur J Clin Invest* 5:397, 1975

538. SASSA S, ZALAR GL, POH-FITZPATRICK MB, KAPPAS A: Studies in porphyria IX: Detection of the gene defect of erythropoietic protoporphyria in mitogen-stimulated human lymphocytes. *Trans Assoc Am Physicians* 92:268, 1979

539. HAEGER-ARONSEN B: Erythropoietic protoporphyria. A new type of inborn error of metabolism. *Am J Med* 35:450, 1963

540. DONALDSON EM, DONALDSON AD, RIMINGTON C: Erythropoietic protoporphyria: A family study. *Br Med J* 1:659, 1967

541. REED WB, WUEPPER KD, EPSTEIN JH, REDEKER A, SIMONSON RJ, MCKUSICK VA: Erythropoietic protoporphyria: A clinical and genetic study. *JAMA* 214:1060, 1970

542. NAYLOR EW, MURPHEY WH, DOMOSZLAI EI, GUTHRIE R: Erythropoietic protoporphyria, heterozygous cystinuria, and reduced peptidase A activity in a patient with 46,XX/46,XX,18q—mosaicism. *J Med Genet* 15:157, 1978

543. CHAPEL TA, STEWART RH, WEBSTER SB: Erythropoietic protoporphyria. Report of a case successfully treated with carotene. *Arch Dermatol* 105:572, 1972

544. SASSA S, SCHWARTZ S, RUTH G: Accumulation of protoporphyrin IX from δ- aminolevulinic acid in bovine skin fibroblasts with hereditary erythropoietic protoporphyria. A gene dosage effect. *J Exp Med* 153:1094, 1981

545. BLOOMER JR: Characterization of deficient heme synthase activity in protoporphyria with cultured skin fibroblasts. *J Clin Invest* 65:321, 1980

546. KRAMER S, VILJOEN JD: Erythropoietic protoporphyria: Evidence that it is due to a variant ferrochelatase. *Int J Biochem* 12:925, 1980

547. BRUN A, SANDBERG S, HØVDING G, BJORDAL M, ROMSLO I: Zinc as an oral photoprotective agent in erythropoietic protoporphyria? *Int J Biochem* 12:931, 1980

548. SASSA S, ZALAR GL, POH-FITZPATRICK MB, ANDERSON KE, KAPPAS A: Studies in porphyria X: Functional evidence for a partial deficiency of ferrochelatase activity in mitogen-stimulated lymphocytes from patients with erythropoietic protoporphyria. *J Clin Invest*, in press

549. KUSHNER JP, CARTWRIGHT GE: Sideroblastic anemia. *Adv Intern Med* 22:229, 1977

550. BOTTOMLEY SS: Porphyrin and iron metabolism in sideroblastic anemia. *Semin Hematol* 14:169, 1977

551. LUZZATTO L, USANGA EA, BIENZLE U, ESAN GFJ, FASUAN FA: Imbalance in X-chromosome expression: Evidence for a human X-linked gene affecting growth of hemopoietic cells. *Science* 205:1418, 1979

552. CRIPPS DJ, GOLDFARB SS: Erythropoietic protoporphyria: Hepatic cirrhosis. *Br J Dermatol* 98:349, 1978

553. SCHWARTZ S, RAUX WA, SCHACTER BA, STEPHENSON BD, SHOFFNER RN: Loss of hereditary uterine protoporphyria through chromosomal rearrangement in mutant Rhode Island red hens. *Int J Biochem* 12:935, 1980

554. TAKAKU F, YANO Y, AOKI Y, NAKAO K, WADA O: δ-Aminolevulinic acid synthetase activity of human bone marrow erythroid cells in various hematological disorders. *Tohoku J Exp Med* 107:217, 1972

555. MATHEWS-ROTH MM, PATHAK MA, FITZPATRICK TB, HARBER LC, KASS EH: Beta-carotene as a photoprotective agent in erythropoietic protoporphyria. *N Engl J Med* 282:1231, 1970

556. MATHEWS MM, SISTROM WR: The function of the carotenoid pigments of sarcina lutea. *Arch Microbiol* 35:139, 1960

557. MATHEWS MM: Protective effect of β-carotene against lethal photosensitization by haematoporphyrin. *Nature* 203: 1092, 1964

558. FRITSCH P, GSCHNAIT F, HÖNIGSMANN H, WOLFF K: Protective action of beta-carotene against lethal photosensitization of fibroblasts *in vitro*. *Br J Dermatol* 94:263, 1976

559. MATHEWS-ROTH MM, PATHAK MA, FITZPATRICK TB, HARBER LC, KASS EH: β-Carotene as an oral photoprotective agent in erythropoietic protoporphyria. *JAMA* 228:1004, 1974

560. MATHEWS-ROTH MM, PATHAK MA, FITZPATRICK TB, HARBER LC, KASS EH: Beta carotene therapy for erythropoietic protoporphyria and other photosensitivity diseases. *Arch Dermatol* 113:1229, 1977

561. THOMSEN K, SCHMIDT H, FISCHER A: Beta-carotene in erythropoietic protoporphyria: 5 years' experience. *Dermatologica* 159:82, 1979

562. ZALAR GL, POH-FITZPATRICK M, KROHN DL, JACOBS R, HARBER LC: Induction of drug photosensitization in man after parenteral exposure to hematoporphyrin. *Arch Dermatol* 113:1392, 1977

563. SUURMOND D: Some aspects of erythropoietic protoporphyria in the Netherlands. *Dermatologica* 138:303, 1969

564. FUSARO RM, RUNGE WJ: Erythropoietic protoporphyria. IV. Protection from sunlight. *Br Med J* 1:730, 1970

565. KNIFFEN JC: Protoporphyrin removal in intrahepatic porphyrastasis. *Gastroenterology* 58:1027, 1970

566. LISCHNER HW: Cholestyramine and porphyrin-binding (letter). *Lancet* ii:1079, 1966

567. MUELLER MN, KAPPAS A: Estrogen pharmacology. I. The influence of estradiol and estriol on hepatic disposal of sulfobromophthalein (BSP) in man. *J Clin Invest* 43: 1905, 1964

568. GOLDBERG A, RIMINGTON C: *Diseases of Porphyrin Metabolism*. Springfield, Ill, Charles C Thomas, 1962

569. WETTERBERG L: *A Neuropsychiatric and Genetical Investigation of Acute Intermittent Porphyria*. Svenska Bokfölaget, Norstedts, Scandinavian University Books, 1967

570. ROMEO G: The hepatic porphyrias, in Steinberg AG, Bearn AG, Motulsky AG, Childs B (eds): *Progress in Medical Genetics: Genetics of Gastrointestinal Disease*, vol 4. Philadelphia, Saunders, 1980, p 169

571. KREIMER-BIRNBAUM M, MOSOVICH LL, BANNERMAN RM: Acute intermittent porphyria: A clinical, biochemical and family study. *J Med (Basel)* 2:149, 1971

572. BARCLAY N: Acute intermittent porphyria in childhood. A neglected diagnosis? *Arch Dis Child* 49:404, 1974

573. WHITELAW, AGL: Acute intermittent porphyria, hypercholesterolaemia, and renal impairment. *Arch Dis Child* 49:406, 1974

574. WALDENSTRÖM J: The porphyrias as inborn errors of metabolism. *Am J Med* 22:758, 1957

575. GOLDBERG A: Acute intermittent porphyria: A study of 50 cases. *Q J Med* 28:183, 1959

576. STEIN JA, TSCHUDY DP: Acute intermittent porphyria: A clinical and biochemical study of 46 patients. *Medicine* 49:1, 1970

577. BEATTIE AD, GOLDBERG A: Acute intermittent porphyria: Natural history and prognosis, in Doss M (ed): *Porphyrins and Human Disease*. Basel, Switzerland, S Karger, 1976, p 245

578. WALDENSTRÖM J: Neurological symptoms caused by so-called acute porphyria. *Acta Psychiatr Neurol* 14:375, 1939

579. TSCHUDY DP, VALSAMIS M, MAGNUSSEN CR: Acute intermittent porphyria: Clinical and selected research aspects. *Ann Intern Med* 83:851, 1975

580. RIDLEY A: Porphyric neuropathy, in Dyck PJ, Thomas PK, Lambert EH (eds): *Peripheral Neuropathy*, vol 2. Philadelphia, Saunders 1975, p 942

581. DE FRANCISCO M, SAVINO PJ, SCHATZ NJ: Optic atrophy in acute intermittent porphyria. *Am J Opthalmol* 87:221, 1979

582. LAI CW, HUNG T, LIN WSJ: Blindness of cerebral origin in acute intermittent porphyria. *Arch Neurol* 34:310, 1977

583. KAELBLING R, CRAIG JB, PASAMANICK B: Urinary porphobilinogen: Results of screening 2500 psychiatric patients. *Arch Gen Psychiatry* 5:494, 1961

584. SCHUMAKER HM, TISHLER PV, KNIGHTON DJ: A spot test for uroporphyrinogen I synthase, the enzyme that is deficient in intermittent acute porphyria. *Clin Chem* 22:1991, 1976

585. MAGNUSSEN CR, DOHERTY JM, HESS RA, TSCHUDY DP: Grand mal seizures and acute intermittent porphyria: The problem of differential diagnosis and treatment. *Neurology (Minneap)* 25:1121, 1975

586. BIAGINI R, TIGNANI R, FIFI M, NAPPINI L: Acute intermittent porphyria and epilepsy. *Arch Dis Child* 54:644, 1979

587. BONKOWSKY HL, SINCLAIR PR, EMERY S, SINCLAIR JF: Seizure management in acute hepatic porphyria: Risks of valproate and clonazepam. *Neurology (Minneap)* 30:588, 1980

588. NIELSEN B, THORN NA: Transient excess urinary excretion of antidiuretic material in acute intermittent porphyria with hyponatremia and hypomagnesemia. *Am J Med* 38: 345, 1965

589. PERLROTH MG, TSCHUDY DP, MARVER HS, BERARD CW, ZEIGEL RF, RECHCIGL M, COLLINS A: Acute intermittent porphyria: New morphologic and biochemical findings. *Am J Med* 41:149, 1966

590. BLOOMER JR, BERK PD, BONKOWSKY HL, STEIN JA, BERLIN NI, TSCHUDY DP: Blood volume and bilirubin production in acute intermittent porphyria. *N Engl J Med* 284:17, 1971

591. STEIN JA, CURL FD, VALSAMIS M, TSCHUDY DP: Abnormal iron and water metabolism in acute intermittent porphyria with new morphologic findings. *Am J Med* 53:784, 1972

592. EALES L, DOWDLE EB, SWEENEY GD: The electrolyte disorder of the acute porphyric attack and the possible role of delta-amino-laevulinic acid. *S Afr J Lab Clin Med* 17 (special issue):89, 1971

593. EALES L, DAY RS, BLEKKENHORST GH: The clinical and biochemical features of variegate porphyria: An analysis of 300 cases studied at Groote Schuur Hospital, Capt Town. *Int J Biochem* 12:837, 1980

594. BAROIS A, GAJDOS P, LIENHART A, GOULON M: Hypercalcémie au cours de la porphyrie aiguë intermittente: A propos de 3 observations. *Sem Hôp Paris* 53:1115, 1977

595. SØRENSEN AWS, WITH TK: Persistent paresis after porphyric attacks. *S Afr J Lab Clin Med* 17 (special issue): 101, 1971

596. BECKER DM, KRAMER S: The neurological manifestations of porphyria: A review. *Medicine* 56:411, 1977

597. ANZIL AP, DOZIC S: Peripheral nerve changes in porphyric neuropathy: Findings in a sural nerve biopsy. *Acta Neuropathol* 42:121, 1978

598. GIBSON JB, GOLDBERG A: The neuropathology of acute porphyria. *J Pathol* 71:495, 1956

599. CAVANAGH JB, MELLICK RS: On the nature of the peripheral nerve lesions associated with acute intermittent porphyria. *J Neurol Neurosurg Psychiatry* 28:320, 1965

600. SWEENEY VP, PATHAK MA, ASBURY AK: Acute intermittent porphyria: Increased ALA-synthetase activity during an acute attack. *Brain* 93:369, 1970

601. WOCHNIK-DYJAS D, NIEWIADOMSKA M, KOSTRZEWSKA E: Porphyric polyneuropathy and its pathogenesis in the light of electrophysiological investigations. *J Neurol Sci* 35: 243, 1978

602. ALBERS JW, ROBERTSON WC, DAUBE JR: Electrodiagnostic findings in acute porphyric neuropathy. *Muscle and Nerve* 1:292, 1978

603. FLÜGEL KA, DRUSCHKY KF: Electromyogram and nerve conduction in patients with acute intermittent porphyria. *J Neurol* 214:267, 1977

604. MUSTAJOKI P, SEPPÄLÄINEN AM: Neuropathy in latent hereditary hepatic porphyria. *Br Med J* 2:310, 1975

605. FELDMAN DS, LEVERE RD, LIEBERMAN JS, CARDINAL RA, WATSON CJ: Presynaptic neuromuscular inhibition by porphobilinogen and porphobilin. *Proc Natl Acad Sci USA* 68:383, 1971

606. HUBBARD JI, QUASTEL DMJ: Micropharmacology of vertebrate neuromuscular transmission. *Annu Rev Pharmacol Toxicol* 13:199, 1973

607. SHANLEY BC, PERCY VA, NEETHLING AC: Pathogenesis of neural manifestations in acute porphyria. *S Afr Med J* 51:458, 1977

608. MAINES MD: Regional distribution of the enzymes of haem biosynthesis and the inhibition of 5-aminolaevulinate synthase by manganese in the rat brain. *Biochem J* 190:315, 1980

609. OMIECINSKI CJ, NAMKUNG MJ, JUCHAU MR: Mechanistic aspects of the hematin-mediated increases in brain monooxygenase activities. *Mol Pharmacol* 17:225, 1980

609a. DE MATTEIS F, ZETTERLUND P, WETTERBERG L: Brain 5-aminolaevulinate synthase. Developmental aspects and evidence for regulatory role. *Biochem J* 196:811, 1981

610. SHANLEY BC, NEETHLING AC, PERCY VA, CARSTENS M: Neurochemical aspects of porphyria: Studies on the possible neurotoxicity of delta-aminolaevulinic acid. *S Afr J Lab Clin Med* 49:576, 1975

611. MCGILLION FB, MOORE MR, GOLDBERG A: The effect of δ-aminolaevulic acid on the spontaneous activity of mice. *Scott Med J* 18:133, 1973

612. MCGILLION FB, THOMPSON GG, MOORE MR, GOLDBERG A: The passage of δ-aminolaevulinic acid across the blood-brain barrier of the rat: Effect of ethanol. *Biochem Pharmacol* 23:472, 1974

613. MCGILLION FB, THOMPSON GG, GOLDBERG A: Tissue uptake of δ-aminolaevulinic acid. *Biochem Pharmacol* 24:299, 1975

614. BECKER DM, KRAMER S, VILJOEN JD: Delta-aminolevulinic acid uptake by rabbit brain cerebral cortex. *J Neurochem* 23:1019, 1974

615. PERCY VA, SHANLEY BC: Porphyrin precursors in blood, urine and cerebrospinal fluid in acute porphyria. *S Afr Med J* 52:219, 1977

616. PERCY VA, SHANLEY BC: Lack of effect of phenobarbitone treatment on metabolism and brain uptake of delta-aminolaevulinic acid in rats. *Biochem Pharmacol* 26:802, 1977

617. GOLDBERG A, PATON WDM, THOMPSON JW: Pharmacology of the porphyrins and porphobilinogen. *Br J Pharmacol* 9:91, 1954.

618. GOLDBERG A: Fate of porphobilinogen, administered enterally or parenterally, in the rat. *Biochem J* 59:37, 1955

619. GRANICK S, VANDEN SCHREIECK HG: Porphobilinogen and δ-aminolevulinic acid in acute porphyria. *Proc Soc Exp Biol Med* 88:270, 1955

620. JARRETT A, RIMINGTON C, WILLOUGHBY DA: δ-Aminolaevulic acid and porphyria. *Lancet* i:125, 1956

621. MARCUS RJ, WETTERBERG L, YUWILER A, WINTERS WD: Electroencephalographic and behavioral effects of experimental porphyria in the rat. *Electroencephalogr Clin Neurophysiol* 29:602, 1970

622. PIERACH CA, GUIDON L, PETRYKA ZJ, BAUR HR, WATSON CJ: Effect and fate of intravenously administered porphobilin in rats. *Experientia* 33:873, 1977.

623. BIEMPICA L, KOSOWER NS, NOVIKOFF AB: Cytochemical and ultrastructural changes in rat liver in experimental porphyria. I. Effects of a single injection of allylisopropylacetamide. *Lab Invest* 17:171, 1967

624. YUWILER A, WETTERBERG L, GELLER E: Tryptophan pyrrolase, tryptophan and tyrosine transaminase changes during allylisopropylacetamide-induced porphyria in the rat. *Biochem Pharmacol* 19:189, 1970

625. KOSOWER NS, ROCK RA: Seizures in experimental porphyria. *Nature* 217:565, 1968

626. MOORE MR, MEREDITH PA: The association of delta-aminolaevulinic acid with the neurological and behavioral effects of lead exposure, in Hemphill DD (ed): *Trace Substances in Environmental Health X. A Symposium*, Columbia, Mo, University of Missouri, 1976, p 363

627. SHANLEY BC, PERCY VA, NEETHLING AC: Neurochemistry of acute porphyria: Experimental studies on δ-aminolaevulinic acid and porphobilinogen, in Doss M (ed): *Porphyrins in Human Disease*. Basel, Switzerland, S Karger, 1976, p 155

628. PIERACH CA, EDWARDS PS: Neurotoxicity of δ-aminolevulinic acid and porphobilinogen. *Exp Neurol* 62:810, 1978

629. SCOTT JJ: The metabolism of δ-aminolaevulinic acid, in Wolstenholme GWE, Miller ECP (eds): *Ciba Foundation Symposium on Porphyrin Biosynthesis and Metabolism*. London, Churchill, 1955, p 55

630. FELDMAN DS, LEVERE RD, LIEBERMAN JS: Presynaptic neuromuscular

inhibition by delta-aminolevulinic acid, a porphyrin precursor. *Trans Am Neurol Assoc* 93:206, 1968

631. BORNSTEIN JC, PICKETT JB, DIAMOND I: Inhibition of the evoked release of acetylcholine by the porphyrin precursor δ-aminolevulinic acid. *Ann Neurol* 5:94, 1979

632. NICOLL RA: The interaction of porphyrin precursors with GABA receptors in the isolated frog spinal cord. *Life Sci* 19:521, 1976

633. MÜLLER WE, SNYDER SH: δ-Aminolevulinic acid: Influences on synaptic GABA receptor binding may explain CNS symptoms of porphyria. *Ann Neurol* 2:340, 1977

634. BRENNAN MJW, CANTRILL RC: δ-Aminolaevulinic acid is a potent agonist for GABA autoreceptors. *Nature* 280:514, 1979

635. BECKER D, VILJOEN D, KRAMER S: The inhibition of red cell and brain ATPase by δ-aminolevulinic acid. *Biochim Biophys Acta* 225:26, 1971

636. ISAACSON LC, DOUGLAS R, EALES L: Inhibition of sodium and water transport by δ-aminolevulinic acid. *S Afr J Lab Clin Med* 17:97, 1971

637. EALES L, DOUGLAS R, ISAACSON LC: The effects of △-aminolaevulinic acid on sodium and water movement across frog skin. *Experientia* 27:276, 1971

638. BECKER DM, GOLDSTUCK N, KRAMER S: Effect of delta-aminolevulinic acid on the resting membrane potentiál of frog sartorius muscle. *S Afr J Lab Clin Med* 49:1790, 1975

639. CUTLER MG, DICK JM, MOORE MR: Effect of delta-aminolevulinic acid on frog nerve-muscle function. *Life Sci* 23:2233, 1978

640. LOOTS JM, BECKER DM, MEYER BJ, GOLDSTUCK N, KRAMER S: The effect of porphyrin precursors on monosynaptic reflex activity in the isolated hemisected frog spinal cord. *J Neural Transmission* 36:71, 1975

641. CUTLER MG, MOORE MR, DICK JM: Effects of δ-aminolaevulinic acid on contractile activity of rabbit duodenum. *Eur J Pharmacol* 64:221, 1980

642. BRENNAN MJW, CANTRILL RC: The effect of delta-aminolaevulinic acid on the uptake of efflux of [³H]GABA in rat brain synaptosomes. *J Neurochem* 32:1781, 1979

643. BRENNAN MJW, CANTRILL RC, KRAMER S: Effect of δ-aminolaevulinic acid on GABA receptor binding in synaptic plasma membranes. *Int J Biochem* 12:833, 1980

644. IRVINE DG, BAYNE W, MIYASHITA H: Identification of kryptopyrrole in human urine and its relation to psychosis. *Nature* 224:811, 1969

645. IRVINE DG: Pyrroles in neuropsychiatric and porphyric disorders: Confirmation of a metabolite structure by synthesis. *Life Sci* 23:983, 1978

646. MOORE MR, GRAHAM DJM: Monopyrroles in porphyria, psychosis and lead exposure. *Int J Biochem* 12:827, 1980

647. GRAHAM DJM, THOMPSON GG, MOORE MR, GOLDBERG A: The effects of selected monopyrroles on various aspects of heme biosynthesis and degradation in the rat. *Arch Biochem Biophys* 197:132, 1979

648. GORCHEIN A: Urine concentration of 3-ethyl-5-hydroxy-4,5-dimethyl-△³-pyrrolin-2-one ('mauve factor') is not causally related to schizophrenia or to acute intermittent porphyria. *Clin Sci* 58:469, 1980

649. SEARS WG, EALES L: Urinary dipyrrylmethenes in patients with porphyria: A preliminary study of the brown pigments in the urine of a case of acute intermittent porphyria. *Enzyme* 17:11, 1974

650. SCHLEY G, BOCK KD, HOCEVAR V, MERGUET P, SCHRÖDER JGRS, SCHÜMAN HJ: Hochdruch und Tachykardie bei der akuten inter-mittierenden Porphyrie. *Klin Wochenschr* 36, 1970

651. BEAL MF, ATUK NO, WESTFALL TC, TURNER SM: Catecholamine uptake, accumulation, and release in acute porphyria. *J Clin Invest* 60:1141, 1977

652. KEZDI P: Neurogenic hypertension in man in porphyria. Transient hypertension and tachycardia caused by disruption of the carotid sinus. Review of buffer nerve mechanism. *Arch Intern Med* 94:122, 1954

653. HELD H, PRZERWA M: Effect of the female sexual cycle on the activity of δ-aminolaevulinate synthase in rat liver. *Eur J Clin Invest* 6:411, 1976

654. MERCKE C, LUNDH B: Erythrocyte filterability and heme catabolism during the menstrual cycle. *Ann Intern Med* 85:322, 1976

655. DELIVORIA-PAPADOPOULOS M, COBURN RF, FORSTER RE: Cyclic variations of rate of carbon monoxide production in normal women. *J Appl Physiol* 36:49, 1974

656. KAPPAS A, BRADLOW HL: Metabolism of progesterone and etiocholanolone in patients with acute intermittent porphyria, in Doss M (ed): *Porphyrins in Human Disease*. Basel, Switzerland, S Karger, 1976, p 271

657. ANDERSON KE, BRADLOW HL, KAPPAS A: Unpublished observations

658. LEVIT EJ, NODINE JH, PERLOFF WH: Progesterone-induced porphyria. *Am J Med* 22:831, 1957

659. WELLAND FH, HELLMAN ES, COLLINS A, HUNTER GW JR, TSCHUDY DP: Factors affecting the excretion of porphyrin precursors by patients with acute intermittent porphyria. II. The effect of ethynyl estradiol. *Metabolism* 13:251, 1964

660. WATSON CJ, RUNGE W, BOSSENMAIER I: Increased urinary porphobilinogen and uroporphyrin after administration of stilbesterol in a case of latent porphyria. *Metabolism* 11:1129, 1962

661. ORTIZ DE MONTELLANO PR, KUNZE KL, YOST GS, MICO BA: Self-catalyzed destruction of cytochrome P-450: Covalent binding of ethynyl sterols to prosthetic heme. *Proc Natl Acad Sci* 76:746, 1979

662. KAPPAS A, BRADLOW HL, GILLETTE PN, LEVERE RD, GALLAGHER TF: A defect of steroid hormone metabolism in acute intermittent porphyria. *Fed Proc* 31:1293, 1972

663. KAPPAS A, BRADLOW HL, GILLETTE PN, GALLAGHER TF: Studies in porphyria. I. A defect in the reductive transformation of natural steroid hormones in the hereditary liver disease, acute intermittent porphyria. *J Exp Med* 136:1043, 1972

664. BRADLOW HL, GILLETTE PN, GALLAGHER TF, KAPPAS A: Studies in porphyria. II. Evidence for a deficiency of steroid Δ^4-5α-reductase activity in acute intermittent porphyria. *J Exp Med* 138:754, 1973

665. ANDERSON KE, BRADLOW HL, SASSA S, KAPPAS A: Studies in porphyria. VIII. Relationship of the 5α-reductive metabolism of steroid hormones to clinical expression of the genetic defect in acute intermittent porphyria. *Am J Med* 66:644, 1979

666. BRADLOW HL, ANDERSON KE, KAPPAS A: Differences between cutaneous and hepatic steroid Δ-5α-reductase in patients with acute intermittent porphyria, in Doss M (ed): *Porphyrins in Human Disease*, Basel, S Karger, 1976, p 173

667. PAXTON JW, MOORE MR, BEATTIE AD, GOLDBERG A: 17-Oxosteroid conjugates in plasma and urine of patients with acute intermittent porphyria. *Clin Sci Molec Med* 46:207, 1974

668. KAPPAS A, GALLAGHER TF: Study of the genetic and extragenetic determinants of alpha-ketosteroid production in man. *J Clin Invest* 39:620, 1960

669. BURSTEIN S: Determination of initial rates of cortisol 2α- and 6β-hydroxylation by hepatic microsomal preparations in guinea pigs: Effect of phenobarbital in two genetic types. *Endocrinology* 82:547, 1968

670. EVERSON RB, LI FP, FRAUMENI JF JR: Familial male breast cancer. *Lancet* i:9, 1976

671. PETERSON RE, IMPERATO-MCGINLEY J, GAUTIER T, STURLA E: Male pseudohermaphroditism due to steroid 5α-reductase deficiency. *Am J Med* 62:170, 1977

672. GROSS SR, HUTTON JJ: Induction of hepatic δ-aminolevulinic acid synthetase activity in strains of inbred mice. *J Biol Chem* 246:606, 1971

673. BECKER B, SHIN DH, PALMBERG PF, WALTMAN SR: HLA antigens and corticosteroid response. *Science* 194:1427, 1976

674. ANDERSON KE, KAPPAS A: Unpublished observations

675. PFAFFENBERGER CD, HORNING EC: Additional data supporting sexual differences in human urinary steroid metabolic profiles. *Anal Biochem* 88:689, 1978

676. KAPPAS A, BRADLOW HL, BICKERS DR, ALVARES AP: Induction of a deficiency of steroid Δ^4-5α-reductase activity in liver by a porphyrinogenic drug. *J Clin Invest* 59:159, 1977

677. BRODIE MJ, BEATTIE AD, MOORE MR, GOLDBERG A: Pregnancy and hereditary hepatic porphyria, in Doss M (ed): *Porphyrins in Human Disease*, Basel, S Karger, 1976, p 251

678. PETERS HA, CRIPPS DJ, REESE HH: Porphyria. Theories of etiology and treatment. *Int Rev Neurobiol* 16:301, 1974

679. ANDERSON KE, KAPPAS A: Hormones and liver function, in Schiff L (ed): *Diseases of the Liver*. Philadelphia, Lippincott, 1981, in press

680. LAATIKAINEN T, KARJALAINEN O: Excretion of conjugates of neutral steroids in human bile during late pregnancy. *Acta Endocrinol (Copenh)* 69:775, 1972

681. ALTMAN K, GORDON GG, SOUTHREN AL, VITTEK J, WILKER S: Induction of hepatic testosterone A-ring reductase by medroxyprogesterone acetate. *Endocrinology* 90:1252, 1972

682. SARDANA MK, SASSA S, KAPPAS A: Differential induction responses of δ-aminolevulinate synthase and haem oxygenase during pregnancy. *Biochem J* 198:403, 1981

683. MUSTAJOKI P, HEINONEN J: General anesthesia in "inducible" porphyrias. *Anesthesiology* 53:15, 1980

684. PETERS PG, SHARMA ML, HARDWICKE DM, PIPER WN: Sulfonamide inhibition of rat hepatic uroporphyrinogen I synthetase activity and the biosynthesis of heme. *Arch Biochem Biophys* 201:88, 1980

685. RIFKIND AB: Drug-induced exacerbations of porphyria. *Primary Care* 3:665, 1976

686. EALES L: Porphyria and the dangerous life-threatening drugs. *S Afr Med J* 56:914, 1979

687. TREECE GL, MAGNUSSEN CR, PATTERSON JR, TSHUDY DP: Exacerbation of porphyria during treatment of pulmonary tuberculosis. *Am Rev Respir Dis* 113:233, 1976

688. PARIKH RK, MOORE MR: Effect of certain anaesthetic agents on the activity of rat hepatic δ-aminolaevulinate synthase. *Br J Anaesth* 50:1099, 1978

689. BLEKKENHORST GH, HARRISON GG, COOK ES, EALES L: Screening of certain anaesthetic agents for their ability to elicit acute porphyric phases in susceptible patients. *Br J Anaesth* 52:759, 1980

690. KOSTRZEWSKA E, GREGOR A, LIPINSKA D: Ketamine in acute intermittent porphyria—dangerous or safe? *Anesthesiology* 49:377, 1978

691. SHANLEY BC, ZAIL SS, JOUBERT SM: Effect of ethanol on liver δ-aminolevulinate synthetase activity and urinary porphyrin excretion in symptomatic porphyria. *Br J Haematol* 17:389, 1969

692. BONKOWSKY HL, POMEROY JS: Human hepatic δ-aminolaevulinate synthase: Requirement of an exogenous system for succinyl-coenzyme A generation to demonstrate increased activity in cirrhotic and anticonvulsant-treated subjects. *Clin Sci Mol Med* 52:509, 1977

693. EALES L, BLEKKENHOSRT GH: The use of the rat in the experimental investigation of the porphyrias. *J S Afr Vet Assoc* 49:249, 1978

694. MAXWELL JD, MEYER UA: Effect of lead on hepatic δ-aminolevulinic acid synthetase activity in rats: A model for drug sensitivity in intermittent acute porphyria. *Eur J Clin Invest* 6:373, 1976

695. BONKOWSKY HL, MAGNUSSEN CR, COLLINS AR, DOHERTY JM, HESS RA, TSCHUDY DP: Comparative effects of glycerol and dextrose on porphyrin precursor excretions in acute intermittent porphyria. *Metabolism* 25:405, 1976

696. ROSE JA, HELLMAN ES, TSCHUDY DP: Effect of diet on the induction of experimental porphyria. *Metabolism* 10:514, 1961

697. TSCHUDY DP: The influence of hormonal and nutritional factors on the regulation of liver heme biosynthesis, in De Matteis F, Aldridge WN (eds): *Heme and Hemoproteins*. Berlin, Springer-Verlag, 1978, p 255

698. BONKOWSKY HL, COLLINS A, DOHERTY JM, TSCHUDY DP: The glucose effect in rat liver: Studies of δ-aminolevulinate synthetase and tyrosine aminotransferase. *Biochim Biophys Acta* 320:561, 1973

699. BIEMPICA L, KOSOWER N, MA MH, GOLDFISCHER S: Hepatic porphyrias: Cytochemical and ultrastructural studies of liver in acute intermittent porphyria and porphyria cutanea tarda. *Arch Pathol* 98:336, 1974

700. BRADLOW HL, KAPPAS A: Alterations in cortisol metabolism in patients with acute intermittent porphyria, in Doss M (ed): *Porphyrins in Human Disease*. Basel, S Karger, 1976, p 266

701. STEIN JA, BLOOMER JR, BERK PD, CORCORAN PL, TSCHUDY DP: The kinetics of organic anion excretion by the liver in acute intermittent porphyria. *Clin Sci* 38:677, 1970

702. EDWARDS PM, FRANCIS JE, DE MATTEIS F: The glutathione-linked metabolism of 2-allyl-2-isopropylacetamide in rats: Further evidence for the formation of a reactive metabolite. *Chem Biol Interact* 23:233, 1978

703. MAINES MD: Effect of allylisopropylacetamide on glutathione metabolism in the rat liver. *Biochem J* 196:285, 1981

704. KOBZA K, GYR K, NEUHAUS K, GUDAT F: Acute intermittent porphyria with relapsing acute pancreatitis and unconjugated hyperbilirubinemia without overt hemolysis. *Gastroenterology* 71:494, 1976

705. JONES EA, BLOOMER JR, BERLIN NI: The measurement of the synthetic rate of bilirubin from hepatic hemes in patients with acute intermittent porphyria. *J Clin Invest* 50:2259, 1971

706. TADDEINI L, NORDSTROM KL, WATSON CJ: Hypercholesterolemia in experimental and human hepatic porphyria. *Metabolism* 13:691, 1964

707. LEES RS, SONG CS, LEVERE RD, KAPPAS A: Hyper β-lipoproteinemia in acute intermittent porphyria: Preliminary report. *N Engl J Med* 282:432, 1970

708. GOLDBERG A, RIMINGTON C, FENTON JCB: Experimentally produced porphyria in animals. *Proc R Soc London [Biol]* 143:257, 1955

709. PINELLI A, FAVALLI L, FORMENTO M: Antiporphyric activity of 3,5-dimethylpyrazole in allylisopropylacetamide-treated rats. *Life Sci* 12:117, 1973

710. PAZDEROVA-VEJLUPKOVÁ J, NĚMCOVA M, PÍCKOVÁ J, JIRÁSEK L, LUKÁŠ E: The development and prognosis of chronic intoxication by tetrachlorodibenzo-p-dioxin in men. *Arch Environ Health* 36:5, 1981

711. HAUST HL, HEAGY FC: Abnormal perchlorate-induced radio-iodide loss from the thyriod gland in porphyrinopathies. *Int J Biochem* 12:981, 1980

712. WAXMAN AD, SCHALCH DS, ODELL WD, TSCHUDY DP: Abnormalities of carbohydrate metabolism in acute intermittent porphyria. *J Clin Invest* 46:1129, 1967

713. PERLROTH MG, TSCHUDY DP, WAXMAN A, ODELL WD: Abnormalities of growth hormone regulation in acute intermittent porphyria. *Metabolism* 16:87, 1967

714. HELLMAN ES, TSCHUDY DP, ROBBINS J, RALL JE: Elevation of the serum protein-bound iodine in acute intermittent porphyria. *J Clin Endocrinol Metab* 23:1185, 1963

715. HOLLANDER CS, SCOTT RL, TSCHUDY DP, PERLROTH M, WAXMAN A, STERLING K: Increased protein-bound iodine and thyroxine-binding globulin in acute intermittent porphyria. *N Engl J Med* 277:995, 1967

716. MANN JG, DE NARDO GL: Acute intermittent porphyria associated with hyperthyroidism. *J Clin Endocrinol Metab* 25:1151, 1965

717. BRODIE MJ, GRAHAM DJM, GOLDBERG A, BEASTALL GH, RATCLIFFE WA, RATCLIFFE JG, YEO PPB: Thyroid function in acute intermittent porphyria: A neurogenic cause of hyperthyroidism? *Horm Metab Res* 10:327, 1978

718. WAXMAN AD, BERK PD, SCHALCH D, TSCHUDY DP: Isolated adrenocorticotrophic hormone deficiency in acute intermittent porphyria. *Ann Intern Med* 70:317, 1969

719. BASILIERE J, NEWCOMER AD: Primary aldosteronism associated with acute intermittent porphyria: Report of a case. *N Engl J Med* 285:595, 1971

720. HARRIS MY, MILLS GC, LEVIN WC: Coexistent systemic lupus erythematosus and porphyria. *Arch Intern Med* 117:425, 1966

721. HEDGER RW, HARDISON WGM: Transient macroamylasemia during an exacerbation of acute intermittent porphyria. *Gastroenterology* 60:903, 1971

722. ACKNER B, COOPER JE, GRAY CH, KELLY M, NICHOLSON DC: Excretion of porphobilinogen and δ-aminolaevulinic acid in acute porphyria. *Lancet* i:1256, 1961

723. DOSS M, SCHERMULY E: Urinary porphyrin excretion pattern and isomer distribution of I and III in human porphyrin disorders, in Doss M (ed): *Porphyrins and Human Disease*. Basel, S Karger, 1976, p 189

724. GILBERTSEN AS, LOWRY PT, HAWKINSON V, WATSON CJ: Studies of the dipyrrylmethene ("fuscin") pigments. I. The anabolic significance of the fecal mesobilifuscin. *J Clin Invest* 38:1166, 1959

725. WETTERBERG L, HAEGER-ARONSEN B, STATHERS G: Faecal porphyrins as a diagnostic index between acute intermittent porphyria and porphyria variegata. *Scand J Clin Lab Invest* 22:131, 1968

726. REIO L, WETTERBERG L: False porphobilinogen reactions in the urine of mental patients. *JAMA* 207:148, 1969

727. WATSON CJ, SCHWARTZ S: A simple test for urinary porphobilinogen. *Proc Soc Exp Biol Med* 47:393, 1941

728. WATSON CJ, TADDEINI L, BOSSENMAIER I: Present status of the Ehrlich aldehyde reaction for urinary porphobilinogen. *JAMA* 190:501, 1964

729. LAMON J, WITH TK, REDEKER AG: The Hoesch test: Bedside screening for urinary porphobilinogen in patients with suspected porphyria. *Clin Chem* 11:1438, 1974

730. LAMON JM, FRYKHOLM BC, TSCHUDY DP: Screening tests in acute porphyria. *Arch Neurol* 34:709, 1977

731. PIERACH CA, CARDINAL R, BOSSENMAIER I, WATSON CJ: Comparison of the Hoesch and the Watson-Schwartz tests for urinary porphobilonogen. *Clin Chem* 23:1666, 1977

732. SASSA S, GRANICK S, KAPPAS A: Effect of lead and genetic factors on heme biosynthesis in the human red cell. *Ann NY Acad Sci* 244:419, 1975

733. ANDERSON PM, REDDY RM, ANDERSON KE, DESNICK RJ: Characterization of the PBG-deaminase deficiency in acute intermittent porphyria. I. Immunologic evidence for heterogeneity of the genetic defect. *J Clin Invest* 68:1, 1981

734. TONGIO MM, MAYER S, HAUPTMANN G, NORTH ML, KOEHL C, ABECASSIS J, MANDEL P, WERTENSCHLAG J: Lack of linkage between acute intermittent porphyria and the A and B loci of the HLA system. *Tissue Antigens* 13:273, 1979

735. DEAN KS, CONNEALLY PM, SASSA S, ANDERSON KE: Absence of close linkage between acute intermittent porphyria and the ABO, Rh, P, acid phosphatase, Pr, orosomucoid and pepsinogen loci. *Hum Genet* 1982, in press

736. TSCHUDY DP, PERLROTH MG, MARVER HS, COLLINS A, HUNTER G JR, RECHCIGL M JR: Acute intermittent porphyria: The first "overproduction disease" localized to a specific enzyme. *Proc Natl Acad Sci USA* 53:841, 1965

737. NAKAO K, WADA O, KITAMURA T, UONO K: Activity of aminolaevulinic acid synthetase in normal and porphyric human livers. *Nature* 210:838, 1966

738. DOWDLE EB, MUSTARD P, EALES L: δ-Aminolevulinic acid synthetase activity in normal and porphyric human livers. *S Afr Med J* 41:1093, 1967

739. DOWDLE E, MUSTARD P, SPONG N, EALES L: The metabolism of [5-14C]δ-aminolevulinic acid in normal and porphyric human subjects. *Clin Sci* 34:233, 1968

740. ANDERSON KE, ALVAREZ AP, SASSA S, KAPPAS A: Studies in porphyria V: Drug oxidation rates in hereditary hepatic porphyria. *Clin Pharmacol Ther* 19:47, 1976

741. BRENNER DA, BLOOMER JR: Heme content of normal and porphyric cultured skin fibroblasts. *Biochem Genet* 15:1061, 1977

742. SONG CS, BONKOWSKY HL, TSCHUDY DP: Salicylamide metabolism in acute intermittent porphyria. *Clin Pharmacol Ther* 15:431, 1974

743. ANDERSON KE, CONNEY AH, KAPPAS A: Nutrition and oxidative drug metabolism in man: Relative influence of dietary lipids, carbohydrate, and protein. *Clin Pharmacol Ther* 26:493, 1979

744. PIPER WN, VAN LIER RBL, HARDWICKE DM: Pteridine regulation of uroporphyrinogen I synthetase activity, in Kisliuk, Brown (eds): *Chemistry and Biology of Pteridines*. Amsterdam, Elsevier North Holland, 1979, p 329

745. SCHWARTZ S, EDMONDSON P, STEPHENSON B, SARKAR D, FREYHOLTZ H: Direct spectrofluorometric determination of porphyrin in diluted urine. *Ann Clin Res* 8:156, 1976

746. RIMINGTON C: Investigation of porphyria: Qualitative tests. *Assoc Clin Pathol Broadsheet* No. 20, November 1958

747. BLUM M, KOEHL C, ABECASSIS J: Variations in erythrocyte uroporphyrinogen I synthetase activity in non porphyrias. *Clin Chim Acta* 87:119, 1978

748. ANDRIOLO A, MOCELIN AJ, STELLA SR, AJZEN H, RAMOS OL: Determination of erythrocyte uroporphyrinogen I synthetase activity in chronic renal failure. *Clin Chim Acta* 104:241, 1980

749. O'FLAHERTY EJ, HAMMOND PB, LERNER SI, HANENSON IB, RODA SMB: The renal handling of δ-aminolevulinic acid in rat and in the human. *Toxicol Appl Pharmacol* 55:423, 1980

750. MACGEE J, RODA SMB, ELIAS SV, LINGTON A, TABOR MW, HAMMOND PB: Determination of δ-aminolevulinic acid in blood plasma and urine by gas-liquid chromatography. *Biochem Med* 17:31, 1977

751. LAMON JM, FRYKHOLM BC, TSCHUDY DP: Family evaluations in acute intermittent porphyria using red cell uroporphyrinogen I synthetase. *J Med Genet* 16:134, 1979

752. ASTRUP EG: Family studies on the activity of uroporphyrinogen I synthase in diagnosis of acute intermittent porphyria. *Clin Sci Mol Med* 54:251, 1978

753. NORDMANN Y, GRANDCHAMP B, GRELIER M, PHUNG NG, DE VERNEUIL H: Detection of intermittent acute porphyria trait in children. *Lancet* ii:201, 1976

754. RICHARDS FF, SCOTT JJ: Glycine metabolism in acute porphyria. *Clin Sci* 20:387, 1961

755. BRODIE MJ, MOORE MR, THOMPSON GG, GOLDBERG A: The treatment of acute intermittent porphyria with laevulose. *Clin Sci Mol Med* 53:365, 1977

756. DHAR GJ, BOSSENMAIER I, PETRYKA ZJ, CARDINAL R, WATSON CJ: Effects of hematin in hepatic porphyria: Further studies. *Ann Intern Med* 83:20, 1975

757. PETERSON A, BOSSENMAIER I, CARDINAL R, WATSON CJ: Hematin treatment of acute porphyria: Early remission of an almost fatal relapse. *JAMA* 235:520, 1976

758. LAMON JM, FRYKHOLM BC, BENNETT M, TSCHUDY DP: Prevention of acute porphyric attacks by intravenous haematin. *Lancet* ii:492, 1978

759. LAMON JM, FRYKHOLM BC, HESS RA, TSCHUDY DP: Hematin therapy for acute porphyria. *Medicine* 58:252, 1979

760. PIERACH CA, BOSSENMAIER I, CARDINAL R, WEIMER M, WATSON CJ: Hematin therapy in porphyric attacks. *Klin Wochenschr* 58:829, 1980

761. PETRYKA ZJ, DHAR GJ, BOSSENMAIER I: Hematin clearance in porphyria, in Doss M (ed): *Porphyrins in Human Disease*. Basel, S Karger, 1976, p 259

762. MULLER-EBERHARD U, MORGAN WT: Porphyrin-binding proteins in serum. *Ann NY Acad Sci* 244:624, 1975

763. LIEM HH, SPECTOR JI, CONWAY TP, MORGAN WT, MULLER-EBERHARD U: Effect of hemoglobin and hematin on plasma clearance of hemopexin, photo-inactivated hemopexin and albumin. *Proc Soc Exp Biol Med* 148:519, 1975

764. McCOLL KEL, THOMPSON GT, MOORE MR, GOLDBERG A: Haematin therapy and leucocyte δ-aminolaevulinic-acid-synthase activity in prolonged attack of acute porphyria. *Lancet* i:133, 1979

765. PETRYKA ZJ, PIERACH CA, SMITH A, GOERTZ MN, EDWARDS PS: Biliary excretion of exogenous hematin in rats. *Life Sci* 21:1015, 1977

766. DHAR GJ, BOSSENMAIER I, CARDINAL R, PETRYKA ZJ, WATSON CJ: Transitory renal failure following rapid administration of a relatively large amount of hematin in a patient with acute intermittent porphyria in clinical remission. *Acta Med Scand* 203:437, 1978

767. LAMON JM, FRYKHOLM BC, TSCHUDY DP: Hematin administration to an adult with lead intoxication. *Blood* 53:1007, 1979

768. ANDERSON KE, PETERSON CM, ALVARES AP, KAPPAS A: Oxidative drug metabolism and inducibility by phenobarbital in sickle cell anemia. *Clin Pharmacol Ther* 22:580, 1977

769. PERLROTH MG, MARVER HS, TSCHUDY DP: Oral contraceptive agents and the management of acute intermittent porphyria. *JAMA* 194:1037, 1965

770. SCHLEY G, ANLAUF M, BOCK KD: Orale Kontrazeptiva zur Prophylaxe akuter Schübe der intermittierenden Porphyrie. *Dtsch Med Wschr* 101:1901, 1976

771. ZIMMERMAN TS, McMILLIN JM, WATSON CJ: Onset of manifestations of hepatic porphyria in relation to the influence of female sex hormones. *Arch Intern Med* 118:229, 1966

772. RIFKIND AB, GILLETTE PN, SONG CS, KAPPAS A: Induction of hepatic δ-aminolevulinic acid synthetase by oral contraceptive steroids. *J Clin Endocrinol Metab* 30:330, 1970

773. HUGHES MJ, RIFKIND AB: Danazol, a new steroidal inducer of δ-aminolevulinic acid synthetase. *J Clin Endocrinol Metab* 52:549, 1981

774. LAMON JM, FRYKHOLM BC, HERRERA W, TSCHUDY DP: Danazol administration to females with menses. Associated exacerbations of acute intermittent porphyria. *J Clin Endocrinol Metab* 48:123, 1979

775. ATSMON A, BLUM I, FISCHL J: Treatment of an acute attack of porphyria variegata with propranolol. *S Afr Med J* 46:311, 1972

776. BEATTIE AD, MOORE MR, GOLDBERG A, WARD RL: Acute intermittent porphyria: Response of tachycardia and hypertension to propranolol. *Br Med J* 3:257, 1973

777. BLUM I, ATSMON A: Reduction of porphyrin excretion in porphyria variegata by propranolol: A case report. S Afr Med J 50:898, 1976

778. DOUER D, WEINBERGER A, PINKHAS J, ATSMON A: Treatment of acute intermittent porphyria with large doses of propranolol. JAMA 240:766, 1978

779. BONKOWSKY HL, TSCHUDY DP: Hazard of propranolol in treatment of acute porphyria. Br Med J 4:47, 1974

780. BLUM I, SCHOENFELD N, ATSMON A: The effect of DL-propranolol on δ-aminolevulinic acid synthetase activity and urinary excretion of porphyrins in allylisopropylacetamide-induced experimental porphyria. Biochim Biophys Acta 320:242, 1973

781. SCHOENFELD N, EPSTEIN O, ATSMON A: The effect of beta-adrenergic blocking agents on experimental porphyria induced by 3,5-diethoxycarbonyl-1,4-dihydrocollidine (DDC) in vivo and in vitro. Biochim Biophys Acta 444:286, 1976

782. SCHOENFELD N, EPSTEIN O, ATSMON A: Inhibitory effect of membrane active compounds on the uptake of ^{14}C-α-aminoisobutyric acid (AIB) in cultured chick embryo liver cells. Life Sci 21:329, 1977

783. EASTON JD, SHERMAN DG: Somatic anxiety attacks and propranolol. Arch Neurol 33:689, 1976

784. KAPPAS A, BRADLOW HL: Enhancement of 5α-steroid hormone metabolism in patients with acute intermittent porphyria following treatment with triiodothyronine, in Doss M (ed): Porphyrins in Human Disease. Basel, S Karger, 1976, p 274

785. OLSSON RA, TICKTIN HE: Zinc metabolism in acute intermittent porphyria. J Lab Clin Med 60:48, 1962

786. ROMAN W: Zinc in porphyria. Am J Clin Nutr 22:1290, 1969

787. HAMFELT A, WETTERBERG L: Pyridoxal phosphate in acute intermittent porphyria. Ann NY Acad Sci 166:361, 1969

788. GAJDOS A, GAJDOS-TÖRÖK M: Studies on the porphyrias in France. S Afr J Lab Clin Med 9:295, 1963

789. WATSON CJ, BOSSENMAIER I, CARDINAL R: Lack of significant effect of vitamin E on porphyrin metabolism. Arch Intern Med 131:698, 1973

790. REES HA, GOLDBERG A, COCHRANE, AL, WILLIAMS MJ, DONALD KW: Renal haemodialysis in porphyria. Lancet i:919, 1967

791. HAEGER-ARONSEN B, STATHERS G, SWAHN G: Hereditary coproporphyria. Study of a Swedish family. Ann Intern Med 69:221, 1968

792. BRODIE MJ, THOMPSON GG, MOORE MR, BEATTIE AD, GOLDBERG A: Hereditary coproporphyria. Demonstration of the abnormalities in haem biosynthesis in peripheral blood. Q J Med 46:229, 1977

793. DEAN G, KRAMER S, LAMB P: Coproporphyria. S Afr Med J, 43:138, 1969

794. JAEGER A, TEMPE JD, GEISLER F, NORDMANN Y, MANTZ JM: La coproporphyrie héréditaire. Sept observations. Nouv Presse Med 4:2783, 1975

795. PAXTON JW, MOORE MR, BEATTIE AD, GOLDBERG A: Urinary excretion of 17-oxosteroids in hereditary coproporphyria. Clin Sci Mol Med 49:441, 1975

796. HUNTER JAA, KHAN SA, HOPE E, BEATTIE AD, BEVERIDGE GW, SMITH AWM, GOLDBERG A: Hereditary coproporphyria. Photosensitivity, jaundice and neuropsychiatric manifestations associated with pregnancy. Br J Dermatol 84:301, 1971

797. BERGER H, GOLDBERG A: Hereditary coproporphyria. Br Med J 2:85, 1955

798. CARLSON RE, DOLPHIN D, BERNSTEIN M: Copper coproporphyrin excretion in familial coproporphyria. Clin Chem 24:2009, 1978

799. NORDMANN Y, GRANDCHAMP B: Hereditary coproporphyria: Demonstration of a genetic defect in coproporphyrinogen metabolism. Monogr Hum Genet 10:217, 1978

800. KAUFMAN K, MARVER HS: Biochemical defects in two types of human hepatic porphyria. N Engl J Med 283:954, 1970

801. SASAKI H, KANEKO K, TSUNEYAMA H: Activities of δ-aminolevulinic acid synthetase in the liver and bone marrow of hepatic coproporphyria (hereditary coproporphyria). Acta Med Biol (Niigata) 17:97, 1969

802. MCINTYRE N, PEARSON AJG, ALLAN DJ, CRASKE S, WEST GML, MOORE MR, BEATTIE AD, PAXTON J, GOLDBERG A: Hepatic δ-aminolaevulinic acid synthetase in an attack of hereditary coproporphyria and during remission. Lancet i:560, 1971

803. SMITH SG, EL-FAR MA: The effect of fasting and protein calorie malnutrition on the liver porphyrins. Int J Biochem 12:979, 1980

804. DEAN G: The Porphyrias: A Study of Inheritance and Environment. Great Britain, Pitman Medical, 1963

805. DEAN G: The Porphyrias: A Study of Inheritance and Environment, 2d ed. Great Britain, Pitman Medical, 1971

806. MUSTAJOKI P: Variegate porphyria: Twelve years' experience in Finland. Q J Med 44:191, 1980

807. MACALPINE I, HUNTER R, RIMINGTON C, BROOKE J, GOLDBERG A: Porphyria: A Royal Malady. London, British Medical Association, 1968

808. EARLES L: Porphyria as seen in Cape Town: A survey of 250 patients and some recent studies. S Afr J Lab Clin Med 9:151, 1963

809. MUSTAJOKI P: Variegate porphyria. Ann Intern Med 89:238, 1978

810. BRADLOW HL, KAPPAS A: Metabolism of testosterone in variegate porphyria and porphyria cutanea tarda, in Doss M (ed): Porphyrins in Human Disease. Basel, S Karger, 1976, p 179

811. PERLROTH MG, TSCHUDY DP, RATNER A, SPAUR W, REDEKER A: The effect of diet in variegate porphyria. Metabolism 17:571, 1968

812. TU J-B, BLACKWELL RQ, FENG Y-S: Clinical and biochemical studies of hereditary hepatic porphyria in Chinese subjects in Taiwan. Metabolism 20:629, 1971

813. HUSQUINET H, NOIRFALISE A, PARENT, M-T: Porphyria variegata (Etude d'une grande famille). J Genet Hum 26:367, 1978

814. RIMINGTON C, LOCKWOOD WH, BELCHER RV: The excretion of porphyrin-peptide conjugates in porphyria variegata. Clin Sci 35:211, 1968

815. ELDER GH, MAGNUS IA, HANDA F, DOYLE M: Faecal "X porphyrin" in the hepatic porphyrias. Enzyme 17:219, 1974

816. RIMINGTON C: Patterns of porphyrin excretion and their interpretation. S Afr J Lab Clin Med 9:255, 1963

817. DAY RS, PIMSTONE NR, EALES L: The diagnostic value of blood plasma porphyrin methyl ester profiles produced by quantitative TLC. Int J Biochem 9:897, 1978

818. DAY RS, BLEKKENHORST GH, EALES L: Hepatic porphyrins in variegate porphyria. N Engl J Med 303:1368, 1980

819. PIMSTONE NR, BLEKKENHORST G, EALES L: Enzymatic defects in hepatic porphyria: Preliminary observations in patients with porphyria cutanea tarda and variegate porphyria. Enzyme 16:354, 1973

819a. DEYBACH JC, DE VERNEUIL H, NORDMANN Y: The inherited enzymatic defect in porphyria variegata. Hum Genet 58:425, 1981

820. BRODIE MJ, MOORE MR, GOLDBERG A: Enzyme abnormalities in the porphyrias. Lancet ii:699, 1977

821. JACKSON AH, GAMES DE, COUCH P, JACKSON JR, BELCHER RB, SMITH SG: Conversion of coproporphyrinogen III to protoporphyrin IX. Enzyme 17:81, 1974

822. SMITH SG, JACKSON AH, JACKSON TR: Incubation of double labelled coproporphyrinogen with chicken red cell hemolysates: Chemical and TLC fractionation of extracts. Ann Clin Res 8(Suppl):53, 1976

823. BLEKKENHORST GH, PIMSTONE NR, WEBBER BL, EALES L: Hepatic haem metabolism in porphyria cutanea tarda (PCT): Enzymatic studies and their relation to liver ultrastructure. Ann Clin Res 8:108, 1976

824. WATSON CJ, CARDINAL RA, BOSSENMAIER I, PETRYKA ZJ: Porphyria variegata and porphyria cutanea tarda in siblings: chemical and genetic aspects. Proc Natl Acad Sci USA 72:5126, 1975

825. WATSON CJ, CARDINAL RA, BOSSENMAIER I, PETRYKA ZJ: Porphyria variegata and porphyria cutanea tarda in siblings: Chemical and genetic aspects, addendum. Proc Natl Acad Sci USA 73:1323, 1976

826. BARNES HD: Porphyria in South Africa: The faecal excretion of porphyrin. S Afr Med J 32:680, 1958

827. CRAMERS M, JEPSEN LV: Porphyria variegata: Failure of chloroquin treatment. Acta Derm Venereol (Stockh) 60:89, 1980

828. PERROT H, THIVOLET J, BOUCHERAT M, GERVEZ F: La Porphyrie variegata (à propos de 4 cas). Lyon Medical 235:905, 1976

829. BARNES HD: Porphyria in the Bantu races on the Witwatersrand. S Afr Med J 29:781, 1955

830. MALINA L, CHLUMSKY J, CHLUMSKA A: Porphyria Cutanea Tarda. New Facts on Aetiology, Pathogenesis, Clinical Manifestations and Treatment. Czechoslovakia, Universita Karlova, 1974

831. BEHM AR, UNGER WP: Oral contraceptives and porphyria cutanea tarda. Can Med Assoc J 110:1052, 1974

832. GROSSMAN ME, BICKERS DR, POH-FITZPATRICK MB, DE LEO VA, HARBER LC: Porphyria cutanea tarda: Clinical features and laboratory findings in 40 patients. Am J Med 67:277, 1979

833. CRUCES PRADO MJ, DE SALAMANCA ER, VEREA HERNANDO M, PEÑA PAYERO ML, CATALAN BELTRAN T, ROBLEDO AGUILAR, A: Two cases of infantile and familial porphyria cutanea tarda. Dermatologica 161:205, 1980

834. DAY RS, EALES L, PIMSTONE NR: Familial symptomatic porphyria in South Africa. S Afr Med J 56:909, 1979.

835. FRANKS AG, PULINI M, BICKERS DR, RAYFIELD EJ, HARBER LC: Carbohydrate metabolism in porphyria cutanea tarda. Am J Med Sci 277:163, 1979

836. HETERINGTON GW, JETTON RL, KNOX JM: The association of lupus erythematosus and porphyria. Br J Dermatol 82:118, 1970

837. CRAM DL, EPSTEIN JH, TUFFANELLI DL: Lupus erythematosus and porphyria: Coexistence in seven patients. Arch Dermatol 108:779, 1973

838. GORDON W: The cutaneous lesions of systemic and chronic discoid lupus erythematosus and porphyria symptomatica in the same patient. Br J Dermatol 78:53, 1966

839. HOXTELL E, MANICK KP, FISHER I: Coexistence of discoid lupus erythematosus and porphyria cutanea tarda. Cutis 17:83, 1976

840. EALES L, SEARS WG, KING KB, LEVEY MJ, RIMINGTON C: Symptomatic porphyria in a case of Felty's syndrome. I. Clinical and routine biochemical studies. Clin Chem 18:459, 1972

841. RIMINGTON C, SEARS WG, EALES L: Symptomatic porphyria in a case of Felty's syndrome. II. Biochemical investigations. *Clin Chem* 18:462, 1972

842. POH-FITZPATRICK MB, BELLET N, DE LEO VA, GROSSMAN ME, BICKERS DR: Porphyria cutanea tarda in two patients treated with hemodialysis for chronic renal failure. *N Engl J Med* 299:292, 1978

843. POH-FITZPATRICK MB, MASULLO AS, GROSSMAN ME: Porphyria cutanea tarda associated with chronic renal disease and hemodialysis. *Arch Dermatol* 116:191, 1980

844. GROSSMAN ME, POH-FITZPATRICK MB: Porphyria cutanea tarda: Diagnosis and management. *Med Clin North Am* 64:807, 1980

845. ENERBÄCH L, LUNDVALL O: Properties and distribution of liver fluorescence in porphyria cutanea tarda (PCT). *Virchow Arch (Pathol Anat)* 350:293, 1970

846. CORTÉS JM, OLIVA H, PARADINAS FJ, HERNANDEZ-GUIO C: The pathology of the liver in porphyria cutanea tarda. *Histopathology* 4:471, 1980

847. JAMES KR, CORTES JM, PARADINAS FJ: Demonstration of intracytoplasmic needle-like inclusions in hepatocytes of patients with porphyria cutanea tarda. *J Clin Pathol* 33:899, 1980

848. WALDO ED, TOBIAS H: Needle-like cyotplasmic inclusions in the liver in porphyria cutanea tarda. *Arch Pathol* 96:368, 1973.

849. KORDAC V: Frequency of occurrence of hepatocellular carcinoma in patients with porphyria cutanea tarda in long-term followup. *Neoplasma* 19:135, 1972

850. TIMME AH: The ultrastructure of the liver in human symptomatic porphyria: A preliminary communication. *S Afr J Lab Clin Med* 17 (special issue):58, 1971

851. DE SALAMANCA RE, LADERO JM, CATALAN T, MAS B, RICO R, OLMOS A: Hepatic metabolism of bromosulphthalein in porphyria cutanea tarda. *Int J Biochem* 12:855, 1980

852. UTHEMANN H, KOTITSCHKE R, LISSNER R, GOERZ G: Serologische hepatitis-B-marker bei porphyria cutanea tarda. *Dtsch Med Wochenschr* 105:1718, 1980

853. TURNBULL A: Iron metabolism in the porphyrias (comment). *Br J Dermatol* 84:380, 1971

854. KRAMER S: Iron metabolism in the porphyrias. *S AFr J Lab Clin Med* 9:283, 1963

855. LUNDVALL O, WEINFELD A, LUNDIN P: Iron storage in porphyria cutanea tarda. *Acta Med Scand* 188:37, 1970

856. REIZENSTEIN P, HÖGLUND S, LANDEGRENN J, CARLMARK B, FORSBERG K: Iron metabolism in porphyria cutanea tarda. *Acta Med Scand* 198:95, 1975

857. FRENCH TJ, WEIR H, DOWDLE E: Ferrokinetics in symptomatic porphyria. *S Afr J Lab Clin Med* 17 (special issue):62, 1971

858. BRISSOT P, PHUNG N, AUBREE A, DE VERNEUIL H, SIMON M, NORDMANN Y, BOUREL M: Porphyries et hémochromatose idiopathique: Étude de 32 cas. *Gastroenterol Clin Biol* 2:603, 1978

859. SHANLEY BC, ZAIL SS, JOUBERT SM: Porphyrin metabolism in experimental hepatic siderosis in the rat. *Br J Haematol* 18:79, 1970

860. WATSON CJ: The problem of porphyria: Some facts and questions. *N Engl J Med* 263:1205, 1960

861. VAIL JT: Porphyria cutanea tarda and estrogens. *JAMA* 20:671, 1967

862. ROENIGK HH, GOTTLOB ME: Estrogen-induced porphyria cutanea tarda: Report of three cases. *Arch Dermatol* 102:260, 1970

863. STEIN KM, RAQUE CJ, ZEIGERMAN JH, SHRAGER JD: Porphyria cutanea tarda induced by natural estrogens: A case report. *Obstet Gynecol* 38:755, 1971

864. TAYLOR JS, ROENIGK HH Jr: Estrogen-induced porphyria cutanea tarda symptomatica, in Doss M (ed): *Porphyrins in Human Disease*. Basel, S Karger, 1976, p 328

865. SAEED-UZ-ZAFAR M, GRONEWALD WR, BLUHM GB: Co-existent Klinefelter's syndrome, acquired cutaneous hepatic porphyria and systemic lupus erythematosus. *Henry Ford Hosp Med J* 18:227, 1970

866. STERN R, FISHMAN J, BRUSMAN H, KUNKEL HG: Systemic lupus erythematosus associated with Klinefelter's syndrome. *Arthritis Rheum* 19:18, 1977

867. OCKNER RK, SCHMID R: Acquired porphyria in man and rat due to hexachlorobenzene intoxication. *Nature* 189:499, 1961

868. DE MATTEIS F, PRIOR BE, RIMINGTON C: Nervous and biochemical disturbances following hexachlorobenzene intoxication. *Nature* 191:363, 1961

869. STONARD MD: Experimental hepatic porphyria induced by hexachlorobenzene as a model for human symptomatic porphyria. *Br J Haematol* 27:617, 1974

870. ELDER GH, EVANS JO, MATLIN SA: The effect of the porphyrogenic compound, hexachlorobenzene, on the activity of the hepatic uroporphyrinogen decarboxylase in the rat. *Clin Sci Mol Med* 51:71, 1976

871. CAM C, NIGOGOYSAN G: Acquired toxic porphyria cutanea tarda due to hexachlorobenzene. *JAMA* 183:88, 1963

872. DOĞRAMACI I: Porphyrias and porphyrin metabolism, with special reference to porphyria in childhood. *Adv Pediatr* 13:11, 1964

873. SCHMID R: Cutaneous porphyria in Turkey. *N Engl J Med* 263:397, 1960

874. CRIPPS DJ, GOCMEN A, PETERS HA: Porphyria turcica. Twenty years after hexachlorobenzene intoxication. *Arch Dermatol* 116: 46, 1980

875. CRIPPS DJ: Experimental pembe yara. *Clin Res* 29:591A, 1981

876. BLEIBERG J, WALLEN M, BRODKIN R, APPLEBAUM I: Industrially acquired porphyria. *Arch Dermatol* 89:793, 1964

877. JIRÁSEK L, KALENSKÝ J, KUBEC K, PAZDEROVÁ J, LUKÁŠ E: Chlorakne, Porphyria cutanea tarda and andere Intoxikationen durch Herbizide. *Hautarzt* 27:328, 1976

878. LYNCH RE, LEE GR, KUSHNER JP: Porphyria cutanea tarda associated with disinfectant misuse. *Arch Intern Med* 135:549, 1975

879. POLAND AP, SMITH D: A health survey of workers in a 2,4-D and 2,4,5-T plant with special attention to chloracne, porphyria cutanea tarda, and psychologic parameters. *Arch Environ Health* 22:316, 1971

880. KOSTER P, DEBETS FMH, STRIK JJTWA: Porphyrinogenic action of fire retardant. *Bull Environ Contam Toxicol* 25:313, 1980

881. GOLDSTEIN JA, HICKMAN P, BERGMAN H, VOS JG: Hepatic porphyria induced by 2,3,7,8-tetrachlorodibenzo-*p*-dioxin in the mouse. *Res Commun Chem Pathol Pharmacol* 6:919, 1973

882. GOLDSTEIN JA, HICKMAN P, JUE DL: Experimental hepatic porphyria induced by polychlorinated biphenyls. *Toxicol Appl Pharmacol* 27:437, 1974

883. GOLDSTEIN JA, FRIESEN M, SCOTTI TM, HICKMAN P, HASS JR, BERGMAN H: Assessment of the contribution of chlorinated dibenzo-p-dioxins and dibenzofurans to hexachlorobenzene-induced toxicity, porphyria, changes in mixed function oxygenases, and histopathological changes. *Toxicol Appl Pharmacol* 46:633, 1978

884. DAY RS, EALES L: Porphyrins in chronic renal failure. *Nephron* 26:90, 1980

885. PARRILLA JG, ORTEGA R, PENA ML, RODICIO JL, DE SALAMANCA RE, OLMOS A, ELDER GH: Porphyria cutanea tarda during maintenance haemodialysis. *Br Med J* 280:1358, 1980

886. TOPI GC, D'ALESSANDRO GANDOLFO L, DE COSTANZA F, CANCARINI GC: Porphyria and pseudo-porphyria in hemodialyzed patients. *Int J Biochem* 12:963, 1980

887. FIEL RJ, HOWARD JC, MARK EH, DATTA GUPTA N: Interaction of DNA with a porphyrin ligand: Evidence for intercalation. *Nucleic Acids Res* 6:3093, 1979

888. VORON DA, TONKENS SW: Lupus erythematosus coexisting with porphyria cutanea tarda: Lysosomal photoreactivity as a common denominator. *Cutis* 15:69, 1975

889. TIO TH, LEYNSE B, FELTKAMP TEW, NEUMANN H: Auto-immunity and cutaneous porphyria. *S Afr J Lab Clin Med* 17 (special issue): 199, 1971

890. CHRISTENSEN NK, WITH TK: Latent cutaneous porphyria, type PCT, in a caucasian woman. *Am J Med* 53:517, 1972

891. ELDER GH: Porphyrin metabolism in porphyria cutanea tarda. *Semin Hematol* 14:227, 1977

892. BORUP P, KORDAC V, PEDERSEN JS, WITH TK: The porphyrin pattern in normal urine. *Int J Biochem* 12:1075, 1980

893. NACHT S, SAN MARTIN DE VIALE LC, GRINSTEIN M: Human porphyria cutanea tarda: Isolation and properties of the urinary porphyrins. *Clin Chim Acta* 27: 445, 1970

894. DOWDLE E, GOLDSWAIN P, SPONG N, EALES L: The pattern of porphyrin isomer accumulation and excretion in symptomatic porphyria. *Clin Sci* 39:147, 1970

895. KALIVAS J: Urinary clues to the pathogenesis of porphyria cutanea tarda. *Clin Biochem* 2:417, 1969

896. ELDER GH: The metabolism of porphyrins of the isocoproporphyrin series. *Enzyme* 17:61, 1974

897. SMITH SG: Porphyrins found in urine of patients with symptomatic porphyria. *Biochem Soc Trans* 5:1472, 1977

898. DOSS VM, LOOK D, HENNING H, LÜDERS CJ, DÖLLE W, STROHMEYER G: Chronische hepatische porphyrien. *J Clin Chem Clin Biochem* 9:471, 1971

899. MOORE MR, THOMPSON GG, ALLEN BR, HUNTER JAA, PARKER S: Plasma porphyrin concentrations in porphyria cutanea tarda, short communication. *Clin Sci Mol Med* 45:711, 1973

900. ALLEN BR, PARKER S, THOMPSON GG, MOORE MR, DARBY FJ, HUNTER, JAA: The effect of treatment on plasma uroporphyrin levels in cutaneous hepatic porphyria. *Br J Dermatol* 93:37, 1975

901. RUNGE W, WATSON CJ: Experimental production of skin lesions in human cutaneous porphyria. *Proc Soc Exp Biol Med* 109:809, 1962

902. MALINA L, MILLER VL, MAGNUS IA: Skin porphyrin assay in porphyria. *Clin Chim Acta* 83:55, 1978

903. BERK PD, BLASCHKE TF, SCHARSCHMIDT BF, WAGGONER JG, BERLIN NI: A new approach to quantitation of the various sources of bilirubin in man. *J Lab Clin Med* 87:767, 1976

904. GRINSTEIN M, FERRAMOLA DE SANCOVICH AM, SANCOVICH HA: The isolation of a new compound from urine of humans with porphyria cutanea tarda. *Biochim Biophys Acta* 500:433, 1977

905. TOPI G, D'ALESSANDRO GANDOLFO L: Inheritance of porphyria cutanea tarda: Analysis of 14 cases in 5 families. *Br J Dermatol* 97:617, 1977

906. DAHLIN O, ENERBÄCK L, LUNDVALL O: Porphyria cutanea tarda: A genetic disease? A biochemical and fluorescence microscopical study in four families. *Acta Med Scand* 194; 265, 1973

907. BENEDETTO AV, KUSHNER JP, TAYLOR JS: Porphyria cutanea tarda in three generations of a single family. *N Engl J Med* 298:358, 1978

907a. DE VERNEUIL H, NORDMANN Y: Porphyrie cutanée symptomatique. Type familial et type sporadique. *Nouv Pr Med* 10:3541, 1981

908. TOMIO JM, GARCIA RC, SAN MARTIN DE VIALE LC, GRINSTEIN M: Porphyrin biosynthesis. VII. Porphyrinogen carboxylase from avian erythrocytes: Purification and properties. *Biochim Biophys Acta* 198:353, 1970

909. SANTOIANNI P, DE FELICE M, AYALA F, BUDILLON G, ZAPPACOSTA S: A novel association between HLA and disease: Porphyria cutanea tarda and HLA-AW32. *Dermatologica* 160:371, 1980

910. LLORENTE L, DE SALAMANCA RE, CAMPILLO F, PEÑA ML: HLA and porphyria cutanea tarda. *Arch Dermatol Res* 269:209, 1980

911. DOSS M, VON TIEPERMANN R, LOOK D, HENNING H, NIKOLOWSKI J, RYCKMANNS F, BRAUN-FALCO O: Hereditäre and nicht-hereditäre Form der chronischen hepatischen Porphyrie: unterschiedliches verhalten der uroporphyrinogen-decarboxylase in Leber und Erythrozyten. *Klin Wochenschr* 58:1347, 1980

912. SAN MARTIN DE VIALE LC, RIOS DE MOLINA M, BATTLE DEL C AM, WAINSTOK DE, CALMANOVICI R, TOMIO JM: Porphyrins and porphyrinogen carboxy-lyase in hexachlorobenzene induced porphyria. *Biochem J* 168:393, 1977

913. BRODIE MJ, THOMPSON GG, MOORE MR, McCOLL KEL, GOLDBERG A, HARDIE RA, HUNTER JAA: Haem biosynthesis in cutaneous hepatic porphyria: Comparison with alchoholism and liver disease. *Acta Hepato-Gastroenterologica (Stuttg)* 26:122, 1979

914. MOORE MR, McCOLL KEL, GOLDBERG A: The activities of the enzymes of haem biosynthesis in the porphyrias and during treatment of acute intermittent porphyrias. *Int J Biochem* 12:941, 1980

915. PARERA VE, STELLA AM, WIDER DE XIFRA EA, FUKUDA H, BATTLE DEL C AM: Porphyrin biosynthesis and enzymic studies in erythrocytes from normals and porphyric humans. *Int J Biochem* 12:947, 1980

916. STONARD MD, NENOV PZ: Effect of hexachlorobenzene on hepatic microsomal enzymes in the rat. *Biochem Pharmacol* 23:2175, 1974

917. JONES KG, SWEENEY GD: Dependence of the porphyrogenic effect of 2,3,7,8-tetrachlorodibenzo(p)dioxin upon inheritance of aryl hydrocarbon hydroxylase responsiveness. *Toxicol Appl Pharmacol* 53:42, 1980

918. KOSS G, SEUBERT S, SEUBERT A, KORANSKY W, KRAUS P, IPPEN H: Conversion products of hexachlorobenzene and their role in the disturbance of the porphyrin pathway in rats. *Int J Biochem* 12:1003, 1980

919. DEBETS FMH, HAMERS WJHMB, STRIK JJTW: Metabolism as a prerequisite for the porphyrinogenic action of polyhalogenated aromatics, with special reference to hexachlorobenzene and polybrominated biphenyls (Firemaster BP-6). *Int J Biochem* 12:1019, 1980

920. TAIRA MC, SAN MARTIN DE VIALE LC: Porphyrinogen carboxylase from chick embryo liver: In vivo effect of heptachlor and lindane. *Int J Biochem* 12:1033, 1980

921. IBRAHIM NG, HOFFSTEIN ST, FREEDMAN ML: Induction of liver cell haem oxygenase in iron-overloaded rats. *Biochem J* 180:257, 1979

922. IPPEN H, AUST D: Über den Einfluss von Steroid-hormonen auf die experimentelle Porphyrie der Ratte durch Hexachlorobenzol. *Klin Wochenschr* 50:793, 1972

923. DOSS M, VON TIEPERMANN R, STUTZ G, TESCHKE R: Uroporphyrinogen decarboxylase inhibition in rat liver after alcohol ingestion. *Pharmacology* 8:562, 1980

924. STEIN JA, TSCHUDY DP, CORCORAN PL, COLLINS A: δ-Aminolevulinic acid synthetase. III. Synergistic effect of chelated iron on induction. *J Biol Chem* 245:2213, 1970

925. JONES KG, SWEENEY GD: Association between induction of aryl hydrocarbon hydroxylase and depression of uroporphyrinogen decarboxylase activity. *Res Commun Chem Pathol Pharmacol* 17:631, 1977

926. ELDER GH: Identification of a group of tetracarboxylate porphyrins, containing one acetate and three propionate β-substituents, in faeces from patients with symptomatic cutaneous hepatic porphyria and from rats with porphyria due to hexachlorobenzene. *Biochem J* 126:877, 1972

927. JACKSON AH, LASH TD, RYDER DJ, SMITH SG: Synthetic and biosynthetic studies on porphyrins. V. Evidence for an alternative pathway in the biosynthesis of haem. *Int J Biochem* 12:775, 1980

928. FELSHER B, KUSHNER JP: Hepatic siderosis and porphyria cutanea tarda: Relation of iron excess to the metabolic defect. *Semin Hematol* 14:243, 1977

929. KUSHNER JP, LEE GR, NACHT S: The role of iron in the pathogenesis of porphyria cutanea tarda: An *in vitro* model. *J Clin Invest* 51:3044, 1972

930. LEVIN EY: Enzymatic properties of uroporphyrinogen III cosynthetase. *Biochemistry* 10:4669, 1971

931. RASMUSSEN GL, KUSHNER JP: The enzymatic decarboxylation of the naturally occurring isomers of uroporphyrinogen by human erythrocytes. *J Lab Clin Med* 93:54, 1979

932. SAN MARTIN DE VIALE LC, ARÁGONES A, TOMIO JM: Tetrapyrroles as substrates and inhibitors of porphyrinogen carboxy-lyase from rat liver. *Acta Physiol Lat Am* 26:403, 1976

933. KAPLOWITZ N, JAVITT N, KAPPAS A: Coproporphyrin I and III excretion in bile and urine. *J Clin Invest* 51:2895, 1972

934. RAMSAY CA, MAGNUS IA, TURNBULL A, BARKER H: The treatment of porphyria cutanea tarda by venesection. *Q J Med* 43:1, 1974

935. WALDENSTRÖM J, HAEGER-ARONSEN B: The porphyrias: A genetic problem. *Prog Med Genet* 5:58, 1967

936. DE SALAMANCA RE, CATALAN T, CRUCES MJ, PEÑA ML, OLMOS A, MAS V: The inheritance of porphyria cutanea tarda. *Int J Biochem* 12:869, 1980

937. MAGNIN PH, WIDER DE XIFRA EA, LENCZNER M, STELLA AM, BATLLE DEL C AM: Studies on the excretion pattern of porphyrins and its use as a tool for diagnosing both symptomatic and asymptomatic cases of porphyria cutanea tarda. *Int J Biochem* 12:873, 1980

938. DOSS M: Pathobiochemical transition of secondary coproporphyrinuria to chronic hepatic porphyria in humans. *Klin Wochenschr* 58:141, 1980

939. LEVERE RD: Stilbestrol-induced porphyria: Increase in hepatic δ-aminolevulinic acid synthetase. *Blood* 28:569, 1966

940. MOORE MR, TURNBULL AL, BARNARDO D, BEATTIE AD, MAGNUS IA, GOLDBERG A: Hepatic δ-aminolaevulinic acid synthetase activity in porphyria cutanea tarda. *Lancet* ii:97, 1972

941. ZAIL SS, JOUBERT SM: Hepatic δ-aminolaevulinic acid synthetase activity in symptomatic porphyria. *Br J Haematol* 15:123, 1968

942. LEVERE RD: Porphyrin synthesis in hepatic cirrhosis: Increase in δ-aminolevulinic acid synthetase. *Biochem Med* 1:92, 1967

943. JAVITT NB, RIFKIND A, KAPPAS A: Porphyrin-heme pathway: Regulation by intermediates in bile acid synthesis. *Science* 182:841, 1973

944. BLEKKENHORST G, PIMSTONE NR, EALES L: Porphyria cutanea tarda in South Africa. Metabolic basis of disordered haem biosynthesis, in Doss M (ed): *Porphyrins in Human Disease.* Basel, S Karger, 1976, p 299

945. BLEKKENHORST GH, EALES L, PIMSTONE NR: The nature of hepatic cytochrome P-450 induced hexachlorobenzene-fed rats. *Clin Sci Mol Med* 55:461, 1978

946. GRAEF V, GOLF SW, GOERZ G: The involvement of porphyrogenic steroids in the development of experimental porphyria. *Experientia* 36:1090, 1980

947. ELDER GH: Differentiation of porphyria cutanea tarda symptomatica from other types of porphyria by measurement of isocoproporphyrin in faeces. *J Clin Pathol* 28:601, 1975

948. POH-FITZPATRICK MB, LAMOLA AA: Direct spectrofluorometry of diluted erythrocytes and plasma: A rapid diagnostic method in primary and secondary porphyrinemias. *J Lab Clin Med* 87:362, 1976

949. LONGAS MO, POH-FITZPATRICK MB: High-pressure liquid chromatography of plasma free acid porphyrins. *Anal Biochem* 104:268, 1980

950. LUNDVALL O: The effect of replenishment of iron stores after phlebotomy therapy in porphyria cutanea tarda. *Acta Med Scand* 189:51, 1971

951. DE SALAMANCA RE, RICO R, PEÑA ML, ROMERO F, OLMOS A, JIMENEZ J: Patterns of porphyrin excretion in porphyria cutanea tarda under venesection treatment. *Int J Biochem* 12:861, 1980

952. ADJAROV D, IVANOV E: Clinical value of serum γ-glutamyl transferase estimation in porphyria cutanea tarda. *Br J Dermatol* 102:541, 1980

953. CHLUMSKÝ J, MALINA L, CHLUMSKÁ A: The effect of venesection therapy on liver tissue in porphyria cutanea tarda. *Acta Hepato-Gastroenterol (Stuttg)* 20:124, 1973

954. LINDEN LH, STEFFEN CT, NEWCOMER VD: Development of porphyria during chloroquin therapy for chronic discoid lupus erythematosus. *Calif Med* 81:235, 1954

955. CRIPPS DJ, CURTIS AC: Toxic effect of chloroquine on porphyria hepatica. *Arch Dermatol* 86:575, 1962

956. DAVIS MJ, VANDER PLOEG DE: Acute porphyria and coproporphyrinuria following chloroquine therapy: A report of two cases. *Arch Dermatol* 75:796, 1957

957. MARSDEN CW: Porphyria during chloroquine therapy. *Br J Dermatol* 71:219, 1959

958. THORNSVARD CT, GUIDER BA, KIMBALL DB: An unusual reaction to chloroquine-primaquine. *JAMA* 235:1719, 1976

959. SWEENEY GD, SAUNDERS SJ, DOWDLE EB, EALES L: Effects of chloroquine on patients with cutaneous porphyria of the "symptomatic" type. *Br Med J*:128, 1965

960. FELSHER BF, REDEKER AG: Effects of chloroquine on hepatic uroporphyrin metabolism in patients with porphyria cutanea tarda. *Medicine* 45:575, 1966

961. KOWERTZ MJ: The therapeutic effect of chloroquine: Hepatic recovery in porphyria cutanea tarda. *JAMA* 223:515, 1973

962. TALJAARD JJF, SHANLEY BC, STEWART-WYNNE EG, DEPPE WM, JOUBERT SM: Studies on low dose chloroquine therapy and the action of chloroquine in symptomatic porphyria. *Br J Dermatol* 87:261, 1972

963. MALKINSON FD, LEVITT L: Hydroxychloroquine treatment of porphyria cutanea tarda. *Arch Dermatol* 116:1147, 1980

964. COHEN SN, PHIFER KO, YIELDING KL: Complex formation between chloroquine and ferrihaemic acid *in vitro*, and its effect on the antimalarial action of chloroquine. *Nature* 202:805, 1964

965. SCHOLNICK PL, EPSTEIN J, MARVER HS: The molecular basis of the action of chloroquine in porphyria cutanea tarda. *J Invest Dermatol* 61:226, 1973

966. WISE RD, MALKINSON FD: Ferrous iron and porphyria cutanea tarda. *Arch Dermatol* 113:850, 1977

967. VIZETHUM W, DAHLMANN D, BOLSEN K, GOERZ G: Influence of chloroquine (Resochin^R) on hexachlorobenzene (HCB) induced porphyria of the rat. *Arch Dermatol Res* 264:125, 1979

968. SALTZER EI, REDEKER AG, WILSON JW: Porphyria cutanea tarda. Remission following chloroquine administration without adverse effects. *Arch Dermatol* 98:496, 1968

969. KORDAČ V, SEMRÁDOVÁ M: Treatment of porphyria cutanea tarda with chloroquine. *Br J Dermatol* 90:95, 1974

970. KORDAČ V, PAPEŽOVÁ R, SEMRÁDOVÁ M: Chloroquine in the treatment of porphyria cutanea tarda, correspondence. *N Engl J Med* 296:949, 1977

971. ROLLER JA, ANDERSON PC: Chloroquine in the treatment of porphyria cutanea tarda. *J Mo State Med Assoc* 74:167, 1977

972. CHLUMSKA A, CHLUMSKY J, MALINA L: Liver changes in porphyria cutanea tarda patients treated with chloroquine. *Br J Dermatol* 102:261, 1980

973. DE SALAMANCA RE, PEÑA ML, OLMOS A, MOLINA C, LADERO JM: Follow-up studies of porphyrin excretion in porphyria cutanea tarda treated with *p*-aminobenzoic acid. *Ann Clin Res* 12:279, 1980

974. TIO TH, LEIJNSE B, JARRETT A, RIMINGTON C: Acquired porphyria from a liver tumor. *Clin Sci Mol Med* 16:517, 1961

975. BERMAN J, BRAUN A, VOLEK V: Jaterni biopsie a jeji klinicke hodnoceni u porphyria cutanea tarda, *Acta Univ Carol [Med] (Praha)* 8:589, 1959

976. THOMPSON RPH, NICHOLSON DC, FARNAN T, WHITMORE DN, WILLIAMS R: Cutaneous porphyria due to a malignant primary hepatoma. *Gastroenterology* 59:779, 1970

977. KECZKES K, BARKER DJ: Malignant hepatoma associated with acquired hepatic cutaneous porphyria. *Arch Dermatol* 112:78, 1976

978. BELCHER RV, SMITH SG, NICHOLSON DC, WILLIAMS R: Study of porphyrins present in hepatoma tissue. *Biochem J* 119:16, 1970

979. HEILMEYER L, CLOTTEN R: Die kongenitale erythropoietische Coproporphyrie. *Dtsch Med Wochenschr* 89:649, 1964

980. ANDERSON KE, FISCHBEIN A, KESTENBAUM D, SASSA S, ALVARES AP, KAPPAS A: Plumbism from airborne lead in a firing range. An unusual exposure to a toxic heavy metal. *Am J Med* 63:306, 1977

981. DAGG JH, GOLDBERG A, LOCHHEAD A, SMITH JA: The relationship of lead poisoning to acute intermittent porphyria. *Q J Med* 34:163, 1965

982. BERK PD, TSCHUDY DP, SHEPLEY LA, WAGGONER JG, BERLIN NI: Hematologic and biochemical studies in a case of lead poisoning. *Am J Med* 48:137, 1970

983. DOWDLE EB, WILSON E, BURGER P: Symptomatic porphyria. I. The effects of lead on the synthesis of porphyrin and haem. *S Afr J Lab Clin Med* 17 (special issue):38, 1971

984. ALVARES AP, FISCHBEIN A, SASSA S, ANDERSON KE, KAPPAS A: Lead intoxication: Effects on cytochrome P-450-mediated hepatic oxidations. *Clin Pharmacol Ther* 19:183, 1976

985. SASSA S: Toxic effects of lead, with particular reference to porphyrin and heme metabolism, in De Matteis F, Aldridge WN (eds): *Heme and Hemoproteins*. Berlin, Springer-Verlag, 1978, p 333

986. VALENTINE WN, PAGLIA DE, FINK K, MADOKORO G: Lead poisoning. Association with hemolytic anemia, basophilic stippling, erythrocyte pyrimidine 5'-nucleotidase deficiency, and intraerythrocytic accumulation of pyrimidines. *J Clin Invest* 58:926, 1976

987. STRIFE CF, ZUROWESTE EL, EMMETT EA, FINELLI VN, PETERING HG, BERRY HK: Tyrosinemia with acute intermittent porphyria: Aminolevulinic acid dehydratase deficiency related to elevated urinary aminolevulinic acid levels. *J Pediatr* 90:400, 1977

988. AOKI Y, MURANAKA S, NAKABAYASHI K, UEDA Y: δ-Aminolevulinic acid synthetase in erythroblasts of patients with pyridoxine-responsive anemia. Hypercatabolism caused by the increased susceptibility to the controlling protease. *J Clin Invest* 64:1196, 1979

989. PASANEN AVO, SALMI M, VUOPIO P, TENHUNEN R: Heme biosynthesis in sideroblastic anemia. *Int J Biochem* 12:969, 1980

990. AOKI Y: Multiple enzymatic defects in mitochondria in hematological cells of patients with primary sideroblastic anemia. *J Clin Invest* 66:43, 1980

991. SUTHERLAND DA, WATSON CJ: Studies of coproporphyrin. VI. The effect of alcohol on the per diem excretion and isomer distribution of the urinary coproporphyrins. *J Lab Clin Med* 37:29, 1951

992. ORTEN JM, DOEHR SA, BOND C, JOHNSON H, PAPPAS A: Urinary excretion of porphyrins and porphyrin intermediates in human alcoholics. *Q J Med* 24:598, 1963

993. WATSON CJ: Porphyrin metabolism in the anemias. *Arch Intern Med* 99:323, 1957

994. BANNERMAN RM, KEUSCH G, KRIEMER-BIRNBAUM M, VANCE VK, VAUGHAN S: Thalassemia intermedia, with iron overload, cardiac failure, diabetes mellitus, hypopituitarism and porphyrinuria. *Am J Med* 42:476, 1967

995. AZIZ MA, SCHWARTZ S, WATSON CJ: Studies of coproporphyrin. VII. Adaptation of the Eriksen paper chromatographic method to the quantitative analysis of the isomers in normal human urine. *J Lab Clin Med* 63:585, 1964

996. SMITH SG, RAO KRN, JACKSON AH: The porphyrins of normal urine, with a comparison of the excretion pattern in porphyria cutanea tarda. *Int J Biochem* 12:1081, 1980

997. KOSKELO P, TOIVONEN I, ADLERCREUTZ H: Urinary coproporphyrin isomer distribution in the Dubin-Johnson syndrome. *Clin Chem* 13:1006, 1967

998. BEN-EZZER J, RIMINGTON C, SHANI M, SELIGSOHN U, SHEBA CH, SZEINBERG A: Abnormal excretion of the isomers of urinary coproporphyrin by patients with Dubin-Johnson syndrome in Israel. *Clin Sci* 40:17, 1971

999. WOLKOF AW, COHEN LE, ARIAS IM: Inheritance of the Dubin-Johnson syndrome. *N Engl J Med* 288:113, 1973

1000. KONDO T, KUCHIBA K, SHIMIZU Y: Coproporphyrin isomers in Dubin-Johnson syndrome. *Gastroenterology* 70:1117, 1976

1001. SHIMIZU Y, KONDO T, KUCHIBA K, URATA G: Uroporphyrinogen III cosynthetase in liver and blood in the Dubin-Johnson syndrome. *J Lab Clin Med* 89:517, 1977

1001. SHIMIZU Y, IDA S, NARUTO H, URATA G: Excretion of porphyrins in urine and bile after the administration of delta-aminolevulinic acid. *J Lab Clin Med* 92:795, 1978

1003. KONDO T, KUCHIBA K, SHIMIZU Y: Metabolic fate of exogenous delta-aminolevulinic acid in Dubin-Johnson syndrome. *J Lab Clin Med* 94:421, 1979

1004. KOSKELO P, MUSTAJOKI P: Altered coproporphyrin-isomer excretion in patients with the Dubin-Johnson syndrome. *Int J Biochem* 12:975, 1980

1005. WOLKOFF AW, ARIAS IM: Coproporphyrin excretion in amniotic fluid and urine from premature infants: A possible maturation defect. *Pediatr Res* 8:591, 1974

1006. WITH TK: Toxic porphyria after treatment with sulphonal and trional. *S Afr J Lab Clin Med* 17 (special issue):133, 1971

1007. COWGER ML, LABBE RF: Contraindications of biological oxidation inhibitors in the treatment of porphyria. *Lancet* i:88, 1965

1008. RIFKIND AB, GILLETTE PN, SONG CS, KAPPAS A: Drug stimulation of δ-aminolevulinic acid synthetase and cytochrome P-450 *in vivo* in chick embryo liver. *J Pharmacol Exp Ther* 185:214, 1973

1009. DE MATTEIS F: Drugs and porphyria. *S Afr J Med* 17:126, 1971

1010. LARSON AW, WASSERSTROM WR, FELSHER BF, SHIH JC: Posttraumatic epilepsy and acute intermittent porphyria. Effects of phenytoin, carbamazepine, and clonazepam. *Neurology* 28:824, 1978

1011. GARCIA MERINO JA, LOPEZ-LOZANO JJ: Risks of valproate in porphyria. *Lancet* ii:856, 1980

1012. BLEKKENHORST GH, COOK ES, EALES L: Drug safety in porphyria. *Lancet* i:1367, 1980

1013. TSCHUDY DP, BONKOWSKY HL: Experimental porphyria. *Fed Proc* 31:147, 1972

1014. FISCHER PWF, FERIZOVIC A, NEILSON IR, MARKS GS: Porphyrin-inducing activity of alfaxolone and alfadolone acetate in chick embryo liver cells. *Anesthesiology* 50:350, 1979

1015. BRODIE MJ: Drug safety in porphyria. *Lancet* ii:86, 1980

1016. EISEMAN JL, ALVARES AP: Alterations induced in heme pathway enzymes and monooxygenases by gold. *Mol Pharmacol* 14:1176, 1978

1017. ZIMAN MR, BRADSHAW JJ, IVANETICH KM: The effect of fluroxene [(2,2,2-trifluoroethoxy)ethane] on haem biosynthesis and degradation. *Biochem J* 190:571, 1980

1018. HARBER LC: Porphyria cutanea tarda, in Dennis J, Crounse R, Dobson R, McGuire J (eds): *Clinical Dermatology*, vol 2, New York, Harper and Row, 1980, p 2

1019. SMITH SG: The use of thin layer chromatography in the separation of free porphyrins and porphyrin methyl esters. *Br J Dermatol* 93:291, 1975

61

HEREDITARY JAUNDICE AND DISORDERS OF BILIRUBIN METABOLISM

ALLAN W. WOLKOFF

J. ROY CHOWDHURY

IRWIN M. ARIAS

1. Bilirubin is an orange pigment which is derived from the degradation of heme proteins, particularly the hemoglobin of mature circulating erythrocytes.

2. Bilirubin is a waste product which is normally excreted into bile by the liver. With the exception of patients with profound unconjugated hyperbilirubinemia, who are at risk for bilirubin encephalopathy (kernicterus), bilirubin is harmless. Its accumulation in plasma and tissues results in jaundice, which has attracted the attention of patients and clinicians since antiquity.

3. Following its formation in the reticuloendothelial system, bilirubin is released into the circulation where it avidly binds to serum albumin and is rapidly cleared by the liver. Extraction of bilirubin from the circulation under physiologic conditions appears to be a specific hepatic function and has carrier-mediated kinetics. Within the liver cell, bilirubin binds to cytosolic proteins, the most abundant of which is ligandin. The water-insoluble bilirubin molecule is transformed sequentially into water-soluble bilirubin mono- and diglucuronides which are excreted into the bile canaliculus.

4. Inheritable disorders of bilirubin metabolism result in hyperbilirubinemia. Their study provides much of our basic understanding of hepatic bilirubin transport and metabolism. These disorders include those resulting in predominantly unconjugated hyperbilirubinemia (Gilbert's syndrome; Crigler-Najjar syndrome, types I and II) and those resulting in predominantly conjugated hyperbilirubinemia (Dubin-Johnson syndrome, Rotor's syndrome, benign recurrent intrahepatic cholestasis). Deficient activity of bilirubin UDP-glucuronyltransferase has been described in each of the three unconjugated hyperbilirubinemias (complete absence in Crigler-Najjar syndrome, type I; partial deficiency in type II and Gilbert's syndrome), although an uptake defect for bilirubin has also been suggested in Gilbert's syndrome. The pathogenesis of the conjugated hyperbilirubinemias is less well understood. The Dubin-Johnson syndrome is associated with a characteristic abnormality of porphyrin metabolism in which over 80 percent of urinary coproporphyrin is coproporphyrin I, as compared to less than 35 percent in normal individuals. Although phenotypically similar to Dubin-Johnson syndrome, Rotor's syndrome differs with respect to urinary coproporphyrin excretion and hepatic metabolism of sulfobromophthalein (BSP).

5. Family studies reveal that Crigler-Najjar syndrome, type I, has an autosomal recessive pattern of inheritance. Inheritance patterns of Crigler-Najjar syndrome, type II, and Gilbert's syndrome have not been established, and differentiation of these two syndromes from each other may be arbitrary. Studies of urinary coproporphyrin excretion reveal autosomal recessive pat-

terns of inheritance for Dubin-Johnson and Rotor's syndromes.

6. *Several animal models of inheritable disorders of bilirubin metabolism are important in understanding the pathophysiology of their human counterparts. These models include the Gunn rat (Crigler-Najjar syndrome, type I), mutant Southdown sheep (? Gilbert's syndrome), and mutant Corriedale sheep (Dubin-Johnson syndrome).*

Bilirubin is an orange pigment derived from the degradation of heme proteins, particularly the hemoglobin of mature circulating erythrocytes. It is a waste product which has no deleterious effect except in patients with profound unconjugated hyperbilirubinemia, who are at risk for bilirubin encephalopathy (kernicterus). Studies of bilirubin chemistry, synthesis, transport, metabolism, distribution, and excretion have attracted the attention of generations of chemists, biologists, and clinical investigators. Because bilirubin is an organic anion of limited aqueous solubility, it has proved to be a model for the study of the transport, metabolism, and excretion of other more biologically important organic anions.

Defects in bilirubin formation or disposal are usually manifested by hyperbilirubinemia and jaundice. A number of inherited disorders affecting these pathways have been described in both humans and animals. Study of these disorders has provided important information regarding normal and abnormal metabolic pathways. In a few of the inherited disorders specific forms of treatment have been discovered.

BILIRUBIN

Formation of Bilirubin

In humans 250 to 400 mg of bilirubin is formed daily by breakdown of hemoglobin and other hemoproteins. Approximately 75 percent is derived from the hemoglobin of senescent erythrocytes, and the remainder originates from other hemoproteins [1]. After injection of radiolabeled glycine or δ-aminolevulinic acid in humans or rats, radioactivity is incorporated into bile pigments in two peaks [2, 3, 4, 5] (Fig 61-1). The first peak ("early-labeled peak" of bilirubin, ELB) appears within 3 days and contains an initial component and a slow later phase. The initial component comprises two-thirds of the ELB in humans and is derived from nonhemoglobin heme [6]. Myoglobin has a relatively long half-life and is an unlikely source. Hepatic hemoproteins, particularly cytochrome P_{450} and catalase, may be important sources [4]. Induction of hepatic cytochrome P_{450} enhances the ELB [7]. The hepatic pool of free heme has a rapid turnover rate and may also contribute [8]. The slower phase of the ELB is derived from erythroid and nonerythroid sources and is enhanced in conditions associated with "ineffective erythropoiesis," such as congenital dyserythropoietic anemias, megaloblastic anemias, iron-deficiency anemia, and lead poisoning [6]. The ELB is also increased in erythropoietic porphyria [5] but not in porphyria cutanea tarda [9] or acute intermittent porphyria [10]. The erythroid phase is increased in accelerated erythropoiesis, probably due to intramedullary

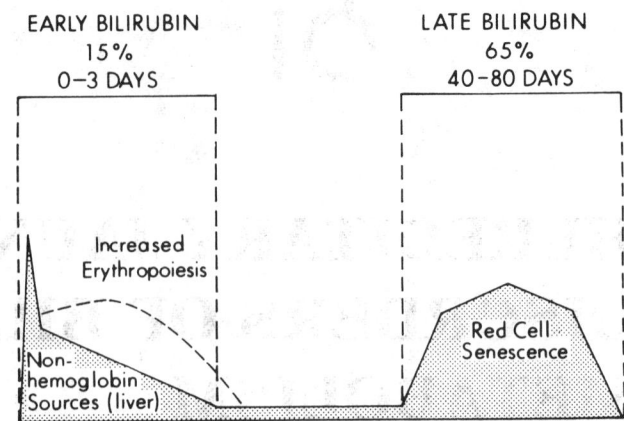

Figure 61-1 Labeling of plasma bilirubin in UDP-glucuronosyltransferase-deficient rats (Gunn strain) after the injection of glycine-2-[¹⁴C]. The early (0 to 3 days) peak has an initial "sharp" and a slower component (see text for details). (*Reprinted from S.H. Robinson in* Hemopoetic Cellular Proliferation, *ed. F. Stohlman Jr., Grune and Stratton, New York, 1970, p. 180.*)

destruction of normoblasts, destruction of reticulocytes in the peripheral circulation [11, 12], and injury to reticulocytes during maturation [13]. δ-Aminolevulinic acid is preferentially incorporated into hepatic hemoproteins. When labeled δ-aminolevulinic acid is used as a precursor, the slow component of the ELB does not include radioactivity [4]. A late-labeled peak appears approximately at 50 days in rats and 110 days in humans and is derived from the hemoglobin of senescent erythrocytes [4].

Mechanism of Opening of the Heme Ring Ferroprotoporphyrin IX is the heme prosthetic group (Fig. 61-2) in mammalian hemoproteins. The porphyrin ring is selectively cleaved at the α-methene bridge. The first step requires an electrophilic attack, Fe(II), and a reducing agent, such as NADPH and oxygen, and forms α-oxyheme (Fig. 61-2). Several explanations have been offered to account for the specificity of oxidation at the α-methene bridge. Microsomal heme oxygenase catalyzes oxidation of the α-bridge carbon [14]. Enzyme activity is highest in organs that are involved in sequestration of senescent erythrocytes and is enhanced in hemolytic states [15]. Heme oxygenase appears to be rate-limiting in conversion of heme to bilirubin, and the adaptive increase in enzyme activity may aid in catabolizing heme. An enzyme that catalyzes oxidation of the α-methene bridge of heme has been purified from pig spleen [16] and rat liver [17]. Alternatively, a quasienzymatic mechanism has been suggested in which heme combines with a microsomal apoenzyme to produce a holoenzyme (cytochrome P_{450} or its variant). In this model, oxygen bound to the heme-apoprotein complex undergoes reductive activation in the presence of NADPH and may react with an external substrate or "accidentally" with the α-methene carbon of heme [18].

The second step in opening the heme ring involves autooxidation by molecular oxygen and probably occurs nonenzymatically [19, 20]. Carbons at the angular positions of the porphyrin ring neighboring the α-methene bridge are oxidized; carbon monoxide and iron are eliminated, and the porphyrin ring is opened (Fig. 61-2), resulting in formation of the green pigment biliverdin. In mammals and fish which excrete bilirubin, biliverdin is converted to bilirubin by a soluble enzyme, biliverdin reductase, which requires NADH or NADPH for activity [21, 22].

Although bilirubin IXα is the most abundant isomer in

nature, small amounts of non-α isomers (Fig. 61-3) have been detected in human and animal bile [23, 24, 25, 26]. Bilirubin IXβ may be the predominant isomer in the bile of fetal primates [27]. The mechanism of formation of non-α bilirubins is not known.

Quantitation of Bilirubin Production

Since bilirubin production reflects the turnover of biologically important hemoproteins, its quantitation is important in physiologic investigations. Bilirubin production can be quantitated in biliary excretions in animals, but this is not practical in humans. Bilirubin is converted to urobilinogen by bacteria in the gastrointestinal tract (see below), and fecal urobilinogen excretion approximates daily bilirubin production [28, 29, 30], although conversion to urobilinogen may not be quantitative [30]. In humans bilirubin production is conveniently quantitated from the turnover of radioisotopically labeled bilirubin. Radiolabeled bilirubin bound to albumin is injected intravenously, blood samples are collected at frequent intervals, and plasma bilirubin concentration and radioactivity are measured [31]. Plasma bilirubin clearance (the fraction of plasma from which bilirubin is irreversibly extracted) is proportional to the reciprocal of the area under the radiobilirubin disappearance curve [32]. Bilirubin removal is quantitated as the product of plasma bilirubin concentration and clearance. When plasma bilirubin concentrations remain steady, removal of bilirubin equals the amount of newly synthesized bilirubin entering the plasma pool.

Bilirubin formation can also be quantitated from carbon monoxide production. The subject is placed in a closed rebreathing system to prevent CO excretion. CO production is calculated from the CO concentration in the breathing chamber or from an increment in blood carboxyhemoglobin saturation [33–36]. This method assumes that body CO stores rapidly equilibrate, blood carboxyhemoglobin reflects total body CO, and metabolism of CO is insignificant compared to its rate of production. Under certain circumstances, such as anoxia, assumption of a steady equilibrium of body stores of CO with blood carboxyhemoglobin may not be correct [37]. CO production exceeds plasma bilirubin turnover by 12 to 18 percent. This discrepancy is partly due to a small portion of bilirubin which is produced in the liver and excreted into bile

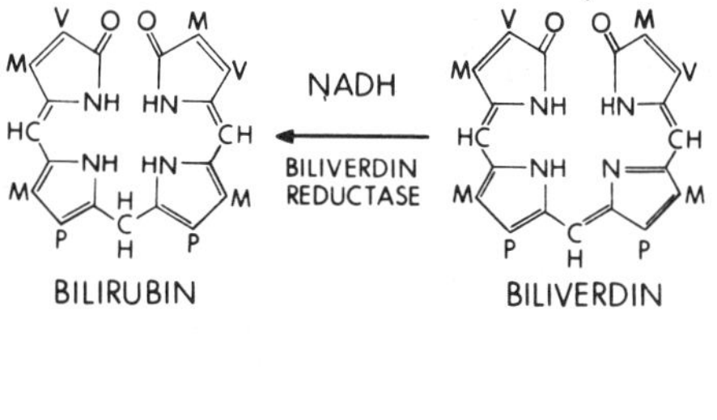

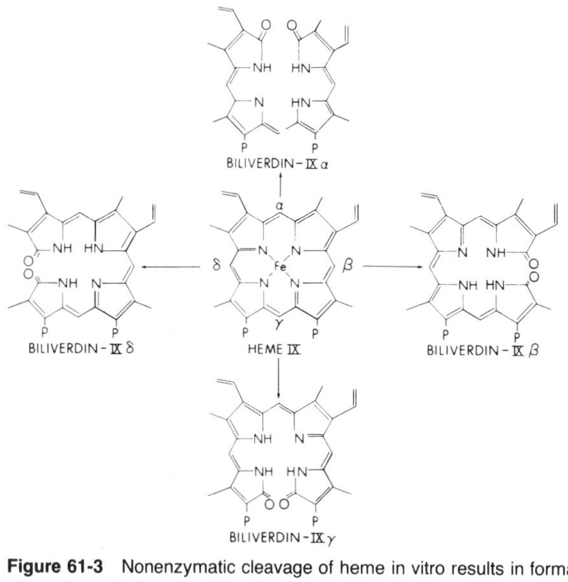

Figure 61-3 Nonenzymatic cleavage of heme in vitro results in formation of four isomeric forms of biliverdin owing to nonequivalence of the four methene bridge positions (α, β, γ, and δ). P = CH_2CH_2COOH.

without appearing in the serum. A portion of CO in expired air may be produced from nonheme sources, such as halogenated methane [38] and polyphenolic compounds, including catecholamines [39]. A small fraction of the CO may be formed by intestinal bacteria [40].

Chemistry of Bilirubin

The systematic name given bilirubin IXα is 1'8'-dioxo-1,3,6, 7-tetramethyl-2,8-divinylbiladiene-a,c-dipropionic acid(4,5) [41]. The gross chemical structure (Fig. 61-3) assigned to bilirubin by Fischer [42] has been confirmed by analysis of x-ray diffraction data (Fig. 61-4) [43]. The bonds between pyrrolenone rings A and B (C_4 to C_5) and C and D (C_{15} to C_{16}) are in the Z or transconfiguration. The oxygen attached to the outer pyrrolenone ring is in a lactam rather than lactim configuration. Titration of bilirubin in aqueous solutions suggests a pK value of 7 to 8 [44, 45]. Since bilirubin tends to form insoluble aggregates below pH 8.0, determination of pK by titration of aqueous solutions of bilirubin is misleading [46]. Recent studies utilizing ^{13}C nuclear magnetic resonance (nmr) spectra, and potentiometric and spectrophotometric titrations in aqueous solutions indicate that bilirubin has four acidic groups. The pK value of the two carboxyl groups is 4.4 and that of the two lactam groups is 13.0 [46].

Solubility of Bilirubin IXα   Accurate measurement of solubility of bilirubin IXα at physiologic pH is difficult because the pigment is unstable in aqueous solutions and tends to form colloids or surface films [47]. Solubility studies using crystalline bilirubin and organic solvents of various degrees of polarity suggest that bilirubin is relatively polar [48]. At acidic, neutral, or mildly alkaline pH, bilirubin partitions from aqueous solutions to water-immiscible solvents such as chloroform, ethyl acetate, or methylethyl ketone. Binding of bilirubin to polar lipids may be important in its deposition in brain and other tissues. A comparison of solubility in various solvents indicates that bilirubin IXα is less polar than is biliverdin IXα at physiologic pH [48]. Since both pigments have two propi-

Figure 61-2 Mechanism of heme ring opening and subsequent reduction of biliverdin to bilirubin.

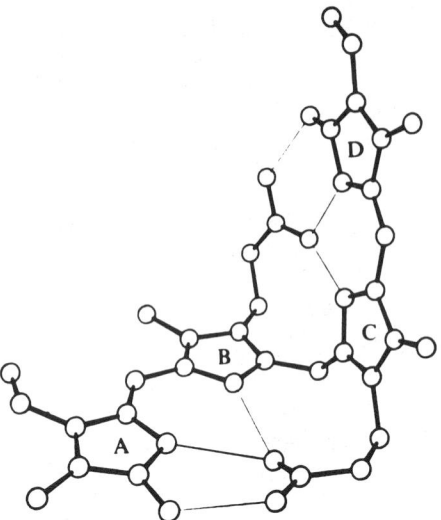

Figure 61-4 X-ray crystallographic structure of bilirubin showing a ridge-tile configuration caused by internal hydrogen bonding of the propionic acid carboxyls to the amino groups and the lactam oxygen of the pyrrolenone rings of the opposite half of the molecule. The bonds between the pyrrolenone rings A and B and C and D are in the Z (trans) configuration.

onic acid side chains, the difference in polarity is difficult to explain from the linear structure of bilirubin (Fig. 61-2). A possible explanation for this apparent inconsistency was suggested by Fog and Jellum [49] and Kuenzle et al. [50, 51], who proposed that bilirubin IXα may be internally stabilized by hydrogen bonding between the carboxyl and the two external pyrrolenone rings (Fig. 61-5). X-ray diffraction studies of crystalline bilirubin reveal hydrogen bonding between each propionic acid side chain and the pyrrolic and lactam sites in the opposite half of the molecule [43]. The molecule takes the form of a "ridge tile" (Fig. 61-4). In nonpolar solvents, the structure of bilirubin oscillates between that shown in Fig. 61-3 and its mirror image [52]. A similar conformation has been proposed for bilirubin dianions in aqueous solutions [53]. The preferred conformation of bilirubin in body fluids is uncertain. The hydrogen bonded structure may explain many of its physicochemical properties. Both carboxylic groups, all NH groups, and the two lactam oxygens are engaged by hydrogen bonding, rendering the molecule insoluble in water. Esterification of the propionic acid side chains interferes with hydrogen bonding and makes the molecule labile [50, 51], water-soluble, and reactive with diazo reagents. Addition of methanol, ethanol, or 6 M urea interferes with hydrogen bonding and results in an immediate diazo reaction. Biliverdin and bilirubin IXβ, IXγ, and IXδ isomers lack hydrogen-bonded structure and are more polar. Following injection of these unnatural isomers in rats, they were readily excreted in bile in unconjugated form [54]. In contrast, bilirubin IXα binds to lipid membranes, circulates bound to albumin, and is removed from the body only after conversion to a polar molecule. Bilirubin IXα dissolved in organic solvents has a strong absorption band (max 454 to 458 nm) and a molar extinction coefficient of 54,300 to 63,000 [55, 56].

Effect of Light on Bilirubin   (1) Fluorescence: Pure bilirubin does not fluoresce. When it is dissolved in detergent, albumin solution, or alkaline methanol, an intense fluorescence is observed at 510 to 530 nm [57, 58, 59]. Determination of fluorescence of bilirubin shows promise as a rapid method

for detection of blood bilirubin concentrations and unsaturated bilirubin binding capacity of albumin (see below). (2) Photooxidation and degradation: Whether in aqueous solution or protein or lipid bound, bilirubin undergoes gradual bleaching in the presence of light and oxygen [59]. Bleaching results in formation of colorless fragments, chiefly maleimides and propentdyopent adducts, due to a self-sensitized reaction involving singlet oxygen. A small amount of biliverdin is also formed by mechanisms that are not established [59]. (3) Geometric isomerization: As mentioned earlier (Fig. 61-4), the 5 and 15 bridges of bilirubin are in a *trans-* or Z configuration. On exposure to light (453 nm), one or both bridges may undergo *cis-* or E configuration, forming ZE, EZ, or EE isomers (Fig. 61-6). These geometric isomers rapidly attain a steady state, are relatively stable at room temperature in the absence of light, and revert to bilirubin IXαZZ isomer [60]. The EZ isomerization may interfere with intramolecular hydrogen bonding. Each geometric isomer is more polar than is bilirubin IXαZZ. When injected in rats, non-ZZ isomers are readily excreted in bile, where they promptly revert to bilirubin IXαZZ. Geometric isomerization may be responsible for excretion of unconjugated bilirubin during phototherapy of babies with unconjugated hyperbilirubinemia [61]. (4) Dipyrrolic scrambling: When bilirubin IXα is irradiated in deoxygenated aqueous solution, free radical disproportionation results in formation of bilirubin IIIα and bilirubin XIIIα (Fig. 61-6), which are non-

Figure 61-5   Ionic species of bilirubin. *A.* Internally hydrogen bonded form; *B.* bilirubin acid with hydrogen bonds disrupted; *C.* bilirubin dianion.

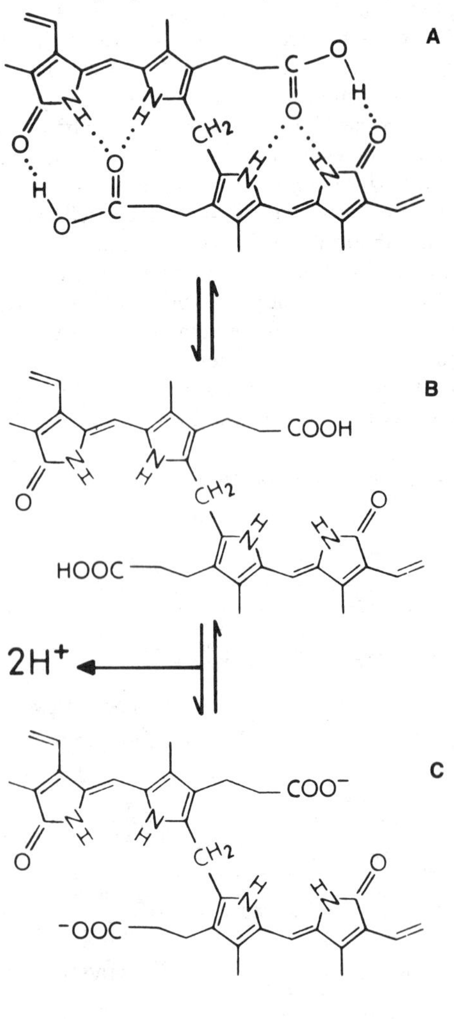

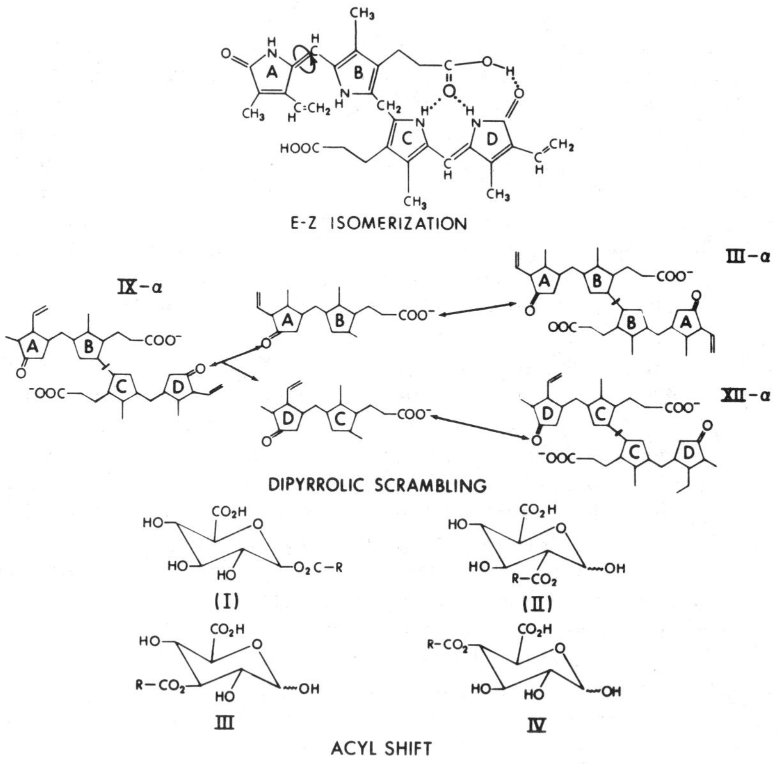

Figure 61-6 Isomerization of unconjugated and conjugated bilirubin. *Upper panel:* Geometric isomerization: the bond between the pyrrolenone rings A and B or C and D can change into an E (cis) configuration, as shown here on the left half of the bilirubin molecule, resulting in the EZ, ZE, or EE isomers. E configuration of the bond between the pyrrolenone rings interferes with hydrogen bonding and renders the molecule relatively polar. *Middle panel:* Non-enzymatic dipyrrolic scrambling involves formation of dipyrrolic free radicals and their random reassembly into asymmetrical (bilirubin IXα) and symmetrical (bilirubin IIIα and XIIIα) tetrapyrroles. *Lower panel:* Acylshifting of bilirubin glucuronides occurs on nonenzymatic incubation, resulting in conversion of the normal 1-*O*-acylglucuronide to 2-, 3- or 4-*O*-acyl forms (see text). R = propionyl side chain of bilirubin.

physiologic symmetrical isomers of bilirubin [62]. The reaction is faster in the presence of oxygen and is catalyzed by acid [63].

Dimerization and Aggregation of Bilirubin λ_{max} of bilirubin in dilute alkaline aqueous solution is 440 nm. With increasing concentration, a shoulder appears around 520 nm and is due to dimerization of bilirubin. Dimer formation is rapid, reversible, and independent of pH in the range of 7.5 to 9.0 [64]. The equilibrium is shifted toward dissociation with increasing temperature and toward dimerization at high salt concentrations. In contrast, at near neutral pH, when the bilirubin concentration exceeds the limit of solubility, there is a slow decrease in absorbance and gradual appearance of a shoulder at 490 nm. This is followed by an abrupt increase in light scattering caused by the self-aggregation of bilirubin. The temporary stability of the colloid solution may be explained by persistence of a negative charge at the surface of the aggregated particles [46]. A single crystal may initiate crystallization, which proceeds until equilibrium is reached between aggregation and dissolution. Lee and Gartner propose that bilirubin toxicity may result from interaction of the colloidal sol of bilirubin with the surface of cells [65].

Toxicity of Bilirubin

Studies in intact animals, perfused tissues, and in vitro indicate that bilirubin is potentially toxic. In mutant rats (Gunn strain) with congenital nonhemolytic hyperbilirubinemia (see below), bilirubin inhibits RNA synthesis, protein synthesis and carbohydrate metabolism in brain, and protein synthesis in liver [66, 67, 68, 69, 70]. Bilirubin also decreases respiration of isolated brain mitochondria, uncouples oxidative phosphorylation, inhibits ATPase activity, and induces swelling [70, 71, 72, 73,

74]. Bilirubin releases glyceraldehyde-3-phosphate dehydrogenase from erythrocyte membranes and eventually results in hemolysis [75, 76]. Bilirubin damages several tissues in vivo and in culture by inhibition of protein synthesis and tissue respiration [77, 78, 79, 80, 81]. In vitro bilirubin inhibits many enzymes, including hydrolytic enzymes [82], dehydrogenases [83, 84, 85], and enzymes involved in the electron transport system [84, 86]. The toxic effects of bilirubin are reduced or reversed by albumin in vivo and in vitro. Increased plasma concentrations of bilirubin increase the risk of bilirubin encephalopathy in newborn babies. A serum concentration of 20 mg/dl is generally accepted as the highest limit of safety [87], although kernicterus can occur at lower serum bilirubin concentrations [88]. Serum albumin concentrations, pH, and substances which compete for albumin binding are important in the pathogenesis of bilirubin encephalopathy [89].

Binding of Bilirubin to Albumin

Bilirubin circulates in blood bound to albumin. The physiologic importance of albumin binding was emphasized by Benhold in 1929 [90]. Albumin protects against an otherwise lethal dose of unconjugated bilirubin following intravenous injection in puppies [91]. Toxicity of bilirubin on isolated brain mitochondria is abolished by an equimolar amount of albumin [92]. Prophylactic use of sulfonamides in newborn babies enhances bilirubin encephalopathy [93], probably as a result of dissociation of bilirubin by sulfonamide from its binding to albumin [94]. Infusion of albumin increases the plasma bilirubin concentration because of transfer of bilirubin from tissues to plasma [95, 96, 97].

When bilirubin binds to albumin, two complexes may form: (1) In normal plasma, bilirubin is present bound almost exclusively as the dianion to a primary binding site on albumin, while smaller amounts are located at one or two secondary sites [46]. The reaction is fast and reversible. The binding affinity is high, and equilibrium is independent of pH. (2) The second type of binding occurs slowly at pH 7.4 or below, involves aggregation of albumin molecules with nonionized bilirubin acid [98], and depends critically on a low pH. In hyperbilirubinemic states and acidosis the plasma is supersaturated with respect to bilirubin, and there is a tendency to form bilirubin acid-albumin aggregates [46]. Binding isotherms indicate that there is a primary and a secondary binding site on albumin for bilirubin [99, 100]. Spectrophotometric studies provide evidence for a third binding site. When delipidated albumin is used, a fourth binding site becomes apparent [101].

The binding of bilirubin to albumin has been evaluated by separating bound from free bilirubin by ultrafiltration, ultracentrifugation, gel chromatography, affinity chromatography on albumin agarose polymers, dialysis, and electrophoresis. Unbound bilirubin is rapidly destroyed by treatment with H_2O_2 and horseradish peroxidase, as compared with bound bilirubin. Binding of bilirubin to albumin induces bilirubin fluorescence, circular dichroism, quenching of protein fluorescence, and shift in absorbance spectra. Each of these effects has been used to quantitate the binding of bilirubin to albumin [46]. The equilibrium constant for bilirubin binding to the primary site has been investigated (see Table 61-1 for results). In most studies, the value of the primary binding constant at physiologic pH and temperature is slightly below 10^8 M^{-1}. The binding constant for the secondary site is believed to be 10 times less than the primary constant [46].

Peptides derived by enzymatic hydrolysis or cyanogen bromide cleavage of albumin have also been studied. Fragments containing amino acid residues 186 to 248 [102], 1 to 386, 49 to 307 [103], and 182 to 585 [104] bind bilirubin. Affinity labeling studies indicate that bilirubin is primarily bound to a fragment containing residues 124 to 297 and, to a lesser extent, to residues 446 to 547 [105]. Enzymatic hydrolysis and

analysis of albumin covalently bound to bilirubin indicate that bilirubin is bound to lysine 240 in human albumin and to lysine 238 in bovine serum albumin [106].

Binding of other ligands to albumin plays a major role in determining bilirubin binding capacity. The other ligand may bind at the same site as does bilirubin, resulting in competitive displacement or noncompetitive displacement at a different site. Noncompetitive binding may not affect bilirubin binding or may produce conformational changes which enhance (cooperative binding) or decrease (anticooperative) bilirubin binding. Sulfonamides, anti-inflammatory drugs, and contrast media for cholangiography displace bilirubin competitively from albumin and increase the risk of kernicterus in jaundiced newborn babies [107]. Some benzodiazepine drugs and long-chain fatty acids in low concentrations bind to human albumin without affecting bilirubin binding [108, 109, 110]. Albumin binding of medium-chain fatty acids, such as laureate and myristate, increases the binding constant for bilirubin [111]. Short-chain fatty acids bind to albumin anticooperatively with bilirubin [112]. When large amounts of fatty acid bind to albumin, major conformational changes occur which generally decrease the binding of other ligands, including bilirubin. Acidosis increases the risk of brain damage in neonatal jaundice [113, 114] but does not influence bilirubin binding to the primary site of albumin. The increased risk of kernicterus may result from increased transport of bilirubin from plasma to selected areas of the central nervous system [46].

Because of the influence of many metabolites and drugs on albumin binding of bilirubin and its transfer from plasma to the central nervous system, measurement of plasma bilirubin concentration does not accurately estimate the risk of brain damage from unconjugated bilirubin. It is generally believed, although not experimentally verified, that unbound bilirubin is transferred from plasma to the central nervous system [94]. Efforts have been made to quantitate unbound bilirubin in serum by gel chromatography [115], peroxidase treatment

Table 61-1 Principal differential characteristics of chronic unconjugated hyperbilirubinemias

	Crigler-Najjar syndrome, type I	Crigler-Najjar syndrome, type II	Gilbert's syndrome
Histology of liver	Normal	Normal	Normal
Serum bilirubin concentration	20–50 mg/dl	< 20 mg/dl	Usually < 3 mg/dl
Routine liver function test results	Normal	Normal	Normal
45-minute plasma BSP retention	Normal	Normal	Usually normal, may be elevated in some patients
Bile	Usually pale; contains trace of unconjugated bilirubin and monoconjugates	Increased proportion of bilirubin monoglucuronide	Increased proportion of bilirubin monoglucuronide
Hepatic bilirubin UDP-glucuronyltransferase activity	Absent	Reduced	Reduced
Effect of phenobarbital on serum bilirubin concentration	None	Reduction	Reduction
Mode of inheritance	Autosomal recessive	Autosomal recessive?	Autosomal dominant?
Prevalence	Rare	Uncommon	Common (≤ 5% of the population)
Prognosis	Kernicterus	Usually benign	Benign
Animal model	Homozygous Gunn rat	Heterozygous Gunn rat?	Mutant Southdown sheep?

[116], electrophoresis on cellulose acetate [117], and fluorimetry of serum with or without detergent treatment [118]. Free bilirubin concentration is determined from the equilibrium equation

$$[F] = [B]([RA]\cdot K)$$

where $[F]$ is the free bilirubin concentration, $[B]$ is albumin-bound bilirubin concentration, $[RA]$ is the concentration of reserve bilirubin binding sites on albumin, and K is the association constant for bilirubin. Equilibrium between free and bound bilirubin is assumed, and binding of bilirubin to tissues and secondary binding sites on albumin are ignored. The numerical values for binding constants as determined from experiments with pure albumin and bilirubin are assumed to be valid in serum. These assumptions may not be valid with icteric serum, and, therefore, it is not possible to calculate reliably the concentration of unbound bilirubin [46]. The alternative approach is to determine the amount of unoccupied bilirubin binding sites on albumin. Titration of serum with bilirubin or a dye which binds to albumin has been used to estimate unoccupied bilirubin binding sites. Binding to secondary binding sites occurs before primary sites are saturated, and some dyes bind at sites other than the bilirubin binding site. Binding of bilirubin to erythrocytes depends on the albumin/bilirubin ratio in serum and indirectly reflects reserve bilirubin binding sites on albumin [119]. Competitive binding by a ^{14}C-labeled ligand (monoacetyl-4,4′-diaminodiphenyl sulfone) [120] or a spin-labeled ligand ([1-N-(2,2,6,6-tetramethyl-1-oxyl-4-piperidinyl)5-N-(1-aspartate)-2,4-dinitrobenzene]) [121] has been used to determine reserve binding capacity. A recently developed fluorimetric method for determination of bound albumin and reserve bilirubin binding capacity [118] in small quantities of whole blood is simple and promising. Despite inaccuracies, several empirical tests for determination of reserve bilirubin binding capacity of serum albumin correlate clinically with brain damage [122] and may be useful in assessing the risk of bilirubin toxicity. The newer methods are more accurate and theoretically sounder, but clinical experience is needed for their evaluation.

Uptake of Bilirubin by the Liver

Although bilirubin is tightly bound to albumin in plasma, it is rapidly removed from the circulation by the liver (Fig. 61-7). The ability to extract bilirubin from the circulation under physiologic conditions appears to be a specific hepatic function [123, 126]. Kinetic studies of bilirubin uptake in isolated perfused liver of dog [127] and rat [128, 129] and in rats in vivo [123] reveal that the process is saturable. A preloading effect on transport of bilirubin in rat liver has been described [123] (i.e., following an intravenous loading dose of bilirubin, the plasma disappearance of a subsequent tracer dose of ^{3}H-labeled bilirubin is enhanced). Countertransport of bilirubin (i.e., efflux of radiolabeled ligand from liver after subsequent infusion with unlabeled ligand) has been claimed [123], but the data may represent efflux of ligand from intracellular binding sites. Mutual competition for hepatic uptake in vivo has been described with respect to bilirubin and other organic anions, such as indocyanine green (ICG) [123, 130], sulfobromophthalein (BSP) [123, 130], and conjugated bilirubin [131]. Bile

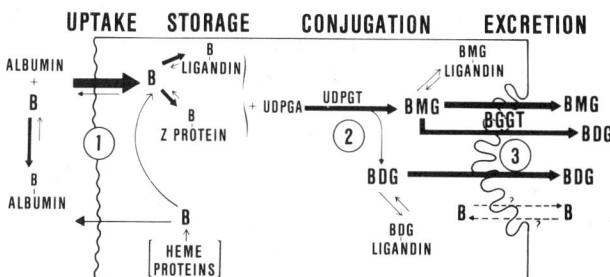

Figure 61-7 Schematic summary of hepatic transport and metabolism of bilirubin (B). In the circulation, bilirubin is bound avidly to albumin. This complex dissociates, and bilirubin alone enters the liver cell by a process with characteristics of facilitated diffusion (1). A fraction of bilirubin within the liver cell is derived from breakdown of hepatic heme proteins. Bilirubin inside the hepatocyte binds to cytosolic proteins (ligandin and Z protein) which prevents its efflux from the cell. Bilirubin is conjugated with glucuronic acid (2) in the presence of bilirubin UDP-glucuronyltransferase (UDPGT) and UDP-glucuronic acid (UDPGA) to form bilirubin monoglucuronide (BMG) and bilirubin diglucuronide (BDG), both of which may bind to ligandin in the cytosol. Normally, conjugation is virtually obligatory for biliary excretion of bilirubin (3), although small amounts of unconjugated bilirubin are found in bile in some circumstances. The hepatocyte plasma membrane is enriched in an enzyme, bilirubin glucuronoside glucuronosyltransferase (BGGT), which dismutates BMG to BDG and unconjugated bilirubin. The relationship of BGGT to biliary excretion is unknown. Canalicular excretion is thought to be an energy-requiring process which is normally rate limiting in bilirubin throughput and may be shared by other organic anions except bile salts.

acids do not compete with these compounds for hepatic uptake [123, 128, 131].

Bilirubin is extracted from albumin before entering the liver cell, and albumin does not accompany bilirubin into the hepatocyte. In intact rats, 5 min after injection of [3H]bilirubin and ^{131}I-labeled albumin, approximately 60 percent of injected bilirubin is in the liver, whereas only 10 percent of injected albumin is in liver, probably in the vascular space [126]. In isolated perfused rat and dog liver, simultaneous injection of ^{125}I-albumin and [3H]bilirubin discloses rapid bilirubin uptake, with no removal of albumin from the perfusate [127, 128, 132, 133]. Similar results occur in rat liver tissue slices [134] and in humans, judging from plasma disappearance rates of labeled bilirubin and albumin [96]. The potential role of the albumin-bilirubin complex in hepatic uptake of bilirubin is controversial. It is not clear whether free or albumin-bound bilirubin interacts with the hepatocyte. Weisiger et al. [135, 136] hypothesized on the basis of kinetic studies that the albumin-bilirubin complex interacts directly with an albumin receptor on the liver cell surface, but additional studies to quantitate free and bound bilirubin are necessary and there are alternative explanations of the data. In studies of isolated rat liver which was perfused with protein-free fluorocarbon, uptake of bilirubin proceeded equally well whether injected as a complex with albumin, ligandin, or with fluorocarbon alone [137]. These results suggest that albumin binding does not facilitate hepatic bilirubin uptake. In other studies, organic anion uptake rates in isolated perfused liver varied inversely with the albumin concentration in the perfusate [138, 139]. Oie and Levy demonstrated a strong correlation between plasma clearance of bilirubin in rats and the free fraction of bilirubin [140]. In studies performed in four hypoalbuminemic patients, a similar inverse relationship between the plasma albumin concentration and hepatic BSP removal was described [141]. These studies suggest that albumin binding may prevent bilirubin from diffusing nonspecifically into other tissues without playing a direct role in the hepatic uptake mechanism.

Based on these studies, bilirubin uptake by the liver has been postulated to be a carrier-mediated mechanism. The biochemistry of this mechanism is not known, although it does not appear to require energy or the presence of Na^+ [128]. A variety of seemingly unrelated organic anions compete with bilirubin and other organic anions for hepatic uptake. These include ICG and BSP, which have been noted above, and others such as probenecid [142–145], rifampicin [145–148], flavispidic acid [149, 150], and cholecystographic agents [151, 152]. Recent studies have suggested that uptake of some of these compounds may be, at least in part, independent of bilirubin [148, 153, 154].

One hypothesis was that ligandin, an abundant intrahepatocellular organic anion-binding protein (see below), mediates hepatic bilirubin uptake. This was tested in isolated perfused rat liver [133]. Bilirubin influx and efflux rates were quantitated using a multiple indicator dilution technique in normal and thyroidectomized rats before and after treatment with phenobarbital. Because ligandin is induced after phenobarbital administration and stabilized in the absence of thyroid hormone, these treatments increase liver ligandin levels two- to threefold [155]. Analysis revealed no positive correlation between hepatic ligandin concentration and the influx rate of bilirubin. The efflux rate of bilirubin from liver back to plasma varied inversely with hepatic ligandin concentration [133, 156]. This study suggests that intracellular protein binding of bilirubin plays no role in the extraction of bilirubin from serum albumin and subsequent transport into the hepatocyte. Intracellular binding to ligandin influences net uptake of bilirubin. Once ligand enters the hepatocyte, it is less available for efflux into plasma.

A specific interaction of bilirubin with the plasma membrane of the hepatocyte prior to uptake has been hypothesized. Several studies have measured the binding of bilirubin and other organic anions to rat liver cell plasma membrane preparations (LPM). Cornelius et al. [157] demonstrated saturable binding of BSP to rat LPM and found 200 nmol bound per milligram of protein. Bilirubin had no effect on binding of BSP. Reichen et al. [158] determined K_d of BSP binding to LPM as 390 to 650 μM, with saturation at 230 to 440 nmol per milligram of protein. Although the results of these two studies are in agreement, the number of binding sites is high, and the affinity of BSP for LPM is lower by two orders of magnitude than is the affinity of BSP for albumin. Tiribelli et al. [159] studied BSP binding to rat LPM and described high affinity binding with K_d of 4.88 to μM and saturation at 40.4 nmol per milligram of BSP protein. Bilirubin (0.5 mM) competetively inhibited BSP binding, resulting in an apparent K_d of 10.5 μM and indicating an approximately 100-fold lower affinity of membrane for bilirubin. Subsequently a protein was isolated by gel chromatography from an acetone powder of LPM [160]. This 170,000-dalton protein binds over 100 nmol of BSP per milligram, implying at least 17 binding sites for BSP. Whether these 17 binding sites represent only high affinity binding sites is not clear. Wolkoff and Chung [161] also studied interaction of BSP with rat LPM, and described high affinity ($K_a = 0.27 \mu M^{-1}$) saturable (6.3 nmol per milligram of protein) binding of [^{35}S]BSP which was eliminated after preincubation of membrane with trypsin. To identify specific membrane binding proteins, a photoaffinity probe was devised in which [^{35}S]BSP was covalently bound to LPM after exposure to ultraviolet light.

Subsequent SDS polyacrylamide gel electrophoresis and fluorography revealed radioactivity predominantly associated with a single 55,000-dalton protein. A protein with identical electrophoretic mobility was purified from deoxycholate-solubilized LPM after affinity chromatography on GSH(glutathione)-BSP-agarose gel. This protein is immunologically distinct from rat serum albumin and ligandin and binds bilirubin with a K_d of 20 μM, as determined by tryptophan fluorescence quenching. The relationship of this protein to that isolated by Tiribelli and colleagues is unknown. A protein of similar molecular weight was purified by Reichen and Berk [162], following affinity chromatography of Triton X-100 solubilized liver cell plasma membranes on bilirubin agarose gel. Although these proteins avidly bind organic anions, their role as liver cell plasma membrane receptors for organic anions and their relationship to transmembrane transport of these compounds await additional study.

Further evidence in support of carrier-mediated hepatic uptake of bilirubin comes from study of uptake in regenerating rat liver. The normal rat hepatocyte divides approximately once per year [163]. Following two-thirds hepatectomy, rapid cellular replication occurs throughout the liver remnant and is associated with expression of oncofetal antigens [164]. These findings suggest that hepatic regeneration is accompanied by transient "retrodifferentiation" of hepatocytes. With use of a multiple-indicator dilution technique, single-pass transport of [^{3}H]bilirubin was determined in isolated perfused rat liver from 6 h to 6 days after two-thirds hepatectomy or sham surgery [165]. In this procedure influx of bilirubin is independent of liver mass. Within 6 h of two-thirds hepatectomy, influx of bilirubin decreased by 50 percent as compared to that in sham-operated controls, and returned to normal 4 days later. The fact that influx of both bilirubin and asialoorosomucoid reached a nadir at the time of greatest cellular proliferation and subsequently returned to normal suggests "maturation" of liver cell function for restoration of a specific hepatocyte function.

Intrahepatocellular Storage of Bilirubin

Fifteen minutes after the intravenous injection of [^{3}H]bilirubin into rats, plasma [^{3}H]bilirubin declines by over 90 percent and 25 to 30 percent of the injected dose remains in liver [124–126]. Radioactivity does not appear in bile until 3 to 4 min after injection and subsequently appears at a rate of approximately 3 percent of the injected dose per minute [124]. Thus, from the time bilirubin is cleared from plasma and subsequently excreted into bile, it is accumulated, or stored, within the hepatocyte.

At all times after intravenous injection, a large proportion of [^{3}H]bilirubin is associated with the 100,000 × g cytosol of liver homogenates [124–126]. Bilirubin is only slightly soluble in aqueous solutions at physiologic pH and is presumably bound to protein in cytosol. Gel filtration of cytosol containing [^{3}H]bilirubin or [^{35}S]BSP reveals that radioactivity is associated with two protein peaks, termed Y and Z (Fig. 61-8) [166]. These proteins differ from albumin and each other with respect to biochemical and immunologic characteristics [167]. When a tracer quantity of radiolabeled anion is added to liver homogenate, binding is almost exclusively to the Y protein, whereas with larger amounts binding to the Z protein becomes more apparent [166]. This suggests that under physiologic condi-

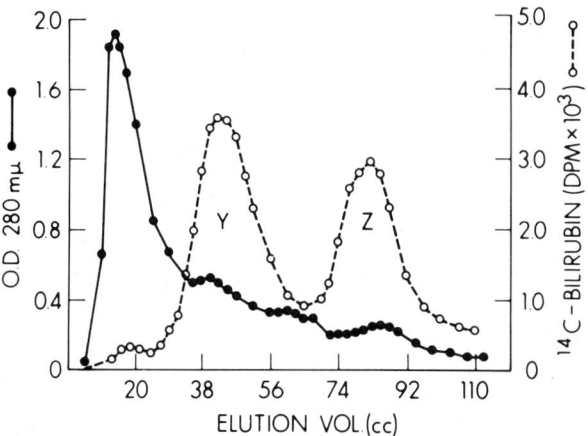

Figure 61-8 Binding of bilirubin to cytosolic proteins. Sephadex G75 gel chromatography of 110,000 × g rat liver supernatant to which [^{14}C]-bilirubin has been added reveals association of radioactivity with two protein peaks, Y and Z. Y protein was determined to be quantitatively more important in organic anion binding and has subsequently been named ligandin.

tions Y protein is the principal cytoplasmic protein to which organic anions bind.

Y protein has been purified to homogeneity [167], and further study revealed that it avidly binds many compounds, including various drugs, hormones, and organic anions [166, 168–171]. Similar proteins have been identified by other investigators. Morey and Litwack [172] identified a protein by its ability to bind a cortisol metabolite, while Ketterer et al. [173] identified a protein that bound an azo-dye carcinogen. These three proteins proved to be identical by structural and immunologic techniques and were termed *ligandin* [174]. Ligandin accounts for approximately 5 percent of liver cytosol protein [167, 175] and also has GSH-transferase [176–178], ketosteroid isomerase [179], and GSH-peroxidase activities [180, 181]. In the rat ligandin is identical to GSH transferase B, the major member of a class of six distinct basic GSH transferases which were purified from rat liver cytosol [177, 178, 182, 183]. Five GSH transferases have been isolated from human liver, but unlike the comparable rat proteins, the human proteins have identical amino acid composition and cross-react immunologically [184]. Each of the rat and human GSH transferases avidly binds bilirubin and other organic anions as nonsubstrate ligands [124, 169, 184, 185–187].

The high affinity of these proteins for organic anions suggested that they may play a role in transport by the liver [188–190]. Circumstantial evidence for this hypothesis was provided by studies of ontogeny and phylogeny. Addition of BSP to liver cytosol followed by Sephadex G75 chromatography revealed that in elasmobranchs, teleosts, and the gill-breathing amphibia, there was no detectable Y peak; the Z peak was either undetectable or present in trace amounts. Prominent Y and Z peaks were found in lung-breathing amphibians, reptiles, birds, and mammals [191].

An ontogenic study to determine the developmental pattern of the soluble organic anion binding proteins in three species of frog during metamorphosis failed to reveal Y and Z peaks in the youngest forms. With partial development, a prominent Z peak was seen, and both Y and Z peaks were present in adults [191]. Similar results were obtained in guinea pigs [192] and monkeys [193]; "maturation" of ligandin coincided with normalization of hepatic organic anion transport. Additional studies of organic anion transport in elasmobranchs revealed that the relationship of ligandin and other GSH transferases to

hepatic organic anion transport may be complex [194, 195]. These animals have low but detectable levels of GSH transferase activity in liver, [196] but 24 h after injection, 75 to 85 percent of [^{35}S]BSP was recovered in bile and liver.

Although many organic anions bind to ligandin following their uptake by the liver, the ability to bind to ligandin does not imply that a given compound will be removed from the circulation by the liver. An example is Evans blue which is slowly excreted by the liver in vivo. After intravenous injection of Evans blue into a rat, no binding to the Y and Z fractions of rat liver cytosol occurs, whereas addition of the dye to liver cytosol in vitro reveals binding to the Y peak to a similar degree as with BSP or ICG [166].

Although bilirubin and other organic anions are stored in the liver primarily bound to ligandin, the selectivity of organic anion uptake by the liver cell is probably a function of the plasma membrane (see preceding section). Studies showing that serum albumin has a greater affinity for bilirubin than does purified ligandin have challenged its transport role [197]. One suggestion is that affinity of ligandin for bilirubin decreases during purification [198]. That this view is incorrect was demonstrated in a circular dichroism study of bilirubin ligandin interactions in rat liver cytosol and fractions obtained at various stages during purification of ligandin [199]. Ligandin retained its capacity to bind bilirubin in the presence of components of liver supernatant, but albumin lost the capacity to bind bilirubin in liver supernatant. In their respective physiologic milieus, albumin and ligandin are structurally adapted to bind ligands: albumin in serum, and ligandin in the cytosol of the liver cell. With respect to organic anion transport, ligandin may function within the hepatocyte much as albumin does in the circulation, binding bilirubin and preventing efflux from the hepatocyte back into the circulation, [133] and nonspecific diffusion of bilirubin into compartments of the hepatocyte in which it may do harm. This hypothesis is supported by the finding that bilirubin inhibits mitochondrial respiration in vitro, an effect that is completely prevented by ligandin [200]. The relationship of ligandin binding of bilirubin and its conjugates to the processes of conjugation and biliary excretion is not known.

Conjugation of Bilirubin

Before bilirubin is excreted across the bile canaliculus, it is rendered polar by esterification of the propionic acid carboxyl groups. Esterification of one or both propionic acid side chains forms mono- or diconjugates, respectively. Studies of human T-tube bile [201, 202] and bile from dogs [203, 204, 205], alligators, cats, chickens, horses, opossums, rabbits, and snakes [206] reveal xylosyl and glucosyl conjugates. More complex conjugating sugar groups, including glucuronosyl-glucosyl, glucuronosyl-glucuronosyl, and glucosyl-glucosyl-glucuronosyl, were characterized in human T-tube bile by Kuenzle [207]. Glucuronic acid is the major conjugating group in normal mammalian bile [208].

Although the existence of bilirubin monoglucuronide as a chemical entity was questioned for many years [209, 210], bilirubin glucuronides are now known to be present as mono- and diconjugates (Fig. 61-9) [211, 212]. Bilirubin IXα is an asymmetrical molecule, and, therefore, bilirubin IXα monoglucuronide exists as two isomers, depending on where the glucuronyl group is attached. The two isomers have been sep-

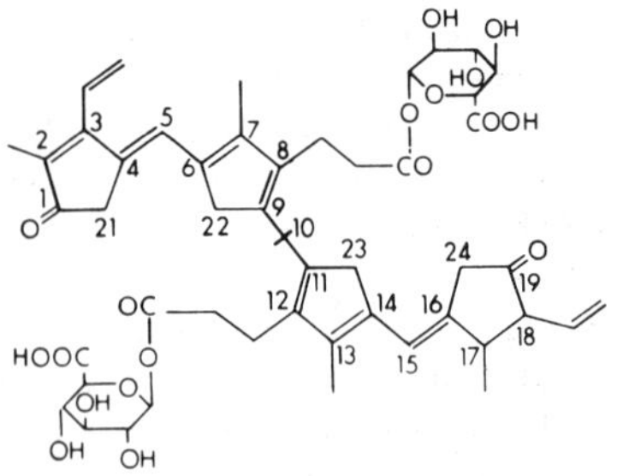

Figure 61-9 Bilirubin glucuronides. Both propionic acid side chains are glucuronidated in bilirubin diglucuronide. Bilirubin monoglucuronide can exist as two molecular species, depending on whether the C_{12} or C_8 propionic acid is conjugated.

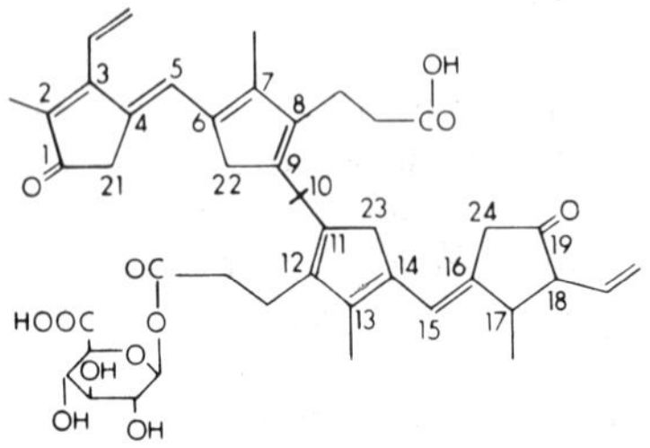

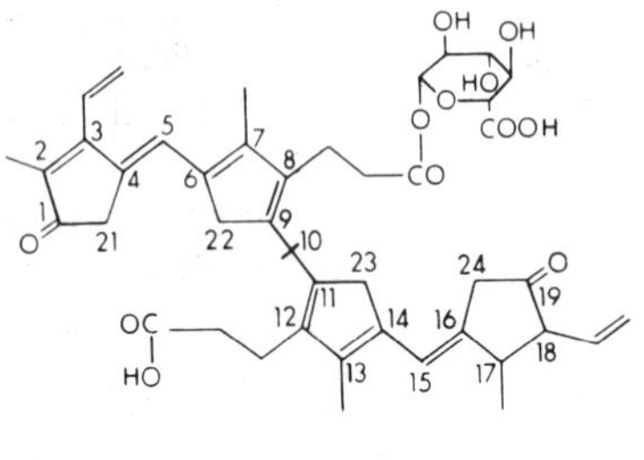

arated by thin-layer chromatography or high performance liquid chromatography after substitution of the conjugating group by NH_2 [213] or CH_3 groups [214].

Quantitation of Bilirubin and Its Conjugates Since bilirubin conjugates are structurally unstable and easily undergo oxidation, quantitation and structural characterization of bilirubin glucuronides have been primarily performed with the two dipyrrolic derivatives formed by the diazo reaction of bilirubin. The diazo reaction is a multistep process which begins with electrophilic attack by a diazonium ion at the 9 and 11 positions of bilirubin [215] and converts the tetrapyrrole to diazotized azopyrroles and formaldehyde (Fig. 61-10). Unconjugated bilirubin is converted to two unconjugated dipyrroles, bilirubin diglucuronide forms two conjugated azodipyrroles, and bilirubin monoconjugates form one conjugated and one unconjugated azodipyrrole (Fig. 61-10). In 1916 van den Bergh and Muller [216] discovered that serum contains two species of bilirubin. One type reacts with sulfanilic acid diazo reagent within minutes, while the other reacts as rapidly only when accelerator substances such as methanol or caffeine are present [216]. The first type of reaction is called "direct" and the second type is the "indirect" diazo reaction. Later it was realized that indirect reacting bilirubin represents unconjugated bilirubin, and that direct reacting bilirubin largely represents conjugated bilirubin [217]. The direct diazo reaction overestimates the levels of conjugated bilirubin. For example, solutions of crystalline bilirubin may show as much as 10 percent of total pigment as direct reacting. In most clinical laboratories, a direct-reacting bilirubin concentration which is less than 15 percent of total is normal [6]. Various modifications of the van den Bergh reaction are commonly used for clinical determination of bilirubin conjugates. More recently, ethylanthranilate and p-iodoaniline diazo reagents were used in place of the sulfanilic acid diazo reagent. These methods are more sensitive, accurate, and selective, and the azodipyrroles formed can be extracted and analyzed by thin-layer [205] and high pressure liquid chromatography (Fig. 61-11). The conjugated azopyrrole formed by reaction of bilirubin conjugates with ethylanthranilate diazonium reagent has been

characterized as the 1-O-acylglucopyranuric acid glycoside [208, 218]. When bile flow is impeded, bilirubin IXα-1-O-acylglucuronides rearrange with formation of 2-, 3- and 4-acylglucuronides (Fig. 61-6) [218]. This sequential migration of the bilirubin O-acyl group from position 1 to positions 2, 3, and 4 of glucuronic acid is catalyzed by base and occurs on incubation of bile or isolated bilirubin IXα-glucuronides at 37°C [205, 218].

Although it is convenient to quantitate and characterize bilirubin and its conjugates from their azoderivatives, this method cannot be applied to quantitate accurately the parent tetrapyrroles in a complex mixture of mono- and diconjugates. The azopigments are usually analyzed by thin-layer chromatography, which may lead to incomplete pigment recovery and inaccurate quantitation. For these reasons methods for separation and quantitation of intact bilirubin tetrapyrroles have been developed. In 1954 Cole et al. separated serum bile pigment into unconjugated bilirubin and two direct reacting components, pigment I and pigment II, by column chromatography [219]. Pigment II was characterized as bilirubin diglucuronide. The exact nature of pigment I, which yielded equimolar amounts of conjugated and unconjugated azodipyrroles on diazo reaction, remained controversial. Subsequently, Heirwegh and associates developed highly resolving thin-layer chromatographic systems for separation of bilirubin and its conjugates. Analysis of azoderivatives of each tetrapyrrole revealed predominantly bilirubin IXα conjugates in the bile of various species. In addition, small amounts of bilirubin IXβ, IXγ, and IXδ occur in dog bile [25, 220]. Small amounts of sulfate, phosphate, and taurine conjugates of bilirubin have also been described in bile [48, 221–224]. Although separation of intact bilirubin tetrapyrroles by thin-layer chromatography has led to better understanding of bilirubin conjugates, the methods are tedious and quantitative pigment recovery after thin-layer chromatography is not possible. High performance liquid chromatography (HPLC) offers high resolution and quantitative recovery of bile pigments. Methyl esters formed by alkaline methanolysis of bilirubin mono- and diconjugates have been separated and quantitated by HPLC [225]. In this method, the conjugating moieties are replaced by methyl groups, and the pigments cannot be separated on the basis of their conjugating moieties. Methods for separation and quantitation of intact bilirubin tetrapyrrole conjugates by HPLC have been recently developed [226, 227, 228, 229] and offer accurate and sensitive means to identify and quantitate bilirubin conjugates in body fluids and in vitro (Fig. 61-12).

Bilirubin diglucuronide is the major pigment in human, dog, and rat bile [230, 231, 232]. Conjugation of bilirubin with glucuronic acid is catalyzed by the microsomal enzyme, uridine:diphosphoglucuronate glucuronosyltransferase (UDP-glucuronyltransferase, EC 2.4.1.17), which catalyzes transfer of the glucuronyl moiety of UDP-glucuronate to a variety of aglycones, forming ether, ester, thiol, and N-glucuronides [233]. UDP-glucuronyltransferase plays an important role in glucuronidation and disposition of many endogenous substances in addition to bilirubin, such as thyroxine, tetrahydrocortisol, and steroid hormones, and various exogenous compounds [234]. The enzyme activity is present in mammalian liver [234] and in the liver of many salt- and freshwater fish [235, 236]. Highest specific enzyme activity is in the microsomal fraction of liver homogenates [234], and the enzyme is also present in renal cortex, gastrointestinal mucosa, epidermis, and adrenal tissue. Activities in these tissues are lower than in liver [234, 237, 238].

UDP-glucuronyltransferase is an integral part of the microsomal membrane, and function depends on its lipid environment. Treatment of microsomes with phospholipase A inactivates the enzyme, and activity is restored on addition of phospholipid micelles [239]. Delipidation of deoxycholate-solubilized enzyme inactivates the enzyme. Virtually complete reactivation was obtained following dialysis of the delipidated enzyme preparation with lecithin [240].

The activity of UDP-glucuronyltransferase in vitro is influenced by membrane-perturbing agents. Detergents, such as Triton X-100 [241], Lubrol [242], digitonin [243], Tween [244], and low concentrations of deoxycholate [245] enhance enzyme activity. An increase in enzyme activity occurs after sonication of microsomal preparations [246], storage at 0°C in potassium chloride solution [247], and brief incubation with phospholipase A [248]. Two models have been proposed to explain the activation of UDP-glucuronyltransferase activity by membrane-perturbing agents. In the compartmental model, the catalytic site of the enzyme is partially separated from its substrates by the lipid membranes. Membrane perturbation enhances enzyme activity in vitro by increasing accessibility of substrates to the catalytic site [249]. In the allosteric model, enzyme activity is constrained by the membrane. Activating agents release the enzyme from constraint and increase enzyme activity [250].

UDP-glucuronyltransferase appears to consist of a group of related enzymes. Following treatment of rats with methyl cholanthrene, hepatic UDP-glucuronyltransferase activity is influenced differently toward different aglycone substrates [251]. Attempts to solubilize enzyme activity from rat liver microsomes with detergents yield different results with bilirubin and p-nitrophenol as substrates [252, 253]. UDP-glucuronyltransferase activity toward o-aminophenol and other xenobiotics develops in late fetal rat liver, whereas bilirubin and steroid hormone glucuronidating activity develops postnatally [254]. Treatment of pregnant rats with glucocorticoids results in precocious development of fetal UDP-glucuronyltransferase activity with phenolic substrates but not with bilirubin [254]. A similar effect occurs in cultured liver cells. Homozygous Gunn rats cannot form bilirubin glucuronides but form acyl- and N-glucuronides and glucuronides of several phenolic substrates, such as thyroxine and tetrahydrocortisol [255, 256, 257]. Glucuronidating activity toward o-aminophenol is deficient in vitro but is restored to normal by pretreatment of microsomes with diethylnitrosamine [257]. The effect of diethylnitrosamine does not depend on microsomal membranes, since the effect persists in UDP-glucuronyltransferase purified from Gunn rat liver. These studies suggest functional heterogeneity of UDP-glucuronyltransferase. Recently, at least two functionally different UDP-glucuronyltransferases have been purified to apparent homogeneity from rat liver microsomes [258, 259, 260]. 1-Naphthol, p-nitrophenol, and 3-hydroxybenzo(a)pyrene are substrates for one class of UDPglucuronyltransferase which is inducible by methylcholanthrene in rats [261]. Bilirubin and several steroid hormones represent a second class of UDP-glucuronyltransferase which is inducible by

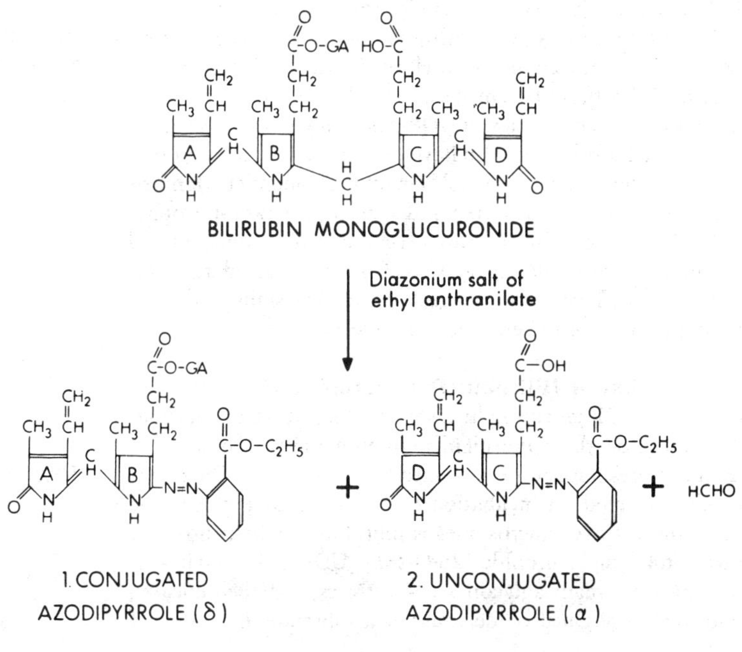

Figure 61-10 Reaction of bilirubin tetrapyrrole with the diazonium salt of ethylanthranilate results in the formation of equimolar amounts of two azodipyrroles. The central methenyl bridge is converted to formaldehyde. GA = glucuronic acid.

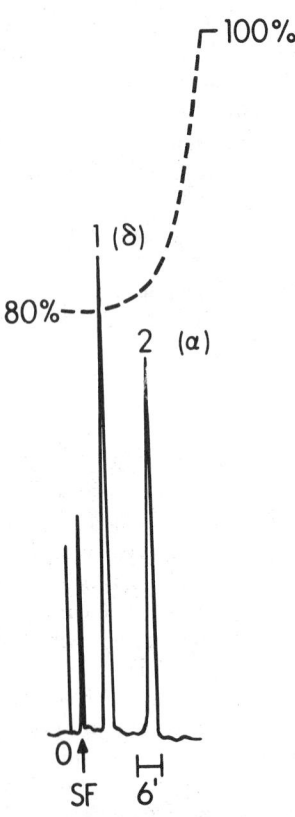

Figure 61-11 Separation of ethylanthranilate azodipyrroles by HPLC. Wistar rat bile was diazotized with ethylanthranilate diazo reagent, azodipyrroles were extracted [205], organic solvents were eliminated in reduced pressure, the pigments were dissolved in methanol and separated by reverse phase HPLC (μ-Bondapak C-18 column, Waters') using a concave gradient (interrupted line) of methanol (80 to 100 percent) in sodium acetate (0.1 M, pH 4.0) containing 5 mM 1-heptane sulfonic acid in 30 min, at 1 ml/min. SF = solvent front. Peak 1 (OD, 530 nm) represents glucuronidated azodipyrrole, which was designated δ by Heirwegh and his associates [205] and peak 2 represents the unconjugated azodipyrrole, designated [205] α (see Fig. 61-10).

phenobarbital [261]. There may be other functional classes and subclasses. Classification on the basis of inducibility may be species-specific. For example, methylcholanthrene induces UDP-glucuronyltransferase activity toward bilirubin in mice [262] but not in rats [261]. Although much evidence suggests heterogeneity of UDP-glucuronyltransferase, there are similarities between the different classes of the enzyme. Gunn rats have not only a deficiency in UDP-glucuronyltransferase activity toward bilirubin but also have defective glucuronidation of p-nitrophenol, o-aminophenol, 1-naphthol, and methylumbelliferone [263]. Antibody prepared against pure rat p-nitrophenol UDP-glucuronyltransferase precipitates p-nitrophenol and bilirubin glucuronidating activity from solubilized rat liver microsomes. This result suggests structural similarity of at least a portion of the enzyme molecule.

Formation of Bilirubin Diglucuronide Since the discovery of UDP-glucuronyltransferase, formation of bilirubin diglucuronide, the major pigment in human, rat, and dog bile, has been presumed to be catalyzed by this enzyme. The major product formed on incubation of bilirubin, UDP-glucuronic acid, and rat liver microsomes is bilirubin monoglucuronide, rather than diglucuronide [264–266]. UDP-glucuronyltransferase accepts many aglycones as substrates, and, theoretically, bilirubin monoglucuronide could be a substrate. In studies of

the separate conversion of bilirubin to bilirubin monoglucuronide and bilirubin monoglucuronide to bilirubin diglucuronide by cat liver microsomes, the two reactions differed in pH optima, inhibition by competitive substrates, and the effect of albumin [267]. UDP-glucuronic acid dependent conversion of bilirubin monoglucuronide to diglucuronide has been shown in a rat liver microsomal system [268]. A second enzyme catalyzing conversion of bilirubin monoglucuronide to diglucuronide was purified from plasma membrane–enriched fractions of rat liver homogenate [269]. The enzyme catalyzes dismutation of 2 mol of bilirubin monoglucuronide to 1 mol of bilirubin diglucuronide and 1 mol of unconjugated bilirubin [270]. The mechanism may involve either transesterification or enzyme-catalyzed rearrangement of dipyrroles. Neither mechanism has been established. The product of the reaction retains the IXα configuration, which is the configuration of bilirubin conjugates in bile [270]. The highest specific activity of the enzyme is in the canalicular-enriched subfraction of rat liver plasma membrane preparations. Enzyme activity is normal in Gunn rat liver and in patients with Crigler-Najjar syndrome who lack UDP-glucuronyltransferase activity toward bilirubin [271]. The function of the enzyme has been tested in vivo. The major bilirubin conjugate in the liver cell is almost exclusively bilirubin monoglucuronide, even in rats which excrete predominantly bilirubin diglucuronide in bile [124]. When unconjugated bilirubin is infused intravenously in rats at rates exceeding the maximum excretory capacity, conjugated bilirubin accumulates in blood. Bilirubin conjugates in serum are mostly bilirubin monoglucuronide, whereas bilirubin diglucuronide is the predominant pigment in bile [270]. Bilirubin monoglucuronide infused in Gunn rats was excreted in bile partly as bilirubin diglucuronide [269, 271]. When bilirubin monoglucuronide with ^{3}H label on bilirubin and ^{14}C label on glucuronic acid was infused in Gunn rats, the bilirubin diglucuronide excreted in bile had twice the ^{14}C/^{3}H ratio compared to the injected pigment. When double-labeled bilirubin monoglucuronide was infused in normal rats, the ^{14}C/^{3}H ratio in the bilirubin diglucuronide

Figure 61-12 Separation of bilirubin diglucuronide (1), bilirubin monoglucuronide C₁₂ (2), and C₈ (3) and unconjugated bilirubin (4) (see Fig. 61-10) on HPLC of Wistar rat bile. Bile (0.025 ml) was chromatographed on a reverse phase (μ-Bondapak C-18, Waters') column. Pigments were eluted with a concave gradient (interrupted line) of methanol (50 to 100 percent in 60 min) in sodium acetate (0.1 M, pH 4.0) containing 5 mM 1-heptane sulfonic acid at 1 ml/min. SF = solvent front.

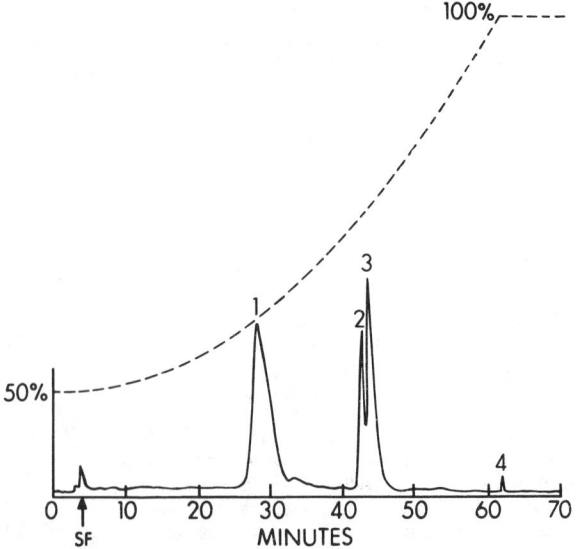

excreted in bile was greater than the ratio in injected bilirubin monoglucuronide, but not double. This may be due to partial conversion of [3H]bilirubin produced in the dismutation reaction to bilirubin diglucuronide. When an excess of unconjugated bilirubin is injected with the double-labeled bilirubin monoglucuronide, the $^{14}C/^3H$ ratio in bilirubin diglucuronide in bile is the same as the ratio in the injected pigment. This suggests that dismutation of bilirubin monoglucuronide is inhibited by a high intrahepatic unconjugated bilirubin concentration [272]. Others have infused double-labeled bilirubin monoglucuronide with an excess of unconjugated bilirubin and found no difference in the $^{14}C/^3H$ ratio in bilirubin diglucuronide excreted in bile and in the injected bilirubin monoglucuronide. Conversion of bilirubin monoglucuronide to bilirubin diglucuronide has also been observed in isolated perfused Gunn rat liver in which the intrahepatic bilirubin concentration was depleted by perfusion with an albumin-containing solution. Conversion to diglucuronide was reduced when the intrahepatic bilirubin was repleted by perfusion with a solution containing bilirubin. These results suggest that bilirubin monoglucuronide is converted to bilirubin diglucuronide by both UDP-glucuronyltransferase and enzymatic dismutation. When the intrahepatic concentration of unconjugated bilirubin is high, dismutation is inhibited, UDP-glucuronyltransferase mechanism persists, and bilirubin diglucuronide formation proceeds at a slower rate than normal.

Biliary Excretion of Bilirubin

Canalicular excretion of bilirubin is thought to be an energy-dependent process which transports the pigment against a concentration gradient. In fish, unconjugated bilirubin can be excreted in bile. In mammals, conjugation is essential in bilirubin excretion. For example, Gunn rats and patients with the Crigler-Najjar syndrome, type I, lack UDP-glucuronyltransferase activity and manifest life-long unconjugated hyperbilirubinemia (see below). Accumulation of conjugated bilirubin in serum following intravenous infusion of unconjugated bilirubin at a rate exceeding the maximal excretory capacity of bilirubin suggests that canalicular transport, rather than conjugation, is rate-limiting in bilirubin excretion [270, 273]. When UDP-glucuronyltransferase activity is partially or totally deficient, conjugation may be rate-limiting in bilirubin excretion [274].

Patients with the Dubin-Johnson syndrome and mutant Corriedale sheep with an analogous hepatic defect have reduced capacity to transport conjugated bilirubin, BSP, indocyanine green (ICG), iopanoic acid, phylloerythrin, and metanephrine glucuronide into the bile. Affected patients and sheep have normal transport maximum for infused taurocholate [275, 276, 277, 278]. A dissociation between bilirubin and bile salt excretory capacity also occurs in the primate fetus [279]. These observations indicate that there are at least two mechanisms for organic anion excretion by the liver, one for bile salts and another for other organic anions.

Maximal bilirubin excretory capacity (T_{max}) depends on bile flow. Flow is increased by infusion of bile salts, [280] or phenobarbital treatment which enhances bile flow rate by a non-bile salt–dependent mechanism [281]. T_{max} of bilirubin is enhanced in both cases. Several other bile salt–independent choleretics increase bile flow, but not the T_{max} for organic anions [282].

It has been proposed that incorporation of bilirubin conjugates in bile salt mixed micelles in bile reduces the concentration of bilirubin in bile and results in canalicular excretion of bilirubin down a gradient into a "micellar sink" [283]. Infusion of non-micelle-forming bile salts also enhances bilirubin excretory capacity [284]. The relationship of bile salt excretion, bile flow, and bilirubin excretion has been studied in patients with gallstones [285]. Approximately one-third of bilirubin excretion has been calculated to be bile salt–independent. This suggests that bile salt micelles are not essential for canalicular transport of conjugated bilirubin in man. Excretion of unconjugated bilirubin, which comprises about 3 percent of bilirubin excreted in humans, may depend on interaction with mixed micelles [286]. Kinetic studies of taurocholate and BSP excretion suggest that there may be an interaction of bile salt receptors and receptors for other organic anions at the level of canalicular excretion [287]. Self-aggregation and incorporation of bilirubin in mixed micelles [283] may occur in bile and decrease the bilirubin concentration in the aqueous phase; the functional significance of this phenomenon is uncertain [6].

Bilirubin, BSP, and ICG apparently compete for biliary excretion. Since these anions compete for hepatic uptake and share intracellular binding proteins, it cannot be assumed that they share a common receptor in the bile canaliculus. Combined bilirubin and BSP infusion studies in rats indicate that BSP is excreted by two canalicular pathways. Bilirubin competes for only one of these [286].

The enzyme-catalyzing dismutation of bilirubin monoglucuronide is concentrated in the canalicular subfraction of rat liver plasma membrane preparations [271]. Since bilirubin diglucuronide is not found within the hepatocyte, despite a high affinity for ligandin [124], a possible linkage may exist between bilirubin monoglucuronide dismutase and biliary secretion of diglucuronide [6].

Fate of Bilirubin in the Gastrointestinal Tract Bilirubin reaches the intestinal tract mainly conjugated and is not substantially absorbed [288]. In some circumstances, there may be enhanced excretion of unconjugated bilirubin into the intestine. Absorption of unconjugated bilirubin from the intestine may contribute to neonatal hyperbilirubinemia [289]. Absorption of bilirubin from the gallbladder occurs in animals [290].

Bilirubin is degraded by intestinal bacteria into a series of urobilinogen and related products [291, 292]. The specific products may relate to strains of bacteria present in the intestine [293]. Urobilinogens are present in deconjugated states. It is not known whether deconjugation precedes or follows bilirubin degradation, but bacterial β-glucuronidase plays a role in the deconjugation [289, 294]. Most of the urobilinogen reabsorbed from the intestine is reexcreted in the bile. A small fraction is excreted by the kidney. Enhanced tubular absorption and instability of the pigment in acid urine makes urobilinogen excretion in urine an unreliable indicator of the status of bilirubin metabolism. Absence of urobilinogen in stool and urine indicates complete obstruction of the bile duct. In liver disease and increased bilirubin production, urinary urobilinogen excretion is increased. Urobilinogen is colorless. Oxidation leads to formation of urobilin, which contributes to the color of normal urine and stool.

Alternate Pathways of Bilirubin Elimination After injection of labeled unconjugated bilirubin only 3 percent of radioactivity is normally excreted by the kidney in humans [295]. Even in the presence of marked hyperbilirubinemia, bile remains the main route of bilirubin excretion [6].

In patients with Crigler-Najjar syndrome and in Gunn rats, a small amount of unconjugated bilirubin is secreted in bile. Additional unconjugated bilirubin may reach the intestinal lumen by passage across the intestinal wall or by desquamation of intestinal epithelial cells [296]. Ambient light or phototherapy forms geometric isomers of bilirubin (EE, EZ, or ZE forms), which are excreted in unconjugated form and converted to bilirubin IXα-ZZ in the bile [297, 298, 60]. Considerable bilirubin is degraded to polar diazo-negative compounds which are excreted in both bile and urine [296]. A fraction of pigment is converted to tetrapyrrole dihydroxyl derivatives and dipyrroles [299, 300]. Bilirubin catabolism in the liver is enhanced by induction of mixed function oxidases [301].

In intrahepatic or extrahepatic cholestasis, the plasma-conjugated bilirubin concentration increases. After injection of radiolabeled bilirubin in animals with experimentally ligated bile ducts [302] and in children with biliary atresia [303], 50 to 90 percent of injected radioactivity is excreted in urine. In total biliary obstruction, urinary excretion becomes the major pathway of bilirubin excretion [304]. Renal excretion of conjugated bilirubin depends on glomerular filtration of a small non-protein-bound fraction of conjugated bilirubin [304, 305]. There is evidence for tubular reabsorption but none for tubular secretion of bilirubin [305].

DISORDERS OF BILIRUBIN METABOLISM

The hepatic transport of bilirubin involves four distinct but probably interrelated stages: (1) uptake from the circulation; (2) intracellular binding or storage; (3) conjugation, largely with glucuronic acid; and (4) biliary excretion. Abnormalities in any of these processes may result in hyperbilirubinemia. Complex clinical disorders, such as hepatitis or cirrhosis, may affect multiple processes. In several inheritable disorders, the transfer of bilirubin from blood to bile is disrupted at a specific step. Study of these disorders has permitted better understanding of bilirubin metabolism in health and disease. Each disorder is characterized by varied degrees of hyperbilirubinemia of the unconjugated or conjugated type.

Disorders of Bilirubin Metabolism Resulting in Predominantly Unconjugated Hyperbilirubinemia

Neonatal Hyperbilirubinemia By adult standards, every newborn baby has hyperbilirubinemia, and about half of all neonates become clinically jaundiced during the first 5 days of life. Serum bilirubin is predominantly unconjugated. Exaggeration of this "physiologic jaundice" can result in marked hyperbilirubinemia with an attendant risk of kernicterus (see "Bilirubin Toxicity"). In 4000 consecutive infants, 16 percent had maximal serum bilirubin concentrations of 10 mg/dl or above, and in 5 percent, bilirubin concentrations exceeded 15 mg/dl [306]. In the normal, full-term human neonate, the

serum bilirubin concentration increases rapidly from 1–2 to 5–6 mg/dl in approximately 72 h and subsequently decreases until normal levels are attained in 7 to 10 days [307]. Physiologic jaundice of the newborn appears to result from a combination of increased bilirubin production and delayed maturation in the capability of the liver to dispose of bilirubin. Severe neonatal unconjugated hyperbilirubinemia results from exaggeration in one or more of the regularly occurring developmental restrictions which are characteristic of the newborn period or superimposition of additional mechanisms.

BILIRUBIN PRODUCTION Increased bilirubin production in the newborn period is evidenced by increased endogenous carbon monoxide production [308], early-labeled peak from erythroid and nonerythroid sources [309], and decreased erythrocyte half-life [310]. The meconium contains unconjugated bilirubin which is primarily derived from hydrolysis of conjugated bilirubin by intestinal β-glucuronidase [311]. As compared to adults, newborns lack intestinal bacteria which degrade bilirubin to urobilinogen and have a greater surface to volume ratio of the bowel. As a result, intestinal absorption of unconjugated bilirubin in neonates may be increased [311, 312]. Hemolytic diseases of the fetus increases bilirubin production and may lead to severe neonatal unconjugated hyperbilirubinemia. Rh incompatibility between mother and fetus was formerly a common cause of severe neonatal unconjugated hyperbilirubinemia and kernicterus ("erythroblastosis fetalis"). This disease can be prevented by treatment of the mother with anti-Rh immunoglobulins [313, 314]. Major blood group (ABO) incompatibility remains a common cause of exaggerated neonatal hyperbilirubinemia, which often requires treatment [315, 316].

HEPATIC BILIRUBIN UPTAKE Cumulative hepatic bilirubin uptake capacity is reduced during the first 24 h of life in the rhesus monkey. Relative hepatic uptake deficiency extends beyond the second day of life and correlates with maturation of hepatic ligandin [317, 318, 319] which influences the "net" hepatic uptake of bilirubin (see "Bilirubin Uptake"). Delayed closure of the ductus venosus may permit portal blood, which is enriched in unconjugated bilirubin from the intestine, to bypass the liver [320]. Reduced caloric intake, which reduces hepatic bilirubin clearance in adults (see "Gilbert's Syndrome"), may have a similar effect in neonates.

HEPATIC BILIRUBIN CONJUGATION In many mammals, including humans, UDP-glucuronyltransferase activity toward bilirubin is deficient in fetal liver and rapidly develops to adult levels during the first few days of life [321]. In fetal dog liver, UDP-glucuronyltransferase activity toward bilirubin is relatively mature, and newborn puppies do not have unconjugated hyperbilirubinemia [322]. Deficiency in bilirubin conjugation is not the only defect in the newborn; BSP clearance [323] and T_{max} for conjugated bilirubin [324] are also reduced. Deficiency of UDP-glucuronyltransferase activity may be prolonged and exaggerated in some inheritable disorders due to inhibitory factor(s) in maternal milk or serum (see below).

CANALICULAR EXCRETION OF BILIRUBIN During the late newborn period, hepatic bilirubin uptake, conjugation, and canalicular excretion attain adult levels, while the bilirubin load remains increased. In this period of life, as in adults, canalicular excretion appears to be rate-limiting in the hepatic disposition of bilirubin. Consequently, when the bilirubin load is further increased, conjugated bilirubin accumulates in serum [325].

Transient Nonhemolytic Unconjugated Hyperbilirubinemia Associated with Breast-feeding   Plasma bilirubin concentrations tend to be higher in breast-fed infants as compared with formula-fed babies [326] and occasionally rise to maximum concentrations of 15 to 24 mg/dl within 10 to 19 days of life [327]. Discontinuation of breast-feeding promptly ameliorates jaundice, which otherwise disappears within 1 month. No infant with this syndrome has developed kernicterus [327].

Neonatal unconjugated hyperbilirubinemia related to breast-feeding is associated with an inhibitor of UDP-glucuronyltransferase activity in maternal milk but not maternal serum [327, 328, 329]. A progestational steroid, 3α,20β-pregnanediol, was isolated from the milk of mothers of infants who had the syndrome. The steroid inhibited o-aminophenol glucuronidation by guinea pig liver microsomes [327] and bilirubin glucuronidation by rat and rabbit liver [327, 328], but not by human liver [330]. Experimental feeding of the steroid to healthy infants yielded contradictory results [331, 332]. Women whose infants have prolonged jaundice associated with breast-feeding have increased amounts of 3α,20β-pregnanediol in their urine [333].

The free fatty acid concentration in maternal milk correlates positively with its inhibitory effect on human hepatic glucuronyltransferase activity [331], and free fatty acids inhibit UDP-glucuronyltransferase activity in vitro in proportion to the number of double bonds in unsaturated fatty acids and in inverse proportion to the chain lengths of saturated fatty acids (C_{10} to C_{18}) [334]. Odievre and associates postulate that a lipolytic enzyme which is present in some maternal milk samples may be responsible for the increased concentration of free fatty acids in the milk. The inhibitory effect of maternal milk on UDP-glucuronyltransferase increases on storage and is destroyed by heating at 56°C [334]. Prolonged neonatal jaundice in breast-fed infants appears to result from multiple causes.

Transient Familial Neonatal Hyperbilirubinemia   In this syndrome, which was described by Lucey, Arias, and their associates in 1965 [335, 336], jaundice occurs within the first 4 days of life. In 24 infants [336], peak serum bilirubin concentrations of 8.9 to 65 mg/dl were reached within 7 days. An unidentified inhibitor of UDP glucuronyltransferase was found in the serum of mothers of these infants [336]. Kernicterus was observed at autopsy in three infants. One died at 36 h. This condition is clinically distinguished from jaundice associated with digestion of maternal milk by earlier onset of severe hyperbilirubinemia and occasional kernicterus.

Management of Neonatal Unconjugated Hyperbilirubinemia   Although a plasma bilirubin concentration of 20 mg/dl is usually considered dangerous, kernicterus occurs at lower concentrations of bilirubin (see "Toxicity of Bilirubin"). The goal of treatment is to decrease serum bilirubin concentrations to an acceptable level until the capacity of the liver to dispose of bilirubin matures. Exchange transfusion and phototherapy are the two most commonly used modes of management (see "Treatment of Crigler-Najjar Syndrome, Type I"). Although phototherapy is useful and safe, concern persists

about its potential side effects. Ingestion of agar to bind unconjugated bilirubin in the intestine also decreases serum bilirubin concentrations [312], but the efficacy of this treatment is not certain [311].

Increased Bilirubin Production   Hyperbilirubinemia in the presence of normal liver function often occurs in disorders associated with increased bilirubin production. The serum bilirubin is unconjugated and rarely exceeds 3 to 4 mg/dl. Higher levels usually indicate hepatobiliary dysfunction in addition to bilirubin overproduction [6, 337]. The most common cause of increased bilirubin production is hemolysis such as occurs in sickle-cell anemia, hereditary spherocytosis, and toxic or idiosyncratic drug reactions in susceptible individuals. These disorders are associated with premature destruction of erythrocytes, and, consequently, determinations of red cell life span and red cell morphology are abnormal. Rarely, in acute massive hemolysis the rate of bilirubin production may transiently exceed the excretory transport maximum for biliary excretion of conjugated bilirubin, and conjugated hyperbilirubinemia may result [338, 339]. Ineffective erythropoiesis occurs in thalassemia and other hematologic disorders and is often associated with hyperbilirubinemia [340]. Congenital dyserythropoietic anemias are a group of rare hereditary anemias that are characterized by ineffective erythropoiesis, intramedullary normoblastic hyperplasia, secondary hemochromatosis, and unconjugated hyperbilirubinemia [341–344].

Crigler-Najjar Syndrome, Type I

CLINICAL FINDINGS   Crigler-Najjar syndrome, type I, is a rare disorder in which hepatic bilirubin UDP glucuronyltransferase is absent (Table 61-1). The syndrome was described by Crigler and Najjar in 1952 in six infants in three related families [345]. All infants manifested severe nonhemolytic icterus within the first few days of life. Jaundice was characterized by increased plasma concentration of indirect-reacting bilirubin and was lifelong. Five of the six infants died of kernicterus by the age of 15 months. Although icteric, the single surviving infant was free of neurologic disease until 15 years of age, when he suddenly developed kernicterus and died 6 months later [346, 347]. A female cousin also had Crigler-Najjar syndrome with neurologic symptoms developing at 18 years of age. She died at the age of 24 [6, 348, 349]. This family has increased consanguinity and several other recessively inherited traits, such as Morquio's syndrome, homocystinuria, metachromatic leukodystrophy, and bird-headed dwarfism [350].

Since 1952, approximately 60 other patients with Crigler-Najjar syndrome, type I, have been described, almost all of whom died with kernicterus during the neonatal period [6, 351, 352]. Survival past the neonatal period is uncommon, but several individuals have survived only to succumb to kernicterus later in life [346, 348, 249, 352–354]. With the advent of better treatment of neonatal hyperbilirubinemia, individuals with this disorder survive into childhood. The syndrome occurs in all races, is transmitted as an autosomal recessive trait (Fig. 61-13) [347, 355, 356], and is often associated with consanguinity.

LABORATORY EXAMINATION   Laboratory test results in Crigler-Najjar syndrome, type 1, are normal except for the serum bilirubin level, which is usually 20 to 25 mg/dl, but may be as high as 50 mg/dl [345–349, 351–353, 355, 356]. Virtu-

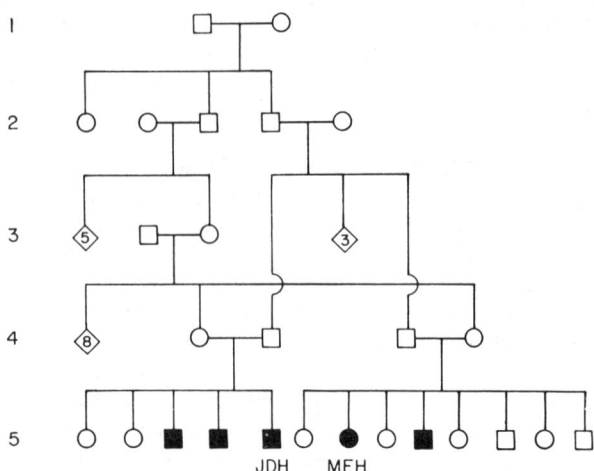

Figure 61-13 Inheritance of Crigler-Najjar syndrome, type I. This family, originally described by Crigler and Najjar in 1952, is unique in that two cousins, JDH and MEH, escaped kernicterus in infancy only to die at ages 16 and 24, respectively. (*From Blaschke et al. [348]. Used by permission.*)

ally all of the serum bilirubin is unconjugated, and no serum conjugated bilirubin has been found. There is no bilirubinuria, but the urine may be yellow due to a chloroform-soluble pigment of unknown structure [357]. The level of icterus in a given patient may vary and is lower in summer, and on exposure to sun, and is higher during intercurrent illness [296, 348, 352, 358]. The bile may be pale [356] (see below). Stool color is normal, and fecal urobilinogen excretion is reduced [345, 356, 359]. Bilirubin production [296, 348, 359], hematocrit, bone marrow morphology, and red cell survival [348, 356, 358] are normal. Results of routine liver function tests are normal, including studies of plasma disappearance of BSP [345, 348] and ICG [348] and radiologic visualization of the biliary tree by cholecystographic agents. The patients have normal physical examinations, apart from jaundice and neurologic impairment, and lack hepatosplenomegaly. Liver biopsy reveals normal histology. In several patients, canalicular and bile ductular cholestasis were described (Fig. 61-14) [345, 348, 352]. This probably results from biliary excretion of unconjugated bilirubin as an effect of phototherapy, with subsequent precipitation of bilirubin in the bile canaliculi. Electron microscopy of the liver reveals no specific pathologic change [360–364].

Gunn Rat The description by Gunn in 1938 of mutant Wistar rats with nonhemolytic unconjugated hyperbilirubinemia [365] and the wisdom of the late Professor William E. Castle, emeritus professor of genetics at Berkeley, who maintained the mutants for over 15 years, have resulted in major advances in understanding bilirubin metabolism, transport, and encephalopathy. Jaundice in these animals is inherited as an autosomal recessive trait [365]. Heterozygotes are anicteric. Homozygous rats have bilirubin levels that range from 3 to 20 mg/dl, depending upon the rat strain. All serum bilirubin is unconjugated [366], there is no bilirubinuria, and bile is virtually colorless, although small amounts of nonglucuronide and glucuronide conjugates of bilirubin have been detected [300]. Liver histology is normal by light microscopy [366] and shows minor nonspecific structural modifications of the endoplasmic reticulum on electron microscopy [360].

Homozygous Gunn rats are prototypes of Crigler-Najjar syndrome, type I, and frequently develop kernicterus [352,

367, 368]. Before studies in the Gunn rat, investigation of the pathogenesis of bilirubin encephalopathy was hampered by lack of a good experimental model [352]. Regional staining of the brain and selective necrosis of gray matter nuclei could not be produced in experimental animals by infusion of bilirubin, unless there was superimposed asphyxia. The Gunn rat is the only experimental model in which endogenously produced bilirubin results in neuropathologic lesions and neurologic deficits. These rats develop cytoplasmic neuronal changes on the third day of life, and by 2 weeks, degeneration of Purkinje cells and other neurons occurs. These degenerative changes begin by enlargement of mitochondria and formation of membranous cytoplasmic bodies. By 8 days of age many mitochondria contain glycogen [369, 370]. Although all Gunn rats have degenerative lesions of the brain, only half have gross disturbances of gait [352]. When a healthy Gunn rat is killed and rapidly perfused with saline or formalin, the brain does not show yellow staining. Administration of sulfadimethoxine, a drug that competes with bilirubin for binding to albumin, to 14-day-old animals results in neurologic deterioration and yellow staining in the brain [371]. The basis of selectivity of bilirubin for certain types of neurons is unknown [113]. Whether these neurons specifically bind bilirubin or depend on metabolic processes that are specifically inhibited by bilirubin cannot be answered at the present time [92, 372].

Gunn rats are unable to concentrate urine and do not tolerate water deprivation [373, 374]. The renal medullary bilirubin concentration in these animals is high and interferes with sodium and water transport [373–375]. Occasionally, renal papillary necrosis occurs [375]. Treatment of rats with agents designed to lower serum bilirubin, such as cholestyramine, agar, or phototherapy, may ameliorate the renal lesion [374, 376]. Similar concentrating problems have not been described in patients with Crigler-Najjar syndrome, type I, although bilirubin is deposited in the kidney [133, 377]. Hereditary hydronephrosis and renal cysts occur in some Gunn rat colonies but are unrelated to the disorder in bilirubin metabolism and reflect a concomitant genetic abnormality [378].

Figure 61-14 High power view (hematoxylin and eosin; magnification ×650) of a liver biopsy obtained from a patient with Crigler-Najjar syndrome, type I, during phototherapy. A portal area is shown with portal vein (PV) and a bile ductule B containing amorphous material, which appeared to be bilirubin. (*From Wolkoff et al. [352]. Used by permission.*)

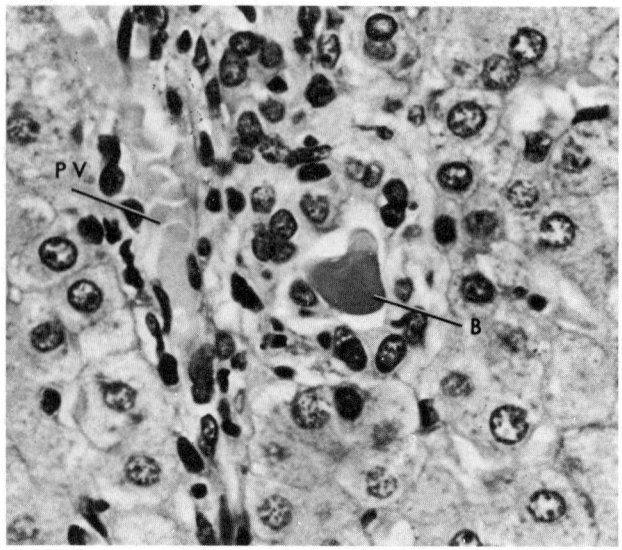

BIOCHEMICAL DEFECT   Similar to patients with Crigler-Najjar syndrome, type I, Gunn rats have virtually no bilirubin conjugates in bile [296, 300, 366]. Although they can excrete many organic anions, including BSP [300], phenol red [379], and conjugated bilirubin [131, 273], little if any exogenously administered unconjugated bilirubin is excreted in bile [54, 366, 274]. Aside from impaired formation of bilirubin glucuronides, conjugation of other xenobiotics with glucuronic acid is also reduced in vivo and in vitro. Study of the biochemistry and physiology of the conjugation defect in these rats has led to much of our current understanding of hepatic bilirubin glucuronidation, which is described in further detail in the section on conjugation.

TREATMENT OF CRIGLER-NAJJAR SYNDROME, TYPE I
Unconjugated hyperbilirubinemia in Crigler-Najjar syndrome, type I, is usually associated with bilirubin encephalopathy ("kernicterus"). Treatment is designed to reduce serum bilirubin levels and is often ineffective or impractical on a long-term basis. Unlike results in patients with Crigler-Najjar syndrome, type II, and Gilbert's syndrome, the serum bilirubin level and hepatic bilirubin glucuronidation activity do not respond to phenobarbital administration [348, 356, 358, 380, 381]. Plasmapheresis is the most efficient means for reducing serum bilirubin concentration acutely (Fig. 61-15) [348, 349, 352]. This procedure takes advantage of the fact that bilirubin is tightly bound to serum albumin and may be quantitatively removed from the body by removal of albumin. Phototherapy has received widespread acceptance and is the major treatment for icteric newborns whose serum bilirubin concentrations place them at risk for kernicterus [297, 348, 349, 352, 380–383]. Experience with phototherapy in older children and adults is limited to patients with Crigler-Najjar syndrome, type I. After children reach 3 or 4 years of age, phototherapy becomes relatively less effective due to thickening of the skin, increased skin pigmentation, and decreased surface area in relation to body mass [352]. The mechanisms whereby phototherapy reduces serum bilirubin concentrations are complex and are described in the section on chemistry of bilirubin.

Chronic phlebotomy in Crigler-Najjar syndrome, type I, was employed in one patient to reduce the average age of circulating erythrocytes and hence to reduce bilirubin production [384]. As expected, bilirubin production fell significantly but was accompanied by an unexpected and unexplained reduction in plasma bilirubin clearance. The plasma bilirubin level remained unaffected. Affinity chromotography of bilirubin-containing blood on albumin-conjugated agarose gel has also been suggested as treatment for this disorder [349, 385, 386]. While effective in reducing hyperbilirubinemia in Gunn rats, difficulties due to removal of formed elements are encountered with simian or human blood [387, 388].

Because Crigler-Najjar syndrome, type I, results from deficiency of a single enzyme, enzyme replacement may be a realistic means of therapy in the future. In the rat, bilirubin UDP-glucuronyltransferase is present in kidney and liver. Transplantation of kidney from a normal rat into a Gunn rat reduces hyperbilirubinemia [271, 389]. Enzyme activity in the human kidney is below the limit of detectability and, therefore, renal transplantation in Crigler-Najjar syndrome, type I, cannot be recommended. Following subcutaneous transplantation of cells from a clonal strain of rat hepatoma, Gunn rats developed the capacity to conjugate bilirubin, which was excreted subsequently into bile [390]. Transplantation of small pieces of

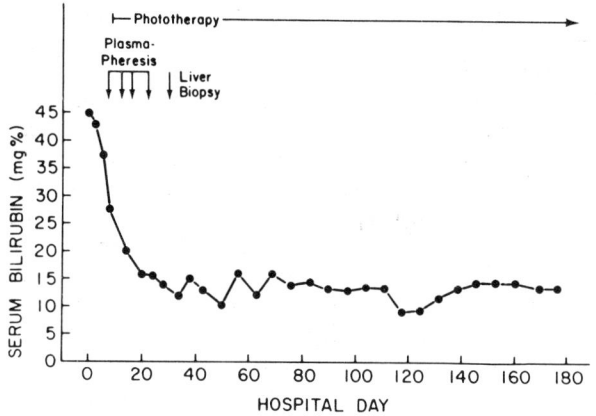

Figure 61-15 Summary of the hospital course of a 19-year-old patient with Crigler-Najjar syndrome, type I, who was admitted with acute bilirubin encephalopathy. Before hospitalization, the patient's serum bilirubin ranged between 35 and 45 mg/dl. After an initial course of plasmapheresis and maintenance phototherapy, serum bilirubin was maintained between 10 and 15 mg/dl. (*From Wolkoff et al. [352]. Used by permission.*)

normal Wistar rat liver into the liver of Gunn rats reduced serum bilirubin concentrations and produced normal hepatic UDP-glucuronyltransferase activity [391], but an attempt to confirm these results [392] was unsuccessful. Serum bilirubin levels were reduced in immunosuppressed Gunn rats 2 months after portal vein infusion of hepatocytes isolated from heterozygous Gunn rats [393]. Similar results were obtained in another study in which iron-labeled hepatocytes from normal rats were infused into the portal vein of Gunn rats, with subsequent appearance of bilirubin conjugates in bile and UDP-glucuronyltransferase activity in liver [394]. Enzyme activity remained even after apparent degeneration of transplanted hepatocytes. As experience with enzyme replacement therapy for other disorders accumulates, it is hoped that treatment will become available for patients with Crigler-Najjar syndrome, type I.

Crigler-Najjar Syndrome, Type II

CLNICAL FINDINGS   Crigler-Najjar syndrome, type II, is phenotypically similar to Crigler-Najjar syndrome, type I, except that it is almost always clinically benign, and the serum bilirubin concentration is usually below 20 mg/dl (Table 61-1) [337]. This disorder was first described in 1962 [353] in a study of chronic unconjugated hyperbilirubinemia in 8 patients between 14 and 52 years of age. Although half the patients were known to be icteric before the age of 1 year, one patient was 30 years old before jaundice was noted. In these patients, serum bilirubin concentration ranged from 8 to 18 mg/dl; each had reduced hepatic glucuronyltransferase activities using bilirubin, o-aminophenol, or 4-methylumbelliferone as glucuronide acceptor. [^{51}Cr] Red cell survival was normal. All patients were clinically normal, apart from icterus, except for a 43-year-old female with a neurologic syndrome resembling kernicterus. The patient died at the age of 44. Autopsy revealed a histologically normal liver. The brain was small and lacked bilirubin staining but demonstrated the typical histology of kernicterus.

Other cases have been described subsequently. Three brothers had Crigler-Najjar syndrome, type II, for over 50 years [395]. Two were neurologically normal, while the third had a slight bilateral intention tremor and nonspecific abnormalities on electroencephalogram. These nonspecific neurologic changes had not been noted previously. The third patient was a 15-year-old male who was icteric from the second day of life [396]. Total serum bilirubin was 24 mg/dl at 10 months and averaged approximately 15 mg/dl thereafter. Development was normal, although psychological testing revealed a perceptual deficit and slightly subnormal intelligence. At age 13, following surgery for acute appendicitis, the serum bilirubin rose to 40 mg/dl, and the patient developed diplopia, generalized seizures, confusion, and an abnormal electroencephalogram. He was treated for hyperbilirubinemia and, after recovering from surgery, resumed a bilirubin level of 15 mg/dl. His neurologic status returned to baseline and he has remained well.

LABORATORY EXAMINATION As in Crigler-Najjar syndrome, type I, laboratory examination is normal except for elevated serum bilirubin, which is usually less than 20 mg/dl but may be as high as 40 mg/dl during fasting [395] or intercurrent illness [396]. Serum bilirubin is unconjugated and there is no bilirubinuria. The bile is pigmented, although less than 50 percent of estimated daily bilirubin production was excreted into the bile [356, 396]. While over 90 percent of conjugated bilirubin in normal bile is bilirubin diglucuronide, the major pigment in this syndrome is bilirubin monoglucuronide [396, 397]. The biochemical reason for this change in biliary conjugates is not known. The liver has virtually no bilirubin UDP-glucuronyltransferase activity [353, 356].

EFFECT OF PHENOBARBITAL The reduced levels of hepatic bilirubin UDP-glucuronyltransferase activity in Crigler-Najjar syndrome, type II, suggested that an inducer of microsomal enzymes could ameliorate the hyperbilirubinemia [398–400]. Subsequent study revealed that hyperbilirubinemia is reduced following treatment with phenobarbital [356]. Similar results were obtained with other liver microsomal enzyme inducers [401–405]. The response to phenobarbital treatment differentiates Crigler-Najjar syndrome, type I, in which there is no response, from Crigler-Najjar syndrome, type II (Fig. 61-16) [356]. Although phenobarbital may act by inducing bilirubin UDP-glucuronyltransferase activity, increased enzyme activity has only rarely been demonstrated (Fig. 61-17) [395, 404]. Assay for this enzyme is relatively insensitive, and a small increase in activity could ameliorate hyperbilirubinemia.

INHERITANCE Crigler-Najjar syndrome, type II, commonly occurs in families [353, 356]. There is neither sex predilection nor evidence of consanguinity. The pattern of inheritance is not certain. Both autosomal dominant transmission with incomplete penetrance [353, 356] and autosomal recessive transmission [405, 406] have been suggested. In one study of three families, parents and sibs of affected individuals had mild unconjugated hyperbilirubinemia consistent with Gilbert's syndrome [405, 406], and it was suggested that Crigler-Najjar syndrome, type II, might represent a homozygous form of Gilbert's syndrome [407]. Whether Crigler-Najjar syndrome, type II, differs from Gilbert's syndrome or represents a more severe form is conjectural. More detailed biochemical analysis of bilirubin conjugates in patients and their families may clarify the inheritance of this disorder [396, 397].

Gilbert's Syndrome

CLINICAL FINDINGS This syndrome, described by Gilbert in 1901, has also been called constitutional hepatic dysfunction and familial nonhemolytic jaundice [408, 409]. It is characterized by mild, chronic, unconjugated hyperbilirubinemia (Table 61-1). Familial occurrence is common [401], and a dominant mode of inheritance has been suggested [411], although most patients present as isolated cases.

Typically, Gilbert's syndrome is diagnosed in young adults who present with mild, predominantly unconjugated hyperbilirubinemia [412]. Serum bilirubin levels are usually less than 3 mg/dl, fluctuate with time, and rise to higher levels during intercurrent illness. Aside from icterus, physical examination is normal. Some patients complain of vague constitutional symptoms, including fatigue and abdominal discomfort [412]. These patients usually have seen many physicians and have undergone many diagnostic tests. Their symptoms are probably manifestations of anxiety. Newly presenting patients are rarely symptomatic. Results of routine laboratory tests in Gilbert's syndrome are normal except for elevated serum bilirubin concentrations. There is no elevation of serum alkaline phosphatase or aminotransferase activities. Oral cholecystography allows visualization of the gallbladder. Although percutaneous liver biopsy is not routinely indicated in patients with Gilbert's syndrome, liver histology is normal. Often, a nonspecific accumulation of lipofuscin pigment is seen in the centrilobular

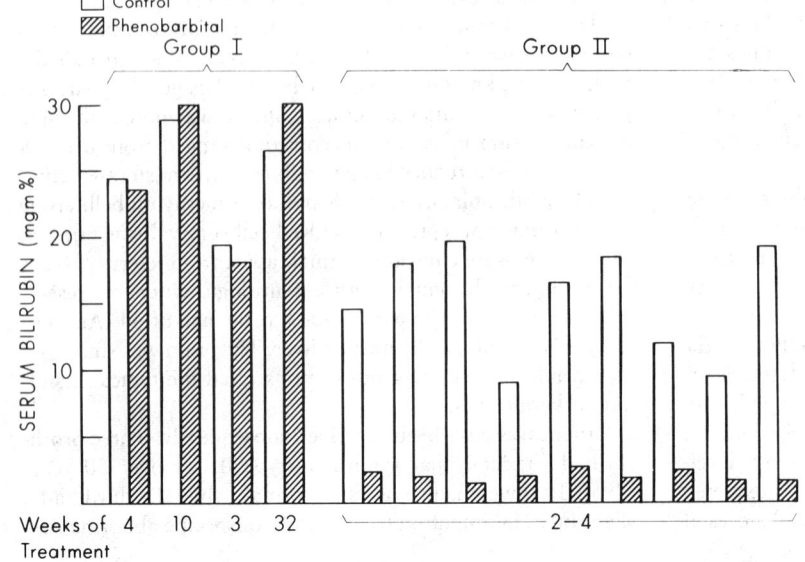

Figure 61-16 Differentiation of types I and II Crigler-Najjar syndrome on the basis of response to phenobarbital. All patients had chronic unconjugated hyperbilirubinemia and were treated for at least several weeks with phenobarbital. (*From Arias et al.* [356]. *Used by permission.*)

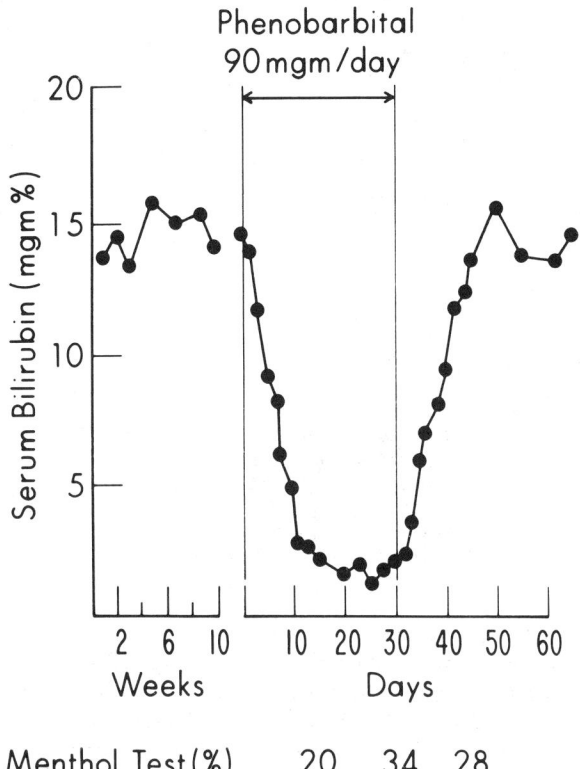

Menthol Test (%)   20   34   28

Fecal Urobilinogen   40   125   65
(mgm/day)

Figure 61-17 The effect of phenobarbital administration on serum bilirubin concentration, menthol tolerance test, and fecal urobilinogen excretion in a patient with Crigler-Najjar syndrome, type II. (*From Arias et al.* [356]. *Used by permission.*)

zones [360, 413, 413]. Electron-microscopic studies have not revealed consistent ultrastructural alterations [415–417].

ORGANIC ANION TRANSPORT   The pathogenesis of unconjugated hyperbilirubinemia in Gilbert's syndrome is not known. Several studies of the disappearance of plasma bilirubin after intravenous injection into patients with Gilbert's syndrome have demonstrated reduced clearance (Fig. 61-18) [404, 418–423]. Multicompartmental analysis suggests that reduced plasma clearance results from reduction in hepatic bilirubin uptake as well as bilirubin conjugation [418, 419, 421, 422]. Because the hepatic uptake of bilirubin is independent of intracellular events, such as protein binding [133], the presence of defects in uptake and conjugation in Gilbert's syndrome suggests coexistence of two seemingly unrelated biochemical abnormalities. Goresky et al. [424] determined the initial plasma disappearance of radiolabeled bilirubin and then determined an initial space of distribution by dividing the injected dose by the plasma volume as determined after radiolabeled albumin injection. The initial plasma disappearance of bilirubin was as rapid in patients with Gilbert's syndrome as in normal subjects. These results suggest that uptake of bilirubin is normal in Gilbert's syndrome [424, 425]. Reduced activity of hepatic bilirubin UDP-glucuronyltransferase has been described in Gilbert's syndrome (Fig. 61-19) [353, 356, 404, 426–429]. Its relationship to hyperbilirubinemia is not clear, since the remaining enzyme activity exceeds by tenfold that necessary to conjugate normal daily bilirubin production. Because of low intrinsic activity this membrane-bound enzyme

is assayed after activation with detergents [426]. Consequently the measured enzyme activity may not truly reflect that which is physiologically available. Administration of phenobarbital or other microsomal enzyme inducers reduces the hyperbilirubinemia in Gilbert's syndrome and increases the plasma clearance of bilirubin [404, 405, 430, 431]. Hepatic bilirubin UDP-glucuronyltransferase activity does not increase in these patients [349, 404, 428, 432].

It is likely that Gilbert's syndrome represents a heterogeneous group of disorders, some of which have an anion uptake defect. Although plasma disappearance of organic anions other than bilirubin is usually normal in Gilbert's syndrome (Fig. 61-20), two subsets have been described in which BSP [433–435] and ICG [436] plasma disappearance is abnormal (Fig. 61-21). In one group reduced BSP and ICG plasma disappearance suggests reduced hepatic uptake. In the second group compartmental analysis revealed a defect in BSP transport at a later stage in the transport process. BSP is conjugated in the liver with glutathione, whereas ICG is excreted into bile intact. Excretion of neither of these compounds depends on bilirubin UDP-glucuronyltransferase activity, since their plasma disappearance is normal in Crigler-Najjar syndrome, type I, and in Gunn rats.

The serum bilirubin level in a patient with Gilbert's syndrome fluctuates for unknown reasons [412]. Factors such as intercurrent illness, physical exertion, and stress have been implicated, and a relationship to the menstrual cycle has been reported in two women [437]. A 48-h fast exaggerates the unconjugated hyperbilirubinemia of Gilbert's syndrome [423, 432, 438–444]. Serum bilirubin levels in normal individuals [432, 438–444] and in individuals with other hepatobiliary disorders also rise with fasting [432, 440]. Although serum bilirubin response following a 48-h fast has been claimed to be diagnostic of Gilbert's syndrome, this is controversial. The fasting test appears to be of limited use in the differential diagnosis of Gilbert's syndrome.

The mechanism of fasting-induced hyperbilirubinemia is not understood. It results from reduced hepatic clearance of bilirubin from plasma rather than increased production of bilirubin [404, 431, 444]. Studies in normal rats revealed no change in hepatic bilirubin UDP-glucuronyltransferase activity during fasting [445], although there was reduced activity of UDP-glucose dehydrogenase resulting in reduced hepatic content of UDPGA [446]. Fasting must also affect hepatic disposition of bilirubin at a step other than conjugation, because fasting exacerbates hyperbilirubinemia in homozygous Gunn rats [444, 445, 447, 448]. It may be a result of several factors, and roles for increased serum nonesterified fatty acids [449] and reduced hepatic content of the cytosolic ligandin and Z protein [450] have been suggested.

Intravenous nicotinic acid administration has also been proposed as a provocative test for the diagnosis of Gilbert's syndrome [451, 452]. Like fasting, its diagnostic value is controversial, and it does not clearly separate patients with Gilbert's syndrome from normal subjects or those with hepatobiliary disease [452, 453]. Unconjugated hyperbilirubinemia following nicotinic acid administration does not occur after splenectomy [451], and nicotinic acid–induced unconjugated hyperbilirubinemia is probably the result of increased erythrocyte fragility, increased splenic heme oxygenase activity, and increased splenic bilirubin formation [454].

The diagnosis of Gilbert's syndrome has conventionally been applied to individuals with mild unconjugated hyperbilirubinemia without evidence of hemolysis or structural liver

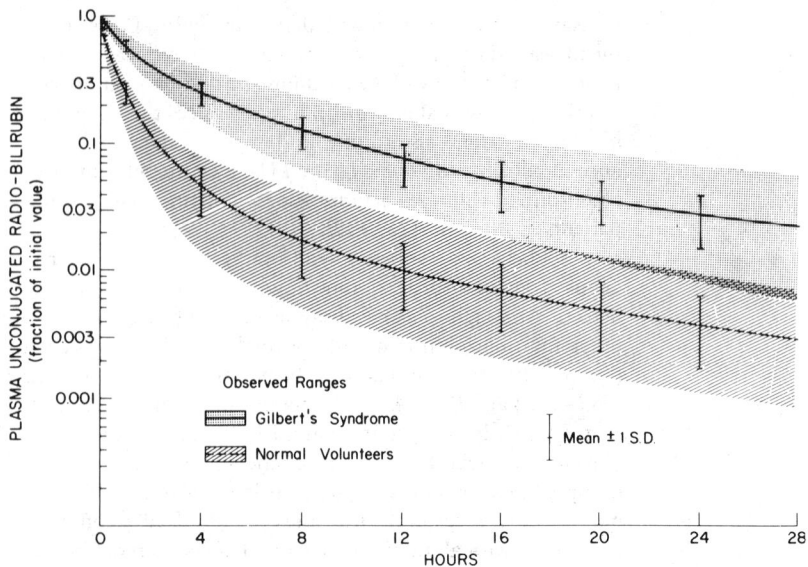

Figure 61-18 Plasma disappearance of a tracer dose of [³H]bilirubin after intravenous administration to patients with Gilbert's syndrome and normal volunteers. There is no overlap between the two groups for the first 16 h after injection. (*From Berk et al. [419]. Used by permission.*)

disease. By determining plasma clearance of radiolabeled bilirubin in hyperbilirubinemic patients with hemolysis, individuals with reduced clearance, as is characteristic of Gilbert's syndrome, were described [419, 420, 455]. Gilbert's syndrome may be more frequently seen in chronic hemolysis [456], because the combination of both factors results in higher, more clinically apparent bilirubin levels than in individuals with either abnormality alone. In a recent investigation radiolabeled bilirubin clearance studies were performed in patients with chronic hemolysis due to hereditary spherocytosis [457]. Following elective splenectomy, which normalized the hemolytic state, the studies were repeated. In seven patients, initially normal values for bilirubin clearance were unaltered by surgery. In another seven patients, low preoperative bilirubin clearance values uniformly improved following splenectomy and became normal in five patients. Family studies and reduced activity of hepatic bilirubin UDP-glucuronyltransferase supported the initial diagnosis of Gilbert's syndrome. These patients may represent a latent form of Gilbert's syndrome which is unmasked by increased bilirubin production during hemolysis.

The relative content of bilirubin mono- and diglucuronide in bile may be of great potential use in the diagnosis of Gilbert's syndrome. Similar to findings in patients with Crigler-Najjar syndrome, type II, and heterozygous Gunn rats, bile from patients with Gilbert's syndrome has an increased proportion of bilirubin monoglucuronide (Table 61-2) [396, 397, 424, 458]. The relationship of reduced hepatic bilirubin UDP-glucuronyltransferase activity to this abnormal pattern of biliary bilirubin conjugates is not known. The findings suggest that Crigler-Najjar syndrome, type II, may represent a more pronounced phenotypic expression than does Gilbert's syndrome of a common biochemical defect. Although the specificity of elevated bilirubin monoglucuronide in bile for these two syndromes is not known, it may serve as a useful marker for diagnosis and for studies of inheritance.

INHERITANCE   Although it is a relatively common disorder, the incidence of Gilbert's syndrome is not known, primarily because a uniform definition for diagnosis has not been established. It is commonly accepted that the *sine qua non* of Gilbert's syndrome is unconjugated hyperbilirubinemia without overt hemolysis. The normal upper limit of serum bilirubin is

not always apparent in a given laboratory, and serum bilirubin levels in the general population have been described as following a skewed [459–462] rather than a Gaussian distribution. Others have suggested a bimodal distribution [411, 463]. Serum bilirubin levels in the male population are significantly higher than in the female population [463–465], which may account, in part, for the reported higher incidence of Gilbert's syndrome in males [411, 412]. Because of these difficulties in diagnosis, mild Gilbert's syndrome may go unrecognized. A clinically inapparent latent form of the disorder has been described [457]. In contrast, unconjugated hyperbilirubinemia to levels of 5 to 8 mg/dl occurs in Gilbert's syndrome and in patients with Crigler-Najjar syndrome, type II. Differentiation

Figure 61-19 Hepatic bilirubin UDP-glucuronyltransferase activity in patients with hepatitis, cirrhosis, and Gilbert's syndrome. The hatched area indicates the normal range. (*From Black and Billing [426]. Used by permission.*)

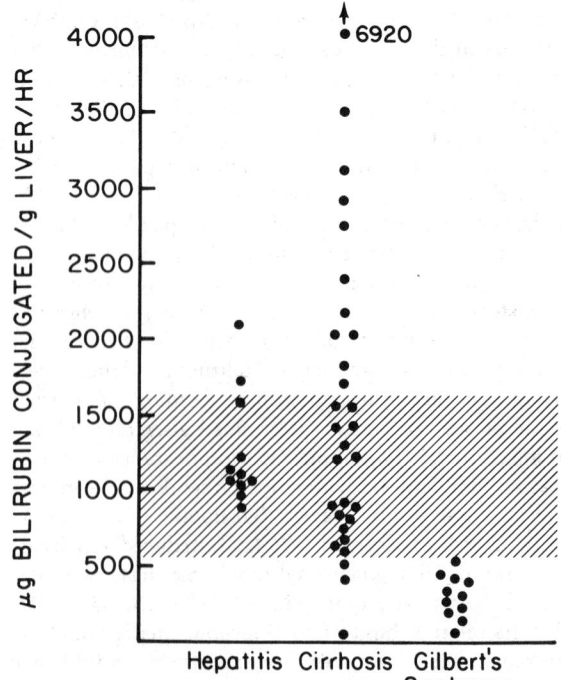

Table 61-2 Distribution of bile pigments in biliary aspirates from normal control subjects and patients with Gilbert's syndrome

	Relative content (%) mean $\pm$ SD	
Bilirubin tetrapyrrole	*Normal subjects, n = 13*	*Patients with Gilbert's syndrome, n = 16*
Bilirubin diglucuronide	87.6 $\pm$ 4.3	67.8 $\pm$ 9.3*
Bilirubin monoglucoside monoglucuronide diester	2.2 $\pm$ 3.7	3.6 $\pm$ 3.4
Bilirubin monoglucuronide	6.8 $\pm$ 4.7	23.4 $\pm$ 9.4*
Bilirubin	4.4 $\pm$ 3.5	5.0 $\pm$ 2.7

* p <0.001
SOURCE: From Goresky et al. [424]. Used by permission.

of these disorders based upon serum bilirubin levels, hepatic bilirubin UDP-glucuronyltransferase activity, and bilirubin monoglucuronide content of bile may be arbitrary.

That Gilbert's syndrome is an inheritable disorder, although one sometimes difficult to diagnose, is clear. Its familial occurrence has been repeatedly documented [409–411, 461, 466–469]. Whether Gilbert's syndrome and Crigler-Najjar syndrome, type II, represent distinct pathophysiologic disorders, or a spectrum of a single disorder, is not clear. Although an autosomal dominant inheritance has been suggested for Gilbert's syndrome [411, 461, 466], the difficulties inherent in diagnosing the disorder make this conclusion tenuous. Additional family studies using markers such as bilirubin monoglucuronide content of bile may provide more conclusive information as to inheritance.

Mutant Southdown Sheep Congenital photosensitivity in Southdown sheep was first observed in New Zealand in 1942 [470]. It is inherited as an autosomal recessive trait [471] and is characterized by unconjugated hyperbilirubinemia and photodermatitis resulting from retention of phylloerythrin, the end product of chlorophyll metabolism that is normally excreted by the liver into bile [472]. The original mutant line of sheep was destroyed, but similar photosensitive mutants were later found in California [473]. These sheep have reduced plasma disappearance of intravenously administered bilirubin, BSP, ICG and ^{131}I-labeled rose bengal [473], and reduced BSP transport maximum (T_m) and relative storage capacity (S) [473, 474]. It has been suggested that mutant sheep have increased bilirubin production from nonerythroid sources, and overproduction of bilirubin from hepatic heme has been postulated [475]. Plasma disappearance of intravenously administered [14C]bilirubin has been studied, and it was suggested that on the basis of compartmental analysis, the results resembled those obtained during similar studies in patients with Gilbert's syndrome [476], but there was a similarity only in reduced hepatic influx of bilirubin. As distinct from patients with Gilbert's syndrome, mutant sheep had significantly increased efflux from liver to plasma and normal hepatic sequestration rates. Bilirubin UDP-glucuronyltransferase activity is normal in mutant sheep [476]. The mechanism of unconjugated hyperbilirubinemia in these animals most likely differs from that in patients with Gilbert's syndrome. In addition to hyperbilirubinemia, mutant sheep demonstrate chronic interstitial nephritis manifested by polyuria, increased sodium excretion, and

reduced renal plasma flow, glomerular filtration rate, and urea clearance [477, 478]. The relationship of these findings to the hyperbilirubinemia is unknown.

Disorders of Bilirubin Metabolism Resulting in Predominantly Conjugated Hyperbilirubinemia

Dubin-Johnson Syndrome

CLINICAL FINDINGS   In 1954, Dubin and Johnson [479] and Sprinz and Nelson [480] described patients with chronic nonhemolytic jaundice. The liver was grossly black, but the histology was normal except for an unidentified pigment in hepatocytes. Subsequently this disorder has been described in both sexes in virtually all nationalities and races [351, 481–492]. Dubin-Johnson syndrome occurs frequently (1:1300) in Persian Jews [493] in whom it is associated with clotting factor VII deficiency [494–496].

The syndrome is clinically characterized by mild, predominantly conjugated hyperbilirubinemia (Table 61-3). Except for jaundice, physical examination is normal. An occasional patient may have hepatosplenomegaly. Mild constitutional complaints such as vague abdominal pains and weakness occur, but for the most part patients are asymptomatic [481, 493]. Pruritus is absent in Dubin-Johnson syndrome, and serum bile acid levels are normal [491, 497]. The degree of icterus is increased by intercurrent illness, oral contraceptives, and pregnancy (Fig. 61-22) [491]. The Dubin-Johnson syndrome is rarely detected before puberty, although cases have been reported in neonates [498–500]. Often the disorder is not noted until a woman becomes pregnant or receives oral contraceptives, which convert mild chemical hyperbilirubinemia into overt jaundice [491].

Figure 61-20 Plasma concentration of BSP 45 min after intravenous administration of 5 mg/kg to normal individuals and patients with Gilbert's syndrome. There is a subset of patients in whom BSP retention is elevated. (*From Berk et al. [433]. Used by permission.*)

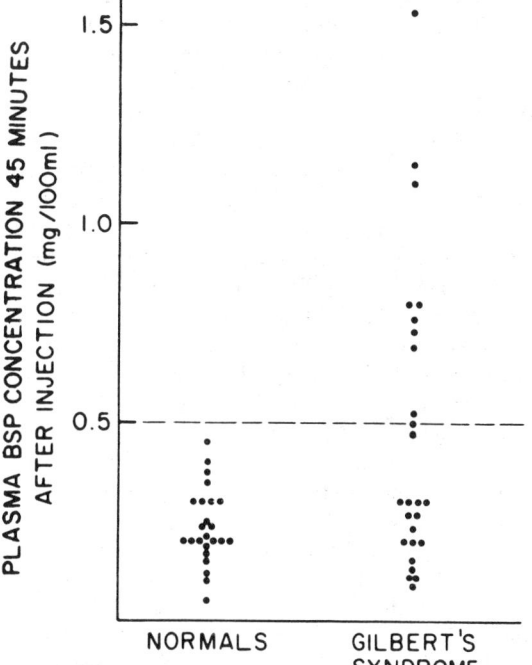

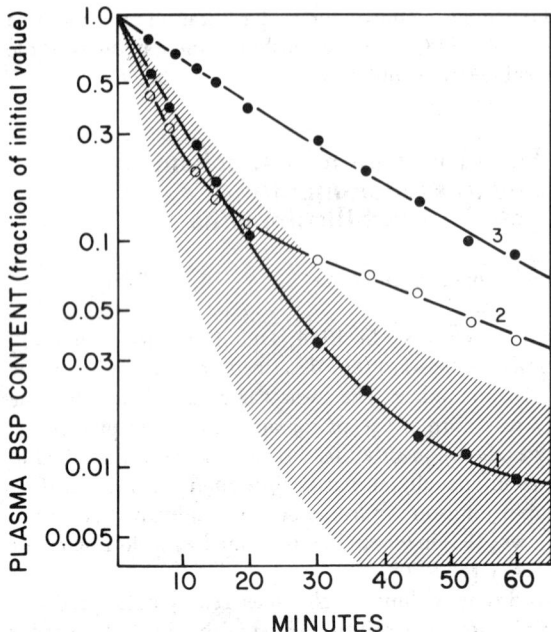

Figure 61-21 Plasma BSP disappearance curves in three patients with Gilbert's syndrome. The shaded area indicates the normal range. Curve 1 is indistinguishable from normal. Curves 2 and 3 are representative of the two subtypes of abnormal BSP disappearance seen in some patients with otherwise typical Gilbert's syndrome. (*From Berk et al. [433]. Used by permission.*)

LABORATORY EXAMINATION   Routine laboratory examination [481, 483, 488, 491–493] reveals normal complete blood count, serum albumin, cholesterol, transaminases, alkaline phosphatase, and prothrombin time. Serum bilirubin is usually between 2 and 5 mg/dl but can be as high as 20 to 25 mg/dl. Bilirubinuria is frequent and 50 percent or more of total serum bilirubin is conjugated. The serum bilirubin level fluctuates, and frequently individual determinations may be normal. Oral cholecystography, even using a "double dose" of contrast material, usually does not visualize the gallbladder, although visualization may occur 4 to 6 h after intravenous injection of iodipamide [501–503]. On direct inspection, the liver is black. Light microscopy reveals normal histology except for accumulation of a dense pigment, which on electron microscopy appears to be contained within lysosomes [504, 505].

Several investigators have suggested that these pigment granules are composed primarily of poorly defined lipofuscins [506–508]. On the basis of histochemical staining characteristics and physicochemical properties of extracted pigment, other investigators suggested that the Dubin-Johnson pigment resembled melanin [509–512]. The mutant Corriedale sheep is an animal model of Dubin-Johnson syndrome (see below) in which the hepatic pigment has also been shown to resemble melanin histochemically [513]. Studies performed in mutant Corriedale sheep infused with [³H]epinephrine revealed reduced biliary excretion of radioactivity and demonstrated incorporation of the isotope into the hepatic pigment [514–516], which is consistent with the pigment being a melanin-like derivative. A recent study of Dubin-Johnson pigment by electron spin resonance (ESR) spectroscopy suggests differences from authentic melanin [517]. The nature of the pigment was not defined, and the study was consistent with the pigment being composed of polymers of epinephrine metabolites [518, 519]. The degree of hepatic pigmentation may be variable in

individuals with the Dubin-Johnson syndrome [483, 485]. Some variability in pigmentation may be due to occurrence of coincidental disease such as acute viral hepatitis, in which the pigment is cleared from the liver only to reaccumulate slowly after recovery [520–524].

ORGANIC ANION TRANSPORT   In the Dubin-Johnson syndrome, initial plasma disappearance of bilirubin [418, 525], BSP [491–493, 525–527], dibromsulphalein (DBSP) [527], ICG [525, 527], and ¹²⁵I-labeled rose bengal [527] following intravenous administration are usually normal, although plasma BSP concentration at 45 min may be normal or may show mild retention [491–493, 525]. Of diagnostic significance is that in approximately 90 percent of patients, the plasma BSP concentration is higher 90 min after intravenous administration than at 45 min (Fig. 61-23) [491–493, 501, 528]. This is due to reflux of conjugated BSP from the liver cell into the circulation [501, 528]. This secondary rise is not seen following intravenous administration of other organic anions such as a DBSP, ¹²⁵I-labeled rose bengal, and ICG, which are not conjugated prior to excretion by the hepatocyte [525, 527]. A similar secondary rise has been described following intravenous administration of unconjugated bilirubin [517, 525]. Administration of conjugated BSP (GSH-BSP) to two patients with Dubin-Johnson syndrome resulted in markedly delayed plasma disappearance without the appearance of a secondary rise [526]. Although the secondary rise of plasma BSP is char-

Table 61-3   Principal differential characteristics of chronic conjugated hyperbilirubinemias

	Dubin-Johnson syndrome	*Rotor's syndrome*
Appearance of liver	Grossly black	Normal
Histology of liver	Dark pigment; predominantly in centrilobular areas. Otherwise normal	Normal; no increase in pigmentation
Serum bilirubin	Elevated–usually between 2–5 mg/dl; occasionally as high as 20 mg/dl. Predominantly direct reacting	Elevated–usually between 2–5 mg/dl; occasionally as high as 20 mg/dl. Predominantly direct reacting
Routine liver function tests	Normal except for bilirubin	Normal except for bilirubin
45-min plasma BSP retention	Normal or elevated; secondary rise at 90 min	Elevated; no secondary rise at 90 min
BSP infusion studies	T_m virtually 0; S normal	T_m and S both reduced
Oral cholecystogram	Usually does not visualize the gall bladder	Usually visualizes the gallbladder
Urinary coproporphyrin	Normal total; >80% as coproporphyrin I	Elevated total; elevated proportion of coproporphyrin I but <80%
Mode of inheritance	Autosomal recessive	Autosomal recessive
Prevalence	Uncommon (1:1300 in Persian Jews)	Rare
Prognosis	Benign	Benign
Animal model	Mutant Corriedale sheep	None

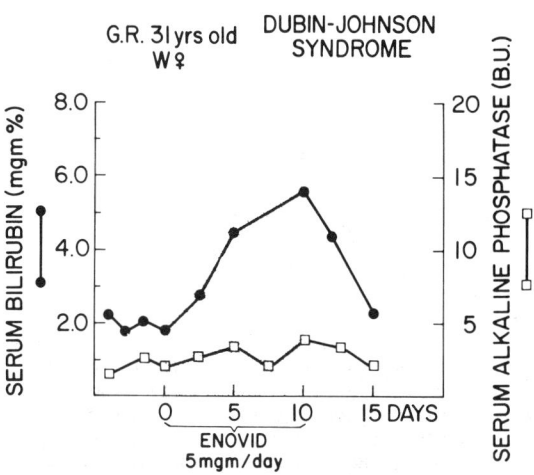

Figure 61-22 Exacerbation of conjugated hyperbilirubinemia by oral contraceptive administration in a patient with Dubin-Johnson syndrome. Similar findings may be seen in pregnancy.

acteristic of Dubin-Johnson syndrome, it is not diagnostic and occurs in other hepatobiliary disorders [529].

Studies of BSP transport during constant intravenous infusion reveal that T_m is reduced to only 10 percent of normal, and the relative hepatic storage capacity is normal [275, 491, 530]. This finding was also demonstrated directly in a patient with Dubin-Johnson syndrome who had a biliary fistula [276]. In this patient, dehydrocholate choleresis did not augment biliary BSP excretion. Similar studies of BSP transport have been performed in phenotypically normal parents and children (i.e., carriers) of Dubin-Johnson syndrome patients and were normal [275, 491].

INHERITANCE AND URINARY COPROPORPHYRIN EXCRETION
The familial nature of Dubin-Johnson syndrome was noted in its initial descriptions, but its mode of inheritance was unclear. The available genetic data did not fit an autosomal dominant pattern, and investigators were unable to detect carriers for the syndrome, even with constant infusion studies of BSP transport [275, 491]. In 1967, Koskelo et al. observed that urinary coproporphyrin I excretion is increased in patients with Dubin-Johnson syndrome to a greater degree than in patients with other hepatobiliary disorders [531]. These results were confirmed in Israel [532], the United States [533], and Japan [534]. Coproporphyrin exists in two isomeric forms, coproporphyrin I and coproporphyrin III. Isomer III porphyrins are precursors of heme, whereas isomer I porphyrins are metabolic by-products without known function and are excreted into urine and bile [535].

Coproporphyrin isomers I and III are normally found in urine, where 75 percent of total urinary coproporphyrin is coproporphyrin III. In Dubin-Johnson syndrome, total urinary coproporphyrin excretion is normal, but over 80 percent is coproporphyrin I [532–534]. Urinary coproporphyrin excretion has been determined in phenotypically normal relatives of patients with Dubin-Johnson syndrome (Fig. 61-24) [533, 534, 536]. In obligate heterozygotes (i.e., unaffected parents and children of patients with Dubin-Johnson syndrome) total urinary coproporphyrin excretion was reduced by 40 percent as compared to normal control subjects [533, 534, 536]. This was due to a 50 percent reduction in coproporphyrin III excretion. The proportion of coproporphyrin I in urine was intermediate between results in controls and in patients with Dubin-

Johnson syndrome. Analysis of data from studies revealed that with respect to urinary coproporphyrin excretion Dubin-Johnson syndrome is inherited as an autosomal recessive characteristic (Fig. 61-24, Table 61-4). A similar mode of inheritance was determined in a study of BSP and bilirubin metabolism in 173 sibs of 44 patients with Dubin-Johnson syndrome [537]. No other hepatobiliary disorder or porphyria has been described in which total urinary coproporphyrin excretion is normal, with over 80 percent of the total as coproporphyrin I. In the presence of a consistent history and physical examination, urinary coproporphyrin excretion appears to be diagnostic of this disorder.

The significant overlap of results in carriers with those in controls [533, 534, 536] makes determination of urinary coproporphyrin excretion less useful in deciding whether an individual carries the gene for the syndrome, although in this benign disorder genetic counseling is rarely required. Urinary coproporphyrin excretion has proved useful in diagnosing Dubin-Johnson syndrome in two neonates [498, 500]. Although neonates normally have elevated urinary content of coproporphyrin I as compared to adults, levels are not as high as seen in Dubin-Johnson syndrome [538].

The pathogenesis of the abnormal urinary coproporphyrin excretion in this syndrome is unknown, as is its relationship to conjugated hyperbilirubinemia. In addition to being present in urine, coproporphyrins are also found in bile, where isomer I constitutes approximately 65 percent of the total [535]. Normally, total daily biliary coproporphyrin excretion is approximately three times that of total daily urinary excretion. In most hepatobiliary disorders, including cholestasis, coproporphyrin levels are increased in urine [532, 539]. In these disorders, total urinary coproporphyrin excretion is elevated and the proportion of isomer I in urine is usually less than 65 percent. Dubin-Johnson syndrome is unique in that total urinary coproporphyrin is normal, but the proportion of isomer I is over 80 percent. It seems unlikely that the abnormal pattern of coproporphyrin isomers seen in the Dubin-Johnson syndrome results simply from reduced biliary excretion, and an alteration in hepatic porphyrin biosynthesis has been postulated (Fig. 61-25) [533, 538]. Reduced coproporphyrin III formation

Figure 61-23 Typical BSP plasma disappearance curve in a patient with Dubin-Johnson syndrome. A secondary rise occurs 45 min after the intravenous injection of the dye. (*From Erlinger et al.* [527]. *Used by permission.*)

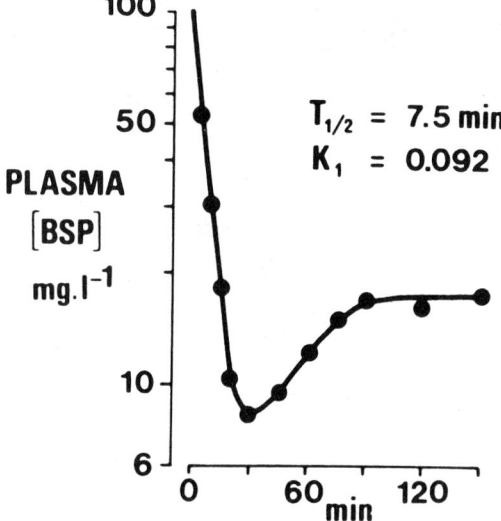

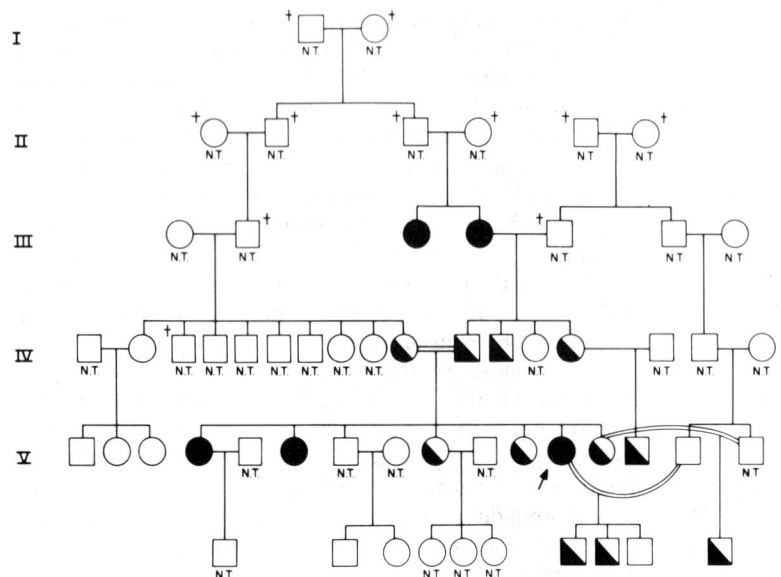

Figure 61-24 Pedigree of a family in which consanguinity resulted in three children with Dubin-Johnson syndrome (generation V). Solid symbols indicate individuals with Dubin-Johnson syndrome. Partial symbols indicate phenotypically normal individuals with urinary coproporphyrin excretion in the heterozygous range. Clear symbols represent phenotypically normal individuals with normal urinary coproporphyrin excretion. N.T. indicates those individuals who were not tested. In this family, the defect was detected in four generations. (*From Wolkoff et al. [533]. Used by permission.*)

could result from decreased activity of hepatic uroporphyrin III cosynthetase [533]. Enzyme activity as determined in blood cells and liver from four patients did not differ from normal [540]. Following an intravenous load of δ-aminolevulinic acid (ALA), coproporphyrin III content of urine and bile changed very little in patients with Dubin-Johnson syndrome, as compared with results in normal control subjects [541, 542]. Further study of porphyrin biosynthesis is required to elucidate the mechanism of abnormal coproporphyrin excretion and the relationship of the porphyrin abnormality to the conjugated hyperbilirubinemia which characterizes the syndrome.

Mutant Corriedale Sheep In 1965, Cornelius et al. described a mutant strain of Corriedale sheep showing photosensitivity, mild conjugated hyperbilirubinemia, hepatic pigmentation, and reduced biliary excretion of conjugated bilirubin, BSP, ICG, phylloerythrin, iodopanoic acid and ^{125}I-labeled rose bengal [474, 513–516, 543–545]. Taurocholate excretion is normal, and infusion of taurocholate does not increase biliary excretion of BSP [278, 516]. Biliary excretion of the organic cation procainamide ethobromide is normal in mutant sheep, as is renal excretion of PAH [278]. Studies suggesting that the hepatic pigment granules are related to mela-

nin have been discussed above. The photosensitivity manifested by the sheep results from retention of phylloerythrin [277, 544]. The disorder is transmitted as an autosomal recessive trait, and the organic anion excretory defect in the mutant sheep is indistinguishable morphologically and functionally from Dubin-Johnson syndrome in humans. Whether these two disorders represent similar metabolic defects remains to be determined.

Rotor's Syndrome

CLINICAL FINDINGS In 1948, Rotor, Manahan, and Florentin described several individuals from two families in whom there was chronic predominantly conjugated hyperbilirubinemia [546]. Serum alkaline phosphatase and cholesterol values were normal. Plasma disappearance of BSP was greatly delayed. Liver histology was normal. For many years, Rotor's and Dubin-Johnson syndromes were considered to be variants of a single pathophysiologic disorder [485, 547–549]. Recently, it has become evident that these disorders differ from each other (Table 61-3) [550, 551]. Rotor's syndrome is benign and is characterized by chronic predominantly conjugated hyperbilirubinemia without evidence of hemolysis [546–556]. The liver is normal on histologic examination and does not have excess pigmentation. Although it has been described in several nationalities and races, Rotor's syndrome is rare.

ORGANIC ANION EXCRETION Oral cholecystographic agents usually do not visualize the gallbladder in the Dubin-Johnson syndrome, whereas roentgenologic visualization usually is possible in Rotor's syndrome [548, 549]. In Dubin-Johnson syndrome, plasma retention of BSP 45 min after the intravenous injection of a 5 mg/kg dose is inconstant and rarely exceeds 15 percent whereas in Rotor's syndrome dye retention is a regular occurrence and invariably exceeds 25 percent [547–549, 551, 557, 558]. In Dubin-Johnson syndrome, the plasma BSP level is higher 90 min after BSP injection than at 45 min due to reflux of conjugated BSP from the liver (Fig. 61-23). This secondary rise of BSP does not occur in Rotor's syndrome, and conjugated BSP is not found in plasma (Fig. 61-26) [526, 551, 557]. Following their intravenous administration, there is also marked plasma retention of unconjugated bilirubin [552,

Figure 61-25 Pathway of porphyrin biosynthesis. δ-Aminolevulinic acid (δ-ALA) condenses to form porphobilinogen (PBG). In the presence of uroporphyrinogen synthetase, PBG forms the isomer I porphyrins, which are excretory products without known function. On addition of uroporphyrinogen cosynthetase, PBG forms the isomer III porphyrins which are precursors of heme. (*From Wolkoff et al. [533]. Used by permission.*)

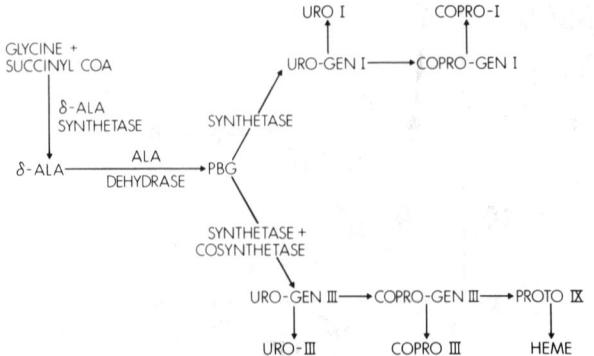

Table 61-4   Analysis of urinary coproporphyrin excretion in relatives of Dubin-Johnson syndrome patients from five families,* chi square = 4.3[†]

Subjects	Expected	Observed
Dubin-Johnson syndrome	5	9
Heterozygote	40	34
Normal	19	21

* Observed results are compared to those expected if Dubin-Johnson syndrome is inherited as an autosomal recessive characteristic.

† There is no significant difference (p >0.10) between the observed inheritance pattern and an autosomal recessive inheritance.

SOURCE: From Wolkoff et al. [533]. Used by permission.

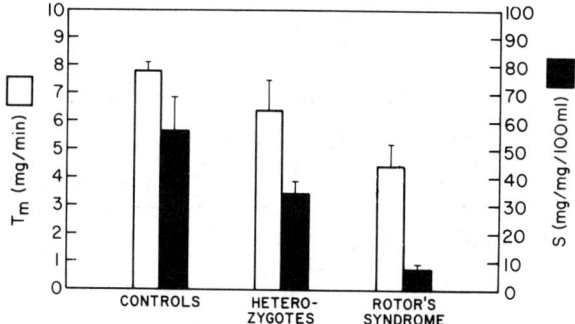

Figure 61-27   Hepatic relative storage capacity (S) and transport maximum (T_m) for BSP in six patients with Rotor's syndrome, five phenotypically normal heterozygotes, and six normal controls. (*From Wolpert et al. [551]. Used by permission.*)

557] and ICG [557]. Phenotypically normal obligate heterozygotes for Rotor's syndrome have mildly abnormal BSP retention at 45 min, which is intermediate between results in affected patients and normal controls [551].

With the use of a constant infusion technique, BSP T_m and relative hepatic storage capacity (S) have been determined in patients with Rotor's syndrome (Fig. 61-27) [551, 557]. In Dubin-Johnson syndrome T_m is virtually zero while S is normal. In Rotor's syndrome, S was reduced by 75 to 90 percent and T_m was reduced by 50 percent [551, 557]. Determination of T_m and S in phenotypically normal obligate heterozygotes revealed results intermediate between those in patients with Rotor's syndrome and controls [551]. The modest reduction in T_m accompanied by a larger reduction in S is similar to observations in "hepatic storage disease," a familial disorder manifested by predominantly conjugated hyperbilirubinemia and normal liver histology [559, 560]. Since there is little to differentiate Rotor's syndrome from hepatic storage disease, they may represent a single pathophysiologic entity.

URINARY COPROPORPHYRIN EXCRETION   As occurred in Dubin-Johnson syndrome, the familial nature of Rotor's syndrome was initially recognized, but the mode of inheritance remained unclear. The finding of abnormal BSP transport in obligate heterozygotes suggested an autosomal recessive pattern of inheritance [551]. A more complete genetic analysis was performed following determination of urinary coproporphyrin excretion in patients with Rotor's syndrome and phenotypically normal relatives (Fig. 61-28) [550, 558]. Unlike results for Dubin-Johnson syndrome, total urinary coproporphyrin is increased by 250 to 500 percent as compared to control subjects, and the proportion of coproporphyrin I in urine is approximately 65 percent of total [550, 558]. These results are similar to those seen in many other hepatobiliary disorders [531, 532, 539, 561–563]. Phenotypically normal obligate heterozygotes have a coproporphyrin excretory pattern which is intermediate between that of control subjects and patients with Rotor's syndrome. Statistical analysis reveals that, with respect to urinary coproporphyrin excretion, Rotor's syndrome is inherited as an autosomal recessive characteristic and is distinct from Dubin-Johnson syndrome (Table 61-5, Fig. 61-29) [550, 558]. The urinary coproporphyrin abnormality in Rotor's syndrome, unlike that in Dubin-Johnson syndrome, is most likely caused by a reduced biliary excretion of coproporphyrins, with concomitant increased filtration and excretion by the kidney. The nature of the organic anion transport defect in Rotor's syndrome is unknown.

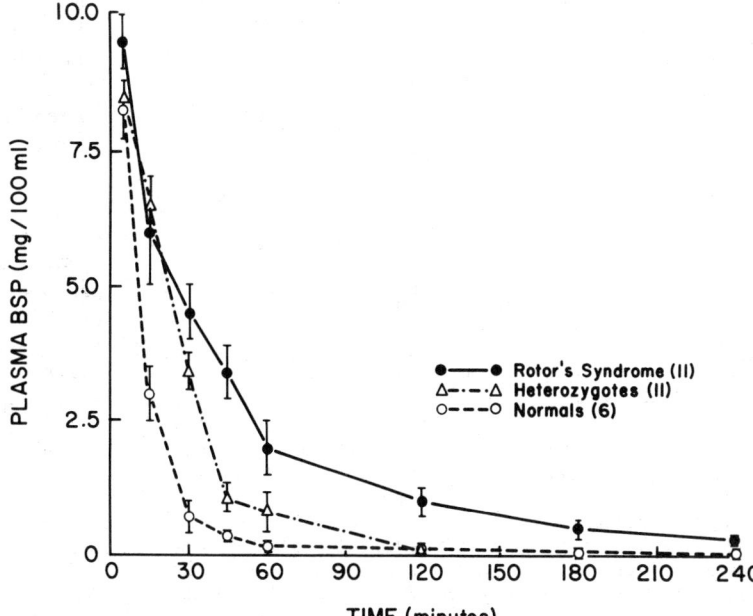

Figure 61-26   Plasma disappearance of BSP after intravenous injection of a 5 mg/kg dose into 11 patients with Rotor's syndrome, 11 phenotypically normal first-degree relatives defined as heterozygotes for the syndrome on the basis of urinary coproporphyrin administration, and 6 normal controls. There is no secondary rise of plasma BSP, and conjugated BSP is not found in plasma. (*From Wolpert et al. [551]. Used by permission.*)

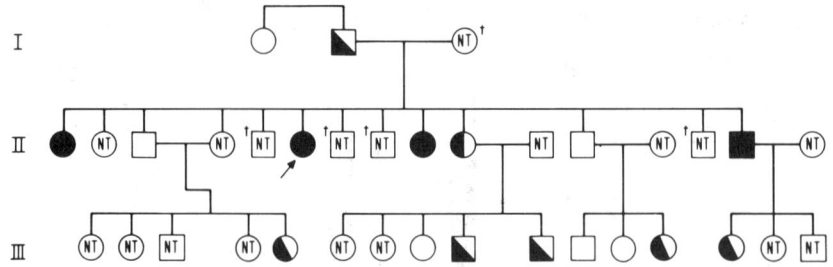

Figure 61-28 Pedigree of a Philippine family originally described by Rotor in 1948. Solid symbols indicate individuals with Rotor's syndrome. Partial symbols indicate phenotypically normal individuals with urinary coproporphyrin excretion in the heterozygous range. Clear symbols represent phenotypically normal individuals with normal urinary coproporphyrin excretion. NT indicates those individuals who were not tested. (*From Wolkoff et al. [550]. Used by permission.*)

Benign Recurrent Intrahepatic Cholestasis

CLINICAL FINDINGS   Benign recurrent intrahepatic cholestasis is a rare disorder first described in 1959 by Summerskill and Walshe [564]. The disorder is characterized by recurrent attacks of cholestasis. Generally, there is a preicteric phase lasting 2 to 4 weeks in which patients experience malaise, anorexia, and pruritus [565–568]. Subsequently, patients become icteric and may have an enlarged tender liver. There is no splenomegaly and patients are afebrile [564–573]. The clinical presentation may suggest biliary obstruction, and in the past, many of these patients underwent one or more exploratory laparotomies. The onset of symptoms is usually in adolescence or early adulthood [568], although this disorder has been described as presenting in infancy [567–569, 573] as well as in middle age [572]. Typically, episodes of cholestasis last from a few weeks to several months [568], and intervals between attacks may range from several months to years. In a given patient, recurrent attacks resemble each other as to symptoms and duration. Because of the prolonged cholestasis, patients may develop malabsorption characterized by steator-

Table 61-5   Analysis of urinary coproporphyrin excretion in relatives of Rotor's syndrome patients from three families,* chi square = 1.34†

Subjects	Expected	Observed
Rotor's syndrome	7.	10
Heterozygote	13.2	14
Normal	8.8	9

* Observed results are compared to those expected if Rotor's syndrome is inherited as an autosomal recessive characterisitc.
† There is no significant difference ($p = 0.50$) between the observed inheritance pattern and an autosomal recessive inheritance.
SOURCE: From Wolkoff et al. [550]. Used by permission.

rhea and weight loss, and may require parenteral administration of fat-soluble vitamins. Between episodes of cholestasis patients are clinically normal, and this disorder is termed benign because no negative influence on longevity has been noted. The familial nature of this disorder has been clearly documented, but the mode of inheritance is not known [568].

LABORATORY FINDINGS   Early in the course of cholestatic episodes, serum bile acids rise to abnormal levels [566, 574–577]. This is accompanied by elevated serum alkaline phosphatase activity and conjugated hyperbilirubinemia. Serum transaminases may be mildly elevated, and the prothrombin time may be elevated because of malabsorption of vitamin K. During the cholestatic episode, plasma disappearance of unconjugated bilirubin is normal, but conjugated bilirubin rises in serum as it refluxes from liver [565, 578–580]. Light-microscopic examination of the liver during episodes reveals typical features of intrahepatic cholestasis [564–575, 580–583]. Electron-microscopic examination reveals markedly altered bile canaliculi with distorted and reduced microvilli, almost complete disappearance of nucleoside phosphatase activity, and reduction in the number of acid phosphatase–rich lysosomes [567, 575, 583]. These changes are not specific for this disorder and may be seen nonspecifically in cholestasis. Between attacks, biochemical studies are normal in these patients, and histology of the liver is normal both by light microscopy and electron microscopy [567, 575, 583]. The pathogenesis of this rare disorder is unknown, and there is no specific treatment to prevent or shorten the occurrence of cholestatic episodes.

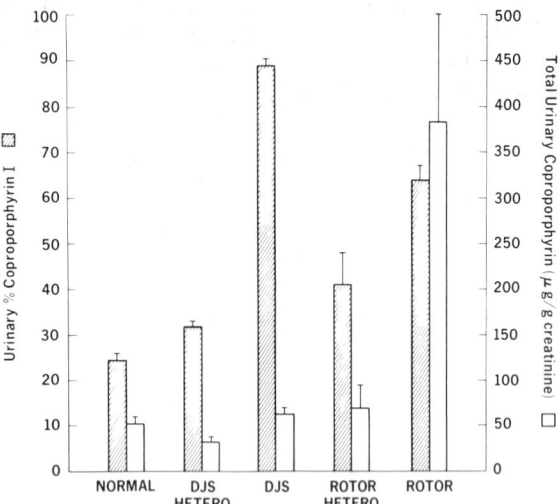

Figure 61-29 Urinary coproporphyrin excretion in Dubin-Johnson and Rotor's syndromes. The shaded bars represent the percentage of total urinary coproporphyrin excreted as coproporphyrin I. The open bars represent total urinary coproporphyrin excretion. Vertical bars represent 1 SEM. Total urinary coproporphyrin excretion is normal in the Dubin-Johnson syndrome (DJS) with a markedly elevated proportion of coproporphyrin I (>80 percent). Both variables are elevated in Rotor's syndrome, and with respect to urinary coproporphyrin excretion, the two disorders are distinct. Results in obligate heterozygotes for each of these disorders (DJS Hetero, Rotor Hetero) lie intermediate between results in normal individuals and in individuals manifesting the respective disorder. (*From Berk et al. [337]. Used by permission.*)

REFERENCES

1. BERK PD, HOWE RB, BLOOMER JR, BERLIN NI: Studies of bilirubin kinetics in normal adults. *J Clin Invest* 48:2176, 1969
2. LONDON IM, WEST R, SHEMIN D, RITTENBERG D: On the origin of bile pigment in normal man. *J Biol Chem* 184:351, 1950

3. GRAY CH, NEUBERGER A, SNEATH PHA: Studies in congenital porphyria. 2. Incorporation of ^{15}N in the stercobilin in the normal and in the porphyric. *Biochem J* 47:87, 1950

4. ROBINSON SH: Origins of the early-labeled peak, in Berk PD, Berlin NI (eds): *The Chemistry and Physiology of Bile Pigments.* Washington, USDEW, MIH, 1977, p 175

5. SCHWARTZ S, JOHNSON JA, STEPHENSON BD, ANDERSON AS, EDMONDSON PR, FUSARO RM: Erythropoietic defects in protoporphyria: A study of factors involved in labelling of porphyrins and bile pigments from ALA^{3}H and glycine-^{14}C. *J Lab Clin Med* 78:411, 1971

6. BERK PD, JONES EA, HOWE RB, BERLIN NI: Disorders of bilirubin metabolism, in Bondy PK, Rosenberg LE (eds): *Metabolic Control and Disease,* 8th ed. Philadelphia, Saunders, 1980, p 1009

7. LEVITT M, SCHACTER BA, ISRAELS LG: The nonerythropoietic component of early bilirubin. *J Clin Invest* 47:1281, 1968

8. YANNONI CZ, ROBINSON SH: Early-labelled heme synthesis in normal rats and rats with iron deficiency anemia. *Biochim Biophys Acta* 428:533, 1976

9. GRAY CH, SCOTT JJ: The effect of haemorrhage on the incorporation of [^{14}C]glycine into stercobilin. *Biochem J* 71:38, 1959

10. BUTLER RC: The early life cycle of red blood cells. *J Biol Chem* 249:7491

11. HAMER JW, FITZGERALD PH: Disturbed marrow cell proliferation in primary shunt hyperbilirubinemia. *Blood* 41:539, 1973

12. ROBINSON SH, TSONG M: Hemolysis of "stress" reticulocytes: A source of erythropoietic bilirubin formation. *J Clin Invest* 49:1025, 1970

13. COME SE, SHOHET SB, ROBINSON SH: Surface remodeling vs. whole-cell hemolysis of reticulocytes produced with erythroid stimulation or iron deficiency anemia. *Blood* 44:817, 1974

14. TENHUNEN R, MARVER HS, SCHMID R: Microsomal heme oxygenase: Characterization of the enzyme. *J Biol Chem* 244:6388, 1969

15. TENHUNEN R, MARVER HS, SCHMID R: The enzymatic catabolism of hemoglobin: Stimulation of microsomal heme oxygenase by hemin. *J Lab Clin Med* 75:410, 1970

16. YOSHIDA T, KIKICHI G: Heme oxygenase purified to apparent homogeneity from pig spleen microsomes. *J Biochem* 81:265, 1977

17. MAINES MD, IBRAHIM NG, KAPPAS A: Solubilization and partial purification of heme oxygenase from rat liver. *J Biol Chem* 252:5900, 1977

18. O'CARRA P, COLLERAN E: Nonenzymic and quasienzymatic models for catabolic heme cleavage, in Berk PD, Berlin NI (eds): *The chemistry and Physiology of Bile Pigments.* Washington, USDHEW, NIH, 1977, p 26

19. JACKSON AH, KENNER W: Recent developments in porphyrin chemistry, in Goodwin TW (ed): *Porphyrins and Related Compounds.* London and New York, Academic, 1968, p 5

20. LEMBERG R: The chemical mechanism of bile pigment formation. *Rev Pure Appl Chem* 6:1, 1956

21. COLLERAN E, O'CARRA P: Enzymology and comparative physiology of biliverdin reduction, in Berk PD, Berlin NI (eds): *The Chemistry and Physiology of Bile Pigments.* Washington, USDEW, NIH, 1977, p 69

22. TENHUNEN R, ROSS ME, MARVER HS, SCHMID R: Reduced nicotinamide-adenine dinucleotide phosphate dependent bilverdin reductase: partial purification and characterization. *Biochemistry* 9:298, 1970

23. BLUMENTHAL SG, TAGGART DB, IKEDA RM, RUEBNER B, BERGSTROM DE: Conjugated and unconjugated bilirubins in bile of humans and rhesus monkeys. Structure of adult human and rhesus-monkey bilirubins compared with dog bilirubin. *Biochem J* 167:535, 1977

24. HEIRWEGH KPM, BLANCKAERT N, COMPERNOLLE F, FEVERY J, ZAMAN Z: Detection and properties of the non-α-isomers of bilirubin-IX. *Biochem Soc Trans* 5:316, 1977

25. BLANCKAERT N, FEVERY J, COMPERNOLLE F, HEIRWEGH, KPM: Presence of bilirubin IXβ, γ and δ in bile of man and various animals. *Gastroenterology* 69:A-10/810, 1975

26. BLANCKAERT N, HEIRWEGH KPM, COMPERNOLLE F: Synthesis and separation by thin-layer chromatography of bilirubin-IX isomers. Their identification as tetrapyrroles and dipyrrol anthranilate azo derivatives. *Biochem J* 155:405, 1976

27. BLUMENTHAL SG, STUCKER T, RASMUSSEN RD, IKEDA RM, RUEBNER BH, BERGSTROM DE, HANSON FW: Changes in bilirubin in human prenatal development. *Biochem J* 186:693, 1980

28. HOWE RB, BERLIN NI, BERK PD: Estimation of bilirubin production in man, in Berk PD, Berlin NI (eds): *Chemistry and Physiology of Bile Pigments.* Washington, USDEW, NIH, 1977, p 105

29. DHAR GJ: Enterohepatic circulation and plasma transport of urobilinogen, in Berk PD, Berlin NI (eds): *The Chemistry and Physiology of Bile Pigments.* Washington, USDEW, NIH, 1977, p 526

30. BLOOMER JR, BERK PD, HOWE RB, WAGGONER JG, BERLIN NI: Comparison of fecal urobilinogen excretion with bilirubin production in normal volunteers and patients with increased bilirubin production. *Clin Chim Acta* 29:463, 1970

31. JONES EA, SHRAGER R, BLOOMER JR, BERK PD, HOWE RB, BERLIN NI: Quantitative studies of the delivery of hepatic synthesized bilirubin to plasma utilizing δ-aminolevulinic acid-4-^{14}C and bilirubin-^{3}H in man. *J Clin Invest* 51:2450, 1972

32. JONES EA, BLOOMER JR, BERK PD, CARSON ER, OWENS D, BERLIN NI: Quantitation of hepatic bilirubin synthesis in man, in Berk PD, Berlin NI (eds): *The Chemistry and Physiology of Bile Pigments.* Washington USDEW, NIH, 1977, p 189

33. COBURN RF, BLAKEMORE WS, FORSTER RE: Endogenous carbon monoxide production in man. *J Clin Invest* 42:1172, 1963

34. BERK PD, RODKEY FL, BLASCHKE, COLLISON HA, WAGGONER JG: Comparison of plasma bilirubin turnover and carbon monoxide production in man. *J Lab Clin Med* 83:29, 1974

35. BENSINGER TA, MAISELS MJ, MAHMOOD L, McCURDY PR, CONRAD MD: Effect of intravenous urea in invert sugar on heme catabolism in sickle cell anemia. *N Eng J Med* 285:995, 1971

36. LYNCH SR, MOEDE AL: Variation in the rate of endogenous carbon monoxide production in normal human beings. *J Lab Clin Med* 79:85, 1972

37. COBURN RF, GONDRIE P, ABBOUD F, PLOEGMAKERS E: Myocardial myoglobin oxygen tension. *Am J Physiol* 224:870, 1973

38. STEWART RD, FISHER TN, HOSKO MJ, PETERSON JE, BARETTA ED, DODD HC: Carboxyhemoglobin elevation after exposure to dichloromethane. *Science* 176:295, 1972

39. ENGEL RR: Alternative sources of carbon monoxide, in Berk PD, Berlin NI (eds): *Chemistry and Physiology of Bile Pigments.* Washington, DHEW, NIH, 1977, p 148

40. WESTLAKE DWS, ROXBURGH JM, TALBOT G: Microbial production of carbon monoxide from flavinoids. *Nature (London)* 189:510, 1961

41. RUDIZER W: In Herz W, Grischback H, Kirby GW (eds): *Progress in the Chemistry of Organic Natural Compounds.* Wien, New York, Springer Verleg, 1972, vol 29

42. FISCHER H, PLIENINGER H: Synthese des biliverdins (uteroverdins) und bilirubins der biliverdine XIII, und III, sowie der Vinulneoxanthosaure. Hoppe-Seylers A. *Physiol Chem* 274:231, 1942

43. BONNET RJ, DAVIS E, HURSTHOUSE MB: Structure of bilirubin. *Nature* 262:326, 1976.

44. GRAY CH, KULCZYCKA A, NICHOLSON DC: The chemistry of bile pigments. IV. Spectrophotometric titration of the bile pigments. *J Chem Soc* 442:2276, 1961

45. KRASNER J, YAFFE SJ: The automatic titration of bilirubin. *Biochem Med* 7:128, 1973

46. BRODERSON R: Binding of bilirubin to albumin. CRC critical reviews in Clinical Laboratory *Sciences* p. 305, 1980

47. GANZONI A, HILLMAN RS, FINCH CA: Maturation of the macroreticulocyte. *Br H Haematol* 16:119, 1969

48. McDONAGH AF; In *The Porphyrins,* Vol. VI. Bile Pigments. Bilatrienes and 5, 15-Biladiences. *Academic Press, Inc.,* 1979

49. FOG J, JELLUM E: Structure of bilirubin. *Nature (London)* 198:88, 1963

50. KUENZLE CC, WEIBEL MH, PELLONI RR: A proposed novel structure for the metal chelates of bilirubin. *Biochem J* 130:1147, 1973

51. KUENZLE CC, WEIBEL MH, PELLONI RR: The reaction of bilirubin with diazomethane. *Biochem J* 133:357, 1973

52. MARITTO P, MONTI D: Free energy barrier of conformational inversion in bilirubin. *J Chem Soc Chem Commun* 122, 1976

53. KNELL AJ, HANCOCK F, HUTCHINSON DW: In Bakken AF, Fog J (eds): *Bilirubin and Related Tetrapyrroles.* Oslo, Norway, Pediatr Res Inst, Rikshospitalet 1975, p 234

54. BLANCKAERT N, HEIRWEGH KPM, ZAMAN Z: Comparison of the biliary excretion of the four isomers of bilirubin-IX in Wistar and homozygous Gunn rats. *Biochem J* 164:229, 1977

55. KUENZLE CC: Bilirubin conjugates of human bile. Nuclear magnetic resonance, infrared and optical spectra of model compounds. *Biochem J* 119:395, 1970

56. FATIADI AJ, SCHAFFER R: Periodic acid as a new oxidant for the degradation of bile pigments. Isolation of a biliverdin type of reaction intermediate on oxidation of bilirubin with periodic acid. *Experientia* 27:1139, 1971

57. CU A, BELLAH GG, LIGHTNER DA: On the fluorescence of bilirubin. *J Am Chem Soc* 97:2579, 1975

58. KRASNER J, YAFFE SJ: Birth defects. *Orig Art Ser* 12, No 2, 168, 1976

59. McDONAGH AF, PALMA LA: In Berlin NI, Berk PD, Watson CJ (eds): *Chemistry and Physiology of Bile Pigments.* Washington, DHEW, NIH, 1977 p 81

60. LIGHTNER DA, WOOLDRIDGE TA, McDONAGH AF: Photobilirubin. An early bilirubin photoproduct detected by absorbance difference spectroscopy. *Proc Natl Acad Sci USA* 76:29, 1979

61. McDONAGH AF: Phototherapy of neonatal jaundice. *Soc Trans* 4:219, 1976

62. McDONAGH AF: Thermal and photochemical reactions of bilirubin IX. *Ann NY Acad Sci* 244:553, 1975

63. MANITO P, MONTI D: In Bakken AF, Fog J (eds): *Metabolism and Chemistry of Bilirubin and Related Tetrapyrroles.* Oslo, Norway, Pediatr Res Inst, Rikshospitalet, 1975, p 191

64. BRODERSEN R: Dimerisation of bilirubin anion in aqueous solution. *Acta Chem Scand* 20:2895, 1966

65. LEE KS, GARTNER LM: Spectrophotometric characteristics of bilirubin. *Pediatr Res* 10:782, 1976

66. KATOH R, KASHIWAMATA S, NIWA F: Studies on cellular toxicity of bilirubin. Effect on the carbohydrate metabolism in the young rat brain. *Brain Res* 83:81, 1975

67. GREENFIELD S, NANDI MAJUMDAR AP: Bilirubin encephalopathy. Effect on protein synthesis in the brain of the Gunn rat. *J Neurol Sci* 22:83, 1974

68. NANDI MAJUMDAR AP: Bilirubin encephalopathy. Effect on RNA polymerase activity and chromatin template activity in the brain of the Gunn rat. *Neurobiology* 4:425, 1974

69. NANDI MAJUMDAR AP, GREENFIELD S: Evidence of defective protein synthesis in liver in rats with congenital hyperbilirubinemia. *Biochim Biophys Acta* 335:260, 1974

70. MUSTAFA MG, COWGER ML, KING TE: Effects of bilirubin on mitochondrial reactions. *J Biol Chem* 244:6403, 1969

71. DIAMOND I, SCHMID R: Oxidative phosphorylation in experimental bilirubin encephalopathy. *Science* 155:1288, 1967

72. MENKEN M, WAGGONER JG, BERLIN NI: The influence of bilirubin on oxidative phosphorylation and related reactions in brain and liver mitochondria. Effects of protein binding. *J Neurochem* 13:1241, 1966

73. VOGT MT, BASFORD RE: The effect of bilirubin on the energy metabolism of brain mitochondria. *J Neurochem* 15:1313, 1968

74. ZETTERSTROM R, ERNSTER L: Bilirubin, an uncoupler of oxidative phosphorylation in isolated mitochondria. *Nature (London)* 178:1335, 1956

75. KAPPOR CL, KRISHNA MURTI CR, BAJPAI PC: Toxic effect of bilirubin on human red blood cells and its reversal by RBC lipids. *Indian J Med Res* 60:918, 1972

76. GIROTTI AW: Glyceraldehyde-3-phosphate dehydrogenase in the isolated human erythrocyte membrane. Selective displacement by bilirubin. *Biophys* 173:210, 1976

77. COWGER ML, IGO P, LABBE RF: The mechanism of bilirubin toxicity studied with purified respiratory enzyme and tissue culture systems. *Biochemistry* 4:2763, 1965

78. DAY R: In Sass-Kortsak A (ed): *Kernicterus*. Toronto Univ. of Toronto Press, 1959, p 167

79. KIKICHI K: Effects of bilirubin on the multiplication of animal cells in tissue culture. *Jap J Exp Med* 31:71, 1961

80. RASMUSSEN LF, WENNBERG RP: Pharmacologic modification of bilirubin toxicity in tissue culture cells. *Res Commun Chem Pathol Pharmacol* 3:567, 1972

81. PARADISI F, GRAZIANO L, DE RITIS F: The action of unconjugated bilirubin on some enzyme activities of in vitro cultured cells. *Res Exp Med* 161:224, 1973

82. STRUMIA E: Effect of bilirubin on some hydrolases. *Boll Soc Ital Biol Sper* 35:2160, 1959

83. FLITMAN R, WORTH NH: Inhibition of hepatic alcohol dehydrogenase by bilirubin. *J Biol Chem* 241:669, 1966

84. NOIR BA, BOVERIS A, GARAZO PEREIPA AM, AND STOPPANI AOM: Bilirubin: A multi-site inhibitor of mitochondrial respiration. *FEBS Lett* 27:270, 1972

85. OGASAWARE N, WATANABE T, GOTO H: Bilirubin: A potent inhibitor of NAD$^+$ linked isocitrate dehydrogenase. *Biochim Biophys Acta* 327:233, 1973

86. HADDOCK JH, NADLER HL: Bilirubin toxicity in human cultivated fibroblasts and its modification by light treatment. *Proc Soc Exp Biol Med* 134:45, 1970

87. HSIA D Y-Y, ALLEN FH, GELLIS SS, DIAMOND LK: Erythroblastosis fetalis. VIII. Studies on serum bilirubin in relation to kernicterus. *N Engl J Med* 247:668, 1952

88. ODELL GB: Influence of binding on the toxicity of bilirubin. *Ann NY Acad Sci* 226:225, 1973

89. LEE KS, GARTNER LM, EIDELMAN AI, EZHUTHACHAN S: Unconjugated hyperbilirubinemia in very low birth weight infants. *Clin Perinatol* 4:305, 1977

90. BENHOLD H: The transport of bilirubin in the circulating blood and its pathogenic importance. *Acta Med Scand Suppl* 445:223, 1966

91. BOWEN WR, PORTER E, WATERS WF: The protective action of albumin in bilirubin toxicity in newborn puppies. *Am J Dis Child* 98:568, 1959

92. MUSTAFA MG, COWGER ML, KING TE: Effects of bilirubin on mitochondrial reactions. *J Biol Chem* 244:6403, 1969

93. SILVERMANN WA, ANDERSEN DH, BLANC WA, CROZIER DN: A difference in mortality rate and incidence of kernicterus among premature infants allotted to two prophylactic antibacterial regimens. *Pediatrics* 18:614, 1956

94. ODELL GB: The dissociation of bilirubin from albumin and its clinical implications. *J Pediatr* 55:268, 1959

95. SCHMID R, DIAMOND I, HAMMAKER I, GUNDERSEN CB: Interaction of bilirubin with albumin. *Nature (London)* 204:1041, 1965

96. BLOOMER JR, BERK PD, VERGALLA J, BERLIN NI: Influence of albumin on the extravascular distribution of unconjugated bilirubin. *Clin Sci Mol Med* 45:517, 1973

97. ODELL GB, COHEN SN, GORDES EH: Administration of albumin in the management of hyperbilirubinemia by exchange transfusion. *Pediatrics* 30:613, 1962

98. BRODERSEN R, FUNDING L, PEDERSEN AO, ROJGAARD-PETERSEN H: Binding of bilirubin to low-affinity sites of human serum albumin in vitro followed by co-crystallization. *Scand J Clin Lab Invest* 29:433, 1972

99. JACOBSEN J: Binding of bilirubin to human serum albumin. Determination of the dissociation constants. *FEBS Lett* 5:112, 1969

100. BRODERSEN R: Bilirubin solubility and interaction with albumin and phospholipid. *J Biol Chem* 254:2364, 1979

101. BERDE CB, HUDSON BS, SIMONI RD, SKLAR LA: Human serum albumin: Spectroscopic studies of binding and proximity relationships for fatty acid and bilirubin. *J Biol Chem* 254:391, 1979

102. REED RG, FELDHOFF RC, CLUTE OL, PETERS T: Fragments of bovine serum albumin produced by limited proteolysis. Conformation and ligand binding. *Biochemistry* 14:4578, 1975

103. GEISOW MJ, BEAVEN GH: Large fragments of human serum albumin. *Biochem J* 161:619, 1977

104. SJODIN T, HANSSON R, SJOHOLM I: Isolation and identification of a trypsin-resistant fragment of human serum albumin with bilirubin- and drug-binding properties. *Biochim Biophys Acta* 494:61, 1977

105. GITZELMANN-CUMARASAMY N, KUENZLE CC, WILSON KJ: Mapping of the primary bilirubin binding site of human serum albumin. *Experientia* 32:768, 1976

106. JACOBSEN C: Lysine residue 240 of human serum albumin is involved in high-affinity binding of bilirubin. *Biochem J* 171:453, 1978

107. BRODERSEN R: Free bilirubin in blood plasma of the newborn. Effects of albumin, fatty acids, pH, displacing drugs and phototherapy. Appendix: A provisional survey of the bilirubin-displacing effect of 150 drugs, in Stern L (ed.): *Intensive Care in the Newborn*. New York, Masson, 1978, vol 2, p 331

108. BRODERSEN R, SJODIN T, SJOHOLM I: Independent binding of benzodiazepines and bilirubin to human serum albumin. *J Biol Chem* 252:5067, 1977

109. ODELL GB: The distribution of bilirubin between albumin and mitochondria. *J Pediatr* 68:164, 1966

110. WOOLLEY PW, HUNTER M: Binding and circular dichroism data on bilirubin-albumin in the presence of oleate and salicylate. *Arch Biochem Biophys* 140:197, 1970

111. BRODERSEN R: Binding of bilirubin and other ligands of human serum albumin, in Peters T, Sjoholm I (eds): *Albumin, Structure, Biosynthesis, Function*. FEBS 11th Meeting, Copenhagen, 1977. Oxford, Pergamon, 1978, p 61

112. RUDMAN D, BIXLER TJ, DEL RIO AE: Effect of free fatty acid on binding of drugs by bovine serum albumin, by human serum albumin and by rabbit serum. *J Pharmacol Exp Ther* 176:261, 1971

113. DIAMOND I, SCHMID R: Experimental bilirubin encephalopathy. The mode of entry of bilirubin-^{14}C into the central nervous system. *J Clin Invest* 45:678, 1966

114. STERN L, DENTON RL: Kernicterus in small premature infants. *Pediatrics* 35:483, 1965

115. KAPITULNIK J, VALAES T, KAUFMANN NA, BLONDHEIM SH: Clinical evaluation of Sephadex gel filtration in estimation of bilirubin binding in serum in neonatal jaundice. *Arch Dis Child* 49:886, 1974

116. BRODERSEN R, CASHORE W, WENNBERG RP, AHLFORS CE, RASMUSSEN LF, SHUSTERMAN D: Kinetics of bilirubin oxidation with peroxidase, as applied to studies of bilirubin-albumin binding. *Scand J Clin Lab Invest* 39:143, 1979

117. ATHANASSIADIS S, CHOPRA DR, FISHER M, McKENNA J: An electrophoretic method for detection of unbound bilirubin and reserve bilirubin binding capacity in serum of newborns. *J Lab Clin Med* 83:968, 1974

118. LAMOLLA AA, EISINGER J, BLUMBERG WE, PALET SC, FLORES J: Fluorometric study of the partition of bilirubin among blood components: basis for rapid microassays of bilirubin and bilirubin binding capacity in whole blood. *Anal Biochem* 15:25, 1979

119. BRATLID D: Reserve albumin binding capacity salicylate saturation index, and red cell binding of bilirubin in neonatal jaundice. *Arch Dis Child* 48:393, 1973

120. BRODERSEN R: Determination of the vacant amount of high affinity bilirubin binding site on serum albumin. *Acta Pharmacol Toxicol* 42:153, 1978

121. HSIA JC, KWAN NH, ER SS, WOOD DJ, CHANCE GW: Development of a spin assay for reserve bilirubin loading capacity of human serum. *Proc Natl Acad Sci USA* 75:1542, 1978

122. PORTER EG, WATERS WJ: A rapid micromethod for measuring the reserve albumin binding capacity in serum for newborn infants with hyperbilirubinemia. *J Lab Clin Med* 67:660, 1966

123. SCHARSCHMIDT BF, WAGGONER JG, BERK PD: Hepatic organic anion uptake in the rat. *J Clin Invest* 56:1280, 1975

124. WOLKOFF AW, KETLEY JN, WAGGONER JG, BERK PD, JAKOBY W: Hepatic accumulation and intracellular binding of conjugated bilirubin. *J Clin Invest* 61:142, 1978

125. BERNSTEIN LH, BEN-EZZER JB, GARTNER L, ARIAS IM: Hepatic intracellular distribution of tritium-labeled unconjugated and conjugated bilirubin in normal and Gunn rats. *J Clin Invest* 45:1194, 1966

126. BROWN WR, GRODSKY GM, CARBONE JV: Intracellular distribution of tritiated bilirubin during hepatic uptake and excretion. *Am J Physiol* 207:1237, 1964

127. GORESKY CA: The hepatic uptake process: Its implications for bilirubin transport, in Goresky CA, Fisher MM (eds): *Jaundice*. New York, Plenum, 1975, p 159

128. PAUMGARTNER G, REICHEN J: Kinetics of hepatic uptake of unconjugated bilirubin. *Clin Sci Mol Med* 51:169, 1976

129. BLOOMER JR, ZACCARIA J: Effect of graded bilirubin loads on bilirubin transport by perfused rat liver. *Am J Physiol* 230:736, 1976

130. HUNTON DB, BOLLMAN JL, HOFFMAN HN II: The plasma removal of indocyanine green and sulfobromophthalein: Effect of dosage and blocking agents. *J Clin Invest* 40:1648, 1961

131. SHUPECK M, WOLKOFF AW, SCHARSCHMIDT BF, WAGGONER JG, BERK PD: Studies of the kinetics of purified conjugated bilirubin-3H in the rat. *Am J Gastroenterol* 70:259, 1978

132. GORESKY CA: The hepatic uptake and excretion of sulfobromophthalein and bilirubin. *Can Med Assoc J* 92:851, 1965

133. WOLKOFF AW, GORESKY CA, SELLIN J, GATMAITAN Z, ARIAS IM: Role of ligandin in transfer of bilirubin from plasma into liver. *Am J Physiol* 236:E638, 1979

134. BLOOMER JR, BERK PD, VERGALLA J, BERLIN NI: Influence of albumin on the hepatic uptake of unconjugated bilirubin. *Clin Sci Mol Med* 45:505, 1973

135. WEISIGER R, GOLLAN J, OCKNER R: Receptor for albumin on the liver cell surface may mediate uptake of fatty acids and other albuminbound substances. *Science* 211:1048, 1981

136. WEISIGER R, GOLLAN J, OCKNER R: An albumin receptor on the liver cell may mediate hepatic uptake of sulfobromophthalein and bilirubin: bound ligand, not free, is the major uptake determinant. *Gastroenterology* 79:1065, 1980 (abstract)

137. WOLKOFF AW, OHMI N, GARTNER U: Uptake of bilirubin by the liver does not require an albumin receptor. *Gastroenterology* 79:1068, 1980 (abstract)

138. CLARENBURG R, BARNHART JL: Interaction of serum albumin and bilirubin at low concentrations. *Am J Physiol* 225:493, 1973

139. BARNHART JL, CLARENBURG R: Factors determining clearance of bilirubin in perfused rat liver. *Am J Physiol* 225:497, 1973

140. OIE S, LEVY G: Effect of plasma protein binding on elimination of bilirubin. *J Pharm Sci* 64:1433, 1975

141. GRAUSZ H, SCHMID R: Reciprocal relation between plasma albumin level and hepatic sulfobromophthalein removal. *N Engl J Med* 284:1403, 1971

142. BLONDHEIM SH: Effect of probenecid on excretion of bromosulphthalein. *J Appl Physiol* 7:529, 1955

143. GOETZEE AE, RICHARDS TG, TINDALL VR: Experimental changes in liver function induced by probenecid. *Clin Sci* 19:63, 1960

144. VOGIN EE, SCOTT W, BOYD J, BEAR WT, MATTIS PA: Effect of probenecid on indocyanine green clearance. *J Pharm Exp Ther* 152:509, 1966

145. KENWRIGHT S, LEVI AJ: Impairment of hepatic uptake of rifamycin antibiotics by probenecid, and its therapeutic implications. *Lancet* 2:1401, 1973

146. ACOCELLA G, NICOLIS FB, TENCONI LT: The effect of an intravenous infusion of rifamycin SV on the excretion of bilirubin, bromsulphalein, and indocyanine green in man. *Gastroenterology* 49:521, 1965

147. ACOCELLA G, BILLING BH: The effect of rifamycin SV on bile pigment excretion in rats. *Gastroenterology* 49:526, 1965

148. LAPERCHE Y, GRAILLOT C, ARONDEL J, BERTHELOT P: Uptake of rifampicin by isolated rat liver cells. Interaction with sulfobromophthalein uptake and evidence for separate carriers. *Biochem Pharm* 28:2065, 1979

149. NOSSLIN B, MORGAN EH: The effect of phloroglucinol derivatives from male fern on dye excretion by the liver in the rabbit and rat. *J Lab Clin Med* 65:891, 1965

150. HAMMAKER I, SCHMID R: Interference with bile pigment uptake in the liver by flavaspidic acid. *Gastroenterology* 53:31, 1967

151. BERTHELOT P, BILLING BH: Effect of bunamiodyl on hepatic uptake of sulfobromophthalein in the rat. *Am J Physiol* 211:395, 1966

152. BOLT RJ, DILLON RS, POLLARD HM: Interference with bilirubin excretion by a gall bladder dye (bunamiodyl). *N Engl J Med* 265:1043, 1961

153. GARTNER U, LEVINE WG, WOLKOFF AW: Evidence for independent hepatic uptake mechanisms for BSP and bilirubin. *Gastroenterology* 79:1019, 1980 (abstract)

154. CLARENBURG R, KAO CC: Shared and separate pathways for biliary excretion of bilirubin and BSP in rats. *Am J Physiol* 225:192, 1973

155. REYES H, LEVI AJ, GATMAITAN Z, ARIAS IM: Studies of Y and Z, two hepatic cytoplasmic anion-binding proteins: Effect of drugs, chemicals, hormones and cholestasis. *J Clin Invest* 50:2242, 1971

156. WOLKOFF AW: The glutathione S-transferases: Their role in the transport of organic anions from blood to bile, in Javitt NB (ed): *Liver and Biliary*

157. CORNELIUS CE, BEN-EZZER J, ARIAS IM: Binding of sulfobromophthalein sodium (BSP) and other organic anions by isolated hepatic cell plasma membranes in vitro. *Proc Soc Exp Biol Med* 124:665, 1967

158. REICHEN J, BLITZER BL, BERK PD: The binding of anionic dyes to hepatocellular plasma membranes. *Clin Res* 25:468, 1976 (abstract)

159. TIRIBELLI C, PANFILI E, SANDRI G, FREZZA M, SOTTOCASA GL: Liver bromsulphonphthalein transport as a carrier mediated process, in Leevy CM (ed): *Diseases of the Liver and Biliary Tract*. Basel, S Karger AG, 1976, p 55

160. TIRIBELLI C, LUNAZZI G, LUCIANI GL, PANFILI E, GASSIN B, LIUT G, SANDRI G, SOTTOCASA G: Isolation of a sulfobromophthalein-binding protein from hepatocyte plasma membrane. *Biochim Biophys Acta* 532: 105, 1978

161. WOLKOFF AW, CHUNG CT: Identification, purification, and partial characterization of an organic anion binding protein from rat liver cell plasma membrane. *J Clin Invest* 65:1152, 1980

162. REICHEN J, BERK PD: Isolation of an organic anion binding protein from rat liver plasma membrane fractions by affinity chromatography. *Biochem Biophys Res Commun* 91:484, 1979

163. STEINER JW, PERZ ZM, TAICHMAN LB: Cell population dynamics in the liver. A review of quantitative morphological techniques applied to the study of physiological and pathological growth. *Exp Mol Pathol* 5:146, 1966

164. BUCHER NL, MALT RA: *Regeneration of Liver and Kidney*, Boston, Little, Brown, 1971

165. GARTNER U, STOCKERT RJ, MORELL AG, WOLKOFF AW: Modulation of the transport of bilirubin and asialoorosomocoid during liver regeneration. *Hepatology* 1:99, 1981

166. LEVI AJ, GATMAITAN Z, ARIAS IM: Two hepatic cytoplasmic protein fractions, Y and Z, and their possible role in the hepatic uptake of bilirubin, sulfobromophthalein, and other anions. *J Clin Invest* 48:2156, 1969

167. FLEISCHNER G, ROBBINS J, ARIAS IM: Immunological studies of Y protein: a major cytoplasmic organic anion binding protein in rat liver. *J Clin Invest* 51:677, 1972

168. LICHTER M, FLEISCHNER G, KIRSCH R, LEVI AJ, KAMISAKA K, ARIAS IM: Ligandin and Z protein in binding of thyroid hormones by the liver. *Am J Physiol* 230:1113, 1976

169. KAMISAKA K, LISTOWSKY I, GATMAITAN Z, ARIAS IM: Interactions of bilirubin and other ligands with ligandin. *Biochemistry* 14:2175, 1975

170. KIRSCH R, KAMISAKA K, FLEISCHNER G, ARIAS IM: Structural and functional studies of ligandin, a major renal organic anion binding protein. *J Clin Invest* 55:1009, 1975

171. GOLDSTEIN EJ, ARIAS IM: Interaction of ligandin with radiographic contrast media. *Invest Radiol* 11:594, 1976

172. MOREY KS, LITWACK G: Isolation and properties of cortisol metabolite binding proteins of rat liver cytosol. *Biochemistry* 8:4813, 1969

173. KETTERER B, ROSS-MANSELL P, WHITEHEAD JK: The isolation of carcinogen-binding protein from livers of rats given 4-dimethylaminoazobenzene. *Biochem J* 103:316, 1967

174. LITWACK G, KETTERER B, ARIAS IM: Ligandin: An abundant liver protein which binds steroids, bilirubin, carcinogens and a number of exogenous anions. *Nature* 234:466, 1971

175. FLEISCHNER GM, ROBBINS JB, ARIAS IM: Cellular localization of ligandin in rat, hamster, and man. *Biochem Biophys Res Commun* 74:992, 1977

176. KAPLOWITZ N, PERCY-ROBB IW, JAVITT NB: Role of hepatic anion-binding protein in bromsulphthalein conjugation. *J Exp Med* 138:483, 1973

177. HABIG WH, PABST MJ, JAKOBY WB: Glutathione S-transferases. The first enzymatic step in mercapturic acid formation. *J Biol Chem* 249:7130, 1974

178. HABIG WH, PABST MJ, FLEISCHNER G, GATMAITAN Z, ARIAS IM, JAKOBY WB: The identity of glutathione S-transferase B with ligandin, a major binding protein of liver. *Proc Nat Acad Sci USA* 10:3879, 1974

179. BENSON AM, TALALAY P, KEEN JH, JAKOBY WB: Relationship between the soluble glutathione-dependent Δ5-3-ketosteroid isomerase and the glutathione S-transferases of the liver. *Proc Natl Acad Sci USA* 74:158, 1977

180. PROHASKA JR, GANTHER HE: Glutathione peroxidase activity of glutathione S-transferase purified from rat liver. *Biochem Biophys Res Commun* 76:437, 1977

181. LAWRENCE RA, PARKHILL LK, BURK RF: Hepatic cytosolic non selenium-dependent glutathione peroxidase activity: Its nature and the effect of selenium deficiency. *J Nutr* 108:981, 1978

182. HABIG WH, PABST MJ, JAKOBY WB: Glutathione S-transferase AA from rat liver. *Arch Biochem Biophys* 175:710, 1976

183. PABST MJ, HABIG WH, JAKOBY WB: Glutathione S-transferase A: a novel kinetic mechanism in which the major reaction pathway depends on substrate concentration. *J Biol Chem* 249:7140, 1974

184. KAMISAKA K, HABIG WH, KETLEY JN, ARIAS IM, JAKOBY WB: Multiple forms of human glutathione S-transferase and their affinity for bilirubin. *Eur J Biochem* 60:153, 1975

Tract Physiology I. Baltimore, Baltimore University Park Press, 1980, p 151

185. KETLEY JN, HABIG WH, JAKOBY WB: Binding of non-substrate ligands to the glutathione transferases. *J Biol Chem* 250:8670, 1975

186. BHARGAVA MM, LISTOWSKY I, ARIAS IM: Ligandin: Bilirubin binding and glutathione S-transferase activity are independent processes. *J Biol Chem* 253:4112, 1978

187. BHARGAVA MM, OHMI N, LISTOWSKY I, ARIAS IM: Structural, catalytic, binding, and immunological properties associated with each of the two subunits of rat liver ligandin. *J Biol Chem* 255:718, 1980.

188. JAKOBY WB: The glutathione S-transferases: A group of multifunctional detoxification proteins, in Meister A (ed): *Advances in Enzymology and Related Areas of Molecular Biology.* New York, Wiley, 1978, p 383

189. WOLKOFF AW, WEISIGER RA, JAKOBY WB: The multiple roles of the glutathione transferases (Ligandins), in Popper H, Schaffner F, (eds): *Progress in Liver Diseases.* New York, Grune and Stratton, 1979, vol 6, p 213

190. ARIAS IM: Ligandin: A review and update of a multifunctional protein. *Med Biol* 57:328, 1979

191. LEVINE RI, REYES H, LEVI AJ, GATMAITAN Z, ARIAS IM: Phylogenetic study of organic anion transfer from plasma into the liver. *Nature (New Biol)* 231:277, 1971

192. LEVI AJ, GATMAITAN Z, ARIAS IM: Deficiency of hepatic organic anion-binding protein as a possible cause of nonhaemolytic unconjugated hyperbilirubinemia in the newborn. *Lancet* 2:139, 1969

193. LEVI AJ, GATMAITAN Z, ARIAS IM: Deficiency of hepatic organic anion-binding protien, impaired organic anion uptake by liver and "physiologic" jaundice in newborn monkeys. *N Engl J Med* 283:1136, 1970

194. BOYER JL, SCHWARZ J, SMITH N: Biliary secretion in elasmobranchs. I. Bile collection and composition. *Am J Physiol* 230:970, 1976

195. BOYER JL, SCHWARZ J, SMITH N: Biliary secretion in elasmobranchs. II. Hepatic uptake and biliary excretion of organic anions. *Am J Physiol* 230:974, 1976

196. BEND JR, FOUTS JR: Glutathione S-transferase: Distribution in several marine species and partial characterization in hepatic soluble fractions from little skate, *Raja erinaces,* liver. *Bull Mt Desert Island Biol Lab* 13:4, 1973

197. KAMISAKA K, LISTOWSKY I, FLEISCHNER G, GATMAITAN Z, ARIAS IM: The binding of bilirubin and other organic anions to serum albumin and ligandin (Y protein), in *Bilirubin Metabolism in the Newborn (II).* Excerpta Medica International Congress Series No. 380, Amsterdam, Excerpta Medica, 1976, p 156

198. KETTERER B, TIPPING E, BEALE D, MEUWISSEN JATP: Ligandin, glutathione transferase, and carcinogen binding, in Arias IM, Jakoby WB (eds): *Glutathione: Metabolism and Function.* New York, Raven, 1976, p 243

199. LISTOWSKY I, GATMAITAN Z, ARIAS IM: Ligandin retains and albumin loses bilirubin binding capacity in liver cytosol. *Proc Natl Acad Sci USA* 75:1213, 1978

200. KAMISAKA K, GATMAITAN Z, MOORE CL, ARIAS IM: Ligandin reverses bilirubin inhibition of liver mitochondrial respiration in vitro. *Pediatr Res* 9:903, 1975

201. HEIRWEGH KPM, VAN HEES GP, LEROY P, VAN ROY FP, JANSEN FH: Heterogeneity of bile pigment conjugates as revealed by chromatography of their ethyl anthranilate azopigments. *Biochem J* 120:877, 1970

202. FEVERY J, VAN DAMME B, MICHIELS R, DE GROOTE J, HEIRWEGH KPM: Bilirubin conjugates in bile of man and rat in the normal state and in liver disease. *J Clin Invest* 51:2482, 1972

203. BLANCKAERT N, CAMPERNOLLE F, LEROY P, VAN HOURTTE R, FEVERY J, HEIRWEGH KPM: The fate of bilirubin 1Xα glucuronide in cholestasis and during storage in vitro. *Biochem J* 171:203, 1978

204. COMPERNOLLE F, VAN HEES GP, FEVERY J, HEIRWEGH KPM: Mass-spectrometric structure elucidation of dog bile azopigments as the acyl glycosides of glucopyranose and xylopyranose. *Biochem J* 125:811, 1971

205. FEVERY J, VAN HEES GP, LEROY P, COMPERNOLLE F, HEIRWEGH KPM: Excretion in dog bile of glucose and xylose conjugates of bilirubin. *Biochem J* 125:803, 1971

206. CORNELIUS CE, KELLY KC, HIMES JA: Heterogeneity of bilirubin conjugates in several animal species. *Cornell Vet* 65 (1):90, 1975

207. KUENZLE CC: Bilirubin conjugates of human bile. *Biochem J* 119:411, 1970

208. GORDON ER, GORESKY CA, CHAN TH, PERLIN AS: The isolation and characterization of bilirubin diglucuronide, the major bilirubin conjugate in dog and human bile. *Biochem J* 155:477, 1976

209. WEBER A, SCHALM L, WITMANS J: Bilirubin monoglucuronide (pigment I): A complex. *Acta Med Scand* 173:19, 1963

210. NOSSLIN B: The direct diazo reaction of bile pigments in serum. Experimental and clinical studies. *Scand J Clin Lab Invest* 12:(suppl 49)1, 1960

211. OSTROW JD, MURPHY NH: Isolation and properties of conjugated bilirubin and bile. *Biochem J* 120:311, 1970

212. JANSEN FH, BILLING BH: Separation and structural analysis of vinyl and isovinyl azobilirubin derivatives. *Biochem J* 125:585, 1971

213. JANSEN FH, BILLING BH: The identification of mono-conjugates of bilirubin in bile as amide derivatives. *Biochem J* 125:917, 1971

214. BLANCKAERT N: Analysis of bilirubin and bilirubin mono and diconjugates. Determination of their relative amounts in biological fluids. *Biochem J* 185:115, 1980

215. HUTCHINSON DW, JOHNSON B, KNELL AJ: The reaction between bilirubin and aromatic diazo compounds. *Biochem J* 127:907, 1972

216. VAN DEN BERGH AAH, MULLER P: Ueber eine direkte und eine indirekte Diazoreaktion auf Bilirubin. *Biochem Z* 77:90, 1916

217. TALAFANT E: Properties and composition of bile pigment giving direct diazo reaction. *Nature (London)* 178:312, 1956

218. COMPERNOLLE F, VAN HEES GP, BLANCKAERT N, HEIRWEGH KPM: Glucuronic acid conjugates of bilirubin 1Xα in normal bile compared with post-obstructive bile. *Biochem J* 171:185, 1978

219. COLE PG, LATHE GH, BILLING BH: Separation of the bile pigments of serum, bile and urine. *Biochem J* 57:514, 1954

220. HEIRWEGH KPM, FEVERY J, MICHIELS R, VAN HEES GP, COMPERNOLLE F: Separation by thin layer chromatography and structure elucidation of bilirubin conjugates isolated from dog bile. *Biochem J* 145:185, 1975

221. ISSELBACHER KJ, MCCARTHY EA: Studies on bilirubin sulfate and other non-glucuronide conjugates. *J Clin Invest* 38:645, 1959

222. NOIR BA, DE WALZ AT, RODRIGUEZ G: Studies on the bilirubin sulfate conjugate excreted in human bile. *Biochim Biophys Acta* 222:15, 1970

223. TENHUNEN R: Studies on bilirubin and its metabolism. *Ann Med Exp Biol Fein Suppl* 6:1, 1965

224. ETTER-KJELSAAS H, KUENZLE CC: A polypeptide conjugate of bilirubin from human bile. *Biochim Biophys Acta* 400:83, 1975

225. BLANCKAERT N, KABRA PM, FARINA FA, STAFFORD BE, MARTON LJ, SCHMIDT R: Measurement of bilirubin and its mono- and diconjugates in human serum by alkaline methanolysis and high performance liquid chromatography. *J Lab Clin Med* 96:198, 1980

226. ONISHI S, ITOH S, KAWADE N, ISOBE K, SUGIYAMA S: An accurate and sensitive analysis by high pressure liquid chromatography of conjugated and unconjugated bilirubin 1Xα and in various biological fluids. *Biochem J* 185:281, 1980

227. JANSEN PLM: β-Glucuronidase resistant bilirubin glucuronide isomers in cholestatic liver disease-Determination of bilirubin metabolites in serum by means of high-pressure liquid chromatography. *Clin Chim Acta,* 110:309, 1981

228. JANSEN PLM, TANGERMAN A: Separation and characterization of bilirubin conjugates by high performance liquid chromatography. *J Chromat* 182:100, 1980

229. ROY CHOWDHURY J, ARIAS IM: Dismutation of bilirubin, in Colowick SP, Kaplan NO (eds): *Methods in Enzymology* vol. 77 (in press)

230. FEVERY JB, VAN DAMME R, MICHIELS R, DE GROOTE J, HEIRWEGH KPM: Bilirubin conjugates in bile of man and rat in the normal state and in liver disease. *J Clin Invest* 51:2482, 1972

231. GORDON ER, DADOUN M, GORESKY CA, CHAN TH, PERLIN AS: The isolation of an azobilirubin β-D monoglucoside from dog gall bladder bile. *Biochem J* 143:97, 1974

232. BILLING BH, COLE PG, LATHE GH: The excretion of bilirubin as a diglucuronide giving the direct Van den Bergh reaction. *Biochem J* 65:774, 1957

233. DUTTON GJ, BURCHELL B: Newer aspects of glucuronidation. *Prog Drug Metab* 2:1, 1977

234. DUTTON GJ: The biosynthesis of glucuronides, in Dutton GJ (ed): *Glucuronic Acid Free and Combined.* New York, Academic, 1966, p 185

235. ROY CHOWDHURY J, ROY CHOWDHURY N, ARIAS IM: Bilirubin conjugation in the spiny dog fish, *Squalus acanthias,* the small skate, *Raja erinaeca* and the winter flounder, *Pseudopleuronectes americanas. Comp Biochem Physiol* 66B:523, 1979

236. CHAMBERS JE, YARBOROUGH JD: Xenobiotic transformation systems in fishes. *Comp Biochem Physiol* 55C:77, 1976

237. DUTTON GJ, STEVENSON IH: The stimulation by 3,4-benzpyrene of glucuronide synthesis in skin. *Biochim Biophys Acta* 58:633, 1962

238. AITTIO A: Academic dissertation, Turku, Finland, 1973

239. GRAHAM AB, PECHEY DT, TOOGOOD KC, THOMAS SB, WOOD GC: The phospholipid dependence of uridine diphosphate glucuronyl transferase. *Biochem J* 163:117, 1977

240. JANSEN PLM, ARIAS IM: Delipidation and reactivation of UDP glucuronosyl transferase from rat liver. *Biochim Biophys Acta* 391:28, 1975

241. MULDER GJ: The effect of phenobarbital on the submicrosomal distribution of uridine diphosphate glucuronyl transferase from rat liver. *Biochem J* 117:319, 1970

242. GREGORY DH, STRICKLAND RD: Solubilization and characterization of hepatic bilirubin UDP glucuronyl transferase. *Biochim Biophys Acta* 327:36, 1973

243. HEIRWEGH KPM, MEUWISSEN JATP: Activation in vitro and solubilization of glucuronyl transferase (assay with bilirubin as acceptor) with digitonin. *Biochem J* 110:31, 1968

244. JANSEN PLM: Studies on UDP glucuronyl transferase. Ph.D dissertation. University of Nijmegen, the Netherlands, 1972

245. ADLARD BFP, LATHE GH: The effect of steroids and nucleotides on solu-

bilized bilirubin uridine diphosphate glucuronyl transferase. *Biochem J* 119:437, 1970

246. HENDERSON P: Activation in vitro rat hepatic UDP glucuronyl transferase by ultra sound. *Life Science* part II, 9:511, 1970

247. GRAHAM AB, WOOD GC: Factors affecting the response of microsomal UDP-glucuronyltransferase to membrane perturbants. *Biochim Biophys Acta* 311:45, 1973

248. VESSEY DA, ZAKIM D: Regulations of microsomal enzymes by phospholipids. *J Biol chem* 246:4649, 1971

249. HEIRWEGH KPM, CAMPBELL M, MEUWISSEN JATP: Compartmentation of membrane bound enzymes. Some basic concepts and consequences for kinetic studies, in Aitio A (ed): *Conjugation Reactions in Drug Biotransformation*. Amsterdam, Elsevier/North-Holland, 1978, p 191

250. TERENCE H: In Aitio A (ed):*Conjugation Reactions in Drug Biotransformation*. Amsterdam, Elsevier/North-Holland, 1978, p 257

251. BOCK KW, FROHLING W, REMMER H, REXER B: Effects of phenobarbital and 3 methyl cholanthrene on substrate specificity of rat liver microsomal UDP glucuronyl transferase. *Biochim Biophys Acta* 327:46, 1973

252. TOMLISON GA, YAFFE SJ: The formation of bilirubin and *p*-nitrophenyl glucuronides by rabbit liver. *Biochem J* 99:507, 1966

253. HALAC E, REFF A: Studies on bilirubin UDP glucuronyl transferase. *Biochim Biophys Acta* 139:328, 1967

254. WISHART GJ: Functional heterogeneity of UDP glucuronosyl transferase as indicated by its differential development and inducibility by glucocorticoids. *Biochem J* 174:485, 1978

255. VAN LEUSDEN HAIM, BAKKEREN JAJM, ZILLIKEN F, STOLTE LAM: Nitrophenyl glucuronide formation by homozygous adult Gunn rats. *Biochem Biophys Res Commun* 7:67, 1962

256. DRUCKER WD: Glucuronic acid conjugation of tetrahydrocortisone *p*-nitrophenol in the homozygous Gunn rats. *Proc Soc Exp Biol Med* 129:308, 1968

257. MOWAT AP, ARIAS IM: Observations of the effect of diethyl nitrosamine on glucuronide formation. *Biochim Biophys Acta* 212:175, 1970

258. GORSKI JP, KASPER CB: Purification and properties of microsomal UDP glucuronyl transferase from rat liver. *J Biol Chem* 252:1336, 1977

259 BURCHELL B: Purification of UDP glucuronyl transferase from untreated rat liver. *FEBS Lett* 78:101, 1977

260. BOCK KW, JOSLING D, LILENBLUM WM, PFEIL H: Purification of rat liver glucuronyl transferase—Separation of two enzyme forms inducible by 3-methylcholanthrene or phenobarbital. *Eur J Biochem* 98:19, 1979

261. BOCK KW, KITTEL J, JOSTING D: Purification of rat liver UDP glucuronyl transferase: Separation of two enzyme forms with different substrate specificity and differential inducibility, in Aitio A (ed): *Conjugation Reactions in Drug Biotransformation*. Amsterdam, Elsevier/North Holland, 1978, p 357

262. MALIK N, OWENS IS: Induction of bilirubin UDP glucuronosyl transferase (T'ase) activity in mice by 3-methylcholanthrene (MC) and 2,3,7,8,-tetrachlorodibenzo-p-dioxin (TCDD). *Pharmacologist* 20:200, 1978 (abstract)

263. NAKATA D, ZAKIM D, VASSEY DA: Defective function of a microsomal UDP glucuronyl transferase in Gunn rats. *Proc Natl Acad Sci USA* 73:289, 1976

264. FEVERY J, LEROY P, VAN DE VIJVER M, HEIRWEGH KPM: Structures of bilirubin conjugates synthesized *in vitro* from bilirubin and uridine diphosphate glucuronic acid, uridine diphosphate glucose or uridine diphosphate xylose by preparations from rat liver. *Biochem J* 129:635, 1972

265. BLACK M, BILLING BH, HEIRWEGH KPM: Determination of bilirubin UDP-glucuronyl transferase activity in needle biopsy specimens of human liver. *Clin Chim Acta* 29:27, 1970

266. HEIRWEGH KPM, VAN DE VIJVER M, FEVERY J: Assay and properties of digitonin-activated bilirubin uridine diphosphate glucuronyl transferase from rat liver. *Biochem J* 129:605, 1972

267. JANSEN PLM: Mono and diglucuronidation of bilirubin. *Fol Med Neur* 15:205, 1972

268. BLANCKAERT N, GOLLAN J, SCHMID R: Bilirubin diglucuronide synthesis by a UDP glucuronic acid dependent enzyme system in rat liver microsomes. *Proc Natl Acad Sci* 76:2037, 1979

269. ROY CHOWDHURY J, ROY CHOWDHURY N, BHARGAVA M, ARIAS IM: Purification and partial characterization of rat liver bilirubin glucuronoside glucuronosyl transferase. *J Biol Chem* 254:8336, 1979

270. JANSEN PLM, ROY CHOWDHURY J, FISCHBERG EB, ARIAS IM: Enzymatic conversion of bilirubin monoglucuronide to diglucuronide by rat liver plasma membranes. *J Biol Chem* 252:2710, 1977

271. ROY CHOWDHURY J, FISCHBERG EB, DANILLER A, JANSEN PLM, ARIAS IM: Hepatic conversion of bilirubin monoglucuronide to bilirubin diglucuronide in uridine diphosphate glucuronyl transferase deficient man and rat by bilirubin glucuronoside glucuronosyl transferase. *J Clin Invest* 21:191, 1978

272. ROY CHOWDHURY J, ROY CHOWDHURY N, GARTNER U, WOLKOFF AW, ARIAS IM: Bilirubin diglucuronide formation in intact rats and in isolated Gunn rat liver. *J Clin Invest* (in press)

273. ARIAS IM, JOHNSON L, WOLFSON S: Biliary excretion of injected conjugated and unconjugated bilirubin by normal and Gunn rats. *Am J Physiol* 200:1091, 1961

274. ROBINSON SH, YANNONI C, NAGASAWA S: Bilirubin excretion in rats with normal and impaired bilirubin conjugation. Effect of phenobarbital. *J Clin Invest* 50:2606, 1971

275. SHANI M, GILON E, BEN-EZZER J, SHEBA C: Sulfobromophthalein tolerance test in patients with the Dubin-Johnson syndrome and their relatives. *Gastroenterology* 59:842, 1970

276. GUTSTEIN S, ALPERT S, ARIAS IM: Studies of hepatic excretory function. IV. Biliary excretion of sulfobromophthalein in a patient with Dubin-Johnson syndrome and a biliary fistula. *Isr J Med Sci* 4:46, 1968

277. CORNELIUS CE: Organic anion transport in mutant sheep with congenital hyperbilirubinemia. *Arch Environ Health* 19:852, 1969

278. ALPERT S, MOSHER M, SHANSKE A, ARIAS IM: Multiplicity of hepatic excretory mechanism for organic anions. *J Gen Physiol* 53:238, 1969

279. BERNSTEIN RB, NOVY MJ, PIASECKI GJ, LESTER R, JACKSON BT: Bilirubin metabolism in the fetus. *J Clin Invest* 48:1678, 1969

280. UPSON DW, GRONWALL RR, CORNELIUS CE: Maximal hepatic excretion of bilirubin in sheep. *Proc Soc Exp Biol Med* 134:9, 1970

281. KLAASSEN CD, PLAA GL: Studies on the mechanism of phenobarbital-enhanced sulfobromophthalein disappearance. *J Pharmacol Exp Ther* 161:361, 1968

282. BARNHART J, RITT S, WARE A, COOMBES B: A comparison of the effects of taurocholate and theophylline on BSP excretion in dogs, in Paumgartner G, Preisig R (eds): *The Liver: Quantitative Aspects of Structure and Function*. Basel, S Karger, 1973, p 315

283. SCHARSCHMIDT BF, SCHMID R: The "micellar sink". *J Clin Invest* 62:1122, 1978

284. BINET S, DELAGE Y, ERLINGER S: Influence of taurocholate, taurochenodeoxycholate and taurodehydrocholate on sulfobromophthalein transport into bile. *Am J Physiol* 236:E10, 1979

285. SHULL SD, WAGNER CI, TROTMAN BW, SOLOWAY RD: Factors affecting bilirubin excretion in patients with cholesterol or pigment gallstones. *Gastroenterology* 72:625, 1977

286. CLARENBURG R, KAO CC: Shared and separate pathways for biliary excretion of bilirubin and BSP in rats. *Am J Physiol* 225:192, 1973

287. FORKER EL: Canalicular anion transport. Effect of bile acid-independent choleretics, in Berk PD, Berline NI (eds): *Bile Pigments, Chemistry and Physiology*. Washington, USDEW, NIH, 1977, Chap 38, p 383

288. LESTER R, SCHMID R: Intestinal absorption of bile pigments. II. Bilirubin absorption in man. *N Engl J Med* 269:178, 1963

289. BRODERSEN R, HERMAN LS: Intestinal reabsorption of unconjugated bilirubin: A possible contributing factor in neonatal jaundice. *Lancet* 1:1242, 1963

290. OSTROW JD: Absorption of bile pigments by the gall bladder. *J Clin Invest* 46:2035, 1967

291. WATSON CJ: The urobilinoids: Milestones in their history and some recent developments, Berk PD, Berlin NI (eds): *The Chemistry and Physiology of Bile Pigments*. Washington, USDEW, NIH, 1977, p 469

292. STOLL MS, LIM CK, GRAY CH: Chemical variants of the urobilins, in, PD Berk, NI Berlin (eds): *The Chemistry and Physiology of Bile Pigments*. Washington, USDEW, NIH, 1977, p 483

293. MOSCOWITZ A, WEIMER M, LIGHTNER DA, PETRYKA ZJ, DAVIS H, WATSON CJ: The *in vitro* conversion of bile pigments to the urobilinoids by a rat clostridia species as compared with the human fecal flora. III. Natural *d*-urobilin, synthetic *i*-urobilin, and synthetic *i*-urobilinogen. *Biochem Med* 4:149, 1970

294. ELDER G, GRAY CH, NICHOLSON DG: Bile pigment fate in gastrointestinal tract, in Schmid R, Jaffe ER, Miescher PA (eds): *Physiology and Disorders of Hemoglobin Degradation. Seminars in Hematology*. New York, Grune and Stratton, 1972, p 71

295. BERK PD: Personal communication

296. SCHMID R, HAMMAKER L: Metabolism and disposition of C^{14}-bilirubin in congenital nonhemolytic jaundice. *J Clin Invest* 42:1720, 1963

297. LUND HT, JACOBSEN J: Influence of phototherapy on the biliary bilirubin excretion patterns in newborn infants with hyperbilirubinemia. *J Pediatr* 85:262, 1974

298. OSTROW JD: Photocatabolism of labeled bilirubin in the congenitally jaundiced (Gunn) rat. *J Clin Invest* 50:707, 1971

299. BERRY CS, ZAREMBO JE, OSTROW JD: Evidence for conversion of bilirubin to dihydroxyl derivatives in the Gunn rat. *Biochem Biophys Res Commun* 49:1366, 1972

300. BLANKAERT N, FEVERY J, HEIRWEGH KPN, COMPERNOLLE F: Characterization of the major diazopositive pigments in bile of homozygous Gunn rats. *Biochem J* 164:237, 1977

301. KAPITULNIK J, OSTROW JD: Stimulation of bilirubin catabolism in jaundiced Gunn rats by an inducer of microsomal mixed function monooxygenases. *Proc Natl Acad Sci USA* 75:682, 1978

302. CAMERON JL, PULASKI EJ, ABEL T, IBER FL: Metabolism and excretion of bilirubin ^{14}C in experimental obstructive jaundice. *Ann Surg* 163:330, 1966

303. CAMERON JL, FILLER RM, IBER FL, ABEL T, RANDOLPH JG: Metabolism and excretion of ^{14}C labeled bilirubin in children with biliary atresia. N Engl J Med 274:231, 1966

304. FULOP M, SANDSON J, BRAZEAU P: Dialyzability, protein binding, and renal excretion of plasma conjugated bilirubin. J Clin Invest 44:666, 1965

305. GOLLAN JL, DALLINGER KJC, BILLING BH: Excretion of conjugated bilirubin in the isolated perfused rat kidney. Clin Sci Mol Med 54:381, 1978

306. HARDY JB, PEEPLES MO: Serum bilirubin levels in newborn infants. Distributions and associations with neurological abnormalities during the first year of life. Johns Hopkins Med J 128:265, 1971

307. GARTNER LM, LEE K, VAISMAN S, LANE D, ZARAFU I: Development of bilirubin transport and metabolism in the newborn Rhesus monkey. J Pediatr 90:513, 1977

308. MAISELS MJ, PATHAK A, NELSON NM, NATHAN DG, SMITH CA: Endogenous production of carbon monoxide in normal and erythroblastic newborn infants. J Clin Invest 50:1, 1971

309. VEST M, STREBEL L, HAUENSTEIN D: The extend of "shunt" bilirubin and erythrocyte survival in the newborn infant measured by the administration of (^{15}N) glycine. Biochem J 95:11c, 1965

310. PEARSON HA: Life-span of the fetal red blood cell. J Pediatr 70:166, 1967

311. BRODERSEN R, HERMAN LS: Intestinal reabsorption of unconjugated bilirubin: A possible contributing factor in neonatal jaundice. Lancet 1:1242, 1963

312. POLAND RL, ODELL GB: Physiologic jaundice: The enterohepatic circulation of bilirubin. N Engl J Med 284:1, 1971

313. FREDA VJ, GORMAN JG, POLLACK W: Successful prevention of experimental Rh sensitization in man with an anti Rh gamma 2 globulin antibody preparation. Transfusion 4:26, 1964

314. CLARKE CA, DONOHOE WTA, FINN R, LEHANE D, McCONNELL RB, SHEPPARD PM, TOWERS SH, WOODROW JC, BOWLEY CC, TOVEY LAD, BIAS WB, KREVANS JR: Combined study: Prevention of Rh hemolytic disease: Final results of the "high risk" clinical trial. A combined study from centers in England and Baltimore. Brit Med J 2:607, 1971

315. HABERMAN S, KRAFFT EJ, LEUCKE PE, PEACH RO: ABO isoimmunization: The use of the specific Coombs and best elution tests in the detection of hemolytic disease. J Pediatr 56:471, 1960

316. HSIA D Y-Y, GELLIS SS: Studies on erythroblastosis fetalis due to ABO incompatibility. Pediatrics 13:503, 1954

317. LEVI AJ, GATMAITAN Z, ARIAS IM: Deficiency of hepatic organic anion-binding protein as a possible cause of nonhaemolytic unconjugated hyperbilirubinemia in the newborn. Lancet 2:139, 1969

318. GRODSKY GM, KOLB HJ, FANSKA RE, NEMECHEK C: Effect of age of rat on development of hepatic carriers for bilirubin: A possible explanation for physiologic jaundice and hyperbilirubinemia in the newborn. Metabolism 3:246, 1970

319. LEVI AJ, GATMAITAN Z, ARIAS IM: Deficiency of hepatic organic anion-binding protein, impaired organic anion uptake by liver and "physiologic" jaundice in newborn monkeys. N Engl J Med 283:1136, 1970

320. ODELL GB: "Physiologic" hyperbilirubinemia in the neonatal period. N Engl J Med 277:193, 1967

321. BROWN AK, ZUELZER WW: Studies on the neonatal development of the glucuronide conjugating system. J Clin Invest 37:332, 1958

322. BERNSTEIN RB, NOVY MJ, PIASECKI GJ, LESTER R, JACKSON BT: Bilirubin metabolism in the fetus. J Clin Invest 48:1678, 1969

323. MARTIUS G, HUBER W: Bromsulphalein clearance and bilirubin levels in the newborn. Ger Med Mon 10:192, 1965

324. GARTNER LM, ARIAS IM: The transfer of bilirubin from blood to bile in the neonatal guinea pig. Pediatr Res 3:171, 1969

325. HSIA D Y-T, PATTERSON P, ALLEN FH, DIAMOND LK, GELLIS SS: Prolonged obstructive jaundice in infancy: General Survey of 156 cases. Pediatrics 10:243, 1952

326. ARTHUR LJH, BEVAN BR, HOLTON JB: Neonatal hyperbilirubinemia and breast feeding. Dev Med Child Neurol 8:279, 1966

327. ARIAS IM, GARTNER LM, SEIFTER S, FURMAN M: Prolonged neonatal unconjugated hyperbilirubinemia associated with breast feeding and a steroid, pregnane-3(alpha), 20(beta)-diol, in maternal milk that inhibits glucuronide formation in vitro. J Clin Invest 43:2037, 1964

328. HARGREAVES T, PIPER RF: Breast milk jaundice: Effect of inhibitory breast milk and 3(alpha), 20(beta) pregnanediol on glucuronyl transferase. Arch Dis Child 46:195, 1971

329. HOLTON JB, LATHE GH: Inhibitors of bilirubin conjugation in newborn infant serum and male urine. Clin Sci 25:499, 1963

330. ADLARD BPF, LATHE GH: Breast milk jaundice: Effect of 3(alpha), 20(beta)-pregnanediol on bilirubin conjugation by human liver. Arch Dis Child 45:186, 1970

331. ARIAS IM, GARTNER LM: Production of unconjugated hyperbilirubinaemia in full-term new born infants following administration of pregnane-3(alpha), 20(beta)-diol. Nature 203:1292, 1964

332. RAMOS A, SILVERBERG M, STERN I: Pregnanediols and neonatal hyperbilirubinemia. Am J Dis Child 111:353, 1966

333. JOHNSON JD: Neonatal nonhemolytic jaundice. N Engl J Med 292:194, 1975

334. FOLIOT A, PLOUSSARD JP, HOUSETT E, CHRISTOFOROV B, LUZEAN R, ODIEVRE M: Breast milk jaundice: In vitro inhibition of rat liver bilirubin-uridine diphosphate glucuronyltransferase activity and Z protein-bromosulphophthalein binding by human breast milk. Pediatr Res 10:594, 1976

335. LUCEY JF, DRISCOL JJ: Physiological jaundice re-examined, in Sass-Kortsak A, (ed): Kernicterus. Toronto, University of Toronto Press, 1961, p 29

336. ARIAS IM, WOLFSON S, LUCEY JF, McKAY RJ JR: Transient familial neonatal hyperbilirubinemia. J Clin Invest 44:1442, 1965

337. BERK PD, WOLKOFF AW, BERLIN NI: Inborn errors of bilirubin metabolism. Med Clin NA 59:803, 1975

338. SCHALM L, WEBER AP: Jaundice with conjugated bilirubin in hyperhaemolysis. Acta Med Scand 176:549, 1964

339. SNYDER AL, SATTERLEE W, ROBINSON SH, SCHMID R: Conjugated plasma bilirubin in jaundice caused by pigment overload. Nature (London) 213:93, 1967

340. ROBINSON S, VANIER T, DESFORGES JF, SCHMID R: Jaundice in thalassemia minor: A consequence of "ineffective erythropoiesis". N Engl J Med 267:523, 1962

341. ISRAELS LG, ZIPURSKY A: Primary shunt hyperbilirubinemia due to an alternate path of bilirubin production. Am J Med 27:693, 1959

342. BERENDSOHN S, LOWMAN J, SUNDBERG D, WATSON CJ: Idiopathic dyserythropoietic jaundice. Blood 24:1, 1964

343. VERWILGHEN R, VERHAEGEN H, WAUMANNS P, BEERT J: Ineffective erythropoiesis with morphologically abnormal erythroblasts and unconjugated hyperbilirubinemia. Brit J Haematol 17:27, 1969

344. VERWILGHEN R, LEWIS S, DACIE J, CROOKSTON J, CROOKSTON M: Hempas: Congenital dyserythropoietic anaemia (type II). Quart J Med 42:257, 1973

345. CRIGLER JF, NAJJAR VA: Congenital familial non-hemolytic jaundice with kernicterus. Pediatrics 10:169, 1952

346. CHILDS B, NAJJAR VA: Familial nonhemolytic jaundice with kernicterus: A report of two cases without neurological damage Pediatrics 18:369, 1956

347. CHILDS B, SIDBURY JB, MIGEON CJ: Glucuronic acid conjugation by patients with familial non-hemolytic jaundice and their relatives. Pediatrics 23:903, 1959

348. BLASCHKE TF, BERK PD, SCHARSCHMIDT BF, GUYTHER JR, VERGALLA J, WAGGONER JG: Crigler-Najjar syndrome: An unusual course with development of neurologic damage at age eighteen. Pediatr Res 8:573, 1974

349. BERK PD, MARTIN JF, BLASCHKE TF, SCHARSCHMIDT BF, PLOTZ PH: Unconjugated hyperbilirubinemia: Physiological evaluation and experimental approaches to therapy. Ann Intern Med 82:552, 1975

350. SLEISENGER MH, KAHN I, BARNIVILLE H, RUBIN W, BEN-EZZER J, ARIAS IM: Nonhemolytic unconjugated hyperbilirubinemia with hepatic glucuronyl transferase deficiency: a genetic study in four generations. Trans Assoc Am Phys 80:259, 1967

351. SCHMID R: Hyperbilirubinemia, in Stanbury JB, Wyngaarden JB, Fredrickson DS (eds): The Metabolic Basis of Inherited Disease, 3d ed New York, McGraw-Hill, 1972, p 1141

352. WOLKOFF AW, CHOWDHURY JR, GARTNER LA, ROSE AL, BIEMPICA L, GIBLIN DR, FINK D, ARIAS IM: Crigler-Najjar syndrome (Type I) in an adult male. Gastroenterology 76:3380, 1979

353. ARIAS IM: Chronic unconjugated hyperbilirubinemia without overt signs of hemolysis in adolescents and adults. J Clin Invest 41:2233, 1962

354. JERVIS GA: Constitutional nonhemolytic hyperbilirubinemia with findings resembling kernicterus. Arch Neurol Psychiatr 81:55, 1959

355. SZABO L, EBREY P: Studies on the inheritance of Crigler-Najjar syndrome by the menthol test. Acta Paediatr Hung 4:153, 1963

356. ARIAS IM, GARTNER LM, COHEN M, BEN-EZZER J, LEVI AJ: Chronic nonhemolytic unconjugated hyperbilirubinemia with glucuronyl transferase deficiency: Clinical, biochemical, pharmacologic, and genetic evidence for heterogeneity. Am J Med 47:395, 1969

357. KAPITULNIK J, KAUFMANN NA, GOITEIN K, CIVIDALLI G, BLONDHEIM SH: A pigment found in the Crigler-Najjar syndrome and its similarity to an ultrafilterable photo-derivative of bilirubin. Clin Chim Acta 57:231, 1974

358. BLOOMER JR, BERK PD, HOWE RB, BERLIN NI: Bilirubin metabolism in congenital nonhemolytic jaundice. Pediatr Res 5:256, 1971

359. BILLING GH, GRAY CH, KULCYCKA A, MANFIELD P, NICHOLSON DC: The metabolism of ^{14}C-bilirubin in congenital nonhaemolytic hyperbilirubinaemia. Clin Sci 27:163, 1964

360. NOVIKOFF AB, ESSNER E: The liver cell. Am J Med 29:102, 1960

361. DE BRITO T, BORGES MA, DASILVA LC: Electron microscopy of the liver in nonhemolytic acholuric jaundice with kernicterus (Crigler-Najjar) and in idiopathic conjugated hyperbilirubinemia (Rotor). Gastroenterologia 106:325, 1966

362. MINIO-PALUELLO, GAUTIER A, MAGNENAT P: L'ultrastructure du foie humain dans un cas de Crigler-Najjar. *Acta Hepatosplenol* 15:65, 1968

363. HUANG PWH, ROZDILSKY B, GERRARD JW, GOLUBOFF N, HOLMAN CH: Crigler-Najjar syndrome in four of five siblings with post-mortem findings in one. *Arch Pathol* 90:536, 1970

364. ROTHMALER G, LOWE H: Elektroneoptische untersuchungen der lever bei einem fall von kongenitalem nichthamolytischen ikterus (morbus Crigler-Najjar). *Padiatr Radol* 7:135, 1972

365. GUNN CH: Hereditary acholuric jaundice in a new mutant strain of rats. *J Hered* 29:137, 1938

366. SCHMID R, AXELROD J, HAMMAKER L, SWARM RL: Congenital jaundice in rats due to a defective glucuronide formation. *J Clin Invest* 37:1123, 1958

367. JOHNSON L, SARMIENTO F, BLANC WA, DAY R: Kernicterus in rats with an inherited deficiency of glucuronyl transferase. *Am J Dis Child* 97:591, 1959

368. BLANC WA, JOHNSON L: Studies on kernicterus. *J Neuropathol Exp Neurol* 18:165, 1959

369. SCHUTTA HS, JOHNSON L: Bilirubin encephalopathy in the Gunn rat: a fine structure study of the cerebrellar cortex. *J Neuropathol Exp Neurol* 26:377, 1967

370. ROSE AL, JOHNSON A: Bilirubin encephalopathy: Neuropathological and histochemical studies in the Gunn rat model. *Neurology* 22:420, 1972

371. SCHUTTA HS, JOHNSON L: Clinical signs and morphologic abnormalities in Gunn rats treated with sulfadiethoxine. *J Pediatr* 75:1070, 1969

372. COWGER ML: Bilirubin encephalopathy, in Gaull G (ed): *Biology of Brain Dysfunction*. New York, Plenum, 1973, vol 2, p 265

373. ODELL GB, NATZSCHKA JC, STOREY G: Bilirubin nephropathy in the Gunn strain of rat. *Am J Physiol* 212:931, 1967

374. CALL NB, TISHER CC: The urinary concentrating defect in the Gunn strain of rat. Role of bilirubin. *J Clin Invest* 55:319, 1975

375. AXELSEN RA: Spontaneous renal papillary necrosis in the Gunn rat. *Pathology* 5:43, 1973

376. ODELL GB, BOLEN JL, POLAND RL, SEUNGDAMBONG S, CUKIER JD: Protection from bilirubin nephropathy in jaundiced Gunn rats. *Gastroenterology* 66:1218, 1974

377. GARDNER WA, KONIGSMARK B: Familial nonhemolytic jaundice: bilirubinosis and encephalopathy. *Pediatrics* 43:365, 1969

378. LOZZIO BB, CHERNOFF AL, MACHEDO ER, LOZZIO SH: Hereditary renal disease in a mutant strain of rats. *Science* 156:1742, 1967

379. HOMAN ER, GUARINO AM: Biliary excretion of phenol red by Wistar and Gunn rats. *Proc Soc Exp Biol Med* 146:46, 1974

380. GORODISCHER R, LEVY G, KRASNER J, YAFFE SJ: Congenital nonobstructive, nonhemolytic jaundice: effect of phototherapy. *N Engl J Med* 282:375, 1970

381. KARON M, IMACH D, SCHWARTZ A: Effective phototherapy in congenital nonobstructive, nonhemolytic jaundice. *N Engl J Med* 282:377, 1970

382. BEHRMAN RE, BROWN AK, CURRIE MR, HARBER LC, HASTINGS JW, ODELL GB, SCHAFFER R, SETLOW RB, VOGL TP, WURTMAN RJ: Committee on phototherapy in the newborn. *Final report of the committee*. Division of Medical Sciences, Assembly of Life Sciences, National Research Council, National Academy of Sciences, Washington, D.C., 1974

383. CALLAHAN EW, THALER M, KARON M, BAUER K, SCHMID R: Phototherapy of severe unconjugated hyperbilirubinemia: Formation and removal of labeled bilirubin derivatives. *Pediatrics* 46:841, 1970

384. BERK PD, SCHARSCHMIDT BF, WAGGONER JG, WHITE SC: The effect of repeated phlebotomy on bilirubin turnover, bilirubin clearance and unconjugated hyperbilirubinaemia in the Crigler-Najjar syndrome and the jaundiced Gunn rat: Application of computers to experimental design. *Clin Sci Mol Med* 50:333, 1976

385. PLOTZ PH, BERK PD, SCHARSCHMIDT BF, GORDON JK, VERGALLA J: Removing substances from blood by affinity chromatography. I. Removing bilirubin and other albumin-bound substances from plasma and blood with albumin-conjugated agarose beads. *J Clin Invest* 53:778, 1974

386. SCHARSCHMIDT BF, PLOTZ PH, BERK PD, WAGGONER JG, VERGALLA J: Removing substances from blood by affinity chromatography. II. Removing bilirubin from the blood of jaundiced rats by hemoperfusion over albumin-conjugated agarose beads. *J Clin Invest* 53:786, 1974

387. SCHARSCHMIDT BF, MARTIN JF, SHAPIRO LJ, PLOTZ PH, BERK PD: Hemoperfusion through albumin-conjugated agarose gel for the treatment of neonatal jaundice in Rhesus monkeys. *J Lab Clin Med* 89:101, 1977

388. SCHARSCHMIDT BF, MARTIN JF, SHAPIRO LJ, PLOTZ PH, BERK PD: The use of calcium chelating agents and prostaglandin El to eliminate platelet and white blood cell losses resulting from hemoperfusion through uncoated charcoal, albumin-agarose gel, and neutral and cation exchange resin. *J Lab Clin Med* 89:110, 1977

389. FOLIOT A, CHRISTOFOROV B, PETITE JP, ETIENNE JP, HOUSSET E, DUBOIS M: Bilirubin UDP-glucuronyltransferase activity of Wistar rat kidney. *Am J Physiol* 229:340, 1975

390. RUGSTAD HE, ROBINSON SM, YANNONI C, TASJIA AH: Transfer of bilirubin uridine diphosphate glucuronyl transferase to enzyme deficient rats. *Science* 170:553, 1970

391. MUKHERJEE AB, KRASNER J: Induction of an enzyme in genetically deficient rats after grafting of normal liver. *Science* 183:68, 1973

392. VAN HOUWELINGEN CAJ, ARIAS IM: Attempts to induce hepatic uridine diphosphate glucuronyl transferase in genetically deficient Gunn rats by grafting of normal liver tissue. *Pediatr Res* 10:830, 1976

393. MATAS AJ, SUTHERLAND DER, STEFFES MW, MAVES SM, LOWE A, SIMMON RL, NAJARIAN JS: Hepatocellular transplantation for metabolic deficiencies. Decrease of plasma bilirubin in Gunn rats. *Science* 192:892, 1976

394. SEBROW O, GATMAITAN Z, ORLANDI F, CHOWDHURY JR, ARIAS IM: Replacement of hepatic UDP glucuronyl transferase activity in homozygous Gunn rats. *Gastroenterology* 78:1332, 1980 (abstract)

395. GOLLAN JL, HUANG SM, BILLING B, SHERLOCK S: Prolonged survival in three brothers with severe type II Crigler-Najjar syndrome. Ultrastructural and metabolic studies. *Gastroenterology* 68:1543, 1975

396. GORDON ER, SHAFFER EA, SASS-KORTSAK A: Bilirubin secretion and conjugation in the Crigler-Najjar syndrome type II. *Gastroenterology* 70:761, 1976

397. FEVERY J, BLANCKAERT N, HEIRWEGH KPM, PREAUX A-M, BERTHELOT P: Unconjugated bilirubin and an increased proportion of bilirubin monoconjugates in the bile of patients with Gilbert's syndrome and Crigler-Najjar syndrome. *J Clin Invest* 60:970, 1977

398. ARIAS IM, GARTNER L, FURMAN M, WOLFSON S: Studies of the effect of several drugs on hepatic glucuronide formation in newborn rats and humans. *Ann New York Acad Sci* 111:274, 1963

399. CATZ C, YAFFE SJ: Pharmacological modification of bilirubin conjugation in the newborn. *Am J Dis Child* 104:516, 1962

400. YAFFE SJ, LEVY G, MATSUZAWA T, BALIAH T: Enhancement of glucuronide-conjugating capacity in a hyperbilirubinemic infant due to apparent enzyme induction by phenobarbital. *N Engl J Med* 275:1461, 1966

401. THOMPSON RPH, PILCHER CWT, ROBINSON J, STRATHERS GM, MCLEAN AEM, WILLIAMS R: Treatment of unconjugated jaundice with dicophane. *Lancet* 2:4, 1969

402. HUNTER J, THOMPSON RPH, RAKE MO, WILLIAMS R: Controlled trial of phetharbital, a non-hypnotic barbiturate, in unconjugated hyperbilirubinaemia. *Brit Med J* 2:497, 1971

403. ORME MLE: Increased glucuronidation of bilirubin in men and rat by administration of antipyrine (phenazone). *Clin Sci Mol Med* 46:511, 1974

404. BLACK M, FEVERY J, PARKER D, JACOBSON J, BILLING BH, CARSON ER: Effect of phenobarbitone on plasma (^{14}C) bilirubin clearance in patients with unconjugated hyperbilirubinaemia. *Clin Sci Mol Med* 46:1, 1974

405. BLASCHKE TF, BERK PD, RODKEY FL, SCHARSCHMIDT BF, COLLISON HA, WAGGONER JG: Effects of glutethimide and phenobarbital on hepatic bilirubin clearance, plasma bilirubin turnover, and carbon monoxide production in man. *Biochem Pharmacol* 23:2795, 1974

406. HUNTER JO, THOMPSON RPH, DUNN PM, WILLIAMS R: Inheritance of type II Crigler-Najjar hyperbilirubinemia. *Gut* 14:46, 1973

407. SMITH PM, MIDDLETON JE, WILLIAMS R: Studies on the familial incidence and clinical history of patients with chronic unconjugated hyperbilirubinemia. *Gut* 8:449, 1967

408. GILBERT A, LEREBOULLET P: La cholemie simple familiale. *Sem Med* 21:241, 1901

409. GILBERT A, LEREBOULLET P, HERSCHER M: Les trois cholemies congenitales. *Bull Mem Soc Med Hop Paris* 24:1203, 1907

410. THOMPSON RPH: Genetic transmission of Gilbert's syndrome, in Okolicsanyi L (ed): *Familial Hyperbilirubinemia*. New York, Wiley, 1981, p 91

411. POWELL LW, HEMINGWAY E, BILLING BH, SHERLOCK S: Idiopathic unconjugated hyperbilirubinemia (Gilbert's syndrome): A study of 42 families. *N Engl J Med* 277:1108, 1967

412. FOULK WT, BUTT HR, OWEN CA, WHITCOMB FF: Constitutional hepatic dysfunction (Gilbert's disease): Its natural history and related syndrome. *Medicine* 38:25, 1959

413. SAGILD U, DALGAARD OZ, TYGSTRUP N: Constitutional hyperbilirubinemia with unconjugated bilirubin in the serum and lipochrome-like pigment granules in the liver. *Ann Intern Med* 56:308, 1962

414. BARTH RF, GRIMLEY PM, BERK PD, BLOOMER JR, HOWE RB: Excess lipofuscin accumulation in constitutional hepatic dysfunction (Gilbert's syndrome). *Arch Pathol* 91:41, 1971

415. SIMON G, VAVONIER HS: Etude au microscope electronique du foie de deux cans d'ictere non-hemolytique congenital de type Gilbert. *Schweiz Med Wochenschr* 93:459, 1963

416. FELDMANN G, ONDEA P, DOMART-ONDES MC, MOLAS G, FAUVERT R: L'ultrastructure hepatique au cours de la maladie de Gilbert. *Pathol Biol (Paris)* 16:943, 1968

417. MCGEE JOD, ALLAN JG, RUNEL RL, PATRICK RS: Liver ultrastructure in Gilbert's syndrome. *Gut* 16:220, 1975

418. BILLING BH, WILLIAMS R, RICHARDS TG: Defects in hepatic transport of bilirubin in congenital hyperbilirubinaemia. An analysis of plasma bilirubin disappearance curves. *Clin Sci* 27:245, 1964

419. BERK PD, BLOOMER JR, HOWE RB, BERLIN NI: Constitutional hepatic dysfunction (Gilbert's syndrome): A new definition based on kinetic studies with unconjugated radiobilirubin. *Am J Med* 49:296, 1970

420. FREZZA M, PERONA G, CORROCHER R, CELLERINO R, BASSETTO MA, DESANDRE G: Bilirubin H³ kinetic studies: Pattern of normals, Gilbert's syndrome and hemolytic state. *Acta Hepato-Gastroenterol* 20:363, 1973

421. COBELLI C: Modeling, identification and parameter estimation of bilirubin kinetics in normal, hemolytic and Gilbert's states. *Comp Biomed Res* 8:522, 1975

422. OKOLICSANYI L, GHIDINI O, ORLANDO R, CORTELLAZZO S, BENEDETTI G, NACCARATO R, MANITTO P: An evaluation of bilirubin kinetics with respect to the diagnosis of Gilbert's syndrome. *Clin Sci Mol Med* 54:535, 1978

423. OKOLICSANYI L, ORLANDO R, VENUTI M, DALBRUN G, COBELLI C, RUGGERI A, SALVAN A: A modeling study of the effect of fasting on bilirubin kinetics in Gilbert's syndrome. *Am J Physiol* 240:266, 1981

424. GORESKY CA, GORDON ER, SHAFFER EA, PARIE P, CARASSAVAS D, ARONOFF A: Definition of a conjugation dysfunction in Gilbert's syndrome: Studies of the handling of bilirubin loads and of the pattern of bilirubin conjugates secreted in bile. *Clin Sci Mol Med* 1:63, 1978

425. SCHARSCHMIDT BF: Bilirubin kinetics in Gilbert's syndrome: Clinical applications and pathophysiological implications, in Okolicsanyi L (ed): *Familial Hyperbilirubinemia* New York, Wiley, 1978, p 99

426. BLACK M, BILLING BH: Hepatic bilirubin UDP glucuronyltransferase activity in liver disease and Gilbert's syndrome. *N Engl J Med* 280:1266, 1969

427. AUCLAIR C, HAKIM J, BOIVIN P, TROUBE H, BOUCHERROT J: Bilirubin and paranitrophenol glucuronyl transferase activity of the liver in patients with Gilbert's syndrome. *Enzyme* 21:97, 1976

428. FELSHER BF, CRAIG JR, CARPIO N: Hepatic bilirubin glucuronidation in Gilbert's syndrome. *J Lab Clin Med* 81:829, 1973

429. BELLET H, RAYNAND A: An assay of bilirubin UDP glucuronyl transferase on needle biopsies applied to Gilbert's syndrome. *Clin Chim Acta* 53:51, 1974

430. BLACK M, SHERLOCK S: Treatment of Gilbert's syndrome with phenobarbitone. *Lancet* 1:1359, 1970

431. KIRSHENBAUM G, SHAMES DM, SCHMID R: An expanded model of bilirubin kinetics: effect of feeding, fasting, and phenobarbital in Gilbert's syndrome. *J Pharmacokinet Biopharm* 2:115, 1976

432. FELSHER BR, CARPIO NM: Caloric intake and unconjugated hyperbilirubinemia. *Gastroenterology* 69:42, 1975

433. BERK PD, BLASCHKE TF, WAGGONER JG: Defective BSP clearance in patients with constitutional hepatic dysfunction (Gilbert's syndrome). *Gastroenterology* 63:472, 1972

434. CARTEL GVM, CHISESI T, CAZZAVILLIAN M, BARBUI T, BATTISTA R, DINI E: Bromsulphthalein-Ausscheidung und Hyperbilirubinamia beim Gilbert Syndrome. *Dtsch Z Verdau Stoffwechselkr* 35:169, 1975

435. COBELLI C, RUGGERI A, TOFFOLO G, OKOLICSANYI L, VENUTI M, ORLANDO R: BSP vs bilirubin kinetics in Gilbert's syndrome, in Okolicsanyi L (ed): *Familial Hyperbilirubinemia*. New York, Wiley, p 121, 1981

436. MARTIN JF, VIERLING JM, WOLKOFF AW, SCHARSCHMIDT BF, VERGALLA J, WAGGONER JG: Abnormal hepatic transport of indocyanine green in Gilbert's syndrome. *Gastroenterology* 70:385, 1976

437. YAMAGUCHI K, OKUDA K, YANEMITSU H, TSUKADA Y, SHIGATA H: Cyclic premenstrual unconjugated hyperbilirubinemia. Report of two cases. *Ann Intern Med* 83:514, 1975

438. FELSHER BF, RICKARD D, REDEKER AG: The reciprocal relation between caloric intake and the degree of hyperbilirubinemia in Gilbert's syndrome. *N Engl J Med* 283:170, 1970

439. BARRETT PVD: The effect of diet and fasting on the serum bilirubin concentration in the rat. *Gastroenterology* 4:572, 1971

440. OWENS D, SHERLOCK S: Diagnosis of Gilbert's syndrome: Role of reduced caloric intake test. *Br Med J* 3:559, 1973

441. BENSINGER TA, MAISELS MJ, CARLSON DE, CONRAD ME: Effect of low caloric diet on endogenous carbon monoxide production: Normal adults and Gilbert's syndrome. *Proc Soc Exp Biol Med* 144:417, 1973

442. GOLLAN JL, BATEMAN C, BILLING BH: Effect of dietary composition on the unconjugated hyperbilirubinamia of Gilbert's syndrome. *Gut* 5:335, 1976

443. FELSHER BF: Effect of changes in dietary components on the serum bilirubin in Gilbert's syndrome. *Am J Clin Nutr* 7:705, 1976

444. BLOOMER JR, BARRETT PV, RODKEY FL, BERLIN NI: Studies on the mechanism of fasting hyperbilirubinemia. *Gastroenterology* 61:479, 1971

445. BARRETT PVD: Hyperbilirubinemia of fasting. *J Am Med Assoc* 217:1349, 1971

446. FELSHER BF, CARPIO NM, VAN COUVERING K: Effect of fasting and phenobarbital on hepatic UDP-glucuronic acid formation in the rat. *J Lab Clin Med* 93:414, 1979

447. GOLLAN JL, HATT KJ, BILLING BH: The influence of diet on unconjugated hyperbilirubinemia in the Gunn rat. *Clin Sci Mol Med* 49:229, 1975

448. GOLLAN JL, HOLE DR, BILLING BH: The role of dietary lipid in the regulation of unconjugated hyperbilirubinemia in Gunn rats. *Clin Sci* 57:327, 1979

449. COWAN RE, THOMPSON RPH, KAYE JP, CLARK GM: The association between fasting hyperbilirubinaemia and serum non-esterified fatty acids in man. *Clin Sci Mol Med* 53:155, 1977

450. STEIN LB, MISHKIN S, FLEISCHNER G, GATMAITAN Z, ARIAS IM: Effect of fasting on hepatic ligandin, Z protein, and organic anion transfer from plasma in rats. *Am J Physiol* 231:1371, 1976

451. FROMKE VL, MILLER D: Constitutional hepatic dysfunction (CHD: Gilbert's disease): a review with special reference to a characteristic increase and prolongation of the hyperbilirubinemic response to nicotinic acid. *Medicine* 51:451, 1972

452. DAVIDSON AR, ROJAS-BUENO A, THOMPSON RPH, WILLIAMS R: Reduced caloric intake and nicotinic acid provocation tests in diagnosis of Gilbert's syndrome. *Br Med J* 2:480, 1975

453. FEVERY J, VERWILGHEN R, TAN TG, DE GROOTE J: Glucuronidation of bilirubin and the occurrence of pigment gallstones in patients with chronic haemolytic diseases. *Eur J Clin Invest* 10:219, 1980

454. OHKUBO H, MUSHA H, OKUDA K: Studies on nicotinic acid interaction with bilirubin metabolism. *Dig Dis Sci* 24:700, 1979

455. BERK PD, BLASCHKE TF: Detection of Gilbert's syndrome in patients with hemolysis, using radioactive chromium. *Ann Intern Med* 77:527, 1972

456. POWELL LW, BILLING BH, WILLIAMS HS: An assessment of red cell survival in idiopathic unconjugated hyperbilirubinemia (Gilbert's syndrome) by the use of radioactive diisopropyl-fluorophosphate and chromium. *Austr Ann Med* 16:221, 1967

457. BERK PD, BERMAN MD, BLITZER BL, CHRETIEN P, MARTIN JF, SCHARSCHMIDT BF, VIERLING JM, WOLKOFF AW, VERGALLA J, WAGGONER JG: Effect of splenectomy on hepatic bilirubin clearance in patients with hereditary spherocytosis: Implications for the diagnosis of Gilbert's syndrome. *J Lab Clin Med.* 98:37, 1981

458. VAN STEENBERGEN W, KUTZ K, FEVERY J: Effects of conjugation, bile flow and bile acid load on the apparent maximal excretion of bilirubin ("Tm"), in Preisig R, Paumgartner G (eds): *The Liver. Proc 3rd Gstaad Symposium.* 1979, p 208

459. VAUGHAN JM, HASLEWOOD GAD: The normal level of plasma bilirubin. *Lancet* i:133, 1938

460. ALWALL N, LAURELL CB, NILSBY I: Studies on heredity in cases of "Non-hemolytic hyperbilirubinemia without direct van den Bergh reaction" (hereditary, non-hemolytic bilirubinemia). *Acta Med Scand* 124:114, 1946

461. O'HAGEN JE, HAMILTON T, DE BRETON EG, SHAW AE: Human serum bilirubin. *Clin Chem* 3:609, 1957

462. BAILEY A, ROBINSON D, DAWSON AM: Does Gilbert's disease exist? *Lancet* 1:931, 1977

463. OWENS D, EVANS J: Population studies on Gilbert's syndrome. *J Med Genet* 12:152, 1975

464. WERNER M, TOLLS RE, HULTIN JV, MELLECKER J: Influence of sex and age on the normal range of eleven serum constituents. *Z Klin Chem u Klin Biochem* 8:105, 1970

465. WILDING P, ROLLASON JG, ROBINSON D: Patterns of change for various biochemical constituents detected in well population screening. *Clin Chim Acta* 41:375, 1972

466. DAMASHEK W, SINGER K: Familial nonhemolytic jaundice. Constitutional hepatic dysfunction with indirect van den Bergh reaction. *AMA Arch Intern Med* 67:259, 1941

467. ALWALL N: On hereditary non-hemolytic bilirubinemia. *Acta Med Scand* 123:560, 1946

468. MEULENGRACHT E: A review of chronic intermittent juvenile jaundice. *Quart J Med* 16:83, 1947

469. BAROODY WG, SHUGART RT: Familial nonhemolytic icterus. *Am J Med* 20:314, 1956

470. CUNNINGHAM IJ, HOPKIRK CSM, FILMER JF: Photosensitivity diseases in New Zealand. I. Facial eczema: Its clinical pathological and biochemical characteristics. *N Z J Sci Tech* 24A:185, 1942

471. HANCOCK J: Congenital photosensitivity in Southdown sheep. A new sublethal factor in sheep. *N Z J Sci Tech* 32A:16, 1950

472. CLARE NT: Photosensitivity diseases in New Zealand. IV. Photosensitizing agent in Southdown photosensitivity. *N Z J Sci Tech* 27A:23, 1945

473. CORNELIUS CE, GRONWALL RR: Congenital photosensitivity and hyperbilirubinemia in Southdown sheep in the United States. *Am J Vet Res* 29:291, 1968

474. GRONWALL R: Sulfobromophthalein sodium excretion and hepatic storage in Corriedale and Southdown sheep with inherited hepatic dysfunction. *Am J Vet Res* 31:2131, 1970

475. MIA AS, CORNELIUS CE, GRONWALL RR: Increased bilirubin production from sources other than circulating erythrocytes in mutant Southdown sheep. *Proc Soc Exp Biol Med* 136:227, 1970

476. MIA AS, GRONWALL RR, CORNELIUS CE: Bilirubin ¹⁴C turnover in normal and mutant Southdown sheep with congenital hyperbilirubinemia. *Proc Soc Exp Biol Med* 133:955, 1970

477. MIA AS, GRONWALL RR, MCGAVIN MD, CORNELIUS CE: Renal function defect in mutant Southdown sheep with congenital hyperbilirubinemia. *Proc Soc Exp Biol Med* 137:1237, 1971

478. MCGAVIN MD, GRONWALL RR, CORNELIUS CE, MIA AS: Renal radial fibrosis in mutant Southdown sheep with congenital hyperbilirubinemia. *Am J Pathol* 67:601, 1972

479. DUBIN IN, JOHNSON FB: Chronic idiopathic jaundice with unidentified pigment in liver cells: A new clinicopathologic entity with a report of 12 cases. *Medicine (Baltimore)* 33:155, 1954

480. SPRINZ H, NELSON RS: Persistent nonhemolytic hyperbilirubinemia associated with lipochrome-like pigment in liver cells: Report of four cases. *Ann Intern Med* 41:952, 1954

481. DUBIN IN: Chronic idiopathic jaundice: A review of fifty cases. *Am J Med* 24:268, 1958

482. BEKER S, READ AE: Familial Dubin-Johnson syndrome. *Gastroenterology* 35:387, 1958

483. WOLF RL, PIZETTE M, RICHMAN A, DREILING DA, JACOBS W, FERNANDEZ O, POPPER H: Chronic idiopathic jaundice: A study of two afflicted families. *Am J Med* 28:32, 1960

484. BERKOWITZ D, ENTINE J, CHUNN L: Dubin-Johnson syndrome: Report of a case occurring in a Negro male. *N Engl J Med* 262:1028, 1960

485. ARIAS IM: Studies of chronic familial non-hemolytic jaundice with conjugated bilirubin in the serum with and without an unidentified pigment in the liver cells. *Am J Med* 31:510, 1961

486. HISLOP DMC: A case of Dubin-Johnson syndrome in a North American Cree Indian with suggestive evidence of familial occurrence. *Can Serv Med J* 20:61, 1964

487. BURNS-COX CJ: The Dubin-Johnson syndrome in a Timorese. *Med J Malaya* 19:311, 1965

488. BUTT HR, ANDERSON VE, FOULK WT, BAGGENSTOSS AH, SCHOENFIELD LJ, DICKSON ER: Studies of chronic idiopathic jaundice (Dubin-Johnson syndrome). II. Evaluation of a large family with the trait. *Gastroenterology* 51:619, 1966

489. BANERJEE AK: Dubin-Johnson syndrome: a family study. *Med J Malaya* 25:21, 1970

490. VAUGHAN JP, MARUBBIO AT, MADDOCKS I, COOKE RA: Chronic idiopathic jaundice in Papua and New Guinea: A report of nine patients with Dubin-Johnson's syndrome or Rotor's syndrome. *Trans R Soc Trop Med Hyg* 64:287, 1970

491. COHEN L, LEWIS C, ARIAS IM: Pregnancy, oral contraceptives, and chronic familial jaundice with predominantly conjugated hyperbilirubinemia (Dubin-Johnson syndrome). *Gastroenterology* 62:1182, 1972

492. KONDO T, KUCHIBA K, OHTSUKA Y, YANAGISAWA W, SHIOMURA T, TAMINATO T: Clinical and genetic studies on Dubin-Johnson syndrome in a cluster area in Japan. *Jap J Hum Genet* 18:378, 1974

493. SHANI M, SELIGSOHN U, GILON E, SHEBA C, ADAM A: Dubin-Johnson syndrome in Israel. I. Clinical laboratory, and genetic aspects of 101 cases. *W J Med* 39:549, 1970

494. SELIGSOHN U, SHANI M, RABOT B, ADAM A, SHEBA C: Hereditary deficiency of blood clotting factor VII and Dubin-Johnson syndrome in an Israeli family. *Israel J Med Sci* 5:1060, 1969

495. SELIGSOHN U, SHANI M, RAMOT B, ADAM A, SHEBA C: Dubin-Johnson Syndrome in Israel. II. Association with factor-VII deficiency. *Quart J Med* 39:569, 1970

496. LEVANON M, RIMON S, SHANI M, RAMOT B, GOLDBERG E: Active and inactive factor-VII in Dubin-Johnson syndrome with factor-VII deficiency, hereditary factor-VII deficiency and on coumadin administration. *Br J Haematol* 23:669, 1972

497. JAVITT NB, KONDO T, KUCHIBA K: Bile acid excretion in Dubin-Johnson syndrome. *Gastroenterology* 75:931, 1978

498. KONDO T, YAGI R, KUCHIBA K: Dubin-Johnson syndrome in a neonate. *N Engl J Med* 292:1028, 1975

499. IVICIC L, SOSOVEC V: Vrodena benigni konjugovena hyperbilirubinemia S pigmentom peceni (Dubin-Johnson syndrom) u novorodenca. *Cs Pedict* 30:287, 1975

500. NAKATA F, OYANAGI K, FUJIWARA M, SOGAWA H, MINANI R, HORINO K, NAKAO K, KONDO T: Dubin-Johnson syndrome in a neonate. *Eur J Pediatr* 132:299, 1979

501. MANDEMA E, DE FRAITURE WH, NIEWEG HO, ARENDS A: Familial chronic idiopathic jaundice (Dubin-Sprinz disease), with a note on bromsulphalein metabolism in this disease. *Am J Med* 28:42, 1960

502. DITTRICH H, SEIFERT E: Uber das verhalten des pigmentes sowie der biligrafin ausscheidung bei einem patienten mit Dubin-Johnson syndrom. *Acta Hepatosplen* 9:45, 1962

503. MORITA M, KIHAVA T: Intravenous cholecystography and metabolism of meglumin iodipamide (biligrafin) in Dubin-Johnson syndrome. *Radiology* 99:57, 1971

504. ESSNER E, NOVIKOFF AB: Human hepatocellular pigments and lysosomes. *J Ultrastruct Res* 3:374, 1960

505. MUSCATELLO U, MUSSINI I, AGNOLUCCI MT: The Dubin-Johnson syndrome: An electronmicroscopic study of the liver cell. *Acta Hepatosplen* 14:162, 1967

506. OPPERMANN A, CARBILLET J-P, GISSELBRECHT H, PAGEANT G, CLEMENT D: Syndrome de Dubin-Johnson: Donnees ultrastructurales. *Sem Hop Paris* 47:2721, 1971

507. CALLARD P, GANTER P, KALIFAT SR, DUPUY-COIN AM, DELARUE J: Etude cytochimique et ultrastructurale du pigment d'un cas de maladie de Dubin-Johnson. *Virchows Archt Abt B Zellpath* 7:63, 1971

508. KERMAREC J, DUPLAY H, DANIEL R: Etude histochimique et ultrastruturale comparative des pigments de la melanose colique et du syndrome de Dubin-Johnson. *Ann Biol Clin* 30:567, 1972

509. EHRLICH JC, NOVIKOFF AB, PLATT R, ESSNER E: Hepatocellular lipofuscin and the pigment of chronic idiopathic jaundice. *Bull NY Acad Med* 36:488, 1960

510. WEGMANN R, RANGIER M, ETEVE J, CHARBONNIER A, CAROLI J: Melanose hepato-splenique avec ictere chronique a bilirubine directe: maladie de Dubin-Johnson? Etude clinique et biologique de la maladie. Etude histochimique, chimique et spectrographique du pigment anormal. *Sem Hop Paris* 26:1761, 1960

511. DE SARAM WG, GALLAGHER CH, GOODRICH BS: Melanosis of sheep liver. I. Chemistry of the pigment. *Aust Vet J* 45:105, 1969

512. SONNET J, STEICHEN-DE FALQUE M, BRISBOIS P: Isolement et proprietes d'une melanine obtenue a partir de melanogenes urinaires dans un cas de maladie de Dubin-Johnson. *Clin Chim Acta* 24:325, 1969

513. ARIAS IM, BERNSTEIN L, TOFFLER R, CORNELIUS C, NOVIKOFF AB, ESSNER E: Black liver disease in Corriedale sheep: A new mutation affecting hepatic excretory function. *J Clin Invest* 43:1249, 1964

514. ARIAS IM, BERNSTEIN L, TOFFLER R, BEN EZZER J: Biliary and urinary excretion of metabolites of 7-H³-epinephrine in mutant Corriedale sheep with hepatic pigmentation. *Gastroenterology* 48:495, 1965

515. ARIAS IM, BERNSTEIN L, TOFFLER R, BEN EZZER J: Black liver disease in Corriedale sheep: Metabolism of tritiated epinephrine and incorporation of isotope into the hepatic pigment *in vivo*. *J Clin Invest* 44:1026, 1965

516. ARIAS IM: Chronic idiopathic jaundice, in Beck K (ed): *Ikterus*. Stuttgart, FK Schattauer Verlag, 1968, p 65

517. SWARTZ HM, SARNA T, VARMA RR: On the nature and excretion of the hepatic pigment in the Dubin-Johnson syndrome. *Gastroenterology* 76:958, 1979

518. ARIAS IM, BLUMBERG W: The pigment in Dubin-Johnson syndrome. *Gastroenterology* 77:820, 1979 (letter)

519. SWARTZ HM, SARNAT T, VARMA RR: The pigment in Dubin-Johnson syndrome. *Gastroenterology* 77:821, 1979 (letter)

520. HUNTER FM, SPARKS RD, FLINNER RL: Hepatitis with resulting mobilization of hepatic pigment in a patient with Dubin-Johnson syndrome. *Gastroenterology* 47:631, 1964

521. MASUDA M: On the relation between Dubin-Johnson syndrome and Rotor type; a case of Dubin-Johnson syndrome complicated with serum hepatitis. *Rev Intern Hepatol* 15:1227, 1965

522. VARMA RR, GRAINGER JM, SCHEUER PJ: A case of the Dubin-Johnson syndrome complicated by acute hepatitis. *Gut* 11:817, 1970

523. WARE AJ, EIGENBRODT EH, SHOEY J, COMBES B: Viral hepatitis complicating the Dubin-Johnson syndrome. *Gastroenterology* 63:331, 1972

524. WARE A, EIGENBRODT E, NAFTALIS J, COMBES B: Dubin-Johnson syndrome and viral hepatitis. *Gastroenterology* 67:560, 1974

525. SCHOENFIELD LJ, MCGILL DB, HUNTON DB, FOULK MT, BUTT HR: Studies of chronic idiopathic jaundice (Dubin-Johnson syndrome). I. Demonstration of hepatic excretory defect. *Gastroenterology* 44:101, 1963

526. ABE H, OKUDA K: Biliary excretion of conjugated sulfobromophthalein (BSP) in constitutional conjugated hyperbilirubinemias. *Digestion* 13:272, 1975

527. ERLINGER S, DHUMEAUX D, DESJEUX JF, BENHAMON JP: Hepatic handling of unconjugated dyes in the Dubin-Johnson syndrome. *Gastroenterology* 64:106, 1973

528. CHARBONNIER A, BRISBOIS P: Etude chromatographique de la BSP au cours de l'epreuve clinique d'epuration plasmatique de ce colorant. *Rev Intern Hepatol* 10:1163, 1960

529. RODES J, ZUBIZARRETA A, BRUGUERA M: Metabolism of the bromsulphalein in Dubin-Johnson syndrome. Diagnostic value of the paradoxical in plasma levels of BSP. *Dig Dis* 17:545, 1972

530. WHEELER HO, MELTZER JI, BRADLEY SE: Biliary transport and hepatic storage of sulfobromophthalein sodium in the unanesthetized dog, in normal man, and in patients with hepatic disease. *J Clin Invest* 39:1131, 1960

531. KOSKELO P, TOIVONEN I, ADLERCREUTZ H: Urinary coproporphyrin isomer distribution in Dubin-Johnson syndrome. *Clin Chem* 13:1006, 1967

532. BEN-EZZER J, RIMINGTON C, SHANI M, SELIGSOHN U, SHEBA C, SZEINBERG A: Abnormal excretion of the isomers of urinary coproporphyrin by patients with Dubin-Johnson syndrome in Israel. *Clin Sci* 40:17, 1971

533. WOLKOFF AW, COHEN LE, ARIAS IM: Inheritance of the Dubin-Johnson syndrome. *N Engl J Med* 288:113, 1973

534. KONDO T, KUCHIBA K, SHIMIZU Y: Coproporphyrin isomers in Dubin-Johnson syndrome. *Gastroenterology* 70:1117, 1976

535. KAPLOWITZ N, JAVITT N, KAPPAS A: Coproporphyrin I and III excretion in bile and urine. *J Clin Invest* 51:2895, 1972

536. BEN-EZZER J, BLONDER J, SHANI M, SELIGSOHN U, POST CA, ADAM A, SZEINBERG A: Dubin-Johnson syndrome. Abnormal excretion of the isomers of urinary coproporphyrin by clinically unaffected family members. *Isr J Med Sci* 9:1431, 1973

537. EDWARDS RH: Inheritance of the Dubin-Johnson-Sprinz syndrome. *Gastroenterology* 68:734, 1975

538. WOLKOFF AW, ARIAS IM: Coproporphyrin excretion in amniotic fluid and urine from premature infants: A possible maturation defect. *Pediatr Res* 8:591, 1974

539. AZIZ MA, SCHWARTZ S, WATSON CJ: Studies of coproporphyrin. VIII. Reinvestigation of the isomer distribution in jaundice and liver diseases. *J Lab Clin Med* 63:596, 1964

540. SHIMIZU Y, KONDO T, KUCHIBA K, URATA G: Uroporphyrin III cosynthetase in liver and blood in the Dubin-Johnson syndrome. *J Lab Clin Med* 89:517, 1977

541. SHIMIZU Y, IDA S, NARUTO H, URATA G: Excretion of porphyrins in urine and bile after the administration of delta-aminolevulinic acid. *J Lab Clin Med* 92:795, 1978

542. KONDO T, KUCHIBA K, SHIMIZU Y: Metabolic fate of exogenous delta-aminolevulinic acid in Dubin-Johnson syndrome. *J Lab Clin Med* 94:421, 1979

543. CORNELIUS CE, ARIAS IM, OSBURN BI: Hepatic pigmentation with photosensitivity: a syndrome in Corriedale sheep resembling Dubin-Johnson syndrome in man. *J Am Vet Med Assoc* 146:709, 1965

544. CORNELIUS CE, OSBURN BI, GRONWALL RR, CARDINET GH: Dubin-Johnson syndrome in immature sheep. *Am J Dig Dis* 13:1072, 1968

545. MIA AS, GRONWALL RR, CORNELIUS CE: Unconjugated bilirubin transport in normal and mutant Corriedale sheep with Dubin-Johnson syndrome. *Proc Soc Exp Biol Med* 135:33, 1970

546. ROTOR AB, MANAHAN L, FLORENTIN A: Familial nonhemolytic jaundice with direct van den Bergh reaction. *Acta Med Phil* 5:37, 1948

547. PECK OC, REY DF, SNELL AM: Familial jaundice with free and conjugated bilirubin in the serum and without liver pigmentation. *Gastroenterology* 39:625, 1960

548. PORUSH JG, DELMAN AJ, FEUER MM: Chronic idiopathic jaundice with normal liver histology. *Arch Intern Med* 109:102, 1962

549. PEREIRA-LIMA JE, UTZ E, AND ROSENBERG I: Hereditary nonhemolytic conjugated hyperbilirubinemia without abnormal liver cell pigmentation. A family study. *Am J Med* 40:628, 1966

550. WOLKOFF AW, WOLPERT E, PASCASIO FN, ARIAS IM: Rotor's syndrome: A distinct inheritable pathophysiologic entity. *Am J Med* 60:173, 1976

551. WOLPERT E, PASCASIO FM, WOLKOFF AW, ARIAS IM: Abnormal sulfobromophthalein metabolism in Rotor's syndrome and obligate heterozygotes. *N Engl J Med* 296:1099, 1977

552. SCHIFF L, BILLING BH, OIKAWA Y: Familial nonhemolytic jaundice with conjugated bilirubin in the serum. *N Engl J Med* 260:1315, 1959

553. HAVERBACK BJ, WIRTSCHAFTER SK: Familial nonhemolytic jaundice with normal liver histology and conjugated bilirubin. *N Engl J Med* 262:113, 1960

554. POBLETE PF, REYES M, MANAHAN L, DALMACIO-CRUZ A: Rotor's syndrome: A family study. *Acta Med Phil* 4:64, 1967

555. PASCASIO FM, DE LA FUENTE D: Rotor-Manahan-Florentin syndrome: Clinical and genetic studies. *Phil J Med* 7:151, 1969

556. PASCASIO FM, DE LA FUENTE D: Rotor-Manahan-Florentin syndrome: The mode of inheritance of a family included in the report of Rotor et al. *Acta Med Phil* 5:127, 1969

557. KAWASAKI H, KINWA N, IRISA T, HIRAYAMA C: Dye clearance studies in Rotor's syndrome. *Am J Gastroenterol* 71:380, 1979

558. SHIMIZU Y, NARUTO H, IDA S, KOHAKURA M: Urinary coproporphyrin isomers in Rotor's syndrome. A study in eight families. *Hepatology* 1:173, 1981

559. HADCHOUEL P, CHARBONNIER A, LAGERON A, LEMONNIER F, RAUTUREAU M, SCOTTO J, CAROL J: A Propos d'une Nouvelle forme d'ictere chronique idiopathique. Hypothese physio-pathologic. *Rev Med Chir Mal Foie* 46:61, 1971

560. DHUMEAUX D, BERTHELOT P: Chronic hyperbilirubinemia associated with hepatic uptake and storage impairment: A new syndrome resembling that of the mutant Southdown sheep. *Gastroenterology* 69:988, 1975

561. LOCALIO SA, SCHWARTZ MS, GANNON CF: The urinary/fecal coproporphyrin ratio in liver disease. *J Clin Invest* 20:7, 1941

562. KOSKELO P, EISALA A, TOIVONEN I: Urinary excretion of porphyrin precursors and coproporphyrin in healthy females on oral contraceptives. *Brit Med J* 1:652, 1966

563. KOSKELO P, TOIVONEN I: Urinary excretion of coproporphyrin isomers I and III and aminolaevulinic acid in normal pregnancy and obstetric hepatosis. *Acta Obstet Gynecol Scand* 47:292, 1968

564. SUMMERSKILL WHJ, WALSHE JM: Benign recurrent intrahepatic obstructive jaundice. *Lancet* 2:686, 1959

565. WILLIAMS R, CARTTER MA, SHERLOCK S, SCHEUER PJ, HILL KR: Idiopathic recurrent cholestasis: A study of the functional and pathological lesions in four cases. *Q J Med* 33:387, 1964

566. SPIEGEL EL, SCHUBERT W, PERRIN E, SCHIFF L: Benign recurrent intrahepatic cholestasis with response to cholestyramine. *Am J Med* 39:682, 1965

567. RUYMANN FB, TAKEUCHI A, BOYCE HW: Idiopathic, recurrent cholestasis. *Pediatrics* 45:812, 1970

568. DE PAGTER AGF, VAN BERGE HENEGOUWEN GP, BOKKEL-HUINNUK JA, BRANDT K-H: Familial benign recurrent intrahepatic cholestasis. *Gastroenterology* 71:202, 1976

569. TYGSTRUP N: Intermittent possibly familial intrahepatic cholestatic jaundice. *Lancet* 1:1171, 1960

570. KUHN HA: Intrahepatic cholestasis in two brothers. *German Med Monthly* 8:185, 1963

571. SCHAPIRO RH, ISSELBACHER KJ: Benign recurrent intrahepatic cholestasis. *N Engl J Med* 268:708, 1963

572. SUMMERSKILL WHJ: The syndrome of benign recurrent cholestasis. *Am J Med* 38:298, 1965.

573. TYGSTRUP N, JENSEN B: Intermittent intrahepatic cholestasis of unknown etiology in five young males from the Faroe Islands. *Acta Med Scand* 185:523, 1969

574. SCHUBERT WK, GARANCIS J, PERRIN E: Idiopathic benign recurrent cholestasis: Biochemical and histologic changes induced by cholestyramine therapy (abstract). *Clin Res* 13:409, 1965

575. BIEMPICA L, GUTSTEIN S, ARIAS IM: Morphological and biochemical studies of benign recurrent cholestasis. *Gastroenterology* 52:521, 1967

576. VAN BERGE HENEGOUWEN GP, BONNDT K-H, DE PAGTER AGF: Is an acute disturbance in hepatic transport of bile acids the primary cause of cholestasis in benign recurrent intrahepatic cholestatis? *Lancet* 1:1249, 1974

577. ENDO T, UCHIDA K, AMURO Y, HIGASHINO K, YAMAMURA Y: Bile acid metabolism in benign recurrent intrahepatic cholestasis. Comparative studies on the icteric and anicteric phases of a single case. *Gastroenterology* 76:1002, 1979

578. BLOOMER JR, BERK PD, HOWE RB: Hepatic clearance of unconjugated bilirubin in cholestatic liver diseases. *Am J Dig Dis* 19:9, 1974

579. BRODERSEN R, TYGSTRUP N: Serum bilirubin studies in patients with intermittent intrahepatic cholestasis. *Gut* 8:46, 1967

580. SUMMERFIELD JA, SCOTT J, BERMAN M, GHENT C, BLOOMER JR, BERK PD, SHERLOCK S: Benign recurrent intrahepatic cholestasis: studies of bilirubin kinetics, bile acids, and cholangiography. *Gut* 21:154, 1980

581. DICKSON ER, FLETCHER J, SUMMERSKILL WHJ: Ultrastructural changes of the liver in benign recurrent cholestasis. *Proc Mayo Clin* 40:288, 1965

582. LESSER PB: Benign familial recurrent intrahepatic cholestasis. *Am J Dig Dis* 18:259, 1973

583. BEAUDOIN M, FELDMANN G, ERLINGER S, BENHAMOU J-P: Benign recurrent cholestasis. *Digestion* 9:49, 1973

62

ACATALASEMIA

This summary is adapted from the summary written by Hugo E. Aebi and Sonja R. Wyss for the fourth edition of this book [1].

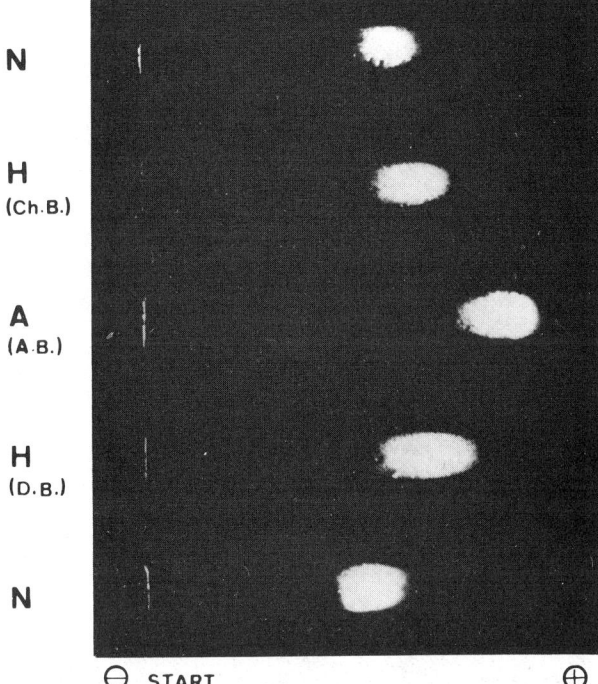

N

H
(Ch.B.)

A
(A.B.)

H
(D.B.)

N

$\ominus$ START $\oplus$

Starch-gel electrophoresis of erythrocyte catalase preparations from normal (N), heterozygous (H), and homozygous (A) individuals from a family with the Swiss-type of acatalasemia. Leukocyte catalase preparations reveal an identical pattern. Note that the mutant homozygote catalase moves faster than the normal enzyme.

1. Acatalasemia *is a rare hereditary deficiency of erythrocyte catalase which has been found in Japanese, Swiss, Peruvian, and Israeli people. Erythrocyte catalase deficiency is transmitted as an autosomal recessive trait and may be combined with a lack of tissue catalase, the extent of which depends on the type of enzyme mutant.*

2. *The disorder was discovered by Takahara in 1946 in a patient with ulcerating gangrenous lesions of the oral cavity. Addition of hydrogen peroxide to the operative site resulted in no foaming and caused the tissues to turn black. Takahara's disease, formerly observed in about 50 percent of children homozygous for the acatalasemia gene, has become considerably less frequent in recent years. Affected persons whose teeth are removed and whose lesions have healed may remain entirely well thereafter.*

3. *Most individuals homozygous for the acatalasemia gene are asymptomatic but can be detected by screening tests for blood catalase activity. Hypocatalasemia, the heterozygous carrier state, can be detected by screening or by specific identification techniques (electrophoresis, heat stability tests). The genes for*

acatalasemia apparently have a worldwide distribution, but the gene frequency varies considerably, being most common in Koreans living in Japan.

4. *At least five different classes of mutant enzymes can be distinguished in different families, indicating considerable genetic heterogeneity. These variant types differ in respect to the level of residual catalase activity in red cells (0 to 8 percent) and tissues as well as in their chemical nature. No differences in antigenic properties have been detected. In most families, blood catalase values show a trimodal distribution with no overlap between groups. In others, the range of normal and that of heterozygotes merge.*

5. *Analogous disorders of catalase activity with similar genetic characteristics have been observed in dogs, guinea pigs, and mice. In each of these species the level of blood catalase has a wide range of variation. This is due in part to polymorphism and in part to the existence of nonfunctional or silent alleles. By systematic inbreeding of mice with subnormal catalase levels, five different mutant strains have been obtained.*

6. *The presence of small amounts of catalase activity in the blood of individuals with acatalasemia as well as*

1421

mice is due to the synthesis of an enzyme variant of poor stability or of low specific activity. Evidence for both alternatives was obtained by means of heat stability tests, by in vitro analysis of the cellular distribution of residual catalase in blood fractions, and by a study of the enzyme turnover in various organs.

REFERENCES

1. AEBI HE, WYSS SR: Acatalasemia, in Stanbury JB, Wyngaarden JB, Fredrickson DS (eds): *The Metabolic Basis of Inherited Disease*, ed 4. New York, McGraw-Hill Book Co, 1978, p 1792
2. DELSADO W, CALDERION R: Acatalasia in two Peruvian siblings. *J Oral Pathol* 8:358, 1979
3. OGATA M, MIZUGAKI J: Properties of residual catalase in the erythrocytes of Japanese-type acatalasemia. *Hum Genet* 48:329, 1979

PART 10

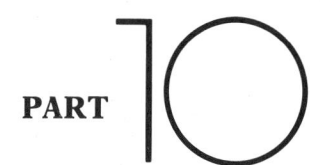

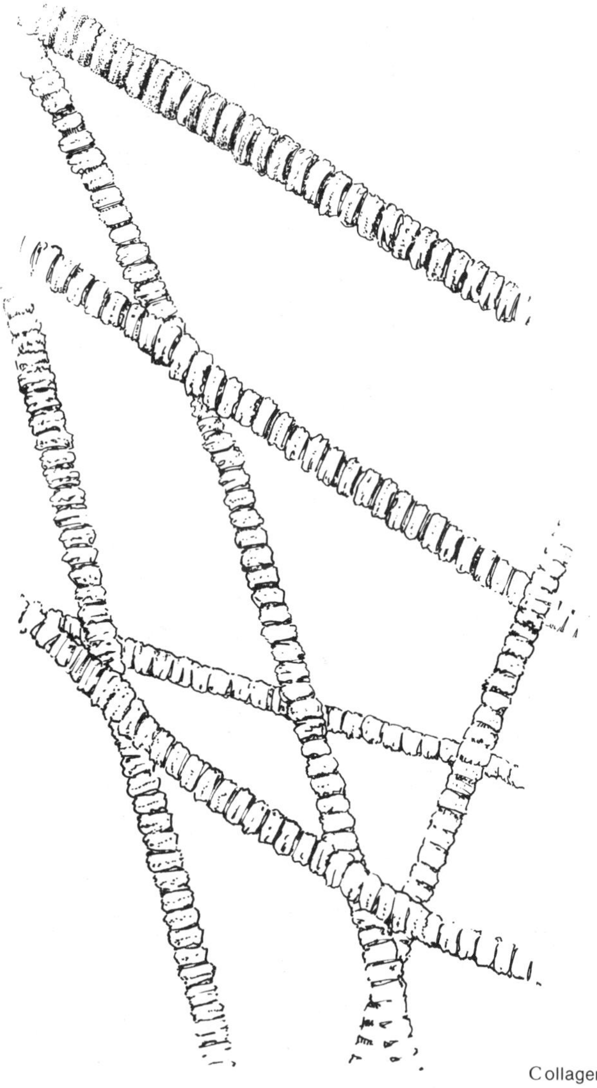

Collagen fibrils

DISORDERS INVOLVING CONNECTIVE TISSUE, MUSCLE, AND BONE

63

DISORDERS OF COLLAGEN

SHELDON R. PINNELL

SAOOD MURAD

1. Collagen is a family of related molecules each composed of three polypeptide chains called α chains wrapped ropelike around each other. Eight separate alpha chains, each a distinct gene product, have been identified (see Table 63-1). Following synthesis on ribosomes, procollagen chains are modified in the endoplasmic reticulum by prolyl hydroxylase, lysyl hydroxylase, and two hydroxylysyl glycosyl transferases. Following helix formation, procollagen is secreted from the cell through Golgi vacuoles. In the extracellular space, specific proteases cleave extension peptides from both ends of the molecule. Following fibrillogenesis, crosslinking occurs. Lysyl oxidase converts specific lysyl and hydroxylsyl residues to reactive aldehydes which form aldimine linkages joining adjacent molecules. Eventually polyfunctional crosslinks form, leading to fiber stability. Collagen biosynthesis is complex, with multiple postribosomal enzymatic modifications. Alterations at any one of these steps might be expected to result in disease.

2. Many forms of the Ehlers-Danlos syndrome (EDS) have been recognized by biochemical and clinical criteria (see Table 63-2). Increased collagen fiber diameters have been recognized in EDS-I, EDS-II, and EDS-III, but no biochemical defects have been described. In EDS-IV, type III collagen synthesis is diminished. An additional form has been described with an apparent

structural mutation in pro $\alpha_1(III)$, which results in intracellular accumulation. One form of EDS-V as well as X-linked cutis laxa is deficient in lysyl oxidase activity. EDS-VI results from deficiency of lysyl hydroxylase activity. Two mutant forms of the enzyme have been characterized. EDS-VII results from procollagen aminoprotease deficiency. A second form has been described with an apparent structural mutation in pro $\alpha_2(I)$ which prevents cleavage of the aminoterminal extension peptide.

3. Several clinical and biochemical forms of osteogenesis imperfecta (OI) have been described (see Table 63-4). OI-II has been associated with decreased type I procollagen synthesis. Hydroxylysine-enriched collagens have been isolated from OI-II tissues which may relate to excessive hydroxylation associated with delayed helix formation. OI-III has been described with deficient pro $\alpha_2(I)$ synthesis. Another form of OI-III has an apparent structural mutation in type I procollagen associated with excess mannose in the carboxyterminal propeptide, resulting in delayed secretion.

4. Deficient type I collagen synthesis in the aorta has been described in the Marfan syndrome. Another form has been reported with an apparent structural mutation in pro $\alpha_2(I)$.

5. Connective tissue disease in homocystinuria and alkaptonuria results from interference with collagen

1425

crosslinking resulting from accumulation of homocysteine and homogentisic acid. In Menkes' syndrome altered copper metabolism apparently results in diminished lysyl oxidase activity.

6. *Recessive dystrophic epidermolysis bullosa results from enhanced synthesis of a structurally altered collagenase. Generalized epidermolysis bullosa simplex has been described, associated with deficient galactosylhydroxylysine glucosyltransferase activity.*

This chapter deals with genetic disorders involving abnormalities in the structure or metabolism of collagen. Diseases that are discussed include the nine types of Ehlers-Danlos syndrome, cutis laxa, osteogenesis imperfecta, Marfan's syndrome, and epidermolysis bullosa. In order to understand the molecular basis of these diseases, an examination of the structure, biosynthesis, and regulation of collagen is necessary. Because of the voluminous literature that has accumulated, no effort is made here to review the subject exhaustively. Rather, important concepts are presented, and where possible references are made to review articles and recent publications. Several recent reviews on collagen have appeared [1–6].

THE COLLAGEN MOLECULE

Molecular Structure

Collagen is the most abundant protein in the human body. It is found in the extracellular matrix of connective tissues, often in association with proteoglycans, glycoproteins, and elastin. It is a family of related molecules whose composition, organization, and amount relative to other matrix components govern the characteristic properties of connective tissues, such as the unidirectional strength of tendons, the flexibility of skin, the elasticity of large arteries, and the rigidity of bone. Collagen is largely a fibrous protein. Its major function is to provide structural support for almost all tissues and organs of the body. The physical strength of collagen is inherent in its molecular and fibrillar structure (Fig. 63-1). The basic unit has a molecular weight of about 300,000 and is a tightly assembled molecule, approximately 3000 Å in length and 15 Å in diameter. Each molecule is composed of three polypeptide chains coiled around each other in a triple helix. This helical conformation is made possible because of the unusual amino acid sequence, with glycine in every third position of each chain. Being the smallest amino acid, glycine fits in the restricted space where the three chains come together [7]. The general structure of the polypeptide chain comprising about 1000 amino acid residues can be represented as $[Gly-X-Y-]_{333}$ where X and Y are a variety of amino acids. Here, X is frequently proline and Y is the characteristic imino acid 4-hydroxyproline. A small amount of 3-hydroxyproline is found in collagen in the X position but only next to 4-hydroxyproline. Another distinctive amino acid of collagen is hydroxylysine, which occurs in the Y position. The proportion of hydroxyproline in collagen is about 10 percent; that of hydroxylysine varies from 0.5 to 5.0 percent [8]. Collagen is also relatively rich in alanine; the only natural amino acid not present in collagen is tryptophan.

The driving force for triple helix formation is the hydrogen

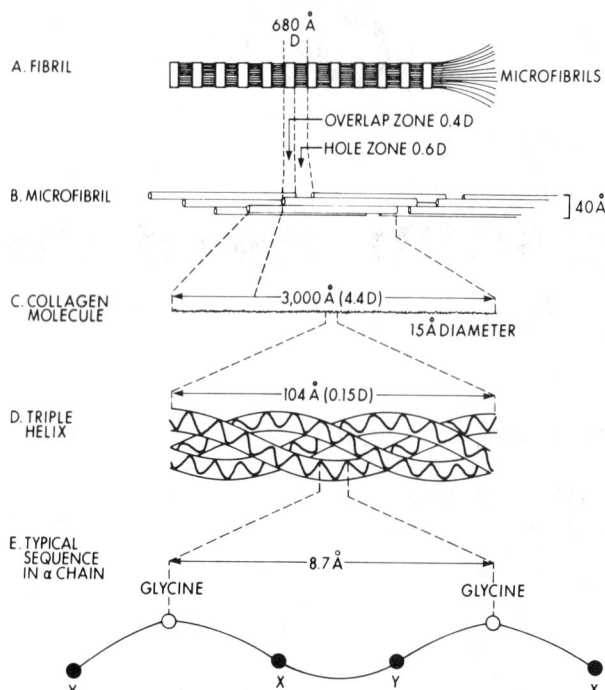

Figure 63-1 Structure of collagen. The collagen fiber is composed of fibrils, each of which is composed of microfibrils. The microfibril is a pentafibril with individual molecules quarter-staggered one to another by a distance (D) of 680 Å. The molecule itself consists of three polypeptide chains called α *chains* that wrap around each other in a triple helix. The helix is made possible because each third amino acid in the polypeptide chain is glycine. (*Modified by permission of the publisher from* Rheumatology and Immunology, A. Cohen (ed.), vol. 4, p. 46, 1979.)

bonding that can occur between the NH group of a glycine residue in one chain and the CO group of a proline residue or some other amino acid in the X position of an adjacent chain [7]. With proline, hydrogen bonding occurs directly, whereas with an amino acid other than proline, hydrogen bonding may occur through a water-bridged structure, which is believed to be stabilized by additional hydrogen bonding with the OH group of the trans-4-hydroxyproline [9]. Because of their five-membered ring, proline and hydroxyproline confer upon the collagen molecule special stereochemical properties, i.e., they hinder the free rotation of the N—C bond where these imino acids occur. Because proline and hydroxyproline are present in relatively large amounts in collagen, the restriction comes very close to the value required for the triple helix. Studies with synthetic polypeptides have shown that not only the amount of proline in collagen but also its position in the triplet is important. Thus, the thermal stability decreases in the following order of repeating sequence: Gly-Pro-Hyp > Gly-Pro-Pro > Gly-Pro-Y > Gly-X-Pro > Gly-X-Y [10–12].

As a consequence of the triple helical structure, and unlike most globular proteins, the amino acid side chains in the collagen molecule are outside the semirigid structure, thus allowing ionic and hydrophobic interactions between molecules. These interactions result in spontaneous aggregation of collagen molecules, first into insoluble microfibrils, then larger fibrils, and finally fibers [13–16]. The interactions must be highly specific and ordered since in the fibril each molecule is shifted from the nearest neighbor by a repeating distance of 680 Å, or about one-fourth of the molecular length. This packing arrangement is responsible for the alternating light and dark zones observed by electron microscopy of collagen fibers after negative staining. The dark zones correspond to the space left between the end of one molecule and the beginning of another in the same direction, where stain deposition occurs. The fibrillar structure is stabilized by enzyme-catalyzed covalent interactions involving lysyl and hydroxylysyl side chains brought in apposition by the quarter-stagger. The resulting cross links impart tensile strength to collagen fibers and prevent slippage of molecules past one another when under tension. The arrangement of the fiber bundles depends on the tissue. This is parallel in tendon, right angle in cornea, tubular in blood vessels, and random in bone and skin.

Although the triple helix extends throughout most of the collagen molecule, there are nonhelical peptides comprising 10 to 20 amino acid residues at both the amino and carboxy termini. Hydroxylysine occurs in both the helical and nonhelical regions of the collagen molecule, where it plays an important role in intermolecular cross-link formation.

In addition to its role in collagen crosslinking, hydroxylysine provides sites for attachment of galactose and α1,2-glucosylgalactose. These sugars are linked to hydroxylysine side chains through a β-glycosidic bond. Like hydroxylysine, the total carbohydrate content as well as the ratio of monosaccharide to disaccharide residues is highly variable [8]. The sugar residue may have a role in determining fibril diameter.

Structural Heterogeneity

Several genetically distinct types of collagen are known which differ in amino acid composition of their constituent polypeptides called α *chains* [17] (Table 63-1). They are identified by Roman numerals in the chronological order of their discovery. Each collagen type is composed of either three identical chains or two identical chains and one nonidentical chain. The chains are identified by a subscript preceding the type designation.

Type I collagen is a heterotrimer of $\alpha_1(I)$ and $\alpha_2(I)$ chains in a 2:1 ratio. It is the most ubiquitous of all collagen types and is

predominant in tendon, ligament, bone, dentin, and adult dermis. It tends to form long, thick fibers. A homotrimer consisting of $\alpha_1(I)$ chain is a minor component of dermal collagen [18].

Type II collagen is a homotrimer of $\alpha_1(II)$ chain and is found almost exclusively in cartilage. It forms short, thin fibers.

Type III collagen is a homotrimer of $\alpha_1(III)$ chain and is invariably associated with type I collagen. It is most abundant in blood vessels and uterus and is absent in bone and tendon. Fetal or infant dermis and fresh scars are relatively rich in this type [19–21]. Type III collagen contains interchain disulfide bonds not found in types I and II collagen and forms a fine reticular network [5, 22].

Type IV collagen is composed of $\alpha_1(IV)$ and $\alpha_2(IV)$ chains and is the characteristic collagen of basement membranes [23, 24]. Morphologically, it is unique in that it is not fibrillar in structure and is susceptible to proteolytic enzymes. It is the largest of all collagen types and contains cysteine. A distinguishing feature of its amino acid composition is the relatively large amount of 3-hydroxyproline.

Type V collagen is a heterotrimer of $\alpha_1(V)$ and $\alpha_2(V)$ chains in a 2:1 ratio [25–29]. It is generally found in association with cell surfaces and basement membranes. A homotrimer consisting of $\alpha_1(V)$ chain occurs as a minor component in hyaline cartilage [30].

In addition to differences in primary structure, variations in the content of hydroxylysine and hydroxylysine glycosides occur between different collagen types. Thus, types IV and V collagen are generally most extensively hydroxylated and glycosylated, followed by type II and then types I and III collagen. This heterogeneity also occurs within the same genetic type, particularly type I [8].

The tissue specificity of various collagen types is also reflected in cells in culture. Thus, fibroblasts, osteoblasts, and odontoblasts synthesize type I collagen. Cultured human skin fibroblasts and smooth muscle cells synthesize types I and III collagen. Chondroblasts synthesize type II collagen, and epithelial or endothelial cells synthesize type IV collagen.

Collagen Synthesis

Collagen is synthesized in a precursor form which is substantially larger (about 50 percent) than the collagen molecule [3, 5, 31] (Fig. 63-2). The procollagen has peptide extensions at both the amino and carboxy termini. These propeptides are believed to enhance solubility and thus facilitate transport. The

Table 63-1 Collagen molecules

Type	Composition	Characteristics
I	$[\alpha_1(I)]_2\alpha_2(I)$	Predominant structural collagen of the body; prominent in tendon, bone, and dentin; constitutes 80–85 percent of dermal collagen
$\alpha_1(1)$ trimer	$[\alpha_1(I)]_3$	Minor component of dermal collagen
II	$[\alpha_1(II)]_3$	Found in cartilage and vitreous humor; not present in skin; rich in hydroxylysine and hydroxylysine glycosides
III	$[\alpha_1(III)]_3$	Prominent in vascular and visceral structures; constitutes 15–20 percent of dermal collagen; interchain disulfide bridges in the helical region near the carboxy terminus
IV	Unknown; contains $\alpha_1(IV)$ and $\alpha_2(IV)$	Found in basement membranes; rich in 3-hydroxyproline, hydroxylsine, and hydroxylysine glycosides
V or AB$_2$	$[\alpha_1(V)]_2\alpha_2(V)$	Prominent in fetal membrane, cornea, and heart valve; minor component of skin
$\alpha_1(V)$ trimer or B$_3$	$[\alpha_1(V)]_3$	Minor component of cartilage

Figure 63-2 Structure of type I procollagen. The type I procollagen molecule is composed of two pro $\alpha_1(I)$ chains and one pro $\alpha_2(I)$ chain. See the text for structural details. Procollagen is converted to collagen by extracellular enzymatic cleavage of amino and carboxy terminal propeptides. *(Modified by permission from Grant et al. [35].)*

TYPE I PROCOLLAGEN

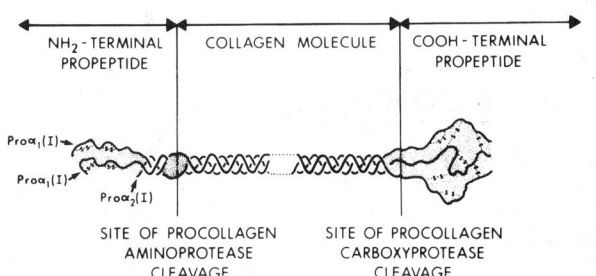

carboxy terminal propeptide consists entirely of nonhelical sequences and contains mannose and N-acetylglucosamine, whereas the amino terminal propeptide consists of a hydroxy-proline-containing helical region flanked by two nonhelical regions. Both peptides contain intrachain disulfide bonds. The carboxy terminal propeptide contains in addition interchain disulfide bonds, the formation of which is considered important in chain selection and alignment necessary for helix formation.

Translation of Procollagen mRNA   The translation of procollagen mRNA occurs by the usual steps of protein synthesis involving membrane-bound polyribosomes. Synthesis of molecules consisting of nonidentical chains seems to occur by simultaneous translation of separate mRNAs [32]. From the size of procollagen-synthesizing polysomes sedimenting at 28 to 30 S, the molecular weight of the mRNA has been estimated to be 1.7 to 1.8×10^6 [33–35]. This is somewhat higher than the expected minimum molecular weight of 1.5×10^6 based on 1500 amino acid residues in a pro α chain. This difference appears to be due to the presence of about 150 nontranslatable polyadenylate sequences [34, 35] and the fact that procollagen mRNA codes for a prepro α chain with an amino terminal signal peptide [35, 36]. In addition to being one of the largest mRNAs in eukaryotic cells, the procollagen mRNA must have an unusually high content of guanosine and cytosine, bases that occur at least twice in each of the triplets that code for glycine and proline. The synthesis of pro α chains takes an unusually long time, i.e., 6 to 7 min [32, 37]. The slow rate of translation may be related to the abnormal demand for glycyl- and prolyl-tRNAs or the unfolding of the secondary structure of procollagen mRNA.

Hydroxylation and Glycosylation   The pro α chains that are synthesized under the direction of mRNA do not contain hydroxyproline or hydroxylysine. These amino acids are synthesized posttranslationally as the growing polypeptide chain penetrates the rough endoplasmic reticulum. The hydroxylation reactions are essential for secretion and maturation of collagen and thus are of paramount importance.

The synthesis of peptidyl 4-hydroxyproline is catalyzed by prolyl 4-hydroxylase [38] (Fig. 63-3). The enzyme requires molecular oxygen, ferrous ions, α-ketoglutarate, and ascorbate [39–41]. Although ascorbate can be replaced by other reducing agents [38, 42, 43], it appears to be the functional reductant for the reaction in vivo. During the reaction α-ketoglutarate is decarboxylated, and one atom of oxygen is incorporated into the hydroxyl group and the other into succinate [38]. The

enzyme is capable of catalyzing a partial reaction in which the decarboxylation occurs in the absence of substrate or in the presence of polypeptides containing no susceptible prolyl residues [44, 45]. The enzyme does not hydroxylate free proline and hydroxylates only that present in the sequence Gly-X-Pro; the best substrates are those in which X is proline [46]. The enzyme has an unusually high affinity for unhydroxylated collagen. The minimum substrate requirement is a triplet, and the affinity of the enzyme for polypeptide substrates is directly related to chain length [47]. The hydroxylation of prolyl residues is not always complete, as judged from the presence in the Y position of a small number of prolyl residues in collagen [48].

It is now generally believed that prolyl hydroxylation occurs prior to release of the nascent polypeptides from ribosomes. Immunocytochemical studies with ferritin-labeled antibodies against prolyl hydroxylase indicate that the enzyme is located within the cisternae of the rough endoplasmic reticulum [49]. Prolyl 4-hydroxylase has been purified from several sources and extensively characterized [39, 50]. It exists in an active form and an inactive but immunologically reactive form. The active form is a tetramer with a molecular weight of about 240,000 and is composed of two dissimilar subunits. The inactive form has a molecular weight of 85,000 to 105,000 and has been detected in all sources thus far examined, but whether it is a precursor of prolyl hydroxylase or a degradation product is not clear.

The synthesis of peptidyl 3-hydroxyproline is catalyzed by a separate enzyme, prolyl 3-hydroxylase, which appears to have the same cofactor requirement as prolyl 4-hydroxylase. The substrate must have the sequence Gly-Pro-4 Hyp [51, 52]. The enzyme does not act on helical substrate [53], and recent studies suggest that the time for helix formation may in part determine the extent of prolyl 3-hydroxylation in the cell [54]. Levels of prolyl 3-hydroxylase are particularly high in kidney cortex, in accord with the relative abundance of 3-hydroxy-proline in kidney basement membrane collagen [55].

The synthesis of peptidyl hydroxylysine is catalyzed by lysyl hydroxylase, an enzyme similar to prolyl 4-hydroxylase with respect to cofactor requirement [56, 57] (Fig. 63-4). The enzyme recognizes the sequence Gly-X-Lys. The sequence requirement appears to be relatively less stringent, and the enzyme can hydroxylate lysine residues in noncollagenous sequences [58–60]. This may explain the presence of hydroxy-lysine in short, nonhelical sequences at both ends of the collagen molecule. In these sequences the extent of lysyl hydroxylation is relatively high in embryonic and neonatal tissues but decreases during subsequent development [61, 62]. In collagen a relatively large number of lysyl residues in the Y position are not hydroxylated [63], but some of these residues can be hydroxylated if the denatured collagen is incubated with lysyl hydroxylase. This suggests that helix formation may be one of the factors limiting the extent of lysyl hydroxylation in the cell [64]. The enzyme activity appears to be virtually absent in skin fibroblasts from patients with Ehlers-Danlos type VI (see below). In this connective tissue, disease hydroxylysine levels are reduced in most tissues but are normal in cartilage. This suggests the possibility that tissue-specific lysyl hydroxylases exist [65]. Further evidence for the presence of isoenzymes comes from recent studies in which the enzyme activity in diseased cultured fibroblasts was measured with substrates corresponding to various genetic types of collagen [66]. The enzyme is associated almost exclusively with the microsomal fractions

Figure 63-3   Prolyl hydroxylase reaction. Certain prolyl residues in the Y position of the repeating Gly-X-Y amino acid sequence are converted to 4-hydroxyproline by prolyl 4-hydroxylase. The enzyme acts on the growing polypeptide chain in the endoplasmic reticulum.

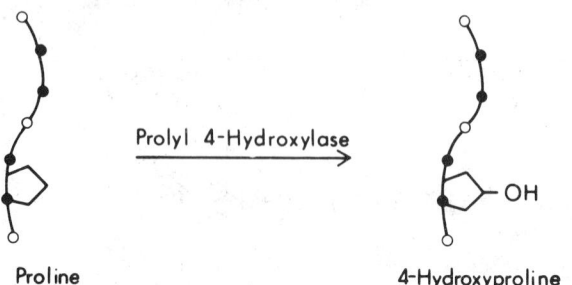

Proline   4-Hydroxyproline

Prolyl 4-Hydroxylase

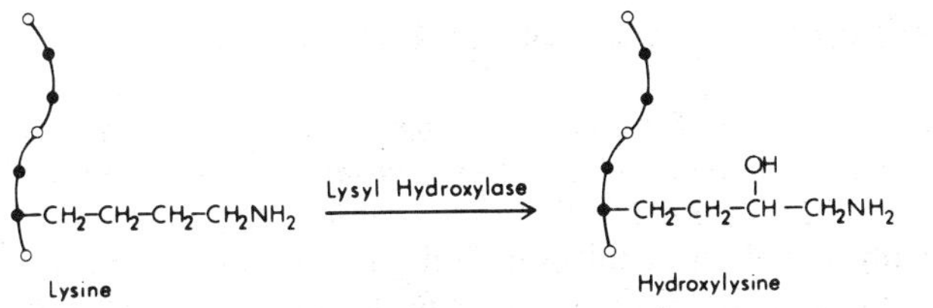

Figure 63-4 Lysyl hydroxylase reaction. Certain lysyl residues in the Y position of the repeating Gly-X-Y amino acid sequence are converted to hydroxylysine by lysyl hydroxylase. The enzyme acts on the growing polypeptide chain in the endoplasmic reticulum.

[67]. Purified chick embryo lysyl hydroxylase is a dimer composed of 85,000-dalton subunits [68].

After hydroxylation, glycosylation of peptidyl hydroxylysine occurs, catalyzed by two specific glycosyl transferases [69] (Fig. 63-5). Hydroxylysyl galactosyltransferase transfers galactose from UDP-galactose to some hydroxylysyl residues. Next, galactosylhydroxylysyl glucosyltransferase transfers glucose from UDP-glucose to some galactosylhydroxylysyl residues. Both enzymes require Mn^{2+} for optimal activity [69, 70]. The enzymes act only on nonhelical substrates; high molecular weight acceptors appear to be better substrates than low molecular weight acceptors [69]. Whether a given hydroxylysyl residue will be diglycosylated, monoglycosylated, or remain unglycosylated may depend on the amino acid sequence surrounding the triplet Gly-X-Hyl. Galactosylation as well as glycosylation appears to begin at the level of nascent polypeptides still attached to ribosomes. Both enzymes are associated with microsomal fractions [71, 72]. The glucosyltransferase has been purified and has a molecular weight of 72,000 to 78,000 [73]. The galactosyltransferase has been only partially purified [69]. Recently, a deficiency of the glucosyltransferase has been found in some members of one family with a dominantly inherited form of epidermolysis bullosa (see below).

Relatively little is known about the incorporation of sugars more typical of glycoproteins. Mannose and N-acetylglucosamine appear to be added in the rough endoplasmic reticulum through a dolichol intermediate [69, 74–77].

Assembly and Secretion   The process by which pro α chains are assembled into procollagen is now believed to be initiated by formation of interchain disulfide bonds in the carboxy terminal propeptide [78–82]. The formation of disulfide bonds seems to begin in the rough endoplasmic reticulum soon after the polypeptides are released from ribosomes and is rapidly followed by triple helix formation [78, 79]. Disruption of the disulfide bonds by chemical reduction leads to reduced rates of helix formation at low temperatures; formation of these bonds may determine the rate of helix formation [80]. The rate of disulfide bond formation and helix formation varies considerably among various cell types [54] and may be responsible for varying levels of hydroxylation and glycosylation, because the extent of these modifications depends not only on the levels of enzymes but also on the time available to act on nonhelical substrates. The time differences in procollagen secretion among various cell types [34, 54] may also be related to the time required to achieve triple helical conformation.

The first step in secretion of procollagen polypeptides after their synthesis on polysomes is transfer through the membrane of the endoplasmic reticulum into the cisternal space. This translocation is believed to be directed by the hydrophobic sig-

nal peptide acting as a marker for membrane recognition. The nature of the interaction of the signal peptide with the membrane and the driving force for insertion are not known. Soon after translocation, the signal peptide is apparently removed by a specific peptidase. Once assembled into procollagen, the molecules traverse the smooth endoplasmic reticulum, including the Golgi apparatus [83], where they are packaged into membranous vesicles for release into the extracellular space by exocytosis [84–86]. The exact mechanism of secretion is unknown but may involve microtubules [87–89].

Extracellular Modifications   The conversion of procollagen to the functional protein occurs extracellularly and is initiated by two neutral proteases which require Ca^{2+} for best activity and show a preference for helical conformation of the substrates [90] (Fig. 63-2). The amino terminal propeptide is cleaved off the molecule by procollagen aminoprotease, leaving procollagen with only the carboxy terminus [91–95]. The carboxy terminal propeptide in turn is removed by procollagen carboxyprotease [93, 96]. In dermatosparaxis, a connective tissue disease of cattle and sheep, accumulation of procollagen containing only the amino terminal propeptide occurs as a result of a deficiency of procollagen aminoprotease (see below). Type IV procollagen does not seem to undergo cleavage of its propeptides.

Removal of propeptides results in insoluble collagen molecules which subsequently undergo self-assembly into fibrils. The next step is the formation of crosslinks [97, 98]. The initial stage of crosslink formation involves the oxidative deamination of the εNH_2 group of certain lysyl or hydroxylysyl residues in short nonhelical peptides at both ends of the collagen molecule (Fig. 63-6). The reaction is catalyzed by lysyl oxidase [99, 100], an extracellular copper-dependent enzyme [101]. Purified lysyl oxidase has a molecular weight of 30,000 [100, 102, 103] and requires pyridoxal phosphate for full activity [104, 105]. The enzyme acts only on native collagen fibrils [106].

The aldehydes thus formed react spontaneously with other aldehydes in the adjacent chain of the same molecule and certain strategically located hydroxylysyl or glycosylated hydroxylysyl residues in the helical region of adjacent molecules [98]. Two allysyl residues react to form the intramolecular aldol condensation product [107, 108] (Fig. 63-7A). This reaction results in a β component in which two α chains are linked

Figure 63-5 Structure of hydroxylysine glycosides. Galactose and α1, 2-glucosylgalactose are linked to certain hydroxylysyl side chains through a β-glycosidic bond. The glycosides are formed by sequential addition of galactose and glucose catalyzed by specific transferases which act on the growing polypeptide chain in the endoplasmic reticulum.

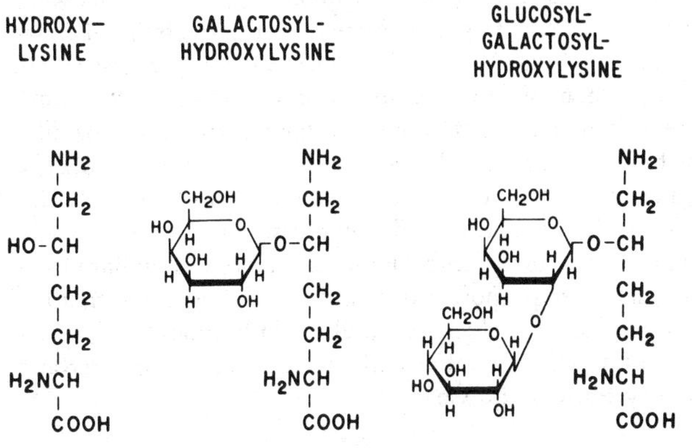

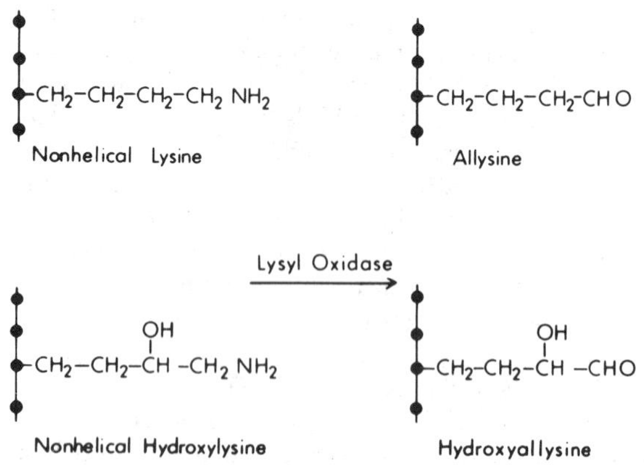

Figure 63-6 Lysyl oxidase reaction. Lysyl or hydroxylysyl residues located in short nonhelical regions at both the amino and carboxy termini of the collagen molecule are converted to corresponding aldehydes by lysyl oxidase. The enzyme acts extracellularly on the collagen fibril.

together. One allysyl residue and one hydroxylysyl residue condense to form an intermolecular aldimine crosslink dehydro-hydroxylsinonorleucine (Fig. 63-7B). One hydroxyallysyl residue and one hydroxylysyl residue condense to form another intermolecular aldimine corsslink, which rearranges to form the ketoamine crosslink hydroxylysino-5-ketonorleucine (Fig. 63-7C). The last two crosslinks may also occur in the glycosylated form [109, 110]. The type of crosslink present depends on the tissue and appears to be governed by the degree of hydroxylation of lysyl residues in nonhelical peptides. Thus, dehydro-hydroxylysinonorleucine is predominant in collagen of soft tissues such as skin, whereas hydroxylysino-5-ketonorleucine is predominant in collagen of hard tissues such as bone. Both of these crosslinks are present in tendon. Related to the degree of hydroxylation of lysyl residues in nonhelical peptides is a shift in crosslink from hydroxylysino-5-ketonorleucine to the more labile dehydro-hydroxylysinonorleucine during postnatal development [111]. All of these crosslinks are reducible and as such are best detected in young tissues. As tissues get older, collagen solubility decreases and stability increases [112, 113]. Asssociated with these changes is a decrease in reducible crosslinks which suggests their conversion to nonreducible forms [114]. One such form is a pyridinium derivative which appears to be derived from ketoamine crosslinks [115] and joins two hydroxyallysyl residues with one hydroxylysyl residue [116, 117] (Fig. 63-7D). Pyridinoline is present in bone, cartilage, and tendon [118] but not in skin [119]. Other polyfunctional crosslinks containing histidine have been proposed [120–122], but their natural occurrence has been questioned [123].

Crosslink formation can be inhibited by administration of lathyrogens such as β-aminopropionitrile, which inactivates lysyl oxidase, resulting in an increase in the solubility of collagen and consequently extremely fragile connective tissue (see below) (Fig. 63-8). Another inhibitor of crosslink formation is D-penicillamine, which may block the reactive aldehyde allysine by forming a thiazolidine ring (see below) (Fig. 63-8). The formation of this complex does not seem to occur with hydroxyallysine, and accordingly crosslinking in bone would not be affected by D-penicillamine. By analogy, a similar mechanism has been proposed for inhibition of crosslink formation by homocysteine, which accumulates in homocystinuria as a result of a deficiency of cystathionine synthetase in liver and brain (see below and Chap. 25).

Collagen Degradation and Turnover

The catabolism of insoluble collagen found in the connective tissue matrix is accomplished by a group of enzymes termed *collagenases* [124–127] (Fig. 63-9). The initial reaction may be depolymerization of collagen fibrils. The depolymerization is possible because of the presence in the collagen molecule of short nonhelical regions from which both intra- and intermolecular crosslinks originate. These regions are susceptible to proteolytic enzymes which can remove crosslinked peptides, thus converting a β or γ component to α chains and consequently dismantling the fibrillar structure. The primary degradation is catalyzed by the rate-limiting enzyme collagenase, a remarkably specific extracellular metalloprotease which in vertebrates cleaves the triple helix at a single point, about threefourths the length of the collagen molecule from its amino terminus [128]. In type I collagen the enzyme cleaves a specific Gly-Ile bond of the α_1 chain and a Gly-Leu bond of the α_2 chain [129, 130]. Type III collagen appears to be the best substrate for human skin collagenase, followed in order by type I and type II [131]; homologous substrates are better than heterologous substrates of the same collagen type. Types IV and V collagen are not degraded by fibroblast collagenase [132]. Denatured collagen is generally a poor substrate for collagenase. The enzyme acts on both collagen molecules and collagen fibrils, preferably uncrosslinked, a property consistent with the accumulation of insoluble collagen during aging [131, 133–135]. Collagenase is normally found in a partially inactive form which can be activated by proteolytic enzymes or chemical treatments, and there is no general agreement as to whether it is a precursor or an enzyme-inhibitor complex [136–139]. How the latent enzyme is activated in vivo is an open question.

Further degradation of collagen is believed to occur through the action of gelatinase in conjunction with extracellular peptidases [140, 141]. Gelatinase is another extracellular metalloprotease specific for denatured collagen, which is also called *gelatin*. Collagen is not normally denatured under physiologic conditions, but the fragments derived from collagenase action can undergo denaturation at physiologic temperature and thus become susceptible to gelatinase. Recent studies suggest that newly synthesized collagen, like other proteins, undergoes intracellular degradation [141], which may be an important mechanism for regulating the amount of collagen produced [142] as well as for getting rid of any abnormal or defective collagen that might be formed [143]. It has been estimated that 20 to 40 percent of procollagen may be degraded within minutes of synthesis [144]. This degradation appears to take place in lysosomes.

Measurements of hydroxyproline in urine have often been used as an index of collagen turnover [145]. Collagen contains large amounts (9 to 13 percent) of this unique amino acid, which can be easily measured colorimetrically. Since hydroxyproline is not reutilized in collagen biosynthesis, its presence in urine has been taken to indicate collagen breakdown. Unfortunately, such studies do not reflect true rates of collagen degradation, for the released hydroxyproline is rapidly metabolized by hydroxyproline oxidase. The hydroxyproline that is excreted in urine is 95 percent peptide bound.

Collagen turnover has been difficult to measure in animals and even more so in humans. In 12-week-old rats, the half-life of skin collagen was estimated to be 60 to 70 days [146]. The

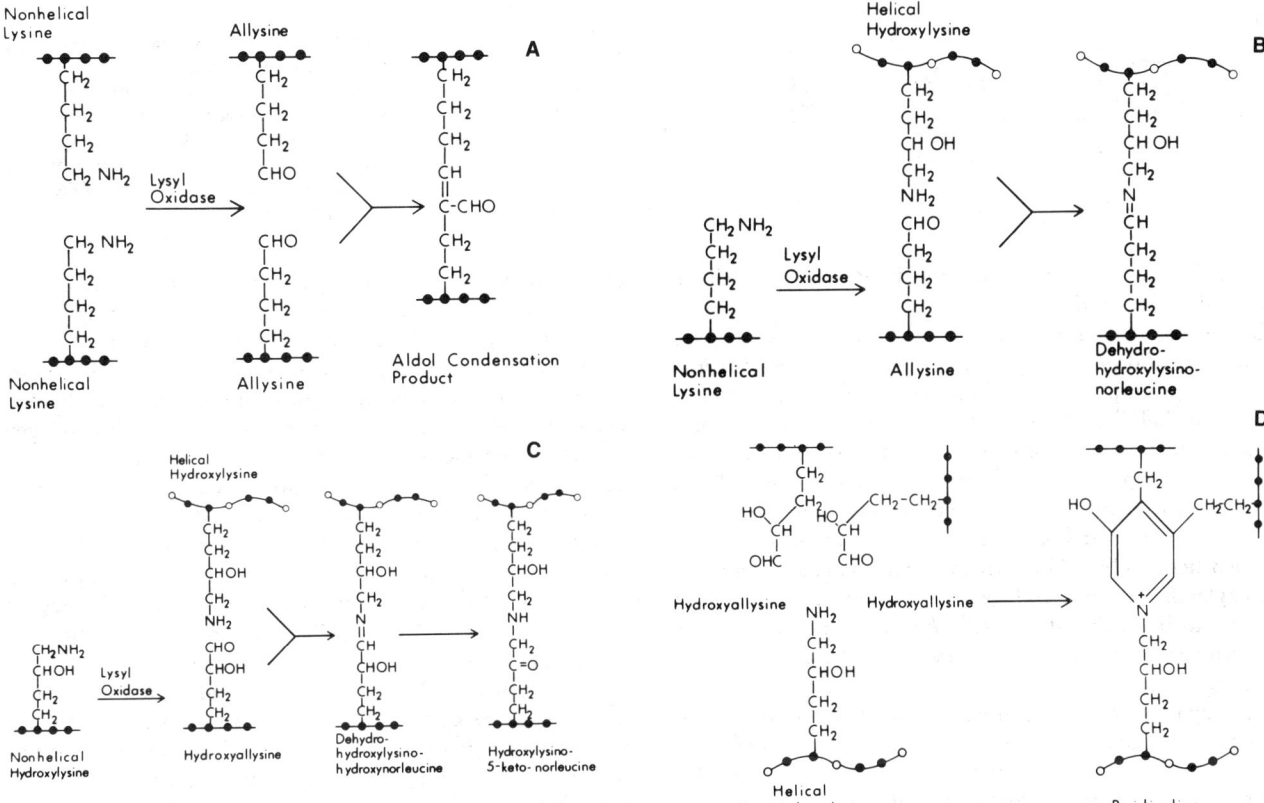

Figure 63-7 *A.* Collagen crosslink formation. The aldol condensation product is an intramolecular interchain crosslink derived from allysyl residues formed in the nonhelical region of the collagen molecule. *B.* Collagen crosslink formation. Dehydro-hydroxylysinonorleucine is an aldimine crosslink derived from an allysyl residue formed in the nonhelical region of the collagen molecule and a hydroxylysyl residue in the helical region of an adjacent molecule. If the hydroxylysyl residue is glycosylated, the resulting crosslink will be glycosylated. *C.* Collagen crosslink formation. Dehydro-hydroxylysinohydroxynorleucine is an aldimine crosslink derived from a hydroxyallysyl residue formed in the nonhelical region of the collagen molecule and a hydroxylysyl residue in the helical region of an adjacent molecule. This crosslink can rearrange to form a more stable ketoamine linkage. If the hydroxylysyl residue is glycosylated, the resulting crosslink will be glycosylated. *D.* Collagen crosslink formation. Pyridinoline is a polyfunctional crosslink which joins two hydroxyallysyl residues formed in the nonhelical region of the collagen molecule with a hydroxylysyl residue in the helical region of an adjacent molecule. The unglycosylated form of the crosslink is shown.

best data on collagen turnover in humans come from patients with hereditary deficiency of hydroxyproline oxidase [147–149]. This condition is familial and probably inherited as an autosomal recessive trait. It has been found in apparently normal persons and in association with mental deficiency. These patients excrete about 300 mg hydroxyproline per day, which is equivalent to about 2.25 g collagen. Some undoubtedly represents metabolism of the C1q component of complement, which has a synthetic rate of about 4.5 mg/kg per day [150]. An appreciable amount may result from intracellular degradation of newly synthesized collagen [151]. In a normal person who catabolizes 50 to 60 g protein per day, collagen contributes only a small amount to total body protein metabolism. Urinary hydroxyproline in patients with hydroxyproline oxidase deficiency is 85 to 93 percent free and 7 to 15 percent peptide bound.

Hydroxylysine or its glycosides have also been measured in urine as an indicator of collagen turnover [152, 153]. The hydroxylysine content in most collagens is less than 10 percent that of hydroxyproline, and only one-third of these hydroxylysine residues are glycosylated in human skin and bone [154]. The determinations are cumbersome, and interpretation is difficult because hydroxylysine and its glycosides are also present in the C1q component of complement. Furthermore, free hydroxylysine is metabolized through hydroxylysine kinase found in liver and kidney [155]. Although most glycosylated hydroxylysine is excreted as such, glycosidases which can cleave these linkages apparently exist [156, 157].

Regulation of Collagen Production

Regulation of collagen production hypothetically could occur at the level of transcription, translation, posttranslation, or degradation. Factors that determine selection of collagen genes and production of appropriate mRNAs are largely unknown. The marked increase in collagen synthesis during periods of rapid growth [158] suggests that developmental factors are important for genetic expression. The genetic expression can be modified by cell culture conditions. For example, chondrocytes synthesize type II collagen in suspension culture but type I collagen in monolayer culture [159–161]. The relative amounts of collagen types may also be influenced by culture conditions. Thus, in human skin fibroblasts the ratio of type III to type I collagen synthesis is increased at high cell density [162], and in human gingival fibroblasts this ratio is decreased by serum [163]. In lung culture, type III collagen synthesis appears to be preferentially increased in a hyperoxic environment [164]. Some of these factors may be responsible for dif-

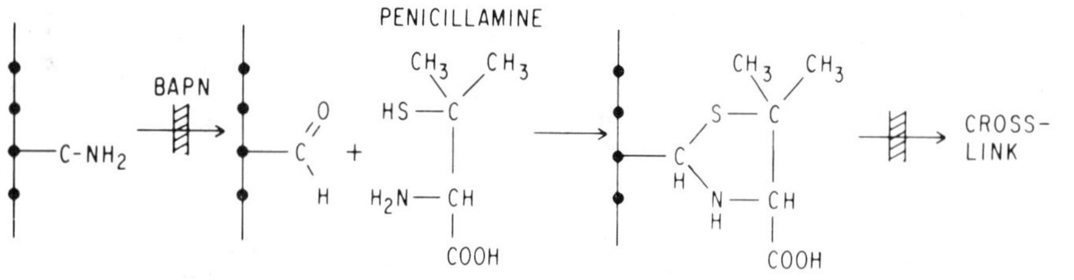

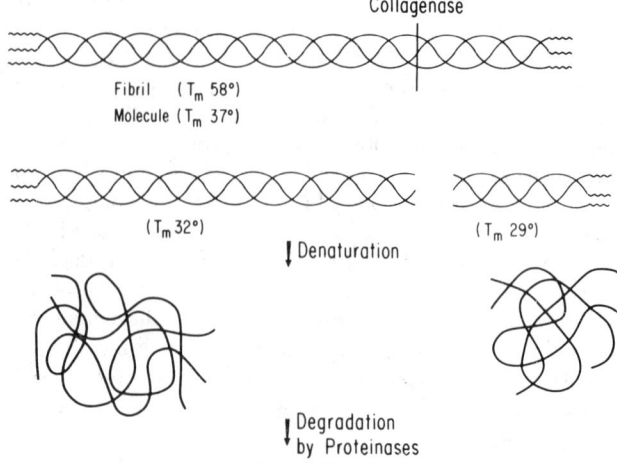

Figure 63-8   Inhibition of collagen crosslinking. β-aminopropionitrile interferes with collagen crosslinking by irreversibly inactivating lysyl oxidase. Penicillamine interferes with collagen crosslinking by reacting with allysyl residues. The thiazolidine ring thus formed makes the aldehyde unavailable for collagen crosslinking. BAPN, β-aminopropionitrile.

ferences in the collagen-synthesizing ability between cells in vivo and in vitro [165].

There is increasing evidence that hormones may be involved in the regulation of collagen synthesis. In fetal rat calvaria, parathyroid hormone reduced collagen synthesis by approximately one-half, and this effect was accompanied by a proportionate reduction in the level of mRNA for type I procollagen [166]. Other hormones implicated in regulation of collagen production are somatomedins, which increase collagen synthesis [167], and growth hormone [167], progesterone [168], and glucocorticoids [169–171], which decrease collagen synthesis. Prostaglandins inhibit collagen production, and this effect appears to be mediated by cyclic AMP, which increases the intracellular degradation of newly synthesized collagen [141].

The capacity of cells in culture to produce collagen can also be modified by matrix components, serum factors, and factors derived from other cells. Thus, proteoglycans [172], β-xylosides which stimulate proteoglycan production [173], and certain glycoproteins have been found to inhibit collagen synthesis in human skin fibroblasts [174]. Hyperlipidemic rat serum increases collagen synthesis in chick embryo and chick tendon fibroblasts [175, 176]. Mononuclear cells stimulated by phytohemagglutinin have been found both to stimulate [177] and to inhibit [178] collagen synthesis in human skin fibroblasts. Viral transformation of human and animal fibroblasts is accompanied by a decrease in collagen synthesis, concomitant with a diminution in the level of procollagen mRNA [179–181].

Abnormal collagen metabolism is well known in scleroderma [182, 183] and keloids [184]. Skin fibroblasts from affected persons exhibit high rates of collagen synthesis compared to the controls, but the factors leading to or the level at which this derangement occurs are not known. Increased collagen synthesis has also been noted in hypertensive rats [185], and this condition was reversed by reserpine or hypophysectomy [186].

Because of the unusually high demand for glycine and proline in collagen synthesis, the levels of these amino acids may exert translational control [187]. Experiments with organ culture and human cirrhotic liver suggest a direct relationship between collagen synthesis and tissue levels of free proline [188–190]. An additional mechanism seems to involve the amino terminal propeptides, which have been shown to inhibit procollagen synthesis in intact cells as well as in a cell-free system [191, 192]. That this negative feedback may be a physiologically important mechanism is supported by the observation that skin fibroblasts from patients with Ehlers-Danlos type VII, characterized by a deficiency of procollagen aminoprotease, exhibit significantly high rates of collagen synthesis compared to controls [193]. It is not known how these peptides might enter the cell and affect intracellular synthesis.

Since prolyl hydroxylation appears to be the first and critical reaction in the posttranslational modification, collagen pro-

duction may be specifically regulated at this level. Support for this concept is derived from experiments in which hydroxylation of prolyl residues has been inhibited by anaerobiosis [194] or chelation of iron with α,α'dipyridyl [195]. Under these conditions protein synthesis continues normally, but the collagen synthesized is underhydroxylated [47]. This collagen is not secreted and is retained in the cells. The small portion of the material that is secreted apparently consists of small peptides derived from degradation of underhydroxylated collagen. The failure of cells to secrete underhydroxylated collagen is attributed to an inability to retain triple helical conformation under physiologic conditions because of the deficiency of hydroxyproline [47, 196, 197]. This hypothesis is supported by the observation that underhydroxylated collagen can be secreted normally when in the triple helical conformation, i.e., at temperatures below 24°C [198]. Furthermore, experiments with proline analogues such as 3,4-dehydroproline, cis-4-hydroxyproline, and azetidine-2-carboxylic acid suggest that triple helical conformation is a requirement for optimal procollagen secretion [199, 200]. These analogues can be incorporated into pro α chains instead of proline and are believed to prevent triple helix formation, resulting in reduced rates of procollagen secretion [47].

A more natural situation leading to the formation of underhydroxylated procollagen is ascorbate deficiency. This can be experimentally produced in animals such as guinea pigs, for which ascorbic acid is a vitamin. An easily manageable system for studying the influence of ascorbic acid on collagen synthesis consists of fibroblasts, cells that cannot synthesize ascorbic

Figure 63-9   Collagen degradation. Under physiologic conditions the collagen molecule is resistant to most proteases except collagenases, which cleave the molecule into 75 percent and 25 percent fragments. These fragments denature at body temperature and are degraded by tissue proteinases.

Collagenase

Fibril   (T_m 58°)
Molecule (T_m 37°)

(T_m 32°)   (T_m 29°)

↓ Denaturation

↓ Degradation by Proteinases

PEPTIDES AND AMINO ACIDS

acid and therefore become deficient when cultured in its absence. Procollagen that is synthesized under these conditions is deficient in hydroxyproline only [201–203], a fact which may be related to the relative affinities of prolyl and lysyl hydroxylases for ascorbate and the presence of reducing factors that might replace ascorbate [202]. Alternatively, it has been suggested that inhibition of prolyl hydroxylation in ascorbate deficiency retards helix formation and thus provides more time for the lysyl hydroxylase reaction [2]. Whatever the explanation, the result is decreased secretion of procollagen in ascorbate-deficient cultures. The underhydroxylated procollagen that accumulates intracellularly might eventually inhibit further synthesis, and this may be the basis for defective wound healing in scurvy [204].

The studies described above suggest that prolyl hydroxylation is the rate-limiting factor in collagen production. Measurement of prolyl hydroxylase levels under a variety of experimental and clinical conditions further supports the notion that the activity of this enzyme may control the rate of collagen production [205]. Recent studies indicate that prolyl hydroxylase activity, hydroxyproline formation, and collagen production may not always be coordinated. In these studies ascorbate stimulated total collagen synthesis in human skin fibroblasts without affecting noncollagen protein synthesis [203] (Fig. 63-10). Maximal stimulation occurred at as little as 25 μM L-ascorbate, a level found in serum of healthy young adults. D-Ascorbate and D-isoascorbate also produced similar effects, but at about 10 times higher concentrations, in accord with their antiscorbutic potencies. The effect appeared unrelated to the known cofactor function of ascorbate [206]. A direct effect at the level of translation is suggested from the ability of ascorbate to aggregate collagen-synthesizing ribosomes specifically [207, 208].

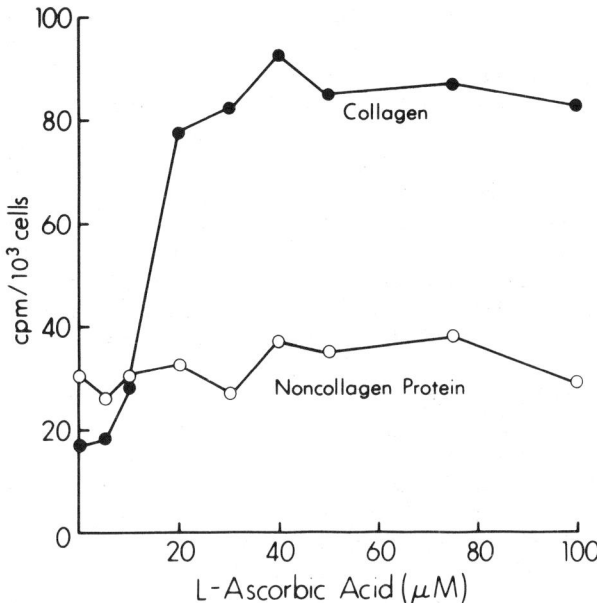

Figure 63-10 Specific stimulation of collagen synthesis in human skin fibroblasts by ascorbic acid. Confluent cells were labeled with tritiated proline for 6 h following 18-h exposure to ascorbic acid. Radioactivity incorporated into collagen and noncollagen protein was determined after digestion with purified clostridial collagenase. Total radioactivity (cells plus medium) is plotted.

ANIMAL MODELS OF CONNECTIVE TISSUE DISORDERS

Lathyrism

Lathyrism is a connective tissue disorder produced when β-aminopropionitrile is administered to experimental animals during active growth [209, 210]. The condition results in marked weakening of supporting tissues, and the animals have decreased tensile strength [211], and collagen [212] as well as elastin [213–215] is abnormally soluble. Lathyrism results from abnormal crosslinking of both collagen and elastin through inhibition of lysyl oxidase, the enzyme responsible for the initial step in crosslinking of both proteins [216] (Fig. 63-8). β-Aminopropionitrile binds tightly to purified lysyl oxidase at 37°C, and this binding cannot be disrupted by subsequent dialysis or ion-exchange and molecular-sieve chromatography.

Copper Deficiency

Animals deprived of dietary copper develop skeletal and cardiovascular abnormalities [217–219], including osteoporosis, abnormal bone development, spontaneous fractures, and unstable joints. Cardiovascular abnormalities result in "falling disease," in which the animal develops sudden rupture of the aorta or a large artery [220].

Tissues from copper-deficient animals have deficient elastin [221] and collagen [222] crosslinks; indeed, copper-deficient animals are the best source of soluble elastin. Since lysyl oxidase is a copper-dependent enzyme, its activity is reduced in copper deficiency.

Penicillamine

Administration of penicillamine to animals causes fragile skin and delayed wound healing [223]. Since soft tissues are predominantly involved, this condition has been called *dermatolathyrism*, in contrast to osteolathyrism, produced by β-aminopropionitrile. Penicillamine interferes with crosslinking of collagen [224–226] and elastin [221, 227] apparently by forming a thiazolidine complex with allysine, thus rendering it unavailable for crosslink formation [228] (Fig. 63-8). More recent evidence suggests a predominant effect on formation of polyfunctional crosslinks [229].

In addition, penicillamine and other thiol compounds may solubilize collagen by cleaving existing aldimine crosslinks [230, 231]. Since aldimine crosslinks in collagen from hard tissues are mostly stabilized to ketoamine crosslinks, the resistance of these tissues to penicillamine may reflect a lack of susceptible aldimines. Penicillamine at 10^{-4} to $10^{-2} M$ inhibits lysyl oxidase and subsequent aldehyde formation, probably by chelating copper [232, 233]. At these levels skeletal lesions similar to those seen in osteolathyrism are produced [234].

Mottled Mice

Mice with certain alleles for coat color at the mottled locus on the X chromosome have connective tissue changes similar to those seen in lathyrism. These mice have fragile skin with reduced tensile strength and bone abnormalities, and they often die from aortic rupture [235].

The connective tissue defect is apparently related to abnormal crosslinking of collagen and elastin due to deficient lysine to allysine conversion [236]. Lysyl oxidase levels in the skin of affected males were 5 to 30 percent of normal, and carrier females had an intermediate level of activity [237]. No serum inhibitor of the enzyme was detected [236], and the abnormality could be demonstrated in fibroblast culture.

Evidence has been presented for defective copper transport in mottled mice [238]. The serum ceruloplasmin level in mutant mice was two-thirds of normal. Tissue copper levels were 60 percent of normal in brain and 40 percent of normal in liver but about twice normal in intestine. Copper may actually accumulate in some tissues, but in a form that is unavailable because of tight association with specific cellular binding proteins [239]. Brain noradrenaline activity was 30 to 45 percent of normal [240], and dopamine β-hydroxylase activity [241], which was diminished in vivo, could be restored in vitro by copper supplementation [238]. Many similarities exist between these mice and patients with Menkes' disease (see Chap. 58).

Dermatosparaxis

Dermatosparaxis is a connective tissue disorder of calves [242], sheep [243], and cats [244]. It is inherited as an autosomal recessive trait [245]. Clinically, it is characterized by extremely fragile skin. Affected animals lose skin after minor trauma, and this may result in wound infection, septicemia, and death. When birth is particularly difficult, affected animals may be born without skin. In Belgium the gene was selected in cattle because heterozygotes produced tender meat.

Electron microscopy of the skin has disclosed sparse, disorganized collagen fibers [246] with a characteristic "hieroglyphic" appearance in cross section [247]. The mechanical stability of collagen is diminished [242]. Chemical studies have revealed the presence of elongated α chains with polypeptide extensions at the amino terminus of the molecule [248]. These extensions interfere with proper fibril and crosslink formation [249]. The defect results from deficient procollagen aminoprotease activity [91].

Other animals models for the Ehlers-Danlos syndrome have been described in mink and dogs [250–255]. These are inherited as an autosomal dominant trait, but the biochemical defect is unknown.

HUMAN INHERITED DISORDERS OF CONNECTIVE TISSUE

Ehlers-Danlos Syndrome

The *Ehlers-Danlos syndrome* is a group of disorders sharing phenotypic features such as hyperextensible skin and joints, easy bruisability, friability of tissues with poor wound healing, and a notable lack of bone fragility [3, 256, 257] (Table 63-2) (Fig. 63-11). Life-threatening complications include spontaneous arterial rupture and gastrointestinal perforation; these

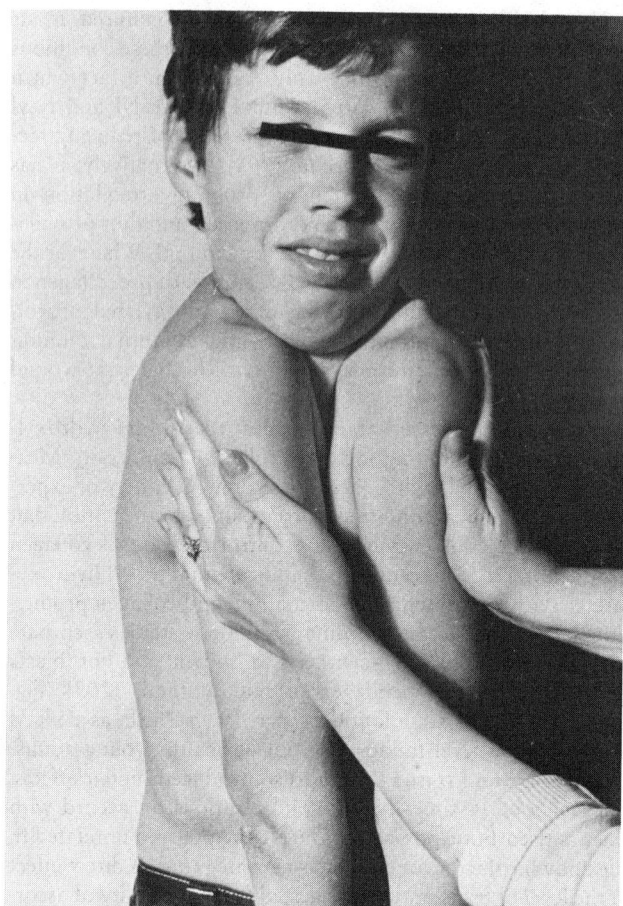

Fig 63-11 Ehlers-Danlos syndrome (hydroxylysine deficient). Marked hyperextensibility allows approximation of shoulders without discomfort. *(Courtesy of L. D. Elsas.)*

occur most commonly in the ecchymotic form (type IV). Several disorders of collagen biosynthesis have been found in patients with the Ehlers-Danlos syndrome.

Clinical Features   Birth is often premature [258] and frequently associated with premature rupture of fetal membranes. Since fetal membranes are mostly derived from the fetus, they share the connective tissue fragility of the rest of the body. The poor neuromuscular tone in affected infants may suggest a primary neuromuscular disorder such as amyotonia congenita. Common facial features include epicanthal folds, a flat nasal bridge, and ears which stick out from the side of the head and point downward.

The skin is unusually soft and feels like chamois. It may be thin and is often strikingly hyperextensible. Its response to stretching is usually rubberlike. With aging the skin may sag, particularly over the elbows. In contrast to the rest of the body, the skin over the palms and soles is often wrinkly and redundant. Fragile skin may split with blunt trauma, resulting in gaping wounds which often require taping to repair because the tissue is too friable to hold stitches. Wound healing is prolonged, and scar tissue is of poor quality. Wide "fish mouth" scars result from poor retraction of the atrophic scar tissue. So-called molluscoid pseudotumors are common over the elbows and knees and apparently result from repeated trauma, hemorrhage, connective tissue organization, fatty degeneration, and calcification. Pea-sized, freely movable calcified spherules can sometimes be palpated subcutaneously over the

Table 63-2 Ehlers-Danlos syndrome

Type	Inheritance	Major clinical features	Ultrastructural defect	Biochemical defect
I (gravis)	Autosomal dominant	Prematurity associated with premature rupture of fetal membranes; marked skin fragility and poor wound healing; marked joint and skin hyperextensibility; easy bruisability	Increased collagen fibril diameter	Unknown
II (mitis)	Autosomal dominant	Mild manifestations; joint hypermobility limited to digits	Increased collagen fibril diameter	Unknown
III (benign, hypermobile)	Autosomal dominant	Marked large joint hypermobility	Increased collagen fibril diameter	Unknown
IV (ecchymotic)	A. Autosomal dominant	Marked bruisability; thin, fragile skin; arterial rupture; intestinal perforation	Not determined	Unknown
	B. Autosomal recessive	Similar to IV(A)	Not determined	Diminished type III collagen synthesis
	C. Unknown	Marked bruisability; thin skin	Small collagen fibril diameter; massive dilatation of rough endoplasmic reticulum	Intracellular accumulation of collagen (? type III)
V (X-linked)	A. X-linked recessive	Short stature, hernias, mitral and tricuspid valve prolapse, moderate joint hypermobility	Not determined	Lysyl oxidase deficiency
	B. X-linked recessive	Extensible skin; mild to moderate joint hypermobility	Increased collagen fibril diameter	Unknown
VI (hydroxylysine deficient)	Autosomal recessive	Marked joint hypermobility; kyphoscoliosis; ocular fragility	Small collagen fibril diameter	Lysyl hydroxylase deficiency
VII (arthrochalasis multiplex congenita)	A. Autosomal recessive	Marked joint hypermobility; hip dislocation; short stature	Not determined	Procollagen aminoprotease deficiency
	B. Probable sporadic heteozygote	Marked joint hypermobility; hip dislocation	Not determined	Probable structural mutation of pro $\alpha_2(I)$
VIII (periodontitis)	Autosomal dominant	Severe generalized periodontitis; marked skin fragility	Not determined	Unknown
IX (mental retardation)	Autosomal recessive	Hernias; protuberant ears; fragile skin	Not determined	Unknown

arms and legs. Varicosities are often prominent under the thin skin. Easy bruisability may be the most striking clinical manifestation of the disease.

Clotting is usually normal [259]. The ecchymoses are thought to be related to friable blood vessels and to dissection of blood through planes of tissue that are poorly held together. Isolated clotting factor deficiencies [260] and qualitative platelet abnormalities have been described [261, 262]. Collagen prepared from patients with Ehlers-Danlos syndrome has been reported to cause deficient [263] or normal [264] platelet aggregation. Abnormal platelet aggregation in a family with mild Ehlers-Danlos syndrome (probably type II) was corrected with fibronectin [265].

Joints may be remarkably hyperextensible. Chronic dislocations of patellae, shoulders, hips, clavicles, and temporomandibular joints may require surgical intervention. Hypermobile joints make motor control difficult during early life. Repeated falls, coupled with friable skin and poor wound healing, often result in appreciable cosmetic disfigurement. With time, joint hypermobility may lead to "wear and tear" arthritis and joint effusion [266]. Although there is notable lack of bone fragility in Ehlers-Danlos syndrome, kyphoscoliosis is frequent; joint looseness and hypotonic musculature may contribute to this complication. Pes planus is common, and leg cramps may be severe during childhood. Teeth may be carious, and severe periodontitis occasionally occurs. Some patients are able to touch the tip of the nose with the tongue (Gorlin sign) [267].

Ophthalmologic features consist of epicanthal folds, myopia, microcornea, and blue scleras. The upper eyelids can sometimes be easily everted (Metenier's sign). Ocular fragility, including keratoconus, dislocated lens, and retinal detachment, has been described [268–275].

Rupture of large arteries is a dramatic and often catastrophic manifestation [276–278]. This commonly results from mild to moderate trauma and is not usually associated with aneurysm.

Angiography is risky [279] and should be avoided whenever possible.

Mitral valve prolapse is common [280] and occasionally is symptomatic. Congenital heart defects including bicuspid aortic valve, pulmonary valvular stenosis, ventricular septal defect, atrial septal defect, tetrology of Fallot, and aortic arch abnormalities have been described [280–283].

Emphysema as well as lung rupture and pneumothorax can occur. Inguinal, hiatal, and umbilical hernias occur at all ages and frequently recur after repair. Diverticulas of the gastrointestinal and genitourinary tract are common. Visceral perforation may be life-threatening [284]. Surgery must be undertaken with caution, otherwise serious bleeding as well as persistent oozing and hematoma formation may follow. The friable tissues are difficult to work with, and sometimes with poor healing, wound dehiscence may prove disastrous.

Pregnancy is risky; perinatal lacerations and hemorrhage regularly occur. Forceps delivery should be avoided. Striae gravidarum are uncommon. Uterine prolapse is a frequent complication [285].

Genetics   The Ehlers-Danlos syndrome has been classified into nine types according to clinical manifestations and inheritance patterns. A molecular basis for each of the types is not established.

TYPE I (GRAVIS) EDS-I   This type is characterized by striking hyperextensibility of skin and joints, fragile skin which bruises easily, poor wound healing, hernias, and prematurity associated with premature rupture of fetal membranes. Inheritance is autosomal dominant.

TYPE II (MITIS) EDS-II   This type has only mild manifestations and often goes undiagnosed. Joint hypermobility is usually limited to hands and feet; skin hyperextensibility and bruisability are mild. Inheritance is autosomal dominant. Although EDS-II shares many clinical features with other types, the degree of clinical involvement within a family remains similar and appears to be unique.

TYPE III (BENIGN HYPERMOBILE) EDS-III   The major manifestations of this type are marked hyperextensibility of joints which occasionally become arthritic. Large joint hypermobility is particularly striking. Skin hyperextensibility is variable. Inheritance is autosomal dominant.

TYPE IV (ECCHYMOTIC) EDS IV   This type is associated with impressive bruising. Joint and skin hyperextensibility are minimal. Serious internal manifestations including arterial rupture and intestinal perforation are often life-threatening. This disorder is associated with diminished tissue levels of type III collagen. Both autosomal dominant and autosomal recessive forms occur. In addition, an apparent defect in type III collagen secretion has been identified in a sporadic case (see below).

TYPE V (X-LINKED) EDS-V   This type has only moderate involvement of skin and joints. Subtypes have been described with [286] and without lysyl oxidase deficiency [287]. Inheritance is X-linked recessive.

TYPE VI (HYDROXYLYSINE-DEFICIENT) EDS-VI   In this type joint hypermobility is extreme, and dislocated joints and kyphoscoliosis are common. Skin hyperextensibility, easy bruisability, and poor wound healing are usual, and ocular fragility may occur. The disorder is associated with lysyl hydroxylase deficiency. Severe ocular disease without hydroxylysine deficiency has been suggested as a subtype [274, 275]. Inheritance is autosomal recessive.

TYPE VII (ARTHROCHALASIS MULTIPLEX CONGENITA) EDS-VII   Patients with this type have short stature; their joints are lax, and hip dislocation is frequent. The disorder is associated with procollagen aminoprotease deficiency. Inheritance is autosomal recessive. A sporadic case with incomplete procollagen-to-collagen conversion has been described which probably represents an $\alpha_2(I)$ structural gene mutation.

TYPE VIII (PERIODONTITIS) EDS-VIII   Patients with this type have exteme, generalized absorptive periodontitis associated with fragile skin and poor wound healing [288]. Bruising and skin hyperextensibility are minimal, and joint hypermobility is limited to fingers. Inheritance is autosomal dominant.

TYPE IX (MENTAL RETARDATION) EDS-IX   This type is associated with severe mental deficiency and is characterized by hypermobile joints, fragile skin with poor wound healing, inguinal hernias, and protuberant ears [289, 290]. Inheritance is autosomal recessive.

Pathology   Light microscopy is not a useful diagnostic technique in Ehlers-Danlos syndrome [291]. No differences have been detected in collagen, elastin, or dermal thickness, with the exception of a single EDS-IV dermis which was thin. Transmission electron microscopy revealed enlarged collagen fiber diameters in EDS-I, -II, -III, and -V [292, 293]. Approximately 5 percent of collagen fibers were two to five times normal and irregular in diameter; these have been called *collagen flowers* [294]. Scanning electron microscopy revealed disordered collagen fiber bundles with an inability to aggregate. Progressive disarray had been observed in the order: mitis (type II) to X-linked (type IV) to gravis (type I) [295]. In EDS-IV [296] and -VI [297] collagen fiber diameters are about two-thirds normal, and one patient with EDS-IV had massive dilatation of the rough endoplasmic reticulum and an apparent type III collagen secretory defect [296].

Connective Tissue Defect   The many varieties of Ehlers-Danlos syndrome are the best studied molecular disorders of collagen. Hydroxylysine-deficient collagen disease which results from lysyl hydroxylase deficiency was the first recognized and well-understood human collagen disorder [65, 298]. Diagnosis can be made by amino acid analysis of skin. Hydroxylysine levels are markedly diminished, but in one family the levels were only moderately reduced [297]. Inheritance is autosomal recessive, and clinically normal heterozygotes can be detected by altered skin fibroblast lysyl hydroxylase activity [299]. At least two types of mutant lysyl hydroxylase have been recognized. One of these had an altered affinity for ascorbic acid and altered thermal stability [300]. The other had normal affinity for ascorbate and normal thermal stability but, maximum activity was only 25 percent of normal [299]. The latter mutant enzyme was derived from a patient who improved clinically with ascorbic acid therapy [301], a response which may be related to stimulation of collagen synthesis by ascorbate (see above).

Hydroxylysine-deficient collagen appeared to be normally secreted from the cell [65] but was unable to form intermolecular crosslinks [302]. Skin collagen was more hydroxylysine deficient than collagen of other tissues, whereas cartilage collagen was normally hydroxylated [65]. Preliminary studies show that types I and III collagen are hydroxylysine deficient but that type II collagen (cartilage) is not [303]. This suggests the existence of isoenzymes for lysyl hydroxylase. Studies on the Clq component of complement in hydroxylysine-deficient collagen disease have revealed slightly deficient [304] or normal [305] hydroxylation of lysine with no evidence of functional impairment.

In EDS-VII the biochemical defect is an incomplete conversion of procollagen to collagen. In most patients the disorder appears to be due to procollagen aminoprotease deficiency and is probably autosomal recessive [193, 306]. A similar enzyme defect is known to occur in dermatosparaxis, a disease of cattle and sheep (see above). The cutaneous manifestations are quite different, however, in that the marked fragility of skin characteristic of dermatosparaxis is absent in the human disease. The reason for this striking clinical difference is unclear. In one patient with EDS-VII, normal cleavage of the amino terminal peptide of the pro α_2(I) chain was apparently prevented by a structural defect. The patient's defect may be due to a sporadic mutation, with one normal and one abnormal gene coding for pro α_2(I) [306].

Lysyl oxidase deficiency has been detected in a family with X-linked Ehlers-Danlos syndrome (EDS-V) [286]. The patients had clinical similarities to those with X-linked cutis laxa, which also manifests lysyl oxidase deficiency [307] (see below). Two other families with X-linked Ehlers-Danlos syndrome had normal lysyl oxidase levels and collagen crosslinking [287].

In the ecchymotic form of Ehlers-Danlos syndrome (EDS-IV), tissue levels of type III collagen were markedly diminished [308, 309]. Skin and lung fibroblasts from patients with the disorder synthesized deficient levels of type III procollagen [308–312]. In another form of the disorder in which tissue levels of type III collagen were low, the rough endoplasmic reticulum of skin fibroblasts was massively dilated, presumably with an abnormal type III procollagen [296]. In still another form of the disorder, tissue levels of type III collagen were low but type III procollagen synthesis in skin fibroblasts was apparently normal [3].

Cutis Laxa

Cutis laxa is a rare group of disorders in which loose, inelastic skin appears to be too large for the body (Table 63-3) (Fig. 63-12). Redundant facial skin may give the appearance of premature aging [257].

Clinical Findings   The skin is poorly tethered to the underlying subcutaneous tissue and feels doughy and thin. Although it is slightly hyperextensible, recoil is slow, unlike the skin in Ehlers-Danlos syndrome. In addition, other characteristic features of Ehlers-Danlos syndrome, including fragile skin, easy bruising, and hypermobile joints, are not usually found in cutis laxa. Characteristic facial features have been noted in many patients with cutis laxa. These include a long upper lip and a hooked nose with a short columella. The voice may be deep due to lax vocal cords. Hernias, rectal and vaginal prolapse, and diverticula of the gastrointestinal and genitourinary tract are quite common. Arteries may be tortuous, with distal spiraling, peripheral pulmonary stenosis, and aortic dilatation [313, 314]. The most serious complication of cutis laxa

is emphysema. This may begin early and lead to eventual death from cor pulmonale [315, 316]. A particularly severe form of the disease with joint laxity, congenital hip dislocation, and intrauterine growth retardation has been found in six girls and one boy [317, 318].

Genetics   Autosomal dominant [319], autosomal recessive [319–321], and X-linked recessive [307] forms of cutis laxa have been described. The autosomal dominant form may appear at any age from infancy to midlife; it is associated with few systemic abnormalities, with normal growth, and usually with normal life expectancy. Systemic involvement is often severe in the autosomal recessive form. Early death may occur from severe pulmonary involvement and cor pulmonale. Only one family with X-linked cutis laxa has been reported. These patients had some clinical features of Ehlers-Danlos syndrome, i.e., joint hypermobility and skeletal abnormalities [322]. An acquired form of cutis laxa has been reported which often follows an inflammatory skin disorder [323, 324]. Many of these patients have facial features characteristic of cutis laxa and may represent late onset of the autosomal dominant form.

Pathology   Elastic fibers are reduced in number, and individual fibers are short, fragmented, and clumped and appear to be undergoing granular degeneration [325, 326]. Individual collagen fibril abnormalities have been detected in autosomal dominant cutis laxa [327], and collagen fibril diameters are increased in both X-linked [307] and dominant forms [327].

Connective Tissue Defect   Lysyl oxidase activity was diminished in whole skin and cultured skin fibroblasts from two patients with X-linked cutis laxa [307]. In addition, collagen crosslinks were diminished and collagen solubility was increased in fibroblasts. The patients had low levels of serum copper and ceruloplasmin and may have had a disorder of copper metabolism similar to that seen in the mottled mouse animal model described above. Abnormal collagen crosslinking was noted in a brother and sister with autosomal recessive cutis laxa [304] but lysyl oxidase levels in their fibroblasts were normal [328].

Osteogenesis Imperfecta

Osteogenesis imperfecta is a generalized disorder of connective tissue involving bone but also affecting tendon, ligament, fascia, sclera, and dentin [329, 330] (Table 63-4).

Clinical Characteristics   The clinical hallmark of osteogenesis imperfecta is fragile or brittle bones which are osteoporotic and easily fractured. The amount of trauma necessary to produce a fracture is often trivial. Fractures are usually transverse and subperiosteal, with minimal displacement. The most striking clinical manifestations of the disease are usually skeletal deformities produced from repeated fractures and weight bearing. The long bones of the upper and lower extremities are often severely bowed. Kyphoscoliosis is common. The skull is frequently a mosaic of bone islands (Wormian bones). Vertebrae undergo biconcave deformities caused by pressure from the intervertebral disk on the soft bone of the vertebral body. The disk may actually perforate the vertebral body, producing a characteristic radiologic density (Schmorl's node). The head of the femur may erode through the acetabulum (protrusio acetabuli), and the skull often has a characteristic

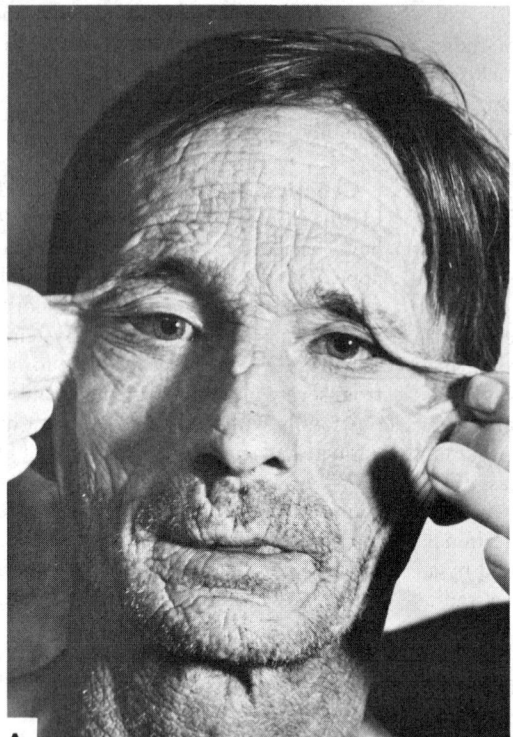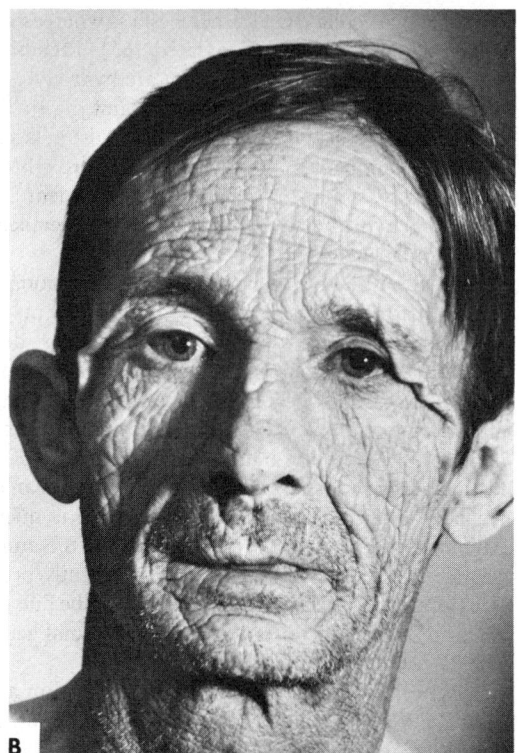

Figure 63-12 Cutis laxa. *A.* Hyperextensible skin and marked facial wrinkling. *B.* Following release, skin fails to return to its previous contour.

frontal and parietal bossing and an overhanging of the occiput ("helmet head" or "mushroom" deformity). Skeletal involvement often leads to shortened stature, which is often incorrectly diagnosed as achondroplasia. The tendency for fracturing diminishes after puberty. Healing usually takes place normally, but a hyperplastic response with hypertrophic callus may suggest osteogenic sarcoma [*331*].

The joints, especially the fingers and toes, are hypermobile, and tendons may be fragile and may rupture easily. Hernias are frequent.

The skin is thin and atrophic but not hyperelastic or fragile.

Scar formation may be abnormal; both atrophic and hypertrophic scars have been noted [*332, 333*]. Easy bruisability is common, and the Rumpel-Leede test and other tests of platelet function may be abnormal [*261, 333, 334*].

Teeth are often involved in osteogenesis imperfecta. They may be hypoplastic, misshapen, or anomalously positioned. The color is often amber to opalescent gray. The dentin may be hypoplastic (dentinogenesis imperfecta), and root canals are sometimes obliterated [*335*]. The teeth may be brittle and may chip easily but are often resistant to cavities.

An outstanding feature of the disease is the blue color of the

Table 63-3 Cutis Laxa

	Lax skin	Characteristic facies	Pulmonary involvement	Hernias	Special features	Connective tissue defects
1. Autosomal dominant	+	+	+	+	Onset may be delayed until middle age; cosmetic problems	Unknown; ultrastructural abnormalities of collagen and elastic tissue
2. Autosomal recessive	++	+	++	++	May be rapidly progressive and fatal	Decreased elastic tissue; short, fragmented elastic fibers
3. X-linked recessive	+	+	−	+	Joint laxity; pectus deformity	Lysyl oxidase deficiency; abnormal copper metabolism
4. Acquired	+	±	+	+	Often occurs following an inflammatory skin disease	Unknown

Symbols: − absent; + present; ++ severe.

Table 63-4 Osteogenesis Imperfecta

Type	Inheritance	Fractures	Sclera	Dentinogenesis imperfecta	Hearing loss	Special features	Biochemical abnormality
IA	Autosomal dominant	+	Blue	−	+	Birth and perinatal fractures are rare; joint hypermobility and easy bruisibility	Decreased ratio of type I to type III collagen in skin
IB	Autosomal dominant	+	Blue	+	+	Same as IA.	Unknown
II	Autosomal recessive	+++	Blue			Intrauterine or early infant death; intrauterine growth retardation; marked tissue fragility; broad, crumpled thighs; beaded ribs; poor cranial calcification	1. Decreased type I collagen synthesis 2. Hydroxylysine-rich collagen
III	Autosomal recessive	++	Blue at birth but less blue with age	+	Rare	May have congenital fractures; marked postnatal growth retardation; wormian bones; marked kyphoscoliosis	1. Decreased secretion of type I procollagen associated with excess mannose in carboxyterminal propeptide 2. Absence of $\alpha_2(I)$ synthesis
IVA	Autosomal dominant	+	White	−	Rare	Kyphoscoliosis; postnatal growth retardation	Unknown
IVB	Autosomal dominant	+	White	+	Rare	Same as IVA	Unknown

sclera. Several hues of blue are seen. This is present in up to 90 percent of patients. The color is caused by choroid pigment showing through thin scleras [336]. The cornea is thin, and keratoconus and megalocornea have been noted.

Otosclerosis eventually leading to deafness may begin during the second or third decade. The growth of new spongy bone may eventually impede the movement of the foot plate of the stapes on the oval window. A perceptible hearing loss may also occur, and tinnitus is frequent. The tympanic membrane may be blue.

Cardiovascular lesions consist of dilated aortic and mitral valve rings with associated functional regurgitation [337–339]. Valve cusps may be redundant and floppy, and chordae tendineae often rupture [340]. Cystic medionecrosis of the aorta has been reported [341].

Pulmonary function studies have revealed no evidence of abnormalities in ventilation or perfusion [342]. Generalized hypermetabolism has been described [343].

Pregnancy is risky for both the mother and the fetus. The trauma of delivery is often more than fragile bones can withstand, and cesarean section is recommended [344].

Genetics Osteogenesis imperfecta is a common genetic disorder occurring at a frequency of 1 in 15,000 [329]. On the basis of clinical characteristics and inheritance patterns, six forms of the disease have been proposed (see Table 63-4). Abbreviations designate each type and are used for identification in the text.

OSTEOGENESIS IMPERFECTA TYPE I (OI I) This is the most common form and is inherited as an autosomal dominant disorder. Fractures may occur at any time, and in 10 percent of the cases they are present at birth. Body weight and length at birth are normal, and short stature occurs as a postnatal event. Variability in clinical severity is great within a family. Kyphoscoliosis and small joint hypermobility are common. Blue sclerae

are a constant feature, and arcus corneae is frequent. Hearing loss is present in 40 percent of the cases and may be conductive or sensorineural in nature [345]. This type is subdivided into two depending on the presence of dental changes. Dentinogenesis imperfecta is uncommon but in some families segregates as an independent trait (type IB). Type IA is without dentinogenesis imperfecta but otherwise has similar clinical features.

OSTEOGENESIS IMPERFECTA TYPE II (OI II) Inherited as an autosomal recessive disease, this is a severe form resulting in intrauterine or early infant death. The infants are small and the tissues are extremely fragile; limbs or head may be torn from the trunk during delivery. Extreme bone fragility is evident, with beaded ribs and crumpled long bones. The skull is poorly ossified, and multiple bone plates are detected by palpation.

OSTEOGENESIS IMPERFECTA TYPE III (OI-III) This rare form is inherited as an autosomal recessive condition. Congenital and early infant fractures may occur. Birth size is usually normal. Ossification of the calvarium is more complete, and limb deformity is less severe than in type II. The scleras are usually blue at birth but become progressively lighter. Prenatal growth failure may be severe, with marked deformity of bones because of repeated fractures.

OSTEOGENESIS IMPERFECTA TYPE IV (OI IV) This form is inherited as an autosomal dominant disorder. Bone fragility is variable, scleras are white, and hearing loss is unusual. Dentinogenesis imperfecta may be absent (type IVA) or present (type IVB). Without a family history, this type is difficult to distinguish from type III.

Pathology The cortex of the bone is thin and the number of trabeculae diminished [346, 347]. Bone remodeling and production of haversian systems do not occur in the normal manner [348]. Bone turnover and osteoclastic resorption may be normal [349] or increased [350]. Scanning electron microscopy of bone collagen has revealed diminished size of fiber bundles [351]. Electron microscopy of scleral collagen has disclosed disruption of the normal lamellar, plywoodlike architecture [347]. The fiber diameters of corneal collagen were appreciably smaller than those in controls [347]. Skin thickness was diminished, and dermal collagen fibrils were thin and decreased in number [352, 353]. The morphology of skin fibroblasts in culture was abnormal; the cells had a rough, irregular shape that was different from that of normal skin fibroblasts [354]. Scanning electron microscopy of opalescent teeth from osteogenesis imperfecta type IB revealed few dentin tubules and abnormal calcification fronts [355].

Connective Tissue Defect   Several alterations in collagen structure and synthesis have been detected in osteogenesis imperfecta. Dermal fibroblasts derived from a patient with type II produced diminished amounts of type I procollagen [144, 356], probably as a result of defective synthesis. Since bone is composed almost entirely of type I collagen, its deficiency would be expected to have profound effects. Type III collagen has been detected in type II bone but not normal bone [357]; its presence may reflect tissue immaturity.

Collagen isolated from several tissues from an infant with type II had increased hydroxylation of lysine in different collagen chains including $\alpha_1(I)$, $\alpha_2(I)$, and $\alpha_1(II)$ [358]. Levels of hydroxylysine glycosides were also increased. Hydroxylysine enrichment has been found in bone [359] and dentin [360] in other cases of osteogenesis imperfecta.

Skin fibroblasts from a patient with osteogenesis imperfecta who had multiple fractures at birth (probably type III) secreted type I procollagen with excess mannose in the carboxy terminal propeptide. The structural alteration was associated with slightly diminished collagen secretion and abnormal aggregation [361].

Dermal fibroblasts from a patient with moderately severe osteogenesis imperfecta (probably type III) born to normal consanguine parents produced a single species of α chain which may have been $[\alpha_1(I)]_3$ collagen; no $\alpha_2(I)$ chain was detected [362]. A similar defect was found in a patient with clinical features of both osteogenesis imperfecta and Marfan's syndrome [363].

Several strains of osteogenesis imperfecta dermal fibroblasts have been found to synthesize type I collagen in decreased amounts relative to type III collagen [364–367]. In addition, skin from type I as well as other probable types may contain reduced amounts of type I relative to type III collagen [368]. Type III collagen has been detected in bone [369] and dentin [370] from patients with osteogenesis imperfecta; these tissues ordinarily do not contain type III collagen. Collagen crosslink abnormalities have been detected in skin [371] and bone [372] in type I. The changes may relate to altered type-specific collagen content, increased levels of hydroxylysine, or decreased conversion to nonreducible forms. In other studies, the collagen content was found to be diminished in demineralized bone [359] and skin [373] from patients with osteogenesis imperfecta.

Marfan's Syndrome

The *Marfan's syndrome* is a generalized disorder of connective tissue characterized by skeletal, ocular, and cardiovascular

manifestations [257, 374]. The inheritance pattern is autosomal dominant.

Clinical Features   The affected person is usually tall and thin, with long extremities. The arm span is greater than the height, and the floor-to-pubis measurement (lower segment) exceeds the pubis-to-crown measurement (upper segment). The fingers are long and thin (arachnodactyly) (Fig. 63-13). Small joints of the hands and feet tend to be lax, but dislocation is uncommon. Kyphoscoliosis is frequent and may be rapidly progressive during the adolescent growth spurt [374]. Sternal deformities are thought to result from excessive longitudinal rib growth. Pectus excavatum is more common than pectus carinatum [374]. Abnormal palatal growth results in a high, narrow palate with crowding of the incisors. Musculature is often poorly developed and hypotonic. Spontaneous pneumothorax as well as emphysema may occur. Inguinal hernias are common and may recur after repair.

The ocular hallmark is ectopia lentis, which is nearly always bilateral. Ectopia lentis is present early and probably occurs in utero [374]. The lens is displaced upward and zonules remain intact, permitting excellent vision. The elongated globe often results in myopia.

Degeneration of the media of the aorta causes the most dangerous manifestations of the disorder and is the usual cause of death. Aortic enlargement begins at the root of the vessel and may involve the coronary sinuses. When the valve ring is stretched, aortic regurgitation occurs. Aortic aneurysm is common, and rupture is often terminal. Mitral valve prolapse frequently occurs and may aggravate aortic disease. The average age of 72 patients at death was 32 years [375].

Several marfanoid syndromes have been described. A marfanoid hypermobility syndrome has crossover features with the Ehlers-Danlos syndrome. Inherited as an autosomal dominant disorder, it is characterized by generalized joint hypermobility, hyperextensible skin, muscular hypotonia, and aortic regurgitation [376]. A marfanoid habitus is seen in patients with hydroxylysine-deficient collagen disease, a subtype of the Ehlers-Danlos syndrome. Ectopia lentis and cardiovascular manifestations are not present, and inheritance is autosomal re-

Figure 63-13   Marfan's syndrome. Arachnodactyly of fingers and toes.

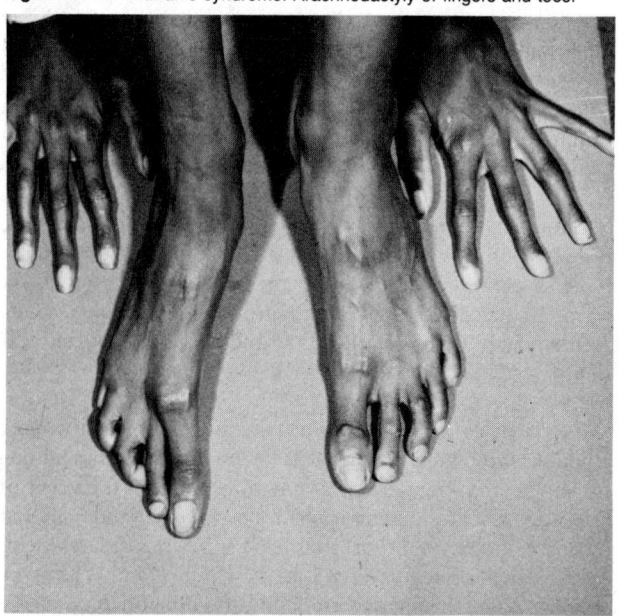

cessive [65]. Congenital contractural arachnodactyly is a dominantly inherited syndrome with arachnodactyly, kyphoscoliosis, contractures, abnormally shaped ears, and osteopenia. Cardiovascular or eye involvement is absent [377]. Patients with homocystinuria characteristically have a marfanoid habitus, kyphoscoliosis, ectopia lentis, and sternal deformity. In addition, they may have osteoporosis, mental deficiency, accelerated arteriosclerosis, and a malar flush. They excrete excessive homocystine in the urine. The disease is inherited as an autosomal recessive condition and results from a deficiency of cystathionine synthetase [378] (see Chap. 25). A marfanoid syndrome occurs with mucosal neuromas, pheochromocytoma, and medullary carcinoma of the thyroid [379].

Genetics   Marfan's syndrome is inherited as an autosomal dominant trait. Marked variability of expression of the disease may occur within a family [380]. Prevalence is estimated at 40 to 60 per million population [374]. There is neither sexual nor racial predilection. Fifteen percent of cases are sporadic and may represent new mutations. Paternal age averages 7 years older in sporadic cases [381].

Pathology   The aortic media is disrupted by intercellular deposition of a metachromatic myxoid substance with disruption of elastic fibers [382]. Pulmonary elastic fibers may also be abnormal [383].

Connective Tissue Defect   Abnormal type I collagen synthesis has been found in tissue culture of Marfan aorta [384, 385]. Another patient has been described with an apparent structural mutation in $proα_2(I)$ [386]. Other studies have revealed increased hyaluronic acid synthesis in skin fibroblast culture [387, 388]. How these observations are related is not clear.

Homocystinuria

Homocystinuria results from several inborn errors of methionine metabolism, the most common of which is deficiency of cystathionine synthase (see Chap. 25). Clinical features include an appearance similar to that of Marfan's syndrome, with arachnodactyly, kyphoscoliosis, and ectopia lentis. Other manifestations include osteoporosis, arterial and venous thrombosis, mental retardation, and malar flush. Connective tissue manifestations are thought to result from accumulation of the metabolic intermediate homocysteine, which intereferes with collagen crosslinking [389] in a manner similar to that of penicillamine. Thus, reactive aldehydes necessary for collagen crosslinking may be blocked [389] or formation of polyfunctional crosslinks may be impeded by homocysteine [229].

Menkes' Kinky Hair Syndrome

Menkes' kinky hair syndrome is an X-linked recessive disorder with neurologic, connective tissue, pigmentary, and hair abnormalities. The disorder is associated with abnormal copper metabolism and is considered in detail in Chap. 58. Many of the clinical features appear to result from deficiencies of copper-dependent enzymes. Since lysyl oxidase requires copper, the connective tissue disorder has been presumed to be related to lysyl oxidase activity. Tissue activities of lysyl oxidase in this disease are not known.

Alkaptonuria

In *alkaptonuria* homogentisic acid accumulates due to a deficiency of homogentisic acid oxidase. Homogentisic acid oxidizes readily to benzoquinone acetic acid, which polymerizes and has a special affinity for collagen-containing tissues [390–392]. Eventual connective tissue breakdown leads to the most serious clinical manifestation of the disorder, which is degenerative joint disease. Homogentisic acid inhibits lysyl hydroxylase activity, hydroxylysine formation, and subsequent collagen crosslink formation in chick calvaria [393]. The effect appears at levels known to occur in serum of patients with alkaptonuria. The predilection of the disease for cartilage which contains hydroxylysine-rich collagen may be related to this effect on lysyl hydroxylase.

Epidermolysis Bullosa

Epidermolysis bullosa is the designation of a group of inherited disorders characterized by blister formation in response to minimal skin trauma. At least six forms have been described which differ in mode of inheritance, clinical characteristics, and anatomic level of separation in the skin [394]. In two types, recessive dystrophic epidermolysis bullosa and generalized epidermolysis bullosa simplex, available information suggests an underlying connective tissue abnormality. Only these two forms of the disorder will be considered.

Clinical Features   Recessive dystrophic epidermolysis bullosa is characterized by blisters and erosions that may or may not result from previous trauma and may occur anywhere on the surface of the body. Repeated cycles of blistering with slow healing associated with secondary infection and scarring lead to most of the manifestations of the disorder (Figs. 63-14, 63-15). Bullae or erosions may be present at birth, and milia are usually evident. Repeated blistering and scarring of digits lead to eventual fusion, flexion deformity, and encasement in a mitt of epidermis. Scarring frequently results in loss of hair and nails. The ears may be deformed and bound to the scalp. Mucous membranes may be involved with bullae. Chronic blisters and erosions of the oral mucosa often result in severe

Figure 63-14   Recessive dystrophic epidermolysis bullosa. Scarring and alopecia of scalp and face. *(Courtesy of R. A. Briggaman.)*

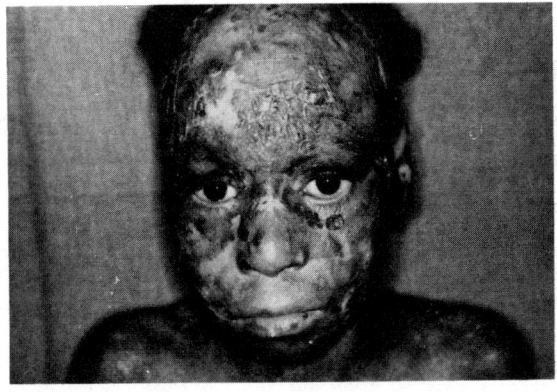

feeding problems and require soft diets. The tongue may become bound to the oral mucosa so that it cannot be protruded, and the mouth may be "puckered" from scarring. Bullae in the esophagus may cause stenosis [395, 396]. Abnormal dentition, with focal hypoplasia of the enamel and carious teeth, is common. Conjunctival involvement is unusual.

Pyodermas are frequent, and there is increased incidence of glomerulonephritis. Amyloidosis may appear in long-standing cases. Squamous cell carcinoma of the skin or mouth occurs and may metastasize [397, 398]. Anemia, impaired growth, and poor nutrition are related to the severity of the disease.

In generalized epidermolysis bullosa simplex, blisters occur following frictional trauma. Although most blistering occurs on the hands and feet, any area of the body may be involved. Blisters heal without scarring.

Genetics Recessive dystrophic epidermolysis bullosa is inherited as an autosomal recessive condition and generalized epidermolysis bullosa simplex as an autosomal dominant condition.

Pathology In recessive dystrophic epidermolysis bullosa, blister formation occurs just below the basal lamina [399]. Macrophages gather at the dermal-epidermal junction, and abnormal collagen fibers of varying diameters can be detected. There is a striking absence of anchoring fibrils, i.e., small fibrillar structures which connect the underside of the basal lamina to the upper dermis [400] (Fig. 63-16). These changes can be seen in affected newborns in apparently normal skin which has never blistered. The anchoring fibrils are synthesized by dermis, but their nature is unknown. Recombination experiments utilizing separated dermis and epidermis from normal and epidermolysis bullosa skin revealed an inability of the diseased dermis to synthesize anchoring fibrils [401].

In generalized epidermolysis bullosa simplex, cleavage occurs predominantly through basal cells of the epidermis. Early changes include edema and degeneration within the cytoplasm, following by disruption of cells. The blister base is composed of disrupted basal cells attached by plasma membrane and hemidesmosomes to normal lamina lucida and basal lamina [394].

Connective Tissue Defect Collagenase levels are elevated in involved and clinically normal skin from patients with recessive dystrophic epidermolysis bullosa [402–404]. Skin fibroblasts from patients with the disorder synthesize more

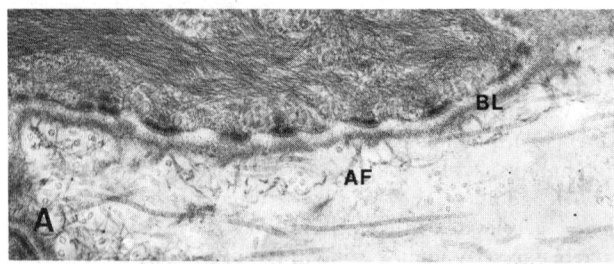
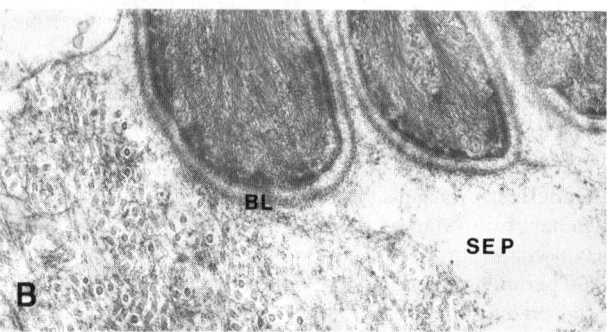
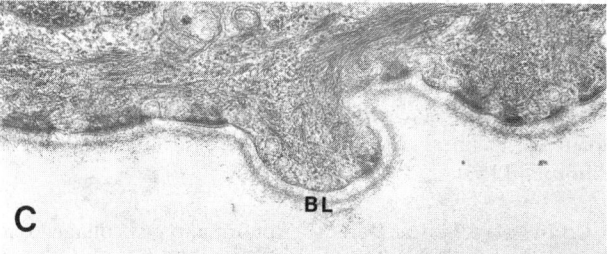

Figure 63-16 Electron micrographs of epidermal-dermal junction in a patient with recessive dystrophic epidermolysis bullosa and in normal skin. *A.* Normal epidermal-dermal junction showing basal lamina (BL) and anchoring fibrils (AF). *B.* Recessive dystrophic epidermolysis bullosa of the epidermal-dermal junction. Note absence of anchoring fibrils beneath the basal lamina (BL) and area of epidermal-dermal separation (SEP). *C.* Recessive dystrophic epidermolysis bullosa epidermis mechanically separated from dermis. Separation has occurred beneath the basal lamina (BL). *(Reproduced by permission from R. A. Briggaman and C. Wheeler [400].)*

collagenase than control cells [405]. Collagenase with altered thermal stability, lowered affinity for calcium, and diminished catalytic efficiency has been found in the disease [406]. Treatment with phenytoin, which inhibits collagenase production in fibroblast culture, has been clinically effective in some patients with the disorder [407].

Decreased levels of galactosylhydroxylysyl glucosyltransferase in a large family with generalized epidermolysis bullosa simplex have been reported [408]. The enzyme activity was low in serum, skin, and cultured skin fibroblasts. Eleven of 12 affected family members had deficient enzyme levels. Two of 15 clinically normal family members also had deficient enzyme levels. How this enzyme deficiency may relate to pathogenesis of the disease is not clear.

Supported in part by grants 5 RO1 AM17128 and 1 RO1 AM 28304 from the National Institutes of Health and a grant from the National Foundation.

Figure 63-15 Recessive dystrophic epidermolysis bullosa. Mitten-like epidermal encasement of hands. *(Courtesy of R. A. Briggaman.)*

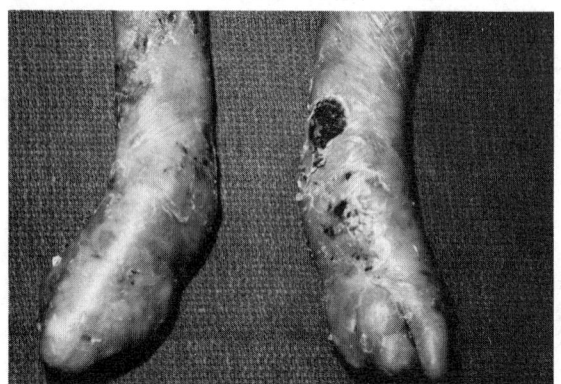

REFERENCES

1. RAMACHANDRAN GN, REDDI AH (eds): *Biochemistry of Collagen.* New York, Plenum Publishing Corp, 1976

2. PROCKOP DJ, KIVIRIKKO KI, TUDERMAN L, GUZMAN NA: The biosynthesis of collagen and its disorders. *N Engl J Med* 301:13, 1979
3. BORNSTEIN P, TRAUB W: The chemistry and biology of collagen, in Neurath H, Hill RL, Boeder C-L (eds): *The Proteins*, ed 3. New York, Academic Press, Inc, 1979, vol 4, p 411
4. BORNSTEIN P, BYERS PH: Disorders of collagen metabolism, in Bondy PK, Rosenberg LE (eds): *Metabolic Control and Disease*, ed 8. Philadelphia, WB Saunders Co, 1980, p 1089
5. BAILEY AJ, ETHERINGTON DJ: Metabolism of collagen and elastin, in Florkin M, Nueberger N, Van Deenen LLM (eds): *Comprehensive Biochemistry*. Amsterdam, Elsevier/North-Holland Biomedical Press, 1980, p 229
6. MINOR RR: Collagen metabolism. A comparison of diseases of collagen and diseases affecting collagen. *Am J Pathol* 98:227, 1980
7. TRAUB W, PIEZ KA: The chemistry and structure of collagen. *Adv Protein Chem* 25:243, 1971
8. SCHOFIELD JD, FREEMAN IL, JACKSON DS: The isolation, and amino acid and carbohydrate composition of polymeric collagens prepared from various human tissues. *Biochem J* 124:467, 1971
9. RAMACHANDRAN GN, BANSAL M, RAMAKRISHNAN C: Hydroxyproline stabilizes both intrafibrillar structure as well as inter-protofibrillar linkages in collegen. *Curr Sci* 44:1, 1975
10. SEGAL DM: Polymers of tripeptides as collagen models. VII. Synthesis and solution properties of four collagen-like polyhexapeptides. *J Mol Biol* 43:497, 1969
11. BROWN FR III, HOPFINGER AJ, BLOUT ER: The collagen-like triple helix to random-coil transition: Experiment and theory. *J Mol Biol* 63:101, 1972
12. SAKAKIBARA K, INOUYE K, SHUDO K, KISHIDA Y, KOBAYASHI Y, PROCKOP DJ: Synthesis of (Pro-Hyp-Gly)n of defined molecular weights. Evidence for the stabilization of collagen triple helix by hydroxyproline. *Biochim Biophys Acta* 303:198, 1973
13. BAILEY AJ, LIGHT ND, ATKINS EDT: Chemical cross-linking restrictions on models for the molecular organization of the collagen fibre. *Nature* 288:408, 1980
14. TRUS BL, PIEZ KA: Compressed microfibril models of the native collagen fibril. *Nature* 286:300, 1980
15. GELMAN RA, PIEZ KA: Collagen fibril formation in vitro. *J Biol Chem* 255:8098, 1980
16. SILVER FH, TRELSTAD RL: Type I collagen in solution. *J Biol Chem* 255:9427, 1980
17. BORNSTEIN P, SAGE H: Structurally distinct collagen types. *Ann Rev Biochem* 49:957, 1980
18. UITTO J: Collagen polymorphism: Isolation and partial characterization of α1(I)-trimer molecules in normal human skin. *Arch Biochem Biophys* 192:371, 1979
19. EPSTEIN EJ JR: [α1(III)]3 Human skin collagen. Release by pepsin digestion and preponderance in fetal life. *J Biol Chem* 249:3225, 1974
20. BAILEY AJ, BAZIN S, SIMMS TJ, LE LOUS M, NICOLETIS C, DELAUNAY A: Characterization of the collagen of human hypertrophic and normal scars. *Biochim Biophys Acta* 405:412, 1975
21. MEIGEL WN, GAY S, WEBER L: Dermal architecture and collagen type distribution. *Arch Derm Res* 259:1, 1977
22. GAY S, FIETZEK PP, REMBERGER K, EDER M, KUHN K: Liver cirrhosis: Immunofluorescence and biochemical studies demonstrate two types of collagen. *Wochenschr Klin W* 53:205, 1975
23. TRYGGVASON K, ROBEY PG, MARTIN GR: Biosynthesis of type IV procollagens. *Biochemistry* 19:1284, 1980
24. ALITALO K, VAHERI A, KRIEG T, TIMPL R: Biosynthesis of two subunits of type IV procollagen and of other basement membrane proteins by a human tumor cell line. *Eur J Biochem* 109:247, 1980
25. BURGESON RE, ADLI FAE, KAITILA II, HOLLISTER DW: Fetal membrane collagens: Identification of two new collagen alpha chains. *Proc Natl Acad Sci USA* 73:2579, 1976
26. BENTZ H, BACHINGER HP, GLANVILLE R, KUHN K: Physical evidence for the assembly of A and B chains of human placental collagen in a single triple helix. *Eur J Biochem* 92:563, 1978
27. MADRI JA, FURTHMAYR H: Isolation and tissue localization of type AB2 collagen from normal lung parenchyma. *Am J Pathol* 94:323, 1979
28. KUMAMOTO CA, FESSLER JH: Biosynthesis of A,B procollagen. *Proc Natl Acad Sci USA* 77:6434, 1980
29. WELSH C, GAY S, RHODE RK, PFISTER R, MILLER EJ: Collagen heterogeneity in normal rabbit cornea. I. Isolation and biochemical characterization of the genetically-distinct collagens. *Biochim Biophys Acta* 625:78, 1980
30. RHODES PK, MILLER EJ: Physicochemical characterization and molecular organization of the collagen A and B chains. *Biochemistry* 17:3442, 1978
31. FESSLER JH, FESSLER LI: Biosynthesis of procollagen. *Ann Rev Biochem* 47:129, 1978
32. VUUST J, PIEZ KA: A kinetic study of collagen biosynthesis. *J Biol Chem* 247:856, 1972
33. BOEDTKER H, CRKVENJAKOV RB, LAST JA, DOTY P: The identification of collagen messenger RNA. *Proc Natl Acad Sci USA* 71:4208, 1974
34. GRANT ME, JACKSON DS: The biosynthesis of procollagen. *Essays Biochem* 12:77, 1976
35. GRANT ME, HEATHCOTE JG, CHEAH KSE: The synthesis and processing of collagen precursors, in Rapoport S, Schewe T (eds): *Processing and Turnover of Proteins and Organelles in the Cell*. Elmsford, NY, Pergamon Press, Inc, 1978, FEBS Symposia, vol 53, p 29
36. PALMITER RD, DAVIDSON JM, GAGNON J, ROWE DW, BORNSTEIN P: NH2-terminal sequence of the chick pro α1(I) chain synthesized in the reticulocyte lysate system. *J Biol Chem* 254:1433, 1979
37. MILLER EJ, WOODALL DI, VAIL MS: Biosynthesis of cartilage collagen: Use of pulse labelling to order the cyanogen bromide peptides in the α1(II) chain. *J Biol Chem* 248:1666, 1973
38. CARDINALE GJ, UDENFRIEND S: Prolyl hydroxylase. *Adv Enzymol* 41:245, 1974
39. TUDERMAN L, MYLLYLA R, KIVIRIKKO KI: Mechanism of the prolyl hydroxylase reaction. I. Role of co-substrates. *Eur J Biochem* 80:341, 1977
40. MYLLYLA R, TUDERMAN L, KIVIRIKKO KI: Mechanism of the prolyl hydroxylase reaction. 2. Kinetic analysis of the reaction sequence. *Eur J Biochem* 80:349, 1977
41. MYLLYLA R, KUUTTI-SAVOLAINEN E-R, KIVIRIKKO KI: The role of ascorbate in the prolyl hydroxylase reaction. *Biochem Biophys Res Commun* 83:441, 1978
42. NOLAN JC, CARDINALE GJ, UDENFRIEND S: The formation of hydroxyproline in collagen by cells grown in the absence of serum. *Biochim Biophys Acta* 543:116, 1978
43. PETERKOFSKY B, KALWINSKY D, ASSAD R: Substance in L-929 cell extracts which replaces the ascorbate requirement for prolyl hydroxylase in a tritium release assay for reducing cofactor; correlation of its concentration with the extent of ascorbate-independent proline hydroxylation and the level of prolyl hydroxylase activity in these cells. *Arch Biochem Biophys* 199:362, 1980
44. RAO NV, ADAMS E: Partial reaction of prolyl hydroxylase (GLY-PRO-ALA)n stimulates α-ketoglutarate decarboxylation without prolyl hydroxylation. *J Biol Chem* 253:6327, 1978
45. COUNTS DF, CARDINALE GJ, UDENFRIEND S: Prolyl hydroxylase half reaction: Peptidyl prolyl-independent decarboxylation of α-ketoglutarate. *Proc Natl Acad Sci USA* 75:2145, 1978
46. RAPAKA RS, RENUGOPALAKRISHNAN V, URRY DW, BHATNAGAR RS: Hydroxylation of proline in polytripeptide models of collagen: Stereochemistry of polytripeptide-prolyl hydroxylase interaction. *Biochemistry* 17:2892, 1978
47. PROCKOP DJ, BERG RA, KIVIRIKKO KI, UITTO J: Intracellular steps in the biosynthesis of collagen, in Ramachandran GN, Reddi AH (eds): *Biochemistry of Collagen*. New York, Plenum Publishing Corp, 1976, p 163
48. BORNSTEIN P: Comparative sequence studies of rat skin and tendon collagen. I. Evidence for incomplete hydroxylation of individual prolyl residues in the normal proteins. *Biochemistry* 6:3082, 1967
49. OLSEN BR, BERG RA, KISHIDA Y, PROCKOP DJ: Collagen synthesis: Localization of prolyl hydroxylase in tendon cells detected with ferritin-labeled antibodies. *Science* 182, 825, 1973
50. BERG RA, KEDERSHA NL, GUZMAN NA: Purification and partial characterization of the two nonidentical subunits of prolyl hydroxylase. *J Biol Chem* 254:3111, 1979
51. ADAMS E, FRANK L: Metabolism of proline and the hydroxyprolines. *Ann Rev Biochem* 49:1005, 1980
52. RISTELI J, TRYGGVASON K, KIVIRIKKO KI: A rapid assay for prolyl 3-hydroxylase activity. *Anal Biochem* 84:423, 1978
53. RISTELI J, TRYGGVASON K, KIVIRIKKO KI: Prolyl 3-hydroxylase: Partial characterization of the enzyme from rat kidney cortex. *Eur J Biochem* 73:485, 1977
54. MAJAMAA K: Effect of prevention of procollagen triple-helix formation on proline 3-hydroxylation in freshly isolated chick embryo tendon cells. *Biochem J* 196:203, 1981
55. TRYGGVASON K, MAJAMAA K, KIVIRIKKO KI: Prolyl 3-hydroxylase and 4-hydroxylase activities in certain rat and chick-embryo tissues and age-related changes in their activities in the rat. *Biochem J* 178:127, 1979
56. PUISTOLA U, TURPEENNIEMI-HUJANEN TM, MYLLYLA R, KIVIRIKKO KI: Studies on the lysyl hydroxylase reaction. I. Initial velocity kinetics and related aspects. *Biochim Biophys Acta* 611:40, 1980
57. PUISTOLA U, TURPEENNIEMI-HUJANEN TM, MYLLYLA R, KIVIRIKKO KI: Studies on the lysyl hydroxylase reaction. II. Inhibition kinetics and the reaction mechanism. *Biochim Biophys Acta* 611:51, 1980
58. FIETZEK PP, KUHN K: The primary structure of collagen. *Int Rev Connect Tissue Res* 7:1, 1976
59. STIMLER NP, TANZER ML: Isolation and characterization of a double chain intermolecular cross-linked peptide from insoluble calf bone collagen. *J Biol Chem* 254:666, 1979
60. RYHANEN L, MYLLYLA R, KIVIRIKKO KI: Hydroxylation of lysyl residues

in lysine-rich and argine-rich histones by lysyl hydroxylase *in vitro*. *Biochim Biophys Acta* 397:50, 1977

61. MILLER EJ, MARTIN GR, PIEZ KA, POWER MJ: Characterization of chick bone collagen and compositional changes associated with maturation. *J Biol Chem* 242:5481, 1967

62. BARNES MJ, CONSTABLE BJ, MORTON LF, ROYCE PM: Age related variations in hydroxylation of lysine and proline in collagen. *Biochem J* 139:461, 1974

63. BUTLER WT: Partial hydroxylation of certain lysines in collagen. *Science* 161:796, 1968

64. KIVIRIKKO KI, RYHANEN L, ANTTINEN H, BORNSTEIN P, PROCKOP DJ: Further hydroxylation of lysyl residues in collagen by protocollagen lysyl hydroxylase *in vitro*. *Biochemistry* 12:4966, 1973

65. PINNELL SR, KRANE SM, KENZORA JE, GLIMCHER MJ: A heritable disorder of connective tissue: Hydroxylysine-deficient collagen disease. *N Engl J Med* 286:1013, 1972

66. RISTELI L, RISTELI J, IHME A, KRIEG T, MULLER PK: Preferential hydroxylation of type IV collagen by lysyl hydroxylase from Ehlers-Danlos syndrome type VI fibroblasts. *Biochem Biophys Res Commun* 96:1778, 1980

67. PETERKOFSKY B, ASSAD R: Localization of chick embryo limb bone microsomal lysyl hydroxylase at intracisternal and intramembrane sites. *J Biol Chem* 25:4714, 1979

68. TURPEENNIEMI-HUJANEN TM, PUISTOLA U, KIVIRIKKO KI: Isolation of lysyl hydroxylase, an enzyme of collagen synthesis, from chick embryos as a homogenous protein. *Biochem J* 189:247, 1980

69. KIVIRIKKO KI, MYLLYLA R: Collagen glycosyltransferases, in Hall DA, Jackson DS (eds): *International Review of Connective Tissue Research*. New York, Academic Press, Inc, 1979, vol 8, p 23

70. MYLLYLA R, ANTTINEN H, KIVIRIKKO KI: Metal activation of galactosylhydroxylysyl glucosyltransferase, an intracellular enzyme of collagen biosynthesis. *Eur J Biochem* 101:261, 1979

71. SPIRO RG, SPIRO MJ: Studies on the biosynthesis of the hydroxylysine-linked disaccharide unit of basement membranes and collagens. III. Tissue and subcellular distribution of glycosyltransferases and the effect of various conditions on the enzyme levels. *J Biol Chem* 246:4919, 1971

72. HARWOOD R, GRANT ME, JACKSON DS: The association of collagen galactosyl and glucosyl transferases with subcellular fractions of embryonic chick tendon cells. *Biochem Soc Trans* 3:136, 1975

73. MYLLYLA R, ANTTINEN H, RISTELI L, KIVIRIKKO KI: Isolation of collagen glucosyltransferase as a homogeneous protein from chick embryos. *Biochim Biophys Acta* 480:113, 1977

74. GUZMAN NA, GRAVES PN, PROCKOP DJ: Addition of mannose to both the amino- and carboxy-terminal propeptides of type II procollagen occurs without formation of a triple helix. *Biochem Biophys Res Commun* 84:691, 1978

75. ANTTINEN H, OIKARINEN A, RYHANEN L, KIVIRIKKO KI: Evidence for the transfer of mannose to the extension peptides of procollagen within the cisternae of the rough endoplasmic reticulum. *FEBS Lett* 87:222, 1978

76. DUKSIN D, BORNSTEIN P: Changes in surface properties of normal and transformed cells caused by tunicamycin, an inhibitor of protein glycosylation. *Proc Natl Acad Sci USA* 74:3433, 1977

77. HOUSLEY TJ, ROWLAND FN, LEDGER PW, KAPLAN J, TANZER ML: Effects of tunicamycin on the biosynthesis of procollagen by human fibroblasts. *J Biol Chem* 255:121, 1980

78. SCHOFIELD JD, UITTO J, PROCKOP DJ: Formation of interchain disulfide bonds and helical structure during biosynthesis of procollagen by embryonic tendon cells. *Biochemistry* 13:1801, 1974

79. UITTO J, PROCKOP DJ: Biosynthesis of cartilage procollagen: Influence of chain association and hydroxylation of prolyl residues on the folding of the polypeptides into the triple-helical conformation. *Biochemistry* 13:4586, 1974

80. UITTO J, PROCKOP DJ: Rate of helix formation by intracellular procollagen and protocollagen. Evidence for a role of disulfide bonds. *Biochem Biophys Res Commun* 55:904, 1973

81. FESSLER LI, RUDD C, FESSLER JH: Renaturation of disulfide-linked procollagen. *J Supramol Struct* 2:103, 1974

82. HARWOOD R, MERRY AH, WOOLLEY DE, GRANT ME, JACKSON DS: The disulphide-bonded nature of procollagen and the role of the extension peptides in the assembly of the molecule. *Biochem J* 161:405, 1977

83. HARWOOD R, GRANT ME, JACKSON DS: The route of secretion of procollagen. The influence of α,α'-bipyridyl, colchicine and antimycin A on the secretory process in embryonic chick tendon and cartilage cells. *Biochem J* 156:81, 1976

84. TRELSTAD RL: Vacuoles in the embryonic chick corneal epithelium, an epithelium which produces collagen. *J Cell Biol* 48:689, 1971

85. OLSEN BR, PROCKOP DJ: Ferritin-conjugated antibodies used for labeling of organelles involved in the cellular synthesis and transport of procollagen. *Proc Natl Acad Sci USA* 71:2033, 1974

86. WEINSTOCK M, LEBLOND CP: Synthesis, migration, and release of precursor collagen by odontoblasts as visualized by radioautography after [³H]proline administration. *J Cell Biol* 60:92, 1974

87. DEHM P, PROCKOP DJ: Time lag in the secretion of collagen by matrix-free tendon cells and inhibition of the secretory process by colchicine and vinblastine. *Biochim Biophys Acta* 264:375, 1972

88. DIEGELMANN RF, PETERKOFSKY B: Inhibition of collagen secretion from bone and cultured fibroblasts by microtubular disruptive drugs. *Proc Natl Acad Sci USA* 69:892, 1972

89. EHRLICH HP, ROSS R, BORNSTEIN P: Effects of antimicrotubular agents on the secretion of collagen. *J Cell Biol* 62:390, 1974

90. MORRIS NP, FESSLER LI, FESSLER JH: Procollagen propeptide release by procollagen peptidases and bacterial collagenase. *J Biol Chem* 254:11024, 1979

91. LAPIERE CM, LENAERS A, KOHN LD: Procollagen peptidase: An enzyme excising the coordination peptides of procollagen. *Proc Natl Acad Sci USA* 68:3054, 1971

92. TUDERMAN L, KIVIRIKKO KI, PROCKOP DJ: Partial purification and characterization of a neutral protease which cleaves the N-terminal propeptides from procollagen. *Biochemistry* 17:2948, 1978

93. LEUNG MKK, FESSLER LI, GREENBERG DB, FESSLER JH: Separate amino and carboxyl procollagen peptidases in chick embryo tendon. *J Biol Chem* 254:224, 1979

94. NUSGENS B, LAPIERE CM: A simplified procedure for measuring aminoprocollagen peptidase type I. *Anal Biochem* 95:406, 1979

95. NUSGENS BV, GOEBELS Y, SHINKAI H, LAPIERE CM: Procollagen type III N-terminal endopeptidase in fibroblast culture. *Biochem J* 191:699, 1980.

96. KESSLER E, GOLDBERG B: A method for assaying the activity of the endopeptidase which excises the nonhelical carboxyterminal extensions from type I procollagen. *Anal Biochem* 86:463, 1978

97. TANZER ML: Cross-linking, in Ramachandran GN, Reddi AH (eds): *Biochemistry of Collagen*. New York, Plenum Publishing Corp, 1976, p 137

98. LIGHT ND, BAILEY AJ: Molecular structure and stabilization of the collagen fibre, in Viidik A, Vuust J (eds): *Biology of Collagen*. New York, Academic Press, Inc, 1980, p 15

99. PINNELL SR, MARTIN GR: The cross-linking of collagen and elastin: Enzymatic conversion of lysine in peptide linkage to α-aminoadipic-δ-semialdehyde (allysine) by an extract from bone. *Proc Natl Acad Sci USA* 61:708, 1968

100. SIEGEL RC: Lysyl oxidase, in Hall DA, Jackson DS (eds): *International Review of Connective Tissue Research*. New York, Academic Press, Inc, 1979, vol 8, p 73

101. SIEGEL RC, PINNELL SR, MARTIN GR: Crosslinking of collagen and elastin: Properties of lysyl oxidase. *Biochemistry* 9:4486, 1970

102. STASSEN FLH: Properties of highly purified lysyl oxidase from embryonic chick cartilage. *Biochim Biophys Acta* 438:49, 1976

103. JORDAN RE, MILBURY R, SULLIVAN KA, TRACKMAN PC, KAGAN HM: Studies on lysyl oxidase of bovine ligamentum nuchae and bovine aorta, in Sandberg LB, Gray WR (eds): *Elastin and Elastic Tissue*. New York, Plenum Publishing Corp, 1976, p 531

104. MURRAY JC, FRASER DR, LEVENE CI: The effect of pyridoxine deficiency on lysyl oxidase activity in the chick. *Exp Mol Pathol* 28:301, 1978

105. FUJII K, KAJIWARA T, KUROSU H: Effect of vitamin B6 deficiency on the crosslink formation of collagen. *FEBS Lett* 97:193, 1979

106. SIEGEL RC: Biosynthesis of collagen crosslinks: Increased activity of purified lysyl oxidase with reconstituted collagen fibrils. *Proc Natl Acad Sci USA* 71:4826, 1974

107. BORNSTEIN P, PIEZ KA: The nature of the intramolecular cross-links in collagen. The separation and characterization of peptides from the crosslink region of rat skin collagen. *Biochemistry* 5:3460, 1966

108. EYRE DR, GLIMCHER MJ: Evidence for intramolecular crosslinks in chicken bone collagen: The isolation of peptides containing allysine aldol. *Biochim Biophys Acta* 295:301, 1973

109. EYRE DR, GLIMCHER MJ: Analysis of a crosslinked peptide from calf bone collagen: Evidence that hydroxylysyl glycoside participates in the crosslink. *Biochem Biophys Res Commun* 52:663, 1973

110. ROBINS SP, BAILEY AJ: Isolation and characterization of glycosyl derivatives of the reducible cross-links in collagens. *FEBS Lett* 38:334, 1974

111. BAILEY AJ, SIMS TJ: Chemistry of the collagen cross-links. Nature of the cross-links in the polymeric forms of dermal collagen during development. *Biochem J* 153:211, 1976

112. KOHN RR, ROLLERSON E: Relationship of age to swelling properties of human diaphragm tendon in acid and alkaline solutions. *J Gerontol* 13:241, 1958

113. BANFIELD WG: Age changes in the acetic-acid soluble collagen in human skin. *Arch Pathol* 68:680, 1959

114. ROBINS SP, SHIMOKOMAKI M, BAILEY AJ: Age-related changes in the reducible components of intact bovine collagen fibres. *Biochem J* 131:771, 1973

115. EYRE DR, OGUCHI H: The hydroxypyridinium crosslinks of skeletal collagens: Their measurement, properties and a proposed pathway of formation. *Biochem Biophys Res Commun* 92:403, 1980

116. FUJIMOTO D, MORIGUCHI T, ISHIDA T, HAYASHI H: The structure of pyridinoline, a collagen crosslink. *Biochem Biophys Res Commun* 84:52, 1978

117. FUJIMOTO D: Evidence for natural existence of pyridinoline crosslink in collagen. *Biochem Biophys Res Commun* 93:948, 1980

118. FUJIMOTO D, MORIGUCHI T: Pyridinoline, a non-reducible crosslink of collagen. Quantitative determination, distribution, and isolation of a crosslinked peptide. *J Biochem* 83:863, 1978

119. MORIGUCHI T, FUJIMOTO D: Crosslink of collagen in hypertrophic scar. *J Invest Dermatol* 72:143, 1979

120. HOUSLEY TANZER ML, HENSON E, GALLOP PM: Collagen crosslinking: Isolation of hydroxyaldol-histidine, a naturally-occuring crosslink. *Biochem Biophys Res Commun* 67:824, 1975

121. TANZER ML, HOUSLEY T, BERUBE L, FAIRWEATHER R, FRANZBLAU C, GALLOP PM: Structure of two histidine-containing cross-links from collagen. *J Biol Chem* 248:393, 1973

122. BERNSTEIN PH, MECHANIC GL: A natural histidine-based imminium cross-link in collagen and its location. *J Biol Chem* 255:10414, 1980

123. ROBINS SP, BAILEY AJ: The chemistry of the collagen cross-links—the characterization of fraction C, a possible artifact produced during the reduction of collagen fibres with borohydride. *Biochem J* 135:657, 1973

124. HARRIS ED, KRANE SM: Collagenases. *N Engl J Med* 291:557, 605, 625, 1974

125. GROSS J: Aspects of the animal collagenases, in Ramachanchran GN, Reddi AH (eds): *Biochemistry of Collagen*. New York, Plenum Publishing Corp, 1976, p 275

126. HARPER E: Collagenases. *Ann Rev Biochem* 49:1063, 1980

127. BAUER EA, STRICKLIN GP, WELGUS HG, JEFFREY JJ, SELTZER JL, EISEN AZ: Collagenase, in Goldsmith LA (ed): *The Biochemistry and Physiology of the Skin*. New York, Oxford University Press, 1982, in press

128. GROSS J, NAGAI Y: Specific degradation of the collagen molecule by tadpole collagenolytic enzyme. *Proc Natl Acad Sci USA* 54:1197, 1965

129. GROSS J, HARPER E, HARRIS ED, MCCROSKERY PA, HIGHBERGER JH, CORBETT C, KANG AH: Animal collagenases: Specificity of action, and structures of the substrate cleavage site. *Biochem Biophys Res Commun* 61:555, 1974

130. HIGHBERGER JH, CORBETT C, KANG AH, GROSS J: The amino acid sequence of chick skin collagen α1-CB7: The presence of a previously unrecognized triplet. *Biochem Biophys Res Commun* 83:43, 1978

131. WELGUS HG, JEFFREY JJ, STRICKLIN GP, EISEN AZ: Specificity of human skin collagenase on collagen types of various species. *Clin Res* 28:477A, 1980

132. LIOTTA LA, ABE S, ROBEY PG, MARTIN GR: Preferential digestion of basement membrane collagen by an enzyme derived from a metastatic murine tumor. *Proc Natl Acad Sci USA* 76:2268, 1979

133. WELGUS HG, JEFFREY JJ, STRICKLIN GP, ROSWIT WT, EISEN AZ: Characteristics of the action of human skin fibroblast collagenase on fibrillar collagen. *J Biol Chem* 255:6806, 1980

134. HARRIS ED, MCCROSKERY PA: The influence of temperature and fibril stability on degradation of cartilage collagen by rheumatoid synovial collagenase. *N Engl J Med* 290:1, 1974

135. VATER CA, HARRIS ED, SIEGEL RC: Native cross-links in collagen fibrils induce resistance to human synovial collagenase. *Biochem J* 181:639, 1979

136. STRICKLIN GP, BAUER EA, JEFFREY JJ, EISEN AZ: Human skin collagenase: Isolation of precursor and active forms from both fibroblast and organ cultures. *Biochemistry* 16:1607, 1977

137. SHINKAI H, NAGAI Y: A latent collagenase from embryonic human skin explants. *J Biochem* 81:1261, 1977

138. REYNOLDS JJ, SELLERS A, MURPHY G, CARTWRIGHT E: A new factor that may control collagen resorption. Lancet 2:333, 1977

139. SELLERS A, CARTWRIGHT E, MURPHY G, REYNOLDS J: Evidence that latent collagenase are enzyme-inhibitor complexes. *Biochem J* 163:303, 1977

140. SOPATA I, DANCEWICZ AM: Presence of a gelatin-specific proteinase and its latent form in human leucocytes. *Biochim Biophys Acta* 370:510, 1974

141. BIENKOWSKI RS, COWAN MJ, MCDONALD JA, CRYSTAL RG: Degradation of newly synthesized collagen. *J Biol Chem* 253:4356, 1978

142. BAUM BJ, MOSS J, BREUL SD, BERG RA, CRYSTAL RG: Effect of cyclic AMP on the intracellular degradation of newly synthesized collagen. *J Biol Chem* 255:2843, 1980

143. BERG RA, SCHWARTZ ML, CRYSTAL RG: Regulation of the production of secretory proteins: Intracellular degradation of newly synthesized "defective" collagen. *Proc Natl Acad Sci USA* 77:4746, 1980

144. STEINMANN BU, MARTIN GR, BAUM BI, CRYSTAL RG: Synthesis and degradation of collagen by skin fibroblasts from controls and from patients with osteogenesis imperfecta. *FEBS Lett* 101:269, 1979

145. LAITINEN O: Applications of urinary hydroxyproline determination. *Acta Med Scand Suppl* 577:8, 1974

146. NISSEN R, CARDINALE GJ, UDENFRIEND S: Increased turnover of arterial collagen in hypertensive rats. *Proc Natl Acad Sci USA* 75:451, 1978

147. EFRON ML, BIXBY EM, PRYLES CV: Hydroxyprolinemia. II. A rare metabolic disease due to a deficiency of the enzyme "hydroxyproline oxidase". *N Engl J Med* 272:1299, 1965

148. EFRON ML, BIXBY EM, HOCKADAY TDR, SMITH LH JR, MESHORER E: Hydroxyprolinemia. III. The origin of free hydroxyproline in hydroxyprolinemia. Collagen turnover, evidence for a biosynthetic pathway in man. *Biochim Biophys Acta* 165:238, 1968

149. PELKONEN R, KIVIRIKKO KI: Hydroxyprolinemia, an apparently harmless familial metabolic disorder. *N Engl J Med* 283:451, 1970

150. KOHLER PF, MULLER-EBERHARD HJ: Metabolism of human Clq. Studies in hypogammaglobulinemia, myeloma, and systemic lupus erythematosus. *J Clin Invest* 51:868, 1972

151. SAKAMOTO M, SAKAMOTO S, BRICKLEY-PARSONS D, GLIMCHER MJ: Collagen synthesis and degradation in embryonic chick-bone explants. *J Bone Joint Surg* 61A:1042, 1979

152. KRANE SM, KANTROWITZ FG, BRYNE M, PINNELL SR, SINGER FR: Urinary excretion of hydroxylysine and its glycosides as an index of collagen degradation. *J Clin Invest* 59:819, 1977

153. KELLEHER PC: Urinary excretion of hydroxyproline, hydroxylysine and hydroxylysine glycosides by patients with Paget's disease of bone and carcinoma with metastases in bone. *Clin Chim Acta* 92:373, 1979

154. PINNELL SR, FOX R, KRANE SM: Human collagens: Differences in glycosylated hydroxylysines in skin and bone. *Biochim Biophys Acta* 229:119, 1971

155. HILES RA, HENDERSON LM: The partial purification and properties of hydroxylysine kinase from rat liver. *J Biol Chem* 247:646, 1972

156. POTT G, HENKEL W, WERRIES E: Stereospezifischer enzymatischer abbau von glucopyranosylgalaktopyranosylhydroxylysin aus aortenkollagen. *Hoppe-Seyler's Z Physiol Chem* 355:787, 1974

157. HAMAZAKI H, HOTTA K: Purification and characterization of an α-glucosidase specific for hydroxylysine-linked disaccharide of collagen. *J Biol Chem* 254:9682, 1979

158. MOEN RC, ROWE DW, PALMITER RD: Regulation of procollagen synthesis during the development of chick embryo calvaria. Correlation with procollagen mRNA content. *J Biol Chem* 254:3526, 1979

159. HANDLEY CJ, BATEMAN JF, OAKES BW, LOWTHER DA: Characterization of the collagen synthesized by cultured cartilage cells. *Biochim Biophys Acta* 386:444, 1975

160. DESHMUKH K, KLINE WG: Characterization of collagen and its precursors synthesized by rabbit-articular-cartilage cells in various culture system. *Eur J Biochem* 69:117, 1976

161. NORBY DP, MALEMUD CJ, SOKOLOFF L: Differences in the collagen types synthesized by lapine articular chondrocytes in spinner and monolayer culture. *Arthritis Rheum* 20:709, 1977

162. ABE S, STEINMANN BU, WAHL LM, MARTIN GR: High cell density alters the ratio of type III to I collagen synthesis by fibroblasts. *Nature* 279:442, 1979

163. NARAYANAN AS, PAGE RC: Serum modulates collagen types in human gingiva fibroblasts. *FEBS Lett* 80:221, 1977

164. BHATNAGAR RS, HUSSAIN MZ, STREIFEL JA, TOLENTINO M, ENRIQUEZ B: Alteration of collagen synthesis in lung organ cultures by hyperoxic environments. *Biochem Biophys Res Commun* 83:392, 1978

165. ROWE DW, NOEN RC, DAVIDSON JM, BYERS PH, BORNSTEIN P, PALMITER RH: Correlation of procollagen mRNA levels in normal and transformed chick embryo fibroblasts with different rates of procollagen synthesis. *Biochemistry* 17:1581, 1978

166. KREAM BE, ROWE DW, GWOREK SC, RAISZ LG: Parathyroid hormone alters collagen synthesis and procollagen mRNA levels in fetal rat calvaria. *Proc Natl Acad Sci USA* 77:5654, 1980

167. CANALIS EM, HINTZ RL, DIETRICH JW, MAINA DM, RAISZ LG: Effect of somatomedin and growth hormone on bone collagen synthesis in vitro. *Metabolism* 26:1079, 1977

168. CANALIS E, RAISZ LG: Effect of sex steroids on bone collagen synthesis in vitro. *Calcif Tissue Res* 25:105, 1978

169. PONEC M, KEMPENAAR JA, VAN DERM NEULEN-VAN HARSKAMP GA, BACHRA BN: Effects of glucocorticosteroids on cultured human skin fibroblasts. IV. Specific decrease in the synthesis of collagen but not effect on its hydroxylation. *Biochem Pharmacol* 28:2777, 1979

170. PONEC M, HASPER I, VIANDEN GDNE, BACHRA BN: Effects of glucocorticosteroids on primary human skin fibroblasts. II. Effects on total protein and collagen biosynthesis by confluent cell cultures. *Arch Dermatol Res* 259:125, 1977

171. MCCOY BJ, DIEGELMANN RF, COHEN IK: *In vitro* inhibition of cell growth, collagen synthesis, and prolyl hydroxylase activity by triamcinolone acetonide (40750). *Proc Soc Exp Biol Med* 163:216, 1980

172. HANDLEY CJ, BROOKS PR, LOWTHER DA: Extracellular matrix metabolism by chondrocytes. VI. Concomitant depression by exogenous levels of proteoglycan of collagen and proteoglycan synthesis by chondrocytes. *Biochim Biophys Acta* 544:441, 1978

173. SCHWARTZ NB, DORFMAN A: Effect of β-D-xylosides on collagen synthesis in cultured fibroblasts. *Biochem Biophys Res Commun* 67:1108, 1975

174. AALTO M, POTILA M, KULONEN EL: Glycoproteins from experimental granulation tissue and their effects on collagen synthesis in embryonic chick tendon cells. *Biochim Biophys Acta* 587:606, 1979

175. RONNEMAA T, JUVA K, KULONEN E: Effect of hyperlipidemic rat serum on the synthesis of collagen by chick embryo fibroblasts. *Atherosclerosis* 21:315, 1975

176 RONNEMAA T, DOHERTY NS:Effect of serum and liver extracts from hypercholesterolemic rats on the synthesis of collagen by isolated aortas and cultured aortic smooth muscle cells. *Atherosclerosis* 26:261, 1977

177. SPIELVOGEL RL, KERSEY JH, GOLTZ RW: Mononuclear cell stimulation of fibroblast collagen synthesis. *Clin Exp Dermatol* 3:25, 1978

178. JIMENEZ SA, MCARTHUR W, ROSENBLOOM J: Inhibition of collagen synthesis by mononuclear cell supernates. *J Exp Med* 150:1421, 1979

179. ADAMS SL, SOBEL ME, HOWARD BH, OLDEN K, YAMADA KM, DE CROMBRUGGHE B, PASTAN I: Levels of translatable mRNAs for cell surface protein, collagen precursors, and two membrane proteins are altered in rous sarcoma virus-transformed chick embryo fibroblasts. *Proc Natl Acad Sci USA* 74:3399, 1977

180. PARKER I, FITSCHEN W: Procollagen mRNA metabolism during the fibroblast cell cycle and its synthesis in transformed cells. *Nucleic Acids Res* 8:2823, 1980

181. KRIEG T, AUMAILLEY M, DESSAU W, WIESTNER M, MULLER P: Synthesis of collagen by human fibroblasts and their SV40 transformants. *Exp Cell Res* 125:23, 1980

182. LEROY EC, MCGUIRE M, CHEN N: Increased collagen synthesis by scleroderma skin fibroblasts in vitro. *J Clin Invest* 54:880, 1974

183. UITTO J, BAUER EA, EISEN AZ: Scleroderma. Increased biosynthesis of triple-helical type I and type III procollagen associated with unaltered expression of collagenase by skin fibroblasts in culture. *J Clin Invest* 64:921, 1979

184. DIEGELMANN RF, COHEN IK, MCCOY BJ: Growth kinetics and collagen synthesis of normal skin, normal scar and keloid fibroblasts in vitro. *J Cell Phys* 98:341, 1979

185. IWATSUKI K, CARDINALE GJ, SPECTOR S, UDENFRIEND S: Hypertension: Increase of collagen biosynthesis in arteries but not in veins. *Science* 198:403, 1977

186. OOSHIMA A, FULLER GC, CARDINALE GJ, SPECTOR S, UDENFRIEND S: Reduction of collagen biosynthesis in blood vessels and other tissues by reserpine and hypophysectomy. *Proc Natl Acad Sci USA* 74:777, 1977

187. CARPOUSIS A, CHRISTNER P, ROSENBLOOM J: Preferential usage of tRNA isoaccepting species in collagen synthesis. *J Biol Chem* 252:8023, 1977

188. FINERMAN GAM, DOWNING S, ROSENBERG LE: Amino acid transport in bone. II. Regulation of collagen synthesis by perturbation of proline transport. *Biochim Biophys Acta* 135:1008, 1967

189. ROJKIND M, DE LEON LD: Collagen biosynthesis in cirrhotic rat liver slices. A regulatory mechanism. *Biochim Biophys Acta* 217:512, 1970

190. KERSHENOBICH D, FIERRO FJ, ROJKIND M: The relationship between the free pool of proline and collagen content in human liver cirrhosis. *J Clin Invest* 49:2246, 1970

191. WIESTNER M, KRIEG T, HORLEIN D, GLANVILLE RW, FIETZEK P, MULLER PK: Inhibiting effect of procollagen peptides on collagen biosynthesis in fibroblast cultures. *J Biol Chem* 254:7016, 1979

192. PAGLIA L, WILCZEK J, DE LEON LD, MARTIN GR, HORLEIN D, MULLER P: Inhibition of procollagen cell-free synthesis by amino-terminal extension peptides. *Biochemistry* 18:5030, 1979

193. LICHTENSTEIN JR, MARTIN GR, KOHN LD, BYERS PH, MCKUSICK VA: Defect in conversion of procollagen to collagen in a form of the Ehlers-Danlos syndrome. *Science* 182:298, 1973

194. JUVA K, PROCKOP DJ, COOPER GW, LASH JW: Hydroxylation of proline and the intracellular accumulation of a polypeptide precursor of collagen. *Science* 152:92, 1966

195. JIMENEZ SA, DEHM P, OLSEN BR, PROCKOP DJ: Intracellular collagen and protocollagen from embryonic tendon cells. *J Biol Chem* 248:720, 1973

196. JIMENEZ SA, HARSH M, ROSENBLOOM J: Hydroxyproline stabilizes the triple helix of chick collagen. *Biochem Biophys Res Commun* 52:106, 1973

197. BURJANADZE TV: Hydroxyproline content and location in relation to collagen thermal stability. *Biopolymers* 18:931, 1979

198. JIMENEZ SA, HARSCH M, MURPHY L, ROSENBLOOM J: Effects of temperature on conformation, hydroxylation, and secretion of chick tendon procollagen. *J Biol Chem* 249:4480, 1974

199. SALVADOR RA, TSAI I, MARCEL RJ, FELIX AM, KERWAR SS: The *in vivo* inhibition of collagen synthesis and the reduction of prolyl hydroxylase activity by 3,4-dehydroproline. *Arch Biochem Biophys* 174:381, 1976

200. UITTO J, PROCKOP DJ: Incorporation of proline analogs into procollagen. Assay for replacement of imino acids by *cis*-4-hydroxy-L-proline and *cis*-4-fluoro-L-proline. *Arch Biochem Biophys* 181:293, 1977

201. BATES J, PRYNNE CJ, LEVENE CI: The synthesis of underhydroxylated collagen by 3T6 mouse fibroblasts in culture. *Biochim Biophys Acta* 263:397, 1972

202. QUINN RS, KRANE SM: Collagen synthesis by cultured skin fibroblasts

203. MURAD S, GROVE D, LINDBERG KA, REYNOLDS G, SIVARAJAH A, PINNELL SR: Regulation of collagen synthesis by ascorbic acid. *Proc Natl Acad Sci USA* 78:2879, 1981

204. BARNES MJ, KODICEK E: Biological hydroxylations and ascorbic acid with special regard to collagen metabolism. *Vitam Horm* 30:1, 1972

205. RISTELI J, KIVIRIKKO KI: Intracellular enzymes of collagen biosynthesis in rat liver as a function of age and in hepatic injury induced by dimethylnitrosamine. Changes in prolyl hydroxylase, lysyl hydroxylase, collagen galactosyltransferase and collagen glucosyltransferase activity. *Biochem J* 158:361, 1976

206. MURAD S, SIVARAJAH A, PINNELL SR: Unpublished observation

207. FERNANDEZ-MADRID F, PITA J JR: Mechanism of action and ascorbic acid in the biosynthesis of collagen, in Balazs EA (ed): *Chemistry and Molecular Biology of the Intracellular Matrix*. London and New York, Academic Press, Inc, 1970, vol 1, p 439

208. HARWOOD R, GRANT ME, JACKSON DS: Influence of ascorbic acid on ribosomal patterns and collagen biosynthesis in healing woulds of scorbutic guinea pigs. *Biochem J* 142:641, 1974

209. SELYE H: Lathyrism. *Rev Can Biol* 16:1, 1957

210. TANZER MI: Experimental lathyrism. *Int Rev Connect Tissue Res* 3:91, 1965

211. FRY P, HARKNESS MLR, HARKNESS RD, NIGHTINGALE M: Mechanical properties of tissues and lathyritic animals. *J Physiol* 164:77, 1962

212. LEVENE CI, GROSS J: Alterations in state of molecular aggregation of collagen induced in chick embryos by β-aminopropionitrile (lathyrus factor). *J Exp Med* 110:771, 1959

213. SYKES BC, PARTRIDGE SM: Isolation of a soluble elastin from lathyritic chicks. *Biochem J* 130:1171, 1972

214. NARAYANAN AS, PAGE RC, MARTIN GR: On the preparation of tropoelastin from embryonic chick aorta. *Biochim Biophys Acta* 351:126, 1974

215. FOSTER JA, RICH CB, BERGLUND N, HUBER S, MECHAM RP, LANGE G: The anti-proteolytic behavior of lathyrogens. *Biochim Biophys Acta* 587:477, 1974

216. NARAYANAN NS, SIEGEL RC, MARTIN GR: On the inhibition of lysyl oxidase by β-aminopropionitrile. *Biochem Biophys Res Commun* 46:745, 1972

217. CARNES WH: Copper and connective tissue metabolism. *Int Rev Connect Tissue Res* 197:995, 1968

218. CARNES WH: Role of copper in connective tissue metabolism. *Fed Proc* 30:995, 1971

219. COULSON WF: Copper deficiency with special reference to the cardiovascular system. *Methods Achiev Exp Pathol* 6:111, 1972

220. SHIELDS GS, COULSON WF, KIMBALL DA, CARNES WH, CARTWRIGHT GE, WINTROBE MM: Studies on copper metabolism. 32. Cardiovascular lesions in copper-deficient swine. *Am J Pathol* 41:603, 1962

221. MILLER EJ, MARTIN GR, MECCA CE, PIEZ KA: The biosynthesis of elastin crosslinks: The effect of copper deficiency and a lathyrogen. *J Biol Chem* 240:3623, 1965

222. CHOU WS, SAVAGE JE, O'DELL BL: Role of copper in biosynthesis of intramolecular cross-links in chick tendon collagen. *J Biol Chem* 244:5785, 1969

223. HOFFBRAND BI (ed): Penicillamine: Recent work. *Postgrad Med J* (suppl 2):50, 1974

224. NIMNI ME, BAVETTA LA: Collagen defect induced by penicillamine. *Science* 150:905, 1965

225. NIMNI ME: A defect in the intramolecular and intermolecular cross-linking of collagen caused by penicillamine. I. Metabolic and functional abnormalities in soft tissues. *J Biol Chem* 243:1457, 1968

226. DESHMUKH K, NIMNI ME: A defect in the intramolecular and intermolecular cross-linking of collagen caused by penicillamine. II. Functional groups involved in the interaction process. *J Biol Chem* 244:1787, 1969

227. PINNELL SR, MARTIN GR, MILLER EJ: Desmosine biosynthesis: Nature of inhibition by D-penicillamine. *Science* 161:475, 1968

228. NIMNI ME, DESHMUKH K, DESHMUKH A: Mechanism of inhibition of collagen crosslinking and depolymerization of an incompletely crosslinked form of insoluble collagen caused by D-penicillamine, in Balazs EA (ed): *Chemistry and Molecular Biology of the Intracellular Matrix*. London and New York, Academic Press, Inc, 1970, vol 1, p 417

229. SIEGEL RC: Collagen cross-linking. Effects of D-penicillamine on crosslinking *in vitro*. *J Biol Chem* 252:254, 1977

230. NIMNI ME: Extraction of α and β components from insoluble collagen by thiol compounds. *Biochim Biophys Res Commun* 25:434, 1966

231. BAILEY AJ: Intermediate labile intermolecular crosslinks in collagen fibres. *Biochim Biophys Acta* 160:447, 1968

232. DESHMUKH A, DESHMUKH K, NIMNI ME: Synthesis of aldehydes and their interactions during the *in vitro* aging of collagen. *Biochemistry* 10:2337, 1971

233. NIMNI ME, DESHMUKH GN: Collagen defect induced by penicillamine. *Nature (New Biol)* 240:220, 1972

234. JACOBUS D, GRENAN M, WAGNER B, MARGOLIS C, JAFFE I: Osteolathyrogenic effect of penicillamine. *Am J Pathol* 54:21, 1969

235. ANDREWS EJ, WHITE WJ, BULLOCK LP: Spontaneous aortic aneurysms in *blotchy* mice. *Am J Pathol* 78:199, 1975

236. ROWE DW, McGOODWIN EB, MARTIN GR, SUSSMAN MD, GRAHN D, FARIS B, FRANZBLAU C: A sex-linked defect in the cross-linking of collagen and elastin associated with the mottled locus in mice. *J Exp Med* 139:180, 1974

237. ROWE DW, McGOODWIN EB, MARTIN GR, GRAHN D: Lysyl oxidase activity in the aneurysm-prone mottled mouse. *J Biol Chem* 252:939, 1977

238. HUNT DM: Primary defect in copper transport underlies mottled mutants in the mouse. *Nature* 249:852, 1974

239. PORT AE, HUNT DM: A study of the copper-binding proteins in liver and kidney tissue of neonatal normal and mottled mutant mice. *Biochem J* 183:721, 1979

240. HUNT DM, JOHNSON DR: Aromatic amino acid metabolism in brindled (Mo^{br}) and viable-brindled (Mo^{vbr}), two alleles at the mottled locus in the mouse. *Biochem Genet* 6:31, 1972

241. HUNT DM, JOHNSON DR: An inherited deficiency in noradrenaline biosynthesis in the brindled mouse. *J Neurol* 19:2811, 1972

242. HANSET R, ANSAY M: Dermatosparaxie (peau dechiree) chez le veau: Un defaut general du tissu conjonctif, de nature hereditaire. *Ann Med Vet* 111:451, 1967

243. HELLE O, NES NN: A hereditary skin defect in sheep. *Acta Vet Scand* 13:443, 1972

244. COUNTS DF, BYERS PH, HOLBROOK KA, HEGREBERG GA: Dermatosparaxis in a Himalayan cat: I. Biochemical studies of dermal collagen. *J Invest Dermatol* 74:96, 1980

245. HANSET R, LAPIERE CM: Inheritance of dermatosparaxis in the calf. *J Hered* 65:356, 1974

246. SIMAR LJ, BETZ EH: Dermatosparaxis of the calf: A genetic defect of the connective tissue. 2. Ultrastructural study of the skin. *Hoppe Seyler's Z Physiol Chem* 352:13, 1971

247. FJOLSTAD M, ODDVAR H: A hereditary dysplasia of collagen tissues in sheep. *J Pathol* 112:183, 1974

248. LENAERS A, ANSAY M, NUSGENS BV, LAPIERE CM: Collagen made of extended α-chains: Procollagen in genetically-defective dermatosparaxic calves. *Eur J Biochem* 23:533, 1971

249. BAILEY AJ, LAPIERE CM: Effect of an additional peptide extension of the N-terminus of collagen from dermatosparactic calves on the crosslinking of the collagen fibers. *Eur J Biochem* 34:91, 1973

250. HEGREBERG GA, PADGETT GA, GORHAM JR, HENSON JB: A connective tissue disease of dogs and mink resembling the Ehlers-Danlos syndrome of man. II. Mode of inheritance. *J Hered* 60:249, 1969

251. HEGREBERG GA, PADGETT GA, HENSON JB: Connective tissue disease of dogs and mink resembling Ehlers-Danlos syndrome of man. III. Histopathologic changes of the skin. *Arch Pathol* 90:159, 1970

252. HEGREBERG GA, PADGETT GA, OTT RL, HENSON JB: A heritable connective tissue disease in dogs and mink resembling Ehlers-Danlos syndrome of man. I. Skin tensile strength properties. *J Invest Dermatol* 54:377, 1970

253. GETHING MA: Suspected Ehlers-Danlos syndrome in the dog. *Vet Rec* 89:638, 1971

254. COUNTS DF, KNIGHTEN P, HEGREBERG G: Biochemical changes in the skin of mink with Ehlers-Danlos syndrome: Increased collagen biosynthesis in the dermis of affected mink. *J Invest Dermatol* 69:521, 1977

255. COUNTS DF: Isolation of collagen from the skins of Ehlers-Danlos syndrome-affected dogs by acetic acid extraction and pepsin digestion. *Biochim Biophys Acta* 626:208, 1980

256. BEIGHTON P (ed): *The Ehlers-Danlos Syndrome.* London, William Heinemann Medical Books Ltd, 1970

257. McKUSICK VA (ed): *Heritable Disorders of Connective Tissue,* ed 4. St. Louis, CV Mosby Co, 1972

258. BARABAS AP: Ehlers-Danlos syndrome: Associated with prematurity and premature rupture of foetal membranes: Possible increase in incidence. *Br Med J* 2:682 1966

259. DAY HJ, ZARAFONETIS CJD: Coagulation studies in four patients with Ehlers-Danlos syndrome. *Am J Med Sci* 86:565, 1961

260. FANTL P, MORRIS KN, SAWERS RJ: Repair of cardiac defect in patient with Ehlers-Danlos syndrome and deficiency of Hageman factor. *Br Med J* 1:1202, 1961

261. ESTES JW: Platelet abnormalities in heritable disorders of connective tissue. *Ann NY Acad Sci* 201:445, 1972

262. ONEL D, ULUTIN SB, ULUTIN ON: Platelet defect in a case of Ehlers-Danlos syndrome. *Acta Haematol* 50:238, 1973

263. KARACA M, CRONBERG L, NILSSON IM: Abnormal platelet-collagen reaction in Ehlers-Danlos syndrome. *Scand J Haematol* 9:465, 1972

264. DELIYANNIS AA, KONTOPOULOU-GRIVA I, TSEVRENIS HV: Normal platelet aggregating properties of Ehlers-Danlos syndrome "collagen". *Thromb Diath Haemorrh* 32:203, 1974

265. ARNESON MA, HAMMERSCHMIDT DE, FURCHT LT, KING RA: A new form of Ehlers-Danlos syndrome. Fibronectin corrects defective platelet function. *JAMA* 244:144, 1980

266. BEIGHTON P, HORAN F: Orthopaedic aspects of the Ehlers-Danlos syndrome. *J Bone Joint Surg* 51B:444, 1969

267. GORLIN RJ, PINDBORG JJ (eds): *Syndromes of the Head and the Neck.* New York, McGraw-Hill Book Co, 1964, p 96

268. BRUNO MS, NARASIMHAN P: The Ehlers-Danlos syndrome: A report of four cases in two generations of a Negro family. *N Engl J Med* 264:274, 1961

269. PEMBERTON JW, FREEMAN HM, SCHEPENS CL: Familial retinal detachment and the Ehlers-Danlos syndrome. *Arch Ophthalmol* 76:817, 1966

270. MOESTRUP B: Tenuity of cornea with Ehlers-Danlos syndrome. *Acta Ophthalmol* 47:704, 1969

271. HYAMS SW, DAR H, NEUMANN E: Blue sclerae and keratoglobus. *Br J Ophthalmol* 53:53, 1969

272. FUXA G, BRANDT HP: Beitrag zum Ehlers-Danlos syndrom. *Klin Monatsbl Augenheilkd* 166:247, 1975

273. ROBERTSON I: Keratoconus and the Ehlers-Danlos syndrome: A new aspect of Keratoconus. *Med J Aust* 1:571, 1975

274. JUDISCH GF, WAZIRI M, KRACHMER JH: Ocular Ehlers-Danlos syndrome with normal lysyl hydroxylase activity. *Arch Ophthalmol* 94:1489, 1976

275. BARD LA: Genetic counseling of families with Marfan syndrome and other disorders showing a marfanoid body habitus. *Ophthalmology* 86:1764, 1979

276. BEIGHTON P: Lethal complications of the Ehlers-Danlos syndrome. *Br Med J* 3:656, 1968

277. DALES HC, O'NEILL JJ: Management of arterial complications in a case of the arterial type of Ehlers-Danlos syndrome. *Br J Surg* 57:476, 1970

278. BARABAS AP: Vascular complications in the Ehlers-Danlos syndrome. *J Cardiovasc Surg* 12:160, 1972

279. BEIGHTON P, THOMAS ML: The radiology of the Ehlers-Danlos syndrome. *Clin Radiol* 20:354, 1969

280. LEIER CV, CALL TD, FULKERSON PK, WOOLEY CF: The spectrum of cardiac defects in the Ehlers-Danlos syndrome, types I and III. *Ann Intern Med* 92:171, 1980

281. ANTANI J, SRINIVAS HV: Ehlers-Danlos syndrome and cardiovascular abnormalities. *Chest* 63:214, 1973

282. SIMON AP, STEIN PD: Aortic insufficiency in Ehlers-Danlos syndrome. *Angiologia* 25:290, 1974

283. BEIGHTON P: Cardiac abnormalities in the Ehlers-Danlos syndrome. *Br Heart J* 31:227, 1969

284. BEIGHTON P, MURDOCH JL, VOTTELER T: Gastrointestinal complications of the Ehlers-Danlos syndrome. *Gut* 10:1004, 1969

285. BEIGHTON P: Obstetric aspect of the Ehlers-Danlos syndrome. *J Obstet Gynaecol Br Commonw* 76:97, 1969

286. DI FERRANTE N, LEACHMAN RD, ANGELINI P, DONNELLY PV, FRANCIS G, ALMAZAN A: Lysyl oxidase deficiency in Ehlers-Danlos syndrome type V. *Connect Tissue Res* 33:49, 1975

287. SIEGEL RC, BLACK CM, BAILEY AJ: Cross-linking of collagen in the X-linked Ehlers-Danlos type V. *Biochem Biophys Res Commun* 88:281, 1979

288. STEWART RE, HOLLISTER DW, RIMOIN DL: A new variant of Ehlers-Danlos syndrome: An autosomal dominant disorder of fragile skin, abnormal scarring, and generalized periodontitis. *Birth Defects* 13:85, 1977

289. HERNANDEZ A, AGUIRRE-NEGRETE MG, RAMIREZ-SOLTERO S, GONZALES-MENDOZA A, MARTINEZ Y MARTINEZ R, VELAZQUEZ CABRERA A, CANTU JM: A distinct variant of the Ehlers-Danlos syndrome. *Clin Genet* 16:335, 1979

290. BEASLEY RP, COHEN MM JR: A new presumably autosomal recessive form of the Ehlers-Danlos syndrome. *Clin Genet* 16:19, 1979

291. SULICA VI, COOPER PH, POPE M, HAMBRICK GW JR, GERSON BM, McKUSICK VA: Cutaneous histological features in Ehlers-Danlos syndrome. *Arch Dermatol* 115:40, 1979

292. VOGEL A, HOLBROOK KA, STEINMANN B, GITZELMANN R, BYERS PH: Abnormal collagen fibril structure in the gravis form (type I) of Ehlers-Danlos syndrome. *Lab Invest* 40:201, 1979

293. SEVENICH M, SCHULTZ-EHRENBURG U, ORFANOS CE: Ehlers-Danlos Syndrom: Eine fibroblasten- und kollangenkrankheit. Typisierung und elektronenmorskopische befunde bei funf kranken. *Arch Dermatol Res* 267:237, 1980

294. VOLPIN D, PASQUALI-RONCHETTI I, CASTELLANI I, GIRO MG, PESERICO A, MORI G: Ultrastructural and biochemical studies on a case of elastosis perforans serpiginosa. *Dermatologica* 156:209, 1978

295. BLACK CM, GATHERCOLE LJ, BAILEY AJ, BEIGHTON P: The Ehlers-Danlos syndrome: An analysis of the structure of the collagen fibres of the skin. *Br J Dermatol* 102:85, 1980

296. BYERS PH, HOLBROOK KA, McGILLIVRAY BA, MacLEOD PM, LOWRY RR: Clinical and ultrastructural heterogeneity of type IV Ehlers-Danlos syndrome. *Hum Genet* 47:141, 1979

297. STEINMANN B, GITZELMANN R, VOGEL A, GRANT ME, HARWOOD R, SEAR CHJ: Ehlers-Danlos syndrome in two siblings with deficient lysyl hydrox-

ylase activity in cultured skin fibroblasts but only mild hydroxylysine deficit in skin. *Helv Paediatr Acta* 30:255, 1975

298. KRANE SM, PINNELL SR, ERBE RW: Lysyl-protocollagen hydroxylase deficiency in fibroblasts from siblings with hydroxylysine-deficient collagen. *Proc Natl Acad Sci USA* 69:2899, 1972

299. MILLER RL, ELSAS LJ III, PRIEST RE: Ascorbate action on normal and mutant human lysyl hydroxylases from cultured dermal fibroblasts. *J Invest Dermatol* 72:241, 1979

300. QUINN RS, KRANE SM: Abnormal properties of collagen lysyl hydroxylase from skin fibroblasts of siblings with hydroxylysine-deficient collagen. *J Clin Invest* 57:83, 1976

301. ELSAS LJ, MILLER RL, PINNELL SR: Inherited human collagen lysyl hydroxylase deficiency—ascorbic acid response. *J Pediatr* 92:378, 1978

302. EYRE DR, GLIMCHER MJ: Reducible cross-links in hydroxylysine-deficient collagens of a heritable disorder of connective tissue. *Proc Natl Acad Sci USA* 69:2594, 1972

303. IHME A, KRIEG T, RISTELI J, RISTELI R, GLANVILLE J, RAUTERBERG PK, MÜLLER MPI: Heterogeneity of ED type VI. *J Invest Dermatol* 75:455, 1980

304. PINNELL SR: Abnormal collagens in connective tissue diseases. *Birth Defects* 11:23, 1975

305. HANAUSKE-ABEL HM, ROHM KH: The collagenous part of Clq is unaffected in the hydroxylysine-deficient collagen disease. *FEBS Lett* 110:73, 1980

306. STEINMANN B, TUDERMAN L, PELTONEN L, MARTIN GR, McKUSICK VA, PROCKOP DJ: Evidence for a structural mutation of procollagen type I in a patient with the Ehlers-Danlos syndrome type VII. *J Biol Chem* 255:8887, 1980

307. BYERS PH, SIEGEL RC, HOLBROOK KA, NARAYANAN AS, BORNSTEIN P, HALL JC: X-Linked cutis laxa: Defective cross-link formation in collagen due to decreased lysyl oxidase activity. *N Engl J Med* 303:61, 1980

308. POPE FM, MARTIN GR, LICHTENSTEIN JR, PENTTINEN R, GERSON B, ROWE DW, McKUSICK VA: Patients with Ehlers-Danlos syndrome type IV lack type III collagen. *Proc Natl Acad Sci USA* 72:1314, 1975

309. CLARK JG, KUHN C III, UITTO J: Lung collagen in type IV Ehlers-Danlos syndrome: Ultrastructural and biochemical studies. *Am Rev Respir Dis* 122:971, 1980

310. GAY S, MARTIN GR, MULLER PK, TIMPL R, KUHN K: Simultaneous synthesis of types I and III collagen by fibroblasts in culture. *Proc Natl Acad Sci USA* 73:4037, 1976

311. POPE FM, MARTIN GR, McKUSICK VA: Inheritance of Ehlers-Danlos type IV syndrome *J Med Genet* 14:200, 1977

312. AUMAILLEY M, KRIEG T, DESSAU W, MULLER PK, TIMPL R, BRICAUD H: Biochemical and immunological studies of fibroblasts derived from a patient with Ehlers-Danlos syndrome type IV. Demonstrate reduced type III collagen synthesis. *Arch Dermatol Res* 269:169, 1980

313. WAGSTAFF LA, FIRTH JC, LEVIN SE: Vascular abnormalities in congenital generalized elastolysis (cutis laxa): Report of a case. *S Afr Med J* 44:1125, 1970

314. MEINE F, GROSSMAN H, FORMAN W, JACKSON D: Radiographic findings in congenital cutis laxa. *Radiology* 113:687, 1974

315. HAJJAR BA, JOYNER EN III: Congenital cutis laxa with advanced cardiopulmonary disease. *J Pediatr* 73:116, 1968

316. MERTEN DF, ROONEY R: Progressive pulmonary emphysema associated with congenital generalized elastolysis (cutis laxa). *Radiology* 113:691, 1974

317. PHILIP ACS: Cutis laxa with intrauterine growth retardation and hip dislocation in a male. *J Pediatr* 93:150, 1978

318. REISNER SH, SEELENFREUND M, BEN-BASSAT M: Case report. Cutis laxa associated with severe intrauterine growth retardation and congenital dislocation of the hip. *Acta Paediatr Scand* 60:357, 1971

319. BEIGHTON P: The dominant and recessive forms of cutis laxa. *J Med Genet* 9:216, 1972

320. MEHREGAN AH, LEE SC, NABAI H: Cutis laxa (generalized elastolysis), a report of four cases with autopsy findings. *J Cutan Pathol* 5:116, 1978

321. AGHA A, SAKATI NO, HIGGINBOTTOM MC, JONES KL, BAY C, NYHAN WL: Two forms of cutis laxa presenting in the newborn period. *Acta Paediatr Scand* 67:775, 1978

322. BYERS PH, NARAYANAN AS, BORNSTEIN P, HALL JG: An X-linked form of cutis laxa due to deficiency of lysyl oxidase. *Birth Defects* 12:293, 1976

323. REED WB, HOROWITZ RE, BEIGHTON P: Acquired cutis laxa: Primary generalized elastolysis. *Arch Dermatol* 103:661, 1971

324. NANKO H, JEPSEN LV, ZACHARIAE H, SØGAARD H: Acquired cutis laxa (generalized elastolysis): Light and electron microscopic studies. *Acta Derm (Stockh)* 59:315, 1979

325. GOLTZ RH, HULT AM, GOLDFARB M, GORLIN RJ: Cutis laxa: A manifestation of generalized elastolysis. *Arch Dermatol* 92:373, 1965

326. HASHIMOTO K, KANZAKI T: Cutis laxa. Ultrastructural and biochemical studies. *Arch Dermatol* 111:861, 1975

327. MARCHASE P, HOLBROOK K, PINNELL SR: A familial cutis laxa syndrome with ultrastructural abnormalities of collagen and elastin. *J Invest Dermatol* 75:399, 1980

328. LINDBERG KA, PINNELL SR: Unpublished results

329. SILLENCE DO, SENN A, DANKS DM: Genetic heterogeneity in osteogenesis imperfecta. *J Med Genet* 16:101, 1979

330. SILLENCE DO, RIMOIN DL, DANKS DM: Clinical variability in osteogenesis imperfecta—Variable expressivity or genetic heterogeneity. *Birth Defects* 15:113, 1979

331. KREPLER R, ZHUBER K: Hyperplastische kallusbildung bei osteogenesis imperfecta. *Z Orthop* 112:306, 1974

332. SCOTT D, STIRIS G: Osteogenesis imperfecta tarda: A study of 3 families with special reference to scar formation. *Acta Med Scand* 145:237, 1953

333. BERGSTROM L: Osteogenesis imperfecta: Otologic and maxillofacial aspects. *Laryngoscope* 87(suppl 6):1, 1977

334. HATHAWAY WE, SOLOMONS CC, OTT JE: Platelet function and pyrophosphates in osteogenesis imperfecta. *Blood* 39:500, 1972

335. RUSHTON MA: The structure of the teeth in a late case of osteogenesis imperfecta. *J Pathol Bacteriol* 48:591, 1939

336. RUEDEMANN AD JR: Osteogenesis imperfecta congenita and blue scleotics. A. Clinicopathologic study. *Arch Ophthalmol N S* 49:6, 1953

337. CAREY MC, FITZGERALD O, McKIERNAN E: Osteogenesis imperfecta in twenty-three members of a kindred with heritable features contributed by a non-specific skeletal disorder. *Q J Med* 37:437, 1968

338. HEPPNER RI, BABITT HI, BIACHINE JW, WARBASSE JR: Aortic regurgitation and aneurysm of sinus of valsalva associated with osteogenesis imperfecta. *Am J Cardiol* 31:654, 1973

339. WEISINGER B, GLASSMAN E, SPENCER FC, BERGER A: Successful aortic valve replacement for aortic regurgitation associated with osteogenesis imperfecta. *Br Heart J* 37:475, 1975

340. WOOD SJ, THOMAS J, BRAIMBRIDGE MW: Mitral valve disease and open heart surgery in osteogenesis imperfecta tarda. *Br Heart J* 35:103, 1973

341. CRISCITIELLO MG, RONAN JA Jr, BESTERMAN EMM, SCHOENWETTER W: Cardiovascular abnormalities in osteogensis imperfecta. *Circulation* 31:255, 1965

342. FALVO KA, KLAIN DB, KRAUSS AN, ROOT L, AULD PAM: Pulmonary function studies in osteogenesis imperfecta. *Am Rev Respir Dis* 108:1258, 1973

343. CROPP GJA, MYERS DN: Physiological evidence of hypermetabolism in osteogenesis imperfecta. *Pediatrics* 49:375, 1972

344. ROBERTS JM, SOLOMONS CC: Management of pregnancy in osteogenesis imperfecta: New perspectives. *Obstet Gynecol* 45:168, 1975

345. QUISLING RW, MOORE GE, JAHRSDOERFER RA, CANTRELL RW: Osteogenesis imperfecta. *Arch Otolaryngol* 105:207, 1979

346. FALVO KA, BULLOUGH PG: Osteogenesis imperfecta: A histometric analysis. *J Bone Joint Surg* 55A:275, 1973

347. RILEY GC, JOWSEY J: Osteogenesis imperfecta: Morphologic and biochemical studies of connective tissue. *Pediatr Res* 9:757, 1973

348. ENGFELDT B, ENGSTROM A, ZETTERSTROM R: Biophysical studies of the bone tissue in osteogenesis imperfecta. *J Bone Joint Surg* 36B:654, 1954

349. DOTY SB, MATHEWS RS: Electron microscopic and histochemical investigation of osteogenesis imperfecta tarda. *Clin Orthop* 80:191, 1971

350. ALBRIGHT JP, ALBRIGHT JA, CRELIN ES: Osteogenesis imperfecta tarda. *Clin Orthop* 108:204, 1975

351. TEITELBAUM SL, KRAFT WJ, LANG R, AVIOLI LV: Bone collagen aggregation abnormalities in osteogensis imperfecta. *Calcif Tissue Res* 17:75, 1974

352. FOLLIS RH JR: Maldevelopment of the corium in the osteogenesis imperfecta syndrome. *Bull Johns Hopkins Hosp* 93:225, 1953

353. FURNESS ET, WHITE TA: A case of osteogenesis imperfecta, diagnosed in utero. *Med J Aust* 1:390, 1973

354. LANCASTER G, GOLDMAN H, SCRIVER CR, GOLD RJM, WONG I: Dominantly inherited osteogensis imperfecta in man: An examination of collagen biosynthesis. *Pediatr Res* 9:83, 1975

355. LEVIN LS, BRADY JM, MELNICK M: Scanning electron microscopy of teeth in dominant osteogenesis imperfecta: Support for genetic heterogeneity. *Am J Med Genet* 5:189, 1980

356. PENTTINEN RP, LICHTENSTEIN JR, MARTIN GR, McKUSICK VA: Abnormal collagen metabolism in cultured cells in osteogenesis imperfecta. *Proc Natl Acad Sci USA* 72:586, 1975

357. POPE FM, NICHOLLS AC, EGGLETON C, NARCISSI P, HEY EN, PARKIN JM: Osteogenesis imperfecta (lethal) bones contain types III and V collagens. *J Clin Pathol* 33:534, 1980

358. TRELSTAD RL, RUBIN D, GROSS J: Osteogenesis imperfecta congenita. Evidence for a generalized molecular disorder of collagen. *Lab Invest* 36:501, 1977

359. BLECKMANN H, KRESSE H, WOLLENSAK J, BUDDECKE E: Glykosaminoglykan- und kollagenanalysen bei osteogenesis imperfecta. *Z Kinderheilkd* 110:74, 1971

360. EASTOE JE, MARTENS P, THOMAS NR: The amino-acid composition of human hard tissue collagens in osteogenesis imperfecta and dentinogenesis imperfecta. *Calcif Tissue Res* 12:91, 1973

361. PELTONEN L, PALOTIE A, PROCKOP DJ: A defect in the structure of type I procollagen in a patient who had osteogenesis imperfecta: Excess mannose

in the COOH-terminal propeptide. *Proc Natl Acad Sci USA* 77:6178, 1980

362. NICHOLLS AC, POPE FM, SCHLOON H: Biochemical heterogeneity of osteogenesis imperfecta: New variant. *Lancet* 1:1193, 1979

363. MEIGEL WN, MULLER PK, PONTZ BF, SORENSEN N, SPRANGER J: A constitutional disorder of connective tissue suggesting a defect in collagen biosynthesis. *Klin Wochenschr* 52:906, 1974

364. MULLER PK, LEMMEN C, GAY S, MEIGEL WN: Disturbance in the regulation of the type of collagen synthesized in a form of osteogenesis imperfecta. *J Biochem* 59:97, 1975

365. KRIEG T, KIRSCH E, MATZEN K, MULLER PK: Osteogenesis imperfecta: Biochemical and clinical evaluation of 13 cases. *Klin Wochenschr* 59:91, 1981

366. MATZEN K, MULLER PK, KRIEG T: Osteogenesis imperfecta: Biochemische charakterisierung verschiedener Gruppen. *Z Orthop* 116:585, 1978

367. TURAKAINEN H, LARJAVA H, SAARNI H, PENTTINEN R: Synthesis of hyaluronic acid and collagen in skin fibroblasts cultured from patients with osteogenesis imperfecta. *Biochim Biophys Acta* 628:388, 1980

368. SYKES B, FRANCIS MJO, SMITH R: Altered relation of two collagen types in osteogenesis imperfecta. *N Engl J Med* 296:1200, 1977

369. MULLER PK, RAISCH K, MATZEN K, GAY S: Presence of type III collagen in bone from a patient with oteogenesis imperfecta. *Eur J Pediatr* 125:29, 1977

370. SAUK JJ, GAY R, MILLER EJ, GAY S: Immunohistochemical localization of type III collagen in the dentin of patients with osteogenesis imperfecta and hereditary opalescent dentin. *J Oral Pathol* 9:210, 1980

371. FUJII K, KAJIWARA T, KUROSU H: Osteogenesis imperfecta: Altered content of type III collagen and proportion of the crosslinks in skin. *FEBS Lett* 82:251, 1977

372. FUJII K, TANZER ML: Osteogenesis imperfecta: Biochemical studies of bone collagen. *Clin Orthop* 124:271, 1977

373. STEVENSON CJ, BOTTOMS E, SHUSTER S: Skin collagen in osteogenesis imperfecta. *Lancet* 1:860, 1970

374. PYERITZ RE, MCKUSICK VA: Current concepts: The Marfan syndrome. *N Engl J Med* 300:772, 1979

375. MURDOCH JL, WALKER BA, HALPERN BL, KUZMA JW, MCKUSICK VA: Life expectancy and causes of death in the Marfan syndrome. *N Engl J Med* 286:804, 1972

376. WALKER BA, BEIGHTON PH, MURDOCH JL: The marfanoid hypermobility syndrome. *Ann Intern Med* 71:349, 1969

377. BEALS RK, HECHT F: Congenital contractural arachnodactyly: A heritable disorder of connective tissue. *J Bone Joint Surg* 53A:987, 1971

378. BRENTON DP, DOW CJ, JAMES JIP, HAY RL, WYNNE-DAVIES R: Homocystinuria and Marfan's syndrome. A comparison. *J Bone Joint Surg* 54B:277, 1972

379. GORLIN RJ, MIRKIN BL: Multiple mucosal neuromas, phenochromocytoma, medullary carcinoma of the thyroid and marfanoid body build with muscle wasting. *Z Kinderheilk* 113:313, 1972

380. PYERITZ RE, MURPHY EA, MCKUSICK VA: Clinical variability in the Marfan syndrome(s). *Birth Defects* 15:155, 1979

381. MURDOCH JL, WALKER BA, MCKUSICK VA: Parental age effects on the occurrence of new mutations for the Marfan syndrome. *Ann Hum Genet (Lond)* 35:331, 1972

382. BOLANDE RP: The nature of the connective tissue abiotrophy in the Marfan syndrome. *Lab Invest* 12:1987, 1963

383. SAYERS CP, GOLTZ RW, MOTTAZ J: Pulmonary elastic tissue in generalized elastolysis (cutis laxa) and Marfan's syndrome. A light and electron microscopic study. *J Invest Dermatol* 65:451, 1975

384. KRIEG T, MULLER PK: The Marfan syndrome: 'In vitro' study of collagen metabolism in tissue specimens of the aorta. *Exp Cell Biol* 45:207, 1977

385. HALBRITTER R, AUMAILLEY M, RACKWITZ R, KRIEG T, MULLER PK: Case report and study of collagen metabolism in Marfan's syndrome. *Klin Wochenschr* 59:83, 1981

386. SCHECK M, SIEGEL RC, PARKER J, CHANG Y-H, FU JCC: Aortic aneurysm in Marfan's syndrome; changes in the ultrastructure and composition of collagen. *J Anat* 129:654, 1979

387. LAMBERG SI: Stimulatory effect of exogenous hyaluronic acid distinguishes cultured fibroblasts of Marfan's disease from controls. *J Invest Dermatol* 71:391, 1978

388. APPEL A, HORWITZ AL, DORFMAN A: Cell-free synthesis of hyaluronic acid in Marfan syndrome. *J Biol Chem* 254:12199, 1979

389. KANG AH, TRELSTAD RL: A collagen defect in homocystinuria. *J Clin Invest* 52:2571, 1973

390. MILCH RA: Biochemical studies on the pathogenesis of collagen tissue changes in alcaptonuria. *Clin Orthop* 24:213, 1962

391. MILCH RA, TITUS ED, LOO TL: Atmospheric oxidation of homogentisic acid: Spectrophotometric studies. *Science* 126:209, 1957

392. ZANNONI VG, MALAWISTA SE, LA DU BN: Studies on ochronosis. II. Studies on benzoquinone-acetic acid, a probable intermediate in the connective tissue pigmentation of alcaptonuria. *Arthritis Rheum* 5:547, 1962

393. MURRAY JC, LINDBERG KA, PINNELL SR: *In vitro* inhibition of chick embryo lysyl hydroxylase by homogentisic acid. *J Clin Invest* 59:1071, 1977

394. BRIGGAMAN RA: The epidermal dermal junction and genetic disorders of this area, in Goldsmith LA (ed): *Biochemistry and Biophysiology of the Skin.* New York, Oxford University Press, 1982, in press

395. MARSDEN RA: Epidermolysis bullosa of the oesophagus with oesophageal web formation. *Thorax* 29:287, 1974

396. ORLANDO RC, BOZYMSKI EM, BRIGGAMAN RA, BREAM CA: Epidermolysis bullosa: Gastrointestinal manifestations. *Ann Intern Med* 81:203, 1974

397. WESCHSLER HL, KRUGH FJ, DOMONKOS AN, SCHEEN R, DAVIDSON CL: Polydysplastic epidermolysis bullosa and development of epidermal neoplasma. *Arch Dermatol* 102:374, 1970

398. REED WB, COLLEGE J JR, FRANCIS MJO, ZACHARIAE H, MOHS F, SHER MA, SNEDDON IB: Epidermolysis bullosa dystrophica with epidermal neoplasms. *Arch Dermatol* 110:894, 1974

399. PEARSON RW: Studies on the pathogenesis of epidermolysis bullosa. *J Invest Dermatol* 39:551, 1962

400. BRIGGAMAN RA, WHEELER CE JR: Epidermolysis bullosa dystrophica-recessive: A possible role of anchoring fibrils in the pathogenesis. *J Invest Dermatol* 65:203, 1975

401. BRIGGAMAN RA, DALLDORF FG, WHEELER CE: Formation and origin of basal lamina and anchoring fibrils in adult human skin. *J Cell Biol* 51:384, 1971

402. EISEN AZ: Human skin collagenase: Relationship to the pathogenesis of epidermolysis bullosa dystrophica. *J Invest Dermatol* 52:449, 1969

403. LAZARUS GS: Collagenase and connective tissue metabolism in epidermolysis bullosa. *J Invest Dermatol* 58:242, 1972

404. BAUER EA, EISEN AZ: Recessive dystrophic epidermolysis bullosa: Evidence for increased collagenase as a genetic characteristic in cell culture. *J Exp Med* 148:1378, 1978

405. VALLE K-J, BAUER EA: Enhanced biosynthesis of human skin collagenase in fibroblast cultures from recessive dystrophic epidermolysis bullosa. *J Clin Invest* 66:176, 1980

406. BAUER EA: Recessive dystrophic epidermolysis bullosa: Evidence for an altered collagenase in fibroblast cultures. *Proc Natl Acad Sci USA* 74:4646, 1977

407. BAUER EA, COOPER TW, TUCKER DR, ESTERLY NB: Phenytoin therapy of recessive dystrophic epidermolysis bullosa. Clinical trial and proposed mechanism of action on collagenase. *N Engl J Med* 303:776, 1980

408. SAVOLAINEN E-R, KERO M, PIHLAJANIEMI T, KIVIRIKKO KI: Deficiency of galactosylhydroxylysyl glucosyltransferase, an enzyme of collagen synthesis, in a family with dominant epidermolysis bullosa simplex. *N Engl J Med* 304:197, 1981

64

α_1-ANTITRYPSIN DEFICIENCY

JAMES E. GADEK

RONALD G. CRYSTAL

1. α_1-Antitrypsin, the principal serum protease inhibitor, is a single polypeptide glycoprotein with a molecular weight of 52,000. It is produced in the hepatocyte and secreted at a rate that maintains serum concentrations of 150 to 200 mg/dl. This macromolecule demonstrates a remarkable degree of genetic heterogeneity; at least 33 variants have been identified by isoelectric focusing. These variants form the basis for the Pi system of α_1-antitrypsin phenotypes. A single autosomal allele is inherited from each parent, and the phenotype is expressed in an autosomal codominant pattern. The clinical relevance of this genetic diversity is seen in certain phenotypes in which a profound serum deficiency of α_1-antitrypsin is associated with the development of emphysema in the fourth to fifth decades of life and, less frequently, with liver disease in children and adults.

2. The most common form of α_1-antitrypsin is type M; approximately 95 percent of the U.S. population is PiMM. The best studied α_1-antitrypsin variant is type Z, which is estimated to affect 1 in 2000 U.S. Caucasians. Whereas PiMM individuals have serum α_1-antitrypsin levels of 150 to 250 mg/dl, those with PiZZ have α_1-antitrypsin levels that are 10 to 15 percent of normal. This profound serum deficiency results from a substitution of a lysine for a glutamic acid residue at position 53 from the C terminus of the molecule. This single amino acid substitution significantly affects release of α_1-antitrypsin from the hepatocyte, resulting in the markedly decreased serum levels seen in the PiZZ homozygote.

3. The pathogenesis of the emphysema associated with the PiZZ state is related to the fact that α_1-antitrypsin is the major inhibitor of neutrophil elastase in the human lower respiratory tract. In experimental animals, instillation of this protease produces a lesion closely resembling emphysema in humans. In the case of serum α_1-antitrypsin deficiency, individuals have little α_1-antitrypsin in their alveolar structures, thus rendering them vulnerable to progressive destruction by neutrophil elastase. In this context, bronchoalveolar lavage studies demonstrate that PiZZ individuals with emphysema have free neutrophil elastase and little α_1-antitrypsin in their alveolar structures, thus supporting this "elastase-antielastase" theory of emphysema in α_1-antitrypsin deficiency. The pathogenesis of the liver disease associated with α_1-antitrypsin deficiency remains unclear, except that development of hepatitis and cirrhosis occurs only in association with the sequestration of large quantities of α_1-antitrypsin in the hepatocyte.

4. It is logical to predict that the specific therapy of α_1-antitrypsin-deficient lung disease will depend on the successful augmentation of α_1-antitrypsin levels in serum and lung. One therapeutic approach involves the use of the anabolic steroid danazol. Administration of

this drug results in modest (50 percent above baseline) increases in endogenous serum α₁-antitrypsin. More promising is the use of parenteral α₁-antitrypsin replacement therapy to reestablish the balance between protease and antiprotease within the α₁-antitrypsin-deficient lung. Pilot studies using this approach have shown that weekly infusions of 4 g of α₁-antitrypsin result in maintenance of serum and lung α₁-antitrypsin levels thought to be sufficient to protect against attack by neutrophil elastase.

α₁-Antitrypsin is a glycoprotein that accounts for 90 percent of the α₁ globulins of human serum. Its major physiologic role is that of an antiprotease, a molecule that combines with proteolytic enzymes to render them inactive [1–5]. While α₁-antitrypsin inhibits a variety of proteases, including trypsin, thrombin, chymotrypsin, and plasmin, its most specific function is to inhibit neutrophil elastase, a broad-spectrum protease capable of degrading most structural proteins comprising the extracellular matrix of tissues [6–10].

The clinical importance of α₁-antitrypsin was recognized in 1963 by Laurell and Eriksson, who observed that individuals with markedly deficient serum levels of α₁-antitrypsin also had emphysema [11, 12]. It soon became apparent that this deficiency in serum α₁-antitrypsin was inherited as an autosomal recessive trait and that the responsible genetic locus was extremely polymorphic [13, 14]. In the context of the physiologic role of α₁-antitrypsin, the result of a reduction in serum α₁-antitrypsin is that the serum of individuals has very little antielastase activity [15]. While this seems to have minor significance for most organs, it has dire consequences for the lung, an organ that, if insufficiently protected, is particularly vulnerable to elastolytic attack [16, 17]. The concept of the vulnerability of the lung to elastases was strengthened by studies demonstrating that proteases with elastolytic activity produce a lesion resembling human emphysema when instilled into the lungs of experimental animals [18–21].

Together, these clinical and experimental observations have led to what is commonly called the *protease-antiprotease theory* (or the *elastase-antielastase theory*) of destructive lung disease [16, 18, 21, 22]. This theory, for which there is overwhelming support, holds that the lung is constantly under a burden of elastase activity but under normal circumstances is adequately protected by an antielastase screen, supplied primarily by α₁-antitrypsin as it diffuses through the alveolar structures. When this balance is shifted in favor of elastase activity, such as occurs in humans who are deficient in α₁-antitrypsin or in animals when overwhelming amounts of elastase are instilled into the lower respiratory tract, the result is destruction of the lung parenchyma, i.e., emphysema [23, 24]. This theory goes far beyond explaining the pathogenesis of α₁-antitrypsin deficiency; it is also central to the current concepts of the pathogenesis of emphysema in the destructive lung disease resulting from cigarette smoking.

The progress of research in this field has been rapid. The structure, source, and function of α₁-antitrypsin and its variants have been defined. The likely cause of the reduction in serum levels of α₁-antitrypsin in this disease is understood, and the population genetics and epidemiology of α₁-antitrypsin deficiency have been evaluated worldwide. Besides destructive lung disease, it is now recognized that α₁-antitrypsin-deficient individuals, particularly children, have a high incidence of liver disease [2–5]. Furthermore, it has been demonstrated that the antielastase-elastase balance of the lower respiratory tract can be reestablished in α₁-antitrypsin-deficient individuals by intermittent parenteral administration of the deficient protein [24, 25].

STRUCTURE OF α₁-ANTITRYPSIN AND ITS VARIANTS

The α₁-antitrypsin molecule consists of a single polypeptide chain with a molecular weight of 47,000 to 52,000, 10 to 15 percent of which is composed of carbohydrate side chains. Many variants of α₁-antitrypsin are known. It is thought that most of this polymorphism results from single amino acid substitutions [2, 5, 26–29].

Classification of the α₁-Antitrypsin Variants: The Pi System

The variants of α₁-antitrypsin are classified by the Pi (protease inhibitor) system, which is based on the differences in charge among the different α₁-antitrypsin molecules. The most useful electrophoretic systems used to distinguish Pi variants are acid-starch gels (either alone or combined with crossed electrophoresis into agarose containing anti-α₁-antitrypsin antibody) and isoelectric focusing in polyacrylamide gels [26–29].

Acid-starch gels resolve purified α₁-antitrypsin obtained from a homozygote into five to eight bands, two of which are major and three to six are minor (Fig. 64-1A) [27]. The reasons for this heterogeneity in the homozygote are unknown. Current concepts suggest that it reflects heterogeneity of the carbohydrate side chains attached to identical polypeptide chains, i.e., there is only one structural gene for α₁-antitrypsin inherited from each parent [30].

The Pi nomenclature assigns a letter to the electrophoretic variants depending on the relative mobility of the major bands in acid-starch gels (Fig. 64-1A). These differences in mobility in acid-starch gels reflect the difference in isoelectric points of the variants resulting from their dissimilar primary sequences. Those variants that migrate close to the anode (i.e., those with a lower isoelectric point) are assigned the letters at the beginning of the alphabet. The normal or most common form of α₁-antitrypsin has an intermediate mobility in acid-starch gels and is designated the *M protein* [26].

Higher resolution of α₁-antitrypsin variants can be achieved with isoelectric focusing in polyacrylamide gels (Fig. 64-1B) [28, 29]. With this method, a total of 33 variants have been described, several of which cannot be distinguished with acid-starch gels. Thus isoelectric focusing is now the procedure of choice in evaluating α₁-antitrypsin phenotypes, [26, 28, 29]. Similar to the results obtained with acid-starch gels, isoelectric focusing of each variant demonstrates two major and two to six minor bands. The serum of the original patients described by Laurell and Eriksson contained the Z type of α₁-antitrypsin [11, 12]. By coincidence, this is the variant that moves most slowly toward the anode (i.e., it has the least net negative charge of all known variants).

Kindred studies have unequivocally shown that α₁-antitrypsin variants are inherited as codominant alleles, with both parental haplotypes expressed equally [31–33]. By convention

A. ACID STARCH GEL ELECTROPHORESIS

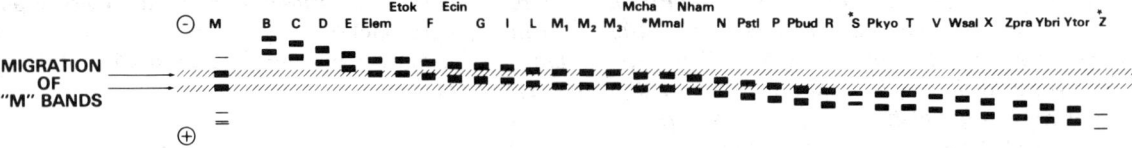

B. POLYACRYLAMIDE GEL ISOELECTRIC FOCUSING

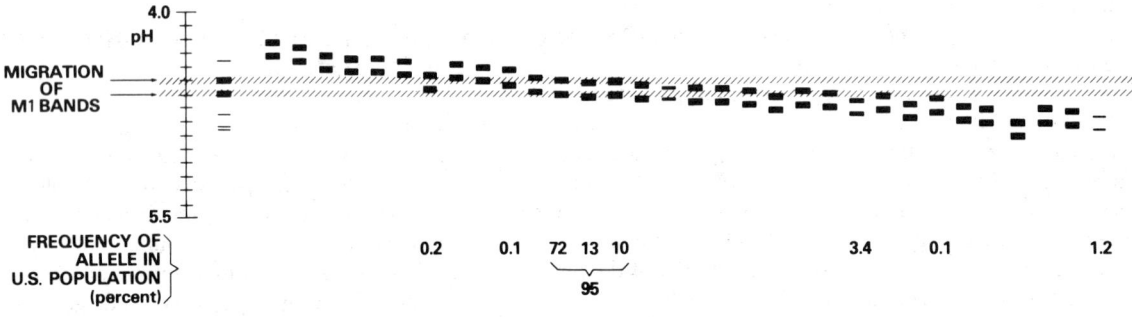

C. CLINICALLY IMPORTANT Pi PHENOTYPES

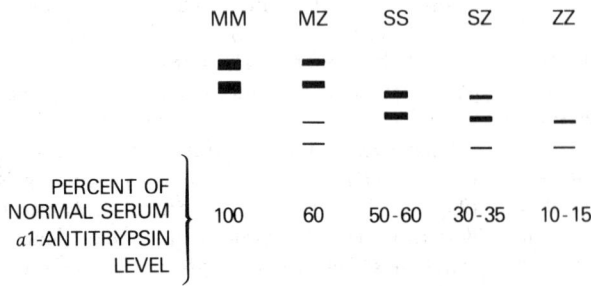

Figure 64-1 The phenotyping system of α₁-antitrypsin variants. *A.* Acid-starch gel electrophoresis. The relative mobility toward the anode (B through Z, respectively) of the known 33 α₁-antitrypsin variants is shown. Typically, two major and four minor bands are seen for each variant; this can be seen in the far left pattern labeled "M." For clarity, only the two major bands of the other variants are seen. This microheterogeneity seen with each variant is thought to result from differences in side chain oligosaccharides among a population of α₁-antitrypsin molecules with the same amino acid sequence. The *M* variant is the most common; for comparison, the electrophoretic mobility of the two major bands of the *M* variant are shown by crosshatching. Actually, the variant recognized as the *M* type on acid-starch gel electrophoresis is really a superimposition of three variants (M_1, M_2, M_3). Of these, M_1 is the most common. Those alleles associated with a significant reduction in serum α₁-antitrypsin concentration are indicated as * and include M_{mal}, *S*, and *Z. B.* Polyacrylamide isoelectric focusing. This technique provides greater reproducibility of phenotyping and permits identification of all 33 variants, including the M subtypes that cannot be distinguished by acid-starch gel electrophoresis. The frequency of the most common alleles is indicated [37]. All others have an allelic frequency of < 0.1 percent. *C.* Clinically important Pi phenotypes. Shown are the isoelectric focusing patterns of the major bands of Pi phenotypes associated with a marked reduction in serum α₁-antitrypsin concentration relative to the pattern obtained in individuals homozygous for the common M_1 protein (indicated as MM) [26].

the variant alleles are designated by superscript (e.g., Pi^M), and the phenotype expressed in serum is referred to by capital letters (e.g., PiM or M type) [26, 27]. In this nomenclature, heterozygous phenotypes are expressed as PiMZ or PiSZ. Rare individuals have been described with no detectable α₁-antitrypsin in their serum; they are designated Pi null (or Pi⁻⁻) [32]. A heterozygote for the null allele would be designated PiM⁻. The recognition of the existence of a null allele has added a level of complexity to the Pi system of classification, since it demands that a kindred analysis be carried out to exclude its presence from a serum sample that displays a single Pi variant. Thus, PiZ⁻ cannot be distinguished from PiZZ without study of the pattern of transmission of the PiZ allele within the family [26, 27]. In this context, if a kindred analysis is not available, the phenotype is designated as a single symbol (i.e., PiZ, rather than the presumed PiZZ) in recognition of the fact that the Pi^- allele cannot be excluded.

Population Genetics of the Pi Variants

The most common α₁-antitrypsin allele is the M type (Fig. 64-1) [33, 34]. In most populations Pi^M is found in greater than 85 percent. In Caucasians of northern European extraction it is present in at least 95 percent. In some populations the frequency is even higher. Non-Pi^M alleles are very rare (<1 percent) in black Africans, Asians, Finns, Lapps, Greenland eskimos, and Easter Island natives [35–40]. The single M pattern detected by acid-starch gels (Fig. 64-1A) is actually one of at least three different alleles: M1, M2, and M3 (Fig. 64-1B). Of these, M1 is the most frequent [34].

After the M type, the most common alleles are Pi^S, Pi^Z, and Pi^F [2–5]. Pi^S is most commonly found in the Iberian peninsula (11 to 12 percent) [35], rarely in northern Europe (<1 percent) [36], but more frequently in the United States (3 to 4 percent) [37]. Pi^Z is found with a frequency of 1 to 2 percent in Caucasians of northern European ancestry [36, 37]. The highest frequencies of Pi^Z are in Maoris in New Zealand (8.2 percent) [38] and in Iranians (2.2 percent) [39] and the lowest in black Africans (0 percent in studies from Mozambique and Zaire) [40]. Pi^F, an allele rarely found in the United States, is relatively frequent in Iranians [39], Hungarians, and Germans (6 to 9 percent). Some studies suggest that the PiM protein can give a PiF pattern if stored under unsuitable conditions [2]; thus, the frequency of PiF in various populations is still under investigation. A few alleles are prevalent in specific populations (Pi^X in 1.3 percent of Malaysians [41] and Pi^L in 3 percent of black Africans [40]), but most alleles other than M, S, Z, and F are very rare, representing far less than 1 percent of those tested [2–5]. The null allele has been described in only about 20 cases [26, 32].

As expected from the allelic distribution, the most common Pi phenotypes are MM, MZ, and MS (Fig. 64-1C) [2–5].

While it is clear that α₁-antitrypsin is expressed as an autosomal gene, the Pi locus has not been definitively established. Family studies suggest that it is linked to the Gm locus coding for the heavy chain of IgG, i.e., on human chromosome 6 [42], but evaluations of mouse-human hybrids have not confirmed this concept [43].

The importance of the α₁-trypsin variants is related to the association of some phenotypes with reduced serum levels of α₁-antitrypsin. In normal MM individuals, the concentration of α₁-antitrypsin in the serum is usually reported in the range of 180 to 240 mg/dl [2–5], but it has recently been recognized

that many of the reference standards used in the past have been impure. When purified material is used as a reference, the actual serum concentration is found to be in the 130 to 150 mg/dl range [44]. The α₁-antitrypsin alleles associated with reduced serum concentration of α₁-antitrypsin include Pi^Z, Pi^S, Pi^-, Pi^P and $Pi^{M\ duarte}$ (Pi^M-like and $Pi^{M\ malton}$ as well, but these alleles are probably identical to $Pi^{M\ duarte}$) [26]. If we consider the phenotype MM as associated with 100 percent of the normal serum levels, then the serum levels for the most common phenotypes associated with reduced serum levels are: SS (54 percent), ZZ (12 percent), MS (80 percent), and MZ (60 percent) [2, 5] (Fig. 64-1C). In addition, there have been reports of reduction of serum α₁-antitrypsin levels associated with the SZ (35 percent), MM duarte (55 percent), MP (80 percent), M⁻ (50 percent), and ⁻⁻ (0 percent) phenotypes [2–5, 26, 27]. Not enough of theses individuals have been studied to know whether these levels are typical for each phenotype. It is estimated from these allelic frequencies that 1 in 3000 to 1 in 4000 U.S. Caucasians are ZZ and 1 in 800 are SZ, consistent with approximately 50,000 Z homozygotes and 250,000 SZ heterozygotes [1–5, 26, 27, 37].

Structure of the M Protein Most of the structural knowledge of α₁-antitrypsin comes from study of the common M protein. The most frequently occurring amino acid residues are leucine, lysine, glutamic acid, and asparagine. The dominance of acidic residues gives the molecule an isoelectric point of 4.6 to 4.8 [46].

PiM α₁-antitrypsin has not been completely sequenced, but the sequences of several important fragments are known, including 33 N-terminal [47] and 152 C-terminal residues [48, 49] (Fig. 64-2A). In addition, the sequence of the active protease inhibitory site is known [50, 51] (Fig. 64-2B). α₁-Antitrypsin interacts with different proteases in slightly different ways, but it is generally agreed that it centers its interaction with human neutrophil elastase through a methionine residue [51, 52]. Evidently seven residues centered on this methionine are important for recognition and reaction of α₁-antitrypsin with elastase [52]. Although the sequence of the active site is known, its location in the molecule is unclear [50, 51]. Johnson et al. [51] and Kress et al. [53] have suggested that it is centered approximately 50 residues from the N terminus, while Carrell et al. [50] and Koide et al. [54] have evidence placing it 35 residues from the C terminus.

There is striking homology between the C-terminal sequence of α₁-antitrypsin and the C-terminal sequence of antithrombin III [50, 54], a human serum antiprotease that functions to inhibit thrombin. In addition, sequence similarities of both of these antiproteases to chicken ovalbumin suggest that there may be families of antiproteases derived from a common ancestral gene [55].

The oligosaccharide side chains of PiM α₁-antitrypsin are of the N-glycosidic type, contain N-acetylneuraminic acid (a common form of sialic acid at the terminal position), galactose, mannose, and N-acetylglucosamine, and are linked to the protein through asparaginyl residues [56, 57] (Fig. 64-2C). The oligosaccharides exist in two forms. The more complex A form contains two branch points, while the B form contains one. The A structure has features similar to those of thyroglobulin, and the B structure is identical to that in human transferrin. The number of oligosaccharide side chains present on each PiM polypeptide is not clear. Most workers believe that there are three or four, with B chains predominating [56, 57]. Importantly, analysis of the oligosaccharides of the PiM protein

A. PRIMARY STRUCTURE

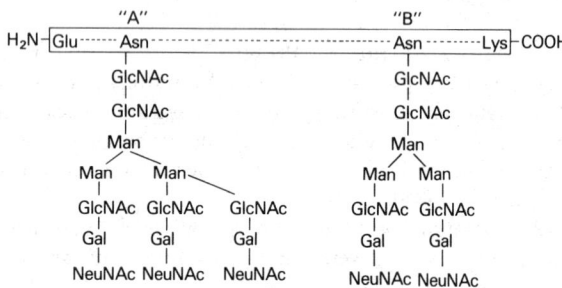

33 RESIDUES   ~300 RESIDUES   152 RESIDUES

B. ACTIVE (PROTEASE-COMBINING) SITE

Leu—Glu—Ala—Ile—Pro—Met—Ser/Thr—Ile—Pro—Pro—Glu—Val

P_6 P_5 P_4 P_3 P_2 P_1 P_1' P_2' P_3' P_4' P_5' P_6'

C. STRUCTURE OF OLIGOSACCHARIDE SIDE CHAINS

"A"   "B"

H₂N—Glu------Asn------------------------Asn--------Lys—COOH

| | |
GlcNAc   GlcNAc
GlcNAc   GlcNAc
Man   Man
Man Man   Man Man
GlcNAc GlcNAc GlcNAc   GlcNAc GlcNAc
Gal Gal Gal   Gal Gal
NeuNAc NeuNAc NeuNAc   NeuNAc NeuNAc

Figure 64-2 The structure of human α_1-antitrypsin. A. α_1-Antitrypsin consists of a single polypeptide chain to which three or four carbohydrate side chains (CHO) are attached through asparaginyl residues (the uncertainty regarding the fourth side chain is indicated by the broken circle). The amino acid sequence of 33 N-terminal residues and 152 C-terminal residues of the common M protein is known. The sequence of the intervening approximately 300 amino acids is uncertain. The abnormality of the Z protein is found at a position 53 residues from the C terminus, where a lysine is substituted for the glutamic acid found in the M protein. The S variant contains a valine substituted for the normal glutamic acid at a position 131 residues from the C terminus. B. The active (protease-combining) site of α_1-antitrypsin consists of a methionine at the center. The methionine binds to the protease. This critical methionine is flanked by small aliphatic amino acids (P_6 through P_2 and P_1' through P_6', respectively). The location of this active combining sequence within the α_1-antitrypsin molecule is unclear. It is situated either 35 residues from the C terminus or within the approximately 300 unsequenced residues, proximal to the N terminus. Both of these regions are indicated by shading in (A). Current evidence suggests that there is only one functional protease combining site per α_1-antitrypsin molecule. C. Structure of the oligosaccharide side chains of α_1-antitrypsin. The α_1-antitrypsin molecule contains two types of oligosaccharides, designated A and B. These carbohydrate chains differ in the number of branch points at a mannose residue. The oligosaccharides are attached to asparagine residues within the polypeptide chain through an N-glycosidic linkage. The B oligosaccharide is found more commonly than the A chain. The Z variant of α_1-antitrypsin protein probably contains one less complete oligosaccharide side chain than does the M or S variant.

bands shows variable numbers of side chains in each band [30]. This incomplete glycosylation may be a random process giving rise to a heterogeneous population of α_1-antitrypsin molecules, or it may occur only at specific sites. In any case, it may explain the multiple bands seen when various electrophoretic techniques are used [30] (Fig. 64-1).

There is little information on the higher-order structure of α_1-antitrypsin. Circular dichroism and fluorescent quenching studies suggest that 16 to 50 percent is in the form of an α helix and 15 to 50 percent is in the form of a β-pleated sheet [58, 59].

Structure of the Z Variant The Z protein differs from the M protein in a single amino acid substitution [60, 61] and in carbohydrate composition [62, 63]. The amino acid substitution is the primary abnormality.

Early structural studies of the Z protein demonstrated that it has fewer sialic acid residues than the M variant [63]. In this context the initial hypothesis used to explain the different electrophoretic mobilities of the M and Z proteins suggested that the entire difference could be explained on the basis of differences in the carbohydrate side chains only, e.g., secondary to inherited deficiency of sialytransferase in the cells that synthesize α_1-antitrypsin [64]. In support of this premise was the observation that removal of sialic acid residues from the M protein produced a shift in the electrophoretic mobility of the protein toward that of the cathodal Z position [30]. However, it was soon recognized (1) that removal of sialic acid residues from both the M and Z proteins produced a commensurate cathodal shift in the electrophoretic position of both the M and Z forms [30] and (2) that sialytransferase activity was similar

in the M and Z patients [65]. Thus, the striking difference in the electrophoretic behavior of the variants could not be attributed to discrepancies in the carbohydrate moiety alone.

The true molecular basis of the Z protein variant was uncovered by detailed peptide mapping of the constituent peptide fragments of the α_1-antitrypsin polypeptide. Yoshida et al. [61] and Jeppsson [60] independently used tryptic and cyanogen bromide fragments, respectively, of the purified M and Z α_1-antitrypsin to provide a comparative analysis of the primary structure of these proteins. These studies demonstrated that the Z protein differed from the M protein by the substitution of a lysine residue for a glutamic acid residue [60, 61] at position 53 from the C terminus of the molecule [48, 49]. This substitution is consistent with the alteration of C → T at the gene level and results in the incorporation of a basic amino acid for an acidic one. This produces a shift in the isoelectric point of the protein and explains the differences in electrophoretic behavior of the two proteins.

Although it is clear that there is a primary sequence difference in the Z and M proteins, it is also clear that the initial observations of differences in the carbohydrate compositions of the two molecules were also correct [62, 63]. The Z protein has 30 percent less carbohydrate, including two sialic acid residues, one basic sugar, and several neutral sugars [62]. Taken together, this implies that compared to the M variant, the Z variant has one less complete oligosaccharide side chain [5].

Structure of the S and Other Variants Besides the Z protein, the S protein is the only other α₁-antitrypsin variant to be studied in detail. Like the Z protein, the S differs from the M in a single amino acid (residue 131 from the C terminus, glu → val, T → A) [66, 67]. However, unlike the Z variant, current data suggest that the carbohydrate content of the S protein is identical to that of the M protein. Presumably, the S substitution of a valine residue does not have the same effect on the addition of carbohydrates as does the Z substitution of a lysine 78 residues distant [5].

At this time, the molecular basis of the other α₁-antitrypsin variants is unknown. It is presumed, however, that like the Z and S proteins, they differ from the M protein in a single amino acid, with or without concomitant changes in carbohydrate composition. [2, 5, 68, 69].

PHYSIOLOGY OF α₁-ANTITRYPSIN

Source

The primary source of serum α₁-antitrypsin is the hepatocyte [70–73]. Small pieces of human liver [70], heterogeneous populations of human liver cells [71], perfused rat liver [72], and cultured human fetal hepatocytes [73] all synthesize α₁-antitrypsin *de novo*. α₁-Antitrypsin is also present in other cell types, including platelets [74, 75], megakaryocytes [74], blood monocytes [76] alveolar macrophages [77], pancreatic islet cells [78, 79], lymphocytes [80], and polymorphonuclear leukocytes [81], but it is generally conceded that these cells contribute little, if any, to α₁-antitrypsin serum levels. Definitive demonstration of this concept has been provided by the study of individuals who received a liver transplant for advanced cirrhosis. In all cases, the phenotype of the recipients changed to that of the allograft donor [82, 83].

Catabolism

Metabolic studies utilizing labeled α₁-antitrypsin have estimated that PiM individuals produce 34 mg/kg body weight per day and catabolize 33 percent intravascular pool per day [84–86]. The observed half-life for the M protein in PiM individuals is approximately 5 days, as is the half-life for the Z protein in PiM individuals [85]. The latter observation is important since it suggests that increased catabolism is not the cause of the reduced serum α₁-antitrypsin levels in PiZ individuals. In addition, the half-life of the M protein in PiZ individuals is known to be normal. This is a critical fact in assessing the feasibility of direct replacement therapy for α₁-antitrypsin-deficient individuals.

The factors controlling the catabolism of α₁-antitrypsin are not understood. Unlike IgG [87], serum α₁-antitrypsin catabolism is independent of its serum concentration [84]. Some studies suggest that α₁-antitrypsin catabolism may be partially regulated by the status of the terminal sugars of the oligosaccharide side chains [88]. Evaluation of labeled M and Z proteins injected into animals or humans demonstrates that when

α₁-antitrypsin has been partially or completely desialyated (i.e., making galactose the terminal sugar; Fig. 64-2C), the serum half-life is changed from days to minutes and there is rapid uptake of radioactivity in the liver [84–86, 88]. These observations are compatible with the concept that hepatocytes have surface receptors that bind and clear desialyated glycoproteins [88]. PiM individuals are heterogeneous in the oligosaccharide side chains, and accordingly, there may be heterogeneity in the half-life of circulating α₁-antitrypsin molecules. Desialyzation may be one mechanism which initiates the process of catabolism of circulating α₁-antitrypsin.

Synthesis and Secretion

Like other glycoproteins destined for secretion, α₁-antitrypsin is likely synthesized on the rough endoplasmic reticulum, moves into the Golgi apparatus, and is exported via Golgi-formed secretory vesicles. The addition of oligosaccharide side chains to α₁-antitrypsin probably occurs in the cisterna of the endoplasmic reticulum [5]. Since in vitro labeling studies with liver explants have shown that newly synthesized α₁-antitrypsin is found mostly in the medium the process of synthesis and export of α₁-antitrypsin must occur rapidly [70–73].

The mechanisms modulating the synthesis of α₁-antitrypsin are not known. It is found in the serum at 4 weeks of gestation, and adult levels are reached by 26 weeks [89]. Except for a mild reduction for a few weeks following birth [90], the serum levels are held relatively constant thereafter [2–5]. It is an acute phase reactant, and levels rise with bacterial infection, pregnancy, malignancy, severe burns, or administration of typhoid vaccine [2–5]. Feedback inhibition by extracellular α₁-antitrypsin has been shown in vitro, but whether this occurs in vivo is not known [70].

Once it was recognized that the Z variant had fewer carbohydrate side chians than the M protein, it was hypothesized that α₁-antitrypsin deficiency was a disorder of secretion, i.e., the Z molecule could not be exported because it lacked the proper oligosaccharide "signals" for secretion. This hypothesis is supported by the finding that α₁-antitrypsin accumulates within the liver of PiZ individuals [70, 91, 92]. Hepatocytes of these individuals contain eosinophilic globules, which stain with anti-α₁-antitrypsin antibody. The cisternae of these hepatocytes are filled with fibrillar material that cross-reacts with α₁-antitrypsin antibody [93]. In addition, direct isolation of inclusions from the PiZ liver shows that the major component is α₁-antitrypsin [91, 92]. It is likely that this accumulation of α₁-antitrypsin in the endoplasmic reticulum of the PiZ hepatocyte occurs over a very long period. Short-term in vitro labeling studies of liver explants of PiZ individuals have failed to demonstrate any buildup of newly synthesized α₁-antitrypsin within the cell [70].

The mechanism responsible for the carbohydrate side chain abnormalities of the Z variant (and secondarily, the secretory defect) has been the subject of several investigations. It was once thought that PiZ individuals were deficient in sialyltransferase, an enzyme that adds terminal sialic acid residues to oligosaccharide side chains [64]. However, even though the PiZ state can be associated with reduced serum sialyltransferase, it is now recognized that this results from coexistent liver disease and is not a reflection of a generalized defect [65]. Most workers now believe that the Z protein has one less complete oligosaccharide side chain as a consequence of a conformational change in the molecule resulting from the single amino acid substitution in the primary sequence [5, 62, 63]. It seems likely that the basic, relatively bulky lysine residue of the Z protein alters the molecule, thereby preventing addition of a normal carbohydrate side chain. This concept is particularly attractive because it combines multiple observations into a unified hypothesis, i.e., that the serum deficiency of α_1-antitrypsin in the PiZ individual results from a single amino acid-base substitution that prevents normal glycosylation and hence normal secretion of the Z molecule. It should be remembered that the rate of synthesis of α_1-antitrypsin by the PiZ liver is not known. There may also be a reduction in synthesis of α_1-antitrypsin, perhaps secondary to negative feedback by the α_1-antitrypsin that accumulates within the endoplasmic reticulum [70].

Little information is available concerning synthesis or secretion of the other α_1-antitrypsin variants. Consistent with the hypothesis of the serum deficiency associated with the PiZ homozygote is the fact that α_1-antitrypsin accumulates in the liver in the MZ and SZ individuals, albeit to a much lesser extent than the Z homozygote [2–5, 24, 93]. Also, evaluation of the livers of Pi^{--} individuals reveals no α_1-antitrypsin. This is consistent with the concept that the serum deficiency in these patients results from a deletion in the expression of the α_1-antitrypsin gene [93]. Interestingly, small amounts of α_1-antitrypsin have been reported in the serum of Pi^{--} individuals [94]. Since the Pi^{--} liver does not accumulate α_1-antitrypsin, it is conceivable that the small quantity in serum is derived from sources such as circulating monocytes, cells that produce small amounts of α_1-antitrypsin in vitro.

Distribution

Because of its molecular mass, α_1-antitrypsin has the capacity to diffuse through most tissues and as such is found on serosal surfaces (pleural [95], peritoneal [96], articular [97]), epithelial surfaces (alveolar [98], cervical [99], ocular [100], intestinal [101]), cerebrospinal fluid [102], and amniotic fluid [103]. Approximately 54 percent of total body α_1-antitrypsin is extravascular and 45 percent intravascular [85].

Immunofluorescent studies have confirmed the presence of α_1-antitrypsin in the alveolar structures and within alveolar macrophages [98, 104]. With the flexible fiberoptic bronchoscope and bronchoalveolar lavage, lower respiratory tract fluid can be sampled independently from that of the trachea and segmental bronchi. This allows quantitative assessment of the α_1-antitrypsin present on the epithelial surface of the human lower respiratory tract. The concentration of α_1-antitrypsin obtained from the lower respiratory tract of PiM individuals is 51 ± 10 µg/mg albumin recovered (albumin is used to correct for the variable amount of dilution consequent to the lavage process) (Fig. 64-3A). This is in close agreement with that of serum (52 ± 11 µg/mg albumin) and implies that the majority of lung α_1-antitrypsin is derived by diffusion from the intravascular pool [105].

In contrast, α_2-macroglobulin, the other principal antielastase of serum, is severely restricted in its diffusion to the lower respiratory tract. While the serum concentration of α_2-macroglobulin is 254 ± 30 µg/mg albumin, the lower respiratory tract concentration is < 3 µg/mg albumin [105]. This is not surprising, since the molecular weight of α_2-macroglobulin of 725,000 severely limits the ability of this molecule to diffuse into tissues.

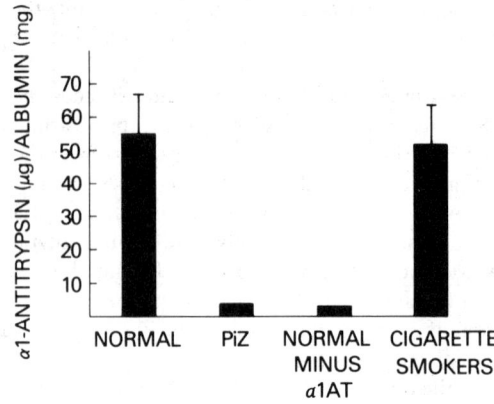

A. AMOUNT OF LUNG α1-ANTITRYPSIN

B. FUNCTION OF LUNG α1-ANTITRYPSIN

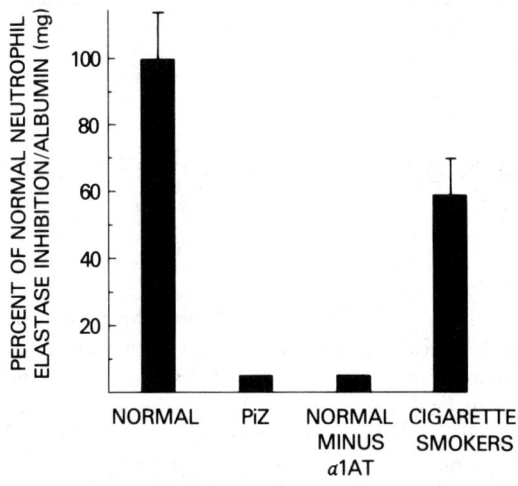

Figure 64-3 Amount and function of α_1-antitrypsin within the alveolar structures. A. Immunochemical quantification of the amount of α_1-antitrypsin recovered from the lower respiratory tract by bronchoalveolar lavage. Shown are data from normals (PiM), PiZ homozygotes, normals in whom α_1-antitrypsin has been removed by antibody precipitation, and asymptomatic normals who are cigarette smokers. The amount of lower respiratory tract α_1-antitrypsin is expressed as a function of the albumin recovered in the lavage, a convention that corrects for differences in dilution by the lavage fluid. B. Function of lung α_1-antitrypsin. Shown is the inhibition of human neutrophil elastase by the lavage fluid recovered from the lungs of the same groups shown in (A). α_1-Antitrypsin accounts for > 95 percent of the elastase inhibitory capacity of PiM lavage fluid. Note that although asymptomatic PiM cigarette smokers have normal amounts of α_1-antitrypsin in lavage fluid, the population of α_1-antitrypsin molecules present will inhibit only about 50 percent as much as that of the nonsmoker.

The concept of the pathogenesis of the destructive lung disease associated with α_1-antitrypsin deficiency rests on the hypothesis that a reduction in serum α_1-antitrypsin deficiency connotes a reduction in lung α_1-antitrypsin levels [1–5, 16, 105, 106]. Direct evaluation of the lower respiratory tract of PiZ individuals with the lavage technique has validated this concept: PiZ individuals have < 3µg α_1-antitrypsin/albumin on their alveolar epithelial surface (compared to 5 µg α_1-antitrypsin/albumin in PiZ serum) [105] (Fig. 64-3A). In addition, the PiZ individual, like the PiM individual, has little α_2-macroglobulin in the lower respiratory tract.

Studies with labeled PiM and PiZ proteins have shown that both diffuse into the lower respiratory tract (of PiM or PiZ individuals) at approximately the same rate. This is an important observation. It implies that the Z lung does not have a selective barrier against α_1-antitrypsin, and thus if PiZ individuals should be treated with parenteral α_1-antitrypsin, the infused material could be expected to reach the lower respiratory tract [105a].

Function of α_1-Antitrypsin

α_1-Antitrypsin is a multipurpose protease inhibitor [1–5, 107–112]. While it derives its name from its trypsin inhibitory activity, this is because trypsin was the protease used in early studies. α_1-Antitrypsin inhibits a variety of serine proteases, including the neutrophil proteases elastase [14] and cathepsin G [107], pancreatic elastase, human pancreatic trypsin (cathodal and anodal variants) [107], pancreatic chymotrypsin [107], factor XI [108], factor XIII, plasmin [109, 111], and thrombin [112]. Because of its broad specificity for human proteases, it has been argued that the term α_1-antitrypsin should be replaced by α_1-antiprotease or α_1-proteinase inhibitor. Nevertheless, in the interest of establishing a common terminology, an international committee on nomenclature recommended retention of the original term, α_1-antitrypsin [26].

Although α_1-antitrypsin is a broad-spectrum protease inhibitor, its major function as an antiprotease is to inhibit neutrophil elastase. This concept evolved out of several observations.

First, it is well established that destructive lung disease is the major disease associated with α_1-antitrypsin deficiency and that the only type of protease that can produce emphysema in experimental animals are those with elastaselike activity [16–22]. In this context, human neutrophil elastase is very effective in inducing experimental emphysema.

Second, relevant to the pathogenesis of emphysema, there are two potential sources of elastase in the human lung: neutrophils and alveolar macrophages. α_1-Antitrypsin is an effective inhibitor of the former but not the latter [6, 107, 110].

Third, while α_1-antitrypsin exhibits antiprotease activity against proteases that function in coagulation and fibrinolytic cascades, individuals with α_1-antitrypsin deficiency exhibit no abnormalities associated with either system. Thus, this part of the antiprotease spectrum of α_1-antitrypsin is not as critical to normal function as is its antielastase activity. α_1-Antitrypsin provides approximately 90 percent of the antielastase activity of serum [110], but only a small proportion of the serum's activity against proteases such as plasmin or thrombin, enzymes that are more effectively dealt with by serum antiproteases such as antiplasmin [111] and antithrombin III [112], respectively.

Fourth, kinetic analysis of the interaction of α_1-antitrypsin with various proteases demonstrates that the association rate constant for the interaction of α_1-antitrypsin with neutrophil elastase is 500 times that with bovine trypsin, 10 times that with human chymotrypsin, 100 times that with human trypsin, 6000 times that with human cationic trypsin, 3×10^5 times that with human plasmin, and 10^6 times that with human thrombin [107, 113]. It has been estimated that in the presence of saturating amounts of α_1-antitrypsin, neutrophil elastase is inactivated, with a half-life of 420 μs compared to 9.6 min for the inactivation of thrombin [107]. These data are relevant to the in vivo role of α_1-antitrypsin, since if it plays a primary role in maintaining the protease-antiprotease balance, it must have

the capacity to inhibit the protease prior to its interaction with the substrate to be conserved [113].

The major site of action of α_1-antitrypsin as an antielastase is in tissues, not in the blood. There is no evidence of any adverse intravascular consequences of α_1-antitrypsin deficiency, even in Pi^{--} individuals who have essentially no serum α_1-antitrypsin. This fact further substantiates the concept that regulation of serologic effector systems, such as the coagulation and fibrinolytic pathways, is not an important function of α_1-antitrypsin.

Interaction of α_1-Antitrypsin with Neutrophil Elastase
α_1-Antitrypsin inhibits neutrophil elastase by interacting with the protease to form a tight, "pseudoirreversible" complex with a low dissociation constant ($K_i < 10^{-9}$/M) [107, 110, 113, 114]. Although it has been suggested that α_1-antitrypsin is a multivalent inhibitor with more than one inhibitory site, it is now generally accepted that α_1-antitrypsin inhibits neutrophil elastase in a 1:1 molar ratio [107, 110]. Once α_1-antitrypsin combines with a protease, there is limited proteolytic cleavage of α_1-antitrypsin at the methionine-serine (or threonine) bond within the active site. The α_1-antitrypsin molecule is then unable to function again as an antiprotease [114]. Although the elastase is nonfunctional while bound to the α_1-antitrypsin, the complex can dissociate, albeit slowly [62, 110, 115]. If this does occur, the dissociated elastase is free to act on its true substrates. Ohlsson et al. have proposed that while α_1-antitrypsin is an effective antielastase, its role is to pick up the protease and transfer it to α_2-macroglobulin, which is then "cleared" by receptors on the surface of the reticuloendothelial system [115]. It is now believed that this so-called transfer process is simply a reflection of the random interaction of the protease with α_2-macroglobulin; that is, elastase that dissociates from α_1-antitrypsin randomly interacts with molecules in its vicinity. It could just as well combine with another α_1-antitrypsin molecule as with α_2-macroglobulin. Furthermore, this controversy is probably irrelevant for the lung since α_2-macroglobulin is present in such small amounts [105].

On a molar basis, purified Z-type α_1-antitrypsin is equally as effective as an antielastase as is the M variant [62]. The explanation for this is that the lysine for glutamic acid substitution in the Z molecule is sufficiently distant from the active site of the molecule that it does not affect its antiprotease function [5, 50]. This fact reemphasizes the concept that the major problem in α_1-antitrypsin deficiency is a reduction in the number of α_1-antitrypsin molecules in serum (and hence lung), not in the antielastase activity of each molecule.

It is critical that each α_1-antitrypsin molecule functions properly. When α_1-antitrypsin comes in contact with elastase, the methionine in the active site of α_1-antitrypsin must be in a reduced form. If this methionine residue is oxidized, the association constant of α_1-antitrypsin with neutrophil elastase is reduced by a factor of 2000, while the measured rate constant for normal α_1-antitrypsin is 6.5×10^7 M/s, and the rate constant for oxidized α_1-antitrypsin is 3.1×10^4 M/s [107, 113]. Since the protective role of α_1-antitrypsin depends on its ability to prevent elastase from attacking the alveolar structures in vivo, this function is critical to the role of α_1-antitrypsin in the lung. This concept is particularly relevant to situations in which the alveolar structures are exposed to oxidants such as those produced by cigarette smoke.

Other Functions of α_1-Antitrypsin   Besides its function as an antielastase, α_1-antitrypsin binds to IgA [116] and influences a variety of physiologic processes, including the response of macrophages to lymphokines [117], the production of immunoglobulins [118], and the response of polymorphonuclear leukocytes to chemotactic stimuli [119]. The last is relevant to α_1-antitrypsin deficiency, because these individuals have neutrophils in their lower respiratory tract (see below) [120]. The data concerning these nonelastase functions of α_1-antitrypsin have been conflicting and at present are considered to be in vitro curiosities.

DESTRUCTIVE LUNG DISEASE ASSOCIATED WITH α_1-ANTITRYPSIN DEFICIENCY

Emphysema is a chronic condition defined as a permanent enlargement of the air spaces distal to the terminal bronchioles consequent to destruction of the alveolar walls [23]. Because the destructive process is at the center of the pathogenesis of emphysema, many clinicians now refer to this disorder as *destructive lung disease*. An understanding of the pathogenesis of this disease requires an understanding of what is destroyed, what effects the destruction, and why this process can occur.

What Is Destroyed?

The alveolar structures are composed of four major cell types (epithelial type I and type II, endothelial, fibroblasts) and a connective tissue framework [17, 121]. While all of the alveolar structures are destroyed in this disease, the principal target is the connective tissue matrix [16]. This matrix is composed of four classes of macromolecules: collagen (60 percent), elastic fibers (30 percent), proteoglycans (5 percent), and other glycoproteins, including fibronectin, laminin, and noncollagen basement membrane components (together about 5 percent) [121]. Many of these classes have subclasses. For example, the alveolar structures contain four types of collagen and six glycosaminoglycan components of proteoglycans [121]. While each of these is affected in emphysema, it is now recognized that for destructive lung disease to occur, the destruction of elastic fibers is of primary importance [18, 21]. The reason elastic fibers are a more important target than the other connective tissue components is not known, but it is recognized that (1) elastic fibers turn over very slowly [122], i.e., if destroyed they cannot be easily replaced; (2) elastic fibers play a critical role in normal lung function, particularly in modulating elastic recoil [18, 21, 123]; and (3) when proteases are instilled into the lungs of experimental animals, only when the protease possesses elastase-like activity will the animal develop emphysema [18–22]. In view of these considerations, for destructive lung disease to occur in association with the α_1-antitrypsin deficiency state, there must be destruction of the elastic fibers of the alveolar structures.

What Effects the Destruction? Elastic fibers are composed of two components: elastin and microfibrils [17, 121]. While the latter is sensitive to a variety of proteases, elastin is a unique matrix component in that only one protease, elastase, is capable of destroying it in the physiologic milieu [110]. Thus, an understanding of the mechanisms of lung destruction in

α_1-antitrypsin deficiency first requires insight into the sources of elastase in the α_1-antitrypsin-deficient lung.

Several lines of evidence suggest that the neutrophil, rather than the macrophage, is the major source of this elastase. First, while the alveolar macrophage produces an elastase, α_1-antitrypsin cannot inhibit this enzyme [6]; hence a deficiency of α_1-antitrypsin would not be relevant to the macrophage enzyme. Second, there is no evidence that macrophages in the α_1-antitrypsin-deficient lung are activated and produce large quantities of elastase. Third, while the normal lung does not contain neutrophils, there are neutrophils in the lower respiratory tract of patients with α_1-antitrypsin deficiency [120]. Finally, neutrophil elastase can be recovered by lavage of the lower respiratory tract of α_1-antitrypsin-deficient patients [120].

Neutrophil elastase is a basic protein (isoelectric point 9.6) with a molecular weight of 29,500 [110, 124]. Besides elastin, it cleaves a variety of proteins, including all the major classes of macromolecules comprising the connective tissue matrix of human alveolar structures [6, 8–10, 16]. It is not surprising, therefore, that free elastase can wreak havoc in the alveolar structures. In the neutrophil elastase is stored in the primary (azurophilic) granules as an active enzyme [6, 16]. Since the neutrophil is a short-lived cell, the presence of a neutrophil outside the vascular space implies that within a short time, elastase is released. Alternatively, neutrophils can be stimulated by a variety of mechanisms to discharge their elastase upon arrival at a tissue site [16]. Once discharged from the neutrophil, elastase rapidly adsorbs to its connective tissue substrates via electrostatic interactions. Elastin is a favored target because it is negatively charged and elastase is positively charged [110].

While there is clear evidence of neutrophils in the lower respiratory tract of α_1-antitrypsin-deficient individuals [120], the mechanisms underlying this fact are diverse. Since neutrophils are not normally found in the alveolar structures, there must exist within the α_1-antitrypsin-deficient lung an attractive force(s) that induces neutrophils to leave the pulmonary capillaries and migrate into the alveolar structures. Currently, there are two hypotheses to explain this phenomenon:

1. It is known that individuals who are deficient in serum α_1-antitrypsin are also deficient in a serum chemotactic factor inhibitor [125]. It is not clear if this deficiency in chemotactic factor inhibitor is inherited concomitant with the Pi^Z allele or is acquired. The alveolar structures may have a constant low-level source of chemotactic stimuli, but in normal individuals this chemotactic activity may be prevented from recruiting neutrophils by chemotactic factor inhibitors. In the setting of chemotactic factor inhibitor deficiency, the low level of chemotactic activity may be unopposed, and neutrophils may be attracted to the alveolar structures [16, 125].

2. Under the influence of various stimuli (e.g., cigarette smoke or environmental particulates), alveolar macrophages release a low molecular weight lipid chemotactic factor that selectively recruits neutrophils to the lower respiratory tract [126–128]. Preliminary evidence suggests that α_1-antitrypsin-deficient individuals who smoke cigarettes have larger numbers of neutrophils in their alveolar structures than those who do not [120].

Why Is the Destruction Allowed to Occur? The presence of neutrophils in the lungs of individuals with α_1-antitrypsin deficiency would have little consequence if the alveolar structures possessed protective mechanisms against the potentially devastating effects of neutrophil elastase. α_1-Antitrypsin is of critical importance to the lung not only because it functions as an antielastase but because the alveolar structures have no alternative antielastase. In the absence of α_1-antitrypsin the lower respiratory tract is completely devoid of protection against neutrophil elastase [105]. The evidence for this comes from two observations: (1) while PiM lavage fluid inhibits neutrophil elastase on a 1:1 molar basis with the amount of α_1-antitrypsin present, removal of α_1-antitrypsin from lower respiratory tract fluid obtained from a PiM individual renders that fluid unable to inhibit neutrophil elastase (Fig. 64-3B); and (2) comparable quantities of lavage fluid (based on albumin content) from a PiZ individual do not inhibit neutrophil elastase (Fig. 64-3B).

These observations provide direct confirmation of the antiprotease aspect of the α_1-antitrypsin deficiency hypothesis, namely, that α_1-antitrypsin deficiency in serum implies antielastase deficiency in the lower respiratory tract [16, 105]. In addition, the demonstration that the alveolar structures have no alternative antielastase other than α_1-antitrypsin serves to minimize the importance of the observation that alveolar macrophages produce α_2-macroglobulin in vitro [126] and confirms that serum α_2-macroglobulin, the other serum antielastase, does not reach the extravascular alveolar structures. Furthermore, these observations point out that the "bronchomucus inhibitor" (a potent inhibitor of neutrophil elastase produced by epithelial cells of the upper respiratory tract) [129, 130] does not function as an alternative to α_1-antitrypsin as an antielastase of the lower respiratory tract [16, 105].

Determinants of Destructive Lung Disease in α_1-Antitrypsin Deficiency   A reduced serum level of α_1-antitrypsin is not synonymous with the development of destructive lung disease. Two factors, serum (and hence lung) levels of α_1-antitrypsin and cigarette smoking, play major roles in determining the extent of destructive lung disease in these individuals [131].

While the risk of developing emphysema in the PiZ homozygote is 20 times that of the PiM homozygote [132], there is considerable argument as to whether the risk for the MZ heterozygote (serum level 60 percent that of MM individuals) is any different from that of the PiM homozygote [133]. It seems likely that there is a threshold level of serum α_1-antitrypsin below which the development of destructive lung disease is likely and above which it is not. The phenotypes associated with destructive lung disease have levels 35 percent or less than normal, e.g., "null" (0 percent normal levels), ZZ (10 to 15 percent normal), and SZ (30 to 35 percent). In contrast, those phenotypes that are not at higher risk have levels above 35 percent of normal, e.g., SS (50 to 60 percent), MZ (60 percent), and MS (80 percent). Thus, the 35 percent level (approximately 70 to 80 mg/dl) seems to be the threshold above which enough α_1-antitrypsin can diffuse through the alveolar structures and protect them from elastolytic attack [16].

Given a serum α_1-antitrypsin level of less than 35 percent of normal, a major determinant of the extent of disease is cigarette smoking. The evidence for this concept is overwhelming. For example, in a study of 246 adults with severe α_1-antitrypsin deficiency, Larsson showed that independent of sex, 70 percent of smoking PiZ individuals were dead at age 50 compared to 20 percent of those who did not smoke [131]. Consistent with this concept, the average PiZ smoker developed dyspnea at age 40, while the average PiZ nonsmoker does not develop dyspnea until age 54.

The influence of cigarette smoking on the lung in the setting of α_1-antitrypsin deficiency is not the superimposition of two diseases. Rather, all available evidence suggests that smoking accelerates the development of destructive disease in α_1-antitrypsin deficiency, i.e., it is the same disease but it occurs 10 to 15 years earlier and, for a given level of α_1-antitrypsin, the destructive processes are more extensive.

Several observations help to explain why the effect of cigarette smoking is simply to accelerate the same destructive processes (i.e., elastase-antielastase imbalance) rather than to superimpose a second disease on a background of α_1-antitrypsin deficiency. First, alveolar macrophages of cigarette smokers spontaneously produce a neutrophil chemotactic factor that attracts neutrophils to the alveolar structures, thus increasing the elastase burden [128]. Consistent with this concept, direct evaluation of the lower respiratory tract of PiZ smokers shows that they have more neutrophils than PiZ nonsmokers. Second, it is known that cigarette smoke renders α_1-antitrypsin functionally impotent as an antielastase [134, 135]. The mechanism for this phenomenon is that cigarette smoke oxidizes the methionine residue at the active elastase inhibitory site of α_1-antitrypsin [136]. Although PiZ individuals have not been evaluated in this regard, it is known that while α_1-antitrypsin levels in the lungs of PiM smokers are normal (Fig. 64-3A), the functional α_1-antitrypsin activity in the lungs of these individuals is only 60 percent that in the lungs of PiM nonsmokers [134] (Fig. 64-3B). Thus, it is likely that the cigarette-smoking α_1-antitrypsin-deficient individual has multiple processes that interact to shift the elastase-antielastase balance in the lung strongly in favor of elastase, and hence, lung destruction ensues.

Although α_1-antitrypsin serum levels and cigarette smoking are clearly the major determinants of the development of destructive lung disease in α_1-antitrypsin deficiency, there is still a wide spectrum in the incidence and extent of disease in the α_1-antitrypsin-deficient population, i.e., there is no quantitative correlation between the extent of disease and the absolute serum α_1-antitrypsin level or the smoking history. In addition, there are cases in which other factors are clearly operating. For example, Stableforth has described two sisters with phenotype ZZ who had comparable serum α_1-antitrypsin levels and a similar smoking history, yet one sister had advanced destructive disease while the other was symptom-free with mild lung functional abnormalities [137]. In addition, there are probably many individuals with severe α_1-antitrypsin deficiency in the general population who are never identified as such. The reports on the prevalence of severe α_1-antitrypsin deficiency are almost entirely based on populations evaluated at medical centers. While many unreported (and mostly unidentified) individuals may be nonsmokers, it is more likely that factors other than serum levels and smoking influence disease expression.

The variability of expression is probably related to factors that modulate the elastase-antielastase burden of the lung [140], including (1) the number of neutrophils that migrate to the alveolar structures per unit time, which in turn is influenced by the levels of chemotactic factors for neutrophils within the alveolar structures and the response of neutrophils to these chemotactic factors; (2) the elastase burden created by the neutrophils, i.e., different individuals may have different quantities of elastase/neutrophil [138, 139]; and (3) the functional state of the α_1-antitrypsin within the alveolar structures [134]. In addition, it is conceivable that the relative resistance of the alveolar structures to destruction may play a role in modulating disease susceptibility.

These considerations are also relevant to the question of whether the MZ heterozygote is at increased risk for the development of destructive lung disease. While it seems clear that the risk is not great [133], the MZ state implies a shift in the elastase-antielastase balance of the lung. The MZ individual is poised at the edge of disaster. Cigarette smoking and the other factors discussed above may conspire to shift the balance in favor of the destructive processes, with resulting disease.

CLINICAL MANIFESTATIONS OF THE DESTRUCTIVE LUNG DISEASE ASSOCIATED WITH α_1-ANTITRYPSIN DEFICIENCY

Although there is broad variability in the extent of disease, 80 to 90 percent of PiZZ individuals with α_1-antitrypsin deficiency have panacinar emphysema, most prominently in the lower lung zones [1–5, 141]. Unfortunately, except for scattered case reports, there is not much detailed clinical information available concerning the lung disease that occurs with the other phenotypes that are associated with serum levels of ≤ 35 percent of normal. All available evidence suggests that the destructive disease in those individuals is indistinguishable from that which occurs in the PiZZ state [142].

The classic α_1-antitrypsin-deficient patient develops symptoms referable to the lungs between ages 30 and 40. The earliest symptom usually is dyspnea on exertion [1–5, 141–144]. Although it is infrequent as an initial symptom, approximately 50 percent eventually develop a cough and recurrent pulmonary infections [141–144]. Physical examination reveals a thin individual with decreased breath sounds, particularly at the bases. The chest film shows flattened diaphragms and hyperinflated lungs with reduced peripheral vasculature, particularly in the lower lobes (Fig. 64-4A). Pulmonary function test results are consistent with severe emphysema. These indicate increased total lung capacity, increased ratio of residual volume to total lung capacity, evidence of limitation to airflow, reduced diffusing capacity, decreased maximum transpulmonary pressure, reduced coefficient of retraction (i.e., for a given total lung capacity, less negative pleural pressure necessary to expand the lungs fully), increased lung compliance, mild hypoxemia at rest which may worsen with exercise, mild hypocarbia with a compensated respiratory alkalosis, and mild pulmonary artery hypertension which worsens with exercise [141–144]. The ECG is consistent with a chronic strain on the right heart, commonly with right axis deviation, right atrial hypertrophy, and right bundle branch block.

The limitation to airflow in approximately 50 percent of the PiZ population is related entirely to the loss of lung elastic recoil. This is consistent with the concept that the lung disease associated with α_1-antitrypsin deficiency is a destructive process affecting primarily the alveolar structures [145]. Interestingly, approximately 50 percent of PiZ individuals also develop chronic bronchitis, as evidenced by their history and by increased airway resistance secondary to intrinsic airway disease [141, 143].

The major feature that distinguishes the destructive lung disease of the classic α_1-antitrypsin-deficient individual from the common acquired form of emphysema is the lower lung zone predilection of the disease in the former compared to the upper zone distribution in the latter [1–5, 144]. This can be seen on a routine chest film (Fig. 64-4A) and has been confirmed by a variety of techniques, including ventilation-perfusion scanning and angiography [146, 147]. Scintigraphic studies of α_1-antitrypsin-deficient individuals demonstrate markedly decreased perfusion of the lower zones, with a compensatory shift of blood flow upward. Angiographic studies of the pulmonary vasculature confirm these findings. There is sparsity of arborization and decreased capillary filling, particularly in the lower zones [147], with the bases clearing the gas much slower than the apex [146].

The few morphologic studies of the lungs of individuals with severe α_1-antitrypsin deficiency are consistent with the concept that the primary disease is panacinar emphysema, more prominently in the lower lung zones [144, 145] (Fig. 64-4B).

There is little long-term follow-up information on the causes of death in individuals with severe α_1-antitrypsin deficiency and destructive lung disease, but as in the study of 56 such individuals by Larsson, respiratory insufficiency is probably responsible in most [148].

Clinical Syndromes Other Than Destructive Lung Disease Associated with α_1-Antitrypsin Deficiency

The allelic variants of α_1-antitrypsin are so common that it is not surprising that there are a number of other clinical disorders associated with the deficiency state. The most important of these associations are with various forms of hepatocellular disease, joint disease, and nondestructive lung disease. In addition, there is a growing list of other conditions that seem to be associated with certain α_1-antitrypsin phenotypes [1–5].

Hepatic Disease   The association of hepatic disease with the PiZ phenotype was first observed by Sharp et al. in 1969 [149]. It is now recognized that severe α_1-antitrypsin deficiency is associated with neonatal hepatitis, cryptogenic cirrhosis in children and adults, and non-B chronic active hepatitis [149–152].

Neonatal hepatitis occurs in approximately 20 percent of PiZ infants. These infants account for as many as one-third of all cases of nonsurgical infantile obstructive jaundice [151]. In addition, larger numbers of PiZ infants have subclinical neonatal hepatocellular inflammation, as evidenced by elevated serum transaminase levels.

The clinical syndrome of neonatal hepatitis associated with α_1-antitrypsin deficiency is marked by evidence of cholestasis. The lesion is characterized by hepatocyte necrosis, neutrophils, bile duct proliferation, mild portal fibrosis, and the presence of diastase-resistant, PAS-positive granules composed of immunoreactive α_1-antitrypsin within the hepatocytes [152]. The hepatocellular damage remits with the return of normal hepatic function in the majority of infants, but in approximately 10 percent of those affected, there is subsequent development of cirrhosis, progressing to portal hypertension and hepatic failure by the second decade of life [151].

The pathogenesis of neonatal hepatitis associated with α_1-antitrypsin deficiency remains obscure. A causal relationship between the intracytoplasmic inclusions of α_1-antitrypsin

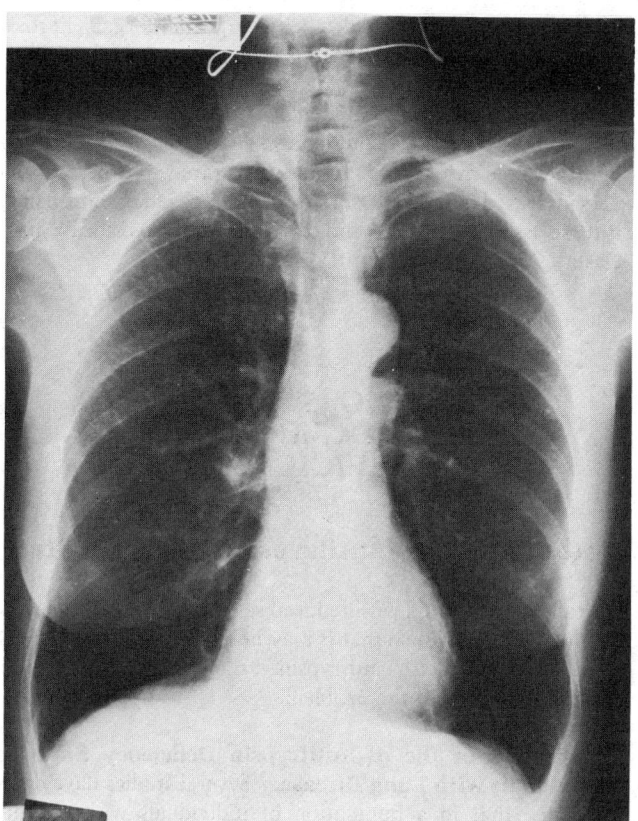

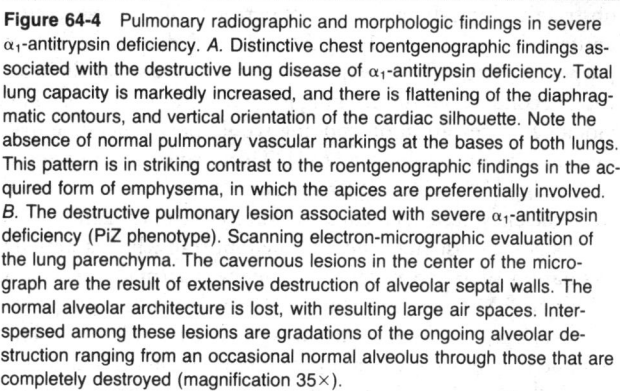

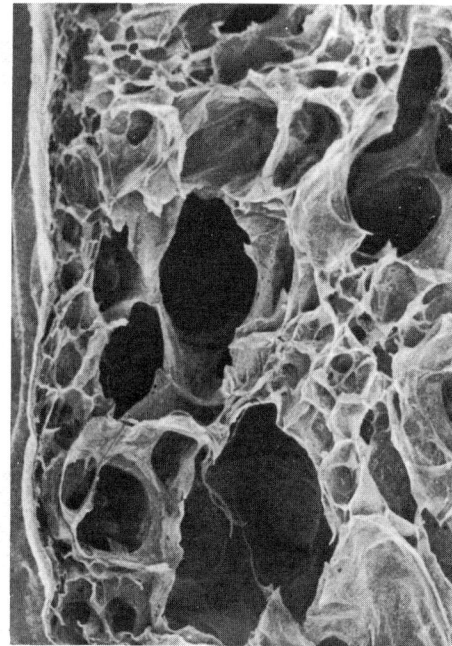

Figure 64-4 Pulmonary radiographic and morphologic findings in severe α₁-antitrypsin deficiency. *A.* Distinctive chest roentgenographic findings associated with the destructive lung disease of α₁-antitrypsin deficiency. Total lung capacity is markedly increased, and there is flattening of the diaphragmatic contours, and vertical orientation of the cardiac silhouette. Note the absence of normal pulmonary vascular markings at the bases of both lungs. This pattern is in striking contrast to the roentgenographic findings in the acquired form of emphysema, in which the apices are preferentially involved. *B.* The destructive pulmonary lesion associated with severe α₁-antitrypsin deficiency (PiZ phenotype). Scanning electron-micrographic evaluation of the lung parenchyma. The cavernous lesions in the center of the micrograph are the result of extensive destruction of alveolar septal walls. The normal alveolar architecture is lost, with resulting large air spaces. Interspersed among these lesions are gradations of the ongoing alveolar destruction ranging from an occasional normal alveolus through those that are completely destroyed (magnification 35×).

within the hepatocyte and the neonatal hepatic inflammation has been suggested; i.e., sequestered α₁-antitrypsin results in damage to the hepatocyte or renders it more susceptible to injury from hepatic toxins or virus [5]. This hypothesis is supported by the fact that the Pi null state, the most severe form of serum α₁-antitrypsin deficiency, is not associated with the presence of these inclusions or with neonatal hepatitis [93]. An alternative hypothesis is that a protease-antiprotease imbalance exists within the liver similar to that postulated to underlie the destructive lung disease. However, evidence in support of this postulate is lacking save for the observation that, in some cases, protease-bearing neutrophils participate in the inflammatory lesion [152].

In the adult, cryptogenic cirrhosis has been associated with the α₁-antitrypsin phenotypes ZZ, MZ, and SZ, and non-B chronic active hepatitis has been associated with phenotype MZ [149, 150, 152, 153]. Cirrhosis is said to occur in 10 to 20 percent of homozygotes, but the incidence of liver disease in adults with α₁-antitrypsin deficiency is not well established. The diagnosis depends on finding the characteristic intracytoplasmic granules in hepatocytes. Otherwise these disorders

cannot be distinguished from those not associated with α₁-antitrypsin deficiency [149]. The pathogenesis of these adult liver diseases is no less an enigma than the mechanisms underlying the neonatal hepatitis.

Although there was initial speculation that emphysema and liver disease in α₁-antitrypsin-deficient individuals were mutually exclusive, it is now clear that both adults and children with hepatic involvement can also have destructive lung disease [154]. Unfortunately, there are no long-term data on what happens to α₁-antitrypsin-deficient neonates who develop liver disease. Presumably, they are as much at risk for the development of destructive lung disease as α₁-antitrypsin-deficient individuals who do not develop liver disease.

Hepatocellular carcinomas have been described in a variety of α₁-antitrypsin phenotypes, most commonly in MZ and ZZ individuals [155, 156]. The true incidence is not known, and even the validity of the association has been questioned [155]. It has been suggested that compared to PiMM individuals, α₁-antitrypsin-deficient patients with cirrhosis have an increased incidence of hepatic malignancy, but hepatomas have also been described in deficient individuals without coexistent cirrhosis [155, 156].

Joint Disease In some studies the Pi^Z allele has been found in increased frequency in patients with adult rheumatoid arthritis and juvenile chronic polyarthritis [1–5]. The most convincing argument linking α₁-antitrypsin deficiency to the development of joint disease is the study of Cox and Huber, who demonstrated an association between Pi^Z heterozygosity and erosive joint destruction [157]. From a theoretical standpoint this is reasonable, since inheritance of a deficient allele with consequent reduction of antiprotease activity might influence the severity of an inflammatory process. The pathogenesis of the joint disorders associated with the α_1-antitrypsin deficiency has not been determined.

Lung Disease   The association of destructive lung disease with the inherited deficiency of α_1-antitrypsin is so frequent that it is unusual for a PiZ adult not to develop this disorder. Other respiratory disorders have also been noted with α_1-antitrypsin deficiency.

The original case reports of α_1-antitrypsin deficiency included diffuse bronchiectasis [158]. Since then scattered case reports have appeared, as have reports of α_1-antitrypsin deficiency associated with pulmonary cavitation following pneumonia [159]. Presumably, all of these conditions may be exacerbated by the lack of a lung antiprotease screen, but there are so few cases that the pathogenesis of these conditions has not been determined. Geddes et al. have noted an increased incidence of the MZ phenotype in idiopathic pulmonary fibrosis [160]. This is appealing from a pathophysiologic standpoint, since this disease is characterized by the chronic influx of neutrophils into the alveolar structures [161]. There are also reports of decreased α_1-antitrypsin levels associated with the respiratory distress syndrome of the newborn [162] and with nonatopic, steroid-dependent asthma [163]. The latter is of interest because a high proportion of PiZ adults with destructive disease also have reactive airways. In contrast, studies of individuals with pulmonary cancer show no association with α_1-antitrypsin, except perhaps an increase in serum levels [164].

Hemorrhagic Disorders   Various clotting abnormalities have been associated with α_1-antitrypsin deficiency, including platelet dysfunction, disseminated intravascular coagulation, and clotting system disturbances in infants [5]. A notable exception is the single report of an α_1-antitrypsin variant in which the abnormality caused the α_1-antitrypsin molecule to have greatly magnified protease-inhibitory effects on thrombin. The α_1-antitrypsin acted like heparin, blocking the coagulation cascade, particularly at the thrombin-fibrinogen reaction [165].

Fertility   There are a number of observations that link α_1-antitrypsin deficiency to increased fertility. It is known that the sperm-egg interaction requires proteolytic action and α_1-antitrypsin levels in cervical mucus decrease before ovulation [101] (independent of serum levels). There are reports of increased numbers of children in families with α_1-antitrypsin variants, a greater number of pregnancies in MZ, MS, and SS phenotypes compared to the MM phenotype, and an increased incidence of twins in α_1-antitrypsin variants [166].

Miscellaneous Associations   A variety of other associations have been proposed with the α_1-antitrypsin-deficient state, including membranoproliferative glomerulonephritis [167], acute anterior uveitis [168], acute and chronic pancreatitis [169], pancreatic fibrosis [170], C4 deficiency [171], paraproteinemia (e.g., myeloma) [172], prealbumin deficiency [173], Down's syndrome [174, 175], sex chromosome mosaicism [176], severe combined immunodeficiency disease [177], persistent cutaneous vasculitis [178], familial hypercholesterolemia [179], growth hormone deficiency [180], duodenal ulcer [181], Hashimoto's thyroiditis [182], cystathioninuria and renal iminoglycinuria [183], polypoid gastric heterotopy and primary hyperparathyroidism in a family with multiple endocrine adenomatosis [184], Weber-Christian disease [185],

an Ehler-Danlos-like syndrome [186], multiorgan fibrosis [187], and diabetes mellitus [188]. The relevance of these associations to the α_1-antitrypsin deficiency state is not clear. Most reports involve a small number of patients, and for many of these reports there are conflicting studies that have failed to find the same association. In addition, rarely are these disorders increased in incidence in the PiZ homozygous state. Thus, if these associations are valid, they are not linked to the anti-elastase function of α_1-antitrypsin.

DETECTING, STAGING, AND TREATING α_1-ANTITRYPSIN DEFICIENCY

Detecting the α_1-Antitrypsin Deficiency State

The alleles associated with reduced serum α_1-antitrypsin levels are frequent enough so that it may be useful to screen various populations for the α_1-antitrypsin variants. The following is a general approach to the problem.

Detection of the α_1-Antitrypsin Deficiency State in Individuals with Lung Disease.   Several studies have demonstrated that in a population of individuals with chronic obstructive lung disease, 5 to 10 percent will have severe α_1-antitrypsin deficiency [1–5]. Such knowledge serves several purposes. First, it helps explain the pathogenesis of their disease. Second, cigarette smoking is so devastating to these individuals that cessation of smoking would have a major impact on outcome of the disease [131]. Third, since all offspring of such individuals will carry at least one Pi allele associated with the deficiency state, screening of family members can be used for genetic counseling. There is one report in which a prenatal evaluation of α_1-antitrypsin deficiency was made in a fetus with two PiMZ parents. Thus, the fetus had a 25 percent risk of severe α_1-antitrypsin deficiency. Analysis of fetal blood obtained by fetoscopy demonstrated that the fetus had at least one Pi^M gene. The pregnancy was continued, and at birth a PiMZ phenotype was found [189]. Fourth, since rational approaches to the reestablishment of the antielastase screen of the lung in α_1-antitrypsin deficiency are now becoming available (see below), detection of the severe deficiency state may permit direct therapeutic intervention.

Detection of the α_1-Antitrypsin Deficiency State in Individuals with Liver Disease   Since there is no convincing evidence that therapeutic intervention is helpful to these patients, detection of the deficiency state is useful only in terms of categorizing the cause of the liver disease in a given patient. In addition, although it is rational to suggest that such individuals should avoid circumstances that may potentiate liver injury (e.g., alcohol, halothane anesthesia) [5], there is no convincing evidence of the validity of this concept.

Detection of the α_1-Antitrypsin Deficiency State in the General Population   With phenotypic frequencies in the U.S. population of only 0.025 percent and 0.12 percent for the ZZ and SZ states, respectively, it is difficult to argue that screening the general population for α_1-antitrypsin deficiency would be cost-effective. Nevertheless, the significance of cigarette smoking to individuals with these phenotypes is so great that some investigators have recommended screening all smokers for the deficiency state [190].

Available Screening Methods The simplest method for detecting α_1-antitrypsin deficiency is radial immunodiffusion with α_1-antitrypsin antibody. The current method of choice for determining the α_1-antitrypsin phenotype is isoelectric focusing of serum [27], but for general clinical purposes this should be reserved for the evaluation of individuals with pre-existing disease and their families.

Staging α₁-Antitrypsin-deficient Patients with Lung or Liver Disease

Since the lung disease associated with α_1-antitrypsin deficiency is destructive disease of the alveolar structures, a patient with this disorder is best staged with those tests that directly evaluate the structure and function of the lung parenchyma [191]. While certain chest film abnormalities are characteristic of the disease, it is doubtful that the chest film accurately gauges progression of the disease. Diffusion capacity, static deflation volume-pressure curves, airflow measurements, gas-exchange parameters (particularly with exercise), and ventilation-perfusion scans are all sensitive to changes in the status of the structure and function of the alveoli.

There are few data on the long-term consequences of the liver disease associated with α_1-antitrypsin deficiency. Routine liver function parameters are used to follow these patients.

Therapy for the Destructive Lung Disease

In the context of the elastase-antielastase theory, there are several obvious points at which therapeutic intervention might reestablish the dominance of the antielastase side of the equation. The elastase burden of the lung might be reduced by decreasing the traffic of neutrophils to the alveolar structures or suppressing the ability of the neutrophils to release their preformed elastase. Alternatively, the deficiency of lung antielastase resulting from a deficiency of serum α_1-antitrypsin could be reestablished by increasing the output of α_1-antitrypsin from the liver or by directly replacing the missing antiprotease with naturally occurring or synthetic antielastases. While most of these approaches remain theoretical or in the realm of experimental animal models, two approaches, danazol therapy and direct α_1-antitrypsin replacement therapy, have been evaluated in PiZ individuals with destructive lung disease.

Danazol Therapy The concept that the liver could be induced to produce or secrete more α_1-antitrypsin is not new. For example, α_1-antitrypsin levels have been shown to rise transiently in PiZ individuals after administration of typhoid vaccine [2]. In order to treat α_1-antitrypsin deficiency successfully, it is necessary to use an agent that can be administered chronically so that high serum levels can be maintained. One such agent is danazol (2,3-isoxazol-17 α-ethinyl testosterone), an anabolic steroid classified as an "impeded" androgen that has been used successfully in the treatment of another serum antiprotease deficiency, hereditary angioedema [192, 193]. When it is administered to PiZ individuals, the serum levels of α_1-antitrypsin increase approximately 40 percent and remain at this level [194]. Long-term studies of danazol therapy in

severe α_1-antitrypsin deficiency have not been carried out, but preliminary studies suggest that danazol therapy is safe. It may afford the lung more α_1-antitrypsin molecules and hence help protect the alveolar structures against elastolytic attack. Thus, even though danazol therapy does not induce the liver to release sufficient α_1-antitrypsin to raise the serum levels above the theoretical threshold of 80 mg/dl which is thought to protect the lung, it represents one approach to reestablishing the antielastase screen in the lower respiratory tract.

Direct Replacement Therapy The definitive approach to the lung disease associated with α_1-antitrypsin deficiency would be the quantitative replacement of the missing antielastase via parenteral administration of α_1-antitrypsin obtained from plasma of blood donors [195]. Unfortunately, this creates several formidable problems not encountered in the replacement therapy of disorders such as hemophilia [196]. The destructive lung disease in PiZ individuals is a chronic, progressive problem (unlike the episodic expression of hemophilia), thus requiring continuous maintenance therapy with α_1-antitrypsin. In addition, in contrast to the replacement therapy of hypogammaglobulinemia [197], in which the plasma half-life of the missing protein is 30 days, the half-life of plasma α_1-antitrypsin is 4 to 5 days. Thus, while replacement therapy in hypogammaglobulinemia can be administered at intervals as long as 1 month, effective maintenance therapy of α_1-antitrypsin deficiency would require infusions at intervals no longer than 1 week. This also implies that a successful program of α_1-antitrypsin replacement therapy would necessitate harvesting the normal plasma α_1-antitrypsin at a very high yield. This requirement has been met by sequential polyethylene glycol precipitations that permit the preparation of an α_1-antitrypsin concentrate suitable for intravenous administration.

Preliminary studies in PiZ individuals with destructive lung disease have shown that infusion of 4 g α_1-antitrypsin concentrate once each week results in establishment of an elastase-antielastase balance within the lower respiratory tract. Serum α_1-antitrypsin levels were maintained above the theoretical threshold level (Fig. 64-5A), lung α_1-antitrypsin levels increased to 60 percent of normal (Fig. 64-5B), lung antielastase levels increased to 60 percent of normal (Fig. 64-5C), and the result was the disappearance of active elastase from the lower respiratory tract [198] (Fig. 64-5D). As with danazol therapy, there have been no long-term trials of direct replacement therapy in individuals with severe α_1-antitrypsin deficiency. Nevertheless, the evidence is overwhelming that the decreased serum level of this protein is responsible for the destructive lung disease. Thus it is generally assumed that if such a therapeutic approach could be applied on a large-scale basis to young individuals with severe α_1-antitrypsin deficiency, the destructive disease would be prevented.

Other Therapeutic Approaches Another promising approach to reestablishing the normal elastase-antielastase balance in the α_1-antitrypsin-deficient lung is the use of synthetic inhibitors of neutrophil elastase such as chloromethyl ketone peptides [199] or short chain fatty acids [200]. Not only are such agents effective in vitro inhibitors of neutrophil elastase, but studies with experimental models of emphysema have demonstrated that chloromethyl ketone methoxysuccinyl-alanyl-alanyl-prolyl-valine administered parenterally will prevent subsequent lung destruction secondary to intratracheal instillation of elastase [201, 202]. Unfortunately, although

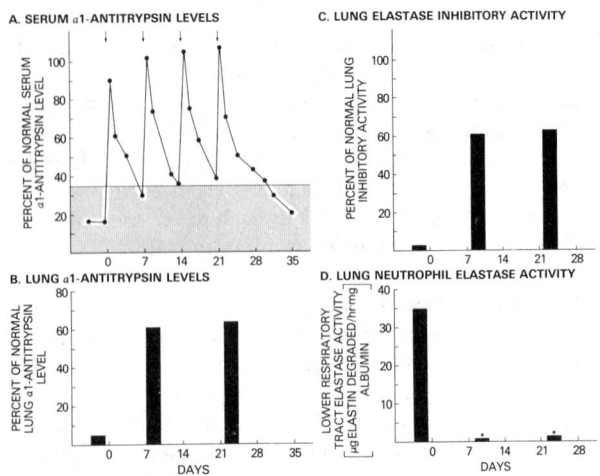

Figure 64-5 Parenteral replacement therapy for α_1-antitrypsin deficiency. *A.* Serum α_1-antitrypsin levels following the intravenous administration of 4 g of α_1-antitrypsin (arrows) at weekly intervals for 4 consecutive weeks in a PiZ individual. The estimated threshold serum level necessary to provide protection against progressive alveolar destruction is denoted by the shaded area of the graph. *B.* Lung α_1-antitrypsin levels expressed as a percent of that of normals. Bronchoalveolar lavage was performed before therapy and then 2 days following the second and fourth infusions. *C.* Lung elastase inhibitory activity following parenteral α_1-antitrypsin replacement. The fluid recovered from the lower respiratory tract 2 days following replacement therapy inhibited neutrophil elastase at 60 percent of the normal inhibitory level. *D.* Lung neutrophil elastase activity. Lower respiratory tract elastase activity was quantified as μg [^{3}H]elastin degraded per hour per milligram lavage fluid albumin before replacement therapy and following the second and fourth infusions of α_1-antitrypsin. Following the initiation of replacement therapy, free lung neutrophil elastase activity was no longer detectable (indicated by *).

chloromethyl ketones specific for elastase can be made easily in large quantities, they are quite toxic, and thus considerable work will be necessary to develop similar compounds that are safe for human use [202].

Symptomatic Therapy   Like patients with the common form of emphysema, patients with destructive lung disease secondary to α_1-antitrypsin deficiency do not respond as well to symptomatic therapy as do patients with the more bronchitic form of chronic obstructive lung disease. Oxygen therapy can induce lower pulmonary artery pressure and increase oxygen delivery and may be useful late in the course of the disease. Broncho-dilators may help some of these patients, although the pathogenesis of the bronchial disease is unclear.

Therapy for the Liver Disease   Since there is no consensus regarding the pathogenesis of the various forms of liver disease associated with α_1-antitrypsin deficiency, it is not surprising that there are no convincing therapeutic prospects for the hepatic manifestations of the disorder. Glucocorticoids have been employed in children with hepatitis, with no apparent beneficial effect. Liver transplantation represents the only definitive approach to the hepatocellular failure consequent to α_1-antitrypsin deficiency, but experience with this approach is discouraging, and at present it is not recommended [83].

REFERENCES

1. KUEPPERS F, BLACK LF: α-Antitrypsin and its deficiency. *Am Rev Respir Dis* 110:176, 1974
2. KUEPPERS F: Inherited differences in alpha $_1$-antitrypsin, in Litwin SD (ed): *Genetic Determinants of Pulmonary Disease.* New York, Marcel Dekker, Inc, 1978, p 23
3. LIEBERMAN J: Alpha $_1$-antitrypsin deficiency. *Curr Pulmonol* 2:41, 1980
4. MORSE JO: Alpha $_1$-antitrypsin deficiency. *N Engl J Med* 299:1045, 1099, 1978
5. CARRELL RW, OWEN MC: α_1-Antitrypsin: Structure, variation and disease. *Essays Med Biochem* 4:83, 1980
6. JANOFF A, WHITE R, CARP H, HAREL S, DEARING R, LEE E: Lung injury induced by leukocytic proteases. *Am J Pathol* 97:111, 1979
7. HARRIS ED, CARTWRIGHT EC: Mammalian collagenases, in Barrett AJ (ed): *Proteinases in Mammalian Cells and Tissues.* Amsterdam, North Holland, 1977, p 249
8. MacDONALD J, BAUM B, ROSENBERG D, KELMAN J, SENIOR R, CRYSTAL RG: Fibronectin, the major cell surface protein of cultured human lung fibroblasts: Destruction of structure and biological function by human neutrophil proteinases. *Am Rev Respir Dis* 117:170, 1978
9. GADEK JE, FELLS GA, WRIGHT DH, CRYSTAL RG: Neutrophil elastase functions as a type III collagenase. *Biochem Biophys Res Commun* 95:1815, 1980
10. MAINARDI CL, DIXIT SN, KANG AH: Degradation of type IV (basement membrane) collagen by a proteinase isolated from human polymorphonuclear leukocyte granules. *J Biol Chem* 255:5435, 1980
11. LAURELL CB, ERIKSSON S: The electrophoretic α_1-globulin pattern of serum in α_1-antitrypsin deficiency. *Scand J Clin Lab Invest* 15:132, 1963
12. ERIKSSON S: Pulmonary emphysema and alpha $_1$-antitrypsin deficiency. *Acta Med Scand* 177:175, 1964
13. FAGERHOL MK, LAURELL CB: The polymorphism of "prealbumins" and α_1-antitrypsin in human sera. *Clin Chim Acta* 16:199, 1967
14. FAGERHOL MK, LAURELL CB: The Pi system. Inherited variants of serum alpha $_1$-antitrypsin. *Prog Med Genet* 7:96, 1970
15. TURINO GM, SENIOR RM, GARG BD, KELLER S, LEVI MM, MANDL I: Serum elastase inhibitor deficiency and α_1-antitrypsin deficiency in patients with obstructive emphysema. *Science* 165:709, 1969
16. GADEK JE, HUNNINGHAKE GW, FELLS GA, ZIMMERMAN RL, KEOGH BA, CRYSTAL RG: Evaluation of the protease-antiprotease theory of human destructive lung disease. *Bull Eur Physiopathol Respir* 16:27, 1980
17. HANCE AJ, CRYSTAL RG: The connective tissue of lung. *Am Rev Respir Dis* 112:657, 1975
18. KARLINSKY JB, SNIDER GL: State of the art. Animal models of emphysema. *Am Rev Respir Dis* 117:1109, 1978
19. SENIOR RM, TEGNER H, KUHN C, OHLSSON K, STARCHER BC, PIERCE JA: The introduction of pulmonary emphysema with human leukocyte elastase. *Am Rev Respir Dis* 116:469, 1977
20. JANOFF A, SLOAN B, WEINBAUM G, DAMIANO V, SANDHAUS RA, ELIAS J, KIMBEL P: Experimental emphysema induced with purified human neutrophil elastase. Tissue localization of the instilled protease. *Am Rev Respir Dis* 115:461, 1977
21. KUHN C, SENIOR RM: The role of elastases in the development of emphysema. *Lung* 155:185, 1978
22. LIEBERMAN J: Elastase, collagenase, emphysema and alpha $_1$-antitrypsin deficiency. *Chest* 70:62, 1976
23. Chronic bronchitis, asthma, and pulmonary emphysema. Statement of the American Thoracic Society by the Committee on Diagnostic Standards for Nontuberculous Respiratory Diseases. *Am Rev Respir Dis* 85:762, 1962
24. BEARN AG: Alpha $_1$-antitrypsin deficiency: A biological enigma. *Gut* 19:470, 1978
25. GADEK JE, KLEIN H, HOLLAND P, CRYSTAL RG: Replacement therapy of alpha $_1$-antitrypsin deficiency. *Clin Res* 28:528A, 1980
26. COX DW, JOHNSON AM, FAGERHOL MK: Report of nomenclature meeting for alpha $_1$-antitrypsin. *Hum Genet* 53(3):429, 1980
27. TALAMO RC, BRUCE RM, LANGLEY CE, BERNINGER RW, PIERCE JA, BRANT LJ, DUNCAN DB: *Alpha $_1$-Antitrypsin Laboratory Manual, Maryland and Missouri.* Washington, DC, Dept of Health, Education and Welfare, Publication No. (NIH) 78-1420, 1978
28. ALLEN RC, HARLEY RA, TALAMO RC: A new method for determination of alpha $_1$-antitrypsin phenotypes using isoelectric focusing on polyacrylamide gel slabs. *Am J Clin Pathol* 62:732, 1974
29. ARNAUD P, CREYSSEL R, CHAPUIS-CELLIER C: The detection of α_1-antitrypsin variants (Pi system) by analytical thin-layer electrofocusing in polyacrylamide gel. *LKB Application Note* 185, 1975
30. YOSHIDA A, WESSELS M: Origin of the multiple components of human α_1-antitrypsin. *Biochem Genet* 16:641, 1978
31. FAGERHOL MK: Acid starch gel electrophoresis for detection of α_1-antitrypsin variants (Pi types). Outline of techniques employed currently, in Mittman C (ed): *Pulmonary Emphysema and Proteolysis.* New York, Academic Press, Inc, 1972, p 145
32. TALAMO RC, LANGLEY CE, REED CE, MAKINO S: α_1-Antitrypsin. *Science* 181:70, 1973
33. FAGERHOL MK, GEDDE-DAHL T: Genetics of the Pi serum types. Family study of the inherited variants of serum α_1-antitrypsin. *Hum Hered* 19:354, 1969
34. GENZ TH, MARTIN JP, CLEVE H: Classification of alpha $_1$-antitrypsin (Pi)

phenotypes by isoelectric focusing—distinction of six subtypes of the PiM phenotype. *Hum Genet* 38:325, 1977

35. FAGERHOL MK, TENFJORD OW: Serum Pi types in some European, American, Asian and African populations. *Acta Pathol Microbiol Scand* 72:601, 1968

36. FAGERHOL MK: Serum Pi types in Norwegians. *Acta Pathol Microbiol Scand* 70:421, 1967

37. PIERCE JA, ERADIO B, DEW TA: Antitrypsin phenotypes in St. Louis. *JAMA* 231:609, 1975

38. JANUS ED, JOYCE PR, SHEAT JM, CARRELL RW: Alpha ₁-antitrypsin variants in New Zealand. *N Z Med J* 82:289, 1975

39. KELLERMAN G, WALTER H: Investigations on the population genetics of alpha ₁-antitrypsin polymorphism. *Humangenetik* 10:145, 1970

40. VANDEVILLE D, MARTIN JP, ROPARTZ C: Alpha ₁-antitrypsin polymorphism in a Bantu population. *Humagenetik* 21:33, 1974

41. FAGERHOL MK: The serum alpha ₁-antitrypsin polymorphism, in deGrouchy J, Ebling FJG, Henderson IW (eds): *Human Genetics. Proceedings of the 4th International Congress of Human Genetics.* Amsterdam, Excerpta Medica, 1972, p 277

42. GEDDE-DAHL T, FAGERHOL MK, COOK PJL, NOADES J: Autosomal linkage between the Gm and Pi loci in man. *Ann Hum Genet* 35:393, 1972

43. TURNER BM, TURNER VS: Secretion of α₁-antitrypsin by an established human hepatoma cell line and by human/mouse hybrids. *Somatic Cell Genet* 6:1, 1980

44. TRAVIS J: Discussion of serum alpha ₁-antitrypsin levels. *Bull Eur Physiopathol Respir* 16(suppl):40, 1980

45. HEIMBURGER N, HAUPT H, SCHWICK HG: Proteinase inhibitors in human plasma, in Fritz H, Tschesche H (eds): *Proceedings of the International Research Conference on Proteinase Inhibitors.* New York, Walter de Gruyter, Inc, 1971, p 1

46. CHAN SK, LUBY J, WU YC: Purification and chemical composition of human α₁-antitrypsin of the MM type. *FEBS Lett* 35:79, 1973

47. MORII M, ODANI S, KOIDE T, IKENAKA T: Human alpha ₁-antitrypsin. Characterization and the N- and C-terminal sequences. *J Biochem (Tokyo)* 83(1):269, 1979

48. SHOCHAT D, STAPLES S, HARGROVE K, KOZEL JS, CHAN SK: Primary structure of human α₁-protease inhibitor. The complete amino acid sequence of cyanogen bromide fragment II. *J Biol Chem* 253:5630, 1978

49. OWEN MC, LORIER M, CARRELL RW: α₁-Antitrypsin structural relationships of the substitutions of the S and Z variants. *FEBS Lett* 88:234, 1978

50. CARRELL RW, BOSWELL D, BRENNAN SO, OWEN MC: Active site of α₁-antitrypsin: Homologous site in antithrombin-III. *Biochem Biophys Res Commun* 93:399, 1980

51. JOHNSON D, TRAVIS J: Structural evidence for methionine at the reactive site of human α₁-proteinase inhibitor. *J Biol Chem* 253:7142, 1978

52. NAKAJIMA K, POWERS JC, ASHE BM, ZIMMERMAN M: Mapping the extended substrate binding site of cathepsin G and human leukocyte elastase. *J Biol Chem* 254:4027, 1979

53. KRESS LF, KURECKI T, CHAN SK, LASKOWSKI M SR: Characterization of the inactive fragment resulting from limited proteolysis of human α₁-proteinase inhibitor by crotalus adamanteus proteinase II. *J Biol Chem* 254:5317, 1979

54. KOIDE T, OHTA Y, ONO T: The C-terminal sequence of human and porcine antithrombin III and its homology with human α₁-proteinase inhibitor. *Experientia* 36:516, 1980

55. CARRELL RW, BOSWELL DR, BRENNAN SO, OWEN MC: Active site of alpha ₁-antitrypsin: Homologous site in antithrombin III. *Biochem Biophys Res Commun* 93(2):399, 1980

56. HODGES LC, LAINE R, CHAN SK: Structure of the oligosaccharide chains in human α₁-protease inhibitor. *J Biol Chem* 254:8208, 1979

57. MARGA T, LUJAN E, YOSHIDA A: Studies on the oligosaccharide chains of human α₁-protease inhibitor. II. Structure of oligosaccharides. *J Biol Chem* 255:4057, 1980

58. GLASER CB, KARIC L: Spectral studies on two genetic forms of the human serum proteinase inhibitor, alpha ₁-antitrypsin. *Int J Pep Protein Res* 12:284, 1978

59. JIRGENSONS B: Circular dichroism and conformation of human α₁-antitrypsin. *Biochim Biophys Acta* 473:352, 1977

60. JEPPSSON J: Amino acid substitution Glu→Lys in α₁-antitrypsin PiZ. *FEBS Lett* 65:195, 1976

61. YOSHIDA A, LIEBERMAN J, GAIDULIS L, EWING C: Molecular abnormality of human α₁-antitrypsin variant (PiZ) associated with plasma activity deficiency. *Proc Natl Acad Sci USA* 73:1324, 1976

62. MILLER RR, KUHLENSCHMIDT MS, COFFEE CJ, KUO I, GLEW RH: Comparison of the chemical, physical, and survival properties of normal and Z-variant α₁-antitrypsins. *J Biol Chem* 251:4751, 1976

63. CHAN SK, REES DC: Molecular basis for the α₁-protease inhibitor deficiency. *Nature* 255:240, 1975

64. KUHLENSCHMIDT MS, YUNIS EJ, IAMMARINO RM, TURCO SJ, PETERS SP, GLEW RH: Demonstration of sialyltransferase deficiency in the serum of a

65. ERIKSSON S, LARSSON C: The serum sialyltransferase activity in α₁-antitrypsin deficiency. *Biochim Biophys Acta* 445:67, 1976

66. JEPPSSON JO, LAURELL CB, FAGERHOL M: Properties of isolated α₁-antitrypsins of Pi types M, S and Z. *Eur J Biochem* 83:143, 1978

67. OWEN MC, CARRELL RW: Alpha ₁-antitrypsin: Molecular abnormality of S variant. *Br Med J* 1:130, 1976

68. ROLL D, AGUANNO JJ, COFFEE CF, GLEW RH, IMMARINO RM: Comparison of the carbohydrate and amino acid composition of normal and S-variant alpha ₁-antitrypsin. *Biochim Biophys Acta* 532(1):171, 1978

69. YOSHIDA A, WESSELS M: Origin of the multiple components of alpha ₁-antitrypsin. *Biochem Genet* 16:641, 1978

70. BHAN AK, GRAND RJ, COLTEN HR, ALPER CA: Liver in α₁-antitrypsin deficiency: Morphologic observations and *in vitro* synthesis of α₁-antitrypsin. *Pediatr Res* 10:35, 1976

71. GAUTIER M, MARTIN JP, POLINI G: In vitro synthesis of alpha ₁-antitrypsin in long term monolayer human liver cell cultures. *Biomedicine* 27:116, 1977

72. KOJ A, REGOECZI E, TOEWS CJ, LEVEILLE R, GAULDIE J: Synthesis of antithrombin III and alpha ₁-antitrypsin by the perfused rat liver. *Biochim Biophys Acta* 539:496, 1978

73. ERIKSSON S, ALM R, ASTEDT B: Organ cultures of human fetal hepatocytes in the study of extra- and intracellular α₁-antitrypsin. *Biochim Biophys Acta* 542:496, 1978

74. NACHMAN RL, HARPEL PC: Platelet α₂-macroglobulin and α₁-antitrypsin. *J Biol Chem* 251:4514, 1976

75. BAGDASARIAN A, COLMAN RW: Subcellular localization and purification of platelet α₁-antitrypsin. *Blood* 51:139, 1978

76. WILSON GB, WALKER JH, WATKINS JH, WOLGROCH D: Determination of subpopulations of leukocytes involved in the synthesis of α₁-antitrypsin *in vitro* (40832). *Proc Soc Exp Biol Med* 164:105, 1978

77. COHEN AB: Interrelationships between the human alveolar macrophage and alpha ₁-antitrypsin. *J Clin Invest* 52:2793, 1973

78. RAY MB, DESMET VJ, GEPTS W: Alpha ₁-antitrypsin immunoreactivity in islet cells of adult human pancreas. *Cell Tiss Res* 185:63, 1977

79. MCELRATH MJ, GALBRAITH RM, ALLEN RC: Demonstration of alpha ₁-antitrypsin by immunofluorescence on paraffin-embedded hepatic and pancreatic tissue. *J Histochem and Cytochem* 27:794, 1979

80. LIPSKY JJ, BERNIGER RW, HYMAN LR, TALAMO RC: Presence of alpha ₁-antitrypsin on mitogen-stimulated human lymphocytes. *J Immunol* 122:24, 1979

81. BENITEZ-BRIBIESCA L, FREYRE-HORTA R: Immunofluorescent localization of alpha ₁-antitrypsin in human polymorphonuclear leukocytes. *Life Sci* 21:99, 1978

82. ALPER CA, RAUM D, AWDEH ZL, PETERSEN BH, TAYLOR PD, STARZL TE: Studies of hepatic synthesis *in vivo* of plasma proteins, including orosomucoid, transferrin, α₁-antitrypsin, C8, and factor B¹. *Clin Immunol Immunopathol* 16:84, 1980

83. PUTNAM CW, PORTER KA, PETERS RL, ASHCAVAI M, REDEKER AG, STARZL TE: Liver replacement for alpha ₁-antitrypsin deficiency. *Surgery* 81:258, 1977

84. JONES EA, VERGALLA J, STEER CJ, BRADLEY-MOORE PR, VIERLING JM: Metabolism of intact and desialylated α₁-antitrypsin. *Clin Sci Mol Med* 55:139, 1978

85. LAURELL CB, NOSSLIN B, JEPSSON JO: Catabolic rate of α₁-antitrypsin of Pi type M and Z in man. *Clin Sci Mol Med* 52:457, 1977

86. GLASER CB, KARIC L, FALLAT RJ, STOCKERT R: Plasma survival studies in the rat of the normal and homozygote deficient forms. *Biochim Biophys Acta* 495:87, 1977

87. WALDMANN TA, STROBER W: Metabolism of immunoglobulins. *Prog Allergy* 13:1, 1969

88. YU SD, GAN JC: The role of sialic acid and galactose residues in determining the survival of human plasma α₁-antitrypsin in the blood circulation. *Arch Biochem Biophys* 179:477, 1977

89. SINGER AD, THIBEAULT DW, HOBEL CJ, HEINER DC: Alpha ₁-antitrypsin in amniotic fluid and cord blood of preterm infants with the respiratory distress syndrome. *J Pediatr* 88:87, 1976

90. PIANTELLI M, POZZUOLI R, AUCONI P, MUSIANI P: Alpha ₁-antitrypsin in umbilical cord serum: Pi phenotypes and relationships with idiopathic respiratory distress syndrome. *Eur J Pediatr* 127:101, 1978

91. JEPPSSON JO, LARSSON C, ERIKSSON S: Characterization of α₁-antitrypsin in the inclusion bodies from the liver in α₁-antitrypsin deficiency. *N Engl J Med* 293:576, 1975

92. ERIKSSON S, LARSSON C: Purification and partial characterization of pas-positive inclusion bodies from the liver in alpha ₁-antitrypsin deficiency. *N Engl J Med* 292:176, 1975

93. SRINGE P, BENHAMOU JP: The ultrastructure of hepatocytes in alpha ₁-antitrypsin deficiency with the genotype Pi⁻. *Gut* 16:796, 1975

94. MARTIN JP, SESBOUE R, CHARLIONET R: Does alpha ₁-antitrypsin null phenotype exist? *Humangenetik* 30:121, 1975

95. HAVEMAN K, JANOFF A (eds): *Neutral Proteases of Human Polymorphonuclear Leukocytes.* Munich, Urban and Schwarzenberg, 1978, p 1

96. OHLSSON K: Collagenase and elastase released during peritonitis are complexed by plasma protease inhibitors. *Surgery* 79:652, 1976

97. SWEDLUNG HA, HUNDER GG, GLEICH GJ: α_1-Antitrypsin in serum and synovial fluid in rheumatoid arthritis. *Ann Rheum Dis* 33:162, 1974

98. OLSEN GN, HARRIS JO, CASTLE JR, WALDMAN RH, KARMGARD HJ: Alpha $_1$-antitrypsin content in the serum, alveolar macrophages, and alveolar lavage fluid of smoking and nonsmoking normal subjects. *J Clin Invest* 55:427, 1975

99. GALVEZ S, FARCAS A, MONARI M: The concentration of alpha $_1$-antitrypsin in cerebrospinal fluid and serum in a series of 40 intracranial tumors. *Clin Chim Acta* 91(2):191, 1979

100. BERMAN MB, BARBER JC, TALAMO RC, LANGLEY CE: Corneal ulceration and the serum antiproteases I. α_1-Antitrypsin. *Invest Ophthalmol Vis Sci* 12:759, 1973

101. SCHUMACHER GFB, PEARL MJ: Alpha $_1$-antitrypsin in cervical mucus. *Fertil Steril* 19:91, 1968

102. PRICE P, CUZNER ML: Proteinase inhibitors in cerebrospinal fluid in multiple sclerosis. *J Neurol Sci* 42(2):251, 1979

103. GUIBAUD S, BONNET M, THOULON JM, DUMONT M: Alpha $_1$-antitrypsin in amniotic fluid. *Obstet Gynecol* 45:35, 1975

104. TUTTLE WC, JONES RK: Fluorescent antibody studies of alpha $_1$-antitrypsin in adult human lung. *Am J Clin Pathol* 64:477, 1975

105. GADEK JE, ZIMMERMAN RL, FELLS GA, CRYSTAL RG: Antielastases of the human alveolar structures: Assessment of the protease-antiprotease theory of emphysema. *J Clin Invest* 68:889, 1981

105a. JONES EA, GADEK JG, VERGALLA J, CRYSTAL RG: Unpublished observations

106. ERIKSSON S: Proteases and protease inhibitors in chronic obstructive lung disease. *Acta Med Scand* 203:449, 1978

107. BEATTY K, BIETH J, TRAVIS J: Kinetics of association of serine proteinases with native and oxidized α_1-proteinase inhibitor and α_1-antichymotrypsin. *JBC* 255:3931, 1980

108. HECK LW, KAPLAN AP: Substrates of Hageman factor. I. Isolation and characterization of human factor XI (PTA) and inhibition of the activated enzyme by α_1-antitrypsin. *J Exp Med* 140:1615, 1974

109. HABAL FM, BURROWES CE, MOVAT HZ: Generation of kinin by plasma kallikrein and plasmin and the effect of α_1-antitrypsin and antithrombin III on the kininogenases. *Adv Exp Med Biol* 70:23, 1976

110. BIETH J: Elastases: Structure, function and pathological role. *Front Matrix Biol* 6:1, 1978

111. COLLEN D, DE COCK F, VERSTRAETE M: Immunochemical distinction between antiplasmin and alpha $_1$-antitrypsin. *Thrombosis Research* 7:245, 1975

112. LEARNED LA, BLOOM JW, HUNGER MJ: The antithrombin activity of α1-protease inhibitor: The antitrypsin activity of antithrombin III. *Thromb Res* 8:99, 1976

113. BIETH JG: Pathophysiological interpretation of kinetic constants of protease inhibitors. *Bull Eur Physiopathol Resp* 16:183, 1980

114. JOHNSON DA, TRAVIS J: Human alpha $_1$-proteinase inhibitor mechanism of action: Evidence for activation by limited proteolysis. *Biochem Biophys Res Commun* 72:33, 1976

115. OHLSSON K, LAURELL CB: The disappearance of enzyme-inhibitor complexes from the circulation of man. *Clin Sci Mol Med* 51:87, 1976

116. TOMASI TB, HAUPTMAN SP: The binding of α_1-antitrypsin to human IgA. *J Immunol* 112:2274, 1974

117. REMOLD HG, ROSENBERG RD: Enhancement of migration inhibitory factor activity by plasma esterase inhibitors. *J Biol Chem* 250:6608, 1975

118. ARORA PK, MILLER HC, ARONSON LD: α_1-Antitrypsin is an effector of immunological stasis. *Nature* 274:589, 1978

119. GOETZL EJ: Modulation of human neutrophil polymorphonuclear leucocyte migration by human plasma alpha-globulin inhibitors and synthetic esterase inhibitors. *J Immunol* 29:163, 1975

120. GADEK JE, HUNNINGHAKE GW, FELLS GA, ZIMMERMAN RL, KEOGH BA, CRYSTAL RG: Validation of the α-1-antitrypsin hypothesis: Recovery of active connective tissue-specific proteases from the lung of PiZ patients and reversal with α-1-antitrypsin replacement therapy. *Clinical Research* 29:550A, 1981

121. RENNARD SI, FERRANS VJ, BRADLEY KH, CRYSTAL RG: Lung connective tissue, in Witchi H (ed): *CRC Reviews, Pulmonary Toxicology* (in press), 1982

122. KEELEY FW, FAGEN DG, WEBSTER SI: Quantity and character of elastin in developing human lung parenchymal tissues of normal infants and infants with respiratory distress syndrome. *J Lab Clin Med* 90:981, 1977

123. STARKEY PM, BARRETT AJ: Human lysosomal collagenase. Catalytic and immunological properties. *Biochem J* 155:265, 1976

124. OHLSSON K: Granulocyte collagenase and elastase and their interactions with alpha $_1$-antitrypsin and alpha $_2$-macroglobulin, in Reich E, Rifkin D, Shaw E (eds): *Proteases and Biological Control.* Cold Spring Harbor, NY, Cold Spring Harbor Laboratory, 1975, p 591

125. WARD PA, TALAMO RC: Deficiency of the chemotactic factor inactivator in human sera with α_1-antitrypsin deficiency. *J Clin Invest* 52:516, 1973

126. HUNNINGHAKE GW, GADEK JE, FALES HM, CRYSTAL RG: Human alveolar macrophage-derived chemotactic factor for neutrophils: Stimuli and partial characterization. *J Clin Invest* 66:473, 1980

127. GADEK JE, HUNNINGHAKE GW, ZIMMERMAN RL, CRYSTAL RG: Regulation of release of alveolar macrophage-derived neutrophil chemotactic factor. *Am Rev Respir Dis* 121:723, 1980

128. HUNNINGHAKE GW, GADEK JE, CRYSTAL RG: Mechanism by which cigarette smoke attracts polymorphonuclear leukocytes to lung. *Chest* 77:237A, 1980

129. FRITZ H, SCHIESSLER H, GEIGER R, OHLSSON K, HOCHSTRASSER K: Naturally occurring low molecular weight inhibitors of neutral proteinases from PMN-granulocytes and of kallikreins. *Agents Actions* 8:57, 1978

130. TEGNER H: Quantitation of human granulocyte protease inhibitors in nonpurulent bronchial lavage fluids. *Acta Ottolaryingol* 85:282, 1978

131. LARSSON C: Natural history and life expectancy in severe, alpha $_1$-antitrypsin deficiency, PiZ. *Acta Med Scand* 204:345, 1978

132. HUTCHISON DCS: Homozygous and heterozygous alpha $_1$-antitrypsin deficiency: Prevalence in pulmonary emphysema. *Proc R Soc Med* 69:130, 1976

133. MITTMAN C: The PiMZ phenotype: Is it a significant risk factor for the development of chronic obstructive lung disease? *Am Rev Respir Dis* 118:649, 1978

134. GADEK JE, FELLS G, CRYSTAL RG: Cigarette smoking induces functional antiprotease deficiency in the lower respiratory tract in humans. *Science* 206:1315, 1979

135. JANOFF A, CARP H: Possible mechanisms of emphysema in smokers. Cigarette smoke condensate suppresses protease inhibition *in vitro. Am Rev Respir Dis* 116:65, 1977

136. JOHNSON D, TRAVIS J: The oxidative inactivation of human alpha $_1$-proteinese inhibitor. Further evidence for methionine at the reactive center. *J Biol Chem* 254(10):4022, 1979

137. Stableforth DE: Lung function in alpha $_1$-antitrypsin deficient sisters. *Br J Dis Chest* 72:125, 1978

138. GALDSTON M, MELNICK EL, GOLDRING RM, LEVYTSKA V, CURASI CA, DAVID AL: Interactions of neutrophil elastase, serum trypsin inhibitory activity, and smoking history as risk factors for chronic obstructive pulmonary disease in patients with MM, MZ and ZZ phenotypes for alpha $_1$-antitrypsin. *Am Rev Respir Dis* 116:837, 1977

139. KIDOKORO Y, KRAVIS TC, MOSER KM, TAYLOR JC, CRAWFORD IP: Relationship of leukocyte elastase concentration to severity of emphysema in homozygous α_1-antitrypsin-deficient persons. *Am Rev Respir Dis* 115:793, 1977

140. EDITORIAL: The pathogenesis of pulmonary emphysema. *Lancet* 1:743, 1980

141. BLACK LF, HYATT RE, STUBBS SE: Mechanism of expiratory airflow limitation in chronic obstructive pulmonary disease associated with α_1-antitrypsin deficiency. *Am Rev Respir Dis* 105:891, 1972

142. LARSSON C, BIRKSEN H, SUNDSTROM G, ERIKSSON S: Lung function studies in asymptomatic individuals with moderately (Pi SZ) and severely (Pi Z) reduced levels of α_1-antitrypsin. *Scand J Respir Dis* 57:267, 1976

143. RAWLINGS W JR, KREISS P, LEVY D, COHEN B, MENKES H, BRASHEARS S, PERMUTT S: Clinical, epidemiologic, and pulmonary function studies in alpha $_1$-antitrypsin-deficient subjects of Pi Z type. *Am Rev Respir Dis* 114:945, 1976

144. GUENTER CA, WELCH MH, RUSSELL TR, HYDE RM, HAMMARSTEN JF: The pattern of lung disease associated with alpha $_1$-antitrypsin deficiency. *Arch Intern Med* 122:254, 1968

145. THURLBECK WM, HENDERSON JA, FRASER RG, BATES DV: Chronic obstructive disease. A comparison between clinical, roentgenologic, functional and morphologic criteria in chronic bronchitis, emphysema, asthma and bronchiectasis. *Medicine* 49:81, 1970

146. FALLAT RJ, POWELL MR, KUEPPERS F, LILKER E: ^{133}Xe ventilatory studies in α_1-antitrypsin deficiency. *J Nucl Med* 14:5, 1972

147. STEIN PD, LEU JD, WELCH MH, GUENTER CA: Pathophysiology of the pulmonary circulation in emphysema associated with alpha $_1$-antitrypsin deficiency. *Circulation* 43:227, 1971

148. LARSSON C: Natural history and life expectancy in severe α_1-antitrypsin deficiency, PiZ. *Acta Med Scand* 204:345, 1978

149. SHARP HL, BRIDGES RA, KRIVIT W, FREIER EF: Cirrhosis associated with alpha $_1$-antitrypsin deficiency: A previously unrecognized inherited disorder. *J Lab Clin Med* 73:934, 1969

150. HODGES JR, MILLWARD-SADLER GH, BARBATIS C, WRIGHT R: Heterozygous MZ alpha $_1$-antitrypsin deficiency in adults with chronic active hepatitis and cryptogenic cirrhosis. *N Engl J Med* 304:557, 1981

151. SVEGER T: Liver disease in α_1-antitrypsin deficiency detected by screening of 200,000 infants. *N Engl J Med* 294:1316, 1976

152. YUNIS EJ, AGOSTINI RM JR, GLEW RH: Fine structural observations of the liver in α_1-antitrypsin deficiency. *Am J Pathol* 82:265, 1976

153. PALMER PE, GHERARDI GJ, BALDWIN JM, WOLFE HJ: Adult liver disease in SZ phenotype alpha ₁-antitrypsin deficiency. *Ann Intern Med* 88:59, 1978

154. GLASGOW JFT, LYNCH M, HERCZ A, LEVISON H, SASS-KORTSAK A: Alpha ₁-antitrypsin deficiency in association with both cirrhosis and chronic obstructive lung disease in two sibs. *Am J Med* 54:181, 1973

155. REINTOFT I, HAGERSTRAND IE: Does the Z gene variant of alpha ₁-antitrypsin predispose to hepatic carcinoma? *Hum Pathol* 10(4):419, 1979

156. SCHLEISSNER LA, COHEN AH: Alpha ₁-antitrypsin deficiency and hepatic carcinoma. *Am Rev Respir Dis* 111:863, 1975

157. COX DW, HUBER O: Association of severe rheumatoid arthritis with heterozygosity for alpha ₁-antitrypsin deficiency. *Clin Genet* 17(2):153, 1980

158. LONGSTRETCH GF, WEITZMAN MD, BROWNING RJ, LIEBERMAN J: Bronchiectasis and homozygous alpha ₁-antitrypsin deficiency. *Chest* 67:233, 1975

159. ROSENFELD S, GRANOFF DM: Pulmonary cavitation and Pi SZ alpha ₁-antitrypsin deficiency. *J Pediatr* 94:768, 1979

160. GEDDES DM, WEBLEY M, BREWERTON DA: α₁-Antitrypsin phenotypes in fibrosing alveolitis and rheumatoid arthritis. *Lancet* 1:1049, 1977

161. CRYSTAL RG, GADEK JE, FERRANS VJ, FULMER JD, LINE BR, HUNNINGHAKE GW: Interstitial lung disease: Current concepts of pathogenesis, staging and therapy. *Am J Med* 70:542, 1981

162. EVANS HE, KELLER S, MANDL I: Serum trypsin inhibitory capacity and the idiopathic respiratory distress syndrome. *J Pediatr* 81:588, 1972

163. SCHWARTZ RH, VAN ESS JD, JOHNSTONE DE, DREYFUSS EM, ABRISHAMI MA, CHAI H: Alpha ₁-antitrypsin in childhood asthma. *J Allergy Clin Immunol* 59:31, 1977

164. HARRIS CC, COHEN MH, CONNOR R, PRIMACK A, SACCOMANNO G, TALAMO RC: Serum alpha ₁-antitrypsin in patients with lung cancer or abnormal sputum cytology. *Cancer* 38:1655, 1976

165. LEWIS JH, IAMMARINO RM, SPERO JA, HASIBA U: Antithrombin Pittsburgh: An α₁-antitrypsin variant causing hemorrhagic disease. *Blood* 51:129, 1978

166. LIBERMAN J, BORHANI NO, FEINLEIB M: α₁-Antitrypsin deficiency in twins and parents-of-twins. *Clin Genet* 15:29, 1979

167. MOROZ SP, CUTZ E, BALFE JW, SASS-KORTSAK A: Membranoproliferative glomerulonephritis in childhood cirrhosis associated with alpha ₁-antitrypsin deficiency. *Pediatrics* 57:232, 1976

168. BREWERTON DA, WEBLEY M, MURPHY AH, WARD AM: The α₁-antitrypsin phenotype MZ in acute anterior uveitis. *Lancet* 1:1103, 1978

169. LANKISCH PG, KOOP H, WINCKLER K, KABOTH U: α₁-Antitrypsin in pancreatic diseases. *Digestion* 18:138, 1978

170. FREEMAN HJ, WEINSTEIN WM, SHNITKE TK, CROCKFORD PM, HERBERT FA: α-₁-Antitrypsin deficiency and pancreatic fibrosis. *Ann Intern Med* 85:73, 1976

171. PREVOST CL, FROMMEL D, DUPUY JM: Complement studies in alpha ₁-antitrypsin deficiency in children. *J Pediatr* 87:571, 1975

172. ANANTHAKRISHNAN R, BIEGLER B, DENNIS PM: Alpha ₁-antitrypsin phenotypes in paraproteinaemias. *Lancet* 1:561, 1979

173. PREMACHANDRA BN, YU SY: Association of prealbumin deficiency with alpha ₁-antitrypsin deficiency. *Metabolism* 28:890, 1979

174. GUANTI G, DI LORETO M: α₁-Antitrypsin quantitative and qualitative (Pi phenotyping) characterization in the Down syndrome subjects and in their parents. *Am J Hum Genet* 32:174, 1980

175. MCPHEE H, ANANTHAKRISHNAN R, TAFT LI: Antiproteases and Down's syndrome in an Australian population. *J Med Genet* 17:170, 1980

176. FINEMAN RM, KIDD KK, JOHNSON AM, BREG WR: Increased frequency of heterozygotes for α₁-antitrypsin variants in individuals with either sex chromosome mosaicism or trisomy 21. *Nature* 260:320, 1976

177. GELFAND EW, COX DW, LIN MT, DOSCH HM: Severe combined immunodeficiency disease in patient with alpha ₁-antitrypsin deficiency (letter). *Lancet* 2:593, 1979

178. BRANDRUP F, OSTERGAARD PA: α₁-Antitrypsin deficiency associated with persistent cutaneous vasculitis. *Arch Dermatol* 114:921, 1978

179. VICTORINO R, SILVEIRA JCB, GEADA H, MOURA MC: Familial hypercholesterolaemia with alpha ₁-antitrypsin deficiency. *Br Med J* 1:413, 1978

180. SCHYLDLOWER M, WAXMAN SH, PATTERSON PH: Coexistence of deficiency in alpha ₁-antitrypsin and in growth hormone. *N Engl J Med* 300:366, 1979

181. ANDRE F, ANDRE C, LAMBERT R, DESCOS F: Prevalence of alpha ₁-antitrypsin deficiency in patients with gastric or duodenal ulcer. *Biomedicine* 21:222, 1974

182. NICHOLLS MG, JANUS ED: Hashimoto's thyroiditis and homozygous alpha ₁-antitrypsin deficiency. *Aust N Z J Med* 3:516, 1973

183. HALAL F, SCHRIVER CR, COX DW, JABER L, VARSANO I: Cystathioninuria, renal iminoglycinuria and α₁-antitrypsin deficiency in the same family: Relevance in medical practice. *Can Med Assoc J* 121:64, 1979

184. EBERLE VF, ADLER G, KERN HF, MARTINI GA: Polypoid gastric heterotopy of the small intestine in a patient with primary hyperparathyroidism and alpha ₁-antitrypsin deficiency belonging to a MEA-family. With particular reference to the ultrastructure of the epithelial cells. *Z Gastroenterol* 17:354, 1979

185. RUBINSTEIN HM, JAFFER AM, KUDRNA JC, LERTRATANAKUL Y, CHANDRASEKHAR AJ, SLATER D, SCHMID FR: Alpha ₁-antitrypsin deficiency with severe panniculitis. *Ann Intern Med* 86:742, 1977

186. LEDOUX-CORBUSTER M, ACHTEN G: α₁-Antitrypsin deficiency and skin abnormalities. *J Cutan Pathol* 2:25, 1975

187. PALMER PE, WOLFE HJ, KOSTAS CI: Multisystem fibrosis in alpha ₁-antitrypsin deficiency. *Lancet* 1:221, 1978

188. AMBRUS CM, AMBRUS JL, COUREY N, MOSOVICH L, BRUCK E, ALLEN J, JUNG O, MIRAND E, NISWANDER K: Inhibitors of fibrinolysis in diabetic children, mothers, and their newborn. *Am J Hematol* 7:245, 1979

189. JEPPSON A: Use of amniocentesis to establish the Pi phenotype in utero. *N Engl J Med* 300:1441, 1979

190. FAGERHOL MK: Clinical relevance of PI typing and estimation of α₁-antitrypsin. *Inserm* 40:15, 1975

191. BOUSHY SF, ABOUMRAD MH, NORTH LB, HELGASON AH: Lung recoil pressure, airway resistance, and forced flows related to morphologic emphysema. *Am Rev Respir Dis* 104:551, 1971

192. GELFAND JA, SHERINS RJ, ALLING DW, FRANK MM: Treatment of hereditary angioedema with danazol: Reversal of clinical and biochemical abnormalities. *N Engl J Med* 295:1444, 1976

193. GADEK JE, HOSEA SW, GELFAND JA, FRANK MM: Response of variant hereditary angioedema phenotypes to danazol therapy. Genetic implications. *J Clin Invest* 64:280, 1979

194. GADEK JE, FULMER JD, GELFAND JA, FRANK MM, PETTY TH, CRYSTAL RG: Danazol-induced augmentation of serum alpha ₁-antitrypsin levels in individuals with marked deficiency of this antiprotease. *J Clin Invest* 66:82, 1980

195. GADEK JE, KLEIN H, HOLLAND PV, CRYSTAL RG: Replacement therapy of α-₁-antitrypsin deficiency: Reversal of protease-antiprotease imbalance within the alveolar structures of PiZ subjects. *J Clin Invest* 68:1158, 1981

196. JOHNSON AJ, KARPATKIN MH, NEWMAN J: Preparation of and clinical experience with antihemophilic factor concentrates. *Thromb Diath Haemorrh* 35 (suppl):49, 1969

197. JANEWAY CA, ROSEN FS: The gamma globulins. IV. Therapeutic uses of gamma globulin. *N Engl J Med* 275:826, 1966

198. GADEK JE, HOSEA SW, GELFAND JA: Replacement therapy in hereditary angioedema. Successful therapy in hereditary angioedema with partially purified CI inhibitor. *N Engl J Med* 302:542, 1980

199. POWERS JC, GUPTON BF, HARLEY AD, NISHINO N, WHITLEY RJ: Specificity of porcine pancreatic elastase, human leukocytes elastase and cathepsin-G. Inhibition with chloromethyl ketone peptides. *Biochim Biophys Acta* 485:156, 1977

200. ASHE BM, ZIMMERMAN M: Specific inhibition of human granulocyte elastase by cis-unsaturated fatty acids and activation by the corresponding alcohols. *Biochem Biophys Res Commun* 75:194, 1977

201. JANOFF A, DEARING R: Prevention of elastase-induced experimental emphysema by oral administration of synthetic elastase inhibitor. *Am Rev Respir Dis* 121:1025, 1980

202. KLEINERMAN J, RANGA V, RYNBRANDT D, IP MPC, SORENSEN J, POWERS JC: The effect of the specific elastase inhibitor alanyl alanyl prolyl alanine chloromethyl ketone, on elastase-induced emphysema. *Am Rev Respir Dis* 121:381, 1980

65

THE HEREDITARY AMYLOIDOSES

This summary is adapted from the summary written by George
C. Glenner, Thomas E. Ignaczak, and David L. Page for the 4th
edition of this book [1].

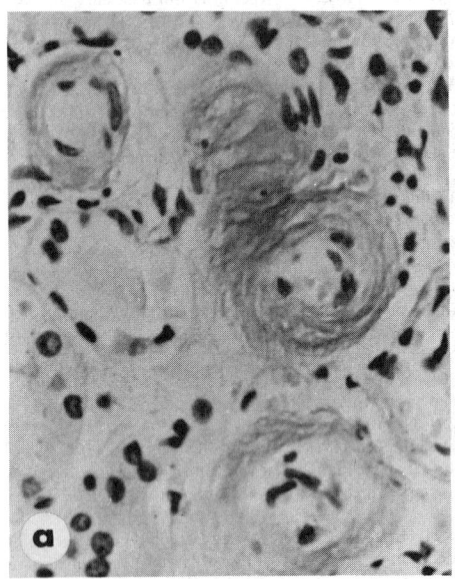
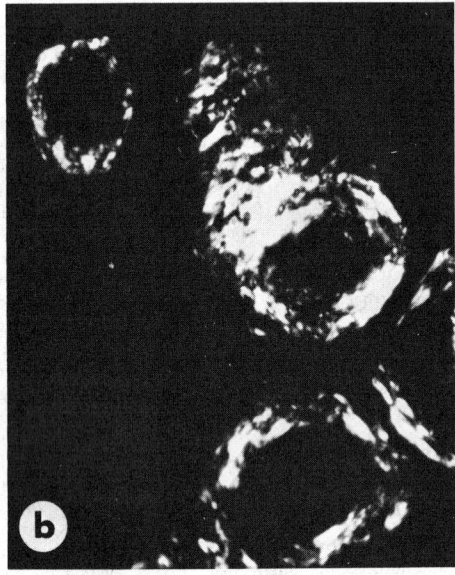

A. Congo red-stained section of renal
arterioles infiltrated with amyloid deposits
in a patient with the Portuguese neuropathic form of hereditary amyloidosis. *B.*
The same section viewed under polarized
light, demonstrating the birefringence of
amyloid. × 450.

1. The systemic amyloidoses are a group of diseases
caused by the extracellular deposition of twisted β-
pleated protein fibrils. These inert amyloid fibrils are
formed from various proteins by several different
pathogenic mechanisms. Their accumulation in tissues leads to pressure atrophy and cellular death,
causing interference with the normal metabolic functions of affected vital organs such as the heart and kidneys. The systemic amyloidoses occur in both acquired
and genetic forms.

2. In acquired systemic amyloidosis associated with multiple myeloma, patients have monoclonal immunoglobulin components in serum and urine. Almost
invariably, their amyloid fibrils are composed solely of
homogeneous light polypeptide chains of immunoglobulins (Bence Jones protein) or their amino terminal variable fragments, or both. In acquired systemic
amyloidosis associated with chronic inflammatory or
infectious processes (such as osteomyelitis, tuberculosis, or leprosy), patients almost invariably deposit
amyloid fibrils composed of a major protein, AA, having a molecular weight of 5000 to 9000 and a minor
lambda light polypeptide chain component. The serum
of these patients contains a protein, SAA, with a molecular weight of 180,000, which shares antigenic determinants with the AA protein. The AA protein is an

amino terminal fragment of SAA and is derived from it
by proteolysis.

3. The hereditary amyloidoses are a collection of familial
diseases that have in common the systemic deposition
of amyloid fibrils. Syndromes with predominantly neuropathic, nephropathic, or cardiopathic involvement
are recognized, but there is considerable overlap of
organ involvement in these diseases. Several neuropathic syndromes have been described: (1) a lower
limb neuropathy, characterized by progressively severe
neuronal degeneration with marked autonomic nervous system involvement and occurring in patients
from Portugal, Japan, and a family of Greek origin in
the United States; (2) a milder disease, characterized
by a carpal tunnel syndrome and vitreous opacities
and occurring in families of Swiss origin in Indiana
and of German origin in Maryland; and (3) a more
severe variety of generalized neuropathy, characterized
by the presence of renal amyloidosis and occurring in a
family of English-Irish-Scottish ancestry in Iowa. The
most common form of nephropathic amyloidosis
occurs in patients with familial Mediterranean fever.
Several large families with cardiopathic involvement
have been reported, one in a Danish family and another
in a family of Mexican-American origin.

4. All of the hereditary forms of amyloidosis are inherited

as autosomal dominant traits, with one exception. The exception is the amyloidosis of familial Mediterranean fever, which is inherited as an autosomal recessive trait and which occurs predominantly in people of Mediterranean ancestry, especially Sephardic Jews.

5. Among the genetically determined amyloidoses, only the proteins of the amyloid fibrils of familial Mediterranean fever and the Portuguese neuropathy have been defined. In familial Mediterranean fever, a major AA protein component and a minor light chain constituent are found, while in the Portuguese neuropathy a third class of amyloid fibril protein, FAP, also having an antigenically related serum component, has been detected. The "amyloidogenic" protein in each of the different heritable amyloidoses may, therefore, be a specific protein characteristic of the disease process.

6. There are no specific biochemical tests that enable the differentiation of one type of hereditary amyloidosis from the other. Thus, the diagnosis rests on the specific clinical pattern together with the demonstration of amyloid infiltration on biopsy specimens and historical evidence of familial involvement. The prognosis for the different syndromes is variable. There is no specific treatment.

REFERENCES

1. GLENNER G, IGNACZAK TE, PAGE DL: The inherited systemic amyloidoses and localized amyloid deposits, in Stanbury JB, Wyngaarden JB, Fredrickson DS (eds): *The Metabolic Basis of Inherited Disease*, ed 4. New York, McGraw-Hill Book Co, 1978, p 1308

2. GLENNER G: Amyloid deposits and amyloidosis. *N Engl J Med* 302:1282, 1333, 1980

3. MEYERHOFF J: Familial Mediterranean fever: Report of a large family, review of the literature, and discussion of the frequency of amyloidosis. *Medicine* 59:66, 1980

66

THE MUSCULAR DYSTROPHIES

STANLEY H. APPEL

ALLEN D. ROSES

1. The muscular dystrophies are genetically determined diseases with progressive muscular weakness as the most prominent clinical manifestation and with evidence of muscle degeneration on biochemical, histologic, and electromyographic examination. The most important types of muscular dystrophy are Duchenne's, limb girdle, facioscapulohumeral, and myotonic muscular dystrophy.

2. Each type of muscular dystrophy has a distinct clinical and genetic expression and is probably a separate inborn error of metabolism. The expression of these disorders is not limited to muscle but may involve several organ systems. Patients with myotonic muscular dystrophy, which is inherited as an autosomal dominant trait, may demonstrate functional defects of smooth, skeletal, and cardiac muscle, as well as functional defects of lens, retina, brain, pancreas, testis, ovary, skin, bone, gamma globulin, and red blood cells. Patients with Duchenne's muscular dystrophy, which is inherited as an X-linked recessive trait, have abnormalities of cardiac and skeletal muscle, as well as of brain and red blood cells.

3. Creatinuria is characteristic of the muscular dystrophies and is most pronounced in Duchenne's dystrophy. Serum creatine phosphokinase activity is similarly elevated in several of the muscular dystrophies but is most significantly increased early in the course of Duchenne's dystrophy.

4. The specific metabolic defect has not been defined in any of these disorders. Despite the lack of definitive data as to the primary biochemical defect, experimental evidence suggests that the muscular dystrophies represent genetically induced alterations, with prominent defects in the structure and function of the cellular membranes. Studies of red blood cells as well as skeletal muscle have contributed valuable information on the metabolic abnormalities.

5. There is no specific treatment for these dystrophic conditions.

The muscular dystrophies are genetically determined diseases with progressive muscular weakness as the most prominent clinical manifestation and evidence of characteristic muscle degeneration on electrical, biochemical, and histologic examination. They represent more than one clinical syndrome, each of which represents a separate inborn error of metabolism, with clinical expression in several organ systems in addition to muscle. The specific metabolic defect has not been defined in any of these disorders; as a result, their classification is primarily clinical. The grouping is based upon the mode of inheritance, the age of onset, the muscle groups involved, the rate of progression, and the clinical course (Table 66-1). Such a classification has been useful for determining prognosis and for genetic counseling (primarily in Duchenne muscular dystro-

Table 66-1 Classification of the major muscular
dystrophies

1. Sex-linked muscular dystrophies
   a. Duchenne's muscular dystrophy (DMD)
   b. Becker's muscular dystrophy
   c. Emery-Dreifuss dystrophy

2. Autosomal dominant muscular dystrophies
   a. Facioscapulohumeral muscular dystrophy (FSH)
   b. Myotonic muscular dystrophy (MyD)
   c. Distal muscular dystrophy
   d. Ocular muscular dystrophy (a heterogeneous array of cases,
      some with widespread systemic defects, others sporadic)
   e. Oculopharyngeal muscular dystrophy

3. Autosomal recessive muscular dystrophy
   a. Limb girdle (LG) muscular dystrophy (many varieties; some
      sporadic, others inherited as autosomal dominant)

phy), but it is still not completely satisfactory because of the
many clinical subvarieties which have been described. In the
discussion to follow, the major clinical syndromes are presented (Table 66-2). A short discussion of some of the recently
described lipid metabolic abnormalities is also included. Space
does not permit a detailed description of the wide range of less
common clinical syndromes associated with progressive and
nonprogressive degenerations of muscle.

Recent research advances in the muscular dystrophies have
led to a broadening of theories of pathogenesis. Considerable
effort has been expended to prove that the muscular dystrophies do not represent primary myopathies, but rather are the
result of either neuronal abnormalities which cause denervation and muscle degeneration or vascular lesions which compromise the blood supply to muscle. Both theories emphasize
the secondary nature of the deficits in muscle. These notions
are a modern recapitulation of the discussions on the neuropathic versus the myopathic etiology of the dystrophies first
presented in the nineteenth century, when the dystrophies were
described [1]. The available evidence is insufficient to support
either a primary neurogenic or a primary vascular hypothesis.

The clinical, pathologic, and biochemical data support a
widespread expression of the metabolic defects in many organ

systems, with muscle as the most prominent target organ. The
biochemical data suggest that the muscular dystrophies represent genetically induced primary as well as secondary alterations in the structure and function of cellular membranes. The
critical question, then, is not whether nerve or muscle is the
primary target of the genetic defect, but how and to what
extent the inherited metabolic disorder is expressed in all tissues, including nerve and muscle.

DUCHENNE'S MUSCULAR DYSTROPHY (DMD)

Genetics

Duchenne's muscular dystrophy (DMD) is the most widely
known of the muscular dystrophies and possesses the best-
defined and least variant clinical features and patterns of inheritance [2]. It is inherited as an X-linked recessive trait. Penetrance is complete, and no cases of partial expression have
been reported in known DMD families. Women carriers are
usually asymptomatic, but careful examination may reveal
physical signs and laboratory evidence of the carrier state (discussed below).

Severe dystrophy in young girls has been reported as indicating an autosomal recessive form of the disease. These latter
cases are sporadic, clinical signs develop later, and the disease
progresses more slowly [3]. One female with DMD whose case
has been well documented is an identical twin whose mother is
a definite carrier of DMD [4]. Several true cases of DMD in
females have also been reported in Turner's syndrome or in
other individuals with an X/O sex chromosome composition.
Recent cytogenetic findings in young affected females indicate
that the gene for DMD is located on the short arm of the X
chromosome at X (p 21) [4a, 4b].

A high spontaneous mutation rate has been postulated for
DMD [5] since affected males do not reproduce. Recent studies
suggest that many apparently isolated cases may involve sons
of carrier mothers rather than new mutations [6, 7]. Similar
data have been reported for other X-linked diseases in which

Table 66-2 The major muscular dystrophy syndromes

Disease	Mode of inheritance	Age at clinical onset	Usual distribution	Rate of progression	Mental retardation	Distinguished findings
Duchenne's dystrophy (DMD)	X-linked recessive	About 3 years	Hips and shoulders, quadriceps femoris, gastrocnemius (pseudohypertrophy)	Rapid	Frequent	Elevated serum enzymes (CPK, LDH, SGOT, aldolase)
Facioscapulo-humeral (FSH) dystrophy	Autosomal dominant	In first or second decade	Shoulder girdle, neck, face, pelvic girdle (late)	Moderate	Occasional	Several distinct muscle pathologies
Limb girdle (LG) dystrophy	Poorly defined or recessive	Variable	Pelvic and shoulder girdles	Variable	Variable	Collection of several diseases
Oculopharyngeal dystrophy	Autosomal dominant	In second or third decade	External ocular, pharynx, neck, pelvic	Slow	Unusual	
Myotonic dystrophy (MyD)	Autosomal dominant	Variable—birth to fifth decade	Distal extensor muscle, eyelids, face, neck, hands, pharynx	Slow, related to age at clinical onset, faster with younger patients	Frequent	Percussion myotonia, cataracts, diabetic GTT despite increased insulin, testicular atrophy, decreased IgG

better carrier detection tests are available, such as Lesch-Nyhan disease and hemophilia A [8, 9]. Until the inborn error in DMD is delineated, whether the new mutation took place in the ovum of the mother of an affected sporadic case will remain unresolved and give rise to diverse opinions with respect to genetic counseling.

Clinical Features

Muscle Abnormalities The symptoms of DMD are remarkably constant. Kinnier Wilson's description can hardly be improved [10] (Fig. 66-1). "Beginning in childhood or youth, the onset is so stealthy and the course so gradual that initial symptoms are often overlooked or misunderstood. Slight trouble in going upstairs or lifting the lower limbs is combined with a habit of keeping the back very straight. A keen eye will note how the knee is advanced in walking to neutralize weakness of extension of that joint. The child is not as sprightly on his or her feet as usual, and a trivial push may result in an unexpected fall. Rising from a seat, the child is observed to have a little trick of putting the hands on the thighs or on the sides of the chair to gain the erect position. In getting up from the floor, the child turns on the face and uses the arms to keep the legs and trunk successively fixed, thereby taking weight off affected muscles and disclosing weakness in the thighs, pelvis, girdle, and back. Lordosis follows progressive enfeeblement, forward tilting of the pelvis and protuberance of the abdomen being counteracted by bracing back of the shoulders and upper trunk. The cautious, slow, and slightly rocking gait, with head thrown back and arms a little abducted, gives the impression that insecure body segments are being carried in a kind of balancing act. To cite the alliterative phrase of an eminent neurologist, 'he straddles as he stands and waddles as he walks.' Should dystrophy first affect the upper limbs, 'looseness' of the shoulders will be noted. They are said to be 'growing out,' become visibly prominent through the child's clothing. Muscles fixing the scapulae to the thorax weaken, allowing the vertebral borders of the blades to stand out link wings. Lifted by the armpits, the child's shoulders come almost to the ears; at rest, upper scapular angles are in sight above the line of the neck."

As the disease advances, trunk muscle wasting becomes general, until the back looks almost like that of a skeleton. Pectoral atrophy hollows the chest *(thorax en bateau)*, throwing the inner ends of the collarbones into relief. Falling away of abdominal recti and obliques narrows the body between the lower ribs and iliac crests (the *wasp waist* or *taille de guepe*).

Progression of the disease is more rapid than in other forms of dystrophy. Initial signs are usually apparent as early as the child can be adequately tested. Most cases are diagnosed when the patient is between 3 and 6 years of age, although in retrospect, an earlier history of weakness can usually be obtained. Affected children are reported by mothers to have been easy to care for in infancy; they are not "wiggly" babies and stay in one place better than sibs. Subsequent patients in the same family can be detected by concerned parents and experienced observers within the first 2 years. As activity increases with running, climbing stairs, and interaction with other children, motor difficulties become more obvious (Fig. 66-2).

Following diagnosis there is usually a period when the rate of progression appears to be slower or halted. It is unfortunate that during this period many patients are followed up less frequently or even lost to follow-up until the child can no longer walk. The gait difficulties appear to stabilize for several years during periods of rapid growth, but subtle substitutions and adjustments are made by the patient that lead to delicately balanced ambulation. Later, deterioration seems rapid. During this period the pelvic musculature becomes progressively weaker. Patients gradually walk more on their toes due to contractures of the heel cord. Lordosis that had been mild now becomes more striking. The center of gravity shifts; patients have difficult maintaining their sense of balance and frequently fall. Any intercurrent illness that takes patients off their feet for even short periods of time hastens the development of contractures. The falls are produced by instability, rather than overt weakness, and may result in injuries that put these patients in bed. Some patients never walk again. The rate of heel cord contracture can be slowed by the use of lightweight plastic heel splints that can be worn in shoes and in bed. Treatment of contractures after they have developed is surgical (see below). A more helpful approach is to slow the development of contractures, thereby slowing the rate of the secondary changes in posture and prolonging the period of ambulation.

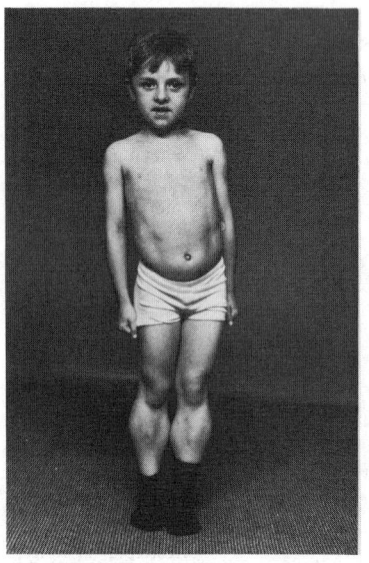
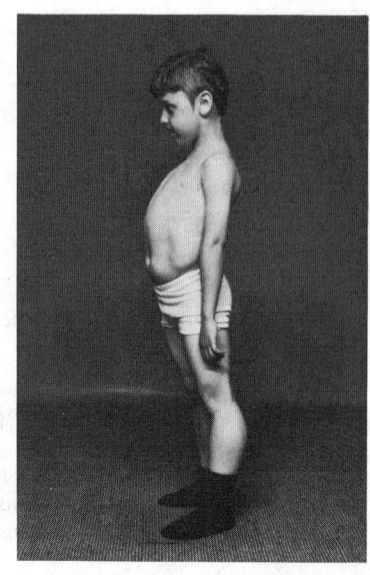

Figure 66-1 Seven-year-old patient with DMD. Note lordotic posture, distinct pseudohypertrophy of the calves, prominence of the shoulders, indication of winging of the scapula (lateral), and the prominence and narrowing of distance between the lower ribs and the iliac crests. This patient was able to maintain posture with feet together but demonstrates a marked waddling gait.

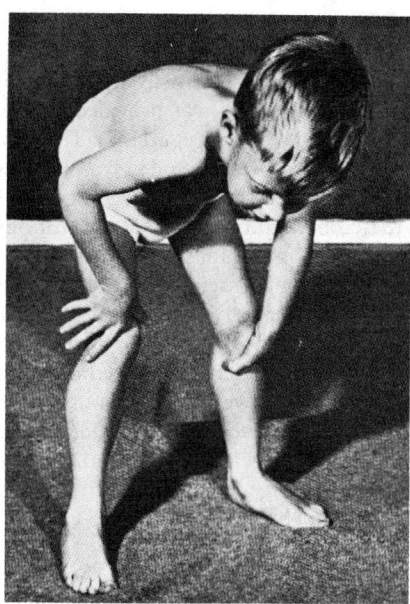

Figure 66-2 Proximal weakness in a 5-year-old boy with DMD, demonstrating hypertrophy of the calves and the characteristic method of attempting to assume the erect posture. (*Courtesy of Dr. J. D. Spillane.*)

The disease process can be remarkably specific, involving the sternocostal portions of the pectoralis muscle but sparing the clavicular portion. Similarly, the middle and lower trapezius may be affected and the upper trapezius relatively spared. The gastrocnemius muscles usually become enlarged because of infiltration by fat and connective tissue (pseudohypertrophy). Enlarged muscle fibers are also present early, so that true hypertrophy and pseudohypertrophy exist together [11]. Macroglossia may occur. Facial weakness may appear late. Proximal muscles become wasted before distal muscles, but advanced cases demonstrate both proximal and distal dystrophy. Deep-tendon reflexes are diminished and occasionally lost in the upper extremities and at the knees relatively early. Ankle jerks may persist. Contractures of the hip flexors, hamstrings, and biceps brachii develop later in the course of the disease, especially when the patient is no longer ambulatory. Hand, jaw, laryngeal, pharyngeal, and ocular muscles are relatively spared.

Cardiac Abnormalities   Cardiac involvement occurs in almost all patients [12–14]. Characteristic electrocardiographic (ECG) abnormalities of tall R waves in the right precordial leads and deep Q waves in the left precordial and limb leads are present early but do not seem to change significantly until late in the course [14, 15]. Tachycardia is common, and sudden death may occur. Chronic cardiac failure is uncommon, and presentation with congestive heart failure and acute pulmonary edema is rare. Careful cardiac examination may allow early detection of slight changes in cardiac function that are asymptomatic. New murmurs or gallop arrhythmias may develop insidiously. Cardiac enlargement on chest x-rays also occurs. Even though gross failure is not apparent, it may occur suddenly so that early therapy with digitalis may be helpful later in the course of the disease.

Mental Retardation   Recent studies have indicated a high frequency of mental retardation in DMD. In 30 percent of boys, the IQ is less than 75 [16]. This may be overemphasized by the motor and social effects of this severely crippling disease

[17]. The majority of patients are obviously slower mentally than their unaffected sibs. There appears to be no relationship between the severity and rate of progression of the dystrophy and the state of retardation. The mental defect is not progressive. A small minority of patients may be severely crippled but have normal or even superior intelligence.

Emery et al. attempted to separate DMD into several different clinical entities according to the degree of intellectual impairment and the rate of progression of the weakness [18]. In DMD patients with normal intelligence the onset of weakness and disease progression were more rapid than in those with impaired intelligence. However, the sample was too small to justify clinical characterization of distinct forms of the disease, and more specific biochemical markers than were provided in this report will be required to define the degree of disease heterogeneity.

Laboratory Findings

Diagnosis is facilitated by laboratory examination. The history and physical examination combined with elevated serum enzyme levels are virtually diagnostic. Aldolase (ALD), serum glutamic oxaloacetic transaminase (SGOT), lactic dehydrogenese (LDH), and creatine phosphokinase (CPK) activities may be increased (see below). CPK levels are especially elevated early in the course [19]. In addition, the previously described ECG findings are commonly present.

Electromyography (EMG) and muscle biopsy are usually performed to rule out Kugelberg-Welander disease [20] and lysosomal acid maltase deficiency (Pompe's disease). Reduction in the mean duration of motor unit potentials, increase in polyphasic forms, and a normal interference pattern on EMG may be present in DMD. Similar findings occur in other myopathies and thus are not specific for DMD [21]. Kugelberg-Welander disease presents with EMG features of neurogenic involvement. These include fibrillations, fasciculations, reduced number of motor unit potentials on voluntary effort, and an increase in the area of motor unit territory with the presence of high-voltage, long-duration potentials [20, 21]. Since a mild to moderate elevation of CPK may occur in Kugelberg-Welander disease [22] and a moderate CPK increase may occur in Pompe's disease, pathologic confirmation is needed in the first case in any pedigree.

Pathologic examination of muscle from a patient with DMD yields distinctive myopathic changes which permit differentiation from the neuropathic findings in Kugelberg-Welander disease and the evidence of abnormal glycogen storage in Pompe's disease [11]. Grossly, the muscle is pale, with obvious fat infiltration even early in the disease. The disappearance of muscle fibers and the great variation in the size of individual fibers are striking under the microscope [11a] (Fig. 66-3). Slightly affected muscle may demonstrate many hypertrophic fibers that appear swollen and rounded on cross section. Occasional contraction bands are noted. Hyalinization of large fibers with loss of striations occurs. Splitting of muscle fibers into daughter fibers is common. Each daughter fiber has a distinct sarcolemma within the same endomysial tube. Nuclei are usually increased in number, occur intracellularly, and vary in shape and staining characteristics. Bands of connective tissue and fat cells separate the atrophic muscle fibers. Grouped lesions, found in Kugelberg-Welander disease and other neuropathic syndromes, do not occur in DMD. Recent studies on nonne-

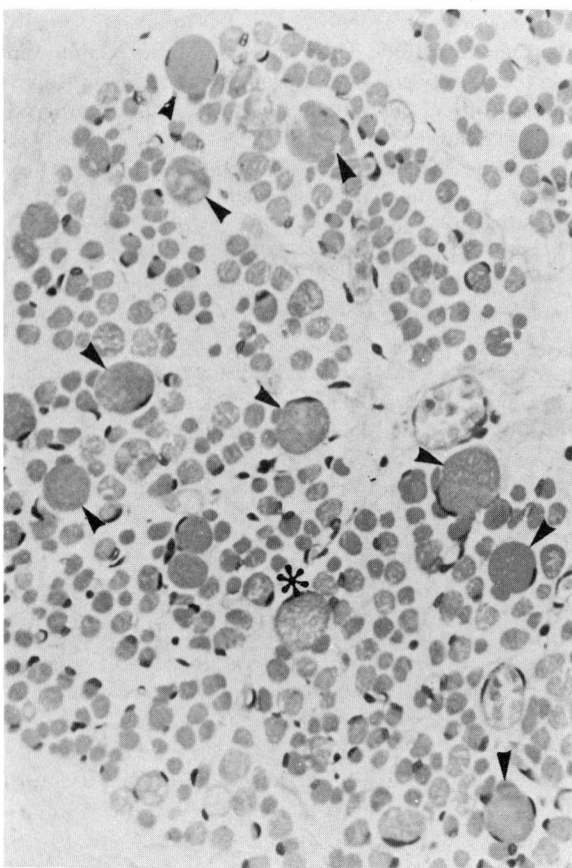

Figure 66-3 Quadriceps biopsy from the 2½-week-old affected son of a proven DMD carrier, who had been diagnosed at birth on the basis of a grossly elevated CPK activity in cord blood. This section shows considerable endomysial and perimysial fibrosis with scattered "hyaline" or hypercontracted fibers (arrows). Large normal fiber indicated by star. There was no evidence of phagocytosis of regeneration at this stage, although these features were abundant in a second biopsy that was done at age 28 months, when the child's CPK was markedly elevated. Hemotoxin and eosin stain magnified ×320 [11A]. (Courtesy of Dr. P. Hudgson.)

crotic muscle fibers with high-resolution phase microscopy demonstrate focal wedge-shaped lesions. Electron microscopy demonstrates the absence or disruption of the plasma membrane overlying the lesion, with preservation of the basement membrane (Fig. 66-4). An early, basic abnormality in the plasma membrane, possibly resulting in an ineffective cellular barrier, has been suggested by these studies [23].

The application of freeze fracture techniques to muscle obtained at biopsy has provided evidence for a decrease in the number of protoplasmic-face (P face) as well as extracellular-face (E face) intramembranous particles in skeletal muscle plasma membranes [24, 25]. The most dramatic change was in the number of orthogonal arrays. DMD biopsy specimens demonstrated 0 to 0.5 arrays per square micrometer, whereas control tissue demonstrated 13.2 arrays per square micrometer, with a mid-range of 6 to 22. Intramembranous particles were not decreased in the P or E face of muscle specimens from patients with facioscapulohumeral dystrophy or myotonic muscular dystrophy. However, alterations in membrane particles are not specific for DMD and the number of orthogonal arrays was decreased in facioscapulohumeral dystrophy, but not to the extent noted in DMD [24, 25]. Schotland's laboratory has demonstrated an alteration in the binding of lectins,

specifically concanavalin A, to muscle surface membranes in DMD [26].

An attempt to confirm the involvement of plasma membranes from different organs was provided by the studies of lymphocyte capping by Pickard et al. [27]. These investigators reported a decreased rate of capping in lymphocytes from carriers as well as patients with DMD. Several groups have failed to confirm these observations [28–31]. One of our laboratories (SHA) was able to demonstrate a slight but significant decrease in mean capping rate in DMD patients and carriers. The considerable overlap between control and DMD populations precludes the usefulness of this test for either diagnosis or further definition of the pathogenesis of this disorder.

Wakayama et al. [32] have reported that an increased number of satellite cells are present in DMD biopsy specimens and that the cells have an increased amount of euchromatin content. These changes were more evident in later stages of the disease, suggesting ineffective regenerative activity [32].

Treatment

A goal of research in DMD is the detection of carriers and the elimination of new cases by prenatal diagnosis. Affected males may be helped if the inborn error is amenable to intervention, but at present there is no treatment that slows the relentless progression of muscle destruction. Many drugs, including steroids, vitamins, and minerals, have been suggested, but none has met the test of time, safety, and experience [2, 23]. In fact, the side effects of several agents have complicated the course.

There are two avenues of therapeutic intervention that may help these patients. The course is characterized by rapid development of contractures, especially during periods of immobilization of intercurrent illnesses or surgery. Even without immobilization, contracture of calf muscles frequently results in toe walking, which, combined with pelvic girdle weakness, impairs balance and frequently leads to early confinement to a wheelchair. Prophylactic lightweight plastic splints allow contractures to be delayed and may prolong ambulation. Properly timed percutaneous heel cord lengthenings, ileotibial tract releases, and posterior-tibial tendon transfers combined with insistence on immediate postoperative ambulation and splints can significantly prolong walking [34]. Surgery alone without appropriate postoperative care can cause increased weakness and contractures in other areas, such as the hip flexors, and result in earlier wheelchair confinement.

Detection of Carriers

Approximately a third of DMD cases occur in families in which there is no history of any other affected males or any serum CPK elevation in the patient's mother. These cases have been presumed to result from spontaneous new mutations. A very high mutation rate (10×10^{-5} genes per generation) has been estimated [5]. Recent biological and clinical studies have suggested that spontaneous new mutations in mothers of patients are uncommon and that isolated cases of DMD may be the result of nondetection of genetic carriers [6, 7, 35].

The genetic studies suggesting this high mutation rate are based on analysis of DMD pedigrees. Three basic assumptions are made in the analysis: (1) the mutation rate is equal in males and females, (2) no heterozygote advantage exists, and (3) ascertainment of the pedigrees by clinical presentation is complete (no fetal wastage or preclinical deaths account for the lack of family history in previous generations).

Whether or not a sporadic case of DMD represents a new mutation or the first ascertained genetic case may not be answered until the inborn error is defined and carrier females can be accurately detected. The current implications for genetic counseling, including prenatal detection of male fetuses in carriers, make this question a real concern. The authors are not unbiased in this area [36].

There is suggestive evidence that more mothers of DMD sons are genetic carriers than would be estimated by the indirect method [6]. Since there are no independent corroborating experimental studies, this remains controversial. Mothers of DMD patients underwent careful manual muscle tests, and a surprisingly large proportion (90 percent) of carriers from DMD kindreds, as well as the same proportion of mothers of isolated cases, demonstrated weakness of muscle groups similar to the characteristic pattern of weakness and dystrophy in DMD patients [37, 38]. It should be emphasized that less than 10 percent of these women had symptomatic weakness, but they could be distinguished from controls by specific manual muscle-testing techniques. Increased erythrocyte membrane phosphorylation of a particular membrane protein under well-controlled experimental conditions was found in a group of mothers of isolated cases whose sons would have been expected to be new mutations, as well as in known carriers.

These experimental studies could not identify individual carriers but suggested that the group of carriers "expected" to be normal had biochemical data which in fact were different from those of matched controls but similar to those of known carriers [6].

Extensive testing of females in DMD pedigrees have demonstrated elevations of nonspecific but relatively sensitive serum enzymes such as CPK in relatives who usually do not undergo investigation if a large proportion of cases are assumed to result from new mutations [39]. Recent data concerning the effect of age on serum CPK make older studies in the literature difficult to evaluate [40–43], but we have demonstrated clearly elevated CPK levels in females tested solely because they were relatives of DMD patients, particularly cousins. There are statistical programs for evaluating pedigree and biochemical data, and it is clear that more complete studies of pedigrees from many clinics are necessary [44, 45]. It is hoped that an understanding of the specific inborn error will allow the development of more direct, specific, and sensitive carrier detection tests.

Prenatal Detection

It was recently postulated that fetoscopy might permit the use of fetal blood samples for measurement of CPK levels, and that prenatal detection of DMD in the male child might be possible as early as 20 weeks of gestation [46]. This has proved not to be a practical means of detection [45–49]. In a series of 24

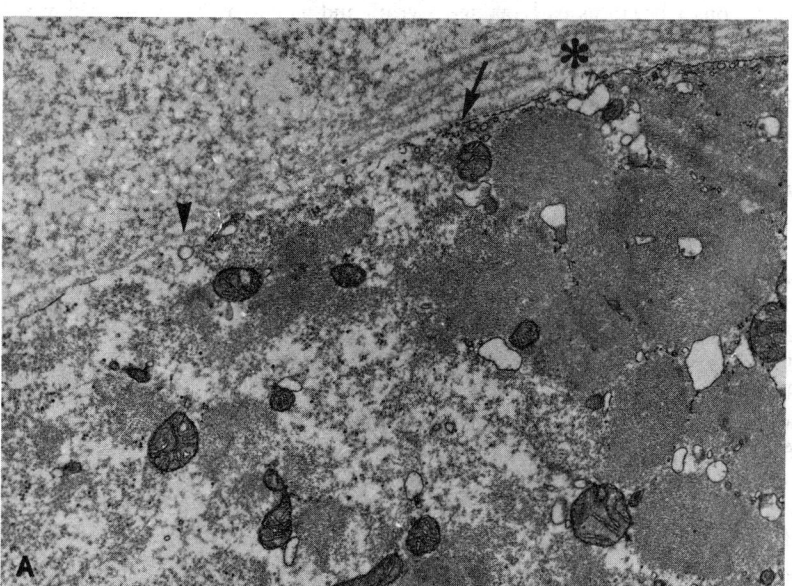

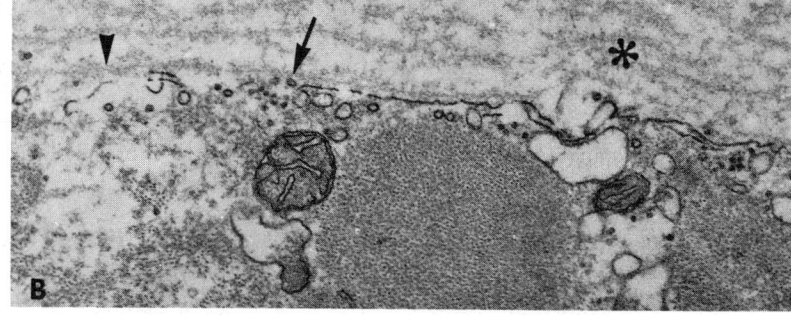

Figure 66-4 Electron micrograph of a superficially located lesion. Myofilaments are abnormally sparse in the affected region. Mitochondria are intact, while sarcotubular profiles are dilated in and around the abnormal region. There is an extensive defect in the plasma membrane over the lesion (to the left of the arrow). The transitional zone between the preserved and absent plasma membrane is shown at higher magnification in B. The basal lamina is preserved (arrowhead) in a sector from which plasma membrane is absent and is replicated over the right upper part of the fiber (asterisk). A, ×25,500; B, ×56,600. (*Courtesy of Drs. B. Mokri and A. G. Engel* [23].)

cases, blood samples of fetuses at risk were obtained through fetoscopy at or about the twentieth week of pregnancy. In three instances, the fetal serum CPK levels were considered to be normal, but at delivery cord blood CPK levels were abnormally high in two. A diagnosis was confirmed in one of these three cases by subsequent muscle biopsy and an elevated serum CPK level. In the second case, confirmatory studies were not done. In the third case, although the fetal CPK levels were normal, the pregnancy was terminated and the fetal muscle was judged to be dystrophic [48]. In another series of seven fetuses at risk, fetal blood was obtained by fetoscopy or prior to delivery by hysterotomy. In three fetuses the muscle was considered to be dystrophic, but only one of these had a raised serum CPK level [49].

The best methods at present are obviously inadequate for determining involvement or noninvolvement of a male fetus, and the false negatives are too frequent to justify fetal CPK as an effective diagnostic tool.

BECKER'S DYSTROPHY

Becker's dystrophy, inherited as an X-linked recessive trait, resembles DMD in its proximal weakness, calf enlargement, and elevated serum enzyme assay values [50]. Becker's dystrophy may account for approximately 10 percent of all X-linked dystrophies. Clinical symptoms usually begin between the ages of 5 and 10 years but in some families may begin earlier. In one series, onset began as early as age 3 years and as late as 21 years [51]. Since the presentation of symptoms may overlap with the age range of DMD, it may be difficult to give an accurate prognosis unless previous pedigree members were affected. Some authors have found quite similar clinical patterns within a pedigree, while others have noted some families with more phenotypic variation. We and others have found families in which two brothers have strikingly different clinical courses. In one of our sibships, in which the mother immigrated from Germany, and was the sister of one of Becker's patients, the older son is still able to walk with difficulty at age 20, while the younger son has been in a wheelchair since age 11. They were diagnosed at age 7 and 5 years, respectively. Thus, there appears to be a wider range of disease expression in the Becker form of X-linked dystrophy than in DMD. Affected boys without a family history may be diagnosed as having DMD until their clinical pattern has been followed up for a number of years. Whether or not DMD and Becker's dystrophy are allelic or represent different gene mutations has been discussed in the literature, but these analyses have been based on clinical criteria. It is possible that each clinical group may consist of several distinct biochemical defects. For the present, care must be exercised in diagnosing DMD without considering the more favorable prognosis of Becker's dystrophy.

The early presymptomatic signs of Becker's dystrophy include large calves and a tendency to toe-walk. Early symptoms include an abnormal gait with difficulty in climbing stairs. With some differences in detail, the pattern of progression is quite similar to that of DMD, but with an extended time frame. The abnormalities of the ECG found in DMD have been found with less constancy in Becker's dystrophy. Mabry et al. reported a genetic isolate with late onset, slow progression,

and frequent ECG abnormalities; it is unclear whether this family is distinct from Becker's dystrophy [52].

Most pathologists find the histologic changes of Becker's dystrophy to be essentially identical to those of DMD. Some authors have suggested clues to differentiate these conditions, but it is difficult to do so prospectively, selectively, and accurately.

EMERY-DREIFUSS DYSTROPHY

Emery-Dreifuss X-linked humeroperoneal dystrophy, with early neck, elbow, and ankle contractions and cardiomyopathy, probably warrants a distinct designation [53]. Affected individuals are relatively rare, and there is confusion as to whether or not particular families in the literature belong in this classification. Contractions at the elbows with proximal arm weakness, onset between the ages of 2 and 10 years, toe walking and distal leg weakness appearing later, and a prolonged clinical course characterize this disease. Cardiac abnormalities may be asymptomatic, or palpitations and syncope may occur. Cardiac arrhythmias are thought to be a common cause of death in affected males, who usually, but not always, had previously been symptomatic.

The patients have a distinct clinical presentation. They are usually thin and have restricted neck flexion, contractures at the elbows and knees, and wasting of the upper arms. Biceps and triceps are weaker and more wasted than the scapular and deltoid muscles. This finding may be useful in separating this group from the scapuloperoneal atrophies and dystrophies. Distal leg muscles are usually affected before proximal muscles.

FACIOSCAPULOHUMERAL (FSH) MUSCULAR DYSTROPHY

Genetics

Facioscapulohumeral (FSH) muscular dystrophy is inherited as an autosomal dominant trait. Variation of clinical expression within families is common. In some patients, the disease may be mild and relatively asymptomatic. FSH patients present with relatively uniform symptoms and signs, although with a significant variation in the degree and age of onset of clinical manifestations. For many years FSH was considered one of the better examples (like DMD) of a muscular dystrophy which probably was a single disease entity. Widespread application of EMG and muscle pathology to patients with FSH has shown that families who have virtually identical clinical disease have an array of differing pathologic and EMG features. Thus, there may be a number of distinct biochemical defects responsible for the phenotypic clinical expression of FSH [54].

Clinical Features

Symptoms of facial or shoulder girdle weakness usually appear in adolescence, but signs of the disease may be apparent in early childhood. The first difficulties may be in whistling or closing the eyes; weakness of the shoulder girdle, apparent during lifting or raising the arms overhead, is also a common initial complaint. Facial weakness may be prominent, but ocular and tongue muscles and those of mastication are spared. Dour faces with protuberant lower lips, prominent eyes, and winged scapulas are frequent. Specific portions of muscles are involved in FSH dystrophy. The sternal head of the pectoral muscle is usually much weaker and more wasted than the clavicular head. In addition, the lower trapezius is more severely involved that the upper. These patterns are common to DMD and FSH dystrophy but are not invariable in either. The supraclavicular triangle appears enlarged, with the clavicles parallel to the floor and the superior margins of the scapula visible from the front. The course and progression of the disease are exceedingly variable, but patients continue to walk because of the relative sparing of the pelvic girdle. Lordosis may develop as the disease progresses, and anterior tibial involvement may also occur early in the course.

Considerable pathologic variation segregates some families with FSH from others with clinically indistinguishable presentations. Figure 66-5 presents the pedigree of a family first reported by Hudgson et al. [55]. Muscle mitochondria demonstrated bizarre structural abnormalities. Multiple members of this family presented with the clinical picture of FSH, and all had similar mitochondrial abnormalities [56]. Other families have had inflammatory changes similar to those of polymyositis associated with hypertrophy of type 2 fibers. This suggests that an inflammatory phase may exist in some patients and in some families with FSH [57]. Patients from other families may show only occasional small, rounded type 1 fibers scattered throughout the biopsy specimen, while others may demonstrate small angular fibers reminiscent of denervations [58]. One of our clinics (ADR) has identified a family in which all affected individuals have absence of muscle phosphorylase activity. Distinctive pathologic changes seem to run true within members of families, while similar nonspecific alterations may be seen in most cases. This generalization seems to suggest that FSH consists of a number of distinct pathologic entities that no doubt represent heterogeneity of genetic defects.

Adding further confusion to this group of diseases are the scapuloperoneal syndromes. There may be considerable overlap with FSH with respect to clinical presentation. These patients usually have weakness of the scapular suspension muscles and the anterior tibial and peroneal muscles. Facial weakness may be present but is usually not prominent. There has been great difficulty in classifying these families as having dystrophies or neurogenic atrophies. Whether or not the patients represent a variant of FSH, or whether they are dystrophic or atrophic, are probably moot points. Affected individuals in different families may show considerable variation of phenotypic expression, suggesting that this group of syndromes consists of a number of genetic entities. This possibility is also supported by the finding of an X-linked form of the scapuloperoneal syndromes [59].

LIMB GIRDLE (LG) SYNDROMES

Limb girdle (LG) syndromes, a variety of muscular dystrophy, have an extremely variable clinical expression [60, 61]. Undoubtedly, many separate diseases have been clinically assigned to this group because they did not fit the clinical picture of DMD or FSH dystrophy. In the absence of definitive biochemical data, the classification of LG dystrophy serves as a repository for many proximal myopathies of unknown causes and variable patterns of inheritance. Nevertheless, there are several large genetic isolates with well-documented LG dystrophy inherited as an autosomal recessive trait [62].

Genetics

Autosomal dominant and recessive varieties of LG dystrophy have been reported. Many patients have no positive family history, and autosomal recessive inheritance has been assumed. Muscular dystrophy in young girls that has been labeled *DMD with autosomal recessive inheritance* probably belongs to this category. When examined in isolation from any known DMD relative, these patients may be classified as having LG dystrophy [63]. Female carriers of DMD, who are mosaics because of X inactivation (Chap.1), would be expected to show symp-

Figure 66-5 Pedigree of a family with facioscapulohumeral (FSH) muscular dystrophy. *(Courtesy of Dr. P. Hudgson [56].)*

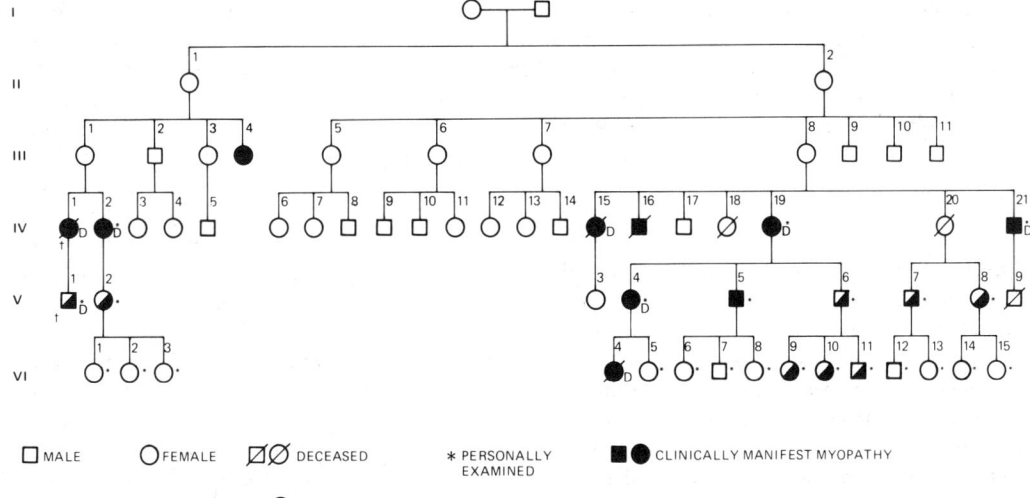

toms and signs of dystrophy dependent on the proportion of cells expressing the X chromosome bearing the DMD gene. Pedigree testing in our clinic (ADR) has demonstrated X-linked inheritance in several cases of so-called LG dystrophy who are probably "manifesting carriers" of DMD with no affected male relatives. In brief, LG dystrophy represents a variety of diseases that remain to be adequately delineated.

Clinical Features

The majority of patients classified as having LG dystrophy initially show involvement of either shoulder or pelvic girdle muscles, but both sites eventually become involved. Hypertrophy of the calves, lateral vasti muscles, or deltoids may occur. Distribution of weakness may be similar to that in DMD, but occasionally involvement is asymmetric, and progression is much slower. The tendency to contractures is less, although if a patient is in bed for an extended period, they do occur. Cardiac involvement and mental retardation are uncommon.

It is necessary to differentiate LG dystrophy from nonprogressive myopathies such as nemaline and central core disease or from muscle glycogenoses, polymyositis, Kugelberg-Welander disease, and metabolic myopathies such as those secondary to thyrotoxicosis and steroid therapy. Myopathic EMG and muscle biopsy findings are helpful in this respect. Serum enzyme levels are usually normal or moderately (polymyositis) elevated. No inborn error of metabolism has been described in any clinical subvariety. The uncertainties concerning LG syndromes have been recently reviewed [60].

MYOTONIC DYSTROPHY (MyD)

Genetics

Myotonic dystrophy (MyD) is inherited as an autosomal dominant trait with high penetrance and variable expression. The MyD gene is known to be closely linked to the ABH-secretor locus and loosely to the Lutheran blood group locus. The MyD-secretor-Lutheran linkage has been provisionally assigned to chromosome 19 [63a]. Severely affected infants and children are usually the products of affected mothers. Cases due to new mutations are uncommon. Studies of many large kindreds have demonstrated greater apparent expression of the disease in subsequent generations. The biochemical basis for such apparent "anticipation" is not known and it is thought to be an artifact of ascertainment and observation.

Clinical Features

The clinical presentation of MyD is extremely variable [64–67]. A diffuse constellation of symptoms and signs may be expressed fully in some individuals, while in others the clinical picture consists only of cataracts or a symptom such as dysphagia (Table 66-3). The completely developed pattern of muscular involvement distinguishes MyD from other dystrophies. The age at onset in Thomasen's series was 18 years [64]. The cranial musculature is prominently affected. Weakness

and atrophy of temporal, facial, and masticatory muscles give the face an elongated, lean appearance that has been called *hatchet facies* (Fig. 66-6). Weakness may occur in the levator palpebrae, pharyngeal, laryngeal, esophageal, and cervical musculature. Wasting of the sternocleidomastoid muscles and weakness of neck flexion are especially prominent. In the extremities the weakness is characteristically distal rather than proximal, and extensor muscles are more involved than flexor muscles. Fine movements of the hands are impaired by both wasting and myotonia. Bilateral incomplete foot drop is common. Gradually proximal weakness occurs, and the patient becomes unable to walk. Respiratory muscle weakness may lead to alveolar hypoventilation [68].

Myotonia, the sustained contraction of muscle, has been the focus of many investigations. It may be seen in patients with very little weakness or prior to the development of weakness, or it may be prominent in patients with the full spectrum of clinical involvement [64–67]. As the disease progresses and the extent of dystrophy increases, the myotonia tends to diminish, especially in the most severely affected muscles. Difficulties with handwriting, releasing door handles or bottle caps, and releasing after shaking hands are frequent complaints. Myotonia is usually demonstrated by percussion of the thenar eminence or tongue (percussion myotonia) or by asking the patient to release after forced grasp (action myotonia). Action myotonia may be present in the levator palpebrae muscles, as well as in hand, facial, pharyngeal, and esophageal musculature. Percussion myotonia is usually most prominent in the thenar eminence and tongue, but is also occasionally elicited from proximal musculature. Myotonia increases in cold weather and decreases with repetitive use. The latter is called the *warm up* phenomenon.

When MyD occurs in childhood, it is associated with early feeding problems, facial diplegia, dysphagia, dysphonia, and mental retardation [69, 70]. Children with congenital MyD are almost always the offspring of affected mothers [71]. The weakness begins proximally and then gradually involves distal musculature. Myotonia and cataracts are less prominent in these young patients than in those with adult onset. Agenesis of the diaphragm with diffuse myopathic muscle disease led to death within hours after birth in a child of an affected mother [72].

Abnormalities appear in many organ systems as well as in muscle, and they suggest a defect of membranes. Mental retardation is common in affected family members [64–67, 73, 74]. Personality changes make it difficult to provide good medical follow-up and care. The patients appear reticent, suspicious, and relatively unconcerned about their degree of deficit and the rate of progression of the disorder. Cardiac involvement is present in a high percentage of cases and may explain the sudden death in family members [75–78]. Bony abnormalities occur in the skull [65]. These include hyperostosis, large sinuses, small sella turcica, and a large jaw. IgG levels are decreased secondary to increased catabolism [79, 80]. Endocrine changes are frequently noted. These include testicular atrophy in approximately 80 percent of males after the attainment of sexual maturity [64], reduced 17-ketosteroid excretion in the urine, atrophy and hyalinization of the seminiferous tubules, and hyperplasia of interstitial cells [65, 81]. Ovarian fibrosis and dysfunction are present in many females. Decreased basal metabolic rate without evidence of thyroid dysfunction is frequently noted [64–67, 81, 82], as are abnor-

Table 66-3 Clinical and laboratory findings in myotonic dystrophy

Organ or system	Clinical findings	Laboratory findings
Muscle	Myotonia, weakness, dystrophy	Electromyography: decreased resting membrane potential; repetitive depolarization ("dive bomber" sound) Pathology: sarcoplasmic masses, ringed fibers, internal nuclei, frequent; nuclei often in chains; large variation in fiber size
Heart	Bradycardia common; complete heart block frequent; prolonged P-R interval	First-degree heart block, bradycardia on ECG; abnormal vectorcardiogram; SA node, right and left bundle branch dysfunction, and increased His-Purkinje conduction (His bundle studies)
Lens	Post- or subcapsular, scintillating cataracts	Dustlike cataracts (possibly visible only on slit lamp examination)
Eye	Decreased vision (independent of cataracts and diabetic retinopathy)	Pigmentary disorders of macula, keratosis, sicca; decreased intraocular pressure
CNS	Mental retardation, distinctive personalities	Possible neuronal heterotopias
Endocrine system	Diabetes mellitus; testicular (and ovarian) atrophy	Abnormal glucose tolerance with elevated insulin levels; gonadal fibrosis (pathology), decreased 17-ketosteroids (occasional); decreased metabolic rate, normal thyroid hormone levels
Integument	Frontal balding	
Gastrointestinal system	Dysphagia, abdominal pain	Disordered esophageal and gastric peristalsis; dilation of intestine
Skeletal system	Cranial and facial abnormalities; malocclusion of dentition	Cranial bony abnormalities, hyperostosis of skull (localized or diffuse), small sella turcica, large sinuses
Blood	None	Abnormal erythrocyte-scanning electron microscopy; decreased phosphorylation of erythrocyte protein peak III; decreased ouabainresponsive sodium efflux; increased fluidity of membrane (electron spin resonance spectroscopy)

malities of glucose tolerance [81, 83, 84]. Loss of hair resembling male pattern baldness occurs in most males and some females [64]. Eye findings include stellate opacities of the posterior lens, pigmentary disorders of the macula, keratosis sicca, decreased intraocular pressure, and abnormal iris vasculature [64–67, 90]. Smooth muscle of the gastrointestinal tract is clearly involved [78, 85, 86]. Difficulty in swallowing, impairment of esophageal motility, and gastric peristalsis and dilation of the colon have been reported in numerous cases [66, 67].

Cataracts Posterior subcapsular iridescent, dustlike cataracts are found in over 90 percent of adult patients and may often be the only clinical expression of the disease [64 67]. Furthermore, they are so characteristic that they may be considered pathognomonic of MyD. These cataracts do not often interfere with vision. They are usually apparent only upon slit lamp examination. When the patient complains of visual disturbances, physicians should be alerted to the possible complication of diabetic cataracts or macular degeneration. Lens opacification has been linked to an alteration of the cation pump in the epithelial cell layer in hereditary cataracts in mice. The opacification was thought to be due to membrane alterations which cause an imbalance of Na^+ and K^+ and an accumulation of calcium inside the lens [87]. Similar structural and functional abnormalities of the membrane may help explain cataract formation in MyD [88, 89].

Abnormal Glucose Tolerance In many patients with MyD, oral glucose tolerance test results are abnormal [83]. Fasting blood sugar values are normal, but the peak glucose values occur 2 h after glucose administration. Intravenous glucose tolerance tests show glucose disappearance constants significantly lower than in normal subjects. Fasting plasma

insulin levels are elevated. Insulin secretion is markedly exaggerated in response to glucose, glucagon, and tolbutamide [84]. Following tolbutamide administration, the excessive insulin secretion reduces blood sugar to only 65 percent of the fasting level. These observations suggest the possibility that endogenously secreted insulin is either structurally different from normal human insulin or has an abnormal peripheral action. The immunologic properties of plasma insulin from patients with MyD are no different from those of normal human insulin; responses to exogenous nonhuman insulin are normal in MyD patients. Recent data have demonstrated that insulin binding by monocytes is altered in MyD [91, 92]. Changes in both number and affinity of receptor binding sites have been reported and may reflect the down regulation of the receptor secondary to increased circulating insulin rather than a primary abnormality in the receptor itself. Nevertheless, these data do add to the evidence demonstrating diverse membrane involvement [93].

It is of interest that in MyD both muscle and pancreas have exaggerated responses of their normal physiologic functions. In muscle, repetitive depolarization of the surface membrane follows normal nerve stimulation and leads to tetanic contraction. A similar membrane abnormality in pancreatic cells might convert a normal glucose signal into an excessive insulin release.

Recent studies in experimental animals demonstrate that the plasma membranes of pancreatic β cells possess a high potassium permeability (P_K) in the absence of glucose [94, 95]. This permeability appears to be activated by calcium. Quinine blocks the calcium-activated P_K, depolarizes the β cell membrane, and increases input resistance. Inhibitors of mitochondrial energy metabolism raise intracellular calcium and stimulate the P_K. Glucose appears to act like quinine, and insulin release is associated with decreased P_K and membrane depo-

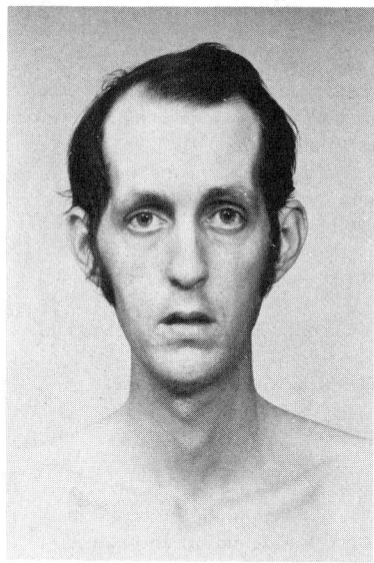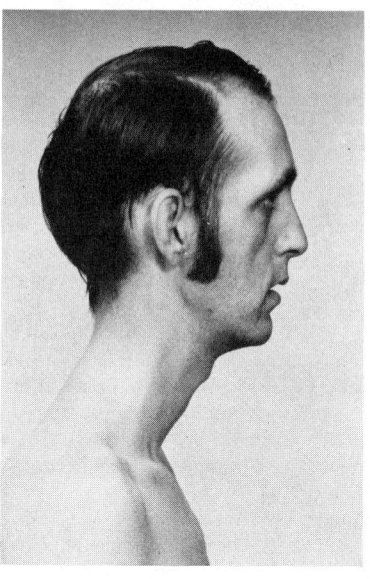

Figure 66-6 Patient P.P. with MyD, age 26 years. The patient has frontal balding, wasting of temporalis and sternocleidomastoid muscles, and weakness of facial musculature.

larization. The enhanced insulin release in MyD may thus reflect an impairment of calcium-activated P_K.

Heart Cardiac involvement occurs in about two-thirds of patients [66, 67, 75–78]. Variable expression characterizes heart involvement, and it is possible to have syncope and laboratory evidence of conduction defects before skeletal muscle myotonia or dystrophy are symptomatic. Sudden death, not only in symptomatic patients but particularly in undiagnosed or preclinical relatives, is fairly common in pedigrees. Episodic presyncopal symptoms in MyD patients or relatives should be taken more seriously than such complaints in the general population [78].

Progressive disease in the His-Purkinje system has been demonstrated in MyD patients who were free of any symptoms of cardiac involvement. Serial electrophysiologic studies (His bundle electrograms) of nine patients over a 3-year (mean) period demonstrated progression of conduction disease [78]. The His-ventricular (HV) interval was prolonged in three patients at the initial study and in seven patients at the final study. Of the nine patients, only the two with a normal PR interval had a normal HV interval. Thus, presyncopal symptoms in an MyD patient or relative at risk who has an increased PR interval on an ECG should be thoroughly evaluated. In addition, pedigree studies should include careful cardiac histories and ECG examination in order to detect preclinical MyD patients at risk for conduction defects and possible sudden death. Evidence of disease in the conduction system has also been demonstrated by histopathologic studies of cardiac biopsy specimens [96–98]. Pacemakers have been implanted in several presyncopal patients with abnormal electrophysiologic studies to protect against complications of complete heart block. During the follow-up period, several demand pacemakers have become operational.

Several other techniques have been used to identify MyD patients and relatives at risk for cardiac complications, including long-term ambulatory monitoring, ECG, vectorcardiography, and radionuclide angiography. In one recent series nine MyD patients who had no cardiac symptoms (mean age 35 years) were investigated with radionuclide angiography at rest and with exercise. All patients had abnormal results [99]. Three patients demonstrated asyneresis in the inferior, apical, or anterior left ventricular wall motion at rest, and five patients had normal left ventricular wall motion at rest but demonstrated asyneresis with exercise. Six of eight patients who achieved an adequate exercise performance demonstrated an abnormal drop in their left ventricular ejection fraction with exercise, including the single patient who had normal left ventricular wall motion [99]. Family members at risk are being tested to determine if cardiac complications can be anticipated before overt clinically diagnostic manifestations of MyD appear.

Laboratory Tests

Diagnosis of MyD is relatively straightforward in the presence of a positive family history and full clinical expression of the disorder. Many diagnostic procedures are of considerable help when the clinical presentation is more limited. The slit lamp examination, EMG studies, ECG studies (including His bundle examination), elevated insulin levels in response to a glucose load, and decreased serum IgG all aid in the diagnosis. Serum enzyme values of CPK, SGOT, and LDH are usually normal. As in the other muscular disorders, EMG and muscle biopsy have been extremely useful as diagnostic procedures.

In families with no history of parental involvement, the disease has been diagnosed in affected individuals by combinations of physical examinations, laboratory examinations (including slit lamp and EMG studies), and genetic mapping. Research blood tests have been evaluated in these genetic studies. Family S illustrates the pleiotropic expression of the disease (Fig. 66-7).

Patients IIIa and IIIb were investigated during a research study in 1968. Both have typical MyD with myotonia, dystrophy, cataracts, IgG abnormalities, and abnormal muscle biopsy specimens. Patient IIb and his wife were investigated clinically (including EMG studies), and neither could be documented as the genetic carrier. At the time, a "negative" family history was obtained. Patient Ia was living, had cataracts (not typical) and decreased IgG, and no other physical signs. He subsequently died from alcoholic liver disease and bleeding esophageal varices. His brother, patient Ib, had died suddenly years earlier but was diagnosed as having Parkinson's disease, with stiff hands, an abnormal gait, and no tremor. A visit to the home of patient IIc revealed a man with typical MyD complete with a fully developed reticence and suspicion of physicians.

When first examined in 1971, when the oldest patient, IVa,

was 11 years old, the six children in generation IV had no symptoms. Clinical examination and EMG were normal at that time. Examination in 1975 revealed percussion myotonia, early cataracts, and increased insertional activity on EMG examination. Subsequent examinations have documented myotonia in two additional children, patients IVc and IVe, with signs appearing in asymptomatic individuals during the teenage years.

Early diagnosis of affected individuals is an important goal since cardiac difficulties with sudden death may be the first indication of MyD in a small number of active, young family members who were otherwise asymptomatic. Individuals at risk may be suspected early by finding a prolonged PR interval and prolongation of the HV conduction interval.

Prenatal prediction of the inheritance of MyD is possible in a small minority of patients when analysis of linkage to the secretor gene (determining ABH substances) can be performed. This method requires complicated genetic testing of the affected spouse and the unaffected mate and their families. As a practical matter, prenatal prediction is presently feasible in only 5 to 10 percent of families.

Pathology of Muscle

Muscle biopsy specimens from patients with MyD demonstrate characteristic myopathic changes which are helpful in diagnosis, although they are not totally specific [11, 100, 101]. Variation in fiber size, increased numbers of internal nuclei, evidence of degeneration and regeneration, the presence of connective tissue and fat replacement, and sarcoplasmic masses and ring fibers are commonly described by light microscopy. Characteristically, type I fibers show more atrophy than other types [102]. By electron microscopy, alterations are noted in the Z line and there is a general myofibrillar degeneration [103, 104]. The sarcoplasmic masses on light microscopy consist of myofibrils, vesicles, mitochondria, and other cytoplasmic constituents which presumably represent evidence of regeneration [105, 106]. Ringbinden appear as normal myofibrils in an altered orientation [107]. Abnormalities in muscle membranes have also been described. Enlargement of sarcoplasmic reticulum has been noted [104, 106]. The presence of tubules arrayed in a honeycomb formation and increasing branching have been described in the T system, and the plasma membranes as well as the T system appear abundant and excessively folded [104] (Fig. 66-8). Ultrastructural abnormalities of the muscle spindle, including the intrafusal muscle fibers, sensory, and motor terminals, have been described [108]. All of these changes have been observed in other disor-

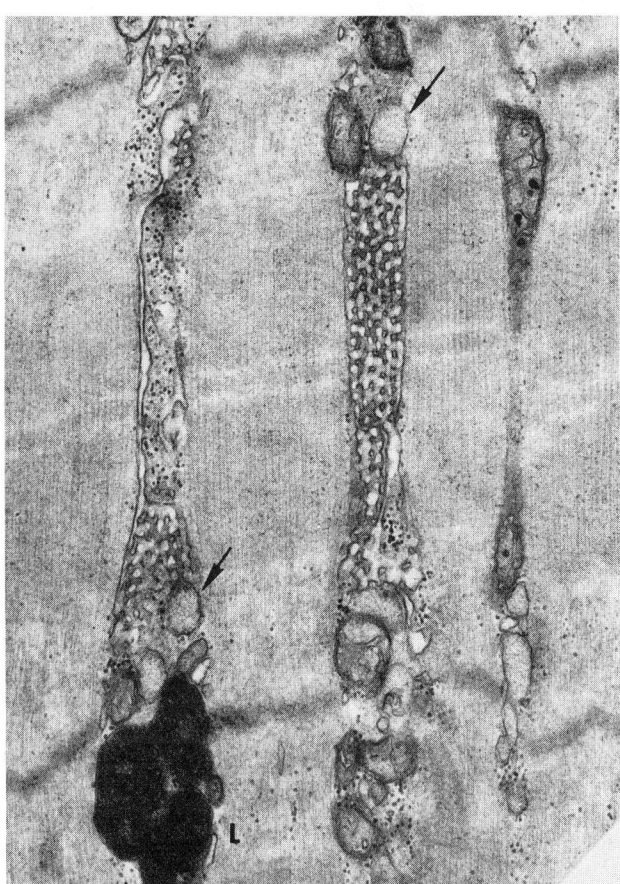

Figure 66-8 Muscle from a patient with MyD. Elongated tubular networks are adjacent to elements of the sarcoplasmic reticulum (single arrows) and, in one instance, to a lysosomelike body (L). ×37,300. (*Courtesy of Dr. Donald L. Schotland* [104].)

ders. These changes cannot explain the altered electrical properties of the muscle fiber in MyD.

Pathophysiology of Myotonic Dystrophic Muscle

Myotonia represents an abnormal tendency of the muscle membrane to discharge trains of repetitive action potentials in response to depolarization. This leads to a tetanic contraction of the individual fibers. The abnormal electrical activity persists after nerve block or following administration of curare and is a property of the muscle fiber membrane per se, not of the nerve or the neuromuscular junction [109–111]. The myotonia is readily detected by EMG. Upon insertion of the needle, prolonged trains of spikes and positive waves in great profusion appear, sometimes synchronized in unusual forms. They are evoked by the slightest movement of the needle. The discharges occur at high frequency up to 120/s, and have a characteristic quality of waxing and waning in both frequency and amplitude. Sound produced over the loudspeaker has been compared to that of a World War II dive bomber. The fibers continue to fire repetitively long after mechanical stimulation ceases. The EMG findings of myotonia are not specific for MyD but appear as well in myotonia congenita and chondrodystrophic myotonia and bear a resemblance to the "pseudomyotonic discharges" occurring in several glycogen storage diseases. These disorders are all readily distinguished from

Figure 66-7 Pedigree of the S family.

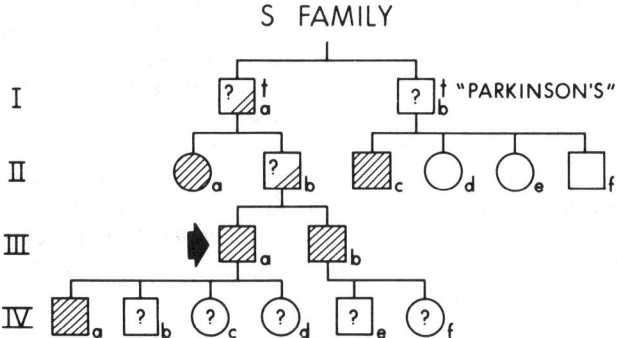

MyD by the clinical picture as well as by laboratory examination. The most helpful factor in distinguishing MyD from myotonia congenita is the absence of weakness and atrophy in the latter. Furthermore, EMG findings of myopathy are present in MyD but not in myotonia congenita.

More detailed evaluation of the pathophysiology of MyD has been reported from several laboratories. The major findings are a decreased resting membrane potential of -62 to -68 mV [112]. Membrane resistance appears to be normal and membrane conductance, 80 percent of which is explained by chloride conductance, is also normal. An increased membrane capacitance has been described [113]. Since membrane capacitance is primarily a property of the tubular membranes, its increase in MyD is readily attributed to the proliferation of T-tubular membranes noted on pathologic studies (Fig. 66-8).

The physiologic properties of the intercostal muscles of patients with MyD are considerably different from those reported in human congenital myotonia. A normal resting membrane potential, a threefold increase in membrane resistance, and a decreased chloride conductance have been reported in human myotonia congenita [114]. Similar findings have been reported in goat myotonia, as well as in drug-induced myotonias [115]. Although a complete understanding of the molecular events responsible for muscle myotonia in any of these disorders is not at hand, the experiments of Adrian and Bryant [116] with goat myotonia suggest a possible mechanism for the repetitive depolarization in that disorder. An action potential spreading into the transverse tubular system is thought to raise the potassium concentration in the lumen of the tubules under normal circumstances. The passage of several action potentials and the increased tubular potassium would result in a cumulative afterdepolarization which would be offset by the entry of chloride into the muscle fiber. If chloride conductance is decreased and cannot counterbalance the depolarizing effect of increased tubular potassium, repetitive action potentials would result.

The same scheme cannot be employed to explain the myotonia of MyD, since membrane resistance and chloride conductance appear to be normal. Tissue cultures obtained from biopsy specimens of patients with MyD have been used to study the possible electrophysiologic abnormalities [117]. Hyperexcitability was observed in MyD myotubes, as demonstrated by an increased tendency to fire repetitive action potentials. In addition, the resting membrane potential was depolarized by approximately 10 mV, and there was a diminution in the action potential afterhyperpolarization. These changes are similar to those noted in MyD biopsy specimens studied directly, with the exception of the afterhyperpolarization, which is not usually noted in adult fibers. Although a molecular explanation for these alterations is not available, an abnormality in outgoing potassium current provides a reasonable hypothesis to account for the in vitro studies [117]. This impairment in a slow outgoing current could also be related to an abnormality of transmembrane movements of calcium. It is of interest that abnormalities of calcium release from the sarcoplasmic reticulum have been noted in skinned muscle fibers from patients with MyD [118]. Thus abnormalities of calcium movements across the surface membrane could be associated with the repetitive activity, and abnormalities of calcium movements across the sarcoplasmic reticulum could be associated with the muscle stiffness and the impaired relaxation.

Treatment

There is no treatment for the dystrophic process in MyD. The myotonia appears to respond to a number of agents, including quinidine, procainamide, and phenytoin [119]. These drugs relieve symptomatic myotonia but do not affect any of the other complaints. They may have not effect whatsoever on the severe disabling dysphagia, gastrointestinal problems, cardiac difficulties, and muscle weakness which may be present. Weight reduction and lightweight splints may prolong ambulation for considerable periods of time in some patients.

An important aspect of treatment is the prevention of cardiac catastrophies in MyD patients and their relatives. As discussed above, a thorough cardiac history, physical examination, and laboratory examination can frequently identify individuals at risk. Quinidine and procainamide may increase the potential for heart block in these patients.

Another area of therapeutic concern is ocular and visual difficulties. The pathognomonic cataracts of MyD do not interfere with vision. When vision becomes impaired, other possibilities should be evaluated, including macular degeneration, glaucoma, and diabetic retinopathy, as well as cataracts.

OTHER TYPES OF MUSCULAR DYSTROPHY

There are a number of patients with muscle involvement who cannot be easily classified in any of the aforementioned categories. *Distal myopathy* was first described by Gowers in 1902 [120]. More recently, an extensive series was reported from Sweden by Welander [121]. The disease is inherited as an autosomal dominant trait and is clinically manifested between the ages of 40 and 60 years. The small muscles of the hand and anterior tibialis and calf muscles are affected first. This condition is rare in Great Britain and the United States. It is extremely difficult to distinguish this disorder from spinal muscular atrophy, and the characterization of possible neuronal defects has been incomplete. Within families there may be relative homogeneity, but some of the patients may have had MyD.

Positive ptosis with external ophthalmoplegia was originally described by Von Graefe [122]. Kiloh and Nevin [123] suggested that progressive external ophthalmoplegia should be regarded as a muscular dystrophy rather than a degeneration of muscle secondary to oculomotor nuclear involvement. Some of the patients with ocular myopathy were dysphagic. Victor et al. [124] described patients with progressive ptosis and dysphagia; they considered them to have a separate disease, oculopharyngeal muscular dystrophy. Whether these are distinct entities is unclear. Progressive external ophthalmoplegia has now been described in association with a wide variety of other disorders, including deafness, cerebellar ataxia and periphal neuropathy, pyramidal and extrapyramidal signs, mental retardation and endocrine dysfunction, retinitis pigmentosa, and proximal myopathy with abnormal mitochondria [125–129]. Since the inherited biochemical defects in these disorders are not known, their classification is presently uncertain. Many of these patients clearly demonstrate morphologic abnormalites of mitochondria, with "ragged red" fibers and the involvement of many organ systems [128, 129]. The presence of ragged red fibers with morphologic alterations in mitochondria is not specific for progressive external ophthalmoplegia. Furthermore, syndromes with demonstrated metabolic alterations in mitochondrial function do not necessarily present with ocular dysfunctions (see below).

Oculopharyngeal muscular dystrophy is inherited as an autosomal dominant trait. Clinical expression is variable within families. In addition, the syndrome varies among families. Onset of symptoms begins in middle age, Blepharoptosis with paralysis of the external ocular muscles may be the predominant presentation [130]. Other families may have severe pharyngeal symptoms but only mild ocular muscle paresis. In severe cases, death has occurred from starvation. These patients can now be fed by gastrostomy. Other families may have symptomatic proximal muscle weakness associated with ocular and pharyngeal difficulties. EMG and muscle biopsy of symptomatic patients suggest myopathy. The serum enzyme values are usually normal, and no definitive tests are available to sort out the heterogeneous syndromes included in this category of muscular dystrophies. These disorders have many similarities to myotonic dystrophy.

One typical patient with oculopharyngeal muscular dystrophy was reported to have abnormal mitochondria and "fingerprint" inclusions on electron microscopic examination of a deltoid muscle biopsy specimen [131]. The inclusions were composed of concentric lamellae of short, electron-dense linear elements. Structures identical to these have been reported in other diffuse myopathic disorders and accordingly cannot be regarded as a specific morphologic feature of oculopharyngeal dystrophy. Furthermore, without biochemical analysis of mitochondrial function it is not possible to ascertain whether the mitochondrial involvement is primary or secondary.

An unusual X-linked humeroperoneal neuromuscular disease that has features of neuropathy and myopathy has recently been described. This disease affects the distal leg and proximal arm muscle groups and is associated with electrocardiographic atrial disease. As in MyD, early recognition is important, since ventricular pacing may be indicated in many of these patients to prevent serious sequellae [132].

THE BIOCHEMICAL ABNORMALITIES IN THE MUSCULAR DYSTROPHIES

The clinical patterns described in the preceeding sections suggest that the muscular dystrophies must be considered separate entities, each with a distinctive inborn error of metabolism and with a variable expression in different organ systems. At present the primary metabolic defect cannot be defined. Nevertheless, alterations in the structure and function of cellular membranes are the hallmark of these disorders. For example, a selective increase of membrane permeability is quite pronounced in DMD and helps explain the increased urinary excretion of creatine and the dramatic elevation of normal skeletal muscle enzymes in the serum. The myotonia of MyD can also be attributed to a surface membrane defect in which repetitive depolarization leads to tetanic contraction even after nerve or neuromuscular blockade. Alterations in membrane

function could lead to a wide range of deleterious effects in muscle, and most biochemical analyses of muscle probably reflect secondary consequences rather than the initiating cause of the dystrophic process. The specificity of biochemical changes in any of the muscular dystrophies could be obscured by the many different causes which lead to a similar end stage of muscle degeneration. For example, an increased cellular permeability to calcium could induce contractures, activate proteolytic enzymes, impair energy production, and enhance muscle deterioration. Thus any metabolic error which raises intracellular calcium could lead to a similar end stage, namely, dystrophic muscle.

Creatine and Creatinine

An increase in the urinary excretion of creatine associated with an increased plasma level of creatine was one of the earliest noted concomitants of myopathy [133]. Creatine is normally synthesized in liver by transmethylation of guanidoacetate (glycocyamine) from S-adenosyl methionine. The guanidoacetate is formed from arginine and glycine by a transaminidase in kidney, pancreas, and liver [134, 135]. This reaction is subject to feedback inhibition by creatine [136]. Creatine circulates in plasma and is taken up by muscle, where it is converted into the high-energy phosphate compound creatine phosphate by CPK. The urine of normal individuals contains little or no creatine (0 to 40 mg/24 h in males and 0 to 100 mg/24 h in females) [137]. Excretion of creatine is elevated in children and in women during pregnancy.

If muscle mass is reduced, creatine is removed less rapidly from the blood, leading to higher plasma levels and a greater excretion by the kidneys. Also, a decreased transport of creatine into muscle or an increased leak of creatine from muscle would be expected to increase the urinary excretion of creatine. Many of these factors appear to contribute to the creatinuria of the muscular dystrophies, poliomyelitis, neuropathies, and diffuse muscle atrophy [138–140].

Creatinine, the anhydride of creatine, is formed in muscle from creatine at a constant rate of 2 percent per day by a nonenzymatic reaction. It diffuses back into the plasma and is excreted by the kidney. The daily urinary excretion of creatinine is 0.6 to 1.5 g/24 h in women and 1.0 to 2.0 g/24 h in men [141]. Though creatine excretion is increased in DMD, creatinine excretion is reduced. Creatinine excretion is reduced in many of the muscular dystrophies and is a nonspecific reflection of the diminution in total body creatine stores and total muscle mass. Thus, any myopathic or neurogenic condition which decreases muscle mass also decreases creatinine excretion.

Serum Enzymes

Certain enzymes of muscle origin are present in high concentrations in the serum of patients with muscle disease. Their quantification has been extremely useful in the diagnosis of skeletal muscle damage. The first observation of increased serum enzyme levels in muscular dystrophy was made by Sibley and Lehninger [142], who found an increased level of serum ALD in two patients with progressive muscular dystrophy. Later studies demonstrated that other intramuscular enzymes, such as glutamic oxaloacetic transaminase (GOT), glutamic pyruvic transaminase (GPT), LDH, and especially CPK, appear in increased amounts in the serum of patients with muscular dystrophy [143–152].

Increased CPK enzyme activity is not specific for muscular dystrophy, since activity is also increased in patients with neuromuscular disorders [146, 148, 153, 156], myocardial infarction [154, 155], hypothyroidism [156], cerebrovascular disease [157], and epilepsy [158]. Nevertheless, the most striking elevations of serum CPK occur in DMD [152]. Serum enzyme levels are less elevated in those with chronic, slowly progressive adult forms such as FSH. They may be significantly elevated in the serum in inflammatory and traumatic lesions of muscles, although the rise is usually less sustained.

In DMD, serum CPK activity is a more sensitive index of muscle involvement than any other serum enzyme [152]. The serum enzyme levels tend to be highest early in the disease, and the rise is observed even before any clinical manifestations are present. In the study by Munsat et al. [152], the mean CPK activity was 27 times normal in the late stages (Fig. 66-9). The mean activity of the other enzymes was three to six times normal in the late stages. CPK activity showed a definite inverse relationship with age. Although the clinical disease progressed in a linear fashion, Munsat et al. noted an abrupt drop in enzyme activity just after age 10 years.

Both CPK and ALD activities, as well as other elevated enzyme levels in serum, are predominantly of skeletal muscle origin. In fact there is relatively little CPK activity in many other tissues, including liver and kidney. Human tissues contain three isoenzymes of CPK. The fraction migrating in the albumin range on electrophoresis is BB (brain type), the intermediate fraction in the alpha globulin region is MB (hybrid type), and the fraction migrating cathodally in the region of gamma globulin is MM (muscle type). In the study of Goto [159], the MB/MM ratio averaged less than 0.34 in normal skeletal muscle at biopsy or autopsy. The ratio in cardiac muscle always exceeded 0.38. Normal serum contained primarily the MM form, whereas 80 percent of the patients with DMD, 75 percent of patients with congenital muscular dystrophy, and 20 percent of patients with LG dystrophy had both MM

and MB types in their serums, as did patients with myocardial infarction. The appearance of the MB form did not relate to the extent of rise of CPK activity or the age of the patient. Since skeletal muscle of patients with DMD and LG dystrophy has normal MB/MM ratios, the elevated MB in the serum was interpreted as evidence of cardiac muscle involvement in these disorders. The elevated MB/MM ratios in skeletal muscle of patients with polymyositis and FSH dystrophy suggested that the presence of the MB isoenzyme in the serums of these patients need not always indicate heart muscle involvement but may be a reflection of the skeletal muscle involvement. Somer et al. [160] obtained an even higher percent of dystrophic serums with MB isoenzyme (91 percent), and they cite the reports of elevated MB in skeletal muscle [161, 162] as evidence that serum enzyme changes are solely a relfection of skeletal muscle involvement. Pathologic studies definitely indicate cardiac involvement in DMD, and the MB isoenzyme in serum is probably a reflection of both skeletal muscle and cardiac involvement.

Two factors may contribute to the selective elevation of serum CPK so frequently encountered in patients with early cases of DMD. (1) The particular muscle fiber type involved in DMD may itself possess high levels of CPK. Support for this derives from histochemical studies which localize CPK to type 2 fibers [163]. In DMD, type 2A fibers are selectively depleted and a new type 2 fiber (type 2C, ATPase dark, NADH dark) appears [164]. (2) Synthesis of CPK may be increased in DMD muscle. No direct evidence supports this, but ribosomes isolated from DMD and DMD carrier muscle tissue demonstrate enhanced protein synthesis in vitro [165, 166].

The simplest way to explain an increase in serum enzymes in DMD is to assume that the permeability of muscle membranes is altered. The defect cannot merely reflect a nonspecific necrotizing lesion of muscle membranes, since CPK levels are highest in young children with minimal but definite evidence of muscle necrosis [167]. Also, the leakage is selective and must depend upon the shape, charge, and size of the molecules as well as other factors. For example, CPK, with a molecular weight of 80,000, shows a greater tendency to leak from muscle in DMD than does myoglobin, which has a molecular weight of 17,000 [168]. Amino acid excretion is variable but is probably not elevated in DMD, although earlier reports had suggested significant increases [169]. In MyD there is no elevation of serum CPK, but the excretion of several amino acids (threonine, glycine, glutamate, serine, and ornithine) is increased [169, 170]. In DMD, plasminogen activator may also leak out of muscle and result in an increase of fibrin split products [171]. Serum carnitine concentration increases significantly in conditions of acute muscle necrosis but is not increased in DMD [172]. Urinary excretion of carnitine appears to be decreased in DMD, whereas it is normal in FSH and LG dystrophy and may be increased in progressive spinal muscle atrophy [173].

The simultaneous elevation in levels of serum CPK, myoglobin, and carnitine, as well as other constituents, could reflect (1) altered plasma membrane permeability, leading to increased extracellular calcium, enhanced proteolysis, and enhanced leakage of protein constituents, and (2) a failure of energy production and depletion of ATP necessary to maintain the integrity of the sarcolemma [174]. The latter situation is exemplified by syndromes with impaired glycogen metabolism in which ATP levels might decline in vigorous exercise because of a block in anaerobic glycolysis [175–178]. Impaired lipid

Figure 66-9 A comparison of relative elevation of serum enzymes in DMD before and after age 10 years. (*Modified from Munsat et al. [152].*)

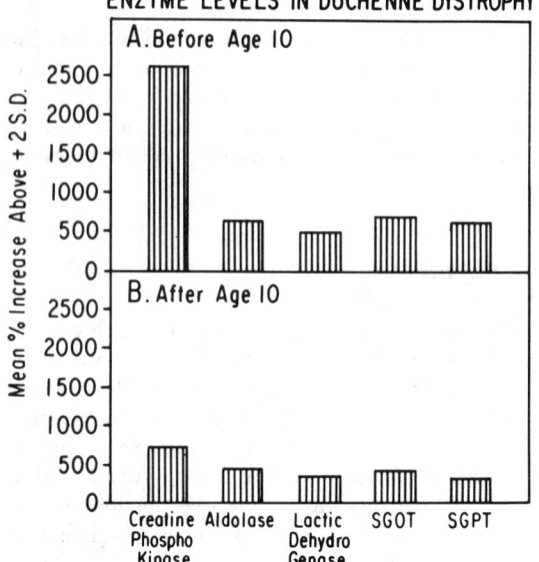

ENZYME LEVELS IN DUCHENNE DYSTROPHY

and purine metabolism also depletes energy reserves, because lipid provides more than 50 percent of muscle energy requirements [179–183]. Alteration in both these metabolic pathways in humans may result in a sarcolemmal leak of myoglobin in preference to or in addition to CPK. In DMD, there is a rather different profile of serum changes, in which considerable CPK activity and very little myoglobin are present. The pattern in DMD is, therefore, less likely to result from a general depletion of energy and more likely to reflect a primary membrane defect or a more specific effect of raised intracellular calcium. Similarly, energy depletion would not be anticipated in MyD, in which serum constitutents are normal in spite of muscle atrophy.

Biochemical Analyses of Muscle

The direct biochemical analysis of muscle constituents has been generally unproductive in the muscular dystrophies and has failed to yield significant information about the primary inborn errors of metabolism. The major difficulty is the extensive range of responses of muscle to injury. These include increased connective tissue, fatty infiltration, infiltration of inflammatory cells, muscle nuclear proliferation, membrane proliferation, changes in membrane permeability, changes of denervation, and variable patterns of degeneration and regeneration. Such changes make the selection of an appropriate reference base and an adequate control extremely difficult. Noncollagen protein nitrogen has recently gained acceptance as a reference, since it appears to correlate with the severity of muscle involvement as assessed histologically [165]. With this reference, many values previously considered abnormal now fall within the normal range, but many other enzyme activities still show dramatic changes from normal [173, 184].

Muscle Proteins Many of the muscle structural proteins appear to be decreased in DMD. The contractile material of muscle consists of long series of partially overlapping arrays of actin and myosin filaments which form myofibrils. The actin-combining ability and ATP activity are associated with the heavy meromyosin subunit of the myosin molecule. In DMD the actomyosin ATPase activity is decreased, whether activated by magnesium, calcium, or EDTA-potassium chloride [185, 186]. Furthermore, the initial rate of superprecipitation of actomyosin, which correlates with ATPase activity, is also slowed. These results in vitro may relate to the slowing of mean contraction times in DMD [187]. The content of tropomyosin and that of troponin are also reduced in DMD [188, 189], but no qualitative changes are present in any of these constituents. The pH stability of the actomyosin ATPase is normal [186], the electrophoretic properties of tropomyosin and troponin are normal [188], and myosin exhibits normal immunoelectrophoretic behavior [190]. More detailed biochemical studies of human contractile proteins are still necessary.

A diminution in the content of myoglobin has been reported in the muscular dystrophies, but no reproducible changes in the myoglobin molecule [191]. The specific function of muscle myoglobin is unknown, although it has been proposed as a short- and long-term oxygen store [192]. Several different groups have analyzed human myoglobin from patients with DMD. Peptide mapping [193] and immunoelectrophoretic [194] and sequence analysis [192] have given results within normal limits. Earlier reported abnormalities in DMD myoglobin are readily explained by preparative artifacts, such as the presence of degraded hemoglobin, the binding of myoglobin to proteins of small molecular weight, and the variable deamidation of myoglobin [192].

Muscle Enzymes A vast array of muscle enzymes has been analyzed, especially in DMD, and no specific insight into the inborn error of metabolism has been revealed. Activity of several glycolytic enzymes (phosphorylase, phosphoglucomutase, and aldolase) is reduced in muscle from patients with DMD [195, 196], as is CPK [151] and AMP deaminase [184, 197]. Hexokinase [198], fructose-1,6-diphosphatase [199], and LDH [198] are reported as normal; and glucose-6-phosphate dehydrogenase, isocitrate dehydrogenase, and phosphogluconate dehydrogenase are increased [200]. ATP, ADP, and creatine phosphate are also decreased [201]. A variety of hydrolytic activities, many of which are obviously of lysosomal origin, are clearly increased in DMD and probably reflect the nonspecific tissue response to diseases with diverse causes. Increases of proteolytic activity [202], ribonucleases [203], arylsulfatase [204], and alkaline phosphatase [205] activity have been reported. The more severely the muscle fiber is affected, the more predictable the elevation, regardless of whether denervation, inflammation, or primary myopathy is the inciting factor. Some of these changes must be related to changes in the structure and function of skeletal muscle membranes; others, such as LDH and CPK isoenzymes, resemble enzyme activity seen in immature or fetal muscle and may reflect the presence of regeneration. The increase in 5′-nucleotidase has been specifically attributed to an increase in connective tissue [206].

Lipids

Many of the limitations of enzymatic analyses are also applicable to the lipid changes reported in dystrophic muscle. The presence of atrophy, fatty infiltration, membrane changes, and muscle regeneration reflect changes in lipid metabolism. Hughes [207] demonstrated a change in the composition of phospholipids in DMD muscle toward a pattern which resembled that of immature normal muscle. Sphingomyelin and cholesterol were increased, while phosphatidylcholine and choline plasmalogens were decreased. Such changes are clearly not specific, since measurements on biopsy specimens from patients with peripheral neuropathy gave similar values. No change in total lipid phosphorus was noted per gram wet weight, but noncollagen protein was not used as a reference. Lin et al. [208] observed a decrease in fatty acid oxidation by skeletal muscle mitochondria from DMD patients with a family history of X-linked recessive inheritance, as well as in definite female carriers of the disorder. In two isolated cases the rate of palmitate oxidation was normal. These findings suggested that isolated cases may represent a metabolic disorder different from that of the familial cases. However, recent studies of the DMD carrier state suggest that isolated cases are far less common than previously reported. If all the cases represent merely a variable expression of the same genetic defect, the different levels of fatty acid oxidation might reflect a variable clinical muscle involvement. Normal values of fatty acid oxidation might reflect minimal myographic involvement in isolated cases, and the dramatic decreases of fatty acid oxidation of familial cases might reflect a more severe involvement. The changes would represent not necessarily the primary metabolic error but perhaps some secondary and possibly nonspecific responses to an alteration either in the structure and function of the mitochondrial membranes or in other muscle constituents.

Further evidence against the etiologic significance of a primary lipid abnormality in DMD comes from the recent descriptions of disorders of lipid metabolism in muscle. Bradley et al. [209] provided the first morphologic observations of excessive lipid accumulation in muscle fibers associated with myopathy. A defect in the utilization of long-chain fatty acids by muscle was described in twin girls with recurrent myoglobinuria [179]. In 1973 Engel and Angelini identified the first patient with carnitine deficiency [182], and DiMauro and DiMauro described muscle carnitine palmityltransferase (CPT) deficiency in two brothers with recurrent myoglobinuria [210]. Additional patients have been described, and DiMauro et al. have recently reviewed disorders of lipid metabolism in muscle [211].

CPT is apparently required to catalyze the transfer of fatty acids across the mitochondrial membranes by formation of palmityl carnitine on the outer face of the inner mitochondrial membrane and the formation of palmityl coenzyme A and carnitine on the inner face of the same membrane (Fig. 66-10). Two forms of this enzyme may exist, each of which may catalyze one of these steps [181]. In these patients a probable lack of a mitochondrial outer membrane enzyme impaired long-chain fatty acid utilization and resulted in increased content of plasma-free fatty acids and plasma triglycerides. The two original cases with CPT deficiency appeared to be asymptomatic when they maintained a high carbohydrate diet. Twenty-one patients have now been reported [211].

Carnitine deficiency was described in a patient with muscle weakness but no cramps or myoglobinuria [182]. In this disorder the concentration of muscle carnitine was dramatically decreased, while lipid content was increased. The enzyme defect has not been delineated, but the disorder appears to be distinctly different from CPT deficiency. Nine cases have been reviewed [211]. Eight patients complained of progressive weakness, which in three began during adult life. All had abnormal EMG examinations, normal or very slightly decreased serum carnitine levels, and pathologic evidence of lipid storage in muscle. Six patients responded well to treatment with carnitine or prednisone.

Several additional clinical syndromes associated with lipid accumulation in muscle have been described in which muscle carnitine and CPT are normal. The metabolic abnormalities in these syndromes of abnormal lipid metabolism have yet to be defined, but they clearly differ from the muscular dystrophies described in this chapter.

MEMBRANE ALTERATIONS

Biologic membranes are important cellular constitutents modulating a wide range of specialized functions. They are intimately involved in the formation of cell-to-cell contacts and the development of complex and precise cellular networks. They represent a point for the translation of environmental stimuli into intracellular metabolic events. They are important for regulation of the ionic composition of the cell and the extracellular space. The membranes of excitable tissues such as nerve and muscle have additional specialization for generation of action potentials and for intercellular communication. The entire cycle of muscle function, starting with the arrival of a nerve signal, can be divided into four events, three of which intimately involve muscle membranes: (1) excitation (sarcolemma and transverse tubules); (2) coupling (transverse tubule and sarcoplasmic reticulum); (3) contraction; and (4) relaxation (sarcoplasmic reticulum) [212].

Neuromuscular Junction and Sarcoplasmic Reticulum

Acetylcholine receptors at the neuromuscular junction are activated by the arrival of the nerve impulse at the nerve terminal and the release of the neurotransmitter acetylcholine (Fig. 66-11). The resulting end plate potential gives rise to an action potential which spreads along the sarcolemma and into the transverse tubule membranes, presumably to the point of contact between the T-tubule membrane and the membrane of the sarcoplasmic reticulum. At this point there is a functional cou-

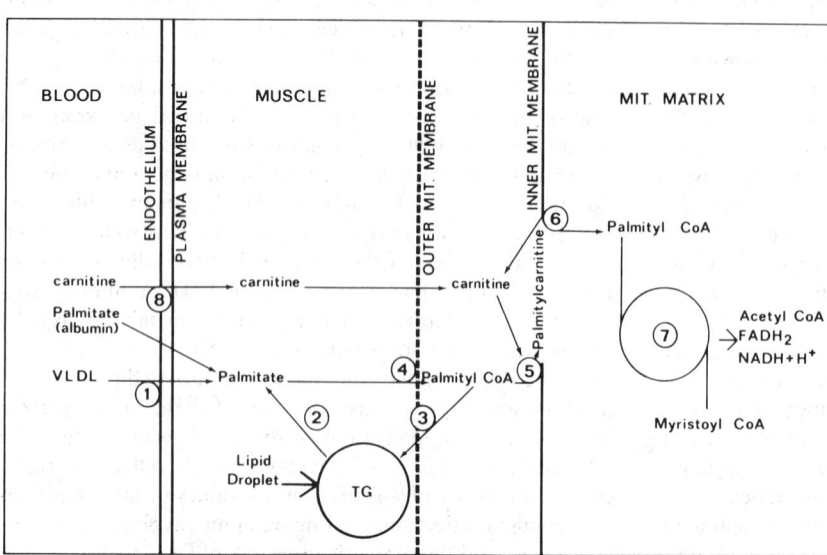

Figure 66-10 Schematic representation of the principal pathways of lipid metabolism in muscle. Palmitate is used as a typical long-chain fatty acid. Exogenous, blood-borne substrates are represented by fatty acids bound to albumin and by triglycerides in the form of very low density lipoproteins (VLDL). Endogenous lipid stores are triglycerides (TG) in lipid droplets. Enzymes or enzyme complexes are indicated by circled numbers adjacent to the membranes to which they are bound. MIT = mitochondrial. 1 = lipoprotein lipase; 2 = tri-, di-, and monoglyceride lipase; 3 = synthesis of triglycerides from long-chain acyl-CoA requiring glycerol-1-phosphate and three enzymes: glycerol-phosphate acyltransferase, phosphatidate phosphatase, and diglyceride acyltransferase; 4 = palmityl-CoA synthetase; 5 = carnitine palmityltransferase (CPT) 1; 6 = CPT 11; 7 = β oxidation pathway, including acyl-CoA dehydrogenase, enoyl-CoA hydratase, β-hydroxyacyl-CoA dehydrogenase, and β-keto-acyl-CoA thiolase; 8 = active transport system of carnitine into muscle. (Reprinted with permission of Dr. S. DiMauro [211].)

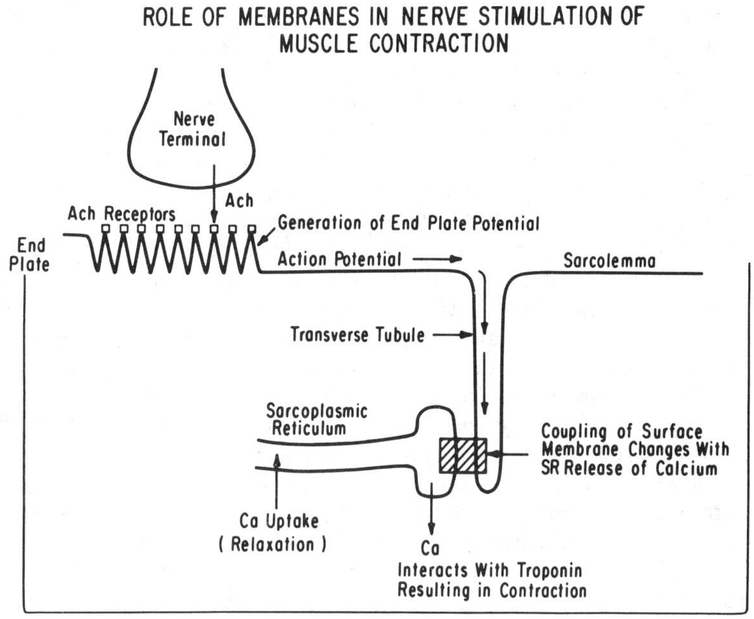

ROLE OF MEMBRANES IN NERVE STIMULATION OF
MUSCLE CONTRACTION

Figure 66-11 Scheme of the flow of information from nerve to muscle resulting in contraction.

pling of T-tubule and sarcoplasmic reticulum which results in the release of calcium from the sarcoplasmic reticulum. The exact mechanism for coupling is unknown, although there are three prominent theories: (1) a direct [213] electrical coupling to a low-resistance pathway by which ionic current could flow and result in the release of calcium from sarcoplasmic reticulum; (2) a transient "extra" current [214] generated at the transverse tubule with a voltage-dependent movement of charge within or across the T-tubule membrane and a sensing of this regulatory current by molecules which cross the junctional gap and regulate the release of calcium [215]; (3) the release of a "trigger" substance from the T-tubule membrane—possibly calcium itself—which diffuses across the junctional gap and excites the release of more calcium from the sarcoplasmic reticulum [216].

Following the release of calcium by the sarcoplasmic reticulum, the subsequent events in the mechanism of contraction are well characterized. The released calcium binds to troponin. Troponin is inhibitory to actin in the troponin-tropomyosin system. Removal of the inhibition of actin permits the interaction with myosin to take place. The splitting of ATP supplies the energy for the development of tension. Relaxation is brought about by removal of calcium from its interaction with troponin and uptake into the sarcoplasmic reticulum.

The leakage of enzymes as well as creatine from muscle fibers has directed attention to the surface membrane of muscle as the most significant change in muscular dystrophy. The leakage of these constituents is not specific and is not sufficient to implicate an inherited defect in membrane structure as the cause of any of the dystrophies. Mokri and Engel [23] have demonstrated disruption of the plasma membrane as an early abnormality in the muscle of seven patients with DMD. The lesions in the plasma membrane readily permitted the entry of peroxidase-containing extracellular fluid. These findings appear to be specific, since they were only rarely observed in control specimens or biopsy specimens of patients with other muscular dystrophies.

Other evidence suggesting structural or functional abnormalities of the plasma membrane has come from freeze fracture analyses of sarcolemma showing a decrease in intra-

membranous particles in DMD [24, 25] and from studies demonstrating an alteration in concanavalin A binding to DMD surface membranes [26].

Analysis of muscle membrane, including intrinsic enzyme activities, has provided the major biochemical evidence for primary membrane involvement. These studies themselves have a major limitation, viz., the yield and purity of various membranes isolated from muscle biopsy specimens is not known and probably varies considerably with the degree of pathologic change. Most techniques for subcellular membrane fractionation depend on both particle and membrane density, and disease-induced changes could be expected to alter the membrane density and obscure the appropriate reference base for any specific biochemical assay.

Techniques for the isolation of sarcoplasmic reticulum in humans are advanced, and considerable attention has been directed to the lipid and protein composition as well as biologic function of this fraction. Takagi and his colleagues [217] reported that the phospholipid and cholesterol content of these membranes from DMD muscle was normal but that the proportion of individual phospholipids was altered and that there was a decrease in phosphatidylcholine. The polypeptide profile of such membranes was normal. But, as pointed out by the authors, their fractions of sarcoplasmic reticulum may well have been contaminated by sarcolemmal membranes, microsomes, and adipose and connective tissue.

Four different laboratories have reported a decreased ability of fragmented sarcoplasmic reticulum to accumulate calcium ions in DMD [217–220]. Both the rate and extent of calcium uptake appear to be decreased in vesicles from DMD muscle. Although contamination of this fraction by other membrane fragments could explain these results, this could not easily explain the altered K_m for calcium transport [221]. If this defect were present in vivo, then the cytoplasmic concentration of calcium might be elevated and result in delayed relaxation of muscle [222]. Impairment in calcium transport could be attributed either to an increased passive permeability of the sarcoplasmic reticulum to calcium or to a decreased activity of the calcium pump. No consistent alteration has been seen in ATPase activity in DMD, but studies of the pertinent ATPase activity associated with the calcium pump viz., the "extra ATPase," defined as the difference between the activities of calcium-magnesium-ATPase and magnesium-ATPase [223] have not been carried out in parallel with the calcium transport studies. In MyD calcium uptake by fragmented sarcoplasmic reticulum has been described as reduced [224, 225], normal [225], or high [219, 225]. The reduced uptake appears in severe, advanced disease. Of interest is the increased rate of uptake, which may be an early change in the muscle sarcoplasmic reticulum membrane. Nevertheless, these studies did not measure the extra ATPase activity, and one cannot be certain whether the increased calcium transport was related to an enhanced calcium pump or a decreased calcium leak.

The alterations in calcium transport of the sarcoplasmic reticulum are clearly not specific for DMD and MyD, since other processes such as denervation and polymyositis may produce similar results. Brody [226] has described a patient with impaired muscle relaxation whose sarcoplasmic reticulum fragments demonstrated a decreased rate of calcium uptake. This patient had no clinical or laboratory features of muscular dystrophy.

Recent studies using the skinned fiber technique have demonstrated a defective regulation of calcium by the sarcoplasmic reticulum in DMD [227]. The consequence of increased myoplasmic calcium could lead to (1) myofibrillar contractures, (2) activation of a neutral protease and breakdown of myofibrils, and (3) impairment of mitochondrial energy production and subsequent cell death [228]. Evidence for the increased calcium content of DMD muscle fibers has come from histochemical [229], electrocytochemical [230], and x-ray microanalytical studies [231]. All of these data suggest that enhanced membrane permeability to calcium may play a key role in the pathogenesis of the dystrophic process, even if such abnormalities in calcium transport are secondary rather than primary.

Erythrocyte Changes

Although muscle has been the principal target organ of study of the muscular dystrophies, a number of artifacts and nonspecific changes have clouded the interpretation of data derived solely from analysis of muscle biopsy specimens. For at least two of the dystrophies (DMD and MyD), there is sufficient clinical involvement of different organ systems to suggest that the inborn error of metabolism may be expressed in tissues other than muscle. Erythrocytes are an easily accessible source of membrane preparations for testing the hypothesis that the genetic defect is diffusely expressed in many organ systems and that cellular membranes are a principal locus of the metabolic error. It has now been over a decade since publication of the original reports of abnormalities in red blood cells from patients with muscular dystrophy. Although not all lines of evidence are free from criticism, the overall results in these years from red blood cell studies do support the concept that membrane defects are widespread in DMD and MyD. The use of the red blood cells had not defined the specific inborn error of metabolism, nor has it permitted the conclusion that defects are intrinsic to the membrane. The reported observations would be equally consistent with abnormalities in membranes being secondary to biochemical lesions either inside or outside the cells under study.

Enzymatic Investigations No differences have been demonstrated in polypeptide profiles on polyacrylamide gel electrophoresis of erythrocyte membrane proteins from patients with MyD or DMD as compared with those from normal subjects. In DMD, altered activities have been reported for the sodium-potassium-ATPase, calcium-magnesium-ATPase, protein kinase, and adenylate cyclase. In MyD, there are reports of abnormal activities for both the sodium-potassium-ATPase and protein kinase.

Brown et al. [232] initiated the interest in the ouabain-sensitive ATPase by reporting that ouabain stimulated rather than inhibited ATP hydrolysis in red blood cell ghosts prepared from patients with DMD, MyD, and myotonia congenita. This stimulation was detected only in the presence of low concentrations of sodium and potassium. Optimal activation of ATPase by physiologic concentrations of sodium and potassium resulted in the expected ouabain inhibition of both ATP hydrolysis and active transport of sodium and potassium [233, 234]. Other laboratories, including our own, have failed to confirm the reported alterations even at the low ion concentrations [233]. Two reports claim to confirm the findings of Brown and suggest that a plasma factor is responsible for the specific effects [235, 236]. An explanation for the variability of results from different laboratories is not readily at hand. However, it is known that slight differences in the preparation of erythrocyte membranes can result in vast differences in enzymatic activities in vitro. Thus, the variability from different laboratories may reflect differential effects of tissue preparation on membrane abnormalities rather than the failure of certain laboratories to detect specific enzymatic defects.

Hull and Roses [237] reported an alteration in the stoichiometry of ouabain-sensitive sodium-potassium exchange in MyD. The normal ratio of sodium efflux to potassium influx is 1.5, but in MyD this ratio was reduced to 1.0. This finding awaits confirmation since one other group was not able to confirm this difference using different techniques [238].

Although the calcium-magnesium-ATPase activity of red blood cell membranes from DMD patients is normal, kinetic studies suggest that the apparent affinity of the enzyme for its magnesium-ATP substrate is higher in DMD red blood cells [239]. No further studies have documented whether this apparent affinity shift is a consequence of the protein itself or of other abnormalities which influence the enzyme. One potential activator of the enzyme is calmodulin, a ubiquitous calcium-binding protein which influences many calcium-dependent enzymes. Luthra et al. [240] attempted to assess the effect of calmodulin in DMD and MyD red blood cells by adding crude hemolysates, presumably containing calmodulin, and measuring calcium-magnesium-ATPase activities. Since the effect of the hemolysates was the same whether DMD, MyD, or controlled preparations were employed, they concluded that the differences in activation involved inherent membrane properties. However, no calmodulin measurements were made, and it is possible that the levels differ in different tissues.

Studies of protein phosphorylation in red cell membranes have demonstrated a decrease in MyD and an increase in DMD, with different specific polypeptides affected in the two conditions. In MyD red cell membranes, the decrease in protein phosphorylation was first demonstrated with membrane ghosts frozen at $-20°C$ for 7 days [241] and subsequently in fresh erythrocyte ghosts that had been prepared in the absence of magnesium [242]. In the latter study, decreased phosphorylation of a protein moiety of band 3 (90,000 to 100,000 daltons) was observed. More recently, Wong and Roses [243] fractionated band 3 glycoproteins into three components using affinity chromatography on a Ricin-Sepharose column. Phosphorylation of two of the fractions by an endogenous protein kinase was normal. The third fraction, which represented only 3 percent of the total red blood cell membrane protein, was phosphorylated 50 percent less in membranes from seven MyD patients than in control material. These results have suggested a possible structural abnormality in half the molecules of this fraction of band 3 protein [244].

Other investigators have obtained different results in studies of protein phosphorylation in red blood cell membranes obtained from patients with various muscular dystrophies. Iyer et al. [245] observed an increase in total phosphorylation in MyD, while Vickers et al. found no differences in phosphorylation of band 3 protein in MyD, using red blood cell membranes at 30°C but found lower activities in MyD than in control membranes at 37°C [246].

When similar studies were carried out with red blood cell ghosts from patients with DMD, a different pattern of altered phosphorylation was noted [247]. Both the initial rate of phosphorylation and the maximal extent of phosphorylation of band 2 (spectrin, 220,000 daltons) were increased in DMD patients and in groups of possible, probable, and definite carriers. Increased ^{32}P phosphorylation was also demonstrated in both tryptic and cyanogen bromide cleavage products of purified spectrin in DMD [248, 249], and altered extractability of spectrin was noted in DMD cell membranes [250, 251]. Three groups have been unable to confirm increased band 2 phosphorylation in DMD [245, 252, 253], but in each instance the methodologies were different from the original ones employed [254].

Alterations in the activity of adenylate cyclase have been reported in red blood cells from patients with DMD [255]. The major changes were increased basal activity and an insensitivity to epinephrine. These results, like those of other enzymes mentioned above, could be explained either by a nonspecific alteration in the structure of the membrane or the presence in the membrane of some circulating factor which is normally not found in control human erythrocytes. For example, certain abnormalities of erythrocytes in DMD can be duplicated in normal cells by increasing their calcium content [256]. Osmotic fragility was found to be reduced and the cellular content of potassium twofold greater than in control cells when DMD cells were exposed to the ionophore A23187, which enhances uptake of calcium. Plishker and Appel [257] found no difference in the uptake of calcium in DMD compared to control values. However, erythrocytes from patients with MyD had both an increased accumulation and an increased efflux of calcium [258]. Thus, it is possible that the intracellular concentration of calcium rather than alterations of specific membrane proteins may give rise to the range of disturbances in membrane structure and function which have been reported in red blood cells from patients with various dystrophies.

Membrane Lipids   Theoretically, the change in enzymatic activities, cell morphology, membrane biophysics, and ion transport in the muscular dystrophies could be explained by primary defects in lipid metabolism. The relative proportion of different phospholipids, the chain length and degree of saturation of the fatty acid constituents of various lipids, and the sterol content of the plasma membrane make a major contribution to membrane structure and function. However, no reproducible alteration in red blood cell membrane lipids have been reported in the dystrophies. Kunze et al. [259] reported a change in the phospholipid composition as well as the fatty acid pattern in red blood cells from patients with DMD and

suggested a decreased incorporation of linoleic acid into phosphatidylcholine as the primary metabolic error. Several laboratories, including our own, have not been able to confirm these results [246]. Neither studies by Godin et al. [260], McLaughlin and Engel [261], Coski et al. [262] nor those presented by Plishker and Appel [257] can document any difference in red blood cell lipids between normal and DMD membranes. One explanation for the findings in those studies which report alterations in phospholipids may be that the membrane lipids have undergone autoxidation in vitro. Furthermore, although diazacholesterol induces myotonia in humans, goats, and rats, there is no evidence that desmosterol, which accumulates in the experimental myotonias, can be detected in human MyD [257, 263].

Biophysical Studies of Red Blood Cell Membranes
To investigate possible structural alterations of the red blood cell membrane, electron spin resonance spectroscopy has been utilized. The magnetic measurements of a spin-labeled probe intercallated into the membrane provide a measure of membrane fluidity and polarity [264]. By the use of stearic acid with nitroxide groups on the alkyl chain, MyD membranes were found to be more fluid and less polar than control membranes [264]. The fluidity difference was most apparent near the surface of the membrane, while the polarity difference was approximately constant at various depths within the membrane. Similar changes were noted in myotonia congenita and in drug-induced myotonias but not in DMD. With the use of nitroxide-labeled maleimide, which has a high affinity for sulfhydryl groups of membrane proteins, similar alterations were noted in MyD red blood cells [265].

Wilkerson et al. [266] demonstrated a difference between erythrocytes from patients with DMD and control cells employing saturation transfer electron paramagnetic resonance. Their studies with this extremely sensitive technique suggested that fatty acid labels take a longer time to reach equilibrium in red blood cells from a DMD patient compared to a normal individual. Comparable reports on increased rigidity have been previously demonstrated by Percy and Miller [267] employing a simple technique in which red blood cells are aspirated into a micropipette to determine membrane elasticity.

Scanning Electron Microscopy of Erythrocytes   Matheson and Howland [268] first demonstrated an alteration in morphologic characteristics of red blood cells of mouse and specific echinocytic changes in human DMD using scanning electron microscopy. Our own studies of unmanipulated cells from patients with DMD demonstrated no such specificity [269]. A large increase in stomatocytes could be demonstrated, but similar stomatocytes could be produced in normal cells by adverse conditions such as washing before fixation or extreme pH, although the changes noted in red blood cells from patients with myopathy were more marked. The stomatocytic changes of MyD were not specific for this condition but were also noted in other muscular disorders, including DMD, the DMD carrier state, LG dystrophy, and myotonia congenita, as well as in a person with no clinical evidence of muscle disease. There is no evidence that erythrocytes of any of these patients were misshapen in vivo. Thus, the changes observed appear to be artifacts produced in vitro by the fixation procedure and are insufficient to establish or confirm a specific diagnosis, although they do confirm the presence of a membrane defect.

Summary of Biochemical Studies

Each type of muscular dystrophy has a distinct clinical and genetic expression and is probably a separate inborn error of metabolism. The experimental evidence obtained to date suggests that these metabolic defects may be expressed in membranes of many different tissues. The data derived solely from muscle are limited by the extensive secondary biochemical consequences of connective tissue and fat infiltration and muscle degeneration and regeneration.

The most critical questions still to be answered are: (1) What is the molecular defect responsible for the dystrophic process? (2) What is the molecular defect responsible for the myotonias? (3) What is the inborn error of metabolism in each of the disorders, and how does it relate to the functional alterations, including muscle weakness? To date, none of the research data provide a specific insight into whether the genetic defects responsible for membrane abnormalities are primarily in lipid metabolism or in the structure of membrane protein constituents. Further investigations should help clarify the pathogenesis of these membrane disorders as well as shed light on normal membrane structure and function.

THEORIES OF PATHOGENESIS

Investigations of the muscular dystrophies have the unique distinction of having been sidetracked from the main task of determining the inborn errors of metabolism by theories which emphasize the exclusive etiologic importance of one or another organ system. Clearly, the severe and progressive degeneration of muscle is the most striking clinical and pathologic change in muscular dystrophy in humans. Yet impairment of motor neuron function may significantly influence many functional and metabolic properties of muscle. McComas and his colleagues [270–275] proposed a neurogenic theory of muscular dystrophy based upon the demonstration of a decreased number of motor units in the extensor digitorum brevis muscle in DMD or other muscular dystrophies in humans. Their techniques of motor unit recording have been criticized by several groups [276–280], and their findings could not be confirmed in any of the dystrophies except MyD [280]. Their conclusions have also been weakened by their own demonstration that McArdle's syndrome, known to be caused by a phosphorylase deficiency limited to muscle, also shows a decrease in motor units [274]. The variable reports of myopathic or neuropathic alterations in murine muscular dystrophy [280] cannot be used to strengthen the case for a neurogenic hypothesis, since there is no evidence that any of these animal dystrophies is an exact model for any of the human muscular dystrophies.

In 1961 Demos [281] advanced a vascular hypothesis as the cause of muscular dystrophy, claiming that ischemia was responsible for muscle fiber degeneration. Patients with DMD were reported to have a prolonged arm-to-arm circulation time very early in the disease and a shortened circulation time late in the disease. Furthermore, a similarity was noted in the pathologic picture between the early stages in DMD and that experimentally produced in rabbits by microembolization with dextran particles [282] or by aortic ligation and administration of 5-hydroxytryptamine (serotonin) [283]. Evidence against the vascular theory is convincing [284–286]. With the use of

^{133}Xe, muscle blood flow at rest and after ischemic exercise was found to be normal in DMD and LG muscular dystrophy, and a significantly higher muscle blood flow after histamine injection was reported in DMD [285]. Studies with the Falck-Hillarp histochemical technique demonstrate no abnormality of the catecholamine content of adrenergic nerves around small arterioles in skeletal muscle of patients with DMD [287]. Finally, morphologic analysis of the early stages of DMD reveals subtle pathologic alterations of the muscle surface membrane [23] but no changes compatible with vascular insufficency [23, 288].

It is unlikely that either the neurogenic or the vascular etiologic theories will totally explain the defect in any of the muscular dystrophies. The clinical, pathologic, and biochemical data suggest that many organ systems are involved. Even if nerve involvement is firmly established, the myopathic changes need not be secondary but may be a separate expression of the disease process, as are the mental changes, the red blood cell involvement, cardiac involvement, etc. The most likely explanation in these, as in other genetic disorders, is a widespread expression of the metabolic defect in many organ systems rather than a limited expression of the defect in nerve or muscle. This approach suggests that cells cultured from various tissues from dystrophic patients may be extremely useful in demonstrating the expression in different organs. Tissue culture may, as pointed out by Huxley [289], have great potential for carrier detection, antenatal diagnosis, and perhaps identification of the primary defect. In fact, the ability to demonstrate alterations of electrical parameters in cultured myotubes from patients with MyD suggests that the inborn error of metabolism can be expressed independently in muscle, and neither nerve nor blood vessels are required for disease expression in at least one of these disorders [117].

REFERENCES

1. ERB W: Dystrophic muscularis progressive: Klinische and pathologischanatomische Studien. *Dtsch Z Nervenkeilkd* 1:13, 1981
2. ROWLAND LP, LAYZER RB: X-linked muscular dystrophies, in Vinken PJ, Bruyn GW (eds): *Handbook of Clinical Neurology.* Amsterdam, Elsevier North-Holland 1979, vol 40, p 349
3. PENN AS, LISAK RP, ROWLAND LP: Muscular dystrophy in young girls. *Neurology (Minn)* 20:147, 1970
4. GOMEZ MR, ENGEL AG, DEWALD C: Failure of inactivation of Duchenne dystrophy X-chromosome in one of female identical twins. *Neurology* 26:371, 1976
4a. LINDENBAUM RH, CLARKE G, PATEL C, MONCRIEFF M, HUGHES JT: Muscular dystrophy in an X;1 translocation female suggests that Duchenne locus is on the X chromosome short arm. *J Med Genet* 11: 389, 1979
4b. VERELLEN CH, FREUND M, DEMEYER R, LATERRE CH, SCHOLBERG B, FREDERIC J: Progressive muscular dystrophy of the Duchenne type in a young girl associated with an aberration of chromosome X. Excerpta Medica, Int Congr Ser 92
5. GARDNER-MEDWIN D: Mutation rate in Duchenne type of muscular dystrophy. *J Med Genet* 7:334, 1970
6. ROSES AD, ROSES MJ, MILLER SE, HULL KL, APPEL SH: Carrier detection in Duchenne muscular dystrophy. *N Engl J Med* 294:193, 1976
7. FISHER ER, WISSINGER HA, GERNETH JA, DANOWSKI TS: Ultrastructural changes in skeletal muscle of muscular dystrophy carriers. *Arch Pathol* 94:546, 1972
8. FRANCKE U, FELSENSTEIN J, GARTLER SM, MIGEON BR, DANCIS J, SEEGMILLER JE, BAKAY B, NYHAN WL: The occurrence of new mutants in the X-linked recessive Lesch-Nyhan disease. *Am J Hum Genet* 28:123, 1976
9. GRAHAM JB: Genotype assignment (carrier detection) in the haemophilias. *Clin Haematol* 8:115, 1979
10. WILSON SAK: *Neurology.* London E. Arnold, Ltd, 1947, vol 2, pp 975–976
11. DUBOWITZ V, BROOKE MH: *Muscle Biopsy: A Modern Approach.* Philadelphia, WB Saunders Co, 1973

11a. Bradley WG, Hudgson P, Larson PF, Papatetropoulos TA, Jenkison U: Structural changes in the early stages of Duchenne muscular dystrophy. *J Neurol Neurosurg Psychiatry* 35:451, 1972

12. Zatuchni J, Aegerter EE, Molthan L, Schuman C: The heart in progressive muscular dystrophy. *Circulation* 3:846, 1951

13. Perloff JK, Roberts WC, deLeon AC, O'Doherty D: The distinctive electrocardiogram of Duchenne progressive muscular dystrophy. *Am J Med* 42:179, 1967

14. Farah MG, Evans EB, Vignos PJ: Echocardiographic evaluation of left ventricular function in Duchenne's muscular dystrophy. *Am J Med* 69:298, 1980

15. Schott J, Jacobi M, Wald MA: Electrocardiographic patterns in the differential diagnosis of progressive muscular dystrophy. *Am J Med Sci* 229:517, 1955

16. Dubowitz, V: Mental retardation in Duchenne muscular dystrophy, in Rowland LP (ed): *Pathogenesis of the Human Muscular Dystrophies.* Amsterdam, Excerpta Medica, 1977, p 205

17. Cohen HJ, Molnar GE, Taft LT: The genetic relationship of progressive muscular dystrophy (Duchenne type) and mental retardation. *Dev Med Child Neurol* 10:754, 1968

18. Emery AEH, Skinner R, Holloway S: A study of possible heterogeneity in Duchenne Muscular Dystrophy. *Clin Genet* 15:444, 1979

19. Ebashi S, Toyokura Y, Momoi H, Sugita H: High creatine phosphokinase activity of sera of progressive muscular dystrophy patients. *J Biochem (Tokyo)* 46:103, 1959

20. Kugelberg E, Welander M: Heredofamilial juvenile muscular atrophy stimulating muscular dystrophy. *Arch Neurol Psychiatr* 75:500, 1950

21. Buchthal F: Diagnostic significance of the myopathic EMG, in Rowland LP (ed): *Pathogenesis of the Human Muscular Dystrophies.* Amsterdam, Excerpta Medica, 1977, p 205

22. Meadows JC, Marsden CD, Harriman DGF: Chronic spinal muscular atrophy in adults. II. Other forms. *J Neurol Sci* 9:551, 1969

23. Mokri B, Engel AG: Duchenne dystrophy: Electron microscopic findings, pointing to a basic or early abnormality in the plasma membrane of the muscle fiber. *Neurology* 25:1111, 1975

24. Schotland DL, Bonilla E, Van Meter M: Duchenne dystrophy: Alterations in plasma membrane structure. *Science* 196:1005, 1977

25. Schotland DL, Bonilla E, Wakayama Y: Ultrastructural studies of muscle membrane in neuromuscular disease in Angelini, C Danieli GA, Fontaneri D (eds): *Muscular Dystrophy Research.* Amsterdam, Excerpta Medica, 1980, p 70

26. Bonilla E, Schotland DL, Wakayama Y: Duchenne dystrophy: Focal alterations in the distribution of concanavalin A binding sites at the muscle cell surface. *Ann Neurol* 4:117, 1978

27. Pickard NA, Gruemer H, Verrill HL, Isaacs ER, Robinow M, Nance WF, Myers FC, Goldsmith B: Systemic membrane defect in the proximal muscular dystrophies. *N Engl J Med* 299:841, 1978

28. Stem CMM, Kaban MC, Dubowitz V: Lymphocyte capping in Duchenne muscular dystrophy. *Lancet* 1:1300, 1979

29. Hauser S, Weiner H, Ault K, Unanue E: Lymphocyte capping in Duchenne muscular dystrophy. *N Engl J Med* 300:861, 1979

30. Sybert VP, Kadim ME: Lymphocyte capping in carriers of Duchenne muscle dystrophy. *N Engl J Med* 301:724, 1979

31. Bader PL: Lymphocyte capping in carriers of Duchenne muscular dystrophy. *N Engl J Med* 301:725, 1979

32. Wakayama Y, Schotland DL, Bonilla E, Orecchio E: Quantitative ultrastructural study of muscle satellite cells in Duchenne dystrophy. *Neurology* 29:401, 1979

33. Drachman DB, Toyka KV, Myer E: Prednisone in Duchenne muscular dystrophy. *Lancet* 2:1409, 1974

34. Eyring EJ, Johnson EW, Burnett C: Surgery in muscular dystrophy. *JAMA* 222:1056, 1977

35. Harper PS: Critical evaluation of carrier detection, in Schotland DL (ed): *Diseases of the Motor Unit.* New York, Wiley, 1982, p 821

36. Roses AD, Emery AEH, Harper PS, Thompson MW, Walton JN: Carrier Detection Panel Discussion in Schotland DL (ed): See reference 35, p 847

37. Roses MS, Nicholson MT, Kircher CS, Roses AD: Evaluation and detection of Duchenne's and Becker's muscular dystrophy carriers by manual muscle testing. *Neurology* 27:20, 1977

38. Lane RJ, Muskrey P, Nicholson GA, Siddiqui PQ, Nicholson M, Gascoigne P, Pennington RJ, Gardner-Medwin D, Walton JN: An evaluation of some carrier detection techniques in Duchenne muscular dystrophy. *J Neurol Sci* 43:377, 1979

39. Roses AD, Roses MJ, Metcalf BS, Hall KL, Nicholson GA, Hartwig GB, Roe CR: Pedigree testing in Duchenne muscular dystrophy. *Ann Neurol* 2:271, 1977

40. Nicholson GA, Gardner-Medwin D, Pennington RJ, Walton JN: Carrier detection in Duchenne muscular dystrophy: Assessment of the effect of age on detection rate with serum creatine kinase activity. *Lancet* 1:692, 1979

41. Smith I, Elton RA, Thomson WH: Carrier detection in X-linked recessive (Duchenne) muscular dystrophy: Serum creatine phosphokinase values in premenarchal, menstruating, postmenopausal and pregnant normal women. *Clin Chim Acta* 98:207, 1979

42. Davie AM, Emery AEH: Estimation of proportion of new mutants among cases of Duchenne muscular dystrophy. *J Med Genet* 15:249, 1978

43. Lane RJM, Roses AD: Variation of serum creatine kinase (CK) levels with age in normal females: Implications for genetic counseling in Duchenne muscular dystrophy. *Clin Chim Acta* 113:75, 1981

44. Conneally PM, Heuch I: A computer program to determine genetic risks: A simplified version of PEDIG (Heuch and Li, 1972). *Am J Hum Genet* 26:773, 1975

45. Winter RM: Estimation of male to female ratio of mutation rates from carrier-detection tests on X-linked disorders. *Am J Hum Genet* 32:582, 1980

46. Mahoney MJ, Haseltine FP, Hobbins JC, Banker BQ, Caskey CT, Golbus MS: Prenatal diagnosis of Duchenne's muscular dystrophy. *N Engl J Med* 297:968, 1977

47. Ionasescu V, Zelleger H, Cancilla P: Fetal serum-creatine-phosphokinase: Not a valid predictor of Duchenne muscular dystrophy. *Lancet* 2:1250, 1978

48. Globus MS, Stephens VD, Mahoney MJ, Hobbins JC, Haseltine FP, Caskey CT, Banker BQ: Failure of fetal creatine phosphokinase as a diagnostic indicator of Duchenne muscular dystrophy. *N Engl J Med* 300:860, 1979

49. Emery AEH, Burt D, Dubowitz V, Rocker I, Donnai D, Harris R, Donnai P: Antenatal diagnosis of Duchenne muscular dystrophy. *Lancet* 1:847, 1979

50. Becker PE, Keiner F: Eine neue X chromosomale Muskeldystrophie. *Z Neurol* 193:427, 1955

51. Emery AEH, Skinner R: Clinical studies in benign (Becker type) X-linked muscular dystrophy. *Clin Genet* 10:189, 1976

52. Mabry CC, Roeckel JE, Munich RI, Robertson D: X-linked pseudohypertrophic muscular dystrophy with a late onset and slow progression. *N Engl J Med* 273:1062, 1965

53. Emery AEH, Dreifuss FE: Unusual type of benign X-linked muscular dystrophy. *J Neurol Neurosurg Psychiatry* 29:338, 1966

54. Carroll JE: Facioscapuloperoneal and scapuloperoneal syndromes, in Vinken, PJ, Bruyn GW (eds): *Handbook of Clinical Neurology.* Amsterdam, Elsevier North-Holland, 1979, vol 40, p 349

55. Hudgson P, Bradley WG, Jenkison J: Familial mitochondrial myopathy. I. Clinical, electrophysiological and pathological findings. *J Neurol Sci* 16:343, 1972

56. Mechler F, Fawcett PRW, Mastaglia FL, Hudgson P: Mitochondrial myopathy. A study of clinically affected and asymptomatic members of a six generation family. *J Neurol Sci,* 50:191, 1981

57. Munsat TL, Piper D, Cancilla P, Mednick J: Inflammatory myopathy with facioscapulohumeral distribution. *Neurology (Minn)* 22:335, 1972

58. Brooke MH, Engel WK: The histologic diagnosis of neuromuscular diseases: A review of 79 biopsies. *Arch Phys Med* 47:99, 1966

59. Thomas PK, Calne DB, Elliott CF: X-linked scapuloperoneal syndromes. *J Neurol Neurosurg Psychiatry* 35:208, 1972

60. Bradley WG: The limb-girdle syndromes, in Vinken PJ, Bruyn GW (eds): *Handbook of Clinical Neurology.* Amsterdam, Elsevier North-Holland, 1979, vol 40, p 349

61. Walton JN, Nattrass FJ: On the classification, natural history and treatment of the myopathies. *Brain* 77:170, 1954

62. Jackson CE, Stoehler DA: Limb girdle muscular dystrophy: Clinical manifestation and detection of preclinical disease. *Pediatrics* 41:495, 1968

63. Moser H, Emery AEF: The manifesting carrier in Duchenne muscular dystrophy. *Clin Genet* 5:271, 1974

63a. McKusick VA: Human gene map, Personal communication, 1982

64. Thomasen E: *Myotonia. Thomsen's Disease (Myotonia Congenita), Paramyotonia and Dystrophia Myotonica.* Aarhus, Universitetsforlaget, 1948, p 251

65. Caughey JE, Myrianthopoulos NC: *Dystrophia Myotonica and Related Disorders.* Springfield, Ill, Charles C Thomas, Publisher, 1963, p 282

66. Harper PS: *Myotonic Dystrophy.* Philadelphia, WB Saunders Co, 1979

67. Roses AD, Harper PS, Bossen EH: Myotonic mucular dystrophy, in Vinken PJ, Bruyn GW (eds): *Handbook of Clinical Neurology.* 1979, vol 40, p 485

68. Kilburn K II, Eagen JT, Heyman A: Cardiopulmonary insufficiency associated with myotonic dystrophy. *Am J Med* 26:929, 1959

69. Dodge PR, Gamstorp I, Byers RK, Russel P: Myotonic dystrophy in infancy and childhood. *Pediatrics* 35:3, 1965

70. Watters GV, Williams TW: Early onset myotonic dystrophy: Clinical and laboratory findings in five families and a review of the literature. *Arch Neurol* 17:137, 1967

71. Harper PS: Congenital myotonic dystrophy in Britain. II. Genetic basis. *Arch Dis Child* 50:514, 1975

72. Bossen EH, Shelburne JD, Verkauf BS: Respiratory muscle involvement in infantile myotonic dystrophy. *Arch Pathol* 97:250, 1974

73. Maas O, Paterson AS: Mental changes in families affected by dystrophia myotonica. *Lancet* 232:21, 1937

74. Pruzanski W: Myotonic dystrophy—a multisystem disease: Report of 67 cases and a review of the literature. *Psychiatr Neurol* 149:302, 1965

75. Kohn NH, Faires JS, Rodman T: Unusual manifestations due to involvement of involuntary muscle in dystrophia myotonica. *N Engl J Med* 271:1179, 1964

76. Church SC: The heart in myotonica atrophica. *Arch Intern Med* 119:176, 1967

77. Bache RJ, Sarosi GA: Myotonia atrophica: Diagnosis in a patient with complete heart block and Stokes-Adams syncope. *Arch Intern Med* 121:369, 1968.

78. Prystowsky EN, Pritchett EL, Roses AD, Gallagher JJ: The natural history of conduction system disease in myotonic muscular dystrophy as determined by serial electrophysiologic studies. *Circulation* 60:1360, 1979

79. Wochner DR, Drews B, Strober W, Waldman TA: Accelerated breakdown of immunoglobulin G (IgG) in myotonic dystrophy: A hereditary error of immunoglobulin catabolism. *J Clin Invest* 45:321, 1966

80. Jensen H, Jensen KB, Jarnum S: Turnover of IgG and IgM in myotonic dystrophy. *Neurology* 21:68, 1971

81. Drucker WD, Rowland LP, Sterling K, Christy NP: On the function of the endocrine glands in myotonic muscular dystrophy. *Am J Med* 31:941, 1961

82. Kuhl WJ, Halper IS, Dowben RM: Thyroxine and triiodothyronine turnover studies in dystrophia myotonica. *J Clin Endocrinol* 21:1592, 1961

83. Huff TA, Horton ES, Lebovitz HE: Abnormal insulin secretion in myotonic dystrophy. *N Engl J Med* 277:837, 1967

84. Huff TA, Lebovitz HE: Dynamics of insulin secretion in myotonic dystrophy. *J Clin Endocrinol* 28:992, 1969

85. Hughes DTD, Swann JC, Gleeson JA, Lee FI: Abnormalities in swallowing associated with dystrophia myotonica. *Brain* 88:1037, 1965

86. Harvey JC, Sherbourne DH, Siegel CI: Smooth muscle involvement in myotonic dystrophy. *Am J Med* 39:81, 1965

87. Iwata S: Process of lens opacification and membrane function: A review. *Ophthalmic Res* 6:138, 1974

88. Dark AJ, Streeter BW: Ultrastructural study of cataract in myotonic dystrophy. *Am J Ophthalmol* 84:666, 1977

89. Ginsberg J, Hamblet J, Menefee M: Ocular abnormality in myotonic dystrophy. *Ann Ophthalmol* 10:1021, 1978

90. Stern LE, Cross HE, Crebo AR: Abnormal iris vasculature in myotonic dystrophy. An anterior segment angiographic study. *Arch Neurol* 35:224, 1978

91. Tevarrwerk GJ, Strickland KP, Lin CH, Hudson AJ: Studies on insulin resistance and insulin receptor binding in myotonia dystrophica. *J Clin Endocrinol Metab* 49:216, 1979

92. Festoff BW, Moore WV: Evaluation of insulin receptor in myotonic dystrophy. *Ann Neurol* 6:60, 1979

93. Roses AD, Appel SH: Protein kinase activity in erythrocyte ghosts of patients with myotonic muscular dystrophy. *Proc Natl Acad Sci USA* 70:1855, 1973

94. Atwater I, Ribalet B, Rojas E: Mouse pancreatic B-cells: Tetraethylammonium blockage of the potassium permeability increase induced by depolarization. *J Physiol* 288:561, 1979

95. Atwater I, Dawson CM, Ribalet B, Rojas E: Potassium permeability activated by intracellular calcium ion concentration in the pancreatic B-cell. *J Physiol* 288:575, 1979

96. Motta J, Guilleminault C, Billingham M, Barry W, Mason J: Cardiac abnormalities in myotonic dystrophies. Electrophysiologic and histopathologic studies. *Am J Med* 67:467, 1979

97. Casanova G, Jerusalem F: Myopathology of myotonic dystrophy. A morphometric study. *Acta Neuropathol (Berl).* 45:231, 1979

98. Ladatschen RM, Kerner H, Amikam S, Gellei B: Myotonia dystrophia with heart involvement: An electron microscopic study of skeletal, cardiac and smooth muscle. *J Clin Pathol* 31:1057, 1978

99. Hartwig GB, Roses AD, Rao KR, Jones RH: Radionuclide angiocardiography in myotonic dystrophy. *Neurology,* 31:116, 1981

100. Wohlfart G: Dystrophia myotonica and myotonia congenita: Histopathological studies with special reference to changes in the muscles. *J Neuropathol Exp Neurol* 10:109, 1951

101. Adams RD: Pathological reactions of the skeletal muscle fibre in man, in Walton J (ed): *Disorders of Voluntary Muscle,* ed3. Edinburgh, Churchill Livingstone, Ltd, 1974, p 168

102. Brooke MH, Engel WK: The histographic analysis of human muscle biopsies with regard to fiber types. 3. Myotonias, myasthenia gravis and hypokalemic periodic paralysis. *Neurology* 19:469, 1969

103. Johnson AG: Alterations of the Z-lines and I-band myofilaments in human skeletal muscle. *Acta Neuropathol* 12:218, 1969

104. Schotland DL: An electron microscopic investigation of myotonic dystrophy. *J Neuropathol Exp Neurol* 29:241, 1970

105. Klinkerfuss GH: An electron microscopic study of myotonic dystropy. *Arch Neurol* 16:181, 1967

106. Mussini I, DiMauro S, Angelini C: Early ultrastructural and biochemical changes in muscle in dystrophia myotonica. *J Neurol Sci* 10:585, 1970

107. Schotland DL, Spiro D, Carmel P: Ultrastructural studies of ring fibers in human muscle disease. *J Neuropathol Exp Neurol* 25:431, 1966

108. Stranock SD, Davis JN: Ultrastructure of the muscle spindle in dystrophia myotonia. I. The intrafusal muscle fibres. II. The sensory and motor nerve terminals. *Neuropathol Appl Neurobiol* 4:393, 407, 1978

109. Brown GL, Harvey AM: Congenital myotonia in the goat. *Brain* 62:341, 1939

110. Floyd K, Kent P, Page F: An electromyographic study of myotonia. *Electroencephalogr Clin Neurophysiol* 7:621, 1955

111. Hofman WW, Alston W, Rowe G: A study of individual neuromuscular junctions in myotonia. *Electroencephalogr Clin Neurophysiol* 21:521, 1966

112. Hofman WW, DeNardo GL: Sodium flux in myotonic muscular dystrophy. *Am J Physiol* 214:330, 1968

113. Lipicky RJ: Studies in human myotonic dystrophy, in Rowland LP (ed): *Pathogenesis of the Human Muscular Dystrophies.* Amsterdam, Excerpta Medica, 1977, p 729

114. Lipicky RJ, Bryant SH, Salmon JH: Cable parameters, sodium, potassium, chloride, and water content and potassium efflux in isolated external intercostal muscle of normal volunteers and patients with myotonia congenita. *J Clin Invest* 50:2091, 1971

115. Lipicky RJ, Bryant SH: Sodium, potassium, and chloride fluxes in intercostal muscle from normal goats and goats with hereditary myotonia. *J Gen Physiol* 50:2091, 1966

116. Adrian RH, Bryant SH: On the repetitive discharge in myotonic muscular fibers. *J Physiol* 240:505, 1974

117. Merickel M, Gray R, Chauvin P, Appel SH: Cultured muscle from myotonic muscular patients: Altered membrane electrical properties. *Proc Natl Acad Sci USA* 78:648, 1981

118. Wood DS, Lipicky RJ, Bryant SH: Myotonic dystrophy: In vitro physiologic analysis of intact and skinned fibers. *Neurology* 30:423, 1980

119. Munsat TL: Therapy of myotonia: A double blind comparison of diphenylhydantoin, procainamide and placebo. *Neurology* 17:359, 1967

120. Gowers WR: A lecture on myopathy and a distal form. *Br Med J* 2:89, 1902

121. Welander L: Myopathia distalis tarda hereditaria. *Acta Med Scand (Suppl)* 265:1, 1951

122. Von Graefe A: Verhandlungen arztlicher Gesellschaften. Berliner medicinische Gesellschaft. *Klin Wochenschr* 5:127, 1902

123. Kiloh LG, Nevin S: Progressive dystrophy of the external ocular muscles (ocular myopathy). *Brain* 74:115, 1951

124. Victor M, Hayes R, Adams RD: Oculopharyngeal muscular dystrophy. *N Engl J Med* 267:1267, 1962

125. Kearns TP, Sayre GP: Retinitis pigmentosa, external ophthalmoplegia and complete heart block. *Arch Ophthalmol* 60:280, 1958

126. Drachman DA: Ophthalmoplegia plus: The neurodegenerative disorders associated with progressive external ophthalmoplegia. *Arch Neurol* 18:654, 1968

127. Rosenberg RN, Schotland DL, Lovelana RE, Rowland LP: Progressive ophthalmoplegia: Report of cases. *Arch Neurol* 19:362, 1968

128. Olson W, Engel WK, Walsh GO, Einaugler R: Oculocraniosomatic neuromuscular disease with "ragged red" fibers: Histochemical and ultrastructural changes in limb muscles of a group of patients with idiopathic progressive external ophthalmoplegia. *Arch Neurol* 26:193, 1972

129. Morgan-Hughes JA, Mair WG: A typical muscle mitochondria in oculoskeletal myopathy. *Brain* 96:215, 1973

130. John OC, Kuwabara T: Oculopharyngeal muscular dystrophy. *Am J Ophthalmol* 77:872, 1974

131. Julieu J, Vital U, Vallat JM, Vallat M, LeBlanc M: Oculopharyngeal muscular dystrophy: A case with abnormal mitochondria and "fingerprint" inclusions. *J Neurol Sci* 21:165, 1974

132. Waters DD, Nutter DO, Hopkins LC, Dorrey ER: Cardiac features of an unusual X-linked humeroperoneal neuromuscular disease. *N Engl J Med* 293:1017, 1975

133. Milhorat AT: Creatine and creatine metabolism and diseases of the neuromuscular system. *Assoc Res Nerv Ment Dis Proc* 32:400, 1953

134. Sandberg AA, Hecht HH, Tyler FH: Studies in disorders of muscle. X. The site of creatine synthesis in the human. *Metabolism* 2:22, 1953

135. Hoberman HD, Sims EAH, Peter JH: Creatine and creatine metabolism in normal male adult studies with the aid of isotopic nitrogen. *J Biol Chem* 172:45, 1948

136. Walker JB: Metabolic control of creatine biosynthesis. II. Restoration of transamidinase activity following creatine regression. *J Biol Chem* 236:493, 1961

137. BEESON P, McDERMOTT W (eds): *Textbook of Medicine*. Philadelphia, WB Saunders Co, 1975, p 1888

138. VAN PILSUM JF, WOLIN EA: Guanidinium compounds in blood and urine of patients suffering from muscle disorders. *J Lab Clin Med* 51:219, 1958

139. BENEDICT JP, KALINSKY HJ, SCARRONE LA, WERTHEIM AR, STETTEN DeW JR: The origin of urinary creatine in progressive muscular dystrophy. *J Clin Invest* 34:141, 1955

140. FITCH CC, SINTON DW: A study of creatine metabolism in diseases causing muscle wasting. *J Clin Invest* 43:444, 1964

141. DAVIDSOHN I, HENRY JB (ed): *Todd-Sanford Clinical Diagnosis by Laboratory Methods*. Philadelphia, WB Saunders Co, 1974

142. SIBLEY JA, LEHNINGER AL: Aldolase in the serum and tissues of tumor-bearing animals. *J Natl Cancer Inst* 9:303, 1949

143. SIEKART RG, FLEISHER GA: Serum glutamic oxaloacetic transaminase in certain neurologic and neuromuscular diseases. *Proc Staff Meet Mayo Clin* 31:459, 1956

144. PEARSON CM: Serum enzymes in muscular dystrophy and certain other muscular and neuromuscular diseases: I. Serum glutamic oxaloacetic transaminase. *N Engl J Med* 256:1069, 1957

145. THOMPSON WHS, LEYBURN P, WALTON JN: Serum enzyme activity in muscular dystrophy. *Br Med J* 2:1276, 1960

146. OKIUMAHA S, KUMAGIA N, EBASHI S, SUGITA H, MOMOI H, TOYOKURA Y, FUJIE Y: Serum creatine phosphokinase activity in progressive muscular dystrophy and neuromuscular disorders. *Arch Neurol* 4:520, 1961

147. SWAIMAN KE, SANDLER B: The use of serum creatine phosphokinase and other serum enzymes in the diagnosis of progressive muscular dystrophy. *J Pediatr* 63:1116, 1963

148. GOTO I, PETERS HA, REESE HH: Creatine phosphokinase in neuromuscular disease. *Arch Neurol* 16:529, 1967

149. NICHOL CJ: Serum creatine phosphokinase measurements in muscular dystrophy studies. *Clin Chim Acta* 2:404, 1965

150. PEARCE JMS, PENNINGTON RJ, WALTON JN: Serum enzyme studies in muscle diseases: Part II. Serum creatine kinase activity in muscular dystrophy and in other myopathic and neuropathic disorders. *J Neurol Neurosurg Psychiatry* 27:96, 1964

151. BRAY GM, FERENDELLI JA: Serum creatine phosphokinase in muscle disease: An evaluation of two methods of determination and comparison with serum aldolase. *Neurology* 18:480, 1968

152. MUNSAT TL, BALCH R, PEARSON CM, FOWLER W: Serum enzyme alterations in neuromuscular disorders. *JAMA* 226:1536, 1973

153. HUGHES BP: A method for the estimation of serum creatine kinase and its use in comparing creatine kinase and aldolase activity in normal and pathological sera. *Clin Chim Acta* 7:597, 1962

154. HESS JW, MacDONALD RP, FREDERICK RJ, JONES RN, NEELY J, GROSS D: Serum creatine phosphokinase (CPK) activity in disorders of heart and skeletal muscle. *Ann Intern Med* 61:1015, 1964

155. DUMA RJ, SIEGAL AL: Serum creatine phosphokinase in acute myocardial infarctions: Diagnostic value. *Arch Intern Med* 115:443, 1965

156. GRIFFITHS PD: Creatine phosphokinase levels with hypothyroidism. *Lancet* 1:894, 1963

157. ACHESON J, JAMES DC, HUTCHINSON EC, WESTHEAD R: Serum creatine kinase level in cerebral vascular disease. *Lancet* 1:1306, 1965

158. BELTON NR, BACKUS RE, MILLICHAP JG: Serum creatine phosphokinase activity in epilepsy: Clinical and experimental studies. *Neurology* 17:1073, 1967

159. GOTO I: Creatine phosphokinase isoenzymes in neuromuscular disorders. *Arch Neurol* 31:116, 1974

160. SOMER H, DONNER M, MURROS J, KONTTINEN A: A serum isoenzyme study in muscular dystrophy. *Arch Neurol* 29:343, 1973

161. TZVETANOVA E: Creatine kinase isoenzyme in muscle tissue of patients with neuromuscular diseases in human fetuses. *Enzyme* 12:279, 1971

162. CAO A, DeVIRGILIS S, LIPPI C, COPPA G: Serum and muscle creatine kinase isoenzymes and serum aspartate aminotransferase isoenzymes in progressive muscular dystrophy. *Enzyme* 12:49, 1971

163. SHERWIN AL, KARPATI G, BULCHE JA: Immunohistochemical localization of creatine phosphokinase in skeletal muscle. *Proc Natl Acad Sci USA* 64:171, 1969

164. BALOH R, CANCILLA PA: An appraisal of histochemical fiber types in Duchenne muscular dystrophy. *Neurology* 22:243, 1972

165. IONASESCU V, ZELLWEGER H, CONWAY TW: Ribosomal protein synthesis in Duchenne muscular dystrophy. *Arch Biochem Biophys* 144:51, 1971

166. IONASESCU V, ZELLWEGER H, SHIRK P, CONWAY TW: Identification of carriers of Duchenne muscular dystrophy by muscle protein synthesis. *Neurology* 23:497, 1973

167. PEARSON CM: Histopathological features of muscle in the preclinical stages of muscular dystrophy. *Brain* 85:109, 1962

168. ROWLAND LP, LAYZER RB, KAGEN LJ: Lack of some muscle proteins in serum of patients with Duchenne dystrophy. *Arch Neurol* 18:272, 1968

169. BANK WJ, ROWLAND LP, IPSEN J: Amino acids of plasma and urine in diseases of muscle. *Arch Neurol* 24:176, 1971

170. EMERY AE, BURT D: Amino acid, creatine and creatinuria studies in myotonic dystrophy. *Clin Chim Acta* 39:361, 1972

171. BERMAN PH, NIGRO MA, HARRIS MB, OSKI FA: Activation of fibrinolysis in muscular dystrophy. *Arch Neurol* 29:65, 1973

172. DiMAURO S, SCOTT C, PENN AS, ROWLAND LP: Serum carnitine: An index of muscle destruction in man. *Arch Neurol* 28:186, 1973

173. MARBASHI M, KAWAMURA N, YOSHINAGA K: Urinary excretion of carnitine in progressive muscular dystrophy. *Nature (Lond)* 249:173, 1974

174. ROWLAND LP, PENN AS: Myoglobinuria. *Med Clin North Am* 56:1233, 1972

175. McARDLE B: Myopathy due to a defect in muscle glycogen breakdown. *Clin Sci* 10:13, 1951

176. SCHMID R, MAHLER R: Chronic progressive myopathy with myoglobinuria: Demonstration of a glycogenolytic defect in the muscle. *J Clin Invest* 38:2044, 1959

177. TARUI S, OKUNO G, IKURA Y, TANAKA J: Phosphofructokinase deficiency in skeletal muscle: A new type of glycogenosis. *Biochem Biophys Res Commun* 19:517, 1965

178. LAYZER RB, ROWLAND LP, RANNEY HM: Muscle phosphofructokinase deficiency. *Arch Neurol* 17:517, 1967

179. ENGEL WK, VICK NA, GLUECK CJ, LEVY RI: A skeletal-muscle disorder associated with intermittent symptoms and a possibile defect in lipid metabolism. *N Engl J Med* 282:697, 1970

180. BANK WJ, DiMAURO S, BONILLA E, CAPUZZI DM, ROWLAND LP: A disorder of muscle lipid metabolism and myoglobinuria. *N Engl J Med* 292:443, 1975

181. HOPPEL CL, TOMEC RJ: Carnitine palmityltransferase: Location of two enzymatic activities in rat liver mitochondria. *J Biol Chem* 247:832, 1972

182. ENGEL AG, ANGELINI C: Carnitine deficiency of human skeletal muscle with associated lipid storage myopathy: A new syndrome. *Science* 179:899, 1973

183. SABINA RL, SWAIN JL, PATTEN BM, ASHIZAWA T, O'BRIEN WE, HOLMES EW: Disruption of the purine nucleotide cycle. *J Clin Invest* 66:1419–1423, 1980

184. KAR NC, PEARSON CM: Muscle adenylic acid deaminase activity: Selective decrease in early-onset Duchenne muscular dystrophy. *Neurology* 23:478, 1973

185. FURAKOWA T, PETERS JB: Superprecipitation and adenosine triphosphatase activity of myosin B in Duchenne muscular dystrophy. *Neurology* 21:920, 1971

186. SAMAHA FJ: Actomyosin alterations in Duchenne muscular dystrophy. *Arch Neurol* 28:405, 1973

187. BUCHTHAL F, SCHMALBRUCH H, KAMIENIECKA Z: Contraction times and fiber types in patients with progressive muscular dystrophy. *Neurology* 21:131, 1971

188. SAMAHA FJ: Tropomyosin and troponin in normal dystrophic human muscle. *Arch Neurol* 26:547, 1972

189. FURUKAWA T, PETER JB: Muscular dystrophy and other myopathies. *Arch Neurol* 28:385, 1972

190. PENN AS, CLOAK RA, ROWLAND LP: Myosin from normal and dystrophic human muscle: Immunochemical and electrophoretic studies. *Arch Neurol* 27:159, 1972

191. PERKOFF GT: Studies of human myoglobin in several muscle disease. *N Engl J Med* 270:263, 1964

192. ROMERO-HERRERA AE, LEHMAN H, TOMLINSON BE, WALTON JN: Myoglobin in primary muscle disease. I. Duchenne muscular dystrophy. II. Muscular dystrophy of distal type. *J Med Genet* 10:309, 1973

193. KOSSMAN RJ, FAINER DC, BOYER SH: Study of myoglobin in disease with comments concerning the myoglobin minor components. *Cold Spring Harbor Symp Quant Biol* 29:375, 1964

194. ROWLAND LP, DUNNE PB, PENN AS, MAHER E: Myoglobin and muscular dystrophy. *Arch Neurol* 18:141, 1968

195. SCHAPIRA G, DREYFUS JC, SCHAPIRA F, KRUH J: Glycogenolytic enzymes in human progressive muscular dystrophy. *Am J Phys Med* 34:313, 1955

196. VIGNOS PJ JR, KIFTOWITZ M: A biochemical study of certain skeletal muscle constituents in human progressive muscular dystrophy. *J Clin Invest* 38:873, 1959

197. PENNINGTON RJT: Some enzyme studies in muscular dystrophy. *Proc Assoc Clin Biochem* 2:17, 1962

198. RONZONI E, BERG L, LANDAU W: Enzyme studies in progressive muscular dystrophy. *38th Annual Meeting ARNMD, NY Assoc Res Nerv Ment Dis* 38:721, 1960

199. KAR NC, PEARSON CM: Fructose 1-6-diphosphatase in normal and diseased human muscle. *Clin Chim Acta* 38:252, 1972

200. HEYCK H, LAUDALAN G, LUDERS CJ: Fermentaktivitats besturmunger in der gesunden, menschlichen Muskulator und bei Myopathien. II. Mitteilung. Enzymaktivitatsveranderungen in Muskel bei Dystrophia musculorum progressiva. *Klin Wochenschr* 41:500, 1963

201. STENGEL-RUTKOWSKI L, BARTHELMAI W: Uber den Musdel-Energic-Stoff-

wechsel bei Kindern mit progressiver muskeldystrophie Typ Duchenne. *Klin Wochenschr* 51:957, 1973

202. PENNINGTON RJ, ROBINSON JE: Cathepsin activity in normal and dystrophic human muscle. *Enzymol Biol Clin* 9:175, 1968

203. ABDULLAH F, PENNINGTON RJ: Ribonucleases in normal and dystrophic human muscle. *Clin Chim Acta* 20:365, 1968

204. HOOFT C, DELACY P, LAMBERT Y: Etude comparative de l'activite enzymatique du tissue musculaine de l'enfant normal et d'enfants atteints de dystrophic musculaire progressive aux differents stages de la maladie. *Rev Fr Etud Clin Biol* 2:510, 1966

205. KAR NC, PEARSON CM: Alkaline phasphatase in normal and diseased human muscle. *Proc Soc Exp Biol Med* 141:4, 1972

206. KAR NC, PEARSON CM: 5' Nucleotidase activity of normal and dystrophic human muscle. *Proc Soc Exp Biol Med* 143:1125, 1973

207. HUGHES BP: Lipid changes in Duchenne muscular dystrophy. *J Neurol Neurosurg Psychiatry* 35:658, 1972

208. LIN CH, HUDSON AJ, STRICKLAND KP: Fatty acid oxidation by skeletal muscle mitochondria in Duchenne muscular dystrophy. *Life Sci* 2:355, 1972

209. BRADLEY WG, HUDGSON P, GARDNER-MEDWIN D, WALTON JN: Myopathy associated with abnormal lipid metabolism in skeletal muscle. *Lancet* 1:495–598, 1969

210. DIMAURO S, DIMAURO PMM: Muscle carnitine palmityltransferase deficiency and myoglobinuria. *Science* 182:929–931, 1973

211. DIMAURO S, TREVISAN C, HAYS A: Disorders of lipid metabolism in muscle. *Muscle Nerve* 3:369–388, 1980

212. WEBER A, MURRAY JM: Molecular control mechanisms in muscle contraction. *Physiol Rev* 53:612, 1973

213. FRANZINI-ARMSTRONG C: Membrane particles and transmission at the triad. *Fed Proc* 34:1382, 1975

214. EBASHI S, ENDO M: Calcium ion and muscle contraction. *Prog Biophys Mol Biol* 18:123, 1968

215. SCHNEIDER MF, CHANDLER WK: Voltage dependent charge movement of skeletal muscle: A possible step in excitation-contraction coupling. *Nature (Lond)* 242:244, 1973

216. BIANCHI CP, BOLTON TC: Action of local anesthetics on coupling systems in muscle. *J Pharmacol Exp Ther* 157:388, 1967

217. TAKAGI A, SCHOTLAND DL, ROWLAND LP: Sarcoplasmic reticulum in Duchenne muscular dystrophy. *Arch Neurol* 28:380, 1973

218. SUGITA H, OKIMOTO K, EBASHI S, OKINAKA S: Biochemical alterations in progressive muscular dystrophy with special reference to the sarcoplasmic reticulum, in Milhorat AT (ed): *Exploratory Concepts in Muscular Dystrophy and Related Disorders*. Amsterdam, Excerpta Medica, 1967, p 147

219. SAMAHA FJ, GERGELY J: Biochemical abnormalities of the sarcoplasmic reticulum in muscular dystrophy. *N Engl J Med* 280:184, 1969

220. PETER JB, WORSFOLD M: Muscular dystrophy and other myopathies: Sarcotubular vesicles in early disease. *Biochem Med* 2:364, 1969

221. WORSFOLD M, PETER JB, DUNN RF: Duchenne muscular dystrophy: Distinctive biochemical and electron microscopic abnormalities of the sarcotubular vesicle fraction, in Walton JN (ed): *Muscle Disease*. Amsterdam, Excerpta Medica, 1970, p 303

222. ROE RD, YAMAJI KY, SANDOW A: Contractile responses in dystrophic muscle of mouse and man, in Milhorat AT (ed): *Exploratory Concepts in Muscular Dystrophy and Related Disorders*. Amsterdam, Excerpta Medica, 1967, p 299

223. HASSELBACH W, MAKINOSE M: Die Calcium Pumpe der Erschlaffungsgrana "des Muskels und ihre Abhangigkeit von der ATP-Spaltung." *Biochem Z* 333:518, 1960–1961

224. RADU H, GODRI I, ABU E, RADU A, ROBU R: Calcium uptake and bioelectrical activity of denervated and myotonic muscle. *J Neurol Neurosurg Psychiatry* 33:294, 1970

225. MUSSINI I, DIMAURO S, ANGELINI C: Early ultrastructural and biochemical changes in muscle in dystrophic myotonica. *J Neurol Sci* 10:585, 1970

226. BRODY IA: Muscle contracture induced by exercise. *N Engl J Med* 281:187, 1969

227. WOOD DS, SORENSON MM, EASTWOOD AB, CHERAPH WE, REUBEN JP: Duchenne dystrophy: Abnormal generation of tension and Ca^{++} regulation in single skinned fibers. *Neurology* 28:447, 1978

228. WROGEMANN K, PENA SD: Mitochondrial calcium overload: A general mechanism for cell-necrosis in muscle diseases. *Lancet* 1:672, 1976

229. BODENSTEINER JB, ENGEL AG: Intracellular calcium accumulation in Duchenne dystrophy and other myopathies: A study of 567,000 muscle fibers in 114 biopsies. *Neurology* 28:439, 1978

230. OBERC MA, ENGEL WK: Ultrastructural localization of calcium in normal and abnormal skeletal muscle. *Lab Invest* 36:566, 1977

231. MAUNDER-SEWRY CA, DUBOWITZ V: Myonuclear calcium in carriers of Duchenne muscular dystrophy. *J Neurol Sci* 42:337, 1979

232. BROWN HD, CHATTOPADHYAY SK, PATEL AB: Erythrocyte abnormality in human myopathy. *Science* 157:1577, 1967

233. KLASSON GA, BLOSTEIN R: Adenosine triphosphatase and myopathy. *Science* 163:492, 1969

234. SONWEINE G, BERNARD JC, LANCE Y, LACHANAT J: The sodium pump of erythrocytes from patients with Duchenne muscular dystrophy: Effect of ouabain on the active sodium flux and on (Na, K) ATPase. *J Neurol* 217:287, 1978

235. PETER JB, WORSFOLD M, PEARSON CM: Erythrocyte ghost adenosine triphosphatase (ATPase) in Duchenne dystrophy. *J Lab Clin Med* 74:103, 1969

236. SIGGIQUI PQ, PENNINGTON RJ: Effect of ouabain upon erythrocyte membrane adenosine triphosphatase in Duchenne muscular dystrophy. *J Neurol Sci* 34:365, 1977

237. HULL KL, ROSES AD: Stoichiometry of sodium and potassium transport in erythrocytes from patients with myotonic muscular dystrophy. *J Physiol* 254:160, 1976

238. HOBBS AS, BRUMBACK RA, FESTOFF BW: Monovalent cation transport in myotonic dystrophy. Na-K pump ratio in erythrocytes. *J Neurol Sci* 41:299, 1979

239. HODSON A, PLEASANT D: Erythrocyte cation-activated adenosine triphosphatase in Duchenne muscular dystrophy. *J Neurol Sci* 32:361, 1977

240. LUTHRA MG, STEM LZ, KIM HD: (Ca + Mg)-ATPase of red cells in Duchenne and myotonic cystrophy: Effect of soluble cytoplasmic activator. *Neurology* 29:835, 1979

241. ROSES AD, APPEL SH: Protein kinase activity in erythrocyte ghosts of patients with myotonic muscular dystrophy. *Proc Natl Acad Sci USA* 70:1855, 1973

242. ROSES AD, APPEL SH: Phosphorylation of component a of the human erythrocyte membrane in myotonic muscular dystrophy. *J Membrane Biol* 20:51, 1975

243. WONG P, ROSES AD: Isolation of an abnormally phosphorylated erythrocyte membrane band 3 glycoprotein from patients with myotonic muscular dystrophy. *J Membr Biol* 45:147, 1979

244. ROSES AD, HARTWIG GB, MABRY M, NAGANO Y, WONG P, MILLER SE: On membrane proteins in Duchenne and myotonic muscular dystrophy: Erythrocyte and fibroblast studies. *Muscle Nerve* 3:36, 1980

245. IYER SL, HOEINING PA, SHERBLOM AP, HOWLAND JL: Membrane function affected by genetic muscular dystrophy. I. Erythrocyte ghost protein kinase. *Biochem Med* 18:384, 1977

246. VICKERS JD, RATHBONE MP, ROSES AD: Alterations of erythrocyte ghost protein phosphorylation in the Duchenne and myotonic muscular dystrophies. *Biochem Med* 20:434, 1978

247. ROSES AD, HERBSTREITH MH, APPEL SH: Membrane protein kinase alteration in Duchenne muscular dystrophy. *Nature* 254:350, 1975

248. ROSES AD, SHILE PE, HERBSTREITH MH, BALAKRISHNAN CV: Identification of abnormally (^{32}P)-phosphorylated cyanogen bromide cleavage product of erythrocyte membrane spectrin in Duchenne muscular dystrophy. *Neurology* 31:1026, 1981

249. MABRY ME, ROSES AD: Increased (^{32}P)-phosphorylation of tryptic peptides of erythrocyte spectrin in Duchenne muscular dystrophy. *Muscle Nerve* 4:489, 1981

250. NAGANO Y, WONG P, ROSES AD: Altered erythrocyte spectrin extractability in Duchenne muscular dystrophy. *Clin Chim Acta* 108:469, 1980

251. TSUCHIYA Y, SUGITA H, ISHURA S, IMAHORI K: Spectrin extractability from erythrocyte in Duchenne muscular dystrophies and the effect of proteases on erythrocyte ghosts. *Clin Chim ACta* 109:285, 1981

252. FALK RS, CAMPION D, GUTHRIE D, SPARKE RS, FOX CF: Phosphorylation of the red cell membrane proteins in Duchenne muscular dystrophy. *N Engl J Med* 5:258, 1979

253. FISCHER S, TORTOLERO M, PIAU JP, DELAUNAY J, SCHAPIRA G: Protein kinase and adenylate cyclase of erythrocyte membrane from patients with Duchenne muscular dystrophy. *Clin Chim Acta* 88:437, 1978

254. ROSES AD, MABRY ME, HERBSTREITH MH, SHILE PV, BALAKRISHNAN CV: Increased ^{32}P-phosphorylation of spectrin peptides in Duchenne muscular dystrophy, in Schotland (see reference 35), p 414

255. MAWATARV S, SCHONBERG M, OLARTE M: Biomedical abnormalities of erythrocyte membranes in Duchenne dystrophy: Adenosine triphosphatase and adenyl cyclase. *Arch Neurol* 33:489, 1976

256. DISE CA, GOODMAN DB, LAKE WC, HODSON A, RASMUSSEN H: Enhanced sensitivity to calcium in Duchenne muscular dystrophy. *Biochem Biophys Res Commun* 79:1286, 1977

257. PLISHKER GA, APPEL SH: Red blood cell alteration in muscular dystrophy: The role of lipids. *Muscle Nerve* 3:70, 1980

258. PLISHKER GA, GITELMAN WJ, APPEL SH: Myotonic muscular dystrophy: Altered calcium transport in erythrocytes. *Science* 200:323, 1978

259. KUNZE D, REICHMANN G, EGGER E, LEUSCHNER G, ECKHARDT H: Erythrozytenlipide bei progressiver Muskel Dystrophie. *Clin Chim Acta* 43:333, 1973

260. GODIN DV, BRIDGE MA, MACLEOD PJ: Chemical compositional studies of erythrocyte membranes in Duchenne muscular dystrophy. *Res Commun Chem Pathol Pharmacol* 20:331, 1978

261. MCLAUGHLIN J, ENGEL WK: Lipid composition of erythrocytes. Findings

in Duchenne's muscular dystrophy and myotonic atrophy. *Arch Neurol* 36:351, 1979

262. KOSKI CL, JUNGALWALA FB, KOLODNY EH: Normality of erythrocyte phospholipids in Duchenne muscular dystrophy. *Clin Chim Acta* 85:295, 1978

263. ANDIMAN RM, PETER JB, DHOPESHWARKAR G: Myotonic dystrophy and myotonia congenita: ATPase and lipid composition of erythrocyte membranes and serum lipids with special reference to desmosteral. *Neurology* 24:352, 1974

264. BUTTERFIELD DA, ROSES AD, COOPER ML, APPEL SH, CHESTNUT DB: A comparative ESR study of the erythrocyte membrane in myotonic muscular dystrophy. *Biochemistry* 13:5078, 1974

265. BUTTERFIELD DA, ROSES AD, APPEL SH, CHESTNUT DB: Electron spin resonance studies of membrane proteins in erythrocytes in myotonic muscular dystrophy. *Arch Biochem Biophys* 177:226, 1976

266. WILKERSON LS, PERKINS RC, ROELOFS R, SWIFT L, DALTON LR, PARK JH: Erythrocyte membrane abnormalities in Duchenne muscular dystrophy monitored by saturation transfer electron paramagnetic resonance spectroscopy. *Proc Natl Acad Sci USA* 75:838, 1978

267. PERCY AK, MILLER ME: Reduced deformability of erythrocyte membranes from patients with Duchenne muscular dystrophy. *Nature* 258:147, 1975

268. MATHESON DW, HOWLAND JL: Erythrocyte deformation in human muscular dystrophy. *Science* 184:165, 1974

269. MILLER SE, ROSES AD, APPEL SH: Scanning electron microscopy studies in muscular dystrophy. *Arch Neurol* 33:172, 1976

270. McCOMAS AJ, CAMPBELL MJ, SICA REP: Electrophysiological study of dystrophia myotonica. *J Neurol Neurosurg Psychiatry* 34:132, 1971

271. McCOMAS AJ, SICA REP, CURRIE S: An electrophysiological study of Duchenne dystrophy. *J Neurol Neurosurg Psychiatry* 34:461, 1971

272. SICA REP, McCOMAS AJ: An electrophysiological investigation of limb-girdle and fascioscapulohumeral dystrophy. *J Neurol Neurosurg Psychiatry* 34:469, 1971

273. McCOMAS AJ, SICA REP, CAMPBELL MJ: "Sick motoneurones": A unifying concent of muscle disease. *Lancet* 1:321, 1971

274. UPTON ARM, McCOMAS AJ, BIANCHI FA: Neuropathy in McArdle's syndrome. *N Engl J Med* 289:750, 1973

275. McCOMAS AJ, SICA REP, CURRIE S: Muscular dystrophy: Evidence for a neural factor. *Nature (Lond)* 226:1263, 1970

276. PANAYIOTOPOULOS CP, SCARPALEZOS S, PAPAPETROPOULOS TA: Electrophysiological estimation of motor units in Duchenne muscular dystrophy. *J Neurol Sci* 23:89, 1974

277. SCARPALEZOS S, PANAYIOTOPOULOS CP: Duchenne muscular dystrophy: Reservations to the neurogenic hypothesis. *Lancet* 2:458, 1973

278. BALLANTYNE JP, HANSEN S: Myopathies: The neurogenic hypothesis? *Lancet* 1:1060, 1974

279. BALLANTYNE JP, HANSEN S: New method for the estimation of the number of motor units in a muscle. 2. Duchenne, limb-girdle and fascioscapulohumeral, and myotonic muscular dystrophies. *J Neurol Neurosurg Psychiatry* 37:1195, 1974

280. BRADLEY WG: State of play in the neural hypothesis of muscular dystrophy. *Nature (Lond)* 250:285, 1974

281. DEMOS J: Un nouveau problem pose per la myopathie humaine: Les troubles des temps de circulation et leur liaison avec l'activite enzymatique serique. *Soc Med Hop Paris* 77:636, 1961

282. HATHAWAY PW, ENGEL WK, ZELLWEGER H: Experimental myopathy after microarterial embolization: Comparison with childhood X-linked pseudohypertrophic muscular dystrophy. *Arch Neurol* 22:365, 1970

283. MENDELL JR, ENGEL WK, DERRER EC: Duchenne muscular dystrophy: Functional ischemia reproduces its characteristic lesions. *Science* 172:1143, 1971

284. PAULSON OB, ENGEL AG, GOMEZ MR: Muscle blood flow in Duchenne type muscular dystrophy, limb-girdle dystrophy, polymyositis and in normal controls. *J Neurol Neurosurg Psychiatr* 37:685, 1974

285. JERUSALEM F, ENGEL AG, GOMEZ MR: Duchenne dystrophy. I. Morphometric study of the muscle microvasculature. *Brain* 97:115, 1974

286. BRADLEY WG, O'BRIEN MD, WALDER DN, MURCHISON D, JOHNSON M, NEWELL DJ: Failure to confirm a vascular cause of muscular dystrophy. *Arch Neurol* 32:466, 1975

287. WRIGHT TL, O'NEILL JA, OLSON WH: Abnormal intravibrillar monoamines in sex-linked muscular dystrophy. *Neurology* 23:510, 1973

288. JERUSALEM F, ENGEL AG, GOMEZ MR: Duchenne dystrophy. II. Morphometric study of motor end plate fine structure. *Brain* 97:123, 1974

289. HUXLEY AF: Future prospects. *Br Med Bull* 36:199, 1980

67

FAMILIAL PERIODIC PARALYSIS

This summary is adapted from a summary written by Carl M. Pearson and Krishna Kalyanaraman for the third edition of this book [1].

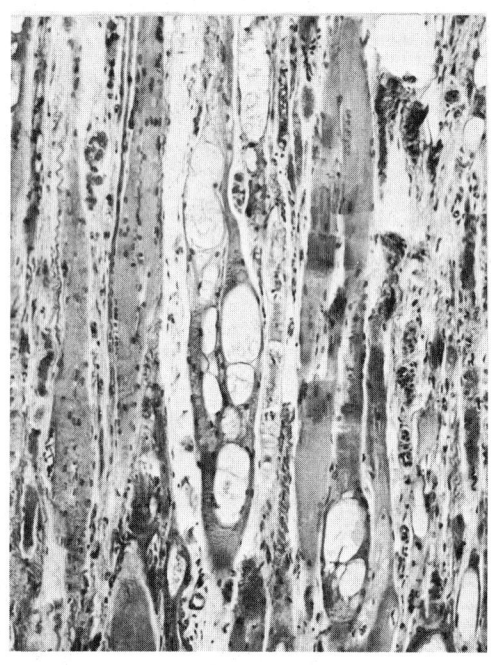

Severe vacuolization and myopathic changes in muscle and interstitial tissue from a patient with hypokalemic periodic paralysis and permanent myopathic weakness. X 162. (*From CM Pearson, by permission [1].*)

1. *The familial periodic paralyses are a group of disorders characterized by attacks of flaccid paralysis. The paralysis rarely involves the bulbar and cranial musculature, and there are no sensory or sphincter changes. Three varieties of the disorder are recognized, one with reduced plasma concentrations of potassium during attacks, another with increased concentrations, and a third with normal plasma potassium. All are inherited as autosomal dominant traits. Periodic paralysis may also occur secondary to thyrotoxicosis and other metabolic disorders.*

2. *Hypokalemic periodic paralysis occurs more frequently and severely in males than in females. Attacks occur on rest after exertion, after a high-carbohydrate diet, or on exposure to cold or other stress. They may be induced by insulin with glucose, ACTH, adrenal cortical steroids, and epinephrine. Characteristic vacuoles appear within the myofibrils. During attacks the plasma potassium falls, but there is a net positive total body balance of potassium before the attack commences. Sodium is retained as well. The muscle membranes are depolarized during attacks. The pathogenesis of the disease remains undetermined.*

3. *Hyperkalemic periodic paralysis is also more severe in* males. Attacks are precipitated by rest after exertion, by cold and hunger, and may be induced by administration of potassium. During seizures the muscle content of potassium falls. The pathogenesis of this disorder is unknown. Paramyotonia congenita is a related syndrome.

4. *Normokalemic periodic paralysis has been described in a single large kindred. Duration of paralytic attacks is much longer than in the other two types. Muscle biopsy findngs are indistinguishable from those of the other types.*

5. Periodic paralysis *which occurs in association with thyrotoxicosis is not familial. This disorder has been seen mostly but not exclusively in Japanese. It disappears with correction of the thyrotoxicosis. The clinical pattern is indistinguishable from that of hypokalemic periodic paralysis.*

REFERENCE

1. PEARSON CM, KALYANARAMAN K: The periodic paralyses, in Stanbury JB, Wyngaarden JB, Fredrickson DS (eds): *The Metabolic Basis of Inherited Disease,* ed 3. New York, McGraw-Hill Book Co, 1972, p 1181

68

HYPOPHOSPHATASIA

HOWARD RASMUSSEN

1. *Hypophosphatasia is a familial disease in which severe skeletal defects resembling rickets result from a failure of deposition of bone mineral in osteoid and in epiphyseal cartilage. The serum and bone alkaline phosphatase activities are low, and the urinary excretion and plasma concentrations of phosphorylethanolamine and inorganic pyrophosphate are elevated. This rickets is resistant to treatment with vitamin D.*

2. *Three clinical types of hypophosphatasia have been recognized: (a) infantile, (b) childhood, and (c) adult. This classification is based upon the time of diagnosis and the clinical severity of the disease. Death may occur early in life, but some patients may develop signs and symptoms in adult life. There may be premature synostosis of the cranial vault, premature loss of deciduous teeth, somatic retardation, spontaneous fractures, hypercalcemia, and nephrocalcinosis.*

3. *Diagnosis is based on radiologic and histologic changes in bone indistinguishable from those of rickets, high concentrations of pyrophosphate and phosphorylethanolamine in plasma or urine, and low serum alkaline phosphatase activity. Renal clearance of phosphorylethanolamine is high.*

4. *Cases of so-called pseudohypophosphatasia have been described in kindreds containing clearly defined cases of hypophosphatasia. These patients have all or many of the clinical, radiologic, and biochemical signs of the disease but have normal concentrations of serum alkaline phosphatase.*

5. *The cardinal pathologic feature of the disease is inadequate or total lack of calcification of bone matrix and of cartilage. It seems likely that this is due to a deficiency or abnormality of bone alkaline phosphatase. In the normal process of mineralization, both in membranous bone and in epiphyseal cartilage, initial mineral crystal deposition takes place in extracellular, membrane-enclosed matrix vesicles. The membranes of these vesicles contain large amounts of alkaline phosphatase (pyrophosphatase), and it is currently believed that the activity of this enzyme on pyrophosphate and other phosphate esters leads to the accumulation of inorganic phosphate by the matrix vesicles, leading in turn to the nucleation of the first bone mineral crystals within the vesicles. The relationship between phosphorylethanolamine, alkaline phosphatase, and the mineralization process is not known.*

6. *The disease appears to be inherited as an autosomal recessive trait. Heterozygotes may have low serum alkaline phosphatase concentrations, high urinary excretion of phosphorylethanolamine, or both, without bone disease. In some instances an autosomal dominant mode of inheritance has been suggested.*

7. *The only treatment that may be effective is a continuous high oral phosphate intake.*

8. Prenatal diagnosis of the severe disease is possible by measurement of the extent of fetal skull calcification by ultrasonography.

Hypophosphatasia is a familial disease characterized by disturbances of the normal sequence of bone mineralization (Fig. 68-1), premature loss of deciduous teeth, subnormal serum and tissue alkaline phosphatase activities, and excessive quantities of phosphorylethanolamine (PEA) in the plasma and urine. Hypercalcemia, renal damage, and occasionally premature synostosis of the cranial vault may also be found. It is probably transmitted as an autosomal recessive trait.

HISTORICAL ASPECTS

Although the disease was first given its present name by Rathbun [1] in 1948, there are scattered reports of what is undoubtedly the same entity going back 20 years before that time. The historical aspects are covered in detail in the reviews by Fraser [2], by Currarino and associates [3], and by Rasmussen [4]. The following reports are of special interest in the development of currently accepted concepts of the disease: Huhne and Schonfeld [5], in 1929, described a patient with a syndrome clearly recognizable in retrospect as hypophosphatasia. Chown [6], in 1935, described two similar patients who at autopsy were found to have nephrocalcinosis. Kubatsch [7], in 1938, described "islands" of bone in the skull of a patient whose father had evidence of premature synostosis. Alkaline phosphatase values were not reported. Anspach and Clifton [8], in 1939, noted hypercalcemia in a child with pathognomonic changes in the bones, including premature synostosis.

Serum alkaline phosphatase concentrations were very low, except for one value in early infancy. Macey [9], in 1940, described two brothers (one 36 years of age) with hypophosphatasia who gave a history of severe rickets in childhood and of numerous fractures in adult life. Rathbun, in his classic description, reported that alkaline phosphatase activity was low in bone, intestinal mucosa, and kidney. In 1953 Sobel and associates [10] first described premature loss of deciduous teeth as part of the syndrome. They also found low alkaline phosphatase activity in plasma, bone, cartilage, liver, and a tooth; their data suggested hypersensitivity to vitamin D.

Fraser and associates [11] and McCance [12] discovered simultaneously, in 1955, that the urinary excretion of phosphorylethanolamine (PEA) is an integral feature of the disease. They showed also that the parents of patients might have abnormally low serum alkaline phosphatase values. Fraser et al. [11] found that PEA might appear in the plasma of patients and in the urine of the otherwise normal parents of patients with hypophosphatasia. Fraser and Yendt [13] also showed that the cartilage of rachitic rats would calcify in the serum of patients with hypophosphatasia but that costochondral cartilage and osteoid from a patient would not calcify in the serum of normal persons or in a synthetic medium containing appropriate concentrations of calcium and phosphate ions. Scaglione and Lucey [14] reported, in 1956, that a patient with abnormally low phosphatase activity in bone might nevertheless have normal phosphatase activity in the liver, duodenal juice, and, indeed, in osteoblasts in tissue culture. In 1958 Kretchmer and associates [15] reported alkaline phosphatase activity absent from the leukocytes of a patient and normal in the leukocytes of the mother (whose serum phosphatase activity was low).

Pimstone et al. [16] showed that the serum alkaline phosphatase activity could be normal in patients known on genetic grounds to have hypophosphatasia—including even one patient with bone disease, excessive urinary PEA, and premature loss of deciduous teeth. In an adult patient with the full syndrome [17] they showed reciprocal fluctuations of serum alkaline phosphatase and urinary PEA values over a 5-year period, although each was normal on several occasions. This patient also excreted phosphorylcholine in excessive amounts. The significance of serum alkaline phosphatase values in hypophosphatasia can be clarified only when the source of the phosphatase can be identified. Scriver and Cameron [18] reported that in a patient with normal total values the only significant abnormality appeared to be a decrease in affinity of the plasma phosphatase (isoenzyme) for PEA. Likewise, Méhes et al. [19] have reported five patients with clinical signs of the disease in whom serum alkaline phosphatase assay values proved to be normal upon repeated examination. Rasmussen [4] showed that the renal clearance of PEA varies directly with plasma PEA, approaching the creatinine clearance in homozygotes with the highest plasma values. His elegant chemical studies by refined techniques establish for the first time *normal* urinary, plasma, and clearance values for PEA.

CLINICAL FINDINGS

On the basis of clinical information and, in particular, the estimated time of development of bone lesions, three clinical types of hypophosphatasia have been recognized [2, 19–21]:

Figure 68-1 The proposed sequence of events in normal calcification at the epiphyseal plate or in membranous bone. Step I involves the formation of extracellular matrix vesicles, probably by a process of budding from the plasma membrane of the cartilage or bone cells. Step II involves the movement of calcium accumulated in the mitochondria of the cells out of the cell into the vesicles. Step III (note magnification is changed so that vesicles appear larger) involves the hydrolysis of inorganic pyrophosphate, and probably other phosphate esters, by the alkaline phosphatase   in the vesicle membrane, with accumulation of inorganic phosphate within the vesicle. Step IV involves the nucleation of the first mineral crystals within the vesicles. Step V involves mineral crystal growth with eventual rupture of vesicle membrane.

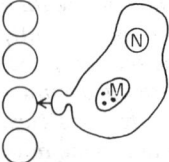

I Vesicle Formation

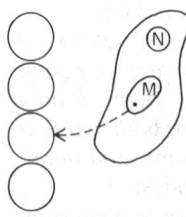

II Calcium Uptake

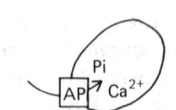

III Pyrophosphate Hydrolysis

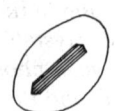

IV Hydroxyapatite Crystal Formation

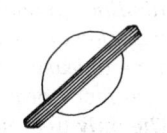

V Mineral Crystal Growth

(1) infantile, (2) childhood, and (3) adult. In the infantile type, severe rickets, hypercalcemia, failure to thrive, and severe bony abnormalities exist, and the condition is lethal in over 50 percent of affected subjects. The childhood type is characterized by premature shedding of the deciduous teeth [22, 23], increased susceptibility to infection, somatic retardation, and radiologically by irregular epiphyses and irregular islands of radiolucency in the shafts of the bones. The adult form may include spontaneous fractures, often a history of "rickets" in childhood, and radiolucent zones in the skeleton. Some adult subjects have been recognized by chance measurement of plasma alkaline phosphatase. In spite of the utility of this classification, there is no sharp division between the different forms. A fourth, clearly distinguishable type, pseudohypophosphatasia, has been described in which the usual signs and symptoms of the infantile, childhood, or adult type of disease were present but in which the plasma alkaline phosphatase concentration was normal. The appearance of patients with hypophosphatasia and pseudohypophosphatasia in the same kindred [19] argues that they represent variations of the same basic disease state.

The clinical findings in hypophosphatasia are probably all attributable to the defect in formation of true bone, to premature synostosis of the skull, or to the hypercalcemia which is a frequent but not constant feature. Since the essential feature of the generalized bone disease is inadequacy of mature bone mineralization, the earlier the appearance of the disorder, the more severe the clinical manifestations. When the disease appears in utero, infants are often stillborn and lack adequate bony support for cranial and thoracic cavities. When it appears in adult life, patients may be asymptomatic or have only the symptoms attendant upon an occasional fracture. The disease of bone includes the gross changes of true rickets, with beading of costochondral junctions, bowing of the legs, and widening of the ends of the long bones. It may resemble the disorder *congenital bowing of the long bones,* in which the histologic and biochemical defects of hypophosphatasia are not found

[24]. Genu valgum is commonly seen in hypophosphatasia. The ends of the long bones may assume a characteristic "notched" appearance by x-ray that clearly differs from the smooth "cupping' of untreated rickets and resembles that of the metaphyseal dysplasia. Figure 68-2 shows such lesions in a child of 39 months with hypophosphatasia.

Premature synostosis may be suspected in infancy by the *absence* of radiologically demonstrable bone over large areas of skull. As in the syndrome of oxycephaly or acrocephalosyndactyly [25, 26], these areas represent, in fact, uncalcified osteoid without fibrous septums [27]. As they calcify, exophthalmos and an increase in intracranial pressure may appear. The skull may take on a "beaten silver" appearance by x-ray [28, 29]. Convulsions, serious brain damage, and death may ensue if surgical decompression is not performed. The late manifestations are those of oxycephaly. The sutures may show characteristic prominent bony ridges.

Subperiosteal new bone formation, not normally seen in rickets, has been reported in three patients [1, 2, 30]. Premature loss of the anterior deciduous teeth occurs frequently. Indeed, this sign, which may appear without other evidence of bone disease [16, 22, 23], may be a valuable genetic marker for patients with a minimal expression of the syndrome.

Hypercalcemia is common, especially in infants, and hypercalcuria results. The nausea and vomiting of some patients are clearly attributable to the hypercalcemia.

Some patients have come to medical attention for the first time as adults [9, 17–19, 29, 31–37]. In some, rickets was said to have been present in childhood, followed by an interim period of apparently normal health. They were later found in adulthood to have radiolucent bones and, in most instances, pseudofractures. In some, the rib cage still showed the classic deformities of infantile rickets [29]. One patient had "osteoporosis," hypophosphatasia, and phosphorylethanolaminuria, but no evidence of earlier disease. It thus appears that spontaneous, virtually complete remissions may occur and that new manifestations may not appear for a number of years.

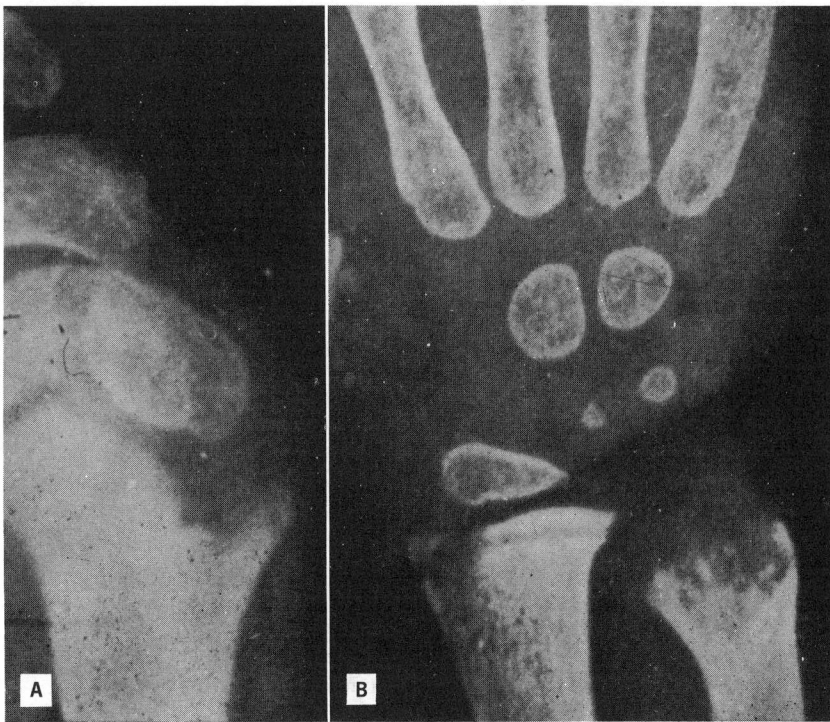

Figure 68-2 X-ray of the shoulder (*A*) and wrist (*B*) of a 39-month-old female with hypophosphatasia. Note defects in epiphyseal ossification. (*By permission of Dr. Edna Sobel.*)

Recent studies emphasize that the adult form of the disease is more common than previously supposed. Whyte et al. [38] investigated the kindred of a 58-year-old female with the adult form of the disease who presented with recurrent fractures. Twelve persons (out of 44 examined) in three generations were found with subnormal serum alkaline phosphatase activity. All 12 were clinically well, but a majority had either a history of severe caries or early loss of permanent teeth. On bone biopsy at least four had an increase in osteoid volume, and several, particularly the females, had osteopenia as measured by bone densitometry.

LABORATORY DIAGNOSIS

Laboratory diagnosis consists of (1) demonstration of serum alkaline phosphatase values below normal for the patient's age, (2) histologic characterization of the bone lesions, and (3) demonstration of abnormal quantities of PEA in the urine and plasma. PEA is found in small quantities in normal urine and plasma and is found in such large quantities in the urine of patients with other metabolic bone diseases that its use as a "marker" for subjects heterozygous for hypophosphatasia is of limited value [39].

Rasmussen [4] provided the first quantitative values for urinary excretion, plasma concentration, and renal clearance of PEA in normal control subjects, as well as in patients. The normal values were 17 to 99 μmol/24 h, 0.21 to 0.33 μmol/dl, and 4 to 12 ml/min, respectively. Heterozygotes for hypophosphatasia (see below) showed urinary values three to eight times those of normal controls, plasma values about twice normal, and clearances about four times normal. Patients with hypophosphatasia showed urinary values from 10 to 50 times normal, and plasma values about twice those of heterozygotes (0.75 to 0.85 μmol/dl). The renal clearance of PEA in these patients approached the creatinine clearance.

Rasmussen also studied the fate of "loads" of PEA in normal persons, in heterozygous carriers of hypophosphatasia, and in patients with the full syndrome. All the results show an apparent "tubular maximum" for reabsorption of PEA of about 3 μmol/min. Normal subjects, filtering only slightly more than this, excrete very little (about 7 percent of the load), whereas homozygous patients, filtering three to four times as much, reabsorb the same absolute amount and excrete about 90 percent of the load. Rasmussen's experiments showed also that patients, as compared to normal subjects, achieved higher plasma concentrations of PEA for a given load (e.g., 16 μmol/dl following a load of 21 μmol/kg body weight in patients, versus 10 μmol/dl in a normal subject) and showed a lower rate of decline in spite of the higher renal clearance.

Licata et al. [39] have reported on measurements of the urinary excretion of PEA in a variety of diseases other than hypophosphatasia. They found that children under 15 excreted approximately 130 μmol/g creatinine per day, but adults excreted approximately half this value (70 to 76 μmol/g creatinine per day). Patients with a variety of metabolic bone diseases and different endocrine disorders all excreted amounts 1.5 to 2.0 times greater than the control subjects, values close to those previously reported for some heterozygotes.

Hydroxyproline excretion, which serves as an index of collagen metabolism, may be extremely low in hypophosphatasia [40], whereas it is high in vitamin D–resistant rickets. This suggests that hydroxyproline excretion in hypophosphatasia reflects bone destruction (which is clearly decreased in the syndrome), rather than osteoid formation (which is clearly increased).

The histologic picture is generally indistinguishable from that of true rickets. The defect in ossification of cartilage appears, as in rickets, as a widening of the zones of provisional calcification, disruption of the normal columnar arrangement of cells, and failure of calcification of degenerating cartilage. Figure 68-3 shows a section from a costochondral junction of a child with the disorder [10]. The defect in appositional and subperiosteal bone formation appears as wide zones of uncalcified osteoid lined with osteoblasts. There is virtually no osteoclast, nor is there fibrosis of the marrow or other evidence of bone destruction. As in osteomalacia, the total mass of bone plus matrix may appear greater than normal [27]. The defect in membranous bone, which may be so extensive as to leave only plaques of true bone in the skull [1], is histologically similar, showing wide areas of uncalcified osteoid. As observed in microradiologic studies, the true bone in this disease may have a relatively primitive structure for the patient's age, and the collagen fibrils may be correspondingly poorly arranged [41]. The primitive structure may result from the relative absence of remodeling of osteoid as compared with that in true bone.

THE CALCIFICATION PROCESS

Within the past decade our views of the calcification process and the role of alkaline phosphatase have undergone a marked change, primarily because of the identification of extracellular membrane-bound vesicles [42]. Apparently playing a central role in the initiation of the mineralization process, these vesicles contain significant amounts of alkaline phosphatase, pyrophosphatase, and ATPase. Matrix vesicles were first identified in calcifying cartilage [43–45], but have since been found in membranous and cortical bone [44–47], fracture callus [48], dentin [49–53], deer antler [54], and even in calcifying arteriosclerotic aortic valves [55–56]. Hence, it appears that they are found in all mammalian systems undergoing calcification.

All matrix vesicles are enveloped by a membrane that appears trilaminar by electron microscopy (Fig. 68-4). They vary in size from 300 Å to 1 μm but are usually 1000 Å in diameter. They contain osmium-staining material that is yet to be completely characterized, but may be a mixture of polysaccharide [45], phospholipids and glycolipids [57–59], and amorphous calcium phosphate [60–62]. The source of these vesicles is not established. The three most probable sites of origin are the cell membrane [45], the mitochondria [62, 63], and the lysosomes [64]. It seems clear that the vesicles exist as separate entities, not connected by any processes to the cartilage or bone cells. Present evidence [42, 45, 57–59, 65–68], consisting principally of the nature of the lipid and enzyme, favors the view that these matrix vesicles arise by budding off of the plasma membranes of the appropriate cells, but verification of this sequence awaits further research.

Over 30 percent of the total alkaline phosphatase in a crude homogenate of calcifying cartilage sediments with the matrix vesicle fraction. A similar distribution of bone pyrophospha-

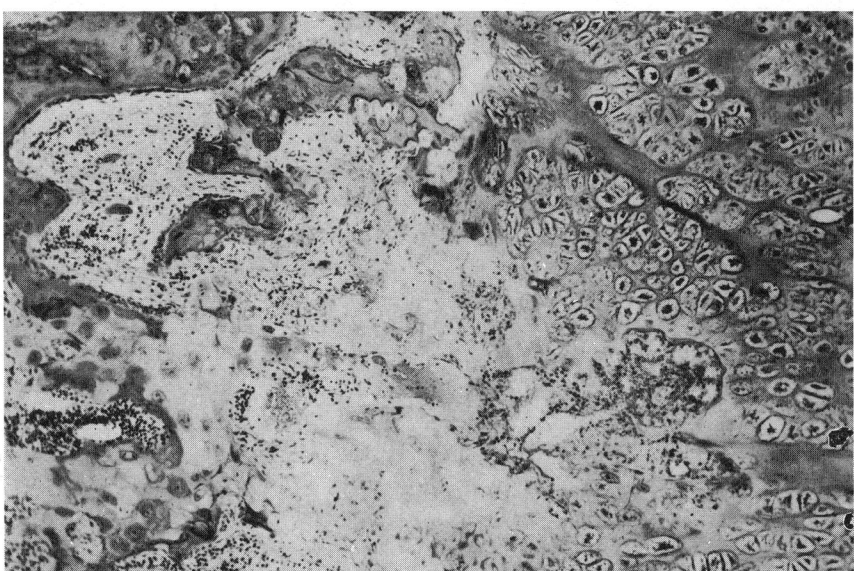

Figure 68-3 Costochondral junction of a rib of a 39-month-old girl with hypophosphatasia. Note the disorganization of cartilage and osteoid seams lined with osteoblasts. Undecalcified. (*By permission of Dr. Edna Sobel.*)

tase is found. There is increasing evidence that bone alkaline phosphatase and bone pyrophosphatase are one and the same enzyme [69, 70]. These observations shed new light on the role of this enzyme in the calcification process.

Almost 50 years ago Robison [71] first proposed a role of phosphatase in calcification. This theory was based upon three facts: (1) phosphatase is omnipresent in calcifying areas; (2) calcification in vitro of epiphyseal cartilage slices is improved when they are incubated with ester phosphates; and (3) there is a close correlation between calcification of rachitic cartilage slices in vitro and glycolysis. In spite of a great deal of effort, it was never possible to identify the biologic substrate for this enzyme, nor to define precisely how it would induce calcification. As more became known about the initiation of mineralization, the Robison theory was rejected in favor of the view that the organic matrix (collagen and possibly other components) serves as the template for the nucleation of bone mineral crystals [72, 73]. However, a point of continuing conflict with this latter view has been evidence pointing to amorphous calcium phosphate as the initial mineral phase in bone.

Another more recent proposal, which in a sense updates the Robison theory, is that alkaline phosphatase serves as a pyrophosphatase and that the concentration of its substrate, pyrophosphate, controls the mineralization process [74]. Pyrophosphate is known to inhibit apatite formation and dissolution. In this view the hydrolysis of pyrophosphate at local sites within the bone would allow mineralization to proceed at those sites while blocking it elsewhere. More recent studies by Anderson [42] and Anderson and Reynolds [47] have shown that small quantities of pyrophosphate actually promote matrix vesicle calcification. They have proposed that initial mineralization is promoted by the enzymatic hydrolysis of pyrophosphate by the pyrophosphatase in the matrix vesicle membrane, yielding inorganic phosphate that is accumulated by the vesicle, and thereby promoting initial bone mineral crystal formation.

On the basis of these studies it is possible to propose a five-step scheme for the events in the initiation of bone or cartilage mineralization (Fig. 68-1): (1) the budding off of matrix vesicles from the plasma membrane and their appearance as separate entities in the extracellular matrix; (2) the movement of calcium from the mitochondria of the cartilage or bone cells to the vesicles (this uptake of calcium by the vesicles may be an active process or may occur because there are phospholipids, amorphous phosphates, and polysaccharides with high calcium-binding capacity within the vesicles); (3) the hydrolysis of pyrophosphate, and probably other phosphate esters, by vesicle-bound phosphatase and the uptake of the product, inorganic phosphate, by the vesicles; (4) the nucleation of the first hydroxyapatite crystals within the vesicles; (5) the growth of these crystals until they rupture the vesicle membrane and cause its dissolution.

BIOCHEMICAL DEFECT IN HYPOPHOSPHATASIA

Although slices of rachitic cartilage from vitamin D–deficient rats or humans calcify readily in vitro in normal serum or in solutions containing physiologic concentrations of calcium and phosphate ions, cartilage slices from patients with hypophosphatasia do not calcify either in these solutions or when incubated in normal human serum [11, 13]. Conversely, rat rachitic slices will calcify in the serum obtained from patients with hypophosphatasia. Furthermore, no inhibitor of alkaline phosphatase is found in the plasma of such patients [10, 11, 27, 41]. These data show that the defect is a local one at the site of mineralization and is not due to some plasma factor.

The scheme depicted in Fig. 68-1 is a newer version of the old Robison phosphatase theory of mineralization put into a proper structural framework. From the point of view of the disease hypophosphatasia, its importance is that it implies that alkaline phosphatase has a crucial role in the initiation of mineralization. Thus, there is a direct connection between the lack of this enzyme and the defect in mineralization that is evident in the bones of affected individuals. An important question not yet answered is whether or not matrix vesicles appear in calcifying sites in this disease.

It is known, for example, that in ordinary vitamin D–deficiency rickets, normal-appearing matrix vesicles with their

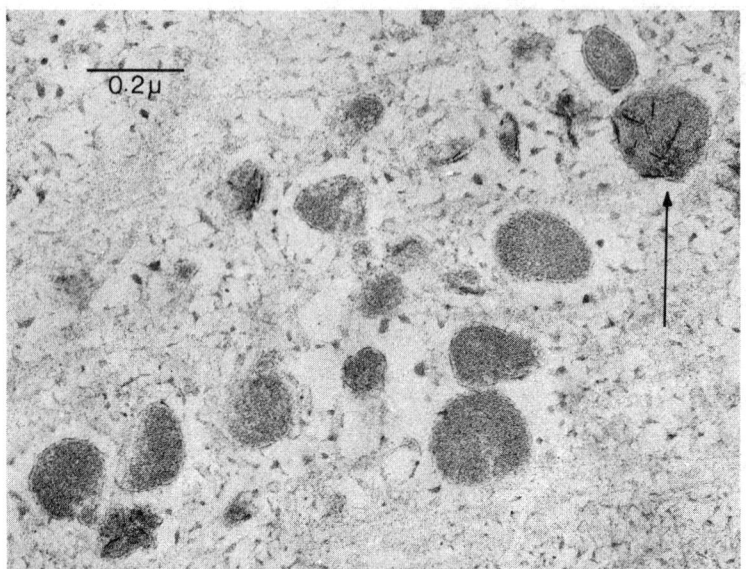

Figure 68-4 Calcifying matrix vesicles in the growth plate cartilage of a rachitic rat 8 h after intraperitoneal injection of a 0.1 M NaH$_2$PO$_4$ solution to reestablish calcification. At this point in the healing of rickets early mineral deposition is seen as electron-dense needles of apatite (arrow), mostly within the matrix vesicles. Later, heavy deposition of apatite occurs at the surfaces of the vesicles, with mineral accumulating by appositional crystal proliferation. Electron micrograph. Section stained with uranyl acetate and lead citrate. × 88,000. (*From Am J Pathol 79:237, 1975. Kindly supplied by Dr. H Clarke Anderson.*)

normal content of alkaline phosphatase are found within the longitudinal cartilage septums [75–79]. Furthermore, when such slices are incubated in vitro in a simple calcifying solution, apatite accumulation is found to occur specifically and selectively within the matrix vesicles [75–77]. Repeated freezing and thawing or pretreatment of cartilage slices with deoxycholate inhibits this calcification in vitro. The effect of low concentrations of deoxycholate is apparently that of solubilizing but not inactivating the matrix vesicle alkaline phosphatase (pyrophosphatase) [80] without totally disrupting the vesicle membrane [65]. This indicates that the membrane must apparently retain the phosphatase in order to function. Also, beryllium, an inhibitor of alkaline phosphatase [81], inhibits vesicle calcification of rachitic rat cartilage slices in vitro. This further establishes a direct link between the enzyme, the vesicles, and the initial steps in the calcification process.

In view of this evidence and the fact that cartilage slices taken from patients with hypophosphatasia do not calcify even in normal serum, it appears possible that the vesicles do not form in this disease, because alkaline phosphatase is a necessary structural component of the matrix vesicle membrane, or that the vesicles form but, because of an inability to hydrolyze phosphate esters and pyrophosphate, they do not accumulate phosphate and thus do not mineralize.

A major problem is that of accounting for the normal concentrations of plasma alkaline phosphatase in some patients with the bony manifestations of hypophosphatasia [18, 19]. In the patient studied by Scriver and Cameron [18], two features of the plasma alkaline phosphatase were noteworthy: (1) the enzyme was more heat labile than normal bone alkaline phosphatase; and (2) the enzyme had a higher K_m for phosphorylethanolamine. Unfortunately, the K_m for pyrophosphate was not determined. These data suggest that there may be cases in which the disease presents with a normal amount of an abnormal enzyme, rather than with a reduced amount of a normal enzyme. This structural abnormality might take at least two forms: (a) a decrease in substrate affinity, i.e., increased K_m; or (b) a reduction in the ability of the enzyme to bind to vesicle membrane.

One feature of the biochemical abnormality that has not been fully explored concerns the possibility that in some patients an abnormal enzyme is made with little or no hydrolytic activity but with immunologic properties similar to those of normal alkaline phosphatase. An immunologic assay for bone alkaline phosphatase could be a useful tool in the further characterization of the biochemical abnormalities associated with this condition.

Although major emphasis has been placed on the increase in urinary excretion of PEA, excretion of inorganic pyrophosphate is also increased in patients with hypophosphatasia and their kindred [82, 83]. This finding further supports the concept that inorganic pyrophosphate is a natural substrate for the enzyme, alkaline phosphatase. Administration of a high phosphate diet to such a patient led to an increase in pyrophosphate excretion and improved bone mineralization [83].

One of the major difficulties is in characterizing plasma alkaline phosphatase and relating it directly to the bone enzyme. Several different methods have been employed to distinguish the bone enzyme from the liver and intestinal enzymes in plasma [18, 84–88]. The most recent studies have employed acrylamide-slab-disk gel electrophoresis [86]. In a study of serum from 10 subjects with hypophosphatasia, the concentration of small-intestinal isoenzyme was found to be normal or high, the liver enzyme either reduced or absent, and the bone enzyme reduced or absent, but the pattern of change was not consistent, i.e., patients were found with reduced liver and absent bone isoenzymes, others with reduced bone and absent liver isoenzymes, and yet others with reduced liver and bone isoenzymes [86]. In addition, the alkaline phosphatase of polymorphonuclear leukocytes is reduced in some patients [13, 35, 89].

Another approach to classifying this disease has employed analysis of alkaline phosphatase activity from different tissues [90–93]. Unfortunately, as with the serum enzymes, there is still considerable confusion. Bone, liver, kidney, and intestinal alkaline phosphatases have different electrophoretic mobilities [91]. However, different organs contain multiple isoenzymes of alkaline phosphatase, and by immunologic methods liver, bone, spleen, and one of the kidney isoenzymes are found to be immunologically identical [92]. Intestinal alkaline phosphatase is primarily in a second immunologic group, and the placental enzyme in a third.

Using the combination of heat inactivation, 1-phenylalanine inhibitor, and electrophoresis of the alkaline phosphatase isoenzymes on polyacrylamide gel and cellulose acetate membrane, together with specific antiserums against the liver-bone, intestinal, and placental isoenzymes, Millán and coworkers [94] quantitated the different isoenzymes in the serums of 23 adult members of a kindred affected by the adult form of hypophosphatasia. Nine subjects had values of total alkaline phosphatase activity two standard deviations below the normal mean for age- and sex-matched controls. The activity of the bone enzyme was reduced in the serums of all nine subjects, but the liver enzyme was reduced in only four. There was a small but variable amount of the intestinal isoenzyme. The excretion of both phosphoethanolamine and phosphoserine in the urine was studied in eight of these nine patients. The rate of urinary excretion of these two substances was inversely correlated with the amount of the liver enzyme but did not correlate with the amount of the bone enzyme. The authors suggest that the increase in the urinary excretion of these substances is not related as previously supposed to a change in bone metabolism, but to a change in liver metabolism.

Greater than normal amounts of PEA have been isolated from the urine and plasma of patients and of some of their parents. Although alkaline phosphatase readily hydrolyzes this ester, there is no reasonable explanation for the association of the two biochemical defects in the disease. It has been suggested that PEA is the "true substrate" for bone alkaline phosphatase [32]. Thus, a hereditary defect resulting in a block in the reaction

$$NH_2CH_2CH_2-O-\overset{\overset{\displaystyle OH}{|}}{\underset{\underset{\displaystyle OH}{|}}{P}}=O + H_2O \xrightarrow[\text{phosphatase}]{\text{alkaline}}$$

$$H_3PO_4 + NH_2CH_2CH_2OH$$

would lead to an excess of plasma and urinary PEA. In any case, in some patients with fluctuating levels of serum alkaline phosphatase, an inverse relationship between serum alkaline phosphatase and PEA excretion has been reported. These findings support the concept that PEA is a substrate for alkaline phosphatase.

PEA is normally found in serum and urine in small quantities [4] and is a normal constituent of brain tissue. It may appear in excess in the urine of patients with liver disease [95], celiac disease, and erythroblastosis fetalis [96], and in patients with a wide variety of bone diseases [38].

PEA may be formed by (1) phosphorylation of ethanolamine, (2) hydrolysis of phosphatidyl ethanolamine, (3) hydrolysis of an α-PEA-plasmalogen, and (4) the aldolase cleavage of phosphorylsphingosine.

Phosphorylcholine (PC) has also been found in the urine of a patient with hypophosphatasia [17]. PC is formed by a series of reactions analogous to those by which PEA is formed. Indeed, phosphatidyl ethanolamine (itself readiy converted to phosphatidyl choline) and phosphatidyl choline are converted to PEA and PC, respectively, by identical enzymes, i.e., lecithinase, lysolecithinase, and glycerophosphorylcholine diesterase, followed by choline kinase—requiring ATP. Finally, both may lose the phosphate radical through the action of alkaline phosphatase. PEA may also be formed from phosphorylsphingosine through the action of an aldolase. Since the origin of the excessive PEA in hypophosphatasia is as obscure as its function, these observations do not clarify the question of whether excessive production or decreased utilization (or degradation) of PEA is the ultimate defect.

Hypercalcemia and hypercalcuria occur frequently but not constantly in hypophosphatasia. When they do occur there may be nitrogen retention and nephrocalcinosis. The serum calcium may undergo wide fluctuations without apparent cause, and hypercalcemia may result from therapy with moderate doses of vitamin D. It may also occur in subjects who have never received supplemental vitamin D. Thus, one patient developed a serum calcium concentration of 17 mg/dl after 10 days on 50,000 IU/day [10]; another, who had a serum calcium concentration of 12 to 15 mg/dl before therapy with the vitamin, showed a return of serum calcium values to normal while receiving 50,000 IU/day [30].

The cause of the hypercalcemia is not known. No measurements of plasma parathyroid hormone (PTH) or 1,25-dihydroxyvitamin D_3 have been reported. It is possible that during periods of rapid bone growth and mineralization a factor from bone is involved in regulating intestinal calcium absorption and renal calcium retention, but no studies of this possibility have been made. On the other hand, reduced tubular reabsorption of phosphate (TRP) has been reported [19] in both homo- and heterozygotes; this suggests that plasma PTH level may be elevated.

GENETICS

The reliability of a genetic analysis depends upon the number of markers available and the precision with which each can be analyzed: the less sensitive the chemical method, the poorer the penetrance will appear to be for the marker. In hypophosphatasia, for which the propositus always has bone disease, such markers include premature shedding of deciduous teeth, urinary and plasma PEA concentrations, and, of course, a low serum alkaline phosphatase activity. With the development of sensitive tests for urinary and plasma PEA [4], the detection of heterozygotes and the differentiation of hetero- from homozygotes appeared to rest upon quantitative measurements, but newer evidence that patients with various bone diseases excrete large amounts of PEA [38] has cast doubt upon the value of this marker. Furthermore, normal values of serum alkaline phosphatase activity are not infrequently found in subjects who are clearly affected [16, 18, 19]; indeed, in one patient, values fluctuated from normal to very low at different times, with reciprocal variations in urinary PEA [17].

Nearly all the published data are consistent with the inheritance of hypophosphatasia as an autosomal recessive trait [4, 13, 16, 19, 27, 83, 97, 98]. This conclusion has been reached most clearly by measurement of urinary PEA excretion, urinary pyrophosphate excretion, the premature shedding of deciduous teeth, the presence of bone disease, and the measurement of serum alkaline phosphatase (Fig. 68-5). The use of alkaline phosphatase alone gives less clear results, and it has even been suggested that the defect in PEA excretion and that of phosphatase may not be carried by the same gene. Until the nature of tissue isoenzyme distribution is clearly worked out, and until the relationship of increased PEA excretion to the bone disease is discovered, this seems to be an unwarranted conclusion.

The studies of Silverman [28] and some of the data reported by Pimstone et al. [16] suggest that an autosomal dominant mode of transmission may occur in some instances (Fig. 68-5). Silverman reported hypophosphatasia in a father and two of his sons in a family in which there was no evidence of heterozygosity, as measured by serum phosphatase and urinary PEA, in the mother or two other children. Likewise, Poland et al.

[93] refer to a family of Trygstad's in whom a mother, her two daughters, and two sons of the one daughter all had the disease without evidence of any biochemical changes indicative of heterozygosity in any of the marriage partners. Likewise, Whyte et al. [38] have reported on a kindred spanning three generations in whom the adult-onset disease displayed an autosomal dominant mode of inheritance.

Figure 68-5 *A.* Pedigree of Patient L.B., an adult with hypophosphatasia. *B.* Pedigrees of the three patients with childhood form of hypophosphatasia. (*From Pimstone et al. [16], with permission.*)

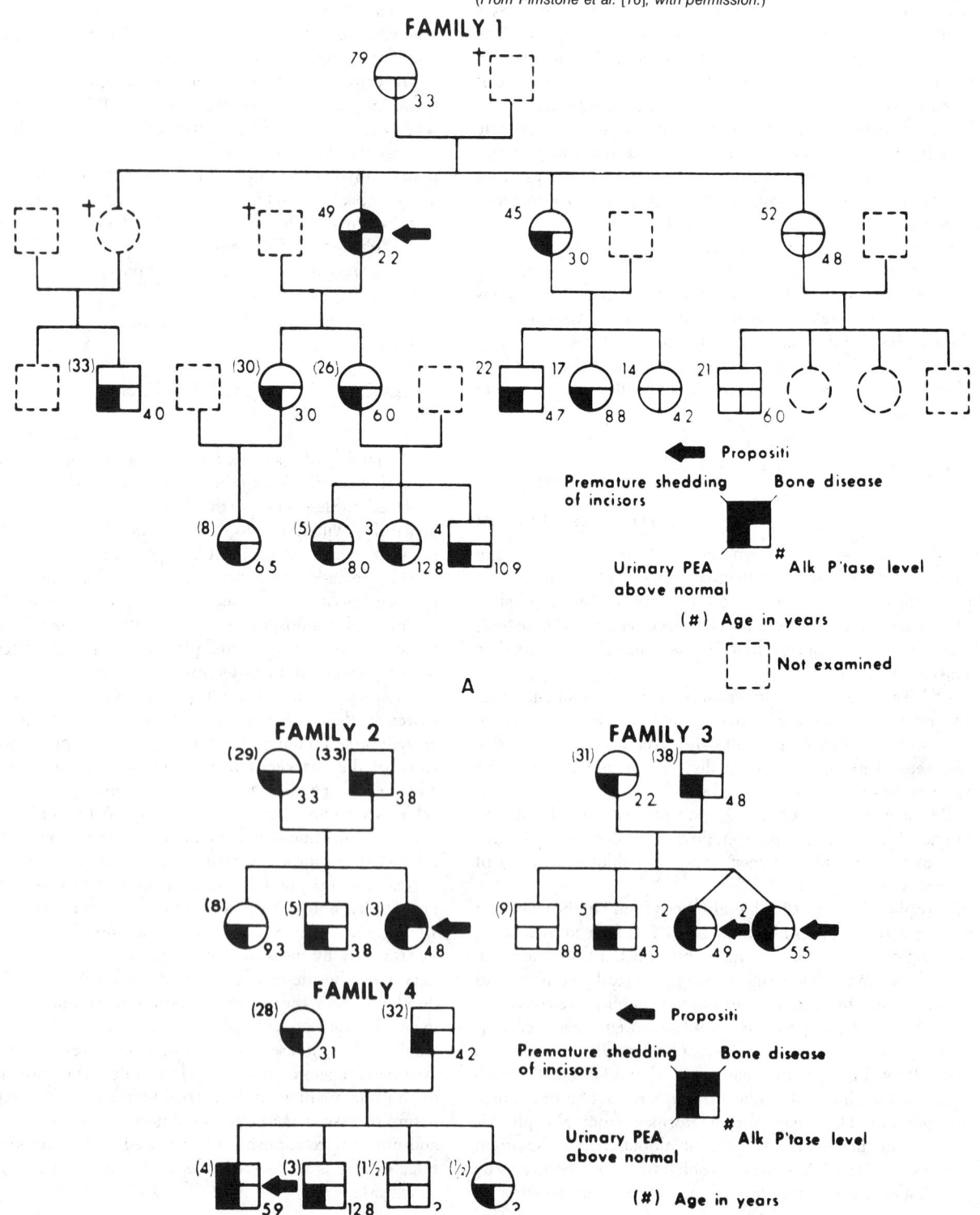

PRENATAL DIAGNOSIS

A combination of two methods has proven useful in the prenatal diagnosis of severe hypophosphatasia: ultrasound evaluation of intrauterine skeletal calcification, and alkaline phosphatase activity in amniotic fluid or cells derived from this fluid.

In all reports [99, 103], the use of ultrasonography has proven valuable. By 16 weeks in a normal pregnancy, sufficient mineralization of the fetal skull has taken place so that this structure is easily detected by routine ultrasonic examination. Its absence in a fetus in a mother with a known offspring with hypophosphatasia, or in one with a strong family history, is presumptive evidence of the diagnosis. The major differential diagnosis is anencephaly, but this differential can be easily made by analysis of α-fetoprotein in amniotic fluid. It is high in fetuses with anencephaly and normal in those with hypophosphatasia.

The measurement of alkaline phosphatase in amniotic fluid has also been evaluated [99, 103]. The total activity is an unreliable guide because most of the activity is derived from the fetal intestinal isoenzyme, and the disease affects the bone/liver enzymes. Estimation of the activity of this isoenzyme in amniotic fluid reveals that its content varies considerably in the fluid from normal control, and low values are common; hence this approach also does not seem promising. The most promising biochemical approach has been the measurement of alkaline phosphatase activity in cultured cells from the amniotic fluid [100]. These cells produce the bone/liver isoenzyme. In two studies the activity was 3 to 4 percent of the mean of a number of control cultures, or approximately 40 percent lower than the lowest control value. Because of the rarity of the disease, it is not possible to obtain data on large numbers of patients in a short time. For the present, the best approach to the diagnosis of the severe form of the disease is ultrasonography and measurement of the alkaline phosphatase activity of cultured amniotic fluid cells. Whether either approach is of value in the diagnosis of the milder forms of the disease is not known.

TREATMENT

Treatment of patients with hypophosphatasia with vitamin D has not been successful [2, 10]. In some instances improvement in the rickets has been reported concomitant with the appearance of vitamin D intoxication, and this healing may represent a combination of a rise in plasma phosphate and an inhibition of longitudinal growth. At present there is no reason to believe that the use of the newer vitamin D metabolites offers any therapeutic advantage in the treatment of this condition. Cortisone has also been tried without notable success [2].

Perhaps the most rational treatment to date is that reported by Bongiovanni et al. [83] and by Trygstad (quoted in [83]), who have described the treatment of three patients with high oral phosphate intakes. Treatment with 1.25 to 3.0 g phosphate, as neutral sodium phosphate, given in four to five divided doses throughout the day, caused a slight rise in plasma phosphate concentration, an increased excretion of pyrophosphate in the urine, and a significant improvement in the calcification of bone as assessed radiologically. These results suggest that sustained oral phosphate supplements may be of significant therapeutic value in patients with hypophosphatasia. Unfortunately, in several other patients this therapy has not proven of value.

Recently, Kolb [104] has found that a combination of vitamin D and fluoride has caused a healing of the osteomalacia and a rise in alkaline phosphatase in two patients. In our similar adult patient with significant osteomalacia there was no positive therapeutic response to the same program. One must conclude that at present there is no effective treatment for this condition.

REFERENCES

1. RATHBUN JC: Hypophosphatasia, a new developmental anomaly. *Am J Dis Child* 75:822, 1948
2. FRASER D: Hypophosphatasia. *Am J Med* 22:730, 1957
3. CURRARINO G, NEUHAUSER E, REYERSBACK G, SOBEL E: Hypophosphatasia. *Am J Roentgenol* 78:392, 1957
4. RASMUSSEN K: Phosphorylethanolamine and hypophosphatasia. *Dan Med Bull* 15:1, 1968
5. HUHNE T, SCHONFELD E: Eine eigenartige Wachstumstorung in Kindesalter. *Monatsschr Kinderheilkd* 42:267, 1929
6. CHOWN B: Renal rickets and dwarfism: A pituitary disease. *Br J Surg* 23:552, 1935–1936
7. KUBATSCH H: Über eine seltene Knochenerkrankung. *Monatsschr Kinderheilkd* 75:253, 1938
8. ANSPACH WE, CLIFTON WM: Hyperparathyroidism in children. *Am J Dis Child* 58:540, 1939
9. MACEY HB: Multiple pseudofractures: Report of case. *Proc Staff Meet Mayo Clin* 15:789, 1940
10. SOBEL EH, CLARK LC, FOX RP, ROBINOW M: Rickets, deficiency of "alkaline" phosphatase activity and premature loss of teeth in childhood. *Pediatrics* 11:309, 1953
11. FRASER D, YENDT ER, CHRISTIE FH: Metabolic abnormalities in hypophosphatasia. *Lancet* 1:286, 1955
12. McCANCE RA: The excretion of phosphoethanolamine and hypophosphatasia. *Lancet* 1:131, 1955
13. FRASER D, YENDT ER: Metabolic abnormalities in hypophosphatasia. *Am J Dis Child* 90:552, 1955
14. SCAGLIONE PR, LUCEY JF: Further observations on hypophosphatasia. *Am J Dis Child* 92:493, 1956
15. KRETCHMER N, STONE M, BAUER C: Hereditary enzymatic effects as illustrated by hypophosphatasia. *Ann NY Acad Sci* 75:279, 1958
16. PIMSTONE B, EISENBERG E, SILVERMAN S: Hypophosphatasia: Genetic and dental studies. *Ann Intern Med* 65:722, 1966
17. EISENBERG E, PIMSTONE B: Hypophosphatasia in an adult. *Clin Orthop* 52:199, 1967
18. SCRIVER CR, CAMERON D: Pseudohypophosphatasia. *N Engl J Med* 281:604, 1969
19. MÉHES K, KLUJBER L, LASSU G, KAJTÁR P: Hypophosphatasia: Screening and family investigations in an endogamous Hungarian village. *Clin Genet* 3:60, 1972
20. STERNBERG R, LIAPPIS N, GIFFELS G: Über die freien Aminosäuren um Serum und im Harn bei einem Fall von infantiler Hypophosphatsie. *Monatsschr Kinderheilkd* 122:127, 1974
21. POURFAR M, BORUSU B, SCHNECK R: Childhood hypophosphatasia: Clinical and cytogenetic studies. *NY State J Med* Sept 15, 1972, p 2341
22. WITKOP CJ, RAO S: Inherited defects in tooth structure. *Birth Defects* 7(7):153, 1971
23. BEUMER J III, TROWBRIDGE HO, SILVERMAN S Jr, EISENBERG E: Childhood hypophosphatasia and the premature loss of teeth: A clinical and laboratory study of seven cases. *Oral Surg* 35(5):631, 1973
24. KELLSEY DC: Hypophosphatasia and congenital bowing of long bones. *JAMA* 179:187, 1962
25. PARK EA, POWERS CF: Acrocephaly and scaphocephaly with symmetrically distributed malformation of the extremities. *Am J Dis Child* 20:235, 1920
26. BARTTER FC: Oxycephaly, in Beeson PB, McDermott W (eds): *Textbook of Medicine*, ed 11. Philadelphia, WB Saunders Co, 1963, p 1517
27. McCANCE RA, FAIRWEATHER DVI, BARRETT AM, MORRISON AB: Genetic, clinical, biochemical and pathological features of hypophosphatasia. *Q J Med* ns 25:523, 1956
28. SILVERMAN JL: Apparent dominant inheritance of hypophosphatasia. *Arch Intern Med* 110:191, 1962
29. BETHUNE J, DENT CE: Hypophosphatasia in the adult. *Am J Med* 28:615, 1960
30. SCHLESINGER B, LUDER J, BODIAN M: Rickets with alkaline phosphatase deficiency: An osteoblastic dysplasia. *Arch Dis Child* 30:265, 1955

31. FAAS FH, WADKINS CL, DANIELS JR, DAVIS GR, CARTER WJ, WYNN JO: Hyperparathyroidism in an elderly adult with hypophosphatasia. *Clin Orthop* 101:216, 1974

32. DENT CE: In *Bone Structure and Metabolism, CIBA Foundation Symposium.* London, Churchill, Livingstone, Inc, 1956, p 266

33. OWEN JA, PESKIN H: Clinical study of an adult with hypophosphatasia. *Clin Res* 6:249, 1958

34. RYSSING E: 2 Tilfaelde of hypophosphatasia. *Ugeskr Laeger* 124:1997, 1962

35. BEISEL WR, BENJAMIN N, AUSTEN KF: Absence of leucocyte alkaline phosphatase activity in hypophosphatasia. *Blood* 14:975, 1959

36. SCRIVER CR, DAVIES E: Endogenous renal clearance rates of free amino acids in prepubertal children. *Pediatrics* 36:592, 1965

37. BIRTWELL VM JR, RIGGS BL, PETERSON LFA, JONES JD: Hypophosphatasia in an adult. *Arch Intern Med* 120:90, 1967

38. WHYTE MP, TEITELBAUM SL, MURPHY WA, BERGFELD MA, AVIOLI LV: Adult hypophosphatasia. *Medicine* 58:329, 1979

39. LICATA AA, RADFOR N, BARTTER FC, BOU E: The urinary excretion of phosphoethanolamine in diseases other than hypophosphatasia. *Am J Med* 64:133, 1978

40. TEREE RM, KLEIN L: Hypophosphatasia: Clinical and metabolic studies. *Pediatrics* 72:41, 1968

41. ENGFELDT B, ZETTERSTROM R: Osteodysmetamorphosis fetalis: Clinical pathological study of congenital skeletal disease with retarded growth (hypophosphatasemia) and renal damage. *J Pediatr* 45:125, 1954

42. ANDERSON HC: Matrix vesicles of cartilage and bone, in Bourne GH (ed): *Biochemistry and Physiology of Bone.* New York, Academic, 1976, vol. 5, p 232

43. ANDERSON HC: Electron microscopic studies of induced cartilage development and calcification. *J Cell Biol* 35:81, 1967.

44. ANDERSON HC: Vesicles associated with calcification in the matrix of epiphyseal cartilage. *J Cell Biol* 41:59, 1969

45. BONUCCI E: Fine structure and histochemistry of "calcifying globules" in epiphyseal cartilage. *Z Zellforsch Mikrosk Anat* 103:192, 1970

46. BERNARD GW, PEASE E: An electron microscopic study of initial intramembranous osteogenesis. *Am J Anat* 125:271, 1969

47. ANDERSON HC, REYNOLDS JJ: Pyrophosphate stimulation of calcium uptake into cultured embryonic bones. Fine structure of matrix vesicles and their role in calcification. *Develop Biol* 34:211, 1973

48. SCHENK AK, MILLER J, ZINKERNAGEL A, WILLENEGGER H: Ultrastructure of normal and abnormal bone repair. *Calcif Tissue Res* 4(suppl):110, 1970

49. BERNARD GW: Ultrastructural observations of initial calcification in dentine and enamel. *J Ultrastruct Res* 41:1, 1972

50. EISENMAN DR, GLICK PN: Ultrastructure of initial crystal formation in dentin. *J Ultrastruct Res* 41:18, 1972

51. LARSSON A, BLOOM GD: Studies on dentinogenesis in the rat: Fine structure of developing odontoblasts and predentin in relation to the mineralization process. *Z Anat Entwicklungsgesch* 139:227, 1973

52. SISCA AF, PROVENZA DY: Initial dentin formation in human deciduous teeth: An electron microscope study. *Calcif Tissue Res* 9:1, 1972

53. SLAVKIN HC, BRINGAS P JR, CROISSANT R, BAVETTA LA: Epithelial-mesenchymal interactions during odontogenesis. II. Intercellular matrix vesicles. *Mech Ageing Dev* 1,2:139, 1972

54. NEWBERRY JW, BANKS WJ: Characterization of developing antler cartilage matrix. *Calcif Tissue Res* 17:289, 1975

55. KIM KM, HUANG SN: Ultrastructural study of calcification of human aortic valve. *Lab Invest* 26:481, 1972

56. KIM KM: Calcification of vesicles in matrix of human aortic valves, abstracted. *Fed Proc* 31:621, 1972

57. PERESS NS, SAJDERA SW, ANDERSON HC: Lipid analysis of vesicles isolated from the matrix of calcifying cartilage, abstracted. *Fed Proc* 30:1244, 1971

58. PERESS NS, ANDERSON HC, SAJDERA SW: The lipids of matrix vesicles from bovine fetal epiphyseal cartilage. *Calcif Tissue Res.* 14:275, 1974

59. WUTHIER RE: Enzymatic, lipid, and electrolyte composition of epiphyseal cartilage subcellular fractions, abstracted. *J Dent Res* 52(special):175, 1973

60. ANDERSON HC, MATSUZAWA T, SAJDERA SW, AU SY: Membranous particles in calcifying cartilage matrix. *Trans NY Acad Sci* 32:619, 1970

61. OZAWA H, YAJIMA T, KOBAYASHI S: Ultrastructure and cytochemistry of matrix vesicles in mineralizing tissues, abstracted. *J Dent Res* 52:1002, 1973

62. BRIGHTON CJ, HUNT RM: Mitochondrial calcium and its role in calcification: Histochemical localization of calcium in electron micrographs of the epiphyseal growth plate with K-pyroantimonate. *Clin Orthop* 100:406, 1974

63. LEHNINGER AL: Mitochondria and calcium ion transport. *Biochem J* 119:129, 1970

64. THYBERG J, FRIBERG V: Ultrastructure and acid phosphate activity of matrix vesicles and cytoplasmic dense bodies in the epiphyseal plate. *J Microsc (Oxf.)* 97:83, 1970

65. MATSUZAWA T, ANDERSON HC: Phosphates of epiphyseal cartilage studies by electron microscopic cytochemical methods. *J Histochem Cytochem* 19:801, 1971

66. AU SY, SAJDERA SW, ANDERSON HC: Isolation and characterization of calcifying matrix vesicles from epiphyseal cartilage. *Proc Natl Acad Sci USA* 67:1513, 1970

67. ALI, SY: Analysis of matrix vesicles and their role in the calcification of epiphyseal cartilage. *Fed Proc* 35:135, 1976

68. BRIGHTON CT, HUNT RM: Histochemical localization of calcium in growth plate mitochondria and matrix vesicles. *Fred Proc* 35:143, 1976

69. EATON RH, MOSS DW: Inhibition of the orthophosphatase and pyrophosphatase activities of human alkaline-phosphatase preparations. *Biochem J* 102:917, 1967

70. EATON RH, MOSS DW: Kinetic studies on the orthophosphatase and inorganic pyrophosphatase activities of human alkaline phosphatase. *Enzymologia* 35:31, 1968

71. ROBISON R: Possible significance of hexosephosphoric esters in ossification. *Biochem J* 17:286, 1923

72. NEUMAN WF, NEUMAN MW: *The Chemical Dynamics of Bone Mineral.* Chicago, University of Chicago Press, 1958

73. GLIMCHER MJ, HODGE AJ, SCHMITT FO: Macromolecular aggregation states in relation to mineralization: The collagen hydroxyapatite system as studied *in vitro. Proc Natl Acad Sci USA* 43:860, 1957

74. FLEISCH H: Role of nucleation and inhibition in calcification. *Clin Orthop* 32:170, 1964

75. ANDERSON HC: in Slavin HC (ed): *Remarks on Cartilage Calcification to the Santa Catalina Colloquium on Comparative Molecular Biology to Extracellular Matrices.* New York, Academic, 1972, p 199

76. ANDERSON HC, CECIL R, SAJDERA SW: Calcification of rachitic cartilage *in vitro* as mediated by extracellular matrix vesicles. *Isr J Med Sci* 10:1462, 1974

77. ANDERSON HC, CECIL R, SAJDERA SW: Calcification of rachitic cartilage by extracellular matrix vesicle. *Am J Pathol* 79:237, 1975

78. SIMON OR, BERMAN I, PITA JC, HOWELL DS: Evidence for the role of extracellular matrix vesicles in the calcification of rat epiphyseal cartilage. *Clin Res* 20:519, 1972

79. SIMON DR, BERMAN I, HOWELL DS: Relationship of extracellular matrix vesicles to calcification in normal and healing rachitic epiphyseal cartilage. *Anat Rec* 176:167, 1973

80. FRANKLIN S, FORTUNA R: Matrix vesicles of bovine fetal cartilage. *Fed Proc* 35:154, 1976

81. THOMAS M, ALDRIDGE WN: The inhibition of phosphoglucomutase by beryllium. *Biochem J* 98:94, 1966

82. RUSSEL RGG: Excretion of inorganic pyrophosphate in hypophosphatasia. *Lancet* 2:461, 1965

83. BONGIOVANNI AM, ALBUM MM, ROOT AW, HOPE JW, MARINO J, SPENCER DM: Studies on hypophosphatasia and response to high phosphate intake. *Am J Med Sci* March, p 163, 1968

84. POSEN S, NEALE FC, CLUBB JS: Heat inactivation in the study of human alkaline phosphatases. *Ann Intern Med* 62, 1234, 1965

85. FISHMAN WH, GREEN S, INGLIS NI: L-Phenylalanine: An organ specific stereospecific inhibitor of human intestinal alkaline phosphatase. *Nature (Lond)* 198:685, 1963

86. DANOVITCH GH, BAER PN, LASTER L: Intestinal alkaline phosphatase activity in familial hypophosphatasia. *N Engl J Med* 278:1253, 1968

87. HOFFMANN V, HOSENFLED D: Eine neue Methode zur Darstellung zur Isoenzyme der alkalischen Serumphosphatase mit Hilfe der Flachdiskelektrophorese. *Med Welt* 22:749, 1971

88. HOSENFELD D, HOSENFELD A: Qualitative and quantitative Untersuchungen der Isoenzyme der alkalischen Serumphosphatase bei der Hypophosphatasie. *Klin Paediatr* 185:437, 1973

89. JUSTUS VON J, RUPPECHT E, RECKNAGEL R, JUSTUS B: Morphologischer und klinischer Beitrag zur Hypophosphatasia congenita letalis. *Kinderaerztl Prax* 4:148, 1974

90. HOSENFELD, D: Über die Isoenzyme der alkalischen Serumphosphatase und ihre selektive Abhängigkeit von verschiedenen Faktoren. *Klin Wochenschr* 51:290, 1973

91. YONG, JM: Origins of serum alkaline phosphatase. *J Clin Pathol* 20:647, 1967

92. BOYER SH: Human organ alkaline phosphatases: Discrimination by several means including starch gel electrophoresis of antienzyme-enzyme supernatant fluids. *Ann NY Acad Sci* 103:938, 1963

93. POLAND C III, EVERSOLE IR, BIXLER D, CHRISTIAN JC: Histochemical observations of hypophosphatasia. *J Dent Res* 51:333, 1972

94. MILLÁN JL, WHYTE MP, AVIOLI LV, FISHMAN WH: Hypophosphatasia (adult form): Quantitation of serum alkaline phosphatase isoenzyme activity in a large kindred. *Clin Chem* 26:840, 1980

95. WALSHE JM: Disturbances of amino acid metabolism following liver injury: A study by means of paper chromatography. *Q J Med* ns, 22:483, 1953

96. FISHER OD, NEILL DW: Excretion of ethanolamine phosphoric acid in coeliac disease. *Lancet* 1:334, 1955

97. Rubecz I, Méhes K, Klujber L, Bozzay L, Weisenbach J, Fenyvesi J: Hypophosphatasia: Screening and family investigation. *Clin Genet* 6:155, 1974

98. Harris H, Robson EB: A genetical study of ethanolamine phosphate excretion in hypophosphatasia. *Hum Genet* 23:421, 1958

99. Rudd NL, Miskin M, Hoar DI, Benzie R, Doran TA: Prenatal diagnosis of hypophosphatasia. *N Engl J Med* 295:146, 1976

100. Mulivor RA, Mennoti M, Zackai EH, Harris H: Prenatal diagnosis of hypophosphatasia, genetics, biochemical, and clinical studies. *Am J Hum Genet* 30:271–282, 1978

101. Clark PJ, Pryse-Davies J, Sandler M, Blank, Rattenbury JM, Pooley PJ: Prenatal diagnosis of hypophosphatasia. *Lancet* 1:306, 1976

102. Benzie R, Doran TA, Escoffery W, Gardner HA, Hoar DI, Hunter A, Malone R, Miskin M, Rudd NL: Prenatal diagnosis of hypophosphatasia. *Birth Defects: Orig Art Ser* 12(6):271–282, 1976

103. Beratis NG, Kaffe S, Aron AM, Hirschhorn K: Alkaline phosphatase activity in cultured skin fibroblasts from fibrodysplasia ossificans progressiva. *J Med Genet* 13:307–309, 1976

104. Kolb F: Personal communication

69

PSEUDOHYPOPARATHYROIDISM

MARC K. DREZNER

FRANCIS A. NEELON

1. *Pseudohypoparathyroidism is a clinical disorder characterized by hypocalcemia and hyperphosphatemia, which are present in spite of increased circulating levels of parathyroid hormone.*

2. *The associated clinical features of this disorder are short stature, round face, brachydactyly, and decreased mental function. These are collectively referred to as Albright's hereditary osteodystrophy. These features may be absent, or present without hypocalcemia or hyperphosphatemia. In the latter case the disorder is referred to as pseudo-pseudohypoparathyroidism.*

3. *The primary abnormality underlying the pathogenesis of pseudohypoparathyroidism is target organ resistance to parathyroid hormone.*

4. *Discrete subtypes of the disease, discriminated by the mechanisms underlying the renal resistance, have been recognized. Pseudohypoparathyroidism type 1 is due to an abnormality in the parathyroid hormone-receptor-adenylate cyclase moiety in the renal cell membranes and results in deficient production of cyclic AMP. Pseudohypoparathyroidiasm type 2 results from an inability of intracellular cyclic AMP to initiate parathyroid hormone-directed metabolic events.*

5. *The molecular defect underlying pseudohypoparathyroidism type 1 in some but not all patients is a defect in the nucleotide-binding protein moiety of the adenylate cyclase unit.*

6. *The hypocalcemia of pseudohypoparathyroidism* *arises from defective mobilization of calcium from bone. This defect is secondary either to an innate abnormality in bone, similar to that in kidney, or to decreased renal production of 1,25-dihydroxyvitamin D, or to both.*

7. *Although there is no doubt that pseudohypoparathyroidism is a genetic disease, the inheritance pattern remains unclear. This obscurity is due to the biochemical heterogeneity typical of the disease, which has precluded adequate clinical characterization, and to genetic heterogeneity.*

Pseudohypoparathyroidism is a term representing a heterogeneous group of disorders characterized by end-organ unresponsiveness to parathyroid hormone. In its prototypic form, the disease is a hereditary syndrome of short stature, mental retardation, distinctive skeletal abnormalities, hypocalcemia, and hyperphosphatemia, which are present despite excessive secretion of parathyroid hormone. These manifestations occur in different combinations in various forms of the disorder, reflecting both biochemical and genetic heterogeneity.

The biochemical hallmark of the disease is renal resistance to parathyroid hormone. This can be due to several mechanisms. These mechanisms form the basis for segregating the disease into discrete subtypes. Thus, pseudohypoparathyroidism type 1 is due to a defect in the interaction of parathyroid hormone with specific renal cell hormone receptors or in adenylate cyclase, resulting in deficient production of cyclic AMP. Pseudohypoparathyroidism type 2 results from an inability of normally generated renal cyclic AMP to initiate parathyroid hormone-directed metabolic events. These abnormalities lead to defective transcellular phosphate transport in the kidney and consequent hyperphosphatemia. Additional hypothetical mechanisms which may underlie the renal resistance include production of abnormal parathyroid hormone that blocks hormone receptors, the presence of antibodies to parathyroid hormone or its receptors, and excessive destruction of intracellular cyclic AMP; insufficient data are available to substantiate these possibilities.

HISTORICAL DEVELOPMENT

In 1942 Albright et al. [1] described three patients with the clinical and biochemical stigmata of hypoparathyroidism in whom administration of parathyroid hormone evoked neither a phosphate diuresis nor an increase in serum calcium concentration. These patients exhibited a number of developmental abnormalities, including round facies, short stature, brachydactyly, ectopic calcification, and ectodermal anomalies. The diminished response to parathyroid hormone administration contrasted sharply to the brisk responses of patients with surgical or idiopathic hypoparathyroidism. Albright et al. attributed the condition to end organ unresponsiveness to parathyroid hormone. In view of the biochemical similarities to hypoparathyroidism, they termed the disorder *pseudohypoparathyroidism*.

Ten years later, Albright et al. [2] described a young woman who had the physical stigmata of pseudohypoparathyroidism but whose serum calcium and phosphorus were normal. Such individuals have normal metabolic responses to administered parathyroid hormone [3, 4]. Since they do not show the true syndrome of pseudohypoparathyroidism, Albright et al. used the sobriquet *pseudo-pseudohypoparathyroidism* to denote those individuals with the structural anomalies (collectively called *Albright's hereditary osteodystrophy* or AHO) but without biochemcial abnormalities.

Aside from observations on the coexistence of both pseudohypoparathyroidism and pseudo-pseudohypoparathyroidism in single families [5], there was little progress in understanding the biochemical basis for parathyroid hormone resistance in pseudohypoparathyroidism until 1966, when Tashjian et al. [6] demonstrated increased concentrations of circulating parathyroid hormone in patients with this disorder. They also found increased amounts of calcitonin in the thyroid gland of one patient with pseudohypoparathyroidism [7] and wondered whether excessive secretion of calcitonin conferred resistance to parathyroid hormone action. Shortly thereafter, this hypothesis was eliminated by two independent studies [8, 9] which showed no alleviation of hypocalcemia by thyroid ablation in patients with pseudohypoparathyroidism.

In 1967 Chase and Aurbach [10] reported an increased urine excretion of cyclic adenosine 3',5'-monophosphate (cyclic AMP) as the earliest manifestation of parathyroid hormone administration. In 1969, Chase et al. [3] found no such cyclic AMP response in patients with pseudohypoparathyroidism and implicated a defective renal parathyroid hormone receptor-cyclic AMP generating system in the pathogenesis of this

disorder. Bell and his coworkers [11] added further support for this theory when they showed that circumvention of the block in cyclic AMP formation (by giving the dibutyryl derivative of cyclic AMP intravenously) produced a phosphate diuresis in patients with pseudohypoparathyroidism. Subsequent studies have concentrated on defining the nature of the biochemical lesion which impairs cyclic AMP formation and on elucidating the biochemical abnormalities associated with pseudohypoparathyroidism.

NORMAL PHYSIOLOGY OF PARATHYROID HORMONE FUNCTION

The abnormalities underlying the pathogenesis of pseudohypoparathyroidism include defects in parathyroid hormone action on phosphorus and calcium homeostasis, and in regulation of vitamin D metabolism. Many aspects of the proposed sequence of the pathophysiologic events remain unexplained. In order to appreciate the basic formulation of the pathogenesis of pseudohypoparathyroidism, it is necessary to understand the physiology of parathyroid hormone function.

Parathyroid Hormone Control of Phosphorus Metabolism

The renal mechanisms which maintain phosphate homeostasis include filtration and reabsorption. Under conditions of normal diet and parathyroid hormone activity the mammalian kidney reabsorbs more than 80 percent of the filtered load of phosphate. This reabsorption occurs by an active transport process which is markedly inhibited by parathyroid hormone [12]. An increase in parathyroid hormone concentration inhibits phosphate reabsorption, resulting in increased net urinary phosphate excretion and eventually in a decreased serum phosphate concentration. Indeed, parathyroid hormone effects on phosphate reabsorption are the major determinants of the plasma phosphate levels [13].

Phosphate reabsorption occurs primarily in the distal segments of the proximal convoluted tubule and in the pars recta, but there is probably also a distal tubular component which may be small in magnitude but physiologically important [14–16]. The mechanism that mediates parathyroid hormone-sensitive phosphate reabsorption along the nephron is uncertain. Since parathyroid hormone also diminishes proximal tubular reabsorption of sodium, bicarbonate, and water, the phosphaturic action of parathyroid hormone was once thought to be due to the effects of the hormone on sodium and bicarbonate reabsorption. Recent data indicate that phosphate reabsorption is largely independent of parathyroid hormone effects on other ions [17].

Parathyroid Hormone Control of Calcium Metabolism

The maintenance of normocalcemia in humans is almost entirely a function of parathyroid hormone. Persistent hypocalcemia occurs only in the absence of parathyroid hormone or with resistance to its action(s) [18]. Parathyroid hormone raises the serum calcium by (1) mobilizing calcium from bone; (2) reducing the renal clearance of calcium; and (3) increasing calcium absorption from the intestine (mediated by enhanced formation of 1,25-dihydroxyvitamin D [$1,25(OH)_2D$]). Although the relative contribution of each of these actions remains incompletely defined, there is little doubt that the effect on bone is the one primarily responsible for calcium homeostasis. The effects of parathyroid hormone on renal calcium excretion and intestinal absorption complement this activity.

Action of Parathyroid Hormone on Bone   Bone contains more than 90 percent of the calcium in the body. Therefore, changes in calcium balance depend on the net movement of calcium in and out of bone. At present two distinct cellular systems have been identified in bone which regulate the mobilization of calcium—the remodeling system and the homeostatic system [19]. The remodeling system, consisting primarily of osteoclasts and osteoblasts, is engaged in the reabsorption and removal of old bone and its replacement with newly formed tissue. The homeostatic system, composed of both "inactive" surface osteocytes and osteocytes lodged in lacunar spaces deep within the bone, regulates movement of calcium between the bone fluid and the extracellular fluid. These two independent systems govern calcium replacement and bone remodeling, and each is modulated by parathyroid hormone [19–21].

Bone remodeling is an ordered and predictable process characterized by osteoclast-mediated resorption of old bone and osteoblast-mediated formation of an equal volume of new bone [22, 23]. Parathyroid hormone increases the number and activity of osteoclasts, thereby increasing the rate of bone remodeling. This action involves increased protein synthesis and lasts for several hours after stimulation by parathyroid hormone has ceased. Long-standing parathyroid hormone excess results in extensive bone remodeling and the radiographic and histologic picture of osteitis fibrosa cystica [24]. In spite of calcium mobilization during remodeling, parathyroid hormone stimulation of this process does not affect the long-term, steady state plasma calcium concentration. Because bone resorption and formation are coupled, within 4 to 6 weeks after the onset of parathyroid hormone stimulation, the mobilization of calcium by resorption is precisely balanced by the uptake of calcium for bone formation. Thus, the effects of parathyroid hormone on bone remodeling produce only minimal and transient changes in plasma calcium [23].

Although plasma calcium concentration is not regulated by bone resorption and bone turnover, it is controlled by the exchange of calcium between a surface fluid compartment of bone and the extracellular fluid, i.e., by the homeostatic system [23, 25–28]. Variations in the flux of calcium alter the equilibrium between plasma and bone fluid. Thus, a decrease in movement of calcium from the bone surface compartment results in equilibrium at a lower plasma calcium level and a net gain of calcium by bone (and vice versa). Since the concentration of calcium in plasma is greater than in bone fluid, an active process must facilitate calcium transport from the bone surface compartment to the plasma. Whether or not this process is a calcium pump is unknown, but facilitation of calcium transport is under parathyroid hormone control, and this serves as the primary mechanism setting the steady state plasma calcium level [29].

The homeostatic system also responds to acute changes in the plasma calcium level. In the face of sudden hypocalcemia, bone calcium is mobilized by increased transport of calcium from the surface compartment as well as by increased removal of mineral from the osteocyte perilacunar sites and by increased osteoclast activity [29].

Both the homeostatic and bone remodeling systems require one or more metabolites of vitamin D in order to function normally [29–31]. Under physiologic circumstances, $1,25(OH)_2D$ appears to be the metabolite which augments the action of parathyroid hormone. In the presence of $1,25(OH)_2D$ deficiency, the blood-bone equilibrium of calcium is reduced, recovery from acute hypocalcemia is impaired, and bone turnover is depressed. A sufficiently great increase in parathyroid hormone concentration can sometimes overcome the effects of $1,25(OH)_2D$ deficiency and restore plasma calcium or bone turnover to normal or supranormal levels [18]. The remodeling system is less dependent on $1,25(OH)_2D$ than the homeostatic system, and accordingly, osteitis fibrosa cystica may develop in spite of persistent hypocalcemia [18].

In addition to parathyroid hormone, hyperphosphatemia itself has been implicated in the control of serum calcium by several mechanisms, including enhanced bone formation. This potential cause of hypocalcemia is important when considering certain abnormalities in pseudohypoparathyroidism. However, it is clear that the effects of hyperphosphatemia on serum calcium levels are transient and cannot explain sustained hypocalcemia. Indeed, in most instances of chronic elevation of plasma phosphate (other than hypoparathyroidism) the plasma calcium is normal, due to correction of the steady state plasma calcium level by parathyroid hormone [32].

Action of Parathyroid Hormone on Kidney and Intestine   Parathyroid hormone stimulates renal reabsorption of calcium. Acute parathyroidectomy increases calcium excretion, although the calciuria declines as the plasma calcium concentration falls below 7 mg/dl. Administration of parathyroid hormone decreases urinary calcium excretion [13]. Micropuncture studies indicate that parathyroid hormone has a dual effect on renal calcium reabsorption, inhibiting sodium and calcium reabsorption in the proximal tubule and selectively enhancing calcium reabsorption at more distal loci, so that the net effect is one of increased reabsorption [33, 34]. Preliminary data indicate that the collecting duct may be the distal site of calcium reabsorption. Hence the terminal nephron is the final parathyroid hormone-responsive regulator of urinary calcium excretion. The increased net tubular reabsorption of calcium complements parathyroid hormone action on bone by conserving the mobilized bone calcium, but the precise interrelationship by which these processes maintain a steady state plasma calcium concentration remains unclear.

Parathyroid hormone increases intestinal absorption of calcium, and parathyroid hormone deficiency results in calcium malabsorption. In addition, parathyroid hormone increases sodium-dependent calcium transport across the basolateral pole of the intestinal mucosal cell in vitro [35]. Neither of these actions results from a direct effect of parathyroid hormone on the intestine; both are due principally to increased production of $1,25(OH)_2D$ in the parathyroid hormone-stimulated kidney.

Action of Parathyroid Hormone on Vitamin D Metabolism   Vitamin D undergoes a series of hydroxylations which culminate in the production of $1,25(OH)_2D$ by the kidney

[36]. This dihydroxylated derivative appears to be the form of vitamin D primarily responsible for the renal, osseous, and intestinal actions of the vitamin. A series of control factors modulate renal production of this active metabolite from 25-hydroxyvitamin D (25(OH)D). Parathyroid hormone (possibly via cyclic AMP production), hypocalcemia, and hypophosphatemia all stimulate 1,25(OH)$_2$D synthesis, while lack of parathyroid hormone, hypercalcemia, hyperphosphatemia, and 1,25(OH)$_2$D itself suppress formation of the active metabolite [36]. In pseudohypoparathyroidism the absence of parathyroid hormone function leads to a reduced circulating level of 1,25(OH)$_2$D and to the decreased gastrointestinal absorption of calcium which is characteristic of the hypoparathyroid state [37].

Mechanism of Parathyroid Hormone Action

The first known effect of parathyroid hormone on kidney cells and bone cells is stimulation of adenylate cyclase activity. Parathyroid hormone binds to specific plasma membrane receptors, activating adenylate cyclase. As a result of this enzyme activation, intracellular cyclic AMP content increases. Considerable evidence points to the rapid rise in cyclic AMP as the initial biochemical event underlying all the physiologic actions of parathyroid hormone [38]. After injection of parathyroid hormone into humans, there is an abrupt and transient increase in urinary cyclic AMP excretion. The peak occurs shortly after the maximum rise in plasma cyclic AMP but precedes any measureable effect on urinary excretion of phosphate (an event previously considered the earliest action of the hormone) [10]. In addition, administration of dibutyryl cyclic AMP to parathyroidectomized animals effectively simulates the actions of parathyroid hormone on kidney and bone [39]. Moreover, theophylline and imidazole (which alter the intracellular destruction of cyclic AMP) produce effects which support the hypothesis that cyclic AMP is the mediator of parathyroid hormone action [39].

The precise, parathyroid-hormone responsive, biochemical processes that are directly influenced by cyclic AMP remain unknown. By analogy to systems in which the sequence of biochemical events is better known, we might suppose that parathyroid hormone-induced cyclic AMP activates an intracellular protein kinase, thereby initiating a cascade of specific protein phsophorylations that are ultimately responsible for the effects of parathyroid hormone on kidney and bone.

The ability of parathyroid hormone to increase intracellular cyclic AMP depends on the binding of the hormone to specific membrane receptors, resulting in the activation of adenylate cyclase. This is a more complex process than originally appreciated, since the receptor-adenylate cyclase membrane unit consists of not only a specific hormone receptor and the catalytic moiety of the enzyme but, in addition, a distinct regulatory component of the system, called the *guanine nucleotide regulatory protein* (*N protein*). Rodbell et al. [40, 41] showed that under appropriate conditions polypeptide hormone stimulation of adenylate cyclase has an absolute requirement for guanosine triphosphate (GTP). These observations suggested that a specific guanine nucleotide binding site was associated with the adenylate cyclase complex. This binding activity resides in the N protein. It consists of three polypeptide chains with molecular weights of 52,000, 45,000, and 35,000 [42]. Each of the subunits appears to be needed for activity.

The proposed role of the N protein in modulating adenylate cyclase activity may be summarized as follows (Fig. 69-1). Interaction of parathyroid hormone with its receptor leads to the formation of a low affinity, freely reversible complex (PTH·R). A conformational change is induced in the receptor which permits it to couple to the guanine nucleotide regulatory protein, establishing a complex of hormone-receptor and N protein (PTH·R·N). Formation of this complex is associated with a loss of tightly bound guanosine diphosphate (GDP) from the N protein, thereby facilitating the binding of GTP to the nucleotide regulatory site. Bound GTP destabilizes the complex, freeing the hormone receptor and releasing N protein charged with GTP. The GTP·N protein complex then interacts with the catalytic moiety, resulting in the synthesis of cyclic AMP from adenosine triphosphate [43]. Abnormalities at any of these steps may impair hormone activation of the adenylate cyclase system.

Several lines of evidence indicate that not all of the physiologically important actions of parathyroid hormone require activation of adenylate cyclase. Modest increases of the hormone can elevate plasma calcium without measurably raising the bone cyclic AMP content [44]. Parathyroid hormone increases cell membrane permeability to calcium and the uptake of calcium by bone cells apparently without affecting cyclic AMP [45]. The resulting increase in intracellular calcium concentration may well participate in the sequence of cyclic AMP-directed events. Dibutyryl cyclic AMP does not mimic the effects of parathyroid hormone on renal distal tubular reabsorption of calcium, nor are these effects temporally related to renal production of cyclic AMP [17, 46]. Nevertheless, it remains likely that cyclic AMP mediates the most characteristic actions of parathyroid hormone.

Regulation of Parathyroid Hormone Biosynthesis and Secretion

The homeostatic role of parathyroid hormone has been clarified by examining the mode of control of hormone production in relation to physiologic need. There is no doubt that calcium plays a dominant role in controlling the secretion of parathyroid hormone. Indeed, a decrement of only 0.1 mg/dl in the ionized calcium concentration stimulates parathyroid hormone release, apparently by altering parathyroid gland adenylate cyclase activity [47, 48]. Adrenergic receptors are part of the receptor-adenylate cyclase unit of the parathyroid gland. This suggests that adrenergic stimulation may modify calcium-induced changes in hormone secretion [49, 50].

The intracellular signal that couples hormone secretion with hormone synthesis is unknown. Nevertheless, hormone biosynthesis must be closely linked to secretory activity since parathyroid hormone stores are sufficient to meet the needs of a hypocalcemic state for only 1 to 2 h without a coordinate increase in hormone biosynthesis [51]. There are many potential sites for control of parathyroid hormone biosynthesis. Transcription of the complete polypeptide information encoded in the "parathyroid hormone" gene results in the synthesis of preproparathyroid hormone, a 115 amino acid precursor which is converted to an intermediate product, proparathyroid hormone (90 amino acids in length), in the endoplasmic reticulum. The final 84 amino acid product, parathyroid hormone, is formed in the Golgi apparatus and stored in secretory granules [51]. Calcium concentration does not affect

PROPOSED MECHANISM OF ADENYLATE CYCLASE ACTIVATION

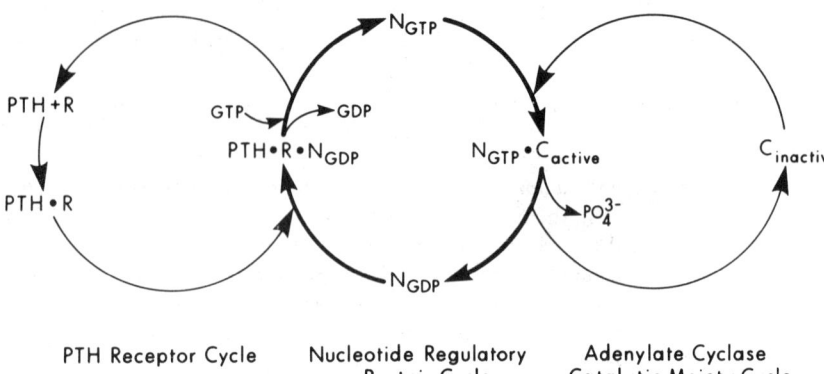

PTH Receptor Cycle   Nucleotide Regulatory   Adenylate Cyclase
                        Protein Cycle   Catalytic Moiety Cycle

Figure 69-1 Proposed mechanism of adenylate cyclase activation by parathyroid hormone and guanosine triphosphate. Together with the parathyroid hormone receptor and the catalytic moiety of the adenylate cyclase enzyme, the interaction of guanosine triphosphate with the guanine nucleotide regulatory protein determines the function of the enzyme. PTH, parathyroid hormone; R, receptor; N, nucleotide regulatory protein; C, catalytic moiety; GTP, guanosine triphosphate; GDP, guanosine diphosphate. *(Adapted from Lefkowitz and Hoffman [43] by permission of Trends in Pharmaceutical Science.)*

either the translation of parathyroid hormone-specific messenger RNA or the rate at which hormone precursors are processed to the final hormone product. It is most likely that regulation of biosynthesis occurs at the transcriptional level and that calcium concentration controls the number of messenger RNA molecules synthesized.

PATHOPHYSIOLOGY OF PSEUDOHYPOPARATHYROIDISM

End-organ resistance to the effects of parathyroid hormone results in (1) phosphate retention and hyperphosphatemia secondary to deficient renal phosphate excretion; and (2) defective calcium homeostatis, including inadequate flow of calcium from bone into the extracellular fluid, calcium malabsorption, and renal calcium wasting. Pseudohypoparathyroidism is heterogeneous, and the molecular bases underlying the various forms of the disorder are distinctly different.

Pseudohypoparathyroidism Type 1

The failure of parathyroid hormone to promote phosphate excretion by the kidney has been demonstrated by assessing urinary phosphate excretion in response to both acute and chronic administration of exogenous parathyroid hormone or to treatment with EDTA (which induces acute hypocalcemia and secondary hyperparathyroidism). Carefully controlled studies show an inadequate increase in phosphate excretion in affected subjects as compared to normal subjects or to patients with idiopathic or surgical hypoparathyroidism [4, 52]. On occasion a "normal" phosphaturic response has been seen in patients with pseudohypoparathyroidism, and this has been interpreted as indicating partial resistance to parathyroid hormone effects [4]. This explanation remains plausible, but the absence of control studies or of analysis of variation in phosphate excretion in the reported cases precludes our being certain.

The intrarenal site of parathyroid hormone resistance is the proximal tubule, where the major portion of hormone-dependent phosphate reabsorption occurs. In addition, some degree of proximal tubular resistance to hormone-stimulated bicarbonate and potassium excretion occurs in pseudohypo-

parathyroidism [53, 54]. Indeed, circumstantial evidence indicates that hormone unresponsiveness may be limited to the proximal tubule since hypercalciuria does not occur after treatment of pseudohypoparathyroid patients with vitamin D, as it does in patients with idiopathic or surgical hypoparathyroidism [4]. This lack of hypercalciuria is most likely due to normal effects of parathyroid hormone on renal distal tubular calcium reabsorption.

Mechanism of Hormone Resistance Insight into the mechanism(s) underlying renal resistance to parathyroid hormone in pseudohypoparathyroidism type 1 was provided by the demonstration that affected patients did not appreciably increase urinary cyclic AMP excretion or renal vein cyclic AMP concentration after parathyroid hormone administration (Fig. 69-2) [3]. Nevertheless, many subjects show detectable but subnormal increments in urinary cyclic AMP, the variability of which may reflect the nature of the defect in parathyroid hormone interaction with the kidney.

The defective cyclic AMP response suggests that it is a lack of renal cell cyclic AMP that results in a failure of the intracellular actions necessary to decrease phosphate reabsorption. This hypothesis is supported by studies in which administration of dibutyryl cyclic AMP to patients with pseudohypoparathyroidism type 1 reproduced the renal effects of parathyroid hormone [11]. This finding indicated that the renal cellular response mechanism to cyclic AMP is intact. Renal resistance therefore appears to be an inability of parathyroid hormone to produce cyclic AMP, but several alternative mechanisms must be considered. It is possible that cyclic AMP, formed normally within the renal tubular cell, is destroyed at an increased rate by phosphodiesterases. The inability of theophylline (a potent phosphodiesterase inhibitor) to alter significantly the parathyroid hormone responsiveness of affected subjects makes this unlikely [55, 55a]. Defective transport of cyclic AMP across the renal tubular cell membranes might account for the deficiency of urinary cyclic AMP. This also seems unlikely since the intracellular concentration would (presumably) be normal and the ability of dibutyryl cyclic AMP to bypass the physiologic defect would be unexplained. These arguments highlight the crucial role of the parathyroid hormone-sensitive adenylate cyclase system in the pathogenesis of the renal tubular resistance.

Apparent defects in hormone-sensitive adenylate cyclase activity may, in theory, result from an abnormality in any component of the parathyroid hormone receptor-enzyme complex

(Fig. 69-1). Marcus et al. [56] and Drezner and Burch [57], in separate studies of renal cortical plasma membranes from single patients with pseudohypoparathyroidism type 1, found no evidence for either a defective parathyroid hormone receptor or an abnormal caytalytic moiety. In both studies adenylate cyclase was normally stimulated by parathyroid hormone when the plasma membranes were incubated with 1mM ATP (sufficient nucleotide to saturate enzyme requirements for ATP and to substitute for GTP in the interaction with the N protein). Drezner and Burch concluded that N protein function was defective since parathyroid hormone stimulation of adenylate cyclase at subsaturating concentrations of ATP (0.1 mM) was diminished in the pseudohypoparathyroid kidney membranes and could be restored to normal by addition of GTP to the incubation medium (Fig. 69-3). These observations suggested that this pseudohypoparathyroid type 1 kidney had an N protein with an altered affinity or capacity for binding GTP.

These studies did not address the possible heterogeneity of the biochemical abnormality or whether the defect in N protein affects not only kidney (and perhaps bone) but all cells in which cyclic AMP is a second messenger. Bourne [58–60, 60a] and Spiegel [61, 61a] and their coworkers have clarified these issues by measuring the N protein component of adenylate cyclase in erythrocytes from patients with pseudohypoparathyroidism type 1 (Fig. 69-4). In approximately 60 percent of patients (type 1A) N protein activity was decreased by 50 percent. This implicated by extrapolation a defect in the N protein of parathyroid hormone target tissues as the primary abnormality in these patients. Almost all of these patients (32/33) manifested the features of AHO.

In contrast, the remaining patients (type 1B) had normal N protein activity. Thus, the primary biochemical abnormality is heterogeneous. In this group the majority of patients had normal somatic features. Measurements of N protein activity in platelet and fibroblast membranes confirm these observations [62, 62a].

The ubiquity of N protein in animal cells and its essential role in activation of adenylate cyclase suggest that the defective N protein activity observed in pseudohypoparathyroidism type 1A represents the kidney abnormality which limits cyclic AMP responsiveness to parathyroid hormone. Nevertheless, there is no reason to suspect that hormone unresponsiveness should be limited to parathyroid hormone target tissues. Rather, resistance to the action of other hormones that act via cyclic AMP might be expected. It is noteworthy that abnormal thyroid responsiveness to thyroid-stimulating hormone has been reported in patients with pseudohypoparathyroidism type 1 [62] and that abnormal ovarian and testicular response to gonadotropin stimulation has been found occasionally [63, 64] (see below). Further, glucagon infusion caused a markedly reduced increment in hepatic-derived plasma cyclic AMP in three of four patients with pseudohypoparathyroidism type 1A [62]. These data favor the hypothesis that decreased N protein activity does impair many cyclic AMP-mediated hormone responses. The reason parathyroid hormone response is so severely affected remains unsettled. Possibly the hormone-sensitive phosphate transport system is more critically dependent on even minor fluctuations in cyclic AMP generation, in which case a 50 percent reduction in N protein activity (Fig. 69-4) would severely disturb renal phosphate transport while minimally or not detectably altering other hormonal systems with greater "reserve." Acceptance or rejection of this hypothesis awaits greater understanding of the deranged biochemistry of pseudohypoparathyroidism.

The precise nature of the defect underlying pseudohypoparathyroidism type 1B remains obscure. The abnormality is apparently not due to aberrant N protein activity. Defects in other elements of the adenylate cyclase enzyme complex may account for the disorder, although abnormal N protein function, undetectable by current methodology, cannot be excluded. A variety of alternative defects unrelated to the adenylate cyclase moiety per se have also been suggested. Fisher [65] reported a bioinactive parathyroid hormone in several patients with pseudohypoparathyroidism type 1B. The end-organ resistance was attributed to occupancy of parathyroid hormone receptor sites by inert hormone or to down regulation of the number of parathyroid hormone receptors due to increased

Figure 69-2 Effect of parathyroid hormone infusion on urinary cyclic AMP excretion in patients with pseudohypoparathyroidism type 1 and type 2. In the baseline state (A) patients with pseudohypoparathyroidism type 1 excrete low normal levels of urinary cyclic AMP. In contrast, patients with pseudohypoparathyroidism type 2 have frankly elevated urinary cyclic AMP excretion. Intravenous infusion of parathyroid hormone (B) in patients with pseudohypoparathyroidism type 1 causes either no increase of urinary cyclic AMP or an increase to values less than 20 μmol/g creatinine. Patients with pseudohypoparathyroidism type 2 have a brisk ten- to fiftyfold increase in cyclic AMP excretion from baseline values. *(Adopted from Drezner et al. [111].)*

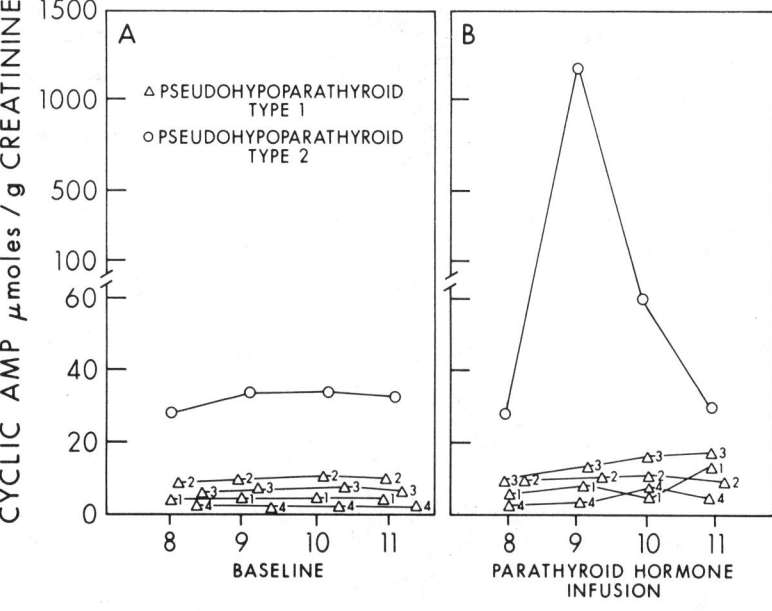

TIME

hormone levels. These possibilities cannot be dismissed even though parathyroid hormone has been demonstrated to be bioactive in a few cases [6] because such counterarguments ignore the remarkable heterogeneity of pseudohypoparathyroidism.

Nature of the Hypocalcemic Defect   In spite of progress in unraveling the renal pathophysiology of pseudohypoparathyroidism type 1, the nature of the metabolic defect(s) underlying the characteristic hypocalcemia remains uncertain. In patients with pseudohypoparathyroidism type 1 hypocalcemia results from defective parathyroid hormone-driven mobilization of bone calcium. Diminished hormone effects on renal and intestinal handling of calcium further deplete circulating calcium.

The bone resistance to parathyroid hormone has usually been ascribed to an innate defect in bone similar to that in the kidney. The observations concerning defective N protein activity in type 1A disease reinforce this hypothesis, but it is not yet known whether parathyroid hormone resistance is accompanied by a failure to increase cyclic AMP in bone [18]. Indeed, the conclusion that bone cells are innately unresponsive has been largely one of inference based on the systemic hypocalcemia and a subnormal rise in serum calcium when parathyroid hormone is administered to patients with pseudohypoparathyroidism. Even from the time of the earliest clinical investigations of this syndrome, there has been evidence that bone may respond to parathyroid hormone. Approximately 5 percent of reported cases of pseudohypoparathyroidism type 1 have shown normocalcemia [4, 5, 53, 62, 66–74], which may be intermittent (commensurate parathyroid hormone levels may be normal [66, 67] or elevated [68]. The fact that often the normocalcemic subjects are infants suggests that hypocalcemia is acquired and that bone resistance is due, at least in part, to factors other than innate abnormalitites of bone cell function

[66, 67, 70]. Support for this possibility is found in a study of the effects of parathyroidectomy in a patient with pseudohypoparathyroidism type 1. Removal of all four parathyroid glands resulted in a marked worsening of hypocalcemia. Thus, a significant fraction of the extracellular fluid calcium depended upon parathyroid hormone mobilization of bone stores [4].

Moreover, hypocalcemia does not necessarily indicate complete osseous resistance to parathyroid hormone. In 21 reported patients with pseudohypoparathyroidism type 1 there has been a paradoxical coexistence of hypocalcemia (and hyperphosphatemia) with osteitis fibrosa cystica, severe bone demineralization, or other evidence of excessive parathyroid hormone-directed bone remodeling (Fig. 69-5) [53, 74–88]. These observations imply that the homeostatic system in bone is more resistant to parathyroid hormone than is the remodeling system. It has been suggested [75, 81] that these patients have an atypical form of pseudohypoparathyroidism in which a renal defect is the sole abnormality and the hypocalcemia is secondary to hyperphosphatemia. As noted previously, however, the effects of hyperphosphatemia on serum calcium are transient and cannot underlie the persistent hypocalcemia. The sum of data indicates that bone resistance in pseudohypoparathyroidism is not complete and that parathyroid hormone may act differently on the homeostatic and remodeling systems. These observations do not exclude an innate abnormality in bone cells but do make it likely that an acquired and variable abnormality contributes to the defect.

Role of 1,25(OH)$_2$D in the Hypocalcemic Defect   One possible contribution to the variable bone resistance to parathyroid hormone is a deficiency of 1,25(OH)$_2$D. Competitive binding assays of serum 1,25(OH)$_2$D levels have revealed a marked decrease in concentration in untreated hypocalcemic patients with pseudohypoparathyroidism type 1 (Fig. 69-6) [82, 85, 89–91, 91a–91c]. Values ranging from 3 to 26 pg/ml in hypocalcemic subjects, both youths and adults, are substantially below the normal range. Levels determined by bioassay have been likewise decreased, although the magnitude of the deficiency is less striking [92]. The decreased serum 1,25(OH)$_2$D levels are not unexpected since kidney resistance to parathyroid hormone can be anticipated to compromise the stimulatory effects of this hormone on renal 25(OH)D-1α-hydroxylase enzyme activity. This hypothesis is supported by the recent observation that exogenous parathyroid hormone administration to patients with pseudohypoparathyroidism type 1 fails to increase the serum 1,25(OH)$_2$D level, while similar treatment in normal subjects increases the serum 1,25(OH)$_2$D more than twofold [90, 93, 94].

A role for the 1,25(OH)$_2$D deficiency in modulating bone resistance in pseudohypoparathyroidism type 1 is suggested by several observations. First, treatment with pharmacologic amounts of vitamin D restores the calcemic responsiveness of some patients to normal [81, 82, 95, 96]. The improved response generally occurs after prolonged treatment (>4 months) when the serum parathyroid hormone levels have returned toward normal. Calcemic responsiveness has not been restored by vitamin D treatment which produced short periods of normocalcemia. This observation suggests that a critical level or duration of inhibition of parathyroid hormone secretion and consequent alteration in bone dynamics are essential to the restoration of function [95, 97]. Second, administration of physiologic amounts of 1,25(OH)$_2$D normalizes calcium homeostasis (serum calcium; gastrointestinal

Figure 69-3   Effect of guanosine triphosphate (GTP) on parathyroid hormone-stimulated adenylate cyclase activity in control (C) and pseudohypoparathyroid (P) kidney membrane preparations. Adenylate cyclase activity was compared in the renal plasma membranes from three controls and a single patient with pseudohypoparathyroidism type 1. Basal and parathyroid hormone-stimulated activity was significantly less in the preparation from the pseudohypoparathyroid kidney compared to controls when GTP was excluded from the incubation medium. In contrast, addition of GTP to the incubation medium normalized the adenylate cyclase activity in the pseudohypoparathyroid kidney membranes. Hatched bars represent basal activity and open bars hormone stimulated activity. *(Adapted from Drezner and Burch [57].)*

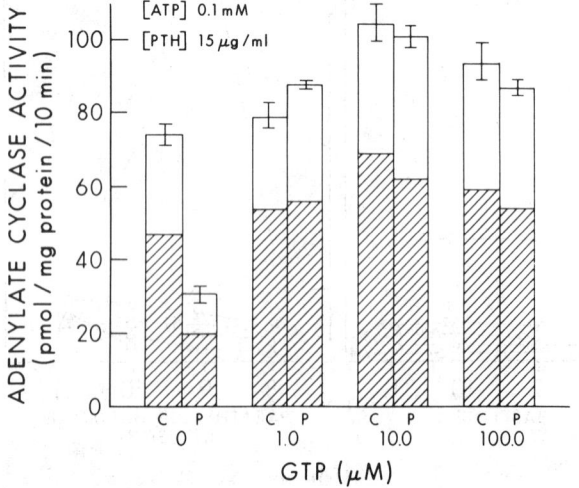

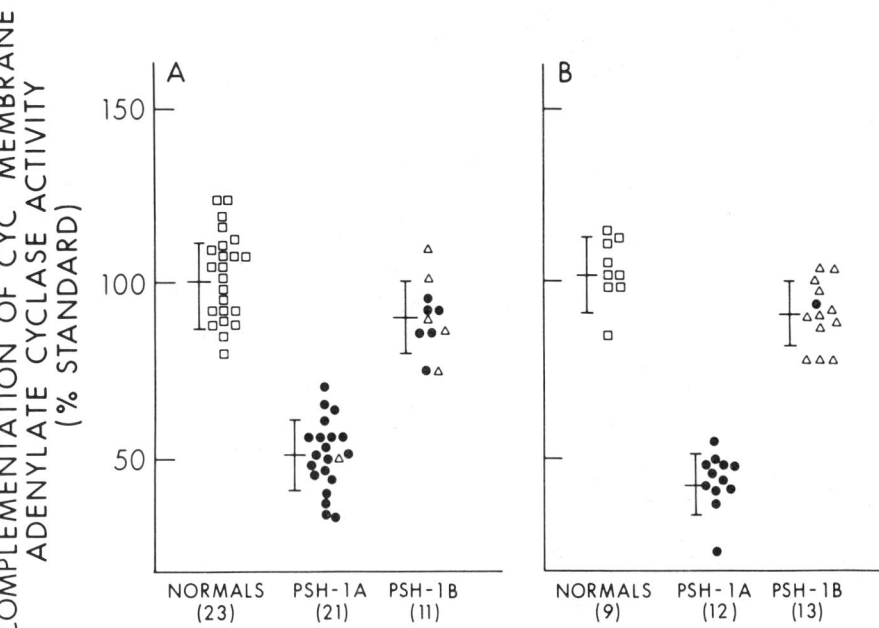

Figure 69-4 Measurement of erythrocyte nucleotide regulatory protein (N protein) activity by the ability of membrane extracts to augment adenylate cyclase activity in cyc^- membranes. Panel A shows the N protein activity (normalized by comparison with a standard membrane preparation) determined by Bourne and his associates in normal individuals (□), subjects with pseudohypoparathyroidism type 1 and Albright's hereditary osteodystrophy (●), and subjects with pseudohypoparathyroidism type 1 without skeletal abnormalities (△). Panel B shows similar data obtained by Spiegel and his associates. Vertical bars represent means ± 1 SD. *(Courtesy of Dr. HR Bourne, University of California, San Francisco, and Dr. AM Spiegel, Metabolic Disease Branch, NIADDK, NIH, Bethesda, Md.)*

absorption of calcium) in affected patients [98–101]. Third, patients with normocalcemic pseudohypoparathyroidism type 1 have a normal bone response to parathyroid hormone, and the serum 1,25(OH)₂D levels, when measured, are normal (Fig. 69-6) [66, 66a]. In contrast, in patients without pseudohypoparathyroidism but with an isolated deficiency of serum 1,25(OH)₂D there is an absent calcemic response to parathyroid hormone [102, 103]. Moreover, when administration of pharmacologic amounts of parathyroid extract does increase serum 1,25(OH)₂D levels, as reported in one patient with pseudohypoparathyroidism [93], calcemic responsiveness is normal. Finally, the lesser dependence of the remodeling system on 1,25(OH)₂D, compared with the homeostatic system, provides an explanation for the concurrence of hypocalcemia and osteitis fibrosa cystica in patients with pseudohypoparathyroidism type 1 [18, 29]. Parathyroid hormone overproduction secondary to hypocalcemia may eventually override the dependence on 1,25(OH)₂D for remodeling while failing to overcome the inhibition that 1,25(OH)₂D deficiency imparts to hormone-directed calcium mobilization. A similar explanation has been offered for the analogous paradox of hypocalcemia and osteitis fibrosa cystica in chronic renal failure [104].

Analysis of bone histomorphometric findings in patients with pseudohypoparathyroidism type 1 lends further credence to the vitamin D hypothesis. Bone biopsy specimens in six patients with radiographic evidence of increased parathyroid hormone activity demonstrate osteitis fibrosa cystica and excess unmineralized osteoid (Fig. 69-5). Moreover, bone biopsy specimens from hypocalcemic subjects without roentgenographic evidence of osteitis fibrosa cystica or excessive bone demineralization show a gradient in parathyroid hormone activity on bone remodeling and early evidence of vitamin D deficiency as well (Fig. 69-7) [82, 92, 101, 105–107]. Bone resorption and periosteocytic lacunar size vary from decreased to flagrantly increased levels, while increased osteoid tissue and abnormal mineralization dynamics are occasionally present. Indeed, radioactive calcium kinetic studies have confirmed an increased bone turnover rate in six patients [86, 101, 108, 109]. These observations suggest that a balance

between 1,25(OH)₂D deficiency and parathyroid hormone overproduction sets the rate of bone remodeling in pseudohypoparathyroidism type 1. The observation that 1,25(OH)₂D treatment restores bone histology to normal supports this hypothesis [92]. This does not necessarily imply that an N protein defect (or another innate abnormality) is not present in the osteoclast or osteocyte. It does indicate that 1,25(OH)₂D modulates events central to remodeling and calcium mobilization.

Control of Parathyroid Hormone Secretion Most observations indicate that calcium regulation of parathyroid hormone secretion is normal in pseudohypoparathyroidism type 1. Secondary hyperparathyroidism develops in response to the persistent hypocalcemia in untreated subjects with pseudohypoparathyroidism. All patients in whom measurements have been made have markedly increased peripheral concentrations of parathyroid hormone [3, 6, 8, 73, 82, 84, 110]. As is consistent with secondary hyperparathyroidism, hormone concentrations are lowered by calcium infusion and raised by disodium-EDTA infusion [4, 9, 82]. The presumably universal abnormality in N protein in type 1A patients raises the possibility that the integrated effects of calcium on parathyroid hormone secretion may be abnormal. Several observations support this speculation. Parfitt [32] has reported that the serum parathyroid hormone concentration and parathyroid gland mass in patients with pseudohypoparathyroidism are significantly less than in patients with renal failure who have similar degrees of hypocalcemia. The disparity in the circulating hormone concentration cannot be attributed merely to increased retention of parathyroid hormone metabolites due to decreased renal clearance. This apparent impairment of parathyroid hormone secretion may play a role in the steady state hypocalcemia. Furthermore, in patients studied by the authors [110a] and by Brinkman [110b], the serum parathyroid hormone concentration remains elevated despite long-term restoration of normocalcemia. The suppressive effects of calcium on parathyroid hormone secretion therefore seem incomplete. It seems essential to study carefully calcium effects on parathyroid hormone synthesis and secretion in order to determine if

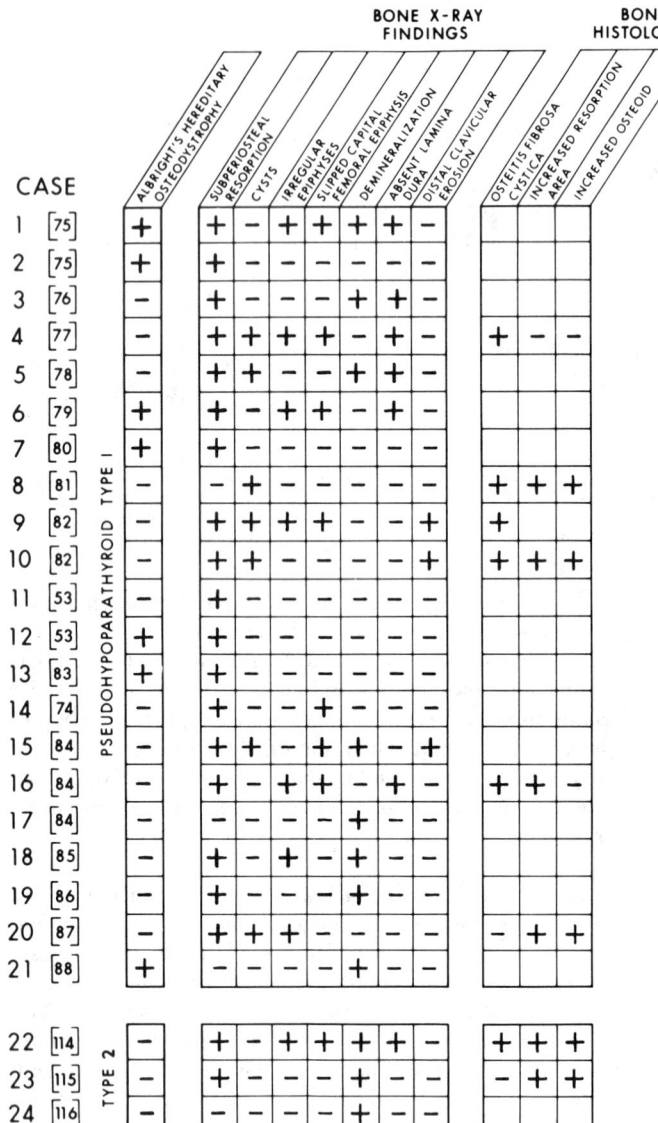

SUMMARY OF BONE ABNORMALITIES IN PATIENTS WITH PSUEDOHYPOPARATHYROIDISM AND "HYPERPARATHYROID" BONE DISEASE

Figure 69-5 Summary of bone abnormalities in patients with pseudohypoparathyroidism and "hyperparathyroid" bone disease. The apparently paradoxical occurrence of radiographic and histologic bone abnormalities characteristic of increased parathyroid hormone activity has been reported in hypocalcemic patients with both pseudohypoparathyroidism type 1 and type 2. The various findings reported are indicated by a + when present, a − if absent, and a blank space when information is not available.

abnormal regulation of hormone availability contributes to the abnormalities of calcium homeostasis or bone remodeling.

Pseudohypoparathyroidism Type 2

In 1973 Drezner et al. [111] reported studies performed on a 22-month-old male with symptomatic hypocalcemia and an elevated serum parathyroid hormone level. The infant had no phosphaturic response to a single intraveous injection of parathyroid extract, nor did he demonstrate a calcemic or hypophosphatemic response to parathyroid extract administered intramuscularly for 4 days. Since he was small in stature (10th percentile) and mentally retarded (IQ 51), the diagnosis of pseudohypoparathyroidism seemed likely. However, an elevated basal urinary cyclic AMP excretion and a normal increase in urinary cyclic AMP after intravenous administration of parathyroid extract (Fig. 69-2) appeared to exclude the diagnosis of pseudohypoparathyroidism (type 1) in spite of the undeniable evidence of end-organ resistance to the phosphaturic action of parathyroid hormone. The dilemma was resolved by postulating normal parathyroid hormone-receptor-adenylate cyclase activity in the renal cell membrane and attributing the defect to an inability of intracellular cyclic AMP to initiate the hormone-specific chain of events at the kidney (and perhaps the bone). Drezner et al. termed the new disorder *pseudohypoparathyroidism type 2.*

Since the initial description, 19 additional patients with pseudohypoparathyroidism type 2 have been recognized [112–122, 122a]. Each presented with hypocalcemia, hyperphosphatemia, and diminished urinary phosphate excretion. Parathyroid hormone infusion has uniformly provoked a normal rise in urinary cyclic AMP, but the increase in phosphate excretion has been blunted or absent. Although these data reinforce the supposition that pseudohypoparathyroidism type 2 results from a defect in initiating or completing the events directed by cyclic AMP in the renal cell, a recent observation challenges this interpretation. In a single affected patient the intravenous infusion of dibutyryl cyclic AMP generated a phosphaturia identical to that observed in normal subjects and patients with pseudohypoparathyroidism type 1 [113]. It seems unlikely that inhibition of phosphodiesterase, a known effect of dibutyryl cyclic AMP, is the property that explains the inactivity of endogenous cyclic AMP in the face of responsiveness to its dibutyryl derivative. At present this observation remains unexplained. Whether it implies further biochemical heterogeneity of pseudohypoparathyroidism remains to be determined.

Some insight into the mechanism(s) underlying the renal resistance to parathyroid hormone in pseudohypoparathyroidism type 2 has been provided by the recent demonstration that renal phosphaturic response is restored by normalization of the serum calcium (employing acute or chronic calcium infusions or long-term vitamin D_2 therapy). These observations suggest that the metabolic defect may be due to an inability of parathyroid hormone to increase renal cell membrane permeability to calcium. The resultant failure to activate postulated calcium (or calcium and cyclic AMP)-dependent enzymatic reactions would then lead to the loss of hormone-specific physiologic effects. The fact that these patients have a normal sodium and bicarbonate excretory response to parathyroid hormone suggests that such a defect in calcium transport would affect only phosphate transport in the renal tubule. We need a better understanding of the physiologic interdependence of renal cyclic AMP and calcium before the nature of the metabolic defect can be ascertained.

The cause of the hypocalcemia in pseudohypoparathyroid-

Figure 69-6 Measurement of serum 1,25-dihydroxyvitamin D [1,25(OH)$_2$D] levels in patients with pseudohypoparathyroidism type 1. Values for 1,25(OH)$_2$D, determined by competitive protein-binding assays, are low in affected youths and adults who are hypocalcemic. In contrast, serum 1,25(OH)$_2$D levels in normocalcemic patients with pseudohypoparathyroidism are near the upper limit of the normal range. The data shown reflect previously reported observations from several laboratories [82, 85, 89–91] as well as personal communications from Dr. Mark Haussler (University of Arizona, Tucson), Dr. Jacob Lemann (The Medical College of Wisconsin, Milwaukee), and Dr. Russel Chesney (University of Wisconsin, Madison). The assays utilized for these measurements had normal ranges for adults of 19 to 50, 16 to 56, 19 to 49, 20 to 48, 17 to 58, 15 to 48, and 20 to 45 pg/ml, values essentially identical. Normal ranges for youths 5 to 18 years of age are higher, averaging 23 to 70 pg/ml. The distribution of values in normal individuals shown in this figure is a representative normal range [82]. Vertical bars are the mean ± SD (excluding data from the normocalcemic patients with pseudohypoparathyroidism).

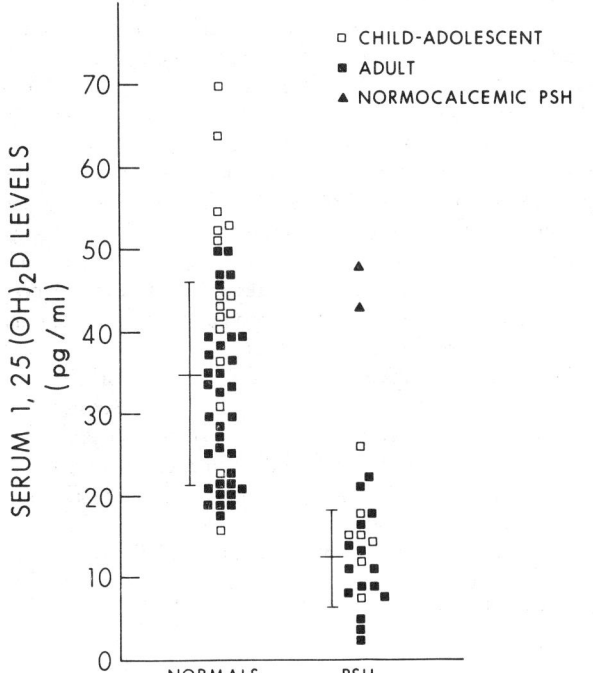

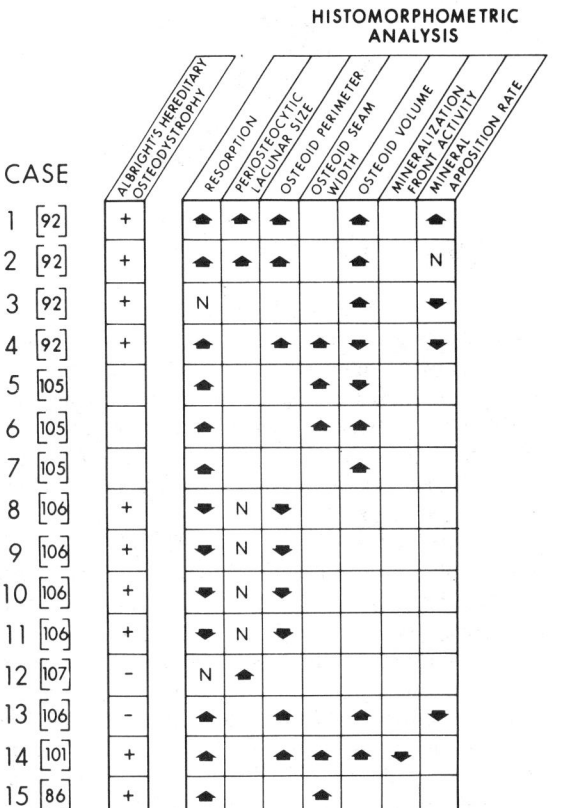

Figure 69-7 Summary of histomorphometric data from bone biopsy specimens in patients with pseudohypoparathyroidism type 1. Biopsy specimens obtained from patients without radiographic evidence of bone disease were evaluated for evidence of parathyroid hormone effects. A spectrum of abnormalities indicating decreased to excessive parathyroid action is evident (+, present; −, absent; ↑, increased; ↓, decreased; N, normal; blank, data not available).

ism type 2 is likewise uncertain. The ability of normal serum calcium (and the subsequent normalization of serum parathyroid hormone levels) to restore bone response to parathyroid hormone has not been determined. Hence, the presence of a biochemical defect of the bone (similar to that hypothesized at the kidney) is inferential. Moreover, no measurements of serum 1,25(OH)$_2$D levels are available in affected subjects, and the potential role of vitamin D deficiency in the genesis of the hypocalcemia and bone resistance remains speculative. Patients with pseudohypoparathyroidism type 2 occasionally do develop bone demineralization, osteitis fibrosa cystica, or osteomalacia (Fig. 69-5). This suggests, as in type 1 disease, some persistent responsiveness of the bone remodeling system to parathyroid hormone. Further studies are necessary to establish this relationship.

In an effort to confirm that the defect in pseudohypoparathyroidism type 2 is not related to an abnormality of the parathyroid hormone-receptor-adenylate cyclase complex, Farfel and his associates [59] have measured N protein activity in a single patient. They found normal N protein activity, consistent with the hypothesis that this variant of pseudohypoparathyroidism results from a defect in cyclic AMP action rather than in cyclic AMP formation.

In pseudohypoparathyroidism type 2 the absence of skeletal anomalies of AHO emphasizes the difference between this condition and pseudohypoparathyroidism type 1. Furthermore, the variable age of onset of this disease (22 months to 70 years) and the absence of any evidence for familial transmission testify to the distinction of type 2 from type 1 disease and even raise the question of whether pseudohypoparathyroidism type 2 may be an acquired defect.

CLINICAL FEATURES

Signs and Symptoms

The clinical expression of pseudohypoparathyroidism is referable either to the hypoparathyroidism per se or to the associated skeletal and developmental defects. Most patients with pseudohypoparathyroidism present with hypocalcemia and hyperphosphatemia. Serum calcium values are rarely above 7.5 mg/dl or the serum phosphorus levels less than 5.0 mg/dl in adults (7.0 mg/dl in children). Serum levels of parathyroid hormone (as measured by radioimmunoassay) are elevated in virtually all untreated subjects [3, 6, 8, 73, 82, 84, 110–112]. Normalization of serum calcium by treatment with vitamin D or its metabolites results in lowered circulating levels of parathyroid hormone. Alkaline phosphatase activity is usually normal except when osteitis fibrosa cystica or excessive parathyroid hormone-mediated bone remodeling exists.

The multiple skeletal and developmental defects found in pseudohypoparathyroidism type 1 include round or moon-shaped facies, depressed nasal bridge, a thickset, stocky, or obese body habitus (Fig. 69-8), and multiple discrete abnormalities in bones (including shortness of the metacarpals or metatarsals and sometimes of the phalanges as well) (Table 69-1) [1, 2]. The metacarpal and metatarsal defects arise from early closure of the epiphyses preceded by a decrease in longitudinal growth. The fifth and especially the fourth digits are most often involved, while the second digit is most often spared and is never the only one involved [123, 124]. When the hand is closed, the knuckles on the affected fingers are replaced by dimples (Fig. 69-8), although this sign may be absent when multiple digits are affected. Additional features of the osteochondrodystrophy include radius curvus, cubitus valgus, coxa vara, coxa valga, genu varum, and genu valgum deformities. The radius curvus is not uncommon. It may be a mild curvature or extreme bowing with epiphyseal displacement [4, 124, 125].

The average age at onset of symptoms in pseudohypoparathyroidism type 1 is 8.5 years, but the duration of symptoms prior to establishment of the diagnosis averages 9 to 12 years [126, 127]. Some patients have been reported who, although symptomatic, remained undiagnosed for 30 to 40 years [126, 128].

Most of the symptoms of pseudohypoparathyroidism reflect increased neuromuscular excitability resulting from the abnormally low calcium level in the blood and extracellular fluid. Curiously, neither the severity nor the frequency of the symptoms correlates with the degree of the hypocalcemia. Tetany, manifest as carpopedal spasm, tetanic convulsions, paresthesias, or stridor, has been observed in almost all reported cases [4]. The most striking clinical manifestation is convulsions, which occur in 60 percent of affected subjects. These resemble grand mal seizures except that a preceding aura, loss of consciousness, and sphincter incontinence are often absent. Rarely, the seizures may resemble those of petit mal epilepsy. The electroencephalogram is often abnormal, and therefore

Table 69-1 Incidence of signs and symptoms in pseudohypoparathyroidism type 1

Signs and symptoms	%	(n)
Biochemical		
Hypocalcemia	96	(175)
Elevated alkaline phosphatase activity	20	(134)
Body habitus		
Short stature (<1.55 m)*	80	(87)
Round face	92	(158)
Thickset, stocky, or obese	50	(40)
Ocular		
Lenticular opacities	44	(144)
Strabismus	10	(40)
Dental		
Hypoplasia, enamel defects	51	(67)
Unerupted teeth	56	(93)
Root defects	17	(7)
Soft tissue calcification		
Subcutaneous	55	(33)
Ectopic ossification	56	(155)
Basal ganglia	50	(140)
Choroid plexus, falx, cerebellum, cerebrum	15	(8)
Extremities		
Brachymetacarpia	68	(169)
Brachymetatarsia	43	(105)
Brachyphalangia	50	(38)
Neurologic		
Mental retardation	75	(161)
Seizures	59	(114)
Muscle cramps, twitching	38	(40)
Skeletal		
Thickened calvaria	62	(68)
Decreased density	15	(75)

* Patients older than 16 years.

patients may be labeled epileptic. Antiepileptic therapy invariably fails to control the seizures since relief depends on normalizing the serum calcium concentration.

Mental derangements varying from depression to acute or chronic psychosis, paranoia, dementia, schizophrenic behavior, hallucinations, and delusions have all been encountered, and all have been reversed by normalization of the serum calcium. In addition, impairment of memory and emotional lability have been reported [4]. Mental retardation is common in patients with pseudohypoparathyroidism type 1, but it is not known whether the mental deficiency is a consequence of the hypocalcemia or is an associated heritable defect. When the hypocalcemia is prenatal in onset and continues through the first few months of life, brain functioning may be permanently impaired. When the hypocalcemia begins after the critical developmental period, the symptoms of mental deficit are often at least partially reversible [126, 129].

Subcapsular cataracts are a relatively common complication of pseudohypoparathyroidism type 1 [4, 126]. The typical lenticular opacity is located in one or more cortical layers which are separated from each other and from the lens capsule by zones of clear cortex. The pathogenesis of the cataracts is not known but, although the opacities are irreversible, their progression can be stopped by normalization of the serum calcium. The eye may also show ectopic calcification in the sclera and choroid [130].

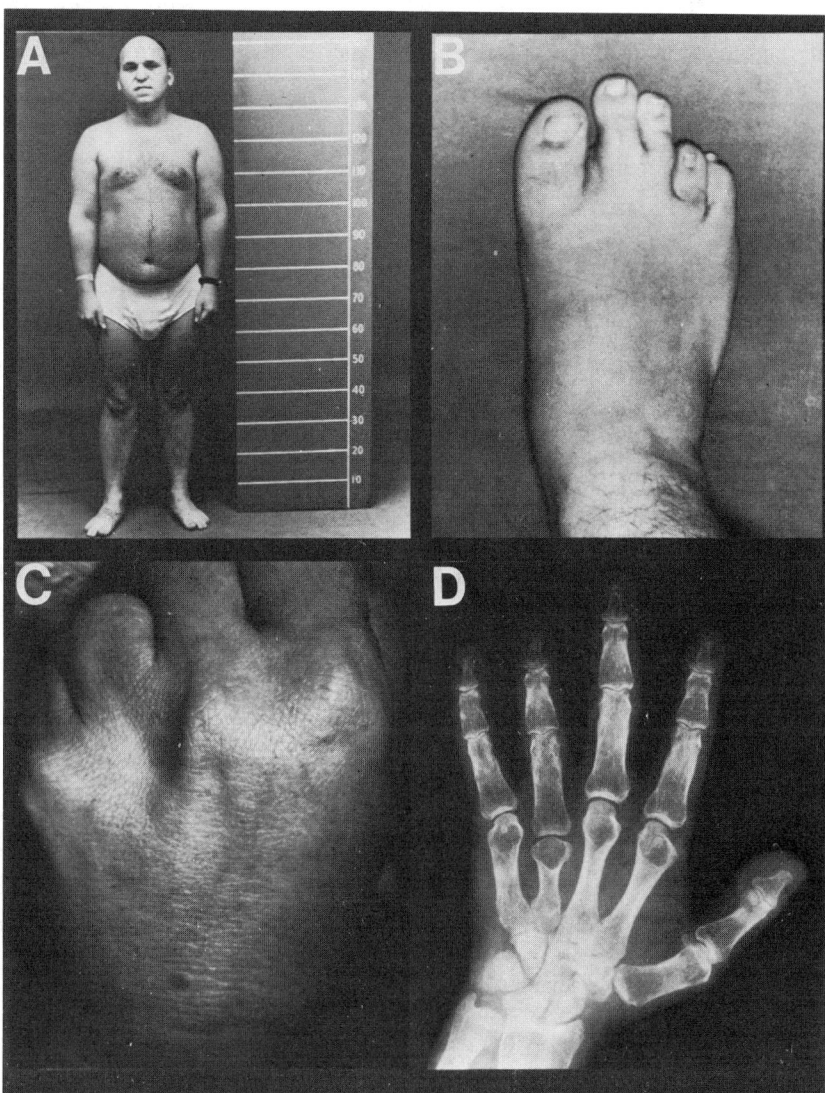

Figure 69-8 *A.* A middle-age patient with pseudohypoparathyroidism exhibiting short stature, obesity, and rounded facies. *B.* A close-up view of the right foot demonstrates shortened first, fourth, and fifth metatarsals. *C.* The left hand of another patient with pseudohypoparathyroidism shows the classic "dimple" replacing the absent fourth knuckle. *D.* An x-ray of the same left hand illustrates the shortened left fourth metacarpal.

Enamel hypoplasia (pitting or defects, depending upon the age at onset and duration of the hypocalcemia) is commonly present in patients with pseudohypoparathyroidism, along with dentin defects, short and blunted tooth roots, and delay or absence of tooth eruptions [131, 132]. Hypoplastic teeth are prone to caries, and many patients lose all their teeth. These dental defects can sometimes be used to date the age of onset of hypocalcemia [133].

Soft tissue calcification is common, especially in the subcutaneous tissues and the brain, particularly the basal ganglia. The subcutaneous calcium deposits are associated with ectopic bone formation, which usually appears early in life and preferentially in the extremities and around large joints [134]. Calcification of the basal ganglia has been observed in 50 percent of patients, and extrapyramidal symptoms (chorea, dystonia, tremors) can occur [4, 135]. Occasionally the symptoms improve with correction of the hypocalcemia, but the calcification is irreversible [136].

Some degree of bone change is usual in pseudohypoparathyroidism, although x-ray examination is usually normal or even shows increased bone density, particularly of the skull. Severe demineralization, including frank osteitis fibrosa cystica, and occasionally rickets or osteomalacia has been observed in 24

patients, 21 with type 1 disease and 3 with type 2 (Fig. 69-5). In eight subjects bone disease has been confirmed by bone biopsy. Many of the type 1 subjects with severe bone disease are atypical in that they do not have the classic physical stigmata or a family history of the disease. Eight subjects do have classic AHO, and three of them are from families with the disease [53, 80]. The occurrence of osteitis fibrosa cystica has led to speculation that these subjects may represent a variant form of pseudohypoparathyroidism. Bone biopsy specimens from 15 additional subjects with pseudohypoparathyroidism (Fig. 69-7) show a spectrum of abnormalities indicative of excessive parathyroid hormone activity [82, 92, 101, 105–107]. Resorptive activity was normal in six subjects but increased in the remaining nine, and unmineralized osteoid excess was seen in at least eight additional patients. These observations indicate that osteitis fibrosa cystica may be simply the extreme end of a continuum which balances differing degrees of bone responsiveness on the one hand with parathyroid hyperactivity on the other.

Recently, a distinctive impairment in olfaction and the ability to taste sour and bitter substances has been reported in the majority of patients with pseudohypoparathyroidism type 1 [137]. The reason is not known. Another unexplained phenomenon is the finding of unusual dermatoglyphic abnormalities, including frequent hypothenar patterns and distally located triradii [138].

Associated Endocrinopathies

Hypothyroidism has frequently been associated with pseudohypoparathyroidism type 1. In initial reports [139–141] the hypothyroidism was ascribed to a selective thyrotropin (TSH) deficiency (an observation still to be documented with the sensitive TSH assays presently available). More recently, patients have had elevated levels of TSH [142, 143], which in a single case was shown to be biologically active.

A recent extensive study [62] of the hypothalamic-pituitary-thyroid axis in 10 patients with pseudohypoparathyroidism revealed 8 who had laboratory findings consistent with subtle hypothyroidism, but with mild or absent clinical signs. Each patient had a slightly decreased serum T_4 and free T_4 concentration but only modestly elevated basal TSH values (range 7.6 to 15 μu/ml; normal <5.0). Thyrotropin-releasing hormone (TRH) stimulation resulted in an exaggerated TSH response and an abnormally small increment in the serum T_3 concentration. The eight subjects had pseudohypoparathyroidism type 1A, while the two unaffected subjects had pseudohypoparathyroidism type 1B. Whether the abnormality will be restricted to those patients with N protein deficiency (type 1A) remains unclear. Patients with pseudohypoparathyroidism deserve a careful clinical and full thyroid function assessment.

Gonadal dysfunction has also been found in association with pseudohypoparathyroidism. Wolfsdorf et al. [63] described a woman with pseudohypoparathyroidism type 1 and partial ovarian insufficiency, elevated levels of gonadotropins, and an exaggerated gonadotropin response to gonadotropin-releasing hormone (GnRH). Similarly, Shapiro et al. [64] have studied a male subject with pseudohypoparathyroidism type 1 in whom basal testosterone levels were normal but gonadotropins were elevated and GnRH infusion caused an inordinate increase in both leutinizing hormone (LH) and follicle-stimulating hormone (FSH). These data suggest a defect in the hypothalamic-pituitary-gonadal axis similar to that observed in the hypothalamic-pituitary-thyroidal axis, but other studies have not confirmed this [62]. Thus, a strong association between gonadal dysfunction and pseudohypoparathyroidism appears lacking, although an N protein deficiency might account for impaired function.

Carlson and his associates [144] found deficient prolactin responses to chlorpromazine or thyrotropin-releasing hormone (TRH) in pseudohypoparathyroid patients with or without dysmorphic features or deficient N protein concentration. These data imply that impaired prolactin secretion is common in pseudohypoparathyroidism. In contrast, Levine et al. [62] found normal basal and TRH-stimulated prolactin levels. The reason(s) for the difference is not clear, and the prevalence of decreased prolactin secretion in pseudohypoparathyroidism remains to be established.

There is an increased prevalence of diabetes mellitus in patients with pseudohypoparathyroidism and in their families [4]. The severity varies from mild glucose intolerance to frank diabetes with its associated complications. The significance of this association is unknown.

Other endocrinopathies associated with pseudohypoparathyroidism are probably chance occurrences. Those reported include acromegaly, diabetes insipidus, multiple pheochromocytomas, and hyperthyroidism [4].

DIAGNOSIS AND DIFFERENTIAL DIAGNOSIS

A diagnosis of pseudohypoparathyroidism must be entertained in all patients who have hypocalcemia and hyperphosphatemia in the presence of normal renal function. Finding the characteristic skeletal and developmental defects in the patient or a family history of short stature and skeletal anomalies in first-order relatives increases the likelihood of the diagnosis. Pseudohypoparathyroidism must also be considered in patients with unexplained increases in alkaline phosphatase and in all patients with ill-defined metabolic bone disease, particularly children with slipped capital femoral epiphyses (see Fig. 69-5), whether hypocalcemia is present or not. Application of specific tests permits diagnosis as well as definition of subtypes of the disease by demonstrating the characteristic lack of responsiveness to parathyroid hormone at the kidney (and less often bone) and the presence of secondary hyperparathyroidism.

Diagnostic Methods

Patients with hypocalcemia should have secondary hyperparathyroidism. When no parathyroid hormone is detectable by either amino- or carboxyterminal immunoassays, idiopathic or surgical (if the history is appropriate) hypoparathyroidism is the likely diagnosis. If elevated levels of hormone are present, the hypocalcemia probably is due to end-organ resistance, although the presence of bioinactive hormone remains a theoretical possibility.

Renal resistance to parathyroid hormone is demonstrated by measuring the urinary excretion of cyclic AMP and phosphate following the injection of parathyroid hormone [3, 111]. The procedure is performed on a control and test day. Patients are fasted after midnight on both days of study and are given water (20 ml per kilogram of body weight) to drink from 7 to 8 A.M. From 8 A.M. until noon, water is ingested in a volume equal to the volume of voided urine. Urine collections are made from 8 to 9 A.M.; 9 to 9:30 A.M.; 9:30 to 10 A.M.; 10 to 11 A.M., and 11 A.M. to 12 noon. On the test day, 200 to 300 USP units of parathyroid hormone are infused in 50 ml of 0.45 percent saline from 9 to 9:15 A.M. The rise in cyclic AMP is generally maximal in the 9 to 9:30 A.M. collection. Patients with pseudohypoparathyroidism type 1 have a blunted urinary cyclic AMP response (Fig. 69-2) which does not exceed 20 μmol/g creatinine. In comparison, patients with idiopathic or surgical hypoparathyroidism have a brisk, ten- to fiftyfold increase in cyclic AMP excretion from a basal value of 1.5 to 5.0 μmol/g creatinine.

The segregation of pseudohypoparathyroidism type 1 from type 2 requires evaluation of parathyroid hormone effects on phosphate as well as cyclic AMP excretion. Unfortunately, there are serious difficulties in interpretation of the phosphaturic response [111]. While the mean values of the parathyroid hormone-induced decrement in tubular reabsorption of phosphate (TRP), of the increase in phosphate excretion, or of the decrement in plasma phosphate clearly distinguish pseudo-hypoparathyroidism from other hypoparathyroid states, variation among individual determinations (reflected by large standard deviations) creates an element of uncertainty in any given patient. Since the excretion of phosphate (as well as TRP) varies nonlinearly until the tubular maximum is reached, enhanced discrimination of parathyroid hormone responsiveness can be achieved by determining changes in the renal tubular maximum for the reabsorption of phosphate per liter of glomerular filtrate (TmP/GFR). Infusion of parathyroid hormone decreases the TmP/GFR (mean $\pm$ SD) by 0.95 ± 0.33 ($n = 18$), 1.92 ± 0.33 ($n = 5$), and 0.61 ± 0.30 ($n = 8$) in normals, patients with idiopathic hypoparathyroidism, and patients with pseudohypoparathyroidism, respectively [111]. The test procedure requires measurement of phosphate and creatinine in the same urine collections used to test the cyclic AMP response, and determination of serum phosphate and creatinine at the midpoint of each collection. Subsequently, TmP/GFR is determined by the method of Bijvoet [145], and the maximum fall from the mean of control periods is calculated.

Measurement of plasma cyclic AMP after infusion of parathyroid hormone may also be used to demonstrate hormone unresponsiveness [146–148]. In normal subjects and patients with surgical or idiopathic hypoparathyroidism, intravenous infusion of 200 units of parathyroid hormone increases plasma cyclic AMP four- to tenfold within 10 min of injection. Patients with pseudohypoparathyroidism do not respond. This method simplifies testing procedures, but the inability to assess renal phosphate handling limits its discriminant value.

The serum calcium response to intramuscularly administered parathyroid hormone has been employed to assess the response of bone. Relatively few patients have been tested in this way, and adequate comparative data from normal subjects are not available. Nevertheless, a rise in serum calcium of <1.0 mg/dl after 3 to 10 days of stimulation (200 to 800 units every 6 h) is considered to indicate parathyroid hormone unresponsiveness [4, 149]. On several occasions increments in serum calcium as large as 3 mg/dl have been observed in patients with pseudohypoparathyroidism type 1 [97, 139]. The increment occurs only after prolonged stimulation and probably represents the transient effects of a responsive remodeling system on calcium homeostasis rather than the effect of parathyroid hormone on the homeostatic system in bone.

Recently, the measurement of N protein activity has been used to characterize the biochemical basis underlying pseudohypoparathyroidism. Currently available assays can be performed using plasma membranes from any conveniently available tissue. At present this measurement remains a research tool, and its potential clinical utility is uncertain.

Parathyroid extract for human use is no longer in commercial production. It seems likely that a suitable product will become available shortly, but until that time the diagnosis of pseudohypoparathyroidism must rely solely on determination of elevated serum parathyroid hormone levels.

Differential Diagnosis

The differential diagnosis of pseudohypoparathyroidism involves two principal categories of illness: (1) the various causes of hypocalcemia, and (2) syndromes with skeletal anomalies simulating those of pseudohypoparathyroidism.

The hyperphosphatemia distinguishes this disease from many other conditions in which hypocalcemia and hypophosphatemia are present.

Common Causes of Hypocalcemia with Hyperphosphatemia Hypocalcemia and hyperphosphatemia are manifestations of parathyroid hormone deficiency (true hypoparathyroidism). Parathyroid hormone deficiency may be classified into three major divisions: idiopathic, acquired, and reversible.

Idiopathic hypoparathyroidism refers to all cases not due to surgery or other well-defined causes. It is a relatively rare disorder in which parathyroid hormone deficiency is an isolated entity. When present at birth, the disorder usually is due to congenital absence of the parathyroid glands [150]. Most cases are sporadic, but familial occurrence with both X-linked recessive and autosomal recessive modes of inheritance have been reported. Idiopathic hypoparathyroidism in children often begins between 2 and 10 years of age, in which case females are affected twice as frequently as males and three of four cases are sporadic. In affected subjects there is a high prevalence of parathyroid antibodies [151]. In contrast, when idiopathic hypoparathyroidism occurs in adult life, it is invariably sporadic and without antiparathyroid antibodies, and onset may be at any age up to the eighth decade.

Idiopathic hypoparathyroidism may occur as part of the polyglandular failure syndrome type 1 and the Di George syndrome. The major components of the polyglandular failure syndrome type 1 are hypoparathyroidism, hypoadrenalism, and mucocutaneous candidiasis, at least two of which are present in each affected subject. An autoimmune basis has been inferred from the presence of organ-specific autoantibodies. Antibodies are often absent, and there is no association of the disease with specific HLA haplotypes [152, 153]. Symptoms of hypoparathyroidism in this syndrome generally develop in the first two decades of life and follow the onset of candidiasis by an average of 4 years. Adrenal failure, when present, usually develops after the hypocalcemia.

The Di George syndrome includes congenital absence of the parathyroids and the thymus, organs embryologically derived from the third and fourth branchial pouches [154, 155]. Affected infants, in addition to having tetany, are subject to repeated infections because of abnormalities in cell-mediated immunity. Associated abnormalities, due to maldevelopment of the first and fifth branchial clefts, include low set and notched, asymmetrical ears, hyperteleorism, macrognathia, right-sided aortic arch, and Fallot's tetralogy. Although most patients die in infancy, survival into adolescence is possible, and the syndrome should be considered in the diagnosis of hypoparathyroid states.

Surgical hypoparathyroidism is by far the most common variety of hypoparathyroidism. Generally the onset of disease follows thyroidectomy but may occur after resection of adenomatous or hyperplastic parathyroid glands. Since the parathyroid glands are not always found in the excised specimen, the injury most likely results from parathyroid ischemia [151, 156].

Additional causes of acquired parathyroid hormone deficiency include the infrequent occurrence of radiation damage [151]. Although the parathyroid glands are unusually resistant to irradiation, hypoparathyroidism has been observed after radioiodine treatment of hyperthyroidism. Moreover, the functional reserve of the parathyroid glands may be compromised by radioiodine treatment. Occasionally, iron overload (e.g., hemochromatosis) and neoplastic infiltration may impair parathyroid gland function [151].

Reversible causes of parathyroid deficiency include delayed maturation of parathyroid function, suppression of normal glands by systemic hypercalcemia, and impaired hormone synthesis because of magnesium depletion. Delayed onset of normal parathyroid function is accompanied by neonatal hypocalcemia and tetany. In all infants the serum calcium falls after birth to a level 1 to 2 mg/dl below normal, the nadir occurring within 24 to 48 h, after which there is spontaneous recovery. Early neonatal tetany represents an exaggeration of this normal phenomenon and may be associated with maternal diabetes or with prematurity, low birth weight, or respiratory distress in the infant.

Suppression of normal parathyroid function by hypercalcemia occurs in infants born to mothers with primary hyperparathyroidism, presumably because of transmission of maternal hypercalcemia to the fetus via the placenta. Symptoms begin in the first 2 weeks of life, and recovery occurs within 3 months. Hypocalcemia resulting from suppressed parathyroid function may also occur after removal of a hyperfunctioning parathyroid adenoma, although reversal of hyperparathyroid bone disease with resultant uptake of serum calcium ("bone hunger") is more often the precipitating factor.

Magnesium depletion of any cause may result in hypocalcemia. The mechanism includes impaired synthesis of parathyroid hormone, presumably due to a deficiency of a magnesium-dependent enzyme. Parathyroid hormone deficiency is central to the pathogenesis of the hypocalcemia in the childhood disease, primary congenital hypomagnesemia [157], but the cause is not so certain in adults [158]. In any case, replacement of magnesium quickly reverses the hypocalcemia.

Additional causes of hypocalcemia are listed in Table 69-2. Hypophosphatemia distinguishes vitamin D–deficient states from pseudohypoparathyroidism. Many other causes of hypocalcemia are extremely rare or associated with easily recognized primary diseases (e.g., renal failure, acute pancreatitis); often the cause of the hypocalcemia remains unknown. See the chapter by Parfitt [151] for a detailed and useful review of these hypocalcemic conditions.

Skeletal Abnormalities   Patients with a variety of developmental and skeletal anomalies, including Gardner's syndrome [159], Turner's syndrome [160], basal cell nevus syndrome [161], and familial calcification of the basal ganglia [4], share certain physical features with pseudohypoparathyroidism. Generally, the similarity is limited to short metacarpals or metatarsals, but occasional reports that these patients are resistant to the phosphaturic effects of parathyroid hormone have led to speculation that these disorders are related to pseudohypoparathyroidism. Serum calcium and phosphorus are invariably normal, and studies by Aurbach et al. [162] have established that these patients have normally responsive urinary cyclic AMP excretion. Thus, these syndromes do not share the characteristic metabolic defects of pseudohypoparathyroidism. Whether the skeletal defects have a common genetic basis with AHO is not clear, and this raises the question of how to diagnose *pseudo-pseudohypoparathyroidism*. We have applied this term only to the eumetabolic but skeletally affected members of kindreds containing other individuals with unequivocal pseudohypoparathyroidism.

TREATMENT

Treatment of pseudohypoparathyroidism is directed at normalizing the serum calcium concentration and thus controlling the neuromuscular symptoms. Conventional therapy is based on use of vitamin D, usually as ergocalciferol (D_2), administered in a dose of 50,000 to 100,000 units/day. From 1 to 2 g elemental calcium may also be given orally. The beneficial effect of vitamin D depends on enhanced gastrointestinal absorption of calcium as well as on increased bone resorption. Dosage of medication is adjusted to maintain the serum calcium level between 8.7 and 10.0 mg/dl. In general, the daily dose of vitamin D is less than that required in postsurgical or idiopathic hypoparathyroidism. Nevertheless, vitamin D intoxication may develop without any apparent change in a dosage of vitamin D that has long been optimal. In our experience the incidence of intoxication is remarkably decreased when control of the serum calcium is achieved using vitamin D alone. If hypercalcemia does occur, the long duration of vitamin D action may result in an elevated serum calcium for weeks or months, and corticosteroid therapy may be required to temporize the abnormality.

The decreased serum $1,25(OH)_2D$ concentration observed in patients with pseudohypoparathyroidism (Fig. 69-6) and the role of $1,25(OH)_2D$ in restoring bone responsiveness to parathyroid hormone indicate that improved therapy might be achieved by using physiologic replacement doses of $1,25(OH)_2D_3$. Indeed, recent reports [98–101, 163–166] have described an excellent response to therapy with this active vitamin D metabolite or its synthetic analogue, $1\alpha(OH)D$. These compounds bypass the renal hydroxylation step in vitamin D metabolism which is defective in pseudohypoparathyroidism. In addition, they have a short half-life, so that any hypercalcemia is reversible within hours after cessation of therapy. Despite these advantages $1,25(OH)_2D_3$ has not yet been approved for use in pseudohypoparathyroidism, but it is com-

Table 69-2   Causes of hypocalcemia other than hypoparathyroidism

Vitamin D deficiency
Vitamin D dependency
Chronic renal failure*
Intestinal malabsorption (of vitamin D/calcium)
Osteoblastic metastases
Drug induced
    Calcitonin
    Mithramycin
    Ethanol
    Phosphate
    Citrate (in massive transfusions)
Acute pancreatitis
Fall in protein-bound calcium
    Hemodilution
    Hypoalbuminemia
Bone healing
    After surgery for hyperparathyroidism
    After surgery for hyperthyroidism
    Upon treatment of rickets/osteomalacia
Malignant hyperthermia*

* Accompanied by hyperphosphatemia.

mercially available and can be used (after appropriate informed consent of the patient) if the condition proves difficult to manage by conventional means.

Therapy with 1,25(OH)$_2$D$_3$ alone normalizes the serum calcium within days. The serum parathyroid hormone concentration falls toward or into the normal range. The usual dose of 1,25(OH)$_2$D$_3$ is 1 to 2 µg/day, an amount significantly less than that necessary in the true hypoparathyroid disorders. The initial dose is 0.25 µg orally per day and, provided hypercalcemia or hypercalciuria does not develop, the dose is increased by 0.25 µg/day at weekly intervals until normocalcemia is achieved. The drug is given in a divided dose every 12 h. Blood and urine calcium values should be monitored periodically to detect inadequate or excessive therapy. A decline in dose requirement may be seen after long periods of therapy. This reinforces the necessity for close observation [167]. Moreover, the occasional report of deteriorating renal function in association with 1,25(OH)$_2$D$_3$ treatment indicates that the serum creatinine concentration should be measured periodically.

GENETICS

We believe that no definitive statement can be made regarding the genetics of pseudohypoparathyroidism. Several factors contribute to this impasse.

1. *Incomplete recording.* Although pseudohypoparathyroidism occurs in familial patterns and is no doubt a heritable disease, family trees are incompletely recorded in the literature available for analysis [5, 53, 58, 59, 62, 67, 79, 95, 101, 124, 132, 149, 168–174]. This has led to an apparent preponderance of affected to unaffected offspring (83/28). Many of these reports describe only a single parent and single offspring, without mention of other family members. Consequently, it is often impossible to determine whether there are unaffected sibs or not.

2. *Incomplete investigation.* Few studies rely on more than one or two metabolic variables (hypocalcemia; lack of phosphaturic, calcemic, or cyclic AMP response to parathyroid hormone stimulation; elevated serum parathyroid hormone concentration) to establish the diagnosis of pseudohypoparathyroidism. As a result, some family members may be misclassified. Furthermore, the recent ability to measure the N protein concentration has demonstrated subgroups (type 1A and type 1B) of pseudohypoparathyroidism. It is conceivable that these subtypes are inherited by different mechanisms, but only the most recently studied pedigrees include N protein data. It is quite possible, therefore, that the genetic patterns have been confused by the indiscriminate inclusion of different genotypes of the disorder.

3. *Incomplete observation.* Few of the recorded family pedigrees include more than two generations. Since detection of the metabolic abnormalities of pseudohypoparathyroidism may require careful laboratory documentation and observation on multiple occasions, some family members may have been misclassified as normal because they are asymptomatic. In any case, the pattern of inheritance, even within single families, is not well documented over multiple generations.

4. *Uncertainty in the diagnosis of Albright's hereditary osteodystrophy (AHO).* We have already discussed the difficulties in discriminating AHO with certainty from other phe-

notypically similar disorders. Confusion is introduced if we assume that families demonstrating only AHO without evidence of parathyroid hormone unresponsiveness represent the same genetic lesion as those with pseudo-pseudohypoparathyroidism. Such families have been described [5, 173] and show a clearly autosomal dominant mode of inheritance. We exclude these pedigrees from our analysis since we restrict the definition of pseudo-pseudohypoparathyroidism to metabolically normal individuals (with AHO) who are members of families with definite pseudohypoparathyroidism.

5. *Apparent infertility of pseudohypoparathyroid men.* Thirty-one affected parents (pseudohypoparathyroid or pseudo-pseudohypoparathyroid) have been noted to produce affected offspring. Only four of these parents are males, three of whom are pseudo-pseudohypoparathyroid. This unexplained decrease in male fertility may bias certain genetic analyses. For example, no instances of male-male transmission of the complete syndrome have been recorded (indeed, there is only one recorded instance [53] of female-male transmission), but this may be due to diminished male fertility rather than to chromosome linkage of the pseudohypoparathyroid gene(s).

6. *Lack of familial occurrence of pseudohypoparathyroidism type 2.* There are no known examples of families having more than one member with pseudohypoparathyroidism type 2. Therefore, we cannot say that it represents a genetic disorder rather than an acquired defect. Thus, none of our subsequent discussion on genetics should be applied to pseudohypoparathyroidism type 2.

In spite of these deficiencies, a review of published pedigrees does allow us to draw some conclusions about the patterns of inheritance in pseudohypoparathyroidism; at least certain possibilities can be excluded. The following discussion refers only to pseudohypoparathyroidism type 1 considered in the general sense. Too few data exist to permit a separate analysis of whether types 1A and 1B have different genetic bases, likely as that possibility seems. Restriction of genetic analysis to pedigrees with N protein measurement is a project for the future which may clarify some of our confusion. For the present, we will consider in turn whether pseudohypoparathyroidism type 1 results from an X-linked dominant, an autosomal dominant or recessive, or a multifactorial mode of inheritance.

X-linked Dominant Inheritance

For many years pseudohypoparathyroidism has been considered to exemplify an X-linked dominant pattern of inheritance. This belief stems from two observations [5, 173]: (1) affected females outnumber affected males by nearly 2:1 (the anticipated ratio for X-linked dominance); (2) there are no known examples of male-male transmission of the complete syndrome. This latter observation may result from the diminished fertility of pseudohypoparathyroid men, but in the absence of established male-male transmission of the syndrome, X-linked dominant inheritance remains a possibility. However, this possibility is lessened by the reports of Levine et al. [62] and Weinberg and Stone [168], which show that affected males produced unaffected daughters, a finding inconsistent with X-linked dominance.

The most compelling argument against X-linked dominant inheritance comes from a consideration of the published pedigrees. Mann et al. [5] postulated sex linkage because their search of the literature showed that pseudohypoparathyroid females outnumbered affected males by 2:1. This ratio still persists and is unexplained; our review of acceptable cases [5, 53, 58, 59, 62, 67, 79, 95, 101, 124, 132, 149, 168–174] shows 50 affected females and 32 affected males. Spranger [173] suggested that this female preponderance might result from a discovery bias which more commonly brings affected females to medical attention (the incomplete recording of family trees might accentuate this bias). We have examined the sex ratios of affected sibs of the affected propositus in all cases in which nontwin sibs and a propositus were recorded. Of the pseudohypoparathyroid sibs, 15 are male and 9 are female. On the other hand, only 7 of the propositi are male, as compared to 13 females. These data suggest that Spranger is right: Females are more likely to be propositi, but there is no female preponderance among either the affected (15 males to 9 females) or unaffected (11/9) sibs in these families. The *total* number of affected children (propositi and sibs) in these families is 44, of whom 22 are male and 22 female. This analysis gives no support to the X-linked dominant hypothesis, which appears untenable at present.

Autosomal Dominant or Recessive Inheritance

The analysis in the preceding section reveals a ratio of affected to unaffected sibs of 22:20. This observation is consistent with autosomal dominant inheritance, as is the frequent observation of the disorder in consecutive generations [67, 174]. In addition, the biochemical data that show a 50 percent reduction in N protein concentration in affected individuals favor a dominant mode of inheritance. Nevertheless, there have been several instances [79, 172, 174] in which normal parents produced affected offspring, suggesting autosomal recessive inheritance (assuming no error in paternity). These conflicting observations suffer from the defects noted at the beginning of this section, but they do permit some conclusions: Pseudohypoparathyroidism type 1 is either biochemically heterogeneous (some forms inherited in dominant, others in recessive fashion), or the inheritance is complex and not due to simple segregation of alleles. Both explanations may be correct.

Multifactorial Inheritance

The confusing patterns of inheritance of pseudohypoparathyroidism (even excluding the possibility of different phenocopies, each having different modes of inheritance) may be explained by assuming that the defect results from the simultaneous inheritance of two or more characteristics which must be present in the appropriate combination(s) to produce the syndrome. Certainly the genetic lesion which produces AHO appears to be separate from (but closely linked with) that which produces loss of parathyroid hormone responsiveness. It is intriguing that offspring of families with pseudohypoparathyroidism may have the complete syndrome, may have only AHO (i.e., pseudo-pseudohypoparathyroidism), or may be normal. In these families the metabolic lesion does not segregate from AHO, although AHO does occur without the metabolic lesion. On the other hand, entire families have been described that have the metabolic defect but no AHO. The genetic bases of these observations is unknown but surely not Mendelian.

Johnson [175] has proposed a form of inheritance (meta-

bolic interference) which is neither recessive nor dominant and in which only the heterozygote is affected. This scheme postulates, for example, mutations in the subunit genes of multisubunit enzyme or structural proteins. Certain combinations of subunits produce normal function, while other combinations of the same mutant subunits are inactive. Inheritance patterns can be quite complex, at times appearing dominant, at others recessive (depending on the frequency with which subunit combinations are functional or not). Johnson cites pseudohypoparathyroidism as a candidate disorder to be explained by such metabolic interference. His hypothesis appeals to us, but we cannot be certain whether his or some other explanation is correct. We can conclude, however, that pseudohypoparathyroidism appears not to be inherited by an X-linked dominant mechanism; that it does have certain characteristics of autosomal dominant inheritance; and that there is reason to postulate a complex rather than simple form of genetic transmission.

REFERENCES

1. ALBRIGHT E, BURNETT CH, SMITH PH, PARSON W: Pseudo-hypoparathyroidism, an example of Seabright-Bantam Syndrome. Report of three cases. *Endocrinology* 30:922, 1942
2. ALBRIGHT F, FORBES AP, HENNEMAN H: Pseudo-pseudohypoparathyroidism. *Trans Assoc Am Phys* 65:337, 1952
3. CHASE LR, MELSON GL, AURBACH GD: Pseudohypoparathyroidism: Defective excretion of 3',5'-AMP in response to parathyroid hormone. *J Clin Invest* 48:1832, 1969
4. NAGANT DE DEUXCHAISNES C, KRANE SM: Hypoparathyroidism, in Avioli LV, Krane SM (eds): *Metabolic Bone Disease*. New York, Academic Press, Inc, 1978, p 218
5. MANN JB, ALTERMAN S, HILLS AG: Albright's hereditary osteodystrophy comprising pseudohypoparathyroidism and pseudopseudohypoparathyroidism. *Ann Intern Med* 56:315, 1962
6. TASHJIAN AH JR, FRANTZ AG, LEE JB: Pseudohypoparathyroidism: Assays of parathyroid hormone and thyrocalcitonin. *Proc Natl Acad Sci USA* 56:1138, 1966
7. ALIAPOULIOS MA, VOELKEL EF, MUNSON PL: Assay of human thyroid glands for thyrocalcitonin activity. *J Clin Endocrinol Metab* 26:897, 1966
8. LEE JB, TASHJIAN AH JR, STREETO JM, FRANTZ AG: Familial pseudohypoparathyroidism. *N Engl J Med* 279:1179, 1968
9. SUH SM, KOOH SW, CHAN AM, FRASER D, TASHJIAN AH JR: Pseudohypoparathyroidism: No improvement following total thyroidectomy. *J Clin Endocrinol Metab* 29:429, 1969
10. CHASE LR, AURBACH GD: Parathyroid function and the renal excretion of 3',5'-adenylic acid. *Proc Natl Acad Sci USA* 58:518, 1967
11. BELL NH, AVERY S, SINHA T, CLARK LC JR, ALLEN DO, JOHNSTON C JR: Effects of dibutyryl cyclic adenosine 3',5'-monophosphate and parathyroid extract on calcium and phosphorus metabolism in hypoparathyroidism and pseudohypoparathyroidism. *J Clin Invest* 51:816, 1972
12. EGAWA J, NEUMAN WF: Effect of parathyroid extract on the metabolism of radioactive phosphate in kidney. *Endocrinology* 74:90, 1964
13. BIJVOET OLM: Kidney function in calcium and phosphate metabolism, in Avioli LV, Krane SM (eds): *Metabolic Bone Disease*. New York, Academic Press, Inc, 1978, p 50
14. AMIEL CH, KUNTZIGER H, RICHET G: Micropuncture study of handling of phosphate by proximal and distal nephron in normal and parathyroidectomized rat. Evidence for distal reabsorption. *Pfleugers Arch* 317:93, 1970
15. DENNIS VW, BELLO-REUSO E, ROBINSON RR: Response of phosphate transport to parathyroid hormone in segments of rabbit nephron. *Am J Physiol* 233:F29, 1977
16. PASTORIZA-MUNOZ E, COLINDRES RE, LASSITER WE, LECHENE C: Effect of parathyroid hormone on phosphate reabsorption in rat distal convolution. *Am J Physiol* 235:F321, 1978
17. GOLDBERG M, AGUS ZS, GOLDFARB S: The renal handling of phosphate, calcium and magnesium, in Brenner BM, Rector FC (eds): *The Kidney*, Philadelphia, WB Saunders, Co, 1976
18. PARFITT AM, KLEERKOPER M: Clinical disorders of calcium, phosphorus, and magnesium metabolism, in Maxwell MH, Kleeman CR (eds): *Clinical Disorders of Fluid and Electrolyte Metabolism*. New York, McGraw-Hill Book Co, 1980, p 947
19. PARFITT AM: The actions of parathyroid hormone on bone: Relation to bone remodeling and turnover, calcium homeostasis, and metabolic bone

diseases. II. PTH and bone cells: Bone turnover and plasma calcium regulation. *Metabolism* 25:909, 1976

20. BIDDULPH DM, GALLIMORE LB: Sensitivity of the kidney to parathyroid hormone and its relationship to serum calcium in the hamster. *Endocrinology* 94:1241, 1974

21. TALMADGE RV: Studies on the maintenance of serum calcium levels by parathyroid hormone action on bone and kidney. *Ann NY Acad Sci* 64:326, 1956

22. HARRIS WH, HEANEY RP: Skeletal renewal and metabolic bone disease. *N Engl J Med* 280:183, 253, 303, 1969

23. PARFITT AM: The actions of parathyroid hormone on bone: Relation to bone remodeling and turnover, calcium homeostasis, and metabolic bone disease. I. Mechanisms of calicum transfer between blood and bone and their cellular basis: Morphologic and kinetic approaches to bone turnover. *Metabolism* 25:809, 1976

24. PARFITT AM: The actions of parathyroid hormone on bone. Relation to bone remodeling and turnover, calcium homeostasis and metabolic bone disease. III. PTH and osteoblasts, the relationship between bone turnover and bone loss, and the state of the bones in primary hyperparathyroidism. *Metabolism* 25:1033, 1976

25. TALMAGE RV, GRUBB SA: A laboratory model demonstrating osteocyte-osteoblast control of plasma calcium concentration. *Clin Orthop* 122:299, 1977

26. GROER PG, MARSHALL JH: Mechanism of calcium exchange at bone surfaces. *Calcif Tissue Res* 12:175, 1973

27. NEUMAN WF, BAREHAM BJ: Evidence for the presence of secondary calcium phosphate in bone and its stabilization by acid production. *Calcif Tissue Res* 18:161, 1975

28. TALMAGE RV: Morphological and physiological considerations in a new concept of calcium transport in bone. *Am J Anat* 129:467, 1970

29. PARFITT AM, KLEERKOPER M: The divalent ion homeostatic system—physiology and metabolism of calcium, phosphorus, magnesium, and bone, in Maxwell MH, Kleeman CR (eds): *Clinical Disorders of Fluid and Electrolyte Metabolism*. New York, McGraw-Hill Book Co, 1980, p 269

30. NICHOLS G JR, SCHARTUM S, VAES GM: Some effects of vitamin D and parathyroid hormone on the calcium and phosphorus metabolism of bone in vitro. *Acta Physiol Scand* 57:51, 1963

31. MASSRY SG, STEIN R, GARTY J, ARIEFF AI, COBURN JW, NORMAN AW, FRIEDLER RM: Skeletal resistance to the calcemic action of parathyroid hormone in uremia: Role of 1,25(OH)₂D₃. *Kidney Int* 9:467, 1976

32. PARFITT AM: Target cell resistence in pseudohypoparathyroidism: single or multiple?, in Norman AW, Schaefer K, Herrath DV, Grigoleit HG, Coburn JW, DeLuca HF, Mawer EB, Suda T (eds): *Vitamin D Basic Research and Its Clinical Application*. Berlin, Walter de Gruyter and Co., 1979, p 949

33. SUTTON RAL, WONG NLM, DIRKS JH: Effects of parathyroid hormone on sodium and calcium transport in the dog nephron. *Clin Sci Mol Med* 51:345, 1976

34. AGUS ZS, CHUI PJS, GOLDBERG M: Regulation of urinary calcium excretion in the rat. *Am J Physiol* 1:F545, 1977

35. BIRGE SJ, SWITZER SC, LEONARD DR: Influence of sodium and parathyroid hormone on calcium release from intestinal mucosal cells. *J Clin Invest* 54:702, 1974

36. HAUSSLER MR, McCAIN TA: Basic and clinical concepts related to vitamin D metabolism and action. *N Engl J Med* 297:974, 1977

37. NORMAN AW: Vitamin D metabolism and calcium absorption. *Am J Med* 67:989, 1979

38. SLATOPOLSKY E, HRUSKA K, MARTIN K, FREITAG J: Physiologic and metabolic effects of parathyroid hormone, in Brenner BM, Stein JH (eds): *Hormonal Function and the Kidney*. New York, Churchill Livingstone, Inc., 1979, p 167

39. RASMUSSEN H, PECHET M, FAST D: Effect of dibutyryl cyclic adenosine 3′,5′-monophosphate, theophylline, and other nucleotides upon calcium and phosphate metabolism. *J Clin Invest* 47:1843, 1968

40. RODBELL M, LIN M, SALOMON Y, LONDOS C, HARWOOD JP, MARTIN BR, RENDELL M, BERMAN M: Role of adenosine and guanine nucleotides in the activity and response of adenylate cyclase systems to hormones. Evidence for multisite transition states, in Drummond GI, Greengard P, Robinson GA (eds): *Advances in Cyclic Nucleotide Research*. New York, Raven Press, 1975, vol 5, p 3

41. RODBELL M, LIN MC, SALOMON Y: Evidence for independent action of glucagon and nucleotides on the hepatic adenylate cyclase system. *J Biol Chem* 249:59, 1974

42. NORTHUP JK, STERNVEIS PC, SMIGEL MD, SCHLEIFER LS, ROSS EM, GILMAN AG: Purification of the regulatory component of adenylate cyclase. *Proc Natl Acad Sci USA* 77:6516, 1980

43. LEFKOWITZ RJ, HOFFMAN BB: New directions in adrenergic receptor research. *Trends Pharmaceut Sci* 1:314, 1980

44. NAGATA N, SASAKI M, KIMURA N, NAKANE K: The hypercalcemic effect of parathyroid hormone and skeletal cyclic AMP. *Endocrinology* 96:725, 1975

45. DZIAK R, STERN PH: Calcium transport in isolated bone cells III. Effects of parathyroid hormone and cyclic 3′,5′-AMP. *Endocrinology* 97:1281, 1975

46. FROELING PGAM, BIJVOET OLM: Kidney mediated effects of parathyroid hormone on extracellular homeostasis of calcium phosphate and acid-base balance in man. *Neth J Med* 17:174, 1974

47. MATSUZAKI S, DUMONT JE: Effect of calcium ion on horse parathyroid gland adenyl cyclase. *Biochim Biophys Acta* 284:227, 1972

48. SHERWOOD LM, ABE M, RODMAN JS, LUNDBERG WB JR, TARGOVNIK JH: Parathyroid hormone: Synthesis, storage and secretion in Talmage RV, Munson PL (eds): *Calcium, Parathyroid Hormone and the Calcitonins*. International Congress Ser No 243, Amsterdam, Excerpta Medica, p 183

49. WILLIAMS GA, HARGIS GK, BOWSER EN, HENDERSON WJ, MARTINEZ NJ: Evidence for a role of adenosine 3′,5′-monophosphate in parathyroid hormone release. *Endocrinology* 92:687, 1973

50. WILLIAMS GA, KUKREJA SC, HARGIS GK, BOWSER EN, HENDERSON WJ: Role of adrenergic stimuli and cyclic AMP in the physiological control of parathyroid hormone secretion in man. *Clin Res* 22:652A, 1974

51. HABENER JF, POTTS JT: Biosynthesis of parathyroid hormone. *N Engl J Med* 299:580, 635, 1978

52. COULSON R, MOSES AM: Effect of chlorpropamide on renal response to parathyroid hormone in normal subjects and in patients with hypoparathyroidism and pseudohypoparathyroidism. *J Pharmacol Exp Ther* 194:603, 1975

53. MOSES AM, BRESLAU N, COULSON R: Renal responses to PTH in patients with hormone-resistant (pseudo) hypoparathyroidism. *Am J Med* 61:184, 1976

54. BRESLAU N, MOSES AM: Renal calcium reabsorption caused by bicarbonate and by chlorthiazide in patients with hormone resistant (pseudo) hypoparathyroidism. *J Clin Endocrinol Metab* 46:389, 1978

55. WERTZNIAN R, MURAD F: Effects of aminophylline, chlorpropamide and parathyroid extract on plasma and urinary cyclic AMP in pseudohypoparathyroidism. *Clin Res* 21:89, 1973

55a. DREZNER MK, NEELON FA: Unpublished observations

56. MARCUS R, WILBER, JF, AURBACH GD: Parathyroid hormone-sensitive adenyl cyclase from the renal cortex of a patient with pseudohypoparathyroidism. *J Clin Endocrinol Metab* 33:537, 1971

57. DREZNER MK, BURCH WM JR: Altered activity of the nucleotide regulatory site in the parathyroid hormone-sensitive adenylate cyclase from the renal cortex of a patient with pseudohypoparathyroidism. *J Clin Invest* 62:1222, 1978

58. BOURNE HR, BRICKMAN AS, FARFEL Z: Molecular basis of pseudohypoparathyroidism in Cohn DV, Talmage RV, Matthews LJ (eds): *Hormonal Regulation of Calcium Metabolism*. Amsterdam, Excerpta Medica, 1981

59. FARFEL Z, BRICKMAN AS, KASLOW HR, BROTHERS VM, BOURNE HR: Defect of receptor-cyclase coupling protein in pseudohypoparathyroidism. *N Engl J Med* 303:237, 1980

60. FARFEL Z, BOURNE HR: Deficient activity of receptor-cyclase coupliing protein in platelets of patients with pseudohypoparathyroidism. *J Clin Endocrinol Metab* 51:1202, 1980

60a. Bourne HR: Personal communication

61. LEVINE MD, DOWNS RW JR, SINGER M, MARX SJ, AURBACH GD, SPIEGEL AM: Deficient activity of guanine nucleotide regulatory protein in erythrocytes from patients with pseudohypoparathyroidism. *Biochem Biophys Res Commun* 94:1319, 1980

61a. Spiegel AM: Personal communication

62. LEVINE MA, DOWNS RW JR, MARX SJ, LASKER RD, AURBACH GD, SPIEGEL AM: Clinical and biochemical features of pseudohypoparathyroidism. *Proceedings of the VIIth Parathyroid Conference* In Press

62a. BOURNE HR: Personal communication

63. WOLFSDORF JI, ROSENFIELD RL, FANG VS, KABAYASHI R, RAZDON AK, KIM MH: Partial gonadotrophin resistance in pseudohypoparathyroidism. *Acta Endocrinol* 88:321, 1978

64. SHAPIRO MS, BERNHEIM J, GUTMAN A, ARBER I, SPITZ IM: Multiple abnormalities of anterior pituitary hormone secretion in association with pseudohypoparathyroidism. *J Clin Endocrinol Metab* 51:483, 1980

65. FISCHER JA: Biologically inactive parathyroid hormone in pseudohypoparathyroidism—Type I (PHP-1), in Cohn DV, Talmage RV, Matthews LJ (eds): *Hormonal Control of Calcium Metabolism Proceedings of the Seventh International Conference on Calcium Regulating Hormones*. Amsterdam, Excerpta Medica, 1981

66. DREZNER MK, HAUSSLER MR: Normocalcemic pseudohypoparathyroidism: Association with normal vitamin D₃ metabolism. *Am J Med* 66:503, 1979

66a. DREZNER MK, NEELON FA: Unpublished observations

67. MONN E, BJORN ASNES J, OYL L, WEFRING KW: Pseudohypoparathyroidism, a difficult diagnosis in early childhood. *Acta Paediatr Scand* 65:487, 1976

68. BALACHANDER V, PAHUJA J, MADDAIAH VT, COLLIPP PJ: Pseudohypopar-

athyroidism with normal serum calcium levels. *Am J Dis Child* 129:1092, 1975

69. COHEN ML, DONNEL GN: Pseudohypoparathyroidism with hypothyroidism. *J Pediatr* 56:369, 1960

70. RAY EW, GARDNER LI: Pseudopseudohypoparathyroidism in a child: Report of the youngest case. *Pediatrics* 23:520, 1959

71. MOUTALEN CA, DYMLING JF, HORWITH M: Pseudohypoparathyroidism 1942–1966, a negative progress report. *Am J Med* 42:977, 1967

72. HINKLE DO, TRAVIS LB, DODGE WF: Albright's hereditary osteodystrophy in a mother and daughter. *Tex Rep Biol Med* 23:463, 1965

73. WERDER EA, FISCHER JA, ILLIG R, KIND HP, BERNASCONI S, FANCONI A, PRADER A: Pseudohypoparathyroidism and idiopathic hypoparathyroidism: Relationship between serum calcium and parathyroid hormone levels and urinary cyclic adenosine-3′,5′-monophosphate response to parathyroid extract. *J Clin Endocrinol Metab* 46:872, 1978.

74. GERTNER JM, TOMLINSON S, GONZALEZ-MACIAS J: Normocalcemic pseudohypoparathyroidism with unusual phenotype. *Arch Dis Child* 53:312, 1978

75. KOLB FO, STEINBACH HL: Pseudohypoparathyroidism with secondary hyperparathyroidism and osteitis fibrosa. *J Clin Endocrinol Metab* 22:59, 1962

76. SINGLETON EB, TENG CT: Pseudohypoparathyroidism with bone changes simulating hyperparathyroidism: Report of a case. *Radiology* 78:388, 1962

77. COSTELLO JM, DENT CE: Hypo-hyper-parathyroidism. *Arch Dis Child* 38:397, 1963

78. BELL NH, GERARD ES, BARTTER FC: Pseudohypoparathyroidism with osteitis fibrosa cystica and impaired absoption of calcium. *J Clin Endocrinol Metab* 23:759, 1963

79. FANCONI A, HEINRICH HG, PRADER A: Klinischer and biochemischer hypoparathyreoidismus mit radiologischem hyperparathyriochismus. *Helv Paediatr Acta* 19:181, 1964

80. CHRISTIAENS L, FONTAINE G, FARRIAUX JP, BISEITE G: Le pseudohypopara-thyroidisme chronique: aprapos de 3 cas familiaux. *Acta Paediatr Belg* 21:5, 1967

81. FRAME B, HANSON CA, FROST HM, BLOCK M, ARNSTEIN AR: Renal resistance to parathyroid hormone with osteitis fibrosa: "Pseudohypohyperparathyroidism." *Am J Med* 52:311, 1972

82. DREZNER MK, NEELON FA, HAUSSLER M, McPHERSON HT, LEBOVITZ HE: 1,25-Dihydroxycholecalciferol deficiency: The probable cause of hypocalcemia and metabolic bone disease in pseudohypoparathyroidism. *J Clin Endocrinol Metab* 42:621, 1976

83. FLATMAN JG: What is your diagnosis? Pseudohypoparathyroidism with bone changes typical of hyperparathyroidism. *Rev Interam Radiol* 2:243, 1977

84. KIDD GS, SCHAAF M, ADLER RA, LASSMAN MN, WRAY HL: Skeletal responsiveness in pseudohypoparathyroidism: A spectrum of clinical disease. *Am J Med* 68:772, 1980

85. WILSON JD, HADDEN DR: Pseudohypoparathyroidism presenting with rickets. *J Clin Endocrinol Metab* 51:1184, 1980

86. CONNORS MH, IRIAS JJ, GOLABI M: Hypo-hyperparathyroidism: Evidence for a defective parathyroid hormone. *Pediatrics* 60:343, 1977

87. ALLEN EH, MILARD FJC, NASSIM JR: Hypo-hyperparathyroidism. *Arch Dis Child* 43:295, 1968

88. OKANO K, FUJITA T, ORIMO H, YOSHIKAWA M: A case of pseudohypoparathyroidism with increased bone turnover and demineralization. *Endocrinol Jap* 16:423, 1969

89. LAWOYIN S, NORMAN DA, ZERWEKH JE, BRESLAU NA, PAK CYC: A patient with pseudohypoparathyroidism with increased serum calcium and 1α25-dihydroxyvitamin D after exogenous parathyroid hormone administration. *J Clin Endocrinol Metab* 49:783, 1979

90. LAMBERT PW, HOLLIS BW, BELL NH, EPSTEIN S: Demonstration of a lack of change in serum 1α,25-dihydroxyvitamin D in response to parathyroid extract in pseudohypoparathyroidism. *J Clin Invest* 66:782, 1980

91. ISHIDA M, SEINO Y, SIMOTSUJI T, ISHII T, YAMAOKA K, HRADA T, YABUNCHI H, NISHIMURA K: Differential diagnosis of hypoparathyroid disorders during childhood. *Calcif Tissue Int* 31:203, 1980

91a. HAUSSLER MR: Personal communication

91b. LEMANN J: Personal communication

91c. CHESNEY R: Personal communication

92. BELL NH, KHAIR NH, JOHNSTON CC JR: Effects of 1,25-dihydroxyvitamin D$_3$ on calcium metabolism and quantitative bone histology in pseudohypoparathyroidism. *Excerpta Med* 421:33, 1978

93. MASON RS, LISSNER D, POSEN S: Parathyroid hormone effect on 1,25-dihydroxyvitamin D in hypoparathyroidism. *Ann Intern Med* 92:260, 1980

94. AKSNES L, AARSKOG D: Effect of parathyroid hormone on 1,25-dihydroxyvitamin D formation in type 1 pseudohypoparathyroidism. *J Clin Endocrinol Metab* 51:1223, 1980

95. STÖGMANN W, FISCHER JA: Pseudohypoparathyroidism. Disappearance of the resistance of parathyroid extract during treatment with vitamin D. *Am J Med* 59:140, 1975

96. KIND HP, PARKINSON DK, SUH SM, FRASER D, KOOH SW: Parathyroid hormone response and effects of vitamin D in hypoparathyroidism and pseudohypoparathyroidism. *Abstracts of the Endocrine Society* 55:164, 1973

97. BIRKENHAGER JC, SALDENRATH HJ, HACKENG WHL, SCHELLEKENS APM, VAN DER VEER ALJ, ROELFSEMA F: Calcium and phosphorus metabolism, parathyroid hormone, calcitonin and bone histology in pseudohypoparathyroidism. *Eur J Clin Invest* 3:27, 1973

98. KOOH SW, FRASER D, DELUCA HF, HOLIICK MF, BELSEY RE, CLARK MB, MURRAY TM: Treatment of hypoparathyroidism and pseudohypoparathyroidism with metabolites of vitamin D: Evidence for impaired conversion of 25-hydroxyvitamin D to 1α,25-dihydroxyvitamin D. *N Engl J Med* 293:840, 1975

99. WERDER WA, KIND HP, EGERT F, FISCHER JA, PRADER A: Effective long term treatment of pseudohypoparathyroidism with oral 1α-hydroxy- and 1,25-dihydroxyvitamin D in pseudohypoparathyroidism. *J Pediatr* 89:266, 1976

100. SINHA TK, DELUCA HF, BELL NH: Evidence for a defect in the formation of 1α25-dihydroxyvitamin D in pseudohypoparathyroidism. *Metabolism* 26:731, 1977

101. DAVIES M, HILL LF, TAYLOR CM, STANBURY SW: 1,25-Dihydroxycholecalciferol in hypoparathyroidism. *Lancet* 1:55, 1977

102. METZ SA, BAYLINK DJ, HUGHES MR, HAUSSLER MR, ROBERTSON RP: Selective deficiency of 1,25-dihydroxycholecalciferol: A cause of isolated skeletal resistance to parathyroid hormone. *N Engl J Med* 297:1084, 1977

103. DREZNER MK, FEINGLOS MN: Osteomalacia due to 1α,25 dihydroxycholecalciferol deficiency: Association with a giant cell tumor of bone: *J Clin Invest* 60:1046, 1977

104. PRIEN EL JR, PYLE EB, KRANE SM: Secondary hyperparathyroidism, in Greep RO Astwood EB (sec eds), Aurbach GD, (vol ed), Geiger SR (book ed): *Handbook of Physiology, 7: Endocrinology, vol 7: Parathyroid Gland.* Washington, DC, American Physiological Society, 1976, p 383

105. JOWSEY J: Bone in parathyroid disorders in man, in Talmage RV, Belanger LE (eds): *Parathyroid Hormone and Thyrocalcitonin.* Amsterdam, Excerpta Medica, 1968, vol 159, p 137

106. TAKAHASHI H, FROST HM, KUHN T: Bone tissue and cell dynamics determined by tetracycline labeling in a case of pseudohypoparathyroidism (and in the patient's mother). *Clin Orthop* 49:163, 1966

107. NAGANT DE DEUXCHAISNES C, DEVOGELAER JP, DOCQUIER C, CRABBE J: Physio-pathologie du pseudohypoparathyroidisme. *Ann Endocrinol (Paris)* 40:159, 1979

108. FANCONI J-P, VAINSEL M, SIX R, CORVILAIN J, LEFEBVRE J: Le pseudohypoparathyroidisme: resultats complementaires a propos de 4 cas familaux. *Arch Ped* 33:445, 1976

109. MAZZUOLI GF, COEN C, ANTONOZZI I: Study on calcium metabolism, thyrocalcitonin assay and effect of thyroidectomy in pseudohypoparathyroidism. *Isr J Med Sci* 3:627, 1967

110. DEFTOS LJ, POTTS JT JR: Parathyroid hormone, calcitonin, vitamin D, bone and bone mineral metabolism, in Bondy PK, Rosenberg LE (eds): *Duncan's Diseases of Metabolism,* ed 7. Philadelphia, WB Saunders Co, 1974, p 1225

110a. DREZNER MK, NEELON FA: Unpublished observations

110b. BRINKMAN AS: Personal communication

111. DREZNER MK, NEELON FA, LEBOVITZ HE: Pseudohypoparathyroidism type II: A possible defect in the reception of the cyclic AMP signal. *N Engl J Med* 289:1056, 1973

112. RODRIGUEZ HJ, VILLARREAL H, KLAHR S, SLATOPOLSKY E: Pseudohypoparathyroidism type II: Restoration of normal renal responsiveness to parathyroid hormone by calcium administration. *J Clin Endocrinol Metab* 39:693, 1974

113. YAMADA K, TAMURA Y, YAMAMATO M, KUMAGAI R: Effect of calcium administration on renal responsiveness to parathyroid hormone in pseudohypoparathyroidism type I and II—in comparison with normals, idiopathic and surgical hypoparathyroidism. *Endocrinol Jpn* 26:147, 1979

114. MILGRAM JW, ENGH CA, HAMILTON CR, KAMMER GM: Renal resistance to parathyroid hormone with hyperphosphatemic osteomalacia and osteitis fibrosa. *J Bone Joint Surg* 56A:1493, 1974

115. DUCK SC, ROSENBERG EM, RATZAN SK, HAYMOND MW: Renal resistant hormonoplethoric hypoparathyroidism with evidence for a defective response to cAMP. *J Clin Endocrinol Metab* 47:640, 1978

116. BRICKMAN AS, NORMAN AW, COBURN JW: Vitamin D and pseudohypoparathyroidism, in Norman AW, Schaefer, K, Coburn JW, DeLuca HF, Fraser D, Grigoleit HG, Herrath DV (eds): *Vitamin D Biochemical, Chemical and Clinical Aspects Related to Calcium Metabolism* Berlin, Walter de Gruyter and Co, 1977, p 867

117. SCHWILLE PO, VOLLMAR D, SCHOLZ D, SCHMIDT-GAYK H: Failure of intravenous calcium to restore PTH-induced phosphaturia in pseudohypoparathyroidism type II, in Norman AW, Schaefer K, Coburn JW, DeLuca HF, Fraser D, Grigoleit HG, Herrath DV (eds): *Vitamin D Biochemical, Chemical and Clinical Aspects Related to Calcium Metabolism* Berlin, Walter de Gruyter and Co, 1977, p 447

118. Pallardo-Sanchez LF, Montero A, Vid LO, Sanchez-Sicilia L, Cerdan A: Familial form of type II pseudohypoparathyroidism. *Rev Clin Esp* 145:369, 1977

119. Kind HP, Parkinson DK, Suh SM, Fraser D: A classification of the hypoparathyroid syndrome based on the PTH response test. *Pediatr Res* 7:324, 1973

120. Suh SM, Fraser C, Kooh SW: Pseudohypoparathyroidism: Responsiveness to parathyroid extract induced by vitamin D₂ therapy. *J Clin Endocrinol Metab* 30:609, 1970

121. Frame B, Fruchtman M, Smith RW Jr: Chronic hypocalcemia in a patient with parathyroid clear-cell hyperplasia. *N Engl J Med* 267:1112, 1962

122. Garceau GJ, Miller WE: Osteochondrodystrophy as a result of or in relation to pseudohypoparathyroidism. *J Bone Joint Surg* 38A:134, 1956

122a. Fukami T: Personal communication

123. Spech HJ, Olah AJ: Symptoms and recent findings in pseudo-hypoparathyroidism. *Med Klin* 69:387, 1974

124. Steinbach HL, Young DA: The roentgen appearance of pseudohypoparathyroidism (PH) and pseudopseudohypoparathyroidism (PPH). *Am J Roentgenol Radium Ther Nucl Med* 97:49, 1966

125. Eyre WG, Reed WB: Albright's Hereditary Osteodystrophy with cutaneous bone formation. *Arch Derm* 104:635, 1971

126. Bronsky D, Kushner DS, Dubin A, Snapper I: Idiopathic hypoparathyroidism and pseudohypoparathyroidism: Case reports and review of the literature. *Medicine (Balt)* 37:317, 1958

127. Aurbach GD, Potts JT Jr: The parathyroids, in Levine R, Luft R (eds): *Advances in Metabolic Disorders*. New York, Academic Press Inc, 1964, vol 1 p 45

128. Gsell O: Chronische idiopathische Tetanie (mit Psoriasis) (Hypoparathyreoider Kretinismus). *Deutsche Med Wchnschr* 35:117, 1950

129. Money J, Ehrhardt AA: Correlation of mental functioning and calcium regulation in a rare case of pseudohypoparathyroidism. *Johns Hopkins Med J* 123:276, 1968

130. Wong S, Zakov ZN, Albert DM: Scleral and choroidal calcifications in a patient with pseudohypoparathyroidism. *Br J Ophthalmol* 63:177, 1979

131. Ritchie GM: Dental manifestations of pseudohypoparathyroidism. *Arch Dis Child* 40:565, 1965

132. Croft LK, Witkop CJ Jr, Glas JE: Pseudohypoparathyroidism. *Oral Surg* 20:758, 1965

133. Nikiforuk G, Frasier D: Etiology of enamel hypoplasia and interglobular dentin: The roles of hypocalcemia and hypophosphatemia. *Metab Bone Dis* 2:17, 1979

134. Barranco VP: Cutaneous ossification in psed{uohypoparathyroidism. *Arch Dermatol* 104:643, 1971

135. Korn-Lubetzki I, Lubinger D, Siew F: Visualization of basal ganglia calcification by cranial computed tomography in a patient with pseudohypoparathyroidism. *Isr J Med Sci* 16:40, 1980

136. Dudley AW Jr, Hawkins H: Mineralization of the central nervous system in pseudopseudohypoparathyroidism (PPH). *J Neurol Neurosurg Psychiatry* 33:147, 1970

137. Henkin RI: Impairment of olfaction and of the tastes of sour and bitter in pseudohypoparathyroidism. *J Clin Endocrinol Metab* 28:624, 1968

138. Forbes AP: Fingerprints and palmprints (Dermatoglyphics) and palmar flexion creases in gonadal dysgenesis, pseudohypoparathyroidism and Kleinfelter's syndrome. *N Engl J Med* 270:1268, 1964

139. Zisman E, Lotz M, Jenkins ME, Bartter FC: Studies of pseudohypoparathyroidism. Two new cases with a probable selective deficiency of thyrotropin. *Am J Med* 46:464, 1969

140. Winnacker JL, Becker KL, Moore CF: Pseudohypoparathyroidism and selective deficiency of thyrotropin: An interesting association. *Metabolism* 16:644, 1967

141. Turner RW, Takamura T: Pseudohypoparathyroidism and hypothyroidism. *Ann Intern Med* 56:276, 1962

142. Marx SJ, Hershman JM, Aurbach GD: Thyroid ddysfunction in pseudohypoparathyroidism. *J Clin Endocrinol Metab* 33:822, 1971

143. Werder EA, Illig R, Bernasconi S, Kind H, Prader A, Fisher JA, Fanconi A: Excessive thyrotropin response to thyrotropin-releasing hormone in pseudohypoparathyroidism. *Pediatr Res* 9:12, 1975

144. Carlson HE, Brickman AS, Botazzo GF: Prolactin deficiency in pseudohypoparathyroidism. *N Engl J Med* 296:140, 1977

145. Bijvoet OLM: Renal phosphate excretion in man. *Folia Med Neerl* 15:84, 1972

146. Mallet E, Basuyau JP, Brunelle P, De Menisbus CH: Plasma cyclic nucleotide determination in the investigation of hypocalcemia. *Pediatr Res* 13:647, 1979

147. Tomlinson S, Hendy GN, O'Riordan JH: A simplified assessment of response to parathyroid hormone in hypoparathyroid patients. *Lancet* 1:62, 1976

148. Ashby JP, Renton WB, MacPherson JN, Price WH, Abbot SR: Plasma cyclic-AMP response to parathyroid hormone in Turner's syndrome and Albright's hereditary osteodystrophy. *Clin Endocrinol (Oxf)* 10:553, 1979

149. McDonald KM: Responsiveness of bone to parathyroid extract in siblings with pseudohypoparathyroidism. *Metabolism* 21:521, 1972

150. Barr DGD, Prader A, Esper U, Rampini S, Marrian VJ, Forfar JO: Chronic hypoparathyroidism in two generations. *Helv Paediatr Acta* 26:507, 1971

151. Parfitt AM: Surgical, idiopathic and other varieties of parathyroid hormone deficient hypoparathyroidism, in DeGroot LJ, Cahill GF Jr, Odell WD, Martini L, Potts JT Jr, Nelson DH, Steinberger E, Winegrad AI (eds): *Endocrinology*. New York, Grune & Stratton, Inc, 1979, p 755

152. Eisenbarth GS, Jackson RA: Immunogenetics of polyglandular failure and related diseases, in Farid NR (ed): *Endocrine and Metabolic Disorders*. New York, Academic Press, Inc, 1981, p 835

153. Eisenbarth GS, Wilson PW, Ward F, Buckley C, Lebovitz H: The polyglandular failure syndrome: Disease inheritance, HLA type and immune function. *Ann Intern Med* 91:528, 1979

154. Freedom RM, Rosen FS, Nadas AS: Congenital cardiovascular disease and anomalies of the third and fourth pharyngeal pouch. *Circulation* 46:165, 1972

155. Taitz LS, Zarati-Salvador C, Schwartz E: Congenital absence of the parathyroid and thymus gland in an infant (III and IV pharyngeal-pouch syndrome). *Pediatrics* 38:412, 1966

156. Girling JA, Murley RS: Parathyroid insufficiency after thyroidectomy. *Br Med J* 1:1323, 1967

157. Suh SM, Tashjian AH, Mutuso N: Pathogenesis of hypocalcemia in primary hypomagnesemia: Normal end-organ responsiveness to parathyroid hormone, impaired parathyroid gland function. *J Clin Invest* 52:153, 1973

158. Medalle R, Waterhouse C: A magnesium-deficient patient presenting with hypocalcemia and hyperphosphatemia. *Ann Intern Med* 79:76, 1972

159. Witkop CJ Jr: Gardner's syndrome and other osteognathodermal disorders with defects in parathyroid functions. *J Oral Surg* 26:639, 1968

160. Van Der Werfften Bosch JJ: The syndrome of brachymetacarpal dwarfism ("pseudo-pseudohypoparathyroidism"). *Lancet* 1:69, 1959

161. Chopra IJ, Nugent CA: Concurrence of features of pseudohypoparathyroidism, pseudopseudohypoparathyroidism and basal cell nevus syndrome. *Am J Med Sci* 260:171, 1970

162. Aurbach GD, Marcus R, Winickoff RN, Epstein EH Jr, Nigra TP: Urinary excretion of 3′×5′-AMP in syndromes considered refractory to parathyroid hormone. *Metabolism* 19:799, 1970

163. Beale MG, Chan JC, Oldham SB, DeLuca HF: Vitamin D: The discovery of its metabolites and their therapeutic applications. *Pediatrics* 57:729, 1976

164. Kind HP, Prader A, DeLuca HF, Gugler E: Letter: 1,25-dihydroxycholecalciferol in hypoparathyroidism and pseudohypoparathyroidism. *Lancet* 1:1145, 1975

165. Sinha TK, Bell NH: Letter: 1,25-dihydroxyvitamin D₃ and pseudohypoparathyroidism. *N Engl J Med* 294:612, 1976

166. Furukawa Y, Sohn H, Unakami H, Yumita S: Treatment of pseudohypoparathyroidism with 1α-hydroxyvitamin D₃. *Contrib Nephrol* 22:68, 1980

167. Bell NH, Stern PH: Hypercalcemia and increases in serum hormone value during prolonged administration of 1α,25-dihydroxyvitamin D. *N Engl J Med* 298:1241, 1978

168. Weinberg AG, Stone RT: Autosomal dominant inheritance in Albright's hereditary osteodystrophy. *J Pediatr* 79:996, 1971

169. Williams AJ, Wilkinson JL, Taylor WH: Pseudohypoparathyroidism. Variable manifestations within a family. *Arch Dis Child* 52:798, 1977

170. Winter JSD, Hughes IA: Familial pseudohypoparathyroidism without somatic anomalies. *Can Med Assoc J* 123:26, 1980

171. Farriaux JP, Delmas Y, Rapartz C, Fontaine G: Letter: Brachymetacarpia. HL-A group. Linkage in a family with pseudohypoparathyroidism. *Nouv Presse Med* 4:589, 1975

172. Cederbaum SD, Lippe BM: Probable autosomal recessive inheritance in a family with Albright's Hereditary Osteodystrophy and an evaluation of the genetics of the disorder. *Am J Hum Genet* 25:638, 1973

173. Spranger JW: Skeletal dysplasias and the eye: Albright's Hereditary Osteodystrophy, in Bergsma D (ed): *Part IV "Skeletal Dysplasias"*. Baltimore, Williams & Wilkins Co, 1966, p 126

174. Farfel Z, Brothers VM, Brickman AS, Conte F, Neer R, Bourne HR: Pseudohypoparathyroidism: Inheritance of deficient receptor-cyclase coupling activity. *Proc Natl Acad Sci USA*, 78: 3098, 1981

175. Johnson WG: Metabolic interference and the + − heterozygote. A hypothetical form of simple inheritance which is neither dominant nor recessive. *Am J Hum Genet* 32:374, 1980

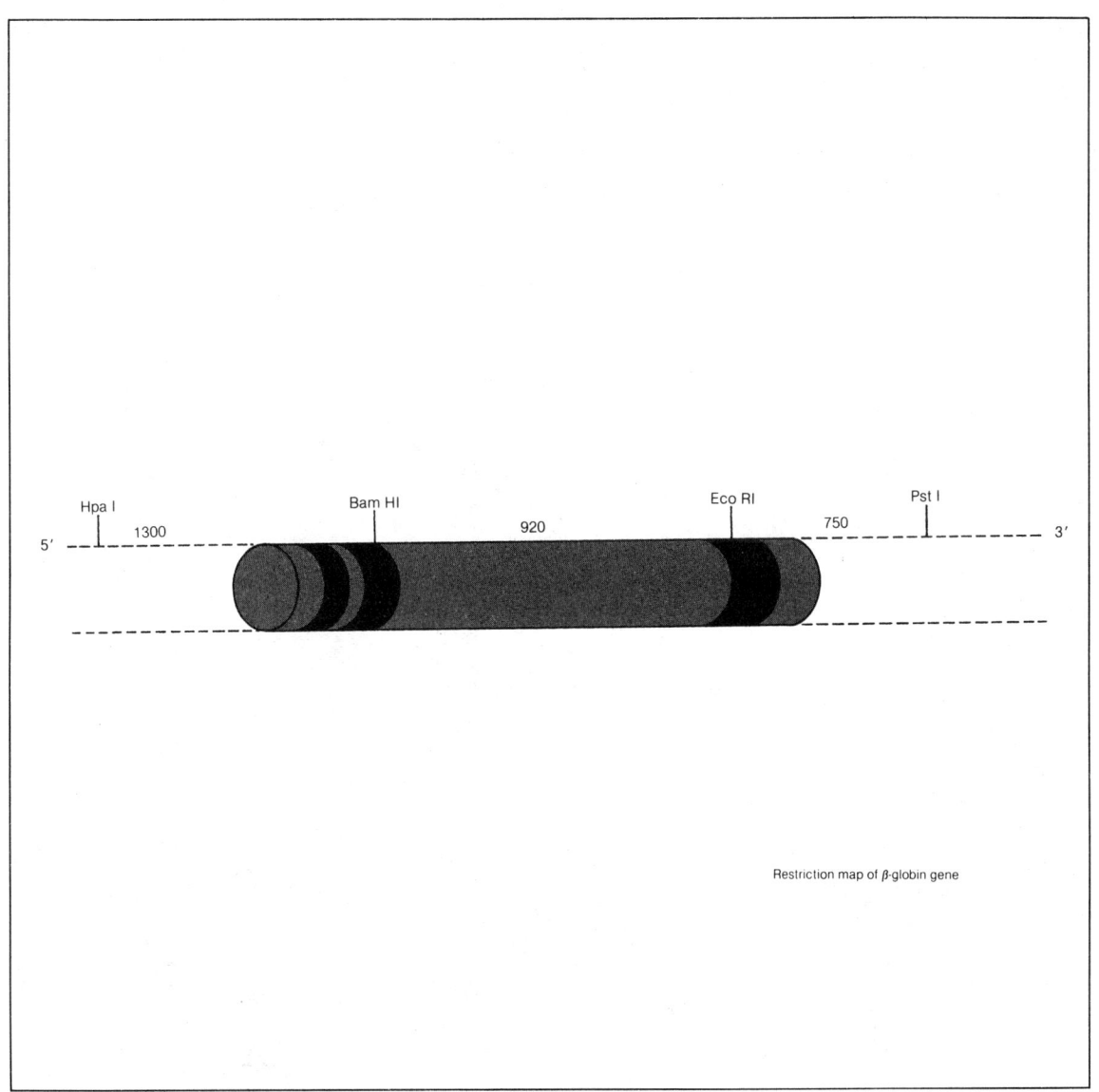

PART 11

Restriction map of β-globin gene

DISORDERS OF THE BLOOD AND BLOOD-FORMING TISSUES

70

HEMOSTASIS AND DISORDERS OF BLOOD COAGULATION

PATRICK A. McKEE

1. Blood coagulation occurs as a sequence of complicated, extraordinarily well-controlled enzymatic reactions, many of which are enhanced greatly by surfaces containing phospholipids. The precise events which trigger blood coagulation remain obscure. The most popular formulation is that platelets tend to stick to an abnormal surface, and the platelet membranes then become distorted as a consequence of platelet-surface and platelet-platelet interactions. Concomitantly, the intrinsic pathway of blood coagulation is triggered as factor XII becomes activated. Prekallikrein, which is concentrated on the surface as a complex with a high molecular weight kininogen, becomes activated to kallikrein and continues to activate factor XII. The enzymatic form of factor XII then activates factor XI, which is bound to altered surfaces in a complex with a high molecular weight kininogen. Activated factor XI converts factor IX to its serine proteinase form, which then forms a complex with factor VIII to activate factor X to an activated form. The coagulation scheme can also be initiated through the extrinsic pathway when tissue factor, a lipoprotein, forms an active complex with the plasma protein, factor VII. This complex also activates factor X to its enzymatic form, which converts prothrombin to thrombin. In the final step of blood coagulation, thrombin converts fibrinogen to fibrin simultaneously with the activation of factor XIII that catalyzes formation of covalent isopeptide bonds between fibrin monomers. The series of blood coagulation reactions is regulated by various plasma proteinase inhibitors. Finally, the fibrinolytic system also plays a role in blood coagulation, since it appears to be required for dissolving fibrin and recanalizing blood vessels in the area of wounds.

2. Hereditary disorders have been described in which the plasma is deficient in one or more of the factors involved in hemostasis, with the exception of calcium ion or phospholipids.

3. The clinical presentations of the various hereditary hemorrhagic disorders lack specificity. Although a differential diagnosis may be proposed from the family history, the precise diagnosis still depends upon laboratory studies.

4. A variety of screening tests such as the clotting time, the partial thromboplastin time, and the prothrombin time are useful in identifying most clotting abnormalities. Differential diagnoses continue to depend on determining whether the patient's plasma will correct the clotting defect in plasma from another patient known to have the specific deficiency under consideration.

5. Classic hemophilia, factor VIII deficiency, and factor IX deficiency are inherited as X-linked recessive traits. Most of the other clotting factor deficiencies are inher-

ited as autosomal recessive traits with the possible exceptions of factor V and factor XIII deficiencies, which have been suspected of being autosomal dominant and X-linked, respectively. Antithrombin III deficiency and the dysfibrinogenemias occur as autosomal dominant traits.

6. *Most of the hemorrhagic disorders are due to true deficiency of a clotting factor. Nonfunctional variants of the missing factors may also be the cause of disease.*

7. *The blood coagulation system contains a vast array of positive and negative feedback reactions, some of which account for the frequently observed discordance between the degree of the coagulation defect and the severity of the patient's symptoms.*

8. *As perhaps best exemplified by recent work on von Willebrand's disease and antithrombin III deficiency, rigorous study of clinical problems of bleeding or thrombosis will expand our understanding of normal mechanisms.*

The importance of genetics in understanding blood coagulation mechanisms may be unparalleled when compared to most other inherited human disorders. The various inherited bleeding and thrombotic disorders have clearly led to the identification and definition of the biochemical events that culminate in the generation of a fibrin clot. Over the past decade the continuous expansion of biochemical knowledge has permitted close ties to be developed with the genetics of each disorder. New proteins and new reactions of blood coagulation components continue to be discovered. Fortunately, the expansion of knowledge has been accompanied by considerable clarification and simplification of many mechanisms that occur in human blood coagulation [1, 2].

Hemostasis is the spontaneous arrest of bleeding when the circulatory system is disrupted. It seems certain that platelet-vessel wall and platelet-platelet interactions are the first steps in hemostasis (see Chap. 71). Platelets initially adhere to an abnormal surface, whether this be damaged endothelium, a severed vessel with exposure of blood to the surrounding tissues, or an artificial surface. Platelet adhesion somehow promotes the release of certain constituent components that alter platelet surfaces, so that other platelets aggregate to those already adherent. The platelet changes that occur as a consequence of these reactions allow membrane phospholipids to become available for participation in many of the clotting reactions. Both the exposure of certain binding sites on the altered platelet membrane and the availability of membrane phospholipid then provide the sort of surface on which certain of the blood-clotting plasma proteins become concentrated and activated. Normal blood coagulation continues as a tightly modulated, ordered series of chemical events which begins with the activation of a few molecules and culminates in the formation of the insoluble protein fibrin. There are about 20 substances that are critical for normal blood coagulation. Most of these are plasma proteins that circulate as zymogens in microgram per milliliter concentrations and undergo proteolytic cleavage to become active serine proteinases. Certain of the clotting proteins are not enzymes and serve instead as cofactors that facilitate protein-protein interactions.

Because the nomenclature of the blood-clotting factors became confusing, with each factor seeming to have several names, Roman numerals were assigned to achieve some degree of uniformity. Ordinarily, the activated form of a clotting factor is designated by appending a subscript a to the appropriate Roman numeral. It is unfortunate that the Roman numerals bear little chronologic relationship to the step at which a clotting factor participates in the series of chemical reactions leading to fibrin formation. For example, in the last step of coagulation, fibrinogen (factor I) is converted to fibrin in a reaction in which the enzyme, fibrin stabilizing factor (factor XIII), plays an important role. Table 70-1 lists the factors by Roman numeral and also gives their trivial names, some of which are surnames of the index patient with the clotting factor deficiency. Over the past several years, additional plasma proteins important to the generation of thrombin have been discovered; these have not yet received a Roman numeral. Figure 70-1 is a representation of the scheme of blood coagulation reactions.

BIOCHEMISTRY OF HUMAN BLOOD COAGULATION AND FIBRINOLYSIS

Intrinsic Coagulation Pathway—Contact Activation Phase

The constituent plasma proteins of this portion of the blood coagulation scheme include factor XII (Hageman factor), prekallikrein (Fletcher factor), factor XI (plasma thromboplastin antecedent), and high molecular weight kininogen (Fitzgerald factor) [3, 4]. The first three of these are zymogens of serine proteinases, while high molecular weight kininogen serves as a cofactor that augments certain of the reactions of factor XI_a and kallikrein with their substrates. Neither phospholipid nor calcium ion is required for the interactions of the contact phase of blood coagulation. Three important physiologic events occur as a consequence of contact activation: (1) initiation of blood coagulation; (2) generation of kinins; and (3) activation of the fibrinolytic system.

Factor XII (Hageman Factor) Factor XII zymogen, a single-chain glycoprotein of about 74,000 daltons, is present in human plasma in an average concentration of about 35 μg/ml [5]. Human and bovine factor XII have closely similar physicochemical properties [6–8]. As a zymogen in solution, it has no amidase or esterase activity and does not bind naturally occurring inhibitors such as antithrombin III, or chemical inhibitors such as diisopropyl fluorophosphate [9, 10]. Factor XII develops enzymatic activity by one or more of three mechanisms. The most important of these is probably the binding of zymogen factor XII to certain negatively charged surfaces such as glass [11, 12]. Kaolin, celite, urate crystals [13, 14], vascular subendothelial elements, collagen and, more recently, endotoxin [15], large polymers of dextran sulfate [10], and sulfatide [10] are other examples of negatively charged surfaces on which factor XII is readily activated. The net electronegativity of a given surface is clearly critical to binding since positively charged substances inhibit the absorption of factor XII [16, 17]. Upon binding, the conformation of factor XII becomes altered [18] so that amidase activity and the ability to cleave certain protein macromolecules develop [19–22]. These substrates include prekallikrein and factor XI zymogen, each of which circulates in plasma as a bimolecular complex with the

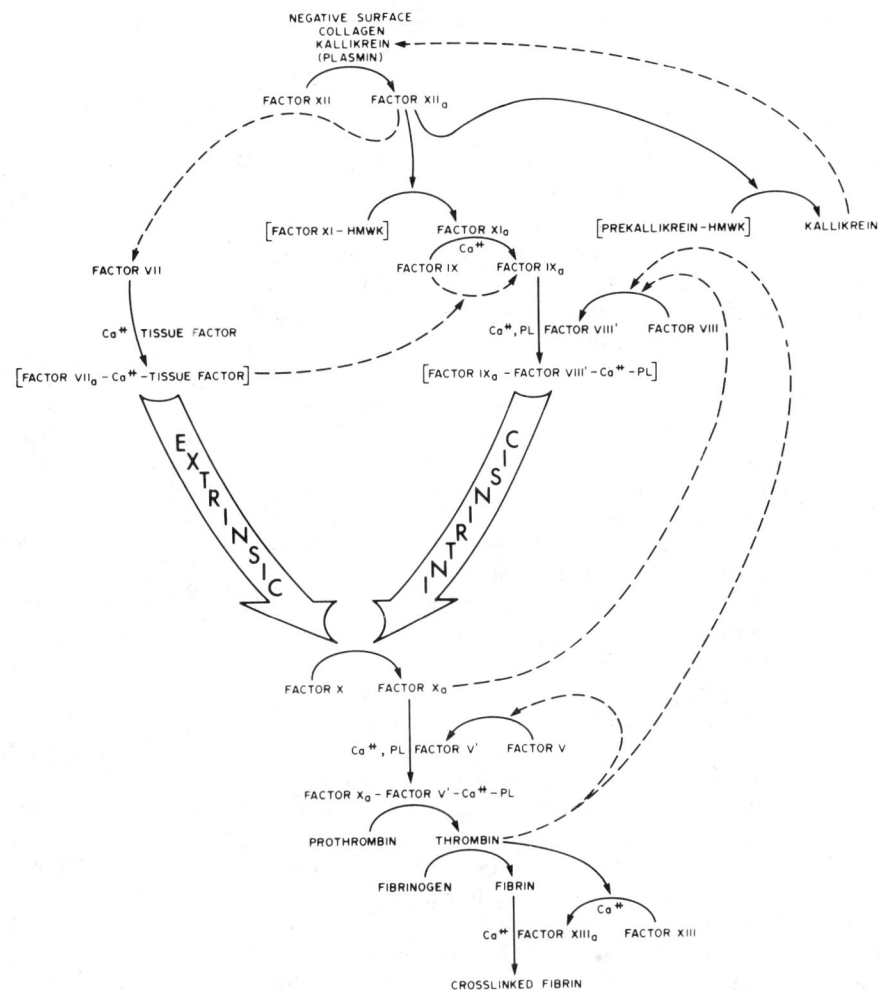

Figure 70-1 Blood coagulation scheme depicting forward and feedback reactions. High molecular weight kininogen is abbreviated HMWK. Reactive complexes are enclosed by brackets. Phospholipid is indicated as PL. The subscript a designates the activated, or enzyme form, of the clotting factor. The dashed lines indicate pathways which may be important in vivo but are not yet completely proven. Both factors V and VIII are cleaved by thrombin to produce forms that have enhanced activity, as indicated by the superscript prime. Neither is an enzyme.

high molecular weight kininogen. Recent experiments, in which bovine proteins were used, show that surface-bound factor XII zymogen readily activates prekallikrein in the presence of high molecular weight kininogen [23]. In separate experiments, in which factor XII_a was purposely substituted for factor XII zymogen, the initial rates of conversion of prekallikrein to kallikrein were about the same. Hence, the surface-bound factor XII and soluble factor XII_a appear essentially equally potent in converting prekallikrein to kallikrein. In the instance of factor XI different results were obtained. While the surface-bound zymogen factor XII can activate factor XI in the presence of high molecular weight kininogen, the activation rate is twofold greater when factor XII_a is used [22]. In the latter situation, the activation of factor XI to XI_a proceeds at approximately the same rate as when prekallikrein is converted to kallikrein by surface-bound factor XII zymogen or factor XII_a.

In other studies, ellagic acid, which tends to form surface-active aggregates in aqueous media, was used, and as with other negatively charged surfaces, human factor XII zymogen activated factor XI in the presence of high molecular weight kininogen [19]. There was no indication that human factor XII became cleaved to lower molecular weight fragments during this reaction. Results from several laboratories now support the concept that in the initial phase of the activation, single-chain factor XII converts prekallikrein to kallikrein in the presence of high molecular weight kininogen and a negatively

charged surface. Consequently, a popular view is that the enzymatic activity displayed by single-chain factor XII on binding to a surface is the event that initiates the cascade of reactions which flow through the intrinsic limb of blood coagulation.

The second method for generating factor XII_a occurs by reciprocal activation between prekallikrein and factor XII [23–27]. Compared to factor XII in solution, surface-bound factor XII zymogen is cleaved to XII_a 30 to 500 times more rapidly by several enzymes [25, 27–30]. Kallikrein cleaves surface-bound factor XII within a disulfide loop to form a two-chain serine proteinase, composed of a 47,000-dalton heavy chain and a 28,000-dalton light chain. Factor XII_a then not only cleaves prekallikrein to kallikrein but also has the ability to activate factor XI about four times faster than single-chain, surface-bound factor XII [22]. Prekallikrein does not undergo autocatalysis, nor is it activated by factor XI_a. In contrast, factor XI_a can activate factor XII, but this is probably not a very significant reaction in whole plasma since kallikrein is generated much more rapidly and is about four times more efficient in cleaving XII to XII_a [10]. Interestingly, when plasma deficient in prekallikrein is incubated with kaolin for about 10 min before the addition of kallikrein, it has a normal clotting time [29]. Presumably, factor XI_a is slowly generated by surface-bound, single-chain factor XII. Once formed, factor XI_a augments the initiation of the clotting process by converting factor XII to XII_a. If the level of single-chain factor XII is increased substantially, factor XI can be easily activated in the absence of prekallikrein and the kaolin clotting time can be normalized [6, 31]. Nevertheless, in spite of these demonstrations in vitro it remains likely that factor XI$_a$ is not very significant for the activation of factor XII in vitro.

Other mechanisms of factor XII activation have been suggested. Most of these reactions are controversial and remain to be convincingly established as physiologically important. Rabbit factor XII zymogen is said to be activated by factor XII$_a$ [32]. Prekallikrein and factor XII have also been proposed to possess weak enzymatic activity as zymogens [33], but this is probably not a necessary mechanism in vivo in view of the reactions described above. Recent data have also been interpreted as showing that trace factor XII$_a$ or perhaps surface-bound factor XII is capable of activating zymogen XII [34, 35], but a concern remains about the absolute exclusion of a few molecules of kallikrein. Purified human factor XII is activated relatively slowly by factor XI$_a$ [10], plasmin [36], or kallikrein [23] in solution, whereas the inclusion of a surface such as kaolin accelerates by thirtyfold, a hundredfold, and five hundredfold, respectively, the formation of factor XII$_a$ [27].

The portion of single-chain factor XII which binds to surfaces ultimately becomes the heavy chain of the two-chain factor XII$_a$ enzyme; the light chain contains the active site and is not involved in surface binding [37]. On exposure to trypsin, factor XII zymogen is cleaved on the amino-terminal side of a disulfide loop to yield a large fragment that contains only a small portion of the heavy chain, but all of the light chain, and hence the active site [37]. If kallikrein is used to activate zymogen factor XII, a mixture of factor XII$_a$ and the active site containing factor XII$_a$ fragment is formed [35]. Both factor XII$_a$ and the factor XII$_a$ fragment hydrolyze a variety of substrates and have about the same specific activities [35], but only factor XII$_a$ readily corrects the deficiency in factor XII-deficient plasma. The factor XII$_a$ fragment does not activate zymogen factor XII, nor is it a very efficient activator of zymogen factor XI [35, 38].

Recently, factor XII$_a$ has been shown to activate factor VII [39, 40]. The formation of factor XII$_a$ occurs by a peptide bond cleavage, the rate of which appears increased at low temperature [41]. To some extent the activation of factor VII by factor XII$_a$ broadens the notion that the intrinsic and extrinsic pathways do not function independently. The fact that results of tests of the intrinsic system are normal in factor VII deficiency suggests that the contribution of factor VII$_a$ to the overall integrity of the intrinsic pathway is not very significant.

Prekallikrein The plasma concentration of human prekallikrein in about 15 to 45 μg/ml [3, 42]. It circulates as a complex with high molecular weight kininogen [43, 44], the latter protein readily binding to negatively charged surfaces. This allows prekallikrein to become concentrated on the same surface to which factor XII becomes bound, so that the active-site serine of surface-bound factor XII zymogen or factor XII$_a$ can cleave prekallikrein to the serine proteinase, kallikrein [25, 28]. Most likely, surface-bound, single-chain factor XII activates prekallikrein as the initial step of the contact activation pathway [23]. In contrast to factor XI, which is also surface-bound through complex formation with high molecular weight kininogen and remains so after conversion to factor XI$_a$, kallikrein is released into the circulation or surrounding tissues [30]. Purified human prekallikrein exists in two forms, each with an apparent molecular weight of about 85,000, but one probably has a slightly higher content of the intramolecular

Table 70-1 Blood coagulation factors

Roman numeral assigned	Substance	Normal plasma conc. (μg/ml)
I*	Fibrinogen Hypofibrinogenemia Afibrinogenemia Dysfibrinogenemia	1500–4000
II*	Prothrombin	150
III*	Tissue thromboplastin; tissue factor	—
IV*	Calcium ion	—
V	Proaccelerin; labile factor	10
(VI)	Not assigned	—
VII	Proconvertin; stable factor	<1
VIII	Antihemophilic factor	<.05
IX	Christmas factor; plasma thromboplastin component (PTC)	5
X	Stuart factor or Stuart-Prower factor	8
XI	Plasma thromboplastin antecedent (PTA)	5
XII	Hageman factor	35
XIII	Fibrin-stabilizing factor	20
—*	Prekallikrein (Fletcher factor)	30
—*	High molecular weight kininogen (Fitzgerald, Williams or Flaujeac factor)	80
—*	von Willebrand factor	16
—*	Protein C	5
—*	Protein S	5
—*	Antithrombin III	240
—*	α$_2$-antiplasmin	70
—*	Inhibitor to protein C	?
—*	Plasminogen	150

N = normal. ↑ = prolonged.
* Not usually referred to by Roman numeral or not assigned a number.
† Ability of plasma to correct plasma from a patient with known deficiency or by assay using specific synthetic substrate.

disulfide bonds [45]. On exposure to factor XII$_a$, both forms of prekallikrein undergo a cleavage of a single peptide bond within a disulfide loop to form a 42,000-dalton light chain and a 52,000-dalton heavy chain. With continued incubation, the 42,000-dalton subunit is cleaved to 37,000 daltons. As a zymogen, prekallikrein is inactivated by diisopropyl fluorophosphate with a second-order rate constant of 0.59 M^{-1} min^{-1}, whereas the active enzyme, kallikrein, is inhibited by DFP with a second-order rate constant of 500 M^{-1} min^{-1} [45]. For many years a link has been evident between the con-

Table 70-1 Blood coagulation factors *(Continued)*

Deficiency inheritance pattern	Estimated frequency per million	Laboratory assessment				Selected tests
		Thrombin time	Prothrombin time	Partial thromboplastin time	Bleeding time	
Autosomal recessive	<0.5	↑ (⇔)	↑ (∞)	↑ (∞)	N	Fibrinogen <100 mg/dl
Autosomal recessive	<0.5	∞	∞	∞	N(↑)	Fibrinogen absent immunologically
Autosomal recessive	<0.5	± ↑	± ↑	± ↑	N	Delayed fibrinopeptide release or impaired fibrin monomer aggregation
Autosomal recessive	<0.5	N	↑	↑	N	Specific assay†
No deficiency known	—	—	—	—	—	—
Autosomal recessive	<0.5	N	↑	↑	N	Specific assay†
Autosomal recessive	<0.5	N	↑	N(↑)	N	Specific assay†
X-linked recessive	60–80	N	N	↑	N	Specific assay†. Normal ristocetin-platelet aggregation
X-linked recessive	15–20	N	N	↑	N	Specific assay†
Autosomal recessive	<.05	N	↑	↑	N	Specific assay†
Autosomal recessive	1.0	N	N	↑	N(↑)	Specific assay†
Autosomal recessive	1.0	N	N	↑	N	Specific assay†
Autosomal recessive	<0.5	N	N	N	N	Plasma clots soluble in 5 *M* urea or 1 percent monochloroacetic acid
Autosomal recessive	<0.5	N	N	↑	N	Specific assay†
Autosomal recessive	<0.5	N	N	↑	N	Specific assay†
Autosomal codominant	5–10	N	N	↑	↑	Von Willebrand protein decreased (~75 percent of patients) or normal (~20 percent of patients) by immunologic studies; ristocetin-platelet aggregation decreased with rare exceptions; factor VIII procoagulant activity decreased
No deficiency known	—	—	—	—	—	—
No deficiency known	—	—	—	—	—	
Autosomal dominant	<0.5	N	N	N	N	Specific assay†
Autosomal recessive	One report	N	N	N	N	Euglobulin and whole blood clot lysis times shortened
Autosomal recessive	<0.5	N	↑	↑	N	Combined factors V and VIII deficiency by specific assays
Autosomal recessive	<0.5	N	N	N	N	Euglobulin lysis time prolonged; decreased activation by streptokinase

tact activation system and the initiation of fibrinolysis, yet this was not precisely established until recently, when it was shown that the conversion of prekallikrein to kallikrein coincides with the cleavage of plasminogen to plasmin in a synthetic system [45]. Since monospecific antiprekallikrein antiserum or Cl⁻ inhibitor simultaneously abolishes kallikrein activity and the factor XII-dependent plasminogen activator activity, it appears that kallikrein and the previously described plasminogen proactivator are identical [45, 46]. Whether or not this is biologically significant remains controversial since urokinase is almost 2000 times more potent on a molar basis than kallikrein in the activation of plasminogen. Kallikrein, besides activating factor XII, also cleaves both high molecular weight and low molecular weight kininogens to generate peptides known as *kinins*, the best known of which is bradykinin [42, 47, 48]. These peptides have diversified effects such as increasing vascular permeability, contracting smooth muscle, stimulating pain, and influencing the migration of leukocytes [42]. Recently, kallikrein has also been shown to convert plasma prorenin to renin, followed by the generation of angiotensin I from angiotensinogen [49, 50], but the physiologic significance of this reaction is uncertain.

High Molecular Weight Kininogen   Human high molecular weight kininogen has a plasma concentration of 70 to 90 μg/ml [3]. It is a single polypeptide chain of 120,000 daltons [51] and readily forms soluble complexes with prekallikrein or human factor XI [43, 44, 52]. As noted earlier, when the high molecular weight kininogen-prekallikrein complex binds to a surface in close approximation to surface-bound, activated factor XII, cleavage of prekallikrein to kallikrein occurs [25, 28]. Similarly, high molecular weight factor XI complexes become adsorbed to the same surface, presumably facilitating the ability of activated factor XII to convert XI to XI$_a$ [30]. Once kallikrein is formed, it is released from the complex and activates additional molecules of surface-bound factor XII zymogen. Hence, a prime function of high molecular weight kininogen may be to enhance the concentration of two zymogen blood-clotting proteins, prekallikrein and factor XI, on damaged vascular endothelium or artificial surfaces. Free plasma kallikrein cleaves two peptide bonds in a disulfide loop of high molecular weight kininogen to release bradykinin and other peptides totaling about 15,000 daltons [51]. Hence, kinin-free kininogen is a two-chain molecule having a 66,000-dalton heavy chain disulfide-linked to a 37,000-dalton light chain [51]. The single-chain precursor form of high molecular weight kininogen and the cleaved, two-chain form have about the same level of accelerating effects on activation of factor XII [51, 53]. The new amino terminus of the light chain is contiguous with a region of amino acid sequence that is especially rich in histidine residues and is therefore positively charged. This region of the molecule is involved in the binding to negatively charged surfaces. In bovine high molecular weight kininogen, a second cleavage is made by kallikrein to release a peptide termed *fragment 1·2* which contains about 20 percent histidine and is clearly responsible for the binding of high molecular weight kininogen to negatively charged surfaces [53]. So long as fragment 1·2 is present, the light chain of high molecular weight kininogen functions as a procoagulant [53]. In addition, bovine fragment 1·2 inhibits the binding of intact bovine high molecular weight kininogen to surfaces. The fact that isolated human light chain alone possesses procoagulant function suggests that the human counterpart of fragment 1·2 is not cleaved from the light chain by plasma kallikrein [52].

The requirement of high molecular weight kininogen for the binding of factor XI to a surface has recently been challenged [54]. Factor XI was found to bind to glass surfaces in purified solution in the absence of high molecular weight kininogen. With increasing concentrations of high molecular weight kininogen, less factor XI was bound. On the other hand, factor XI did not bind in Fitzgerald-deficient plasma, which lacks high molecular weight kininogen. With the addition of high molecular weight kininogen, factor XI was noted to bind, but this could be inhibited if the high molecular weight kininogen concentration was increased above normal. It is possible that high molecular weight kininogen functions as a modulating protein in the contact phase by augmenting the binding of factor XI to surfaces as well as preventing inappropriate surface binding of factor XI. An alternative suggestion is that high molecular weight kininogen overcomes a plasma inhibitor of factor XI surface adsorption so that factor XI can then freely adhere, the evidence being that factor XI adsorption from plasma is far less than from plasma-free solutions [54]. These

issues continue to be uncertain, but it is safe to assume that human plasma contains an intricate system that controls the surface availability of both prekallikrein and factor XI for reactions with other plasma proteins.

Factor XI   The concentration of factor XI in normal human plasma is about 5 μg/ml [55]. Factor XI is present in plasma in a complex with high molecular weight kininogen [30, 52], the latter modulating the binding and activation of factor XI on negatively charged surfaces. Factor XI circulates in zymogen form as two polypeptide chains held together by disulfide bonds, the native molecular weight being reported as 163,000 to 124,000 [55, 56]. It contains about 5 percent carbohydrate. The two polypeptide chains are identical, and when exposed to enzymatic levels of surface-bound factor XII$_a$, two cleavages occur within disulfide loops to form factor XI$_a$, now composed of a pair of identical heavy chains and a pair of identical light chains, all held together by disulfide bonds. The molecular weights of the heavy and light chains are reported as 50,000 to 35,000 and 33,000 to 25,000, respectively [55, 56]. The basis for the different values is not clear, but it does seem apparent that factor XI activation is not accompanied by a loss of mass. Each of the light chains has an active-center serine. Unlike kallikrein, when factor XI$_a$ enzyme is formed, it remains bound to high molecular weight kininogen and does not circulate [30]. In the presence of divalent cation, factor XI$_a$ readily cleaves zymogen factor IX to its activated form [57]; it is uncertain whether both active sites function in the activation of factor IX. In accord with the presence of two active sites, factor XI$_a$ reacts with diisopropyl fluorophosphate, and 1 mol of factor XI$_a$ combines with 2 mol of the plasma proteinase inhibitor, antithrombin III [56]. Both α_1-antitrypsin and Cl$^-$ inhibitor are naturally occurring plasma inhibitors of factor XI$_a$ [58, 59]. α_2-Macroglobulin does not inhibit factor XI$_a$ [60]. Antithrombin III inhibits XI$_a$ slowly, but in the presence of heparin, the inhibition is instantaneous [61]. Factor XI$_a$ is a weak plasminogen activator, having a specific activity several thousandfold less than that of urokinase [62]. This low level of plasminogen activator activity, combined with that of kallikrein, probably accounts for the previously described plasminogen proactivator activity of the contact activation phase of blood clotting. Trypsin has also been found to activate factor XI but yields a somewhat more fragmented pattern [63]. Kallikrein has no effect on factor XI.

Factor IX   Factor IX is a glycoprotein that has a molecular weight of about 57,000 and contains about 17 percent carbohydrate [64–67]. It circulates in plasma in a concentration of about 5 μg/ml [67]. Factor IX is synthesized in the hepatocyte, where certain glutamic acid residues in its amino-terminal portion undergo a post-ribosomal modification that is dependent upon oxygen and bicarbonate, a carboxylase enzyme, and vitamin K [68]. The γ-carboxylation of these specific glutamic acid residues is required for calcium-dependent phospholipid binding. Coumarin-type drugs prevent the posttranslational γ-carboxylation by interfering with the conversion of stored vitamin K epoxide to its active reduced form. The polypeptide structure of factor IX continues to be synthesized but is non-functional since it lacks γ-carboxylated glutamic acids. This form of nonfunctional factor IX cannot interact fully with calcium and phospholipid to form a complex that, in concert with factor VIII$_a$, activates factor X to factor X$_a$.

In the presence of calcium ion, but not requiring phospholipid, factor XI$_a$ cleaves factor IX zymogen to factor XI$_a$ [57, 67, 69]. An initial cleavage occurs between an arginyl-alanyl peptide bond within a disulfide loop to form an intermediate, inactive procoagulant factor IX composed of disulfide-linked heavy and light polypeptide chains. Next, the scission of an arginyl-valyl bond occurs, with the release of a carbohydrate-rich 11,000-dalton peptide from the amino terminus of the heavy chain of the intermediate factor IX [64, 65, 67]. This second cleavage results in the formation of factor IX$_a$, which now possesses full procoagulant activity. The active-site serine is in the 27,000-dalton heavy chain, while the γ-carboxylated glutamic acid groups are in the 17,000-dalton light chain [65, 67]. Except for the rates of cleavage, a similar two-step mechanism is observed for the activation of bovine factor IX by activated factor XI [70].

The reaction product of tissue thromboplastin and factor VII (extrinsic pathway) can activate factor IX (intrinsic pathway) provided calcium ion is also present [71]. Only catalytic amounts of factor VII are needed to demonstrate that factor IX$_a$ clotting activity is generated concomitantly with the appearance of the heavy and light chains of IX$_a$. Thus, contact of blood with tissue thromboplastin results in the formation of a product that can activate factor IX and bypass the need for activated factor XI. Clearly, the extrinsic and intrinsic pathways are not mechanistically distinct, but instead merely represent operationally convenient outlines. Factor IX$_a$ is inactivated slowly by diisopropyl fluorophosphate but fairly rapidly by benzamidine or antithrombin III-heparin mixtures [65, 70]. Factor IX is also activated by Russell's viper venom, but only one cleavage is made, the activation peptide being retained in the two-chain structure [70]. This activated factor IX species has only about half the procoagulant activity as when factor IX$_a$ is formed by factor XI$_a$ in the presence of calcium ion. Factor X$_a$ [72], thrombin [73], and kallikrein [67] have been said to activate factor IX, although some disagreement exists about the reproducibility and significance of these reactions, especially since factor X$_a$, for example, cleaves prothrombin far more rapidly than factor IX [70, 71].

Both calcium and phospholipid are required to attain a maximal rate of factor X activation by factor IX$_a$. In addition, the presence of factor VIII that has been modified by thrombin or a thrombinlike enzyme markedly potentiates the rate of factor X$_a$ generation by IX$_a$ [73, 74]. Factor IX$_a$, thrombin-cleaved factor VIII, phospholipid, and calcium are presumed to form a complex that activates factor X; however, the physicochemical details of this complex are unknown [75]. A hypothetical model of the interactions of factors IX$_a$, X, VIII, phospholipid, and calcium ion is shown in Fig. 70-2.

Factor VIII/von Willebrand Protein (Antihemophilic Factor/von Willebrand Protein) Both factor VIII (antihemophilic factor) activity and von Willebrand factor activity appear to be properties of a complex glycoprotein that circulates in plasma in a concentration of about 16 μg/ml [76]. Factor VIII somehow accelerates the rate of factor X$_a$ formation by factor IX$_a$, whereas von Willebrand factor activity is necessary for platelets to interact with damaged vessel surfaces as well as perhaps for platelets to interact with other platelets. The two activities will be considered together since they either circulate in plasma as a complex of two different moieties or are both properties of the same molecule, or simply copurify. Three recent reviews analyze in detail the problems of structure-function relationships of the two activities [77–79]. When

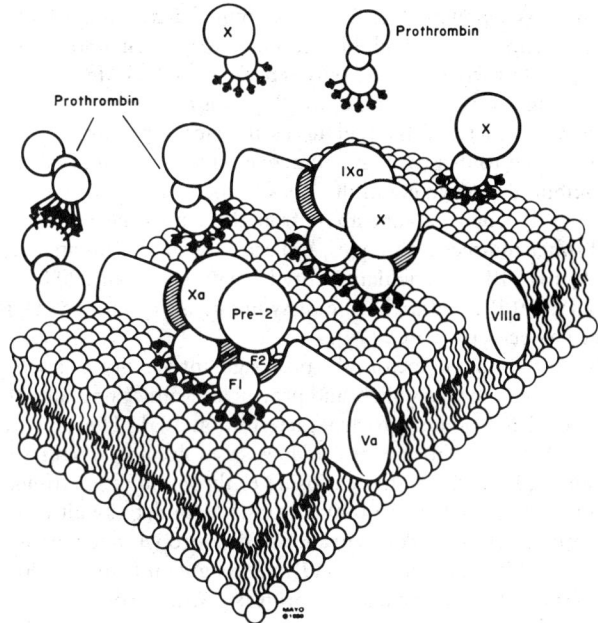

Figure 70-2 Model of two collected blood coagulation reactions: conversion of factor X to factor X$_a$, and conversion of prothrombin to thrombin. Their respective catalysts are bound adjacent to one another on their respective cofactors on the platelet membrane. The scheme for the factor IX$_a$-X-VIII$_a$ interaction is hypothetical, and it is made analogous to the factor X$_a$-prothrombin-factor V$_a$ interaction, for which more experimental evidence exists. A molecule of factor V$_a$ is embedded in the lipid surface and is in 1:1 stoichiometry with factor X$_a$. Activation of factor V by proteolysis is suggested by the concavity in its structure. Prothrombin molecules, each with its fragment 1 (F1), fragment 2 (F2), and prethrombin domains, are shown in solution and on the vesicle surface. Binding of prothrombin to the phospholipid surface occurs by Ca$^+$ bridging mediated by the γ-carboxy-glutamate residues of the fragment 1 domain. A prothrombin dimer is shown in solution with the interaction between the two molecules through Ca$^+$ and γ-carboxy-glutamate residues. (*Used with permission of KG Mann* [374].)

the factor VIII/von Willebrand protein complex is purified, it has a molecular weight ranging from 1 to 14 million [80–82]. In the presence of reducing reagents the complex consists of subunits which have a molecular weight of about 200,000 by sodium dodecyl sulfate gel electrophoresis or analytical ultracentrifugation [80, 83]. The inability to demonstrate other protein bands in such preparations has been used as an argument that both activities are present on a single molecule. Nevertheless, under peculiar solvent conditions such as buffers of high ionic strength and especially those containing 0.25 M CaCl$_2$, the factor VIII and von Willebrand activities can be separated by agarose gel filtration chromatography [84–87]. The separated factor VIII procoagulant activity lacks von Willebrand factor activity, and similarly the peak of protein with von Willebrand factor activity contains little or no factor VIII procoagulant activity. With this method the amount of protein in the factor VIII procoagulant peak is less than 1 percent by weight of the factor VIII/von Willebrand protein complex [86, 88]. Based on indirect estimates from purification yields, the concentration of factor VIII procoagulant activity in normal plasma may be as little as 50 ng/ml. Essentially all of the glycoprotein of the complex elutes in the void volume with the von Willebrand activity [87]. If the human factor VIII/von Willebrand glycoprotein is exposed to trace amounts of thrombin before chromatography on 2 to 4 percent agarose in 0.25 M CaCl$_2$, the separation of the two activities is strikingly potentiated [87, 98]. Conversely, if blood is collected with a minimum of venepuncture trauma and immediately mixed with several serine protease inhibitors, only a very small amount of factor VIII procoagulant activity separates on 0.25 M CaCl$_2$ 4 percent agarose chromatography [90]. This has led to the speculation that factor VIII circulates as an inactive precursor that is converted to its procoagulant active form by thrombin or a thrombin-like enzyme. On the basis of the elution position of factor VIII procoagulant activity from the agarose gel columns and other indirect techniques, molecular weight estimates of the factor VIII procoagulant entity have ranged from 100,000 to 285,000 [91–93]. The site of synthesis is not known. The liver has been proposed [94].

Recently, bovine factor VIII procoagulant activity was separated from the von Willebrand protein and sufficient material recovered for preliminary characterization [95]. The bovine factor VIII protein appears to have a molecular weight of about 93,000, which after exposure to thrombin yields triplet peptides of 80,000 to 55,000 daltons. These data await confirmation. At high concentrations, diisopropyl fluorophosphate inhibited bovine factor VIII procoagulant activity. This suggests that it may be a serine protease [95]. In contrast, diisopropyl fluorophosphate has no effect on human factor VIII or VIII$_a$ [90]. Similarly, other naturally occurring proteinase inhibitors do not affect the activity of factor VIII. Exposure to low concentrations of EDTA causes an immediate loss of factor VIII procoagulant activity that cannot be reversed by the addition of divalent cation [87, 96]. A high concentration of calcium ion, 1 percent albumin, or the addition of the separated von Willebrand protein partially stabilizes factor VIII procoagulant activity [87, 97, 98]. Data in vivo suggest that the von Willebrand protein acts to stabilize and protect the factor VIII moiety from inactivation [98].

Factor VIII activity is extraordinarily sensitive to proteases. Thrombin and trypsin initially enhance procoagulant activity, after which it is progressively lost. Trace amounts of plasmin rapidly destroy factor VIII activity [99, 100]. The effect of thrombin on the factor VIII activity in the factor VIII/von Willebrand factor entity is complex and may be stoichiometric rather than enzymatic [97]. Exposure to thrombin increases factor VIII procoagulant activity four- to tenfold and appears to occur by proteolysis [97]. In part, this phenomenon is used to support the notion that factor VIII must be cleaved by thrombin or a thrombinlike enzyme to maximize the velocity of the conversion of factor X to X$_a$ by the factor IX$_a$-phospholipid-calcium ion complex [74, 75, 80, 90]. In purified systems the rapid activation of factor VIII by thrombin is followed immediately by a slow loss of activity which may not be due to a proteolytic cleavage, but instead to a conformational change in an unstable, yet highly active factor VIII species [97]. Others disagree with this and have reported that thrombin initially cleaves factor VIII from a 285,000-dalton protein to one of 116,000 daltons coincident with factor VIII activation, after which the activated factor VIII is inactivated by a succession of cleavages by thrombin [93].

Heterologous antibodies to factor VIII/von Willebrand factor readily inhibit and precipitate the von Willebrand protein, but usually only partially inhibit factor VIII procoagulant activity. Most likely the latter occurs as an indirect steric effect on the factor VIII protein in the factor VIII/von Willebrand complex. On the other hand, spontaneous or acquired homologous antibodies to factor VIII procoagulant activity inhibit factor VIII activity only, do not form precipitin lines, and have no significant effect on von Willebrand factor activity [101].

Advantage has been taken of this latter phenomenon for developing radioimmunoassays for factor VIII procoagulant protein [102].

The synthesis of the von Willebrand protein occurs in endothelial cells in all parts of the circulation [103]. Direct evidence of synthesis has been obtained in vitro from cultures of umbilical vein endothelial cells [104]. Von Willebrand protein is also synthesized by megakaryocytes [105] and is found in platelets [106]. That found in or on platelets does not seem to occur as a consequence of exchange with plasma von Willebrand factor [107, 108]. Factor VIII procoagulant activity has not been found in endothelial cell cultures [109, 110]. As already noted, factor VIII/von Willebrand glycoprotein exists in plasma as a population of multimeric forms (1 to 14 million daltons) [81, 82, 111], the higher molecular weight species having the most von Willebrand factor activity as defined by ristocetin-induced platelet aggregation or by the ability to adhere to subendothelium [112–115]. The carbohydrate side chains of the von Willebrand glycoprotein appear to be important for its interactions with platelets [116–119]. Removal of terminal sialic acid residues reduces von Willebrand factor activity by about 50 percent and results in the asialo-factor VIII/von Willebrand glycoprotein being cleared from plasma by the liver about 50 times faster than normal factor VIII/von Willebrand factor [116]. Modification of the penultimate galactose residue further reduces von Willebrand factor activity to about 12 percent of normal, yet this form of carbohydrate-modified von Willebrand factor has no increased affinity for the hepatocyte receptor [117, 119]. In both of the carbohydrate-modified forms of factor VIII/von Willebrand factor, full factor VIII procoagulant activity is retained [117]. Ristocetin or certain other positively charged substances [120] appear to reduce the net surface charge on platelets [121], thereby making specific binding sites accessible on platelet membranes for the factor VIII/von Willebrand glycoprotein [122]. Since binding of factor VIII/von Willebrand factor can be closely correlated with ristocetin-induced platelet aggregation, these sites have been termed *receptors* [122]. The presence of factor VIII/von Willebrand receptors on the platelet membrane is supported by the finding that heterologous antibody to platelet membrane glycoprotein I inhibits ristocetin-induced factor VIII/von Willebrand factor-dependent aggregation [123]. In addition, platelets from patients with the Bernard-Soulier syndrome (see Chap. 71) are deficient in platelet membrane glycoprotein I and show little or no aggregation in response to ristocetin and added factor VIII/von Willebrand protein [124]. Modification of the carbohydrate on factor VIII/von Willebrand factor is accompanied by marked reduction in its ability to bind to platelets or to stimulate ristocetin-induced platelet aggregation [125]. Interestingly, the activity of the von Willebrand protein in the ristocetin assay is not very sensitive to either proteolysis or denaturing solvents, which is in marked contrast to factor VIII activity [99, 100]. Additional carbohydrate studies have revealed that each 200,000-dalton subunit in the factor VIII/von Willebrand complex has approximately one of the ABO blood group structures covalently linked, probably to asparagine [126]. The significance of this latter observation is unknown.

Extrinsic Coagulation System

Factor VII Human blood-clotting factor VII is present in plasma in a concentration of about 0.5 µg/ml. It is synthesized by the liver, being a vitamin K–dependent coagulation factor with at least two γ-carboxyglutamic acid residues in its amino-terminal portion [127]. Both bovine and human factor VII are single-chain proteins that have molecular weights of about 48,000 [127–129]. On exposure to factor X_a in the presence of calcium ion and phospholipid, bovine factor VII is cleaved to an active serine proteinase composed of two chains joined by disulfide bonds [127, 129]. The active-center serine is in the 29,500-dalton heavy chain, while the γ-carboxyglutamic acid groups are in the 23,500-dalton light chain [129, 130]. The activity of factor VII_a in the modified prothrombin time assay is increased twenty-five to thirtyfold over that of its single-chain zymogen form [127, 130]. Morever, factor VII_a incorporates diisopropyl fluorophosphate about two and a half times faster than factor VII zymogen [127]. In the presence of tissue factor and $CaCl_2$, the inhibition by diisopropyl fluorophosphate occurred about five times more rapidly than for either factor VII_a enzyme or factor VII zymogen alone. This suggests that complexing with tissue factor exposes the active site in factor VII zymogen [127]. Recent results show that antithrombin III inhibits factor VII_a only in the presence of relatively high concentrations of heparin [127]; at lower heparin concentrations inhibition is not observed [131]. Under these conditions the rate of inhibition of factor VII_a is about 25 times faster than for zymogen factor VII, but even this does not approach the rates at which other serine proteinase coagulation factors are inhibited by antithrombin III and heparin. The presence of tissue factor and $CaCl_2$ does not prevent the inhibition of factor VII or factor VII_a by antithrombin III-heparin mixtures, which is in accord with the diisopropyl fluorophosphate incorporation data. Antibody to the apoprotein of tissue factor appears to block binding of factor VII, but if the tissue factor-factor VII complex is formed first, the antibody has little or no effect on factor VII activity [132]. This suggests that the expression of factor VII activity indeed depends on its binding to tissue factor or that the factor VII in the tissue factor-factor VII complex becomes modified to its active form and then no longer depends on the tissue factor apoprotein binding site for activating factor X [132]. Most investigators presume that factor VII forms a complex with a tissue factor such that its active site becomes available for cleaving factor X to factor X_a. In the absence of phospholipid and calcium ion, enzymatic levels of factor XII_a or factor XII_a fragments will activate factor VII to VII_a without causing additional cleavages that inactivate factor VII_a [127, 130, 133]. This suggests that initiation of coagulation by the contact activation phase may indeed flow through both the intrinsic and extrinsic pathways. Thrombin alone will catalyze the formation of factor VII_a, but only at a fraction of the rate observed with factor X_a, phospholipid, and calcium [129].

The tissue factor-factor VII complex is also a potent factor IX activator in purified systems [71]. The evidence that this is a mechanism that bypasses the contact activation pathway appears to establish another important link between the extrinsic and intrinsic coagulation pathways. The fact that factor XI deficiency usually results in only a mild bleeding disorder may be explained by the ability of the tissue factor-factor VII complex to function as an alternative pathway for activating factor IX. Patients who lack factor IX activity or other clotting factors beyond this level usually have a more severe form of bleeding disorder.

Tissue Factor Tissue factor (thromboplastin) functions as a cofactor with factor VII in the conversion of factor X to X_a. It is present in the membranes of most tissues, especially lung, brain, subintimal layers of blood vessels, and placenta [134, 135]. Based on dry weight, brain and lung tissue factors consist of 72 and 36 percent lipid and 11 and 54 percent protein, respectively [136]. Interestingly, the apoprotein of each appears to be closely similar with respect to molecular weight, amino acid composition, and lipid binding properties [136]. Each apoprotein is a single polypeptide chain which contains about 5 to 10 percent carbohydrate and has a molecular weight of about 50,000 to 56,000 [136, 137]. In dilute buffers the apoprotein forms aggregates with molecular weights of 1.5 million. The purified protein lacks any clotting activity, but the lipid fraction behaves functionally as a partial thromboplastin. When recombined, full thromboplastic activity is observed. Tissue factor hybrids formed by combining lung lipids with the brain apoprotein or brain lipids with the lung apoprotein have about the same activities as when the lipid and protein are from the same tissue source [136]. The phospholipid content of tissue factor is about 35 percent phosphatidylcholine, 35 percent sphingomyelin, and 18 percent phosphatidylethanolamine; the remainder is phosphatidylinositol, phosphatidylserine, and lysophosphatidylcholine [138]. The specific phospholipids vary in their ability to restore procoagulant function when combined with the protein. Phosphatidylethanolamine and phosphatidylcholine are consistently more active than the others, but a phospholipid mixture combined with the apoprotein gives the highest procoagulant activity, especially if a small amount of phosphatidylserine is included [137]. So far there have been no described deficiencies or inherent abnormalities of tissue factor. In clotting reactions, tissue factor is usually supplied as a suspension of lyophilized brain or lung that is standardized for its ability to shorten the prothrombin time.

The Common Pathway for the Intrinsic and Extrinsic Systems

Factor X Factor X circulates as a zymogen in a plasma concentration of about 8 μg/ml and is dependent on vitamin K for its synthesis by the liver [68]. In its precursor form, it has a two-chain subunit structure that is joined by disulfide bonds. It contains about 15 percent carbohydrate and has a molecular weight of 59,000 [66]. Its complete amino acid sequence has been determined [139]. The 43,000-dalton heavy chain possesses an active-site serine, and the 17,000-dalton light chain contains 12 γ-carboxyglutamic acid residues that bind to acidic phospholipids through calcium bridges [66, 139]. Factor X is converted to its active form, factor X_a, by either factor IX_a or factor VII_a, each of which forms a complex with phospholipid and calcium ion that then cleaves factor X at an arginyl-isoleucyl bond of the heavy chain. Trace quantities of thrombin-activated factor VIII greatly enhance the rate of conversion of factor X to X_a by the factor IX_a-phospholipid-calcium complex [75]. As a final step, a carboxyl-terminal peptide is autolytically cleaved from the heavy chain of X_a without discernible biochemical effect [66]. Once formed, factor X_a is an enzyme with a high degree of specificity, cleaving at the carboxyl end of two specific arginine residues to form thrombin [140]. Similarly, factor X_a will cleave at the carboxyl end of certain substituted arginine esters, anilides, and some peptides [140]. Factor X_a is especially sensitive to inhibition by antithrombin III-heparin or diisopropylfluorophosphate [141, 142].

Factor V   Factor V has a plasma concentration of about 10 μg/ml and circulates in a precursor form that must be proteolytically cleaved in order to function optimally as a cofactor in the conversion of prothrombin to thrombin. Factor V is not an enzyme. There is some controversy about the molecular weight of native factor V. Most investigators estimate it to be about 330,000 [143, 144], but one group suggests that factor V exists in plasma with a molecular weight greater than 800,000 [145]. In purified systems thrombin cleaves several peptide bonds in factor V to give factor V_a, which has a thirtyfold increase in activity and consists of 150,000-, 121,000-, and 95,000- to 91,000-dalton fragments plus smaller peptides [143, 144, 146]. Of these, the 121,000- and 95,000- to 91,000-dalton components bind to platelets, but the 150,000-dalton peptide fragment does not [144]. Factor V has one high affinity calcium ion binding site that appears critical for maintaining the tertiary structure of the protein [147, 148] and several weaker calcium binding sites that join in the formation of the factor X_a-prothrombin-phospholipid complex [147]. Factor V_a interacts stoichiometrically with factor X_a to augment the generation of thrombin from prothrombin [146]. Precursor factor V initially participates in this reaction, which goes very slowly, as manifested by a lag phase in the generation of thrombin. Then, as factor V is converted to factor V_a by the first few molecules of generated thrombin, the formation of thrombin is greatly accelerated. Factor X_a and prothrombin appear to bind to factor V_a through the low affinity calcium binding regions of the V_a molecule [147], but the binding of factor V_a to phospholipid is independent of calcium [149]. Whether or not phospholipid is present, the second cleavage of prothrombin to yield thrombin occurs at about the same rate, providing factor V_a is present [150]. Based on this finding, it seems likely that the intermediate form of prothrombin binds directly to the V_a molecule. With continued exposure to thrombin, factor V_a is cleaved further, and its accelerating effects on the generation of thrombin from prothrombin are then lost. Platelets possess about 900 high affinity ($Kd = 3 \times 10^{-10}$ M) sites for factor V_a and about 3500 lower affinity ($Kd = 3 \times 10^{-9}$ M) sites [151]. Precursor factor V will bind only to the lower affinity sites. Recently, it has been shown that platelet-bound factor V must be converted to factor V_a in order for factor X_a to become bound to platelets [152]. Figure 70-2 shows the interaction of factor V_a with the platelet surface as well as with factor X_a and prothrombin during the activation of prothrombin.

Prothrombin   The blood clotting factor, prothrombin, circulates in plasma in a concentration of 70 to 100 μg/ml. It is synthesized by the liver as a single-chain glycoprotein that contains 10 percent carbohydrate and has a molecular weight of 72,500 [153]. It is dependent on vitamin K for the γ-carboxylation of the 10 to 12 glutamic acid residues in its amino-terminal portion [154–156]. Either thrombin or factor X_a can cleave prothrombin to generate active thrombin [157]. Two recent reviews provide detailed descriptions of prothrombin activation to thrombin [2, 153]. Thrombin initially cleaves the amino-terminal peptide, termed *fragment 1,* to generate "prethrombin 1" and then cleaves a second contiguous peptide, termed *fragment 2,* to generate "prethrombin 2." Factor X_a cleaves prothrombin slightly differently; the initial two amino-terminal peptides, fragments 1 and 2, are cleaved as a single unit, referred to as *fragment 1·2.* The remainder of the parent

molecule, or prethrombin 2, can then be cleaved within a disulfide loop by thrombin or factor X_a to give the two-chain molecule, thrombin. Hence, during the conversion of prothrombin to thrombin, about half of the amino-terminal mass of prothrombin is lost, thrombin being derived from the carboxyl-terminal half. Recent experiments in whole blood indicate that prothrombin activation occurs primarily by factor X_a and not to any significant extent by thrombin [158]. Figure 70-2 schematically depicts the activation of prothrombin by factor X_a.

In the presence of calcium ion, acidic phospholipid accelerates prothrombin activation about a hundredfold, but for this to occur, the amino-terminal peptide, fragment 1, of native prothrombin must be present [159]. This peptide region of the prothrombin molecule contains the γ-carboxyglutamic acid residues which are believed responsible for the calcium-mediated binding of prothrombin to phospholipid [154–156]. The binding of prothrombin and factor X_a to phospholipid optimizes the generation of thrombin by concentrating the enzyme and substrate in the same locale, perhaps by as much as ten thousandfold [160]. In animals fed vitamin K antagonists, the amino-terminal γ-carboxyglutamic acid groups are not present in the fragment 1 region of prothrombin, and its ability to bind to phospholipid is impaired and the generation of thrombin is slowed [68].

The fragment 2 region of prothrombin appears to bind factor V_a specifically, lipid not being required for this interaction. For example, if fragment 1·2 is removed from prothrombin to form prethrombin 2, the ability of factor V_a to accelerate the conversion of this prothrombin intermediate to thrombin is lost [161]. If, however, fragment 2 is added back to prethrombin 2, then the ability of factor V_a to enhance the rate of thrombin formation is restored [161]. The presence of factor V_a increases the rate of thrombin generation by three hundredfold. Thrombin then presumably feeds back into this reaction and inactivates factor V_a by proteolytic cleavages. Disulfide bridges do not connect the fragment 1·2 peptide with the region of the prothrombin molecule that gives rise to thrombin. Fragment 1·2 remains bound to the phospholipid surface through the γ-carboxyglutamic acid-calcium ion bridges, and thrombin readily dissociates from the site of activation and can then approximate its several substrates—factor V, factor VIII, factor XIII, and fibrinogen. This differs significantly with respect to the other vitamin K–dependent serine proteinase enzymes since they remain attached to phospholipid surfaces by γ-carboxyglutamic acid-calcium bridges.

Platelet membranes serve as the source of phospholipid in the various lipid-dependent clotting reactions; serum phospholipid appears to have little or no function in blood clotting. Certain coagulation factors, such as factor V_a and factor X_a, can be concentrated on platelet membrane surfaces [151, 152]. The demonstration that factor V_a is the binding site for factor X_a requires that platelets be treated initially with thrombin or that the platelet membrane become altered by agents that promote the "release reaction" such that platelet membrane factor V is converted to V_a [152, 162] (see Chap. 71). Recent findings show that factor V-deficient patients have diminished factor X_a binding to their platelets, and it now appears fairly conclusive that the factor X_a receptor on platelets is indeed factor V_a [163]. In the presence of platelets and sufficient calcium ion, the conversion of prothrombin to thrombin by X_a is accelerated about a hundred thousandfold when compared to the rate of thrombin generation in a strictly plasma system [164]. Most likely, this is explained by the exposed negatively charged phospholipids in altered platelet membranes serving as the surface on which several of the clotting factors become concentrated for participation in this series of reactions.

Conversion of Fibrinogen to Fibrin

Thrombin Thrombin does not circulate, being the end product of the succession of cleavages of prothrombin as described above. Three recent reviews provide in-depth information about this proteinase [165–167]. The primary enzymatic product of prothrombin activation, α-thrombin, has a molecular weight of 39,000 and is composed of a 28,500-dalton heavy chain (B′ chain) disulfide-linked to a 3500-dalton light chain (A chain) that contains the active site serine [168, 169]. α-Thrombin undergoes autolysis to β-thrombin and then γ-thrombin, neither of which has much fibrinogen clotting activity, although both cleave small synthetic substrates. Although thrombin hydrolyzes a variety of synthetic substrates, it has a fairly restricted specificity and cleaves relatively few proteins. The proteolytic activity of thrombin does not depend on other cofactors, such as calcium ion or phospholipid. Thrombin functions in the clotting system in several ways. (1) It directly promotes platelet aggregation and generates specific binding sites on platelet surfaces, an example being the conversion of membrane-bound factor V to factor V_a, which then binds factor X_a. (2) It cleaves both plasma factor V and factor VIII, initially enhancing and subsequently leading to inactivation of both activities. (3) It cleaves the amino-terminal peptide from the catalytic subunit of zymogen factor XIII. (4) It cleaves two pairs of arginyl-glycyl bonds to allow the release of amino-terminal peptides from the fibrinogen molecule to form fibrin monomer, which then polymerizes into a gel. (5) Finally, a more recent function for thrombin, the physiologic importance of which is not yet understood, is the cleavage of the precursor form of the plasma protein, protein C, to its active serine proteinase form when bound to endothelial cell surfaces (see the section "Protein C and Protein S").

The activity of thrombin is readily inhibited by diisopropyl fluorophosphate and even more rapidly and specifically by dansylarginine-4-ethylpiperidine amide [170]. Hirudin, a naturally occurring basic protein derived from leech saliva, virtually instantaneously inhibits thrombin by binding to regions of the thrombin molecule other that the active site [171]. Similarly, certain physiologic plasma inhibitors, most notably antithrombin III, inactivate thrombin by forming a 1:1 stoichiometric complex that is essentially irreversible; this reaction is potentiated by heparin (see the section "Antithrombin III"). Thrombin is also inhibited to some extent by α_2-macroglobulin [172]. In this reaction, two molecules of thrombin are presumed to bind per one molecule of α_2-macroglobulin [173]. Lastly, thrombin activity is also restricted due to its removal from the plasma milieu by binding to polymerizing fibrin [174].

Fibrinogen Fibrinogen is made by the liver, each polypeptide chain being synthesized by the hepatocyte [175]. Since the plasma level of fibrinogen responds to a variety of stimuli, fibrinogen is considered an acute phase reactant. The content of fibrinogen in human plasma is about 1.5 to 4.0 mg/ml. It has a molecular weight of 340,000 and is composed of three pairs of identical subunit polypeptides, termed Aα *chain* (68,000 daltons), Bβ *chain* (57,000 daltons), and γ *chain* (47,000 daltons) [176]. Virtually all of the amino acid sequence is now completed, including placement of disulfide bonds [177]. The

subunit chains are joined by disulfide bonds such that the fibrinogen molecule has a dimeric structure, the two halves also being disulfide-linked; its subunit formula may be written as $[A\alpha B\beta\gamma]_2$. As is evident in Fig. 70-3, electron-microscopic studies show fibrinogen to be composed of three nodular structures that are arranged linearly to form a molecule about 45 nm long [178, 179]. Following incubation with plasmin, the isolated terminal digestion products of fibrinogen show that the central nodule, which contains the amino-terminal region of fibrinogen, is fragment E, and that the outer two nodules constitute the fragment D regions [179].

Thrombin initially cleaves fibrinopeptide A from each of the two Aα chains, giving rise to a fibrin monomer with the subunit formula $[\alpha B\beta\gamma]_2$. This intermediate form of fibrin monomer aligns in a two-molecule-thick, staggered half-overlap arrangement, the net effect of which is the production of an elongated fibrin strand termed a *protofibril* [180, 181]. During this process, the cleavage of fibrinopeptide B by thrombin is facilitated, presumably by making a specific arginyl-glycyl bond more accessible [180]. This results in a fibrin monomer with the subunit formula $[\alpha\beta\gamma]_2$. The cleavage of fibrinopeptide B allows a rapid alignment of the protofibrils into large fibers that quickly form a gel [182]. Figure 70-4 provides a schematic of fibrin polymerization as deduced by electron microscopy. At this stage, the polymerized fibrin is soluble in a variety of dispersing reagents, such as 1 percent monochloroacetic acid or 5 M urea [183]. Under normal conditions in vivo, thrombin simultaneously cleaves a pair of amino-terminal fibrinopeptides from factor XIII (see the section "Factor XIII"), which, in the presence of calcium ion, catalyzes the formation of ε-lysyl-γ-glutamyl isopeptide bonds between spe-

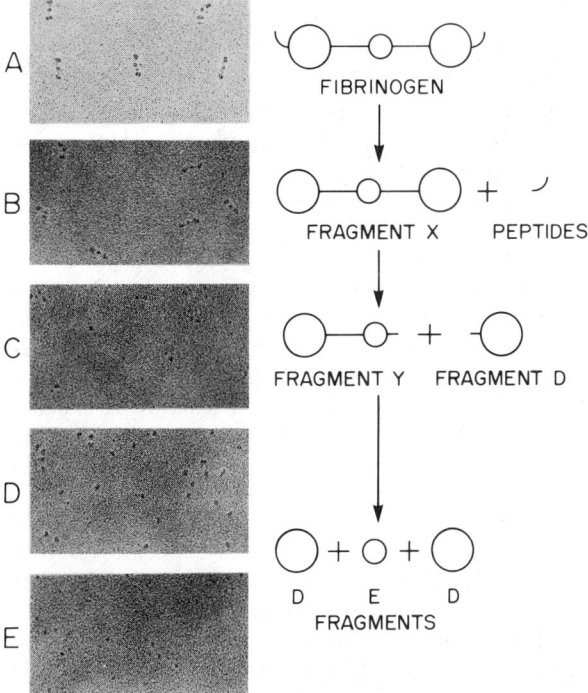

Figure 70-3 Electron microscopy of fibrinogen (panel A) and the order of its cleavage by plasmin. The first product, fragment X (panel B), retains the trinodular structure since the initial plasmic cleavages remove only carboxyl terminal peptides, as depicted in the accompanying schematic diagram. An asymmetric cleavage then occurs to produce fragment Y (panel C) and fragment D (panel D). Lastly, fragment Y is cleaved to yield another fragment D and the central nodule, fragment E (panel E). Magnification × 150,000. (*Adapted from Fowler et al.* [179].)

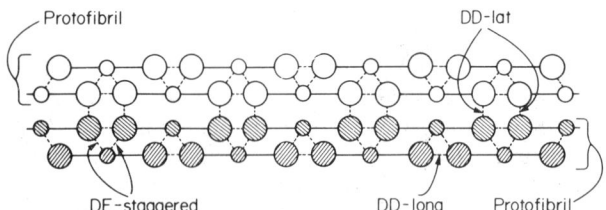

Figure 70-4 Model of fibrin polymerization. Each fibrin monomer is represented by a trinodular rodlike structure (see Fig. 70-3). Two protofibrils are indicated, each consisting of two strands with a twofold screw symmetry. The two contacts that give rise to protofibril formation are identified as *DD-long*, indicating end-to-end elongation, and *DD-staggered*, the latter being the stronger bond. These two types of contacts are completely saturated within the protofibril except for the two ends. The interaction of two protofibrils occurs by lateral association and probably involves binding between D nodules, as indicated by *DD-lat*. The two protofibrils are not coplanar, but instead are arranged around three- or fourfold axes to form a three-dimensional lattice. (*Adapted with permission of HP Erickson [375].*)

cific lysine donor and glutamine acceptor groups of different fibrin monomers. The first intermolecular crosslinks are catalyzed between glutamine and lysine residues that are 14 and 6 residues, respectively, from the carboxyl terminus of neighboring γ chains of fibrin monomers abutting end-to-end in the protofibril [176, 181]. This crosslinking reaction results in a pair of ε-lysyl-γ-glutamyl crosslinks between two fibrin monomers. The γ chain crosslinking reaction occurs very rapidly, while the second series of crosslinks forms more slowly between specific glutamine and lysine groups on the α chains of different fibrin monomers [183]. At least one, but sometimes two, pairs of crosslinks are formed per α chain as α polymerization proceeds [184]. The spatial arrangement of the donor and acceptor groups within the γ chain do not allow for more than dimerization; but in the α chain, the one or two donor groups are much farther from the one or two acceptor groups so that each α chain crosslinks with more than one fibrin monomer [184]. The total of four to six pairs of ε-amino-γ-glutamyl crosslinks shared by each fibrin monomer with other fibrin monomers adds to the tensile strength of fully polymerized fibrin and simultaneously makes it resistant to proteolysis by enzymes such as plasmin [185]. As fibrin forms, some thrombin becomes adsorbed to it, and this may be one of the mechanisms for removing thrombin from solution [174].

Fibrinogen is also contained in platelets, but its precise function remains unknown. As discussed elsewhere (see Chap. 71), fibrinogen binds to activated platelets and probably is the agent most responsible for platelets sticking to each other in many of the platelet aggregation reactions [186].

Factor XIII   The total content of blood factor XIII is about evenly divided between plasma and platelets [187]. The exact site of synthesis of factor XIII has not been established. Human plasma factor XIII has a concentration of about 20 μg/ml [188]. Factor XIII has been the subject of two recent extensive reviews [188, 189]. The zymogen form has a molecular weight of 320,000 and is composed of two pairs of noncovalently bound subunits, termed a and b, to give the subunit formula a_2b_2 [185]. The molecular weight of the a subunit is 75,000, while that of the b subunit is 88,000 [185]. Each of the a chains contains a catalytically active-site cysteine [190]. The b chains, which do not participate in the reactions of factor XIII$_a$, appear to prolong the survival of the a_2 dimer in the circulation. Thrombin converts factor XIII zymogen to an intermediate, preactivated form by cleaving an amino-terminal peptide of about 4000 daltons from each of the a chains. The

thrombin-modified factor XIII now has the subunit formula a'_2b_2 and is designated *factor XIII'*. Calcium is required for the expression of enzymatic activity of factor XIII' [191]. It binds to the catalytically active a' subunits and causes the dissociation of the a'_2 and b_2 dimers with the simultaneous exposure of the active-site cysteine in each a' subunit. Since the rate of this conversion is maximal at 10 mM calcium, it is conjectured that the normal plasma concentration of ionized calcium of 1.5 mM is partially responsible for controlling the expression of factor XIII activity. Recently, plasma fibrinogen has been identified as modulating the activity of factor XIII' by reducing the amount of calcium ion required for the a'_2b_2 to a'_2 (factor XIII$_a$) transition [192]. A specific domain on the Aα chain of the fibrinogen molecule appears responsible for this regulatory function [193]. Factor XIII$_a$ (a'_2) reacts with the γ-carboxyl of specific glutamine residues (acceptor groups) in fibrin monomer to form a γ-glutamyl-S-ester bond which undergoes amino lysis and reacts with the ε-amino group of specific lysine residues (donor groups). Ammonia is released and ε-(γ-glutamyl) lysyl peptide crosslinks are formed. As a consequence of this reaction, a variety of radiolabeled or fluorescent amino compounds have been used as synthetic donor groups for developing quantitative assays for factor XIII activity [194].

Platelet factor XIII zymogen has a molecular weight of 179,000 and consists of two a subunits that are identical to the subunits of plasma factor XIII [185]. Platelet factor XIII is made in megakaryocytes and is found in the platelet cytosol, but not in the various granules [195]. Platelet and plasma factor XIII do not exchange. The latter is not secreted during the platelet release reaction [196]. Just as with plasma factor XIII, thrombin cleaves the amino-terminal peptide from each a chain, and calcium ion is required for exposure of the active-site sulfhydryl group on each a' chain in the resultant factor XIII$_a$.

Besides catalyzing the formation of fully stabilized, crosslinked fibrin (see the section "Fibrinogen"), factor XIII$_a$ catalyzes ε-lysyl-γ-glutamyl crosslinks between fibrin and other proteins. For example, the resistance of fully stabilized fibrin to plasmin digestion may be due in part to the crosslinking of α$_2$-antiplasmin into the fibrin network without affecting its plasmin-inhibiting activity [197]. Platelet myosin and actin are also substrates for factor XIII$_a$ and become crosslinked to fibrin, thereby providing a mechanism for the covalent attachment of disrupted platelet masses to the fibrin clot [198, 199]. Fibronectin, the protein on the surface of several cell types, is also a substrate for factor XIII$_a$, leading to the suggestion that the crosslinking of fibrin to fibronectin on fibroblast membranes is important for normal wound healing [200]. Factor XIII$_a$ also catalyzes ε-lysyl-γ-glutamyl crosslinks between fibronectin and collagen [201]. There are a variety of transglutaminases in other tissues, most notably the skin and liver, which will also crosslink fibrin in vitro [202]. These are not important to blood clotting and have no identity with factor XIII other than their activity.

New Blood Coagulation Proteins

Protein C and Protein S   Protein C is a vitamin K–dependent protein that contains γ-carboxyglutamic acid groups in its amino-terminal portion [203, 204]. It is present in normal plasma as a two-chain, disulfide-linked zymogen in a concentration of about 5 μg/ml. Activation of protein C by thrombin occurs by proteolytic cleavage of a small peptide from its heavy chain [205]. During normal blood clotting, little protein C becomes activated [205], Recent data suggest that thrombin binds to a specific site on endothelial cells such that it retains activity toward protein C [206]. Once activated, protein C behaves in blood as an anticoagulant due to its ability to inactivate factor V and factor VIII [207, 208]. Interestingly, the activated forms of factors V and VIII are inactivated more rapidly [95, 207, 208]. It now seems apparent that another plasma protein, protein S, participates in these reactions as a cofactor. Protein S, which is also a vitamin K–dependent protein, but lacking in serine proteinase activity, markedly accelerates the proteolysis of factor V_a by activated protein C [209]. Activated protein C also inactivates the platelet-bound factor V_a unless it is occupied by its ligand, factor X_a [210]. Assays of plasma samples from two different families with combined factor V and VIII deficiencies indicate that their plasma lacks a normally occurring specific inhibitor to activated protein C [211] (see the section "Combined Deficiencies of Factor V and Factor VIII"). The series of reactions involving protein C and protein S are proposed to be important for inhibiting in vivo the effects of factor V_a and factor VIII_a, thereby providing a control mechanism for confining the clotting process to the site of vascular damage.

Fibrinolysis

The fibrinolytic system consists of (1) the plasma protein plasminogen, (2) a variety of activators which convert plasminogen to plasmin, (3) inhibitors of the active enzyme plasmin (see the next section), and (4) fibrin. The biochemistry of fibrinolysis has been extensively reviewed [212, 213]. Native human plasminogen circulates as a single-chain protein with a molecular weight of about 92,000 and has two states of glycosylation which result in two forms of plasminogen with slightly different molecular weights [214]. The different carbohydrate content and the minor differences in amino acid sequence probably account for the several isoelectric forms of plasminogen [215]. All forms have glutamic acid as the amino-terminal group (referred to as *Glu-plasminogen*) and asparagine as the carboxyl-terminal group [216, 217]. The complete amino acid sequence of plasminogen is known [213, 218]. Native circulating Glu-plasminogen has a plasma concentration of about 20 mg percent. Plasmin rapidly cleaves the amino-terminal 76 residues from Glu-plasminogen to give an intermediate form of plasminogen with lysine as its new amino terminus, which is referred to as *Lys-plasminogen*. This latter molecule differs significantly in many of its physical properties from Glu-plasminogen, having a molecular weight of 83,000 and a considerably looser, more open conformation [219]. In contrast to Glu-plasminogen, Lys-plasminogen binds to fibrin [220] and is activated by plasminogen activators about ten- to twentyfold more rapidly [221].

A number of proteins are known to convert either Glu-plasminogen or Lys-plasminogen to the active enzyme, plasmin. As mentioned earlier, fibrinolysis may be initiated as a consequence of factor XII (Hageman factor)-dependent activation of the contact system of blood coagulation. It is through this pathway that kallikrein and factor XI_a are generated, either of which slowly converts plasminogen to plasmin [45, 62]. Urokinase, an enzyme synthesized in the human kidney and excreted in the urine, is a serine protease which rapidly catalyzes the cleavage of an arginyl-valinyl bond within a disulfide loop

of Glu-plasminogen or Lys-plasminogen to give a disulfide-linked heavy- and light-chain enzyme [214, 222]. The active-site serine is contained in the light chain of plasmin. Initially, Glu-plasmin autocatalytically cleaves the amino-terminal peptide bond in the Glu-plasmin heavy chain to give Lys-plasmin. Either Glu-plasmin or Lys-plasmin can cleave the amino-terminal peptide in any Glu-plasminogen not yet activated to yield intermediate Lys-plasminogen, which is then more rapidly activated to Lys-plasmin [221]. Plasmin will not cleave the arginyl-valinyl activation bond in either Glu-plasminogen or Lys-plasminogen to form plasmin.

Streptokinase (SK), a product of β-hemolytic streptococci, also promotes conversion of plasminogen to plasmin, but through distinctly novel biochemical interactions. SK itself has no proteolytic activity and does not cleave any synthetic substrate. There are two important steps in the series of reactions between plasminogen and SK [223, 224]. Initially plasminogen forms a 1:1 stoichiometric complex with SK so that the conformation of plasminogen is altered and its active site exposed. The complex, now possessing enzyme activity, can intramolecularly cleave the activation peptide bond within the SK·Glu-plasminogen complex to generate SK Glu-plasmin complexes. This small amount of plasmin cleaves the amino-terminal peptide of Glu-plasminogen in the SK·Glu-plasminogen complex to SK·Lys-plasminogen, which then undergoes intramolecular activation and yields SK·Lys-plasmin. The most stable form of plasminogen activator is the SK·Lys-plasmin complex. Only catalytic levels of the equimolar complexes—SK·Lys-plasmin, SK·Glu-plasmin, or SK·Glu-plasminogen—are required to convert either form of free plasminogen to plasmin. While in the SK-plasmin complex, plasmin proteolytically degrades SK, but this reaction is relatively slow [225].

Plasminogen contains five very similar disulfide loops within the region of the molecule that eventually becomes the heavy chain of plasmin. These loops are highly homologous in sequence and have been termed *kringles* [218]. The first kringle, which is the most amino-terminally placed, contains a site that binds L-lysine or its analogues, ε-amino caproic acid or tranexamic acid, fairly strongly ($Kd = 320$ μM, 9 μM, and 1 μM, respectively) [226, 227]. There are also four or five weaker L-lysine binding sites with considerably lower Kd values spread among the other kringle structures. Occupancy of the weaker binding sites by lysine or its analogues causes a pronounced conformational change in Glu-plasminogen to that of the more flexible, asymmetric, Lys-plasminogen, and as a consequence, its rate of activation to plasmin is enhanced ten- to twentyfold [228]. The strong lysine binding site has little or no influence on the gross conformation of Glu-plasminogen or on its activation rate. Nevertheless, this binding site appears to be important in the binding of Lys-plasminogen to fibrin as well as for interacting with the α_2-antiplasmin inhibitor [220, 227].

Fibrin itself can stimulate the conversion of plasminogen to plasmin, presumably because plasminogen activators present in a variety of human tissues (e.g., endothelium, uterus, myocardium, prostate) have a strong affinity for fibrin [229, 230]. Consequently, when Lys-plasminogen becomes bound to the fibrin, it is juxtaposed to the tissue-derived activator so that plasmin formation as well as fibrin degradation is enhanced [230]. Plasmin degrades a variety of proteins besides fibrin. With respect to the clotting proteins, it readily digests fibrinogen in an orderly sequence to form a progression of cleavage products (termed *fibrinogen/fibrin split products*) [231]. Some of these interfere with normal fibrin formation. Similarly, plasmin proteolytically cleaves factors V and VIII to destroy quickly their procoagulant activities [99, 100]. The effects of plasmin on fibrinogen, factor V, and factor VIII become manifest only in vivo during diffuse intravascular coagulation syndromes, primary fibrinolysis, or with intravenous administration of urokinase or SK.

Plasma Proteinase Inhibitors of Blood Coagulation and Fibrinolysis

About 750 to 1000 mg/dl of human plasma protein consists of serine proteinase inhibitors such as α_1-antitrypsin, α_1-antichymotrypsin, inter-α-trypsin inhibitor, Cl^- inactivator, antithrombin III, and α_2-plasmin inhibitor [232]. Inherited deficiencies of antithrombin III or α_2-antiplasmin have been associated with thrombotic or bleeding tendencies, respectively (see the sections "Inherited Deficiency of Antithrombin III" and "α_2-Antiplasmin Deficiency"). The other proteolytic enzyme inhibitors are less specific and have a secondary role in inhibiting various blood-clotting serine proteinases or the fibrinolytic proteinase, plasmin. Probably there are other specific serine proteinase inhibitors, such as the one suggested for activated protein C [211]

Antithrombin III   Antithrombin III has a normal plasma concentration of about 23 mg/dl. It is a 63,000-dalton, single-chain polypeptide that contains 13 percent carbohydrate [142, 233]. it inhibits thrombin, factor IX_a, factor X_a, factor XI_a, factor XII_a, kallikrein, and plasmin by forming 1:1 stoichiometric proteinase-inhibitor complexes [142]. Heparin potentiates the rate of inhibition by antithrombin III of these clotting factors by several hundredfold [142, 234]. Factor VII_a is inhibited by antithrombin III only in the presence of heparin [127]. High molecular weight fractions of heparin are reported to have higher anticoagulant activities than low molecular weight heparin [235]. Others have observed that the anticoagulant activity of heparin fractions seems to depend on their anionic densities [236]. In keeping with this observation, the repeating unit of the heparin molecule that has the highest affinity for antithrombin III is an octasaccharide unit in which the glucosamine residues at positions 4 and 6 are N-sulfated [237]. The absence of either one of these N-sulfate groups results in a decreased binding affinity and anticoagulant activity. The mechanism by which heparin facilitates the inhibitory potential of antithrombin III is probably by binding to one or more positively charged lysine residues in the carboxylterminal region of antithrombin III to cause a rapid conformational change in antithrombin III [142]. A tryptophan residue is also in this region, and its availability is critical for heparin binding [238]. A covalent bond forms between a reactive-site arginine in the antithrombin III molecule and the active-center serine of the proteinase. This bond is essentially irreversible in vitro. The fact that hydroxylamine or dilute sodium hydroxide will reverse the proteinase-antithrombin III interaction suggests that the bond is a carboxylic ester linkage [239]. Indirect evidence from animal experiments suggests that the proteinase-antithrombin III complexes are cleared slightly faster than antithrombin III alone. In these same studies, it was evident that proteinase-antithrombin III complexes became dissociated in vivo, but not without loss of activity and structural changes in both the enzyme and antithrombin III [240].

α_2-Antiplasmin   This proteinase inhibitor has a concentration of about 7 mg/dl in plasma and circulates as a single-chain glycoprotein of 70,000 daltons [213, 231, 242]. It binds plasmin extraordinarily rapidly and strongly, having a rate constant of $3 \times 10^7 \ M^{-1} \ s^{-1}$ and a dissociation constant of about 10^{-9} [243]. Since it inhibits plasmin almost instantaneously, α_2-antiplasmin is believed to be the primary plasmin inhibitor in blood, with α_2-macroglobulin or α_2-antitrypsin participating only when α_2-antiplasmin is saturated. Plasmin reacts with α_2-antiplasmin in a two-step sequence. Initially, plasmin forms a reversible complex with α_2-antiplasmin by binding to the high affinity lysine binding site on plasmin. Then in an irreversible reaction, plasmin becomes bound to α_2-antiplasmin in a 1:1 molar ratio, concomitantly cleaving a nondisulfide-linked polypeptide of 8000 daltons. Then an ester bond forms between the new carboxyl-terminal leucine α_2-antiplasmin and the active-center serine of plasmin [244]. Plasmin activity cannot be regenerated when the ester bond is cleaved with ammonium hydroxide. Removing or blocking the high affinity lysine binding site of plasmin [228] decreases its rate of inhibition by α_2-antiplasmin about fiftyfold [220]. The adsorption of plasmin onto fibrin during fibrinolysis appears to be mediated through the same high affinity lysine binding site; hence if the lysine binding sites on plasmin are involved in binding to fibrin, then plasmin may be protected to some extent from inactivation by α_2-antiplasmin [245, 246]. At normal plasma concentrations, α_2-antiplasmin readily binds the intermediate form of plasminogen, Lys-plasminogen (see the previous section "Fibrinolysis") and inhibits about 50 percent of the binding of Lys-plasminogen to fibrin [246]. α_2-Antiplasmin has little affinity for the proteolytically active plasmin SK complex [247] (see the previous section "Fibrinolysis"). α_a-antiplasmin becomes crosslinked into fibrin as a result of catalysis by factor XIII_a, and this may be another control mechanism for modulating plasmin activity, since the crosslinked α_2-antiplasmin can still inhibit active plasmin [197]. While α_2-antiplasmin appears fairly specific for plasmin, it also inhibits trypsin. Heparin has no effect on the reactions of α_2-antiplasmin.

CLINICAL ASSESSMENT OF PATIENTS PRESENTING WITH BLEEDING

History and Physical Examination

Clearly, the medical history is important for determining if a familial bleeding pattern exists. The age of onset, type of bleeding, and sites of bleeding are important aspects. These are described further under each of the individual clotting factor deficiencies. Whether or not bleeding occurs spontaneously and whether joints are involved is helpful. Most often when the bleeding tendency is inherited, the defect is noted in infancy and recurent bleeding continues to be a problem with relatively minimal trauma. These historical data vary considerably among patients with proven blood clotting disorders. The physical examination allows assessment of whether petechiae, purpura, hematomas, or hemarthroses are present. Platelet abnormalities are more apt to be associated with petechiae and purpura, while in general, certain clotting factor deficiencies commonly cause hematomas and joint bleeding.

Laboratory Assessment

Routine coagulation screens, which include the prothrombin time and partial thromboplastin time, usually segregate the clotting defects to either the intrinsic, extrinsic, or common pathways of blood coagulation. Details of these assays are fully described elsewhere [248]. The patient's plasma must contain an adequate fibrinogen level so that fibrin endpoints can be observed in the coagulation assays. A normal thrombin time, calculated by determining the time required for the clotting of a plasma sample to which thrombin has been added, indicates an adequate fibrinogen level and a normal rate of fibrinogen conversion to fibrin. The prothrombin time assesses the extrinsic pathway and is prolonged with deficiencies of factor VII, factor X, factor V, and prothrombin, assuming a normal level of fibrinogen and the lack of a specific inhibitor to any of these factors. The partial thromboplastin time is often calculated as an activated partial thromboplastin time, kaolin or celite powder being added to provide maximal activation of the contact components. In general, the partial thromboplastin time assesses the intrinsic pathway and is prolonged with deficiencies of factors XII, XI, IX, VIII, X, V, or prothrombin. If there are deficiencies common to both the extrinsic and intrinsic systems, then both the prothrombin time and the partial thromboplastin time will be prolonged, although this is not invariable. If the clotting factor deficiency can be localized to one of the pathways in the coagulation scheme, further identification can be carried out by determining whether fresh normal plasma (containing all factors), barium sulfate-adsorbed normal plasma (lacking vitamin K–dependent clotting factors), or normal serum (containing activated factors IX, X, XI, and XII, but not factors V or VIII) will correct the defect in the patient's plasma when tested by the prothrombin time or partial thromboplastin time. By various assays which contain permutations of mixtures of these reagents, the patient's defect can usually be pinpointed. In practice, clinical laboratories usually identify specific clotting factor deficiencies by testing the patient's plasma against commercially available plasmas known to have well-defined deficiencies. The prothrombin time or partial thromboplastin time is then modified slightly so that test dilutions of the patient's plasma can be compared with those of normal control plasma for the ability to correct the clotting time of a plasma with the known factor deficiency. The patient's values are then expressed as a percentage of normal control values to give an estimation of the level of clotting factor activity. Usually the levels of the clotting factors in the individual normal patients vary from 40 to 180 percent of the amount found in a plasma pool from individuals with no history of bleeding or thrombotic diseases. Additional specific laboratory assays will be mentioned as each of the inherited deficiencies is discussed.

CLINICAL ASPECTS OF INHERITED CLOTTING FACTOR DEFICIENCIES

Classic Hemophilia

Clinical Manifestatons *Classic hemophilia* is caused by a deficiency of antihemophilic factor or, officially, factor VIII [249, 250]. It afflicts 1 out of every 10,000 males and is the most frequently encountered inherited bleeding disorder. The frequency and severity of hemorrhage in hemophilic patients correlate roughly with the level of factor VIII activity in the plasma and tend to be fairly similar in family members. Approximately half of the men with hemophilia have recurrent, severe joint hemorrhages that eventually result in deformity and crippling. These patients ordinarily have factor VIII levels less than 5 percent of normal, often less than 1 percent. The other half of hemophilic patients have factor VIII levels 5 to 20 percent of the average normal individual and have a less severe bleeding tendency. Some have virtually no clinical problems unless they require surgery or sustain significant trauma. Bleeding is unusual at birth, even from the umbilical cord, since the extrinsic pathway of clotting is intact. Bleeding may follow circumcision—a fact noted in the third century A.D. Talmud by a rabbi who advised that boys whose brothers bled from circumcision might be exempted from this ritual [251]. If the hemophilic defect is particularly severe, soft tissue hematomas may occur during infancy, but usually the bleeding episodes are more obvious and disturbing as the child becomes physically active and progresses from crawling to walking. Bleeding occurs frequently in the large joints, such as the elbows, knees, and ankles. The joints of the wrists and hands are less often involved but sometimes do become severely deformed by recurrent hemarthrosis. The patient experiences considerable pain with hemarthroses, mostly as a consequence of joint capsule expansion. Eventually the ends of long bones become eroded and periosteal pain, necrosis, and pseudocyst formation become chronic problems. Intraosseous hemorrhage or intramuscular hemorrhage immediately adjacent to long bones can give rise to firm, laminated fibrous masses that erode bone and are essentially inseparable from contiguous tissue. These are called *pseudotumors*, and sometimes the pain and tissue destruction associated with them require that they be removed surgically [249]. Fairly severe hematomas may occur in any of the muscles and soft tissues. This is of particular concern when they occur in the thigh muscles or retroperitoneal musculature, where blood loss may be difficult to diagnose. Essentially any anatomic area can be involved with hemorrhage in the hemophilic patient. All varieties of gastrointestinal hemorrhage have been observed. Hematuria is common. Central nervous system hemorrhage occurs occasionally, but usually following trauma. Much of the bleeding in these patients seems to develop spontaneously and appears in clusters, the patient frequently being unable to associate trauma as a cause. Often he is aware that the tendency to hemorrhage spontaneously is associated with periods of mental stress. All types of surgery, including dental extractions, can be accompanied by significant blood loss, even in those with a mild to moderate deficiency.

Diagnosis The bleeding pattern of the patient, the family history, and the physical examination can give important information for establishing the diagnosis. Except for the partial thromboplastin time, other laboratory tests of coagulation are normal. The whole blood clotting time is usually prolonged in moderate to severe classic hemophilia but may be normal despite a clinically significant deficiency of factor VIII. The prothrombin time is normal, but the partial thromboplastin time is prolonged. The definitive diagnosis is made by showing that dilutions of the patient's plasma do not correct the defect in the plasma from persons with known classic hemophilia. Hemophilia can be confused with von Willebrand's disease, but the latter can be excluded if both bleeding time and ristocetin-induced platelet aggregation are normal [252]. The performance of laboratory tests on other family members may help define the inheritance pattern. At the time of diagnosis the presence of a circulating factor VIII inhibitor should be excluded as an explanation for deficient factor VIII function.

Treatment Depending on the medical history, the degree of physical impairment, and the plasma level of factor VIII, the patient is guided into a lifestyle commensurate with the severity of his disease. Therefore the patient and his family must be educated about hemophilia, the immediate management of bleeding episodes, the overall prognosis with respect to future lifestyle, and the genetics of the disorder. As a child, the patient requires more than the usual protection from accidental trauma until he understands the constraints imposed upon him by his disease. Often the parents seem to vacillate between overprotection and, perhaps as a denial mechanism, unwitting encouragement for participation in dangerous activities by their child. Despite knowing better, the adolescent or child sometimes insists on indulging in risk-taking behavior [253]. Patients who have only mild to moderate hemophilia may participate in noncontact sports and lead a fairly normal, active existence. By adulthood, the patient is usually familiar with all the nuances of his disease and understands better his own behavior. He should be encouraged to develop his education and interests as fully as possible and should not be limited in career choice so long as he is not exposed to unnecessary risks.

Bleeding episodes are managed by administering commercially prepared lyophilized factor VIII concentrates or factor VIII-rich plasma cryoprecipitate [250]. The latter is prepared by freezing fresh normal plasma at −90°C followed by thawing at 4°C [254]. About 30 to 50 percent of the factor VIII contained in the plasma forms a mucoid precipitate which is collected by centrifugation and stored frozen at −20 to −90°C. The supernatant plasma is returned to the cells for transfusions when red cell administration is the primary goal. Just before use, the cryoprecipitate, which now contains factor VIII concentrated five- to tenfold compared to plasma, is thawed at 37°C and given intravenously. The use of cryoprecipitate or other forms of factor VIII concentrate avoids overtransfusing with large volumes of plasma that would be required to attain therapeutic levels of factor VIII activity. The extent of replacement therapy depends on (1) the severity and site of hemorrhage; (2) the plasma level of factor VIII estimated to be needed for halting the hemorrhage; (3) the content of factor VIII in the concentrate to be given; (4) the half-life of the infused factor VIII; and (5) whether or not the patient has an inhibitor to factor VIII. Early hemarthrosis or hematuria can be managed by maintaining a plasma factor VIII level at 25 to 50 percent of normal for 2 to 3 days. Muscle hematomas need a longer period of sustained factor VIII levels, usually about 40 percent of normal for 4 to 6 days. Serious trauma requires factor VIII levels in excess of 40 percent for about 2 weeks. Major surgery should be performed only after sufficient factor VIII concentrate has been given to raise the level to 70 percent of normal. Then, postoperatively, a level of about 50 percent of normal is maintained for 2 to 3 weeks. It is difficult to establish firm guidelines about when factor VIII therapy can be stopped following a bleeding episode or after major surgery, but usually factor VIII concentrates are continued for about 2 days after cessation of any evidence of bleeding.

The amount of factor VIII concentrate to be given is esti-

mated by knowing that a normal plasma volume is about 40 ml per kilogram of body weight; that 1 ml normal plasma contains 1 unit of factor VIII activity; and that the factor VIII protein has a half-life in the circulation of about 10 to 12 h [255]. Infusions are usually given twice a day, and calculations are made to ensure that the plasma level before the next infusion will be adequate to maintain hemostasis. The factor VIII activity units on vials of commercially prepared lyophilized concentrates of factor VIII can be used to guide therapy. If bleeding persists despite replacement therapy, the patient may not be receiving sufficient factor VIII, or the factor VIII concentrate may have less activity than usual, or the patient has developed an inhibitor to factor VIII.

Joint bleeding poses a continuing problem with respect to both acute and chronic consequences [249]. Acutely, it is helpful to apply ice packs to decrease swelling and discomfort of the joint. An immediate infusion of factor VIII concentrate is given to raise the level to about 50 percent of normal, which is sometimes sufficient to stop the bleeding. Hemarthroses are not aspirated unless such acute pain and tension are present that pressure necrosis becomes a major possibility. Importantly, factor VIII concentrates must be given prior to any efforts at aspiration. Splinting or wrapping a hemarthrosis with elastic bandages makes the patient more comfortable and helps position the joint so that maintenance of function is optimized. In some medical centers synovectomies and artificial joint replacement are being done on patients who have severe chronic joint deformities. These are usually performed by an orthopedist who specializes in such procedures and then only in conjunction with a physician who is an expert in managing replacement therapy.

The patient must receive regular dental examinations by a dentist familiar with the care of hemophilic patients. As a rule, all dental procedures, including the filling of dental caries, should be done only after giving factor VIII concentrates. In severe hemophilia, the administration of one bag of cryoprecipitate for each 4 kg body weight, followed by oral administration of 4 g ε-aminocaproic acid every 4 h for 10 days is recommended [256]. In patients who have only mild to moderate hemophilia, minimal dental manipulations have been performed after giving ε-aminocaproic acid by mouth just before the procedure and afterward [257]. This is usually done in centers specializing in the care of hemophilia or by dentists who are particularly knowledgeable about the disorder.

Pain is a frequent complaint, especially joint pain. It is essential that aspirin be avoided because of its effects on platelet interactions. Acetaminophen and codeine are probably the best choice of analgesic drugs. Narcotics should be used as infrequently as possible because of the risk of addiction in those patients who have regular bouts of joint pain.

Home treatment programs have been developed in many university medical centers or clinics in large cities [249]. In 1980, the 22 comprehensive hemophilia centers in the United States treated about 5,500 hemophiliacs, or half the known total. The average annual cost of health care for each patient in a center was approximately $5,300. Unemployment among patients treated at the centers has been reduced from 36 to 13 percent [258]. These programs clearly allow the patient a fuller life with far less hospitalization and requirement for acute medical care [249]. The patient and his family are taught how to give intravenous infusions of lyophilized factor VIII concentrates on any suspicion or evidence of bleeding, particularly into joints. Whenever possible, it is essential that the patient be introduced to and encouraged to participate in home- or self-care programs.

The major complications of moderately severe and severe hemophilia are progressive joint deformity and crippling, the development of inhibitors to factor VIII activity, and hepatitis [259]. The latter two complications probably correlate loosely with the frequency of replacement therapy. Factor VIII inhibitors occur in about 15 percent of patients with severe hemophilia and have no known cause [260, 261]. In most instances, these patients have been the recipients of numerous infusions of cryoprecipitate or other factor VIII concentrates and have manifested the inhibitor since childhood. Once developed, the inhibitor usually continues as a periodic problem throughout life. Replacement therapy may become so ineffective that catastrophic hemorrhage results. Factor VIII inhibitors are IgG immunoglobulins that do not fix complement. The presence of an inhibitor is detected by mixing the patient's plasma with an equal quantity of normal plasma and observing that the partial thromboplastin time remains prolonged, since the capacity of normal plasma to correct the deficiency of factor VIII is blocked by the patient's inhibitor. For minor bleeding episodes, efforts are made to effect hemostasis without requiring factor VIII replacement. When hemorrhaging is severe, large amounts of factor VIII concentrate must be given to overcome the inhibitor. If the inhibitor level is so high that the amount of factor VIII is prohibitive, then plasmapheresis or exchange transfusion may lower the inhibitor level so that it can be neutralized by factor VIII replacement therapy. In countries where they are approved for use, porcine factor VIII concentrates have been used since some human inhibitors have no activity toward them. Immunosuppressive therapy has not been very successful.

In general, even patients with severe hemophilia can now expect a fairly bright future, especially with the availability of home-care treatment programs and factor VIII concentrates. Life expectancy has been prolonged, but to what extent is not clear. Hemorrhage continues to be a major cause of death.

Genetics   The inheritance pattern of the disorder is X-linked, with about 70 percent of patients having a positive family history. Hence, hemophilia occurs only in males except in the remote event that a homozygous female results from the mating of a hemophilic male and female carrier or in the case of extreme lyonization [262]. The locus for the hemophilic gene is near those determining deuteran color blindness [263] and glucose-6-phosphate dehydrogenase synthesis [264]. Both CRM$^+$ and CRM$^-$ forms of hemophilia have been described. It appears that factor VIII deficiency is a true deficiency since about 90 percent of patients have less than 10 percent of the expected level of factor VIII coagulant antigen by immunoradiometric assay [265–267]. Patients with mild disease tend to have antigen values that are normal and, in some instances, higher than normal. The exact definition of the breakdown between CRM$^+$ and CRM$^-$ hemophilia remains somewhat open to question since normal factor VIII protein has not been isolated and characterized, nor has its structural relationship in vivo with the large, complex von Willebrand protein been defined. The latter must be considered with respect to the accessibility of a specific antibody to the factor VIII procoagulant protein.

The daughters of the patient with hemophilia will be carriers, but all his sons will be normal. A carrier woman is a true genetic mosaic, having a 50 percent chance of producing a hemophilic son and 50 percent chance of producing a normal son. Ordinarily her cells will consist of two populations, one containing a normal and the other an abnormal X chromosome. Since one X chromosome is randomly and irreversibly inactivated in each cell prior to implantation of the embryo, most carrier women should have about 50 percent of the normal level of factor VIII activity. In fact, the broad range of factor VIII levels found among carriers must reflect a disproportionate inactivation of one X chromosome, perhaps earlier than usual, so that its frequency in the developing zygote is much less than the frequency of the other X chromosome. This presumably accounts for the finding of essentially normal factor VIII levels in some carriers, while others have levels low enough to be commensurate with the diagnosis of hemophilia [262].

Obligate carriers of the hemophilic gene are daughters of men with the disorder, mothers of more than one hemophiliac, or mothers who have a hemophilic son and another hemophilic male relative in their pedigree. Since only about 15 percent of the instances of hemophilia are estimated to occur by spontaneous mutation, detection of carriers assumes importance. The measurement of factor VIII procoagulant activity is not sensitive enough to identify more than about one-half of proven carriers [268, 269]. Potential carriers of the hemophilic gene can be identified with approximately 90 percent accuracy by applying logarithmic discriminate analysis to the results of simultaneously performed measurements of factor VIII procoagulant level, and the concentration of factor VIII-like protein detected by heterologous antiserum from the Laurell method of semiquantitative immunoelectrophoresis [268]. In the carrier state, the ratio of factor VIII procoagulant activity and the concentration of factor VIII-like antigen are disproportionately lower when compared to the same values in normal women. Surprisingly, few women at risk for being a carrier seek this information; even more surprising is the number of proven carriers who continue to risk conception or choose to complete their pregnancy [270]. The intrauterine diagnosis of hemophilia appears possible. This method requires a fetal blood sample obtained from the umbilical vein by a skilled fetoscopist. Then, by the use of an immunoradiometric measurement of factor VIII coagulant antigen, the diagnosis appears possible most of the time since the majority of severe hemophilia patients are CRM$^-$ [79, 271, 272].

von Willebrand's Disease

This bleeding disorder, described in 1926 by the physician Erik Adolph von Willebrand [273], is due to a deficiency of the plasma glycoprotein known as *von Willebrand factor*. This glycoprotein is required for the normal adherence of platelets to sites of vascular injury and possibly for the aggregation of platelets to surface-adherent platelets. The disorder is inherited as an autosomal codominant defect, and for reasons unknown, it is observed more frequently in women than men. As indicated in the section dealing with the biochemistry of this clotting factor, poorly understood structural relationships exist between factor VIII and the von Willebrand protein that cause these two activities to circulate in normal plasma as a complex protein. Von Willebrand's disease has a broad spectrum of clinical and laboratory features which include low levels of factor VIII procoagulant activity. Hence the diagnosis of von Willebrand's disease must be considered in the differential diagnosis of classic hemophilia, and vice versa. Unlike hemophilia, the severity of symptoms in von Willebrand's disease varies considerably among afflicted family members. Usually only homozygotes manifest severe bleeding. In heterozygotes, the hemorrhagic tendency is often asymptomatic or so mild that it becomes manifest only with trauma, surgery, or dental extractions. Women with the disorder experience excessive menses and postpartum bleeding. Gastrointestinal bleeding is common, whereas joint hemorrhage occurs rarely. The frequency and severity of bleeding in patients with this disorder tend to lessen with age, but the reason for this is unknown.

Genetics   For some time it has been proposed that as many as five variant forms of von Willebrand's disease exist, but recently this notion has been challenged. Serial laboratory tests in over 50 persons from 27 families with von Willebrand's disease suggest strongly that variability in test values over time probably accounts for the proposed "variant" forms of the disease [252, 274]. Only in the homozygous state were the bleeding time, factor VIII procoagulant activity, von Willebrand factor antigen level, and von Willebrand factor-ristocetin cofactor activity consistently below normal. These patients have clinically severe bleeding and essentially no detectable von Willebrand antigen. Factor VIII procoagulant activity and factor VIII procoagulant antigen are always detectable [265, 266, 275]. Consanguinity is often present in the families of these patients. The von Willebrand protein is not present in endothelial cells of these patients [276]. Occasionally after replacement infusions, the homozygote with von Willebrand's disease will develop antibodies that precipitate von Willebrand factor and inhibit both ristocetin cofactor activity and factor VIII procoagulant activity [227].

The clearest and most readily accepted laboratory criterion for von Willebrand's disease in the heterozygote is the combination of a prolonged bleeding time, a low level of factor VIII procoagulant activity, decreased factor VIII/von Willebrand antigen, and impaired platelet aggregation in response to ristocetin. About 80 percent of von Willebrand patients manifest abnormalities in these four laboratory values. In addition, the sodium dodecyl sulfate-agarose electrophoresis of plasma shows a generalized decrease in the concentration of all sizes of the von Willebrand protein multimers [79, 114]. This form of the disease is termed *type I*.

Most agree that about 15 percent of patients with symptoms of von Willebrand's disease have a second form of the disorder that is characterized by slightly low or normal factor VIII procoagulant activity, normal levels of factor VIII/von Willebrand antigen, a prolonged bleeding time, and impaired ristocetin-induced platelet aggregation. These patients lack the large forms of the von Willebrand protein and have an increased amount of the small antigenic forms [79, 278]. These patients are classified as type IIA. Other combinations and permutations of abnormal laboratory assays are less frequently encountered in patients who present with bleeding and most probably represent variability in the manifestations of the two forms of the disease. A few patients with clinical features of von Willebrand's disease have been noted to have the unusual combination of a prolonged bleeding time and low factor VIII procoagulant activity, but an increased platelet aggregation response to ristocetin [279]. These are categorized as type IIB. Whether they truly have von Willebrand's disease has been challenged by data suggesting that they may have both an abnormal factor VIII/von Willebrand protein and a platelet membrane defect [280]. These observations require further definition.

Interestingly, intravenous infusions of small amounts of normal plasma, cryoprecipitate, hemophilic plasma, or normal serum into the von Willebrand patient cause a delayed increase in factor VIII procoagulant activity that is out of proportion to the content of factor VIII in the transfused plasma or serum [281, 282]. The transfused factor VIII/von Willebrand protein disappears with the usual half-life of 10 to 14 h, and despite the prolonged elevation in the level of factor VIII procoagulant activity that follows, there is no concomitant increase in the level of factor VIII/von Willebrand protein. These observations have been repeated numerous times but still are not understood. They have been interpreted as suggesting the presence of a tropinlike substance in the transfused plasma or serum that stimulates the production or release of factor VIII procoagulant activity independent of the von Willebrand entity.

Therapy   Cryoprecipitate is used to treat clinically severe bleeding. More highly purified factor VIII/von Willebrand protein concentrates such as the commercially available glycine-precipitated preparations do not correct the bleeding time defect, as will cryoprecipitate [282]. Hence, despite the fact that the lyophilized concentrates will correct the factor VIII procoagulant deficiency, bleeding may persist. The main goal of therapy should be the attainment of a normal bleeding time, but in practice this is highly variable. Most often, if bleeding is present, the amount of cryoprecipitate to be given (approximately 10 bags twice daily) is based on the restoration of acceptable levels of factor VIII procoagulant activity in the patient's plasma as well as the correction of the patient's Duke bleeding time [283]. In three patients with heterozygous von Willebrand's disease, the attainment of normal factor VIII procoagulant activity and normal levels of von Willebrand antigen in response to stress did not cause the bleeding time to become normal [284]. This suggests that the von Willebrand protein made by these patients is abnormal with respect to its role in the bleeding time. In contrast to hemophilia, the patient with von Willebrand's disease who is to have surgery should receive cryoprecipitate several hours before the operation so that a maximal rise of factor VIII procoagulant activity is achieved. Although rare, the development of antibodies to the platelet cofactor activity of the von Willebrand protein has been reported in patients with homozygous von Willebrand's disease, but not in the heterozygous forms [277]. In women with von Willebrand's disease, excessive menstrual blood loss can be managed with hormonal suppression. Levels of factor VIII procoagulant activity, von Willebrand platelet cofactor activity, and factor VIII/von Willebrand antigen may become normal during pregnancy in women with this disorder, and in spite of a prolonged bleeding time, obstetrical delivery may be performed without excessive hemorrhage [285]. Postpartum blood loss may become severe and require replacement infusions of cryoprecipitate.

Coagulation Factor Deficiencies of the Contact Activation System

Factor XII Deficiency (Hageman Trait)   This deficiency is typically found serendipitously, often as a consequence of preoperative blood coagulation screens. It is usually asymptomatic, although on occasion mild bleeding with trauma has been attributed to the lack of factor XII activity. No defects exist in the inflammatory or fibrinolytic responses. The whole blood glass clotting time and partial thromboplastin time are prolonged. Other tests of bleeding and coagulation are entirely normal. The specific diagnosis is made by observing that the unknown or test plasma will not readily correct the defect in plasma from a patient with known factor XII deficiency. Since patients with this deficiency have no bleeding diathesis, no therapy is required. The disorder is mostly a curiosity since if contact activation is lacking, one would surmise that a bleeding disorder should occur. This probably does not result because factor XI can be activated by a different mechanism [see the sections "Factor XII (Hageman Factor)" and "Factor XI"]. The level of factor XII varies from approximately 35 to 185 percent of a pool of normal plasma samples [286]. The defect is autosomal recessive [287], and about 10 percent of the patients are from consanguine matings [288]. The heterozygote has an intermediate level of factor XII activity [288, 289]. In one family the inheritance pattern appeared to be autosomal dominant [290]. The diminished factor XII activity in all patients studied so far appears to result from a true deficiency of factor XII protein since immunologic assays indicate a lack of cross-reacting material in plasma [291, 292]. Interestingly, the index patient, John Hageman, died of pulmonary embolism after pelvic fracture [293].

Prekallikrein Deficiency (Fletcher Trait) This disorder is a rare defect in blood coagulation and, like factor XII, is not accompanied by any clinical bleeding disorder. It is essentially a laboratory diagnosis that becomes suspected when the whole blood glass clotting time and partial thromboplastin time are inexplicably prolonged. If the patient's plasma is incubated with kaolin and phospholipid prior to recalcification, the activated partial thromboplastin time is restored to normal, presumably because factor XI itself gradually becomes activated as a consequence of surface contact with kaolin powder (see the section "Factor XI") [29]. The definitive diagnosis is established if the patient's plasma corrects the defect in commercially available prekallikrein-deficient plasma. Impairments of all the reactions of prekallikrein or kallikrein have been described. These include delayed clotting through the extrinsic [294] and intrinsic [295] pathway, decreased generation of bradykinin [296, 297], lessened fibrinolytic activity [295, 296], and diminished chemotactic activity [298]. Additionally, the property of plasma that is said to enhance vascular permeability is reduced [295, 296]. These defects can all be corrected by the addition of prekallikrein or kallikrein to the deficient plasma. Despite these in vitro abnormalities, the patient suffers no apparent consequences of the deficiency. Prekallikrein deficiency is inherited as an autosomal recessive disorder and appears to be a true deficiency since immunologic assays have not suggested the presence of an abnormal prekallikrein protein [297, 299].

High Molecular Weight Kininogen Deficiency (Fitzgerald, Williams, or Flaujeac Trait) This disorder is also asymptomatic and must be considered if both the glass clotting time and partial thromboplastin time are prolonged. Other clotting assays, including specific tests of factors XI, IX, and VIII activities, are normal. The diagnosis is made if the patient's plasma corrects the defects in plasma deficient in high molecular weight kininogen. Just as with the prekallikrein deficiency (see the previous section), all the functions of the contact activation pathway are diminished in patients lacking high molecular weight kininogen. Also, like patients deficient in factor XII or prekallikrein, patients who lack high molecular weight kininogen do not have a bleeding tendency as a consequence of their deficiency. The deficiency is rare and appears to be inherited as an autosomal recessive trait. The Fitzgerald trait [31, 300, 301] appears due to a functional absence of high molecular weight kininogen alone, while the index patients with Williams trait [302] or Flaujeac trait [303] are also deficient in low molecular weight kininogen. The high and low molecular weight kininogens are distinct and are not precursor-product related but, as suggested by the characterizations of the two bovine kininogens [53], low molecular weight kininogen may be similar to, if not identical with, the heavy-chain portion of high molecular weight kininogen.

Factor XI Deficiency This disorder is commonly observed in Jews of European descent and also appears to have a higher frequency in Japanese. The deficiency is inherited as an autosomal recessive trait. The heterozygous state occurs in about 2 percent of European Jews, while the homozygous state has a prevalence of 0.01 percent [304]. The homozygote usually has less than 20 percent of the average normal level of factor XI activity and may have a mild bleeding disorder that becomes evident after dental procedures, slight trauma, and surgery [304, 305]. Serious, life-threatening bleeding is seldom a problem. The heterozygote has about 50 percent of the normal level of factor XI activity and does not have a bleeding tendency [304, 305]. Laboratory tests show a prolonged whole blood glass clotting time and a prolonged partial thromboplastin time. Other blood clotting studies are usually normal, although in a few cases the bleeding time has been prolonged. The diagnosis is made by observing that the patient's plasma will correct other plasma samples with known specific deficiencies, but not plasma from factor XI-deficient patients. The management of clinically significant bleeding is relatively simple, requiring fresh plasma. Usually 1 unit is sufficient since the half-life of this factor is about 60 h.

Vitamin K–dependent Clotting Factors

Factor IX Deficiency (Christmas Disease) This disorder, also occasionally termed *hemophilia B*, is encountered about one-fifth as frequently as classic hemophilia *(hemophilia A)*. Clinically, the manifestations of the two hemophilias are indistinguishable. Both are inherited as X-linked recessive traits. Hence the disorder essentially occurs only in males. Those rare instances of females appearing to have clinically significant deficiencies of factor IX may occur as a consequence of an abnormal gene being inherited from both parents or extreme lyonization. Interestingly, a patient with Turner's syndrome has factor IX deficiency, presumably because she is a carrier who lacks a normal X chromosome [306]. Just as in classic hemophilia, patients with severe factor IX deficiency suffer frequent hemarthroses that eventually result in crippling and joint deformity. Since the prothrombin time is normal and the partial thromboplastin time is prolonged, the deficiency can be localized to the intrinsic pathway and can be further defined by showing that the patient's plasma will not correct plasma known to be deficient in factor IX. The range of factor IX activity in normal plasma is about 50 to 180 percent [64, 307]. Patients with mild factor IX deficiency have levels 5 to 30 percent of normal and are usually not bothered with joint hemorrhage. Factor IX activity levels of 1 to 5 percent may be accompanied by a history of moderate bleeding, whereas patients with less than 1 percent of factor IX activity have frequent bouts of soft tissue bleeding and hemarthroses, some of which appear to occur spontaneously [307].

GENETICS   More than half of the patients have a family history of bleeding. Occasionally the heterozygote may have a bleeding tendency, but usually she is asymptomatic [308]. The gene on the X chromosome for the synthesis of factor IX is near that for serum protein Xm and is fairly distant from that for antihemophilic factor or deuteran color blindness [309, 310]. Until recently, factor IX deficiency was thought to be due to an absence (CRM$^-$) of the factor IX protein, but now it is estimated that about 10 percent of factor IX–deficient patients have normal (CRM$^+$) levels of immunoreactive factor IX protein [64]. A few patients, designated as CRM^r, have been reported as having reduced levels of immunologically cross-reacting protein and no clotting factor activity. One of the CRM$^+$ mutants does not interact normally with phospholipid [311]. Another CRM$^+$ mutant has a prolonged partial thromboplastin time if ox brain is used as the source of lipid [312]. This abnormal factor IX has been characterized [313]. Another CRM$^+$ mutant has been shown to have delayed activation by factor XI$_a$ in the presence of calcium ion [314]. This abnormal factor IX, termed *factor IX Chapel Hill,* appears to have an amino acid substitution in the region of its second cleavage by factor XI$_a$ [315]. In the CRM^r subclass, mild factor VII deficiency has been noted [316]. In one kindred, the levels of immunoreactive factor IX increase with the patient's age but never attain normal levels.

TREATMENT   The general care of the patient and treatment of hemarthroses are the same as outlined in the section dealing with the treatment of patients with factor VIII deficiency. Replacement therapy differs substantially from that of classic hemophilia. In instances of mild bleeding, fresh frozen plasma may be used, but, due to the low concentration of factor IX in normal plasma the patient's factor IX level is seldom raised above 25 percent of normal [64]. For moderate to severe hemorrhage, such as large hemarthroses or muscle hematomas, treatment with commercially prepared factor IX concentrates should be given with the intent of raising the level of the patient's factor IX activity to 100 percent of normal [317]. Although factor IX has a half-life of 20 h, replacement therapy is given twice daily to ensure therapeutic plasma levels. Potential complications of repeated replacement therapy include hepatitis and the rare development of an antibody inhibitor to factor IX procoagulant activity [318]. Commercial lyophilized concentrates of factor IX remain relatively crude and carry a 30 to 70 percent risk for development of hepatitis [259]. Because of their variable content of factors IX$_a$ and X$_a$ and the potential for generating thrombin, these concentrates place the patient at risk for thromboembolism or diffuse intravascular coagulation [319]. It is recommended that the use of the commercial concentrates be reserved for instances in which large volumes of plasma become a major risk. Ordinarily, women who are carriers of this disorder have factor IX levels that are sufficient to effect normal hemostasis, but depending on the degree of lyonization, some carriers may bleed following trauma or surgery. Laboratory definition of the carrier state remains unreliable.

Hereditary Deficiency of Prothrombin   This disorder may occur because of either decreased or absent synthesis (hypoprothrombinemia) or the synthesis of an abnormal prothrombin that has reduced or absent activity (dysprothrombinemia). Approximately 10 patients have been reported to have hereditary hypoprothrombinemia, and all lack immunochemical evidence of prothrombin [167]. The inheritance pattern is that of an autosomal recessive trait. Consanguinity is frequently present. Heterozygotes have approximately 50 percent of the normal level of prothrombin and do not show bleeding. The severity of bleeding parallels approximately the level of prothrombin activity. Homozygotes usually have prothrombin levels about 5 to 16 percent of normal. The tendency for severe bleeding appears to develop at prothrombin levels of 1 to 2 percent of normal. Minor bleeding may occur at prothrombin values 5 to 25 percent of normal. Bleeding symptoms include subcutaneous hemorrhage, mucous membrane bleeding, and hemorrhage following trauma and surgery. Hemarthroses have been noted in patients with 1 to 6 percent of the normal prothrombin level. The diagnosis is established by specific functional and immunologic assays for prothrombin.

In the dysprothrombinemias, normal levels of immunologically reactive material are usually present [167]. In seven families, one or more members have had an abnormal prothrombin that could be separated from normal prothrombin by electrophoretic, chromatographic, or immunologic methods as well as by a variety of functional assays. Normal amounts of thrombin are not generated from these prothrombins in activation systems that contain homologous clotting factors. Other proteins and proteases, such as staphylocoagulase, trypsin, or an enzyme from *Echis carinatus* snake venom cleave different bonds in the abnormal prothrombin molecule and yield normal levels of thrombin activity. Treatment consists of transfusions of fresh frozen plasma or infusions of commercial concentrates of the vitamin K–dependent factors. The biologic half-life of prothrombin is 3 to 5 days.

Factor VII Deficiency   This disorder is the subject of two recent reviews [320, 321]. Factor VII deficiency has been reported in about 60 to 75 patients, most of whom have a history of bleeding in infancy or early childhood. The bleeding pattern varies considerably from patient to patient. Occasionally, even with marked factor VII deficiency, the bleeding tendency is barely manifest, but in some, bleeding may be severe and resemble that of classic hemophilia. Mucous membrane bleeding, epistaxis, intramuscular hemorrhage, hemarthrosis, and menorrhagia are common. Gastrointestinal bleeding occurs in about 20 percent of factor VII-deficient patients; hematuria and central nervous system bleeding are observed only occasionally. Over time the clinical manifestations of bleeding may vary from mild to severe in the same patient. Of interest are the patients who have undergone surgery without abnormal hemorrhage as well as those factor VII-deficient patients who have suffered thromboembolism [322]. Laboratory assays show the prothrombin time to be prolonged, whereas the partial thromboplastin time is normal. The latter finding need not be absolute, but the observation of a normal partial thromboplastin time excludes the possibility of factor X deficiency. In instances of a slightly lengthened partial thromboplastin time and a prolonged prothrombin time, if the clotting time of the patient's plasma in response to Russell's viper venom (directly activates factor X; called the *Stypven time*) is normal, factor X deficiency can be ruled out except in the rare instance of the abnormal factor X Friuli [323]. The definitive diagnosis is made by the inability of the patient's plasma to correct the prothrombin time defect in plasma from a person known to have factor VII deficiency. The hereditary deficiency of factor VII occurs in both women and men and is an autosomal recessive trait. The heterozygote has 25 to 75 percent of the expected normal range of factor VII activity and does not have a tendency to bleed. In homozygotes the concentration of factor VII is less than 10 percent. Patients have been reported who appear to synthesize an abnormally functioning factor VII molecule [324], while in other patients a true deficiency is present [325]. Isolated deficiencies of factor VII have been described in patients with the Dubin-Johnson, Gilbert, or Rotor hereditary defects of bilirubin metabolism [326, 327]. Treatment of bleeding is with normal plasma, not necessarily stored frozen, since factor VII activity is very stable. Commercially available concentrates of the vitamin K–dependent clotting factors obviate vascular volume overload but carry the attendant risks for thromboembolism [319] or hepatitis [259]. The half-life of factor VII is short, about 1 to 5 h, and therefore replacement infusion must be given frequently during bleeding episodes. Excessive blood loss during menses may be controlled by oral contraceptive agents.

Factor X (Stuart-Prower) Deficiency This deficiency has essentially the same clinical manifestations as factor VII deficiency, but it occurs less frequently. Consanguinity is often present in family pedigrees that show the deficiency to be inherited as an autosomal recessive trait [328, 329]. Heterozygotes do not tend to bleed, but minimal abnormalities may be noted in their clotting assays. Ordinarily, they have 20 to 50 percent of normal factor X activity levels [328]. In patients who are homozygous for factor X deficiency, the level of factor X activity is less than 10 percent of normal [330]. In some patients the disorder appears to be a true deficiency [331], while in others, protein which cross-reacts with heterologous antibody to factor X is present [332]. An abnormal factor X, termed *factor X Fruili*, has been reported in a large kindred, several members of which have a bleeding disorder [323]. Their factor X activity is low when tissue thromboplastin is used in tests to assess factor X activity, but when Russell's viper venom is used, their factor X activity is normal. Factor X antigen is present in normal levels in these patients.

The diagnosis of factor X deficiency can be suspected when both the prothrombin time and partial thromboplastin time are prolonged. Both tests become corrected when normal serum is added, but not with barium sulfate-adsorbed plasma, the latter excluding factor V deficiency. In the Stypven clotting time, Russell's viper venom, which specifically activates factor X, will clot normal plasma more quickly than factor X-deficient plasma. The latter assay distinguishes the deficiency from a lack of factor VII. The diagnosis is established definitively by the inability of plasma to correct factor X-deficient plasma. Significant hemorrhage is usually treated with fresh plasma transfusions that can be spaced somewhat since factor

X has a 2- to 3-day half-life in the circulation. Concentrates of the vitamin K–dependent factors should be avoided because of the risk of hepatitis [259] and thrombotic [319] disorders associated with their use.

Conversion of Prothrombin to Thrombin

The inherited deficiencies of this part of the coagulation scheme include both the deficiencies of factor X and prothrombin as well as the cofactor protein required for this conversion, factor V (see the section "Factor V"). This latter factor is not a vitamin K–dependent clotting factor and does not fit well in other sections. Accordingly, it will be considered alone.

Factor V Deficiency (Parahemophilia) This can be a moderately severe bleeding disorder which has clinical manifestations essentially the same as those of classic hemophilia, except that joint bleeding is rare [286, 333]. The incidence of this disorder is less than 1 in 1 million. About 60 families have been reported. All ethnic groups are affected, and males and females are affected with about equal frequency. Intermarriage in several families with factor V deficiency has been noted. Factor V deficiency is most likely inherited as an autosomal recessive trait [333, 334], but suggestions of an autosomal dominant transmission [333, 335] have been made. Immunologic results are consistent with decreased or absent synthesis of factor V protein [336, 337]. As with other clotting factor deficiencies, hemorrhage may occur in any anatomic area [333]. The severity of bleeding does not necessarily correlate with the level of factor V activity present. Bleeding may vary from mild to severe, and death from hemorrhage is known to occur. Mucous membrane bleeding is common, especially epistaxis and oropharyngeal hemorrhage after relatively minor injuries or following dental extractions. Ecchymoses are often present. Menorrhagia may be particularly troublesome, and death from hemorrhage has occurred during the first menstrual period. Some women with this deficiency have normal menses or only mild menorrhagia. In general, the tendency to have large losses of blood during menses lessens with age. Obstetrical deliveries may occur with little or no bleeding, but postpartum hemorrhage is frequent and requires replacement therapy. The laboratory diagnosis of this disorder shows that the prothrombin time is prolonged but can be corrected by the addition of fresh normal plasma from which factors IX, X, prothrombin, and factor VII have been adsorbed by barium sulfate. Normal serum lacks factor V and will not correct the deficient plasma. Because factor V functions in the reactions common to both the intrinsic and extrinsic pathways, the partial thromboplastin time may also be prolonged. A prolonged bleeding time has been reported in factor V deficiency, but it is unclear why this should occur [337].

Factor V is normally present on the surface of platelets, and when platelets are exposed to thrombin, platelet membrane-bound factor V is cleaved and becomes a specific ligand for activated factor X [152, 163]. Factor V–deficient patients lack platelet-bound factor. Evidence favors the interpretation that factor V on platelets is simply adsorbed from plasma [338].

Because of the extreme lability of human factor V in stored blood, fresh frozen plasma is used for treatment of hemorrhage. The attainment of in vivo factor V activity levels between 10 and 25 percent of normal are believed necessary to achieve adequate hemostasis during bleeding episodes or following surgery. Acceptable levels of factor V persist in fresh frozen plasma for several months. The half-life of infused factor V is estimated to be 12 to 36 h [338]. Cryoprecipitate or other commercially available lyophilized plasma concentrates are not useful since they contain little or no factor V. Circulating acquired inhibitors have been noted in a few patients after multiple transfusions [336, 338].

Conversion of Fibrinogen to Fibrin

Congenital Afibrinogenemia This disorder has been reported in approximately 130 patients and is characterized by either a total absence of plasma fibrinogen or levels less than 10 percent of normal [339, 350]. Throughout life, severe bleeding may occur and involve almost any organ system. Hemarthroses occur in 20 percent of patients [341]. Central nervous system bleeding is common. Bleeding is particularly severe following trauma and dental extractions. Although the inability to form a fibrin clot seems virtually lethal early in life, if not in utero, these patients may sometimes have long intervals between bleeding episodes. They may develop pseudocysts of bone, as occurs in hemophilia [342]. The onset of menses in girls who have afibrinogenemia may be characterized by abnormal bleeding, but instances of normal menarche are known [342]. The laboratory diagnosis of this disorder is easy since fibrin endpoints are absent in all coagulation tests. The erythrocyte sedimentation rate is zero. Defective platelet adhesion to glass and abnormalities of platelet aggregation in response to adenosine diphosphate, epinephrine, thrombin, or collagen have been reported [343–345]. Presumably fibrinogen is not available for binding to specific sites that develop on platelet membranes when exposed to added or released adenosine diphosphate (see Chap. 71). Probably as a consequence of the lack of fibrinogen to participate in platelet interactions, the bleeding time is often prolonged. Occasionally it may be normal, but the hemostatic plug is not very stable and bleeding frequently recurs. The disorder is distributed about equally between the sexes and appears to be inherited as an autosomal recessive trait [286, 339, 340]. Consanguine unions have been noted in about half the families with this disorder.

The disorder appears to be a true deficiency state. In a few instances trace amounts of fibrinogen have been observed by immunologic methods. In addition to patients classified as afibrinogenemic, there are those who have profoundly decreased fibrinogen, i.e., levels between 20 and 100 mg/dl. These patients, categorized as having hypofibrinogenemia, have milder problems with bleeding. The inheritance pattern appears to be the same as in afibrinogenemia. Occasionally the diagnosis of hypofibrinogenemia is confused with that of dysfibrinogenemia (see the next section). Some have proposed that afibrinogenemia represents the homozygous state, while hypofibrinogenemia is the heterozygous one. Definitive family studies have not been done.

The treatment of bleeding episodes is primarily with cryoprecipitate which diminishes the risk of hepatitis that accompanies the use of commercial fibrinogen concentrates from plasma pools. Ordinarily, sufficient cryoprecipitate is given to raise the plasma fibrinogen level to about 100 mg/dl, the normal range being about 200 to 400 mg/dl. Fibrinogen has a biphasic half-life in plasma. Initially, about 50 percent disappears in 2 days, and then only 15 percent disappears each day.

The prognosis for these patients is probably not very good, since they are always at risk for life-threatening hemorrhage from even modest trauma. Interestingly, three patients with afibrinogenemia died from pulmonary emboli made up of platelet masses [346, 347]. Instances of inhibitors to fibrinogen developing after transfusion therapy are known [346].

Congenital Dysfibrinogenemia In this disorder the patient has a normal or slightly depressed level of immunologically detectable fibrinogen. The clinical features are highly variable [340]. The majority of patients found to have abnormal fibrinogen are without significant histories of bleeding, and many have been recognized because of mild to moderate bleeding after surgery or trauma. The current policy is to name an abnormal fibrinogen after the city in which it was first discovered. In virtually all patient pedigrees, the defect appears to be an autosomal dominant trait. In several patients with different abnormal fibrinogens, significant normal fibrinogen has also been found, and this has led to the conclusion that dysfibrinogenemias reflect a heterozygous state [340]. Detailed laboratory studies have revealed unique molecular structural defects in some of these abnormal fibrinogens. Patients with abnormal fibrinogens characterized by a slow release of fibrinopeptides have bleeding or thrombotic tendencies [348]. Those with defective fibrin monomer gelation are usually asymptomatic. Patients with abnormal fibrinogens that do not cross-link normally when converted to fibrin sometimes have defective wound healing [349, 350]. Fibrinogen Detroit [351] has an amino acid substitution in the fibrinopeptide A Region, while fibrinogen Paris I has an extended γ-chain carboxyl-terminal sequence and does not cross-link when converted to fibrin (see the section "Fibrinogen") [352]. Several abnormal fibrinogens are cleaved extraordinarily slowly by thrombin to release the amino-terminal fibrinopeptides A and B. Other abnormal fibrinogens, despite a normal cleavage rate of fibrinopeptides, do not polymerize into a fibrin gel at a normal rate. Some are suspected of having an abnormally short half-life [353]. The majority of dysfibrinogenemic patients do not require treatment. In instances in which bleeding is occurring or can be anticipated, e.g., in surgery, it is useful to use cryoprecipitate infusions as outlined in the management of congenital afibrinogenemia.

Factor XIII (Fibrin-stabilizing Factor) Deficiency This is a rare bleeding disorder. About 100 patients have been reported [188, 354]. It occurs with equal frequency in males and females. The bleeding tendency of inherited factor XIII deficiency is often serious and can be life-threatening. The anatomic location and pattern of hemorrhage give important historical clues to the diagnosis. Bleeding is often said to be delayed, commonly occurring several hours after trauma. Initially, the ability to form normal fibrin clots does not seem to be impaired, but later these same clots become friable and dissolve at the site of injury, with attendant re-bleeding. This sequence of events is probably due to increased susceptibility of these clots to digestion by plasmin. Delayed, abnormal bleeding is usually noted from the umbilical stump during the first day of life in about 80 percent of patients with this disorder. In decreasing order, superficial bruising, subcutaneous hematomas, oral cavity hemorrhage, intracranial bleeding, muscle hematomas, and hemarthroses are sites of bleeding in 24 to 60 percent of patients with this disorder [188]. Other anatomic sites appear to be involved less frequently. Bleeding is common after trauma and must be anticipated with any surgery. About 14 percent of patients are said to have delayed and defective wound healing. This may relate to the lack of fibrin becoming cross-linked to the fibronectin which coats fibroblast membranes or to collagen itself (see the section "Factor XIII"). Women who have inherited this deficiency frequently suffer spontaneous abortion and are unable to achieve a term pregnancy. Male homozygotes seem to be sterile. Laboratory tests show no impairment of thrombin formation, and the rate of conversion of fibrinogen to a fibrin gel is normal in all assays. Platelet function tests are normal. The diagnosis of factor XIII deficiency is proven by observing that the fibrin made by recalcifying the plasma dissolves overnight at room temperature in 5 M urea or 1 percent monochloroacetic acid. Normal fibrin clots remain intact indefinitely at room temperature in these solvents. The finding of fibrin solubility in dispersing reagents such as 5 M urea suggest a factor XIII level of less than 1 percent and indicates a propensity to hemorrhage.

In one study, 37 percent of reported patients resulted from consanguine unions [188]. The disorder is most probably inherited as an autosomal recessive trait, but this is not certain since 20 families are reported to have only males with the disorder. The lack of maternal uncles with inherited factor XIII deficiency in these families is evidence against X-linked inheritance. Although the mode of inheritance remains uncertain, other data suggest that two forms of factor XIII deficiency exist [133]. In the majority of the presumed homozygotes tested, the a subunit, which contains the active site of the enzyme, is lacking. Most of these patients also have subnormal plasma levels of the b subunit, usually being about 30 percent of normal. There are isolated reports of patients who lack both a and b subunits. In another report, two patients were found to have normal plasma concentrations of the a subunit, but no factor XIII activity. These findings suggest both quantitative and qualitative defects in the synthesis of factor XIII, and therefore two inherited forms of factor XIII deficiency.

The treatment of this disorder is simple, since less than 200 ml fresh plasma promotes normal hemostasis with tooth extraction [354]. A plasma factor XIII level less than 10 percent of normal will catalyze normal fibrin crosslinking. Cryoprecipitate contains 15 to 30 percent of the factor XIII activity in the initial volume of plasma and can be used in the therapy of factor XIII deficiency. Commercially prepared factor XIII concentrates are also available and useful. The half-life of infused factor XIII in vivo is about 12 days, which simplifies the management of this disorder and allows prophylactic approaches to be developed. Because central nervous system hemorrhage is a major risk in these patients, factor XIII-deficient patients may be given 500 ml fresh frozen normal plasma or four to six bags of cryoprecipitate every 3 weeks. With adequate prophylaxis these patients can lead normal lives and participate in most activities, although contact sports should be avoided. There is one report of an antibody developing to factor XIII, presumably as a consequence of repeated transfusions [355].

Miscellaneous Inherited Disorders of Blood Coagulation

Combined Deficiencies of Factor V and Factor VIII

This combination of deficiencies has been reported in over a dozen families, consanguinity being present in about half [356]. The inheritance pattern appears to be autosomal recessive with variable expressivity in heterozygotes, and males and females are affected with equal frequency. Except in one instance, isolated factor V or factor VIII deficiencies have not been observed in parents or relatives. A popular explanation of this deficiency is that a single gene plays a major role in controlling the synthesis of precursory material common to both factor V and factor VIII [357]. Since these patients are CRM$^+$ for both factor V and factor VIII, it appears likely that the abnormality occurs as a posttranscriptional event. A slightly different view is that a single gene somehow controls the blood level of these two factors. Some variation of this hypothesis now seems more likely. Recently, plasma from 13 different families with this disorder has been shown to lack or have reduced amounts of an inhibitor to protein C (see the section "Protein C and Protein S") [211, 358]. The activated form of protein C, a vitamin K–dependent serine protease, destroys factor V and factor VIII and, even more rapidly, their activated forms, V_a and VIII$_a$ [207, 208]. In one report, the transfusion of normal plasma caused a rise in factor VIII that was greater than could be explained by the amount in the transfused plasma [359]. It now seems possible to explain this observation if a sufficient amount of the inhibitor of activated protein C was supplied by the transfused plasma. Other than the finding of a disproportionate increase in factor VIII procoagulant activity following transfusion, this disorder has no other features of von Willebrand's disease.

Combined Deficiency of Factor VII, Factor IX, Factor X, and Prothrombin

Only one patient, a female, has been reported with this combination of deficiencies. She has had a bleeding disorder since infancy. Vitamin K deficiency secondary to malabsorption, liver disease, or coumarin administration has been excluded. It appears that the defect in this disorder probably involves the proteins responsible for the vitamin K–dependent γ-carboxylation of certain glutamic acid residues in factors VII, IX, X, and prothrombin. The immunoreactive levels of the four vitamin K–dependent factors were greater than 50 percent of normal concentrations, but the functional activity of each was less than 1 percent [360]. Both parents were found to have normal activity levels of the four factors involved.

Passovoy Factor

This is a bleeding disorder that has been described in four members of a family over three generations and in a fifth unrelated individual [361]. The deficient function in this disorder has not been identified but is postulated to be in the intrinsic system. The disorder resembles factor XI deficiency.

Other Deficiencies

A variety of other inherited coagulation disorders in plasma factors have been proposed. Most are not sharply defined or lack confirmation. These include a combined deficiency of factor VIII and XI as well as other deficiencies, such as Nishimine factor, Tatsumi factor, Dynia factor, and Flood factor [286].

Inherited Deficiency of Antithrombin III

Several families have been described with this disorder [362–365]. Clinically, these patients have thromboembolic disease that usually begins in the late teenage period or the early twenties. The tendency to form clots spontaneously occurs mostly on the venous side of the circulation, although there are scattered reports of arterial thromboses. Poorly healing necrotic skin ulcers on the lower extremities may be a problem. The high frequency of recurrent venous thromboembolism among family members, despite antithrombin III concentrations about 50 percent of normal, establishes the disorder as an autosomal dominant trait. Specific functional and immunochemical assays are available for quantitating the level of antithrombin III in plasma. Most patients with this disorder lack cross-reacting material and appear to have a true deficiency, but recently patients have been identified with normal immunologic levels of the protein [365, 367]. In these patients the antithrombin III protein can be separated into two fractions, half of which has reduced affinity for heparin. In the absence of heparin both fractions inhibit factor X_a and thrombin normally, but the inhibitory activity of the abnormal antithrombin III in these reactions cannot be increased by heparin [366, 368].

Since the effect of heparin in vivo depends on the presence of a normal concentration of antithrombin III, heparin is not useful in the treatment of this disorder. In fact, some patients have developed thromboses while on heparin. Management usually consists of giving coumarin-type anticoagulants, which, for inapparent reasons, significantly increase the levels of antithrombin III in some patients [362]. The onset of symptoms in most patients occurs between 10 and 30 years of age. Debate continues about when to start anticoagulation medication. In women, estrogen-containing contraceptives should be avoided since estrogen decreases antithrombin III concentration in normal people. Progesterone does not have this effect. During acute thrombotic episodes, a combination of heparin and transfusions of fresh normal plasma may be useful, the goal being to raise the patient's circulating levels of antithrombin III. Then, in the presence of the heparin, antithrombin III should rapidly inactivate those serine protease clotting factors for which it has an affinity (see the section "Antithrombin III").

Inherited Disorders of the Fibrinolytic System

Plasminogen Abnormal plasminogen has been described in one patient who exhibited a propensity for thrombosis since the teens. Normal levels of immunoreactive plasminogen were present and could be converted to the two-chain enzyme plasmin, the activity of which was virtually nil. The inheritance pattern seems to be autosomal recessive [369, 370]. The abnormal plasminogen showed a different pattern of isoelectric forms compared to normal plasminogen. Other instances of abnormal plasminogens are reported to have impaired binding of activators and plasmin active-site formation [371]. It has not been clearly established that these are associated with clinically defective fibrinolysis.

α₂-Antiplasmin Deficiency Recurrent severe hemorrhage has been described in a patient with congenital deficiency of α₂-antiplasmin (see the section "Plasma Proteinase Inhibitors of Blood Coagulation and Fibrinolysis") [372, 373]. Neither parent was affected, and other family members were normal. The deficiency seemed quantitative since the patient lacked immunologically identifiable α₂-antiplasmin. The

bleeding tendency in the patient was proposed to be due to ineffective opposition of the effects of plasmin on factors V, VIII, prothrombin, fibrinogen, and fibrin at sites of injury.

REFERENCES

1. DAVIE EW, FUJIKAWA K, KURACHI K, KISIEL W: The role of serine proteases in the blood coagulation cascade. *Adv Enzymol* 48:277, 1979
2. JACKSON CM, NEMERSON Y: Blood coagulation. *Ann Rev Biochem* 49:767, 1980
3. KAPLAN AP: Initiation of the intrinsic coagulation and fibrinolytic pathways of man: The role of surfaces, Hageman factor, prekallikrein, high molecular weight kininogen and factor XI. *Prog Hemost Thromb* 4:127, 1978
4. COCHRANE CH, GRIFFIN JH: Molecular assembly in the contact phase of the Hageman factor system. *Am J Med* 67:657, 1979
5. REVAK SD, COCHRANE CG, JOHNSTON AR, HUGHI TE: Structural changes accompanying enzymatic activation of human Hageman factor. *J Clin Invest* 54:619, 1974
6. FUJIKAWA K, WALSH K, DAVIE EW: Isolation and characterization of bovine factor XII (Hageman factor). *Biochemistry* 16:2270, 1977
7. CLAEYS H, COLLEN D: Purification and characterization of bovine factor XII. *Eur J Biochem* 87:69, 1978
8. GRIFFIN JH, COCHRANE CG: Human factor XII (Hageman factor), in Lorand L (ed): *Methods in Enzymology*. New York, Academic Press, Inc, 1976, vol 45, p 56
9. FUJIKAWA K, KURACHI K, DAVIE EW: Characterization of bovine factor XIIₐ (activated Hageman factor). *Biochemistry* 16:4182, 1977
10. FUJIKAWA K, HEIMARK RL, KURACHI K, DAVIE EW: Activation of bovine factor XII (Hageman factor) by plasma kallikrein. *Biochemistry* 19:1322, 1980
11. RATNOFF OD, ROSENBLUM JM: Role of Hageman factor in the initiation of clotting by glass. Evidence that glass frees Hageman factor from inhibition. *Am J Med* 25:160, 1958
12. MARGOLIS J: Activation of a permeability factor in plasma by contact with glass. *Nature* 181:635, 1959
13. KELLERMEYER RW, BRECKENRIDGE RT: The inflammatory process in acute gouty arthritis. I. Activation of Hageman factor by sodium urate crystals. *J Lab Clin Med* 65:307, 1965
14. GINSBERG MH, JACQUES B, COCHRANE CG, GRIFFIN JH: Urate crystal-dependent cleavage of Hageman factor in human plasma and synovial fluid. *J Lab Clin Med* 95:497, 1980
15. MORRISON DC, COCHRANE CG: Direct evidence for Hageman factor (factor XII) activation by bacterial lipopoly-saccharides (endotoxins). *J Exp Med* 140:797, 1974
16. EISEN V: Effect of hexadimethrine bromide on plasma kinin formation, hydrolysis of *p*-tosyl-*l*-arginine methyl ester and fibrinolysis. *Br J Pharmacol* 22:87, 1964
17. NOSSEL HL, RUBIN H, DRILLINGS M, HSIEH R: Inhibition of Hageman factor activation. *J Clin Invest* 47:1172, 1968
18. FAIR BD, SAITO H, RATNOFF OD, RIPPON WB: Detection by fluorescence of structural changes accompanying the activation of Hageman factor (factor XII). *Proc Soc Exp Biol Med* 155:199, 1977
19. SAITO H: Purification of high molecular weight kininogen and the role of this agent in blood coagulation. *J Clin Invest* 60:584, 1977
20. RATNOFF OD, SAITO H: Amidolytic properties of single-chain activated Hageman factor. *Proc Natl Acad Sci USA* 76:958, 1979
21. RATNOFF OD: The relative amidolytic activity of Hageman factor (factor XII) and its fragments. The effect of high molecular weight kininogen and kaolin. *J Lab Clin Med* 96:267, 1980
22. KURACHI K, FUJIKAWA K, DAVIE EW: Mechanism of activation of bovine factor XI by factor XII and factor XIIₐ. *Biochemistry* 19:1330, 1980
23. HEIMARK RL, KOTOKU K, FUJIKAWA K, DAVIE EW: Surface activation of blood coagulation, fibrinolysis and kinin formation. *Nature* 286:456, 1980.
24. COCHRANE CG, REVAK SD, WUEPPER KD: Activation of Hageman factor in solid and fluid phases. A critical role of kallikrein. *J Exp Med* 138:1564, 1973
25. GRIFFIN JH, COCHRANE CG: Mechanism for involvement of high molecular weight kininogen in surface-dependent reactions of Hageman factor (coagulation factor XII). *Proc Natl Acad Sci USA* 73:2554, 1976
26. REVAK SD, COCHRANE CG, GRIFFIN JH: The binding and cleavage characteristics of human Hageman factor during contact activation. A comparison of normal plasma with plasmas deficient in factor XI, prekallikrein or high molecular weight kininogen. *J Clin Invest* 59:1167, 1977
27. GRIFFIN JH: The role of surface in the surface-dependent activation of Hageman factor (factor XII). *Proc Natl Acad Sci USA* 75:1998, 1978
28. LIU CY, SCOTT CF, BAGDASARIAN A, PIERCE JV, KAPLAN AP, COLMAN

RW: Potentiation of the function of Hageman factor fragments by high molecular weight kininogen. *J Clin Invest* 60:7, 1977

29. MEIER HK, WEBSTER ME, MANDLE R, COLMAN RW, KAPLAN AP: Activation and function of human Hageman factor. The role of high molecular weight kininogen and prekallikrein. *J Clin Invest* 60:18, 1977

30. WIGGINS RC, BOUMA BN, COCHRANE CG, GRIFFIN JH: Role of high molecular weight kininogen in surface-binding and activation of coagulation factor XI and prekallikrein. *Proc Natl Acad Sci USA* 74:4636, 1977

31. SAITO H, RATNOFF OD, WALDMANN R, ABRAHAM JP: Fitzgerald trait. Deficiency of a hitherto unrecognized agent, Fitzgerald factor, participating in surface-mediated reactions of clotting, fibrinolysis, generating of kinins, and the property of diluted plasma enhancing vascular permeability (pf/dil). *J Clin Invest* 55:1082, 1975

32. WIGGINS RC, COCHRANE CG: The autoactivation of rabbit Hageman factor. *J Exp Med* 150:1122, 1979

33. GRIFFIN JH, COCHRANE CG: Recent advances in the understanding of contact activation reactions. *Semin Thromb Hemostas* 5:254, 1979

34. SILVERBERG M, KETTNER C, SHAW E, KAPLAN AP: Enzymatic activities of native and activated Hageman factor, abstract, *Circulation* 62(suppl 2):57, 1980

35. SILVERBERG M, DUNN JT, GAREN L, KAPLAN AP: Autoactivation of human Hageman factor: Demonstration utilizing a synthetic substrate. *J Biol Chem* 255:7281, 1980

36. KAPLAN AP, AUSTEN KF: A prealbumin activator of prekallikrein: II. Derivation of activators of prekallikrein from native Hageman factor by digestion with plasmin. *J Exp Med* 133:696, 1971

37. REVAK SD, COCHRANE CG: The relationship of structure and function in human Hageman factor. The association of enzymatic and binding activities with separate regions of the molecule. *J Clin Invest* 57:852, 1976

38. KAPLAN AP, AUSTEN KF: A prealbumin activator of prekallikrein. *J Immunol* 105:802, 1970

39. KISIEL W, FUJIKAWA K, DAVIE EW: Activation of bovine factor VII (proconvertin) by factor XII$_a$ (activated Hageman factor). *Biochemistry* 19:4189, 1977

40. RADCLIFFE R, BAGDASSARIAN A, COLMAN R, NEMERSON Y: Activation of bovine factor VII by Hageman factor fragments. *Blood* 50:611, 1977

41. SELIGSOHN U, ØSTERUD B, GRIFFIN JH, RAPAPORT SI: Evidence for the participation of both activated factor XII and activated factor IX in the cold-promoted activation of factor VII. *Thromb Res* 13:1049, 1978

42. PISANO JJ: Chemistry and biology of the kallikrein-kinin system, in Reich E, Rifkin DB, Shaw E (eds): in *Proteases and Biological Control.* Cold Spring Harbor, NY, Cold Spring Harbor Laboratory, 1975, p 199

43. MANDLE R JR, COLMAN RW, KAPLAN AP: Identification of prekallikrein and HMW kininogen as a circulating complex in human plasma. *Proc Natl Acad Sci USA* 73:4179, 1976

44. THOMPSON RE, MANDLE R JR, KAPLAN AP: Studies of binding of prekallikrein and factor XI to high molecular weight kininogen and its light chain. *Proc Natl Acad Sci USA* 76:4862, 1979

45. BOUMA BN, MILES LA, BERETTA G, GRIFFIN JH: Human plasma prekallikrein. Studies of its activation by activated factor XII and its inactivation of diisopropyl phosphofluoridate. *Biochemistry* 19:1151, 1980

46. MANDLE R JR, KAPLAN AP: Hageman factor substrates. Human plasma prekallikrein: Mechanism of activation by Hageman factor and participation in Hageman factor dependent fibrinolysis. *J Biol Chem* 252:6097, 1977

47. ROCH E SILVA M, BERALDO WT, ROSENFIELD G: Bradykinin, a hypotensive and smooth muscle stimulating factor released from plasma by snake venoms and by trypsin. *Am J Physiol* 156:261, 1949

48. WUEPPER KD: Biochemistry and biology of components of the plasma kinin-forming system, in Lepow IH, Ward PA (eds): *Inflammation: Mechanisms and Control.* New York: Academic Press, Inc, 1972, p 93

49. DERKX FHM, BOUMA BN, SCHALEKAMP MPA, SCHALEKAMP MADH: An intrinsic factor XII-prekallikrein-dependent pathway activates the human plasma renin-angiotensin system. *Nature* 280:315, 1979

50. SEALEY JE, ATLAS SA, LARAGH JH, SILBERBERG M, KAPLAN AP: Initiation of plasma prorenin activation by Hageman factor dependent conversion of plasma prekallikrein to kallikrein. *Proc Natl Acad Sci USA* 76:5914, 1979

51. THOMPSON RE, MANDLE R JR, KAPLAN AP: Characterization of human high molecular weight kininogen: Procoagulant activty associated with the light chain of kinin-free high molecular weight kininogen. *J Exp Med* 147:488, 1978

52. THOMPSON RE, MANDLE R JR, KAPLAN AP: Association of factor XI and high molecular weight kininogen in human plasma. *J Clin Invest* 60:1376, 1977

53. KATO H, SUGO T, IKARI N, HASHIMOTO N, MARUYAMA I, HAN YN, IWANAGA S, FUJII S: Role of bovine high molecular weight kininogen in contact-mediated activation of bovine factor XIII, in Fujii S, Moriya H, Suzuki T (eds): *Kinins II: Systemic Proteases and Cellular Function,* New York: Plenum Publishing Corp, 1979, p 19

54. MARGALIT R, SCHIFFMAN S: Factor XI adsorption to surface: Interaction of high molecular weight kininogen (HMWK) and a plasma adsorption inhibitor. *Blood* 56:168, 1980

55. BOUMA BN, GRIFFIN JH: Human blood coagulation factor XI. Purification, properties and mechanism of activation by activated XII. *J Biol Chem* 252:6432, 1977

56. KURACHI K, DAVIE EW: Activation of human factor XI (plasma thromboplastin antecedent) by factor XII$_a$ (activated Hageman factor). *Biochemistry* 16:5831, 1977

57. RATNOFF OD, DAVIE EW: The activation of Christmas factor (factor IX) by activated plasma thromboplastin antecedent (activated factor XI). *Biochemistry* 1:667, 1962

58. HECK LW, KAPLAN AP: Substrates of Hageman isolation and charactization of human factor XI (PTA) and inhibition of the activated enzyme by α_1-antitrypsin. *J Exp Med* 140:165, 1974

59. FORBES CD, PENSKY J, RATNOFF OD: Inhibition of activated Hageman factor and activated plasma thromboplastin antecedent (factor XI). *J Lab Clin Med* 80:786, 1972

60. HARPEL PC: Separation of plasma thromboplastin antecedent from kallikrein by the plasma α_2-macroglobulin kallikrein inhibitor. *J Clin Invest* 50:2084, 1971

61. DAMUS PS, HICKS M, ROSENBERG RD: Anticoagulant action of heparin. *Nature* 246:355, 1973

62. MANDLE RJ JR, KAPLAN AP: Hageman factor-dependent fibrinolysis: Generation of fibrinolytic activity by the interaction of human activated factor XI and plasminogen. *Blood* 54:850, 1979

63. MANNHALTER C, SHIFFMAN S, JACOBS A: Trypsin activation of human factor XI. *J Biol Chem* 255:2667, 1980

64. CHUNG KS, GOLDSMITH JC, ROBERTS HR: Factor IX: Genetic, chemical and biophysical characteristics, in Seligson D, Schmidt RM (eds): *Handbook Series in Clinical Laboratory Science,* Section I: *Hematology.* Boca Raton, Fla, CRC Press, Inc, 1980, vol 3, p 85

65. ROSENBERG JS, MCKENNA PW, ROSENBERG RD: Inhibition of human factor IX$_a$ by human antithrombin. *J Biol Chem* 250:8883, 1975

66. DISCIPIO RG, HERMODSON MA, YATES SG, DAVIE EW: A comparison of human prothrombin, factor IX (Christmas factor), factor X (Stuart factor) and factor S. *Biochemistry* 16:1698, 1977

67. ØSTERUD B, BOUMA BN, GRIFFIN JH: Human blood coagulation factor IX. Purification, properties and mechanism of activation by activated factor XI. *J Biol Chem* 253:5946, 1978

68. SUTTIE JW: Oral anticoagulant therapy: The biosynthetic basis. *Semin Hematol* 14:365, 1977

69. BYRNE R, AMPHLETT GW, CASTELLINO FJ: Metal ion specificity of the conversion of bovine factors IX, IX$_a$ and IX$_{a\alpha}$ to IX$_{a\beta}$. *J Biol Chem* 255:1430, 1980

70. LINDQUIST PA, FUJIKAWA K, DAVIE EW: Activation of bovine factor IX (Christmas factor) by factor XI$_a$ (activated plasma thromboplastin antecedent) and a protease from Russell's viper venom. *J Biol Chem* 253:1902, 1978

71. ØSTERUD B, RAPAPORT SI: Activation of factor IX by the reaction product of tissue factor and factor VII: Additional pathway for initiating blood coagulation. *Proc Natl Acad Sci USA* 74:5260, 1977

72. KALOUSEK F, KONIGSBERG W, NEMERSON Y: Activation of factor IX by activated factor X: A link between the extrinsic and intrinsic coagulation systems. *FEBS Lett* 50:382, 1975

73. IRWIN JF, MAMMEN EF: Activation of factor IX by thrombin preparations in the absence of factor XI. *Thromb Res* 8:141, 1976

74. RAPAPORT SI, SCHIFFMAN S, PATCH MJ, AMES SB: The importance of activation of antihemophilic globulin and proaccelerin by traces of thrombin in the generation of intrinsic prothrombinase activity. *Blood* 21:221, 1963

75. VAN DIEIJEN G, TANS G, ROSING J, HEMKER HC: The role of phospholipid and factor VIII$_a$ in the activation of bovine factor X. *J Biol Chem* 256:3433, 1980

76. KAO K-J, PIZZO SV, MCKEE PA: A radioreceptor assay for quantitating plasma factor VIII/von Willebrand's protein. *Blood* 57:579, 1981

77. COOPER HA: The factor VIII complex and its associated activities, in Seligson D, Schmidt RM (eds): *Handbook Series in Clinical Laboratory Science,*Section I: *Hematology.* Boca Raton, Fla, CRC Press, Inc, 1980, vol 3, p 61

78. MCKEE PA: Observations on structure-function relationships of human antihemophilic/von Willebrand factor protein. *Ann NY Acad Sci* 370:210, 1981

79. HOYER LW: The factor VIII complex: Structure and function. *Blood* 58:1, 1981

80. LEGAZ ME, WEINSTEIN MJ, HELDEBRANT CM, DAVIE EW: Isolation and characterization of human factor VIII (antihemophilic factor). *J Biol Chem* 248:3946, 1973

81. FASS DN, KNUTSON GJ, BOWIE EJW: Porcine Willebrand factor: A population of multimers. *J Lab Clin Med* 91:307, 1978

82. HOYER LW, SHAINOFF JR: Factor VIII-related protein circulates in normal

human plasma as high molecular weight multimers. *Blood* 55:1056, 1980

83. McKEE PA, ANDERSEN JC, SWITZER ME: Molecular structural studies of human factor VIII. *Ann NY Acad Sci* 240:8, 1975

84. THELIN GM, WAGNER RH: Sedimentation of plasma antihemophilic factor. *Arch Biochem Biophys* 95:70, 1961

85. OWEN WG, WAGNER RH: Antihemophilic factor. A new method of purification. *Thromb Res* 1:71, 1972

86. SWITZER ME, McKEE PA: Studies on human antihemophilic factor. Evidence for a covalently linked subunit structure. *J Clin Invest* 57:925, 1976

87. SWITZER ME, McKEE PA: Some effects of calcium on the activation of human factor VIII/von Willebrand factor protein. *J Clin Invest* 60:819, 1977

88. WAGNER RH, COOPER HA: Current concepts of the antihemophilic factor (factor VIII) molecule, in Ultin ON, Peake IR (eds): *Hemophilia.* Amsterdam, Excerpta Medica, 1975, p 13

89. COOPER HA, REISNER FF, HALL M, WAGNER RH: The effects of thrombin treatment on preparations of factor VIII and the Ca²⁺-dissociated small active fragment. *J Clin Invest* 56:751, 1975

90. SWITZER MEP, PIZZO SV, McKEE PA: Is there a precursive, relatively procoagulant-inactive form of normal antihemophilic factor (factor VIII)? *Blood* 54:916, 1979

91. COOPER HA, GRIGGS TR, WAGNER RH: Factor VIII recombination after dissociation by CaCl₂. *Proc Natl Acad Sci USA* 70:2326, 1973

92. RICK ME, HOYER LM: Molecular weight of human factor VIII procoagulant activity. *Thromb Res* 7:909, 1975

93. HOYER LW, TRABOLD NC: The effect of thrombin on human factor VIII. Cleavage of the factor VIII procoagulant protein during activation. *J Lab Clin Med* 97:50, 1981

94. SHAW E, GIDDINGS JC, PEAKE IR, BLOOM AL: Synthesis of procoagulant factor VIII, factor VIII related antigen and other coagulation factors by the isolated perfused rat liver. *Br J Haematol* 41:585, 1979

95. VEHAR GA, DAVIE EW: Preparation and properties of bovine factor VIII (antihemophilic factor). *Biochemistry* 19:401, 1980

96. WEISS HJ: A study of the cation- and pH-dependence of factors V and VIII in plasma. *Thromb Diath Haemorrh* 14:32, 1965

97. SWITZER MEP, McKEE PA: Reactions of thrombin with human factor VIII/von Willebrand factor protein. *J Biol Chem* 255:10606, 1980

98. WEISS HJ, SUSSMAN II, HOYER LW: Stabilization of factor VIII in plasma by von Willebrand factor—studies on posttransfusion and dissociated factor VIII and in patients with von Willebrand's disease. *J Clin Invest* 60:390, 1977

99. ATICHARTAKARN V, MARDER VJ, KIRBY EP, BUDZYNSKI AZ: Effects of enzymatic digestion on the subunit composition and biologic properties of human factor VIII. *Blood* 51:281, 1978

100. ANDERSEN JC, SWITZER MEP, McKEE PA: Support of ristocetin-induced platelet aggregation by procoagulant-inactive and plasmin-cleaved forms of human factor VIII/von Willebrand factor. *Blood* 55:101, 1980

101. HOYER LW: Immunologic properties of antihemophilic factor. *Prog Hematol* 8:191, 1974

102. LAZARCHICK J, HOYER LW: Immunoradiometric measurement of the factor VIII procoagulant antigen. *J Clin Invest* 62:1048, 1978

103. HOYER LW, DE LOS SANTOS R, HOYER JR: Antihemophilic factor antigen. Localization in endothelial cells by immunofluorescent microscopy. *J Clin Invest* 52:2737, 1973

104. JAFFE EA, HOYER LW, NACHMAN RL: Synthesis of von Willebrand factor by cultured human endothelial cells. *Proc Natl Acad Sci USA* 71:1906, 1974

105. NACHMAN R, LEVINE R, JAFFE EA: Synthesis of factor VIII antigen by cultured guinea pig megakaryocytes. *J Clin Invest* 60:914, 1977

106. NACHMAN RL, JAFFE EA: Subcellular platelet factor VIII antigen and von Willebrand factor. *J Exp Med* 141:1101, 1975

107. HOWARD MA, MONTGOMERY DC, HARDISTY RM: Factor VIII-related antigen in platelets. *Thromb Res* 4:617, 1974

108. SULTAN Y, JEANNEAU C, LAMAZIERE J: Absence of factor VIII-related antigen penetration and binding to von Willebrand's platelets after transfusion. *Circulation* 53(suppl 2):115, 1976

109. STEAD NW, McKEE PA: Destruction of factor VIII procoagulant activity in tissue culture media. *Blood* 52:408, 1978

110. TUDDENHAM EGD, LAZARCHICK J, HOYER LW: Synthesis and release of factor VIII by cultured human endothelial cells. *Br J Haematol* 47:617, 1981

111. ZIMMERMAN TS, ROBERTS J, EDGINGTON TS: Factor VIII-related antigen: Multiple molecular forms in human plasma. *Proc Natl Acad Sci USA* 72:5121, 1975

112. DOUCET-DEBRUINE MHM, SIXMA JJ, OVER J, BEESER-VISSER NH: Heterogeneity of human factor VIII. II. Characterization of forms of factor VIII binding to platelets in the presence of ristocetin. *J Lab Clin Med* 92:96, 1978

113. TSCHOPP TB, WEISS HJ, BAUMGARTNER HR: Decreased adhesion of plate-

lets to subendothelium in von Willebrand's disease. *J Lab Clin Med* 83:276, 1974

114. MEYER D, OBERT B, PIETU G, LAVERGNE JM, ZIMMERMAN TS: Multimeric structure of factor VIII/von Willebrand factor in von Willebrand's disease. *J Lab Clin Med* 95:590, 1980

115. BAUMGARTNER HR, TSCHOPP TB, MEYER D: Shear rate dependent inhibition of platelet adhesion and aggregation on collagen surfaces by antibodies to human factor VIII/von Willebrand factor. *Br J Haematol* 44:127, 1980

116. SODETZ JM, PIZZO SV, McKEE PA: Relationship of sialic acid to function and *in vivo* survival of human factor VIII/von Willebrand factor protein. *J Biol Chem* 252:5538, 1977

117. SODETZ JM, PAULSON JC, PIZZO SV, McKEE PA: Carbohydrate on human factor VIII/von Willebrand factor. Impairment of function by removal of specific galactose residues. *J Biol Chem* 253:7202, 1978

118. GRALNICK HR, SULTAN Y, COLLER BS: von Willebrand's disease. Combined qualitative and quantitative abnormalities. *N Engl J Med* 296:1024, 1977

119. GRALNICK HR: Factor VIII/von Willebrand factor protein. Galactose, a cryptic determinant of von Willebrand factor activity. *J Clin Invest* 62:496, 1978

120. ROSEBOROUGH TK: von Willebrand factor, polycations and platelet agglutination. *Thromb Res* 17:481, 1980

121. COLLER BS: The effects of ristocetin and von Willebrand factor on platelet electrophoretic mobility. *J Clin Invest* 61:1168, 1978

122. KAO K-J, PIZZO SV, McKEE PA: Platelet receptors for human factor VIII/von Willebrand protein: Functional correlation of receptor occupancy and ristocetin-induced platelet aggregation. *Proc Natl Acad Sci USA* 76:5317, 1979

123. NACHMAN RL, JAFFE EA, WEKSLER BB: Immunoinhibition of ristocetin-induced platelet aggregation. *J Clin Invest* 59:143, 1977

124. JENKINS CSP, PHILIPS DR, CLEMETSON KJ, MEYER D, LARRIEU M-J, LÜSCHER EF: Platelet membrane glycoproteins implicated in ristocetin-induced aggregation. *J Clin Invest* 57:112, 1976

125. KAO K-J, PIZZO SV, McKEE PA: Factor VIII/von Willebrand protein. Modification of its carbohydrate causes reduced binding to platelets. *J Biol Chem* 255:10134, 1980

126. SODETZ JM, PAULSON JC, McKEE PA: Carbohydrate composition and identification of blood group A, B and H oligosaccharide structures on human factor VIII/von Willebrand factor. *J Biol Chem* 254:10754, 1979

127. BROZE GJ, MAJERUS PW: Purification and properties of human coagulation factor VII. *J Biol Chem* 255:1242, 1980

128. KISIEL W, DAVIE EW: Isolation and characterization of bovine factor VII. *Biochemistry* 14:4928, 1975

129. RADCLIFFE R, NEMERSON Y: Activation and control of factor VII by activated factor X and thrombin. *J Biol Chem* 250:388, 1975

130. KISIEL W, FUJIKAWA K, DAVIE EW: Activation of bovine factor VII (proconvertin) by factor XIIₐ (activated Hageman factor). *Biochemistry* 16:4189, 1977

131. JESTY J: The inhibition of activated bovine coagulation factors X and VII by antithrombin III. *Arch Biochem Biophys* 185:165, 1978

132. ØSTERUD B, BJØRKLID E, BROWN SF: The interaction of human blood coagulation factor VII and tissue factor: The effect of anti factor VII, anti tissue factor and diisopropylfluorophosphate. *Biochem Biophys Res Commun* 88:59, 1979

133. RADCLIFFE R, BAGDASARIAN A, COLMAN R, NEMERSON Y: Activation of bovine factor VII by Hageman factor fragments. *Blood* 50:611, 1977

134. ZELDIS S, NEMERSON Y, PITLICK FA, LENTZ TL: Tissue factor (thromboplastin): Localization to plasma membranes by peroxidase conjugated antibodies. *Science* 175:766, 1972

135. ZACHARSKI LR, McINTYRE OR: Membrane-mediated synthesis of tissue factor (thromboplastin) in cultured fibroblasts. *Blood* 41:679, 1973

136. LIU DTH, McCOY L: Tissue extract thromboplastin: Quantitation, fractionation and characterization of protein components. *Thromb Res* 7:199, 1975

137. BJØRKLID E, STORM E: Purification and some properties of the protein component of tissue thromboplastin from human brain. *Biochem J* 165:89, 1977

138. LIU DTH, McCOY L: Phospholipid requirements of tissue thromboplastin in blood coagulation. *Thromb Res* 7:213, 1975

139. THØGERSEN HC, PETERSEN TE, SOTTRUP-JENSEN L, MAGNUSSON S, MORRIS HR: The N-terminal sequences of blood coagulation factor X₁ and X₂ light chains. Mass-spectrometric identification of twelve residues of γ-carboxyglutamic acid in their vitamin K–dependent domains. *Biochem J* 175:613, 1978

140. HENRIKSEN RA, JACKSON CM: The chemistry and enzymology of bovine factor X. *Semin Thromb Hemostas* 1:284, 1975

141. YIN ET, WESSLER S, STOLL PJ: Rabbit plasma inhibitor of the activated species of blood coagulation factor X: Purification and some properties. *J Biol Chem* 246:3694, 1971

142. HARPEL PC, ROSENBERG RD: α_2-Macroglobulin and antithrombin-heparin cofactor: Modulators of hemostatic and inflammatory reactions, in Spaet TH (ed): *Progress in Hemostasis and Thrombosis*. New York, Grune & Stratton, Inc, 1976, p 145

143. DAHLBACK B: Human coagulation factor V purification and thrombin-catalyzed activation. *J Clin Invest* 66:583, 1980

144. KANE WH, MAJERUS PW: Purification and characterization of human coagulation factor V. *J Biol Chem* 256:1002, 1981

145. BARTLETT S, LATSON P, HANAHAN DJ: High molecular weight factor V of bovine and human plasma. *Biochemistry* 19:273, 1980

146. NESHEIM ME, MANN KG: Thrombin-catalyzed activation of single chain bovine factor V. *J Biol Chem* 254:1326, 1979

147. HIBBARD LS, MANN KG: The calcium-binding properties of bovine factor V. *J Biol Chem* 255:638, 1980

148. ESMON CT: The subunit structure of thrombin-activated factor V. Isolation of activated factor V, separation of subunits, and reconstitution of biological activity. *J Biol Chem* 254:964, 1979

149. BLOOM JW, NESHEIM ME, MANN KG: Phospholipid-binding properties of factor V and factor V_a. *Biochemistry* 18:4419, 1979

150. BAJAJ SP, BUTKOWSKI RJ, MANN KG: Prothrombin fragments. Ca^{2+} binding and activation kinetics. *J Biol Chem* 250:2150, 1975

151. TRACY PB, PETERSON MJ, NESHEIM ME, McDUFFIE FC, MANN KG: Interaction of coagulation factor V and factor V_a with platelets. *J Biol Chem* 254:10354, 1979

152. KANE WH, LINDHOUT MJ, JACKSON CM, MAJERUS PW: Factor V_a-dependent binding factor of X_a to human platelets. *J Biol Chem* 255:1170, 1980

153. MANN KG, ELION J: Prothrombin, in Seligson D, Schmidt RM (eds): *Handbook Series in Clinical Laboratory Science*, Section I: Hematology. Boca Raton, Fla, CRC Press, Inc, 1980, vol 3, p 15

154. STENFLO J, FERNLUND P, EGAN W, ROEPSTORFF P: Vitamin K dependent modifications of glutamic acid residues in prothrombin. *Proc Natl Acad Sci USA* 71:2730, 1974

155. NELSESTUEN GL, ZYTKOVICZ T, HOWARD JB: Identification of γ-carboxy glutamic acid as a component of prothrombin. *J Biol Chem* 249:6347, 1974

156. MAGNUSSON S, SOTTRUP-JENSEN L, PETERSEN T-E: Primary structure of the vitamin K–dependent part of prothrombin. *FEBS Lett* 44:189, 1974

157. STENN KS, BLOUT ER: Mechanism of bovine prothrombin activation by an insoluble preparation of bovine factor X_a (thrombokinase). *Biochemistry* 11:4502, 1972

158. ARONSON DL, STEVAN L, BALL AP, FRANZA BR JR, FINLAYSON JS: Generation of the combined prothrombin activation peptide (Fl·2) during the clotting of blood and plasma. *J Clin Invest* 60:1410, 1977

159. DOMBROSE FA, GITEL SN, ZAWALICH K, JACKSON CM: The association of bovine prothrombin fragment 1 with phospholipid. *J Biol Chem* 254:5027, 1979

160. SUTTIE JW, JACKSON CM: Prothrombin structure, activation and biosynthesis. *Physiol Rev* 57:1, 1977

161. ESMON CT, JACKSON CM: The conversion of prothrombin to thrombin. IV. The function of the fragment 2 region during activation in the presence of factor V. *J Biol Chem* 249:7791, 1974

162. DAHLBÄCK B, STENFLO J: The activation of prothrombin by platelet-bound factor X_a. *Eur J Biochem* 104:549, 1980

163. MILETICH JP, KANE WH, HOFMANN SL, STANFORD N, MAJERUS PW: Deficiency of factor X_a-factor V_a binding sites on the platelets of a patient with a bleeding disorder. *Blood* 54:1015, 1979

164. MILETICH JP, JACKSON CM, MAJERUS PW: Properties of the factor X_a binding site on human platelets. *J Biol Chem* 253:6908, 1978

165. WORKMAN EF JR, LUNDBLAD RL: Thrombin, in Seligson D, Schmidt RM (eds): *Handbook Series in Clinical Laboratory Science*, Section I: Hematology. Boca Raton, Fla, CRC Press, Inc, 1980, vol 3, p 149

166. LUNDBLAD RL, KINGDON HS, MANN KG: Thrombin, in Lorand L (ed): *Methods in Enzymology*. New York, Academic Press, Inc, 1976, vol 45, p 156

167. SHAPIRO SS, McCORD S: Prothrombin, in Spaet TH (ed): *Progress in Hemostasis*. New York, Grune & Stratton, Inc, 1978, vol 4, p 177

168. LANCHANTIN GF, FRIEDMAN JA, HART DW: Two forms of human thrombin. *J Biol Chem* 248:5956, 1973

169. BUTKOWSKI RJ, ELION J, DOWNING MR, MANN KG: Primary structure of human prethrombin 2 and α-thrombin. *J Biol Chem* 252:4942, 1977

170. OKAMOTO S, HIJIKATA A, KINJO K, KIKUMOTO R, OHKUBO K, TONOMURA S, TAMAO Y: A novel series of synthetic thrombin inhibitors having extremely potent and selective action. *Kobe J Med Sci* 21:43, 1975

171. MARKWARDT F: Hirudin as an inhibitor of thrombin, in Perlmann GE, Lorand L (eds): *Methods in Enzymology*. New York, Academic Press, Inc, 1970, vol 19, p 924

172. VOGEL CN, KINGDON HS, LUNDBLAD RL: Correlation of in vivo and in vitro inhibition of thrombin by plasma inhibitors. *J Lab Clin Med* 93:661, 1979

173. POCHON F, FAVAUDON V, TOURBEZ-PERRIN M, BIETH J: Localization of

174. LIU CY, KAPLAN KL, MARKOWITZ AH, NOSSEL HL: Thermodynamic characterization of thrombin binding by crosslinked and noncrosslinked fibrin in the presence and absence of Ca^{2+}. *J Biol Chem* 255:7627, 1980

175. FULLER GM, NICKERSON JM: Fibrinogen biosynthesis: In vitro translation, glycosylation and translocation of fibrinogen peptide chains. *Thromb Haemost* 46:252, 1981

176. DOOLITTLE RF: Structural aspects of the fibrinogen to fibrin conversion. *Adv Protein Chem* 27:1, 1973

177. DOOLITTLE RF: Fibrinogen, in Seligson D, Schmidt RM (eds): *Handbook Series in Clinical Laboratory Science*, Section I: Hematology. Boca Raton, Fla, CRC Press, Inc, 1980, vol 3, p 3

178. HALL CE, SLAYTER HS: The fibrinogen molecule: Its size, shape and mode of polymerization. *J Biophys Biochem Cytol* 5:11, 1959

179. FOWLER WE, FRETTO LJ, ERICKSON HP, McKEE PA: Electron microscopy of plasmic fragments of human fibrinogen as related to trinodular structure of the intact molecule. *J Clin Invest* 66:50, 1980

180. HANTGAN RR, HERMANS J: Assembly of fibrin. A light scattering study. *J Biol Chem* 254:11272, 1979

181. FOWLER EW, ERICKSON HP, HANTGAN RR, McDONAGH J, HERMANS J: Crosslinked fibrinogen dimers demonstrate a feature of the molecular packing in fibrin fibers. *Science* 211:287, 1981

182. BLOMBÄCK B, HESSEL B, HAGG D, THERKILDSEN L: 2-Step fibrinogen-fibrin transition in blood coagulation. *Nature* 275:501, 1978

183. McKEE PA, SCHWARTZ ML, PIZZO SV, HILL RL: Crosslinking of fibrin by fibrin-stabilizing factor. *Ann NY Acad Sci* 202:127, 1972

184. FRETTO LJ, McKEE PA: Structure of α-polymer from in vitro and in vivo highly crosslinked human fibrin. *J Biol Chem* 253:6614, 1978

185. SCHWARTZ ML, PIZZO SV, HILL RL, McKEE PA: Human factor XIII from plasma and platelets. Molecular weights, subunit structures, proteolytic activation and crosslinking of fibrinogen and fibrin. *J Biol Chem* 248:1395, 1973

186. MARGUERIE GA, EDGINGTON TS, PLOW EF: Interaction of fibrinogen with its platelet receptor as part of a multistep reaction in ADP-induced platelet aggregation. *J Biol Chem* 254:154, 1979

187. LOPACIUK S, LOVETTE KM, McDONAGH J, CHUANG HYK, McDONAGH RM: Subcellular distribution of fibrinogen and factor XIII in human blood platelets. *Thromb Res* 8:453, 1976

188. LORAND L: Human factor XIII: Fibrin-stabilizing factor, in Spaet TH (ed): *Progress in Hemostasis and Thrombosis*. New York, Grune & Stratton, Inc, 1980, vol 5, p 245

189. FOLK JE, CHUNG SI: Blood coagulation factor XIII: Relationship of some biological properties to subunit structure, in Reich E, Rifkin DB, Shaw E (eds): *Proteases and Biological Control*. Cold Spring Harbor, NY, Cold Spring Harbor Laboratory, 1975, p 157

190. CURTIS CG, STENBERG P, CHOU CHJ, GRAY A, BROWN KL, LORAND L: Titration and subunit localization of active center cysteine in fibrinoligase (thrombin-activated fibrin stabilizing factor). *Biochem Biophys Res Commun* 52:51, 1973

191. CURTIS CG, BROWN KL, CREDO RB, DOMANIK RA, GRAY A, STENBERG P, LORAND L: Calcium dependent unmasking of active center cysteine during activation of fibrin-stabilizing factor. *Biochemistry* 13:3774, 1974

192. CREDO RB, CURTIS CG, LORAND L: Ca^{2+}-related regulatory function of fibrinogen. *Proc Natl Acad Sci USA* 75:4234, 1978

193. CREDO RB, CURTIS CG, LORAND L: α-Chain domain of fibrinogen controls generation of fibrinoligase (coagulation factor XIIIa). Calcium ion regulatory aspects. *Biochemistry* 20:3770, 1981

194. CURTIS CG, LORAND L: Fibrin stabilizing factor (factor XIII), in Lorand L (ed): *Methods in Enzymology*. New York, Academic Press, Inc, 1976, vol 45, p 177

195. McDONAGH J, WAGNER RH: Site of synthesis of plasma and platelet factor XIII. *Ann NY Acad Sci* 202:31, 1972

196. JOIST JH, NIEWIAROWSKI S: Retention of platelet fibrin stabilizing factor during the platelet release reaction and clot retraction. *Thromb Diath Haemorrh* 29:679, 19773

197. SAKATA Y, AOKI N: Crosslinking of α_2-plasmin inhibitor to fibrin by fibrin stabilizing factor. *J Clin Invest* 65:290, 1980

198. COHEN I, YOUNG-BANDALA L, BLANKENBERG TA, SIEFRING GE, BRUNER-LORAND J: Fibrinoligase-catalyzed crosslinking of myosin from platelet and skeletal muscle. *Arch Biochem Biophys* 192:100, 1979

199. COHEN I, BLANKENBERG TA, BORDEN D, KAHN DR, VEIS A: Factor XIII catalyzed crosslinking of platelet and muscle actin. Regulation by nucleotides. *Biochim Biophys Acta* 628:365, 1980

200. KESKI-OJA J, MOSHER DF, VAHERI A: Crosslinking of a major fibroblast surface-associated glycoprotein (fibronectin) catalyzed by blood coagulation factor XIII. *Cell* 9:29, 1976

201. MOSHER DF, SCHAD PE, VANN JM: Crosslinking of collagen and fibronectin by factor XIII_a: Localization of participating glutaminyl residues to a tryptic fragment of fibronectin. *J Biol Chem* 255:1181, 1980

202. CHUNG SI: Comparative studies on tissue transglutaminase and factor XIII. *Ann NY Acad Sci* 202:240, 1972

203. STENFLO J: A new vitamin K–dependent protein: Purification from bovine plasma and preliminary characterization. *J Biol Chem* 251:355, 1976

204. KISIEL W: Human plasma protein C. Isolation, characterization and mechanism of activation by α-thrombin. *J Clin Invest* 64:761, 1979

205. KISIEL W, ERICSSON LH, DAVIE EW: Proteolytic activation of protein C from bovine plasma. *Biochemistry* 15:4893, 1976

206. OWEN WG, ESMON CT: Functional properties of an endothelial cell cofactor for thrombin-catalyzed activation of protein C. *J Biol Chem* 256:5532, 1981

207. WALKER FJ, SEXTON PW, ESMON CT: The inhibition of blood coagulation by activated protein C through the selective inactivation of activated factor V. *Biochim Biophys Acta* 571:333, 1979

208. MARLAR RA, KLEISS AJ, GRIFFIN JH: Anticoagulation action of human protein C, in H Peeters (ed): *Protides of the Biological Fluids*. New York, Pergamon Press, Inc, 1980, p 341

209. WALKER FJ: Regulation of activated protein C by a new protein. *J Biol Chem* 255:5521, 1980

210. DAHLBACK B, STENFLO J: Inhibitory effect of activated protein C on activation of prothrombin by platelet-bound factor X_a. *Eur J Biochem* 107:331, 1980

211. MARLAR RA, GRIFFIN JH: Deficiency of protein C inhibitor in combined factor V/VIII deficiency disease. *J Clin Invest* 66:1186, 1980

212. CASTELLINO FJ: Recent advances in the chemistry of the fibrinolytic system. *Chem Rev* 81:431, 1981

213. KLINE DL, REDDY KNN: *Fibrinolysis*. Boca Raton, Fla, CRC Press, Inc, 1980

214. VIOLAND BN, CASTELLINO FJ: Mechanism of the urokinase-catalyzed activation of human plasminogen. *J Biol Chem* 251:3906, 1976

215. SUMMARIA L, SPITZ F, ARZADON L, BOREISHA IG, ROBBINS KC: Isolation and characterization of the affinity chromatography forms of human Glu- and Lys-plasminogen and plasmins. *J Biol Chem* 251:3693, 1976

216. WALLÉN P, WIMAN B: Characterization of human plasminogen. II. Separation and partial characterization of different molecular forms of human plasminogen. *Biochim Biophys Acta* 257:122, 1972

217. ROBBINS KC, SUMMARI AL, HSIEH B, SHAH RJ: The peptide chains of human plasmin. Mechanism of activation of human plasminogen to plasmin. *J Biol Chem* 242:2333, 1967

218. SOTTRUP-JENSEN L, CLAEYS H, ZAJDEL M, PETERSEN TE, MAGNUSSON S: The primary structure of human plasminogen: Isolation of two lysine-binding fragments and one "mini"-plasminogen (MW 38,000) by elastase-catalyzed-specific limited proteolysis, in Davidson JF, Rowan RM, Samama MM, Desnoyers PC (eds): *Progress in Chemical Fibrinolysis*. New York, Raven Press, 1978, vol 3, p 191

219. VIOLAND BN, SODETZ JM, CASTELLINO FJ: The effects of ε-aminocaproic acid on the gross conformation of plasminogen and plasmin. *Arch Biochem Biophys* 170:300, 1975

220. THORSEN S: Differences in the binding to fibrin of native plasminogen and plasminogen modified by proteolytic degradation. Influence of ω-amino-carboxylic acids. *Biochim Biophys Acta* 393:55, 1975

221. CLAEYS H, VERMYLEN J: Physicochemical and proenzyme properties of NH_2-terminal glutamic acid and NH_2-terminal lysine human plasminogen. Influence of 6-aminohexanoic acid. *Biochim Biophys Acta* 342:351, 1974

222. SUMMARIA L, ARZADON L, BERNABE P, ROBBINS KC: The activation of plasminogen to plasmin by urokinase in the presence of the plasmin inhibitor Trasylol. *J Biol Chem* 250:3988, 1975

223. REDDY KNN, MARKUS G: Mechanism of activation of human plasminogen by streptokinase. Presence of active center in streptokinase-plasminogen complex. *J Biol Chem* 247:1683, 1972

224. SCHICK LA, CASTELLINO FJ: Interaction of streptokinase and rabbit plasminogen. *Biochemistry* 12:4315, 1973

225. BROCKWAY WJ, CASTELLINO FJ: Characterization of native streptokinase isolated from a human plasminogen activator complex. *Biochemistry* 13:2063, 1974

226. MARKUS G, DEPASQUALE JL, WISSLER FC: Quantitative determination of the binding of ε-aminocaproic acid to native plasminogen. *J Biol Chem* 253:727, 1978

227. LERCH PG, RICKLI EE, LERGIER W, GILLESSEN D: Localization of individual lysine-binding regions in human plasminogen and investigations on their complex-forming properties. *Eur J Biochem* 107:7, 1980

228. MARKUS G, PRIORE RL, WISSLER FC: The binding of tranexamic acid to native (Glu) and modified (Lys) human plasminogen and its effect on conformation. *J Biol Chem* 254:1211, 1979

229. THORSEN S, GLAS-GREENWALT S, ASTRUP T: Difference in the binding of fibrin by urokinase and tissue activator. *Thromb Diath Haemorrh* 28:65, 1972

230. LLOYD DA, CEDERHOLM-WILLIAMS SA, SHARP AA: Binding of plasminogen and vascular plasminogen activator to fibrin and the fibrin alpha-chain. *Thromb Haemost* 46(1):163, 1981

231. FERGUSON EW, FRETTO LJ, McKEE PA: A re-examination of the cleavage of fibrinogen and fibrin by plasmin. *J Biol Chem* 250:7210, 1975

232. HEIMBURGER N: Proteinase inhibitors of human plasma—their properties and central functions, in Reich E, Rifkin DB, Shaw E (eds): *Proteases and Biological Control*, Cold Spring Harbor, NY, Cold Spring Harbor Laboratory, 1975 p 367

233. DAMUS PS, ROSENBERG RD: Antithrombin-heparin cofactor, in Lorand L (ed): *Methods in Enzymology*. NY, Academic Press, Inc, 1976, vol 45, p 653

234. WESSLER S, GITEL SN: Heparin, in Seligson D, Schmidt RM (eds): *Handbook Series in Clinical Laboratory Science, Section I: Hematology*. Boca Raton Fla, CRC Press, Inc, 1980, vol 3, p 289

235. MacGREGOR IR, LANE DA, KAKKAR VV: Evidence for a plasma inhibitor of the heparin accelerated inhibition of factor X_a by antithrombin III. *Biochim Biophys Acta* 586:584, 1979

236. HURST RE, MENTER JM, WEST SS, SETTINE JM, COYNE EH: Structural basis for the anticoagulant activity of heparin. 1. Relationship to the number of charged groups. *Biochemistry* 18:4283, 1979

237. RIESENFELD J, THUNBERG L, HÖÖK M, LINDAHL U: The antithrombin-binding sequence of heparin. Location of essential N-sulfate groups. *J Biol Chem* 256:2389, 1981

238. BLACKBURN MN, SIBLEY CC: The heparin binding site of antithrombin III. *J Biol Chem* 255:824, 1980

239. OWEN WG: Evidence for the formation of an ester between thrombin and heparin cofactor. *Biochim Biophys Acta* 405:380, 1975

240. LAM LSL, REGOECZI E, HATTON MWC: In vivo behaviour of some antithrombin III-protease complexes. *Br J Exp Pathol* 60:151, 1979

241. MOROI M, AOKI N: Isolation and characterization of alpha α_2-plasmin inhibitor in human plasma. A novel proteinase inhibitor which inhibits activator-induced clot lysis. *J Biol Chem* 251:5956, 1976

242. WIMAN B, COLLEN D: Purification and characterization of human antiplasmin, the fast acting plasmin inhibitor in plasma. *Eur J Biochem* 78:19, 1977

243. WIMAN B, BOMAN L, COLLEN D: On the kinetics of the reaction between human antiplasmin and a low molecular weight form of plasmin. *Eur J Biochem* 87:143, 1978

244. WIMAN B, COLLEN D: On the mechanism of the reaction between human α_2-antiplasmin and plasmin. *J Biol Chem* 254:9291, 1979

245. AOKI N, SAKATA Y: Influence of α_2-plasmin inhibitor on adsorption of plasminogen to fibrin. *Thromb Res* 19:149, 1980

246. MOROI M, AOKI N: Inhibition of plasminogen binding to fibrin by α_2-plasmin inhibitor. *Thromb Res* 10:851, 1977

247. CEDERHOLM-WILLIAMS SA, DeCOCK F, LIJNEN HR, COLLEN D: Kinetics of the reactions between streptokinase, plasmin and α_2-antiplasmin. *Eur J Biochem* 100:125, 1979

248. OWEN CA JR, BOWIE EJW, THOMPSON JH JR: *The Diagnosis of Bleeding Disorders*. Boston, Little, Brown and Co, 1975

249. ALEDORT LM: *Recent Advances in Hemophilia*, New York, Annals of the New York Academy of Sciences, vol 240, 1975

250. RATNOFF OD: Antihemophilic factor (factor VIII). *Ann Intern Med* 88:403, 1978

251. EPSTEIN I: *The Babylonian Talmud*. London, Soncino Press, Yebamoth sec 64B vol 1, 1936

252. ABILDGAARD CF, SUZUKI Z, HARRISON J, JEFCOAT K, ZIMMERMAN TS: Serial studies in von Willebrand's disease: Variability versus "variants." *Blood* 56:712, 1980

253. AGLE DP, MATTISON A: Psychiatric and social care of patients with hereditary hemorrhagic disease, in Ratnoff OD (ed): *Treatment of Hemorrhagic Disorders*. New York, Harper & Row, Publishers, Inc, 1968, p 111

254. POOL JG, SHANNON AE: Production of high potency concentrates of antihemophilic globulin in a closed-bag system. *N Engl J Med* 273: 1443, 1965

255. SHULMAN NR: Surgical care of patients with hereditary disorders of blood coagulation, in Ratnoff OD, *Treatment of Hemorrhagic Disorders*. New York, Harper & Row, Publishers, Inc, 1968, p 61

256. WALSH PN, RIZZA CR, MATTHEWS JM, EIPE J, KERNOFF PBA, COLES MD, BLOOM AL, KAUFMAN BM, BECK P, HANAN CM, BIGGS R: Epsilon-aminocaproic acid therapy for dental extractions in haemophilia and Christmas disease: A double blind controlled trial. *Br J Haematol* 20:463, 1971

257. WEBSTER WP, ROBERTS HR, PENICK GD: Dental care of patients with hereditary disorders of blood coagulation, in Ratnoff OD (ed): *Treatment of Hemorrhagic Disorders*. New York, Harper & Row, Publishers, Inc, 1968, p 93

258. *Blood Services Bulletin*. Washington DC, American National Red Cross, June 8, 1981

259. WHITE GC II, BLATT PM, McMILLAN CW, WEBSTER WP, LESESNE HR, ROBERTS HR: Medical complications of hemophilia. *South Med J* 73:155, 1980

260. FEINSTEIN DI, RAPAPORT SI: Acquired inhibitors of blood coagulation, in Spaet TH (ed): *Progress in Hemostasis and Thrombosis*. New York, Grune & Stratton, Inc, 1972, vol 1, p 75

261. SHAPIRO SS: Acquired anticoagulants, in Williams WJ, Beutler E, Erslev AJ, Rundles RW (eds): *Hematology.* New York, McGraw-Hill Book Co, 1977, p 1447

262. GRAHAM JB, BARROW ES, ELSTON RC: Lyonization in hemophilia: A cause of error in direct detection of heterozygous carriers. *Ann NY Acad Sci* 240:141, 1975

263. WHITTACKER DL, COPELAND DL, GRAHAM JB: Linkage of color blindness to hemophilias A and B. *Am J Hum Genet* 14:492, 1962

264. McKUSICK VA: On the X chromosome of man. *Q Rev Biol* 37:69, 1962

265. LAZARCHICK J, HOYER LW: Immunoradiometric measurement of the factor VIII procoagulant antigen. *J Clin Invest* 62:1048, 1978

266. PEAKE IR, BLOOM AL, GIDDINGS JC, LUDLAM CA: An immunoradiometric assay for procoagulant factor VIII antigen: Results in hemophilia, von Willebrand's disease and fetal plasma and serum. *Br J Haematol* 42:269, 1979

267. REISNER HM, PRICE WA, BLATT PM, BARROW ES, GRAHAM JB: Factor VIII coagulant antigen in hemophilic plasma: A comparison of five allo-antibodies. *Blood* 56:615, 1980

268. RATNOFF OD, JONES PK: The laboratory diagnosis of the carrier state for classic hemophilia. *Ann Intern Med* 86:521, 1977

269. RATNOFF OD, JONES PK: The art of betting: Which of a bleeder's female relatives is a carrier? *Ann Intern Med* 89:281, 1978

270. RATNOFF OD: Implications of the identification of carriers of chronic disease. *J Chronic Dis* 30:543, 1977

271. FIRSHEIN SI, HOYER LW, LAZARCHICK J, FORGET BG, HOBBINS JC, CLYNE LP, PILICK FA, MUIR WA, MERKATZ IR, MAHONEY MJ: Prenatal diagnosis of hemophilia. *N Engl J Med* 300:937, 1979

272. MIBASHAN RS, RODECK CH, FURLONG RA, BAINES L, PEAKE IR, THUMPSTON JK, GORER R, BLOOM AL: Dual diagnosis of prenatal haemophilia by measurement of fetal VIIIC and VIIIC antigen (VIIICAg). *Lancet* 2:904, 1980

273. von WILLEBRAND EA: Uber hereditare pseudohamophilie. *Acta med Scand* 76:521, 1931

274. MILLER CH, GRAHAM JB, GOLDIN LR, ELSTON RC: Genetics of classic von Willebrand's disease. I. Phenotypic variation within families. *Blood* 54:117, 1979

275. ITALIAN WORKING GROUP: Spectrum of von Willebrand's disease: A study of 100 cases. *Br J Haematol* 35:101, 1977

276. HOLMBERG L, MANNUCCI PM, TURESSON I, RUGGERI ZM, NILSSON IM: Factor VIII antigen in the vessel walls in von Willebrand's disease and haemophilia A. *Scand J Haematol* 13:33, 1974

277. RUGGERI ZM, CIAVARELLA N, MANNUCCI PM, MOLINARI A, DAMMACCO F, LAVERGNE JM, MEYER D: Familial incidence of precipitating antibodies in von Willebrand's disease. A study of four cases. *J Lab Clin Med* 94:60, 1979

278. RUGGERI ZM, ZIMMERMAN TS: Variant von Willebrand disease. Characterization of two subtypes by analysis of multimeric composition of factor VIII/von Willebrand factor in plasma and platelets. *J Clin Invest* 65:1318, 1980

279. RUGGERI ZM, PARETI FI, MANNUCCI PM, CIAVARELLA N, ZIMMERMAN TS: Heightened interaction between platelets and factor VIII/von Willebrand factor in a new subtype of von Willebrand's disease. *N Engl J Med* 302:1047, 1980

280. TAKAHASHI H: Studies on the pathophysiology and treatment of von Willebrand's disease. IV. Mechanism of increased ristocetin-induced platelet aggregation in von Willebrand's disease. *Thromb Res* 19:857, 1980

281. BOWIE EJW, FASS DN, OLSON JD, OWEN CA Jr: Transfusion and autotransfusion of plasma in von Willebrand's disease. *Thromb Res* 5:479, 1974

282. BLATT PM, BRINKHOUS KM, CULP HR, KRAUSS JS, ROBERTS HR: Antihemophilic concentrate therapy in von Willebrand disease. Dissociation of bleeding-time factor and ristocetin-cofactor activities. *JAMA* 236:2770, 1976

283. NILSSON IM: *Haemorrhagic and Thrombotic Diseases.* New York, John Wiley & Sons, Inc, 1971, p 96

284. RATNOFF OD, BENNETT B: Clues to the pathogenesis of bleeding in von Willebrand's disease. *N Engl J Med* 289:1182, 1973

285. NOLLER KL, BOWIE EJW, KEMPERS RD, OWEN CA Jr: Von Willebrand's disease in pregnancy. *Obstet Gynecol* 41:865, 1973

286. RATNOFF OD: Hereditary disorders of hemostasis, in Stanbury JB, Wyngaarden JB, Fredrickson DS (eds): *The Metabolic Basis of Inherited Disease,* 4th ed. New York, McGraw-Hill Book Co, 1978, p 1755

287. RATNOFF OD, STEINBERG AG: Further studies on the inheritance of Hageman trait. *J Lab Clin Med* 59:980, 1962

288. VELTKAMP JJ, DRION EF, LOELIGER EA: Detection of the carrier state in hereditary coagulation disorders II. *Thromb Diath Haemorrh* 19:403, 1968

289. VELTKAMP JJ, HEMKER HC, LOELIGER EA: Detection of heterozygotes for factors VIII, IX and XII deficiency. *Thromb Diath Haemorrh* 12(17):181, 1965

290. BENNETT B, RATNOFF OD, HOLT JB, ROBERTS HR: Hageman trait (factor XII deficiency): A probable second genotype inherited as an autosomal dominant characteristic. *Blood* 40:412, 1972

291. SAITO H, RATNOFF OD, PENSKY J: Radioimmunoassay of human Hageman factor (factor XII). *J Lab Clin Med* 88:506, 1976

292. SMINK M McL, DANIEL TM, RATNOFF OD, STAVITSKY AB: Immunological demonstration of a deficiency of Hageman factor-like material in Hageman trait. *J Lab Clin Med* 69:819, 1967

293. RATNOFF OD, BUSSE RJ Jr, SHEON RP: The demise of John Hageman. *N Engl J Med* 279:760, 1968

294. STORMORKEN H, ABILDGAARD CF: The Fletcher factor-prekallikrein deficiency: A diagnostic test which identifies heterozygotes. *Thromb Res* 5:375, 1974

295. SAITO H, RATNOFF OD, DONALDSON VH: Defective activation of clotting, fibrinolysis, and permeability-enhancing systems in human Fletcher trait plasma. *Circ Res* 34:641, 1974

296. WUEPPER KD: Prekallikrein deficiency in man. *J Exp Med* 138:1345, 1973

297. DONALDSON VH, SAITO H, RATNOFF OD: Defective esterase and kinin-forming activity in human Fletcher trait plasma: A fraction rich in kallikrein-like activity. *Circ Res* 34:652, 1974

298. WEISS AS, GALLIN JI, KAPLAN AP: Fletcher-factor deficiency: A diminished rate of Hageman factor activation caused by the absence of prekallikrein with abnormalities of coagulation, fibrinolysis, chemotactic activity and kinin generation. *J Clin Invest* 53:622, 1974

299. SAITO H, RATNOFF OD: Inhibition of normal clotting and Fletcher factor activity by rabbit antikallikrein antiserum. *Nature* 248:597, 1974

300. WALDMAN R, ABRAHAM J: Fitzgerald factor: A heretofore unrecognized coagulation factor. *Blood* 46:761, 1975

301. SAITO H, GOLDSMITH C, RATNOFF OD: Fletcher factor activity in plasmas of various species. *Proc Soc Exp Biol Med* 147:519, 1974

302. COLMAN RW, BAGDASARIAN A, TALAMO RC, SCOTT CF, SEAVEY M, GUIMARAES JA, PIERCE JV, KAPLAN AP: Williams trait: Human kininogen deficiency with diminished levels of plasminogen proactivator and prekallikrein associated with abnormalities of the Hageman factor-dependent pathways. *J Clin Invest* 56:1650, 1975

303. WUEPPER KD, MILLER DR, LaCOMBE MJ: Flaujeac trait. Deficiency of human plasma kininogen. *J Clin Invest* 56:1663, 1975

304. MUIR WA, RATNOFF OD: The prevalence of plasma thromboplastin antecedent (PTA, factor XI deficiency). *Blood* 44:569, 1974

305. RAPAPORT SI, PROCTOR RP, PATCH MJ, YETTRA M: The mode of inheritance of PTA deficiency: Evidence for the existence of major PTA deficiency. *Blood* 18:149, 1961

306. BITHELL TC, PIZARA A, MacDIARMID WD: Variant of factor IX deficiency in a patient with 45,X Turner's syndrome. *Blood* 36:169, 1979

307. BARROW EM, BULLOCK WR, GRAHAM JB: A study of the carrier state for plasma thromboplastin component (PTC, Christmas factor) deficiency, utilizing a new assay procedure. *J Lab Clin Med* 55:936, 1960

308. MOOR-JANKOWSKI JK, HUSER HF, ROSIN S, TROUG G, SCHNEER-BERGER M, GEIGER M: *Hemophilia B: Genetics, Hematology and Clinical Aspects.* Basel, S Karger, 1958

309. WALL RL, McCONNELL J, MOORE D, MacPHERSON CR, MARSON A: Christmas disease, color-blindness and blood group Xgᵃ. *Am J Med* 43:214, 1967

310. BERG K, BEARN A: Common X-linked serum marker and its relation to other loci on the X chromosome. *Trans Assoc Am Physicians* 79:165, 1966

311. ROBERTS HR, CHUNG KS, GOLDSMITH JC: Mutant forms of factor IX. *Thromb Haemost* 38:338, 1977

312. HOUGIE C, TWOMEY JJ: Haemophilia Bₘ: a new type of factor IX deficiency. *Lancet* 1:698, 1967

313. ØSTERUD B, LAVINE K, KASPER CK, RAPAPART SI: Isolation and properties of the abnormal factor IX molecule of hemophilia Bₘ. *Thromb Haemost* 38:51, 1977

314. CHUNG KS, GOLDSMITH JC, ROBERTS HR: Purification and characterization of factor IX Chapel Hill. *Blood* 48:974, 1976

315. BRAUNSTEIN KM, GRIFFITH MJ, BRIËT E, ROBERTS HR: The molecular defect of factor IX Chapel Hill. *Thromb Haemost* 46(1):256, 1981

316. GIROLAMI A, STICCHI A, BURUL A, DAL BO ZANON R: An immunological investigation of hemophilia B with a tentative classification of the disease into five variants. *Vox Sang* 32:230, 1977

317. ZAUBER NP, LEVIN J: Factor IX levels in patients with hemophilia B (Christmas disease) following transfusion with concentrates of factor IX or fresh plasma. *Medicine* 56:213, 1977

318. BLATT PM, ROBERTS HR: Immunology of inhibitors to clotting factors, in Rose NR, Friedman H (eds): *Manual of Clinical Immunology.* Washington, DC, American Society for Microbiology, 1976, p 542

319. WHITE GC, ROBERTS HR, KINGDON HS, LUNDBLAD RL: Prothrombin complex concentrates: Potentially thrombogenic materials and clues to the mechanism of thrombosis *in vitro. Blood* 49:159, 1977

320. SEELER RA: Congenital "hypoprothrombinemias." Deficiency of factors II, VII, and X. *Med Clin North Am* 56(1):127, 1972

321. JESTY J: Coagulation factor VII, in Seligson D, Schmidt RM (eds): *Handbook Series in Clinical Laboratory Science, Section I:, Hematology.* Boca Raton, Fla, CRC Press, Inc, 1980, vol 3, p 41

322. GERSHWIN ME, GUDE JK: Deep vein thrombosis and pulmonary embolism in congenital factor VII deficiency. *N Engl J Med* 288:141, 1973

323. GIROLAMI A, MOLARO G, LAZZARIN M, SCARPA R, BRUNETTI A: A "new" haemorrhagic condition due to the presence of an abnormal factor X (factor X Friuli). A study of a large kindred. *Br J Haematol* 21:695, 1971

324. GOODNIGHT SH, FEINSTEIN DI, ØSTERUD B, RAPAPORT SI: Factor VII antibody-neutralizing material in hereditary and acquired factor VII deficiency. *Blood* 38:1, 1971

325. PRYDZ H: Studies on proconvertin (factor VII). VI. The production in rabbits of an antiserum against factor VII. *Scand J Clin Lab Invest* 17:66, 1965

326. SELIGSOHN U, SHANI M, RAMOT B, ADAM A, SHEBA C: Dubin-Johnson syndrome in Israel. II. Association with factor-VII deficiency. *Q J Med* 39:569, 1970

327. SELIGSOHN U, SHANI M, RAMOT B: Gilbert syndrome and factor-VII deficiency. *Lancet* 1:1398, 1970

328. GRAHAM JB, BARROW EM, HOUGIE C: Stuart factor defect. II. Genetic aspects of a "new" hemorrhagic state. *J Clin Invest* 36:497, 1957

329. ROOS J, VAN ARKEL C, VERLOOP MC, JORDAN FLJ: A "new" family with Stuart-Prower deficiency. *Thromb Diath Haemorrh* 3:59, 1959

330. RABINER SF, KRETCHMER N: The Stuart-Prower factor: Utilization of clotting factors obtained by starch-block electrophoresis for genetic evaluation. *Br J Haematol* 7:99, 1961

331. RATNOFF OD: The molecular basis of hereditary clotting disorders, in Spaet TH (ed): *Progress in Hemostasis and Thrombosis.* New York, Grune & Stratton, Inc, 1972, vol 1, p 39

332. DENSON KWE, LURIE A, DECATALDO F, MANNUCCI PM: The factor-X defect: Recognition of abnormal forms of factor X. *Br J Haematol* 18:317, 1970

333. SEELER RA: Parahemophilia. Factor V deficiency. *Med Clin North Am* 56:119, 1972

334. KINGSLEY CS: Familial factor V deficiency: The pattern of heredity. *Q J Med* 23:323, 1954

335. OWEN CA JR: Parahemophilia. *Arch Intern Med* 95:194, 1955

336. FRATANTONI JC, HILGARTNER M, NACHMAN RL: Nature of the defect in congenital factor V deficiency: Study in a patient with an acquired circulating anticoagulant. *Blood* 39:751, 1972

337. BREEDERVELD K, VAN ROYEN EA, TEN CATE JW: Severe factor V deficiency with prolonged bleeding time. *Thromb Diath Haemorrh* 32:538, 1974

338. COLMAN RW: Factor V, in Spaet TH (ed): *Progress in Hemostasis and Thrombosis.* New York, Grune & Stratton, Inc, 1976, vol 3, p 109

339. MAMMEN EF: Congenital abnormalities of the fibrinogen molecule. *Semin Thromb Hemostas* 1:184, 1974

340. GRALNICK HR: Congenital disorders of fibrinogen, in Williams WJ, Beutler E, Erslev AJ, Rundles RW (eds): *Hematology*, ed 2. New York: McGraw-Hill Book Co, 1977, p 1423

341. EGBRING R, ANDRASSY K, EGLI H, MEYER-LINDENBERG J: Diagnostische und therapeutische probleme bei congenitaler afibrinogenämie. *Blut* 22:175, 1971

342. BRÖNNIMANN R: Kongenital afibrinogenämie. *Acta Haematol* 11:41, 1954

343. SOLUM N, STORMORKEN H: Influence of fibrinogen on the aggregation of washed human platelets induced by adenosine diphosphate, thrombin, collagen and adrenaline. *Scand J Clin Lab Invest* 84 (suppl):170, 1966

344. INCEMAN S, CAEN J, BERNARD J: Aggregation, adhesion, and viscous metamorphosis of platelets in congenital fibrinogen deficiencies. *J Lab Clin Med* 68:21, 1966

345. GIROLAMI A, DEMARCO L, VIRGOLINI L, PERUFFO R, FABRIS F: Platelet adhesiveness and aggregation in congenital afibrinogenemia: An investigation of three patients with post-transfusion cross-correction studies between two of them. *Blut* 30:87, 1975

346. DE VRIES A, ROSENBERG T, KOCHWA S, BOSS JH: Precipitation antifibrinogen antibody appearing after fibrinogen infusions in a patient with congenital afibrinogenemia. *Am J Med* 30:486, 1961

347. INGRAM GIC, MCBRIEN DJ, SPENCER H: Fatal pulmonary embolus in congenital fibrinopenia. Report of two cases. *Acta Haematol* 35:56, 1966

348. MAMMEN EF, PRASAD AS, BARNHART MI, AU CC: Congenital dysfibrinogenemia: Fibrinogen Detroit. *J Clin Invest* 48:235, 1969

349. MÉNACHÉ D: Constitutional and familial abnormal fibrinogen. *Thromb Diath Haemorrh* 13:173, 1964

350. FORMAN WB, RATNOFF OD, BOYER MH: An inherited qualitative abnormality in plasma fibrinogen: Fibrinogen Cleveland. *J Lab Clin Med* 72:455, 1968

351. BLOMBÄCK M, BLOMBÄCK B, MAMMEN EF, PRASAD AS: Fibrinogen Detroit—a molecular defect in the N-terminal disulphide knot of human fibrinogen. *Nature* 218:134, 1968

352. MOSESSON MW, AMRANI DL, MÉNACHÉ D: Studies on the structural abnormality of fibrinogen Paris I. *J Clin Invest* 57:782, 1976

353. MARTINEZ J, HOLBURN RR, SHAPIRO S, ERSLEV AJ: Fibrinogen Philadelphia: A hereditary hypodysfibrinogenemia characterized by fibrinogen hypercatabolism. *J Clin Invest* 53:600, 1974

354. KITCHENS CS, NEWCOMB TF: Factor XIII. *Medicine* 58:413, 1979

355. LORAND L, URAYAMA T, DE KIEWET J: Diagnostic and genetic studies on fibrin stabilizing factor with a new assay based on amine incorporation. *J Clin Invest* 48:1054, 1969

356. OERI J, MATTER M, ISENSCHMID H, HAUSER F, KOLLER F: Angeborener Mangel an Faktor V (Parahaemophilie) verbunden mit echter Haemophilia A bei zwei Brüdern. *Bibl Paediatr (Mod Probl Paediatr)* 1:575, 1954

357. GRAHAM JM: Genetic control of factor VIII. *Lancet* 1:340, 1980

358. GIDDINGS JC, BLOOM AL: Inhibition of activated protein C in combined factor V/VIII deficiency. *Thromb Haemost* 46(1):61, 1981

359. SAITO H, SHIOYA M, KOIE K, KAMIYA T, KATSUMI O: Congenital combined deficiency of factor V and factor VIII: A case report and the effect of transfusion of normal plasma and hemophilia blood. *Thromb Diath Haemorrh* 22:316, 1969

360. CHUNG K-S, BEZEAUD A, GOLDSMITH JC, MCMILLAN CW, MÉNACHÉ D, ROBERTS HR: Congenital deficiency of blood clotting factors II, VII, IX, and X. *Blood* 53:776, 1979

361. HOUGIE C, MCPHERSON RA, ARONSON L: Passovoy factor: A hitherto unrecognized factor necessary for hemostasis. *Lancet* 2:290, 1975

362. MARCINIAK E, FARLEY CH, DESIMONE PA: Familial thrombosis due to antithrombin III deficiency. *Blood* 43:219, 1974

363. MACKIE M, BENNETT B, OGSTON D, DOUGLAS AS: Familial thrombosis: Inherited deficiency of antithrombin III. *Br Med J* 1:136, 1978

364. FILIP DJ, ECKSTEIN JD, VELTKAMP JJ: Hereditary antithrombin III deficiency and thromboembolic disease. *Am J Hematol* 2:343, 1976

365. SAS G, BLASKÓ G, BÁNHEGYI D, JÁKÓ J, PÁLOS LA: Abnormal antithrombin III (Antithrombin III 'Budapest') as a cause of a familial thrombophilia. *Thromb Diath Haemorrh* 32:105, 1974

366. SAS G, PETÖ I, BÁNHEGYI D, BLASKÓ G, DOMJÁN G: Heterogeneity of the "classical" antithrombin III deficiency. *Thromb Haemost* 44:133, 1980

367. TRAN TH, BOUNAMLAUX H, BONDELI C, HORKANEN H, MARBET GA, DUCKERT F: Purification and partial characterization of a hereditary abnormal antithrombin III fraction of a patient with recurrent thrombophlebitis. *Thromb Haemost* 44:87, 1980

368. TRAN TH, BONDELI C, MARBET GA, DUCKERT F: Reactivity of a hereditary abnormal antithrombin III fraction in the inhibition of thrombin and factor Xa. *Thromb Haemost* 44:92, 1980

369. AOKI N, MOROI M, SAKATA Y, YOSHIDA N, MATSUDA M: Abnormal plasminogen. A hereditary molecular abnormality found in a patient with recurrent thrombosis. *J Clin Invest* 61:1186, 1978

370. SAKATA Y, AOKI N: Molecular abnormality of plasminogen. *J Biol Chem* 255:5442, 1980

371. WOHL RC, SUMMARIA L, ROBBINS KC: Physiological activation of the human fibrinolytic system. Isolation and characterization of human plasminogen variants, Chicago I and Chicago II. *J Biol Chem* 254:9063, 1979

372. AOKI N, SAITO H, KAMIYA T, KOIE K, SAKATA Y, KOBAKURA M: Congenital deficiency of α_2-plasmin inhibitor associated with severe hemorrhagic tendency. *J Clin Invest* 63:877, 1979

373. AOKI N, SAKATA Y, MATSUDA M, TATENO K: Fibrinolytic states in a patient with congenital deficiency of α_2-plasmin inhibitor. *Blood* 55:483, 1980

374. MANN KG, NESHEIM ME, HIBBARD LS, TRACY PB: The role of factor V in the assembly of the prothrombinase complex. *Ann NY Acad Sci* 370:378, 1981

375. FOWLER WE, HANTGAN RR, HERMANS J, ERICKSON HP: The structure of the fibrin protofibril. *Proc Natl Acad Sci USA* 78:4872, 1981

71

INHERITED DISORDERS OF PLATELETS

RODGER P. McEVER

PHILIP W. MAJERUS

1. *Glanzmann's thrombasthenia and Bernard-Soulier disease are inherited defects of the platelet membrane. Both diseases are characterized by autosomal recessive transmission. In both thrombasthenia and Bernard-Soulier disease, the absence of a platelet membrane glycoprotein is associated with a serious impairment in platelet function which results in clinically significant bleeding.*

2. *Platelets from patients with Glanzmann's thrombasthenia do not aggregate in response to physiologic agonists such as ADP or thrombin, and they fail to support normal clot retraction. The platelet membranes lack a glycoprotein known as IIb-IIIa. Current evidence suggests that the lack of this glycoprotein prevents the platelet membrane from interacting with extracellular fibrinogen and intracellular contractile proteins, a process required for normal platelet aggregation and clot retraction.*

3. *Bernard-Soulier platelets (like platelets from patients with von Willebrand's disease) do not adhere normally to exposed subendothelial surfaces of blood vessels. Membranes from Bernard-Soulier platelets lack glycoprotein Ib, which is probably the receptor for plasma von Willebrand Factor (vWF). The absence of this receptor prevents platelets from binding vWF, which is required for platelet adhesion to subendothelium.*

4. *Inherited platelet abnormalities associated with defects in platelet secretion have also been described. Some of these appear to represent abnormalities in the synthesis of, or response to, prostaglandins. Others are associated with deficiencies in platelet storage granules. The inheritance patterns and the pathogenetic mechanisms of these disorders require further clarification.*

The enormous progress that has been made in the investigation of disorders of hemostasis can be illustrated by a statement from the original chapter on blood clotting factors written for this book 20 years ago: "The clotting factors are not known as specific chemical species (excepting Ca^{++}) and the reactions which they undergo or catalyze are known only phenomenologically" [1, p 1145]. There was no mention of platelet disorders in that chapter. With the recent isolation of all of the known human coagulation factors (except antihemophilic factor) and with the development of methods for studying the biology of platelets, a much clearer picture is emerging. In this chapter we present in detail two genetic disorders of platelets and mention a few others that await clear definition. Future editions of this text will undoubtedly contain descriptions of many more inherited disorders of platelet function.

ROLE OF PLATELETS IN NORMAL HEMOSTASIS

The initial response to injury of a vessel is the adherence of platelets to a surface, such as collagen, in the tissues beneath the endothelium. Platelets do not adhere to intact endothelium because of unique properties of endothelial cell membranes [2] and also because endothelial cells can produce the platelet inhibitory substance, prostacyclin [3, 4]. The adherence of platelets to nonendothelial surfaces depends on a plasma protein that has been designated *von Willebrand Factor (vWF)*. Lack of this protein produces a bleeding disorder, von Willebrand's disease, that is described in Chap. 70. Following the initial adherence of platelets to the wound surface, the hemostatic plug enlarges as other platelets attach to the initial layer in a process known as *aggregation*. This process requires that fibrinogen bind to the platelet surface [5–14].

As platelets aggregate, they also secrete the contents of granules, a response referred to as the *release reaction*. The substances secreted include calcium ions, adenosine diphosphate (ADP), fibrinogen, coagulation factor V, a growth factor that participates in wound healing, a heparin-neutralizing protein called *platelet factor 4*, and many other substances [15]. In addition, arachidonic acid is released from phosphatidylinositol [16, 17] and is metabolized to form thromboxane A_2, a labile compound that is a potent stimulus for further platelet aggregation and secretion [18]. Although thromboxane A_2 stimulates platelet aggregation and secretion, it is not required for these processes since thrombin can activate platelets that cannot synthesize thromboxane [19]. This has been shown by treatment of platelets with aspirin, which covalently acetylates a serine residue in the active site of cyclooxygenase [20], the first enzyme in the synthesis of thromboxane from arachidonic acid. Its inactivation results in the absence of thromboxane production.

It is likely that the most important physiologic stimulant of platelets is thrombin. Early in hemostasis a minute amount of thrombin forms by an unknown pathway [21], binds to specific receptors on the platelet surface, and triggers the events of platelet activation outlined above [22]. In addition, the interaction of platelets with coagulation factors is important in promoting reactions leading to fibrin formation. The best-studied reaction is the conversion of prothrombin to thrombin. Platelets possess about 200 receptor sites per cell, where factors X_a, V_a, and prothrombin interact very efficiently to produce thrombin [23, 24]. Finally, platelets are able to contract, and because they are bound to the fibrin network, they can consolidate the hemostatic plug into a tight mass.

Platelet function can be assessed by measurement of in vitro aggregation in response to various agonists, or by measurement of the secretion of granule contents. The products of arachidonate metabolism can also be measured. Clot retraction in vitro is a measure of the ability of platelets to contract. The test of platelet function which best predicts the likelihood of abnormal bleeding is measurement of the bleeding time after a standard 1-mm cutaneous incision [25].

GLANZMANN'S THROMBASTHENIA

In 1918 Glanzmann described a heterogeneous group of disorders, including some characterized by abnormal clot retrac-

tion, which were ascribed to a platelet defect [26]. Other early workers noted that the disease, designated *Glanzmann's thrombasthenia*, was also characterized by a prolonged bleeding time, the lack of any clumped platelets, and the appearance of isolated platelets on the peripheral blood smear [27, 28]. In 1964 Hardisty et al. demonstrated decreased aggregation of thrombasthenic platelets in response to physiologic agonists [29]. Since that report numerous patients with similar abnormalities have been described, and an autosomal recessive pattern of inheritance has been clearly documented [30–36]. The incidence of the disease has not been determined, in part because the molecular defect has only recently been elucidated. Glanzmann's thrombasthenia is probably the most common inherited disorder of platelet function.

Diagnosis

A diagnosis of Glanzmann's thrombasthenia can be made on the basis of the following criteria:

1. Mucocutaneous bleeding of variable severity which is usually present from birth.
2. History of bleeding in sibs compatible with autosomal recessive transmission.
3. Normal platelet count and morphology in the presence of
   a. Prolonged bleeding time.
   b. Absent or diminished clot retraction.
   c. Absent platelet aggregation by ADP, epinephrine, collagen, and thrombin, but normal aggregation by ristocetin and human vWF.
4. Normal coagulation factors (prothrombin time and partial thromboplastin time both normal.)

The diagnosis can be confirmed specifically by demonstration of the decrease or absence of membrane glycoprotein IIb-IIIa (discussed below). Other abnormalities are a decrease in total platelet fibrinogen, failure of platelets to bind fibrinogen, and absence of the Pl^{A1} alloantigen.

Clinical Manifestations

The pattern of bleeding in thrombasthenia is characteristic of that in patients with thrombocytopenia or qualitative platelet defects. Purpura, epistaxis, gingival bleeding, and menorrhagia are common. Gastrointestinal hemorrhages and hematuria are also seen. Unlike coagulation factor deficiencies, such as hemophilia A, hemarthroses are unusual. The severity of bleeding varies widely among patients but is frequently severe enough to require transfusion. Some patients die of hemorrhage during childhood, but most survive to adulthood and several have had unexplained amelioration as they grew older. Some virtually asymptomatic homozygous patients have been discovered in the course of family studies undertaken after the diagnosis of a more severely affected proband. Heterozygotes for the disease are always asymptomatic.

Laboratory Studies

Plasma coagulation factors and platelet counts are normal. The appearance of platelets by light microscopy is normal, except for their occurrence as isolated elements, rather than aggregates on a smear. Electron microscopy shows no specific structural abnormalities [30]. The morphology of the bone marrow is unremarkable. Survival of ^{51}Cr-labeled platelets is normal [30]. Total platelet fibrinogen is usually reduced [30, 31, 33]. The bleeding time is invariably prolonged, usually markedly. Clot retraction is absent in most patients but may be seen to a reduced extent in some [30].

The most striking functional defect is the failure of thrombasthenic platelets to aggregate in response to any physiologic agonist, including ADP, epinephrine, collagen, and thrombin [29–36]. Unlike Bernard-Soulier platelets, thrombasthenic platelets do aggregate when exposed to normal plasma and the antibiotic ristocetin [15]. Thrombasthenic platelets bind thrombin normally and respond with shape change and the release reaction [37]. This suggests that the aggregation defect in thrombasthenic platelets is due to an abnormality occurring at a stage subsequent to initial platelet activation.

Human platelets which are washed free of plasma require exogenous fibrinogen in order for aggregation to occur after stimulation with ADP, epinephrine, or collagen [5–7]. Thrombin causes release of intracellular fibrinogen, so that exogenous fibrinogen is not required for aggregation when thrombin is the stimulus. Several recent studies have helped to clarify the role of fibrinogen in platelet aggregation with the demonstration that platelets possess specific, saturable receptors for fibrinogen [8–14]. Fibrinogen binding requires exposure of platelets to an agonist, and maximal binding occurs with the same concentrations of fibrinogen and calcium ions required for optimal platelet aggregation [8–14]. Although two groups have suggested that there are two classes of fibrinogen receptor [13, 14], three others have presented evidence for the presence of a single class of receptors with approximately 45,000 fibrinogen molecules bound per platelet under optimal conditions [8–11]. One fascinating observation arising from these experiments is that thrombasthenic platelets are unable to bind fibrinogen [9, 13, 14, 38, 39]. This suggests that the defect in platelet aggregation may be caused by the absence of the membrane receptor for fibrinogen. The relationship of the fibrinogen binding defect to the deficiency in intracellular fibrinogen is not clear, but it suggests that the platelet surface fibrinogen receptor is involved in the process by which platelet granules acquire fibrinogen.

Membrane Glycoprotein Defect in Thrombasthenia

Nurden and Caen studied platelet membrane proteins by sodium dodecyl sulfate polyacrylamide gel electrophoresis and first noted a deficiency in a major glycoprotein in thrombasthenia [40]. Phillips and Agin, using two-dimensional sodium dodecyl sulfate gel electrophoresis of radioiodinated platelets, found that two membrane polypeptides, now known as *IIb* and *IIIa*, are decreased in the disease [41]. This finding has since been confirmed in other studies of thrombasthenic platelet proteins [42, 43]. It now seems clear that the polypeptides IIb and IIIa are subunits of a single membrane protein. When normal platelet membranes are solubilized in Triton X-100 and examined by crossed immunoelectrophoresis, a number of immunoprecipitates are found, as shown in Fig. 71-1A [44]. One of these proteins, designated *16* in Fig. 71-1A, is absent in extracts from thrombasthenic platelets (Fig. 71-1B). This immunoprecipitate, eluted from agarose and further analyzed by sodium dodecyl sulfate polyacrylamide gel electrophoresis, contains both polypeptides IIb and IIIa, suggesting that they are subunits of a single protein designated *glycoprotein IIb-IIIa*.

We have developed a monoclonal hybridoma antibody,

called *Tab*, that is directed against platelet glycoprotein IIb-IIIa [45]. The glycoprotein has been isolated from solubilized normal platelet membranes by affinity chromatography on a column of *Tab* coupled to agarose. When analyzed by gel electrophoresis, the purified protein consists only of polypeptides IIb and IIIa, along with traces of a Mr = 43,000 peptide which may be platelet actin (Fig. 71-2). Studies with ^{125}I-*Tab* indicate that the antibody binds to ~40,000 sites per platelet (Fig. 71-3). Assuming that one *Tab* molecule binds per glycoprotein, there are ~40,000 IIb-IIIa molecules per normal platelet. *Tab* binding sites are absent from the platelets of thrombasthenic patients, indicating absence of glycoprotein IIb-IIIa in the membrane. Family members who are heterozygotes for the disease have intermediate levels of glycoprotein IIb-IIIa, a finding consistent with the autosomal recessive pattern of inheritance. Crossed immunoelectrophoresis studies [46] and experiments with an alloantibody from a transfused thrombasthenic patient [55] also show that heterozygotes have intermediate levels of glycoprotein IIb-IIIa.

The degree of deficiency of glycoprotein IIb-IIIa may vary among patients. Caen originally noted that the majority of patients, designated *type I*, had absent clot retraction and undetectable platelet fibrinogen, while *type II* patients had some clot retraction and detectable, although reduced, platelet fibrinogen [47]. Crossed immunoelectrophoresis demonstrates that type I patients lack the IIb-IIIa immunoprecipitate and an arc representing fibrinogen [44], while type II patients have detectable, although markedly decreased, arcs for IIb-IIIa and fibrinogen.

We have isolated glycoprotein IIb-IIIa using the *Tab* antibody and have then separated the subunits and analyzed them [48]. The amino acid compositions, although not identical, are similar, suggesting some sequence homology. However, tryptic peptide maps are entirely different, which indicates that the structural relationship of the two subunits does not arise from conversion of one subunit into the other [48]. Both IIb and IIIa contain ~15 percent carbohydrate by weight, but the relative proportions of individual sugars differ between the two glycoproteins. It has been proposed on the basis of immunologic evidence that glycoprotein IIIa may be identical to α-actinin, a protein in muscle and nonmuscle cells that can bind actin [49]. This hypothesis is not supported by the amino acid composition of IIIa, which differs markedly from that of α-actinin [50, 51].

The Pl^{A1} antigen is a platelet-specific alloantigen present in 98 percent of the normal population [52]. It is absent or reduced in all patients with thrombasthenia [53], and recent studies have established that the antigen resides on the IIIa subunit of glycoprotein IIb-IIIa [54]. Individuals who lack Pl^{A1} but are otherwise normal have normal levels of glycoprotein IIb-IIIa [53]. The Pl^{A1} antigen is not required for normal function of the protein. The antigen is absent in thrombasthenic platelets because glycoprotein IIb-IIIa is missing. A family study of thrombasthenic homozygotes and heterozygotes in which glycoprotein IIb-IIIa levels and Pl^{A1} antigen levels were simultaneously measured indicates that the genes for inheritance of Pl^{A1} and expression of glycoprotein IIb-IIIa segregate independently [46].

Pathophysiology of Thrombasthenia

Several studies point to a relationship between the functional abnormalities in thrombasthenic platelets and the deficiency in glycoprotein IIb-IIIa. An antibody obtained from the serum of

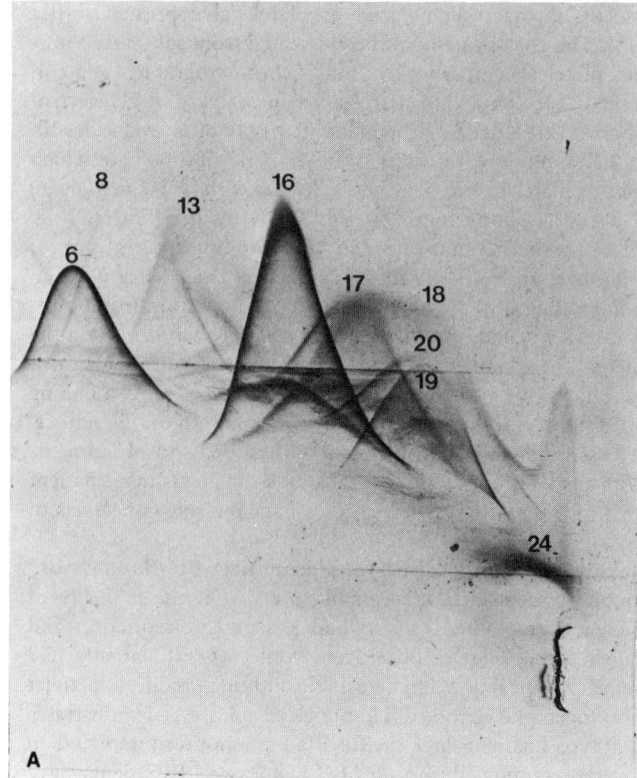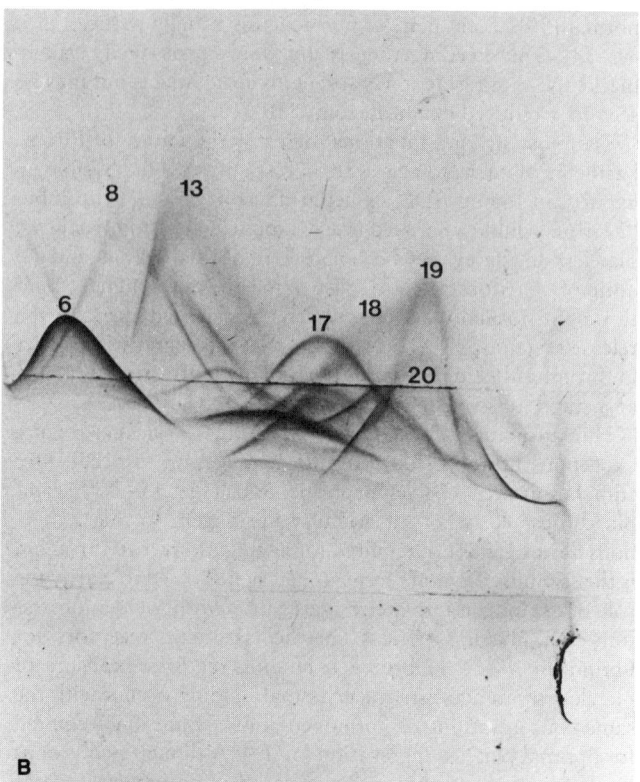

Figure 71-1 Crossed immunoelectrophoresis of Triton X-100 solubilized proteins from (A) normal platelets and (B) thrombasthenic platelets. Electrophoresis in the vertical second dimension was performed in agarose gel containing rabbit antibodies to whole platelets. The thrombasthenic platelets lack two immunoprecipitates: peak 16, which represents membrane glycoprotein IIb-IIIa, and peak 24, which is platelet fibrinogen. (*From [44], with permission of the author and publisher.*)

a multiply transfused thrombasthenic patient reacted with normal platelets but not thrombasthenic platelets [55]. The antibody presumably arose from the fact that the patient was not tolerant to the normal platelet glycoprotein IIb-IIIa. The antibody precipitated glycoprotein IIb-IIIa [44] and inhibited aggregation of normal platelets by ADP, epinephrine, collagen, and thrombin [56]. These data suggest that glycoprotein IIb-IIIa is required for normal platelet aggregation. The estimated 45,000 fibrinogen receptors on normal platelets [9–11] equal the 40,000 IIb-IIIa molecules estimated from ^{125}I-*Tab* binding to platelets [45]. This information, plus the finding that thrombasthenic platelets, which lack IIb-IIIa, cannot bind fibrinogen, suggests that glycoprotein IIb-IIIa is necessary for platelet aggregation because it is the fibrinogen receptor.

Evidence for an interaction of glycoprotein IIb-IIIa with intracellular contractile proteins has also been presented [57]. The residue remaining after solubilizing unstimulated platelets in Triton X-100 consists primarily of actin, actin binding protein, and myosin when examined by sodium dodecyl sulfate polyacrylamide gel electrophoresis. When platelets are stimulated with thrombin and then solubilized in Triton X-100, a larger residue is obtained, which on analysis contains increased amounts of myosin and actin as well as glycoprotein IIb-IIIa. These experiments suggest that exposure of platelets to thrombin allows membrane glycoprotein IIb-IIIa to interact with platelet contractile proteins. Our finding of traces of a protein which may represent actin associated with the glycoprotein IIb-IIIa purified by *Tab* affinity chromatography is also consistent with an interaction of contractile elements with IIb-IIIa [45].

These lines of evidence suggest that platelet stimulation allows membrane glycoprotein IIb-IIIa to bind fibrinogen on the cell exterior and contractile proteins in the cell interior (Fig. 71-4). The former allows platelet aggregation, the latter clot retraction. The absence of this critical linking glycoprotein in thrombasthenic platelets accounts for the failure of platelet aggregation and clot retraction. Direct demonstration of binding of fibrinogen and of contractile protein(s) to glycoprotein IIb-IIIa is needed to verify this model.

Further information is required to define the molecular pathology in thrombasthenia since no structural studies on glycoprotein IIb-IIIa from thrombasthenic mutants have been completed. Our studies on the normal protein imply that the subunits IIb and IIIa are the products of separate genes. It is not clear whether thrombasthenia can result from mutations in either subunit, although theoretically that is possible. By analogy with other inherited defects, it is likely that apparently homozygous subjects have defects in both alleles for the same subunit. This could result in defective combination with the other subunit or defective insertion into the membrane. Type II thrombasthenia could result from partial incorporation of an abnormal protein into the platelet membrane. It is even conceivable that thrombasthenia results from an abnormality in a yet undiscovered protein required for insertion of IIb-IIIa into the platelet membrane.

Treatment

Treatment of this disease is limited to supportive measures. Chronic or acute hemorrhage may require blood transfusions or supplemental iron therapy. Platelet transfusions should be reserved for serious or life-threatening bleeding since patients may develop antibodies to normal platelets and become refractory to future transfusion [35, 55]. Hormonal control of menses is usually effective in controlling menorrhagia.

BERNARD-SOULIER DISEASE

In 1948 Bernard and Soulier reported a 5-month-old infant with a history of spontaneous mucocutaneous bleeding beginning shortly after birth [58]. The patient had a prolonged bleeding time, and his platelets appeared abnormally large on the peripheral blood smear. The parents and one sib had no history of abnormal bleeding, but a sister died of hemorrhage at age 3 years. In 1964 a review in the French literature described 14 symptomatic patients who had prolonged bleeding times, large platelets, and normal clot retraction [59]. Autosomal recessive inheritance was demonstrated. Since then, 28 patients who meet these criteria have been reported in the English literature [60–72]. Nineteen of them [64–72] were shown to have the platelet aggregation defect or membrane

Figure 71-2 Sodium dodecyl sulfate polyacrylamide gel electrophoresis of purified glycoprotein IIb-IIIa, isolated by affinity chromatography from platelet membrane proteins solubilized in Triton X-100. The affinity resin was made by crosslinking the monoclonal antibody, *Tab*, to agarose. 2-Mercaptoethanol (2ME) was added to some samples to reduce disulfide bands prior to electrophoresis. Lanes left to right: lane 1, molecular weight standards; lane 2, Triton X-100 solubilized platelet membranes before application to the affinity column, reduced; lane 3, glycoprotein IIb-IIIa eluate from *Tab*-agarose, reduced; lane 4, glycoprotein IIb-IIIa eluate, unreduced. After reduction of disulfide bonds, the apparent molecular weight of IIb decreases because of release of a small disulfide-linked polypeptide chain which can be seen at the bottom of the gel. The apparent molecular weight of IIIa increases, presumably because of cleavage of intrachain disulfide bonds, which allows the molecule to unfold. In lane 3, a faint band of Mr = 43,000 is also seen, which may represent platelet actin. (*From [45], with permission of the publisher.*)

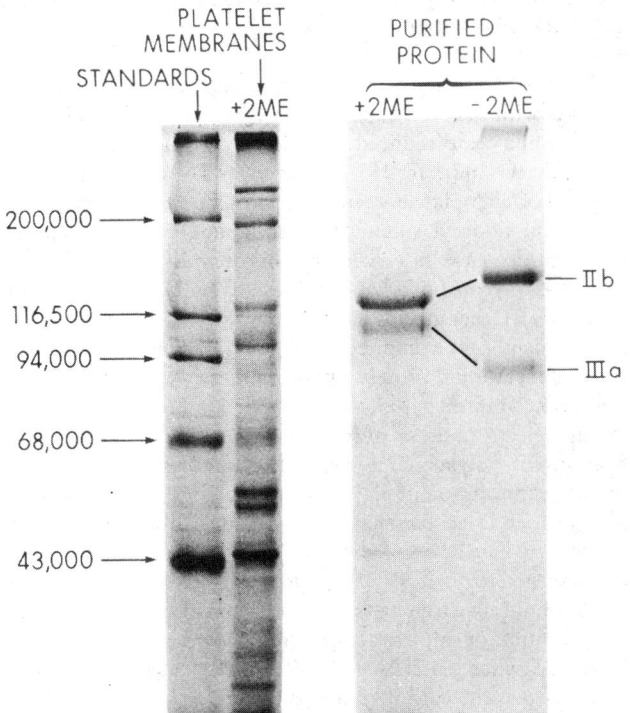

glycoprotein deficiency (described below) considered specific for the disease. The incidence of the disorder, now known as *Bernard-Soulier disease*, is unknown, in part because it has only recently been precisely defined. It probably occurs less frequently than thrombasthenia.

Diagnosis

Bernard-Soulier disease can be diagnosed by applying the following criteria:

1. Mucocutaneous bleeding.
2. History of bleeding in sibs compatible with autosomal recessive transmission.
3. Normal or moderately decreased platelet count with:
   a. Giant platelets on peripheral blood smear.
   b. Normal clot retraction.
   c. Absent platelet aggregation with human vWF plus ristocetin or with bovine vWF alone.
   d. Normal platelet aggregation with ADP, epinephrine, collagen, and thrombin.
4. Normal coagulation factors (prothrombin time and partial thromboplastin time both normal).

An unequivocal diagnosis can be made by demonstrating the absence of membrane glycoprotein Ib (see below). Other abnormalities are failure to bind vWF, absence of receptors for drug-dependent antibodies to platelets, and an abnormal serum prothrombin time.

Clinical Manifestations

The degree of bleeding varies among patients, even within a family, but most experience episodes severe enough to require transfusion. The nature of the bleeding is similar to that seen in patients with thrombasthenia. Purpura, gingival bleeding, epistaxis, and menorrhagia are common. Gastrointestinal hemorrhage, hematuria, and cerebral hemorrhage have been reported. Unlike patients with coagulation factor abnormalities, these patients do not suffer from hemarthroses.

Laboratory Features

Morphology   On peripheral blood smear, Bernard-Soulier platelets appear large (Fig. 71-5). Electron micrographs have also demonstrated large platelets, but no other consistent ultrastructural abnormalities [66, 67, 69]. One group has claimed that circulating Bernard-Soulier platelets are actually of normal size and shape and appear large on smear because of an abnormal shape change occurring during smear preparation [73]. It is difficult to reconcile this observation with the finding that the total protein content of Bernard-Soulier platelets ranges from 2 to 5 times normal [62, 66, 72]. Normal or increased numbers of megakaryocytes are found in the bone marrow, and their morphology appears normal [60–62, 66].

Aggregation and Adhesion Studies   Bernard-Soulier platelets aggregate normally in response to ADP, collagen, and epinephrine [64–71]. Aggregation in response to thrombin has also been reported to be normal [64, 65, 71], although one study suggests that the rate of aggregation in response to low

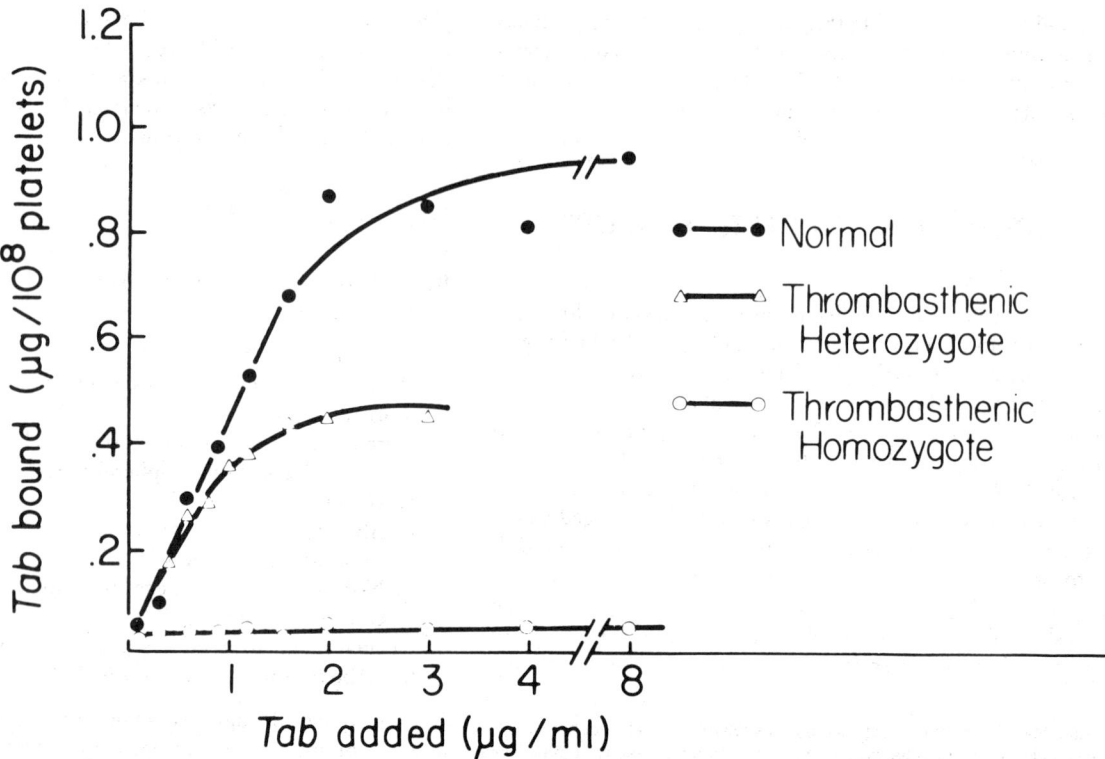

Figure 71-3 Steady state binding of [125]I-*Tab* to normal and thrombasthenic platelets. At saturation, the *Tab* antibody, which recognizes membrane glycoprotein IIb-IIIa, binds to ~40,000 sites on normal platelets. *Tab* does not bind to platelets of thrombasthenic homozygotes and has reduced binding to platelets of thrombasthenic heterozygotes. (*From* [45], *with permission of the publisher.*)

thrombin concentrations is reduced [74]. Bernard-Soulier platelets fail to aggregate in the presence of autologous plasma and the antibiotic ristocetin [65, 66, 69–75]. The same abnormality is seen in von Willebrand's disease, which results from a deficiency of plasma vWF (Chap. 70). The aggregation defect in von Willebrand's disease platelets is corrected by the addition of normal plasma or plasma from a Bernard-Soulier patient. However, Bernard-Soulier platelets fail to aggregate with ristocetin even in the presence of plasma from a normal subject [65, 75]. This observation suggests that Bernard-Soulier platelets lack a receptor for a plasma component, most likely vWF. Recent binding studies with purified, radiolabeled vWF have confirmed the presence of receptors for human vWF on normal platelets [76, 77] but not on Bernard-Soulier platelets [78]. The vWF binding, as does vWF-induced aggregation, requires the antibiotic ristocetin. Absence of either the vWF receptor in Bernard-Soulier disease or plasma vWF in von Willebrand's disease results in failure of aggregation of platelet-rich plasma in the presence of ristocetin.

Although ristocetin-induced aggregation is an in vitro phenomenon, it is a manifestation of a more physiologic interaction of platelets with exposed subendothelial surfaces. Baumgartner and Muggli [79] have described a method to measure this interaction, in which anticoagulated blood is circulated through a perfusion chamber containing segments of rabbit aorta in which the subendothelium has been exposed. The segments are fixed and examined microscopically, and the percentage of surface to which platelets have become adherent is measured. Platelets from Bernard-Soulier patients [68, 70], like those from von Willebrand's disease patients [80, 81], show a decreased adherence to subendothelium. In vivo, some element in exposed subendothelium may promote the binding of vWF to platelets and the interaction of platelets with the vessel wall. Thus the functional defect in vivo in Bernard-Soulier disease is

a failure of adherence of platelets to exposed subendothelium.

Membrane Glycoprotein Defect in Bernard-Soulier Disease

In 1969 Gröttum and Solum reported that platelets from three patients with Bernard-Soulier disease had reduced electrophoretic mobility and reduced sialic acid, and suggested a membrane defect [62]. In 1975 Nurden and Caen fractionated Bernard-Soulier platelet membrane proteins by electrophoresis in sodium dodecyl sulfate polyacrylamide gels and demonstrated a decrease in a major glycoprotein of $Mr = 155,000$ [82]. This glycoprotein has been designated *Glycoprotein I* or Ib [83, 84]. Other groups have also shown a discrete reduction in this membrane component [43, 71]. Claims of additional platelet membrane protein abnormalities in the disease have not been confirmed [63, 85]. Recent studies using crossed immunoelectrophoresis of solubilized platelets [44] and modifications of polyacrylamide gel electrophoresis that provide improved resolution of platelet glycoproteins [72] suggest that glycoprotein Ib is absent in Bernard-Soulier platelets (Fig. 71-6). Intermediate levels of glycoprotein Ib have been reported in obligate heterozygotes [71]. Glycocalicin, a glycoprotein of similar molecular weight, is liberated from platelet membranes by sonication or salt extraction [86–88] and is also missing in Bernard-Soulier platelets [42–44]. Purified glycocalicin contains 60 percent carbohydrate, including a large amount of sialic acid [87]. Although glycocalicin was originally thought to be a distinct protein, it now appears most likely that it arises from proteolysis of glycoprotein Ib. Crossed immunoelectrophoresis has shown that glycocalicin and glycoprotein Ib are immunologically related [88]. Moreover, since the liberation of glycocalicin from platelets can be inhibited with EDTA, glycocalicin may be cleaved from integral membrane glycoprotein Ib by a calcium-dependent platelet protease [88].

Pathophysiology of Bernard-Soulier Disease

The relationship of the absence of membrane glycoprotein Ib to the functional abnormalities in Bernard-Soulier platelets has been the subject of several studies. Two antiserums that produce a Bernard-Soulier-like platelet-adhesion defect in vitro have been described [89, 90]. One was derived from a Bernard-Soulier patient who had received numerous transfusions [89]. The other was a rabbit antihuman platelet antiserum [90]. Both antiserums precipitate a protein of Mr ≃ 155,000 from solubilized normal platelet membranes. This suggests that they contain antibodies to glycoprotein Ib and that binding of antibody to the glycoprotein interferes with its interaction with vWF and subendothelium. In other studies, a glycoprotein migrating in the glycoprotein I region on sodium dodecyl sulfate polyacrylamide gel electrophoresis has been purified from detergent-solubilized platelets by wheat germ agglutinin chromatography [91, 92]. This glycoprotein inhibits ristocetin-induced platelet aggregation in human plasma [91] or vWF-induced aggregation in bovine plasma [92]. At least three glycoproteins migrate in the glycoprotein I region on polyacrylamide gels [84], and therefore the studies described above could not establish that the protein in each case is the one that is absent from Bernard-Soulier platelets [72]. Nevertheless, the evidence is consistent with a model in which glycoprotein Ib acts as the receptor for vWF. The binding of vWF to Ib promotes the adherence of platelets to exposed subendothelial structures. The absence of glycoprotein Ib in Bernard-Soulier platelets accounts for their inability to interact with vWF and subendothelial surfaces. Thus the pathogenesis of von Willebrand's disease and Bernard-Soulier disease is related.

Role of Glycoprotein Ib in Drug-induced Purpura Certain drugs, such as quinine and quinidine, are capable of causing immune thrombocytopenia in susceptible individuals [93, 94]. Platelet damage requires the presence of the drug, antibody, and plasma [94]. Lymphocytes from sensitized patients proliferate (as determined by [3H]thymidine incorporation) when exposed to platelet membranes, drug, and normal plasma [95] but fail to respond if von Willebrand's disease plasma is used [96]. The addition of purified vWF to the mixture restores lymphocyte proliferation [96]. This suggests that the plasma factor necessary for drug-induced antibody formation and subsequent platelet damage is vWF. Bernard-Soulier platelets, unlike normal platelets, do not react with these drug-dependent antibodies and do not stimulate [3H]thymidine incorporation in lymphocytes from sensitized patients [95, 97]. These observations are consistent with previously cited evidence that Bernard-Soulier platelets fail to bind vWF and suggest that the platelet component required for antigenic stimulus is glycoprotein Ib. Thus the antigenic moiety in these patients appears to be drug bound to vWF, which in turn is bound to platelet glycoprotein Ib.

Other Reported Abnormalities Glycocalicin inhibits thrombin binding to platelets [98]. Moreover, platelets from two Bernard-Soulier patients were reported to have approximately one-third the normal number of thrombin receptors and a decreased rate of aggregation at low levels of thrombin [74]. These authors proposed that glycoprotein Ib and glycocalicin function as the receptor for thrombin as well as for vWF. However, since thrombin does not inhibit the binding of vWF to platelets, there may be separate receptors for the two proteins [76]. Other investigators have noted normal aggregation responses to thrombin [64, 65, 71]. Most importantly, since glycoprotein Ib is totally absent in Bernard-Soulier platelets [44, 72], a complete lack of thrombin binding and thrombin response would be expected if this glycoprotein is the

Figure 71-4 Model for the function of platelet membrane glycoprotein IIb-IIIa. When platelets are activated, IIb-IIIa binds to fibrinogen on the cell exterior and to one or more contractile proteins on the cell interior, thereby promoting platelet aggregation and, subsequently, clot retraction. The model explains how the structural abnormality, absence of glycoprotein IIb-IIIa, leads to the platelet functional defects in Glanzmann's thrombasthenia.

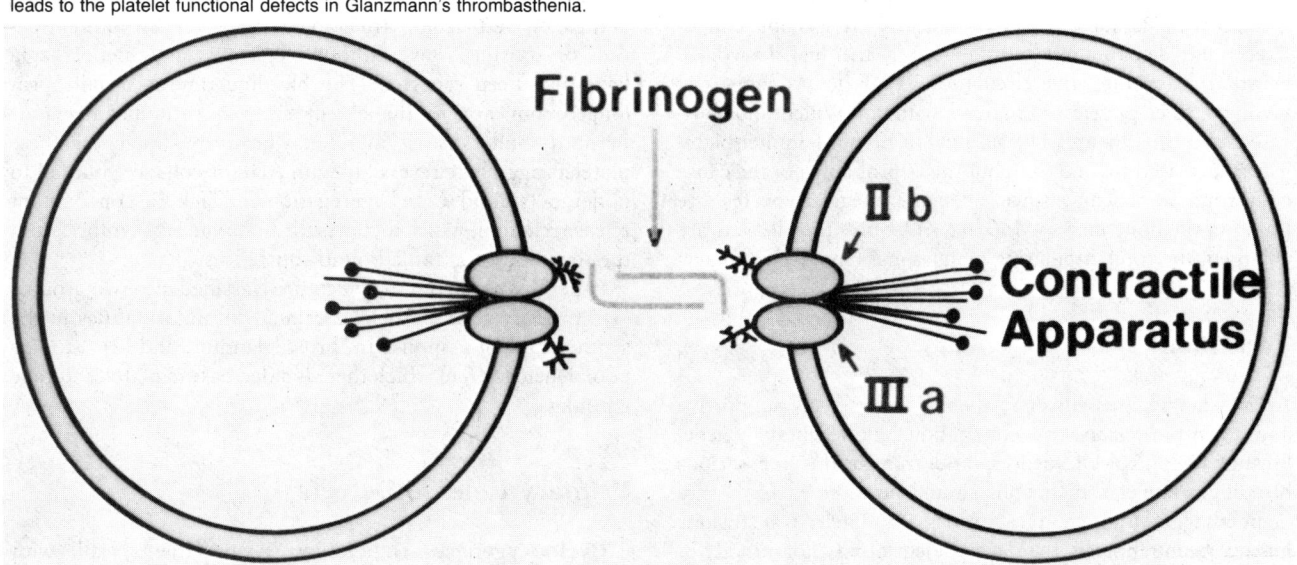

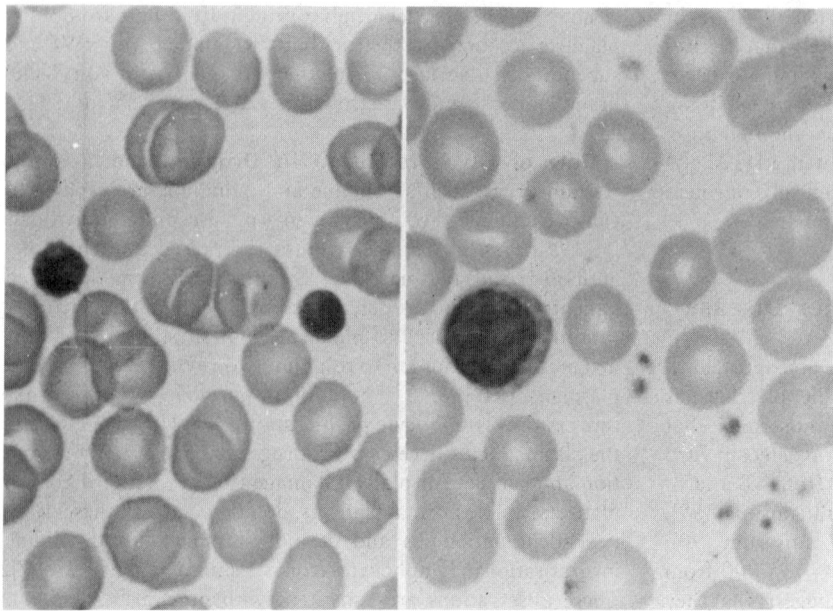

Figure 71-5 *Left,* peripheral blood smear from a patient with Bernard-Soulier disease (C.L. from Ref. 71), containing two characteristically enlarged platelets. *Right,* normal peripheral blood smear, showing a lymphocyte and several normal-size platelets.

thrombin receptor. We conclude that glycoprotein Ib is not the thrombin receptor.

The shortened prothrombin time measured in serum from Bernard-Soulier patients [60, 64, 65, 67, 69] indicates decreased prothrombin consumption during the clotting of whole blood and therefore possibly defective conversion of prothrombin to thrombin at the platelet surface. The reason for this interesting defect is not understood. It has been proposed that defective binding of vWF may result in failure to activate the coagulant activity of factor VIII [75]. If so, deficiency of activated factor VIII might result in generation of less factor Xa, which in turn is required for prothrombin activation. It would be of interest to measure the binding of factors Xa and Va [23, 24] to Bernard-Soulier platelets to determine if this receptor is directly affected by the Bernard-Soulier defect. Decreased adsorption of the clotting activities of factors V, VIII, and XI to washed Bernard-Soulier platelets has been described [69], but the specificity of this adsorption and its physiologic significance are unclear.

The mechanism for formation of large platelets in the disease is unknown. Perhaps the lack of membrane glycoprotein Ib affects the demarcation of platelets in the megakaryocyte before release into the circulation. vWF is probably not involved, since platelets in patients with von Willebrand's disease are normal in size. The survival of Bernard-Soulier platelets is decreased [61, 62, 99], but this is probably not the cause of thrombocytopenia, since adequate megakaryocytes are found in the bone marrow [60, 62, 66]. Since the platelets are enlarged, the total circulating platelet mass may be normal.

Treatment

As in Glanzmann's thrombasthenia, treatment is supportive and consists of iron supplementation, good dental hygiene, hormonal control of menses, and transfusions for serious bleeding. Platelet transfusions should be reserved for severe hemorrhage. Although refractoriness to platelet transfusions has not been reported, the development of an alloantibody in one patient [89] suggests that this could become a clinical

problem. Splenectomy has been attempted in some patients because of thrombocytopenia [64, 66, 70]. This may produce a transient increase in platelet count but no reduction in bleeding, because the basic platelet defect remains. Corticosteroids have been tried without benefit [65].

SECRETION DEFECTS

In the past 15 years there have been many reports describing patients with congenital defects in agonist-induced platelet secretion. These patients represent an extremely heterogeneous group of disorders. In some cases hereditary transmission of the platelet defect is evident, but in others only isolated patients are described.

Patients with secretion defects usually have less severe bleeding symptoms than those with thrombasthenia or Bernard-Soulier disease. The most frequent symptoms are easy bruising and excessive bleeding after operations such as tooth extraction or tonsillectomy, although epistaxis and menorrhagia have also been reported. The bleeding time is usually prolonged, but not to the extent seen in thrombasthenia or Bernard-Soulier disease, and it may be normal. In general these platelets aggregate reversibly with ADP or collagen, but fail to undergo "second wave" aggregation and lack the concomitant release reaction, which includes thromboxane A_2 synthesis and the secretion of granule-bound substances.

Patients with secretion defects are classified into two groups: (1) "primary release" defects related to abnormalities in the synthesis of, or response to, prostaglandins, and (2) "storage pool deficiency," in which there is a decrease in platelet storage granules.

Primary Release Defects

Cyclooxygenase Deficiency Five patients, all with mildly abnormal bleeding, have been reported to lack the enzyme cyclooxygenase [100–103]. This enzyme catalyzes the conversion of arachidonic acid to cyclic endoperoxide, which is an intermediate in the production of thromboxane A_2. Thromboxane A_2, in turn, stimulates platelet aggregation and secretion [18], although it is not required for thrombin activation. In these patients exogenous arachidonic acid fails to induce platelet aggregation and secretion, but addition of cyclic endoperoxide is effective. There are insufficient genetic data to determine whether any of these cases have an inherited enzyme deficiency. The same functional defect is seen in individuals who ingest aspirin, which permanently acetylates cyclooxygenase [19]. Although the reported patients are said to have abstained from aspirin, it is difficult to prove this in view of the extremely low levels of aspirin required to inactivate the enzyme [104]. Measurement of cyclooxygenase levels by radioimmunoassay [105] should make it possible to detect patients who definitely lack the enzyme.

Platelet Unresponsiveness to Thromboxane A_2 Recently, a family with a mild autosomal dominant bleeding disorder has been described in which platelets of affected members do not undergo secretion and second-wave aggregation in response to ADP and epinephrine [106, 107]. Platelets of the propositus fail to aggregate or undergo the release reaction in response to either arachidonic acid or a cyclic endoperoxide analogue. Thromboxane A_2 formation from added arachi-

donic acid is normal, as determined by levels of thromboxane B_2, a stable metabolite of thromboxane A_2. Rapid addition of arachidonate-stimulated normal platelet-rich plasma (which contains thromboxane A_2) fails to aggregate the patient's platelets. Thus the defect in platelets from this family appears to be due to a failure of the platelets to respond to thromboxane A_2. The mechanism for this lack of responsiveness remains to be defined.

Storage Pool Deficiency

Patients in this heterogeneous group have platelets with diminished numbers of electron-dense granules when examined by electron microscopy [108]. Deficiencies in other structures known as α *granules* are sometimes seen in the same platelets [108]. Only two patients (gray platelet syndrome) have been reported with an isolated deficiency in α granules [109]. The relation between the usually minor functional abnormalities of the platelets and the decrease in storage granules is not understood. Two families with storage pool deficiency have been described in which the defect is transmitted in an autosomal dominant manner [110, 111]. Morphologic abnormalities of platelet granules have been associated with other inherited disorders, including the Hermansky-Pudlak syndrome [112, 113], Wiskott-Aldrich syndrome [114], syndrome of thrombocytopenia with absent radius [115], and Chediak-Higashi syndrome [116, 117]. The relationship of the platelet abnormalities to the other congenital defects is unknown.

We thank Drs. Stephen Prescott and Douglas Tollefsen for helpful criticisms of this chapter. We also thank Dr. James

Figure 71-6 Gel electrophoresis of normal (top) and Bernard-Soulier platelets. Electrophoresis in polyacrylamide gels which contain sodium dodecyl sulfate was performed without reduction of disulfide bonds. The gel was stained with periodic acid-Schiff and scanned by densitometry. Bernard-Soulier platelets lack the peak representing glycoprotein Ib, indicated by the heavy arrow. (From [72], *with permission of the author and publisher.*)

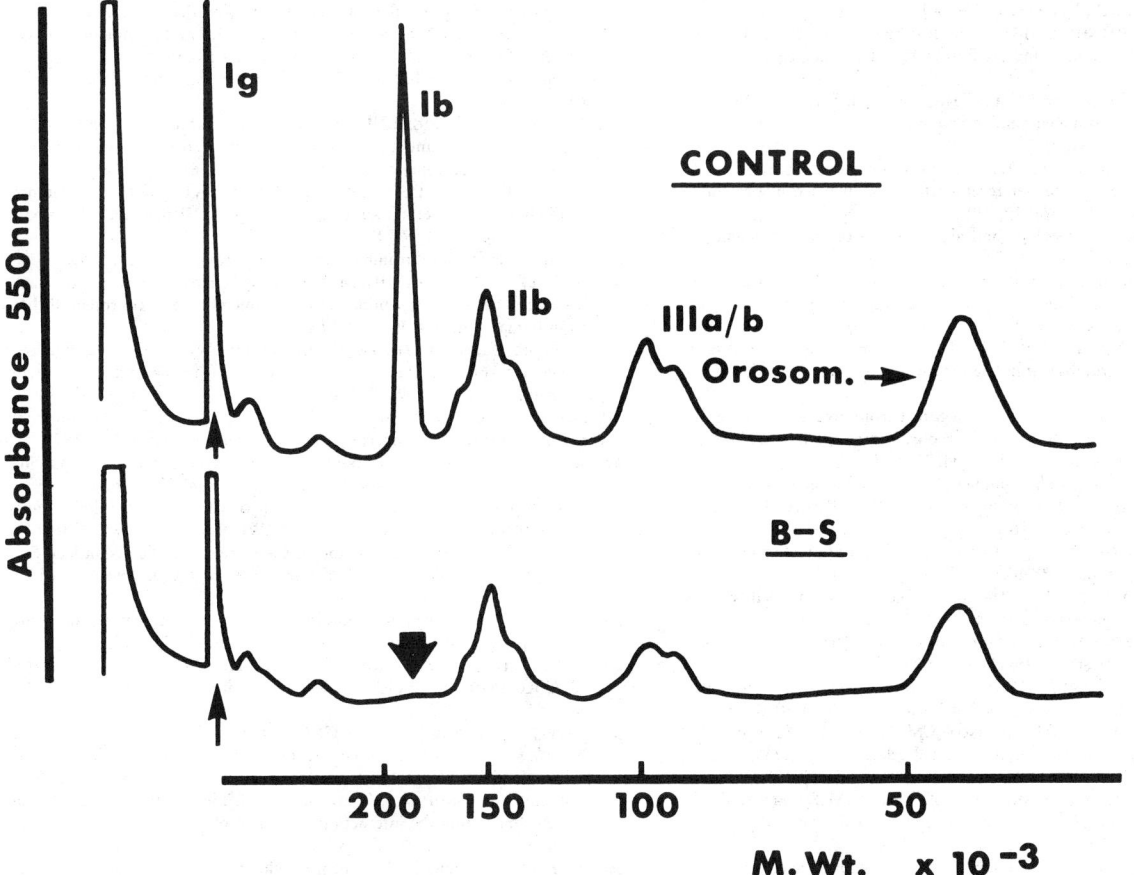

George for providing the blood smear of the Bernard-Soulier patient and Virginia Minnich for preparing the photomicrograph. This research was supported by Grants HLBI 14147 (Specialized Center in Thrombosis Research), HL 07088, and HL 16634 from the National Institutes of Health.

REFERENCES

1. BIGGS R, GASTON LW: The blood clotting factors, in Stanbury JB, Wyngaarden JB, Fredrickson DS (eds): *The Metabolic Basis of Inherited Disease.* New York, McGraw-Hill Book Co, 1960, p 1145

2. CZERVIONKE RL, SMITH JB, FRY GL, GOAK JC, HAYCRAFT DL: Inhibition of prostacyclin by treatment of endothelium with aspirin. Correlation with platelet adherence. *J Clin Invest* 63:1089, 1979

3. MONCADA S, HERMAN EA, VAN JR: Human arterial and venous tissues generate prostacyclin, a potent inhibitor of platelet aggregation. *Lancet* 1:18, 1977

4. MONCADA A, HERMAN HG, HIGGS EA, VANE JR: Differential formation of prostacyclin by layers of the arterial wall. An explanation for the antithrombotic properties of vascular endothelium. *Thromb Res* 11:323, 1977

5. SOLUM NO, STORMORKEN H: Influence on the aggregation of washed human blood platelets induced by adenosine diphosphate, thrombin, collagen, and adrenalin. *Scand J Clin Lab Invest* 17 (suppl 84):170, 1965

6. BRINKHOUS KM, READ MS, MASON RG: Plasma thrombocyte-agglutinating activity and fibrinogen. Synergism with adenosine diphosphate. *Lab Invest* 14:335, 1965

7. CROSS MJ: Effect of fibrinogen on the aggregation of platelets by adenosine phosphate. *Thromb Diath Haemorrh* 12:524, 1964

8. MARGUERIE GA, PLOW EF, EDGINGTON TS: Human platelets possess an inducible and saturable receptor specific for fibrinogen. *J Biol Chem* 254:5357, 1979

9. BENNETT JS, VILAIRE G: Exposure of platelet fibrinogen receptors by ADP and epinephrine. *J Clin Invest* 64:1393, 1979

10. HAWIGER J, PARKINSON S, TIMMONS S: Prostacyclin inhibits mobilization of fibrinogen-binding sites on human ADP- and thrombin-treated platelets. *Nature (Lond)* 283:195, 1980

11. MARGUERIE GA, EDGINGTON TS, PLOW EF: Interaction of fibrinogen with its platelet receptor as part of the multistep reaction in ADP-induced platelet aggregation. *J Biol Chem* 255:154, 1980

12. MUSTARD JF, PACKHAM MA, KINLOUGH-RATHBONE RL, PERRY DN, REGOECZI E: Fibrinogen and ADP-induced platelet aggregation. *Blood* 52:453, 1978

13. PEERSCHKE EI, ZUCKER MB, GRANT RA, EAGAN JJ, JOHNSON MM: Correlation between fibrinogen binding to human platelets and platelet aggregability. *Blood* 55:841, 1980

14. NIEWAROWSKI S, BUDZYNSKI AZ, MORINELLI TA, BUDZYNSKI TM, STEWART GJ: Exposure of fibrinogen receptor on human platelets by proteolytic enzymes. *J Biol Chem* 256:917, 1981

15. WEISS HJ: Platelet physiology and abnormalities of platelet function *N Engl J Med* 293:531, 580, 1975

16. BELL RL, KENNERLY DA, STANFORD N, MAJERUS PW: Diglyceride lipase: The pathway for arachidonate release from human platelets. *Proc Natl Acad Sci USA* 76:3238, 1979

17. PRESCOTT DM, MAJERUS PW: The fatty acid composition of phosphatidylinositol from thrombin-stimulated platelets. *J Biol Chem* 256:579, 1981

18. HAMBERG M, SVENSSON J, SAMUELSSON B: Thromboxanes: A new group of biologically active compounds derived from prostaglandin endoperoxides. *Proc Natl Acad Sci USA* 72:2994, 1975

19. SALZMAN EW: Prostaglandins and platelet function, in Samuelsson B, Paoletti R (eds): *Advances in Prostaglandins and Thromboxane Research 2.* New York, Raven Press, 1976

20. ROTH GJ, STANFORD N, MAJERUS PW: Acetylation of prostaglandin synthase by aspirin. *Proc Natl Acad Sci USA* 72:3073, 1975

21. SHUMAN MA, MAJERUS PW: The measurement of thrombin in clotting blood by radioimmunoassay. *J Clin Invest* 58:1249, 1976

22. MAJERUS PW, MILETICH JP: Relationships between platelets and coagulation factors in hemostasis. *Ann Rev Med* 29:41, 1978

23. MILETICH JP, JACKSON CM, MAJERUS PW: Interaction of coagulation Factor X_a with human platelets. *Proc Natl Acad Sci USA* 74:4033, 1977

24. KANE WH, LINDHOUT MJ, JACKSON CM, MAJERUS PW: Factor V_a-dependent binding of Factor X_a to human platelets. *J Biol Chem* 255:1170, 1980

25. MIELKE CH, KANESHIRO MM, MAHER IA, WEINER JM, RAPAPORT SI: The standardized normal Ivy bleeding time and its prolongation by aspirin. *Blood* 34:204, 1969

26. GLANZMANN E: Hereditäre hämorrhagische thrombasthenie: ein beitrag zur pathologie der blutplättchen. *J Kinderk* 88:113, 1918

27. NAEGELI D: *Blut krankheiten und blut diagnostik.* Berlin, Springer-Verlag, Vol 1, 1931

28. FONIO A, SCHWENDENER J: *Die thrombocyten des menschlichen blutes.* Bern, H. P. Huber Co, 1942

29. HARDISTY RM, DORMANDY KM, HUTTON RA: Thrombasthenia. Studies on three cases. *Br J Haematol* 10:371, 1964

30. CAEN JP, CASTALDI PA, LECLERC JC, INCEMAN S, LARRIEU MJ, PROBST M, BERNARD J: Congenital bleeding disorders with long bleeding time and normal platelet count I. Glanzmann's thrombasthenia (report of fifteen patients). *Am J Med* 41:4, 1966

31. ZUCKER MB, PERT JH, HILGARTNER MW: Platelet function in a patient with thrombasthenia. *Blood* 28:524, 1966

32. WALSH PN: Platelet coagulant activities in thrombasthenia. *Br J Haematol* 23:553, 1972

33. WEISS HJ, KOCHWA S: Studies of platelet function and proteins in 3 patients with Glanzmann's thrombasthenia. *J Lab Clin Med* 71:153, 1968

34. ROSSI EC, GREEN D: Disorders of platelet function. *Med Clin North Am* 56:35, 1972

35. BROWN CH III, WEISBERG RJ, NATELSON EA, ALFREY CP JR: Glanzmann's thrombasthenia: Assessment of the response to platelet transfusions. *Transfusion* 15:124, 1975

36. LUSHER JM, BARNHARD MI: congenital disorders affecting platelets. *Semin Thromb Haemost* 4:123, 1977

37. WHITE GC II, WORKMAN EF JR, LUNDBLAD RL: Thrombin binding to thrombasthenic platelets. *J Lab Clin Med* 91:76, 1978

38. MUSTARD JF, KINLOUGH-RATHBONE RL, PACKHAM MA, PERRY DW, HARFENIST EI, PAI KRM: Comparison of fibrinogen association with normal and thrombasthenic platelets on exposure to ADP or chymotrypsin. *Blood* 55:169, 1979

39. COLLER BS: Interaction of normal, thrombasthenic and Bernard-Soulier platelets with immoblized fibrinogen: Defective platelet interaction in thrombasthenia. *Blood* 55:169, 1980

40. NURDEN AT, CAEN JP: An abnormal platelet glycoprotein pattern in three cases of Glanzmann's thrombasthenia. *Br J Haematol* 28:253, 1978

41. PHILLIPS DR, AGIN PP: Platelet membrane defects in Glanzmann's thrombasthenia. Evidence for decreased amounts of two major glycoproteins. *J Clin Invest* 60:535, 1977

42. NURDEN AT, CAEN JP: The different glycoprotein abnormalities in thrombasthenic and Bernard-Soulier platelets. *Semin Hematol* 16:234, 1979

43. JAMIESON GA, OKUMURA T, FISHBACK C, JOHNSON MM, EGAN JJ, WEISS HJ: Platelet membrane glycoproteins in thrombasthenia, Bernard-Soulier syndrome, and storage pool disease. *J Lab Clin Med* 93:652, 1979

44. HAGEN I, NURDEN A, BJERRUM OJ, SOLUM NO, CAEN J: Immunochemical evidence for protein abnormalities in platelets from patients with Glanzmann's thrombasthenia and Bernard-Soulier syndrome. *J Clin Invest* 65:722, 1980

45. MCEVER RP, BAENZIGER NL, MAJERUS PW: Isolation and quantitation of the platelet membrane glycoprotein deficient in thrombasthenia using a monoclonal hybridoma antibody. *J Clin Invest* 66:1311, 1980

46. KUNICKI TJ, PICARD D, CAZENAVE J-P, NURDEN AT, CAEN JP: Inheritance of the human platelet alloantigen, Pl^{A1}, in type I Glanzmann's thrombasthenia. *J Clin Invest* 67:717, 1981

47. CAEN J: Glanzmann thrombasthenia. *Clin Haematol* 1:383, 1972

48. MCEVER RP, BAENZIGER JU, MAJERUS PW: Isolation and structural characterization of the polypeptide subunits of membrane glycoprotein IIb-IIIa from human platelets. *Blood* 59:80, 1982

49. GERRARD JM, SCHOLLMEYER JV, PHILLIPS DR, WHITE JG: α-Actinin deficiency in thrombasthenia. Possible identity of α-actinin and glycoprotein III. *Am J Pathol* 94:509, 1979

50. SUZUKI A, GOLL DE, STROMER MH, SINGH I, TEMPLE J: α-Actinin from red and white porcine muscle. *Biochim Biophys Acta* 295:188, 1973

51. ROBSON RM, ZEECE MG: Comparative studies of α-actinin from porcine cardiac and skeletal muscle. *Biochim Biophys Acta* 295:208, 1973

52. VAN LOGHEM JJ JR, DORFMEIJER H, VAN DER HART M: Serological and genetical studies on a platelet antigen (ZW). *Vox Sang* 4:161, 1959

53. KUNICKI TJ, ASTER RH: Deletion of the platelet-specific alloantigen Pl^{A1} from platelets in Glanzmann's thrombasthenia. *J Clin Invest* 61:1225, 1978

54. KUNICKI TJ, ASTER RH: Isolation and immunologic characterization of the human platelet alloantigen, Pl^{A1}. *Mol Immunol* 16:353, 1979

55. DEGOS L, DAUTIGNY A, BROUET JC, COLOMBANI M, ARDAILLOU N, CAEN JP, COLOMBANI J: A molecular defect in thrombasthenic platelets, *J Clin Invest* 56:326, 1975

56. LEVY-TOLEDANO S, TOBELEM G, LEGRAND C, BREDOUX R, DEGOS L, NURDEN A, CAEN JP: Acquired IgG antibody occurring in a thrombasthenic patient: Its effect on human platelet function. *Blood* 51:1065, 1978

57. PHILLIPS DR, JENNINGS LK, EDWARDS HH: Identification of membrane proteins mediating the interaction of human platelets. *J Cell Biol* 86:77, 1980

58. BERNARD J, SOULIER JP: Sur une nouvelle varieté de dystrophie thrombocytaire haémorragiparre congénitale. *Sem Hop Paris* 24:3217, 1948

59. ALAGILLE D, JOSSO F, BINET JL, BLIN ML: La dystrophie thrombocytaire hémorragipare. Discussion nosologique. *Nouv Rev Fr Hematol* 4:755, 1964

60. KAŃSKA B, NIEWIAROWSKI S, OSTROWSKI L, PROPLAWSKI A, PROKOPOWICZ J: Macrothrombocytic thrombopathia. Clinical, coagulation and hereditary aspects. *Thromb Diath Haemorrh* 10:88, 1963

61. CULLUM C, COONEY DP, SCHRIER SL: Familial thrombocytopenic thrombocytopathy. *Br J Haematol* 13:147, 1967

62. GRÖTTUM KA, SOLUM NO: Congenital thrombocytopenia with giant platelets: A defect in the platelet membrane. *Br J Haematol* 16:277, 1969

63. JENKINS CSP, PHILLIPS DR, CLEMENTSON KJ, MEYER D, QARRIEU M-I, LÜSCHER EF: Platelet membrane glycoproteins implicated in ristocetin-induced aggregation. Studies of the proteins on platelets from patients with Bernard-Soulier syndrome and von Willebrand's disease. *J Clin Invest* 57:112, 1976

64. BITHELL TC, PAREKH SJ, STRONG RR: Platelet function studies in the Bernard-Soulier syndrome. *Ann NY Acad Sci* 201:145, 1972

65. HOWARD MA, HUTTON RA, HARDISTY RM: Hereditary giant platelet syndrome: A disorder of a new aspect of platelet function. *Br Med J* 2:586, 1973

66. EVENSEN SA, SOLUM NO, GRÖTTUM KA, HOVIG T: Familial bleeding disorder with a moderate thrombocytopenia and giant blood platelets. *Scand J Haematol* 13:203, 1974

67. MALDONADO JE, GILCHRIST GS, BRIGDEN LP, BOWIE EJW: Ultrastructure of platelets in Bernard-Soulier syndrome. *Mayo Clin Proc* 50:402, 1975

68. WEISS HJ, TSCHOPP TB, BAUMGARTNER HR, SUSSMAN II, JOHNSON MM, EGAN JJ: Decreased adhesion of giant (Bernard-Soulier) platelets to subendothelium. Further implications on the role of the von Willebrand Factor in hemostasis. *Am J Med* 57:920, 1974

69. WALSH PN, MILLS DCB, PARETI FI, STEWARD GJ, MACFARLANE DE, JOHNSON MM, EGAN IJ: Hereditary giant platelet syndrome. Absence of collagen induced coagulant activity and deficiency of Factor-XI binding to platelets. *Br J Haematol* 29:639, 1975

70. CAEN JP, NURDEN AT, JEANNEAU C, MICHEL H, TOBELEM G, LEVY-TOLEDANO S, SULTAN Y, VALENSI F, BERNARD J: Bernard-Soulier syndrome: A new platelet glycoprotein abnormality. Its relationship with platelet adhesion to subendothelium and with the Factor VIII von Willebrand protein. *J Lab Clin Med* 87:586, 1976

71. GEORGE JN, REIMANN TA, MOAKE JL, MORGAN RK, CIMO PL, SEARS DA: Bernard-Soulier disease: A study of four patients and their parents. *Br J Haematol* 48:459, 1981

72. NURDEN AT, DUPUIS D, KUNICKI TJ, CAEN JP: Analysis of the glycoprotein and protein composition of Bernard-Soulier platelets by single and two-dimensional SDS-polyacrylamide gel electrophoresis. *J Clin Invest* 67:1431, 1981

73. FROJNOVIC MM, MILTON JG, CAEN JP, TOBELEM G: Platelets from "giant platelet syndrome (BBS)" are discocytes and normal sized. *J Lab Clin Med* 91:109, 1978

74. JAMIESON GA, OKUMURA T: Reduced thrombin binding and aggregation in Bernard-Soulier platelets. *J Clin Invest* 61:861, 1978

75. CAEN JP, LEVY-TOLEDANO S: Interaction between platelets and von Willebrand factor provides a new scheme for primary haemostasis. *Nature New Biol* 244:159, 1973

76. KAO K-J, PIZZO SV, MCKEE PA: Demonstration and characterization of specific binding sites for Factor VIII/von Willebrand factor on human platelets. *J Clin Invest* 63:656, 1979

77. MOAKE JL, OLSON JD, TROLL JA JR, WEINGER RS, PETERSON DM: Interaction of platelets, von Willebrand factor, and ristocetin during platelet agglutination. *J Lab Clin Med* 96:168, 1980

78. MOAKE JL, OLSON JD, TANG SS, FUNICELLA T, PETERSON DM: Binding of radioiodinated human von Willebrand factor to Bernard-Soulier, thrombasthenic, and von Willebrand's disease platelets. *Thromb Res* 19:21, 1980

79. BAUMGARTNER HR, MUGGLI R: Adhesion and aggregation: Morphological demonstration and quantitation in vivo and in vitro, in Gordon JL (ed): *Platelets in Biology and Pathology*, Amsterdam, Elsevier/North Holland 1976, p 23

80. TSCHOPP T, WEISS HJ, BAUMGARTNER H: Decreased adhesion of platelets to subendothelium in von Willebrand's disease. *J Lab Clin Med* 83:296, 1974

81. WEISS HJ, BAUMGARTNER HR, TSCHOPP TB, TURITTO VT, COHEN D: Correction by Factor VIII of the impaired platelet adhesion to subendothelium in von Willebrand disease. *Blood* 51:267, 1978

82. NURDEN AT, CAEN JP: Specific roles for platelet surface glycoproteins in platelet function. *Nature* 255:720, 1975

83. PHILLIPS DR: Effect of trypsin on the exposed polypeptides and glycoproteins in the human platelet membrane. *Biochemistry* 11:4582, 1972

84. PHILLIPS DR, AGIN PP: Platelet plasma membrane glycoproteins. Evidence for the presence of nonequivalent disulfide bonds using non-reduced-reduced two-dimensional gel electrophoresis. *J Biol Chem* 252:2121, 1977

85. SHULMAN S, KARPATKIN S: Crossed immunoelectrophoresis of human platelet membranes. Diminished major antigen in Glanzmann's thrombasthenia and Bernard-Soulier syndrome. *J Biol Chem* 255:4320, 1980

86. OKUMURA T, JAMIESON GA: Platelet glycocalicin I. Orientation of glycoproteins of the human platelet surface. *J Biol Chem* 251:5944, 1976

87. OKUMURA T, LOMHART C, JAMIESON GA: Platelet glycocalicin II. Purification and characterization. *J Biol Chem* 251:5950, 1976

88. SOLUM NO, HAGEN I, FILION-MYKLEBUST C, STABACK T: Platelet glycocalicin. Its membrane association and solubilization in aqueous media. *Biochim Biophys Acta* 597:235, 1980

89. TOBELEM G, LEVY-TOLEDANO S, BREDOUX R, MICHEL H, NURDEN A, CAEN JP, DEGOS L: New approach to determination of specific functions of platelet membrane sites. *Nature* 263:427, 1976

90. NACHMAN RL, JAFFE EA, WEKSLER BB: Immune inhibition of ristocetin-induced platelet aggregation. *J Clin Invest* 59:143, 1977

91. NACHMAN RL, TARASOV E, WEKSLER BB, FERRIS B: Wheat germ agglutinin affinity chromatography of human platelet membrane glycoproteins. *Thromb Res* 12:91, 1977

92. COOPER HA, CLEMENTSON KJ, LÜSCHER EF: Human platelet membrane receptor for bovine von Willebrand factor (platelet aggregating factor): An integral membrane glycoprotein. *Proc Natl Acad Sci USA* 76:1069, 1979

93. ACKROYD JF: Allergic purpura, including purpura due to food, drugs and infections. *Am J Med* 14:605, 1953

94. BOLTON FG: Thrombocytopenic purpura due to quinidine. II. Serologic mechanisms. *Blood* 11:547, 1956

95. HOSSEINZADEH PK, FIRKIN BG, PFUELLER SL: Study of the factors that cause specific transformation in cultures of lymphocytes from patients with quinine- and quinidine-induced immune thrombocytopenia. *J Clin Invest* 66:638, 1980

96. PFUELLER SL, HOSSEINZADEH PK, FIRKIN BG: Quinine- and quinidine-dependent anti-platelet antibodies. Requirement of Factor VIII-related antigen for platelet damage and for *in vitro* transformation of lymphocytes from patients with drug-induced thrombocytopenia. *J Clin Invest* 67:907, 1981

97. KUNICKI TJ, JOHNSON MM, ASTER RH: Absence of the platelet receptor for drug-dependent antibodies in the Bernard-Soulier syndrome. *J Clin Invest* 62:716, 1978

98. OKUMURA T, HASITZ M, JAMIESON GA: Platelet glycocalicin. Interaction with thrombin and role as thrombin receptor of the platelet surface. *J Biol Chem* 253:3435, 1978

99. NAJEAN Y, ARDAILLOU N, CAEN JP, LARRIEU MJ, BERNARD J: Survival of radiochromium-labeled platelets in thrombocytopenias. *Blood* 22:718, 1963

100. MALMSTEN C, HAMBER M, SVENSSON J, SAMUELSSON B: Physiological role of an endoperoxide in human platelets: Haemostatic defect due to platelet cyclooxygenase deficiency. *Proc Natl Acad Sci USA* 72:1446, 1975

101. WEISS HJ, LAGES BA: Possible congenital defect in thromboxane synthetase. *Lancet* 1:760, 1977

102. LAGARDE M, BYRON PA, VARGAFTIG BB, DECHAVENUE M: Impairment of platelet thromboxane A2 generation and of the platelet release reaction in two patients with congenital deficiency of platelet cyclo-oxygenase. *Br J Haematol* 38:251, 1978

103. PARETI FI, MANNUCCI PM, D'ANGELO A: Congenital deficiency of thromboxane and prostacyclin. *Lancet* 1:898, 1980

104. BURCH JW, STANFORD N, MAJERUS PW: Inhibition of platelet prostaglandin synthetase by oral aspirin. *J Clin Invest* 61:314, 1978

105. ROTH GJ, MACHUGA ET: Radioimmune assay of human platelet prostaglandin synthetase. *J Lab Clin Med* 99:187, 1982

106. WU KK, MINKOFF IM, ROSSI EC, CHEN Y-C: Hereditary bleeding disorder due to a primary defect in platelet release reaction. *Br J Haematol* 47:241, 1981

107. WU KK, LE BRETON GC, TAI H-H, CHEN Y-C: Primary release disorders due to an abnormal platelet response to thromboxane A2. *J Clin Invest* 67:1801, 1981

108. WEISS HJ, WITTE LD, KAPLAN KL, QAGES BA, CHERNOFF A, NOSSEL HL, GOODMAN DS, BAUMGARTNER HR: Heterogeneity in storage pool deficiency: Studies on granule-bound substance in 18 patients including variants deficient in α-granules, platelet factor 4, β-thromboglobulin, and platelet-derived growth factor. *Blood* 54:1296, 1979

109. GERRARD JM, PHILLIPS DR, RAO GHR, PLOW EF, WALZ DA, ROSS R, HARKER LA, WHITE JG: Biochemical studies of two patients with the gray platelet syndrome. *J Clin Invest* 66:102, 1980

110. WEISS HJ, CHERVENICK PA, ZALUSKY R: Factor A: A familial defect in platelet function associated with impaired release of adenosine diphosphate. *N Engl J Med* 281:1264, 1969

111. INGERMAN CM, SMITH JB, SHAPIRO S, SEDAR A, SILVER MJ: Hereditary abnormality of platelet aggregation attributable to nucleotide storage pool deficiency. *Blood* 52:332, 1978

112. WHITE JG, EDSON JR, DESNICK SJ, WITKOP CJ: Studies of platelets in a variant of the Hermansky-Pudlak syndrome. *Am J Pathol* 63:319, 1971

113. Hardisty RM, Mills DCB, Ketsa-Ard K: The platelet defect associated with albinism. *Br J Haematol* 23:679, 1972

114. Gröttum KA, Hoving T, Holmsen H: Wiskott-Aldrich syndrome: Qualitative platelet defects and short platelet survival. *Br J Haematol* 17:373, 1969

115. Day HJ, Holmsen H: Platelet adenine nucleotide "storage pool deficien-

cy" in thrombocytopenic absent radius syndrome. *JAMA* 221:1053, 1972

116. Buchanan GR, Handin RI: Platelet function in the Chediak-Higashi syndrome. *Blood* 47:941, 1976

117. Costa JL, Fauci AS, Wolff SM: A platelet abnormality in the Chediak-Higashi syndrome of man. *Blood* 48:517, 1976

72

DISORDERS OF THE RED CELL MEMBRANE SKELETON:
Hereditary Spherocytosis and Hereditary Elliptocytosis

SAMUEL E. LUX

1. The red blood cell membrane is composed of a bilayer of lipids and integral membrane proteins laminated to an underlying skeleton. The skeleton is a two-dimensional meshwork of spectrin tetramers cross-linked by protein 4.1 and short actin filaments. It is joined to the membrane by interactions with ankyrin and the integral membrane protein 3. The skeleton is a major determinant of membrane shape, strength, and flexibility and helps to control integral protein mobility and topography, endocytosis, membrane fusion, and lipid organization.

2. Hereditary spherocytosis (HS) is a congential hemolytic anemia caused by an intrinsic red cell defect that is manifest in heterozygotes. The primary molecular lesion appears to reside in the membrane skeleton and, in some patients, is expressed as an increased susceptibility to membrane fragmentation and a loss of membrane surface. In one family an abnormal spectrin has been identified that binds protein 4.1 poorly and, as a consequence, interacts only weakly with actin. The progressive loss of membrane surface causes the HS red cell to become increasingly spheroidal, osmotically fragile, and rigid and subjects it to detention in the splenic cords where the metabolically inhospitable environment and the high concentration of macrophages combine, in a still uncertain manner, to accentuate the basic membrane defect and enhance

spheroidicity. This process is known as splenic conditioning. Conditioned red cells appear as microspherocytes in the peripheral circulation and are particularly susceptible to recapture and destruction in the spleen and other parts of the reticuloendothelial system.

3. Patients with HS typically have mild to moderate anemia, modest splenomegaly, and intermittent mild jaundice. Individuals with compensated hemolysis and no anemia are common, and occasionally severe, transfusion-dependent anemia occurs. Although the disease is inherited as an autosomal dominant trait, in about 25 percent of families neither parent is discernibly abnormal. The explanation of these exceptions is currently uncertain. Common complications include neonatal jaundice, gallbladder disease, and intermittent aplastic crises. In all cases red cell conditioning and hemolysis abate following splenectomy, although the basic defect and its principal secondary consequences (membrane loss and spherocytosis) persist.

4. Hereditary elliptocytosis (HE) is a heterogeneous group of congenital red cell disorders characterized by elliptically shaped cells and, in its more severe forms, by spherocytes, fragmented red cells, and other bizarre poikilocytes. At least five distinct phenotypes are discernible: mild HE, mild HE with poikilocytosis in infancy, spherocytic HE, stomatocytic HE, and hereditary pyropoikilocytosis (HPP). Mild HE, the most com-

mon form, is a dominant condition with prominent elliptocytosis. Usually there is little or no hemolysis, but significant red cell destruction may appear in patients who develop splenomegaly in response to exogenous stimuli. In some families the primary genetic defect is linked to the Rh gene on chromosome 1. A subgroup of Italian patients with mild HE and anemia due to dysplastic and ineffective erythropoiesis has recently been reported. Rare patients with homozygous mild HE and severe hemolysis are also observed. Mild HE with poikilocytosis in infancy occurs primarily in black populations and is similar to typical mild HE after the first year of life. Neonates with this disease have moderate hemolytic anemia and marked red cell fragmentation which apparently reflects a special instability of fetal red cells. Spherocytic HE is clinically and pathophysiologically similar to HS. Patients usually have a moderate hemolytic anemia, with both spherocytosis and elliptocytosis, increased osmotic fragility, and glucose-responsive autohemolysis. Stomatocytic HE is a newly discovered, possibly recessive, variant of HE, observed so far only in Melanesian peoples. It is characterized by a unique erythrocyte morphology, increased cation permeability, decreased expression of blood group antigens, and little or no hemolysis. Hereditary pyropoikilocytosis is a rare recessive disorder manifested by severe hemolysis, marked poikilocytosis, and a characteristic sensitivity of the red cells to heat-induced fragmentation. In this and other forms of HE associated with hemolysis, red cell destruction responds well to splenectomy.

5. *Recent evidence indicates that all forms of HE are probably caused by defects in the membrane skeleton. Isolated skeletons retain the elliptocytic or poikilocytic shape of the parent red cells, and specific skeletal protein defects have been identified in a number of HE kindreds, including a deficiency of protein 4.1 and diminished spectrin-spectrin and ankyrin-protein 3 interactions.*

During its 4-month life span the average human red blood cell travels around the circulation 500,000 times, a distance of several hundred miles. To complete this journey, it must be durable enough to withstand strong circulatory shearing forces and flexible enough to negotiate repetitively the narrow portals connecting the splenic cords and sinuses. The flexibility and durability of the intact red cell are largely determined by the shape, strength, and pliancy of its membrane, and these, in turn, are controlled by a submembranous meshwork of proteins termed the *red cell membrane skeleton* (or, less accurately, the red cell cytoskeleton[1]). This structure has been intensively studied during the past 5 years. All the major skeletal proteins have been purified and most of their interconnections have been defined. Recently, the first of what will probably be a large number of defects in these proteins has been identified. This chapter focuses on the structure of the normal

membrane skeleton and on two groups of disorders that are believed to be caused by genetic alterations of this structure: hereditary spherocytosis (HS) and hereditary elliptocytosis (HE).

For the interested reader good reviews covering other aspects of normal and abnormal red cell membrane structure are available including: membrane lipids [1–4], integral membrane proteins [4–8], disorders of red cell permeability [4, 9, 10], and acquired or secondary membrane disorders [4]. Red cell membrane defects also contribute to the pathophysiology of abetalipoproteinemia (Chap. 29), lecithin-cholesterol acyltransferase deficiency (Chap. 31), Wilson's disease (Chap. 58), the porphyrias (Chap. 60), the muscular dystrophies (Chap. 66), pyruvate kinase deficiency (Chap. 73), glucose-6-phosphate dehydrogenase deficiency (Chap. 74), the hemoglobinopathies (Chap. 76), and the thalassemias (Chap. 77).

STRUCTURE OF THE NORMAL RED CELL MEMBRANE SKELETON

General Aspects of Membrane Structure

The red cell membrane contains approximately equal parts of proteins and lipids (Table 72-1). Phospholipids and cholesterol predominate and are present in nearly equal proportions (C/PL = 0.8). These and the other lipids are organized in an asymmetric planar bilayer. The glycolipids and most of the choline phospholipids (phosphatidylcholine and sphingomyelin) are located in the outer half of the bilayer, while phosphatidylinositols and the amino phospholipids (phosphatidylethanolamine and phosphatidylserine) are concentrated in the inner half [11, 12, 15–17] (Table 72-1). The 10 to 12 major membrane proteins are conventionally separated and classified by polyacrylamide gel electrophoresis in sodium dodecyl sulfate (SDS-PAGE) (Fig. 72-1) and fall into two general classes: integral and peripheral (Table 72-2).

Integral membrane proteins penetrate or traverse the lipid bilayer and interact with the hydrophobic lipid core [20, 21].

Figure 72-1 Schematic illustration of the SDS polyacrylamide gel electrophoresis patterns of the proteins of red cell membranes (M) and membrane skeletons (S) stained for proteins with Coomassie Blue (CB) and for sialoglycoproteins with periodic acid Schiff (PAS). The two gel systems in common use are shown: Fairbanks-Steck gels containing 5 percent acrylamide and Laemmli gels containing 11.5 percent acrylamide. GPA, GPB, and GPC refer to glycophorins A, B, and C, respectively. (GPA)₂ and (GPB)₂ are the dimers and GPA-GPB is the heterodimer of GPA and GPB.

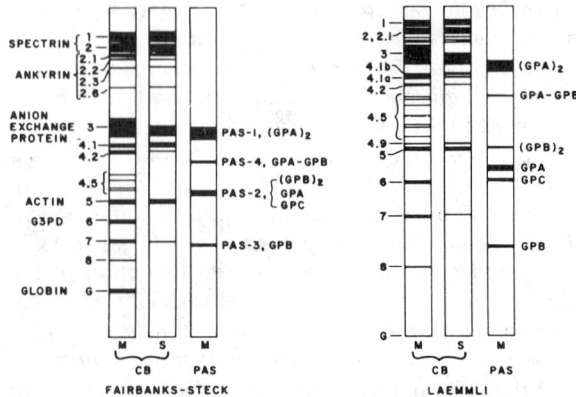

---

[1] In nucleated cells the term *cytoskeleton* refers to a structure composed of microtubules, microfilaments, and intermediate filaments that is not found in mature red cells. There is some evidence that nucleated cells also have a *membrane skeleton*, analogous to the red cell skeleton, but it is less well characterized than the more prominent cytoskeleton.

Table 72-1 Composition of normal human erythrocyte membranes (ghosts)

Component	Wt %	Gm/ghost($\times 10^{13}$)	Approximate number of molecules/ghost($\times 10^6$)	% in outer half of bilayer[a]	% in inner half of bilayer[a]
Proteins + glycoproteins	55	5.7[b]	3.7[c]		
Lipids					
Phospholipids[d]	28	3.0	250[e]		
Sphingomyelin	7.1	0.76	65	80	20
Phosphatidylcholine	7.9	0.85	70	75	25
Phosphatidylethanolamine	7.8	0.84	70	20	80
Phosphatidylserine	3.8	0.41	35	0	100
Phosphatidylinositols	0.4	0.04	3	20	80
Phosphatidic acid	0.4	0.04	3	Unknown	Unknown
Other	0.6	0.06	5	Unknown	Unknown
Cholesterol[d]	13	1.3	195	~50	~50
Glycolipids[f]	3	0.3	10	100	0
Free fatty acids[g]	1	0.1	20	Unknown	Unknown
	100	10.4	480		

[a] Based on data in Refs. 11 and 12.
[b] An average of three reported values compiled in Ref. 13.
[c] Based on an average molecular weight of 93,000/molecule calculated from the data in Table 72-2.
[d] Based on compiled data in Tables I and II of Ref. 2.
[e] Number of phospholipids per ghost based on an average molecular weight of 723 calculated from the average red cell phospholipid polar head group and fatty acid side chain composition [2].
[f] Based on data in Ref. 14.
[g] An average of two reported values compiled in Ref. 1.

They characteristically have hydrophobic surfaces exposed at such contact points and tend to aggregate or denature in aqueous solution. In the red cell protein 3, which forms the anion exchange channel, and the sialic acid-bearing glycophorins are the major examples of this class (Table 72-2). These proteins have an external carbohydrate-bearing region, a membrane-spanning hydrophobic portion, and an internal, hydrophilic domain. It is likely that all integral proteins have similar amphipathic properties. Integral membrane proteins form the intramembranous particles (IMP) seen on freeze-cleave electron microscopy of membranes. In the red cell the 80 to 100-Å IMP are randomly distributed and are believed to be protein 3 tetramers [22] or a complex of protein 3 tetramers and glycophorin molecules [23, 24].

Peripheral proteins are bound to the membrane by interactions with integral proteins or the polar portions of the lipid bilayer. In the red cell the major peripheral proteins are located on the cytoplasmic membrane surface and include enzymes such as glyceraldehyde-3-phosphate dehydrogenase (G3PD, protein 6) and the structural proteins of the membrane skeleton.

Components of the Membrane Skeleton

Operationally, the red cell membrane skeleton is the insoluble proteinaceous residue that remains after extraction of red cells [25, 26] or their ghosts [27, 28] with the nonionic detergent Triton X-100. It comprises 55- to 60 percent of the membrane protein mass and includes all the spectrin, actin, ankyrin, protein 4.1, and protein 4.9, and a portion of the proteins designated 3, 4.2, and 7 (Fig. 72-1) [25–28]. Spectrin, actin, and proteins 4.1 and 4.9 form the core of the structure since the skeleton retains its shape when other components are eluted with hypertonic KC1 [26] but disintegrates if spectrin or actin is removed [25, 26]. When the skeleton is isolated in relatively low concentrations of detergent, it contains some residual phospholipid, particularly sphingomyelin [25–27], but this is

not an integral part of the structure since it is absent when higher concentrations of detergent are used [25, 26].

Spectrin Spectrin is the major skeletal protein and accounts for about 50 to 75 percent of the skeletal mass, depending on the method of preparation [25–28]. It contains two enormous polypeptide chains that are structurally and functionally distinct: protein bands 1 (α chain; 240,000 daltons) and 2 (β chain; 220,000 daltons) [30, 31]. These chains are linear arrays of organized helical domains linked by short protease-sensitive regions [32, 33]. They are aligned side by side in the heterodimer, forming a long (97 nm), slender, twisted wormlike molecule (Fig. 72-2) [34]. The association between the chains appears to be relatively weak, except at the ends, since they are often partially separated from each other (Fig. 72-2). The protein is highly flexible [34–37] and assumes a variety of conformations, an unusual property that may be critical for normal membrane pliancy.

Spectrin heterodimers (αβ) join head to head to form heterotetramers (αβ)$_2$ (Fig. 72-2) [34]. These are structurally identical to the heterodimers but are twice as long (194 nm). Under certain circumstances spectrin also forms higher-order oligomers in which each molecule joins to two others in a circular ("daisy chain") arrangement [38, 39]. The proportion of spectrin that exists as tetramers and higher oligomers in the membrane is unknown. In solution complex oligomers form readily [39], but cross-linking studies [40] and direct analysis of spectrin released from the membrane at low ionic strength [41] suggest that the tetramer is the predominant species in vivo. This may be because membrane-bound spectrin molecules have much more limited access to each other than do molecules in solution.

In vitro spectrin dissociates into dimers at low concentrations, low ionic strengths, and higher temperatures (e.g., 37°C) [41]. Tetramers are favored at higher ionic strengths and lower temperatures (e.g., 25 to 30°C). At low temperatures (e.g., 0 to 4°C) the equilibrium is kinetically frozen because of its high activation energy [41]. Thus, it is possible to extract spectrin

Table 72-2 Major erythrocyte membrane proteins

Protein band[a]	Approximate molecular weight	Identification	Integral or peripheral	Approximate proportion, wt %[b]	Approximate copies/ghost[c]
1	240,000 ⎫	Spectrin[d]	P	25	200,000[d]
2	220,000 ⎬				
2.1	210,000 ⎫				
2.2	195,000 ⎪	Ankyrin (or syndeins)[e]	P	5	100,000
2.3	175,000 ⎬				
2.6	145,000 ⎭				
3	93,000	Anion exchange protein	I	25	1,000,000
4.1	80,000	Unnamed	P	4–5	200,000
4.2	72,000	Unnamed	P	4–5	200,000
4.9	45,000	Unnamed	P	0.5–1	50,000
5	43,000	Actin	P	4–5	400,000
6	35,000	Glyceraldehyde-3-phosphate dehydrogenase	P	4–5	500,000
7	29,000	Unnamed	P	4–5	500,000
8	23,000	Unnamed	P	1.2	150,000
GPA	31,000	Glycophorin A	I	1.5	400,000[f]
GPB	~23,000[g]	Glycophorin B	I	0.5	150,000[f]
GPC	~29,000[g]	Glycophorin C (glycoconnectin)	I	0.3	100,000[f]

[a] Numbering system of Fairbanks [13] and Steck [18] for proteins 1 to 8. GPA, GPB, and GPC refer to glycophorins A, B, and C [7, 19], respectively.
[b] Proteins 1 to 8 estimated from Ref. 13 and unpublished studies of the author. Estimates of the glycophorins are from Refs. 7 and 19 and include weight of the carbohydrate.
[c] Based on an estimate of 5.7×10^{-13} g protein per ghost [13].
[d] Spectrin is a heterodimer of protein bands 1 and 2. These bands are also referred to as α and β chains of spectrin, respectively. The number of copies per ghost shown refers to the αβ dimer. The native spectrin species is the $\alpha_2\beta_2$ tetramer (100,000 copies per ghost).
[e] Protein 2.1 is intact ankyrin. Proteins 2.2, 2.3, and 2.6 are proteolytic degradation products of ankyrin that are probably present in the native erythrocyte.
[f] Assumes 60% carbohydrate for all three glycophorins. This figure is accurately known only for glycophorin A [7, 19]; hence, the numbers of glycophorins B and C shown are only rough estimates.
[g] Estimated from migration in SDS gels relative to glycophorin A and from Refs. 7 and 19.

from the membrane at low temperatures and analyze its state of association directly or to manipulate it in vitro to produce any desired oligomeric species [39, 41, 42].

In addition to interactions with itself, spectrin also binds to ankyrin, protein 4.1, and actin. These associations are discussed in succeeding sections.

Spectrin is synthesized very early in erythroid development. It is plentiful in pronormoblasts [43] and is detectable in undifferentiated erythroleukemia cells [44] and possibly in mature committed erythroid stem cells (CFU-E) [45]. Small amounts may also be present in other cell types [46], although this is controversial [47, 48]. It is ubiquitous in both vertebrate [49] and invertebrate [50] red cells. Interestingly, even in the most primitive organisms regions of the molecule are immunochemically (and hence structurally) similar to the human protein [50]. This evolutionary conservation suggests that some spectrin function is critical for the survival of the erythrocyte.

Actin (Protein Band 5) Red cell actin is very similar to other actins, both structurally [51] and functionally [51–54]. Most is of the β type [55, 56], although some γ-actin may also be present [55]. These actin subtypes are found in a variety of other nonmuscle cells [57]. Unlike the actin in other cells, red cell actin appears to be organized as *short*, double helical F-actin filaments ("protofilaments") about 10 to 20 monomers long [58]. This is not rigorously proved, but it is quite likely for a number of reasons. First, spectrin binds only to F-actin [58–60]. Second, ADP is the predominant nucleotide in red cell actin [60a] as it is in F-actin. Third, spectrin-actin complexes extracted from red cell membranes stimulate G-actin polymer-

ization like F-actin nuclei; and cytochalasin D, which blocks the polymerizing ends of actin filaments, prevents this stimulation [58, 61, 62]. These observations suggest that most red cell actin is in the F form. The relatively small amount of actin [400,000 monomers/ghost] and the large number of cytochalasin D binding sites [30,000 to 40,000/ghost] [62, 63] indicate that the filaments are, on average, relatively short. It is not clear whether these short filaments are stabilized simply by their interactions with spectrin and protein 4.1 (see below) or whether a specific "capping" protein is present. Protein 4.9 is associated with spectrin, actin, and 4.1 in the core skeletal structure and is present in amounts that are compatible with a capping function (~1 mole per 8 moles actin), but there is currently no direct evidence that it actually functions in this capacity.

There is some evidence that the state of actin polymerization is functionally important to the red cell since compounds that inhibit actin polymerization increase membrane flexibility, while compounds that promote its polymerization rigidify the membrane [55]. Spectrin dimers bind to the side of actin filaments at a site near the tail end of the spectrin molecule [59, 64] (Fig. 72-3). Spectrin tetramers are therefore bivalent and can cross-link actin filaments; binding is weak ($K_d \sim 10^{-4}$ M) and ineffectual in the absence of protein 4.1 [59, 64–68].

Protein 4.1 This globular protein (78,000 daltons, 5.7-nm sphere) [69] is a core skeletal component and is necessary for normal skeletal stability [59, 64–68]. It binds tightly ($K_d \sim 10^{-7}$ M) to spectrin at the tail end of the molecule, very near the actin binding site [69] (Fig. 72-3), and cooperatively

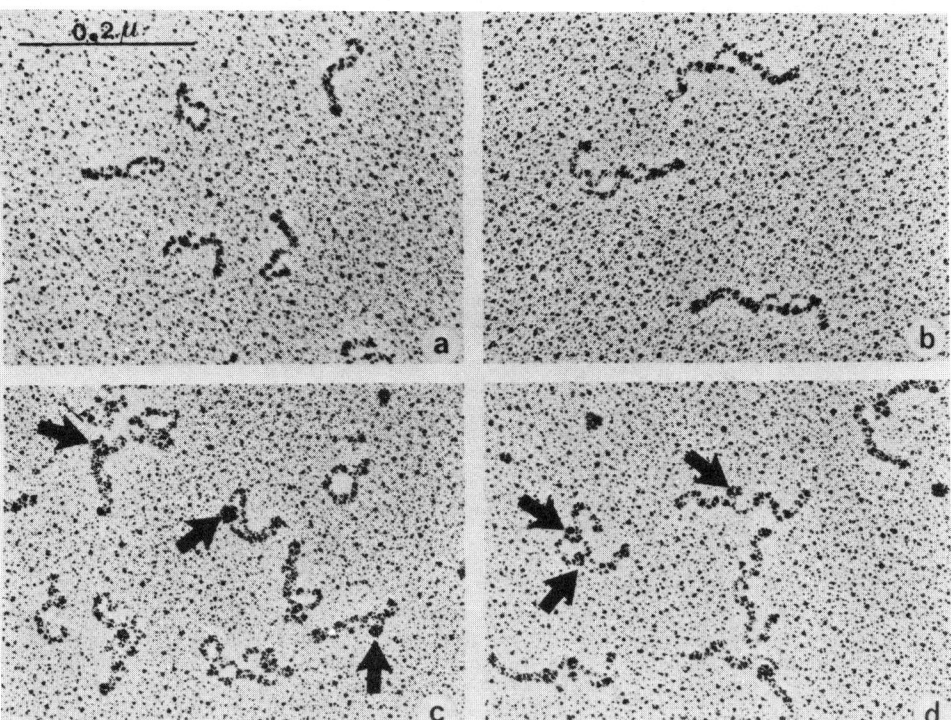

Figure 72-2 Electron micrographs of rotary-shadowed specimens of red cell membrane skeletal proteins: (A) Spectrin dimers; (B) spectrin tetramers; (C) spectrin dimers with bound ankyrin (arrows); (D) spectrin tetramers with bound ankyrin (arrows). *(By permission of D Branton, Cell, 24: 24, 1981.)*

strengthens the otherwise weak spectrin-actin interaction [68]. Little is known about this complex interaction or about the physical properties of protein 4.1. In the Laemmli SDS gel system the protein splits into two bands: 4.1a and 4.1b [29, 70] (Fig. 72-1). The proportion of these two components changes slightly with red cell age, 4.1b being more prominent in younger erythrocytes [70]. It is not known whether these subcomponents are synthesized by different genes or arise by posttranslational processing.

The relative amounts of spectrin dimer, protein 4.1, and actin in the red cell (Table 72-2) suggest that the stoichiometry is S_D:4.1:A = 1:1:2. If actin is present as short filaments, then this interaction will join several spectrin molecules at a kind of molecular junction. Spectrin-actin-4.1 complexes produced in vitro or extracted from ghosts show such a structure. Spectrin molecules radiate from a dense central core, presumably composed of actin and protein 4.1 (Fig. 72-3).

Protein 4.1 probably also binds to membrane lipids or to another membrane protein since most of it remains attached to the membrane when spectrin and actin are extracted at low ionic strength [13]. The binding site has not been identified, although there is some evidence that one of the minor glycophorins (glycophorin C or PAS-2) may be involved [71].

Ankyrin (Protein Bands 2.1, 2.2, 2.3, and 2.6) Ankyrin is a large, pyramidal-shaped (8.3 × 10 nm) protein [69] that serves as the high affinity ($K_d \sim 10^{-7}$ M) binding site for the attachment of spectrin to the inner membrane surface [72–75]. Ankyrin binds to spectrin at a site 20 nm from the end of the molecule involved in dimer-tetramer interactions [69] (Fig. 72-2). Proteolytic fragments of spectrin and ankyrin containing the respective binding sites have been isolated and partially characterized [33, 75, 76]. Judging from its relative abundance

(Table 72-2), each spectrin tetramer probably binds on average only one ankyrin molecule, even though two binding sites are available. Ankyrin, in turn, is bound to the cytoplasmic portion of protein 3, the true anchor for the membrane skeleton [77–79].

Ankyrin is very sensitive to proteolysis and is easily pared from its native 210,000-dalton size to a number of lower molecular weight forms (protein bands 2.2, 2.3, and 2.6) [80]. It is probable, but unproved, that these peptides form normally during the red cell life-span since they are present in freshly isolated ghosts. No direct tests of their function have been made, but the fact that they partition with the parent molecule (protein 2.1) during the preparation of skeletons or spectrin-depleted ghosts suggests that they are able to bind to both spectrin and protein 3.

Anion Exchange Protein (Protein 3) Protein 3, the major red cell membrane protein ($\sim 1 \times 10^6$ copies/cell), is a 93,000-dalton transmembrane glycoprotein that probably exists in the membrane as a noncovalently linked tetramer [22, 79, 81]. Six to seven percent of the population is heterozygous for a slightly larger ($\sim 96,000$ daltons), but apparently functionally normal, variant [82]. Like other integral proteins, protein 3 contains several structurally and functionally unique domains [5, 83, 84]. The external (C-terminal) domain is glycosylated and bears concanavalin A receptors [85] and the I,i blood group antigens [86]. The glycosylation is heterogeneous, which accounts for the diffuse electrophoretic mobility of protein 3 on SDS gels [87, 88]. The hydrophobic intramembranous domain forms the physiologically important anion exchange channel [6, 84] that enables the red cell to exchange Cl^- for HCO_3^- and transport CO_2 from the tissues to the lungs.

The cytoplasmic (N-terminal) domain functions as a binding site for a large number of red cell proteins including: hemoglobin [89, 90]; protein 4.2 [91]; ankyrin [77–79]; and the gly-

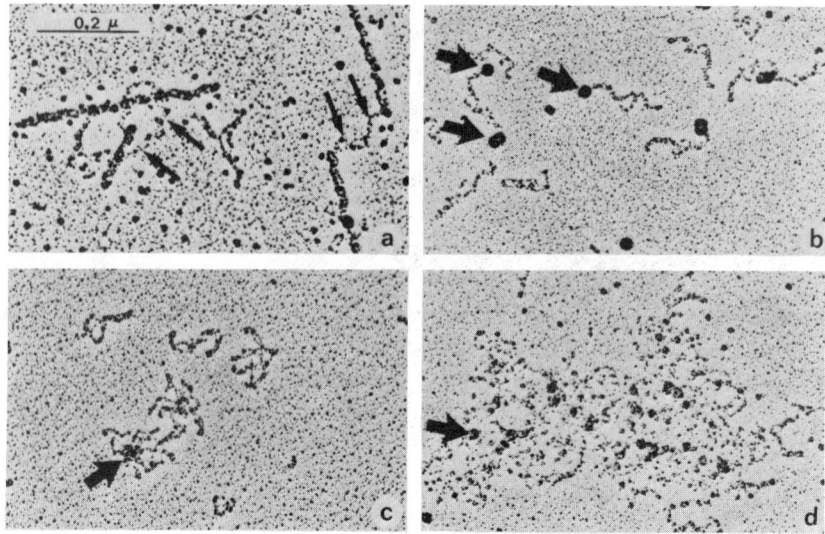

Figure 72-3 Electron micrographs of rotary-shadowed specimens of red cell membrane skeletal proteins: (A) spectrin tetramers bound to actin filaments in the presence of protein 4.1; (B) ferritin-labeled protein 4.1 (arrows) bound to spectrin tetramers; (C) complexes of spectrin dimer, actin, and protein 4.1 formed at molar ratios close to those found in the normal red cell (arrow indicates putative actin protofilament); (D) complexes formed as in (C) except that spectrin tetramer was used instead of dimer, leading to the formation of an extended network (arrow indicates putative actin protofilament). (By permission of D Branton, Cell 24:24, 1981.)

colytic enzymes glyceraldehyde-3-phosphate dehydrogenase [91], phosphofructokinase [92], and aldolase [93]. Recent studies suggest that normally one ankyrin molecule binds avidly ($K_d \sim 10^{-9}\,M$) to each protein 3 tetramer [79]. With this stoichiometry approximately 30 to 40 percent of the protein 3 molecules will be bound to ankyrin and the membrane skeleton. So far no differences have been detected in the protein 3 molecules that are bound to ankyrin and those that are not [77, 79]. There is little information about what proportion of protein 3 interacts with the other proteins noted above or what purpose these binding reactions serve. There is some evidence that the kinetics of the various glycolytic enzymes are altered by binding [92, 93], but it is not clear that this is a physiologically significant phenomenon.

As noted earlier, protein 3 may also interact with glycophorin A, the other major integral membrane protein [23, 24]. If so, the interaction is weak since glycophorin and protein 3 are not associated when they are extracted (and diluted) in nonionic detergents [77].

Organization of the Membrane Skeleton

Electron micrographs of the membrane skeleton show an anastomosing network of twisted, relatively unordered microfilaments (Fig. 72-4) [25, 27, 28, 94, 95]. Judged by their appearance and abundance, these filaments must be spectrin or a complex of spectrin and other skeletal proteins. In some cases they seem to be arranged centripetally around a dense central core [96] (Fig. 72-5), a structure which closely resembles isolated spectrin-actin-4.1 complexes (Fig. 72-3). In cross-sectional views (Fig. 72-5), vertical components can be seen attaching the filaments to the underside of the lipid bilayer. Presumably these structures are the cytoplasmic portion of a protein 3 tetramer and its attached ankyrin molecule. The average thickness of the skeletal protein layer has been estimated to be 3 to 6 nm from x-ray diffraction data [97, 97a] and 7 to 10 nm from electron micrographs [96, 98]. These dimensions suggest that the skeleton is only one or two molecules thick on average, which means that it must cover about 25 to 35 percent of the inner membrane surface area.

A scale model of the red cell membrane skeleton based on the available evidence is shown in Fig. 72-6. The upper portion

Figure 72-4 Scanning electron micrographs of the membrane skeleton in a torn, flattened ghost (Top) Low-power view (bar = 2 μm). Five regions are shown: α, the outer surface of the membrane; β, the torn margin; γ, a nonadherent region of the skeleton that is raised from the underlying membrane bilayer; δ, the inner (cytoplasmic) surface of the floor of the ghost with the skeleton adherent to the membrane; ε, a raised portion of the inner surface of the membrane. (Bottom) High-power view (bar = 0.5 μm) of the transition zone between the γ and δ regions in another ghost. (From Hainfeld and Steck [94] by permission of the Journal of Supramolecular Structure.)

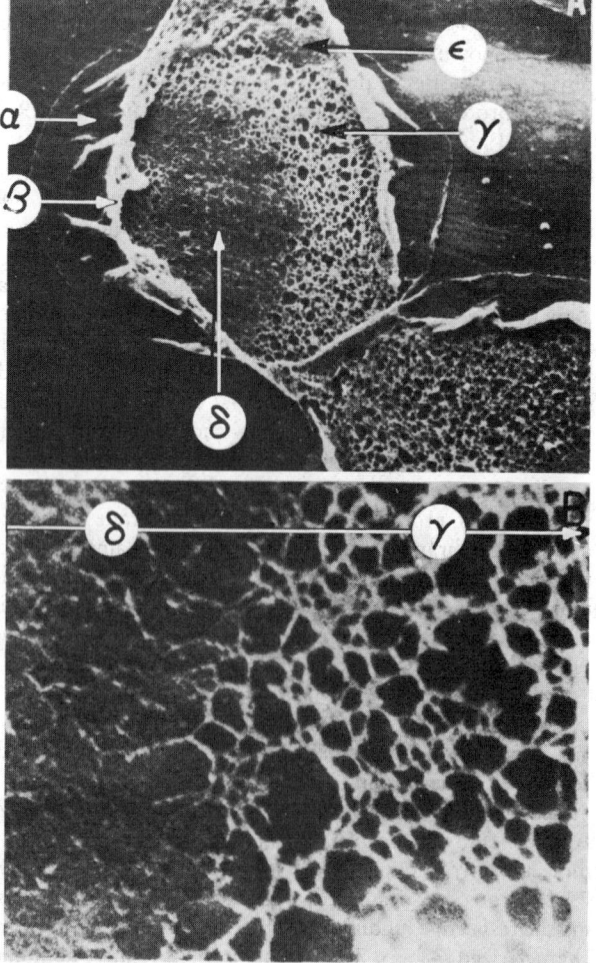

of the figure shows the various skeletal proteins and their interactions. The lower portion of the figure covers an area of 0.01 μ^2 (one fourteen-thousandth of the total membrane area) and shows these proteins at their physiologic density. Spectrin dimer is depicted as a twisted, flexible polymer of protein bands 1 and 2 that joins head to head to form the tetramer. An 80,000-dalton domain at one end of protein band 1 (the α subunit) contains one of the two interacting sites [33]; location of the complementary site is unknown, but it may lie in the phosphorylated region at the C-terminal end of the β subunit since spectrin phosphorylated sites (see below) have tentatively been localized to this end of the molecule [99, 99a]. As noted earlier, the state of spectrin association on the membrane is controversial. Most investigators believe that the tetramer predominates [40, 41], although small amounts of dimers (Fig. 72-6, asterisk) and higher-order oligomers (Fig. 72-6, small arrowheads) may also be present. Others contend that most of the spectrin is organized as complex oligomers [39].

Spectrin molecules are linked into a two-dimensional network by interactions with actin protofilaments and protein 4.1 [59, 64–68]. These associations occur at the tail ends of the bifunctional spectrin tetramer. The predicted complexes (large arrow in Fig. 72-6) are morphologically similar to isolated spectrin-actin-4.1 complexes (Fig. 72-3) and to structures observed *in situ* in normal ghosts (Fig. 72-5). They appear to serve as a kind of molecular junction or branch point in skeletal construction.

Individual spectrin tetramers are attached to the overlying lipid bilayer through high affinity interactions with ankyrin and protein 3 [72–75, 77–79]. Current evidence suggests that protein 3 is a tetramer in the membrane [22, 79, 81] and that this tetramer probably binds only one molecule of ankyrin [79]. If so, about 40 percent of the protein 3 molecules are involved in anchoring the membrane skeleton. The ankyrin binding site on spectrin is located 20 nm from the end of the molecule that participates in dimer-dimer binding [69]. Although the spectrin tetramer contains two such sites, on average only one site per tetramer can be filled. As shown at the bottom of Fig. 72-6 the density of spectrin in the skeleton is such that there is considerable overlap and intertwining of the long, floppy molecules. Interestingly, this is exactly the type of skeletal structure predicted from biomechanical analyses of red cell membranes [100–102].

Modulation of Membrane Skeletal Structure

Polyanions   It has recently been discovered that physiologic concentrations of organic polyanions such as 2,3-diphosphoglycerate (2,3-DPG) and adenosine triphosphate (ATP) dissociate the membrane skeleton [103] and increase the lateral mobility of protein 3 in ghosts [104]. At the molecular level these compounds dramatically inhibit spectrin-actin interactions, even in the presence of protein 4.1 [68]. Whether these or other anions (e.g., polyphosphorylated phosphoinositides) are "physiologic" mediators in vivo is unknown.

Phosphorylation   Almost all the membrane skeletal proteins are phosphorylated by either cAMP-independent (spectrin, protein 3) or cAMP-dependent (ankyrin, proteins 4.1, and 4.9) protein kinases [105–109], but with the exception of spectrin little is known about these reactions. Spectrin is phosphorylated at four sites in a small region (<10,000 daltons) at the

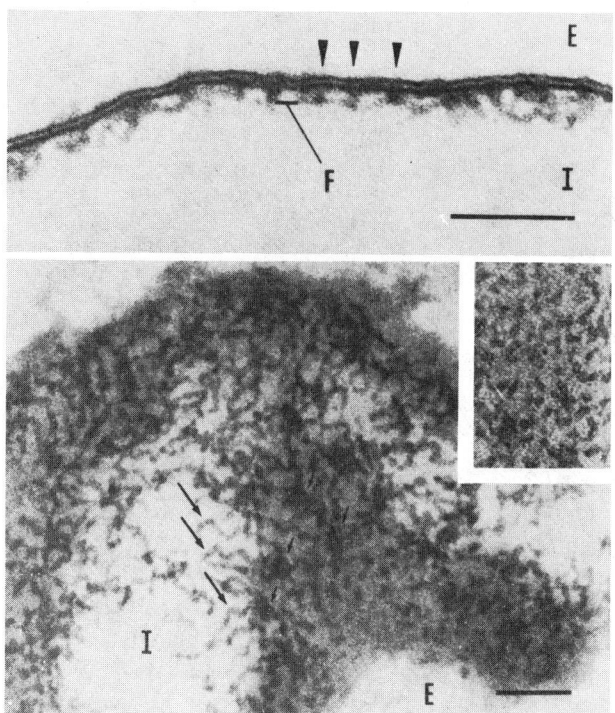

Figure 72-5   Thin-section electron micrographs of normal red cell membranes stained with tannic acid-glutaraldehyde to enhance the membrane skeleton. *(Top)* Cross-sectional view from exterior (E) to interior (I) of the membrane. The skeletal network is visible on the cytoplasmic surface and appears to be composed of two components: vertical granular components (arrowheads) and horizontal filaments (F). Bar = 0.1 μm. *(Bottom)* Obliquely cut section extending from exterior (E) to interior (I) of the membrane. The granular components are visible near the exterior surface (better seen in the inset). Near the interior surface filamentous components (large arrows) are seen that closely resemble spectrin molecules in size and configuration (see Fig. 72-2). Note that the filaments are organized centripetally around a dense, round, central core (small arrows) and that the resulting complexes closely resemble spectrin-actin-4.1 complexes formed in vitro (Fig. 72-3C). Bar = 0.1 μm. *(From Tsukita, Tsukita, and Ishikawa [96], by permission of the* Journal of Cell Biology.)

C-terminal end of the β-subunit [99]. Normally 90 to 95 percent of the sites are occupied, indicating that their turnover (which occurs randomly) is regulated by a phosphoprotein phosphatase rather than by the spectrin kinase [110]. Recent peptide mapping studies suggest that these sites are located near the dimer-dimer binding sites (Fig. 72-6) [110a]. So far, no direct effect of phosphorylation on this [41] or other [59, 60, 111] spectrin binding interactions has been detected, and their function remains a mystery.

Functions of the Membrane Skeleton

Membrane Flexibility and Durability   Biochemical analyses of the red cell membrane predict that the structural properties of the membrane are almost entirely determined by the membrane skeleton. The best evidence for this hypothesis comes from studies of four mouse mutants with very severe, inherited hemolytic anemias [112, 113]. The red cells of these mice are spherocytic and fragile and spontaneously vesiculate in the circulation (Fig. 72-7). All the mutants lack spectrin [112, 113], and the degree of spectrin deficiency correlates with the apparent clinical severity [113]. Red cells from the more deficient mutants lack elasticity, show marked plastic deformation (see following section), and mechanically resem-

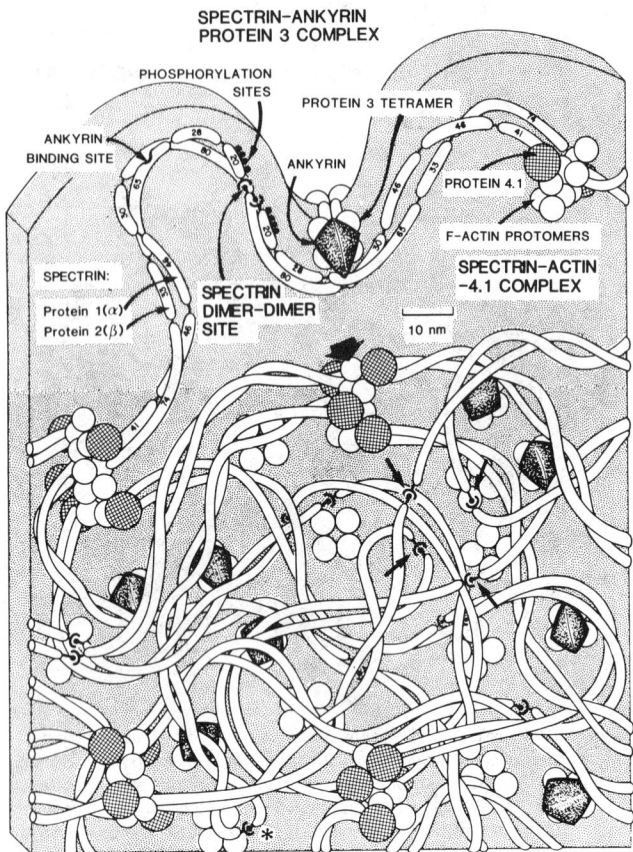

SPECTRIN-ANKYRIN PROTEIN 3 COMPLEX

PHOSPHORYLATION SITES

PROTEIN 3 TETRAMER

ANKYRIN BINDING SITE

ANKYRIN

PROTEIN 4.1

SPECTRIN:
Protein 1(α)
Protein 2(β)

SPECTRIN DIMER-DIMER SITE

F-ACTIN PROTOMERS

SPECTRIN-ACTIN -4.1 COMPLEX

10 nm

Figure 72-6 Schematic illustration of the organization of the red cell membrane skeleton.

ble lipid bilayers [114]. Reconstitution of mutant ghosts with normal spectrin restores normal membrane stability [115].

Numerous other observations attest to the structural importance of the skeleton. In intact red cells denaturation of spectrin by exposure to heat [116–118] or low pH [117, 119, 120] destabilizes and rigidifies the membrane and promotes membrane fragmentation and spherocytosis. In isolated membranes vesiculation occurs when spectrin is extracted at low ionic strength [121] or even when spectrin-actin bonds are weakened by 2,3-DPG [103]. Similarly, isolated skeletons become mechanically fragile when spectrin tetramers are converted to dimers by in vitro manipulations of temperature and ionic strength [42]. In contrast, cross-linking of membrane skeletal proteins by a variety of mechanisms increases membrane rigidity [117, 122–126].

Red Cell Shape In general isolated membrane skeletons retain the shape of the ghosts from which they are derived [28, 113]. This and other observations [125, 127–130] confirm the shape-maintaining role of the skeleton. It is widely believed that spectrin phosphorylation is a critical element in this process since conditions that promote biconcavity also promote spectrin phosphorylation [131] and conditions that induce dephosphorylation generate echinocytes [116, 132–134]. Nevertheless, recent experiments clearly show that spectrin phosphorylation and membrane shape are not causally related [111, 135].

Biomechanical analyses and modeling studies [100–102] suggest that a membrane formed by a phospholipid bilayer bonded to a membrane skeletal network will assume a bicon-

cave shape spontaneously to minimize mechanical strain. Normally the red cell rapidly regains this shape if it is temporarily deformed, but if the distortion is maintained for some time, the cell will remain misshapen. This phenomenon, known as *plastic deformation*, is probably due to realignment of dynamic skeletal interactions in response to the stress of distortion [136, 137]. Diminished skeletal interactions would presumably accelerate this process and foster poikilocytosis. More severe skeletal weakness would permit membrane budding and fragmentation and, in the most extreme cases, lead to the spherical shape characteristic of isolated phospholipid vesicles and spectrin-deficient mouse red cells [113].

Integral Protein Distribution and Mobility Perturbations that cause spectrin molecules to precipitate or aggregate on the inner membrane surface immobilize integral proteins in clusters directly over the spectrin aggregates [138–141]. Conversely, congenital absence of spectrin in mice, partial displacement of spectrin from the membrane by a proteolytic fragment of ankyrin, or weakening of spectrin-actin interactions with 2,3-DPG enhances the lateral diffusion of integral proteins in the bilayer plane [104, 142, 143]. These experiments clearly show that the membrane skeleton normally restricts the mobility of some integral membrane proteins. The mechanism of this restriction is uncertain. Presumably it is at least partially due to the association between protein 3 and the spectrin-ankyrin complex, but because only 30 to 40 percent of the protein 3 molecules participate in this interaction [79], other constituents are probably also involved. Perhaps the cytoplasmic domains of many integral proteins are simply trapped in the skeletal meshwork. Alternatively, poorly described interactions between the skeleton and membrane lipids or between the skeleton and other integral proteins may be important.

There is some evidence that the distribution of integral membrane proteins influences the interaction of red cells with other cells they encounter in the circulation. The only well-studied example is the abnormal adherence of sickle cells and cultured human umbilical vein endothelial cells [144, 145]. This adherence appears to be related to surface charge topography since it is normalized by desialylation and since negative charges on the sickle-cell surface (presumably sialic acids on glycophorin molecules) are abnormally clustered [145]. Sialic acids are also clustered on thalassemic red cells [146], but the interaction of

Figure 72-7 Spectrin-deficient mutant mice. *(Left)* Scanning electron micrograph of *sph/sph* red cells. Note the intense spherocytosis and membrane budding. Bar = 3 μm. *(Right)* Polyacrylamide gel electrophoresis in sodium dodecyl sulfate of mouse red cell membranes from normal (N) and high reticulocyte control (HR) mice and from the "normoblastosis," *nb/nb* (Nb); "hemolytic anemia," *ha/ha* (Ha); "spherocytosis," *sph/sph* (Sph); and "jaundiced," *ja/ja* (Ja) mutants. *(From Lux [113], by permission of Seminars in Hematology.)*

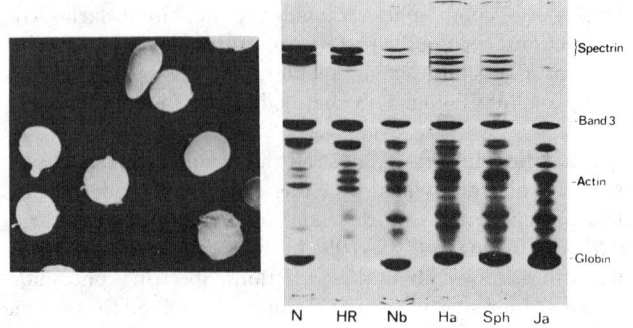

Spectrin
Band 3
Actin
Globin

N   HR   Nb   Ha   Sph   Ja

these cells with endothelial cells has not been tested. It is not known whether the charge clustering in either type of cell is due to a defect in the membrane skeleton, although this is a likely possibility.

Membrane Endocytosis and Fusion In addition to its probable importance in cell-cell interactions, skeletal control of integral protein topography appears to help regulate membrane endocytosis and fusion. Recent studies have shown that endocytic vacuoles in red cells and ghosts are spectrin-depleted and arise from spectrin-free areas of the membrane, produced by rearrangement of the membrane skeleton [147, 148]. Pretreatment of ghosts with alkaline phosphatase blocks endocytosis and spectrin rearrangement, suggesting that phosphorylation of some membrane component is required [147]. The identity of this component has not been established.

It appears that a similar process occurs during membrane fusion. Recent studies emphasize that the first step in fusion is the clustering of integral membrane proteins to produce areas of protein-free lipid bilayer [149, 150]. Apparently fusion results when such bare areas contact each other if the lipids are in a proper configuration [150]. It is known that spectrin is involved in this process [115, 151–154]. Antispectrin antibodies inhibit the fusion of red cell membranes induced by Sendai virus [152], and crude spectrin extracts prevent Ca^{2+}-induced fusion of phosphatidylserine vesicles [153, 154]. In addition spectrin-deficient mouse red cells readily fuse with one another in the absence of any inducing agent [115], a defect that is corrected by reconstituting the cells with normal mouse spectrin [115]. Thus, by immobilizing integral proteins in a diffuse distribution, the membrane skeleton protects red cells from fusing with the many other cells they encounter in the circulation.

Membrane Lipid Asymmetry In model systems spectrin interacts with negatively charged phospholipids such as phosphatidylserine (PS) and alters their physical properties and responses to divalent cations [154, 155]. It is unclear whether similar interactions occur in the red cell membrane. In the cell inner membrane phospholipids such as PS and phosphatidylethanolamine (PE) can be cross-linked to spectrin [17] in a close spatial relationship. However, little or no spectrin binds to ankyrin-depleted inside-out vesicles [38]. Thus, if spectrin-phospholipid binding occurs, it must have a relatively low affinity. This is possible since the apparent concentration of spectrin at the membrane surface (100 to 200 mg/ml for a skeleton 4.5 to 9 nm thick [113]) is four to five orders of magnitude greater than that used in the reported binding studies. Unfortunately it is difficult to test directly since very high concentrations of spectrin are difficult to prepare.

Indirect evidence suggests that functionally significant interactions do occur. Haest and his associates [156] report that 30 to 50 percent of the inner membrane PS and PE becomes accessible at the outer membrane surface when intact red cells are oxidized with agents that selectively cross-link spectrin. This implies that spectrin normally interacts with these phospholipids and stabilizes their orientation toward the inner membrane surface. Damage to spectrin releases this constraint and allows PS and PE to flip to the outer lipid layer. Obviously such studies are limited by the inability to be certain that only spectrin is damaged by oxidation. Nevertheless, since half of the PS and PE appear on the outer membrane surface within 2 hours in oxidized red cells [156], it is clear that some specific constraints must exist to maintain normal phospholipid asymmetry throughout the red cells' 120-day life span.

HEREDITARY SPHEROCYTOSIS

Hereditary spherocytosis (HS), or *congenital hemolytic jaundice*, is an important, dominantly inherited hemolytic anemia in which an incompletely characterized defect of the membrane skeleton leads to spheroidal, osmotically fragile cells that are selectively trapped in the spleen and that survive almost normally after splenectomy.

Early History

Hereditary spherocytosis was first described more than 100 years ago by the Belgian physicians Vanlair and Masius [157]. They portrayed a young woman who developed recurrent abdominal pain over her enlarged spleen associated with prostration, vomiting, jaundice, anemia, aphonia, and marked muscular weakness. At the time of this attack (presumably a hemolytic crisis), the authors noted that the majority of the red cells were spherical and much smaller than normal (4 μm diameter!). They termed these cells *microcytes* and named the disease *microcythemia*. The unstained cells were illustrated in a beautiful lithograph drawn and tinted by Vanlair (Fig. 72-8). The drawing clearly shows spherocytosis [although the relatively large number of elliptocytes (19 percent of the evaluable cells) raises the question whether the true diagnosis may not have been spherocytic elliptocytosis]. Later when the patient had improved, her red cells were somewhat larger, but still abnormal, and her spleen remained enlarged.

Vanlair and Masius thought the mircrocytes were senile normal cells ("globules atrophiques") and that the spleen assisted in their aging. They argued that when red cells are sequestered in the pulp of the spleen, they are removed from the active circulation, lose volume, and become dense, spherical, and microcytic. They believed an enlarged spleen produces even more of such cells than a normal spleen and that the liver completes the work of the spleen by destroying the microcytes it receives via the splenic vein. They suggested that the large number of microcytes in their patient was due in part to splenomegaly and in part to atrophy of the liver. Finally, they noted that the patient's older sister had suffered from an identical illness and had died during an apparent crisis. The mother was also subject to jaundice.

This remarkable paper must rank among the most prescient in hematology. Not only did the authors describe the first example of a hereditary hemolytic anemia well before the microscope was in general use in the analysis of blood diseases, but their deductions concerning the pathophysiology, particularly the role of the spleen, predated Ham and Castle's concept of erythrostasis [158] by more than two-thirds of a century! Their analysis is placed in better perspective when one realizes that 40 to 65 years later HS was ascribed to causes as diverse as hereditary syphilis [159] and splenic hemolysins [160].

Unfortunately, Vanlair and Masius's report and a subsequent description of the disease by Wilson and Stanley in 1890s [161, 162] went largely unnoticed. The latter authors clearly recognized the hereditary nature of the disease and were

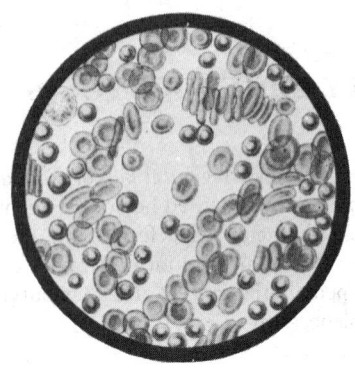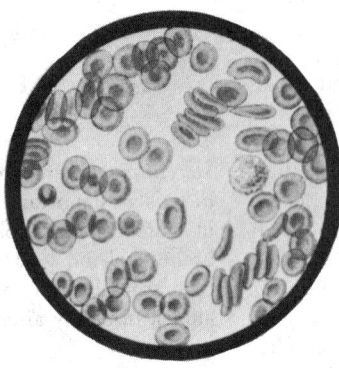

Figure 72-8 Lithograph of normal red cells *(right)* and cells from a patient *(left)* with "microcythemia" described by Vanlair and Masius in 1871 [*157*].

the first to describe the pathology of the spleen, which, at autopsy, was grossly firm and dark and microscopically engorged with red cells. A report by Minkowski in 1900 [*163*] received wide attention, and many additional papers soon appeared [*164, 165*], including Chauffard's historic definition of osmotic fragility [*166*] and reticulocytosis [*167*] as hallmarks of the disease.

At about the same time, Widal [*168, 169*] differentiated an acquired form of "congenital hemolytic jaundice" (now recognizable as Coombs' test–positive immunohemolytic anemia). Because Hayem had previously reported similar cases [*170*], the acquired form of the disease soon became the Hayem-Widal type, while the congenital form was given the eponym Minkowski-Chauffard.

The use of splenectomy was soon advocated, and in 1911 Michaeli [*171*] removed the spleen from a patient with acquired hemolytic jaundice. The fortunately brilliant result, combined with the subsequent success of splenectomy in the congenital disease [*172, 173*], soon led to widespread acceptance of the procedure. Actually, the first successful splenectomy for HS was unintentionally performed by Spencer Wells in England in 1887 (3 years before Wilson's description of the disease in that country!) [*174*]. Operating on a jaundiced woman for a supposed uterine fibroid, he instead encountered and removed an enormous spleen. The patient recovered and the jaundice disappeared. Forty years later Dawson restudied the woman and her son and found the characteristic osmotic fragility [*174*].

Thus by the time of Tileston's [*175*] and Gänssler's [*176*] reviews in 1922, almost all the major clinical features of HS were documented, the spleen was thought to be involved in the hemolysis, and splenectomy was known to be curative. Nevertheless, with the exception of Vanlair and Masius's farsighted (and still unrecognized) premonitions, nothing substantive was known about the basic mechanism of the disorder or its pathogenesis. These aspects of the disease will be discussed in the sections that follow. Readers interested in more details of the history of HS should consult the superb chapters by Dacie, Wintrobe, and Crosby in *Blood, Pure and Eloquent,* a delightful account of the history of hematology, edited by Wintrobe [*177*].

Prevalence and Genetics

HS is the most common hemolytic anemia in people of North-

ern European extraction. In this population the prevalence is roughly 1:5000 [*178*]. The disease occurs, but is less frequent, in other races and ethnic groups.

Most families exhibit classic autosomal dominant inheritance [*178, 179*], but there are exceptions that continue to evade precise genetic definition. In particular, both parents of the propositus are apparently normal in 20 to 25 percent of HS families [*178*], and in some studies a deficiency of affected sibs has been noted [*179*]. It is unclear whether these variants are due to reduced penetrance, new mutations, or a recessive form of the disease. The arguments for reduced penetrance are that mildly affected patients are commonly found in careful family studies [*178, 180*] and that the common diagnostic tests are presumably less than optimally sensitive since they are based on secondary manifestations of the disease such as spherocytosis or hemolysis and do not detect the primary molecular defect(s). The major argument against reduced penetrance (and for new mutations) is that affected individuals have the expected proportion of affected children [*179*]. Nevertheless, the existence of families with multiple affected children and seemingly normal parents [*181–184*] suggests that reduced penetrance cannot be ignored. These families could also be examples of recessive inheritance, but, with the exception of a probably unique recessive form of HS observed in Japan [*185*], there is little support for this concept. In particular, HS has never been described in consanguine matings of normal individuals. A recessive disease that is clinically similar to human HS exists in deer mice [*186*], but the biochemical relationship of the two disorders is unknown. It is hoped that current studies of the interactions between HS membrane proteins will soon lead to the specific tests needed to resolve these uncertainties.

No definite homozygotes for HS have ever been identified, which suggests that homozygosity for the typical dominant disease may be incompatible with life. A family reported by Race [*179*] supports this supposition. He described a mating between first cousins in which both parents and three children were affected, one child was normal, and two miscarriages had occurred. A French family with 13 successive affected children [*187*] is sometimes said to be an example of homozygosity, but the mother was normal and the father was not clinically worse than his offspring (as his productivity attests).

There is little information regarding the degree of genetic heterogeneity of HS, although biochemical evidence that the disease is heterogeneous is beginning to emerge [*185, 188, 189*]. Recent genetic studies suggest that in some families the defective gene is linked to the Gm locus, possibly on chromosome 12 [190, 191].

Etiology

Cross-transfusion experiments clearly show that hereditary spherocytes are intrinsically defective [192–194], but despite decades of intensive and often ingenious research the precise molecular defect is still uncertain. Some of the many abnormalities identified in HS red cells are listed in Table 72-3. A membrane lesion seems most likely since no serious derangements of hemoglobin or red cell metabolism have been identified. Studies of glycolysis mostly show a mild increase in glycolysis and ATP turnover [201–203] required to support increased cation pumping [201], and a mild decrease in 2,3-DPG concentrations [206, 207], probably due to activation of 2,3-DPG phosphatase [206] by the acidic intracellular pH of the HS red cell [208, 209]. The latter abnormalities are at least partly attributable to splenic detention since both the acidosis and DPG deficiency improve following splenectomy [206–208].

Loss of Membrane Surface The membrane lesion is expressed as a loss of surface area, but whether this is due to an actual physical loss (i.e., fragmentation) or to contraction of the membrane surface is not completely clear. Most of the evidence favors fragmentation.[2] Careful biomechanical measurements show that the force required to fragment HS membranes is only one-third as great as normal [212]. The force required to deform them is also reduced, but to a lesser degree. These results, obtained in a single patient, may not be extrapolatable to all patients. In addition, HS red cells lose membrane much more readily than normal when metabolically deprived [213–216]. This has not been shown to occur in metabolically maintained spherocytes, but the surface loss probably occurs slowly under these conditions (~1 to 2 percent/day), and none of the reported studies have been conducted for long periods of time. The phospholipid and cholesterol contents of isolated spherocytes are decreased by 15 to 20 percent, consistent with the loss of surface area [213, 218–220]. Presumably integral membrane proteins are also lost [250], but no quantitative measurements have been made. Since budding red cells are only rarely observed in HS blood smears, membrane loss either occurs fairly rapidly (i.e., in seconds to minutes) or occurs in bywaters of the circulation such as the reticuloendothelial system.

The major evidence that surface loss involves more than simple fragmentation is that the surface deficit exceeds the measured lipid loss. After splenectomy HS red cells are deficient in lipid compared with *splenectomized* controls, but their lipid content is similar to that of normal cells from unsplenecto-

---

[2] Some authors [249] have argued that the surface loss of the HS red cell cannot be due to fragmentation because the amount of cytoplasmic contents [i.e., mean corpuscular hemoglobin (MCH)] is normal. In a spherical red cell:

$$\frac{\text{Volume of vesicles lost}}{\text{Volume of red cell}} \Big/ \frac{\text{surface area of vesicles lost}}{\text{surface area of red cell}} = \frac{\text{average diameter of vesicles}}{\text{diameter of cell}}$$

Thus, even if fragmentation involves moderately large vesicles (e.g., 0.5 μm diameter), the decrease in MCH associated with a 20 to 30 percent decrease in surface area (the estimated surface loss of an HS red blood cell) would be approximately only 1.5 to 2 percent, an immeasurably small change.

Table 72-3 Reported abnormalities of hereditary spherocytes

Findings	References
Cellular properties	
Stomatocytic to spherocytic shape	[195]
Decreased deformability and filterability	[195–199]
Hemoglobin	
Increased MCHC	[200]
Metabolism	
Increased ATP turnover[a]	[201–203]
Increased glycolysis[b]	[201, 202]
Decreased 2,3-DPG[c]	[206, 207]
Decreased intracellular pH	[208, 209]
Membrane	
General	
Wrinkled and pitted membrane surface	[210, 211]
Decreased tension required for membrane fragmentation	[212]
Increased membrane loss during ATP depletion	[213–216]
Diminished endocytosis	[217]
Lipids	
Decreased phospholipids and cholesterol per cell[d]	[213, 218–220]
Decreased long-chain fatty acids in some phospholipids[d]	[221]
Increased lipid viscosity[e]	[223, 224]
Cations and transport	
Increased Na+ permeability	[201, 226, 227]
Increased Ca2+ content[f]	[228]
Decreased Ca2+ efflux[f]	[230]
Decreased Ca2+-ATPase[f]	[231, 232]
Phosphorylation	
Abnormal membrane protein phosphorylation[g]	[189, 233–237]
Proteins	
Increased membrane skeletal dissociation[h]	[242]
Increased membrane-bound hemoglobin and catalase	[243]
Decreased cation-induced aggregation of solubilized proteins	[244–246]
Decreased binding of protein 4.1 to HS spectrin[i]	[247, 248]
Absence of protein 4.2[i]	[185, 210]
Inextractable spectrin[i]	[188]

[a] Not confirmed by other investigators [204].
[b] Not confirmed by other investigators [205].
[c] Not confirmed by other investigators [203].
[d] Not confirmed by other investigators [222].
[e] Not confirmed by other investigators [225].
[f] Not confirmed by other investigators [229].
[g] It should be noted that the various investigators referenced have reported an extraordinary range of different phosphorylation defects. Other investigators have found no phosphorylation defect in HS red cells [238–241].
[h] But more recent studies have shown that this effect is dependent on preparation of the skeletons with aged Triton X-100.
[i] Defect observed only in a subset of HS kindreds.

mized individuals, despite the fact that they are more spherical and more osmotically fragile [218]. The explanation of this discrepancy is unknown. It is possible that red cell lipids are more tightly packed in hereditary spherocytes or that the surface is contracted in some other way; it is not easy to understand how this could occur. Alternatively, integral proteins may be disproportionately lost during fragmentation or HS red cells may undergo internal as well as external fragmentation. The latter process would decrease surface area without causing a measurable loss of membrane lipid. Thin-section electron micrographs do not show cytoplasmic vesicles in hereditary spherocytes [217], but a careful search has not been reported.

Membrane Lipids   The relative proportions of cholesterol and the various phospholipids are normal in HS red cells [251], and the phospholipids show the usual transmembrane asymmetry [252]. It has been reported that very long chain fatty acids are missing from certain classes of phospholipids [221], but this has not been confirmed [222]. Controversy also exists over whether membrane lipid fluidity is [223] or is not [224] normal. At the present time it is unclear whether these differences are due to technical factors or to genetic heterogeneity of the disease. Even if real, it seems likely that in the affected patients the changes in fatty acid composition and membrane fluidity are secondary to an underlying membrane protein defect.

Cations and Transport   It has been known for many years that HS red cells are intrinsically leaky to sodium but not potassium ions [201, 226, 227]. The resulting sodium influx activates $Na^+ - K^+$ ATPase, and the monovalent cation pump and the accelerated pumping, in turn, increase ATP turnover and glycolysis [201]. At one time it was believed that this modest sodium leak was responsible for the hemolysis of red cells [201], particularly those cells trapped in the unfavorable metabolic environment of the spleen (see "Erythrostasis" later), but it now appears that this is incorrect, since the magnitude of the sodium flux does not correlate with the extent of hemolysis in HS [194]. In addition, patients with hereditary stomatocytosis who have a much greater defect in sodium permeability do not develop microspherocytes and sometimes have a very mild hemolytic process [253].

Attention has also focused on a possible role of calcium ions in the pathophysiology of HS. Published reports that red cell calcium is increased [228] and that Ca^{2+}-dependent ATPase activity is diminished in hereditary spherocytes [231, 232] have not been confirmed [229].

Phosphorylation   Almost all the major membrane skeletal proteins are phosphorylated, and it is generally assumed, though unproven, that some of these phosphates may modulate skeletal protein interactions and skeletal function. This supposition has spawned intensive investigation of membrane protein phosphorylation in a number of hemolytic processes, particularly HS [189, 233–241]. Unfortunately, the widely varied results have produced considerable confusion. Much of the variability can be explained by the nature of the reactions. Unlike typical soluble enzyme systems, in isolated membranes both the enzymes (cAMP-dependent and cAMP-independent protein kinases [105, 106, 109] and one or more poorly characterized phosphoprotein phosphatases [254]) and their substrates are immobilized, so that the reactions depend on topographic factors affecting the accessibility of the reactants as well as on the reactions themselves. Not surprisingly, this complex system is sensitive to a variety of environmental parameters (pH, ionic strength, buffer composition, etc.) [105, 106, 238, 241], and experiments conducted under different incubation conditions have given very different results. In general, these can be summarized as follows: (1) Defective phosphorylation of HS membranes is evident only when the reaction is performed at *low ionic strength* for relatively long periods of time [233–236, 241]. (2) Even under these conditions the results are variable and are not specific for HS [234]. (3) The defect is not limited to a single protein; all the major phosphorylated proteins are affected (spectrin, protein 3, and protein 4.9), in both the presence and absence of cAMP [233, 234, 241]. (4) The defect is manifest only after a period of incubation at low ionic strength; *initial rates* of phosphorylation are *normal* [234, 238, 241]. (5) Phosphorylation of HS membranes is normal at higher ionic strenghs [239–241], including ionic strengths in the physiologic range [241]. (6) The protein kinase activities of HS erythrocytes are normal when assayed under a variety of conditions against exogenous substrates [239, 240, 255]. These observations strongly suggest that the phosphorylation defect detected in isolated HS membranes is not the primary membrane lesion responsible for the disease. This is confirmed by the fact that membrane protein phosphorylation is entirely normal in *intact* hereditary spherocytes if the incubations are performed in physiologic buffer systems [241]. Curiously, even in intact cells differences between HS and control erythrocytes are observed under certain nonphysiologic conditions [237].

There is one possible exception to this conclusion—a family with an unusual form of HS that *did not respond to splenectomy* [189]. In the absence of cAMP the affected members of this kindred had a selective decrease in spectrin phosphorylation under assay conditions in which typical HS patients showed no defect. In the presence of cAMP, protein 4.9 also incorporated less phosphate than normally. The relationship of these abnormalities to the pathophysiology of HS in this kindred is unknown.

Membrane Proteins   The structural instability of HS membranes suggests a defect in the membrane skeleton. As noted earlier (see "Functions of the Membrane Skeleton"), this structure is the major determinant of membrane strength and durability. There is no evidence for a quantitative deficiency of any membrane skeletal protein in HS. In all but a few unique cases described below, the membrane protein composition is normal [220, 236, 241, 256] except for a subtle increase in membrane-associated catalase and hemoglobin [243]. There is now increasing evidence for a qualitative skeletal defect.

In 1971 Jacob and his coworkers reported that solubilized but unfractionated HS membrane proteins aggregate less than normally in the presence of cations or vinblastine [244, 245]. Subsequently they discovered that many of the characteristics of hereditary spherocytes can be induced in *normal* red cells by treatment with vinblastine or colchicine [257] and that these deleterious effects are blocked by high concentrations of cyclic nucleotides but not by their noncyclic analogues [258]. Studies of isolated ghosts and spectrin extracts suggest that vinblastine selectively precipitates spectrin and inhibits spectrin phosphorylation and that these actions are prevented by cyclic nucleotides [258]. Although these findings are difficult to interpret in terms of modern concepts of skeletal structure, they imply that spectrin may function abnormally in HS red cells.

Other observations also suggest a defect in spectrin and the membrane skeleton. For example: (1) HS skeletons prepared with aged (but not fresh) Triton X-100 reproducibly dissociate at concentrations of urea much lower than those required to dissociate normal skeletons [242]. (2) Homogenized suspensions of HS skeletons gel poorly or not at all when treated with a crude preparation of spectrin kinase, while normal skeletons gel firmly under the same conditions [259]. (3) Water-solubilized HS membrane proteins precipitate at a butanol-water interface less well than normally in response to an increase in cation concentrations or a decrease in pH [246]. Unfortunately these complex effects have provided little insight into the primary molecular defect in HS, but they have given impetus to more specific studies of skeletal protein interactions. The results of this work are now beginning to emerge.

SPECTRIN-4.1 INTERACTIONS   We have recently observed a defect in the binding of protein 4.1 by spectrin in all four affected members of one family with typical HS [247], and Goodman and his coworkers have detected a similar abnormality in two other HS families [248]. In our patients (Fig. 72-9, left), purified spectrin dimer binds only 61 ± 4 percent as much 4.1 as normal. Other spectrin functions, such as the equilibrium between spectrin dimer and tetramer and the interactions of spectrin with ankyrin and actin, are unaffected. The abnormal binding does not correlate with red cell age or with splenic function. This implies that it may be the primary molecular defect rather than a secondary phenomenon. This implication is supported by Scatchard analysis (Fig. 72-9, right), which suggests that the faulty binding is due to two populations of spectrin: a subpopulation (~40 percent) of defective molecules with reduced binding capacity and a second subpopulation with normal binding affinity. Chromatography of the spectrin dimers from this family on a column of immobilized normal protein 4.1 separates these subpopulations: 40 percent of the spectrin molecules do not adhere to the column and have no detectable 4.1 binding capacity; 60 percent adhere normally and, following elution, have normal binding activity [247a]. Because HS is expressed in the heterozygous state, the data strongly suggest that the abnormal molecules are the

product of the HS gene and that, at least in this family, HS arises from defective spectrin 4.1 interactions. Attempts to characterize the molecular abnormality in the imperfect subpopulation are currently in progress.

The proportion of HS patients with this defect is unknown, but the work to date [247, 247a, 248] suggests that it is only present in a fraction of HS families. The possibility that other families may have the complementary binding defect in protein 4.1 is currently under investigation. As discussed later in this chapter, patients with a quantitative deficiency of protein 4.1 have the *spherocytic* form of hereditary elliptocytosis [260], a disease that is clinically and pathophysiologically similar to HS.

INEXTRACTIBLE SPECTRIN   Two Australian HS patients have been reported whose spectrin is very tightly bound to the red cell membrane and is not released at 37°C under the usual low ionic strength conditions [188]. Clinical details are not given in the brief report, but apparently the patients have an atypical form of HS (excessive poikilocytosis and an unusual autohemolysis reaction) [261]. Unfortunately more extensive studies of this interesting condition have not been possible.

PROTEIN 4.2   Japanese investigators have reported a few families with clinically typical HS in which affected patients lack the red cell membrane protein 4.2 [185, 210]. The available information suggests that this defect may be inherited in a *recessive* fashion [185]. A small, but statistically significant, deficiency of protein 4.2 was also noted in other types of HS [185]. The relationship of this defect to the pathophysiology of HS is presently obscure. Virtually nothing is known about protein 4.2 other than the fact that it binds to the cytoplasmic domain of protein 3 [91]. It seems unlikely that the absence of protein 4.2 is directly responsible for HS since it is also missing (apparently reversibly) in Japanese patients with biliary obstruction [262]. Such patients have the typical lipid-laden target cells observed in other patients with obstructive liver disease [263, 264] and do not develop spherocytosis or hemolysis.

Pathophysiology

The major problems of the hereditary spherocyte are the rheologic consequences of its decreased surface-to-volume ratio. The red cell membrane is very flexible, but it can expand its surface area only about 3 percent before rupturing [265]. Consequently, as the red cell becomes more and more spherical, it becomes less and less deformable, an impairment that Jandl has likened to "an obese man attempting to bend at the waist" [196]. In the case of HS red cells this poor deformability is a hindrance only in the spleen, since hereditary spherocytes survive well after splenectomy [266, 267].

The Spleen   In the spleen most of the arterial blood empties directly into the cords: a narrow, honeycombed maze of passages formed by reticular cells and lined by phagocytes [211, 268, 269]. Histologically this is an "open" circulation, but apparently most of the blood that enters the cords travels in fairly direct (i.e., functionally "closed") pathways [269, 270]. If flow through these passages is impeded, red cells are diverted deeper into the labyrinthine portions of the cords where blood flow is slow and the cells may be detained for

Figure 72-9 Defective binding of normal ^{125}I-labeled protein 4.1 by spectrin in one family with HS. *(Left)* Binding curves obtained by the method of Tyler et al. [69]. The complete curve is shown for one normal (0) and one HS (□) patient, and the binding at saturation (60 µg/ml of free protein 4.1) is shown for the other three affected family members and two additional controls. The binding curves for the controls are very similar to those previously reported [69]. As shown at the bottom, in this family all four family members with HS had abnormal spectrin. *(Right)* Scatchard plots of binding data indicate that the number of binding sites is diminished (normal = 2.1 mol 4.1 bound/mol spectrin dimer, HS = 1.3 mol/mol), but that the binding affinity of HS spectrin is equivalent to normal ($K_d = 2.5 \times 10^{-7}$ M). This is compatible with the existence of two populations of spectrin in the presumably heterozygous HS patients: a population (~40 percent) of defective molecules with reduced binding capacity and a population (~60 percent) of normal molecules. *(Wolfe LC, John KM, Falcone J, Lux SE, unpublished observations).*

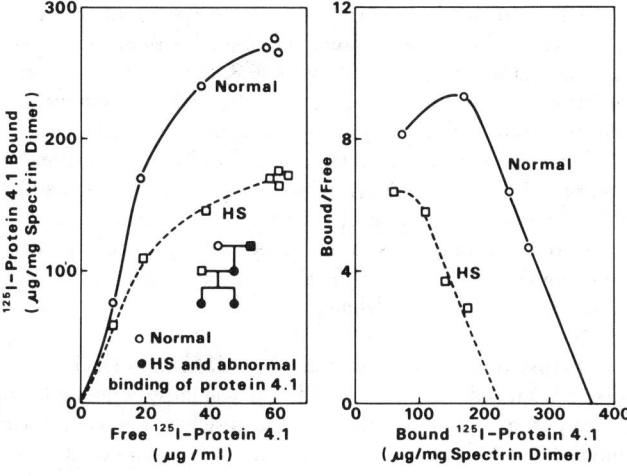

minutes to hours. To exit and return to the venous circulation, red cells must squeeze between the endothelial cells that form the walls of the venous sinusoids. Even when maximally distended, these narrow, elliptical fenestrations are much smaller than red cells (Fig. 72-10) [269], which must undergo considerable contortion during their passage [268, 269, 271].

It is clear that spherocytic red cells are considerably hindered at this point in the circulation. Isolated hereditary spherocytes are poorly deformable and pass 3- to 5-μm filters with difficulty [196, 199, 272], sometimes bursting in the process [199]. HS red cells are trapped in the cords during in vitro perfusion through spleens removed from patients with idiopathic thrombocytopenic purpura [273], and ^{51}Cr-labeled spherocytes are selectively sequestered in the spleen in vivo [274–279]. As a consequence HS spleens characteristically show massively congested cords and relatively empty venous sinuses on light microscopy [211, 280–282], and electron micrographs show

Figure 72-10 *(Top)* Schematic illustration of the anatomy of the spleen. Note that blood entering the splenic cords must pass through the walls of the splenic sinuses to reenter the venous circulation. *(Bottom)* Scanning electron micrograph of a splenic sinus wall viewed from a splenic cord. A portion of the overlying cordal structure has been removed. The narrow transmural slits between the endothelial (END) and adventitial (ADV) cells of the sinus wall are easily seen. It is likely that these cells are normally opposed and that the slits are "potential" structures rather than fixed pores [269]. They are evident here because of a drying artifact. Note that the adjacent erythrocytes (E₁ and E₂) are considerably larger than these slits and must be flexible to pass through them into the splenic sinus. *(From Lux and Glader [4], by permission of W. B. Saunders Co.)*

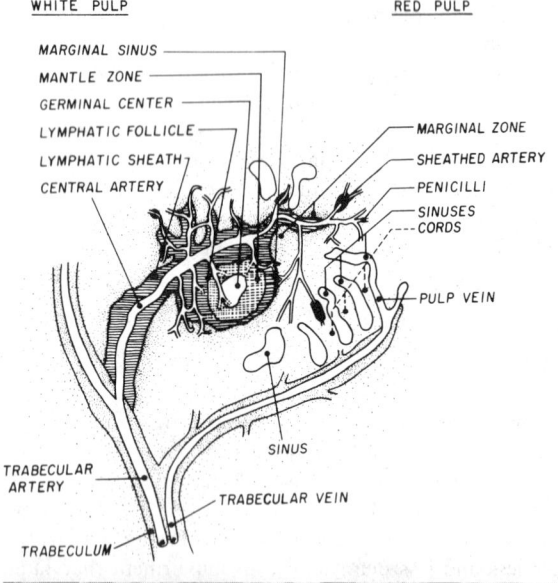

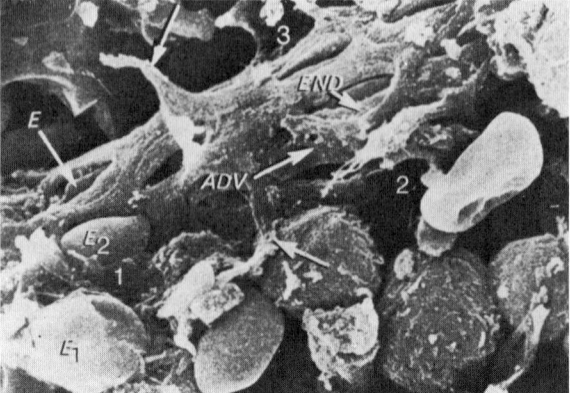

relatively few spherocytes traversing the sinus wall [211, 282, 283], in contrast to normal spleens where such cells are easily found [269].

It is also clear that spherocytes are damaged by their detention in the cords. In unsplenectomized HS patients two populations of spherocytes are detectable—a minor population of hyperchromic "microspherocytes" that form the "tail" of very fragile cells on unincubated osmotic fragility tests and a major population of cells that may be only slightly more spheroidal than normal. Although it was known as early as 1913 that red cells obtained from the splenic vein were more osmotically fragile than those in the peripheral circulation [284], the significance of this observation was not fully appreciated until the classic studies of Emerson [192] and Young [273] and their colleagues published in the early 1950s. These investigators clearly showed that the osmotically fragile microspherocytes are concentrated in and apparently emanate from the splenic pulp (Fig. 72-11). After splenectomy the tail of hyperfragile cells is no longer evident, although the major population of moderately fragile spherocytes persists [192, 273, 280]. These and other data led to the conclusion that the spleen detains and *conditions* circulating HS red cells in a way that increases their spheroidicity and hastens their demise [192, 273]. The kinetics of this process were beautifully illustrated in vivo by Griggs and his coworkers [278], who showed that a cohort of ^{59}Fe-labeled HS red cells gradually shifted from the major, less fragile, population to the minor, more fragile, population during their circulation in vivo. Although most conditioned HS red cells are probably recaptured and destroyed in the spleen, the damage incurred is sufficient to permit their recognition and destruction in extrasplenic sites since conditioned spherocytes isolated from the spleen at the time of splenectomy and reinfused postoperatively are rapidly destroyed [278, 285].

The mechanism of splenic conditioning is less clear. It is difficult to obtain precise information about the cordal environment, but the data that exist suggest the climate is inhospitable. Arteries supplying the white pulp skim off plasma and dramatically increase congestion in the cords where the crowded red cells must compete with metabolically voracious phagocytes for very limited supplies of glucose [286]. Even if glucose were available it is questionable whether the red cell could use it effectively. Because of the stagnant circulation, lactic acid accumulates [272] and the extracellular pH falls, probably to between 6.5 and 7.0 [192, 272, 287]. Intracellular pH must also decline, inhibiting hexokinase [288] and phosphofructokinase [289], the rate-limiting enzymes of glycolysis, and retarding glucose utilization. Under these conditions stores of 2,3-DPG will be metabolized to provide energy for the cell. The loss of this polyvalent anion, combined with the decreased anionic charge on hemoglobin (pI = 6.8) that occurs in an acid environment, is compensated for by the entry of monovalent chloride ions [290]. The resulting increase in osmolarity will cause water to enter the HS red cell and will worsen its already compromising spheroidicity. Thus the spherocyte, detained in the splenic cords because of its surface deficiency, is severely stressed by erythrostasis in a metabolically threatening environment. Whether this is sufficient to cause its demise has been a matter of continuing debate.

Erythrostasis   As Ham and Castle [158] and Dacie [291] first recognized, the HS red cell is particularly vulnerable to erythrostasis. When incubated in the absence of glucose, their physiologic substrate, all red cells undergo a series of changes

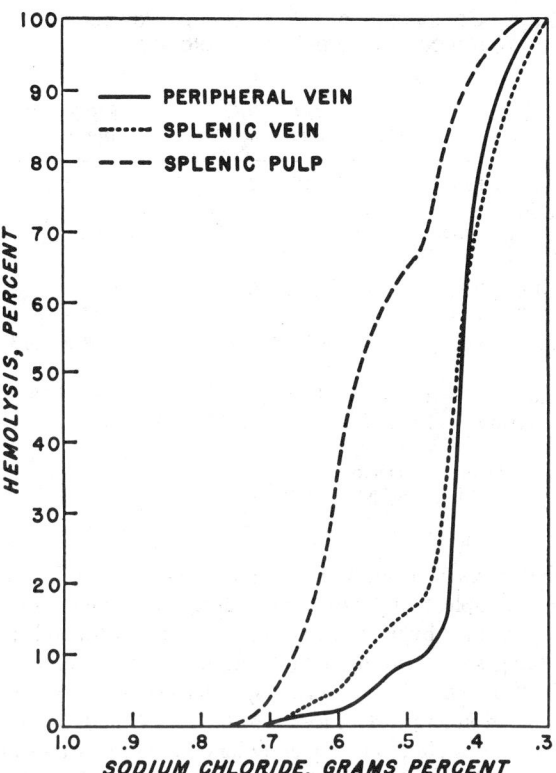

Figure 72-11 Influence of the spleen on the osmotic fragility of hereditary spherocytes. In this example, drawn from the work of Emerson and his co-workers [192], the majority of the red cells in the peripheral blood (solid line) are only slightly more spherical (i.e., osmotically fragile) than normal. A small proportion (~10 percent) are decidedly more spherical and produce a "tail" on the osmotic fragility curve. A slightly higher proportion of the hyperspherical cells are present in blood from the splenic vein (dotted line), whereas in the splenic pulp (dashed line) the majority of the cells are highly spherical. Observations such as this indicate that hereditary spherocytes trapped in the spleen undergo an additional spherical transformation or "conditioning."

that culminate in autohemolysis. As shown in Fig. 72-12, these changes are accelerated in HS red cells. They are initially jeopardized by an increase in the permeability of their membranes to sodium [201, 226]. This is normally balanced by increased ATP-dependent sodium pumping and increased glycolysis [201], a response that is impaired in erythrostasis where substrate is limited. Consequently HS red cells exhaust serum glucose and become ATP-depleted more rapidly than normal (Fig. 72-12, panel A). As ATP levels fall, cation pumps fail and the cells gain sodium and water and swell (Fig. 72-12, panel B). Later, when ATP reaches very low levels, intracellular calcium also rises owing to failure of the calcium pump. This leads to a selective efflux of red cell potassium, the so-called Gardos phenomenon [292, 293]. The molecular mechanism of this permeability change is not well understood, but its consequences are well defined: as intracellular potassium declines, water exits in response to the change in osmolality and the cells shrink (Fig. 72-12, panel B). The sodium gain is accelerated in HS red cells but is insufficient by itself to induce hemolysis in vitro since cation-mediated cell swelling peaks at 12 to 16 h (Fig. 72-12, panel B), long before autohemolysis occurs (Fig. 72-12, panel D). HS red cells are doubly jeopardized. As noted earlier, they are inherently unstable and fragment excessively during metabolic depletion [213–216]. Membrane lipids are lost at more than twice the normal rate (Fig. 72-12, panel C) [215]. It is not known whether a proportional loss of integral membrane pro-

teins occurs, although this seems likely. At first this surface loss is balanced by cell dehydration (as shown by stabilization of the calculated volume/surface ratio between 20 and 30 h in Fig. 72-12, panel E), but eventually membrane loss predominates, the cells exceed their critical hemolytic volume (volume/surface ratio >100), and autohemolysis ensues (Fig. 72-12, panel D).

Dynamics of Splenic Trapping   One of the major unanswered issues about the pathophysiology of HS is whether the events that lead to conditioning and destruction of HS red cells in the spleen are the same as those that lead to increased spheroidicity and autohemolysis during erythrostasis in vitro. During the past several decades many investigators have assumed they are, and argument has focused on the relative importance of membrane leakiness [201, 294] versus membrane fragility [213, 214, 216, 295, 296] in the spherocytes' demise. Estimates of the dynamics of splenic blood flow in HS [4] and measurements of the metabolic status of HS red cells trapped in the splenic cords raise questions about this assumption.

In the first place it appears that most HS red cells are not

Figure 72-12 The effects of erythrostasis on normal (---) and HS (——) red cells incubated at 37°C in their own serum at hematocrit values of 25 to 45 percent. Because HS red cells are more permeable to sodium than normal, they require excess ATP for sodium transport and exhaust available serum glucose and red cell ATP more rapidly than normal (panel A). This leads to cell swelling, which is followed by cell shrinkage due to calcium accumulation and potassium loss (Gardos phenomenon) (panel B). The relatively more rapid loss of membrane fragments (panel C) gradually increases the volume/surface ratio (panel E) until the critical hemolytic volume is reached (volume/surface ratio = 100) and autohemolysis ensues (panel D). (From Lux and Glader [4], by permission of W. B. Saunders Co.)

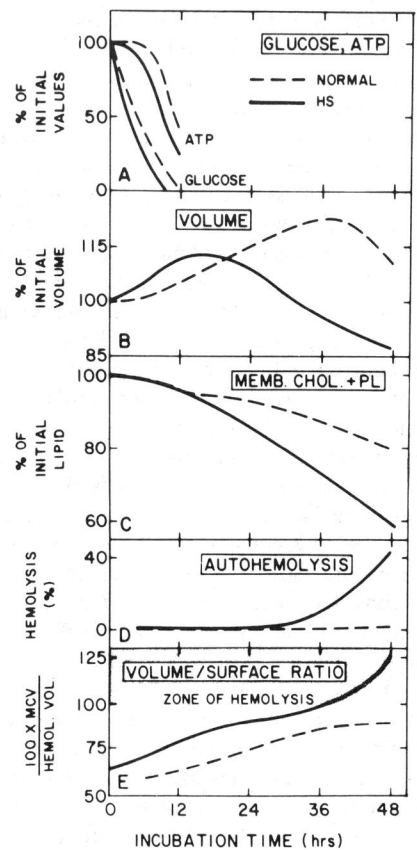

ERYTHROSTASIS OF
NORMAL AND HS RBC's

detained in the splenic cords long enough for damage to occur by simple erythrostasis. The normal adult spleen has a red cell volume of about 30 to 40 ml [4] and normally receives about 3 percent of the resting cardiac output [297, 298]. As noted earlier, most of this blood probably travels through relatively direct channels in the red pulp and is diverted into the more stagnant portions of the cords only if flow through this pathway is impeded. One can calculate (see Table 16-7 of Ref. 4) that the average normal red cell, traveling the direct pathway, will spend only 30 to 40 s in the splenic cords, a time that corresponds closely to measured transit times in isolated perfused canine spleens [286].

The average spleen of an adult patient with HS contains a much larger red cell volume (~450 to 500 ml) but also receives a larger share of the cardiac output (~8 to 10 percent) [297]. Mixing experiments with labeled HS red cells indicate that 90 to 99 percent of this blood is shunted rapidly through the spleen, presumably via the direct cordal pathways, and only 1 to 10 percent [275–277, 299] is detained in the congested cords. Even so, the calculated residence time of the average HS red cell in the splenic cords is only 10 to 100 min [4]—far too short a time for any significant metabolic depletion to occur at the rates shown in Fig. 72-12. One could argue that a completely stagnant cordal subpopulation exists that is not detected in such mixing experiments, but if such a compartment were large enough to account for the turnover of HS red cells (4 to 8 percent per day), by simple erythrostasis (i.e., over the 36- to 48-h period required for autohemolysis) it would have to occupy 30 to 80 percent of the splenic red cell volume [4]. There is no evidence for such a large static compartment.

Thus if HS red cells are conditioned by metabolic deprivation, the damage must occur repetitively. This is conceivable since under conditions in which the *average* red cell spends 1 h in the splenic cords a small fraction of the cells will be trapped for a considerably longer time and may become significantly ATP-depleted. It is often assumed that if such cells escape the spleen, they will return to the cords within minutes, but their actual recirculation time may be much longer. When splenic cordal flow is low (1 percent of splenic blood flow) and cordal residence time is greatest (~100 min), one can calculate that the average red cell will not reenter the stagnant part of the cordal circulation for nearly 400 min [4]. Judged from in vitro studies [300], this should be more than enough time to rejuvenate even moderately ATP-depleted cells. Some consequences of ATP depletion (e.g., potassium and lipid loss) are not reversible. These changes would promote longer detention and more rapid recapture and could eventually lead to irreversible splenic sequestration and hemolysis.

This scenario is supported by direct analysis of splenic red cells. As shown in Table 72-4, HS red cells obtained from the splenic pulp immediately after splenectomy and containing approximately *90 percent conditioned cells* are moderately cation-depleted and show changes in ADP and 2,3-DPG concentrations consistent with metabolism in an acidic environment, but their ATP levels are *normal* [301]. Others have reported similar findings [276, 277]. Thus if splenic conditioning is caused by metabolic depletion, it must occur by an intermittent process which allows most of the cells to recover and maintain normal or near-normal concentrations of ATP.

The data in Table 72-4 may also be taken to indicate that splenic conditioning is *not* caused by ATP depletion. The effects of other aspects of the splenic environment on heredi-

Table 72-4   Comparison of splenic cordal and circulating red cells in hereditary spherocytosis

	*Peripheral RBCs, 30% conditioned**	*Splenic cordal RBCs, 90% conditioned**
Na$^+$, meq/liter RBC	10 ± 2	17 ± 3
K$^+$, meq/liter RBC	78 ± 7	58 ± 12
Na$^+$ + K$^+$, meq/liter RBC	89 ± 9	75 ± 13
ATP, mM/liter RBC	1.48 ± 0.16	1.46 ± 0.18
ADP, mM/liter RBC	0.40 ± 0.08	0.85 ± 0.14
2,3-DPG, mM/liter RBC	4.72 ± 0.35	3.02 ± 0.57
ATP turnover, relative specific activity	102 ± 9%	93 ± 7%

* As measured by osmotic fragility tests.
SOURCE: Data from Mayman and Zipursky [301].

tary spherocytes have not been carefully investigated. It is possible, for example, that potassium loss and membrane instability are aggravated by the low pH of the splenic cords and lead to the changes depicted in the table. Alternatively, membrane damage of hereditary spherocytes by macrophages may contribute to cation and surface loss. The latter possibility is supported by the careful, but frequently ignored, observations of Coleman and Finch [302]. These investigators found that large doses of cortisone (400 mg/day) markedly ameliorated HS in nonsplenectomized patients. The effects were similar to those produced by splenectomy. Hemoglobin production, reticulocytosis, and fecal urobilinogen declined, red cell life span doubled, and hyperspheroidal, conditioned red cells *disappeared* from the circulation. It is well known that similar doses of corticosteroids inhibit splenic processing and destruction of IgG- or C3b-coated red cells in patients with immunohemolytic anemias, probably by suppressing macrophage-induced red cell sphering and phagocytosis [303, 304]. Early light microscopic studies showed little evidence for splenic erythrophagocytosis in HS [280, 281], but recent electron microscopy indicates that this is common, particularly in the splenic cords [282, 283]. In addition, phagocytes expressed from the cords of HS patients contain "bits of ghost-like membrane debris" [305], presumably resulting from membrane fragmentation. These observations suggest that macrophage processing may be a critical factor in splenic conditioning. It should be noted that no direct evidence for this speculation is presently available, and other explanations for the improvement induced by corticosteroids, such as changes in splenic size or alterations in the membrane properties of hereditary spherocytes, cannot be excluded.

In summary, it is clear that HS red cells are selectively detained by the spleen and that this custody is detrimental, leading to a loss of membrane surface that fosters further splenic trapping and eventual destruction (Fig. 72-13). It appears likely that splenic trapping is initially promoted by membrane skeletal instability, but details of the process of surface loss and the molecular nature of the basic skeletal defect remain to be defined. Some progress is being made in these areas, as indicated by the discovery of the defect in spectrin-4.1 binding described earlier (Fig. 72-9) [247, 248]. The mechanisms of splenic conditioning and red cell destruction are also uncertain. Kinetic considerations make it unlikely that red cells are continuously trapped within the cords for the long periods

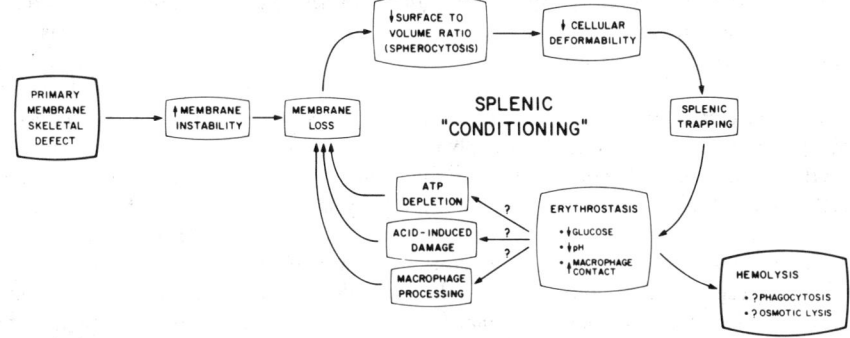

Figure 72-13 Pathophysiology of the splenic conditioning and destruction of red cells observed in hereditary spherocytosis. *(From Lux and Glader [4], by permission of W. B. Saunders Co.)*

required to induce passive sphering and autohemolysis by metabolic depletion. Repetitous metabolic damage remains a possibility. A special susceptibility of the HS red cell to the acidic environment of the spleen and active intervention of macrophages in the processing of erythrostatically damaged spherocytes must also be considered, but direct evidence for these two hypotheses remains to be established.

Clinical Features

The characteristic clinical features of HS are anemia, jaundice, and splenomegaly. The disease frequently presents as jaundice in the first few days of life [306–309]. The combination of hemolysis and the reduced capacity of the neonatal liver to conjugate bilirubin can cause serum concentrations of unconjugated bilirubin to rise rapidly, and, because kernicterus is a risk [308], exchange transfusions are sometimes necessary. Mild anemia is common at this time, but severe anemia is rare. There is no evidence that patients with HS who are symptomatic as neonates have a more severe form of the disease. Indeed most become asymptomatic within the first few weeks of life. Subsequently the course of the disease depends on the equilibrium established between the rates of red cell production and destruction.

Mild HS In a surprisingly large number of patients (~20 to 30 percent), red cell production and destruction are balanced, and no anemia is present [180, 200]. These individuals are said to have "compensated hemolysis." They are often asymptomatic, and in some cases diagnosis may be difficult since hemolysis, spherocytosis, and splenomegaly are usually mild. Hemolysis may become severe with illnesses that cause the spleen to enlarge, such as infectious mononucleosis [310]. Many of these patients are diagnosed during family studies or are discovered as adults when splenomegaly or gallstones are noticed or transient episodes of jaundice appear. Although mild HS may be familial [311], it also develops sporadically in families with more severely affected members [200]. Presumably this is due to the inheritance of modifying genes, such as those affecting splenic function.

One of the interesting mysteries about HS and other hemolytic anemias is why these "compensated" patients continue to have erythroid hyperproduction when their hemoglobin levels are normal. The phenomenon is difficult to reconcile with the generally accepted theory that erythropoiesis is controlled by tissue hypoxia. As noted earlier, the concentration of 2,3-DPG in hereditary spherocytosis is low [206, 207], which should increase oxygen affinity and promote erythropoiesis, but this effect is apparently balanced by the high intracellular hemoglobin concentration (which enhances oxygen delivery) [312] since the P_{50} of HS blood is normal [207].

Typical HS The majority of HS patients (~60 to 75 percent) have incompletely compensated hemolysis and mild to moderate anemia. Intermittent subtle jaundice is common and is sometimes associated with mild viral infections, presumably due to reticuloendothelial stimulation and an increase in hemolysis. The spleen is palpable in about 50 percent of these patients during infancy and in 75 to 95 percent during later childhood and adult life [200, 313, 314]. Splenomegaly is usually modest, but it may be massive [174, 175, 315, 316]. There is no published evidence that the size of the spleen correlates with the severity of HS, although such a correlation probably exists, considering the pathophysiology of the disease (Fig. 72-13).

Severe HS A small proportion of HS patients (~5 to 10 percent) have severe and sometimes transfusion-dependent anemia. These individuals may present diagnostic difficulties if tranfusions are begun before HS is diagnosed, since in the most severe cases the abnormal cells may be destroyed so rapidly that, except for a few spherocytic reticulocytes, only transfused cells are available for testing [4]. In addition to the risks of recurrent transfusions, these patients often suffer from aplastic crises (to be discussed) and may develop growth retardation [315, 316], delayed sexual maturation [315], and frontal bossing or other changes in the facial bones similar to those observed in thalassemia [315].

Laboratory Features

The major laboratory findings are those common to all hemolytic processes: hyperplasia of erythroid precursors in the bone marrow, an increased concentration of reticulocytes, a slight to moderate rise in unconjugated (indirect) bilirubin in the plasma, and an elevated fecal excretion of urobilinogens [200, 314, 317]. Plasma hemoglobin is normal [318], and haptoglobin is only variably reduced [319], because most of the hemoglobin that is released from destroyed hereditary spherocytes is catabolized to bilirubin at the site of destruction (so-called extravascular hemolysis).

Red Cell Morphology and Indices Spherocytosis is the hallmark of HS and, with reticulocytosis, is the most reliable finding. In 20 to 25 percent of patients the typical hyperchromic, conditioned microspherocytes are relatively sparse [200, 314]. Peripheral blood smears from these patients may sometimes mistakenly be considered normal, even by relatively experienced observers [200]. Interestingly, although hereditary spherocytes, and particularly the conditioned cells, appear spherical in conventional dried smears, most are actually thickened discocytes or spherostomatocytes when examined by scanning electron microscopy [195] (Fig. 72-14). Because the morphologic defect is acquired gradually in the circulation, HS erythroblasts are morphologically and rheologically normal [197], and circulating reticulocytes are only slightly spheroidal [320].

The mean corpuscular hemoglobin concentration (MCHC) of HS red cells is increased owing to mild cellular dehydration and exceeds the upper limit of normal (36 percent) in about half of the patients [200]. Red cell sodium concentrations are normal or slightly elevated, but cell potassium and water are low [295, 301, 321], particularly in cells removed from the splenic pulp [301]. The mean corpuscular hemoglobin (MCH) and mean corpuscular volume (MCV) fall within the normal range [200], but because young red cells normally have a high cell volume, the MCV in HS is actually relatively low.

Fragility and Autohemolysis Tests   The *osmotic fragility* (OF) *test*, particularly its incubated variant, is the most sensitive test generally available for the diagnosis of HS. The unincubated OF provides interesting information on the proportion of conditioned cells in the circulation [192, 273, 280], information that is lost in the incubated OF. The test is performed by suspending the cells in aqueous solutions containing various concentrations of sodium chloride [192]. Since there is almost no exchange of cations during the short duration of the test, osmotic equilibrium is achieved almost entirely by the rapid movement of water across the membrane. In hypotonic solutions, red cells swell until they become spheres and then burst. Cells with a decreased surface-to-volume ratio, such as hereditary spherocytes, can tolerate less swelling than normal and are termed *osmotically fragile*. From 20 to 25 percent of HS patients have a normal or near-normal unincubated OF test prior to splenectomy—particularly the mildly affected patients who are most difficult to diagnose [181, 313]. The incubated OF, in contrast, is more often positive [313] since, during the period of preincubation (24 h at 37° C), hereditary spherocytes become metabolically depleted and lose membrane surface more rapidly than normal cells (Fig. 72-12), which accentuates their spheroidicity and enhances the sensitivity of the test. Occasional patients with normal incubated OFs have been reported [322, 323], and it seems likely that such patients are even more common than these rare reports suggest, since the OF test detects a secondary property of HS red cells (their loss of membrane surface) rather than the primary molecular defect.

The *autohemolysis test* was first described by Ham and Castle [158] and was carefully standardized by Dacie [291, 295] and Young [313, 324] and their coworkers. The principle of the test is illustrated in Fig. 72-12. Autohemolysis of HS red cells, incubated in their own plasma in the absence of added glucose, is increased at 48 h. In most HS patients much less autohemolysis is observed if supplemental glucose is added [295, 311, 313, 324]. This is not true in patients with large numbers of conditioned spherocytes [325], an exception that can lead to considerable diagnostic confusion since autohemolysis that is unresponsive in glucose is a common feature of a number of hemolytic anemias [311, 324].

Other tests for HS are available including the mechanical fragility test [192, 313], the rate of hemolysis in acidified glycerol [323, 326, 327], and the ouabain osmotic fragility test [328]. The former test lacks specificity and has no proven diagnostic benefit, but the latter two procedures appear to be somewhat more sensitive than the standard OF and autohemolysis tests [323, 328] and should be diagnostically useful if further studies confirm this increased sensitivity.

Complications

Crises   Patients with HS, like patients with other hemolytic processes, are subject to various "crises." Mild *hemolytic crises* are probably most frequent [200], although this is controversial [329]. They usually occur with common viral syndromes and are characterized by a mild, transient increase in jaundice, splenomegaly, anemia, and reticulocytosis. Severe hemolytic crises are rare but have been reported [315, 330].

Aplastic crises, on the other hand, are less frequent but are often more serious, since severe anemia and even death [174, 315] can result. They also develop in association with apparent viral infections and typically present with fever, vomiting, abdominal pain, headache, pallor, and symptoms of anemia [329, 331, 332]. Sometimes multiple family members are affected simultaneously [331]. During the aplastic phase the hematocrit level and reticulocyte count fall, marrow erythroblasts disappear, and unused iron accumulates in the serum [329]. Mild granulocytopenia and thrombocytopenia are common but are not invariably present. Since production of new HS red cells is halted, the cells that remain age, and microspherocytosis and osmotic fragility increase [311, 333]. The bilirubin level declines owing to a decrease in the number of abnormal red cells that have to be destroyed. Since the usual aplastic crisis lasts 10 to 14 days [329] (about half the life span of HS red cells), the hemoglobin concentration typically falls to about half its usual value before recovery ensues. The return of marrow function is heralded by a fall in serum iron concentration, a rise in granulocytes and platelets to normal levels, and reticulocytosis [329].

Megaloblastic crises result when the dietary intake of folic acid is insufficient for the increased needs of the erythroid HS bone marrow. They are usually observed during pregnancy [334, 335] when the need for folic acid is particularly high.

Gallbladder Disease   The most common complication of HS from its first reports [161, 162] to the present day has been

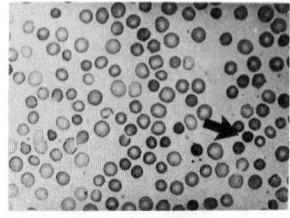 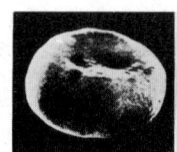 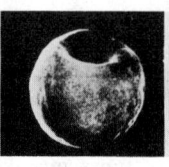 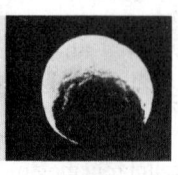

A   B   C

Figure 72-14 Morphology of hereditary spherocytes. *(Left)* Peripheral blood smear of a patient with HS prior to splenectomy. Numerous dense, hyperchromic, conditioned microspherocytes (arrow) are evident. *(Right)* Scanning electron micrographs of HS red cells show only a small number of true spherocytes (C). Most cells are thickened discoytes (A) or spherostomatocytes (B).

gallbladder disease. Pigment gallstones have been detected in patients as young as 3 years [333] but are most prevalent in adolescents and adults [336]. The available data indicate that 55 to 85 percent of untreated HS patients will eventually acquire stones [313, 336, 337] and that roughly half of these individuals will have symptoms of cholecystitis or, less commonly, biliary obstruction [174, 330, 337].

Other Complications Rare patients with HS develop gout [175, 338], indolent leg ulcers [164, 339], or a chronic erythematous dermatitis on the legs [340]. Occasionally patients also develop extramedullary masses of hematopoietic tissue, particularly alongside the posterior thoracic or lumbar spine [174, 338, 341]. These gradually enlarge with time and may be mistaken for neoplasms [338]. Interestingly, Schaeffer and his colleagues have suggested that untreated HS may predispose patients to a true neoplasm—multiple myeloma [342]. Three patients with HS and myeloma have been reported [342, 343]. None was splenectomized and two had gallbladder disease. They argue that the association may be due to chronic reticuloendothelial stimulation since splenic clearance of abnormal red cells induces proliferation of lymphocytes and plasma cells as well as macrophages [344]. HS patients have a mild, polyclonal hypergammaglobulinemia [342, 345], and there is evidence favoring the association of myeloma and chronic gallbladder disease [342, 346]. Untreated HS has also been associated with hemochromatosis, and several of eight reported patients subsequently died of liver failure or hepatoma [341, 347, 348]. The cause of this complication is unclear. None of the patients had received blood transfusions or chronic iron administration, and it is unlikely that they had coincidental idiopathic hemochromatosis. It is possible that they represent an extreme consequence of increased iron absorption associated with HS, but it is controversial whether iron absorption is [349] or is not [350] increased in this disease. If the relationship of untreated HS to myeloma and hemochromatosis proves valid, it will certainly provide additional impetus for splenectomy.

Diagnostic Problems

In general, HS is easily diagnosed and differentiated from other causes of spherocytosis, but there are several situations in which diagnosis can be difficult. In the neonatal period it may be hard to differentiate HS from ABO incompatibility since microspherocytosis is prominent in both and the Coombs' test is frequently negative in ABO disease [351]. Fortunately, in most affected infants with ABO incompatibility, anti-A (or −B) antibodies can be eluted from the red cells, and free anti-A (or −B) IgG antibodies can be detected in the infant's serum. Occasionally older patients with immunohemolytic anemias and spherocytosis also have so few antibody molecules attached to their red cells that the Coombs' test is negative and differentiation of the disease from HS is possible only with the use of radioactive antiglobulin reagents [352].

Diagnostic difficulties also arise in patients who present during an aplastic crisis. Early in the crisis the acute nature of the symptoms may suggest an acquired process, and the absence of reticulocytes may divert the physician from a diagnosis of hemolytic anemia. Later, as marrow function returns, the physician may be misled by the fact that the emerging young HS red cells are initially much less spherocytic and osmotically fragile than usual [320] and acquire their typical microspherocytic form only with age and reticuloendothelial conditioning.

HS may also be camouflaged by association with disorders that increase the surface-to-volume ratio of the red cells, such as iron deficiency [353] or obstructive jaundice [4, 218]. Iron deficiency corrects the abnormal shape and fragility of hereditary spherocytes but does not improve their life span [353], whereas obstructive jaundice improves both shape and survival [218].

The rare patients with "atypical" HS may also cause diagnostic confusion. Most such patients actually represent combinations of typical HS and diseases affecting other organ systems [354, 355], Coombs-negative immunohemolytic anemias (see above), or typical severe HS in which large numbers of very defective spherocytes remain in the circulation owing to saturation of the reticuloendothelial system [356, 357]. A few families have been described with unusual forms of hereditary spherocytic hemolytic anemias that resemble HS in some respects but not in others. For example, Boivin and his colleagues have reported a family with a dominantly inherited hemolytic anemia characterized by spherocytosis, decreased spectrin phosphorylation, and failure to improve following splenectomy [189]. Brain, Belin, and Dacie also studied a patient with a congenital spherocytic hemolytic anemia who responded poorly to splenectomy [358]. Her small, contracted, osmotically fragile red cells were excessively permeable to potassium ions and, as a consequence, were deficient in potassium and total red cell cations. Finally Zail and his coworkers have described a family with a dominantly inherited disorder characterized by spherocytosis and mild compensated hemolysis in which fresh red cells had a normal or *decreased* osmotic fragility and ^{51}Cr-labeled red cells lacked the characteristic pattern of splenic sequestration that is typical of HS [359]. The relationship of these patients to each other and to typical HS is unclear.

Splenectomy

It is one of the rare absolutes in medicine that patients with true, uncomplicated HS always respond dramatically to splenectomy. The major issues today are who should be splenectomized and how they should be treated postoperatively. These topics are beyond the scope of the present chapter but are covered in detail in recent hematology textbooks (e.g., see Ref. 4).

Following splenectomy spherocytosis persists, but conditioned microspherocytes disappear, and changes typical of the postsplenectomy state, including Howell-Jolly bodies, target cells, acanthocytes, and siderocytes, appear in the peripheral smear [280, 311]. Reticulocyte counts fall to normal or near-normal levels, although red cell life span, if carefully measured, remains slightly shortened (96 ± 13 days) [266]. In all cases anemia and jaundice remit and do not recur except in the rare case of regrowth of a missed accessory spleen. This is the only proven cause of postsplenectomy failure in HS and is sometimes overlooked since it may not become evident for years [360] or even decades [361].

HEREDITARY ELLIPTOCYTOSIS

Hereditary elliptocytosis (HE) is a relatively common, clinically and genetically heterogeneous disorder characterized by the presence of a large number of elliptically shaped red cells in the peripheral blood. These cells are sometimes called *ovalocytes*, but *elliptocytes* and *elliptocytosis* are the more accurate designations as the cells are elliptical rather than egg-shaped. In the more severe forms of the disease spherocytes or bizarre poikilocytes are also present, and sometimes these shapes predominate. *Hereditary pyropoikilocytosis* (HPP) is an example of the latter situation. Although HPP is usually considered to be a separate entity, emerging biochemical and genetic information suggests it is related to HE, at least in some families, and the two disorders will be considered together here.

History

According to Lambrecht [362], elliptocytosis was first observed by Goltz in Königsburg, Germany, in 1860, but no written report of this observation is known. The disease was first reported in 1904 by Dresbach, a physiologist at Ohio State University, in one of his histology students during a laboratory exercise in which the students were examining their own blood [363]. His brief report elicited some controversy as the student died soon thereafter, leading the prominent American physician Austin Flint to suggest that he had actually had incipient pernicious anemia [364]. Dresbach replied that the student died of acute rheumatic carditis and took his slides to Germany where famous pathologists such as Ewing, Ehrlich, and Arneth supported his view that the red cell disorder was primary [365]. This was substantiated during the next two decades by the reports of Bishop [366], Sydenstricker [367] and Huck and Bigelow [368]. Hunter's demonstration of elliptocytosis in three generations of one family firmly established the hereditary nature of the disease [369, 370].

In the 1930s and early 1940s there was considerable debate about whether HE was a disease or simply a morphologic curiosity. In retrospect, this is surprising since a number of individuals with hemolytic HE were described during this interval [362, 371–375] and some authors had clearly differentiated hemolytic and nonhemolytic forms [362, 371, 372]. In fact as early as 1928 van den Bergh even reported that anemia and jaundice cleared following splenectomy in one patient [374]. Early on, some confusion also existed in differentiating HE from sickle-cell anemia [376, 377] and "hypochromic elliptocytosis" (probably thalassemia) [378] and later in differentiating hemolytic HE from hereditary spherocytosis [379]. These reports illustrate a point that will be emphasized later—namely, that HE, particularly its hemolytic variants, can sometimes be morphologically deceptive.

For the reader interested in the historical and clinical features of the disease, the reports of Wyandt and her coworkers [379], Wolman and Özge [380], Dacie [381], Josephs and Avery [382], Weiss [383], and Cutting and his coworkers [384] are particularly recommended.

Prevalence and Genetics

HE is clearly heterogeneous from a clinical, genetic, or biochemical point of view. This was not appreciated by early investigators, and recent workers have not classified subtypes of the disease in a consistent way. In most papers all patients with HE are simply lumped together. Accordingly it is difficult to relate much of the available information to the different clinical forms of the disease.

The prevalence of all forms of HE in the United States is about 250 to 500 per million [379, 385]. Elliptocytic red cells have been observed in all racial and ethnic groups, but the distribution of some of the clinical phenotypes is clearly restricted. With the exception of HPP and possibly stomatocytic HE, the disease is inherited as an autosomal dominant trait. Unlike hereditary spherocytosis, penetrance of the more common forms is complete. No instance of a spontaneous mutation has been recorded in the past 50 years.

Genetic studies show that one of the elliptocytosis genes (El$_1$) is closely linked to the Rh locus on the short arm of chromosome 1 (1p33) [386–389]. The location of the other genes is unknown.

Clinical Syndromes

Most of the reported cases of HE can be classified into one of five clinical syndromes: mild HE, mild HE with poikilocytosis in infancy, spherocytic HE, stomatocytic HE, and hereditary pyropoikilocytosis (HPP). It must be emphasized that these appelations denote clinical phenotypes and *not* specific molecular or genetic etiologies. Defects in the membrane proteins of hereditary elliptocytosis are currently being identified at a rapid rate, but at the present time the relationship between these abnormalities and the different clinical phenotypes is only beginning to be defined.

Mild HE This is the most common form of HE. It is inherited as an autosomal dominant and is observed in all races.

COMPENSATED MILD HE As implied by the name, this form of the disease is mild [379, 390–394]. Typically patients have no anemia and no splenomegaly (Table 72-5). Sometimes red cell survival is normal [391, 421], but more often there is very mild, compensated hemolysis with a slight reticulocytosis and a decreased haptoglobin level [379, 393, 394]. In these patients HE is little more than a morphologic curiosity. The peripheral blood smear shows prominent elliptocytosis with little red cell budding or fragmentation and no spherocytosis. Elliptocytes almost always exceed 30 percent of the red cells and sometimes approach 100 percent (Fig. 72-15A) [379, 390, 393]. Very elongated elliptocytes (rod forms) are common (>10 percent). In contrast, normal individuals have less than 15 percent elliptocytes and less than 5 percent rod-shaped cells [379, 390, 393]. Somewhat higher proportions are seen in patients with anemia, particularly megaloblastic and hypochromic-microcytic anemias, but even in these individuals elliptocytes and rod forms do not exceed 35 percent and 15 percent, respectively [390]. Hence the morphologic diagnosis of mild HE is rarely difficult. This may not be true in the neonatal period. Some investigators have noted that elliptocytes are infrequent in the cord blood of infants with mild HE and become more prominent with time [370, 379, 422]. For example, Wyandt and coworkers detected only 11 percent elliptocytes at birth in one infant, whereas by 4 months of age 80 percent of the cells were elliptical [379]. These observations, although few, suggest that the disease may be expressed differently in fetal red cells, a point that will be discussed in more detail in the following section. Early workers used a complex system for quantitating ellipticity [423], but the method is time-consuming and has not proven more useful in diagnosing HE than simple subjective estimation [390]. In addition it is not prognostically useful since there is no correlation between

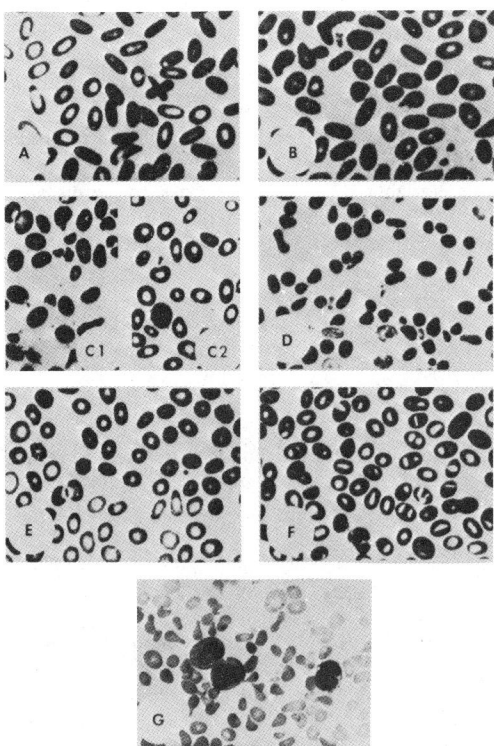

Figure 72-15 Peripheral blood morphology in the various types of hereditary elliptocytosis. (A) Mild HE, compensated form; (B) mild HE, uncompensated form; (C) mild HE with poikilocytosis in infancy: C1 = at birth, C2 = at 1 year; (D) homozygous mild HE; (E) spherocytic HE; (F) stomatocytic HE; (G) hereditary pyropoikilocytosis.

the proportion of elliptocytes or their ellipticity and the severity of the disease.

Phenotypically identical mild HE is caused by more than one molecular lesion since in some families mild HE is linked to the Rh gene and in other families it is not [388, 424]. The best example of the Rh-linked disease is the large Dutch-American family first described by Hunter [369, 370] and van den Bergh [425] and their associates and more recently restudied by Geerdink et al. [393, 424].

UNCOMPENSATED MILD HE   In many large kindreds with typical compensated mild HE, a minority (5 to 20 percent) of the patients have more severe hemolysis and anemia [393, 394]. The etiology of this variation is not always clear. In some instances it is a transient acquired state due to hyperplasia of the spleen in response to a variety of stimuli (e.g., cirrhosis [426], infectious mononucleosis [394, 396], bacterial infections [394], or malaria [427, 428]). For unknown reasons pregnancy may also transiently aggravate the disease [394]. In other, apparently sporadic, cases chronic hemolysis exists in the absence of any detectable disease process. It is generally assumed that the latter individuals have inherited one or more modifier genes that aggravate the basic membrane defect or improve the performance of the spleen, but this hypothesis remains to be proved. If true, such genes must be relatively common to explain how a mother with compensated mild HE bore two children with the uncompensated disease from unrelated fathers [429].

Except for signs of increased hemolysis and anemia, patients with uncompensated mild HE are similar to their less severely affected relatives. Splenomegaly and morphologic evidence of red cell destruction (e.g., fragmentation and poikilocytosis) are

somewhat more prevalent in this group but are not reliable differentiating features. It appears that most of these patients respond well to splenectomy, although extensive data are not available [395, 430].

MILD HE WITH ABNORMAL ERYTHROPOIESIS   In a small number of families with otherwise typical mild HE, the sporadic occurrence of hemolysis and anemia is at least partially due to the development of dysplastic and ineffective erythropoiesis. All the reported patients [397] are from central and southern Italy, have somewhat less elongated red cells than is typical for mild HE, and show the characteristic findings of ineffective erythropoiesis (high bilirubin, serum iron, and plasma iron turnover; relatively low reticulocyte count; and low incorporation of iron into circulating erythroid cells) [397]. Their bone marrows are hyperplastic, with excessive intermediate erythroblasts, and have some dysplastic features including asynchrony of nuclear-cytoplasmic maturation, binuclearity, and small numbers of ringed sideroblasts. Anemia and presumably erythroid dysplasia usually commence during adolescence or early adult life and advance gradually over a number of years. Because dysplasia persists after splenectomy, response to the operation is incomplete. The available data suggest that dysplasia and elliptocytosis cosegregate since no individuals with dysplasia have been observed who did not also carry the elliptocytosis gene. If so, these families must represent a unique subtype of mild HE. The numbers are small, and it is not clear that the nonelliptocytic members of the reported kindreds have been thoroughly examined [397].

HOMOZYGOUS MILD HE   A few patients with apparently homozygous mild HE have been reported [379, 398–401]. Most have had a very severe or even fatal [401] transfusion-dependent hemolytic anemia (Hb = 2 to 5 g/dl) with marked fragmentation, poikilocytosis, spherocytosis, and elliptocytosis (Table 72-5, Fig. 72-15D), but in a few patients hemolysis was less rampant (Hb = 7 to 11 g/dl) [379, 399]. In all cases the parents were related. Clinically the disease is very similar to hereditary pyropoikilocytosis (to be described). All patients have responded dramatically to splenectomy.

Mild HE with Poikilocytosis in Infancy   In contrast to those described in the previous section, infants with this form of "mild" HE often begin life with moderately severe hemolytic anemia and neonatal jaundice (Table 72-5), characterized by marked red cell budding, fragmentation, and poikilocytosis (Fig. 72-15C1) [382, 402, 403]. In most cases sufficient elliptocytes are present to suggest the diagnosis, but sometimes this is not so and the disorder may be mistaken for infantile pyknocytosis, hereditary pyropoikilocytosis, or a microangiopathic or oxidant-induced hemolytic anemia [402, 403]. The correct diagnosis is easily made if the parents' smears are examined, since one will have mild HE. With time, fragmentation and hemolysis decline, and the clinical picture of mild HE emerges (Fig. 72-15C2). This transition requires from 4 months to 2 years. The change in morphology often occurs somewhat faster than the decline in hemolysis [413]. Subsequently the disease is clinically indistinguishable from typical mild HE. The unusual neonatal course and the fact that most of the patients are black strongly suggest that this is a unique clinical entity. The prevalence is unknown, but in our experience [431] this is the most common form of HE in black families and is not rare (approximately 30 percent of the kindreds with HE seen at Children's Hospital Medical Center, Boston,

Table 72-5 Clinical phenotypes of hereditary elliptocytosis

Phenotype	Hemolysis	Anemia	Splenomegaly	Blood smear
Mild HE				
Compensated form	Mild or none	None	None	Prominent elliptocytes, rod forms
Uncompensated form	Mild to moderate	Mild to moderate	Variable	Elliptocytes, rod forms, variable poikilocytes and fragments
Mild HE with abnormal erythropoiesis	Mild to moderate	Moderate	Usual	Rounded elliptocytes
Homozygous mild HE	Severe	Moderate to severe	Usual	Elliptocytes, budding red cells, fragments, spherocytes, bizarre poikilocytes
Mild HE with poikilocytosis in infancy				
Infants (<6 mo)	Moderate	Mild to moderate	Variable	Budding, fragments, bizarre poikilocytes
Older children and adults (>1 yr)	Mild or none	Mild or none	None	Elliptocytes, variable mild budding, and fragmentation
Spherocytic HE	Mild to moderate	Mild	Usual	Rounded elliptocytes, spherocytes Variable morphology within kindred
Stomatocytic HE	Mild or none	None	None	Rounded elliptocytes with transverse bars (stomatocytic elliptocytes)
Hereditary pyropoikilocytosis	Moderate to severe	Moderate to severe	Usual	Budding, fragments, spherocytes, elliptocytes, triangular RBCs, bizarre poikilocytes

in the past 5 years). The disorder is not restricted to blacks. We have observed it in one Puerto Rican family, and a possible example in an Italian kindred is recorded [432].

The fragmenting neonatal red cells are very sensitive to heat, like hereditary pyropoikilocytes (see below), but unlike pyropoikilocytes this sensitivity lessens as the patients mature [404]. The dense poikilocytic red cells are rich in hemoglobin F [431], which suggests that the change in the course of the disease is due to the conversion from fetal to adult erythropoiesis. If so, interactions between the genetically defective protein, and other skeletal proteins, must differ in fetal and adult red cells. Whether this is due to the presence of unique fetal skeletal proteins or other secondary effects is unknown. Such differences could also explain the paucity of elliptocytes in the neonatal period in mild HE, described earlier, and the variations in other, presumably "skeletal," properties observed in normal fetal erythrocytes [148, 433, 434].

Spherocytic HE This form of HE is a phenotypic hybrid of mild HE and hereditary spherocytosis. It has been reported only in white families of European descent, is not linked to the Rh gene, and appears to be a unique subtype (Table 72-5) [371, 383, 384, 405–407]. Its prevalence is unknown, but, judged from the number of published reports and our own experience, it may constitute as much as 15 to 25 percent of the HE cases in this population. Unlike mild HE, almost all the affected patients have some hemolysis. This is usually mild to moderate and is often incompletely compensated. The elliptocytes are less prominent and less elongated than in mild HE, and some spherocytes, microspherocytes, and microelliptocytes are usually present (Fig. 72-15E). Red cell morphology varies greatly, even within the same family. Some family members may have relatively prominent spherocytes and as few as 15 to 25 percent elliptocytes, while in others elliptocytes pre-

dominate and spherocytes are rare [371, 384]. This may cause diagnostic confusion initially, particularly if the propositus has few elliptocytes. Family studies will almost always reveal some members with obvious elliptocytosis.

As in HS, the red cells in spherocytic HE are osmotically fragile, particularly after incubation [383, 384, 406]. Increased autohemolysis that responds to glucose and excessive mechanical fragility are also characteristic [383, 384, 405, 535]. Gallbladder disease is common [384, 406], and aplastic crises are a risk. The splenic pathology also mimics HS [436, 437]. Splenic sequestration is evident [384], red cells are conditioned during splenic passage [405], and hemolysis abates following splenectomy [381, 383, 384, 405, 406, 436].

Stomatocytic HE This fascinating condition has only recently been discovered and is still incompletely defined. So far it has been reported only in the aboriginal populations of Melanesia [408–410, 412] and in one Philippino family [411]. The gene is very common in Melanesia, particularly in lowland tribes where malaria is endemic, and there is some evidence that it may provide protection against this disease [409]. In these tribes 10 to 15 percent of the natives are affected. Genetic studies suggest an autosomal recessive inheritance [410], although autosomal dominance with incomplete penetrance has not been excluded.

The morphology is unique and is characterized by roundish elliptocytes traversed by one or two transverse bars. This gives the cells the appearance of double stomatocytes (Fig. 72-15F) [410–412]. Hemolysis is apparently mild [412] or absent [411], although extensive hematologic data have not been published. In one well-studied patient red cell Na^+ and K^+ permeability was increased, glucose consumption was elevated to compensate for increased cation pumping, autohemolysis was increased, and the cells were osmotically resistant [411]. Curi-

Table 72-5 Clinical phenotypes of hereditary elliptocytosis (*Continued*)

Osmatic fragility	Genetics	Other	Selected references
N or ↓	AD, all races	Significant hemolysis with diseases producing splenomegaly	379, 399, 390–394
N or ↓	Sporadic in families with mild HE	Responds well to splenectomy	372, 393–396
N	Sporadic in some Italian families with mild HE	Gradual onset of erythroid dysplasia and ineffective erythropoiesis; incomplete response to splenectomy	397
↑↑	Both parents with mild HE	Low MCV; responds well to splenectomy	379, 398–401
N		↑Thermal sensitivity of RBCs; neonatal jaundice	
	AD, especially blacks		382, 402–404
N		Thermal sensitivity normal or near normal	
↑	AD, especially whites	↑Glucose-responsive autohemolysis; responds well to splenectomy	371, 383, 384, 405–407
N or ↓	?AR, ?AD with incomplete penetrance; Melanesians	↑Monovalent cation permeability; ↓expression of blood groups; ?protection against malaria	408–412
↑↑	?AR, ?double heterozygote of mild HE and unknown gene; especially blacks	↑Thermal sensitivity of RBCs; low MCV; responds well to splenectomy	413–420

ously, many blood group antigens are poorly expressed on the surface of these cells [410]. This remarkable finding is totally unexplained, but it may prove to be the most important property of the cells because recent work [438, 439] indicates that specific blood group antigens are required for the attachment and invasion of red cells by malarial parasites.

Hereditary Pyropoikilocytosis This interesting, rare, apparently recessive disease presents in infancy or early childhood as a severe hemolytic anemia (Table 72-5) characterized by extreme poikilocytosis with budding red cells, fragments, spherocytes, elliptocytes, triangulocytes, and other bizarre-shaped cells [413–416, 418] (Fig. 72-15G). The morphology is similar to that observed in homozygous mild HE and mild HE with poikilocytosis in infancy. Most [413, 415, 416, 418] but not all [375, 414, 419] of the probable cases have occurred in blacks. Complications of severe anemia including growth retardation [415], frontal bossing [415], and early gallbladder disease [413] are reported. Osmotic fragility tests are very abnormal, particularly after incubation [413–415], and autohemolysis is greatly elevated [413–415]. The MCV is very low (25 to 55 μm³) because of the large number of red cell fragments [414, 415].

Another characteristic feature of these cells is their remarkable thermal sensitivity. Hereditary pyropoikilocytes fragment at 45° to 46°C (normal = 49°C) after short periods of heating (10 to 15 min) [413, 416]. With prolonged heating (>6 h) they fragment even at body temperatures [413]. Presumably this property is responsible for the rampant hemolysis evident in most unsplenectomized patients. Following splenectomy, hemolysis is greatly lessened by not eliminated [413, 415].

Although HPP is often considered as a separate disease, there is accumulating evidence for a relationship with some forms of HE. First, as noted above, the disease is clinically and

morphologically similar to the more severe forms of hemolytic elliptocytosis and shares the characteristic of red cell heat sensitivity observed in infants with mild HE and poikilocytosis. In addition, in at least 4 of the 13 reported cases one of the parents or sibs has had typical mild HE (or possibly mild HE with poikilocytosis in infancy) [413, 414]. Several other similar families are currently under study [414a]. In some of the latter kindreds an apparently identical functional defect in spectrin (see the following section) is observed in sibs with phenotypically different diseases (i.e., HPP and mild HE). In other families, all the first-degree relatives are phenotypically normal. These findings suggest that HPP is genetically heterogeneous. At present the best hypothesis is that the HPP phenotype can be produced by homozygosity for an HPP gene, homozygosity for one of the elliptocytosis genes, or double heterozygosity for HPP and HE. The molecular nature of the HPP gene and the mechanism of its interaction with the HE gene are totally unknown.

Etiology

Recent evidence clearly shows that HE is a red cell membrane disorder. In all HE patients studied so far isolated ghosts and membrane skeletons retain the elliptocytic or poikilocytic shape of the parent red cells [440] (Fig. 72-16). HE ghosts and membrane skeletons are also intrinsically fragile. Isolated skeletons disintegrate much more readily than normal when subjected to simple mechanical shaking [441], and intact elliptocytes fragment more rapidly than normal under shear stress [442]. These observations imply that the basic membrane defects lie in the membrane skeleton. Studies of the composition of HE skeletons and the interactions between HE skeletal proteins are currently ongoing in a number of laboratories, and

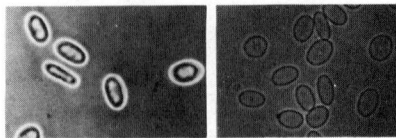 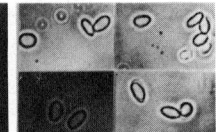

Figure 72-16 The morphology of HE red cells *(left)*, ghosts *(center)*, and membrane skeletons *(right)*. Essentially all the elliptocytic ghosts form elliptocytic membrane skeletons. *(From Tomaselli, John, and Lux [440], by permission of the* Proceedings of the National Academy of Science of the United States of America.)

results are emerging at a rapid rate. At the present time there are insufficient data to correlate all these structural studies with the various clinical phenotypes, but it is already clear that defects in a variety of skeletal protein interactions are observed in patients with HE.

Thermal Sensitivity of Spectrin   It has been known for more than a century that red cells heated to temperatures approaching 50°C for short periods of time become unstable and fragment spontaneously [443]. Recent work shows that this phenomenon is due to denaturation of spectrin [116–118]. Normal spectrin denatures at 49°C (10-min exposure) [440], and normal red cells fragment at the same temperature [440]. As noted earlier, all patients with HPP and some patients with other forms of HE have thermally sensitive red cells. Hereditary pyropoikilocytes and red cells from infants with mild HE and poikilocytosis fragment after 10 min at 44 to 46°C [404, 413]. Red cells from some but not all patients with mild HE fragment at 47 to 48°C [440]. As expected, purified spectrin from these red cells is also heat-sensitive [417, 440]. The thermal instability of HE red cells and spectrin is either present or absent in all the affected patients in a kindred [413, 440]. These patients must have a molecular abnormality of spectrin, but it is not known whether this is a primary sequence defect or a posttranslational modification of the protein. There is preliminary evidence that some of the families with thermally sensitive spectrin also have defective dimer-tetramer-oligomer association (see the following section), but it is not clear that this correlation holds in all cases or that the two phenomena are related in a cause-and-effect manner.

Abnormalities of Spectrin Dimer-Tetramer-Oligomer Association   Spectrin dimers bind head to head to form tetramers or higher-order oligomers [34, 39, 41]. The exact state of oligomerization on the membrane is currently a matter of dispute, although most evidence favors the tetramer form [40, 41]. The interaction is regulated by simple equilibrium thermodynamics [41] and can be shifted on the membrane [42] or in solution [41] by simple manipulations of temperature and ionic strength. At 0°C the reaction is kinetically frozen because of its high activation energy, and no association or dissociation occurs [41].

Approximately 95 percent of the spectrin extracted from normal red cells at 0°C is in the form of tetramers and higher-order oligomers [41, 42]. In contrast, Liu and Palek and their associates find that low temperature spectrin extracts of hereditary pyropoikilocytes contain increased amounts of dimer (20 to 40 percent), implying a defect in dimer-tetramer association [420, 441] (Fig. 72-17, *left*). They have demonstrated this directly in two patients by analyzing the conversion of purified spectrin dimers to tetramers in solution. As expected, HPP dimer forms tetramers poorly ($Ka \simeq 1 \times 10^5 \ M^{-1}$) compared

with normal ($Ka \simeq 8 \times 10^5 \ M^{-1}$) [420] (Fig. 72-17, *right*). In preliminary studies, Knowles, Morrow, and Marchesi [444] have observed a similar (but more severe) defect in another family with HPP. In their patients all of the extracted spectrin was in the form of dimers, and no conversion to tetramers occurred in solution. The defect was traced to an 80,000-dalton tryptic fragment of the α chain by peptide mapping. This peptide is known to contain one of the two binding sites involved in the dimer-tetramer-oligomer interaction [33] (Fig. 72-6). There is indirect evidence that spectrin structure may also be disturbed in the region of the complementary binding site on the β chain. Preliminary peptide mapping studies suggest that spectrin phosphorylation sites are located in this area [444a] (Fig. 72-6). Spectrin phosphorylation is markedly depressed in HPP ghosts in spite of normal spectrin kinase activity [416], which implies a defect in the structure or accessibility of the phosphorylated end of the molecule.

As noted earlier, isolated membrane skeletons are mechanically unstable in all forms of HE tested, including HPP [441]. Similar instability can be induced in *normal* skeletons by preincubating the parent ghosts under conditions that dissociate approximately half of the spectrin tetramers into dimers [42]. Reassociation of these dimers restores normal stability. Together these results strongly suggest that the dimer-tetramer interaction is crucial for normal membrane skeletal stability and that its derangement is responsible for the mechanical instability of red cells and skeletons in many, and perhaps all, patients with HPP.

Liu and his colleagues [441] and, more recently, others [431, 444] have observed that dimer-tetramer association is also defective in some patients with mild HE (or possibly mild HE with poikilocytosis in infancy). The number of individuals examined is too small to assess the prevalence of this defect, but it does not appear to be rare (5 of 11 patients tested) [441]. As in HPP, many of but not all the affected patients have been black. Preliminary mapping studies of the defective HE spectrin show an anomalous tryptic peptide [431], but it is not yet certain that this is the same peptide that is abnormal in HPP. Nevertheless, it appears likely that the two diseases are related

Figure 72-17 Abnormality in spectrin dimer-tetramer equilibrium in hereditary pyropoikilocytosis. *(Left)* Nondenaturing polyacrylamide gel electrophoresis of spectrin extracts from normal, HPP, and HPP carrier red cell membranes. The positions of high molecular weight spectrin complexes (complex), spectrin tetramers (Sp-T), and spectrin dimers (Sp-D) are indicated. Note the increased proportion of spectrin dimer in the HPP patient (38 percent) and his asymptomatic mother (20 percent) (HPP carrier) compared with normal (5 percent). *(Right)* Kinetics of dimer to tetramer conversion at 30°C of normal, HPP, and HPP carrier spectrin. *(From Liu, Palek, Prochal, and Castelberry [420], by permission of the* Journal of Clinical Investigation.)

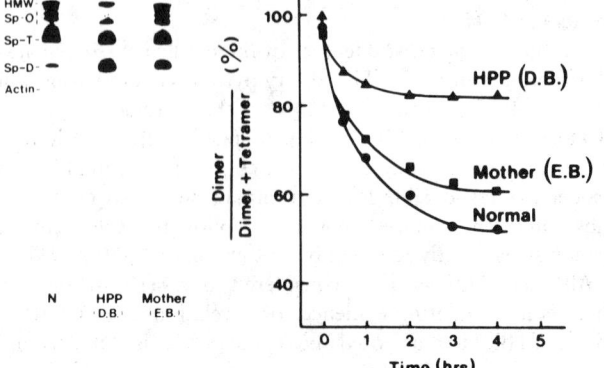

since, as noted earlier, both may appear in the same kindred. For example, Liu, Chilcotte, and Palek have investigated a family in which the mother is normal, the father and son have mild HE, and the daughter has typical HPP [444]. The three affected individuals have decreased dimer-tetramer association and skeletal stability, but, contrary to expectation, the magnitude of the defects is the same in all three patients. In other words, the severity of the clinical and presumed molecular defects do not correlate in this family. The available information in other patients with defects in dimer-tetramer association, although still preliminary, supports this conclusion. The shift in dimer-tetramer equilibrium in many patients with HPP is similar to that observed in HE [441, 444], although in some patients it may be more severe [444]. The most likely explanation of these findings is that many HPP patients are double heterozygotes inheriting one gene for mild HE (or mild HE with poikilocytosis in infancy) that affects the dimer-tetramer equilibrium and a second mutation that affects skeletal stability in some other way.

Abnormalities of Spectrin-Actin-Protein 4.1 Interactions. Recently Tchernia [407] and Feo [445] and their associates have studied a consanguine Algerian family in which HE is associated with a deficiency of protein 4.1 [Fig. 72-18]. The heterozygotes have approximately 50 percent of the normal amount of protein 4.1; no 4.1 is detected in the presumed homozygotes. Clinically the heterozygotes have a mild form of *spherocytic* HE (positive osmotic fragility test, relatively rounded elliptocytes, and little or no hemolysis). In contrast the homozygotes have a severe, transfusion-dependent hemolytic anemia with marked osmotic fragility, normal thermal stability, bizarre red cell morphology (elliptocytosis, spherocytosis, and red cell fragmentation), and a very good response to splenectomy [407]. The homozygous-deficient red cells fragment much more rapidly than normal at moderate shear stresses, an indication of their intrinsic instability [407]. Cells from the partially deficient heterozygotes show intermediate stability.

Mueller and Morrison have described a similar patient in several preliminary reports [71, 446]. In addition to protein 4.1, the red cell membranes of their patient also lack glycophorin C (also called *PAS-2* or *glycoconnectin*). This minor sialoglycoprotein (Table 72-2) is not resolved with the standard Fairbanks gel system (Fig. 72-1), and relatively little is known about its structural properties and function. There is preliminary evidence that it interacts with the membrane skeleton [72] which, combined with its absence in this patient, raises the possibility that it may serve as a binding site for protein 4.1. This has not been proved, since a direct interaction between purified glycophorin C and protein 4.1 has not been demonstrated. It is not known whether glycophorin C is present or absent in the Algerian family with 4.1 deficiency, and it is not clear in this patient whether the glycophorin C deficiency or the deficiency of protein 4.1 is the primary molecule defect. Nevertheless these patients clearly show that either protein 4.1 or glycophorin C or both are necessary for normal membrane stability. It is also interesting that these patients manifest the form of HE that is most like hereditary spherocytosis since, as noted earlier, some patients with HS have a defect that also involves protein 4.1 (i.e., diminished binding of normal protein 4.1 to a defective HE spectrin molecule) (Fig. 72-9) [247].

Abnormalities of the Spectrin-Ankyrin-Protein 3 Interaction Agre, Orringer, Chui, and Bennett have recently

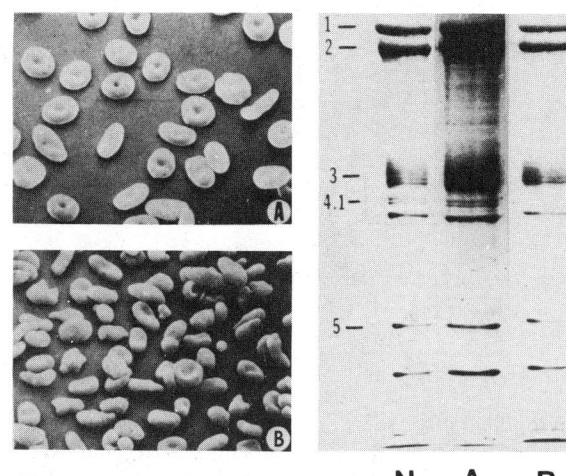

Figure 72-18 Deficiency of protein 4.1 in spherocytic HE. *(Right)* SDS polyacrylamide gels (Laemmli system, see Fig. 72-1) of red cell membranes from a normal individual (N), a heterozygous parent with 50 percent of the normal amount of protein 4.1 (A), and a homozygous-deficient daughter (B). Note that both components of protein 4.1 (4.1a and 4.1b) are decreased (relative to protein 3) in the parent and missing in the daughter and that other proteins are present in normal concentrations. *(Left)* Scanning electron micrographs of red cells from the parent (A) and daughter (B). Note that the homozygous-deficient daughter shows marked fragmentation, spherocytosis, elliptocytosis, and bizarre poikilocytosis, while the heterozygous-deficient parent displays only modest elliptocytosis and slightly spheroidal discocytes. *(From Tchernia, Mohandas, and Shohet [407], by permission of the* Journal of Clinical Investigation.)

reported a defect in ankyrin binding in two unrelated families with a form of hemolytic elliptocytosis that is difficult to classify [444, 447]. The four affected patients have moderate hemolysis and anemia, marked fragmentation and poikilocytosis, positive osmotic fragility and autohemolysis tests, and normal red cell thermal stability, and have had an excellent response to splenectomy. The patients' spectrin and ankyrin function normally in the various interactions between spectrin, ankyrin, and protein 3, but the number of high affinity ankyrin binding sites (protein 3 molecules) on the patients' ankyrin-depleted membrane vesicles is reduced by 50 to 60 percent [447]. Low affinity ankyrin binding is normal. Surprisingly the 43,000-dalton ankyrin-binding fragment of protein 3, obtained from the patients' abnormal vesicles, functions normally in solution. Thus the isolated ankyrin binding sites are normal, but they do not function correctly on the membrane. This may be due to an abnormal arrangement of protein 3 molecules or to defective modulation of the binding portion of protein 3 by neighboring proteins or lipids.

Other Studies As expected from the observations cited above, there is no evidence of an abnormality of hemoglobin or metabolism in hereditary elliptocytes [384, 406, 448]. Reports that ATP utilization [435] and cation pumping [449] are accelerated in hemolytic HE overlook the fact that these are changes characteristic of young red cells. Membrane lipid composition [251] is also normal. There is some evidence that lipid arrangement is altered and, in particular, that cholesterol is concentrated at the apices of HE red cells [450], but this has never been confirmed. The permeability of the membrane to monovalent cations is increased in stomatocytic elliptocytosis [411] but is normal in at least some of the other forms of HE [449]. Divalent cation permeability has been examined only in hered-

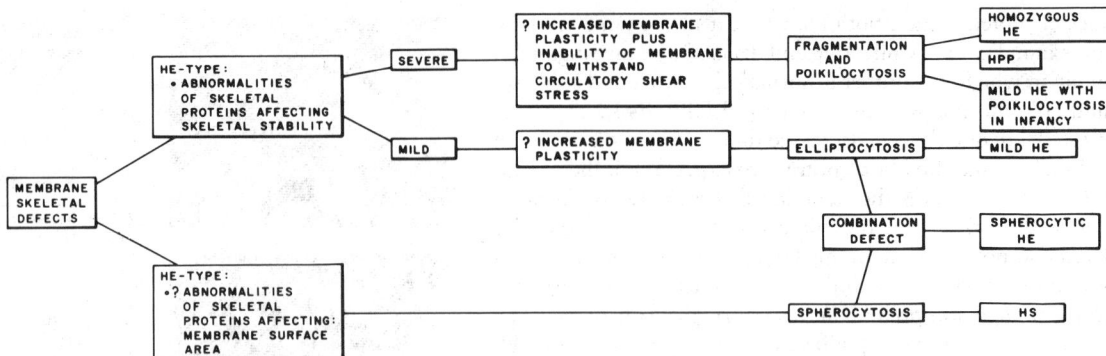

Figure 72-19 Hypothetical pathophysiology of the changes in red cell shape in the various forms of hereditary elliptocytosis (excluding stomatocytic HE).

itary pyropoikilocytosis. HPP red cells have an elevated calcium influx [415], a blunted calcium efflux [416], and excessive membrane-bound calcium [415]. The relationship of these findings to the observed defect in dimer-tetramer interactions is unknown.

Pathophysiology

Any explanation of the various forms of HE must consider the fact that nucleated elliptocytic precursors are round and elongate or fragment only gradually as they circulate [451]. This process resembles the gradual development of spherocytosis in hereditary spherocytes [197, 320] and aging normal cells [452] and is consistent with the concept that the change in shape is secondary to the intrinsic structural instability of the skeleton. According to this hypothesis (Fig. 72-19), *mild* skeletal defects lead to elliptocytosis by increasing membrane plasticity (i.e., *plastic deformation*). As noted earlier, normal red cells rapidly regain their shape if they are transiently deformed, but they remain misshapen if the distortion is maintained for long periods of time (minutes to hours) [136, 137]. Presumably, dynamic skeltal interactions realign in response to stress. In a cell with weakened skeletal interactions, like the hereditary elliptocyte, this process would be accelerated. In vivo red cells are deformed into a stable elliptical or torpedo shape in very small capillaries [453] and are sometimes detained for short periods of time. It is easy to imagine how this distortion, repeated hundreds or thousands of times per day, could cause red cells to gradually elongate and assume their characteristic shape in typical mild HE and in adults with the form of mild HE characterized by poikilocytosis in infancy. Whether this is, in fact, the pathophysiologic mechanism in these diseases remains to be proved.

Red cells with more *severe* skeletal defects would also tend to elongate, but if skeletal instability were sufficiently compromised, they would be unable to withstand the shear stresses experienced in the normal circulation, and fragmentation or combinations of fragmentation and shape change induced by plastic deformation (i.e., bizarre-shaped poikilocytes) would predominate (Fig. 72-19). This process would explain the nearly identical morphology observed in homozygous HE and hereditary pyropoikilocytosis, and in neonates with mild HE and poikilocytosis. In patients with spherocytic HE the pathophysiology is presumably a combination of that observed in HS and typical mild HE.

In spite of the uncertainties about the molecular mechanisms involved in the different subtypes of HE, the available information suggests that red cell death in the various hemolytic forms follows a similar pathway. In all cases hemolysis is markedly ameliorated by splenectomy, and, where examined, splenic pathology shows cordal congestion essential identical to that observed in HS [395, 436, 437, 454]. As in HS, the specific pathophysiologic mechanism(s) responsible for splenic sequestration and red cell destruction remain to be defined.

REFERENCES

1. COOPER RA: Lipids of human red cell membranes: Normal composition and variability in disease. *Semin Hematol* 7:296, 1970
2. VAN DEENAN LLM, DE GIER J: Lipids of the red cell membrane, in Surgenor D Mac N (ed): *The Red Blood Cell*, 2d ed. New York, Academic, 1974, vol 1, p 148
3. COOPER RA: Abnormalities of cell-membrane fluidity in the pathogenesis of disease. *N Engl J Med* 297:371, 1977
4. LUX SE, GLADER BE: Disorders of the red cell membrane, in Nathan DG, Oski FA (eds): *Hematology of Infancy and Childhood*, 2d ed. Philadelphia, Saunders, 1981, p 456
5. STECK TL: The band 3 protein of the human red cell membrane: A review, in Lux SE, Marchesi VT, Fox CF (eds): *Normal and Abnormal Red Cell Membranes*. New York, Alan R. Liss, 1979, p 33
6. ROTHSTEIN A, KNAUF DA, GRINSTEIN S, SHAMI Y: A model for the action of the anion exchange protein of the red blood cell, in Lux SE, Marchesi VT, Fox CF (eds): *Normal and Abnormal Red Cell Membranes*. New York, Alan R. Liss, 1979 p 483
7. FURTHMAYR H: Structural comparison of glycophorins and immunochemical analysis of genetic variants. *Nature* 271:519, 1978
8. MARCHESI VT: Functional proteins of the human red cell membrane. *Semin Hematol* 16:3, 1979
9. NATHAN DG, SHOHET SB: Erythrocyte ion transport defects and hemolytic anemia: "Hydrocytosis" and "desiccytosis." *Semin Hematol* 7:381, 1970
10. PARKER JC, WELT LG: Pathological alterations of cation movements in red blood cells. *Arch Intern Med* 129:320, 1972
11. VERKLEIJ AJ, ZWAAL RFA, ROELOFSEN B, COMFURIUS P, KASTELIJN D, van DEENAN LLM: The asymmetric distribution of phospholipids in the human red cell membrane. A combined study using phospholipase and freeze-etch electron microscopy. *Biochim Biophys Acta* 323:178, 1973
12. LOW MG, FINEAN JB: Modification of erythrocyte membranes by a purified phosphatidylinositol-specific phospholipase C (*Staphylococcus aureus*). *Biochem J* 162:235, 1972
13. FAIRBANKS G, STECK TL, WALLACH DFH: Electrophoretic analysis of the major polypeptides of the human erythrocyte membrane. *Biochemistry* 10:2606, 1971
14. SWEELEY CC, DAWSON G: Lipids of the erythrocyte, in Jamieson GA, Greenwalt TJ (eds): *Red Cell Membrane Structure and Function*. Philadelphia, Lippincott, 1969, p 172
15. ROTHMAN JE, LENARD J: Membrane asymmetry. *Science* 195:743, 1977
16. BERGELSON LD, BARSUKOV LI: Topological asymmetry of phospholipids in membranes. *Science* 197:224, 1977
17. MARINETTI GV, CRAIN RC: Topology of amino-phospholipids in the red cell membrane, in Lux SE, Marchesi VT, Fox CF (eds): *Normal and Abnormal Red Cell Membranes*. New York, Alan R. Liss, 1979 p 1
18. STECK TL: The organization of proteins in the human red cell membrane. *J Cell Biol* 62:1, 1974

19. FURTHMAYR H: Glycophorins A, B, and C: A family of sialoglycoproteins. Isolation and preliminary characterization of trypsin derived peptides, in Lux SE, Marchesi VT, Fox CF (eds): *Normal and Abnormal Red Cell Membranes.* New York, Alan R. Liss, 1979, p 195

20. BERCOVICI T, GITLER C: 5-[125I]iodonaphthyl azide, a reagent to determine the penetration of proteins into the lipid bilayer of biological membranes. *Biochemistry* 17:1484, 1978

21. KAHANE I, GITLER C: Red cell membrane glycophorin labelling from within the lipid bilayer. *Science* 201:351, 1978

22. WEINSTEIN RS, KHODADAD JK, STECK TL: The band 3 protein intramembrane particle of the human red blood cell, in Lassen UV, Ussing HH, Wieth JO (eds): *Membrane Transport in Erythrocytes.* Copenhagen, Munksgaard, 1980, p 35

23. GAHMBERG CG, TAURÉN G, VIRTANEN I, WARTIOVAARA J: Distribution of glycophorin on the surface of human erythrocyte membranes and its association with intramembrane particles: An immunochemical and freeze-fracture study of normal and En(a-) erythrocytes, in Lux SE, Marchesi VT, Fox CF (eds): *Normal and Abnormal Red Cell Membranes.* New York, Alan R. Liss, 1979, p 59

24. NIGG EA, BRON C, GIRARDET M, CHERRY RJ: Band 3-glycophorin A association in erythrocyte membranes demonstrated by combining protein diffusion measurements with antibody-induced cross-linking. *Biochemistry* 19:1887, 1980

25. SHEETZ MP, SAWYER D: Triton shells of intact erythrocytes, in Lux SE, Marchesi VT, Fox CF (eds): *Normal and Abnormal Red Cell Membranes.* New York, Alan R. Liss, 1979, p 121

26. SHEETZ MP: Integral membrane protein interaction with Triton cytoskeletons of erythrocytes. *Biochim Biophys Acta* 557:122, 1979

27. YU J, FISCHMAN DA, STECK TL: Selective solubilization of proteins and phospholipids of red blood cell membranes by nonionic detergents. *J Supramol Struct* 1:233, 1973

28. LUX SE, JOHN KM, KARNOVSKY MJ: Irreversible deformation of the spectrin-actin lattice in irreversibly sickled cells. *J Clin Invest* 58:955, 1976

29. THOMPSON S, RENNIE CM, MADDY A: A re-evaluation of the surface complexity of the intact erythrocyte. *Biochim Biophys Acta* 600:756, 1980

30. DUNN MJ, KEMP RB, MADDY AH: The similarity of the two high-molecular weight polypeptides of erythrocyte spectrin. *Biochem J* 173:197, 1978

31. ANDERSON JM: Structural studies on human spectrin. Comparison of subunits and fragmentation of native spectrin. *J Biol Chem* 254:939, 1979

32. SPEICHER DW, MORROW JS, KNOWLES WJ, MARCHESI VT: Identification of proteolytically resistant domains of human erythrocyte spectrin. *Proc Natl Acad Sci USA* 77:5673, 1980

33. MORROW JS, SPEICHER DW, KNOWLES WJ, HSU CJ, MARCHESI VT: Identification of functional domains of human erythrocyte spectrin. *Proc Natl Acad Sci USA* 77:6592, 1980

34. SHOTTON DM, BURKE BE, BRANTON D: The molecular structure of human erythrocyte spectrin. Biophysical and electron microscopic studies. *J Mol Biol* 131:303, 1979

35. BØE A, ELGSAETER A, OFTEDAL G, STRAND KA: Human spectrin. III. A study based on dynamic and static light scattering. *Acta Chem Scand* A33:245, 1979

36. STOKKE BT, ELGSAETER A: Human spectrin. VI. A viscometric study. *Biochim Biophys Acta* 640:640, 1981

37. DUNBAR JC, RALSTON GB: Hydrodynamic characterization of the heterodimer of spectrin. *Biochim Biophys Acta* 667:177, 1981

38. TYLER JM, HARGREAVES WR, BRANTON D: Purification of two spectrin-binding proteins: Biochemical and electron microscopical evidence for site specific reassociation between spectrin and bands 2.1 and 4.1 *Proc Natl Acad Sci USA* 76:5192, 1979

39. MORROW JS, MARCHESI VT: Self-assembly of spectrin oligomers in vitro: A basis for a dynamic cytoskeleton. *J Cell Biol* 88:463, 1981

40. JI TH, KIEHM DJ, MIDDAUGH CR: Presence of spectrin tetramer on the erythrocyte membrane. *J Biol Chem* 255:2990, 1980

41. UNGEWICKELL E, GRATZER W: Self-association of human spectrin. A thermodynamic and kinetic study. *Eur J Biochem* 88:379, 1978

42. LIU SC, PALEK J: Spectrin tetramer-dimer equilibrium and the stability of erythrocyte membrane skeletons. *Nature* 285:586, 1980

43. GEIDUSCHEK JB, SINGER SJ: Molecular changes in the membranes of mouse erythroid cells accompanying differentiation. *Cell* 16:149, 1979

44. EISEN H, BACH R, EMERY R: Induction of spectrin in erythroleukemic cells transformed by Friend virus. *Proc Natl Acad Sci USA* 74:3898, 1977

45. HASTHORPE S: Quantification of spectrin-containing erythroid precursor cells in normal and pertured erythropoiesis. *Exp Hematol* 8:1001, 1980

46. GOODMAN SR, KULIKOWSKI RR: Identification of spectrin in nonerythroid cells. *J Supramol Struct Cell Biochem (Suppl)* 5:261, 1981

47. PAINTER RG, SHEETZ M, SINGER SJ: Detection and ultrastructural localization of human smooth muscle myosin-like molecules in human non-muscle cells by specific antibodies. *Proc Natl Acad Sci USA* 72:1359, 1975

48. HILLER G, WEBER K: Spectrin is absent in various tissue culture cells. *Nature* 266:181, 1977

49. TILLACK TW, MARCHESI SL, MARCHESI VT, STEERS E JR: A comparative study of spectrin: A protein isolated from red blood cell membranes. *Biochim Biophys Acta* 200:125, 1970

50. PINDER JC, PHETHEAN J, GRATZER WB: Spectrin in primitive erythrocytes. *FEBS Lett* 97:278, 1978

51. PUSZKIN S, PUSZKIN E, MAIMON J, ROUAULT C, SCHOOK W, ORES C, KOCHWA S, ROSENFIELD R: α-Actinin and tropomyosin interaction with a hybrid complex of erythrocyte actin and muscle myosin. *J Biol Chem* 252:5529, 1977

52. TILNEY LG, DETMERS P: Actin in erythrocyte ghosts in its association with spectrin: Evidence for a nonfilamentous form of these two molecules *in situ. J Cell Biol* 66:508, 1975

53. SHEETZ MP, PAINTER RG, SINGER SJ: Relationships of the spectrin complex of human erythrocyte membranes to the actomyosins of muscle cells. *Biochemistry* 15:4486, 1976

54. OHNISHI T: Isolation and characterization of an actin-like protein from membranes of human red cells. *Br J Haematol* 35:453, 1977

55. NAKASHIMA K, BEUTLER E: Comparison of structure and function of human erythrocyte and human muscle actin. *Proc Natl Acad Sci USA* 76:935, 1979

56. PINDER JC, UNGEWICKELL E, BRAY D, GRATZER WB: The spectrin-actin complex and erythrocyte shape, in Lux SE, Marchesi VT, Fox CF (eds): *Normal and Abnormal Red Cell Membranes.* New York, Alan R. Liss, 1979, p 161

57. KORN ED: Biochemistry of actomyosin-dependent cell motility (A review). *Proc Natl Acad Sci USA* 75:588, 1978

58. BRENNER SL, KORN ED: Spectrin/actin complex isolated from sheep erythrocytes accelerates actin polymerization by simple nucleation. Evidence for oligomeric actin in the erythrocyte cytoskeleton. *J Biol Chem* 255:1670, 1980

59. UNGEWICKELL E, BENNETT PM, CALVERT R, OHANIAN V, GRATZER WB: In vitro formation of a complex between cytoskeletal proteins of the human erythrocyte. *Nature* 280:811, 1979

60. BRENNER SL, KORN ED: Spectrin-actin interaction. Phosphorylated and dephosphorylated spectrin tetramer cross-link F-actin. *J Biol Chem* 254:8620, 1979

60a. PINDER J: Personal communication.

61. COHEN CM, BRANTON D: The role of spectrin in erythrocyte membrane-stimulated actin polymerization. *Nature* 279:163, 1979

62. LIN DC, LIN S: Actin polymerization induced by a motility-related high-affinity cytochalasin binding complex from human erythrocyte membrane. *Proc Natl Acad Sci USA* 76:2345, 1979

63. LIN DC, LIN S: A rapid assay for actin-associated high-affinity cytochalasin binding sites based on isoelectric precipitation of soluble proteins. *Anal Biochem* 103:316, 1980

64. COHEN CM, TYLER JM, BRANTON D: Spectrin-actin associations studied by electron microscopy of shadowed preparations. *Cell* 21:875, 1980

65. COHEN CM, FOLEY SF: Spectrin-dependent and -independent association of F-actin with the erythrocyte membrane. *J Cell Biol* 86:694, 1980

66. FOWLER VM, LUNA EJ, HARGREAVES WR, TAYLOR DL, BRANTON D: Spectrin promotes the association of F-actin with the cytoplasmic surface of the human erythrocyte membrane. *J Cell Biol* 88:388, 1981

67. COHEN CM, KORSGREN C: Band 4.1 causes spectrin-actin gels to become thixotropic. *Biochem Biophys Res Commun* 97:1429, 1980

68. WOLFE LC, LUX SE, OHANIAN V: Spectrin-actin binding in vitro; effect of protein 4.1 and polyphosphates. *J Supramol Struct Cell Biochem (Suppl)* 5:123, 1981 (abstract)

69. TYLER JM, REINHARDT BN, BRANTON D: Associations of erythrocyte membrane proteins. Binding of purified bands 2.1 and 4.1 to spectrin. *J Biol Chem* 255:7034, 1980

70. SAUBERMAN N, FORTIER NL, FAIRBANKS G, O'CONNOR RJ, SNYDER LM: Red cell membranes in hemolytic disease. Studies on variables affecting electrophoretic analysis. *Biochim Biophys Acta* 556:292, 1979

71. MUELLER TJ, MORRISON M: Glyconnectin (PAS2), a component of the cytoskeleton of the human erythrocyte membrane. *J Cell Biol* 87:202a, 1980 (abstract)

72. BENNETT V, STENBUCK PJ: Identification and partial purification of ankyrin, the high affinity membrane attachment site for human erythrocyte spectrin. *J Biol Chem* 254:2533, 1979

73. LUNA EJ, KIDD GH, BRANTON D: Identification by peptide analysis of the spectrin-binding protein in human erythrocytes. *J Biol Chem* 254:2526, 1979

74. YU J, GOODMAN S: Syndeins: The spectrin-binding protein(s) of the human erythrocyte membrane. *Proc Natl Acad Sci USA* 76:2340, 1979

75. BENNETT V, STENBUCK PJ: Human erythrocyte ankyrin. Purification and properties. *J Biol Chem* 255:2540, 1980

76. BENNETT V: Purification of an active proteolytic fragment of the membrane attachment site for human erythrocyte spectrin. *J Biol Chem* 253:2292, 1978

77. BENNETT V, STENBUCK PJ: The membrane attachment protein for spectrin is associated with band 3 in human erythrocyte membranes. *Nature* 280, 468, 1979

78. BENNETT V, STENBUCK PJ: Association between ankyrin and the cytoplasmic domain of band 3 isolated from the human erythrocyte membrane. *J Biol Chem* 255:6424, 1980

79. HARGREAVES WR, GIEDD KN, VERKLEIJ A, BRANTON D: Reassociation of ankyrin with band 3 in erythrocyte membranes and in lipid vesicles. *J Biol Chem* 255:11965, 1980

80. SIEGEL DL, GOODMAN SR, BRANTON D: The effect of endogenous proteases on the spectrin binding proteins of human erythrocytes. *Biochim Biophys Acta* 598:517, 1980

81. NIGG EA, CHERRY RJ: Anchorage of a band 3 population at the erythrocyte cytoplasmic membrane surface. Protein rotational diffusion measurements. *Proc Natl Acad Sci USA* 77:4702, 1980

82. MUELLER TJ, MORRISON M: Detection of a variant of protein 3, the major transmembrane protein of the human erythrocyte. *J Biol Chem* 252:6573, 1977

83. STECK TL, RAMOS B, STRAPAZON E: Proteolytic dissection of band 3, the predominant transmembrane polypeptide of the human erythrocyte membrane. *Biochemistry* 15:1154, 1976

84. DRICKAMER LK: Fragmentation of the band 3 polypeptide from human erythrocyte membranes. *J Biol Chem* 252:6909, 1977

85. WEST CM, McMAHON D, MOLDAY RS: Identification of glycoproteins, using lectins as probes, in plasma membranes from Dictyostelium discoideum and human erythrocytes. *J Biol Chem* 253:1716, 1978

86. CHILDS RA, FEIZI T, FUKUDA M, HAKAMORI S: Blood group I activity associated with band 3, the major intrinsic membrane protein of human erythrocytes. *Biochem J* 173:333, 1978

87. YU J, STECK TL: Isolation and characterization of band 3, the predominant polypeptide of the human erythrocyte membrane. *J Biol Chem* 250:9170, 1975

88. MUELLER TJ, LI Y-T, MORRISON M: Effect of endo-β-galactosidase on intact human erythrocytes. *J Biol Chem* 254:8103, 1979

89. SHAKLAI N, YGUERABIDE J, RANNEY JM: Interaction of hemoglobin with red blood cell membranes as shown by a fluorescent chromophore. *Biochemistry* 16:5585, 1977

90. SHAKLAI N, YGUERABIDE J, RANNEY HM: Classification and localization of hemoglobin binding sites on the red blood cell membrane. *Biochemistry* 16:5593, 1977

91. YU J, STECK TL: Associations of band 3, the predominant polypeptide of the human erythrocyte membrane. *J Biol Chem* 250:9176, 1975

92. KARADSHEH NS, UYEDA K: Changes in the allosteric properties of phosphofructokinase bound to erythrocyte membranes. *J Biol Chem* 252:7418, 1977

93. STRAPAZON E, STECK TL: Interaction of the aldolase and the membrane of human erythrocytes. *Biochemistry* 16:2966, 1977

94. HAINFELD JF, STECK TL: The submembrane reticulum of the human erythrocyte: A scanning electron microscope study. *J Supramol Struct* 6:301, 1977

95. LIU SC, PALEK J: Protein-protein interactions in red cell membranes, in Cokelet GR, Meiselman HJ, Brooke DE (eds): *Erythrocyte Mechanics and Blood Flow*. New York, Alan R. Liss, 1980, p 15

96. TSUKITA S, TSUKITA S, ISHIKAWA H: Cytoskeletal network underlying the human erythrocyte membrane. Thin-section electron microscopy. *J Cell Biol* 85:567, 1980

97. PAPE EH, KLOTT K, KREUTZ W: The determination of the electron density profile of the human erythrocyte ghost membrane by small-angle X-ray diffraction. *Biophys J* 19:141, 1977

97a. PAPE EH: Personal communication.

98. McCAUGHAN L, KRIMM S: X-ray and neutron scattering density profiles of the intact human red blood cell membrane. *Science* 207:1481, 1980

99. HARRIS HW JR, LUX SE: Structural characterization of the phosphorylation sites of human erythrocyte spectrin. *J Biol Chem* 255:115122, 1980

99a. SPEICHER D: Personal communication.

100. BULL BS, BRAILSFORD JD: The biconcavity of the red cell: An analysis of several hypotheses. *Blood* 41:833, 1973

101. BULL B: The implications of rheology for the red cell membrane structure. *Blood Cells* 3:431, 1977

102. EVENS EA, HOCHMUTH RM: A solid-liquid composite model of the red cell membrane. *J Membr Biol* 30:357, 1977

103. SHEETZ MP, CASALY J: 2,3-Diphosphoglycerate and ATP dissociate erythrocyte membrane skeletons. *J Biol Chem* 255:9955, 1980

104. SCHINDLER M, KOPPEL D, SHEETZ MP: Modulation of membrane protein lateral mobility by polyphosphates and polyamines. *Proc Natl Acad Sci USA* 77:1457, 1980

105. AVRUCH J, FAIRBANKS G: Phosphorylation of endogenous substrates by erythrocyte membrane protein kinases. I. A monovalent cation-stimulated reaction. *Biochemistry* 13:5507, 1974

106. FAIRBANKS G, AVRUCH J: Phosphorylation of endogenous substrates by erythrocyte protein kinases. II. Cyclic adenosine monophosphate-stimulated reactions. *Biochemistry* 13:5514, 1974

107. PLUT DA, HOSEY MM, TAO M: Evidence for the participation of cytosolic protein kinases in membrane phosphorylation in intact erythrocytes. *Eur J Biochem* 82:333, 1978

108. THOMAS EL, KING LE JR, MORRISON M: The uptake of cyclic AMP by human erythrocytes and its effect on membrane phosphorylation. *Arch Biochem Biophys* 196:459, 1979

109. TAO M, CONWAY R, CHETA S: Purification and characterization of a membrane-bound protein kinase from human erythrocytes. *J Biol Chem* 255:2563, 1980

110. HARRIS HW JR, LEVIN N, LUX SE: Comparison of the phosphorylation of human erythrocyte spectrin in the intact red cell and in various cell-free systems. *J Biol Chem* 255:11521, 1980

110a. SPEICHER D: Personal communication.

111. ANDERSON JM, TYLER JM: State of spectrin phosphorylation does not affect erythrocyte shape or spectrin binding to erythrocyte membranes. *J Biol Chem* 255:1259, 1980

112. GREENQUIST AC, SHOHET SB, BERNSTEIN SE: Marked reduction of spectrin in hereditary spherocytosis in the common house mouse. *Blood* 51:1149, 1978

113. LUX SE: Spectrin-actin membrane skeleton of normal and abnormal red blood cells. *Semin Hematol* 16:21, 1979

114. SMITH B, PEASE B, LUX SE, LACELLE P: Manuscript submitted for publication

115. SHOHET SB: Reconstruction of spectrin-deficient spherocytic mouse erythrocyte membranes. *J Clin Invest* 64:483, 1979

116. MOHANDAS N, GREENQUIST AC, SHOHET SB: Effects of heat and metabolic depletion on erythrocyte deformability, spectrin extractability, and phosphorylation, in Brewer GJ (ed): *The Red Cell*. New York, Alan R Liss, 1978, p 435

117. LUX SE, JOHN KM, UKENA TE: Diminished spectrin extraction from ATP-depleted human erythrocytes. Evidence relating spectrin to changes in erythrocyte shape and deformability. *J Clin Invest* 61:815, 1978

118. DEELEY JDT, CRUM LA, COAKLEY WT: The influence of temperature and incubation time on deformability of human erythrocytes. *Biochim Biophys Acta* 556:90, 1979

119. SMITH BD, LACELLE PL: Parallel decrease of erythrocyte membrane deformability and spectrin solubility at low pH. *Blood* 53:15, 1979

120. CRANDALL ED, CRITZ AM, OSHER AS, KELJO DJ, FORSTER RE: Influence of pH on elastic deformability of the human erythrocyte membrane. *Am J Physiol* 235:c269, 1978

121. MARCHESI VT, STEERS E JR: Selective solubilization of a protein component of the red cell membrane. *Science* 159:203, 1968

122. PALEK J, LIU SC, SNYDER LM: Metabolic dependence of protein arrangement in human erythrocyte membranes. I. Analysis of spectrin-rich complexes in ATP-depleted red cells. *Blood* 51:385, 1978

123. NAKASHIMA K, BEUTLER E: Effect of antispectrin antibody and ATP on deformability of resealed erythrocyte membranes. *Proc Natl Acad Sci USA* 75:3823, 1978

124. FISCHER TM, HAEST CWM, STÖHR M, KAMP D, DEUTICKE B: Selective alteration of erythrocyte deformability by SH-reagents. Evidence for an involvement of spectrin in membrane shear elasticity. *Biochim Biophys Acta* 510:270, 1978

125. HAEST CWM, FISCHER TM, PLASA G, DEUTICKE B: Stabilization of erythrocyte shape by a chemical increase in membrane shear stiffness. *Blood Cells* 6:539, 1980

126. JOHNSON GJ, ALLEN DW, FLYNN TP, FINKEL B, WHITE JG: Decreased survival in vivo of diamide-incubated dog erythrocytes. A model of oxidant-induced hemolysis. *J Clin Invest* 66:955, 1980

127. BIRCHMEIER W, SINGER SJ: Muscle G-actin is an inhibitor of ATP-induced erythrocyte ghost shape changes and endocytosis. *Biochem Biophys Res Commun* 77:1354, 1977

128. SHEETZ MP, SINGER SJ: On the mechanism of ATP-induced shape changes in human erythrocyte membranes. I. The role of the spectrin complex. *J Cell Biol* 73:638, 1977

129. LIN DC, LIN S: High affinity binding of [³H]-dihydrocytochalasin B to peripheral membrane proteins related to the control of cell shape in the human red cell. *J Biol Chem* 253:1415, 1978

130. JOHNSON RM, TAYLOR G, MEYER DB: Shape and volume changes in erythrocyte ghosts and spectrin-actin networks. *J Cell Biol* 86:371, 1980

131. FAIRBANKS G, AVRUCH J, DINO JE, PATEL VP: Phosphorylation and dephosphorylation of spectrin, in Lux SE, Marchesi VT, Fox CF (eds): *Normal and Abnormal Red Cell Membranes*. New York, Alan R Liss, 1979, p 213

132. BIRCHMEIER W, SINGER SJ: On the mechanism of ATP-induced shape changes in human erythrocyte membranes. II. The role of ATP. *J Cell Biol* 73:647, 1977

133. HUI DY, HARMONY JAK: Interaction of plasma lipoproteins with erythrocytes. I. Alteration of erythrocyte morphology. *Biochim Biophys Acta* 550:407, 1979

134. HUI DY, HARMONY JAK: Interaction of plasma lipoproteins with erythrocytes. II. Modulation of membrane-associated enzymes. *Biochim Biophys Acta* 550:425, 1979

135. PATEL VP, FAIRBANKS G: Spectrin phosphorylation and shape change of human erythrocyte ghosts. *J Cell Biol* 88:430, 1981

136. HOCHMUTH RM, EVANS EA, COLVARD DF: Viscosity of human red cell membranes in plastic flow. *Microvasc Res* 11:155, 1976

137. CHIEN S, SUNG K-LP, SKALAK R, USAMI S, TÖZEREN A: Theoretical and experimental studies on viscoelastic properties of erythrocyte membranes. *Biophys J* 24:463, 1978

138. NICOLSON GL, PAINTER RG: Anionic sites of human erythrocyte membranes. II. Anti-spectrin-induced transmembrane aggregation of the binding sites for positively charged colloidal particles. *J Cell Biol* 59:395, 1973

139. ELGSAETER A, BRANTON D: Intramembrane particle aggregation in erythrocyte ghosts. I. The effects of protein removal. *J Cell Biol* 63:1018, 1974

140. ELGSAETER A, SHOTTON DM, BRANTON D: Intramembrane particle aggregation in erythrocyte ghosts. II. The influence of spectrin aggregation. *Biochim Biophys Acta* 426:101, 1976

141. SHOTTON D, THOMPSON K, WOFSY L, BRANTON D: Appearance and distribution of surface proteins of the human erythrocyte membrane. An electron microscope and immunochemical labeling study. *J Cell Biol* 76:512, 1978

142. SHEETZ MP, SCHINDLER M, KOPPEL DE: Lateral mobility of integral membrane proteins is increased in spherocytic erythrocytes. *Nature* 285:510, 1980

143. FOWLER V, BENNETT V: Association of spectrin with its membrane attachment site restricts lateral mobility of human erythrocyte integral membrane proteins. *J Supramol Struct* 8:215, 1978

144. HOOVER R, RUBIN R, WISE G, WARREN R: Adhesion of normal and sickle erythrocytes to endothelial monolayer cultures. *Blood* 54:872, 1979

145. HEBBEL RP, YAMADA O, MOLDOW CF, JACOB HS, WHITE JG, EATON JW: Abnormal adherence of sickle erythrocytes to cultured vascular endothelium. Possible mechanism for microvascular occlusion in sickle cell disease. *J Clin Invest* 65:154, 1980

146. KAHANE I, POLLIACK A, RACHMILEWITZ EA, SKUTELSKY E: Distribution of sialic acids on the red blood cell membrane in β-thalassaemia. *Nature* 271:674, 1978

147. HARDY B, BENSCH KG, SCHRIER SL: Spectrin rearrangement early in erythrocyte ghost endocytosis. *J Cell Biol* 82:654, 1979

148. TOKUYASU KT, SCHEKMAN R, SINGER SJ: Domains of receptor mobility and endocytosis in the membranes of neonatal human erythrocytes and reticulocytes are deficient in spectrin. *J Cell Biol* 80:481, 1979

149. ZAKAI N, KULKA RG, LOYTER A: Fusion of human erythrocyte ghosts by the combined action of calcium and phosphate ions. *Nature* 263:696, 1976

150. CULLIS PR, HOPE MJ: Effects of fusogenic agents on membrane structure of erythrocyte ghosts and the mechanism of membrane fusion. *Nature* 271:672, 1978

151. SEKIGUCHI K, ASANO A: Participation of spectrin in Sendai virus-induced fusion of human erythrocyte ghosts. *Proc Natl Acad Sci USA* 75:1740, 1978

152. LALAZAR A, LOYTER A: Involvement of spectrin in membrane fusion: Induction of fusion in human erythrocyte ghosts by proteolytic enzymes and its inhibition by antispectrin antibody. *Proc Natl Acad Sci USA* 76:318, 1979

153. PORTIS A, NEWTON C, PANGBORN W, PAPAHADJOPOULOS D: Studies on the mechanism of membrane fusion: Evidence for an intermembrane Ca²⁺-phospholipid complex, synergism with Mg²⁺, and inhibition by spectrin. *Biochemistry* 18:780, 1979

154. MOMBERS C, VERKLEIJ AJ, DE GIER J, VAN DEENAN LLM: The interaction of spectrin-actin and synthetic phospholipids. II. The interaction with phosphatidyl serine. *Biochim Biophys Acta* 551:279, 1979

155. MOMBERS C, DE GIER J, DEMEL RA, VAN DEENAN LLM: Spectrin-phospholipid interaction. A monolayer study. *Biochim Biophys Acta* 603:52, 1980

156. HAEST CWM, PLASA G, KAMP D, DEUTICKE B: Spectrin as a stabilizer of the phospholipid asymmetry in the human erythrocyte membrane. *Biochim Biophys Acta* 509:21, 1978

157. VANLAIR CF, MASIUS JB: De la microcythémie. *Bull R Acad Méd Belg* 5:515, 1871

158. HAM TH, CASTLE WB: Studies on destruction of red cells. *Proc Am Phil Soc* 82:411, 1940

159. CHAUFFARD A: Pathogénie de l'ictère hémolytique congénitale. *Ann Méd* 1:3, 1914

160. DAMESHEK W, SCHWARTZ SO: Hemolysins as the cause of clinical and experimental hemolytic anemias. With particular reference to the nature of spherocytosis and increased fragility. *Am J Med Sci* 196:769, 1938

161. WILSON C: Some cases showing hereditary enlargement of the spleen. *Trans Clin Soc (London)* 23:162, 1890

162. WILSON C, STANLEY D: A sequel to some cases showing hereditary enlargement of the spleen. *Trans Clin Soc (London)* 26:163, 1893

163. MINKOWSKI O: Ueber eine hereditäre, unter dem Bilde eines chronischen Ikterus mit Urobilinurie, Splenomegalie und Nierensiderosis ver laufende Affection. *Verh Dtsch Kongr Inn Med* 18:316, 1900

164. BARLOW T, SHAW HB: Inheritance of recurrent attacks of jaundice and of abdominal crises, with hepatosplenomegaly. *Trans Clin Soc (London)* 35:155, 1902

165. GILBERT A, CASTAIGNE J, LEREBOULLET P: De l'ictère familial. Contribution a l'étude de la diathèse biliaire. *Bull Mém Soc Méd d'Hôp Paris* 17:948, 1900

166. CHAUFFARD MA: Pathogéne de l'ictère congenital de l'adulte. *Sem Méd (Paris)* 27:25, 1907

167. CHAUFFARD MA: Les ictères hémolytique. *Sem Méd* 28:49, 1908

168. WIDAL F, ABRAMI P, BRULÉ M: Différenciation de plusieurs types d'ictères hémolytiques par le procédé des hématies deplasmatisées. *Presse Méd* 15:641, 1907

169. WIDAL F, ABRAMI P, BRULÉ M: Les icterus d'origine hémolytique. *Arch Mal Coeur* 1:193, 1908

170. HAYEM G: Sur une variété particulière d'ictère chronique. Ictère infectieux chronique splénomégalique. *Presse Méd* 6:121, 1898

171. MICHELI F: Unmittelbare Effecte der Splenektomie bei einem Fall von erworbenem hämolytischen Splenomegalischen Ikterus Typus Hayem-Widal (Splenohämolytischer Ikterus). *Wien Klin Wochenschr* 24:1269, 1911

172. WYNTER WE: Case of acholuric jaundice after splenectomy. *Proc R Soc Med (Clin Sec)* 6:80, 1912–1913

173. GIFFIN HZ: Haemolytic jaundice: A review of 17 cases. *Surg Gynecol Obstet* 25:152, 1917

174. DAWSON of PENN: The Hume Lectures on haemolytic icterus. *Br Med J* i:921 and i:1963, 1931

175. TILESTON W: Hemolytic jaundice. *Medicine* 1:355, 1922

176. GÄNSSLEN M: Über hämolytischen Ikterus. *Dtsch Arch Klin Med* 140:210, 1922

177. WINTROBE MM: *Blood, Pure and Eloquent.* New York, McGraw-Hill, 1980

178. MORTON NE, MACKINNEY AA, KOSOWER N, SCHILLING RF, GRAY MP: Genetics of spherocytosis. *Am J Hum Genet* 14:170, 1962

179. RACE RR: On the inheritance and linkage relations of acholuric jaundice. *Ann Eugenics* 11:365, 1942

180. JENSSON Ó, JÓNASSON JL, MAGNÚSSON S: Studies on hereditary spherocytosis in Iceland. *Acta Med Scand* 201:187, 1977

181. YOUNG LE: Observations on inheritance and heterogeneity of chronic spherocytosis. *Trans Assoc Am Phys* 68:141, 1955

182. MACKINNEY AA JR: Hereditary spherocytosis. Clinical family studies. *Arch Intern Med* 116:257, 195

183. BISCHEL MGD: Inheritance of familial spherocytosis. *J Am Med Wom Assoc* 19:214, 1964

184. ROZIER JC: Sporadic cases of hereditary spherocytosis. *NC Med J* 32:136, 1971

185. HAYASHI S, KOOMOTO R, YANO A, ISHIGAMI S, ISUJINO G, SAEKI S, IANAKA T: Abnormality in a specific protein of the erythrocyte membrane in hereditary spherocytosis. *Biochem Biophys Res Commun* 57:1038, 1974

186. ANDERSON R, HUESTIS RR, MOTULSKY AG: Hereditary spherocytosis in the deer mouse. Its similarity to the human disease. *Blood* 15:491, 1960

187. BERNARD J, BOIRON M, ESTAGER J: Une grand famille hémolytique. Treize cas de maladie de Minkowski-Chauffard observés dans la même fratne. *Sem Hôp Paris* 28:3741, 1952

188. SHEEHY R, RALSTON GB: Abnormal binding of spectrin to the membrane of erythrocytes in some cases of hereditary spherocytosis. *Blut* 36:145, 1978

189. BOIVIN P, DELAUNAY J, GALAND C: Altered erythrocyte membrane protein phosphorylation in an unusual case of hereditary spherocytosis. *Scand J Haematol* 23:251, 1979

190. KIMBERLING WJ, FULBECK T, DIXON L, LUBS HA: Localization of spherocytosis to chromosome 8 or 12 and report of a family with spherocytosis and a reciprocal translocation. *Am J Hum Genet* 27:586, 1975

191. KIMBERLING WJ, TAYLOR RA, CHAPMAN RG, LUBS HA: Linkage and gene localization of hereditary spherocytosis (HS). *Blood* 52:859, 1978

192. EMERSON CP JR, SHEN SC, HAM TH, FLEMING EM, CASTLE WB: Studies on the destruction of red blood cells. IX. Quantitative methods for determining the osmotic and mechanical fragility of red cells in the peripheral blood and splenic pulp; the mechanism of increased hemolysis in hereditary spherocytosis (congenital hemolytic jaundice) as related to the function of the spleen. *Arch Intern Med* 97:1, 1956

193. DACIE JV, MOLLISON PL: Survival of normal erythrocytes after transfusion to patients with familial haemolytic anaemia (acholuric jaundice). *Lancet* i:550, 1943

194. WILEY JS: Red cell survival in hereditary spherocytosis. *J Clin Invest* 49:666, 1970

195. LeBlond PF, de Boisfleury A, Bessis M: La forme des érythrocytes dans la sphérocytose héréditaire. Étude au microscope à balayage. Relation avec leur déformabilité. *Nouv Rev Fr Hematol* 13:873, 1973

196. Jandl JH, Simmons RL, Castle WB: Red cell filtration and the pathogenesis of certain hemolytic anemias. *Blood* 18:133, 1961

197. LeBlond PF, LaCelle PL, Weed RI: Rhéologie des érythroblastes et des érythrocytes dans la sphérocytose congénitale. *Nouv Rev Fr Hematol* 11:537, 1971

198. LaCelle PL: Pathologic erythrocytes in the capillary microcirculation. *Blood Cells* 1:269, 1975

199. Johnsson R, Vuopio P: Studies on red cell flexibility in spherocytosis using a polycarbonate membrane filtration method. *Acta Haematol* 60:329, 1978

200. MacKinney AA, Jr, Morton NE, Kosower NS, Schilling RF: Ascertaining genetic carriers of hereditary spherocytosis by statistical analysis of multiple laboratory tests. *J Clin Invest* 41:554, 1962

201. Jacob HS, Jandl JH: Cell membrane permeability in the pathogenesis of hereditary spherocytosis (HS). *J Clin Invest* 43:1704, 1964

202. Mohler DN: Adenosine triphosphate metabolism in hereditary spherocytosis. *J Clin Invest* 44:1417, 1965

203. Loder PB, Babarczy G, de Gruchy GC: Red cell metabolism in hereditary spherocytosis. *Br J Haematol* 13:95, 1967

204. Reed CF, Young LE: Erythrocyte energy metabolism in hereditary spherocytosis. *J Clin Invest* 46:1196, 1967

205. Dunn I, Ibsen KH, Coe EL, Schneider AS, Weinstein IM: Erythrocyte carbohydrate metabolism in hereditary spherocytosis. *J Clin Invest* 42:1535, 1963

206. Palek J, Mirčevová L, Brabec V: 2,3-Diphosphoglycerate metabolism in hereditary spherocytosis. *Br J Haematol* 17:59, 1969

207. Fernandez LA, Erslev AJ: Oxygen affinity and compensated hemolysis in hereditary spherocytosis. *J Lab Clin Med* 80:780, 1972

208. Bromberg PA, Theodore J, Robin ED, Jensen WN: Human erythrocyte pH with special reference to intracellular acidosis in hereditary spherocytosis. *J Clin Invest* 41:1349, 1962 (abstract)

209. Kagimoto T, Hayashi F, Yamasaki M, Morino Y, Akasaka K, Kishimoto S: Phosphorus-31-NMR study on nucleotides and intracellular pH of hereditary spherocytes. *Experientia* 34:1092, 1978

210. Nozawa Y, Noguchi T, Iida H, Fukushima T, Sekiya T, Ito Y: Erythrocyte membranes of hereditary spherocytosis: Alteration in surface ultrastructure and membrane proteins, as inferred by scanning electron microscopy and SDS-disc gel electrophoresis. *Clin Chim Acta* 55:81, 1974

211. Barnhart MT, Lusher JM: The human spleen as revealed by scanning electron microscopy. *Am J Hematol* 1:243, 1976

212. Waugh RE, LaCelle PL: Abnormalities in the membrane material properties of hereditary spherocytes. *J Biomech Eng* 102:240, 1980

212a.Waugh RE: Personal communication

213. Reed CF, Swisher SN: Erythrocyte lipid loss in hereditary spherocytosis. *J Clin Invest* 45:777, 1966

214. Weed RI, Bowdler AJ: Metabolic dependence of the critical hemolytic volume of human erythrocytes: Relationship to osmotic fragility and autohemolysis in hereditary spherocytosis and normal red cells. *J Clin Invest* 45:1137, 1966

215. Cooper RA, Jandl JH: The selective and conjoint loss of red cell lipids. *J Clin Invest* 48:906, 1969

216. Snyder LM, Lutz HU, Sauberman N, Jacobs J, Fortier NL: Fragmentation and myelin formation in hereditary xerocytosis and other hemolytic anemias. *Blood* 52:750, 1978

217. Schrier SL, Ben-Bassat I, Bensch K, Seeger M, Junga I: Erythrocyte membrane vacuole formation in hereditary spherocytosis. *Br J Haematol* 26:59, 1974

218. Cooper RA, Jandl JH: The role of membrane lipids in the survival of red cells in hereditary spherocytosis. *J Clin Invest* 48:736, 1969

219. Langley GR, Felderhof CH: Atypical autohemolysis in hereditary spherocytosis as a reflection of two cell populations: Relationship of cell lipids to conditioning by the spleen. *Blood* 32:569, 1968

220. Johnsson R: Red cell membrane proteins and lipids in spherocytosis. *Scand J Haematol* 20:341, 1978

221. Zail SS, Pickering A: Fatty acid composition of erythrocytes in hereditary spherocytosis. *Br J Haematol* 42:399, 1979

222. Kuiper PJC, Livne A: Differences in fatty acid composition between normal erythrocytes and hereditary spherocytosis affected cells. *Biochim Biophys Acta* 260:755, 1972

223. Aloni B, Shinitzky M, Moses S, Livne A: Elevated microviscosity in membranes of erythrocytes affected by hereditary spherocytosis. *Br J Haematol* 31:117, 1975

224. Jansson S-E, Johnsson R, Gripenberg J, Vuopio P: The fluidity gradient in erythrocyte membranes in hereditary spherocytosis: A spin label study. *Br J Haematol* 46:73, 1980

225. Cooper RA, Sawyer WH, Leslie MH, Hill JS, Gill FM, Wiley JS: Normal fluidity of red cell membranes in hereditary spherocytosis. *Br J Haematol* 46:299, 1980

226. Bertles JE: Sodium transport across the surface membrane of red blood cells in hereditary spherocytosis. *J Clin Invest* 36:816, 1957

227. Zipursky A, Israels LG: Significance of erythrocyte sodium flux in the pathophysiology and genetic expression of hereditary spherocytosis. *Pediatr Res* 5:614, 1971

228. Feig SA, Bassilan S: Increased erythrocyte Ca^{2+} content in hereditary spherocytosis. *Pediatr Res* 9:928, 1975

229. Zail SS, van den Hoek AK: Studies on calcium transport and calcium-dependent adenosine triphosphatase activity of erythrocyte membranes in hereditary spherocytosis. *Br J Haematol* 34:605, 1976

230. Johnsson R, Santaholma S, Saris NE: Calcium transport and adenosine triphosphatase activities of erythrocyte membranes in congenital spherocytosis. *Scand J Clin Lab Invest* 38:121, 1978

231. Feig SA, Guidotti G: Relative deficiency of Ca^{2+}-dependent adenosine triphosphatase activity of red cell membranes in hereditary spherocytosis. *Biochem Biophys Res Commun* 58:487, 1974

232. Kirkpatrick FH, Woods GM, LaCelle PL: Absence of one component of spectrin adenosine triphosphatase in hereditary spherocytosis. *Blood* 46:945, 1975

233. Greenquist AC, Shohet SB: Phosphorylation in erythrocyte membranes from abnormally shaped cells. *Blood* 48:877, 1976

234. Beutler E, Guinto E, Johnson C: Human red cell protein kinase in normal subjects and patients with hereditary spherocytosis, sickle cell disease, and autoimmune hemolytic anemia. *Blood* 48:887, 1976

235. Matsumoto N, Yawata Y, Jacob HS: Association of decreased membrane protein phosphorylation with red blood cell spherocytosis. *Blood* 49:233, 1977

236. Yawata Y, Koresawa S, Miyashima K: Membrane protein phosphorylation and protein kinases in normal and hereditary spherocytosis red cells. *Hemoglobin* 4:717, 1980

237. Nakao M, Fujii Y, Hara Y, Nomura T, Nakao T, Kanatsu Y: Membrane protein phosphorylation in intact normal and hereditary spherocytic human erythrocytes. *J Biochem* 88:327, 1980

238. Boivin P, Delaunay J: Altered erythrocyte membrane protein phosphorylation in an unusual case of hereditary spherocytosis. *Scand J Haematol* 23:251, 1979

239. Zail SS, van den Hoek AK: Studies of protein kinase activity and the binding of adenosine 3′5′-monophosphate by membranes of hereditary spherocytosis erythrocytes. *Biochem Biophys Res Commun* 66:1078, 1975

240. Boivin P, Galand G: Erythrocyte membrane phosphorylation in hereditary spherocytosis. *Biomedicine* 27:34, 1977

241. Wolfe LC, Lux SE: Membrane protein phosphorylation of intact normal and hereditary spherocytic erythrocytes. *J Biol Chem* 253:3336, 1978

242. Wolfe LC, Lux SE: Diminished stability of red cell membrane skeletons in hereditary spherocytosis. *Blood* 52 (*Suppl* 1):106, 1978 (abstract)

243. Allen DW, Cadman S, McCann SR, Finkel B: Increased membrane binding of erythrocyte catalase in hereditary spherocytosis and in metabolically stressed normal cells. *Blood* 49:113, 1977

244. Jacob HS, Ruby A, Overland ES, Mazia D: Abnormal membrane protein of red blood cells in hereditary spherocytosis. *J Clin Invest* 50:1800, 1971

245. Jacob HS: The abnormal red cell membrane in hereditary spherocytosis: Evidence for the causal role of mutant microfilaments. *Br J Haematol* 23:35, 1972

246. Engelhardt R: Impaired reassemblance of red blood cell membrane components in hereditary spherocytosis, in Bolis L, Hoffman JF, Leaf A (eds): *Membranes and Disease*. New York, Raven, 1976, p 75

247. Wolfe LC, John KM, Falcone J, Lux SE: Identification of the molecular defect in some kindreds with hereditary spherocytosis (HS): Defective binding of protein 4.1 by its spectrin. *Blood* (*Suppl* 1):50a, 1981

247a.Wolfe LC, John KM, Falcone J, Lux SE: Manuscript submitted for publication

248. Goodman SR, Eyster EM: Alteration of the spectrin-protein 4.1 interaction in hereditary spherocytosis. *Blood* (*Suppl* 1):42a, 1981 (abstract)

249. Jandl JH, Cooper RA: Hereditary spherocytosis, in Stanbury JB, Wyngaarden JB, Fredrickson DS (eds): *The Metabolic Basis of Inherited Disease*, 4th ed. New York, McGraw-Hill, 1978, p 1396

250. Lutz HU, Liu S, Palek J: Release of spectrin-free vesicles from human erythrocytes during ATP depletion. *J Cell Biol* 73:548, 1977

251. de Gier J, van Deenan LLM: Phospholipid and fatty acid characteristics of erythrocytes in some cases of anaemia. *Br J Haematol* 10:246, 1964

252. Zail SS, van den Hoek AK: The topology of red cell membrane lipids in hereditary spherocytosis. *S Afr J Med Sci* 40:67, 1975

253. Oski FA, Naiman JL, Blum SF, Zarkowsky HS, Whaun J, Shohet SB, Green A, Nathan DG: Congenital hemolytic anemia with high-sodium, low-potassium red cells: Studies of three generations of a family with a new variant. *N Engl J Med* 280:909, 1969

254. Fischer S, Tortolero M, Piau J-P, Delaunay J, Schapira G: Phosphorylation and dephosphorylation reactions by erythrocyte plasma membrane enzymes. *Biochim Biophys Acta* 598:463, 1980

255. MICHIELIN E, CLARI G, FALEZZA GC: Partial characterization of cytosol and membrane-bound protein kinases in hereditary spherocytosis erythrocytes. *Clin Chim Acta* 92:41, 1979

256. BOIVIN P, GALAND C: Protéines de la membrane érythrocytaire. I. Étude électrophorétique des protéines solubilisées des membranes d'érythrocytes humains normaux et pathologiques. *Nouv Rev Fr Hematol* 14:355, 1974

257. JACOB H, AMSDEN T, WHITE J: Membrane microfilaments of erythrocytes: Alteration in intact cells reproduces the hereditary spherocytosis syndrome. *Proc Natl Acad Sci USA* 69:471, 1972

258. JACOB HS, YAWATA Y, MATSUMOTO N, AHMAN S, WHITE J: Cyclic nucleotide-membrane proteins interaction in the regulation of erythrocyte shape and survival: Defect in hereditary spherocytosis, in Brewer GJ (eds): *Erythrocyte Structure and Function.* New York, Alan R Liss, 1975, p 235

259. PINDER JC, LUX SE, GRATZER WB: Unpublished observations

260. TCHERNIA G, MOHANDAS N, SHOHET SB: Deficiency of cytoskeletal membrane protein band 4.1 in homozygous hereditary elliptocytosis: Implications for red cell membrane stability. *J Clin Invest,* in press

261. RALSTON G: Personal communication

262. IIDA H, HASEGAWA I, NOZAWA Y: Biochemical studies on abnormal erythrocyte membranes. Protein abnormality of erythrocyte membrane in biliary obstruction. *Biochim Biophys Acta* 443:394, 1976

263. COOPER RA, JANDL JH: Bile Salts and cholesterol in the pathogenesis of target cells in obstructive jaundice. *J Clin Invest* 47:809, 1968

264. COOPER RA, DILOY-PURAY M, LANDO P, GREENBERG MS: An analysis of lipoproteins, bile acids, and red cell membranes associated with target cells and spur cells in patients with liver disease. *J Clin Invest* 51:3182, 1972

265. EVANS EA, WAUGH R, MELNIK C: Elastic area compressibility modulus of red cell membranes. *Biophys J* 16:585, 1976

266. CHAPMAN RG: Red cell life span after splenectomy in hereditary spherocytosis. *J Clin Invest* 47:2263, 1968

267. BAIRD RN, McPHERSON AS, RICHMOND J: Red blood cell survival after splenectomy in congenital spherocytosis. *Lancet* 1:1060, 1971

268. CHEN L-T, WEISS L: Electron microscopy of red pulp of human spleen. *Am J Anat* 134:425, 1972

269. WEISS L: A scanning electron microscopic study of the spleen. *Blood* 43:665, 1974

270. KNISELY MH: Spleen studies. I. Microscopic observations of the circulating system of living unstimulated mammalian spleen. *Anat Rec* 65:23, 1936

271. CHEN L-T, WEISS L: The role of the sinus wall in the passage of erythrocytes through the spleen. *Blood* 41:529, 1973

272. MURPHY JR: The influence of pH and temperature on some physical properties of normal erythrocytes and erythrocytes from patients with hereditary spherocytosis. *J Lab Clin Med* 69:758, 1967

273. YOUNG LE, PLATZER RF, ERVIN DM, IZZO MJ: Hereditary spherocytosis. II. Observations on the role of the spleen. *Blood* 6:1099, 1951

274. JANDL JH, GREENBERG MS, YONEMOTO RH, CASTLE WB: Clinical determination of the sites of red cell sequestration in hemolytic anemias. *J Clin Invest* 35:842, 1956

275. HARRIS IM, McALISTER J, PRANKERD TAJ: Splenomegaly and the circulating red cell. *Br J Haematol* 4:97, 1958

276. MOTULSKY AG, CASSERD F, GIBLETT ER, BROUN GO Jr, FINCH CA: Anemia and the spleen. *N Engl J Med* 259:1164, 1215, 1958

277. PRANKERD TAJ: Studies on the pathogenesis of haemolysis in hereditary spherocytosis. *Q J Med (New Series)* 24:199, 1960

278. GRIGGS RC, WEISMAN R Jr, HARRIS JW: Alterations in osmotic and mechanical fragility related to *in vivo* erythrocyte aging and splenic sequestration in hereditary spherocytosis. *J Clin Invest* 39:89, 1960

279. PRANKERD TAJ: The spleen and anaemia. *Br Med J* 2:517, 1963

280. DACIE JV: Familial haemolytic anaemia (acholuric jaundice), with particular reference to changes in fragility produced by splenectomy. *Q J Med (New Series)* 12:101, 1943

281. WILAND OK, SMITH EB: The morphology of the spleen in congenital hemolytic anemia (hereditary spherocytosis). *Am J Clin Pathol* 26:619, 1956

282. MOLNAR Z, RAPPAPORT H: Fine structure of the red pulp of the spleen in hereditary spherocytosis. *Blood* 39:81, 1972

283. MATSUMOTO N, ISHIHARA T, SHIBATA M, UCHINO F, NAKASHIMA K, MIWA S: Electron microscopic studies of the spleen and liver in hereditary spherocytosis. *Acta Pathol Jap* 23:507, 1973

284. BANTI G: Splénomégalie hémolytique au hémopoïétique: Le rôle de la rate dans l'hémolyse. *Sem Méd* 33:313, 1913

285. MacPHERSON AIS, RICHMOND J, DONALDSON GWK, MUIR AR: The role of the spleen in congenital spherocytosis. *Am J Med* 50:35, 1971

286. JANDL JH, ASTER RH: Increased splenic pooling and the pathogenesis of hypersplenism. *Am J Med Sci* 253:383, 1967

287. LaCELLE PL: pH in the mouse spleen and its effect on erythrocyte flow properties. *Blood* 44:910, 1974 (abstract)

288. RAKITZIS ET, MILLS GC: Relation of red cell hexokinase activity to extracellular pH. *Biochim Biophys Acta* 192:157, 1969

289. MINAKAMI S, YOSHIKAWA H: Studies on erythrocyte glycolysis. III. The effects of active cation transport, pH and inorganic phosphate concentration on erythrocyte glycolysis. *J Biochem (Tokyo)* 59:145, 1966

290. PARKER JC: Ouabain-insensitive effects of metabolism on ion and water content in red blood cells. *Am J Physiol* 221:338, 1971

291. DACIE JV: Observations on autohemolysis in familial acholuric jaundice. *J Pathol Bacteriol* 52:331, 1941

292. GARDOS G: The role of calcium in the potassium permeability of human erythrocytes. *Acta Physiol Acad Sci Hung* 15:121, 1959

293. SACHS JR, KNAUF PA, DUNHAM PB: Transport through red cell membranes, in Surgenor D MacN (ed): *The Red Blood Cell,* 2d ed. New York, Academic, 1975, vol 2, p 613

294. JANDL JH: Hereditary spherocytosis, in Beutler E (ed): *Hereditary Disorders of Erythrocyte Metabolism.* New York, Grune & Stratton, 1968, p 209

295. SELWYN JG, DACIE JV: Autohemolysis and other changes resulting from the incubation *in vitro* of red cells from patients with congenital hemolytic anemia. *Blood* 9:414, 1954

296. LANGLEY GR, AXELL M: Changes in erythrocyte membranes and autohaemolysis during *in vitro* incubation. *Br J Haematol* 14:593, 1968

297. BLENDIS LM, BANKS DC, RAMBOER C, WILLIAMS R: Spleen blood flow and splanchic haemodynamics in blood dyscrasia and other splenomegalies. *Clin Sci* 38:73, 1970

298. HUCHZERMEYER H, SCHMITZ-FEUERHAKE T, RABLIN T: Determination of splenic blood flow by inhalation of radioactive rare gases. *Eur J Clin Invest* 7:345, 1977

299. TOGHILL PJ: Red cell pooling in enlarged spleens. *Br J Haematol* 10:347, 1964

300. PALEK J, LIU PA, LIU SC: Polymerization of red cell membrane protein contributes to spheroechinocyte shape irreversibility. *Nature* 274:505, 1978

301. MAYMAN D, ZIPURSKY A: Hereditary spherocytosis: The metabolism of erythrocytes in the peripheral blood and in the splenic pulp. *Br J Haematol* 27:201, 1974

302. COLEMAN DH, FINCH CA: Effect of adrenal steroids in hereditary spherocytic anemia. *J Lab Clin Med* 47:602, 1956

303. ATKINSON JP, SCHREIBER AS, FRANK MM: Effects of corticosteroids and splenectomy on the immune clearance and destruction of erythrocytes. *J Clin Invest* 52:1509, 1973

304. SCHREIBER AD, PARSONS J, McDERMOTT P, COOPER RA: Effect of corticosteroids on the human monocyte IgG and complement receptors. *J Clin Invest* 56:1189, 1975

305. BOWMAN HS, OSKI FA: Splenic macrophage interaction with red cells in pyruvate kinase deficiency and hereditary spherocytosis. *Vox Sang* 19:168, 1970

306. TRUCCO JI, BROWN AK: Neonatal manifestations of hereditary spherocytosis. *Am J Dis Child* 113:263, 1967

307. STAMEY CC, DIAMOND LK: Congenital hemolytic anemia in the newborn. *Am J Dis Child* 94:616, 1957

308. BURMAN D: Congenital spherocytosis in infancy. *Arch Dis Child* 33:335, 1958

309. ERLANDSON ME, HILGARTNER M: Hemolytic disease in the neonatal period and early infancy. *J Pediatr* 54:566, 1959

310. GEHLBACH SH, COOPER BA: Haemolytic anaemia in infectious mononucleosis due to inapparent congenital spherocytosis. *Scand J Haematol* 7:141, 1970

311. DACIE JV: Hereditary spherocytosis, in *The Hemolytic Anemias Congenital and Acquired,* p l. *The Congenital Anemias,* 2d ed. New York, Grune & Stratton, 1960, p 82

312. BELLINGHAM AJ, DELTEN JC, LENFANT C: Regulatory mechanism of hemoglobin oxygen affinity in acidosis and alkalosis. *J Clin Invest* 50:700, 1971

313. YOUNG LE, IZZO MJ, PLATZER RF: Hereditary spherocytosis. I. Clinical, hematologic and genetic features in 28 cases, with particular reference to the osmotic and mechanical fragility of incubated erythrocytes. *Blood* 6:1073, 1951

314. KRUEGER HC, BURGERT EO: Hereditary spherocytosis in 100 children. *Mayo Clin Proc* 41:821, 1966

315. DEBRÉ R, LAMY M, SÉE G, SCHRAMECK G: Congenital and familial hemolytic disease in children. *Am J Dis Child* 56:1189, 1938

316. DIAMOND LK: Indications for splenectomy in childhood. Results in fifty-two operated cases. *Am J Surg (NS)* 39:400, 1938

317. WATSON CJ: Studies of urobilinogen. III. The per diem excretion of urobilinogen in the common forms of jaundice and disease of the liver. *Arch Intern Med* 59:206, 1937

318. SEARS DA, ANDERSON PR, FOY AL, WILLIAMS HL, CROSBY WH: Urinary iron excretion and renal metabolism of hemoglobin in hemolytic disease. *Blood* 28:708, 1966

319. MÜLLER-EBERHARD U, JAVID J, LIEM HH, HANSTEIN A, HANNA M: Plasma concentrations of hemopexin, haptoglobin and heme in patients with various hemolytic diseases. *Blood* 32:811, 1968

320. PAOLINO W: Variations of the mean diameter in the ripening of the erythrocyte. *Acta Med Scand* 136:141, 1949

321. MAIZELS M: The anion and cation content of normal and anaemic bloods. *Biochem J* 30:821, 1936

322. JACOB HS: Hereditary spherocytosis: A disease of the red cell membrane. *Semin Hematol* 2:139, 1965

323. ZANELLA A, IZZO C, REBULLA P, ZANUSO F, PERRONI L, SIRCHIA G: Acidified glycerol lysis test: A screening test for spherocytosis. *Br J Haematol* 45:481, 1980

324. YOUNG LE, IZZO MJ, ALTMAN KI, SWISHER SN: Studies on spontaneous in vitro autohemolysis in hemolytic disorders. *Blood* 11:977, 1956

325. LANGLEY GR, FELDERHOF CH: Atypical autohemolysis in hereditary spherocytosis as a reflection of two cell populations: Relationship of cell lipids to conditioning by the spleen. *Blood* 32:569, 1968

326. GOTTFRIED EL, ROBERTSON NA: Glycerol lysis time of incubated erythrocytes in the diagnosis of hereditary spherocytosis. *J Lab Clin Med* 84:746, 1974

327. GOTTFRIED EL: Acidified glycerol lysis test (correspondence), *Br J Haematol* 47:323, 1981

328. JOHNSSON R, SALMINEN S: Effect of ouabain on osmotic resistance and monovalent cation transport of red cells in hereditary spherocytosis. *Scand J Haematol* 29:323, 1980

329. OWREN PA: Congenital hemolytic jaundice. The pathogenesis of the "hemolytic crisis." *Blood* 3:231, 1948

330. BARKER K, MARTIN FRR: Splenectomy in congenital microspherocytosis. *Br J Surg* 56:561, 1969

331. ROBINS MM: Familial crisis in hereditary spherocytosis: Report of six affected siblings. *Clin Pediatr* 4:210, 1965

332. CONKLIN GT, GEORGE JN, SEARS DA: Transient erythroid aplasia in hemolytic anemia: A review of the literature with two case reports. *Tex Rep Biol Med* 32:391, 1974

333. GAIRDNER D: The association of gall-stones with acholuric jaundice in children. *Arch Dis Child* 14:109, 1939

334. DELAMORE IW, RICHMOND J, DAVIES SH: Megaloblastic anaemia in congenital spherocytosis. *Br Med J* 1:543, 1961

335. KOHLER HG, MEYNELL MJ, COOKE WT: Spherocytic anaemia, complicated by megaloblastic anaemia of pregnancy. *Br Med J* 1:779, 1960

336. BATES GC, BROWN CH: Incidence of gallbladder disease in chronic hemolytic anemia (spherocytosis). *Gastroenterology* 21:104, 1952

337. LAWRIE GM, HAM JM: The surgical treatment of hereditary spherocytosis. *Surg Gynecol Obstet* 139:208, 1974

338. HANFORD RB, SCHNEIDER GF, MACCARTHY JD: Massive thoracic extramedullary hemopoieses. *N Engl J Med* 263:120, 1960

339. TAYLOR ES: Chronic ulcer of the leg associated with congenital jaundice. *JAMA* 112:1574, 1939

340. BEINHAUER LG, GRUHN JG: Dermatologic aspects of congenital spherocytic anemia. *Arch Dermatol* 75:642, 1957

341. BARRY M, SCHEUER PJ, SHERLOCK S, ROSS CF, WILLIAMS R: Hereditary spherocytosis with secondary haemochromatosis. *Lancet* 2:481, 1968

342. SCHAFER AI, MILLER JB, LESTER EP, BOWERS TK, JACOB HS: Monoclonal gammopathy in hereditary spherocytosis: A possible pathogenic relation. *Ann Intern Med* 88:45, 1978

343. LEMPERT KD: Gammopathy and spherocytosis. *Ann Intern Med* 89:145, 1978

344. JANDL JH, FILES NM, BARNETT SB, MACDONALD RA: Proliferative response of the spleen and liver to hemolysis. *J Exp Med* 122:299, 1965

345. SCHILLING RF: Hereditary spherocytosis; a study of splenectomized persons. *Semin Hematol* 13:169, 1976

346. ISOBE T, OSSERMAN EF: Pathologic conditions associated with plasma cell dyscrasias: A study of 806 cases. *Ann NY Acad Sci* 190:507, 1971

347. LAWRENCE RD: Haemochromatosis in three families and in a woman. *Lanct* 1:736, 1949

348. WILSON JD, SCOTT PJ, NORTH JDK: Hemochromatosis in association with hereditary spherocytosis. *Arch Intern Med* 120:701, 1967

349. PARKIN JD, RUSH B, DEGROOT RJ, BUDD RS: Iron absorption after splenectomy in hereditary spherocytosis. *Aust NZ J Med* 4:58, 1974

350. BENDER-GÖLZE CH, HEINREICH HC, GABBE EE, OPPITZ KH, SCHÄFER KH, SCHRÖTER W, WHANG DH: Intestinal absorption under the influence of available storage iron and erythroblastic hyperplasia. *Z Kinderheilkd* 118:283, 1975

351. ZIPURSKY A: Isoimmune hemolytic diseases, in Nathan DG, Oski FA (eds): *Hematology of Infancy and Childhood,* 2d ed. Philadelphia, Saunders, 1981, p 50

352. GILLILAND BC, BAXTER E, EVANS RS: Red cell antibodies in acquired hemolytic anemia with negative antiglobulin serum tests. *N Engl J Med* 285:252, 1971

353. CROSBY WH, CONRAD ME: Hereditary spherocytosis: Observations on hemolytic mechanisms and iron metabolism. *Blood* 15:662, 1960

354. MCCANN SR, JACOB HS: Spinal cord disease in hereditary spherocytosis: Report of two cases with a hypothesized common mechanism for neurologic and red cell abnormalities. *Blood* 48:259, 1976

355. ZETTERSTRÖM R, STRINDBERG B: Sporadic congenital spherocytosis associated with congenital hypoplastic thrombocytopenia and malformations. *Acta Paediatr* 47:14, 1958

356. WILEY JS, FIRKIN BG: An unusual variant of hereditary spherocytosis. *Am J Med* 48:63, 1970

357. GARWICZ S: Atypical spherocytosis, a disease of spleen as well as of red blood cells. *Lancet* 1:956, 1975

358. BRAIN MC, BEILIN LJ, DACIE JV: Atypical congenital spherocytosis: Evidence of abnormal permeability of K^+. *Br J Haematol* 15:323, 1968 (abstract)

359. ZAIL SS, KRAWITZ P, VILJOEN E, METZ J: Atypical hereditary spherocytosis: Biochemical studies and sites of erythrocyte destruction. *Br J Haematol* 13:323, 1967

360. MACKENZIE FAF, ELLIOT DH, EASTCOTT HHG, HUGHES-JONES NC, BARKHAN P, MOLLISON PL: Relapse in hereditary spherocytosis with proven splenunculus. *Lancet* 1:1102, 1962

361. BART JB, APPEL MF: Recurrent hemolytic anemia secondary to accessory spleens. *South Med J* 71:608, 1978

362. LAMBRECHT K: Die Elliptocytose (Ovalocytose) und ihre klinische Bedeutung. *Ergeb Inn Med Kinderheilkd* 55:295, 1938

363. DRESBACH M: Elliptical human red corpuscles. *Science* 19:469, 1904

364. FLINT A: Elliptical human erythrocytes. *Science* 19:796, 1904

365. DRESBACH M: Elliptical human erythrocytes. *Science* 21:473, 1905

366. BISHOP FW: Elliptical human erythrocytes. *Arch Intern Med* 14:388, 1914

367. SYDENSTRICKER VP: Elliptic human erythrocytes. *JAMA* 81:113, 1923

368. HUCK JG, BIGELOW RM: Poikilocytes in otherwise normal blood (elliptical human erythrocytes). *Bull Johns Hopkins Hosp* 34:390, 1923

369. HUNTER WC, ADAMS RB: Hematologic study of three generations of a white family showing elliptical erythrocytes. *Ann Intern Med* 2:1162, 1929

370. HUNTER WC: Further study of a white family showing elliptical erythrocytes. *Ann Intern Med* 6:775, 1932

371. GIFFIN HZ, WATKINS CH: Ovalocytosis with features of hemolytic icterus. *Trans Assoc Am Physicians* 54:355, 1939

372. PENFOLD J, LIPSCOMB JM: Elliptocytosis in man, associated with hereditary haemorrhagic telangiectasis. *Q J Med* 12:157, 1943

373. GRZEGORZEWSKI H: Ueber familiäres Vorkommennis elliptische Erythrozyten beim Menschen. *Folia Haematol* 50:260, 1933

374. VAN DEN BERGH AAH: Elliptische rote Blutköperchen, (Addendum). *Dtsch Med Wochenschr* 54:1244, 1928

375. MASON VR: Ovalocytosis (elliptical human erythrocytes), in Downey H (ed): *Handbook of Hematology,* New York, Paul B Hoeber, 1938, vol III, p 2351

376. LAWRENCE JS: Elliptical and sickle-shaped erythrocytes in the circulating blood of white persons. *J Clin Invest* 5:31, 1927

377. POLLOCK LH, DAMESHEK W: Elongation of red blood cells in a Jewish family. *Am J Med Sci* 188:822, 1934

378. INTROZZI P: Anaemia ipocromica splenomegalica emolitica con ovalocitosi (ellipticitosi), poichilocitosi ed aumento della resistenza osmotica der globuli rossi, Splenectomia. *Haematologica* 16:525, 1935

379. WYANDT H, BANCROFT PM, WINSHIP TO: Elliptic erythrocytes in man. *Arch Intern Med* 68:1043, 1941

380. WOLMAN IJ, ÖZGE A: Studies on elliptocytosis. I. Hereditary elliptocytosis in the pediatric age period: a review of recent literature. *Am J Med Sci* 234:702, 1957

381. DACIE JV: Hereditary elliptocytosis, in *The Hemolytic Anemias, Congenital and Acquired, pt I. The Congenital Anemias,* 2d ed. New York, Grune & Stratton, 1960, p 151

382. JOSEPHS HW, AVERY ME: Hereditary elliptocytosis associated with increased hemolysis. *Pediatrics* 16:741, 1955

383. WEISS HJ: Hereditary elliptocytosis with hemolytic anemia. *Am J Med* 35:455, 1963

384. CUTTING HO, MCHUGH, CONRAD FG, MARLOW AA: Autosomal dominant hemolytic anemia characterized by ovalocytosis. A family study of seven involved members. *Am J Med* 39:21, 1965

385. MCCARTY SH: Elliptical red blood cells in man. A report of eleven cases. *J Lab Clin Med* 19:612, 1934

386. GOODALL HB, HENDRY DWW, LAWLER SD, STEPHEN SA: Data on linkage in man: Elliptocytosis and blood groups. II. Family 3. *Ann Eugenet (London)* 17:272, 1953

387. MORTON NE: The detection and estimation of linkage between the genes for elliptocytosis and the Rh blood type. *Am J Hum Genet* 8:80, 1956

388. BANNERMAN RM, RENWICK JH: The hereditary elliptocytoses: Clinical and linkage data. *Ann Hum Genet (London)* 26:23, 1962

389. COOK PJL, NOODES JE, NEWTON MS, DE MEY R: On the orientation of the Rh El_1 linkage group. *Ann Hum Genet (London)* 41:157, 1977

390. FLORMAN AL, WINTROBE MM: Human elliptical red corpuscles. *Bull Johns Hopkins Hosp* 63:209, 1938

391. MOTULSKY AG, SINGER K, CROSBY WH, SMITH V: The life span of the elliptocyte. Hereditary elliptocytosis and its relationship to other familial hemolytic diseases. *Blood* 9:57, 1954

392. GARRIDO-LECCA G, MERINO C, LUNA G: Hereditary elliptocytosis in a Peruvian family. *N Engl J Med* 256:311, 1957

393. GEERDINK RA, HELLEMAN PW, VERLOOP MC: Hereditary elliptocytosis and hyperhaemolysis. A comparative study of 6 families with 145 patients. *Acta Med Scand* 179:715, 1966

394. JENSSON Ó, JÓNASSON TH, ÓLAFSSON Ó: Hereditary elliptocytosis in Iceland. *Br J Haematol* 13:844, 1967

395. BLACKBURN EK, JORDAN A, LYTLE WJ, SWAN HT, TUDHOPE GR: Hereditary eliptocytic haemolytic anaemia. *J Clin Pathol* 11:316, 1958

396. MCCURDY PR: Clinical, genetic and physiological studies in hereditary elliptocytosis, in *Proc IX Cong Int Soc Hematol*. Universidad Nacional Autónoma de Mexico, 1964, vol 1, p 155

397. TORLONTANO G, FIORITONI G, SALVATI AM: Hereditary haemolytic ovalocytosis with defective erythropoiesis. *Br J Haematol* 43:435, 1979

398. LIPTON EL: Elliptocytosis with hemolytic anemia; the effects of splenectomy. *Pediatrics* 15:67, 1955

399. GRECH JL, CACHIA EA, CALLEJA F, PULLICINO F: Hereditary elliptocytosis in two Maltese families. *J Clin Pathol* 14:365, 1961

400. PRYOR DS, PITNEY WR: Hereditary elliptocytosis: A report of two families from New Guinea. *Br J Haematol* 13:126, 1967

401. NIELSEN JA, STRUNK KW: Homozygous hereditary elliptocytosis as a cause of haemolytic anaemia in infancy. *Scand J Haematol* 5:486, 1968

402. AUSTIN RF, DESFORGES JF: Hereditary elliptocytosis: An unusual presentation of hemolysis in the newborn associated with transient morphologic abnormalities. *Pediatrics* 44:196, 1969

403. CARPENTIERI U, GUSTAVSON LP, HAGGARD ME: Pyknocytosis in a neonate: An unusual presentation of hereditary elliptocytosis. *Clin Pediatr* 16:76, 1977

404. ZARKOWSKY HS: Heat-induced erythrocyte fragmentation in neonatal elliptocytosis. *Br J Haematol* 41:515, 1979

405. DAVIDSON RJL, STRAUSS WT: Hereditary elliptocytic anaemia. *J Clin Pathol* 14:615, 1961

406. GREENBERG LH, TANAKA KR: Hereditary elliptocytosis with hemolytic anemia—a family study of five attracted members. *Calif Med* 110:389, 1969

407. TCHERNIA G, MOHANDAS N, SHOHET SB: Deficiency of cytoskeletal membrane protein band 4.1 in homozygous hereditary elliptocytosis: Implications for red cell membrane stability. *J Clin Invest* 1981, in press

408. AMATO D, ANDREWS S: Elliptocytosis in Papua, New Guinea. *Proc Int Soc Haematol, Asian-Pacific Div*, Jakarta, 1975, p 124

409. SERJEANTSON S, BRYSON K, AMATO D, BABONA D: Malaria and hereditary ovalocytosis. *Hum Genet* 37:161, 1977

410. BOOTH PB, SERJEANTSON S, WOODFIELD DG, AMATO D: Selective depression of blood group antigens associated with hereditary ovalocytosis among Melanesians. *Vox Sang* 32:99, 1977

411. HONIG GR, LACSON PS, MAURER HS: A new familial disorder with abnormal erythrocyte morphology and increased permeability of the erythrocytes to sodium and potassium. *Pediatr Res* 5:159, 1971

412. HARRISON KL, COLLINS KA, MCKENNA HW: Hereditary elliptical stomatocytosis; a case report. *Pathology* 8:307, 1976

413. ZARKOWSKY HS, MOHANDAS N, SPEAKER CB, SHOHET SB: A congenital haemolytic anaemia with thermal sensitivity of the erythrocyte membrane. *Br J Haematol* 29:537, 1975

414. DACIE JV, MOLLISON PL, RICHARDSON N, SELWYN JG, SHAPIRO L: Atypical congenital haemolytic anaemia. *J Med (New Series)* 22:79, 1953

414a. LIU SC, PALEK J: Personal communication.

415. WILEY JS, GILL FM: Red cell calcium leak in congenital hemolytic anemia with extreme microcytosis. *Blood* 47:197, 1976

416. WALTER T, MENTZER W, GREENQUIST A, SCHRIER S, MOHANDAS N: RBC membrane abnormalities in hereditary pyropoikilocytosis. *Blood* 50 (Suppl 1):98, 1977 (abstract)

417. CHANG K, WILLIAMSON JR, ZARKOWSKI HS: Effect of heat on the circular dichroism of spectrin in hereditary pyropoikilocytosis. *J Clin Invest* 64:326, 1979

418. PALEK J, LIU SC, LIU PY, PROCHAL J, CASTLEBERRY RP: Altered assembly of spectrin in red cell membranes in hereditary pyropoikilocytosis. *Blood* 57:130, 1981

419. COETZER T, ZAIL SS: Tryptic digestion of spectrin in variants of hereditary elliptocytosis. *J Clin Invest* 67:1241, 1981

420. LIU SC, PALEK J, PROCHAL J, CASTELBERRY RP: Altered spectrin dimer-dimer association and red cell membrane skeleton instability in hereditary pyropoikilocytosis. *J Clin Invest* 1981, in press

421. TRINICK RH: Elliptocytosis (letter). *Lancet* 1:963, 1948

422. HELZ MK, MENTEN ML: Elliptocytosis, a report of two cases. *J Lab Clin Med* 29:185, 1944

423. GÜNTHER H: Die Klinische Bedeutung der Ellipsenformen der Erythrozyten. *Dtsch Arch Klin Med* 162:215, 1928

424. GEERDINK RA, NIJNHUIS LE, HUIZINGA J: Hereditary elliptocytosis: Linkage data in man. *Ann Hum Genet* 30:363, 1967

425. VAN DEN BERGH AAH, REHORST K: A propos des hématies elliptiques (ovalocytose). *Rev Belg Sci Méd* 3:683, 1931

426. ÖZER L, MILLS GC: Elliptocytosis with haemolytic anaemia, *Br J Haematol* 10:468, 1964

427. NKRUMAH FK: Hereditary elliptocytosis associated with severe haemolytic anaemia and malaria. *Afr J Med Sci* 3:131, 1972

428. PANICH V, NA-NAKORN S: Hemolytic anemia in elliptocytosis. Report of two cases. *J Med Assoc Thai* 55:367, 1972

429. PEARSON HA: The genetic basis of hereditary elliptocytosis with hemolysis. *Blood* 32:972, 1968

430. BAKER SJ, JACOB E, RAJAN KT, GAULT EW: Hereditary haemolytic anaemia associated with elliptocytosis: A study of three families. *Br J Haematol* 7:210, 1961

431. LUX SE, JOHN KM: Unpublished observations

432. SCHOLNIK AP, VAN TILBURG CP, HOFFMAN GC: Hereditary elliptocytosis. *Cleve Clin Q* 41:23, 1974

433. SCHEKMAN R, SINGER SJ: Clustering and endocytosis of membrane receptors can be induced in mature erythrocytes of neonatal but not adult humans. *Proc Natl Acad Sci USA* 73:4075, 1976

434. GROSS GP, HATHAWAY WE: Fetal erythrocyte deformability. *Pediatr Res* 6:593, 1972

435. DE GRUCHY GC, LODER PB, HENNESSY IV: Haemolysis and glycolytic metabolism in hereditary elliptocytosis. *Br J Haematol* 8:168, 1962

436. WILSON HE, LONG MJ: Hereditary ovalocytosis (elliptocytosis) with hypersplenism. *Arch Intern Med* 95:438, 1955

437. MATSUMOTO N, ISHIHARA T, TAKAHASHI M, UCHINO F, ONO J, MIWA S, KIYOMITSU Y: Fine structure of the spleen in hereditary elliptocytosis. *Acta Pathol Jap* 26:533, 1976

438. MILLER LH, MASON SJ, DVORAK JA, MCGINNISS MLT, ROTHMAN IK: Erythrocyte receptors for (*Plasmodium knowlesi*) malaria: Duffy blood group determinants. *Science* 189:561, 1975

439. MILLER LH, MCAULIFFE FM, JOHNSON JG: Invasion of erythrocytes by malaria merozoites in Lux SE, Marchesi VT, Fox CF (eds): *Normal and Abnormal Red Cell Membranes*. New York, Alan R Liss, 1979, p 497

440. TOMASELLI MB, JOHN KM, LUX SE: Elliptical erythrocyte membrane skeletons and heat-sensitive spectrin in hereditary elliptocytosis. *Proc Natl Acad Sci USA* 78:1911, 1981

441. LIU SC, PALEK J, PRCHAL J, CASTLEBERRY RP: Self-association of spectrin in abnormal red blood cells. *J Supramol Struct Cell Biochem (Suppl)* 5:131, 1981 (abstract)

442. CLARK MR, MOHANDAS N, SHOHET SB: The red cell membrane in hemolytic anemias, in Fairbanks VF (ed): *Current Hematology*. New York, Wiley, 1981, vol 2, in press

443. SCHULTZE M: Ein heizbarer Objecthisch und seine Verwendung bei Untersuchungen des Blutes. *Arch Mikrobiol Anat* 1:1, 1865

444. LUX SE: Report of workshop on the cytoskeleton of abnormal red blood cells, in Marchesi VT, Gallo R, Majerus P (eds): *Differentiation and Function of Hematopoietic Cell Surfaces*. New York, Alan R Liss, 1981, in press

444a. SPEICHER D: Personal communication.

445. FEO CJ, FISCHER S, PIAU JP, GRONGE MJ, TCHERNIA G: Première observation de l'absence d'une proteine de la membrane érythrocytaire (band 4.1) dans un cas anémie elliptocytaire familiale. *Nouv Rev Fr Hématol* 22:315, 1981

446. MUELLER TJ, MORRISON M: Cytoskeletal alterations in hereditary elliptocytosis. *J Supramol Struct Cell Biochem (Suppl)* 5:131, 1981 (abstract)

447. AGRE P, BENNETT V: A molecular defect in hemolytic elliptocytosis. *J Supramol Struct Cell Biochem (Suppl)* 5:130, 1981 (abstract)

448. TORLONTANO G, FONTANA L, DELAURENZI A, PAPA G, PROLETTI M: Hereditary elliptocytosis. Haematological and metabolic findings. *Acta Haematol* 48:1, 1972

449. PETERS JC, ROWLAND M, ISRAELS LG, ZIPURSKY A: Erythrocyte sodium transport in hereditary elliptocytosis. *Can J Physiol Pharmacol* 44:817, 1966

450. MURPHY JR: Erythrocyte metabolism. VI. Cell shape and the location of cholesterol in the erythrocyte membrane. *J Lab Clin Med* 65:756, 1965

451. SCHARTUM-HANSEN H: Die Genese der Ovalozyten. *Acta Med Scand* 86:348, 1935

452. COHEN NS, EKHAM JE, LUTHRA MG, HANAHAN DJ: Biochemical characterization of density-separated human erythrocytes. *Biochim Biophys Acta* 419:229, 1976

453. GAEHTGENS P, DÜHRSSEN C, ALBRECHT KH: Motion, deformation, and interaction of blood cells and plasma during flow through narrow capillary tubes. *Blood Cells* 6:799, 1980

454. SCHNEIDMAN D, KIESSLING P, ONSTAND J, WOLF P: Red pulp of the spleen in hereditary elliptocytosis. *Virchows Arch [Pathol Anat Histol]* 372:337, 1977

73

PYRUVATE KINASE AND OTHER ENZYME DEFICIENCY DISORDERS OF THE ERYTHROCYTE

WILLIAM N. VALENTINE

KOUICHI R. TANAKA

DONALD E. PAGLIA

1. *Pyruvate kinase deficiency hemolytic anemia is the first-described, best-studied, and most common of the hemolytic anemias resulting from an enzyme defect in the Embden-Meyerhof pathway. The disorder occurs worldwide but predominantly in patients of northern European ancestry. It is characterized clinically by hemolytic anemia of variable, but often severe, degree and partial improvement after splenectomy. Metabolically, the main abnormalities in the deficient red cells are decreased ATP and increased 2,3-DPG concentrations compared with normal red blood cells of the same age.*

2. *PK deficiency is transmitted as an autosomal recessive trait. Heterozygotes are clinically and hematologically normal. Most often conventional assay reveals about half-normal PK activity, but mutant enzymes may also exhibit qualitative abnormalities in terms of kinetics and behavior toward cofactors and allosteric modifiers. In the absence of consanguinity, the clinically affected patients are usually doubly heterozygous for two defective mutant genes. On a molecular basis, there is strong evidence that most, if not all, mutations involve the structural gene coding for L-type PK. Characterization of the abnormal products of the mutant genes is increasing our understanding of the relationship of the defective enzyme and clinical symptoms.*

3. *Severe deficiencies of certain other glycolytic en-*

zymes—hexokinase, glucosephosphate isomerase, phosphofructokinase, aldolase, triosephosphate isomerase, phosphoglycerate kinase, 2,3-diphosphoglyceromutase and phosphatase, and lactate dehydrogenase—have been identified. LDH deficiency is not associated with hemolysis. Deficiencies of 2,3-DPGM and 2,3-DPGP (both activities reside in a single protein) are associated with mild erythrocytosis secondary to near absence of 2,3-DPG, but not with a hemolytic disorder.

4. *Three basic subunit types of PFK are recognized, with the erythrocyte enzyme consisting of a heterogeneous mixture of five tetrameric proteins reflecting all combinations of M (muscle type) and L (liver type) isozymes. One phenotype of PFK deficiency is characterized by severe myopathy, compensated hemolysis, and diminished 2,3-DPG and is due to severe deficiency of subunit M, the sole subunit in muscle. A second phenotype exhibits hemolytic anemia, no or minimal myopathy, and could result from absent or unstable L subunits or unstable M subunits.*

5. *Aldolase deficiency has been recognized in but a single kindred. PGK deficiency is X-chromosome linked and associated with neurologic abnormalities. TPI deficiency is a generalized disorder with severe neurologic and other systemic manifestations as well as hemolytic anemia.*

6. *Enzyme deficiencies of the PP shunt and related GSH*

metabolism are also recognized. Deficiency and genetic variation of 6-PGD are documented, but not clearly causative of a hemolytic disorder. Severe deficiency of GSSG-R apoenzyme has been firmly documented in a single kindred where an affected subject had a hemolytic episode on ingesting fava beans but did not experience chronic hemolysis. Numbers of reports of GSSG-R deficiency in a wide variety of clinical settings now appear secondary to nutritional deficiency of the flavin cofactor rather than of the apoenzyme. GSH-P$_x$ deficiency has been reported to cause hemolytic anemia. This association must be cautiously evaluated in light of the demonstration of genetically determined reductions in GSH-P$_x$ activity in apparently healthy subjects in certain ethnic groups to levels only one-half those usually found.

7. *The first enzyme of GSH synthesis, γ-glutamyl cysteine synthetase, when severely deficient in activity, is associated with chronic hemolysis and spinocerebellar degeneration. The second, GSH synthetase, is characterized, when deficient, by two phenotypes. In one of the latter, hemolytic anemia is the only manifestation, presumably owing to the fact that the molecular lesion results in an unstable gene product which can be continuously renewed in nucleated tissues. A second phenotype, presumably due to generalized deficiency of the enzyme, is associated with variable hemolysis, the excretion of large amounts of pyroglutamate in the urine, and metabolic acidosis.*

8. *Disturbances in erythrocyte nucleotide metabolism that are clearly associated with shortened cell life spans and hemolytic anemia of variable severity include: (a) overproduction of adenosine deaminase, a dominantly inherited disorder characterized by decreases in erythrocyte adenine nucleotide concentrations (less than half normal means), elevations in pyrimidine nucleotidase activity (three- to fourfold), and forty- to one hundredfold elevations in adenosine deaminase activity; (b) severe deficiency of adenylate kinase, inherited as an autosomal recessive trait; and (c) severe deficiency of pyrimidine nucleotidase, transmitted as an autosomal recessive disorder or acquired secondary to lead toxicity. This is characterized by ineffective clearance of RNA degradation products from the maturing reticulocyte, with consequent accumulation of pyrimidine ribonucleotides, prominent basophilic stippling on the stained blood film, an increase in cell GSH up to twofold, and decreases in ribosephosphate pyrophosphokinase activity.*

9. *The pathogenesis of hemolysis in enzymopathies of the PP shunt is associated with increased susceptibility of Hb to oxidant damage, denatured Hb in the form of Heinz bodies, GSH instability, and damage to the plasma membrane of the red cell. There is no universal consensus as to the primary pathogenic event in enzymopathies of anaerobic glycolysis. We favor metabolic depletion secondary to block of glycolysis as a result of a wide variety of structural gene mutations and gene products as the dominant factor in pathogenesis. Secondary, but important, phenomena would then be accumulation of glycolytic intermediates, diminished ATP, translocation of Ca^{2+}, loss of membrane deformability, shape alterations and loss of*

membrane by budding, and increased susceptibility to phagocytosis by macrophages.

10. *The pathogenesis of hemolysis in pyrimidine nucleotidase deficiency is speculative, but the accumulated pyrimidine ribonucleotides conjecturally interfere with normal glycolysis by virtue of their demonstrated ability to bind to sites on crucial enzymes where adenosine phosphates are preferred and far more efficient. The hemolytic syndrome, associated with great increases in the activity of red cell adenosine deaminase and greatly diminished ATP, presumably results from removal of an important substrate, adenosine, from a salvage pathway for renewal of the adenine nucleotide pool of the red cell. ATP depletion results.*

11. *Erythrocyte enzymopathies may also have hematologic expression other than hemolysis, may have no obvious deleterious consequences, or may be associated with clinical disorders affecting other than hematopoietic tissue.*

The mature erythrocyte is deprived of many metabolic options through its lack of a nucleus, mitochondria, or other organelles. While the reticulocyte retains deteriorating capacities for oxidative phosphorylation and for a modicum of protein and lipid synthesis, the akaryote mature red blood cell supports itself energetically by primitive and universal metabolic pathways converting glucose to lactate and stores a portion of the energy generated in the form of ATP. Fortunately, oxygen transport by hemoglobin (Hb) requires no expenditure of energy, for only 5 percent of red cell constituents other than water are available to form the plasma membrane and to carry out functions essential to survival. Figure 73-1 depicts certain important metabolic pathways available to the human erythrocyte.

Energy requirements, while limited, must nonetheless be met if the normal 120-day life span of the circulating erythrocyte is to be achieved. The biconcave discoidal shape of the red cell, and the ready deformability of its plasma membrane, must be preserved. ATP fuels the phosphorylations of the early stages of glycolysis, the synthesis of glutathione (GSH), the pumping of cations against electrochemical gradients, the phosphorylations, acetylations and acylations of membrane protein, lipid, and phospholipid constituents; it is also required in certain salvage pathways of adenine nucleotide metabolism. Hb must be protected against oxidative denaturation, and its iron maintained in the functional ferrous form. Certain enzymes of nucleotide metabolism are also essential for normal erythrocyte survival. For example, the maturing reticulocyte must possess the enzymatic machinery to degrade its ribosomes and to rid itself of end products of RNA degradation.

Anaerobic glycolysis (the Embden-Meyerhof pathway) permits net generation of ATP and the cycling of oxidized and reduced nicotinamide adenine dinucleotide (NAD, NADH). NADH is required for enzymatic reduction of methemoglobin. The Rapoport-Luebering shunt [1] permits the generation of 2,3-diphosphoglycerate (2,3-DPG), the most abundant phosphorylated intermediate of glycolysis and one which has important effects on the oxygen dissociation curve of Hb [2]. The mutase responsible for 2,3-DPG formation and the phosphatase returning it to the mainstream of glycolysis as 3-phosphoglycerate (3-PG) are activities residing in the same enzyme protein [3, 4]. The shunt bypasses the phosphoglycerate kinase

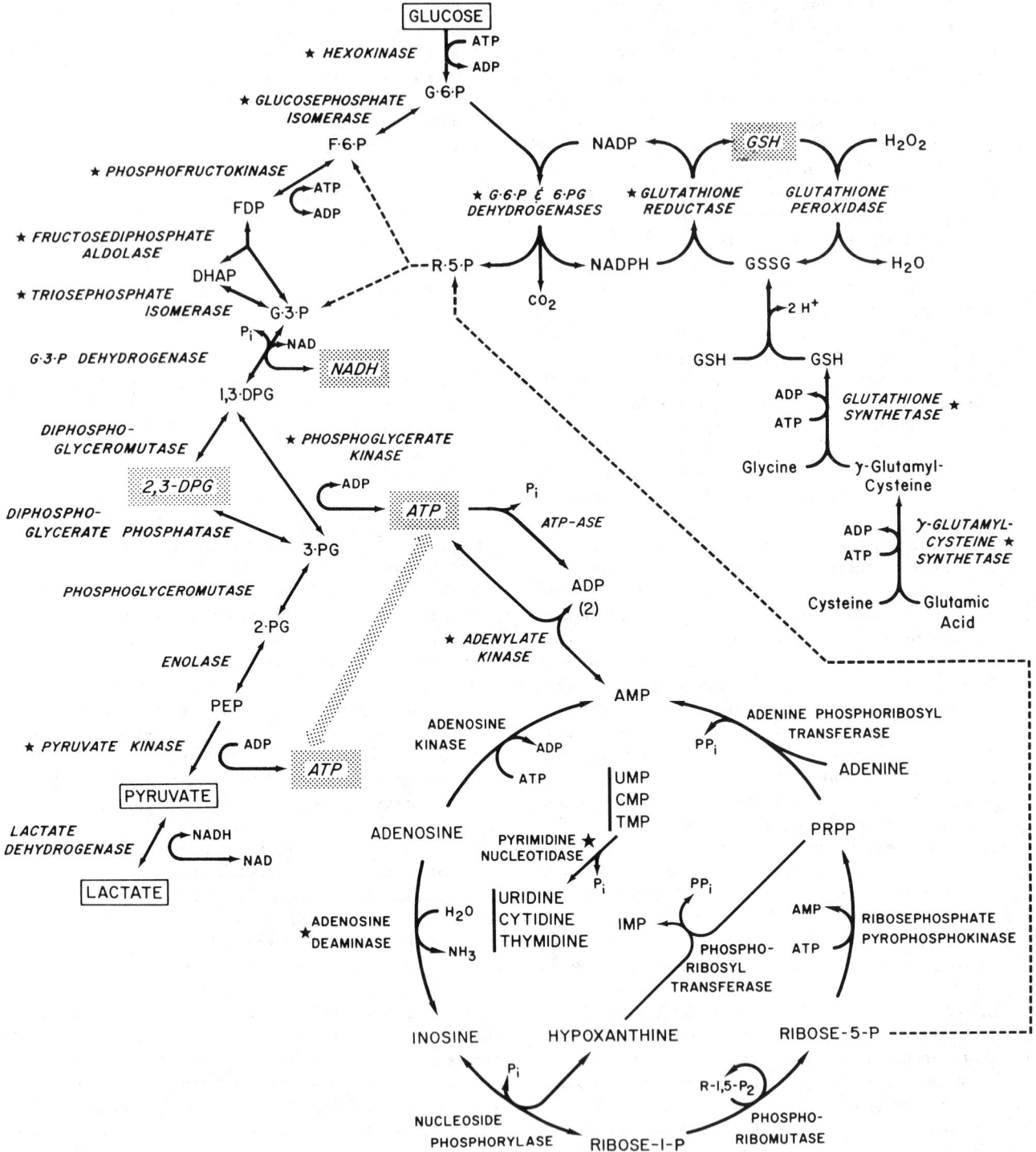

Figure 73-1 Pathways of energy metabolism in human erythrocytes. Glucose-6-phosphate (G-6-P) may be degraded anaerobically to two moles of lactate via the Embden-Meyerhof pathway on the left, or oxidatively via the dehydrogenases of the pentose phosphate pathway. Ribose-5-phosphate (R-5-P) can reenter anaerobic glycolysis as fructose-6-phosphate (F-6-P) and glyceraldehyde-3-phosphate (G-3-P), after conversion by enzymes of the terminal pentose phosphate pathway, and is also a product of adenosine or inosine degradation. 2,3-Diphosphoglycerate (2,3-DPG) may be generated instead of ATP by diversion of triose through the Rapoport-Luebering shunt. Glutathione may be directly synthesized from constituent amino acids, and its cycling from oxidized (GSSG) to reduced form (GSH) is dependent upon reduced pyridine cofactor (NADPH) generation. Stars indicate those enzymes found defective in association with hereditary hemolytic anemia.

(PGK)-mediated ATP generating step in glycolysis, and the variable proportion of glucose traversing it helps fine-tune ATP production in accordance with fluctuating needs. The 2,3-DPG also provides a reservoir for glycolysis capable of supporting ATP generation for a time during periods of relative glucose deprivation.

The aerobic pentose phosphate (PP) shunt is another available metabolic sequence whose importance lies in the production of pentose from glucose and in the generation of reduced nicotinamide adenine dinucleotide phosphate (NADPH). Function of the PP pathway depends not only upon its two dehydrogenases, but also upon the enzymatic mechanisms by which GSH is synthesized, by which it converts peroxides to water or the corresponding alcohol, and by which its oxidized form (GSSG) is reduced. The PP shunt is the only significant red cell source of NADPH and constitutes the major mechanism of protection against Hb damage by noxious oxidants. The proportion of glucose traversing the shunt varies widely since it is dependent upon the rate of GSH oxidation. The latter, in turn, reflects the magnitude of oxidant stresses in the environment of the moment. Glucose metabolized aerobically or anaerobically traverses the same terminal pathway to lactate (Fig. 73-1).

Given the relative metabolic impoverishment of the normal erythrocyte and the inevitable deterioration of nonrenewable enzymatic machinery as it ages, it is not surprising that severe genetically imposed handicaps involving its limited metabolic resources should result in shortened life span and, hence, in hemolytic anemia. The definition of hemolytic syndromes secondary to enzyme deficiencies had roots in studies culminating in the recognition of glucose-6-phosphate dehydrogenase (G-6-PD) deficiency [5], as well as in the investigations initiated by Dacie and his colleagues [6, 7] and extended by others [8–10] of certain hereditary anemias termed *nonspherocytic* to distinguish them from the better-defined disorder of hereditary spherocytosis. The first enzyme deficiency of anaerobic glycolysis incriminated in the pathogenesis of hereditary hemolytic anemia was pyruvate kinase (PK) [11, 12]. Since then, deficiencies of other glycolytic enzymes, of enzymes of the PP shunt and closely related GSH metabolism, and of enzymes of nucleotide metabolism have emerged as causes of hemolytic anemia (see reviews since 1976 [13–19]).

PYRUVATE KINASE DEFICIENCY

Clinical Aspects

Prevalence Pyruvate kinase deficiency is the most common glycolytic enzyme defect associated with chronic hemolysis [13, 19–22]. Over 300 cases of PK deficiency hemolytic anemia have been reported [14, 22–24] since its original description in 1961 [11, 12]. PK deficiency and G-6-PD deficiency together account for most of the patients in whom an enzymatic abnormality has been defined as the cause of their hereditary nonspherocytic hemolytic anemia. Other inborn errors of the Embden-Meyerhof pathway as well as those involving glutathione and pyrimidine metabolism, which have been described subsequently and are discussed later in this chapter, are comparatively rare.

Patients with this disorder have been found primarily in the United States, Europe, and Japan but have also been noted in Canada, Australia, New Zealand, Hong Kong, and Venezuela [22]. There is increasing evidence for worldwide distribution, but its prevalence in many parts of the world is still unknown. The disease is clearly most common in people of North European ancestry but has also been reported from the Mediterranean area, for example, Spain [25], Italy, Syria, and Arabia [22]. PK deficiency has also been noted in Filipinos, Mexicans, and American Negroes and in patients with part American-Indian ancestry [20, 22]. A particularly high prevalence of this disorder has been identified in the Mifflin County (Pennsylvania) Amish deme [26]. Both sexes are affected equally [12, 22].

Clinical Features Patients with PK deficiency hemolytic anemia have no distinguishing or pathognomonic clinical features. They have the usual hallmarks of most chronic hemolytic processes, such as variable degrees of jaundice, slight to moderate splenomegaly, and an increased incidence of gallstones. The spectrum of clinical disease varies considerably, ranging from severe neonatal anemia requiring exchange or multiple transfusions to sustain life to a fully compensated hemolytic process in apparently healthy adults [20, 22]. On the whole, PK deficiency is a more severe disease than hereditary spherocytosis [27].

In most cases, anemia or jaundice or both are noted in infancy or early childhood, but some patients apparently escape detection until adulthood, even to age 72 [28]. Typically, the early-onset form of the disease is severe or moderate in nature, requiring numerous transfusions or often culminating in splenectomy during the first years of life. Thereafter, most of these patients have a stable but moderately low hemoglobin level and can be maintained usually without transfusions [29]. Patients having a later onset of symptoms generally have a milder form of the disease. They are often asymptomatic and are frequently diagnosed during investigations of an intercurrent acute illness [20, 22]. PK-deficient patients may have greater tolerance for their anemia because of the right shift in the oxygen dissociation curve as a result of the characteristic elevation of red cell 2,3-DPG levels [30].

Slight to moderate splenomegaly is the rule but is not invariable. Hepatomegaly is inconstant. Chronic leg ulcers occur but are rare [25, 31–33]. General development is usually normal, but growth retardation and prominent frontal bosses have been observed in some of the severely affected children [22]. Kernicterus is a rare complication [26]. Acute pancreatitis secondary to biliary tract disease has been seen in a boy [34]. Several adult patients have developed iron overload [25, 35, 36].

The chronic hemolytic process may be exacerbated by various types of acute illnesses as well as by pregnancy [12, 20, 22, 37] and possibly by oral contraceptives [38]. Aplastic crises have also been observed [39]. Women with PK deficiency have tolerated pregnancy with no unusual complications, although blood transfusions were required at the time of delivery in almost all these patients who otherwise had not previously been transfused or who rarely needed transfusions [20, 22, 40].

Most PK deficiency patients survive to adulthood, but a particularly severe form found in the Amish kindreds is often fatal in early childhood unless splenectomy is performed [41]. Only individuals homozygous or doubly heterozygous for the red cell PK defect manifest clinical disease [22, 42]. Although certain erythrocyte biochemical abnormalities may be demonstrable in heterozygotes, clinical manifestations do not develop except in rare instances [22, 43].

Hematologic Findings Red cell morphologic abnormalities are not a prominent feature of PK deficiency anemia. The erythrocytes are normochromic with only an occasional spiculated or irregularly contracted cell, except in some infants or young children with severe anemia. Nonspecific changes reflecting the existence of an increased erythroid output are present; macrocytosis, for instance, is related to the degree of reticulocytosis and not due to folic acid or vitamin B_{12} deficiency [22]. Certain features such as Pappenheimer bodies, siderocytes, Howell-Jolly bodies, and target cells may appear following splenectomy but are not specific for this disorder. The presence of many crenated red cells of unusual form (shrunken echinocytes) on a postsplenectomy blood smear is suggestive of PK deficiency [44]. The levels of hemoglobin and packed red cell volumes vary widely among patients but generally fall in the range of 6 to 12 g/dl and 0.17 to 0.37 liter/liter, respectively [22]. Extremely low hemoglobin values have been noted in some instances during infancy and the first few years of life, with subsequent stabilization at a higher level either following splenectomy or even without splenectomy. The frequent paradoxical rise in the percentage of circulating reticulocytes after splenectomy is characteristic of PK deficiency; very high values (40 to 70 percent range) are observed only after splenectomy [20, 21, 40, 44–46]. The white blood count and platelet count are normal or slightly increased.

There is usually modest to moderate elevation of the serum bilirubin, which is mostly indirect reacting. As expected, serum haptoglobin may be decreased or absent, and fecal urobilinogen excretion is increased [20, 22]. The serum iron is normal or slightly increased, with a normal total iron-binding capacity. The osmotic fragility of fresh red cells is usually normal, but the incubated osmotic fragility test may show varying degrees of abnormality [22].

The Coombs' test and acid serum (Ham's) test results are negative. Donath-Landsteiner antibody and cold agglutinins are also absent. Hemoglobin is of the normal adult type (AA); fetal hemoglobin and hemoglobin A_2 are within normal limits. The glutathione stability test result is normal. No Heinz bodies are observed by supravital staining, except for rare instances [22].

Other Laboratory Findings PK deficiency is not associated with specific organ dysfunction other than hemolytic anemia and its manifestations and complications. Routine urinalysis is normal, but urobilinogen may be increased. Liver function test results are normal except for the bilirubinemia already mentioned. Bone changes consistent with a hyperplastic marrow as seen in other chronic hemolytic anemias may be demonstrated roentgenologically in some of the severe cases [22, 47].

Erythrokinetics Ferrokinetic studies utilizing ^{59}Fe show a short plasma clearance time, before or after splenectomy. A rapid maximal or near maximal appearance of radioiron in circulating erythrocytes is usually seen. ^{59}Fe organ scans indicate that the spleen and liver are major sites of destruction of the newly formed PK-deficient red cells [48].

Red cell life span as determined with the ^{51}Cr procedure for erythrocyte labeling is moderately to severely shortened in most instances, but there is considerable variability among patients. Biphasic ^{51}Cr survival curves obtained in some studies suggest that two populations of cells are present, one doomed to almost immediate destruction and the other with a more favorable outlook for survival [22, 49, 50].

Although the ^{51}Cr data in regard to splenic sequestration are conflicting, there is now substantial evidence to indicate that PK-deficient poorly deformable reticulocytes may be selectively sequestered in the spleen, where they undergo irreversible damage and ultimately premature destruction [22, 51]. Splenectomy permits longer survival of newly formed cells, and hence the reticulocyte count usually rises after removal of the spleen in this disorder.

Pathology The bone marrow, as expected, undergoes normoblastic hyperplasia and usually shows hemosiderin in increased quantities. Chromosome aberrations have been observed in bone marrow cells but not in cultured lymphocytes [52]. There are no specific histologic findings in the spleen by light microscopy; reticuloendothelial hyperplasia, variable degrees of congestion and deposits of hemosiderin, erythrophagocytosis, and foci of extramedullary hematopoiesis have been noted [22]. The frequent presence of reticulocytes in the sinuses and their phagocytosis by cordal macrophages as demonstrated by electron microscopy are characteristic of PK deficiency [49, 53, 54]. Histologic examination of the liver is normal or shows only minimal changes; rarely, iron overload has been noted [22, 35, 36]. As in any chronic hemolytic disease, cholelithiasis is common and may occur at an early age. To date, there is little autopsy information [26, 36].

Diagnosis

The diagnosis of PK deficiency hemolytic disease depends on the specific demonstration of quantitatively reduced activity or qualitative abnormalities of the erythrocyte enzyme. This is readily achieved by spectrophotometric assay of a hemolysate prepared from red cells carefully freed of white cells [55, 56]. Contaminating leukocytes may obscure proper results since the white cell/red cell PK activity is about 300:1 on a per cell basis and leukocytes are not affected in PK deficiency. The assay procedure uses phosphoenolpyruvate (PEP) as substrate for PK, crystalline lactate dehydrogenase, and NADH and is quantitated in terms of the linked reaction by which pyruvate formed is transformed to lactate with the conversion of NADH to NAD.

The quantitative procedure has proved a fairly reliable index for separating homozygous, heterozygous, and normal subjects [22]. More sophisticated examination of the enzyme in a dialyzed hemolysate at low concentrations of PEP with and without the allosteric effector fructose-1,6-diphosphate (F-1,6-P_2) may be necessary whenever a variant form of PK is suspected. Recommended methods for the characterization of PK variants have been published [57]. Two screening methods [58, 59] have been described but have not been employed exclusively.

A review of the clinical reports and our experience indicate that most PK-deficient patients have about 5 to 25 percent of the normal (mean) red cell enzyme level, and heterozygotes have about half of the normal activity. Although assayed activity varies considerably within the homozygous and heterozygous ranges, the values usually do not overlap. Family studies may be helpful in difficult cases. The possibility of a kinetically aberrant mutant PK should be considered whenever clinically affected patients have PK values in the heterozygous, normal, or even increased range [22]. The poor qualitative correlation between PK activity and clinical severity and the fact that some asymptomatic heterozygotes have PK values within the homozygous range [22] indicate that the assay, although useful, does not provide a precise quantitative measure of the metabolic derangement in the intact cell. This is discussed further in the sections on pyruvate kinase enzyme and pathogenesis of hemolysis in erythroenzymopathies.

Red cell PK activity is elevated in reticulocytes. Thus, various hemolytic anemias other than PK deficiency or conditions characterized by young red cell populations have slight to marked elevation of PK activity [22]. Acquired PK deficiency is discussed later.

The autohemolysis test demonstrates that erythrocytes of many cases of PK deficiency have increased hemolysis after 48 h of sterile incubation, which is not corrected by glucose (type II as originally defined by Selwyn and Dacie [7]). The autohemolysis pattern is variable [22], and the test is no longer useful in the diagnosis of this disorder.

Genetics

Erythrocyte PK deficiency is inherited in an autosomal reces-sive manner [11, 12, 22]. Clinically overt disease requires the inheritance of a mutant gene from each parent. In most cases the parents are not consanguine, and thus the usual patient with PK deficiency will have inherited two different mutant genes rather than being homozygous for a single mutant gene. It is therefore not surprising that PK deficiency is a heterogeneous disorder. Figure 73-2 is an illustrative example. Heterozygotes most commonly demonstrate about half the normal PK activity on assay and are not anemic.

To date no linkage of PK deficiency with serum or blood group antigens has been observed [22]. Geographic distribution of the mutant genes appears to be worldwide, with a preponderance among peoples of northern European descent. In Germany, the prevalence of apparent heterozygosity for PK deficiency is about 1 percent [60, 61]. We have found a similar prevalence [20]. In Spain, 4 deficient individuals were detected in examination of 1636 normal blood samples by Beutler's screening procedure, or a frequency of 0.24 percent [62]. An animal model for this disorder exists in Basenji dogs in which PK deficiency is common [63, 64].

Biochemistry and Metabolism

Normal and Mutant Pyruvate Kinase   Pyruvate kinase (ATP: pyruvate phosphotransferase, EC 2.7.1.40) is one of the rate-limiting key enzymes of the glycolytic pathway [65]. PK catalyzes the conversion of phosphoenolpyruvate (PEP) to pyruvate with regeneration of ATP (Fig. 73-1). Initial observations that hereditary deficiency of pyruvate kinase was restricted to erythrocytes suggested that this enzyme might exist in more than one molecular form. Subsequent studies have shown that in human tissues there are three distinct isozymes [66, 67], often designated as M_1, M_2, and L. Muscle contains M_1-type PK, and leukocytes and platelets contain M_2-type PK.

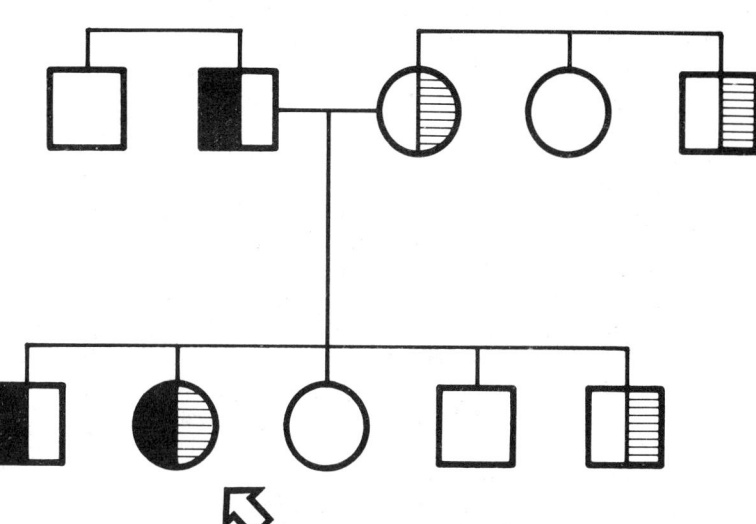

Figure 73-2 Genealogy of a typical family with PK deficiency. Cross-hatching indicates heterozygosity for a mutant enzyme with impaired kinetics. Solid areas indicate heterozygosity for an unstable mutant enzyme. The proband, indicated by the arrow, is a genetic compound harboring both mutations and is clinically affected, whereas the heterozygotes are not.

Liver possesses two isozymes, M_2 and L. Electrophoretically, erythrocytes show two PK bands with different migration from L-type PK of liver [68–70]. These interconvertible isozymes, designated R_1 and R_2 [69], are closely related to the L protein of liver and almost certainly coded by the same gene [66, 71–73]. PK-R_1, predominant in erythroblasts [73] and young red cells [14, 69, 73, 74], is composed of four identical L' units. The major form of erythrocyte enzyme, PK-R_2, is a heterotetramer designated L_2L_2', while liver (L-type) pyruvate kinase is composed of four identical L subunits according to a model proposed by Kahn et al. [73]. In vitro, a mild proteolytic attack on L_4' results in the formation first of L_2L_2' and then of L_4. This L_4 enzyme is similar to the liver enzyme electrophoretically, immunologically, and kinetically. It has been postulated that in the erythroblasts L-type PK is synthesized initially as an L_4' form (each subunit about 62,000 daltons) and that red cell maturation and aging are accompanied by partial proteolysis of two subunits resulting in the heterotetramer L_2L_2'. The L subunit is about 58,000 daltons [14, 73]. The intracellular enzyme(s) responsible for this transition in the erythrocyte is unknown. In the adult liver a very active proteolytic system presumably causes total transformation of L_4' into L_4 pyruvate kinase. This is consistent with the reports of defective L-type PK in the liver of PK deficiency patients [43, 70, 75–77].

The postsynthetic maturation of L_4' into L_4 favorably influences the molecular behavior and improves the regulatory properties of the PK enzyme [73, 78]. For instance, L_4' is less stable and has a lower affinity for PEP than L_4. In the reticulocytes of hereditary deficiency of PK activity, the mutated L_4' form is predominant and may be responsible for the marked sensitivity to hemolysis of the PK-deficient reticulocyte [48]. Furthermore, in some patients with PK deficiency, the mutant protein has been found to be resistant to the favorable effects of proteolysis [23, 79].

Neither the model of Kahn and associates [73] discussed above nor a simpler model in which both R_1 and R_2 are tetramers of identical subunits is entirely adequate [80]. Other "immature" bands have been observed in electrophoretic patterns of mutant PK enzymes [80–82].

Recently, 40,000-fold purification of human erythrocyte PK has been achieved with a yield of 30 percent [66]. Active proteolytic substances liberated from stroma and leukocytes during purification may be responsible for the appearance in purified preparations of L_4 with its different properties. It is to be recalled that in vivo L_4 is absent even in old red cells [73].

In vitro studies of activation and inhibition of human erythrocytic PK suggest that the in vivo regulation of the enzyme is likely to be complex and will depend on the cellular environment. The data for PK [83, 84] are consistent with the two-state conformational model for allosteric enzymes of Monod, Wyman, and Changeux [85]. The R conformation is characterized by hyperbolic kinetics, a decreased sensitivity for the positive allosteric effector, F-1,6-P_2, and an increased affinity for substrate PEP. The T conformation is characterized by increased sensitivity to F-1,6-P_2, decreased affinity for PEP, and increased sensitivity to the inhibitor ATP [83, 84]. Phosphorylation of L' subunits of erythrocyte PK by endogenous cyclic 3',5' AMP-dependent protein kinases has been demonstrated, but whether it occurs in vivo and whether it plays any physiologic role remains uncertain [86, 87].

A wide range of clinical severity was recognized with the first descriptions of PK deficiency [11, 12]. It soon became

evident that the severity of hemolysis did not always correlate with residual PK activity as assayed conventionally [20, 22]. These observations are now explained in large part by the realization that phenotypically normal heterozygotes harbor many different mutant genes which code for mutant PK enzyme proteins differing in catalytic capacity, thermostability, kinetics, electrophoretic mobility, pH optima, and behavior toward allosteric modifiers and nucleotide cofactors, as well as in other ways [20, 22–25, 46, 76, 80, 82, 88–97]. While amino acid sequencing data are lacking, it appears that in most instances a structural gene mutation is involved. Thus, in the absence of consanguinity, most patients are genetic compounds with two different mutant structural genes, and hence their erythrocytes contain two separate mutant proteins within each cell. Figure 73-2 is an illustrative example. Figure 73-3 depicts an erythrocyte PK isoenzyme with markedly defective kinetics. While catalytic activity was demonstrable in the red cells of the proband by in vitro assay at high substrate (PEP) concentrations, half maximal activity was achieved only at a substrate concentration some 10 times greater than normally required. This means that proband PK was virtually ineffectual at PEP concentrations attainable in vivo. The mother and certain maternal relatives, while hematologically normal, also demonstrated aberrant kinetics of red cell PK which were intermediate between normal and patient and were consistent with the coexistence in their erythrocytes of normal and mutant protein. The kinetics of PK in the father's erythrocytes were normal, but there was decreased activity. The patient, inheriting a kinetically aberrant enzyme protein from his mother, coupled with a catalytically useless protein from his father, had red cells with insufficient PK activity for normal survival.

Most variants were identified initially by using crude hemolysates, a variety of techniques, and inadequate parameters; thus, interpretation of data is difficult [13, 19, 22]. Standard methods for the identification of PK variants have now been developed [57]. By utilization of these recommended methods,

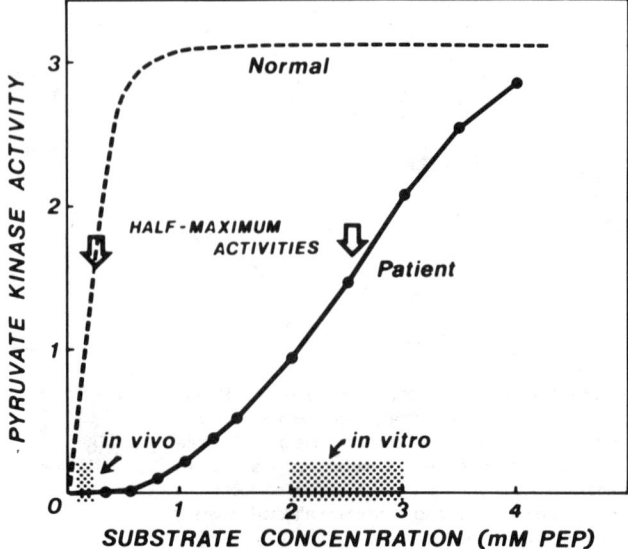

Figure 73-3 An example of erythrocyte PK isoenzyme with severely defective kinetics. PK activity at different substrate (phosphoenolypyruvate, PEP) concentrations in normal subjects and in a patient with hemolytic anemia. $K_{0.55}$ (PEP) and PEP concentrations present in vivo and used in vitro as indicated.

seven true homozygotes from consanguine marriages have been characterized in Japan and designated PK Tokyo, PK Nagasaki, PK Sapporo, PK Maebashi, PK Itabashi, PK Fukushima, and PK Aizu [46]. From our laboratories 12 presumed genetic compounds [82] and an additional 13 from Japan [24] have been characterized using the recommended methods. These reports, as well as other studies utilizing partially purified enzymes [14, 23, 80, 94, 95, 97, 98], indicate that there is a definite relationship between properties of the defective PK enzymes and the severity of hemolysis. The important characteristics of mutant PK enzymes involved in clinical expression of red cell PK deficiency appear to be very low residual activity, decreased affinity for PEP, thermal instability, increased inhibition by ATP, and decreased activation by F-1,6-P$_2$.

Red Cell Metabolism in Pyruvate Kinase Deficiency

The specific deficiency of red cell PK occurs near the final step of glycolysis (Fig. 73-1). All other reactions of the Embden-Meyerhof and pentose phosphate pathways, as well as a number of nonglycolytic reactions, are normally active. In fact, as expected in erythrocyte populations of young mean cell age, the activities of other age-related enzymatic activities are increased. PK-deficient red cells have a normal content of reduced glutathione [12, 20, 22].

Pyruvate kinase deficiency results in impaired glycolysis and diminished capacity to generate ATP and to cycle NAD. Red cell ATP is often low in PK deficiency, but patients with high reticulocyte counts usually have normal or even elevated ATP levels [20, 22, 40, 45]. The latter finding is explained by the observation that PK-deficient reticulocytes depend almost entirely on mitochondrial oxidative phosphorylation rather than on glycolysis to maintain ATP levels [45]. The reliance of such cells on oxidative phosphorylation is supported further by the increased oxygen consumption of PK-deficient reticulocytes compared with normal reticulocytes [48]. Upon loss of oxidative phosphorylation during maturation, the subsequent obligatory dependence on glycolytic ATP synthesis dooms the PK-deficient erythrocytes. Less severely affected red cells are able to survive maturation long enough to demonstrate their impaired glycolytic energy production. As a consequence, ATP levels in mild cases may be anomalously lower than in severe cases [45].

If oxidative phosphorylation in PK-deficient reticulocytes is inhibited in vitro or possibly compromised in the splenic environment, ATP levels decline rapidly, producing alterations in the red cell membrane which result in marked loss of potassium and water. The result is a shrunken, spiculated, viscous cell whose rheologic properties would favor its sequestration by the reticuloendothelial system [48].

Glycolytic intermediates proximal to the PK enzyme defect are usually increased substantially, whereas pyruvate and lactate levels are generally normal or occasionally decreased [20, 22]. Even glucose-6-phosphate, which is near the beginning of the glycolytic sequence, may be increased to over twice the normal level [22, 99]. The concentration of 2,3-DPG is consistently increased and may reach two to three times the normal range. The content of NAD and NADH is reduced, and the level of red cell NAD falls markedly during incubation in vitro [22].

Glucose utilization is defective in PK deficiency in spite of the increased percentage of reticulocytes with their extremely high capacity for glucose consumption [12, 22, 45]. Pyruvate

kinase is normally operating far below saturation with respect to phosphoenolpyruvate. PK-deficient cells reach much higher and even saturating levels of PEP in order to utilize a larger proportion of their enzyme [100]. The accumulation of fructose diphosphate and dihydroxyacetone phosphate may be due to glyceraldehyde phosphate dehydrogenase becoming rate limiting as a result of an increased ratio of reduced to oxidized nicotinamide adenine dinucleotide and increased 1,3-diphosphoglyceric acid. In vivo, complex regulatory mechanisms control glycolysis in the PK-deficient and normal red cell [100].

Although the PK heterozygote has a normal hemogram, some metabolic impairment of the red cells may result from the partial reduction in PK activity. ATP content may be low or unstable on incubation [22]. Occasionally, the content of 2,3-DPG may be slightly increased or PEP level may be elevated [99]. Red cell life span is usually normal but may perhaps be decreased minimally in heterozygotes [22].

Therapy

Specific therapy is not available. The usual hematopoietic agents as well as steroids are ineffective [22]. Supportive treatment has consisted primarily of blood transfusions as deemed necessary. Beyond the early childhood period, most PK patients maintain a tolerable hemoglobin level without transfusions except during exacerbations.

Splenectomy is not curative but is frequently of distinct value, especially in infants and young children with severe disease. Packed cell volume levels increase slightly, and transfusion requirements may decrease or be eliminated. Growth and development in severely affected children may be accelerated after splenectomy. In the severely affected Amish patients splenectomy may be lifesaving [41]. On the other hand, anemia in the mild cases may be unchanged by the procedure.

In contrast to splenectomy in hereditary spherocytosis, hemolysis clearly persists, and aplastic or hemolytic crises may still occur [22]. Erythrocyte survival and sequestration studies utilizing ^{51}Cr-labeled cells are not often useful in selecting patients for surgery.

Experimental approaches with agents which either modify enzyme activity or circumvent the metabolic aberrations induced by the defective enzyme have been attempted. The administration of AMP [101], magnesium [102], riboflavin [103], methylene blue and ascorbic acid [21], oral mannose, galactose, and fructose [104], and infusion of adenine, inosine, and guanosine [105], mostly in single cases, have yielded negative results or no convincing clinical improvement and should be considered experimental.

Hereditary Pyruvate Kinase Deficiency in Combination with Other Disorders

Partial deficiency of PK has been observed in combination with β thalassemia, hereditary spherocytosis, hereditary elliptocytosis, and G-6-PD deficiency [22, 106]. There is some [107, 108], but as yet insufficient, evidence to implicate interaction between PK deficiency and other disorders of the red cell. In a case of Gaucher's disease, however, cerebroside storage was probably enhanced by the hemolysis due to homozygous PK deficiency [109]. An accelerated level of hemolysis was observed when an acute Coombs-positive hemolytic anemia developed during the course of infectious mononucleosis in a patient with PK deficiency anemia [110].

Acquired Pyruvate Kinase Deficiency

Acquired PK deficiency is much more frequent than the hereditary form, but its clinical significance is unclear. Reduced PK activity is the most frequent finding among multiple enzymatic aberrations of the erythrocyte described in a wide variety of hematologic disorders, particularly acute or smoldering leukemia, refractory anemia with or without sideroblasts, and pancytopenia [111–115]. Decreased activity of PK is also common following chemotherapy [116, 117] but occurs occasionally prior to treatment of cancer [116]. In most instances of acquired deficiency, PK values are only slightly to moderately reduced but on occasion may be markedly decreased. Accumulation of glycolytic intermediates prior to the PK step may occur but probably does not result in shortened red cell survival [115].

The cause of acquired enzyme defects remains to be elucidated, but the molecular abnormalities likely are heterogeneous in nature [118–121]. In some cases decreased concentration of PK-related antigen has been noted; in others, normal concentrations of antigen with restoration of activity by dialysis, treatment with sulfhydryl reagents, or partial purification

has suggested postsynthetic modifications [112, 123]. A probable explanation is an injury of the bone marrow stem cells inducing the production of abnormal clones and disturbance of protein synthesis [111, 117].

Differentiation between acquired and hereditary PK deficiency (usually the heterozygous state) is occasionally difficult; family studies or follow-up after therapy for the underlying disorder may be necessary.

OTHER ENZYMOPATHIES OF ANAEROBIC GLYCOLYSIS

Severe deficiencies of six Embden-Meyerhof pathway enzymes in addition to PK have been firmly documented in association with hemolytic anemia (Fig. 73-1 and Table 73-1).

Hexokinase (HK)

Of all the glycolytic enzymes of the erythrocyte, HK is lowest in activity. Moreover, the activity in the oldest red blood cells is but one-tenth that of reticulocytes [124–127]. As a consequence, HK activity is characteristically increased up to several-fold in young, reticulocyte-rich red cell populations, and its deficiency must be evaluated in this context [126, 127].

Table 73-1 Erythrocyte enzymopathies

Expression	Category of metabolism	Enzyme abbreviation, name, and gene locus*			Reference†
Severe deficiency documented					
Hemolytic syndrome	Anaerobic glycolysis (Embden-Meyerhof pathway)	HK	Hexokinase	10q	
		GPI	Glucosephosphate isomerase	19	
		PFK	Phosphofructokinase		
		Ald	Aldolase		
		TPI	Triosephosphate isomerase	12p	
		PGK	Phosphoglycerate kinase	Xq	
		PK	Pyruvate kinase		
	Aerobic glycolysis (pentose phosphate shunt)	G-6-PD	Glucose-6-phosphate dehydrogenase	Xq	
	Glutathione	GSSG-R	Glutathione reductase	8p	
			γ-Glutamyl cysteine synthetase		
			GSH synthetase		
	Nucleotide	AK	Adenylate kinase	9q	
		Pyr-5'-N	Pyrimidine 5'-nucleotidase		
	Porphyrin		Ferrochelatase		[300]
Hemolytic syndrome reported, relation to enzymopathy doubtful or controversial	Aerobic glycolysis	6-PGD	6-Phosphogluconate dehydrogenase	1p	
	Glutathione	GSH-Px	Glutathione peroxidase		
	Nucleotide	ATPase	Adenosine triphosphatase		[301, 302]
Erythrocytosis	Anaerobic glycolysis	2,3-DPGM	2,3-Diphosphoglycerate mutase		
(no hemolysis)	(Rapoport-Luebering shunt)	2,3-DPGP	2,3-Diphosphoglycerate phosphatase		
Hereditary methemoglobinemia	Methemoglobin		NADH-cytochrome b$_5$ reductase		[303]

Table 73-1 Erythrocyte enzymopathies (*continued*)

Expression	Category of metabolism		Enzyme abbreviation, name, and gene locus*		Reference†
Megaloblastic anemia	Nucleotide	RPK	Ribosephosphate pyrophosphokinase (PRPP synthetase)		[304]
			Orotate phosphoribosyltrans-ferase		[305]
			Orotidine-5-phosphate decarboxylase		[305]
Clinical disease, no hematologic expression					
Lesch-Nyhan syndrome	Nucleotide	HGPRTase	Hypoxanthine-guanine phosphoribosyltrans-ferase	Xq	[306]
Dihydroxyadenine urolithiasis		APRTase	Adenine phosphoribosyltrans-ferase	16q	[307]
Immunodeficiency		ADA	Adenosine deaminase	20q	[308]
Immunodeficiency		NP	Nucleoside phosphorylase	14q	[309]
Galactosemia	Carbohydrate		Galactose-1-phosphate uridyltransferase	9p	[310]
Argininosuccinic aciduria	Amino acid		Argininosuccinase	7	[311]
Acatalasemia	Peroxide		Catalase		[312]
No known disease	Carbohydrate		Glyoxalase II		[313]
	Nucleotide	ITPase	Inosine triphosphatase	20p	[314]
	Acetylcholine		Acetylcholinesterase		[315, 316]
	Anaerobic glycolysis	LDH	Lactate dehydrogenase		
Markedly increased enzyme activity documented					
Hemolytic syndrome	Nucleotide	ADA	Adenosine deaminase		
Precise nature of enzymopathy uncertain					
Erythropoietic porphyria	Porphyrin	Uro-S Uro-CoS	Uroporphyrinogen I synthetase and cosynthetase		[317]

* Gene loci are those assigned in Ref. 142. Numbers after enzyme name are chromosome numbers. p = short arm, q = long arm, X = X-chromosome.

† References given only for enzymes not discussed in detail in text.

NOTE: 2,3-DPGM and 2,3-DPGP are separate activities of same enzyme protein. When an abbreviation precedes enzyme name, it is the one employed in text.

HK is inhibited by its product, glucose-6-phosphate (G-6-P), by glucose-1,6-diphosphate, and by 2,3-DPG and is stimulated by inorganic phosphorus (P_i) [128, 129]. Three families have been reported in which HK deficiency was but one of a galaxy of multiple malformations, latent diabetes mellitus, and, in some, the classic Fanconi syndrome and panmyelopathy [130]. A total of 12 cases of severe red cell HK deficiency associated only with hemolytic anemia have been documented in 10 unrelated families of European, peri-Mediterranean, Scandinavian, and Oriental ancestry [126, 127, 129, 131–138]. Characteristically, HK activity has assayed within or well below that of red cells of normal mean age and far below that expected in comparably reticulocyte-rich blood. On the HK scale of aging, proband reticulocytes were approaching physiologic senility and, hence, lacked the capacity for normal survival. Dominantly transmitted hereditary hemolytic anemia has recently been reported in association with defective HK which, however, exhibited increased activity by assay. The conclusion that hemolysis was related to defective HK was based, indirectly,

on glycolytic intermediate patterns and enzyme ratios. The conflict with HK assay data requires resolution [139].

In the first reported case, glucose and fructose were converted to lactate at rates substantially below those of other populations of young mean cell age [126]. Splenectomy at age 5 months appeared to result in partial benefit, but fluctuating anemia and reticulocytosis of 7 to 21 percent persisted. In a number of HK-deficient subjects, diminished glucose consumption has been mirrored by subnormal concentrations of red cell 2,3-DPG. Despite its rarity, HK deficiency has proved to be genetically polymorphic with variably normal or abnormal Michaelis-Menton constants for glucose and Mg-ATP^{2+}, electrophoretic migration of HK isoenzymes, and enzyme stability documented in different combinations and permutations or, indeed, with no abnormality in these parameters identified [138]. While heterozygotes in affected kindreds have usually been clinically and hematologically normal, some are identifiable in terms of partial decrements in red cell HK or increased erythrocyte concentrations of G-6-P. In two kindreds, however, there has been evidence that a single copy of a defective gene may have been sufficient to induce a hemolytic syndrome [132, 137]. The presence of at least two and perhaps four normal isoenzymes of HK and possible variations in isoenzyme patterns as a function of cell age [140, 141] give rise to many possible combinations of normal and defective isoenzymes and render evaluations difficult, particularly when lack of consanguinity dictates a probability of compound heterozygosity for two separate mutant genes. In one reported case in which homozygosity appears highly probable in view of parental consanguinity, the patient's red cells showed decreased affinity for the HK inhibitor glucose-1,6-diphosphate and insensitivity to P_i which normally is able to overcome partially this inhibition as well as that of G-6-P [129]. The gene for HK is carried on chromosome 10 [142].

Glucosephosphate Isomerase (GPI)

Of glycolytic enzymopathies associated with hemolytic syndromes, GPI deficiency is second in frequency only to that of PK [143–173]. The hemolytic disorder is transmitted in an autosomally recessive manner and is associated with variably severe anemia with or without transfusion requirements [143, 163]. In severely anemic patients, splenectomy may be of partial—but only partial—benefit. Tissue-specific isoenzymes of GPI do not exist in either normal or deficient states [174, 175]. GPI is a dimeric molecule, and its structural gene is located on autosome 19 [142]. Thus, GPI deficiency is not confined to erythrocytes, but clinical manifestations are nonetheless limited to those accompanying hemolytic anemia. Most mutant variants have been characterized by prominent enzyme instability, a feature for which continuous enzyme synthesis, possible in most nucleated tissues but not in the red cell, is compensatory. Many variant GPI mutant alleles have been demonstrated in terms of altered electrophoretic migration, catalytic activity, stability, and other parameters [143–173]. Red cell G-6-P is sometimes demonstrably increased in concentration. Evolution of $^{14}CO_2$ from glucose labeled in the second-carbon position depends upon recycling of pentose through the PP shunt following its conversion to fructose-6-phosphate (F-6-P) by transketolase and transaldolase. Since F-6-P must traverse the GPI step in order to be isomerized to G-6-P and reenter the PP shunt, this recycling capacity may be as low as 0.2 to 10 percent of normal in severe GPI deficiency [163]. In a few cases, GPI-deficient subjects have been true homozygotes; in the majority the inheritance of two different abnormal structural genes is probable [163–173].

Phosphofructokinase (PFK)

PFK, a key enzyme of the glycolytic pathway, is an oligomeric protein whose smallest active form is a tetramer [176, 177]. Together with HK and PK it constitutes one of three enzymes of anaerobic glycolysis whose actions are thermodynamically essentially irreversible. It is subject to complex allosteric regulation by metabolites such as $F-1,6-P_2$, ATP, ADP, AMP, citrate, NH_4^+, and SO_4^{2-} [177]. Three basic subunit types are recognized in humans: M, muscle type; L, liver type; and F (or P) type, found in fibroblasts, platelets, brain, lymphocytes, and kidney. Normal muscle contains only type M; mature granulocytes possess largely type L subunits; erythrocyte PFK consists of a heterogeneous mixture of five tetrameric isoenzymes—M_4, M_3L, M_2L_2, ML_3, and L_4 [176, 178–183]. A total of 12 cases of inherited PFK deficiency in 10 unrelated families have been described [181, 184–194]. One phenotype is essentially identical to that initially reported by Tarui et al. [184, 185] and Layzer et al. [186, 187] and characterized by profound myopathy, fully compensated, clinically insignificant hemolysis, and sometimes even by mild erythrocytosis. Erythrocyte PFK activity is reduced to approximately 50 percent of normal. Such patients are homozygously deficient in subunit M, the sole subunit in muscle [178, 180]. A recent study of such a patient utilizing high-resolution chromatography revealed total absence of the four M-containing isoenzymes and persistence only of isoenzyme L_4 in red cells [181]. Despite red cell PFK activity approximating 50 percent, there was (as initially reported by Tarui et al. [185] and Layzer [186]) a clear element of hemolysis, but also a compensatory mild erythrocytosis. Residual PFK activity of 50 percent or less results in significant impairment of glycolysis and diminished concentrations of intermediates such as $F-1,6-P_2$ and 2,3-DPG distal to the defective enzyme in patient cells [181, 195]. Compensatory erythrocytosis presumably results from unfavorable shifts in the oxygen dissociation curve of Hb secondary to the diminished levels of 2,3-DPG. A second group of PFK-deficient patients have presented with hemolysis but with no or minimal myopathic manifestations. Though not precisely characterized thus far, such cases could be the result of absent or highly unstable L subunits or unstable M subunits. In the latter instance, ongoing synthesis of M subunits in muscle, but not in red cells, could explain lack of myopathic features. Thus varying clinical phenotypes may stem from differing defects in PFK subunits as a result of inheritance of different genetic lesions [180, 181].

Aldolase (ALD)

Severe deficiency of erythrocyte ALD has been reported in but one patient, was transmitted as an autosomal recessive trait, and was associated with hemolysis and mental retardation [196].

Triosephosphate Isomerase (TPI)

Deficiency of TPI [197–207], first described in 1965 [197], is a severe, generalized disorder [199]. In addition to hemolytic anemia, all patients documented thus far have had a severe, progressive neurologic deficit beginning in the first few months of life. Cardiac-type sudden deaths have also occurred in three children, and cardiac muscle is believed to share the deficiency that has been documented in leukocytes, plasma, spinal fluid, skeletal muscle, and cultured skin fibroblasts, as well as in red cells [199]. Usually the hemolytic anemia is fairly severe, but expressions of the deficiency in nervous and other tissues are more ominous. Death in childhood has been the general rule, but one patient with severe neurologic dysfunction has lived into the third decade [203]. Deficient erythrocytes incubated with glucose accumulate large amounts of dihydroxyacetone phosphate [198, 199]. TPI deficiency in one kindred has coexisted with that of G-6-PD and with a sickle-cell trait [198]. In two females, triply heterozygous for all three inborn errors, clinical manifestations were absent when no oxidant drugs were being administered. The structural gene for one subunit of TPI has been assigned by regional mapping to chromosome 12 [208].

Phosphoglycerate Kinase (PGK)

Deficiencies of PGK [209, 210] and G-6-PD are the only enzymopathies of the Embden-Meyerhof and PP shunt pathways which are X-chromosome-linked [210–213]. PGK deficiency was first demonstrated in an unmarried woman without known family [209]. In a large Chinese kindred, X-chromosome linkage was strongly suggested by clinical abnormalities in two severely affected male third cousins, mild hemolytic anemia in the mother and grandmother of the proband, and a highly suggestive history of early deaths associated with anemia and neurologic symptoms in a number of male relatives [210, 213]. X-chromosome linkage for the PGK structural gene was later confirmed [211, 212], and the PGK locus assigned to the long arm [142]. Erythrocyte PGK deficiency [209–224] is severe in red cells of affected males. Exacerbations in hemolytic anemia may necessitate transfusions during periods of crises often brought on by intercurrent infections, as was the case in the proband and his third cousin in the first kindred studied. PGK deficiency is shared by leukocytes [210] and, presumably, by certain other body tissues. Mild mental retardation, behavioral aberrations, and neurologic symptoms are clearly associated with the deficiency [210]. Although rare, several affected kindreds are now known. Splenectomy has appeared to alleviate partially the severity of hemolysis in one patient.

The complete amino acid sequence of normal PGK which has a molecular weight of 50,000 has been determined [220, 225]. Specific amino acid substitutions have now been identified in three PGK variants. PGK-II, an electrophoretic variant in southern Pacific populations with normal activity, has an asparagine for threonine substitution at position 352 [220]. PGK-München [222], a variant with diminished activity and thermal instability, but without associated hemolysis, has an asparagine for aspartic acid substitution at position 268 [220]. PGK-Uppsala, a mutant associated with severe deficiency and hemolytic anemia, exhibits kinetic abnormalities, and at the 206th position arginine is replaced by proline [220, 226].

OTHER ENZYMOPATHIES

Two enzymes of anaerobic glycolysis, 2,3-DPG mutase (2,3-DPGM) and lactate dehydrogenase (LDH), when severely deficient, are not associated with hemolytic syndromes. Autosomally transmitted, severe deficiency of 2,3-DPGM was manifested in the proband by nearly undetectable levels of red blood cell 2,3-DPG or of the activities of 2,3-DPGM or 2,3-DPG phosphatase (2,3-DPGP), confirming that both enzymic activities of the Rapoport-Luebering shunt reside in the same protein [3]. Sufficient trace amounts of 2,3-DPG to support catalytically the interconversion of the monophosphoglycerates presumabably remained. Lack of 2,3-DPG resulted in increased oxygen affinity of Hb, diminished delivery of O_2 to tissues at any given partial pressure, and a compensatory modest increase in the circulating red cell mass, but there was no hemolysis, and clinical manifestations were absent. Both par-

ents had partial deficiencies of 2,3-DPGM and 2,3-DPGP. Although 2,3-DPGM deficiency has been inferred in certain patients with hemolysis [22, 227], puzzling features and the indirect nature of evidence in some cases have demanded reservations. The kindred described above [3], however, appears to document unequivocally the biochemical and hematologic characteristics of severe, nearly complete 2,3-DPGM and 2,3-DPGP deficiency, and hemolysis is notably absent. The Rapoport-Luebering shunt is not directly related to energy generation per se.

A severe deficiency of LDH due to genetically determined inability to form the normal H subunit of the enzyme has been well documented in a Japanese kindred [228, 229]. Interestingly, no hemolysis was present. While pyruvate and lactate formed within the erythrocyte are diffusible, and hence can be disposed of elsewhere, it might have been surmised that LDH deficiency would impair NADH oxidation and produce significant derangement in NAD/NADH ratios. While the latter were not entirely normal, sufficiently rapid cycling of NAD/NADH to maintain glycolysis occurred (probably by way of a multiplicity of reactions), and overt hemolysis was absent.

ENZYMOPATHIES INVOLVING THE PENTOSE PHOSPHATE SHUNT AND RELATED GSH METABOLISM

6-Phosphogluconate Dehydrogenase (6-PGD)

While G-6-PD deficiency is the first-described and most common red blood cell enzymopathy associated with hemolytic anemia in humans, deficiency of 6-PGD, the second dehydrogenase of the PP shunt, has never been clearly documented as pathogenetic for a hemolytic syndrome [19, 22]. Numerous variants, some with greatly reduced activity, have been recognized [230–233]. Since NADPH can still be generated via G-6-PD in such patients, there may not be a crucial role of the second dehydrogenase.

Glutathione Peroxidase (GSH-Pₓ)

GSH is oxidized when peroxides are enzymatically destroyed through the action of GSH-P_x [234–237]. The subsequent NADPH-dependent reduction of GSSG is mediated by glutathione reductase. While a number of patients with hemolytic anemia associated with partial, moderate GSH-P_x deficiency have been reported [238–244], cause-and-effect relationship still requires confirmation. Genetically determined GSH-P_x activities approximately half-normal have been documented in large numbers of entirely healthy persons of Jewish and Mediterranean origin [245]. The possibility exists that reported hemolytic syndromes could represent the fortuitous association of an unrelated hemolytic process with a not too uncommon enzyme variant in a healthy population. Additional studies are required to resolve the dilemma [19, 22, 233, 245].

Glutathione Reductase (GSSG-R)

A wide diversity of syndromes, including neurologic disorders, hemolytic anemias, and panmyelopathies, have been reported in association with diminished GSSG-R activity in red cells [19, 233, 246–248]. Beutler's observations that apparent reductase deficiency in many such patients, and even in some normal subjects, was in reality a reflection of inadequate synthesis of cofactor flavin adenine dinucleotide (FAD) clarified this confusing state of affairs [249, 250]. FAD synthesis depends on dietary riboflavin and its metabolism [250–252]. It is now clear that moderate GSSG-R deficiency is not associated with hemolysis. When GSSG-R activity is substantially diminished by assay, the latter must be repeated after preincubation of hemolysate with FAD. The administration of 5 mg of riboflavin daily corrects this spurious enzymopathy in most cases within a few days [250]. However, virtually complete absence of GSSG-R apoenzyme activity, not correctible by FAD, has now been firmly documented in three sibs, with partial deficiency demonstrable in the presumably heterozygous parents [253]. In the sibs, GSH was markedly unstable in red cells during incubation with acetylphenylhydrazine. One sib had a hemolytic crisis after ingesting fava beans, and in two of the sibs cataracts were a possibly related concomitant of the GSSG-R deficiency. Leukocytes shared the deficiency. GSSG-R consists of two identical subunits and is coded for by a single gene residing on the short arm of chromosome 8 [142].

γ-Glutamylcysteine and GSH Synthetases

GSH is synthesized in two ATP-requiring enzymatic steps [254, 255]. In the first, γ-glutamylcysteine is formed from constituent amino acids; in the second, glycine is added to complete the tripeptide. Deficiencies of both γ-glutamylcysteine synthetase [256, 257] and GSH synthetase [259–268] have been clearly associated with moderate hemolytic anemia and virtually total lack of red cell GSH. Both are autosomally transmitted. In the former, leukocytes share the deficiency, and hemolytic anemia, spinocerebellar degeneration, and generalized aminoaciduria were present in both homozygous sibs [256, 257]. In the latter, GSH synthetase deficiency, two clinically distinct syndromes are recognized. In one, hemolytic anemia is the sole manifestation [258–263]. In the other, GSH synthetase deficiency is associated with variable hemolysis, marked pyroglutamic aciduria (or 5-oxoprolinuria), and chronic metabolic acidosis in affected children [264–267]. In many mammalian tissues, though not in red cells, GSH is synthesized and destroyed via the γ-glutamyl cycle described by Orlowski and Meister [268, 269]. In the near absence of GSH synthetase activity, the feedback inhibition of γ-glutamyl cysteine by GSH [270] is removed and the dipeptide accumulates in large amounts. An intermediate of the cycle, 5-oxoproline, is formed at a rate outstripping the capacity of oxoprolinase to degrade it, accounting for its accumulation and urinary excretion in large amounts. The syndrome with oxoprolinuria is believed to occur when GSH synthetase deficiency is generalized; when hemolysis alone is present, the deficiency is severe only in red cells presumably by virtue of their inability (in contrast to nucleated tissues) to renew by ongoing synthesis the enzymatic activity of an unstable, but initially catalytically active, mutant variant [267]. Generalized GSH deficiency can be ascribed to diminished enzyme synthesis or to synthesis of an inactive or very highly labile GSH synthetase. All hemolytic syndromes due to enzymopathies of the PP shunt are believed susceptible to exacerbation by the same drugs and oxidant stresses producing crises in G-6-PD deficient patients. In all, hemolysis is associated with oxidative denaturation of Hb with Heinz body formation.

DISTURBANCES IN ENZYMES OF NUCLEOTIDE METABOLISM

The metabolic reactions outlined in Fig. 73-1 are delicately balanced to provide optimal concentrations of high energy compounds. Because so many crucial cell functions depend upon ATP, perturbations affecting its generation via glycolysis or its maintenance via salvage pathways may have deleterious effects on erythrocyte longevity and function. Within the adenine nucleotide pool, AMP is in particular jeopardy, since its deamination either before or after dephosphorylation yields inosine monophosphate or diffusible inosine, and mechanisms do not exist in mature erythrocytes to retrieve the purine moiety from these compounds. This may be especially important in older cells where salvage mechanisms probably assume greater relative metabolic roles as glycolytic capacity diminishes with age.

Disorders of purine and pyrimidine metabolism in erythrocytes include both deficient and hyperactive enzymes (Table 73-1) [271]. Severe deficiencies of adenosine deaminase, nucleoside phosphorylase, adenine and hypoxanthine-guanine phosphoribosyl transferases, and hyperactive ribosephosphate pyrophosphokinase usually have no discernible detrimental effects on erythrocytes. A few cases of ribosephosphate pyrophosphokinase and hypoxanthine-guanine phosphoribosyl transferase deficiencies have been noted to have megaloblastic changes. The anemia in these patients does not respond to exogenous folate but does respond to adenine. Severe deficiencies of orotate phosphoribosyl transferase and orotidine 5'-decarboxylase in hereditary orotic aciduria have also been associated with megaloblastic changes, perhaps reflecting broader disturbances in purine and pyrimidine biosynthesis.

Three principal disorders are associated with shortened erythrocyte life span and hemolytic anemia of varying severity: hereditary hyperactivity of adenosine deaminase, hereditary deficiency of adenylate kinase, and severe hereditary or acquired deficiencies of pyrimidine nucleotidase.

The rare disorder caused by hyperactive adenosine deaminase (adenosine aminohydrolase, E.C. 3.5.4.4) has been studied extensively in an American family and a Japanese kindred [272–275]. Affected individuals may be asymptomatic with well-compensated chronic hemolysis, but they can be identified by slight to moderate reticulocytosis, decrements in erythrocyte ATP to less than half expected concentrations, three- to fourfold increases in pyrimidine nucleotidase activity, and markedly hyperactive adenosine deaminase. The latter may range from 40 to 100 times the activities found in normal erythrocytes, in those from unaffected family members, or in reticulocyte-rich blood. The enzyme protein itself appears normal by all conventional biochemical criteria including electrophoresis, kinetics for various substrates and inhibitors, heat stability, specific activity, pH optimum, immunologic reactivity, amino acid composition, and peptide patterns. The basic abnormality thus appears to result from overproduction of structurally normal adenosine deaminase, presumably through an alteration of genetic control mechanisms for switching off enzyme synthesis in erythroid precursors.

The defect is transmitted as a genetic dominant and appears confined to erythroid elements, since granulocytes, lymphocytes, and cultured skin fibroblasts from affected individuals exhibit normal activities. If increased activity were somehow due to alterations in molecular structure, as may occur with hyperactive ribosephosphate pyrophosphokinase, then specific activity would be increased and other tissues with the same isoenzyme would be expected to share the anomaly. In adenosine deaminase deficiency associated with immune incompetence, all tissues exhibit decreased activities. This is consistent with evidence that tissue-specific isoenzymes of adenosine deaminase share a common protein [276, 277], the production of which is governed by a single genetic locus on chromosome 20 [278].

Even though the elevated pyrimidine nucleotidase activities associated with this disorder were the highest ever recorded, there was no evidence that this enzyme could dephosphorylate AMP to cause the observed reductions in total adenine nucleotides. Pronounced hyperactivity of adenosine deaminase, however, could account for reduced concentrations of cellular ATP, if the adenosine kinase pathway were normally necessary for replenishing and maintaining the adenine nucleotide pool by generating AMP from adenosine. Adenosine is present in the plasma in low concentrations and is available to erythrocytes by diffusion and facilitated transport. The direction of adenosine flow within the erythrocyte is influenced by the relative activities and substrate affinities of adenosine kinase and deaminase. Under certain conditions adenosine may be preferentially deaminated because this enzyme is normally much more active than the kinase [279] and also is in close physical association with the membrane components responsible for adenosine transport [280]. At very low adenosine concentrations, however, phosphorylation may predominate, because kinase has a much greater substrate affinity than the deaminase.

Deaminase activity in the affected cells, increased almost two orders of magnitude over normal cells and perhaps even more in subpopulations, might effectively divert ambiently available adenosine away from the kinase-mediated pathway despite the greater substrate affinity of adenosine kinase. The defective cells therefore might not be able to compensate for random nucleotide losses, and low concentrations of adenine nucleotides could result.

In support of this hypothesis, the converse situation has been observed in some cases of severe immunodeficiency disease associated with absent adenosine deaminase activity. These cases may exhibit markedly increased concentrations of cellular adenine nucleotides or deoxynucleotides [281–285]. The absence of deaminase activity apparently allows an inordinate amount of adenosine or deoxyadenosine to be phosphorylated to AMP or dAMP, and the cell's nucleotide pool is consequently expanded. The biochemical abnormalities in these two distinct genetic anomalies strongly suggest that the availability of adenosine and a balanced competition for it between adenosine kinase and deaminase are necessary for normal maintenance of the adenine nucleotide pool in mature erythrocytes.

An equally rare disorder, hereditary deficiency of adenylate kinase (myokinase) (ATP:AMP phosphotransferase, E.C. 2.7.4.3), has been detected in an Israeli Arab [286, 287] and a French family [288]. Adenylate kinase activities in the range of 10 percent or less of normal means were observed in subjects from both kindreds who had moderate to severe hemolytic anemia. In one case, anemia was associated with partial G-6-PD deficiency and in the other with psychomotor retardation. Parents in each kindred possessed the common AK-1 electrophoretic phenotype. Family studies suggested an autosomal recessive mode of transmission with nonanemic heterozygotes identifiable by enzyme activities approximately half the normal mean.

Ineffective use of the salvage pathway mediated by adenosine kinase may be the primary pathogenetic mechanism of premature hemolysis both in instances of adenosine deaminase hyperactivity and in adenylate kinase deficiency. Since AMP formed from plasma adenosine by adenosine kinase cannot be phosphorylated to ADP (and eventually to ATP) without adenylate kinase, adenosine could not be effectively incorporated into the adenine nucleotide pool in the absence of this enzyme. Additionally, severely deficient adenylate kinase might be expected to result in increased concentrations of AMP, secondarily enhancing losses from the adenine nucleotide pool by potential AMP deamination or dephosphorylation.

The most common enzyme defect within the category of nucleotide anomalies in red cells is that of pyrimidine nucleotidase deficiency [289]. Nucleotidases are widely distributed throughout nature as a heterogeneous group of isoenzymes, all of which react with both purine and pyrimidine substrates with variable affinities. Catalytic capability of erythrocyte nucleotidase, however, is sharply limited to pyrimidine substrates [290], an almost mandatory adaptation in erythrocytes, since a nucleotidase also capable of dephosphorylating AMP would impose a constant drain on the adenine nucleotide pool, requiring compensation by other salvage pathways if the red cells were to survive normally.

Severe hereditary deficiency states have been identified in a relatively large number of individuals with wide geographic distribution [289]. Those of peri-Mediterranean, Jewish, or African ancestry may be especially susceptible. The genetic defect is transmitted as an autosomal recessive trait. Heterozygotes exhibit partial decrements in nucleotidase activity but are otherwise hematologically and biochemically normal.

This nucleotidase probably functions only during reticulocyte maturation, serving to dephosphorylate the pyrimidine products of RNA degradation without jeopardizing the purine components [291]. Nucleotidase deficiency, therefore, may result in accumulation of pyrimidines which cannot diffuse from the cells so long as they remain phosphorylated.

Impaired degradation of RNA results in aggregates of intact or partially degraded ribosomal nucleoprotein. This provides the most distinctive hematologic finding in this disease, which is pronounced basophilic stippling on the Wright's-stained peripheral smears (Fig. 73-4). The diagnosis is established by demonstration of significantly decreased nucleotidase activities, generally to about 5 percent of that observed in comparably young cell populations, or the identification of intracellular pyrimidine compounds, which normally are not present in erythrocytes in detectable amounts. Chromatographic techniques are required to identify specific pyrimidines, but a simple determination of the ultraviolet absorption spectrum can readily detect their presence and establish the diagnosis, since pyrimidines accumulate in no other known erythrocyte condition (Fig. 73-5). In subjects with severe hereditary or acquired nucleotidase deficiency, the presence of significant intracellular concentrations of pyrimidine compounds produces shifts in absorption peaks from the usual 257 nm often up to 265 to 270 nm. Since these nucleotides are often as much as 80 per-

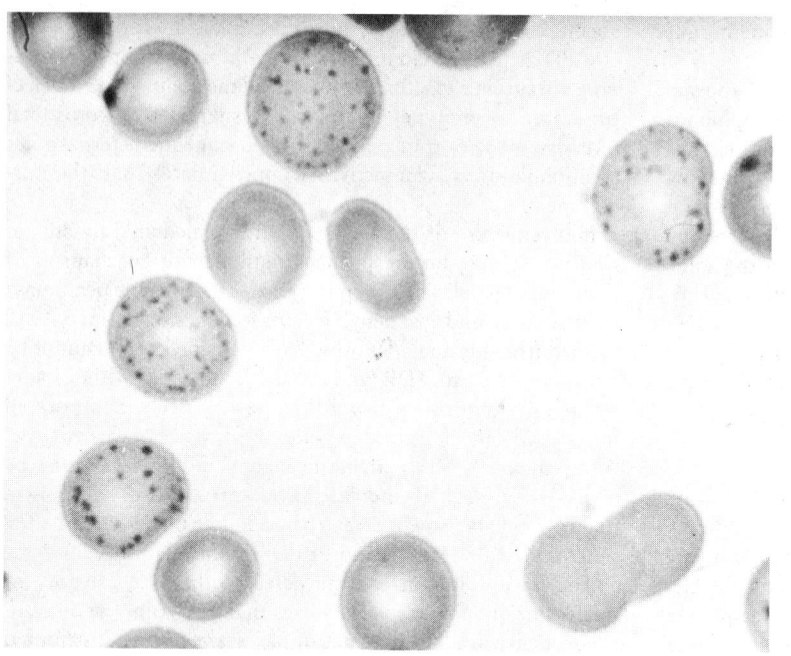

Figure 73-4 Basophilic stippling in peripheral erythrocytes from patient with severe hereditary deficiency of pyrimidine nucleotidase (Wright's stain).

cent pyrimidine compounds, the adenine nucleotide pool is actually diminished on an absolute scale, and this may be at least partially responsible for premature hemolysis.

Two epiphenomena that have been consistent concomitants in this disorder are twofold elevations in erythrocyte glutathione concentrations and decreases in ribosephosphate pyrophosphokinase activities to about one-fourth expected values. No adequate explanations have been proffered for their etiology or pathophysiologic significance, if any.

Deficiencies of pyrimidine nucleotidase may also occur on an acquired basis secondary to lead toxicity. The remarkable sensitivity of this enzyme to inactivation by lead and certain other heavy metals [290] and the common feature of basophilic stippling led to elucidation of its role in the pathogenesis of lead-induced hemolytic anemia. Concentrations of lead that totally obliterate nucleotidase activity have minimal effects on most glycolytic and many other erythrocyte enzymes, although they may have perceptible effects on heme biosynthesis. Humans exposed to chronic low-level overburden of industrial lead insufficient to cause anemia or basophilic stippling may still exhibit significant depressions of nucleotidase activity with otherwise normal glycolytic enzyme profiles [292]. When blood lead levels approach 200 μg per deciliter of packed cells, pyrimidine nucleotidase activity is depressed to levels comparable to those found in homozygous deficiency states. Basophilic stippling then becomes apparent, and pyrimidine nucleotides begin to accumulate to detectable levels within the erythrocytes [293–295].

The three conditions reviewed here, hyperactivity of adenosine deaminase and deficiencies of adenylate kinase and of pyrimidine nucleotidase, all induce hemolytic anemias of variable severities. The first two are very rare, but studies of the two affected kindreds suggest that the anemia of hyperactive adenosine deaminase may be subclinical or totally compensated, whereas that of adenylate kinase deficiency can be life-threatening. Pyrimidine nucleotidase deficiency is one of the more common erythroenzymopathies, having been reported in 33 homozygotes from 24 kindreds, and is associated with hemolytic anemia of intermediate severity, infrequently neces-

sitating transfusions. Acquired deficiencies of nucleotidase activity induced by lead overburden, if sufficiently severe, almost completely recapitulate the syndrome associated with homozygous deficiency states. Splenectomy has not been demonstrably effective, and therapy is restricted to supportive measures.

Studies of cellular perturbations resulting from these defects have provided a broader understanding of normal erythrocyte metabolism, as well as the pathophysiology of underlying hemolytic mechanisms.

PATHOGENESIS OF HEMOLYSIS IN ERYTHROENZYMOPATHIES

In hemolytic syndromes involving G-6-PD deficiency and dysfunction of other constituents of the PP shunt, there is a large measure of general agreement that oxidant denaturation of Hb is the dominant factor in pathogenesis. Denatured Hb in the form of Heinz bodies often is observed closely attached to the plasma membrane whose function is secondarily damaged. An increased loss of potassium is one concomitant. The "pitting" of Heinz bodies by the spleen contributes to red blood cell fragmentation. While nonspherocytic hemolytic anemia dominates the clinical picture in some cases, prominent intravascular hemolysis with hemoglobinuria or hemosiderinuria or both is the frequent manifestation, particularly in crises induced by drugs, ingestion of fava beans, or certain infections.

In the case of enzymopathies of anaerobic glycolysis, a consensus is lacking [298, 299]. In early investigations, often quoted, a disparity was frequently noted between clinical severity of hemolysis and activity as assayed in vitro in the presence of unphysiologic concentrations of substrate and cofactors. The extensive literature on PK deficiency is particularly pertinent, and lack of correlation of clinical and metabolic data has often been cited. However, (1) heterozygotes with 50 percent reductions in PK activity are ordinarily devoid of clinical manifestations; (2) most severe hemolytic syndromes occur with severe PK deficiency of 5 to 20 percent by assay; and (3), most importantly, the apparent discrepancies are greatly narrowed when the now-recognized wide variation in kinetic properties, stability, pH optima, and behavior with cofactors and inhibitors among the many documented mutant enzyme proteins are considered. Most mutant proteins are relatively unstable, but there is great difficulty in quantitating this parameter since apparent instability is influenced by rate of red cell turnover, and since the available thermostability test cannot be extrapolated quantitatively into stability in vivo.

It is now universally agreed that the vast majority of inherited enzymopathies are associated with structural gene mutations and with an astonishingly wide array of variant enzymes recognizable by immunologic or other means as gene products. Usually the transmission of the molecular lesion in terms of Mendelian genetics is readily demonstrable. Such being the case, the primary event initiating hemolysis should be directly related to the mutant gene product. Absent or severely impaired activity of an enzyme of anaerobic glycolysis has two inevitable counterparts, both of which have been demonstrated in many of the severe deficiency states. The first is an interruption of the smooth flow of glycolytic intermediates frequently detectable in terms of less than expected glycolytic rates and ATP concentrations and, more subtly, by accumulations of glycolytic intermediates proximal to or by their diminution distal to a point of metabolic block. The second is that the altered pattern of glycolytic intermediates varies with the site of the molecular lesion. Theoretically, the altered pattern of intermediates could in some way be pathogenetic in the hemolytic anemia. Mechanisms for this are entirely unclear. The fact is that severe deficiencies in glycolytic enzyme activities identified with hemolytic syndromes have remarkably similar clinical and hematologic manifestations despite different molecular lesions and widely disparate patterns of intermediates.

We favor the concept that the dominant event triggering premature cell destruction in the enzymopathies of the Embden-Meyerhof pathway is metabolic depletion and failure of energy generation in the erythrocyte. This is considered to result from progressive deterioration of a nonrenewable, often unstable, often kinetically or otherwise catalytically impaired mutant enzyme, incapable of maintaining a smooth flow of metabolites even in the reticulocyte-rich, young erythrocyte population available for assay. By definition, a cell population still circulating is sufficiently compensated to be still surviving. Mean activities of such populations derived from assay may reflect poorly the metabolic states of the small subpopulation which at any one moment is approaching the brink of destruction.

A primary event involving metabolic depletion does not deny the pathogenetic impact of secondary phenomena: diminished ATP/ADP ratios, altered cation fluxes, translocation of Ca^{2+}, loss of membrane plasticity, budding of plasma membrane constituents without initial loss of Hb, disk-echinocyte-spherocyte transformation, and increased susceptibility to phagocytosis by the macrophage. Neither is a role for possible deleterious effects secondary to altered intermediate patterns in special cases regarded as ruled in or out. A lack of consensus, however, demands that future investigations define precisely and unequivocally events now subject to divergent views [298, 299].

Certain enzymes of purine and pyrimidine nucleotide metabolism are also associated with hemolytic anemia. In adenylate kinase (AK) deficiency, the hemolytic syndrome appears essentially identical with those accompanying severe deficiencies of anaerobic glycolytic enzymes. AK catalyzes the interconversion of ATP, ADP, and AMP and, hence, is basically an integral cog in the glycolytic machinery. The pathogenesis of hemolysis in pyrimidine 5'-nucleotidase deficiency is speculative. The enormous accumulation in severely deficient erythrocytes of pyrimidine-containing nucleotides capable of binding to sites where adenosine phosphates are preferred and much more efficient provides a conjectural mechanism for impaired glycolysis and energy generation in this syndrome. The pyrimidine nucleotides may well have other, less evident, deleterious effects. In the syndrome characterized by hemolysis and enormously increased ADA activity, ATP levels are 50 percent or less of those expected. Presumably, the greatly enhanced deamination of adenosine largely removes an important substrate of a pathway permitting replenishment of the adenine nucleotide pool in the erythrocyte, with ATP depletion a concomitant. The red cell relies on salvage pathways as it cannot synthesize adenosine phosphates de novo from small molecules. Progressive diminution in ATP concentration presumably leads ulti-

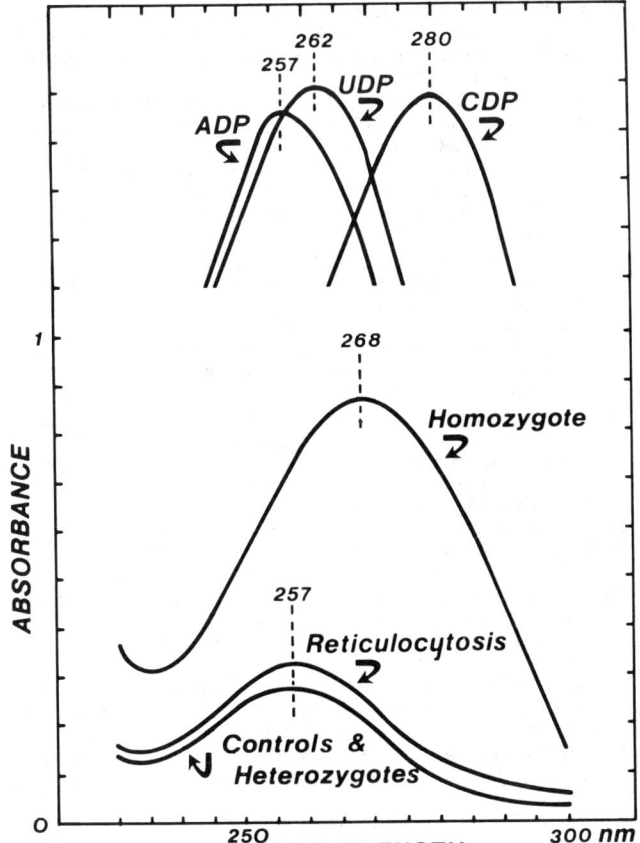

Figure 73-5 Absorption spectra of equimolar concentrations of pure ADP, uridine diphosphate and cytidine diphosphate compared with spectra of neutralized perchloric acid extracts of whole blood from normal subjects, patients with homozygous or heterozygous deficiency of pyrimidine nucleotidase, and individuals with reticulocytosis due to other causes. Curves are normalized to comparable cell quantities, and so their relative amplitudes demonstrate that young cells have increased concentrations of adenine nucleotides relative to normal samples, and total nucleotides in the homozygous deficiency state are markedly increased. Absorption peak shifts occur only in severe nucleotidase deficiency, reflecting intracellular accumulation of pyrimidine compounds.

mately to metabolic depletion and shortened red cell survival.

RED CELL ENZYMOPATHIES WITH HEMATOLOGIC EXPRESSION OTHER THAN HEMOLYSIS OR WITHOUT HEMATOLOGIC EXPRESSION

Erythrocyte enzymopathies may or may not have clinical expression in hematologic abnormalities. The latter, when they occur, may be expressed as hemolytic syndromes, as mild erythrocytosis without hemolysis, as megaloblastic anemia, or as congenital methemoglobinemia. In some instances, association with clinical and laboratory abnormalities may be absent or doubtful and controversial. In still others, the freely floating red cell may provide convenient diagnostic biopsy material for enzymopathies producing clinical disease without hematologic expression, but resulting from impaired function of body tissues other than the blood. In enzymopathies with hematologic expression, there may be or may not be associated disorders of nonhematopoietic origin. Table 73-1 summarizes data relative to these varied manifestations. Representative references are given only for enzymopathies not extensively discussed in the text and are not exhaustive. The list of documented enzymopathies is also limited to these receiving major attention in the literature and is not intended to be all-inclusive.

Certain reported studies from the authors' laboratories were supported by United States Public Health Service Research Grants HLB 12944 and AM 14898 from the National Heart, Lung and Blood Institute and the National Institute of Arthritis, Metabolism and Digestive Diseases.

REFERENCES

1. RAPOPORT S, LUEBERING J: The formation of 2,3-diphosphoglycerate in rabbit erythrocytes: The existence of a diphosphoglycerate mutase. *J Biol Chem* 183:507, 1950
2. BENESCH R, BENESCH RE: Intracellular organic phosphates as regulators of oxygen release by haemoglobin. *Nature* 221:618, 1969
3. ROSA R, PREHIC M-P, REUZAID Y, ROSA J: The first case of a complete deficiency of diphosphoglycerate mutase in human erythrocytes. *J Clin Invest* 62:907, 1978
4. ROSA R, GAILLARDON J, ROSA J: Diphosphoglycerate mutase and 2,3-diphosphoglycerate phosphatase activities of red cells: Comparative electrophoretic study. *Biochem Biophys Res Comm* 51:536, 1973
5. BEUTLER E: Glucose-6-phosphate dehydrogenase activity, in Stanbury JB, Wyngaarden JB, Fredrickson DS, Goldstein JL, Brown MS (eds): *The Metabolic Basis of Inherited Disease*, 5th ed. New York, McGraw-Hill, 1982
6. DACIE JV, MOLLISON PL, RICHARDSON N, SELWYN JG, SHAPIRO L: Atypical congenital haemolytic anaemia. *Q J Med* 22:79, 1953
7. SELWYN JG, DACIE JV: Autohemolysis and other changes resulting from the incubation in vitro of red cells from patients with congenital hemolytic anemia. *Blood* 9:414, 1954
8. DE GRUCHY GC, CRAWFORD H, MORTON D: Atypical (nonspherocytic) congenital haemolytic anaemia. *Proc VII Congr Internat Soc Hematol, Rome,* Il Pensiero Scientifico, 1958, vol 2, pt 1, p 425
9. DE GRUCHY GC, SANTAMARIA JN, PARSONS IC, CRAWFORD H: Nonspherocytic congenital hemolytic anemia. *Blood* 16:1371, 1960
10. ROBINSON MA, LODER PB, DE GRUCHY GC: Red-cell metabolism in nonspherocytic congenital haemolytic anaemia. *Br J Haematol* 7:327, 1961
11. VALENTINE WN, TANAKA KR, MIWA S: A specific erythrocyte glycolytic enzyme defect (pyruvate kinase) in three subjects with congenital nonspherocytic hemolytic anemia. *Trans Assoc Am Physicians* 74:100, 1961

12. TANAKA KR, VALENTINE WN, MIWA S: Pyruvate kinase (PK) deficiency hereditary non-spherocytic hemolytic anemia. *Blood* 18:784, 1961 (abstract); *Blood* 19:267, 1962
13. PIOMELLI S, CORASH L: Hereditary hemolytic anemia due to enzyme defects in glycolysis. *Adv Hum Genet* 6:165, 1976
14. KAHN A, KAPLAN J-C, DREYFUS J-C: Advances in hereditary red cell enzyme anomalies. *Hum Genet* 50:1, 1979
15. BEUTLER E: Red cell enzyme defects as nondiseases and as diseases. *Blood* 54:1, 1979
16. VALENTINE WN: The Stratton lecture: Hemolytic anemia and inborn errors of metabolism. *Blood* 54:549, 1979
17. MIWA S: Significance of the determination of red cell enzyme activities. *Am J Hematol* 6:163, 1979
18. VALENTINE WN, PAGLIA DE: Genetic defects of the human red cell and hemolytic anemia, in Atkinson DE, Fox CF (eds): *Modulation of Protein Function.* New York, Academic, 1979, p 423
19. BEUTLER E: Hemolytic anemia in disorders of red cell metabolism, in Wintrobe MM (ed): *Topics in Hematology.* New York, Plenum, 1978
20. TANAKA KR, PAGLIA DE: Pyruvate kinase deficiency. *Semin Hematol* 8:367, 1971
21. MENTZER WC JR: Pyruvate kinase deficiency and disorders of glycolysis, in Nathan DG, Oski FA (eds): *Hematology of Infancy and Childhood.* Philadelphia, Saunders, 1974, p 328
22. VALENTINE WN, TANAKA KR: Pyruvate kinase and other enzyme deficiency hemolytic anemias, in Stanbury JB, Wyngaarden JB, Fredrickson DS (eds): *The Metabolic Basis of Inherited Disease*, 4th ed. New York, McGraw-Hill, 1978, p 1410
23. MARIE J, ZANELLA A, VIVES-CORRONS JL, NAJMAN A, KAHN A: Significance of the electrophoretic modifications of defective pyruvate kinase variants. Study of six new observations. *Clin Chim Acta* 93:61, 1979
24. ISHIDA Y, MIWA S, FUJII H, FUJINAMI N, TAKEGAWA S, YAMATO K: Thirteen cases of pyruvate kinase deficiency found in Japan. *Am J Hematol* 10:239, 1981
25. VIVES-CORRONS JL, MARIE J, PUJADES MA, KAHN A: Hereditary erythrocyte pyruvate-kinase (PK) deficiency and chronic hemolytic anemia: Clinical, genetic and molecular studies in six new Spanish patients. *Hum Genet* 53:401, 1980
26. BOWMAN HS, MCKUSICK VA, DRONAMRAJU KR: Pyruvate kinase deficient hemolytic anemia in an Amish isolate. *Am J Hum Genet* 17:1, 1965
27. DACIE JV: Recent advances in knowledge of the hereditary haemolytic anaemias. *Schweiz Med Wochenschr* 98:1624, 1968
28. SCHRÖTER W, TILLMANN W: Membrane-localized pyruvate kinase of red blood cells in hemolytic anemia associated with pyruvate kinase deficiency. *Klin Wochenschr* 53:1101, 1975
29. VAN EYS J, GARMS P: Pyruvate kinase deficiency hemolytic anemia: A model for correlation of clinical syndrome and biochemical anomalies. *Adv Pediatr* 18:203, 1971
30. DELIVORIA-PAPADOPOULOS M, OSKI FA, GOTTLIEB AJ: Oxygen-hemoglobin dissociation curves: Effect of inherited enzyme defects of the red cell. *Science* 165:601, 1969
31. TANAKA KR, VALENTINE WN, SCHNEIDER AS: Pyruvate kinase deficiency in hereditary nonspherocytic hemolytic anemia: An inborn error of metabolism, in *Proc IX Cong Europ Soc Haematol, Lisbon, 1963.* Basel, S Karger, 1963, vol 2, pt 1, p 739
32. MÜLLER-SOYANO A, DE ROURA ET, DUKE PR, DE ACQUATELLA GC, ARENDS T, GUINTO E, BEUTLER E: Pyruvate kinase deficiency and leg ulcers. *Blood* 47:807, 1976
33. CURIEL CARIAS D, VALASQUEZ GA, PAPA R, SOMOZA DE MARTINEZ R, LINARES F, SMITH P, RIOS DE VIELMA H, DE ACQUATELLA G: Hemolytic anemia and leg ulcers due to pyruvate kinase deficiency. Report of the second Venezuelan family. *Sangre* 22:64, 1977
34. MAHOUR GH, LYNN HB, HILL RW: Acute pancreatitis with biliary disease in erythrocyte pyruvate-kinase deficiency. *Clin Pediatr* 8:608, 1969
35. SALEM HH, VAN DER WEYDEN MB, FIRKIN BG: Iron overload in congenital erythrocyte pyruvate kinase deficiency. *Med J Aust* 1:531, 1980
36. TANAKA KR: Unpublished data
37. IGLEWSKI BH, IGLEWSKI WJ, BIGLEY RH, KOLER RD: Virus-induced hemolysis in erythrocytes deficient in pyruvate kinase. *Clin Res* 23:131A, 1975
38. KENDALL AG, CHARLOW GF: Red cell pyruvate kinase deficiency: Adverse effect of oral contraceptives. *Acta Haematol* 57:116, 1977
39. NIXON AD, BUCHANAN JG: Haemolytic anaemia due to pyruvate kinase deficiency. *N Z Med J* 66:859, 1967
40. TANAKA KR, VALENTINE WN: Pyruvate kinase deficiency, in Beutler E (ed): *Hereditary Disorders of Erythrocyte Metabolism,* City of Hope Symposium Series. New York, Grune & Stratton, 1968, vol 1, p 229
41. BOWMAN HS, PROCOPIO F: Hereditary non-spherocytic hemolytic anemia of the pyruvate-kinase deficient type. *Ann Intern Med* 58:567, 1963
42. PAGLIA DE, VALENTINE WN, RUCKNAGEL DL: Defective erythrocyte pyruvate kinase with impaired kinetics and reduced optimal activity. *Br J Haematol* 22:651, 1972

43. KAHN A, MARIE J, GALAND C, BOIVIN P: Chronic haemolytic anaemia in two patients heterozygous for erythrocyte pyruvate kinase deficiency. Electrofocusing and immunological studies of erythrocyte and liver pyruvate kinase. *Scand J Haematol* 16:250, 1976

44. LEBLOND PF, LYONNAIS J, DeLAGE J-M: Erythrocyte populations in pyruvate kinase deficiency anaemia following splenectomy. I. Cell morphology. *Br J Haematol* 39:55, 1978

45. KEITT AS: Pyruvate kinase deficiency and related disorders of red cell glycolysis. *Am J Med* 41:762, 1966

46. MIWA S, FUJII H, TAKEGAWA S, NAKATSUJI T, YAMATO K, ISHIDA Y, NINOMIYA N: Seven pyruvate kinase variants characterized by the ICSH recommended methods. *Br J Haematol* 45:575, 1980

47. BECKER MH, GENIESER NB, PIOMELLI S, DOVE D, MENDOZA RD: Roentgenographic manifestations of pyruvate kinase deficiency hemolytic anemia. *Am J Roentgenol Radium Ther Nucl Med* 113:491, 1971

48. MENTZER WC JR, BAEHNER RL, SCHMIDT-SCHONBEIN H, ROBINSON SH, NATHAN DG: Selective reticulocyte destruction in erythrocyte pyruvate kinase deficiency. *J Clin Invest* 50:688, 1971

49. BOWMAN HS, OSKI FA: Laboratory studies of erythrocytic pyruvate kinase deficiency. *Am J Clin Pathol* 70:259, 1978

50. WAZEWSKA-CZYZEWSKA M, GUMÍNSKA M: Congenital non-spherocytic haemolytic anaemia variants with primary and secondary pyruvate kinase deficiency. I. Erythrokinetic patterns. *Br J Haematol* 41:115, 1979

51. LEBLOND PF, LYONNAIS J, DeLAGE J-M: Erythrocyte populations in pyruvate kinase deficiency anaemia following splenectomy. II. Cell deformability. *Br J Haematol* 39:63, 1978

52. MIWA S: Hereditary hemolytic anemia due to erythrocyte enzyme deficiency. *Acta Haematol Jap* 36:573, 1973

53. MATSUMOTO N, ISHIHARA T, NAKASHIMA K, MIWA S, UCHINO F, KONDO M: Sequestration and destruction of reticulocyte in the spleen in pyruvate kinase deficiency hereditary nonspherocytic hemolytic anemia. *Acta Haematol Jap* 35:525, 1972

54. MATSUMOTO N, ISHIHARA T, MIWA S, UCHINO F: The mechanism of mitochondrial extrusion from reticulocytes in the spleen from patients with erythrocyte pyruvate kinase (PK) deficiency. *Acta Haematol Jap* 37:25, 1974

55. TANAKA KR: Pyruvate kinase, in Yunis JJ (ed): *Biochemical Methods in Red Cell Genetics*. New York, Academic, 1969, p 167

56. BEUTLER E: *Red Cell Metabolism. A Manual of Biochemical Methods*, 2d ed. New York, Grune & Stratton, 1975, pp 10, 60

57. MIWA S, BOIVIN P, BLUME KG, ARNOLD H, BLACK JA, KAHN A, STAAL GEJ, NAKASHIMA K, TANAKA KR, PAGLIA DE, VALENTINE WN, YOSHIDA A, BEUTLER E: Recommended methods for the characterization of red cell pyruvate kinase variants. International Committee for Standardization in Haematology. *Br J Haematol* 43:275, 1979

58. BRUNETTI P, NENCI G: A screening method for the detection of erythrocyte pyruvate kinase deficiency. *Enzymol Biol Clin* 4:51, 1964

59. BEUTLER E: A series of new screening procedures for pyruvate kinase deficiency, glucose-6-phosphate dehydrogenase deficiency, and glutathione reductase deficiency. *Blood* 28:553, 1966

60. BLUME KG, LÖHR GW, PRAETSCH O, RÜDIGER HW: Beitrag zur populations-genetik der pyruvatkinase meschlicher erythrocyten. *Humangenetik* 6:261, 1968

61. HELBIG W, JACOBASCH G: Sippenuntersuchung bei pyruvatkinasemangel anämie. *Folia Haematol* 91:65, 1969

62. GARCIA SC, MORAGÓN AC, LÓPEZ-FERNÁNDEZ ME: Frequency of glutathione reductase, pyruvate kinase and glucose-6-phosphate dehydrogenase deficiency in a Spanish population. *Hum Hered* 29:310, 1979

63. SEARCY GP, MILLER DR, TASKER JB: Congenital hemolytic anemia in the Basenji dog due to erythrocyte pyruvate kinase deficiency. *Can J Comp Med* 35:67, 1971

64. SEARCY GP, TASKER JB, MILLER DR: Animal model of human disease: Pyruvate kinase deficiency in dogs. *Am J Pathol* 94:689, 1979

65. MINAKAMI S, YOSHIKAWA H: Studies on erythrocyte glycolysis. II. Free energy changes and rate limiting steps in erythrocyte glycolysis. *J Biochem* 59:139, 1966

66. MARIE J, KAHN A, BOIVIN P: Human erythrocyte pyruvate kinase. Total purification and evidence for its antigenic identity with L-type enzyme. *Biochim Biophys Acta* 481:96, 1977

67. IBSEN KH: Interrelationships and functions of the pyruvate kinase isozymes and their variant forms: A review. *Cancer Res* 37:341, 1977

68. BLUME KG, LÖHR GW, RÜDIGER HW, SCHALHORN A: Pyruvate kinase in human erythrocytes. *Lancet* i:529, 1968

69. NAKASHIMA K: Further evidence of molecular alteration and aberration of erythrocyte pyruvate kinase. *Clin Chim Acta* 55:245, 1974

70. IMAMURA K, TANAKA T, NISHINA T, NAKASHIMA K, MIWA S: Studies on pyruvate kinase (PK) deficiency. II. Electrophoretic, kinetic, and immunological studies of pyruvate kinase of erythrocytes and other tissues. *J Biochem* 74:1165, 1973

71. MARIE J, GARREAU H, KAHN A: Evidence for a postsynthetic proteolytic transformation of human erythrocyte pyruvate kinase into L-type enzyme. *FEBS Letters* 78:91, 1977

72. KAHN A, MARIE J, BOIVIN P: Pyruvate kinase isozymes in man. II. L-type and erythrocyte type isozymes. Electrofocusing and immunologic studies. *Hum Genet* 33:35, 1976

73. KAHN A, MARIE J, GARREAU H, SPRENGERS ED: The genetic system of the L-type pyruvate kinase forms in man. Subunit structure, interrelation and kinetic characteristics of the pyruvate kinase enzymes from erythroctyes and liver. *Biochim Biophys Acta* 523:59, 1978

74. ODA S, ODA E, TANAKA KR: Relationship of density distribution and pyruvate kinase electrophoretic pattern of erythrocytes in sickle cell diseases and other disorders. *Acta Haematol* 60:201, 1978

75. BIGLEY RH, KOLER RD: Liver pyruvate kinase (PK) isozymes in a PK-deficient patient. *Ann Hum Genet* 31:383, 1968

76. NAKASHIMA K, MIWA S, ODA S, TANAKA T, IMMAMURA K, NISHINA T: Electrophoretic and kinetic studies of mutant erythrocyte pyruvate kinases. *Blood* 43:537, 1974

77. NAKASHIMA K, MIWA S, FUJII H, SHINOHARA K, YAMAUCHI K, TSUJI Y, YANAI M: Characterization of pyruvate kinase from the liver of a patient with aberrant erythrocyte pyruvate kinase, PK Nagasaki. *J Lab Clin Med* 90:1012, 1977

78. SPRENGERS ED, STAAL GEJ: Functional changes associated with the sequential transformation of L′₄ into L₄ pyruvate kinase. *Biochim Biophys Acta* 570:259, 1979

79. KAHN A, MARIE J: Postsynthetic maturation of erythrocyte pyruvate kinase in patients with hereditary defect in this enzyme, in Hommes FA (ed): *Model for the Study of Inborn Errors of Metabolism*. Amsterdam, Elsevier/North Holland, 1979, p 191

80. BLACK JA, RITTENBERG MB, BIGLEY RH, KOLER RD: Hemolytic anemia due to pyruvate kinase deficiency: Characterization of the enzymatic activity from eight patients. *Am J Hum Genet* 31:300, 1979

81. KAHN A, DREYFUS JC: Molecular basis of the hereditary defects of enzyme activity, in Schewe T, Rapoport S (eds): *Molecular Diseases*. New York, Pergamon Press, 1979, vol 56, p 1

82. SHINOHARA K, TANAKA KR: Pyruvate kinase deficiency hemolytic anemia: Enzymatic characterization studies in twelve patients. *Hemoglobin* 4:611, 1980

83. STAAL GEJ, KOSTER JF, KAMP H, van MILLIGEN-BOERSMA L, VEEGER C: Human erythrocyte pyruvate kinase. Its purification and some properties. *Biochim Biophys Acta* 227:86, 1971

84. BLACK JA, HENDERSON MH: Activation and inhibition of human erythrocyte pyruvate kinase by organic phosphates, amino acids, dipeptides and anions. *Biochim Biophys Acta* 284:115, 1972

85. MONOD J, WYMAN J, CHANGEUX JP: On the nature of allosteric transitions: A plausible model. *J Mol Biol* 12:88, 1965

86. MARIE J, TICHONICKY L, DREYFUS J-C, KAHN A: Endogenous, cyclic 3′-5′ AMP-dependent phosphorylation of human red cell pyruvate kinase. *Biochem Biophys Res Comm* 87:862, 1979

87. MARIE J, BUC H, SIMON M-P, KAHN A: Phosphorylation of human erythrocyte pyruvate kinase by soluble cyclic-AMP-dependent protein kinases. Comparison with human liver-L-type enzyme. *Eur J Biochem* 108:251, 1980

88. PAGLIA DE, VALENTINE WN, BAUGHAN MA, MILLER DR, REED CF, McINTYRE OR: An inherited molecular lesion of erythrocyte pyruvate kinase. Identification of a kinetically aberrant isozyme associated with premature hemolysis. *J Clin Invest* 47:1929, 1968

89. PAGLIA DE, KONRAD PN, WOLFF JA, VALENTINE WN: Biphasic reaction kinetics in an anomalous isozyme of erythrocyte pyruvate kinase. *Clin Chim Acta* 73:395, 1976

90. MIWA S, NAKASHIMA K, ARIYOSHI K, SHINOHARA K, ODA E, TANAKA T: Four new pyruvate kinase (PK) variants and a classical PK deficiency. *Br J Haematol* 29:157, 1975

91. SHINOHARA K, MIWA S, NAKASHIMA K, ODA E, KAGEOKA T, TSUJINO G: A new pyruvate kinase variant (PK Osaka) demonstrated by partial purification and condensation. *Am J Hum Genet* 28:474, 1976

92. STAAL GEJ, CEERDINK RP, VLUG AMC, HAMELINK ML: Defective erythrocyte pyruvate kinase. *Clin Chim Acta* 68:11, 1976

93. KAHN A, MARIE J, GALAND C, BOIVIN P: Molecular mechanism of erythrocyte pyruvate kinase deficiency. *Humangenetik* 29:271, 1975

94. MARIE J, VIVES-CORRONS JL, KAHN A: Hereditary erythrocyte pyruvate kinase deficiency: Molecular and functional studies of four mutant PK variants detected in Spain. *Clin Chim Acta* 81:153, 1977

95. SPRENGERS ED, MARIE J, KAHN A, PUNT K, STAAL GEJ: Human erythrocyte pyruvate kinase deficiency: The use of a kinetic study of mutant enzymes for the detection of heterozygotes. *Hum Genet* 41:61, 1978

96. PAGLIA DE, VALENTINE WN, WILLIAMS KO, KONRAD PN: An isozyme of erythrocyte pyruvate kinase (PK-Los Angeles) with impaired kinetics corrected by fructose-1, 6-diphosphate. *Am J Clin Pathol* 68:229, 1977

97. ZANELLA A, REBULLA P, IZZO C, ZANUSO F, SIRCHIA G: Concomitance of an active and an inactive mutant of red cell pyruvate kinase (PK). *Scand J Haematol* 22:145, 1979

98. SPRENGERS ED, BEEMER FA, STAAL GEJ: A new pyruvate kinase variant: PK-WOUW. *J Mol Med* 3:271, 1978

99. MIWA S, NISHINA T: Studies on pyruvate kinase (PK) deficiency. I. Clinical, hematological and erythrocyte enzyme studies. *Acta Haematol Jap* 37:1, 1974

100. ROSE IA, WARMS JVB: Control of glycolysis in the human red blood cell. *J Biol Chem* 241:4848, 1966

101. TEITEL P, BRATU V, XENAKIS A, BUTOIANU E: Favourable therapeutic effect of adenosine-5-monophosphate in a case of chronic compensated haemolytic disease with an impaired erythrocyte energy metabolism, in *Proceedings 10th Congress International Society of Blood Transfusion,* 1964, p 557, 1965

102. WAZEWSKI-CZYZEWSKA M, GUMINSKA M: The influence of magnesium ions on pyruvate kinase-deficient red blood cells. *Folia Haematol* 102:576, 1975

103. BLUME KG, ARNOLD H, HASSLINGER K, LÖHR GW: Effect of riboflavin treatment on human red cell pyruvate kinase deficiency. *Clin Chim Acta* 71:331, 1976

104. STAAL GEJ, SYBESMA JPHB, CAMERON ARE, van MILLIGEN-BOERSMA L, MOES M: Familial haemolytic anaemia due to pyruvate kinase deficiency. *Folia Med Neerl* 14:72, 1971

105. BUSCH D, HOFFBAUER RW, BLUME KG, LÖHR GW: Kinetic properties of pyruvate kinase and problems of therapy in different types of pyruvate kinase deficiency, in Ramot B (ed): *Red Cell Structure and Metabolism.* New York, Academic, 1971, p 193

106. NEUMANN VE, SCHWARZMEIER J, HONETZ H: Hereditare elliptozytose und pyruvatkinasemangel der erythrozyten. *Wien Klin Wochenschr* 84:712, 1972

107. OSKI FA, NATHAN DG, SIDEL VW, DIAMOND LK: Extreme hemolysis and red-cell distortion in erythrocyte pyruvate kinase deficiency. I. Morphology, erythrokinetics, and family enzyme studies. *N Engl J Med* 270:1023, 1964

108. BROOK J, TANAKA KR: Combination of pyruvate kinase (PK) deficiency and hereditary spherocytosis (HS) (abstract). *Clin Res* 18:176, 1970

109. EULDERINK F, CLETON FJ: Gaucher's disease with severe renal involvement combined with pyruvate-kinase deficiency. *Pathol Eur* 5:409, 1970

110. DHARMKRONG-AT A, BLOOM GE: Acquired hemolytic anemia associated with infectious mononucleosis in a patient with congenital pyruvate kinase deficiency. *Clin Pediatr* 12:119, 1973

111. VALENTINE WN, KONRAD PN, PAGLIA DE: Dyserythropoiesis, refractory anemia, and "preleukemia": Metabolic features of the erythrocytes. *Blood* 41:857, 1973

112. BOIVIN P, GALAND C, HAKIM J, KAHN A: Acquired red cell pyruvate kinase deficiency in leukemias and related disorders. *Enzyme* 19:294, 1975

113. TANPHAICHITR VS, van EYS J: Erythrocyte pyruvate kinase activity in patients with hematological malignancies. *Scand J Haematol* 15:10, 1975

114. LOPEZ G, MURO M: Disminución de actividad PK eritrocitaria y aparición de HbF en las pancitopenias. *Sangre* 21:467, 1976

115. ABE S: Secondary red cell pyruvate kinase deficiency. I. Study of 30 subjects of malignant hematological disorders. *Acta Haematol Jap* 39:247, 1976

116. RENOUX M, BERNARD JF, TORRES M, SCHLEGEL N, AMAR M, LOPEZ M, BOIVIN P: Erythrocyte abnormalities induced by chemotherapy and radiotherapy: Induction of preleukaemic states? *Scand J Haematol* 21:323, 1978

117. ETIEMBLE J, BERNARD JF, PICAT C, BELPOMME D, BOIVIN P: Red blood cell enzyme abnormalities in patients treated with chemotherapy. *Br J Haematol* 42:391, 1979

118. ARNOLD H, BLUME KG, LÖHR GW, BOULARD M, NAJEAN Y: "Acquired" red cell enzyme defects in hematological diseases. *Clin Chim Acta* 57:187, 1974

119. ARNOLD H, BLUME KG, LÖHR GW: Mechanisms for acquired red cell enzyme defects. *Blood* 49:1022, 1977

120. ABE S: Secondary red cell pyruvate kinase deficiency. II. Biochemical studies for the mechanism of pyruvate kinase deficiency in erythroleukemia. *Acta Haematol Jap* 39:255, 1976

121. ETIEMBLE J, PICAT C, BOIVIN P: Studies on the mechanism of the erythrocyte enzyme abnormalities induced by chemotherapy. *Scand J Haematol* 25:394, 1980

122. KAHN A, MARIE J, BERNARD JF, COTTREAU D, BOIVIN P: Mechanisms of the acquired erythrocyte enzyme deficiencies in blood diseases. *Clin Chim Acta* 71:379, 1976

123. KAHN A, COTTREAU D, BOYER C, MARIE J, GALAND C, BOIVIN P: Causal mechanisms of multiple acquired red cell enzyme defects in a patient with acquired dyserythropoiesis. *Blood* 48:653, 1976

124. BROK F, RAMOT B, ZWANG E, DANON D: Enzyme activities in human red blood cells of different age groups. *Israel J Med Sci* 2:291, 1966

125. SEAMAN C, WYSS S, PIOMELLI S: The decline in energetic metabolism with aging of the erythrocyte and its relationship to cell death. *Am J Haematol* 8:31, 1980

126. VALENTINE WN, OSKI FA, PAGLIA DE, BAUGHAN MA, SCHNEIDER AS, NAIMAN JL: Hereditary hemolytic anemia with hexokinase deficiency. Role of hexokinase in erythrocyte aging. *N Engl J Med* 276:1, 1967

127. VALENTINE WN, OSKI FA, PAGLIA DE, BAUGHAN MA, SCHNEIDER AS, NAIMAN JL: Erythrocyte hexokinase and hereditary hemolytic anemia, in Beutler E (ed): *Hereditary Disorders of Erythrocyte Metabolism.* New York, Grune & Stratton, 1968, p 288

128. RIJKSEN G, STAAL GEJ: Regulation of human erythrocyte hexokinase. The influence of glycolytic intermediates and inorganic phosphate. *Biochim Biophys Acta* 485:75, 1977

129. RIJKSEN G, STAAL GEJ: Human erythrocyte hexokinase deficiency. Characterization of a mutant enzyme with abnormal regulatory properties. *J Clin Invest* 62:294, 1978

130. LÖHR GW, WALLER HD, ANSCHÜTZ F, KNOOP A: Biochemische defekte in den blutzellen bei familiärer panmyelopathie (Typ Fanconi). *Humangenetik* 1:383, 1965

131. KEITT AS: Hemolytic anemia with impaired hexokinase activity. *J Clin Invest* 48:1997, 1969

132. NECHELES TF, RAI US, CAMERON D: Congenital nonspherocytic hemolytic anemia associated with an unusual erythrocyte hexokinase abnormality. *J Lab Clin Med* 76:593, 1970

133. MOSER K, CIRESA M, SCHWARZMEIER J: Hexokinasemangel bei hämolytischer anämie. *Med Welt* 46:1977, 1970

134. GILSANZ F, MEYER E, PAGLIA DE, VALENTINE WN: Congenital hemolytic anemia due to hexokinase deficiency. *Am J Dis Child* 132:637, 1978

135. BOARD PG, TRUEWORTHY R, SMITH JE, MOORE K: Congenital nonspherocytic hemolytic anemia with an unstable hexokinase variant. *Blood* 51:111, 1978

136. BEUTLER E, DYMENT PG, MATSUMOTO F: Hereditary nonspherocytic hemolytic anemia and hexokinase deficiency. *Blood* 51:935, 1978

137. SIIMES MA, RIHIALA E-L, LEISTI J: Hexokinase deficiency in erythrocytes: A new variant in 5 members of a Finnish family. *Scan J Haematol* 22:214, 1979

138. PAGLIA DE, SHENDE A, LANZKOWSKY P, VALENTINE WN: Hexokinase "New Hyde Park." A low activity erythrocyte isozyme in a Chinese kindred. *Am J Hematol* 10:107, 1981

139. NEWMAN P, MUIR A, PARKER AC: Nonspherocytic haemolytic anaemia in mother and son associated with hexokinase deficiency. *Br J Haematol* 46:537, 1980

140. CHAPMAN RG, SCHAUMBURG L: Glycolysis and glycolytic enzyme activity of aging red cells in man. Changes in hexokinase, aldolase, glyceraldehyde-3-phosphate dehydrogenase, pyruvate kinase and glutamic-oxalacetic transaminase. *Br J Haematol* 13:665, 1967

141. ROGERS PA, FISHER RA, HARRIS H: An examination of the age-related patterns of decay of the hexokinases of human red cells. *Clin Chim Acta* 65:291, 1975

142. MCKUSICK VA: The anatomy of the human genome. *Am J Med* 69:267, 1980

143. BAUGHAN MA, VALENTINE WN, PAGLIA DE, WAYS PO, SIMONS ER, deMARSH QB: Hereditary hemolytic anemia associated with glucosephosphate isomerase (GPI) deficiency—a new enzyme defect of human erythrocytes. *Blood* 32:236, 1968

144. PAGLIA DE, HOLLAND P, BAUGHAN MA, VALENTINE WN: Occurrence of defective hexosephosphate isomerization in human erythrocytes and leukocytes. *N Engl J Med* 280:66, 1969

145. CARTIER P, TEMKINE H, GRISCELLI C: Etude biochimique d'une anémie hémolytique avec déficit familial en phosphohexoisomérase. *Enzymol Biol Clin* 10:439, 1969

146. ARNOLD H, BLUME KG, BUSCH D, LENKEIT U, LÖHR GW, LÜBS E: Klinische und biochemische untersuchungen zur glucosephosphatisomerase normaler menschlicher erythrocyten und bei glucosephosphatisomerasemangel. *Klin Wochenschr* 48:1299, 1970

147. TARIVERDIAN G, ARNOLD H, BLUME KG, LENKEIT U, LÖHR GW: Zur formalgenetik der phosphoglucoseisomerase (EC 5.3.1.9). Untersuchung einer sippe mit PGI-defizienz. *Humangenetik* 10:218, 1970

148. SCHRÖTER W, BRITTINGER G, ZIMMERSCHMITT E, KÖNIG E: A new haemolytic syndrome with glucosephosphate isomerase (GPI) and glucose-6-phosphate dehydrogenase (G6PD) deficiency of the erythrocytes. Biochemical studies. *Eur J Clin Invest* 1:145, 1970 (abstract)

149. SCHRÖTER W, BRITTINGER G, ZIMMERSCHMITT E, KÖNIG E, SCHRADER D: Combined glucophosphate isomerase and glucose-6-phosphate dehydrogenase deficiency of the erythrocytes: A new haemolytic syndrome. *Br J Haematol* 20:249, 1971

150. OSKI F, FULLER E: Glucose-phosphate isomerase (GPI) deficiency associated with abnormal osmotic fragility and spherocytes. *Clin Res* 19:427, 1971 (abstract)

151. BLUME KG, HRYNIUK W, POWARS D, TRINIDAD F, WEST C, BEUTLER E: Characterization of two new variants of glucose-phosphate-isomerase deficiency with hereditary nonspherocytic hemolytic anemia. *J Lab Clin Med* 79:942, 1972

152. ARNOLD H, ENGELHARDT R, LÖHR GW, JACOBI H, LIEBOLD I: Glucose-

phosphate-isomerase Typ Recklinghausen: Eine neue defektvariante mit hämolytischer anämie. *Klin Wochenschr* 51:1198, 1973

153. LÖHR GW, ARNOLD H, BLUME KG, ENGELHARDT R, BEUTLER E: Hereditary deficiency of glucosephosphate isomerase as a cause of nonspherocytic hemolytic anemia. *Blut* 26:393, 1973

154. MATSUMOTO N, ISHIHARA T, ODA E, MIWA S, NAKASHIMA K, UCHINO F, FUKUMOTO Y: Fine structure of the spleen and liver in glucose-phosphate isomerase (GPI) deficiency hereditary nonspherocytic hemolytic anemia—Selective reticulocyte destruction as a mechanism of hemolysis. *Acta Haematol Jap* 36:46, 1973

155. MIWA S, NAKASHIMA K, ODA S, ODA E, MATSUMOTO N, OGAWA H, FUKUMOTO Y: Glucosephosphate isomerase (GPI) deficiency hereditary nonspherocytic hemolytic anemia. Report of the first case found in Japanese. *Acta Haematol Jap* 36:65, 1973

156. MIWA S, NAKASHIMA K, ODA S, MATSUMOTO N, OGAWA H, KOBAYASHI R, KOTANI M, HARATA A, ONAYA T, YAMADA T: Glucosephosphate isomerase (GPI) deficiency hereditary nonspherocytic hemolytic anemia. Report of the second case found in Japan. *Acta Haematol Jap* 36:70, 1973

157. NAKASHIMA K, MIWA S, ODA S, ODA E, MATSUMOTO N, FUKUMOTO Y, YAMADA T: Electrophoretic and kinetic studies of glucose-phosphate isomerase (GPI) in two different Japanese families with GPI deficiency. *Am J Hum Genet* 25:294, 1973

158. ARNOLD H, BLUME KG, ENGELHARDT R, LÖHR GW: Glucosephosphate isomerase deficiency: Evidence for in vivo instability of an enzyme variant with hemolysis. *Blood* 41:691, 1973

159. ARNOLD H, BLUME KG, LÖHR GW, SCHRÖTER W, KOCH HH, WONNEBERGER B: Glucose phosphate isomerase deficiency with congenital nonspherocytic hemolytic anemia: A new variant (type Nordhorn). II. Purification and biochemical properties of the defective enzyme. *Pediatr Res* 8:26, 1974

160. SCHRÖTER W, KOCH HH, WONNEBERGER B, KALINOWSKY W, ARNOLD H, BLUME KG, HÜTHER W: Glucose phosphate isomerase deficiency with congenital nonspherocytic hemolytic anemia: A new variant (type Nordhorn): I. Clinical and genetic studies. *Pediatr Res* 8:18, 1974

161. CHILICOTE RR, BAEHNER RL: Red cell (RBC) glucose phosphate isomerase deficiency (GPI): Clinical and laboratory evidence of increased blood viscosity. *Pediatr Res* 8:398, 1974

162. HUTTON JJ, CHILICOTE RR: Glucose phosphate isomerase deficiency with hereditary nonspherocytic hemolytic anemia. *J Pediatr* 85:494, 1974

163. PAGLIA DE, VALENTINE WN: Hereditary glucophosphate isomerase deficiency. A review. *Am J Clin Pathol* 62:740, 1974

164. PAGLIA DE, PAREDES R, VALENTINE WN, DORANTES S, KONRAD PN: Unique phenotypic expression of glucosephosphate isomerase deficiency. *Am J Hum Genet* 27:62, 1975

165. ARNOLD H, DODINVAL-VERSIE J, LAMBOTTE C, LÖHR GW, VAN DER HOFSTADT J: Glucosephosphate isomerase deficiency type Liège: A new variant with congenital nonspherocytic hemolytic anemia. *Blut* 35:187, 1977

166. KAHN A, BUC HA, GIROT R, COTTREAU D, GRISCELLI C: Molecular and functional anomalies in two new mutant glucose-phosphate-isomerase variants with enzyme deficiency and chronic hemolysis. *Hum Genet* 40:293, 1978

167. SCHRÖTER W, TILLMAN W: Congenital nonspherocytic hemolytic anemia associated with glucose-phosphate isomerase deficiency: Variant Paderborn. *Klin Wochenschr* 55:393, 1977

168. BIERVLIET VAN JPGM, MILLIGEN-BOERSMA VAN L, STAAL GEJ: A new variant of glucosephosphate isomerase deficiency: GPI Utrecht. *Clin Chim Acta* 65:157, 1975

169. BIERVLIET VAN JPGM, VLUG A, BARSTRA H, ROTTEVEEL JJ, DE VAAN GAM, STAAL GEJ: A new variant of glucosephosphate isomerase deficiency. *Hum Genet* 30:35, 1975

170. KAHN A, VIVES-CORRONS JL, BERTRAND O, COTTREAU D, MARIE J, BOIVIN P: Glucosephosphate isomerase deficiency due to a new variant (GPI Barcelona) and to a silent gene: Biochemical, immunological, and genetic studies. *Clin Chim Acta* 66:145, 1976

171. STAAL GEJ, AKKERMAN JWN, EGGERMONT E, BIERVLIET VAN JPGM: A new variant of glucosephosphate isomerase: G.P.I.-Kortrijk. *Clin Chim Acta* 78:121, 1977

172. GALAND C, TORRES M, BOIVIN P, BOURGEAUD JP: A new variant of glucosephosphate isomerase deficiency with mild haemolytic anaemia (GPI-Mytho). *Scand J Haematol* 20:77, 1978

173. ZANELLA A, IZZO C, REBULLA P, PERRONI L, MARIANI M, CANESTRI G, SANSONE G, SIRCHIA G: The first stable variant of erythrocyte glucosephosphate isomerase associated with severe hemolytic anemia. *Am J Hematol* 9:1, 1980

174. CARTER ND, YOSHIDA A: Purification and characterization of human phosphoglucose isomerase. *Biochim Biophys Acta* 181:12, 1969

175. PAYNE DM, PORTER DW, GRACY RW: Evidence against the occurrence of tissue-specific variants and isoenzymes of phosphoglucose isomerase. *Arch Biochem Biophys* 151:122, 1972

176. COTTREAU D, LEVIN MJ, KAHN A: Purification and partial characterization of different forms of phosphofructokinase in man. *Biochim Biophys Acta* 568:183, 1979

177. STAAL GEJ, KOSTER JF, BÄNZIGER CJM, VAN MILLIGEN-BOERSMA L: Human erythrocyte phosphofructokinase: Its purification and some properties. *Biochim Biophys Acta* 276:113, 1972

178. MEIENHOFER M-C, LAGRANGE J-L, COTTREAU D, LENOIR G, DREYFUS J-C, KAHN A: Phosphofructokinase in human blood cells. *Blood* 54:389, 1979

179. KAHN A, COTTREAU D, MEIENHOFFER M-C: Purification of F4 phosphofructokinase from human platelets and comparison with the other phosphofructokinase forms. *Biochim Biophys Acta* 611:114, 1980

180. VORA S, SEAMAN C, DURHAM S, PIOMELLI S: Isozymes of human phosphofructokinase: Identification and subunit structural characterization of a new system. *Proc Natl Acad Sci USA* 77:62, 1980

181. VORA S, CORASH L, ENGEL WK, DURHAM S, SEAMAN C, PIOMELLI S: The molecular mechanism of the inherited phosphofructokinase deficiency associated with hemolysis and myopathy. *Blood* 55:629, 1980

182. KAHN A, MEIENHOFFER M-C, COTTREAU D, LAGRANGE J-L, DREYFUS J-C: Phosphofructokinase (PFK) isozymes in man. *Hum Genet* 48:93, 1979

183. VORA S, DURHAM S, PIOMELLI S: Isozymes of phosphofructokinase in human blood cells: Molecular and genetic evidence for a multigenic system. *Blood* 54(Suppl 1):35a, 1979 (abstract)

184. TARUI S, OKUNO G, IKURA Y, TANAKA T, SUDA M, NISHIKAWA M: Phosphofructokinase deficiency in skeletal muscle. A new type of glycogenosis. *Biochem Biophys Res Commun* 19:517, 1965

185. TARUI S, KONO N, NASU T, NISHIKAWA M: Enzymatic basis for the coexistence of myopathy and hemolytic disease in inherited muscle phosphofructokinase deficiency. *Biochem Biophys Res Commun* 34:77, 1969

186. LAYZER RB, ROWLAND LP, RANNEY HM: Muscle phosphofructokinase deficiency. *Arch Neurol* 17:512, 1967

187. LAYZER RB, ROWLAND LP, BANK WJ: Physical and kinetic properties of human phosphofructokinase from skeletal muscle and erythrocytes. *J Biol Chem* 244:3823, 1969

188. SERRATRICE G, MONGES A, ROUX H: Forme myopathique due déficit en phosphofructokinase. *Rev Neurol* 120:271, 1969

189. TOBIN WE, HUIJING F, PORRO RS, SALZMAN RT: Muscle phosphofructokinase deficiency. *Arch Neurol* 28:128, 1973

190. WATERBURY L, FRANKEL EP: Hereditary nonspherocytic hemolysis with erythrocyte phosphofructokinase deficiency. *Blood* 39:415, 1972

191. MIWA S, SATO T, MURAO H: A new type of phosphofructokinase deficiency: Hereditary non-spherocytic hemolytic anemia. *Acta Haematol Jap* 35:113, 1972

192. BOULARD MR, MEIENHOFFER MC, BOIS M, REVIRON M, NAJEAN Y: Red cell phosphofructokinase deficiency. *N Engl J Med* 291:978, 1974

193. KAHN A, ETIEMBLE J, MEIENHOFFER MC, BOIVIN P: Erythrocyte phosphofructokinase deficiency associated with an unstable variant of muscle phosphofructokinase. *Clin Chim Acta* 61:415, 1975

194. ODA S, ODA E, TANAKA KR: Erythrocyte phosphofructokinase (PFK) deficiency: Characterization and metabolic studies. *Clin Res* 25:344A, 1977 (abstract)

195. TAURI S, KONO N, KUWAJIMA M, KITANI T: Hereditary and acquired abnormalities in erythrocyte phosphofructokinase activity: The close association with altered 2,3-diphosphoglycerate levels. *Hemoglobin* 4:581, 1980

196. BEUTLER E, SCOTT S, BISHOP A, MARGOLIS N, MATSUMOTO F, KUHL W: Red cell aldolase deficiency and hemolytic anemia: A new syndrome. *Trans Assoc Am Physicians* 86:154, 1973

197. SCHNEIDER AS, VALENTINE WN, HATTORI M, HEINS HL JR: Hereditary hemolytic anemia with triosephosphate isomerase deficiency. *N Engl J Med* 272:229, 1965

198. VALENTINE WN, SCHNEIDER AS, BAUGHAN MA, PAGLIA DE, HEINS HL JR: Hereditary hemolytic anemia with triosephosphate isomerase deficiency. Studies in kindreds with co-existent sickle cell trait and erythrocyte glucose-6-phosphate dehydrogenase deficiency. *Am J Med* 41:27, 1966

199. SCHNEIDER AS, VALENTINE WN, BAUGHAN MA, PAGLIA DE, SHORE NA, HEINS HL JR: Triosephosphate isomerase deficiency. A.A multi-system inherited enzyme disorder. Clinical and genetic aspects, in Beutler E (ed): *Hereditary Disorders of Erythrocyte Metabolism*. New York, Grune & Stratton, 1968, p 265

200. SCHNEIDER AS, DUNN I, IBSEN KH, WEINSTEIN IM: Triosephosphate isomerase deficiency. B. Inherited triosephosphate isomerase deficiency. Erythrocyte carbohydrate metabolism and preliminary studies of the erythrocyte enzyme, in Beutler E (ed): *Hereditary Disorders of Erythrocyte Metabolism*. New York, Grune & Stratton, 1968, p 273

201. KAPLAN JC, TEEPLE L, SHORE NA, BEUTLER E: Electrophoretic abnormality in triosephosphate isomerase deficiency. *Biochem Biophys Res Commun* 31:768, 1968

202. ANGELMAN H, BRAIN MC, MACIVER JE: A case of triosephosphate isomerase deficiency with sudden death. *Abstr XIIIth Int Congr Hematol*, Munich, Germany, 1970, p 122

203. HARRIS SR, PAGLIA DE, JAFFÉ ER, VALENTINE WN, KLEIN RL: Triosephosphate isomerase deficiency in an adult. *Clin Res* 18:529, 1970 (abstract)

204. EBER SW, DÜNWALD M, BELOHRADSKY BH, BIDLINGMAIER F, SCHIEVELBEIN H, WEINMANN HM, KRIETSCH WKG: Hereditary deficiency of triosephosphate isomerase in four unrelated families. *Eur J Clin Invest* 9:195, 1979

205. VIVES-CORRANS JL, RUBINSON-SKALA H, MATEO M, ESTELLA J, FELIN E, DREYFUS J-C: Triosephosphate isomerase deficiency with hemolytic anemia and severe neuromuscular disease. Familial and biochemical studies of a case found in Spain. *Hum Genet* 42:171, 1978

206. SKALA H, DREYFUS J-C, VIVES-CORRONS JL, MATSUMOTO F, BEUTLER E: Triosephosphate isomerase deficiency. *Biochem Med* 18:226, 1977

207. FREYCON F, LAURAS B, BOVIER-LAPIERRE F, DORCHE CL, GODDON R: Anémie hémolytique congénitale par déficit en triosephosphate isomerase. *Pédiatrie* 30:55, 1975

208. JONGSMA APM, HAGMEIJER J, MIERALHAN P: Regional mapping of TPI, LDH-B and PEP-B on chromosome 12 of man, in *Second International Workshop on Human Gene Mapping, Rotterdam Conference*. Basel, National Foundation, 1974, p 189

209. KRAUS AP, LANGSTON MF JR, LYNCH BL: Red cell phosphoglycerate kinase deficiency. A new cause of non-spherocytic hemolytic anemia. *Biochem Biophys Res Commun* 30:173, 1968

210. VALENTINE WN, HSIEH H-S, PAGLIA DE, ANDERSON HM, BAUGHAN MA, JAFFÉ ER, GARSON OM: Hereditary hemolytic anemia: Association with phosphoglycerate kinase deficiency in erythrocytes and leukocytes. *Trans Assoc Am Physicians* 81:49, 1968

211. CHEN S-H, MALCOLM LA, YOSHIDA A, GIBLETT ER: Phosphoglycerate kinase: An X-linked polymorphism in man. *Am J Hum Genet* 23:87, 1971

212. KHAN PM, WESTERVELD A, GRZESCHIK KH, DEYS BF, GARSON OM, SINISCALCO M: X-linkage of human phosphoglycerate kinase confirmed in man-mouse and man-Chinese hamster somatic cell hybrids. *Am J Hum Genet* 23:614, 1971

213. VALENTINE WN, HSIEH H, PAGLIA DE, ANDERSON HM, BAUGHAN MA, JAFFÉ ER, GARSON OM: Hereditary hemolytic anemia associated with phosphoglycerate kinase deficiency in erythrocytes and leucocytes. A probable X-chromosome-linked syndrome. *N Engl J Med* 280:528, 1969

214. MAZZA U, ARESE P, BOSIA A, GALLO E, PESCARMONA GP: Red cell metabolism in a case of 3-phosphoglycerate kinase deficiency. *Abstr XIIIth Int Congr Hematol*, Munich, Germany, p 121, 1970

215. HJELM M, WADMAN B: Nonspherocytic haemolytic anaemia with phosphoglycerate kinase deficiency. *Abstr XIIIth Int Congr Hematol*, Munich, Germany, p 121, 1970

216. MIWA S, NAKASHIMA K, ODA S, OGAWA H, NAGAFUJI H, ARIMA M, OKUNA T, NAKASHIMA T: Phosphoglycerate kinase (PGK) deficiency hereditary nonspherocytic hemolytic anemia: Report of a case found in Japanese family. *Acta Haematol Jap* 35:571, 1972

217. ARESE P, BOSIA A, GALLO E, MAZZA U, PESCARMONA GP: Red cell glycolysis in a case of 3-phosphoglycerate kinase deficiency. *Eur J Clin Invest* 3:86, 1973

218. KONRAD PN, MCCARTHY DJ, MAUER AM, VALENTINE WN, PAGLIA DE: Erythrocyte and leukocyte phosphoglycerate kinase deficiency with neurologic disease. *J Pediatr* 82:456, 1973

219. CARTIER P, HABIBI B, LEROUX JP, MARCHAD JC: Anémie hémolytique congénitale associée a un déficit en phosphoglycerate kinase dans les globules rouges, les polynucléaires, et les lymphocytes. *Nouv Rev Fr Hematol* 11:565, 1971

220. HUANG I-Y, FUJII H, YOSHIDA A: Structure and function of normal and variant human phosphoglycerate kinase. *Hemoglobin* 4:601, 1980

221. BOIVIN P, HAKIM J, MANDEREAU J, GALAND G, DEGOS F, SCHAISON G: Déficit en 3-phosphoglycerate kinase érythrocytaire et leucocytaire. Etude des propriétés de l'enzyme, de la fonction phagocytaire des polynucléaires et revise de la litteratura. *Nouv Rev Fr Hematol* 14:495, 1974

222. KRIETSCH WKG, KRIETSCH H, KAISER W, DÜNNWALD M, KUNTZ GWK, DÜHM J, BÜCHER T: Hereditary deficiency of phosphoglycerate kinase: A new variant in erythrocytes and leucocytes, not associated with haemolytic anaemia. *Eur J Clin Invest* 7:427, 1977

223. ROSA R, GEORGE CL, ROSA J: Severe deficiency of red cell phosphoglycerate kinase (PGK) without concomitant hemolysis. *Blood* 54:35a, 1979 (suppl 1) (abstract)

224. KAHN A, COTTREAU O, GALAND C, BOIVIN P: Human erythrocyte phosphoglycerate kinase deficiency. Presence in a deficient patient of a stable variant with lowered catalytic activity. *Clin Chim Acta* 69:21, 1976

225. YOSHIDA A, WATANABE S: Human phosphoglycerate kinase. I Crystallization and characterization of normal enzyme. *J Biol Chem* 247:440, 1972

226. FUJII H, YOSHIDA A: Molecular abnormality of phosphoglycerate kinase-Uppsala associated with chronic nonspherocytic hemolytic anemia. *Proc Natl Acad Sci USA* 77:5461, 1980

227. SCHRÖTER W: 2,3-Diphosphoglyceratstoffwechsel und 2,3-diphosphoglyceratmutase-mangel in erythrozyten. *Blut* 20:311, 1970

228. MIWA S, NISHINA T, KAKEHASHI Y, KITAMURA M, HIRATSUKA A, SHIZUME K: Brief notes. Studies on erythrocyte metabolism in a case with

229. KITAMURA M, IIJIMA N, HASHIMOTO F, HIRATSUKA A: Hereditary deficiency of subunit H of lactate dehydrogenase. *Clin Chim Acta* 34:419, 1971

230. PARR CW, FITCH LI: Inherited quantitative variations of human phosphogluconate dehydrogenase. *Ann Hum Genet* 30:339, 1967

231. BREWER GJ, DERN RJ: A new inherited enzymatic deficiency of human erythrocytes: 6 Phosphogluconate dehydrogenase deficiency. *Am J Hum Genet* 16:472, 1964

232. DERN RJ, BREWER GJ, TASHIAN RE, SHOWS TB: Hereditary variation of erythrocytic 6-phosphogluconate dehydrogenase. *J Lab Clin Med* 67:255, 1966

233. BEUTLER E: Red cell enzyme defects as nondiseases and as diseases. *Blood* 54:1, 1979

234. MILLS GC: The purification and properties of glutathione peroxidase of erythrocytes. *J Biol Chem* 234:502, 1959

235. MILLS GC: Glutathione peroxidase and the destruction of hydrogen peroxide in animal tissues. *Arch Biochem Biophys* 86:1, 1960

236. COHEN G, HOCHSTEIN P: Glutathione peroxidase: The primary agent for the elimination of hydrogen peroxide in erythrocytes. *Biochemistry* 2:1420, 1963

237. PAGLIA DE, VALENTINE WN: Studies on the quantitative and qualitative characterization of erythrocyte glutathione peroxidase. *J Lab Clin Med* 70:158, 1967

238. BOIVIN P, GALAND C, HAKIM J, ROGÉ J, GÚEROULT N: Anémie hémolytique avec déficit en glutathion-peroxydase chez un adulte. *Enzymol Biol Clin* 10:68, 1969

239. BOIVIN P, GALAND C, HAKIM J, BLERY M: Déficit en glutathionperoxydase érythrocytaire et anémie hémolytique médicamenteuse. *Presse Med* 78:171, 1970

240. HOPKINS J, TUDHOPE GR: Glutathione peroxidase in human red cells in health and disease. *Br J Haematol* 25:563, 1973

241. NECHELES TF, MALDONADO N, BARQUET-CHEDIAK A, ALLEN DM: Homozygous erythrocyte glutathione-peroxidase deficiency: Clinical and biochemical studies. *Blood* 33:164, 1969

242. NECHELES TF, STEINBERG MH, CAMERON D: Erythrocyte glutathione-peroxidase deficiency. *Br J Haematol* 19:605, 1970

243. STEINBERG MH, BRAUER MJ, NECHELES TF: Acute hemolytic anemia associated with erythrocyte glutathione-peroxidase deficiency. *Arch Intern Med* 125:302, 1970

244. STEINBERG MH, NECHELES TF: Erythrocyte glutathione peroxidase deficiency. *Am J Med* 50:542, 1971

245. BEUTLER E, MATSUMOTO F: Ethnic variation in red cell glutathione peroxidase activity. *Blood* 46:103, 1975

246. WALLER HD: Glutathione reductase deficiency, in Beutler E (ed): *Hereditary Disorders of Erythrocyte Metabolism*. New York, Grune & Stratton, 1968, p 185

247. BLUME KG, GOTTWIK M, LÖHR GW, RUDIGER HW: Familienuntersuchungen zum glutathionreduktase-mangel menschlicher erythrocyten. *Humangenetik* 6:163, 1968

248. BEUTLER E: Drug-induced hemolytic anemia. *Pharmacol Rev* 21:73, 1969

249. BEUTLER E: Glutathione reductase: Stimulation in normal subjects by riboflavin supplementation. *Science* 165:613, 1969

250. BEUTLER E: Effect of flavin compounds on glutathione reductase activity: In vivo and in vitro studies. *J Clin Invest* 48:1957, 1969

251. BAMJI MS: Glutathione reductase activity in red blood cells and riboflavin nutritional status in humans. *Clin Chim Acta* 26:263, 1969

252. BEUTLER E, SRIVASTAVA SK: Relationship between glutathione reductase activity and drug-induced haemolytic anaemia. *Nature* 226:759, 1970

253. LOOS H, ROOS D, WEENING R, HOUWERZIJL J: Familial deficiency of glutathione reductase in human blood cells. *Blood* 48:53, 1976

254. MOOZ ED, MEISTER A: Tripeptide (glutathione) synthetase. Purification properties, and mechanism of action. *Biochemistry* 6:1722, 1967

255. MAJERUS PW, BRAUNER MJ, SMITH MB, MINNICH V: Glutathione synthesis in human erythrocytes. II. Purification and properties of the enzymes of glutathione biosynthesis. *J Clin Invest* 50:1637, 1971

256. KONRAD PN, RICHARDS F II, VALENTINE WN, PAGLIA DE: γ-Glutamylcysteine synthetase deficiency. A cause of hereditary hemolytic anemia. *N Engl J Med* 286:557, 1972

257. RICHARDS F, COOPER MR, PEARCE LA, COWAN RJ, SPURR CL: Familial spinocerebellar degeneration, hemolytic anemia, and glutathione deficiency. *Arch Intern Med* 134:534, 1974

258. OORT M, LOOS JA, PRINS HK: Hereditary absence of reduced glutathione in the erythrocytes—a new clinical and biochemical entity? *Vox Sang* 6:370, 1961

259. PRINS HK, OORT M, LOOS JA, ZÜRCHER C, BECKERS T: Congenital nonspherocytic hemolytic anemia, associated with glutathione deficiency of the erythrocytes. Hematologic, biochemical and genetic studies. *Blood* 27:145, 1966

260. PRINS HK, LOOS JA, ZÜRCHER C: Glutathione deficiency, in Beutler E (ed): *Hereditary Disorders of Erythrocyte Metabolism*. New York, Grune & Stratton, 1968, p 165

261. BOIVIN P, GALAND C, ANDRÉ R, DEBRAY J: Anémies hémolytiques congénitales avec déficit isolé en glutathion réduit par déficit en glutathion synthétase. *Nouv Rev Fr Hematol* 6:859, 1966

262. BOIVIN P, GALAND C: La synthése du glutathion au cours de l'anémie hémolytique congénitale avec déficit en glutathion réduit. Déficit congénital en glutathion-synthétase érythrocytaire. *Nouv Rev Fr Hematol* 5:707, 1965

263. MOHLER DN, MAJERUS PW, MINNICH V, HESS CE, GARRICK MD: Glutathione synthetase deficiency as a cause of hereditary hemolytic disease. *N Engl J Med* 283:1253, 1970

264. LARSSON A, ZETTERSTROEM R: Pyroglutamic aciduria (5-oxoprolinuria), an inborn error in glutathione metabolism. *Pediatr Res* 8:852, 1974

265. WELLNER VP, SEKURA R, MEISTER A, LARSSON A: Glutathione synthetase deficiency, an inborn error of metabolism involving the gamma-glutamyl cycle in patients with 5-oxoprolinuria (pyroglutamic aciduria). *Proc Natl Acad Sci USA* 71:2505, 1974

266. MARSTEIN S, JELLUM E, HALPERN B, ELDJARN L, PERRY TL: Biochemical study of erythrocytes in a patient with pyroglutamic acidemia (5-oxoprolinemia). *N Engl J Med* 295:406, 1976

267. SPIELBERG SP, GARRICK MD, CORASH LM, BUTLER JD, TIETZE F, ROGERS L, SCHULMAN JD: Biochemical heterogeneity in glutathione synthetase deficiency. *J Clin Invest* 61:1417, 1978

268. ORLOWSKI M, MEISTER A: The γ-glutamyl cycle: A possible transport system for amino acids. *Proc Natl Acad Sci USA* 67:1248, 1970

269. MEISTER A: Glutathione and the γ-glutamyl cycle, in Arias IM, Jacoby WB (eds): *Glutathione: Metabolism and Function*. New York, Raven, 1976, p 35

270. RICHMAN P, MEISTER A: Regulation of γ-glutamyl-cysteine synthetase by nonallosteric feedback inhibition by glutathione. *J Biol Chem* 250:1422, 1975

271. PAGLIA DE, VALENTINE WN: Haemolytic anemia associated with disorders of the purine and pyrimidine salvage pathways. *Clin Haematol* 10:81, 1981.

272. VALENTINE WN, PAGLIA DE, TARTAGLIA AP, GILSANZ F: Hereditary hemolytic anemia with increased red cell adenosine deaminase (45- to 70-fold) and decreased adenosine triphosphate. *Science* 195:783, 1977

273. PAGLIA DE, VALENTINE WN, TARTAGLIA AP, GILSANZ F, SPARKES RS: Control of red blood cell adenine nucleotide metabolism. Studies of adenosine deaminase, in *The Red Cell*. New York, AR Liss, 1978, p 319

274. MIWA S, FUJII H, MATSUMOTO N, NAKATSUJI T, ODA S, ASANO H, ASANO S, MIURA Y: A case of red-cell adenosine deaminase overproduction associated with hereditary hemolytic anemia found in Japan. *Am J Hematol* 5:107, 1978

275. FUJII H, MIWA S, SUZUKI K: Purification and properties of adenosine deaminase in normal and hereditary hemolytic anemia with increased red cell activity. *Hemoglobin* 4:693, 1980

276. HIRSCHHORN R, LEVYTSKA V, POLLARA B, MEUWISSEN HJ: Evidence for control of several different tissue-specific isozymes of adenosine deaminase by a single genetic locus. *Nature [New Biol]* 246:200, 1973

277. HIRSCHHORN R: Conversion of human erythrocyte-adenosine deaminase activity to different tissue-specific isozymes. Evidence for a common catalytic unit. *J Clin Invest* 55:661, 1975

278. TISCHFIELD JA, CREAGAN RP, NICHOLS EA, RUDDLE FH: Assignment of a gene for adenosine deaminase to human chromosome 20. *Hum Hered* 24:1, 1974

279. PARKS RE JR, BROWN PR: Incorporation of nucleosides into the nucleotide pools of human erythrocytes. Adenosine and its analogs. *Biochemistry* 12:3294, 1973

280. AGARWAL RP, PARKS RE JR: A possible association between the nucleoside transport system of human erythrocytes and adenosine deaminase. *Biochem Pharmacol* 24:547, 1975

281. AGARWAL RP, CRABTREE GW, PARKS RE JR, NELSON JR, KEIGHTLEY R, PARKMAN R, ROSEN FS, STERN RS, POLMAR SH: Purine nucleoside metabolism in the erythrocytes of patients with adenosine deaminase deficiency and severe combined immunodeficiency. *J Clin Invest* 57:1025, 1976

282. SCHMALSTIEG FC, GOLDMAN AS, MILLS GC, MONAHAN TM, NELSON JA, GOLDBLUM RM: Nucleotide metabolism in adenosine deaminase deficiency. *Pediatr Res* 10:393, 1976

283. COHEN A, HIRSCHHORN R, HOROWITZ SD, RUBENSTEIN A, POLMAR SH, HONG R, MARTIN DW JR: Deoxyadenosine triphosphate as a potentially toxic metabolite in adenosine deaminase deficiency. *Proc Natl Acad Sci USA* 75:472, 1978

284. COLEMAN MS, DONOFRIO J, HUTTON JJ, HAHN L: Identification and quantitation of adenine deoxynucleotides in erythrocytes of a patient with adenosine deaminase deficiency and severe combined immunodeficiency. *J Biol Chem* 253:1619, 1978

285. NELSON JA, KUTTESCH JF, GOLDBLUM RM, GOLDMAN AS, SCHMALSTIEG FC: Analysis of adenosine and adenine nucleotides in severe combined immunodeficiency disease, in Baer HP, Drummond GI (eds): *Physiological and Regulatory Functions of Adenosine and Adenine Nucleotides*. New York, Raven, 1979, p 417

286. SZEINBERG A, GAVENDO S, CAHANE D: Erythrocyte adenylate-kinase deficiency. *Lancet* 1:315, 1969

287. SZEINBERG A, KAHANA D, GAVENDO S, ZAIDMAN J, BEN-EZZER J: Hereditary deficiency of adenylate kinase in red blood cells. *Acta Haematol* 42:111, 1969

288. BOIVIN P, GALAND C, HAKIM J, SIMONY D, SELIGMAN M: Un nouvelle érythroenzymopathie. Anémie hémolytique congénitale non sphérocytaire et déficit héréditaire en adénylate-kinase érythrocytaire. *Presse Med* 79:215, 1971

289. PAGLIA DE, VALENTINE WN: Hereditary and acquired defects in the pyrimidine nucleotidase of human erythrocytes. *Curr Top Hematol* 3:75, 1980

290. PAGLIA DE, VALENTINE WN: Characteristics of a pyrimidine-specific 5'-nucleotidase in human erythrocytes. *J Biol Chem* 250:7973, 1975

291. VALENTINE WN, FINK K, PAGLIA DE, HARRIS SR, ADAMS WS: Hereditary hemolytic anemia with human erythrocyte pyrimidine 5'-nucleotidase deficiency. *J Clin Invest* 54:866, 1974

292. PAGLIA DE, VALENTINE WM, DAHLGREN JG: Effects of low-level lead exposure on pyrimidine 5'-nucleotidase and other erythrocyte enzymes. Possible role of primidine 5'-nucleotidase in the pathogenesis of lead-induced anemia. *J Clin Invest* 56:1164, 1975

293. VALENTINE WN, PAGLIA DE, FINK K, MADOKORO G: Lead poisoning. Association with hemolytic anemia, basophilic stippling, erythrocyte pyrimidine 5'-nucleotidase deficiency, and intraerythrocytic accumulation of pyrimidines. *J Clin Invest* 58:926, 1976

294. PAGLIA DE, VALENTINE WN, FINK K: Lead poisoning. Further observations on erythrocyte pyrimidine-nucleotidase deficiency and intracellular accumulation of pyrimidine nucleotides. *J Clin Invest* 60:1362, 1977

295. BUC HA, KAPLAN J-C: Red-cell pyrimidine 5'-nucleotidase and lead poisoning. *Clin Chim Acta* 87:49, 1978

296. MEISTER A: Glutathione and the γ-glytamyl cycle, in Arias IM, Jacoby WB (eds): *Glutathione: Metabolism and Function*. New York, Raven, 1976, p 34

297. RICHMAN P, MEISTER A: Regulation of γ-glutamyl-cysteine synthetase by nonallosteric feedback inhibition by glutathione. *J Biol Chem* 250:1422, 1975

298. VALENTINE WN, PAGLIA DE: The primary cause of hemolysis in enzymopathies of anaerobic glycolysis: A viewpoint. *Blood Cells* 6:819, 1980

299. BEUTLER E: A commentary. *Blood Cells* 6:827, 1980

300. BONKOWSKY HO, BLOOMER JR, EBERT PS, MAHONEY MJ: Heme synthetase deficiency in human protoporphyria: Demonstration of the defect in liver and cultured skin fibroblasts. *J Clin Invest* 56:1139, 1975

301. HARVALD B, HANEL KH, SQUIRES R, TRAP-JENSEN J: Adenosine-triphosphatase deficiency in patients with non-spherocytic haemolytic anaemia. *Lancet* 2:18, 1964

302. COTTE J, KISSIN C, MATHIEU M, PONCET J, MONNET P, SALLE B, GERMAIN D: Observation d'un cas de déficit partiel en ATPase intraérythrocytaire. *Rev Fr Etud Clin Biol* 13:284, 1968

303. SCHWARTZ JM, JAFFÉ ER: Hereditary methemoglobinemia with deficiency of NADH dehydrogenase, in Stanbury JB, Wyngaarden JB, Fredrickson DS (eds): *The Metabolic Basis of Inherited Disease*, 4th ed. New York, McGraw-Hill, 1978, p 1452

304. WADA Y, NISHIMURA Y, TANABU M, YOSHIMURA I, IINUMA K, YOSHIDA T, ARAKAWA T: Hypouricemic, mentally retarded infant with a defect of 5-phosphoribosyl-1-pyrophosphate synthetase of erythrocytes. *Tohoku J Exp Med* 113:149, 1974

305. KELLEY WN, SMITH LH JR: Hereditary orotic aciduria, in Stanbury JB, Wyngaarden JB, Fredrickson DS (eds): *The Metabolic Basis of Inherited Disease*, 4th ed. New York, McGraw-Hill, 1978, p 1045

306. SEEGMILLER JE, ROSENBLOOM FM, KELLEY WN: An enzyme defect associated with a sex-linked human neurological disorder and excessive purine synthesis. *Science* 155:1682, 1967

307. VAN ACKER KJ, SIMMONDS HA, POTTER C, CAMERON JS: Complete deficiency of adenine phosphoribosyltransferase. *N Engl J Med* 297:127, 1977

308. GIBLETT ER, ANDERSON JE, COHEN F, POLLARA B, MEUWISSEN HJ: Adenosinedeaminase deficiency in two patients with severely impaired cellular immunity. *Lancet* 2:1067, 1972

309. GIBLETT ER, AMMANN AJ, WARA DW, SANDMAN R, DIAMOND LK: Nucleoside phosphorylase deficiency in a child with severely defective T-cell immunity and normal B-cell immunity. *Lancet* 1:1010, 1975

310. ISSELBACHER KJ, ANDERSON EP, KURAHASHI K, KALCKAR HM: Congenital galactosemia, a single enzymatic block in galactose metabolism. *Science* 123:635, 1956

311. SHIH VE: Urea cycle disorders and other congenital hyperammonemic syndromes, in Stanbury JB, Wyngaarden JB, Fredrickson DS (eds): *The Met-*

abolic Basis of Inherited Disease, 4th ed. New York, McGraw-Hill, 1978, p 362

312. TAKAHARA S: Acatalasemia and hypocatalasemia in the Orient. *Semin Hematol* 8:397, 1971

313. VALENTINE WN, PAGLIA DE, NEERHOUT RC, KONRAD PN: Erythrocyte glyoxalase II deficiency with coincidental hereditary elliptocytosis. *Blood* 36:797, 1970

314. VANDERHEIDEN BS: Genetic studies of human erythrocyte inosine triphosphatase. *Biochem Genet* 3:289, 1969

315. JOHNS R: Familial reduction in red cell cholinesterase. *N Engl J Med* 267:1344, 1962

316. SHINOHARA K, TANAKA KR: Hereditary deficiency of erythrocyte acetylcholinesterase. *Am J Hematol* 7:313, 1979

317. MIYAGI K, KANESHIMA M, KAWAKAMI J, NAKADA F, PETRYKA ZJ, WATSON CJ: Uroporphyrinogen I synthase from human erythrocytes: Separation purification, and properties of isozymes. *Proc Natl Acad Sci USA* 76:6172, 1979

74

GLUCOSE-6-PHOSPHATE DEHYDROGENASE DEFICIENCY

ERNEST BEUTLER

1. *Glucose-6-phosphate dehydrogenase (G-6-PD) deficiency was discovered as a result of investigation of the hemolytic effect of the antimalarial drug primaquine. G-6-PD-deficient persons also develop hemolytic anemia when exposed to certain sulfonamides, acetanilid, phenacetin, Furadantin, and a variety of other drugs. Hemolysis may occur during infection, diabetic acidosis, in the neonatal period, or, in some persons, upon ingestion of fava beans.*

2. *In the absence of an efficient NADPH-generating system erythrocytes are unable to maintain GSH in the reduced state when subjected to an oxidative stress. As a consequence the enzyme-deficient cells are unable to reduce peroxides by way of the glutathione peroxidase system. Accumulating peroxide and GSSG may produce the cellular damage which ultimately leads to shortening of red blood cell life span.*

3. *The gene for G-6-PD is sex linked. Female heterozygotes for G-6-PD deficiency have two populations of red cells, cells with normal enzyme activity and those with deficient enzyme activity.*

4. *G-6-PD deficiency can readily be detected in red cells through an NADP-linked assay or through a variety of screening tests. G-6-PD deficiency is widely distributed in the populations of the world. One of the factors that may cause the high incidence of this abnormality*
to be maintained in some populations is its protective effect against falciparum malaria.

5. *There are many genetic variants of G-6-PD. Some have normal activity and are of interest primarily as genetic markers. The more common of the deficient variants include G-6-PD A− (found in African populations), G-6-PD Mediterranean (found in Greeks, Sephardic Jews, and other Mediterranean populations), and G-6-PD Canton (found in Chinese subjects). Less common are the functionally severely deficient variants of G-6-PD that cause nonspherocytic hereditary hemolytic anemia. Two mutant forms of G-6-PD have been fingerprinted, and amino acid substitutions identified. The partial amino acid sequence of normal G-6-PD has been established. The clinical manifestations of G-6-PD deficiency are almost entirely confined to its effect on the erythrocytes.*

Glucose-6-phosphate dehydrogenase (G-6-PD) deficiency is the most common disease-producing enzyme deficiency of human beings. G-6-PD is subject to many different mutations. Some of these cause a deficiency of enzyme activity in erythrocytes, leading to hemolytic anemia. Others are electrophoretically detectable mutations, without significant deficiency or clinical effect. Because the gene for G-6-PD is X-linked, the product of a single gene can be isolated in pure form from the tissues of males, facilitating its biochemical characterization. This favorable combination of circumstances not only has caused G-6-PD mutations to be of great interest to the clinician, but also has made them an important tool of the cell biologist, the biochemist, and the population geneticist.

HISTORY

G-6-PD deficiency was discovered as a result of investigations of the hemolytic anemia induced in some individuals by the antimalarial drug primaquine (see [1] for references). Hemolytic anemia following the administration of the 8-aminoquinoline antimalarial pamaquine was first reported in 1926. In the subsequent quarter century, many additional reports were published. Characteristically, the patient developed dark, often black, urine a few days after pamaquine therapy was begun. Jaundice appeared, and the red blood cell count and hemoglobin level fell abruptly. The patient usually recovered but sometimes succumbed to massive destruction of red blood cells. Early attempts to understand why some individuals developed severe hemolytic anemia when they received pamaquine while others suffered no untoward hematologic effects were unsuccessful. Immunologic investigations and fragility studies failed to shed any light on the origin of pamaquine sensitivity. Nor did in vitro incubations of red cells of susceptible individuals with pamaquine or with plasma of patients who had recently received the drug clarify the cause of the sensitivity. Nevertheless, some observations were made which in retrospect were significant. As early as 1928, Heinz bodies, which consist largely of hemoglobin denaturation products, were noted in the red cells of a patient with pamaquine-induced hemolysis (Fig. 74-1). Attention was called to the familial nature of pamaquine sensitivity, and by 1948 analogies had been drawn between this disorder and favism. Many observers recognized the differences in susceptibility to pamaquine-induced hemolysis of persons of different racial origin.

It was not until the introduction of primaquine, a therapeutically more effective 8-aminoquinoline antimalarial, that it became possible to study intensively the hemolytic anemia induced by these compounds. The demonstration that sensitivity to primaquine was due to an intrinsic abnormality of the red blood cell was the starting point for these investigations. The biochemistry of primaquine-sensitive cells suggested that their susceptibility to hemolysis was related in some way to the content and stability of their glutathione (GSH). Examination of the pathways of GSH metabolism in drug-sensitive red cells disclosed the primary defect, a deficiency of G-6-PD. Subsequent observations established that the red cells of patients with favism and of some patients with nonspherocytic hemolytic anemia also were deficient in G-6-PD activity. It gradually became apparent that there were many different varieties of G-6-PD deficiency, which could be distinguished from one another by biochemical examination of the residual enzyme. Standardization of techniques for characterization of G-6-PD variants has been established by a World Health Organization scientific group [2], and the recommendations of this group have been generally adopted. There has also been international agreement about the nomenclature of G-6-PD variants. In general, they are designated by geographical names based on the place of origin. Exceptions were made in the case of variants

such as A− and A, the names of which had already become well-ingrained in the literature. All of the variants are divided into five classes according to degree of enzyme deficiency and clinical manifestations, class I representing the most severely deficient variants, associated with nonspherocytic hemolytic anemia, and class V designating variants with increased activity. The most common types are the relatively mild deficiency found in persons of African ancestry (the A− type), the more severe deficiency found in persons of Mediterranean origin (the Mediterranean type), and the Canton and Hong Kong-Pokfulam types found in Asia. Less common deficiency variants have been described in laboratories throughout the world.

CLINICAL ASPECTS

G-6-PD Deficiency without Nonspherocytic Hemolytic Anemia

Mild G-6-PD Deficiency The common A− type of G-6-PD deficiency found in persons of African origin may be considered the prototype of "mild" G-6-PD deficiency. Individuals with this type of G-6-PD deficiency are essentially asymptomatic except under stress, such as that imposed by drug administration, infection, diabetic acidosis, and, possibly, the neonatal period. A somewhat anomalous finding is that the deformability of G-6-PD-deficient red cells seems to be greater than that of normal cells. Moreover, incubation with acetylphenylhydrazine, while decreasing the deformability of G-6-PD-deficient red cells, has less effect on these cells than it does on normal erythrocytes. [3]

The clinical course of primaquine-induced hemolysis has been studied under carefully controlled conditions [4] in males with the A− type of G-6-PD deficiency. When 30 mg primaquine is given daily, there is little or no evidence of hemolysis during the first 2 or 3 days. Then the urine begins to turn dark. In mild cases, the patient commonly observes no other abnormality; in more severe cases the patient complains of weakness

Figure 74-1 Heinz bodies in erythrocytes from a G-6-PD-deficient person. These particles of denatured protein, adhering to the red cell membrane and staining with basic dyes, are found in the red cells of G-6-PD-deficient individuals after drug exposure. They are found in normal or G-6-PD-deficient red cells after incubation with certain "oxidant" chemicals in vitro. The pattern shown is characteristic of G-6-PD-deficient red cells which have been incubated with acetylphenylhydrazine.

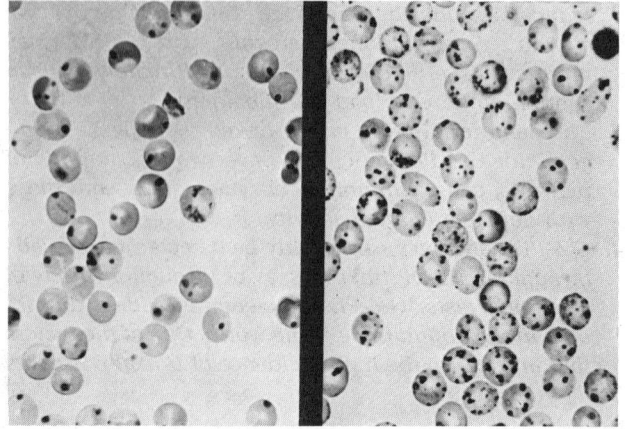

and of abdominal and back pain and develops icterus and black urine. Heinz bodies appear in many of the red cells [5]; the hemoglobin, red blood count, and hematocrit levels fall rapidly, and the number of reticulocytes increases. This "acute hemolytic phase" ends spontaneously in about 1 week, even when drug administration is continued, and the "recovery phase" begins. The patient feels better, the color of the urine becomes normal, and the hemoglobin, red cell, and hematocrit values begin to rise. The reticulocyte count remains high at first and then declines. Throughout the period of drug administration the Coombs' test result is negative, and red cell fragility remains unaltered. The main morphologic changes in the blood are polychromasia and the appearance of Heinz bodies in the red cells during the first stages of hemolysis. Finally, the peripheral blood picture returns to normal, and the symptoms vanish, even when administration of the drug is continued in the same dosage that initially caused hemolysis. The refractory state which develops in G-6-PD deficiency is not due to altered metabolism of the drug but rather to an alteration in reactivity of the red cell population [4].

Sensitivity to the hemolytic action of primaquine is a function of red cell age [5]. There is a marked decrease in red cell G-6-PD activity with increasing cell age, even in normal cells, and the decline in activity is accelerated in red cells with the A− type enzyme [6–8]. The relatively normal enzyme levels in younger cells of G-6-PD A− subjects [6–8] provide some degree of protection against drug-induced hemolysis.

Acetanilid, sulfanilamide, diaphenylsulfone, and a number of other drugs [9, 10] have also been given under controlled laboratory conditions to subjects known to be G-6-PD-deficient. In addition, there are many case reports of hemolytic anemia induced accidentally by various other chemicals [1] in Afro-Americans who were G-6-PD-deficient or who, on clinical grounds, may be presumed to have been. The hemolytic anemia induced by these drugs is similar to that induced by primaquine. Hemolysis induced by thiazolsulfone may vary greatly in intensity. Studies of the mechanism of this variability suggest that it is due to differences in absorption or metabolism of the drug [9]. Many lists of drugs purported to produce hemolytic anemia in persons with G-6-PD deficiency have been published. These lists generally include innocuous drugs which have been erroneously implicated for various reasons. For example, dipyrine has been mentioned [11] as one of the several components of a proprietary drug ingested by a patient who developed hemolytic anemia. As a consequence, it was commonly included in the tabulations of hemolytic drugs. Aspirin, too, is usually included in lists which are proscribed in patients with a G-6-PD deficiency. Yet, the administration of 3.6 g of aspirin daily did not produce hemolysis of G-6-PD A−
[51]chromium-labeled cells [12], and doses ranging from 4 to 12 g a day produced only very mild destruction of G-6-PD A− cells [13]. Extensive analysis of clinical data [14] exonerates aspirin as a hemolytic agent in the severe Mediterranean type of deficiency. Why, then, is aspirin so frequently included as a hemolytic agent? Probably because of a misinterpretation of the clinical significance of data in which huge doses of aspirin were administered and because of cases in which hemolysis associated with aspirin administration [15] was probably actually a consequence of infection rather than of drug administration. Critical analysis makes it possible to list drugs that do (Table 74-1) and do not (Table 74-2) produce clinically significant hemolytic anemia when given to G-6-PD-deficient subjects in normal therapeutic doses.

Infections and diabetic acidosis also can precipitate hemo-

Table 74-1 Drugs and chemicals that have clearly been shown to cause clinically significant hemolytic anemia in G-6-PD deficiency*

Acentanilid	Primaquine
Methylene blue	Sulfacetamide
Nalidixic acid (NeGram)	Sulfamethoxazole (Gantanol)
Naphthalene	Sulfanilamide
Niridazole (Ambilhar)	Sulfapyridine
Nitrofurantoin (Furadantin)	Thiazolesulfone
Pamaquine	Toluidine blue
Pentaquine	Trinitrotoluene (TNT)
Phenylhydrazine	

* References given in Beutler [16].

lytic reactions in those with the A− type of G-6-PD deficiency [17–21]. It has been suggested that neonatal icterus may be due to G-6-PD A− [22–29], but this has not been observed uniformly [30, 31] and appears to be most common in the black population outside the United States. Severe azotemia has been reported to occur in patients who undergo hemolysis when they also have renal infection [32].

Severe G-6-PD Deficiency The Mediterranean type of G-6-PD deficiency may be considered to be the prototype of severe G-6-PD deficiency without nonspherocytic hemolytic anemia. Most patients with G-6-PD deficiency of the Mediterranean type also do not manifest clinical signs or symptoms unless exposed to drugs. Contact with the fava bean [33–36] and infections [37, 38] also induce hemolytic crises. Jaundice is particularly severe when G-6-PD-deficient subjects contract hepatitis [39–47]. On occasion, hemolysis occurs in persons with the Mediterranean defect even when there is no known inciting cause [48–51], and hemolysis has occurred in the course of a surgical procedure [52]. Renal failure may result from hemolysis [53, 54]. Neonatal icterus occurs in G-6-PD-deficient infants among several Mediterranean and Oriental populations [55–64] and is not necessarily associated with evidence of hemolytic anemia [64]. It may lead to fatal kernicterus.

In general, the clinical course of hemolysis is similar to that in subjects with the A− type of deficiency, but it may be somewhat more severe [65–67] and is not self-limited [36, 68]. At least one drug, chloramphenicol, which failed to cause hemolysis in persons with the A− type of G-6-PD deficiency [12] and the Canton type of deficiency [69], has produced hemolysis in some Caucasians with G-6-PD deficiency [70–72]. The spectrum of drugs which cause hemolysis in subjects with the Mediterranean type of deficiency is broader than that affecting individuals with the A− type of defect. Fava bean-induced hemolysis does not seem to occur with the A− type of defect but may occur within hours of contact with fava beans in Mediterranean [35], Chinese [73], and Thai [74] subjects with G-6-PD deficiency and is often more severe than primaquine-induced hemolysis.

G-6-PD Deficiency with Hereditary Nonspherocytic Hemolytic Anemia

In contrast to patients with the common forms of G-6-PD deficiency, some patients with rare and usually unstable or kinetically grossly abnormal variants of G-6-PD have the clinical syndrome of hereditary nonspherocytic hemolytic anemia.

Table 74-2 Drugs that can probably be given safely in normal therapeutic doses to G-6-PD-deficient subjects without nonspherocytic hemolytic anemia*

Acetaminophen (paracetamol, Tylenol, Tralgon, hydroxyacetanilid)	p-Aminobenzoic acid
	Phenylbutazone
	Phenytoin
Acetophenetidine (phenacetin)	Probenecid (Benemid)
Acetylsalicylic acid (aspirin)	Procainamide hydrochloride (Pronestyl)
Aminopyrine (Pyramidon, amidopyrine)	Pyrimeythamine (Daraprim)
Antazoline (Anistine)	Quinidine
Antipyrine	Quinine
Ascorbic acid (vitamin C)	Streptomycin
Benzhexol (Artane)	Sulfacytine
Chloramphenicol	Sulfadiazine
Chlorguanide (Proguanil, Paludrine)	Sulfaguanidine
	Sulfamerazine
Chloroquine	Sulfamethoxypyridazine (Kynex)
Colchicine	Sulfisoxazole (Gantrisin)
Diphenylhydramine (Benedryl)	Trimethoprim
Isoniazide	Tripelennamine (Pyribenzamine)
L-Dopa	Vitamin K
Menadione sodium bisulfite (Hykinone)	
Menapthone	

* References given in Beutler [16].

These patients manifest varying degrees of anemia and reticulocytosis, even in the absence of drug administration. The osmotic fragility of red cells is normal, and the appearance of the erythrocytes on the blood film does not suggest the presence of spherocytosis. In most cases, the anemia is mild. Often, neonatal jaundice is present, and increased hemolysis is commonly associated with drug administration and infections. Favism was observed in one patient [75]. The spleen is often somewhat enlarged, but splenectomy does not usually appear to be beneficial.

The degree of enzyme deficiency in some of these patients may be very severe, but hereditary nonspherocytic hemolytic anemia due to G-6-PD deficiency has also been noted in some instances when the residual G-6-PD activity, assayed under standard conditions, has exceeded the level of residual enzyme found in the A− type of deficiency. In some instances the enzyme is presumably much less effective metabolically than it appears to be from assays in vitro. This may be because of abnormal kinetic properties of the enzyme, such as increased sensitivity to inhibition by NADPH (see "Biochemistry of G-6-PD-Deficient Erythrocytes" below).

RED CELL METABOLISM

Overall Erythrocyte Glucose Metabolism

Glucose serves as the primary energy source of the erythrocyte. After phosphorylation of glucose to glucose-6-phosphate in the hexokinase reaction, two alternate pathways of further metabolism are available. The major metabolic route is the Embden-Meyerhof pathway, discussed in greater detail in Chap. 73. This pathway serves to supply the erythrocyte with

ATP to power the ion pumps and to phosphorylate membrane proteins and with NADH to maintain hemoglobin in the reduced form. It is also the pathway in which 2,3-diphosphoglycerate, an important physiologic modulator of the oxygen dissociation curve of hemoglobin, is formed. The second metabolic pathway that glucose-6-phosphate may traverse is the hexose monophosphate (HMP) shunt. This pathway serves to supply the erythrocyte with NADPH, maintaining glutathione in the reduced state, and with five carbon sugars required for the synthesis of nucleotides.

Reactions of the Hexose Monophosphate Pathway

G-6-PD catalyzes the first step in the HMP pathway, the oxidation of glucose-6-phosphate to 6-phosphogluconolactone by NADP, which is reduced to NADPH. The 6-phosphogluconolactone hydrolyzes spontaneously to 6-phosphogluconate, which serves as substrate for 6-phosphogluconate dehydrogenase and NADP. 6-Phosphogluconate is oxidized to ribulose-6-phosphate and carbon dioxide, with the reduction of NADP to NADPH. Further steps in the pathway include isomerization of ribulose-5-phosphate to ribose-5-phosphate and to xylulose-5-phosphate and a series of intermolecular rearrangements, catalyzed by transketolase and transaldolase. Finally, fructose-6-phosphate and glyceraldehyde-3-phosphate, intermediates in the Embden-Meyerhof pathway, are produced.

Regulation of the HMP Pathway

In the unstressed, normal erythrocyte approximately 10 percent of the glucose-6-phosphate is metabolized by way of the HMP pathway, while the other 90 percent follows the Embden-Meyerhof pathway of anaerobic glycolysis [76]. The main regulatory step of HMP metabolism is the G-6-PD reaction. The rate of metabolism by way of the HMP pathway can vary greatly, depending principally upon the rate of NADPH oxidation, on the one hand, and on the activity of G-6-PD (in the case of deficient mutants), on the other.

When assayed under optimal conditions, normal erythrocyte G-6-PD has the capacity to oxidize approximately 3 μmol glucose-6-phosphate per milliliter of red cells per minute, a rate which is about 100 times that at which red cells normally metabolize glucose. The G-6-PD reaction obviously proceeds at a rate much lower than the maximal one within the intact erythrocyte. When assayed under optimal conditions, even mildly or moderately deficient variants, such as G-6-PD A−, can oxidize glucose-6-phosphate much more rapidly than the rate observed in maximally stimulated normal cells. The kinetic properties of G-6-PD explain the relatively low rate of oxidation of glucose-6-phosphate in intact red cells. In resting cells the enzyme is markedly inhibited by NADPH [77–80], and the normal level of NADP is well below the K_m of the enzyme even if the competitive inhibitor, NADPH, were not present. Furthermore, the level of glucose-6-P in normal erythrocytes is under that required for maximal G-6-PD activity, and ATP, at physiologic concentrations, is a competitive inhibitor of G-6-PD with respect to glucose-6-phosphate [81, 82].

Because of the manner in which the intracellular G-6-PD reaction is regulated, the rate of metabolism by way of the HMP is easily altered. This is accomplished primarily by circumstances that result in the oxidation of NADPH to NADP, such as the oxidation of GSH to GSSG, relieving inhibition of G-6-PD and increasing the availability of one of the two limiting substrates. It appears that even if the NADP/NADPH ratio and other inhibitory effects on the rate of G-6-PD activity are taken into account, the G-6-PD reaction occurs more slowly in intact cells than predicted from the known kinetic properties of the enzyme [83]. The reason for this discrepancy is unknown, but the effect is greatest at low NADP concentrations and is observed, although to a limited extent, in resealed erythrocytes [84].

Red cells contain the enzyme NADPH diaphorase, which catalyzes the oxidation of NADPH when a suitable receptor, such as methylene blue, toluidine blue, Nile blue, or brilliant cresyl blue, is available. The physiologic role of this pathway is unclear, since the absence of NADPH diaphorase, demonstrated in a single subject, was not accompanied by any clinical abnormality [85]. However, this pathway of NADPH oxidation can be useful because the reduced dye reacts nonenzymatically [86] with methemoglobin, reducing it to hemoglobin. Thus, catalytic amounts of these dyes, either injected intravenously into patients or placed in in vitro systems, greatly hasten the rate of methemoglobin reduction in normal red cells. This phenomenon is the basis of the treatment of toxic methemoglobinemia with methylene blue and the use of methylene blue in various screening tests for G-6-PD deficiency (see below). However, methylene blue precipitates hemolytic anemia in G-6-PD-deficient subjects [87] because the oxidation of NADPH, which is mediated by NADPH diaphorase in the presence of dyes, deprives the G-6-PD-deficient cells of much-needed NADPH.

Very high concentrations of glucose are known to increase metabolism by way of the hexose monophosphate pathway [88]. This is achieved through the enzyme L-hexonate dehydrogenase, which catalyzes the oxidation of NADPH and the reduction of glucose to sorbitol [89]. Pyruvate exerts a similar effect through lactic dehydrogenase which, particularly at low pH levels and high pyruvate levels, is not entirely specific for the NAD/NADH system, but can also function with the NADP/NADPH system [90, 91].

Pyrroline-5-carboxylate also stimulates the HMP of intact red cells [92]. It exerts this effect through the NADPH-linked enzyme pyrroline-5-carboxylase reductase which reduces it to proline, oxidizing NADPH in the process.

Glutathione

The maintenance of glutathione in the reduced state (GSH) is probably the most important function of the HMP pathway.

Structure and Function Glutathione is a tripeptide of glutamic acid, cysteine, and glycine. It differs from most other oligopeptides in that the bond between the glutamic acid and cysteine involves the γ-carboxyl group of glutamic acid, rather than the α-carboxyl group.

Almost all the nonprotein sulfhydryl groups of erythrocytes are in the form of glutathione [93]. In the steady state, about 99.8 percent of the glutathione is reduced (GSH); only about 0.2 percent is in the oxidized form (GSSG) [94-96]. A number of red cell enzymes, such as hexokinase, glyceraldehyde-phosphate dehydrogenase, and glutathione reductase, have active sulfhydryl groups, and hemoglobin has an exposed sulfhydryl

group at the β-93 position. These -SH groups are maintained in the reduced form, at least in part, by the action of red cell GSH. How GSH performs this function is not entirely clear, but it may do so either by reducing mixed disulfides which have formed or by forming mixed disulfides (protein-S-SG) which can subsequently be reduced by the action of glutathione reductase and NADPH (see below).

The red cell has the enzymatic apparatus for the two steps required for the synthesis of glutathione: γ-glutamyl synthetase and glutathione synthetase [94-96]. Deficiencies of each of these enzymes have been described [95, 97, 98]. They result in marked deficiency of red cell GSH and in a mild hemolytic anemia which resembles in many respects that observed in G-6-PD deficiency. Although it has been proposed [99] that the other enzymes of the γ-glutamyl cycle (described in Chap. 17) exist in erythrocytes, careful investigations of leukocyte-free erythrocyte preparations have failed to disclose the presence of at least one of the key enzymes of this cycle, γ-glutamyl transpeptidase [100, 101]. Moreover, treatment of red cells with a substrate for this enzyme fails to result in the hydrolysis of GSH [102].

Glutathione is rapidly synthesized in mature erythrocytes. Since its level in circulating erythrocytes remains constant, the erythrocyte must possess a means for disposal of glutathione. Indeed, human erythrocyte glutathione has been found to turn over with a half-time of approximately 4 days [103]. The in vivo turnover of red cell glutathione can be accounted for by the energy-dependent outward transport of GSSG from the erythrocyte [104-107]. Evidence has been presented that in tissues other than the erythrocyte GSH may be transported from one cell to another, presumably through the blood plasma [108]. The enzyme γ-glutamyl transpeptidase may be involved in such transport; when this enzyme is inhibited or genetically absent, glutathione is excreted in the urine [109, 110].

Oxidation and Reduction Probably the most important role of NADPH in erythrocytes is the reduction of oxidized glutathione to reduced glutathione by way of the glutathione reductase (GR) reaction:

$$\text{GSSG} + \text{NADPH} + \text{H}^+ \xrightarrow{\text{GR}} 2 \text{ GSH} + \text{NADP}^+$$

and the reduction of mixed disulfides of glutathione and proteins (Pr), particularly hemoglobin [111], by the same enzyme:

$$\text{Pr-S-SG} + \text{NADPH} + \text{H}^+ \xrightarrow{\text{GR}} \text{Pr} + \text{GSH} + \text{NADP}^+$$

GSSG and protein-S-SG disulfides are therefore important regulators of the hexose monophosphate pathway [112]. Indeed, red cell GSH is constantly being oxidized in the glutathione peroxidase (GSH-Px) reaction,

$$2 \text{ GSH} + \text{R-O-OH} \xrightarrow{\text{GSH-Px}} \text{GSSG} + \text{H}_2\text{O} + \text{R-OH}$$

in which GSH rids the erythrocyte of potentially damaging hydrogen and organic peroxides. Hydrogen peroxide may arise in the erythrocyte through the action of superoxide dismutase [113] acting upon superoxide radicals formed from oxyhemoglobin:

$$\text{O}_2^- + 2\text{H}_2\text{O} \xrightarrow{\text{superoxide dismutase}} 2\text{H}_2\text{O}_2 + e^-$$

Glutathione may also be oxidized by peroxihemoglobin formed by the reaction of hemoglobin with the drug [114-116].

In vitro, compounds such as primaquine, phenylhydrazine,

and ascorbic acid greatly increase the rate of HMP metabolism of normal erythrocytes. They do so by increasing the rate of oxidation of GSH to GSSG, probably by generating peroxides [117]. The availability of GSSG as substrate for the glutathione reductase reaction results in formation of NADP. With the lowering of NADPH levels and the increase of NADP levels, the inhibition of G-6-PD is relieved, and glucose-6-phosphate is oxidized at a higher rate.

Normal G-6-PD

Erythrocyte G-6-PD has been prepared in highly purified form [77, 78, 118–126] and has been crystallized and fingerprinted [127, 128]. The G-6-PD molecule appears to consist of several identical [129] subunits, each with a molecular weight of 55,000. The enzyme polymer contains tightly bound NADP [130, 131], and, when this is removed, G-6-PD dissociates into monomeric units, which are enzymatically inactive [119, 132]. Activity can be restored by incubating with traces of NADP. Hybridization of the enzyme has been accomplished with rat and human [133, 134], rat and cow [133], and different

human variants [135]. The molecular weight of G-6-PD has been estimated variously at 190,000 [121], 105,000 [119], and 240,000 [118]. It apparently exists in several different aggregational states [130], but in vivo it is probably a dimer with a molecular weight in the range of 105,000 to 120,000 [136]. The amino acid composition of the enzyme has been determined [128], and most of the sequence has been determined (Fig. 74-2). The enzyme contains approximately 18 sulfhydryl groups per dimer and probably contains no S-S bridges. The exposed sulfhydryl groups are essential for enzyme activity [137]. A histidine residue may be important in the catalytic activity of G-6-PD [138].

The Michaelis constant (K_m) of red cell G-6-PD for glucose-6-phosphate is 35 to 60 μM [2, 139, 140]. The K_m for NADP is very low, and therefore difficult to measure accurately, but seems to be in the range of 2 to 4 μM. On the basis of equilibrium dialysis studies using ^{14}C-labeled NADP and NADPH [79], it was concluded that the dimeric enzyme associated with one molecule of NADP with a dissociation constant 1.7 × 10^{-7} M at 37°C. The same binding site can be occupied, instead, by a molecule of NADPH, which is bound with a dissociation constant of 4.9 × 10^{-7} M. Although it has been

Figure 74-2 The amino acid sequence of normal human glucose-6-phosphate dehydrogenase. Residues enclosed in parentheses require sequencing. Sequences enclosed in brackets require confirmation.

1   10   20

Pyro-Glu-Met-Asn-Ala-Leu-His-Lei-Gly-Ser-Glu-Ala-Asn-Arg-Leu-Phe-Tyr-Leu-Ala-Leu-Pro-Pro-Thr-Val-Tyr-Glu-Ala-Val-Thr-
  30   40   50

Lys-Asn-Ile-Glu-(His,Cys,Asp,Ser,Ser,Glu,Gly)-Arg-Ile-Val-Glu-Lys-Pro-Phe-Gly-Arg-Lys-Ser-Arg-Lys-Asp-Leu-Gln-Ser-Ser-
  60   70   80

Asp-Arg-Leu-Asp-Phe-Glu-His-Ser-Glu-Lys-Asp-Ser-Tyr-Val-Ala-Gly-Gln-Tyr-Asp-Ser-Ala-Ser-Tyr-Gln-Arg-Leu-Ser-Asn-His-
  90   100   110

Ile-Ser-Ser-Leu-Phe-Arg-Ile-Asp-His-Tyr-Leu-Gly-Lys-Glu-Asp-Glu-Ile-Tyr-Arg-Leu-Lys-Leu-Glu-Asp-Phe-Phe-Ala-Arg-Ala-
  120   130   140

Arg-Ala-Thr-Pro-Glu-Glu-Trp-Lys-[His-Asp-Leu-Cys-Ser-Met-Val-Gln-Gly-Asn-Leu-Met-Thr-Pro-Gly-Phe-His-Glu-Ile-Ser-Gly-
                      160

(Asx,Thr,Glx, Glx,Glx,Ala,Ala,Val,Ile,Phe)-Lys]-Val-Gly-Val-Gly-Pro-Gly-Met-Val-Cys-Thr-Ser-Arg-
                    180   190

(Cys,Arg,Thr,Thr,Glx,Glx,Pro,Pro,Val,Val,Ile,Leu)-Met-Gly-Ala-Ser-Gly-Asp-Leu-Ala-Lys-Ile-Leu-Arg-Ala-Glu-Val-Arg-Val-
  200   210   220

Leu-Lys-Leu-Arg-Gly-Tyr-Leu-Asp-Asp-Pro-Thr-Val-Pro-Arg-Tyr-Lys-Val-Lys-Gly-Gly-Cys-Lys-Ala-Val-Val-Leu-Gly-Gln-Tyr-
  230   240   250

Val-Gly-Asn-Pro-Asp-Gly-Glx-Gly-Glx-Ala-Lys-Gly-Gly-Tyr-Phe-Asp-Gln-Phe-Gly-Ile-Ile-Arg-[Trp-Phe-Ala-Thr-Asn-Glu-Pro-
  260   270   280

Glu-Gln-Leu-Ala-Asp-Val-Ala-Met-Cys-Lys-Pro-Ala-Ser-Gly-Asn-Gly-Lys]-Leu-Gln-Phe-His-Asp-Ala-Val-Gly-Asp-Ile-Phe-His-
  290   300   310

Gln-Gln-Cys-Lys-Ala-Glu-Val-Asp-Leu-Glu-Arg-Glu-Pro-Phe-Gly-Thr-Glu-Gly-Arg-Val-Val-Lys-Ala-Leu-Glu-Glu-Asp-Arg-
  320   330   340

Glu-Leu-Ser-Arg-Glu-Ala-Val-Tyr-Thr-Lys-Asp-Glu-Lys-Ser-Ser-Leu-Lys-Met-Met-Thr-Lys-Lys-Pro-Gly-Met-Phe-Phe-Asn-Pro-
  350   360

Glu-Glu-Ser-Glu-Leu-Asp-Leu-Thr-Tyr-Gly-Gly-Arg-Val-Ile-Leu-Ser-Gly-Cys-Glu-Met-Gln-Asp-His-Leu-Leu-Met-Pro-Arg-Pro-
370   380   390

-Asp-Ala-Asp-Leu-Ser-Gly-(Cys,Thr,Ser,Glx,Ala,Val,Tyr,Phe,Phe)-Lys-Asn-Gln-Leu-Val-Ile-Arg-Asp-Val-Leu-Leu-Arg-Pro-Lys-
400   420

Phe-Ala-Asn-Arg-Ala-Ser-Glu-Gly-Lys-(His,Cys,Asx,Asx,Thr,Thr,Ser,Ser,Glx,Glx,Pro,Pro,Ala,Ala,Val,Ile,Leu,Leu,Tyr)-Met-
  430   440   450

His-Phe-Val-Arg-Ser-Arg-Glu-Leu-Arg-Glu-Ala-Trp-Arg-Ile-Phe-Thr-Pro-Leu-His-Ile-Glu-Leu-Lys-Leu-Pro-Asp-Ala-Tyr-Glu-
  460   470   480

Arg-Asn-Val-Lys-Tyr-Lys-Ile-Tyr-Gly-Ser-Arg-Gly-Pro-Thr-Glu-Ala-Asp-Glu-Leu-Met-Lys-Arg-Val-Gly-Phe-Glu-Tyr-Glu-Gly-
  490

Thr-Thr-Lys-Leu-Trp-Val-Asp-Pro-His-Gly-COOH.

suggested that the enzyme has allosteric properties with respect to NADP [80, 141], it has also been alleged that such properties are found only in the presence of borate buffers [79]. The enzyme is strongly inhibited by NADPH [78–80], the inhibition being competitive with NADP. This strong product inhibition may account for some of the difficulty in accurately appraising the kinetics at low NADP levels. The enzyme is also inhibited by ATP, the inhibition being competitive with glucose-6-phosphate [81, 82], and by cyanate [142].

In addition to utilization of its natural substrates, glucose-6-P and NADP, red cell G-6-PD can also utilize substrate analogues such as glucose [143], 2-deoxyglucose-6-phosphate, galactose-6-P, deamino NADP, and NAD [139]. The use of such analogues has been helpful in studying differences between various genetic variants of G-6-PD. G-6-PD does not have an absolute requirement for divalent ions, but activity is increased by 0.01 M magnesium chloride, 0.1 M sodium chloride, and 0.1 M potassium chloride [122].

The primary structure of red cell G-6-PD is determined by the same gene that determines the structure of G-6-PD in other tissues. This is readily apparent from the fact that genetic mutations involving the electrophoretic mobility of G-6-PD seem to affect the mobility of the enzyme in all tissues [144]. A microsomal enzyme, hexose-6-phosphate dehydrogenase [145] present in liver and in many other tissues [146], can readily be distinguished from glucose-6-phosphate dehydrogenase on the basis of its greater capacity to oxidize galactose-6-phosphate, as well as by its capacity to oxidize glucose with NAD as a coenzyme. Although G-6-PD in all tissues seems to be under the same genetic control, subtle differences in charge can be appreciated by use of isoelectric focusing. Some post-transcriptional changes are related, at least in part, to the age of the enzyme [147]. The kinetic properties of the fibroblast enzyme appear to be the same as those of the red cell enzyme, and fibroblast cultures can therefore be useful in characterization of G-6-PD mutants.

BIOCHEMISTRY OF G-6-PD-DEFICIENT ERYTHROCYTES

Alterations in G-6-PD

The basic abnormality in G-6-PD deficiency is the decreased G-6-PD activity in mature red cells. The existence of different variants of G-6-PD has been established on the basis of the following measurements: (1) Red cell enzyme activity; (2) electrophoretic mobility; (3) the Michaelis constant for its substrates, glucose-6-P and NADP; (4) capacity to utilize 2-deoxyglucose-6-phosphate, galactose-6-phosphate, and deamino NADP and NAD; (5) heat stability; and (6) pH optimum. In addition, certain variants can be distinguished by measuring susceptibility to inhibition by sulhydryl reagents [148], chromatographic mobility on ion-exchange columns [149–151], transition temperatures [150], and heat sensitivity in tissue culture [152].

The normal enzyme is designated G-6-PD B. G-6-PD A is an electrophoretically fast variant which has normal or nearly normal catalytic activity and properties. G-6-PD A− has an electrophoretic mobility indistinguishable from G-6-PD A in the usual electrophoretic systems but manifests a moderate

degree of enzyme deficiency. Even within the group of patients considered to have "normal" G-6-PD, on the basis of activity and electrophoretic mobility, some kinetic and electrophoretic heterogeneity has been uncovered [153]. It has been proposed that, at least within the Nigerian population, two isoalleles of G-6-PD B exist, B_1 and B_2, and that alleles designated as A_1 and A_2 might also exist within what has previously been designated as G-6-PD A. It has been suggested that simple thermal stability also reveals many otherwise unsuspected variants [154]. Table 74-3 lists those variants that have been characterized. Although standardized methods have been used for the characterization of the variants listed in Table 74-3, minor differences in technique, aging of enzyme preparations with consequent change in properties, and variability in commercially available reagents make it difficult to be certain that variants from two laboratories which appear to be distinct are, in reality, different. A striking example of this recently came to light when it was found that an enzyme which had previously been designated as G-6-PD Cornell [250] and which had generally been accepted as being a distinct variant came from a member of a family which had previously been characterized as G-6-PD Chicago [162]. Moreover, computerized comparison of the characteristics of all the variants listed in Table 74-3 reveals that the characteristics of some are very similar. For example, G-6-PD Helsinki [175] and G-6-PD Mahidol [229] are virtually identical with respect to all their biochemical characteristics. Yet, Mahidol occurred in Thai subjects, while Helsinki was discovered in Finland. Moreover, G-6-PD Helsinki occurred in a person with nonspherocytic hemolytic anemia and is therefore characterized as a class 1 variant, while G-6-PD Mahidol was not associated with hemolysis and is therefore categorized as a class 3 variant. Attention is also drawn to the close similarity between the characteristics of G-6-PD San Diego [159] and G-6-PD Tahta [200], class 1 and class 3 variants, respectively, arising from black and Egyptian subjects. Helsinki and Kamiube, a Finnish and a Japanese variant [222], are also very similar. It is not presently possible to determine whether such variants represent the same mutations occurring by happenstance in the same population or whether they are, in reality, distinct. With currently available technology it must be admitted that variants which appear to be distinct may actually be identical, while clearly variants with different amino acid substitutions may, when characterized by the standard techniques available, appear to be identical.

A deficiency of G-6-PD activity can occur because of decreased production of enzyme molecules, formation of enzyme molecules with decreased catalytic activity, or production of enzyme molecules with reduced stability. These mechanisms appear to be operative in various combinations. Enzyme stability seems to be particularly important. Since human red cells are devoid of the capacity to synthesize protein, they are particularly susceptible to the effects of stability mutants. Age fractionation studies of normal red cells show that there is a substantial decrease in the activity of G-6-PD with aging [6, 8, 251–253]. This disparity is accentuated in many deficient G-6-PD variants in which the mutant enzyme has impaired stability in vivo [6–8, 254]. In the A− type of deficiency, production of the enzyme appears to be normal; i.e., activity of the enzyme in bone marrow cells and reticulocytes is not appreciably diminished [8]. In the peripheral red cells, however, electrophoretic studies on the purified enzyme [255], fluorescence studies on enzymes titrated with NADPH [255], and immunologic investigations [149, 151, 254, 256]

Table 74-3 Variants of G-6-PD

CLASS I VARIANTS (ASSOCIATED WITH NONSPHEROCYTIC
HEMOLYTIC ANEMIA)

Electrophoretically fast variants
  Baudelocque[b, h, i, q, u] [155]
  Lincoln Park[b, f, h, i, p, x] [156]
  Hotel Dieu[b, f, h, k, p, v] [157]
  Charleston[b, f, h, k, q] [158]
  San Diego[b, g, o, u] [159]
  East Harlem[c, f, g, i, p] [160]
  Jackson[b, f, g, k, o, u] [161]
  Pea Ridge[a, f, g, i, q, u] [162]

Electrophoretically normal variants
  Chinese[a, g, i, o, u] [163]
  Bat-Yam[b, h, q, v] [164]
  Albuquerque[c, f, g, q, x] [50]
  Bangkok[a, f, h, q, x] [165]
  Oklahoma[c, f, g, p, x] [166]
  Duarte[a, f, h, q, w] [167]
  Hong Kong[b, f, h, o, u] [168]
  Boston[b, e, h, k, p, w] [169]
  Englewood[a, e, h, p, v] [170]
  New York[a, d, h, p, w] [170]
  Hawaii[b, f, i, q, v] [171]
  Tokushima[a, f, g, i, q, u] [172]
  Hayem[b, h, k, p, u] [173]
  Aarau[b, f, h, k, q, v] [174]
  Helsinki[b, d, g, i, o, u] [175]
  Kremenchug[b, e, h, k, o, u] [176]
  Ogikubo[b, d, h, i, q, u] [177]
  Yokohama[a, f, g, k, p, u] [177]
  Akita[b, d, g, i, p, u] [177]
  Dothan[a, f, g, i, q, u] [178]

Electrophoretically slow variants
  Long Prairie[b, d, h, k, q, x] [179]
  Grand Prairie[b, d, g, k, q, u] [180]
  Chicago[a, d, g, q, u] [181, 162]
  Panama[b, e, h, k, p, v] [182]
  Arlington Heights[c, f, g, i, q, x] [156]
  Tripler[b, g, k, q, v] [183]
  Alhambra[a, e, g, p, x] [184]
  Hong Kong Pokfulam[a, g, k, o, u] [163]
  Santa Barbara[a, f, g, i, q, w] [185]
  Ashdod[c, h, p, v] [164]
  Ramat Gan[b, h, q, v] [164]
  Manchester[a, f, h, k, p, v] [186]
  West Town[a, f, h, k, q, u] [156]
  Atlanta[a, f, g, i, q, u] [187]
  Worcester[b, f, g, i, q, w] [188]
  San Francisco[c, f, g, k, q, u] [189]
  Tokyo[a, f, g, i, q, u] [172]

CLASS 2 VARIANTS (SEVERELY DEFICIENT, LESS THAN
10% RESIDUAL ACTIVITY)

Electrophoretically fast variants
  Huanlien-Chi[b, h, o, v] [190]
  San Jose[a, d, h, i, o] [191]
  Union[b, d, h, k, p, v] [192]
  Ankara[a, f, g, k, p, v] [193]
  Ferrara[b, d, h, k, q, u] [194]
  Lublin[b, f, g, o] [195]
  Taiwan-Hakka[b, h, o, v] [196]
  Markham[b, h, p, v] [6]
  Hualien[b, h, q, v] [190]
  Teheran[b, g, o, v] [190]

Electrophoretically normal variants
  Campbellpore[b, h, q, v] [197]
  Mediterranean[b, e, h, k, p, v] [198]
  Corinth[b, h, i, p, v] [199]
  El Fayoum[b, h, k, p, v] [200]
  Matam[b, e, h, k, p, v] [201]
  Abrami[b, f, h, k, p, v] [202]
  Hamm[b, f, h, k, q, x] [203]
  Tarsus[b, f, h, k, p, x] [203]
  Petrich[b, h, k, p, v] [204]
  Gotze Delchev[b, h, k, q, v] [204]
  Blida[b, h, i, p, v] [205]
  Ogori[b, f, g, k, o, v] [206]

Electrophoretically slow variants
  Jammu[a, f, g, i, o, u] [207]
  Toulouse[a, e, h, k, q, v] [208]
  Panay[b, f, g, p, v] [209]
  Zakataly[b, d, h, k, p, v] [210]
  Salata[c, f, h, i, o, u] [211]
  Poznan[b, e, h, p, v] [212]
  Okhut I[b, d, h, k, p, v] [210]
  Aachen[a, f, g, i, q, u] [213]
  Shirin-Bulakh[b, e, h, k, q, x] [210]
  Kurume[b, f, h, k, q, v] [214]
  Lifta[b, h, q] [164]
  Zhitomir[b, e, h, k, p, v] [215]
  West Bengal[b, f, g, o, u] [216]
  Alger[b, h, i, q, v] [205]
  Bideiz[b, d, h, k, q, v] [210]
  Fukushima[b, f, g, i, p, u] [214]
  Wakayama[b, f, g, k, q, u] [214]
  Shekii[b, e, h, k, q, v] [210]
  Yamaguchi[b, f, h, k, q, x] [214]

CLASS 3 VARIANTS (MODERATELY DEFICIENT, 10-60%
RESIDUAL ACTIVITY)

Electrophoretically fast variants
  Puerto Rico[b, g, p] [217]
  A−[a, d, g, i, o, u] [139, 149, 218]
  Debrousse[b, e, h, o, u] [219]
  Lozere[b, f, g, i, p, v] [220]
  Ube[a, f, g, i, o, u] [221]
  Castilla[a, f, h, k, p, u] [206]
  Konan[b, f, g, i, o, u] [222]
  Chibuto[b, f, g, p, u] [221]
  Chiapas[b, e, g, i, p, w] [223]
  San Juan[b, h, q, v] [217]
  Kabyle[a, g, o, u] [224]
  Laghouat[b, h, i, o, u] [205]
  Toronto[b, f, h, k, p, u] [225]
  Canton[b, h, p, v] [226]
  Bukitu[c, f, h, k, p, u] [211]
  Tahta[b, g, o, u] [200]
  Velletri[c, d, h, k, q, v] [227]
  Gallura[b, f, g, k, p, u] [228]

Electrophoretically normal variants
  Mahidol[b, g, i, o, u] [229]
  El Morro[b, h, k, p, v] [217]
  Siriraj[b, h, k, p, v] [230]
  Hofu[b, f, h, k, o, u] [231]
  El Kharga[a, h, i, p, x] [200]
  Kamiube[b, d, g, i, o, u] [222]

Electrophoretically slow variants
  Intanon[a, e, g, i, o, v] [232]
  Athens[b, f, h, k, p, v] [233]
  Siwa[b, h, k, p, v] [200]
  Bogia[a, f, h, k, o, u] [211]

Table 74-3   Variants of G-6-PD *(Continued)*

Kaluan[c, f, h, i, q, u] [211]
Vientiane[b, f, h, k, o, u] [234]
Washington[a, g, o, u] [190]
Benevento[b, h, p, v] [217]
Los Angeles[b, f, h, i, o, v] [235]
Titteri[b, h, i, o, x] [205]
Trinacria[b, e, h, k, p, v] [236]
Okhut II[b, f, h, k, p, u] [210]
Camperdown[b, e, h, k, o, v] [199]
Thenia[a, g, i, o, v] [205]
Seattle[b, e, h, o, v] [237]
Kerala[b, e, h, o, v] 216]
Carswell[b, f, g, o, u] [238]
Anant[b, g, k, o, u] [239]

CLASS 4 VARIANTS (NORMAL ACTIVITY, 60–150%)

Electrophoretically fast variants
Inhambane[b, f, g, o, v] [240]
Luz Saint Sauveur[b, d, g, o, u] [241]
A[a, d, g, i, o, u] [139, 218, 242]
Steilacom[a, d, g, o, u] [243]
Laurenzo Marquez[a, d, g, o, u] [221]
Kiwa[b, f, h, k, o, u] [222]

Electrophoretically normal variants
B[a, d, g, i, o, u] [16, 118, 119, 244]

Electrophoretically slow variants
Alexandra[b, d, g, i, o, u] [199]
Baltimore-Austin[a, d, g, o, u] [245]
Manjacase[c, d, g, o, u] [245]
Pinar del Rio[b, d, g, p, v] [246]
Port Royal[b, h, i, p] [247]
Ibadan-Austin[a, d, g, o, u] [245]
Porbandar[b, e, h, k, o, u] [248]

CLASS 5 VARIANTS (INCREASED ACTIVITY)

Electrophoretically fast variants
Hektoen[a, d, g, i, o, u] [249]

[a] Normal K_m G-6-P (50–70 μM).
[b] Low K_m G-6-P.
[c] High K_m G-6-P.
[d] Normal K_m NADP (2.9–4.4 μM).
[e] Low K_m NADP.
[f] High K_m NADP.
[g] Normal 2-deoxy G-6-P utilization (<4% of G-6-P).
[h] High 2-deoxy G-6-P utilization.
[i] Normal deamino NADP utilization (55–60% of NADP).
[j] Low deamino NADP utilization.
[k] High deamino NADP utilization.
[l] Normal K_i NADPH (19.22 ± 5.82).
[m] Low K_i NADPH.
[n] High K_i NADPH.
[o] Heat-stable (normal).
[p] Labile.
[q] Very labile.
[r] Normal pH optimum.
[s] Slightly biphasic pH optimum.
[t] Biphasic.
[u] pH activity curve, monobasic, abnormal.
[v] Thermal stability—abnormal, activity increased with heating.
[w] No clear pH optimum.
[x] Electrophoretic mobility TEB and phosphate, 98%, on TRIS 105%.

have established that the number of enzyme molecules is decreased. It has been suggested that the enzyme may be more susceptible than normal to oxidation [257]. In the Mediterranean type of enzyme defect a decreased amount of enzyme is present even in very young red cells [8]. In addition, each enzyme molecule has decreased catalytic activity [254, 256].

Mixtures of normal and G-6-PD-deficient hemolysates reveal no evidence of enzyme inhibition [258].

The extent to which deficient G-6-PD variants result in impaired cell function depends largely on kinetic alterations manifested by the mutant enzyme. In the case of the A− variant, in the absence of stress red cell survival is normal, or nearly so, even though old red cells contain very low levels of enzyme. But the residual type A− enzyme has an increased resistance to inhibition by NADPH [79, 80, 259]. The lowered K_m for NADP and for G-6-P [198, 260] of the G-6-PD Mediterranean may play a role in the relatively normal survival of red cells with this variant enzyme. On the other hand, variants that have relatively high levels of G-6-PD activity when measured under optimal conditions in vitro may manifest impaired red cell survival because of increased sensitivity to inhibition by NADPH [79].

Highly purified normal G-6-PD (G-6-PD B) from 20 units of blood has been fingerprinted, and the fingerprints have been compared with those from G-6-PD A. A single amino acid substitution, a change from asparagine to aspartic acid, was found [127, 128], (Fig. 74-2). Similarly, the purified enzyme from G-6-PD Hektoen has proved to have a single amino acid substitution, in this case histidine to tyrosine [261]. The development of newer methods for purifying G-6-PD with higher yields will make possible the molecular characterization of many other G-6-PD variants.

In Vitro Response of G-6-PD-Deficient Red Cells to Oxidative Challenge

Incubation of G-6-PD-deficient red cells with acetylphenylhydrazine results in rapid loss of GSH [114] and an increase in red cell GSSG levels [262]. The same effect is produced on incubation with primaquine, phenylhydrazine, ascorbic acid nitrofurantoin, α- and β-naphthoquinone, and certain vitamin K derivatives. Such agents appear to oxidize GSH in the presence of oxyhemoglobin by forming either free radicals [116] or hydrogen peroxide [117]. GSH is undoubtedly oxidized by these agents in normal, as well as in G-6-PD-deficient, red cells. Normal red cells, however, have the capacity to reduce the GSSG formed with NADPH through the glutathione reductase reaction, whereas G-6-PD-deficient cells, being unable to reduce NADP to NADPH, lack this capacity. The ability of red cells to reduce GSSG can be demonstrated more directly by oxidizing GSH with agents such as methylphenylazoformate [263], diamide [264], t-butylhydroperoxide, or cumene hydroperoxide [265]. The latter two agents act as substrates for the glutathione peroxidase reaction and, as such, are effective in oxidizing GSH selectively, exerting very few other effects on the erythrocyte. After GSH has been oxidized by any of these agents, the rate of reduction can be followed by measuring its reappearance. The lack of capacity of G-6-PD-deficient cells to reduce GSSG is in sharp contrast to that of normal cells which, in the presence of glucose, will regenerate virtually all the GSH originally present within about $\frac{1}{2}$ h.

Methemoglobin Formation and Reduction

Reduction of methemoglobin in the presence of methylene blue, largely a NADPH-linked process, is diminished in G-6-

PD-deficient red cells [266]. In the absence of such an auxiliary dye, the rate of methemoglobin reduction in deficient cells is normal [266, 267]. There is much less methemoglobin formation in G-6-PD-deficient cells than in normal cells when they are exposed to nitrosobenzol. Presumably, nitrosobenzol is reduced to phenylhydroxylamine by NADPH in order to form methemoglobin [268]. Similarly, the inhibition of glutathione reductase by chromate occurs in normal cells but not in G-6-PD-deficient cells [269]. The process requires NADPH [269, 270], presumably to expose -S11 groups of the glutathione reductase molecule.

CO_2 Production and Oxygen Consumption

The HMP shunt is the only known pathway of oxygen consumption and CO_2 production in the mature red cell [271]. Measurement of these parameters is a direct reflection of metabolic flow along this pathway. It is of interest that red cells with the relatively mild A− type of deficiency are able to oxidize glucose at a normal rate in the resting state. When the rate of NADPH oxidation is hastened either by the addition of agents such as methylene blue or by the oxidation of GSH to GSSG, the enzyme-deficient cells are unable to increase adequately the rate of glucose oxidation and CO_2 production [272].

NADP/NADPH Ratio

The ratio of NADP to NADPH is increased in G-6-PD-deficient red cells [273]. Since the rate of HMP metabolism of resting G-6-PD A− cells is the same as that of normal cells, even though the V_{max} of the G-6-PD of these cells is only some 10 percent of normal, the residual A− G-6-PD is functioning at a rate closer to its V_{max} than is the normal enzyme. This would be the natural consequence of a higher NADP level (greater saturation with NADP) and lower NADPH level (less NADPH inhibition of G-6-PD). The degree of distortion of the NADP/NADPH ratio would necessarily be even greater in the case of variants in which the resting rate of HMP metabolism is diminished or in G-6-PD-deficient cells under conditions of oxidative stress. For example, if most of the GSH has been oxidized to GSSG and the cell is unable to reduce the GSSG, one may presume that since available NADPH already has been oxidized by the GSSG in the glutathione reductase reaction, most of the coenzyme is in the NADP form.

Other Biochemical Abnormalities

The activities of many different enzymes have been measured in G-6-PD-deficient red cells [1]. Although conflicting results have been obtained in a number of cases, the existence of some alterations has been confirmed. The increased activity of glutathione reductase [274–277] is well established; it may be due to the presence of less "active" FAD-containing glutathione reductase in G-6-PD-deficient red cells [275.]. The decrease of NADPH diaphorase activity in G-6-PD-deficient cells [267, 276] is quite consistent but remains unexplained. We have found the glutathione peroxidase activity of G-6-P deficiency red cells to be consistently increased [278] in spite of reports to the contrary [28, 279].

Although the structure of G-6-PD-deficient erythrocytes as seen with a light microscope is normal [5], abnormalities of the stroma resembling changes found in normal aging [280] have been detected wth the aid of electron microscopy. The membranes of red cells from patients with G-6-PD deficiency and hereditary nonspherocytic hemolytic anemia, but not from those who have G-6-PD A−, contain large molecular weight aggregates of proteins cross-linked by disufide bonds [281, 282]. Similar high molecular weight aggregates are also found in patients with nonspherocytic hemolytic anemia due to other enzyme defects [283], and it is possible that this change represents a common pathway of red cell damage in a number of metabolic abnormalities. The significance of minor differences in the results of chemical modification and fluorescence studies carried out on membranes from G-6-PD A− and G-6-PD A red cells is doubtful [284]. It has been suggested that the life span of red cells with G-6-PD A− [285] and G-6-PD Mediterranean [286] variants is slightly less than normal, but the significance of these observations is in doubt, normal values having been observed by a number of investigators [16].

EFFECT OF DRUG ADMINISTRATION ON G-6-PD-DEFICIENT RED CELLS

Biochemical Changes

When primaquine is administered to an individual with G-6-PD A−, only the older and therefore more severely enzyme-deficient members of the red cell population are destroyed [287] (see above). Hence, during an episode of drug-induced hemolysis, a rise in average erythrocyte G-6-PD levels toward normal is observed [288, 289].

The administration of primaquine to a G-6-PD A− subject initially results in a rapid fall in the average GSH level of the red cells. This change precedes major episodes of red cell destruction. Hemolysis is accompanied by a return of the average red cell GSH to the same level or a slightly higher level than that measured prior to administration of the drug [288]. Similar observations have been made in patients with favism and sulfonamide-induced hemolytic anemia [1]. Apparently, the GSH in the older red cells is initally almost completely destroyed, and its level in the blood rises as the depleted cells are removed from the circulation [114]. Some of the GSH lost from the red cells may form mixed disulfides with hemoglobin [290–292], particularly with the exposed sulfhydryl group of the cysteine residue in the ninety-third position of the β chain. There is probably also some loss of GSSG from the enzyme-deficient cells by outward transport [104]. The levels of methemoglobin found in the blood of G-6-PD subjects given hemolytic drugs are not greater than those observed with normal subjects, and may even be less [12].

Mechanism of Red Cell Destruction

Primaquine and related drugs do not preferentially lyse G-6-PD-deficient red cells in vitro [5]. Indeed, there is some evidence that G-6-PD-deficient cells may be less susceptible to lysis in vitro [293]. It appears, rather, that hemolytic drugs damage G-6-PD-deficient red cells in such a way that they are selected for removal by the reticuloendothelial system. Such changes might include the charge on the surface of the cell or alterations in its shape or deformability.

As primaquine-induced hemolysis begins to develop, Heinz bodies are formed [5, 288]. Heinz bodies (Fig. 74-1) consist largely of hemoglobin denaturation products, such as verdoglobin, choleglobin, and possibly other hemichrome derivatives [294–296]. They are attached to the red cell membrane, but the mode of their attachment has been the subject of some disagreement. It has been suggested that they are covalently bound with disulfide bridges [297], but evidence has also been presented that the mode of attachment is quite different, consisting perhaps of hydrophobic bonds [298].

The sequence of reactions which begins with the exposure of the red cell to a drug or a product of drug metabolism remains poorly understood. It seems probable that the formation of hydrogen peroxide plays an important role since peroxides produce rapid oxidation of GSH to GSSG through the glutathione peroxidase reaction [299]. Lacking a mechanism for the regeneration of GSH from GSSG, G-6-PD-deficient cells would be expected to accumulate peroxide which could then oxidize other red cell components. Direct covalent interaction between heme of hemoglobin and various phenolic compounds has been demonstrated [300]. If such complexes are formed in vivo, they might also lead to the denaturation of hemoglobin. The role of methemoglobin formation in the subsequent irreversible degradation of hemoglobin remains unclear. Methemoglobin increases the tendency for heme to dissociate from globin [301], and heme-free globin is particularly unstable [302]. Under some circumstances the oxidation of iron seems to precede the formation of hemichromes [296]. While many of the drugs which cause hemolytic anemia in G-6-PD deficiency also have the capacity to induce methemoglobinemia, Heinz bodies may be formed without perceptible methemoglobinemia [303, 304], and the formation of large amounts of methemoglobin in experimental animals does not produce and may even protect against hemolysis by drugs such as phenylhydrazine [305–308]. It seems quite likely that the oxidative denaturation of hemoglobin is a consequence not primarily of heme oxidation, but rather of the oxidation of the β93 cysteine, with the subsequent unfolding of the hemoglobin molecule and oxidation of its hidden sulfhydryl groups [290]. Acetylphenylhydrazine has been shown to produce hemoglobin chain separation [309].

Electron microscopic studies have shown that though normal red cells move readily from the splenic cords to sinusoids through small openings, Heinz bodies are held up when red cells containing these inclusions follow the same route [310]. Presumably the rigid Heinz bodies are removed from the cell, along with attached membrane, rendering the cells vulnerable to destruction, particularly if another Heinz body forms. A somewhat anomalous finding is that the deformability of G-6-PD-deficient red cells seems to be greater than that of normal cells. Moreover, incubation with acetylphenylhydrazine, while decreasing the deformability of G-6-PD-deficient red cells, has less effect on these cells than it does on normal erythrocytes [3].

Other biochemical alterations may also play a role in the destruction of G-6-PD-deficient red cells. The possible interference of GSSG with glycolysis, resulting in decreased ATP levels, has been suggested [268, 311], as has the inhibition of the enzyme directly by drugs [312–314].

The mechanism of hemolysis after ingestion of fava beans has attracted the attention of many investigators. In every case of favism in which the red cells have been studied, the erythrocyte defect has been demonstrated, but subjects known to have G-6-PD deficiency have eaten fava beans with impunity [33, 315]. In addition, ^{51}Cr-labeled G-6-PD-deficient red cells are not necessarily destroyed in vivo when fava beans are eaten [34, 316, 317]. It seems likely that another genetic defect in addition to G-6-PD deficiency is required to cause sensitivity to the hemolytic effect of fava beans [318]. The nature of the additional defect is obscure. It has been proposed that the second defect may be an inability to form glucuronides [319], and data have been presented to show that glucaric acid excretion [320], an indirect measure of glucuronide formation, and salicylamide-glucuronide formation [321] are decreased in persons with a history of favism. A thorough search for antibodies to bean components has failed to implicate immune mechanisms in favism [322]. Certain fractions of fava beans, divicine and isouremil, have the capacity to destroy the GSH of G-6-PD deficiency red cells [323, 324] and to damage G-6-PD-deficient red cells so that they are quickly destroyed in vivo [324]. Attention has been drawn to the high L-dopa content of fava beans, and it has been suggested that oxidation of this compound to dopaquinone might be responsible for the hemolysis which accompanies fava bean ingestion in persons with favism [325, 326]. However, no evidence directly supporting this hypothesis is available, and G-6-PD-deficient individuals in general tolerate L-dopa without untoward effects [327]. Indeed, it has been suggested that L-dopa may act as a free-radical trap and may protect against hemolysis of G-6-PD-deficient cells by drugs [328]. The reported correlation between acid phosphatase phenotype and sensitivity to fava bean hemolysis [329] is not likely to represent a cause-and-effect relationship.

In the case of infection, too, the mechanism of hemolysis is unknown. It has been proposed that the generation of hydrogen peroxide observed when leukocytes phagocytose bacteria might be the source of damage to G-6-PD-deficient cells [330]. Influenza virus preferentially lyses G-6-PD-deficient red cells in vitro [331]. Similar effects may occur in vivo.

Diabetic acidosis may impair the supplies of red cell NADPH through several different mechanisms. Hexokinase, the rate-limiting enzyme of glucose metabolism, is very pH-sensitive, and if the pH of the red cell falls to sufficiently low levels, its energy supplies may be choked off. High glucose levels have the capacity to drain NADPH from the cell through the action of L-hexonate dehydrogenase [89]. Pyruvate, too, can act as a hydrogen acceptor for NADPH providing that the level of pyruvate is sufficiently high and the pH sufficiently low [90]. It is not clear whether any of these changes alone, or in combination, can account for the severe hemolysis that is sometimes seen in patients with G-6-PD deficiency.

The cause of neonatal icterus in G-6-PD deficiency is also unknown. The activities of some enzymes, particularly NADH diaphorase [332], catalase [333], and glutathione peroxidase [334], are decreased in red cells of the newborn. Perhaps the level of vitamin E, too, may be of some importance; it has been suggested that vitamin E may protect G-6-PD-deficient red cells against premature destruction [335]. The relatively lower levels of these potential protectors against oxidative damage may make the red cell more vulnerable to the destructive influence of hydrogen peroxide, which is generated spontaneously in vivo. Similarly, red cells with functionally severe deficits of G-6-PD in patients with nonspherocytic congenital hemolytic anemia may be destroyed even at naturally occurring levels of peroxide.

GENETICS OF G-6-PD DEFICIENCY

X Linkage of G-6-PD

Analysis of pedigrees of G-6-PD-deficient subjects has shown a lack of male-to-male transmission [33, 65, 336]. Further evidence for the sex linkage of G-6-PD deficiency has come from observations of linkage with color blindness [337–340] and from studies with hybrid cells [341].

The recombination fraction between the gene for G-6-PD and deuteranopia has been estimated to be 5 percent [340]. In a study from Sardinia the two genes were most frequently in the coupling phase [337], while in other studies from Israel [338] occurrence in the repulsion phase was significantly more frequent. It has been suggested that the genes for deuteranopia and proteranopia may be relatively far apart on the X chromosome and that the gene for G-6-PD lies between their loci [342]. A map of four X-linked genes that was produced by the study of fused hamster-human genes suggested that they are arranged in the order: phosphoglycerate kinase—α-galactosidase—hypoxanthine-guanine-phosphoribosyl transferase—G-6-PD [498]. A maximum likelihood estimate of the recombination fraction between Becker's muscular dystrophy and G-6-PD is reported to be 0.27 [343]. No linkage has been found to exist between the locus for G-6-PD and the loci for Xg [344–346], Duchenne's muscular dystrophy [343], or anhydrotic ectodermal dysplasia [347]. A human gene which may be that for G-6-PD has recently been cloned [499] but the nucleotide sequence data from this gene are not yet available for comparison with the amino acid sequence of the enzyme.

G-6-PD and the X-Inactivation Hypothesis

Though a large proportion of females heterozygous for G-6-PD deficiency have intermediate levels of enzyme activity, numerous exceptions are found. For example, as indicated in Fig. 74-3, affected subjects have been found in whom the defect could be demonstrated in neither parent (cf. family 12, LA: 111-7,8 produced IV-12). The fact that neither parent of some propositi has a demonstrable defect indicates that the gene can be carried without causing a detectable disorder in the red cell. Conversely, some females with marked G-6-PD deficiency are proven heterozygotes because they have borne boys who are not affected (cf. Fig. 74-3, family K.: 11-A, K. and E. K. have produced four negative sons—III. J. K., P. K., Go. K., and G. K.). In some such cases it has been shown that the heterozygote had a normal female chromosomal complement [348]. Females, who possess two X chromosomes, have no more G-6-PD activity [7, 349] or only very slightly more [350] than males possessing only one X chromosome, and persons with more than two X chromosomes do not have greater than normal red cell G-6-PD activity [349]. These findings, the markedly variable expression of G-6-PD activity in heterozygotes and the cytologic findings of Ohno [351], originally led us to suggest that one of the X chromosomes of human females was inactive [352–354]. The same proposal was made also by Lyon [355] on the basis of study of coat color genes in mice.

X-inactivation would require that heterozygotes with intermediate enzyme activity have two red cell populations—red cells with normal activity and red cells that are grossly deficient in G-6-PD activity. This was first shown to be the case by demonstrating that the curve of reduction of methemoglobin in the presence of Nile blue sulfate has two components when red cells of heterozygotes for G-6-PD deficiency are studied [352]. These curves resemble exactly those obtained from artificial mixtures of cells obtained from normal subjects and from hemizygotes for G-6-PD deficiency. Similarly, the disappearance of GSH from the red cells of heterozygotes when challenged in vitro with acetylphenylhydrazine, or the regeneration of GSH in azoester-treated cells, takes place in two components, just as in artificial mixtures from normal subjects and hemizygotes [263, 352]. Separation of enzyme-deficient cells from the blood of heterozygous subjects has been accomplished [356]. The bimodality of the red cell population with respect to G-6-PD deficiency has also been confirmed by microspectrophotometric measurement of individual red cell methemoglobin levels [357] using a tetrazolium-linked technique [358] and by the finding of two populations in red cell survival studies [359]. Mosaicism in heterozygotes for G-6-PD deficiency has also been demonstrated using the methemoglobin elution technique [360–365]. Since it is possible to produce mosaicism or pseudomosaicism in preparations made from normal cells or from males hemizygous for mild G-6-PD deficiency, only limited weight can be given to these findings [366–368].

The fact that only one gene for G-6-PD is active in each somatic cell has been confirmed by cloning studies [369] and in naturally occurring clones, i.e., tumors [144, 358, 370]. Thus, investigations of uterine myomas in women heterozygous for G-6-PD A and B revealed that each tumor manifested only a single G-6-PD phenotype, although intervening normal myometrium contained both G-6-PD A and B [370]. Extension of this technique to a variety of other neoplasms [371] revealed that most were clonal in origin, although there were certain exceptions, particularly with respect to genetically determined neoplasms such as trichoepithelioma. The use of G-6-PD as a clonal marker provided confirmation of the fact that not only the leukocytes but also erythrocytes were part of the neoplastic process in chronic myeloid leukemia [372] and acute myeloid leukemia [373, 374] and that patients with polycythemia vera had both a clone of erythropoietin-independent cells and nonclonal erythropoietin-sensitive precursors [375]. By use of G-6-PD as a marker, it was demonstrated [376] that paroxysmal nocturnal hemoglobinuria is a clonal disorder. The possible clonal origin of atheromata is of particular interest [377, 378], but the validity of this observation has recently been challenged [379].

Population Genetics of G-6-PD Deficiency

G-6-PD deficiency has a worldwide distribution (see Beutler [16] for references). It has been found in virtually all racial groups. The A and A− types are found chiefly in Africa and in areas to which Africans have migrated. G-6-PD A− has also been found in Sicily. The gene frequency is approximately 11 percent among black Americans. A high prevalence of G-6-PD deficiency is also found around the Mediterranean basin and in East Indians, Orientals, and Filipinos. Sporadic cases are reported from northern Europe. The geographic distribution of G-6-PD deficiency led to the suggestion that this gene may confer some degree of resistance to falciparum malaria. The most convincing evidence that this is the case comes from ele-

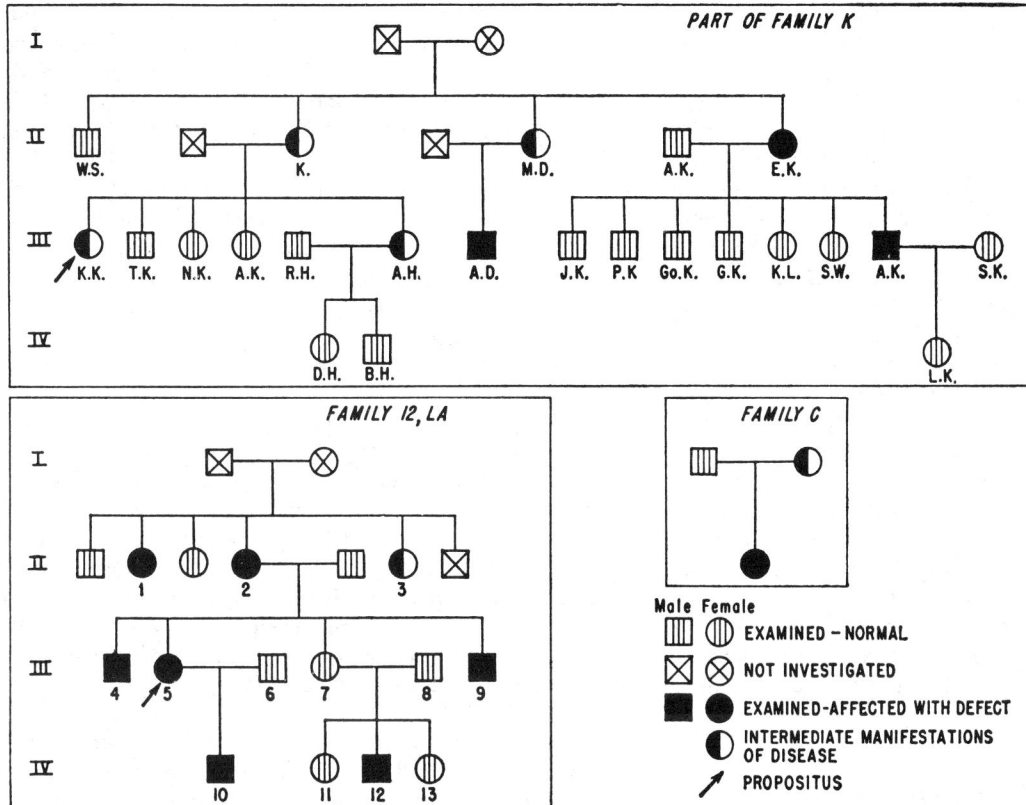

Figure 74-3 Some revealing pedigrees of families with G-6-PD deficiency. The K. family, only a part of which has been presented, and the C. family were studied by Gross et al. [65]; family 12 was studied by Childs et al. [336].

gant studies [380] of the distribution of malaria parasites in the blood of heterozygotes for G-6-PD A−. Deficient cells were found to be less frequently parasitized than were normal cells. It was suggested that the infected red cell either serves as an unsuitable host for the malaria parasite or behaves as a "suicide package," being rapidly sequestered in the spleen once it is infected. In either case, the host would benefit. It has been pointed out that because young red cells are preferentially invaded by falciparum malaria parasites, the apparent predilection of the parasite for G-6-PD-normal cells might be more apparent than real [381]. Even G-6-PD A− reticulocytes would presumably appear normal on the methemoglobin elution test [366] and might therefore be misinterpreted as being G-6-PD-normal cells. Very recent analyses of population data have been interpreted as indicating that the effect of G-6-PD on malaria incidence may be a secondary phenomenon [382]. The weight of evidence seems to favor the view that G-6-PD deficiency protects against falciparum malaria, but this protection appears to occur in heterozygotes, not in hemizygotes or homozygotes [383]. It has also been proposed that the nondeficient G-6-PD A variant confers some degree of immunity to malaria in hemizygotes [384].

The relationship between hemoglobin S and G-6-PD A− has received considerable attention. Earlier studies that purported to show an increased incidence of G-6-PD deficiency in patients with sickle-cell anemia [385] failed to be supported by other investigations [386]. More recent studies using more sophisticated methods seemed also to show an increased incidence of G-6-PD deficiency in patients with sickle-cell disease [387]. Studies by a number of investigators, however, in both

the United States [388, 389] and Africa [390] have failed to support this finding. The incidence of G-6-PD deficiency in patients with sickle-cell disease was either the same as in normal controls [389, 390] or somewhat elevated [388] but no more elevated than among nonsickling sibs of patients with sickle-cell disease.

It has been suggested that age stratification with respect to G-6-PD deficiency is present in the United States black population [391]. These results may be spurious, since they are based on the study of heterogeneous populations with different representations of African genes at various age levels. No stratification of the sickle gene was observed. The study of a homogeneous Mediterranean population showed no stratification over the relatively narrow age range of 6 to 20 years [392] and no age effect was noted in Africa [393]. It has been proposed that there is a negative association between G-6-PD deficiency and cancer [394, 395], but no convincing evidence to support this view has been presented.

Variability of G-6-PD appears to be much more limited in nonhuman species than it is in humans. Partial deficiency has been observed in isolated cases in the rat [396] and the dog [397], and an electrophoretic polymorphism exists in the chimpanzee [398, 399].

DIAGNOSIS OF G-6-PD DEFICIENCY

The detection of male hemizygous G-6-PD-deficient subjects is a relatively simple matter which can be achieved either by the use of a quantitative assay or by application of one of the many available screening procedures. Immediately following an episode of hemolysis the detection of G-6-PD deficiency is more difficult in the hemizygous G-6-PD A− subject because the older, more enzyme-deficient erythrocytes have been removed from the circulation. Under these circumstances, a quantitative G-6-PD assay is more likely to yield accurate results, particularly when combined with the assay of another age-dependent enzyme, such as hexokinase or glutamic oxalocetic-transaminase. Assaying the more dense, older erythrocytes has been found to be useful [289, 400]. Similar measures must be employed to detect the G-6-PD-deficient phenotype in an individual who has hemolytic anemia due to some other cause, such as sickle-cell anemia. Detection of G-6-PD deficiency in heterozygotes may also be difficult, because varying proportions of enzyme-deficient cells coexist in the peripheral circulation (see "The Genetics of G-6-PD Deficiency" above). The usual screening tests are not very satisfactory under these circumstances [401]. A quantitative G-6-PD assay will usually yield an intermediate result when approximately equal numbers of deficient and normal cells are present in the circulation. When the proportion of deficient cells present is small, quantitative assay of the hemolysate will not detect the abnormality; special techniques designed to detect small numbers of deficient erythrocytes must be utilized under these circumstances.

Quantitative Enzyme Assays

Quantitative assay for G-6-PD is carried out by measuring the rate of NADP reduction in the presence of glucose-6-phosphate, by estimating either the increase in optical density at 340 μm or the fluorescence of the reduced pyridine nucleotide. The 6-phosphogluconic acid that is formed in the G-6-PD reaction will be partially oxidized by phosphogluconic dehydrogenase yielding additional NADPH. Thus, the simple one-step assay does not measure G-6-PD activity alone. This difficulty may be overcome by determining the phosphogluconic dehydrogenase (6-PGD) activity in a cuvette containing no glucose-6-phosphate but containing a saturating quantity of 6-phosphogluconic acid. Subtraction of the 6-PGD activity from the system in which both activities are being measured gives an accurate appraisal of the G-6-PD activity [402]. This technique is not suitable when G-6-PD activity is very low, since it is then necessary to subtract a large value from a value that is only slightly greater. Alternatively, purified 6-PGD may be added to the system to make certain that the second reaction proceeds at maximum velocity [402], or a potent inhibitor of 6-PGD such as 2,3 diphosphoglycerate [403] or maleimide [404] may be used to provide accurate measurement of G-6-PD alone. There has been agreement on a standard procedure for the measurement of G-6-PD activity [2] in order to facilitate the comparison of results from different laboratories.

Further Qualitative Characterization of G-6-PD

Detailed consideration of the techniques for further characterization of G-6-PD mutants is beyond the scope of this chapter. Standardized techniques have been adopted for the determination of the Michaelis-Menten constants of the enzyme for glu-

cose-6-P and for NADP, for measuring its relative rate of utilization of 2-deoxyglucose-6-phosphate, and for determining its electrophoretic mobility [2]. In addition to the standard systems, many other electrophoretic methods [233, 405, 406], isoelectric focusing [398, 407, 408], chromatography [148, 150, 151, 409], estimation of pH activity curves, sensitivity to inhibition by NADPH, and the utilization of deamino-NADP, NAD, and glucose have had a place in characterizing new variants. Unless the standard techniques [2] have been carried out in addition, it is impossible to compare a putative new variant with those that have been characterized previously.

Screening Tests

Heinz Body Formation   When G-6-PD-deficient erythrocytes are incubated with a variety of reducing agents (such as acetylphenylhydrazine, phenylhydrazine, primaquine, or ascorbic acid), the pattern of Heinz body formation observed differs from that which occurs when normal cells are incubated under identical conditions [410]. The sensitivity of the test to changes in oxygen tension and hematocrit [410] was a significant disadvantage, and this procedure has now been superseded by more specific screening methods.

GSH Stability Test   Largely of historical interest, the incubation of red cells with acetylphenylhydrazine and the measurement of GSH stability are a reliable method for the detection of the red cell defect of drug sensitivity [411, 412]. This method provides clear separation of enzyme-deficient from normal males but is less reliable for the detection of heterozygotes. Correlation between G-6-PD assays is usually good [65, 413–416], but occasionally discrepancies are observed [415–418]. False positive results are obtained in Hb E thalassemia disease [419], probably because of the participation of hemoglobin in the destruction of GSH [114, 420]. The GSH content of red cells and its stability are decreased without any decrease in G-6-PD activity in renal insufficiency [421]. Red cells obtained from infants up to the age of 74 h have unstable GSH [65, 418, 422, 423] as a result of the rapid depletion of already reduced quantities of blood glucose [418]. Addition of glucose to the system reverses the apparent defect in all but those infants who have a deficiency of G-6-PD [418, 424].

Dye-linked Screening Methods   A number of screening tests have been described in which NADP reduction is measured indirectly by the reduction of a dye that absorbs in the visible spectrum. Decolorization of brilliant cresyl blue is the most widely used of these tests. Hemolysate is added to a buffered mixture of dye, NADP, and glucose-6-P [258]. Some lots of dye are unsatisfactory [425], but, in general, this method has been useful [415, 425, 426]. The reaction is light-sensitive when methylene blue is used as the receptor [427]. Other useful dyes include dichloroindophenol [428, 429] and 3(4,5-dimethylthiazolyl-1-2)2,5-diphenyltetrazolium bromide (MTT) [430].

Methemoglobin Reduction Test   This test [431] takes advantage of the fact that methemoglobin reduction in the presence of methylene blue proceeds largely through the hexose monophosphate shunt. When G-6-PD activity is impaired, the rate of methemoglobin reduction is diminished. The test is relatively simple and requires no expensive reagents, but the blood used must be fresh. False positive tests occur with some frequency [432].

Methylene Blue Absorption Test Leukomethylene blue becomes tightly bound to red cells. The absorption of methylene blue by erythrocytes has formed the basis of two tests [433, 434]. Relatively fresh blood must be used.

Ascorbate Cyanide Test This test [435, 436] depends upon the generation of H_2O_2 when red cells are incubated with ascorbate. If the decomposition of H_2O_2 by catalase is inhibited by cyanide, the hemoglobin in G-6-PD-deficient cells is denatured because they are unable to utilize efficiently the glutathione peroxidase system. The test is simple and requires no expensive reagents, but 2 ml of fresh blood is required. Many conditions other than G-6-PD deficiency will produce positive results. These include glutathione deficiency [437], hemoglobinopathies with unstable hemoglobins, and pyruvate kinase deficiency [401].

Fluorescent Spot Test This test is highly specific, is exceedingly simple to perform, requires only a small volume of blood, and is inexpensive. It is based upon the fact that reduced pyridine nucleotides fluoresce, while oxidized pyridine nucleotides do not. Incubation of a blood sample for 5 to 10 min suffices. The screening reagent contains glucose-6-phosphate, NADP, buffer, and saponin [438]. The incorporation of GSSG into the test reagent makes it sufficiently sensitive to detect mild G-6-PD deficiency by reoxidation through the glutathione reductase reaction of the small amounts of NADP, which may have been reduced to NADPH [439]. The mixture is spotted on filter paper and inspected under long-wave ultraviolet light. If the spot fluoresces, the blood is not G-6-PD deficient. This method has been widely used [400, 440, 441], is the most satisfactory screening test for detecting G-6-PD deficiency, and has been recommended by the International Committee for Standardization in Hematology. This test is also quite suitable for quantitation [442]. Reliable tests may be obtained even on blood which has been stored for a month or more, or dried on filter paper [443, 444].

By centrifuging a blood sample in a microhematocrit tube and applying the fluorescent spot test to the lowest portion of the packed red cell column, it is possible to diagnose G-6-PD deficiency even in acute hemolytic crisis [289, 400].

Heterozygote Detection

The detection of heterozygotes poses serious problems that have been described in considerable detail elsewhere [401, 445]. Since the red cells of the heterozygote are a mixture of normal and enzyme-deficient erythrocytes, a cell lysate may not reveal the fact that it was prepared from a heterozygous individual if the proportion of enzyme-deficient cells is relatively small. Methods that depend upon the activity of individual red cells, such as the methemoglobin elution test [362], the tetrazolium-linked cytochemical method [446], or the ascorbate-cyanide test, have proved to be more sensitive in the detection of small populations of G-6-PD-deficient cells than has a quantitative enzyme assay.

G-6-PD ACTIVITY IN CELLS OTHER THAN ERYTHROCYTES

The synthesis of G-6-PD in most or all other tissues is under the same genetic control as that in the red blood cells. Another form of G-6-PD (hexose-6-PD) has been found in microsomes of mammalian liver [145]. This enzyme is inherited through an autosomal gene [447, 448] and has broad substrate specificity [145, 449]. It is found in many tissues, including kidney, heart, lung, testis, and adrenal, but not in erythrocytes, leukocytes, brain, or breast [146]. This enzyme is identical to an enzyme formerly known as glucose dehydrogenase [145] and is immunologically [450] and structurally distinct from the sex-linked form of G-6-PD.

Leukocyte G-6-PD activity has been found to be nearly normal in G-6-PD-deficient subjects of African ancestry [451] but is decreased in leukocytes from persons of Mediterranean [452, 453] and Chinese ancestry [454] and from persons who inherit variants associated with hereditary nonspherocytic hemolytic anemia [455]. In some families with severe G-6-PD deficiency a total absence of enzyme in leukocytes has been associated with impaired phagocytic function [456, 457].

The leukocyte enzyme and the red cell enzyme are genetically and structurally very similar [458–460]. However, some minor differences in the isoelectric point of leukocyte, erythrocyte, platelet, and fibroblast G-6-PD have been noted [147, 461], presumably because of posttranscriptional alterations such as deamidation of the enzyme with aging. The C-terminal end of leukocyte and erythrocyte G-6-PD differ in that the C-terminus of the leukocyte enzyme is lysine-leucine, while glycine was found as the C-terminus of erythrocyte G-6-PD [462]. In G-6-PD deficiency a decrease in enzyme activity has also been described in lens tissue [463], kidney [454], platelets [250, 454, 464, 465], skin fibroblast culture [454, 466], saliva [467], breast milk [468], sperm [469], and liver [58, 454, 470–472]. The magnitude of decrease in other tissues, particularly those with nucleated cells, is generally less than in erythrocytes. The inability to synthesize protein and relatively long life span of the red cell allow the defect to reach its maximum extent there.

There is some evidence to suggest that G-6-PD deficiency may have effects in tissues other than the erythrocyte. Severe G-6-PD deficiency may cause cataracts, although very few such instances have been reported [473, 474]. An alteration in glucose tolerance curves has been found [475] but not confirmed [476]. Conflicting data have been published regarding steroid metabolism in G-6-PD deficiency [477, 478]. A decline in level of serum cholesterol upon primaquine administration was observed in G-6-PD-deficient subjects but not in normal ones [479]. Liver biopsies of patients with hemolysis induced by lobar pneumonia showed the presence of cholestasis [480], and the jaundice which may occur in the newborn seems out of keeping with the degree of hemolysis [481]. A slight decrease in glucuronide formation by G-6-PD-deficient newborns has been reported [482]. Although the overall incidence of G-6-PD deficiency is approximately average in schizophrenic patients, the suggestion has been made that those subjects with a diagnosis of catatonic schizophrenia have a much higher than normal incidence of the deficiency and those with paranoid schizophrenia a greatly decreased incidence [483]. This was not confirmed in another study [484].

In spite of the possible effects of G-6-PD deficiency, its overall clinical impact, at least on the adult Afro-American population, is so slight that it cannot be detected in population studies. In an investigation of 65,154 consecutive black male patients admitted to hospitals, no difference in the incidence of any clinical disorder was found between those who were enzyme-deficient and those who were not [485].

TREATMENT OF G-6-PD DEFICIENCY

Fortunately, most persons with G-6-PD deficiency require no therapy. The vast majority do not experience even a single hemolytic episode during their life span. When hemolytic anemia does occur, hemolysis promptly abates upon removal of the inciting agent. Indeed, in the mild A− type, hemolysis abates even when drug administration is continued, because the remaining young erythrocytes are resistant to destruction. Phototherapy has been advocated [486] for G-6-PD deficient, icteric infants, and the suggestion has been made that G-6-PD deficient blood should not be transfused [487, 488]. The single report of hemolysis following blood transfusion with G-6-PD-deficient blood [487] has not been confirmed in nearly two decades. Indeed subsequent study of the donor by an experienced laboratory [489] showed that he was not even G-6-PD-deficient. Except for use in exchange transfusions for infants with neonatal icterus, there is no compelling evidence to suggest that G-6-PD-deficient blood is unsuitable.

If anemia in G-6-PD deficiency is very severe, transfusion may be required. This occurs at times in patients with favism or after particularly severe drug- or infection-induced episodes of hemolytic anemia. Patients with nonspherocytic congenital hemolytic anemia due to G-6-PD deficiency generally are only mildly anemic and do not require transfusion. Splenectomy has been carried out in some patients with this type of hemolytic disease, but usually without any benefit.

Hyperbilirubinemia in infants with G-6-PD deficiency has sometimes required exchange transfusion. It has been suggested that the need for exchange transfusions can be diminished by the administration of barbituric acid [490]. The oral administration of agar had no effect [491]. A number of attempts have been made to modify the hemolytic effect of drugs in G-6-PD deficiency by the administration of various chemicals. EDTA was suggested as a possible agent but was found to be ineffective in influencing phenylhydrazine hemolysis in rats [308]. L-Dopa influences Heinz body formation in G-6-PD-deficient red cells and has been proposed as a possible free-radical trap in the treatment of G-6-PD-deficient hemolysis [328]. An attempt to favorably influence chronic hemolysis in patients with unstable G-6-PD variants by achieving the increase of erythrocyte pyridine nucleotide levels through administration of large doses of nicotinic acid has been found to be unsuccessful [492]. It has also been proposed that alternate substrates for NADP reduction such as xylitol [493] or isocitrate [494] be used, but no successful trials of these agents have been carried out. Administration of vitamin E to patients with G-6-PD variants associated with hereditary nonspherocytic hemolytic anemia has been reported to produce a slight, but significant, improvement in red cell life span and hemoglobin levels of blood [335, 495]. In one other study, no beneficial effect of vitamin E was detected [496].

Thus, the mainstay of management of G-6-PD-deficient patients is the avoidance of drugs known to be hemolytic or their administration in essentially subhemolytic doses. Community-wide screening of ethnic groups in which the frequency of G-6-PD deficiency is high has sometimes been considered. One would anticipate the occurrence of many of the same problems that have been encountered in connection with sickle-cell screening [497] as a result of such programs. Genetic counseling for G-6-PD deficiency is likely to be ineffectual since the disorder is sex-linked and unnecessary since it is benign. For these reasons such screening programs cannot be recommended. The responsibility for the administration of drugs should rest with physicians, and it is they who must evaluate the risk of unusual susceptibility to toxic effects of a drug. Fortunately, in the case of drugs that produce hemolysis in persons with G-6-PD deficiency, the determination of who is sensitive can now be readily made.

REFERENCES

1. BEUTLER E: Glucose-6-phosphate dehydrogenase deficiency, in Stanbury JB, Wyngaarden JB, Fredrickson DS (eds): *The Metabolic Basis of Inherited Disease* 3d ed. New York, McGraw-Hill, 1972, pp 1358–1388
2. BETKE K, BEUTLER E, BREWER GJ, KIRKMAN HN, LUZZATTO L, MOTULSKY AG, RAMOT B, SINISCALCO M: Standardization of procedures for the study of glucose-6-phosphate dehydrogenase. Report of a WHO Scientific Group. Who Tech Rep Ser no. 366, 1967
3. TILLMANN W, LABITZKE N, SCHRÖTER W: Günstige rheologische Eigenschaften der Erythrozyten beim Glucose-6-phosphatdehydrogenase-mangel. *Klin Wochenschr* 55:385, 1977
4. DERN RJ, BEUTLER E, ALVING AS: The hemolytic effect of primaquine, II. The natural course of the hemolytic anemia and the mechanism of its self-limited character. *J Lab Clin Med* 44:171, 1954
5. BEUTLER E, DERN RJ, ALVING AS: The hemolytic effect of primaquine. III. A study of primaquine-sensitive erythrocytes. *J Lab Clin Med* 44:177, 1954
6. KIRKMAN HN, KIDSON C, KENNEDY M: Variants of human glucose-6-phosphate dehydrogenase. Studies of samples from New Guinea, in Beutler E (ed): *Hereditary Disorders of Erythrocyte Metabolism*, City of Hope Symposium Series, vol I. New York, Grune & Stratton, 1968, pp 126–145
7. MARKS PA, GROSS RT: Erythrocyte glucose-6-phosphate dehydrogenase deficiency: Evidence of differences between Negroes and Caucasians with respect to this genetically determined trait. *J Clin Invest* 38:2253–1959
8. PIOMELLI S, CORASH LM, DAVENPORT DD, MIRAGLIA J, AMOROSI EL: In vivo lability of glucose-6-phosphate dehydrogenase in Gd^A and Gd^{Mediterranean} deficiency. *J Clin Invest* 47:940, 1968
9. DERN RJ, BEUTLER E, ALVING AS: The hemolytic effect of primaquine. V. Primaquine sensitivity as a manifestation of a multiple drug sensitivity. *J Lab Clin Med* 45:30, 1955
10. DEGOWIN RL, EPPES RB, POWELL RD, CARSON PE: The haemolytic effects of diaphenylsulfone (DDS) in normal subjects and in those with glucose-6-phosphate-dehydrogenase deficiency. *Bull WHO* 35:165, 1966
11. KIMBRO EL JR, SACHS MV, TORBERT JV: Mechanism of the hemolytic anemia induced by nitrofurantoin (Furadantin). *Johns Hopkins Med J* 101:245, 1957
12. BEUTLER E: The hemolytic effect of primaquine and related compounds. A review. *Blood* 14:103, 1959
13. KELLERMEYER RW, TARLOV AR, BREWER GJ, CARSON PE, ALVING AS: Hemolytic effect of therapeutic drugs. Clinical considerations of the primaquine-type hemolysis. *JAMA* 180:388, 1962
14. HERMAN J, BEN-MEIR S: Overt hemolysis in patients with glucose-6-phosphate dehydrogenase deficiency. *Isr J Med Sci* 2:340, 1975
15. SZEINBERG A, KELLERMANN J, ADAM A, SHEBA C, RAMOT B: Haemolytic jaundice following aspirin administration to a patient with a deficiency of glucose-6-phosphate dehydrogenase in erythrocytes. *Acta Haematol* 23:58, 1960
16. BEUTLER E: *Hemolytic Anemia in Disorders of Red Cell Metabolism*. New York, Plenum, 1978
17. BURKA ER, WEAVER Z III, MARKS PA: Clinical spectrum of hemolytic anemia associated with G-6-PD deficiency. *Ann Intern Med* 64:817, 1966
18. MENGEL CE, METZ E, YANCEY WS: Anemia during acute infections. Role of glucose-6-phosphate dehydrogenase deficiency in Negroes. *Arch Intern Med* 119:287, 1967

19. BERRY DH, VIETTI TJ: Clinical manifestations of primaquine-sensitive anemia. *Am J Dis Child* 110:166, 1965

20. TUGWELL P: Glucose-6-phosphate-dehydrogenase deficiency in Nigerians with jaundice associated with lobar pneumonia. *Lancet* 1:968, 1973

21. GELLADY A, GREENWOOD RD: G-6-PD hemolytic anemia complicating diabetic ketoacidosis. *J Pediatr* 80:1037, 1972

22. KARAYALCIN G, KIM KY, ABALLI AJ, LANZKOWSKY P: Glucose-6-phosphate dehydrogenase (G-6-PD) deficiency and hyperbilirubinemia in black American term infants. *Am Soc Hematol* (abstract 165) p 92, 1973

23. IFEKWUNIGWE AE, LUZZATTO L: Kernicterus in G-6-PD-deficiency, *Lancet* 1:667, 1966

24. ESHAGHPOUR E, OSKI FA, WILLIAMS M: The relationship of erythrocyte glucose-6-phosphate dehydrogenase deficiency to hyperbilirubinemia in Negro premature infants. *J Pediatr* 70:595, 1967

25. GILLES HM, TAYLOR BG: The existence of the glucose-6-phosphate dehydrogenase deficiency trait in Nigeria and its clinical implications. *Ann Trop Med Parasitol* 55:64, 1961

26. HENDRICKSE RG: In discussion of paper by Motulsky A: Theoretical and clinical problems of glucose-6-phosphate dehydrogenase deficiency. Its occurrence in Africans and its combination with hemoglobinopathy. *Abnormal Haemoglobins in Africa* (Symposium) Jonxis JHP (Ed) 208, Oxford, Blackwell, 1965

27. LOPEZ R, COOPERMAN JM: Glucose-6-phosphate dehydrogenase deficiency and hyperbilirubinemia in the newborn. *Am J Dis Child* 122:66, 1971

28. BIENZLE U, EFFIONG CE, AIMAKU VE, LUZZATTO L: Erythrocyte enzymes in neonatal jaundice. *Acta Haematol* 55:10, 1976

29. GIBBS WN, GRAY R, LOWRY M: Glucose-6-phosphate dehydrogenase deficiency and neonatal jaundice in Jamaica. *Br J Haematol* 43:263, 1979

30. O FLYNN MED, HSIA DY: Serum bilirubin levels and glucose-6-phosphate dehydrogenase deficiency in newborn American Negroes. *J Pediatr* 63:160, 1963

31. ZINKHAM WH: Peripheral blood and bilirubin values in normal full-term primaquine-sensitive negro infants: Effect of vitamin K. *Pediatrics* 31:983, 1963

32. OWUSU SK, FOLI AK, KONOTEY HULU FID, ADDY JH, JANOSI M, LARBI EB: Acute reversible renal failure associated with glucose-6-phosphate dehydrogenase deficiency. *Lancet* 2:1255, 1972

33. SANSONE G, PIGA AM, SEGNI G: Il favismo. *Minerva Med* Torino, 1958

34. DAVIES P: Favism: A family study. *Q J Med* 31:157, 1962

35. KATTAMIS CA, KYRIAZAKOU M, CHAIDAS S: Favism. Clinical and biochemical data. *J Med Genet* 6:34, 1969

36. GEORGE JN, SEARS DA, McCURDY P, CONRAD ME: Primaquine sensitivity in Caucasians: Hemolytic reactions induced by primaquine in G-6-PD deficient subjects. *J Lab Clin Med* 70:80, 1967

37. SZEINBERG A, ASHER Y, SHEBA C: Studies on glutathione stability in erythrocytes of cases with past history of favism or sulfa-drug-induced hemolysis. *Blood* 13:348, 1958

38. HERSKO C, VARDY PA: Haemolysis in typhoid fever in children with G-6-PD deficiency. *Br Med J* 1:214, 1967

39. BERRY E, MELMED RN: Infectious hepatitis and glucose-6-phosphate dehydrogenase deficiency. *Isr J Med Sci* 13:600, 1977

40. CHOREMIS C, KATTAMIS CHA, KYRIAZAKOU M, GAVRIILIDOU E: Viral hepatitis in G-6-PD deficiency. *Lancet* 1:269, 1966

41. BOON WH: Viral hepatitis in G-6-PD deficiency. *Lancet* 1:882, 1966

42. SUTTON RNP: Viral hepatitis in G-6-PD deficiency. *Lancet* 1:550, 1966

43. SALEN G, GOLDSTEIN F, HAURANI F, WIRTS CW: Acute hemolytic anemia complicating viral hepatitis in patients with glucose-6-phosphate dehydrogenase deficiency. *Ann Intern Med* 65:1210, 1966

44. PHILLIPS SM, SILVERS NP: Glucose-6-phosphate dehydrogenase deficiency, infectious hepatitis, acute hemolysis, and renal failure. *Ann Intern Med* 70:99, 1969

45. CLEARFIELD HR, BRODY JI, TUMEN HJ: Acute viral hepatitis, glucose-6-phosphate dehydrogenase deficiency, and hemolytic anemia. *Arch Intern Med* 123:689, 1969

46. KATTAMIS CA, TJORTJATOU F: The hemolytic process of viral hepatitis in children with normal or deficient glucose-6-phosphate dehydrogenase activity. *J Pediatr* 77:422, 1970

47. FRIED D, GOTLIEB A, ROITMAN A: Infectious hepatitis with excessive hyperbilirubinemia and a hemolytic crisis in an 8-year-old boy. *Clin Pediatr* 16:482, 1977

48. LISKER R, LORIA A, STRYGLER I: Hemolytic anemia associated to instability of the reduced glutathione of the erythrocyte. Family affected with this defect. *Prensa Med Mex* 25:2, 1960

49. BEN-ISHAY D, IZAK G: Chronic hemolysis associated with glucose-6-phosphate deficiency. *J Lab Clin Med* 63:1002, 1964

50. BEUTLER E, MATHAI CK, SMITH JE: Biochemical variants of glucose-6-phosphate dehydrogenase giving rise to congenital nonspherocytic hemolytic disease. *Blood* 31:131, 1968

51. SCHETTINI F, MELONI T: Characterization of glucose-6-phosphate dehydrogenase in Sardinian children with congenital nonspherocytic haemolytic anaemia. *Acta Haematol* 37:198, 1967

52. SAZAMA K, KLEIN HG, DAVEY RJ, CORASH L: Intraoperative hemolysis. *Arch Intern Med* 140:845, 1980

53. ROECKEL IE: Transfusion requirements of patients with enzyme deficient red cells. *Ann Clin Lab Sci* 7:511, 1977

54. GULATI PD, RIZVI SNA: Acute reversible renal failure in G-6-PD-deficient siblings. *Postgrad Med J* 52:83, 1976

55. JIM RTS, CHU FK: Hyperbilirubinemia due to glucose-6-phosphate dehydrogenase deficiency in a newborn Chinese infant. *Pediatrics* 31:1046, 1963

56. SCHAERER K, HERZKA H, MARTI HR: Kernicterus bei mangel an Glukose-6-phosphat-dehydrogenase der Erythrocyten. *Helv Paediatr Acta* 2:148, 1963

57. DOXIADIS SA, FESSAS P, VALAES T, MASTROKALOS N: Glucose-6-phosphate dehydrogenase deficiency. *Lancet* 1:297, 1961

58. PANIZON F: Dimostrazione della anomalia enzimatica nel fegato di soggetti con difetto eritrocitario di glucose-6-fosfato deidrogenasi. *Boll Soc Ital Biol Sper* 36:106, 1960

59. DOXIADIS SA, FESSAS P, VALAES T: Erythrocyte enzyme deficiency in unexplained kernicterus. *Lancet* 2:44, 1960

60. SMITH G, VELLA F: Erythrocyte enzyme deficiency in unexplained kernicterus. *Lancet* 1:1133, 1960

61. WEATHERALL, DJ: Enzyme deficiency in haemolytic disease of the newborn. *Lancet* 2:835, 1960

62. PANIZON F: L'Ictere grave du nouveau-ne associe a une deficience en glucose-6-phosphate dehydrogenase. *Biol Neonate* 2:167, 1960

63. LU TC, WEI H, BLACKWELL RQ: Increased incidence of severe hyperbilirubinemia among newborn Chinese infants with G-6-PD deficiency. *Pediatrics* 37:994, 1966

64. MILBAUER B, PELED N, SVIRSKY S: Neonatal hyperbilirubinemia and glucose-6-phosphate dehydrogenase deficiency. *Isr J Med Sci* 9:1547, 1973

65. GROSS RT, HURWITZ RE, MARKS PA: An hereditary enzymatic defect in erythrocyte metabolism: Glucose-6-phosphate dehydrogenase deficiency. *J Clin Invest* 37:1176, 1958

66. SZEINBERG A, PRAS M, SHEBA C, ADAM A, RAMOT B: The hemolytic effect of various sulfonamides on subjects with a deficiency of glucose-6-phosphate dehydrogenase of erythrocytes. *Isr J Med Sci* 18:176, 1959

67. BERNARD J, DREYFUS JC: Hemolyse aigue familiale et deficit de la glucose-6-phosphate desy- drogenase des erythrocytes. *Nouv Rev Fr Hematol* 2:135, 1962

68. LARIZZA P, BRUNETTI P, GRIGNANI F, VENTURA S: I fabici sono sensibili alla primachina. *Minerva Med* 49:3769, 1958

69. CHAN TK, CHESTERMAN CN, McFADZEAN AJS, TODD D: The survival of glucose-6-phosphate dehydrogenase-deficient erythrocytes in patients with typhoid fever on chloramphenicol therapy. *J Lab Clin Med* 77:177, 1971

70. McCAFFREY RP, HALSTED CH, WAHAB MFA, ROBERTSON RP: Chloramphenicol-induced hemolysis in Caucasian glucose-6-phosphate dehydrogenase deficiency. *Ann Intern Med* 74:722, 1971

71. LARIZZA P, BRUNETTI P, GRIGNANI F: Anemie emolitiche enzimopeniche. *Haematologica (Pavia)* 45:1, 129, 1960

72. CHATTERJI SC, DAS PK: Chloramphenicol induced haemolytic anaemia due to enzymatic deficiency of erythrocytes. *J Indian Med Assoc* 40:172, 1963

73. VELLA F: Favism in Asia. *Med J Aust* 2:196, 1959

74. PANICH V, NA NAKORN S: Acute hemolysis in G-6-PD Union (Thai). Report on four cases. *J Med Assoc Thai* 56:241, 1973

75. WITT I, YOSHIOKA S: Biochemical characterization of a glucose-6-phosphate dehydrogenase variant with favism: G-6-PD Zaehringen. *Klin Wochenschr* 50:205, 1972

76. MURPHY JR: Erythrocyte metabolism. II. Glucose metabolism and pathways. *J Lab Clin Med* 55:286, 1960

77. KIRKMAN HN: Glucose-6-phosphate dehydrogenase from human erythrocytes. I. Further purification and characterization. *J Biol Chem* 237:2364, 1962

78. SOLDIN SJ, BALINSKY D: The kinetic properties of human erythrocyte glucose-6-phosphate dehydrogenase. *Biochemistry* 7:1077, 1968

79. YOSHIDA A: Hemolytic anemia and G-6-PD deficiency. *Science* 179:532, 1973

80. AFOLAYAN A, LUZZATTO L: Genetic variants of human erythrocyte glucose-6-phosphate dehydrogenase. I. Regulation of activity by oxidized and reduced nicotinamide adenine dinucleotide phosphate. *Biochemistry* 10:415, 1971

81. AVIGAD G: Inhibition of glucose-6-phosphate dehydrogenase by adenosine-5-triphosphate. *Proc Natl Acad Sci USA* 56:1543, 1966

82. BEN-BASSAT I, BEUTLER E: Inhibition by ATP of erythrocyte glucose-6-phosphate dehydrogenase variants. *Proc Soc Exp Biol Med* 142:410, 1973

83. GAETANI GD, PARKER JC, KIRKMAN HN: Intracellular restraint: A new basis for the limitation in response to oxidative stress in human erythro-

cytes containing low-activity variants of glucose-6-phosphate dehydrogenase. *Proc Natl Acad Sci USA* 71:3584, 1974

84. WILSON WG, KIRKMAN HN, CLEMONS EH: Regulation of glucose-6-phosphate dehydrogenase. *J Lab Clin Med* 95:888, 1980

85. SASS MD, CARUSO CJ, FARHANGI M: TPNH-methemoglobin reductase deficiency: A new red-cell enzyme defect. *J Lab Clin Med* 70:760, 1967

86. BEUTLER E, BALUDA MC: Methemoglobin reduction. Studies of the interaction between cell populations and of the role of methylene blue. *Blood* 22:323, 1963

87. ROSEN PJ, JOHNSON C, MCGEHEE WG, BEUTLER E: Failure of methylene blue treatment in toxic methemoglobinemia. Association with glucose-6-phosphate dehydrogenase deficiency. *Ann Intern Med* 75:83, 1971

88. TRAVIS SF, MORRISON AD, CLEMENTS JR RS, WINEGRAD AI, OSKI FA: Metabolic alterations in the human erythrocyte produced by increases in glucose concentration. The role of the polyol pathway. *J Clin Invest* 50:2104, 1971

89. BEUTLER E, GUINTO E: The reduction of glyceraldehyde by human erythrocytes. L-Hexonate dehydrogenase activity. *J Clin Invest* 53:1258, 1264, 1974

90. BEUTLER E, GUINTO E: Mechanism of stimulation of the hexose monophosphate shunt of erythrocytes by pyruvate. *Enzyme* 18:7, 1974

91. MEISTER A: Reduction of alpha, gamma-diketo and alpha-keto acids catalyzed by muscle preparations and by crystalline lactic dehydrogenase. *J Biol Chem* 184:117, 1950

92. YEH GC, PHANG JM: The function of pyrroline-5-carboxylate reductase in human erythrocytes. *Biochem Biophys Res Commun* 94:450, 1980

93. WOODWARD GE: Glyoxalase III. Glyoxalase as a reagent for the quantitative micro-estimation of glutathione. *J Biol Chem* 109:1, 1935

94. MINNICH V, SMITH MB, BRAUNER MJ, MAJERUS PW: Glutathione biosynthesis in human erythrocytes I. Identification of the enzymes of glutathione synthesis in hemolysates. *J Clin Invest* 50:507, 1971

95. BOIVIN P, GALAND C, ANDRE R, DEBRAY J: Anemies hemolytiques congenitales avec deficit isole en glutathion reduit par deficit en glutathion synthetase. *Nouv Rev Fr Hematol* 6:859, 1966

96. BOIVIN P, GALAND C, BERNARD JF: Deficiencies in G-SH biosynthesis, in Flohe L, Benöhr HC, Sies H, Waller HD, Wendel A (eds): *Glutathione.* New York, Academic, 1974, pp 146–157

97. MOHLER DN, MAJERUS PW, MINNICH V, HESS CE, GARRICK MD: Glutathione synthetase deficiency as a cause of hereditary hemolytic disease. *N Engl J Med* 283:1253, 1970

98. KONRAD PN, RICHARDS II F, VALENTINE WN, PAGLIA DE: Gamma-glutamyl-cysteine synthetase deficiency. *N Engl J Med* 286:557, 1972

99. MEISTER A: On the enzymology of amino acid transport. *Science* 180:33, 1973

100. SRIVASTAVA SK, AWASTHI YC, MILLER SP, YOSHIDA A, BEUTLER E: Studies on gamma-glutamyl transpeptidase in human and rabbit erythrocytes. *Blood* 47:645, 1976

101. BOARD PG, SMITH JE: Erythrocyte gamma-glutamyl transpeptidase. *Blood* 49:667, (letter to the editor), 1977

102. YOUNG JD, ELLORY JC, WRIGHT PC: Evidence against the participation of the gamma-glutamyltransferase-gamma-glutamylcyclotransferase pathway in amino acid transport by rabbit erythrocytes. *Biochem J* 152:713, 1975

103. DIMANT E, LANDBERG E, LONDON IM: The metabolic behavior of reduced glutathione in human and avian erythrocytes. *J Biol Chem* 213:769, 1955

104. SRIVASTAVA SK, BEUTLER E: The transport of oxidized glutathione from human erythrocytes. *J Biol Chem* 244:9, 1969

105. SRIVASTAVA SK, BEUTLER E: The transport of oxidized glutathione from the erythrocytes of various species in the presence of chromate. *Biochem J* 114:833, 1969

106. PRCHAL J, SRIVASTAVA SK, BEUTLER E: Active transport of GSSG from reconstituted erythrocyte ghosts. *Blood* 46:111, 1975

107. SMITH JE: Relationship of in vivo erythrocyte glutathione flux to the oxidized glutathione transport system. *J Lab Clin Med* 83:444, 1974

108. GRIFFITH OW, MEISTER A: Glutathione: Interorgan translocation, turnover, and metabolism. *Proc Natl Acad Sci USA* 76:5606, 1979

109. SCHULMAN JD, GOODMAN SI, MACE JW, PATRICK AD, TIETZE F, BUTLER EJ: Glutathionuria: Inborn error of metabolism due to tissue deficiency of gamma-glutamyl transpeptidase. *Biochem Biophys Res Commun* 65:68, 1975

110. GRIFFITH OW, MEISTER A: Excretion of cysteine and gamma-glutamyl-cysteine moieties in human and experimental animal gamma-glutamyl transpeptidase deficiency. *Proc Natl Acad Sci USA* 3384, 1980

111. SRIVASTAVA SK, BEUTLER E: Glutathione metabolism of the erythrocyte. The enzymic cleavage of glutathione-haemoglobin preparations by glutathione reductase. *Biochem J* 119:353, 1970

112. JACOB HS, JANDL JH: Effects of sulfhydryl inhibition on red blood cells. III. Glutathione in the regulation of the hexose monophosphate pathway. *J Biol Chem* 241:4243, 1966

113. FRIDOVICH I: Oxygen: Boon and bane. *Am Sci* 63:54, 1975

114. BEUTLER E, ROBSON M, BUTTENWIESER E: The mechanism of glutathione destruction and protection in drug-sensitive and non-sensitive erythrocytes. In vitro studies. *J Clin Invest* 36:617, 1957

115. KOSOWER NS, SONG KR, KOSOWER EM, CORREA W: Glutathione II. Chemical aspects of azoester procedure for oxidation to disulfide. *Biochim Biophys Acta* 192:8, 1969

116. KOSOWER ND: Discussion of "Glutathione deficiency" by Prins HK, Loos JA, Zürcher C, in Beutler E (ed): *Hereditary Disorders of Erythrocyte Metabolism,* New York, City of Hope Symp Series, Grune & Stratton, 1968, vol I, pp 176–178

117. COHEN G, HOCHSTEIN P: Generation of hydrogen peroxide in erythrocytes by hemolytic agents. *Biochemistry* 3:895, 1964

118. YOSHIDA A: Glucose-6-phosphate dehydrogenase of human erythrocytes. I. Purification and characterization of normal (B+) enzyme. *J Biol Chem* 241:4966, 1966

119. KIRKMAN HN, HENDRICKSON EM: Glucose-6-phosphate dehydrogenase from human erythrocytes. II. Subactive states of the enzyme from normal persons. *J Biol Chem* 237:2371, 1962

120. MARKS PA, SZEINBERG A, BANKS J: Erythrocyte glucose-6-phosphate dehydrogenase of normal and mutant human subjects: Properties of the purified enzyme. *J Biol Chem* 236:10, 1961

121. CHUNG AE, LANGDON RG: Human erythrocyte glucose-6-phosphate dehydrogenase I. Isolation and properties of the enzyme. *J Biol Chem* 238:2309, 1963

122. BALINSKY D, BERNSTEIN RE: The purification and properties of glucose-6-phosphate dehydrogenase from human erythrocytes. *Biochim Biophys Acta* 67:313, 1963

123. RATTAZZI MC: Isolation and purification of human erythrocyte glucose-6-phosphate dehydrogenase from small amounts of blood. *Biochim Biophys Acta* 181:1, 1969

124. DE FLORA A, MORELLI A, BENATTI U, GIULIANO F: An improved procedure for rapid isolation of glucose 6-phosphate dehydrogenase from human erythrocytes. *Arch Biochem Biophys* 169:362, 1975

125. DE FLORA A, GIULIANO F, MORELLI A: Rapid purification of glucose 6-phosphate dehydrogenase from human erythrocytes by means of affinity chromatography. *Ital J Biochem* 22:258, 1973

126. KAPLAN NO, EVERSE J, DIXON JE, STOLZENBACH FE, LEE C, LEE CLT, TAYLOR SS, MOSBACH K: Purification and separation of pyridine nucleotide-linked dehydrogenases by affinity chromatography techniques. *Proc Natl Acad Sci USA* 71:3450, 1974

127. YOSHIDA A: A single amino acid substitution (asparagine to aspartic acid) between normal (B+) and the common Negro variant (A+) of human glucose-6-phosphate dehydrogenase. *Proc Natl Acad Sci USA* 57:835, 1967

128. YOSHIDA A: Human glucose-6-phosphate dehydrogenase: Purification and characterization of Negro type variant (A+) and comparison with normal enzyme (B+). *Biochem Genet* 1:81, 1967

129. YOSHIDA A: Subunit structure of human glucose-6-phosphate dehydrogenase and its genetic implication. *Biochem Genet* 2:237, 1968

130. BONSIGNORE A, CANCEDDA R, NICOLINI A, DAMIANI G, DE FLORA A: Metabolism of human erythrocyte glucose-6-phosphate dehydrogenase VI. Interconversion of multiple molecular forms. *Arch Biochem Biophys* 147:493, 1971

131. MORELLI A, BENATTI U, GIULIANO F, DE FLORA A: Human erythrocyte glucose-6-phosphate dehydrogenase. Evidence for competitive binding of NADP and NADPH. *Biochem Biophys Res Commun* 70:600, 1976

132. CHUNG AE, LANGDON RG: Human erythrocyte glucose 6-phosphate dehydrogenase. II. Enzyme-coenzyme interrelationship. *J Biol Chem* 238:2317, 1963

133. BEUTLER E, COLLINS Z: Hybridization studies in the further characterization of erythrocyte glucose-6-phosphate dehydrogenase. *Experientia* 22:827, 1966

134. ROSA R, DREYFUS JC: Hybridation de la glucose-6-phosphate deshydrogenase des globules rouges et des globules blancs humains avec l' enzyme de differents tissus de rat. *Clin Chim Acta* 24:199, 1969

135. YOSHIDA A, STEINMANN L, HARBERT P: In vitro hybridization of normal and variant human glucose-6-phosphate dehydrogenase. *Nature* 216:275, 1967

136. RATTAZZI MC: Glucose-6-phosphate dehydrogenase from human erythrocytes: Molecular weight determination by gel filtration. *Biochem Biophys Res Commun* 31:16, 1968

137. YOSHIDA A: Change of activity and substrate specificity of human glucose-6-phosphate dehydrogenase by oxidation. *Arch Biochem Biophys* 159:82, 1973

138. KAHN A, LAGNEAU J, BOIVIN P, HAKIM J: Importance et role des groupes imidazole et sulfhydrile dans L'activite catalytique de la glucose 6 phosphate deshydrogenase erythrocytaire humaine. *Biochimie* 54:997, 1972

139. KIRKMAN HN, MCCURDY PR, NAIMAN JL: Functionally abnormal glucose-6-phosphate dehydrogenases. *Cold Spring Harbor Symp, Quant Biol* 29:391, 1964

140. KIRKMAN HN, RILEY HD JR, CROWELL BB: Different enzymic expressions

of mutants of human glucose-6-phosphate dehydrogenase. *Proc Natl Acad Sci USA* 46:938, 1960

141. LUZZATTO L: Regulation of the activity of glucose-6-phosphate dehydrogenase by NADP+ and NADPH. *Biochim Biophys Acta* 146:18, 1967

142. GLADER BE, CONRAD ME: Cyanate inhibition of erythrocyte glucose-6-phosphate dehydrogenase. *Nature* 237:336, 1972

143. KISSIN C, BEUTLER E: The utilization of glucose by normal glucose-6-phosphate dehydrogenase and by glucose-6-phosphate dehydrogenase Mediterranean. *Proc Soc Exp Biol Med* 128:595, 1968

144. BEUTLER E, COLLINS Z, IRWIN L: Value of genetic variants of glucose-6-phosphate dehydrogenase in tracing the origin of malignant tumors. *N Engl J Med* 276:389, 1967

145. BEUTLER E, MORRISON M: Localization and characteristics of hexose-6-phosphate dehydrogenase (glucose dehydrogenase). *J Biol Chem* 242:5289, 1967

146. MANDULA B, SRIVASTAVA SK, BEUTLER E: Hexose-6-phosphate dehydrogenase: Distribution in rat tissues and effect of diet, age and steroids. *Arch Biochem Biophys* 141:155, 1970

147. KAHN MA, MEIENHOFER MC, VIBERT M, DREYFUS JC: Vieillissement moleculaire de la glucose 6 phosphate deshydrogenase humaine. *C R Acad Sci (D) (Paris)* 278:1265, 1974

148. LUZZATTO L, AFOLAYAN A: Different types of human erythrocyte glucose-6-phosphate dehydrogenase, with characterization of two new genetic variants. *J Clin Invest* 47:1833, 1968

149. YOSHIDA A, STAMATOYANNOPOULOS G, MOTULSKY A: Negro variant of glucose-6-phosphate dehydrogenase deficiency (A−) in man. *Science* 155:97, 1967

150. LUZZATTO L, ALLAN NC: Different properties of glucose-6-phosphate dehydrogenase from human erythrocytes with normal and abnormal enzyme levels. *Biochem Biophys Res Commun* 21:547, 1965

151. YOSHIDA A: The structure of normal and variant human glucose-6-phosphate dehydrogenase, in Beutler E (ed): *Hereditary Disorders of Erythrocyte Metabolism* City of Hope Symp Series, New York, Grune & Stratton, 1968, vol I, pp 146–164

152. DE MARS R: A temperature-sensitive glucose-6-phosphate dehydrogenase in mutant cultured human cells. *Proc Natl Acad Sci USA* 61:562, 1968

153. MODIANO G, BATTISTUZZI G, ESAN GJF, TESTA U, LUZZATTO L: Genetic heterogeneity of "normal" human erythrocyte glucose-6-phosphate dehydrogenase: An isoelectrophoretic polymorphism. *Proc Natl Acad Sci USA* 76:852, 1979

154. BERNSTEIN SC, BOWMAN JE, NOCHE LK: Genetic variation in Cameron: Thermostability variants of hemoglobin and of glucose-6-phosphate dehydrogenase. *Biochem Genet* 18:21, 1980

155. JUNIEN C, KAPLAN JC, MEIENHOFER MC, MAIGRET P, SENDER A: G 6 PD Baudelocque: A new unstable variant characterized in cultured fibroblasts. *Enzyme* 18:48, 1974

156. HONIG GR, HABACON E, VIDA LN, MATSUMOTO F, BEUTLER E: Three new variants of glucose-6-phosphate dehydrogenase associated with chronic nonspherocytic hemolytic anemia: G-6-PD Lincoln Park, G-6-PD Arlington Heights, and G-6-PD West Town. *Am J Hematol* 6:353, 1979

157. KAHN A, DAO C, COTTREAU D, BILSKI SQUIER G: "GD (−) Hotel Dieu": A new G-6-PD variant with chronic hemolysis in a Negro patient from Senegal. *Hum Genet* 39:353, 1977

158. BEUTLER E, GROOMS AM, MORGAN SK, TRINIDAD F: Chronic severe hemolytic anemia due to G-6-PD Charleston: A new deficient variant. *J Pediatr* 80:1005, 1972

159. HOWELL EB, NELSON AJ, JONES OW: A new G-6-PD variant associated with chronic non-spherocytic haemolytic anaemia in a Negro family. *J Med Genet* 9:160, 1972

160. FELDMAN R, GROMISCH DS, LUHBY AL, BEUTLER E: Congenital nonspherocytic hemolytic anemia due to glucose-6-phosphate dehydrogenase East Harlem: A new deficient variant. *J Pediatr* 90:89, 1977

161. THIGPEN JT, STEINBERG MH, BEUTLER E, GILLESPIE GT JR, DREILING BJ, MORRISON FS: Glucose-6-phosphate dehydrogenase Jackson. A new variant associated with hemolytic anemia. *Acta Haematol* 51:310, 1974

162. FAIRBANKS VF, NEPO AG, BEUTLER E, DICKSON ER, HONIG G: Glucose-6-phosphate dehydrogenase variants: Reexamination of G6PD Chicago and Cornell and a new variant (G6PD Pea Ridge) resembling G6PD Chicago. *Blood* 55:216, 1980

163. CHAN TK, LAI MCS: Glucose-6-phosphate dehydrogenase: Identity of erythrocyte and leukocyte enzyme with report of a new variant in Chinese. *Biochem Genet* 6:119, 1972

164. RAMOT B, BEN-BASSAI I, SHCHORY M: New glucose-6-phosphate dehydrogenase variants observed in Israel and their association with congenital nonspherocytic hemolytic disease. *J Lab Clin Med* 74:895, 1969

165. TALALAK P, BEUTLER E: G-6-PD Bangkok: A new variant found in congenital nonspherocytic hemolytic disease (CNHD). *Blood* 33:772, 1969

166. KIRKMAN HN, RILEY HD JR: Congenital nonspherocytic hemolytic anemia. *Am J Dis Child* 102:313, 1961

167. NANCE WE: Turner's syndrome, twinning, and an unusual variant of glucose-6-phosphate dehydrogenase. *Am J Hum Genet* 16:380, 1964

168. WONG PWK, SHIH LY, HSIA DYY: Characterization of glucose-6-phosphate dehydrogenase among Chinese. *Nature* 208:1323, 1965

169. NECHELES TF, SNYDER LM, STRAUSS W: Glucose-6-phosphate dehydrogenase Boston. A new variant associated with congenital nonspherocytic hemolytic disease. *Humangenetik* 13:218, 1971

170. RATTAZZI MC, CORASH LM, VAN ZANEN GE, JAFFE ER, PIOMELLI S: G6PD deficiency and chronic hemolysis: Four new mutants—relationships between clinical syndrome and enzyme kinetics. *Blood* 38:205, 1971

171. BEUTLER E, MATSUMOTO F: Unpublished data, 1975

172. MIWA S, ONO J, NAKASHIMA K, ABE S, KAGEOKA T, SHINOHARA K, ISOBE J, YAMAGUCHI H: Two new glucose 6-phosphate dehydrogenase variants associated with congenital nonspherocytic hemolytic anemia found in Japan: GD(−) Tokushima and GD(−) Tokyo. *Am J Hematol* 1:433, 1976

173. KAHN A, BOULARD M, HAKIM J, SCHAISON G, BOIVIN P, BERNARD J: Anemie hemolytique congenitale non spherocytaire par deficit en glucose-6-phosphate-deshydrogenase erythrocytaire. Description de deux nouvelles variantes: GD(−) Saint Louis (Paris) et GD (−) Hayem. *Nouv Rev Fr Hematol* 14:587, 1974

174. GAHR M, SCHRÖTER W, STURZENEGGER M, BORNHALM D, MARTI HR: Glucose-6-phosphate dehydrogenase (G-6-PD) deficiency in Switzerland. *Helv Paediatr Acta* 31:159, 1976

175. VUOPIO P, HARKONEN R, JOHNSON R, NUUTINEN M: Red cell glucose-6-phosphate dehydrogenase deficiency in Finland. *Ann Clin Res* 5:168, 1973

176. CHERNYAK NB, BATISCHEV AI, LAMZINA NV, TOKAREV YN, ALEXEEV GA: Electrophoretic and kinetic properties of glucose-6-phosphate dehydrogenase from erythrocytes or patients with hemolytic anemia, related to deficiency of the enzyme activity. *Vopr Med Khim* 23:166, 1977

177. MIWA S, FUJII H, NAKASHIMA K, MIURA Y, YAAMADA K, HAGIWARA T, FUKUDA M: Three new electrophoretically normal glucose-6-phosphate dehydrogenase variants associated with congenital nonspherocytic hemolytic anemia found in Japan: G6PD Ogikubo, Yokohama, and Akita. *Hum Genet* 45:11, 1978

178. PRCHAL J, MORENO H, CONRAD M, VITEK A: G-6-PD Dothan: A new variant associated with chronic hemolytic anemia. *IRCS* 7:348, 1979

179. JOHNSON GJ, KAPLAN ME, BEUTLER E: G-6-PD Long Prairie: A new mutant exhibiting normal sensitivity to inhibition by NADPH and accompanied by nonspherocytic hemolytic anemia. *Blood* 49:247, 1977

180. CEDERBAUM AI, BEUTLER E: Nonspherocytic hemolytic anemia due to G-6-PD Grand Prairie. *IRCS* 3:579, 1975

181. KIRKMAN HN, ROSENTHAL IM, SIMON ER, CARSON PE, BRINSON AG: "Chicago I" variant of glucose-6-phosphate dehydrogenase in congenital hemolytic disease. *J Lab Clin Med* 63:715, 1964

182. BEUTLER E, MATSUMOTO F, DIABER A: Nonspherocytic hemolytic anemia due to G-6-PD Panama. *IRCS* 2:1389, 1974

183. ENGSTROM PF, BEUTLER E: G-6-PD Tripler: A unique variant associated with chronic hemolytic disease. *Blood* 36:10, 1970

184. BEUTLER E, ROSEN R: Nonspherocytic congenital hemolytic anemia due to a new G-6-PD variant: G-6-PD Alhambra. *Pediatrics* 45:230

185. KIDDER WR, BEUTLER E: Unpublished data, 1979

186. MILNER G, DELAMORE IW, YOSHIDA A: G-6-PD Manchester: A new variant associated with chronic nonspherocytic hemolytic anemia. *Blood* 43:271, 1974

187. BEUTLER E, KELLER JW, MATSUMOTO F: A new glucose-6-P dehydrogenase (G-6-PD) variant associated with nonspherocytic hemolytic anemia: G-6-PD Atlanta. *IRCS* 4:579, 1976

188. SNYDER LM, NECHELES TF, REDDY WJ: G-6-PD Worcester: A new variant, associated with X-linked optic atrophy. *Am J Med* 49:125, 1970

189. MENTZER WC JR, WARNER R, ADDIEGO J, SMITH B, WALTER T: G6PD San Francisco: A new variant of glucose-6-phosphate dehydrogenase associated with congenital nonspherocytic hemolytic anemia. *Blood* 55:195, 1980

190. MCCURDY PR: Unpublished data, 1975

191. CASTRO GAM, SNYDER LM: G6PD San Jose: A new variant characterized by NADPH inhibition studies. *Humangenetik* 21:361, 1974

192. YOSHIDA A, BAUR EW, MOTULSKY AG: A Philippino glucose-6-phosphate dehydrogenase variant (G6PD Union) with enzyme deficiency and altered substrate specificity. *Blood* 35:506, 1970

193. KAHN A, NORTH ML, MESSER J, BOIVIN P: G-6-PD "Ankara," a new G-6-PD variant with deficiency found in a Turkish family. *Humangenetik* 27:247, 1975

194. CARANDINA G, MORETTO E, ZECCHI G, CONIGHI C: Glucose-6-phosphate dehydrogenase Ferrara. A new variant of G-6-PD identified in northern Italy. *Acta Haematol* 56:116, 1976

195. PAWLAK AL, ZAGORSKI Z, ROZYNKOWA D, HORST A: Polish variant of glucose-6-phosphate dehydrogenase (G-6-PD Lublin). *Humangenetik* 10:340, 1970

196. MCCURDY PR, BLACKWELL PQ, TODD D, TSO, SC, TUCHINDA S: Further studies on glucose-6-phosphate dehydrogenase deficiency in Chinese subjects. *J Lab Clin Med* 75:788, 1970

197. McCurdy PR, Mahmood L: Red cell glucose-6-phosphate dehydrogenase deficiency in Pakistan. *J Lab Clin Med* 76:943, 1970

198. Kirkman HN, Schettini F, Pickard BM: Mediterranean variant of glucose-6-phosphate dehydrogenase. *J Lab Clin Med* 63:726, 1964

199. Yoshida A: Unpublished data, 1975

200. McCurdy PR, Kamel K, Selim O: Heterogeneity of red cell glucose-6-phosphate dehydrogenase (G-6-PD) deficiency in Egypt. *J Lab Clin Med* 84:673, 1974

201. Kahn A, Hakim J, Cottreau D, Boivin P: GD (−) Matam, an African glucose-6-phosphate dehydrogenase variant with enzyme deficiency. Biochemical and immunological properties in various hemopoietic tissues. *Clin Chim Acta* 59:183, 1975

202. Kahn A, Bernard J-F, Cottreau D, Marie J, Boivin P: GD(−) Abrami. A deficient G-6-PD variant with hemizygous expression in blood cells of a woman with primary myelofibrosis. *Humangenetik* 30:41, 1975

203. Gahr M, Bornhalm D, Schröter W: Haemolytic anaemia due to glucose-6-phosphate dehydrogenase (G6PD) deficiency: Demonstration of two new biochemical variants, G6PD Hamm and G6PD Tarsus. *Br J Haematol* 33:363, 1976

204. Shatskaya TL, Krasnopolskaya KD, Tzoneva M, Mavrudieva M, Toncheva D: Variants of erythrocyte glucose-6-phosphate dehydrogenase (G6PD) in Bulgarian populations. *Hum Genet* 54:115, 1980

205. Benabadji M, Merad F, Benmoussa M, Trabuchet G, Junien C, Dreyfus JC, Kaplan JC: Heterogeneity of glucose-6-phosphate dehydrogenase deficiency in Algeria. *Hum Genet* 40:177, 1978

206. Lisker R, Briceno RP, Zavala C, Navarrete JI, Wessels M, Yoshida A: A glucose 6-phosphate dehydrogenase GD(−) Castilla variant characterized by mild deficiency associated with drug induced hemolytic anemia. *J Lab Clin Med* 90:754, 1977

207. Beutler E: Glucose-6-phosphate dehydrogenase deficiency: A new Indian variant. G 6 PD Jammu, in Sen NN, Basu AK (eds): *Trends in Haematology.* Calcutta, NN Sen, 1975, pp 279–283

208. Vergnes H, Yoshida A, Gourdin D, Gherardi M, Bierme R, Ruffie J: Glucose-6-phosphate dehydrogenase Toulouse. A new variant with marked instability and severe deficiency discovered in a family of Mediterranean ancestry. *Acta Haematol* 51:240, 1974

209. Fernandez M, Fairbanks VF: Glucose-6-phosphate dehydrogenase deficiency in the Phillipines: Report of a new variant—G 6 PD Panay. *Mayo Clin Proc* 43:645, 1968

210. Krasnopolskaya KD, Shatskaya TL, Filippov IK, Annenkov GA, Zakharova TV, Mekhtiev NK, Movsum-Zade KM: Genetic heterogeneity of G 6 PD deficiency: Study of mutant alleles in Shekii district of Azerbaijan. *Genetika* 13:1455, 1977

211. Chockkalingam K, Board PG: Further evidence for heterogeneity of glucose-6-phosphate dehydrogenase deficiency in Papua New Guinea. *Hum Genet* 1981, in press

212. Pawlak AL, Mazurkiewicz CA, Ordynski J, Rozynkowa D, Horst A: G-6-PD Poznan, variant with severe enzyme deficiency. *Humangenetik* 28:163, 1975

213. Kahn A, Esters A, Habedank M: GD(−)Aachen, a new variant of deficient glucose-6-phosphate dehydrogenase. *Hum Genet* 32:171, 1976

214. Miwa S, Fujii H, Nakatsuji T, Ishida Y, Oda E, Kaneto A, Motokawa M, Ariga Y, Fukuchi S, Sasai S, Hiraoka K, Kashii H, Kodama T: Four new electrophoretically slow-moving glucose 6-phosphate dehydrogenase variants associated with congenital nonspherocytic hemolytic anemia found in Japan: Gd(−) Kurume, Gd(−) Fukushima, Gd(−) Yamaguchi and Gd(−) Wakayama. *Am J Hematol* 5:131, 1978

215. Shatskaya TL, Krasnopolskaya KD, Idelson LJ: Mutant forms of erythrocyte glucose-6-phosphate dehydrogenase in Ashkenazi. Description of two new variants: G6PD Kirovograd and G6PD Zhitomir. *Hum Genet* 33:175, 1976

216. Azevedo E, Kirkman HN, Morrow AC, Motulsky AG: Variants of red cell glucose-6-phosphate dehydrogenase among Asiatic Indians. *Ann Hum Genet* 31:373, 1968

217. McCurdy PR, Maldonado N, Dillon DE, Conrad ME: Variants of glucose-6-phosphate dehydrogenase (G-6-PD) associated with G-6-PD deficiency in Puerto Ricans. *J Lab Clin Med* 82:432, 1973

218. Kirkman HN, Hendrickson EM: Sex-linked electrophoretic difference in glucose-6-phosphate dehydrogenase. *Am J Hum Genet* 15:241, 1963

219. Kissin C, Cotte J: Etude d'un variant de glucose-6-phosphate deshydrogenase: Le type Constantine. *Enzyme* 11:277, 1970

220. Vergnes H, Gherardi M, Yoshida A: G6PD Lozere and Irinacria-like. Segregation of two non hemolytic variants in a French family. *Hum Genet* 34:293, 1976

221. Nakashima K, Ono J, Abe S, Miwa S, Yoshida A: G6PD Ube, a glucose-6-phosphate dehydrogenase variant found in four unrelated Japanese families. *Am J Hum Genet* 29:24, 1977

222. Nakatsuji T, Miwa S: Incidence and characteristics of glucose-6-phosphate dehydrogenase variants in Japan. *Hum Genet* 51:297, 1979

223. Lisker R, Briceno RP, Agrilar L, Yoshida A: A variant glucose-6-phosphate dehydrogenase Gd(−) Chiapas associated with moderate

enzyme deficiency and occasional hemolytic anemia. *Hum Genet* 43:81, 1978

224. Kaplan JC, Rosa R, Seringe P, Höffel JC: Le polyorphisme genetique de la glucose-6-phosphate deshydrogenase erythrocytaire chez l'homme. *Enzyme* 8:332, 1967

225. Crookston JH, Yoshida A, Lin M, Booser DJ: G 6 PD Toronto. *Biochem J* 8:259, 1973

226. McCurdy PR, Kirkman HN, Naiman JL, Jim RTS, Pickard BM: A Chinese variant of glucose-6-phosphate dehydrogenase. *J Lab Clin Med* 67:374, 1966

227. Mandelli F, Amadori S, De Laurenzi A, Kahn A, Isacchi G, Papa G: Glucose-6-phosphate dehydrogenase Velletri. *Acta Haematol* 57:121, 1977

228. Sansone G, Perroni L, Yoshida A: Glucose-6-phosphate dehydrogenase variants from Italian subjects associated with severe neonatal jaundice. *Br J Haematol* 31:159, 1975

229. Panich V, Sungnate T, Wasi P, Na Nakorn S: G-6-PD Mahidol. The most common glucose-6-phosphate dehydrogenase variant in Thailand. *J Med Assoc Thai* 55:576, 1972

230. Panich V, Sungnate T, Na Nakorn S: Acute intravascular hemolysis and renal failure in a new glucose-6-phosphate dehydrogenase variant: G-6-PD Siriraj. *J Med Assoc Thai* 55:726, 1972

231. Miwa S, Nakashima K, Ono J, Fujii H, Suzuki E: Three glucose 6-phosphate dehydrogenase variants found in Japan. *Hum Genet* 36:327, 1977

232. Panich V: G-6-PD Intanon. A new glucose-6-phosphate dehydrogenase variant. *Humangenetik* 21:203, 1974

233. Stamatoyannopoulos G, Yoshida A, Bacopoulos C, Motulsky A: Athens variant of glucose-6-phosphate dehydrogenase. *Science* 157:831, 1967

234. Kahn A, North ML, Cottreau D, Giron G, Lang JM: G6PD Vientiane: A new glucose-6-phosphate dehydrogenase variant with increased stability. *Hum Genet* 43:85, 1978

235. Beutler E, Matsumoto F: A new glucose-6-phosphate dehydrogenase variant: G-6-PD (−) Los Angeles. *IRCS* 5:89, 1977

236. Sansone G, Perroni L, Yoshida A, Dave V: A new glucose-6-phosphate dehydrogenase variant (GD Trinacria) in two unrelated families of Sicilian ancestry. *Ital J Biochem* 26:44, 1977

237. Kirkman HN, Simon ER, Pickard BM: Seattle variant of glucose-6-phosphate dehydrogenase. *J Lab Clin Med* 66:834, 1965

238. Siegel NH, Beutler E: Hemolytic anemia caused by G-6-PD Carswell, a new variant. *Ann Intern Med* 75:437, 1971

239. Panich V, Sungnate T: Characterization of glucose-6-phosphate dehydrogenase in Thailand. *Humangenetik* 18:39, 1973

240. Reys L, Manso C, Stamatoyannopoulos G: Genetic studies on southeastern Bantu of Mozambique. I. Variants of glucose-6-phosphate dehydrogenase. *Am J Hum Genet* 22:203, 1970

241. Vergnes H, Gherardi M, Quilici JC, Yoshida A, Giacardy R: G6PD Luz-Saint-Sauveur: A new variant with abnormal electrophoretic mobility mild enzyme deficiency and absence of haematological disorders. *IRCS* (73-7) 3-1-14 (abstract), 1973

242. Hurwic M: Dziedziczny Niedobor Dehydrogenazy Glukozo-6-fosforanowej w krwince czerwonej. *Postepy Hig Med Dosw* 24:497, 1970

243. Yoshida A, Baur E, Voigtlander B: Unpublished data, 1975

244. Boyer SH, Porter IH, Weilbacher RG: Electrophoretic heterogeneity of glucose-6-phosphate dehydrogenase and its relationship to enzyme deficiency in man. *Proc Natl Acad Sci USA* 48:1868, 1962

245. Long WK, Kirkman HN, Sutton HE: Electrophoretically slow variants of glucose-6-phosphate dehydrogenase from red cells of Negroes. *J Lab Clin Med* 65:81, 1965

246. Gonzalez R, Wade M, Estrada M, Svarch E, Colombo B: G6PD Pinar Del Rio: A new variant discovered in a Cuban family. *Biochem Genet* 15:909, 1977

247. Kaplan JC, Hanzlickova Leroux A, Nicholas AM, Rosa R, Weiler C, Lepercq G: A new glucose-6-phosphate dehydrogenase variant (G6PD Port-Royal). *Enzyme* 12:25, 1970

248. Nurse GT, Balinsky D: Unpublished data, 1975

249. Dern RJ, McCurdy PR, Yoshida A: A new structural variant of glucose-6-phosphate dehydrogenase with a high production rate (G6PD). *J Lab Clin Med* 73:283, 1969

250. Miller DR, Wollman MR: A new variant of glucose-6-phosphate dehydrogenase deficiency hereditary hemolytic anemia, G6PD Cornell: Erythrocyte, leukocyte, and platelet studies. *Blood* 44:323, 1974

251. Rubinstein D, Ottolengthi P, Denstedt OF: The metabolism of the erythrocyte XIII. Enzyme activity in the reticulocyte. *Can J Biochem* 34:222, 1956

252. Marks PA, Johnson AB, Hirschberg E: Effect of age on the enzyme activity in erythrocytes. *Proc Natl Acad Sci USA* 44:529, 1958

253. Löhr GW, Waller HD, Karges O, Schlegel B, Müller AA: Zur Biochemie der Alterung Menschlicher Erythrozyten. *Klin Wochenschr* 36:1008, 1958

254. MORELLI A, BENATTI U, GAETANI GF, DE FLORA A: Biochemical mechanisms of glucose-6-phosphate dehydrogenase deficiency. *Proc Natl Acad Sci USA* 75:1979, 1978

255. KIRKMAN H, CROWELL BB: Molecular deficiency of glucose-6-phosphate dehydrogenase in primaquine sensitivity. *Nature* 197:286, 1963

256. MARKS PA, TSUTSUI EA: Human Glucose-6-P dehydrogenase: studies on the relation between antigenicity and catalytic activity—the role of TPN. *Ann NY Acad SCI* 103:903, 1963

257. BABALOLA O, CANCEDDA R, LUZZATTO L: Genetic variants of glucose 6-phosphate dehydrogenase from human erythrocytes: Unique properties of the A− variant isolated from "deficient" cells. *Proc Natl Acad Sci USA* 69:946, 1972

258. MOTULSKY AG, CAMPBELL-KRAUT JM: Population genetics of glucose-6-phosphate dehydrogenase deficiency of the red cell, in Blumberg BS (ed): *Proc Conf Genetic Polymorphisms and Geographic Variations in Disease.* New York, Grune & Stratton, 1961, pp 159–180

259. LUZZATTO L, AFOLAYAN A: Genetic variants of human erythrocyte glucose-6-phosphate dehydrogenase. II. In vitro and in vivo function of the A− variant. *Biochemistry* 10:420, 1971

260. RAMOT B, BAUMINGER S, BROK F, GAFNI D, SHWARTZ J: Characterization of glucose-6-phosphate dehydrogenase in Jewish mutants. *J Lab Clin Med* 64:895, 1964

261. YOSHIDA A: Amino acid substitution (histidine to tyrosine) in a glucose-6-phosphate dehydrogenase variant (G6PD Hektoen) associated with overproduction. *J Mol Biol* 52:483, 1970

262. SRIVASTAVA SK, BEUTLER E: Formation and cleavage of mixed disulfide of hemoglobin-glutathione in intact erythrocytes. *Haematologia (Budap)* 8:121, 1975

263. KOSOWER NS, VANDERHOFF GA, LONDON IM: The regeneration of reduced glutathione in normal and glucose-6-phosphate dehydrogenase deficient human red blood cells. *Blood* 29:313, 1967

264. KOSOWER NS, KOSOWER EM, WERTHEIM B: Diamide, a new reagent for the intracellular oxidation of glutathione to the disulfide. *Biochem Biophys Res Commun* 37:593, 1969

265. SRIVASTAVA SK, AWASTHI YO, BEUTLER E: Useful agents for the study of glutathione metabolism in erythrocytes. Organic hydroperoxides. *Biochem J* 139:289, 1974

266. DAWSON JP, THAYER WW, DESFORGES JF: Acute hemolytic anemia in the newborn infant due to naphthalene poisoning. Report of two cases with investigation into the mechanism of the disease. *Blood* 13:1113, 1958

267. JAFFE ER: The reduction of methemoglobin in erythrocytes of a patient with congenital methemoglobinemia, subjects with erythrocyte glucose-6-phosphate dehydrogenase deficiency, and normal individuals. *Blood* 21:561, 1963

268. LÖHR GW, WALLER HD: Biochemie und Pathogenese der enzymopenischen haemolytischen Anaemien. *Dtsch Med Wochenschr* 86:27, 1961

269. KOUTRAS GA, SCHNEIDER AS, HATTORI M, VALENTINE WN: Studies on chromated erythrocytes. Mechanisms of chromate inhibition of glutathione reductase. *Br J Haematol* 11:360, 1965

270. KOUTRAS GA, HATTORI M, SCHNEIDER AS, EBAUGH FG JR, VALENTINE WN: Studies on chromated erythrocytes. Effect of sodium chromate on erythrocyte glutathione reductase. *J Clin Invest* 43:323, 1964

271. BRIN M, YONEMOTO RH: Stimulation of the glucose oxidative pathway in human erythrocytes by methylene blue. *J Biol Chem* 230:307, 1958

272. DAVIDSON WD, TANAKA KR: Continuous measurement of pentose phosphate pathway activity in erythrocytes. An ionization chamber method. *J Lab Clin Med* 73:173, 1969

273. KIRKMAN HN, GAETANI GD, CLEMONS EH, MARENI C: Red cell NADP+ and NADPH in glucose-6-phosphate dehydrogenase deficiency. *J Clin Invest* 55:875, 1975

274. SCHRIER SL, KELLERMEYER RW, CARSON PE, ICKES CE, ALVING AS: The hemolytic effect of primaquine (IX. Enzymatic abnormalities in primaquine-sensitive erythrocytes). *J Lab Clin Med* 52:109, 1958

275. FLATZ G: Enhanced binding of FAD to glutathione reductase in G-6-PD deficiency. *Nature* 226:755, 1970

276. BONSIGNORE A, FORNAINI G, SEGNI G, FANTONI F: Glutathione-reductase and methaemoglobin-reductase in erythrocytes of human subjects with a case history of favism. *Ital J Biochem* 9:345, 1960

277. WASSERZUG O, SZEINBERG A, SPERLING O: Erythrocyte glutathione reductase in gout and in glucose-6-phosphate dehydrogenase deficiency. *Monogr Hum Genet* 9:16, 1978

278. BEUTLER E: Glucose-6-phosphate dehydrogenase deficiency and red cell glutathione peroxidase. *Blood* 49:467, 1977

279. SWARUP-MITRA S: Activity of glutathione peroxidase and glutathione reductase in G-6-PD deficient subjects. *Indian J Med Res* 66:253, 1977

280. LÖHR GW, WALLER HD: Haemolytische Erythrocytopathie durch Fehlen von Glukose-6-Phosphat- Dehydrogenase in roten blutzellen als dominant verbliche Krankheit. *Klin Wochenschr* 36:865, 1958

281. ALLEN DW, JOHNSON GJ, CADMAN S, KAPLAN ME: Membrane polypeptide aggregates in glucose-6-phosphate dehydrogenase deficient and in vitro aged red blood cells. *J Lab Clin Med* 91:321, 1978

282. JOHNSON GJ, ALLEN DW, CADMAN S, FAIRBANKS VF, WHITE JG, LAMPKIN BC, KAPLAN ME: Red-cell-membrane polypeptide aggregates in glucose-6-phosphate dehydrogenase mutants with chronic hemolytic disease. *N Engl J Med* 301:522, 1979

283. COETZER T, ZAIL SS: Erythrocyte membrane proteins in hereditary glucosephosphate isomerase deficiency. *J Clin Invest* 63:552, 1979

284. AFOLAYAN A: Plasma membrane of human erythrocyte with different levels of glucose-6-phosphate dehydrogenase. *Int J Biochem* 10:361, 1979

285. BREWER GJ, TARLOV AR, KELLERMEYER RW: The hemolytic effect of primaquine. XII. Shortened erythrocyte life span in primaquine-sensitive male Negroes in the absence of drug administration. *J Lab Clin Med* 58:217, 1961

286. BERNINI L, LATTE B, SINISCALCO M, PIOMELLI S, SPADA U, ADINOLFI M, MOLLISON PL: Survival of 51 Cr-labelled red cells in subjects with thalassemia-trait or G6PD deficiency or both abnormalities. *Br J Haematol* 10:171, 1964

287. BEUTLER E, DERN RJ, ALVING AS: The hemolytic effect of primaquine. IV. The relationship of cell age to hemolysis. *J Lab Clin Med* 44:439, 1954

288. FLANAGAN CL, SCHRIER SL, CARSON PE, ALVING AS: The hemolytic effect of primaquine VIII. The effect of drug administration on parameters of primaquine sensitivity. *J Lab Clin Med* 51:600, 1958

289. HERZ F, KAPLAN E, SCHEYE ES: Diagnosis of erythrocyte glucose-6-phosphate dehydrogenase deficiency in the Negro male despite hemolytic crisis. *Blood* 35:90, 1970

290. JACOB HS, BRAIN MC, DACIE JV, CARRELL RW, LEHMANN H: Abnormal haem binding and globin SH group blockade in unstable haemoglobins. *Nature* 218:1214, 1968

291. ALLEN DW, JANDL JH: Oxidative hemolysis and precipitation of hemoglobin. II. Role of thiols in oxidant drug action. *J Clin Invest* 40:454, 1961

292. BIRCHMEIER W, TUCHSCHMID PE, WINTERHALTER H: Comparison of human hemoglobin A carrying glutathione as a mixed disulfide with the naturally occurring human hemoglobin A3. *Biochemistry* 12:3667, 1973

293. GEORGE JN, O'BRIEN RL, POLLACK S, CROSBY WH: Studies of in vitro primaquine hemolysis: Substrate requirement for erythrocyte membrane damage. *J Clin Invest* 45:1280, 1966

294. WEBSTER SH: Heinz body phenomenon in erythrocytes—a review. *Blood* 4:479, 1949

295. FERTMAN MH, FERTMAN MD: Toxic anemias and Heinz bodies. *Medicine (Baltimore)* 34:131, 1955

296. RACHMILEWITZ EA, PEISACH J, BLUMBERG WF: Studies on the stability of oxyhemoglobin A and its constituent chains and their derivatives. *J Biol Chem* 246:3356, 1971

297. JACOB HS: Mechanisms of Heinz body formation and attachment to red cell membrane. *Semin Hematol* 7:341, 1970

298. WINTERBOURN CC, CARRELL RW: The attachment of Heinz bodies to the red cell membrane. *Br J Haematol* 25:585, 1973

299. COHEN G, HOCHSTEIN P: Glutathione peroxidase: The primary agent for the elimination of hydrogen peroxide in erythrocytes. *Biochemistry* 2:1420, 1963

300. ITANO HA, HIROTA K, VEDVICK TS: Ligands and oxidants in ferrihemochrome formation and oxidative hemolysis. *Proc Natl Acad Sci USA* 74:2556, 1977

301. BUNN HF, JANDL JH: Exchange of heme among hemoglobins and between hemoglobin and albumin. *J Biol Chem* 243:465, 1968

302. ROSSI-FANELLI A, ANTONINI E, CAPUTO A: Studies on the structure of human hemoglobin. I. Physicochemical properties of human globin. *Biochim Biophys Acta* 30:608, 1958

303. RENTSCH G: Genesis of Heinz bodies and methemoglobin formation. *Biochem Pharmacol* 17:423, 1967

304. MARTIN H, WÖRNER W, RITTMEISTER B: Haemolytische Anaemie durch inhalation von Hydroxylaminen. *Klin Wochenschr* 42:725, 1964

305. BEUTLER E, BALUDA MC: The role of methemoglobin in oxidative degradation of hemoglobin. *Acta Haematol* 27:321, 1962

306. MAGOS L: Effect of the methemoglobinemia on Heinz body formation. *Experientia* 16:197, 1960

307. BEUTLER E: Drug-induced haemolytic anaemias and the mechanism and significance of Heinz body formation in red blood cells. *Nature* 196:1095, 1962

308. BEUTLER E, BALUDA MC, KELLY BM: The role of methemoglobin in the mechanism of drug-induced hemolytic anemia. *Proc IX Cong Int Soc Hematol* Mexico City, 1962, p 233

309. RACHMILEWITZ EA, HARARI E, WINTERHALTER KH: Separation of alpha- and beta-chains of hemoglobin A by acetylphenylhydrazine. *Biochim Biophys Acta* 371:402, 1974

310. RIFKIND RA: Heinz body anemia: An ultrastructural study. II. Red cell sequestration and destruction. *Blood* 26:433, 1965

311. MOHLER DN, WILLIAMS WJ: The effect of phenylhydrazine on the adenosine triphosphate content of normal and glucose-6-phosphate dehydrogenase-deficient human blood. *J Clin Invest* 40:1735, 1961

312. DESFORGES JF, KALAW E, GILCHRIST P: Inhibition of glucose-6-phosphate dehydrogenase by hemolysis inducing drugs. *J Lab Clin Med* 55:757, 1960

313. SHAHIDI NT, WESTRING DW: Acetylsalicylic acid-induced hemolysis and its mechanism. *J Clin Invest* 49:1334, 1970

314. COTTON DWK, SUTORIUS AHM: Inhibiting effect of some antimalarial substances on glucose-6-phosphate dehydrogenase. *Nature* 233:197, 1971

315. SZEINBERG A, SHEBA C, ADAM A: Selective occurrence of glutathione instability in red blood corpuscles of the various Jewish tribes. *Blood* 13:1043, 1958

316. GREENBERG MS, WONG H: Studies on the destruction of glutathione-unstable red blood cells. The influence of fava beans and primaquine upon such cells in vivo. *J Lab Clin Med* 57:733, 1961

317. PANIZON F, VULLO C: The mechanism of haemolysis in favism. *Acta Haematol* 26:337, 1961

318. STAMATOYANNOPOULOS G, FRASER GR, MOTULSKY AG, FESSAS P, AKRIVAKIS A, PAPAYANNOPOULOU T: On the familial predisposition to favism. *Am J Hum Genet* 18:253, 1966

319. CASSIMOS CHR, TSIURES I, DANIELIDES B: Disturbances of salicylamide glucuronide formation in normal and G-6-PD deficient children. *IRCS Hematology* (73-3) 17-3-1, 1973

320. CASSIMOS CHR, MALAKA ZAFIRIU K, TSIURES J: Urinary D-glucaric acid excretion in normal and G-6-PD deficient children with favism. *J Pediatr* 84:871, 1974

321. CUTILLO S, COSTA S, VINTULEDDU MC, MELONI T: Salicylamide-glucuronide formation in children with favism and in their parents. *Acta Haematol* 55:296, 1976

322. FIORELLI G, PODDA M, CORRIAS A, FARGION S: The relevance of immune reactions in acute favism. *Acta Haematol* 51:211, 1974

323. MAGER J, GLASER G, RAZIN A, IZAK G, BIEN S, NOAM M: Metabolic effects of pyrimidines derived from fava bean glycosides on human erythrocytes deficient in glucose-6-phosphate dehydrogenase. *Biochem Biophys Res Commun* 20:235, 1965

324. PANIZON F, ZACCHELLO F: The mechanism of haemolysis in favism. Some analogy in the activity of primaquine and fava juice. *Acta Haematol* 33:129, 1965

325. BEUTLER E: L-Dopa and favism. *Blood* 36:523, (editorial), 1970

326. KOSOWER NS, KOSOWER EM: Does 3,4-dihydroxyphenylalanine play a part in favism? *Nature* 215:285, 1967

327. GAETANI G, SALVIDIO E, PANNACCIULLI I, AJMAR F, PARAVIDINO G: Absence of haemolytic effects of L-Dopa on transfused G6PD-deficient erythrocytes. *Experientia* 26:785, 1970

328. SNYDER LM, EDELSTEIN L, FORTIER N, CARIGLIA N, JACOBS J, CIPRO D: The protective effect of L-Dopa on Heinz body formation in G6PD deficient red cells. *Experientia* 30:85, 1974

329. BOTTINI E, LUCARELLI P, AGOSTINO R, PALMARINO R, BOSINCO L, ANTOGNONI G: Favism: Association with erythrocyte acid phosphatase phenotype. *Science* 171:409, 1971

330. BAEHNER RL, NATHAN DG, CASTLE WB: Oxidant injury of Caucasian glucose-6-phosphate dehydrogenase-deficient red cells by phagocytosing leukocytes during infection. *J Clin Invest* 50:2466, 1971

331. NECHELES TF, GORSHEIN D: Virus-induced hemolysis in erythrocytes deficient in glucose-6-phosphate dehydrogenase. *Science* 160:535, 1968

332. ROSS JD: Deficient activity of DPNH-dependent methemoglobin diaphorase in cord blood erythrocytes. *Blood* 21:51, 1963

333. JONES PEH, MCCANCE RA: Enzyme activities in the blood of infants and adults. *Biochem J* 45:464, 1949

334. NECHELES TF, BOLES TA, ALLEN DM: Erythrocyte glutathione-peroxidase deficiency and hemolytic disease of the newborn infant. *J Pediatr* 72:319, 1968

335. SPIELBERG SP, BOXER LA, CORASH LM, SCHULMAN JD: Improved erythrocyte survival with high dose vitamin E in chronic hemolyzing G6PD and glutathione synthetase deficiencies. *Ann Intern Med* 90:53, 1978

336. CHILDS B, ZINKHAM W, BROWNE EA, KIMBRO EL, TORBERT JV: A genetic study of a defect in glutathione metabolism on the erythrocyte. *Johns Hopkins Med J* 102:21, 1958

337. SINISCALCO M, MOTULSKY AG, LATTE B, BERNINI L, MONTALENTI G: Indagini genetiche sulla predisposizione al favismo. II. Dati familiari: Associazione genica con il daltonismo. *Accad Naz Dei Lincei* 28:1, 1960

338. ADAM A: Linkage between deficiency of glucose-6-phosphate dehydrogenase and colour-blindness. *Nature* 189:686, 1961

339. SINISCALCO M, FILIPPI G: Recombination between protan and deutan genes; data on their relative positions in respect of the G6PD locus. *Nature* 204:1062, 1964

340. PORTER IH, SCHULZE J, MCKUSICK VA: Genetical linkage between the loci for glucose-6-phosphate dehydrogenase deficiency and colour-blindness in American Negroes. *Ann Hum Genet* 26:107, 1962

341. NABHOLZ M, MIGGIANO V, BODMER W: Genetic analysis with human-mouse somatic cell hybrids. *Nature* 223:358, 1969

342. KALMUS H: Distance and sequence of the loci for protan and deutan defects and for glucose-6-phosphate dehydrogenase deficiency. *Nature* 194:214, 1962

343. ZATZ M, ITSKAN SB, SANGER R, FROTA-PRESSOA O, SALDANHA PH: New linkage data for the X-linked types of muscular dystrophy and G6PD variants, colour blindness, and Xg blood groups. *J Med Genet* 11:321, 1974

344. ADAM A, SHEBA C, SANGER R, RACE RR: The linkage relation of G6PD to XG. *Am J Hum Genet* 18:110 (letters to the editor), 1966

345. BOWMAN JE, CARSON PE, FRISCHER H: The segregation in one family of three alleles at the glucose-6-phosphate dehydrogenase locus. *Hum Hered* 19:25, 1969

346. SINISCALCO M, FILIPPI G, LATTE B, PIOMELLI S, RATTAZZI M, GAVIN J, SANGER R, RACE RR: Failure to detect linkage between Xg and other X-borne loci in Sardinians. *Ann Hum Genet* 29:231, 1966

347. FILIPPI G, RINALDI A, CRISPONI G, DANIELS GL, SINISCALCO M: X-mapping in man: Evidence against measurable linkage between anhidrotic ectodermal dysplasia and G6PD deficiency. *J Med Genet* 16:223, 1979

348. TRUJILLO J, FAIRBANKS VF, OHNO S, BEUTLER E: Chromosomal constitution in glucose-6-phosphate-dehydrogenase deficiency. *Lancet* 2:1454, 1961

349. GRUMBACH MM, MARKS PA, MORISHIMA A: Erythrocyte glucose-6-phosphate dehydrogenase activity and X-chromosome polysomy. *Lancet* 1:1330, 1962

350. DAVIDSON RG, MIGEON BR, BORDEN M, CHILDS B: Dosage compensation in the regulation of erythrocyte glucose-6-phosphate dehydrogenase activity. *Johns Hopkins Med J* 112:318, 1963

351. OHNO S, KAPLAN WD, KINOSITA R: Formation of the sex chromatin by a single X-chromosome in liver cells of *Rattus norvegicus. Exp Cell Res* 18:415, 1959

352. BEUTLER E, YEH M, FAIRBANKS VF: The normal human female as a mosaic of X-chromosome activity: Studies using the gene for G-6-PD deficiency as a marker. *Proc Natl Acad Sci USA* 48:9, 1962

353. BEUTLER E: Biochemical abnormalities associated with hemolytic states, in Weinstein I, Beutler E (eds): *Mechanisms of Anemia in Man.* New York, McGraw-Hill, 1962, p 195

354. LYON MF: Sex chromatin and gene action in the mammalian X-chromosome. *Am J Hum Genet* 14:135, 1962

355. LYON MF: Gene action in the X-chromosome of the mouse (*Mus musculus* L.). *Nature* 190:372, 1961

356. BEUTLER E, BALUDA MC: The separation of glucose-6-phosphate dehydrogenase-deficient erythrocytes from the blood of heterozygotes for glucose-6-phosphate dehydrogenase deficiency. *Lancet* 1:189, 1964

357. KAPLAN JC, DREYFUS JC, BESSIS M: La structure en mosaique du chromosome X chez la femme. *Nouv Rev Fr Hematol* 5:835, 1965

358. FIALKOW PJ: The origin and development of human tumors studied with cell markers. *N Engl J Med* 291:26, 1974

359. SARTORI E, PANIZON F, ZACCHELLO F: Bimodal distribution of erythrocytes in heterozygotes for strong Mediterranean glucose-6-phosphate dehydrogenase deficiency. *J Med Genet* 3:42, 1966.

360. SANSONE G, RASORE QUARTINO A, VENEZIANO G: Two red-cell populations in the human female heterozygous for G-6-PD deficiency. *Lancet* 1:329, 1964

361. TÖNZ O, ROSSI E: Morphological demonstration of two red cell populations in human females heterozygous for glucose-6-phosphate dehydrogenase deficiency. *Nature* 202:606, 1964

362. GALL JR JC, BREWER GJ, DERN RJ: Studies of glucose-6-phosphate dehydrogenase activity of individual erythrocytes: The methemoglobin-elution test for identification of females heterozygous for G6PD deficiency. *Am J Hum Genet* 17:359, 1965

363. TÖNZ O: The problem of defining the heterozygous carrier in glucose-6-phosphate dehydrogenase deficiency. *Ann Paediat* 204:24, 1965

364. KATTAMIS CA: Glucose-6-phosphate dehydrogenase deficiency in female heterozygotes and the X-inactivation hypothesis. *Acta Paediatr Scand (Suppl)* 172:103, 1967

365. STAMATOYANNOPOULOS G, PAPAYANNOPOULOU TH, BAKOPOULOS CHR, MOTULSKY AG: Detection of glucose-6-phosphate dehydrogenase deficient heterozygotes. *Blood* 29:87, 1967

366. BEUTLER E, COLLINS Z: Pseudo-mosaicism in males with mild glucose-6-phosphate dehydrogenase deficiency. *Lancet* 1:552, 1965

367. PAPAYANNOPOULOU T, STAMATOYANNOPOULOS G: Pseudo-mosaicism in males with mild glucose-6-phosphate dehydrogenase deficiency. *Lancet* 2:1215, 1964

368. BETKE K, KLEIHAUER E, KNOTEK Z: Zytologische Untersuchungen zur frage des Zellmosaiks bei heterozygoten Frauen mit Glukose-6-phosphat-dehydrogenase-mangel. *Acta Paediatr Scand (Suppl)* 172:30, 1967

369. DAVIDSON RG, NITOWSKY HM, CHILDS B: Demonstration of two populations of cells in the human female heterozygous for glucose-6-phosphate dehydrogenase variants. *Proc Natl Acad Sci USA* 50:481, 1963

370. LINDER D, GARTLER SM: Glucose-6-phosphate dehydrogenase mosaicism: Utilization as cell marker in the study of leiomyomas. *Science* 150:67, 1965

371. FIALKOW PJ: Clonal origin of human tumors. *Biochim Biophys Acta* 458:283, 1976

372. FIALKOW PJ, GARTLER SM, YOSHIDA A: Clonal origin of chronic myelocytic leukemia in man. *Proc Natl Acad Sci USA* 58:1468, 1967

373. WIGGANS RG, JACOBSON RJ, FIALKOW PJ, WOOLLEY PV, MAC DONALD JS, SCHEIN PS: Probable clonal origin of acute myeloblastic leukemia following radiation and chemotherapy of colon cancer. *Blood* 52:659, 1978

374. BEUTLER E, WEST C, JOHNSON C: Involvement of the erythroid series in acute myeloid leukemia. *Blood* 53:1203, 1979

375. ADAMSON JW, FIALKOW PJ, MURPHY S, PRCHAL JF, STEINMANN L: Polycythemia vera: Stem-cell and probable clonal origin of the disease. *N Engl J Med* 295:913, 1976

376. ONI SB, OSUNKOYA BO, LUZZATTO L: Paroxysmal nocturnal hemoglobinuria: Evidence for monoclonal origin of abnormal red cells. *Blood* 36:145, 1970

377. PEARSON TA, KRAMER EC, SOLEZ K, HEPTINSTALL RH: The human atherosclerotic plaque. *Am J Pathol* 86:657, 1977

378. PEARSON TA, WANG A, SOLEZ K, HEPINSTALL RH: Clonal characteristics of fibrous plaques and fatty streaks from human aortas. *Am J Pathol* 81:379, 1975

379. THOMAS WA, REINER JM, JANAKIDEVI K, FLORENTIN RA, LEE KT: Population dynamics of arterial cells during atherogenesis. *Exp Mol Pathol* 31:367, 1979

380. LUZZATTO L, USANGA EA, REDDY S: Glucose 6-phosphate dehydrogenase deficient red cells: Resistance to infection by malarial parasites. *Science* 164:839, 1969

381. MARTIN SK, MILLER LH, ALLING D, OKOYE VC, ESAN GJF, OSUNKOYA BO, DEANE M: Severe malaria and glucose-6-phosphate-dehydrogenase deficiency: A reappraisal of the malaria/G-6-PD hypothesis. *Lancet* 1:524, 1979

382. GLORIA-ROTTINI F, FALSI AM, MORTERA J, BOTTINI E: The relations between G-6-PD deficiency, thalassemia and malaria. Further analysis of data from Sardinia and the Po Valley. *Experientia* 36:541, 1980

383. LUZZATTO L: Genetics of red cells and susceptibility to malaria. *Blood* 54:961, 1979

384. BIENZLE U, LUCAS AO, AYENI O, LUZZATTO L: Glucose-6-phosphate dehydrogenase and malaria. Greater resistance of females heterozygous for enzyme deficiency and of males with non-deficient variant. *Lancet* 1:107, 1972

385. LEWIS R, HATHORN M: Correlation of S hemoglobin with glucose-6-phosphate dehydrogenase deficiency and its significance. *Blood* 26:176, 1965

386. NAYLOR J, ROSENTHAL I, GROSSMAN A, SCHULMAN I, HSIA DYY: Activity of glucose-6-phosphate dehydrogenase in erythrocytes of patients with various abnormal hemoglobins. *Pediatrics* 26:285, 1960

387. PIOMELLI S, REINDORF CA, ARZANIAN MT, CORASH LM: Clinical and biochemical interactions of glucose-6-phosphate dehydrogenase deficiency and sickle-cell anemia. *N Engl J Med* 287:213, 1972

388. BEUTLER E, JOHNSON C, POWARS D, WEST C: Prevalence of glucose-6-phosphate dehydrogenase deficiency in sickle cell disease. *N Engl J Med* 290:826, 1974

389. STEINBERG MH, DREILING BJ: Glucose-6-phosphate dehydrogenase deficiency in sickle cell anemia. *Ann Intern Med* 80:217, 1974

390. LUZZATTO L: New developments in glucose-6-phosphate dehydrogenase deficiency. *Isr J Med Sci* 9:1484, 1973

391. PETRAKIS NL, WIESENFELD SL, SAMS BJ, COLLEN MF, CUTLER JL, SIEGELAUB AB: Prevalence of sickle-cell trait and glucose-6-phosphate dehydrogenase deficiency. *N Engl J Med* 282:767, 1970

392. KATTAMIS C, KARAMBULA K, METAXOTOU-MAVROMATI A, MATSANIOTIS N: G-6-PD deficiency and age. *Lancet* 1:235, 1971

393. BERNSTEIN SC, BOWMAN JE, NOCHE LK: Population studies in Cameroon. *Hum Hered* 30:251, 1980

394. BEACONSFIELD P, RAINSBURY R, KALTON G: Glucose-6-phosphate dehydrogenase deficiency and the incidence of cancer. *Oncology* 19:11, 1965

395. NAIK SN, ANDERSON DE: The association between glucose-6-phosphate dehydrogenase deficiency and cancer in American Negroes. *Oncology* 25:356, 1971

396. WERTH G, MÜELLER G: Vererbbarer Glucose-6-phosphatdehydrogenasemangel in Den Erythrocyten von Ratten. *Klin Wochenschr* 45:265, 1967

397. SMITH JE, RYER K, WALLACE L: Glucose-6-phosphate dehydrogenase deficiency in a dog. *Enzyme* 21:379, 1976

398. BEUTLER E, WEST C: Glucose-6-phosphate dehydrogenase variants in the chimpanzee. *Biochem Med* 20:364, 1978

399. KHAN PM, VAN SOMEREN H, DE JONG WW, VERVLOET M: Red cell enzyme polymorphisms in rhesus monkeys and chimpanzees. *Transplant Proc* 4:137, 1972

400. RINGELHAHN B: A simple laboratory procedure for the recognition of A− (African type) G6PD deficiency in acute haemolytic crisis. *Clin Chim Acta* 36:272, 1972

401. FAIRBANKS VF, FERNANDEZ, MN: The identification of metabolic errors associated with hemolytic anemia. *JAMA* 208:316, 1969

402. GLOCK GE, MCLEAN P: Further studies on the properties and assay of glucose-6-phosphate dehydrogenase, and 6-phosphogluconate dehydrogenase of rat liver. *Biochem J* 55:400, 1953

403. CATALANO EW, JOHNSON GF, SOLOMON HM: Measurement of erythrocyte glucose-6-phosphate dehydrogenase activity with a centrifugal analyzer. *Clin Chem* 21:134, 1975

404. DEUTSCH J: Maleimide as an inhibitor in measurement of erythrocyte glucose-6-phosphate dehydrogenase activity. *Clin Chem* 24:885, 1978

405. RATTAZZI MC, BERNINI LF, FIORELLI G, MANNUCCI PM: Electrophoresis of glucose-6-phosphate dehydrogenase: A new technique. *Nature* 213:79, 1967

406. DER KALOUSTIAN VM, IDRISS-DAOUK SH, HALLAL RT, AWDEH ZL: Analysis of human erythrocyte glucose-6-phosphate dehydrogenase isozymes by isoelectric focusing in polyacrylamide gel. *Biochem Genet* 12:51, 1974

407. VERGNES H, BRUN H: Characterization of some erythrocyte G6PD variants by isoelectric focusing. *Hum Genet* 53:43, 1979

408. KAHN A, BERTRAND O, COTTEREAU D, BOIVIN P, DREYFUS JC: Studies on the nature of different molecular forms of glucose-6-phosphate dehydrogenase purified from human leukocytes. *Biochim Biophys Acta* 445:537, 1976

409. LUZZATTO L, OKOYE VCN: Resolution of genetic variants of human erythrocyte glucose-6-phosphate dehydrogenase by thin layer chromatography. *Biochem Biophys Res Commun* 29:705, 1967

410. BEUTLER E, DERN RJ, ALVING AS: The hemolytic effect of primaquine. VI. An in vitro test for sensitivity of erythrocytes to primaquine. *J Lab Clin Med* 45:40, 1955

411. BEUTLER E: In vitro studies of the stability of red cell glutathione: A new test for drug sensitivity. *J Clin Invest* 35:690 (abstract), 1956

412. BEUTLER E: The glutathione instability of drug-sensitive red cells. A new method for the in vitro detection of drug-sensitivity. *J Lab Clin Med* 49:84, 1957

413. ZINKHAM WH, LENHARD RE Jr, CHILDS B: A deficiency of glucose-6-phosphate dehydrogenase activity in erythrocytes from patients with favism. *Johns Hopkins Med J* 102:169, 1958

414. SANSONE G, BORRONE C, ROVEI S: Suscettibilita degli eritrociti a formare corpi di Heinz in vitro in condizioni normali (neonati e lattanti) e patologiche (favismo e talessemia). *Boll Soc Ital Biol Sper* 34:1561, 1958

415. KRAUS AP, NEEL YCL, CAREY FT, KRAUS LM: Detection of deficient erythrocyte regeneration of reduced triphosphopyridine nucleotide from glucose-6-phosphate. Evaluation of a rapid screening test. *Ann Intern Med* 56:765, 1962

416. SALVIDIO E, PANNACCIULLI I, TIZIANELLO A: Evaluation experimentale de quelques methodes biochimiques permettant de deceler la susceptibilite a l'hemolyse due aux medicaments. *Nouv Rev Fr Hematol* 3:233, 1963

417. SZEINBERG A, SHEBA C, ADAM A: Enzymatic abnormality in erythrocytes of a population sensitive to *Vicia faba* or drug induced hemolytic anemia. *Nature* 181:1256, 1958

418. ZINKHAM WH: An in vitro abnormality of glutathione metabolism in erythrocytes from normal newborns: Mechanism and clinical significance. *Pediatrics* 23:18, 1959

419. SWARUP S, GHOSH SK, CHATTERJEA JB: Glutathione stability test in haemoglobin E-thalassemia disease. *Nature* 188:153, 1960

420. BALINSKY D, BERNSTEIN RE: Oxidation of reduced glutathione by acetylphenylhydrazine. *Nature* 199:187, 1963

421. THEIL GE, BRODINE CE, DOOLAN PD: Red cell glutathione content and stability in renal sufficiency. *J Lab Clin Med* 58:736, 1961

422. SZEINBERG A, RAMOT B, ADAM A, SHEBA C: Glutathione metabolism in cord blood and in the newborn infant. *Am J Dis Child* 96:542, 1958

423. GROSS RT, HURWITZ RE: The pentose phosphate pathway in human erythrocytes. Relationship between age of the subject and enzyme activity. *Pediatrics* 22:453, 1958

424. SZEINBERG A, RAMOT B, SHEBA C, ADAM A, HALBRECHT I, RIKOVER M, WISHNIEVSKY S, RABAU E: Glutathione metabolism in cord and newborn infant blood. *J Clin Invest* 37:1436, 1958

425. BERNSTEIN RE: Brilliant cresyl blue screening test for demonstrating glucose-6-phosphate dehydrogenase deficiency in red cells. *Clin Chim Acta* 8:158, 1963

426. LEE TC, SHIH LY, HUANG PC, LIN CC, BLACKWELL BN, BLACKWELL RQ, HSIA DY: Glucose-6-phosphate dehydrogenase deficiency in Taiwan. *Am J Hum Genet* 15:126, 1963

427. TOENZ O, BETKE K: Einfacher Farbtest zur bestimmung der Glucose-6-phosphatdehydrogenase in Menschlichen Erythrocyten. *Klin Wochenschr* 40:649, 1962

428. ELLS HA, KIRKMAN HN: A colorimetric method for assay of erythrocytic glucose-6-phosphate dehydrogenase. *Proc Soc Exp Biol Med* 106:607, 1961

429. BERNSTEIN RE: A rapid screening dye test for the detection of glucose-6-phosphate dehydrogenase deficiency in red cells. *Nature* 194:192, 1962

430. FAIRBANKS VF, BEUTLER E: A simple method for detection of erythrocyte glucose-6-phosphate dehydrogenase deficiency (G-6-PD spot test), *Blood* 20:591, 1962

431. BREWER GJ, TARLOV AR, ALVING AS: The methemoglobin reduction test for primaquine-type sensitivity of erythrocytes. *JAMA* 180:386, 1962

432. BAPAT JP, BAXI AJ, BHATIA HM: Is methemoglobin reduction test a true index of G-6-PD deficiency? *Indian J Med Res* 64:1687, 1976

433. OSKI FA, GROWNEY PM: A simple micromethod for the detection of erythrocyte glucose-6-phosphate dehydrogenase deficiency. *J Pediatr* 66:90, 1965

434. SASS MD, CARUSO CJ, AXELROD DR: Rapid screening for D-glucose-6-phosphate: NADP oxidoreductase deficiency with methylene blue. *J Lab Clin Med* 68:156, 1966

435. RAKITZIS ET: Test for glucose-6-phosphate dehydrogenase deficiency. *Lancet* 2:1182, 1964

436. JACOB H, JANDL JH: A simple visual screening test for G-6-PD deficiency employing ascorbate and cyanide. *N Engl J Med* 274:1162, 1966

437. PRINS HK, LOOS JA, ZUERCHER C: Glutathione deficiency, in Beutler E (ed): *Hereditary Disorders of Erythrocyte Metabolism.* City of Hope Series, New York, Grune & Stratton, 1968, vol I, pp 165–184

438. BEUTLER E: A series of new screening procedures for pyruvate kinase deficiency, glucose-6-phosphate dehydrogenase deficiency, and glutathione reductase deficiency. *Blood* 28:553, 1966

439. BEUTLER E, MITCHELL M: Special modifications of the fluorescent screening method for glucose-6-phosphate dehydrogenase deficiency. *Blood* 32:816, 1968

440. WHITE PA: Special modifications of the fluorescent screening test for glucose-6-phosphate dehydrogenase deficiency. *Aust J Med Technol* 3:133 [cited in *Excerpta Med* 10.2:(502)], 1972

441. YEUNG CY, LAI HC, LEUNG NK: Fluorescent spot test for screening erythrocyte glucose-6-phosphate dehydrogenase deficiency in newborn babies. *J Pediatr* 76:931, 1970

442. BENI A, FIORITONI G, SALVATI AM, TENTORI L, TORLONTANO G: Quantitation of the ultraviolet light test for erythrocyte glucose-6-phosphate dehydrogenase, pyruvate kinase and glutathione reductase. *Clin Chim Acta* 49:41, 1973

443. PENTON E, PASCUAL C, LLANES A, THIELMANN K: The activity of glucose-6-phosphate dehydrogenase in whole blood samples dried and stored on filter paper. *Acta Biol Med Ger* 28:177, 1972

444. DOW PA, PETTEWAY MB, ALPERIN JB: Simplified method for G6PD screening using blood collected on filter paper. *Am J Pathol* 61:333, 1974

445. BEUTLER E: G-6-PD activity of individual erythrocytes and X-chromosomal inactivation, in Yunis JJ (ed): *Biochemical Methods in Red Cell Genetics.* New York, Academic, 1969, pp 95–113

446. FAIRBANKS VF, LAMPE LT: A tetrazolium-linked cytochemical method for estimation of glucose-6-phosphate dehydrogenase activity in individual erythrocytes: Applications in the study of heterozygotes for glucose-6-phosphate dehydrogenase deficiency. *Blood* 31:589, 1968

447. SHAW CR, BARTO E: Autosomally determined polymorphism of glucose-6-phosphate dehydrogenase in *Peromyscus. Science* 148:1099, 1965

448. TAN SG, ASHTON GC: An autosomal glucose-6-phosphate dehydrogenase (hexose-6-phosphate dehydrogenase) polymorphism in human saliva. *Hum Hered* 26:113, 1976

449. OHNO S, PAYNE HW, MORRISON M, BEUTLER E: Hexose-6-phosphate dehydrogenase found in human liver. *Science* 153:1015, 1966

450. BLUME KG, SRIVASTAVA SK, BEUTLER E, YOSHIDA A: Biochemische und immunologische Unterschiede zwischen Glucose-6-phosphat-Dehydrogenase und Hexose-6-phosphat-Dehydrogenase aus menschlicher Leber. *Hoppe Seylers Z Physiol Chem* 354:213, 1973

451. MARKS PA, GROSS RT, HURWITZ RE: Gene action in erythrocyte deficiency of glucose-6-phosphate dehydrogenase: Tissue enzyme-levels. *Nature* 183:1266, 1959

452. SCHILIRO G, RUSSO A, MAURO L, PIZZARELLI G, MARINO S: Leukocyte function and characterization of leukocyte glucose-6-phosphate dehydrogenase in Sicilian mutants. *Pediatr Res* 10:739, 1976

453. RAMOT B, FISHER S, SZEINBERG A, ADAM A, SHEBA C, GANNI D: A study of subjects with erythrocyte glucose-6-phosphate dehydrogenase deficiency. II. Investigation of leukocyte enzymes. *J Clin Invest* 38:2234, 1959

454. CHAN TK, TODD D, WONG CC: Tissue enzyme levels in erythrocyte glucose-6-phosphate dehydrogenase deficiency. *J Lab Clin Med* 66:937, 1965

455. KAHN A, HAKIM J, BOIVIN P, BOUCHEROT J, DURAND D, TROUBE H: Leucocytes et deficits en G-6-PD erythrocytaire. *Nouv Rev Fr Hematol* 14:291, 1974

456. GRAY GR, KLEBANOFF SJ, STAMATOYANNOPOULOS G, AUSTIN T, NAIMAN SC, YOSHIDA A, KLIMAN MR, ROBINSON GCF: Neutrophil dysfunction, chronic granulomatous disease, and nonspherocytic haemolytic anaemia caused by complete deficiency of glucose-6-phosphate dehydrogenase. *Lancet* 2:530, 1973

457. COOPER MR, DE CHATELET LR, MCCALL CE, LA VIA JF, SPURR CL, BAEHNER RL: Complete deficiency of leukocyte glucose-6-phosphate dehydrogenase with defective bactericidal activity. *J Clin Invest* 51:769, 1972

458. CHAN TK, TODD D, LAI MCS: Glucose 6-phosphate dehydrogenase: Identity of erythrocyte and leukocyte enzyme with report of a new variant in Chinese. *Biochem Genet* 6:119, 1972

459. JUSTICE P, SHIH LY, GORDON J, GROSSMAN A, HSIA D: Characterization of leukocyte glucose-6-phosphate dehydrogenase in normal and mutant human subjects. *J Lab Clin Med* 68:552, 1966

460. YOSHIDA A, STAMATOYANNOPOULOS G, MOTULSKY AG: Biochemical genetics of glucose-6-phosphate dehydrogenase variation. *Ann NY Acad Sci* 155:868, 1968

461. COTTREAU D, KAHN A, BOIVIN P: Human platelet glucose-6-phosphate dehydrogenase: Total purification, kinetic studies and relationship with enzyme from other blood cells. *Enzyme* 21:142, 1976

462. KAHN A, BERTRAND O, COTTREAU D, BOIVIN P, DREYFUS JC: Evidence for structural differences between human glucose-6-phosphate dehydrogenase purified from leukocytes and erythrocytes. *Biochem Biophys Res Commun* 77:65, 1977

463. ZINKHAM WH: Enzyme studies on lenses from persons with primaquine-sensitive erythrocytes. *Am J Dis Child* 100:525, 1960

464. RAMOT B, SZEINBERG A, ADAM A, SHEBA C, GAFNI D: A study of subjects with erythrocyte glucose-6-phosphate dehydrogenase deficiency: I. Investigation of platelet enzymes. *J Clin Invest* 38:1659, 1959

465. GRAY GR, NAIMAN SC, ROBINSON GCF: Platelet function and G-6-PD deficiency. *Lancet* 1:997 (letter), 1974

466. GARTLER SM, GANDINI E, CEPPELLINI R: Glucose-6-phosphate dehydrogenase deficient mutant in human cell culture. *Nature* 193:602, 1962

467. RAMOT B, SHEBA C, ADAM A, ASHKENASI I: Erythrocyte glucose-6-phosphate dehydrogenase deficient subjects: Enzyme-level in saliva. *Nature* 185:931, 1960

468. SKLAVUNU-ZURUKZOGLU S, MAMELETZIS C, KATRIU D: Observations on the glucose-6-phosphate dehydrogenase of the breast milk. *Helv Paediatr Acta* 20:193, 1965

469. SARKAR S, NELSON AJ, JONES OW: Glucose-6-phosphate dehydrogenase (G6PD) activity of human sperm. *J Med Genet* 14:250, 1977

470. PANIZON F: Erythrocyte enzyme deficiency in unexplained kernicterus. *Lancet* 2:1093, 1960

471. BRUNETTI P, ROSSETTI R, BROCCIA G: New findings on the bioenzymology of icteric hemoglobinuric favism. III. The activity of glucose-6-phosphate dehydrogenase in the liver parenchyma. *Clin Ter* 32:338, 1960

472. OLUBOYEDE OA, ESAN GJF, FRANCIS TI, LUZZATTO L: Genetically determined deficiency of glucose-6-phosphate dehydrogenase (type A−) is expressed in the liver. *J Lab Clin Med* 93:783, 1979

473. WESTRING DW, PISCIOTTA AV: Anemia, cataracts, and seizures in patient with glucose-6-phosphate dehydrogenase deficiency. *Arch Intern Med* 118:385, 1966

474. HELGE H, BORNER K: Kongenitale nichtsphaerozytaere haemolytische anaemie, Katarakt und Glucose-6-phosphat-dehydrogenase-mangel. *Dtsch Med Wochenschr* 91:1584, 1966

475. CHANMUGAM D, FRUMIN AM: Abnormal oral glucose tolerance response in erythrocyte glucose-6-phosphate dehydrogenase deficiency. *N Engl J Med* 271:1202, 1964

476. EPPES R, BREWER G, DE GOWIN R, MC NAMARA J, FLANAGAN C, SCHRIER S, TARLOV A, POWELL R, CARSON P: Oral glucose tolerance in Negro men deficient in G-6-PD. *N Engl J Med* 275:855, 1966

477. BORKOWSKI AJ, MARKS PA, KATZ FH, CHRISSTY NP: An abnormal pathway of steroid metabolism in patients with glucose-6-phosphate dehydrogenase deficiency. *J Clin Invest* 41:1346 (abstract), 1962

478. SO PL, CHAN TK, LAM SK, TENG CS, YEUNG RT, TODD D: Cortisol metabolism in glucose-6-phosphate dehydrogenase deficiency. *Metabolism* 22:1443, 1973

479. TARLOV AR, BREWER GJ, SWANSON SH: The effect of primaquine administration on the serum cholesterol in drug-sensitive Amer. Negroes. *Clin Res* 9:190, 1961

480. WILLIAMS AO, TUGWELL P, EDINGTON GM: Glucose-6-phosphate dehydrogenase deficiency and lobar pneumonia. *Arch Pathol Lab Med* 100:25, 1976

481. MELONI T, COSTA S, CUTILLO S: Haptoglobin, hemopexin, hemoglobin and hematocrit in newborns with erythrocyte glucose-6-phosphate dehydrogenase deficiency. *Acta Haematol* 54:284, 1975

482. MELONI T, COSTA S, CORTI R, CUTILLO S: Salicylamide glucuronide formation in newborn babies with G-6-PD deficiency. *Biol Neonate* 33:189, 1978

483. DERN RJ, GLYNN MF, BREWER GJ: Studies on the correlation of the genetically determined trait, glucose-6-phosphate dehydrogenase deficiency, with behavioral manifestations in schizophrenia. *J Lab Clin Med* 62:319, 1963

484. BOWMAN JE, BREWER GJ, FRISCHER H, CARTER JL, EISENSTEIN RB, BAYRAKCI C: A re-evaluation of the relationship between glucose-6-phosphate

dehydrogenase deficiency and the behavioral manifestations of schizophrenia. *J Lab Clin Med* 65:222, 1965

485. HELLER P, BEST WR, NELSON RB, BECKTEL J: Clinical implications of sickle-cell trait and glucose-6-phosphate dehydrogenase deficiency in hospitalized black male patients. *N Engl J Med* 300:1001, 1979

486. TAN KL: Phototherapy for neonatal jaundice in erythrocyte glucose-6-phosphate dehydrogenase-deficient infants. *Pediatrics* 59:1023, 1977

487. VAN DER SAR A, SCHOUTEN H, STRUYKER BOUDIER AM: Glucose-6-phosphate dehydrogenase deficiency in red cells. Incidence in the Curacao population, its clinical and genetic aspects. *Enzyme* 27:289, 310, 1964

488. CARSON PE, TARLOV AR: Biochemistry of hemolysis. *Annu Rev Med* 13:105, 1962

489. McCURDY PR, MORSE EE: Glucose-6-phosphate dehydrogenase deficiency and blood transfusion. *Vox Sang* 28:230, 1975

490. MELONI T, DORF A, CUTILLO S: Effect of barbituric acid on hyperbilirubinemia in newborn infants with glucosephosphate dehydrogenase deficiency in the erythrocytes. *Helv Paediatr Acta* 27:197, 1972

491. MELONI T, COSTA S, CORTI R, CUTILLO S: Agar in control of hyperbilirubinemia of full-term newborn infants with erythrocyte G-6-PD deficiency. *Biol Neonate* 34:295, 1978

492. BEUTLER E: Red cell metabolism. A. Defects not causing hemolytic disease. B. Environmental modification. *Biochimie* 54:759, 1972

493. WANG YM, PATTERSON HJ, VAN EYS J: The potential use of xylitol in glucose-6-phosphate dehydrogenase deficiency anemia. *J Clin Invest* 50:1421, 1971

494. WANG YM, KING SM, VAN EYS J: Isocitrate metabolism in normal and glucose-6-phosphate dehydrogenase deficient red cells. *Biochem Med* 11:327, 1974

495. CORASH L, SPIELBERG S, BARTSOCAS C, BOXER L, STEINHERTZ R, SHEETZ M, EGAN M, SCHLESSLEMAN J, SCHULMAN JD: Reduced chronic hemolysis during high-dose vitamin E administration in Mediterranean-type glucose-6-phosphate dehydrogenase deficiency. *N Engl J Med* 303:416, 1980

496. NEWMAN JG, NEWMAN TB, BOWIE LJ, MENDELSOHN J: An examination of the role of vitamin E in glucose-6-phosphate dehydrogenase deficiency. *Clin Biochem* 12:149, 1979

497. BEUTLER E, BOGGS DR, HELLER P, MAURER A, MOTULSKY AG, SHEEHY TW: Hazards of indiscriminate screening for sickling. *N Engl J Med* 285:1485 (letter), 1971

498. GOSS SJ, HARRIS H: Gene transfer by means of cell fusion. I. Statistical mapping of the human X-chromosome by analysis of radiation-induced gene segregation. *J Cell Sci* 25:17, 1977

499. PERSICO MG, TONIOLO D, NOBILE C, D'URSO M, LUZZATTO L: CDNA sequences of human glucose-6-phosphate dehydrogenase cloned in pBR322. *Nature* 294:778, 1981

75

HEREDITARY METHEMOGLOBINEMIA WITH DEFICIENCY OF NADH CYTOCHROME b5 REDUCTASE

JOEL M. SCHWARTZ

ALLAN L. REISS

ERNST R. JAFFÉ

1. A balance between the oxidation and reduction of heme iron determines the level of methemoglobin in erythrocytes. Less than 1 percent of the total hemoglobin present in normal cells is in the ferric or methomoglobin form, because the capacity of normal cells to reduce ferric heme exceeds the spontaneous rate of heme oxidation by several hundredfold.

2. One form of hereditary methemoglobinemia results from homozygous deficiency of NADH cytochrome b5 reductase. Normally methemoglobin is reduced nonenzymatically by the ferrous form of cytochrome b5. The ferric cytochrome b5 which is generated is reduced, in turn, by NADH cytochrome b5 reductase of the erythrocyte cytosol. Severe deficiency of the enzyme permits intracellular accumulation of the methemoglobin spontaneously formed by the release of superoxide from oxyhemoglobin (auto-oxidation). Some 10 percent of patients additionally display deficient activity of cytochrome b5 reductase embedded in the endoplasmic reticulum (microsomes) of many tissues. Failure of the enzymatic reduction of cytochrome b5 in brain microsomes is associated with neurologic dysfunction, mental retardation, and premature death.

3. The cytochrome b5 and NADH cytochrome b5 reductase, which compose the methemoglobin-reducing system in the cytosol of mature human erythrocytes, originate from the endoplasmic reticulum of nucleated red cell precursors. The respective proteins represent the polar catalytic segments of amphipathic parent polypeptide chains embedded in microsomes which are solubilized during erythroid maturation through proteolytic cleavage of their hydrophobic tails. The microsomal cytochrome b5 reductase system is known to participate in the desaturation of fatty acids to give 9,10 unsaturated derivatives such as oleic acid. It has been suggested that impaired biosynthesis of unsaturated fatty acids by brain microsomes may be responsible for the coexisting neurologic syndrome in some patients with hereditary methemoglobinemia.

4. NADH cytochrome b5 reductase is determined by a gene located on human chromosome 22. Multiple electrophoretic phenotypes in erythrocytes which contain normal enzyme activity occur with an overall incidence of about 1 in 100; they signify allelism at the gene locus. Inheritance of a pair of abnormal alleles which specify an enzyme with decreased activity occurs only rarely and leads to hereditary methemoglobinemia. Uncomplicated methemoglobinemia results from a mutation in paired alleles which primarily influences the stability, function, or, possibly, solubilization of the polar segment of the enzyme. Methemoglobinemia with neurologic dysfunction, on the other hand, is thought to represent either gene deletions or a mutation in paired alleles determining the function, stabil-

ity, or attachment to the endoplasmic reticulum of the enzyme polypeptide chain as a whole: i.e., polar plus hydrophobic segments.

5. *In spite of the decreased oxygen-carrying capacity and the presence of partially oxidized hemoglobin tetramers (valence hybrids) in the erythrocytes of patients with hereditary methemoglobinemia, the disorder is surprisingly well tolerated, and treatment is rarely necessary. The physiologic mechanisms which function to compensate for the hypoxemia and for the tendency of valence hybrids to hold fast to oxygen are poorly understood. The benign nature of the disorder in some patients is explained, at least in part, by sequestration of methemoglobin within a small population of older cells. This serves to minimize the opportunities for interaction between ferric and ferrous hemes.*

6. *When nitrates, aniline derivatives, or other chemical agents markedly accelerate the oxidation of heme, the formation of methemoglobin can outstrip the reducing capacity of the normal erythrocytes. The propensity to display cyanosis after exposure to chemicals which form methemoglobin is increased in individuals with impaired capacity to reduce methemoglobin such as newborn infants and persons homozygous or heterozygous for cytochrome b5 reductase deficiency. Toxic methemoglobinemia that develops suddenly is poorly tolerated, and the outcome may be fatal. Administration of methylene blue activates the dormant NADPH dehydrogenase pathway for methemoglobin reduction and can rapidly relieve the symptoms and cyanosis.*

Oxyhemoglobin has traditionally been considered a ferrous-oxy compound, but there are compelling reasons to believe that the heme iron atoms in oxyhemoglobin are in the ferric state, with partial transfer of an electron to oxygen to form the superoxide anion [1].[1] Although oxygen usually returns the acquired electron before leaving the heme pocket, liberation of superoxide and formation of methemoglobin (ferrihemoglobin, hemiglobin) occur at a slow, predictable rate. Since methemoglobin cannot bind oxygen, erythrocyte-reducing mechanisms must restore the lost electrons in order to preserve normal hemoglobin function. Less than 1 percent of the total hemoglobin present in red blood cells is in the methemoglobin form because the capacity of normal cells to reduce ferric heme exceeds the spontaneous rate of heme oxidation by several hundredfold [2]. Accumulation of methemoglobin within erythrocytes (methemoglobinemia) occurs when the rate of oxidation of heme accelerates sufficiently to outstrip the reducing capacity (acute toxic methemoglobinemia), when an alteration in the globin moiety stabilizes methemoglobin and renders it resistant to metabolic reduction (hemoglobin M disorders), or when there is a significant deficiency in the reducing capabilities of the erythrocyte.

Of several metabolic pathways for the reduction of methemoglobin, the most important involves an NADH dehydrogenase enzyme, more precisely named NADH cytochrome b5

reductase (EC 1.6.2.2). This chapter will examine the reactions which regulate the methemoglobin level in the cytosol of mature erythrocytes, the critical importance of NADH cytochrome b5 reductase to the regulatory process, the origin of this enzyme protein from endoplasmic reticulum, and the biologic consequences of inherited deficiency of the enzyme.

HISTORY

Methemoglobinemia in humans was first recognized in individuals who were exposed to chemicals that increased the rate of hemoglobin oxidation. In 1891, Dittrich [3] produced toxic methemoglobinemia in dogs by administering nitroglycerine and acetanilid. He noted that the methemoglobin in dogs, as in humans, tended to disappear without hemolysis of the red cells, and he suggested that erythrocytes possessed the capacity to reduce the oxidized pigment.

Congenital cyanosis without obvious cardiac or pulmonary disease was reported by François [4] in 1845, and the familial clusters of idiopathic congenital cyanosis were described by Hitzenberger [5] in 1932. The idiopathic cases were initially ascribed to the endogenous production of a substance capable of oxidizing hemoglobin [6] and later to impaired reduction of methemoglobin formed continuously in red cells [7]. The classic investigations of Gibson in 1948 [8] provided experimental evidence for deficiency of an NADH-dependent reducing system in the erythrocytes of patients with idiopathic methemoglobinemia. In 1959, Scott and Griffith identified an enzyme which catalyzed the reduction of methemoglobin by NADH [9]. They reported severe deficiency of the enzyme in the erythrocytes of native Alaskans with methemoglobinemia and intermediate activity in the cells of their acyanotic parents and children [10, 11]. They reasoned that the affected individuals inherited one gene for NADH methemoglobin reductase deficiency from each parent. In this way, they accounted for the typically recessive inheritance of idiopathic methemoglobinemia suggested by the family histories of many patients with this disorder.

Deficient activity of an NADH-dependent enzyme required for methemoglobin reduction has been reported in at least 150 cases of chronic idiopathic methemoglobinemia from all parts of the world. Another 150 patients are presumed to have the same disorder because of apparent recessive inheritance of the methemoglobinemia or the prompt disappearance of cyanosis after the intravenous injection of methylene blue. An unusually high incidence of hereditary methemoglobinemia of the enzyme-deficiency type has been reported among Alaskan Eskimos and Indians [12], Navajo Indians [11], Puerto Ricans [13, 14], Mediterraneans [15], and the natives of the Yakutsk region of Siberia 1000 miles west of the Bering Sea [16].

Methemoglobinemia in some families is transmitted as a dominant trait from generation to generation. Hörlein and Weber [17] demonstrated an abnormality in the globin in one such family; the abnormal hemoglobin was later designated *hemoglobin M.* The several types of hemoglobins M are each characterized by specific alterations in the amino acid sequence of the heme pocket of globin peptide chains which impede the normal reduction of methemoglobin. The hemoglobin M disorders are discussed in Chap. 76.

---

[1] The limitations of space and the need to include newer information have forced the authors to restrict their discussion and documentation. Fuller treatment of certain themes and a more complete list of references to the older literature are available in Stanbury JB, Wyngaarden JB, Fredrickson DS (eds): *The Metabolic Basic of Inherited Disease*, 4th ed. New York, McGraw-Hill, 1978, chap 65.

DEFINITION AND PROPERTIES OF METHEMOGLOBIN

The definition of methemoglobin and some structural characteristics which distinguish it from oxyhemoglobin are clarified by analogy with the structure of myoglobin as defined by x-ray crystallography at 2.8Å resolution or less. The sixth coordination position of the iron atom of deoxymyoglobin is vacant [18] and is, therefore, available to bind oxygen reversibly. The corresponding position in metmyoglobin, on the other hand, is occupied either by a water molecule or by a hydroxyl ion, depending on the pH [19]. The dissociation of the coordinated water with change in pH occurs according to the following scheme:

$$Hgb(Fe^{3+}) \cdot H_2O \rightleftharpoons Hgb(Fe^{3+}) \cdot OH^- + H^+$$

Because the optical spectra of heme proteins at the visible wavelengths reflect the structure of the heme sites, the spectrum of the ferric (but not of the deoxy- or oxy-) derivatives of myoglobin and of hemoglobin varies with pH. The wavelengths of maximum absorption for acid methemoglobin, which is the predominant species present at physiologic pH, are 631 and 500 nm, and the color of the pigment is brown. The wavelengths of maximum absorption for the alkaline form are 575 and 540 nm, and the color of the pigment is dark red. Methemoglobin may therefore be defined as an oxidation product of hemoglobin in which the sixth coordination position of ferric heme is bound to a water molecule (acid form) or to a hydroxyl ion (alkaline form), each with its characteristic optical spectrum.

Spontaneous transformation of oxyhemoglobin into methemoglobin (auto-oxidation) occurs slowly in vitro. The relative stability of oxyhemoglobin may be understood in terms of the asymmetric sharing of electrons between the iron atoms and the coordinated oxygen: the unlike charges of the ferric iron and the superoxide radical tend to hold the molecule together and to discourage dissociation [20]. Fridovich and his collaborators have suggested that the spontaneous, slow auto-oxidation, which occurs normally, is a consequence of the complete liberation of superoxide [21, 22]. The reaction may involve nucleophilic displacement of superoxide from the heme irons by chloride [23], which ultimately is replaced by water. Hydrogen peroxide is formed subsequently by the reaction of superoxide with itself [22] (in the presence of superoxide dismutase) and with oxyhemoglobin [24–26]:

$$O_2^- + O_2^- + 2H^+ \longrightarrow H_2O_2 + O_2$$
$$2H^+ + O_2^- + Hgb(Fe^{3+})\text{—}O_2^- \longrightarrow H_2O_2 + O_2 + Hgb(Fe^{3+})$$

The hydrogen peroxide which is generated can also oxidize hemoglobin [26].

Alpha chains auto-oxidize more rapidly than beta chains [27], and half-oxidized hemoglobin intermediates (valence hybrids) are produced [28]. Auto-oxidation of oxyhemoglobin is accelerated at low pH, in the presence of salts and metal atoms, and when the solution of hemoglobin is partially deoxygenated. The increased concentration of methemoglobin in the blood of abortuses, newborns, and individuals who live at high altitude may result, in part, from the hypoxemia and the consequent unsaturation of the hemoglobin [1].

Various chemicals or their metabolites increase the rate of oxidation of hemoglobin 100 to 1000 times by their reaction as (1) direct oxidants of ferrous heme (e.g., ferricyanide) or (2) reducing agents of molecular oxygen or of oxyhemoglobin which generate superoxide anion, hydroperoxy radical, hydrogen peroxide, or an intermediate peroxyhemoglobin complex [1, 29–31]. Aniline dyes, primaquin, sulfonamides, acetylphenylhydrazine, phenacetin, and benzocaine are among the agents thought to form methemoglobin by the second mechanism. The unimpeded generation of toxic oxygen and drug-derived radicals in erythrocytes whose antioxidant defenses are compromised by deficiency of glucose-6-phosphate dehydrogenase (G-6-PD) can denature their hemoglobin and damage their membranes, leading to splenic trapping and destruction [31]. The mechanism of methemoglobin formation by nitrites, often incriminated in toxic methemoglobinemia of infants and children, is complicated and ill-defined but may involve the formation of intermediate complexes between hemoglobin and nitrite redox products [29]. Regardless of how or by what agent methemoglobin is produced, its essential spectral and metabolic properties appear to be the same or very similar [32].

Methemoglobin forms complexes with a number of ligands which affect its physical and functional properties. Reaction with cyanide abolishes the absorption peak at 631 nm and converts acid methemoglobin to an unreactive derivative. On the other hand, reaction with ferrocyanide or organic phosphates enhances both the enzymatic and nonenzymatic reduction of methemoglobin [7, 33–35].

REGULATION OF METHEMOGLOBIN LEVELS IN ERYTHROCYTES

Protection Against Oxidation of Hemoglobin

The heme moiety attached to each globin chain lies within a hydrophobic pocket formed of proximal and distal histidines and of amino acids with nonpolar side chains that shield the heme iron from oxidation. The critical role of globin in stabilizing the iron-oxygen complex is emphasized by the contrast between the relative stability of oxyhemoglobin and the rapid oxidation of free ferrous heme. Structural alterations in and around the heme pocket in certain unstable hemoglobin variants result in a marked increase in their rate of spontaneous oxidation.

In addition to the inherent protection provided by the structure of the normal heme pocket, active metabolic processes within human erythrocytes provide some safeguards against methemoglobin formation. The superoxide produced during physiologic or accelerated oxidation of hemoglobin might oxidize other hemoglobin molecules [24–26] were it not destroyed by superoxide dismutase. Since dismutation converts superoxide anion to hydrogen peroxide which can also oxidize hemoglobin [26], the protective effect of superoxide dismutase requires coupling with a second reaction to remove the peroxide. Erythrocytes possess two enzymatic mechanisms for the destruction of hydrogen peroxide: (1) glutathione peroxidase plus reduced glutathione (GSH) which reduces hydrogen peroxide to water at the expense of NADPH generated by the pentose phosphate pathway [36] and (2) catalase, a low affinity enzyme which operates most effectively at high concentrations of peroxide [37, 38]. Patients with acatalasemia do not ordinarily have increased concentrations of methemoglobin

[39], but they are placed at risk by high rates of formation of hydrogen peroxide which exceed the peroxidative capacity of GSH and the pentose phosphate pathway [37]. Transient deficiencies of GSH peroxidase and of the NADH-dependent methemoglobin reducing enzyme account for the susceptibility of newborn infants to toxic methemoglobinemia.

Reduction of Methemoglobin to Hemoglobin

Less than 1 percent of the total hemoglobin present in normal human erythrocytes is in the methemoglobin form. The relatively constant concentration may be looked upon as the expression of an equilibrium between the slow, spontaneous oxidation of hemoglobin and the rate of its metabolic reduction. Several pathways for the reduction of methemoglobin have been described: NADH- and NADPH-dependent enzymatic pathways and direct reducing pathways involving ascorbic acid, reduced glutathione, and tetrahydropterin. Together these provide the erythrocyte with a reducing capacity 250 times greater than the rate at which methemoglobin is normally formed [2]. The most important of the reducing pathways is enzymatic and is linked to the oxidation of NADH. The enzyme involved has been variously named erythrocyte NADH dehydrogenase I, NADH methemoglobin reductase, and, most recently, NADH cytochrome b5 reductase.

NADH-dependent Reducing Pathway When normal human erythrocytes, treated with sufficient sodium nitrite to convert most of the hemoglobin to methemoglobin, are washed thoroughly and incubated with substances that can be metabolized by the cell to generate NADH, reduction of methemoglobin occurs (Fig. 75-1). Erythrocytes from patients with hereditary methemoglobinemia who are severely deficient in NADH dehydrogenase reduce methemoglobin very slowly, if at all. Erythrocytes from obligatory heterozygotes with inter-

mediate activity of the enzyme display an intermediate rate of methemoglobin reduction [40]. Although the degree of impairment in the ability of intact erythrocytes to reduce methemoglobin tends to parallel the level of enzyme activity, a precise correlation has not been found [40, 41]. The rate is enhanced when the concentration of NADH in normal erythrocytes is increased by preincubation with nicotinic acid; this manipulation has no effect in the cells of patients with hereditary methemoglobinemia [42]. Recent studies of methemoglobin reduction in erythrocyte hemolysates fortified selectively and in systems reconstituted from purified components indicate that, under conditions which approximate those in vivo, the rate is influenced by the concentration of cytochrome b5 and methemoglobin in addition to the concentration of enzyme [43–45]. In theory, therefore, severe deficiency of either NADH or cytochrome b5 might lead to methemoglobinemia. Such disorders have not yet been described.

The reduction of methemoglobin in intact cells requires an active anaerobic glycolytic pathway forming NADH at one or the other of the two NAD/NADH-linked reactions: glyceraldehyde phosphate dehydrogenase (GAPD) and lactate dehydrogenase (LDH) (Fig. 75-2). During normal steady state glycolysis, NADH produced by the former is consumed in the latter, and there is no net accumulation. Several lines of evidence suggest that the GAPD reaction is the major source of the NADH utilized for the enzymatic reduction of methemoglobin. (1) When nitrite-treated normal erythrocytes are incubated with glucose, pyruvate accumulates in an amount nearly equivalent stoichiometrically to the amount of methemoglobin which is reduced. This suggests diversion of NADH away from the LDH reaction for the enzymatic reduction of methemoglobin [8]. (2) Inhibition of glycolysis by iodoacetate diminishes methemoglobin reduction with glucose as substrate, whereas inhibition by fluoride stimulates the reduction of methemoglobin [8]. Iodoacetate probably inactivates GAPD, whereas fluoride blocks the more distal enolase step and markedly increases the level of 2,3-diphosphoglycerate (2,3-DPG). The diversion of glucose metabolism to 2,3-DPG and away from lactate may make more NADH available for the reduction of methemoglobin [46]. (3) Human erythrocytes may generate NADH through utilization of NADPH in the pentitol [47] and the sorbitol [48, 49] transhydrogenase pathways (Fig. 75-2), but the amounts of glucose metabolized and NADPH formed through the pathways are probably small. Moreover, the functioning of the pentitol pathway in its entirety in erythrocytes has not been clearly established.

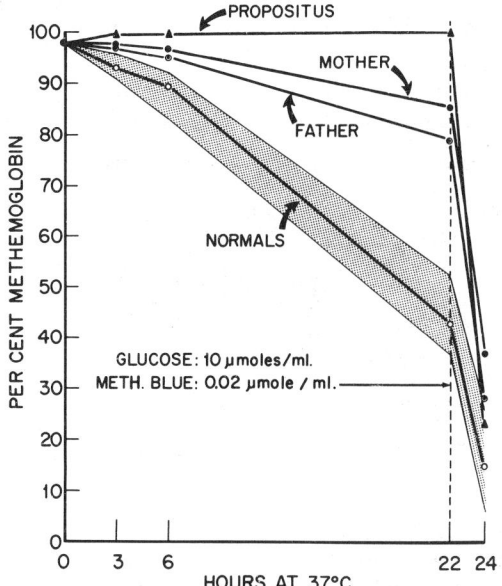

Figure 75-1 Reduction of methemoglobin by nitrite-treated washed erythrocytes utilizing glucose as substrate. Propositus was a child with homozygous deficiency of NADH diaphorase (cytochrome b5 reductase). (*From Jaffé et al.* [40]. *Reproduced with permission of the* American Journal of Medicine.)

NADPH-dependent Reducing Pathway Methylene blue dramatically accelerates oxygen consumption and methemoglobin reduction in intact erythrocytes incubated in solutions containing glucose as substrate (Fig. 75-1). These catalytic effects, which are observed both in normal erythrocytes and in the cells of patients deficient in NADH dehydrogenase, led Kiese [29, 50] and Gibson [8] to postulate a second enzymatic pathway for the reduction of methemoglobin—one which is dependent upon the generation of NADPH. The flow of electrons through the system is believed to occur as follows:

$$NADPH \xrightarrow{\ \ e\ \ } NADPH\ dehydrogenase \xrightarrow{\ \ e\ \ } methylene\ blue \xrightarrow{\ \ e\ \ } methemoglobin$$

NADPH dehydrogenase rapidly reduces methylene blue to leucomethylene blue which, in turn, spontaneously reduces met-

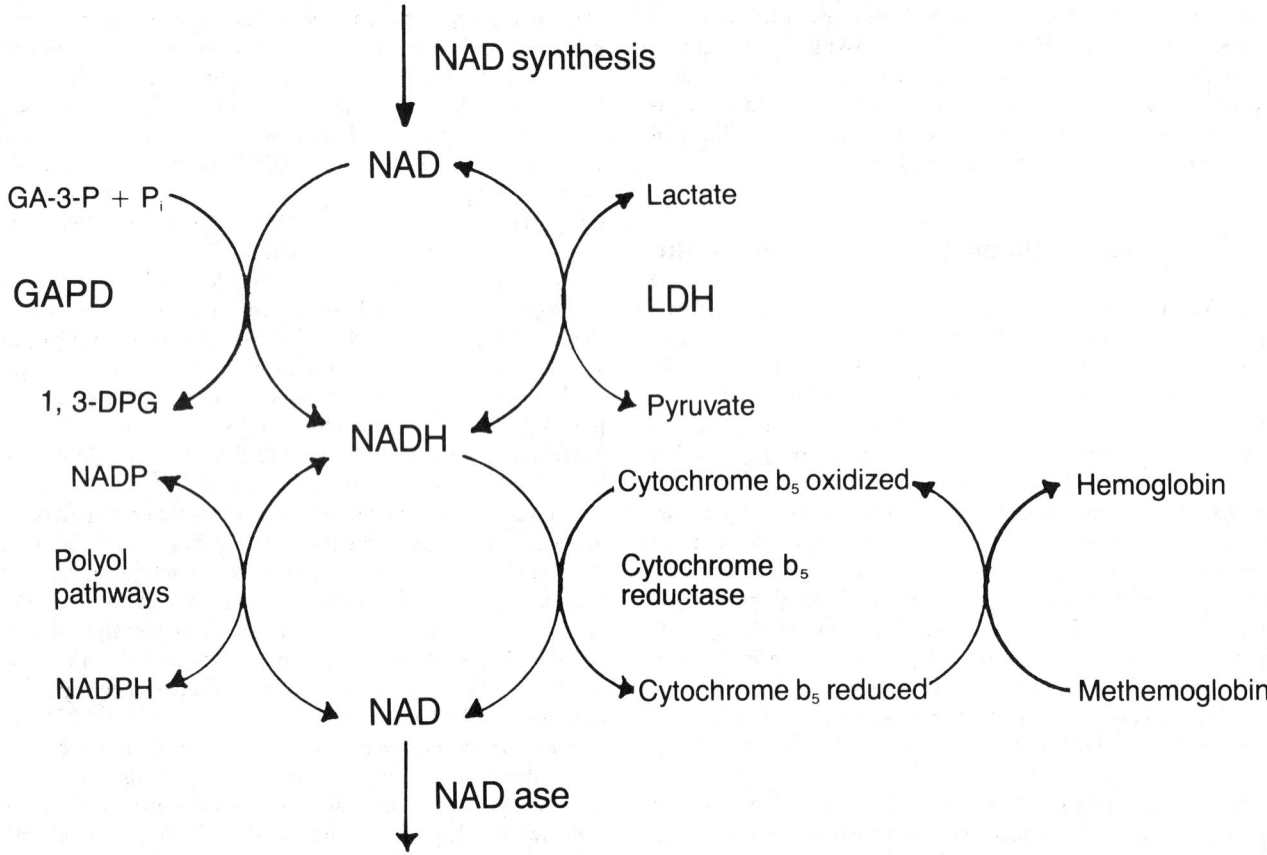

Figure 75-2 Metabolic pathways for generation and utilization of NADH in erythrocytes. Polyol (pentitol and sorbitol) pathways catalyze the interconversion of reduced pyridine nucleotides, but the amount of glucose metabolized and NADPH formed via these pathways is probably small. Glyceraldehyde phosphate dehydrogenase (GAPD) supplies most of the NADH used for the enzymatic reduction of cytochrome b5. Methemoglobin is reduced nonenzymatically by cytochrome b5. (*Modified from Brewer [125]. Reproduced with the permission of the author and Academic Press.*)

hemoglobin (or oxygen) with the regeneration of methylene blue. The required NADPH is provided by G-6-PD of the pentose phosphate pathway. Cells deficient in G-6-PD fail to show the normal acceleration of methemoglobin reduction and oxygen consumption in the presence of methylene blue. The stimulatory effect of methylene blue also fails in erythrocytes deficient in NADPH dehydrogenase [51, 52]. Recent studies by Yubisui, Matsuki, and coworkers indicate that riboflavin can substitute for methylene blue in activating this system [53–55].

Although the activation of the NADPH-reducing pathway by methylene blue dramatically relieves the cyanosis in patients with hereditary or toxic methemoglobinemia, it is unlikely that this pathway plays a significant role under physiologic conditions. The one known patient deficient in erythrocyte NADPH dehydrogenase [51] and patients deficient in G-6-PD do not have methemoglobinemia, and the reduction of methemoglobin in their nitrite-treated cells proceeds normally in the absence of methylene blue. Conversely, the increased level of methemoglobin in the erythrocytes of patients with hereditary methemoglobinemia has no effect on the activity of the pentose phosphate pathway, which is normal and which does not decrease when methemoglobin is rendered unavailable for reduction by binding with cyanide [56]. Finally, the affinity constant of NADPH dehydrogenase for flavins is relatively high (50 μM), and the concentration of free flavin in normal erythrocytes is low. This suggests that the enzyme cannot ordinarily reduce methemoglobin through the reduction of flavin [53].

Direct Reduction of Methemoglobin   Ascorbic acid, reduced glutathione, and tetrahydropterin [57] slowly reduce

methemoglobin in vitro, probably without the intervention of enzymes. The dehydroascorbic acid or oxidized glutathione formed by these reactions can be converted back to the parent compounds by specific reductases. Tetrahydropterin may be regenerated through glutathione-induced reduction of the dihydro form [57]. The reactions can be represented as follows:[2]

$$
\begin{array}{l}
\text{Methb}\!\!\smile\!\!\text{ascorbic acid} \longleftarrow \text{GSSG} \longrightarrow \text{NADPH} \\
\hspace{3.5cm} E_1 \hspace{2.0cm} E_2 \\
\text{Hb}\!\!\smile\!\!\text{dehydroascorbic acid} \longrightarrow \text{GSH} \longleftarrow \text{NADP}
\end{array}
$$

$$
\begin{array}{l}
\text{Methb}\!\!\smile\!\!\text{GSH} \longleftarrow \text{NADP} \\
\hspace{2.5cm} E_2 \\
\text{Hb}\!\!\smile\!\!\text{GSSG} \longrightarrow \text{NADPH}
\end{array}
$$

$$
\begin{array}{l}
\text{Methb}\!\!\smile\!\!\text{tetrahydropterin} \!\!\smile\!\! \text{GSSG} \longrightarrow \text{NADPH} \\
\hspace{5.5cm} E_2 \\
\text{Hb}\!\!\smile\!\!\text{dihydropterin} \!\!\smile\!\! \text{GSH} \longleftarrow \text{NADP}
\end{array}
$$

2 KEY:
E_1 = dehydroascorbic acid reductase.
E_2 = glutathione reductase.
GSH and GSSG = reduced and oxidized glutathione.

Methemoglobinemia is not a feature of scurvy [58] or of severe deficiency of erythrocyte glutathione [59, 60]. Further, depletion of glutathione by binding with N-ethylmaleimide does not impair the reduction of methemoglobin in nitrite-treated cells [42, 56]. The above observations and the slow rate of methemoglobin reduction which is supported by physiologic concentrations of these substrates make it doubtful that any of them normally contributes in more than a very minor way to the maintenance of ferrous hemoglobin in vivo.

ENZYMATIC MEDIATORS OF METHEMOGLOBIN REDUCTION

The search for the physiologically important methemoglobin-reducing enzyme has spawned a bewildering array of erythrocyte enzyme activities. The main reason for the confusion is that none of the isolated enzyme preparations reduces unmodified methemoglobin at a significant rate. In order to improve the efficiency of methemoglobin reduction, investigators have added methylene blue, ferrocyanide, ferrous EDTA, cytochromes, flavin, and other substances to their assay systems. Alternatively, they have substituted 2,6-dichloroindophenol (DCIP) dye, ferricyanide, or cytochromes for methemoglobin as the terminal electron acceptor. The purified enzymes are variably named *methemoglobin, DCIP dye, cytochrome* or *flavin reductases* (depending on the preferred electron acceptor), and *NADH-* or *NADPH-linked dehydrogenases* (depending on the preferred electron donor). The diaphorase activity of NADH- and NADPH-linked dehydrogenases refers to their capacity to reduce DCIP dye.

That an NADH-dependent enzyme system is primarily responsible for the reduction of methemoglobin in intact cells emerged most clearly from the studies of Gibson in 1948 [8]. This hypothesis was subsequently confirmed by Scott and Griffith [9] and thereafter by Hegesh et al. [61] and Kitao et al. [62], who demonstrated deficient activity of NADH-linked enzymes capable of methemoglobin reduction in hemolysate of patients with hereditary methemoglobinemia. Current evidence suggests that the activities studied by the three research groups—NADH dehydrogenase I, NADH methemoglobin ferrocyanide reductase, and NADH cytochrome b5 reductase, respectively—are different manifestations of a single enzyme protein which is separate and distinct from the NADPH-linked methemoglobin-reducing activity of human erythrocytes.

NADH Dehydrogenase Enzymes (NADH Cytochrome b5 Reductase)

Scott and his associates isolated two NADH dehydrogenases (I and II) from normal erythrocytes [63, 64]. The major form, NADH dehydrogenase I, was absent in an Eskimo with hereditary methemoglobinemia [65]. The enzyme specifically required NADH as electron donor, the rate with NADPH being only 1.5 percent of that with NADH, but reduced a number of different electron acceptors. The reduction of methemoglobin or DCIP dye catalyzed by NADH dehydrogenase I appeared to proceed in two steps: Rapid reduction of the enzyme by NADH, followed, in turn, by rate-limiting reduction of the final electron acceptor by the reduced enzyme.

Because the rate with DCIP dye was 9000 times faster than with methemoglobin, the reduction of the dye has been utilized to measure the NADH diaphorase activity of the enzyme in erythrocyte hemolysate [10].

The flavin content of the purified NADH dehydrogenase was very low. Yet Scott considered flavin an essential component since the kinetics of the diaphorase reaction are of a double displacement type which is characteristic of the dehydrogenation reactions catalyzed by some flavoproteins. Kuma and Inomata found 1 mole of flavin adenine dinucleotide (FAD) per mole of enzyme protein purified 129,000 times [66]. The presence of an FAD prosthetic group has been confirmed [67], and its reported absence in one preparation [68] may reflect modification of the enzyme induced by the isolation procedure.

Although the specific diaphorase activity of the various enzyme preparations increased with purification, the isolated enzymes reduced methemoglobin at a rate which was hardly, if at all, faster than in intact red cells. This slow reduction, even in the presence of excess NADH and methemoglobin, implied that additional factors influence the catalyzed reduction of methemoglobin, e.g., (1) the conformation of the methemoglobin molecule and (2) the presence of a carrier substance in the cells capable of transferring electrons from the reduced enzyme to methemoglobin.

Hegesh and Avron observed that the addition of potassium ferrocyanide to erythrocyte hemolysate markedly increased NADH-dependent methemoglobin reduction [33]. Activation reached a maximum at a molar ratio of ferrocyanide to methemoglobin of 4:1, and the added ferrocyanide was tightly bound. The authors proposed that a complex, formed between ferrocyanide and methemoglobin, had altered the conformation of methemoglobin, allowing closer access of the reducing enzyme to the heme groups. Recent studies of the mechanism of the activation of methemoglobin reduction by ferrocyanide, conducted in our own laboratory, indicate that ferrocyanide reduces methemoglobin directly and that the ferricyanide which is formed is reconverted to ferrocyanide by the action of NADH dehydrogenase [69]. These observations are consistent with the idea that the ferrocyanide utilized in the Hegesh and Avron system serves as an intermediate electron carrier between the reduced enzyme and methemoglobin:

$$\text{NADH} \xrightarrow{e} \text{NADH dehydrogenase} \xrightarrow{e} \text{ferricyanide} \xrightarrow{e} \text{methemoglobin}$$

Organic phosphates, such as 2,3-DPG, adenosine triphosphate, and inositol hexaphosphate, bind to methemoglobin, change its conformation [70, 71], and enhance the rate of methemoglobin reduction in the presence of enzyme [35] or vitamin C [34]. Matteson and Taketa have attributed the enhancement of methemoglobin reduction to allosteric interaction between the phosphate polyanions and the methemoglobin substrate [72]. They have suggested that when the level of methemoglobin is raised, binding of 2,3-DPG may activate the methemoglobin substrate through a conformational change and in this way help to regulate the rate of enzymatic reduction of methemoglobin in vivo. However, the enhancement by organic phosphate seemed to require methemoglobin ferrocyanide as substrate and was minimal when the methemoglobin was prepared by nitrition [35, 44]. It is thus likely that the conformational change in methemoglobin induced by organic phosphate enhances the rate of the direct reduction of methemoglobin by ferrocyanide and that the action of NADH dehydrogenase in this system is to reduce ferricyanide rather than methemoglobin.

Passon and his colleagues recently isolated cytochrome b5 from human erythrocytes [73] and an NADH diaphorase enzyme which catalyzes the reduction of cytochrome b5 [67]. Many of the properties of the heme protein and of the enzyme which reduced it were similar to those of corresponding proteins present in microsomes and mitochondria of nonerythroid tissues [74]. The enzyme rapidly reduced human erythrocyte cytochrome b5, DCIP dye, and potassium ferricyanide; these reactions were specific for NADH. The enzyme reduced methemoglobin very slowly, but the addition of cytochrome b5 in concentrations comparable to those in vivo stimulated methemoglobin reduction more than seventyfold [75]. Hultquist and Passon proposed that methemoglobin is reduced nonenzymatically by cytochrome b5, which is reduced by the action of NADH cytochrome b5 reductase (Fig. 75-12). They visualized the flow of electrons as follows:

$$\text{NADH} \xrightarrow[1]{e} \text{cytochrome b5 reductase} \xrightarrow[2]{e} \text{cytochrome b5} \xrightarrow[3]{e} \text{methemoglobin}$$

Studies by Sugita et al. [68], using enzymes from human erythrocytes and microsomal cytochrome b5 solubilized from rat liver, confirmed the feasibility of the suggested mechanism and validated the renaming of the enzyme. Further, their enzyme, purified 44,000 times, catalyzed efficient NADH-specific reduction of DCIP dye and methemoglobin ferrocyanide in addition to cytochrome b5. A recent examination of the elution behavior of the three activities from a calibrated column of Sephadex gel suggested that all three resided in a single protein with a molecular weight of about 33,000 [76] (see Ref. 1, Fig. 61-3). Each activity was absent or proportionally reduced in crude extracts prepared from the erythrocytes of patients with hereditary methemoglobinemia [62, 76, 77]. Identity of the activities and their catalysis by a single protein was further suggested by immunologic studies in which antiserums developed in chickens against human NADH methemoglobin ferrocyanide reductase neutralized the NADH diaphorase and cytochrome b5 reductase activities extracted from human erythrocytes [78, 79].

The kinetics of methemoglobin reduction have recently been studied in selectively fortified erythrocyte hemolysates, and in systems reconstituted from purified human erythrocyte components [43–45], in order to clarify the function of this reducing system in vivo. The concentrations of cytochrome b5 (0.22 to 0.5 μmol per liter of cells, i.e., 0.22 to 0.5 μM) [44, 45] and NADH (circa 0.04 μM) [45, 80] which are available in human erythrocytes did not fully saturate the reducing enzyme (the apparent K_m of cytochrome b5 at neutral pH was 7 μM and K_m of NADH was 0.022 μM). The reduction of cytochrome b5 in vivo would therefore be expected to be sluggish, limited at step 1 and especially at step 2 of the electron flow diagram above by the concentration of each substrate and by that of the enzyme (circa 0.05 μM) [44, 66]. At the normal methemoglobin concentration of 0.15 to 0.2 mM (in globin monomer), the nonenzymatic reduction of methemoglobin by cytochrome b5 (depicted in step 3) is also rate-limiting. An increase in the concentration of methemoglobin above normal would thus increase reduction of methemoglobin in vivo somewhat, but the enzymatic reduction of cytochrome b5 would remain bottlenecked by a concentration of this substrate which is far below the K_m of the enzyme.

The overall model of methemoglobin reduction which emerges from these findings can account for (1) the observed rate of methemoglobin reduction in nitrite-treated normal red cells (1 mM/h), (2) the inability of the normal system to reduce rapidly toxic accumulations of methemoglobin, (3) the incapability of a system with severe enzyme deficiency to reduce even physiologic formations of the oxidized pigment, and (4) the propensity of infants and of individuals with heterozygous deficiency of the enzyme to acquire toxic methemoglobinemia.

Righetti, Gacon, et al. [81, 82] have provided a direct visual demonstration of the binding of cytochrome b5 to methemoglobin, utilizing a novel isoelectric focusing-electrophoresis technique. Maximum interaction between the proteins occurred in the 6 to 8 pH range, suggesting that the stability of the complex formed depended mainly on electrostatic interactions between surface lysine residues in methemoglobin and acidic residues in cytochrome b5. Substitution of glutamic acid for lysine at positions 66 (E 10) or 95 (FG 2) of β hemoglobin chain variants weakened the stability of the cytochrome b5-methemoglobin complex and impaired the reduction of the methemoglobin variants by a cytochrome b5–dependent reducing system. Lysine residues E 10 and FG 2 are located near the heme crevice in both α and β chains, and the authors postulated that these sites, together with lysine residues E5 and E9 of α and β chains, compose the main part of the cytochrome b5 binding domain. By analogy with the mechanism observed with other heme proteins, the authors have proposed that interactions between complementary charged domains around the heme groups bring the heme moieties of the interacting proteins close together, allowing transfer of electrons to take place.

NADPH Dehydrogenase Enzymes

Erythrocyte NADPH dehydrogenase enzymes transfer electrons to free flavins [53–55] or to methylene blue [64, 83]; these, in turn, can reduce methemoglobin nonenzymatically. Since an increase in the methemoglobin content of intact red cells does not stimulate the activity of the pentose phosphate pathway [56], there is apparently no endogenous substrate capable of transferring electrons between NADPH and methemoglobin. Flavin nucleotides tightly bound to enzyme proteins apparently cannot serve as electron acceptors.

Neithammer and Huennekens have contended that erythrocyte NADH and NADPH dehydrogenase activities could represent a single enzyme protein capable of using either NADH or NADPH as electron donor [83]. There is abundant evidence which argues against this view. The two proteins are readily separated electrophoretically [84, 85] and by gel filtration [1, 76, 85]. In sharp contrast to NADH dehydrogenase, NADPH dehydrogenase does not reduce methemoglobin ferrocyanide or cytochrome b5 [1, 76], is not neutralized by antiserums developed in chickens against methemoglobin ferrocyanide reductase [78], and is present in normal quantity in the erythrocytes of patients with hereditary methemoglobinemia. These physical, functional, and immunologic differences as well as their independent genetic transmission are more consistent with the thesis that the NADH- and NADPH-linked reducing enzymes reside in separate and distinct enzyme proteins.

ORIGIN OF THE METHEMOGLOBIN-REDUCING SYSTEM OF MATURE ERYTHROCYTES

The cytochrome b5 and NADH cytochrome b5 reductase, which constitute the methemoglobin reducing system of mature human erythrocytes, originate from the endoplasmic reticulum of nucleated red blood cell precursors where they subserve entirely different functions. The conversion of a redox system of the endoplasmic reticulum into a soluble system in the mature erythrocyte is a remarkable example of conservation of cellular material during cell maturation.

The chemistry of cytochrome b5 and cytochrome b5 reductase has been studied extensively in the microsomal fraction of mammalian liver homogenates [86–91]. Each protein consists of a single polypeptide chain folded into two functionally distinct domains: A polar segment which contains the prosthetic heme (in cytochrome b5) or FAD (in cytochrome b5 reductase) group and a hydrophobic segment which composes about one-third of the total peptide chain length and is embedded in the endoplasmic reticulum membrane. The system is known to participate in two types of reactions: (1) Desaturation of fatty acids to give 9,10 unsaturated derivatives [92–96], e.g., the conversion of stearic to oleic acid, and (2) some cytochrome P450-mediated monooxygenase reactions yielding a hydroxylated lipid-soluble metabolite (steroid or drug) and water [96–99]. Ozols has proposed that the polar segments of cytochrome b5 and its reductase, each bearing their respective catalytic moieties, are oriented toward the cytosol, which provides the NADH required to reduce the enzyme [100]. Interaction between the polar segments of the reduced enzyme and cytochrome b5 [101] results in the rapid reduction of the latter's heme iron to the ferrous form. The reduced cytochrome b5, in turn, tunnels electrons via its hydrophobic tail [94, 95] to the fatty acid desaturase or cytochrome P450 submerged within the lipid bilayer of the endoplasmic reticulum adjacent to their respective lipid-soluble substrates.

Nucleated mouse erythrocyte precursors have endoplasmic reticulum containing cytochrome b5 and cytochrome b5 reductase [102]. The concentration of these proteins decreases as the cell matures, but small quantities of the water-soluble forms can be recovered in the cytoplasm even after all the organelles have disappeared [67, 73, 102, 103]. Comparison of the structures of cytochrome b5 and cytochrome b5 reductase in mature erythrocytes [1, 103–105] and in liver microsomes [86, 87, 89, 90, 103–105] indicates that the former represent the polar peptide segments which have presumably arisen by proteolytic processing of the parent molecules in the endoplasmic reticulum.

If particulate cytochrome b5 and cytochrome b5 reductase are solubilized during erythroid maturation by removal of their hydrophobic tails, what is the solubilizing agent? One possibility is a protease provided by lysosomes of the immature red cell. Indeed, in vitro extraction of bovine microsomes with proteases derived from liver lysosomes (cathepsins D and B) or rabbit reticulocyte membrane has yielded soluble forms of cytochrome b5 and of enzyme which closely resemble those found in mature bovine erythrocytes [105]. Further, the molecular weights of lysosome-extracted bovine microsomal enzyme [87] and human erythrocyte enzyme [1] are the same (33,000).

Additional support for the hypothesis that the methemoglobin-reducing enzyme of mature erythrocytes originates from a redox system of the endoplasmic reticulum is provided by (1) immunologic studies which indicate antigenic similarity between microsomal and soluble forms of cytochrome b5 [106–108] and of cytochrome b5 reductase [106–109] and (2) concomitant deficiency of both soluble and microsomal cytochrome b5 reductase in hereditary methemoglobinemia with mental retardation [15, 77].

GENETIC HETEROGENEITY OF NADH CYTOCHROME b5 REDUCTASE

The diaphorase activity of NADH cytochrome b5 reductase permits visualization of the enzyme after electrophoresis of hemolysate or tissue extract in starch or polyacrylamide gels [84] (Fig. 75-3). A survey of 2783 healthy persons for variants of erythrocyte NADH diaphorase revealed five electrophoretic phenotypes with normal staining intensity; the overall prevalence of the variants was about 1 in 100 [110]. Similar studies in the rare patients with hereditary methemoglobinemia have revealed at least 10 additional phenotypes [1]. The pattern of segregation of the phenotypes within families is consistent with allelism at the enzyme's gene locus.

The gene which codes for soluble NADH cytochrome b5 reductase has recently been assigned to human chromosome 22. The assignment is based upon studies of the electrophoretic mobility and isoelectric focusing patterns of soluble enzyme in the cytosol of rodent-human fibroblast hybrids, together with concurrent cytogenetic analysis [111, 112]. The same gene locus is assumed to code for the full length of the enzyme polypeptide chain (i.e., polar plus membranous segments) embedded in the endoplasmic reticulum.

The fully expressed neurologic syndrome which accompanies 10 to 15 percent of cases with hereditary methemoglobinemia consists of opisthotonus and generalized hypertonia, strabismus, attacks of bilateral athetoid movements, severe mental retardation, microcephaly, and retarded growth [15, 40, 113]. The clinical signs first become apparent at 2 to 3 months of age; death may occur as early as 1 year. Kaplan, Leroux, and their associates have demonstrated nearly total deficiency of microsomal cytochrome b5 reductase in the leukocytes, muscle, liver, fibroblasts, and brain of one such patient [77] and in the fibroblasts and leukocytes of six others [15, 114]. Methemoglobin ferrocyanide reductase activity in leukocytes was extremely low in all 8 patients with the neurologic syndrome and was normal or only moderately reduced in 14 patients with normal neurologic function. On the strength of these observations, the authors postulated that the neurologic syndrome represented either gene deletions or a mutation in paired alleles determining the activity or stability of the enzyme polypeptide chain as a whole (polar plus hydrophobic segments), or the attachment of its hydrophobic segment to the endoplasmic reticulum. By contrast, uncomplicated methemoglobinemia was attributed to a mutation in paired alleles which primarily influenced the stability or function of the soluble form of the enzyme, or its proteolytic cleavage from the parent molecule in the endoplasmic reticulum [15]. Cerebral lipids have not been analyzed in methemoglobinemia patients who have died with severe neurologic abnormalities. Normal

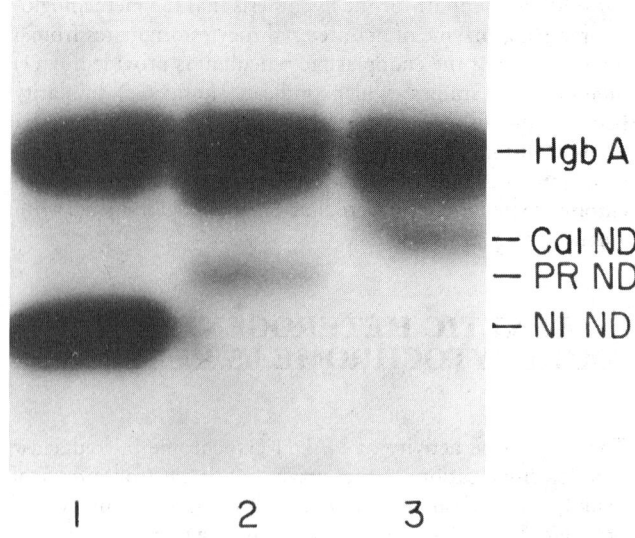

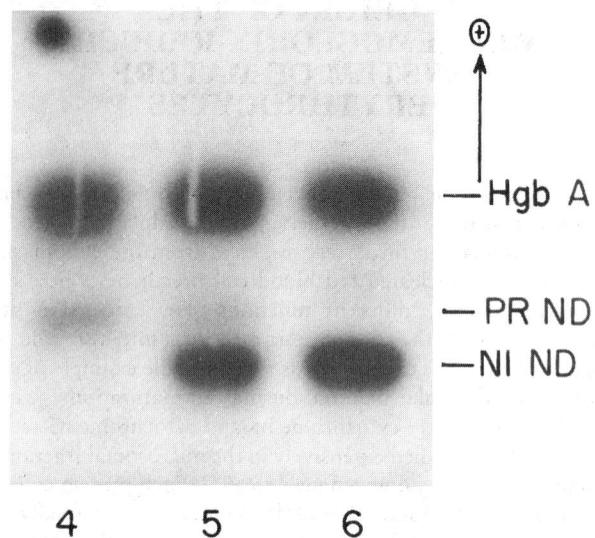

Figure 75-3 Erythrocyte hemolysates of normal and hereditary methemo-globinemia subjects after electrophoresis in starch gel at pH 8.6 and stain-ing for NADH diaphorase (tetrazolium method). Purple enzyme bands con-trast with hemoglobin spots. Hemolysate in positions 1 and 6, normal; 2 and 4, Puerto Rico homozygote; 3, California homozygote; 5, mother of Puerto Rico homozygote. ND is NADH diaphorase. (*From Schwartz et al.* [126]. *Reproduced with the permission of the* Israel Journal of Medical Sciences.)

myelin phospholipid is rich in oleic acid, and the suggestion has been made that impaired biosynthesis of unsaturated fatty acids due to deficient cytochrome b5 reductase in brain micro-somes may account for the central nervous system disease [77].

Lability in vivo is a property of the normal erythrocyte enzyme which loses about one-sixth of its activity as red cells age [14, 115]. Exaggerated lability characterizes at least five enzyme variants [1]. In the case of the Puerto Rico and Boston slow enzymes, the lability was considered to be of a sufficient degree to account for both the deficient enzyme activity in vivo and the tendency of the methemoglobin to accumulate in erythrocytes of increasing cell age [14, 115]. That neither of the two patients with exaggerated erythrocyte enzyme lability was mentally retarded could result from the inability of mature erythrocytes (but not brain microsomes) to renew their pro-teins through synthesis.

CLINICAL FEATURES OF NADH CYTOCHROME b5 REDUCTASE DEFICIENCY

Patients with hereditary methemoglobinemia characteristically have persistent slate-gray cyanosis, often dating from birth. There is no evidence of cardiac or pulmonary disease, nor any clubbing of the fingers. Hardly any adverse effects are discern-ible when the methemoglobin level is 25 percent or less, and even at levels up to 40 percent the only complaints may be those of fatigability and of dyspnea after vigorous exercise. The great majority of patients do not have an associated neu-rologic disorder, and their life expectancy is normal. Pregnan-cies are not compromised, and there is no erythrocyte hemoly-sis. As these patients are really more blue than sick, treatment is rarely necessary. Nevertheless, psychologic considerations may sometimes justify decreasing the methemoglobin level with medicinal supplements of ascorbic acid (0.5 g/day) or riboflavin (20 mg/d) [116] or by intravenous injection of meth-ylene blue (1 mg/kg). The effectiveness of oral riboflavin in the treatment of methemoglobinemia is based upon its ability to

penetrate intact red cells and activate the NADPH dehydroge-nase pathway for methemoglobin reduction [53, 54]. The side effects of the long-term administration of large doses of ribo-flavin are not known, but similar usage of ascorbic acid has been associated with hyperoxaluria and stone formation [117]. Following intravenous treatment with methylene blue, methe-moglobin reaccumulates at a rate of 1 to 3 percent each day and levels off at the pretreatment value after 10 to 14 days.

Partial oxidation of the hemes in a hemoglobin tetramer increases the affinity for oxygen of the remaining ferrohemes [118] and interferes with oxygen unloading. Since valence hybrids are present in hereditary methemoglobinemia [28], the resulting tissue anoxia should trigger the elaboration of eryth-ropoietan and the development of compensatory erythrocyto-sis. Thus it is puzzling that significant erythrocytosis is found only occasionally and that the position of the oxygenation curve is normal or shifted only slightly to the left [119]. Seg-regation of methemoglobin within a discrete population of older cells has been invoked to account for the normal position of the oxygenation curve in some cases [56]. Additionally, the normal or nearly normal position could be an expression of simultaneous interactions which tend to shift the curve in opposite directions: e.g., (1) interactions between ferric and ferrous hemes in partially oxidized tetramers which increase oxygen affinity and (2) interactions between fully functional tetramers and 2,3-DPG which facilitate oxygen release [1].

Systemic deficiency of microsomal NADH cytochrome b5 reductase has been discussed above. The symptoms seem to be limited to the central nervous system.

Infants below the age of 3 months and heterozygous carriers of an allelic gene which specifies the formation of deficient soluble enzyme have intermediate levels of erythrocyte activity. The rate of reduction of methemoglobin in their intact cells is decreased [40, 120] (Fig. 75-1), and they tend to develop cya-nosis after exposure to chemicals and drugs which form met-hemoglobin. Diapers labeled with inks or washed in disinfec-tants which contain aniline, and milk formulas constituted with nitrate-rich water, have caused epidemics of methemoglobinemia in nurseries; the mortality rate has been as high as 10 percent. (Nitrates in water are reduced to nitrites by the action of bacteria in the intestinal tract.) Malaria chemoprophylaxis is generally harmless, but primaquin, chloroquine, and diaminodiphenylsulfone have provoked toxic methemoglobinemia when given to adults with heterozygous enzyme deficiency [121].

The opportunity for physiologic compensation of the chronic cyanosis in patients with hereditary methemoglobinemia may explain, to a certain extent, the benign nature of the condition. On the other hand, cyanosis which develops rapidly, as in toxic methemoglobinemia, abruptly decreases the oxygen-carrying capacity of the blood and shifts the oxygenation curve to the left [118]. Direct effects of the toxic agent can add to the patient's disability. Symptoms of headache, vomiting, dyspnea, fatigue, and syncope appear at toxic methemoglobin levels of 20 to 30 percent, and there is danger of coma and death when more than half the total hemoglobin is oxidized [122]. The frequency and severity of toxic methemoglobinemia have increased markedly in the last decade owing to the ready availability of butyl and related nitrites in commercial preparations sold as "room odorizers" and the abuse of these products by drug culture enthusiasts [123]. Although a single injection of methylene blue is generally sufficient therapy for the symptomatic subject who has inhaled liquid nitrite, repeated injections, and even exchange transfusions or hemodialysis, may be required to relieve the coma and profound cyanosis which can follow ingestion of these chemicals. Hemodialysis to remove offending chemicals and red cell transfusion to improve oxygen-carrying capacity may be required in patients with coincident G-6-PD deficiency and alarming symptoms attributable to a high concentration of methemoglobin. Subjects with G-6-PD deficiency cannot respond to methylene blue [124], the effectiveness of which depends on the capacity of the red cell to regenerate the reduced NADP consumed by activation to NADPH dehydrogenase.

DIAGNOSIS

Comparable degrees of clinical cyanosis are produced by deoxyhemoglobin, methemoglobin, or sulfhemoglobin in concentrations of 5, 1.5, and 0.5 g per deciliter of blood, respectively. Methemoglobinemia is often first suspected when the administration of oxygen and other measures aimed at relieving cardiac and pulmonary causes of hemoglobin unsaturation do not remove the cyanosis, and when the purple or brown color of shed blood persists after vigorous shaking with air. The presence of methemoglobin A may be confirmed by recording spectral absorption peaks at 500 and 631 nm at pH 6.5, and methemoglobin may be quantified by measuring the rapid decrease of the latter upon the addition of neutralized cyanide. Methemoglobin M should be suspected if the peaks are shifted toward lower wavelengths and if their disappearance upon the addition of cyanide is slow and incomplete.

A careful history often helps distinguish the various forms of methemoglobinemia. Recent onset of unexplained cyanosis is most compatible with toxic methemoglobinemia. Parent-to-child transmission of long-standing cyanosis suggests the possibility of hemoglobin M, whereas congenital cyanosis in sibs

and a history of consanguinity are more consistent with deficiency of NADH cytochrome b5 reductase. Definitive diagnosis of hereditary methemoglobinemia rests on the demonstration of markedly deficient erythrocyte enzyme activity by direct assay of NADH methemoglobin ferrocyanide reductase (Hegesh assay) [61], NADH diaphorase (Scott assay) [10], or NADH cytochrome b5 reductase (Strittmatter assay) [67].

The Hegesh assay is preferred for routine use because it is accurate at low levels of activity, does not require repeated washing of test cells or extraction of hemoglobin from test hemolysate, and is not influenced by the simultaneous presence of NADPH dehydrogenase. The Hegesh procedure may also be used to measure microsomal enzyme activity in leukocytes and, in this way, to predict the risk of the neurologic dysfunction syndrome in newly diagnosed infants [15, 77]. The diaphorase reaction, linked to the reduction of tetrazolium, finds its greatest applicability in staining the enzyme after electrophoresis [84] in order to discover variants with altered mobility and to assist in the detection of heterozygous carriers (Fig. 75-3).

Support in part by grants HL 13585 and AM 7294 from the National Institutes of Health.

REFERENCES

1. SCHWARTZ JM, JAFFÉ ER: Hereditary methemoglobinemia with deficiency of NADH dehydrogenase, in Stanbury JB, Wyngaarden JB, Fredrickson DS (eds): *The Metabolic Basis of Inherited Disease*, 4th ed. New York, McGraw-Hill, 1978, p 1452
2. SCOTT EM: Congenital methemoglobinemia due to DPNH-diaphorase deficiency, in Beutler E (ed): *Hereditary Disorders of Erythrocyte Metabolism*. New York, Grune & Stratton, 1968, p 102
3. DITTRICH P: Uber methämoglobinbildende Gifte. *Naunyn-Schmiedebergs Arch Exp Pathol Pharmacol* 29:247, 1891
4. FRANCOIS: Cas de cyanose congénitale sans cause apparente, *Bull Acad R Med Belg* 4:698, 1845
5. HITZENBERGER K: Autotoxische Cyanose (intraglobuläre methämoglobinamie). *Wein Arch Intern Med* 23:85, 1932
6. DIECKMANN WJ: Methemoglobinemia. *Arch Intern Med* 50:574, 1932
7. GIBSON QH: The reduction of methemoglobin by ascorbic acid. *Biochem J* 37:615, 1943
8. GIBSON QH: The reduction of methemoglobin in red blood cells and studies on the cause of idiopathic methaemoglobinemia. *Biochem J* 42:13, 1948
9. SCOTT EM, GRIFFITH IV: The enzymic defect of hereditary methemoglobinemia: Diaphorase. *Biochim Biophys Acta* 134:584, 1959
10. SCOTT EM: The relation of diaphorase of human erythrocytes to inheritance of methemoglobinemia. *J Clin Invest* 39:1176, 1960
11. BALSAMO P, HARDY WR, SCOTT EM: Hereditary methemoglobinemia due to diaphorse deficiency in Navaho Indians. *J Pediatr* 65:928, 1964
12. SCOTT EM, HOSKINS DD: Hereditary methemoglobinemia in Alaskan Eskimos and Indians. *Blood* 13:795, 1958
13. HSIEH HS, JAFFÉ ER: Electrophoretic and functional variants of NADH methemoglobin reductase in hereditary methemoglobinemia. *J Clin Invest* 50:196, 1971
14. SCHWARTZ JM, PARESS PS, ROSS JM, DIPILLO F, RIZEK R: Unstable variant of NADH methemoglobin reductase in Puerto Ricans with hereditary methemoglobinemia. *J Clin Invest* 51:1594, 1972
15. KAPLAN JC, LEROUX A, BEAUVAIS P: Formes cliniques et biologiques du déficit en cytochrome b5 réductase. *Comptes Rendus Séances Soc Biologie* 173:368, 1979
16. JAFFÉ ER: Methemoglobinemia. *Clin Haematol*, 10:99, 1981
17. HÖRLEIN H, WEBER G: Über chronische familiäre Methämoglobinamie und eine neu Modifikation des Methämoglobins. *Dtsch Med Wochenschr* 73:476, 1948
18. NOBBS CL, WATSON HC, KENDREW JC: Structure of deoxymyoglobin: A crystallographic study. *Nature (London)* 209:339, 1966
19. STRYER L, KENDREW JC, WATSON HC: The mode of attachment of the azide ion to sperm whale metmyoglobin. *J Mol Biol* 8:96, 1964
20. GRIMES AJ: *Human Red Cell Metabolism*. Oxford, Blackwell Scientific Publications, 1980, p 225

21. MISRA HP, FRIDOVICH I: The generation of superoxide radicals during the autooxidation of hemoglobin. *J Biol Chem* 247:6960, 1972

22. FRIDOVICH I: The biology of oxygen radicals. *Science* 201:875, 1978

23. WALLACE WJ, MAXWELL JC, CAUGHEY WS: The mechanism of hemoglobin autooxidation. Evidence for proton-assisted nucleophilic displacement of superoxide by anions. *Biochem Biophys Res Commun* 57:1104, 1974

24. SUTTON HC, ROBERTS PB, WINTERBOURN CC: The rate of reaction of superoxide radical ion with oxyhemoglobin and methemoglobin. *Biochem J* 155:503, 1976

25. LYNCH RE, LEE GR, CARTWRIGHT GE: Inhibition by superoxide dismutase of methemoglobin formation from oxyhemoglobin. *J Biol Chem* 251:1015, 1976

26. LYNCH RE, THOMAS JE, LEE GR: Inhibition of methemoglobin formation from purified oxyhemoglobin by superoxide dismutase. *Biochemistry* 16:4563, 1977

27. MANSOURI A, WINTERHALTER KH: Nonequivalence of chains in hemoglobin oxidation. *Biochemistry* 12:4946, 1973

28. TOMODA A, IMOTO M, HIRANO M, YONEYAMA Y: Analysis of met-form hemoglobin in human erythrocytes of normal adults and of a patient with hereditary methemoglobinemia due to deficiency of NADH cytochrome b5 reductase. *Biochemistry J* 181:505, 1979

29. KIESE M: *Methemoglobinemia: A Comprehensive Treatise.* Cleveland, CRC Press, 1974

30. CASTRO CE, WADE RS, BELSER NO: Conversion of oxyhemoglobin to methemoglobin by organic and inorganic reductants. *Biochemistry* 17:225, 1978

31. BABIOR BM: Oxidizing radicals and red cell destruction, in Wallach, DFH (ed): *The Function of Red Blood Cells: Erythrocyte Pathobiology,* New York, Alan R. Liss, 1981, p 173

32. ANTONINI E, BRUNORI M: Hemoglobin and methemoglobin, Surgenor DMN (ed): *The Red Blood Cell,* 2d ed. New York, Academic, 1975, vol II p 753

33. HEGESH E, AVRON M: The enzymatic reduction of ferrihemoglobin. I. The reduction of ferrihemoglobin in red blood cells and hemolysates. *Biochim Biophys Acta* 146:91, 1967

34. TOMODA A, MATSUKAWA S, TAKESHITA M, YONEYAMA Y: Effect of organic phosphates on methemoglobin reduction by ascorbic acid. *J Biol Chem* 251:7494, 1976

35. TAKETA F, CHEN JY: Activation of the NADH methemoglobin reductase reaction by inositol hexaphosphate. *Biochem Biophys Res Commun* 75:389, 1977

36. COHEN G, HOCHSTEIN P: Glutathione peroxidase: The primary agent for the elimination of hydrogen peroxide in erythrocytes. *Biochemistry* 2:1420, 1963

37. AEBI H, BOSSI E, CANTZ M, MATSUBARA S, SUTER H: Acatalas(em)ia in Switzerland, in Beutler E (ed): *Hereditary Disorders of Erythrocyte Metabolism.* New York, Grune & Stratton, 1968, p 41

38. NICHOLLS P: Contributions of catalase and glutathione peroxidase to red cell peroxide removal. *Biochim Biophys Acta* 279:306, 1972

39. JACOB HS, INGBAR SH, JANDL JH: Oxidative hemolysis and erythrocyte metabolism in hereditary acatalasia. *J Clin Invest* 44:11, 1965

40. JAFFÉ ER, NEUMANN G, ROTHBERG H, WILSON FT, WEBSTER RM, WOLFF JA: Hereditary methemoglobinemia with and without mental retardation: A study of three families. *Am J Med* 41:42, 1966

41. KANAZAWA Y, HATORI M, KOSAKA K, NAKAO K: The relationship of NADH-dependent diaphorase activity and methemoglobin reduction in human erythrocytes. *Clin Chim Acta* 19:524, 1968

42. JAFFÉ ER, NEUMANN G: Hereditary methemoglobinemia, toxic methemoglobinemia and the reduction of methemoglobin. *Ann NY Acad Sci* 151:795, 1968

43. SANNES LJ, HULTQUIST DE: Effects of hemolysate concentration, ionic strength and cytochrome b5 concentration on the rate of methemoglobin reduction in hemolysates of human erythrocytes. *Biochim Biophys Acta* 544:547, 1978

44. SANNES LJ, HULTQUIST DE: Personal communication

45. ABE K, SUGITA Y: Properties of cytochrome b5 and methemoglobin reduction in human erythrocytes. *Eur J Biochem* 101:423, 1979

46. KEITT AS: Hereditary methemoglobinemia with deficiency of NADH methemoglobin reductase, in Stanbury JM, Wyngaarden JB, Fredrickson DS (eds): *The Metabolic Basis of Inherited Diseases,* 3d ed. New York, McGraw-Hill, 1972, p 1389

47. EATON JW, BREWER GJ: Pentose phosphate metabolism, in Surgenor DMN (ed): *The Red Blood Cell,* 2d ed. New York, Academic, vol I 1974, p 435

48. MORRISON AD, CLEMENTS RS, TRAVIS SB, OSKI F, WINEGRAD AI: Glucose utilization by the polyol pathway in human erythrocytes. *Biochem Biophys Res Commun* 40:199, 1970

49. TRAVIS SF, MORRISON AD, CLEMENTS RS, WINEGRAD A, OSKI FA: The role of the polyol pathway in methemoglobin reduction in human red cells. *Br J Hematol* 27:597, 1974

50. KIESE M: Die Reduktion des Hämiglobins. *Biochem Z* 316:264, 1944

51. SASS MD, CARUSO CJ, FARHANGI M: TPNH-methemoglobin reductase deficiency: A new red-cell enzyme defect. *J Lab Clin Med* 70:760, 1967

52. SASS MD: Observations on the role of TPNH dehydrogenase in human red cells. *Clin Chim Acta* 21:101, 1968

53. YUBISUI T, MATSUKI T, TANISHIMA K, TAKESHITA M, YONEYAMA Y: NADH-flavin reductase in human erythrocytes and the reduction of methemoglobin through flavin by the enzyme. *Biochem Biophys Res Commun* 76:174, 1977

54. MATSUKI T, YUBISUI T, TOMODA A, YONEYAMA Y, TAKESHITA M, HIRANO M, KOBAYASHI K, TANI Y: Acceleration of methaemoglobin reduction by riboflavin in human erythrocytes. *Br J Haematol* 39:523, 1978

55. YUBISUI T, MATSUKI T, TAKESHITA M, YONEYAMA Y: Characterization of the purified NADPH-flavin reductase of human erythrocytes. *J Biochem* 85:719, 1979

56. KEITT AS, SMITH TW, JANDL JH: Red cell "pseudomosaicism" in congenital methemoglobinemia. *N Engl J Med* 275:398, 1966

57. TAYLOR D, HOCHSTEIN P: Reduction of methemoglobin by tetrahydropterin and glutathione. *Arch Biochem Biophys* 179:456, 1977

58. WALLERSTEIN RO, WALLERSTEIN RO JR: Scurvy. *Semin Hematol* 13:211, 1976

59. MOHLER DN, MAJERIES PW, MINNICH V, HESS CE, GARRICK MD: Glutathione synthetase deficiency as a cause of hereditary hemolytic disease. *N Engl J Med* 283:1253, 1970

60. KONRAD PN, RICHARDS F, VALENTINE WN, PAGLIA DW: Gamma-glutamylcysteine synthetase deficiency: A cause of hereditary hemolytic anemia. *N Engl J Med* 286:557, 1972

61. HEGESH E, CALMANOVICI N, AVRON M: New method for determining ferrihemoglobin reductase (NADH-methemoglobin reductase) in erythrocytes. *J Lab Clin Med* 72:339, 1968

62. KITAO T, SUGITA Y, YONEYAMA Y, HATTORI K: Methemoglobin reductase (cytochrome b5 reductase) deficiency in congenital methemoglobinemia. *Blood* 44:879, 1974

63. SCOTT EM, MCGRAW JC: Purification and properties of diphosphopyridine nucleotide diaphorase of human erythrocytes. *J Biol Chem* 237:249, 1962

64. SCOTT EM, DUNCAN IW, EKSTRAND V: The reduced pyridine nucleotide dehydrogenases of human erythrocytes. *J Biol Chem* 240:481, 1965

65. SCOTT EM: Purification of diphosphopyridine nucleotide diaphorase from methemoglobinemic erythrocytes. *Biochem Biophys Res Commun* 9:59, 1962

66. KUMA F, INOMATA H: Studies of methemoglobin reductase. II. The purification and molecular properties of reduced nicotinamide adenine dinucleotide-dependent methemoglobin reductase. *J Biol Chem* 247:556, 1972

67. PASSON PG, HULTQUIST DE: Soluble cytochrome b5 reductase from human erythrocytes. *Biochim Biophys Acta* 275:62, 1972

68. SUGITA Y, NOMURA S, YONEYAMA Y: Purification of reduced pyridine nucleotide dehydrogenase from human erythrocytes and methemoglobin reduction by the enzyme. *J Biol Chem* 246:6072, 1971

69. REISS AL, SCHWARTZ JS, PATEL S: Mechanism of the enzyme dependent reduction of methemoglobin in the presence of NADH and ferrocyanide. *Blood* 50, *Suppl* 1:84, 1977

70. PERUTZ MF, FERSHT AR, SIMON SR, ROBERTS GCK: Influence of globin structure on the state of heme. II. Allosteric transitions in methemoglobin. *Biochemistry* 13:2174, 1974

71. HENSLEY P, EDELSTEIN SJ, WHARTON DC, GIBSON QH: Conformation and spin state in methemoglobin. *J Biol Chem* 250:952, 1975

72. MATTESON KJ, TAKETA F: Inhibition of NADH methemoglobin reductase by organic phosphates. *Biochem Biophys Acta* 571:112, 1979

73. PASSON PG, REED DW, HULTQUIST DE: Soluble cytochrome b5 from human erythrocytes. *Biochim Biophys Acta* 275:51, 1972

74. HULTQUIST DE: Methemoglobin reduction system of erythrocytes, in Fleisher S, Packer L (eds): *Methods in Enzymology,* vol 52, *Biomembranes.* New York, Academic, 1978, p 463

75. HULTQUIST DE, PASSON PG: Catalysis of methemoglobin reduction by erythrocyte cytochrome b5 and cytochrome b5 reductase. *Nature [New Biol]* 229:252, 1971

76. SCHWARTZ JM, REISS AL: Erythrocyte diaphorases: Their identity and role. *Program of the American Society of Hematology, 17th Annual Meeting* (abstract 192) 1974

77. LEROUX A, JUNIEN C, KAPLAN JC, BAMBERGER J: Generalized deficiency of cytochrome b5 reductase in congenital methaemoglobinemia with mental retardation. *Nature* 258:619, 1975

78. LEROUX A, KAPLAN JC: Presence of red cell type NADH-methemoglobin reductase (NADH-diphorase) in human non-erythroid cells. *Biochem Biophys Res Commun* 49:945, 1972

79. SCHWARTZ JM, PATEL SM, REISS AL: Erythrocyte diaphorase enzymes: Their number and significance. Submitted for publication

80. JACOBASCH G, MINAKAMI S, RAPOPORT SM: Glycolysis of the erythrocyte, in Yoshikawa H, Rapoport SM (eds): *Cellular and Molecular Biology of Erythrocytes.* Baltimore, University Park Press, 1974, p 55

81. RIGHETTI PG, GACON G, GIANAZZA E, LOSTANLEN D, KAPLAN JC: Titration curves of interacting cytochrome-b5 and hemoglobin by isoelectric focusing-electrophoresis. *Biochem Biophys Res Commun* 85:1575, 1978

82. GACON G, LOSTANLEN D, LABIE D, KAPLAN JC: Interaction between cytochrome b5 and hemoglobin: Involvement of β 66 (E10) and β 95 (FG2) lysyl residues of hemoglobin. *Proc Natl Acad Sci USA* 77:1917, 1980

83. NEITHAMMER D, HUENNEKENS FM: DPNH- and TPNH-dependent methemoglobin reducing systems from human erythrocytes. *Blood* 38:831, 1971

84. KAPLAN JC, BEUTLER E: Electrophoresis of red-cell NADH- and NADPH-diaphorases in normal subjects and patients with congenital methemoglobinemia. *Biochem Biophys Res Commun* 29:605, 1967

85. HEGESH E, CALMANOVICI N, LUPO M, BOCHKOWSKY R: Diaphorases of human erythrocytes, in Ramot B (ed): *Red Cell Structure and Metabolism.* New York, Academic, 1971, p 113

86. TAKESUE S, OMURA T: Purification and properties of NADH cytochrome b5 reductase solubilized by lysosomes from rat liver microsomes. *J Biochem* 65:267, 1970

87. SPATZ L, STRITTMATTER P: A form of reduced nicotinamide adenine dinucleotide cytochrome b5 reductase containing both the catalytic site and an additional hydrophobic membrane-binding segment. *J Biol Chem* 248:793, 1973

88. MIHARO K, SATO R: Purification and properties of the intact form of NADH-cytochrome b5 reductase from rat liver microsomes. *J Biochem* 78:1057, 1975

89. OZOLS J, GERARD C, NOBREGA FG: Proteolytic cleavage of horse liver cytochrome b5. Primary structure of the heme-containing moiety. *J Biol Chem* 251:6767, 1976

90. OZOLS J, GERARD C: Covalent structure of membranous segment of horse cytochrome b5: Chemical cleavage of the native hemoprotein. *J Biol Chem* 252:8549, 1977

91. MIHARO K, SATO R, SAKAKIBARA R, WADA H: Reduced nicotinamide adenine dinucleotide cytochrome b5 reductase: Location of the hydrophobic, membrane-binding region at the carboxyl-terminal end and the masked amino terminus. *Biochemistry* 17:2829, 1978

92. HOLLOWAY PW, KATZ JT: A requirement for cytochrome b5 in microsomal stearyl coenzyme A desaturation. *Biochemistry* 11:3689, 1972

93. OSHINO N, OMURA T: Immunochemical evidence for the participation of cytochrome b5 in mitochondrial stearyl-CoA desaturation reaction. *Arch Biochem* 157:395, 1973

94. STRITTMATTER P, SPATZ L, CORCORAN D, ROGERS MJ, SETLOW B, REDLINE R: Purification and properties of rat liver microsomal stearyl coenzyme A desaturase. *Proc Natl Acad Sci USA* 71:4565, 1974

95. ENOCH HG, CATALA A, STRITTMATTER P: Mechanism of rat liver microsomal stearyl-CoA desaturase. Studies of the substrate specificity, enzyme substrate interactions, and the function of lipid. *J Biol Chem* 251:5095, 1976

96. SCHENKMAN JB, JANSSON I, ROBIE-SUH KM: The many roles of cytochrome b5 in hepatic microsomes. *Life Sci* 19:611, 1976

97. HILLEBRANDT A, ESTABROOK RW: Evidence for the participation of cytochrome b5 in hepatic microsomal mixed-function oxidation reaction. *Arch Biochem Biophys* 143:66, 1971

98. LU AYH, WEST SW, VORE M, RYAN D, LEVIN W: Role of cytochrome b5 in hydroxylation by a reconstituted cytochrome P-450-containing system. *J Biol Chem* 249:6701, 1974

99. MANNERING GJ, KUWANARA S, OMURA T: Immunochemical evidence for the participation of cytochrome b5 in the NADH synergism of the NADPH dependent monooxidase system of hepatic microsomes. *Biochem Biophys Res Commun* 57:476, 1974

100. OZOLS J: The role of microsomal cytochrome b5 in the metabolism of ethanol, drugs and the desaturation of fatty acids. *Ann Clin Res* 8: Suppl 17:182, 1976

101. DAILEY HA, STRITTMATTER P: Modification and identification of cytochrome b5 carboxyl groups involved in protein-protein interaction with cytochrome b5 reductase. *J Biol Chem* 254:5388, 1979

102. SLAUGHTER SR, HULTQUIST DE: Membrane-bound redox proteins of the murine Friend virus-induced erythroleukemia cell. *J Cell Biol* 83:231, 1979

103. HULTQUIST DE, DEAN RT, DOUGLAS RH: Homogeneous cytochrome b5 from human erythrocytes. *Biochem Biophys Res Commun* 60:28, 1974

104. DOUGLAS RH, HULTQUIST DE: Evidence that two forms of bovine erythrocyte cytochrome b5 are identical to segments of microsomal cytochrome b5. *Proc Natl Acad Sci USA* 75:3118, 1978

105. HULTQUIST DE, SANNES LJ, SCHAFER DA: The NADH/NADPH-methemoglobin reduction system of erythrocytes, Brewer GJ (ed): *Proc Fifth Int Conf Red Cell Metab Function.* New York, Alan R. Liss, 1981 p 291

106. KUMA F, PROUGH RA, MASTERS BSS: Studies on methemoglobin reductase: Immunochemical similarity of soluble methemoglobin reductase and cytochrome b5 of human erythrocytes with NADH cytochrome b5 reductase and cytochrome b5 of rat liver microsomes. *Arch Biochem Biophys* 172:600, 1976

107. LEROUX A, TORLINSKI L, KAPLAN JC: Soluble and microsomal forms of NADH-cytochrome b5 reductase from human placenta: Similarity with NADH-methemoglobin reductase from human erythrocytes. *Biochim Biophys Acta* 481:50, 1977

108. LOSTANLEN D, DEBARROS AV, LEROUX A, KAPLAN JC: Soluble NADH cytochrome b5 reductase from rabbit liver cytosol: Partial purification and characterization. *Biochim Biophys Acta* 526:42, 1978

109. GOTO-TOMURA R, TAKESUE Y, TAKESUE S: Immunological similarity between NADH-cytochrome b5 reductase of erythrocytes and liver microsomes. *Biochim Biophys Acta* 423:293, 1976

110. HOPKINSON DA, CORNEY G, COOK PJL, ROBSON EB, HARRIS H: Genetically determined electrophoretic variants of human red-cell NADH diaphorase. *Ann Hum Genet* 34:1, 1970

111. FISHER RA, POVEY S, BOBROW M, SOLOMON E, BOYD Y, CARRETT B: Assignment of the DIA₁ locus to chromosome 22. *Ann Hum Genet* 41:151, 1977

112. JUNIEN C, VIBERT M, WEIL D, VAN-CONG N, KAPLAN JC: Assignment of NADH cytochrome b5 reductase (DIA₁ locus) to human chromosome 22. *Hum Genet* 42:233, 1978

113. FIALKOW PJ, BROWDER JA, SPARKES RS, MOTULSKY AG: Mental retardation in methemoglobinemia due to diaphorase deficiency. *N Engl J Med* 273:840, 1965

114. BEAUVAIS P, KAPLAN JC: La méthémoglobinémie congénitale récessive: Étude de huit cas avec encephalopathie. Nouvelle conception nosalogique. *Journ Parisiennes Pédiatrie,* p 145, 1978

115. FEIG SA, NATHAN DG, GERALD PS, ZARKOWSKI HS: Congenital methemoglobinemia—the result of age-dependent decay of methemoglobin reductase. *Blood* 39:407, 1972

116. KAPLAN JC, CHIROUZE M: Therapy of recessive congenital methaemoglobinaemia by oral riboflavine. *Lancet* 2:1043, 1978

117. TISELIUS HG, ALMGARD LE: The diurnal urinary excretion of oxalate and the effect of pyridoxine and ascorbate on oxalate excretion. *Eur Urol* 3:41, 1977

118. DARLING RC, ROUGHTON FJW: The effect of methemoglobin on the equilibrium between oxygen and hemoglobin. *Am J Physiol* 137:56, 1942

119. JAFFÉ ER: Hereditary methemoglobinemias associated with abnormalities in the metabolism of erythrocytes. *Am J Med* 41:786, 1966

120. LEE WM, BRAGG FE, JAFFÉ ER: Reduction of methemoglobin in human adult and cord blood erythrocytes incubated with glucose or inosine. *Proc Soc Exp Biol Med* 124:214, 1967

121. COHEN RJ, SACHS JR, WICKER DJ, CONRAD M: Methemoglobinemia provoked by malarial chemoprophylaxis in Vietnam. *N Engl J Med* 279:1127, 1968

122. FINCH CA: Methemoglobinemia and sulfhemoglobinemia. *N Engl J Med* 239:470, 1948

123. SHARP CW, STILLMAN RC: Blush not with nitrites. *Ann Intern Med* 92:700, 1980

124. ROSEN PJ, JOHNSON C, MCGEHEE WG, BEUTLER E: Failure of methylene blue treatment in toxic methemoglobinemia: Association with glucose-6-phosphate dehydrogenase deficiency. *Ann Intern Med* 75:83, 1971

125. BREWER GJ: General red cell metabolism in Surgenor DMN (ed): *The Red Blood Cell,* 2d ed. New York, Academic, 1974, vol I, p 387

126. SCHWARTZ JM, ROSS JM, PARESS PS, FAGELMEN K, FOGEL L: Electrophoretic and kinetic characterization of NADH-diaphorase variant in a methemoglobinemic subject, in Ramot B (ed): *Red Cell Structure and Metabolism.* New York, Academic, 1971, p 135

76

THE HEMOGLOBINOPATHIES

ROBERT M. WINSLOW

W. FRENCH ANDERSON

1. The function of the hemoglobin molecule is the transport of oxygen from the lung to respiring tissues. The tetrameric structure is essential to the efficiency of this process and is the basis for cooperativity and the Bohr effect. Many of the abnormal properties of the mutant hemoglobins can be explained in terms of the known structure-function relationships.

2. During development from fetus to adult, there is an orderly progression of synthesis of several different hemoglobin polypeptide chains. At birth, fetal hemoglobin predominates and is rapidly replaced by hemoglobin A by about 6 months of age. Hemoglobin A_2 constitutes about 2.5 percent of the total in adults.

3. The known hemoglobin mutants can be explained by point mutations, deletions, insertions, frameshifts, and unequal crossing-overs.

4. Hemolytic anemia can result from substitutions affecting the heme pocket or the $\alpha_1\beta_1$ interface, or by disruption of α-helix formation. When such mutations occur, heme iron can be more easily oxidized, and a sequence of events occurs that leads to the formation of Heinz bodies.

5. Mutations in the immediate environment of heme iron can lead to its oxidation (the M, or methemoglobins). Except for the mild cyanosis that results from reduced oxygen-carrying capacity, no serious consequences follow.

6. Mutations that affect the equilibrium between the high affinity (R) and low affinity (T) structures of hemoglobin usually shift the equilibrium toward R. Because of high oxygen affinity, these hemoglobins release oxygen poorly, and polycythemia can result.

7. Hemoglobin S has the most severe clinical consequences (sickle-cell anemia) of all the hemoglobinopathies. As a result of this mutation, deoxygenated hemoglobin molecules aggregate and form fibers which cause cells to become rigid and to "sickle," leading to capillary occlusion and "crisis."

In 1908 Sir William Osler wrote, "Given a haemoglobin of poor quality, incapable of combining normally with O_2 a greater number of erythrocytes would have to be manufactured to meet the usual demands of the system" [1]. Thus, the suspicion of a relation between an abnormal hemoglobin molecule and its clinical manifestations was born, but the proof of such a relation was provided much later. In 1948, Horlein and Weber described a family in which cyanosis was transmitted as a dominant characteristic, and they demonstrated that the affected family members carried a hemoglobin molecule whose globin was abnormal [2]. This was subsequently proved to be the first example of an inherited *methemoglobin*, and its tendency to oxidation of heme accounted for its striking clinical manifestations. The most severe hemoglobinopathy, however, is *hemoglobin S*, which in homozygous form causes *sickle-cell anemia*, a disease with severe clinical consequences. Pauling first demonstrated an electrophoretic difference between hemoglobins A and S [3], and Ingram showed that the substitution in hemoglobin S was valine for glutamic acid at position 6 of the β chain [4]. This was the first demonstration of a specific amino acid substitution in an inherited abnormal protein. It came at a time when little was known about the molecular mechanism of inheritance and introduced the concept that a "mutation" could involve the substitution of a single amino acid for another.

Since Ingram identified the structural alteration of hemoglobin S, over 300 additional variants arising by a number of different genetic mechanisms and with various clinical effects have been described. Some mutant hemoglobins have no clinical consequences and are therefore not properly called *hemoglobinopathies;* true hemoglobinopathies are those disorders in which a set of clinical abnormalities can be directly attributed to the properties of a genetically altered hemoglobin molecule. The study of these variants has yielded important contributions to medicine, genetics, biochemistry, and physiology. In no area of human biology do such detailed correlations exist between molecular, cellular, and physiologic levels as in hemoglobin structure and function.

The clinical consequences of hemoglobin mutations can be understood only in the light of the known mechanisms of normal hemoglobin structure and function. Many of the mutations affect multiple properties of the molecule and therefore cannot be uniquely classified as *high affinity* or *unstable* hemoglobins, for example. In this chapter, after review of normal hemoglobin structure, function, synthesis, and genetics, the hemoglobinopathies will be classified according to their principal clinical manifestations: hemolysis, cyanosis, polycythemia, and sickling.

NORMAL HEMOGLOBIN

Structure

Hemoglobin is a globular protein whose molecular weight is 68,000. It is composed of four subunit polypeptide chains of about 140 amino acids each (Fig. 76-1). Each chain has a molecular weight of 16,100 and carries a tetrapyrrole iron-containing prosthetic group, heme. The protein from which heme has been removed is called *globin*. In humans several hemoglobins occur normally, all containing four subunits; the differences are limited to the primary structure (amino acid sequence) of the globin (Fig. 76-2). Each polypeptide chain is designated by a Greek letter, and each is the product of a specific genetic locus. For example, hemoglobin A, the major component of adult human red blood cells, is $\alpha_2\beta_2$; i.e., it contains two α chains and two β chains in a tetrameric arrangement.

Primary Structure Hemoglobin was one of the first proteins whose sequence, or primary structure, was determined (Fig. 76-2). This achievement was the result of the cumulative effort of many investigators who applied the techniques developed by Sanger and coworkers in their pioneering work on the sequence of insulin. A by-product of this effort was the

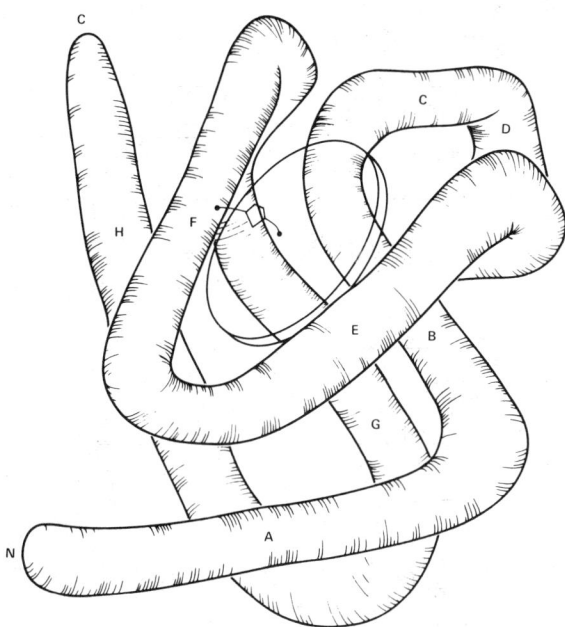

Figure 76-1 Schematic diagram of a globin chain. Any of the globin chains (or myoglobin) could fit the diagram with only minor alteration. The α-helical regions are lettered (cf. Fig. 76-2), and heme is shown as a disk. The only covalent link between heme and globin is between the iron atom and His F8, the "proximal" histidine.

remarkable advance in the methods in protein chemistry; today, elucidation of a sequence which would have taken years three decades ago is a relatively trivial matter. Moreover, the high-resolution x-ray crystallographic analysis by Perutz and coworkers [6] has allowed an extensive integration of sequence and functional data. This integration leads to an appreciation of structure-function relationships so delicate that substitution of 1 amino acid in 280 can lead to disastrous clinical consequences.

Secondary Structure About two-thirds of the residues of each chain are arranged in coiled structures called helices. There are 7 and 8 of these in the α and β chains, respectively, designated from A to H, and they vary from 7 to 20 residues in length. There are 3.6 residues per turn of helix, and the coils are stabilized by hydrogen bonds which form between the coils longitudinally along their axes. The remaining one-third of the residues are distributed over corners or nonhelical regions of the chain. In these regions no regular pattern can be distinguished.

Myoglobin and all the various hemoglobin chains resemble each other to a remarkable degree. To emphasize this resemblance and to facilitate comparison between chains, residues are given designations according to their position in or between helical regions. For example, residue 10 of the α chain is Val A7(10) because it occupies position 7 from the beginning of the A helix. Although the corresponding residue in the β chain is valine [Val A7(11)β], it occupies the eleventh position from the N-terminus of that chain. Similarly, the residues in the interhelical regions are designated by letters of adjacent helices: The third residue in the C-D region of the α chain is His CD3(45)α, and in the β chain Ser CD3(44)β.

Tertiary Structure The three-dimensional folding of a globin chain is shown in Fig. 76-1. The similarity between the various chains is sufficient that the figure could represent any

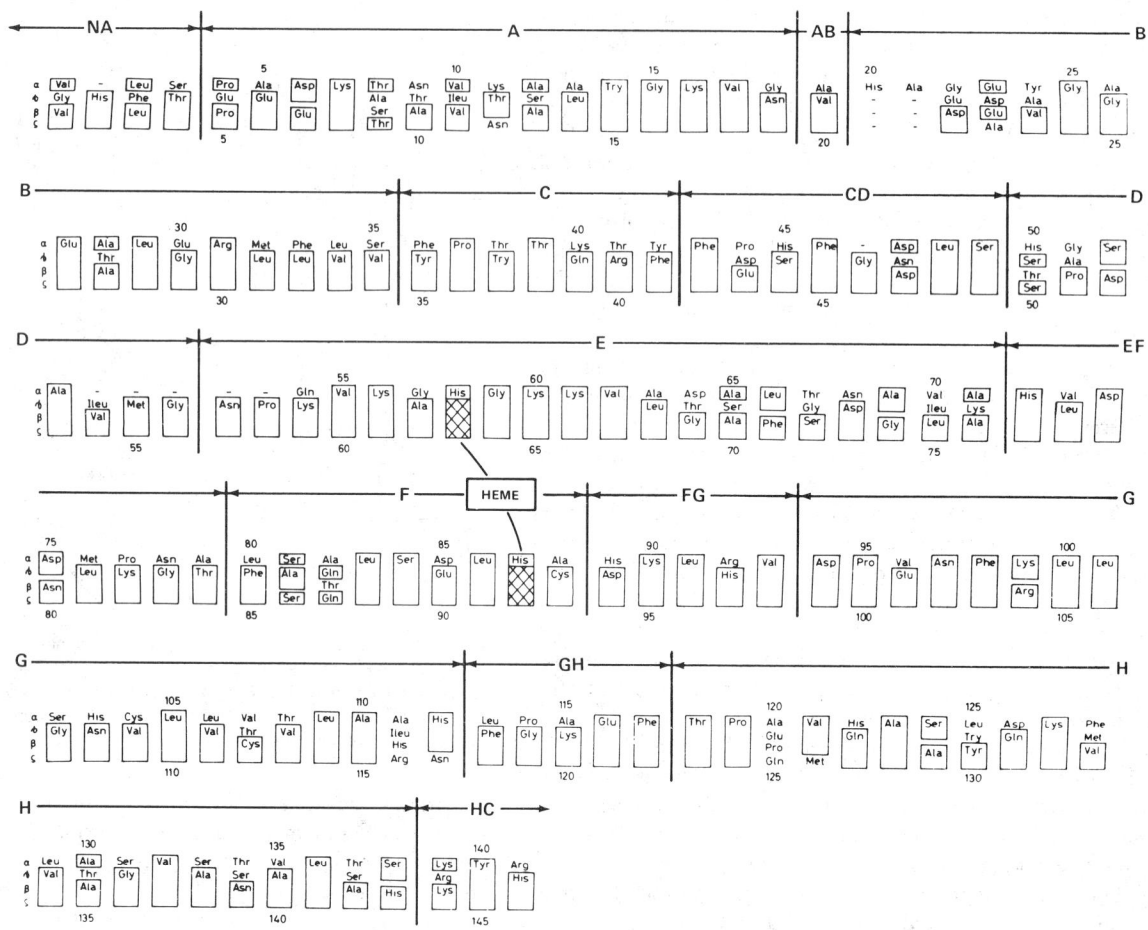

Figure 76-2 The sequences of the normal adult human globin chains. Helical regions are designated by letters A to H. The numbers above each row refer to residues of the α chain, those below the rows to the non-α chains. Residues which are common to more than one chain are enclosed in boxes. (*From Lehmann and Huntsman [5].*)

of them, with only minor alterations. Heme is represented as a flat ring between the E and F helices.

Proline does not fit into a helix because of its pyrrolidine ring; it cannot form hydrogen bonds with the next coil in the helix. Therefore, it is likely to occur at corners and interhelical regions. Other corners are stabilized by a variety of stereochemical mechanisms, some of which involve portions of chains which lie nearby. Interactions can also occur between helical segments which lie in proximity to one another. For example, the B and E helices are stabilized by glycine residues in each helix which afford a compact fit at their crossing.

A very important force stabilizing the globin chain structure is the presence of heme itself. Free globin is much less soluble than the molecule containing heme. It is embeddded firmly into a "pocket" in the chain as shown in Fig. 76-1. It has a polar and a nonpolar end, one formed by propionic acid groups and the other by vinyl and methyl groups, respectively. The amino acid side groups which line the heme pocket are largely nonpolar and allow the heme to enter, vinyl-end first. It is then anchored there by a large number of interactions between the pyrrole ring and amino acids of the heme pocket. In addition, it is covalently linked to histidine F8, which is called the *proximal* histidine. The *distal* histidine, E7, is not covalently linked to the heme group, but its presence in the heme pocket is important in maintaining spatial relationships. The hydrophobic nature of the heme pocket is extremely important in the maintenance of the heme iron in its reduced (Fe^{2+}) state, which is required for oxygenation. As discussed below, a num-

ber of mutations in the environment of the heme pocket can lead to the entry of water, oxidation of the iron, and, as a result, methemoglobin formation.

Quaternary Structure The hemoglobin molecule is tetrameric. Hemoglobin A contains two α and two β chains. It is this association of chains which leads to cooperativity, the Bohr effect, the DPG effect, and suitable oxygen affinity so that tissue oxygen requirements can be met. The molecule has a twofold axis of symmetry, each half containing one α and one β chain, which are held tightly together by a large number of atomic interactions. There are four areas of contact between the subunits: $\alpha_1\beta_1$, $\alpha_2\beta_2$, $\alpha_1\beta_2$, $\alpha_2\beta_1$. The $\alpha_1\beta_2$ and $\alpha_2\beta_1$ regions are somewhat weaker than the $\alpha_1\beta_1$ and $\alpha_2\beta_2$ contacts and allow movement during oxygenation (Table 76-1, Fig. 76-3) [7, 8]. Isolated hemoglobin chains are less stable than the fully associated tetramers. Thus, the regions of contact between them are important in maintaining normal solubility. Several unstable mutants that involve the $\alpha_1\beta_1$ and, to a lesser degree, the $\alpha_1\beta_2$ contacts will be discussed.

The complete molecule is somewhat akin to a doughnut in shape: it is globular with a central "cavity." This cavity is filled with water and allows the entrance of charged molecules that affect molecular function, such as 2,3-DPG and salts. Most of

Table 76-1 The $\alpha_1\beta_1$ and $\alpha_1\beta_2$ contacts in normal hemoglobin

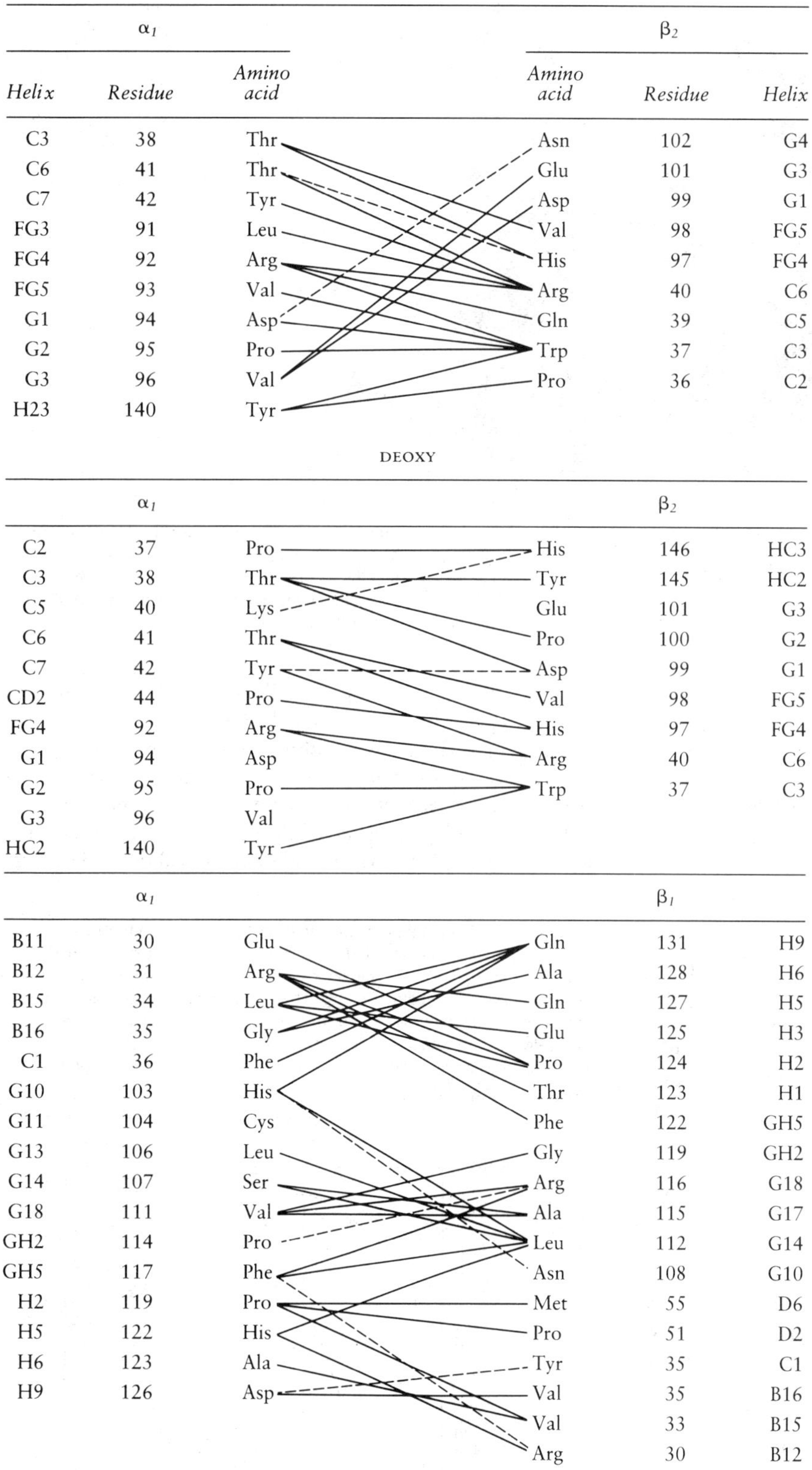

Oxy

	α_1			β_2	
Helix	Residue	Amino acid	Amino acid	Residue	Helix
C3	38	Thr	Asn	102	G4
C6	41	Thr	Glu	101	G3
C7	42	Tyr	Asp	99	G1
FG3	91	Leu	Val	98	FG5
FG4	92	Arg	His	97	FG4
FG5	93	Val	Arg	40	C6
G1	94	Asp	Gln	39	C5
G2	95	Pro	Trp	37	C3
G3	96	Val	Pro	36	C2
H23	140	Tyr			

DEOXY

	α_1			β_2	
C2	37	Pro	His	146	HC3
C3	38	Thr	Tyr	145	HC2
C5	40	Lys	Glu	101	G3
C6	41	Thr	Pro	100	G2
C7	42	Tyr	Asp	99	G1
CD2	44	Pro	Val	98	FG5
FG4	92	Arg	His	97	FG4
G1	94	Asp	Arg	40	C6
G2	95	Pro	Trp	37	C3
G3	96	Val			
HC2	140	Tyr			

	α_1			β_1	
B11	30	Glu	Gln	131	H9
B12	31	Arg	Ala	128	H6
B15	34	Leu	Gln	127	H5
B16	35	Gly	Glu	125	H3
C1	36	Phe	Pro	124	H2
G10	103	His	Thr	123	H1
G11	104	Cys	Phe	122	GH5
G13	106	Leu	Gly	119	GH2
G14	107	Ser	Arg	116	G18
G18	111	Val	Ala	115	G17
GH2	114	Pro	Leu	112	G14
GH5	117	Phe	Asn	108	G10
H2	119	Pro	Met	55	D6
H5	122	His	Pro	51	D2
H6	123	Ala	Tyr	35	C1
H9	126	Asp	Val	35	B16
			Val	33	B15
			Arg	30	B12

KEY: Solid lines are hydrophobic bonds; dashed lines are hydrogen bonds. Note that there are two sets of interactions at the $\alpha_1\beta_2$ interface, one for oxyhemoglobin (top) and one for deoxyhemoglobin (middle). The $\alpha_1\beta_1$ interface (bottom) (or $\alpha_2\beta_2$ interface) involves more bonds and does not change with oxygenation. From Perutz et al. [7].

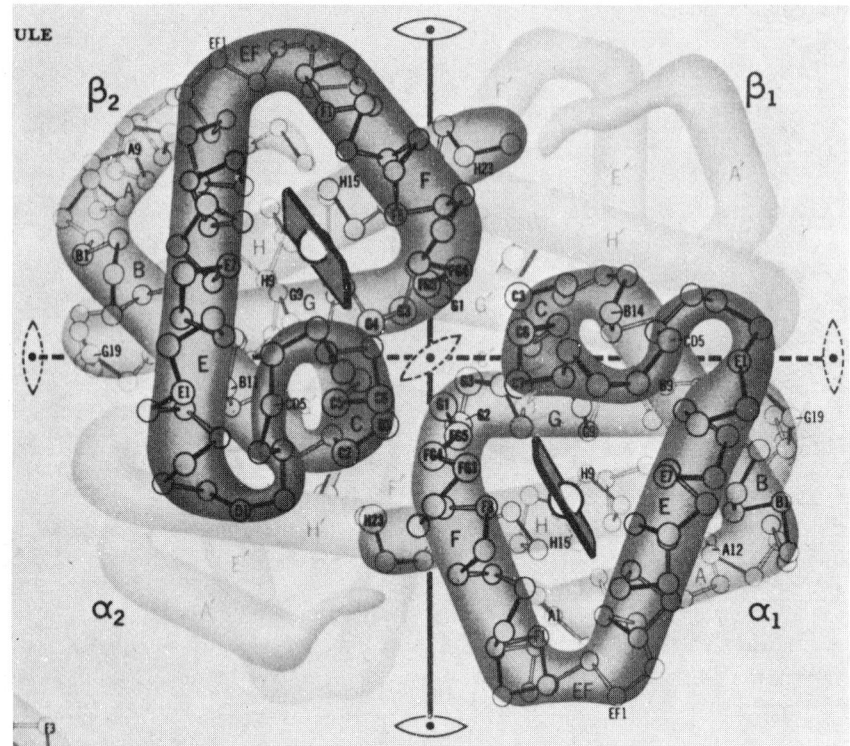

Figure 76-3 The quaternary structure of hemoglobin. The α_1 and β_2 chains are in the foreground, and the α_2 and β_1 chains are behind them. The contact is at the center of the figure. (*From Dickerson and Geis* [8]*.*)

the charged amino acid side groups are directed toward the outside of the molecule and enter into electrostatic relations with solvents, allowing very high solubility within the red blood cells. Buried in the midst of the globin chains are the four heme groups containing ferrous iron, protected against oxidation by a hydrophobic environment.

Function

The reciprocal transport of the respiratory gases, O_2 and CO_2, between tissues and lungs is the raison d'être of hemoglobin. The molecular properties that underlie these characteristics are the cooperative binding of oxygen to heme sites, the Bohr effect, and the interactions of small molecules (2,3-DPG, salts, and CO_2) which alter oxygen binding. All these properties are closely interrelated with extraordinary intricacy, and only in recent years have structural, functional, and theoretical concepts been reconciled to form a unified picture of hemoglobin function.

Oxygen Equilibrium Curve (OEC) The shape of the hemoglobin oxygen equilibrium curve (OEC) is sigmoid (Fig. 76-4). This property is of great importance because it allows the normal loading and unloading of oxygen under physiologic conditions. Myoglobin and single hemoglobin subunits bind oxygen with an affinity which is so high that no effective oxygen release could occur at tissue sites. This is illustrated in Fig. 76-4, which shows the equilibrium curves for hemoglobin and myoglobin under identical conditions. The oxygen tension in the lung is about 100 mmHg and at tissue sites in resting humans is an average of 40 mmHg. It is apparent from the figure that at 40 mmHg, hemoglobin has given up 30 percent of its oxygen load. If myoglobin were the respiratory pigment

in blood, P_{O_2} in the tissues would have to reach about 4 mmHg before 30 percent of its O_2 could be released. Since the oxygen affinity of individual hemoglobin chains is approximately that of myoglobin, we can see that the tetrameric structure of hemoglobin leads to its suitably low oxygen affinity.

Early physiologists observed the sigmoid nature of the OEC and concluded that oxygen binding increased during progres-

Figure 76-4 Oxygen equilibrium curves of hemoglobin and myoglobin. Arterial oxygen tension is about 100 mmHg; mixed venous oxygen tension is about 40 mmHg; and the minimum oxygen tension required for the cytochrome enzymes is about 5 mmHg. The figure illustrates that association of chains into a tetrameric structure (hemoglobin) results in much greater oxygen delivery than would be possible with single chains. Myoglobin and hemoglobin chains have about the same oxygen affinity. (*From Hill* [9]*.*)

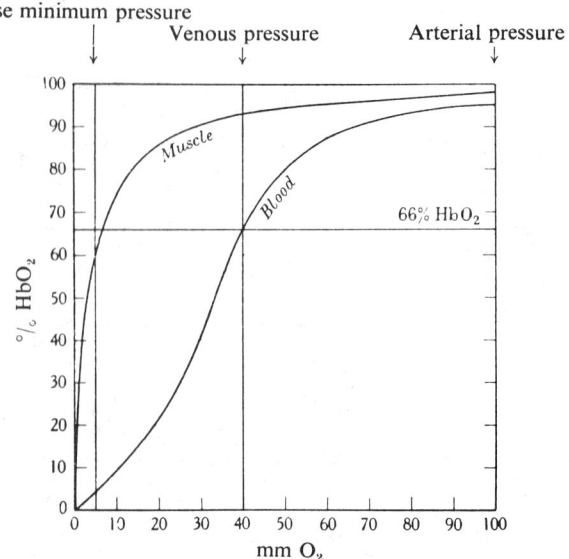

sive oxygenation. They felt that this reflected interaction between heme sites so that oxygen binding to one site made binding at the next site more likely. Thus, they called this phenomenon *cooperativity*.

Hill derived an empirical equation,

$$\text{Log}\ \frac{Y}{1 - Y} = n\ \log\ p + K$$

that relates hemoglobin saturation *(Y)* to oxygen tension *(p)* for oxygen equilibrium curves [10]. When plotted according to this equation, the major portion of the OEC falls on a straight line with slope *(n)* proportional to the degree of cooperativity. It was found that *n* for hemoglobin was about 3 and for myoglobin, devoid of cooperativity, 1.

The first significant attempt at quantitation of the oxygenation of hemoglobin was made by G. S. Adair, whose paper in 1925 [11] is a classic in protein chemistry. He began with equations for the stepwise oxygenation of hemoglobin:

$$Hb(O_2)_i + O_2 = Hb(O_2)_{i + 1}$$

where *i* ranges from 1 to 3 and the equilibrium constants could be represented:

$$k = \frac{Hb(O_2)_i}{[Hb(O_2)_{i + 1}]\ [O_2]}$$

Combining the four resulting equations, we have

$$Y = \frac{k_1 p + k_1 k_2 p^2 + k_1\ k_2 k_3 p^3 + k_1 k_2 k_3 k_4 p^4}{1 + 4\ (k_1 p + k_1 k_2 p^2 + k_1 k_2 k_3 p^3 + k_1 k_2 k_3 k_4 p^4)}$$

where *Y* = fractional saturation of hemoglobin with oxygen *k* = equilibrium constant for each individual combination of O_2 with hemoglobin *p* partial pressure of O_2. Combining the *k*'s, we have

$$Y = \frac{a_1 p + a_2 p^2 + a_3 p^3 + a_4 p^4}{1 + 4(a_1 p + a_2 p^2 + a_3 p^3 + a_4 p^4)}$$

The *a*'s are usually referred to as the *Adair constants* and have been estimated for hemoglobin and, more recently, for whole blood.

The difficulty with the Adair scheme is that it is too general; unique values of the *a*'s are difficult to determine, and therefore the *k*'s nearly impossible, because of the high degree of dependence among the parameters. The scheme was based only on the phenomenologic observation of oxygenation before the structure of hemoglobin was known. More information was needed about the molecular details of the reaction before the model could be restricted to few parameters. Nevertheless, it is possible to describe the OEC by the Adair parameters, and this has some utility even if the values are not unique.

Allosteric Model   Since the elucidation of the exact structure of hemoglobin, several theories for the molecular mechanics of function have been proposed [12], but the work of Monod, Wyman, and Changeaux [13] and of Perutz [14] is the basis of the most widely applicable model. According to the MWC model, hemoglobin can exist in either of two conformations called *relaxed* (R) and *tense* (T).

In the absence of ligand (oxygen), molecules can exist in either of the two conformations, each with its unique oxygen affinity. The equilibrium constants for their reactions with oxygen are K_R and K_T. The ratio of these constants, $C = K_R/K_T$, is about 0.01 for hemoglobin A; i.e., the affinity of mole-

cules in the R conformation is much greater than of those in the T conformation. The constant *C* is characteristic of a given hemoglobin. The essence of the allosteric theory is that the equilibrium between the two conformations in the deoxy state, $Hb^R = Hb^T$, given by the allosteric constant, $L = Hb^T/Hb^R$, is influenced by any of a number of other molecules or allosteric effectors, such as H^+ or 2,3-DPG. These small molecules react with hemoglobin at nonheme sites in such a way as to stabilize one conformation or the other (T, in the case of H^+ and 2,3-DPG). Thus, the overall reactivity of a mixture of R and T hemoglobin molecules toward oxygen will depend on the position of the R-T equilibrium (or *L*). Monod, Wyman, and Changeaux related the allosteric constant *L* to P_{O_2} *(p)* and fractional saturation of hemoglobin with oxygen *(Y)*:

$$Y = \frac{LC\ (1 - C\alpha)^{n - 1} + \alpha(1 + \alpha)^{n - 1}}{L(1 + C)^n + (1 + \alpha)^n}$$

where $\alpha = p/K_R$ and $n = 4$, the number of oxygen binding sites.

Of fundamental importance in this model is that the T state is physically constrained to a much greater degree than the R state. With successive oxygenation of the heme groups of molecules in the T conformation, the stability of that conformation decreases, and, as a result, they undergo a transition to the R state with the release of the constraints and an increase in oxygen affinity. For deoxyhemoglobin the equilibrium is almost entirely on the T side. It is the shift from T to R during oxygenation which accounts for cooperativity. For normal hemoglobin, most of the molecules probably shift from T to R between binding of the second and third oxygen molecules; hence the OEC is steepest in the middle portion.

Although the MWC model may not apply in all circumstances, it has been very useful in explaining certain properties of some abnormal hemoglobins. Many of them can be viewed as structural alterations which affect the value of *L* by favoring either the T (low affinity hemoglobins) or R (high affinity hemoglobins) conformation.

Structural Basis of the Allosteric Model   The structural basis of the model presented above is provided by the work of Perutz and associates, who found different structures of oxy- and deoxyhemoglobin, corresponding to the R and T states, respectively [14]. Their data are from x-ray diffraction studies of human and horse hemoglobins crystallized in the oxy and deoxy conformations. They found that combination of deoxyhemoglobin with oxygen produced shifts of the helical regions of 2 to 3 Å and a change in the tilt of the heme group relative to the globin chain. These are accompanied by shifts of the iron group within the porphyrin and of the heme-linked histidine. In the β subunit, the γ-methyl group of valine E11 blocks the heme pocket. In the oxy form (R), this pocket widens, making room for the binding of an oxygen molecule. There is little difference at the $\alpha_1\beta_1$ (and $\alpha_2\beta_2$) contact, but a significant change at the $\alpha_1\beta_2$ (and $\alpha_2\beta_1$) contact occurs (Table 76-1). The region is dovetailed so that the CD α region of one chain fits into the FGβ region of the other. During transition from T to R, the dovetailing between CDα and FGβ changes so that the hydrogen bond linking Asp G1(94)α to Asn G4(102)β is replaced by another between Tyr C7(42)α and Asp G1(99)β (see Fig. 76-18).

Finally, large differences occur in the areas of the C-terminal residues. In deoxyhemoglobin the tyrosines (HC2) occupy pockets between helices F and H, and their phenolic groups are hydrogen-bonded to valines FG5. The C-terminal residues are constrained by participation in salt bridges:

$$\begin{array}{c} \text{Val NA1(1)}\alpha_2 \\ \text{Arg HC3(141)}\alpha_1 \Big\langle \\ \text{Asp H9(126)}\alpha_2 \end{array}$$

$$\begin{array}{c} \text{Lys C6(40)}\alpha_2 \\ \text{His HC3(146)}\beta_1 \Big\langle \\ \text{Asp FG1(94)}\beta_2 \end{array}$$

In oxyhemoglobin, the phenolic groups of Tyr HC2 are ejected from their pockets, and the salt bridges are broken.

Perutz and coworkers proposed a model that relates these molecular changes to the two-state MWC theory (Figs. 76-5 [15] and 76-6). The first, or "trigger," step results from the combination of iron with oxygen. When this occurs, the atomic radius of iron decreases (high-to-low spin transition), allowing it to move closer to the plane of the porphyrin ring. This movement is less than 1Å, but it is sufficient to change the distance between the heme-linked histidine and the plane of the prophyrin ring, initiating the sequence of changes leading to the T-R transition. This description applies to the α chain; but in β, the hydrophobic side group of valine E11 is in the heme pocket, providing an additional block to heme binding. Movement of the porphyrin ring relative to the heme-linked histidine results in a narrowing of the pocket between helices F and H into which the phenolic group of Tyr HC2 fits, which leads to its ejection. Rotation of this group distorts the C-terminal amino acids so that the salt bridges are no longer possible and they rupture (Fig. 76-5).

Figure 76-5 The changes in tertiary structure produced by transition from oxy- to deoxyhemoglobin. In oxyhemoglobin (A), iron is in the plane of the heme, pulling His F8 upward. Arg HC3 rotates freely. When oxygen moves out (B), the E helix moves in and the F helix moves down, forming a pocket between it and the H helix. The phenolic group of Tyr HC2 can occupy this pocket (C), and its entry pulls Arg HC3 into position so that it can form the salt bridges described in the text. (*From Charache [15].*)

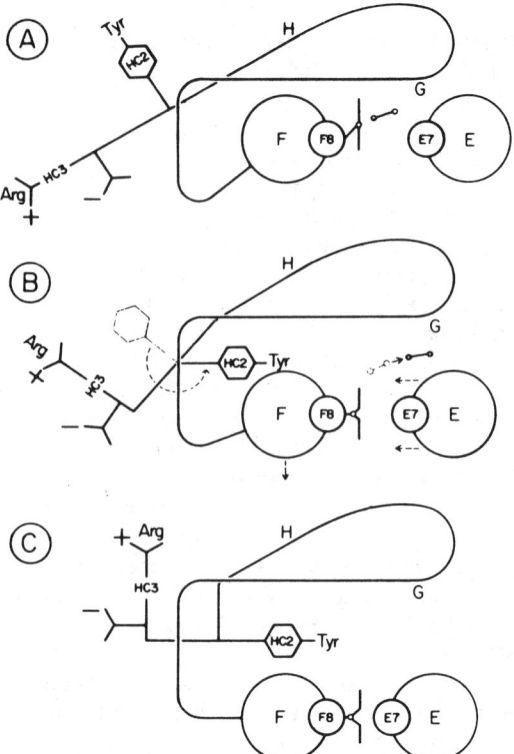

Each subunit undergoes change in the tertiary structure with successive oxygenation, as described above. After two or three of them have done so, there is a change in the quaternary structure. This change involves a rotation of the two halves of the molecules (αβ subunits) relative to one another, and a "sliding" occurs at the $\alpha_1\beta_2$ and $\alpha_2\beta_1$ interfaces (Fig. 76-6).

Bohr Effect   Bohr observed that the position of the blood OEC along the abscissa was affected by changes in P_{CO_2} [16]. That is, when pH was lowered (or P_{CO_2} raised), the oxygen affinity of the blood was decreased. According to convention, the value P50 is used to designate the oxygen tension at which blood or hemoglobin saturation is 50 percent. Thus, decreased pH would increase P50. Recently, the separate effects of H^+ and CO_2 have been elucidated [17]. They are qualitatively similar, but the effect of H^+ (now properly called the pH Bohr effect) is much stronger than the CO_2 effect in lowering oxygen affinity.

Hydrogen ion decreases oxygen affinity and, according to the MWC theory, does so by shifting the R-T equilibrium toward T, stabilizing that structure. The stereochemical interpretation of this phenomenon is that it arises from the opening and closing of salt bridges involving the C-terminal residues. The pKs of the imidazoles of His (HC3(146)β and of Val Na1(1)α are lowered in oxyhemoglobin as a result of the rupture of the salt bridges in which they participate. This change in pK leads to a release of protons during the transition T to R. Experiments with mutant and chemically modified hemoglobins suggest that these groups account for about two-thirds of the alkaline Bohr effect [18].

2,3-DPG   The normal intracellular constituent 2,3-DPG (and, to a lesser extent, ATP) are very important in the regulation of the blood OEC [19]. 2,3-DPG is present in normal human red blood cells and is a metabolic intermediate in the glycolytic pathway. Under conditions of diminished oxygen availability (such as anemia), its concentration increases, and the blood OEC is moved to the right. If arterial oxygenation is normal, this facilitates transfer of oxygen to the tissues. The regulatory mechanisms which govern the concentration of 2,3-DPG are not completely understood, but alkalosis in response to hyperventilation is probably an important factor.

2,3-Diphosphoglycerate can bind to deoxyhemoglobin in a molar ratio of 1:1 and, by doing so, increases the constraints on the T state, leading to a further shift of the R-T equilibrium toward T and lowering of oxygen affinity. Salt bridges involving the free amino groups of Val NA1(1)β and the imidazoles of His H21(143)β are probably the most important binding sites [20]. In deoxyhemoglobin, 2,3-DPG lies in the central cavity of the molecule and is coordinated to the groups mentioned above, plus the ε-amino groups of Lys EF6(82)β. On transition to the R structure, the valines move apart, the H helices move together, and 2,3-DPG drops out. In agreement with the effects of the other salt bridges in the deoxy structure, 2,3-DPG increases the alkaline Bohr effect.

CO₂ Binding   Finally, CO_2 can bind to the α-amino groups of the N-terminal amino acids with a resultant decrease of oxygen affinity [21]. This binding is diminished in the presence of 2,3-DPG, since both 2,3-DPG and CO_2 can bind to the β-chain N-terminal amino group. Such competition does not occur for the α-chain N terminus, since 2,3-DPG binding does not require it.

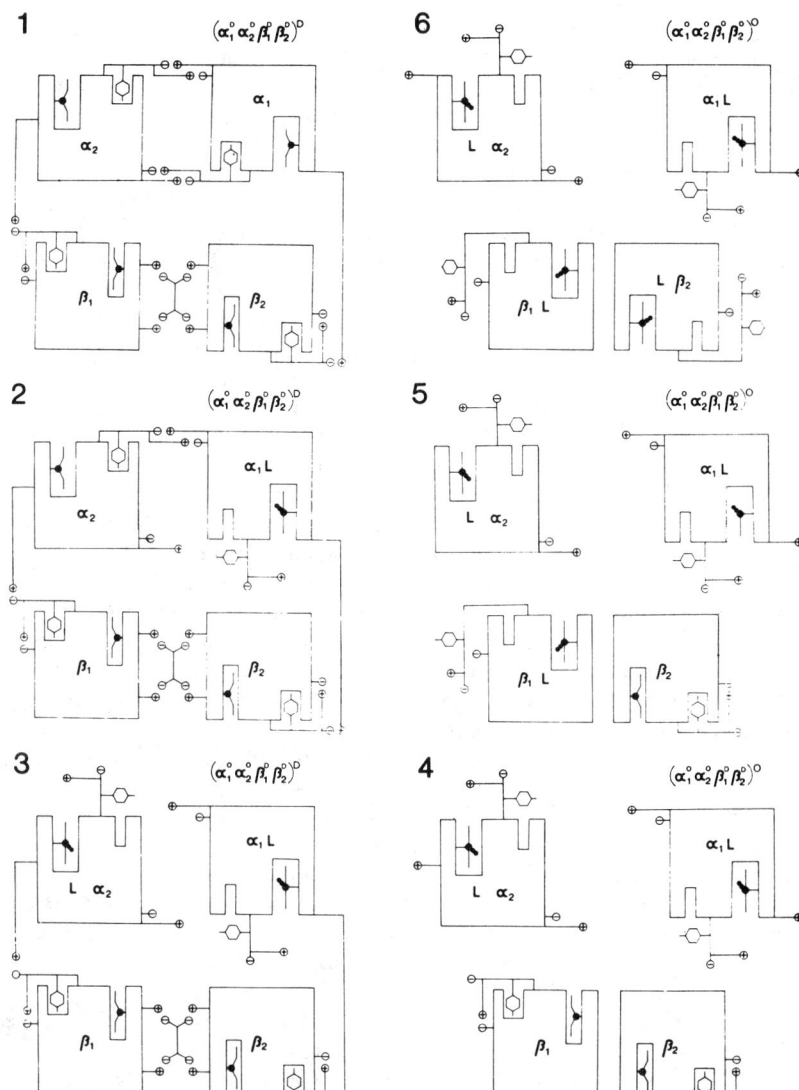

Figure 76-6 Schematic representation of the sequential reaction of hemoglobin with oxygen. (1) Deoxyhemoglobin with all salt bridges intact and one DPG molecule clamped between the β chains. In steps 1-2 and 2-3, the α chains are oxygenated, ejecting the phenolic groups of Tyr HC2 from their pockets. Between steps 3 and 4, the quaternary structure switches from deoxy to oxy (T to R) with expulsion of DPG and rupture of the intersubunit salt bridges. At steps 4-5 and 5-6, β chains react with oxygen, and the remaining intrasubunit salt bridges rupture. Note that the quaternary transition (T → R) could occur at any stage of oxygenation and that the sequence in which subunits react might be other than that shown, without affecting the cooperative mechanism. (*From Perutz* [14].)

Cellular Function Although the structure and function of hemoglobin in a purified state are understood to a remarkable degree, only broad correlations can be made with function within the red blood cell. Development of experimental methods such as x-ray crystallography, nmr studies, stopped-flow analysis, flash photolysis, and precise techniques for the measurement of hemoglobin OEC [22] has led to this understanding. In contrast, the development of methods to study the properties of red cells and whole blood is in its infancy. Precise methods for the measurement of whole blood OEC are now emerging [23], and laser flash photolysis of whole blood [24] offers the possibility of understanding its kinetic properties. Still needed are methods for the accurate measurement of intracellular pH and kinetic and oxygen equilibrium measurements in single cells. Because the physiologic and medical consequences of these studies are important, development of such methods should take place in the coming decade and may lead to an understanding of the function of the red cell that matches the sophistication of the theories describing the function of purified hemoglobin.

Synthesis

More is known about the mechanism of synthesis of hemoglobin than of any other protein. In bacteria, the processes of transcription (synthesis of messenger RNA from DNA) and translation (synthesis of protein from messenger RNA) occur together. In eukaryotic cells the two are distinct: mRNA is synthesized in the nucleus and is then transported to the cytoplasm where it is translated into protein. A detailed account of what is known about globin gene organization and structure, the transcription and translation of globin messenger RNA, and the regulatory mechanisms at the transcriptional, posttranscriptional, translational, and posttranslational levels, is beyond the scope of this text. A description of the organization, structure, and expression of globin genes is presented in Chap. 77, "The Thalassemias." Here we will summarize what is known about the mechanism and regulation of hemoglobin (protein) synthesis.

Overview The mechanism of globin messenger RNA translation has been investigated extensively for a number of years. The primary system used for study is the immature red blood cell, the reticulocyte. This enucleated cell is essentially a bag of protein-synthesizing machinery that makes primarily one protein, hemoglobin. Synthesis of globin chains (and all other proteins) can be divided into three processes. (1) Initiation: The attachment of ribosomal subunits and other necessary components to the 5' end of the coding sequence of mRNA, leading to a series of events that ensure the recognition of the initiator AUG codon of mRNA and the decoding of the template in the correct reading frame. (2) Elongation: The stepwise addition of amino acids, in an order determined by the nucleotide sequence of mRNA, to produce a growing polypeptide chain. (3)Termination: The final stage, in which the ribosome and the newly synthesized polypeptide are released from the mRNA. Initiation is the rate-limiting step and is the one subject to sophisticated control mechanisms.

It has been known for over 25 years that a lysate of reticulocyte cells could still synthesize hemoglobin. This lysate preparation has been steadily improved until it is now almost as efficient as the intact reticulocyte in hemoglobin synthesis. Schweet and his colleagues [25] successfully separated the lysate into polysomes and a supernatant fraction, thus producing the first "fractionated" cell-free protein-synthesizing system. The activity of their system was, however, very low. Ronald Miller, a graduate student with Schweet, attempted to fractionate this cell-free system further. He tried to isolate messenger RNA from the reticulocyte polysomes by washing the polysomes in a high salt solution (0.5 M KCl). He could not identify messenger RNA, but he did discover a protein fraction which greatly stimulated protein synthesis in the fractionated system [26]. Initiation factors had been discovered in bacteria at that time, but no evidence had been found for initiation factors in any eukaryotic system. Anderson and his colleagues at NIH began a systematic examination of all components required for the synthesis of hemoglobin in rabbit and human reticulocyte cell-free systems. They discovered that the protein fraction of Miller and Schweet was, in fact, composed of a number of different initiation factors [27], and these have been systematically purified to homogeneity and characterized by a number of laboratories (for reivew, see Ref. 28; Table 76-2 lists the various initiation factors as of February 1981). Marcker and his colleagues demonstrated in 1970 that the initiator tRNA for eukaryotic systems was Met-tRNA$_f$ [29]. Their original observation was quickly confirmed, and it is now clear that Met-tRNA$_f$ initiates all eukaryotic systems, including hemoglobin. After a number of papers from various laboratories presented suggestive evidence for the existence of eukaryotic mRNA, the first conclusive data were published by Lingrel and his colleagues in 1971 when they successfully isolated globin mRNA from mouse reticulocytes [30].

From this brief historical review it is clear that the reticulocyte can be fractionated into a number of components which can be individually purified and then recombined in order to study the separate steps of hemoglobin synthesis. We will examine the initiation process in detail below. Elongation is catalyzed by two elongation factors, EF-1, and EF-2, and termination by at least on protein factor, called *release factor*. Elongation and termination of the human α-globin chain can be described as follows. Valine tRNA combines with EF-1 and GTP to form a ternary complex which then allows the Val-tRNA to be placed at the appropriate site on the 80S initiation complex (this 80S complex is composed of the ribosome, mRNA, Met-tRNA$_f$, various initiation factors, and GTP). A peptide bond is then formed between methionine and valine catalyzed by peptidyl transferase, an enzyme located in the 60S ribosomal subunit. The next step, translocation, is catalyzed by EF-2. At this point, a new cycle begins with the addition of the next aminoacyl-tRNA, Leu tRNA (for α globin) as part of an [EF-1:GTP:aminoacyl-tRNA] complex. This cycle contin-

ues until the termination code word UAA is reached, at which point release factor (and perhaps other factors) cause the release of the completed polypeptide chain. When the nascent globin chain is between 15 and 30 amino acids long, the N-terminal methionine (contributed by the initiator tRNA) is cleaved by a specific peptidase. The completed globin chain, therefore, has valine as the N-terminal amino acid in most species. The globin chain combines with heme, an α and a β chain combine to form a dimer, two dimers associate to form a tetramer, and the final hemoglobin molecule is completed.

In order to translate globin messenger RNA in vitro (for example, in studying the synthesis of an abnormal hemoglobin), it is not necessary to use a totally fractionated system. Several crude cell-free protein-synthesizing systems are available which are very effective. These include the message-dependent reticulocyte lysate, the Krebs ascites system, the wheat germ system, and amphibian oocytes (via microinjection of the mRNA). In each case, the protein synthesis machinery of the cytoplasm is utilized to translate the globin messenger RNA, and then the hemoglobin product is analyzed by column chromatography or other analytical procedures. A simple technique for examining globin synthesis in bone marrow cells or in peripheral blood is to incubate the intact blood cells with a radiolabeled amino acid (usually ^{3}H-leucine or ^{35}S-methionine). The total hemoglobin fraction is then analyzed by chromatography or electrophoresis. Examples of this approach are given later in this chapter (see "Hemolysis: The Unstable Hemoglobins") and in the following chapter where globin synthesis in the various thalassemia syndromes is discussed.

Initiation of Globin Synthesis The sequence of events composing the initiation of protein synthesis in mammalian systems can be divided into four major steps, depicted schematically in Fig. 76-7. (1) A native ribosomal subunit (called 43S$_N$) is generated from a previously used 40S ribosomal subunit. (2) The initiator tRNA (Met-tRNA$_f$) then binds to the 43SN to form the 43$_S$ preinitiation complex. (3) This is followed by mRNA binding to form an intermediate preinitiation complex, which sediments at 48S. (4) The final step is the joining of a 60S ribosomal subunit to complete the formation of an 80S initiation complex.

Assembly of the 80S initiation complex is catalyzed by specific initiation factors (see Table 76-2). Five of these factors are required (eIF-2, -3, -4A, -4B, -5); one other, eIF-4E, may be required; two have only stimulatory effects (eIF-1 and eIF-4C); and one, recycling factor (RcF), appears to be involved in recycling the factor eIF-2. The remaining two (eIF-2A and eIF-4D) are active only in model assay systems with artificial templates. Their physiologic function is unclear. In addition to ribosomal subunits, Met-tRNA$_f$, mRNA, and the initiation factors, GTP and ATP, are required for the initiation of protein synthesis. For detailed analysis of the initiation process, see Ref. 28.

Production of Native 43S Ribosomal Subunits (43S$_N$) The first step in the formation of the 80S initiation complex is the generation of native, small ribosomal subunits. During polypeptide chain termination, 80S ribosomes transiently dissociate into free subunits upon release of the messenger RNA. Mammalian ribosomal subunits possess a high affinity for each other in vivo, with the equilibrium favoring the formation of nonfunctional 74S ribosomal couples. Dissociation of 74S nonfunctional couples to 40S and 60S subunits by nonribosomal proteins is an obligatory first step for all subsequent stages

Table 76-2 Mammalian initiation factors*

| Factor | | Molecular weight, $\times 10^{-3}$ | | Function (where known) |
| | | Dodecyl sulfate | Native | |
Nomenclature†	Other names‡			
eIF-1	IF-El	15	15	Stabilization of initiation complex
eIF-2	IF-MP, IF-E2, IFL3, IF1, IF-1, EIF3, EIF2	α 32 β 35 γ 55	125	Met-tRNA$_f$ binding to 43S
eIF-2A	IF-M1	65	65	Uncertain
eIF-3	IF-M5, IF-E3, IF-3, EIF-3	35 39 43 49 69 110 130	700	Formation of 43S
eIF-4A	IF-M4, IF-E4, IF-EMC	50	50	mRNA binding
eIF-4B	IF-M3, IF-E6	80	80	mRNA binding
eIF-4C	IF-M2Bβ, IF-E7	19	17	Stimulates 43S formation and 60S subunit joining
eIF-4D	IF-M2Bα	17	15	Uncertain
eIF-4E (postulated)§		24	24	? Cap-binding protein
eIF-5	IF-M2A, IF-E5, IF-L2, IF-3, IF-11, F-0.25, IF-S2	150	125	60S subunit joining
RcF¶	Anti-HRI sRF, ESP	32 40 57 65 80	250	eIF-2 recycling

* Adapted from Refs. 28 and 31.
† Adopted at International Symposium on Protein Synthesis, 1976 [32].
‡ Under which factor has been described.
§ Containment of eIF-3 and eIF-4B; may be a new factor.
¶ Proposed name [31].

of initiation complex formation. The specific initiation factor responsible for formation of active 43S$_N$ ribosomal subunits appears to be eIF-3, a large polypeptide complex (Table 76-2). Native eIF-3 has a molecular weight of approximately 700,000, corresponding to a sedimentation coefficient of 15-17S. Electrophoresis in the presence of dodecyl sulfate reveals nine major polypeptide components ranging in mass from 35,000 to 160,000 daltons. There is one eIF-3 complex per 43S$_N$ ribosomal unit.

The exact mechanism by which eIF-3 interacts with 40S ribosomal subunits is not known, although it does so independently of ATP or GTP and does not require other initiation factors. Electron-microscopic observations of 43S$_N$ ribosomal subunits indicate that eIF-3 binds to the 40S subunit in the region that interfaces with the 60S ribosomal subunit in a functional ribosome. The binding of eIF-3 may sterically inhibit nonspecific ribosomal subunit association. Since the interfacing region is considered to be a functional site in the initiation process, as well as the region of mRNA localization during translation, it is possible that eIF-3 serves to organize the interaction of other initiation factors at the active site of translation.

Another factor, eIF-4C, appears to be involved in the pro-

duction of 43S$_N$ ribosomal subunits in conjunction with eIF-3. In the presence of eIF-3, it stimulates the dissociation of 74S ribosomal couples and can be found in amounts equivalent to eIF-2, eIF-3, and Met-tRNA$_f$ in 43S preinitiation complexes (see below). The entire initiation sequence can occur in the absence of eIF-4C, but the efficiency of the overall reaction is considerably lower.

Met-tRNA$_f$ Binding to 43S$_N$ Ribosomal Subunits The second step of initiation is the binding of the specific initiator tRNA (Met-tRNA$_f$) to 43S$_N$ ribosomal subunits. This is accomplished by means of the initiation of factor eIF-2. The biologic form of eIF-2 has a molecular weight of 122,000 and is composed of three subunits, α, β, and γ, with molecular weights of α, 32,000; β, 35,000; γ, 55,000 (see Table 76-2). eIF-2 forms a stable ternary complex with Met-tRNA$_f$ and GTP. Met-tRNA$_f$ binding to 43S$_N$ ribosomal subunit occurs exclusively via this ternary complex. The resulting 43S preinitiation complex has the form eIF-2·GTP·Met-tRNA$_f$·3S$_N$.

It has been suggested that the subunit of eIF-2 binds guanine nucleotides (i.e., GTP), while the subunit possesses the Met-tRNA$_f$ binding activity. More recent studies indicate the possibility that it is the γ subunit which possesses Met-tRNA$_f$

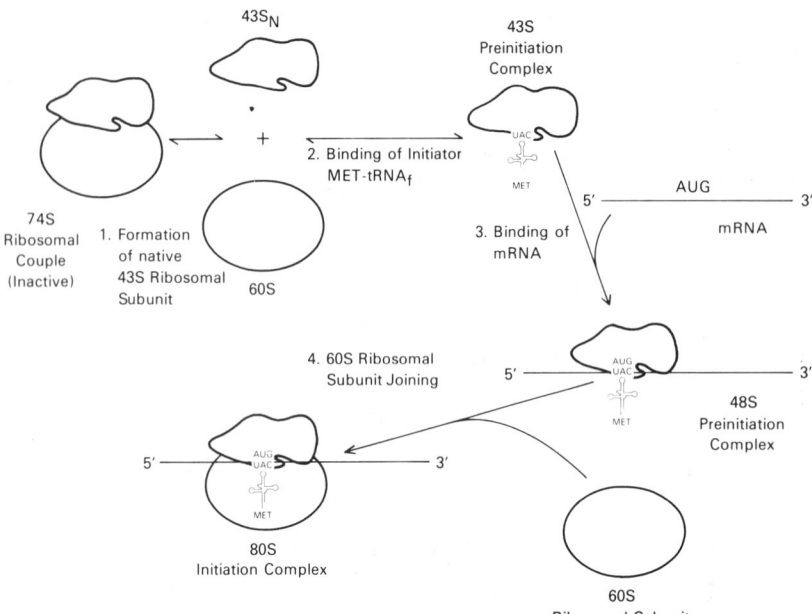

Figure 76-7 Initiation of protein synthesis in mammalian cells. The four basic steps in the pathway of 80S initiation complex are shown. The small ribosomal subunit is depicted according to the model shown in Ref. 33.

binding activity and the β subunit is important for the recycling of the eIF-2 after each round of initiation. The recycling factor, RcF, is postulated to play a critical role here.

Although eIF-2 is sufficient for the binding of Met-tRNA$_f$ to 43S$_N$ ribosomal subunits, the binding takes place more readily in the presence of eIF-3. eIF-1 and eIF-4C have also been reported to possess stimulatory effects. Met-tRNA$_f$ binding is independent of mRNA; in reticulocyte lysate, Met-tRNA$_f$ is normally found in association with 43S ribosomal subunits in which no mRNA can be detected.

Binding of mRNA to 43S Preinitiation Complex Binding of mRNA to the 43S preinitiation complex is the third major step in the initiation of protein synthesis. Work on reconstituted, fractionated, and unfractionated systems has demonstrated that mRNA binding to 40S ribosomal subunits is totally dependent on boung Met-tRNA$_f$ and eIF-2. In fractionated, reconstituted systems, three initiation factors (eIF-3, eIF-4A, and eIF-4B) are required for the step, together with ATP. Factor eIF-3, which binds first to 40S subunits together with eIF-4C, is discussed above. The role of eIF-4A and -4B appears to be related to characteristic structural features of eukaryotic mRNAs. Most eukaryotic cell and viral mRNAs have a 5'-terminal structure of the form $m^7G(5')ppp(5')Nm$-N'..., in which the terminal 7-methylguanosine is linked by a 5'-5' triphosphoric bridge to an adjacent methylated nucleotide. Several roles for such "caps" have been proposed, but a major one is their influence on the initiation of translation. The efficiency of ribosome binding and translation of mRNA in cell-free protein-synthesizing systems appears to depend on the presence of cap structures. However, the presence of a cap is not mandatory; it appears to increase the affinity of mRNA for the small ribosomal subunit, and it is recognized during initiation.

Eukaryotic initiation factors have been assayed in fractionated systems for "cap-binding activity." From these studies it appears that the cap-binding activity is associated with a 24,000-dalton polypeptide present as a minor contaminant in eIF-3 and eIF-4B. It is not yet clearly established whether the predominant peptide in eIF-4B has mRNA binding properties

of its own, or whether that activity resides solely in the contaminating 24,000-dalton peptide. Because this polypeptide is present in less than stoichiometric amounts, it should be regarded as a distinct initiation factor and perhaps classified as eIF-4E.

ATP is required during mRNA binding to the 43S preinitiation complex. During mRNA binding, ATP is hydrolyzed. Nonhydrolyzable ATP analogues do not sustain mRNA binding.

Messenger RNA molecules are found in cell cytoplasm as ribonucleoprotein complexes (mRNPs). It is uncertain whether some mRNPs might be initiation factors.

Suggestions that there are mRNA specificity factors altering the rates of translation of specific mRNAs have provoked considerable controversy. Current understanding favors the view that the existence of mRNA-specific factors is not proved and that such explanations are not necessary to account for observed differences in the translation of different mRNAs. Differences in affinities between various mRNAs for 43S preinitiation complexes or initiation factors, or both, can lead to changes in relative translational efficiencies. For example, β-globin mRNA has a fiftyfold greater affinity than α-globin mRNA for eIF-4B. Thus, differences in the affinity of eIF-4B for different mRNAs may provide a mechanism for the differential control of protein synthesis.

60S Ribosomal Subunit Joining The fourth step during formation of the 80S initiation complex is the joining of the 60S ribosomal subunit to the 48S preinitiation complex. This step is mediated by eIF-5 and is accompanied by loss of eIF-2 and eIF-3. The initiation factor of eIF-5 is a large, single polypeptide of molecular weight 125,000 (Table 76-2).

Immediately before 60S subunit joining, the 48S preinitiation complex contains equimolar amounts of 40S ribosomal subunits, eIF-2, eIF-3, eIF-4C, Met-tRNA$_f$, GTP, and mRNA; stable binding of eIF-4A and -4B has not been demonstrated. Although initiation can proceed as far as the formation of the 48S preinitiation complex with nonhydrolyzable GTP analogues, both initiation factor release and 60S ribosomal subunit joining require GTP hydrolysis.

GENETICS OF THE HEMOGLOBINS

Normal Inheritance

During fetal development at least three different non-α-hemoglobin chains are produced, and each is a product of a separate gene. The ζ and ε chains are found in very early fetuses, and γ chains later and in newborns. The quantities of these vary (Fig. 76-8). They associate to form the hemoglobins shown in Table 76-3.

Early in embryonic life there may be a relative lack of α-chain synthesis, as suggested by the presence of three hemoglobins which do not contain α chains. These are hemoglobins Gower 1 [35] and Portland 1 and 2 [36]. The α and β chains then appear, as ζ- and ε-chain synthesis declines (Fig. 76-8). Very small amounts of ε and ζ chains may be found in newborns and larger amounts in infants with certain chromosomal anomalies [37]. It has been suggested, largely on the basis of comparisons with other animals, that the chains are produced by a separate line of erythropoietic cells of yolk sac origin, while δ and other non-α chains are produced by cells of hepatic origin which later populate the bone marrow. The waxing and waning of these gene products provide an excellent model for the study of gene activation. Presumably, environmental stimuli trigger their exposure. But whether they exist because of their suitability for gas exchange during fetal life or whether they are merely indications of phylogenetic links to lower organisms (like gill slits and aortic arches) is unknown. Isolation of these hemoglobins is difficult, and they are in short supply. Little is known about their structure and function. Hemoglobin Portland is known to have very low oxygen affinity and a cooperative oxygen binding curve [38]. By about 6 months of postnatal life, the quantitative distribution of the hemoglobins has assumed the adult pattern: Hemoglobin F is less than 1 percent, hemoglobin A_2 is 2.5 to 3.5 percent, and hemoglobin A constitutes the balance.

The existence of the various hemoglobin genes illustrates the principles of molecular evolution. Ingram [39] suggested that the hemoglobin genes have arisen by a series of duplications and subsequent evolution. The temporal relations between the points of divergence of the various genes can be deduced by

Table 76-3 Ontogeny of human hemoglobins

Stage	Hemoglobin	Formula
Embryo	Hb Portland 1	$\gamma_2\zeta_2$
	Hb Portland 2	ζ_4
	Hb Gower 1	ϵ_4
	Hb Gower 2	$\alpha_2\zeta_2$
Fetus	Hb F	$\alpha_2\gamma_2$
Adult	Hb A	$\alpha_2\beta_2$
	Hb A2	$\alpha_2\delta_2$

analysis of the number of differences among their amino acid sequences. For example, the greatest number of differences exists between α chains and all non-α chains (Fig. 76-9). Therefore, it is likely that their divergence was one of the first events. Similarly, one amino acid difference is known between the two γ chains (position 136 can be either Gly or Ala), and therefore their divergence must have been relatively recent. A third γ gene is suggested by the finding of a fetal hemoglobin with γ75 (E19) Ile → Thr in a large number of normal newborns [41]. The two α loci probably have identical structures, and they are not even found in all populations [40].

That α and non-α genes are carried on separate chromosomes was deduced from the study of the inheritance of two different abnormal hemoglobins in a single family: Hemoglobin S (a β-chain variant) and hemoglobin Hopkins-2 (an α-chain variant), segregated independently [42]. More recently, α and non-α genes have been assigned separate chromosomal locations by experimentation (see "Synthesis" earlier in this chapter). Close linkage between β, δ, and γ chains has been inferred from the lack of recombination in matings between family members with variants involving more than one non-α gene [43] and from the study of "fusion" peptides involving the β, δ, and γ loci. The probable chromosomal arrangements of the non-α genes is γG-γA-δ-β [44].

The existence of multiple α-chain loci in humans was suspected because α-chain variants usually constitute about 25 percent of the hemoglobin in a heterozygote, while β-chain variants usually account for 40 to 50 percent. Thus, an individual heterozygous for an α-chain variant might have three normal functional α genes and one that makes the altered gene product [45]. In support of this concept are the observations of two α-chain variants in addition to hemoglobin A in certain individuals. For example, examination of a Hungarian family revealed that three brothers each had three structurally different α chains [46]. The three were present in the ratio 24 G Pest:54A:22 J Buda. Note that these proportions are those expected in the presence of $\alpha^{G\ Pest}$:α^A:$\alpha^{J\ Buda}$ genes in the same ratio. Similarly, individuals carrying α^A, α^{Rampa}, and $\alpha^{Koya\ Dora}$ chains [47] and α^A, $\alpha^{Hopkins-2}$, and $\alpha^{Hopkins-2\ (odd)}$ simultaneously [48] have been observed. In contrast with these findings, however, is the observation that individuals homozygous for hemoglobin J Tongariki contain only $\alpha^{J\ Tongariki}$ globin chains and no others [49]. Moreover, carriers of hemoglobin Anantharaj, A8(11) αLys→Glu, have 41 to 47 percent of the variant in their hemolysates [50]. Thus, the duplication of the α gene may not be present in all populations.

Point Mutations To date, approximately 315 human hemoglobin variants have been discovered (Table 76-4). Most of them are caused by single amino acid substitutions which are called *point mutations*. With the exception of hemoglobin Bristol, E11(67) β Val → Asp [52], all are consistent with the

Figure 76-8 Ontogeny of the human globin chains. The earliest detectable globins are the chains of hemoglobins Gower 1 and 2. The ζ chain of hemoglobins Portland 1 and 2 appear only transiently. By 3 months of gestational age, F is the predominant hemoglobin; by 6 months of adult life, hemoglobin A constitutes about 97 percent of the total. The δ chains are synthesized starting relatively late in fetal life. (*Based on data from Refs. 34 and 36.*)

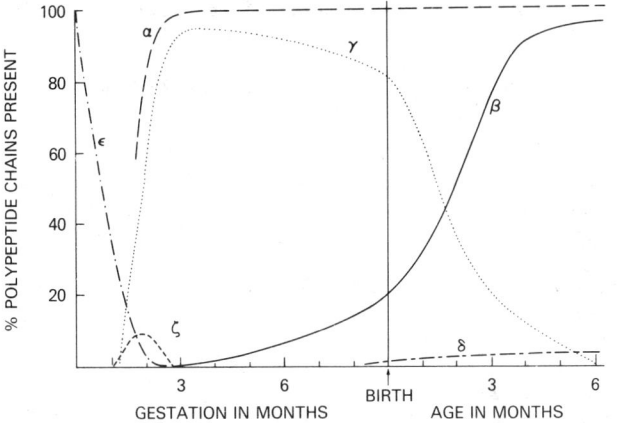

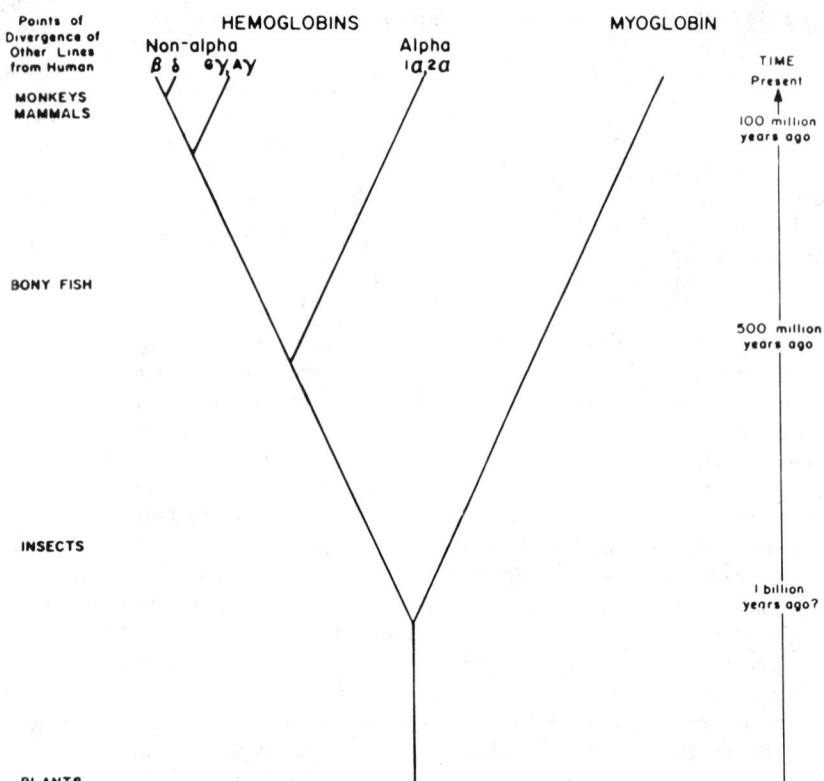

Figure 76-9 Evolution of the globin genes. Points of divergence are deduced by the number of amino acid differences between the sequences of the gene products. For example, the differences between α and non-α chains are greater than between β and δ chains. (*From Dayhoff [40].*)

genetic code. In the case of hemoglobin Bristol, a different mechanism must be postulated, possibly a two-step mutation.

Most of the variants have been detected because of alteration of their electrophoretic mobility, but some have been discovered because of alterations of other properties, such as oxygen affinity or solubility. Replacements of neutral amino acids by other neutral amino acids which do not result in clinical consequences (silent mutations) tend to be overlooked. Therefore, the true mutation rate for the hemoglobin genes is unknown. Nevertheless, in the interval since the previous edition of this text was published, the list of point mutations in the α and β chains has increased from 212 to 282. The list is too long to reproduce here. Complete lists of these mutants can be found in Refs. 41 and 53.

Table 76-4 lists the phenotypic expression of the point mutants. Fewer α-chain than β-chain variants are known, and they tend to have milder consequences. This is probably a result of the fact that α chains participate in the formation of all postembryonic hemoglobins (Table 76-3), while β-chain synthesis is not expressed in fetal life (Fig. 76-8). Therefore, an α-chain variant will affect hemoglobin F, while a β-chain variant will not appear until after birth.

A few instances are known in which more than one substitution has occurred in the same peptide chain (Table 76-5). These can be explained only by supposing that two completely independent genetic events have occurred. Now that determination of the sequence of globin chains is more readily available than previously, description of new variants is usually accompanied by amino acid analysis of the entire chain in which the substitution has occurred. As more data of this type are collected, a more accurate estimation of the true mutation rate of the globin genes will be possible.

Deletions, Insertions, and Additions   As might be

expected, mutations that change the length of the globin chains tend to have more serious consequences and are therefore relatively rare. Again, more of these mutants affect the β chain [*14*] than the α chain [*6*], but these values are probably too small to allow any conclusions. These mutants are listed in Tables 76-6 and 76-7.

Addition or removal of amino acids from the globin chains can arise by a number of mechanisms. A single base substitution in the normal code word "terminate" can give rise to a code word for an amino acid instead, and the chain can be extended until the next terminate code word is encountered in the mRNA. Hemoglobins Constant Spring, Icaria, Koya Dora, and Tak are probably examples of this type of substitution. Similarly, a triplet that normally specifies an animo acid can be altered by a single base substitution to one which specifies termination. Hemoglobin McKees Rocks, which lacks the two C-terminal amino acids from the β chain, has probably arisen by such a mechanism.

Deletion of one or two nucleotide bases can shift the reading frame of all code words that follow. Such an event observed in

Table 76-4   Major physical properties of the abnormal hemoglobins

Chain	α	β	δ	γ	δβ	γβ	Total
Normal function	64	68	10	16	6	1	165
Unstable	14	58					72
Oxidation (M)	2	3					5
Increased O₂ affinity	11	40					51
Decreased O₂ affinity	1	14					15
Dimerization	3	1					4
Sickling		1					1
Crystallization		1					1
Polymerization		1					1
Total	95	187	10	16	6	1	315

Table 76-5 Hemoglobins with more than one point mutation in the same chain

Hemoglobin	Substitution	Reference
C-Harlem	β6 (A3) Glu→Val	54
(G-Georgetown)	β73 (E17) Asp→Asn	55
Arlington Park	β6 (A3) Glu→Lys	56
	β95 (FG2) Lys→Glu	
C-Ziguinchor	β6 (A3) Glu→Val	57
	β58 (E2) Pro→Arg	
S-Travis	β6 (A3) Glu→Val	58
	β142 (H20) Ala→Val	
J-Singapore	β78 (EF2) Asn→Asp	59
	β79 (EF3) Ala→Gly	

microorganisms was called a *frameshift mutation*, and this mechanism is presumed to account for hemoglobins Wayne in the α chain and Cranston in the β chain (Fig. 76-10).

The hemoglobins with alterations at the C-terminal end allow deductions of portions of the nucleotide sequence in that region. Figure 76-10 illustrates this by aligning the sequences of the mutants with base compositions derived experimentally. The combined results allow, for example, the conclusion that the normal termination codon for the α chain is UAA. One further example of the extension of the globin chain is hemoglobin Grady, in which residues α139–141 have been repeated. Presumably this has occurred by duplication of the genetic material coding for that sequence.

Several deletions of amino acids have been observed (Table 76-7) and can involve the removal of one or more amino acids. The exact genetic mechanism for such deletions is not known, but enough of the gene has been deleted in these instances so that a frameshift does not occur. Many of these mutations lead to unstable hemoglobin molecules because they cause a severe disruption of structure.

Unequal Crossing-over The mechanism most often invoked to explain deletions, duplications, and fusion peptides is unequal, or nonhomologous, crossing-over of adjacent genes. Such a mechanism has also been called upon to explain the proliferation of the immunoglobulin genes [78]. As an example, hemoglobin Lepore contains a non-α chain that is β-like at its N terminus and δ-like at its C terminus. Baglioni proposed that this could occur by a process of unequal crossing-over (Fig. 76-11) [79]. Since the hemoglobins Lepore were first described, other examples have been found (Table 76-8). In addition, the opposite (anti-Lepore) fusion product, hemoglobin Miyada, has been found [82].

Removal of larger segments of genetic material by this mechanism is possible, and hemoglobin Kenya and the hereditary persistence of fetal hemoglobin (HPFH) are possible examples. The HPFH was first described in black families which had an average of 28 percent hemoglobin F in the heterozygous state and 100 percent in the homozygous state [85]. Heterozygotes had decreased hemoglobin A₂, and homozygotes had none. The presumed mechanism for this situation of β and δ genes on one chromosome; it is illustrated in Fig. 76-11. Several varieties of HPFH are now known (see Chap. 77, "The Thalassemias"). Once again, this condition suggests that the β and δ loci are very closely linked; deletion of both of them has occurred simultaneously.

Hemoglobin Kenya is a fusion peptide which is δ-like at its N-terminus and β-like at its C-terminus [44]. Carriers have diminished hemoglobin A₂, and heterozygotes for both hemo-

globins Kenya and S have no hemoglobin A synthesis. Therefore, this is an example of the deletion of the δ and β genes with unequal crossing-over, as shown in Fig. 76-12. In contrast with HPFH, a fusion peptide results. Presumably this occurs because the exact alignment of chromosomes at the time of meiosis is slightly different in the two conditions. The hemoglobin Kenya mutation provides further evidence for the close linkage between β and δ genes and, in addition, suggests that the δ loci are also very closely linked with them.

Thus, analysis of these interesting hemoglobin mutants has provided evidence for the universality of the genetic code, has suggested some actual base sequences of mRNA, and has shown that the β, δ, and γ genes are carried on the same chromosome and are very closely linked.

Variants of Hemoglobin A₂ and F In addition to the mutations of hemoglobin A, variants of hemoglobins F and A₂ have also been observed. These have been detected by routine screening. As far as is known, they are all point mutations. Tables 76-9 and 76-10 give the known mutations of the γ and δ chains. With the single exception of the F-Poole, an unstable fetal hemoglobin causing hemolytic disease in the newborn, they are without known consequences.

HEMOLYSIS: THE UNSTABLE HEMOGLOBINS

History

In 1890 Heinz described inclusion bodies in red blood cells which, for the next 60 years, were thought to be the result of damage by toxins [112]. In the 1950s these inclusions were believed to be associated with primaquine-induced hemolysis, but in 1952 they were observed in a patient who had no history of exposure to toxins [113]. In 1958 a family was reported in which Heinz body anemia was clearly present in father and son, both of whom had dark brown urine [114]. In 1960 such a

Table 76-6 Extended chains

Residue	Name	Inserted residue	Reference
α142–172	Constant Spring	Glu-Ala-Gly-Ala-Ser Val-Ala-Val-Pro-Pro Ala-Arg-Trp-Ala-Ser Gln-Arg-Ala-Leu-Leu-Pro Ser-Leu-His-Arg-Pro Phe-Leu-Val-Phe-Glu	60
α115–118	Grady	Gly-Thr-Phe repeated	61
α139–146	Wayne	Asn-Thr-Val-Lys-Leu Glu-Pro-Arg	62
α142–172	Icaria	Identical to Constant Spring except Lys instead of Gln at 142	63
α142–157	Koya Dora	(Ser,Ala,Gly,Ala,Ser, Val,Ala,Val,Pro,Pro, Ala)-Arg-(?,Ala,Ser,Gln)- Arg	47
β145–155	Cranston	Ser-Ile-Thr-Lys-(Leu, Asn,Ala,Ser)-Leu-Phe- Tyr	64
β146–157	Tak	Thr-Lys-Leu-Ala-Phe- Leu-Leu-Ser-Asn-Phe-Tyr	65

Table 76-7 Shortened chains

Residue	Name	Alteration	Reference
β6 or 7	Leiden	Glu→0	66
β17–18	Lyon	(Lys-Val)→0	67
β23	Freiburg	Val→0	68
β42–44	Niteroi	(Phe-Glu-Ser)→0	69
or β43–45		or (Glu-Phe-Ser)→0	
β56–59	Tochigi	(Gly-Asn-Pro-Lys)→0	70
β74–75	St. Antoine	(Glu-Leu)→0	71
β75	Vicksburg	Leu→0	72
β87	Tours	Thr→0	71
β91–95	Gun Hill	(Leu-His-Cys-Asp-Lys)→0	73
β131	Leslie	Gln→0	74
β141	Coventry	Leu→0	75
β145	McKees Rocks	(Tyr-His)→0	76

case was associated with an electrophoretically abnormal hemoglobin [115], but in 1962 Grimes and Meisler [116] found that a portion of the hemoglobin from a patient with congenital Heinz body hemolytic anemia precipitated on heating. Dacie et al. [117] showed that such "unstable hemoglobins" were not necessarily electrophoretically abnormal.

Hemoglobin Köln was the first unstable hemoglobin whose amino acid substitution was determined [118]. In the years that followed, several additional mutants were described by Carrell, Lehmann, and their coworkers. This laid the groundwork for the present concepts of the structure-function relations in the unstable hemoglobin diseases. Over 75 such mutants have been described, and the disease is more common than was initially thought. Although *congenital Heinz body hemolytic anemia* is the name that has been applied to this entity for many years, *unstable hemoglobin disease* is more precise and should supplant it.

Recently a clearer picture of the mechanism of Heinz body formation has begun to emerge, and rather precise correlations

between amino acid substitutions and instability are now possible. An area that remains puzzling is the correlation between instability and clinical expression. Undoubtedly, many environmental and genetic factors influence the degree of clinical severity in the unstable hemoglobin disorders.

Prevalence

A large number of unstable variants have been reported (Table 76-11). Nevertheless, they are still considered rare, and many of the reported cases appear to be sporadic; i.e., mutation *de novo* is considered to have occurred when authenticated parents of an affected individual do not carry the mutation. As can be seen from Table 76-11, the mutants with the most severe clinical consequences are most likely to have arisen by such mutation. This probably attests to the deleterious nature of the disease and to the fact that subjects with severe hemolysis are less likely to reproduce than those with mild disease.

Hemoglobin Köln is the most common of all the unstable hemoglobins. At least 43 patients in 11 different families have been reported [198]. The true prevalence of the unstable hemoglobins cannot be estimated because discovery of cases is still haphazard.

Most of the known mutations involve the α or β chains, but an interesting γ-chain variant, hemoglobin F-Poole [H8(130)

Figure 76-10 Nucleotide sequence changes underlying some mutations of the carboxyl ends of the α and β chains. The base sequences from direct sequencing of mRNA [77] are underlined; others are inferred from the genetic code. A U → C change in the normal α-termination code word is responsible for hemoglobin Constant Spring. Deletion of an A in the code word for Lys 139α leads to a shift in the reading frame in hemoglobin Wayne 1. Note that this hypothesis is an agreement with the amino acid sequence of hemoglobin Constant Spring. Duplication of an AG dinucleotide in the code word for Lys 144β might explain the observed sequence in hemoglobin Cranston. The substitution U → A in the code word for Tyr 145β can account for the premature shortening in hemoglobin McKees Rocks.

α Chain

				140								
A	...	Thr	Ser	Lys	Tyr	Arg	Term					
		ACC	UCC	AAA	UAC	CGU	UAA –					
Constant Spring	...	Thr ..	Ser ..	Lys ..	Tyr ..	Arg ..	Gln ..	Ala ..	Gly ..	Ala ..	Ser ..	Val .. Ala ...
		ACU	UCU	AAA	UAC	CGU	CAA	GCU	GGA	GCC	UCG	GUA GCU –
Wayne 1	...	Thr	Ser	Asn	Thr	Val	Lys	Leu	Glu	Pro	Arg	Term
		ACC	UCC	AAU	ACG	GUU	AAG	CUG	GAG	CGU	CGG	UAG –

β Chain

		144						
A	...	His	Lys	Tyr	His	Term		
		CAC	AAG	UAU	CAC	UAA	GC –	
Cranston	...	His	Lys	Ser	Ile	Thr	Lys	Leu ...
		CAC	AAG	AGU	AUC	ACU	AAG	CU –
McKees Rocks	...	His	Lys	Term				
		CAC	AAG	UAA –				

Table 76-8 Fusion polypeptides

Helical segment	A6	A9	B4	D1	F2	F3	G18	G19	H2	H4
Residue number	9	12	22	50	86	87	116	117	124	126
α	Thr	Asn	Ala	Ser	Ser	Gln	Arg	Asn	Gln	Met
β	Ser	Thr	Glu	Thr	Ala	Thr	His	His	Pro	Val

		Reference
Lepore-Hollandia	δ ———— β	80
Lepore-Baltimore	δ ———— β	81
Lepore-Washington, Baltimore	δ ———— β	79
Miyada	β ———— δ	82
P Congo	β ———— δ	83
P Nilotic	β ———— δ	84

Helical segment	NA1	EF4	EF5	F2	F3
Residue number	1	80	81	86	87
α	Gly	Asp	Leu	Ala	Gln
β	Val	Asn	Leu	Ala	Thr

		Reference
Kenya	δ ———— β	44

NOTE: The amino acid sequence differences between the globin chains are shown. When δβ or αβ fusions are isolated, those residues can be examined to determine whether they are β-like, or δ-like, or α-like or β-like, respectively.

Try → Gly], causes hemolytic disease in the newborn [111], and Hb Coventry is also associated with hemolysis [75].

Molecular Pathology

Amino acid replacements (or deletions) that disrupt the coherence of the hemoglobin molecule might be expected to lead to its instability. The various features of the molecule which contribute to its stability are outlined at the beginning of this chapter in "Normal Hemoglobin." Such alterations would be those that insert polar residues into the interior of the molecule (which is mainly hydrophobic), interfere with α-helix formation, disrupt heme binding, or alter the $\alpha_1\beta_1$ or the $\alpha_2\beta_2$ contact. All these share in common the final effect of increasing the flexibility of the heme pocket that leads to denaturation (see "The Mechanism of Heinz Body Formation" later in this chapter). This classification is necessarily artificial, since many mutants have more than one defect in the molecule. The locations of some of these mutants are shown in Fig. 76-12.

Insertion of Polar Residues in the Interior of the Molecule The insertion of a polar amino acid side chain into the hydrophobic interior of the hemoglobin molecule can lead to the entry of water, disruption of the tertiary structure, heme oxidation, and precipitation. In some cases the new polar group is forced to the surface of the molecule, causing widespread distortion of globin structure. Examples of this type of mechanism are hemoglobins Ann Arbor, Riverdale-Bronx, Zurich, Boros, and Olmsted. In some instances, the new polar group can be partially neutralized by neighboring groups as with hemoglobins Bristol and Wein. In hemoglobin M-Milwaukee, the new group is neutralized by the ferric heme iron, and the stability is almost normal (see "Cyanosis: The Methemoglobins" later in this chapter.)

Interference with Interchain Contacts Isolated hemoglobin chains or αβ dimers have a high propensity for denaturation by oxidation and hemichrome formation [199]. Therefore, these mutants that tend to dissociate are often unstable. In general, those that dissociate along the $\alpha_1\beta_1$ interface are less stable than those that dissociate along the $\alpha_1\beta_2$ interface.

Figure 76-11 Unequal (nonhomologous) crossing-over. Misalignment of chromosomes at meiosis with subsequent crossing-over from one DNA strand to the other during synthesis (dashed lines) can lead to abnormal gene products. This mechanism has been invoked to explain the fusion peptides and HPFH. In A, both predicted gene products have been found, but the abnormal segments predicted in B and C have not yet been detected. It is possible that the fitness of these products (labeled ?) might be so low that they have been eliminated.

NON-HOMOLOGOUS CROSSINGOVER

Table 76-9 δ-Chain point mutations

Residue	Substitution	Name	Reference
2 (NA2)	His→Arg	A₂-Sphakia	86
12 (A9)	Asn→Lys	A₂-NYV	87
16 (A13)	Gly→Arg	A₂-(B2)	88
20 (B2)	Val→Glu	A₂-Roosevelt	89
22 (B4)	Ala→Glu	A₂-Flatbush	90
43 (CD2)	Glu→Lys	A₂-Melbourne	91
51 (D2)	Pro→Arg	A₂-Adria	92
69 (E13)	Gly→Arg	A₂-Indonesia	93
116 (G18)	Arg→His	A₂-Coburg	94
136 (H14)	Gly→Asp	A₂-Babinga	95

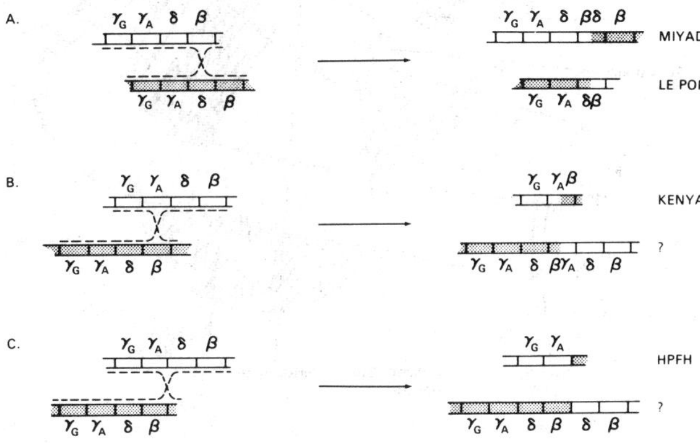

UNSTABLE MUTANTS OF THE α CHAIN

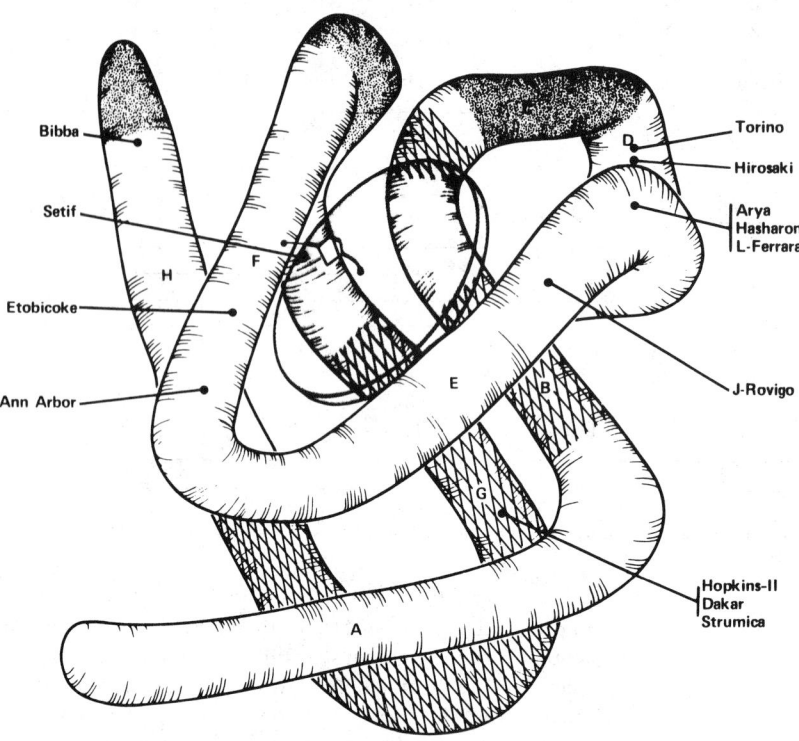

UNSTABLE MUTANTS OF THE β CHAIN

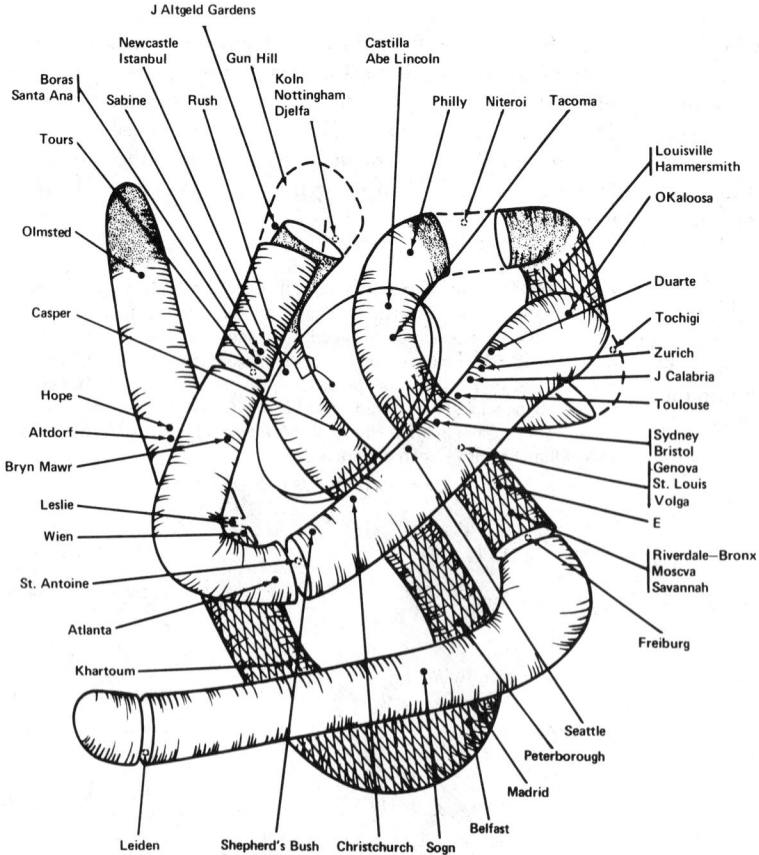

Figure 76-12 Locations of some unstable hemoglobin mutations. The various mutants of the α (A) and β (B) chains are placed on the chain in their approximate positions. Regions of the molecule which participate in the α₁β₂ contacts are shown with a dotted area behind them. The α₁β₁ contacts have a cross-hatched area behind them. Deletions are indicated; they have been detected only in β chains.

Table 76-10 γ-Chain point mutations

Residue	Name	Substitution	Reference
1 (NA1)	F-Malaysia	Gly→Cys (136 Gly)	96
5 (A2)	F-Texas-I	Glu→Lys (136 Ala)	97
6 (A3)	F-Texas-II	Glu→Lys	98
7 (A4)	F-Auckland	Asp→Asn (136 Gly)	99
12 (A9)	F-Alexandria	Thr→Lys	100
16 (A13)	F-Melbourne	Gly→Arg (136 Gly)	101
22 (B4)	F-Kuala Lumpur	Asp→Gly (136 Ala)	102
61 (E5)	F-Jamaica	Lys→Glu (136 Ala)	103
80 (EF4)	F-Victoria-Jubilee	Asp→Tyr (136 Ala)	104
97 (FG4)	F-Dickinson	His→Arg (136 Ala)	105
108 (G10)	F-Ube	Asn→Lys	106
117 (G19)	F-Malta I	His→Arg (136 Gly)	107
121 (GH4)	F-Hull	Glu→Lys (136 Gly)	108
121 (GH4)	F-Carlton	Glu→Lys (136 Ala)	109
125 (H3)	F-Port Royal	Gly→Ala (136 Gly)	110
130 (H8)	F-Poole	Try→Gly (136 Gly)	111

Examples of hemoglobins that affect the $\alpha_1\beta_1$ contacts are Philly, Tacoma, and Khartoum [200]. This explanation is not completely satisfying, however, because other mutants of the $\alpha_1\beta_1$ interface do not display instability. Hemoglobins G Chinese, 11βGlu→Gln, and Chiapas, 114α Pro→Arg, for example, are not unstable, and others require the postulation of complex mechanisms to explain their instability (e.g., hemoglobins Hopkins-II and E).

Many of the mutants that occur at the $\alpha_2\beta_1$ interface have altered oxygen affinity (see "Polycythemia: Hemoglobins with Increased Oxygen Affinity" later in this chapter), but only hemoglobins Rush, Köln, Nottingham, Djelfa, and Setif are unstable. Some hemoglobins dissociate extensively into $\alpha\beta$ dimers under physiologic conditions. Examples are hemoglobins G Georgia [201], Richmond [202, 203], and Kansas [204, 205], which are not highly unstable. Finally, hemoglobin McKees Rocks, in which the last two amino acids of the chain are deleted, cannot form some of the interchain salt bridges characteristic of the deoxy conformation, yet it is not unstable [76].

The bulk of this evidence suggests that the $\alpha_1\beta_1$ interface is much more important in maintaining normal hemoglobin stability than is the $\alpha_1\beta_2$ interface. The former contact is tight, ensuring that $\alpha\beta$ dimers function as a single subunit. The latter is loose, allowing movement which is necessary in allosteric transition (see "Function" under "Normal Hemoglobin" earlier in the chapter). Unstable mutants that affect the $\alpha_1\beta_2$ contact probably require ancillary explanations for the instability. Examples are hemoglobins Rush, Köln, and Nottingham, in which the substitutions also affect heme contacts.

Hemoglobins Bibba and Savannah are unstable and also extensively dissociated. These mutations are not at the site of either of the interchain contacts listed by Perutz (Table 76-1), and their disruptive effects might be multiple, including decreased heme binding as well as increased subunit dissociation [200].

Defective Heme Binding Many unstable hemoglobins have been shown to be heme-depleted either in solution or as precipitates (e.g., hemoglobins Bushwick, Tours, Santa Ana, Sabine, St. Etienne, Gun Hill, Köln, and Hammersmith). Whether heme loss is an artifact of isolation or representative of the condition in vivo is not clear in all cases, but it never-

theless emphasizes that the bonding of heme to globin is important to normal hemoglobin solubility. Moreover, most of the unstable hemoglobins listed in the first category in Table 76-11 involve alterations in regions of heme contacts.

Most of these mutant proteins lose heme because of alterations of the residues that enter into hydrophobic bonds with heme. Hemoglobin Bushwick is an interesting exception. Its substitution, Gly→Val at position E18(74)β, forces the EF corner apart because the side chain of valine is larger than that of glycine and is not easily accommodated there. This might result in the loosening of several heme contacts [200].

The hemoglobins M are additional exceptions. Although their substitutions involve the heme pocket, the nature of those substitutions adds additional stabilizing forces so that they do not precipitate (see "Cyanosis: The Methemoglobins" later in the chapter).

Interference with α-Helix Formation As discussed earlier (see "Normal Hemoglobin"), insertion of proline will cause disruption of an α helix unless the insertion is at one of the first three positions of the helix or at the end of it. Accordingly, hemoglobins Bibba (H1), Sabine (F7), Abraham Lincoln (B14), Casper (G8), Santa Ana (F4), Duarte (E6), Madrid (G17), Atlanta (E19), and Genova (B10) are all unstable. On the other hand, hemoglobins Singapore, HC3(141)α Arg→Pro (171), and Syracuse, H21(143)β His→Pro (206), are not. In hemoglobin Singapore, substitution occurs at an interhelical region, while in hemoglobin Syracuse, it is at the last residue of the H helix.

Some of the mutants that disrupt α-helix formation have other effects. For example, in hemoglobins Bibba, Santa Ana, and Casper the substitutions involve the heme contact, while in hemoglobin Abraham Lincoln the substitution is adjacent to the heme contact and may influence it. Hemoglobin Zurich is apparently stabilized somewhat in the liganded state. Thus subjects who smoke and have elevated COHb also have a reduced hemolytic rate [207].

Mechanism of Heinz Body Formation The traditional view of the mechanism of hemoglobin precipitation in the unstable hemoglobin disorders involves the following sequence: the oxidation of Cys β 93, the formation of mixed disulfides with glutathione, the dissociation of heme from globin, the association of the precipitates with red cell membranes by disulfide bridges, leading to increased membrane permeability, and lysis [208]. In recent years this view has been modified considerably because of progress in the understanding of hemoglobin derivatives found during precipitation and the correlation of the effects of an increasing number of unstable mutants which underscore various features of the hemoglobin degradative pathway. The current hypothesis that is finding the widest acceptance is that the hemoglobins are oxidized to methemoglobin and converted to compounds known as hemichromes that precipitate to form Heinz bodies and are attached to red cell membranes by hydrophobic bonds [209], leading to increased membrane permeability and lysis.

Oxidation of Heme Iron

Reversible oxygenation of hemoglobin results in the partial transfer of an electron from ferrous iron to the oxygen mole-

Table 76-11 A clinical classification of the unstable hemoglobin diseases

Hemoglobin	Substitution	%[a]	Electrophoretic identification[b]	Oxygen affinity[c]	Sporadic[d]	Splenomegaly	Hb[e]	Reticulocytes[e]	Reference
I. Severe hemolysis, no improvement after splenectomy									
Bibba	α136(H19)Leu→Pro	10	+	NA	NA	NA	6.5*–7.5	6*–16	120
Savannah	β24(]36)Gly→Val	30	+	NA	+	+	3.7–5.5	50	121
Abraham Lincoln (Perth)	β32(B14)Leu→Pro	33	0	N1	+	+	8.5	27	122, 123
Castilla	β32(B14)Leu→Arg	22	+	NA	+	+	9.6		124
Hammer-smith	β42(CD1)Phe→Ser	30	0	↓	+	+	6–6.2	46–71	125
Bristol	β67(E11)Val→Asp	36	0	↓	+	+	7	37	52
Sabine	β91(F7)Leu→Pro	8–12	+	NA	+	+	8.5–10.5*	35–67*	126
Nottingham	β98(GF5)Val→Gly	NA	NA	↑	+	+	5–6.7	50	127
Indiana-polis	β112(G14)Cys→Arg	NA	0	NA	0	+	4.0*	10.6*	128
Olmsted	β141(H19)Leu→Arg	NA	NA	NA	+	+	4.8	7	129
II. Severe hemolysis with improvement after splenectomy									
Torino	α42(CD1)Phe→Val	8	0	↓	0	+	7–9.5	4–12	130
Ann Arbor	α80(F1)Leu→Arg	14	+	NA	0	+	12*	10*	131
Volga	β27(B9)Ala→Asp	15–20	0	NA	+	+	10–13	20–40	131a
Genova	β28(B10)Leu→Pro	15–20	0	NA	0	+	10.2	9–16	133
St. Louis	β28(B10)Leu→Gln	30	NA	↑	+	+	10	28.3	134
Christ-church	β71(E15)Phe→Ser	NA	NA	NA	+	+	5.5–10.5	8–15	135
Shepherd's Bush	β74(E18)Gly→Asp	24	+	↑	0	+	13*	5–8*	136
Santa Ana	β88(F4)Leu→Pro	NA	+	NA	+	+	6.9–9	16–21	137
Boras	β88(F4)Leu→Arg	NA	+	↑	0	NA	8.1	NA	138
Istanbul (St. Etienne)[f]	β92(F8)His→Gln	25	+	N1	+	+	9.1	4	139–141
Newcastle	β92(F8)His→Pro	17	+	NA	NA	NA	7.6	18	142
Köln	β98(FG5)Val→Met	22	+	↑	+	+	9–12.4	7–16	118,143
Casper[g]	β106(G8)Leu→Pro	15	0	↑	+	+	4.5–11	22–94	119,144, 145
Wien	β130(H8)Tyr→Asp	24.2	+	NA	+	+	10.5*	43*	146
III. Mild hemolysis with intermittent exacerbations									
Hirosaki	α43(CE1)Phe→Leu		0	NA	0	+	8–14	2.9–17.6	147
L. Ferrara	α47(CD5)Asp→Gly	30	+	N1	0	+	13	9.4	148
Hasharon	α47(CD5)Asp→His	16–19	+	N1	0	0	No	1–4	149–151
Strumica (Serbia)	α112(G19)His→Arg	16	+	NA	0	NA	10–11	NA	152
Leiden	β6(or7)Glu→deleted	25	+	↓	0	NA	11.3–13.6	3–6	66
Belfast	β15(A12)Trp→Arg	27.5	+	↑	0	+	13.7	13	153
Freiburg	β23(B5)Val→deleted	27–32	+	↑	NA	+	11–12	9	68
Riverdale-Bronx	β24(B6)Gly→Arg	30	+	NA	NA	+	11–12	10	154
Lufkin	β29(B11)Gly→Asp	NA	+	N1	NA	NA	12	6–8	155
Philly	β35(C1)Tyr→Phe	30–35	0	NA	0	0	12.6–14.6	12	156, 157
Louisville (Bucuresti)	β42(CD1)Phe→Leu	30–35	0	↓	0	+	11.5–13.5	9	158
Niteroi	β42–44 or 43–45 deleted	NA	+	NA	0	NA	6.8	12–20	69
Duarte	β63(E6)Ala→Pro	NA	0	↓	0	+	15.1	10–4	159
Zurich	β63(E7)His→Arg	25	+	↑	0	0	11–14.7	2–8	160
Toulouse	β66(10)Lys→Glu	40	+	N1	+	+	12–14	1–4	161
Sydney	β67(E11)Val→Ala	NA	0	NA	0	0	10	4–10	162
Seattle	β70(E14)Ala→Asp	43	+	↓	0	0	9.5–10.4	3	163, 164
Bushwick	β74(E18)Gly→Val	1–2	+	NA	0	NA	10.5–11.1	2–5.7	165
Atlanta	β75(E19)Leu→Pro	NA	0	NA	0	+	11.6	32	166
Bryn Mawr (Buenos Aires)	β85(F1)Phe→Ser	25	+	↑	+	+	12–15	5–18	167, 168
J Altgeld Gardens	β92(F8)His→Asp	NA	+	N1	0	NA	9.5	NA	169
Gun Hill	β91–95 F7–GF2 92–96 F8–FG3 (deleted)	30–35	+	↑	0	+	12.6–14.5	4–10	73

Table 76-11 A clinical classification of the unstable hemoglobin diseases (*Continued*)

Hemoglobin	Substitution	%[a]	Electrophoretic identification[b]	Oxygen affinity[c]	Sporadic[d]	Splenomegaly	Hb[e]	Reticulocytes[e]	Reference
Burke	β107(G9)Gly→Arg	30	+	↓	NA	NA	6	50	170
Peterborough	β111(G13)Val→Phe	33.4	0	↓	0	0	11.9	4	171
Madrid	β115(G17)Ala→Pro	NA	NA	NA	+	+	9.7	33.5	172
North Shore	β134(H12)Val→Glu	30	+	N1	0	0	11.7–13.5	n1	173
Altdorf	β135(1113)Ala→Pro	35	0	↑	0	NA	9–12	2–17	174
IV. No disease									
Prato	α31(B12)Arg→Σεθ	20–29	+	N1	0	NA	13.2	1.4	175
Arya	α47(CD5)Asp→Asn	22	+	NA	0	0	N1	NA	176
J-Rovigo	α53(E2)Ala→Asp	33–50	+	NA	0	0	N1	NA	177
Etobicoke	α84(F5)Ser→Arg	15	+	NA	0	0	11.1–14.1	1–3	178
Hopkins	α112(G19)His→Asp	17–27	+	↑	0	0	N1	1–2	48
Dakar	α112(G19)His→Gln	10	+	NA	0	0	N1	NA	179
Sögn	β14(A11)Leu→Arg	30	+	NA	0	0	12–13	4	180
Saki	β14(A11)Leu→Pro	41	NA	NA	0	NA	12.2	NA	181
E	β26(B8)Glu→Lys	22–48	+	N1	0	0	8.2–14.1		182, 183
Tacoma	β30(B12)Arg→Ser	43	+	NA	0	0	13–13.8	4	184
Okaloosa	β48(CD7)Leu→Arg	32–36	+	↓	0	0	13–17.9	4.3	185
J Calabria	β64(E8)Gly→Asp	38	+	↑	0	NA	12.8	39	186
Rush	β101(G3)Glu→Gln	35	+	N1	0	0	12	NA	187
Leslie	β131(119)Gl→deleted	30	+	NA	0	0	10–14	3–4	74
Coventry	β141(H19)→deleted	<10	NA	↑	0	+	10.0	10.0	75
Cranston	β chain elongated	35	+	NA	NA	NA	15–17	5–8	64, 188
V. Insufficient data for classification									
Port Phillip	α91(FG3)Leu→Pro	7	+	NA	NA	NA	10.7	34	189
Steif	α94(G1)Asp→Tyr	12	+	NA	NA	NA	NA	NA	190
Moscva	β24(B6)Leu→Gln	17	+	NA	NA	NA	NA	NA	191
Henri Mandor	β26(B8)Glu→Val	37.5	NA	NA	NA	NA	7.5	20	192
Bicetre	β63(E7)His→Pro	NA	NA	NA	NA	+	NA	1.4	193
St. Antoine	β74–75(E18–19) deleted	NA	0	N1	NA	NA	NA	NA	71
Tours	β87(F3) deleted	25	+	↑	NA	NA	NA	NA	71
Djelfa	β98(FG5)Val→Ala	5	+	↑	NA	NA	NA	NA	194
Tubingen	β106(G8)Leu→Glu	41	+	↑	NA	NA	NA	NA	195
Khartoum	β124(H2)Pro→Arg	30	0	NA	NA	NA	NA	NA	196
J Guantanamo	β128(H6)Ala→Asp	36–38	+	NA	NA	NA	10–11	3–4	197

[a] Percentage of abnormal hemoglobin in hemolysate.
[b] +: Abnormal band (not free chains) seen after electrophoresis.
0: No abnormality in any electrophoretic system.
[c] Oxygen affinity of blood or red cell suspensions.
[d] +: Authentic parents free of mutation.
0: Mutation found in other family members.
[e] Hemoglobin and reticulocyte counts before spenectomy. Values marked by an asterisk are after splenectomy.
[f] Hemoglobin St. Etienne: Identical substitution appears not to be sporadic.
[g] The subject was noted to have chronic hemolysis with cyanosis.
NOTE: NA Indicates the information is not available.
SOURCE: Modified from Koler et al. [*119*].

cule, which is bound as a superoxide anion (.0-0⁻) [*210*]. Upon dissociation of oxygen from the iron atom, oxidation to the ferric state can occur in the presence of water. Normal red blood cells contain powerful mechanisms for safeguarding against the oxidation of heme iron. A DPNH-dependent methemoglobin reductase system reduces methemoglobin. The highly reactive superoxide anion is detoxified by superoxide dismutase (also called *erythrocuperin*), and H_2O_2 is reduced by catalase and glutathione reductase. The reducing capacity of the normal red cell is about 250 times its oxidizing capacity [*211*]. This margin of safety is sufficient in the normal red cell, even in the presence of drugs which are strong oxidizing agents. If any reducing mechanism breaks down, then oxidation of heme iron may occur and hemolysis can follow.

Precipitation of hemoglobin and Heinz body formation do not necessarily follow methemoglobin formation. Individuals with hereditary deficiencies of the methemoglobin reductase (diaphorase) system [*212*] or with one of the abnormal methemoglobins (see "Cyanosis: The Methemoglobins" later in this chapter) can have up to 40 percent methemoglobin without significant hemolysis. Nevertheless, methemoglobin is probably a first step in the precipitation of the unstable hemoglobins.

Hemichrome Formation Hemichromes are derivatives of methemoglobin in which the fifth coordination position of the iron remains bound to His F8, but the sixth position is free and available for reaction with other ligands. One such ligand is the imidazole group of the "distal" His (E7), which lies in close proximity to the heme. Some of these derivatives are reversible and some are not (Fig. 76-13).

Hemichromes can be detected because of their unique spectral properties. They have been observed during the degradation of many unstable hemoglobins [199]. Moreover, in some instances methemoglobin can be clearly identified as an intermediate found during the formation of hemichromes from oxyhemoglobin. This supports the concept that methemoglobin is a necessary prerequisite for hemichrome formation.

A second requirement for hemichrome formation would appear to be a high degree of flexibility of the portions of the globin chain forming the heme pocket. Irreversible hemichromes are formed when iron is liganded to groups that require considerable distortion of the heme pocket. Perhaps methemoglobins are not unstable, even though they are easily oxidized, because they do not display such distortion. This flexibility could explain the instability of certain mutants that do not affect the heme contacts, such as hemoglobins Riverdale-Bronx, Freiberg, and St. Louis [200].

Subunit Dissociation Separated globin chains form hemichromes much more rapidly than tetramers in vitro [213]. The tendency of these chains to form hemichromes is $\alpha > \beta > \gamma$. Therefore, those mutations that affect the $\alpha_1\beta_1$ interface might be unstable because of the ease of hemichrome formation of the resultant subunits. Also, it might explain why α chains appear to precipitate very early in the life of a red blood cell for an individual with β thalassemia, while in α thalassemia the precipitates are often seen in older cells. Similarly, precipitates containing γ chains have not been reported.

Dissociation of the globin subunits has been thought to be a prerequisite for Heinz body formation [208], but recent evidence suggests that while Heinz bodies for some unstable hemoglobins may contain a predominance of one type of chain, this is not a feature common to all of them [214].

Role of Sulfhydryl Groups The oxidation of sulfhydryl groups of hemoglobin is probably not a fundamental cause of precipitation and may be the result of the oxidizing influence of the superoxide radical which is released upon conversion of oxyhemoglobin to methemoglobin [215]. Furthermore, complex formation with glutathione is not necessary for the binding of Heinz bodies to membranes; rather, such bonds are probably hydrophobic [209]. The oxidation of GSH to GSSG which occurs during the precipitation of unstable hemoglobins is probably also the result of the superoxide generated from the conversion of methemoglobin to hemichrome [216]. Glutathione peroxidase is one of the enzyme systems which detoxifies the H_2O_2 formed from the superoxide metabolism.

The loss of heme during precipitation has been inferred by the finding of a reduced ratio of heme to globin in hemoglobin precipitates and Heinz bodies [200]. Such observations have suggested that heme loss might be the cause of the instability of some mutants (Köln and Bushwick). On the other hand, other mutants (e.g., Christchurch and Sydney) precipitate with their heme intact. Thus, heme loss does not appear to be a necessary prerequisite for precipitation.

Hemoglobin Köln is present in cells as the substantially β-heme-depleted derivative and probably precipitates after formation of a hemichrome by the chain [215]. It can be stabilized

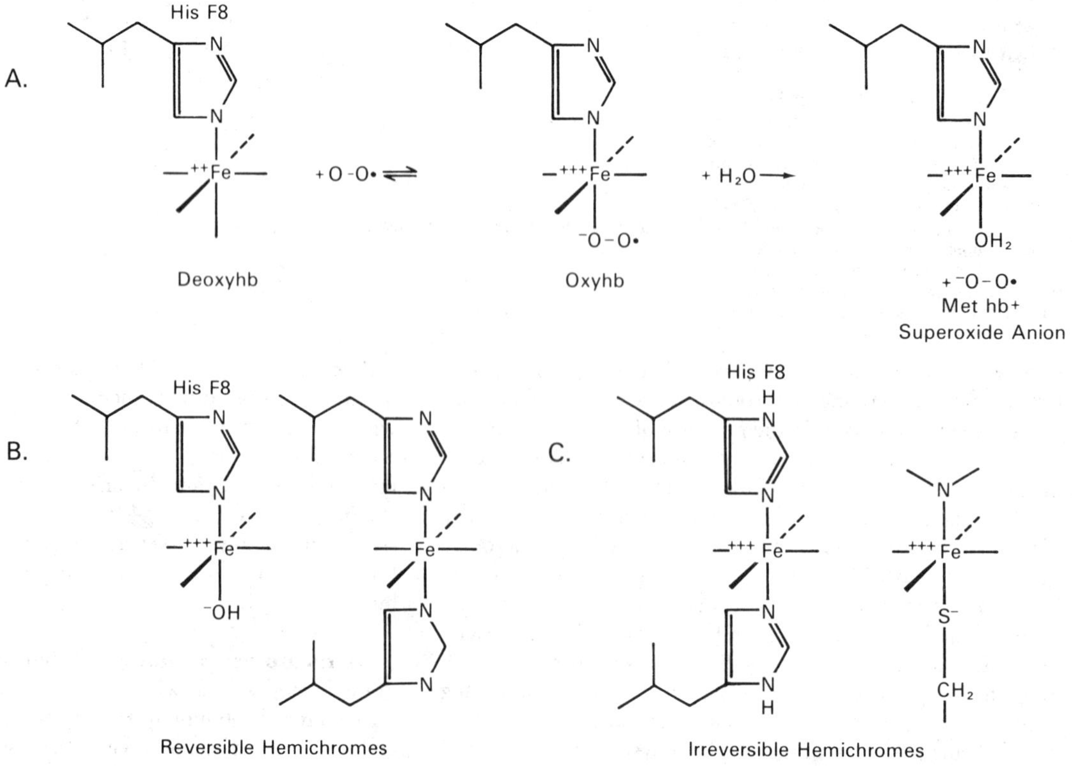

Figure 76-13 Heme oxidation and hemichrome formations. In deoxyhemoglobin, ferrous iron can combine with one molecule of oxygen. In doing so, it partially donates an electron, resulting in a formal change to the ferric state. Oxygen is bound as a superoxide anion. In the presence of water, methemoglobin can form upon dissociation of oxygen, preventing further oxygen binding (*A*). The hemichromes are derivatives of methemoglobin in which the sixth coordination position is bound either reversibly (e.g., with a hydroxyl group of His E7) β (*B*) or irreversibly (e.g., with a protonated histidine or a mercaptide and nitrogenous base) (*C*). (*Modified from Rachmilewitz [199].*)

by the presence of heme ligands that prevent oxidation [217]. Since the α chain is especially susceptible to hemichrome formation, this could be an additional factor in the instability of other variants which undergo loss of β heme.

A Model

The above considerations, based largely on the recent work of Winterbourn, Carrell, and Rachmilewitz, allow a tentative model (Fig. 76-14):

1. The mutations of the unstable hemoglobins all have in common increased flexibility in the heme pocket. This may be the result of a variety of disturbances including the dissociation into αβ dimers by alterations at the intersubunit interfaces.

2. Increased flexibility can lead to the entry of water into the heme pocket of oxyhemoglobin with subsequent generation of methemoglobin and superoxide free radicals. The latter are detoxified by superoxide dismutase, catalase, and glutathione peroxidase, leading to increased amounts of oxidized glutathione.

3. Methemoglobin, again because of disturbances of tertiary structure, can form reversible or irreversible hemichromes in which distortion can lead to exposure of hydrophobic residues which are ordinarily internally oriented. Precipitation follows.

4. Aggregates of precipitated protein can be hydrophobically bonded to the red cell membrane, with subsequent permeability changes, splenic sequestration, and hemolysis.

5. This model further accommodates subunit dissociation and loss of heme as possible concomitants (but not causes) of precipitation.

Synthesis of the Unstable Hemoglobins

An old observation, which is still incompletely explained is, that the various abnormal hemoglobins are present in amounts other than those predicted from their supposed gene doses. For example, sickle-trait blood contains 20 to 45 percent hemoglobin S instead of the expected 50 percent. In general, α-chain variants tend to be present in lower amounts, but this may be explicable on the basis of multiple α-chain genes (see "Genetics of the Hemoglobins" above). Furthermore, the role of interacting α-thalassemia genes has not yet been fully elucidated.

The unstable hemoglobins represent a striking variability in the proportions of hemoglobins present, and some of them have been studied in an effort to discover whether this is due to variable rates of synthesis, destruction, or both. Literature on this subject is confusing because early experiments incorporating radioactive amino acids did not take into account such problems as the existence of pools of free α chains in β-chain disorders, exchange of subunits between completed tetramers, and rapid postsynthetic destruction [218].

Hemoglobins Riverdale-Bronx [219], Bristol [220], Hammersmith [221], Bushwick [165], and Sabine [222] are all synthesized to an extent approximately equal to hemoglobin A in the red blood cells of carriers, but each of these is present in reduced amounts in peripheral blood (Table 76-11). Therefore, preferential loss of these hemoglobins might occur by Heinz body formation and subsequent removal by the reticuloendothelial system. Hemoglobin Bushwick is present in red cells as only 1 to 2 percent of the total hemoglobin, and hemo-

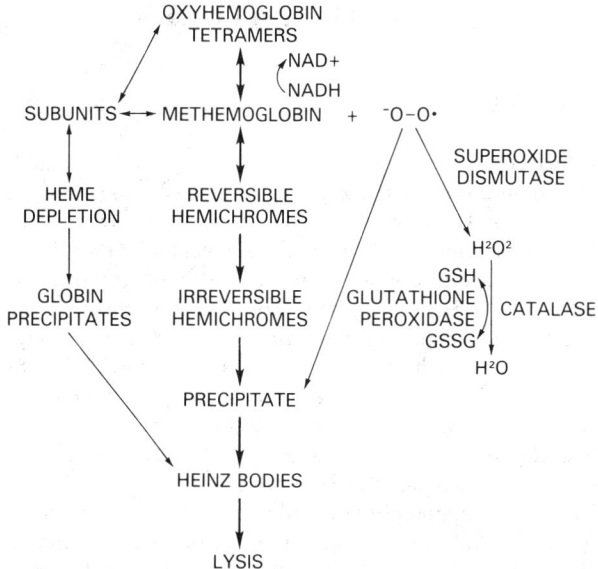

Figure 76-14 Model for the intracellular denaturation of the unstable hemoglobins. The principal pathway is shown by bold arrows. Other pathways which may affect certain mutants are shown by light arrows. (*Modified from Winterbourn and Carrell [215].*)

globin Indianapolis is so unstable that it can be detected only by pulse-labeling techniques [128]. A further hypothesis is suggested in regard to hemoglobin Bushwick because the cells are not hypochromic: Compensation by the normal globin genes might occur. The means for such compensation remains a mystery. Hemoglobins Köln [223] and Hasharon [224] might be reduced in carriers because of a combination of decreased synthesis of the hemoglobin variant and preferential loss in the peripheral blood.

Additional synthetic variations have been postulated for individual unstable hemoglobins. Hemoglobin Ann Arbor [225], an α-chain variant, occurs as about 14 percent of the total hemoglobin of carriers. Studies of hemoglobin labeling with radioactive amino acids suggested the unique possibility that the release of $β^A$ chains from precipitates within the cell effect a feedback inhibition of further $β^A$-chain synthesis, reducing the imbalance between α- and β-chain production in this disorder. Studies with marrow of subjects with hemoglobin Leiden [226] have suggested increased $α^A$-chain synthesis with a resulting pool of free α chains and normal red cell hemoglobin content, in spite of precipitation of the unstable hemoglobin Leiden. Finally, the $β^{Gun Hill}$ chain appears to be synthesized 20 to 50 percent faster than $β^A$ chains in the same cells, in spite of the finding of only 32 percent hemoglobin Gun Hill in peripheral blood [227].

These observations are difficult to reconcile. The general pattern which seems to emerge is that the unstable hemoglobins are synthesized in amounts equal to their gene dose (or slightly less) and their final proportion in the peripheral blood is further regulated by their rate of Heinz body formation and removal. The possibilities of accelerated synthesis of $β^{Gun Hill}$ and the possible feedback inhibition of $β^A$ chains, in hemoglobin Ann Arbor, would appear to be the mechanisms most in need of further investigation. The question of the quantitative control of the amount of hemoglobin synthesized per cell, as illustrated by the compensation of $β^A$ chains in the subjects with hemoglobin Bushwick, might be relevant to the question of regulation of hemoglobin synthesis in the thalassemias (see Chap. 77, "The Thalassemias").

CLINICAL FEATURES

Presentation

The final common pathway in the pathogenesis of the unstable hemoglobin disorders is the precipitation of hemoglobin, the formation of Heinz bodies, which may be removed in the spleen, and hemolysis. Heinz bodies are metabolized by mechanisms that are incompletely understood. One group of byproducts is a variety of dipyrrole compounds of the mesobilifuscin type which may appear in the urine [228]. A wide range in the severity of hemolysis may be seen. Before 1970 the majority of the variants were found in subjects with severe hemolysis who had been under clinical observation for many years. Recently, increased awareness of these diseases has resulted in the diagnosis of less severe cases.

The most common physical and historical findings are those associated with hemolytic anemia: weakness, pallor, jaundice, and splenomegaly. Dusky cyanosis has been described in association, for example, with hemoglobins Shepherd's Bush, Hammersmith, Freiberg, and Sydney. It is probably due to the presence of methemoglobin and sulfhemoglobin, derivatives which cannot be oxygenated [229]. Pigmenturia is a helpful clue, but it is not present in all the patients with unstable hemoglobin disorders. Furthermore, in some instances (e.g., hemoglobins Köln and Zurich) it may be present episodically in association with acute hemolysis. In the most severe cases, marrow expansion can be seen, with bossing of the skull, as in a young patient with hemoglobin Nottingham [127]. Hemoglobin Indianapolis is so unstable that it is detectable only in pulse-labeling experiments with bone marrow. Carriers therefore have a clinical syndrome identical to that of β thalassemia [128]. Chronic leg ulcers have been reported in hemoglobin Köln disease [229].

Clinical Classification

The grouping of the disorders in Table 76-11 has been suggested by Koler et al. [119]. It is based on clinical considerations and is intended to aid in therapy and prognosis.

In the first group the disease is considered *severe*. These patients came to clinical attention early in life, some in infancy, with almost all the signs and symptoms listed above. Except for hemoglobins Bibba and Indianapolis, all appeared to be new mutations. They all have low hemoglobin values and high reticulocyte counts. The latter might be spurious in some cases, because hemoglobin precipitates can be confused with reticulin in reticulocyte stains. Splenectomy in these patients did not lead to clinical improvement.

In the second category of disorders, patients also exhibit severe hemolysis but with improvement after splenectomy. The distinction between these two groups is not easy to make but carries therapeutic importance because the decision for splenectomy can often be difficult, particularly in young patients. In general, the degree of anemia or reticulocytosis or the amount of pigmenturia was not helpful in distinguishing group II patients. They tended to be discovered in late childhood or adolescence, and in about one-half the cases a family history of hemolytic disease was present. Cholelithiasis, intermittent jaundice, splenomegaly, or hemolytic crises were often the presenting complaints. After splenectomy, anemia was mild or absent, but reticulocytosis persisted.

The third category, which embraces the majority of the mutants, is associated with *mild* hemolysis. Many of these patients are detected because of "crisis" associated with sulfonamide ingestion (e.g., hemoglobins Zurich, Shepherd's Bush, Torino, and Peterborough). A more common cause of crisis, however, is mild infection, usually viral upper respiratory infection. These subjects are asymptomatic between crises. They seldom have splenomegaly. Affected family members have been detected in all but three instances (hemoglobins Toulouse, Bryn Mawr, and Madrid).

The fourth category is made up of hemoglobins that are found to be unstable as an incidental matter. All these are distinguishable electrophoretically, and most were discovered by routine screening. They are of no particular clinical importance when present in the heterozygous form. An exception is hemoglobin E, which is extremely common in Southeast Asia and may cause mild hemolysis when occurring with thalassemia genes or in the homozygous form. It is slightly unstable in the presence of oxidant drugs [183].

Thus, the important factors in the classification of a given unstable hemoglobin disorder would seem to be the presence or absence of the mutation in the parents, splenomegaly, age at presentation, degree of anemia, and a history of episodic hemolysis with pigmenturia.

Role of Blood Oxygen Affinity

The hemoglobin level correlates poorly with the severity of clinical symptoms in the unstable hemoglobin diseases. In these patients, "anemia" must be redefined. *Functional anemia* exists when tissue oxygen demands are not met. The amount of oxygen that can be delivered to tissue sites depends on many factors besides hemoglobin concentration, including blood oxygen affinity. For example, blood with low oxygen affinity can give up as much oxygen as blood with normal oxygen affinity, but with higher hemoglobin concentration. Conversely, blood with high oxygen affinity requires a high hemoglobin concentration in order to give up as much oxygen as blood with normal hemoglobin concentration and normal oxygen affinity. Of course, this is a simplified formulation because cardiovascular and pulmonary factors, 2,3-DPG, and acid-base status are also involved, but it has some utility in an approach to clinical problems.

Considerations such as these prompted Bellingham and Huehns to examine the oxygen affinity of red blood cells from patients with a variety of unstable hemoglobins [230]. They found that "compensated" hemolysis could occur when, for example, the high oxygen affinity of hemoglobin Köln was associated with a relatively high, almost normal, hemoglobin level (see "Polycythemia: Hemoglobins with Increased Oxygen Affinity" later in this chapter). Many of the unstable hemoglobins are now known to have altered oxygen affinity, and these alterations are probably important in regulating the clinical expression of the disorder. For example, patients with hemoglobins Casper, Boras, Köln, St. Louis, and Shepherd's Bush are all in the second category (severe hemolysis improved by splenectomy; see Table 76-11). Their oxygen affinities are high, resulting in poorer oxygen delivery than would be expected on the basis of their hemoglobin values alone. In contrast, patients with hemoglobins Louisville, Leiden, Seattle, and Peterborough (third category, mild hemolysis) are less severely affected in spite of equally low hemoglobin levels and equally rapid hemolysis. Their oxygen affinities are low, resulting in better oxygen delivery than would be predicted on the basis of their hemoglobin concentrations.

A striking contrast due to differences in oxygen affinity is illustrated by patients with hemoglobins Hammersmith and Nottingham [229]. Both are in category I (severe hemolysis not improved by splenectomy). The patient with hemoglobin Hammersmith, a low affinity hemoglobin, had a hemoglobin of 6 to 7 g per deciliter of blood but developed normally with no evidence of marrow expansion. The patient with hemoglobin Nottingham, a high affinity hemoglobin, had a similar hemoglobin concentration and degree of hemolysis but showed signs of marrow expansion and required maintenance transfusion.

The question of blood oxygen affinity is also important in a consideration of splenectomy. If a young patient with unstable hemoglobin disease is shown to have low blood oxygen affinity, splenectomy can probably be delayed. If oxygen affinity is high, however, tissue oxygen delivery may not be adequate in spite of a minimal reduction of hemoglobin concentration. In the latter patients, splenectomy can lead to significant erythrocytosis.

Laboratory Findings Mean corpuscular hemoglobin concentration (MCHC) is usually low, presumably because of loss of hemoglobin as Heinz bodies. Reticulocytosis is a constant finding unless complicating iron or folate deficiency is present. Platelets may be low if there is significant splenic sequestration. In patients who have had splenectomy, Heinz bodies can usually be found in fresh blood; in others, incubation at 37°C for 24 h is required. They can also be generated by incubation with oxidant dyes such as cresyl blue, methylene blue, or new methylene blue, stains which are used for reticulocytes. Care must be taken to distinguish reticulin from precipitated protein. When there is serious difficulty, determination of red blood cell RNA, present in reticulin but not Heinz bodies, can be helpful [231]. The red cells often show poikilocytosis, basophilic stippling, polychromatophilia, and hypochromia. The bone marrow is usually intensely erythroid but shows normal maturation. In severely affected patients such as those with hemoglobins Nottingham and Hammersmith, a bone marrow picture not unlike that of congenital dyserythropoietic anemia has been observed [232].

Although many of the variants are electrophoretically "silent" (Table 76-11), electrophoresis should be done in all instances in which an unstable hemoglobin is suspected. Even in some mutant hemoglobins in which there is no change in charge, electrophoretic mobility can be altered because of the extreme distortions in tertiary structure that can occur. Although the use of Mylar-backed cellulose thin-layer sheets has virtually replaced the more tedious starch gel for electrophoresis at pH 8.6, the latter can be especially useful to detect mutants occurring in small amounts, such as hemoglobin Bushwick, or free α chain (where β chains precipitate disproportionately) because they can be loaded very heavily.

The heat denaturation test is the single most important procedure in establishing a diagnosis of unstable hemoglobin disease. Other tests which use oxidant dyes can also be positive in deficiencies of those enzymes required to prevent oxidation of hemoglobin (see "The Mechanism of Heinz Body Formation" earlier in this chapter). Most simply, a fresh hemolysate (made by freezing and thawing equal volumes of water and packed cells) is diluted into 50 volumes of 0.15 M Tri-Cl, pH 7.4. This is heated at 60°C. At intervals the precipitates are removed from samples by centrifugation, and the optical density of the supernatant is measured. A simple and rapid test, involving dilution of the hemolysate into a buffered isopropanol solution, appears to be quite sensitive and specific and is also a convenient method for the isolation of unstable hemoglobins [233].

Altered blood oxygen affinity is a common finding in the unstable hemoglobin disorders [229]. Such a finding has important therapeutic as well as diagnostic implications, as discussed above. The various methods for measuring blood oxygen affinity which are in common use are described briefly later (see "Polycythemia: Hemoglobins with Increased Oxygen Affinity").

Complications and Treatment

Few deaths have been reported that could be linked to unstable hemoglobins. A 6-year-old patient with hemoglobin Hammersmith died of pneumococcal septicemia following splenectomy [229], and two patients with hemoglobin Duarte died after splenectomy of thromboembolic disease which might have been related to erythrocytosis [159]. Other complications include hemolytic crises (as a result of either infection or oxidant drugs), cholelithiasis, and chronic anemia.

Until one has evidence that the blood of a patient in whom the diagnosis is suspected does not hemolyze in response to oxidant drugs in vitro, it is prudent to warn the patient against taking such drugs.

The question of transfusion is a difficult one, and the course undertaken must be a compromise between alleviating symptoms of anemia and the risk of iron overload and transfusion reactions. The problem is much like that of the thalassemias. Fortunately, few of the unstable hemoglobins lead to severe chronic hemolysis, and transfusion is required only during hemolytic crises.

If indications for splenectomy are present (refractory anemia, pancytopenia) in a patient who appears to fit into category I or II (see Table 76-11), the decision for surgery must be based on the degree of pancytopenia. When splenectomy is considered because of anemia alone, placing the patient in category I or II before surgery may be helpful. This requires a detailed family study and the determination of the structure and oxygen affinity of the abnormal hemoglobin. It has been suggested that the hemoglobins that are most unstable may also be removed by the liver, and therefore splenectomy may be of little use to Group I patients [229]. At any rate, one can probably expect that the result of splenectomy will not be dramatic, and, if done, it should be carried out under circumstances that minimize complications. These would include waiting until the patient is 6 years of age or older and using appropriate antibiotic coverage during and after surgery.

CYANOSIS: THE METHEMOGLOBINS

For hundreds of years a strange disease called *kuchikuro* (black mouth) was endemic in the Iwate prefecture of northern Japan [234]. In 1937 it was shown to be a hereditary disorder and was called *black blood disease* because the blood of carriers was said to be the color of Japanese soy sauce [235]. Horlein and Weber [2] first demonstrated that the hemoglobin from members of a German family with similar physical findings existed mainly as methemoglobin because of an abnormal globin moiety. In 1955 Singer suggested that these "congenital methemoglobins" be designated the M hemoglobins [236], and in 1961 Gerald and Efron determined the structural alterations of several of them [237].

There are five different abnormal hemoglobins whose primary consequence is congenital cyanosis (Table 76-12). These are the methemoglobins (M hemoglobins). Some of the unstable hemoglobins also oxidize abnormally rapidly, but their primary clinical consequence is hemolysis (see "Hemolysis: The Unstable Hemoglobins" earlier in this chapter).

All the M hemoglobins have amino acid substitutions in the heme pocket that directly affect the heme-globin bond. New bonds are formed between the inserted amino acid and the heme iron and are sufficiently strong that molecular instability is *not* an important property. Instead, the abnormal chains are maintained in the ferric (methemoglobin, Fig. 76-13) form and are incapable of reversible oxygenation. Two of the mutations involve the proximal histidine [hemoglobins M_{Iwate}, F8(87)αTyr, and $M_{Hyde Park}$, F8(92)β Tyr] and two the distal histidine [hemoglobins M_{Boston}, E7(58)αTyr, and $M_{Saskatoon}$, E7(63)βTyr]. In each case, the phenolic side chain of the new Tyr is bonded with the heme iron. A fifth mutant, $M_{Milwaukee-1}$, contains a substitution [E11(67)β Val→Glu] sufficiently close to the heme iron that a stable bond between it and the carboxyl group of the new glutamate can be formed. Finally, increased methemoglobin has been observed in a carrier of hemoglobin Wood, FG4(97)β His→Leu, following ingestion of oxidizing drugs. In this special case, the abnormal hemoglobin is probably a poor substrate for enzymatic reduction [248, 249].

Molecular Pathology

Although carriers (i.e., heterozygotes) suffer no functional impairment, the study of these hemoglobins has provided valuable insight into the mechanisms of interaction of the globin chains. Only half the purified hemoglobin M molecule is capable of binding oxygen, since two of its four chains carry mutations that prevent oxygenation. Although never observed, the homozygous state would be expected to be lethal.

The unusual functional properties of the M hemoglobins (Table 76-12) are (1) low oxygen affinity of hemoglobins M_{Boston} and M_{Iwate} (α-chain variants) with almost no Bohr effect, (2) normal oxygen affinity of hemoglobins $M_{Saskatoon}$ and $M_{Hyde Park}$ (β-chain variants) with a normal Bohr effect, and (3) low oxygen affinity of hemoglobin $M_{Milwaukee-1}$ with a normal Bohr effect. All the mutants show decreased cooperativity. The properties are summarized in Ref. 238. Recently, studies using a variety of physical and chemical methods have somewhat clarified the mechanisms underlying these properties, but some questions remain.

In hemoglobin M_{Boston}, the phenolic group of Tyr E7(58)α is aligned with the heme iron and forms a ferric complex with it (Fig. 76-15) [250]. This bond is stronger than the ferrous iron bond with His E7(58)α of hemoglobin A. The latter bond is under tension, and its absence in hemoglobin M_{Boston} means that the F helix can rotate and move slightly away from the heme. This rotation and movement are similar to those associated with the R-T transition in hemoglobin A (see Fig. 76-5). As a result the F and H helices move slightly apart, allowing entry of Tyr HC2 into its pocket. This stabilizes the C terminus and favors interchain salt bridges [251–253]. Thus, because the abnormal α chains cannot undergo the tertiary changes required for a quaternary T-R switch, the molecules are found to be "locked" in the lower-affinity T conformation. Since the Bohr effect and cooperativity are manifestations of such a switch, these features are nearly absent (see "Function of Normal Hemoglobin" earlier in this chapter).

The crystal structure of hemoglobin M_{Iwate} has also been studied [254] but at lower resolution. In that mutant, the E helix is slightly shifted toward the heme, and the phenolic group of Tyr F8α is probably bonded to the ferric iron. Nuclear magnetic resonance studies suggest that it does not undergo a T-R transition [255], and therefore the explanation for its abnormal properties is probably similar to that for hemoglobin M_{Boston} [250].

Crystallographic study of hemoglobin $M_{Hyde Park}$ was made difficult by loss of heme for the abnormal chains when they crystallized [254], but accommodation of the new Tyr causes disturbances of the F helix and the FG corner. Hemoglobins $M_{Hyde Park}$ and $M_{Saskatoon}$ are probably capable of an R-T transformation that results in a Bohr effect and relatively normal oxygen affinity.

Table 76-12 Functional properties of the M hemoglobins

Name	Substitution	O_2 Affinity	n	Bohr effect	Heat labile	Hemolysis	Present at birth	Hb	Reference
M_{Boston}*	αE7(58)His→Tyr		1.2		0	0	+	14.2	237–239
M_{Iwate}†	αF8(87)AB→Tyr		1.1		0	0	+	15.5	237, 238, 241, 242
$M_{Saskatoon}$‡	βE7(63)His→Tyr	nl	1.2	nl	+	+	0	12	237, 238, 243–245
$M_{Hyde Park}$§	βF8(92)His→Tyr	nl	1.3	nl	+	+	0	12.8	237, 238, 243–246
$M_{Milwaukee-1}$	βE11(67)Val→Glu		1.2	nl	0	+	0	13.2	237, 238, 247

* Also hemoglobins M-Kishunhalas, Osaka, Gothenberg.
† Also hemoglobins M-Kankakee, Oldenberg.
‡ Also hemoglobins M-Emory, Kurume, Chicago, Radom, Hida, Arthus, Leipzig, Novi Sad, Erlangen, Horlein-Weber.
§ Also hemoglobin M-Akita.
NOTE: Values for oxygen affinity, cooperativity (*n*), and the Bohr effect are for purified hemoglobins. Average hemoglobin (Hb) concentrations in carriers are given.

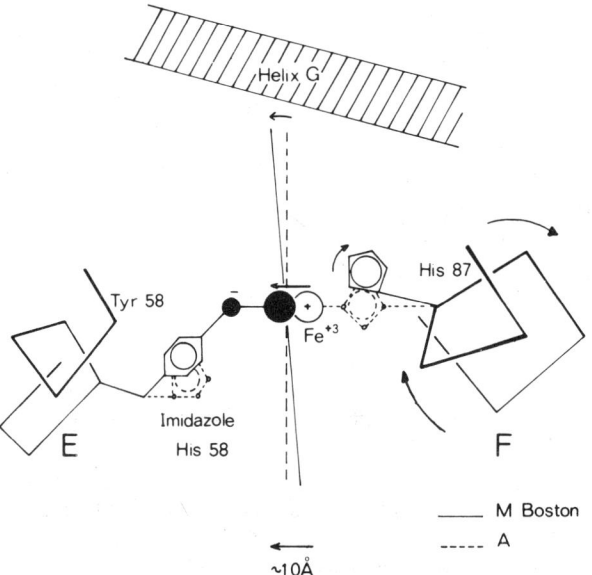

Figure 76-15 Stereochemical interpretation of hemoglobin M$_{Boston}$. Introduction of a Tyr at E7 introduces a tight bond between its phenolic group and ferric iron. The normal bond between ferrous iron and histidine F8 cannot form, and the result is a rotational movement of the F helix. This change in tertiary structure favors the T quaternary structure. (*From Pulsinelli et al.* [250].)

Hemoglobin M$_{Milwaukee-1}$ has been studied in great detail [252, 256]. The sixth coordination site of the ferric heme is bonded to the carboxyl group of Glu E11(67)β. The ferric subunits take up the deoxy tertiary conformation and cause the quaternary structure to favor T. Low oxygen affinity results. In contrast with the α-substitued hemoglobins M, the ferric subunits of M$_{Milwaukee-1}$ do undergo a change in their tertiary structure upon oxygenation of the α chains, allowing a change to the quaternary R structure. Thus, a Bohr effect is present.

In all the M hemoglobins, a structural defect can be viewed as the insertion of new amino acid groups which at once stabilize the heme groups and hold the iron in its ferric state. In the α-substituted hemoglobins, the R-T equilibrium is pushed so far in favor of T that oxygen affinity is very low and essentailly no Bohr effect is seen. In the β-substituted variants, R-T transition occurs and a Bohr effect is present. In hemoglobin M$_{Milwaukee-1}$ the R-T equilibrium favors T, reducing oxygen affinity, but a transition *does* occur (although late during the oxygenation reaction) so that a Bohr effect is seen. In all these mutants, cooperativity is reduced because only two oxygen binding sites are available per hemoglobin tetramer.

Clinical Manifestations

Presentation Cyanosis is the presenting feature of patients with the M hemoglobins. This bluish discoloration can also occur from capillary oxygen desaturation, as in congenital heart disease. In the latter instance, about 5 g deoxygenated hemoglobin per deciliter of blood is required before cyanosis is noted. Only 1.5 to 2 g methemoglobin per deciliter of blood is required for the same level of discoloration. This is because the M hemoglobins have unique visible spectra, and the blood of affected subjects has a characteristic "chocolate-brown" appearance.

The inheritance of the M hemoglobins is said to be "dominant," and that feature serves to distinguish it from congenital deficiencies of methemoglobin reductase ("recessive inheritance"). The heterozygote for an M hemoglobin has detectable clinical signs (e.g., cyanosis), while the heterozygote for methemoglobin reductase deficiency appears normal. M hemoglobins arising as mutations *de novo* have been observed [240]. Subjects carrying the α-substituted M hemoglobins are usually cyanotic at birth, while in carriers of the β-chain mutants, cyanosis does not appear until 6 months to 1 year of age [244]. This is because the synthesis of the β chain is not fully developed until 6 months after birth (Fig. 76-8).

Carriers of the M hemoglobins usually come to medical attention because of their color, although they are quite healthy. They are normally active unless they have been erroneously diagnosed as having congenital heart disease and their activity restricted.

In Japan, where a large number of patients with M hemoglobins have been studied, a clinical classification has been proposed which distinguishes between the α- and β-substituted variants [234]. The carriers of the α-substituted M hemoglobins are not anemic and are normal except for the presence of cyanosis. The carriers of the β-substituted variants have signs of mild hemolysis: anemia, splenomegaly, reticulocytosis, and hyperbilirubinemia. This classification is helpful only in a general sense because hemolysis in the β variants is variable [5, 246] and in some cases has been associated with oxidant drugs [244]. Increased oxygen affinity and reduced oxygen-carrying capacity could result in a compensatory increase in red blood cell mass in the carriers of α-chain variants, but insufficient evidence exists to prove the point. Thus, the clinical distinction between α and β variants is not clear-cut, but when coupled with the history of the time of onset of cyanosis after birth, it may have some validity.

Diagnosis

Although the M hemoglobins do not produce significant clinical consequences, diagnosis is important because of the seriousness of the alternative causes of cyanosis. These include congenital heart disease, methemoglobinemia due to red blood cell enzyme deficiency, and drug abuse (particularly phenacetin).

Confusion about diagnosis of these patients has led to unnecessary cardiac catheterization in at least one instance [245], and in another a woman was denied surgery for ovarian carcinoma and later died because of it [257]. A member of the family studied by Horlein and Weber was rejected from the military during the Franco-Prussian War because of cyanosis [2].

The clinical history reveals no exercise intolerance, as seen with congenital heart disease, and clubbing of the fingers is not found on examination. The blood appears chocolate-brown (in contrast with the purple color of deoxygenated normal blood) and remains so after mixing with air. Arterial oxygen tension is normal.

Measurement of methemoglobin by the widely used method of Evelyn and Malloy [258] leads to confusion. This method depends on the characteristic spectra of met- and cyanomethemoglobins, but in the M hemoglobins these spectra are altered (Fig. 76-16). Therefore, the amount of methemoglobin determined in this way can be normal or low, depending on the particular variant in question. In the red cell enzyme deficiencies, however, this method will always reveal a high level of methemoglobin.

Hemoglobin electrophoresis should be done in all cases, but the results can be difficult to interpret unless the hemoglobin has first been oxidized with potassium ferricyanide [240]. Abnormal bands are seen with the M hemoglobins. Exact identification of a particular hemoglobin variant must be done by peptide analysis, although examination of the spectrum and electron spin resonance patterns [259] can be helpful, if available.

Treatment

No treatment is indicated. The only consequences appear to be cosmetic annoyance and intermittent mild hemolysis in β-variant carriers. Hemolysis has never been reported to be a serious problem. Both methylene blue and ascorbic acid have been given to reduce the discoloration, but without success.

An Exception: Hemoglobin Kansas

A family has been discovered in which cyanosis was present in a 14-year-old boy who was normal except for mild exercise intolerance [260]. In this instance no methemoglobin was present, and the abnormality was found to be due to hemoglobin Kansas, G4(102)βAsn→Thr, a variant with exceedingly low oxygen affinity. Patients with hemoglobin Beth Israel, G4(102)βAsn→Ser, present a similar clinical syndrome [261]. These hemoglobins have been studied intensively, and the defect in their function can probably be attributed to markedly reduced oxygen affinity of the R conformer [204]. Thus, T-R transition occurs, but late in the oxygenation sequence relative to hemoglobin A. As a result, oxygen affinity and cooperativity are reduced [262, 263]. The stereochemical basis for these effects probably involves a disturbance at the $\alpha_1\beta_2$ interface, since G4(102)β forms the only hydrogen bond in that region in the oxy structure (see "Function of Normal Hemoglobin" earlier in this chapter).

POLYCYTHEMIA: HEMOGLOBINS WITH INCREASED OXYGEN AFFINITY

In 1965 a 78-year-old man came to the medical clinic of the Johns Hopkins Hospital because of chest pain. He was found to have a packed cell volume of 58 percent and an electrophoretically abnormal hemoglobin [264]. This hemoglobin was named *Chesapeake* after the area in which the man had spent his life. It was found to have a high affinity for oxygen and an amino acid substitution, Arg → Leu at position FG4(92), in the α chain [265]. Since the observation of hemoglobin Chesapeake, 28 additional examples of polycythemia caused by abnormal hemoglobins have been described (Table 76-13). Although these disorders are rare, they are clinically important because of the diagnoses with which they can be confused, physiologically important because they allow insight into the mechanism of oxygen delivery, and biochemically important because they confirm and extend the model for hemoglobin function.

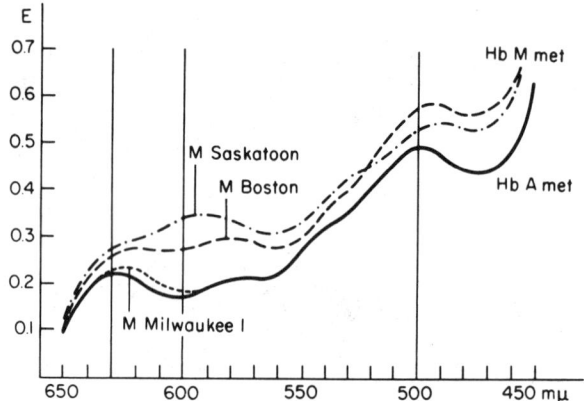

Figure 76-16 Methemoglobin spectra of hemolysates from subjects with some M hemoglobins. (*From Tonz [240].*)

Hemoglobins with high oxygen affinity (reduced P50, the oxygen tension at half saturation) lead to polycythemia because they do not give up as much oxygen as normal hemoglobin under the same conditions. For example, consider two blood samples, each with a total oxygen capacity of 20 ml O_2 per deciliter of blood, but with different P50 values, 28 mmHg and 14mmHg. The first sample will give up 50 percent of its oxygen or 10 ml per deciliter of blood at 28 mmHg tissue P_{O_2}, but for the second sample a tissue level of 14 mmHg must be reached before an identical amount will be delivered. Thus, the kidney in the latter patient must function at an abnormally low P_{O_2} and responds by elaborating the hormone erythropoietin, which stimulates bone marrow activity. The resulting increase in red blood cell mass (hence, greater oxygen capacity of the blood) means that more oxygen can be delivered to tissue sites per volume of blood, and the tissue hypoxia is partially relieved. This mechanism is only part of the response to hypoxia, but it is an important one [301].

Molecular Pathology

Allosteric Model The mutants that cause polycythemia because of increased oxygen affinity can be interpreted according to the two-state allosteric model. According to this model, cooperativity (as measured by Hill's parameter, n) is maximal at just greater than 50 percent saturation, corresponding to the point at which most of the molecules "switch" from the T to R quaternary conformation. If the point at which such a switch occurs is either earlier or later in the oxygenation sequence, the apparent n value will diminish. Thus, the relation of n to the allosteric constant L is a bell-shaped curve, with maximum value of about 3 for n [302, 303].

X-ray crystallographic studies of some mutants, such as hemoglobin Chesapeake [304], demonstrate that they favor the R conformation. Therefore, the T-R switch would occur very early in oxygenation, with resulting high oxygen affinity and loss of cooperativity. The prediciton that the oxygen affinity of hemoglobin Chesapeake can be lowered by adding allosteric effectors which tend to stabilize the T conformation (and therefore ensure cooperativity) has been demonstrated [269].

Mutation at the $\alpha_1\beta_2$ Interface Of the 28 mutants causing polycythemia, 14 occur at the $\alpha_1\beta_2$ interface. In both R and T states, this interface is made up of many nonpolar bonds, plus one hydrogen bond (Table 76-1). That bond is between Asp G1(99)β_2 and Tyr C7(42)α_1 in T and Asn G4(102)β_2 and

Table 76-13 High affinity hemoglobins associated with polycythemia

Name	Substitution	Electrophoresis 6.0	Electrophoresis 8.6	Blood Hb	Blood P50	Hemoglobin P50	Hemoglobin n	Bohr effect	DPG effect	References
α-Chain variants										
Sawara	A4(6)Asp→Ala	NA	Slow	NA	NA	↓	0	0	0	266
Chapel Hill	EF3(F4)Asp→Gly	NA	Slow	15.5	23(28)	0.9(1.5)	NA	NA	NA	267
Chesapeake	FG4(92)Arg→Leu	0	Fast	16.9(15.6)	20.3(23.8)	0.39(2.4)	1.22	0	0	265, 268, 269
J-Cape Town	FG4(92)Arg→Gln	NA	Fast	15.2(13.5)	↓	1.33(3.42)	2.23	0	NA	270, 271
β-Chain variants										
Olympia	B2(20)Val→Met	0	0	19.5(14.6)	18.6(26.8)	*	0	0	0	272
Malmö	FG4(97)His→Gln	0	0	18.9	↓	*	1.58	0	NA	273, 274
Wood	FG4(97)His→Leu	0	0	21.5	9(26)	3(11)	1.5	0	0	248
Kempsey	G1(99)Asp→Asn	NA	Slow	19.3(15.1)	13.5(33)	4(23)	↓	0	NA	275
Yakima	G1(99)Asp→Asn	NA	Slow	17.9(12.8)	12(26)	5(26)	1.0	0	NA	276, 277
Ypsilanti	G1(99)Asp→Tyr	NA	Slow	16.6	17(27)	NA	NA	NA	NA	278, 279
Brigham	G2(100)Pro→Leu	0	0	16.5	19(26)	NA	NA	0	0	280
British Columbia	G3(101)Glu→Lys	Slow	Slow	16.8	15.7	↓	↓	0	NA	281
Alberta	G3(101)Glu→Gly	NA	Slow	21.0	10.3	↓	↓	0	0	282
Potomac	G3(101)Glu→Asp	0	0	17.5	12.6(20)	↓	↓	0	0	283
Heathrow	G5(103)Phe→Leu	NA	0	17.2(13.3)	9.5(23)	NA	NA	NA	NA	284
San Diego	G11(109)Val→Met	0	0	17.3(14.1)	NA	NA	NA	0	0	285
Ty Gard	H2(124)Pro→Gln	NA	0	19.2	21(26)	NA	0	NA	NA	286
Ohio	H20(142)Ala→Asp	NA	NA	19.7	16.8(28)	↓	↓	0	0	287
Abruzzo	H21(143)His→Arg	NA	Slow	17.7(11.7)	NA	↓	0	0	0	288, 289
Little Rock	H21(143)His→Gln	Fast	0	NA	↓	1.9(5.2)	2.5–3	0	NA	290
Syracuse	H21(143)His→Pro	0	0	19.2–23.8	↓	0.35(3)	1.1	↓	↓	291
Andrew-Minneapolis	HC1(144)Lys→Asn	NA	Fast	19.8	15(30)	3.3(18.5)	2.4	↓	0	292
Bethesda	HC2(145)Tyr→His	Fast	0	19.3(16.9)	12.8(26.5)	0.18(3.9)	1.1	↓	↓	293
Rainier	HC2(145)Tyr→Cys	Slow	NA	16.8(11.8)	13(27)	0.18(2.38)	1.09	↓	0	294
Osler	HC2(145)Tyr→Asp	NA	Slow	17.6(13.8)	↓	0.14(3.10)	1.1	↓	↓	295–297
McKees Rocks	HC2(145)Tyr→Term	Fast	0	18.6(14.6)	9.8(26.3)	0.66(10)	1.04	↓	↓	76
Hiroshima	HC3(146)His→Asp	Slow	Fast	15.6(12.2)	5(10.3)	0.31(2.38)	1.4	↓	0	298
York	HC3(146)His→Asp	Fast	0	NA	NA	0.62(9.7)	1.8	↓	0	299
Cowtown	HC3(146)His→Leu	Fast	0	19.5	17.0	1.7(4.7)	0	↓	↓	300

NOTES: Normal control values, when available, are given in parentheses.
* Indicates that hemoglobin could not be isolated in pure form. NA means data not available. 0 means normal.

Asp G1(94)α_1 in R (Fig. 76-17). In hemoglobins Yakima, Kempsey, and Ypsilanti, replacement of Asp G1(99)β means that the hydrogen bond cannot form in the T structure. This shifts the equilibrium toward R. Increased oxygen affinity and decreased cooperativity are the result [305].

Substitutions in hemoglobins Chesapeake and J-Capetown occur at the same location in the α chain, but the oxygen affinity of the former is much higher than that of the latter. Erythrocytosis is definitely present in carriers of hemoglobin Chesapeake, but carriers of hemoglobin J-Capetown have hemoglobin levels only slightly higher than those of unaffected family members (Table 76-13). The crystallographic structure of hemoglobin Chesapeake shows mild disturbances in oxy but none in the deoxy states [304]. Therefore, its increased oxygen affinity is presumed to be due to stabilization of the R structure. The crystal structure of oxyhemoglobin J-Capetown has not been studied. Hemoglobin Malmo involves the β-chain amino acid homologous to that of hemoglobins Chesapeake and J-Capetown mutation (FG4). Its oxygen affinity is high also, but the details of the mechanism are not known.

C Terminus The mutants with highest oxygen affinities are those which affect the C-terminal region of the β chains. As

described earlier, the role of Tyr HC2 is extremely important in the R-T equilibrium (Fig. 76-5). When it is absent (hemoglobin McKees Rocks) or replaced by another residue (hemoglobins Bethesda, Rainier, and Osler), or when its function is influenced by nearby mutations (hemoglobins Abruzzo, Little Rock, Syracuse, Andrew-Minneapolis, Hiroshima, Cowtown, or York), the T conformation is destabilized. Consequently, oxygen affinity is high and cooperativity is low. This region of the molecule is also important in 2,3-DPG binding and the Bohr effect (see "Structure and Function of Normal Hemoglobin" earlier in this chapter). Thus, these hemoglobins all have reduced Bohr effects because the interchain salt bonds involving His HC3(146)β either are not formed at all or are weakened. DPG binding is reduced in several of these hemoglobins, but since other sites are also involved in its binding, this property is only partially reduced.

$\alpha_1\beta_1$ Interface Hemoglobin San Diego is interesting because it is the only mutation in the $\alpha_1\beta_1$ interface that results in high oxygen affinity and erythrocytosis. The stereochemical interpretation of its effects is that an important hydrogen bond at the interface [Asp H9(126)α_1-Tyr C1(35)β_1] is weakened as is a salt bond [Asp H9(126)α_1-Arg HC3(141)α_2], and a new

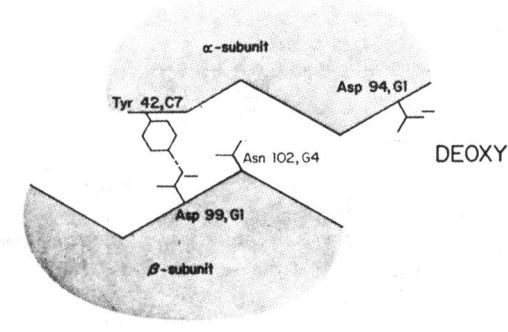

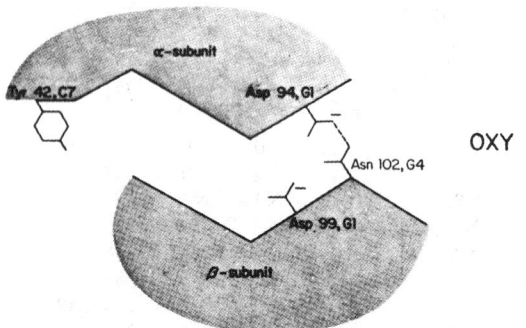

Figure 76-17 Changes at the $\alpha_1\beta_1$ contact on oxygenation. The contact "clicks" from one dovetailing area to another, involving a switch from one hydrogen bond to a second. The other bonds are nonpolar (see Table 76-1). (*From Morimoto et al. [305].*)

intrasubunit bond is formed [Arg H9(126)α_1-His G5(122)α_1]. The net result is thought to be a change in the tertiary structure which destabilizes the deoxy tetramer, resulting in high oxygen affinity and low cooperativity [306].

A Surface Mutation Hemoglobin Olympia would appear to be unique in that it has high oxygen affinity, but the site of its mutation does not correlate in any obvious way with its properties. The mutation, B2(20)β Val→Met, occurs on the surface of the β subunit, and it has been suggested that the effects of the alteration must somehow be propagated into the interior of the molecule [272].

Subunit Dissociation A number of mutants dissociate into $\alpha\beta$ subunits along the interface when they are oxygenated. This can lead to instability (see "Hemolysis: The Unstable Hemoglobins" earlier in this chapter), but it can also lead to increased oxygen affinity. The latter is so because $\alpha\beta$ subunits have "R" properties, and dissociation of oxy tetramers will pull the T-R equilibrium toward R. Thus, hemoglobins G Georgia and Rampa have slightly increased affinity [201]. Hemoglobin Richmond is an interesting example of the interaction of various effectors of oxygen affinity [202]. Its mutation, G4(102)β Asn→Lys occurs at the $\alpha_1\beta_2$ interface and results in increased dissociation to $\alpha\beta$ dimers, resulting in increased oxygen affinity. For reasons that are not clear, the dissociation is pH-dependent and greater at low pH. Thus, hydrogen ion both increases affinity by promoting dissociation and reduces affinity by stabilizing the T conformation (the Bohr effect). The net result is a markedly reduced dependence of oxygen affinity on pH. The α-chain residue with which

G4(102) interacts is G1(94)Asp (Fig. 76-18). Hemoglobin Titusville, G1(94)Asp→Asn, has similar properties [307].

High Affinity Unstable Hemoglobins Some mutant hemoglobins whose primary clinical consequence is hemolysis also have increased oxygen affinity (see "Hemolysis: The Unstable Hemoglobins"). Many of the changes affect the heme pocket [305]. For example, in hemoglobin Zurich, His E7(63)β is replaced by Arg, which cannot be accommodated in the heme pocket and therefore is excluded. This facilitates entry of oxygen into the heme pocket, and high oxygen affinity results. In hemoglobin Shepherd's Bush, the new Asp E8(74)β does not fit in the deoxy structure, and therefore the R-T equilibrium favors R. High oxygen affinity of hemoglobin Duarte indicates that the effect of the mutation, which is on the surface of the E helix, is probably transmitted into the heme pocket, facilitating entry of oxygen.

Clinical Aspects

Many of the patients with polycythemia due to abnormal hemoglobins have been under investigation for other possible diseases, such as polycythemia vera, tumors, or renal and cardiovascular disease. It is important to establish the diagnosis in these cases because misdiagnosis can lead to particularly harmful diagnostic or therapeutic procedures.

The normal range for hemoglobin concentration is 14 to 18 g per deciliter of blood for men and 12 to 16 g per deciliter of blood for women [198]. Therefore, an occasional normal subject will have a hemoglobin concentration at the upper limit of normal. At the same time, the hemoglobin value might be altered by a host of environmental and nutritional factors. Therefore, the next step is to establish the familial presence of polycythemia by measuring hemoglobin and hematocrit values of as many family members as possible. Heterozygotes for hemoglobins J-Capetown and Hiroshima have normal hemoglobin values, but they are significantly higher than those of noncarrier family members (Table 76-13). Many of the carriers of other high affinity hemoglobins have hemoglobin concentrations at the upper limit of normal. A familial pattern is helpful when present but not necessary; hemoglobin Bethesda is apparently a spontaneous mutation [293].

Differential Diagnosis

The high affinity hemoglobins are rare. Cigarette smoking (the presence of carboxyhemoglobin), cardiopulmonary disease, neoplasm (e.g., solid tumors of the kidney), polycythemia vera, and vascular malformations are much more common and should be considered first in all cases. Spurious polycythemia can be excluded by appropriate measurement of plasma volume and red blood cell mass.

Laboratory Diagnosis

When a high affinity hemoglobin is being considered, the critical test is measurement of blood oxygen affinity. If a red blood cell abnormality leads to polycythemia, it must do so by decreased oxygen delivery. Therefore, if blood oxygen affinity is normal, an abnormal hemoglobin as the *cause of polycythe-*

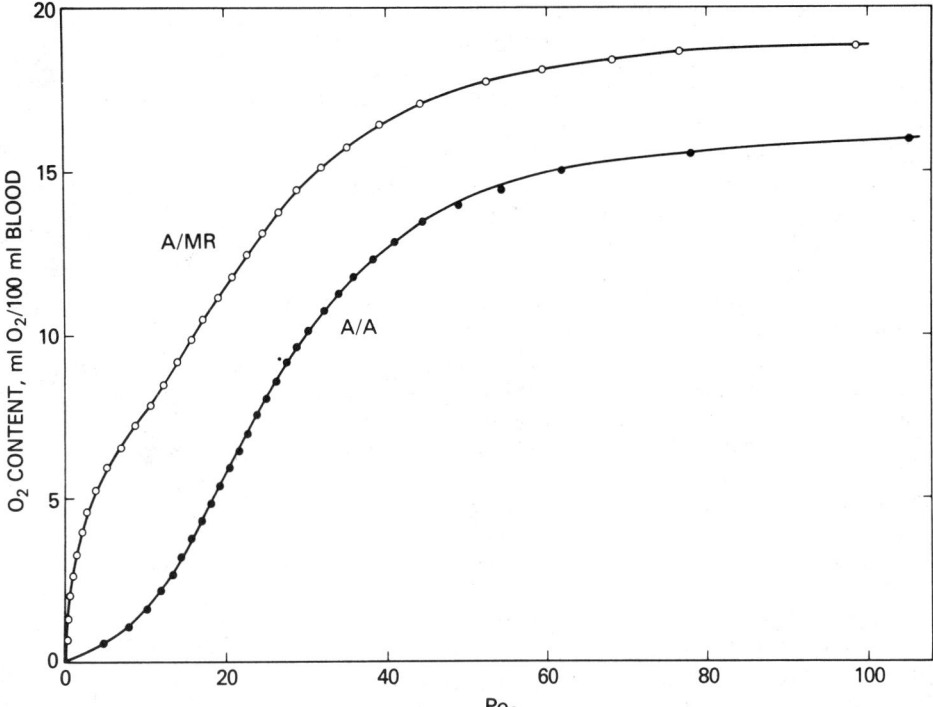

Figure 76-18 Blood OEC in a patient with a high affinity hemoglobin (McKees Rocks). Note that the McKees Rocks curve is biphasic: A component is present which oxygenates rapidly at low P_{O_2}. As P_{O_2} is increased, hemoglobin A oxygenates. The studies are done at pH 7.4, 37°C, P_{CO_2} 40 mmHg. (*From Winslow et al.* [76].)

mia has been excluded (note that an *abnormal hemoglobin* has not been excluded). Several methods are available for measurement of blood oxygen affinity. The new automated procedures [23] are the most convenient and accurate. The OEC must be determined under standard conditions (pH 7.4, P_{CO_2} 40 mmHg, 37°C), and a control sample from a subject who does not smoke should be examined at the same time. One must be aware that the presence of carboxyhemoglobin and methemoglobin can increase oxygen affinity, and they should be measured. Normal blood P50 is about 27 mmHg under these conditions, and a deviation of 2 to 3 mm from that value is probably significant. When a component is present which has increased oxygen affinity (Fig. 76-18), it leads to a biphasic oxygen equilibrium curve. The high affinity component oxygenates first, followed by hemoglobin A, and saturation is much higher than normal at low oxygen tensions.

If a biphasic curve such as the one in Fig. 76-18 is found, this is strong evidence for the presence of an abnormal hemoglobin. In order to exclude the possibility of the influence of intracellular pH or 2,3-DPG, the oxygen equilibrium of a hemolysate should also be measured. If the oxygen affinity of the hemolysate is abnormal, the structural alteration should be sought. If it is normal, an abnormality in 2,3-DPG metabolism or intraerythrocytic pH should be considered. Other possibilities might be the alteration of the 2,3-DPG-binding sites, which could lead to a relative increase of blood oxygen affinity in the presence of 2,3-DPG but to normal oxygen affinity in its absence. This is seen in blood which contains hemoglobin F [308] and in carriers of hemoglobins Providence [309] and Rahere [310].

Electrophoresis should always be done, but the results cannot be used to exclude the diagnosis of a hemoglobinopathy. Table 76-13 lists seven variants in which no electrophoretic abnormality could be detected. Three could be seen only by isoelectric focusing (hemoglobins Syracuse, Potomac, and Wood), and six were abnormal in one system but normal in another.

Treatment

Polycythemia due to a hemoglobinopathy appears to be benign. In a family with hemoglobin Malmo, sudden death in the fourth and fifth decades was reported, but this family also had hypercholesterolemia [273]. In a patient who is symptomatic with dizziness or headaches, cautious phlebotomy may be used as a trial, but one should keep in mind that polycythemia in these patients is a mechanism which compensates for reduced oxygen-delivering capacity. The main role of the physician in these cases is to protect the patient from treatment with antimetabolites, ^{32}P, or vigorous phlebotomy.

Genetic and Physiologic Considerations

Most of the high affinity variants that cause polycythemia are β-chain variants. As pointed out earlier ("Genetics of the Hemoglobins"), this might indicate that α variants are less fit. Moreover, the α-chain variants with extremely high affinity represent instances in which the oxygen affinity of a pregnant woman carrier would be higher than that of the fetus. Since, in all mammals, fetal blood has higher oxygen affinity than maternal blood, this would indeed be unusual. Nevertheless, no deleterious effects upon the fetus are known in these situations.

THE SICKLING DISORDERS

For centuries West Africans have been aware of a disease that caused relentless, gnawing pain in the long bones and joints. One afflicted family has been traced through nine generations to 1670 [311]. In 1910 a Chicago cardiologist, James Herrick, published the first account of "a large number of thin, elongated, sickle-shaped and crescent-shaped forms" in the blood smear of an ailing West Indian student [312]. Although he could have had little insight into the pathophysiology of the disease, he wrote that it was caused by "some unrecognized change in the composition of the corpuscle itself."

In 1915 Cook and Myer [313] thought the disease might be familial, but it was Emmel in 1917 who demonstrated that the red blood cells of the father of an affected male sickled after incubation for 24 h [314]. Hahn and Gillespie in 1927 [315] discovered that sickling was dependent on the removal of oxygen and that it was reversible. They also observed that sickling was promoted by high temperature and low pH. In the same year Hahn [316] proposed the term *sickle-cell trait* to describe the subjects who were not anemic but whose cells could be made to sickle in vitro. In 1932 Diggs [317] showed a quantitative difference between the rates and degree of erythrocyte sickling in subjects who were anemic (sickle-cell anemia) and those who were not (sickle-cell trait). Sherman, in 1940, suggested that this difference was due to an abnormality of the red cell [318].

Although Herrick, Hahn, and Sherman all thought the abnormality of sickle-cell anemia was located within the red cell, it remained for Pauling in 1949 to show that hemoglobin from subjects with sickle-cell anemia was electrophoretically altered and that cells from subjects with sickle-cell trait contained both the altered and the normal hemoglobins [3]. In 1956 Ingram localized the electrophoretic charge difference of sickle hemoglobin (hemoglobin S) to a small peptide fragment by his "fingerprinting" technique [4] and then demonstrated that valine had replaced glutamic acid at position 6 of the β chain of this hemoglobin (Fig. 76-19) [319].

Sickle-cell anemia is thus the prime example of a "molecular disease." A single amino acid substitution in the hemoglobin molecule leads to severe disease in homozygous individuals. Although understanding of genetic mechanisms grew explosively after the findings of Pauling, Ingram, and others, understanding of the manner in which this substitution causes disease has advanced painfully slowly. Nearly three decades after Pauling's paper was published, there still is no effective therapy for sickle-cell anemia.

Incidence and Genetics of the Sickling Syndromes

The S gene occurs throughout tropical Africa as well as in blacks in the United States and other countries to which Africans were exported during the slave trade. In addition, it is found in the Middle East and may occur in some Caucasians [320]. Lehmann has proposed that the gene arose in the Middle East among the Veddoids and spread from there into Africa and India [321]. There are approximately 50,000 patients with sickle-cell anemia in the United States. The other common syndromes that give rise to the sickling phenomenon are hemoglobin SC disease and hemoglobin S-thalassemia disease. The approximate frequencies of these disorders is given in Table 76-14. Less common sickling disorders will be discussed below.

In some parts of Africa, up to 45 percent of the population are carriers of the sickle-cell gene [320]. This extraordinarily high frequency may be due to a balanced polymorphism. Thus, the loss of the deleterious S gene in homozygotes is balanced by the selective advantage for the heterozygous state [323, 324].

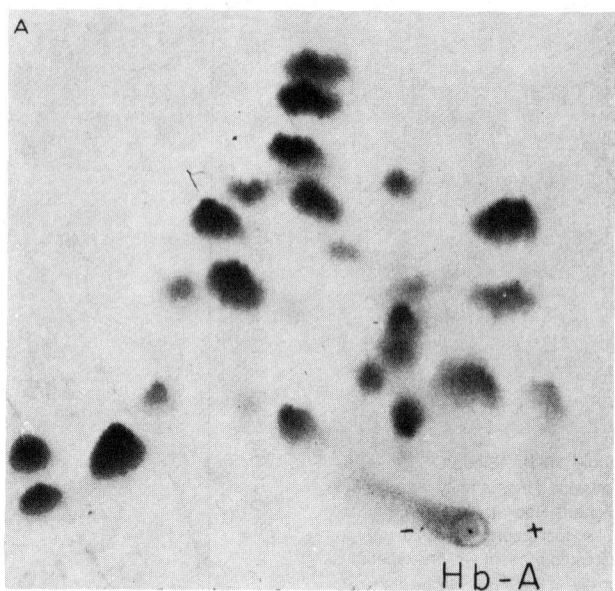

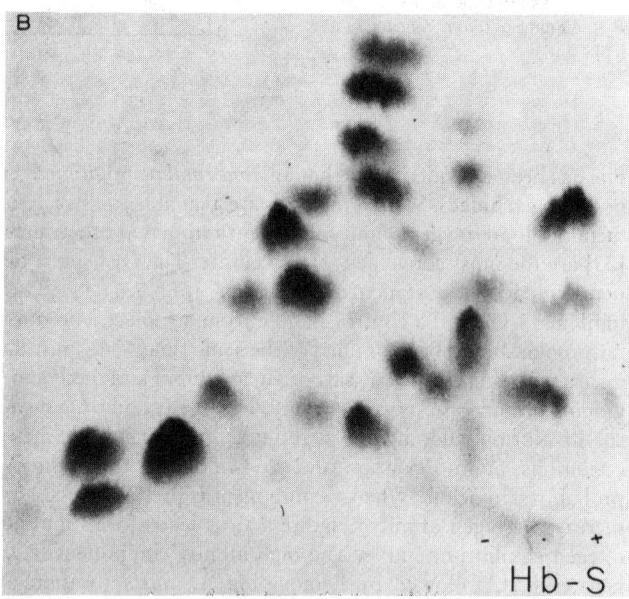

Figure 76-19 Fingerprints of hemoglobins A and S. The hemoglobin was digested with trypsin; the resulting peptides were separated by electrophoresis (*horizontal direction*) and then chromatography (*vertical direction*). Peptide β T-1 has been displaced in the hemoglobin S fingerprint because of the Glu→Val mutation (lower right portions of figures). (*From Baglioni [319].*)

This selective advantage appears to be resistance to *Plasmodium falciparum* malaria, which individuals with the sickle-cell trait enjoy [325, 326]. This resistance is due to an alteration of the interior of the red cell containing hemoglobin S which results from abnormal K+ transport across the cell membrane [329]. Inbreeding in some African tribes is high, and it is possible that other factors might also contribute to the balanced polymorphism [327]. About 8 percent of American Negroes are carriers [328], but whether a balanced polymorphism exists in America is uncertain.

Pathophysiology of Sickle-Cell Anemia

Structure of Hemoglobin S Fiber   The fibers of hemo-

Table 76-14 Frequency of some sickling disorders

Disorder	Frequency at birth (per 10^5)
SS	160
SC	120
S and β-thalassemia	60
S and HPFH	40

SOURCE: Motulsky [322].

globin S that cause the distortion of cells (i.e., sickling) are long, tubular structures. Each is made up of six filaments which turn about a hollow core with a pitch of about 3000Å (about 45 hemoglobin molecules). Alternatively, the fiber can be viewed as a series of "disks," each made up of six hemoglobin molecules. Each disk is slightly rotated with respect to its neighbors, giving rise to the rotation about the central core (Fig. 76-20) [330].

The means by which the substitution at A2(6)β Glu→Val leads to fiber formation is still unclear. These positions are on the surface of the molecule and are accessible for intermolecular contact. Since fiber formation does not occur in oxyhemoglobin S, the spatial changes associated with the R-T transition (see "Normal Hemoglobin Structure and Function" earlier in this chapter) must allow specific interaction between molecules. The strongest bonds between hemoglobin molecules and the fibers are along the axis of the filaments (vertical in Fig. 76-20), because when fibers disintegrate, they fray out as monofilaments [330]. There are several possibilities for the orientation of the A2(6)β valines [331], and there are probably multiple other stabilizing interactions among the hemoglobin S molecules [332].

Kinetics of Fiber Formation   Sickling of red cells is not instantaneous. When cells containing hemoglobin S are suddenly deoxygenated, a short delay occurs before the cells begin to transform gradually into the typical sickle and holly leaf shapes [333]. This cellular delay is probably related to a "molecular delay" [334] which is due to condensation of molecules prior to fiber formation, a situation similar to crystallization after nucleus formation (Fig. 76-21). The magnitude of this delay time is highly dependent on the hemoglobin concentration, and it is also sensitive to oxygen saturation and temperature. Although there is probably great variability in the capillary transit times among organs, among individuals, and in individuals under different conditions, these delay times may be of sufficient magnitude to be physiologically important.

Sickle-Cell Formation   When hemoglobin S polymerizes, cells assume their typical sickle shapes (Fig. 76-22). A given cell can undergo reversible sickling several times, but during each "sickle-unsickle" cycle, it probably loses a small portion of membrane [335]. This loss of membrane leads to the loss of cell water, an increase in intracellular hemoglobin concentration, and, consequently, an increased tendency to sickle. Finally, it is no longer able to unsickle and becomes an "irreversibly sickled cell."

Irreversibly sickled cells can be found by examining an oxygenated blood smear. The actual number varies widely among individuals, but it is remarkably consistent in an individual over time [336, 337]. The role of these cells in the pathophysiology of sickle-cell anemia is not yet clear, but it is known that they are associated with a short red blood cell survival [338] and contain the least amounts of hemoglobin F and 2,3-DPG

[339]. They have very low oxygen affinity [339], which is probably a result of their very high hemoglobin concentration [340].

The irreversibly sickled cells raise many questions of theoretical and clinical importance. Is their low oxygen affinity a result of an interaction between hemoglobin S gelling and oxygenation, or of low intracellular pH? Are they useful in delivering oxygen to tissue because of their low oxygen affinity, or are they unable to oxygenate in the pulmonary capillaries because of this low affinity? Are they more likely to occlude capillaries because of their shape, or are they excluded from such vessels because of their shape? Finally, what factors determine the rate at which a cell will become irreversibly sickled? The answers to these questions need to be known in order to understand the pathogenesis of sickle-cell anemia.

Molecular Interaction of Hemoglobin S with Other Hemoglobins   Hemoglobin F, when present in the cells of persons carrying hemoglobin S, is beneficial. Thus, a newborn with sickle-cell anemia is little affected by this disease until hemoglobin F synthesis declines. Similarly, subjects with hemoglobin S and HPFH (see "Genetics of the Hemoglobins" above), who have about 25 percent hemoglobin F, have a benign clinical course in spite of the presence of nearly 75 percent hemoglobin S in their red blood cells [341]. Moreover, there is variable elevation of hemoglobin F in red cells of patients with sickle-cell anemia, and it is thought that the unusually high levels (about 18 percent) found in the Middle East offer a protective effect. Homozygous S patients in that region have few symptoms [342]. Similarly, subjects with sickle-cell trait are essentially symptom-free. The explanation for these findings is that hemoglobins A and F dilute the hemoglobin S within the cell and do not enter into the fibers when the cells sickle [343].

Double heterozygotes for hemoglobins S and C [A2(6)βGlu

Figure 76-20 Structure of a hemoglobin S fiber. (From *Finch* [330].)

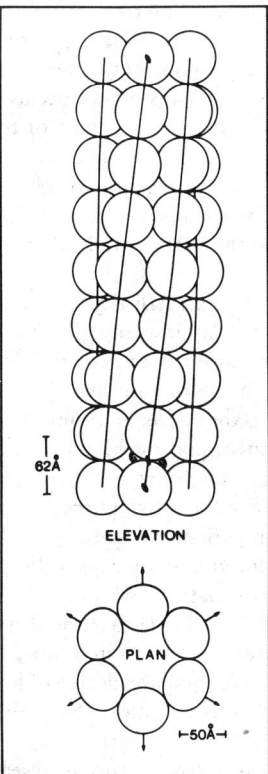

62Å

ELEVATION

PLAN

50Å

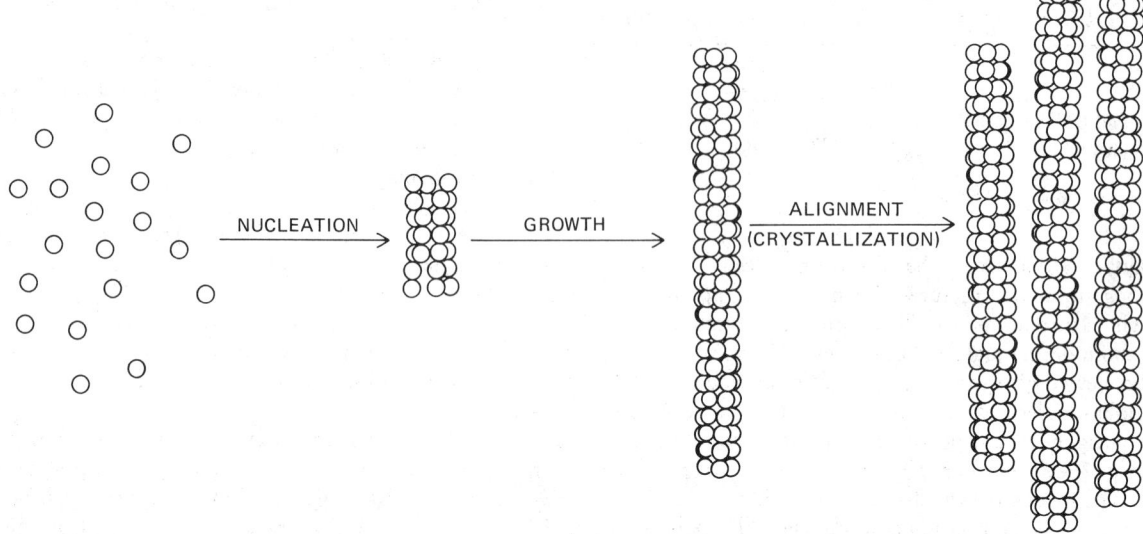

Figure 76-21 A possible mechanism for hemoglobin S fiber formation. Aggregation of molecules (about 30 molecules) is probably rate-limiting and accounts for the "delay time" observed in gelation and sickling. This mechanism is dependent on hemoglobin S concentration, among other factors. *(From Hofrichter et al. [334].)*

→Lys], D$_{Punjab}$ [GH4(121)βGlu→Gln], and O$_{Arab}$ [GH4(121) βGlu→Lys] do not usually have clinically significant symptoms, but these hemoglobins do copolymerize with hemoglobin S (344). An α-chain variant, hemoglobin Memphis [B4(23)αGlu→Gln], is of interest because, when it is present in a patient who is homozygous for the S gene, it seems to confer a relatively mild clinical course. The molecular basis for this observation is not clear, but it does raise the possibility that modification of the hemoglobin molecule at a site distant from β6 can have a beneficial effect [345, 346].

Pathogenesis of the Sickle Crisis   There are, unfortunately, large gaps in our knowledge between the molecular, cellular, and clinical levels in the pathogenesis of sickle-cell crises and organ damage. There is great variability among individuals in the degree of involvement of various organs and the severity of symptoms. A myriad of environmental factors probably modulates the molecular events outlined above, but the basic pathologic phenomenon appears to be deformation of red blood cells which leads to vasoocclusion, pain, and tissue death. Figure 76-23 outlines some of the important features of the pathogenesis of sickle-cell crises in Ghana [311]. In addition to simple vasoocclusion, red cells seem to adhere to endothelial cells abnormally [347], and this adherence may have importance in the pathogenesis of crisis.

Role of Blood Oxygen Affinity   Since polymerization of hemoglobin S occurs at low oxygen tensions, it probably depends on the presence of the deoxy (T) conformation (see "Normal Hemoglobin Structure and Function"). Therefore, any factor that shifts the R-T equilibrium should affect sickling [348]. It is well known that the blood of patients with sickle-cell anemia has very low oxygen affinity (Fig. 76-24) [344]. This does not serve an adaptive purpose, since oxygen transport is improved in patients after exchange transfusion, demonstrating that reduced flow of sickle cells is a limiting property [350]. Blood from patients with sickle cell anemia contains a high level of 2,3-DPG [351], but the degree of increase of oxygen affinity is out of proportion to the 2,3-DPG elevation. The factors which determine the degree of lowering of oxygen affinity in sickle cell anemia (intracellular pH, gelation, hemoglobin concentration, or other factors) are poorly understood but are the subject of intensive current research.

Clinical Description and Natural History

Until recently, the sickle-cell diseases have not usually been diagnosed until after the onset of "crisis." Now that newer methods for diagnosis are available, the early spectrum of clinical manifestations is more widely recognized [352]. Reticulocytosis, sickling, and the indicators of uncompensated hemolysis are seen by 10 to 12 weeks of age. By 5 to 6 months of age, splenomegaly is usually detectable. Typically, the spleen remains enlarged for about 6 to 8 years, when it shrinks because of scarring from repeated infarction. Concurrent with the enlargement of the spleen, there is generalized exuberant reticuloendothelial proliferation, including lymphadenopathy. Such proliferation is associated with the *sequestration crisis:* sudden massive enlargement of the liver and spleen with entrapment of red blood cells, and hemolysis.

The hand-foot syndrome is an initial complication in about one-third of patients with sickle-cell disease. This is swelling of the dorsum of the hands and feet with periostitis and osteolysis of the small bones. Infection is a serious problem in children with sickle-cell disease. Enlarged and functionally abnormal reticuloendothelial systems [353], decreased efficiency of polymorphonuclear leukocyte phagocytosis and chemotaxis [354], and diminished opsonization of pneumococci [355] probably all contribute to the unusual incidence of pneumococcal and *Salmonella* infections. Pneumococcal pneumonia and meningitis can lead to a cataclysmic downhill course and sudden death in children [352].

The *sickle-cell crisis* is a clinical entity which at present has no objective parameters. It is the sudden, dramatic change in the course of the disease which is accompanied by recognizable clinical signs and symptoms. Konotey-Ahulu [311] recognizes four main types of crisis in African patients: (1) Vasoocclusive *infarctive crisis.* This often has no warning and is characterized by sudden, severe pain, usually in the long bones but also in the joints or in the chest. The pain can mimic many other causes of pain such as pulmonary embolus or myocardial infarction. (2) *Hemolytic crisis:* Sudden hemolysis associated with underlying illness, such as viral illness. (3) *Sequestration syndrome:* Sudden massive enlargement of the liver and spleen with acute decrease in hematocrit. This occurs in patients who have functional spleens and is therefore seen most often in childhood. (4) *Aplastic or hypoplastic crisis:* Very low reticulocyte counts in the face of hemolysis. This is usually associated with underlying infection and may be a feature of the other types of crisis listed above. This classification is necessarily arbitrary, since there is often considerable overlap between the types of crisis.

Other Sickling Disorders

Milner [356] lists the known genetic disorders in which the sickling phenomenon can be demonstrated. Homozygous sickle-cell disease, hemoglobin SC disease, and S thalassemia are relatively common, but most of the others are rare. They consist of instances in which the affected individuals are double heterozygotes with two abnormal hemoglobins, one of which is S.

Hemoglobin SC Disease Hemoglobin SC disease is the second most frequent sickling disorder. Its clinical manifestations are qualitatively similar to those of sickle-cell anemia but quantitatively less severe. Because hemolysis is milder in hemoglobin SC subjects, their hematocrits, and therefore blood viscosity, tend to be higher than corresponding values in sickle-cell anemia. This leads to the predominance of certain complications which are related to blood viscosity: aseptic necrosis of the femoral heads, retinal hemorrhages, acute pulmonary episodes, and hematuria [356]. Patients with hemoglobin SC disease have mild anemia, but diagnosis is often not made until adulthood. The commonest complaint is musculoskeletal pain, often localized in the joints. The spleen is frequently palpable, but icterus is usually absent. Target cells are common in the blood smear, but sickled forms also appear. There is no specific treatment, but phlebotomy has been employed to reduce blood viscosity in patients in whom retinal hemorrhage is considered a high risk.

Hemoglobin S and β Thalassemia The doubly heterozygous state for hemoglobin S and β thalassemia can be either very mild or as severe as sickle-cell anemia. In general, the clinical manifestations parallel the amount of hemoglobin A present. Those with no hemoglobin A can be severely affected, while those with 20 to 30 percent hemoglobin A are intermediate between sickle-cell trait and sickle-cell anemia. Patients with hemoglobin β° thalassemia can resemble those with sickle-cell anemia, and the differentiation between the two disorders can be difficult. A complete family study is always indicated. In black patients, splenomegaly is present in about 60 percent of cases, regardless of whether hemoglobin A is present [356]. Most have symptoms relating to the spleen, and sequestration crises are common. Splenectomy is sometimes indicated for such patients.

Hemoglobins S and HPFH Double heterozygotes for hemoglobins S and HPFH (see Chap. 77, "The Thalassemias") have about 80 percent hemoglobin S and 20 percent hemoglobin F. In spite of the high amount of hemoglobin S, these subjects are usually asymptomatic, although splenomegaly and occasional painful crises have been reported in Africans [357]. The life span of their cells is normal when infused into normal recipients [85]. A presumed explanation for this protective effect is that hemoglobin F is evenly distributed among cells because it arises from a genetic deletion. In contrast, the patient with homozygous hemoglobin S with elevated hemoglobin F has hemoglobin F unevenly distributed among the cells, thereby affording protection for only a portion of them. This heterogeneous distribution is not completely understood but serves as an important tool for distinguishing between the two disorders.

Diagnosis of the Sickling Disorders

Exact diagnosis of the sickling disorders is important because of the implications for medical care and genetic counseling. Despite popular exposure to the consequences of sickle-cell anemia and trait, confusion persists among the public as to their difference. Moreover, distinction from the many other sickling disorders can be difficult. The clinical features given above can be regarded only as generalizations because the range in clinical involvement is astonishingly wide.

Electrophoresis Hemoglobin electrophoresis should be done in any case in which a hemoglobinopathy is suspected. This is especially important in the sickling disorders because, in contrast with the unstable hemoglobins and those with altered oxygen affinity, all the known variants give rise to altered electrophoretic mobility. Cellulose acetate electrophoresis at pH 8.6 and agar-citrate electrophoresis at pH 6.2 are the most widely used methods, although starch gel has certain advantages when hemoglobin components are present in small amounts. Some common electrophoretic patterns are shown in Fig. 76-25 [358]. It should be noted that hemoglobins S and D_{Punjab} are indistinguishable on cellulose acetate, as are hemoglobins C, E, and O_{Arab}. All these hemoglobins are relatively common and can occur with hemoglobin S in double heterozygotes. They can be distinguished on agar-citrate.

Other Tests for Sickling Disorders The most reliable evidence for the presence of a sickling disorder is the direct visualization of sickled cells after the addition of sodium metabisulfite. By definition, the presence of hemoglobin S cannot definitely be established unless both sickling and its typical electrophoretic pattern have been obtained. For example, a patient with hemoglobin A/D_{Punjab} may erroneously be informed that he or she has sickle trait, unless his or her blood has been examined by the metabisulfite test. Recently, solubility tests for the presence of hemoglobin S have become popular. These tests rely on the decreased solubility of hemoglobin S in buffers of high phosphate concentrations and are especially useful for screening programs. There are pitfalls in all the tests [359]. Combined clinical, laboratory, and family studies are always necessary when diagnosis of sickling disorders is undertaken. Family studies are particularly useful, especially when the possibility of hemoglobin S and β° thalassemia is considered, or when the presence of a hemoglobin which migrates with hemoglobin S in electrophoresis is suspected.

Antenatal Diagnosis of Sickle-Cell Anemia The antenatal diagnosis of homozygous sickle-cell anemia would be of great importance for couples at risk because, with such knowledge, the parents could consider whether to continue their pregnancy [360]. Many couples at risk are presently discouraged from having any children, even though only one-fourth of

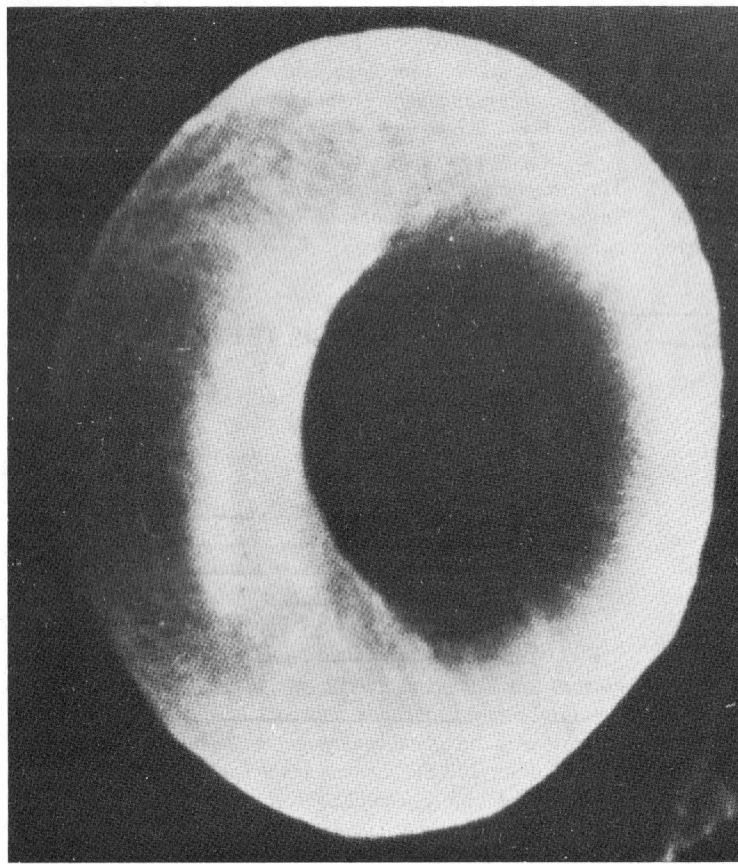

A

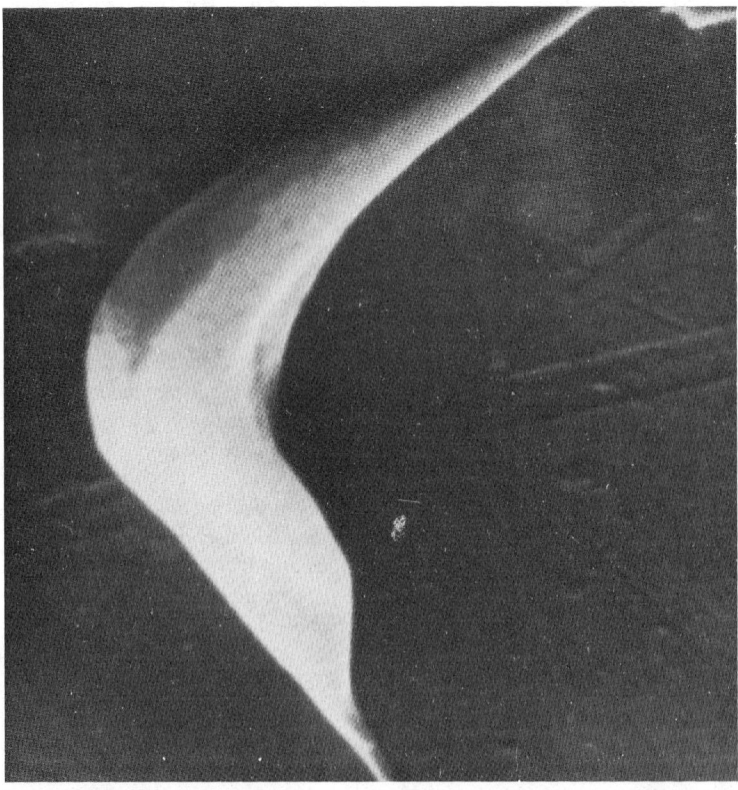

B

Figure 76-22   Scanning electron micrographs of normal and sickle red cells. *A.* A normal red cell magnified ×20,000. *B.* A deoxygenated sickle cell ×15,000. *C.* Oxygenated sickle cells ×2000. Note that some of them do not return to their normal shape. These are "irreversibly sickled cells." *D.* Deoxygenated sickle cells ×2000. (*Courtesy of Dr. Panpit Klug and Dr. Lawrence Lessin.*)

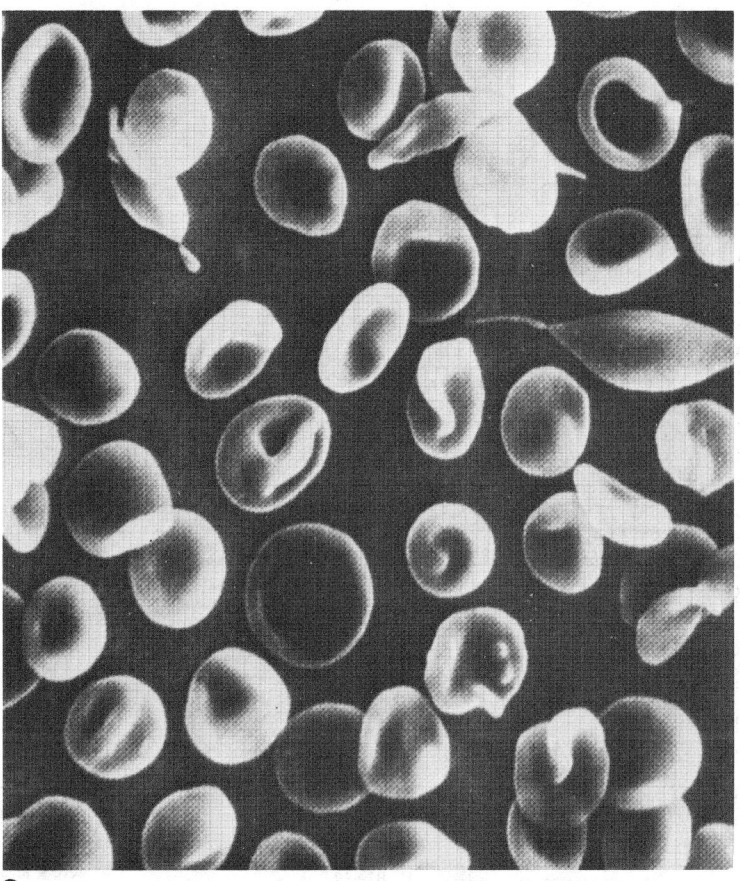

C

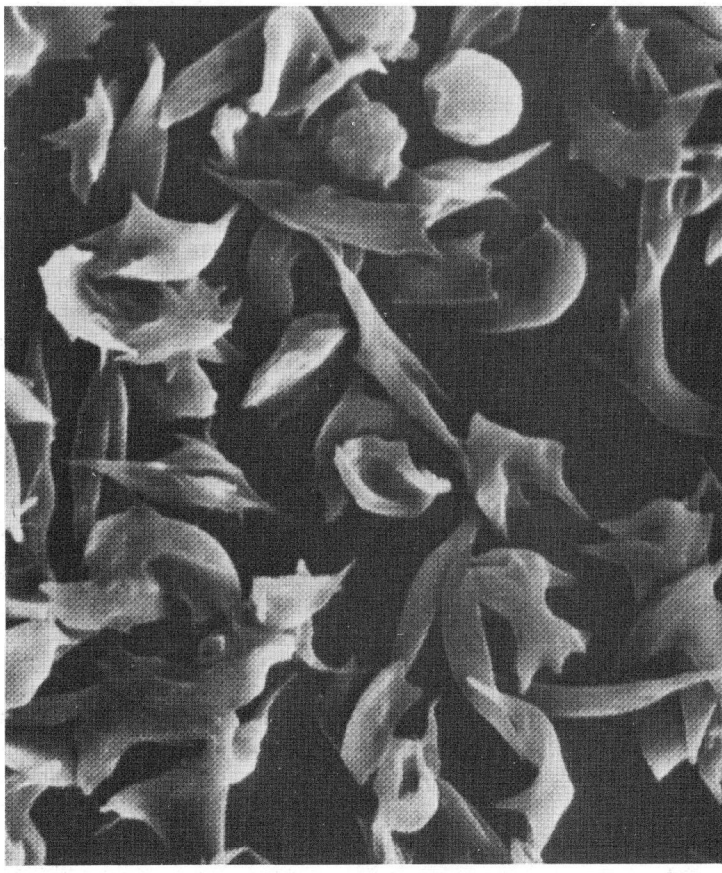

D

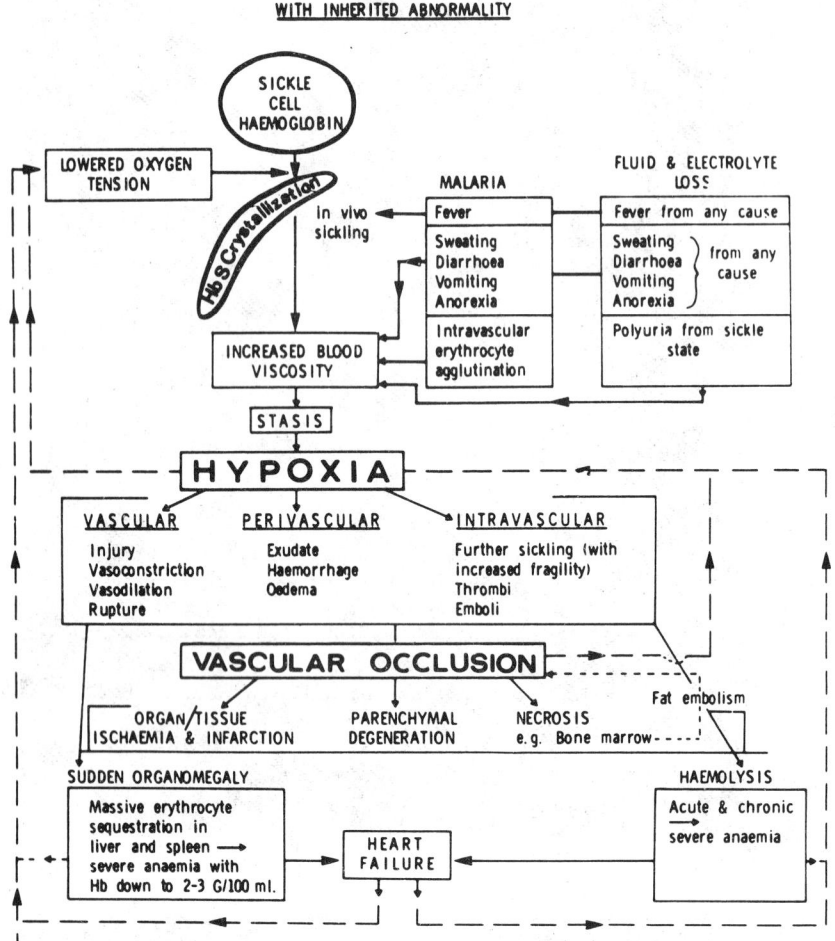

Figure 76-23 Some features of the pathogenesis of sickle-cell crises in Ghana. (*From Konotey-Ahulu* [*311*].)

the children from sickle-trait parents would be expected to have sickle-cell anemia. Antenatal diagnosis of sickle-cell anemia has not been accomplished, although it is theoretically possible. Synthesis of hemoglobins A and S can be detected by 13 weeks of gestation [361], and the difference between sickle-cell anemia and hemoglobin S and β⁺ thalassemia can probably be observed by 20 weeks [362].

Treatment

There is no effective treatment for sickle-cell anemia. Furthermore, much of the clinical research in modes of therapy has been hampered by the unpredictable nature of the disease. Many uncontrolled clinical trials of specific therapeutic agents have given early promise, only to be shown ineffective in the light of properly controlled observations. Crises can occur suddenly, and there appears to be little a patient can do to prevent them or to reduce their severity. In addition to recurrent crises, patients must frequently cope with the problems of chronic anemia, leg ulcers, priapism, aseptic necrosis of femoral and humeral heads, and infection, as well as the cosmetic problems of chronic jaundice. Furthermore, severe psychologic problems can develop in regard to school, work, pregnancy, and fear of death [363].

General Measures Good nutrition and personal hygiene, early diagnosis and treatment of infections, prophylaxis

against malaria where appropriate, and folic acid administration are measures which should be employed for any patient with chronic hemolysis [364]. While it has been fashionable to consider sickle-cell anemia a molecular disease, these simple measures of improving the patient's environmental and social well-being are important [357].

Crisis In the event of a crisis, it is of paramount importance to search for infection and to suspect bone marrow aplasia. The latter is indicated by low or absent reticulocytes and should be treated by transfusion until the marrow recovers. Such aplastic episodes may be megaloblastic but can also occur during infection or in pregnancy. Because red blood cell survival is short in sickle-cell anemia, the hematocrit can fall dramatically. Sequestration crises can also be associated with a rapid decrease in hematocrit and should be treated by transfusion.

Pain is probably the result of sickling in the microvasculature and infarction of tissue. Therefore, even if sickling during a crisis could be reversed, tissue damage and presumably pain might not be alleviated. During the pain crisis, supportive measures include hydration and analgesia, although oxygen administration may be helpful when arterial oxygenation is impaired. Sodium bicarbonate therapy may be of use [365], and alkalization with sodium citrate might decrease requirements for analgesia [366].

Other Problems Requiring Special Attention Leg

ulcers, priapism, pregnancy, and anesthesia all require special attention. Leg ulcers and priapism can be especially difficult to treat [320], but pregnancy and anesthesia can be managed when necessary by judicious transfusion or exchange transfusion [317].

Molecular Therapy   Urea was suggested as a possible therapeutic agent because of its known effect of inhibiting gelling of hemoglobin S in vitro. The rationale was that hydrophobic bonds are involved in hemoglobin S fiber formation and that urea would inhibit such bonding [368]. Although the blood urea levels which were required to achieve a therapeutic effect were too high to be practicable [369], the suggestion has stimulated a great flurry of effort in recent years in discovering ways to manipulate hemoglobin S structure and function in a beneficial way.

Sodium cyanate administration was another significant landmark [370] because the agent acts, in part, by increasing hemoglobin oxygen affinity and decreasing 2,3-DPG binding, thereby decreasing the likelihood of gelation at a given oxygen tension. The clinical results with the orally administered drug were disappointing [371], and neurologic complications appeared in a few patients [372]. Extracorporeal carbamylation of blood is still entertained as an approach with some utility [373], but limited venous access in patients with severest disease still poses an important obstacle.

Many antisickling agents are currently under extensive experimental investigation. These include zinc [374], alkylating agents [375], dimethyladipimidate [376], carbamyl phosphate [377], and androgens [378], among others. It must be kept clearly in mind that reduction of sickling by whatever means might increase red blood cell life span and improve the anemia of sickle-cell anemia, but at the same time it would be expected to increase blood viscosity, with ensuing impairment of the microcirculation. Similarly, an agent or treatment which increases blood oxygen affinity might also reduce tissue oxygen delivery, with resulting tissue hypoxia, cardiovascular stress, and erythropoietic stimulation.

In the light of these considerations, it is important that

Figure 76-24   Oxygen equilibrium curves in sickle-cell anemia. Curves for hemolysates of normal blood and blood containing sickle hemoglobin are very similar, but the whole blood curves are dramatically different. This is probably due partly to low intracellular pH of the sickle cells and partly to the effect of intracellular gelling, which does not occur at the low hemoglobin concentration found in the hemolysates or in normal cells. (*From Winslow* [349].)

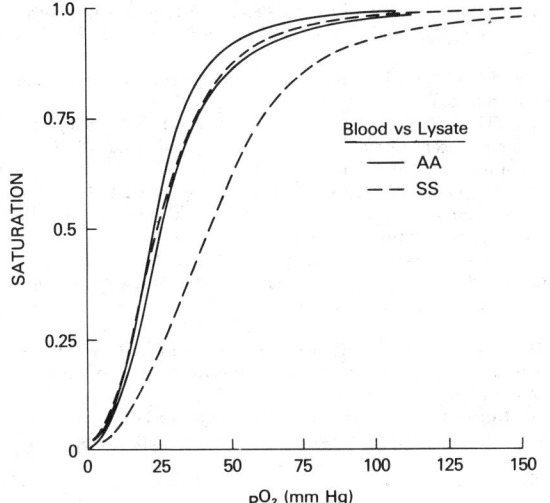

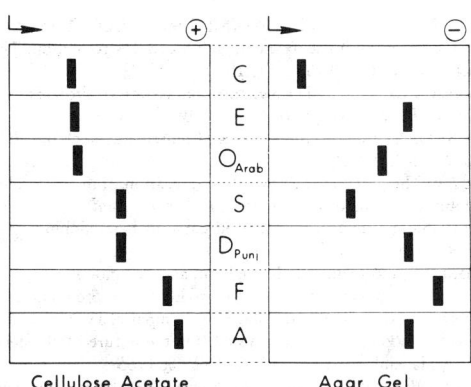

Figure 76-25   Electrophoretic patterns of some abnormal hemoglobins which are involved in the sickling disorders. Note that citrate-agar electrophoresis at pH 6.2 distinguishes between hemoglobins S and D_{Punjab} and between hemoglobins C, E, and O_{Arab}, which can be confused on cellulose acetate at pH 8.6. (*From Jamshid* [358].)

future research efforts not become completely preoccupied with the development of specific "agents" for clinical trials. A deeper understanding of the molecular, cellular, and physiologic mechanisms which operate in patients with sickle-cell anemia is essential because these mechanisms may serve adaptive ends. The alteration of any given variable may lead to far-reaching and unpredictable consequences. As Claude Bernard wrote, "All the vital mechanisms, however varied they may be, have only one object, that of preserving constant the conditions of life in the inner environment" [379].

THE FUTURE

Genetic Manipulation

The enormous progress made recently in the field of molecular genetics, resulting in part from the advent of recombinant DNA technology, has made gene therapy in humans a potential therapeutic approach. Indeed, an attempt at gene therapy was made in July 1980 when human β-globin genes, obtained by molecular cloning, were inserted into the bone marrow cells of two patients with β thalassemia. Unfortunately, considerable knowledge must still be gained, and several technical problems still overcome, before gene therapy in humans will be a viable alternative to present treatment regimens. For an analysis of the scientific, technical, and ethical considerations involved in gene therapy, see Ref. 380.

REFERENCES

1. OSLER W: A clinical lecture on erythraemia (polycythemia with cyanosis, maladie de Vaquez). *Lancet* Jan 18, 143, 1908
2. HORLEIN H, WEBER G: Chronic familial methemoglobinemia and a new modification of methemoglobin. *Dtsch Med Wochenschr* 73:475, 1948
3. PAULING R, ITANO HA, SINGER SJ, WELLS IC: Sickle cell anemia: A molecular disease. *Science* 110:543, 1949
4. INGRAM VM: Abnormal human hemoglobins. III. The chemical difference between normal and sickle cell hemoglobins. *Biochim Biophys Acta* 36:402, 1959
5. LEHMANN H, HUNTSMAN RG: *The Hemoglobinopathies*. New York, McGraw-Hill, 1972, p 1401
6. BOLTON W, PERUTZ MF: Three dimensional fourier synthesis of horse deoxyhaemoglobin at 2.8 Å resolution. *Nature (Lond)* 228:551, 1970

7. PERUTZ MF, MUIRHEAD H, COX JM, GOAMAN LCG: Three-dimensional fourier synthesis of horse oxyhemoglobin at 2.8 Å resolution: The atomic model. *Nature (Lond)* 219:131, 1968

8. DICKERSON RE, GEIS I: *The Structure and Action of Proteins.* New York, Harper & Row, 1961, pp 16 ff

9. HILL R: Oxygen dissociation curves of muscle haemoglobin. *Proc R Soc Lond, Ser B* 120:472, 1936

10. HILL AV: The possible effects of the aggregation of the molecules of haemoglobin on its dissociation curves. *J Physiol (Lond)*40:IV, 1910

11. ADAIR GS: The oxygen dissociation curve of hemoglobin. *J Biol Chem* 63:529, 1925

12. ANTONINI E, BRUNORI M: Hemoglobin and myoglobin in their reactions with ligands, in Neuberger A, Tatum EL (eds): *Frontiers of Biology.* Amsterdam, North-Holland Publishing Company, 1971, vol 21, p 381

13. MONOD J, WYMAN J, CHANGEAUX J: On the nature of allosteric transitions: A plausible model. *J Mol Biol* 12:88, 1965

14. PERUTZ MF: Stereochemistry of cooperative effects in haemoglobin. *Nature (Lond)* 228:726, 1970

15. CHARACHE S: Hemoglobins with altered oxygen affinity. *Clin Haematol* 3:358, 1974

16. BOHR C, HASSELBALCH K, KROGH A: Ueber einen in biologischer Beziehung wichtigen Einfluss, den die Kohlensaurespannung des Blutes auf dessen Sauerstoff-binding ubt. *Skand Arch Physiol* 16:402, 1904

17. KILMARTIN JV, ROSSI-BERNARDI L: Interaction of hemoglobin with hydrogen ions, carbon dioxide, and organic phosphates. *Physiol Rev* 53:836, 1973

18. KILMARTIN JV, HEWITT JA: The effect of removal of C-terminal residues on cooperative interactions in hemoglobin. *Cold Spring Harbor Symp Quant Biol* 36:311, 1971

19. BENESCH R, BENESCH RE, YU CI: Reciprocal binding of oxygen and diphosphoglycerate by human hemoglobin. *Proc Natl Acad Sci USA* 59:526, 1968

20. ARNONE A: X-ray diffraction study of binding of 2,3-diphosphoglycerate to human deoxyhemoglobin. *Nature (Lond)* 237:146, 1972

21. KILMARTIN JV, FOGG J, LUZZANA M, ROSSI-BERNARDI L: Role of the -aminogroups of the α and β chains of human hemoglobin in oxygen-linked binding of CO_2 *J Biol Chem* 248:7039, 1973

22. IMAI K, MORIMOTO H, KOTANI M, WATARI H, HIRATA W, KURODO M: Studies on the function of abnormal hemoglobins. I. An improved method for automatic measurement of the oxygen equilibrium curve of hemoglobin. *Biochim Biophys Acta* 200:189, 1970

23. ROSSI BERNARDI L, LUZZANA M, SAMAJA M, DAVI M, DARIVA-RICCI D, MINOLI J, SEATON B, BERGER RL: The continuous determination of the oxygen dissociation curve of whole blood. *Clin Chem* 21:1747, 1975

24. PARKHURST JT, GIBBON QH: The reaction of carbon monoxide with hemoglobin in solution, in erythrocytes, and in crystals. *J Biol Chem* 242:5762, 1967

25. ALLEN EH, SCHWEET RS: Synthesis of hemoglobin in a cell-free system. I. Properties of the complete system. *J Biol Chem*237:760, 1962

26. MILLER RL, SCHWEET R: Isolation of a protein fraction from reticulocyte ribosomes required for *de novo* synthesis of hemoglobin *Arch Biochem Biophys* 125:632, 1968

27. PRICHARD PM, GILBERT JM, SHAFRITZ DA, ANDERSON WF: Factors for the initiation of haemoglobin synthesis by rabbit reticulocyte ribosomes. *Nature* 226:511, 1970

28. JAGUS R, ANDERSON WF, SAFER B: The regulation of initiation of mammalian protein synthesis. *Prog Nucleic Acid Res & Mol Biol* 25:127, 1981

29. SMITH AE, MARCKER KA: Cytoplasmic methionine transfer RNAs from eukaryotes. *Nature* 226:607, 1970

30. LOCKARD RE, LINGREL JB: Identification of mouse hemoglobin messenger RNA. *Nature [New Biol]* 233:204, 1971

31. SAFER B, JAGUS R: New developments in the regulation of eIF-2. Manuscript in preparation

32. ANDERSON WF, BOSCH L, COHN WE, LODISH H, MERRICK WC, WEISSBACH H, WITTMANN HG, WOOL IG: International symposium on protein synthesis. Summary of Fogarty Center-NIH workshop held in Bethesda, MD on 18–20 October 1976. *FEBS Lett* 76:1, 1977

33. EMANUILVOV I, SABATINI DD, LAKE JA, FREIENSTEIN C: Localization of eukaryotic initiation factor 3 on native small ribosomal subunits. *Proc Natl Acad Sci USA* 75:1389, 1978

34. LODISH HF: Translational control of protein synthesis. *Annu Rev Biochem* 45:39, 1976

35. HUEHNS ER, DANCE N, BEAVEN GH, HECHT F, MOTULSKY AG: Human embryonic hemoglobins. *Cold Spring Harbor Symp Quant Biol* 29:327, 1964

36. HECHT F, JONES RT, KOLER RD: Newborn infants with hemoglobin Portland I: An indicator of α-chain deficiency. *Ann Hum Genet* 31:215, 1967

37. CAPP AL, RIGAS DA, JONES RT: Hemoglobin Portland I: A new human hemoglobin unique in structure. *Science* 157:65, 1967

38. TUCHINDA S: Oxygen dissociation curve of haemoglobin Portland. *FEBS Lett* 49:390, 1975

39. INGRAM VM: Gene evolution and the haemoglobins. *Nature (Lond)* 189:704, 1961

40. DAYHOFF MO: Atlas of protein sequence and structure. Silver Spring, Md, National Biomedical Research Foundation, 1972

41. RICCO G, MAZZA U, TURI RM, PICK PG, CAMASCHELLA C, SAGLIO G, BERNINI LF: Significance of a new type of human fetal hemoglobin carrying a replacement of isoleucine threonine at position 75 (E19) of the chain. *Hum Genet* 32:305, 1976

42. SMITH EW, TORBERT JV: Study of two abnormal hemoglobins with evidence for a new genetic locus for hemoglobin formation. *Bull Johns Hopkins Hosp* 102:38, 1958

43. BOYER SH, RUCKNAGEL DL, WEATHERALL DJ, WATSON-WILLIAMS EJ: Further evidence for linkage between the β and δ-loci governing haemoglobins and the population dynamics of linked genes. *Am J Hum Genet* 15:438, 1963

44. KENDALL AG, OJWANY PJ, SCHROEDER WF, HUISMAN THJ: Hemoglobin Kenya, the product of a δβ fusion gene: Studies of the family. *Am J Hum Genet* 25:548, 1973

45. LEHMANN H, CARRELL RW: Differences between α and β -chain mutants of human haemoglobin and between α and β -thalassemia: Possible duplication of the α-chain gene. *Br Med J* 4:748, 1968

46. HOLLAN SR, JONES RT, KOLER RD: Duplication of haemoglobin genes. *Biochimie* 54:639, 1972

47. DE JONG WW, MEERA KHAN P, BERNINI LF: Hemoglobin Koya Dora: High frequency of a chain termination mutant. *Am J Hum Genet* 27:81, 1975

48. OSTERTAG W, VON ERHENSTEIN G, CHARACHE S: Duplicated α-chain genes in Hopkins-2 haemoglobin of man and evidence for unequal crossing over between them. *Nature [New Biol]* 237:90: 1972

49. GAJDUSEK DC, GUIART J, KIRK RL, CARRELL RW, IRVINE D, KYNOCH PAM, LEHMANN H: Haemoglobin J Tongariki (α 115 alanine → aspartic acid): The first haemoglobin variant found in a Pacific (Melanesian) population. *J Med Genet* 4:1, 1967

50. POOKTRAKUL S, KEMATORN S, NA-NAKORN S, SUANPAN S: A new haemoglobin variant: Haemoglobin Anantharaj AII(A8)Lys→Glu. *Biochim Biophys Acta* 405:161, 1975

52. STEADMAN JH, YATES A, HUEHNS ER: Idiopathic Heinz body anaemia: Hb-Bristol (β 67(E11)Val→Asp). *Br J Haematol* 18:435, 1970

53. LEHMANN H, HUNTSMAN RG: *Man's Haemoglobins.* Philadelphia, Lippincott, 1974

54. BOOKCHIN RM, NAGEL RL, RANNEY HM: Structure and properties of hemoglobin C_Harlem: A human hemoglobin variant with amino acid substitutions in two residues of the β-polypeptide chain. *J Biol Chem* 242:248, 1967

55. GERALD PS, RATH CE: HbC_Georgetown:First abnormal hemoglobin due to two different mutations in the same gene. *J Clin Invest* 45:1012, 1966

56. ADAMS JG, HELLER P: Hemoglobin Arlington Park (β 6 Glu → Lys, β 95 Lys → Glu): An electrophoretically "silent" hemoglobin variant with two amino acid substitutions in the same polypeptide chain. *Blood* 42:990, 1973

57. GROOSENS M, GAREL MC, ANVINET J, BASSET P, FERREIRA-GOMES P, ROSA J, ARONS N: Hemoglobin C Ziguinchor α $_2β_2$ 6(A3)Glu → Val[58] (E2)Pro → Arg: The second sickling variant with amino acid substitutions in 2 residues of the β polypeptide chain. *FEBS Lett* 58:149, 1975

58. MOO-PENN WF, SCHMIDT RM, JUE DL, BECHTEL C, WRIGHT JM, HORNE MK, HAYCROFT GL, RORTH EF, NAGEL R: Hemoglobin S Travis: A sickling hemoglobin with two amino acid substitutions β6(A3) Glutamic Acid Valine and β142(H20) Alanine Valine]. *Europ J Biochem* 77:561, 1977

59. BLACKWELL RW, BOON WH, LIU CS, WENG MT: Hemoglobin J Singapore: β78 Asn → Asp; β79 Ala → Gly. *Biochim Biophys Acta* 278:482, 1972

60. CLEGG JB, WEATHERALL DJ, MILNER PF: Haemoglobin Constant Spring: A chain termination mutant. *Nature (Lond)* 234:337, 1971

61. HUISMAN THJ, WILSON JB, GRAVELY M, HUBBARD M: Hemoglobin Grady: The first example of a variant with elongated chains due to an insertion of residues. *Proc Natl Acad Sci USA* 71:3270, 1974

62. AKHAVEN MS, WINTER WP, ABRAMSON RK, RUCKNAGEL DL: Hemoglobin Wayne: A frameshift mutation detected in human hemoglobin alpha chains. *Proc Natl Acad Sci USA* 73:882, 1976

63. CLEGG JB, WEATHERALL DJ, CONTOPOLOU-GRIVA I, CAROUTSOS K, POUNGOURAS P, TSEVRENIS H: Haemoglobin Icaria: A new chain-termination mutant which causes α thalassemia. *Nature (Lond)* 251:245, 1974

64. BUNN HF, SCHMIDT GJ: Hemoglobin Cranston: An unstable variant having an elongated beta chain due to unequal crossover between two normal genes. *Ann Clin Res* 23:401A, 1975

65. FLATZ G, KINDERLERER JL, KILMARTIN JV, LEHMANN H: Haemoglobin Tak: A variant with additional residues at the end of the β-chains. *Lancet* 1:732, 1971

66. DEJONG WWW, WENT LN, BERNINI LF: Haemoglobin Leiden: Deletion of β6 or 7 glutamic acid. *Nature (Lond)* 220:788, 1968

67. COHEN-SOLAL M, BLOUQUIT Y, GATEL MC, THILLET J, GAILLARD L, CREYSSEL R, GIBAUD A, ROSA J: Hemoglobin Lyon (β 17-18 (A14-15) Lys-Val → 0). *Biochim Biophys Acta* 351:306, 1974

68. JONES RT, BRIMHALL B, HUISMAN THJ, KLEIHAUER E, BETKE K: Hemoglobin Freiburg: Abnormal hemoglobin due to deletion of a single amino acid residue. *Science* 154:1024, 1966

69. BROSTROM K: Unstable haemoglobin haemolytic anemia. *Acta Paediatr Scand* 65:397, 1976

70. SHIBATA S, MIHAJI T, UEDA S, MATSUOKA M, IUCHI I, YAMADA K, SHINKAI N: Hemoglobin Tochigi (beta 56-59 deleted): A new unstable hemoglobin discovered in a Japanese family. *Proc Jap Acad* 46:440, 1970

71. WAJCMAN H, LABIE D, SCHAPIRA G: Two new hemoglobin variants with deletion: Hemoglobin Tours: Thr β 87(F3) deleted and hemoglobin St. Antoine: Gly-Leu β 74-75 (E18-19) deleted: Consequences for oxygen affinity and protein stability. *Biochim Biophys Acta* 295:495, 1973

72. NEWMAN MV, ADAMS JG III, MORRISON WT, IYER F, STEINBERG MH: Hb Vicksburg: A low yield variant which mimics the phenotype of β-thalassemia. *Clin Res* 27:745A, 1979

73. BRADLEY TB, WOHL RC, RIEDER RF: Hemoglobin Gun Hill: Deletion of five amino acid residues and impaired heme-globin binding. *Science* 157:1581, 1967

74. LUTCHER CL, WILSON TB, GRAVELY ME, STEVENS PD, CHEN CJ, LINDERMAN JG, WONG SC, MILLER A, GOTTLIEB M, HUISMAN THJ: Hb Leslie: An unstable hemoglobin due to deletion of glutamyl residue 131(H9) occurring in association with β°-thalassemia, Hb C, and Hb S. *Blood* 47:99, 1976

75. NOZARI G, RAHBAR S, LEHMANN H: Haemoglobin Coventry (β 141 deleted) in Iran. *FEBS Lett* 95:88, 1978

76. WINSLOW RM, SWENBERG ML, GROSS E, CHERVENICK P, BUCHMAN RR, ANDERSON WF: Hemoglobin McKees Rocks (α₂β₂ 145 Tyr→Term): A human "nonsense" mutation leading to a shortened β chain. *J Clin Invest* 57:772, 1976

77. FORGET BA, BALTIMORE D, BENZ EJ JR, HOUSMAN D, LEBOWITZ P, MAROTTA CA, MCCAFFREY RP, SKOULTCHI A, SWERDLOW DS, VERMA IM, WEISSMAN SM: Globin messenger RNA in the thalassemia syndromes. *Ann NY Acad Sci* 232:76, 1974

78. GALLY JA, EDELMAN GM: The genetic control of immunoglobulin synthesis. *Annu Rev Genet* 6:32, 1972

79. BAGLIONI C: The fusion of two peptide chains in hemoglobin Lepore and its interpretation as a genetic deletion. *Proc Natl Acad Sci USA* 48:1880, 1962

80. BARNABAS J, MULLER CJ: Haemoglobin-Lepore Hollandia. *Nature (Lond)* 194:931, 1962

81. OSTERTAG W, SMITH EW: Hemoglobin-Lepore Baltimore: A third type of δβ crossover (δ 50, β 86). *Eur J Biochem* 10:371, 1969

82. YANASE T, HANADA M, SEITA M, OHYA I, OHTA Y, IMAMURA T, FUJIMARA T, KAWASAKI K, YAMUOKA K: Molecular basis of morbidity: From a series of studies of hemoglobinopathies in western Japan. *Jap J Hum Genet* 13:40, 1968

83. LEHMANN H, CHARLESWORTH D: Observations on haemoglobin P. (Congo type). *Biochem J* 119:43, 1970

84. BADR FM, LORKIN PA, LEHMANN H: Haemoglobin P-Nilotic: Containing a β-δ chain. *Nature [New Biol]* 242:107, 1973

85. CONLEY CL, WEATHERALL DJ, RICHARDSON SJ, SHEPARD MK, CHARACHE S: HPFH: A study of 79 affected persons in 15 Negro families in Baltimore. *Blood* 21:261, 1963

86. JONES RT, BRIMHALL B, HUEHNS ER, BARNICOT NA: Hemoglobin Sphakia: A delta variant of hemoglobin A2 from Crete. *Science* 151:1406, 1966

87. RANNEY HM, JACOBS AS, RAMOT B, BRADLEY TB JR: Hemoglobin NYU: A delta chain variant, α₂δ₂ 12 Lys. *J Clin Invest* 48:2057, 1969

88. BALL EW, MEYNELL MJ, BEALE D, KYNOCH P, LEHMANN H, STRETTON AOW: Haemoglobin A₂:α₂δ₂ 16 glycine→arginine. *Nature (London)* 209:1217, 1968

89. RIEDER RF, CLEGG JB, WEISS HJ, CHRISTY NP, RABINOWITZ R: Hemoglobin A2-Roosevelt: α₂δ₂ 20 Val→Glu: *Biochim Biophys Acta* 439:501, 1976

90. JONES RT, BRIMHALL B, HUISMAN TJJ: Chemical structure of hemoglobin A₂ Flatbush α₂δ₂ 22 Glu. *Ann Clin Res* 14:168, 1966

91. SHARMA RS, HARDING DL, WONG SC, WILSON JB, GRAVELY ME, HUISMAN THJ: A new δ chain variant: Haemoglobin-A₂Melbourne or α₂δ₂ Glu→Lys(CD2). *Biochim Biophys Acta* 359:233, 1974

92. MARIUZZI RA, MARINUCCI M, TENTORI L, BORGHESI V: Hb A2-Adria (δ 51 Pro Arg (D2)): A new δ-chain variant found in association with α-thalassemia in Polesine, Italy: New Istanbul. *Contrib Clin Sci* 12:176, 1978

93. ENG LIL, PRIBADA W, BOERMA FW, EFREMOV GD, WILSON JB, REYNOLDS CA, HUISMAN THJ: Hemoglobin A₂-Indonesia or α₂δ₂ 69(E13)Gly→Arg. *Biochim Biophys Acta* 229:335, 1971

94. SHARMA RS, WILLIAMS L, WILSON JB, HUISMAN THJ: Hemoglobin-A₂: Coburg or α₂β₂116 Arg→His (G18). *Biochim Biophys Acta* 393:373, 1975

95. DEJONG WWW, BERNINI LF: Haemoglobin Babinga (δ136) Glycine→Aspartic acid: A new delta chain varinat. *Nature (Lond)* 219:1360, 1968

96. LUAN ENG LI, KAMUZORA H, LEHMANN H: Haemoglobin F Malaysia: α₂δ₂ I (Nal) Glycine→Cysteine; 136 glycine. *J Med Genet* 11:25, 1974

97. AHERN EJ, WILTSHIRE BG, LEHMANN H: Further characterization of haemoglobin F Texas 185 Glutamic acid-Lysine; 136 alanine. *Biochim Biophys Acta* 271:61, 1972

98. LARKIN ILM, BAKER T, LORKIN PA, LEHMANN H, BLACK AJ, HUNTSMAN RG: Haemoglobin F Texas II (α₂δ₂ 6Glu→Lys): The second of the haemoglobin F Texas variants. *Br. J Haematol* 14:233, 1968

99. CARRELL RW, OWEN MC, ANDERSON R, BERRY E: Haemoglobin F Auckland G δ 7 Asp-Asn: Further evidence for multiple genes for the gamma chain. *Biochim Biophys Acta* 365:323, 1974

100. LOUKOPOULOS D, KALTSOYA A, FESSAS P: On the chemical abnromality of H "Alexandria" a fetal hemoglobin variant. *Blood* 33:114, 1969

101. BRENNAN SO, SMITH MB, CARRELL RW: Haemoglobin F Melbourne Gδ 16 Gly→Arg and Haemoglobin F Carlton Gδ 121 Glu⇌ys. *Biochim Biophys Acta* 490:452, 1977

102. LUAN ENG LI, WILTSHIRE BC, LEHMANN H: Structural identification of haemoglobin F Kuala Lumpur (α₂γ₂ 22(B4) Asp-Gly; 136A1a). *Biochim Biophys Acta* 322:224, 1973

103. AHERN EJ, JONES RT, BRIMHALL B, GRAY RH: Haemoglobin F Jamaica (γ 61 Lys→Glu; 136 Ala). *Br J Haematol* 18:369, 1970

104. AHERN E, HOLDER W, AHERN U, SERJEANT GR, SERJEANT BE, FORBES M, BRIMHALL B, JONES RT: Haemoglobin F Victoria Jubilee (α₂Aγ₂80 Asp-Tyr). *Biochim Biophys Acta* 393:188, 1975

105. SCHNEIDER RG, HAGGARD ME, GUSTAVESTON LP, BRIMHALL B, JONES RT: Genetic haemoglobin abnormalities in about 9000 black and 7000 white newborns: Haemoglobin F. Dickinson (Aγ His→Arg): A new variant. *Br. J Haematol* 28:515, 1974

106. OMURA H, MIYAJI T, SHIBATA S: Hemoglobin F Ube (108 Asn Lys), a new abnormal fetal hemoglobin found in a Japanese baby. *Chem Abstr* 83:266, 1975

107. CAUCHI MN, CLEGG JB, WEATHERALL DJ: Haemoglobin F (Malta): A new foetal hemoglobin variant with a high incidence in Maltese infants. *Nature (Lond)* 223:311, 1969

108. SACKER LS, BEALE D, BLACK AJ, HUNTSMAN RG, LEHMANN H, LORKIN PA: Haemoglobin F Hull (γ 121 Glutamic acid→Lysine), homologous with haemoglobins O and O Indonesia. *Br Med J* 3:531, 1967

109. BRENNAN SO, SMITH MD, CARRELL RW: Haemoglobin F Melbourne Gα 16 Gly→Arg and Haemoglobin F Carlton Gα 121 Glu→Lys. *Biochim Biophys Acta* 490:452, 1977

110. BRIMHALL B, VEDVICK TS, JONES RT, PALOMINO E, AHERN V: Haemoglobin F Port Royal (α₂γ₂ 124 Glu→Ala). *Br J Haematol* 27:313, 1973

111. LEE-POTTER JP, DEACON-SMITH RA, SIMPKISS MJ, KAMUZORA H, LEHAMANN H: A new cause of hemolytic anemia in the newborn: A description of an unstable fetal hemoglobin F. Poole, α₂γ₂130 Tryp-Gly. *J Clin Pathol* 28:317, 1975

112. HEINZ R: Morphologishe Veranderungen der rothen Blutkoperchen durch Gifte. *Virchows Arch [Pathol Anta]* 122:112, 1890

113. CATHIE LAB: Apparent idiopathic Heinz body anemia. *Great Ormond St J* 3:42, 1952

114. SCHMID R: Familial hemolytic anemia with erythrocyte inclusion bodies and a defect in pigment metabolism. *Blood* 14:991, 1958

115. SCOTT JL: Congenital hemolytic disease associated with red cell inclusion bodies, abnormal pigment metabolism and an electrophoretic hemoglobin abnormality. *Blood* 16:1239, 1960

116. GRIMES AJ, MEISLER A: Possible cause of Heinz bodies in congenital Heinz body anemia. *Nature (Lond)* 194:190, 1962

117. DACIE JV, GRIMES AJ, MEISLER A, STEINGOLD L, HEMSTED EH, BEAVEN GH, WHITE JC: Hereditary Heinz-body anemia: A report of studies on 5 patients with mild anemia. *Br J Haematol* 10:388, 1964

118. CARRELL RW, LEHMANN H, HUTCHISON HE: Haemoglobin Köln (β-98 Valine→Methionine): An unstable protein causing inclusion-body anaemia. *Nature (Lond)* 210:915, 1966

119. KOLER RD, JONES RT, BIGLEY RH, LITT M, LOURIEN E, BROOKS R, LAHEY ME, FOWLER R: Hemoglobin Casper: 106(G8)Leu→Pro: A contemporary mutation. *Am J Med* 55:549, 1973

120. KLEIHAUER EF, REYNOLDS CA, DOZY AM, WILSON JB, MOORES RR, BERENSON MP, WRIGHT CS, HUISMAN THJ: Hemoglobin Bibba or α₂ 136 Pro β₂: An unstable α-chain abnormal hemoglobin. *Biochim Biophys Acta* 154:220, 1968

121. HUISMAN THJ, BROWN AK, EFREMOV GD, WILSON JB, REYNOLDS CA, UY R, SMITH LL: Hemoglobin Savannah (B6(24)β-Glycine→Valine): An unstable variant causing anemia with inclusion bodies. *J Clin Invest* 50:650, 1971

122. HONIG GR, GREEN D, SHAMSUDDIN M, VIDA LN, MASON RG, GNARRA DJ, MAURER HS: Hemoglobin Abraham Lincoln, β 32(B14)Leucine→Pro-

line: An unstable variant producing severe hemolytic disease. *J Clin Invest* 52:1746, 1973

123. JACKSON JM, YATES A, HUEHNS ER: Haemoglobin Perth: β32 (B14) Leu→Pro: An unstable haemoglobin causing haemolysis. *Br J Haematol* 25:607, 1973

124. GAREL MC, BLOUQUIT Y, ROSA J, ARONS N: Hemoglobin Castilla β 32(B14) Leu→Arg: A new unstable variant producing severe hemolytic disease. *FEBS Lett* 58:145, 1975

125. DACIE JV, SHINTON NK, GAFFNEY PJ JR, CARRELL RW, LEHMANN H: Haemoglobin Hammersmith (β 42(CDI)Phe-Ser). *Nature (Lond)* 216:663, 1967

126. SCHNEIDER RG, SATOSHI U, ALPERIN JB, BRIMHALL B, JONES RT: Hemoglobin Sabine, beta 91(F7)Leu→Pro: An unstable variant causing severe anemia with inclusion bodies. *N Engl J Med* 280:739, 1969

127. GORDON-SMITH EC, DACIE JV, BLECHER TE, FRENCH EA, WILTSHIRE GB, LEHMANN H: Haemoglobin Nottingham, β FG5(98)Val→Gly: A new unstable haemoglobin producing severe hemolysis. *Proc R Soc Med* 66:507, 1973

128. ADAMS JG, BOXER LA, BAEHNER RL, FORGET BG, TSISTRAKIS GA, STEINBERG MH: Hemoglobin Indianapolis (β112 [G14] Arginine). An unstable β-chain variant producing the phenotype of several β-thalassemia. *J Clin Invest* 63, 1979

129. LORKIN PA, LEHMANN H, FAIRBANKS VF, BERGLUND G, LEONHARDT T: Two new pathological haemoglobins: Olmsted β 141 (H19) Leu→Arg and Malmö β 97 (FG4) His→Gln. *Biochem J* 119:68P, 1970

130. BERETTA A, PRATO V, GALLO E, LEHMANN H: Haemoglobin Torino: α 43(CD1) Phenylalanine→Valine. *Nature (Lond)* 217:1016, 1968

131. SUENSSON B, STRAND L: A Swedish family with hemolytic anaemia, Heinz bodies and an abnormal hemoglobin. *Scand J Haematol* 4:241, 1967

131a. IDELSON LI, DIDKOVSKY NA, FILIPPOVA AV, CASEY R, KYNOCH PAM, LEHMAN H: Haemoglobin Volga, β 27(B9) Ala→Asp: A new highly unstable haemoglobin with a suppressed charge. *FEBS Lett* 58:122, 1975

132. RUCKNAGEL DL, BRANDT NJ, SPENCER HH: Chain mutants of human hemoglobin contributing to the genetics of the α-chain locus. *Proc First Int Symp Hemoglobins*, Caracas, 1969

133. SANSONE G, CARRELL RW, LEHMANN H: Haemoglobin Genova: β28(B10) Leucine → Proline. *Nature (Lond)* 214:877, 1967

134. THILLET J, COHEN-SOLAL M, SELIGMAN M, ROSA J: Functional and physical chemical studies of hemoglobin St. Louis β28 (B10) Leu Gln. *J Clin Invest* 58:1098, 1976

135. CARRELL RW, OWEN MC: A new approach to haemoglobin variant identification: Haemoglobin Christchurch β71(E15) Phenylalanine → Serine. *Biochim Biophys Acta* 236:507, 1971

136. WHITE JM, BRAIN MC, LORKIN PA, LEHMANN H, SMITH M: Mild "unstable haemoglobin haemolytic anaemia" caused by haemoglobin Shepherd's Bush (β74(E18) Gly → Asp). *Nature (Lond)* 225:939, 1970

137. OPFELL RW, LORKIN PA, LEHMANN H: Hereditary nonspherocytic haemolytic anaemia with post-splenectomy inclusion bodies and pigmenturia caused by an unstable haemoglobin Santa Ana-β88(F4) Leucine → Proline. *J Med Genet* 5:292, 1968

138. HOLLENDER A, LORKIN PA, LEHMANN H, SUENSSON B: New unstable hemoglobin Boras: β88(F4)Leu-Arg. *Nature (Lond)* 222:953, 1969

139. ASKOY M, ERDEM S, EFREMOV AD: Hemoglobin Istanbul: Substitution of glutamine for histidine in a proximal histidine (F8(92)). *J Clin Invest* 51:2380, 1972

140. BEUZARD Y, COURVALIN J CL, COHEN-SOLAL M, GAREL MC, ROSA, J: Structural studies of hemoglobin St. Etienne β92(F8)His → Glu: A new abnormal hemoglobin with loss of proximal His and absence of heme on the β chains. *FEBS Lett* 27:76, 1972

141. ROSA J, BRIZARD CP, GIBAUD A, BEUZARD Y, COURVALIN J CL, COHEN-SOLAL M, GAREL MC, THILLET J: L'hemoglobine Saint-Etienne: α2Aβ292 His → Glu(F8): Une nouvelle variete d'hemoglobine instable avec absence d'heme sur les chain. *Nouv Rev Fr Hematol* 12:691, 1972

142. FINNEY R, CASEY R, LEHMANN H, WALKER W: Hb Newcastle: 92 (F8) His → Pro. *FEBS Lett* 60:435, 1975

143. PEDERSON PR, MCCURDY PR, WRIGHTSTONE RN, WILSON JB, SMITH LL, HUISMAN THJ: Hemoglobin Koln in a black: Pre and post splenectomy red cell survival (^{DF32}P and ^{51}Cr) and the pathogenesis of hemoglobin instability. *Blood* 42:771, 1973

144. JONES RT, KOLER RD, DUERST M, STOCKLER Z: Hemoglobin Casper G8 β106 Leu → Pro: Further evidence that hemoglobin mutations are not random, in Brewer GA (ed): *Hemoglobin and Red Cell Structure and Function. Adv Exp Med Biol* 28:79, 1971

145. HYDE RD, HALL MD, WILTSHIRE BG, LEHMANN H: Haemoglobin Southhampton, β106(68) Leu → Pro: An unstable variant producing severe hemolysis. *Lancet* 2:1170, 1972

146. LORKIN PA, PIETSCHMANN H, BRAUNSTEINER H, LEHMANN H: Structure of haemoglobin Wien β130(H8)Tyrosine → Aspartic acid: An unstable haemoglobin variant. *Acta Haematol (Basel)* 51:351, 1974

147. OHBA Y, MIYAJI T, MATSUOKA M, YOKOYAMA M, NUMAKURA H, NAGATA K, TAKEUE Y, IZUMI Y, SHIBATA S: Hemoglobin Hirosaki (A43[CE1]Phe-Leu): A new unstable variant. *Biochim Biophys Acta* 405:155, 1975

148. NAGEL RL, RANNEY HM, BRADLEY TB, JACOBS A, UDEM L: Hemoglobin L. Ferrara in a Jewish family associated with a hemolytic state in the propositus. *Blood* 34:157, 1969

149. OSTERTAG W, SMITH FW: Hemoglobin Sinai: A new α chain mutant 47 His. *Humangenetik* 6:377, 1968

150. VELLA F, ENG AC, MERRY CC: An αTpVI hemoglobin variant in Manitoba. *Clin Biochem* 3:125, 1970

151. ADAMS JG, HELLER P, ABRAMSON RK, VAITHIANATHAN T: Sulfonamide-induced hemolytic anemia and hemoglobin Hasharon. *Ann Intern Med* 137:1449, 1977

152. NIAGI OA, EFREMOV GD, NIKOLOV N, HURTER E JR, HUISMAN THJ: Hemoglobin-Strumica or $α_2$ $^{112(G19)His → Arg}$ $β_2$ [with an addendum: Hemoglobin J-Paris-1, $α_2$$^{12(A10)}$ Ala → Asp$β_2$, in the same population]. *Biochim Biophys Acta* 412:181, 1975

153. KENNEDY CC, BLUNDELL G, LORKIN PA, LANG A, LEHMANN H: Haemoglobin Belfast β15(A12)Tryptophan → Arginine: A new unstable haemoglobin variant. *Br Med J* 4:324, 1974

154. RANNEY HM, JACOBS AS, UDEM L, ZALUSKY R: Hemoglobin Riverdale-Bronx: An unstable hemoglobin resulting from the substitution of arginine for glycine at helical residue B6 of the β polypeptide chain. *Biochem Biophys Res Commun* 33:1004, 1960

155. SCHMIDT RM, BECHTEL KC, JOHNSON MH, THERRELL BL JR, MOO-PENN WF: Hemoglobin Lufkin: β29(b11) Gly → Asp. An unstable hemoglobin variant involving an internal amino acid residue. *Hemoglobin* 1:799, 1977

156. RIEDER RF, OSKI FA, CLEGG JB: Hemoglobin Philly (β35 Tyrosine → Phenylalanine): Studies in the molecular pathology of hemoglobin. *J Clin Invest* 48:1627, 1969

157. ASAKURA T, ADACHI K, WILEY JS, FUNG LW-M, HO C, KILMARTIN JV, PERUTZ MF: Structure and function of haemoglobin Philly (Tyr Cβ(35) → Phe) *J Mol Biol* 104:185, 1976

158. KEELING MM, OGDEN LL, WRIGHTSTONE RN, WILSON JB, REYNOLDS CA, KITCHENS JL, HUISMAN THJ: Hemoglobin Louisville (β42(CDI) Phe → Leu): An unstable variant causing mild hemolytic anemia. *J Clin Invest* 50:2395, 1971

159. BEUTLER E, LANG A, LEHMANN H: Hemoglobin Durate: $α_2β_2$$^{62(E6)Ala → Pro}$: A new unstable hemoglobin with increased oxygen affinity. *Blood* 43:527, 1974

160. MULLER CJ, KINGMA S: Haemoglobin Zurich $α_2β_2$63Arg. *Biochim Biophys Acta* 50:595, 1961

161. ROSA L, LABIE D, WAJCMAN H, BOIGNE JM, CABANNES R, BIERME R, RUFFIE J: Haemoglobin I Toulouse: β66(E10)Lys → Glu: A new abnormal hemoglobin with a mutation localized in the E10 porphyrin surrounding zone. *Nature (Lond)* 223:190, 1969

162. CARRELL RW, LEHMANN H, LORKIN PA, RAIK E, HUNTER E: Haemoglobin Sydney: β67(E11)Valine → Alanine: An emerging pattern of unstable haemoglobins. *Nature (Lond)* 215:626, 1967

163. KURACHI S, HERMODSON M, HORNUNG S, STAMATOYANNOPOULOS G: Structure of hemoglobin Seattle. *Nature [New Biol]* 243:275, 1973

164. HUEHNS ER, HECHT F, TOSHIDA A, STAMATOYANNOPOULOS G, HARTMAN J, MOTULSKY AG: Hemoglobin Seattle ($α_2β_2$^{F6Glu}): An unstable hemoglobin causing chronic hemolytic anemia. *Blood* 36:209, 1970

165. RIEDER RF, WOLF DJ, CLEGG JB, LEE SL: Rapid postsynthetic destruction of unstable hemoglobin Bushwick (β74Gly → Val)E18. *Nature (Lond)* 254:725, 1975

166. HUBBARD M, WINTON EF, LINDEMAN JG, DESSAUER PL, WILSON JB, WRIGHTSTONE RN, HUISMAN THJ: Hemoglobin Atlanta or $α_2β_2$$^{75Leu → Pro(E19)}$; an unstable variant found in several members of a Caucasian family. *Biochim Biophys Acta* 386:538, 1975

167. BRADLEY TB, WOHI RC, MURPHY SB, OSKI EA, BUNN HF: Properties of haemoglobin Bryn Mawr β^{85}Phe → Ser: A new spontaneous mutation producing an unstable haemoglobin with high oxygen affinity. *Blood* 40:947, 1972

168. DEWEINSTEIN BL, WHITE JM, WILTSHIRE BA, LEHMANN H: An unstable hemoglobin: Hb Buenos Aires beta 85 (FI) Phe → Ser. *Acta Haematol. (Basel)* 51:250, 1974

169. ADAMS JG III, PREZYWARA KP, SHAMSUDDIN M, HELLER P: Hemoglobin J. Altgeld Gardens (B92(F8) His-Asp): A new hemoglobin variant involving a substitution of the proximal histidine. *Proc Ash* abstract 87, p 75, 1975

170. TURNER JW, JONES RT, BRIMHALL B, DUVAL, MC, KOLER RD: Characterization of Hemoglobin Burke. [β107 (G9) Gly → Arg]. *Biochem Genet* 14:577, 1976

171. KING MAR, WILTSHIRE BG, LEHMANN H, MORIMOTO H: An unstable haemoglobin with reduced oxygen affinity: Hemoglobin Peterborough β111(G13) Val → Phe: Its interaction with normal haemoglobin and haemoglobin Lepore. *Br J Haematol* 22:125, 1972

172. OUTEIRINO J, CASY R, WHITE JM, LEHMANN H: Haemoglobin Madrid β115 (G17) Alanine → Proline: An unstable variant associated with haemolytic anemia. *Acta Haematol (Basel)* 52:53, 1974

173. BRENNAN SO, JONES KOA, CRETHAR L, ARNOLD BJ, FLEMING PJ, WINTERBOURNE CC: Haemoglobin North Shore, β134 Val → Glu. A new unstable haemoglobin. *Biochim Biophys Acta* 494:464, 1977

174. MARTI HR, WINTERHALTER KH, DI IORIO EE, LORKIN PA, LEHMANN H: Hb Altdorf β135 (H13) Ala → Pro: A new electrophoretically silent unstable haemoglobin variant from Switzerland. *FEBS Lett* 63:193, 1976

175. MARINUCCI M, MAVILO F, MASSA A, GABBIANELLI M, FONTANAROSA PO, CARMAGNA A, IGNESTI C, TENTORI L: A new abnormal hemoglobin: Hb Prato (α31 (B12) Arg-Ser). *Biochim Biophys Acta* 578:534, 1979

176. RAHBAR S, MAHDAVI N, NOWZARI G, MOSTAFAVI I: Haemoglobin Arya: α₂47(CD5), Asp Asn. *Biochim Biophys Acta* 386:525, 1975

177. ALBERTI R, MARIUZZI GM, ARTIBIONI I, BRUNORI F, TENTORI L: A new haemoglobin variant: J. Rovigo alpha α53(E2) Alanine → Aspartic acid. *Biochim Biophys Acta* 342:1, 1974

178. CROOKSTON JH, FARQUAHRSON HA, BEALE D, LEHMANN H: Hemoglobin Etobicoke: α84(F5) Serine replaced by arginine. *Can J Biochem* 47:143, 1969

179. ROSA J, OUDART JL, PAGNIER J, BELKHODJA O, BOIGNE JM, LABIE D: A new abnormal hemoglobin: α₂112 His → Gln: Hb Dakar. *Proc 12th Cong Int Soc Haematol NY* (abstract) p 72, 1968

180. MONN E, GAFFNEY PJ, LEHMANN H: Hemoglobin Sogn (β14 arginine): A new haemoglobin variant. *Scand J Haematol* 5:353, 1968

181. BEUZARD Y, BASET P, BRACONNIER F, GAMMAL H EL, MARTIN L, OUDARD JL, THILLET J, CABURI J: Hemoglobin Saki α₂β₂ 14(Leu-Pro(A11)): Structure and function. *Biochim Biophys Acta* 393:182, 1975

182. HUNT JA, INGRAM VM: Abnormal human hemoglobins. VI. The chemical difference between hemoglobins A and E. *Biochim Biophys Acta* 49:520, 1961

183. FRISCHER H, BOWMAN J: Hemoglobin E: An oxidatively unstable mutation. *J Lab Clin Med* 85:531, 1975

184. BRIMHALL B, JONES RT, BAUR EW, MOTULSKY AG: Structural characterization of hemoglobin Tacoma. *Biochemistry* 8:2125, 1969

185. CHARACHE S, BRIMHALL B, MILNER P, COBB L: Hemoglobin Okaloosa (β48(CD7) Leu → Arg): An unstable hemoglobin with decreased oxygen affinity. *J Clin Invest* 52:2858, 1973

186. BLOUQUIT Y, THILLET J, BEUZARD Y, VERNANT JP, DREYFUS B: Structural and functural studies of Hemoglobin J Calabria: β64 (E8) Gly → Asp. *Biochim Biophys Acta* 492:426, 1977

187. ADAMS JG: Hemoglobin Rush (beta 101(G3)Gln): A new unstable hemoglobin causing mild hemolytic anemia. *Blood* 43:261, 1974

188. BUNN HF, SCHMIDT GJ, HANEY DN, DLUHY RG: Hemoglobin Cranston, an unstable variant having an elongated β chain due to nonhomologous crossing over between two normal β chain genes. *Proc Natl Acad Sci USA* 72:3609, 1975

189. BRENNAN SO, TAURO GP, MELROSE W, CARRELL RW: Haemoglobin Port Phillip, α91 (FG3) Leu → Pro. A new unstable haemoglobin. *FEBS Lett* 81:115, 1977

190. WAJCMAN H, BELKHODJA O, LABIE D: Hb Steif: G1(94)α Asp → Tyr: A new α chain hemoglobin variant with substitution of the residue involved in a hydrogen bond between unlike subunits. *FEBS Lett* 27:298, 1972

191. IDELSON LI, DIDKOWSKY NI, CASEY N, LORKIN PA, LEHMANN H: New unstable hemoglobin (Hb-Moscva, β24(B6) Gly → Asp) found in the U.S.S.R. *Nature (Lond)* 249:768, 1974

192. BLOUQUIT Y, AROUS N, MADIADO PEA, GAREL MC: Hb Henri Mandor: β26 (B8) Glu → Val: A variant with a substitution localized at the same position as that of Hb E (β26 Glu-Lys). *FEBS Lett* 72:5, 1976

193. ALLAR CC, MOHONDAS N, WACJMAN H, KRISNNAMOORTHY R: Un cas d.Instabilite majeure de l.hemoglobine: L.hemoglobin Bicetre. *Nouv Rev Fr Hematol* 16:23, 1976

194. GRACON G, WAJEMAN H, LABIE D, COSSON A: A new unstable hemoglobin mutation in β98(FG5) Val → Ala: Hb Djelfa. *FEBS Lett* 58:238, 1970

195. KOHNE R, KLUG HP, KLEIHAUR E, VERSMOLD H, CH BENOHR, BRAUNITZER G: Structural and functional characteristics of Hb Tubingen: β106(G8) Leu-Gln. *FEBS Lett* 64:443, 1976

196. CLEGG JB, WEATHERALL DJ, BOON WB, MUSTAFA D: Two new haemoglobin variants involving proline substitution. *Nature (Lond)* 222:379, 1969

197. MARTINEZ G, LIMA F, COLOMBO B: Haemoglobin J Guantanamo (α₂β₂^128 (H6) Ala-Asp). A new fast unstable haemoglobin found in a Cuban family. *Biochim Biophys Acta* 491:1, 1977

198. WINTROBE MM: *Clinical Hematology,* 7th ed. Philadelphia, Lea & Febiger, 1974

199. RACHMILEWITZ EA: Denaturation of the normal and abnormal hemoglobin molecule. *Semin Hematol* 11:441, 1974

200. RIEDER RF: Human hemoglobin stability and instability: Molecular mechanisms and some clinical correlations. *Semin Hematol* 11:423, 1974

201. SMITH LL, PLESE CF, BARTON BP, CHARACHE S, WILSON JB, HUISMAN THJ: Subunit dissociation of the abnormal hemoglobin G. Georgia (α95-Leu(G2)β₂) and Rampa (α₂95Ser(G2)β₂). *J Biol Chem* 247:1433, 1972

202. EFFREMOV GD, HUISMAN THJ, SMITH LL, WILSON JB, KITCHENS JL, WRIGHTSTONE RN, ADAMS HR: Hemoglobin Richmond: A human hemoglobin which forms asymmetric hybrids with other hemoglobins. *J Biol Chem* 244:6105, 1969

203. WINSLOW RM, CHARACHE S: Hemoglobin Richmond: Subunit dissociation and oxygen equilibrium properties. *J Biol Chem* 250:6939, 1975

204. GIBSON OH, RIGGS A, IMAMURA T: Kinetic and equilibrium properties of hemoglobin Kansas. *J Biol Chem* 248:5976, 1973

205. BONAVENTURA J, RIGGS A: Hemoglobin Kansas: A human hemoglobin with a neutral amino acid substitution and an abnormal oxygen equilibrium. *J Biol Chem* 242:980, 1968

206. JENSEN W, OSKI FA, NATHAN DG, BUNN HF: Hemoglobin Syracuse (α₂β₂143(H21)His-Pro): A new high-affinity variant detected by special electrophoretic methods. *J Clin Invest* 55:469, 1975

207. ZINKHAM WH, HOUTCHENS RA, CAUGHEY WS: Carboxyhemoglobin levels in an unstable hemoglobin disorder (Hb Zurich): Effect on phenotypic expression. *Science* 209:406, 1980

208. JACOB HS: Mechanisms of Heinz body formation and attachment to red cell membrane. *Semin Hematol* 7:341, 1970

209. WINTERBOURN CC, CARRELL RW: The attachment of Heinz bodies to the red cell membrane. *Br J Haematol* 25:585, 1973

210. WITTENBERG JB, WITTENBERG BA, PEISACH J, BLUMBERG WE: On the state of the iron and the nature of the ligand in oxyhemoglobin. *Proc Natl Acad Sci USA* 67:1846, 1970

211. SCOTT EM: Congenital methemoglobinemia due to DPNH-diaphorase deficiency, in Beutler E (ed): *Hereditary Disorders of Erythrocyte Metabolism*. New York, Grune & Stratton, 1968, p 102

212. JAFFE ER, HSIEH HS: DPNH-methemoglobin reductase deficiency and hereditary methemoglobinemia. *Semin Hematol* 8:417, 1971

213. RACHMILEWITZ EA, HARARI E: Slow rate of haemichrome formation from oxidized hemoglobin Bart's (γ₄): A possible explanation for the unequal quantities of haemoglobins H (β₄) and Bart's in alpha-thalassemia. *Br J Haematol* 22:357, 1972

214. WINTERBOURN CC, CARRELL RW: Characterization of Heinz bodies in unstable haemoglobin haemolytic anaemia. *Nature (Lond)* 240:150, 1972

215. WINTERBOURN CC, CARRELL RW: Studies of hemoglobin denaturation and Heinz body formation in the unstable hemoglobins. *J Clin Invest* 54:678, 1974

216. MISRA HP, FRIDOVICH I: The generation of superoxide radical during autoxidation of hemoglobin. *J Biol Chem* 247:6960, 1972

217. JACOB H, WINTERHALTER K: Unstable hemoglobins: The role of heme loss in Heinz body formation. *Proc Natl Acad Sci USA* 65:697, 1970

218. WHITE JM: The synthesis of abnormal haemoglobins. *Semin Haematol* 4:116, 1971

219. BANK A, O'DONNELL JV, BRAVERMAN AS: Globin chain synthesis in heterozygotes for beta chain mutations. *J Lab Clin Med* 76:616, 1970

220. STEADMAN JH, YATES A, HUEHNS ER: Idiopathic Heinz body anemia: Hb Bristol (β67(E11)Val → Asp). *Br J Haematol* 18:435, 1970

221. WHITE JM, DACIE JV: *In vitro* synthesis of hemoglobin Hammersmith (CDI Phe → Ser). *Nature (Lond)* 225:860, 1970

222. SHAEFFER JR: Structure and synthesis of the unstable hemoglobin Sabine (α₂β₂ 91 Leu → Pro). *J Biol Chem* 248:7473, 1973

223. HUEHNS ER, STEADMAN JH: Peptide chain synthesis in unstable hemoglobin diseases. *Proc 13th Cong Int Soc Haematol* Munich, 1970, p 7

224. CHARACHE S, MONDZAC AM, GRESSNER U, GAYLE EC: Hemoglobin Hasharon (α₂ 47His(CD5)β₂): A hemoglobin found in low concentration. *J Clin Invest* 48:834, 1969

225. ADAMS JG III, WINTER WD, RUCKNAGEL DL, SPENCER HH: Biosynthesis of hemoglobin Ann Arbor: Evidence for catabolic and feedback regulations. *Science* 176:1427, 1972

226. RIEDER RF, JAMES GW III: Imbalance in α and β globin synthesis associated with a hemoglobinopathy. *J Clin Invest* 53:948, 1974

227. RIEDER RF: Synthesis of hemoglobin Gun Hill: Increased synthesis of the heme-free β^GH globin chain and subunit exchange with a free α chain pool. *J Clin Invest* 50:388, 1971

228. KREIMER-BIRNBAUM M, RUSNAK PA, BANNERMAN RM, GLASS U: Urinary pyrrole pigments in thalassemia and unstable hemoglobin diseases. *Ann NY Acad Sci* 232:283, 1974

229. WHITE JM: The unstable haemoglobin disorders, in Weatherall DJ (ed): *Clinics in Haematology: The Abnormal Hemoglobins*. London, Saunders, 1974, vol 3, p 333

230. BELLINGHAM AJ, HUEHNS ER: Compensation in haemolytic anaemias caused by abnormal haemoglobins. *Nature (Lond)* 218:924, 1968

231. BURKA ER: Determination of ribonucleic acid in nonnucleated erythroid cells. *J Lab Clin Med* 68:833, 1966

232. FRISCH B, LEWIS SM, SHERMAN D, WHITE JM, GORDON-SMITH EC: The ultrastructure of eyrthropoiesis in two haemoglobinopathies. *Br J Haematol* 28:109, 1974

233. CARRELL RW, KAY R: A simple method for the detection of unstable haemoglobins. *Br J Haematol* 23:615, 1972

234. SHIBATA S, MIYAJI T, INCHI I, OHBA Y, YAMAMOTO K: Hemoglobin M's of Japanese. *Bull Yamaguchi Med Sch* 14:141, 1967

235. Tamura A, Takahashi M: Study on the hereditary black blood disease. *Tohuku J Exp Med* 54:209, 1951

236. Singer K: Heredity hemolytic disorders associated with abnormal hemoglobins. *Am J Med* 18:633, 1955

237. Gerald PS, Efron ML: Chemical study of several varieties of hemoglobin M. *Proc Natl Acad Sci USA* 47:1758, 1961

238. Udem L, Ranney HM, Bunn HF, Pisciotta A: Some observations on the properties of hemoglobin M$_{Milwaukee-1}$. *J Mol Biol* 48:489, 1970

239. Hayashi A, Suzuki T, Shimizu A: Properties of hemoglobin M: Unequivalent nature of the α and β subunits in the hemoglobin molecule. *Biochim Biophys Acta* 168:262, 1968

240. Tonz O: The congenital methemoglobins. *Bibl Haematol* 28, 1968

241. Tamura A: Black blood disease. *Jap J Hum Genet* 9:183, 1964

242. Heller P, Weinstein HG, Yakulis VJ, Rosenthal IM: Hemoglobin M$_{Kankakee}$, a new variant hemoglobin M. *Blood* 20:287, 1962

243. Staven P, Stromme O, Lorkin PA, Lehmann H: Haemoglobin M Saskatoon with slight constant hemolysis, markedly increased by sulfonamides. *Scand J Haematol* 9:566, 1972

244. Farmer MB, Lehmann H, Raine DN: Two unrelated patients with congenital cyanosis due to a haemoglobinopathy M. *Lancet* 2:786, 1964

245. Josephson AM: A new variant of hemoglobin M disease: Hemoglobin M$_{Chicago}$. *J Lab Clin Med* 59:918, 1962

246. Efremov GD: Haemoglobin M Saskatoon and haemoglobin M Hyde Park in two Yugoslavian families. *Scand J Haematol* 13:48, 1974

247. Pisciotta AV, Ebbe SN, Hinz JE: Clinical and laboratory features of two variants of methemoglobin M disease. *J Lab Clin Med* 54:73, 1959

248. Taketa F, Huang YP, Libnoch JA, Dessel BH: Hemoglobin Wood α97 (FG4) His → Leu: A new high-oxygen affinity hemoglobin associated with familial erythrocytosis. *Biochim Biophys Acta* 400:340, 1975

249. Taketa F, Antholine WE, Mauk AG, Libnoch JA: Nitrosylhemoglobin Wood: Effects of inositol hexaphosphate on thiol reactivity and electron paramagnetic resonance spectrum. *Biochemistry* 14:3229, 1975

250. Pulsinelli PD, Perutz MF, Nagel RL: Structure of hemoglobin M$_{Boston}$: A variant with five-coordinated ferric heme. *Proc Natl Acad Sci USA* 70:3870, 1973

251. Perutz MF: Nature of haem-haem interaction. *Nature (New Biol)* 237:5357, 1972

252. Perutz MF, Pulsinelli PD, Ranney HM: Structure and subunit interaction of haemoglobin M Milwaukee. *Nature (New Biol)* 234:259, 1972

253. Anderson L: Intermediate structures of normal human hemoglobin: Methaemoglobin in the deoxy quaternary conformation. *J Mol Biol* 79:495, 1973

254. Greer J: Three dimensional structure of abnormal hemoglobin M, Hyde Park and Iwate. *J Mol Biol* 59:107, 1971

255. Mayer A, Ogawa S, Shulman RG, Gersonde GK: High-resolution proton nuclear magnetic resonance studies of the quaternary state of hemoglobin M Iwate. *J Mol Biol* 81:187, 1973

256. Lindstrom TR, Ho C, Pisciotta AV: Nuclear magnetic resonance studies of haemoglobin M Milwaukee. *Nature (New Biol)* 237:263, 1972

257. Baltzan DM, Sugarman H: Hereditary cyanosis. *Can Med Assoc J* 62:348, 1950

258. Evelyn K, Malloy H: Microdetermination of oxyhemoglobin, methemoglobin, and sulfhemoglobin in a single sample of blood. *J Biol Chem* 126:655, 1938

259. Hayashi A, Shimizu A, Yamamura Y, Watari H: Hemoglobins M: Identification of Iwate, Boston, and Saskatoon variants. *Science* 152:207, 1966

260. Reissmann KR, Ruth WE, Nomura T: A human hemoglobin with lowered oxygen affinity and impaired heme-heme interaction. *J Clin Invest* 40:1826, 1961

261. Nagel RL, Johnson J, Landau L, Brookchin RM, Harris M, Lynfield J: Hemoglobin Beth Israel (β102 Asn → Ser): A new mutant causing clinically apparent cyanosis. *Am Soc Hematol, Dallas* (abstract) 329, 1975

262. Greer J: Three-dimensional structure of abnormal human haemoglobins Kansas and Richmond. *J Mol Biol* 59:99, 1971

263. Hopfield TJ, Ogawa S, Shulman RG: The rate of carbon monoxide binding to hemoglobin Kansas. *Biochem Biophys Res Commun* 49:1480, 1972

264. Charache S: A manifestation of abnormal hemoglobins of man: Altered oxygen affinity. *Ann NY Acad Sci* 241:449, 1974

265. Charache S, Weatherall DJ, Clegg JB: Polycythemia associated with a hemoglobinopathy. *J Clin Invest* 45:813, 1966

266. Sasaki J, Imamura T, Sumida I, Yanase T, Ohya M: Increased oxygen affinity for hemoglobin Sawara: αA4(6) Aspartic Acid → Alanine. *Biochim Biophys Acta* 495:183, 1977

267. Orringer EP, Wilson JB, Huisman THJ: Hemoglobin Chapel Hill or α2 74 Asp Gly β2. *FEBS Lett* 65:297, 1976

268. Clegg JB, Naughton MA, Weatherall DJ: Abnormal human haemoglobins: Separation and characterization of the α and β chains by chromatography, and the determination of two new variants, HB Chesapeake and Hb-J (Bangkok). *J Mol Biol* 19:91, 1966

269. Imai K: Hemoglobin Chesapeake (92α, Arginine → Leucine): Precise measurements and analysis of oxygen equilibrium. *J Biol Chem* 249:7607, 1974

270. Botha MC, Beale D, Isaacs WA, Lehmann H: Haemoglobin J Cape Town α2$^{92 \text{ arginine} \rightarrow \text{glutamine}}$β2. *Nature (Lond)* 212:792, 1966

271. Nagel RL, Gibson QH, Jenkens T: Ligand binding in hemoglobin J. Cape Town *J Mol Biol* 58:643, 1971

272. Stamatoyannopoulos G, Nute PE, Adamson JW, Bellingham AJ, Funk D, Hornung S: Hemoglobin Olympia (α20 Valine → Methionine): An electrophoretically silent variant associated with high oxygen affinity and erythrocytosis. *J Clin Invest* 52:342, 1973

273. Fairbanks VF, Maldonado JE, Charache S, Boyer SH: Familial erythrocytosis due to an electrophoretically undetected hemoglobin with impaired oxygen dissociation (hemoglobin Malmo, α2β2$^{97(Gln)}$). *Mayo Clin Proc* 46:721, 1971

274. Boyer SH, Charache S, Fairbanks VF, Maldonado JE, Noyes A, Gayle E: Hb Malmo β-97(FG4)His → Glu: A cause of polycythemia. *J Clin Invest* 51:666, 1972

275. Reed CS, Hampson R, Gordon S, Jones RT, Novy MJ, Brimhall B, Edwards MJ, Koler RD: Erythrocytosis secondary to increased oxygen affinity of a mutant hemoglobin, hemoglobin Kempsey. *Blood* 31:623, 1968

276. Jones RT, Osgood EE, Brimhall B, Koler RD: Hemoglobin Yakima. I. Clinical and biochemical studies. *J Clin Invest* 46:1840, 1967

277. Novy MJ, Edwards MJ, Metcalfe J: Hb Yakima. II. Blood O$_2$ affinity associated with compensatory erythrocytosis and normal hemodynamics. *J Clin Invest* 46:1848, 1967

278. Glynn KP, Penner JA, Smith JR, Rucknagel DL: Familial erythrocytosis: Description of three families with hemoglobin Ypsilanti. *Ann Intern Med* 69:769, 1968

279. Rucknagel DL, Glynn KP, Smith JR: Hemoglobin Yspi. characterized by increased oxygen affinity, abnormal polymerization and erythremia. *Ann Clin Res* 15:270, 1967

280. Lokich JJ, Mahoney C, Bunn HF, Bruckheimer SM, Ranney H: Hemoglobin Brigham (α2^{A}β2$^{100Pro \rightarrow Leu}$): Hemoglobin variant associated with familial erythrocytosis. *J Clin Invest* 52:2060, 1973

281. Jones RT, Brimhall B, Gray G: Hemoglobin British Columbia (α2β2$^{101 (G3) Glu-Lys}$): A new variant with high oxygen affinity. *Hemoglobin* 1:171, 1976

282. Maut MJ, Salkie ML, Cope N, Appling F, Bolch K, Jayalakshmi M, Graveley M, Wilson JB, Huisman THJ: Hb Alberta or α2β2$^{101 (G3) Glu-Gly}$, a new high-oxygen affinity variant causing erythrocytosis. *Hemoglobin* 1:183, 1976

283. Charache S, Jacobson R, Brimhall B, Murphy EA, Hathaway P, Winslow R, Jones R, Roth C, Simkovich J: Hemoglobin Potomac (β101 Glu-Asp): Speculations about placental oxygen transport in carriers of high-affinity hemoglobins. *Blood* 51:331, 1978

284. White JM, Szur L, Gillis LDS, Lorkin PA, Lehmann H: Familial polycythaemia caused by a new haemoglobin variant: Hb Heathrow, β103(G5) Phenylalanine → Leucine. *Br Med J* iii:665, 1973

285. Nute PE, Stamatoyannopoulos G, Hermodson MA, Roth D, Hornung S: Hemoglobinopathic erythrocytosis due to new electrophoretically silent variant hemoglobin San Diego (β109 (G11)Val → Met). *J Clin Invest* 53:320, 1974

286. Bursaux E, Blouquit Y, Poyart C, Rosa J: Hemoglobin Ty Gard (α2^{A}β2$^{124 (H2) Pro \rightarrow Gln}$) A stable high 02 affinity variant at the α1 β1 contact. *FEBS Lett* 88:155, 1978

287. Jones RT, Shih T-B: Hemoglobin variants with altered oxygen affinity. *Hemoglobin* 4:243, 1980

288. Tentori L, Carta Sorcini M, Buccella C: Hemoglobin Abruzzo: Beta 143(H21)His → Arg. *Clin Chim Acta* 38:258, 1972

289. Bonaventura J, Bonaventura C, Amiconi G, Tentori L, Brunori M, Antonini E: Hemoglobin Abruzzo (β143(H21) His → Arg): Consequences of altering the 2,3-diphosphoglycerate binding site. *J Biol Chem* 250:6273, 1975

290. Bromberg PA, Alben JO, Bare GH, Balcerzak SP, Jones RT, Brimhall B, Padilla F: Haemoglobin Little Rock (β143 His → Gln; H21): A high oxygen affinity hemoglobin variant unique properties. *Nature (New Biol)* 243:177, 1973

291. Jensen W, Oski FA, Nathan DG, Bunn FH: Hemoglobin Syracuse, (α2β2$^{143(H21)His \rightarrow Pro}$): A new high affinity variant detected by special electrophoretic methods. *J Clin Invest* 55:469, 1975

292. Zak SJ, Brimhall B, Jones RT, Kaplan ME: Hemoglobin Andrew-Minneapolis α2^{A}β2$^{144Lys \rightarrow Asn}$. A new high-oxygen-affinity mutant human hemoglobin. *Blood* 44:543, 1974

293. Bunn HF, Bradley TB, Davis WE, Insdale JW, Burke JF, Beck WS, Laver MB: Structural and functional studies on hemoglobin Bethesda (α2β2^{145His}): A variant associated with compensatory erythrocytosis. *J Clin Invest* 51:2299, 1972

294. Haysahi A, Stamatoyannopoulos G, Yoshida A, Adamson J: Haemoglobin Rainier: α145(HC2)Tyrosine → Cysteine and haemoglobin

Bethesda: β145(HC2)Tyrosine → Histidine. *Nature (New Biol)* 230:264, 1971

295. CHARACHE S, BRIMHALL B, JONES RT: Polycythemia produced by hemoglobin Osler (β145(HC2)Tyr → Asp). *Johns Hopkins Med J* 136:132, 1975

296. KLECKNER HB, WILSON JB, LINDEMAN JG, STEVENS PD, NIAZI G, HUNTER E, CHEN CJ, HUISMAN THJ: Hemoglobin Fort Gordon or α2β2 145 Tyr → Asp: A new high-oxygen-affinity-hemoglobin variant. *Biochim Biophys Acta* 400:343, 1975

297. GACON G, WAJCMAN H, LABIE D: Structural and functional study of Hb Nancy: β145(HC2)Tyr → Asp: A high affinity hemoglobin. *FEBS Lett* 56:39, 1975

298. PERUTZ MF, PULSINELLI P, TEN EYCK L, KILMARTIN JV, SHIBATA S, IUCHI I, MIYAJI T, HAMILTON HB: Haemoglobin Hiroshima and the mechanism of the alkaline Bohr effect. *Nature (New Biol)* 232:147, 1971

299. BARE GH, BROMBERG PA, ALBEN JO, BRIMHALL B, JONES RT, MINTZ S, KOTHER I: Altered C-terminal salt bridges in haemoglobin York causing high oxygen affinity. *Nature (Lond)* 259:155, 1976

300. SCHNEIDER RG, BRENNER JE, BRIMHALL B, JONES PT, SPIH T-B: Hemoglobin Cowtown (β146 HC3 His-Leu). A mutant with high oxygen affinity and erythrocytosis. *Am J Clin Pathol* 72:1028, 1978

301. ADAMSON JW, FINCH CA: Hemoglobin function, oxygen affinity, and erythropoietin. *Annu Rev Physiol* 37:351, 1975

302. RUBIN MM, CHANGEAUX JP: On the nature of allosteric transitions: Implications of non-exclusive ligand binding. *J Mol Biol* 21:265, 1966

303. EDELSTEIN SJ: Extension of the allosteric model for haemoglobin. *Nature (Lond)* 230:224, 1971

304. GREER J: Three-dimensional structure of abnormal human hemoglobins Chesapeake and J. Capetown. *J Mol Biol* 62:241, 1971

305. MORIMOTO H, LEHMANN H, PERUTZ MF: Molecular pathology of human hemoglobin: Stereochemical interpretation of abnormal oxygen affinities. *Nature (Lond)* 232:408, 1971

306. ANDERSON NL: Hemoglobin San Diego (β109(G11) Val → Met): Crystal structure of the deoxy form. *J Clin Invest* 53:329, 1974

307. SCHNEIDER RG, ATKINS RJ, HOSTY TS, TOMLIN G, CASEY R, LEHMANN H, LORKIN PA, NAGAI K: Haemoglobin Titusville: A94 Asp-Asn: A new haemoglobin with a lowered affinity for oxygen. *Biochim Biophys Acta* 400:365, 1975

308. BUNN HF, BRIEHL RW, LARRABEE D, HOBART V: The interaction of 2,3-diphosphoglycerate with various human hemoglobins. *J Clin Invest* 49:1088, 1970

309. CHARACHE S, MCCURDY P, FOX J: Hemoglobin Providence (Hb Prov): A fetal-like hemoglobin. *Proc Ash* (abstract) 89:p 76 1975

310. LORKIN PA, STEVENS AD, BEARD MEJ, WRIGLEY DFM, ADAMS L, LEHMANN H: Haemoglobin Rahere (β82 Lys-Thr): A new high affinity haemoglobin associated with decreased 2,3-diphosphoglycerate binding and relative polycythaemia. *Br Med J* 341:200, 1975

311. KONOTEY-AHULU FLD: The sickle cell diseases. *Arch Intern Med* 133:611, 1974

312. HERRICK JB: Peculiar elongated and sickle-shaped red blood corpuscles in a case of severe anemia. *Arch Intern Med* 6:517, 1910

313. COOK JE, MYER J: Severe anemia with remarkable elongated and sickle-shaped red blood cells and chronic leg ulcer. *Arch Intern Med* 16:644, 1915

314. EMMEL VE: A study of the erythrocytes in a case of severe anemia with elongated and sickle-shaped red blood corpuscles. *Arch Med* 20:586, 1917

315. HAHN EV, GILLESPIE EG: Sickle cell anemia: Report of a case greatly improved by splenectomy: Experimental study of sickle cell formation. *Arch Intern Med* 39:233, 1927

316. HAHN EV: Sickle cell (drepanocytic) anemia with a report of a second case successfully treated by splenectomy and further observations on the mechanism of sickle cell formation. *Am J Med Sci* 175:206, 1928

317. DIGGS LW: The sickle cell phenomenon. *J Lab Clin Med* 7:913, 1932

318. SHERMAN IJ: The sickling phenomenon with special reference to the differentiation of sickle cell anemia from sickle cell trait. *Bull Johns Hopkins Hosp* 67:309, 1940

319. BAGLIONI C: An improvement method for the fingerprinting of human haemoglobin. *Biochim Biophys Acta* 48:392, 1961

320. KONOTEY-AHULU FID: History of sickle cell disease in Africa: Geographical distribution and population dynamics of hemoglobin S and C with special reference to West Africa. *Ghana Med J* 11:397, 1972

321. LEHMANN H: Distribution of variations in human hemoglobin synthesis, in Jonxis JHP, Delafregnage JF (eds): *Abnormal Haemoglobins*. Oxford, Blackwell, 1959, p 202

322. MOTULSKY AG: Frequency of sickling disorders in U.S. blacks. *N Engl J Med* 288:31, 1973

323. NEEL JV: The inheritance of sickle cell anemia. *Science* 110:64, 1949

324. NEEL JV: Data pertaining to the population dynamics of sickle cell disease. *Am J Hum Genet* 5:154, 1953

325. BRAIN P: Sickle cell anemia in Africa. *Br Med J* 2:880, 1952

326. BRAIN P: The sickle-cell disease trait: Its clinical significance. *S Afr Med J* 26:925, 1952

327. KIDSON C, GORMAN JD: A challenge to the concept of selection by malaria in glucose-6-phosphate dehydrogenase deficiency. *Nature (Lond)* 196:49, 1962

328. RUCKNAGEL DL: The genetics of sickle cell anemia and related syndromes. *Arch Intern Med* 133:595, 1974

329. FRIEDMAN MJ, TRAGER W: The biochemistry of resistance to malaria. *Sci Am* March 1980, p 154

330. FINCH JT: Structure of sickled erythrocytes and sickle cell hemoglobin fibers. *Proc Natl Acad Sci USA* 70:718, 1973

331. HOFRICHTER J, HENDRICKS DG, EATON WE: Structure of hemoglobin S fibers: Optical detection of the molecular orientation in sickled erythrocytes. *Proc Natl Acad Sci USA* 70:3604, 1973

332. BERTLES JF: Hemoglobin interaction and molecular basis of sickling. *Arch Intern Med* 133:538, 1974

333. RAMPLING MW, SIRS JA: The rate of sickling of cells containing sickle cell haemoglobin. *Clin Sci Mol Med* 45:655, 1973

334. HOFRICHTER J, ROSE PD, EATON WA: Kinetics and mechanism deoxyhemoglobin S gelation: A new approach to understanding sickle cell disease. *Proc Natl Acad Sci USA* 71:4864, 1974

335. LESSIN LS, JENSEN WN: Sickle cell anemia 1910–1973: An overview. *Arch Intern Med* 133:529, 1974

336. DIGGS LW, BIBB J: The erythrocyte in sickle cell anemia. *JAMA* 112:695, 1939

337. BERTLES JF, MILNER PFA: Irreversibly sickled erythrocytes; a consequence of the heterogeneous distribution of hemoglobin types in sickle cell anemia. *J Clin Invest* 47:1731, 1968

338. SERJEANT GR, SERJEANT BE, MILNER PF: The irreversibly sickled cell: A determinant of hemolysis in sickle cell anemia. *Br J Haematol* 17:527, 1969

339. SEAKINS M, GIBBS WN, MILNER PF, BERTLES JF: Erythrocyte Hb-S concentration: An important factor in the low oxygen affinity of blood in sickle cell anemia. *J Clin Invest* 52:422, 1973

340. MAY A, HUEHNS ER: Mechanism of the low oxygen affinity of red cells in sickle cell disease. *Haematol Bluttransfus* 10:279, 1972

341. CHARACHE S, CONLEY CL: Rate of sickling of red cells during deoxygenation of blood from persons with various sickling disorders. *Blood* 24:25, 1964

342. PERRINE RP, BROWN MJ, WEATHERALL DJ, CLEGG JB, MAY A: Benign sickle cell anemia. *Lancet* 2:1163, 1972

343. BERTLES JF, RABINOWITZ R, DOBLER J: Hemoglobin interaction: Modification of solid phase composition in the sickling phenomenon. *Science* 169:375, 1970

344. BOOKCHIN RM, NAGEL RL: Molecular interactions of sickling hemoglobins, in Abramson H, Bertles JF, Wethers DL (eds): *Sickle Cell Disease*. St. Louis, Mosby, 1973, p 140

345. KRAUS AP, MIYUKI T, INCHI I, KRAUS LM: Memphis: A new variety of sickle cell anemia with clinically mild symptoms due to an α-chain variant of hemoglobin α23GluNH2). *J Lab Clin Med* 66:886, 1965

346. COOPER MK, KRAUS AP, FELTS JH, RANUSEUR WL, MEYERS R, KRAUS LM: A third case of hemoglobin Memphis/sickle cell disease. *Am J Med* 55:535, 1973

347. HEBBEL RP, BOOGAERTS MAB, EATON JW, STEINBERG MH: Erythrocyte adherence to endothelium in sickle cell anemia. *N Engl J Med* 302:992, 1980

348. BEUTLER E: Hypothesis: Changes in the O2 dissociation curve and sickling: A general formulation and therapeutic strategy. *Blood* 43:297, 1974

349. WINSLOW RM: Blood oxygen equilibrium studies in sickle cell anemia. *Proc Symp Mol Cell Aspects Sickle Cell Disease*. DHEW Publication no (NIH) 76-1007, 1976, p 235

350. MILLER DM, WINSLOW RM, KLEIN HG, WILSON KC, BROWN FL, STATHAM NJ: Improved exercise performance after exchange transfusion in subjects with sickle cell anemia. *Blood* 55:1127, 1980

351. CHARACHE S, GRISOLIA S, FIEDLER AJ, HELLEGERS A: Effect of 2,3-diphosphoglycerate on oxygen affinity of blood in sickle cell anemia. *J Clin Invest* 49:806, 1970

352. POWARS DR: Natural history of sickle cell disease: The first ten years. *Semin Hematol* 12:267, 1975

353. FALTER ML, ROBINSON MG, KIM OS: Splenic function and infection in sickle cell anemia. *Acta Haematol (Basel)* 50:154, 1973

354. BOGGS DR, HYDE F, SRODES C: An unusual pattern of neutrophil kinetics in sickle cell anemia. *Blood* 41:59, 1973

355. WINKLESTEIN JA, SHIN HS, SMITH MR: Pneumococcal infection in sickle cell disease: Deficiency of heat labile opsonin activity, in Hercules JI, Schechter AN, Eaton WA, Jackson RE (eds): *Proc 1st Nat Symp Sickle Cell Disease*. DHEW Publication (NIH) 75-723, 1974, p 71

356. MILNER PF: The sickling disorders. *Clin Haematol* 31:209, 1974

357. KONOTEY-AHULU FID: Effect of environment of sickle cell disease in West Africa: Epidemiologic and clinical considerations, in Abramson H, Bertles JF, Wethers DL (eds): *Sickle Cell Disease*. St. Louis, Mosby, 1973, p 20

358. JAMSHID J: Hemoglobin SO$_{Arabia}$ disease in a black American. *Am J Med Sci* 265:266, 1973

359. EFREMOV GD, HUISMAN THJ: The laboratory diagnosis of the haemoglobinopathies. *Clin Haematol* 3:527, 1974

360. NATHAN DG, ALTER BP, FRIGOLETTO FD: Antenatal diagnosis of hemoglobinopathies: Social and technical considerations. *Semin Hematol* 12:305, 1975

361. PATARYAS HA, STAMATOYANNOPOULOS G: Hemoglobin in human fetuses: Evidence for adult hemoglobin production after the 11th gestational week. *Blood* 39:688, 1972

362. KAZAZIAN HH, KABACK MM, WOODHEAD AP, LEONARD CO, NERSESIAN WS: Further studies on the antenatal diagnosis of sickle cell anemia and other hemoglobinopathies. *Adv Exp Med Biol* 38:337, 1972

363. CHARACHE S: The treatment of sickle cell anemia. *Arch Intern Med* 133:698, 1974

364. WHO Tech Rep. Ser: Treatment of haemoglobinopathies and allied disorders. Geneva, 1972, no 509

365. HUNTSMAN RG, LEHMANN H: The treatment of sickle cell disease. *Br J Haematol* 28:437, 1974

366. BARRERAS L, DIGGS LW: Sodium citrate orally for painful sickle cell crises. *JAMA* 215:762, 1971

368. MURAYAMA M, NALBANDIAN RM: *Sickle Cell Hemoglobin: Molecule to Man.* Boston, Little, Brown, 1973

369. Cooperative Urea Trials Group: Clinical trials of therapy for sickle cell vasoocclusive crises. *JAMA* 288:1120, 1974

370. CERAMI A: Cyanate as an inhibitor of red-cell sickling. *N Engl J Med* 287:807, 1972

371. CHARACHE S, DUFFY TP, JANDER N, SCOTT JC, BEDINE M, NORRELL R: Toxic-therapeutic ratio of sodium cyanate. *Arch Intern Med* 135:1043, 1975

372. PETERSON CM, DECIUTIIS AC, CERAMI A: Sodium cyanate and sickle cell disease: Efficacy vs. toxicity, in Hercules JI, Schechter AN, Eaton WA, Jackson RE (eds): *Proc 1st Nat Symp Sickle Cell Disease.* DHEW Publication (NIH) 75-723, 1974, p 34

373. LANGER EE, FINCH CA: Extracorporeal treatment with cyanate in sickle cell disease, in Hercules JI, Schechter AN, Eaton WA, Jackson RE (eds): *Proc 1st Nat Symp Sickle Cell Disease.* DHEW Publication (NIH) 75-723, 1974, p 39

374. PRASAD AS, SCHOOMAKER EB, ORTEGA J, BREWER GJ, OBERLEAS D, OELSHLEGEL F: Deficiency of zinc in sickle cell disease, in Hercules JI, Schechter AN, Eaton WA, Jackson RE (eds): *Proc 1st Nat Symp Sickle Cell Disease.* DHEW Publication (NIH) 75-723, 1974, p 33

375. ELBAUM D, NAGEL RL, BOOKCHIN RM, HERSKOVITS TT: Effect of alkyl ureas on the polymerization of hemoglobin S. *Proc Natl Acad Sci USA* 71:4712, 1974

376. LUBIN BH, PENA V, MENTZER WC, BYMUN E, BRADLEY TB, PARKER L: Dimethyl adipimidate: A new antisickling agent. *Proc Natl Acad Sci USA* 72:43, 1975

377. KRAUS LM, JERNIGAN HM, SONI KS, BLATTEIS CM, ALLEN CM JR, KRAUS AP: Carbamyl phosphate effects on human and dog hemoglobin structure-function relationships are correlated with pharmacological studies, in Hercules JI, Schechter AN, Eaton WA, Jackson RE (eds): *Proc 1st Nat Symp Sickle Cell Disease.* DHEW Publication (NIH) 75-723, 1974, p 335

378. ZANGER B, ALFREY CP, McINTYRE LV, LEVERETT B: The effects of dromostanolone in sickle cell anemia. *J Lab Clin Med* 84:889, 1974

379. VIRTANEN R: *Claude Bernard and His Place in the History of Ideas.* Lincoln, University of Nebraska Press, 1969

380. ANDERSON WF, FLETCHER JC: Gene therapy in human beings: When is it ethical to begin? *N Engl J Med* 303:1293, 1980

77

THE THALASSEMIAS

YUET WAI KAN

1. *The thalassemia syndromes are a group of hereditary anemias characterized by defective globin chain synthesis. Unbalanced globin chain production causes anemia and erythroid cell damage. The two main types of thalassemia are α and β thalassemia. These involve errors in synthesis of the α- and β-globin chains, respectively.*

2. *Four clinical syndromes are recognized in α thalassemia. The clinical severity of the disease is related to the malfunctioning of one to four of the duplicated α-globin genes.*

3. *New therapeutic approaches have improved the outlook for β-thalassemia homozygotes. Hypertransfusion and programs of continuous iron chelation forestall many of the complications associated with β thalassemia and allow normal development. Prenatal diagnosis has also had an impact on the frequency of homozygous births in high-risk areas.*

4. *Heterogeneous molecular lesions result in defective globin synthesis in thalassemia. The lesions that have so far been defined include gene deletion, mRNA processing defects due to intron mutations, nonsense mutations due to single nucleotide mutations or frameshifts, and termination codon mutations.*

The *thalassemias* are a heterogeneous group of hereditary anemias in which the common feature is defective globin chain synthesis [1–4]. Normally, globin chain production is coordinated in such a way that the α- and β-like globin chain production is balanced to form globin tetramers. In thalassemia, the impaired production of one or more of these globin components causes deficient hemoglobinization of the erythroid cells. The unaffected chain continues to be produced in normal amounts, and in the homozygous state the excessive accumulation of the unaffected chain may disrupt erythroid cell maturation and function, causing premature destruction of the red blood cell. As will be discussed later, many different molecular lesions cause thalassemia. These mutations can affect the production of any of the globin chains, but as Hb A ($\alpha_2\beta_2$) is the predominant hemoglobin in postnatal life, the two most important types of thalassemia are the α and the β thalassemias, where α- and β-globin chain synthesis, respectively, is impaired [5].

Thalassemia occurs throughout the world and constitutes one of the most common hereditary disorders. In some human populations the frequency of the α-thalassemia gene exceeds that of the normal genotype; in others, the prevalence of the β-thalassemia gene poses major health care problems. The high frequency of thalassemia is probably due to the protection it offers against falciparum malaria.

The history of the discovery and delineation of the thalassemia syndromes has been superbly reviewed [6, 7]. During the past 10 years, important advances have been made in the understanding, management, and prevention of thalassemia. Recently developed techniques in molecular biology have helped define the precise molecular defects in several thalassemia syndromes; others are rapidly being discovered. These techniques include recombinant DNA methods to isolate human globin genes in bacteria [8–10], DNA sequencing methods [11, 12] to define the nucleotide sequences of the normal and defective genes, and restriction endonuclease digestion of DNA [13] and Southern blotting methods [14] to identify the globin genes in the complex human genome.

A better understanding of the pathophysiology of anemia and its clinical consequences has led to more effective approaches to management. New treatment modalities allow many patients affected by homozygous β thalassemia to develop normally, and it now appears that many clinical complications associated with the anemia and iron overload can be forestalled.

The last decade also saw the development of effective methods of prenatal diagnosis for several forms of thalassemia. In countries with a high frequency of β thalassemia, prenatal diagnosis programs have decreased the incidence of the disease and exerted a positive influence on the reproductive patterns of couples at risk.

NORMAL HUMAN GLOBIN

The Globin Chains

The six normal human hemoglobin molecules are listed in Table 77-1. Normal hemoglobin tetramers are made up of a pair of α-like and a pair of β-like chains. Adult hemoglobin is composed of approximately 97 percent Hb A ($\alpha_2\beta_2$), 2.5 percent Hb A_2 ($\alpha_2\delta_2$), and less than 1 percent Hb F ($\alpha_2\gamma_2$).

The first globin chains synthesized in embryonic life are the α-like ζ-globin chain and the β-like ε-globin chain [15]. These, in combination with the α and γ chains, form Hb Gower I, $\zeta_2\epsilon_2$ [16], Hb Portland, $\zeta_2\gamma_2$ [17], and Hb Gower II, $\alpha_2\epsilon_2$ [18]. The ζ and ε chain production ceases prior to the tenth week of gestation, and Hb F ($\alpha_2\gamma_2$) predominates throughout most of intrauterine life [19]. In certain pathologic conditions, embryonic and fetal chain synthesis persists to a later period. For example, in D_1 trisomy, Hb Gower and Hb Portland are detectable at birth, and the Hb F level is above normal [20]. In homozygous α thalassemia, Hb Portland synthesis persists to birth [21, 22]. The ontogeny of globin chain synthesis in normal fetal and early postnatal life is illustrated in Fig. 77-1.

Beta-globin chain synthesis has been detected as early as the eleventh week of fetal life [23]. By the eighteenth week of gestation it comprises approximately 8 percent of the non-α-globin chain production [24, 25]. Analyzing the amount and type of β-globin chain synthesized in fetal blood has provided an approach to prenatal testing for β thalassemia and sickle-cell anemia. The rate of β-globin synthesis rises sharply prior

Table 77-1 The human hemoglobins

A	$\alpha_2\beta_2$			97.0%
A_2	$\alpha_2\delta_2$	Adult		2.5%
F	$\alpha_2\gamma_2$	Fetal		1.0%
Portland	$\zeta_2\gamma_2$			
Gower II	$\alpha_2\ \epsilon_2$	Embryonic		
Gower I	$\zeta_2\ \epsilon_2$			

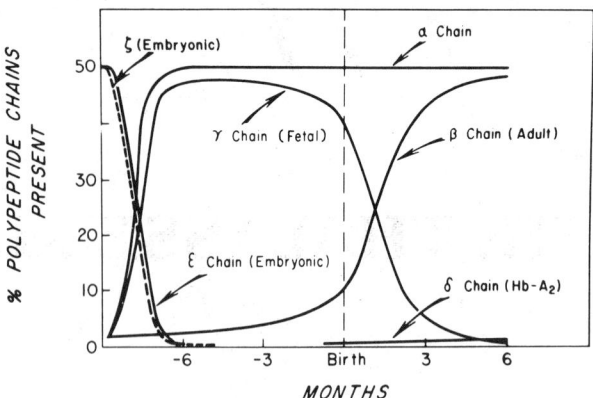

Figure 77-1 The ontogeny of globin chain production. (*Adapted from Bunn, Forget, and Ranney* [2], *with permission.*)

to birth [19] and replaces γ-chain synthesis, which decreases to the adult level by the age of 1 to 2 years.

The γ-globin chain in fetal hemoglobin is heterogeneous. The two forms synthesized by two different γ-chain loci on the DNA differ at amino acid position 136. One contains glycine ($^G\gamma$), the other contains alanine ($^A\gamma$) [26]. The ratio of $^G\gamma$ chain to $^A\gamma$ chain, which is approximately 3:1 in fetal life, changes to 2:3 after birth [27]. Another γ chain, $^T\gamma$, with threonine instead of isoleucine at amino acid number 75, represents a polymorphism of the $^A\gamma$ locus [28–30]. In the adult, low levels of Hb F (< 1 percent) are found in a small percentage of the red blood cells.

When α-globin chain synthesis is severely impaired, as in certain α-thalassemia syndromes, the β chain forms the β_4 tetramer, Hb H [31, 32], and the γ chain forms the γ_4 tetramer, Hb Bart's [33]. Hemoglobin molecules composed of these homotetramers are not useful for oxygen transport as they have a high oxygen affinity (about 10 to 20 times that of Hb A) and lack heme-heme interaction and Bohr effect [34, 35]. Hence, under physiologic conditions they bind the oxygen molecule tightly and do not release it to the tissues.

Globin Gene Arrangement

The location of the α- and β-globin genes on the human chromosome was first determined by constructing hybrid cells, or heterokaryons, composed of mouse erythroleukemia cells that contain different human chromosomes. The human globin genes are detected by use of radioactive probes specific for the α- and β-globin gene sequences. With this method, the α-globin gene complex has been localized to chromosome 16 [36] and the β-globin gene complex to chromosome 11 [37]. Additional studies of cell lines with deletions or translocations that involve different portions of chromosome 11 have placed the β-globin gene complex on the short arm of this chromosome [38, 39].

The arrangement of the β-like globin genes relative to one another was initially deduced from the discovery of fusion hemoglobins such as Hb Lepore and Hb Kenya. The non-α chain in Hb Lepore is a polypeptide chain with δ-globin amino acid sequences at the amino end and β-globin sequences at the carboxyl end [40]. This fusion chain arose from unequal crossing over of chromosomes that were malaligned between the δ- and β-globin genes. Several types of Hb Lepore have been defined on the basis of differences in point of crossover [1]. The δ and β-globin genes are absent from the chromosome homologous to the one which contains the Hb Lepore globin gene. The reciprocal product of the crossover is a chromosome that contains an intact δ-globin gene, a β-δ fusion gene (which produces anti-Lepore hemoglobins such as Hb Miyada and Hb P Congo), and an intact β-globin gene [41, 42]. The arrangement of these two different types of crossover products places the δ-globin gene before (upstream from) the β gene according to the order of transcription. The non-α chain in Hb Kenya is fusion molecule made up of γ-globin sequences on the amino end and β-globin sequences on the carboxyl end [43, 44]. The δ-globin locus apparently is deleted on the homologous chromosome, and fetal hemoglobin production of the Gγ type persists. This chain probably arose from a fusion of the Aγ and β genes, which indicates that the chromosomal arrangement is Aγ-δ-β. The Gγ location could not be ascertained with this method.

Duplication of the two α-globin loci was inferred from analysis of α-globin mutants and α thalassemia [45]. Heterozygotes for an α-globin mutant usually carry 25 percent of the abnormal hemoglobin [46]. Furthermore, the hemoglobin of a double heterozygote for two different α-globin mutants contains 25 percent each of the two abnormal globins as well as 50 percent of the normal Hb A [47]. The existence of duplicated α-globin loci was further confirmed by quantitating the number of α-globin genes in a α thalassemia. Individuals with Hb-H disease have one-quarter the normal number of α-globin genes, indicating that at least four α-globin loci are present in the diploid genome [48].

The arrangement of the α- and β-globin gene complexes has been precisely defined by use of restriction endonuclease analysis and DNA cloning technology [49]. Restriction endonucleases (enzymes that cut DNA at specific sequences) are used to cleave the human DNA into overlapping fragments. These fragments are inserted into lambda bacteriophages and amplified in bacteria. The recombinant phages that contain globin genes will hybridize with radioactive probes specific for those genes and can thus be identified and isolated. By studying overlapping DNA fragments that contain globin genes, the exact order and location of the globin genes on the chromosome and the distances between them have been ascertained [50, 51].

These studies have demonstrated directly that two α-globin loci lie on each chromosome [51]. The distance between the two duplicated α loci is approximately 3700 base pairs [3.7 kilobases (kb)]. The more downstream (rightward) locus according to the order of transcription has been named α1, and the upstream (leftward) locus is known as α2. Further upstream from the α2-gene locus lies a gene that is homologous to the α-globin gene in 75 percent of its sequences. Sequence analysis of this gene shows that it is nonfunctional and does not produce a polypeptide chain; hence, it is called the pseudo-α gene. Further upstream are two α-like genes, ζ1 and ζ2. Recent structural studies show that a termination codon at amino acid position number 6 makes the ζ1 gene nonfunctional, and thus only one functional ζ gene (ζ2) is known [52].

On chromosome 11, the δ-globin structural locus lies approximately 7 kb upstream from the β-globin gene according to the direction of transcription. Further upstream, a pseudo-β gene separates them from the Aγ locus. The distance between the Aγ and δ genes is 15 kb. The Gγ locus is situated about 5 kb upstream from the Aγ locus. Further upstream, the ε-globin locus separates the Gγ gene from another pseudo-β-globin gene [50] (Fig. 77-2).

Thus, both the α- and the γ-globin loci are duplicated. The δ- and β-globin genes can be considered as duplicates, although their structures differ in 10 amino acids. At present, only one functional ζ and one ε chain have been found.

The activation of the α- and β-globin genes from fetal to adult life follows their arrangement according to the direction of transcription. The mechanism of this activation is currently the focus of intense investigation.

Structure and Transcription of the Globin Genes

The entire nucleotide sequences of the duplicated α-globin genes [53–55], the pseudo-α gene [56], the ζ gene [52], as well as the β [57], δ [58], Gγ, Aγ [59], and ε1 [60] genes, have been determined. As with most eukaryotic structural genes, the nucleotide sequences that encode for the globin chains are not continuous but are interrupted by sequences not found in the cytoplasmic messenger RNA (mRNA). The portions of the sequences that are represented in the mature mRNA are called exons, and those that interrupt these sequences are the intervening sequences, or introns. Two introns interrupt the globin gene sequences and divide the exons into three segments. The first intron in both the α- and β-like globin genes lies between amino acids 30 and 31 and is about 130 nucleotides long. The second intron occurs between amino acids 99 and 100 for α-globin and 104 and 105 for the β-like globin chain. It is short (about 150 nucleotides) in the α-globin gene but much longer (850 to 900 nucleotides) in the β-like gene (Fig. 77-3).

The initial transcription product (heterogeneous nuclear RNA or pre-mRNA) contains sequences that correspond to the entire gene, including both exons and introns. Following transcription, several modifications occur to the mRNA: a 7-methyl guanosine triphosphate residue is added to the 5' end of the mRNA in a 5'-to-5' linkage, a process called "capping" [61, 62]; a stretch of adenosine (poly A) is added to the 3' end of the mRNA (polyadenylation) [63]; and certain nucleotide residues are methylated [64]. In the nucleus, the poly A tail is composed of about 150 to 200 residues. The function of capping, polyadenylation, and methylation is not yet clear. They may contribute to the stability of the mRNA and enhance translation. The cap structure promotes binding of the ribosomes to the globin mRNA during the initiation of protein synthesis, but is not absolutely required for this activity [65].

The mRNA then undergoes a process called splicing, in which the sequences corresponding to the intron are excised

Figure 77-2 The arrangement of the α- and β-like globin gene complexes on chromosomes 16 and 11, respectively.

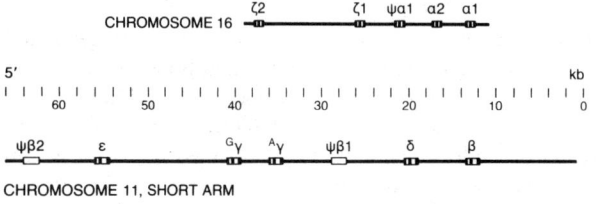

CHROMOSOME 11, SHORT ARM

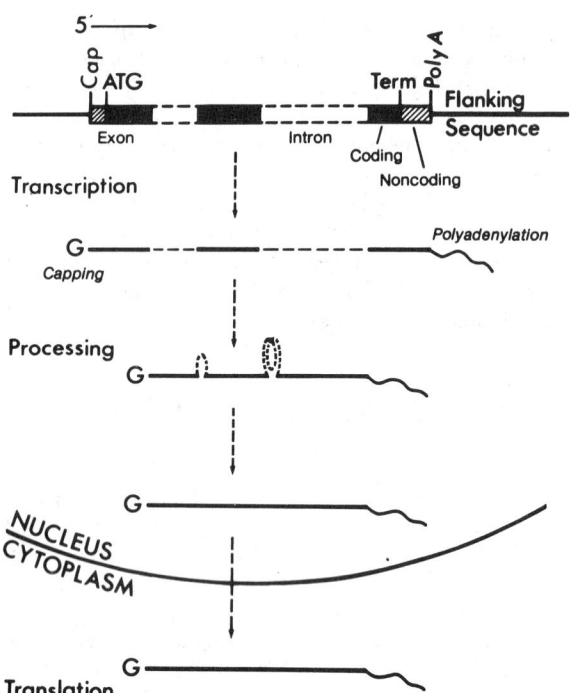

Figure 77-3 Structure and transcription of the globin genes.

and the exons are rejoined [66]. The mechanism of the splicing process has not been defined, although it is known that certain nucleotide sequences are always present at the splice junction. The first two nucleotides at the 5' end of the intron are invariably guanosine (G) and thymidine (T), and the last two nucleotides are adenosine (A) and guanosine [67]. Following splicing, the mRNA is transported from the nucleus to the cytoplasm where protein synthesis occurs. (The process of translation in the cytoplasm has been discussed in detail in Chap. 2.) Improperly spliced messages degrade rapidly in the nucleus, and certain types of thalassemia are due to mutations that affect the splicing process.

Mature cytoplasmic globin mRNA is composed of a cap, nucleotide sequences corresponding to the exon, and a poly A tail about 100 nucleotides long. The initiation codon AUG is preceded by 5' noncoding sequences, and the termination codon (UAA for α- β-, and δ-globin, UGA for γ-globin) is followed by 3' noncoding regions which are not translated into amino acids. Although the amino acid sequences of the α-globin polypeptide chains are identical, the nucleotide sequences of the two loci and the mRNAs differ in several regions, primarily in the intervening sequences and the 3' noncoding region [54, 55]. This is also true for γ-globin where the amino acid sequences of the $^G\gamma$ and $^A\gamma$ chains differ by only one amino acid, but the gene sequences differ in the second intron and the 3' noncoding region [59].

Pseudogenes

The nucleotide sequences of the α- and β-pseudogenes are largely homologous to those of the α- and β-globin genes, but the pseudogenes yield no recognizable globin products. They are probably produced by gene duplication, but subsequent divergence renders them nonfunctional in encoding for globin sequences. The pseudo-α gene has been sequenced in its entirety and bears about 75 percent homology to the α-globin sequences [56]. Certain nucleotide changes render it most

likely nonfunctional. The initiation codon ATG is mutated, some of the consensus sequences of the splice junctions are changed, and deletions and insertions throughout the sequences shift the reading frame. The ζ1 gene, which contains a nonsense mutation, may represent an early stage of a pseudogene [52]. The δ gene may be considered as a β-globin gene duplicate in the process of becoming nonfunctional. For example, this gene exists in the old-world monkeys but produces no δ-globin polypeptide chain [68]. We do not know whether pseudogenes serve other functions in globin gene transcription.

THE THALASSEMIA SYNDROMES

The molecular lesions in thalassemia are extremely diverse, and multiple mutations may depress globin chain synthesis. Some of the mechanisms that have been defined include deletion of stretches of nucleotide sequences of varying lengths and nucleotide mutations which affect mRNA processing or translation. Although defective synthesis of one or more of the α-, β- δ-, and γ-globin chains have been described, the frequency and clinical severity of the α and β thalassemias make them the most important of the thalassemia syndromes.

The α-Thalassemia Syndromes

The α-globin chain defects in α thalassemia range from mild to complete suppression of α-globin chain synthesis. Four clinical syndromes of increasing severity are recognized: the silent-carrier state, α-thalassemia trait, Hb-H disease and homozygous α thalassemia [1].

These four clinical syndromes were originally explained on the basis of two different genetic defects, the α-thalassemia-1 genotype, which severely depresses α-globin chain synthesis, and the α-thalassemia-2 genotype, which mildly affects α-globin chain synthesis [69]. Heterozygotes for the α-thalassemia-2 genotype are known as silent carriers of α thalassemia; heterozygotes for the α-thalassemia-1 genotype and homozygosity for the α-thalassemia-2 genotype both produce the α-thalassemia trait phenotype [70]. Hemoglobin-H disease is due to the compound heterozygous state of α thalassemia-1 and α thalassemia-2. Homozygosity for α thalassemia-1 results in hydrops fetalis. We now know that several different molecular lesions cause the α thalassemia-1 and α-thalassemia-2 genotypes.

The Silent-Carrier State The α-globin chain production is so mildly impaired in this condition that making a firm clinical diagnosis is often impossible. The silent carrier is not anemic, and the red cell morphology is normal. Alpha-globin chain synthesis is mildly imbalanced, with a slightly decreased α/β-globin chain synthetic ratio. Although as a group the mean α/β ratio is below normal, the decrease is too small to be of diagnostic value in individual cases [71]. On electrophoresis the cord blood hemoglobin may show a small amount (trace to 2 percent) of Hb Bart's [70], but hemoglobin electrophoresis of adult blood usually yields normal results. Cord blood analysis underestimates the frequency of this disorder since some silent carriers do not exhibit Hb Bart's [72]. Silent carriers of the type of α thalassemia-2 caused by gene deletion can now be detected with certainty by restriction endonuclease analysis [73].

Hemoglobin Constant Spring is a variation of the silent-carrier state [74]. Here a termination codon mutation of the α-globin locus results in production of a small quantity of an elongated α-globin chain, while the other locus functions normally. Phenotypically this genotype only mildly supresses α-globin chain synthesis and resembles the silent-carrier state.

α-Thalassemia Trait Two of the four α-globin loci malfunction in this carrier state of α thalassemia. Heterozygotes are usually not anemic, although as a group their hemoglobin levels may be slightly below the normal mean. The red cells are characteristically microcytic, and on hemoglobin electrophoresis the percentages of Hb A_2 fall within the normal range.

Alpha-thalassemia trait can be distinguished from iron deficiency by measuring the serum iron levels. Another convenient method of differentiating the two conditions is to compare the degree of anemia relative to the microcytosis [75, 76]. In iron deficiency the microcytosis is usually associated with anemia, whereas in α-thalassemia trait, the hemoglobin level is generally normal. Heterozygous α thalassemia can be diagnosed with certainty in the newborn period since the level of Hb Bart's usually increases to 2 to 10 percent in the cord blood as determined by electrophoresis. It can also be detected by hemoglobin chain synthesis studies which demonstrate a decrease in the α/β synthetic ratio from unity to about 0.7. [71].

When sickle-cell trait occurs in combination with heterozygous α thalassemia, the percentages of sickle hemoglobin present reflect the α thalassemia genotype [77–79]. Nonthalassemic AS heterozygotes have 37 to 44 percent Hb S. When sickle-cell trait is inherited together with the α-thalassemia-2 genotype, the amount of Hb S decreases to 30 to 36 percent. S heterozygotes with α-thalassemia trait have 22 to 29 percent Hb S, and the rare individual with AS combined with the Hb-H genotype has less than 20 percent Hb S [80]. The percentages of Hb S are lower in α thalassemia because the β^S chain has less affinity for the α chain than the β^A chain [81]. Thus, when insufficient α-globin is available, fewer $\alpha_2\beta_2^S$ tetramers are formed than $\alpha_2\beta_2^A$.

Hemoglobin-H Disease In this condition, the more severe defect in α-globin chain synthesis is usually produced by the combination of the α-thalassemia-1 and α-thalassemia-2 genotypes. Hemoglobin-H disease is characterized by a mild to moderate degree of anemia, with hemoglobin levels averaging 10 g/dl. Occasionally the anemia is so mild that the hemoglobin level is nearly normal, but sometimes the anemia is extremely severe, with hemoglobin levels as low as 5 g/dl. The anemia is hemolytic in nature, with a characteristic reticulocytosis of approximately 5 percent. The spleen is often enlarged, although the extent may vary from not palpable to gross enlargement. Occasionally, severe bone marrow expansion results in mild bone abnormalities, but bone changes are more characteristic of the β thalassemias. The anemia can be more severe in young children, during pregnancy, or at times of coincidental infection. Ingestion of oxidant drugs can bring on a hemolytic crisis. In general, the anemia is compensated, and affected individuals lead normal or nearly normal lives.

The red cells in Hb-H disease are characterized by microcytosis and severe aniso- and poikilocytosis. They show the characteristic fine inclusion bodies of Hb H when incubated with the oxidant dye, brilliant cresyl blue. After splenectomy, large inclusions indistinguishable from Heinz bodies are present [82,

83]. The diagnosis can be confirmed by electrophoresis, which demonstrates 5 to 30 percent Hb H and a reduced Hb-A_2 level. In the newborn period, high percentages of Hb Bart's (10 to 20 percent) are demonstrable in the cord blood. Hemoglobin H-Constant Spring is produced by the combination of a Constant Spring carrier with an α-thalassemia-1 gene. Electrophoretic analysis shows up to 5 percent Hb Constant Spring, as well as Hb H [74].

The pathophysiology of the hemolytic anemia in Hb-H disease is well understood. The Hb-H tetramer, β_4, is relatively stable when first produced, but the molecule is so arranged that all eight sulfhydryl groups (two in each β chain) are exposed. In contrast, of the six sulfhydryl groups present in the Hb-A molecule (two in each β chain and one in each α chain), only two (one in each β chain) are exposed [34]. Normally glutathione is the most important reducing agent in the red cell. As the red cell ages and the regeneration of reduced glutathione decreases, the Hb-H molecule acts as a reducing agent and, when oxidized, becomes unstable and precipitates. The precipitates are removed by the reticuloendothelial cells in the spleen and other organs. Often the red cell is also destroyed. Most affected individuals have sufficient Hb A for oxygen transport, and so the fact the Hb H is not useful for this function is less serious than its instability, which causes hemolysis.

Hydrops Fetalis due to Homozygous α Thalassemia In people of southeast Asian origin, homozygous α thalassemia is probably the most common cause of hydrops fetalis [84]. This homozygous condition is invariably lethal. The affected fetus dies either during the third trimester of pregnancy or, if born alive, within hours or at most 1 or 2 days after birth. The fetuses are hydropic, with marked edema and ascites. These changes are sometimes detectable in utero in midtrimester by means of ultrasound. The heart chambers, liver, and spleen are enlarged; the placenta is also grossly swollen and edematous. The condition is associated with severe anemia. The red blood cells are hypochromic and show anisocytosis, poikilocytosis, and extensive normoblastemia. Bone marrow hypertrophy and extramedullary erythropoiesis are evident. Hemoglobin Bart's is the primary hemoglobin component, together with varying amounts (5 to 30 percent) of Hb Portland ($\zeta_2\epsilon_2$) [85], which has a normal oxygen dissociation curve and is believed to help maintain the fetuses to term.

Prenatal diagnosis for homozygous α thalassemia is now possible [86, 87]. The primary indication for the procedure is that termination saves 4 to 5 months of a pregnancy doomed to produce a nonviable fetus. Early termination may also prevent maternal toxemia and postpartum hemorrhage, two complications that often accompany hydropic pregnancies. The technique of amniocentesis is used for prenatal diagnosis. Since the severe form of homozygous α thalassemia is invariably due to deletion of all four α-globin structural genes, DNA from the amniotic fluid cell can be used for restriction endonuclease analysis. The absence of α-globin genes in the fetal DNA confirms the diagnosis. In cases in which the hydropic changes appear prior to the twenty-fourth week of pregnancy, ultrasonograms can also be confirmatory (Fig. 77-4).

Molecular Pathology of the α-Thalassemia Syndromes

The heterogeneous molecular lesions that produce the α thalassemia-1 and α-thalassemia-2 genotypes are summarized in

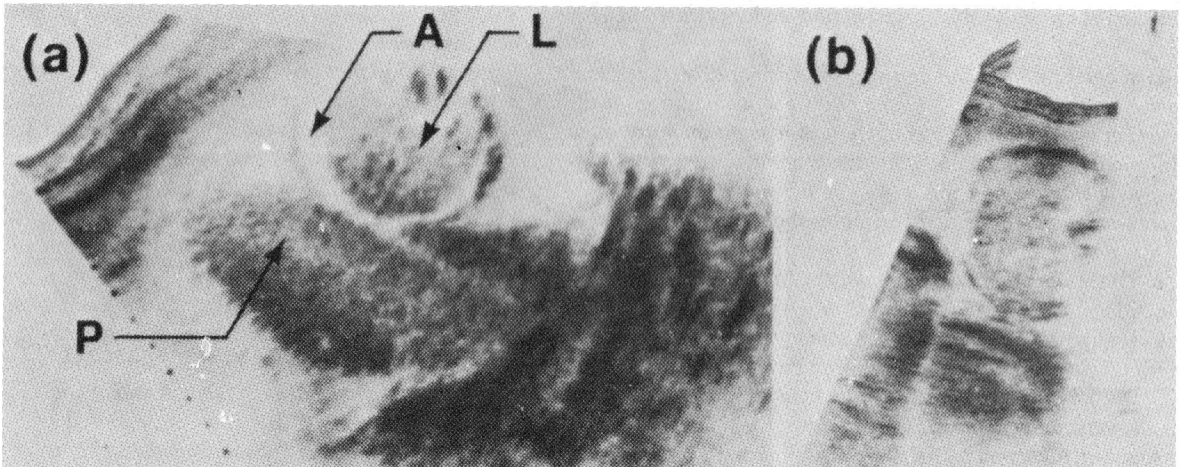

Figure 77-4 Ultrasonogram from a hydropic pregnancy. Ultrasonograms from (A) a hydropic pregnancy and (B) a normal pregnancy. Compare the enlarged placenta (P) and the fetal liver (L) surrounded by ascitic fluid (A) in the hydropic pregnancy with the normal fetus.

Table 77-2. The most common lesions are produced by different deletions which affect various segments of the chromosomes in the α-globin gene cluster. Some α-thalassemia lesions are produced by α-globin genes which are present but do not function properly.

The α-thalassemia-1 genotype is most often caused by deletions that affect both α-globin loci [88, 89]. Several deletions have been characterized. One deletion, which was defined in a Thai individual, affects both α-globin structural genes and the pseudo-α gene. Another, more extensive, gene deletion was identified in a Greek Cypriot and involves both α-globin structural genes, the pseudo-α gene, and the ζ1 gene. Both deletions probably arose from unequal crossing-over events. If, on two homologous chromosomes, the pseudo-α-globin gene on one chromosome malaligns with the ζ2-globin gene on another, the extent of the deletion can be explained by the point of crossover [90]. In the Greek Cypriot, the crossover occurs before the ζ1 gene and removes the ζ, pseudo-α, α1, and α2 genes from one chromosome. In the Thai, the crossover occurs after the ζ1 gene, producing a chromosome with no pseudo-α, α2, or α1 genes. A third deletion, which also renders both ζ-globin genes nonfunctional, involves the entire α2 locus and the 5' portion of the α1 locus up to amino acid 56. Therefore, no intact functional α-globin gene is left on this chromosome [91].

The common cause of the α-thalassemia-2 genotype is a deletion that affects only one of the two α-globin loci [48, 73]. At least two molecular events are known to produce this genotype [92]. In the so-called leftward deletion, a stretch of DNA approximately 4.2 kb long that contains the α2-globin locus is deleted. The so-called rightward deletion removes a 3.7-kb DNA segment which lies downstream from the previous dele-

tion. The two deletions can be distinguished by digesting the DNA with the restriction enzyme *Bgl* II, as they yield fragments of different lengths. Both deletions arose as a result of unequal crossing-over, the leftward deletion by malalignment of the DNA in homologous regions just 3' to the pseudo-α and the α2 loci and the rightward deletion by the malalignment of the α1 and the α2 gene loci [51].

Nondeletion defects can also produce the α-thalassemia-1 genotype, although the molecular lesions responsible for them have not yet been fully characterized. In a Chinese patient [93], both α-globin genes were shown to be intact and active in α-globin mRNA transcription. A single nucleotide mutation in the α2 locus changes the codon 125 from CCT to CGT, changing the amino acid from leucine to proline (Goossens et al., unpublished). This abnormal chain turns over rapidly and causes the thalassemia phenotype.

In the Mediterranean population, an apparent nondeletion α thalassemia is caused by a small deletion at a region vital for mRNA processing [94]. Five base pairs were lost from the 5' end of the first intron of the α2 gene, one nucleotide from the splice junction. This results in defective processing of the α2 transcript and loss of function of that gene. When combined with the deletion type of α-thalassemia-1 gene, this genotype produces Hb-H disease. Other nondeletion α thalassemias have not yet been characterized. The genotype was recently found to be common in Saudi Arabia, where homozygosity also produces Hb-H disease [95].

The α-thalassemia-2 genotype can also arise from a termination codon mutation. If the normal termination codon for the α-globin mRNA (UAA) is mutated so that it encodes for an amino acid rather that a terminator signal, the polyribosomes will continue to assemble the polypeptide chain until the next termination codon is reached. The first example of such a mutation was Hb Constant Spring [74] where the termination codon UAA is mutated to CAA (the codon for glutamine) at the α2-globin gene. Protein synthesis continues through another 31 amino acids until the next UAA termination codon, normally present in the 3' noncoding region of the α-globin mRNA, is reached. The α Constant Spring chain thus contains 172 amino acids rather than the normal 141. We do not yet understand why only small amounts of the α Constant Spring mutant are present in the red cell. Heterozygotes for this con-

Table 77-2   Defined molecular mechanisms in α thalassemia

α *Thalassemia-2 (decreased function of a single α-globin locus)*
1. Deletion of a single α-globin locus (−α)
2. Termination codon mutation in the α2 locus; e.g., Hb Constant Spring (α$^{c.s.}$α)
3. Intron mutation affecting processing of α2 globin mRNA precursor
4. Single amino acid substitution preventing α1β1 formation

α *Thalassemia-1 (decreased function of both α-globin loci in cis)*
Deletion of both α loci (−−); no α-globin chains present in the homozygous state

dition have about 1 percent of the Constant Spring chain, which indicates that the locus is producing much less than the normal 25 percent. Results of globin chain synthesis experiments suggest that the α-globin mRNA from the α Constant Spring locus is unstable [96]. Recently, this was demonstrated directly by detection of the Constant Spring mRNA in the bone marrow but not in the peripheral blood reticulocytes [97].

The α Constant Spring mutant, found in southeast Asia, is the most common termination codon mutation. Other, less common α-globin mutants, hemoglobins Icaria [98], Seal Rock [98a], and Koya Dora [99], have lysine (AAA), glutamic acid (GAA), and serine (UCA), respectively, at amino acid position 142, instead of glutamine as found in Hb Constant Spring.

Population Genetics of α Thalassemia Alpha thalassemia occurs predominantly in people of Mediterranean, African, and Asian origin. The severe homozygous form, hydrops fetalis, occurs almost exclusively in southeast Asia and has been well-characterized in Chinese, Thai, Filipinos, and recently in Vietnamese and Cambodians. Homozygous α thalassemia-1 has rarely been found in people of Greek and Cypriot origin and has never been detected in people of African descent. Hemoglobin-H disease, although common in Asia and the Mediterranean area, is rare in people of African origin.

The differences in geographic distribution of the clinical syndromes in these populations are related to the frequency of the α-thalassemia-1 and α-thalassemia-2 genotypes. Both these genotypes occur with approximately equal frequency in Asians and produce the whole spectrum of α-thalassemia syndromes, including Hb-H disease and hydrops fetalis. In contrast, the α-thalassemia-2 genotype is common in people originating from the Mediterranean region, but the α-thalassemia-1 genotype is rare. Alpha-thalassemia trait in this population is more frequently due to the homozygous state of α thalassemia-2 than to the heterozygous state of α thalassemia-1. Hemoglobin-H disease exists because of the high frequency of the α-thalassemia-2 genotype; homozygous α thalassemia is seldom seen because the α-thalassemia-1 genotype is rare. People of African origin also commonly have the α-thalassemia-2 genotype, but the α-thalassemia-1 genotype is even rarer than in the Mediterranean population. Consequently, Hb-H disease is rare, and hydrops due to homozgous α thalassemia has never been described [72, 100].

In the Saudi Arabian population, the nondeletion form of α thalassemia appears to be the common cause of the α-thalassemia-1 genotype. Since the nondeletion α-thalassemia lesion permits synthesis of reduced amounts of α-globin chain, homozygosity for this gene results in Hb-H disease and not the lethal hydrops fetalis [95].

The α-thalassemia-2 genotype with a single gene deletion occurs frequently throughout the world. For example, the frequency of this genotype is 0.16 in the American black and 0.18 in Sardinians. In some world populations, such as Melanesians and certain East Indians, the frequency of the single α-globin locus exceeds that of the duplicated α loci [78]. The high frequency of the α-thalassemia-2 genotype suggests that it offers a selective advantage. As the geographic distribution of α thalassemia-2 closely parallels that of malaria, it is tempting to suggest that α thalassemia, like the sickle and the β-globin genes, protects against malaria. In vitro studies of malaria cultures indicate a possible disadvantage for the malaria parasite in red blood cells of individuals with α thalassemia [101]. Other environmental factors cannot be ruled out. If, indeed,

the α-thalassemia-2 genotype has a selective advantage, its frequency should exceed that of the sickle and β-thalassemia genotypes since homozygosity for α thalassemia-2 is compatible with normal life and reproductive patterns, whereas homozygosity for β thalassemia or sickle-cell anemia is not. As a consequence, there is a gene pool loss from the latter two conditions but not from α thalassemia-2.

Triplicated α-Globin Loci The high frequency of the single α-globin locus suggests that unequal crossing-over of the two α-globin loci is a common occurrence during the evolutionary process. For this to be true, a reciprocal chromosome that contains three α-globin loci should be present; indeed, gene-mapping studies have uncovered individuals who carry three α-globin loci on one chromosome [102, 103]. In black Americans, the frequency of the triple α locus is 0.004 compared with 0.16 for the single α locus. Chromosomes that carry three α-globin loci have also been found in Caucasians, Greek Cypriots, Israelis, and Malaysians. Triplicated α loci due to both rightward and leftward deletions have been found, although the former are more common [104]. Heterozygosity for the triple α locus produces no apparent clinical effect [102]. Since unequal crossing-over should produce equal numbers of chromosomes with the single locus as with the triple α loci, the fact that more chromosomes with the single α locus have been found again suggests that it has a selective advantage.

The β-Thalassemia Syndromes

Clinical Types Compared with α thalassemia, inheritance of β thalassemia is relatively straightforward. Since there is only one β-globin locus on each chromosome, an individual is either heterozygous or homozygous for the β-thalassemia gene, but different mutations produce many molecular types of β thalassemia. These are broadly classified into several groups according to the degree of involvement of the δ-globin locus, which in turn affects the Hb A_2 level. Fetal hemoglobin levels often increase to a variable extent in the different β-thalassemia syndromes. The most common form of β thalassemia, which does not involve the δ-globin locus, is characterized by an elevated Hb A_2 level [1–3]. This high A_2 type of β thalassemia is divided into two groups, one in which no β-globin is synthesized from the affected locus (β^0) and another where some, albeit a reduced amount, is produced (β^+). The severity of the β^+ type varies. In certain populations it is as severe as the β^0 type, but in others (such as the African) the disease is mild. Usually homozygous β thalassemia is characterized by severe anemia, and the patient is transfusion-dependent. Occasionally the disease is so mild that no transfusions are required in the homozygous state. This milder form of homozygous β thalassemia is called *thalassemia intermedia*.

When both the δ- and β-globin loci are involved, the resultant disorders are classified as δβ thalassemia [105]. Characteristically the Hb A_2 levels are not elevated and, in fact, are often below normal. Homozygous $\delta^0\beta^0$ thalassemia is a very rare disorder in which both δ- and β-globin are absent. The γ-globin locus produces more Hb F than in the high A_2 type of β thalassemia, and this mitigates the severity of the disease. $\delta^+\beta^+$ Thalassemia (the "silent carrier" state of β thalassemia) is a mild lesion, in which β-globin chain synthesis is not completely suppressed, and Hb A_2 levels are normal [106]. It is usually found in combination with high A_2 β thalassemia and produces a mild disease.

γδβ Thalassemia is extremely rare. In the heterozygous state, the absence of γ, δ, and β chain synthesis from the affected chromosome produces hemolytic disease in the newborn period [107, 108].

Hereditary persistence of fetal hemoglobin is not usually classified as thalassemia since no anemia occurs. There is no output from either the δ or β loci, but unlike δβ thalassemia, γ-chain production adequately compensates for the lack of β chain, and few, if any, clinical effects are produced [109, 110].

β-Thalassemia Trait   The carrier, or heterozygous, states of β thalassemia are usually asymptomatic. Hemoglobin levels range from normal to slightly decreased; in the adult, they seldom drop below 10 g/dl. In times of stress precipitated by pregnancy or infection, the patient may become anemic, and in children the hemoglobin levels may fall below 10 g/dl. The peripheral blood is characterized by microcytosis with a variable degree of anisocytosis and poikilocytosis. Occasional coarse basophilic stippling of the red blood cell is found. There are mild hyperplasia of the erythroid series in the bone marrow and defective hemoglobinization of the normoblast. Erythrokinetic studies show mildly ineffective erythropoiesis. Globin chain studies of the peripheral blood reticulocyte give a β/α ratio in the range of 0.5, but in the bone marrow, where the β/α ratio approaches 1, the imbalance is less evident [111]. This may be due to more effective compensation by normal β chains as well as to more efficient proteolysis of the excess α-globin chains in the bone marrow. Occasionally heterozygous β thalassemia is associated with hepatosplenomegaly. Rare instances of severe β-thalassemia trait associated with splenomegaly, gallstones, and leg ulcers have been documented [113, 114].

In high A_2-β-thalassemia trait, the Hb-A_2 level ranges from 3 to 5 percent and occasionally reaches 8 percent. The fetal hemoglobin level varies from less than 1 to about 5 percent. In δβ-thalassemia trait, the Hb A_2 level is normal or slightly decreased, but Hb F composes 5 to 20 percent of the total hemoglobin. Both Hb A_2 and Hb F levels are normal in γδβ-thalassemia trait.

Homozygous β Thalassemia   Of the various thalassemia syndromes, homozygous β thalassemia has the most pronounced medical, social, and economic impact throughout the world. The disease was first described in people of Mediterranean origin, but its distribution extends eastward through the Middle East, the Indian subcontinent, southeast Asia, and Africa [1].

A child affected with homozygous β thalassemia is generally not anemic at birth since the high Hb F levels mask the lack of β-globin chain production. As γ-globin synthesis gradually diminishes during the first few months after birth, the anemia becomes increasingly evident, although sometimes the disease escapes clinical detection until 1 or 2 years after birth. The first signs are pallor, listlessness and failure to thrive. The abdomen becomes enlarged from the hepatosplenomegaly. Bone marrow proliferation produces frontal bossing and maxillary bone enlargement, resulting in the typical mongoloid facies. The outer table of the skull thickens and gives the typical hair-on-end appearance; the ribs expand noticeably owing to bone marrow proliferation, and as the patient gets older many bones

become rarefied and cause pathologic fractures (Fig. 77-5) [115, 116]. The mediastinal and abdominal lymph nodes are markedly hypertrophied from extramedullary erythropoiesis.

Physical and sexual development is retarded. Female patients often have delayed onset of menarche or do not menstruate at all, and male patients have underdeveloped secondary sex characteristics [117, 118]. Ineffective erythropoiesis increases the amount of iron absorbed through the gastrointestinal tract, and this, together with the additional iron load delivered with every blood transfusion, causes hemosiderosis in many organs [119]. Although this sometimes leads to diabetes [120], the most serious effects are on the heart [121]. The severe anemia and hemosiderosis lead to cardiac enlargement, and heart failure usually occurs by the time patients reach their late teens or twenties. Infection is the common cause of childhood mortality, particularly if the patient has undergone splenectomy. Later in life, death occurs from cardiac arrhythmia or cardiac failure. Until recently, few patients with the severe form of homozygous β thalassemia lived beyond their second decade.

Without transfusion the hemoglobin levels can fall to 3 to 5 g/dl. The red cell is severely hypochromic and varies greatly in size and shape. A few normoblasts are visible, and after splenectomy their numbers increase markedly. Splenectomy also elevates the platelet count, sometimes to above 1 million. There is intense bone marrow erythroid hyperplasia, and supervital staining of the bone marrow with crystal violet shows large inclusions of precipitated α-globin chains in the nucleated red cells [122, 123]. These inclusions are also found in the peripheral blood normoblast and red cell following splenectomy. Hemoglobin electrophoresis findings depend on the clinical type; in homozygous $β^+$ thalassemia, the hemoglobin components are F, A_2, and A, while in homozygous $β^0$ thalassemia, only hemoglobins A_2 and F are present. Hemoglobin electrophoresis of the compound heterozygous state of $β^+$ and $β^0$ thalassemia shows hemoglobins A, A_2, and F. Homozygous $δ^0β^0$ thalassemia usually runs a milder clinical course than the homozygous state of high A_2 β thalassemia because of the greater compensatory increase in fetal hemoglobin production. The only hemoglobin present on electrophoresis is Hb F. Compound heterozygosity for $δ^0β^0$ and high A_2 β thalassemia usually produces an intermediate clinical course.

Over the past 10 years, the bleak clinical description associated with homozygous β thalassemia has been markedly altered by changes in therapy. Previously, transfusion was administered sparingly and only when the patient could no longer tolerate the severe anemia. Modern therapy attempts to maintain hemoglobin levels above 10 g/dl to suppress the endogenous erythropoiesis [117, 124, 125]. The rationale is that despite the massive bone marrow expansion in response to the anemia, the erythropoiesis is, for the most part, ineffective and many red cell precursors are destroyed before emerging from the bone marrow. The premature erythroid cell destruction is caused by the vast excess of uncombined α-globin chains which are unstable and precipitate, damaging cell structure and function [126]. The cells that do emerge are grossly abnormal and are destroyed in the reticuloendothelial systems, causing the hepatosplenomegaly. The severe bone marrow proliferation produces the characteristic bone deformities. The resultant anemia and increased iron absorption damage many organs, stunt growth, and produce cardiac abnormalities. Maintaining the hemoglobin level above 10 g/dl suppresses the bone marrow expansion and prevents the bone changes and

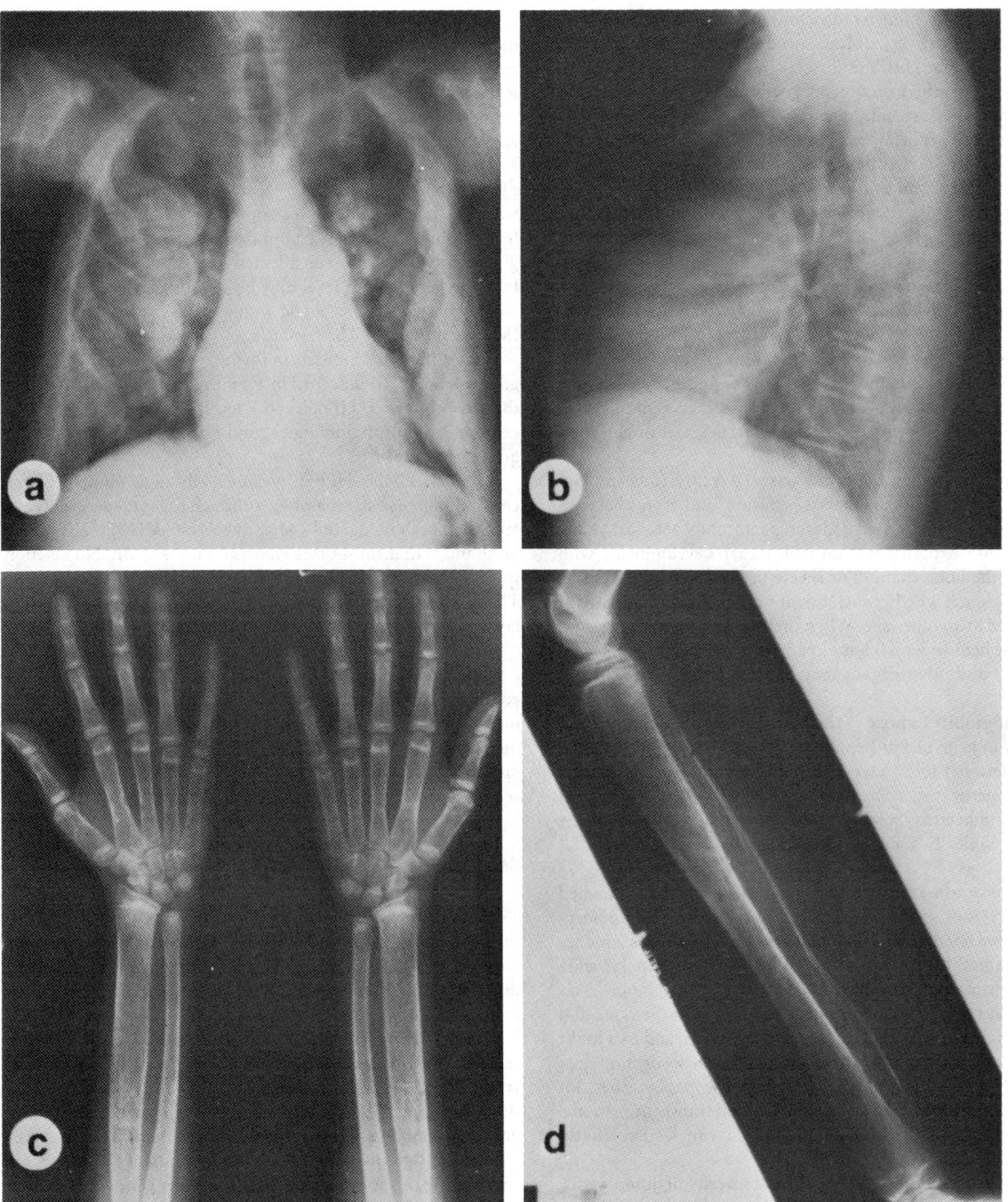

Figure 77-5 X-ray from an adult with homozygous β thalassemia. The changes have not been modified by transfusion. *A* and *B*, PA and lateral view of chest showing massive expansion of the ribs and rarefaction of the vertebrae; *C* and *D*, upper and lower limbs showing extensive rarefaction of bone and linear pseudofractures.

the extramedullary erythropoiesis. The lack of abnormal cells in the blood prevents organ enlargement from hypertrophy of the reticuloendothelial systems. The spleen and liver do not become grossly enlarged, and splenectomy, which previously was commonly required, is now reserved for those patients in whom secondary hypersplenism reduces the life span of the tranfused cells and increases the transfusion requirement [127].

Recently, attempts have been made to maintain the hemoglobin levels above 12 g/dl in order to suppress more effectively the endogenous erythropoiesis [128]. This has not significantly increased the frequency of transfusion. A new technique that uses young red blood cells (neocytes) has reduced the transfusion requirement from once every 4 to 5 weeks to once every 7 to 8 weeks and may further decrease the iron load [128, 129].

An aggressive iron chelation program is now administered in conjunction with the transfusion regimen. The drug deferoxamine, which has been used for many years for iron chelation, was previously administered via intramuscular injection [130]. This mode of delivery did not produce an adequate negative iron balance, and, furthermore, many patients were unable to tolerate the painful injection on a daily basis. It was discovered that the same dose administered by continuous intravenous infusion increased iron excretion severalfold. Continuous subcutaneous infusion has proved to be almost as effective as infusion by the intravenous route and offers the added advantages of sparing vein destruction and enabling at-home administration by parents [131, 132]. Over a 12-h period 1 to 2 g of deferoxamine is infused by a portable battery-operated infusion pump. Infusions are administered 5 to 6 days each week, and during transfusion additional deferoxamine is administered intravenously. The vigorous transfusion regimen achieves a negative iron balance in most cases. Currently, iron chelation therapy commences at 4 years of age, but as the heart and other organs may already have sustained some damage from iron deposit prior to this time, earlier onset of chelation therapy is now being tried [127, 133].

Follow-up studies over the past 10 years indicate that patients who start the hypertransfusion and iron chelation treatment at an early age develop normally. So far, many patients are experiencing normal sexual development, with none of the bone changes or severe hepatosplenomegaly. It is too early to tell whether such therapy alters the cardiac damage evidenced at an older age. When therapy commences after considerable hemosiderosis has already taken place, the damage to the heart and other organs may be irreversible.

Hemoglobin Lepore   The chromosome that contains the δ-β fusion gene of Hb Lepore acts much like a β-thalassemia gene. Heterozygotes have about 15 percent Hb Lepore and typical microcytosis. The homozygous state of Hb Lepore and compound heterozygosity of the Lepore gene with β thalassemia are clinically similar to thalassemia major.

Thalassemia Intermedia   The clinical picture described in the previous section applies to most patients with homozygous β thalassemia. In a few patients, the disease runs a milder course, and this less severe form of homozygous β thalassemia is known as *thalassemia intermedia*. The hemoglobin levels remain at about 9 g/dl without transfusion. All the bone and organ changes occur, although at a slower pace and to a lesser extent. Hemosiderosis from the increased iron absorption does occur, but the effects are delayed since the patient does not receive additional iron from frequent blood transfusions. Some individuals with thalassemia intermedia can lead relatively normal lives [134].

The factors that decrease the clinical severity of homozygous β thalassemia are not completely understood, although several are known. Coinheritance of α thalassemia with homozygous β thalassemia tends to balance the globin chain synthesis and hence reduce the amount of free α-globin chain present. Since it is the excess of free α chain that destroys the red cells, these patients have a milder clinical course [135]. In some instances, continued production of fetal hemoglobin compensates for the lack of β-globin production and ameliorates the severity of the disease, as in homozygous δβ thalassemia. Sometimes a mild defect reduces the level of β-globin chain synthesis, which is probably why $\delta\beta^+$ thalassemia [106] and the African form of β^+ thalassemia are less severe than other types of thalassemia [136].

Hereditary Persistence of Fetal Hemoglobin   In some individuals, fetal hemoglobin synthesis persists into postnatal and adult life. There are two types of hereditary persistence of fetal hemoglobin (HPFH)—pancellular and heterocellular. In the pancellular form, a Kleihauer-Bethke stain shows increased amounts of fetal hemoglobin in all the red cells, although the amounts may vary somewhat among the cells. Red cell morphology and hemoglobin levels are normal in the heterozygous state, and hemoglobin electrophoresis shows elevated fetal hemoglobin levels. In the homozygous state, only fetal hemoglobin is synthesized. The affected individual is not anemic; in fact, the hemoglobin level may be slightly elevated [110]. The red cell is slightly microcytic with a mean corpuscular volume (MCV) in the 70s. The quantity and type of fetal hemoglobin present differs. In the African form, $^G\gamma$-$^A\gamma$ HPFH, a heterozygote has 25 to 30 percent Hb F, with a $^G\gamma/^A\gamma$ ratio of 2:3. In the Greek type, $^A\gamma$ HPFH, Hb F levels are elevated to 15 percent, $^A\gamma$-globin predominates, and only trace amounts of $^G\gamma$ are present [137].

In heterocellular HPFH, an unusually high number of red cells contain fetal hemoglobin, although the total percentage of fetal hemoglobin is only slightly elevated [138, 139]. The mechanism that causes this increase is not known. No deletion in the region of the β-globin cluster has been demonstrated. The genotype is inherited autosomally according to Mendelian laws and appears to be linked to the β locus.

γδβ Thalassemia   Only the heterozygous state of this condition has been described. At birth, the infant exhibits a microcytic hemolytic anemia with normoblastemia. The anemia subsides within a few weeks, but the microcytosis persists, and the clinical picture then resembles heterozygous β thalassemia, except that the Hb A_2 level is normal [107, 108].

Molecular Pathology of β Thalassemia

The lesions that reduce the level of β-globin chain synthesis in the β thalassemias are extremely heterogeneous. The new recombinant DNA technology has facilitated the study of the disease, and a number of molecular defects have now been defined.

Whereas deletion is the most common mechanism in the α thalassemias, it does not often cause β thalassemia. Several types of deletions that affect the β-globin loci have been described (Fig. 77-6). The Lepore hemoglobin can be considered a type of deletion that involves a region of DNA between the δ- and β-globin genes. Reduced amounts of the δ-β-globin fusion gene product are present, giving this genotype an effect similar to a β-thalassemia gene. In the Indian type a deletion involves the 3' portion of the β-globin structural gene and causes β^0 thalassemia [140, 141]. When both the δ- and β-globin loci are absent, the resultant disorder is $\delta^0\beta^0$ thalassemia. Two deletions are known to produce this disorder: one starts at the 3' portion of the δ-globin gene and continues through the entire β-globin gene, leaving only the 5' portion of the δ-globin gene intact [142, 143]. The second, which has been described in Turks, involves the $^A\gamma$, δ, and β loci [142, 144]. Two deletions have also been defined in $^G\gamma$-$^A\gamma$ HPFH. Both extend from a DNA segment downstream from the β-globin gene to a point beyond the δ- and β-globin genes but differ in the extent to which the DNA segment upstream from

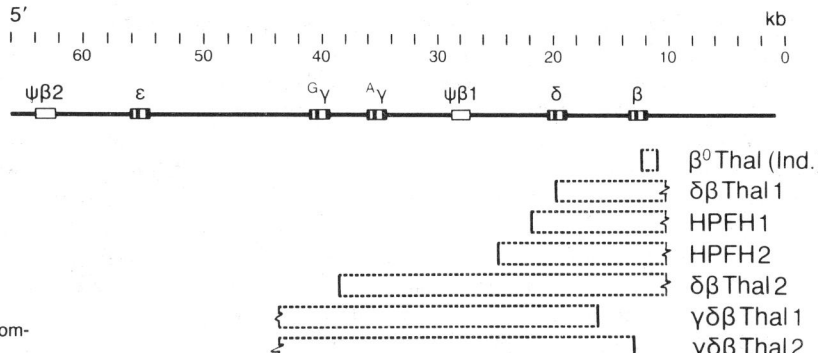

Figure 77-6 Various deletions that affect the β-globin complex. ψβ2 and ψβ1 are the two pseudo-β-globin genes.

the β-globin gene is involved [142–144]. The $^A\gamma$ type of HPFH is not due to any discernible gene deletion [145]. γδβ Thalassemia is also caused by two different gene deletions. One affects the $^G\gamma$, $^A\gamma$, and δ loci and the 5′ portion of the β-globin gene [146]; the other affects the $^A\gamma$-, $^G\gamma$-, and δ-globin genes but stops just before the β-globin gene [108]. β-Globin synthesis from this chromosome is reduced or absent. The reason for the loss of β-globin gene function is not clear. The chromosome may be inactivated by another mutation, or its expression may be regulated by a deleted stretch of DNA considerably upstream from the β-globin gene.

Most commonly, β thalassemia is not due to gene deletion, and only the output from the β locus is affected. Gene mapping studies of high A_2 β thalassemia show that apart from the Indian variety, the β-globin loci are present and intact. In β+ thalassemia, the affected locus produces decreased amounts of β-globin mRNA. Hybridization studies with α- and β-globin-specific probes quantitate higher levels of nuclear β-globin mRNA sequences than cytoplasmic β-globin mRNA sequences in these patients, which suggests a defect in processing of the nuclear pre-mRNA to mature cytoplasmic mRNA [147]. Pulse chase experiments and electrophoretic studies of the newly synthesized β mRNA also show that the large β-globin mRNA is not completely processed to the mature size in some patients [148]. In the cloned and sequenced DNA from one β+ thalassemia patient, a single nucleotide mutation (G to A) occurs in the first intervening sequence on the β-globin gene 22 nucleotides from the normal 3′ splice site (acceptor site) [149, 150]. The mutation produces a stretch of seven nucleotides which resembles the normal 3′ acceptor site and which is utilized as a new acceptor for splicing. Translation along this abnormally spliced mRNA encounters a termination codon about 60 nucleotides downstream and therefore produces no β-globin polypeptide chains. Only rarely does the splicing occur at the normal site and produce a normal mature mRNA. This accounts for the reduced amount of β globin present in such a patient.

The lesions that cause high A_2 β^0 thalassemia are also heterogeneous and β-globin mRNA levels can vary from zero to appreciable quantities. One type of β^0 thalassemia is probably due to abnormal processing. Sequence analysis shows a single base substitution at the 5′ end of the second intervening sequence. The normally invariant GT sequence is mutated to AT [151]. Such a change could affect processing and explain the lack of mature mRNA in the cytoplasm. The molecular lesion in two other types of β^0 thalassemia has been defined as a nonsense mutation where premature termination of the β-globin chain was due to a single nucleotide mutation that pro-

duced a termination codon in the coding region of the β-globin mRNA. In a Chinese patient the codon for the seventeenth amino acid lysine (AAG) was mutated to UAG [152], and in a Sardinian a mutation of the CAG (glutamine) codon to UAG occurred at amino acid number 39 [153]. A fourth lesion has been found where two nucleotides are deleted at a position corresponding to amino acid number 8. The resultant frameshift produces a termination codon UAG at a position corresponding to amino acid number 21 [154].

Thus in both the α and β thalassemias, many mutations can account for the reduced globin chain synthesis. So far, deletions, intron mutations, and nonsense mutations produced by a single nucleotide mutation or a frameshift have been defined. Defective mRNA transcription at a polymerase binding site has recently been found. The mechanism by which this causes β thalassemia is being characterized. Other mutations affecting promoter functions may also exist. Potentially, numerous lesions could produce thalassemia. For instance, a single mechanism, such as the mutation of one nucleotide, could cause nonsense mutations at 29 different positions along the β-globin mRNA [153]. Some mutations that occur in the malarious areas of the world will be more common than others because of selection. For example, the β^{39} $^{CAG} \rightarrow ^{UAG}$ mutation has been found in Sardinia, Morocco, and other Mediterranean populations [153, 154].

Prenatal Diagnosis

Detection of homozygous β thalassemia by prenatal diagnosis has been possible since 1974 [155, 156]. Fetal blood obtained by fetoscopy or placental aspiration is analyzed to quantitate the amount of β-globin chain synthesized relative to γ-globin chain. The β-globin synthesis is quantified by measuring the amount of radioactive amino acid incorporated into the β-globin chain. At the eighteenth week of gestation, when fetal blood sampling is usually performed, the β/α-globin chain synthetic ratio is normally about 0.08. In homozygous β^0 thalassemia, this ratio is 0, while in β+ it is less than 0.02. This method has been adopted by medical centers throughout the world. In areas with a high incidence of β thalassemia, prenatal diagnosis has appreciably reduced the number of homozygotes born and has had a positive influence on the reproductive patterns of parents at risk.

A different method of prenatal diagnosis utilizing amniocentesis can be performed in certain cases of β thalassemia and sickle-cell anemia. This method analyzes DNA from amniotic fluid cells with restriction endonucleases and is based on the principle of linkage analysis using variations in DNA sequence. Such alterations can abolish or create a restriction recognition site and, when they occur in the region of the β-globin gene, can be used for linkage analysis of both normal and mutant β-globin genes.

This technique was first applied to the sickle gene [157]. The restriction enzyme *Hpa* I cleaves DNA whenever the nucleotide sequence GTTAAC occurs. When normal human DNA is digested with this enzyme, the β-globin gene appears in a 7.6-kb DNA fragment. In certain individuals, a polymorphism abolishes the recognition site on the 3' (downstream) side of the β-globin gene, and the length of the DNA fragment containing the gene increases to 13 kb. In the American black population, the normal β^A gene is usually contained in the 7.6-kb fragment, and 70 percent of the time the β^S sickle gene is located in the 13-kb fragment. Therefore, in those families in which the association of the β^S with the 13-kb fragment occurs, the size of the β-globin gene fragment in the amniotic fluid DNA indicates the presence or absence of sickle cell anemia [158].

Another restriction site polymorphism has been used for prenatal diagnosis of β thalassemia [159]. The enzyme *Bam* HI cleaves the coding sequence of the normal β-globin gene into two fragments, each containing a portion of the β-globin gene. One 1.8-kb fragment contains the 5' portion, the other 9.3-kb fragment contains the 3' portion. A polymorphism of this *Bam* HI site on the 3' side of the β-globin gene produces a 22-kb fragment. In most human populations, the 9.3-kb fragment occurs more frequently than the 22-kb fragment. Beta^0 thalassemia in Sardinians and β^0 and β^+ thalassemia in Chinese are always associated with the chromosome containing the 9.3-kb fragment. Therefore, finding a 22-kb fragment excludes the presence of the β-thalassemia gene on that chromosome.

A third restriction endonuclease used for prenatal diagnosis is *Hin* dIII. The *Hin* dIII recognition sites in the intervening sequences of the $^G\gamma$ and $^A\gamma$ gene are polymorphic [160]. Certain individuals have *Hin* dIII sites in both genes (genotype G+A+), some have the site only in the $^G\gamma$ gene (G+A−), and others do not have it in either gene (G−A−). If informative family members are available, one can determine which of these three genotypes is linked to a normal or abnormal β-globin gene. This linkage can be used to diagnose sickle-cell anemia as well as β thalassemia [161, 162].

A more direct method for identifying a genetic disorder consists of analyzing the lesion itself. This can now be done for sickle-cell anemia. The enzyme *Dde* I cleaves normal DNA at the position $\beta^{5\&6}$. This cleavage site is abolished by the sickle mutation, and different-sized DNA fragments are generated [162a]. This test can be used for all pregnancies at risk for sickle-cell anemia [162b].

This direct approach to genetic analysis is only applicable to those few β thalassemias due to gene deletion, or to disorders in which the mutation happens to affect a restriction site. Since the molecular pathology of β thalassemia is so heterogeneous and defining the exact mutation in any given family is not practical, fetal blood sampling remains the mainstay for prenatal diagnosis of these disorders [162c].

CONCLUSION

The thalassemia syndromes have provided an excellent model system for the study of genetic diseases. Because of the ease of

obtaining hemoglobin and globin-specific mRNA, globin-specific genes have been isolated and studied. The molecular lesions in this group of diseases have been defined more precisely than in other genetic disorders. A better understanding of the pathophysiology of thalassemia has provided new and improved management and treatment techniques. The prospects for normal physical development for patients with homozygous β thalassemia have been greatly enhanced by the hypertransfusion and iron chelation therapy. Prenatal diagnosis has enabled many couples at risk to bear healthy children. The use of restriction endonucleases to diagnose thalassemia illustrates how advances in the area of basic science can be applied at a clinical level.

During the next few years, investigations will be directed toward defining the mechanisms that control globin gene expression in order to develop effective gene therapy for thalassemia. One possible strategy involves introducing a normal gene in place of a defective one. Thus far, cloned normal β-globin genes that were introduced into heterologous cells have not been expressed efficiently. Another approach is the maintenance or reactivation of the fetal or embryonic genes. The clinical severity of homozygous β thalassemia or sickle-cell anemia would be considerably ameliorated if γ-globin synthesis could be maintained at a high level after birth. Likewise, continued synthesis of the ζ-globin chain to form the functional Hb Portland ($\zeta_2\gamma_2$) would increase the chance for survival of fetuses affected by homozygous α thalassemia. These approaches may be successful once we gain a better understanding of the mechanisms that control globin gene activation.

REFERENCES

1. WEATHERALL DJ, CLEGG JB: *The Thalassemia Syndromes*, 3d ed. Oxford, Blackwell, 1981
2. BUNN HF, FORGET BG, RANNEY HM: *Human Hemoglobins*. Philadelphia, Saunders, 1977
3. WEATHERALL DJ, CLEGG JB: Recent developments in the molecular genetics of human hemoglobin. *Cell* 16:467, 1979
4. FORGET B: Molecular genetics of human hemoglobin synthesis. *Ann Intern Med* 91:605, 1979
5. INGRAM VM, STRETTON AOW: Genetic basis of the thalassemia diseases. *Nature* 184:1903, 1959
6. BANNERMAN RM: *Thalassemia. A Survey of Some Aspects*. New York, Grune & Stratton, 1961
7. WEATHERALL DJ: Towards an understanding of the molecular biology of some common inherited anemias: The story of thalassemia, in Wintrobe MM (ed): *Blood, Pure and Eloquent*. New York, McGraw-Hill, 1980, p 373
8. MANIATIS T: Recombinant DNA procedures in the study of eukaryotic genes, in Goldstein L, Prescott D (eds): *Comprehensive Cell Biology*. New York, Academic, 1980, vol 3
9. BLATTNER FR, BLECHL AE, DENNISTON-THOMPSON K, FABER HE, RICHARDS JE, SLIGHTOM JL, TUCKER PW, SMITHIES O: Cloning human fetal γ-globin and mouse α-type globin DNA: Preparation and screening of shotgun collections. *Science* 202:1279, 1978
10. LEDER A, MILLER HI, HAMER DH, SEIDMAN JG, NORMAN B, SULLIVAN M, LEDER P: Comparison of cloned mouse α- and β-globin genes: Conservation of intervening sequence locations and extragenic homology. *Proc Natl Acad Sci USA* 75:6187, 1978
11. MAXAM AM, GILBERT W: A new method for sequencing DNA. *Proc Natl Acad Sci USA* 74:560, 1977
12. SANGER F, NICKLEN S, COULSON AR: DNA sequencing with chain-terminating inhibitors. *Proc Natl Acad Sci USA* 74:5463, 1977
13. NATHANS D, SMITH HO: Restriction endonucleases in the analysis and restructuring of DNA molecules. *Ann Rev Biochem* 44:273, 1975
14. SOUTHERN EM: Detection of specific sequences among DNA fragments separated by gel electrophoresis. *J Mol Biol* 98:503, 1975
15. HUEHNS ER, DANCE N, BEAVEN GH, KEIL JV, HECHT F, MOTULSKY G: Human embryonic haemoglobins. *Nature* 201:1095, 1969
16. HUEHNS ER, FAROOQUI AM: Oxygen dissociation properties of human embryonic red cells. *Nature* 254:335, 1975

17. CAPP GL, RIGAS DA, JONES RT: Hemoglobin Portland 1: A new human hemoglobin unique in structure. *Science* 157:65, 1967

18. HUEHNS ER: The structure and function of human haemoglobin: Clinical disorders due to abnormal haemoglobin structure, in Hardesty RM, Weatherall DJ (eds): *Blood and Its Disorders*. Oxford, Blackwell, 1974, p 526

19. WOOD WG: Haemoglobin synthesis during fetal development. *J Med Bul* 32:282, 1976

20. HUEHNS ER, HECHT F, KEIL JV, MOTULSKY AG: Developmental hemoglobin anomalies in a chromosomal triplication: D1 trisomy syndrome. *Proc Natl Acad Sci USA* 51:89, 1964

21. LIE-INJO LE, JO BH: A fast-moving haemoglobin in hydrops foetalis. *Nature* 185:698, 1960

22. TODD D, LAI MCS, BEAVEN GH, HUEHNS ER: The abnormal haemoglobins in homozygous α thalassaemia. *Br J Haematol* 19:27, 1970

23. PATARYAS HA, STAMATOYANNOPOULOS G: Hemoglobins in human fetuses: Evidence for adult hemoglobin production after the 11th gestational week. *Blood* 39:688, 1972

24. KAZAZIAN HH, WOODHEAD AP: Hemoglobin A synthesis in the developing fetus. *N Engl J Med* 289:58, 1973

25. CIVIDALLI G, NATHAN DG, KAN YW, SANTAMARINA B, FRIGOLETTO F: Relationship of beta to gamma synthesis during the first trimester: An approach to prenatal diagnosis of thalassemia. *Pediatr Res* 8:553, 1974

26. SCHROEDER WA, HUISMAN THJ, SHELTON JR, SHELTON JB, KLEIHAUER EF, DOZY AM, ROBBERSON B: Evidence for multiple structural genes for the γ chain of human fetal hemoglobin. *Proc Natl Acad Sci USA* 60:537, 1968

27. SCHROEDER WA, HUISMAN THJ, BROWN AK, UY, R, BOUVER NG, LERCH PO, SHELTON JR, SHELTON JB, APELL G: Postnatal changes in the chemical heterogeneity of human fetal hemoglobin. *Pediatr Res* 5:493, 1971

28. RICCO G, MAZZA U, TURI RM, PICH PG, CAMASCHELLA C, SAGLIO G, BERNINI LF: Significance of a new type of human fetal hemoglobin carrying a replacement isoleucine → threonine at position 75 (E 19) of the γ chain. *Hum Genet* 32:305, 1976

29. SAGLIO G, RICCO G, MAZZA U, CAMASCHELLA C, PICH PG, GIANNI AM, GIANAZZA E, RIGHETTI PG, GIGLIONI B, COMI P, GUZMEROLI C, OTTOLENGHI S: Human Tγ globin chain is a variant of Aγ chain (Aγ Sardinia). *Proc Natl Acad Sci USA* 76:3420, 1979

30. SCHROEDER WA, HUISMAN THJ, EFREMOV GD, SHELTON JR, SHELTON JB, PHILLIPS R, REESE A, GRAVELY M, HARRISON JM, LAM H: Further studies of the frequency and significance of the Tγ-chain of human fetal hemoglobin. *J Clin Invest* 63:268, 1979

31. RIGAS DA, KOLER RD, OSGOOD EE: New hemoglobin possessing a higher electrophoretic mobility than normal adult hemoglobin. *Science* 121:372, 1955

32. GOUTTAS A, FESSAS P, TSEVRENIS H, KEFTERI E: Description d'une nouvelle variete d'anaemia haemolytique congenitale (Etude hematologique, electrophretique et genetique). *Sang* 26:911, 1955

33. AGAR JAM, LEHMANN H: Observations on some "fast" haemoglobins, K, J, N and "Bart's." *Br Med J* 1:929, 1958

34. BENESCH RE, RANNEY HM, BENESCH R, SMITH M: The chemistry of the Bohr effect. II. Some properties of hemoglobin H. *J Biol Chem* 236:2926, 1961

35. HORTON B, THOMPSON RB, DOZY AM, NECHTMAN CM, NICHOLS E, HUISMAN THJ: Inhomogeneity of hemoglobin. VI. The minor hemoglobin components of cord blood. *Blood* 20:302, 1962

36. DEISSEROTH A, NIENHUIS A, TURNER P, VELEZ R, ANDERSON WF, RUDDLE F, LAWRENCE J, CREAGAN R, KUCHERLAPATI R: Localization of the human α-globin structural gene to chromosome 16 in somatic cell hybrids by molecular hybridization assay. *Cell* 12:205, 1977

37. DEISSEROTH A, NIENHUIS A, LAWRENCE J, GILES R, TURNER P, RUDDLE FH: Chromosomal localization of human β globin gene in human chromosome 11 in somatic cell hybrids. *Proc Natl Acad Sci USA* 75:1456, 1978

38. GUSELLA J, KEYS C, VARSANYI-BREINER A, KAO FT, JONES C, PUCK TT, ORKIN S, HOUSMAN D: Precise localization of human β-globin gene complex on chromosome 11. *Proc Natl Acad Sci USA* 76:5239, 1979

39. LEBO RV, CARRANO AV, BURKHART-SCHULTZ K, DOZY AM, YU L-C, KAN YW: Assignment of human β-, γ- and δ-globin genes to the short arm of chromosome 11 by chromosome sorting and DNA restriction enzyme analysis. *Proc Natl Acad Sci USA* 76:5804, 1979

40. BAGLIONI C: The fusion of two peptide chains in hemoglobin Lepore and its interpretation as a genetic deletion. *Proc Natl Acad Sci USA* 48:1880, 1962

41. LEHMANN H, CHARLESWORTH D: Observations of hemoglobin P (Congo type). *Biochem J* 119:43, 1970

42. OHTA Y, KMAOKA K, SUMIDA I, YANASE T: Haemoglobin Miyada, a β-δ fusion peptide (anti-Lepore) type discovered in a Japanese family. *Nature [New Biol]* 234:218, 1971

43. KENDALL AG, OJWANG PJ, SCHROEDER WA, HUISMAN THJ: Hemoglobin Kenya, the product of a gamma-beta fusion gene: Studies of the family. *Am J Hum Genet* 25:548, 1973

44. SMITH DH, CLEGG JB, WEATHERALL DJ, GILES HM: Hereditary persistence of foetal haemoglobin associated with a δβ fusion variant, haemoglobin Kenya. *Nature [New Biol]* 246:184, 1973

45. LEHMANN H, CARRELL RW: Differences between α- and β-chain mutants of human haemoglobin and between α- and β-thalassemia. Possible duplication of the α-chain gene. *Br Med J* 4:748, 1968

46. NUTE PE: Multiple hemoglobin α-chain loci in monkeys, apes and man. *Ann NY Acad Sci* 241:39, 1974

47. HOLLAN SR, SZELENYI JG, BRIMHALL B, DUERST M, JONES RT, KOLER RD, STOCKLEN Z: Multiple alpha chain loci for human haemoglobins: Hb J-Buda and Hb G-Pest. *Nature* 235:47, 1972

48. KAN YW, DOZY AM, VARMUS HE, TAYLOR JM, HOLLAND JP, LIE-INJO LE: Deletion of α-globin genes in haemoglobin-H disease demonstrates multiple α-globin structural loci. *Nature* 255:255, 1975

49. MANIATIS T, FRITSCH EF, LAUER J, LAWN RM: The molecular genetics of human hemoglobins. *Annu Rev Genet* 14:145, 1980

50. FRITSCH EF, LAWN RM, MANIATIS T: Molecular cloning and characterization of the human β-like globin gene cluster. *Cell* 19:959, 1980

51. LAUER J, SHEN C-KJ, MANIATIS T: The chromosomal arrangement of human α-like globin genes: Sequence homology and α-globin gene deletions. *Cell* 20:119, 1980

52. PROUDFOOT N, SHANDER M, WOUDE SV, MANIATIS T: The structure and transcription of normal and abnormal human globin genes. *J Supramol Struct Cell Biochem [Suppl]* 5:381, 1981

53. LIEBHABER SA, GOOSSENS M, KAN YW: Cloning and complete nucleotide sequence of human 5'-α-globin gene. *Proc Natl Acad Sci USA* 77:7054, 1980

54. MICHELSON AM, ORKIN SH: The 3' untranslated regions of the duplicated human α-globin genes are unexpectedly divergent. *Cell* 22:371, 1980

55. LIEBHABER SA, GOOSSENS M, KAN YW: Homology and concerted evolution at the α1 and α2 loci of human α-globin. *Nature* 290:26, 1981

56. PROUDFOOT NJ, MANIATIS T: The structure of a human α-globin pseudogene and its relationship to α-globin gene duplication. *Cell* 21:537, 1980

57. LAWN RM, EFSTRATIADIS A, O'CONNELL C, MANIATIS T: The nucleotide sequence of the human β-globin gene. *Cell* 21:647, 1980

58. SPRITZ RA, DE RIEL JK, FORGET BG, WEISSMAN SM: Complete nucleotide sequence of the human γ-globin gene. *Cell* 21:639, 1980

59. SLIGHTOM JL, BLECHL AE, SMITHIES O: Human fetal Gγ- and Aγ-globin genes: Complete nucleotide sequences suggest that DNA can be exchanged between these duplicated genes. *Cell* 21:627, 1980

60. PROUDFOOT NJ, BARALLE FE: Molecular cloning of the human ε-globin gene. *Proc Natl Acad Sci USA* 76:5435, 1979

61. FURUICHI Y, MORGAN M, MUTHUKRISHNAN S, SHATKIN A: Reovirus messenger RNA contains a methylated blocked 5'-terminal structure: m7G(5')ppp(5')GmpCp-. *Proc Natl Acad Sci USA* 72:362, 1975

62. WEI CM, MOSS B: Methylation of newly synthesized viral messenger RNA by an enzyme in vaccinia virus. *Proc Natl Acad Sci USA* 71:3014, 1974

63. DARNELL JE, JELINEK WR, MOLLOY GR: Biogenesis of mRNA: Genetic regulation in mammalian cells. *Science* 181:1215, 1973

64. LODISH HF: Translational control of protein synthesis. *Annu Rev Biochem* 45:39, 1976

65. KOWALCZEWSKA MZ, BRETNER M, SIERAKOWSKA A, SZCZESNA E, FILIPOWICZ W, SHATKIN AJ: Removal of 5'-terminal m7G from eukaryotic mRNAs by potato nucleotide pyrophosphatase and its effect on translation. *Nucleic Acids Res* 4:3065, 1977

66. LEWIN B: Alternatives for splicing: Recognizing the ends of introns. *Cell* 22:324, 1980

67. BREATHNACH R, BENOIST C, O'HARE K, GANNON F, CHAMBON P: Ovalbumin gene: Evidence for a leader sequence in mRNA and DNA sequences at the exon-intron boundaries. *Proc Natl Acad Sci USA* 75:4853, 1978

68. MARTIN SL, ZIMMER EA, KAN YW, WILSON AC: Silent δ-globin gene in Old World monkeys. *Proc Natl Acad Sci USA* 77:3563, 1980

69. WASI P, NA-NAKORN S, SUINGDUMRONG A: Haemoglobin H disease in Thailand: A genetical study. *Nature* 204:907, 1964

70. LEHMANN H: Different types of alpha-thalassaemia and significance of haemoglobin Bart's in neonates. *Lancet* 2:78, 1970

71. KAN YW, SCHWARTZ E, NATHAN DG: Globin chain synthesis in the alpha thalassemia syndromes. *J Clin Invest* 47:2515, 1968

72. DOZY AM, KAN YW, EMBURY SH, MENTZER WC, WANG WC, LUBIN B, DAVIS JR JR, KOENIG HM: α-Globin gene organisation in blacks precludes the severe form of α thalassaemia. *Nature* 280:605, 1979

73. EMBURY SH, LEBO RV, DOZY AM, KAN YW: Organization of the α-globin genes in the Chinese α-thalassemia syndromes. *J Clin Invest* 63:1307, 1979

74. MILNER PF, CLEGG JB, WEATHERALL DJ: Haemoglobin-H disease due to a unique haemoglobin variant with an elongated alpha-chain. *Lancet* 1:729, 1971

75. ENGLAND JM, FRASER PM: Differentiation of iron deficiency from thalassemia trait by routine blood-count. *Lancet* 1:449, 1973

76. MENTZER WC: Differentiation of iron deficiency from thalassemia trait. *Lancet* 1:882, 1973

77. HUISMAN THJ: Trimodality in the percentages of β chain variants in heterozygotes: The effect of the number of active Hb$_\alpha$ structural loci. Hemoglobin 1:349, 1977

78. BRITTENHAM G: Genetic model for observed distribution of proportions of haemoglobin in sickle-cell trait. Nature 268:635, 1977

79. STEINBERG MH, ADAMS JG, DREILING BJ: Alpha thalassaemia in adults with sickle-cell trait. Br J Haematol 30:31, 1975

80. MATTHAY KK, MENTZER WC, DOZY AM, KAN YW, BAINTON DF: Modification of hemoglobin H disease by sickle trait. J Clin Invest 64:1024, 1979

81. SHAEFFER JR, KINGSTON RE, McDONALD MJ, BUNN HF: Competition of normal β chains and sickle haemoglobin β chains for α chains as a post-translational control mechanism. Nature 276:631, 1978

82. GABUZDA TG, NATHAN DG, GARDNER FH, COUNCIL A, LIMAURO A: The metabolism of the individual C^{14}-labeled hemoglobins in patients with H-thalassemia, with observations of radiochromate binding to the hemoglobins during red cell survival. J Clin Invest 44:315, 1965

83. NATHAN DG, GUNN RB: Thalassemia: The consequences of unbalanced hemoglobin synthesis. Am J Med 41:815, 1960

84. LIE-INJO LE, LIE-HONG G, AGER JAM, LEHMANN H: α Thalassaemia as a cause of hydrops foetalis. Br J Haematol 8:1, 1962

85. TODD D, LAI MCS, BEAVEN GH, HUEHNS ER: The abnormal haemoglobins in homozygous α-thalassaemia. Br J Haematol 19:27, 1970

86. DOZY AM, FORMAN EN, ABUELO DN, BARSEL-BOWERS G, MAHONEY MJ, FORGET BG, KAN YW: Prenatal diagnosis of homozygous α-thalassaemia. JAMA 241:1610, 1979

87. ORKIN SH, ALTER BP, ALTAY C, MAHONEY MJ, LAZARUS H, HOBBINS JC, NATHAN DG: Application of endonuclease mapping to the analysis and prenatal diagnosis of thalassemias caused by globin-gene deletion. N Engl J Med 299:166, 1978

88. OTTOLENGHI S, LANYON WG, PAUL J, WILLIAMSON R, WEATHERALL DJ, CLEGG JB, PRITCHARD J, POOTRAKUL S, WONG HB: The severe form of α thalassaemia is caused by a haemoglobin gene deletion. Nature 251:389, 1974

89. TAYLOR JM, DOZY A, KAN YW, VARMUS HE, LIE-INJO LE, GANESAN J, TODD D: Genetic lesion in homozygous α thalassaemia (hydrops foetalis). Nature 251:392, 1974

90. PRESSLEY L, HIGGS DR, CLEGG JB, WEATHERALL DJ: Gene deletions in α thalassemia prove that the 5' ζ locus is functional. Proc Natl Acad Sci USA 77:3586, 1980

91. ORKIN SH, MICHELSON A: Partial deletion of the α-globin structural gene in human α-thalassaemia. Nature 286:538, 1980

92. EMBURY SH, MILLER JA, DOZY AM, KAN YW, CHAN V, TODD D: Two different molecular organizations account for the single α-globin gene of α-thalassemia-2 genotype. J Clin Invest 66:1319, 1980

93. KAN YW, DOXY AM, TRECARTIN R, TODD D: Identification of a nondeletion defect in α-thalassemia. N Engl J Med 297:1080, 1977

94. ORKIN SH, GOFF SC, HECHTMAN RL: An intervening sequence splice junction mutation in man. Proc Natl Acad Sci USA 78:5041, 1981

95. PRESSLEY L, HIGGS DR, CLEGG JB, PERRINE RP, PEMBREY ME, WEATHERALL DJ: A new genetic basis for hemoglobin-H disease. N Engl J Med 303:1383, 1980

96. KAN YW, TODD D, DOZY AM: Haemoglobin Constant Spring synthesis in red cell precursors. Br J Haematol 28:103, 1974

97. LIEBHABER SA, KAN YW: Differentiation of the mRNA transcripts originating from the α1- and α2-globin gene in normals and α thalassemics. J Clin Invest 68:1012, 1981

98. CLEGG JB, WEATHERALL DJ, CONTOPOULOU-GRIVA I, CAROUTSOS K, POUNGOURAS P, TSEVRENIS H: Haemoglobin Icaria, a new chain-termination mutant which causes α thalassaemia. Nature 251:245, 1974

98a. BRADLEY TB, WOHL RC, SMITH GJ: Elongation of the α chain in a Black family; Interaction with Hb G Philadelphia. Clin Res 23:131, 1975

99. DE JONG WW, KHAN PM, BERNINI LF: Hemoglobin Koya Dora: High frequency of a chain termination mutant. Am J Hum Genet 27:81, 1975

100. HIGGS DR, PRESSLEY L, SERJEANT GR, CLEGG JB, WEATHERALL J: The genetics and molecular basis of alpha thalassaemia in association with Hb S in Jamaican negroes. Br J Haematol 47:43, 1981

101. FRIEDMAN MJ: Oxidant damage mediates variant red cell resistance to malaria. Nature 280:245, 1979

102. GOOSSENS M, DOZY AM, EMBURY SH, ZACHARIADES Z, HADJIMINAS M, STAMATOYANNOPOULOS G, KAN YW: Triplicated α-globin loci in humans. Proc Natl Acad Sci USA 77:518, 1980

103. HIGGS DR, OLD JM, PRESSLEY L, CLEGG JB, WEATHERALL DJ: A novel α-globin gene arrangement in man. Nature 284:632, 1980

104. LIE-INJO LE, HERRERA AR, KAN YW: Two types of triplicated α-globin loci in humans. Nucleic Acids Res 9:3707, 1981

105. STAMATOYANNOPOULOS G, FESSAS P, PAPAYANNOPOULOU TH: F-thalassemia: A study of thirty-one families with simple heterozygotes and combinations of F-thalassemia with A$_2$-thalassemia. Am J Med 47:194, 1969

106. SCHWARTZ E: The silent carrier of beta thalassemia. N Engl J Med 281:1327, 1969

107. KAN YW, FORGET BG, NATHAN DG: Gamma-beta thalassemia: A cause of hemolytic disease of the newborn. N Engl J Med 286:129, 1972

108. VAN DER PLOEG LHT, KONINGS A, OORT M, ROOS D, BERNINI L, FLAVELL RA: γ-β-Thalassaemia studies showing that deletion of the γ- and δ-genes influences β-globin gene expression in man. Nature 283:637, 1980

109. EDDINGTON GM, LEHMANN H: Expression of the sickle gene in Africa. Br Med J 1:1308, 2:1328, 1955

110. WHEELER JT, KREVANS JR: The homozygous state of persistent fetal hemoglobin and the interaction of persistent fetal hemoglobin with thalassemia. Bull Johns Hopkins Hosp 110:217, 1961

111. SCHWARTZ E: Heterozygous beta thalassemia: Balanced globin chain synthesis in bone marrow cells. Science 167:1513, 1970

112. BRAVERMAN AS, BANK A: Changing ratio of globin chain synthesis during erythroid cell maturation in thalassemia. J Mol Biol 42:57, 1969

113. FRIEDMAN SH, OZSOYLU S, LUDDY R, SCHWARTZ E: Heterozygous beta thalassaemia of unusual severity. Br J Haematol 32:65, 1976

114. McCARTHY GM, TEMPERLEY IJ, CLEGG JB, WEATHERALL DJ: Thalassaemia in an Irish family. Ir J Med Sci 1:303, 1968

115. COOLEY TB, WITWER ER, LEE P: Anemia in children with splenomegaly and peculiar changes in bones; report of cases. Am J Dis Child 34:347, 1927

116. BAKER DH: Roentgen manifestations of Cooley's anemia. Ann NY Acad Sci 119:641, 1964

117. WOLMAN IJ, ORTLANI M: Some clinical features of Cooley's anemia patients as related to transfusion schedules. Ann NY Acad Sci 165:407, 1969

118. CANALE VC, STEINHERZ P, NEW M, ERLANDSON M: Endocrine function in thalassemia major. Ann NY Acad Sci 232:333, 1974

119. FINK H: Transfusions hemochromatosis in Cooley's anemia. Ann NY Acad Sci 119:680, 1964

120. McINTOSH N: Endocrinopathy in thalassemia major. Arch Dis Child 51:195, 1976

121. ENGLE MA: Cardiac involvement in Cooley's anemia. Ann NY Acad Sci 119:694, 1964

122. FESSAS P: Inclusions of hemoglobin in erythroblasts and erythrocytes of thalassemia. Blood 21:21, 1963

123. YATAGANAS X, FESSAS P: The pattern of hemoglobin precipitation in thalassemia and its significance. Ann NY Acad Sci 165:270, 1969

124. NECHELES TF, CHUNG S, SABBAH R, WHITTEN D: Intensive transfusion therapy in thalassemia major: An eight-year follow-up. Ann NY Acad Sci 232:179, 1974

125. PIOMELLI S, KARPATKIN MH, ARZANIAN M, ZAMANI M, BECKER MH, GENEISER N, DANOFF SJ, KUHNS WJ: Hypertransfusion regimen in patients with Cooley's anemia. Ann NY Acad Sci 232:186, 1974

126. FESSAS P, LOUKOPOULOS D, THORELL B: Peptide analysis of the inclusions of erythroid cells in β-thalassemia. Biochim Biophys Acta 124:430, 1966

127. PROPPER RD: Current concepts in the overall management of thalassemia. Ann NY Acad Sci 344:375, 1980

128. PROPPER RD, BUTTON LN, NATHAN DG: New approaches to the transfusion management of thalassemia. Blood 55:55, 1980

129. PIOMELLI S, SEAMAN C, REIBMAN J, TYTUN A, GRAZIANO J, TABACHNIK N, CORASH L: Separation of younger red cells with improved survival in vivo: An approach to chronic transfusion therapy. Proc Natl Acad Sci USA 75:3474, 1978

130. MODELL CB, BECK J: Long-term desferrioxamine therapy. Ann NY Acad Sci 232:201, 1974

131. PROPPER RD, SHURIN SB, NATHAN DG: Reassessment of the use of desferrioxamine B in iron overload. N Engl J Med 294:1421, 1976

132. PROPPER RD, COOPER B, RUFO RR, NIENHUIS AW, ANDERSON WF, BUNN HF, ROSENTHAL A, NATHAN DG: Continuous subcutaneous administration of deferoxamine in patients with iron overload. N Engl J Med 297:418, 1977

133. PIOMELLI S, GRAZIANO J, KARPATKIN M, DUDELL GG, HART D, HILGARTNER M, KHANNA K, VALDES-CRUZ LM, VORA S: Chelation therapy, transfusion requirement and iron balance in young thalassemic patients. Ann NY Acad Sci 244:409, 1980

134. PEARSON HA: Thalassemia intermedia: Genetic and biochemical considerations. Ann NY Acad Sci 119:390, 1964

135. KAN YW, NATHAN DG: Mild thalassemia: The result of interactions of alpha and beta thalassemia genes. J Clin Invest 49:635, 1970

136. CHARACHE S, CONLEY CL, DOEBLIN TD, BARTALOS M: Thalassemia in black Americans. Ann NY Acad Sci 232:125, 1974

137. HUISMAN THJ, SCHROEDER WA, STAMATOYANNOPOULOS G, BOUVER N, SHELTON JR, SHELTON JB, APELL G: Nature of fetal hemoglobin in the Greek type of hereditary persistence of fetal hemoglobin with and without concurrent β-thalassemia. J Clin Invest 49:1035, 1970

138. WEATHERALL DJ, CARTER R, CLEGG JB, WOOD WG, MACRAE IA, MACKENZIE A: A form of hereditary persistence of foetal haemoglobin characterized by uneven cellular distribution of haemoglobin F and the production of haemoglobins A and A$_2$ in homozygotes. Br J Haematol 29:205, 1975

139. BOYER SH, MARGOLET L, BOYER ML, HUISMAN THJ, SCHROEDER WA, WOOD WG, WEATHERALL DJ, CLEGG JB, CARTNER R: Inheritance of F cell frequency in heterocellular hereditary persistence of fetal hemoglobin. An example of allelic exclusion. *Am J Hum Genet* 29:256, 1977

140. FLAVELL RA, BERNARDS R, KOOTER JB, DE BOER E: The structure of the human β-globin gene in β-thalassemia. *Nucleic Acids Res* 6:2749, 1979

141. ORKIN SH, KOLODNER R, MICHELSON A, HUSSON R: Cloning and direct examination of a structurally abnormal human β⁰-thalassemia globin gene. *Proc Natl Acad Sci USA* 77:3558,1980

142. FRITSCH EF, LAWN RM, MANIATIS T: Characterization of deletions which affect the expression of fetal globin genes in man. *Nature* 279:598, 1979

143. OTTOLENGHI S, GIGLIONI B, COMI P, GIANNI AM, POLLI E, ACQUAYE CTA, OLDHAM JH, MASERA G: Globin gene deletion in HPFH, δ⁰β⁰ thalassaemia and Hb Lepore disease. *Nature* 278:654, 1979

144. ORKIN SH, ALTER BP, ALTAY C: Deletion of the ᴬγ-globin gene in ᴳγ-δ β thalassemia. *J Clin Invest* 64:866, 1979

145. TUAN D, MURNAME MJ, DE RIEL JK, FORGET B: Heterogeneity in the molecular basis of hereditary persistence of fetal hemoglobin. *Nature* 285:335, 1980

146. ORKIN SH, GOFF SC, NATHAN DG: Heterogeneity of DNA deletion in γδβ-thalassemia. *J Clin Invest* 67:878, 1981

147. KANTOR JA, TURNER PH, NIENHUIS AW: Beta thalassemia: Mutations which affect processing of the β-globin mRNA precursor. *Cell* 21:149, 1980

148. MAQUAT LE, KINNIBURGH AJ, BEACH LR, HONIG GR, LAZERSON J, ERSHLER WB, ROSS J: Processing of the human β-globin mRNA precursor to mRNA is defective in three patients with β⁺ thalassemia. *Proc Natl Acad Sci USA* 77:4287, 1980

149. SPRITIZ RA, JAGADEESWARAN P, CHOUDARY PV, BIRO PA, ELDER JT, DE RIEL JK, MANLEY J, GEFTER ML, FORGET BG, WEISSMAN SM: Base substitution in an intervening sequence of a β⁺-thalassemic human globin gene. *Proc Natl Acad Sci USA* 78:2455, 1981

150. WESTAWAY D, WILLIAMSON R: An intron nucleotide sequence variant in a cloned β⁺-thalassaemia globin gene. *Nucleic Acids Res* 9:1777, 1981

151. MANIATIS T: Personal communication

152. CHANG JC, KAN YW: β⁰ Thalassemia, a nonsense mutation in man. *Proc Natl Acad Sci USA* 76:2886, 1979

153. TRECARTIN RF, LIEBHABER SA, CHANG JC, LEE KY, FURBETTA M, ANGIUS A, CAO A: β⁰ thalassemia in Sardinia is caused by a nonsense mutation. *J Clin Invest* 68:1012, 1981

154. ORKIN SH, GOFF SC: Nonsense and frameshift mutations in β⁰-thalassemia detected in cloned β-globin genes, *J Biol Chem* 256:9782, 1981

155. KAN YW: Prenatal diagnosis of hemoglobin disorders, in Brown EB (ed): *Progress in Hematology*, vol 10. New York, Grune & Stratton, 1977, p 91

156. ALTER BP: Prenatal diagnosis of hemoglobinopathies and other hematologic diseases. *J Pediatr* 95:501, 1979

157. KAN YW, DOZY AM: Polymorphism of DNA sequence adjacent to human β-globin structural gene: Relationship to sickle mutation. *Proc Natl Acad Sci USA* 75:5631, 1978

158. KAN YW, DOZY AM: Antenatal diagnosis of sickle cell anaemia by DNA analysis of amniotic-fluid cells. *Lancet* 2:910, 1978

159. KAN YW, LEE KY, FURBETTA M, ANGIUS A, CAO A: Polymorphism of DNA sequence in the β-globin gene region: Application to prenatal diagnosis of β⁰ thalassemia. *N Engl J Med* 302:185, 1980

160. JEFFREYS AJ: DNA sequence variants in the ᴳγ-ᴬγ-δ- and β-globin genes of man. *Cell* 18:1, 1979

161. LITTLE PFR, ANNISON G, DARLING S, WILLIAMSON R, CAMBA L, MODELL B: Model for antenatal diagnosis of β thalassaemia and other monogenic disorders by molecular analysis of linked DNA polymorphisms. *Nature* 285:144, 1980

162. PHILLIPS JA III, PANNY SR, KAZAZIAN HH JR, BOEHM CD, SCOTT AF, SMITH KD: Prenatal diagnosis of sickle cell anemia by restriction endonuclease analysis: Hin dIII polymorphism in γ-globin genes extend test applicability. *Proc Natl Acad Sci USA* 77:2853, 1980

162a. GEEVER RF, WILSON LB, NALLASETH FS, MILNER PF, BITTNER M, WILSON JT: Direct identification of sickle cell anemia by blot hybridization. *Proc Natl Acad Sci USA* 78:5081, 1981

162b. CHANG JC, KAN YW: Antenatal diagnosis of sickle cell anaemia by direct analysis of the sickle mutation. *Lancet* 2:1127, 1981

162c. ALTER BP: Prenatal diagnosis of haemoglobinopathies: A status report. *Lancet* 2:1152, 1981

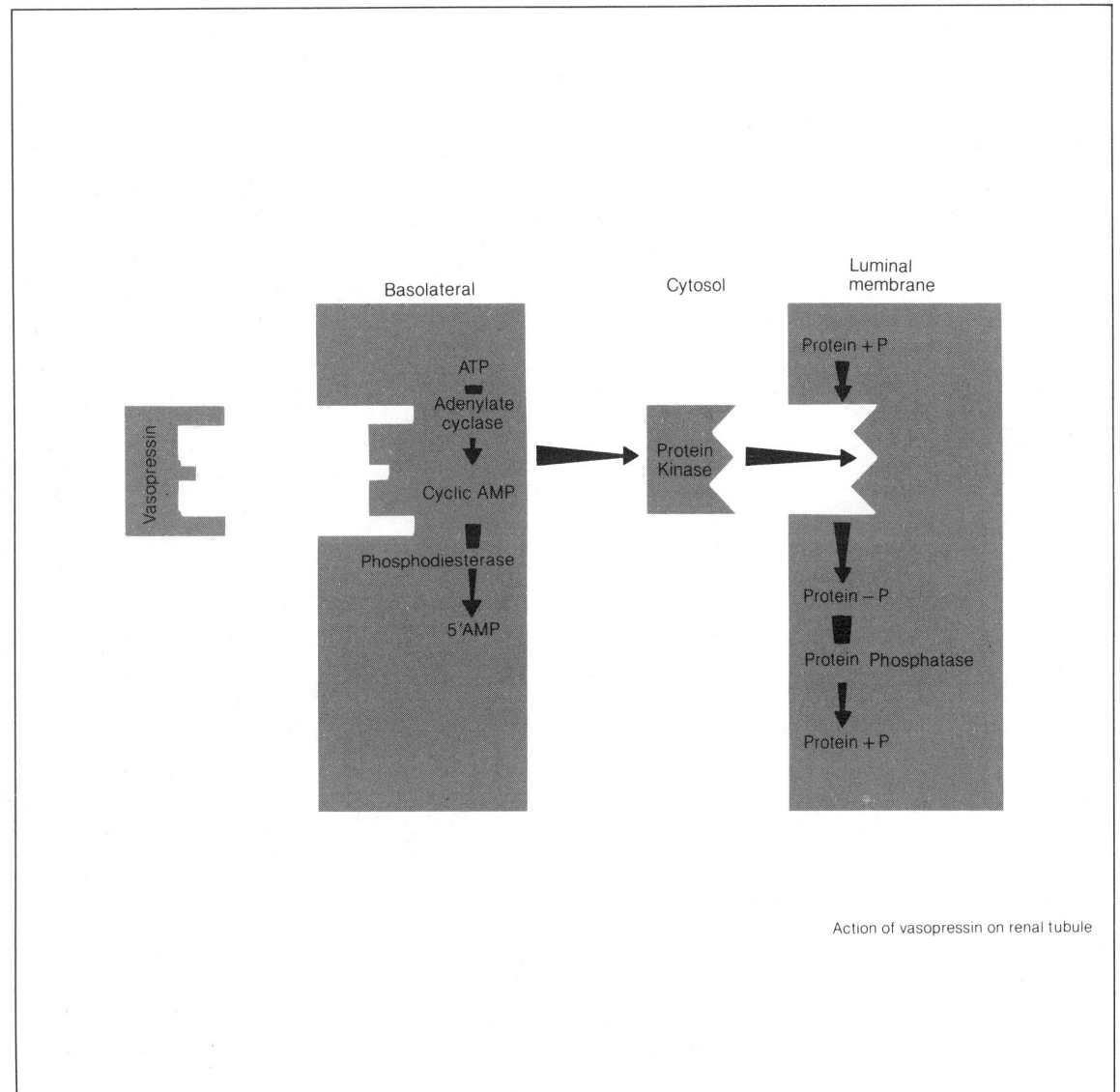

PART 12

Action of vasopressin on renal tubule

DISORDERS OF TRANSPORT

78

INTESTINAL DISACCHARIDASE DEFICIENCIES AND GLUCOSE-GALACTOSE MALABSORPTION

GARY M. GRAY

1. The breakdown products of dietary starch (maltose, maltotriose, and α-dextrins), as well as sucrose and lactose, are hydrolyzed by their specific carbohydrases localized at the luminal border of the small-intestine mucosal cell. After hydrolysis the released monosaccharides are transported by specific mechanisms. Glucose and galactose share an active Na^+-requiring process that accumulates these monosaccharides in the cell against a concentration gradient. Fructose, the other monosaccharide produced in appreciable amounts, is absorbed by facilitated passive diffusion.

2. Clinically, a deficiency of a particular disaccharidase is accompanied by abdominal fullness and bloating, cramping pain, and diarrhea. The unhydrolyzed disaccharide, which is initially unabsorbed, remains free in the intestinal lumen, where it exerts an osmotic effect. Bacteria in the lower ileum and colon metabolize the undigested sugar to monosaccharides and fatty acids. These are poorly absorbed in the more distal intestine and may directly interfere with colonic absorptive processes.

3. Intestinal lactase deficiency occurs in 3 to 19 percent of healthy adult white persons of western European origin and in a majority of Asians, African and American blacks, and Mediterraneans. Intolerance to lactose may appear in childhood or adolescence. The deficiency appears to be inherited as an autosomal reces-

sive characteristic. Environmental factors such as diet, nutrition, and subclinical intestinal disease are also important determinants in some patients.

4. Lactase deficiency in infants is unusual. It has occurred in sibs and is probably inherited as an autosomal recessive. It must be distinguished from a toxic response to ingestion of lactose without enzyme deficiency, a condition which is said to occur rarely in the same age group.

5. Lactase is the intestinal disaccharidase most sensitive to intestinal damage and is uniformly depressed in intestinal disease. Furthermore, it appears to be permanently depressed after some intestinal illnesses. Secondary sucrase and maltase deficiency occurs in a high percentage of patients with malabsorptive disease of the small intestine.

6. Sucrase-α-dextrinase deficiency is a rare malady inherited in an autosomal recessive manner. Intolerance to sugar is discovered in childhood, and the patient and family usually learn to eliminate sucrose from the diet. The α-dextrins released from branched starch, although only partially hydrolyzed, are usually well-tolerated. Radioimmunoassay for sucrase in intestinal tissue from patients with the defect has failed to detect a cross-reacting sucraselike protein.

7. Assay of enzyme activity in small-intestinal biopsy specimens is important for the diagnosis of disaccharidase deficiency. Hydrogen breath tests are superior to

conventional oral tolerance tests for confirmation of disaccharide malabsorption. The dramatic amelioration of symptoms upon withdrawal of the offending sugar from the diet confirms the diagnosis.

8. *Glucose-galactose malabsorption is a rare defect in the transport of these sugars. The clinical syndrome is indistinguishable from disaccharidase deficiency, except that there is intolerance to almost all dietary sugars because most of them contain at least one of these monosaccharides. In contrast to disaccharidase deficiency, the glucose tolerance test produces little or no rise in blood sugar level, and intestinal mucosal biopsy specimens do not accumulate glucose against a concentration gradient. Replacement of all dietary carbohydrate with fructose is successful, since this monosaccharide is absorbed by a different mechanism than glucose or galactose. As estimated from an extensive family study, this disease is a genetic defect with an autosomal recessive pattern of inheritance.*

Intolerance to the dietary disaccharides, sucrose and lactose, and to the hydrolytic products of starch (maltose, maltotriose, and the α-dextrins), results from a deficiency of one or more of the specific intestinal mucosal enzymes responsible for their hydrolysis. Rarely, a patient is identified who is intolerant to all dietary carbohydrate because of an inability to absorb the final hydrolytic products, glucose and galactose. Symptoms of carbohydrate maldigestion or malabsorption include abdominal bloating and distention, nausea, cramping pain, and diarrhea. A secondary malabsorption of other nutrients may develop. The clinician must distinguish these syndromes from "irritable" colon or "spastic" colitis, since treatment of specific carbohydrate maldigestion or malabsorption is very different from that of irritable colon and is often highly successful.

For many years European physicians [1, 2] had observed that certain children develop abdominal distention and diarrhea after ingestion of milk or sugar, but the clinical syndrome lacked a biochemical explanation until methods became available for obtaining [3, 4] and assaying [5] peroral biopsy specimens of the small intestine. An important reason for the slow development of these methods was a general acceptance of the erroneous concept that digestive enzymes are secreted from the intestinal wall into the lumen, but disaccharidases were eventually established to be constituents of the small intestinal brush border membrane [6]. Studies in human beings [7, 8] subsequently demonstrated that these enzymes act at the lumen-cell interface to hydrolyze dietary saccharides to monosaccharide products that can then be taken up by specific hexose transport mechanisms. Since there are no transport processes for disaccharides, failure of their digestion at the intestinal surface produces the syndrome of disaccharide intolerance.

DIGESTION AND ABSORPTION OF CARBOHYDRATES

The mechanisms by which dietary carbohydrates are assimilated by the small intestine are depicted in Fig. 78-1. In essence, there are three sequential stages in the overall process of digestion and absorption: (1) intraluminal hydrolysis of starch and glycogen by α-amylases to oligosaccharides containing from 2 to 10 glucose units; (2) surface hydrolysis of these oligosaccharides and the dietary disaccharides, lactose and sucrose, at the intestinal lumen-cell interface by specific oligosaccharidases integral to the brush border membrane; and (3) transport of the released hexose products (glucose, galactose, fructose) by specific mechanisms.

Luminal Hydrolysis of Starch

Starch constitutes 60 percent of the carbohydrate ingested daily. The branched form (amylopectin) and the straight-chain form (amylose) of starch, as well as glycogen, a minor dietary component having a structure similar to amylopectin, are hydrolyzed extremely rapidly by salivary and pancreatic α-amylase within the duodenal luminal contents. As outlined in Fig. 78-2, α-amylase has high specificity for the $\alpha(1 \rightarrow 4)$ links between adjacent glucose residues in the interior of the straight glucose chain but has no significant specificity for the $\alpha(1,6)$ branching links or $\alpha(1 \rightarrow 4)$ links adjacent to these branching points. Furthermore, it does not cleave the outermost glucose residues in starch or in the released oligosaccharide products. As a result, α-dextrins (branched oligosaccharides averaging five to nine glucose residues) [9, 10], maltose, and maltotriose are the major final products of α-amylase digestion within the intestinal lumen.

Intestinal Membrane Surface Hydrolysis of Oligosaccharides

Figure 78-1 depicts the oligosaccharide substrates in the intestinal lumen and their appropriate surface membrane hydrolases that act to yield the residual monosaccharide products for final transport across the brush border bilayer.

α-Dextrins, the branched oligosaccharide products of α-amylase action on starch, have recently been shown to be cleaved in a specific sequence by a number of different brush border oligosaccharidases. This is shown diagrammatically in Fig. 78-3, where more than one enzyme is capable of acting at all but one of the cleavage steps. On the basis of studies in rats [11], this model α-dextrin can be cleaved only by sequential removal of a single glucose residue from the nonreducing end of the molecule. The glucose attached via the $\alpha(1 \rightarrow 6)$ branching point can be cleaved only after the adjacent, nonreducing $\alpha(1 \rightarrow 4)$-linked glucose unit has been removed. For this "debranching" of the $\alpha(1 \rightarrow 6)$ link there is an absolute requirement for the α-dextrinase moiety of sucrase-α-dextrinase. Glucose is the final product released at the intestinal surface for subsequent assimilation.

The several oligosaccharidases of the brush border possess high specificity for the particular oligosaccharides presented to the intestinal surface, and have their active hydrolytic sites available at the intestinal surface so that saccharides can be hydrolyzed efficiently without requirement for prior translocation to the interior of the cell.

Transport Mechanisms for Released Monosaccharide

Entry of sugar past the hydrophobic brush border lipid bilayer into the interior of the epithelial cell is restricted to those

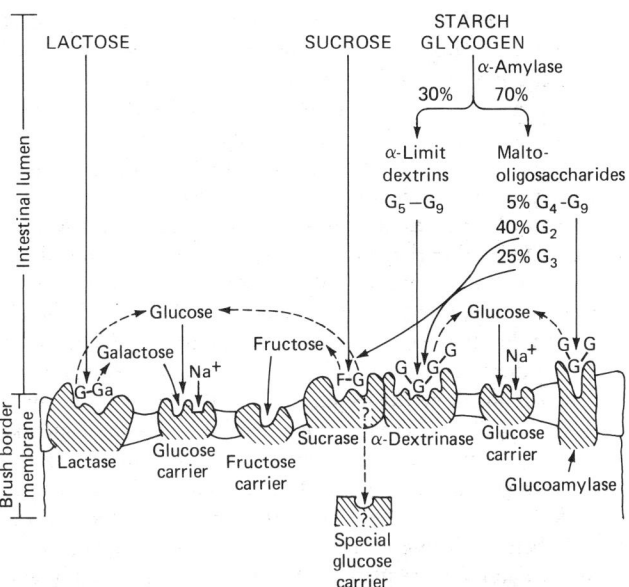

Figure 78-1 Diagrammatic representation of intestinal intraluminal and surface hydrolysis of dietary carbohydrate. The oligosaccharides released from luminal action of α-amylase and the two dietary disaccharides are hydrolyzed by specific enzymes embedded in the brush border membrane so that their active hydrolytic sites (shown as clefts in the molecule) are available at the brush border surface. The released monosaccharides then bind to specific carrier sites in the initial stage of transport. (See Fig. 78-4 for details of glucose transport.) G, glucose, with subscript indicating number of glucose units; Ga, galactose; F, fructose. (*Modified from GM Gray [10] with permission from* The New England Journal of Medicine.)

monosaccharides for which there are specific transport mechanisms. Glucose and galactose, having nearly identical structures, use the same mechanisms of entry, intracellular translocation to the basolateral membrane, and exit from the specialized intestinal cell. The glucose carrier or receptor in the brush border membrane has not yet been isolated, but, judged by kinetic studies of intact intestine [12, 13], isolated cells [14, 15], and membrane vesicles [16, 17], it has precise specificity for hexoses of the glucose configuration with high affinity for both glucose and galactose. Each glucose molecule that binds to the membrane carrier is joined by two molecules of Na+. After the glucose and Na+ are internalized, they enter separate pathways. The glucose binds to a carrier on the basolateral membrane, and the Na+ provides the impetus for active glucose transport by virtue of its ATPase catalyzed transport across the basolateral membrane. The overall mechanism of active glucose and galactose translocation is shown diagramatically in Fig. 78-4.

The only other monosaccharide that is quantitatively important as a nutrient is fructose, a component of sucrose. Because its configuration is appreciably different from that of glucose, it requires its own transport mechanism for intestinal assimilation. Fructose probably has its own surface membrane receptor or transporter; its absorption is efficient but appreciably slower than that for glucose or galactose [18].

Rate-limiting Steps in Digestion and Absorption of Carbohydrate

Figure 78-5 summarizes the dietary contribution of various carbohydrates and considers the rate-limiting steps for the overall assimilation of each type. Intestinal perfusion studies in humans [8, 18] comparing disaccharides to equivalent mono-

saccharide mixtures have demonstrated that hydrolysis is a rapid process which can release sufficient monosaccharide to saturate the glucose-galactose and fructose transport pathways. The sole exception is the hydrolysis of lactose. This proceeds in vivo at only about half the rate of sucrose hydrolysis (Fig. 78-5), and the glucose and galactose released are not sufficient to give maximal rates of active transport [19]. Hence, unlike that for other disaccharides, hydrolysis rather than transport is rate limiting for its overall assimilation [19] (Fig. 78-5). This unique feature of lactose digestion and absorption in normal human beings indicates a relative lack of reserve of lactase activity and helps explain the particular vulnerability of lactose digestion, which is considered in detail below.

Molecular Characteristics of Intestinal Surface Oligosaccharidases

The brush border carbohydrases are most appropriately named *oligosaccharidases* rather than *disaccharidases,* since most of them efficiently hydrolyze saccharides composed of more than two monosaccharide units (Fig. 78-1). As integral constituents of the intestinal cell membrane having physical and biochemical properties similar to one another, the oligosaccharidases have been difficult to isolate and characterize. In Table 64-1 they are considered according to their principal substrates. All are large glycoproteins having pH optima around 6 and apparent K_m values in the low millimolar range. Notably there are several α-glucosidases and a single β-galactosidase in the brush border of villus cells, with highest specific activities in the upper jejunum but with functionally important concentrations persisting at least to midileum. These enzymes complement one another, so that total oligosaccharide digestion encompasses all saccharides of dietary importance. Glucoamylase differs both structurally and functionally from pancreatic or salivary amylases, since it is a much larger molecule that acts as an exoenzyme on $\alpha(1 \rightarrow 4)$malto-oligosaccharides by sequentially removing a single glucose unit from the nonreducing end of the linear oligosaccharide. All the α-glucosidases are capable of hydrolyzing 1,4-glucosyl linkages and therefore are maltases.

Sucrase-α-dextrinase, often called sucrase-isomaltase, is a hybrid enzyme that consists of two distinct polypeptide chains

Figure 78-2 Action of α-amylase on branched starch. A portion of amylopectin and the final hydrolytic products are shown with glucose molecules *(circles)* joined by α-1,4 *(horizontal)* links or α-1,6 *(vertical)* links. (*Reproduced from GM Gray [10] with permission from* The New England Journal of Medicine.)

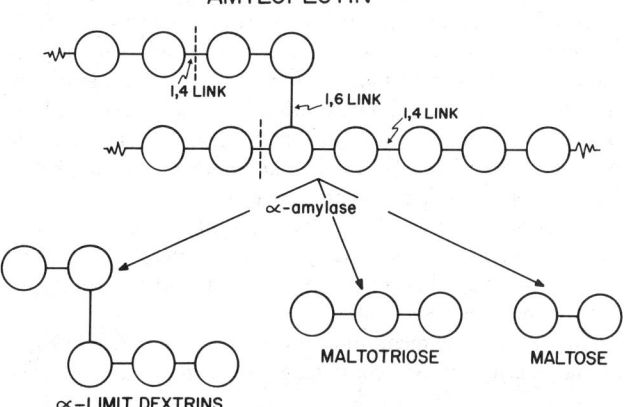

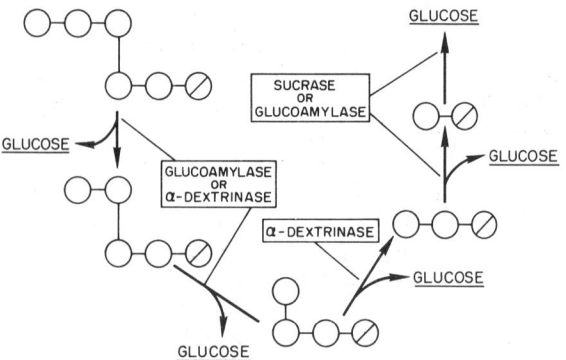

Figure 78-3 Sequence of cleavage of a model α-limit dextrin hexasaccharide to yield glucose by constitutive brush border carbohydrases, based on Ref. 11. Symbols are the same as in Fig. 78-2. The oligosaccharide is attacked only from its nonreducing end by sequential removal of a glucose residue by the action of one or more enzymes at each step. Notably, however, only α-dextrinase can debranch the α(1 → 6)-linked glucose stub from the tetrasaccharide to release maltotriose.

of slightly different mass (sucrase, 125,000 daltons; isomaltase, 115,000 daltons) [22]. Despite the usual nomenclature, both active sites show specificity for a variety of α(1 → 4)-linked glucosyloligosaccharidases (Table 78-1). Sucrase has been shown to be very active against maltose [11]; "isomaltase," although capable of splitting the disaccharide, has higher affinity for larger oligosaccharides and is essential for removal of α(1 → 6)-linked glucosyl units from α-dextrins. It is also the only intestinal carbohydrase that is able to cleave α-dextrins completely to free glucose [11]. Hence, α-dextrinase is the preferred trivial name. Analysis of the specificity and kinetic data in Table 78-1 and Fig. 78-3 reveals that this hybrid enzyme plays an important role in the hydrolysis of many α(1 → 4)-linked glucosyloligosaccharides with maximal specificity for saccharides having greater than two glucose residues.

Development and Regulation of the Oligosaccharidases

The α-glucosidases (see Table 78-1) are acquired by the eleventh week of gestation, but lactase activity remains low until at least the twenty-eighth week of fetal life [23]. All the oligosaccharidases are present at maximal concentrations at birth and, with the exception of lactase in certain population groups as discussed below, are maintained at these high levels throughout life. Little is known about induction or repression of these enzymes by food and drugs. Feeding of sucrose or fructose increases intestinal sucrase in humans after 2 to 5 days [24]. Approximately the same time is required for turnover of the intestinal digestive-absorptive cell. Lactase-deficient patients fed lactose for 6 to 12 months do not increase their intestinal lactase [25, 26], and patients with galactosemia who are kept on a lactose-free diet from birth maintain their lactase activity at normal levels [27]. Thus in humans there is no evidence that lactose has any influence whatsoever on lactase activity. Cortisone promotes precocious acquisition of disaccharidases in the developing rat intestine [28] but has no effect on sucrase or maltase in the adult rat. The effect of corticosteroids on humans has not been studied.

All the intestinal membrane oligosaccharidases (Table 78-1) are large glycoproteins containing one or more subunits con-

sisting of approximately 80 percent protein and 20 percent carbohydrate. The mechanisms whereby they are synthesized within the intestinal cell and then translocated and inserted into the brush border membrane are only beginning to be studied. Examination of other secretory mammalian proteins has clearly shown that there is a steady state level of a particular enzyme protein which is determined by the balance between the zero order rate of synthesis and first order rate of degradation [29]. Rather than being simply synthesized to remain at the intestinal cell membrane, a particular carbohydrase may be turned over repetitively during the cell's life-cycle. Although it is known that the rat intestinal cell exists for only 36 h, recent studies indicate that the half-life of sucrase, even though variable depending upon the feeding state of the animal, is as short as 2.5 to 6 h [30]. There is known diurnal variation of sucrase in rat intestine that can be accounted for by stabilization of the brush border sucrase during fasting, with a half-life as long as 36 h followed by a change to rapid turnover of the enzyme shortly before feeding ensues, resulting in a change of t½ to about 4 h and a consequent decline in sucrase [30]. Although daily variation of sucrase activity with feeding has not been demonstrated in human beings, the known stimulatory effect of sucrose feeding on human sucrase [24] suggests that there may be variation depending upon dietary intake. The regulatory mechanism of rapid change of degradation rate of intestinal disaccharidases is uncertain, but the superficial position of the oligosaccharidases on the surface membrane suggests that pancreatic proteases may be able to cleave them from the membrane under certain circumstances. Thus elastase is capable of removing carbohydrases from intestinal brush border in vitro and the degradation of these enzymes appears to be accelerated when pancreatic enzymes are present in the intestinal lumen [31]. Whether degradation can also be accomplished by endocytic removal and subsequent intracellular protease action, as has been shown in other cell systems, is unknown.

Figure 78-4 Model of glucose or galactose transport by the intestinal cell. The monosaccharide (0) binds to a high affinity site on the brush border surface, and this is greatly facilitated by simultaneous binding of Na⁺ at a separate site on the mucosal carrier. On the basis of recent findings of 2:1 stoichiometry of transport of Na⁺ to glucose, two molecules of Na⁺ appear to bind for each monosaccharide molecule. The glucose may pass through a hydrophobic core of the binding protein to the cytosol side of the membrane where its affinity for the carrier decreases and both glucose and Na⁺ are released. The majority of the glucose then binds to a specific "serosal" carrier on the basolateral membrane and is discharged into the intercellular space. The overall energy for transport is provided by active extrusion of Na⁺ by the Na⁺-K⁺ ATPase at the basolateral surface. The model is based on the original hypotheses of Crane as recently modified [14, 15, 17].

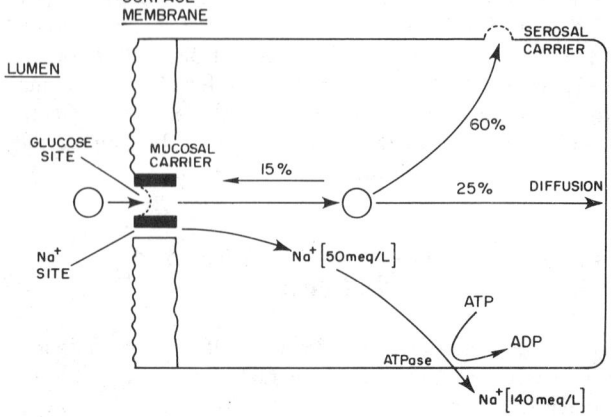

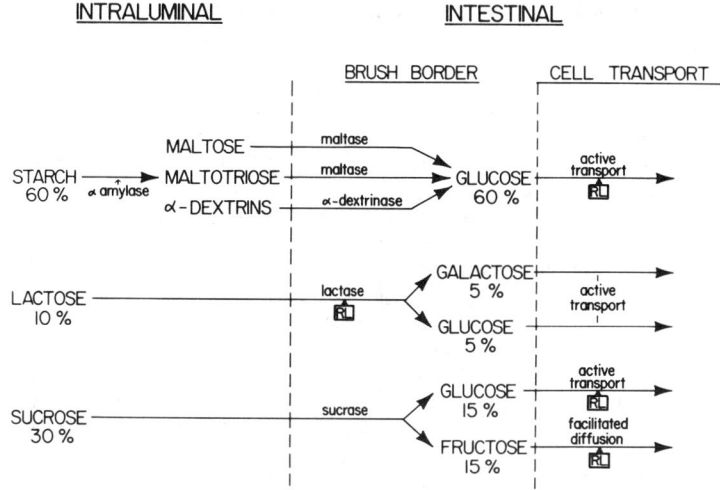

Figure 78-5 Outline of carbohydrate digestion and absorption in human beings. Percentages refer to fraction of total carbohydrate in the diet. *RL,* the rate-limiting step in the overall digestive-absorptive process for each carbohydrate ingested. (*Reproduced from GM Gray [108] with permission of* Gastroenterology.)

Detailed examination of the rates of intracellular synthesis, assembly, and brush border membrane insertion for the oligosaccharidases is only beginning [32, 33]. After an ^{3}H-leucine pulse is given intraluminally to rats, radioactivity can be identified in sucrase within the intestinal cytosol by 5 min and reaches a maximum in 15 min, declining rapidly thereafter [32]. This form of sucrase appears to be devoid of isomaltase activity and has a molecular weight that is 20 percent less than the sucrase moiety subsequently identified in the brush border nearly 3 h later [32]. Whereas the cytosol sucrase does not appear to be a direct precursor of the brush border enzyme, it undoubtedly reflects an early synthetic stage of the specific polypeptide chain containing an active hydrolytic site.

Recently, a single macromolecular polypeptide chain that has both sucrase and isomaltase activity has been identified in Golgi membranes after detergent solubilization and immunoprecipitation by specific antisucrase antiserum [33]. Although the exact molecular size of the sucrase is unknown, it appears large enough to account for both the sucrase and α-dextrinase subunits that subsequently appear in the brush border membrane [34]. This single-chain form of the sucrase-α-dextrinase seems to be transiently identifiable in the brush border but then is later replaced by the sucrase and α-dextrinase molecules. It may constitute a precursor that is subsequently cleaved in the brush border to yield the two-chain hybrid, possibly by action of pancreatic enzymes or integral brush border proteases. The overall synthesis and membrane insertion of a brush border membrane protein such as sucrase-α-dextrinase required a total of 3 to 6 h. Although the peak of the initial intracellular synthesis can be identified in the cytosol in only 15 min and subsequent peaks in endoplasmic reticulum and Golgi body in 30 min, the final movement from Golgi body to the brush border membrane requires an additional 2½ to 5½ h. It appears that the final transport step occurs on membrane-associated vesicles since no cytosolic form of the enzyme can be identified during this period. Recent comparative structural studies of the sucrase and α-dextrinase subunits isolated from protease-treated and detergent-treated membranes have revealed a hydrophobic amino-terminal sequence on the detergent-α-dextrinase subunit that is not present on the corresponding protease subunit [35]. This suggests that the solubilization by non-ionic detergent includes a membrane-imbedded portion of the α-dextrinase molecule that is left behind when proteases such as papain cleave the sucrase-α-dextrinase at the outer membrane surface. In contrast to this specialized hydrophobic amino-terminal region of the α-dextrinase unit, no differences in the detergent-solubilized and papain-solubilized sucrase were found. Thus, the sucrase-α-dextrinase may be anchored in the membrane by virtue of hydrophobic properties of the amino-terminal domain of the α-dextrinase.

Analysis of Intestinal Oligosaccharidases

Peroral small-intestinal biopsy has become a recognized means for evaluating the histologic status in intestinal disease, and as little as 1 to 3 mg of a typical 10 to 25-mg biopsy can be frozen [36] for subsequent oligosaccharidase assay. The assay has been standardized [5] in international enzyme units (U) per gram protein or per gram wet weight, based on specific measurements of glucose released from the disaccharide substrate. Results have been reproducible the world over as long as the biopsy is obtained at the ligament of Treitz or up to 30 cm beyond. The typical range of normal values is shown in Table 78-2. It is of interest that lactase activity, in agreement with in vivo studies described above, is appreciably lower than activity of the other disaccharidases. Activities below those given are usually associated with symptoms of enzyme deficiency.

PATHOGENESIS OF CARBOHYDRATE MALDIGESTION AND MALABSORPTION

Syndrome of Carbohydrate Intolerance

Since dietary carbohydrates are digested and absorbed in a well-defined sequence as outlined above, a defect at any stage will result in accumulation of carbohydrate within the intestinal lumen, where a marked osmotic effect is produced because of the small molecular size of the unabsorbed solute. This in turn induces net fluid secretion in the small intestine [37, 38], a rapid intestinal transit [39], and acid stools (pH < 6.0) due to bacterial metabolism of the carbohydrates to fatty acids in the colon. In addition, the altered intraluminal environment may inhibit absorptive processes in the colon [38]. The net result is

Table 78-1   Characteristics of brush border oligosaccharidases

Enzyme	Principal substrate	Product	$\dfrac{K_m}{mM}$	Mol wt, approximate	Reference
β-Galactosidase					
Lactase	Lactose	Glucose and galactose	18	280,000	70
α-Glucosidase					
Glucoamylase	Nonreducing α(1→4) link of glucosyl-oligosaccharides (including α-dextrins) $(G_2 \to G_a)$*	Glucose; residual oligosaccharide with α(1→6) link	3.8 → 1.1 (G_2) (G_a)	210,000	21
Sucrase†	Sucrose; maltose; maltotriose; α(1→4) end links of α-dextrins	Glucose, fructose; residual oligosaccharide	20 (sucrose) 3.6 (G_3) 2.6 (G_2)	125,000	11,‡ 22
α-Dextrinase†	Nonreducing α(1→4) end links of glucosyl oligosaccharides and α-dextrins; required for removal of nonreducing α(1→6)-linked glucose in α-dextrins	Glucose	5.0 (isomaltose) 1.0 (glucosyl-α-1→6 maltotriose) 11 (G_3) 3.1 (G_2)	115,000	11,‡ 22

* G indicates glucose unit, and subscript denotes the member of the α(1→4)-linked glucose residues in the saccharide.

† Actually present in intestine as the noncovalently linked hybrid enzyme sucrase-α-dextrinase but considered here separately since the hydrolytic sites act independently of each other for all substrates.

‡ Reference 11 describes experiments on rat intestine; human enzymes have nearly identical characteristics.

a profuse watery diarrhea. Secondary malabsorption of fat occurs in about one-third of patients, regardless of whether or not diarrhea is present, and appears to be related to the amount of the offending carbohydrate that is ingested [40]. The mechanisms responsible for the watery diarrhea in patients with lactase deficiency are shown diagrammatically in Fig. 78-6.

Patients with carbohydrate malabsorption complain of abdominal fullness, nausea, distention, and cramping pain within 5 to 60 min after ingesting the offending carbohydrate. Watery diarrhea may occur within a few minutes to as long as 5 h after ingestion of the sugar. Children with lactase deficiency may complain of various types of abdominal pain and yet have no diarrhea [41]. Such complaints are related to the amount of milk taken in, and they disappear when milk products are excluded from the diet.

Disacchariduria

An increase in the excretion of intact disaccharide in the urine may occur in some patients with disaccharidase deficiency. Under normal conditions the intestine is almost impermeable to disaccharides, but trace amounts may be absorbed without hydrolysis. There is little if any metabolism of disaccharides after absorption, and only 50 mg or less of any particular disaccharide is customarily excreted in 24 h in normal humans [42]. This may increase to 300 mg or more in patients with intestinal damage (e.g., celiac sprue [43] or in those who have a

high intraluminal concentration of disaccharide, as may be the case in the disaccharidase deficiencies [44]). Disacchariduria is a nonspecific finding which never accounts for more than 1 percent of the ingested carbohydrate and does not serve as a test for disaccharidase deficiency. In fact there appears to be little reason for undertaking the cumbersome analysis for carbohydrate in the urine in patients suspected of having malabsorption of carbohydrate.

TYPES OF CARBOHYDRATE INTOLERANCE

In essence, there are three broad categories of carbohydrate intolerance: (1) congenital absence of a particular enzyme or transport mechanism; (2) hereditary, delayed-onset deficiency occurring several years after birth; this type of defect accounts for the vast majority of lactase deficiency present in most of the world's population groups; and (3) acquired deficiency of one or more enzymes secondary to intestinal disease. Table 78-3 categorizes the types of carbohydrate intolerance. These will be considered in detail below.

Delayed-Onset Isolated Lactase Deficiency

This is the most common type of isolated lactase deficiency.

The prevalence varies greatly with the particular population group. As shown in Table 78-4, a remarkably high proportion of American blacks, Asians, African Bantus, and Indians have been found to have an isolated deficiency of this one disaccharidase. Even in white North Americans and Western Europeans, a significant percentage of healthy adults have lactase deficiency. Lactose intolerance appears to develop in healthy young children at about 3 years of age in those population groups having a prevalence of lactase deficiency in adult members of greater than 50 percent [67]. Thus, among African (Yoruba, Baganda) and American black groups, American Indians, Thais, and Bangladesh, lactose malabsorption usually develops by age 4. In contrast, North American and Finnish whites do not develop lactose deficiency until about age 13, and even then it occurs in a minority of individuals (see Table 78-4).

Despite the onset of lactose deficiency in early childhood, complaints are often ill-defined because the patient has at least partially eliminated milk from the diet. Occasionally an individual may recall that intolerance began with fever and infection or gastroenteritis, but most lactase-deficient patients cannot relate the onset to a particular illness.

Nearly all lactase-deficient patients in racial groups at high risk for this disorder give a history of appreciable milk ingestion without symptoms as young children. When intolerance does develop, symptoms are often nonspecific and variable. In a study of American black children [68], only 18 percent of those known to be lactose malabsorbers developed clinical symptoms after ingesting lactose (2 g/kg body weight). Furthermore, this low rate of intolerance was no different than the 12 percent found lactose-intolerant among those known to absorb lactose normally. In these black children, 87 percent of lactose malabsorbers and 92 percent of absorbers drank one glass (240 ml) or greater of milk per day. Thus lactose malabsorption and lactose intolerance are certainly not synonymous. Double-blind control studies of a lactose-free versus a lactose-containing (4.5 percent) chocolate drink revealed that no lactase-deficient individuals developed symptoms directly related to the lactose after ingesting 240 ml of milk. Even when two glasses of milk (480 ml) were ingested, the specific lactose intolerance rate was only 16 percent [69, 70]. These studies must be interpreted cautiously because of (1) possible slow gastric emptying of the chocolate drink, (2) a relatively high capillary blood glucose (26 mg/dl) rise that was accepted for normal lactose absorption, and (3) estimation of symptoms by use of a questionnaire rather than by physician interview. Nevertheless, they strongly suggest that the extent of lactose intolerance in lactase deficiency has been overemphasized in the past. This finding may have important implications for the use of milk as a nutritive supplement in groups having a high prevalence of lactase deficiency since milk may be beneficial in symptom-free patients even if they are lactase-deficient. How-

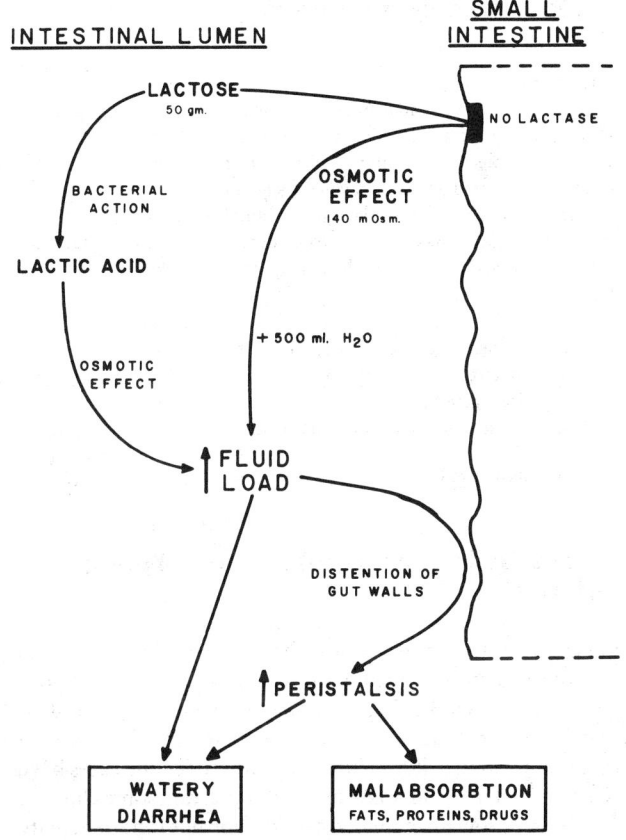

Figure 78-6 Diagrammatic representation of the pathogenesis of the disaccharidase deficiency syndrome. See text for elaboration.

ever, recent studies of Australian aboriginal children given either regular milk or milk in which the lactose was prehydrolyzed to glucose and galactose demonstrated improved growth and weight gain on the lactase-hydrolyzed milk [71, 72] as compared with regular milk. These authors claim that ingestion of regular milk may lead to growth retardation in these children [72].

Often there is a close relationship between the prevalence of lactase deficiency in a particular population group and the quantity of milk ingested. For instance, in Nigeria, those Fulani who are migratory cattle raisers have an even lower prevalence of lactase deficiency (20 percent) than their tribe members who reside within towns (70 percent) [62]. The Yoruba, who live in an adjacent area of Nigeria where there are few cattle and where milk consumption after weaning is nil, are virtually all lactase deficient by age 2 to 4 (Table 78-4).

Since the symptoms of lactose intolerance are similar to those present in many other diseases, it is important to consider an underlying primary illness such as infectious diarrhea, ulcerative colitis, regional enteritis, or irritable colon.

Table 78-2 Normal values of intestinal disaccharidases*

	Lactase	Sucrase	α-Dextrinase†	Maltase	Sucrase/lactase
Units/g protein	45 (15-95)	93 (40-165)	99 (50-160)	262 (128-461)	2.1 (1.0-4.5)
Units/g wet weight	3.5 (1.0-6.5)	8.1 (3.5-14)	8.3 (3.8-14)	20 (10-36)	2.3 (1.0-4.5)

* From combined data on 50 patients from Puerto Rico and the United States. Units = μmoles/min. Mean values with range in parentheses.
† With isomaltose as substrate; this activity is commonly termed isomaltase.

Table 78-3   Carbohydrate intolerance

1 Lactose intolerance
  a Congenital lactase deficiency in infants and children
  b Temporary lactase deficiency in premature infants
  c Severe intolerance in infants without lactase deficiency
  d Delayed-onset lactase deficiency (genetic)
  e Lactase deficiency secondary to intestinal diseases
  f Lactase deficiency secondary to insufficient mucosal contact time (surgically shortened bowel; gastric surgery)
2 Sucrose intolerance
  a Congenital sucrase-α-dextrinase deficiency (genetic)
  b Sucrase-α-dextrinase deficiency in intestinal disease
3 Glucose-galactose malabsorption
  a Congenital (genetic)
  b Acquired; secondary to intestinal disease

SOURCE: Modified from Bayless and Christopher [45].

Lactase Deficiency in Infants and Young Children

Oral lactose tolerance tests show that children have full capacity to digest lactose at birth even if they are members of population groups with a high prevalence of adult lactase deficiency. Though manifest deficiency of intestinal lactase in infants and young children is relatively rare, definite cases have been recorded in the first few months of life, and some children with the syndrome eventually develop normal lactase activity from several months to a year or two after the deficiency is first discovered [73, 74]. Possibly fleeting intestinal injury or the delayed acquisition of lactase may account for these instances. It is important to distinguish this form of lactase deficiency in infants from the peculiar toxic response to lactose without enzyme deficiency which is described next.

Lactose Intolerance in Children without Lactase Deficiency

Occasionally an infant develops overwhelming symptoms of inanition, severe dehydration, and cachexia, sometimes culminating in death, after the ingestion of milk or lactose [2]. In these children the sugar cannot be digested and absorbed normally, at least as estimated from the blood sugar rise after lactose ingestion. Instead, the response to lactose suggests a direct toxic effect on the intestine, and the immediate withdrawal of milk may be lifesaving. Lactosuria is usually a prominent feature. The intestine may be so damaged that it becomes permeable to the disaccharide. Although there appear to be several authenticated cases of this entity [1, 2, 75, 76], there have been few recent reports.

Many pediatricians with whom I have discussed this syndrome say that they have observed an occasional patient who fits the description. Comparative features of lactase deficiency and lactose intolerance without the enzyme deficiency are given in Table 78-5. Until further experimental data are available, pediatricians should carefully attempt to categorize cases of milk intolerance according to clinical criteria, with verification by disaccharidase assay. In this way it may be possible to ascertain whether the apparent toxic response to lactose is still being observed in clinical practice.

Lactase Deficiency in Intestinal Disease

Probably because hydrolysis of lactase is relatively limited in normal persons, milk intolerance due to inadequate digestion of lactose is a fairly frequent secondary manifestation of intestinal disease. Lactase is depressed earlier than the other disaccharidases in nonspecific intestinal injury such as in celiac sprue [77, 78] and is the last of these carbohydrases to return to normal after intestinal disease has subsided. It is not uncommon to find secondary isolated depression of lactase with normal intestinal sucrase, maltase, and α-dextrinase. In fact lactase may be permanently depressed after illnesses such as kwashiorkor [79] and tropical sprue [80] even when these diseases are no longer clinically evident. Deficiency of this enzyme may be the sole legacy of previous or subclinical disease.

Diseases involving the small intestine that are frequently associated with lactase deficiency and other disaccharidase deficiencies appear in Table 78-6. In general all patients with severe surface-cell abnormalities of the intestine due to these diseases will have lactase deficiency, and 50 percent or more will also have sucrase and maltase deficiency. Lactose intolerance may be found after gastrectomy even if enzyme concentrations in the intestine are normal, because patients with a normal concentration of lactase may have so rapid a rate of delivery of ingested lactose that the capacity of the small intestine to hydrolyze it is exceeded. After small-intestine resections the total remaining lactase activity may be insufficient to digest completely the dietary lactose [88, 89].

Table 78-4   Prevalence of lactase deficiency in healthy populations*

Group	No. tested	Percent lactase deficient	Ref.
North American (white)	422	5-20	19, 46–50
North American (black)	44	70-75	46, 48
African Bantu	40	50	51
Puerto Rican	28	21	19
Danish	700	3	52
Finnish	129	10	53
Asians			
Filipino	10	95	54
Indian	22	55	55
Thai	140	97	56
Chinese	15	87	58
Bangladesh		89	58
Eskimo (Greenland)	32	88	59
Canadian	59	73	60
Nigerian			
Yoruba	41	99	61
Fulani	33	58	61
Israeli Jews†	142	61	62
Israeli Arabs	67	81	63
Mexican	401	74	64
American Indian	60	83	65
Pima, Arizona	62	95	66

* Lactase activity below 1 U/g tissue or 15 U/g protein or blood glucose rise less than 20 mg/100 ml after ingestion of 50 g lactose accompanied by abdominal symptoms and diarrhea. In some instances, percentages given may differ from those in the reference.
† Includes Ashkenazi, Sephardi, Iraqis, Yenemite, and Oriental groups with deficiency rates of 44 to 84 percent.

Table 78-5 Lactose intolerance in infancy

Lactase deficiency	Intolerance without lactase deficiency
Failure to gain weight; no severe reaction	Diarrhea, vomiting, toxic state after lactose
Flat lactose tolerance test and lactase deficiency	Normal lactose tolerance or only transient lactase deficiency
Lactosuria (variable)	Lactosuria (characteristic)
Normal absorption of other nutrients	Decreased xylose absorption Aminoaciduria, renal acidosis (common)

Lactase Deficiency in Diseases other than of the Small Intestine

At one time or another claims have been made for an association between lactase deficiency and a variety of diseases in which the small intestine is not directly involved. Ulcerative colitis [90, 91] and duodenal ulcer [92] are but a few of these. In general the associations were made before it was appreciated that there is a high prevalence of lactase deficiency in many racial groups. Nevertheless, two clinical conditions appear to be associated frequently with lactase deficiency. When allowance is made for the background of lactase deficiency in the population group (Table 78-4), chronic alcoholics without malnutrition were found to have a significant increase in lactase deficiency, and one-third of alcoholics were also sucrase deficient [93]. In these same patients 2 weeks after alcohol abstinence, the intestinal oligosaccharidases had increased toward normal. Another recent study [94] extends previous work [95] on the relationship of lactase deficiency to osteoporosis in women. Whereas 3 percent of nonosteoporotic women were lactase deficient, 26 percent of those with osteoporosis were deficient. Although none were aware of lactase intolerance, their intake of milk and calcium was lower than that of the nonosteoporotic controls. Thus isolated lactase deficiency may predispose to osteoporosis because of decreased calcium intake and also perhaps because of a decrease in absorption of ingested calcium from nonmilk sources since lactose is believed to augment intestinal calcium uptake.

Clinical Diagnosis of Lactase Deficiency

Even though there are many excellent specialized tests for disaccharidase deficiency, the diagnosis should be confirmed by the absence of symptoms when the offending carbohydrate is eliminated from the diet.

Assay of Intestinal Biopsy Because of the relatively low prevalence of true lactose intolerance in patients with lactase deficiency and the limited in vivo lactose hydrolysis rates in normal individuals, oral lactose tolerance tests are of limited value in establishing a diagnosis of lactase deficiency. In order to establish a reduction in enzyme concentration in the intestinal surface cells, a peroral intestinal biopsy is necessary. The majority of the specimen can be used for histologic study since 1 to 3 mg will suffice for the oligosaccharidase assays (see "Analysis of Intestinal Oligosaccharidases" above and Table 78-2).

Oral Lactose Tolerance Tests Since smaller medical centers may not have facilities for specialized breath tests (see below) or intestinal mucosal oligosaccharidase assays, the lactose tolerance test has been widely used to confirm suspected lactase deficiency. Unfortunately a false positive test is found in 10 to 30 percent of individuals despite normal lactose absorption [96]. The test can be optimized by giving 1 g/kg body weight of lactose orally followed by capillary blood collection by finger puncture at 0, 15, 30, 60, 90, and 120 min and analysis of plasma glucose for a rise of 20 mg/dl. When severe symptoms such as abdominal cramping pain and diarrhea are observed along with failure of the appropriate plasma glucose rise, a tentative diagnosis of lactose malabsorption due to lactase deficiency can be made. Because such a severe response is unusual in most patients with lactase deficiency and may be associated at times with normal lactose absorption [69, 70, 97], a biopsy assay or one of the more definitive tests discussed below is preferable to establish the diagnosis.

^{14}C-Lactose Breath Test Radioactive breath tests appear to be reliable and safe in the estimation of human intestinal function. The use of only 5 μCi of ^{14}C-lactose along with 50 g lactose carrier has been shown to identify patients with lactase deficiency [98]. In lactose-tolerant control subjects, about 23 percent of the oral dose is excreted in the breath as $^{14}CO_2$ per mole of expired CO_2 over 4 h. The comparable value for lactose-intolerant patients is only 10 percent and reflects the slower rate of hydrolysis and uptake of radioactive sugar for subsequent metabolism in these patients. The test is relatively simple to set up in any nuclear medicine laboratory and appears to be an important noninvasive adjunct to the small-intestine biopsy.

Hydrogen Breath Test Under normal circumstances, small quantities of hydrogen gas are produced by bacterial action on residual carbohydrates in the colon [99], and an insignificant increase occurs after ingestion of an oral lactose load (< 3 ppm in expired air). In patients with disaccharidase deficiency, the residual carbohydrate greatly increases the substrate available to colonic bacteria leading to production of large amounts of hydrogen that can be detected in expired breath by a relatively inexpensive gas chromatographic apparatus (> 50 ppm) 90 min after the ingestion of the sugar [100]. This test was cumbersome in the past because it required a rebreathing bag, but passive collection using nasal prongs has been found to give similar results [100]. This test is now well established and is becoming widely used to identify disaccharidase deficiency. It has the advantages of not requiring a radioisotope and of providing information about total small-bowel digestive-absorptive capacity. Hence, it is more useful that the small-intestinal oligosaccharidase assay in patients with intestinal resection or stasis syndrome where the mucosal enzyme concentration may be normal.

Treatment of Lactase Deficiency

Elimination of lactose from the diet is the only practical way to prevent symptoms, and it is very successful. Addition of crude

Table 78-6 Disaccharidase deficiency in gastrointestinal disorders

Condition	Lactase deficient, %	Sucrase deficient, %	Maltase deficient, %	Ref.
Celiac sprue, untreated				
Severe*	100	100	75	81, 82
Moderate	100	80	20	82
Mild	25	0	0	82
Celiac sprue, treated†				
Excellent response	29	0	0	82
Good response	100	100	43	82
Poor response	100	86	43	82
Kwashiorkor, acute‡	80	50	30	83
Tropical sprue				
Untreated	100	65	68	80
Treated	63	0	0	80
Cholera				
Acute	86	57	20	84
Convalescent	86	0	0	84
Gastroenteritis§				
Acute	100	43	57	84
Convalescent	100	0	0	84
Infant diarrhea, acute	45	27	18	73
Pellagra¶	100	20	30	83
"Irritable" colon	38	0	0	85, 86
Postgastrectomy	36	0	0	87

Note: Most patients were white; there was a presumed prevalence of lactase deficiency in the healthy control group of 5 to 19 percent (see Table 78-4).
* Synonyms: Gluten-sensitive enteropathy, nontropical sprue; categories refer to degree of histologic abnormality.
† Severe disease treated with gluten-free diet.
‡ Patients were 3 to 6 weeks into convalescence period; those with a history of kwashiorkor in the remote past usually have normal enzyme levels [83].
§ Includes nonspecific disease and that caused by bacteria.
¶ African Bantu children; other studies suggest a prevalence of up to 50 percent lactase deficiency in a control group [83].

lactase preparations to food without avoidance of lactose-containing foods also is effective but is an unwieldy and more expensive method than simple substitution of other sources of calories. It is essential that patients with underlying intestinal disease receive appropriate therapy for the primary illness.

Total elimination of lactose is rarely necessary since most patients can tolerate one or even two glasses of milk without symptoms. A minority of patients cannot tolerate a single 4- to 8-oz glass of milk (6 to 12 g lactose) and may require strict elimination of all sources of lactose. Table 78-7 lists some dietary sources of lactose that the patient and physician may not be aware of. Prepackaged and ready-to-eat foods are particularly suspect since lactose is often added as a filler. Individual foods and drug tablets may not contain a large amount of lactose, but, as the list indicates, the varied sources may allow a substantial total intake. It is important that the patient read the statement of contents on the labels of suspect foods.

CAUSES OF LACTASE DEFICIENCY: GENETIC AND ENVIRONMENTAL CONSIDERATIONS

Most mammals other than humans have at birth abundant intestinal lactase, which wanes within days to months with weaning. It has been suggested that loss of lactase occurs with maturation and is probably the normal condition for humans

[104, 105]. If so, white persons of European origin must have somehow maintained their lactase as adults. Possibly an inability to digest lactose was at one time so deleterious for European adults that there was a selective advantage for those who could continue digestion of lactose throughout life. It has been proposed that those groups with a plentiful milk supply that provided an essential food staple have maintained their lactase activity over many generations [106, 107]. There is little evidence that large segments of the world's population were ever dependent on the intake of large amounts of milk to maintain adequate nutrition. On the other hand, milk contains generous amounts of calcium, and lactose appears to augment intestinal calcium absorption. Thus, population groups receiving low ultraviolet radiation or insufficient dietary vitamin D may have been protected against rickets and osteomalacia by virtue of maintenance of intestinal lactose [108]. Also, Finns who have lactase deficiency have lower levels of serum cholesterol and triglyceride than their counterparts whose intestinal lactose is maintained [109]. Although there is a possibility that this may be protective against cardiovascular disease, this has not been established and even then would affect survival only in middle age.

Because of the frequency of lactase deficiency in healthy adults (Table 78-4), it is usually considered to be an inherited condition. There is no doubt that at least half the members of non-European population groups have milk intolerance and lactose intolerance as adolescents or young adults. Furthermore, probability analysis of Finnish [110] and Mexican [111] groups strongly suggests an autosomal recessive inheritance for isolated lactase deficiency. However, in these studies, it is difficult to control other factors such as the peculiar sensitivity of intestinal lactase to intestinal injury (see Table 78-6), persistence of the isolated deficiency state long after any underlying intestinal disease has become quiescent [79, 80], dietary influences, and the unknown residue of subclinical intestinal disease in a given population. In this regard it is interesting that Australian aboriginal [112] and Baganda children [113] have a sudden decline in rate of growth at about 12 months of age that is presumably the result of a high incidence of gastrointestinal and respiratory diseases [112] and suboptimal nutrition [113]. These children begin to have flat lactose tolerance tests at the same age, and nearly all are lactose intolerant by age 4 years [64, 112]. They may develop transitory malnutrition or temporary subclinical disease which leaves them with permanent lactase deficiency. In the individual case, it may be impossible to be certain whether late-onset lactase deficiency is inherited or secondary to subclinical intestinal disease or malnutrition. Hence, the physician should take particular care to rule out an underlying primary intestinal illness.

Though lactase deficiency in infancy is quite rare, it has occurred in sibs [76] and is probably inherited as an autosomal recessive gene. Infant diarrhea of any origin is often associated with transient lactase deficiency [73].

MOLECULAR DEFECT IN LACTASE DEFICIENCY

Various factors may play a role in the lactase deficiency that uniformly develops with intestinal disease (see Table 78-6). In studies of isolated human brush borders, incubation with trypsin-reduced lactase activity in lactase-deficient intestine was relatively greater than in normal intestine; but the actual quantitative loss of lactase was similar in brush borders from both groups [114]. Oral pancreatic enzyme supplements given to patients with exocrine pancreatic insufficiency reduced lactase activity of the jejunal biopsy in both patients who were lactase-normal and lactase-deficient, but no change in the plasma glucose rise after oral lactose tolerance was noted after institution of oral pancreatic enzyme therapy. This suggests that the reduction in lactase may not be of clinical importance [114].

Certain *Bacteroides* species secrete particularly potent proteases that attack human oligosaccharidases, and this mechanism of secondary saccharidase deficiency may be especially important in bacterial overgrowth syndromes [115]. Acute intestinal viral infections of animals appear to produce a dramatic reduction in intestinal oligosaccharidases by invading and destroying mature villus cells approximately 24 h after contact with the mucosal surface. Presumably a specific receptor for the virus is present on the surface membrane of villus cells but absent from crypt cells [116].

Attempts to define the alteration in lactase protein in hereditary late-onset lactase deficiency have been only partially successful. After the initial demonstration that the brush border lactase appeared to be undetectable in patients with lactase deficiency [117], subsequent experiments identified some residual lactase in deficient intestine [118, 119]. This included presence of the lactase protein band on acrylamide electrophoresis [119], a finding verified in recent cross-immunoelectrophoresis experiments in which the correlation between lactase hydrolytic activity and immunoreactivity was similar in normal and deficient intestinal specimens [120]. In these studies, residual activity in lactase-deficient intestine was usually 15 to 20 percent of normal. Definitive study of the precise biochemical defect in lactase-deficient states must await complete purification of the enzyme so that immunologic and structural techniques can be used in the search for an aberrant lactase protein. Nevertheless, the evidence to date points to a depression or absence of lactase protein in both acquired and congenital deficiency. This suggests that a regulatory defect may account for both disorders.

Table 78-7 Foods containing lactose

Food	Source of lactose
Milk (including nonfat, dried, condensed)	Natural
Processed meat (cold cuts, sausage, wieners)	Milk added in processing
Potatoes (French fried or instant)	Lactose filler added in processing
Prepared mixes (muffins, biscuits, cakes, cookies, pancakes, waffles, dry cereals)	Milk added in manufacture
Prepared soups	Lactose added in processing
Canned and frozen fruits	Lactose added in processing
Salad dressings	Lactose added in processing
Instant coffee	Lactose added in processing
Lithium carbonate; fluazepam [102]	Lactose added as filler in tablet

SOURCE: Summarized from Koch et al. [101].

SUCRASE-α-DEXTRINASE DEFICIENCY

Reports of intolerance to sucrose in the diet have come from many areas of the world [121, 122]. Although formerly thought to be a rare disorder, recent studies have suggested that sucrase deficiency may occur in 0.2 percent of North Americans [123] and 10 percent of Greenland Eskimos [124].

The malady appears to be inherited as an autosomal recessive gene. There is no identifying test for heterozygotes. All patients have had low activity not only of sucrase but also of α-dextrinase (isomaltase) in the mucosa of the small intestine. Symptoms occur in early childhood when the offending sugar is ingested and are indistinguishable from those of lactase deficiency, except that they are evoked by table sugar rather than by milk. Starch is usually well tolerated, probably because of several factors: (1) its relatively high molecular weight (1500 average) and less osmotic activity than sucrose, at least in small intestine; (2) the $\alpha(1 \rightarrow 4)$ linkages are hydrolyzed by glucoamylase, and hence about 50 percent of the potential glucose is released for absorption; and (3) only amylopectin contains the nonhydrolizable α(1 → 6) glucosyl linkages; the malto-oligosaccharides released from pancreatic amylase action on the unbranched amylose are readily cleaved by glucoamylase (see Figs. 78-2 and 78-3).

Children usually first develop symptoms at about 4 weeks of age, when fruits and prepared sweetened foods are added to the diet. Families having sucrose-intolerant children often discover the association of symptoms with sugar ingestion and modify the diet accordingly. Tolerance to sucrose may increase with age in some patients but not in others [122, 125]. Elimination of sucrose from the diet prevents the symptoms but may encroach upon the obligate source of calories in some areas of the world.

Even though sucrose exclusion is very effective in preventing symptoms, patients with sucrase deficiency may have recurrent symptoms [125], probably most often because they misunderstand the requirement for permanently avoiding the offending disaccharide.

As in lactase deficiency, diagnosis depends upon a history of intolerance to sucrose, with verification by an oral sucrose tolerance test, the $^{14}CO_2$ breath test after ingestion of ^{14}C-sucrose, or the hydrogen breath test. The definitive diagnosis can be made by assay of the small-intestine biopsy specimen.

Biochemical Defect in Sucrase-α-Dextrinase Deficiency

All patients with sucrase deficiency have intestinal enzyme concentrations that are very low (< 5 U/g protein), but some residual activity is usually present. Preliminary experiments using qualitative immunofluorescence suggested that a cross-reacting protein might be present on the intestinal surface of patients with enzyme deficiency [126]. In one of these patients an additional protein band was found on acrylamide electrophoresis of the brush border preparation, but this protein had no sucrase activity and was not shown to have immunologic cross-reactivity with antisucrase serum [127].

Quantitative radioimmunoassay of sucrase using ^{125}I-labeled human sucrase-α-dextrinase and monospecific antiserum against the enzyme disclosed no evidence of enzymatically inactive cross-reacting material in sucrase-deficient tissues [128]. This was true even though 10 times more intestinal protein was used for deficient tissue than for normal tissue. Hence there does not appear to be an inactive enzyme variant in sucrase deficiency. Instead, the enzyme may have undergone major changes in its three-dimensional structure, or its synthesis may be completely blocked. This can be accounted for either by a no-sense mutation of the structural gene or by complete repression of the regulatory mechanism controlling structural gene function.

GLUCOSE-GALACTOSE MALABSORPTION

More than 20 individuals from different parts of the world have been reported to have a specific defect in intestinal transport of glucose and galactose [129–132]. Children with this abnormality have diarrhea, dehydration, and sugar in the stools after ingestion of almost any dietary carbohydrate,

because all contain at least one of these hexoses. All patients who have been carefully tested have had an associated mild defect in renal tubular reabsorption of glucose. Customarily, they excrete 250 to 1000 mg glucose per dl in the urine. If the disorder is not recognized, the child may die of dehydration and malnutrition. Elimination of all dietary carbohydrate is required, and fructose, with a transport system that is not affected, is substituted as the source of carbohydrate calories. Some patients tolerate sucrose better than other disaccharides because one of its monosaccharide components is the readily absorbed fructose.

The diagnosis should be suspected in a child who tolerates all dietary carbohydrate poorly and who has little or no rise in blood sugar level after a meal. Stools are acid and contain glucose and galactose. Perfusion of the intestine with a solution containing glucose and fructose demonstrates the paradoxical finding of more rapid absorption of the passively transported fructose than of the glucose [133]. In vitro study of a small-intestine biopsy specimen demonstrates loss of normal accumulation of glucose beyond the concentration in the medium [134]. Indeed, tissue concentrations always are less than in the incubation medium. This rare malady may be distinguished from disaccharidase deficiencies because there is no significant rise in blood sugar concentration in the course of a glucose-galactose oral tolerance test.

Supported in part by Grant No. Am-11270 from the National Institute of Arthritis and Metabolic Diseases, National Institutes of Health.

REFERENCES

1. DURAND P: Lattosuria idiopatica in una paziente con diarrea cronica ed acidosi. *Minerva Pediatr* 10:706, 1958
2. HOLZEL A, MEREU T, THOMSON ML: Severe lactose intolerance in infancy. *Lancet* 2:1346, 1962
3. CROSBY WH, KUGLER HW: Intraluminal biopsy of the small intestine. *Am J Dig Dis* 2:236, 1957
4. BRANDBORG LL, RUBIN CE, QUINTON WE: A multipurpose instrument for suction biopsy of the esophagus, stomach, small bowel and colon. *Gastroenterology* 37:1, 1959
5. DAHLQUIST A: Method for assay of intestinal disaccharidases. *Anal Biochem* 7:18, 1964
6. MILLER D, CRANE RK: The digestive function of the epithelium of the small intestine. II. Localization of disaccharide hydrolysis in the isolated brush border portion of intestinal epithelial cells. *Biochim Biophys Acta* 52:293, 1961
7. DAHLQVIST A, BORGSTROM B: Digestion and absorption of disaccharides in man. *Biochem J* 81:411, 1961
8. GRAY GM, INGELFINGER FJ: Intestinal absorption of sucrose in man: The site of hydrolysis and absorption. *J Clin Invest* 44:390, 1965
9. ROBERTS PJP, WHELAN WJ: The mechanism of carbohydrase action. 5. Action of human salivary α-amylase on amylopectin and glycogen. *Biochem J* 76:246, 1960
10. GRAY GM: Carbohydrate digestion and absorption. Role of the small intestine. *N Engl J Med* 292:1225, 1975
11. GRAY GM, LALLY BC, CONKLIN KA: Action of intestinal sucrase-isomaltase and its free monomers on an α-limit dextrin. *J Biol Chem* 254:6038, 1979
12. BARNETT JEG, JARVIS WTS, MUNDAY KA: Structural requirements for active intestinal sugar transport: The involvement of hydrogen bonds at C-1 and C-6 of the sugar. *Biochem J* 109:61, 1968
13. RIKLIS E, QUASTEL JH: Effects of cations on sugar absorption by isolated surviving guinea pig intestine. *Can J Biochem Physiol* 36:347, 1958
14. KIMMICH GA, RANDLES J: Evidence for an intestinal Na$^+$:sugar transport coupling stoichiometry of 2.0. *Biochim Biophys Acta* 596:439, 1980
15. MISFELDT DS, SANDERS MJ: Transepithelial Na$^+$:D-glucose. Stoichiometry is two. *Ann Acad Sci* in press
16. HOPFER U, NELSON K, PERROTTO J, ISSELBACHER KJ: Glucose transport in

isolated brush border membrane from rat small intestine. *J Biol Chem* 248:25, 1973

17. WRIGHT EM, VAN OS CH, MIRCHEFF AK: Sugar uptake by intestinal basolateral membrane vesciesl. *Biochim Biophys Acta* 597:112, 1980

18. FRIDHANDLER L, QUASTEL JH: Absorption of sugars from isolated surviving intestine. *Arch Biochem Biophys* 56:412, 1955

19. GRAY GM, SANTIAGO NS: Disaccharide absorption in normal and diseased human intestine. *Gastroenterology* 51:489, 1966

20. GRAY GM, SANTIAGO NS: Intestinal β-galactosidases. I. Separation and characterization of three enzymes in normal human intestine. *J Clin Invest* 48:716, 1969

21. KELLY JJ, ALPERS DH: Properties of human intestinal glucoamylase. *Biochim Biophys Acta* 315:113, 1973

22. CONKLIN KA, YAMASHIRO KM, GRAY GM: Human intestinal sucrase-isomaltase: Identification of free sucrase and isomaltase and cleavage of the hybrid into active distinct subunits. *J Biol Chem* 250:5735, 1975

23. DAHLQVIST A, LINDBERG T: Development of the intestinal disaccharidase and alkaline phosphatase activities in the human foetus. *Clin Sci* 30:517, 1969

24. ROSENSWIG NS, HERMAN RH: Time response of jejunal sucrase and maltase activity to a high sucrose diet in normal man. *Gastroenterology* 56:500, 1969

25. CUATRECASAS P, LOCKWOOD DH, CALDWELL JR: Lactase deficiency in the adult. A common occurrence. *Lancet* 1:14, 1965

26. GRAY GM: Unpublished observations

27. KOGUT MD, DONNELL GM, SHAW KNF: Studies of lactose absorption in patients with galactosemia. *J Pediatr* 71:75, 1967

28. DOELL RG, KRETCHMER N: Studies of small intestine during development. I. Distribution and activity of β-galactosidase. *Biochim Biophys Acta* 62:353, 1962

29. SCHIMKE RT: Turnover of membrane proteins in animal cells. *Meth Membr Biol* 3:201, 1975

30. KAUFMAN MA, KORSMO HA, OLSEN WA: Circadian rhythm of intestinal sucrase activity in rats. Mechanism of enzyme change. *J Clin Invest* 65:1174, 1980

31. ALPERS DH, TEDESCO FJ: The possible role of pancreatic proteases in the turnover of intestinal brush border proteins. *Biochim Biophys Acta* 401:28, 1975

32. CEZARD J-P, CONKLIN KA, DAS BC, GRAY GM: Incomplete intracellular forms of intestinal surface membrane sucrase-isomaltase. *J Biol Chem* 254:8969, 1979

33. HAURI HP, QUARONI A, ISSELBACHER KJ: Biogenesis of intestinal plasma membrane: Posttranslational route and cleavage of sucrase-isomaltase. *Proc Natl Acad Sci USA* 76:5183, 1979

34. SJÖSTRÖM H, NOREN O, CHRISTIANSEN L, WACKER H, SEMENZA G: A fully active two-active site, single-chain sucrase-isomaltase from pig intestine. Implications for the biosynthesis of a mammalian integral stalked membrane protein. *J Biol Chem* 255:1132, 1980

35. BRUNNER J, HAUSER H, BRAUN H, WILSON KJ, WACKER H, O'NEILL B, SEMENZA G: The mode of association of the enzyme complex sucrase-isomaltase with the intestinal brush border membrane. *J Biol Chem* 254:1821, 1979

36. WALTER WM JR, GRAY GM: Enzyme assay of peroral biopsies. Storage conditions and basis of expression. *Gastroenterology* 54:56, 1968

37. KERN F, STRUTHERS JE: Intestinal lactase deficiency and lactose intolerance in adults. *JAMA* 195:927, 1966

38. CHRISTOPHER ML, BAYLESS TM: Role of the small bowel and colon in lactose-induced diarrhea. *Gastroenterology* 60:845, 1971

39. LAUNIALA K: The effect of unabsorbed sucrose and mannitol on the small intestinal flow rate and mean transit time. *Scand J Gastroenterol* 39:665, 1968

40. RINGROSE RE, THOMPSON JB, WELSH JD: Lactose malabsorption and steatorrhea. *Am J Dig Dis* 17:533, 1972

41. BAYLESS TM, HUANG SS: Recurrent abdominal pain due to milk and lactose intolerance to school-aged children. *Pediatrics* 47:1029, 1971

42. BICKEL H: Mellituria: Paper chromatographic study. *J Pediatr* 59:641, 1961

43. WESER E, SLEISENGER MH: Lactosuria and lactase deficiency in adult celiac disease. *Gastroenterology* 48:571, 1969

44. DURAND P: Lactose intolerance, in Durand P (ed): *Disorders due to Intestinal Defective Carbohydrate Digestion and Absorption.* Rome, Il Pensiero Scientifico Publisher, 1964, p 105

45. BAYLESS TM, CHRISTOPHER ML: Disaccharidase deficiency. *Am J Clin Nutr* 22:181, 1969

46. BAYLESS TM, ROSENSWEIG NS: A racial difference in incidence of lactase deficiency. *JAMA* 197:968, 1966

47. NEWCOMER AD, MCGILL DB: Disaccharidase activity in the small intestine: Prevalence of lactase deficiency in 100 health subjects. *Gastroenterology* 53:881, 1967

48. LITTMAN A, CADY AB, RHODES J: Lactase and other disaccharidase deficiencies in the hospital population. *Isr J Med Sci* 4:110, 1968

49. WELSH JD, ROHRER V, KNUDSEN KB, PAUSTIAN FF: Isolated lactase deficiency: Correlation of laboratory studies and clinical data. *Arch Intern Med* 120:261, 1967

50. SHEEHY TW, ANDERSON PR: Disaccharidase activity in normal and diseased small bowel. *Lancet* 2:1, 1965

51. COOK GC, KAJUBI SK: Tribal incidence of lactase deficiency in Uganda. *Lancet* 1:725, 1966

52. GUDMAND E, DAHLQVIST A, JARNUM S: Specific small-intestinal lactase deficiency in adults. *Scand J Gastroenterol* 4:377, 1969

53. SAHI T, LAUNIALA K: Manifestation and occurrence of selective adult-type lactose malabsorption in Finnish teenagers. A follow-up study. *Dig Dis* 23:699, 1978

54. HUANG SS, BAYLESS TM: Milk and lactose intolerance in healthy Orientals. *Science* 160:83, 1968

55. DESAI HG, CHITRE AV, PAREKH DV, JEEJEEBHOY KN: Intestinal disaccharidases in tropical sprue. *Gastroenterology* 53:375, 1967

56. KEUSCH GT, TRONCALE FJ, THAVARAMARA B, PRINTANONY P, ANDERSON PR, BRAMARAPRAVATHI N: Lactase deficiency in Thailand: Effect of prolonged lactose feeding. *Am J Clin Nutr* 22:638, 1969

57. DAVIS AE, BOLIN T: Lactose intolerance in Asians. *Nature (Lond)* 216:1244, 1967

58. BROWN KH, PARRY L, KHATUN M: Lactose malabsorption in Bangladeshi village children: Relation with age, history of recent diarrhea, nutritional status, and breast feeding. *Am J Clin Nutr* 32:1962, 1979

59. GUDMAN-HØYER AE, JARNUM S: Laktosemalabsorption hos grønlaendere. *Ugeskr Laeger* 131:917, 1969

60. ELLESTAD-SAYED J, HAWORTH JC, HILDES JA: Disaccharide malabsorption and dietary patterns in two Canadian Eskimo communities. *Am J Clin Nutr* 31:1473, 1968

61. KRETCHMER N, HURWITZ R, RANSOME-KUTI O, DUNGY C, ALARIJA W: Intestinal absorption of lactose in Nigerian ethnic groups. *Lancet* 2:392, 1971

62. GILAT T, KUHN R, GELMAN E, MIZRAHY O: Lactase deficiency in Jewish communities in Israel. *Am J Dig Dis* 15:895, 1970

63. GILAT T, MALACHI EG, SHOCHET SB: Lactose tolerance in an Arab population. *Am J Dig Dis* 16:203, 1971

64. LISKER R, LOPEZ-HABIB G, DALTABUTT M, ROSTENBERG I, ARROYO P: Lactase deficiency in a rural area of Mexico. *Am J Clin Nutr* 27:756, 1974

65. CASKEY DA, PAYNE-BOSE D, WELSH JD, GEARHART HL, NANCE MK, MORRISON RD: Effects of age on lactose malabsorption in Oklahoma native Americans as determined by breath H_2 analysis. *Dig Dis* 22:113, 1977

66. JOHNSON JD, SIMOONS FJ, HURWITZ R: Lactose malabsorption among the Pima Indians of Arizona. *Gastroenterology* 73:1299, 1977

67. SIMOONS FJ: Age of onset of lactose malabsorption. *Pediatrics* 66:646, 1980

68. PAIGE DM, BAYLESS TM, MELLITS ED, DAVIS L: Lactose malabsorption in preschool black children. *Am J Clin Nutr* 30:1018, 1977

69. HAVERBERG L, KWON PH, SCRIMSHAW NS: Comparative tolerance of adolescents of differing ethnic backgrounds to lactose-containing and lactose-free dairy drinks. I. Initial experience with a double-blind procedure. *Am J Clin Nutr* 33:17, 1980

70. KWON PH JR, RORICK MH, SCRIMSHAW NS: Comparative tolerance of adolescents of differing ethnic backgrounds to lactose-containing and lactose-free dairy drinks. II. Improvement of a double-blind test. *Am J Clin Nutr* 33:22, 1980

71. BRAND JC, MILLER JJ, VORBACH EA, EDWARDS RA: A trial of lactose hydrolyzed milk in Australian aboriginal children. *Med J Aust (Spec Suppl)* 2:10, 1977

72. MITCHELL JD, BRAND J, HALBISCH J: Weight-gain inhibition by lactose in Australian aboriginal children. *Lancet* 1:500, 1977

73. BURKE V, KERRY KR, ANDERSON CM: The relationship of dietary lactose to refractory diarrhoea in infancy. *Aust Paediatr J* I:147, 1965

74. SUNSHINE P, KRETCHMER N: Studies of small intestine during development. III. Infantile diarrhea associated with intolerance to disaccharides. *Pediatrics* 34:38, 1964

75. DARLING S, MORTENSEN O, SØNDERGAARD G: Lactosuria and amino-aciduria in infancy: A new inborn error of metabolism. *Acta Paediatr (Uppsala)* 49:281, 1960

76. HOZEL A: Sugar malabsorption and sugar intolerance in childhood. *Proc R Soc Med* 61:1095, 1968

77. LIPSHITZ F, KLOTZ AP, HOLMAN GC: Intestinal disaccharidase deficiencies in gluten-sensitive enteropathy. *Am J Dig Dis* 10:47, 1965

78. SHMERLING DH, AURICCHIO S, RUBINO A, HADORN B, PRADER A: Der sekundare Mangel an intestinaler Disaccharidaseaktivitat bei der Coliake: Quantitative Bestimmung der Enzymaktivitat und Klinische Beurtelung. *Helv Paediat Acta* 19:507, 1964

79. COOK GC, LEE FD: The jejunum after kwashiorkor. *Lancet* 2:1263, 1966

80. GRAY GM, WALER WM JR, COLVER EH: Persistent deficiency of intestinal lactase in apparently cured tropical sprue. *Gastroenterology* 54:552, 1968

81. PLOTKIN GR, ISSELBACHER KJ: Secondary disaccharidase deficiency in adult celiac disease (non-tropical sprue) and other malabsorption states. *N Engl M Med* 271:1033, 1964

82. WELSH JD, ZSCHIESCHE OM, ANDERSON J, WALKER A: Intestinal disaccharidase activity in celiac sprue (gluten-sensitive enteropathy). *Arch Intern Med* 123:33, 1969

83. PRINSLOO JG, WITTMANN W, KRUGER H, FREIER E: Lactose absorption and mucosal disaccharidases in convalescent pellagra and kwashiorkor children. *Arch Dis Child* 46:474, 1971

84. HIRSCHHORN N, MOLLA A: Reversible jejunal disaccharidase deficiency in cholera and other diarrheal diseases. *Johns Hopkins Med J* 125:291, 1969

85. MCMICHAEL JB, WEBB J, DAWSON AM: Lactase deficiency in adults: A cause of "functional" diarrhoea. *Lancet* 1:717, 1965

86. WESER E, RUBIN W, ROSS L, SLEISENGER MH: Lactase deficiency in patients with the "irritable-colon syndrome." *N Engl J Med* 273:1070, 1965

87. KOJECKY Z, MATLOCHA Z: Quantitative differences of intestinal disaccharidase activity following the resection of stomach. *Gastroenterologia (Basel)* 104:343, 1965

88. WEIJERS HA, VAN DE KAMER JH: Diarrhoea caused by deficiency of sugar splitting enzymes. II. *Acta Paediatr* 51:371, 1962

89. KERN F, STRUTHERS JE, ARRWOOD WL: Lactose intolerance as a cause of steatorrhea in an adult. *Gastroenterology* 45:477, 1963

90. CADY AB, RHODES JB, LITTMAN A, CRANE RK: Significance of lactase deficit in ulcerative colitis. *J Lab Clin Med* 70:279, 1967

91. NEWCOMER AD, MCGILL DB: Incidence of lactase deficiency in ulcerative colitis. *Gastroenterology* 53:890, 1967

92. AURRICCHIO S, RUBINO S, LANDOLY M, SEMENZA G, PRADER A: Isolated intestinal lactase deficiency in the adult. *Lancet* 2:324, 1963

93. PERLOW W, BARAONA E, LIEBER CS: Symptomatic intestinal disaccharidase deficiency in alcoholics. *Gastroenterology* 72:680, 1977

94. NEWCOMER AD, HODGSON SF, MCGILL DB, THOMAS PJ: Lactase deficiency: Prevalence in osteoporosis. *Ann Intern Med* 89:218, 1968

95. BIRGE SJ JR, KEUTMANN HT, CUATRECASES P, WHEDON GD: Osteoporosis, intestinal lactase deficiency and low dietary calcium intake. *N Engl J Med* 276:445, 1967

96. MCGILL DB, NEWCOMER AD: Comparison of venous and capillary blood samples in lactose tolerance testing. *Gastroenterology* 53:371, 1967

97. LACASSIE Y, WEINBERG R, MÖNCKEBERG F: Poor predictability of lactose malabsorption from clinical symptoms for Chilean populations. *Am J Clin Nutr* 31:799, 1978

98. SASAKI Y, ITO M, KAMEDA H, UEDA H, AOYAGI T, CHRISTOPHER NL, BAYLESS TM, WAGNER NH: Measurement of ^{14}C-lactose absorption in the diagnosis of lactase deficiency. *J Lab Clin Med* 76:824, 1970

99. NEWCOMER AD, MCGILL DB, THOMAS PJ, HOFMANN AF: Prospective comparison of indirect methods for detecting lactase deficiency. *N Engl J Med* 293:1232, 1975

100. PERMAN JA, BARR RG, WATKINS JB: Sucrose malabsorption in children: Noninvasive diagnosis by interval breath hydrogen determination. *J Pediatr* 93:17, 1979

101. KOCH R, ACOSTA P, RAGSDALE N, DONNELL GN: Nutrition in the treatment of galactosemia. *J Am Diet Assoc* 43:216, 1963

102. LIEB J, KAZIENKO DJ: Lactose filler as a cause of "drug-induced" diarrhea. *N Engl J Med* 299:314, 1978

103. DOELL RG, KRETCHMER N: Studies of small intestine during development. I. Distribution and activity of β-galactosidase. *Biochim Biophys Acta* 62:353, 1962

104. FERGUSON A, MAXWELL JD: Genetic aetiology of lactose intolerance. *Lancet* 2:188, 1967

105. COOK GC: Some observations on racial lactase deficiency. *Proc R Soc Med* 61:1102, 1968

106. SIMOONS F: The non-milking area of Africa. *Anthropos* 49:58, 1954

107. JOHNSON JD, KRETCHMER N, SIMOONS FJ: Lactose malabsorption: Its biology and history. *Adv Pediatr* 21:197, 1974

108. FLATZ G, ROTTHAUWE HW: The human lactase polymorphism: Physiology and genetics of lactose absorption and malabsorption. *Prog Med Genet* 2:205, 1977

109. SAHI T: Intestinal lactase polymorphisms and dairy food. *Hum Genet (Suppl 1)* 115, 1978

110. SAHI T, ISOKOSKI M, JUSSILA J, LUANIALA K, PVORALA K: Recessive inheritance of adult-type lactose malabsorption. *Lancet* 2:823, 1973

111. LISKER R, GONZALEZ B, DALTABUTT M: Recessive inheritance of the adult type of intestinal lactase deficiency. *Am J Hum Genet* 27:662, 1975

112. ELLIOTT RB, MAXWELL GM: Lactose maldigestion in Australian aboriginal children. *Med J Aust* 1:46, 1967

113. RUTISHAUSER IHE: Heights and weights of middle class Baganda children. *Lancet* 2:565, 1965

114. SEETHARAM B, PERRILLO R, ALPERS DH: Effect of pancreatic proteases on intestinal lactase activity. *Gastroenterology* 79:827, 1980

115. RIEPE SP, GOLDSTEIN J, ALPERS DH: Effect of secreted *Bacteroides* proteases on human intestinal brush border hydrolases. *J Clin Invest* 66:314, 1980

116. SHEPHERD RW, BUTLER DG, CUTZ E, GALL DG, HAMILTON JR: The musocal lesion in viral enteritis. Extent and dynamics of the epithelial response to virus invasion in transmissible gastroenteritis of piglets. *Gastroenterology* 76:770, 1979

117. GRAY GM, SANTIAGO NA, COLVER EH, GENEL M: Intestinal β-galactosidases. II. Biochemical alteration in human lactase deficiency. *J Clin Invest* 48:729, 1969

118. LEBENTHAL E, TSUBOI K, KRETCHMER N: Characterization of human intestinal lactase and hetero-β-galactosidases of infants and adults. *Gastroenterology* 67:1107, 1974

119. FREIBURGHAUS AU, SCHMITZ J, SCHINDLER M, ROTTHAUWE HW, KUITUNEN P, LAUNIALA K, HADORN B: Protein patterns of brush-border fragments in congenital lactose malabsorption and in specific hypolactasia of the adult. *N Engl J Med* 294:1030, 1976

120. SKOVBJERG H, GUDMAN-HØYER E, FENGER HJ: Immunoelectrophoretic studies on human small intestinal brush border proteins—amount of lactase protein in adult-type hypolactasia. *Gut* 21:360, 1980

121. BURGESS EA, LEVIN B, MAHALANABIS D, TONGE RE: Hereditary sucrose intolerance: Levels of sucrase activity in jejunal mucosa. *Arch Dis Child* 39:431, 1964

122. AMENT ME, PERERA DR, ESTHER LJ: Sucrase-isomaltase deficiency—a frequently misdiagnosed disease. *J Pediatr* 83:721, 1973

123. PETERSON ML, HERBER R: Intestinal sucrase deficiency. *Trans Assoc Am Physicians* 80:275, 1967

124. MCNAIR A, GUDMAN-HØYER E, JARNUM S: Sucrose malabsorption in Greenland. *Br Med J* 2:19, 1972

125. KILBY A, BURGESS A, WIGGLESWORTH S, WALKER-SMITH JA: Sucrase-isomaltase deficiency. A follow-up report. *Arch Dis Child* 53:677, 1978

126. DUBS R, STEINMANN B, GITZELMANN R: Demonstration of an inactive enzyme antigen in sucrase-isomaltase deficiency. *Helv Paediatr Acta* 28:187, 1973

127. FREIBURGHAUS AU, DUBS R, HADORN B, GAZE H, HAURI HP, GITZELMAN R: The brush border membrane in hereditary sucrase-isomaltase deficiency: Abnormal protein pattern and presence of immunoreactive enzyme. *Eur J Clin Invest* 7:455, 1977

128. GRAY GM, CONKLIN KA, TOWNLEY RRW: Sucrase-isomaltase deficiency. Absence of an inactive enzyme variant. *N Engl J Med* 294:750, 1976

129. LINDQUIST B, MEEUWISSE GW: Chronic diarrhoea caused by monosaccharide malabsorption. *Acta Paediatr Scand* 51:674, 1962

130. LAPLANE R, POLONOVSKI C, ETIENNE M, DEBRAY P, LODS J-C, PISSARRO B: L'intolerance au lactose et le syndrome coeliaque. *Arch Fr Pediatr* 19:895, 1962

131. SCHNEIDER AJ, KINTER WB, STIRLING CE: Glucose-galactose malabsorption. *N Engl J Med* 274:305, 1966

132. MEEUWISSE GW, DAHLQVIST A: Glucose-galactose malabsorption. *Acta Paediatr Scand* 57:273, 1968

133. MEEUWISSE G, MELIN K: Glucose-galactose malabsorption. *Acta Paeditr, Scand (Suppl)* 188:3, 1969

134. EGGERMONT E, LOEB H: Glucose-galactose intolerance. *Lancet* 2:343, 1966

135. MELIN K, MEEUWISSE GW: Glucose-galactose malabsorption: A genetic study. *Acta Paediatr Scand (Suppl)* 188:19, 1969

79

FAMILIAL HYPOPHOSPHATEMIC RICKETS AND VITAMIN D–DEPENDENT RICKETS

HOWARD RASMUSSEN

CONSTANTINE ANAST

1. There are two general types of inherited rickets and osteomalacia: familial hypophosphatemic rickets or osteomalacia, and vitamin D–dependent rickets. In each of these there are at least two subtypes. All four probably represent defects in renal tubular function.

2. The predominant type of familial hypophosphatemic rickets is inherited as an X-linked dominant trait and is characterized by hypophosphatemia and decreased renal tubular phosphate reabsorption, normocalcemia, and low normal or low plasma $1,25\text{-}(OH)_2D_3$ concentrations. The patients have slow growth and bowing of the lower extremities with normal muscle tone and an absence of tetany or convulsions, but radiological evidence of rickets and osteomalacia. Intestinal calcium absorption is decreased, as is urinary calcium excretion, but the urinary excretion of amino acids and cyclic AMP are normal, as is plasma immunoreactive parathyroid hormone. This disease appears to result from a defect in tubular (proximal) phosphate transport which leads to a decrease in the Tm_P/GFR. This defect is coupled in some unknown manner with the rate of $1,25\text{-}(OH)_2D_3$ synthesis from $25\text{-}(OH)D_3$ in the kidney tubule which is inappropriately low for the plasma phosphate concentration. The most effective therapy for this condition appears to be a combination or oral phosphate (1.0 to 2.0 g/day in four or five divided doses) and $1,25\text{-}(OH)_2D_3$ (1.0 to 3.0 μg/day).

With optimal therapy normal growth rates are achieved and progressive deformity of the lower extremity is prevented.

3. The rare type of familial hypophosphatemic osteomalacia is also characterized by hypophosphatemia and reduced Tm_P/GFR. This form of the disease is inherited as an autosomal recessive trait. The patients present either in late childhood or adult life with osteomalacia without concomitant or antecedent rickets. Plasma $1,25\text{-}(OH)_2D_3$ and iPTH are both normal. Treatment with $1,25\text{-}(OH)_2D_3$ has been reported to be effective in this condition.

4. Vitamin D–dependent rickets type I is a disorder which presents as classic vitamin D–deficiency rickets with hypotonia, failure to thrive, tetany, convulsions, and radiological evidence of rickets. It is distinguishable from D–deficiency rickets because it is an inherited disease with autosomal recessive transmission which does not respond to usual therapeutic doses of vitamin D. In addition, plasma $25\text{-}(OH)D_3$ concentrations are normal, but $1,25\text{-}(OH)_2D_3$ concentrations are also low. The condition is thought to result from a specific defect in the renal 1-α-hydroxylase responsible for the synthesis of $1,25\text{-}(OH)_2D_3$ from $25\text{-}(OH)D_3$. The fact that in many patients given pharmacological doses of $25\text{-}(OH)D_3$ the plasma $1,25\text{-}(OH)_2D_3$ concentration increases into the normal range suggests that the dis-

ease is caused by an altered enzyme with a higher than normal K_m for the substrate, 25-(OH)D_3, rather than by a complete enzyme deficiency. Specific therapy consists of either large doses of vitamin D (5000 to 40,000 U/day) or small doses of 1,25-(OH)$_2$$D_3$ (1 to 3 μg/day).

5. *Vitamin D–dependent rickets type II is a rare form of inherited rickets in which most of the clinical, radiological, and biochemical findings are similar to those in the type I disease. The disorder also appears to be transmitted as an autosomal recessive trait. Alopecia is often seen in the type II but not in the type I disease. Biochemically, the major difference is that the plasma 1,25-(OH)$_2$$D_3$ concentration is high in patients with type II and low in those with the type I disease. The pathogenesis of the type II disease is not known. End organ resistance to 1,25-(OH)$_2$$D_3$ has been suggested, but an alternative possibility is a lack of some other active metabolite of the vitamin. There is no preferred therapy for the disorder.*

There are two clearly delineated forms of familial or inherited rickets: *hypophosphatemic* (vitamin D–resistant) and *vitamin D–dependency* (pseudo-vitamin D–deficient) *rickets*. These are distinguishable on the basis of their clinical manifestations, their radiologic, histologic, and chemical findings, their underlying pathogenesis, and their modes of inheritance.

In addition to these well-characterized syndromes there are two other recently described syndromes, one called *autosomal hypophosphatemic bone disease* which has some of but not all the features of familial hypophosphatemic rickets, and the other an X-linked condition which presents in adult life as osteomalacia, without prior evidence of rickets in childhood.

Familial hypophosphatemic (vitamin D–resistant) rickets is a specific disorder characterized by

1. Familial inheritance, nearly always due to a single-dose effect of an X-linked gene ("X-linked dominant")
2. Hypophosphatemia, associated with hyperphosphaturia and a decreased renal tubular reabsorption of inorganic phosphate
3. Usually normocalcemia with normal or only slightly elevated plasma parathyroid hormone concentrations
4. Diminished intestinal absorption of calcium and phosphate
5. Decreased growth rate and ultimately shortened stature
6. No known disorder of vitamin D metabolism
7. Rickets and osteomalacia, usually more marked in the lower extremities, that are not responsive to physiologic amounts of vitamin D_3 or D_2, 25-hydroxyvitamin D_3, or 1,25-dihydroxyvitamin D_3, and only partially responsive to combined phosphate and vitamin D therapy.

Vitamin D-dependency or pseudo-vitamin D–deficient rickets is a specific disorder characterized by

1. Inheritance as an autosomal recessive trait
2. Hypocalcemia, with normal, high, or low plasma phosphate concentration
3. Elevated plasma parathyroid hormone concentration
4. Diminished intestinal absorption of calcium and phosphate
5. Usually aminoaciduria

6. Rickets indistinguishable radiologically or histologically from ordinary vitamin D–deficiency rickets
7. A probable specific defect in vitamin D metabolism
8. A decreased responsiveness to both vitamin D and 25-hydroxyvitamin D_3 but probably a normal responsiveness to 1,25-dihydroxyvitamin D_3 (Fig. 79-1)
9. Complete restoration of bone structure, growth rate, and stature following adequate treatment with vitamin D or its metabolites.

HISTORICAL DEVELOPMENTS

Although rickets had been described in antiquity and its clinical manifestations clearly delineated in the seventeenth century, it was not until the second decade of this century that an association between vitamin D and rickets was established. With the work of Mellanby [1], Hess [2], McCollum et al. [3], Steenbock, [4, 5], Askew et al. [6], and Windaus et al. [7], the major cause of rickets in children and osteomalacia in adults was shown to be a deficiency of vitamin D (see Nicolaysen [8]). The only major natural source of this vitamin (vitamin D_3) in humans is its synthesis in the skin in response to an exposure to natural sunlight or artificial ultraviolet radiation. The discovery that certain plant sterols, ergosterols, which in themselves had little or no antirachitic activity, could be endowed with antirachitic potency following brief exposure to ultraviolet radiation led to the eventual isolation of vitamin D_2 and its application to the prevention of rickets and osteomalacia.

Within a few years after the discovery, isolation, and therapeutic use of vitamin D_2, vitamin D–deficiency rickets had largely been eliminated. A small number of rachitic individuals failed to respond in a normal fashion to usual doses of vitamin D. Albright et al. showed in 1937 [9] in one such patient that healing of rickets occurred following the administration of relatively massive doses of vitamin D_2, and they coined the term *vitamin D–resistant rickets* to characterize such individuals.

Christensen [10] first described the familial occurrence of this condition in a mother, her son, and her daughter. Initial genetic classification proposed an autosomal dominant mode of inheritance. However, both Winters et al. [11, 12] and Graham et al. [13] established that the most uniform hallmark of this condition was not rickets but hypophosphatemia and that in many kindreds there were members, particularly females, who had hypophosphatemia without skeletal deformity or rickets. When inheritance was analyzed with hypophosphatemia as the genetic marker, an X-linked inheritance was found with virtually complete generation-to-generation transmission of this abnormality. These studies revealed that a single X-linked gene was sufficient to confer all the usual manifestations of the disease in some affected females, thus strongly suggesting X-linked dominant inheritance.

The clarification of the pattern of inheritance and the emphasis on the biochemical abnormality of hypophosphatemia led to a reconsideration of the possible nature of the underlying defect. As early as 1942, Robertson et al. [14] emphasized that in vitamin D–resistant individuals there was either a primary or secondary decrease in renal tubular phosphate reabsorption, and all later studies have shown this to be a characteristic feature of the disease. On the basis of this type of evidence several groups of workers concluded that the pri-

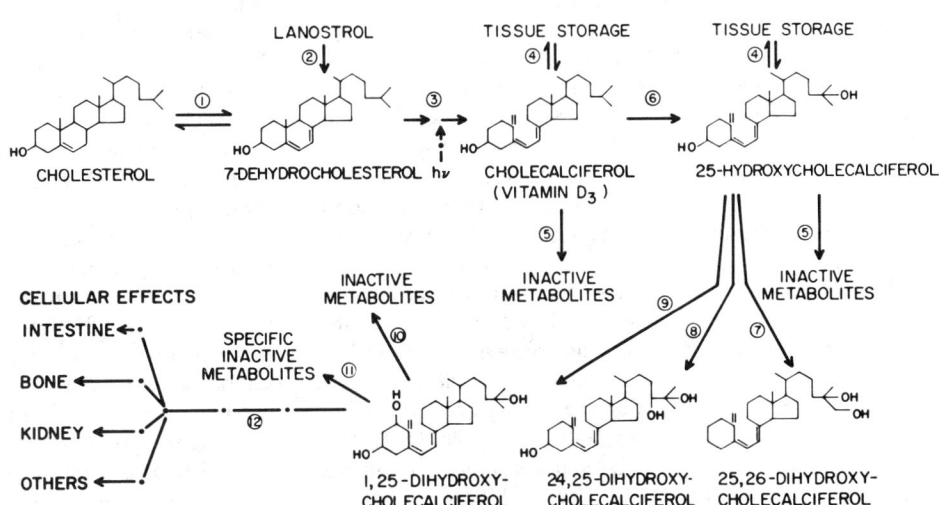

Figure 79-1 The metabolism of vitamin D₃. The immediate precursor of vitamin D₃ is 7-dehydrocholesterol. It is formed either from cholesterol ① or lanosterol ② . Upon exposure to sunlight in the skin, 7-dehydrocholesterol is converted ③ to cholecalciferol (vitamin D₃). Vitamin D₃ is either stored in tissues ④ , converted to inactive metabolites ⑤ , or converted by a hepatic microsomal hydroxylase ⑥ to 25-hydroxycholecalciferol that is either stored ④ , inactivated ⑤ , or converted to one of several metabolites in the kidney ⑧ and ⑨ or elsewhere ⑦ . The major biologically active metabolite is 1,25-dihydroxycholecalciferol that is converted to inactive metabolites ⑩ and ⑪ and that acts on a variety of organs to bring about its biologic effects ⑫

mary defect is a specific phosphate transport defect in the proximal renal tubule, leading to phosphaturia and hypophosphatemia in all individuals and to rickets, osteomalacia, and short stature in some. A proposed alternative theory of pathogenesis was a defect in vitamin D metabolism [15], but evidence does not favor this view.

In spite of advances in our knowledge of calcium and phosphate metabolism, the availability of new techniques for studying these clinical disorders, and the discovery and elucidation of the metabolism of vitamin D and its ionic and hormonal regulation, a number of questions remain. These include:

1. The cause of the phosphaturia, i.e., whether it is an intrinsic renal tubular defect or secondary to the elaboration of some humoral factor

2. A full explanation of the failure of growth in affected children

3. Whether there is any abnormality in the metabolism of vitamin D

4. The role of parathyroid hormone in the pathogenesis of the increased renal phosphate clearance and hypophosphatemia

5. The reason for the lack of correlation between the degree of hypophosphatemia and the appearance and severity of rickets.

As familial hypophosphatemic rickets became more clearly delineated, both genetically and biochemically, a small number of subjects became distinguishable from this general population. The major features of these patients were:

1. A good therapeutic response to 50,000 to 150,000 units vitamin D, in contrast to the limited response of the usual vitamin D–resistant patient to similar doses of vitamin D

2. An autosomal recessive mode of inheritance

3. The possible identification of a specific defect in vitamin D metabolism to account for the pathogenesis of this state.

Fraser and Salter [16] were first to recognize this form of rickets as independent of vitamin D–resistant rickets. The syndrome has been more fully described by Prader et al. [17], as "pseudodeficiency rickets," and by Dent [18] and others [19–21]. In all of its manifestations it is indistinguishable from ordinary vitamin D–deficiency rickets, the only differences being

the requirement for 100 to 1000 times the normal daily dose of vitamin D to effect a cure of the rachitic state.

Most recently Scriver et al. [22] have described an inherited disorder of phosphate homeostasis with osteomalacia without striking rickets, a reduced Tm_P/GFR but normal percent TRP, hypophosphatemia, slightly reduced growth rate, an autosomal dominant mode of inheritance, and a positive therapeutic response to 1,25-$(OH)_2D_3$. Simultaneously, Frymoyer and Hodgkin [23] have described a family with an X-linked disorder characterized by hypophosphatemia and adult onset osteomalacia without prior evidence of rickets. Likewise, a second variety of pseudodeficiency or vitamin D–dependent rickets has recently been identified and will be discussed below.

HORMONAL CONTROL OF CALCIUM AND PHOSPHATE METABOLISM

The major recognized hormonal factors concerned with calcium and phosphate homeostasis are parathyroid hormone (PTH), calcitonin, and vitamin D and its active metabolites (see [24] for more detailed discussion). In this summary we will not discuss the role of calcitonin, because there is no known relationship between this hormone and hypophosphatemic or vitamin D–dependent rickets. However, the metabolism and mode of action of vitamin D, the factors regulating this metabolic pathway, and the metabolism and mode of action of parathyroid hormone are directly related to the pathogenesis and treatment of both forms of rickets.

Vitamin D Metabolism

There are two major sources of vitamin D in the human [25]: the diet and the skin (Fig. 79-1). Nearly all the dietary vitamin D is vitamin D₂, irradiated ergosterol, which is added as a supplement during food processing. The vitamin made in the skin, vitamin D₃, is derived from the photochemical conversion of 7-dehydrocholesterol (Fig. 65-1). This conversion is catalyzed by ultraviolet light of a very specific wavelength

(2967 Å). The subsequent metabolic conversions of vitamins D_2 and D_3 are identical, as far as is known, so that only the pathway of vitamin D_3 metabolism will be discussed.

Once formed, vitamin D_3 is either stored in blood plasma, muscle, or adipose tissue or undergoes conversions by hepatic microsomal enzyme [26] to 25-hydroxy vitamin D_3 [25-$(OH)D_3$] (see Fig. 79-1). 25-$(OH)D_3$ exerts feedback control of its own synthesis but this may not be of great physiologic significance, because the 25-$(OH)D_3$ concentration in blood plasma rises as the intake of vitamin D or the exposure to sunlight is increased [27, 28].

Like vitamin D_3, 25-$(OH)D_3$ is stored in plasma, adipose tissue, and muscle. Both vitamin D and its 25-hydroxy metabolite appear to represent storage or precursor forms of the active vitamin. Once formed, 25-$(OH)D_3$ is either stored or converted to one of three major metabolites [29–37]: 1,25-$(OH)_2D_3$, 24,25-$(OH)_2D_3$, or 25,26-$(OH)_2D_3$ (Fig. 65-1). The site of synthesis of 1,25-$(OH)_2D_3$ appears to be solely in the kidney mitochondria. The site of 25,26-$(OH)_2D_3$ synthesis is not established, and 24,25-$(OH)_2D_3$ is made in both renal and extrarenal sites.

Most attention has been paid to the renal synthesis of 1,25-$(OH)_2D_3$ [29–48], because this compound appears to be the most biologically active form of vitamin D_3. The evidence that 1,25-$(OH)_2D_3$ is the active metabolite of vitamin D_3 is:

1. 1,25-$(OH)_2D_3$ is the major metabolite found in the intestinal mucosa (a major site of vitamin D action)
2. A smaller dose of this metabolite will induce an increase in intestinal calcium transport more rapidly than either 25-$(OH)D_3$ or vitamin D_3
3. This metabolite will induce an increase in calcium transport in nephrectomized animals, but physiologic doses of vitamin D_3 or 25-$(OH)D_3$ will not
4. There is a highly specific 1,25-$(OH)_2D_3$–binding protein in intestinal mucosal cells
5. When animals are fed either 25-$(OH)D_3$ or vitamin D_3 and then adapted to a high calcium diet, intestinal calcium transport decreases, but if fed 1,25-$(OH)_2D_3$ and then fed a high calcium diet, no adaptative change in calcium transport is seen.

1,25-$(OH)_2D_3$ is the major intestinal metabolite of D_3 [34, 35], but whether it accounts for all the biologic effects of vitamin D on other organs, particularly on bone [35, 49], is not certain.

The most striking facts about 1,25-$(OH)_2D_3$ are its rapid turnover and low plasma concentration. The plasma concentration of 1,25-$(OH)_2D_3$ is approximately one three-hundredth that of 25-$(OH)D_3$. It acts within a few hours, and its effects are over in 24 to 48 h [37].

Control of Renal 1-Hydroxylase

Considerable attention has been devoted to the factors that regulate the renal synthesis of 1,25-$(OH)_2D_3$ (Fig.79-1). Control appears to be achieved both by short-term control of the activity of the enzyme present and by longer-term regulation of total enzyme content [37-48]. The major factors that regulate the renal mitochondrial 1-hydroxylase *in situ* in experimental animals are the plasma Ca^{2+}, HPO_4^{2-}, PTH, and 1,25-$(OH)_2D_3$ concentrations. It is assumed but not yet established

that similar factors regulate 1-hydroxylase activity in human beings.

Under most circumstances parathyroid hormone stimulates 1,25-$(OH)_2D_3$ synthesis [39, 41], but, under some conditions inhibition of synthesis has been reported [40]. This difference can be explained by the fact that low-to-moderate concentrations activate the enzyme, whereas high concentrations inhibit its activity [43, 44, 47]. Perhaps the most impressive evidence for the role of PTH in regulating 1,25-$(OH)_2D_3$ synthesis is the fact [50] that the plasma concentration of 1,25-$(OH)_2D_3$ is high in many patients with hyperparathyroidism and low in those with hypoparathyroidism. However, the relationship is not a simple one. Broadus et al. [51] found that approximately 65 percent of patients with proven primary hyperparathyroidism had elevated plasma 1,25-$(OH)_2D$ concentrations, but the remainder had normal values. There was no obvious biochemical difference between the two types in terms of iPTH, serum phosphate or calcium, or nephrogenous cyclic AMP (cAMP). Thus, although an increase in PTH can increase plasma 1,25-$(OH)_2D_3$ concentration, this does not always occur. The other factors determining this PTH-mediated response are not known.

The other major factor controlling 1,25-$(OH)_2D_3$ synthesis is the plasma HPO_4 concentration [43]. The rate of 1,25-$(OH)_2D_3$ synthesis increases in the severely phosphate-depleted rat. Under these circumstances plasma PTH tends to be low, so that the effect of phosphate cannot be accounted for by an indirect effect on PTH secretion. The studies in vitro with chick renal tubules do not lead to the same type of conclusion [44, 45], but this is not surprising. What is more difficult to reconcile with the concept of hypophosphatemia being a physiologic stimulator of 1,25-$(OH)_2D_3$ synthesis is the fact that children with X-linked hypophosphatemic rickets do not have increased intestinal calcium transport [32] and do not have increased amounts of 1,25-$(OH)_2D_3$ in plasma in spite of persistent hypophosphatemia. There are many possible reasons why this human syndrome and the phosphate-depleted rat are not comparable. More work is needed to define the physiologic significance of phosphate control of 1-hydroxylase in human beings. Even so, of adult human subjects presenting with acquired hypophosphatemic syndromes, only some have high 1,25-$(OH)_2D_3$ levels. Again, as in the case of primary hyperparathyroidism, the reason for this lack of uniformity is not known.

Control of Other Steps in Vitamin D Metabolism

As already mentioned, 24,25-$(OH)_2D_3$ is made in kidney and elsewhere. Under experimental circumstances, its rate of synthesis often increases when that of 1,25-$(OH)_2D_3$ decreases [33, 38]. The physiologic role of 24,25-$(OH)_2D_3$ has not been defined. Hence, the significance of this reciprocity of control is not known. Likewise, little is known of the rate, site, or control of 25,26-$(OH)_2D_3$ synthesis, its potential physiologic role, or its further metabolism. These are problems that deserve further attention.

Many pharmacologic agents can profoundly affect vitamin D metabolism. The most general are drugs that induce an increase in the activity of the nonspecific hepatic microsomal hydroxylases. In particular, diphenylhydantoin (Dilantin) and phenobarbital induce these enzymes and cause an increase in the rate of catabolism of vitamin D_3 sufficient to deplete vitamin D stores in the body, with the development of "vitamin D deficiency" [27, 28, 52-55]. Such patients respond to small doses of 25-(OH)D_3. This state has become widely recognized in patients on long-term anticonvulsant therapy and can be minimized by increasing vitamin D intake.

Relationship of PTH and Vitamin D in Calcium and Phosphate Homeostasis

These new discoveries have greatly enhanced our understanding of one of the most important endocrine relationships in the field of calcium and phosphate physiology: the relationship between PTH and vitamin D [23]. Although it has long been known [56] that PTH increases intestinal calcium transport, a direct action of this hormone upon intestinal calcium transport has never been demonstrated [23]. It now seems clear that the fall in intestinal calcium transport in hypoparathyroidism and the rise seen in hyperparathyroidism are due to a PTH-regulated change in the renal synthesis of 1,25-(OH)$_2$D$_3$. In addition, 1,25-(OH)$_2$D$_3$ sensitizes bone to the action of PTH. Thus, the kidney is an endocrine organ of major importance. The renal synthesis of 1,25-(OH)$_2$D$_3$ is a major determinant of bone turnover and of intestinal calcium absorption. Hence the balance of the effects of PTH upon renal tubular calcium and phosphate transport, on the one hand, and upon 1,25-(OH)$_2$D$_3$ synthesis, on the other, determines how the functions of bone, gut, and kidney are integrated to maintain calcium and phosphate homeostasis. These interrelationships can be most easily grasped by considering the respective changes in parathyroid hormone secretion and 1,25-(OH)$_2$D$_3$ synthesis that take place in calcium or phosphate deficiency.

In the presence of normal amounts of vitamin D and 25-(OH)D_3 in the body, a deficiency of dietary calcium leads to a tendency for plasma calcium concentration to fall which is, in turn, a major stimulus for an increase in PTH secretion. The rise in PTH activity leads to an increased distal renal tubular reabsorption of calcium and an increase in renal synthesis of 1,25-(OH)$_2$D$_3$. The rise in 1,25-(OH)$_2$D$_3$ and the rise in PTH act in concert to increase the mobilization of calcium and phosphate from bone. In addition, PTH blocks the proximal tubular reabsorption of phosphate, and the increased 1,25-(OH)$_2$D$_3$ increases intestinal phosphate absorption. Thus, renal phosphate excretion increases. If there is any calcium in the diet, intestinal calcium absorption also increases. Hence, in calcium deficiency the organism adjusts by a renal retention of calcium, a mobilization of calcium from bone mineral, and the renal excretion of the associated phosphate. Long-standing calcium deficiency leads to osteoporosis and growth failure but usually not to rickets or osteomalacia.

By contrast, phosphate deficiency leads to a tendency toward hypercalcemia, low plasma PTH, and decreased distal tubular reabsorption of calcium. Low plasma phosphate also stimulates the synthesis of 1,25-(OH)$_2$D$_3$. The increase in 1,25-(OH)$_2$D$_3$ leads to an increase in the intestinal absorption of calcium and an increase in bone resorption in spite of reduced PTH levels. In addition, low plasma phosphate may enhance intestinal calcium absorption and bone resorption by direct cellular effects independent of its effects upon vitamin D metabolism [57]. The consequences of these physiologic changes are renal retention of phosphate, enhanced absorption of phosphate if any is present in the diet, and enhanced mobilization of phosphate from bone mineral with the simultaneous renal clearance of the calcium mobilized from intestine or bone. In addition, phosphate deficiency, when severe, leads to a delay in the normal process of bone mineralization, so that phosphate deficiency per se, even in the presence of adequate vitamin D stores, can lead to rickets or osteomalacia. This fact is particularly relevant to any discussion of the pathogenesis of hypophosphatemic rickets in humans (see "Pathogenesis" later in this chapter).

VITAMIN D METABOLITES IN THE PATHOGENESIS OF RICKETS AND OSTEOMALACIA

With the discovery that 1,25-(OH)$_2$D$_3$ is the active metabolite of vitamin D that regulates intestinal calcium and phosphate transport, and enhances bone resorption when added directly to bone grown in organ culture, the conclusion was reached that 1,25-(OH)$_2$D$_3$ is *the* active metabolite of vitamin D. One of the predictions resulting from this conclusion is that in simple vitamin D deficiency a fall in the plasma concentration of 1,25-(OH)$_2$D$_3$ should occur. However, when methods were developed for the measurement of plasma 1,25-(OH)$_2$D$_3$, it was found to be normal or elevated in patients with simple D-deficiency [58], in those with anticonvulsant drug-induced osteomalacia [59], and in several other syndromes characterized by the appearance of osteomalacia [60, 61]. In all these patients the plasma concentrations of both 25-(OH)D_3 and 24,25-(OH)$_2$D$_3$ were reduced, and a correlation between low 24,25-(OH)$_2$D$_3$ and bone disease was reported [62, 63]. Conversely, Rasmussen et al. [61] have described a patient with pseudohypoparathyroidism with undetectable levels of 1,25-(OH)$_2$D$_3$ who had normal concentrations of calcium and phosphate in her serum and no histological or radiological evidence of osteomalacia.

This problem has been approached in another way. Bordier et al. [64] reported that human adults with vitamin D–deficiency osteomalacia do not respond to a dose of 0.5 to 1.5 mg/day of 1,25-(OH)$_2$D$_3$ with a healing of their bone disease, even though this dose of 1,25-(OH)$_2$D$_3$ given simultaneously with 5 to 10 μg/day of 24,25(OH)$_2$D$_3$ does result in healing of the bone lesions. Nagant de-Deuxchaisres et al. [65], however, report that the long-term administration of similar doses of 1,25-(OH)$_2$D$_3$ did result in healing of the osteomalacia. There is no ready explanation at present for this difference. Nonetheless, other studies in humans suggest that 24,25-(OH)$_2$D$_3$ has an action qualitatively different than that of 1,25-(OH)$_2$D$_3$. This conclusion is supported by studies of the actions of these metabolites on bone in vivo and in vitro [66–69]. In the absence of any of the D metabolites or of PTH, little calcification of chick limb bud rudiments occurs in vitro. A combination of 1,25-(OH)$_2$D$_3$ plus 24,25-(OH)$_2$D$_3$, but neither alone, promotes calcification to a small extent. If combined with a small dose of PTH which by itself has only a small effect, the two metabolites together have a marked stimulatory effect on bone mineralization [69]. These results are similar to those reported by Bordier et al. [64] in their human studies and suggest that each metabolite has a unique function in regulating bone metabolism. It seems relatively clear that the major effect of 1,25-(OH)$_2$D$_3$ is to increase both osteoclastic and osteocytic osteolysis. Less clear is the effect of 24, 25-(OH)$_2$D$_3$. It appears to act on osteoblasts and possibly osteoid osteocytes to regulate the mineralization process. It is also clear that some metabolite of vitamin D promotes osteoblastic maturation and function, but which metabolite is not known. A particularly interesting clue comes from the studies of Nguyen et al. [63]. They found that plasma 24, 25-(OH)$_2$D$_3$ concentrations were low in patients with D deficiency and rose to values five times normal after initiation of D therapy, then fell gradually as the bone disease healed. Of even greater interest was their study of a child with vitamin D–dependency rickets treated with 1-α-(OH)D$_3$. This disease is thought to result from a specific defect in the renal 25-(OH)D$_3$1-α-hydroxylase, so that 1, 25-(OH)$_2$D$_3$ production is decreased. Although the plasma 24, 25-(OH)$_2$D$_3$ was normal before therapy, it rose dramatically to values 10 times normal and then gradually declined over a period of months while the 1-α-(OH)D$_3$ therapy was continued at a constant dose. The fall in 24, 25-(OH)$_2$D$_3$ concentration paralleled the fall in plasma alkaline phosphatase. These results suggest that the regulation of 24, 25-(OH)$_2$D$_3$ concentration is complex and that this metabolite has an important role in regulating bone formation or mineralization.

Considerably more work is needed before all these facts are fitted into a satisfactory description of the respective roles of the various D metabolites in normal human physiology. It is clear, nonetheless, that 1, 25-(OH)$_2$D$_3$ deficiency per se does not necessarily lead to osteomalacia and, conversely, that rickets or osteomalacia can occur even in the face of normal or even elevated plasma concentrations of 1, 25-(OH)$_2$D$_3$.

ANIMAL MODELS OF THE HUMAN DISEASE

Hypophosphatemic (*Hyp*) Mouse

Discovery and Genetics The discovery and general characteristics of the hypophosphatemic mouse are described by Eicher [70]. In 1966 male mice with shortened trunk and hind limbs were noted in a linkage experiment at the Jackson Laboratory. Low serum phosphate concentrations were observed in the affected mice, and the mutation was named *hypophosphatemia*, with the gene symbol *Hyp*. The mutant *Hyp* allele was transferred to the C57BL/6J inbred strain by repeated matings of *Hyp*/+ females to C57BL/6J+/Y males. This new mutation is dominant and X-linked. Linkage studies place *Hyp* at the distal end of the mouse X chromosome [70]. The disorder in the *Hyp* mouse appears to be similar to X-linked hypophosphatemic rickets in humans. Because both diseases are inherited as X-linked dominants, the human and mouse diseases are probably caused by mutations affecting the homologous gene.

General Phenotype The *Hyp*/+ and *Hyp*/Y mice can be differentiated from their normal littermates at 21 days of age by their shortened hind limbs and tail [70]. The reduced body size persists throughout life. Kyphosis of the thoracic vertebrae, prominent bowing of the femur, and rachitic rosary develop with age in the affected mice. the skeletal abnormalities are more severe in the male than in the female. The mutant mice appear to live a normal life span. The *Hyp*/+ females are

fertile and raise their young. Some *Hyp*/Y males have impaired ability to sire offspring, and those that are able may sire only one or two litters.

Growth as measured by body weight is reduced in the *Hyp* mouse. The body weight of the *Hyp* male as compared with normal male sibs is significantly reduced by 8 days of age, while that of the *Hyp* female as compared with normal female sibs is not significantly reduced until 22 days of age. Thus a single dose of the + allele in the *Hyp*/+ females appears to preserve normal growth up to 22 days of age. A normal sexual dimorphism of body weight between normal female and male mice is observed at 36 days of age, but this dimorphism is not observed in the *Hyp* females and males.

The plasma inorganic phosphate concentrations are lower than normal in both male and female *Hyp* mice by 20 to 49 days of age and remain lower up to and beyond 400 days of age [70,71]. The plasma calcium is slightly but significantly lower, while the plasma alkaline phosphatase is markedly elevated in *Hyp* mice as compared with their normal counterparts [70,72]. The urinary clearance of inorganic phosphate is elevated in *Hyp* mice under various conditions of dietary calcium and phosphorus intake. There are no abnormalities in total or inorganic phosphate content of skeletal muscle [72]. Serum parathyroid hormone levels are not elevated in untreated *Hyp* mice, and there is no histologic evidence of parathyroid gland hyperplasia. The urinary excretion of glucose and amino acids is not increased.

The X-linked mutant genes are associated with hypophosphatemic bone disease in the mouse and humans and are likely to be evolutionary homologues. The phenotypes of the two are similar in time of appearance after birth including the presence of hypophosphatemia without striking hypocalcemia, the high urinary clearance of phosphate, and dwarfism. Hyperparathyroidism is absent in both in the untreated state. Because of the genotypic and phenotypic similarities to X-linked hypophosphatemic rickets in humans, the *Hyp* mouse is a valuable model for elucidation of the basic defect in this disorder. Limited studies to date have been carried out in an effort to characterize the defect in phosphate transport, the abnormalities in bone, possible disturbances in vitamin D metabolism, and the efficacy of therapeutic regimens.

Renal Transport of Phosphate The urinary phosphate excretion of phosphate when expressed as the coefficient of creatinine excretion is similar in *Hyp* mice and normal male sibs [70], but when related to plasma phosphate, is significantly increased. The fractional and absolute tubular reabsorption of phosphate are both decreased in *Hyp* mice [70, 73]. The fractional excretion of phosphate at endogenous plasma phosphate concentrations is 0.20±0.09 (mean ± SEM) in normal mice and 0.35 ± 0.08 in *Hyp* mice [70]. These values are similar to the fractional excretion of phosphate in normal and X-linked hypophosphatemic human subjects, respectively. Micropuncture studies suggest that the defect in phosphate transport in *Hyp* mice is located in the proximal tubule [73, 74]. Sites more distal may also be involved since fractional delivery to the bladder is greater than can be accounted for by failure of reabsorption in the proximal tubule [73].

Studies of renal cortical slices reveal no significant difference in tissue content of phosphate or in the labeling of organic and inorganic phosphate pools in *Hyp* mice and controls [70, 75]. Moreover, there is no significant difference in the net uptake or in the efflux of inorganic phosphate by slices of renal cortex. It is thought that the slice preparation primarily exposes the basolateral membrane of epithelium to the medium. Therefore, these observations indicate that the flux of phosphate across the basolateral membrane is not abnormal in the *Hyp* mouse and that uptake from the peritubular phosphate pool maintains the intracellular pool in the mutant. The results suggest that the defect in the *Hyp* phenotype is not expressed in the basolateral membrane of renal epithelium.

Studies of purified kidney brush border membrane vesicles reveal a specific defect of phosphate transport in the *Hyp* kidney [75–78]. The defect in phosphate transport appears to be limited to the sodium-dependent, arsenate-inhibitable component of phosphate transport. The sodium-independent, nonsaturable mode of transport appears to be intact. The apparent K_m for phosphate cotransport is normal while the U_{max} is approximately half-normal [78]. These observations are in keeping with the partial loss of a saturable component of phosphate transport in X-linked hypophosphatemic humans. The selective localization of the defect to the brush border membrane is consistent with impaired transepithelial transport and diminished net reabsorption in vivo since net flux across the brush border membrane is the primary determinant of net reabsorption. Dennis et al. [79] have described two separate transport systems for phosphate in the mammalian kidney. The defect in the brush border membrane transport of phosphate in the *Hyp* mouse is consistent with an abnormality in one of the transport systems, presumably that controlled by the X-linked gene.

Studies in the *Hyp* mouse [71, 80] demonstrated renal adaptation to phosphorus deprivation in both *Hyp* mice and normal sibs, but the adaptation did not fully correct the mutant phenotype. In the adapted state the *Hyp* mice maintained lower plasma levels and higher urinary excretion of phosphate than their normal sibs. The renal cortex content of phosphate and the net radioisotopic uptake of phosphate by renal cortical slices were not significantly different in the basal state in *Hyp* mice and normal sibs, and no significant changes were observed in either group under conditions of phosphate deprivation. In purified brush border membrane vesicles, on the other hand, the sodium-dependent uptake of phosphate increased by 200 percent in both *Hyp* mice and normal sibs during phosphate deprivation. As indicated earlier, the loss of phosphate transport activity in the *Hyp* mouse is only partial; approximately one-half of the sodium-dependent transport activity is retained in the brush border membranes. The ability of the *Hyp* mouse to adapt to phosphate deprivation suggests that the gene product controlled by the *Hyp* locus does not control the adaptive process [71, 80]. It follows that another membrane component in brush border vesicles is involved in the adaptive response.

Cogwell et al. [73] observed that thyroparathyroidectomy in *Hyp* mice induced a marked decrease in fractional phosphate excretion to identical levels in mutants and controls. The fractional reabsorption in the proximal tubule was enhanced to a greater extent in the thyroparathyroidectomized mutant mice, indicating that parathyroid hormone was necessary for the expression of the reabsorptive defect of the intact mutants. In an effort to determine whether phosphate wasting was the result of an intrinsic tubular defect that was masked by thyroparathyroidectomy, they increased the glomerular fluid phosphate concentration by phosphate infusion in the thyroparathyroidectomized mutants to levels approaching those of the control mice. The fractional phosphate excretion rose markedly with phosphate infusions to values significantly greater than those in noninfused intact mutants. These studies demonstrate the defect in tubular phosphate transport in the absence of parathyroid hormone. The normal tubular response to thyroparathyroidectomy in mutant mice suggests that the physiological action of parathyroid hormone is qualitatively normal in these mice even though the base line level of phosphate reabsorption is abnormally low. Thus, although the defect in phosphate transport is independent of parathyroid hormone, the expression of the defect appears to be influenced by the level of circulating PTH.

The total and fractional excretions of urinary cAMP and cGMP are increased in the *Hyp* mouse in the presence of normal circulating levels of parathyroid hormone [75, 81]. By contrast the urinary excretion of cAMP in human patients with X-linked hypophosphatemic rickets is not increased [82]. Utilizing the technique of nephron microdissection, Brunette et al. [83] showed that the response of adenylate cyclase in *Hyp* mice to parathyroid hormone was decreased in the proximal tubule, while the response to calcitonin was increased in the distal tubule. The apparent K_m for cyclase activation was similar in normal and mutant mice. The physiologic significance of these observations is uncertain.

Gastrointestinal Transport of Phosphate Results of studies of intestinal transport of phosphate in the *Hyp* mouse are at variance. The intestinal transport of phosphate, as studied in isolated jejunal loops [84] and everted gut sacs [85], was reported to be depressed in *Hyp* mice. More recently Tenenhouse et al. [78] observed that the sodium-dependent phosphate transport by intestinal brush border membrane vesicles was not reduced in *Hyp* mice. Moreover, these investigators were unable to demonstrate reduced transport of phosphate in *Hyp* mice by the everted gut sac technique. Contrary to earlier reports, they concluded that the *Hyp* intestine has no apparent defect in phosphate transport. Thus, as in the case of human X-linked hypophosphatemic rickets, the presence or absence of a defect in the intestinal transport of phosphate in *Hyp* mice remains controversial.

Vitamin D Metabolites There is limited information concerning the levels of circulating vitamin D metabolites in the *Hyp* mouse. Normal serum levels of 1, 25-$(OH)_2$D have been observed in the *Hyp* mouse [81, 86, 87], while serum 25-(OH)D levels have variously been reported as normal [87] and depressed [86, 87]. The normal, rather than elevated, circulating 1, 25-$(OH)_2$D levels in the presence of hypophosphatemia suggest that the renal 25-hydroxy vitamin D–1-α-hydroxylase system is defective in the *Hyp* mouse. This is consistent with the finding that, in contrast to normal littermates, *Hyp* mice do not demonstrate an increase in circulating 1, 25-$(OH)_2$D when the serum phosphate concentration is reduced by being fed a low phosphorus diet [86].

Bone Morphology Bone structure is markedly altered in *Hyp* mice. Bone growth failure and defective epiphyseal calcification are reflected in a shorter-than-normal vertebral length associated with a wide epiphyseal growth plate [72]. Microradiography reveals reduced bone density and enlarged osteocyte lacunas. Histological studies of the femur demonstrate reduced mineralization, wide osteoid borders, and wide epiphyseal plates [88]. On stained sections plump osteoblasts line the endosteal and soft tissue spaces of bone of normal mice, whereas in hypophosphatemic animals the osteoblasts are flattened and fibroblastic in appearance. Sections through the knee joint of *Hyp* mice show an abnormal pattern of trabecular bone and irregular areas of unmineralized cartilage; the cartilage of the epiphyseal plate is distorted, and large areas of hypertrophic cells are present in the epiphyses and diaphysis [72].

Histomorphometry reveals impaired endosteal bone mineralization as shown by excessive osteoid surface and thickness and by decreased extent of the mineralization front [88]. Abnormal endochondral calcification is reflected in a wide epiphyseal growth plate. The femur ash weight is less than 50 percent of normal, but the ash has a normal calcium-to-phosphate ratio [72]. The percentage of sodium and potassium is high while that of magnesium is low in bone ash of *Hyp* mice. Bone collagen cross links are quantitatively normal [89].

Magnesium   The *Hyp* mouse has a slight but significantly elevated serum magnesium concentration, increased urinary magnesium excretion, and reduced bone magnesium content [72, 88]. By contrast serum magnesium levels have not been elevated in human X-linked hypophosphatemic rickets [90, 91]. The reason for the abnormalities in serum and urine magnesium is uncertain, but they may be secondary to the deranged phosphate homeostasis in the *Hyp* mouse since correction of serum and urinary magnesium can be achieved by phosphate supplementation [81].

Effects of Treatment   There are scattered reports of treatment of *Hyp* mice with phosphate and vitamin D and vitamin D metabolites [70, 78, 84, 85, 88]. The relative efficacy of the reported regimens is difficult to assess because they were carried out in different laboratories and evaluations varied.

Phosphate supplementation in *Hyp* mice from 3 weeks of age until the time of sacrifice at 14 to 21 weeks of age [70, 88] resulted in an increase in urinary phosphate and a fall in serum calcium while the serum phosphate and urinary cAMP remained unchanged. The serum alkaline phosphatase fell but remained above normal. The elevated serum and urinary magnesium returned to normal while the magnesium content in bone remained depressed.

Phosphate treatment improved but did not normalize growth or the abnormalities in bone. The hind limbs and vertebrae increased in length, and spinal kyphosis did not appear. Histomorphologic studies demonstrated that phosphate treatment corrected endochondral calcification, as reflected in the normalization of the growth plate thickness and of epiphyseal and metaphyseal calcification. On the other hand, endosteal bone mineralization remained abnormal. Osteoblastic and osteoclastic recruitment and activity were increased, probably secondary to increased parathyroid hormone secretion induced by phosphate treatment in *Hyp* mice [75]. These results are in accord with studies in human X-linked hypophosphatemic rickets where phosphate treatment also heals the epiphyseal but not the endosteal defect in bone mineralization [92].

There is a paucity of information regarding the effects of vitamin D metabolites on bone in *Hyp* mice. The administration of 1-α-(OH)D_3 and 1, 25-(OH)$_2D_3$ over a 6-week period reduced tibial head width, improved epiphyseal plate distortions, straightened cartilage cell columns, and increased remodeling of trabecular bone [84]. 1, 25-(OH)$_2$D had no effect on serum calcium and phosphate levels, while 1-α-(OH)D normalized serum phosphate levels and increased serum calcium to above normal.

Results of studies of vitamin D metabolites on renal handling of phosphate in *Hyp* mice are at variance. One group reported that both 1-α-(OH)D_3 and 1, 25-(OH)$_2D_3$ decreased the urinary phosphate excretion index in *Hyp* as well as normal controls [84]. By contrast, no change was observed in either the fractional excretion of phosphate or the sodium-dependent phosphate transport by kidney brush border membranes in either *Hyp* or control mice when treated with 1, 25-(OH)$_2D_3$ at a dose sufficient to increase serum calcium and phosphate levels [78].

As mentioned earlier, the intestinal transport of phosphate has variously been reported as depressed [84, 85] and normal [78] in the *Hyp* mouse. The observations of the effect of 1, 25-(OH)$_2$D on intestinal phosphate transport in *Hyp* mice are equally controversial. 1, 25-(OH)$_2D_3$ stimulated intestinal phosphate transport in the study in which basal transport was normal [78] but not in the study in which it was depressed [84]. In the latter study 1-α-(OH)D reportedly increased both the serum phosphate level and intestinal phosphate transport while treatment with 1, 25-(OH)$_2$D had no effect on either. It was hypothesized that the intestinal phosphate transport system was not genetically deleted in the *Hyp* mouse but instead was able to respond to 1-α-(OH)D but not 1, 25-(OH)$_2$D. Further studies are needed to clarify the disparate results regarding intestinal phosphate transport in *Hyp* mice.

FAMILIAL HYPOPHOSPHATEMIC (VITAMIN D–RESISTANT) RICKETS

Clinical and Radiologic Findings

The most common clinical manifestation is short stature with or without rickets in childhood and osteomalacia in adult life [93]. Striking negative findings are the lack of muscle weakness, tetany, and convulsions which are such common features of both deficiency and pseudodeficiency rickets (Table 79-1).

The mildest abnormality is purely biochemical: hypophosphatemia [11-13, 94]. This may be present at birth, or it may not develop until the age 6 to 12 months [93]. Positive diagnosis cannot be made prenatally or even in the neonatal period in all cases. As long as plasma phosphate concentration is normal, growth rate and skeletal development are usually normal.

When hypophosphatemia appears, skeletal growth decreases, and there is often some retardation of bone age [93]. In affected children who develop rickets, the disease is usually first recognized when the child begins to walk, but if children in a known kindred are followed from birth, x-ray examination may reveal skeletal abnormalities of mild rickets during the first year of life, and within months after the fall in plasma phosphate concentration. These changes in the skeleton are usually associated with a rise in plasma alkaline phosphatase activity, a biochemical marker of active rickets.

Other early manifestations of the disease are late dentition, deformities of the skull, and "sitting" deformities of the legs. Rachitic rosary, deformity of the upper extremities, and active rickets (by x-ray) of spine and pelvis occur less frequently, in contrast to their frequent occurrence in both vitamin D–deficiency and vitamin D–dependency rickets [95–99] The other striking differences are that children with hypophosphatemic rickets usually have normal muscle tone and strength and do

Table 79-1 Comparison of clinical and biochemical changes in childhood rickets and osteomalacia

Type	Clinical and radiologic abnormalities	Concentration in plasma							Concentration in urine		
		Calcium	Phosphate	Alkaline phosphatase	25-(OH)D₃	1,25-(OH)₂D₃	24,25-(OH)₂D₃	iPTH	Calcium	cAMP	HOP
Vitamin D–deficient	Short stature, hypotonia, tetany or convulsions, active rickets	↓	↓ or N	↑	↓	↑, N or ↓	↓	↑	↓	↑	↑
Vitamin D–dependent, type I	Same	↓	↓ or N	↑	N	↓	↓	↑	↓	↑	↑
Type II	Same	↓	↓ or N	↑	N or ↓	↑↑	↓	↑	↓	↑	↑
Familial hypophosphatemic rickets	Short stature, normal muscle tone but fatigability, no tetany or convulsions, active rickets	N	↓	↑	N	↓	↓	N	↓	N	↑
Hypophosphatemic osteomalacia	Bowing, short stature, but no rickets	N	↓	↑	N	N	?	N	↓	N	?

not have tetany or seizures, as may occur in the other two forms of rickets.

As development proceeds in severely affected patients, they may show abnormalities of the maxillofacial region and often have poor dental development and frequent spontaneous tooth abscesses [100, 101]. The two most striking changes are progressive bowing of the lower extremities associated with marked rachitic changes at the distal femoral and proximal tibial metaphyses (Fig. 79-2) and an elevation of plasma alkaline phosphatase concentration [93, 95–99] (see Williams and Winters [90] for a more complete bibliography of the older literature). These changes are associated with an increasingly evident wadding gait and short stature. Patients with rickets of the distal femoral and proximal tibial metaphyses may exhibit either genu varum or valgum.

In hypophosphatemic adults deformities due to rickets in childhood include bowing of the legs and shortening of stature, usually without evidence of continuing active bone disease. A few affected adults have active osteomalacia, as judged by pseudofractures and an elevated serum alkaline phosphatase level. These changes revert toward normal with large doses of vitamin D.

In clinically affected adults, bone overgrowth at the site of major muscular attachments and around joints may cause significant limitation of motion, particularly in elbows, shoulders, and hips [12, 95–99]. Such overgrowth within the spinal canal has produced symptomatic cord compression requiring surgical intervention [90].

Among family members with hypophosphatemia females have a lower incidence of bone disease than males [12, 94], but when present, the disease may be as severe in the female as in the male. Hypophosphatemic males with short stature without rickets have been reported [93], and with or without treatment nearly all hypophosphatemic patients have shorter stature as adults than their unaffected sibs. One of the striking clinical features is the wide variation in growth rate and degree of

skeletal involvement in affected sibs, even of the same sex, and the lack of correlation between the degree of skeletal involvement and the magnitude of the hypophosphatemia.

The growth failure is most manifest in the legs [59, 61–65] but in more severely affected individuals may also involve the upper segment.

Figure 79-2 Anteroposterior view of the knees of a 4-year-old boy (VI-9 of E kindred of Winters et al. [12]), showing marked rachitic changes, with early healing, and lateral curvature of femora and tibias.

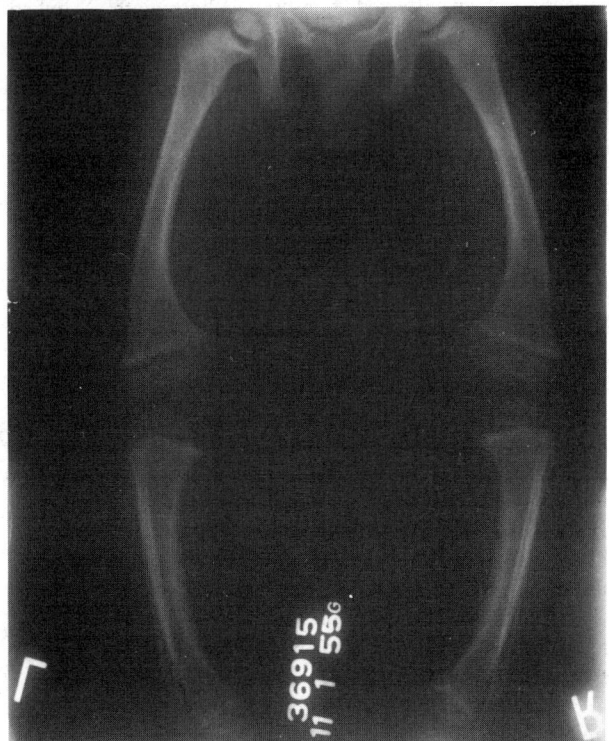

Once epiphyseal closure has occurred, many patients with skeletal deformity and short stature do well with no specific therapy, show no evidence of osteomalacia on radiologic examination, and have no persistent elevation of alkaline phosphatase in spite of continued hypophosphatemia [90]. Other adults may show continued bony changes on x-ray, including pseudofractures, and elevation of alkaline phosphatase. In these patients osteomalacia usually improves with large doses of vitamin D and inorganic phosphate.

Histologic Changes

Examinations of bone and dental tissue from subjects with hypophosphatemic (vitamin D–resistant) rickets show abnormalities that distinguish them from the other forms of rickets. In hypophosphatemic rickets, widened osteoid seams and perilacunar areas of absent mineralization are present, but there is little increase in the extent of bone resorption and minimal elevation of osteoclast counts [90, 102, 103]. Formation and mineralization of postnatal interglobular coronal dentine of teeth is greatly disturbed [100]. Hypomineralization and hypoplasia of the enamel have also been reported [101].

Laboratory Findings

As already noted, the major biochemical abnormality is hypophosphatemia, and the mode of inheritance has been best revealed by using hypophosphatemia as the genetic discriminant [11-13].

In designating a person as hypophosphatemic, allowance must be made for the normal changes in serum phosphorus with age and for differences between the sexes. Greenberg and coworkers [104], using a large number of observations on normal persons, have expressed mathematically and graphically, with limits of statistical confidence, the relationship between serum phosphorus concentration and age for each sex and the changes seen in affected family members with X-linked hypophosphatemia (Fig. 79-3).

The age at which hypophosphatemia first appears is variable. Thus, Harrison et al. [93] have reported normophosphatemia from birth up to the age of 6 months or later in children who then developed hypophosphatemia, growth retardation, and rickets. Harrison et al. suggested that the relatively low glomerular filtration rate characteristic of the first few months of life may result in normal serum phosphorus concentration even though a tubular defect in phosphate reabsorption may already be present. Stickler [105] found consistently low serum phosphorus values from birth. Variability also exists in reported sex differences: Winters et al. [12] found that hypophosphatemic females in affected families had slightly higher values for serum phosphorus than males in the same family, whereas McNair and Stickler [106] found no sex differences, but their studies did not include those who had hypophosphatemia without rickets. The plasma phosphate level is higher in normal males than in normal females, is highest in infancy, is fairly constant between age 4 and puberty, and falls after puberty into the adult range (Fig. 79-3).

The serum alkaline phosphatase level also varies with age and correlates with the rate of bone formation. This level is elevated in affected individuals with evident rickets but is normal in most hypophosphatemic individuals without radiologic signs of rickets.

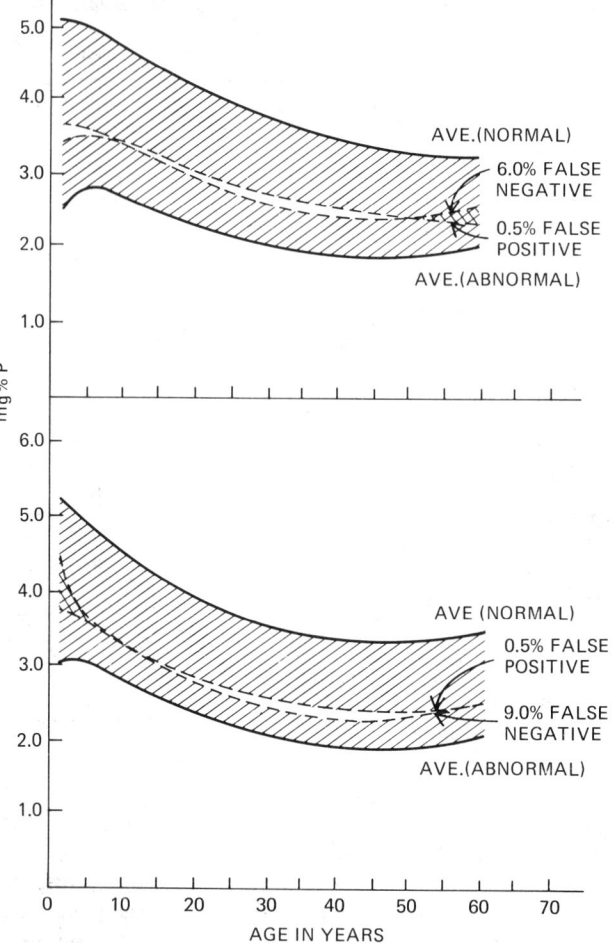

Figure 79-3 The assumed operating characteristics of the lower 99 percent confidence limits for the serum inorganic phosphorus concentration of normal men (top) and women (bottom) as a function of age in the diagnosis of familial hypophosphatemia. The upper solid curves and the upper broken curve are the normal mean values for men (top) and women (bottom) with their 99 percent confidence limits: The lower solid curves are the abnormal curves from the data of Greenberg et al. [104], obtained on 27 males and 41 females in 5 kindreds with this disease. The lower broken curves are the upper confidence limits for the abnormal population of males (top) and females (bottom) in the 5 families studied. (From Greenberg et al. [104], with permission.)

The plasma calcium concentration is usually normal or in the low normal range. Other plasma electrolytes, blood pH, bicarbonate, and BUN are also normal.

Urinary calcium excretion is usually low in the untreated state and urinary phosphate excretion high. Glorieux and Scriver [107] have reported that urinary cAMP concentration is normal in untreated hetero- and homozygotes and that a normal increase in cAMP excretion follows the infusion of bovine PTH. Urinary aminoaciduria, which is common in true vitamin D–deficiency and in vitamin D–dependent rickets, is not seen in untreated subjects with this condition.

The plasma concentration of parathyroid hormone has been measured by a number of investigators. Several groups have reported low [108], normal [109], and high normal values [110], whereas at least two groups have reported slightly elevated concentrations of plasma PTH in untreated subjects [111, 112]. There is general agreement that plasma PTH rises into the abnormally high range in many subjects after the initiation of phosphate therapy. [110]. Secondary hyperparathyroidism varies greatly but may be severe and has required partial parathyroidectomy in an occasional patient. It can usually be reduced or prevented by the simultaneous use of vitamin D or one of its metabolites or supplemental oral calcium. The possible role of parathyroid hormone in the pathogenesis of the syndrome is discussed below.

The plasma concentrations of 25-(OH)D$_3$ are normal in patients with the disease [113]. The plasma concentration of 1,25-(OH)$_2$D$_3$ has been reported to be either low-normal or moderately decreased [114–118] in untreated patients. However, in the face of the persistently low plasma phosphate concentration, and the evidence that under experimental circumstances the 1,25-(OH)$_2$D$_3$ concentration increases as a result of phosphate depletion, all these patients have an inappropriately low 1,25-(OH)$_2$D$_3$ concentration. When normal human subjects are placed on a markedly restricted phosphate intake, their plasma 1,25-(OH)$_2$D$_3$ concentrations rise, but patients with familial hypophosphatemic rickets show no increase in plasma 1,25-(OH)$_2$D$_3$ concentrations, even though they increase tubular phosphate reabsorption as a consequence of phosphate starvation.

There is only one report of plasma 24,25-(OH)$_2$D$_3$ measurements in familial hypophosphatemic rickets [63]. The levels were normal but rose significantly when the patients were given 25-(OH)D$_3$.

Renal Findings

Physiology of Renal Handling of Phosphate   Under normal circumstances, over 85 to 90 percent of plasma phosphate is filtered at the renal glomeruli, and the amount appearing in the urine represents the difference between that filtered and that reabsorbed by the renal tubule. Phosphate reabsorption takes place in both the proximal and distal tubules, the loop of Henle, and probably in the early collecting tubule [119–123].

When the plasma phosphate concentration is increased slowly by the infusion of phosphate salts, the tubular reabsorption of phosphate reaches a maximum value (T$_m$), and further increases in filtered load are excreted quantitatively in the urine. In studies in the isolated nephron, the transport of phosphate also shows saturation kinetics. The most likely mechanism of transcellular phosphate transport involves an active Na$^+$-dependent uptake at the luminal border of the cell and passive diffusion from cell to extracellular fluid, but the fact that a large variety of other substances inhibit tubular phosphate reabsorption has made difficult the elucidation of the underlying transport process.

A significant advance in our understanding of this process has come from the development of methods for the isolation of osmotically intact, right-side-out membrane vesicles from purified brush border membranes prepared from the renal cortex [124, 125]. These are derived primarily from the luminal membranes of the proximal convoluted tubule. When incubated in a phosphate-containing buffer and then exposed to an imposed Na$^+$ gradient (outside>inside), there is a rapid Na$^+$-dependent accumulation of phosphate. Similar vesicles prepared from the brush border membranes of intestinal mucosal cells have been employed in the study of the action of vitamin D on the intestine and are discussed below. There is considerable evidence from studies of phosphate transport in both tissues that a major regulated site in the transcellular transport of phosphate is at the luminal Na$^+$ dependent entry step.

At least three important factors regulate tubular phosphate transport: (1) parathyroid hormone [123], (2) dietary phos-

phate intake [126], and (3) growth hormone [127]. At present there is no evidence that alteration in growth hormone metabolism or action plays any role in the pathogenesis of hypophosphatemic rickets; hence its action will not be considered, but the effects of both dietary phosphate deprivation and PTH will be considered.

When PTH is infused into a normal animal there is a prompt increase in phosphate excretion. Micropuncture data indicate that a major site of reduced phosphate transport is the early proximal nephron [123], and if brush border membrane vesicles are prepared from cortical tissue, there is a reduction in Na$^+$-dependent phosphate transport [128]. A large number of micropuncture studies suggest that when one is dealing with a euparathyroid animal undergoing parathyroidectomy, the major increases in tubular phosphate reabsorption occur distally, i.e., pars recta, distal convoluted tubule, and possibly the collecting duct [123]. To further complicate the issue, PTH also inhibits proximal tubular Na$^+$ and the fluid reabsorption [79]. Although at one time this was considered the primary action of PTH, to account for decreased proximal phosphate reabsorption, the current consensus is that the effects of PTH on Na$^+$ and fluid reabsorption and on proximal phosphate absorption are independent [122, 123].

Dietary phosphate restriction leads to a rapid (1 to 3 days) decrease in urinary phosphate excretion even when plasma phosphate concentration remains normal [126]. It is not known whether this adaptation is due to a local mechanism operating within the nephrons or to the elaboration of some humoral factor. In either case, of particular interest is the result that administration of 1-hydroxyethylidene diphosphoric acid (HEDP), an agent that blocks bone mineralization, leads to a decrease in tubular phosphate reabsorption. This suggests that this renal tubular phosphate transport system can adapt to the phosphate demands of the organism; i.e., a decreased demand leads to a decrease in phosphate reclamation by the tubule.

Micropuncture studies indicate that the adaptation occurs particularly in the early proximal nephron. Whether it involves distal sites as well is a matter of continuing controversy. Studies with isolated brush border membrane vesicles from cortical tissue show a marked increase in the V_{max} of the Na$^+$-dependent phosphate uptake system [126]. This adaptation is due to an increase in the transport capacity of the Na$^+$-phosphate cotransporter and not to a change in Na$^+$ gradient or Na$^+$ permeability [129].

When the response to PTH is compared with that induced by phosphate deprivation, the latter is quantitatively more significant [126]. PTH alters phosphate reabsorption 2 to 5 times, whereas phosphate deprivation and excess can alter this process several hundred times. PTH administration has little effect on phosphate reabsorption in the phosphate-deprived animal even when the filtered load of phosphate is normalized [126] and even though the usual rise in cellular and urinary cAMP concentrations occur after PTH administration. Likewise, the TPX rat alters tubular phosphate reabsorption in response to dietary phosphate restriction. Thus PTH is not necessary for the adaptive process to occur. An unresolved question is whether phosphate deprivation and PTH act on the same or on different phosphate transport systems within the nephron.

An unresolved question is whether vitamin D or its metabolites influence tubular phosphate transport. Some data from rats suggest that both 25-(OH)D$_3$ and 1,25-(OH)$_2$D$_3$ increase proximal tubular reabsorption of phosphate [130]. Data from humans suggest that 25-(OH)D$_3$ but not 1,25-(OH)$_2$D$_3$ has a direct stimulatory effect on tubular phosphate reabsorption

[130]. Finally, in the TPX rat, 1,25-$(OH)_2D_3$ causes a return of tubular phosphate reabsorption to normal but has no effect on the process in a normal, euparathyroid animal [126]. Whether this is a direct renal tubular action of 1,25-$(OH)_2D_3$ or the indirect consequence of some other action of 1,25-$(OH)_2D_3$ is not known.

A major effect of parathyroid hormone upon the renal tubules is the stimulation of adenylate cyclase, which induces a rise in the intracellular concentration and an increase in the urinary excretion of cAMP [131. This evidence, taken in conjunction with the phosphaturia that follows the infusion of cAMP or its dibutyryl analogue [132] has led to this postulated sequence of events in PTH action: (1) activation of adenylate cyclase; (2) a rise in cAMP concentration in the cell; (3) stimulation of the activity of one or more cAMP-dependent protein phosphokinases; (4) phosphorylation of luminal membrane proteins [133]; and (5) a decrease in rate of luminal membrane phosphate flux. Data in support of this concept are that other agents that enhance proximal renal cAMP concentration increase phosphate excretion [119, 120], i.e., reduce the T_m for phosphate; and that a cAMP-dependent protein kinase and a specific substrate have been located on isolated luminal membranes from rat kidneys [134]. On the other hand, the mediation of PTH action may be more complex [22, 23]. A major problem is that when an infusion of cAMP is given, phosphaturia is promptly observed, and upon cessation of the infusion, there is an equally prompt fall in phosphate excretion, while by contrast, when PTH is infused at a slow rate, there is an initial sharp increase in cAMP excretion which then falls off. Its rate of excretion returns to nearly control levels in spite of sustained phosphaturia. Thus, factors other than cAMP may be involved as second messengers in the phosphaturic action of PTH.

One of these other factors may be Ca^{2+}. The effects of calcium ion concentration upon phosphate excretion are complex [119]. Infusion of Ca^{2+} into one renal artery leads to an ipsilateral decrease in urinary phosphate excretion, whereas the chronic infusion of calcium into hypoparathyroid subjects, at a rate sufficient to raise the plasma calcium concentration to normal, leads to a significant increase in phosphate excretion and a fall in plasma phosphate concentration [134]. These latter data, taken in conjunction with the fact that parathyroid hormone stimulates the uptake of calcium into cells [22, 23, 135], raise the possibility that a PTH-mediated increase in intracellular Ca^{2+} concentration may also be a significant factor in PTH-induced phosphaturia. The importance of these conflicting views concerning the mechanism of PTH action to the problem of the role of PTH in the pathogenesis of hypophosphatemic rickets is considered later in "Pathogenesis."

Another aspect of PTH action that has now been clarified is its effects upon distal tubular phosphate reabsorption. Micropuncture data reported by Agus et al. [120] have shown that although both a saline infusion and an increase in PTH decrease proximal tubular phosphate reabsorption to the same extent, only PTH infusion in a normal animal leads to significant phosphaturia. Direct studies of the electrolyte composition of fluid obtained from distal sites in the nephron demonstrate clearly that PTH acts to reduce the distal as well as proximal T_m for phosphate reabsorption. In this regard, PTH appears to be unique; i.e., although several factors other than PTH, such as a saline load or calcitonin, alter proximal phosphate reabsorption, only PTH acts at the distal site.

These findings are also consistent with results of studies of Chabardes et al. [136] on the distribution of PTH-sensitive adenylate cyclase in the rabbit kidney nephron. This hormone was found to stimulate cyclase activity in the proximal convoluted tubule, the pars recta, the cortical portion but not medullary portion of the thick ascending limb, the distal convoluted tubule, and the early branched portion of the collecting tubule. The thin descending limb and the remainder of the collecting tubule did not respond. Thus, both biochemical and physiologic data support the concept of a distal as well as a proximal site of PTH action. (See [24] for further discussion of distal effects of PTH.)

When PTH acts at the proximal site, there is a decrease in tubular reabsorption of Na^+, Ca^{2+}, and HPO_4^{2-}, but at the distal site PTH stimulates calcium reabsorption and inhibits H^+ production and phosphate reabsorption. It is likely that this is also the site at which PTH alters K^+ excretion [23]. An important question is, at which of these sites does PTH regulate the synthesis of 1,25-$(OH)_2D_3$. This question has a direct bearing on the pathogenesis of the decreased intestinal absorption of calcium and phosphate seen in patients with hypophosphatemic rickets. Present evidence indicates that 1,25-$(OH)_2D_3$ synthesis takes place in the latter half of the proximal nephron.

In closing this discussion of the physiology of renal phosphate transport, we reemphasize the major importance of renal tubular transport of phosphate in determining the plasma phosphate concentration. At present two interrelated factors are recognized that are of major importance in determining the rate of tubular phosphate transport. One is the supply of phosphate to the organism which determines the bulk capacity of the nephron to reabsorb phosphate, and the other is parathyroid hormone which fine-tunes the system and relates it to immediate changes in calcium and phosphate intake. The overall process exhibits a transport maximum, which varies as a function of previous phosphate intake and is best assessed clinically by measuring the tubular maximal transport reabsorptive capacity relative to the GFR (Tm_P/GFR) [137].

Renal Abnormality in Hypophosphatemic Rickets   In every instance in which it has been studied, the hypophosphatemia of this disorder has been associated with increased renal excretion and decreased net renal tubular reabsorption of phosphate [10, 14, 90, 138–142]. The most quantitative data have been obtained in studies in which the renal tubular maximum for reabsorption of phosphate (Tm_p) has been measured; in all instances the Tm_p has been low in affected hypophosphatemic persons, with or without demonstrable bone involvement. Values have ranged from 50 to 87μmol phosphate reabsorbed per dl glomerular filtrate, compared with a mean value in normal persons of approximately 130 μmol phosphate reabsorbed per dl glomerular filtrate, with limits of two standard deviations from 90 to 150 μmol. Typical data appear in Figure 79-4.

On rare occasions the administration of large phosphate loads to patients with resistant rickets has produced a calculated net tubular secretion of phosphate [143]. The difficulties of maintaining a steady state in studies of this type raise the possibility that the calculated secretion of phosphate is artifactual.

Except for the low tubular reabsorption of phosphate, renal function is normal. The glomerular filtration rate has been normal in the affected persons in whom it has been measured [90], and the clearance and T_m for the excretion of paraaminohip-

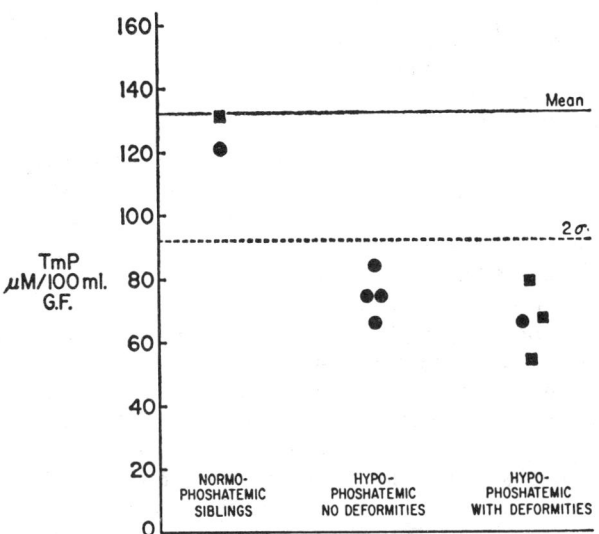

Figure 79-4 Values for maximal tubular reabsorption of phosphate (Tm_p, μmol/100 ml glomerular filtrate) in 10 members of the E kindred of Winters et al. [11, 12]. ■ = male, ● = female. The mean and 2 SD (2σ) for the values of Tm_p of 26 normal subjects are represented by the lines.

purate are reported normal [90]. The carbon dioxide content of the blood is normal with rare exceptions, and the ability to acidify the urine is normal [90]. Concentration and dilution tests are normal.

Amino acid excretion in familial instances of the disorder has been normal [12, 144] with rare exceptions [8, 90], one of which may represent more than simple vitamin D–resistant rickets [139, 140]. Mild glycinuria has been observed in a few families with typical vitamin D–resistant rickets [138]. Observations in patients without a family history have been varied: Some have had no abnormal aminoaciduria [140, 141], while others have had abnormally high excretions of various amino acids which are decreased upon the administration of large doses of vitamin D [145], a response similar to that of the aminoaciduria of vitamin D–deficiency rickets to smaller doses [58, 146, 147] and of vitamin D–dependency rickets to larger doses of vitamin D [58, 110, 111]. The excretory patterns of amino acids after loading with histidine and arginine [146] or methionine [147] are probably abnormal in patients with vitamin D–resistant rickets, but more detailed information is needed including comparable studies of normal persons.

Mild renal glycosuria has been reported rarely in association with vitamin D–resistant rickets in both familial and nonfamilial patients [148]. The large body of negative evidence suggests that an abnormality in glucose reabsorption does not participate in the production of increased phosphate excretion.

The nature of the tubular transport defect has been clarified by the work of Tenenhouse and Scriver [75–78, 80] who showed that the Hyp mouse has a marked reduction in urinary phosphate excretion when placed on a low phosphate diet. Studies of Na^+-dependent phosphate transport in isolated brush border membrane prepared from the renal cortices of these animals (Hyp/y or Hyp/+) show the same adaptive response to phosphate deprivation as in control animals (+/y or +/+). Patients with hypophosphatemic rickets also show a marked decrease in renal phosphate excretion when placed on restricted phosphate intakes [148a]. On the basis of this evidence, earlier studies in hypophosphatemic humans showing a defect in the PTH-sensitive component of phosphate transport

[149], and the occurrence of a hypophosphatemic syndrome inherited as an autosomal dominant trait which shows normal sensitivity to PTH [22], Tenenhouse and Scriver propose that there are two components of tubular phosphate transport: one a PTH-sensitive component which is controlled by a gene on the X-chromosome and another a PTH-insensitive component controlled by an autosomal gene. Support for their conclusion has been provided by Dennis et al. [79], who identified a high capacity, PTH-insensitive component of Pi transport in the early portion of the proximal convoluted tubules of the rabbit nephron and a low capacity, PTH-sensitive component in the later, straight portion of the proximal convoluted tubule.

This is an attractive hypothesis, particularly since the site of 1,25-$(OH)_2D_3$ biosynthesis is in the later or more distal part of the proximal convoluted tubule, i.e., in the same region as the PTH-sensitive component of phosphate transport. There are, however, difficulties. First, many patients with hypophosphatemic rickets demonstrate a normal or even enhanced phosphaturia response to PTH when studied under the proper conditions. Second, data from other animals show clearly that in many the phosphate transport system in the early proximal convoluted tubule is responsive to PTH [123]. It is not known what the distribution of PTH-responsiveness is in the human nephron. Third, when rats, rabbits, or humans are placed on low phosphate diets, there is loss of the PTH-mediated increase in phosphate excretion [126]. One of two interpretations of these findings is possible: One, the capacity of the early transport system has increased so much in response to phosphate deprivation that little or no phosphate is delivered to the more distal site; hence PTH is ineffective. Two, both PTH and phosphate deprivation regulate the same phosphate transport system. Against the former possibility is the finding that when animals previously adapted to low phosphate diets are given a phosphate infusion to raise acutely serum phosphate and therefore filtered load, PTH-responsiveness is not restored [126].

It is possible that there are two separate transport systems, or alternatively that one system is regulated by a number of different regulatory proteins. In either case there is one additional aspect of renal function in this disease that requires discussion, i.e., the control of 1,25-$(OH)_2D_3$ biosynthesis.

As discussed above, the two major, recognized physiological stimuli that enhance 1,25-$(OH)_2D_3$ synthesis are PTH and phosphate restriction. The paradox in patients with familial hypophosphatemic rickets is that they have low or low-normal values of plasma 1,25-$(OH)_2D_3$ at a time when they have marked hypophosphatemia. Furthermore, when placed on phosphate-restricted diets, their plasma 1,25-$(OH)_2D_3$ concentrations do not rise but actually fall, in contrast to normal age-matched controls in whom a rise is observed. A logical supposition is that the intracellular signals that normally regulate 1,25-$(OH)_2D_3$ synthesis in response to phosphate deprivation are not generated in the tubular cells of these patients. The problem is to relate this inappropriate intracellular response to the tubular phosphate transport defect that has been identified in the brush border membrane. Both must be the result of the same mutation, and both most likely relate to a change in cellular phosphate metabolism. If the primary defect resides in the phosphate entry step across the brush border membrane, then the expected result would be intracellular phosphate reduction and stimulation of 1,25-$(OH)_2D_3$ synthesis. Given the likelihood that there is coordination of the transport processes across the brush border and basolateral membranes, it is possible that a primary defect in phosphate egress from the cell across the basolateral membrane could account for the inappropriately low 1,25-$(OH)_2D_3$ synthesis and would lead through some type of feedback mechanism to a reduction in phosphate entry across the brush border membrane. Unfortunately, next to nothing is known about the way phosphate that enters the cell across the brush border membrane is transported out of the cell across the basolateral membrane.

Intestinal Findings

Physiology of Intestinal Calcium and Phosphate Transport A major site in the regulation of calcium and phosphate metabolism is the intestine [8, 23, 34]. Calcium absorption takes place primarily in the duodenum and early jejunum, whereas phosphate absorption is maximal in the mid-jejunum. The absorption of both ions is greatly reduced in all forms of vitamin D deficiency. The major hormonal factor in the regulation of their absorption is 1,25-$(OH)_2D_3$ [23, 30–37, 39, 42]. This is the major intestinal metabolite found in experimental rachitic animals following administration of radioactive vitamin D_3, 25-$(OH)D_3$, or 1,25-$(OH)_2D_3$. It corrects the impaired intestinal absorption of both calcium and phosphate in vitamin D-deficient nephrectomized animals. The biochemical basis for its intestinal actions have not been completely elucidated. A major cellular site of action in regulating intestinal calcium transport is at the location of entry of calcium into the intestinal mucosal cell: the microvillar membrane or brush border of these cells.

The same appears to be the case for phosphate transport. The rate of both calcium uptake and Na^+-dependent phosphate uptake across the brush border membrane is increased by 1,25-$(OH)_2D_3$ treatment [150, 151]. The time courses of these two effects are different, and it appears that this hormone regulates these processes by independent mechanisms. In the case of calcium entry, i.e. transcellular calcium transport, prior administration of cycloheximide (an inhibitor of protein synthesis) or agents that inhibit RNA synthesis, does not block the actions of subsequently administered 1,25-$(OH)_2D_3$ [150, 152]. Recent data suggest strongly that 1,25-$(OH)_2D_3$ mediates its effect on calcium entry by a process that does not require nuclear gene activation and probably involves a primary change in brush order membrane lipid structure [150–155]. The molecular basis for the change in phosphate transport across this membrane is not known, but it appears not to involve changes in membrane lipid structure.

Abnormalities in Intestinal Calcium and Phosphate Absorption in Hypophosphatemic Rickets One of the most striking abnormalities in true vitamin D deficiency is a nearly complete lack of intestinal calcium absorption, so that fecal excretion usually equals calcium intake [8, 32]. In patients with hypophosphatemic rickets intestinal calcium absorption is generally reduced, sometimes to an extent similar to that seen in vitamin D deficiency, but more often the reduction is less marked [68]. As a consequence, urinary calcium excretion is low, but calcium balance is usually slightly positive, although less than the more marked positive calcium balance characteristic of the normally growing child. Using a so-called calcium tolerance test, Condon et al. [156, 157] found that calcium absorption was normal in their subjects with

hypophosphatemic rickets. It is difficult to relate their findings to the many balance studies in which a clear reduction in intestinal calcium absorption was observed.

Treatment of subjects with small doses of 1,25-$(OH)_2D_3$ or 1-α-$(OH)D_3$ (1-α-hydroxyvitamin D_3), a synthetic analogue of 1,25-$(OH)_2D_3$, promotes in nearly all cases a significant increase in intestinal calcium absorption and an increase in urinary calcium excretion [158, 159]. The increase in calcium absorption is a significant aspect of the positive therapeutic effect of these agents.

The question of whether or not intestinal phosphate absorption is altered in this condition is a matter of continuing debate. Older balance studies showed that intestinal phosphate absorption is decreased but not to the extent of reduction of calcium absorption. Recent studies show that 1,25-$(OH)_2D_3$ in small doses induces a marked increase in the rate of intestinal phosphate absorption under conditions in which little or no effect upon renal tubular phosphate reabsorption is seen [158, 159]. These data, plus those of Glorieux et al. [160] showing no abnormality in phosphate uptake in jejunal biopsies from hypophosphatemic subjects, suggest that there is no intrinsic defect in transcellular phosphate transport in the intestine.

Osseous Findings

Physiology of the Calcification Process The mechanism of action of vitamin D and its metabolites upon bone processes is complex [23, 34, 49]. Initial attempts to demonstrate a direct effect of vitamin D upon the mineralization process were either negative or inconclusive [8] and led to the concept that vitamin D had no direct effect upon the mineralization of bone matrix. Nevertheless, one of the major consequences of a lack of vitamin D is the development of rickets or osteomalacia, a failure of the normal process of bone mineralization. This paradox was resolved by postulating that vitamin D deficiency causes a failure of bone mineralization by its actions upon other organs, most notably the intestine, where, by inhibiting the absorption of calcium and phosphate, it induces a fall in plasma calcium and phosphate concentrations and secondary hyperparathyroidism, causing a further fall in plasma phosphate concentration and in the calcium × phosphate product in extracellular fluids [161–163]. This ion product was proposed as the major determinant of mineralization of newly formed bone matrix.

This conclusion was reinforced by two subsequent observations: Carlsson [164] showed that vitamin D did have a direct effect upon bone, that of enhancing bone mobilization; and DeLuca showed that rickets or osteomalacia can be "cured" simply by raising the calcium × phosphate product in the extracellular fluids [165].

Carlsson's experiments demonstrated that the administration of vitamin D to a calcium-deprived, vitamin D–deficient animal was followed by a rise in plasma calcium and phosphate concentration because of a mobilization of calcium and phosphate from old mineralized bone [164]. Subsequent work has shown that vitamin D alters the sensitivity of bone cells to the calcium-mobilizing action of parathyroid hormone [22, 23, 166, 167] and that part of the mobilized mineral is redeposited in previously unmineralized matrix [23]. Although part of the explanation for a lack of bone mineralization in vitamin D deficiency is a fall in the calcium × phosphate ion product in the extracellular fluids, vitamin D or one of its metabolites also has a direct action upon bone to enhance the mineralization of bone matrix (see [23] for a discussion of this evidence). The vitamin D metabolite responsible for this effect has not been identified. Both $1,25\text{-}(OH)_2D_3$ and $24,25\text{-}(OH)_2D_3$ are necessary for the process of mineralization [60]. It seems likely that they act on different cell populations in bone, e.g., $1,25\text{-}(OH)_2D_3$ on osteocytes and osteoclasts and $24,25\text{-}(OH)_2D_3$ on osteoblasts. Considerably more work is needed to sort out their interactions and the ways in which each influences the mineralization processes.

In any form of rickets at least two factors are involved in determining the severity of the bone lesions: the amount of specific vitamin D metabolite(s) available and the calcium × phosphate ion product (or more likely the phosphate concentration per se). The two known causes of rickets are deficiency of vitamin D and deficiency of phosphate.

Abnormalities in Bone in Hypophosphatemic Rickets

Two different types of bone abnormalities have been described in patients with vitamin D–resistant rickets. The first is the characteristic finding which gives the disease its name—the rachitic appearance of the epiphyseal region. There is a markedly expanded zone of proliferating cartilage, with increased osteoid tissue and invasion by wide, tortuous blood vessels [9, 168–170]. These changes are present in patients with and without family histories. The radiologic changes in the epiphyseal area are entirely characteristic of vitamin D–deficiency rickets.

The epiphyseal lesion heals in most instances when the patients are treated with large doses of vitamin D. Healing can also be initiated by supplying large amounts of phosphate, as already noted, and is accelerated by immobilization of patients at the time of osteotomy [141, 144]. Symptomatic improvement has been reported in association with an increased positive balance of calcium and phosphate induced by a large calcium intake [171]. This lack of need for vitamin D itself in order to heal the epiphyseal lesion is also characteristic of vitamin D–deficiency rickets [172]. The healing of the epiphyseal lesion that occurs after administration of large doses of vitamin D usually proceeds without any significant rise in serum phosphorus.

The second type of bony abnormality in familial vitamin D–resistant rickets consists of a distortion of the compact bone of the metaphyses of long bones. Biopsy material (taken before as well as after vitamin D therapy) has shown an abnormal irregular mosaic formation of the haversian systems and trabeculae and probably an increase in osteoblastic borders and areas of active resorption [10, 102, 103, 141, 168]. Other biopsy studies, using fresh, undecalcified sections, have shown perilacunar "halos" of low density bone and slow bone turnover [102, 172, 173]. The bone may appear unusually dense radiologically [174]. The histologic pattern has some features suggestive of Paget's disease or of experimental hyperparathyroidism. In some patients bone from the metaphysis has been almost normal [139, 141]. Finally, Villanueva et al. [102] have reported a normal rate of bone resorption but a decrease in bone formation in biopsy material from subjects with familial hypophosphatemic rickets.

These results are consistent with the conclusion that both hypophosphatemia and some alteration in vitamin D metabolism are involved in the pathogenesis of the bony abnormalities. Vitamin D metabolism in these subjects has been reported

as abnormal [15], but the present clinical methods of studying vitamin D metabolism are open to question and are presently not sufficiently precise to define the possible defect in vitamin D metabolism. As noted above, the plasma concentrations of $1,25\text{-}(OH)_2D_3$ in patients with this disease vary from low to low-normal. Unfortunately, measurements of $24,25\text{-}(OH)_2D_3$ have not been reported in a large number of these patients. At present there is no apparent correlation between the extent of the bone disease and the concentration of phosphate, or of $1,25\text{-}(OH)_2D_3$ in the plasma. Hence, the pathogenesis of the bone lesions remains obscure. To emphasize how difficult it is to define them, one need only realize that Frymoyer and Hodgkins [23] have reported on a kindred with X-linked hypophosphatemic osteomalacia in whom rickets is not apparent during childhood, although hypophosphatemia is, but osteomalacia commonly develops late in life (after the third decade). Likewise, Scriver et al. [22] have described an autosomally-dominant inheritance of hypophosphatemia in children who exhibit osteomalacia but not rickets.

These findings point up the circumstance that the factors responsible for the pathogenesis of rickets (a primary change in the mineralization process at the growth plate) and for the pathogenesis of osteomalacia (a primary change in the mineralization process in true bone) are probably different.

One of the standard biochemical markers for the presence of active rickets and osteomalacia is the serum alkaline phosphatase activity. It is generally elevated in hypophosphatemic patients with rickets. The fact that it fell after puberty in patients with this disease had been taken as evidence for the disappearance of rickets and osteomalacia once the pubertal growth spurt had taken place. Our own recent investigation has shown that most adult subjects with this disease have bone pain and fatigability, and a significant increase in osteoid volume when bone is examined histologically. Osteoid may represent up to 30 percent of the bone volume (normal < 3.0 percent). Even in those adult patients with the most marked degree of osteomalacia, plasma alkaline phosphatase activities were normal. These findings and the positive response of some of these patients to combined therapy with phosphate and $1,25\text{-}(OH)_2D_3$ suggest that lifelong therapy may be necessary.

Growth Retardation

A problem of continuing concern is that most children with resistant rickets never achieve normal height. Several factors contribute:

First, the diagnosis may not be made and effective treatment begun until deformities and growth retardation have already developed.

Second, it is difficult to maintain adequate treatment, and yet avoid hypervitaminosis D, throughout the growing years [175]. As is true with most chronic illnesses requiring continuous treatment, patients with this disorder, their parents, and their physicians frequently let therapy lapse. Or an episode of vitamin D intoxication may require discontinuance of therapy, which is usually not reinstituted until active rickets has reappeared. Thus, any beneficial effect of continuous treatment on growth itself is lost. Stickler et al. [96], for example, recorded at least one episode of hypercalcemia among 23 of 43 treated patients.

Third, the persistence of leg deformities contributes to shortened stature, and in already deformed long bones an improvement in longitudinal growth as a result of treatment adds more to the deformity than to the total height.

Finally, there may be an abnormality in growth of the legs of affected persons which is distinct from active rickets and not corrected by present modes of treatment. In an extensive retrospective evaluation of this problem, McNair and Stickler [106] found that upper-segment growth was not significantly different from normal, but lower-segment growth averaged 15 percent below normal.

It has been suggested that growth deficiency is another result of refractory hypophosphatemia per se. In support of this view is the fact that serum phosphorus levels and growth are often normal for the first 5 to 12 months after birth [176]. The appearance of hypophosphatemia at that time is associated with both a declining growth rate and active rickets. Also, Harrison et al. [176], in a review of experience with 20 patients, found only 1 in whom normal growth rate was achieved. This occurred in association with a rise in serum phosphorus concentration to normal as a result of renal insufficiency from an episode of hypervitaminosis D. Others have reported low serum phosphorus levels as early as the second day after birth [32], and either no or only a poor correlation between serum phosphorus values and degree of shortening [177].

One proposed mechanism for the growth retardation is that phosphate deficiency causes a decrease in the whole blood P_{50}, and this indicates a shift to the left of the oxygen dissociation curve. Depletion of red blood cell phosphate inhibits 2,3-diphosphoglycerate (2,3-DPG) synthesis in red cells, and a fall in 2,3-DPG concentration produces such a shift in the oxygen dissociation curve. It is suggested that release of O_2 from oxyhemoglobin may be impaired in peripheral tissues, and this may account for the impaired growth in these subjects. There is no direct experimental data in support of this hypothesis, and it is hard to see why the growth-inhibiting effect of such a mechanism would be restricted to the skeleton. A more likely alternative is that phosphate deficiency affects bone growth directly. Osteoblastic activity is stimulated by phosphate both in vivo and in vitro [23]. The limiting factor in skeletal growth and mineralization in these hypophosphatemic subjects may well be the availability of phosphate. The predominant localization of the defect to the lower extremities may be accounted for by the fact that this is the skeletal segment with the greatest rate of prepubertal growth.

In keeping with a primary role of phosphate in the pathogenesis of growth retardation are the more recent observations [178] that phosphate therapy combined with vitamin D treatment, when adequate to raise plasma phosphate concentrations into the normal range for a significant part of the day, leads to normal or near-normal rates of linear growth, whereas vitamin D treatment alone, even in doses sufficient to improve the rickets, does not restore growth rates toward normal.

We have found that phosphate alone, even at a dose of 1.5 g/day, does not totally correct either the rickets or the diminished growth, but phosphate alone can stimulate some growth. We and others [115, 118, 159] have found that normal growth rates can be maintained for long periods by the combined use of phosphate and 1-α-(OH)D$_3$ or 1,25-(OH)$_2$D$_3$ (Fig. 79-5).

Pathogenesis

Any discussion of the pathogenesis of familial hypophosphatemic rickets must consider the following facts:

1. Hypophosphatemia and decreased renal tubular phosphate reabsorption are the only abnormalities present in all affected individuals.

2. Plasma parathyroid hormone concentration is normal or only slightly elevated in untreated individuals.

3. There is normal plasma 25-(OH)D$_3$ concentration.

4. There is a decrease in intestinal absorption of calcium that is increased by vitamin D, 25-(OH)D$_3$, 1,25-(OH)$_2$D$_3$, or 1-α-(OH)D$_3$ therapy.

5. There is a reduction in intestinal phosphate absorption that is corrected by 1,25-(OH)$_2$D$_3$ administration.

6. Bone abnormalities occur in many but not all individuals, and the degree of their severity does not correlate with the decrease in plasma phosphate concentration.

7. Administration of either 1,25-(OH)$_2$D$_3$ or 1-α-(OH)D$_3$ does not restore plasma phosphate concentrations to normal or correct the renal tubular defect.

8. An acquired form of vitamin D-resistant osteomalacia has been described in association with certain benign mesenchymal tumors that is totally relieved by removal of such tumors.

9. There is evidence that the parathyroid glands play a permissive role in the pathogenesis of the renal tubular defect in phosphate transport.

Although it was originally suggested that the renal phosphate leak in these patients was due to secondary hyperparathyroidism, present evidence indicates that the defect is intrinsic to the renal tubule. It continues to be evident even in the thyroparathyroidectomized *Hyp* mouse. The weight of evidence also favors the view that the defect is confined to the

Figure 79-5 The growth charts of four children with familial X-linked hypophosphatemic rickets during long-term treatment with combined phosphate and 1-α-(OH)D$_3$. The arrows indicate the time of initiation of treatment in each subject. A and B were females, and C and D are males. (From Rasmussen et al. [115].)

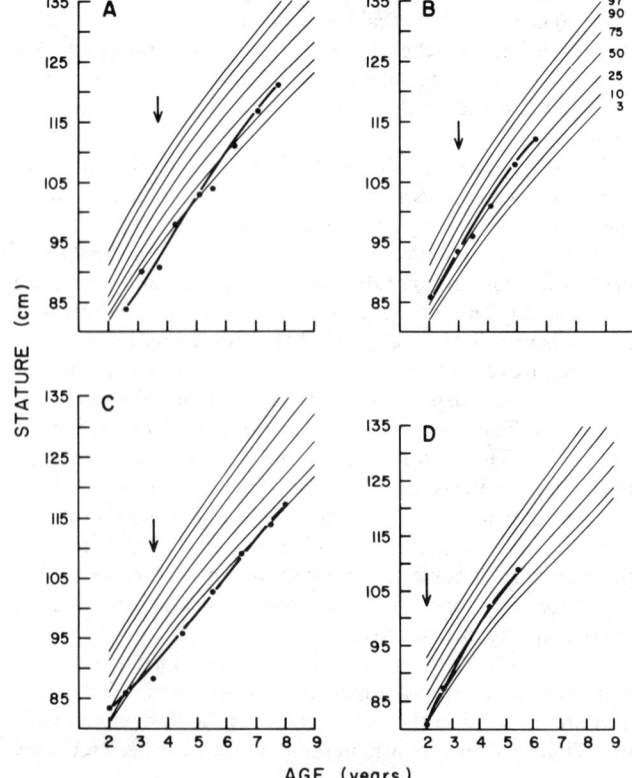

renal tubule and is not simultaneously expressed in the intestinal mucosal cell.

Even though secondary hyperparathyroidism cannot account for the altered renal phosphate excretion, there is evidence that parathyroid hormone plays a 'permissive' role in the altered phosphate Tm. Falls et al. [180] first showed that calcium infusion sufficient to raise plasma calcium concentration to 13 to 14 mg/dl in hypophosphatemic subjects was followed by a complete disappearance of phosphate from the urine. Likewise, Stamp et al. [175] report that calcium infusion leads to an increase in tubular reabsorption of phosphate (TRP) to a normal value when plasma calcium concentration is increased above 13 mg/dl. More recently, Lewy et al. [112] showed that when calcium infusions were given to hypophosphatemic subjects at a slower rate and plasma calcium concentrations rose into the 10.5 to 12 mg/dl range, there was a significant fall in plasma PTH concentration and an associated increase in tubular reabsorption of phosphate to low-normal or near-normal values. Glorieux and Scriver [107] have also reported that PTH infusion caused no increase in urinary phosphate excretion in hypophosphatemic patients, but calcium infusion caused an increase in the renal tubular reabsorption of phosphate, which they concluded was evidence for a calcium-dependent, PTH-independent phosphate transport system in the nephron. They did not infuse PTH into individuals after or during calcium infusion in order to determine whether calcium infusion, by reducing plasma PTH concentration, restored PTH responsiveness.

Acute administration of 1,25-$(OH)_2D_3$ leads to an increase in serum phosphate concentration and to an increase in TRP [181]. Furthermore, after 1,25-$(OH)_2D_3$ treatment, PTH administration leads to a decrease in TRP [181]. Furthermore, Drezner and coworkers [180] have reported that the chronic administration of 1,25-$(OH)_2D_3$ in doses of 2.25 to 3.00 µg/day to two adolescents and two young adults led to a rise in Tm_P/GFR from a mean of 2.12 ± 0.09 to 2.43 ± 0.06, associated with a fall in iPTH. These values of Tm_P/GFR during 1,25-$(OH)_2D_3$ treatment are still below the normal mean value of 3.0 ± 0.3 and indicate that even though renal tubular phosphate transport increased following 1,25-$(OH)_2D_3$ treatment, it did not become normal. The data from both the acute [181] and longer term study [180] are consistent with the conclusion that when 1,25-$(OH)_2D_3$ is given, plasma PTH falls and renal tubular phosphate conservation improves.

Riggs et al. [182] observed that complete parathyroidectomy in a patient with long-standing hypophosphatemia and reduced TRP caused a decrease in renal phosphate loss and a rise in plasma phosphate concentration. Subsequent infusion of parathyroid extract led to a marked increase in urinary phosphate excretion. However, this patient had the adult-onset type of vitamin D-resistant hypophosphatemic rickets and not the X-linked familial disease.

Most recently, Short, Sebastian, Spencer, and Morris [183] showed that PTH infusion in normocalcemic, hypophosphatemic subjects caused a normal increase in urinary cAMP excretion, confirming an earlier report of Glorieux et al. [107], but no increase in urinary phosphate excretion. These subjects were given a massive infusion of calcium, which increased the plasma calcium concentration into the 12 to 14 mg/dl range. Following calcium infusion, phosphate excretion decreased to virtually zero (Fig. 79-6). When parathyroid extract (PTE) was then infused, a striking increase in renal phosphate excretion was observed (Fig. 79-6). This increase in urinary phosphate excretion occurred in affected subjects at a lower dose of PTE

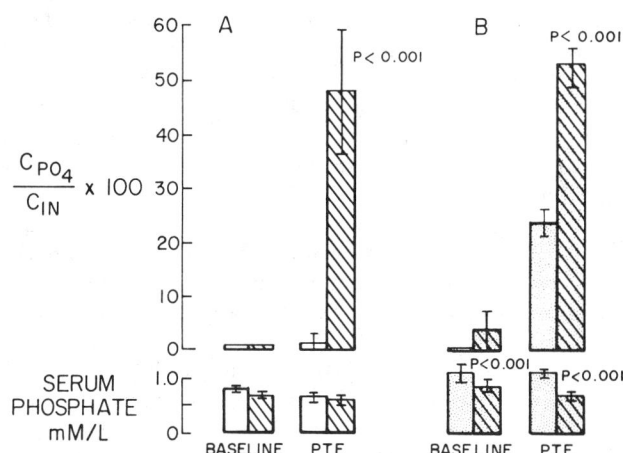

Figure 79-6 A comparison of the fractional excretion of inorganic phosphate and serum inorganic phosphate in hemizygotes and control subjects during temporally comparable post-hypercalcemic periods, before parathyroid extract (PTE) was administered (Baseline) and during the maximal excretion of phosphate that attended its administration (PTE). Bar graphs depict the mean (± 1 SD) of values from three successive clearance periods. *A.* The response of a vitamin D–deficient hypophosphatemic control subject □, and a hemizygotic experimental subject ▨. *B.* The response of normal control subjects (□) and phosphate-primed hemizygotic subjects (▨). Note that in the latter case, when the hemizygote was phosphate-primed but physiologically 'hypoparathyroid,' the fractional excretion of phosphate was low, but upon administration of PTE there was a marked increase. Likewise, PTE infusion induced a marked increase in the fractional excretion of phosphate in the unprimed subject (*A*–▨) but not in the hypophosphatemic control (*A*–□). (*Figure redrawn from Short et al. [183], with permission.*)

than in control subjects, and it was significantly greater in the hypophosphatemic subjects during sustained PTE infusion. By contrast, the increase in urinary cAMP excretion was similar in affected individuals and control subjects. These data provide strong evidence in support of the view that, although PTH elevation is not the primary cause of the reduced tubular reabsorption of phosphate in this syndrome, the presence of PTH is necessary for the expression of the renal tubular defect.

The data from the studies of the *Hyp* mouse indicate that the defect is expressed at least in the proximal tubule and may involve the distal segment as well. As discussed above (see "Animal Models of the Human Disease"), the defect leads both to a decrease in the tubular reabsorption of phosphate and simultaneously to a decrease in the ability of the tubule to synthesize 1,25-$(OH)_2D_3$ in response to a normal hypophosphatemic stimulus. The decreased tubular reabsorption of phosphate is expressed as a decrease in the Na$^+$-dependent entry of phosphate into the cell across the brush border, or luminal membrane. If one assumes this to be the primary site of the defect, then one might logically predict that intracellular phosphate would fall, and this would be a stimulus to 1,25-$(OH)_2D_3$ synthesis, an event which clearly does not occur. The possibility exists that when the transport pool of phosphate falls, the cell compensates by increasing phosphate uptake into the cell across the basolateral membrane. This would restore internal phosphate to normal. However, as phosphate depletion of the organism occurred, the extracellular phosphate concentration would fall, and presumably this would also act as a stimulus to 1,25-$(OH)_2D_3$ synthesis. Hence, it is difficult to link two events in a model in which the primary site of the tubular defect is the luminal membrane. An alternative model could explain this linkage. If the primary defect were in the efflux of phosphate out of the cell across the basolateral membrane, then one could account for the decrease in 1,25-

$(OH)_2D_3$ synthesis in the face of hypophosphatemia, and one could postulate that the raised intracellular phosphate would cause a suppression of luminal phosphate entry by some sort of negative feedback mechanism. Clearly, a more detailed knowledge of the mechanism of transcellular phosphate transport is needed before the mechanism underlying the expression of this gene mutation is elucidated.

Even if this formulation is correct, it leaves unanswered a major question: is the renal defect primary or secondary to the elaboration of some humoral principle? There are two pieces of evidence which suggest that the proposed tubular defect may not be intrinsic to the tubule but results from a humoral factor. The first is the fact that one patient with this syndrome developed renal failure and eventually underwent successful renal transplant [184]. In spite of prior removal of most of his hyperfunctioning parathyroid tissue and a normal circulating PTH 7 months after transplant, his plasma phosphate concentration has remained at 1.4 mg/dl, and his phosphate clearance has remained low. The second is that several patients have been described in whom vitamin D–resistant hypophosphatemic rickets developed in adult life [185–189] or in childhood [190, 191] in association with a mesenchymal tumor. The renal defect, plasma PTH concentrations, the disorder of intestinal function, and the osteomalacia (or rickets) were indistinguishable from the changes seen in patients with the typical X-linked disease. Thus, the possibility exists of the secretion of some humoral factor in the X-linked patients that accounts for their renal tubular defect.

Genetic Aspects

In familial vitamin D–resistant rickets with hypophosphatemia, the inherited trait may vary in the degree of manifestation from severe to mild bone disease associated with hypophosphatemia to hypophosphatemia alone without evidence of active or former rickets. In each of 21 affected families studied by Winters et al. [12, 13] and Burnett et al. [94], when hypophosphatemia was used as the discriminant, transmission was best explained by the presence of a single abnormal gene on an X chromosome. Further, the gene had a single-dose effect, or was dominant, in that it was transmitted from generation to generation without interruption. The segregation ratios in the progeny of affected parents were, with some exceptions discussed below, those to be anticipated with such a gene.

These points are illustrated in Fig. 79-7, which is a part of the original large North Carolina kindred reported by Winters et al. [12, 13]. If individuals were classified as affected solely on the basis of active rickets or postrachitic deformities, there was no clear-cut pattern of inheritance and several instances of "skipping" of a generation occurred. On the other hand, if hypophosphatemia was used as the criterion for the presence of the trait, a clear generation-to-generation transmission emerged.

Studies in 20 additional families in North Carolina and Great Britain are in essential agreement with the original report. These results are summarized in Tables 79-2 and 79-3 and permit the following conclusions:

1. All 97 subjects with active rickets or postrachitic deformities were hypophosphatemic.

2. An additional 49 (47 females and 2 males) were hypophosphatemic with no evidence of active or previous rickets.

3. Included in these 49 were all 13 instances of proved or probable "skipping" when skeletal disease was used as the sole criterion for classification.

4. In 88 of 92 instances in which the requisite data were available, hypophosphatemia was inherited in a predictable fashion in that all hypophosphatemic progeny had one hypophosphatemic parent. A possible explanation of the four exceptions is discussed later in this section.

5. No hypophosphatemic child had more than one hypophosphatemic parent where both parents were examined.

6. Among the progeny of all hypophosphatemic parents, including both normal and affected persons, the total number of brothers was approximately equal to the total number of sisters (86 males and 92 females. Table 79-2).

7. The total number of *affected* male children was half that of *affected* females (31:61) (Table 65-3). A similar ratio for all affected individuals was 46:100 (Table 79-3).

These results strongly suggest that hypophosphatemia is almost uniformly inherited in this disorder, whereas overt bone disease varies considerably. Hypophosphatemia, then, is an important, but not the sole, determinant of bone disease and provides the best discriminant for identifying the trait.

Repeated sampling may be necessary to establish hypophosphatemia. In several instances involving individuals known from previous observations to have been hypophosphatemic, an initial resurvey did not reestablish this biochemical abnormality, but additional multiple sampling did. Provided the samples were drawn more than 2 h after eating, the frequency of demonstration of a low serum or plasma phosphorus level was as great as in those in whom early morning fasting samples were obtained [94]. The reverse problem of false positives, i.e., a single low serum phosphorus with subsequent normal ones, was encountered much less frequently if the 99 percent confidence limit was observed [104].

These results indicate that transmission is due to an abnormal gene on an X chromosome. In Table 65-2 in the classified progeny of 22 affected fathers, all 28 males were normal, while all 31 females were affected. The chance of this distribution occurring on the basis of an autosomal gene is virtually nil. With an abnormal gene residing on an X chromosome, an affected female is therefore heterozygous (X'X), whereas an affected male lacking the normal allele is hemizygous (X'Y). Since the male progeny of an affected male receive the Y chromosome from their fathers, they would all be normal. On the other hand, the female progeny of an affected male receive the single X' chromosome of the father and are, therefore, all affected. This hypothesis also predicts that half the progeny of an affected female should be normal and half affected, without regard to sex. Data on this point are also shown in Table 79-2.

While the pooled data from the North Carolina and British studies meet the expected ratios with a high degree of significance, they do so because of opposite discrepancies in the two series, especially in respect to the female progeny of affected mothers. Thus, in the former (and larger) series there were almost twice as many normal as affected daughters, whereas only 4 of 20 comparable daughters in Great Britain were normal. There is no satisfactory explanation for these discrepancies.

From the 4 families reported by Graham et al. [13] 33 females were resurveyed in 1963 and 1964 by reexamination and by repeating the serum phosphorous measurements 4 to 7 years after their first classification. In 10 of these, originally

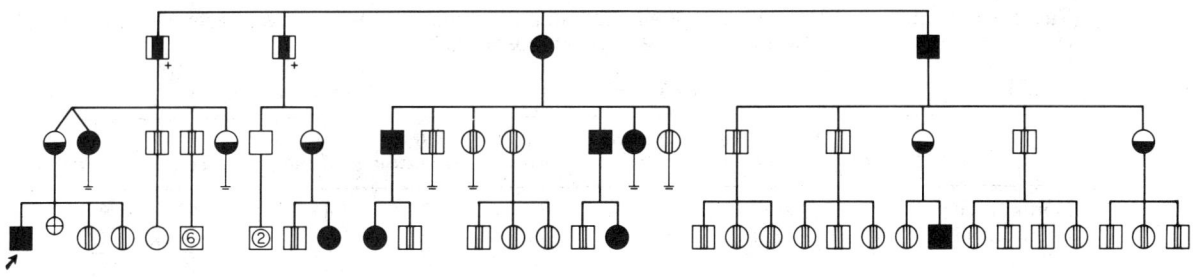

■ *Hypophosphatemia with skeletal disease (examined professionally)*
⬓ *Hypophosphatemia without skeletal disease (examined professionally)*
▯ *Skeletal disease (reliably reported; probably hypophosphatemic)*
▥ *Normophosphatemia and no skeletal disease (examined professionally)*
☐ *Not tested*
+ *Deceased*

Figure 79-7 Portion of original (E) pedigree *[12]*. Note (1) regularity of generation-to-generation transmission, if hypophosphatemia without evidence of skeletal disease is used as a criterion for the presence of the inherited abnormality, and (2) no affected sons but uniformly affected daughters of affected fathers.

normal, there was no change in classification. One child, classified questionably as normal at ages 2 and 3, was found to have hypophosphatemia without evidence of bone disease at age 6. Of 22 hypophosphatemic females without evidence of bone disease, 21 remained hypophosphatemic. The exception was a female classified as hypophosphatemic at age 9 months who was normophosphatemic and clinically normal at age 6 years. It should be noted, in addition, that had single specimens drawn in the field been accepted, 7 of the 22 might have been classified as normal during the resurvey utilizing the curves of Greenberg et al. *[104]* for separating normals from abnormals. Multiple sampling reestablished the presence of hypophosphatemia.

The hypothesis that this trait is transmitted as a single-dose effect by a gene on an X chromosome offers the best explanation of the great majority of the data in other published reports *[17, 143, 176, 192]*. It is possible that some of these were of vitamin D–dependency rickets.

The use of hypophosphatemia as a genetic discriminant has been questioned. Briard-Guillemot et al. *[193]* analyzed 186 subjects from 23 families and concluded that hypophosphatemia was a variable and unreliable index, and that if one based the genetic analysis on bone involvement, the data were compatible with incompletely dominant sex-linked transmission.

In the first kindred studies by Winters et al. *[11, 12]*, a marked difference was observed between heterozygotes and hemizygotes with respect to the severity of bone disease. Hypophosphatemic males nearly always had obvious rickets or postrachitic deformities, while hypophosphatemic females tended to have much less skeletal involvement. In general this difference has been confirmed in the pedigrees subsequently studied *[13, 94]*. Only two males had no demonstrable bone disease. McNair et al. *[13]* have reported no sex difference in severity but their data do not include information about family members with hypophosphatemia alone.

The relative immunity of the female from severe skeletal disease has at least three possible explanations: First, the normal allele may modify the action of the abnormal gene so that the female escapes severe bone disease because of heterozygosity. Second, the relative immunity of the female may be a factor independent of gene dosage. Since there is no proved instance of a homozygous female, this problem remains unresolved. Third, since one of the X chromosomes becomes inactivated, mosaicism and variation in degree of manifestation could result *[194]*.

Table 79-2 Data on 178 classified progeny of hypophosphatemic parents in 21 pedigrees

Pedigree			Classified progeny				
			Male		Female		
Origin	Total	No. of parents	Affected*	Normal	Affected*	Normal	Total
Hypophosphatemic fathers							
North Carolina	5	16	0	19	24	0	43
Great Britain	6	6	0	9	7	0	16
Total	11	22	0	28	31	0	59
Hypophosphatemic mothers							
North Carolina	4	29	21	22	14	27	84
Great Britain	14	16	10	5	16	4	35
Total	18	45	31	27	30	31	119
Grand total	29	67	31	55	61	31	178

* Affected signifies hypophosphatemia with or without skeletal disease. SOURCE: From *[12, 13, 90, 94]*.

Table 79-3 Summary classification of all affected and chemically classified subjects with familial vitamin D–resistant rickets and hypophosphatemia

Pedigree		Hypophosphatemic males			Hypophosphatemic females			
Origin	Total	Bone disease	No bone disease	Total	Bone disease	No bone disease	Total	Grand total
North Carolina	5	30	2	32	19	44	63	95
Great Britain	16	14	0	14	34	3	37	51
Total	21	44	2	46	53	47	100	146

SOURCE: From [12, 13, 90, 94].

Not all cases of vitamin D–resistant rickets are clearly inherited. Sporadic cases could be due to phenocopy, a recessive trait, or new mutations. Winters et al. [195] report one such case and Burnett et al. [94] have described five females and three males in whom the evidence from a fairly extensive study of relatives and sibs indicated that they were the only affected members in their respective kindreds. In the former study an additional four affected mothers, who had borne severely affected children, had apparently normal parents. In two of these repeated examination of the parents and sibs of the affected mother was not possible, and in each of these two there was a possibility that complicating renal disease rendered the normal plasma phosphorus values suspect in the parents. In the two others, a fairly complete survey with resampling of plasma phosphorus was possible.

On the assumption that the last two affected mothers with affected progeny and the eight sporadic cases in the Burnett series were new mutations, rough estimates of mutation rates are possible. For an X-linked gene, the mutation rates per gene per generation were 6.4×10^{-6} and 5.3×10^{-6} for males and females, respectively [94]. These rough estimates are sufficiently similar to those better established in other hereditary diseases to warrant further attempts to ascertain what proportion of sporadic cases represent new mutations.

Differential Diagnosis

The problem of differential diagnosis usually arises in a patient with clinical and chemical evidence of rickets or osteomalacia. Rarely an unexpected finding of asymptomatic hypophosphatemia may be the clue to identifying a new family with this disorder, a step which may have considerable preventive value for potentially affected children.

In general the diagnosis of familial hypophosphatemic (vitamin D–resistant) rickets is arrived at by: (1) a family history of rickets, bony abnormalities, or short stature; (2) a family survey showing hypophosphatemia in members of several generations; and (3) evidence of hypophosphatemia with or without bone disease or short stature or both.

In cases where a new mutant appears or a family survey cannot be done in an infant or young child with rickets, the following may help differentiate this condition from vitamin D–deficient and vitamin D–dependent rickets.

1. The plasma PTH is normal in X-linked hypophosphatemia but usually high in both other states.

2. Often associated with the secondary hyperparathyroidism in these other two conditions is a generalized aminoaciduria or a hyperglycinuria and an increase in urinary cAMP excretion.

3. The plasma 25-(OH)D$_3$ concentration is normal in hypophosphatemic rickets but decreased in the other two.

4. Hypocalcemia and tetany or convulsions do not occur in untreated X-linked patients but are common in both vitamin D–deficiency and vitamin-dependency rickets.

5. Treatment with small (in vitamin D–deficient rickets) or moderate (in vitamin D–dependent rickets) doses of vitamin D leads to a significant rise in plasma phosphate concentration in the other forms, but even massive doses of vitamin D do not restore the plasma phosphate concentration to normal in patients with the X-linked condition.

6. On bone biopsy there is little or no increase in percent of active resorption surface in hypophosphatemic rickets, but there is an increase in both vitamin D–dependent and vitamin D–deficient rickets, in keeping with the presence of secondary hyperparathyroidism in these latter states [23].

As noted earlier in "Pathogenesis," hypophosphatemic rickets, which is indistinguishable clinically, radiologically, and biochemically from the familial X-linked form, may occur in magnesium deficiency [196] and may also occur in association with mesenchymal tumors [185–191]. This last usually results in an adult-onset hypophosphatemic osteomalacia, but at least one case in a child has been described. In these instances the most important information in arriving at the correct diagnosis is a thorough family survey. In searching for other hypophosphatemic family members it is necessary to obtain several blood samples for plasma phosphate analysis from each member. These samples should be obtained preferably in the fasting state or at least 2.5 h after a meal.

At present it is not possible to diagnose reliably by amniocentesis the condition in an affected fetus. As noted before, the plasma phosphate concentration may be normal or low at birth in affected individuals, and a normal plasma phosphate concentration may be found during the first several months of life in individuals who then go on to develop hypophosphatemia, short stature, and rickets.

Treatment

Until recently the cornerstone of treatment of this condition was large doses of vitamin D, 10,000 to 25,000 units/day for infants and up to 300,000 units/day for older children [95–99, 197]. The general results of this mode of therapy have been: (1) no significant effect upon plasma phosphate concentration; (2) usually a significant, although often not complete, healing of rickets; (3) probably a reduced need for, but not the elimination of, osteotomies of tibia or femora to correct bowing; (4) little evidence of improved growth rate; and (5) a significant danger of one or more episodes of vitamin D intoxication with resultant hypercalcemia and renal damage. Treatment with 25-(OH)D$_3$ does not appear to offer any advantage over therapy with the parent vitamin.

All studies in which long-term observations have been made emphasize the failure of vitamin D therapy [12, 16, 95–99, 143, 173, 175, 197] to cure the disease and the serious problem of recurrent vitamin D intoxication and renal damage. Regardless of the diligence and care in administering such therapy, the likelihood is great that in a 10- to 16-year span of therapy nearly every individual will experience at least one episode of intoxication, or if given small doses of vitamin D will experience little therapeutic benefit.

With the advance in our knowledge of this condition, more and more emphasis has been placed upon the importance of phosphate deficiency in the pathogenesis of the rickets and in the decreased rate of skeletal growth (see "Pathogenesis" in this chapter). With this change in emphasis has come a change in therapeutic strategy. The use of oral neutral phosphate has become the cornerstone of therapy [12, 93, 198–200]. To be effective this must be administered at frequent intervals throughout the day. Practically, this is best given in five divided doses at approximately 3.5 to 4.0-h intervals with a total dose of 1 to 4 g/day phosphorus. With this regimen the plasma phosphate concentration can usually be elevated into the normal or low normal range for a significant portion of the day. A major complication of this treatment program is the development of secondary hyperparathyroidism. In a group of six untreated subjects, ranging in age from 3 to 12 years, five of the six showed significant and persistent elevation of plasma immunoreactive parathyroid hormone concentration (iPTH) when given phosphate therapy alone for 6 months [115].

Recent reports indicate that combined therapy with oral phosphate and 1,25-(OH)$_2$D$_3$ is a more effective, and safer, form of therapy than vitamin D and phosphate. Glorieux et al. [118] reported a comparison of vitamin D plus phosphate versus 1,25-(OH)$_2$D$_3$ plus phosphate in 11 patients. They found that with vitamin D plus phosphate mineralization of the growth plate occurred but mineralization of endosteal bone was still greatly impaired. Treatment with 1,25-(OH)$_2$D$_3$ plus phosphate improved both. Treatment with 1,25-(OH)$_2$D$_3$ plus phosphate caused a sustained increase in mean plasma phosphate concentration and an enhanced intestinal absorption of phosphate. In endosteal bone, 1,25-(OH)$_2$D$_3$ administration was associated with a return of the mineralization front to normal and a marked decrease in mean osteoid thickness. Drezner and coworkers reported [180] on the administration of 1,25-(OH)$_2$D$_3$ in doses of 2.25 to 3.00 μg to four patients with X-linked hypophosphatemic rickets. They found increased serum phosphate concentrations, an increase in Tm$_P$/GFR, a fall in alkaline phosphatase activity, and a marked positive balance of both calcium and phosphate with a fall in plasma iPTH. Nonetheless, quantitative morphometric analysis of bone biopsy material in these patients showed that despite the return of the mineralization front to normal, the extent of the osteoid surface did not change, and the osteoid seam width remained increased. These data indicate, therefore, that neither vitamin D$_3$ plus phosphate nor 1,25-(OH)$_2$D$_3$ alone is as effective as a combination of 1,25-(OH)$_2$D$_3$ plus phosphate in the treatment of this disease.

This conclusion is supported by the results of Chan et al. [159]. They treated six patients with combined phosphate and 1,25-(OH)$_2$D$_3$. They found an increase in mean serum phosphate concentration without a change in Tm$_P$/GFR, resulting

from a significant increase in the absorption of both calcium and phosphate. Therapy led to an accelerated growth rate associated with a markedly positive balance of both calcium and phosphate and radiographic evidence of healing of the rickets.

The longest evaluation of combined therapy is that reported by Rasmussen et al. [115] in nine patients treated for a period of 4 to 6 years. All had positive therapeutic responses as judged by radiographic evidence of healing of the rickets, restoration and maintenance of normal growth rates (Fig. 79-5), decrease in plasma alkaline phosphatase activity, and histological evidence of healing of osteomalacia.

The possible problems and complications of this form of therapy have also been discussed [115]. Treatment with phosphate alone can lead to secondary hyperparathyroidism, which may be a particular problem in patients with a history of previous episodes of vitamin D intoxication. Conversely, treatment with 1,25-(OH)$_2$D$_3$ alone can lead to hypercalciuria, hypercalcemia, and reduced creatinine clearance. Hypercalciuria usually develops before hypercalcemia. In employing the two agents, it is necessary to balance their actions so that hyperparathyroidism on the one hand and hypercalciuria on the other are avoided. Our present approach is to begin phosphate therapy and a small dose of 1,25-(OH)$_2$D$_3$ (0.25 to 50 μg/day). Then after 3 weeks we reassess parathyroid function and measure fasting calcium excretion on a spot urine (urinary calcium concentration times serum creatinine/plasma calcium concentration). A normal value is below 0.25 and in untreated subjects is usually below 0.05. If it is below 0.25, the dose of 1,25-(OH)$_2$D$_3$ is increased progressively until parathyroid function is normal and fasting calcium excretion is in the vicinity of 0.25.

There is less experience with combined therapy in adults with this disease, but the results to date suggest that this therapy can be effective in treating the osteomalacia found in these subjects. It is not yet known whether lifelong therapy is necessary.

Preventive Measures

Once the mode of inheritance of the trait has been determined in a particular family (and this will be X-linked dominant in almost all instances), the affected individuals and their spouses should be fully informed of the nature of the transmission of the gene as well as the chances and probable consequences of having a child with the disease. Potentially affected progeny of such a mating should then be studied as early as practicable in order to establish the genotype, with the aim of early institution of therapy to prevent serious degrees of deformity. As already noted, the detection of hypophosphatemia is difficult in the young infant. The diagnosis can be made or excluded with confidence only by obtaining multiple determinations throughout at least the first year of life.

HYPOPHOSPHATEMIC NONRACHITIC BONE DISEASE

In 1977, Scriver and his associates [22] reported a new syndrome of hypophosphatemic nonrachitic bone disease (HBD) associated with persistent hypophosphatemia but distinct from X-linked hypophosphatemic rickets. In five patients an autosomal disorder of renal tubular phosphate handling was associated with hypophosphatemia, osteomalacia with minimal rickets during growth, and a moderate reduction in skeletal growth. Growth retardation and bone disease were both less severe than in patients with the X-linked disease even though the plasma phosphate concentrations were in the same low range in both groups of patients. Metabolic studies in patients with HBD disclosed a normal percent TRP in the fasting state, which is clearly different from patients with the X-linked disease. Also, HBD patients had a normal phosphaturic response to PTH under conditions in which the X-linked patients have a blunted response. Nevertheless, the patients with HBD had a reduced Tm_P/GFR. In a subsequent report, Scriver et al. [181] described additional studies in a 39-month-old female with this disorder in whom administration of 1,25-$(OH)_2D_3$ in a dose of 1 μg/day led to healing of the bone disease, a rise of both plasma phosphate concentration and Tm_P/GFR to normal, and an enhanced rate of growth. This therapeutic response is quite different than in X-linked patients treated with comparable doses of 1,25-$(OH)_2D_3$. The 39-month-old female had a normal plasma 1,25-$(OH)_2D_3$ concentration (30 pg/ml). It is possible that 1,25-$(OH)_2D_3$ therapy in this patient was effective because it reduced plasma PTH levels and hence improved phosphate retention. The father of this subject also had hypophosphatemia but was without radiological or histological evidence of bone disease. Treatment with 1,25-$(OH)_2D_3$ did not correct either the hypophosphatemia or the reduced Tm_P/GFR in the father. Scriver et al. [181] suggest that the component of phosphate transport responsive to sex hormones (renal phosphate reabsorption declines after puberty) may be involved in this differential responsiveness.

These authors point out that it is important to distinguish these patients from those with the X-linked disease because HBD patients can apparently be treated effectively with 1,25-$(OH)_2D_3$ alone and do not require supplemental phosphate.

VITAMIN D–DEPENDENT RICKETS

Vitamin D–dependent rickets was first segregated from other forms of rickets by Fraser and Salter [16] in 1958 and by Prader et al. [17] in 1961. This form of rickets is type III,A,ii in the classification of Fraser and Salter and is also known as *hereditary pseudo-vitamin D–deficiency rickets* (PDR) [147, 201–208], *hypocalcemic, hypophosphatemic rickets with aminoaciduria*, and *autosomal recessive vitamin D–deficiency* (ARVDD) [17–21, 116, 209–213].

Vitamin D–dependent rickets has been categorized into two groups, type I and type II. The clinical features and most of the biochemical findings of the two entities are similar, but the two differ in that the circulating 1,25-$(OH)_2D$ levels are depressed in type I and elevated in type II.

Vitamin D–dependent Rickets Type I

The clinical course of vitamin D–dependent rickets type I is similar to that of ordinary rickets due to vitamin D–deficiency [17–20, 201–203, 209, 210]. The patients appear healthy at

birth. The onset of symptoms is usually within the first year of life and may occur as early as the second to fourth months of age. Hypotonia, weakness, and growth failure are common manifestations. Motor retardation may become apparent with poor head control and failure to stand or walk. Often there is a history of convulsions or tetany, and in some children this may be the presenting clinical feature. Rarely there may be anemia and respiratory difficulties. Pathologic fractures may occur and be the presenting feature. A history of an adequate intake of vitamin D is usually obtained (see Table 79-1 for a comparison of vitamin D–deficient, vitamin D–dependent, and vitamin D–resistant rickets).

Physical examination reveals a small, hypotonic child with signs similar to those found in children with vitamin D–deficient rickets. Included are thickening of the wrists and ankles, frontal bossing with a wide anterior fontanel, rachitic rosary, bony deformities including bowing, and Trousseau and Chvostek signs.

Roentgenograms of the skeleton show classic rickets that may vary in severity from mild to florid changes that are indistinguishable from vitamin D–deficiency rickets. Early abnormalities, which are best visualized in the distal ends of the radius and ulna, include rarefaction, irregular fraying of the provisional zone of calcification, and metaphyseal concavity and widening. Changes in the shaft may not be evident when changes in the metaphyses are first detected, but rarefaction and coarse trabeculation of the shaft usually appear a few weeks later.

The radiologic signs of more advanced stages are similar to those in the early stage, but are more marked. The shadow of the provisional zone of calcification is absent, and the rachitic metaphyses are partially or completely absent; the visible portion of the calcified shaft is therefore shortened longitudinally, and the space between the visible end of the shaft and the epiphyseal ossification center is increased. There may be signs of pathologic or healed fractures.

In contrast to vitamin D–resistant rickets, x-ray evidence of active rickets of spine and pelvis is frequent in vitamin D–dependent rickets type I (see Table 79-1). The enamel of teeth that develop postnatally may be defective [21, 208, 213]. Also, some patients, if not treated early, may have irreversible mental retardation.

Biochemical and Physiologic Studies Hypocalcemia is a cardinal feature of vitamin D–dependent rickets. Plasma calcium concentrations below 8.0 mg/dl are common. The hypocalcemia may give rise to convulsions and tetany and may be present before there is radiographic evidence of rickets. Plasma parathyroid hormone titer is elevated [21, 212, 213]. Urinary calcium content is low, while fecal calcium is high. Metabolic studies have demonstrated grossly impaired intestinal transport of calcium in vitamin D–dependent rickets type I [201, 203, 205, 209]. The intestinal transport of magnesium has been reported normal [209] and reduced [214]. No abnormalities have been demonstrated in the duodenal mucosa by either light or electron microscopy [209].

The plasma phosphate level may be normal or low. Hypophosphatemia, when present, is usually of lesser degree than in vitamin D–resistant rickets. Nonetheless, plasma phosphate levels below 2.2 mg/dl have been reported in a few patients with vitamin D–dependent rickets type I. The net intestinal absorption and retention of phosphate may be reduced to a variable degree [209, 214]. Urinary phosphate excretion is increased when expressed as milligrams phosphate per milligram creatinine [214] or when the 24-h urinary phosphate is examined in relation to serum phosphate concentration. Decreased renal tubular reabsorption of phosphate [21, 204, 213] and of amino acids may be present and has been attributed to an increase in circulating parathyroid hormone [21]. Normal values for renal tubular reabsorption of phosphate [213], phosphate clearance [202], and phosphate excretion index [205, 215] have also been reported.

The plasma alkaline phosphatase level is consistently elevated. As a result of hypocalcemia the circulating level of parathyroid hormone is elevated [21, 212, 213] and probably accounts for the generalized aminoaciduria [202, 210, 216–218] and elevated levels of urinary cAMP [213, 214] that may be found in patients with vitamin D–dependent rickets type I. Increased urinary cAMP is not a consistent finding, and normal levels have been observed in some patients with elevated circulating parathyroid hormone levels [213].

As in vitamin D–deficiency rickets, mild acidosis with hyperchloremia may be observed in vitamin D–dependent rickets.

The calcemic response to parathyroid hormone is usually but not necessarily [214] absent or markedly reduced in vitamin D–dependent rickets type I [202, 206, 208, 215]. This is consistent with the diminished responsiveness of bone to parathyroid hormone that is observed in vitamin D deficiency.

The phosphaturic response to parathyroid hormone is usually impaired [203, 205, 213, 218], although a normal response may be observed [17]. There is limited information regarding the response of urinary cAMP to parathyroid hormone in vitamin D–dependent rickets type I. In two studies in which measurements were made on eight patients, the administration of parathyroid hormone elicited a significant increase in urinary cAMP without a parallel increase in urinary phosphate. In one of the studies the urinary cAMP response to parathyroid hormone was greater and in the other it was less than that observed in the same patients after treatment with 25-(OH)D [214] and 1,25-(OH)$_2$D [213], respectively. The basal levels of urinary cAMP and phosphate were either normal or increased, and, in those patients in whom measurements were made, serum parathyroid hormone levels were elevated [213]. The significance of these observations is uncertain. In vitamin D–deficient rats the urinary cAMP and phosphaturic responses to parathyroid hormone are both impaired [219].

Pathogenesis The clinical and nearly all of the biochemical abnormalities of vitamin D–dependent rickets type I are similar, if not identical, to those of vitamin D–deficient rickets. Both conditions are characterized by hypotonia, muscle weakness, hypocalcemia, convulsions, severe rickets, and growth failure (Table 79-1). These often develop during the first year of life. In both conditions there is evidence of impaired gastrointestinal absorption of calcium. The hypocalcemia is associated with secondary hyperparathyroidism, as shown by elevated plasma immunoreactive parathyroid hormone levels and increased urinary excretion of AMP and amino acids. In both conditions the plasma alkaline phosphatase level is elevated, the plasma phosphate concentration may be normal or moderately depressed, and mild acidosis may be present. The biochemical and clinical manifestations, including growth retardation, are completely reversible in both conditions following treatment with vitamin D, the difference being that pharmacological doses of vitamin D (10 to 300 times the normal require-

ment) are needed to maintain biochemical and radiological healing in patients with vitamin D–dependent rickets type I.

By contrast, there are distinct differences (summarized in Table 79-1) in both the clinical course and the biochemical abnormalities between vitamin D–dependent and vitamin D–resistant rickets (X-linked hypophosphatemia). Unequivocal biochemical and clinical abnormalities may not be seen until the end of the first year or during the second year of life in individuals with X-linked hypophosphatemia. The general condition of such children is good, with normal motor development and absence of muscle hypotonia. Growth retardation and hypophosphatemia are prominent, and both may persist in spite of vitamin D therapy that is adequate for healing of rickets. The plasma calcium level is nearly always within the normal range, and the serum parathyroid hormone level is usually normal or slightly increased (at least in the absence of phosphate therapy). Finally, treatment of X-linked hypophosphatemia with massive doses of vitamin D does not lead to complete healing of the rickets or reestablishment of a normal growth rate (see "Familial Hypophosphatemic Rickets" earlier in this chapter).

Studies of circulating vitamin D metabolites have provided insight into the pathogenesis of vitamin D–dependent rickets type I. Earlier studies demonstrated normal levels of antirachitic activity, as measured by bioassay, in the serum of untreated patients [209, 215]. In more recent studies serum 25-(OH)D levels were normal in untreated patients and elevated in patients receiving therapeutic doses of vitamin D$_3$ (or D$_2$) or 25-(OH)D$_3$ [202, 209, 210, 212, 213]. These results indicate that the intestinal absorption of vitamin D and the production of 25-(OH)D by the liver are not impaired in vitamin D–dependent rickets.

The most significant finding is that circulating levels of 1,25-(OH)$_2$D are low in untreated patients with vitamin D–dependent rickets type I [213, 220, 221]. This observation suggests a defect in the 1-hydroxylase enzyme. In keeping with this hypothesis are the observations that pharmacological doses of vitamin D$_3$ or D$_2$ and 25-(OH)D$_3$ are required to achieve a therapeutic effect in this disorder, while minute, presumably physiologic, amounts of 1,25-(OH)$_2$D$_3$ promote healing of the rachitic lesions and normalization of the biochemical abnormalities [208, 222, 223]. The relative daily doses required to promote healing in two separate studies were (1) 1250 to 2500 μg D$_3$, 200 to 900 μg 25-(OH)D$_3$, and 1 μg 1,25-(OH)$_2$D$_3$; (2) 1000 μg D$_3$, 125 μg 25-(OH)D$_3$; and 1 μg 1,25-(OH)$_2$D$_3$ [210, 222]. The accumulated evidence suggests, therefore, that in vitamin D–dependent rickets type I there is a genetic defect in 25-hydroxylcholecalciferol 1-α-hydroxylase, the enzyme responsible for the conversion of 25-(OH)D to 1,25-(OH)$_2$D.

Serum 1,25-(OH)$_2$D levels remain low or low-normal in D–dependency type I patients successfully treated with vitamin D$_3$ (or D$_2$) or 25-(OH)D$_3$ [116, 212, 220]. These patients have normal serum calcium and phosphorus levels, elevated serum 25-(OH)D levels, and no evidence of active rickets [116, 210, 212]. Moreover, at least in patients treated with 25-(OH)D$_3$, the serum 24,25-(OH)$_2$D level is high [212]. It is uncertain whether elevated circulating levels of 25-(OH)D, 24,25-(OH)$_2$D, or possibly of an unspecified metabolite of vitamin D are responsible for the normal phenotype in these treated patients or whether the low level of 1,25-(OH)$_2$D meets their physiologic requirement for the hormone [116].

Delvin et al. [213] observed that the serum levels of 1,25-

(OH)$_2$D were directly related to the serum concentration of 25-(OH)D in D–dependency type I patients, either untreated or treated with vitamin D. This observation, coupled with the consistent findings of detectable, albeit low, levels of serum 1,25-(OH)$_2$D, indicates that renal 1-α-hydroxylase is not totally absent in D–dependency rickets type I and that the mutation affects its structural integrity, resulting in a modification of its kinetics [213].

As mentioned earlier, D–dependent rickets type I does not become clinically manifest in the neonatal period. Prader et al. [208] had the opportunity to follow an infant from a family with presumed vitamin D–dependent rickets. At birth the infant was normal and was given a routine prophylactic dose of 800 IU of vitamin D daily. The first findings, hyperaminoaciduria and unresponsiveness of serum calcium to intramuscular parathyroid hormone, was observed at 2 months of age. Rickets developed at 4 months, and pharmacologic doses of vitamin D$_3$ were started at 5 months of age. Since it is assumed that the metabolic defect is present at birth, there must be a mechanism that protects the affected fetus and newborn from developing hypocalcemia and rickets. One possibility is the placental transfer of 1,25-(OH)$_2$D from the mother to the fetus [208].

Genetics Vitamin D–dependent rickets type I is inherited as a simple autosomal recessive trait [19, 147, 202]. The mutant gene permits an attenuated response to vitamin D, since normal mineral balance may be maintained in the affected homozygote with 10 to 300 times the normal dose of vitamin D$_2$ or vitamin D$_3$. As discussed earlier, the available evidence, including the presence of low but detectable levels of circulating 1,25-(OH)$_2$D [213, 220, 221], suggests that the apparent deficient activity of renal 25-(OH)D$_3$ 1-α-hydroxylase only partially impairs the synthesis of 1,25-(OH)$_2$D$_3$. No phenotypic signs have been observed in presumed obligate heterozygotes [21].

The incidence of parental consanguinity has been noted to be relatively high in vitamin D–dependent rickets type I [202]. A similar hereditary autosomal recessive disease has been described in pigs [224, 225].

Treatment Vitamin D–dependent rickets type I responds to vitamin D in an appropriate daily dose. The biochemical and clinical abnormalities regress, and normal linear growth is restored. The dose of vitamin D required for adequate treatment varies but usually ranges from 20,000 (500 μg vitamin D) to 100,000 (2500 μg) IU/day. Some patients may require as little as 2500 IU/day and others as much as 150,000 IU/day [14, 21, 208, 209, 211, 215]. The need for relatively large amounts of vitamin D persists throughout childhood and probably for the patient's lifetime.

There have been several reports of the use of 25-(OH)D$_3$ as a therapeutic agent in vitamin D–dependent rickets type I [206, 208, 211, 212, 222, 226]. Balsan et al. [212] made sequential measurements of vitamin D metabolites in two children with vitamin D–dependent rickets type I while they were receiving 500 to 1000 μg of 25-(OH)D$_3$ daily. The children were studied more than 1 year after their skeletal abnormalities had been cured. With continued 25-(OH)D$_3$ therapy over 2½ to 3 years, the serum 25-(OH)D levels were consistently elevated, the serum 24,25-(OH)$_2$D levels were usually elevated, while the serum 1,25-(OH)$_2$D levels were usually in the low-normal range. When 25-(OH)D treatment was discontinued, the

serum calcium fell, the serum parathyroid hormone increased, the serum 25-(OH)D and 24,25-(OH)$_2$D levels rapidly decreased to normal, while the levels of 1,25-(OH)$_2$D remained low-normal and were similar to the levels observed during 25-(OH)D therapy. On the basis of this observation, the authors suggested that the therapeutic action of high doses of 25-(OH)D$_3$ may be related partly, if not totally, to the maintenance of high serum concentrations of 25-(OH)D or 24,25-(OH)$_2$D or both. Published studies suggest that on a weight basis 25-(OH)D$_3$ may be 3 to 8 times more potent than vitamin D in the treatment of vitamin D–dependent rickets/type I [222, 226]. Doses of 100 to 1000 μg/day of 25-(OH)D$_3$ have been reported to result in clinical, biochemical, and radiologic recovery as well as catch-up growth.

1-α-(OH)D$_3$, an analogue of 1,25-(OH)$_2$D$_3$, is effective in the treatment of vitamin D–dependent rickets type I. Excellent results have been reported on the use of oral 1-α-(OH)D$_3$ in doses of 1 to 3 μg/day [208, 210]. The serum calcium increased within 48 h, while the serum phosphate rose slightly later. The alkaline phosphatase activity fell promptly, and rachitic lesions were healed after 7 to 9 weeks of treatment. Balsan et al. [223] also reported good results in treatment of vitamin D–dependent rickets type I with 1-α-(OH)D$_3$, but the required dose in some patients was 4 to 8 μg/day.

Treatment with 1,25-(OH)$_2$D$_3$ seems to be the optimal program in patients with D–dependent rickets type I. Small doses of 1,25-(OH)$_2$D$_3$ have been effective in this disorder [208, 213, 222, 223]. Doses of 1 to 2 μg/day usually produce a prompt rise in serum calcium and phosphate levels. The rise in serum calcium and phosphate is associated with an increase in calcium absorption and increases in calcium and phosphorus balances. The most extensive study of long-term treatment with 1,25-(OH)$_2$D$_3$ is that reported by Delvin et al. [213]. They treated nine children for periods ranging from 4 to 27 months, initially with 0.5 to 1.0 μg/day.

In several the dose was increased to 2 or 3 μg/day because of a lack of biochemical response. Normalization of serum calcium, phosphorus, alkaline phosphatase, and serum immunoreactive parathyroid hormone occurred in all by 4 to 5 months and as early as 1 month after initiation of treatment. Radiologic and histologic improvement paralleled the biochemical improvement. Careful monitoring of the biochemical variables was essential since the 1,25-(OH)$_2$D$_3$ requirements frequently varied during the course of treatment. The dose was reduced after healing or if hypercalcemia supervened. The maintenance doses varied from 0.25 to 2.0 μg/day. During treatment the serum 1,25-(OH)$_2$D levels increased from low to normal or modestly elevated values, while serum 25-(OH)D decreased, frequently from high values (reflecting prior vitamin D therapy) to normal or near-normal values.

A particularly interesting observation made by Nguyen et al. [63] was that patients with type I rickets given 1,25-(OH)$_2$D$_3$ showed a marked rise in plasma 24,25-(OH)$_2$D$_3$ levels. This was followed by a slowly progressive fall in 24,25-(OH)$_2$D$_3$ levels over a period of several months of continuous 1,25-(OH)$_2$D$_3$ treatment, roughly correlated with a progressive fall in plasma alkaline phosphatase activity. These results demonstrate the dynamic nature of plasma 24,25-(OH)$_2$D$_3$ concentration and raise the possibility that this rise in plasma 24,25-(OH)$_2$D$_3$ concentration plays an important role in the positive therapeutic response.

Dihydrotachysterol has a hydroxyl group in position 3 and is rotated 180°, and so this hydroxyl occupies a position analogous to position 1 in 1,25-(OH)$_2$D$_3$. For this reason it was thought that dihydrotachysterol might be of value in treatment of vitamin D–dependent rickets type I. It was, however, found not to be effective in the low-microgram dose range and, therefore, is not equivalent to the 1-α-hydroxy metabolites [208, 210].

Vitamin D–dependent Rickets Type II

The term *vitamin D–dependent rickets type II* has been ascribed to a recently recognized disorder in which the clinical, radiologic, and most of the biochemical findings are similar to those found in vitamin D–dependent rickets type I, but in which the circulating levels of 1,25-(OH)$_2$D are elevated rather than depressed [227]. The increased level of circulating 1,25-(OH)$_2$D is thought to reflect end-organ refractoriness to this metabolite. The clinical features that occur in common with the type I disorder include hypotonia, muscle weakness, growth failure, convulsions, and the bony deformities of classic vitamin D–deficiency rickets. The biochemical findings that occur in common include hypocalcemia, hypophosphatemia, elevated serum alkaline phosphatase activity, elevated serum immunoreactive parathyroid hormone, and increased urinary excretion of amino acids and cAMP. A feature that appears to be unique to vitamin D–dependent rickets type II, in relation to other forms of rickets, is alopecia totalis, which has been reported in several kindreds [212, 228–231]. Because of certain differences as well as incomplete knowledge at this time, vitamin D–dependent rickets type II with and without alopecia will be discussed separately.

Vitamin D–dependent Rickets Type II with Alopecia

Ten patients from five families have been reported with rickets and alopecia totalis [212, 228–231]. Biopsy of the scalp in one patient revealed findings typical of alopecia totalis, with no abnormal lymphocytic infiltration [228]. In six of the patients rickets was noted between 4 and 16 months of age. Three patients, all sibs, died at 2 years of age with severe hypocalcemia and rachitic pneumopathy. The age of onset of rickets was not reported [212]. In one patient widening of the wrists and ankles was observed at birth [230], but x-rays were not obtained until 18 months of age when the diagnosis of rickets was made. The possible occurrence of rickets at birth in vitamin D–dependent rickets type II is in contrast to the findings in vitamin D–dependent rickets type I, where no evidence of rickets at birth has been reported. Alopecia was reported to be congenital in 5 (4 sibs) of the 10 reported cases [212, 230], while in the others alopecia was noted between 4 and 16 months of age at the time when rickets was diagnosed [228, 230, 231].

The serum calcium levels (total or ionized) were low except in one patient who was receiving pharmacologic doses of vitamin D [228]. The serum phosphorus levels were normal or low except for one patient who had high levels [229]. Because of additional biochemical and clinical differences, this patient will be considered separately a little later. The serum alkaline-phosphatase activities and immunoreactive parathyroid hormone levels were elevated. Urinary cAMP and amino acids were increased. In three of four patients tested calcemic, renal phosphate, and AMP responses to parathyroid hormones were elicited.

The circulating 1,25-(OH)$_2$D levels were consistently high

and ranged from 140 to 745 pg/ml. The serum 25-(OH)D levels were normal in the untreated state. In the one patient in whom serum 24,25-(OH)$_2$D was measured in the untreated state, undetectable levels were obtained on multiple occasions [229].

The patient with the low serum 24,25-(OH)$_2$D levels is the same patient who had an elevated serum phosphorus level and who is different from the other patients with rickets and alopecia. At the time of study, this patient, a 13-year-old girl with a history of rickets since infancy, was receiving calcium supplementation but no vitamin D preparation. Her karyotype was normal. She had bilateral cataracts and in the presence of severe hypocalcemia (5.4 to 6.0 mg/dl) and hyperphosphatemia (7.2 to 7.6 mg/dl) had normal or only slightly increased (values not given) serum immunoreactive parathyroid hormone levels. Basal levels of urinary cAMP were only slightly elevated, and, unlike the other patients, hyperaminoaciduria was not present. Brisk calcemic, phosphaturic, and renal cAMP responses to parathyroid hormone were elicited. The laboratory findings suggest that parathyroid hormone secretion, although present, was impaired.

Of the five families reported with alopecia and rickets, consanguinity was present in four, with marriage between first cousins in three and second cousins in one. In the fifth family an aunt was reported to have rickets, but no further details were given. Both males and females are affected, and normal sibs are reported. These findings, including the high incidence of consanguinity, suggest that the defect is transmitted as an autosomal recessive trait.

In comparison with patients with D–dependent rickets type I, patients with D–dependent rickets type II with alopecia are resistant to treatment with pharmocological doses of vitamin D preparations. Thus, there was little or no response to: (1) 50,000 to 1,200,000 IU of vitamin D per day [228–230], (2) 0.8 to 8.0 μg of oral 1,25-(OH)$_2$D$_3$ per day [229–231], (3) 20 μg of intravenous 1,25-(OH)$_2$D per day [229], and (4) 2 mg of A.T.10 per day [229].

In one patient 7 million IU of vitamin D per day restored serum calcium to normal and brought about marked improvement in skeletal radiographs [231]. While on this therapy, the serum 25-(OH)D, 1,25-(OH)$_2$D, and 24,25-(OH)$_2$D levels were 4250, 4.8, and 35 ng/ml. Even with these high serum levels of vitamin D metabolites, the intestinal calcium absorption remained in the lower normal range, and urinary calcium excretion was decidedly low.

There is only one report of treatment of a patient with D–dependent rickets type II with alopecia with 25-(OH)D$_3$ [212]. This patient had previously not responded to 8 μg of 1,25-(OH)$_2$D per day. At doses of 750 to 1500 μg of 25-(OH)D$_3$ there was only partial improvement in the biochemical abnormalities in spite of the fact that the serum levels of 25-(OH)D, 24,25-(OH)$_2$D, and 1,25-(OH)$_2$D were elevated. When this same patient was treated with 5 to 10 μg of 1-α-(OH)D$_3$ per day, there were normalization of the biochemical abnormalities and healing of the bone lesions. This patient, then, had no improvement with 1,25-(OH)$_2$D$_3$, a partial response to 25-(OH)D$_3$, and an excellent response to 1-α-(OH)D$_3$. There appeared to be no correlation between the clinical responses and the circulating levels of 25-(OH)D, 24,25-(OH)$_2$D, and 1,25-(OH)$_2$D that were achieved by the various therapeutic regimens in this patient [212]. In one other patient who received 8.0 μg of 1-α-(OH)D$_3$ per day, there was no improvement [229].

In two patients who failed to heal with 50,000 units of vitamin D daily and 8.0 µg of 1,25-(OH)$_2$D daily, the oral administration of 1.5 g of phosphorus per day led to healing of the rickets with no significant change in serum calcium and parathyroid hormone level, and with only a slight increase in serum phosphate in one of the two patients who initially had a slightly low serum phosphate level [228].

In the patient with low circulating 24,25-(OH)$_2$D levels previously described [229], there was no response to 1,200,000 units of vitamin D, 2 mg of A.T.10 per day, or 5 to 20 µg of 1,25-(OH)$_2$D per day. Treatment with 5 to 10 g of calcium gluconate per day led to healing of the rachitic lesions, but the serum calcium levels remained low. Treatment of this patient with 2 µg of 24,25-(OH)$_2$D$_3$ per day normalized serum calcium, in association with an increase in serum 24,25-(OH)$_2$D and a decrease in serum 1,25-(OH)$_2$D$_3$.

Because of the lack of uniformity in the therapeutic trials reported to date, it is not possible to outline a form of treatment for an individual patient with D–resistant rickets type II with alopecia. It would appear that these patients are resistant to pharmacologic doses of vitamin D preparations, 25-(OH)D$_3$ and 1,25-(OH)$_2$D$_3$. Improvement was observed in one patient who received phosphate supplements, in another who received calcium supplements and subsequently 24,25-(OH)$_2$D$_3$, and in a third who received 1-α-(OH)D$_3$. Further studies are needed to formulate a consistent therapeutic approach to this problem.

Vitamin D–dependent Rickets Type II without Alopecia Three patients from two kindreds have been described with this entity [232, 233]. The clinical and radiologic features were similar to those of the other forms of D–dependent rickets discussed previously. Although the onset of rickets was detected between 5 and 24 months of age, studies of the vitamin D metabolites were carried out when the patients were young adults and after therapy with pharmacologic doses of vitamin D had been discontinued for 3 to 18 months. In all patients there were hypocalcemia, hypophosphatemia, elevated serum alkaline phosphatase, elevated immunoreactive parathyroid hormone, hyperaminoaciduria, and increased urinary cAMP and hydroxyproline. The serum 1,25-(OH)$_2$D levels were elevated in all, ranging from 212 to 280 pg/ml. The serum 25-(OH)D levels were normal, as was the 24,25-(OH)$_2$D level, which was measured in only one patient. In the presence of elevated serum 1,25-(OH)$_2$D and immunoreactive parathyroid hormone levels, the intestinal absorption of calcium was depressed.

During childhood all the patients without alopecia appeared to respond clinically and radiologically to vitamin D in dosages that ranged from 5000 to 40,000 IU/day. In one patient 1,500,000 IU of ergocalciferol was administered IM weekly for 5 months during the second year of life. This produced healing of the rickets, and thereafter the child was successfully maintained on 5000 to 20,000 IU of vitamin D daily by mouth. Upon discontinuation of pharmacologic amounts of vitamin D, relapses occurred in all. In two patients in whom vitamin D therapy was discontinued for varying periods of time during childhood, the adult stature was at or below the first percentile [232].

One of the three patients was maintained on 40,000 IU of vitamin D daily until 18 years of age, when treatment was stopped [232]. At that time she had inactive rickets with only mild bowing. After an uneventful pregnancy at age 20, she had

a relapse with progressive worsening of symptoms until age 27, when she was found to have biochemical, radiologic, and histomorphological evidence of osteomalacia. Whereas she had responded to 40,000 IU of vitamin D per day during childhood, at age 28 years she did not respond to 100,000 to 700,000 IU of vitamin D$_2$ per day. Three months after discontinuing this high dose of vitamin D, the serum vitamin D level was 65 to 100 times greater than normal while the serum 25-(OH)D level was low-normal. On the basis of this observation, it was postulated that this patient had impaired synthesis of 25-(OH)D in addition to end-organ refractoriness to 1,25-(OH)D. Consistent with this postulate was the finding that treatment with 20 to 50 µg of 25-(OH)D$_3$ per day corrected hypocalcemia and secondary hyperparathyroidism, raised intestinal calcium absorption, and reversed the skeletal lesions of osteomalacia. During treatment with 25-(OH)D$_3$, the serum 25-(OH)D levels rose progressively to above normal, while the serum 1,25-(OH)$_2$D levels remained elevated but did not rise further.

The other two patients (brother and sister) with no apparent defect in 25 hydroxylation were apparently able to maintain normal serum calcium and phosphorus levels as adults while taking 20,000 IU of vitamin D$_2$ per day. During this time the serum 25-(OH)D, 24,25-(OH)$_2$D, and 1,25-(OH)$_2$D levels were all elevated. These patients also responded to the daily administration of 200 µg of 25-(OH)D$_3$ over a 1-month period with an increase in intestinal absorption of calcium, normalization of serum phosphorus, and, at least in one patient, a steady rise in serum calcium. In studies of the therapeutic effect of 1,25-(OH)$_2$D$_3$, daily doses of 17 to 20 µg, in addition to calcium supplements, were needed to normalize serum calcium and phosphorus levels and promote resolution of the osteomalacia in these two patients. During treatment with 1,25-(OH)$_2$D$_3$ the serum concentration of 25-(OH)D and 24,25-(OH)$_2$D decreased while the 1,25-(OH)$_2$D levels remained elevated. During pregnancy of the affected sister, the dose of 1,25-(OH)$_2$D$_3$ required to maintain normocalcemia increased from 17 µg/day to 36 µg/day [234]. During pregnancy the serum 1,25-(OH)$_2$D levels ranged from 170 to 680 pg/ml, while the serum 25-(OH)D and 24,25-(OH)$_2$D were normal. After an unremarkable pregnancy, she gave birth to a normal, healthy infant. The cord serum level of 1,25-(OH)$_2$D was elevated (410 pg/ml) while the levels of 25-(OH)D and 24,25-(OH)$_2$D were normal. Except for transient hypercalcemia at 2 h of age, the infant had an uneventful course and was normal at 7 months of age.

The data accumulated to date regarding the responsiveness to vitamin D and vitamin D metabolites of patients with vitamin D–dependent rickets type II with and without alopecia may be summarized as follows: (1) Patients without alopecia were more responsive to pharmacologic doses of vitamin D (responsive to 5000 to 40,000 IU daily) than patients with alopecia (nonresponsive to up to 1,200,000 IU daily); (2) patients without alopecia responded to 17 to 20 µg of 1,25-(OH)$_2$D per day while one patient with alopecia who received 20 µg daily intravenously for 15 days did not respond; and (3) patients without alopecia responded to 20 to 200 µg of 25-(OH)D daily, while doses of 750 to 1500 µg caused an inadequate response in a patient with alopecia. On the basis of available reports, it would appear that patients with D–resistant rickets type II without alopecia are more responsive to vitamin D, 25-(OH)D, and possibly 1,25-(OH)$_2$D than patients with alopecia. Further studies are needed to better document this possibility. In contrast to patients with D–dependent rickets type I, patients with D–dependent rickets type II with or without alopecia do not respond to small physiological doses of 1,25-(OH)$_2$D.

A reasonable conjecture is that vitamin D–dependent rickets type II without alopecia, similar to that with alopecia, is transmitted as an autosomal recessive trait, but there is insufficient evidence to support this thesis at the present time. The reports include an affected brother and sister and a normal brother and sister in one family [232] and the isolated occurrence in a female in another family [233]. There was no previous family history of rickets or bone disease in either family and no known consanguinity in the parents. The latter finding is in contrast to patients with vitamin D–dependent rickets type II with alopecia in whom there was consanguinity in four of the five families. In the family with two affected children the results of skeletal x-rays, and serum chemical, serum immunoreactive parathyroid hormone, and vitamin D metabolite determination were all normal in the two normal sibs and in the parents [232]. Thus, if this disorder proves to be transmitted as an autosomal recessive trait, there is no evidence for an abnormality in mineral homeostasis or vitamin D metabolism in the obligate heterozygotes. Vitamin D–dependent rickets with and without alopecia appear to be clinically distinct, but the relationship between their specific genetic etiologies cannot be stated at the present time.

Pathogenesis of Vitamin D–dependent Rickets Type II

The elevated levels of circulating 1,25-(OH)$_2$D in patients with this disorder suggest an abnormal function in the 1,25-(OH)$_2$D target tissues, such as intestinal mucosa and bone. Similar to other steroid hormones, 1,25-(OH)$_2$D requires nuclear uptake for action. Nuclear uptake is one of a sequence of steps required for steroid hormones to effect a biological response. These steps include entry of hormone into the cell, binding of hormone to a cytosol-receptor protein, entry of cytosol-receptor-hormone complex into the nucleus, and interaction of cytosol-receptor-hormone complex with nuclear acceptor sites, which results in increased transcription of specific structural genes and subsequent appearance of new messenger RNA and protein in the cytoplasm. Studies of an androgen-resistance syndrome in humans have identified defects in the cytosol receptor and possibly at a site distal to the receptor [235]. Similar studies of 1,25-(OH)$_2$D in patients with vitamin D–dependent rickets type II have not been reported, but it seems probable that an abnormality will eventually be detected. It may be pertinent that there was no evidence for an immunoglobulin that binds 1,25-(OH)$_2$D in the circulation of patients with D–dependent rickets type II with alopecia [228].

The occurrence of alopecia in vitamin D–dependent rickets type II is interesting in view of the fact that nuclear uptake of 1,25-(OH)$_2$D has been demonstrated in the outer root sheath cell of the rat hair follicle [236]. Moreover, a vitamin D–dependent calcium-binding protein has been reported in rat skin [237], and possible receptors for 1,25-(OH)$_2$D have been identified in keratinocytes from human epidermis [238]. These findings suggest that 1,25-(OH)$_2$D may have a physiologic role in skin. The finding of alopecia in D–dependent rickets type II may reflect a defect in the physiologic action of 1,25-(OH)$_2$D in skin. As discussed earlier, patients with D–dependent rickets with alopecia appear to be more resistant to pharmacologic actions of vitamin D and D metabolites than patients without

alopecia. Conceivably this difference reflects an abnormality in different steps in the pathway of 1,25-(OH)$_2$D at the cellular level needed to produce a biological response or, alternatively, a difference in severity in the same step in this pathway.

Vitamin D–dependent Rickets in Older Subjects

Three sibs with hypocalcemia have been reported who were considered to have vitamin D–dependent rickets [207] but in none of whom were there severe symptoms during infancy. In one there were no symptoms until age 12 years. The disease was mild, and none of the three sought definitive treatment of metabolic bone disease until adulthood. Serum iPTH levels were normal in spite of hypocalcemia, and the tubular reabsorption of phosphate was relatively high (greater than 95 percent) rather than depressed. Circulating levels of vitamin D metabolites were not determined, and so it is not possible to categorize rickets further in this family. Alopecia was not described, there was no history of parental consanguinity, and all responded to 50,000 to 75,000 IU of vitamin D$_2$ per day.

Rickets accompanied by hypocalcemia, aminoaciduria, and secondary hyperparathyroidism has been reported in a 22-year-old black female with a history of onset at age 15 years [222]. Circulating 25-(OH)D was normal, while 1,25-(OH)$_2$D was elevated consistent with vitamin D–dependent rickets type II. Alopecia was not described. Treatment with 4000 IU of vitamin D$_3$ for 4 weeks normalized serum calcium and immunoreactive parathyroid hormone levels. The patient was lost to follow-up, and so it is not known what effect the vitamin D treatment had on the bony abnormalities. The relationship of these mild and apparently late onset forms of D–dependent rickets to the forms of D–dependent rickets that occur in infancy is unknown.

REFERENCES

1. MELLANBY E: An experimental investigation on rickets. *Lancet* 196:407, 1919
2. HESS AF, WEINSTOCK M, HELMAN FD: The antirachitic value of irradiated phytosterol and cholesterol. I. *J Biol Chem* 63:305, 1925
3. MCCOLLUM EV, SIMONDS N, BECKER JE, SHIPLEY PC: Studies on experimental rickets. XXI. An experimental demonstration of the existence of a vitamin which promotes calcium deposition. *J Biol Chem* 53:229, 1922
4. STEENBOCK H: The induction of growth promoting and calcifying properties in a ration by exposure to light. *Science* 60:224, 1924
5. STEENBOCK H, HERTING DC: Vitamin D and growth. *J Nutr* 57:449, 1955
6. ASKEW FA, BOURDILLON RB, BRUCE HM, JENKINS RG, WEBSTER TA: The distillation of vitamin D. *Proc R Soc Lond [Biol]* b107:76, 1931
7. WINDAUS A, LINSERT O, LUTTRINGHAUS A, WEILDLICH G: Crystalline-vitamin-D$_2$. *Liebigs Ann Chem* 492:226, 1932
8. NICOLAYSEN R, EEG-LARSEN N, MALMO OJ: Physiology of calcium metabolism. *Physiol Rev* 33:242, 1953
9. ALBRIGHT F, BUTLER AM, BLOOMBERG E: Rickets resistant to vitamin D therapy. *Am J Dis Child* 54:529, 1937
10. CHRISTENSEN JF: Three familial cases of atypical late rickets. *Acta Paediatr Scand* 28:274, 1940–1941
11. WINTERS RW, GRAHAM JB, WILLIAMS TF, MCFALLS VW, BURNETT CH: A genetic study of familial hypophosphatemia and vitamin D–resistant rickets. *Trans Assoc Am Physicians* 70:234, 1957
12. WINTERS RW, GRAHAM JB, WILLIAMS TF, MCFALLS VW, BURNETT CH: A genetic study of familial hypophosphatemia and vitamin D–resistant rickets with a review of the literature. *Medicine (Baltimore)* 37:97, 1958
13. GRAHAM JB, MCFALLS VW, WINTERS RW: Familial hypophosphatemia with vitamin D–resistant rickets. II. Three additional kindreds of sex-linked dominant type with a genetic analysis of four such families. *Am J Hum Genet* 11:311, 1959
14. ROBERTSON BR, HARRIS RC, MCCUNE DJ: Refractory rickets: Mechanism of therapeutic action of calciferol. *Am J Dis Child* 64:948, 1942

15. AVIOLO LV, WILLIAMS TF, LUND J, DeLuca HF: Metabolism of vitamin D$_3$-^{3}H in familial hypophosphatemia. *J Clin Invest* 46:1907, 1967

16. FRASER D, SALTER RB: The diagnosis and management of the various types of rickets. *Pediatr Clin North Am* 5:417, 1958

17. PRADER A, ILLIG R, HEIERLI E: Eine besondere form der primären vitamin-D–resistenten rachitis mit hypocalcämie und autosomaldóminantem erbgang: Die hereditäre pseudo-mangelrachitis. *Helv Paediat Acta* 16:452, 1961

18. DENT CE: Rickets (and osteomalacia): Nutritional and metabolic (1919–69). *Proc R Soc Med* 63:401, 1970

19. SCRIVER CR: Vitamin D dependency. *Pediatrics* 45:361, 1970

20. HAMILTON R, HARRISON J, FRASER D, RADDE I, MORECKI R, PAUNIER L: The small intestine in vitamin-D–dependent rickets. *Pediatrics* 45:364, 1970

21. ARNAUD C, MAIJER R, READE T, SCRIVER CR, WHELAN OT: Vitamin D dependency: An inherited postnatal syndrome with secondary hyperparathyroidism. *Pediatrics* 46:871, 1970

22. SCRIVER CR, MACDONALD W, READE T, GLORIEUX FH, NOGRADY BL: Hypophosphatemic nonrachitic bone disease: An entity distinct from X-linked hypophosphatemia in renal defect, bone involvement, and inheritance. *Am J Med Genet* 1:101, 1977

23. FRYMOYER JW, HODGKIN W: Adult-onset vitamin D–resistant hypophosphatemic osteomalacia. *J Bone Joint Surg* 59A:101, 1977

24. RASMUSSEN H, BORDIER P: *The Physiological and Cellular Basis of Metabolic Bone Disease*. Baltimore, Williams & Wilkins, 1974

25. DeLuca HF, BLUNT JW, RIKKERS H: Biogenesis of vitamin D, in Sebrell WH Jr, Harris RS (eds): *The Vitamins*. New York, Academic, 1971, vol III, p 213

26. PONCHON G, KENNAN AL, DeLuca HF: Activation of vitamin D by liver. *J Clin Invest* 48:2032, 1969

27. HADDAD JG JR, KYUNG JC: Competitive protein-binding radioassay for 25-hydroxycholecalciferol. *J Clin Endocrinol Metab* 35:992, 1971

28. HADDAD JG JR, STAMP TCB: Circulating 25-hydroxy-vitamin D in man. *Am J Med* 57, 57, 1974

29. FRASER DR, KODICEK E: Unique biosynthesis by kidney of a biologically active vitamin D metabolite. *Nature (London)*. 228:764, 1970

30. LAWSEN DEM, FRASER DR, KODICEK E, MORRIS HR, WILLIAMS DH: Identification of 1,25-dihydroxychole-calciferol, a new kidney hormone controlling calcium metabolism. *Nature (London)*. 230:228, 1971

31. HOLICK MF, SCHNOES HK, DeLuca HF, SUDA T, COUSINS RJ: Isolation and identification of 1,25-dihydroxycholecalciferol: A metabolite of vitamin D active in intestine. *Biochemistry* 10:2799, 1971

32. AVIOLI LV, HADDAD JG: Vitamin D: Current concepts. *Metabolism* 22:507, 1973

33. DeLuca HF: Vitamin D—1973. *Am J Med* 57:1, 1974

34. DeLuca HF: Vitamin D: The vitamin and the hormone. *Fed Proc* 33:2211, 1974

35. HAUSSLER MR, RASMUSSEN H: Metabolism of vitamin D$_3$ in chick. *J Biol Chem* 273:2328, 1972

36. NORMAN AW: 1,25-Dihydroxy vitamin D$_3$: A kidney-produced steroid hormone essential to calcium homeostasis. *Am J Med* 57:21, 1974

37. HAUSSLER MR, BOYCE DW, LITTLEDIKE ET, RASMUSSEN H: A rapidly acting metabolite of vitamin D. *Proc Natl Acad Sci* 68:177, 1971

38. BOYLE IT, GRAY RW, DeLuca HF: Regulation by calcium of in vivo synthesis of 1,25-dihydroxycholecalciferol and 21,25-dihydroxycholecalciferol. *Proc Natl Acad Sci USA* 68:2131, 1971

39. BOYLE IT, MIRAVET L, GRAY RW, HOLICK MF, DeLuca HF: The response of intestinal calcium transport to 25-hydroxy- and 1,25-dihydroxyvitamin D$_3$ in nephrectomized rats. *Endocrinology* 90:605, 1972

40. RASMUSSEN H, WONG M, BIKLE D, GOODMAN DBP: Hormonal control of the renal conversion of 25-hydroxycholecalciferol to 1,25-dihydroxycholecalciferol. *J Clin Invest* 51:2502, 1972

41. GALANTE L, COLSTON K, MACAULEY S, MACINTYRE I: Effect of parathyroid extract on vitamin D metabolism. *Lancet* 1:985, 1972

42. GARABEDIAN M, TANAKA Y, HOLICK MF, DeLuca HF: Response of intestinal calcium transport and bone calcium mobilization to 1,25-dihydroxyvitamin D$_3$ in thyroparathyroidectomized rats. *Endocrinology* 94:88, 1974

43. TANAKA Y, DeLuca HF: The control of 25-hydroxyvitamin D metabolism by inorganic phosphorus. *Arch Biochem Biophys* 154:566, 1973

44. BIKLE DD, RASMUSSEN H: The metabolism of 25-hydroxycholecalciferol by isolated renal tubules in vitro as studied by a new chromatographic technique. *Biochim Biophys Acta* 362:425, 1974

45. BIKLE ED, RASMUSSEN H: The ionic control of 1,25-dihydroxyvitamin D$_3$ production in isolated chick renal tubules. *J Clin Invest* 55:292, 1975

46. BIKLE ED, RASMUSSEN H: The ionic control of 1,25-dihydroxyvitamin D$_3$ synthesis in isolated chick renal mitochondria: The role of calcium as influenced by inorganic phosphate and hydrogen ion. *J Clin Invest* 55:299, 2975

47. LARKINS RG, MACAULEY SJ, RAPPOPORT A, MARTIN TJ, TULLOCH BR, BYFIELD PGH, MATTHEWS EW, MACINTYRE I: Effects of nucleotides, hor-

mones, ions, and 1,25-dihydroxycholecalciferol on 1,25-dihydroxycholecalciferol production in isolated chick renal tubules. *Clin Sci Mol Med* 46:569, 1974

48. SUDA T, HORIUCHI N, SASAKI S, OGATA E, EZAWA I, NAGATA N, KIMURA S: Direct control by calcium of 25-hydroxycholecalciferol-1-hydroxylase activity in chick mitochondria. *Biochem Biophys Res Commun* 54:512, 1973

49. GRUSON JM, BORDIER PH J, QUEILLE M-L, CARRÉ ML, DEMIGHON JM, MIRAVET LF: Effects of 25-hydroxycholecalciferol and 1,25-dihydroxycholecalciferol on bone resorption, formation, and mineralization in vitamin-D-deficient rats. *IRCS* 2:1154, 1974

50. BRUMBAUGH PF, HAUSSLER DH, BRESSLER R, and HAUSSLER MR: Radioreceptor assay for 1-α,25-dihydroxyvitamin D$_3$. *Science* 183:1089, 1974

51. BROADUS AE, HORST RL, LANG R, LITTLEDIKE ET, RASMUSSEN H: The importance of circulating 1,25-dihydroxyvitamin D in the pathogenesis of hypercalciuria and renal stone formation in primary hyperparathyroidism. *N Engl J Med* 302:421, 1980

52. DENT CE, RICHENS A, ROWE DJF, STAMP TCB: Osteomalacia with long-term anticonvulsant therapy in epilepsy. *Br Med J* 4:69, 1970

53. HAHN TJ, KENDIN BA, SCHARP CR, HADDAD JC JR: Effect of chronic anticonvulsant therapy on serum 25-hydroxycholecalciferol levels in adults. *N Engl J Med* 287:900, 1972

54. HAHN TJ, BIRGE SJ, SCHARP CR, AVIOLI LV: Phenobarbital-induced alterations in vitamin D metabolism. *J Clin Invest* 51:741, 1972

55. STAMP TCB, ROUND JM, ROWE DIF, HADDAD JG JR: Plasma level and therapeutic efficiency of 25-hydro-γ-cholecalciferol in epileptic patients taking anticonvulsant drugs. *Br Med J* 4:9, 1972

56. BIRGE SJ, PECK WA, BERMAN M, WHEDON GD: Study of calcium absorption in man: A kinetic analysis and physiologic model. *J Clin Invest* 48:1705, 1969

57. RIBOVICH ML, DeLuca HF: The influence of dietary calcium and phosphorus on intestinal calcium transport in rats given vitamin D metabolites. *Arch Biochem Biophys* 170:529, 1975

58. EASTWOOD JR, DE WARDENER HE, GRAY RW, LEMANN J JR: Normal plasma 1,25-(OH)$_2$ vitamin D$_3$ concentrations in nutritional osteomalacia. *Lancet* 1:1377, 1979

59. JUBIZ W, HAUSSLER MR, McCAIN TA, TOLMAN KG: Plasma 1,25-dihydroxyvitamin D levels in patients receiving anticonvulsant drugs. *J Clin Endocrinol Metab* 44:617, 1977

60. RASMUSSEN H, BORDIER P: Vitamin D and bone. *Metab Bone Dis Rel Res* 1:7, 1978

61. RASMUSSEN H, BARON R, BROADUS A, DeFRONZO R, LANG R, HORST R: 1,25-(OH)$_2$D$_3$ is not the only D metabolite involved in the pathogenesis of osteomalacia. *Am J Med* 69:360, 1980

62. WEIZMAN T, FATTAL A, EISENBERG Z, HAREL S, SPIRER Z, HARELL A: Decreases serum 24,25-dihydroxyvitamin D concentrations in children receiving chronic anticonvulsant therapy. *Br Med J* 521, 1979

63. NGUYEN TM, GUILLOZO H, GARABEDIAN M, MALLET E, BALSAN S: Serum concentration of 24,25-dihydroxyvitamin D in normal children and in children with rickets. *Pediatr Res* 13:973, 1979

64. BORDIER P, RASMUSSEN H, MARIE P, MIRAVET L, GUERIS J, RYCKWAERT A: Vitamin D metabolites and bone mineralization in man. *J Clin Endocrinol Metab* 46(2):284, 1978

65. DE DEUXCHAISRES DN, ROMBOUTS-LINDEMAN C, HAUX JP, WITHOFS H, MEERSSEMAN F: Healing of vitamin D–deficient osteomalacia by the administration of 1,25-(OH)$_2$D$_3$. *Mol Endo* 375, 1979

66. LIEBERHERR M, GARABEDIAN M, GUILLOZO H, THIL CL, BALSAN S: In vitro effects of vitamin D$_3$ metabolites on rat calvaria cAMP content. *Calcif Tissue Int* 30:209, 1980

67. MALLUCHE HH, HENRY H, MEYER-SABELLEK W, SHERMAN D, MASSRY SG, NORMANN AW: Effects and interactions of 24R,25-(OH)$_2$D$_3$ and 1,25(OH)$_2$D$_3$ on bone. *Am Phys* 5:E495, 1980

68. MASSRY SG, TUMA S, DUA S, GOLDSTEIN DA: Reversal of skeletal resistance to parathyroid hormone in uremia by vitamin D metabolites. *J Lab Clin Med* 94(1):152, 1979

69. ENDO H, KIYOKI M, KANASHIMA K, NARUCHI T, HASHIMOTO Y: Vitamin D$_3$ metabolites and PTH synergistically stimulate bone formation of chick embryonic femur in vitro. *Nature* 286:262, 1980

70. EICHER EM, SOUTHARD JL, SCRIVER, CR, GLORIEUX FH: Hypophosphatemia: Mouse model for human familial hypophosphatemic (vitamin D–resistant) rickets. *Proc Natl Acad Sci* 73:4667, 1976

71. TENENHOUSE HS, SCRIVER CR: Renal adaptation to phosphate derivation in the *Hyp* mouse with X-linked hypophosphatemia. *Can J Biochem* 57:938, 1979

72. MEYER RA JR, JOWSEY J, MEYER MH: Osteomalacia and altered magnesium metabolism in the X-linked hypophosphatemic mouse. *Calcif Tissue Intl* 27:19, 1979

73. COGWELL LD, GOLDFARB S, LAU K, SLATOPOLSKY E, ZALMAN SA: Evidence for an intrinsic renal tubular defect in mice with genetic hypophosphatemic rickets. *J Clin Invest* 63:1203, 1979

74. GIASSON SD, BRUNETTI MG, DANAN G, VIGNEAULT N, CARRIERE S:

Micropuncture study of renal phosphorus transport in hypophosphatemic vitamin D resistant rickets in mice. *Pflügers Arch* 371:33, 1977

75. TENENHOUSE HS, SCRIVER CR, McINNES RR, GLORIEUX FH: Renal handling of phosphate *in vivo* and *in vitro* by the X-linked hypophosphatemic male mouse: Evidence for a defect in the brush border membrane. *Kidney Int* 14:236, 1978

76. TENENHOUSE HS, SCRIVER CR: The defect in transcellular transport of phosphate in the nephron is located in brush-border membranes in X-linked hypophosphatemia (*Hyp* mouse model). *Can J Biochem* 56:640, 1978

77. TENENHOUSE HS, SCRIVER CR, DeLUCA HF: X-linked hypophosphatemia is a disorder of phosphate transport in the renal brush border membrane in the hypophosphatemic (*Hyp*) mouse. Why is serum 1,25-(OH)$_2$D low in the human homologue?, in Norman AW, Schaefer K, Herrath DV (eds): *Vitamin D, Basic Research and Its Clinical Application.* Walter de Gruyter, Berlin, 1979, p 925

78. TENENHOUSE HS, SCRIVER CR: X-linked hypophosphatemia (XLH) in man and the *Hyp* phenotype in mouse. Evidence for homologies. Relevance for treatment of XLH. *J Inherit Metab Dis* (in press)

79. DENNIS VW, BELLO-REUSS E, ROBINSON RR: Response of phosphate transport to parathyroid hormone in segments of rabbit nephron. *Am J Physiol* 233:F29, 1977

80. TENENHOUSE HS, SCRIVER CR: Renal brush border membrane adaptation to phosphorus deprivation in the *Hyp*/Y mouse. *Nature* 281:225, 1979

81. MEUYER RA JR, GRAY RW, KIEBZAK GM, MISH PM: Altered vitamin D, cyclic nucleotide and trace mineral metabolism in the X-linked hypophosphatemic mouse, in Massry SG, Ritz E, Jahn H, (eds): *Phosphate and Minerals in Health and Disease.* New York, Plenum, 1980, p 351

82. GLORIEUX F, SCRIVER CR: Loss of a parathyroid hormone-sensitive component of phosphate transport in X-linked hypophosphatemia. *Science* 175:997, 1972

83. BRUNETTE MG, CHABARDES D, IMBERT-TEBOUL M, CLIQUE A, MONTÉGUT M, MOREL F: Hormone-sensitive adenylate cyclase along the nephron of genetically hypophosphatemic mice. *Kidney Int* 15:357, 1979

84. BEAMER WG, WILSON MC, DeLUCA HF: Successful treatment of genetically hypophosphatemic mice by 1-hydroxyvitamin D$_3$ but not 1,25-dihydroxyvitamin D$_3$. *Endocrinology* 106:1949, 1980

85. O'DOHERTY PJA, DeLUCA HF, EICHER EM: Lack of effect of vitamin D and its metabolites on intestinal phosphate transport in familial hypophosphatemia of mice. *Endocrinology* 101:1325, 1977

86. MEYER RA JR, GRAY RW, MEYER MH: Abnormal vitamin D metabolism in the X-linked hypophosphatemic mouse. *Endocrinology* 107:1577, 1980

87. GLORIEUX F: Personal communication, 1981

88. MARIE PJ, TRAVERS R, GLORIEUX FH: Healing of rickets with phosphate supplementation in the hypophosphatemic male mouse. *J Clin Invest* (in press)

89. VAN DER REST M, DE MIGUEL E, GLORIEUX FH: The collagen crosslinking in the hypophosphatemic male mouse. *Calcif Tissue Int* 33:   , 1981

90. WILLIAMS TF, WINTERS RW: Familial (hereditary) vitamin D–resistant rickets with hypophosphatemia, in Stanbury JB, Wyngaarden JB, Fredrickson DS, (eds): *The Metabolic Basis of Inherited Disease,* 3d ed. New York, McGraw-Hill, 1972, p 1465

91. ANAST CS: Magnesium studies in relation to vitamin D–resistant rickets. *Pediatrics* 40:425, 1967

92. GLORIEUX FH, MARIE PJ, PETTIFOR JM, DELVIN EE: Some response to phosphate salts, ergocaliferol and calcitriol in hypophosphatemic vitamin-D–resistant rickets. *N Engl J Med* 303:1023, 1980

93. HARRISON HE, HARRISON HC, LIPSHITZ F, JOHNSON AD: Growth disturbance in hereditary hypophosphatemia. *Am J Dis Child* 112:290, 1966

94. BURNETT CH, DENT CE, HARPER C, WARLAND BJ: Vitamin D–resistant rickets: Analysis of 24 pedigrees with hereditary and sporadic cases. *Am J Med* 36:222, 1964

95. TAPIA J, STEARNS G, PONSETTI IV: Vitamin-D–resistant rickets. *J Bone Joint Surg* 64-A:935, 1964

96. STICKLER GB, BEABOUT JW, RIGGS BL: Vitamin D–resistant rickets: Clinical experience with 41 typical familial hypophosphatemic patients and 2 atypical nonfamilial cases. *Mayo Clin Proc* 45:197, 1970

97. STEARNS G: A guide to the adequacy of therapy in resistant rickets due to familial or essential hypophosphatemia. *J Bone Joint Surg* 46-A:959, 1964

98. PIERCE DS, WALLACE WM, HERNDON CH: Long-term treatment of vitamin-D–resistant rickets. *J Bone Surg* 46-A:979, 1964

99. STICKLER GB: Familial hypophosphatemic vitamin D–resistant rickets. *Acta Paediatr Scand* 58:213, 1969

100. TRACY WE, CAMPBELL RA: Dento-facial development in children with vitamin-D–resistant rickets. *J Am Dent Assoc* 76:1026, 1968

101. SONI NN, MARKS SC: Microradiographic and polarized-light study of dental tissues in vitamin D–resistant rickets. *Oral Surg* 23:755, 1967

102. VILLANUEVA AR, ILNICKI L, FROST HM, ARNSTEIN R: Measurement of the bone formation rate in a case of familial hypophosphatemic vitamin-D–

103. WITMER G, BALSAN S: Biopsie osseuse dans quatre cas de rachitisme vitamino-résistant idiopathique. *Pathol Biol (Paris)*, 16:421, 1968

104. GREENBERG BG, WINTERS RW, GRAHAM JB: The normal range of serum inorganic phosphorus and its utility as a discriminant in the diagnosis of congenital hypophosphatemia. *J Clin Endocrinol* 20:364, 1960

105. STICKLER GB: Familial hypophosphatemic vitamin D–resistant rickets. *Acta Paediatr Scand* 58:213, 1969

106. McNAIR SL, STICKLER GB: Growth in familial hypophosphatemic vitamin-D rickets. *N Engl J Med* 281:511, 1969

107. GLORIEUX F, SCRIVER CR: Loss of parathyroid-hormone-sensitive component of phosphate transport in X-linked hypophosphatemia. *Science* 173:997, 1972

108. ROOF BS, PIEL CF, GORDAN GS: Nature of defect responsible for familial vitamin D–resistant rickets (VDRR) based on radioimmunoassay for parathormone (PTH) assay. *Trans Assoc Am Physicians* 85:172, 1972.

109. FRANCONI A, FISCHER JA, PRADER A: Serum parathyroid hormone concentrations in hypophosphatemic vitamin D–resistant rickets. *Helv Paediatr Acta* 29:187, 1974

110. ARNAUD C, GLORIEUX F, SCRIVNER CR: Serum parathyroid hormone levels in acquired vitamin D deficiency of infancy. *Pediatrics* 49:837, 1972

111. REITZ RE, WEINSTEIN RL: Parathyroid hormone secretion in familial vitamin-D–resistant rickets. *N Engl J Med* 289:941, 1973

112. LEWY JE, CABANA EC, REPETTO HA, CANTERBURY JM, REISS E: Serum parathyroid hormone in hypophosphatemic vitamin D–resistant rickets. *J Pediatr* 81:294, 1972

113. HADDAD JG, CHYU KJ, HAHN TJ, STAMP TCB: Serum concentrations of 24-hydroxyvitamin D in sex-linked hypophosphatemic vitamin D–resistant rickets. *J Lab Clin Med* 81:22, 1973

114. CHESNEY RW: Tubular defects in phosphate reabsorption in clinical medicine, in *Renal Handling of Phosphate.* New York, Plenum, 1980

115. RASMUSSEN H, PECHET M, ANAST C, MAZUR A, GERTNER J, BROADUS AE: Long term treatment of familial hypophosphatemic rickets with oral phosphate and 1α-hydroxyvitamin D$_3$. *J Pediatr,* 99:16, 1980

116. SCRIVER CR, READE TM, DeLUCA HF, HAMSTRA AJ: Serum 1,25-dihydroxyvitamin D levels in normal subjects and in patients with hereditary rickets or bone disease. *N Engl J Med* 299:976, 1977

117. CHESNEY RW, MAZESS RB, ROSE P, HAMSTRA AJ, DeLUCA HR: Supranormal 25-hydroxyvitamin D and subnormal 1,25-dihydroxyvitamin D their role in X-linked hypophosphatemic rickets. *Am J Dis Child* 134:140, 1980

118. GLORIEUX FH, MARIE PH, PETTIFOR JM, DELVIN EE: Bone response to phosphate salts, ergocalciferol, and calcitriol in hypophosphatemic vitamin D–resistant rickets. *N Engl J Med* 303(18):1023, 1980

119. MASSRY SG, FRIEDLER RM, COBURN JW: Excretion of phosphate and calcium: Physiology of their renal handling and relation to clinical medicine. *Arch Intern Med* 131:828, 1973

120. AGUS ZS, GARDNER LB, BECK LH, GOLDBERG M: Effect of PTH on renal tubular reabsorption of calcium, sodium and phosphorus. *Am J Physiol* 224:1143, 1973

121. AMIEL C: Sites of renal tubular reabsorption of phosphate, in *Renal Handling of Phosphate.* New York, Plenum, 1980

122. KNOX FG, HOPPE A, KEMPSON SA, SHAH SV, DOUSA TP: Cellular mechanisms of phosphate transport, in *Renal Handling of Phosphate.* New York, Plenum, 1980

123. LAU K, GOLDFARB S, GOLDBERG M: The effects of parathyroid hormone on renal phosphate handling, in *Renal Handling of Phosphate.* New York, Plenum, 1980

124. HOPFER U: Isolated membrane vesicles as tools for analysis of epithelial transport. *Am J Physiol* 233:E445, 1977

125. HOFFMAN N, THEES M, KINNE R: Phosphate transport by isolated renal brush border vesicles. *Pflügers Arch* 362:147, 1976

126. BONJOUR JP, FLEISCH H: Tubular adaption to the supply and requirement of phosphate, in *Renal Handling of Phosphate.* New York, Plenum, 1980.

127. RITZ E, KREUSSER W, BOMMER J: Effects of hormones other than parathyroid hormone on renal handling of phosphate, in *Renal Handling of Phosphate.* New York, Plenum, 1980.

128. STEELE TH: Renal resistance to parathyroid hormone during phosphate deprivation. *J Clin Invest* 58:1461, 1976

129. BARRETT PQ, GERTNER JM, RASMUSSEN H: Effect of dietary phosphate on transport properties of pig renal microvillus vesicles. *Am J Physiol* 239:F352, 1980

130. AVIOLI L: Effects of vitamin D and its metabolites on renal handling of phosphate, in *Renal Handling of Phosphate.* New York, Plenum, 1980

131. CHASE LR, AURBACH GD: Parathyroid function and the renal excretion of 3′,5′-adenylic acid. *Proc Natl Acad Sci USA* 58:518, 1967

132. RASMUSSEN H, PECHET M, FAST D: Effect of dibutyryl cyclic adenosine 3′,5′-monophosphate, theophylline, and other nucleotides upon calcium and phosphate metabolism. *J Clin Invest* 47:1843, 1968

133. KINNE R, KINNE-SAFFRAN E, SCHATZ L, SCHWARTZ IL: Mechanism of

action of parathormone on the kidney: Cyclic-AMP-dependent protein kinase in brush border membranes of proximal tubule. *J Memb Biol* 24:145, 1975

134. EISENBERG E: Effects of serum calcium level and parathyroid extracts on phosphate and calcium excretion in hypoparathyroid patients. *J Clin Invest* 44:482, 1965

135. BORLE AB: Calcium metabolism at the cellular level. *Fed Proc* 32:1944, 1973

136. CHABARDES D, IMBERT M, CLIQUE A, MONTEGUT M, MOREL F: PTH-sensitive adenyl cyclase activity in different segments of the rabbit nephron. *Pflügers Arch* 354:229, 1975

137. BIJVOET OLM: Indices for the measurement of the renal handling of phosphate, in *Renal Handling of Phosphate*. New York, Plenum, 1980

138. DENT CE, HARRIS H: Hereditary forms of rickets and osteomalacia. *J Bone Joint Surg (Am)* 38-B:204, 1956

139. FANCONI G, GIRARDET P: Familiärer persistierendes phosphat-diabetes mit D-vitamin resistenter rachitis. *Helv Paediatr Acta* 7:14, 1952

140. SWOBODA W: Die genuine vitamin D-resistente rachitis. *Wein Beitr Kinderheilkd* 6:1, 1956

141. TOBLER R, PRADER A, TAILLARD W: Die familiäre primäre vitamin D-resistant rachitis (phosphat diabetes). *Helv Paediatr Acta* 11:209, 1956

142. DENT CE: Rickets and osteomalacia from renal tubular defects. *J Bone Joint Surg (Br)* 34-B:266, 1952

143. WILSON DR, YORK SE, JAWORSKI ZF, YENDT ER: Studies in hypophosphatemic vitamin D–refractory osteomalacia in adults: Oral phosphate supplements as an adjunct to therapy. *Medicine (Baltimore)* 44:99, 1965

144. CHRISTIANSSON G: Emergence of primary vitamin D–resistant rickets at puberty: Genetic study of primary rickets with familial disposition. *Acta Paediatr Scand* 47:288, 1958

145. JONXIS JHP: Amino-aciduria and rickets. *Helv Paediatr Acta* 10:245, 1955

146. FISHMAN WH: Methionine-induced amino aciduria in vitamin D–resistant rickets. *Metabolism* 4:107, 1955

147. STOOP JW, SCHRAGEN MJC, TIDDENS HAWM: Pseudo-vitamin D–deficiency rickets: Report of four new cases. *Acta Paediatr Scand* 56:607, 1967

148. FREEMAN S, DUNSKY I: Resistant rickets. *Am J Dis Child* 79:409, 1950

148a. GERTNER J: Personal communication

149. GLORIEUX FH, SCRIVER CT: Loss of a parathyroid hormone-sensitive compound of phosphate transport in X-linked hypophosphatemia. *Science* 175:997, 1972

150. RASMUSSEN H, FONTAINE O, MAX EE, GOODMAN DBP: The effect of 1α(OH)D₃ administration on calcium transport in chick intestine brush border membrane vesicles. *J Biol Chem* 254:2993, 1979

151. MATSUMOTO T, FONTAINE O, RASMUSSEN A: Effect of 1,25-dihydroxyvitamin D₃ on phosphate uptake into chick intestinal brush border membrane vesicles. *Biochim Biophys Acta* 599:13, 1980

152. BIKLE DD, ZOLOCK DT, MORRISSEY RL, HERMAN RJ: Independence of 1,25-dihydroxyvitamin D₃-mediated calcium transport from *de novo* RNA and protein synthesis. *J Biol Chem* 253:484, 1978

153. MAX EE, GOODMAN DBP, RASMUSSEN H: Purification and characterization of chick intestine brush border membrane: Effects of 1α(OH)D₃ treatment. *Biochim Biophys Acta* 511:224, 1978

154. FONTAINE O, MATSUMOTO T, GOODMAN DBP, RASMUSSEN H: Lipononic control of Ca²⁺ transport. Relationship to mechanism of action of 1,25-dihydroxyvitamin D₃. *Proc Natl Acad Sci USA* 78:1751, 1981

155. MATSUMOTO T, FONTAINE O, RASMUSSEN H: Effects of 1,25-dihydroxyvitamin D₃ on phosphate uptake into chick intestinal brush border membrane vesicles. *J Biol Chem* 256:3354, 1981

156. CONDON JR, NASSIUM JR, RUTTER A: Defective intestinal phosphate absorption in familial and non-familial hypophosphataemia. *Br Med J* 3:138, 1970

157. CONDON JR, NASSIUM JR, RUTTER A: Pathogenesis of rickets and osteomalacia in familial hypophosphataemia. *Arch Dis Child* 46:269, 1971

158. STEARNS G, OELKE MJ, BOYD JD: Mineral metabolism in late rickets. *Am J Dis Child* 42:88, 1931

159. CHAN JCM, LOVINGER RD, MAMUNES P: Renal hypophosphatemic rickets: Growth acceleration after long-term treatment with 1,25-dihydroxyvitamin D₃. *Pediatrics* 66:445, 1980

160. GLORIEUX FH, MORIN CL, TRAVERS R, DELVIN EE, POIRER R: Intestinal phosphate transport in familial hypophosphatemic rickets. *Pediatr Res* 10:691, 1976

161. HOWLAND J, KRAMER B: Calcium and phosphorous in the serum in relation to rickets. *Am J Dis Child* 22:105, 1921

162. SHIPLEY PG, KRAMER B, HOWLAND J: Calcification of rachitic bones in vitro. *Am J Dis Child* 30:37, 1925

163. SHIPLEY PG, KRAMER B, HOWLAND J: Studies upon calcification in vitro. *Biochem J* 20:379, 1926

164. CARLSSON A: Tracer experiments on the effect of vitamin D on the skeletal metabolism of calcium and phosphorus. *Acta Physiol Scand* 26:212, 1952

165. DELUCA HF: Vitamin D: Part I, in Peters A (ed): Parathyroid Hormone, Thyrocalcitonin, and Related Drugs. *International Encyclopedia of Pharmacology and Therapeutics* (sec 51) Oxford, Pergamon, 1970, vol I, p 10

166. RASMUSSEN H, DELUCA HF, ARNAUD C, HAWKER C, VON STEDINGK M: The relationship between vitamin D and parathyroid hormone. *J Clin Invest* 42:1940, 1963

167. ARNAUD C, RASMUSSEN H, ANAST C: Further studies on the interrelationship between parathyroid hormone and vitamin D. *J Clin Invest* 45:1955, 1966

168. ENGFELDT B, ZETTERSTRÖM R, WINBERG J: Primary vitamin-D resistant rickets. III. Biophysical studies of skeletal tissue. *J Bone Joint Surg (Am)* 38-A:1323, 1956

169. GREGERSEN E: Primary vitamin-resistant rickets. *Acta Pediatr Scand* 44:491, 1955

170. MARIE PJ, GLORIEUX FH: Histomorphometric study of bone remodeling in hypophosphatemic vitamin D–resistant rickets. *Metab Bone Dis Rel Dis* in press

171. FRASER D, GEIGER DW, MUNN JD, SLATER PE, JAHN R, LIU E: Calcification studies in clinical vitamin D–deficiency and in hypophosphatemic vitamin D–refractory rickets: The induction of calcium deposition in rachitic cartilage without the administration of vitamin D. *Am J Dis Child* 96:460, 1958

172. FROST HM: A unique histological feature of vitamin D resistant rickets observed in four cases. *Acta Orthop Scand* 33:220, 1963

173. FRAME B, ARNSTEIN AR, FROST HM, SMITH RW: Resistant osteomalacia: Studies with tetracycline bone labeling and metabolic balance. *Am J Med* 38:134, 1965

174. SILVERMAN FN, CUIRARIANO G: Roentgen manifestations of hereditary metabolic diseases in childhood. *Metabolism* 9:248, 1960

175. STAMP WG, WHITESIDES TE, FIELD MH, SCHEER GE: Treatment of vitamin D–resistant rickets: A long-term evaluation of its effectiveness. *Am J Bone Joint Surg* 46-A:965, 1964

176. HARRISON HE, HARRISON HC, LIFSHITZ F, JOHNSON AD: Growth disturbance in hereditary hypophosphatemia. *Am J Dis Child* 112:290, 1966

177. STEENDIJK R: Growth in vitamin D–resistant rickets. *Calif Tissue Res* 2, suppl 60, 1968

178. GLORIEUX FH, SCRIVER CR, READE TM, GOLDMAN H, ROSEBOROUGH A: Use of phosphate and vitamin D to prevent dwarfism and rickets in X-linked hypophosphatemia. *N Engl J Med* 287:481, 1972

179. GERTNER JM, BRENTON DB, EDWARDS RHT: 1α-hydroxyvitamin D₃ in the treatment of nutritional and metabolic rickets and osteomalacia. *Clin Endocrinol* 7(suppl) 239s, 1977

180. DREZNER MK, LYLES KW, HAUSSLER MR, HARRELSON JM: Evaluation of a role for 1,25-dihydroxyvitamin D₃ in the pathogenesis and treatment of X-linked hypophosphatemic rickets and osteomalacia. *J Clin Invest* 66:1020, 1980

181. SCRIVER CR, READE T, HALAL F, COSTA T, COLE DEC: Autosomal hypophosphatemic bone disease responds to 1,25(OH)₂D₃. *Arch Dis Childhood* in press

182. RIGGS BL, SPRAGUE RG, JOWSEY J, MAHER FT: Adult-onset vitamin D–resistant hypophosphatemic osteomalacia. *N Engl J Med* 281:762, 1969

183. SHORT E, MORRIS RC Jr, SEBASTIAN A, SPENCER M: Exaggerated phosphaturic response to circulating parathyroid hormones in patients with familial x-linked hypophosphatemic rickets. *J Clin Invest* 58:152, 1976

184. MORGAN JM, HAWLEY WL, CHENOWETH AI, RETAN WJ, DIETHELM AG: Renal transplantation in hypophosphatemia with vitamin D–resistant rickets. *Arch Intern Med* 734:549, 1974

185. SALASSA RM, JOWSEY J, ARNAUD CD: Hypophosphatemic osteomalacia associated with "nonendocrine" tumors. *N Engl J Med* 283:65, 1970

186. Case Records of the Massachusetts General Hospital (Case 38, 1968). *N Engl J Med* 273:494, 1965

187. YOSHIKAWA S, KAWABATA M, HATSUYAMA Y, HOSOKAWA O, FUJITA T: A typical vitamin D–resistant osteomalacia: Report of a case. *J Bone Joint Surg (Am)* 46A:998, 1964

188. PRADER A, ILLIG R, ÜHLINGER E, STALDER G: Rachitis infolge knochentumors. *Helv Paediatr Acta* 14:554, 1959

189. OLEFSKY J, KEMPSON R, JONES H, REAVEN G: "Tertiary" hyperparathyroidism and apparent "cure" of vitamin D–resistant rickets after removal of an ossifying mesenchymal tumor of the pharynx. *N Engl J Med* 286:740, 1972

190. POLLOCKS JA, SCHILLER AC, CRAWFORD JD: Rickets and myopathy cured by removal of a nonossifying fibroma of bone. *Pediatrics* 52:364, 1973

191. HARRISON HE: Oncogenous rickets: Possible elaboration by a tumor of a humoral substance inhibiting tubular reabsorption of phosphate. *Pediatrics* 52:432, 1973

192. LIEBE S: Über night heilbare rachitis. *Monatsschr Kinderheilkd.* 78:221, 1939

193. BRIARD-GUILLEMOT ML, RAVERDY E, BALSAN S, REY J, FRÉZAL J: Étude critique de l'hypophosphatémie pour l'étude genetique du rachitisme vitamino-resistant hypophosphatémique familial. *Arch Fr Pediatr* 29:1059, 1972

194. Lyon MF: Sex chromatin and gene action in the mammalian X-chromosome. *Am J Hum Genet* 14:135, 1962

195. Winters RW, McFalls VW, Graham JB: "Sporadic" hypophosphatemia and vitamin D–resistant rickets. *Pediatrics* 25:959, 1960

196. Reddy V, Sivakumar B: Magnesium dependent vitamin D–resistant rickets. *Lancet* 1:963, 1974

197. Stickler GB, Jowsey J, Phil D, Bianco AJ: Possible detrimental effect of large doses of vitamin D in familial hypophosphatemic vitamin D–resistant rickets. *J Pediatr.* 79:68, 1971

198. Menking M, Soros JF: Effect of administration of oral neutral phosphate in hypophosphatemic rickets. *J Pediatr* 75:1001, 1969

199. Stickler GR, Hayles AB, Rosevear JW: Familial hypophosphatemic vitamin D–resistant rickets. *Am J Dis Child* 110:664, 1965

200. West CD: Toward better therapy for resistant rickets. *J Pediatr* 79:181, 1971

201. Dent CE, Friedman M, Watson L: Hereditary pseudo-vitamin D–deficiency rickets. *J Bone Joint Surg* 50B:708, 1968

202. Fanconi A, Prader A: Pseudo-vitamin D–deficiency rickets, in Burland WL, Barltrap D (eds): *Mineral Metabolism in Pediatrics.* Oxford, Blackwell, 1969, p 19

203. Matsuda L, Sugai M, Ohsawa T: Laboratory findings in a child with pseudo-vitamin D–deficiency rickets. *Helv Paediat Acta* 24:329, 1969

204. Suster P, Paala JW: Pseudovitamin D–deficiency rickets. *J Pediatr* 76:937, 1970

205. Birtwell WM, Magsamen BF, Fenn PA, Torg JS, Tourtellotte CD, Martin JH: An unusual hereditary osteomalacic disease—pseudo-vitamin D–deficiency. *Am J Bone Joint Surg* 52A:1222, 1970

206. Balsan S, Garabedian M, LeBouadec L: La rachitisme vitaminoresistant pseudocareitial hypocalcémique. *Arch Fr Pediatr* 29:287, 1972

207. Strewler GJ, Bernstein DS, Pletka, PL: Pseudo-vitamin D–deficiency rickets (PDR) and relative hypoparathyroidism: A report of a family. *J Clin Endocrinol Metab* 37, 1973

208. Prader A, Kind HP, DeLuca HF: Pseudovitamin D deficiency (vitamin D dependency), in Bickel H, Stern J (eds): *Inborn Errors of Calcium and Bone Metabolism,* Baltimore, University Park Press, 1976, p 115

209. Hamilton R, Harrison J, Fraser D, Radde I, Morecki R, Paunier L: The small intestine in vitamin D–dependent rickets. *Pediatrics* 45:364, 1970

210. Reade TM, Scriver CR, Glorieux FH, Nogrady B, Delvin E, Poirier R, Holick F, DeLuca HF: Response to crystalline 1α-hydroxyvitamin D_3 in vitamin D–dependency. *Pediatr Res* 9:593, 1975

211. Fraser D, Scriver CR: Familial forms of vitamin D–resistant rickets revisited. X-linked hypophosphatemia and autosomal recessive vitamin D dependency. *Am J Clin Nutr* 29:1315, 1976

212. Balsan S, Garabedian M, Lieberherr M, Gueris J, Ulmann A: Serum 1,25-dihydroxyvitamin D concentrations in two different types of pseudo-deficiency rickets, in Norman AW, Schaefer K, Herrath DV, Grigoleit H-G, Colburn JW, DeLuca HF, Mawer EB, Suda T (eds): *Vitamin D Basic Research and Its Clinical Application.* Berlin, Walter de Gruyter, 1979, p 1143

213. Delvin EE, Glorieux FH, Marie PJ, Pettifor JM: Vitamin D–dependency: Replacement therapy with calcitriol in press

214. Rosen JF, Finberg L: Vitamin D–dependent rickets: Actions of parathyroid hormone and 25-hydroxycholecalciferol. *Pediatr Res* 6:552, 1972

215. Soriano RR, Einhorn A, Stark H, Edelman CM Jr: Deficiency-type rickets due to decreased sensitivity to vitamin D. *J Pediatr* 68:227, 1966

216. Fraser D, Kooh SW, Scriver CR: Hyperparathyroidism as the cause of hyperaminoaciduria and phosphaturia in human vitamin D deficiency. *Pediatr Res* 1:425, 1967

217. Fanconi A, Prader A: Die hereditare pseudomangel rachitis. *Helv Pediatr Acta* 24:423, 1969

218. Scriver CR: Rickets and the pathogenesis of impaired tubular transport of phosphate and other solutes. *Am J Med* 57:43, 1974

219. Anast CS, Carnes DL, Nickols GA, Forte LR: Interrelationship of parathyroid hormone and vitamin D, in DeLuca HF, Anast CS (eds): *Pediatric Diseases Related to Calcium,* New York, Elsevier, 1980, p 75

220. DeLuca HF: Vitamin D metabolism and function. *Arch Intern Med* 138:836, 1978

221. Haussler MR: Biochemical mechanism of action of 1α-25-dihydroxyvitamin D_3 in the intestine, *Proc. 2d Workshop on Vitamin D.* New York, De Gruyter, 1975

222. Fraser D, Koch SW, Kind HP, Holick MF, Tanaka Y, DeLuca HF: Pathogenesis of hereditary vitamin D–dependent rickets: An inborn error of vitamin D metabolism involving defective conversion of 25-hydroxycholecalciferol to 1α,25-dihydroxyvitamin D. *N Engl J Med* 289:817, 1973

223. Balsan S, Garabedian M, Sorgniard R, Holick MF, DeLuca HF: 1,25-dihydroxyvitamin D_3 and 1,α-hydroxyvitamin D_3 in children: Biologic and therapeutic effects in nutritional rickets and different types of vitamin D resistance. *Pediatr Res* 9:586, 1975

224. Harmeyer J, Plonait H: Generalisierte hyperaminoaciduria mit erblicher rachitis bei schweinen. *Helv Paediatr Acta.* 22:216, 1967

225. Meyer H, Plonait H: Ueber eine erbliche kalziumstoff wechsel storung bein schwein (erbliche rachitis). *Z Vet Med Reihe A* 15:481, 1968

226. Balsan S, Garabedian M: 25-Hydroxycholecalciferol: A comparative study in deficiency rickets and different types of resistant rickets. *J Clin Invest* 51:749, 1972

227. Brooks MH, Bell NH, Love L, Stern PH, Orfei E, Queener SF, Hamstra AJ, DeLuca HF: Vitamin D–dependent rickets type II: Resistance of target organs to 1,25-dihydroxyvitamin D. *N Engl J Med* 298:996, 1978

228. Rosen JF, Fleischman AR, Finberg L, Hamstra A, DeLuca HF: Rickets with alopecia: An inborn error of vitamin D metabolism. *J Pediatr* 94:729, 1979

229. Liberman UA, Halabe A, Samuel R, Kauli R, Edelstein S, Weisman Y, Papapoulos SE, Fraher LJ, Clemens TL, O'Riordan JLH: End-organ resistance to 1,25-dihydroxycholecalciferol. *Lancet* 504, 1980

230. Sockalosky JJ, Ulstrom RA, DeLuca HF, Brown DM: Vitamin D–resistant rickets: End-organ unresponsiveness to 1,25(OH)₂D₃. *J Pediatr* 96:701, 1980

231. Tsuchiya Y, Nobutake M, Cho H, Kumagai M, Yasaka A, Suda T, Orimo H, Shiraki M: An unusual form of vitamin D–dependent rickets in a child: Alopecia and marked end-organ hyposensitivity to biologically active vitamin D. *J Clin Endocrin Metab* 51:685, 1980

232. Marx SJ, Spiegel AM, Brown EM, Gardner DG, Downs RW Jr, Attie M, Hamstra AJ, DeLuca HF: A familial syndrome of decrease in sensitivity to 1,25-dihydroxyvitamin D. *J Clin Endocrinol Metab* 47:1303, 1978

233. Zerwekh JE, Glass K, Jowsey J, Charles YC: An unique form of osteomalacia associated with end organ refractoriness to 1,25-dihydroxyvitamin D and apparent defective synthesis of 25-hydroxyvitamin D. *J Clin Endocrinol Metab* 49:171, 1979

234. Marx SJ, Swart EG Jr, Hamstra AJ, DeLuca HF: Normal intrauterine development of the fetus of a woman receiving extraordinarily high doses of 1,25-dihydroxyvitamin D₃. *J Clin Endocrinol Metab* 51:1138, 1980

235. Griffin JE, Wilson JD: The syndromes of androgen resistance. *N Engl J Med* 302:198, 1980

236. Stumpf WE, Sar M, Reid FA, Tanaka Y, DeLuca HF: Target cells for 1,25-dihydroxyvitamin D₃ in intestinal tract, stomach, kidney, skin, pituitary, and parathyroid. *Science* 206:1188, 1979

237. Laquari D, Pavlovitch H, Deceneux G, Balsan S: A vitamin D–dependent calcium binding protein in rat skin. *FEBS Lett* 111:285, 1980

238. Feldman D, Chen T, Hirst M, Colston K, Karasek M, Cone C: Demonstration of 1,25-dihydroxyvitamin D₃ receptors in human skin biopsies. *J Clin Endocrinol Metab* 51:1463, 1980

80

CYSTINURIA

STANTON SEGAL

SAMUEL O. THIER

1. Cystinuria is a disorder of amino acid transport affecting the epithelial cells of the renal tubule and the gastrointestinal tract. The defective transport of cystine, lysine, arginine, and ornithine is transmitted as an autosomal recessive trait. The heterozygous state may reflect true recessive or incompletely recessive inheritance. In the latter state the affected amino acids are excreted in urine in quantities greater than normal but less than in the homozygous state. By use of the intestinal transport system as a sensitive genetic marker, three types of cystinuric homozygotes can be defined, and the evidence is that these types result from allelic mutations.

2. The intestinal defect can be demonstrated in vivo by oral loading tests and by intestinal perfusion studies. Complementary data showing the defect have also been obtained by incubations in vitro measuring transport into mucosal biopsies. The dibasic amino acids can be absorbed by cystinuric subjects in a normal fashion as dipeptides.

3. The renal lesions for all four amino acids and the mixed disulfide of cysteine-homocysteine can be demonstrated by clearance studies. The clearance of cystine in both humans and dogs with cystinuria frequently exceeds the glomerular filtration rate. This suggests that secretion occurs. Studies in vitro of amino acid transport by renal cortical slices of affected

kidneys demonstrate a defect for dibasic amino acids but not for cystine. There exist, in rat renal tubule fragments and isolated brush border membrane vesicles, multiple systems for cystine and lysine transport. Cystine and the dibasic amino acids appear to share the low K_m, high affinity system which is probably defective in the cystinuric kidney. Microperfusion of rat kidney tubules and studies of rat cortical transport in vivo indicate that there may be an interaction of cystine and dibasic amino acids at the luminal membrane of the renal tubule cells. Cysteine, the intracellular form of cystine, shares a cellular efflux system with dibasic amino acids. This interaction may play an important role in the regulation of cystine transport into renal cortical cells.

4. Cystinuria is expressed clinically as urinary tract calculus disease. Radiopaque cystine stones are formed, and hexagonal cystine crystals appear in the urine. Diagnosis may be pursued by testing urine with nitroprusside, high-voltage electrophoresis, or column amino acid analysis. Stones generally form at cystine excretion rates of greater than 300 mg cystine per gram of creatinine in acid urine. Cystinuric patients are susceptible to all complications of stone disease. Treatment is directed at reducing the concentration of cystine in urine by increasing urine volume, increasing cystine solubility by alkalinizing the urine, and reduc-

ing cystine excretion by use of D-penicillamine. D-Penicillamine, although extremely effective, is not without risk and should be reserved for patients who fail to respond to conservative therapy.

5. *Models of human cystinuria have been described in animals. Studies of these models may help clarify the cellular defect in cystinuria and may provide a system for testing new drug therapy.*

Cystinuria is an inheritable disorder of amino acid transport affecting the epithelial cells of the renal tubules and gastrointestinal tract. The disease is expressed clinically by the formation of calculi in the urinary tract, with the potential for obstruction, infection, and ultimately renal insufficiency. The disease is characterized primarily by the precipitation of cystine, the least soluble of the naturally occurring amino acids; lysine, arginine, ornithine, and cysteine-homocysteine mixed disulfide are also present in excess in the urine. Since this aminoaciduria occurs with a normal or reduced filtered load of cystine and the dibasic amino acids, it was postulated earlier that cystinuria is a disorder of tubular transport in the kidney. The subsequent demonstration of comparably defective transport in the intestine established the present view of this disorder as an inherited defect in a specific transepithelial transport mechanism, which is expressed in two areas, the kidney and the intestine.

HISTORY

The historical development of a theory of the pathogenesis of cystinuria was anything but orderly. Although the data suggesting renal and intestinal lesions appeared in random order, it is easier to trace the history of the renal lesion before that of the intestinal defect.

In 1810 Wollaston analyzed two stones recovered from urinary bladders and discerned that they differed from all previously described calculi. Because of their bladder origin and supposed chemical nature, they were named cystic oxide stones [1]. In 1824 Stromeyer noted hexagonal platelike crystals in the urine of patients with cystinuria [2]. The finding of cystine crystals served for many years as the chief means of diagnosing the disease and remains helpful even today.

In 1833 Berzelius, recognizing that the compound was not an oxide, renamed the substance "cystine," perpetuating the fallacy that it originated in the bladder [3]. Although improved descriptions of the chemistry of cystine were developed over the next 70 years, it was not until 1902 that Friedman defined the chemical structure of cystine [4]. In his 1908 Croonian lectures, Garrod discussed cystinuria among the inborn errors of metabolism and postulated that a defect in the metabolism of cystine was responsible for the disorder [5]. During the next 40 years, in spite of the reports of increased lysine in the urine of cystinuric subjects, there was little advance in our understanding of the disease. The present concepts of cystinuria emerged after the advent of paper chromatography and development of polarographic and microbiologic assays. With these methods, Yeh et al. demonstrated in 1947 that lysinuria and argininuria also occur in cystinuria [6], and Stein found that a

large quantity of ornithine was also present [7]. Subsequently, Dent et al. [8] and Arrow and Westall [9] noted that plasma levels of cystine and of dibasic amino acids were normal or low. Dent and Rose observed that cystine and the dibasic amino acids had structural similarities, i.e., two amino groups separated by four to six chemical bonds. They postulated that there was a single renal transport mechanism shared by these amino acids and proposed that this mechanism was defective or absent in cystinuria [10] (Fig. 80-1). Although defective uptake of lysine and arginine has been demonstrable in tissue slices from cystinuric subjects, cystine uptake was unimpaired, and cystine did not appear to compete with the dibasic amino acids for transport [11].

Recent studies with rat renal cortical tubule fragments [12] and isolated brush border membrane vesicles [13] indicate that there are two transport systems for cystine, one with a high affinity that is shared with dibasic amino acids, another with low affinity that is unshared. It appears that the latter system is the only one observable during in vitro studies with cortical slices and that the results of cystine uptake experiments with slices do not reveal an important aspect of the transport for this amino acid. The data with isolated brush border membranes [13] support the formulation of Dent and Rose and suggest that cystinuria may result from defective function of a common high affinity uptake system for cystine and dibasic amino acids. This explanation for the renal defect in cystinuria is complicated, however, by the occurrence of cystine clearances exceeding creatinine clearances in cystinuric patients. This indicates that cystine secretion may contribute to the aminoaciduria [14–16].

The intestinal defect was not recognized as promptly. Von Udranszky and Baumann in 1889 observed that cadaverine and putrescine, decarboxylation products of lysine and arginine, were present in large amounts in urine of cystinuric subjects [17]. These findings were confirmed by Loewy and Neuberg [18]. Subsequently an increase of urinary cystine excretion was reported in cystinuria in response to protein feeding, but feeding of cystine itself was not observed to increase either serum or urine cystine [19, 20]. After half a century these data were finally interpreted by Milne, who had already recognized the intestinal transport defect asssociated with the renal aminoaciduria in Hartnup disease [21]. Milne performed experiments which demonstrated reduced intestinal absorption of the dibasic amino acids in patients with cystinuria [22, 23]. His findings have been confirmed in vitro by studies of transport in jejunal biopsies [24–26]. The question of why malabsorption of an essential amino acid does not result in more serious problems of growth and development has been answered in part by the observation that oligopeptide absorption from the intestine may account for a significant proportion of amino acid absorption [27, 28]. Lysine absorption from an oligopeptide may be normal in the same cystinuric subject who has poor absorption of free lysine.

CLINICAL ASPECTS

Although cystinuria is thought to be a rare disease because of the estimated prevalence of 1 per 100,000 in Sweden [29] and 1 per 20,000 in England [30, 31], there are populations where homozygous cystinuria is a frequently inherited disorder. The

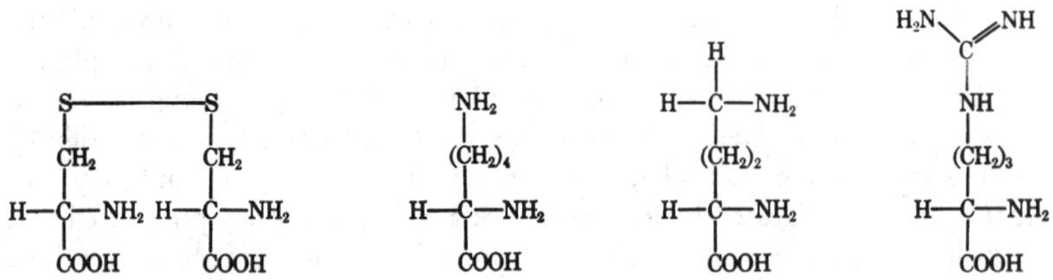

Figure 80-1 Chemical structures of the amino acids excreted in excessive amounts in the urine in cystinuria.

prevalence in Israeli Jews of Libyan origin has been estimated to be 1 in 2500 [32]. Screening programs of newborn babies show the prevalence in England to be 1 in 2000 [33]; in Australia, 1 in 4000 [34]; and in the United States, 1 in 15,000 [35]. According to Levy [36], who summarized the results of newborn screening, the overall prevalence is 1 in 7000, which makes cystinuria one of the most common inherited disorders. The disease occurs equally in both sexes, but males are more severely affected and have a higher mortality rate. The greater severity of the disease in males may be related to urinary tract anatomy, with a greater likelihood of urethral obstruction in males. Although clinical expression of the disease may occur in the first year of life or as late as the ninth decade, the second and third decades appear to be the peak times for expression of cystinuria. Colic, the most common presentation, may be associated with obstruction of the urinary tract, subsequent infection, and eventual loss of function. Infection, hypertension, and renal failure may occur occasionally and cause the patient first to seek medical attention.

Cystine Stones

Both cystine stones and uric acid stones form readily in acid urine, and the two are frequently confused. However, the cystine stone, with its yellow-brown color and maple sugar crystal surface, is much firmer than uric acid and is radiopaque [37, 38]. The radiopacity of cystine is due to the density of the sulfur molecules. On roentgenograms cystine stones appear smooth and are less dense than calcium stones. Cystine calculi tend to occur as staghorn or multiple recurrent stones, frequently necessitating surgery (Fig. 80-2). Calcium stones may also be formed as a result of infection secondary to cystine calculi.

DIAGNOSIS

The diagnosis of cystinuria should be entertained in every patient with urinary calculi or with urinary tract symptoms suggestive of calculi. The simplest diagnostic procedure is the microscopic examination of urinary sediment, preferably in the first voiding in the morning or other concentrated urine, for typical cystine crystals (Fig. 80-3).

The cyanide-nitroprusside test has been widely applied as a chemical screening procedure [39, 40]. It is important that the color obtained be compared with that of a specimen of normal urine to which cystine has been added. Since the lower limit of sensitivity of the reaction is about 75 to 125 mg/g creatinine, the reaction permits easy detection of homozygous stone formers, who usually excrete more than 250 mg/g creatinine [41, 42]. Some but not all of those heterozygotes with

increased urinary cystine may also be detected by this procedure. A positive nitroprusside test may be seen in homocystinuria as well as in patients with acetonuria. Patients with crystalluria or a positive cyanide-nitroprusside test should be further studied for identification of urinary amino acids by such methods as thin-layer chromatography [43] or high-voltage electrophoresis [44]. Quantitation of cystine may be made easily following its electrolytic reduction to the thiol, which can be colorimetrically determined [43]. Quantitative ion-exchange chromatography is the most sophisticated procedure and should be performed whenever possible [45, 46]. By this method the upper limits of normal values for cystine, lysine, arginine, and ornithine in the adult are 18, 130, 16, and 22 mg/g creatinine, respectively [31].

Cystinuria has been associated with hyperuricemia [47], hemophilia [48], retinitis pigmentosa [49], muscular dystrophy [50], muscular hypotonia [51], mongolism [52], and hereditary pancreatitis [53], and it occurs as an isolated aminoaciduria with hypocalcemic tetany [54]. The belief that cystinuric patients are shorter than the general population [55] has not been substantiated [56].

BIOCHEMISTRY OF CYSTINURIA

Consideration of cystinuria as an inborn error of metabolism by Garrod [5] was based on the assumption that an enzyme responsible for cystine catabolism was missing or defective. Although Garrod's concept of a missing enzyme in a metabolic pathway has been substantiated for the other diseases upon which his theory was based, this has not been done for cystinuria. Garrod was not truly incorrect about cystinuria, since the modern view that the disease is an inherited disorder of membrane transport supposes the genetic loss of a mechanism

Figure 80-2 Roentgenogram of the abdomen of a cystinuric patient showing bilateral radiopaque calculi.

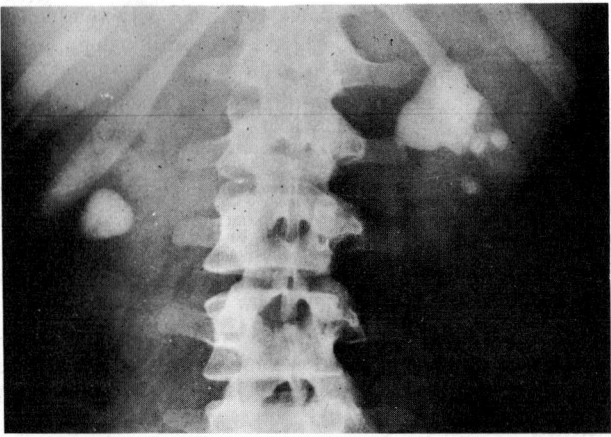

located in the membrane which is responsible for movement of extracellular cystine into the confines of the cell. The concept of a membrane transport mechanism involving an amino acid-binding site and genetic control is consistent with the function of a "carrier" protein. What Garrod did not anticipate was the membrane nature of the disorder and the primary involvement of the kidney and intestine.

Garrod's concept stimulated the elucidation of the transsulfuration metabolic pathway. The feeding experiments of Brand and his colleagues demonstrated that methionine [19] and proteins high in methionine [57] resulted in higher cystine excretion, since methionine is converted to cysteine and then to cystine. Feeding of cystine itself did not give rise to increased amounts of urinary cystine, but giving cysteine did [20]. This can now be interpreted on the basis of an intestinal defect in cystine absorption which does not involve cysteine (see below). The role of cystathionine as an intermediate was shown in du Vigneaud's laboratory when that compound gave rise to cystine [58]. Most recent observations have been concerned with the enzymes of the pathway in relation to homocystinuria [59] and cystathioninuria [60]. The observation that the body can convert methionine or homocystine to cystine by way of the transsulfuration pathway has relegated cystine to the position of a nonessential amino acid, but the demonstration that cystathionase is not active in fetal tissues implies that cystine may be an essential amino acid in fetal development [61].

Relatively less seems to be known of the catabolism of cystine or cysteine to sulfate. Oxidation to cysteinesulfonate, taurine, cysteic acid, and sulfite appears to be involved [62, 63]. Increased urinary sulfate excretion in cystinuric patients fed cystine may involve the oxidation of unabsorbed cystine in the gastrointestinal tract and subsequent absorption of the inorganic ion [64].

These aspects of cystine catabolism may be more appropriately considered with regard to the human cystine storage disease, cystinosis [65], which should not be confused with cystinuria. Although a generalized aminoaciduria is present with cystinosis, the large amounts of cystine and dibasic amino acids found with cystinuria are not found. Cystine storage disease is associated with deposition of cystine in various tissues; in cystinuria there is no tissue deposition, only urinary loss.

Of importance to a basic understanding of both human diseases involving cystine is the fact that the intracellular form of the amino acid is not the disulfide but the free thiol, cysteine [66, 67]. When ^{35}S cystine is incubated with kidney cortex slices or other tissues, the ^{35}S within the cell is mainly in cysteine or glutathione, little or none being maintained as cystine [67] (Table 80-1). Reduction of cystine to cysteine is believed to take place within the cell by a mechanism mediated by glu-

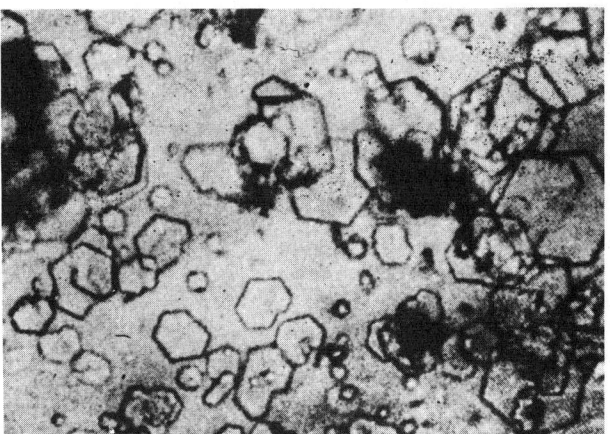

Figure 80-3 Cystine crystals as they appear in the urinary sediment in cystinuria.

tathione cysteine transhydrogenase [68], since cystine taken up by isolated renal brush border membrane vesicles is not reduced to the free thiol [13].

RENAL TRANSPORT DEFECTS

Cystinuria is a classic example of a disorder of renal tubular function. In a discussion of aminoaciduria it should be kept clearly in mind that most aminoacidurias are not disorders of tubular function. Normally amino acids are filtered and are almost entirely reabsorbed in the proximal nephron. There is a maximal capacity to the reabsorptive mechanism which is exceeded in certain disorders. In most cases of aminoaciduria an extrarenal metabolic defect leads to the accumulation of an amino acid in the plasma, which is then filtered in amounts exceeding the normal capacity of the nephron for reabsorption. These are not disorders of tubular function. With normal or low plasma levels and diminished filtered loads of amino acid, if excessive loss still occurs in the urine, then the reabsorptive capacity of the tubule is said to be below normal and tubular dysfunction exists. The latter situation obtains in cystinuria. Excessive urinary losses of cystine and dibasic amino acids occur with normal or less than normal plasma levels of the affected amino acids [8, 9].

Of all amino acids studied, only cystine and the dibasic amino acids are involved in cystinuria. On the basis of this information Dent and Rose postulated a single transport

Table 80-1 Intracellular forms of ^{35}S after incubation of rat kidney cortex slices with labeled L-cystine and L-cysteine

Age of animal	Transported substrate	Concentration, mM	Intracellular form of ^{35}S as percent of intracellular ^{35}S			
			Cystine	Reduced glutathione	Cysteine	Other
5 days	Cystine	0.07	0	25	62	13
5 days	Cysteine	0.07	6	24	62	8
Adult	Cystine	0.07	0	12	68	20
Adult	Cysteine	0.07	14	20	64	8

SOURCE: From Segal and Smith [66].

mechanism shared by cystine and the dibasic amino acids which is defective in cystinuria [10]. Recent reports of clinical disorders in which cystine and dibasic aminoacidurias occur independently have complicated this interpretation and indicate that there may be separate systems for transport of cystine and lysine by the kidney tubule. Brodehl et al. [54] have found isolated cystinuria without dibasic aminoaciduria, and Stephens and Perrett [69] reported a patient with cystine stones who had minimal dibasic aminoaciduria, a finding in many dogs with cystinuria and urolithiasis [70]. Conversely, dibasic aminoaciduria without cystinuria has been observed [71, 72]. Lysinuric protein intolerance is characterized by lysinuria without cystinuria, and defective renal tubular reabsorption of lysine and competition among the dibasic amino acids have been demonstrated [73].

Observations in Vivo

The increase in renal clearance of cystine and the dibasic amino acids reported first by Dent et al. [8] and then by Arrow and Westall [9] has also been found in more recent investigations [74, 75]. Although in many patients the cystine clearance is equal to or somewhat less than the glomerular filtration rate, certain patients with cystinuria have a cystine clearance greater than glomerular filtration, with a $C_{cystine}/C_{inulin}$ ratio ranging between 1 and 2 [14–16]. The clearance of lysine is usually about 50 to 70 percent of the glomerular filtration rate. Arginine and ornithine reabsorption is less defective than that of lysine [75].

The postulate of Dent and Rose that there is a single shared transport mechanism for cystine and dibasic amino acids predicted that increasing the filtered load of one amino acid in the group should reduce the reabsorption of the others. Robson and Rose [76], Lester and Cusworth [74], and Kato [75] demonstrated that this was indeed true in normal humans. Similar data were derived in studies on normal dogs by Webber, Brown, and Pitts [77]. While Robson and Rose did not find that infusion of lysine increased cystine excretion by cystinuric subjects, both Lester and Cusworth [74] and Kato [75] observed such an effect on cystine, ornithine, and arginine excretion. Lester and Cusworth showed that lysine infusion caused the clearance of cystine to increase to a value greater than glomerular filtration, with a $C_{cystine}/C_{creatinine}$ ratio of 1.5. Kato [75] infused increasing amounts of arginine into three patients whose tubular reabsorption of cystine ranged from 10 to 50 percent (normal 99 percent). This reduced the cystine reabsorption to −25 percent.

A careful examination of the data of Webber, Brown, and Pitts [77] indicates that lysine infusion in a normal dog caused the cystine clearance to exceed the glomerular filtration rate. Segal and Bovee [78] have reported that infusion of lysine into a cystinuric dog changed cystine reabsorption from 62 to −210 percent of the filtered load and have found a cystinuric dog whose basal cystine reabsorption was −255 percent of the filtered load [78]. The data are consistent with secretion of cystine under these conditions and raise the question of bidirectional cystine transport. The dibasic amino acid infusion data imply that these amino acids may not only compete with cystine for reabsorption but that by some enigmatic process they induce cystine secretion. The concept of amino acid secretion has been amply supported by experimental findings employing a variety of techniques [79–81].

Additional studies in cystinuric patients have revealed a low

renal threshold for lysine [74]. When homozygous subjects were infused with increasing amounts of lysine, they were unable to reabsorb the amino acid to any extent above the endogenous capacity until the filtered load was seven- to tenfold higher than the basal state. A further increase in the filtered load was associated with a tubular reabsorpton in cystinuric patients that did not differ from the normal rate [75]. These findings are consistent with the function of dual systems for lysine transport, a low capacity system acting at low substrate concentrations which is defective in cystinurics, and a high capacity transport system predominating at high lysine levels which is unaffected. Such a dual transport system for lysine has been described in human renal cortical slices [82]. The occurrence of multiple systems for cystine and dibasic amino acids is also supported by Brodehl, who found that newborn human infants have diminished reabsorption of cystine and dibasic amino acids and that reabsorption capacity matured at different rates for each of the substrates [83].

Examination of the extraction of cystine from blood flowing through the kidneys of cystinuric patients has revealed minimal arteriovenous differences [84, 85] and no alteration from the normal. Assuming that total failure of tubular reabsorption of cystine accounts for cystinuria, a large arteriovenous difference for cystine should be discernible. The inability to demonstrate this has raised the possibility of cystine synthesis de novo or kidney protein catabolism to account for the presence of urinary cystine in the face of normal plasma extraction. Frimpter [86] has attempted to answer this by comparing the specific activity of plasma and urinary cystine after infusing ^{35}S cystine. The fact that these activities were the same argues against an endogenous kidney production of cystine, but it is possible that the long infusion period may have labeled the kidney pools of cystine so that the sought-for specific activity differences would not be detected.

The reduced form of cystine, cysteine, may play an important role in the underlying abnormality. Plasma cysteine in cystinuric patients is decreased proportionally more than cystine or the dibasic amino acids, but little cysteine appears in urine, and no increased conversion of cysteine to cystine has yet been demonstrated [86, 87]. Frimpter [84], having found an arteriovenous difference for cysteine but not for cystine across the kidney of a single patient, postulated that urinary cystine may be derived from plasma cysteine. Rosenberg et al. [85], however, found no increase in cysteine extraction in two patients when compared with controls. An increase in cysteine clearance by the kidney would seem an unlikely source of urinary cystine. The plasma level of cysteine is only about 25 percent of that of cystine, too low to explain the large amounts of urinary cystine on the basis of a total loss of filtered cysteine.

Results of microperfusion experiments with rat kidney tubules [88, 89] show arginine inhibition of cystine and cysteine removal from the lumen of the tubule. Although these data suggest an interaction at the luminal membrane and the possibility of a shared transport system, it must be kept in mind that the cystine in the lumen is a resultant of fluxes and that the effect of arginine may not be a simple inhibition of uptake at the luminal membrane.

A series of in vivo studies of lysine and cystine transport in rats attempted to demonstrate bidirectional transport by examining cellular accumulation after ureteral ligation and cessation of glomerular filtration [90, 91]. The fact that cellular accumulation was maintained in the presence of ureteral ligation suggested that basolateral uptake had occurred, but this interpretation is open to question, since 1 to 2 h after ureteral obstruction in the rat the single nephron glomerular filtration rate is only slightly reduced [92]. The interaction of dibasic amino acids and cystine was also examined in the intact rat kidney [90, 91]. The injection of a large amount of arginine increased the fractional excretion of lysine, while injection of a lysine load increased the excretion of cystine. An unexplained finding was that during the arginine-induced lysinuria, when less lysine would be thought to be entering the tubule cells from the lumen, the tubule cell content of radioactive lysine was greater than in cells of control rats. A similar type of result occurred during lysine induced cystinuria, when an increase in tubule cell cysteine, the intracellular form of cystine, was noted. These increases varied with the depth of the cell from the kidney surface and were greatest in cells of the outer medulla. The significance of these observations is not clear, but they suggest a functional heterogeneity of kidney tubule cells with regard to cystine and dibasic amino acids. Schwartzman, Blair, and Segal [93] have reported that lysine inhibits cysteine efflux from renal tubule cells and have postulated an efflux system shared by lysine and cystine. An elevation of intracellular cysteine could result from an inhibition by lysine of the transfer of cysteine into the peritubular capillary at the basolateral aspect of the cell.

Observations in Vitro

Studies in vitro with slices of human renal cortex have demonstrated that the dibasic amino acids, lysine, arginine, and ornithine, share a common renal transport mechanism [11]. The ability of cortical slices from cystinuric persons to take up lysine and arginine is impaired [11] (Fig. 80–4). The cystinuric tissue has about 50 to 60 percent of the normal capacity to take up lysine. This corresponds to the reabsorptive defect observed

during clearance experiments in vivo [75]. Evidence that the shared dibasic amino acid transport system is only partially defective is that the low uptake of lysine can be further suppressed by the addition of arginine. Rosenberg, Albrecht, and Segal [82] examined the concentration dependence of lysine uptake by normal and cystinuric renal cortex slices. Lineweaver-Burk plots were indicative of the presence of two distinct influx systems, one a high affinity, low capacity system and the other a low affinity, high capacity system. From the observed K_m and V_{max} parameters it appeared that the V_{max} of the high affinity, low K_m system was lower than normal. At a physiologic plasma lysine concentration of 0.1 mM the major lysine transport ability of normal renal tissue would result in the low K_m system, and that system appears to have a limited capacity in cystinuric kidney.

Neither the uptake of cystine [11] nor cysteine [94] is impaired in slices of renal cortex from cystinuric patients. Cystine and the dibasic amino acids did not appear to share a common transport system [11]. Although cysteine transport is effected by dual systems by human cortical slices [94], only one system could be observed for cystine entry into human renal cells [11]. These unexpected findings stimulated an extensive investigation of the characteristics of cystine and dibasic amino acid transport by rat renal cortex slices, isolated tubule fragments, and brush border membrane vesicles.

Numerous experiments have been performed using kidney slice transport techniques. These clearly demonstrate that the transport systems for lysine and cystine in rat kidney cortex are not the same [95–99]. In addition to the lack of mutual inhibition between these two amino acids and their nonparticipation in heteroexchange diffusion, there are certain biochemical differences in their transport characteristics. Lysine transport is only partially dependent on the presence of sodium ion and aerobic conditions, and over a pH range of 6 to 8.5 there is little change of influx in rats [97]. Cystine transport, on the other hand, is completely dependent on sodium and oxygen and shows marked differences in influx with changes in pH,

Figure 80-4 Uptake of lysine and arginine by renal cortex slices from cystinuric and noncystinuric subjects. The distribution ratio is the ratio of radioactivity in counts per milliliter of intracellular fluid to counts per minute per milliliter of incubation media. *(From data in Ref. 11.)*

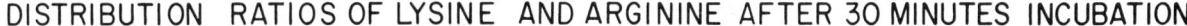

DISTRIBUTION RATIOS OF LYSINE AND ARGININE AFTER 30 MINUTES INCUBATION

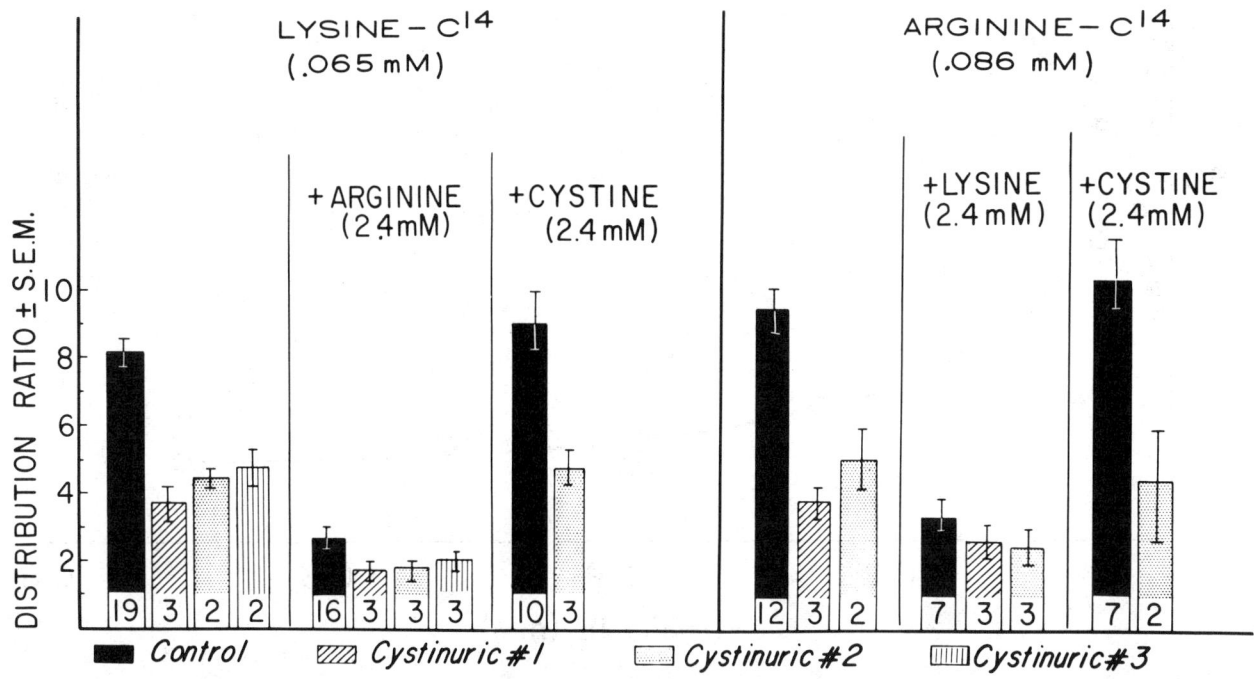

with an optimum of about pH 7.4 [98]. While there is evidence for more than one lysine transport system in rat cortical slices, only one system was evident for cystine, with a K_m of 0.8 mM. Kinetic studies in rat kidney cortex slices have furnished evidence, based on response to alteration of pH, temperature changes, oxygen lack, and sodium deprivation, that the kidney cystine and cysteine transport systems are different [98]. Confirmation of this supposition has come from ontogenetic studies which show a separate developmental time pattern for cystine and cysteine transport in rat kidney cortex [67]. An examination of the transport interaction of cysteine with dibasic amino acids in vitro showed no mutual inhibition of uptake [93]. Even so, incubation of cysteine with lysine causes an enchanced accumulation of the sulfur amino acid by kidney cortex [93, 96]. Schwartzman, Blair, and Segal [93] have explained the lysine-enhanced accumulation of cystine by showing that the dibasic amino acids inhibit the efflux of intracellular cysteine into the incubation fluid. This interaction between the sulfur amino acids and the dibasic amino acids may have physiologic importance since the natural intracellular form is cysteine, even if cystine is the compound being transported [66, 67].

With the recent use of rat tubule fragments [12] and brush border membrane vesicles [13, 100], a more complete picture of cystine and dibasic amino acid transport in the proximal tubule has emerged. Cystine uptake by isolated cortical tubules occurred via two saturable transport systems with K_m values of 0.012 and 0.55 mM. Lysine inhibited cystine uptake via the low K_m system but appeared not to inhibit cystine uptake via the high K_m mechanism. Cystine inhibited the uptake of lysine by the tubules. Figure 80-5 shows the calculated percentages of cystine uptake mediated by the two systems present in tubule

fragments at various cystine concentrations. At the concentration of about 0.05 mM present in plasma, about 50 percent would be handled by each system [12].

With brush border membrane vesicles two comparable transport sytems for cystine were demonstrated with dibasic amino acids inhibiting the low K_m high affinity system [13, 100] (Fig. 80-6). Heteroexchange diffusion of lysine and cystine was demonstrated by the high affinity component [100]. In contrast to tubule fragments, where the cystine entering the cell was reduced to cysteine [12], the intravesicular amino acid was cystine, indicating that the unreduced form was transported across the brush border membrane [13, 100]. Also, unlike the findings in tubule cells where the intracellular cysteine is not bound to proteins, the intravesicular cystine became bound to the membrane. This emphasizes the importance of the intracellular reducing process for maintaining free cysteine within the cell and this facilitates unhampered transcellular movement of the amino acid during the reabsorptive process.

The correlation of the dual cystine transport systems in tubule fragments and in brush border membrane vesicles indicates that transport across the luminal side of the proximal tubule cell can be observed when tubule fragments are studied. With renal cortical slices only one component of cystine transport is demonstrated and that corresponds to the high K_m system observed with both renal cortical tubules and brush border membrane vesicles. Since only the high K_m system is observed in slice experiments, an interaction between cystine and dibasic amino acids would not be expected; this interaction occurs on

Figure 80-5 The percentages of total velocity of cystine uptake by rat renal proximal tubules in vitro mediated by the high (*closed circle*) and low (*open circle*) K_m systems at various cystine concentrations [12]. (*Copyright 1980 by Grune & Stratton, Inc.*)

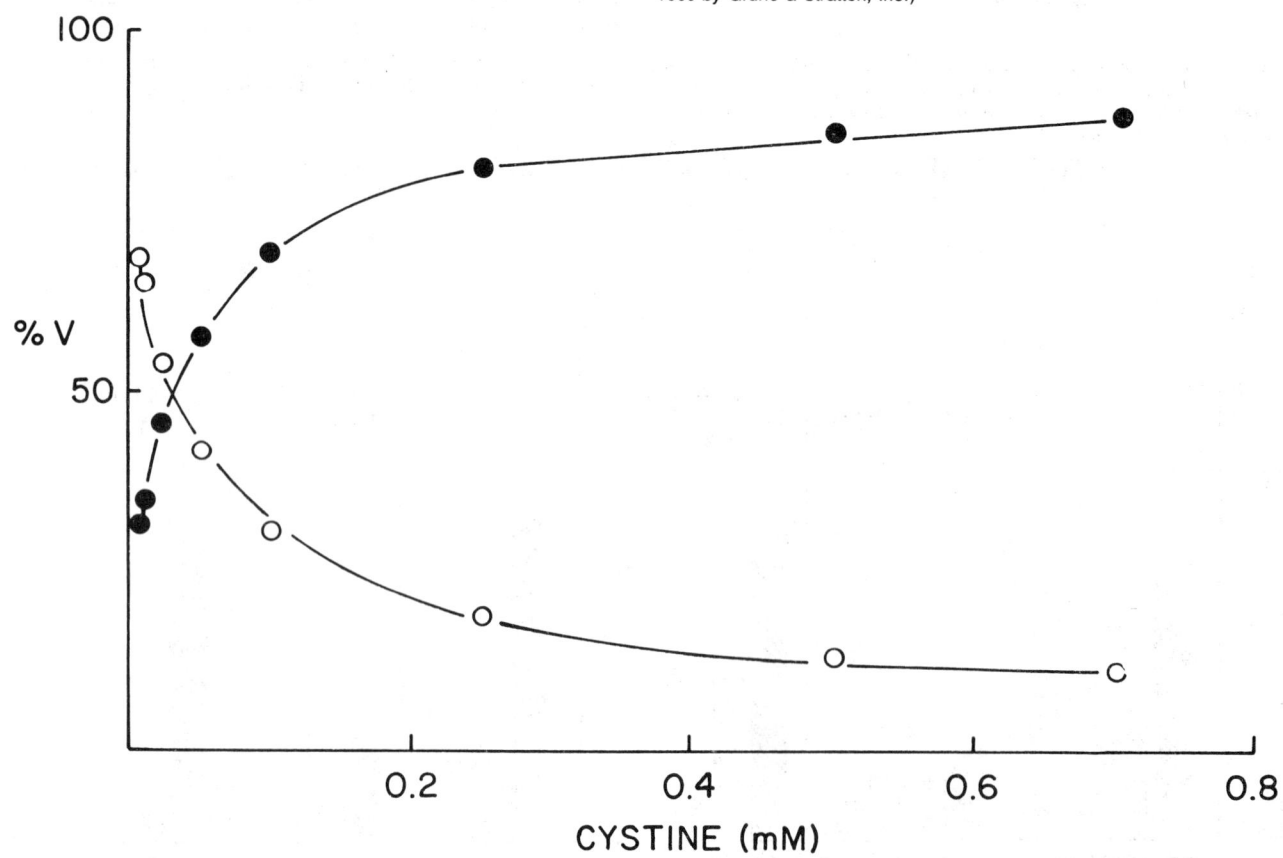

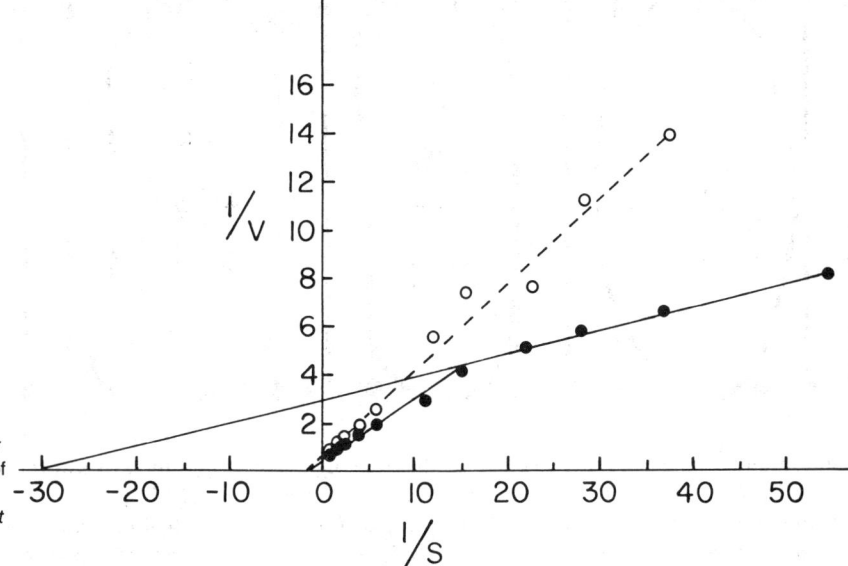

Figure 80-6 Concentration dependence of cystine on the initial rate of uptake by rat renal brush border membrane vesicles. Solid circles represent uptake of ¹⁴L-cystine, and open circles show its uptake in the presence of 1 mmole/liter of L-lysine [13]. (*Copyright 1977 by American Association for Advancement of Science.*)

the low K_m shared system. Why the renal slice experiments give a broad picture of dibasic amino acid transport but only a truncated view of cystine transport is at present enigmatic.

The demonstration of a shared system for cystine and dibasic amino acids in the luminal membrane of the renal tubule cell substantiates the original hypothesis of Dent and Rose [10] that cystinuria results from defective reabsorption by a common transport process. The finding of another unshared system aids in interpreting some of the clinical observations. Figure 80-7 shows a possible model of the carrier systems in the brush border membrane for cystine and dibasic amino acids. A defective low K_m system would result in excessive amounts of cystine, lysine, arginine, and ornithine in urine, as in classic cystinuria. This is the system whose defective function has been observed in human cystinuric kidney slices when lysine was the transported substrate [11], and which was inhibited by infusion of large amounts of lysine in humans and dogs [74–78]. Cystinuric patients, who do not have dibasic aminoaciduria, may have a defect in the high K_m unshared cystine system. Dibasic aminoaciduria without cystinuria [71, 72] may be due to a defect in a dibasic transport system unshared with cystine. Remaining to be explained is the apparent secretion of cystine by some cystinuric patients [14–16] and dogs infused with lysine [78].

URINARY EXCRETION OF OTHER AMINO ACIDS IN CYSTINURIA

Although hyperexcretion of lysine, arginine, ornithine, and cystine in the urine is the hallmark of cystinuria, other amino acids have been found in higher than normal amounts in the urine of some patients. These include glycine [14], methionine [101], cystathionine [102], and homocysteine-cysteine disulfide [103] (Fig. 80-8). The latter is most consistently present in variable amounts up to 224 mg/24 h [84], the amount being related directly to the amount of cystine excreted [104]. This mixed disulfide has also been found in the urine of patients with Fanconi's syndrome on the basis of Wilson's disease, as

well as in dogs with cystinuria [84]. Subsequently, the mixed disulfide was demonstrated in normal plasma and in increased amount in the plasma of a patient with homocystinuria [105]. Although it was thought at first to be uniquely associated with cystinuria, homocysteine-cysteine mixed disulfide probably is a normal plasma constituent which is overexcreted because it participates in the renal tubular defect responsible for the loss of cystine.

INTESTINAL TRANSPORT DEFECTS

When an amino acid is fed, absorption occurs, and the unabsorbed amino acid will be used by the intestinal flora. The less an amino acid is absorbed, the lower the blood levels will be after feeding, and the greater will be the levels of bacterial breakdown products in the stool and perhaps also in plasma and urine. If bacterial flora are suppressed, the nonabsorbed amino acid should be demonstrable in the stool. Lysine, arginine, and ornithine are decarboxylated by bacteria in the intestine to the diamines cadaverine, agmatine, and putrescine. Piperidine is formed from lysine breakdown, and pyrrolidine from arginine and ornithine metabolism (Fig. 80-9). These heterocyclic amines are formed from the diamines. As mentioned earlier, the data suggesting an intestinal transport defect in cystinuric patients were available by the late nineteenth century, when diamines were detected in the urine of these patients [17, 18]. It was only after Milne and coworkers demonstrated defective tryptophan absorption from the intestine of patients with the neutral aminoaciduria, Hartnup disease, in 1960, that the data on cystinuria were finally brought into focus [21]. Milne et al. observed increased putrescine and pyrrolidine in the urine after feeding arginine, and increased cadaverine, piperidine, and pyrrolidine after feeding lysine. Since the pyrrolidine could not have been derived from lysine, it was concluded that lysine was competitively inhibiting arginine transport in the intestine. The role of bacterial degradation in this process was proved in patients treated with oral neomycin; pyrrolidine and putrescine decreased in stool and urine, while

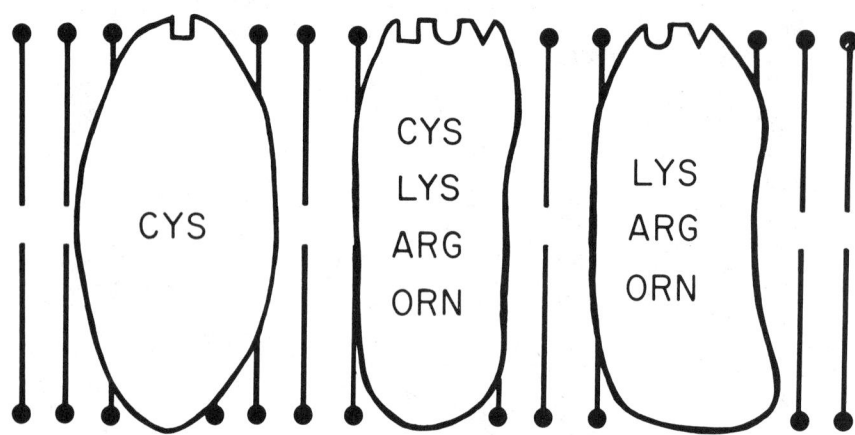

Figure 80-7 Schematic diagram of a membrane from the renal proximal tubule cell showing the possible diversity of carrier proteins for cystine (cys), lysine (lys), arginine (arg), and ornithine (orn).

lysine, arginine, and ornithine increased in the stool of patients so treated [22, 23]. Evidence for a failure of cystine absorption was presented by Brand, Cahill, and Harris [19], by Dent et al. [8], and more recently by London and Foley [64], Rosenberg et al. [85], and Silk et al. [106], using ion-exchange chromatography to measure plasma cystine concentration after oral loading. In all these studies cysteine absorption by cystinuria patients was not impaired [106, 107].

Double-lumen perfusion of the jejunum with low concentrations of lysine demonstrates defective dibasic amino acid transport in vivo, while in the same patient oral administration of a large dose results in a normal increase in the plasma concentration of lysine [108]. The response to a large oral dose of lysine suggests that diffusion or alternate transport routes may protect the cystinuric individuals from amino acid malnutrition. Perhaps a better explanation of why there is little evidence of dibasic amino acid malabsorption in cystinuria derives from recent studies indicating that oligopeptide transport is normal in these patients. In fact, in cystinuria administration of lysylglycine results in a greater increase in plasma lysine than equimolar feeding of free lysine plus glycine. Similarly, casein feeding produces a more rapid increase in plasma arginine and lysine than does a mixture of free amino acids derived from a casein hydrolysate [109–113].

The concept of impaired intestinal amino acid transport derived from feeding experiments received direct confirmation by the demonstration in vitro of defective amino acid accumulation in specimens of jejunal mucosa obtained by peroral biopsy [24–26]. The results of further studies showed that there were some patients who had total impairment of cystine, lysine, and arginine accumulation, others who had small but detectable cystine transport but no dibasic amino acid transport, and still a third group who had normal or only slightly impaired cystine uptake and demonstrable but diminished lysine and arginine accumulation [114] (Fig. 80-10). Later experiments showed that intestinal mucosa from the different types of cystinuria had no impairment of cysteine accumulation in vitro [115]. This finding not only established the independence of the cystine and cysteine transport mechanism but with the results of studies of cystine uptake in vitro explained the many oral feeding experiments previously performed which showed a rise in plasma and urinary cystine after cysteine feeding but not after cystine feeding [64, 107].

Recent work suggests that in mucosal biopsy specimens from cystinuric patients there is diminished lysine permeability at the brush border membrane [116], while in biopsied tissues of patients with lysinuric protein intolerance impaired flux of

lysine exists at the basolateral membrane of the epithelial cells [117].

Differences between the characteristics of intestinal and renal transport of lysine in vitro have been clearly demonstrated in the rat. Lysine uptake by intestinal mucosa is sodium- and oxygen-dependent and sensitive to pH changes; that by the kidney is only minimally affected by changes in sodium, oxygen, or pH [118].

Family studies of cystine excretion alone allowed differentiation of phenotypically identical cystinuric subjects into two genetically different groups [41, 119, 120]. Additional consideration of the intestinal mucosal transport patterns for the dibasic amino acids allows homozygous cystinuric subjects to be differentiated into three groups [114] (Table 80-2). In type I, which includes the majority of patients, there is no accumulation of either cystine or the dibasic amino acids against a gradient, and oral cystine loading fails to raise serum cystine levels (Fig. 80-11). In type II there is detectable active accumulation of cystine but no accumulation of dibasic amino acids; as in type I oral loading fails to raise serum cystine levels. In type III accumulation of cystine and dibasic amino acids does occur but not to the normal extent; oral cystine loading results in normal elevation of plasma cystine levels.

In an elegant study in which urinary excretion of amino acids, renal clearances, intestinal biopsies, and oral cystine loading were performed, Morin et al. [16] obtained data confirming the existence of types I and II cystinuria. They found no patients, however, with a condition corresponding to type III. Disorders suggestive of type III were found in persons produced by the mating of heterozygous carriers of type I and type

Figure 80-8 The structures of cystine and related compounds.

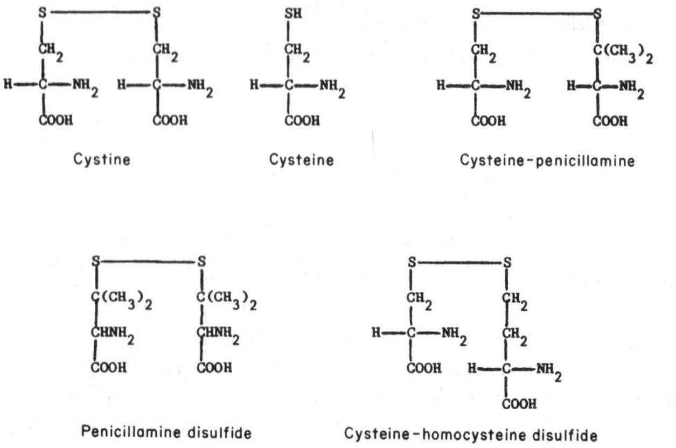

Cystine

Cysteine

Cysteine-penicillamine

Penicillamine disulfide

Cysteine-homocysteine disulfide

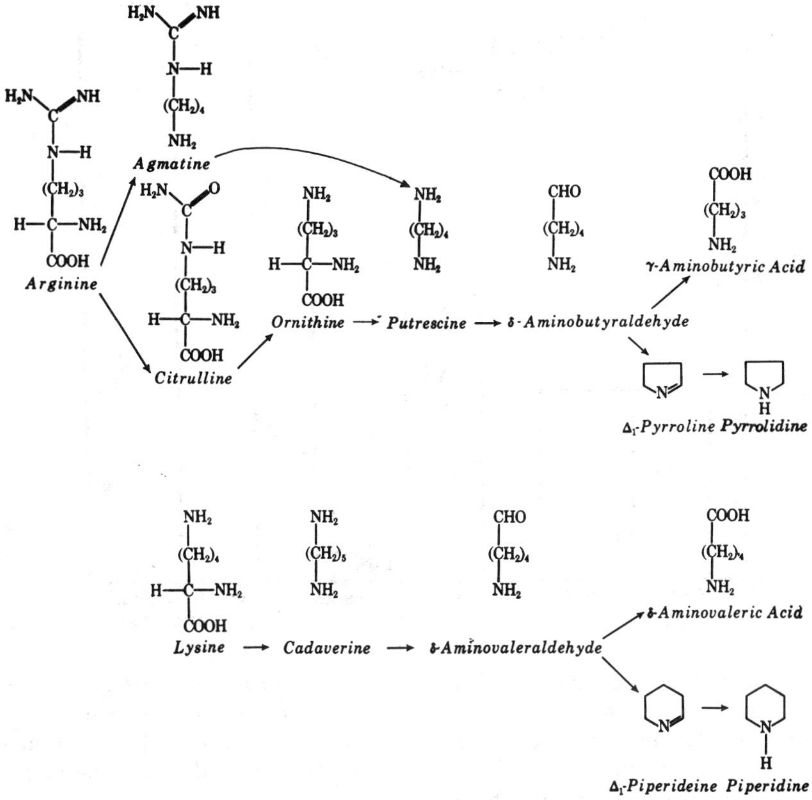

Figure 80-9 Formation of putrescine and pyrrolidine from arginine and cadaverine and of piperidine from lysine. (*After Crawhall and Watts [30].*)

II. The family studies based on this separation will be discussed under "Genetics."

The results of intestinal transport studies in vitro fit the postulate of Dent and Rose that cystine and basic amino acids share a common transport system. In the intestinal mucosa there is evidence of only a single shared system which in many patients is completely defective in its function [26, 114]. That system corresponds to the low K_m, high affinity shared component recently demonstrated in renal brush border membranes [13, 100]. An important difference is that lysine transport by the cystinuric kidney is only partially impaired [11]. Although this intestinal defect may be of little clinical importance, it has served as an extremely sensitive genetic marker and has paved the way for a new genetic classification of cystinuria. The lack of amino acid transport defects in circulating leukocytes of cystinuric patients has precluded their usefulness for discerning genetic aspects of the disease [121].

CYSTINURIA AND THE CENTRAL NERVOUS SYSTEM

There have been numerous reports of an association of cystinuria with central nervous system abnormalities. Scriver et al. [122] reported an increase in the prevalence of cystinuria in a group of mentally disturbed patients, and there have been reports of cystinuria patients with spastic paraplegia [123–125]. Mental retardation has been described occasionally in homozygous patients [126], but testing of a large group of homozygous cystinuric patients for mental deficiency did not reveal an increased prevalence [127]. Smith and Procopis [128] reported a 13 times higher incidence of heterozygous cystinuric subjects than would have been expected in a population of retarded persons in New South Wales, but no instances of homozygous cystinuria were detected. A pertinent question

Table 80-2 Classification of cases of cystinuria

Experimental observations	Type I	Type II	Type III
Intestine:			
In vitro transport	No transport of cystine, lysine, or arginine; normal cysteine transport	No transport of lysine; markedly reduced cystine transport	Transport of cystine reduced but may be normal; lysine variably reduced
Oral cystine administration	No plasma cystine elevation	No plasma cystine elevation	Slow increase in plasma cystine to normal elevation
Kidney:			
In vitro transport cortical slices	Reduced lysine transport		Reduced lysine transport
Urinary amino acid excretion	Increased cystine, lysine, arginine, ornithine excretion	Increased cystine, lysine, arginine, ornithine excretion	Increased cystine, lysine, arginine, ornithine excretion
Urinary amino acid excretion in heterozygotes	Normal	Cystine and lysine above normal	Cystine and lysine above normal

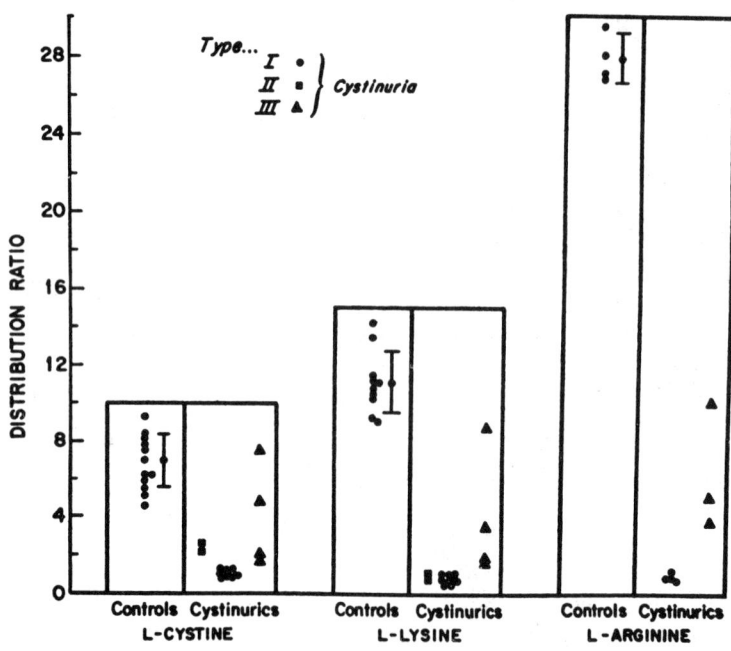

Figure 80-10 Uptake of cystine, lysine, and arginine by jejunal mucosa from control and cystinuric subjects expressed as the distribution ratio, i.e., the ratio of radioactive amino acid inside the cell to that in the medium, after a 45-min incubation [114].

has been whether cystinuric patients are at a greater risk for cerebral dysfunction because there might be defective transport into the brain for an essential amino acid like lysine, or cystine in the neonatal period [61], as has been demonstrated in the intestine or kidney of affected subjects.

The relationship of cystine, cysteine, and lysine transport by isolated rat brain synaptosomes has been examined [129–131]. Dual systems for their uptake were described, but there was no inhibition of either mechanism of cystine entry by dibasic amino acids. Cysteine uptake was only slighly inhibited by lysine but was strongly affected by glycine. The low K_m lysine transport system was shared by other dibasic amino acids but not by cystine, as it is in the kidney or intestines. The uptake of cystine by isolated rat brain capillaries appeared to be independent of dibasic amino acid transport [132]. All the findings in vitro indicate that the systems for entry of these amino acids to brain differ from those of kidney and intestine and make it unlikely that cystinuric subjects are at risk because of transport abnormalities in the central nervous system.

GENETICS

An understanding of the genetics of cystinuria depends on a clear definition of the phenotypically homozygous state. This state is suggested by (1) the excretion of over 250 mg cystine per gram of creatinine, often with formation of urinary calculi, and (2) the presence of an intestinal absorptive defect for cystine and the dibasic amino acids. In the first large-scale genetic studies, Harris and coworkers divided cystinuria into two groups in which phenotypically homozygous subjects were indistinguishable [120]. In one group the disease was transmitted as a true recessive trait; no family members other than the homozygous individual had aminoaciduria. The second group was designated as incompletely recessive; family members frequently excreted excessive amounts of cystine and lysine, although significantly less than homozygotes. The heterozygous incompletely recessive cystinuric subject did not form

stones. On the basis of variable patterns of amino acid excretion in homozygous cystinuric patients Harris and Robson [133] postulated that this group might be under polygenic influences. The exhaustive analysis by Crawhall et al. of urinary cystine, lysine, and arginine excretions by cystine stone formers, their parents, other relatives, and normal persons seems to support this view [31]. After examination of many kindreds these workers emphasized the wide disparities among the amounts of individual amino acids excreted by different heterozygous and homozygous individuals (Figs. 80-12 and 80-13). Thus it appears that multiple genetic factors influence the quantities of the various amino acids excreted in the urine and the final phenotypic expression.

The availability of jejunal mucosa led to the recognition that more than one pattern of cystine and dibasic amino acid transport could be recognized in homozygotes, and that these patterns correlated with different modes of inheritance, as suggested by Harris. Homozygotes can now be differentiated without recourse to family studies. The pattern of jejunal mucosal transport discussed above under "Intestinal Transport Defects" is summarized in Table 80-2. Note that three

Figure 80-11 The change of plasma cystine levels after oral cystine administration of 0.5 μmol/kg [114].

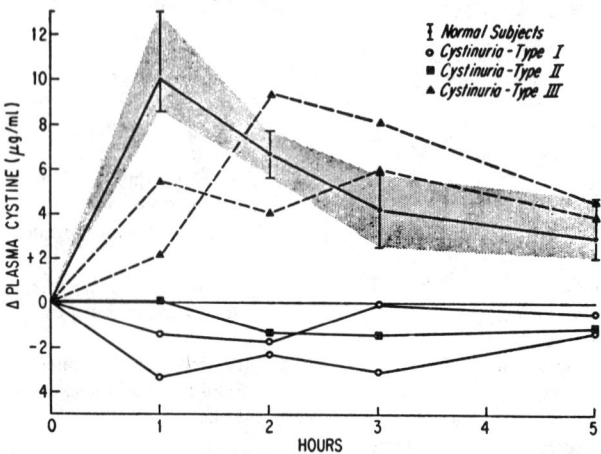

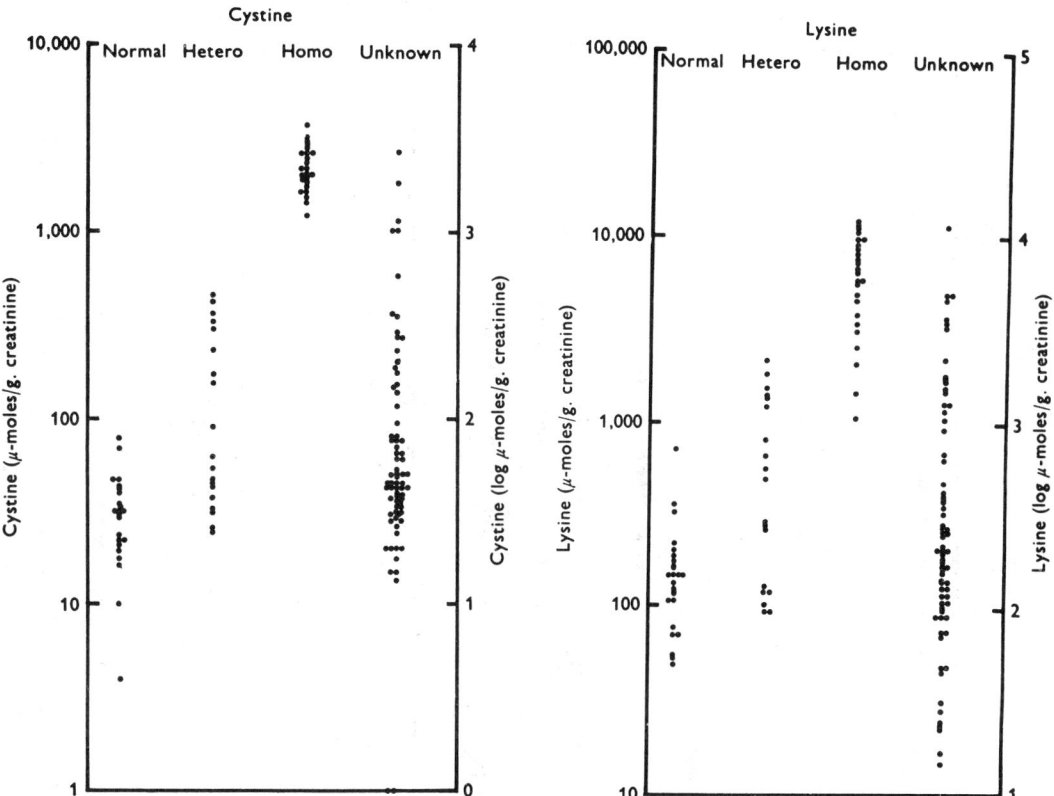

Figure 80-12 The excretion of cystine and lysine by normal subjects, patients with cystinuria, heterozygotes for cystinuria, and relatives of cystinuric patients [31].

classes of cystinuria may now be developed and that the last two were combined in the incompletely recessive group II of Harris.

With the ability to separate homozygous cystinuric subjects into distinct groups based on intestinal transport, Rosenberg restudied the families of these individuals and found distinctive urinary amino acid patterns [134]. Families of type I patients had no abnormal urinary amino acid excretion. Type II and type III heterozygous individuals excreted excessive amounts of cystine and the dibasic amino acids in their urine, and could be distinguished from each other. The quantities excreted were consistently higher in type II heterozygotes. Morin et al. [16], on the other hand, in their study of the urinary amino acid excretion in cystinuric families, did not encounter more than two patterns in heterozygotes. The patterns of excretion that Rosenberg, Durant, and Albrecht [134] considered to indicate type III heterozygotes correspond to that of type I and type II compound heterozygotes (offspring of the mating of type I and type II carriers) found by Morin et al. [16].

The presence of at least three distinct genetic types raised the question of whether cystinuria represented a group of diseases with defects in separate steps of amino acid transport, or different defects in the same genetically controlled step; i.e., were the different types the result of nonallelic or allelic mutations? The results of matings between type I and type II or III heterozygous individuals could provide an answer. If the defects were allelic, a fully expressed homozygous state (a better term is "compound heterozygous state") might appear in the offspring. If the defects were in separate genes, then only the expressed heterozygous state should appear in the offspring, i.e., type II or III. The fact that "homozygous" children were

found suggested that the defects were allelic [135, 136]. Although studies in vitro of intestinal transport have defined what seem to be three phenotypes [108], it should be pointed out that within the third type the cystine uptake by mucosal biopsies ranges from normal to an impairment almost as severe as in the first type (Fig. 80-10). The third type may be an expression of an even greater multiplicity of genetic factors involved in the intestinal transport phenotype.

Thus cystinuria is defined as a genetic disorder with a complex recessive mode of inheritance resulting from allelic mutations. At least some of the mutations may be expressed in the heterozygous state. The most sensitive means for differentiating the three types of homozygous cystinuric subjects is the study of the intestinal transport of cystine and the dibasic amino acids in vitro. Similar differentiation can be attempted from studies of urinary amino acid excretion in families of cystinuric subjects. This approach is neither as sensitive nor as direct as the study of transport in vitro.

ANIMAL MODELS OF CYSTINURIA

Several animal models have been suggested for the study of cystinuria. As a result of studies of amino acid excretion patterns of animals in the London Zoo, Harris thought that the blotched genet excreted large amounts of cystine [137]. The genet appeared to be unique in that "cystine" was excreted without the dibasic amino acids, and was excreted in concentrations far greater than would ordinarily remain in solution.

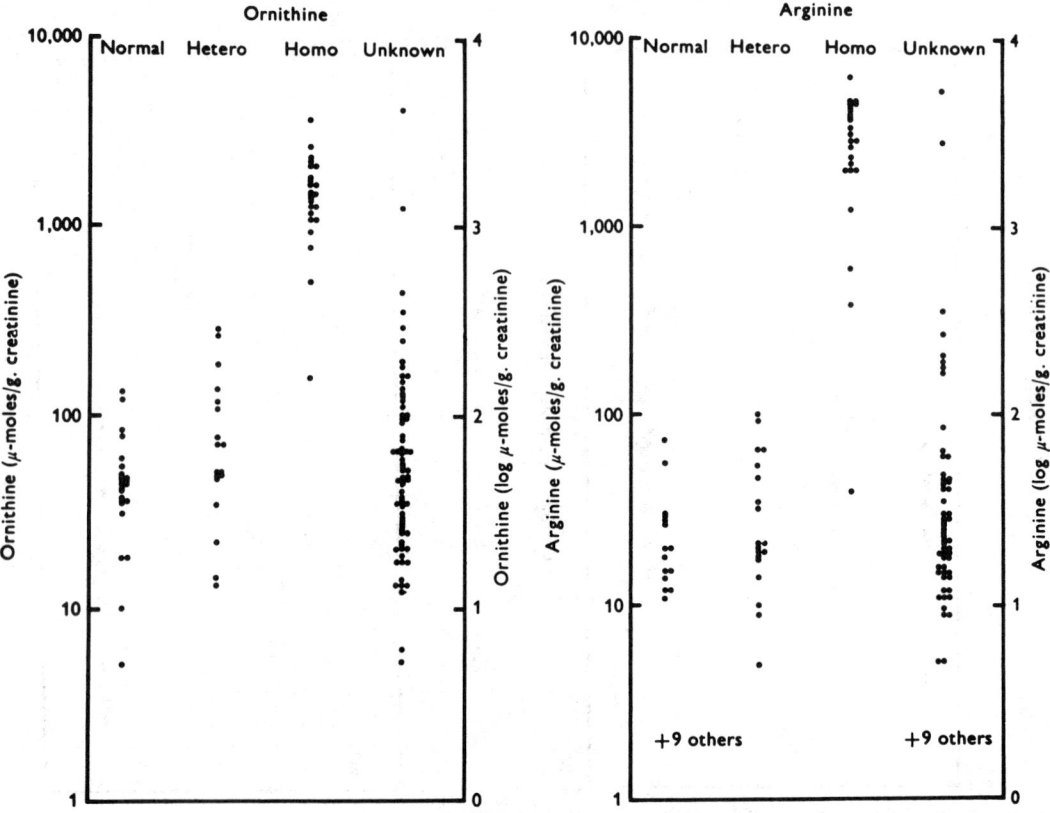

Figure 80-13 The excretion of arginine and ornithine by normal subjects, cystinuric patients, heterozygotes for cystinuria, and relatives of cystinuric patients [31].

Crawhall and Segal subsequently demonstrated that the genet excretes not cystine, but the far more soluble sulfur amino acid, S-sulfo-L-cysteine [138]. There is in fact no abnormality of cystine transport in the genet, and this apparent animal model must be discarded.

In 1956 a male mink with large numbers of apparently pure cystine stones was reported. This was a ranch mink on a higher than usual protein intake but otherwise unremarkable [139]. The presence of cystinuria in an animal group already carefully bred and therefore easily studied bears further investigation, but at present little further information is available.

Canine cystinuria represents potentially the most useful model for study. Although cystine stones in dogs were described as early as 1823, it was not until Brand and Cahill bred a group of Irish terriers with cystinuria that any systematic observations were made [140–144]. The expression of cystinuria corresponded to a sex-linked inheritance pattern. As in human beings, their animals responded with rises in cystine excretion after methionine feeding, and had no change after cystine feeding. Most, if not all, canine cystinuria has appeared in males. Though this may be due to the narrow urethra of male dogs, which brings stone production to clinical attention, amino acid chromatography has not revealed the disease in females to date.

The exact amino acid excretion pattern in canine cystinuria is not clear. Isolated cystinuria, cystinuria plus lysinuria, and the full pattern of cystine and all dibasic amino acids appearing in excess in the urine have been reported [70, 145–148]. An intestinal defect in amino acid transport has been postulated [149].

Recent application of transport techniques in vitro to both intestinal and kidney biopsies of cystine stone-forming dogs has disclosed a defect neither in cystine nor in lysine accumu-

lation by either tissue [70]. The absence of a demonstrable lysine transport defect in these dog tissues is unlike the findings in human biopsies, while the absence of a cystine transport defect is consistent with findings in human beings. It would appear that canine cystinuria is a heterogeneous entity. The presence of large amounts of cystine in the urine of these dogs makes this strain an excellent model for evaluating the nature of hyperexcretion of cystine. Clearance studies have been performed on a group of cystinuric and control dogs [150]. What emerges is a striking cystinuria accompanied by variable degrees of dibasic aminoaciduria. The dibasic aminoaciduria does not correlate well with the degree of cystinuria. The extent of the cystinuria is variable and may reach clearances twice creatinine clearance, documenting the secretion of cystine. Infusion of lysine into cystinuric dogs may cause secretion of cystine [78]. Plasma concentrations of the cystine precursor methionine were elevated and correlated with plasma cystine levels and with fractional reabsorption of cystine. These observations suggest that canine cystinuria may be a metabolic disorder associated with cystine secretion. The cystinuric dog is also an excellent model for assessment of therapeutic approaches for decreasing the amounts of urinary cystine in human beings. To date, fluid intake, alkalinization, and D-penicillamine have all been observed to alter the clinical course favorably [151].

Cystinuria has also been found in the maned wolf of Brazil [152]. Eighty percent of these wolves tested in zoos in the United States and abroad as well as animals whose urine was collected in the Brazilian jungle are affected. Several animals are known to have died in zoos because of cystine stones and urinary tract obstruction. Amino acid clearance studies in five affected wolves revealed variable cystine reabsorptive defects. In one animal there was evidence for secretion not only of cystine but of lysine, arginine, and ornithine as well.

One human experimental model has been described by Brown [153]. He produced increased urinary excretion of several amino acids (principally cystine, lysine, ornithine, and arginine) in amounts similar to homozygous cystinuria in patients fed the nonmetabolizable amino acid, cycloleucine. The rat also shows this response to cycloleucine administration [154]. Holtzapple et al. [155] have shown that cycloleucine is a competitive inhibitor of the transport of both neutral and dibasic amino acid by slices of human kidney cortex. Craan and Bergeron [89] have performed microperfusion experiments with rat renal tubules and have found that cycloleucine inhibits the reabsorption of both cystine and lysine.

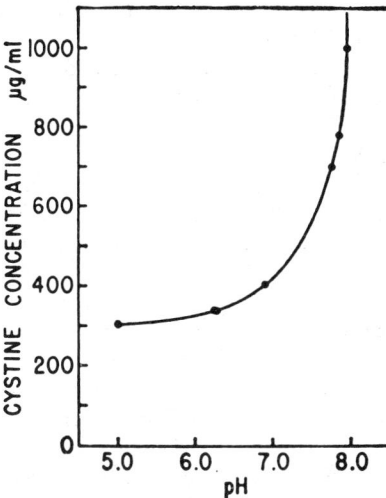

Figure 80-14 The solubility of cystine in relation to urinary pH. (*From Dent and Senior.*)

TREATMENT

Dietary Therapy

Were it not for the insolubility of cystine, cystinuria would be a metabolic oddity of no clinical significance except under conditions of critical limitation of protein intake. Therefore treatment is designed to reduce excretion and increase the solubility of cystine. Therapeutic approaches may be divided into three categories: (1) Dietary restriction aimed at reducing cystine production and excretion, (2) attempts to increase cystine solubility, and (3) attempts to convert cystine to a more soluble compound. Surgical therapy can be divided into three categories: (1) Attempts to dissolve cystine calculi by irrigation, (2) removal of cystine stones by lithotomy, and (3) renal transplantation to replace kidneys destroyed by cystinuria.

Dietary Therapy

Cystine production arises from the essential amino acid methionine. Numerous attempts have been made to design diets low in methionine, yet adequate for nutritional purposes. The results of use of such diets are extremely variable. Disappearance of cystinuria while the patient was on one of these diets has been reported by some investigators, whereas others have been unable to demonstrate any significant reduction in urinary cystine with careful methionine restriction [156, 157]. It is probably reasonable to avoid excessive methionine intake, but it is clear that discomforting diets are not indicated.

Alteration of Cystine Solubility

At urinary pH values below 7.5 about 300 mg cystine per liter of urine will be in solution. Increasing urine volume provides a progressive reduction in urinary cystine concentration and reduces the likelihood of precipitation. Some reports of stone dissolution on high fluid intake programs have appeared [158]. Many cystinuric subjects excrete in the range of 1 g cystine per day and will require a fluid intake of 4 or more liters per day. Cystine solubility can also be enhanced by providing an alkaline pH, but the solubility does not increase significantly until the pH is above 7.5 (Fig. 80-14). Since the maximum urine pH which can be achieved is about 8, there is little leeway in the alkalinizing program. Administration of bicarbonate, citrate,

and carbonic anhydrase inhibitors has been advocated for improving solubility, but while theoretically reasonable it is not clear that much practical benefit occurs. Since varying physical factors, high fluid intake, and alkalinization are logical and simple, they should be included in the first therapeutic program in all cystinuric subjects. In considering high fluid intake therapy, Dent and Senior [159] pointed out the importance of preventing supersaturation of urine with cystine at night when urine flow is low. The intake of two glasses of water at bedtime repeated at 2 or 3 A.M. is recommended. Dent et al. [158] found hydration therapy to be successful in preventing stone formation in about two-thirds of patients who adhered to it, during a 10-year study. Their therapeutic hydration regimen is well outlined in their paper.

Conversion of Cystine to a More Soluble Compound

Penicillamine In spite of the best and most controlled therapeutic efforts, some patients with cystinuria will repeatedly form and pass stones, and a significant number will require surgery for relief of urinary tract obstruction. For those who were apparently not helped by diet, fluid, and alkalinization, there was little to be done until Crawhall, Scowen, and Watts introduced the use of D-penicillamine (ββ-dimethylcysteine). Through a disulfide exchange reaction, this drug can produce the mixed disulfide of cysteine-penicillamine, which is significantly more soluble than cystine [160, 161] (Fig. 80-8). On adequate penicillamine therapy, usually 1 to 2 g/24 h, cystine excretion may be kept below 200 mg/g creatinine, a level at which stone formation is minimal. The reduction of urinary cystine does not appear to be balanced by the amount of cysteine which is combined with penicillamine into the cysteine-penicillamine mixed disulfide. The total molar amount of halfcystine excreted on penicillamine therapy, i.e., the sum of cystine plus the cysteine moiety of the mixed disulfide, is much less than prior to drug treatment. This plus the reduction of plasma cystine levels by the drug suggests another biochemical effect of penicillamine besides disulfide exchange [162–164]. In contrast to the results on cystinuric subjects, the total molar amount of half-cystine in urine of normal individuals given penicillamine is greatly increased [162]. This finding has not been satisfactorily explained.

Although strikingly effective in preventing and dissolving cystine stones [165, 166], penicillamine has certain undesirable side effects. As many as 50 percent of patients receiving the drug will develop allergic reactions, usually fever and rash; rarely arthralgias appear [162]. More severe reactions include development of a nephrotic syndrome [167–169] and of pancytopenia [170]. Proteinuria of more than 500 mg/24 h occurs after several months of therapy in approximately one-third of patients treated with penicillamine. The proteinuria almost invariably clears when the drug is discontinued but usually recurs when the drug is started again [171]. Epidermolysis [172–174], thrombocytosis [175], and loss of taste (hypogeusia) have also been reported [176]. The hypogeusia may be reversed by copper [177]. The chelating property of penicillamine is responsible for increased copper and zinc excretion in the urine. It also has less significant effects on calcium, mercury, and iron excretion [178–180]. Part of the increase in copper excretion is independent of chelation [180] and is as yet unexplained. In addition, a possible problem resulting from inhibition of pyridoxine should be recognized and treated with supplemental pyridoxine phosphate. The possible reaction of penicillamine with pyridoxine to form a thiazolidine led to studies demonstrating a reduced pyridoxal effect in patients on penicillamine therapy (increased kynurenic acid excretion) [181]. The hypogeusia may also be reversed by the administration of pyridoxine [182, 183]. No interference with growth is seen in children, and pregnancies have been successfully completed in women receiving the drug [166, 184]. Most recently the disturbing association of penicillamine therapy with a fatal Goodpasture-like syndrome has been reported [185].

In view of the drawbacks of D-penicillamine therapy, its use should be restricted to patients in whom more conservative therapy has failed or who have lost one kidney from cystine stone disease. Therapy should be started in the hospital in order to monitor reactions of hypersensitivity. In those patients initially sensitive to the drug, adequate results have been obtained by readministering the medication in gradually increasing doses over a period of 1 to 2 months. A related compound, N-acetyl-D-penicillamine, has been developed which is effective in disulfide formation and thus in reducing cystine content; this compound appears to have fewer side effects, perhaps because of the unavailability of an amino group for chemical reaction [31, 186–188]. Cross sensitivity between penicillamine and penicillin has not been a problem.

Mercaptopropionylglycine   Another drug which may be of interest for therapy is mercaptopropionylglycine, which Timmerman et al. [189] suggested would be useful in dissolving renal calculi by renal pelvic perfusion. King first reported the use of mercaptopropionylglycine in cystinuria [190]. Subsequently a number of reports from Japan [191–193], Germany [194], and Greece [195] have suggested that oral mercaptopropionylglycine may substitute for penicillamine in the treatment of cystinuria. Mercaptopropionylglycine has a higher oxidation-reduction potential than penicillamine and may be even more effective in a disulfide exchange reaction leading to the production of a mixed disulfide and cysteine. Mercaptopropionylglycine has a mechanism of action similar to penicillamine and has been effective in cystinuria. Side effects have included skin rash, fever, nausea, and soft feces but not serious hematologic, hepatic, or renal toxicity. It is not

known whether mercaptopropionylglycine will be tolerated by patients sensitive to penicillamine. At present mercaptopropionylglycine is available on an experimental basis in the United States.

Pharmacologic Reduction of Cystine Excretion

Glutamine administered orally or intravenously has been reported to reduce cystine excretion in cystinuria. The original report documented the effectiveness of glutamine in a single patient from Japan [196]. Subsequent studies from the United States failed to demonstrate reduced cystine excretion in patients receiving glutamine orally [197] or intravenously [198]. Therefore the efficiency of glutamine for the treatment of cystinuria remains to be confirmed.

Diazepoxide has been reported to reduce cystine crystalluria [199]. Whether this drug directly alters cystine solubility is not known, but it bears further investigation.

Surgical Approaches

Catheter Irrigation   Reports of dissolution of cystine stones by irrigation of the urinary tract by ureteral catheters placed through supercutaneous nephrostomy have been encouraging [200–202]. Irrigation with alkaline solutions of N-acetylpenicillamine, D-penicillamine, and tromethamine has proved successful in dissolving cystine calculi in 1 week to several months. Although infection may be a complication, if this therapeutic approach is successful, surgery should be avoided.

Lithotomy   Surgical removal of obstructing stones or stones causing intractable pain remains a necessary form of treatment for some cystinuric patients. Correct diagnosis and more effective medical therapy should reduce the need for repeated lithotomies.

Transplantation   Occasionally cystinuria will cause sufficient renal injury to lead to chronic renal failure. In these rare circumstances renal transplantation may be effective. Since the defect in cystinuria resides in the transport epithelium of the genetically affected person, a kidney from a noncystinuric donor should remain disease-free. Normal amino acid excretion has been documented as long as $3\frac{1}{2}$ years after transplantation for cystinuria [203].

Supported by Grant AM 10894 from the National Institutes of Health.

REFERENCES

1. WOLLASTON WH: On cystic oxide: A new species of urinary calculus. *Trans R Soc London* 100:223, 1810
2. NOEHDEN GH: Scientific notices—chemistry, cystic oxide—communicated in a letter from Dr. Noehden to Mr. Children. *Ann Philos* 7:146, 1824
3. BERZELIUS JJ: Calculus urinaries. *Traite Chem* 7:424, 1833
4. FRIEDMAN E: Der Kreislauf des Schwefels in der organischen Natur. *Ergebn Physiol,* 1:15, 1902
5. GARROD AE: Inborn errors of metabolism. *Lancet* 2, 1908. (Lecture I, p. 1; Lecture II, p. 73; Lecture III, p. 142; Lecture IV, p. 214)

6. YEH HL, FRANKL W, DUNN MS, PARKER P, HUGHER B, GYORGY P: The urinary excretion of amino acids by a cystinuric subject. *Am J Med Sci* 214:507, 1947

7. STEIN WH: Excretion of amino acids in cystinuria. *Proc Soc Exp Biol Med* 78:705, 1951

8. DENT CE, SENIOR B, WALSHE JM: The pathogenesis of cystinuria. II. Polarographic studies of the metabolism of sulphur-containing amino-acids. *J Clin Invest* 33:1216, 1954

9. ARROW VK, WESTALL RG: Amino acid clearances in cystinuria. *J Physiol* 142:141, 1958

10. DENT CE, ROSE GA: Amino acid metabolism in cystinuria. *Q J Med* 20:205, 1951

11. FOX M, THIER S, ROSENBERG LE, KISER W, SEGAL S: Evidence against a single renal transport defect in cystinuria. *N Engl J Med* 270:556, 1964

12. FOREMAN JW, HWANG SM, SEGAL S: Transport interactions of cystine and dibasic amino acids in isolated rat renal tubules. *Metabolism* 29:53, 1980

13. SEGAL S, McNAMARA PD, PEPE LM: Transport interaction of cystine and dibasic amino acids in renal brush border vesicles. *Science* 197:169, 1977

14. FRIMPTER GW, HORWITH M, FURTH E, FELLOWS RE, THOMPSON DD: Inulin and endogenous amino acid renal clearances in cystinuria: Evidence for tubular secretion. *J Clin Invest* 41:281, 1962

15. CRAWHALL JC, SCOWEN EF, THOMPSON CJ, WATTS RWE: The renal clearance of amino acids in cystinuria. *J Clin Invest* 46:1162, 1967

16. MORIN CL, THOMPSON MW, JACKSON SH, SASS-KORTSAK A: Biochemical and genetic studies in cystinuria: Observations on double heterozygotes of genotype I/II. *J Clin Invest* 50:1961, 1971

17. VON UDRANSZKY L, BAUMANN E: Ueber das Vorkommen von Diaminen, sogenannten Ptomainen, bei Cystinurie. *Z Physiol Chem* 13:562, 1889

18. LOEWY A, NEUBERG C: Über Cystinurie. *Z Physiol Chem* 43:338, 1904

19. BRAND E, CAHILL GF, HARRIS MM: Cystinuria. II. The metabolism of cysteine, methionine and glutathione. *J Biol Chem* 109:69, 1935

20. BRAND E, CAHILL GF: Further studies on metabolism on sulfur compounds in cystinuria. *Proc Soc Exp Biol Med* 31:1247, 1934

21. MILNE MD, CRAWFORD MA, GIRAO CB, LOUGHRIDGE LW: The metabolic disorder in Hartnup disease. *Q J Med* 29:407, 1960

22. MILNE MD, ASATOOR AM, EDWARDS KDG, LOUGHRIDGE LW: The intestinal absorption defect in cystinuria. *Gut* 2:323, 1961

23. ASATOOR AM, LACEY BW, LONDON DR, MILNE MD: Amino acid metabolism in cystinuria. *Clin Sci* 23:285, 1962

24. THIER S, FOX M, SEGAL S, ROSENBERG LE: Cystinuria: In vitro demonstration of an intestinal transport defect. *Science* 143:482, 1964

25. McCARTHY CF, BORLAND JL, LYNCH HJ, OWEN EE, TYOR MPL: Defective uptake of basic amino acids and L-cystine by intestinal mucosa of patients with cystinuria. *J Clin Invest* 43:1518, 1964

26. THIER S, SEGAL S, FOX M, BLAIR A, ROSENBERG LE: Cystinuria: Defective intestinal transport of dibasic amino acids and cystine. *J Clin Invest* 44:442, 1965

27. HELLIER MD, PERRETT D, HOLDSWORTH CD: Dipeptide absorption in cystinuria. *Br Med J* 4:782, 1970

28. SILK DBA: Progress report—peptide absorption in man. *Gut* 15:494, 1974

29. BOSTROM H, HAMBRAEUS L: Cystinuria in Sweden. VII. Clinical histopathological and medico-social aspect of the disease. *Acta Med Scand* suppl 411, 1, 1964

30. CRAWHALL JC, WATTS RWE: Cystinuria. *Am J Med* 45:736, 1968

31. CRAWHALL JC, PURKISS P, WATTS RWE, YOUNG EP: The excretion of amino acids by cystinuric patients and their relatives. *Ann Hum Genet* 33:149, 1969

32. WEINBERGER A, SPERLING O, RABINOVITZ M, BROSH S, ADAM A, DE VRIES A: High frequency of cystinuria among Jews of Libyan origin. *Hum Hered* 24:568, 1974

33. WOOLF LI: Large-scale screening for metabolic disease in the newborn in Great Britain, in Anderson JA, Swaiman KF (eds): *Phenylketonuria and Allied Metabolic Disorders.* U.S. Department of Health, Education and Welfare (Childrens' Bureau), Washington, 1967, pp 50–59

34. TURNER B, BROWN DA: Amino acid excretion in infancy and early childhood: A survey of 200,000 infants. *Med J Aust* 1:62, 1972

35. LEVY HL, SHIH VE, MADIGAN PM: Massachusetts metabolic disorders screening program. I. Technics and results of urine screening. *Pediatrics* 49:825, 1971

36. LEVY HL: Genetic screening, in Harris H, Hirschhorn K (eds): *Advances in Human Genetics.* New York, Plenum, 1973, vol 4, p 1

37. RENANDER A: The roentgen density of the cystine calculus. *Acta Radiol* suppl 41, 1941

38. HAMBRAEUS L, LAGERGREN C: Cystinuria in Sweden. VI, Biophysical and roentegenological studies of urinary calculi from cystinurics. *J Urol* 88:826, 1962

39. BRAND E, HARRIS MM, BILOON S: Cystinuria: Excretion of a cystine complex which decomposes in the urine with the liberation of free cystine. *J Biol Chem* 86:315, 1930

40. LEWIS HB: Cystinuria: A review of some recent investigations. *Yale J Biol Med* 4:437, 1932

41. HARRIS H, MITTWOCH U, ROBSON EB, WARREN FL: Pattern of amino acid excretion in cystinuria. *Ann Hum Genet* 19:196, 1955

42. HAMBRAEUS L: Comparative studies of the value of two cyanide-nitroprusside methods in the diagnosis of cystinuria. *Scand J Lab Clin Invest* 15:657, 1963

43. CRAWHALL JC, SAUNDERS EP, THOMPSON CJ: Heterozygotes for cystinuria. *Ann Hum Genet* 29:257, 1966

44. SACKETT DL: Adaptation of monodirectional high voltage electrophoresis on long papers to the rapid qualitative identification of urinary amino acids. *J Lab Clin Med* 63:306, 1964

45. STEIN WH: A chromatographic investigation of the amino acid constituents of normal urine. *J Biol Chem* 201:45, 1953

46. SOUPART P: Free amino acids of blood and urine in the human, in *Amino Acid Pools,* edited by JT Holden, p 220. Elsevier, Amsterdam, 1962

47. MELONI CR, CANARY JJ: Cystinuria with hyperuricemia. *JAMA* 200:169, 1967

48. DENT CE, HARRIS H: The genetics of cystinuria. *Ann Hum Genet* 16:60, 1951

49. BROOKS WDW, HEASMAN MA, LOVELL RRH: Retinitis pigmentosa associated with cystinuria: 2 uncommon inherited conditions occurring in family. *Lancet* 1:1096, 1949

50. HURWITZ LJ, CARSON NAJ, ALLEN IV, FANNIN TF, LYTTLE JA, NEILL DW: Clinical, biochemical and histopathological findings in a family with muscular dystrophy. *Brain* 90:799, 1967

51. CLARA R, LOWENTHAL A: Familial and congenital lysine-cystinuria with benign myopathy and dwarfism. *J Neurol Sci* 3:434, 1966

52. TANGUAY RB, GALINDO J: Cystinuria assocated with mongolism and identification of an abnormal pyrrolidine compound in urine. *Am J Clin Pathol* 46:442, 1966

53. GROSS JB, ULRICH JA, JONES JD: Urinary excretion of amino acids in a kindred with hereditary pancreatitis and aminoaciduria. *Gastroenterology* 47:41, 1964

54. BRODEHL J, GALLISSEN K, KOWALEWSKI S: Isolated cystinuria (without lysine-ornithine-argininuria) in a family with hypocalcemic tetany. *Klin Wochenschr* 45:38, 1967

55. COLLIS JE, LEVI AJ, MILNE MD: Stature and nutrition in cystinuria and Hartnup disease. *Br Med J* 1:590, 1963

56. SMITH A, YU JS, BROWN DA: Childhood cystinuria in New South Wales. *Arch Dis Child* 54:676, 1979

57. BRAND E, BLOCK RJ, KASSELL B, CAHILL GF: Cystinuria. V. The metabolism of casein and lactalbumin. *J Biol Chem* 119:669, 1937

58. RACHELE JR, REED LJ, KIDWAL AR, FERGER MF, DU VIGNEAUD V: Conversion of cystathionine labeled with S^{35} to cystine *in vivo. J Biol Chem* 185:817, 1950

59. SCHIMKE RN, McKUSICK VA, WEILBAECHER RG: Homocystinuria, in Nyhan WL (ed): *Amino Acid Metabolism and Genetic Variation.* New York, McGraw-Hill, 1967, pp 297–313

60. FRIMPTER GW: Cystathionuria, in Nyhan WL (ed): *Amino Acid Metabolism and Genetic Variation.* New York, McGraw-Hill, 1967, pp 315–523

61. STURMAN JA, GAULL G, RATHS NCR: Absence of cystathionase in human fetal liver: Is cystine essential? *Science* 169:74, 1970

62. GAITONDE MK, GAULL G: A procedure for the quantitative analysis of the sulphur amino acids of rat tissues. *Biochem J* 102:959, 1967

63. WHELDRAKE JF, PASTERNAK CA: The oxidation of cystine by mast-cell tumor P815, in culture. *Biochem J* 106:437, 1968

64. LONDON DR, FOLEY TH: Cystine metabolism in cystinuria. *Clin Sci* 29:133, 1965

65. CRAWHALL JC, LIETMAN PS, SCHNEIDER JA, SEEGMILLER JE: Cystinosis: Plasma cystine and cysteine concentration and effect of D-penicillamine and dietary treatment. *Am J Med* 44:330, 1968

66. CRAWHALL JC, SEGAL S: The intracellular ratio of cysteine and cystine in various tissues. *Biochem J* 105:891, 1967

67. SEGAL S, SMITH I: Delineation of cystine and cysteine transport systems in rat kidney cortex by development patterns. *Proc Natl Acad Sci USA* 63:926, 1969

68. STATES B, SEGAL S: Distribution of glutathione-cystine transhydrogenase activity in subcellular fractions of rat intestinal mucosa. *Biochem J* 113:443, 1969

69. STEPHENS AD, PERRETT D: Cystinuria: A new genetic variant. *Clin Sci Mol Med* 51:27, 1976

70. HOLTZAPPLE PG, BOVEE K, REA CF, SEGAL S: Amino acid uptake by kidney and jejunal tissue from dogs with cystine stones. *Science* 166:1525, 1969

71. WHELAN DT, SCRIVER CR: Hyperdibasic aminoaciduria: An inherited disorder of amino acid transport. *Pediatr Res* 2:525, 1968

72. OYANGI K, MIURA R, YAMANOUGHI T: Congenital lysinuria: A new inherited transport disorder of dibasic amino acids. *J Pediatr* 77:259, 1970

73. SIMELL O, PERHEENTUPA J: Renal handling of diamino acids in lysinuric protein intolerance. *J Clin Invest* 54:9, 1974

74. LESTER FT, CUSWORTH DC: Lysine infusion in cystinuria: Theoretical renal thresholds for lysine. *Clin Sci* 44:99, 1973

75. KATO T: Renal handling of dibasic amino acids and cystine in cystinuria. *Clin Sci Mol Med* 53:9, 1977

76. ROBSON EB, ROSE GA: The effect of intravenous lysine on the renal clearances of cystine, arginine and ornithine in normal subjects, in patients with cystinuria and Fanconi syndrome and their relatives. *Clin Sci* 16:75, 1957

77. WEBBER WA, BROWN JL, PITTS RF: Interactions of amino acids in renal tubular transport. *Am J Physiol* 200: 380, 1961

78. SEGAL S, BOVEE K: Canine models of human renal transport disorders, in Hommes FA (ed): *Models for the Study of Inborn Errors of Metabolism.* Amsterdam, Elsevier, North Holland, 1979, pp 19–30

79. BERGERON M, VADEBONCOEUR M: Antiluminal transport of L-arginine and L-leucine following microinjections in peritubular capillaries of the rat. *Nephron* 8:355, 1971

80. BERGERON M, VADEBONCOEUR M: Microinjections of L-leucine into tubules and peritubular capillaries of the rat. II. The maleic acid model. *Nephron* 8:367, 1971

81. FOULKES EC: Effects of heavy metals on renal aspartate transport and the nature of solute movement in kidney cortex slices. *Biochim Biophys Acta* 241:815, 1971

82. ROSENBERG LE, ALBRECHT I, SEGAL S: Lysine transport in human kidney: Evidence for two systems. *Science* 155:1426, 1967

83. BRODEHL J: Postnatal development of tubular amino acid reabsorption, in Silbernagel S, Lang F, Greger R (eds): *Amino Acid Transport and Uric Acid Transport.* Stuttgart, Georg Thieme Publishers, 1975, p 128

84. FRIMPTER GW: Cystinuria: Metabolism of the disulfide of cysteine and homocysteine. *J Clin Invest* 42: 1956, 1963

85. ROSENBERG LE, DURANT JL, HOLLAND JM: Intestinal absorption and renal extraction of cystine and cysteine in cystinuria. *N Engl J Med* 273:1239, 1065

86. FRIMPTER GW: Cystinuria: Intravenous administration of S^{35} cystine and S^{35} cysteine. *Clin Sci* 31:207, 1966

87. STEIN WH, MOORE S: The free amino acids of human blood plasma. *J Biol Chem* 211:915, 1954

88. SILBERNAGL S, DEETJEN P: The tubular reabsorption of L-cystine and L-cysteine: A common transport system with L-arginine or not? *Pfluegers Arch* 337:277, 1972

89. CRAAN AG, BERGERON M: Experimental cystinuria: The cycloleucine model. I. Amino acid interactions in renal and intestinal epithelia. *Can J Physiol* 53:1027, 1975

90. AUSIELLO DA, SEGAL S, THIER SO: Cellular accumulation of L-lysine in rat kidney cortex in vivo. *Am J Physiol* 222:1473, 1972

91. GRETH WE, THIER SO, SEGAL S: Cellular accumulation of L-cystine in rat kidney cortex in vivo. *J Clin Invest* 52:454, 1973

92. DAL CANTON A, STANZIALE R, CORRADI A, ANDREUCCI VE, MIGONE L: Effects of acute ureteral obstruction on glomerular hemodynamics in rat kidney. *Kidney Int* 12:403, 1977

93. SCHWARTZMAN L, BLAIR A, SEGAL A: A common renal transport system for lysine, ornithine, arginine and cysteine. *Biochem Biophys Res Commun* 23:220, 1966

94. SEGAL S, CRAWHALL JC: Transport of cysteine by human kidney cortex. *Biochem Med* 1:141, 1967

95. ROSENBERG IE, DOWNING SJ, SEGAL S: Competitive inhibition of dibasic amino acid transport in rat kidney. *J Biol Chem* 237:2265, 1962

96. SCHWARTZMAN L, BLAIR A, SEGAL S: Exchange diffusion of dibasic amino acids in rat-kidney cortex slices. *Biochim Biophys Acta* 135:120, 1967

97. SEGAL S, SCHWARTZMAN L, BLAIR A, BERTOLI D: Dibasic acid transport in rat kidney cortex slices. *Biochim Biophys Acta* 135:127, 1967

98. SEGAL S, CRAWHALL JC: Characteristics of cystine and cysteine transport in rat kidney cortex slices. *Proc Natl Acad Sci USA* 59:231, 1968

99. SEGAL S, SMITH I: Delineation of separate transport systems in rat-kidney cortex for L-lysine and L-cystine by developmental patterns. *Biochim Biophys Res Commun* 35:771, 1969

100. MCNAMARA PD, PEPE LM, SEGAL S: Cystine uptake by renal brush border vesicles. *Biochem J* 194:443, 1981

101. KING JS JR, WAINER A: Cystinuria with hyperuricemia and methioninuria: Biochemical study of a case. *Am J Med* 43:125, 1967

102. FRIMPTER GW: Cystathioninuria in a patient with cystinuria. *Am J Med* 46:832, 1969

103. FRIMPTER GW: The disulfide of L-cysteine and L-homocysteine in urine of patients with cystinuria. *J Biol Chem* 236:651, 1961

104. HAMBRAEUS L: Cystinuria in Sweden. Quantitative studies of urinary amino acid excretion in cystinurics. *Acta Soc Med Ups* 6:1, 1964

105. SCHNEIDER JA, BRADLEY KH, SEEGMILLER JE: Identification and measurement of cysteine-homocysteine mixed disulfide in plasma. *J Lab Clin Med* 71:122, 1968

106. SILK DB, PERRETT D, STEPHENS AD, CLARK ML, SCOWEN EF: Intestinal absorption of cystine and cysteine in normal human subjects and patients with cystinuria. *Clin Sci Mol Med* 47:393, 1974

107. FOLEY TH, LONDON DR: Cysteine metabolism in cystinuria. *Clin Sci* 29:549, 1965

108. HELLIER MD, HOLDSWORTH CD, PERRETT D: Dibasic amino acid absorption in man. *Gastroenterology* 65:613, 1973

109. MAWER GE, NIXON E: The net absorption of amino acid constituents of a protein meal in normal and cystinuric subjects. *Clin Sci* 36:463, 1969

110. MILNE MD: Amino acid metabolism in cystinuria. *Proc Biochem Soc* 122:9P, 1971

111. ASATOOR AM, CROUCHMAN MR, HARRISON AR, LIGHT FW, LOUGHRIDGE LW, MILNE MD, RICHARDS AJ: Intestinal absorption of oligopeptides in cystinuria. *Clin Sci* 41:23, 1971

112. HELLIER MD, PERRETT D, HOLDSWORTH CD, THIRUMALAI C: Absorption of dipeptides in normal and cystinuric subjects. *Gut* 12:496, 1971

113. ASATOOR AM, HARRISON RDW, MILNE MD, PROSSER DI: Intestinal absorption of an arginine-containing peptide in cystinuria. *Gut* 13:95, 1972

114. ROSENBERG LE, DOWNING S, DURANT JL, SEGAL S: Cystinuria: Biochemical evidence for three genetically distinct diseases. *J Clin Invest* 45:365, 1966

115. ROSENBERG LE, CRAWHALL JC, SEGAL S: Intestinal transport of cystine and cysteine in man: Evidence for separate mechanisms. *J Clin Invest* 46:30, 1967

116. COICADAN L, HEYMAN M, GRASSET E, DESJEUX JF: Cystinuria: Reduced lysine permeability at the brush border of intestinal membrane cells. *Pediat Res* 14:109, 1980

117. DESJEUX JF, SIMELL RJ, DUMONTIER AM, PERHEENTUPA J: Lysine fluxes across the jejunal epithelium in lysinuric protein intolerance. *J Clin Invest* 65:1382, 1980

118. SEGAL S, LOWENSTEIN LM, WALLACE A: Comparison of the transport characteristics by rat intestine and kidney cortex. *Gastroenterology* 55:386, 1968

119. HARRIS H, WARREN FL: Quantitative studies on the urinary cystine in patients with cystine stone formation and their relatives. *Ann Eugen* 18:125, 1953

120. HARRIS H, MITTWOCH U, ROBSON EB, WARREN FL: Phenotypes and genotypes in cystinuria. *Ann Hum Genet* 20:57, 1955

121. ROSENBERG LE, DOWNING S: Transport of neutral and dibasic amino acids by human leucocytes: Absence of a defect in cystinuria. *J Clin Invest* 44:1382, 1965

122. SCRIVER CR, WHELAN DT, CLOW CL, DALLAIRE L: Cystinuria: Increased prevalence in patients with mental disease. *N Engl J Med* 283:783, 1970

123. BANERJI NK, MILLAR JHD: Paraplegia associated with cystinuria. *J Neurol Sci* 12:101, 1971

124. DE MYER W, GEBHARD RL: Subacute combined degeneration of the spinal cord with cystinuria. *Neurology* 25:994, 1975

125. BLACKBURN CR, MCLEOD JG: CNS lesions in cystinuria. *Arch Neurol* 32:638, 1977

126. BERRY HK: Cystinuria in mentally retarded siblings with atypical osteogenesis imperfecta. *Am J Dis Child* 97:196, 1959

127. GOLD RJM, DOBRINSKI MJ, GOLD DP: Cystinuria and mental deficiency. *Clin Gen* 12:329, 1977

128. SMITH A, PROCOPIS PG: Cystinuria and its relationship to mental retardation. *Med J Aust* 2:932, 1975

129. HWANG SM, SEGAL S: Developmental and other aspects of [^{35}S]cysteine transport by rat brain synaptosomes. *J Neurochem* 33:1303, 1979

130. SEGAL S, HWANG SM: L-[^{35}S]cystine uptake by rat brain synaptosomes. *J Neurochem* 33:697, 1979

131. HWANG SM, SEGAL S: Developmental and other characteristics of lysine uptake by rat brain synaptosomes. *Biochim Biophys Acta* 557:436, 1979

132. HWANG SM, WEISS S, SEGAL S: Uptake of L-[^{35}S]cystine by isolated rat brain capillaries. *J Neurochem* 35:417, 1980

133. HARRIS H, ROBSON EB: Variation in homozygous cystinuria. *Acta Genet (Basel)* 5:581, 1955

134. ROSENBERG LE, DURANT JL, ALBRECHT I: Genetic heterogeneity in cystinuria: Evidence for allelism. *Trans Assoc Am Phy* 79:284, 1966

135. ROSENBERG LE: Genetic heterogeneity in cystinuria, in *Amino Acid Metabolism and Genetic Variation,* edited by W. L. Nyhan, p. 341. McGraw-Hill, New York, 1967

136. HERSHKO C, BEN-AMI E, PACIORKOVSKI J, LEVIN N: Alleomorphism in cystinuria. *Proc Tel-Hashomer Hosp* 4:21, 1965

137. DATTA SP, HARRIS H: Urinary amino acid patterns of some mammals. *Ann Eugen* 18:107, 1953

138. CRAWHALL JC, SEGAL S: Sulphocysteine in the urine of the blotched Kenya genet. *Nature (Lond)* 208:1320, 1965

139. OLDFIELD JE, ALLEN PH, ADAIR J: Identification of cystine calculi in mink. *Proc Soc Exp Biol Med* 91:560, 1956

140. LASSAIGNE JL: Observation sur l'existence de l'oxide cystique dans un calcul vésical du chien, et essai analytique sur la composition élémentaire de cette substance particulière. *Ann Chim Phys* 2d ser, 23:328, 1823

141. MORRIS ML, GREEN DF, DINKEL JH, BRAND E: Canine cystinuria. *North Am Vet* 16:16, 1935

142. BRAND E, CAHILL GF: Canine cystinuria. III. *J Biol Chem* 114:XV, 1936

143. BRAND E, CAHILL GF, KASSELL B: Canine cystinuria. V. Family history of two cystinuric Irish terriers and cystine determination in dog urine. *J Biol Chem* 133:431, 1940

144. GREEN DG, MORRIS ML, CAHILL GF, BRAND E: Canine cystinuria. II. Analysis of cystine calculi and sulfur distribution in the urine. *J Biol Chem* 114:91, 1936

145. CRANE CW, TURNER AW: Amino acid patterns of urine in blood plasma in a cystinuric Labrador dog. *Nature (Lond)* 177:237, 1956

146. TREACHER RJ: Amino acid excretion in canine cystine-stone disease. *Vet Rec* 74:503, 1962

147. CORNELIUS CE, BISHOP JA, SCHAFFER MH: A quantitative study of amino aciduria in dachshunds with a history of cystine urolithiasis. *Cornell Vet* 177, April 1967

148. GOULDEN BE, LEAVER JL: Low voltage paper electrophoresis as a screening test for the diagnosis of canine cystinuria. *Vet Rec* 80:244, 1967

149. TREACHER RJ: Intestinal absorption of lysine in cystinuric dogs. *J Comp Pathol* 75:309, 1965

150. BOVEE KC, THIER SO, REA C, SEGAL S: Renal clearance of amino acids in canine cystinuria. *Metabolism* 23:51, 1974

151. FRIMPTER GW, THOUIN P, EWALDS BH: Penicillamine in canine cystinuria. *J Am Vet Med Assoc* 151:1084, 1967

152. BOVEE KC, BUSH M, DIETZ J, JEZYK P, SEGAL S: Cystinuria in the maned wolf of South America. *Science* 212:919, 1981

153. BROWN RR: Aminoaciduria resulting from cycloleucine administration in man. *Science* 157:432, 1967

154. GOYER RA, REYNOLDS JO Jr, ELSTON RC: Characteristics of the aminoaciduria resulting from cycloleucine administration in pair fed rats. *Proc Soc Exp Biol Med* 130:860, 1969

155. HOLTZAPPLE P, REA C, GENEL M, SEGAL S: Cycloleucine inhibition of amino acid transport in human and rat kidney cortex. *J Lab Clin Med* 75:818, 1970

156. KOLB FO, EARLL JM, HARRIS HA: Disappearance of cystinuria in a patient treated with prolonged low methionine diet. *Metabolism* 16:378, 1967

157. ZINNEMAN HH, JONES JE: Dietary methionine and its influence on cystine excretion in cystinuric patients. *Metabolism* 15:915, 1966

158. DENT CE, FRIEDMANN M, GREEN H, WATSON LCA: Treatment of cystinuria. *Br Med J* 1:403, 1965

159. DENT CE, SENIOR B: Studies on the treatment of cystinuria. *Br J Urol* 27:317, 1955

160. CRAWHALL JC, SCOWEN EF, WATTS RWE: Effect of penicillamine on cystinuria. *Br Med J* 1:585, 1963

161. CRAWHALL JC, SCOWEN EF, WATTS RWE: Further observations on use of D-penicillamine in cystinuria. *Br Med J* 1:1411, 1964

162. BARTTER FC, LOTZ M, THIER S, ROSENBERG LE, POTTS JT: Cystinuria: Combined clinical staff conference at the National Institutes of Health. *Ann Intern Med* 62:796, 1965

163. CRAWHALL JC, THOMPSON CJ: Cystinuria: Effect of D-penicillamine on plasma and urinary cystine concentrations. *Science* 147:1459, 1965

164. LOTZ M, POTTS JT: Quantitation of the effects of pencillamine therapy in cystinuria. *J Clin Invest* 43:1293, 1964

165. McDONALD JE, HENNEMAN PH: Stone dissolution in vivo and control of cystinuria with D-penicillamine. *N Engl J Med* 273:578, 1965

166. CRAWHALL JC, SCOWEN EF, THOMPSON CJ, WATTS RWE: Dissolution of cystine stones during D-penicillamine treatment of a pregnant patient with cystinuria. *Br Med J* 1:216, 1967

167. FELLERS FX, SHAHIDI NT: The nephrotic syndrome induced by penicillamine therapy. *Am J Dis Child* 98:669, 1959

168. ADAMS DA, GOLDMAN R, MAXWELL MH, LATTA H: Nephrotic syndrome associated with penicillamine therapy of Wilson's disease. *Am J Med* 36:330, 1964

169. ROSENBERG LE, HAYSLETT JP: Nephrotoxic effects of penicillamine in cystinuria. *JAMA* 201:698, 1967

170. CORCOS JM, SOLER-BECHERA J, MAYER K, FREYBERG RH, GOLDSTEIN R, JAFFÉ I: Neutrophilic agranulocytosis during administration of penicillamine. *JAMA* 189:265, 1964

171. HALPERIN EC: The management of cystinuria. Thesis submitted to the Yale University School of Medicine, 1979

172. BEER WE, COOKE KB: Epidermolysis bullosa induced by penicillamine. *Br J Dermatol* 79:123, 1967

173. KATZ R: Penicillamine-induced skin lesions, a possible example of human lathyrism. *Arch Dermatol Syphilol* 95:196, 1967

174. HARRIS ED, SJOERDSMA A: Effect of penicillamine on human collagen and its possible application to treatment of scleroderma. *Lancet* 1:996, 1966

175. FAWCETT NP, NYHAN WL, ANDERSON WW: Thrombocytosis during treatment of cystinuria with penicillamine. *J Pediatr* 69:976, 1966

176. KEISER HR, HENKIN RI, BARTTER FC, SJOERDSMA A: Loss of taste during therapy with penicillamine. *JAMA* 203:381, 1968

177. HENKIN RI, KEISER HR, JAFFE IA, STERNLIEB I, SCHEINBERG IH: Decreased taste sensitivity after D-pencillamine reversed by copper administration. *Lancet* 16:1268, 1967

178. WALSH JM, PATSTON V: Effect of penicillamine on serum iron. *Arch Dis Child* 40:651, 1965

179. BOSTROM H, WESTER PO: Excretion of trace elements in two penicillamine-treated cases of cystinuria. *Acta Med Scand* 181:475, 1967

180. McCALL JT, GOLDSTEIN NP, RANDALL RV, GROSS JB: Comparative metabolism of copper and zinc in patients with Wilson's disease (hepatolenticular degeneration). *Am J Med Sci* 254:35, 1967

181. JAFFE IA, ALTMAN K, MERRYMAN P: The antipyridoxine effect of penicillamine in man. *J Clin Invest* 43:1969, 1964

182. GIBBS K, WALSHE JM: Penicillamine and pyridoxine requirements in man. *Lancet* 175, January 1966

183. HEDDLE JG, METTENRY EW, BEATON GH: Penicillamine and vitamin B₆ interrelationships in the rat. *Can J Biochem Physiol* 42:1215, 1963

184. PRUZANSKI W: Cystinuria and cystine urolithiasis in childhood. *Acta Paediatr Scand* 55:97, 1966

185. STERNLIEB I, BENNETT B, SCHEINBERG IH: D-Penicillamine induced Goodpasture's syndrome in Wilson's disease. *Ann Int Med* 82:673, 1975

186. STOKES GS, POTTS JT, LOTZ M, BARTTER F: A new agent in the treatment of cystinuria: N-acetyl-D-penicillamine. *Br Med J* 1:284, 1968

187. STEPHENS AD, WATTS RWE: The treatment of cystinuria with N-acetyl-D-penicillamine, a comparison with the results of D-penicillamine treatment. *Q J Med* 40:335, 1971

188. MULVANEY WP, QUILTER T, MORTERA A: Experiences with acetylcysteine in cystinuric patients. Abstract. *J Urol* 114:107, 1975

189. TIMMERMAN A, KALLISTRATOS G, FENNER O, SOMMER E: A tentative map suggesting the possible role of urinary minerals for the formation of renal stones, in Hodgkinson A, Nordin BEC (eds): *Renal Stone Research Symposium* (Leeds, 1968). London, J. & A. Churchill, 1969

190. KING JS: Treatment of cystinuria with α-mercaptopropionylglycine: A preliminary report. *Proc Soc Exp Biol Med* 129:927, 1968

191. KINOSHITA K, YACHIKU S, KOTAKE T, TAKEUCHI M, SONODA T: Treatment of cystinuria with 2-mercaptopropionylglycine (MPG), *Proc 2nd Internat Sympos on Thiola.* Osaka, Santen Pharmaceutical Co., 1972, p 50

192. SONODA T, KINOSHITA K, KOTAKE T, YACHIKU S, TAKEUCHI M: Effect of thiola on cystinuria, *Proc Internat Sympos on Thiola.* Osaka, Santen Pharmaceutical Co., 1970, p 231

193. NISHIMURA R, ISHIDO T, TAKAI S: Studies on cystinuria, *Proc 2nd Internat Sympos on Thiola.* Osaka, Santen Pharmaceutical Co., 1972, p 47

194. HAUTMANN R, TERHORST B, STUHLSATZ HW, LUTZEYER W: Mercaptopropionylglycine: A progress in cystine stone therapy. *J Urol* 117:628, 1977

195. KALLISTRATOS G, MITA I, VADALOYKA-KALFAKAKOU V: Management of cystinuric disorders with sulfhydryl drugs, in *The Management of Genetic Disorders.* New York, Alan R. Liss, 1979, pp 255–263

196. MIYAGI K, NAKADA S, OHSHIRO D: Effect of glutamine on cystine excretion in a patient with cystinuria. *N Engl J Med* 301:196, 1979

197. SKOVBY F, ROSENBERG LE, THIER SO: No effect of L-glutamine on cystinuria. Letter to the editor. *N Engl J Med* 302:236, 1980

198. VAN DEN BERG CJ, JONES JD, WILSON DM, SMITH LH: Glutamine therapy of cystinuria. *Invest Urol* 18:155,1980

199. FARISS BL, KOLB FO: Preliminary communications: Factors involved in crystal formation in cystinuria. *JAMA* 205:138,1968

200. SMITH AD, LANGE PH, MILLER RP, REINKE DB: Dissolution of cystine calculi by irrigation with acetylcysteine through percutaneous nephrostomy. *Urology* 13:422, 1979

201. CRISSEY MM, GITTES RF: Dissolution of cystine ureteral calculus by irrigation with tromethamine. *J Urol* 121:811, 1979

202. STARK H, SAVIR A: Dissolution of cystine calculi by pelviocaliceal irrigation with D-penicillamine. *J Urol* 124:895, 1980

203. KELLY S, NOLAN DP: Letter to the editor, *JAMA* 243:1897, 1980

81

FAMILIAL IMINOGLYCINURIA

CHARLES R. SCRIVER

1. Familial iminoglycinuria is a benign inborn error of membrane transport. It is believed to be a deletion or alteration of the membrane transport protein of the renal tubule which selectively binds L-proline, hydroxy-L-proline, and glycine during cellular uptake. The iminoglycinuria phenotype is autosomal recessive.

2. Homozygotes retain significant tubular absorption of the imino acids and glycine. The residual transport system is saturated at endogenous concentrations of substrate, and the normal competitive interactions between the imino acids and glycine during tubular uptake are not observed. These seemingly paradoxical observations can be explained if several species of membrane transport proteins participate in the migration of the imino acids and glycine. Loss of a carrier which is shared by the imino acids and glycine, and retention of other more selective carriers which bind either glycine or imino acids, but not both simultaneously, would account for the homozygous iminoglycinuric phenotype.

3. A variant which only moderately impairs imino acid reclamation but retains a normal T_m proline, and affects glycine reclamation more severely in presumed homozygotes, suggests a further, K_m-variant form of iminoglycinuria.

4. Impaired intestinal transport of L-proline has been demonstrated in some homozygotes. A transport defect has not been demonstrated in the leukocytes or skin fibroblasts of these subjects.

5. Obligate heterozygotes may be "hyperglycinuric" (incompletely recessive) or "silent" (completely recessive) with regard to their phenotypic expression of the mutant allele. Some homozygotes have impaired intestinal absorption of the imino acids and glycine. Thus there is genetic heterogeneity.

6. The different mutations appear to be allelic. Homozygotes with two "silent" mutant alleles, or with two "hyperglycinuric" alleles, or genetic compounds with two mutant alleles of different types, are all of the same renal phenotype.

7. The differential diagnosis of familial iminoglycinuria includes the iminoacidopathies, hyperprolinemia and hydroxyprolinemia, in which iminoglycinuria occurs by a combined saturation-inhibition mechanism; Fanconi's syndrome, in which iminoglycinuria occurs as part of a generalized disturbance of transport; and the newborn, who may have iminoglycinuria as part of the normal hyperaminoaciduria in the first 6 months of life. Neonatal iminoglycinuria involves ontogeny of transport systems not controlled by the gene locus involved in hereditary iminoglycinuria.

8. Several different forms of renal hyperglycinuria are known. These must be distinguished from the hyper-

glycinuric phenotype of the heterozygote with renal iminoglycinuria.

The tools of science are observation, experiment, measurement, and hypothesis. Some observations have a permanent character; others hold a more passing interest until new hypotheses replace old interpretations of earlier data. Such is the case with *iminoglycinuria*. Clinical observations on probands with hereditary renal iminoglycinuria, and on newborn infants with developmental neonatal iminoglycinuria, have a persistent quality. Interpretations of the cellular processes by which the kidney transports proline and glycine change as new methods of measurement and experimentation yield new observations (Fig. 81-1). The phenotypes described in this chapter do not differ from those reported in the fourth edition of this text, and consequently the relevant material in this edition is briefer; there are new data on renal transport of proline and glycine, and consequently they replace the old recorded in the earlier editions.

The initial application by Dent [1] of chromatographic methods to medical investigation fostered an exponential increase in the number of diseases of amino acid metabolism that have been discovered between 1948 and the present time [2]. Interest at first focused primarily on variations in the excretion of the amino acids in the urine [3]. It was soon recognized that urine of young infants normally contains a large quantity of the two imino acids,[1] proline and hydroxyproline, and of the amino acid glycine. Iminoaciduria of the newborn disappears as the infant reaches about 6 months of age, and thereafter urine normally does not contain detectable amounts

of proline or hydroxyproline; the intensity of glycinuria also diminishes at this time.

Several investigators over the years have studied the origin of hyperiminoglycinuria in the human infant [7–10]. Their data indicate that net tubular absorption of several amino acids, including the imino acids and glycine, is impaired in the newborn by comparison with the older subject (Fig. 81-2). The subsequent suppression of iminoglycinuria during the later infantile period is associated with enhanced net tubular absorption of the three solutes.

Persistence of iminoglycinuria beyond early infancy constitutes an abnormality of amino acid metabolism. It occurs under three different circumstances:

1. As a complex "combined" aminoaciduria in the presence of hyperprolinemia [1] or hyperhydroxprolinemia (see Chap. 18 on these diseases)

2. As a specific inborn error of membrane transport of amino acids now usually known as *familial (renal) iminoglycinuria* (the subject of this chapter)

3. As a component of a generalized disturbance of membrane transport, e.g., in Fanconi's syndrome.

It is the second form of iminoglycinuria which concerns us here [12–34]. Joseph and colleagues [12] described familial iminoglycinuria for the first time in 1958 and attributed it to an abnormality of renal tubular transport. Because the trait was associated with a familial convulsive disorder, and because the relation of the one to the other was poorly understood, it was temporarily given the eponym, "Joseph's syndrome" [31]. Shortly thereafter, Jonxis in Holland observed another family with a convulsive disorder in which some members had an iminoglycinuria of renal origin [32]. The second published report appeared in 1965 from Japan [14]. Tada and colleagues [14] described "prolinuria: a new renal tubular defect in transport of proline and glycine," in two unrelated probands. Both patients were mentally retarded, and consanguinity was present in one of the families. A year later Morikawa et al. [15] reported a third Japanese patient with iminoglycinuria and mental retardation. They described a new feature, an associated intestinal transport defect, which also

[1] These compounds are also excreted in bound form as oligopeptides (see Chap. 18, Disorders of Proline and Hydroxyproline Metabolism). Familial iminoglycinuria is a trait affecting only the free forms of proline, hydroxyproline, and glycine. "Imino acid" is a popular term used to distinguish the configuration of the secondary amino group (RC—NHCH—COOH) of the heterocyclic amino acids from the usual primary amine group (NH₂—CHR—COOH) of other amino acids. The term "imino acid" is freely used in standard texts on the biochemistry and metabolism of amino acids [4, 5], but reservations have been expressed about the accuracy of its use in this way [6].

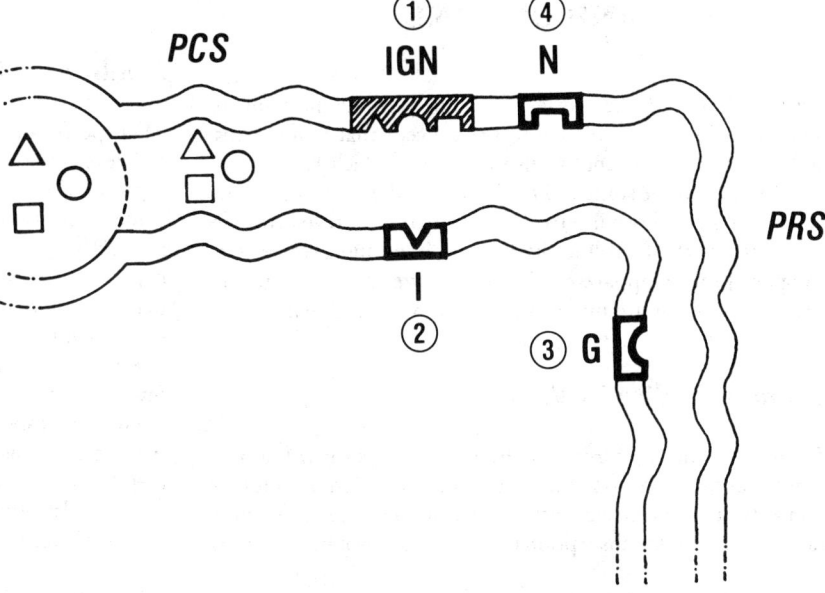

Figure 81-1 Transport sites (membrane carriers) in proximal convoluted segment (PCS) and pars recta segment (PRS) on proximal nephron. *1.* A shared high capacity, low affinity site for imino acids (I) (proline and hydroxyproline), glycine (G), and neutral amino acids (N). *2.* A specific low capacity, high affinity carrier for imino acids. *3.* A specific low capacity, high affinity site for glycine. *4.* Another carrier for neutral amino acids (probably the site involved in the Hartnup phenotype). Familial iminoglycinuria is believed to be a deficiency of carrier 1 activity. Neonatal iminoglycinuria probably reflects ontogeny involving carriers 2 and 3.

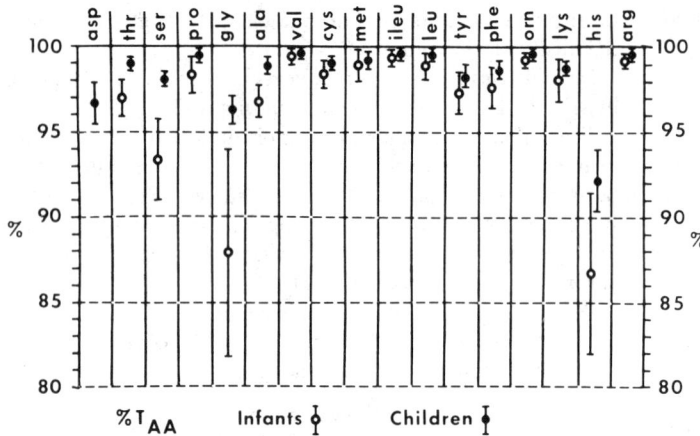

Figure 81-2 Net tubular absorption of amino acids (expressed as percent of filtered load) is less efficient in the newborn human subject than in older subjects. Glycine absorption is particularly impaired, and the presence of imino acids in the urine of the neonate and young infant is noteworthy. (*Redrawn from Brodehl and Gellissen* [10]. *Reproduced from* Pediatrics, *with permission.*)

involved the imino acids and glycine. Familial iminoglycinuria was first reported from North America in an Ashkenazic Jewish pedigree [16]. The proband was a healthy adult male in whom the trait was found incidentally during investigation of the family for the cause of liver cirrhosis in a relative [33]. Other cases of familial iminoglycinuria were then recognized in many different countries. Thus the trait is widely distributed in human beings.

In every reported instance iminoglycinuria has been discovered during investigations carried out for other purposes. In many pedigrees, the proband with iminoglycinuria was initially investigated for an independent medical problem. However, the diversity of the clinical abnormalities in probands with familial iminoglycinuria suggests that there is little or no direct relationship between the inherited disorder of membrane transport and the accompanying illness. Several investigators have proposed that familial iminoglycinuria is indeed a benign inborn error of membrane transport [20–22], a conclusion which is borne out by the occurrence of nine healthy iminoglycinuric sibs of probands and by the prospective discovery of probands through newborn screening programs [28, 30] where follow-up observations indicate no attendant illness.

RENAL TRANSPORT OF IMINO ACIDS AND GLYCINE

Human Studies in Vivo

Titration studies performed on human subjects show that net tubular absorption of L-proline in humans undergoes saturation as the plasma concentration is increased [36]. A maximum rate for net tubular absorption of proline ($T_m$proline) has been

demonstrated [36]. Renal tubular reclamation of hydroxy-L-proline has also been studied in humans by similar titration techniques, and reabsorption of this imino acid can also be saturated [37]. The capacity of the normal human renal tubule to transport proline and hydroxyproline is shown in Table 81-1. A T_m for glycine has not been demonstrated in humans.

Infusion of one imino acid increases urinary excretion of the other and of glycine in humans [36, 37], yet there is little or no influence on the excretion of other amino acids. The same selective interaction between imino acids and glycine is also observed in vivo in the rat [40], mouse, and to some extent in the dog [41], although in the dog the interaction is much less selective. Patients with familial hyperprolinemia have iminoglycinuria [35, 36] which is directly proportional to the concentration of proline in their plasma when the concentration of proline exceeds 1 m*M;* this is the level at which proline itself begins to saturate its own transport system and appears in the urine [36].

Thus, data on imino acid and glycine transport from normal human subjects and from patients with disordered imino acid catabolism complement each other and suggest that the renal tubule transport process is selective in its preference for proline, hydroxyproline, and glycine, and is finite in its capacity; intrarenal oxidation of amino acids may influence net reclamation indirectly. (See the next two sections on metabolic runout.)

Nonhuman Studies in Vivo and *in Situ*

Microperfusion studies of rat nephrons in vivo and *in situ* [42–46] reveal stereospecific, Na$^+$-dependent, net reabsorption of L-proline from lumen to cell in the proximal tubule. There is evidence for two proline transport systems: one with low affinity and high capacity, the other with high affinity and low capacity. The former appears to be an unspecific system for neutral amino acids including glycine; the latter is specific for imino acids and other N-substituted amino acids.

Renal reabsorption of amino acids is a complex process that involves net flux into absorbing epithelium at the brush border membrane followed by metabolic runout into intracellular metabolic pools or permeability runout at the basolateral membrane to peritubular capillaries [47, 48]. The process has been intensively studied for glycine [49, 50] using the isolated perfused rabbit nephron segment technique. Whereas glycine

Investigation

into the cause of iminoglycinuria in familial hyperprolinemia [35, 36] led to the concept that imino acids and glycine share a renal transport system which has preference for these three solutes [11]. Further studies in humans and other mammals, both in vivo and in vitro, have revealed that renal transport of proline, hydroxyproline, and glycine is a complex process apparently involving several reactive membrane sites which are under the control of several genes.

may be a special case and the rabbit nephron not entirely representative of the human nephron, the major findings are of interest. Glycine is actively transported in both proximal convoluted and proximal straight (pars recta) segments. Net flux out of the lumen is active, meaning against a concentration gradient. The unidirectional absorptive flux is saturable and Na^+-dependent. A parallel, nonsaturable, Na^+-independent absorptive component also exists that probably represents a paracellular diffusional flux. Transport of glycine out of the lumen in the proximal convoluted segment has high capacity and low affinity; the capacity of the proximal straight segment cell-to-lumen flux is only about one-tenth that in the convoluted segment, but its affinity for glycine is about fifteenfold greater. These are the characteristics of net transepithelial transport of glycine as they pertain to the transport activity at the luminal membrane *in situ*. A smaller flux from the peritubular space to lumen is also present [49, 50]. Glycine uptake at the basolateral membrane is also active and Na^+-dependent. But, in contrast to the relative magnitude of the brush border flux, the basolateral membrane uptake of glycine is about twofold greater in the straight segment compared with the convoluted segment. The major source of glycine backleak in the proximal nephron is by a paracellular path. It follows that net reabsorption of glycine, as a representative amino acid, is primarily dependent on the activity of carriers in the brush border membrane of the epithelial cell in the proximal segments of the nephron.

Role of Metabolic Runout in Net Reabsorption of Proline

The influence of proline oxidation on its own uptake by kidney has been assessed both in vitro and in vivo [51–53a]. Proline uptake by kidney cortex slices is modified by oxidation, in the sense that the internal pool and therefore the uptake ratio (proline inside/proline outside) are controlled in part by its intracellular metabolism [51]. The latter can be so vigorous as to deplete the internal pool of proline drastically (Fig. 81-3), although this is not the case in human kidney [52].

Intracellular metabolism of solute reclaimed from urine influences its transepithelial reabsorption in vivo. Evidence has been obtained from the mutant homozygous Pro/Re mouse, in which renal oxidation of proline is less than 4 percent of normal. In the Pro/Re mouse the proline concentration of epithelial cells is increased, and although the transport process itself is not affected, equilibrium across the epithelium, and in particular across the brush border membrane, is altered. As a consequence renal clearance of proline is greatly increased (Fig. 81-3) and net tubular reclamation of proline is diminished.

When awareness of the importance of metabolic runout is taken into account, along with knowledge about the character of proline transport on brush border membrane carriers [54–57] (see next section), an interpretation of the T_m phenomenon as it pertains to proline is apparent. Renal oxidation of proline has no influence on binding and translocation of proline on its carriers [51–53a], but it does influence the net reabsorptive flux [51, 53a]. Saturation of net reabsorption is apparently dependent both on the capacity of the oxidative pathway and on the capacity of the carrier. Rodent and murine kidney, with their high oxidative capacity [51, 53], have a high capacity for proline reabsorption [44, 53] relative to humans.

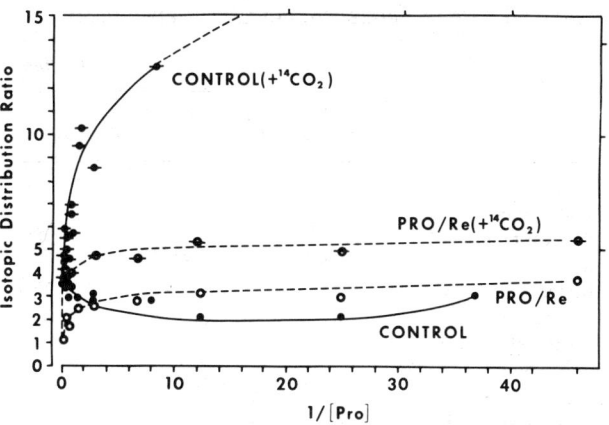

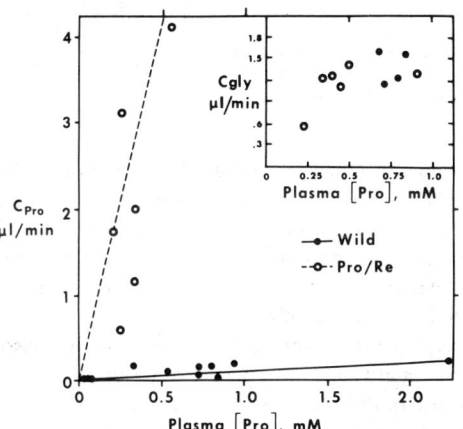

Figure 81-3 The effect of metabolism on proline *uptake* by the kidney cortex slice in vitro and on its net *reabsorption* (transepithelial transport) in vivo in normal mouse and homozygous mutant Pro/Re mouse. The latter retains less than 1 percent of normal proline oxidation in kidney because of deficient proline oxidase activity (sources of evidence cited in [53]. Uptake in vitro (*upper panel*) is influenced by proline oxidase activity. When intact, the soluble pool of proline is kept low and most of the proline taken up is oxidized to CO_2; but when it is deficient, as in Pro/Re kidney, an expanded internal pool is established and the expected saturable uptake kinetics can be observed. The appropriate analysis of uptake kinetics revealed a "high-K_m" and a "low-K_m" process for proline uptake into mouse kidney for which the respective values were similar in Pro/Re and normal kidney and also similar to those reported for human [56] and rat [55] kidney.

Proline transport in vivo (*lower panel*) is dramatically modified by proline oxidase activity. Proline clearance is strikingly elevated in the proline-oxidase deficient mutant (Pro/Re) in which the proline pool of absorbing epithelium is expanded. Back flux from cell to urine can occur so that net transepithelial reabsorption will decrease. Inhibition studies (inset) showing that proline-glycine interaction is normal in Pro/Re kidney indicate normal integrity of the transport system. The failure to observe a T_m for proline in normal (wild-type) mouse kidney (●———●, panel) at markedly elevated levels of proline in plasma indicates that its capacity for proline reabsorption is determined predominantly by the capacity for intracellular oxidation of the substrate. (From Scriver et al. [57] with permission of Proceedings of the National Academy of Sciences of the United States of America.)

Studies with Isolated Brush Border Membrane Vesicles

The brush border membrane vesicle preparation has been used effectively to delineate proline and glycine transport in mammalian kidney [54–57]. This method allows membrane transport to be characterized without concern for metabolic runout or other factors that come to influence the net transcellular

Table 81-1   Renal clearance, net tubular absorption, and T_m of amino acids and glycine in familial iminoglycinuria

	Proline			Hydroxyproline	
Phenotype	Endog. clear., $ml/(min \cdot 1.73\ m^2)$	Reabsorbed, %	T_m, $\mu mol/(min \cdot 1.73\ m^2)$	Endog. clear., $ml/(min \cdot 1.73\ m^2)$	Reabsorbed, %
Normal	0–0.03	>99.8	180–300	0	100
Homozygous mutant* (classical type)					
Mean	6.7			13	
Range	0.5–19.6	77–99.5	10–18	1–33.6	65–99
Heterozygous† ("hyperglycinuric")	0	100	35–117	0	100
Heterozygous‡ ("silent")	0	100	?	0	100
Genetic compound (K_m variant)§	~0.3	>99	Normal with "splay"	2–4	<100

* Compiled from Goodman et al. [18], Scriver [17], Rosenberg et al. [21], Hoefnagel and Pomeroy [19], and Tada et al. [38]; includes genetic compound and homozygous probands.
† Compiled from Goodman et al. [18], Scriver [17], Rosenberg et al. [21], and Hoefnagel and Pomeroy [19].
‡ Compiled from Goodman [39], Scriver [17], and Hoefnagel and Pomeroy [19].
§ Compiled from Greene et al. [27].

flux. Transport of L-proline and glycine is, in both cases, concentrative, Na^+-gradient dependent (Fig. 81-4), and saturable. The partitioning of transport activity is complex and involves several systems. At least one system is shared by the imino acids, glycine, and other neutral amino acids; another serves glycine avidly and selectively; yet another seems to have selective preference for the imino acids [56, 57]. Isolated basolateral membrane preparations have permeability properties that differ from those of the brush border membrane [54] (Fig. 81-4); the specificities of glycine and proline transports have not yet been defined in the basolateral preparation.

Studies in Renal Cortex Slice, Isolated Tubule, and Isolated Glomerulus

The renal cortex slice and collagenase-treated isolated tubule preparations primarily expose the basolateral membrane of epithelial cells to the extracellular medium [58, 59]. Accordingly, observations obtained with such preparations are most informative about events at the antiluminal surface of renal epithelium that come to influence net reabsorption of proline and glycine in vivo.

Transport of L-proline and glycine by renal cortex slices [51–53] and tubules [60, 61] is mediated by membrane carriers. Multiple carriers are involved, at least one of which is shared by L-proline, hydroxy-L-proline, and glycine, others being selective for either the imino acids or glycine. Specificity of transport is exhibited not only toward the chemical structure of the substrate but also its concentration; in general, low quantities of substrate are largely transported on a low-K_m system and large quantities by a high-K_m mediation. L-Proline transport has been studied in the isolated rat glomerulus [62]; high-K_m and low-K_m systems were observed in this preparation also. These findings suggest that membrane gene products serving transport of proline and glycine are comparable in the various plasma membranes of the nephron at which cellular uptake occurs.

Ontogeny of Renal Transport of Imino Acids and Glycine

Hyperiminoglycinuria is characteristic of the normal human newborn infant [3, 7–10]. It reflects transiently reduced net reabsorption of imino acids and glycine [10, 63, 64]. Maturation of tubular transport functions observes independent schedules for proline and glycine [63, 64], suggesting that separate carriers are involved in the ontogeny. This conclusion is supported by studies of probands homozygous for hereditary iminoglycinuria [64]. Such individuals have near total absence of tubular reabsorption for proline and glycine in the early postnatal period. As tubular function matures, some reabsorptive activity for proline appears first, followed by the later appearance of a glycine transport activity. Since the allele for hereditary iminoglycinuria is constantly expressed postnatally, independent ontogeny of proline and glycine transport in the mutant homozygote implies maturing activity of separate carriers not controlled by the gene locus affected by the mutation.

Transient postnatal iminoglycinuria is characteristic of mammals in general [65]. Postnatal maturation of membrane transport activities is believed to involve intensification of specific membrane functions [66]. Although there has been some controversy about the process of ontogeny as it involves renal transport of proline and glycine [67–70], several observations provide an overall insight. First, backflux of amino acids in the immature distal tubule is not a component of postnatal iminoglycinuria [71]. Second, diminished metabolic runout is not a significant cause of dimished net reabsorption [67]. Third, postnatal prolinuria in the rat is associated with low transport activity of the low-K_m, Na^+-dependent proline system in the brush border membrane [72].

Nature of Membrane Transport Sites for Imino Acids and Glycine

The foregoing reveals that the migration and reclamation of imino acids and glycine across the renal tubular cell membrane are mediated by processes that can be saturated, have specificity, and are constitutive in the sense that intracellular metabolism of the solute after its uptake does not modulate the actual process of uptake, even though it may modify transepithelial net reclamation.

Membrane transport proteins comprise a means whereby the cell can achieve specificity in the uptake of metabolites; it

(Continued)

Hydroxyproline	Glycine	
T_m, $\mu mol/(min \cdot 1.73\ m^2)$	Endog. clear., $ml/(min \cdot 1.73\ m^2)$	Reabsorbed, %
60–135	1.2–8.6	93–99
	27	
6	17.0–41.6	61–77
50	14.3	82–95
?	8.6–26.2	
	3.1–6.7	>93
	37–60	65

follows that mutation in the gene which controls a transport protein will modify a specific membrane function; this will be reflected by a phenotype which could be called an inborn error of transport. Familial iminoglycinuria is one of about 30 such traits now known in human beings [73].

MECHANISM OF FAMILIAL IMINOGLYCINURIA

Probands with familial iminoglycinuria are discovered because their urine contains excessive amounts of proline, hydroxyproline, and glycine. The excretion of other amino acids is normal, and the concentration of all the amino acids in the plasma of these subjects is normal. The endogenous renal clearance rates of amino acids and their net tubular absorption rates have been calculated in a number of subjects [17, 19, 21, 38]; only the imino acids and glycine have elevated clearance rates and impaired net absorption rates (Table 81-2). Familial iminoglycinuria is, therefore, the reflection of impaired function of a specific renal tubular transport system. Two related and

important observations emerge from these relatively simple studies:

1. Net tubular absorption of imino acids and glycine is not competely eliminated in homozygotes.

2. The abnormal prolinuria may disappear at low plasma proline concentrations in homozygotes (Fig. 81-5), even though the venous plasma "threshold" for prolinuria is very low in homozygotes (about 0.1 mM) compared with normal subjects (about 0.8 mM).

The ability of homozygotes for hereditary iminoglycinuria to retain a considerable fraction of their specific tubular absorptive function is a feature shared by homozygotes with other inborn errors of membrane transport. For example, the homozygote with classic cystinuria, or with the hypercystinuric trait, or with Hartnup disorder usually retains some capacity to transport the relevant amino acids. A similar characteristic is also observed for hexose transport in glucose-galactose malabsorption in regard to renal tubular absorption of glucose. One interpretation of this phenomenon is that more than one type of transport site serves the migration of a substrate across the cell membrane.

Transport Saturation in the Mutant Phenotype

Mutant homozygotes and obligate heterozygotes have been infused with L-proline and hydroxy-L-proline in order to determine T_m values [16, 17, 21]. These investigations disclosed that imino acid transport is usually saturated in the mutant homozygotes at normal plasma concentration of proline and hydroxyproline (Fig. 81-6). The heterozygote has a T_m which is intermediate between normal and abnormal values (Fig. 81-6); in these subjects imino acid absorption is normal at concentrations below the T_m. This suggests that the affinity of the available imino acid transport sites in the heterozygote is normal. Taken together, these findings indicate that the mutation usually causes deletion of a transport system which has a capacity well above the normal plasma concentration of imino acids. Another modality of uptake with a small but recognizable capacity is retained.

Retention of transport function in the proband reported by Greene et al. [27] reflects, by way of contrast with the aforementioned interpretation, a mutation which does not delete the affected transport function but rather alters its affinity for

Table 81-2 Evidence for allelic mutations in familial renal iminoglycinuria. Phenotype heterogeneity among homozygotes, "genetic compounds," and obligate heterozygotes

Presumed allelic pair	Renal phenotype in		Intestinal phenotype in homozygote (or compound)	Exemplary pedigrees in Fig. 81-8
	Homozygote or compound	Heterozygote		
I-I	IG	N	Present	D
II-II	IG	N	N	B, N
III-III	IG	G	N	E, H, J, M, O
I-III(or II)	IG	N or G	Present	F
	IG	N or G	Not tested	E, G, L
II-IV	iG(K_m)	N or G(K_m)	N	P

KEY: IG = iminoglycinuria (with loss of "high-K_m" system); G = glycinuria alone; iG(K_m) = K_m variant involving "high-K_m" system affecting glycine more than amino acids; N = normal; "Present" implies defective absorption of proline and/or glycine in test procedure.

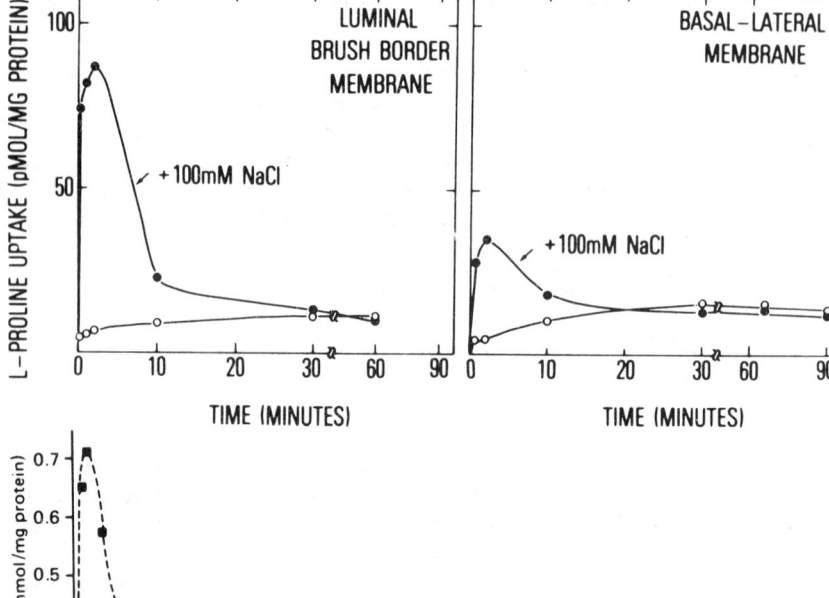

Figure 81-4 *Upper panels:* Transport of L-proline (25 μM) by rabbit kidney brush border and basolateral membranes (●, Na⁺ gradient; ○, Na⁺-free medium, taken from Ref. 54). *Lower panel:* Transport of L-proline and glycine by rat renal brush border membranes (■ □ proline, ● ○ glycine both at 0.06 mM; closed symbols, Na⁺ gradient; open symbols, no Na⁺ gradient, taken from Ref. 56). Graphs show sodium-dependent transport for proline and glycine transport at brush border membrane. Apparent Na⁺ dependence for a small component of proline transport in basolateral membranes reflects contamination of membrane fraction by brush borders during preparation.

its substrates, so that glycine is very poorly bound and proline is less avidly taken up at high concentrations by the mutant carrier (Fig. 81-6)

Interaction between Imino Acids and Glycine in the Mutant Phenotype

Imino acids and glycine normally interact competitively during uptake by the kidney both in vivo and in vitro. These interactions have been studied in subjects with the iminoglycinuric trait, and they are distinctly different from the normal. Though proline or hydroxyproline progressively inhibits tubular absorption of glycine in normal subjects as the concentration in the tubular fluid is increased (Fig. 81-7), neither imino acid inhibits glycine uptake in the mutant homozygote. This can be explained if it is assumed that the persistent glycine transport in the mutant homozygote occurs at a tubular site which is not inhibited by either imino acid [16, 17]. Imino acids are partially effective as competitive inhibitors of glycine transport in heterozygotes (Fig. 81-7), but there is a limit to which glycine transport can be inhibited. Between 8 and 16 μmol/(min · 1.73 m²) it cannot be inhibited in either the normal or the mutant phenotypes. This presumably represents the noninhibitable portion of glycine transport which is not affected by the mutation.

Imino acids also interact competitively with each other during absorption by the normal tubule [35, 36]. Some degree of

interaction is also found in mutant homozygotes [17]. This suggests that the alternate site at which imino acids are transported in the mutant homozygote is shared by these two substrates. It is noteworthy in this context that a specific separate site for hydroxyproline transport has not been identified in bone cells [75] where hydroxyproline is an important constit-

Figure 81-5 Endogenous renal clearance of L-proline related to its concentration in plasma in homozygotes with familial iminoglycinuria. The "venous plasma threshold concentration" at which prolinuria appears is about 0.1 mM; the normal value is about 0.8 mM [36]. Abnormal prolinuria disappears in mutant homozygotes at low plasma proline concentrations, indicating the existence of a small but efficient tubular capacity to transport proline. (*Redrawn from Scriver [17], with permission of* The Journal of Clinical Investigations, *with data (symbol ○) added from Rosenberg and Scriver [74] and other data (symbol ▲) added from Tada et al. [38].*)

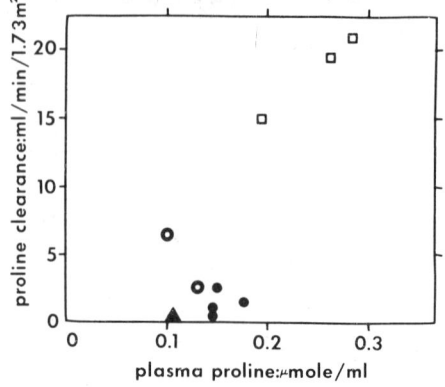

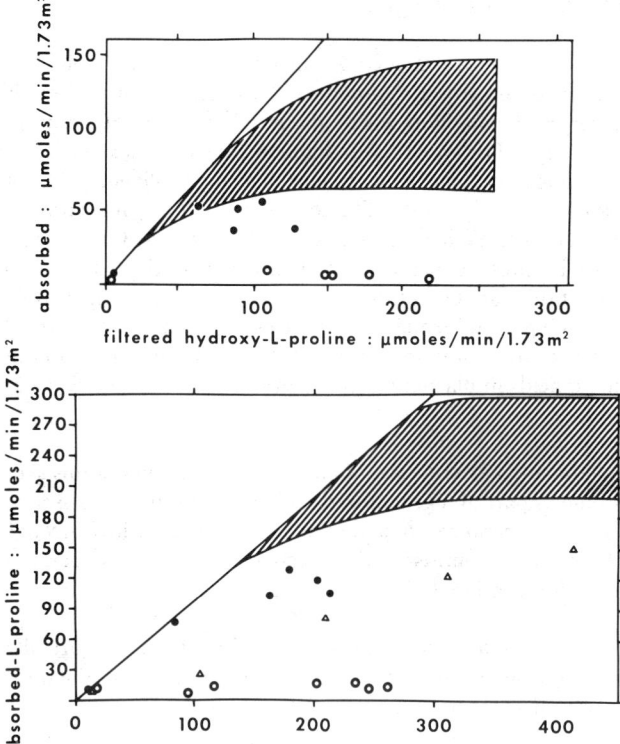

Figure 81-6 Maximum rates of tubular absorption (T_m) of L-proline and hydroxy-L-proline in normal subjects (hatched), heterozygotes (solid circles), and mutant homozygotes (open circles) with classic iminoglycinuria. Data for patient with K_m variant of iminoglycinuria [27], are also shown (△). (Redrawn from Scriver [17] and Greene et al. [27], with permission.)

uent of collagen. There is apparently no advantage to be gained from a separate membrane transport site for hydroxyproline, since hydroxyproline is synthesized in peptide linkage from proline after the latter has been incorporated into a procollagen polypeptide.

Apparent Deployment of Membrane Transport Sites for Uptake of Imino Acids and Glycine in Humans

Calculations have been made of the relative capacities of the systems for transport of imino acids and glycine in mammalian kidney, and something can be said about the preferences and affinities of these systems for their substrates. If the data from human subjects [17] are compared with those obtained from the rat [42–45, 49], there are many similarities in the way in which the kidney of both species reabsorb imino acids and glycine. The membrane sites appear to be deployed with the following characteristics:

1. A site with high capacity which is common to the three substrates.

2. A site with preference for glycine, and which does not transport imino acids but is shared with sarcosine; the capacity of this site is much less than that of the shared site.

3. A site with preference for both imino acids (and sarcosine) and at which proline and hydroxyproline interact; the imino acid capacity of this site is about one-tenth that of the high-capacity shared site.

Expression of Phenotype in Nonrenal Tissues

Intestine   Intestinal transport of imino acids and glycine has been examined in vivo in several homozygotes and in intestinal biopsy material in one subject [21]. Two phenotypes have been identified in vivo in terms of proline absorption (Fig. 81-8). Some homozygotes have normal intestinal transport of L-proline [14, 17, 21], while others have a delayed and depressed uptake of this imino acid into plasma [15, 18]. The association of different intestinal phenotypes with a single renal phenotype suggests that more than one mutant allele is responsible for the iminoglycinuric trait.

Fecal excretion of amino acids has also been examined in homozygotes. In patients with a normal plasma response to oral proline loading [17, 21], the fecal excretion of amino acids is normal. On the other hand, homozygotes with impaired plasma response curves have an elevated concentration of proline in the feces [15, 18]. Morikawa et al. [15] also found a modest excess of glycine in the feces before and after an oral glycine load, even though the plasma glycine response curve was normal after an oral load. It is of interest that the plasma response to glycine loading by mouth is normal in patients with and without demonstrable impairment of proline absorption [15, 18, 21]. This may indicate that the imino-glycine transport systems of the intestine are qualitatively different from those in the kidney.

Leukocytes   Tada and colleagues [76] examined the accumulation of proline in peripheral leukocytes obtained from a mutant homozygote with impaired intestinal and renal transport. The ability of the leukocytes to accumulate proline was normal. Tada [76] proposed that leukocytes do not express the

Figure 81-7 Effect of L-proline and hydroxy-L-proline on net tubular absorption of glycine in normal subjects (hatched), heterozygotes (solid circles), and mutant homozygotes with classic iminoglycinuria. (Redrawn from Scriver [17] and Greene et al. [27], with permission.)

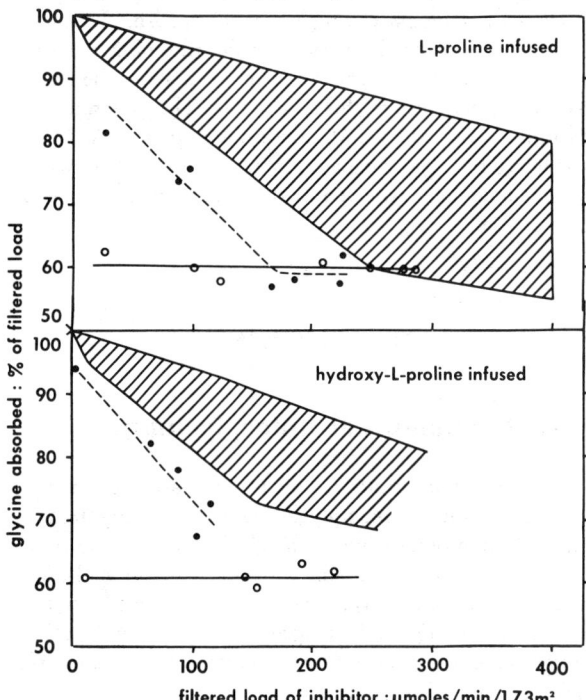

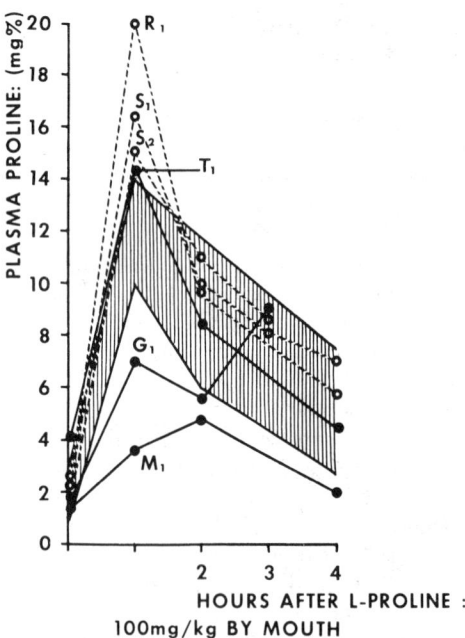

Figure 81-8 Postabsorptive concentration of proline in plasma after an oral load of L-proline (100 mg/kg) in normal subjects (hatched area) and in mutant homozygotes with familial iminoglycinuria. Two types of plasma response are seen in the latter; an increase indicating normal intestinal absorption in subjects S_1 and S_2 [21], R_1 [23], and T_1 [15]; a flattened response indicating impaired absorption in subjects M_1 [16] and G_1 [19].

mutant transport allele for the high-capacity transport system. These leukocyte studies were done at low substrate concentrations (about 0.006 mM), low enough, in fact, that uptake could have occurred almost exclusively on the low-capacity system, which is apparently retained in the mutant trait. Thus, the experiment and its interpretations must be considered inconclusive.

Skin Fibroblasts Tada and his colleagues [76] also studied the incorporation of L-proline into the collagen of fibroblasts from a skin biopsy during incubation for 2 h. The rate of incorporation was not different from the rate obtained with normal skin. The same reservation expressed about the leukocyte studies applies also to this experiment. The substrate concentration was only 0.05 mM, and proline uptake could have been achieved by the low-capacity system, the activity of which would not have been affected in the iminoglycinuric phenotype.

DIAGNOSIS

Criteria for Abnormal Iminoglycinuria

Any degree of *iminoaciduria* after 6 months of age may be considered abnormal. Hyperglycinuria may be recognized on partition chromatograms when the glycine spot is disproportionately intense in comparison with other amino acids. The quantitative criteria for *hyperglycinuria* are urinary excretion exceeding 160 μmol/g total nitrogen [20], or 150 mg/24 h [77], or an endogenous clearance rate exceeding 8.6 ml/(min · 1.73 m²) [78].

Differential Diagnosis

HYPERPROLINEMIA AND HYDROXYPROLINEMIA Iminoglycinuria occurs by a "combined" mechanism when there is hyperprolinemia in excess of about 0.8 mM [36]. Hyperprolinemia, type I or type II (see Chap. 18), is usually accompanied by iminoglycinuria. Patients with hydroxyprolinemia do not exhibit iminoglycinuria. The concentration of hydroxyproline in their plasma has not exceeded 0.4 mM; hydroxyproline must be present in plasma at this concentration at least to inhibit tubular absorption of proline and glycine competitively [37]. Hyperprolinemia and hydroxyprolinemia can be ruled out as a cause of iminoglycinuria if the concentration of both imino acids in plasma is normal in subjects with iminoglycinuria.

FANCONI'S SYNDROME Iminoglycinuria occurs in this syndrome as part of a generalized inhibition of tubular transport. Thus, a generalized hyperaminoaciduria occurs in Fanconi's syndrome, in contrast to the selective nature of the hyperaminoaciduria in familial iminoglycinuria.

NEONATAL IMINOGLYCINURIA The human infant normally has some degree of renal iminoglycinuria until about the third month of postnatal life.

RENAL GLYCINURIA There have been numerous reports of hyperglycinuria without iminoaciduria. Since this phenotype may represent one form of the heterozygote with the iminoglycinuria mutation or the "K_m variant" form of renal iminoglycinuria in the "homozygous" and heterozygous state [27], in addition to the following causes, its differential diagnosis merits some attention.

Pedigrees with dominantly inherited renal hyperglycinuria and nephrolithiasis [79, 80] are discussed below.

Käser and colleagues described autosomal dominant glucoglycinuria. Glucosuria occurred by the type B mechanism of Reubi, i.e., the renal threshold for glucosuria was low (79 mg/dl), but the T_{mG} was normal—386 mg/(min · 173 m²). Of the 44 subjects who were examined, 13 healthy relatives also had glucoglycinuria; no subjects with glucosuria or glycinuria alone were found. Glycinuria apparently occurred through a mechanism similar to that responsible for glucosuria.

Scriver et al. [82] reported a 16-year-old male with hypophosphatemic rickets. Glucoglycinuria was also present. The glucosuria accorded with the Reubi type A mechanism (low T_m). The impairment of glycine transport was apparently a fault of transport, not of binding of glycine to its site. Thus the glucoglycinuria occurred through a mechanism different from that described by Käser et al. [81]. Since the phosphaturia also involved impaired net uptake in this patient, it seems that there was an inhibition of transport analogous to that which is believed to occur in Fanconi's syndrome; but only three metabolites, instead of a great many, were significantly affected. Dent and Harris [83] described patients in whom hypophosphatemic rickets and glycinuria occurred, and further examples are cited by Scriver et al. [82].

These examples indicate that a number of mutant alleles (or, in some cases, perhaps acquired abnormalities) may affect glycine transport in the kidney. All these traits should be distinguished from the "prerenal" form of hyperglycinuria found in hyperglycinemia [see Chap. 27].

GENETICS

Familial renal iminoglycinuria occurs when two mutant autosomal alleles occur at the locus which controls the shared imino-glycine transport site. Consanguinity in parents of iminoglycinuric children in 2 of the 11 pedigrees [14, 22] supports the belief that the trait is recessively inherited. There is no evidence that it is X-linked.

Obligate heterozygotes for the familial iminoglycinuric trait have hyperglycinuria in some pedigrees (Fig. 81-9). Hyperglycinuria might appear as a dominant trait if iminoglycinuric subjects are not also present in the same pedigree. Dominantly inherited hyperglycinuria [79, 80] has been classified in the second edition of the present book as a particular form of "hyperglycinuria." It is more likely that the heterozygous phenotype of familial iminoglycinuria was found in such pedigrees.

Obligate heterozygotes for the iminoglycinuric trait do not always exhibit hyperglycinuria. Pedigrees are known (A, B, C, D, and N, Fig. 81-9) in which neither parent of the iminoglycinuric proband has hyperglycinuria. The presence of two types of heterozygotes for the iminoglycinuric trait suggests that the mutant allele occurs in more than one form. When the mutant allele is expressed (as hyperglycinuria) in the heterozygote, the situation is analogous to the "incompletely recessive" form of cystinuria [84]; when the mutant allele is silent in the heterozygote, the situation is analogous to the "completely recessive" form of cystinuria. A third allele [27] is apparent from observations in pedigree P (Fig. 81-9) in which heterozygote and the "genetic-compound" offspring ("homozygous" affected) have glycinuria because of a mutant transport system with lowered affinity for glycine.

It would be important to know whether the alleles occur at the same gene locus. There are pedigrees (E, F, G, and L, Fig. 81-9) in which one parent of an iminoglycinuric member is hyperglycinuric and the other is not. Nonetheless, the renal phenotype of the presumably "doubly heterozygous" child born to these matings is indistinguishable from that of homozygotes with two hyperglycinuric parents, or with two "silent" parents. Thus, it is likely that such an individual is a "genetic compound" for two different mutant alleles which occur at the same gene locus. Further proof is needed to secure this conclusion and to rule out nonallelism; nonetheless, the circumstances and their interpretation resemble closely those pertaining to the presumably heteroallelic forms of cystinuria which have been described by Rosenberg [85–87].

Yet another feature of the iminoglycinuric phenotype indicates the apparent genetic heterogeneity which underlies this trait. Some mutant homozygotes exhibit impaired intestinal transport of proline (Fig. 81-9), whereas others do not. The phenotype with normal intestinal transport is not consistently associated with one or the other form of the heterozygous phenotypes. In one instance (pedigree B), the parents are of the silent phenotype, while in others (pedigrees E, H, and J) the parents are hyperglycinuric. Interpretation of the various phenotypes, including the K_m variant [27], suggests the presence of four mutant alleles (Table 81-2) which yield obligate heterozygotes, homozygotes, and genetic compounds with a variety of phenotypes.

The prevalence of the iminoglycinuria trait in the general population can be estimated. From data collected by screening newborn infants [27–29], the frequency of the presumed homozygote (or genetic compound) among Caucasians seems to be about 1:15,000 live births; accordingly the frequency of heterozygotes for this autosomal recessive trait could be on the

Figure 81-9 Pedigrees of patients with familial iminoglycinuria.

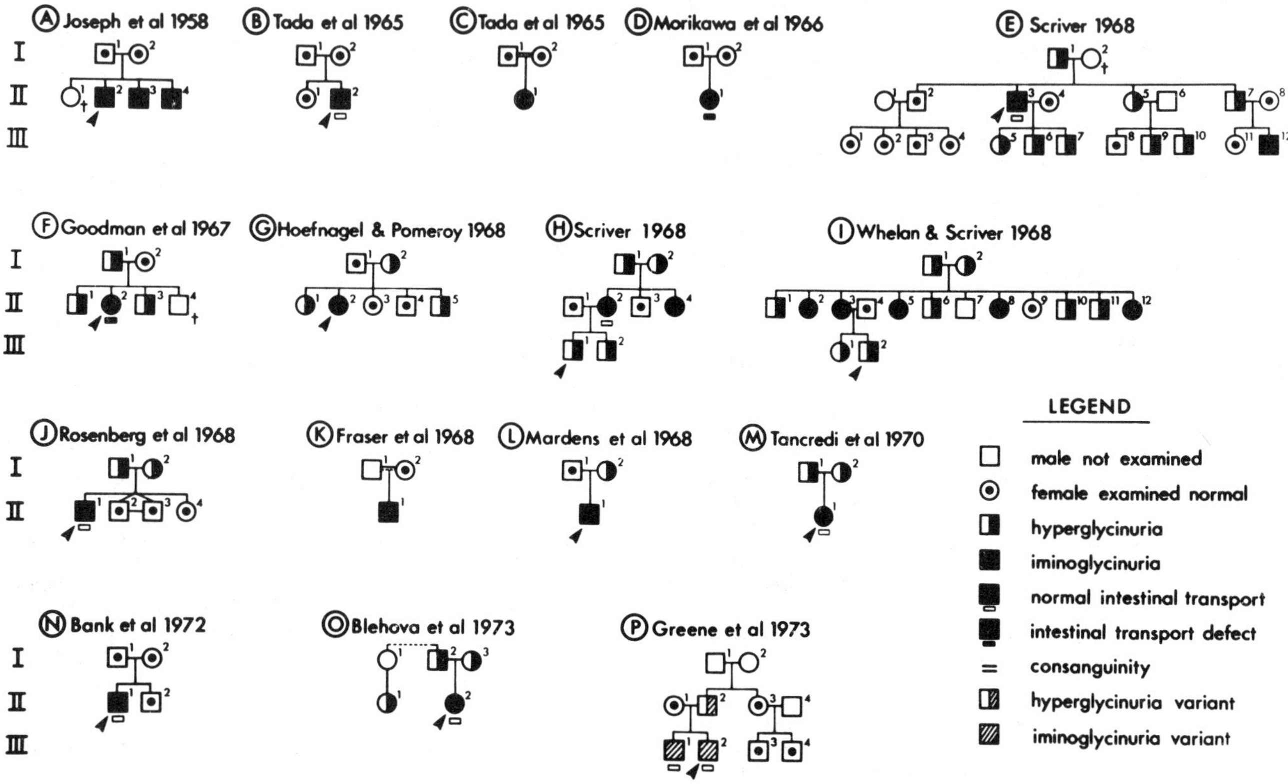

order of 2 percent in the general population. However, pedigree studies (Fig. 81-9) suggest that half the obligate heterozygotes have a "silent" allele, which means that about 1 percent of the general population will be hyperglycinuric because they carry a mutant allele for renal transport of the imino acids and glycine. On the other hand, the newborn heterozygote excretes imino acids and glycine in considerable excess before transport systems mature; thus heterozygotes destined to be recognized by their hyperglycinuria in later life resemble homozygotes by newborn screening [64]. Accordingly, the frequency of the iminoglycinuria homozygote may be 1:15,000 births but is likely to be less.

TREATMENT

Familial iminoglycinuria is a benign condition involving nonessential amino acids, and no treatment is indicated. The considerable number of healthy subjects in whom iminoglycinuria was discovered quite incidentally (viz., pedigree E, subjects II.3 and III.12; pedigree H, subjects II.2 and II.4; and all homozygous members of pedigree I) supports this interpretation. The various illnesses which have been associated with the iminoglycinuric trait apparently served only to bring the transport mutation to attention.

REFERENCES

1. DENT CE: Detection of amino acids in urine and other fluids. *Lancet* 2:637, 1946
2. SCRIVER CR, ROSENBERG LE: *Amino Acid Metabolism and Its Disorders.* Philadelphia, Saunders, 1973
3. SCRIVER CR: Hereditary aminoaciduria, in Bearn A, Steinberg AG (eds): *Progress in Medical Genetics.* New York, Grune & Stratton, 1962, vol 2, p 83
4. GREENSTEIN JP, WINITZ M: *Chemistry of the Amino Acids.* New York, Wiley, 1961
5. MEISTER A: *Biochemistry of the Amino Acids,* 2d ed. New York, Academic, 1965
6. MCMILLAN DE: Letter to the editor. *N Engl J Med* 273:771, 1965
7. SERENI F, MCNAMARA H, SHIBUYA M, KRETCHMER N, BARNETT HL: Concentration in plasma and rate of urinary excretion of amino acids in premature infants. *Pediatrics* 15:575, 1955
8. WOOLF LI, NORMAN AP: The urinary excretion of amino acids and sugars in early infancy. *J Pediatr* 50:271, 1957
9. O'BRIEN D, BUTTERFIELD LJ: Further studies on renal tubular conservation of free amino acids in early infancy. *Arch Dis Child* 38:437, 1963
10. BRODEHL J, GELLISSEN K: Endogenous renal transport of free amino acids in infancy and childhood. *Pediatrics* 42:395, 1968
11. SCRIVER CR, SCHAFER IA, EFRON ML: New renal tubular amino acid transport system and a new hereditary disorder of amino acid metabolism. *Nature (Lond)* 192:672, 1961
12. JOSEPH R, RIBIERRE M, JOB JC, GIRAULT M: Maladie familiale associante des convulsions a début très precoce, une hyperalbuminorachie et une hyperaminoacidurie. *Arch Fr Pediatr* 15:374, 1958
13. MOZZICONACCI P, BOISSE J, LEMONNIER A, CHARPENTIER C: Les maladies métaboliques des acides amines avec arriération mentale (Citation on p. 249) Paris, L'Expansion Scientifique Française, 1968
14. TADA K, MORIKAWA T, ANDO T, YOSHIDA T, MIRAGAWA A: Prolinuria: A new renal tubular defect in transport of proline and glycine. *Tohoku J Exp Med* 87:133, 1965
15. MORIKAWA T, TADA K, ANDO T, YOSHIDA T, YOKOYAMA Y, ARAKAWA T: Prolinuria: Defect in intestinal absorption of imino acids and glycine. *Tohoku J Exp Med* 90:105, 1966
16. SCRIVER CR, WILSON OH: Amino acid transport in human kidney: Evidence for genetic control of two types. *Science* 155:1428, 1967
17. SCRIVER CR: Renal tubular transport of proline, hydroxyproline and glycine. III. Genetic basis for more than one mode of transport in human kidney. *J Clin Invest* 47:823, 1968

18. GOODMAN SI, MCINTYRE CA, O'BRIEN D: Impaired intestinal transport of proline in a patient with familial iminoaciduria. *J Pediatr* 71:246, 1967
19. HOEFNAGEL D, POMEROY J: Personal communication of unpublished data, 1968 and 1969
20. WHELAN DT, SCRIVER CR: Cystathioninuria and renal iminoglycinuria in a pedigree: A perspective on counseling. *N Engl J Med* 278:924, 1968
21. ROSENBERG IE, DURANT JL, ELSAS LJ, II: Familial iminoglycinuria: An inborn error of renal tubular transport. *N Engl J Med* 278:1407, 1968
22. FRASER GR, FRIEDMANN AI, PATTON VM, WADE, DN, WOOLF LL: Iminoglycinuria—a "harmless" inborn error of metabolism? *Humangenetik* 6:362, 1968
23. MARDENS Y, ANDRIAENSSENS K, VAN SANDE M: Glycinurie et iminoacidurie rénales associés à une oligophrénie: Etude clinique et biochimique. *J Neurol Sci* 6:333, 1968
24. TANCREDI F, GUAZZI G, AURICHIO S: Renal iminoglycinuria without intestinal malabsorption of glycine and imino acids. *J Pediatr* 7:386, 1970
25. BANK H, CRISPIN M, EHRLICH D, SZEINBERG A: Iminoglycinuria: A defect of renal tubular transport. *Isr J Med Sci* 8:606, 1972
26. BLEHOVÁ B, PAŽOUTOVÁ, HYÁNEK J, and JIRÁSEK J: Iminoglycinuria in a child in Czechoslovakia. *Humangenetik* 19:207, 1973
27. GREENE ML, LIETMAN PS, ROSENBERG LE, SEEGMILLER JE: Familial hyperglycinuria: New defect in renal tubular transport of glycine and imino acids. *Am J Med* 54:265, 1973
28. LEVY HL: Genetic screening, in Harris H, Hirschhorn K (eds): *Advances in Human Genetics.* New York, Plenum, 1973, vol 4, p 1
29. TURNER B, BROWN DA: Amino acid excretion in infancy and early childhood: A survey of 200,000 infants. *Med J Aust* 1:62, 1972
30. PROCOPIS PG, TURNER B: Iminoaciduria: A benign renal tubular defect. *J Pediatr* 79:419, 1971
31. PAINE RS: Evaulation of familial biochemically determined mental retardation in children, with special reference to aminoaciduria. *N Engl J Med* 262:658, 1966
32. JONXIS JHP: Personal communications, 1962 (cited in [17]) and 1969
33. MILLER M: Familial cirrhosis with hepatoma. *Am J Dig Dis* 12:633, 1967
34. STATTER M, BEN-ZVI A, SHINA A, SCHEIN R, RUSSELL A: Familial iminoglycinuria with normal intestinal absorption of glycine and imino acids in association with profound mental retardation, a possible "cerebral phenotype." *Helv Paediatr Acta* 31:173, 1976
35. SCHAFER IA, SCRIVER CR, EFRON ML: Familial hyperprolinema, cerebral dysfunction and renal anomalies occurring in a family with hereditary nephritis and deafness. *N Engl J Med* 267:51, 1962
36. SCRIVER CR, EFRON ML, SCHAFER IA: Renal tubular transport of proline, hydroxyproline and glycine in health and in familial hyperprolinemia. *J Clin Invest* 43:374, 1964
37. SCRIVER CR, GOLDMAN H: Renal tubular transport of proline, hydroxyproline and glycine. II. Hydroxy-L-proline as substrate and as inhibitor in-vivo. *J Clin Invest* 45:1357, 1966
38. TADA K, HIRONO H, ARAKAWA T: Endogenous renal clearance rates of free amino acids in prolinuric and Hartnup patients. *Tohoku J Exp Med* 93:57, 1967
39. GOODMAN SI: Personal communication, 1969
40. WILSON OH, SCRIVER CR: Specificity of transport of neutral and basic amino acids in rat kidney. *Am J Physiol* 213:185, 1967
41. WEBBER WA: Interactions of neutral and acidic amino acids in renal tubular transport. *Am J Physiol* 202:577, 1962
42. BERGERON M, MOREL F: Amino acid transport in rat renal tubules. *Am J Physiol* 216:1139, 1969
43. DUBORD L, BERGERON M: Multiplicité des systèmes transporteurs à la membrane luminale du néphron chez le rat normal. *Rev Can Biol* 33:99, 1974
44. VOLKL H, SILBERNAGL S, DEETJEN P: Kinetics of L-proline reabsorption in rat kidney studied by continuous microperfusion. *Pflügers Arch* 382:115, 1979
45. VOKL H, SILBERNAGL S: Molecular specificity of tubular reabsorption of L-proline. A microperfusion study in rat kidney. *Pflügers Arch* 387:253, 1980
46. ULLRICH KJ, REIMRICH G, KLOSS S: Sodium dependence of the amino acid transport in the proximal convolution of the rat kidney. *Pflügers Arch* 351:49, 1974
47. SCRIVER CR, CHESNEY RW, MCINNES RR: Genetic aspects of renal tubular transport: Diversity and topology of carriers. *Kidney Int* 9:149, 1976
48. SCHAFER JA, BARFUSS DW: Membrane mechanisms for transepithelial amino acid absorption and secretion. *Am J Physiol* 238:F335, 1980
49. BARFUSS DW, SCHAFER JS: Active amino acid absorption by proximal convoluted and proximal straight tubules. *Am J Physiol* 236(2):F149, 1979
50. BARFUSS DW, MAYS JM, SCHAFER JA: Peritubular uptake and transepithelial transport of glycine in isolated proximal tubules. *Am J Physiol* 238:F324, 1980
51. MOHYUDDIN F, SCRIVER CR: Amino acid transport in mammalian kidney: Identification and analysis of multiple systems for iminoacids and glycine in rat kidney. *Am J Physiol* 219:1, 1970

52. HOLTZAPPLE P, GENE M, REA C, and SEGAL S: Metabolism and uptake of L-proline by human kidney cortex. *Pediatr Res* 7:818, 1973

53. SCRIVER CR, MCINNES RR, MOHYUDDIN F: Role of epithelial architecture and intracellular metabolism in proline uptake and transtubular reclamation in PRO/Re mouse kidney. *Proc Natl Acad Sci USA* 72:1431, 1975

53a. GRETH WE, THIER SO, SEGAL S: The transport and metabolism of L-proline-¹⁴C in the rat and in vivo. *Metabolism* 27:975, 1978

54. SLACK EN, LIANG C-CT, SACKTOR B: Transport of L-proline and D-glucose in luminal (brush border) and contraluminal (basal-lateral) membrane vesicles from the renal cortex. *Biochem Biophys Res Commun* 77:891, 1977

55. HAMMERMAN MR, SACKTOR B: Transport of amino acids in renal brush border membrane vesicles. Uptake of L-proline. *J Biol Chem* 252:591, 1977

56. MCNAMARA PD, OZEGOVIC B, PEPE LM, SEGAL S: Proline and glycine uptake by renal brush border membrane vesicles. *Proc Natl Acad Sci USA* 73:4521, 1976

57. MCNAMARA PD, PEPE LM, SEGAL S: Sodium gradient dependence of proline and glycine uptake in renal brush-border membrane vesicles. *Biochim Biophys Acta* 556:151, 1979

58. WEDEEN RP, WEINER B: The distribution of *p*-aminohippuric acid in rat kidney slices. I. Tubular localization. *Kidney Int* 3:205, 1973

59. ARTHUS MF, SCRIVER CR, BERGERON M: Restriction of exchanges between medium and luminal membrane of nephron during incubation of renal cortex slices. *Clin Res* 28:695A, 1980

60. HILLMAN RE, ALBRECHT I, ROSENBERG LE: Identification and analysis of multiple glycine transport systems in isolated mammalian renal tubules. *J Biol Chem* 243:5566, 1968

61. HILLMAN RE, ROSENBERG LE: Amino acid transport by isolated mammalian renal tubules. II. Transport systems for L-proline. *J Biol Chem* 244:4494, 1969

62. MACKENZIE S, SCRIVER CR: Transport of L-proline and α-aminoisobutyric acid in the isolated rat kidney glomerulus. *Biochim Biophys Acta* 241:725, 1971

63. BRODEHL J: Postnatal development of tubular amino acid reabsorption, in Silbernagl S, Lang F, Greger R (eds): *Amino Acid Transport and Uric Acid Transport*. Symposium Innsbruck, June 1975, Stuttgart, Thieme, 1976, p 128

64. LASLEY L, SCRIVER CR: Ontogeny of amino acid reabsorption in human kidney. Evidence from the homozygous infant with familial renal iminoglycinuria for multiple proline and glycine systems. *Pediatr Res* 13:65, 1979

65. BAERLOCHER K, SCRIVER CR, MOHYUDDIN F: Ontogeny of iminoglycine transport in mammalian kidney. *Proc Natl Acad Sci* 65:1009, 1970

66. CHRISTENSEN HN: On the development of amino acid transport systems. *Fed Proc* 32:19, 1973

67. BAERLOCHER KE, SCRIVER CR, MOHYUDDIN F: The ontogeny of amino acid transport in rat kidney. II. Kinetics of uptake and effect of anoxia. *Biochim Biophys Acta* 249:364, 1971

68. BAERLOCHER KE, SCRIVER CR, MOHYUDDIN F: The ontogeny of amino acid transport in rat kidney. I. Effect on distribution ratios and intracellular

69. ROTH KS, HWANG S-M, LONDON JW, SEGAL S: Ontogeny of glycine transport in isolated rat renal tubules. *Am J Physiol* 233:F241, 1977

70. REYNOLDS R, ROTH KS, HWANG SM, SEGAL S: On the development of glycine transport systems by rat renal cortex. *Biochim Biophys Acta* 511:274, 1979

71. SCRIVER CR, BERGERON M, ARTHUS MF: Ontogeny of amino acid reabsorption in mammalian kidney. The proline model. *Adv Physiol Sci* II, London, Pergamon Press, 1980 in press

72. GOLDMANN DR, ROTH KS, LANGFITT TW JR, SEGAL S: L-Proline transport by newborn rat kidney brush-border membrane vesicles. *Biochem J* 178:253, 1979

73. SCRIVER CR: Inborn errors of membrane transport: Mechanisms and implications for treatment, in Papadotos CJ, Bartsocas C (eds): *Management of Genetic Disorders. Prog Clin Biol Res* 34:231, 1979

74. ROSENBERG LE, SCRIVER CR: Amino acid metabolism, in Bondy PK, Rosenberg LE (eds): *Metabolic Control & Disease*, 8th ed. Saunders, 1980, Philadelphia, p 639

75. FINERMAN GAM, ROSENBERG LE: Amino acid transport in bone: Evidence for separate transport systems for neutral amino and imino acids. *J Biol Chem* 241:1487, 1966

76. TADA K, MORIKAWA T, ARAKAWA, T: Prolinuria: Transport of proline by leukocytes. *Tohoku J Exp Med* 90:189, 1966

77. CARVER MJ, PASKA R: Ion-exchange chromatography of urinary amino acids. I. Normal children. *Clin Chim Acta* 6:721, 1961

78. SCRIVER CR, DAVIES E: Endogenous renal clearance rates of free amino acids in pre-pubertal children. *Pediatrics* 36:592, 1965

79. DEVRIES A, KOCHWA S, LAZEBNIK J, FRANK M, DJALDETTI M: Glycinuria, a hereditary disorder associated with nephrolithiasis. *Am J Med* 23:408, 1957

80. OBERITER V, PURETI CZ, FABE CI, C-SABADI V: Hyperglycinuria with nephrolithiasis. *Eur J Pediatr* 127:279, 1978

81. KÄSER H, COTTIER P, ANTENER I: Glucoglycinuria, a new familial syndrome. *J Pediatr* 61:386, 1962

82. SCRIVER CR, GOLDBLOOM RB, ROY CC: Hypophosphatemic rickets with renal hyperglycinuria, renal glucosuria and glycylprolinuria: A syndrome with evidence for renal tubular secretion of phosphorus. *Pediatrics* 34:357, 1964

83. DENT CE, HARRIS H: Hereditary forms of rickets and osteomalacia. *J Bone Joint Surg* 38B:204, 1956

84. HARRIS H, MITTWOCH U, ROBSON EB, WARREN FL: Pattern of amino acid excretion in cystinuria. *Ann Hum Genet* 19:195, 1955

85. ROSENBERG LE, DURANT JL, ALBRECHT I: Genetic heterogeneity in cystinuria: evidence for allelism. *Trans Ass Am Physicians* 79:284, 1966

86. ROSENBERG LE: Genetic heterogeneity in cystinuria, in Nyhan WL (ed): *Amino Acid Metabolism and Genetic Variation*. New York, McGraw-Hill, 1967, p 341

87. ROSENBERG LE: Cystinuria: genetic heterogeneity and allelism. *Science* 154:1341, 1966

metabolism of proline and glycine. *Biochim Biophys Acta* 249:353, 1971

82

HARTNUP DISEASE

This summary is adapted from the summary written by John B. Jepson for the fourth edition of this text [1].

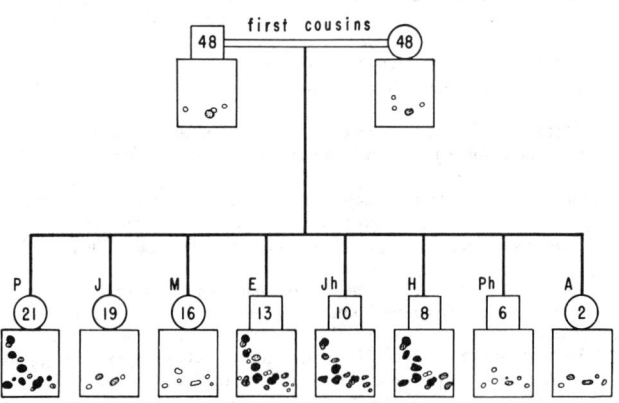

HARTNUP FAMILY - 1953

The genealogy of Hartnup disease as illustrated in the Hartnup family. The parents were first cousins. The age of each subject in 1953 is indicated by the numbers. In the squares are shown the chromatography patterns of urine samples of two-dimensional chromatograms stained for amino acids. Four of the eight sibs (P, E, Jh, and H) show the abnormal aminoaciduria involving neutral monoamino-monocarboxylic amino acids.

1. Hartnup disease is characterized by an intermittent red, scaly, pellagralike rash appearing after exposure to sunlight, by attacks of cerebellar ataxia, and occasionally by psychiatric changes ranging from emotional instability to delirium. A considerble proportion of patients are of somewhat lowered intelligence, but this is not a necessary accompaniment.

2. The disease was originally observed in four out of eight offspring of a first-cousin marriage. Other patients, including at least nine more sets of sibs, have now been described. Present information is consistent with the disease being the homozygous manifestation of a rare autosomal allele, but no test for the heterozygous state is known.

3. The single recognized constant feature of the disease and the only certain diagnostic test is a massive aminoaciduria involving a group of neutral monoamino-monocarboxylic amino acids that share a common renal reabsorption mechanism. The amino acids include: alanine, serine, theonine, asparagine, glutamine, valine, leucine, isoleucine, phenylalanine, tyrosine, tryptophan, histidine, and citrulline.

4. The aminoaciduria arises because patients with the disease have a diminished capacity for the tubular reabsorption of these particular amino acids. The specific defect also applies to intestinal absorption from the jejunum, and so patients retain these specific amino acids in the intestine for abnormally long periods. This allows intestinal bacteria to convert them into decomposition products, some of which are absorbed.

5. The effect of intestinal decomposition is particularly noticeable in the case of tryptophan. Often on a normal diet and always after an oral tryptophan load, patients excrete large quantities of indoxyl sulfate (indican), indolylacetic acid, and indolylacryloylglycine, all of which can be shown by intestinal sterilization to be products of bacterial action.

6. Patients have a lowered ability to convert tryptophan to kynurenine nicotinamide. This is attributed to the deviation of tryptophan from its normal metabolic route because of the absorption defect.

7. In general patients have responded satisfactorily to prolonged oral administration of nicotinamide.

8. Unlike the related condition of cystinuria, the pathologic significance of Hartnup disease does not seem to lie in the aminoaciduria which provides its diagnosis. The accompanying absorption defect in intestine or other nonrenal sites, it has been suggested, has the following effects:

   a. Allows formation of decomposition products that are toxic to the central nervous system.

   b. Diminishes the amount of nicotinamide synthesized from tryptophan, thus causing "pellagra" at times of metabolic strain.

   c. Diminishes somewhat the availability of essential

amino acids, with consequent general or specific malnutrition. Alternative intestinal mechanisms must be responsible for much compensatory absorption.

REFERENCE

1. Jepson JB: Hartnup disease, in Stanbury, JB, Wyngaarden, JB, Fredrickson DS (eds): *The Metabolic Basis of Inherited Disease*, 4th ed. New York, McGraw-Hill, 1978, p 1563

83

RENAL GLYCOSURIA

This summary is adapted from the summary written by Stephen M. Krane for the fourth edition of this text [1].

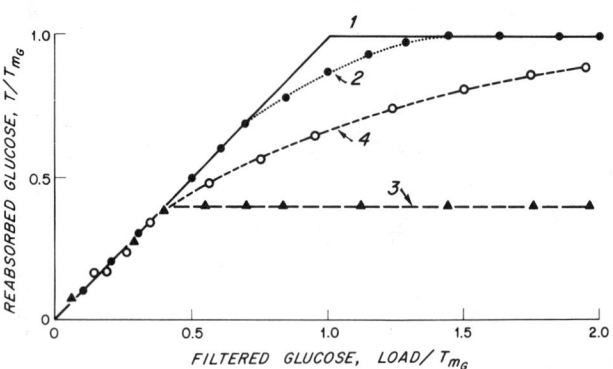

Renal tubular glucose reabsorption is plotted as a function of glucose load presented to the tubule. Curve 1 is a theoretical normal construction. Curve 2 is seen in normal individuals, showing the slight splay from the theoretical Curve 1. Curve 3 is seen in patients with renal glycosuria having a low T_m. Curve 4 is seen in patients with renal glycosuria showing an exaggerated splay.

1. Renal glycosuria is an abnormality in which glucose is excreted in the urine at normal concentrations of blood glucose. The disease is due to an abnormality in the mechanism by which glucose is reabsorbed from the glomerular filtrate and returned to the circulation. In spite of the urinary excretion of large amounts of glucose in some patients, the condition is clinically benign and usually symptomless.

2. It is probable that several different abnormalities are included under the term renal glycosuria. The majority of patients show a decrease in maximal reabsorption rates from glucose and a variable degree of splay of the titration curve. It is possible that those with low maximal reabsorption rates for glucose have a decreased functional capacity of the glucose carrier and those with increased splay have decreased affinity of the carrier for glucose, analogies based on models employing Michaelis-Menten kinetics. Some patients may have mixtures of abnormalities. Others have defects in intestinal absorption of hexoses that accompany the renal defect, although in the so-called intestinal glucose-galactose malabsorption the intestinal defect is severe and the renal abnormality mild.

3. In a few patients careful study has shown structural defects in the renal proximal convoluted tubules; in others no such abnormalities have been detected.

4. Although the pattern of inheritance in some pedigrees is interpreted as autosomal dominant, the pattern in the majority of families is most consistent with that of an autosomal recessive trait.

5. The mechanism of renal tubular transport of glucose is probably similar to that of the intestine. In both systems transport is concentrative and characterized by stereospecific structural requirements, mutual competitive inhibition of transported sugars, saturation kinetics, dependency on aerobic energy generation, and a dependency on Na^+ concentration.

6. In the light of present knowledge of the mechanism of the renal tubular transport of glucose, the excretion of excessive amounts of glucose in the urine at normal levels of blood glucose could result from any of the following: (a) decrease in the anatomic mass of the proximal convoluted tubule relative to the glomerular surface, (b) decrease in the functional capacity of the system responsible for accumulation of glucose against a concentration difference within the tubule cell, (c) abnormal distribution of the transport system relative to glomerular filtration whether on an anatomic or functional basis, (d) reduction in the permeability toward glucose of the luminal membrane of the cell, or (e) decrease in the affinity for glucose of the hypothetical membrane carrier. Success in demon-

strating coupled transport in isolated brush border vesicles and reconstitution of the system after extraction of the vesicles with detergent may provide the means for determining the structural basis of the defects in the future.

REFERENCE

1. KRANE SM: Renal glycosuria, in Stanbury JB, Wyngaarden JB, Fredrickson DS (eds): *The Metabolic Basis of Inherited Disease,* 4th ed. New York, McGraw-Hill, 1978, p 1607

84

RENAL TUBULAR ACIDOSIS AND FANCONI SYNDROME

R. CURTIS MORRIS, JR.

ANTHONY SEBASTIAN

1. Renal tubular acidosis (RTA) is a clinical syndrome of disordered renal acidification characterized by hyperchloremia, reduced plasma bicarbonate concentration (or venous CO_2 content), and, during mild metabolic acidosis, values of urinary pH that are inappropriately high and urinary excretion rates of net acid (titratable acid + ammonium − bicarbonate) that are inappropriately low.

2. In the type of RTA first investigated in detail, the "classic" or type 1 RTA (RTA-1), urinary pH is inappropriately high, and bicarbonaturia occurs during severe as well as mild degrees of acidosis. In affected adult patients, the amount of bicarbonate excreted is a trivial fraction of that filtered by the glomerulus (<5 percent) at normal and reduced plasma bicarbonate concentrations. This finding (1) suggests that reabsorption of bicarbonate by the proximal tubule is not greatly reduced and (2) explains why correction of acidosis is sustained by low-dose alkali therapy (1 to 2 meq/kg per day). In children with RTA-1 the fractional excretion of bicarbonate can be 6 to 14 percent over a broad range of normal and reduced plasma bicarbonate concentrations. Accordingly, sustained correction of acidosis during childhood usually requires high-dose alkali therapy (5 to 14 meq/kg per day). With therapy the genetic potential for somatic growth can be realized.

3. Several kinds of hereditary autosomally transmitted disorders of the renal tubule are expressed as RTA-1. In those affected with those disorders in which acidosis independent hydercalciuria is not a major metabolic phenomenon, hypocitraturia may be a primary expression of the genetic defect causing impaired renal acidification and may be critical in the pathogenesis of nephrocalcinosis and nephrolithiasis. In at least one genotype of RTA-1 (the San Francisco syndrome), the acidification defect is sufficiently severe from early infancy to cause metabolic acidosis without nephrocalcinosis or a reduction in GFR, and in most affected children the amount of bicarbonate excreted at normal plasma bicarbonate concentrations is the major determinant of the occurrence and severity of acidosis. High-dose alkali therapy initiated before 4 years of age can prevent the characteristic occurrence of nephrocalcinosis in childhood and early adulthood.

In another genotype of RTA-1 (the Philadelphia syndrome), the impairment in renal acidification may not be severe enough to cause acidosis unless nephrocalcinosis occurs which is severe enough to reduce renal mass and to be radiographically demonstrable. Nephrocalcinosis may be critical in causing the progression of the nonacidotic or incomplete syndrome of RTA-1 (iRTA-1) to the acidotic or complete syndrome of RTA-1 (cRTA-1). Progression may be prevented by alkali therapy.

In two autosomal dominantly transmitted disorders in which RTA-1 and nephrocalcinosis can be the major clinical findings, hypercalciuria gives rise to Nephrocalcinosis, renal damage, and impairment of renal acidification. In one genotype, (the Atlanta syndrome), the impairment was expressed only as iRTA-1, except in one affected man with acidosis and severe azotemia. In the other genotype in which hypercalciuria is the primarily expressed trait (the Oklahoma City syndrome), both cRTA-1 and iRTA-1 occurred with and without radiographically demonstrable nephrocalcinosis and reduction in GFR.

Hereditary RTA-1 is not rare. cRTA-1 occurs most commonly in women with "autoimmune" diseases, usually Sjögren's syndrome and less commonly "lupoid" hepatitis.

4. Type 2 "proximal" RTA (RTA-2) is characterized by a fractional excretion of at least 15 percent of filtered bicarbonate at normal plasma bicarbonate concentrations and under normal physiologic conditions. This suggests a defect in the acidification process of the proximal tubule. With metabolic acidosis of increasing severity, the magnitude of bicarbonaturia varies directly with the plasma bicarbonate concentration. During severe degrees of acidosis bicarbonaturia disappears, urinary pH decreases to the normal minimum, and acid excretion approaches normal. This suggests that the acidification process of the distal-most nephron is intact. RTA-2 almost always occurs as part of a more complex dysfunction of the proximal tubule and is associated with the Fanconi syndrome. In adult patients, RTA-2 occurs most commonly when intestinal malabsorption gives rise to vitamin D deficiency, hypocalcemia, secondary hyperparathyroidism, and hypophosphatemia. RTA-2 also occurs in children with a dietary deficiency of vitamin D. In both circumstances vitamin D therapy usually corrects the acidification dysfunction and the accompanying aminoaciduria. In patients with myeloma, RTA-2 may precede other manifestations of the disease by several years, and it may occur with explosive suddenness in patients with hereditary fructose intolerance who are given fructose.

5. Type 4 RTA (RTA-4), perhaps the most common type of RTA, is a hyperkalemic form of "distal" RTA characterized by subnormal excretion rates of net acid and reduced renal clearance of potassium. At normal plasma bicarbonate concentrations (during alkali therapy), renal reabsorption of bicarbonate is modestly reduced. During acidosis normal lumen-peritubular H^+ gradients can be attained, but net acid excretion is subnormal and is only in part due to hyperkalemia-mediated suppression of renal ammoniagenesis and the consequent hypoammoniuria. The physiologic characteristics are those that would be predicted from a deficiency of aldosterone in its physiologic effect on the kidney. In studies of aldosterone responsive urinary epithelia, the aldosterone deficiency diminishes the conductance (rate-capacity) of protons through the active transport pathway but does not reduce the protonmotive force (H^+ concen-

tration gradient generating ability) of the H^+ secretory pump.

Although RTA-4 usually occurs in patients with at least moderately severe renal insufficiency, most commonly in patients with diabetes mellitus, and usually as part of the syndrome of hyporeninemic hypoaldosteronism, the disorder occurs in prototype and without reduction in renal mass in familial and acquired states of deficient renal responsiveness to circulating aldosterone.

6. Aldosterone resistant RTA-4 occurs in two distinctly different familial disorders: (1) type 1 pseudohypoaldosteronism (classic pseudohypoaldosteronism of infancy), characterized by hyperkalemia, renal salt wasting, and hypotension, and (2) type 2 pseudohypoaldosteronism, and syndrome of aldosterone resistant hyperkalemia unaccompanied by renal salt wasting or hypotension and frequently associated with hypertension. The primary abnormality in type 2 pseudohypoaldosteronism may be a defect of the distal nephron that increases the reabsorptive avidity of the distal nephron for Cl^-.

7. Fanconi syndrome (FS) consists of two components: (1) a complex dysfunction of the proximal renal tubule characterized by increased renal clearance of phosphate, α-amino acids, usually bicarbonate (RTA-2), and sometimes glucose and uric acid at normal and reduced plasma concentrations of these substances; (2) a metabolic bone disease, which is characteristically rickets in children and osteomalacia in adults. Because all of the substances excessively cleared in FS and in RTA-2 are normally reabsorbed predominantly in the proximal tubule, FS, alone or in combination with RTA-2 (RTA-2/FS), has generally been assumed to reflect dysfunction of the proximal tubule. The clinical picture of FS is dominated by metabolic bone disease and, in affected children, impaired growth and often frank stunting.

8. FS disappears in patients with galactosemia, tyrosinemia, Wilson's disease, and hereditary fructose intolerance (HFI) when disorders are corrected or attenuated by removal of galactose, tyrosine, copper, or fructose, respectively. In these disorders the expression of FS is linked to the abnormal gene product by way of a reversible abnormality of renal metabolism. The renal tubular disorder reversibly induced by fructose in patients with HFI can serve as an experimental model of RTA-2/FS, whose pathogenesis is genetically deficient renal aldolase B and consequent intracellular accumulation of F-1-P. In the model of FS induced by fructose in patients with HFI, and also that induced by maleic acid in rats, renal clearance studies during water diuresis provide strong evidence that disordered function of the proximal tubule underlies RTA-2/FS. In both models a phosphate depletion-dependent disorder of metabolism in cells of the proximal tubule probably underlies the disorder of renal tubular function; in both models, RTA-2/FS is strongly attenuated by phosphate loading.

9. In patients with HFI given fructose and in rats given maleic acid, RTA-2/FS is accompanied by a disorder of the phagolysosomal system expressed as lysozymuria and increased urinary excretion of N-acetylgluco-

saminidase, which is a lysosomal enzyme too large to be filtered by the glomerulus. Similar phenomena occur in cystinosis, the most common cause of RTA-2/FS in children and in which cystine accumulation in lysosomes is well-documented.

10. *Apparently, in a number of patients with RTA-2/FS the renal conversion of 25-OH-vitamin D_3 to 1,25-$(OH)_2D_3$ is impaired and may be important to the pathogenesis of the bone disease of patients with RTA-2/FS and might also be important to the pathogenesis of the renal dysfunction of RTA-2/FS in some patients, including those with the genetically transmitted disorders, vitamin D dependency types 1 and 2.*

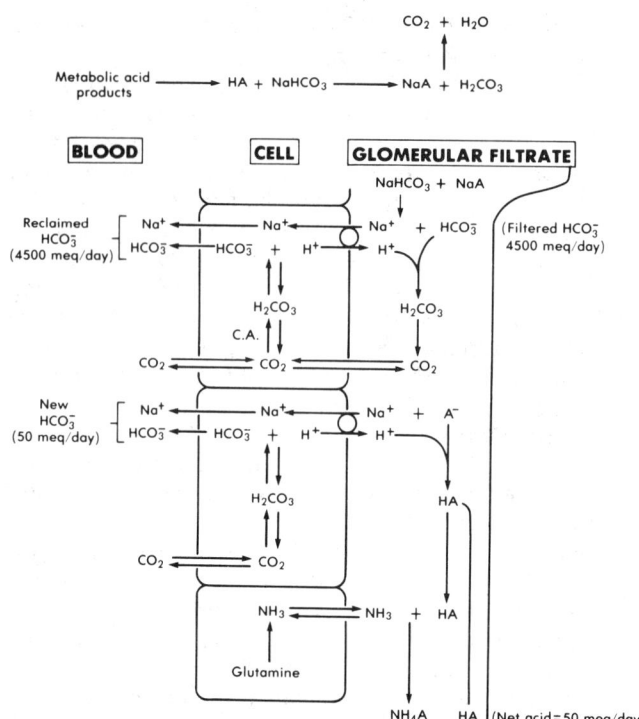

Figure 84-1 Schematic diagram of the normal mammalian renal acidification process. (*Adapted from Seldin and Wilson [2].*)

RENAL TUBULAR ACIDOSIS

Renal tubular acidosis (RTA) is a nonuremic clinical syndrome of disordered renal acidification characterized by hyperchloremic acidosis, inappropriately high urinary pH, bicarbonaturia, and reduced urinary excretion of titratable acid and usually ammonium [1–20]. The syndrome reflects a disorder of renal acidification that can cause acidosis without or with only moderate reduction in renal mass. RTA can reflect several physiologically distinct disorders of renal acidification (Table 84-1). Each of these can occur in a number of specific diseases. In several inherited diseases RTA is the major clinically expressed trait, and in some cases it is the only one.

RENAL ACIDIFICATION

By regulating the concentration of plasma bicarbonate, the renal acidification process of humans and other mammals participates in the regulation of the normal alkalinity of extracellular fluid [2, 21, 26] (Fig. 84-1). In normal humans, under physiologic conditions, the process of renal acidification maintains plasma bicarbonate at normal concentrations both by reclaiming all filtered bicarbonate and by causing the excretion of an amount of acid equal to the net endogenous production of nonvolatile acid, approximately 1 meq/kg of body weight per day in adults [22] and 1 to 3 meq/kg of body weight per day in infants and young children [23]. Both the renal reabsorption of bicarbonate and exretion of acid appear to be mediated by the secretion of H^+ [21, 24–26].

At normal plasma bicarbonate concentrations, and under physiologic conditions, the proximal tubule secretes H^+ at a rate that reclaims 85 to 90 percent of filtered bicarbonate [25, 26] (Fig. 84-1). For each 1 mol of H^+ secreted, 1 mol of cellular HCO_3^- is generated and returned to the blood. Secreted H^+ used in the titration of luminal HCO_3^- is not excreted in the urine as acid. Rather, the H_2CO_3 formed in the titration process dissociates to H_2O and CO_2, which equilibrates with peritubular CO_2. By catalyzing the dissociation, carbonic anhydrase, located at the luminal border of the proximal tubule, acts to reduce the steady-state concentration of luminal H_2CO_3 (and hence luminal H^+) and thereby to facilitate secre-

tion of H^+ [24]. When the catalysis (acetazolamide) of this dissociation is inhibited, H^+ increases in the lumen of the proximal tubule segment and thereby imposes a gradient restriction on the secretion of H^+ in this segment [24]. The normal acidification process of the proximal tubule can be considered to be a high-capacity (rate), low-gradient system [2, 24] and accounts for the great preponderance of H^+ secreted by the renal tubule.

In the distal nephron the H^+ secretory process tritrates to extinction the 10 to 15 percent of filtered bicarbonate unreabsorbed in the proximal tubule, thereby lowering the pH to values less than 6.2. The distal H^+ secretory process further titrates the major urinary buffers, Na_2HPO_4 and NH_3 to NaH_2PO_4 and NH_4^+, a process that begins in the proximal nephron. Usually, "titratable acid" is largely a measure of H^+ excreted as NaH_2PO_4. In the collecting duct the secretory capacity for H^+ is small, but its capacity to generate a large gradient (lumen-peritubular) [24] enables the kidney to reduce urinary pH to normal minima (<5.3) and, by titrating NH_3 and $NaHPO_4$, to excrete ammonium and titratable acid at a combined rate equal to that of the endogenous production of nonvolatile acid. The combined excretion rates of titratable acid and NH_4^+ minus the normally negligible excretion rate of bicarbonate is termed *net acid excretion* [1]. Net acid excretion normally accounts for no more than 3 percent of renal H^+ secretion at normal plasma bicarbonate concentrations. When the rate of excretion of bicarbonate exceeds that of the sum of titratable acid and ammonium, *net base excretion* occurs.

Because the H^+ secretory capacity of the distal nephron is small relative to that of the proximal tubule, relatively small changes in the amount of bicarbonate delivered to the distal nephron can greatly alter urinary pH and net acid (or net base) excretion. And because the amount of bicarbonate delivered to the distal nephron is determined by the amount of bicarbonate rejected by the proximal tubule, the rate at which the proximal

Table 84-1 Physiologic characteristics of clinical disorders of renal acidification

| | RTA (renal tubular acidosis) | | | | | | | |
| | Type 1 (classic, distal) | | | Type 2 (proximal) | | | | |
	Non-HCO$_3^-$ wasting	HCO$_3^-$ wasting	Incomplete	Type 2 RTA	Type 1,2 hybrid	Incomplete	Type 4	Uremic acidosis
Frank acidosis	Present	Present	Absent	Present	Present	Absent	Present	Present
Net renal H$^+$ secretion at normal [HCO$_3^-$]$_p$	Minimally reduced	Moderately reduced	Not reduced	Greatly reduced	Greatly reduced	Not reduced	Moderately reduced	Nearly normal to greatly reduced
Bicarbonaturia, percent of filtered HCO$_3^-$ excreted at normal [HCO$_3^-$]$_p$	<3–5%	5–10%	<1%	>15%	>15%	<2%	<2–15%	<3 to >30%
TA +NH$_4^+$ excretion at normal [HCO$_3^-$]$_p$	Reduced	Reduced	Not reduced	Reduced	Reduced	Not reduced	Reduced	Reduced
Therapeutic alkali requirement, meq of HCO$_3^-$ per kilogram body weight per day	1–3	5–10	None	2 to >10	3 to >10	None	1–2	1–3
Urinary acidification during acidosis	Impaired	Impaired	Impaired	Intact	Impaired	Intact	Intact	Intact
Bicarbonaturia, percent of filtered HCO$_3^-$ excreted	<3%	5–10%	<–1%	None	<3%	None	None	None
TA + NH$_4^+$ excretion during acidosis	Reduced	Reduced	Not reduced or reduced	Not reduced	Reduced	Not reduced	Not reduced or reduced	Reduced
Carbon dioxide tension in HCO$_3^-$-rich urine (UpH >BpH)								
U$_{P_{CO_2}}$ minus B$_{P_{CO_2}}$	<20	<20	<20	>20	<20	>20		
Serum potassium concentration	Normal or reduced	Usually reduced	Normal or reduced	Normal or reduced	Usually reduced	Low to normal	Increased	Normal or increased
Glomerular filtration rate	Normal or slightly	Normal	Normal or slightly reduced	Normal or reduced	Usually reduced	Reduced	Normal to greatly reduced	Greatly reduced

ABBREVIATIONS: [HCO$_3^-$]$_p$, plasma bicarbonate concentration; TA, titratable acid; NH$_4^+$, ammonium; UpH, urine pH; BpH, blood pH; P_{CO_2}, carbon dioxide tension.

tubule secretes H$^+$ and the concentration of plasma bicarbonate (filtered load of bicarbonate) are critical and complementary modulators of urinary pH and net acid (or net base) excretion. The rate at which H$^+$ is secreted by the proximal tubule is increased by K$^+$ depletion [27] and increased arterial P_{CO_2} [28]. The rate at which the distal nephron secretes H$^+$ can be increased by increasing intraluminal negativity (with respect to the peritubular blood), as can be achieved by maneuvers that increase the luminal concentration of poorly reabsorbed anions during states of enhanced distal tubular Na$^+$ reabsorption, i.e., Na$^+$ depletion or the administration of mineralocorticoids [29, 30]. The absence of circulating aldosterone restricts H$^+$ secretion in the distal nephron [31]. It has been generally, if tacitly, assumed that urinary excretion of bicarbonate reflects only bicarbonate that has been rejected by the proximal tubule and unreclaimed by the distal nephron. Since

metabolic alkalosis can enhance HCO$_3^-$ *secretion* by the rabbit collecting tubule [32, 33], urinary excretion of bicarbonate might in some instances reflect secretion of HCO$_3^-$ by the distal nephron.

The net renal secretion of H$^+$, like the net renal reabsorption of sodium, is dampened by expansion of effective extracellular fluid volume [34, 35]. This finding reflects the physiologic interdependence of the two processes.

Hydrogen ion secretion in the proximal tubule is mediated by at least two mechanisms: (1) an electroneutral Na$^+$-H$^+$ exchange across the luminal membrane [36], driven by the lumen-to-cytoplasm Na$^+$ gradient that in turn is generated by the action of (Na$^+$-K$^+$-ATPase) located in the basolateral membrane [37]; (2) an electrogenic H$^+$ "pump" in the luminal membrane that is mediated by a proton-translocating ATPase located in the luminal membrane [38] but is not dependent on luminal Na^+ or creation of a Na^+ gradient. The Na^+-H^+ exchange process could account for as much as 80 percent of proximal resorption of bicarbonate, whereas the electrogenic H^+ secretory process has a lesser capacity but higher $[H^+]$-gradient generating ability [26]. In the mucosa lining the turtle and toad bladder, an epithelium resembling that of the mammalian distal nephron [39–41], the H^+ secretory mechanism is electrogenic, i.e., it is capable of transporting a net positive charge into the lumen [39, 41]; it is not dependent on Na^+ resorption [39, 40], although the rate of H^+ secretion may be influenced by Na^+ resorption. Secretion of H^+ can occur without a favorable transepithelial electrical potential difference and against a transepithelial H^+ concentration gradient until the H^+ concentration in the mucosal fluid is approximately 1000 times greater than that in the serosal fluid [41, 42]. With the attainment of this H^+ gradient, the net rate of H^+ secretion becomes zero. This reflects cessation of unidirectional H^+ secretion from cell to lumen; backleak of H^+ from the mucosal fluid into the cell or serosal fluid is negligible. The magnitude of the transepithelial H^+ concentration gradient required to nullify net H^+ secretion is an index of the *driving force* (protonmotive force) of the H^+ secretory pump. The rate of H^+ secretion when the transepithelial H^+ concentration gradient is nonlimiting is an index of the *conductance* of H^+ through the active transport pathway [41, 42]. In the mucosal border of the turtle bladder, a reversible proton-translocating ATPase can function as an H^+ pump that can account for urinary acidification [43].

TYPE 1 RTA ("CLASSIC" OR "DISTAL")

Physiologic Characteristics

In *type 1 RTA* (RTA-1), urinary pH is inappropriately high during severe as well as mild degrees of acidosis (Fig. 84-2) (usually greater than 6), and there is persistent urinary excre-

Figure 84-2 Relationship between urinary pH and plasma bicarbonate concentration in patients with prototypic type 1 (classic) and type 2 (proximal) renal tubular acidosis (RTA). In patients with type 2 RTA, the urinary pH may be inappropriately high or appropriately low, depending on the severity of systemic acidosis (shaded area represents range of normal plasma bicarbonate concentrations).

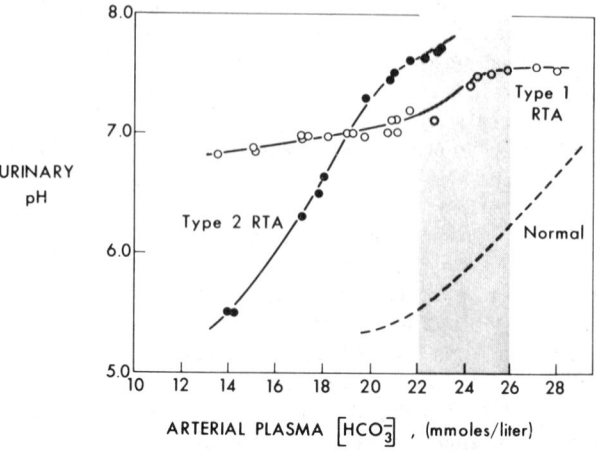

tion of bicarbonate, but the complex dysfunction of the proximal tubule of the Fanconi syndrome (impaired renal reabsorption of glucose, phosphate, and amino acids) is absent [1, 2, 6–18]. RTA-1 can be the expression of a number of disease processes (Table 84-2).

Adults   In adults with RTA-1, the amount of bicarbonate excreted at both normal and reduced plasma bicarbonate concentrations is less than 5 percent of filtered bicarbonate ($C_{HCO_3^-}/C_{in}$) over a broad range of normal and subnormal plasma bicarbonate concentrations (Table 84-1, Fig. 84-3). This finding permits the inference that reabsorption of bicarbonate in the proximal renal tubule (and the distal tubule) is not substantially reduced, and indicates that impaired renal excretion of acid need not be associated with "renal bicarbonate wasting" (see below) [2, 5, 6, 10–18]. In most adult patients with RTA-1, acidosis results principally from a modest urinary excretion of *net base*, HCO_3^- − (titratable acid +

Table 84-2   Clinical spectrum of (classic type 1, distal) renal tubular acidosis

Primary (as part of no obvious systemic diseases)
Hereditary [16, 44–47]
Sporadic [1, 3–7, 10, 11, 14–16, 57]
Autoimmune disorders [58–74]
Dysgammaglobulinemia
    Hyperglobulinemic purpura [58]
    Cryoglobulinemia [59]
Sjögren's syndrome [63–65, 69]
Chronic active hepatitis [60, 70, 71]
Primary biliary cirrhosis [71–73]
Thyroiditis [67]
Fibrosing alveolitis [68]
Disorders causing nephrocalcinosis
Hypercalciuria
    Hereditary [75, 76]
    Sporadic [77, 78]
Primary hyperparathyroidism [79, 80]
Hyperthyroidism [81]
Vitamin D intoxication [82]
Medullary sponge kidney [83, 84]
Hereditary fructose intolerance
    (after chronic fructose ingestion) [85]
Wilson's disease [86]
Fabry's disease [87]
Drug- or toxin-induced nephropathy
Mercury [88]
Amphotericin B [89, 90]
Analgesics [91, 92]
Lithium [93]
Cyclamate [94]
Other renal diseases
Pyelonephritis [95]
Obstructive uropathy [96–99]
Renal transplantation [100, 101]
Leprosy [102]
Genetically transmitted systemic diseases
Ehlers-Danlos syndrome [103]
Hereditary elliptocytosis [104]
Sickle-cell anemia [105, 106]
Marfan's syndrome [107]
Carbonic anhydrase deficiency [108, 109]
Sensorineural deafness [110–113]
Hepatic cirrhosis [114–116]

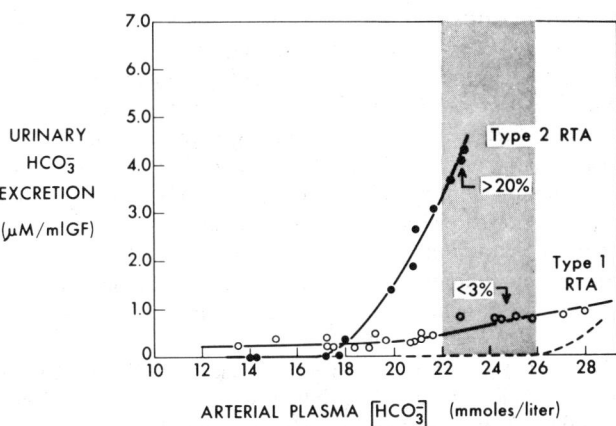

Figure 84-3 The relationship between urinary bicarbonate excretion and plasma bicarbonate concentration in patients with prototypic type 1 (classic) and type 2 (proximal) RTA. In patients with type 1 RTA, bicarbonaturia occurs during severe as well as mild degrees of acidosis, but in affected adult patients the magnitude of bicarbonaturia is invariably small, predictably less than 5 percent of the filtered bicarbonate load. In patients with type 2 RTA, bicarbonaturia is absent during moderately severe acidosis, but of large magnitude at normal plasma bicarbonate concentrations, often mounting to more than 15 percent of the filtered bicarbonate load. (Shaded area represents range of normal plasma bicarbonate concentrations).

ammonium), at normal plasma bicarbonate concentrations [14]. Hence, correction of acidosis is characteristically sustained by an amount of alkali only a fraction more than the normal endogenous production of nonvolatile acid, i.e., a fraction more than 1 meq/kg per day in adults [2, 8, 11, 12, 15].

Children   Renal bicarbonate wasting (RBW) occurs in many prepubertal children with idiopathic or familial RTA-1 who are given alkali therapy in amounts sufficient to sustain correction of acidosis [14, 16, 57]. RBW can be said to occur when the urinary excretion of net base exceeds the rate at which nonvolatile acid is endogenously produced [14, 16]. Since endogenous production of nonvolatile acid may be as high as 3 meq/kg per day in rapidly growing children [23], *renal bicarbonate wasting* can be defined arbitrarily as net base excretion of greater than 3 meq/kg per day at normal (or reduced) plasma bicarbonate concentrations [14]. So defined, RBW is quantitatively more important in the causation of acidosis than reduced excretion of acid per se (which predictably attends RBW because of the inappropriately high urinary pH at which bicarbonate wasting occurs). Reduced excretion of acid leads to acidosis only to the extent that the endogenously produced, nonvolatile acid titrates body buffers, including plasma bicarbonate. Such a loss of base is relatively minor and slowly developing compared to the loss of base which can result from a substantial fractional excretion of filtered bicarbonate. (This statement assumes that endogenous production of nonvolatile acid is not substantially greater than 3 meq/kg per day, as in such conditions as lactic acidosis and diabetic ketoacidosis.)

In infants with RTA-1, RBW can be present from the outset of the disorder [14, 16, 57], but usually occurs a few weeks after alkali therapy has been started [16]. In older affected children RBW usually does not occur until several months after beginning alkali therapy, when growth velocity has greatly increased. The occurrence of RBW in infants and children with RTA-1 does not appear to reflect a qualitative change in the character of the renal acidification defect. Over a broad range of normal and subnormal values of plasma bicarbonate concentration, $C_{HCO_3^-}/C_{in}$ remains relatively fixed but ranges in value from 6 to 14 percent [14, 16, 17, 57]. When RBW occurs in children with RTA-1, the magnitude of RBW at normal plasma bicarbonate concentrations is the major determinant of the amount of alkali required to sustain correction of their acidosis. This amount may range from 5 to 14 meq/kg per day [15, 16, 57], as opposed to an amount of 1 to 3 meq/kg per day, which is sufficient to correct acidosis in the absence of RBW. The persistence of RBW at reduced plasma bicarbonate concentrations accounts for the strikingly severe acidosis both before corrective alkali therapy is begun and soon after it is diminished [14].

Mechanisms and Pathogenesis   The pathophysiological characteristics of RTA-1 are the consequence of a reduced net rate of H^+ secretion in the collecting duct. Such a reduction might result from either of two general mechanisms (Table 84-3): (1) a reduced rate of unidirectional active H^+ secretion (cell-to-lumen), or (2) a "permeability" defect that permits an increased passive backleak of secreted H^+ (lumen-to-cell) or increased luminal entry of HCO_3^- or OH^-. The mechanisms formulated are based to a considerable extent on the results of studies in vitro of the renal acidification process of the mucosa lining the toad and turtle bladder.

Perhaps the best evidence that collecting duct function is impaired in RTA-1 is the finding that the carbon dioxide ten-

Table 84-3   Hypothetical mechanisms of impaired collecting duct function resulting in renal tubular acidosis

I. Reduced cell-to-lumen unidirectional active H^+ secretion
  A. Disorder of H^+ secretory pumps [41, 117–122]
    1. Reduced strength (protonmotive force) of pumps [41, 121]
    2. Reduced proton "conductance" [41, 118, 119]
      a. Decreased number of pumps [41]
      b. Defect in active transport pathway [41, 118, 120]
        (1) Defect in metabolic energy production
        (2) Defect in metabolic energy utilization
        (3) Structural defect of pump
  B. Reduction in electrochemical gradient that ordinarily promotes H^+ secretion [40, 41, 117, 123–125]
    1. Reduced lumen-negative transtubular electrical potential
      a. reduced sodium reabsorption [125]
      b. enhanced potassium secretion
      c. enhanced chloride reabsorption
    2. Reduced availability of cellular H^+
      a. impaired exit of cellular bicarbonate or OH^- to peritubular fluid [126]
      b. carbonic anhydrase defect [41, 127]
    3. Increased luminal H^+ secondary to reduced concentration of luminal proton acceptors
      a. impaired ammoniagenesis [31, 128]
      b. impaired medullary ammonia delivery [129]
      c. hypophosphaturia [130, 131]
II. Impaired luminal acidification despite normal or increased cell-to-lumen unidirectional active H^+ secretion
  A. Permeability defect
    1. Backleak of luminal H^+ through cell membrane or between cells [132, 133]
    2. Increased luminal entry of HCO_3^-, CO_3^{2-}, or OH^-
  B. Abnormal stimulation of active HCO_3^- secretion or $HCO_3^- = Cl^-$ exchange [33, 134]

sion (P_{CO_2}) of the urine does not increase to normally high values during loading with sodium bicarbonate [135, 136]. In normal subjects rendered bicarbonaturic by such loading, urine P_{CO_2} exceeds that of arterial blood by more than 20 mmHg. To a considerable extent, this increment in urine P_{CO_2} arises from the delayed dehydration of carbonic acid (H_2CO_3) generated in the lumen of the collecting duct and formed from the reaction of secreted H^+ with filtered HCO_3^- [138]. In the lumen of the collecting duct, in contradistinction to that of the proximal tubule [24], the dehydration of H_2CO_3 is uncatalyzed. In consequence, dehydration of H_2CO_3 generated in the more proximal segments of the collecting duct (cortex, outer medulla) occurs slowly throughout the more distal segments of the collecting duct (inner medulla). CO_2 so generated in the lumen of these segments does not readily diffuse out, possibly because CO_2 is trapped in the inner medulla owing to its countercurrently arranged, and normally slow, blood flow [138]. Dehydration of H_2CO_3 generated in the collecting duct lumen continues in the renal pelvis and bladder and generates further CO_2. In bicarbonate-loaded patients with RTA-1, the finding that urine P_{CO_2} does not exceed blood P_{CO_2} suggests that dehydration of luminal H_2CO_3 in the collecting duct proceeds to completion and that the CO_2 generated equilibrates with that of the systemic circulation before the luminal fluid enters the inner medullary collecting duct, renal pelvis, or bladder. This circumstance might obtain if the total amount of H_2CO_3 generated in the lumen was greatly reduced because of an abnormally reduced net rate of H^+ secretion. Since it has been found that the pH of the urine exceeds that of the blood during HCO_3^- loading in patients with RTA-1, any reduction in net rate of H^+ secretion in the collecting duct would reflect decreased cell-to-lumen H^+ secretion rather than backleak of luminal H^+ [19, 20, 136].

Reduced generation of H_2CO_3 is not the only mechanism that might restrict the increment in urine P_{CO_2} attained during bicarbonate loading in patients with RTA-1 [15]. Impaired medullary trapping of CO_2 might underlie the same phenomenon. If secretion of H^+ and generation of H_2CO_3 in the lumens of cortical and outer medullary collecting ducts accounts for the major fraction of the normal rise in P_{CO_2} during bicarbonate loading, the generation of urine P_{CO_2} might be reduced if luminal H_2CO_3 were lost at an abnormally rapid rate from these preterminal collecting duct segments, owing either to a permeability abnormality in these segments or to the presence there of abnormal catalysts of H_2CO_3 dehydration [139, 140]. In RTA-1, a single permeability defect of the distal nephron could permit both excessive back-diffusion of H_2CO_3 when the pH of the urine equals or exceeds that of the blood (during bicarbonate loading), and excessive back-diffusion of H^+ when the pH of the urine is less than that of blood (during acidosis) [15].

That an abnormality in permeability of the distal nephron to H^+ could underlie the impairment of urinary acidification in patients with RTA-1 is suggested by the occurrence of apparently typical RTA-1 in patients with the nephropathy induced by amphotericin B [89, 90]. This antifungal antibiotic can alter cell membrane permeability and increase passive H^+ permeability in certain H^+ secreting epithelia [132, 133]. RTA-1 occurs as the major clinical expression of an autosomal dominant genetic trait in patients with medullary sponge kidney (associated with Ehlers-Danlos syndrome) [103]. In adult patients RTA-1 occurs predominantly in women, usually in association with disorders characterized by hypergammaglobulinemia [63–65, 69], most commonly Sjögren's syndrome [62–64, 69, 74] and less commonly chronic active hepatitis

(lupoid hepatitis) [60, 70, 71]. The association of RTA-1 and hypergammaglobulinemia appears to be more than coincidental, but RTA-1 seems not to be caused by hypergammaglobulinemia per se [64, 66]. Rather, RTA-1 could appear to be the functional renal expression of a more general autoimmune disorder (e.g., Sjögren's syndrome) [66, 69] that can give rise to hypergammaglobulinemia. From evidence derived from both experimental models and human disease, a persuasive case can be made that lesions of the renal tubule (and interstitium) can result from immune complexes or autoantibodies directed against constituents of the basement membrane of the renal tubule [141, 142].

Erythrocyte carbonic anhydrase B has recently been found to be deficient in a few children with RTA-1 [108, 109], including three in whom the deficiency might be an autosomal recessive trait (Table 84-4). But while normal renal acidification critically depends on renal carbonic anhydrase, it is not clear that carbonic anhydrase B occurs in the human kidney, except for that present in the circulating erythrocytes [143–145]. Recent studies indicate that membrane-bound carbonic anhydrase in human kidney is an isoenzyme distinct from the B and C isoenzymes, both with respect to amino acid composition and immunoreactivity [146]. Accordingly, the association of deficient erythrocyte carbonic anhydrase B and RTA-1 remains to be clarified.

An impairment in the metabolic generation or transduction of energy in the cells of the distal renal tubule could underlie the acidification dysfunction of RTA-1 (Table 84-2). In most patients with RTA-1 the urinary excretion of citrate is extremely reduced [50, 56, 147–154], and in all but a few patients [50, 56, 152] it increases only modestly with alkali therapy. The hypocitraturia occurs unassociated with hypocitratemia [153], hypokalemia [56, 151], or a recognized basis for an intracellular depletion of potassium that might cause hypocitraturia [155]. Having found in the rat that inhibition of renal carbonic anhydrase with acetazolamide induced renal calcinosis and hypocitraturia [156], Harrison and his coworkers proposed that hypocitraturia in patients with RTA-1 was related to the "fundamental metabolic abnormality of the renal tubule cell" [149]. Dedmond and Wrong found that severe hypocitraturia did not occur in adult patients with nephrocalcinosis associated with renal disorders other than RTA-1 [151]. These workers proposed that hypocitraturia might occur in patients with RTA-1 because "the Krebs cycle is interfered with at one or more points because of a genetic or acquired defect," and that such a defect might be "responsible both for the tubule failure to secrete H^+" and "the reduced urinary excretion of citrate." The prescience of these formulations is suggested by several recent studies of the normal renal mitochondrial metabolism of citrate.

Simpson and Angielski demonstrated that the citrate concentration in mitochondria of rabbit renal cortex was much less at high (40 mM) than at low (10 mM) concentrations of HCO_3^- in the suspending media, and that HCO_3^- per se was determining the phenomenon [157]. They suggested that the concentration of HCO_3^- regulates the transport of citrate across the mitochondrial membrane. Given that an increased renal cortical content of citrate attends metabolic alkalosis [155, 158], they further suggested that such a regulatory mechanism provided an explanation for the greatly increased renal clearance of citrate induced by metabolic alkalosis [155]. In kinetic studies of renal cortical mitochondria, Robinson and his coworkers [159] demonstrated that the concentration of

HCO$_3^-$ in the suspending media regulates not only the rate of citrate efflux from the mitochondrial matrix, but also the activity of pyruvate dehydrogenase. The observed rates of citrate transport in response to bicarbonate were of the same order of magnitude as with other stimulators (L-malate), and the K_m (13.5 mM) determined for HCO$_3^-$ closely approximated its intracellular concentration. On the basis of the results of studies in which specific mitochondrial carriers were individually inhibited, these investigators proposed the following sequence: "Bicarbonate first stimulates phosphate egress from the mitochondria via bicarbonate-phosphate exchange on the phosphate carrier. Phosphate exchanges for malate on the dicarboxylate carrier and the malate then exchanges for citrate on the tricarboxylate carrier." They further proposed that "bicarbonate stimulation of citrate transport, by lowering intramitochondrial citrate concentrations, relieves the constraint placed on the activity of both citrate synthase and pyruvate dehydrogenase by intramitochondrial citrate." One can formulate a genetic defect of the HCO$_3$/PO$_4$ mitochondrial carrier (or of the dicarboxylate or tricarboxylate carriers) such that its K_m for HCO$_3^-$ (or for PO$_4$ or malate) is substantially increased. If, as a consequence, mitochondrial HCO$_3$PO$_4$ exchange in the distal nephron were greatly retarded at normal concentrations of HCO$_3^-$ in the plasma, there could result not only a reduction in the renal production and excretion of citrate, but also an impairment in renal acidification that might be pathogenically linked either to an impairment in mitochondrial pyruvate oxidation or to an increased HCO$_3^-$ concentration in the cytoplasm of the renal tubule cell (Table 84-3).

The genetic defect formulated predicts that the hypocitraturia of RTA-1 could be only *relatively* "alkali resistant." In fact, in a number of patients with genetically transmitted RTA-1 who belonged to a kindred in which the disorder occurred as an autosomal dominant trait, Gyory demonstrated that the urinary excretion of citrate varied directly and linearly with the plasma bicarbonate concentration over a broad range of values including those greatly increased and acutely attained by loading with sodium bicarbonate [50]. Similarly, in patients with apparently genetically transmitted RTA-1, Norman observed that urinary excretion of citrate varied directly with the amount of alkali therapy administered, but increased into the normal range only with an amount twice that found necessary to correct acidosis [56]. Although the data reported by Dedmond and Wrong indicate that alkali therapy only modestly mitigated the hypocitraturia of their patients with RTA-1, the amount of alkali administered was not reported. Whatever its mechanism, hypocitraturia (and reduced renal content of citrate) could be critical to the pathogenesis of nephrocalcinosis and nephrolithiasis [149, 151] that are characteristic of RTA-1, irrespective of whether it is an acquired or a genetic trait. Citrate forms a soluble complex with calcium [160] that could act to prevent the precipitation of calcium in the urinary tract as either calcium phosphate or calcium oxalate [161].

Pathophysiology, Metabolic Derangement, and the Effect of Alkali Therapy (Figs. 84-4 to 84-7)

Calcium and Phosphorus   Hypercalciuria and increased renal clearance of phosphate predictably occur during metabolic acidosis [1, 162, 163]. It is not clear whether the magnitude of either phenomenon is abnormally great in untreated

patients with RTA-1. Medullary nephrocalcinosis and recurrent nephrolithiasis are characteristic and presumably a consequence both of prolonged hypercalciuria [1, 2] and of diminished urinary excretion of citrate (see above) [151, 161, 164]. Calcium phosphate is the major constituent of urinary stones in patients with RTA-1. Hypocalcemia, which may be a consequence of both hypercalciuria and impaired gut absorption of calcium [1, 2, 165], and hypophosphatemia are presumably causally related to the rickets and osteomalacia that can occur [1, 4]. Chronic metabolic acidosis promotes mobilization of skeletal calcium [163] and may inhibit the uniquely renal conversion of 25-OH vitamin D$_3$ to 1,25(OH)$_2$ vitamin D$_3$ [166], the biologically most active metabolite of vitamin D$_3$ with respect to intestinal absorption of calcium, bone resorption, and the healing of rickets [167–170]. It is at present not clear, however, whether chronic, stable metabolic acidosis of mild to moderate severity is attended by an abnormality of vitamin D metabolism that causes physiologically important disturbances of calcium and phosphate metabolism [171, 172]. The combination of nephrocalcinosis and rickets or osteomalacia is nearly specific for RTA-1 when hypervitaminosis D is excluded by the patient's history [173]. In untreated patients with RTA-1 the plasma concentration of parathyroid hormone may be increased, a phenomenon that might be causally related to hypercalciuria as well as to hypocalcemia [174, 175].

With sustained correction of acidosis, hypercalciuria disappears [1, 16], citrate excretion can increase [56, 152, 154], gut absorption of calcium increases [1, 165], the renal clearance of phosphate decreases, and the serum concentrations of both phosphate and calcium become normal [1]. Nephrocalcinosis and nephrolithiasis persist, but stones may be passed less frequently [52, 176]. Rickets and osteomalacia can heal with alkali therapy alone [177, 178], but administration of both alkali and vitamin D would seem prudent in patients with RTA-1 in whom osteomalacia is severe.

In those patients in whom RTA-1 appears to be a late consequence of renal damage caused by genetically determined hypercalciuria and consequent nephrocalcinosis [75, 76], it remains to be determined what effect alkali therapy has had on the magnitude of hypercalciuria, urinary excretion of citrate, or the frequency of stone passage. In one genetically affected boy (hypercalciuria without RTA-1) [75], bilateral nephrocalcinosis became radiographically demonstrable within 4 years of starting alkali therapy.

Growth and Nephrocalcinosis of Children   In infants and young children with untreated RTA-1, impaired growth is characteristic, but normal growth is predictably attained and maintained when correction of acidosis is sustained with alkali therapy, even if frank stunting has occurred [16]. In stunted infants with RTA-1, the velocity of growth predictably increases strikingly within weeks of initiating alkali therapy, and within 3 to 6 months normal stature is predictably attained [16]. Older children may require several years to attain normal height. Renal bicarbonate wasting tends to occur or increase in severity when growth velocity increases sharply. When greatly increased rates of somatic growth are sustained, the external balances of calcium and phosphorus, as well as of sodium and potassium, must perforce become strongly positive. In short and uremic children with renal osteodystrophy, a condition characterized by reduced circulating amounts of 1,25-OH vitamin D$_3$, therapeutic administration of 1,25-(OH)$_2$ vitamin D$_3$ can induce increased rates of

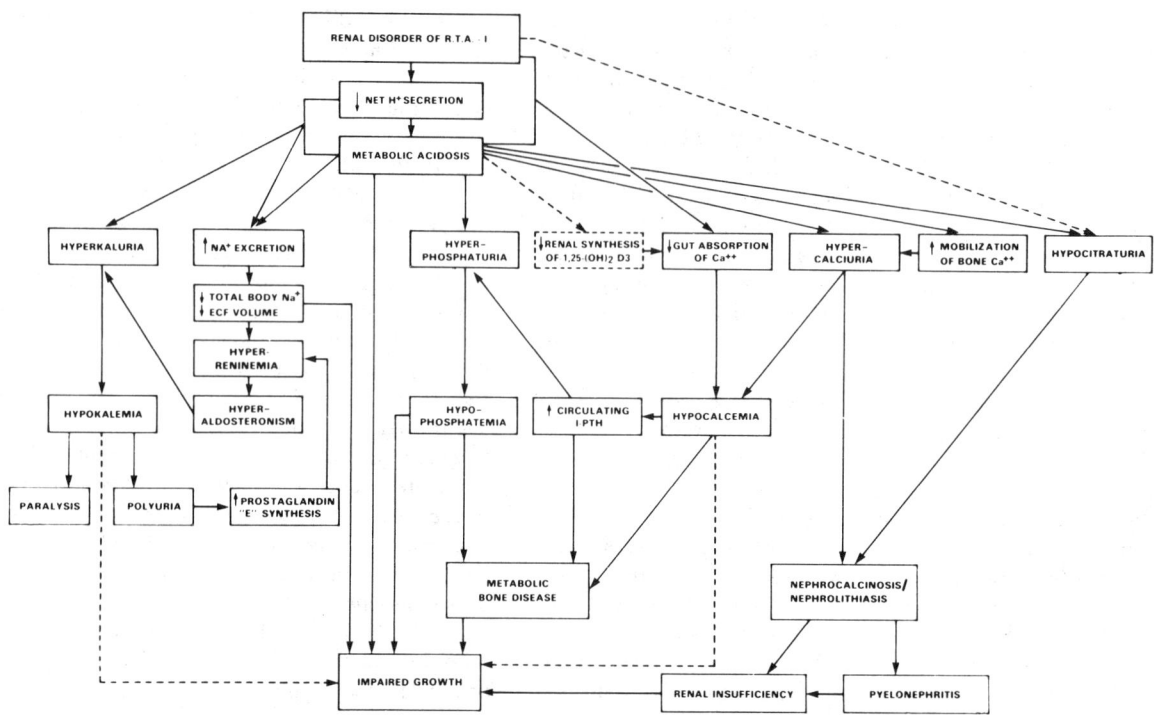

Figure 84-4 Pathogenetic basis of the metabolic and clinical expressions that can occur in patients with type 1 RTA.

growth (as well as healing of rickets) [179]. In short children with RTA-1, alkali induced normalization of growth might depend on a normalization of the metabolism of vitamin D. When initiated before the age of 3 years, alkali therapy sufficient to sustain correction of acidosis (4 mg/kg per day) can prevent nephrocalcinosis [154], possibly by preventing the hypercalciuria and hypocitraturia that are otherwise predictable without alkali therapy [16, 56, 154, 174, 176]. Accordingly, in many and perhaps most children with RTA-1 both impaired growth and nephrocalcinosis can be regarded as preventable.

Potassium and Sodium   Hypokalemia, renal potassium wasting, renal sodium wasting, and secondary hyperaldosteronism are common complications of both RTA-1 and RTA-2 [2, 6–9, 12–15, 81, 180–184]. Renal wasting of potassium can be said to occur when urinary excretion of potassium exceeds 40 meq/day despite hypokalemia (and in the absence of more than moderate metabolic alkalosis) [183] (Fig. 84-5). In patients with RTA-1, but not in patients with RTA-2, correction of acidosis with alkali therapy is predictably attended by a reduction in the urinary excretion rate of potassium, sodium, and aldosterone (Figs. 84-4 to 84-7); with sustained correction of acidosis, the external balances of potassium and sodium may become sufficiently positive to correct hypokalemia and sodium depletion [182]. In most patients with RTA-1, potassium supplements are not required to maintain normokalemia when correction of acidosis is sustained with alkali therapy.

These observations provide the basis for the inference that renal wasting of potassium and sodium in RTA-1 is a consequence of the renal acidification defect and not the consequence of independent abnormalities in renal conservation of sodium and potassium [2, 182]. According to the conventional formulation of the pathogenetic mechanism, the gradient restriction of renal H^+ secretion reduces the rate of renal H^+-Na^+ exchange, which in turn results in a "reciprocal" increase

in renal K^+-Na^+ exchange and urinary loss. Sodium depletion leads to secondary hyperaldosteronism [182]. With correction of acidosis, the attendant increase in intraluminal pH (reflected by the increase in urinary pH) is presumed to remove the inferred gradient restriction on renal H^+ secretion. As a consequence, the rate of H^+-Na^+ exchange increases, the rate of K^+-Na^+ exchange decreases reciprocally, and the urinary excretion rates of sodium and potassium decrease. Correction of sodium depletion would lessen the stimulus to hyperaldosteronism [2, 182].

The observation in patients with RTA-1 that urinary sodium and potassium excretions decrease when acidosis is corrected [81, 182, 183] does not necessarily mean that renal wasting of these cations is a correctable consequence of the acidification defect only. In five of nine patients with RTA-1 studied during sustained correction of acidosis with potassium bicarbonate, a persistent impairment in renal conservation of sodium was observed when dietary intake of sodium was restricted [184] despite values of urinary pH near or greater than those of arterial blood, i.e., no apparent gradient restriction on H^+ secretion. Moreover, in some patients with RTA-1, frank renal potassium wasting persists, in association with persisting hyperaldosteronism, despite sustained correction of acidosis with alkali therapy and the provision of a normal or even supernormal amount of dietary sodium [183]. These disturbances occur unassociated with hypertension and hence are those characteristic of *Bartter's syndrome*, except for the absence of metabolic alkalosis. Such a Bartter's-type syndrome may dominate the clinical picture in patients with RTA-1 [107, 185, 186], particularly in children [185, 186]. In a child with RTA-1 and features of Bartter's syndrome, Rodriquez-Soriano found that the severity of both the renal wasting of potassium and the acidification defect were greatly attenuated by chronic administration of indomethacin, a drug that inhibits prostaglandin synthesis and thereby mitigates hyperreninemia and hyperaldosteronism [185]. As judged from the dramatic attenuation of renal wasting of potassium achieved with indomethacin in two children with a nonacidotic renal disorder that may initially have been expressed as RTA-1 [186], chronically increased renal synthesis of prostaglandin could be an important pathogenic determinant in the evolution of RTA-1 to a renal disorder in children that does not cause acidosis [186].

Genetics of RTA-1

Primary RTA-1 can occur as an autosomal dominant trait that is fully expressed as an unremitting acidosis-causing renal acidification defect in the first months of life [16, 45, 46]. The genetic defect, which apparently can be intrinsic to the kidney [54], can give rise to nephrocalcinosis but does not necessarily compel its occurrence [154] or that of the two phenomena presumably most critical to its pathogenesis, hypercalciuria and hypocitraturia (Table 84-4, Fig. 84-8a, San Francisco syndrome). In all seven affected members of generations I, II, and III of the kindred studied in San Francisco [16, 44–46, 154], and in the one affected member of generation IV who received low-dose alkali therapy (1 to 3 meq/kg per day), nephrocalcinosis was radiographically demonstrable when first sought as early as 5 years of age, even though such alkali therapy had been started as early as 2½ years of age. But, in the four affected members of generation IV [16], and in three other related children with familial, apparently autosomal dominant RTA, in whom high-dose alkali therapy (4 to 12 meq/kg per day) was initiated before 4 years of age [154], neither radiographically demonstrable nephrocalcinosis nor nephrolithiasis has oc-

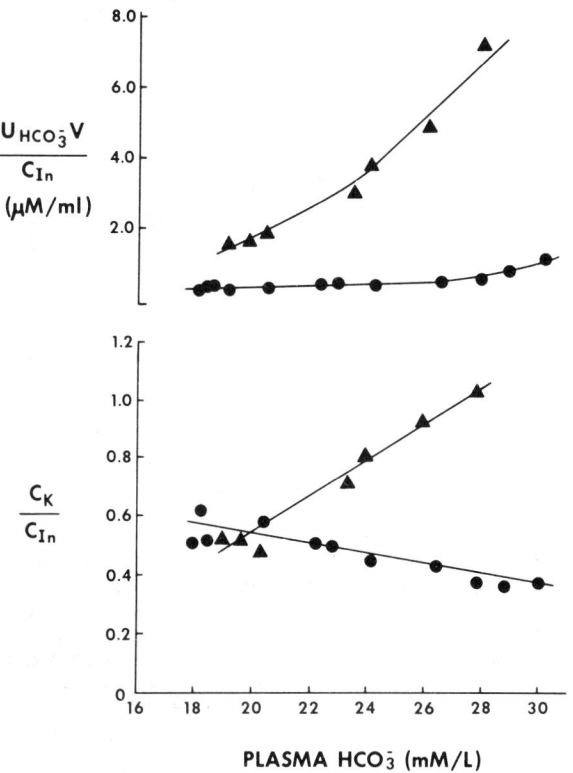

Figure 84-6 Effect of an acute, progressive increase in plasma bicarbonate concentration (intravenous administration of sodium bicarbonate) on the fraction of the filtered load of potassium excreted in the urine (C_K/C_{in}) and on the urinary excretion of bicarbonate ($U_{HCO_3}V/C_{in}$) in a patient with type 1 RTA (circles) and in a patient with type 2 RTA (triangles).

Figure 84-5 Relationship between urinary potassium excretion and serum potassium concentration in patients with RTA in whom correction of acidosis was sustained (◆, ●, ▲, ■) and in normal subjects experimentally depleted of potassium by dietary restriction (O,+,×). Some of the subjects represented by O were mildly alkalotic and were excreting significant amounts of urinary bicarbonate; the subjects represented by + were moderately alkalotic and were excreting more than 50 meq of urinary bicarbonate daily; the subjects represented by X were given large amounts of deoxycorticosterone after hypokalemia had supervened.

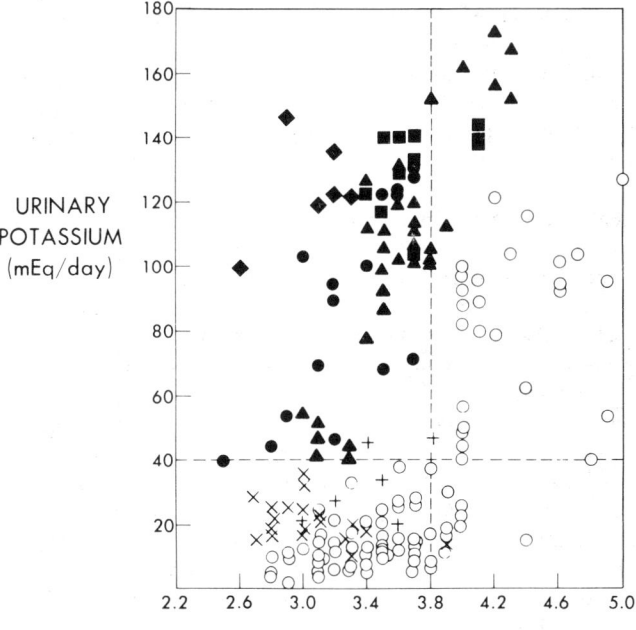

curred over treatment periods ranging from 10 to 20 years, and the glomerular filtration rate has remained normal. In these patients, and in other similarly treated children in whom autosomal dominant, acidosis-causing RTA-1 has been fully expressed in early childhood without radiographically demonstrable nephrocalcinosis or reduction in GFR, hypercalciuria and an otherwise invariable hypocitraturia have been invariably corrected by high-dose alkali therapy [154].

In proposing that a given genotype of RTA-1 could be variably expressed with respect to the severity of dysfunction of renal acidification, Buckalew correctly predicted that the genetically transmitted trait of RTA-1 would occur unaccompanied by frank acidosis in some affected members of some kindreds [92]. Wrong and Davies had earlier introduced the term *incomplete syndrome of RTA* (iRTA) to describe three nonacidotic patients with bilateral nephrocalcinosis who, like patients with the *complete syndrome of RTA* (cRTA-1), failed to decrease urinary pH to normal minima and to increase urinary excretion of titratable acid to normal maxima when they were challenged with NH₄Cl [7]. Wrong and others have proposed that the renal disorder of those with iRTA-1 is a "milder" form of the acidosis-causing renal disorder of patients with cRTA-1, the major difference being that in patients with iRTA-1, functional renal mass and glomerular filtration rate are relatively well-maintained and, as a consequence, excretion of NH₄ is great enough to prevent frank acidosis [7, 164]. This formulation does not always explain why acidosis occurs in some patients with hereditary RTA-1 and not in others. In one nonacidotic child with apparently autosomal dominant RTA-1, the rates of urinary excretion of both ammonium and net acid excretion induced by NH₄Cl were clearly subnormal,

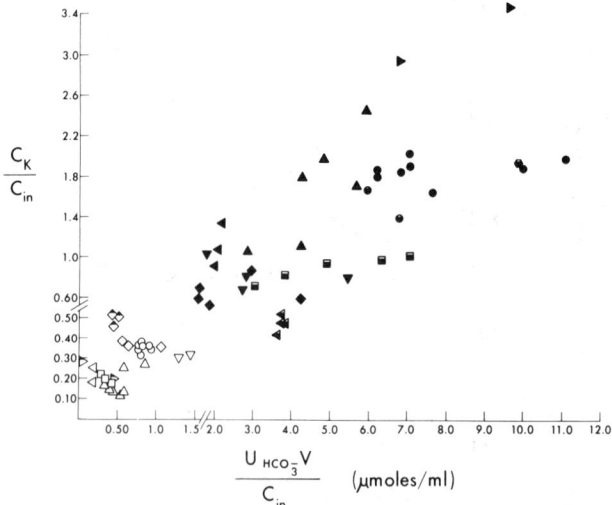

Figure 84-7 Relationship between fractional excretion of filtered potassium (C_K/C_{in}) and urinary excretion of bicarbonate ($U_{HCO_3}V/C_{in}$) in patients with type 2 RTA associated with Fanconi syndrome (closed and three-quarter-closed symbols) in whom plasma bicarbonate concentration was maintained at normal levels [22 to 26 mol/liter for more than 2 months (closed and open symbols)] or was rapidly increased to normal levels (intravenous administration of sodium bicarbonate) (three-quarters-open symbols). Each geometric symbol represents measurements made in a single patient.

whereas in both affected acidotic sibs, the NH_4Cl-induced rates of ammonium excretion were not subnormal; in the sib with the lowest value of plasma bicarbonate before NH_4Cl challenge, the induced rate of net acid excretion was not subnormal [53]. Although bilateral medullary nephrocalcinosis was radiographically demonstrable in one of the acidotic sibs, the glomerular filtration rate was normal in all three, as it has been in acidotic children with autosomal dominant RTA from at least two other affected kindreds, including the San Francisco kindred [16]. In the affected children from these two kindreds, the magnitude of bicarbonate excreted at normal and reduced plasma bicarbonate concentrations was the major determinant of the occurrence and severity of the acidosis.

But in one genotype of RTA-1, iRTA may be the trait initially expressed and may progress to cRTA only when nephrocalcinosis occurs and further restricts the excretion of acid (Table 84-4, Fig. 84-8b, Philadelphia syndrome). In a woman with autosomal dominant RTA-1 in whom Norman and his coworkers documented that cRTA occurred at age 24 in association with radiographically demonstrable nephrocalcinosis and a moderate reduction in GFR, iRTA-1 is reported to have occurred at age 15 without such nephrocalcinosis [56]. cRTA-1 in association with nephrocalcinosis was documented in each of her three affected relatives, father, one sib, and one child [56]. Even though cRTA-1 may have preceded nephrocalcinosis in all members of this kindred, the reported progression of iRTA-1 to cRTA-1 in the affected woman suggests the possibility that an acidosis-causing renal tubular disorder is not a primary expression of the underlying genotype. Of particular interest in this regard are two unrelated 5-year-old girls diagnosed as having iRTA-1 by Norman and his coworkers [56]. Radiographically demonstrable nephrocalcinosis was not present in either girl but occurred in association with cRTA in the mother and aunt of one of the girls and in the father of the other, these three relatives comprising all those found to be affected. In the two girls diagnosed as having iRTA-1, the impairment in renal acidification response to NH_4Cl loading

was clear-cut but much less severe than that in their affected relatives [56].

As described in other patients with hereditary RTA-1, strikingly severe hypocitraturia occurred in all five affected members of these two kindreds and in all four affected members of the kindred that included the woman in whom iRTA progressed to cRTA. In both affected boys in this kindred, in one affected man, and in one of the two girls with iRTA, correction of the hypocitraturia was attained with alkali therapy, although the amount required, 4 meq/kg per day, was twice that said to be required to correct acidosis and hypercalciuria. In the other girl with iRTA, even such high-dose alkali therapy only slightly mitigated the hypocitraturia [56]. Because it seemed likely that cRTA and nephrocalcinosis would occur in both girls with iRTA if they were not treated, and because such progression might depend on continued hypocitraturia that could be mitigated by high-dose alkali therapy, Norman elected to treat both girls with such alkali therapy [56].

In three children with hereditary RTA-1 in whom nephrocalcinosis was radiographically nondemonstrable and in whom acidosis was of quite minimal severity, Coe also found that alkali therapy in amounts that raised plasma bicarbonate concentration to values well within the normal range had little effect on the strikingly severe hypocitraturia but did correct the hypercalciuria and appeared to reduce the frequency of nephrolithiasis [176]. In a nonazotemic 24-year-old man with RTA-1 in whom the combination of nephrocalcinosis, nephrolithiasis, hypercalciuria (on a low calcium diet), and severe hypocitraturia occurred initially in the absence of acidosis, Buckalew and his coworkers described the occurrence over a 1-year period of progressively severe acidosis in association with repeated episodes of renal calculi [92]. Nephrocalcinosis was radiographically demonstrated in the patient's older brother who probably had RTA-1 [92]. Their father had suffered from recurrent renal calculi. Apart from their obvious therapeutic implications, the observations of Norman, Coe, and Buckalew raise the important possibility that in one (or more) genotype(s) of RTA-1, hypocitraturia and hypercalciuria may be not only primary metabolic manifestations but also critical metabolic events in the pathogenesis of nephrocalcinosis and nephrolithiasis and thereby of progression of iRTA to cRTA (Fig. 84-8b).

Buckalew and his coworkers have recently studied a 64-member kindred comprising four successive generations in which hypercalciuria appears to be the primary metabolic manifestation of an autosomal dominant genetic defect (Table 84-4, Fig. 84-8c, Atlanta syndrome) [75]. Radiographic nephrocalcinosis was demonstrated in six affected members from three successive generations, including two children. Four of the six were diagnosed as having RTA-1 on the basis of their urinary pH not decreasing to normal minima after NH_4Cl challenge. In the one affected acidotic patient, a 33-year-old man, the GFR was 6 ml/min and the serum creatinine concentration was 7 mg/dl. Buckalew proposed that the sequence, hypercalciuria—nephrocalcinosis—renal damage was critical to the pathogenesis of the observed impairments in renal acidification. But in two kindred members affected with nephrocalcinosis (and hypercalciuria), an impairment in renal acidification was demonstrably absent. This phenomenon, nephrocalcinosis without impaired renal acidification, appears not to have been documented in other kindreds in which a renal disorder diagnosed as RTA-1 has affected more than one member. In those affected members in whom hypercalciuria

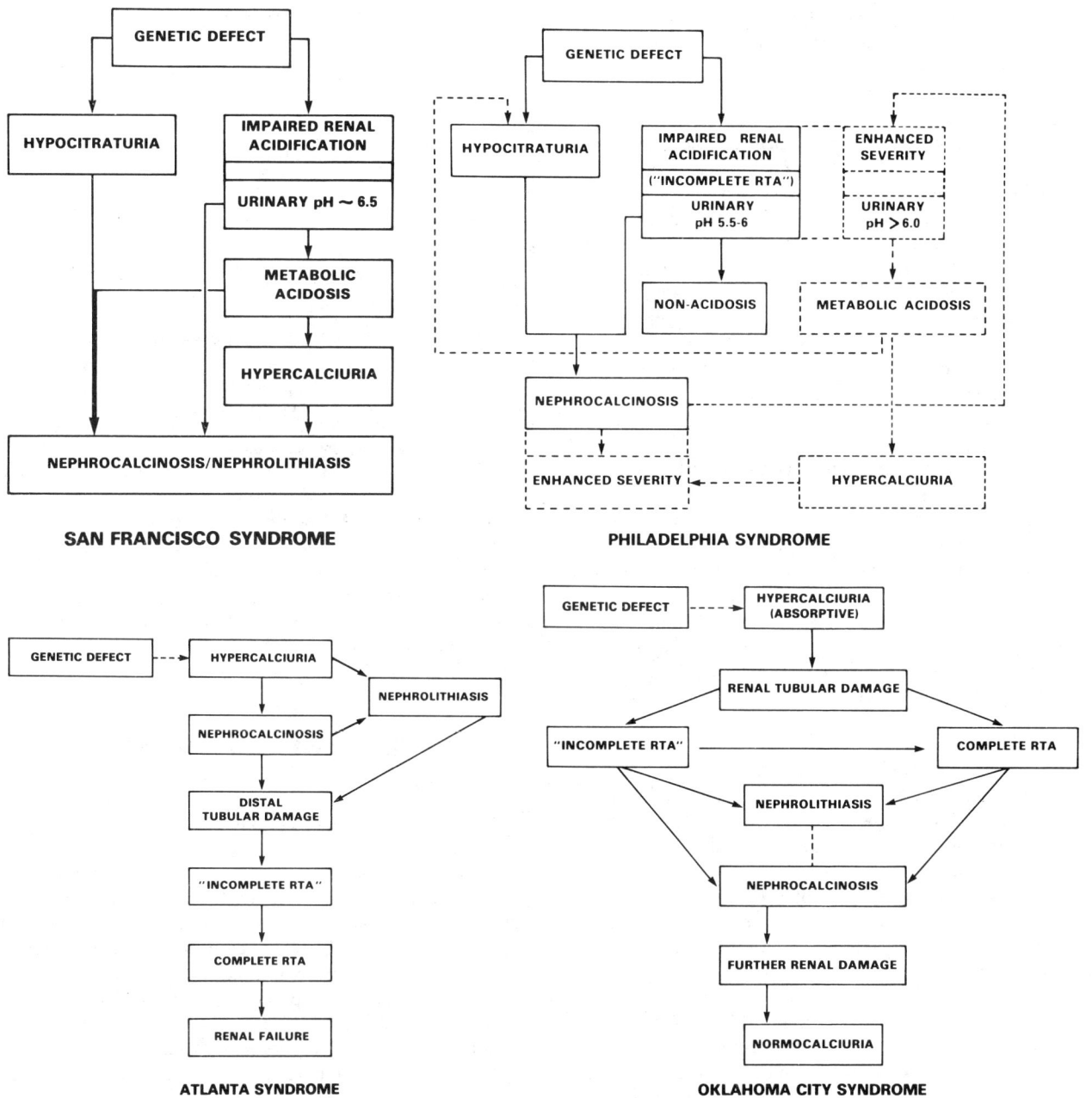

Figure 84-8 Proposed pathogenetic sequence through which genetic defects are pathogenetically linked to impaired renal acidification, nephrocalcinosis, and hypercalciuria (and in two sequences, hypocitraturia) in patients in whom either RTA-1 or hypercalciuria occurs as an autosomal dominant trait. RTA-1 is qualified as *incomplete RTA* (iRTA-1) when the impairment in renal acidification does not give rise to acidosis and *complete RTA-1* (cRTA-1) when it does. As depicted, the physiologic and metabolic consequences of *primary* pathogenetic sequence (uninterrupted line) can be critically enhanced by those of a secondary sequence (interrupted line) whose form is that of a positive feedback "loop." The sequences depicted give rise to clinical syndromes that are separable from each other but variable (and sometimes similar) in physiologic and metabolic expression, depending on the age of those affected and, in at least two of the syndromes (San Francisco and Philadelphia), the likely mitigating effect of alkali therapy on hypercalciuria and hypocitraturia and in one syndrome (Philadelphia), thereby, on the apparently nephrocalcinosis-mediated progression of iRTA-1 to cRTA. The syndromes are named after the city in which they were principally investigated.

was most severe in this kindred studied by Buckalew, there also occurred hyperaminoaciduria, lysozymuria, and immunoglobulin L chainuria, phenomena which implicate the proximal

tubule and rarely accompany RTA-1. The renal disorder of this kindred would thus appear to be unique in the literature.

Hamed and his coworkers have also studied a large kindred in which hypercalciuria appears to occur as an autosomal dominant trait in four successive generations (Table 84-4, Fig. 84-8d, Oklahoma City syndrome) [76]. In this kindred, RTA-1 was diagnosed in eight members of the generations I, II, and III, only in those with hypercalciuria and in none of the 14 children studied (generation IV), including three with hypercalciuria. Nephrocalcinosis was radiographically demonstrated only in the five of seven members of generations I and II in whom RTA-1 was diagnosed. cRTA was diagnosed in four members from generations I and II and in a 17-year-old girl from generation III in whom the GFR was normal. iRTA was diagnosed in three members including two from generation III and a 50-year-old woman from generation II. In those affected in this kindred, Hamed proposed that over time hypercalciuria (which might reflect intestinal hyperabsorption) could damage the renal tubule, impair acidification, and thereby further the pathogenesis of nephrocalcinosis.

In the large kindred recently studied by Buckalew, the relative resistance of the renal acidification process to the potentially disordering effect of nephrocalcinosis may reflect the lack of prior disorder in those nephronal segments affected. It is apparent that the pathogenetic consequences of nephrocalcinosis could depend critically on whether, how, and to what extent the nephronal segments affected were disordered already. A prior disordering might result from a genetic defect either of some component of the renal tubule per se, or of some component of those processes that regulate the synthesis and metabolism of humoral substances that in turn regulate the metabolism of calcium and phosphate by the kidney and gut, e.g., metabolites of vitamin D_3 [168].

Clinical Management of Patients with RTA-1

In patients with previously undiagnosed RTA, hypokalemia, severe acidosis, and hypocalcemia often coexist and may require immediate therapeutic response. Hyperkalemia-mediated respiratory depression and muscle weakness may be life threatening and necessitate hospitalization and careful monitoring of ventilatory rate and depth, as well as facilities for airway maintenance and assisted ventilation. As described above, hypokalemia should be corrected rapidly with intravenously administered potassium—*before* correction of acidosis [2, 17, 18].

Almost all children and infants are able to take $NaHCO_3$ in the amounts necessary to sustain correction of acidosis, even when these amounts are as great as 14 meq/kg per day. In most children with RTA-1, the amount of alkali required will increase, usually when the rate of growth increases sharply. If dietary NaCl is restricted because of a sodium-retaining state, the amount of alkali necessary to correct acidosis is decreased. In some patients, particularly those with autoimmune RTA, potassium supplements of 50 to 100 meq/day may be required to maintain normokalemia even after acidosis has been corrected. One of the frequent complications (and conceivably a cause) of RTA-1 is pyelonephritis, the optimal treatment of which has yet to be determined. Attempted eradication of the causal organism is rarely, if ever, successful and may be unrealistic, particularly in patients with nephrocalcinosis.

Prognosis

The prognosis of most well-managed adult patients with RTA-1 is determined more by the usually accompanying autoimmune disease, Sjögren's syndrome, or chronic liver disorder than by either the functional consequences of the renal disease or its complications, pyelonephritis, nephrocalcinosis, and nephrolithiasis. Morbidity, generally considered to be causally related to the autoimmune state per se, such as Raynaud's phenomenon, recurrent purpura, and even the dry mouth of Sjögren's syndrome, may disappear with alkali therapy. In the great majority of well-managed adult patients with RTA-1, the GFR and the severity of the acidification defect remain unchanged even when the GFR is reduced substantially when alkali therapy is started and despite continuing bacteriologic evidence of chronic pyelonephritis (Fig. 84-9) [187]. For many

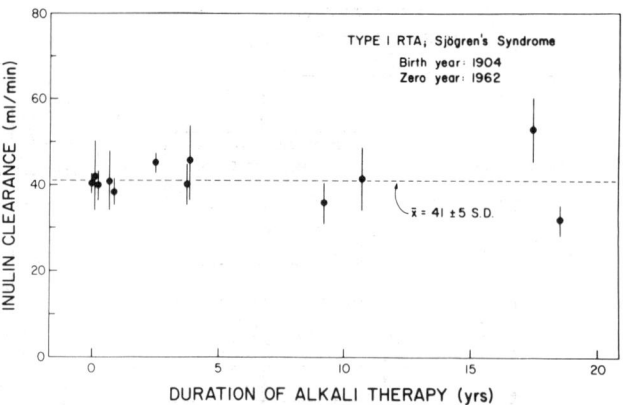

Figure 84-9 Values of renal clearance of inulin throughout a 19-year period in a woman with type 1 RTA, nephrocalcinosis, Sjögren's syndrome, chronic bacteriuria, and recurrent pyelonephritis. The patient was maintained in a nonacidotic and normokalemic state throughout by an unchanging dose of alkali and supplemental potassium.

patients in whom RTA-1 occurs as part of Sjögren's syndrome, life is long and vigorous. In patients in whom RTA-1 occurs as an autosomal dominant trait that is not primarily expressed as hypercalciuria (Table 84-4) (Fig. 84-8c and d) [75, 76], the prognosis is good with continued corrective alkali therapy [187].

TYPE 2 RTA ("PROXIMAL")

Physiologic Characteristics

In patients with *type 2 RTA* (RTA-2) (Table 84-5) (Figs. 84-2, 84-3, 84-5 to 84-7, and 84-10, and 84-11), the identifying observation that tubular reabsorption of bicarbonate ($THCO_3^-$) is reduced by at least 15 percent, at normal plasma bicarbonate concentrations and under normal physiologic conditions, implicates the acidification process of the proximal tubule [11, 13–18]. In prototypic RTA-2, the urine pH is inappropriately high and bicarbonaturia occurs only during moderate or mild degrees of acidosis, the magnitude of bicarbonaturia varying directly with the plasma bicarbonate concentration. During more severe degrees of acidosis, bicarbonaturia disappears, urinary pH decreases to normal minima, and acid excretion is not reduced, suggesting that the acidification process of the distal-most nephron is intact [10–18] (Figs. 84-2, 84-3, 84-6, and 84-10). The physiologic characteristics of RTA-2 are those predicted by the formulation of Worthen and Good [188] and were first demonstrated by Lamy et al. in a child with Fanconi syndrome as part of Lowe's syndrome [189]. RTA-2 almost always occurs as part of a more complex dysfunction of the proximal tubule and is apparently always that type of RTA associated with the Fanconi syndrome [10–13, 190–219] (Table 84-5).

In some patients with a greater than 15-percent reduction in $THCO_3^-$ at normal plasma bicarbonate concentrations, the acidification process of the distal nephron also appears to be impaired; over a broad range of reduced plasma bicarbonate concentrations, $THCO_3^-$ is just less than complete and urinary pH remains inappropriately high. Such findings would appear to reflect a hybrid of RTA-1 and RTA-2 [13, 15, 17, 180].

As in children with bicarbonate wasting RTA-1 [14], in patients with RTA-2 the amount of alkali required to sustain the correction of acidosis is determined principally by the magnitude of bicarbonate wasting at normal plasma bicarbonate concentrations.

Mechanism and Pathogenesis

The subcellular mechanisms of the transport impairment of RTA-2 have not been defined, with the exception of the state of carbonic anhydrase inhibition, in which RTA-2 occurs unassociated with Fanconi syndrome [229, 230]. The occurrence of RTA-2 and the Fanconi syndrome in genetically transmitted disorders of metabolism raises the possibility that in some cases the metabolic production of energy required for active transport may be impaired.

In adult patients, RTA-2 occurs most commonly in the clinical setting of intestinal malabsorption that gives rise to vitamin D deficiency, hypocalcemia, secondary hyperparathyroidism, and hypophosphatemia [180, 200, 202]. RTA-2 also occurs in children with dietary deficiency of vitamin D [199, 201]. In both circumstances, vitamin D therapy corrects the acidification dysfunction and the usually accompanying complex renal tubular dysfunction like that of the Fanconi syndrome. Although circulating parathyroid hormone (PTH) can dampen the normal renal acidification process in humans [234], and primary hyperparathyroidism can *lead to* RTA-2 that persists after surgical correction of hyperparathyroidism [235], it seems unlikely that RTA-2 is caused by the physiologic effect of increased levels of circulating PTH alone [180, 236]. In the rat studied at normal plasma bicarbonate concentrations, systemically administered PTH induces a substantial reduction of bicarbonate reabsorption in the proximal tubule, but bicarbonaturia does not occur, and net acid excretion is not decreased [237]. In the dog and in humans studied at normal plasma bicarbonate concentrations [234, 238–240], experimentally administered PTH induces a reduction in net acid excretion and the occurrence of bicarbonaturia, but the amount of bicarbonate excreted is a trivial fraction of that filtered by the glomerulus. And, when plasma bicarbonate concentration is only minimally decreased (with ammonium chloride), experimentally administered PTH does not induce either bicarbonaturia or a reduction in net acid excretion [234, 240]. Accordingly, one would expect that a disorder of renal acidification caused by PTH alone would not give rise to frank metabolic acidosis, but rather to a slight decrease in plasma bicarbonate concentration. Indeed, a reversible impairment in renal acidification severe enough to cause frank acidosis has been demonstrated in nonazotemic patients with hyperparathyroidism only when the hyperparathyroidism was secondary to hypocalcemia and associated with both vitamin D deficiency and hypophosphatemia. In the otherwise intact dog, prolonged severe hypophosphatemia may be attended by a modest reduction in $THCO_3^-$, at normal plasma bicarbonate concentrations, and a slight decrease in plasma bicarbonate concentration [241]. Emmett and his coworkers reported that in rats rendered chronically hypophosphatemic, a reduction in $THCO_3^-$ gave rise to frank metabolic acidosis only when an otherwise countervailing release of bone buffers (which presumably *required* PTH) [242, 243] was prevented by the administration of colchicine [244]. To the extent that vitamin D–deficient bones are unable to release buffer salts either

because of their depletion of these salts, or because of the extant reduction in the circulating amount of $1,25\text{-}(OH)_2D_3$, the potential for a modest reduction of $THCO_3^-$ to cause acidosis presumably would be enhanced.

Pathophysiology

Potassium, Sodium, and Water In contrast to patients with RTA-1, in patients with RTA-2 renal potassium wasting and polyuria either occur or become more severe when correction of acidosis is sustained with alkali therapy alone [181] (Figs. 84-6 and 84-7). Because the capacity of the proximal tubule to reabsorb bicarbonate is greatly reduced, the distal nephron is swamped with bicarbonate when the plasma bicarbonate concentration is increased from subnormal to normal levels with alkali therapy [181] (Fig. 84-10). Furthermore, expanding an otherwise contracted extracellular fluid volume (ECV) has the effect of further reducing proximal reabsorption of Na^+, HCO_3^-, and Cl^- [245, 246]. In the presence of a continued stimulus for sodium reabsorption in the distal nephron (e.g., hyperaldosteronism), the delivery of greatly supernormal amounts of sodium, bicarbonate, and chloride out of the proximal nephron would be expected to augment net

Figure 84-10 Schematic representation of the proximal renal acidification defect in type 2 RTA. Effect of changes in plasma bicarbonate concentration on delivery of bicarbonate to the distal nephron and, as a consequence, on urinary pH and excretion of bicarbonate. (*a*) In normal subjects, at normal plasma bicarbonate concentrations, approximately 15 percent of the filtered HCO_3 load escapes reabsorption in the proximal tubule and is reabsorbed in the distal nephron; urinary bicarbonate excretion is nil, urinary pH is appropriately low, and net acid excretion is normal. (*b*) In patients with type 2 RTA, bicarbonate excretion may also be nil, urinary pH may be appropriately low, and net acid excretion may not be reduced at reduced plasma bicarbonate concentration (metabolic acidosis). This is because the amount of HCO_3 escaping reabsorption proximally and delivered to the distal nephron is not supernormal when the amount of bicarbonate presented to the proximal tubule for reabsorption is sufficiently reduced. (*c*) When, however, metabolic acidosis is somewhat mitigated (by administration of $NaHCO_3$), supernormal amounts of bicarbonate are delivered out of the proximal tubule because the defective proximal tubule cannot reabsorb the modest increase in filtered load of bicarbonate. As a consequence, some bicarbonate escapes reabsorption in the distal nephron, urinary pH becomes inappropriately high, and net acid excretion becomes reduced. (*d*) If the plasma bicarbonate concentration and filtered bicarbonate load are increased to normal levels, the amount of bicarbonate escaping reabsorption proximally greatly exceeds the reabsorptive capacity of the normal distal nephron and massive bicarbonaturia occurs. In the illustration of type 2 RTA, renal tubular reabsorption of bicarbonate ($T_{HCO_3^-}$) at normal plasma bicarbonate concentration (26 mmol/liter) is reduced by 25 percent.

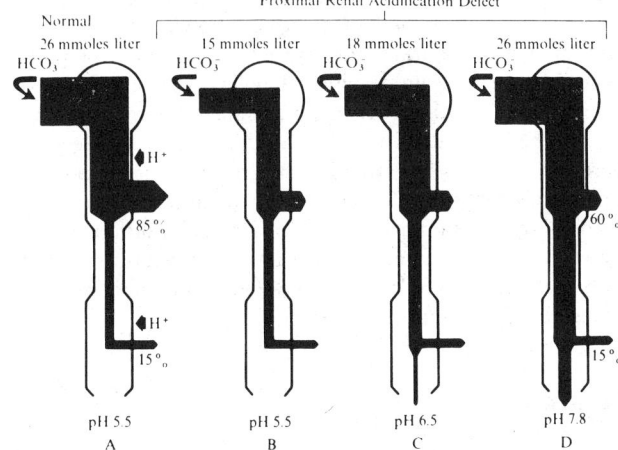

Proximal Renal Acidification Defect

Normal

26 mmoles liter HCO_3^- 15 mmoles liter HCO_3^- 18 mmoles liter HCO_3^- 26 mmoles liter HCO_3^-

85%   60%

15%   15%

pH 5.5   pH 5.5   pH 6.5   pH 7.8

A   B   C   D

Table 84-4 Hereditary autosomally transmitted disorders of the renal tubule expressed as RTA-1 and nephrocalcinosis

Syndrome	Acidification defect (AD)			Nephrocalcinosis (N)		Acidosis	
	Occurs in children	Causes acidosis in children	Causes acidosis with GFR >50 ml/min	Occurs in children	Occurs without AD	Occurs without N	Attends N invariably
1. Dominant							
a. Primary RTA-1							
(1) San Francisco [16,44–46]	+	+	+	+	0	+	+
(2) Philadelphia [9,56]	+	+	+	+	0	0	+
b. Hypercalciuric							
(1) Atlanta [75]	+	0	0	+	+	0	0
(2) Oklahoma City [76]	0	0	+	0	0	+	0
2. Recessive Associated with							
a. Sensorineural deafness	+	+	+	+	0	+	+
b. Deficiency of B isoenzyme of carbonic anhydrase in erythrocytes	+	+	+	+	0	–	–

potassium secretion in the distal nephron [181, 247] and thereby promote renal potassium wasting. During sustained correction of acidosis with alkali therapy, the fraction of the filtered load of potassium excreted frequently exceeds 1.0 (which indicates net renal secretion of potassium) and varies directly with the fractional excretion of filtered bicarbonate [181] (Fig. 84-7). In at least some patients with RTA-2, as in some patients with RTA-1, hyperaldosteronism (and hyperreninemia) persists despite sustained correction of acidosis and the provision of normal or supernormal amounts of dietary sodium [181]. Potassium depletion causes not only an impairment in the renal concentrating function [248, 249] but also thirst and polydipsia as a primary phenomenon [250]. These phenomena, combined with the greatly increased delivery of solute and water out of the proximal tubule, account for what is often strikingly severe polyuria. It is an important clinical point that in patients with RTA-2 (usually as part of the Fanconi syndrome) the urine can be dilute (i.e., hypoosmolar) despite dehydration.

Calcium and Phosphorus In patients diagnosed as having RTA-2, transient [220] and persistent [222], in whom the renal dysfunction of the Fanconi syndrome was absent, hypocalcemia/hypercalciuria and hypophosphatemia/hyperphosphaturia did not occur, despite metabolic acidosis; rickets also did not occur. Furthermore, hypokalemia did not occur either before or during alkali therapy, and potassium supplements were not required. In ways other than the absence of impaired renal reabsorption of glucose, phosphate, and α-amino acids, the renal dysfunction of these patients is clearly different from that of most patients in whom RTA-2 occurs in association with the Fanconi syndrome. (See "Phosphate and Calcium" under "Fanconi Syndrome" below.)

Treatment

The treatment of patients with RTA-2 is directed toward ame-

lioration of their fluid, electrolyte, and acid-base disturbance, and, when possible, correction of the underlying disease process. (Specific treatment of frequently accompanying vitamin D–resistant metabolic bone disease is considered under "Fanconi Syndrome" below.) Sustained correction of acidosis with alkali therapy requires the administration of alkali sufficient to offset the urinary excretion of net base plus the estimated endogenous production of nonvolatile acid, at normal plasma bicarbonate concentrations, net base excretion being essentially equal to bicarbonate excretion. The magnitude of renal bicarbonate excretion at normal plasma bicarbonate concentrations can vary from as little as 2 to 3 meq/kg body weight per day in patients with minimal impairment of proximal bicarbonate reabsorption, or marked reductions in glomerular filtration rate to values greater than 20 meq/kg body weight per day in patients with more marked dysfunction or more nearly normal glomerular filtration rate. The alkali and potassium requirements must then be determined empirically for each patient. When the amount of alkali required to correct acidosis is prohibitively large, hydrochlorothiazide can be a useful therapeutic adjunct [251–253]. This agent may increase proximal bicarbonate reabsorption by inducing contraction of ECV [246, 251–252]; it may, however, increase H^+ secretion directly [254]. With hydrochlorothiazide, the severity of hypokalemia frequently increases. Restriction of dietary NaCl and water may also be useful in reducing the amount of alkali therapy required to correct acidosis, and in reducing the severity of renal potassium wasting and polyuria [246, 255].

TYPE 4 RENAL TUBULAR ACIDOSIS

Metabolic acidosis is commonly associated with hyperkalemia in chronic diseases of the kidney that result in diffuse parenchymal damage and reduced glomerular filtration rate. The severity of acidosis is proportional to the degree of glomerular

(Continued)

	Hypercalciuria		Hypocitraturia
Occurs without acidosis	Corrects with alkali		Corrects with alkali
0	+	+	+
0	+	+	+ and 0
+	−	0	−
+	−	−	−
−	−	−	−
−	−	−	−

insufficiency, whereas hyperkalemia may be absent or of only minimal severity despite even severe glomerular insufficiency. In patients selected because of severe hyperkalemia (serum potassium concentration <5.5 meq/liter), the most common diagnoses of the underlying renal disease are tubulointerstitial nephritis and diabetic nephropathy, and in these patients a characteristic pattern of renal tubular dysfunction has been delineated [128, 256–258]: Renal bicarbonate reabsorption is reduced at normal plasma bicarbonate concentration (sustained by alkali therapy), but the magnitude of the reduction (< 15 percent) is not sufficient to implicate the proximal tubule. The ability of the kidney to establish steep lumen-peritubular H⁺ concentration gradients during spontaneously occurring acidosis is not impaired. But, despite the occurrence of highly acidic urine during metabolic acidosis, net acid excretion remains subnormal. The subnormal excretion reflects in part reduced urinary excretion of ammonium that in part is a consequence of reversibly suppressed renal ammoniagenesis caused by hyperkalemia. Renal ammoniagenesis is impaired even when glomerular filtration rate is reduced only minimally. Renal clearance of potassium is greatly reduced, and the serum concentration of potassium increases strikingly when dietary potassium is increased. Proximal tubular dysfunction does not occur as judged by the absence of hyperaminoaciduria, glycosuria, or increased renal clearance of phosphate. The tubular dysfunction has been designated *type 4 RTA* (RTA-4) (Table 6) [2, 17–20, 128, 324–327].

The physiologic characteristics of RTA-4 are those that would be predicted to occur in patients in whom aldosterone is either deficient in circulating amount of renal physiologic effect. (Table 84-6) [32, 328]. The effect of aldosterone deficiency on the acidification process of the mammalian nephron has been studied in adrenalectomized dogs maintained postoperatively on physiologic replacement doses of glucocorticoid and mineralocorticoid hormones [32]. When the administration of mineralocorticoid hormones is discontinued, net acid excretion decreases, and hyperkalemia and hyperchloremic acidosis occur. The reduction in net acid excretion is accounted

for largely by a reduction in urinary excretion of ammonium, which in turn appears to be due to diminished renal production of ammonia, since it occurs in the absence of an increase in urine pH or a decrease in urine flow. The reduction in ammonia production appears to be due in part to hyperkalemia, since the excretion rate of ammonium varies inversely with the plasma potassium concentration and does not decrease when mineralocorticoid is discontinued if hyperkalemia is prevented from occurring, as by restricting potassium intake.

The results of additional studies in the adrenalectomized dog indicate that aldosterone deficiency impairs the rate-capacity of the distal nephron to secrete H⁺ but does not impair its ability to generate normally steep lumen-to-blood H⁺ concentration gradients. When measured at low luminal buffer concentrations (as when renal production and urine excretion of ammonia are greatly reduced by hyperkalemia), the values of urine pH in mineralocorticoid deficient dogs are not different from those in mineralocorticoid adequate dogs rendered similarly acidotic with exogenous acid (Fig. 84-12). However, when measured at increased luminal buffer concentrations, (as when urine ammonium concentrations and excretion are increased), the urine pH is substantially greater in mineralocorticoid deficient dogs than in mineralocorticoid repleted dogs, a finding indicating that in the former group the H⁺ secretory capacity is blunted. These findings in the dog are consistent with the results of studies in vitro in turtle bladders that indicate that aldosterone deficiency diminishes the conductance of protons through the active transport pathway but not the protonmotive force of the H⁺ secretory pump [117].

In humans, similar studies have been performed in adrenalectomized patients to investigate the renal and systemic acid-base consequences of mineralocorticoid deficiency in the absence of either glucocorticoid deficiency or parenchymal renal disease [238]. Glucocorticoid replacement was provided with dexamethasone, mineralocorticoid replacement with fludrocortisone. Net acid excretion and plasma total CO_2 decreased when mineralocorticoid was discontinued and increased when mineralocorticoid was initiated. The magnitude of the cumulative reduction in net acid excretion correlated with the basal rate of net acid excretion, hence presumably with the basal rate of endogenous acid production. The

Figure 84-11 Relationship between urinary excretion of bicarbonate and plasma bicarbonate concentration during intravenous administration of NaHCO₃ in a patient with type 2 RTA and Fanconi syndrome associated with intestinal malabsorption. Before vitamin D therapy (solid dots) where serum Ca^{2+} was −7.5 mg/dl, 100 $C_{HCO_3^-}/C_{in}$ was 18 percent at arterial plasma [HCO₃] of 23 mmol/ liter; after vitamin D therapy (open dots) where Ca^{2+} was 8.5 mg/dl, 100 $C_{HCO_3^-}/C_{in}$ was 3 percent at arterial plasma [HCO₃] of 23 mmol/liter. Data from normal subjects are represented by the broken line. The shaded area represents the normal range of arterial plasma bicarbonate concentrations.

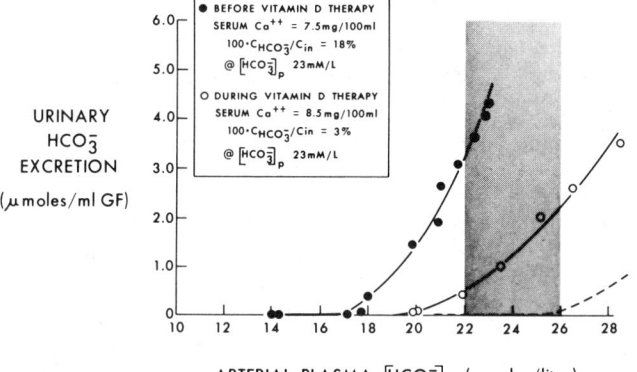

URINARY HCO₃ EXCRETION (μmoles/ml GF)

● BEFORE VITAMIN D THERAPY
SERUM Ca⁺⁺ = 7.5 mg/100ml
100·C_HCO₃/C_in = 18%
@ [HCO₃]_P 23mM/L

○ DURING VITAMIN D THERAPY
SERUM Ca⁺⁺ = 8.5 mg/100ml
100·C_HCO₃/C_in = 3%
@ [HCO₃]_P 23mM/L

ARTERIAL PLASMA [HCO₃] (mmoles/liter)

Table 84-5 Clinical spectrum of type 2 (proximal) renal tubular acidosis

ASSOCIATED WITH MULTIPLE DYSFUNCTION OF PROXIMAL TUBULE
(FANCONI SYNDROME)

Primary (no obvious systemic disease)
Genetically transmitted [190, 191]
Sporadic [192, 193]

Genetically transmitted systemic diseases
Cystinosis [188]
Lowe's syndrome [189]
Wilson's disease [194, 195]
Tyrosinemia [196]
Hereditary fructose intolerance [11]
   (during fructose administration
   or ingestion)
Pyruvate carboxylase deficiency [197]
Metachromatic leucodystrophy [198]

Disorders associated with chronic hypocalcemia and
   secondary hyperparathyroidism
Vitamin D deficiency [15, 199–202]
Vitamin D dependency [203]

Drug- or toxin-induced nephropathy
Outdated tetracycline [204]
Methyl-5-chromone (diacramone) [205]
Streptozotocin [206]
Lead [207]

Other renal diseases
Amyloidosis [208]
Nephrotic syndrome [208–210]
Renal transplantation [211]
Sjögren's syndrome [10]
Medullary cystic disease [212]
Paroxysmal nocturnal hemoglobinuria [213]
Renal vein thrombosis [214]

Multiple myeloma (with monoclonal immunoglobulin L
   chainuria)
Fully expressed [181, 215, 216]
Harrison-Blainey syndrome [217–219]

UNASSOCIATED WITH MULTIPLE DYSFUNCTION OF PROXIMAL TUBULE

Primary
   Sporadic
      Transient [220]
      Persisting [221]
   Genetically transmitted [222]
Osteopetrosis [224]
Carbonic anhydrase deficiency
   Acetazolamide [229, 230]
   Sulfanilamide [231]
York-Yendt syndrome [232]
Cyanotic congenital heart disease [233]

change in plasma total CO_2 correlated with the change in net acid excretion, and the changes in net acid excretion correlated positively with the corresponding changes in sodium balance and negatively with the corresponding changes in potassium balance.

These findings provide strong evidence that renal acidification is under tonic stimulation by mineralocorticoid at circulating levels of mineralocorticoid not exceeding those of normal subjects ingesting typical acid producing diets of normal sodium and potassium content. The extent to which the tonic

stimulation of renal acidification is mediated by a direct effect of mineralocorticoid on renal H^+ transport or by an indirect effect dependent on altered renal sodium or potassium transport or both has not been determined. Nevertheless the findings implicate mineralocorticoid deficiency as (1) an important cause of acidosis-causing impairment of renal acidification that does not depend on the presence of renal disease or glucocorticoid deficiency and (2) one whose potential for causing acidosis would presumably be amplified by increased endogenous acid production.

The role of aldosterone deficiency in the pathogenesis of metabolic acidosis in patients with chronic renal disease and reduced glomerular filtration rate has been investigated in studies in which the potent mineralocorticoid, fludrocortisone, was administered to patients with hyperkalemia and hyporeninemic hypoaldosteronism in the setting of chronic tubulointerstitial nephrisis [128]. With administration of a physiologic replacement dose (0.10 to 0.15 mg/day) of fludrocortisone to a patient so affected with a creatinine clearance 13 ml/min per $1.75m^2$), an already reduced value of urine pH decreased further, net acid excretion increased, and systemic acidosis and hyperkalemia were substantially ameliorated (Fig. 84-13). The reduction in urine pH suggests that mineralocorticoid replacement stimulated H^+ secretion. Presumably the pretreatment values of urine pH would have been considerably higher had the pretreatment rate of renal production of ammonia not been restricted in this patient because of the reduction in renal mass.

When glomerular filtration rate is not greatly reduced (i.e., when creatinine clearance is >25 ml/min), the increase in net acid excretion observed during mineralocorticoid therapy is accounted for predominantly by increased urine titratable acid excretion (Fig. 84-14). Urine pH decreased when mineralocorticoid therapy was initiated, but with continued therapy it increased in parallel with the observed increase in urine ammonium excretion. These findings suggest that the rate of renal production of ammonia increased during mineralocorticoid therapy. A primary increase in ammonia production would result in an increase in the amount of ammonia diffusing into

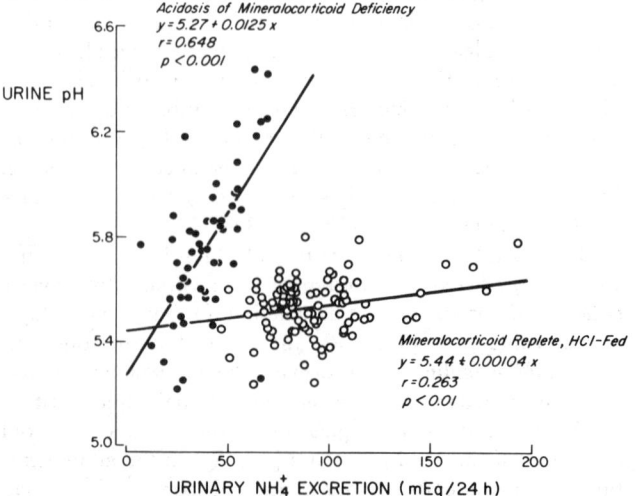

Figure 84-12 Relation between urinary pH and urinary ammonium excretion in glucocorticoid-adequate, mineralocorticoid-deficient adrenalectomized dogs with spontaneously occurring metabolic acidosis (closed circles) and in intact dogs with experimentally induced (HCl-feeding) metabolic acidosis (open circles).

Table 84-6 Clinical spectrum of type 4 renal tubular acidosis

---

Aldosterone deficiency
Combined deficiency of aldosterone and adrenal glucocorticoid
  hormones
    Addisons's disease
    Bilateral adrenalectomy
    Inherited impairment of steroidogensis: 21-hydroxylase deficiency
    ("congenital adrenal hyperplasia") [256, 257]
Selective deficiency of aldosterone
    Inherited impairment of aldosterone biosynthesis: corticosterone
    methyl oxidase deficiency [258–262]
    Secondary to deficient renin secretion [263–269]
      Diabetic nephropathy
      Chronic tubulointerstitial disease with glomerular
      insufficiency
      Indomethacin administration
    Chronic idiopathic hypoaldosteronism in adults and children
      [270–273]
*Pseudohypoaldosteronism (attenuated renal response to aldosterone
with secondary hyperreninemia and hyperaldosteronism)*
    Classical pseudohypoaldosteronism of infancy [258, 274–298]
    Chronic tubulointerstitial disease with glomerular insufficiency
    "saltwasting nephritis" [299]
    Drugs: Spironolactone; amiloride; tiramterene
Attenuated renal response to aldosterone and aldosterone deficiency
Selective tubule dysfunction with impaired renin secretion [300–
309]
Chronic tubulointerstitial disease with glomerular insufficiency
    Associated deficient renin secretion [128, 264, 266, 310]
    Renin status uncertain
Obstructive uropathy with deficient renal secretion [311]
Renal transplantation with deficient renin secretion [312, 313]
Lupus nephritis with deficient renin secretion [314]
Uncertain pathophysiology [315–323]
Chronic pyelonephritis [315, 316]
Lupus nephritis [317]
Renal transplantation [318]
Acute glomerulonephritis [319]
Renal amyloidosis [323]

---

the tubular lumen, which would both augment the excretion of ammonium and, by increasing the amount of luminal buffer, raise urine pH. Urine ammonium excretion correlated inversely with serum potassium concentration and did not decrease on discontinuation of mineralocorticoid therapy when hyperkalemia was prevented by reducing dietary intake of potassium; however, net titratable acid and net acid excretion did decrease (Fig. 84-15). Thus in patients with hypoaldosteronism and chronic renal insufficiency, administration of mineralocorticoid can augment both renal H⁺ secretion and, by correcting hyperkalemia, renal ammonia production as well.

Treatment of patients with RTA-4 and chronic renal insufficiency with mineralocorticoid may not always be indicated. In some patients hypertension occurs and ECV and total exchangeable sodium content are increased. Treatment with mineralocorticoid in these patients, by increasing renal tubular reabsorption of sodium chloride, might increase the severity of hypertension and lead to other deleterious consequences of expansion of ECV. Other therapeutic measures that can be considered include restriction of dietary potassium, administration of potassium-binding resins, sodium bicarbonate, loop diuretics, or some combination thereof.

PSEUDOHYPOALDOSTERONISM

In a wide spectrum of clinical disorders, chronic renal hyperkalemia and RTA-4 occur in the absence of a diffuse renal parenchymal disease and reduced glomerular filtration rate (Table 84-6). In some of these conditions, renal hyperkalemia and RTA-4 can be attributed to a deficiency of aldosterone and can be corrected by administration of exogenous mineralocorticoid hormone in physiologic replacement doses. In other conditions, aldosterone deficiency is not present, and hyperkalemia and acidosis persist despite administration of even superphysiologic doses of mineralocorticoids. Such mineralocorticoid resistant renal hyperkalemia and acidosis occurs in two distinctly different clinical syndromes: (1) classic pseudohypoaldosteronism of infancy, characterized by renal salt

Figure 84-13 Effect of orally administered fludrocortisone on serum carbon dioxide content and potassium concentration, urine pH, urinary titratable acid, ammonium, and net acid excretion in a patient with hyporeninemic hypoaldosteronism and chronic renal insufficiency (creatinine clearance, 13 ml/min per 1.73 m²) (Case 1). Systemic acidosis had not previously been treated. The severity of hyperkalemia had been mitigated before the study was initiated by the provision of a low-normal dietary intake of potassium. In the three bottom panels, the hatched bars represent the difference between the measured value of acid excretion and the mean value before therapy; the magnitude of the difference is indicated by the scale on the left-hand side of the panel. For reference, the mean control value is designated by the numerals within the ellipse. The accumulated values of the daily differences are shown by the solid circles and are indicated by the scale on the right-hand side of the panel.

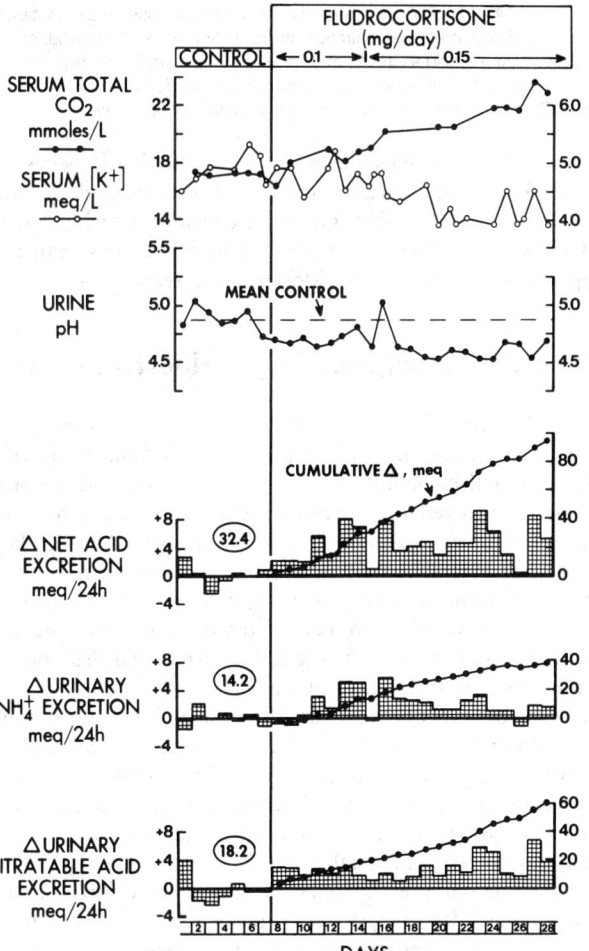

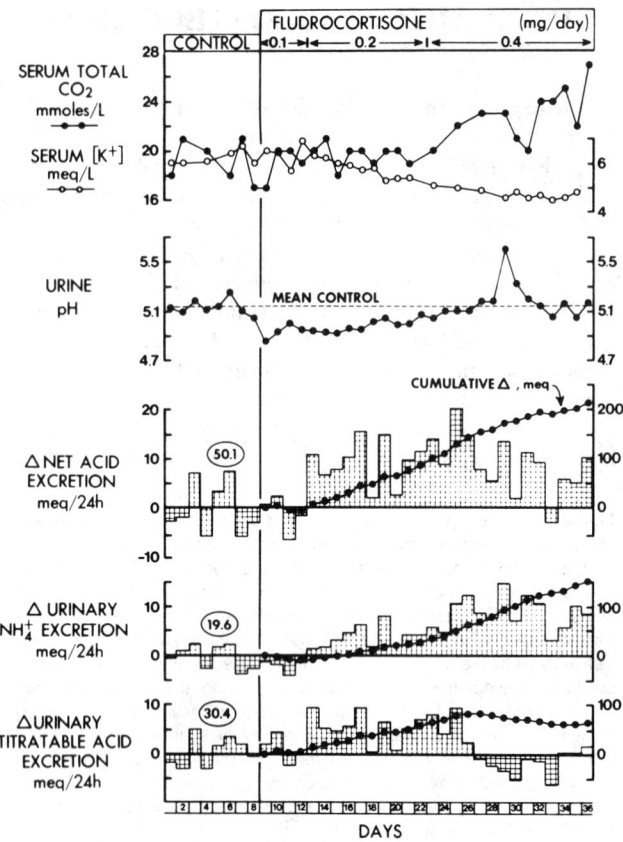

Figure 84-14 Effect of orally administered fludrocortisone on serum carbon dioxide and potassium concentration, urine pH, urinary titratable acid, ammonium, and net acid excretion in a patient with hyporeninemic hypoaldosteronism and chronic renal insufficiency (creatinine clearance 35 ml/min per 1.73 m²). Systemic acidosis had not previously been treated.

wasting and hypotension, and (2) a syndrome of persistent mineralocorticoid resistant acidosis unaccompanied by renal salt wasting or hypotension and frequently associated with hypertension. These two syndromes have been designated as types 1 and 2 pseudohypoaldosteronism, respectively.

Type 1 (Classic) Pseudohypoaldosteronism

Type 1 pseudohypoaldosteronism occurs in infants as an apparently congenital and, in some cases, a familial disorder characterized by failure to thrive, dehydration and hyponatremia due to renal salt wasting, hyperkalemia due to renal potassium retention, and renal tubular acidosis (RTA-4) [258, 274–298]. Plasma renin activity and plasma and urinary aldosterone concentrations are distinctly elevated, whereas plasma deoxycorticosterone and corticosterone concentrations are normal. Renal sodium wasting and reduced renal clearance of potassium persist despite prolonged parenteral administration of large amounts of deoxycorticosterone and aldosterone and oral administration of fludrocortisone. Supplemental sodium chloride can reverse hyponatremia and hyperkalemia, relieve symptoms, and permit normal or improved growth, including catch-up growth in some cases. Characteristically, after infancy the severity of renal dysfunction is sufficiently diminished to permit the supplements of sodium chloride to be discontinued. Renal dysfunction persists, as is evident from recurrence of hyponatremia and hyperkalemia when dietary sodium chloride is restricted [296].

The pathogenesis of classic pseudohypoaldosteronism of infancy has not been elucidated. In the index case reported by Cheek and Perry in 1958, it was postulated "that the defect may be due to a refractory state on the part of the (renal) tubules to endogenous salt-active steroids or mineralocorticoids." [274]. Generalized glomerular and tubular dysfunction does not occur. Examination of renal tissue obtained by biopsy has revealed only the presence of mild hyperplasia of the juxtaglomerular apparatus. Patients with classic pseudohypoaldosteronism of infancy are thus distinguishable from patients with pseudohypoaldosteronism associated with generalized renal parenchymal structural damage (e.g., salt-losing nephritis caused by methicillin nephritis, medullary cystic disease).

In the less than 50 cases of classic pseudohypoaldosteronism of infancy reported in the literature, there has been little study of the pathogenesis of the disease at the cellular level. The pathophysiologic manifestations of the disorder are consistent with a cellular defect that interferes with the action of aldosterone in those segments of the renal tubule normally responsive to aldosterone, specifically the collecting tubules and ducts. In the only study of a patient with pseudohypoaldosteronism in which binding of aldosterone in a target tissue has been investigated, the amount of tritiated aldosterone bound to mucosal cells obtained from the sigmoid colon was similar to that observed in control subjects [296]. In another patient with pseudohypoaldosteronism, mineralocorticoid induced stimulation of transepithelial transport of sodium and potassium was impaired in multiple target organs of aldosterone, including salivary glands, sweat glands, and colon, as well as the kidney [292]. In other patients with pseudohypoaldosteronism, the electrolyte composition of sweat suggests that the sweat glands are deficient in physiologic response to circulating mineralocorticoids [274, 275, 277, 278, 281, 292, 295].

Two groups of investigators have suggested that the renal tubule dysfunction of classic pseudohypoaldosteronism results from a deficiency of Na⁺-K⁺ ATPase [294, 297]. In one patient with classic pseudohypoaldosteronism, renal N⁺-K⁺ ATPase activity was almost undetectable in either proximal or distal nephron segments [294]. This finding may not, however, indicate a primary defect in renal Na⁺-K⁺ ATPase, since the specific activity of renal Na⁺-K⁺ ATPase is known to decrease under a variety of physiologic circumstances that reduce net renal sodium reabsorption. In adrenalectomized animals, net renal sodium reabsorption, as varied by alterations in sodium chloride intake, appears to be a major determinant of the specific activity of Na⁺-K⁺ ATPase, and mineralocorticoid induced increases in Na⁺-K⁺ ATPase activity appear to be secondary to stimulation of tubular sodium transport [329].

In classical pseudohypoaldosteronism the spontaneously occurring apparent amelioration of renal sodium wasting and potassium retention in the postinfancy period is a phenomenon like that described in patients with the salt wasting variant of congenital adrenal hyperplasia (21-hydroxylase deficiency), in whom renal sodium wasting appears to be caused in part by aldosterone deficiency and in part by increased concentrations of adrenal steroid metabolites that function as mineralocorticoid antagonists [330]. In both disorders, clinical remission is associated with persistent supernormal levels of plasma renin and aldosterone. In one patient with classical pseudohypoaldosteronism who was studied at age 9 years, normonatremia and normokalemia were maintained without dietary supplements of sodium chloride, hyperaldosteronism was present, yet hyponatremia and hyperkalemia recurred when the mineralocorticoid antagonist, spironolactone, was administered [296]. By contrast, normal subjects to whom spironolactone is administered chronically do not develop overt hyponatremia or hyperkalemia [331]. Presumably, renal resistance to the physiologic effect of aldosterone can be incomplete in patients with pseudohypoaldosteronism, so that the supernormal levels of circulating aldosterone permit the normokalemia (and normonatremia) to be maintained [296].

It is not known whether the same renal disorder underlies classic pseudohypoaldosteronism of infancy in all those affected, nor is it certain that a genetic abnormality is present in all cases. The familial occurrence of the disorder has been documented in only a small fraction of the reported cases [258, 282, 284–290, 294]. Several families have been described in which asymptomatic older sibs, parents, and grandparents were found to have abnormally increased plasma renin activity or plasma aldosterone concentration or both. This suggests the persistence of a disturbance in renal handling of sodium chloride that might be unmasked by restriction of dietary sodium

Figure 84-15 Effect of discontinuing fludrocortisone on serum carbon dioxide content and potassium concentration, urine pH, urinary titratable acid, ammonium, and net acid excretion in a patient with hyporeninemic hypoaldosteronism and chronic renal insufficiency (creatinine clearance, 35 ml/min per 1.73 m²). In this study dietary intake of potassium was reduced when therapy was discontinued; the serum potassium was reduced when therapy was discontinued; the serum potassium concentration remained constant. The rate of urinary ammonium excretion did not decrease when therapy was discontinued, despite a sustained increase in urine pH.

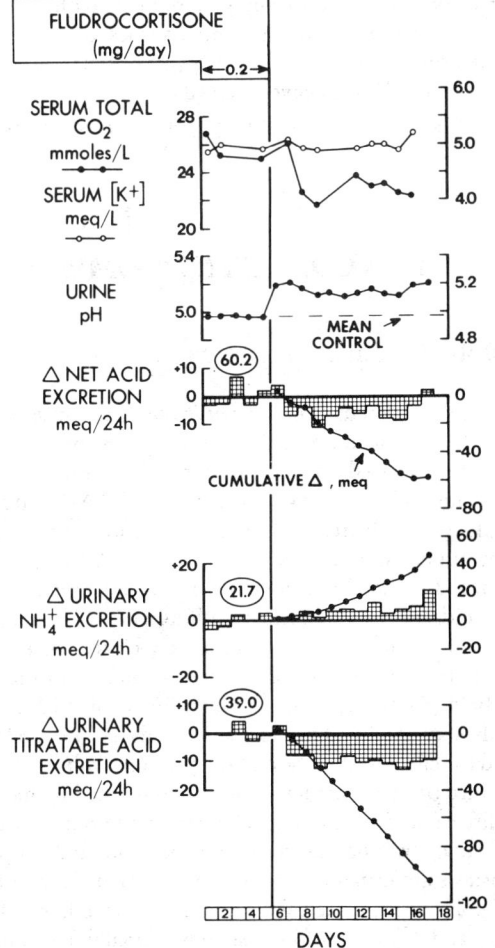

chloride or by administration of an aldosterone antagonist [284, 288, 289]. In these families the disorder appears to be inherited as an autosomal dominant trait.

Type 2 Pseudohypoaldosteronism

The primary abnormality in type 2 pseudohypoaldosteronism has been postulated to be a specific defect of the renal secretory mechanism for potassium, which limits the kaliuretic response to mineralocorticoid hormone but not the sodium and chloride reabsorptive effect of the hormone and which results in acidosis secondary to hyperkalemia. Recent evidence indicates that mineralocorticoid resistant renal hyperkalemia and acidosis in type 2 pseudohypoaldosteronism cannot be attributed to the absence of a renal potassium secretory mechanism, but instead may be dependent upon the amount of chloride available for reabsorption in the distal nephron [309]. The findings suggest that the primary abnormality in this syndrome is a defect of the distal nephron that increases its reabsorptive avidity for chloride, which (1) limits the sodium and mineralocorticoid dependent voltage driving force for potassium and hydrogen secretion, resulting in hyperkalemia and acidosis, and (2) augments distal NaCl reabsorption resulting in hyperchloremia, volume expansion, and hypertension (Fig. 84-16). Such a "chloride shunt" might arise as a result of an abnormal increase in the permeability of the distal nephron to chloride. Restriction of dietary sodium chloride or administration of a chloruretic diuretic (furosemide, thiazide) corrects hyperkalemia and acidosis. Conceivably, a similar kind of chloride shunt might arise as a consequence of diffuse structural damage to the renal parenchyma, as in patients with chronic tubulointerstitial disease or diabetic nephropathy who have RTA-4. This formulation provides an explanation for (1) the frequent concomitance in these patients of hyporeninemic hypoaldosteronism (caused by hyperabsorption of NaCl and consequent ECV expansion) and a diminished acid-excretory and kaliuretic response to mineralocorticoid (caused by chloride shunting of the voltage driving force) [15, 19, 128, 326], and (2) for the favorable therapeutic response to chronic administration of chloruretic diuretics [267, 325, 327].

CLINICAL CONSIDERATIONS APPLICABLE TO MORE THAN ONE TYPE OF RTA

"Autoimmune" RTA

Of 21 patients with "autoimmune" RTA we have studied, all have been women, and all but one have had Sjögren's syndrome [187]. Eighteen have had prototypic RTA-1 and one had a hybrid of RTA-1 and RTA-2. One patient had prototypic RTA-2 in association with the renal dysfunction of the Fanconi syndrome; in this patient evidence of impaired "distal" acidification was demonstrably absent. Joint disease has not been apparent clinically or radiographically, and eye findings are usually minimal. Not all of these patients complained of dry mouth, but histologic changes in salivary ducts diagnostic of Sjögren's syndrome have been invariable in buccal mucosa (except in the patient with autoimmune RTA and in none

CONSEQUENCES OF PROPOSED CHLORIDE SHUNT

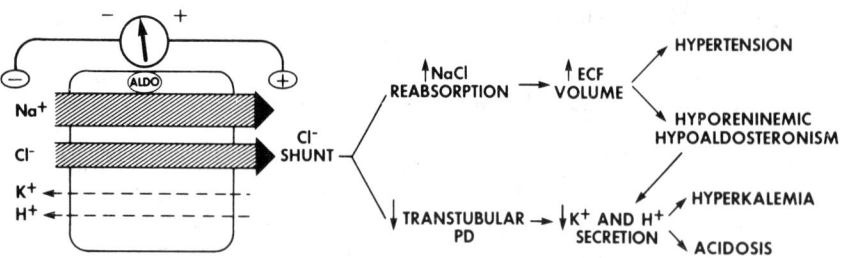

Figure 84-16 Pathophysiological consequences of a defect of the distal nephron characterized by increased reabsorptive avidity for chloride.

of 18 patients with familial, genetically transmitted RTA-1 we have seen). In three patients, autoimmune RTA-1 first became apparent in the immediate postpartum period, when severe proximal muscle weakness occurred acutely in association with striking hypokalemia and renal potassium wasting [187]. Persistent renal potassium wasting (despite alkali therapy) and acute hypokalemic syndromes appear to be much more common in autoimmune RTA-1 than in familial or "idiopathic" RTA-1.

Muscle Weakness and Metabolic Bone Disease

In patients with either RTA-1 or RTA-2, the rapidly occurring, severe muscle weakness of severe hypokalemia is the most dramatic and acutely life-threatening abnormality [332]; in patients with autoimmune RTA-1, it is the all-too-common initial clinical expression. But in patients with RTA-2, muscle weakness is more commonly insidious in onset, less severe, and a consequence of the proximal myopathy that attends metabolic bone disease [333]. In adult patients in whom RTA-2 occurs in the setting of intestinal malabsorption, hypocalcemia, secondary hyperparathyroidism, and hypophosphatemia, chronic weakness (of the proximal muscles) is often the major complaint [1,333–335]. Those affected typically have difficulty rising unassisted from a seated position. The weakness is usually associated with bone pain, symmetrical, often severe bone tenderness, and sometimes radiographic evidence of osteomalacia, most characteristically pseudofractures [1,173]. The metabolic bone disease may be of such striking clinical severity that even modest pretibial pressure elicits excruciating pain. The gait is characteristically slow and waddling (like a duck). All muscular effort may be attended by great discomfort. Deep tendon reflexes remain active [333]. Electromyographic and histologic examination usually reveal little, if any, objective evidence of muscle disease. The weakness is often mistaken as a psychoneurotic symptom. Although its pathogenetic mechanism is undefined, the myopathic disorder is predictably responsive to therapy that heals the associated metabolic bone disease. The myopathy is rare in patients with RTA-1. In affected adults with RTA-1, normal muscle strength returns with alkali therapy alone but often only after several weeks. In affected patients with RTA-2 as part of the malabsorption syndrome, the myopathy responds dramatically and usually rapidly to therapy with alkali and vitamin D. By disturbing the metabolism of calcium and phosphate in muscles, a deficiency or disordered metabolism of vitamin D [336, 337] might be a pathogenetic factor in the myopathy that attends metabolic bone disease. Hyperparathyroidism and phosphate depletion might also be pathogenic factors. In patients with

renal osteodystrophy, striking and rapid amelioration of muscle weakness has been reported with the administration of 1,25-dihydroxyvitamin D_3 [338].

pH-dependent Urinary Excretion of Drugs

In patients with any type of RTA, corrective alkali therapy is invariably attended by intense alkalinity of the urine; the urinary pH is frequently greater than 8. This has important implications with respect to the clinical pharmacology of certain drugs whose urinary excretion is pH-dependent, and an important mode of their disposition [339, 340]. As a group, the phenylalkylamines, including pseudoephedrine, have a high pK (greater than 8), and intense alkalinity of the urine greatly retards their excretion and acts to increase their blood level [341, 342]. The cinchona alkaloids, quinidine and quinine, which also have a pK greater than 8, and salicylate are affected similarly [343, 344]. Accordingly, in patients with any type of RTA, corrective alkali therapy predisposes them to certain kinds of drug intoxication. Frank psychosis has occurred in children with RTA who have received both a corrective dose of alkali therapy and the usual dose of pseudoephedrine for otitis media.

FANCONI SYNDROME

Physiologic Characteristics

As classically defined, *Fanconi syndrome* (FS) consists of two components: (1) a complex dysfunction of the proximal renal tubule characterized by increased renal clearance of phosphate, α-amino acids, usually bicarbonate (RTA-2), and sometimes glucose and uric acid, at normal and reduced plasma concentrations of these substances [11–14, 17, 188, 189, 345–361], and (2) a metabolic bone disease, characteristically rickets in children, osteomalacia in adults [17, 345–352, 335]. Because all of the substances excessively cleared in FS and in RTA-2 normally are reabsorbed predominantly in the proximal tubule, FS alone, or in combination with RTA-2 (RTA-2/FS), has generally (but not universally) [360, 361] been inferred to reflect dysfunction of the proximal tubule. The clinical picture of FS is characteristically dominated by metabolic bone disease and, in affected children, impaired growth and often frank stunting. Disturbances in fluid and electrolyte homeostasis are usually continuously apparent. Thirst or polydipsia, polyuria, and the signs and symptoms of hypokalemia, acidosis, and depletion of ECV stem principally from impaired reabsorption of Na^+, HCO_3^-, Cl^-, and H_2O in the proximal renal tubule (as detailed in the sections on the pathophysiology of RTA-2). Such disturbances of fluid and electrolyte homeostasis may be explosive in onset and extreme in severity when the renal dysfunction occurs acutely, as with drug toxicity [204, 205], or in association with a systemic disturbance of metabolism, particularly one that also gives rise to lactic acidosis [362, 363].

Mechanism and Pathogenesis of the Renal Disorder

FS is a characteristic feature of several genetically transmitted metabolic diseases (Table 84-5): cystinosis [188, 364–366], Lowe's syndrome [189, 367], a certain kind of tyrosinemia [196, 355] when tyrosine or phenylalanine is not restricted [369], and hereditary fructose intolerance (HFI) when fructose is not restricted [356, 370–372]. In these diseases, FS invariably occurs in association with RTA-2 [12, 13, 17, 347]. FS also occurs in other genetically transmitted metabolic diseases, including Wilson's disease [373–377], galactosemia [378, 379], and a glycogen storage disorder [373–377] characterized by galactose intolerance but not by a demonstrable enzyme deficiency. In each of these metabolic diseases, the occurrence of FS might represent a unit response to a disordering of some component of renal metabolism that is critical to the operation of all affected transport processes such as, for example, a component critical to the production or transduction of the energy required for the transport processes [347].

Reversible Disorders of Renal Metabolism   FS disappears in patients with galactosemia, tyrosinemia, Wilson's disease, and HFI when their systemic disorders of metabolism are corrected or attenuated by maneuvers that act to remove galactose [378], tyrosine [369], copper [376, 377], or fructose [356, 370–372], respectively. The abnormal gene products of these diseases do not then act *directly* to impair the operation of transport processes in the renal tubule. Rather, the expression of FS is pathogenetically linked to the abnormal gene product by way of a reversible abnormality of renal metabolism. The abnormal gene product has not been defined in Wilson's disease or in tyrosinemia of the type capable of causing FS. In patients with this type of tyrosinemia, the apparent rapidity with which the reintroduction of dietary tyrosine can induce the expression of FS [369] strongly suggests that a biochemical event consequent to impaired tyrosine metabolism constitutes, determines, or importantly amplifies an injurious biochemical event closely linked to the expression of FS. In patients with galactosemia, renal dysfunction occurs only after days of exposure to galactose [384], whereas hepatic dysfunction can occur within minutes [385]. This observation suggests that the pathogenic biochemical events that are directly linked to the expression of FS are only remotely related to those which are initially determined by the genetically determined kinetic deficiency of galactose-1-phosphate uridyl transferase. In patients with HFI, the expression of FS is caused by an abnormality of renal metabolism that is a direct consequence of the abnormal gene product [11, 347, 357].

The Experimental Model of Hereditary Fructose Intolerance   The renal tubular disorder reversibly induced by fructose in patients with HFI [11, 342, 356, 357, 370–372, 386, 387] can be both a dramatic clinical cause of RTA-2/FS

[347, 370–372] and, uniquely, an acute experimental model of RTA-2/FS [11, 370, 386, 387] whose pathogenesis is defined both with respect to causal defect and initial biochemical event, which are genetically deficient renal aldolase B [388–392] and consequent intracellular accumulation of fructose-1-phosphate (F-1-P) [388, 389], respectively. Minutes after the experimental administration of fructose to patients with HFI, the multiple renal dysfunctions of FS occur simultaneously and in association with those of prototypic RTA-2 [11]. These dysfunctions persist for as long as fructose is continued. Even when the experimental dysfunction is prolonged, there persists an exquisite dose-dependency that is realized within minutes and evident over a broad range of fructose dosage. When administration of fructose is discontinued, the experimental dysfunction disappears within minutes. In those patients who abstain from fructose, renal function remains normal [11]. The experimental disorder therefore provides a model of FS that is uniquely susceptible to systematic analysis and uncomplicated by whatever secondary phenomena attend chronicity of the clinical disorder. The model affords an opportunity to investigate not only the metabolic pathogenesis of FS, but also the nongenetic determinants of the expression of a genetic renal disease.

In the rat, and presumably in humans, renal aldolase B and fructokinase (which catalyzes the phosphorylation of fructose to F-1-P) are restricted to the proximal tubule [393, 394]. In the fructose loaded rat, Burch and her associates demonstrated that the accumulation of F-1-P and reduction of ATP which occur within minutes in the kidney [395] occur exclusively in the proximal tubule [394]. In the experimental RTA-2/FS of patients with HFI acutely exposed to fructose, the distal nephron retains its capacity to secrete H^+ at greatly increased rates and against normally steep lumen-peritubular H^+ gradients [11, 387]. RTA-2/FS in this instance then might be the dysfunctional expression of an abnormality of renal metabolism that occurs only in cells of the proximal tubule and impairs transepithelial transport only in this segment [347].

Recent studies of Brewer and her associates provide evidence in support of this hypothesis [396]. In two unrelated adult patients with HFI undergoing water diuresis, they administered either fructose or acetazolamide intravenously and examined the relationship between solute-free water clearance (C_{H_2O}), a measure of solute reabsorption in the postproximal nephron, and both urine flow (V), a measure of the total solute rejected by the proximal tubule, and the sum of C_{H_2O} and the renal clearance of Cl^- ($C_{H_2O} + C_{Cl}$), a measure of proximally rejected solute that is potentially reabsorbable by the thick ascending limb. When either fructose or acetazolamide induced bicarbonaturia of substantial and similar magnitude (at normal plasma bicarbonate concentrations), brisk and similar increases in C_{H_2O} occurred. With either agent, the increases in $C_{H_2O} + C_{Cl}$ were only slightly greater than the corresponding increases in C_{H_2O}, but the increases in V were much and similarly greater. The observations made with acetazolamide confirm those made in the dog [397–399] and in humans [400]. This class of agent is known to induce an increased rejection of Cl^-, HCO_3^-, and Na^+ out of the proximal tubule [401]. The normal thick ascending limb, which accounts for most of the C_{H_2O} generated during water diuresis [397, 398] is known to reclaim Cl^- and Na^+ and to reject HCO_3^- [402]. When fructose was administered during hyperchloremic acidosis so that bicarbonaturia was absent or negligible, the increases in C_{H_2O} and V were again brisk but nearly commensurate. When the plasma bicarbonate concentration was abruptly increased to normal levels (by administering $NaHCO_3$), such that brisk bicarbonaturia was induced without changing the severity of either the fructosemia or hyperaminoaciduria, V increased further, C_{H_2O} did not change, and urinary excretion of Cl^- decreased. The $NaHCO_3$ induced increment in filtered load of HCO_3^- closely approximated the corresponding increment in HCO_3^- excreted and the inferred increment in HCO_3^- rejected by the proximal tubule (plasma osmolality × ΔV/2). Brewer concluded that in the RTA-2/FS of patients with HFI acutely exposed to fructose: (1) the proximal tubule rejects greatly increased amounts of Cl^-, HCO_3^- and Na^+; (2) a functionally competent thick ascending limb reabsorbs most of the increment in Cl^- rejected by the proximal tubule but rejects virtually all of the proximally rejected HCO_3^-; and (3) proximally rejected HCO_3^- fully accounts for the bicarbonaturia of the RTA-2 induced by the fructose.

These findings provide a convincing demonstration that RTA-2 can actually be anatomically "proximal" RTA. In light of the biochemical observations of Burch and her coworkers [394, 395], these findings suggest that in the RTA-2/FS of patients with HFI acutely exposed to fructose, the pathogenetic mechanism is uniquely compact, i.e., the entire cause-and-effect complex occurs in cells of the proximal tubule.

When patients with HFI are acutely exposed to fructose, genetically defective aldolase B in the liver and epithelium of the small bowel [403], as well as in the renal cortex, dictates not only the acute cellular accumulation of F-1-P by these tissues, but also, as a consequence, their severe cellular depletion of inorganic phosphate (P_i) [388, 404]. Because the amount of P_i sequestered as F-1-P (and other phosphorylated intermediates) in these tissues is great enough to cause severe and near immediate hypophosphatemia [388], the P_i depletion of one tissue in effect amplifies that of the others [388]. Depletion of P_i activates AMP deaminase [405, 406], a cytoplasmic enzyme that catalyzes the deamination of AMP to IMP, a precursor of uric acid via inosine—hypoxanthine—xanthine [394, 395, 404, 407–411]. The adenine nucleotides, AMP, ADP, and ATP (comprising total adenine nucleotides, TAN) are maintained at or near equilibrium in the cytoplasm of the cell by the action of adenylate kinase. Accordingly, by activating AMP deaminase, acute P_i depletion triggers a massive, almost immediate degradation of preformed adenine nucleotides in both the liver and renal cortex and so accounts for the observed acute reduction in TAN and ATP induced by fructose in these tissues in the rat [394, 395, 404, 407, 411] and in humans [409, 410], and hence, for both the hyperuricemia [404,408] and the great increase in urinary excretion of oxypurines induced by fructose loading in humans [408]. In the liver and renal cortex tissues, P_i depletion then restricts the rate at which ATP can be regenerated, both by the depletion of P_i per se and by the reduction of TAN that depletion entails [411]. In the fructose loaded rat, the severity of the reductions in ATP and TAN in both the liver and renal cortex varies directly with the severity of P_i depletion in these tissues [411]. Prior phosphate loading largely prevents the fructose induced reductions of ATP and TAN in the renal cortex and significantly attenuates them in the liver, even though doubling the concentrations of F-1-P [411]. In the fructose loaded rat, prior P_i loading also greatly increases the rate at which ATP is regenerated in the renal cortex [411], and significantly increases the rate in the liver.

In the isolated rat liver perfused with an unrecirculating solution containing fructose (10 mM) and P_i (either 1.2 or .50

mM) Sestoft found that the oxygen uptake was limited by P_i at the lower concentration [412, 413]. After 40 min of perfusion at the higher concentration of P_i (5.0 mM) the uptake of O_2 was 16 percent greater than at the lower concentrations, and the tissue concentration of ATP was significantly greater, 1.45 vs. 1.15 μmol per gram wet weight. The tissue concentration of TAN at the higher perfusion P_i was not significantly greater than the reduced values obtaining at the lower perfusion P_i. These observations strongly suggest that in the fructose perfused liver the rate at which mitochondria can regenerate ATP can be made to vary directly with cellular P_i and independently of an even greatly reduced pool size of adenine nucleotides.

In patients with HFI, hypophosphatemia, hyperuricemia, and hyperinosinuria occur within 10 min of initiating intravenously administered fructose and just precede the occurrence of RTA-2/FS [414]. Prior phosphate loading significantly attenuates not only the severity of the RTA-2/FS [414], but also that of the hyperuricemia [414] and the hyperinosinuria [414]. In a woman with HFI to whom fructose was administered over two 1-h periods interrupted by an interval lasting 100 min, phosphate loading initiated before the second period attenuated the renal tubular dysfunction and abolished the hyperuricemic response [415]. Phosphate loading only modestly attenuates the fructose-induced hyperuricemia in patients with HFI who have not recently received fructose. Accordingly, and since fructose-induced depletion of hepatic adenine nucleotides in humans persists for at least 2 h [410], it seems likely that phosphate loading attenuated the renal tubular dysfunction (despite continued, severely reduced concentrations of ATP and TAN in the proximal tubule) possibly by enhancing mitochondrial respiration and regeneration of ATP in this segment.

It is tempting to invoke the notion of phosphorylation potential [ATP]/[ADP][P_i], to explain how disturbances of cytoplasmic P_i, ATP, and ADP might be linked to disturbances of mitochondrial respiration and regeneration of ATP [416, 417]. Whatever its theoretical appeal, the results of Tager and his associates [418] show that it is not possible to estimate the cytosolic phosphorylation state from measurements of total cellular amounts of P_i, ATP, and ADP. In isolated liver cells, in which mitochondrial and cytosolic fractions were separated by the digitonin technique, these investigators determined that the mitochondrial fraction contained 40 percent of the TAN, the ATP/ADP ratio in the cytosol is much greater than that in the mitochondria, and the concentration of P_i in the mitochondria is about 5 times that in the cytoplasm. The digitonin technique has recently been used to separate mitochondrial and cytosolic fractions in the renal tubule [419], but measurements of P_i and adenine nucleotides have not been reported.

The Experimental Model Induced by Maleic Acid (MA)

The experimental model of RTA-2/FS acutely induced by fructose in patients with HFI has striking parallels with the experimental model of RTA-2/FS acutely induced by MA in the dog and rat [353, 354, 358–360, 420–423]. In studies performed in trained, unanesthetized dogs given MA during water diuresis, Al-Bander and his colleagues made observations very much like those of Brewer and her coworkers in patients with HFI [424]. When the administration of MA predictably induced the nearly immediate and large increase in fractional excretion of filtered bicarbonate (FEHCO$_3$), V, C_{H_2O}, and $C_{Cl} + C_{H_2O}$ increased strikingly. At any increased value for C_{H_2O}, the corresponding value for $C_{Cl} + C_{H_2O}$ were only slightly greater, but the corresponding value for V was much greater. The increase in FEHCO₃ induced by MA varied directly with that of the urine flow/glomerular filtration rate (V/GFR) ratio and the correlation was highly significant ($p < 0.001$). Al-Bander concluded that in the experimental renal tubular disorder induced by MA in the dog: (1) the proximal tubule rejects greatly increased amounts of HCO_3^-, Cl^-, and Na^+; (2) the increment in the proximally rejected HCO_3^- and Na^+ is largely rejected by the postproximal nephron and largely accounts for the increment in HCO_3^- and Na^+ excreted in the urine; (3) the increment in the proximally rejected Cl^- (and an equivalent amount of Na^+) is largely reclaimed in the postproximal nephron. The findings suggest that the urinary findings of RTA-2/FS induced by MA principally reflect impaired transepithelial transport in the proximal tubule [424]. Other investigators have come to a similar conclusion [358, 359, 420, 421, 425, 426].

On the basis of microperfusion and stop flow studies in the intact rat given MA, Bergeron et al. recently postulated that the physiologic consequences of the demonstrated MA induced dysfunction of the proximal convoluted tubule were corrected in the more distal segment of the proximal tubule and that nephronal dysfunction distal to the proximal tubule accounted for the increased renal clearance of amino acids and phosphate [360]. Further, these investigators postulated that MA induces, as its main physiologic effect, an increased efflux of amino acids into the lumen at proximal and distal sites as a consequence of a "modification of cell membrane permeability." But, in studies of MA induced aminoaciduria by free-flow micropuncture and continuous microperfusion, Gunther and his coworkers concluded that MA inhibits the saturable reabsorption mechanism of amino acids along the proximal tubule; they showed (by microperfusion) that MA does not produce a greater efflux of amino acid (into the lumen) at distal sites of the nephron. In light of these findings and those of Al-Bander, it would seem difficult not to conclude that the dysfunction of the proximal tubule largely accounts for the RTA-2/FS induced by MA.

MA does not appear to affect renal tubular reabsorptive transport at the luminal membrane [361, 427]. MA induces morphologic changes in renal cortical mitochondria [423, 428], impairs mitochondrial oxidative metabolism [429–431], and reduces renal anteriovenous oxygen differences [420] and renal cortical concentration of ATP [422, 428, 432]. In the intact rat and in renal tubules from the chick, MA impairs the hydroxylation of 25-OHD₃ to 1,25-(OH)₂D₃ [433], a reaction catalyzed by 25-hydroxyvitamin D₃-1-hydroxylase, an enzyme apparently restricted to the mitochondria of the cell of the proximal tubule [434]. In light of these observations, Al-Bander's finding (i.e., that the severity of RTA-2/FS induced by MA is strikingly attenuated by prior phosphate loading [435]) suggests that a disturbance in mitochondrial oxidative metabolism, possibly of oxidative phosphorylation, could be critical to the pathogenesis of this renal disorder (including the disturbance of phagolysosomal function see below). The severity of RTA-2/FS induced by MA, like that induced by fructose (in patients with HFI), is exquisitely dose-dependent. In isolated and perfused segments of proximal convoluted tubules from the rabbit, Brazy and his coworkers [436] found that arsenate induced a dose-dependent uncoupling of oxidative phosphorylation as its main metabolic effect, and dose-dependent reductions in fluid absorption and net transport of both sodium and phosphate; glucose transport was slightly inhibited. The dose-dependent, *graded* reductions in fluid absorption (and phosphate absorption) corresponded with the dose-dependent, *graded* reductions in oxidative metabolism.

Lysosomal Enzymes *Lysosomes* are cytoplasmic organelles which are bounded by a single membrane and which contain hydrolases and other enzymes required for a variety of normal degradative processes, including the degrading of proteins and peptides. In the normal proximal convoluted tubule, endocytotic vacuoles formed at the luminal border migrate inward and fuse with lysosomes, thereby completing a phagolysosomal continuum. Lysozyme is a low molecular weight protein (MW = 15,000) that is readily filterable by the normal glomerulus, usually completely reabsorbed by the endocytotic process of the renal tubule, and catabolized principally, if not entirely, by lysosomes in the proximal tubule [437–439]. Lysozyme is then a normal constituent of renal lysosomes [440] but is not synthesized in the kidney [441]. Lysozymuria is generally considered to reflect proximal tubule cell damage [442, 433]. Other circulating low molecular weight proteins, including insulin [444], β₂-microglobulin [445–447], and immunoglobulin light (L) chain [448], appear to be handled by the renal tubule in much the same way as lysozyme and are characteristically excreted in the urine in greatly increased amounts in patients with nephropathic cystinosis and other genetically transmitted diseases that cause FS [444, 447, 449].

Some patients with FS excrete increased amounts of lysosomal enzymes. *N*-Acetylglucosaminidase is a "marker" lysosomal enzyme in hepatocytes [450] and in the renal cortex; the enzyme occurs predominantly in lysosomes [451, 452]. Since the molecular weight of *N*-acetylglucosaminidase is approximately 250,000, increased excretion of this enzyme in patients with FS, in the absence of more than minimal albuminuria or a reduction in glomerular filtration, probably reflects a lysosomal abnormality [453, 454].

In the RTA-2/FS induced by fructose in patients with HFI and that induced by MA, lysozymuria and hyper *N*-acetylglucosaminidasuria occur almost at the same time as the urinary findings of disordered transepithelial transport of the proximal tubule [435, 454, 455, 459, 460]. In the rat, sodium maleate reduces the endocytic uptake by the proximal tubule cells of low molecular weight protein and decreases the transport of protein into lysosomes, thus reducing the catabolism of reabsorbed protein [456]. Also, after exposure to MA, endocytic vacuoles rapidly accumulate in the apical cytoplasm but apical tubules disappear, indicating an altered recycling of membrane [456]. In fibroblasts, agents that decrease the ATP level also decrease the endocytosis of horseradish peroxidase [457]. Because ATP levels are decreased in kidneys from sodium maleate treated rats, Christensen and Maunsbach suggested that the decreased renal tubular uptake of lysozyme by endocytosis resulted from impaired "cellular energy supplies in the form of ATP" [456]. It has been suggested by Maunsbach [444], on the basis of protein tracer studies, that one function of the apical tubules is to return membrane material from the endocytic vacuoles to the luminal plasma membrane. The endocytic vacuoles, however, have a life span of only a few minutes [437, 458] as compared with at least a few weeks for the lysosomes [459]. Therefore most of the membrane material of the endocytic vacuoles is not incorporated into the lysosomal membranes but is probably instead recycled from the endocytic vacuoles to the apical cell membrane [456]. The almost complete disappearance of apical tubules in cells of maleate treated animals suggests that the tubules either change into vacuoles or fuse with the cell membrane [456].

Vesicular transport within protein secreting cells is known to be energy dependent [460]. Christensen and Maunsbach suggest that "lack of energy supply" is also the cause of the decreased transport of protein from endocytic vacuoles to lysosomes in proximal tubule cells exposed to sodium maleate. They point out that accumulations of apical vesicles, similar to the endocytic vesicles observed after sodium maleate infusion, have also been observed in proximal tubule cells after both ischemia [461, 462] and exposure to potassium cyanide or sodium iodoacetate [463].

In the MA treated rat, the pathogenetic relationship between the impairment in the phagolysosomal system of the proximal tubule and that of transepithelial transport, if any, remains to be determined. To the extent that the phagolysosomal system normally participates in the recycling of membrane fragments to the luminal membrane [464, 465], and to the extent that this process participates in regulating the composition and spatial arrangements of the luminal membrane and apical tubule, a disordering of this process might lead to an impairment in membrane transport. In the RTA-2/FS induced by fructose in patients with HFI, under certain experimental circumstances, the occurrence of this dysfunction precedes by some time the occurrence of lysozymuria and hyper N-acetylglucosaminidasuria. This observation suggests that the lysosomal abnormality of the renal tubule is not required in the pathogenesis of FS in HFI. The genetically defective enzyme in HFI is not a lysosomal enzyme but a "soluble" cytoplasmic enzyme [466].

Lysozyme and L-Chain Nephropathy   Increased urinary excretion of substantial amounts of lysozyme and immunoglobulin L chain can also reflect their increased production [467–470]. When immunoglobulin L chain or lysozyme are filtered by the glomerulae at rates that overload the phagolysosomal system of the proximal tubule, structural damage [471] and dysfunction of the renal tubule can occur [467–470]. In patients with monocytic leukemia, the not uncommon syndrome of renal potassium wasting appears to be a consequence of lysozyme induced renal dysfunction [467–470]. In patients ultimately diagnosed as having multiple myeloma, the occurrence of RTA-2 in association with the renal findings of FS may precede by years other evidences of the disease and reflect an immunoglobulin-L-chain-induced nephropathy [217–218]. In this instance the immunoglobulin detected in the urine is presumably produced in excess by a single clone of myeloma cells and hence is of a single subtype, κ [217, 218], although one patient is described as having had only the λ subtype [472]. Thus, when patients with FS excrete but one type of immunoglobulin L chain, monoclonal plasma cell dyscrasia, i.e., multiple myeloma, can be inferred to be causal [218]. When increased urinary excretion of immunoglobulin L chain reflects a renal tubular dysfunction that is unassociated with increased production of L chain, both κ and λ subtypes are characteristically excreted [473, 474].

Cystinosis   In patients with cystinosis, the most common disease causally associated with FS in children, "storage" of cystine in lysosomes of the proximal renal tubule might be a primary pathogenetic event in the renal disorder [366]. In so-called nephropathic or "infantile" cystinosis, FS is expressed within the first 12 months of life, progressive reduction in glo-

merular filtration rate leads to terminal uremia by midchildhood, and the free-cystine content of leukocytes is 80 times normal [475]. In so-called benign cystinosis of adulthood, renal disease is absent [476], and the free-cystine content of leukocytes is 30 times normal [480]. So-called adolescent or "intermediate" cystinosis is intermediate in severity with respect to the renal lesion and cystine content of leukocytes [477].

It remains to be demonstrated that an abnormality in lysosomal structure or function is a primary consequence of the abnormal gene product of cystinosis, or that cystine accumulation in the proximal tubule is primarily involved in or is a requirement for the pathogenesis of either FS or of the progressive reduction in renal mass. The continuously massive urinary excretion of N-acetylglucosaminidase and other lysosomal enzymes is unexplained [453]. The possibility of a relationship between the apparent lysosomal disorder of cystinosis and the characteristically striking blondness, fair skin, and blue eyes of those affected [366] appears not to have been investigated. Eight mouse pigment (dilution) mutants are now known which affect both melanosome and lysosome function [478]. It is conceivable that cystinosis is a syndrome caused by a genetic defect in one of several steps in the processing of lysosomes (and exocytic and endocytic vacuoles) and that cystine accumulation in lysosomes is a consequence of such disordered processing. Portale and his associates [479] have recently studied a young girl with RTA-2/FS, massively increased urinary excretion of N-acetylglucosaminidase, and the classic clinical characteristics of cystinosis, including photophobia and retarded growth. Yet, excessive cystine was demonstrably not present in leucocytes or fibroblasts. Renal biopsy revealed no evidence of cystinosis. One can imagine a genetic defect of lysosomal processing which gives rise to disordered and accelerated exocytosis in the proximal renal tubule cell. The curious hypothyroidism in patients with cystinosis [480, 481] might reflect a disorder of the exocytic/endocytic process in the thyroid follicular cell [482].

Pathophysiology and Metabolic Derangement

Potassium and Sodium   See the discussion of pathophysiology under type 2 RTA above for a description of the potassium and sodium metabolic derangements.

Phosphate and Calcium   In FS, sustained hypophosphatemia is a predictable consequence of the persisting impairment in renal reabsorption of phosphate and has generally been assumed to be the principal if not sole pathogenic determinant of the metabolic bone disease [364, 366]. Phosphate therapy alone can heal the metabolic bone disease [193, 483]. This therapeutic phenomenon would appear to have occurred most frequently in patients with adult-onset FS, but it has been described in children with nephropathic cystinosis [366, 484]. Metabolic bone disease can antedate the occurrence of hypophosphatemia in patients with FS [485, 486] and can heal without measured change either in the severity of hypophosphatemia or in the plasma calcium X phosphorus product when large amounts of vitamin D are administered alone [487, 488]. Furthermore, Dent and Harris found evidence of metabolic bone disease (and debility) in but one of four adult sibs with the renal dysfunction characteristic of FS, although hypophosphatemia (and mild metabolic acidosis) occurred in all and was severe in three (<2.0 mg/dl); hypocalcemia occurred in none [489]. The apparent nonoccurrence of metabolic bone disease despite persistent, severe hypophosphatemia (1.7 mg/dl) and mild acidosis has recently been described in an adult woman with FS as part of "light-chain nephropathy" [219]. It is clear that in some patients with the renal dysfunction of FS, rickets or osteomalacia is not a predictable consequence of plasma calcium-X phosphorus product that is less than 30 [487, 488].

Hypophosphatemia or phosphate depletion has been implicated in the pathogenesis of the proximal myopathy that frequently occurs in FS [193, 483, 490, 491]. The myopathy can be reversed with phosphate therapy alone [193, 483, 490]. Myopathy is by no means predictable in FS, even when hypophosphatemia is severe [219, 489].

The renal dysfunction of FS usually does not give rise to hypocalcemia even after prolonged acidosis. Although hypercalciuria occurs [90, 215, 483] and can disappear with alkali therapy [190, 374], its occurrence is not predictably related to that of acidosis [492]. Hypercalciuria is characteristic of patients with Wilson's disease, irrespective of FS, and may reflect increased absorption of calcium from the gut [193, 374]. In our experience hypercalciuria is usual in patients with cystinosis and its severity is unaffected by alkali therapy.

In patients with FS, nephrocalcinosis (and nephrolithiasis) occurs [194, 374, 483] but is quite uncommon, perhaps because urinary excretion of citrate is not reduced and is often increased in those affected [493, 494].

Vitamin D

Metabolic Bone Disease [Including Vitamin D–dependent Rickets (VDDR)]   FS occurs as part of vitamin D dependency, a rare disorder genetically transmitted as an autosomal recessive trait and characterized by hypocalcemia and secondary hyperparathyroidism but modest (or no) hypophosphatemia [203, 495–498] (see Chap. 79). When pharmacologic amounts of vitamin D_2 are administered to those affected, the rickets heals and the hypocalcemia (and hypophosphatemia) and renal dysfunction disappear [203, 495]. In patients with VDDR, "replacement" amounts of either 1,25-$(OH)_2D_3$ or a synthetic analogue, 1α-OH vitamin D_3, can within days correct the hypocalcemia and renal dysfunction and initiate healing of rickets [497–499]. On the basis of this finding, Fraser and his colleagues proposed that vitamin D dependency was caused by a genetic deficiency of 25-OHD_3-1-hydroxylase and consequent deficiency of circulating 1,25-$(OH)_2D_3$ [497, 500, 501]. This hypothesis is strongly supported by the finding of reduced plasma concentration of 1,25-$(OH)_2D_3$ in those affected [502]. Fraser and Scriver regard VDDR as a prototype of "calciopenic hereditary rickets" [501] and the associated renal dysfunction as a consequence of secondary hyperparathyroidism [501].

The phenomenon of vitamin D "dependency" compels an important question: Can disordered renal production of 1,25-$(OH)_2D_3$ contribute to the phenomenon of vitamin D resistant metabolic bone disease in patients with FS who are not hypocalcemic and in whom the renal dysfunction of FS is not reversed with vitamin D therapy? 1,25-$(OH)_2D_3$ is synthesized exclusively in mitochondria of the renal cortex [503–506] by the 1-hydroxylation of 25-OHD_3, which is synthesized princi-

pally in the liver [507]. By impairing either the 1-hydroxylation reaction per se or the accession of 25-OHD_3 to the mitochondrial site of the reaction, abnormalities of the renal cortical tubule capable of causing persistent FS might greatly reduce the renal synthesis of 1,25-$(OH)_2D_3$, and possibly other metabolites of 25-OHD_3, and thereby contribute to the pathogenesis of the bone disease of FS [433]. In animals, the experimental administration of maleic acid induces a reversible renal tubule dysfunction like that of FS [353, 354] and metabolic and structural changes in the renal cortical tubule, particularly in the mitochondria [423, 428–431]. In the vitamin D deficient rat and chick, maleic acid induces a substantial reduction in the conversion of 25-OHD_3 to 1,25-$(OH)_2D_3$, and this reduction occurs without a significant decrease in GFR, where measured in the rat [433]. In a nonazotemic 5-year-old boy with cystinosis, plasma 1,25-$(OH)_2D_3$ was undetectable [508]. In one young girl with nephropathic cystinosis, treatment with a "physiologic" amount of 1,25-$(OH)_2D_3$ (1 μg/day) was attended by rapid healing of rickets and an increase in linear growth rate [509]. Gertner et al. have also reported healing of rickets in three boys with cystinosis given 1α-OHD_3 [510].

Renal Dysfunction   In addition to its ability to reverse the complex renal tubular dysfunction of patients with either deficiency of vitamin D or vitamin D "dependency," 1,25-$(OH)_2D_3$, when administered in very large amounts, can reverse the RTA-2/FS (and metabolic bone disease) in patients with "1,25-$(OH)_2D_3$ resistant rickets" [511, 512] ("type 2 vitamin D dependent rickets" [513]), a syndrome characterized by hypocalcemia, secondary hyperparathyroidism, osteomalacia, osteitis fibrosa cystia, stunted growth, sometimes alopecia, greatly *elevated* levels of 1,25-$(OH)_2D_3$, and normal levels of 25-$(OH)_2D_3$ [513]. These observations suggest the possibility that an abnormality in the renal metabolism of 25-OHD_3 or of 1,25-$(OH)_2D_3$, or in the capacity of the renal tubule to respond to 1,25-$(OH)_2D_3$, can contribute to the pathogenesis of the renal dysfunction of FS and may be required for its expression in some cases. The renal dysfunction of vitamin D dependency and of vitamin D deficiency, of which hypophosphatemia has been considered to be an expression [496, 499], has usually been attributed to hyperparathyroidism secondary to hypocalcemia [496, 500, 501]. But the demonstration in patients with these disorders that the renal dysfunction can be greatly attenuated by experimental correction of the hypocalcemia [15, 180, 496] and presumed suppression of secondary hyperparathyroidism need only mean that circulating PTH, possibly in increased amounts (and perhaps hypocalcemia), is required for the expression of FS. It would appear that hyperparathyroidism is causally associated with reversible FS (including RTA-2) only when secondary to a deficiency, or disturbed metabolism, of vitamin D (see Type 2 RTA above). In this regard it should be noted that when either vitamin D_2 or 1α-OHD_3 was experimentally discontinued in patients with vitamin D dependency, both the occurrence of hypophosphatemia and aminoaciduria antedated that of hypocalcemia [499]. Conversely, hypophosphatemia and aminoaciduria appeared to persist for several days after hypocalcemia had been corrected with 1α-OHD_3 [499]. Furthermore, in several patients with idiopathic FS unassociated with hypocalcemia [514–516], large-dose vitamin D therapy has been attended by correction of FS; and, in the one patient in whom the measurement was made, the plasma concentration of immunoreactive PTH was not increased [511]. 25-OHD_3 and, to a lesser extent, 1,25-$(OH)_2D_3$ can act to increase renal reabsorption of phosphate, sodium, and calcium [517, 518]. 25-OHD_3 can augment renal reabsorption of bicarbonate [519]. It is not known whether the normal operation of any renal tubular function depends on an effect of, or the renal metabolism of, 25-OHD_3 or 1,25-$(OH)_2D_3$.

Therapy

The therapy of Fanconi's syndrome can be dramatically successful when substances critical to its causation can be removed, as in the case of HFI, galactosemia, Wilson's disease, and tyrosinemia (type 1). But, in each of these diseases, morbidity and mortality may be determined more by extrarenal disorders. In cystinosis, in which the renal disease is the principal determinant of morbidity and mortality, no therapy is known to attenuate the severity of FS or to prevent the inexorably progressive reduction in renal mass. Therapy with cysteamine in five children with nephropathic cystinosis [520] caused a consistent dose-related decline in levels of cystine in leukocytes and in extracellular fluid, but caused no improvement in renal tubular function or growth velocity; creatinine clearance may have increased slightly in some patients, but this effect has been questioned [521].

The therapeutic approach to acidosis and hypokalemia is discussed under Type 2 RTA above.

The approach to vitamin D_2 therapy is much like that already considered in the section on familial X-linked hypophosphatemic rickets. It can be anticipated that the synthetic analogue of 1,25-$(OH)_2D_3$, 1α-OHD_3, will be widely used in the treatment of FS; both compounds have already been successfully used in "replacement" doses of 1 μg/day [509, 510]. The very short biologic half-life of both 1α-OHD_3 and 1,25-OH_2D_3 should minimize the danger of their use inducing vitamin D intoxication, a common and serious problem with the use of vitamin D_2. Oral phosphate therapy would appear to be a useful therapeutic adjunct to vitamin D therapy, particularly in adult patients with idiopathic FS [193, 483].

Many of the studies cited in this work were carried out on the General Clinical Research Center, University of California, San Francisco. Much of this work was supported by grants from the National Institutes of Health: RR-00079, General Clinical Research Center, Division of Research Resources; AM-21354, National Institute of Arthritis, Metabolism, and Digestive Diseases; AM-21605, National Institutes of Arthritis, Metabolism and Digestive Diseases. Support was also provided by a generous gift from the Church and Dwight Corporation. The authors gratefully acknowledge the splendid assistance of Ms. Kathleen R. Peterson and Ms. Patricia Douglass.

REFERENCES

1. ALBRIGHT F, BURNETT CH, PARSON W, REIFENSTEIN EC JR, ROOS A: Osteomalacia and late rickets: The various etiologies met in the United States with emphasis on that resulting in a specific form of renal acidosis, the therapeutic indications for each etiological sub-group, and the relationship between osteomalacia and Milkman's syndrome. *Medicine* 25:399, 1946.
2. SELDIN DW, WILSON JD: Renal tubular acidosis, in Stanbury JB, Wyngaarden JB, Fredrickson DS (eds): *The Metabolic Basis of Inherited Disease*, ed 4. New York, McGraw-Hill, 1978
3. PINES KL, MUDGE GH: Renal tubular acidosis with osteomalacia: Report of three cases. *Am J Med* 11:302, 1951.
4. LIGHTWOOD R, PAYNE WW, BLACK JA: Infantile renal acidosis. *Pediatrics* 12:628, 1953.
5. SMITH LH JR, SCHREINER GE: Studies on renal hyperchloremic acidosis. *J Lab Clin Med* 43:347, 1954.
6. REYNOLDS TB: Observations on the pathogenisis of renal tubular acidosis. *Am J Med* 25:503, 1958.
7. WRONG O, DAVIES HEF: The excretion of acid in renal disease. *Q J Med* 28:259, 1959.
8. RELMAN AS: Renal acidosis and renal excretion of acid in health and disease. *Adv Intern Med* 12:295, 1964.
9. ELKINTON JR, McCURDY DK, BUCKALEW VM JR: Hydrogen ion and the kidney, in Black DAK (ed): *Renal Disease*, ed 2. Philadelphia, Davis, 1967, p 110.
10. RODRIQUEZ-SORIANO J, BOICHIS H, EDELMAN CM JR: Bicarbonate reabsorption and hydrogen ion excretion in children with renal tubular acidosis. *J Pediatr* 71:802, 1967.
11. MORRIS RC JR: An experimental renal acidification defect in patients with hereditary fructose intolerance. II. Its distinction from classic renal acidification defect associated with the Fanconi syndrome of children with cystinosis. *J Clin Invest* 47:1648, 1968.
12. RODRIQUEZ-SORIANO JR, EDELMANN CM JR: Renal tubular acidosis. *Ann Rev Med* 20:363, 1969.
13. MORRIS RC JR: Renal tubular acidosis: Mechanisms, classification and implications. *N Engl J Med* 281:1405, 1969.
14. McSHERRY E, SEBASTIAN A, MORRIS RC JR: Renal tubular acidosis in infants: The several kinds, including bicarbonate-wasting, classic renal tubular acidosis. *J Clin Invest* 51:499, 1972
15. SEBASTAIN A, McSHERRY E, MORRIS RC JR: Metabolic acidosis with special reference to the renal acidoses, in Brenner BM, Rector FC Jr (eds): *The Kidney*. Philadelphia, Saunders, 1976, chap 16.
16. McSHERRY E, MORRIS RC JR: Attainment and maintenance of normal stature with alkali therapy in infants and children with classic renal tubular acidosis. *J Clin Invest* 61:509, 1978.
17. MORRIS RC JR, SEBASTIAN A: Disorders of the renal tubule that cause disorders of fluid, acid-base, and electrolyte metabolism, in Maxwell MH, Kleeman CR (eds): *Clinical Disorders of Fluid and Electrolyte Metabolism*, ed 3. New York, McGraw-Hill, 1980, chap 18, p 883.
18. COGAN MG, RECTOR FC JR, SELDIN DW: Acid-base disorders, in Brenner BM, Rector FC Jr (eds): *The Kidney*, ed 2. Philadelphia, Saunders, 1981, chap 17, p 841.
19. ARRUDA JAL, KURTZMAN NA: Mechanisms and classification of deranged distal urinary acidification. *Am J Physiol* 239:F515, 1980.
20. STINEBAUGH BJ, SCHLOEDER FX, TAM SC, GOLDSTEIN MB, HALPERIN ML: Pathogenesis of distal renal tubular acidosis. *Kidney Int* 19:1, 1981.
21. PITTS RF: Renal regulation of acid-base balance, in *Physiology of the Kidney and Body Fluids: An Introductory Test*, ed 2. Chicago, Year Book, 1968.
22. LENNON EJ, LEMANN J JR, LITZOW JR: The effects of diet and stool composition on the net external acid balance of normal subjects. *J Clin Invest* 45:1601, 1966.
23. ALBERT MS, WINTERS RW: Acid-base equilibrium of blood in normal infants. *Pediatrics* 37:728, 1966.
24. RECTOR FC JR, CARTER NW, SELDIN DW: The mechanism of bicarbonate reabsorption in the proximal and distal tubules of the kidney. *J Clin Invest* 44:278, 1965.
25. BENNETT CM, BRENNER BM, BERLINER RW: Micropuncture study of nephron function in the rhesus monkey. *J Clin Invest* 47:203, 1968.
26. WARNOCK DG, RECTOR FC JR: Renal acidification mechanisms, in Brenner BM, Rector FC JR (eds), *The Kidney*, ed 2. Philadelphia, Saunders, 1981, p 440.
27. KUNAU RT JR, FRICK A, RECTOR FC JR, SELDIN DW: Micropuncture study of the proximal tubular factors responsible for the maintenance of alkalosis during potassium deficiency in the rat. *Clin Sci* 34:223, 1968.
28. JACOBSON HR: Effects of CO_2 and acetazolamide on bicarbonate and fluid transport in rabbit proximal tubules. *Am J Physiol* 9:F54, 1981.
29. SCHWARTZ WB, JENSON RL, RELMAN AS: Acidification of the urine and increased ammonia excretion without change in acid-base equilibrium: Sodium reabsorption as a stimulus to the acidifying process. *J Clin Invest* 34:673, 1955.
30. CLAPP JR, RECTOR FC JR, SELDIN DW: Effect of unreabsorbed anions on proximal and distal transtubular potentials in rats. *Am J Physiol* 202:781, 1962.
31. HULTER HN, ILNICHI LP, HARBOTTLE JA, SEBASTIAN A: Impaired renal H^+ secretion and NH_3 production in mineralocorticoid-deficient glucocorticoid-replete dogs. *Am J Med* 232:F136, 1977.
32. McKINNEY TD, BURG MB: Bicarbonate transport by rabbit cortical collecting tubules. *J Clin Invest* 60:766, 1977.
33. McKINNEY TC, BURG MB: Bicarbonate secretion by rabbit cortical collecting tubules in vitro. *J Clin Invest* 61:1421, 1978.

34. Purkerson ML, Lubowitz H, White RW, Bricker NS: On the influence of extracellular fluid volume expansion on bicarbonate reabsorption in the rat. *J Clin Invest* 48:1754, 1969.

35. Kurtzman NA: Regulation of renal bicarbonate reabsorption by extracellular volume. *J Clin Invest* 49:586, 1970.

36. Murer H, Hopfer U, Kinne R: Sodium/proton antiport in brushborder membrane vesicles isolated from rat small intestine and kidney. *Biochem J* 154:597, 1976.

37. Glynn IM, Karlish SJD: The sodium pump. *Ann Rev Physiol* 37:13, 1975.

38. Kinne-Saffran E, Kinne R: Further evidence for the existence of an intrinsic bicarbonate-stimulated Mg++-ATPase in brush border membranes isolated from rat kidney cortex. *J Membr Biol* 49:235, 1979.

39. Steinmetz PR: Characteristics of hydrogen ion transport in urinary bladder of water turtle. *J Clin Invest* 46:1531, 1967.

40. Ziegler TW, Fanestil DD, Ludens JH: Influence of transepithelial potential difference on acidification in the toad urinary bladder. *Kidney Int* 10:279, 1976.

41. Al-Awqati Q, Mueller A, Steinmetz PR: Transport of H+ against electrochemical gradients in turtle bladder. *Am J Physiol* 233:F502, 1977.

42. Steinmetz PR:: Cellular defects in urinary acidification and renal tubular acidosis, in Andreoli TE, Hoffman JF, Fanestil DD (eds): *Physiology of Membrane Disorders.* New York, Plenum, 1978, p 987.

43. Dixon TE, Al-Awqati A: Urinary acidification in turtle bladder is due to a reversible proton-translocating ATPase. *Proc Natl Acad Sci USA* 76:3135, 1979.

44. Pitts HH, Schulte JW, Smith DR: Nephrocalcinosis in a father and three children. *J Urol* 73:208, 1955.

45. Randall, RE, Targgart WH: Familial renal tubular acidosis. *Ann Intern Med* 54:1108, 1961.

46. Randall RE Jr: Familial renal tubular acidosis revisited. *Ann Intern Med* 66:1024, 1967.

47. Schreiner GE, Smith LH, Kyle LH: Renal hyperchloremic acidosis. *Am J Med* 15:122, 1953.

48. Seedat YK: Some observations of renal tubular acidosis: A family study. *S Afr Med J* 38:606, 1964.

49. Seedat YK: Renal tubular acidosis. *S Afr Med J* 41:1007, 1967.

50. Gyory AZ, Edwards KDG: Renal tubular acidosis: A family with an autosomal dominant genetic defect in renal hydrogen ion transport, with proximal tubular and collecting duct dysfunction and increased metabolism of citrate and ammonia. *Am J Med* 45:43, 1968.

51. Buckalew VM Jr, McCurdy KD, Ludwig GD, Chaykin LB, Elkinson E Jr: The syndrome of incomplete renal tubular acidosis. *Am J Med* 45:32, 1968.

52. Wilansky DL, Schucher R: Familial acidosis of renal tubular origin. *Can Med Ass J* 83:308, 1960.

53. Richards P, Wrong OM: Dominant inheritance in a family with familial renal tubular acidosis. *Lancet* 2:998, 1972.

54. Musgrave JE, Bennett WM, Campbelle RA, Eisembert CS: Letter to the editor. *Lancet* 1:1364, 1972.

55. Nebout Th, Desaine Ch, Weil B, Fournier A, Lagrue G: Acidose tubulaire distale familiale. *Sem Hop Paris* 14:557, 1974.

56. Norman ME, Cohn RM, McCurdy DK: Urinary citrate excretion in the diagnosis of distal renal tubular acidosis. *J Ped* 92:394, 1978.

57. Rodriguez-Soriano J, Vallo A, Garcia-Fuentes M: Distal renal tubular acidosis in infancy: A bicarbonate wasting state. *J Pediatr* 86:524, 1975.

58. Cohen A, Way BJ: The association of renal tubular acidosis with hyperglobulinaemic purpura. *Aust Ann Med* 11:189, 1962.

59. LoSpalluto J, Dorward B, Miller W, Ziff M: Cryoglobulinemia based on interaction between a gamma macroglobulin and 7S gamma globulin. *Am J Med* 32:142, 1962

60. Seedat YK, Rain ER: Active chronic hepatitis associated with renal tubular acidosis and successful pregnancy. *S Afr Med J* 39:595, 1965.

61. McCurdy DK, Cornwell GG II, DePratti VJ: Hyperglobulinemic renal tubular acidosis: Report of the two cases. *Ann Intern Med* 67:110, 1967.

62. Morris FC Jr, Fundenberg HH: Impaired renal acidification in patients with hypergammaglobulinemia. *Medicine* 46:57, 1967.

63. Talal N, Zisman E, Schur PH: Renal tubular acidosis, glomerulonephritis and immunologic factors in Sjögren's syndrome. *Arthritis Rheum* 2:774, 1968.

64. Shioji R, Furuyama T, Onodera S, Saito H, Ito H, Sasaki Y: Sjögren's syndrome and renal tubular acidosis. *Am J Med* 48:456, 1970.

65. Mason AMS, Golding PL: Hyperglobulinaemic renal tubular acidosis: A report of nine cases. *Br Med J* 3:143, 1970.

66. Pasternack A, Linder E: Renal tubular acidosis: An immunopathological study on four patients. *Clin Exp Immunol* 7:115, 1970.

67. Mason AMS, Golding PL: Renal tubular acidosis and autoimmune thyroid disease. *Lancet* 2:1104, 1970.

68. Mason AMS, McIllmurray MB, Golding PL, Hughes DTB: Fibrosing alveoitis associated with renal tubular acidosis. *Br Med J* 4:596, 1970.

69. Talal N: Sjögren's syndrome, lymphoproliferation, and renal tubular acidosis, editorial. *Ann Intern Med* 74:633–634, 1971.

70. Bridi GS, Falcon PW, Brackett NC Jr, Still WJS, Sporn IN: Glomerulonephritis and renal tubular acidosis in a case of chronic active hepatitis with hyperimmunoglobulinemia. *Am J Med* 52:267, 1972.

71. Tsantoulas DC, McFarlane IG, Portman B, Eddleston ALWF, Williams R: Cell-mediated immunity to human Tamm-Horsfall glycoprotein in autoimmune liver disease with renal tubular acidosis. *Br Med J* 4:491, 1974.

72. Golding PL: Renal tubular acidosis in chronic liver disease. *Postgrad Med J* 51:550, 1975.

73. Cochrane AMG, Tsantoulos DC, Moussouros A, McFarlane IG, Eddleston ALW, Williams R: Lymphocyte cytotoxicity for kidney cells in renal tubular acidosis of autoimmune liver disease. *Br Med J* 2:276, 1976.

74. Andrassy K, Gebest J, Tan E, Thoenes W, Ritz E: Interstitial Nephritis in a patient with atypical Sjögren's syndrome. *Klin Wochenschr* 58:563, 1980.

75. Buckalew VM, Purvis ML, Shulman MG et al: Hereditary renal tubular acidosis. *Medicine (Baltimore)* 53:229, 1974.

76. Hamed IA, Czerwinski AW, Coats B, Kaufman C, Altmiller DH: Familial Absorptive hypercalciuria and renal tubular acidosis. *Am J Med* 67:385, 1979.

77. Dent CE, Harper CM, Parfitt AM: The effect of cellulose phosphate on calcium metabolism in patients with hypercalciuria. *Clin Sci* 27:463, 1964.

78. Parfitt AM, Higgins BA, Nassim JR, Collins JA, Hilbs A: Metabolic studies in patients with hypercalciuria. *Clin Sci* 27:463, 1964.

79. Cohen SI, Fitzgerald MG, Fourman P, Griffiths WJ, DeWardener HE: Polyuria in hyperparathyroidism. *Q J Med* 26:423, 1964.

80. Reynolds TB, Bethune JE: Renal tubular acidosis secondary to hyperparathyroidism. *Clin Res* 17:169, 1969.

81. Zisman E, Buccino RA, Gorden P, Bartter FC: Hyperthyroidism and renal tubular acidosis. *Arch Intern Med* 121:118, 1968.

82. Ferris T, Kashgarian M, Levitin H, Brant I, Epstein FH: Renal tubular acidosis and renal potassium wasting required as a result of hypercalcemic nephropathy. *N Engl J Med* 265:924, 1961.

83. Deck MDF: Medullary sponge kidney with renal tubular acidosis: A report of 3 cases. *J Urol* 94:330, 1965.

84. Morris RC Jr, Yamauchi H, Palubinskas AJ, Howenstine J: Medullary sponge kidney. *Am J Med* 38:883, 1965.

85. Mass RF, Smithe WR, Walsh JR: The association of hereditary fructose intolerance and renal tubular acidosis. *Am J Med Sci* 251:516, 1966.

86. Fulop M, Sternlieb I, Scheinberg HH: Defective urinary acidification in Wilson's disease. *Ann Intern Med* 68:770, 1968.

87. Yeoh SA: Fabry's disease with renal tubular acidosis. *Singapore Med J* 8:275, 1967.

88. Husband P, McKellar WJD: Infantile renal tubular acidosis due to mercury poisoning. *Arch Dis Child* 45:264, 1970.

89. McCurdy DK, Frederic M, Elkinton JR: Renal tubular acidosis due to amphotericin. *N Engl J Med* 278:124, 1968.

90. Patterson RM, Ackerman GL: Renal tubular acidosis due to amphotericine B nephrotoxicity. *Arch Intern Med* 127:241, 1971.

91. Steele TW, Edwards KDG: Analgesic nephropathy: Changes in various parameters of renal function following cessation of analgesic abuse. *Med J Aust* 1:181, 1974.

92. Steel TW, Gyory AZ, Edwards KDG: Renal function in analgesic nephropathy. *Br Med J* 2:213, 1969.

93. Perez GO, Oster JR, Vaamonde BA: Incomplete syndrome of renal tubular acidosis induced by lithium carbonate. *J Lab Clin Med* 86:386, 1975.

94. Yong JM, Sanderson KV: Photosensitive dermatitis and renal tubular acidosis after ingestion of calcium cyclamate, *Lancet* 2:1273, 1969.

95. Cochran M, Peacock M, Smith PA, Nordin BEC: Renal tubular acidosis of pyelonephritis with renal stone disease. *Br Med J* 2:721, 1968.

96. Berlyne GM: Distal tubular function in chronic hydronephrosis. *Q J Med* 30:339, 1961.

97. Better OS, Arieff AI, Massry SG, Kleeman CR, Maxwell MH: Studies on renal function after relief of complete unilateral ureteral obstruction of three months' duration in man. *Am J Med* 54:234, 1973.

98. Hutcheon RA, Kaplan BS, Drummond KN: Distal renal tubular acidosis in children with chronic hydronephrosis. *J Pediatr* 89:372, 1976.

99. Wilson DR: Renal function during and following obstruction. *Ann Rev Med* 28:329, 1977.

100. Gyory AZ, Steward JG, George CRO, Miller DJ, Edward KDG: Renal tubular acidosis, acidosis due to hyperkalemia, hypercalcemia, disordered citrate metabolism and other tubular dysfunctions following human renal transplantation. *Q J Med* 38:231, 1969.

101. Wilson DR, Siddigui AA: Renal tubular acidosis after kidney transplantation. *Ann Intern Med* 79:353, 1973.

102. Drutz DJ, Gutman RA: Renal tubular acidosis in leprosy. *Ann Intern Med* 75:475, 1971.

103. LEVINE AA, MICHAEL AF JR: Ehlers-Danlos syndrome with renal tubular acidosis and medullary sponge kidneys. *J Pediatr* 71:107, 1967.

104. BAEHNER RL, GILCHRIST GS, ANDERSON EJ: Hereditary elliptocytosis and primary renal tubular acidosis in a single family. *Am J Dis Child* 115:414, 1968.

105. GOOSSENS JP, VAN EPS LWS, SCHOUTEN H, GITERSON AL: Incomplete renal tubular acidosis in sickle cell disease. *Clin Chim Acta* 41:149, 1972.

106. HO PING KONG H, ALLEYNE GAO: Defect in urinary acidification in adults with sickle-cell anaemia. *Lancet* 2:954, 1968.

107. TAKEDA R, MORIMOTO S, KURODA M, MURAKAMI M: Renal tubular acidosis, presenting as a syndrome resembling Bartter's syndrome, in a patient with arachnodatcyly. *Acta Endocrinol (Kbh)* 73:531, 1973.

108. SHAPIRA E, BEN-YOSEPH Y, EYAL FG, RUSSELL A: Enzymatically inactive red cell carbonic anhydrase B in a family with renal tubular acidosis. *J Clin Invest* 53:59, 1974.

109. KONDO T, TANIGUCHI N, TANIGUCHI K, MATSUDA I, MURAO M: Inactive form of erythrocyte carbonic anhydrase B in patients with primary renal tubular acidosis. *J Clin Invest* 62:610, 1978.

110. ROYER P, BROYER M: L'acidose renale au cours des tubulopathies congenitales, in *Proceedings of Actualites Nephrologiques de l'hopital*, Necker, Paris, Flammarion, 73, 1967.

111. DONCKERWOLCKE JRA, BIERVLIET JP, KOORWAAR G, KUYTEN R, STEKELENBURG GJ: The syndrome of renal tubular acidosis and nerve deafness. *Acta Paediatr Scand* 65:100, 1976.

112. DUNGER DB, BRENTON DP, CAIN AR: Renal tubular acidosis and nerve deafness. *Arch Dis Child* 55:221, 1980.

113. CREMERS WRJ, MONNENS LAH, MARRES EHMA: Renal tubular acidosis and sensorineural deafness. *Arch Otolaryngol* 106:287, 1980.

114. BETTER OS, GOLDSCHMID Z, CHAIMOWITZ C, ALROY GG: Defect urinary acidification in cirrhosis. *Arch Intern Med* 130:77, 1972.

115. OSTER JR, HOTCHKISS JL, CARBON M, VAAMONDE CA: Abnormal renal acidification in alcoholic liver disease. *J Lab Clin Med* 85:987, 1975.

116. SHEAR L, BONKOWSKY HL, GABUZDA GL: Renal tubular acidosis in cirrhosis. *N Engl J Med* 280:1, 1969.

117. AL-AWQATI, Q: H⁺ transport in urinary epithelia. *Am J Physiol* 235:F77, 1978.

118. AL-AWQATI Q, NORBY LH, MUELLER A, STEINMETZ PR: Characteristics of stimulation of H⁺ transport by aldosterone in turtle urinary bladder. *J Clin Invest* 58:351, 1976.

119. LUDENS JH, FANESTIL DD: Aldosterone stimulation of acidification of urine by isolated urinary bladder of the Colombian toad. *Am J Physiol* 226:1321, 1974.

120. SCHWARTZ JH, STEINMETZ PR: Metabolic energy and PCO₂ as determinants of H⁺ secretion by turtle urinary bladder. *Am J Physiol* 233:F145, 1977.

121. ARRUDA JAL, SABATINI S, WESTENFELDER C: Vanadate (V) inhibits H⁺ secretion in the turtle bladder. *Clin Res* 28:746A, 1980.

122. HARMS V, FANESTIL DD: Functions of apical membrane of toad urinary bladder: Effects of membrane impairment reagents. *Am J Physiol* 233:F607, 1977.

123. STEINMETZ PR, LAWSON LR: Effect of luminal pH on ion permeability and flows of Na⁺ and H⁺ in turtle bladder. *Am J Physiol* 220:1573, 1971.

124. BEAUWENS R, AL-AWQATI Q: Active H⁺ transport in the turtle urinary bladder: Coupling of transport to glucose oxidation. *J Gen Physiol* 68:421, 1976.

125. HUSTED RF, STEINMETZ PR: The effects of amiloride and ouabain on urinary acidification by turtle bladder. *J Pharm Exper Therap* 210:264, 1979.

126. COHEN LH, MUELLER A, STEINMETZ PR: Inhibition of the HCO₃ exit step in urinary acidification by a disulfonic stilbene. *J Clin Invest* 61:981, 1978.

127. SCHWARTZ JH, FINN JT, VAUGHN G, STEINMETZ PR: Distribution of metabolic CO₂ and the transported ion species in acidifiation by turtle bladder. *Am J Physiol* 226:283, 1974.

128. SEBASTIAN A, SCHAMBELAN M, LINDENFELD S, MORRIS RC JR: Amelioration of metabolic acidosis with fludrocortisone therapy in hyporeninemic hypoaldosteronism. *N Engl J Med* 297:576, 1977.

129. SONNENBERG H, CHEEMA-DHADLI S, GOLDSTEIN MB, STINEBAUGH BJ, WILSON DR, HALPERIN ML: Ammonia addition into the medullary collecting duct of the rat. *Kidney Int* 19:281, 1981.

130. KURTZ TW, HSU CH: Impaired distal nephron acidification in chronically phosphate depleted rats. *Pflugers Arch* 377:229, 1978.

131. ARRUDA JAL, JULKA NK, RUBINSTEIN H, SABATINI S, KURTZMAN NA: Distal acidification defect induced by phosphate depletion. *Metab* 29:826, 1980.

132. STEINMETZ PR, LAWSON LR: Defect in urinary acidification induced in vitro by amphotericin B. *J Clin Invest* 49:596, 1970.

133. FINN JT, COHEN LH, STEINMETZ PR: Acidifying defect induced by amphotericin B: Comparison of bicarbonate and hydrogen ion permeabilities. *Kidney Int* 11:261, 1977.

134. LESLIE BR, SCHWARTZ JH, STEINMETZ PR: Coupling between Cl⁻ absorption and HCO₃ secretion in turtle urinary bladder. *Am J Physiol* 225:610, 1973.

135. PAK POY RK, WRONG O: The urinary PCO₂ in renal disease. *Clin Sci* 19:631, 1960.

136. HALPERIN ML, GOLDSTEIN MB, HAIG A, JOHNSON MD, STINEBAUGH BJ: Studies on the pathogenesis of type 1 (distal renal tubular acidosis as revealed by the urinary PCO₂ tensions. *J Clin Invest* 53:669, 1974.

137. PITTS RF, AYER JL, SCHEISS W: The renal regulation of acid-base balance in man. III. The reabsorption and excretion of bicarbonate. *J Clin Invest* 28:35, 1949.

138. DUBOSE TD JR: Urine to blood PCO₂ gradient (U-B PCO₂) is an index of hydrogen ion secretion by collecting duct. *Clin Res* 29:460A, 1981.

139. DENNARD AE, WILLIAMS RJP: The catalysis of the reaction between carbon dioxide and water. *J Chem Soc (A)*:812, 1966.

140. BRESLOW E: Catalysis of carbon dioxide hydration by cupric chelates, in Plisach J, Aisen P, Blumberg WE (eds): *The Biochemistry of Copper*, New York, Academic, 1966, p 149.

141. STEBLAY RW, RUDOFSKY UH: Transfer of experimental autoimmune renal cortical tubular and interstitial disease in guinea pigs by serum. *Science* 180:166, 1973.

142. ANDRES GA, McCLUSKEY RT: Tubular and interstitial renal disease due to immunologic mechanisms. *Kidney Int* 7:271, 1975.

143. WISTRAND PJ, LINDAHL S, WAHLSTRAND T: Human renal carbonic anhydrase. *Eur J Biochem* 57:189, 1975.

144. McKINLEY DN, WHITNEY PL: Particulate carbonic anhydrase in homogenates of human kidney. *Biochim Biophys Acta* 445:780, 1976.

145. WISTRAND PJ, KINNE R: Carbonic anhydrase activity of isolated brush border and basal-lateral membranes of renal tubular cells. *Pflugers Arch* 370:121, 1977.

146. WISTRAND PJ: Renal membrane-bound carbonic anhydrase: Purification and properties. *Upsala J Med Sci* 26 (suppl):75, 1979.

147. FOURMAN P, ROBINSON JR: Diminished urinary excretion of citrate during deficiencies of potassium in man. *Lancet* 265 (2):656, 1953.

148. HARRISON HE: Mechanisms of action of vitamin D. *Pediatrics* 14:285, 1954.

149. HARRISON HE, CHISOLM JJ JR, HARRISON HC: Congenital renal tubular acidosis. *Am J Dis Child* 96:588, 1958.

150. FRICK PG, RUBINI ME, MERONEY WH: Recurrent nephrolithiasis associated with an unusual tubular defect and hyperchloremic acidosis. *Am J Med* 25:590, 1958.

151. DEDMON RE, WRONG O: The excretion of organic anion in renal tubular acidosis with particular reference to citrate. *Clin Sci* 22:19, 1962.

152. MORRISEY JF, OCHOA M JR, ZOTSPEICH WD, WATERHOUSE C: Citrate excretion in renal tubule acidosis. *Ann Intern Med* 58:159, 1963.

153. BRODWALL EK, WESTLIE L, MYHRE E: The renal excretion and tubular reabsorption of citric acid in renal tubular acidosis. *Acta Med Scand* 192:137, 1972.

154. McSHERRY EM, POKROY MV, MORRIS RC JR: The nonoccurrence of nephrocalcinosis in children with type 1 RTA given high-dose alkali therapy, in preparation, 1981.

155. CRAWFORD MA, MILNE MD, SCRIBNER BH: The effects of changes in acid-base balance on urinary citrate in the rat. *J Physiol* 149:413, 1959.

156. HARRISON HE, HARRISON HC: Inhibition of urine citrate excretion and the production of renal calcinosis in the rat by acetazoleamide (Diamox) administration. *J Clin Invest* 34(11):1962, 1955.

157. SIMPSON DP: Tissue citrate levels and citrate utilization after socium bicarbonate administration. *Proc Soc Exp Biol Med* 114:263, 1963.

158. SIMPSON DP, ANGIELSKI S: Regulation by bicarbonate ion of intramitochondrial citrate concentration in kidney mitochondria. *Biochim Biophys Acta* 298:115, 1973.

159. ROBINSON BH, OEI J, SHEEMA-DHADLI S, HALPERIN ML: Regulation of citrate transport and pyruvate dehydrogenase in rat kidney cortex mitochondria by bicarbonate. *J Biol Chem* 16:5661, 1977.

160. NEUMAN WF, NEUMAN MW: *The Chemical Dynamics of Bone Mineral*, Chicago, University of Chicago Press, 1958.

161. BISAZ S, FELIX R, NEWMAN WF, FLEISCH H: Quantitative determination of inhibitors of calcium phosphate precipitation in whole urine. *Min Electrol Metab* 1:74, 1978.

162. FARQUHARSON F, SALTER WT, TIBETTS DM: Studies of calcium and phosphorus metabolism. XII. The effect of the ingestion of acid-producing substances. *J Clin Invest* 10:221, 1931.

163. LEMANN J JR, LITZOW JR, LENNON EJ: The effects of chronic acid loads in normal man: Further evidence for participation of bone mineral in the defense against chronic metabolic acidosis. *J Clin Invest* 45:1608, 1975.

164. WRONG OM, FEEST TG: The natural history of distal renal tubular acidosis. *Contr Nephrol* 21:137, 1980.

165. GREENBERG AJ, McNAMARA H, McCRORY WW: Metabolic balance studies in primary renal tubular acidosis: Effects of acidosis on external calcium and phosphorus balances. *J Pediatr* 69:4610, 1966.

166. Lee SW, Russel JE, Avioli LV: 25-OHD$_3$ to 1,25-(OH)$_2$D$_3$ conversion impaired by systemic acidosis. *Science* 195:944, 1977.

167. Raisz LG, Trummel CL, Holick MF, DeLuca HF: 1,25-Dihydroxycholecalciferol: A potent stimulator of bone resorption in tissue culture. *Science* 175:768, 1972.

168. Boyle IT, Miravet L, Gray RW, Holick MF, DeLuca HF: The response of intestinal calcium transport to 25-hydroxy and 1,25-dihydroxy vitamin D in nephrectomized rats. *Endocrinology* 90:605, 1972.

169. Norman HW, Henry H: 1,25-Dihydroxycholecalciferol: A hormonally active form of vitamin D$_3$. *Rec Prog Horm Res* 30:431, 1974.

170. DeLuca HF: Some new concepts emanating from a study of the metabolism and function of vitamin D. *Nutrition Rev* 38: 169, 1980.

171. Weber HP, Gray RW, Dominguez JH, Lemann J Jr: the lack of effect of chronic metabolic acidosis on 25-OH-vitamin D metabolism and serum parathyroid hormone in humans. *J Clin Endocrinol Metab* 43: 1047, 1976.

172. Gafter U, Graut JA, Lee DBN, Silis V, Walling MW, Kurokawa K, Haussler MR, Coburn JW: Effect of metabolic acidosis on intestinal absorption of calcium and phosphorus. *Am J Physiol* 239: G480, 1980.

173. Courey RW, Pfister RC: The radiographic findings in renal tubular acidosis. *Diag Radiol* 105: 497, 1972.

174. Coe FL: Evidence for mild reversible hyperparathyroidism in distal renal tubular acidosis. *Arch Intern Med* 135: 1485, 1975.

175. Coe FL, Firpo JJ, Hollandsworth DL, Segil L, Canterbury JM, Reiss E: Effect of acute and chronic metabolic acidosis on serum immunoreactive parathyroid hormone in man. *Kidney Int* 8: 262, 1975

176. Coe FL, Parks JH: Stone disease in hereditary distal renal tubular acidosis. *Ann Intern Med* 93: 60, 1980.

177. Foss GL, Perry CB, Wood FJY: Renal tubular acidosis. *Q J Med* 98: 185, 1956.

178. Richard P, Wrong OM, Chamberlain MJ: Treatment of osteomalacia of renal tubular acidosis by sodium bicarbonate alone. *Lancet* 2: 994, 1972.

179. Chesney RW, Moorthy AV, Eisman JA, Jax DK, Mazess RB, DeLuca HF: Increased growth after long term oral 1,25-vitamin D$_3$ in childhood renal osteodystrophy. *N Engl J Med* 298: 236, 1978.

180. Morris RC Jr, Sebastian A, McSherry E: Renal acidosis. *Kidney Int* 1:322, 1972.

181. Sebastian A, McSherry E, Morris RC Jr: On the mechanisms of renal potassium wasting in renal tubular acidosis associated with Fanconi syndrome (type 2 RTA). *J Clin Invest* 50: 231, 1971.

182. Gill JR Jr, Bell NH, Bartter FC: Impaired conservation of sodium and potassium in renal acidosis and its correction by buffer anions. *Clin Sci* 33: 577, 1967.

183. Sebastian A, McSherry E, Morris RC Jr: Renal potassium wasting in renal tubular acidosis (RTA): Its occurrence in types 1 and 2 RTA despite sustained correction of systemic acidosis. *J Clin Invest* 50: 667, 1971.

184. Sebastian A, McSherry E, Morris RC Jr: Impaired renal conservation of sodium and chloride during sustained correction of systemic acidosis in patients with type 1, classic renal tubular acidosis. *J Clin Invest* 58: 454, 1976

185. Rodriguez-Soriano J, Vallo A, Oliveros R: Bartter's syndrome presenting with features resembling renal tubular acidosis. *Helv Paediat Acta*, 33: 141, 1978.

186. Dillon MJ, Shah V, Mitchell MD: Bartter's syndrome: 10 cases in childhood: Results of long-term indomethacin therapy. *Q J Med* 48: 429, 1979.

187. Morris RC Jr, Sebastian A, McSherry E: Therapeutic experience in patients with classic renal tubular acidosis. *Proc VII International Cong Nephrol.* Basel, S. Karger, 1978, p. 345.

188. Worthen HG, Good RA: The de Toni-Fanconi syndrome with cystinosis. *Am J Dis Child* 95: 653, 1958.

189. Lamy M, Freza J, Rey J, Larsen C: Etude metabolique due syndrome de Lowe. *Rev Eur Etud Clin Biol* 7: 271, 1962.

190. Saville PD, Nassim JR, Stevenson H, Mulligan L, Carey N: The effect of A.T.10 on calcium and phosphorus metabolism in resistant rickets. *Clin Sci* 14: 489, 1955.

191. Lee DBN, Drinkard JP, Rosen VJ, Gonick HC: The adult Fanconi syndrome. *Medicine (Baltimore)* 51: 107, 1972.

192. Hunt DD, Stearns G, McKinley JB, Foning E, Hicks P, Bonfiglio M: Long-term study of a family with Fanconi syndrome without cystinosis (DeToni-Debre-Fanconi syndrome). *Am J Med* 40: 492, 1966.

193. Smith R, Lindenbaum RH, Walton RJ: Hypophosphateaemic osteomalacia and Fanconi syndrome of adult onset with dominant inheritance. *Q J Med* 179: 397, 1976.

194. Litin RB, Randall RV, Goldstein NP, Power NH, Diessner GR: Hypercalciuria in hepatolenticular degeneration (Wilson's disease). *Am J Med Sci* 238: 614, 1959.

195. Wilson DM, Goldstein NP: Bicarbonate excretion in Wilson's disease (hepatolenticular degeneration). *Mayo Clin Proc* 49: 394, 1954.

196. Gentz J, Jagenburg R, Zetterstron R: Tyrosinemia. *J Pediatr* 66: 670, 1965.

197. Gruskin AB, Patel MS, Lindshaw M, Ettenger R, Huff D, Grover W: Renal function studies and kidney pyruvate carboxylase in subacute necrotizing encephalomyelopathy (Leight's syndrome). *Pediatr Res* 7: 932, 1973.

198. Rodriguez-Soriano J, Rivera JM, Vallo A, Prats-Vinas JM, Castillo G: Proximal renal tubular acidosis in metachromatic leukodystrophy. *Helv Paediat Acta* 33: 45, 1978.

199. Guiganar JP, Torrado A: Proximal tubular acidosis in vitamin D deficient rickets. *Acta Paediatr Scand* 62: 543, 1973.

200. Muldowney FP, Donohoe JF, Freaney R, Kampff C, Swan M: Parathormone-induced renal bicarbonate wastage in intestinal malabsorption and in chronic renal failure. *Ir J Med Sci* 3: 221, 1970.

201. Vainsel M, Manderlier TH, Viss HL: Proximal renal tubular acidosis in vitamin D deficiency rickets. *Biomedicine* 22: 35, 1974.

202. Scott J, Elias E, Moult PJA, Barnes S, Wills MR: Rickets in adult cystic fibrosis with myopathy, pancreatic insufficiency and proximal renal tubular dysfunction. *Am J Med* 63: 488, 1977.

203. Stoop JW, Schraagen MJC, Tiddens HAWM: Pseudo-vitamin D deficiency rickets. *Acta Paediatr Scand* 56: 607, 1967.

204. Wegienka LC, Weller JM: Renal tubular acidosis caused by degraded tetracycline. *Arch Intern Med* 114: 232, 1964.

205. Otten J, Vis HL: Acute reversible renal tubular dysfunction following intoxication with methyl-3-chromone. *J Pediatr* 73: 422, 1968.

206. Sadoff L: Nephrotoxicity of streptozotocin. *Cancer Chemother Rep* 54: 457, 1970.

207. Chisolm JJ, Harrison HC, Eberlein WR, Harrison HE: Amionaciduria, hypophosphatemia, and rickets in lead poisoning. *Am J Dis Child* 89: 159, 1955.

208. Sebastian A, McSherry E, Ueki I, Morris RC Jr: Renal amyloidosis, nephrotic syndrome and impaired renal tubular reabsorption of bicarbonate. *Ann Intern Med* 69: 541, 1968.

209. Stickler GB, Rosevear JW, Ulrich JA: Renal tubular dysfunction complicating the nephrotic syndrome: The disturbance in calcium and phosphorus metabolism. *Mayo Clin Proc* 37:376, 1972.

210. Tegelaers WHH, Tiddens HW: Nephrotic-glucosuric-aminoaciduric dwarfism and electrolyte metabolism. *Helv Paediatr Acta* 10: 269, 1955.

211. Massry SG, Preuss HG, Maher JF, Schreiner GE: Renal tubular acidosis after cadaver kidney homotransplantations. *Am J Med* 42: 284, 1967.

212. Morris RC Jr: The clinical spectrum of Fanconi's syndrome. *Calif Med* 108: 225, 1968.

213. Riley AL, Ryan LM, Roth DA: Renal proximal tubular dysfunction and paroxysmal nocturnal hemoglobinurea. *Am J Med* 62: 125, 1977.

214. Cade R, Spooner G, Juncos L, Fuller T, Tarrant D, Raulerson D, Mahoney J, Pickering M, Grubb W, Marbury T: Chronic renal vein thrombosis. *Am J Med* 63: 387, 1977.

215. Sirota JH, Hamerman D: Renal function studies in an adult subject with the Fanconi syndrome. *Am J Med* 16: 138, 1954.

216. Engle RL, Wallis LA: Multiple myeloma and the adult Fanconi syndrome. I. Report of a case with crystal-like deposits in the tumor cells and in the epithelial cells of the kidney. *Am J Med* 22: 5, 1957.

217. Harrison JF, Blainey JD: Adult Fanconi syndrome with monoclonal abnormality of immunoglobulin light chains. *J Clin Pathol* 20:42, 1967.

218. Maldonado JE, Velosa JE, Kyle RA, Wagoner RD, Halley KE, Salassa RM: Fanconi syndrome in adults: A manifestation of a latent form of myeloma. *Am J Med* 58: 354, 1975.

219. Smithline N, Kassirer JP, Cohen JJ: Light-chain nephropathy: Renal tubular dysfunction associated with the light-chain proteinuria. *N Engl J Med* 291: 71, 1976.

220. Nash MA, Torrado AD, Greifer I, Spitzer A, Edelmann CM Jr: Renal tubular acidosis in infants and children. *J Pediatr* 80: 738, 1972.

221. Donckerwolcke RA, VanStekelenburg GJ, Tiddens HA: a case of bicarbonate-losing renal tubular acidosis with defective carbonic anhydrase activity. *Arch Dis Child* 45: 769, 1970.

222. Brenes LG, Brenes JN, Hernandez MM: Familial proximal tubular acidosis. *Am J Med* 63: 244, 1977.

223. Winsnes A, Monn E, Stokke O, Feyling T: Congenital, persistent proximal type renal tubular acidosis in two brothers. *Acta Paediatr Scand* 68: 861, 1979.

224. Vainsel M, Fondu P, Cadranel S, Rocmans CL, Gepts W: Osteopetrosis associated with proximal and distal tubular acidosis. *Acta Paediatr Scand* 61: 429, 1972.

225. Guibaud P, Larbre F, Freycon M-T, Genoud J: Osteopetrose et acidose renale tubulaire deux cas de cette association dans une fratrie. *Arch Franc Ped* 29: 269, 1972.

226. Ohlsson A, Stark G, Sakati N: Marble brain disease: recessive osteopetrosis, renal tubular acidosis and cerebral calcification in three Saudi Arabian families. *Develop Med Child Neurol* 22: 72, 1980.

227. Whyte MP, Murphy WA, Fallon MD, Sly WS, Teitelbaum SL, McAlister WH, Avioli LV: Osteopetrosis, renal tubular acidosis and basal ganglia calcification in three sisters. *Am J Med* 69: 64, 1980.

228. RECTOR FC JR, SELDIN DW, ROBERTS AD JR, SMITH JS: The role of plasma CO_2 tension and carbonic anhydrase activity in the renal reabsorption of bicarbonate. *J Clin Invest* 39: 1706, 1960.

229. LEAF A, SCHWARTZ WB, RELMAN AS: Oral administration of a potent carbonic anhydrase inhibitor ("Diamox"). *N Engl J Med* 250: 759, 1954.

230. SELDIN DW, PORTWOOD RM, RECTOR FC JR, CADE R: Characteristics of renal bicarbonate reabsorption in man. *J Clin Invest* 38: 1663, 1959.

231. BECKMAN WW, ROSSMEISL EC, PETTINGILL RB, BAUER W: Study of effect of sulfanilamide on acid-base metabolism. *J Clin Invest* 19: 635, 1940.

232. YORK SE, YENDT ER: Osteomalacia associated with renal bicarbonate loss. *Can Med Assoc J* 94: 1329, 1966.

233. RODRIGUEZ-SORIANO J, VALLO A, CHOUZA M, CASSTILLO G: Proximal renal tubular acidosis in tetralogy of fallot. *Acta Paediatr Scand* 64: 671, 1975.

234. HELLMAN DE, AU WYW, BARTTER FC: Evidence of a direct effect of parathyroid hormone on urinary acidification. *Am J Physiol* 209: 643, 1965.

235. SIDDIQUI AA, WILSON DR: Primary hyperparathyroidism and proximal renal tubular acidosis: Report of two cases. *Can Med Assoc J* 106: 654, 1972.

236. COE FL: Magnitude of metabolic acidosis in primary hyperparathyroidism. *Arch Intern Med* 134: 262, 1974.

237. BANK N, AYNEDJIAN HS: A micropuncture study of the effect of parathyroid hormone on renal bicarbonate reabsorption. *J Clin Invest* 58: 336, 1976.

238. CRUMB CK, MARTINEZ-MALDONADO M, EKNOYAN G, SUKI WN: Effects of volume expansion purified parathyroid extract and calcium on renal bicarbonate absorption in the dog. *J Clin Invest* 54: 1287, 1974.

239. KARLINSKY ML, SAGER DS, KURTZMAN NA: Effect of parathormone and cyclic adenosine monophosphate on renal bicarbonate reabsorption. *Am J Physiol* 277: 1226, 1974.

240. HERMKENS H, NAWAR T, CARON C, PLANTE GE: Effect of parathyroid hormone on renal excretion of sodium and hydrogen ions. *Can J Physiol Pharmacol* 55: 628, 1977.

241. GOLD LW, MASSRY SG, ARIEFF AI, COBURN JW: Renal bicarbonate wasting during phosphate depletion: A possible cause of altered acid-base homeostasis in hyperparathyroidism. *J Clin Invest* 52: 2556, 1973.

242. FRALEY D, ADLER S: An extrarenal role for parathyroid hormone in the disposal of acute acid loads in rats and dogs. *J Clin Invest* 63: 985, 1979.

243. ALLA V, RUBINSTEIN H, CRUZ-SOTO M, SABATINI S, ARRUDA JAL, KURTZMAN NA: Extrarenal acid buffering: Role and mechanism of action of PTH in normal and in renal failure. *Abstract Proc Am Soc Neph* 12: 76, 1979.

244. EMMETT M, GOLDFARB S, AGUS ZS, NARINS RG: The pathophysiology of acid-base changes in chronically phosphate-depleted rats. *J Clin Invest* 59: 291, 1977.

245. EDELMANN CM JR, HOUSTON IB, RODRIGUEZ-SORIANO J, BIOCHIS H, STARK H: Renal excretion of hydrogen ion in children with idiopathic growth retardation. *J Pediatr* 72: 443, 1968.

246. ARANT BS, GREIFER I, EDELMANN CM JR, SPITZER A: Effect of chronic salt and water loading on the tubular defects of a child with Fanconi syndrome (cystinosis). *Pediatrics* 58: 3, 1976.

247. GIEBISCH G: Some reflections on the mechanism of renal tubular potassium transport. *Yale J Biol Med* 48: 315, 1975.

248. RUBINI ME: Water excretion in potassium deficient man. *J Clin Invest* 40: 2215, 1961.

249. MANNITIUS A, LEVITIN H, BECK D, EPSTEIN FH: On the mechanism of renal concentrating ability in potassium deficiencies. *J Clin Invest* 39: 684, 1960.

250. BERL T, LINAS SL, AISENBREY GA, ANDERSON RJ: On the mechanism of polyuria in potassium depletion. *J Clin Invest* 60: 620, 1977.

251. RAMPINI S, FANCONI A, ILLIG R, PRADER A: Effect of a hydrochlorothiazide on proximal renal tubular acidosis in a patient with idiopathic "de-Toni-Debre-Fanconi syndrome." *Helv Paediatr Acta* 23: 13, 1967.

252. OETLIKER O, ROSSI E: The influence of extracellular fluid volume on the renal bicarbonate threshold; a study in two children with Lowe's syndrome. *Pediatr Res* 3: 140, 1969.

253. DONCKERWOLCKE RA, VAN STEKELENBURG GJ, TIDDENS HA: Therapy of bicarbonate-losing renal tubular acidosis. *Arch Dis Child* 45: 774, 1970.

254. BEYER KH: The mechanism of action of chlorothiazide. *Ann NY Acad Sci* 71: 363, 1958.

255. VANBIERVLIET JPGM, DONCKERWOLCKE RAMG, VANSTEKELENBURG GL, WADMAN SK: Sodium chloride restriction and extracellular fluid volume contraction in hyperphosphaturic vitamin D resistant rickets in the Lowe syndrome. *Helv Paediatr Acta* 30: 365, 1975.

256. IMAI M, IGARASHI Y, SOKABE H: Plama renin activity in congenital virilizing adrenal hyperplasia. *Pediatrics* 41: 897, 1968.

257. OETLIKER O, ZURBRUGG RP: Renal tubular acidosis in salt-losing syndrome of congenital adrenal hyperplasia (CAH). *J Clin Endocrinol Metab* 31: 447, 1970.

258. ROSLER A, THEODOR R, BOICHIS H, GERTY R, ULICK S, ALAGEM M, TABACHNIK E, COHEN B, RABINOWITZ D: Metabolic responses to the administration of angiotensin II, K and ACTH in two salt-wasting syndromes. *J Clin Endocrinol Metab* 44: 292, 1977.

259. ROSLER A, RABINOWITZ D, THEODOR R, RAMIREZ LC, ULICK S: The nature of the defect in a salt wasting disorder in Jews of Iran. *J Clin Endocrinol Metab* 44: 297, 1977.

260. ULICK S: Diagnosis and nomenclature of the disorders of the terminal portion of the aldosterone biosynthetic pathway. *J Clin Endocrinol Metab* 43: 92, 1976.

261. DAVID R, GOLAN S, DRUCKER W: Familial aldosterone deficiency: Enzyme defect, diagnosis, and clinical course. *Pediatrics* 41: 403, 1968.

262. ROSLER A, GAZIT E, THEODOR R, BIOCHIS H, RABINOWITZ D: Salt wastage, raised plasma-resin activity, and normal or high plasma-aldosterone: A form of pseudohypoaldosteronism. *Lancet* 1: 959, 1973.

263. SCHAMBELAN M, STOCKGIT JR, BIGLIERI EG: Isolated hypoaldosteronism in adults, a renin deficiency syndrome. *N Engl J Med* 287: 573, 1972.

264. PEREZ G, SIEGEL L, SCHREINER GE: Selective hypoaldosteronism with hyperkalemia. *Ann Intern Med* 76: 757, 1972.

265. BROWN JJ, CHINN RH, FRASER R, LEVER AF, MORTON JJ, ROBERTSON JIS, TREE M, WAITE MA, PARK DM: Recurrent hyperkalaemia due to selective aldosterone deficiency: Correction by angiotensin infusion. *Br Med J* 1: 650, 1973.

266. WEIDMANN P, REINHART R, MAXWELL MH, ROWE P, COBURN JW, MASSRY SG: Syndrome of hyporeninemic hypoaldosteronism. *J Clin Endocrinol Metab* 36: 965, 1973.

267. OH MS, CARROLL JH, CLEMMONS JE, VAGNUCCI AH, LEVISON SP, WHANG ESM: A mechanism for hyporeninemic hypoaldosteronism in chronic renal disease. *Metabolism* 23: 1157, 1974.

268. PEREZ GO, OSTER JR, VAAMONDE CA: Renal acidosis and renal potassium handling in selective hypoaldosteronism. *Am J Med* 57: 809, 1974.

269. PEREZ GO, OSTER JR, VAAMONDE CA: Renal acidification in patients with mineralocorticoid deficiency. *Nephron* 17: 461, 1976.

270. MARIEB MJ, MELBY JC, LYALL SS: Isolated hypoaldosteronism associated with idiopathic hypoparathyroidism. *Arch Intern Med* 134: 424, 1974.

271. MELLINGER RC, PETERMANN FL, JURGENSON JC: Hyponatremia with low urinary aldosterone occurring in an old woman. *J Clin Endocrinol Metab* 34: 85, 1972.

272. MCGIFF JC, MUZZARELLI RE, DUFFY PA, GONZALEZ Y, PEIRCE CE, FRAWLEY TF: Interrelationships of renin and aldosterone in a patient with hypoaldosteronism. *Am J Med* 48: 247, 1970.

273. RUSSELL A, LEVIN B, SINCLAIR L, OBERHOLZER VG: A reversible salt-wasting syndrome of the newborn and infant. *Arch Dis Child* 38: 313, 1963.

274. CHEEK DB, PERRY JW: A salt wasting syndrome in infancy. *Arch Dis Child* 33: 252, 1958.

275. DONNELL GN, LITMAN N, ROLDAN M: Pseudohypo-adrenalocortism. *Am J Dis Child* 97: 813, 1959.

276. LELONG M, ALAGILLE D, PHILIPPE A, GENTIL C, GABILAN J-C: Diabete salin par insensibilite congenitale du tubule a l'aldosterone: "pseudo-hypo-adrenocorticisme." *Rev Franc Etudes Clin et Biol* 5: 558, 1960.

277. RAINE DN, ROY J: A salt-losing syndrome in infancy. Pseudohypoadrenocorticalism. *Arch Dis Child* 37: 548, 1962.

278. ROYER P, BONNETTE J, MATHIEU H, GABILAN J-C, KLUTCHKO G, ZITTOUN R: Pseudo-hypoaldosteronisme. *Ann de Pediatrie* 54: 596, 1963.

279. TRUNG PH, PIUSSAN C, RODARY C, LEGRAND S, ATTAL C, MOSSICONACCI P: Etude du taux de secretion de l'aldosterone et de l'activite de la renine plasmatique d'un cas de pseudo-hypoaldosteronisme. *Arch Franc Ped* 27: 603, 1970.

280. BARAKAT AY, PAPADOPOULOU ZL, AUGUST GP: A hyperkalemic, salt-wasting syndrome in infancy. *Pediatr Res* 6: 394, 1972.

281. PROESMANS W, GEUSSENS H, CORBEEL L, EECKELS R: Pseudohypoaldosteronism. *Am J Dis Child* 126: 510, 1973.

282. ALVAREZ MN, BARNES ND, STICKLER GB: Salt wasting nephropathy of "pseudohypoaldosteronism" in twins. *Pediatr Res* 8: 453, 1974.

283. SAVITT H, MOLITCH M, KAWAOKA E, LEAKE R: Pseudohypoaldosteronism. *Clin Res* 23: 165A, 1975.

284. ROY C: Pseudohypoaldosteronisme familial (a propos de 5 cas). *Arch Franc Ped* 34: 37, 1977.

285. BONNICI F: Pseudohypoaldosteronisme familial. A transmission autosomique recessive. *Arch Franc Ped* 34: 915, 1977.

286. KAUFMAN E, HAYEK A, GREENBERG R: Pseudohypoaldosteronism in triplets. *Pediatr Res* 11: 426, 1977.

287. LAURAS B, RAVUSSIN J-J, DAVID M, FREYCON F, JEUNE M: Pseudohypoaldosteronisme chez l'enfant. Apropos de quatre observations dont deux concernant des freres. *Pediatrie* 33: 119, 1978.

288. LIMAL JM, RAPPAPORT R, DECHAUX M, RIFFAUD C, MORIN C: Familial dominant pseudohypoaldosteronism. *Lancet* 1:51, 1978.

289. HANUKOGLU A, FRIED D, GOTLIEB A: Inheritance of pseudohypoaldosteronism. *Lancet* 1:1359, 1978.

290. BLACHER Y, KAPLAN BS, GRIFFEL B, LEVIN S: Pseudohypoaldosteronism. *Clin Neph* 11: 281, 1979.

291. ROSENBERG S, FRANKS RC, ULICK S: Mineralocorticoid unresponsiveness with severe neonatal hyponatremia and hyperkalemia. *J Clin Endo Metab* 50: 401, 1980.

292. OBERFIELD SE, LEVINE LS, CAREY RM, BEJAR R, NEW MI: Pseudohypoaldosteronism: Multiple target organ unresponsiveness to mineralocorticoid hormones. *J Clin Endocrinol Metab* 48: 228, 1979.

293. HOGG RJ, FROLICH J, MARVER D, MARKS JF: The basic defect in pseudohypoaldosteronism. *Clin Res* 26: 828A, 1978.

294. BIERICH JR, SCHMIDT U: Tubular Na, K-ATPase deficiency, the cause of the congenital renal salt-losing syndrome. *Europ J Pediat* 121: 81, 1976.

295. ANAND SK, FROBERG L, NORTHWAY JD, WEINBERGER M, WRIGHT JC: Pseudohypoaldosteronism due to sweat gland dysfunction. *Pediat Res* 10:677, 1976.

296. POSTEL-VINAY M-C, ALBERTI GM, RICOUR C, LIMAL J-M, RAPPAPORT R, ROYER P: Pseudohypoaldosteronism: Persistence of hyperaldosteronism and evidence for renal tubular and intestinal responsiveness to endogenous aldosterone. *J Clin Endocrinol Metab* 39: 1038, 1974.

297. POPOVTZER MM, ROSLER A, CERASI E, SHERZER P, CZACZKES JW: Na$^+$−K−ATPase deficiency: A possible mechanism of renal salt-wasting in a newborn baby with "pseudohypoaldosteronism." *Clin Res* 28: 563A, 1980.

298. PETERSEN S, GIESE J, KAPPELGAARD AM, LUND HT, LUND JO, NIELSEN MD, THOMSEN AC: Pseudohypoaldosteronism: Clinical, biochemical and morphological studies in a long-term follow-up. *Acta Paediatr Scand* 67: 255, 1978.

299. COGAN MG, ARIEFF AI: Sodium wasting, acidosis, and hyperkalemia induced by methicillin interstitial nephritis: Evidence for selective distal tubular dysfunction. *Am J Med* 64: 500, 1978.

300. PAVER WKA, PAULINE GJ: Hypertension and hyperpotassaemia without renal disease in a young male. *Med J Aust* 2: 305, 1964.

301. STOKES GS, GENTLE JL, EDWARDS KDG, STEWARD JH: Syndrome of idiopathic hyperkalaemia and hypertension with decreased plasma renin activity: Effects on plasma renin and aldosterone of reducing the serum potassium level. *Med J Aust* 2: 1050, 1968.

302. ARNOLD JE, HEALY JK: Hyperkalemia, hypertension and systemic acidosis without renal failure associated with a tubular defect in potassium excretion. *Am J Med* 47: 461, 1979.

303. GORDON RD, GEDDES RA, PAWSEY GK, O'HALLORAN MW: Hypertension and severe hyperkalaemia associated with suppression of renin and aldosterone and completely reversed by dietary sodium restriction. *Aust Ann Med* 4: 287, 1970.

304. SPITZER A, EDELMANN CM JR, GOLDBERG LD, HENNEMAN PH: Short stature, hyperkalemia and acidosis: A defect in renal transport of potassium. *Kidney Int* 3: 251, 1973.

305. WEINSTEIN SF, ALLAN DME, MENDOZA SA: Hyperkalemia, acidosis, and short stature associated with a defect in renal potassium excretion. *J Pediatr* 85: 355, 1974.

306. BRAUTBAR N, LEVI J, ROSLER A, LEITESDORF E, DJALDETI M, EPSTEIN M, KLEEMAN CR: Familial hyperkalemia, hypertension, and hyporeninemia with normal aldosterone levels: A tubular defect in potassium handling. *Arch Intern Med* 138: 607, 1978.

307. FARFEL Z, IAINA A, ROSENTHAL T, WAKS U, SHIBOLET S, GAFNI J: Familial hyperpotassemia and hypertension accompanied by normal plasma aldosterone levels: Possible hereditary cell membrane defect. *Arch Intern Med* 138: 1828, 1978.

308. LEE MR, BALL SG, THOMAS TH, MORGAN DB: Hypertension and hyperkalaemia responding to bendrofluazide. *Q J Med* 48: 245, 1979.

309. SCHAMBELAN M, SEBASTIAN A, RECTOR FC JR: Mineralocorticoid-resistant renal hyperkalemia without salt wasting (type II pseudohypoaldosteronism): Role of increased renal chloride reabsorption. *Kidney Int* 19: 716, 1981.

310. SZYLMAN P, BETTER O, CHAIMOWITZ C, ROSLER A: Role of hyperkalemia in the metabolic acidosis of isolated hypoaldosteronism. *N Engl J Med* 294: 361, 1976.

311. BATLLE DC, ARRUDA JAL, KURTZMAN NA: Hyperkalemic distal renal tubular acidosis associated with obstructive uropathy. *N Engl J Med* 304: 373, 1981.

312. DEFRONZO RA, GOLDBERG M, COOKE CR, BARKER C, GROSSMAN RA, AGUS ZS: Investigation into the mechanisms of hyperkalemia following renal transplantation. *Kidney Int* 11: 357, 1977.

313. BATLLE DC, MOZES MF, MANALIGOD J, ARRUDA JAL, KURTZMAN NA: The pathogenesis of hyperchloremic metabolic acidosis associated with kidney transplantation. *Am J Med* 70: 786, 1981.

314. DEFRONZO RA, COOKE R, GOLDBERG M, COX M, MYERS AR, AGUS ZS: Impaired renal tubular potassium secretion in systemic lupus erythematosus. *Ann Intern Med* 86: 268, 1977.

315. CARROLL HJ, FARBER SJ: Hyperkalemia and hyperchloremic acidosis in chronic pyelonephritis. *Metabolism* 13: 808, 1964.

316. LATHEM W: Hyperchloremic acidosis in chronic pyelonephritis. *N Engl J Med* 258: 1031, 1958.

317. HANDLER NM, GILL JR JR, GARDNER JD: Impaired renal tubular secretion of potassium, elevated sweat sodium chloride concentration and plasma inhibition of erythrocyte sodium outflux as complications of systemic lupus erythematosus. *Arthritis Rheum* 15: 515, 1972.

318. GYORY AZ, STEWARD JH, GEORGE CRP, TILLER DJ, EDWARDS KDG: Renal tubular acidosis, acidosis due to hyperkalemia, hypercalcemia, disordered citrate metabolism and other tubular dysfunctions following human renal transplantation. *Q J Med* 38: 231, 1969.

319. RUBINI ME, SANFORD JP, MERONEY WH: Studies of potassium secretion in glomerulonephritis. *Am J Med* Nov.: 790, 1977.

320. POSNER JB, JACOBS DR: Isolated analdosteronism: I. Clinical entity, with manifestations of persistent hyperkalemia, periodical paralysis, salt-losing tendency and acidosis. *Metabolism* 13: 513, 1964.

321. JACOBS DR, POSNER JB: Isolated analdosteronism: II. The nature of the adrenal cortical enzymatic defect, and the influence of diet and various agents on electrolyte balance. *Metabolism* 13: 522, 1964.

322. HILL SR, NICKERSON JF, CHENAULT SB, MCNEIL JH, STARNES WR, GAUTNEY MC: Studies in man on hyper- and hypoaldosterism. *Arch Intern Med* 104: 156, 1959.

323. LUKE RG, ALLISON MEM, DAVIDSON JF, DUGUID WP: Hyperkalemia and renal tubular acidosis due to renal amyloidosis. *Ann Intern Med* 70: 1211, 1969.

324. SCHAMBELAN M, SEBASTIAN A, BIGLIERI EG: Prevalence, pathogenesis, and functional significance of aldosterone deficiency in hyperkalemic patients with chronic renal insufficiency. *Kidney Int* 17: 89, 1980.

325. PHELPS KR, LIEBERMAN RL, OH MS, ET AL: Pathophysiology of the syndrome of hyporeninemic hypoaldosteronism. *Metabolism* 29: 186, 1980.

326. SEBASTIAN A, MORRIS RC JR: Renal tubular acidosis, in EARLEY LE, GOTTSCHALK CW (eds): *Strauss and Welt's Diseases of the Kidney.* Boston, Little Brown, 1979, p. 1029.

327. SCHAMBELAN M, SEBASTIAN A, HULTER HN: Mineralocorticoid excess and deficiency syndromes, in Brenner BM, Stein JH (eds): *Acid-Base and Potassium Homeostasis.* New York, Churchill Livingston, 1978, p 232.

328. SEBASTIAN A, SUTTON JM, HULTER HN ET AL: Effect of mineralocorticoid replacement therapy on renal acid-base homeostasis in adrenalectomized patients. *Kidney Int* 18: 762, 1980.

329. WESTENFELDER C, AREVALO GJ, BARANOWSKI RL, KURTZMAN NA, KATZ AI: Relationship between mineralcorticoids and renal Na$^+$−K$^+$-ATPase: sodium reabsorption. *Am J Physiol* 233: F593, 1977.

330. KEENAN BS, HOLCOMBE JH, KIRKLAND RT: Sodium homeostasis and aldosterone secretion in salt-losing congenital adrenal hyperplasia. *J Clin Endo Metab* 48: 430, 1979.

331. MANUEL MA, BEIRNE GH, WAGNILD JP, WEINER MW: An effect of spironolactone on urinary acidification in normal man. *Arch Int Med* 134: 472, 1974.

332. OWEN EE, VERNER JV JR: Renal tubular diseases with muscle paralysis and hypokalemia. *Am J Med* 28: 8, 1960.

333. VICALE CT: The diagnostic features of a muscular syndrome resulting from hyperparathyroidism, osteomalacia owing to renal tubular acidosis, and perhaps to related disorders of calcium metabolism. *Trans Am Neurol Assoc* 74: 143, 1949.

334. SMITH R, STERN G: Muscular weakness in osteomalacia and hyperparathyroidism. *J Neurol Sci* 8: 511, 1969.

335. MALLETTE LE, PATTEN BM, ENGEL WK: Neuromuscular disease in secondary hyperparathyroidism. *Ann Intern Med* 82: 474, 1975.

336. CURRY OB, BASTEN JF, FRANCIS MJO, SMITH R: Calcium uptake by sarcoplasmic reticulum of muscle from vitamin D-deficient rabbits. *Nature* 249: 83, 1974.

337. BIRGE SJ, HADDAD JG JR: 25-Hydroxycholecalciferol stimulation of muscle metabolism. *J Clin Invest* 56: 1100, 1975.

338. HENDERSON RG, LEDINGHAM JGG, OLIVER DP ET AL.: Effects of 1, 25-dihydroxycholecalciferol on calcium absorption, muscle weakness, and bone disease in chronic renal failure. *Lancet* 1: 379, 1974.

339. PRESCOTT LF: Mechanisms of renal excretion of drugs. *Br J Anaesth* 44: 246, 1972.

340. MUDGE GH, SILVA P, STIBITZ GR: Renal excretion by nonionic diffusion: The nature of disequilibrium. *Med Clin N Am* 59: 681, 1975.

341. BECKETT AH, ROWLAND M: Urinary excretion kinetics of amphetamine in man. *J Pharm Pharmacol* 17: 628, 1965.

342. KUNTZMAN RG, TSAI I, BRAND L, MARK LC: The influence of urinary pH on the plasma half-life of pseudoephedrine in man and dog and a sensitive assay for its determination in human plasma. *Clin Pharmacol Ther* 12: 62, 1971.

343. MACPHERSON CR, MILNE MD, EVANS BM: The secretion of salicylate. *Br J Pharmacol* 10: 484, 1955.

344. GERHARDT RE, KNOUSS RF, THYRUM PT, LUCHI RJ, MORRIS JJ: Quinidine excretion in aciduria and alkaluria. *Ann Intern Med* 71: 927, 1969.

345. Fanconi G: Der frühinfantile nephrotisch-glysurische zwerwuchs mit hypophosphatamischer rachitis. *Jahrb Kinderh* 147:299, 1936.

346. LEAF A: The syndrome of osteomalacia, renal glycosuria, aminoaciduria, and increased phosphorus clearance (the Fanconi syndrome), in Stanbury JB, Wyngaarden JB, Frederickson DS (eds): *The Metabolic Basis of Inherited Disease*, ed 4. New York, McGraw Hill, 1978, p 1205.

347. MORRIS RC JR, MCINNES RR, EPSTEIN CJ, SEBASTIAN A, SCRIVER CR: Genetic and metabolic injury of the kidney, in Brenner BM, Rector FC, (eds): *The Kidney*. Philadelphia, Saunders, 1976, p 1193.

348. LINDER GC, BULL GM, GRAYCE I: Hypophosphatemic glycosuric rickets (Fanconi syndrome). *Clin Proc* 8:1, 1949.

349. BICKEL H, SMALLWOOD WC, SMELLIE JM, HICKMANS EM: Cystine storage disease with aminoaciduria and dwarfism (Lignac-Fanconi Disease): clinical description, factual analysis and treatment of Lignac-Fanconi disease. *Acta Paediat* 42(suppl. 90):27, 1952.

350. MILNE MD, STANBURY SW, THOMSON AE: Observations on the Fanconi syndrome and renal hyperchloremic acidosis in the adult. *Quart J Med* 21:61, 1952.

351. SALASSA RM, POWERS MH, ULRICH JA, HAYLES AB: Observations on the metabolic effects of vitamin D in Fanconi's syndrome. *Proc Staff Meet Mayo Clin* 29:214, 1954.

352. SIROTA JH, HAMERMAN D: Renal function studies in an adult subject with Fanconi syndrome. *Am J Med* 16:138, 1954.

353. BERLINER RW, KENNEDY TJ JR, HILTON JG: Effect of maleic acid on renal function. *Proc Soc Exper Biol Med* 75:791, 1950.

354. HARRISON HE, HARRISON HC: Experimental production of renal glycosuria, phosphaturia, and aminoaciduria by injection of maleic acid. *Science* 120:606, 1954.

355. FRITZELL S, JAGENBURG OR, SCHNURER LB: Familial cirrhosis of the liver, renal tubular defects with rickets and impaired tyrosine metabolism. *Acta Paediatr* 53:18, 1964.

356. LEVIN B, SNODGRASS GJAI, OBERHOLZER VG, BURGESS EA, DOBBS RH: Fructosaemia: Observations on seven cases. *Am J Med* 45:826, 1968.

357. MORRIS RC JR: An experimental renal acidification defect in patients with hereditary fructose intolerance. I. Its resemblance to renal tubular acidosis. *J Clin Invest* 47:1389, 1968.

358. HOPPE A, GMAJ P, METLER M, ANGIELSKI S: Additive inhibition of renal bicarbonate reabsorption by maleate plus acetazolamide, *Am J Physiol* 231:1258, 1976.

359. GOUGOUX A, LEMIEUX G, LAVOIE N: Maleate-induced bicarbonaturia in the dog: A carbonic anhydrase-independent effect. *Am J Physiol* 231:1258, 1976.

360. BERGERON M, DUBORD L, HAUSSER C: Membrane permeability as a cause of transport defects in experimental Fanconi syndrome: A new hypothesis. *J Clin Invest* 57:1181, 1976.

361. REYNOLDS R, MCNAMARA PD, SEGAL S: On the maleic acid induced Fanconi syndrome: Effects on transport by isolated rat kidney brush border membrane vesicles. *Life Science* 22:39, 1977.

362. VAN BIERVLIET JPGM, BRUINVIS L, KETTING D, DE BREE PK, VAN DER HEIDEN C, WADMAN SK, WILLEMS JL, BOOKELMAN H, VAN HAELST V, MONNENS LAH: Hereditary mitochondrial myopathy with lactic acidemia, a DeToni-Fanconi-Debre syndrome, and a defective respiratory chain in voluntary striated muscles. *Pediatr Res* 11:1108, 1977.

363. BONNICI F, SMITH S, DE V HEESE H: Letter to the editor. *Lancet* 1:1304, 1977.

364. LEAF A: The syndrome of osteomalacia, renal glycosuria, aminoaciduria, and increased phosphorus clearance (the Fanconi syndrome), in Stanbury JB, Wyngaarden JB, Frederickson DS, (eds): *The Metabolic Basis of Inherited Disease*, ed 2. New York, McGraw-Hill, 1966, p 1205.

365. BICKEL H, BAAR HS, ASTLEY R, DOUGLAS AA, FINCH E, HARRIS H, HARVEY CC, HICKMANS EM, PHILPOTT MG, SMALLWOOD WC, SMELLIE JM, TEALL CG: Cystine storage disease with aminoaciduria and dwarfism (Lignac-Fanconi disease). *Acta Paediat* 42(Suppl. 90):1, 1952.

366. SCHNEIDER JA, SEEGMILLER JE: Cystinosis and the Fanconi syndrome, in Stanbury JB, Wyngaarden JB, Fredrickson DS, (eds): *The Metabolic Basis of Inherited Disease*, ed 3. New York, McGraw-Hill, 1972, p 1581.

367. ABBASSI V, LOWE CU, CALCAGNO PL: Oculocerebrorenal syndrome. *Am J Dis Child* 115:145, 1968.

368. BABER MD: A case of congenital cirrhosis of the liver with renal tubular defects akin to those in the Fanconi syndrome. *Arch Dis Child* 31:335, 1956.

369. HALVORSEN S, GJESSING LR: Studies on tyrosinosis. I. Effect of low-tyrosine and low-phenylalanine diet. *Br Med J* 2:1171, 1964.

370. LAMEIRE N, MUSSCHE M, BAELE G, KINT J, RINGOIR S: Hereditary fructose intolerance: A difficult diagnosis in the adult. *Am J Med* 65:416, 1978.

371. ODIEVRE M, GENTIL C, GAUTIER M, ALAGILLE D: Hereditary fructose intolerance in childhood. *Am J Dis Child* 132:605, 1978.

372. BAERLOCHER K, GITZELMANN R, STEINMANN B, GITZELMANN-CUMARASAMY N: Hereditary fructose intolerance in early childhood: A major diagnostic challenge. *Helv Paediat Acta* 33:465, 1978.

373. BEARN AG, YU TF, GUTMAN AB: Renal function in Wilson's disease. *J Clin Invest* 36:1107, 1957.

374. MORGAN HD, STEWART WK, LOWE KG, STOWERS JM, JOHNSTONE JH: Wilson's disease and the Fanconi syndrome. *Quart J Med* 31:361, 1962.

375. LITIN RB, RANDALL RV, GOLDSTEIN NP, POWER NH, DIESSNER GR: Hypercalciuria in hepatolenticular degeneration (Wilson's disease). *Am J Med Sci* 238:614, 1959.

376. ELSAS LJ, HAYSLETT JP, SPARGO BH, DURANT JL, ROSENBERG LE: Wilson's disease with reversible renal tubular dysfunction: Correlation with proximal tubular ultrastructure. *Ann Intern Med* 75:427, 1971.

377. HOLL DH, TROELSTRA JA: Renale tubulaire functiestoarnissen bij de ziekte van Wilson. *Ned Tijdshcr Geneeskd* 48:2184, 1968.

378. CUSWORTH DG, DENT CE, FLYNN FV: The aminoaciduria in galactosemia. *Arch Dis Child* 30:150, 1955.

379. KONROWER GM, SCHWARTZ V, HOLZEL A, GOLBERG L: A clinical and biochemical study of galactosemia. *Arch Dis Child* 31:254, 1956.

380. FANCONI G, BICKEL H: Die chronische aminoadurie (amino-saurediebetes oder nephrotisch-glukosurischer zwergwuchs) bei der glykogenose und der cystinkrankheit. *Helv Paediatr Acta* 4:359, 1949.

381. LAMPERT F, MAYER H: Glykogenose der liber mit galaktoseverwertungsstorung und schwerem Fanconi-syndrom. *Arch Kinderheilkd* 98:133, 1967.

382. HERS HG, VAN HOOF F: Glycogen storage diseases, in Dickens F, Randle PJ, Whelan WJ (eds): *Carbohydrate Metabolism and its Disorders*. New York, Academic, 1968, vol II.

383. ODIEVRE M: Glycogenose hepatorenale avec tubulopathie complexe. *Rev Int Hepatol* 16:1, 1966.

384. HOLZEL A, KONROWER GM, SCHWARZ V: Galactosemia. *Am J Med* 22:703, 1957.

385. ISSELBACHER KJ: Galactosemia, in Stanbury JB, Wyngaarden JB, Fredrickson DS (eds): *The Metabolic Basis of Inherited Disease*, ed 2. New York, McGraw-Hill, 1966, p 178.

386. STEINER G, WILSON D, VRANIC M: Studies of glucose turnover and renal function in an unusual case of hereditary fructose intolerance. *Am J Med* 62:150, 1977.

387. RICHARDSON RMA, LITTLE JA, PATTEN RL, GOLDSTEIN MD, HALPERIN ML: Pathogenesis of acidosis in hereditary fructose intolerance. *Metabolism* 28:1133, 1979.

388. FROESCH ER: Essential fructosuria and hereditary fructose intolerance, in Stanbury JB, Wyngaarden JB, Fredrickson DS, (eds): *The Metabolic Basis of Inherited Disease*, ed 2. New York, McGraw-Hill, 1966, p 124.

389. HERS HG, JOASSIN G: Anomalie de l'aldolase hepatique dans l'intolerance au fructose. *Enzymol Biol Clin* 1:4, 1961.

390. SCHAPIRA F, HATZFELD A, GREGORI C: Studies on liver aldolases in hereditary fructose intolerance. *Enzyme* 18:73, 1974.

391. MORRIS RC JR, UEKI I, LOH D, EANES RZ, MCLIN P: Absence of renal fructose-1-phosphate aldolase activity in hereditary fructose intolerance. *Nature* 214:920, 1967.

392. KRANHOLD JF, LOH D, MORRIS RC JR: Renal fructose-metabolizing enzymes: Significance in hereditary fructose intolerance. *Science* 165:402, 1969.

393. WACHSMUTH ED, THÖNER M, PFLEIDERER G: The cellular distribution of aldolase isozymes in rat kidney and brain determined in tissue sections by the immuno-histochemical method. *Histochemistry* 45:143, 1975.

394. BURCH HB, COLE B, CHOI S, ALVEY TR, DENCE C: Diversity of effects of fructose loads on different parts of the nephron. *Int J Biochem* 12:37, 1980.

395. BURCH HB, LOWRY OH, MEINHARDT L, MAX P JR, CHYU K-J: Effect of fructose, dihydroxyacetone, glycerol, and glucose on metabolites and related compounds in liver and kidney. *J Biol Chem* 245:2092, 1970.

396. BREWER ED, KRANHOLD JF, SEBASTIAN A, MCSHERRY E, MORRIS RC JR: *The Experimental Renal Dysfunction of Hereditary Fructose Intolerance (HFI): Evidence That Function of the Thick Ascending Limb Is Intact and* HCO_3 *Reabsorptive Capacity of the Proximal Tubule Is Reduced, abstracted.* American Society of Nephrology, Abstracts, 10th annual meeting, Washington, D.C., 1977, p 10A.

397. ROSIN JM, KATZ MA, RECTOR FC JR: Acetazolamide in studying sodium reabsorption in diluting segment. *Am J Physiol* 219:1731, 1968.

398. SELDIN DW, ROSIN JM, RECTOR FC JR: Evidence against bicarbonate reabsorption in the ascending limb, particularly as disclosed by free-water clearance studies. *Yale J Biol Med* 48:337, 1975.

399. DANOVITCH GM, BRICKER NS: Influence of volume expansion on NaCl reabsorption in the diluting segments of the nephron: A study using clearance methods. *Kidney Int* 10:229, 1976.

400. CHAIMOVITZ C, LEIBOVICH H, BETTER OS: Effect of acetazolamide on sodium reabsorption in the diluting segment in man. *J Lab Clin Med* 87:630, 1976.

401. KANAU RT JR: The influence of the carbonic anhydrase inhibitor, benzolamide (CL-11, 366), on the reabsorption of chloride, sodium, and bicarbonate in the proximal tubule of the rat. *J Clin Invest* 51:294, 1972.

402. BURG MB, GREEN N: Function of the thick ascending limb of Henle's loop. *Am J Physiol* 224:659, 1973.

403. NISELL J, LINDEN L: Fructose-1-phosphate aldolase and fructose-1,6-diphosphate aldolase activity in the mucosa of the intestine in hereditary fructose intolerance. *Scand J Gastroenterol* 3:80, 1968.

404. MAENPAA PH, RAIVIO KO, KEKOMAKI: Liver adenine nucleotides: Fructose-induced depletion and its effect on protein synthesis. *Science* 161:1253, 1968.

405. NIKIFORUK G, COLOWICK SP: The purification and properties of 5-adenylic acid deaminase from muscle. *J Biol Chem* 219:119, 1956.

406. CHAPMAN AG, ATKINSON DE: Stabilization of adenylate energy charge by the adenylate deaminase reaction. *J Biol Chem* 248:8309, 1973.

407. WOODS HF, EGGLESTON LB, KREBS HA: The cause of hepatic accumulation of fructose-1-phosphate on fructose loading. *Biochem J* 119:501, 1970.

408. FOX IH, KELLEY WM: Studies on the mechanism of fructose-induced hyperuricemia in man. *Metab Clin Exp* 21:713, 1972.

409. BODE JC, ZELDER O, RUMPELT HF, WITTKAMP U: Depletion of liver adenosine phosphates and metabolic effects of intravenous infusion of fructose on sorbitol in man and in the rat. *Europ J Clin Invest* 3:436, 1973.

410. HULTMAN E, NILSSON LH, SAHLIN K: Adenine nucleotide content of human liver: Normal values and fructose-induced depletion. *Scand J Clin Lab Invest* 35:245, 1975.

411. MORRIS RC, JR, NIGON K, REED EB: Evidence that the severity of depletion of inorganic phosphate determines the severity of the disturbance of adenine nucleotide metabolism in the liver and renal cortex of the fructose-loaded rat. *J Clin Invest* 61:209, 1978.

412. SESTOFT L: Regulation of fructose metabolism in the perfused rat liver: Interrelation with inorganic phosphate, glucose, ketone body and ethanol metabolism. *Biochim Biophys Acta* 343:1, 1974.

413. Sestoft L: Regulatory processes in rat liver induced by sudden changes in fructose concentration, in Lundquist F, Tygstrup N, (eds): *Regulation of Hepatic Metabolism*. Copenhagen, Munksgaard, 1974, p 285.

414. MORRIS RC JR, BREWER ED, BRATER C: Evidence of a severe phosphate-depletion dependent disturbance of cellular metabolism in patients with hereditary fructose intolerance (HFI). *Clin Res* 28:556A, 1980.

415. MORRIS RC JR: Discussion in Coggins CH, Cummings NB (eds): *Prevention of Kidney and Urinary Tract Diseases*. Bethesda, Fogarty International Center Series on Preventive Medicine, vol 5, p 279.

416. WILSON DF, STUBBS M, VEECH RL, ERECINSKA M, KREBS HA: Equilibrium relations between the oxidation-reduction reactions and the adenosine triphosphate synthesis in suspensions of isolated liver cells. *Biochem J* 140:57, 1974.

417. VEECH RL, LAWSON WR, CORNELL NW ET AL: Cytosolic phosphorylation potential. *J Biol Chem* 254:6538, 1979.

418. AKERBOOM TPM, BOOKELMAN H, ZUURENDONK PF, VAN DER MEER R, TAGER JM: Intramitochondrial and extramitochondrial concentrations of adenine nucleotides and inorganic phosphate in isolated hepatocytes from fasted rats. *Eur J Biochem* 84:413, 1978.

419. GUDER WG, PURSCHEL S: The intracellular compartmentation of metabolites in isolated kidney cortex tubules. *Int J Biochem* 12:63, 1980.

420. GAMJ P, HOPPE A, ANGIELSKI S, ROGULSKI J: Acid base behavior of the kidney in maleate treated rats. *Am J Physiol* 222:1182, 1972.

421. GAMJ P, HOPPE A, ANGIELSKI S, ROGULSKI J: Effect of maleate and arsenite on renal absorption of sodium and bicarbonate. *Am J Physiol* 225:90, 1973.

422. KRAMER HJ, GONICK HC: Experimental Fanconi syndrome. I. Effect of maleic acid on renal cortical Na-K-ATPase activity and ATP level. *J Lab Clin Med* 76:799, 1970.

423. ROSEN WG, KRAMER HJ, GONICK HC: Experimental Fanconi syndrome: Effect of maleic acid on renal tubular ultrastructure. *Lab Invest* 28:446, 1973.

424. AL-BANDER H, WEISS R, MORRIS RC JR, HUMPHREYS MH: *Evidence in the Dog That Maleic Acid Induces Increased Rejection of Na⁺, Cl⁻, and HCO₃⁻ Out of the Proximal Tubules.* American Society of Nephrology, 12th annual meeting, 1979, p 78A.

425. GUNTHER R, SILBERNAGL S, DEETJEN P: Maleic acid induced aminoaciduria: Studied by free flow micropuncture and continuous microperfusion. *Pflugers Arch* 382:109, 1979.

426. KRAMER HJ, GONICK HC: Effect of maleic acid on sodium linked tubular transport in experimental Fanconi syndrome. *Nephron* 10:306, 1973.

427. SILVERMAN M: The mechanism of maleic acid nephropathy: Investigations using brush border membrane vesicles. *Clin Res* 28:698A, 1980.

428. SCHARER K, YOSHIDA T, VOYER L, BERLOW S, PIETRA G, METCOFF J: Impaired renal gluconogenesis and energy metabolism in maleic acid induced nephropathy in rats. *Res Exp Med* 157:136, 1972.

429. ANGIELSKI S, ROGULSKI J: Effect of maleic acid on the kidney. I. Oxidation of Krebs cycle intermediate by various tissue of maleate intoxicated rats. *Acta Biochim Pol* 9:357, 1962.

430. ANGIELSKI S, ROGULSKI J: Metabolic studies in experimental renal dysfunction resulting from maleate administration, in Angielski S, Dubach UC (eds): *Biochemical Aspects of Kidney Function*. Bern, H. Huber, 1975, p 86.

431. ROGULSKI J, PACANIS A, ADAMOWICZ W, ANGIELSKI S: On the mechanism of maleate action on rat kidney mitochondria: Effect on oxidative metabolism. *Acta Biochim Pol* 21:403, 1974.

432. SZCEPANSKA M, ANGIELSKI S: Prevention of maleate induced tubular dysfunction by acetoacetate. *Am J Physiol* 8:F50, 1980.

433. BREWER ED, TSAI HC, SZETO KS, MORRIS RC JR: Maleic acid-induced impaired conversion of 25-(OH)D₃ to 1,25-(OH)₂D₃: Implications for Fanconi's syndrome. *Kidney Int* 12:244, 1977.

434. AKIBA T, ENDOU H, KOSEKI C, SAKAI F: Localization of 25-hydroxyvitamin D₃1α-hydroxylase activity in the mammalian kidney. *Biochem Biophys Res Comm* 94:313, 1980.

435. AL-BANDER H, MOCK DM, PAUKERT T, HUMPHREYS MH, MORRIS RC JR: Phosphate loading attenuates the severity of the renal tubular disorder induced by maleic acid (MA) in the dog. *Clin Res* 29:552A, 1981.

436. BRAZY PC, BALABAN RS, GULLANS SR, MANDEL LJ, DENNIS VW: Inhibition of renal metabolism: Relative effects of arsenate on sodium, phosphate and glucose transport by the rabbit proximal tubule. *J Clin Invest* 66:1211, 1980.

437. MAUNSBACH AB: Ultrastructure of the proximal tubule, in Orloff J, Berliner RW (eds): *Handbook of Physiology*. Washington, D.C., American Physiology Society, 1973, sect 8, p 31.

438. MAACK T, SIGULEM D: Renal handling of lysozyme, in Osserman EF, Canfield RE, Beychok S (eds): *Lysozyme*. New York, Academic, 1974, p 321.

439. MAUNSBACH AB: Cellular mechanisms of tubular protein transport, in Thurau K (ed): *International Review of Physiology, Kidney and Urinary Physiology II*. Baltimore, University Park Press, 1976, vol II, chap 5, p 145.

440. SHIBKO S, TAPPEL AL: Rat kidney lysosomes: Isolation and properties. *Biochem J* 95:731, 1965.

441. OSSERMAN EF: Lysozymuria in renal and nonrenal diseases; in Manuel Y, Revillard JP, Betuel H (eds): *Proteins in Normal and Pathological Urine*. New York, Darger, 1970, p 260.

442. HAYSLETT JP, PERILLE PE, FINCH SC: Urinary muramidase and renal disease. *N Engl J Med* 279:506, 1968.

443. BARRATT TM, CRAWFORD R: Lysozyme excretion as a measure of renal tubular dysfunction in children. *Clin Sci* 39:457, 1970.

444. CHAMBERLAIN MJ, STIMMLER L: The renal handling of insulin. *J Clin Invest* 46:911, 1967.

445. BERGGARD I, BEARN AG: Isolation and properties of a low molecular weight β₂-globulin occurring in human biological fluids. *J Biol Chem* 243:4095, 1968.

446. BERNIER GM, CONRAD ME: Catabolism of human β₂-microglobulin by the rat kidney. *Am J Physiol* 217:1359, 1969.

447. PETERSON PA, EVRIN P-E, BERGGARD I: Differentiation of glomerular, tubular, and normal proteinuria: Determinations of urinary excretion of β₂-microglobulin, albumin, and total protein. *J Clin Invest* 48:1189, 1969.

448. MOGIELNICKI RP, WALDMANN TA, STROBER W: The renal handling of low molecular weight proteins. I. L-chain metabolism in experimental renal disease. *J Clin Invest* 50:901, 1971.

449. WALDMANN TA, STROBER W, MOGIELNICKI RP: The renal handling of low molecular weight proteins. II. Disorders of serum protein catabolism in patients with tubular proteinuria, the nephrotic syndrome, or uremia. *J Clin Invest* 51:2162, 1972.

450. SELLINGER OZ, BEAUFAY H, JACQUES P, DOYEN A, DE DUVE C: Tissue fractionation studies. 15. Beta-*n*-acetylglucosaminidase and beta-galactosidase in rat liver. *Biochem J* 74:450, 1960.

451. PRICE RG, DANCE N: The cellular distribution of some rat-kidney glycosidases. *Biochem J* 105:877, 1967.

452. DANCE N, PRICE RG, ROBINSON D, STIRLING JL: Beta-galactosidase, beta-glucosidase and N-acetyl-beta-glucosaminidase in human kidney. *Clin Chim Acta* 24:189, 1969.

453. DANCE N, PRICE RG, CATTELL WR, LANSDELL J, RICHARDS B: The excretion of beta-glucosaminidase and beta-galactosidase by patients with renal disease. *Clin Chim Acta* 27:87, 1970.

454. Morris RC Jr: The clinical spectrum of Fanconi's syndrome. *Calif Med* 108:225, 1968.

455. MORRIS RC JR, SANDMAN R, MCSHERRY E, SEBASTIAN A: Urinary lysosomal enzymes in renal tubular disorders. *Clin Res* 18:460, 1970.

456. CHRISTENSEN EI, MAUNSBACH AB: Proteinuria induced by sodium maleate in rats: Effects on ultrastructure and protein handling in renal proximal tubule. *Kidney Int* 17:771, 1980.

457. STEINMAN RM, SILVER JM, COHN ZA: Pinocytosis in fibroblasts: Quantitative studies in vitro. *J Cell Biol* 63:949, 1974.

458. MAUNSBACH AB: Absorption of ferritin by rat kidney proximal tubule cells: Electron microscopic observations of the initial uptake phase in cells of microperfused single proximal tubules. *J Ultrastruct Res* 16:1, 1966.

459. DINGLE JT, BARRETT AJ: Uptake of biologically active substances by lysosomes. *Proc R Soc London [Biol]* 173:85, 1969.

460. JAMISON JD, PALADE GE: Intracellular transport of secretory proteins in the pancreatic exocrine cell. IV. Metabolic requirements. *J Cell Biol* 39:589, 1968.

461. REIMER KA, GANOTE CE, JENNINGS RB: Alterations in renal cortex following ischemic injury. III. Ultrastructure of proximal tubules after ischemia or autolysis. *Lab Invest* 26:347, 1972.

462. DONOHOE JF, VENKATACHALAM MA, BERNARD DB, LEVINSKY NG: Tubular leakage and obstruction after renal ischemia: Structural-functional correlations. *Kidney Int* 13:208, 1978.

463. LANGER KH, THOENES W: Zur Genese "optisch leerer Vakuolen" in Epithel des energetisch insuffizienten proximalen Nierentubulus: Untersuchungen an der Rattenniere nach Kaliumcyanidvergiftung und hamorrhagischem Schock. *Ver Disch Ges Pathol* 53:394, 1969.

464. MASUR SK, HOLTZMAN E, WALTER R: Hormone-stimulated exocytosis in the toad urinary bladder. *J Cell Biol* 52:211, 1972.

465. HOLTZMAN E, GRONOWICZ G, MERCURIA A: Notes on the heterogeneity, circulation, and modification of membranes, with emphasis on secretory cells, photoreceptors, and the toad bladder, in Manson LA (ed): *Biomembranes*. New York, Plenum Press, 1979, vol 10, p 77.

466. AMAR-COSTESEC A, WIBO M, THINES-SEMPOUX D, BEAUFAY G, BERTHET J: Analytical study of microsomes and isolated subcellular membranes from rat liver. IV. Biochemical, physical, and morphological modifications of microsomal components induced by digitonin, EDTA, and pyrophosphate. *J Cell Biol* 62:717, 1974.

467. OSSERMAN EF, LAWLOR DP: Serum and urinary lysozyme (muramidase) in monocytic and monomyelocytic leukemia. *J Exp Med* 124:921, 1966.

468. MUGGIA FM, HEINEMANN HO, FARHANGI M, OSSERMAN EF: Lysozymuria and renal tubular dysfunction in monocytic and myelomonocytic leukemia. *Am J Med* 47:351, 1969.

469. PRUZANSKI W, PLATTS ME: Serum and urinary proteins, lysozyme (muramidase), and renal dysfunction in mono- and myelomonocytic leukemia. *J Clin Invest* 49:1694, 1970.

470. RUDDERS RA, BLOCK KJ: Myeloma renal disease: Evaluation of the role of muramidase (lysozyme). *Am J Med Sci* 262:79, 1971.

471. CLYNE DH, BRENDSTRUP L, FIRST MR ET AL.: Renal effects of intraperitoneal kappa chain injection: Induction of crystals in renal tubular cells. *Lab Invest* 31:131, 1974.

472. RAWLINGS W JR, GRIFFIN J, DUFFY T, HUMPHREY R: Fanconi syndrome with lambda light chains in urine, correspondence. *N Engl Med* 299:1351, 1976.

473. WALKER BR, ALEXANDER F, TANNENBAUM PJ: Fanconi syndrome with renal tubular acidosis and light chain proteinuria. *Nephron* 8:103, 1971.

474. KAMM DE, FISCHER MS: Proximal renal tubular acidosis and the Fanconi syndrome in a patient with hypergammaglobulinemia. *Nephron* 9:208, 1972.

475. SCHNEIDER JA, WONG V, BRADLEY KH, SEEGMILLER JE: Biochemical comparisons of the adult and childhood forms of cystinosis. *N Engl J Med* 279:1253, 1968.

476. LIETMAN PS, FRAZIER PD, WONG VG, SHOTTON D, SEEGMILLER JE: adult cystinosis-a benign disorder. *Am J Med* 40:511, 1966.

477. SCRIVER CR, WHELAN DT: Cystinuria: Concepts and new observations, in Carson NAJ, Raine DN (eds): *Inherited Disorders of Sulphur Metabolism*. Edinburgh, Churchill Livingston, 1971, p 70.

478. NOVAK EK, WIELAND F, JAHREIS GP, SWANK RT: Altered secretion of kidney lysosomal enzymes in the mouse pigment mutants ruby-eye, Ruby-eye-2J, and Maroon. *Biochem Genetics* 18:549, 1980.

479. PORTALE A, MOCK D, AL-BANDER H, MORRIS RC JR: Unpublished observations.

480. CHAN AM, LYNCH MJG, BAILEY JD, EZRIN C, FRASER D: Hypothyroidism in cystinosis: A clinical, endocrinologic and histologic study involving sixteen patients with cystinosis. *Am J Med* 48:678, 1970.

481. LUCKY AW, MEGYESI K, SCHULMAN JD: Endocrine studies in cystinosis: compensated primary hypothyroidism. *J Pediatr* 91:204, 1977.

482. ERICSON LE: Exocytosis and endocytosis in the thyroid follicle cell. *Molec Cell Endocrinol* 22:1, 1981.

483. WILSON DR, YENDT ER: Treatment of the adult Fanconi syndrome with oral phosphate supplements and alkali. *Am J Med* 35:487, 1963.

484. STEENDIJK R: The effect of a continuous intravenous infusion of inorganic phosphate on the rachitic lesions in cystinosis. *Arch Dis Child* 36:321, 1961.

485. LINDER CC, BULL CM, GRAYCE I: Hypophosphatemic glycosuric rickets (Fanconi syndrome). *Clin Proc Child Hosp.* 8:1, 1949.

486. DENT CE: Commentary. *Clin Proc Child Hosp* 8:21, 1949.

487. STANBURY SW, LUMB GA: Metabolic studies of renal osteodystrophy. I. Calcium, phosphorus and nitrogen metabolism in rickets, osteomalacia and hyperparathyroidism complicating chronic uremia and in the osteomalacia of the adult Fanconi syndrome. *Medicine* 41:1, 1962.

488. STANBURY SW: Bony complications of renal disease, in Black DAK (ed): *Renal Disease* ed 2. Oxford, Blackwell Scientific Publications, 1962, p 508.

489. DENT CE, HARRIS H: The genetics of "cystinuria." *Ann Eugen* 16:60, 1951.

490. Smith R, Lindenbaum RH, Walton RJ: Hypophosphataemic osteomalacia and Fanconi syndrome of adult onset with dominant inheritance. *Q J Med* 179:387, 1976.

491. MALLETTE LE, PATTEN BM: Neurogenic muscle atrophy and osteomalacia in adult Fanconi syndrome. *Ann Neurol* 1:131, 1977.

492. SORIANO JR, HOUSTON IB, BOICHIS H, EDELMANN CM JR: Calcium and phosphorus metabolism in the Fanconi syndrome. *J Clin Endocrinol Metab* 28:1555, 1968.

493. MILNE MD, STANBURY SW, THOMSON AE: Observations on the Fanconi syndrome and renal hyperchloremic acidosis in the adult. *Q J Med* 21:61, 1952.

494. DE TONI E JR, NORDIO S: The relationship between calcium-phosphorus in metabolism, the "Krebs cycle" and steroid metabolism. *Arch Dis Child* 34:371, 1959.

495. PRADER VON A, ILLIG R, HEIERLI E: Eine besondere form der primaren vitamin-D resistenten rachitis mit hypocalcamie and autosomaldominanten erbgang: Die hereditare pseudo-mangelrachitis. *Helv Paediatr Acta* 16:452, 1961.

496. ARNAUD C, MAIJER R, READE T, SCRIVER CR, WHELAN DT: Vitamin D dependency: An inherited postnatal syndrome with secondary hyperparathyroidism. *Pediatrics* 46:871, 1970.

497. FRASER D, KOOH SW, KIND HP, HOLICK MF, TANAKA Y, DELUCA HF: Pathogenesis of hereditary vitamin D-dependent rickets: An inborn error of vitamin D metabolism involving defective conversion of 25-hydroxyvitamin D to 1α,25-dihydroxy-vitamin D. *N Engl J Med* 289:817, 1973.

498. BALSAN S, GARABEDIAN M, SORGNIAR R, HOLICK MF, DELUCA HF: 1,25-Dihydroxyvitamin D₃ and 1α-hydroxyvitamin D₃ in children: Biologic and therapeutic effects in nutritional rickets and different types of vitamin D resistance. *Pediatr Res* 9:586, 1975.

499. READE TM, SCRIVER CR, GLORIEUX FH, NOGRADY B, DELVIN E, POIRIER R, HOLICK MF, DELUCA HF: Response to crystalline 1α-hydroxyvitamin D₃ in vitamin D dependency. *Pediatr Res* 9:593, 1975.

500. SCRIVER CR, GLORIEUX FH, READE TM, TENEHOUSE HS: X-linked hypophosphataemia and autosomal recessive vitamin D dependency: Models for the resolution of vitamin D refractory rickets, in Bikel H, Stern J (eds): *Inborn Errors of Calcium and Bone Metabolism*. Baltimore, University Park Press, 1976, p 150.

501. FRASER D, SCRIVER CR: Familial forms of vitamin D-resistant rickets revisited: X-linked hypophosphatemia and autosomal recessive vitamin D dependency. *Am J Clin Nutri* 29:1315, 1976.

502. SCRIVER CR, READE TM, DELUCA HF, HAMSTRA AJ: Serum 1,25-dihydroxyvitamin D levels in normal subjects and in patients with hereditary rickets or bone disease. *N Engl J Med* 299:976, 1978.

503. FRASER DR, KODICEK E: Unique biosynthesis by kidney of a biologically active vitamin D metabolite. *Nature* 228:764, 1970.

504. GRAY RW, BOYLE I, DELUCA HF: Vitamin D metabolism, The role of kidney tissue. *Science* 172:1232, 1971.

505. MEDGETT RJ, SPEILVOGEL AM, COBURN JW, NORMAN AW: Studies on calciferol metabolism. VI. The renal production of the biologically active form of vitamin D, 1,25-dihydroxycholecalciferol; species, tissue, and subcellular distribution. *J Clin Endocrinol Metab* 36:1153, 1973.

506. NORMAN HW, HENRY H: 1,25-Dihydroxycholecalciferol-a hormonally active form of vitamin D₃. *Rec Prog Horm Res* 30:431, 1974.

507. OLSON EG, KNUTSON JC, BHATTACHARYYA MH, DELUCA HF: The effect of hepatectomy on the synthesis of 25-hydroxyvitamin D₃. *J Clin Invest* 57:1213, 1976.

508. CHESNEY RW, ROSEN JF, HAMSTRA AJ, DELUCA HF: Serum 1,25-dihydroxyvitamin D levels in normal children and in vitamin D disorders. *Am J Dis Child* 134:135, 1980.

509. ETCHES P, PICKERING D, SMITH R: Cystinotic rickets treated with vitamin D metabolites. *Arch Dis Child* 52:661, 1977.

510. GERTNER JM, BRENTON DP, DENT CE, DEMENECH M: Treatment of the rickets of cystinosis with 1α-hydroxy vitamin D₃ (1976), XII European Symposium on Calcified Tissues. *Calcified Tissue Research* 521:63, 1977.

511. SOCKALOSKY JJ, ULSTROM RA, DELUCA HF, BROWN DM: Vitamin D-resistant rickets: End-organ unresponsiveness to 1,25(OH)₂D₃. *J Pediatr* 96:701, 1980.

512. SOCKALOSKY JJ, ULSTROM RA, DELUCA HF, BROWN DM: Letter to the editor. *J Pediatr* 97:697, 190.

513. BELL NH: Vitamin D-dependent rickets type II. *Calcif Tissue Int* 31:89, 1980.

514. SALASSA RM, POWER MH, ULRICK JA, HAYLES AB: Observations on the metabolic effects of vitamin D in Fanconi's syndrome. *Proc Mayo Clin* 29:214, 1954.

515. BERGSTROM WH: The response of multiple renal tubular dysfunction to calciferol. *Pediatr Res* 2:408, 1968.

516. HUGUENIN M, SCHACHT R, DAVID R: Infantile rickets with severe proximal renal tubular acidosis, responsive to vitamin D. *Arch Dis Child* 49:955, 1974.

517. PUSCHETT JB, MORANZ J, KURNICK WS: Evidence for a direct action of cholecalciferol and 25-hydroxycholecalciferol on the renal transport of phosphate, sodium, and calcium. *J Clin Invest* 51:373, 1972.

518. PUSCHETT JB, FERNANDEZ PC, BOYLE IT, GRAY RW, OMDAHL JL, DeLUCA HF: The acute renal tubular effects of 1,25-dihydroxycholecalciferol (36781). *Proc Soc Exp Biol Med* 141:379, 1972.

519. PERAINO RA, GHAFARY E, ROUSE D, STINEBAUGH BJ, SUKI WN: Effect of 25-hydroxycholecalciferol on renal handling of sodium, calcium, and phosphate during bicarbonate infusion. *Min Electrol Metab* 1:321, 1978.

520. YUDKOFF M, FOREMAN JW, SEGAL S: Effects of cysteamine therapy in nephropathic cystinosis. *N Engl J Med* 304:141, 1981.

521. GRETZ N, MANZ F: Cysteamine therapy in nephropathic cystinosis, letter to the editor. *N Engl J Med* 304:1171, 1981.

85

CYSTINOSIS

JERRY A. SCHNEIDER

JOSEPH D. SCHULMAN

1. Cystinosis is a recessively inherited metabolic disorder characterized biochemically by an abnormally high intracellular content of free cystine which results in cystine crystal deposition in the conjunctiva, bone marrow, lymph nodes, leukocytes, and internal organs. There are at least three forms of this disease. The infantile nephropathic form has been the one most thoroughly studied. Children with this form of cystinosis present in the first year of life with the renal tubular defects characteristic of the Fanconi syndrome and also have progressive renal glomerular damage which leads to end-stage kidney failure, usually before 10 years of age. Other patients have a completely benign form of cystinosis and are discovered only when an ophthalmologic examination is done for another reason and reveals characteristic crystalline opacities in the cornea and conjunctiva. Finally, some patients have an intermediate type of cystinosis characterized by later onset of renal disease and renal failure than occurs in the infantile nephropathic variety.

2. A characteristic lesion in the peripheral retina, a patchy depigmentation, is usually found in the infantile nephropathic form but never in the benign form. It has been noted in some, but not all, patients with the intermediate form of cystinosis. Retinal lesions were detectable in a 5-week-old infant with nephropathic cystinosis as well as in an affected aborted fetus.

3. The renal defects in nephropathic cystinosis are probably caused by the large intracellular accumulation of free cystine. Cystine is known to inhibit many sulfhydryl-requiring enzymes, but the cystinotic cell has some protection because this amino acid is compartmentalized in these cells and thus separated from other cellular enzymes. The intracellular site of the cystine storage is the lysosome. The exact mechanism leading to this storage and the identity of the abnormal gene product are not known.

4. The symptomatic management of patients with nephropathic cystinosis is usually not difficult, but so far attempts at specific therapy have been unsuccessful. Renal transplantation has been lifesaving and is receiving more widespread acceptance. Cysteamine (mercaptoethylamine) depletes cystinotic cells of cystine and is now undergoing clinical trial.

5. Prenatal diagnosis is an established procedure for this condition. Affected fetuses have 20 to 100 times the usual amount of free cystine in most internal organs.

Cystinosis is a recessively inherited metabolic disorder characterized biochemically by a high intracellular content of free (nonprotein) cystine which is compartmentalized within lysosomes. This results in crystal deposition in the cornea, conjunctiva, bone marrow, lymph nodes, leukocytes, and internal organs. The abnormal gene product leading to cystine accumulation remains to be identified.

Genetic heterogeneity of this disease is suggested by the variations in severity among families and the similar degree of severity in clinical expression of the disease within a given family. Several reviews of cystinosis and the Fanconi syndrome have appeared over the years and reflect the changing concepts of the disease [1–8].

Cystinosis is a common cause of the Fanconi syndrome in children, although the essential elements of the Fanconi syndrome appear in a variety of other hereditary and acquired disorders (see Chap. 84).

HISTORICAL RÉSUMÉ

Recognition of the various clinical and pathologic features of cystinosis and the Fanconi syndrome was fragmented in time and confounded by chance association with other disorders. (Further details and exact references may be found elsewhere [1, 2].) This confusion began with the first recognition of the disease by Abderhalden in 1903, when he described cystine crystals in the liver and spleen at autopsy of a 21-month-old infant who died of "inanition." Two additional sibs had died previously of a similar illness. Since the urine of the child's father, paternal grandfather, and two sibs contained excessive quantities of cystine, he called the condition a "familial cystine diathesis." This led to an early and unwarranted view that cystinosis was a more severe expression of cystinuria.

Lignac's report in 1924 of cystine deposits in each of three infants with rickets, dwarfism, renal disease, and wasting provided some delineation of the clinical expression of cystinosis. The finding of ureteral cystine stones in one of these children further compounded the confusion with cystinuria. Subsequent reports of other cases of cystine storage without evidence of cystinuria by Russell and Barrie in 1936 and Beumer in 1937 further delineated the multisystem syndrome of "cystine storage disease." The distinction between cystinosis and cystinuria, first suspected on clinical grounds, was clearly established with the subsequent demonstration by Dent and Harris that patients with cystinuria excreted excessive quantities of other dibasic amino acids (lysine, arginine, and ornithine) in addition to cystine.

Additional aspects of the clinical expression of this disease emerged from the association of rickets and stunted growth in a child with glycosuria and albuminuria reported by Fanconi in 1931. Vitamin D–resistant rickets with spontaneous fractures was described in 1933 by deToni in a dwarfed child who also showed a low serum phosphate concentration, acidosis, proteinuria, and glucosuria. A report of a similar child by Debré in 1934 led Fanconi in 1936 to propose a syndrome of "nephrotic-glycosuric dwarfism with hypophosphatemic rickets."

The possibility that the Fanconi syndrome and cystinosis were but two aspects of the same entity, proposed by Beumer and Wepler in 1937, was supported by the demonstration of cystine crystals in the tissues at necropsy of one of Fanconi's original patients. The detailed study by Bickel in 1952 in a larger series of patients provided further evidence of the association of cystinosis with the Fanconi syndrome and progressive glomerular damage.

CLINICAL AND PATHOLOGIC FEATURES

Nephropathic Cystinosis

The major clinical symptomatology of nephropathic cystinosis can, for the most part, be related to the progressive impairment of initially tubular, then glomerular, function to produce an unremitting course.

Early Stage

CLINICAL COURSE   Children with nephropathic cystinosis appear normal at birth and during the first 6 months of life. The first overt signs of the disease are usually produced by the renal tubular defect in water reabsorption. The resulting polyuria and polydipsia make affected children especially vulnerable to dehydration, and this leads to recurrent fever as one of the most common presenting symptoms. In addition, by 1 year of age they usually show growth retardation, rickets, acidosis, and other chemical evidence of renal tubular abnormalities, such as increased renal excretion of glucose, amino acids, phosphate, and potassium. There usually is some evidence of glomerular damage as well, and the subsequent course is determined by the rate at which glomerular insufficiency progresses. Less overt clinical biochemical evidence of the disease has been found at a much earlier age by careful examination of children known to be at risk because of an older affected sib [9, 10]. Some patients show recurrent episodes of acute prostration, weakness, and cardiovascular collapse which can lead to early and sudden death. This has been observed during intravenous infusion of glucose but can also occur without known precipitating cause. This disturbance is associated with gross changes in serum electrolytes. Most of the symptomatology is thought to be related to profound hypokalemia. Three French-Canadian children from the province of Quebec have presented with clinical features of Bartter's syndrome and were subsequently found to have nephropathic cystinosis [11–13].

Failure to thrive is one of the more prominent features of the disease. Affected children show growth failure within the first year of life and almost always remain below the third percentile in both height and weight throughout life. The serum growth hormone concentration is normal [14], but in the later stage of their disease many patients become hypothyroid and require thyroxine replacement therapy [15–17]. Although mental development appears normal, recently it has become apparent that some patients develop hydrocephalus [18, 19]. It is not yet clear whether this is a sporadic occurrence in cystinosis or whether it is a characteristic of the disease in certain families.

Rickets develops at an early age in most patients even on the usual preventive doses of vitamin D (400 units/day). Frontal bossing, genu valgum, thickening of the wrists and ankles, rachitic rosary, and Harrison's groove are frequently seen. X-rays of the long bones show the broadened and frayed epiphyses characteristic of rickets. The glomerular damage progresses in a sporadic but unremitting manner. Glomerular dysfunction may remain constant for many months or even years, followed by periods of fairly rapid deterioration that seem to be unrelated to any environmental or biochemical factor yet detected.

Cystinotic children show a number of clinical features not

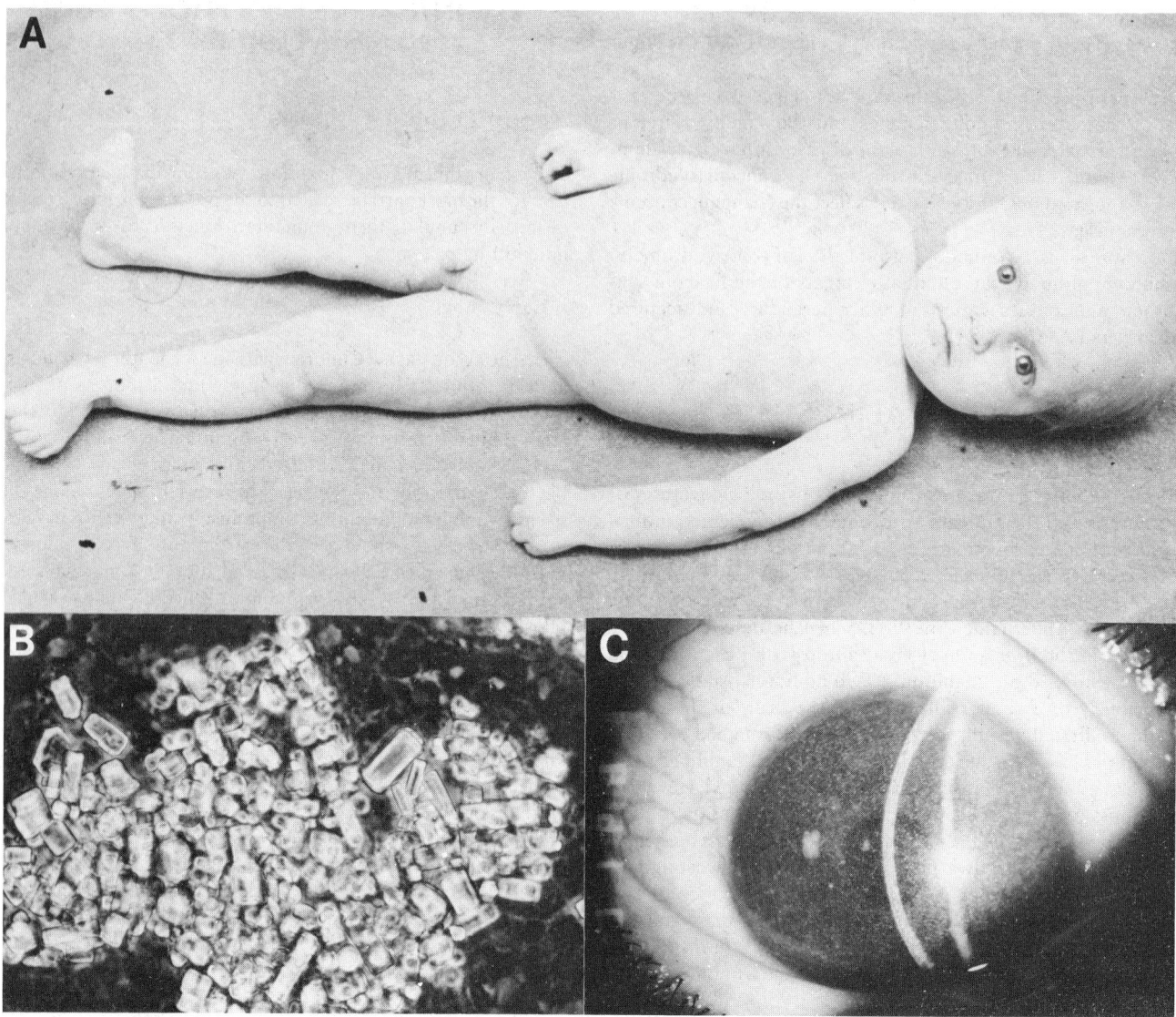

Figure 85-1 *A.* Twenty-month-old child with infantile nephropathic cystinosis showing decreased pigmentation. *B.* Cystine crystals in a bone marrow aspirate from a child with infantile nephropathic cystinosis. This "clump" of crystals is observed with partially crossed polarizing prisms. *C.* Slit-lamp examination of a child with infantile nephropathic cystinosis.

obviously related to the renal abnormalities. The majority have blond hair and a fair complexion, often having substantially lighter pigmentation than their parents (Fig. 85-1A). However, several non-Caucasian children who appear to have typical nephropathic cystinosis have now been identified [20]. In the patients with fair complexion, exposure to sunlight produces skin tanning with far less tendency to sunburn than would be expected from the lack of skin pigment. Cystinotic patients tolerate infections well and show no unusual susceptibility to intercurrent illness.

Severe photophobia develops in most affected children within the first few years of life. Characteristic changes in the eye provide some of the most consistent features of the disease, and a detailed ophthalmologic examination often establishes the clinical diagnosis. The first ophthalmic manifestations were described by Bürki in 1941 [21]. Slit-lamp examination discloses homogeneously dispersed tinsel-like refractile opacities in the cornea and the conjunctiva. Crystalline cystine has been identified by x-ray diffraction in the conjunctival but not in the corneal deposits [22]. The crystalline opacities in the periphery of the cornea occupy the entire corneal thickness. Early in the course of the disease only the anterior one-third to two-thirds

are affected in the central region of the cornea, but with time the entire thickness is involved. These iridescent crystalline particles are so typical as to be virtually diagnostic of all forms of cystinosis; they appear before the full clinical manifestations of nephropathic cystinosis are expressed but are not present at birth [9, 10]. Other disorders are known in which corneal deposits also are found [23].

In addition to the corneal and conjunctival changes, a peripheral retinopathy, which is characteristic only of the nephropathic forms of cystinosis, is present [24]. The pathologic change consists of a generalized pigment disturbance that often assumes a depigmented patchy pattern with superimposed pigment clumps of irregular distribution, varying in size from about one-tenth disk diameter to a fine pepperlike stippling. These changes affect the temporal side more extensively than the nasal and are marked in the peripheral regions of the retina, whereas the central regions are generally devoid of abnormal pigmentation during the first years of life. This retinopathy has permitted a diagnosis of cystinosis to be made in a child as young as 5 weeks of age, even though only a rare crystal was present in the iris at that age [10]. Evidently the retinal changes precede those in the cornea.

LABORATORY FINDINGS   The development of clinical symptoms of the Fanconi syndrome is paralleled by the appearance of laboratory evidence of renal tubular dysfunction. This includes glycosuria, with excretion of from traces to 5 g glucose per 100 ml urine [1, 9], organic aciduria, and amino aciduria. Excessive quantities of multiple amino acids appear in the urine and generally account for about 80 percent of the organic acids. Cystine excretion is generally increased in the same proportion as other amino acids. An increased phosphate excretion is usually found, and a decreased intestinal absorption of phosphate has also been reported [1, 4]. Proteinuria is often present and consists primarily of the so-called tubular protein associated with the Fanconi syndrome. This includes over 50 times the normal excretion of the light chain of gamma globulin [25]. The significance of this characteristic finding remains to be determined. In spite of systemic acidosis, the urine tends to be alkaline and contains increased amounts of ammonium ion. Microscopic examination reveals many granular casts and occasional erythrocytes, as glomerular damage progresses.

The blood sugar concentration is normal. Metabolic acidosis with diminished plasma bicarbonate reflects the renal loss of bicarbonate. Hypophosphatemia is related to the appearance of rickets, the activity of which is reflected in an increased serum concentration of alkaline phosphatase. An increased blood pyruvate concentration has been found in some but not all patients and presumably results from an effect of the cystine on sulfhydryl enzymes [26, 27]. Severe hypokalemia may be present. BUN and serum creatinine are usually in the normal range early in the disease, even though creatinine and urea clearance are substantially diminished. There is often a significant degree of anemia before there is substantial renal failure. The erythrocyte sedimentation rate is usually elevated. The exact reason for this finding is not known but is related to a plasma rather than a red blood cell phenomenon [28].

Late Symptoms and Findings   The clinical course is one of unremitting progression of glomerular damage, leading eventually to end-stage renal failure before puberty. The time course of the progression of glomerular damage is uneven, with periods of apparent stability of renal function interspersed with periods of rapid decline. As in other forms of renal dysfunction, children are able to maintain relatively normal degrees of activity until the renal insufficiency becomes advanced, so that only in the late stages are the children seriously incapacitated.

In some patients advanced renal disease with elevated BUN and creatinine is found as early as 2 years of age. In these patients, the aminoaciduria is often masked by the severely diminished glomerular filtration rate, so that the total amino acid excretion is in the normal range. Other aspects of the Fanconi syndrome may also be obscured in some patients by advanced glomerular damage [27]. In the same manner the hypophosphatemia and hypokalemia are corrected as renal deterioration progresses and are eventually replaced by hyperphosphatemia, hyperkalemia, and a secondary hypocalcemia. The acidosis may then become even more marked. Correction of the acidosis by administration of alkali salts can then result in tetany. Growth failure, progressive renal dysfunction, and

acidosis may also ameliorate the clinical symptoms of rickets. Polyuria and polydipsia also diminish as glomerular insufficiency supervenes. The clinical symptomatology then becomes primarily that associated with severe renal failure and uremia. Weakness and lethargy with edema and congestive cardiac failure result from salt retention and from the profound anemia of renal failure.

The children remain dwarfed throughout life. It is not clear whether this is entirely related to renal failure. Some children have exhibited moderate degrees of "catch-up" growth following renal transplantation (see below). As mentioned, these children have a normal serum growth hormone concentration but often become hypothyroid during the course of their disease. This is presumed to be related to the deposition of cystine crystals in the thyroid gland [14–17]. An abnormal pituitary resistance to thyroid hormone negative feedback also appears to be present in many euthyroid patients [17a].

Now that patients with cystinosis are being kept alive with renal transplants for many additional years, the possibility of impaired function of other organs exists. The organ of most concern is the eye. As these children grow older, both the number of conjunctival and corneal crystals and the degree of retinopathy increase [7, 8, 29]. The retinopathy, which originally is apparent only at the equator of the eye, extends toward the posterior pole. In one study of 10 cystinotic children, aged 11 to 19 years, who had received renal transplants 3 to 9 years previously, none had subjective abnormalities of visual acuity [29]. In another study of 16 cystinotic posttransplant patients, two had marked impairment of vision and another was practically blind [7, 8].

Benign Cystinosis

What appears to be a completely benign variant of cystinosis was first described by Cogan and associates in 1957, and since then many additional cases have been reported [30–35]. This condition has now been diagnosed in a child aged 5 years [36]. The primary clinical distinction between the benign and the nephropathic variants is failure of the former patients to show either retinopathy or renal dysfunction (Table 85-1). Nevertheless, they show crystalline deposits in the cornea, bone marrow, and leukocytes, but these cause no disability. These patients live to adult life, and their cystinosis is usually identified only incidentally during a routine ophthalmologic examination with a slit lamp. This benign variant appears to represent one end of the spectrum of clinical expression. These patients tend to show a somewhat lower concentration of intracellular cystine [32, 37] than do patients with nephropathic cystinosis. Kidney biopsies from two patients demonstrated no cystine crystals [30, 35], and the cystine content of the one biopsy which was measured was not elevated [35]. Thus, it appears that renal function is normal in patients with the benign form of cystinosis because the kidney does not accumulate cystine in these patients.

Intermediate Forms

More recently, a third form of cystinosis has been described [37–47]. This type has been called either *late-onset, intermediate,* or *adolescent cystinosis*. These patients differ from those with benign cystinosis in that they do have renal dysfunction

Table 85-1 Some distinguishing characteristics of the three major types of cystinosis

	Nephropathic		Benign
	Infantile	*Late-onset*	
General symptoms			
Onset of symptoms	6–18 mo	18 mo–17 yr	No symptoms
Growth	Impaired	Variable	Normal
Skin pigmentation	Usually fair*	Variable	Normal
Rickets	Present	Variable	Absent
Bone marrow cystine crystals	Present	Present	Present†
Ocular			
Retinopathy	Present	Variable	Absent
Crystalline deposits in cornea and conjunctiva	Present	Present	Present
Photophobia	Usually present	Variable	Absent‡
Renal			
Tubular dysfunction (Fanconi syndrome)	Present	Often incomplete	Absent
Glomerular failure	Present	Present at a later age than in infantile type	Absent
Inheritance	Autosomal recessive	Autosomal recessive	Autosomal recessive

* Many patients with dark pigmentation have been diagnosed recently [20].
† Cystine crystals could not be demonstrated in bone marrow of two reported cases of benign cystinosis [32 (case 3), 33].
‡ Photophobia occurs in benign cystinosis if it is a part of the ophthalmologic condition which takes the patient to an ophthalmologist.
SOURCE: Adapted from Goldman et al. [37] and Kroll and Lichte [34].

(Table 85-1). They differ from the typical patients with nephropathic cystinosis because their disease is not apparent until an older age, they frequently do not have the complete Fanconi syndrome, and their glomerular insufficiency progresses more slowly. The age at which the first symptoms are noted in these patients has ranged from 18 months [20] to 17 years [41]. When more than one individual in a sibship has this condition, the age of onset and symptomatology are similar. These facts suggest that intermediate cystinosis may represent a range in the spectrum of different types of cystinosis rather than one simply defined disease. It is possible that these patients are either genetic compounds or double heterozygotes who have inherited one gene for the infantile nephropathic form from one parent and a second gene for the benign form from the other parent (see below).

All the patients have shown crystalline material in the cornea and conjunctiva, visible by slit-lamp examination, and have had typical cystine crystals in bone marrow aspirates. Likewise they have all shown abnormally increased concentrations of cystine in leukocytes and cultured skin fibroblasts, although actual values have tended to be lower than generally seen in patients with nephropathic cystinosis [34, 37, 39, 44, 45]. The presence of photophobia and retinopathy has been variable. Unfortunately, most case reports do not comment on skin pigmentation, but a normal skin pigmentation has been reported in one child [37], dark pigmentation in one patient [43], and an extremely fair complexion, typical of patients with nephropathic cystinosis, has been observed in another patient [36]. Growth data on these patients are incomplete. It appears that some patients have near-normal growth, whereas others have delayed growth, but not usually to the extreme degree seen in infantile nephropathic cystinosis.

Genetics

Both the nephropathic and benign forms of cystinosis show autosomal recessive patterns of inheritance. Preliminary evidence indicates that the same is true for the intermediate forms of cystinosis. As a result, consanguine matings such as that shown in Fig. 85-2 appear in greater frequency in families with cystinosis. The frequency of the disease in the general population is difficult to estimate. In a recent French study, the minimum prevalence in the province of Brittany was calculated as 1 per 25,909, but for the rest of France it was calculated as 1 per 326,440 [48]. Although genetic heterogeneity is suggested by the difference in clinical expression of the disease in different families, it is not yet known whether this variation is due to allelic mutations involving one locus or whether several different genetic loci are involved.

Pathology of Cystinotic Tissues

Patients dying of renal failure with cystinosis demonstrate certain pathologic findings typical of uremia, but of greater interest here are the findings unique to cystinosis itself. The specific and characteristic lesion is a striking deposition of cystine crystals in numerous organs, sparing the muscle and brain parenchyma and heavily involving the reticuloendothelial cells of the bone marrow, liver, spleen, and lymphatic system. Cells with a foamy cytoplasm are also frequently found in various tissues and are thought to be cells from which cystine crystals have been removed during preparation of histologic sections. The findings in the kidney and eye will be discussed below.

The solubility of cystine in acid solutions and formalin commonly used as fixatives undoubtedly contributes to the wide variation in the amount of crystal formation observed in histologic preparations. Even in tissues fixed in absolute alcohol or frozen, instances are known in which essentially all crystals were lost during the final exposure to the aqueous solutions used in staining. The cystine crystals are, therefore, best observed in their natural state in frozen or alcohol-fixed tissues before staining, using cross-polarizing filters and phase microscopy. Treatment with organic solvents will remove birefringent lipid materials. The cystine crystals show several different forms including, most frequently, clusters of brick-shaped birefringent crystals, shown in Fig. 85-1B, and less commonly nonbirefringent hexagonal forms. In addition, needle-shaped crystals are also observed in some preparations, but their composition remains to be determined. The medium in which the crystallization occurs can affect the crystal form [49]. Additional points of interest in the histologic preparation of cystinotic tissues are reviewed by Spear [50, 51].

Certain patients given sulfur-restricted diets in attempts to treat cystinosis have developed cirrhosis and osmophilic changes in the lysosomes which are not typical of cystinotic patients not so treated [52].

Kidney Numerous studies describing the pathology of the kidney in cystinosis are reviewed by Spear [50, 51]. Striker and others [53] have analyzed the differences in the pathology of the cystinotic kidney and that of the normal kidney after renal transplantation into a cystinotic host. Their results are discussed in "Renal Transplantation" below.

The morphologic findings vary with the stage of the disease

Figure 85-2 Pedigree showing consanguinity of a family with infantile nephropathic cystinosis.

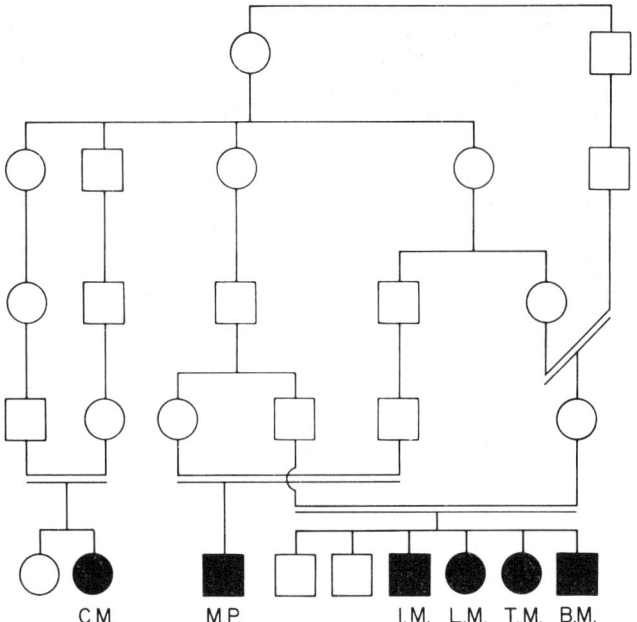

C.M.   M.P.   I.M. L.M. T.M. B.M.

in which the kidneys are studied. A "swan neck" deformity of the proximal convoluted tubule [54] becomes apparent during the first years of life [55] and probably coincides with the clinical onset of the Fanconi syndrome. Although renal lesions may be absent or insignificant early in the disease, the uremic phase of cystinosis has "end-stage" kidneys with glomerular scarring, chronic interstitial nephritis, tubular degeneration, and interstitial fibrosis. There is often a characteristic giant-cell transformation of the visceral glomerular epithelium [40]. Hyperplasia and hypertrophy of the juxtaglomerular apparatus has been described and may correlate with functional alterations of the renin-angiotensin system [56]. Cystine crystals are readily apparent, especially in interstitial cells, but have also been observed in glomerular and tubular cells. Arterial hyperplasia has also been noted.

Kidneys from patients with late-onset nephropathic disease resemble those with advanced changes in the childhood form and, like them, manifest polykaryocytosis of the visceral glomerular cells [39, 47, 57]. A renal biopsy from a single patient considered to have benign cystinosis with hypertensive vascular disease had no crystals by light or electron microscopy, and there was no increase in its cystine content [35].

Electron microscopic studies of cystinotic kidney have been published by several authors [44, 51, 58–60]. Crystalline inclusions, sometimes surrounded by a single limiting membrane, have been observed in a variety of cell types. In an unusual biopsy, Spear observed "dark" cells and cytoplasmic inclusions [61]. Jackson [59] demonstrated by electron diffraction that crystals in a cystinotic kidney sample are L-cystine, while electron probe studies have permitted the conclusion that the dark cells noted by Spear [51] contain an elevated amount of sulfur, in the form of (di)sulfide. Manz and associates described membrane-limited osmophilic structures containing crystal-shaped outlines in podocytes, proximal tubular cells, and mononuclear interstitial cells in a renal biopsy specimen from a patient with late-onset nephropathic cystinosis [47]. Dark cells have also been observed in the liver from a patient with infantile cystinosis [62].

Microscopic examination (light and electron) of the kidney and other tissues of a cystinotic fetus of 23 weeks gestational age [63] failed to reveal cystine crystals, in spite of a marked increase in free cystine content. In contrast, Haynes et al. describe crystals visualized by electron microscopy within Kupffer cell lysosomes in an aborted 22-week cystinotic fetus, although no renal crystals were noted [64].

Eye The striking ocular pathology of cystinosis has been studied by numerous investigators since Bürki [21] first described the corneal crystal deposits in 1941. Several reviews have been published recently [7, 8, 23, 29, 42].

Corneal crystals are present in all forms of cystinosis, although they may be undetectable shortly after birth and are difficult to see without a slit lamp. They are virtually pathognomonic of the disease. The crystals are fusiform or needle shaped in the central cornea where only the anterior portion of the cornea is involved in the early stages. In the peripheral cornea the full thickness may show crystalline deposits which include typical hexagonal or prismatic forms of L-cystine. As in other cystinotic tissues there is no apparent inflammatory reaction to the crystals. The nature of the needle-shaped crystals has not been identified with certainty by electron diffraction nor amino acid analysis. Kenyon and Sensenbrenner have described the electron microscopy of a superficial corneal biopsy in a case of childhood cystinosis [65]. Corneal epithelial cells, histiocytes, and keratocytes showed crystalline inclusions within membrane-limited organelles which the authors considered to have the typical appearance of secondary lysosomes.

Conjunctival cystine crystals (their nature proven by diffraction and amino acid analysis) are prominent in all forms of cystinosis. Electron microscopic studies of several cystinotic variants [35, 65–67] have concluded that these crystals are located within lysosomes in the conjunctival cells. The measurement of the cystine content of conjunctival biopsies has some merit as a rapid method for chemically confirming the diagnosis of cystinosis [68]. Cystine crystals have been described in the entire uveal tract and the sclera, but the lens and vitreous are never involved.

The retinal changes are of help in establishing a diagnosis of cystinosis [24, 42]. They are present usually, and probably invariably if carefully sought, in infantile nephropathic cystinosis. They may be present or absent in late-onset nephropathic cystinosis and have never been observed in patients with benign cystinosis. The retinopathy is of diagnostic significance as it may precede the onset of clinical symptoms or the development of corneal changes by many months, and has been used to make a presumptive diagnosis of cystinosis [10]. A focal and extensive degeneration in the retinal pigment epithelium is most evident near the equator of the eye. An indirect ophthalmoscope may be required for clinical visualization of the patchy depigmentation of the retina. The non-ophthalmologist, with a conventional ophthalmoscope, will often not be able to see these alterations. Cystine crystals are not evident by light microscopy in the retinal pigment epithelium nor in Bruch's membrane, but crystals have been observed in these locations with the electron microscope [69]. It remains to be established whether the retinal changes in crystinosis are related to toxic effects of cysteine [70] or cystine on retinal cells.

In spite of these ocular changes, cystinotic patients demonstrate no consistent abnormality of visual function except a frequently troublesome photophobia, the precise cause of which is undisclosed. The possibility of visual impairment in patients kept alive for many additional years with renal transplants has been discussed earlier in this chapter.

Intracellar Location of Cystine

Cystinotic cells contain large amounts of free cystine in spite of normal activities of the soluble enzyme systems which reduce and further metabolize this amino acid [71]. One explanation for this paradox would be an intracellular compartmentalization of cystine in a location where it is not available to these enzymes.

Lysates of cystinotic leukocytes have been separated into nuclear, granular (acid phosphatase-rich), and soluble fractions, and each fraction assayed for cystine. Most of the total free cystine was found in the granular fraction [72]. Similar results were obtained with lysates of cultured fibroblasts [73] and in both leukocytes and fibroblasts from patients with benign cystinosis [32].

Cystine is released from the granular fraction of cystinotic fibroblasts following treatment with Triton X-100, sodium deoxycholate, or hypotonic solutions [73]. Thus, the cystine in cystinotic cells appears to be separated from the bulk of the cytoplasm by a lipid-containing membrane. Under conditions designed to minimize oxidation-reduction reactions, the compartmentalized cystine of cystinotic fibroblasts was at least fortyfold more concentrated than the cystine detectable in the supernatant cell fraction [74]. Furthermore, this compartmentalized cystine cannot be utilized to supply the cystine requirement of cystinotic fibroblasts grown in cystine-free medium [73], although this cystine pool does have a turnover time of several hours in fibroblasts growing in cystine-containing medium [75].

Compartmentalization of cystine appears to be a primary manifestation of cystinosis, rather than a consequence of prior crystallization of cystine within the cytoplasm. This is shown by several lines of evidence:

1. Cultured cystinotic fibroblasts examined by light or electron microscopy have never shown crystalline deposits. The same is true for cultured cystinotic lymphoblasts, and they, too, have a greatly increased intracellular cystine content [76].

2. Only rare cystine crystals are seen in uncultured cystinotic leukocytes [77, 78], and crystals have not been observed in cystine-rich cystinotic leukocytes prepared from whole blood after using hypotonic saline to disrupt erythrocytes [72].

3. Cystine compartmentalization occurs in the leukocytes and cultured fibroblasts of cystinotic heterozygotes (healthy carriers) in whose cells or tissues cystine crystals have never been observed [79].

Nevertheless, the presence of cytoplasmic osmophilia in cystinotic kidney and liver cells has been interpreted as suggesting that the primary site of cystine "overproduction" is cytoplasmic and that lysosomal "capture" of cystine is secondary [62].

Several morphologic and biochemical approaches have been used to establish the specific type of subcellular organelle involved in the cystinotic process. With the exception of a single unconfirmed report in 1968 [80], all studies have concluded that cystine appears to be stored within the lysosomes. The major evidence for lysosomes being the site of cystine accumulation is as follows:

1. Electron microscopic examination of cystinotic lymph node by Patrick and Lake [81] (Fig. 85-3) revealed crystalline bodies within membrane-limited organelles having the appearance of lysosomes and containing the lysosomal marker enzyme acid phosphatase. Lysosomal location of cystine crystals or noncrystalline amorphous inclusions have also been suggested by others on the basis of electron micrographic study of cystinotic conjunctiva [35, 66, 67, 82], cornea [65], kidney [51], rectal lamina propria, and lymphoctyes [77]. Crystalline outlines have been described within lysosomes of Kupffer cells, but not hepatocytes, in a cystinotic child and fetus [62, 64]. In one study cystinotic conjunctival cells were incubated in vitro with ferritin, an electron-dense protein which upon phagocytosis enters lysosomes. The ferritin was then found within the same membrane-limited organelles as the cystine crystals [82].

2. Cystine and lysosomal marker enzymes were found in the same fractions of sucrose density gradients of the sonicates of washed cystinotic leukocytes [83].

3. Cystinotic fibroblasts cultured in vitro accumulate large

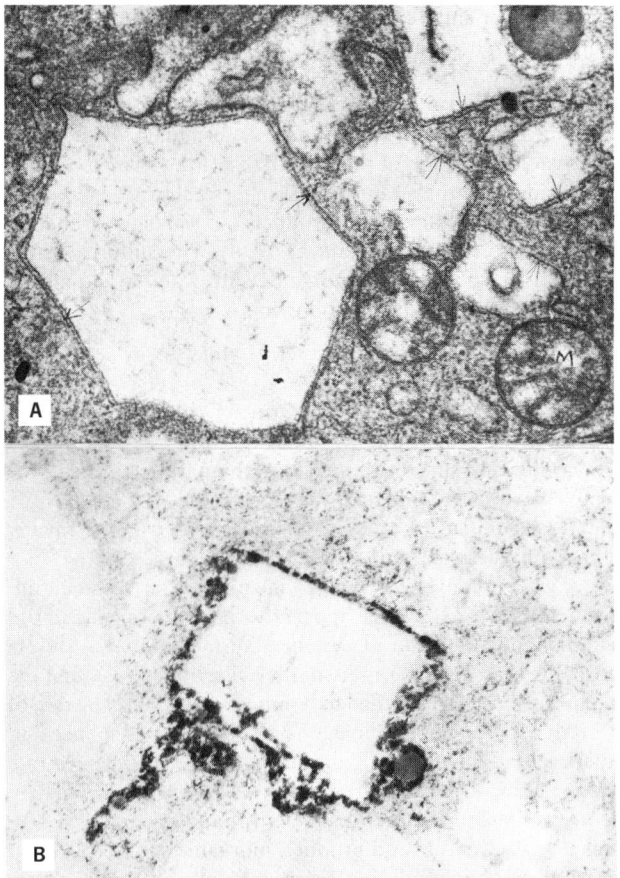

Figure 85-3 Electron photomicrographs of a lymph node biopsy of a patient with cystinosis showing (A) profiles of intracellular cystine crystals within intact limiting membrane as revealed by uranyl acetate stain, and (B) location of acid phosphatase activity at the periphery of a cystine crystal profile as shown by lead deposition after incubation with glycerophosphate. (*Reproduced from Patrick and Lake* [81], *with permission of the Journal of Clinical Pathology.*)

amounts of penicillamine-cysteine disulfide (a cystine analogue) within lysosomelike vacuoles when this compound is added in substantial quantity to the tissue culture medium, while normal fibroblasts under similar conditions do not demonstrate accumulation of this cystinelike compound [84, 85].

4. Highly purified human lysosomes from cystinotic homozygotes and heterozygotes contain abnormally elevated concentrations of cystine [86].

These studies, while seeming to prove the involvement of lysosomes in the cystinotic process, do not definitively exclude the possibility of other organelles being involved to some extent. Even so, it seems reasonable to consider cystinosis as an example of a lysosomal storage disease, differing notably from other such disorders in the small molecular size of the stored metabolite (240 M.W.). Experiments on both human [84, 85] and mouse [87] cells suggest that the lysosomal membrane is relatively impermeable to nonmetabolized amino acids and peptides with a molecular weight greater than approximately 200; thus normal lysosomes presumably have a mechanism permitting the efflux or metabolism of cystine, and the function of this mechanism may well be impaired in cystinosis.

CHEMISTRY OF CYSTINE

Physical and Chemical Properties

L-Cystine crystallizes from water in hexagonal plates that show no birefringence in polarized light. Although hexagonal plates are also found occasionally in bone marrow and other tissues, the most common form is a birefringent rectangular prism. The rectangular birefringent crystals most frequently found in vivo probably represent side views of short hexagonal prisms with two underdeveloped faces [48].

Solubility and pK A saturated aqueous solution contains 112 mg L-cystine per liter at 25°C, 239 mg at 50°C, 523 mg at 75°C, and 1.142 g at 100°C. Cystine is least soluble in the pH range of 3 to 5 [88]. Its solubility rapidly increases as the pH becomes less than 2 or greater than 8 [88]. In aqueous solution, dissociation constants for cystine are: $pK_{a_1} = 8.00$; $pK_{a_2} = 10.25$; $pK_{b_1} = 11.95$; and $pK_{b_2} = 12.96$. Approximately 380 mg cystine per liter (320 μmol half-cystine per 100 ml) [72, 89] can be dissolved in human plasma at 37°C and pH 7.4. Cystine is insoluble in alcohol.

Redox Potential The interconversion of cystine and cysteine constitutes a reversible oxidation-reduction system. Values reported for the absolute redox potential range from −0.21 and −0.23 eV [90, 91] to −0.34 and −0.39 eV [92, 93]. The redox potential for cysteine/cystine relative to GSH/GSSG is + 0.017 to 0.018 eV. The disulfide bond of cystine therefore readily reacts with SH groups of glutathione and a large number of other compounds to form cysteine and the mixed disulfide of cysteine and the original SH compound.

Determination of Cystine and Cysteine The best known method of detecting cyst(e)ine (cystine, cysteine, or both) is with the cyanide-nitroprusside reaction [94]. This reaction is nonspecific and cannot be used for quantitation. There are numerous methods for the measurement of sulfhydryl groups which can be used to measure cystine following its reduction to cysteine [95, 96], but many other thiol compounds interfere with these measurements in physiologic systems. This is especially true in mammalian tissues, which contain a much higher concentration of reduced glutathione than of cyst(e)ine [75]. Older and generally less useful methods for measurement of cysteine and cystine in physiologic samples are referenced in earlier editions of this text [1, 4].

Quantitative amino acid analysis by ion-exchange chromatography is the standard method for measurement of small amounts of cystine or cysteine. Cysteine is usually first stabilized as the adduct with iodoacetate or N-ethylmaleimide. Although accelerated systems of amino acid analysis have become common, physiologic fluids require longer runs than protein hydrolysate [97]. Newer ion-exchange chromatography methods generally have a sensitivity in the subnanomolar range when detection is accomplished with ninhydrin. The use of fluorescamine has made possible the measurement of picomolar quantities of some amino acids following ion-exchange chromatography [98].

A protein-binding assay for cystine has been developed utilizing a cystine-binding protein from *Escherichia coli* [99]. Filtration of a mixture of [14C]cystine and cystine-binding protein through nitrocellulose filters separates the [14C]cystine–cystine-binding protein complex from the unbound cystine. Nonradioactive cystine competes with [14C]cystine, resulting in diminution of bound radioactivity, which permits the direct calculation of the nonradioactive cystine concentrations of unknown samples. The method has substantial specificity and permits measurement of picomolar quantities of cystine. Numerous assays can be performed in a single day. While much simpler and cheaper to perform than quantitative analysis of cystine by ion exchange, the binding protein required for this method is not at present available commercially.

A recurring problem in any biochemical study of sulfur amino acid metabolism is the tendency of sulfhydryl groups to undergo spontaneous oxidation to disulfide groups or sulfonic acids upon exposure to dissolved oxygen. This problem is especially difficult when a determination of the sulfhydryl and disulfide forms of the same compound (cysteine and cystine) is required. The identity of the sulfhydryl group can be maintained by treatment with a reagent that forms a stable compound with sulfhydryl groups, such as iodoacetamide, iodoacetate, or N-ethylmaleimide. The sulfhydryl derivative can then be separated from the disulfide compound and detected with ninhydrin. Separation of such compounds can be achieved with ion-exchange chromatography, high voltage electrophoresis on paper, or by paper or thin-layer chromatography [100–102].

Metabolism of Cystine

Detailed reviews of the metabolic origin and fate of cyst(e)ine have been published [103, 104]. Furthermore, Mudd and Levy in this text (see Chap. 25) have analyzed the reactions involved in the formation of cysteine from methionine. Therefore, in this section we present only a very limited discussion of cyst(e)ine formation and the major features of its degradation and reduction. Most of the reactions referred to are illustrated in Figs. 85-4 and 85-5. The metabolism of cystine in cystinosis is discussed in a subsequent section.

In normal human beings, methionine is an essential amino acid, although cystine, which is not, can replace 80 to 90 percent of the human requirement for methionine [105]. The bulk of ingested methionine is converted to cysteine in normal humans. Children can grow normally on a diet containing adequate methionine but no cystine [106]. Cystine is an essential amino acid for human diploid fibroblasts in culture [107–109] but not for continuous human lymphoid cell lines [110]. Cystine is also required by certain patients deficient in enzymes for methionine-cystine conversion [111] and probably by human fetuses and neonates who normally lack cystathionase [112].

Both glutathione and cellular proteins can serve as cyst(e)ine reservoirs in normal cells [113–115].

Cysteine Synthesis The conversion of methionine to cysteine involves transsulfuration by way of S-adenosyl-L-methionine, S-adenosyl-L-homocysteine, L-homocysteine, and L-cystathionine, as reviewed in Chap. 25. Alternative pathways for cysteine synthesis from methionine have not been elucidated in humans. While there is substantial evidence [111, 116] that the cystathionine pathway is the primary route for cysteine synthesis, animal studies suggest that cysteine can also be synthesized to some extent from sulfide [117, 118], thiosulfate [119, 120], and sulfur [120]. Mammals are unable to synthesize cysteine

from sulfite or sulfate, where the sulfur atom exists in a more highly oxidized state [121].

Cysteine Degradation Known degradative reactions of cyst(e)ine primarily involve cysteine rather than cystine, with the possible exception of the conversion of the latter to cystine disulfoxide and then taurine, as suggested by Medes [122, 123]. The major human end products of cysteine degradation are inorganic sulfate and taurine [124]. The sulfur atom of cysteine is metabolized to inorganic sulfur and eventually to sulfate or thiosulfate in the following ways:

1. Conversion of cysteine to serine and H_2S by serine sulfhydrase [118].
2. Conversion of cysteine to pyruvate, ammonia, and H_2S by cysteine desulfhydrase. A similar reaction can be catalyzed with cystine as substrate, and cystathionase is one enzyme capable of carrying out such reactions [103].
3. Transamination of cysteine to beta-mercaptopyruvate, followed by desulfuration of the latter [125–129].
4. Cysteine conversion by cysteine oxidase to L-cysteinesulfinic acid [130–132]. This appears to be a major reaction in mammalian catabolism of cysteine. Cysteine oxidase (dioxygenase) is present in many tissues (even retina [133]), and the rat enzyme has been purified to homogeneity [134]. The rate of formation of cysteinesulfinate from cysteine is enhanced in experimental animals by high dietary intake of the substrate cysteine [135, 136] or its precursor, methionine [136, 137], by nicotinamide and hydrocortisone [138] and probably by low intake of an eventual end product, inorganic sulfate [139]. In contrast, cysteine oxidase activity is reduced in brain, testis, and seminal vesicles of morphine-treated rats [140], and hepatic cysteine oxidase is decreased in rats injected with glucagon [141]. Cysteinesulfinate may then contribute to formation of inorganic sulfate through sulfite, either by undergoing conversion to alanine and sulfite [142] or by transamination and conversion to pyruvate and sulfite [143–146]. In some tissues, cysteinesulfinate transamination appears to be catalyzed by aspartate aminotransferase [147]. Sulfite is converted irreversibly to sulfate by sulfite oxidase [148], the deficiency of which has been associated with a lethal syndrome in humans [149, 150].

Wainer [151, 152] has described a mitochondrial enzyme system in rat liver which converts cysteine to sulfate. The intermediates in these reaction(s) and their physiologic importance are not established.

Taurine, the most abundant urinary sulfur metabolite, next to sulfate, arises primarily from cysteine by way of cysteine sulfinate (as discussed above) [153–155] but might also be formed from cystine through cystine disulfoxide and from cysteine through cysteamine [138, 156]. Cysteinesulfinate is converted to taurine by way of either hypotaurine or cysteic acid, the former route probably being of greater quantitative significance. The decarboxylases involved in the conversion of cysteinesulfinate to taurine require pyridoxal phosphate, and taurine excretion is reduced in B_6-deficient human beings [157] and rats [138].

Cysteine has additional metabolic fates not discussed above [103, 153]. Of interest are its conversion to the tripeptide glutathione, as elucidated by Block and associates [158, 159], and its oxidation to cystine, which is potentiated by a diverse variety of enzymes and nonenzymatic catalysts [103]. It has recently been shown that human tissues contain pantetheinase

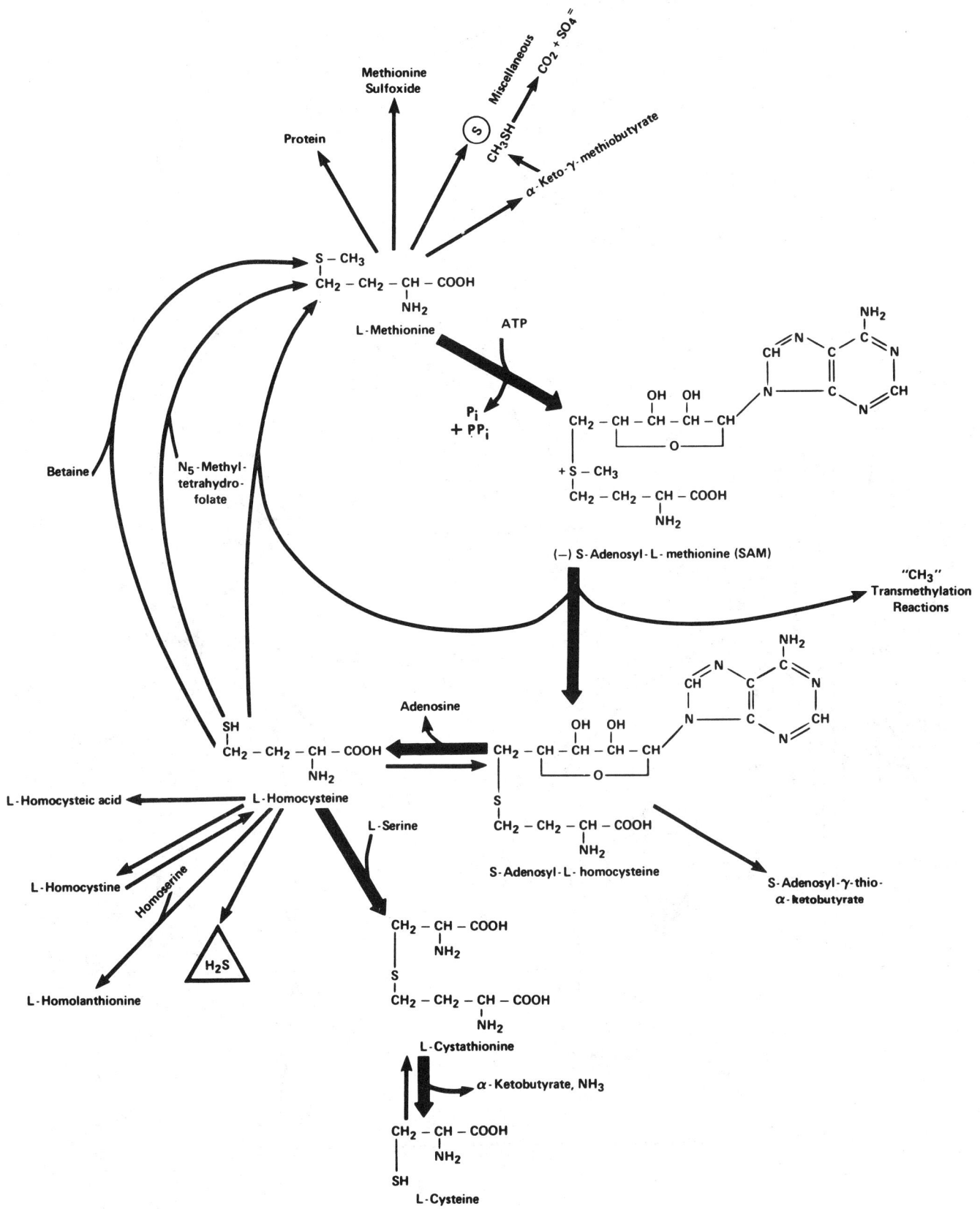

Figure 85-4 Pathways of cysteine synthesis.

activity, considered necessary for the conversion of cysteine to cysteamine [160].

The work of Felten and associates [161] and of Engelhardt et al. [162] suggests that cystine may undergo photochemical degradation in plasma exposed to bright light. Such reaction(s) are of unknown significance in vivo.

Various attempts have been made to identify lysosomal enzymes which might have the ability to catabolize cystine or

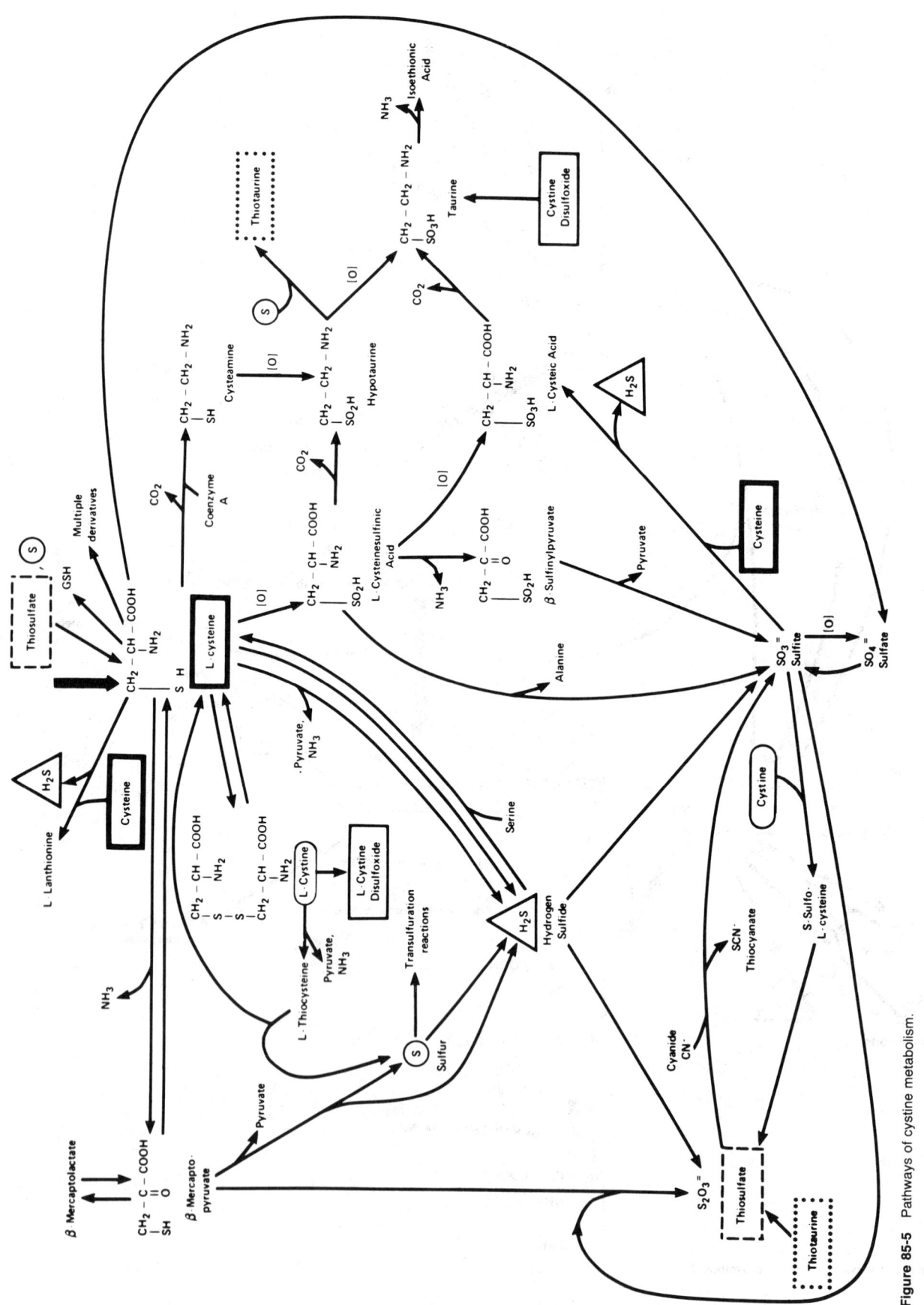

Figure 85-5 Pathways of cystine metabolism.

cysteine, but no lysosomal enzyme of this type has been characterized.

Cystine Reduction   Intracellular cyst(e)ine exists mainly as cysteine [163, 164], in spite of the tendency for aerobic conversion of cysteine to cystine. As summarized by Tietze [104], a number of enzyme systems are presently known which serve to keep cysteine reduced in normal tissues. These form two classes: (1) nucleotide-dependent disulfide reductases, and (2) thiol-disulfide transhydrogenases, which are more correctly regarded as thiol-transferases [165].

Several nucleotide-dependent disulfide reductases include: the NADH-cystine reductases described in yeast, pea seeds, and hog liver by Nickerson and Romano [166, 167] and by Myers and Worthen [168] in tissues of rat, rabbit, and human beings; the NADPH-dependent thioredoxin system [169] studied quantitatively in cultured human fibroblasts by Larsson and associates [170]; the NADPH-dependent disulfide reductase of rat liver [171, 172]; a NADPH-dependent disulfide reductase in yeast and rat liver apparently specific for the mixed disulfide of coenzyme A and glutathione (CoASSG) [173]; and a group of enzyme activities described in several species which catalyze the reduction of protein-bound disulfide groups by reduced nucleotide [104].

The thiol-disulfide transhydrogenases are capable of catalyzing the reduction of disulfides (usually including cystine) by thiols (usually glutathione). The reaction between glutathione and cystine proceeds through formation of the mixed disulfide:

$$GSH + CySSCy \longleftrightarrow CySSG + CySH$$
$$GSH + CySSG \longleftrightarrow GSSG + CySH$$

Reduced glutathione is regenerated from GSSG by the action of glutatione reductase. Many human and mammalian cells contain substantial amounts of both reduced glutathione and a glutathione-disulfide transhydrogenase (or thiol-transferase) which reduces cystine. It is reasonable to suppose that this is a quantitatively significant system for the intracellular reduction of cystine. The extensive literature related to this system has been summarized [104]. Additional thiol-disulfide transhydrogenases, not always unambiguously characterized as distinct from the above system, include: glutathionine-homocystine transhydrogenase of beef liver [174–175]; GSH-CoASSG transhydrogenase of bovine kidney [176]; yeast thiol-disulfide transhydrogenase [177]; GSH-CySSG transhydrogenase of rat liver [178], which also has some activity as a GSH-cystine transhydrogenase; a GSH-thiamine disulfide transhydrogenase [179] unable to reduce cystine (GSH-cystine transhydrogenase of rat liver that can also reduce thiamine disulfide [180]); disulfide-rearranging enzyme [186]; glutathionine-insulin transhydrogenase [182] that may be the same enzyme as the one described by Anfinsen [183]; and a thiol-disulfide transhydrogenase of sea urchin eggs described by Sakai [184].

There is limited and so far unconvincing evidence that lysosomes have enzymatic mechanisms for cystine reduction [185]. There is a report of GSH-insulin transhydrogenase activity in rat liver lysosomes [186], but attempts to confirm this resulted in the conclusion that the assay method was inherently unreliable [187]. Griffiths and Lloyd have published results suggesting the presence of an as yet uncharacterized thiol:protein disulfide oxidoreductase in rat liver lysosomes [187].

Cystine Metabolism in Cystinosis

While the mutant gene product responsible for the development of cystinosis continues to be elusive, substantial progress has been made. Many hypotheses have been proposed only to be discarded because of lack of support by subsequent investigations. The underlying cause of the accumulation of excessive quantities of cystine remains to be identified, but the site of cystine storage has been established as intracellular and has been further localized to the lysosomes, as already noted. Data concerning the intestinal absorption of cyst(e)ine, the plasma concentration and solubility of cyst(e)ine, and the urinary excretion of cyst(e)ine in cystinosis have been presented elsewhere [1, 4]. Suffice it to say that the intestinal absorption, the fasting plasma concentration, and the plasma solubility of cyst(e)ine are normal in cystinotic patients. The urinary excretion of cystine is elevated in cystinosis [27, 49, 188], but to the same degree as other amino acids, and not to the extent which would ever lead to cystine stone formation in the urinary tract as in cystinuria (see Chap. 80.)

Intracellular Concentration of Free Cystine   Since histologic examination of cystinotic tissues shows cystine crystals primarily in reticuloendothelial cells, the simplest explanation is that the crystals are first formed extracellularly and are then phagocytized. On the other hand, Barr concluded 30 years ago, on histologic grounds, that the crystals form inside these cells and are not trapped by phagocytosis [189]. This question was answered definitely by studying the intracellular cystine content of crystal-free cells from patients with cystinosis. An increased intracellular cystine content was found and apparently leads to crystal formation. Earlier measurements of cystine content in cystinotic tissue had merely reflected the presence of cystine crystals [49].

LEUKOCYTE CONTENT OF CYSTINE   Mixed populations of peripheral leukocytes from patients with cystinosis contain much more free cystine than normal cells and thus provided the first meaningful biochemical measurement of cystine accumulation in this disease [72]. Cells containing crystals did not withstand the brief exposure to hypotonic solutions used to lyse erythrocytes during the preparation procedure and were, therefore, never observed in the final leukocyte preparations. Subsequent studies of such leukocyte preparations by electron microscopy have revealed no intracellular crystals [28, 77]. The mean free-cystine (i.e., nonprotein cystine) content of white blood cells from nine children with infantile nephropathic cystinosis was, nevertheless, 80 times normal, and from three patients with benign cystinosis, it was 30 times normal [32, 72] (Fig. 85-6). Patients with intermediate (late-onset) cystinosis tend to have free-cystine content of leukocytes greater than found in patients with benign cystinosis but less than found in patients with infantile nephropathic cystinosis [34, 37, 39]; but many exceptions have been noted [190]. Subsequent studies have demonstrated that cystine stores are primarily in the polymorphonuclear leukocytes and monocytes rather than in lymphocytes [191].

Although cyst(e)ine is known to occur primarily as cysteine within cells [163, 164, 192], an elevation of cysteine (measured as its N-ethylmaleimide adduct) has never been found in cystinotic cells [72]. This may be because only the disulfide form is trapped within cystinotic lysosomes or because the intracellu-

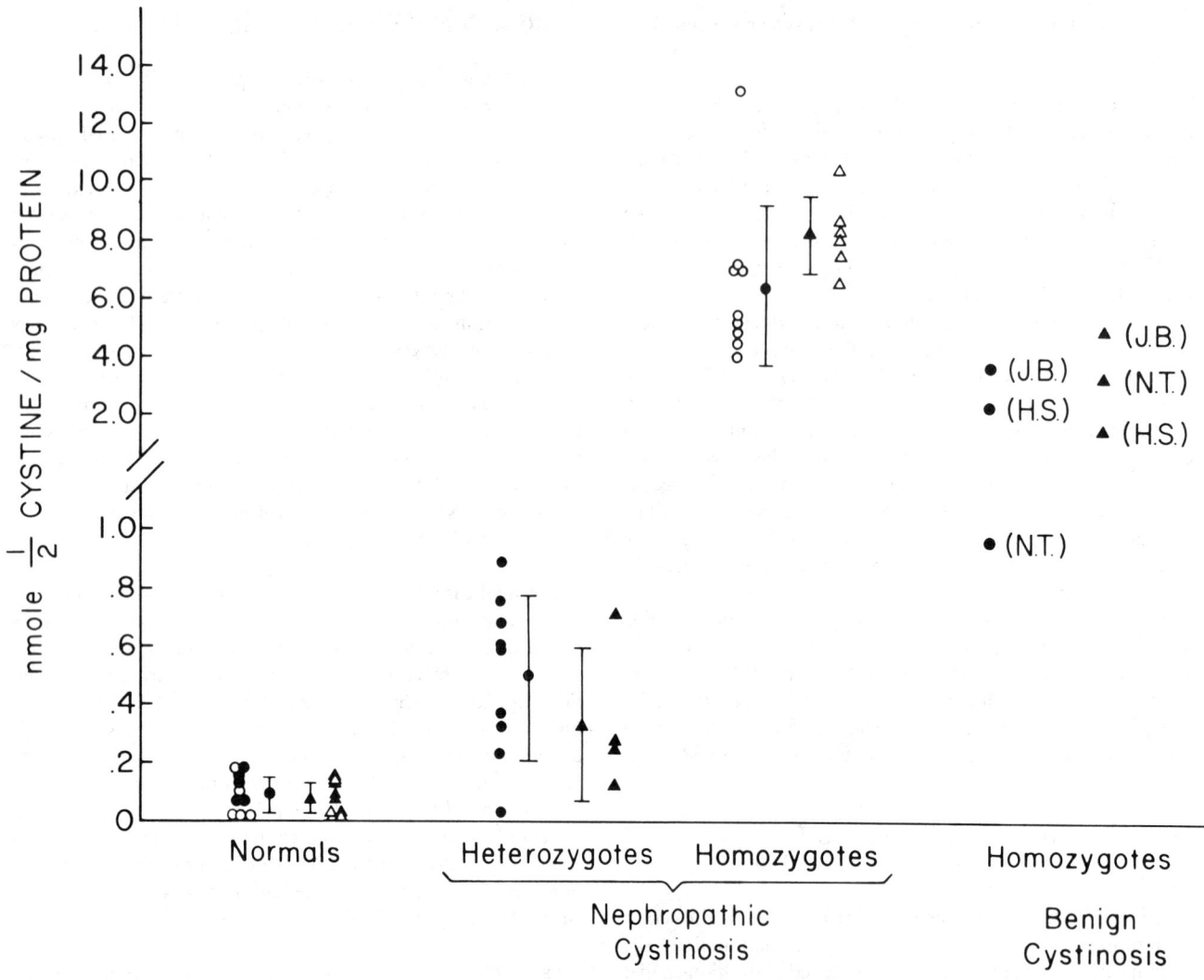

Figure 85-6   Free-cystine content of leukocytes (○,●) and fibroblasts (△, ▲) from patients with infantile nephropathic and benign cystinosis. Open symbols represent children, and closed symbols represent adults. Note the scale change on the ordinate. The brackets indicate ± 1 SD from the mean. (*Reproduced from Schneider et al. [32] with permission of the New England Journal of Medicine.*)

lar cysteine may leak out of the leukocytes during preparation. The content of another reduced sulfhydryl compound of larger molecular weight, glutathione, is normal in leukocytes from patients with cystinosis [75].

CYSTINE CONTENT OF CULTURED CELLS   Fibroblasts cultured in vitro from skin biopsies of patients with cystinosis and maintained in culture through several generations also contain greatly increased amounts of free cystine [73]. Fibroblasts from patients with all types of cystinosis grow normally and appear normal in culture. Cystine crystals have not been seen in these fibroblasts by either phase or electron microscopy [28]. Yet, fibroblasts from patients with infantile nephropathic cystinosis contain over 100 times the normal content of free cystine, and from patients with benign cystinosis about 50 times the normal free-cystine content [32, 73] (Fig. 85-6). Fibroblasts cultured from patients with the intermediate type of cystinosis tend to have a free-cystine content greater than found in patients with benign cystinosis, but less than found in patients with infantile nephropathic cystinosis [34, 37, 39]. Again, many exceptions occur [193].

Continuous lymphoblast cultures (presumably transformed by Epstein-Barr virus) have been established from patients with cystinosis. These cells contain 15 to 20 times more free cystine than continuous lymphoblast cultures from normal

individuals [76]. Cystinotic skin fibroblasts transformed with SV-40 virus [194] contain 30 to 50 times more free cystine per milligram protein than do SV-40 transformed cells from normal control individuals. Both of these cell types should be useful for the study of this disease since they are established lines in which a large number of cells may be produced. Both cells have the disadvantage of containing less free cystine than found in peripheral leukocytes or untransformed skin fibroblasts from cystinotic individuals.

Detection of Heterozygotes   The free-cystine content of peripheral leukocytes and of skin fibroblasts from parents of cystinotic children has provided the first biochemical identification of the heterozygote in this disorder [72, 73], as shown in Fig. 85-6. The mean intracellular content of free cystine in peripheral leukocytes or in fibroblasts from obligate heterozygotes for infantile nephropathic cystinosis is five to six times greater than the mean normal value. Although there is occasional overlap between control and heterozygote values, the differences between these groups is statistically significant

($p<0.001$ for leukocyte values and about 0.01 for fibroblast values). The fact that the cystine content of heterozygote cells is substantially less than half that observed in cells from homozygous patients means that the cystine content is not directly proportional to gene dosage in this recessively inherited disease.

Since these studies [72 , 73] were reported, many more measurements of free cystine have been made in heterozygous leukocytes and fibroblasts. The data in leukocytes have been repeatedly confirmed in many laboratories, but the values in fibroblasts have been erratic, and we cannot recommend this as a method for heterozygote detection [195]. Although only limited data are available, the free cystine content of cells from obligate heterozygotes for both the benign and intermediate types of cystinosis appear to follow the same pattern as in infantile nephropathic cystinosis [27, 190]. Recently, Steinherz et al. have proposed that the retarded rate of clearance of cystine from leukocytes exposed to cystine dimethylester could serve as an additional marker for cystinosis heterozygotes [234].

Source of the Cystine in Cystinotic Cells

Until recently the exact source of the cystine which accumulates in cystinotic cells was not known. The finding that the cystine content of cystinotic cells is somewhat proportional to the cystine content of the medium suggested that some of the accumulated cystine came from extracellular cyst(e)ine [193,196]. On the other hand, Oshima et al. [197] found that after cystinotic fibroblasts are depleted of free cystine with cysteamine, 30 to 50 percent of the cystine reaccumulated in 24 h in the absence of extracelluar cystine. The possibility that the cystine in cystinotic fibroblasts is derived from methionine, cystathionine, or serine was ruled out by experiments with radiolabeled precursors [193,198]. The availability of methods to deplete cystinotic cells of their increased free cystine with either dithiothreitol [199] or cysteamine [200] made the further study of this problem possible. Thoene et al. [198] were able to show that, after depletion of cystine from cystinotic fibroblasts with cysteamine, the cystine which reaccumulates in a cystine-free medium comes from the intracellular degradation of protein. More recently Thoene and Lemons [201] have shown that extracellular protein can also serve as a source of the cystine which accumulates in cystinotic cells. These findings have been misinterpreted to imply that protein degradation is abnormal in cystinotic cells [202]. This is not the case. Protein degradation simply provides a major source of the free cystine which accumulates in the lysosomes of cystinotic cells.

Degradation and Reduction of Cystine in Cystinosis

A working hypothesis to account for the cystine storage in cystinosis is a derangement in lysosomal metabolism or transport of cystine. This view is strengthened by the demonstration that concentrations of reduced glutathione and cysteine are in the normal range in cystinotic cells [75] and that in cystinotic cells and tissues there are normal activities of numerous non-lysosomal enzymes known to use cysteine or cystine as substrates. The mean ratio of reduced to oxidized glutathione (GSH/GSSG) may even be increased in cultured cystinotic fibroblasts [203].

In 1961, Worthen and Good [204] reported decreased activ-

ity of NADH-dependent cystine reductase (to about one-half normal) in the blood of two patients. Mahoney and Trump confirmed this observation [205], but Seegmiller and Howell [206] found that the cysteine-glutathione transhydrogenase of erythrocytes was much more active than cystine reductase in reducing cystine. The transhydrogenase was present in cystinotic liver.

Patrick reported the activity of a large number of enzymes concerned with the degradation of cysteine and cystine in postmortem liver and other organs from children with nephropathic cystinosis and found no evidence for a metabolic block [71]. The enzymes studied included those responsible for the decarboxylation of cysteinesulfinic acid and cysteic acid; the oxidation of cystine and cysteine to inorganic sulfate; and the transamination of cysteinesulfinic acid with alpha-ketoglutarate, yielding beta-sulfinylpyruvic acid which is then desulfinated to pyruvic acid and sulfite.

The bulk of cystine reduction is carried out by soluble cytoplasmic cell fractions [104], although under certain conditions mitochondria [207,208] and possibly lysosomes [185–187] can also carry out cystine reduction. Glutathione reductase, NADH-dependent cystine reductase, and glutathione-cystine transhydrogenase activites were normal in extracts of whole cystinotic kidney and liver [71]. Tietze and associates, after extensive investigations of cystine reduction in cystinotic and normal uncultured and cultured leukocytes, found no differences between cystinotic and normal cells [209]. Glutathione reductase activities were comparable. Granular fraction glutathione-cystine transhydrogenase activities, tested both at acidic and neutral pH, were negligible in comparison with those present in the supernatant cell fractions. Leukocytes, in contrast to liver, demonstrated little or no nucleotide-dependent cystine reductase activity with either NADH or NADPH used as H-donor. Kaye and Nadler [210] reported two isoenzyme forms of cystine-glutathione transhydrogenase but were unable to demonstrate differences in the properties of cystine-glutathione transhydrogenase, cystine reductase, or glutathione reductase in cultured cystinotic and normal skin fibroblasts. States et al. have reported altered patterns of cystine reduction by GSH in extracts of cystinotic fibroblasts and suggest an abnormality in control of cystine reduction in cystinosis. In some cystinotic extracts cystine-reducing activity was actually increased and only a preliminary interpretation of their results was proposed [211].

Orloff et al. examined the possibility that an endogenous cysteamine-generating system was deficient in cystinotic cells. Cysteamine could serve as a "shuttle" between cytoplasmic GSH and intralysosomal cystine, permitting reduction of the latter and its escape from the lysosomes. Pantetheinase activity, however, appeared normal in cystinotic leukocytes and fibroblasts [160].

Waterson and associates [212] considered the possibility that an altered cysteinyl-tRNA synthetase might lead to faulty regulation of cyst(e)ine concentrations in cystinotic cells. In contrast to other investigators [75], these authors found elevated concentrations of both cystine and cysteine in two out of three cystinotic fibroblast lines studied. The cystinotic cells contained normal amounts of tRNAcys and normal activity of cys-tRNA synthetase. The K_m values of the synthetase for cysteine, ATP, and tRNA were also normal.

States and coworkers [213] studied the metabolism of [35S]cyst(e)ine in cystinotic and normal fibroblasts. They found no differences in the conversion of cystine to its acidic sulfur metabolites. This result is compatible with evidence from in vivo and in vitro studies that desulfuration of cysteine and its conversions to cysteine sulfinate, taurine, and sulfate occur at normal rates in cystinosis [71,206,214].

Patrick et al. have studied the properties of the enzyme gamma-glutamyl transpeptidase in cystinotic and normal liver, spleen, leukocytes, and fibroblasts, and in subcellular fractions from the leukocytes [215]. Cystine is an extremely effective amino acceptor of the glutamyl moiety. Meister [159] has postulated a role for this glutathione-catabolizing enzyme in the mediation of amino acid transport. The enzyme was found in lysosomal cell fractions from leukocytes and rat liver. No differences from normal were found in the properties of gamma-glutamyl transpeptidase from several cystinotic tissues and cell fractions [215,216]. Other investigators subsequently reported a mean increase in gamma-glutamyl transpeptidase activity in cultured cystinotic fibroblasts. The relationship of this observation to the fundamental molecular defect in cystinosis is currently unexplained [217]. Butler and Spielberg [218] were able to modify cystine levels in cystinotic cells with transpeptidase inhibitors, and their results may suggest that glutathione catabolism affects the degree of cystinotic cystine storage.

The significance of several other metabolic differences reported in cystinotic tissues is obscure. No direct relation between the aberration of cystine metabolism characteristic of cystinosis and the increased concentration of beta-alanine described by Wenske and Linneweh [219] in cystinotic lymphocytes and platelets is immediately apparent. The selective reduction of arylsulphatase B activity in cystinotic fibroblasts described by Furusho and colleagues [220] has not been confirmed by Scardigli et al., who found instead a moderate reduction in cystinotic beta-galactosidase activity [221].

Transport of [35S]Cystine and [35S]Cysteine by Cystinotic Cells   Since no enzyme defect has yet been identified in cystinosis, a possible defect in cyst(e)ine transport has been postulated [222]. Exploratory studies have been extremely difficult to interpret for several reasons:

1. The cystinotic cells being studied carry a large load of cystine, whereas the control cells do not. Furthermore, although the major portion of the intracellular free cystine in the cystinotic cells is compartmentalized within the lysosome, studies of this compartmentalization [72,73,83] have always shown significant cystine in the cytosol. Whether this is actually the case in vivo or represents an artifact is not clear. Consequently, in studies of cystine transport in a cystinotic cell, the amount of free cystine present in the cytosol compared with the lysosomes is never known.

2. Cystine taken up by the cell is rapidly reduced to cysteine and then incorporated into glutathione [101]. Thus, investigators have been forced to study transport of a compound which is being metabolized rapidly during the study.

3. Fundamental knowledge of the mechanisms of cyst(e)ine transport in cells or subcellular organelles, including lysosomes, is limited [223–227].

[35S]Cystine transport studies in cystinosis were first attempted in peripheral leukocytes [101]. As had been reported previously [228], normal leukocytes do not take up significant amounts of [35S]cystine. The same was found for cystinotic leukocytes. The study was therefore done with [35S] cysteine [101,229]. Cystinotic leukocytes incorporated over 50 percent more [35S] than leukocytes from age-matched controls.

Approximately 30 percent of intracellular [35S] was found in glutathione in both cystinotic and control cells. In the normal leukocytes, approximately two percent of the [35S] was found in the oxidized form, cystine, whereas in the cystinotic cells, 40 percent was found as cystine. When the distribution ratio was recalculated to represent only [35S]cysteine (the form present extracellularly and the form which was actually being transported), the values were not significantly different between the cystinotic and normal control cells.

Similar studies performed in established lines of lymphoblasts cultured from patients with nephropathic cystinosis and normal control individuals showed no significant difference in the uptake of [35S]cystine by these two cell types [76]. The intracellular form of [35S] was not characterized in this study.

The uptake and utilization of cystine have been studied in cystinotic and normal control skin fibroblasts [213]. Although the investigators showed an increased uptake and decreased efflux of cystine from the cystinotic cells, they found that the apparent K_t for cystine entry was the same in both cell types. They were unable to conclude whether the differences in uptake were due to primary changes in membrane function. More recently, these investigators have published preliminary data suggesting that cystinotic fibroblasts have enhanced cystine uptake, compared with normal ones, even when pretreatment with cysteamine has been employed to reduce their intracellular cystine content to normal levels. In these studies transport was assessed under conditions in which cystinotic cystine pool reaccumulation was occurring, which complicated interpretation of the data [230].

If cystinosis is actually caused by a defect in cyst(e)ine transport, it may well be at the level of the lysosomal membrane rather than the plasma membrane. This would explain why cystine accumulates within cystinotic lysosomes. Studies of impure [2] and pure [86] cystinotic lysosomes suggest that other amino acids do not accumulate abnormally at this site. Methods for determining amino acid efflux from isolated lysosomes have been inadequate [231], but evidence has been obtained from studies on whole cells that cystinotic lysosomes are similar to normal in their permeability to nonmetabolizable small molecules [84,85]. Recently, Reeves [232] has described the use of amino acid methylesters for measuring efflux of amino acids from isolated lysosomes. Steinherz et al. [233,234] have applied this method to compare efflux of cystine and other amino acids in normal and cystinotic leucocyte lysosomes. Their results indicate that cystinotic lysosomes have apparently normal efflux of leucine and thus do not have decreased permeability to L-amino acids in general. Cystine efflux was much slower than leucine efflux in both normal and cystinotic lysosomes. The extremely slow normal rate of cystine efflux confounds interpretation of the comparisons. In contrast, when *intact* cystinotic leukocytes were loaded with cystine by exposure to cystine dimethylester, distended lysosomes were observed by electron microscopy. The clearance of cystine from such cells was far slower in cystinotic than in normal overloaded leukocytes, and heterozygotes had, on average, intermediate values [234].

Biochemical Basis of Cystine Toxicity

Effect on Sulfhydryl Enzymes   As a result of the facile sulfhydryl-disulfide interaction occurring between cystine and sulfhydryl groups, cystine can inhibit many sulfhydryl-dependent enzyme systems. The possible inhibition of sulfhydryl enzyme systems as a mechanism involved in the clinical expression of the disease must be considered. The renal tubular defect in cystinosis could very well result from an inhibition of sulfhydryl-dependent enzyme systems presumably involved in tubular reabsorptive processes.

The sulfhydryl-disulfide interaction provides an indirect argument in support of the compartmentalization of the cystine pool in cystinotic cells so that it is not in physical contact with cytoplasmic enzymes. Otherwise the hundredfold increase in cystine concentration, with its consequent inhibition of so many enzymes, would probably be incompatible with life. Such considerations also argue against the mitochondria as the site of cystine storage, since many vital mitochondrial enzymes are inhibited by the oxidized form of this amino acid. Finally, one must evaluate with circumspection any putative primary metabolic defect in cystinosis and be able to prove that a missing enzyme activity is a cause and not a result of the cystine accumulation.

Patrick has reported deficient activities of several sulfhydryl-dependent enzymes in postmortem liver and kidney tissue from patients with nephropathic cystinosis [235]. These enzymes included glucose-6-phosphate dehydrogenase, 6-phosphogluconate dehydrogenase, hexokinase, succinate dehydrogenase, alcohol dehydrogenase, and delta-aminolevulinate dehydrase. Other enzymes not dependent on sulfhydryl groups for activity showed either normal activity in the cystinotic tissue or activities in the range found in other tissues subject to chronic fibrosis from other causes.

Patrick was able to reproduce these decreases in activity of sulfhydryl-requiring enzymes in control tissues by the addition of cystine, but these changes were quickly corrected by the addition of cysteine. The decreased enzyme activities in cystinotic tissue were, in general, only partially restored following the addition of cysteine. It is difficult to evaluate fully the possible significance of such findings, especially since the measurements were made in postmortem tissue that had been chronically involved in the disease process. Activities of glucose-6-phosphate dehydrogenase and 6-phosphogluconate dehydrogenase were virtually absent in leukocyte lysates from patients with nephropathic cystinosis, but both activities were restored to normal following dialysis in a solution of cysteine [236]. Presumably these enzymes have normal activities in the intact cell but are inhibited by cystine following lysis of the cells and partial release of the compartmentalized cystine.

Response of Lysosomes to Cystine Crystals   The predilection of cystinosis to produce selective damage to the kidney remains an enigma. The remarkable tolerance of lysosomes to the presence of cystine crystals is in marked contrast to their response to many other types of crystalline substances. The introduction of crystals of monosodium urate or of sodium orotate into leukocytes by phagocytosis produces a prompt disruption of lysosomes, leading to the death of the phagocytic cell. It also leads to a marked local inflammatory reaction, the acute attack of gouty arthritis representing the most violent spontaneous form (Chap. 50) [237]. The benign tolerance of the lysosome to cystine crystals presumably reflects certain surface features of the crystal that at present remain undefined [238]. Weissman [239, 240] has proposed the hydrogen bonding of monosodium urate crystals to the lysosomal membrane as a major interaction required for lysosome disruption.

TREATMENT

Symptomatic Treatment

The symptomatic treatment of the earlier stages of nephropathic cystinosis consists of providing an adequate fluid intake, correcting the metabolic acidosis and potassium deficit, and healing the rickets. In most patients this is readily accomplished and results in a marked improvement in the child's personality, eating, activity, and "general well-being." As the disease progresses, treatment for renal insufficiency eventually becomes the major concern. Patients with late-onset cystinosis often require treatment similar to that given patients with nephropathic cystinosis. Patients with benign cystinosis, of course, require no therapy.

The significant acidosis and hypokalemia are most easily corrected by the use of a potassium-containing alkalinizing mixture such as a solution of sodium and potassium citrate [241]. We have used the commercially available preparation Polycitra (Willen Drug Co., Baltimore, Maryland) which contains 2.0 g citric acid, 3.0 g sodium citrate, and 3.3 g potassium citrate per 30 ml. This preparation is well tolerated and provides 1 meq sodium and 1 meq potassium per milliliter. The average dose is 45 ml to 60 ml/day. In some patients [242] the serum concentration of bicarbonate cannot be raised above 20 meq/liter regardless of the amount of alkalinizing solution used, but in others the serum bicarbonate concentration can be completely normalized. On this therapy, the serum potassium concentration usually remains at low levels, but no signs of hypokalemia, such as ECG changes, are usually found.

In most patients the rachitic changes are readily corrected with doses of 10,000 to 15,000 units/day of vitamin D (ergocalciferol, vitamin D_2). Some patients are more easily managed with either dihydrotachysterol or 1,25-dihydroxycholecalciferol. Phosphate salts can also be used, either alone or in combination with lower doses of vitamin D to correct rickets [243]. We have seen complete healing of rickets with phosphate salts alone in infants with nephropathic cystinosis. In children whose serum bicarbonate concentration is completely corrected with alkalinizing solutions, the simultaneous administration of phosphate and alkali may produce tetany. Thus, phosphate salts must be used with care. Hydrochlorothiazide has also been used successfully in the treatment of cystinotic rickets [244].

Cystinotic children may have extreme polyuria secondary to their renal tubular damage. Free access to water in large amounts is essential during both day and night. Vigorous intravenous fluid therapy is often necessary for management of viral or other illnesses causing vomiting or diarrhea. When receiving proper treatment, cystinotic children usually tolerate the typical infectious diseases of childhood without difficulty.

Isolated reports of the efficacy of anabolic agents [245–247], ATP, and coenzyme A [248] in cystinotic children have appeared but have not been seriously pursued. Indomethacin has been reported to be helpful in improving the water and electrolyte imbalance in cystinosis [249–251], but this appears to be related to a decrease in glomerular function [250, 251]. We have had no experience with these drugs and feel that patients whose rickets and electrolyte imbalance are controlled often do well for several years without additional agents, although their growth usually is less than normal. It is important to monitor thyroid function in these children since many eventually become hypothyroid.

Specific Therapy

Attempts at specific therapy for nephropathic cystinosis have been difficult to evaluate for three reasons. First, no specific, objective parameter has been available for evaluating therapy. Next, these children often show temporary improvement including improved glomerular function [236] with only symptomatic therapy. Finally, the natural course of the disease is not uniform, and some patients may go several years without a further decrease in glomerular function in the absence of any specific therapy.

Ideally, a successful therapeutic regimen would rid these cystinotic children of their cystine stores. The amounts of free cystine in critical tissues should provide the best objective measurement of cystine accumulation and be helpful in evaluating therapy. Lacking an actual decrease in cystine storage, therapy might still be effective if it protected the actual site of cystine toxicity in the renal tubular and glomerular cells.

Final evaluation of any form of therapy will require prolonged, careful evaluation of renal function while the patient is well-managed symptomatically. As a further complication, nephropathic cystinosis eventually may prove to have more than one cause, and therapy effective for one patient might not be so for all patients.

Three approaches have been suggested for the specific therapy of this disease: specific drugs, low methionine and cystine diet, and renal transplantation [89].

Specific Drugs   One of the first drugs suggested for the specific treatment of cystinosis was penicillamine (beta, beta-dimethylcysteine). Although several investigators thought it was helpful to these patients, two careful studies demonstrated no improvement with this drug [27, 252]. A more recent study has shown that penicillamine (at a concentration of 1.0 mM) is unable to deplete cystinotic fibroblasts of free cystine [200].

A promising new approach to treatment has been suggested by the observation of Goldman et al. that dithiothreitol (DTT) is an effective drug for the lowering of intracellular cystine in fibroblasts cultured from a patient with cystinosis [199]. These workers have reported on the long-term use of DTT in two patients with infantile nephropathic cystinosis [253]. They used an oral dose of 25 mg/kg body weight given every 8 h. The DTT was given in capsule form and caused no harm to the intestine. The free-cystine content of peripheral leukocytes decreased progressively in these children, reaching the heterozygous range after 8 months of therapy. Renal function remained stable during this period but continued to deteriorate when the DTT was discontinued. Obviously, this form of therapy must be evaluated more fully before it can be advocated for general use.

Another thiol compound has recently shown promising results in vitro and in vivo. Cysteamine at concentrations as low as 0.1 mM can remove, within 1 h, all the free cystine from cultured cystinotic fibroblasts [200]. When tested for 1 h at 1.0 mM, pH 7.4, 37°C, cysteamine removed nearly three times as much free cystine from cystinotic fibroblasts as did DTT [200]. This drug has now been used clinically in patients with cystinosis by many investigators [200, 254–257]. As of early 1981, it is still too soon to be certain whether this drug will be help-

ful to children with cystinosis. The drug is available (for experimental use) as cysteamine-HCl. It is given orally in four divided doses at a dose of about 60 mg (expressed as cysteamine-free base) per kilogram of body weight per day. We have monitored each patient's dose individually by maintaining the leukocyte free-cystine content in the heterozygous range [257]. In patients who are slowly brought to full-dose levels over a 3-month period, no toxicity has been observed [258]. The major drawback to this drug is its extremely objectionable smell and taste. Theone and Lemons [259] have shown that a derivative of this drug, phosphocysteamine, is equally effective in depleting cystinotic cells of cystine, both in vitro and in vivo. Phosphocysteamine is odorless and tasteless and may have even less toxicity than cysteamine [259]. It almost certainly is converted to cysteamine, which is the presumed active agent. Unfortunately it is available only in small amounts at present. If cysteamine proves effective for cystinosis, phosphocysteamine will likely become more widely available for use.

In addition to the thiol-containing compounds, another compound with reducing properties, ascorbic acid, showed therapeutic potential in studies in vitro. Over 50 percent of the free cystine can be removed from cultured cystinotic skin fibroblasts by addition of high concentrations of L-ascorbic acid (0.29 to 2.9 mM) to the culture medium. Fresh ascorbic acid must be added to the culture medium daily to produce a progressive decrease of the free-cystine content over a 3-day period [260]. On the basis of this finding, a large double-blind study was done to evaluate the use of high-dose ascorbic acid in these patients. Of 64 patients, 32 received ascorbic acid (200 mg per kilogram of body weight per day) and 32 received placebo. The study was terminated after about two years because there was no evidence that vitamin C was beneficial, and there was accumulating evidence that it might be harmful. The serum creatinine concentration increased 0.53 mg/dl per year in patients receiving ascorbic acid and 0.24 mg/dl per year in patients receiving placebo ($p = 0.08$) [261].

Dietary Therapy   On the basis of information known about cystinosis in the 1960s, it seemed reasonable to attempt treating these children with a diet low in sulfur-containing amino acids. Such diets were derived from either natural proteins which were low in cystine and methionine or from mixtures of free amino acids. Investigators attempted to give just barely adequate amounts of methionine to maintain positive nitrogen balance, with the hope that this would decrease the cystine storage. The subsequent report in 1977 [198] that protein turnover provides a major source of the cystine storage in this disease would lead one to predict the futility of this approach. In fact, Seegmiller and coworkers [89] found that dietary therapy did not reduce intracellular cystine content, and Bickel and coworkers [247] analyzed data from 21 patients so-treated and found no evidence of clinical benefit.

Renal Transplantation   Since the primary abnormality leading to renal failure in cystinosis appears to be a genetically determined defect of the intracellular environment, cells without this genetic defect transplanted into a cystinotic patient should not accumulate cystine. Therefore, in theory, a cystinotic child should be as good a candidate for renal transplantation as any other child with chronic renal disease. Experience with renal transplantation in children is now extensive, and their age and size no longer represent significant barriers to success with the procedure [262]. Hemodialysis is only a palliative approach to end-stage cystinosis, although dialysis permits continued growth [263] and serves as a temporizing measure prior to transplantation. It is not possible to dialyze away the large cystine stores in these children [60, 264].

A report from the Renal Transplant Registry summarized the experience with renal transplantation in 24 cystinotic patients who received 27 kidneys [265]. Of the registry patients 17 received a parental (heterozygous) kidney and 10 received cadaver kidneys, at an average age of 12 years. Nine patients were well more than 3 years after transplant, four others had functioning kidneys but had been followed for a shorter time, and six patients had died of complications of the transplant procedure or immunosuppression. These results are compatible with previously reported series with fewer patients from individual medical centers [53]. More recently Malekzadeh et al. [266] and West and associates [267] have described their experiences with renal transplantation in cystinotic children, and a brief discussion is provided of five cases in Quebec [268]. Broyer et al have reported on 11 cystinotic children who have received kidney transplants [7, 8].

The conclusions from these various studies are concordant. The growth rate of cystinotic patients remains approximately unchanged post transplant [266] and is similar to that of other pediatric renal allograft recipients. Anemia improves, as does renal osteodystrophy. Hepatosplenomegaly may or may not decrease after successful transplantation, but hepatic function does not deteriorate. Corneal crystal deposits and retinopathy tend to progress after transplantation. In the United States' experience, visual function is altered minimally if at all [29, 266], and photophobia may worsen or improve [29]. The French experience with 16 cases over 10 years of age was worse in regard to visual function. One patient was totally blind, two had severe and six had mild impairment of vision [7, 8].

Cystinotic thyropathy can progress after transplantation. Significant degrees of hypothyroidism are not unusual, and thyroid enlargement may be dramatic [267]. Delayed diagnosis of hypothyroidism in a posttransplant cystinotic patient has been associated with death from myxedema coma [269].

Several cystinotics are alive approximately a decade after transplant. Failure of organ function, except for the thyroid and possibly the eye, from cystine accumulation has not so far been observed. Puberty has occurred in the mid or late teens in several patients with whom we are personally familiar.

Transplanted kidneys do not develop the series of functional changes typical of cystinosis, but they may reaccumulate cystine, which electron microscopic studies suggest is largely and perhaps entirely confined to interstitial and mesangial cells, presumably of host origin [53, 60, 266, 267]. This phenomenon occurs in both heterozygous and cadaver donor kidneys. In spite of theoretical concerns that heterozygote donor kidneys might be more prone than cadaver kidneys to cystine reaccumulation [267], there is no evidence that this is of real significance, while it is clearly of importance to have the best possible immunologic match between donor and recipient.

The persistence of crystal-containing cells within the noncystinotic graft tissue suggests that cystinosis is unlikely to be treatable by "corrective factor" therapy and is compatible with the negative results of experiments in vitro in which cystine storage in cystinotic fibroblasts was not corrected by cocultivation with normal fibroblasts [236].

At present, sufficient favorable results from transplantation have accumulated to justify offering this procedure to affected patients in the terminal stages of nephropathic cystinosis, and to their families, with careful explanation of the prospects for success or failure.

PREVENTION OF CYSTINOSIS THROUGH PRENATAL DIAGNOSIS

The prenatal diagnosis of cystinosis by estimation of the free-cystine content of cultured amniotic cells is now a well-established procedure. Since it is often not possible to obtain enough cells for direct cystine measure in sufficient time, a pulse-labeling technique is generally used [101, 270]. The amniotic cells are grown for 24 h in a medium containing [^{35}S]cystine. In normal cells the label is then found in protein, glutathione, cysteine, and to a small extent in cystine. In cystinotic cells the percentage of counts in cystine is much greater [63]. Although it has been reported that cystinotic amniotic fluid cells can be identified after short exposures to [^{35}S]cystine [271], our opinion is that this modification of previously published methods [63, 270] saves little time and complicates the interpretation of the data. The cystine-binding protein method of cystine measurement is a useful alternative if enough cells are available.

In one of the cystinotic fetuses that was studied following surgical hysterotomy, the only tissue that was abnormal by phase, light, or electron microscopy was the retinal pigment epithelium, in which vacuolization was observed [51, 63]. Cystine crystals are generally not seen in cystinotic fetal tissues. Yet, the free-cystine content of the kidney, liver, and spleen has ranged from 20 to 100 times control values [63, 271, 272]. One recent report describes possible cystine crystals in fetal cystinotic liver [64].

REFERENCES

1. SCHNEIDER JA, SEEGMILLER JE: Cystinosis and the Fanconi syndrome, in Stanbury JE, Wyngaarden JE, Fredrickson DS (eds): *The Metabolic Basis of Inherited Disease,* 3d ed. New York, McGraw-Hill, 1972, p 1581
2. SCHULMAN JD: Cystinosis. Washington, D.C., DHEW Publication no (NIH) 72–249. U.S. Government Printing Office, 1973
3. SEEGMILLER JE: Cystinosis, Hers HG, Van Hoof F (eds): *Lysosomes and Storage Diseases.* New York, Academic, 1973, p 485
4. SCHNEIDER JA, SCHULMAN JD, SEEGMILLER JE: Cystinosis and the Fanconi Syndrome, in Stanbury JB, Wyngaarden JB, Fredrickson DS (eds): *The Metabolic Basis of Inherited Disease,* 4th ed. New York, McGraw-Hill, 1978, p 1660
5. SCHNEIDER JA, SCHULMAN JD: Cystinosis: A review. *Metabolism* 26:817, 1977
6. SCHULMAN JD, MUDD SH, SCHNEIDER JA, SPIELBERG SP, BOXER L, OLIVER J, CORASH L, SHIETZ M: Genetic disorders of glutathione and sulfur amino-acid metabolism: New biochemical insights and therapeutic approaches. *Ann Intern Med* 93:330, 1980
7. BROYER M, GUILLOT M, GUBLER M-C, HABIB R: La cystinose infantile, réévaluation des symptômes précoces et tardifs, in Hamburger J, Crosnier J, Funck-Brentano JL (eds): *Actualites Néphrologiques de l'Hôpital Necker.* Paris, Flammarion Médicine-Science, 1980, p 127
8. BROYER M, GUILLOT M, GUBLER M-C, HABIB R: Infantile cystinosis: A reappraisal of early and late symptoms, in Hamburger J, Crosnier J, Grünfeld J-P, Maxwell MH (eds): *Advances in Nephrology.* Chicago, Year Book, 1981, p 137
9. BICKEL H: Die Entwicklung der biochemischen Läsion bei der Lignac-Franconischen Krankheit. *Helv Paediatr Acta* 10:259, 1955
10. SCHNEIDER JA, WONG V, SEEGMILLER JE: The early diagnosis of cystinosis. *J Pediatr* 74:114, 1969

11. LEBEL M, GROSE JH, DELAGE E, CRÉPIN G: Syndrome de Bartter associé a une cystinose. Association des Médicine de la Langue francaise due Canada, Congrès annuel. October 1977

12. LEMIRE J, KAPLAN BS, SCRIVER CR: Presentation of cystinosis as Bartter's syndrome and conversion to Fanconi Syndrome on indomethacin treatment. Pediatr Res 12:544, 1978

13. O'REGAN S, MONGEAU J-G, ROBITAILLE P: A patient with cystinosis presenting with the features of Bartter syndrome. Acta Paediatr Belg 33:51, 1980

14. LUCKY AW, HOWLEY PM, MEGYLESI K, SPIELBERG SP, SCHULMAN JD: Endocrine studies in cystinosis: Compensated primary hypothyroidism. J Pediatr 91:204, 1977

15. CHAN AM, LYNCH MJG, BAILEY JD, EZRIN C, FRASER D: Hypothyroidism in cystinosis. Am J Med 48:678, 1970

16. BURKE JR, EL-BISHTI MM, MAISEY MN, CHANTLER C: Hypothyroidism in children with cystinosis. Arch Dis Child 53:947, 1978

17. CZERNICHOW P, LENOIR G, ROY M-P, RAPPAPORT R, BROYER M: Atteintes thyroidiennes au cours de la cystinose. Arch Fr Pédiatr 35:930, 1978

17a.BERCU BB, ORLOFF S, SCHULMAN JD: Partial pituitary resistance to thyroid hormone in cystinosis. J Clin Endocrinal Metab 5:1262, 1980

18. EHRICH JHH, STOEPPLER L, OFFNER G, BRODEHL J: Evidence for cerebral involvement in nephropathic cystinosis. Neuropädiatrie 10:128, 1979

19. EHRICH JHH, WOLFF G, STOEPPLER L, HEYER R, OFFNER G, BRODEHL J: Psychosozial-intellektuelle Entwicklung bei Kindern mit infantiler Zystinose und Hirnatrophie. Klin Pädiatr 191:483, 1979

20. JONAS A, SCHNEIDER JA: In preparation.

21. BÜRKI VE: Ueber die Cystinkrankheit im Klienkindesalter unter besonderer Berücksichtigung des Augenbefundes. Ophthalmologica 101:257, 1941

22. FRAZIER PD, WONG VG: Cystinosis: Histologic and crystallographic examination of crystals in eye tissues. Arch Ophthalmol (Chicago) 80:87, 1968

23. WONG VG: The eye and cystinosis, in Schulman JD (ed): Cystinosis. Washington, D.C., DHEW Publication no (NIH) 72–249, U.S. Government Printing Office, 1973, p 23

24. WONG VG, LIETMAN PS, SEEGMILLER JE: Alterations of pigment epithelium in cystinosis. Arch Ophthalmol (Chicago) 77:361, 1967

25. WALDMAN TA, MOGIELNICKI RP, STROBER W: The proteinuria of cystinosis: Its pattern and pathogenesis, Schulman JD (ed): Cystinosis. Washington, D.C., DHEW Publication no (NIH) 72–249. U.S. Government Printing Office, 1973, p 55

26. CLAYTON BE, PATRICK AD: Use of dimercaprol or pencillamine in the treatment of cystinosis. Lancet 2:909, 1961

27. CRAWHALL JC, LIETMANN PS, SCHNEIDER JA, SEEGMILLER JE: Cystinosis: Plasma cystine and cysteine concentrations and the effect of D-penicillamine and dietary treatment. Am J Med 44:330, 1968

28. SCHULMAN JD: Unpublished observations

29. YAMAMOTO GK, SCHULMAN JD, SCHNEIDER JA, WONG VG: Long-term ocular changes in cystinosis: Observations in renal transplant recipients. J Pediatr Ophthalmol Strobis 16:21, 1979

30. LIETMAN PS, FRAZIER PD, WONG VG, SHOTTON D, SEEGMILLER JE: Adult cystinosis—a benign disorder. Am J Med 40:511, 1966

31. BRUBAKER RF, WONG VG, SCHULMAN JE, SEEGMILLER JE, KUWABARA T: Benign cystinosis: The clinical, biochemical and morphologic findings in a family with two affected siblings. Am J Med 49:546, 1970

32. SCHNEIDER JA, WONG V, BRADLEY KH, SEEGMILLER JE: Biochemical comparisons of the adult and childhood forms of cystinosis. N Engl J Med 279:1253, 1968

33. KRAUS E, LUTZ P: Ocular cystine deposits in an adult. Arch Ophthalmol (Chicago) 85:690, 1971

34. KROLL WA, LICHTE K-H: Cystinosis: A review of the different forms and of recent advances. Humangenetik 20:75, 1973

35. DODD MG, PUSIN SM, GREEN WR: Adult cystinosis: A case report. Arch Ophthalmol 96:1054, 1978

36. THEONE JG, SCHNEIDER JA: Unpublished data

37. GOLDMAN H, SCRIVER CR, AARON K, DELVIN E, CANLOS Z: Adolescent cystinosis: Comparisons with infantile and adult forms. Pediatrics 47:979, 1971

38. AARON K, GOLDMAN H, SCRIVER CR: Cystinosis; new observations: 1. Adolescent (type III) form. 2. Correction of phenotypes in vitro with dithiothreitol, in Carson NAJ, Raine DN (eds): Inherited Disorders of Sulphur Metabolism. Edinburgh, Churchill Livingstone, 1971, p 150

39. HOOFT C, CARTON D, DE SCHRIJVER F, DELBEKE MJ, SAMIJN W, KINT J: Juvenile cystinosis in two siblings, in Carson NAJ, Raine DN (eds): Inherited Disorders of Sulphur Metabolism. Edinburgh; Churchill Livingstone, 1971, p 141

40. SPEAR GS, SLUSSER RJ, SCHULMAN JD, ALEXANDER F: Polykaryocytosis in the visceral glomerular epithelium in cystinosis with description of an unusual clinical variant. Johns Hopkins Med J 129:83, 1971

41. PITTMAN G, DEODHAR S, SCHULMAN JB, LANDO JE: Nephropathic cystinosis in a young adult—report of a case. Lab Invest 24:442, 1971

42. FRANÇOIS J, HANSSENS M, COPPIETERS R, EVENS L: Cystinosis. A clinical and histopathologic study. Am J Ophthalmol 73:643, 1972

43. ADAMS BK, NAIDOO PM: Cystinosis with Fanconi syndrome: A case report. SA Mediese Tydskrif 53:719, 1978

44. BLANC-BRUNAT N, BERTHOUX F, COLON S, JANIN G: Cystinose a revelation tardive chex deux freres. Arch Fr Pédiatr 35:486, 1978

45. WEBER H-P, HARMS E, KNÖPFLE G: Adoleszenten-Zystinose Literaturübersicht mit eigener Beobachtung. Klin Pädiatr 191:8, 1979

46. VÖLCKER HE, HARMS E, NAUMANN GOH, WEISS G: Cystinosis in two non-infantile patients diagnosed by the ophthalmologist. Metab Pediatr Ophthalmol 3:161, 1979

47. MANZ R, HARMS E, LUTZ P, WALDHERR R, SCHÄRER K: Adolescent cystinosis: Renal function and morphology. Personal communication

48. BOIS E, FEINGOLD J, FRENAY P, BRIARD M-L: Infantile cystinosis in France: Genetics, incidence, geographic distribution. J Med Genet 13:434, 1976

49. BICKEL H, BAAR HS, ASTLEY E, DOUGLAS AA, FINCH E, HARRIS H, HARVEY CC, HICKMANS EM, PHILPOTT MG, SMALLWOOD WC, SMELLIE JM, TEALL, CG: Cystine storage disease with aminoaciduria and dwarfism (Lignac-Fanconi disease). Acta Paediatr 42 (Suppl 90):1, 1952

50. SPEAR GS: The pathology of the kidney, in Schulman JD (ed): Cystinosis. Washington D.C., DHEW Publication no (NIH) 72–249. U.S. Government Printing Office, 1973, p 37

51. SPEAK GS: Pathology of the kidney in cystinosis, Sommers SC (ed): Pathology Annual. New York, Appleton-Century-Crofts, 1974, p 81

52. Feist D, Rossner JA, Stefan M: Indikationen und Ergebnisse der percutanen Leberbiopsie im Kindesalter. Mschr Kinderheilk 120:491, 1972

53. GOODMAN SI, HAMBIDGE KM, MAHONEY CP, STRIKER GE: Renal homotransplantation in the treatment of cystinosis, in Schulman JD (ed): Cystinosis. Washington, D.C., DHEW Publication no (NIH) 72–249, U.S. Government Printing Office, 1973, p 255

54. CLAY RD, DARMADY EM, HAWKINS M: The nature of the renal lesion in Fanconi syndrome. J Pathol Bacterial 65:551, 1953

55. TEREE TM, FRIEDMAN AB, KEST LM, FETTERMAN GH: Cystinosis and proximal tubular nephropathy in siblings. Progressive development of the physiological and anatomical lesion. Am J Dis Child 119:481, 1970

56. GODARD C, VALLOTTON MB, BROYER M, ROYER P: A study of the inhibition of the reninangiotensin system in renal potassium wasting syndromes, including Bartter's syndrome. Helv Pediatr Acta 27:495, 1972

57. ZIMMERMAN TJ, HOOD I, GASSET AR: "Adolescent" cystinosis. A case presentation and review of the recent literatures. Arch Ophthalmol (Chicago) 92:265, 1974

58. SANDERSON PO, KUWABARA T, STARKEV J, WONG VG, COLLINS EM: Cystinosis: A clinical, histopathologic and ultrastructure study. Arch Ophthalmol 91:270, 1974

59. JACKSON JD, SMITH FG, LITMAN NN, YUILE CL, LATTA H: The Fanconi syndrome with cystinosis. Electron microscopy of renal biopsy specimens from five patients. Am J Med 33:893, 1962

60. MAHONEY CP, STRIKER GE, HICKMAN RO, MANNING GB, MARCHIORO TL: Renal transplantation for childhood cystinosis. N Eng J Med 283:397, 1970

61. SPEAR GS, SLUSSER RJ, TOUSIMIS AJ, TAYLOR CG, SCHULMAN JD: Cystinosis: An ultrastructural and electron-probe study of the kidney with unusual findings. Arch Pathol 91:206, 1971

62. SCOTTO JM, STRALIN HG: Ultrastructure of the liver in a case of childhood cystinosis. Virchows Arch [Pathol Anat Hist] 377:43, 1977

63. SCHNEIDER JA, VERROUST FM, KROLL WA, GARVIN AJ, HORGER EO, III, WONG VG, SPEAR GS, JACOBSON C, PELLETT OL, BECKER FLA: Prenatal diagnosis of cystinosis. N Engl J Med 290:878, 1974

64. HAYNES MD, CARTER RF, POLLARD AC, CAREY WF: Light and electron microscopy of infantile and foetal tissues in cystinosis. Micron 11:443, 1980

65. KENYON ER, SENSENBRENNER JA: Electron microscopy of cornea and conjunctiva in childhood cystinosis. Am J Ophthalmol 78:68, 1974

66. WONG VG, KEWABARA T, BRUBAKER R, OLSON W, SCHULMAN J, SEEGMILLER JE: Intralysosomal cystine crystals in cystinosis. Invest Ophthalmol 9:83, 1970

67. VEROUGSTRAETE C, LIBERT J, TOUSSAINT D: Cystinose de l'adolescence-etude clinique et histopathologique. Bull Soc Belge Ophthalmol 180:9, 1978

68. SCHULMAN JD, WONG VG, BRADLEY KH, SEEGMILLER JE: A simple technique for the biochemical diagnosis of cystinosis. J Pediatr 76:289, 1970

69. WONG V: Unpublished data

70. PEDERSEN OO, KARLSEN RL: The toxic effect of L-cysteine on the rat retina: A morphological and biochemical study. Invest Ophthalmol 19:886, 1980

71. PATRICK AD: The degradative metabolism of L-cysteine and L-cystine in vitro by liver in cystinosis. Biochem J 83:248, 1962

72. SCHNEIDER JA, BRADLEY K, SEEGMILLER JE: Increased cystine in leukocytes from individuals homozygous and heterozygous for cystinosis. *Science* 157:1321, 1967

73. SCHNEIDER JA, ROSENBLOOM FM, BRADLEY KH, SEEGMILLER JE: Increased free-cystine content of fibroblasts cultured from patients with cystinosis. *Biochem Biophys Res Commun* 29:527, 1967

74. SCHULMAN JD, BRADLEY KH: *In vitro* studies on cystinosis, Schulman JD (ed): in *Cystinosis*. Washington, D.C., DHEW Publication no (NIH) 72–249, U.S. Government Printing Office, 1973, p 111

75. SCHULMAN JD, SCHNEIDER JA, BRADLEY KH, SEEGMILLER JE: Cystine, cysteine, and glutathione metabolism in normal and cystinotic fibroblasts *in vitro* and in cultured amniotic fluid cells. *Clin Chim Acta* 35:383, 1971

76. SCHULMAN JD, BRADLEY KH, BEREZESKY IK, GRIMLEY PM, DODSON WE, AL-AISH MS: Biochemical, morphologic, and cytogenetic studies of leukocytes growing in continuous culture from normal individuals and from patients with cystinosis. *Pediatr Res* 5:501, 1971

77. HUMMELER K, ZAJAC BA, GENEL M, HOLTZAPPLE PG, SEGAL S: Human cystinosis: Intracellular deposition of cystine. *Science* 168:859, 1970

78. KORN D: Demonstration of cystine crystals in peripheral white blood cells in a patient with cystinosis. *N Engl J Med* 262:545, 1960

79. SCHULMAN JD, SCHNEIDER JA, BRADLEY KH, SEEGMILLER JE: Heterozygote studies in cystinosis. *Clin Chim Acta* 29:73, 1970

80. MORECKI R, PAUNIER L, HAMILTON JR: Intestinal mucosa in cystinosis: A fine structure study. *Arch Pathol* 86:297, 1968

81. PATRICK AD, LAKE BD: Cystinosis: Electron microscopic evidence of lysosomal storage of cystine in lymph node. *J Clin Pathol* 21:571, 1968

82. SCHULMAN JD, WONG V, OLSON WH, SEEGMILLER JE: Lysosomal site of crystalline deposits of cystinosis as shown by ferritin uptake. *Arch Pathol* 90:259, 1970

83. SCHULMAN JD, BRADLEY KH, SEEGMILLER JE: Cystine: Compartmentalization within lysosomes in cystinotic leukocytes. *Science* 166:1152, 1969

84. SCHULMAN JD, BRADLEY KH: Cystinosis: Selective induction of vacuolation in fibroblasts by L-cysteine-D-penicillamine disulfide. *Science* 169:595, 1970

85. SCHULMAN JD, BRADLEY KH: Metabolism of amino acids, peptides and disulfides in the lysosomes of fibroblasts cultured from normal individuals and those with cystinosis. *J Exp Med* 132:1090, 1970

86. HARMS E, SCHNEIDER JA: The lysosomal localization of free-cystine in normal cystinotic cells. *Clin Res* 27:457A, 1979

87. EHRENREICH BA, COHN ZA: The fate of peptides pinocytosed by macrophages *in vitro*. *J Exp Med* 129:227, 1969

88. SANO K: Uber die Loslichkeit der Aminosauren bei variierter Wasserstoffzahl. *Biochem Z* 168:14, 1926

89. SEEGMILLER JE, FRIEDMANN T, HARRISON HE, WONG V, SCHNEIDER JA: Cystinosis. *Ann Intern Med* 68:883, 1968

90. ELDJARN L, PIHL A: Equilibrium constants and oxidation-reduction potentials of some thiol-disulfide systems. *J Am Chem Soc* 79:4589, 1957

91. JOCELYN PC: The standard redox potential of cysteine-cystine from the thiol-disulphide exchange reaction with glutathione and lipoic acid. *Eur J Biochem* 2:327, 1967

92. CLARK WM: *Oxidation-reduction Potentials of Organic Systems*. Baltimore, Williams & Wilkins, 1960, p 471

93. GORIN G, DOUGHTY G: Equilibrium constants for the reaction of glutathione with cystine and their relative oxidation-reduction potentials. *Arch Biochem Biophys* 126:547, 1968

94. BRAND E, HARRIS MM, BILOON S: Cystinuria. The excretion of a cystine complex which decomposes in the urine with the liberation of free cystine. *J Biol Chem* 86:315, 1930

95. ELLMAN GL: Tissue sulfhydryl groups. *Arch Biochem Biophys* 82:70, 1959

96. JOCELYN PC: Assay of thiols and disulfides, in *Biochemistry of the SH Group*. New York, Academic, 1972, p 137

97. LEE PLY: Single-column systems for accelerated amino acid analysis of physiological fluids using five lithium buffers. *Biochem Med* 10:107, 1974

98. UDENFRIEND S, STEIN S, BÖHLEN P, DAIRMAN W, LEIMGRUBER W, WEIGELE M: Fluorescamine: A reagent for assay of amino acids, peptides, proteins, and primary amines in the picomole range. *Science* 178:871, 1972

99. OSHIMA RG, WILLIS RC, FURLONG CE, SCHNEIDER JA: Binding assays for amino acids: The utilization of a cystine binding protein from *Escherichia coli* for the determination of acid-soluble cystine in small physiological samples. *J Biol Chem* 249:6033, 1974

100. SMITH I: *Chromatographic and Electrophoretic Techniques*. New York, Interscience, 1960

101. SCHNEIDER JA, BRADLEY KH, SEEGMILLER JE: Transport and intracellular fate of cysteine-^{35}S in leukocytes from normal subjects and patients with cystinosis. *Pediatr Res* 2:441, 1968

102. STATES B, SEGAL S: Thin-layer chromatographic separation of cystine and the N-ethylmaleimide adducts of cysteine and glutathione. *Anal Biochem* 27:323, 1969

103. SCHULMAN JD: Sulfur metabolism, in Schulman JD (ed): *Cystinosis*. Washington, D.C., DHEW Publication no (NIH) 72–249, U.S. Government Printing Office, 1973, p 67

104. TIETZE F: Enzymic reduction of cystine and other disulfides, in Schulman JD (ed): *Cystinosis*. Washington, D.C., DHEW Publication no (NIH) 72–249, U.S. Government Printing Office, 1973, p 147

105. ROSE WC, WIXOM RL: The amino acid requirements of man. XIII. The sparing effect of cystine on the methionine requirement. *J Biol Chem* 216:763, 1955

106. MCKEAN CM: Growth of phenylketonuric children on chemically defined diets. *Lancet* 1:148, 1970

107. EAGLE H, PIEZ KA, OYAMA VI: The biosynthesis of cystine in human cell cultures. *J Biol Chem* 236:1425, 1961

108. EAGLE H, WASHINGTON C, FRIEDMAN SM: The synthesis of homocystine, cystathionine, and cystine by cultured diploid and heteroploid human cells. *Proc Natl Acad Sci (USA)* 56:156, 1966

109. JACOBY LB, LITTLEFIELD JW: Mutant human fibroblast clones able to grow on homocysteine instead of cyst(e)ine. *Exp Cell Res* 69:447, 1971

110. IGLEHART JD, YORK RM, MODEST AP, LAZARUS H, LIVINGSTON DM: Cystine requirement of continuous human lymphoid cell lines of normal and leukemic origin. *J Biol Chem* 252:7184, 1977

111. BRENTON DP, CUSWORTH DC, DENT DE, JONES EE: Homocystinuria. Clinical and dietary studies. *Q J Med* 35:325, 1966

112. STURMAN JA, GAULL G, RAIHA NCR: Absence of cystathionase in human fetal liver: Is cystine essential? *Science* 169:74, 1970

113. HIGASHI T, TATEISHI N, NARUSE A, SAKAMOTO Y: A novel physiological role of liver glutathione as a reservoir of L-cystine. *J Biochem* 82:117, 1977

114. TATEISHI N, HIGASHI T, NARUSE A, NAKASHIMA K, SHIOZAKI H, SAKAMOTO Y: Rat liver glutathione: Possible role as a reservoir of cysteine. *J Nutr* 107:51, 1977

115. BUTLER JD, SPIELBERG SP: Role of glutathione catabolism by gamma-glutamyl transpeptidase in cystine storage in cystinosis. *Fed Proc* 39:1746, 1980

116. LASTER L, MUDD SH, FINKELSTEIN JD, IRREVERRE F: Homocystinuria due to cystathionine synthase deficiency: The metabolism of L-methionine. *J Clin Invest* 44:1708, 1965

117. BRÜGGEMAN J, SCHLOSSMAN K, MERKENSCHLAGER M, WALDSCHMIDT M: Zur Frage des Vorkommens der Serinsulfhydrase. *Biochem Z* 335:392, 1962

118. BRÜGGEMAN J, WALDSCHMIDT M: Die Serinsulfhydrase aus Hühnerleber: Rückreaktion und Vergleich mit der Cysteindesulfhydrase. *Biochem Z* 335:408, 1962

119. SCHNEIDER JF, WESTLEY J: Direct incorporation of thiosulfate sulfur into cysteine by lysed rat liver mitochondria. *J Biol Chem* 238:PC3516, 1963

120. SCHNEIDER JF, WESTLEY J: Metabolic interrelations of sulfur in proteins, thiosulfate, and cystine. *J Biol Chem* 244:5735, 1969

121. HUOVINEN JA, GUSTAFSSON BE: Inorganic sulfate, sulfite and sulfide as sulfur donors in the biosynthesis of sulfur amino acids in germ-free and conventional rats. *Biochim Biophys Acta* 136:441, 1967

122. MEDES G: Metabolism of sulfur. VI. Oxidation in the body of the sulfur-containing amino-acids and some of their partially oxidized derivatives. *Biochem J* 31:1330, 1937

123. MEDES G, FLOYD N: Metabolism of sulphur. XI. Further investigations of the enzymic oxidation of sulphur-containing amino acids. *Biochem J* 36:259, 1942

124. JACOBSEN JD, SMITH LH JR: Biochemistry and physiology of taurine and taurine derivatives. *Physiol Rev* 48:424, 1968

125. CRAWHALL JC, PARKER R, SNEDDON W, YOUNG EP: Betamercaptolactate-cystine disulfide in the urine of a mentally retarded patient. *Am J Dis Child* 117:71, 1969

126. MEISTER A, FRASER PE, TICE SV: Enzymatic desulfuration of beta-mercaptopyruvate to pyruvate. *J Biol Chem* 206:561, 1954

127. ISHIMOTO Y: Transaminative pathway of cysteine metabolism in rat tissues. *Physiol Chem Phys* 11:189, 1979

128. UBUKA T, UMEMURA S, YUASA S, KINUTA M, WATANABE K: Purification and characterization of mitochondrial cysteine aminotransferase from rat liver. *Physiol Chem Phys* 10:483, 1978

129. IP MPC, THIBERT RJ, SCHMIDT DE: Purification and partial characterization of cysteine-glutamate transaminase from rat liver. *Can J Biochem* 55:958, 1977

130. WAINER A: The production of cysteinesulfinic acid from cysteine *in vitro*. *Biochim Biophys Acta* 104:405, 1965

131. EWETZ L, SORBO B: Characteristics of the cysteinesulfinate-forming enzyme system in rat liver. *Biochim Biophys Acta* 128:296, 1966

132. LOMBARDINI JB, SINGER TP, BOYER PD: Cysteine oxygenase. II. Studies on the mechanism of the reaction with ^{18}oxygen. *J Biol Chem* 244:1172, 1969

133. MACAIONE S, DIGIORGIO RM: Subcellular distribution of cysteine oxidase activity in ox retina. *Life Sci* 20:617, 1977
134. YAMAGUCHI K, HOSOKAWA Y, KOHASHI N, KORI Y, SAKAKIBARA S, UEDA I: Rat liver cysteine dioxygenase (cysteine oxidase): Further purification, characterization, and analysis of the activation and inactivation. *J. Biochem* 83:479, 1978
135. YAMAGUCHI K, SAKAKIBARA S, ASAMIZU J, UEDA I: Induction and activation of cysteine oxidase of rat liver. II. The measurement of cystine metabolism *in vivo* and the activation of *in vivo* activity of cysteine oxidase. *Biochim Biophys Acta* 297:48, 1973
136. KOHASHI N, YAMAGUCHI K, HOSOKAWA Y, KORI Y, FIGII O, UEDA I: Dietary control of cysteine dioxygenase in rat liver. *J Biochem* 84:159, 1978
137. STIPANUK MH: Effect of excess dietary methionine on the catabolism of cysteine in rats. *J Nutr* 109:2126, 1979
138. YAMAGUCHI K, SHIGEHISHA S, SAKAKIBARA S, HOSOKAWA Y, UEDA I: Cysteine metabolism *in vivo* of Vitamin B_6–deficient rats. *Biochim Biophys Acta* 381:1, 1975
139. WHITTLE B, SMITH JT: Effect of dietary sulfur on taurine excretion by the rat. *J Nutr* 104:666, 1974
140. MISRA CH: Effect of morphine on cysteine oxidase activity in the brain and reproductive tract of rats. *Biochem Pharm* 28:1695, 1979
141. HOSOKAWA Y, YAMAGUCHI K, KOHASHI N, KORI Y, UEDA I: Decrease of rat liver cysteine dioxygenase (cysteine oxidase) activity mediated by glucagon. *J Biochem* 84:419, 1978
142. SUMIZU K: Cysteinesulfinic desulfinase in rat liver. *Biochim Biophys Acta* 53:435, 1961
143. CHATAGNER F, BERGERET B, SÉJOURNÉ T, FROMAGEOT C: Transamination et désulfination de l'acide L-cystéinesulfinique. *Biochim Biophys Acta* 9:340, 1952
144. SINGER TP, KEARNEY EB: Enzymatic pathways in the degradation of sulfur-containing amino acids, McElroy WD, Glass HB (eds): in *Amino Acid Metabolism*. Baltimore, Johns Hopkins, 1955, p 588
145. SINGER TP, KEARNEY EB: Intermediary metabolism of L-cysteinesulfinic acid in animal tissues. *Arch Biochem Biophys* 61:397, 1956
146. PALMIERI F, STIPANI I, IACOBOZZI V: The transport of L-cysteinesulfinate in rat liver mitochondria. *Biochim Biophys Acta* 555:531, 1979
147. YAGI T, KAGAMIYAMA H, NOZAKI M: Cysteine sulfinate transamination activity of aspartate aminotransferases. *Biochem Biophys Res Commun* 90:447, 1979
148. FRIDOVICH I, FARKAS W, HANDLER P: Sulfite oxidation in rat liver. *Bull Soc Chim Biol* 40:1795, 1958
149. MUDD SH, IRREVERRE F, LASTER L: Sulfite oxidase deficiency in man: Demonstration of the enzymatic defect. *Science* 156:1599, 1967
150. IRREVERRE F, MUDD SH, HEIZER WD, LASTER L: Sulfite oxidase deficiency: Studies of a patient with mental retardation, dislocated ocular lenses, and abnormal urinary excretion of *S*-sulfo-L-cysteine, sulfite, and thiosulfate. *Biochem Med* 1:187, 1967
151. WAINER A: The production of sulfate from cysteine without the formation of free cysteinsulfinic acid. *Biochem Biophys Res Commun* 16:141, 1964
152. WAINER A: Mitochondrial oxidation of cysteine. *Biochim Biophys Acta* 141:466, 1967
153. MEISTER A: *Biochemistry of the Amino Acids*, 2d ed. New York, Academic, 1965
154. PECK EJ JR, AWAPARA J: Formation of taurine and isethionic acid in rat brain. *Biochim Biophys Acta* 141:499, 1967
155. YOUNG L, MAW A: *The Metabolism of Sulphur Compounds*. New York, Wiley, p 99, 1958
156. CAVALLINI D, DUPRE S, GRAZIANI MT, TINTI MG: Identification of pantethinase in horse kidney extract. *FEBS Lett* 1:119, 1968
157. SWAN P, WENTWORTH J, LINKSWILER H: Vitamin B_6 depletion in man: Urinary taurine and sulfate excretion and nitrogen balance. *J Nutr* 84:220, 1964
158. STRUMEYER DH, BLOCH K: Some properties of gamma-glutamylcysteine synthetase. *J Biol Chem* 235:PC27, 1960
159. MEISTER A: On the enzymology of amino acid transport. *Science* 180:33, 1973
160. ORLOFF S, BUTLER J, TOWNE D, MUKHERGIE AB, SCHULMAN JD: Pantetheinase activity and cysteamine content in cystinotic and normal fibroblasts and leukocytes. *Pediatr Res* 15:1063, 1981
161. FELTEN RP, SYKES SM, LAMANNA A, WAXLER M: Reduced cystine concentration in blood plasma exposed to broad spectrum light. *Photochem Photobiol* 31:273, 1979
162. ENGELHARDT DL, SANTELLA RM, ROSENKRANZ HS, SPECK WT: The effect of illuminated plasma on cell growth. *Photochem Photobiol* 26:53, 1977
163. CRAWHALL JC, SEGAL S: The intracellular cysteine/cystine ratio in kidney cortex. *Biochem J* 99:19c, 1966
164. CRAWHALL JC, SEGAL S: The intracellular ratio of cysteine and cysteine in various tissues. *Biochem J* 105:891, 1967

165. ASKELÖF P, AXELSSON K, ERIKSSON S, MANNERVIK E: Mechanism of action of enzymes catalyzing thiol-disulfide interchange. Thioltransferase rather than trans-hydrogenases. *FEBS Lett* 38:263, 1974
166. NICKERSON WJ, ROMANO AH: Enzymatic reduction of cystine by coenzyme 1 (DPNH). *Science* 115:676, 1952
167. ROMANO AH, NICKERSON WJ: Cystine reductase of pea seeds and yeasts. *J Biol Chem* 208:409, 1954
168. MYERS LT, WORTHEN HG: Cystine reductase in animal tissues. *Fed Prod* 20:218, 1961
169. REICHARD P: The biosynthesis of deoxyribonucleotides. *Eur J Biochem* 3:259, 1968
170. LARSON A, HOLMGREN A, BRATT I: Thioredoxin and glutathione in cultured fibroblasts from human cases with 5-oxoprolinuria and cystinosis. *FEBS Lett* 87:61, 1977
171. TIETZE F: Disulfide reduction in rat liver. I. Evidence for the presence of nonspecific nucleotide-dependent disulfide reductase and GSH-disulfide transhydrogenase activities in the high-speed supernatant fraction. *Arch Biochem Biophys* 138:177, 1970
172. TIETZE F: Disulfide reduction in rat liver. II. Chromatographic separation of nucleotide-dependent disulfide reductase and GSH-disulfide transhydrogenase activities of the high-speed supernatant fraction. *Biochim Biophys Acta* 220:449, 1970
173. ONDARZA RN, ABNEY R: On the active site of the NADPH-dependent CoA-SS-glutathione reductase from yeast and rat liver. *FEBS Lett* 7:227, 1970
174. RACKER E: Metabolism of thiolesters of glutathione. *Fed Proc* 12:711, 1953
175. RACKER E: Glutathione-homocystine transhydrogenase. *J Biol Chem* 217:867, 1955
176. CHANG SH, WILKEN DR: Participation of the unsymmetrical disulfide of coenzyme A and glutathione in an enzymatic sulfhydryl-disulfide interchange. I. Partial purification and properties of the bovine kidney enzyme. *J Biol Chem* 241:4251, 1966
177. NAGAI S, BLACK S: A thiol-disulfide transhydrogenase from yeast. *J Biol Chem* 243:1942, 1968
178. ERIKSSON SA, MANNERVIK R: The reduction of the L-cysteine-glutathione mixed disulfide in rat liver. Involvement of an enxyme catalyzing thiol disulfide interchange. *FEBS Lett* 7:26, 1970
179. KOHNO K, NODA K, MIZOBE M, UTSUMI I: Enzymatic reduction of disulfide-type thiamine derivatives. *Biochem Pharmacol* 18:1685, 1969
180. ERIKSSON S, GUTHENBERG C: The identity of enzymes reducing a thiamine disulfide derivative and cystine derivatives via thioldisulfide exchange. *Biochem Pharmacol* 24:241, 1975
181. ANFINSEN CB: The formation of the tertiary structure of proteins. *Harvey Lect Ser* 61:95, 1966
182. KATZEN HM, TIETZE F, STETTEN DEW JR: Further studies on the properties of hepatic glutathione-insulin transhydrogenase. *J Biol Chem* 238:1006, 1963
183. TIETZE F: Unpublished data
184. SAKAI H: A ribonucleoprotein which catalyzes thioldisulfide exchange in sea urchin eggs. *J Biol Chem* 242:1458, 1967
185. STATES B, SEGAL S: Distribution of glutathione-cystine transhydrogenase activity in subcellular fractions of rat intestinal mucosa. *Biochem J* 113:443, 1969
186. GRISOLIA S, WALLACE R: Insulin degradation by lysosomal extracts from rat liver; model for a role of lysosomes in hormone degradation. *Biochem Biophys Res Commun* 70:22, 1976
187. GRIFFITHS PA, LLOYD JB: Evidence for lysosomal reduction of cystine residues. *Biochem Biophys Res Commun* 89:428, 1979
188. HARRISON HE, HARRISON HC: Aminoaciduria in relation to deficiency disease and kidney function. *JAMA* 164:1571, 1957
189. BARR HS: Pathologie des Aminosäuren-Diabetes. *Mschr Kinderheilk* 99:35, 1951
190. SCHNEIDER JA: Unpublished observations
191. SCHULMAN JD, WONG VG, KUWABARA T, BRADLEY KH, SEEGMILLER JE: Intracellular cystine content of leukocyte populations in cystinosis. *Arch Intern Med* 125:660, 1970
192. ROSENBERG LE, CRAWHALL JC, SEGAL S: Intestinal transport of cystine and cysteine in man: Evidence for separate mechanisms. *J Clin Invest* 46:30, 1967
193. CRAWHALL JC, OSHIMA RG, SCHNEIDER JA: Factors controlling the nonprotein cystine content of cystinotic fibroblasts. *Pediat Res* 11:41, 1977
194. OSHIMA RG, PELLETT OL, ROBB JA, SCHNEIDER JA: Transformation of human cystinotic fibroblasts by SV40: Characteristics of transformed cells with limited and unlimited growth potential. *J Cell Phys* 93:129, 1977
195. KROLL WA, SCHNEIDER JA: Unpublished data
196. SCHULMAN JD, BRADLEY KH: Cystinosis: Therapeutic implications of *in vitro* studies of cultured fibroblasts. *J Pediat* 78:833, 1971
197. OSHIMA RG, RHEAD WJ, THOENE JG, SCHNEIDER JA: Cystine metabolism in human fibroblasts. Comparison of normal, cystinotic and gamma-glutamylcysteine synthetase-deficient cells. *J Biol Chem* 251:4287, 1976

198. THOENE JG, OSHIMA RG, RITCHIE DG, SCHNEIDER JA: Cystinotic fibroblasts accumulate cystine from intracellular protein degradation. *Proc Nat Acad Sci (USA)* 74:4505, 1977

199. GOLDMAN H, SCRIVER CR, AARON K, PINSKY L: Use of dithiothreitol to correct cystine storage in cultured cystonitic fibroblasts. *Lancet* 1:811, 1970

200. THOENE JG, OSHIMA RG, OLSON DL, SCHNEIDER JA: Cystinosis: Intracellular cystine depletion by aminothiols *in vitro* and *in vivo*. *J Clin Invest* 58:180, 1976

201. THOENE JG, LEMONS R: Modulation of the intracellular cystine content of cystinotic fibroblasts by extracellular albumen. *Pediatr Res* 14:785, 1980

202. STATES B, LEE J, SEGAL S: Uptake of cystine by cystine-depleted fibroblasts from patients with cystinosis. *Biochem Biophys Res Comm* 98:290, 1981

203. STATES B, SCARDIGLI K, SEGAL S: Glutathione in fibroblasts from normal and cystinotic children. *Life Sci* 22:31, 1977

204. WORTHEN HG, GOOD RA: The pathogenesis of cystinosis. *Am J Dis Child* 102:494, 1961

205. MAHONEY CP, TRUMP BF: Studies in cystinosis. *Am J Dis Child* 104:563, 1962

206. SEEGMILLER JE, HOWELL RR: Cystine metabolism in deToni-Fanconi syndrome with cystinosis. *Clin Res* 9:189, 1961

207. ELDJARN L, BREMER J: The disulfide-reducing capacity of liver mitochondria. *Acta Chem Scand* 17 (Suppl 1):S59, 1963

208. SKREDE S: The mechanism of disulfide reduction by mitochondria. *Biochem J* 108:693, 1968

209. TIETZE F, BRADLEY KH, SCHULMAN JD: Enzymatic reduction of cystine by subcellular fractions of cultured and peripheral leukocytes from normal and cystinotic individuals. *Pediatr Res* 6:649, 1972

210. KAYE CI, NADLER HL: Enzymic reduction of cystine and glutathione in cultivated human fibroblasts from normal subjects and patients with cystinosis. *J Lab Clin Med* 86:422, 1975

211. STATES B, HARRIS D, SEGAL S: Patterns of cystine reduction by fibroblasts from normal and cystinotic children. *Pediatr Res* 11:685, 1977

212. WATERSON JR, WINTER WP, SCHMICKEL RD: Cysteine activation in cultured cystinotic cells. The specific activity of cysteinyl-tRNA synthetase and tRNA$_{Cys}$ and the determination of the Michaelis-Menten constants for cysteinyl-tRNA synthetase. *J Clin Invest* 54:182, 1974

213. STATES B, HARRIS D, SEGAL S: Uptake and utilization of exogenous cystine by cystinotic and normal fibroblasts. *J Clin Invest* 53:1003, 1974

214. LINNEWEH F, SCHAUMLÖFFEL E, GRAUL EH, HUNDESHAGEN H, KIRSTEN R, Barthelmai W: Über den Cystin-Metabolismus bei der Cystinose. *Klin Wschr* 42:999, 1964

215. PATRICK AD, BERLIN RD, SCHULMAN JD: Gamma-glutamyl transferase: Studies of normal and cystinotic human leukocytes, rabbit neutrophiles, and rat liver. *Pediatr Res* 13:1058, 1979

216. SCHULMAN JD, PATRICK AD, GOODMAN SI, TIETZE F, BULTER J: Gamma-glutamyl transpeptidase (GGTPase): Investigations in normals and patients with inborn errors of sulfur metabolism. *Pediatr Res* 9:355, 1975

217. STATES B, SEGAL S: Levels of gamma-glutamyltranspeptidase in cultured skin fibroblasts from cystinotics and normals. *Life Sci* 27:1985, 1980

218. BUTLER JD, SPIELBERG: Depletion of cystine accumulation in cystinotic cells by inhibitors of gamma-glutamyl transpeptidase. *J Biol Chem* 256:4160, 1981

219. WENSKE G, LINNEWEH F: Beta-Alanin-Vermehrung in Lympho-und Thrombozyten zur biochemischen Diagnose der Cystinose. *Klin Wschr* 50:1082, 1972

220. FURUSHO K, VETRELLA M, LATTA E: Abnormal arysulphatase activities of fibroblasts cultured from patients with mucopolysaccharidosis and cystinosis. *Z Kinderheilkd* 110:324, 1971

221. SCARDIGLI K, KOLDOVSKY O, PALMIERI M, SEGAL S, STATES B: Activities of acid hydrolases in fibroblasts from normal and cystinotic children. *Clin Chim Acta* 75:12, 1977

222. SEGAL S: Disorders of amino acid transport. *Ann Intern Med* 62:847, 1965

223. BANNAI S, KITAMURA I: Transport interaction of L-cystine and L-glutamate in human diploid fibroblasts in culture. *J Biol Chem* 255:2372, 1980

224. FOREMAN JW, HWANG SM, SEGAL S: Transport interactions of cystine and dibasic amino acids in isolated rat renal tubules. *Metabolism* 29:53, 1980

225. WOLOWYK MW, JONES SEM, ELLORY JC: Sodium-dependent cysteine transport in human red blood cells. *Nature* 279:800, 1979

226. SEGAL S, HWANG SM: L-(^{35}S) cystine uptake by rat brain synaptosomes. *J Neurochem* 33:697, 1979

227. KILBERG MS, CHRISTENSEN HN, HANDLOGTEN ME: Cysteine as a system-specific substrate for transport system ASC in rat hepatocytes. *Biochem Biophys Res Comm* 88:744, 1979

228. ROSENBERG LE, DOWNING SJ: Transport of neutral and dibasic amino acids by human leukocytes: Absence of defect in cystinuria. *J Clin Invest* 44:1382, 1965

229. JELLUM E: The prevention of thiol autoxidation in biological systems by means of thiolated sephadex. *Acta Chem Scand* 18:1887, 1964

230. STATES B, LEE J, SEGAL S: Uptake of cystine by cystine depleted fibroblasts from patients with cystinosis. *Biochem Biophys Res Commun* 15:290, 1981

231. REIJNGOUD DJ, TAGER JM: The permeability properties of the lysosomal membrane. *Biochim Biophy Acta* 472:419, 1977

232. REEVES JP: Accumulation of amino acids by lysosomes incubated with amino acid methyl esters. *J Biol Chem* 254:8914, 1979

233. STEINHERZ R, TIETZE F, RAIFORD D, SCHULMAN JD: Amino acid efflux from normal and cystinotic leukocyte lysosomes. *Pediatr Res* 15:570, 1981

234. STEINHERZ R, TIETZE F, SCHULMAN JD: The clearance of cystine from cystinotic, heterozygous and normal leukocytes loaded by exposure to cystine dimethylester. *Am J Hum Genet* (abstract) 1981, in press

235. PATRICK AD: Deficiencies of SH-dependent enzymes in cystinosis. *Clin Sci* 28:427, 1965

236. SCHNEIDER JA, SEEGMILLER JE: Unpublished observation

237. SEEGMILLER JE: Diseases of purine and pyrimidine metabolism, in Bondy PK, Rosenberg LE (eds): *Duncan's Disease of Metabolism*, 7th ed. Philadelphia, Saunders, 1974, p 655

238. SEEGMILLER JE: Acute gout—a study in depth (editorial). *Hosp Pract* 6:9, 1971

239. WEISSMAN G: Acute gout. *Hosp Pract* 6:24, 1971

240. WEISSMAN G, RITA GA: Molecular basis of gouty inflammation: Interaction of monosodium urate crystals with lysosomes and liposomes. *Nature [New Biol]* 240:167, 1972

241. HARRISON HE: The Fanconi syndrome. *J Chronic Dis* 7:346, 1958

242. WORTHEN HG, GOOD RA: The de Toni-Fanconi syndrome with cystinosis. *Am J Dis Child* 95:653, 1958

243. WEST CD, BLANTON JC, SILVERMAN FN, HOLLAND NH: Use of phosphate salts as an adjunct to vitamin D in the treatment of hypophosphatemic vitamin D refractory rickets. *J Pediatr* 64:469, 1964

244. CALLIS L, CASTELLO F, FORTUNY G, VALLO A, BALLABRIGA A: Effect of hydrochlorothiazide on rickets and on renal tubular acidosis in two patients with cystinosis. *Helv Paediat Acta* 25:602, 1970

245. WEBER VH, HAGGE W: Über die erfolgreiche Behandlung der Zystinose mit einem Anabolicum. *Arch Kinderkeilkd* 168:110, 1963

246. BAUER B, ANTENER I: Eine wirksame diätetische und medikamentöse Cystinosebehandlung. *Helv Paediat Acta* 21:19, 1966

247. BICKEL H, LUTZ P, SCHMIDT H: The treatment of cystinosis with diet or drug, in Schulman JD (ed): *Cystinosis*. Washington, D.C., DHEW Publication no (NIH) 72-249, U.S. Government Printing Office, 1973, p 199

248. GENOVA R: Su di un caso di tesaurismosi cistinica. *Minerva Pediatr* 26:1782, 1974

249. BÉTEND B, DAVID L, VINCENT M, HERMIER M, FRANÇOIS R: Successful indomethacin treatment of two pediatric patients with severe tubulopathies. A boy with an unusual hypercalciuria and a girl with cystinosis. *Helv Paediatr Acta* 34:339, 1979

250. HAYCOCK GB, AL-DAHLAN J, CHANTLER C: The effect of indomethacin on renal function in cystinosis. *Pediatr Res* 14:1008, 1980

251. LEMIRE J, KAPLAN BS: Prolonged use of indomethacin in cystinosis. *Pediatr Res* 15:696, 1981

252. HAMBREAUS L, BROBERGER O: Penicillamine treatment of cystinosis. *Acta Paediatr Scand* 56:243, 1967

253. DEPAPE-BRIGGER D, GOLDMAN H, SCRIVER CR, DELVIN E, MAMER O: The *in vivo* use of dithiothreitol in cystinosis. *Pediatr Res* 11:124, 1977

254. ROY LP, POLLARD AC: Cysteamine therapy for cystinosis. *Lancet* 2:729, 1978

255. GIRARDIN EP, DEWOLFE MJ, CROCKER JFS: Treatment of cystinosis with cysteamine. *J Pediatr* 94:838, 1979

256. YUDKOFF M, FOREMAN JW, SEGAL S: Effects of cysteamine therapy in nephropathic cystinosis. *N Engl J Med* 304:141, 1981

257. SCHNEIDER JA, SCHULMAN JD, THOENE JG: Cysteamine therapy in cystinosis. *N Engl J Med* letter to the editor 304:1172, 1981

258. CORDEN BJ, SCHULMAN JD, SCHNEIDER JA, THOENE JG: Adverse reactions to oral cysteamine use in nephropathic cystinosis. *Dev Pharm Therap* 3:25, 1981

259. THOENE JG, LEMONS R: Cystine depletion of cystinotic tissues by phosphocysteamine (WR638). *J Pediatr* 96:1043, 1980

260. KROLL WA, SCHNEIDER JA: Decrease in free-cystine content of cultured cystinotic fibroblasts by ascorbic acid. *Science* 186:1040, 1974

261. SCHNEIDER JA, SCHLESSELMAN JJ, MENDOZA SA, ORLOFF S, THOENE JG, KROLL WA, GODFREY AD, SCHULMAN JD: Ineffectiveness of ascorbic acid therapy in nephropathic cystinosis. *N Engl J Med* 300:756, 1979

262. CERILLI J, EVANS WE, SOTOS JF: Renal transplantation in infants and children. *Transplant Proc* 4:633, 1972

263. BROYER M, KLEINKNECHT C, LOIRAT C, MARTI-HENNEBERG C, ROY MP: Growth in children treated with long term hemodialysis. *J Pediatr* 84:642, 1974

264. MAHONEY CP, MANNING GB, HICKMAN RO: Hemodialysis in a patient with cystinosis. *Am J Dis Child* 112:65, 1966

265. Advisory Committee to the Renal Transplant Registry: Renal transplantation in congenital and metabolic diseases. A report from the ASC/NIH Renal Transplant Registry. *JAMA* 232:148, 1975

266. MALEKZADEH MH, NEUSTEIN HB, SCHNEIDER JA, PENNISI AJ, ETTENGER RB, UITTENBOGAART CH, KOGUT MD, FINE RN: Cadaver renal transplantation in children with cystinosis. *Am J Med* 63:525, 1977

267. WEST JC, GOODMAN SI, SCHROTER GP, BLOUSTEIN PA, HAMBIDGE KM, WEIL R: Pediatric kidney transplantation for cystinosis. *J Ped Surg* 12:651, 1977

268. MONGEAU J-G, ROBITAILLE P, GRALL M-M: Chronic renal failure in children. *CMA* 118:907, 1978

269. HURLEY JK, LIU HM: Myxedema coma in cystinosis. *J Pediatr* 91:341, 1977

270. SCHULMAN JD, FUJIMOTO WY, BRADLEY KH, SEEGMILLER JE: Identification of heterozygous genotype for cystinosis *in utero* using a new pulse-labelling technique: Preliminary report. *J Pediatr* 77:468, 1970

271. STATES B, BLAZER B, HARRIS D, SEGAL S: Prenatal diagnosis of cystinosis. *J Pediatr* 87:558, 1975

272. BOMAN H, SCHNEIDER JA: Prenatal diagnosis of nephropathic cystinosis. *Acta Paediatr Scand* 1981, in press

86

NEPHROGENIC DIABETES INSIPIDUS

R. MICHAEL CULPEPPER

STEVEN C. HEBERT

THOMAS E. ANDREOLI

1. *Nephrogenic diabetes insipidus is a disorder, familial or acquired, characterized by renal tubular insensitivity to the antidiuretic hormone (ADH). Polydipsia, polyuria, and hyposthenuria are the cardinal clinical manifestations of this disease. Nephrogenic diabetes insipidus is distinguished from pituitary diabetes insipidus by a lack of response to exogenous vasopressin and by serum levels of arginine vasopressin that vary appropriately with changes in serum osmolality.*

2. *The familial disorder exhibits a hereditary pattern consistent with X-linked transmission with variable degrees of manifestation in females. All reported males are completely unresponsive to vasopressin. Milder forms of the disease, exhibiting a limited response to vasopressin, may be observed in female members of affected families. Acquired nephrogenic diabetes insipidus may occur either as a consequence of drug therapy with lithium or demethylchlortetracycline or volatile anesthetics such as methoxyflurane, or in association with systemic disorders such as amyloidosis, Sjögren's syndrome, or sarcoidosis.*

3. *The causes for vasopressin unresponsiveness in either the familial or acquired forms of the disorder are not certain. In normal individuals, ADH enhances cAMP accumulation in collecting duct cells; in turn, cAMP enhances the rate of water transport, possibly by increasing the number of water-specific channels in urinary (luminal) membranes. Inferential but not conclusive data in patients and experimental animals sug-*

gest that, in the familial disease, there is an inability of renal tubular cells to accumulate cAMP in response to vasopressin. Demethylchlortetracycline may also produce a defect in vasopressin-stimulated cAMP accumulation by renal tubular cells. In lithium-induced nephrogenic diabetes insipidus, there may be defects both in vasopressin-stimulated cAMP formation and in cAMP enhancement of water transport through urinary (luminal) membranes.

4. *Maintenance of water balance by ingestion of adequate amounts of water is sufficient treatment. When the amount of water required is inconveniently large, this can be reduced by restriction of solute intake and by the administration of chlorothiazide or its congeners. Life expectancy is normal if episodes of dehydration are prevented.*

Nephrogenic diabetes insipidus is a disorder produced by a lack of response of renal tubular cells to antidiuretic hormone (ADH).[1] Polydipsia and polyuria, which are the clinical hall-

---

[1] Details of the chemistry and conformation of ADH will be discussed in "Water Homeostasis." Neurohypophyseal extracts from amphibians, certain reptiles, birds, and mammals contain cyclic octapeptides having antidiuretic activity. In humans and most other mammalian species, the naturally occuring antidiuretic hormone is the octapeptide arginine vasopressin (AVP). Unless otherwise specified, the term *vasopressin* will be used in this chapter to designate AVP. Pitressin is a commercial mammalian neurohypophyseal extract which contains predominantly arginine vasopressin.

marks of the syndrome, are the direct result of this tubular refractoriness to ADH. In normal individuals, the plasma osmolality is maintained remarkably constant, in the range of 285 to 295 mosmol/kg H_2O, despite wide variations in water intake. The major components of the physiologic factors responsible for osmotic homeostasis of the body fluids are illustrated schematically in Fig. 86-1. Slight increments in plasma osmolality or reductions in plasma volume stimulate ADH release from the neurohypophysis. Within collecting duct cells, ADH binding to contraluminal plasma membranes results in activation of the enzyme adenyl cyclase (EC 4.6.1.1), which catalyzes the formation of cyclic AMP (cAMP; cyclic 3',5'-adenosine monophosphate) from ATP. In turn, cAMP-mediated processes increase the water permeability of luminal membranes in collecting duct cells, thereby permitting osmotic equilibration of collecting duct fluid with a medullary interstitium made hypertonic by the renal countercurrent multiplication and exchange systems. Thus, in the presence of circulating ADH, normal individuals can excrete urine that is hypertonic to plasma.

In contrast, an individual having nephrogenic diabetes insipidus excretes urine which is consistently hypotonic to plasma, even when plasma osmolality and plasma ADH concentrations are significantly increased, because the epithelial cells of collecting ducts are insensitive to ADH. Virtually all the clinical manifestations of the disease, including the obligatory requirement for ingesting large volumes of solute-free water, the effects of polyuria on the hydrodynamics of the urinary tract, and the hypertonic dehydration that inevitably attends water restriction, are directly referable to this deficient renal mechanism for water homeostasis.

The first modern descriptions of nephrogenic diabetes insipidus focused on a relatively rare sex-linked hereditary disorder [1–4]. Polyuric disorders due to failure of the renal tubule to respond to ADH may also occur as a complication of either drug therapy or, in rare instances, systemic diseases. Because the clinical and pathophysiologic findings in these conditions resemble closely those occurring in familial nephrogenic diabetes insipidus, this chapter will consider both the familial and acquired forms of nephrogenic diabetes insipidus.

THE FAMILIAL DISEASE: CLINICAL CONSIDERATIONS

History

Observations on familial diabetes insipidus were recorded in 1841 by LaCombe [5] and in 1884 by Weil [6]. In 1892, McIlraith [7] described (Fig. 86-2) three generations of individuals with diabetes insipidus: Males were affected with "extreme thirst," females were "slightly affected," and male offspring of "slightly affected" females suffered from "extreme thirst." He concluded that this form of diabetes insipidus involved "a heredity occurring chiefly in males on the female side of the house." In 1935, de Lange [8], in a report of a family with hereditary diabetes insipidus involving four generations, observed no male-to-male transmission and noted that injections of posterior pituitary lobe extracts did not reduce urine volume or increase urine specific gravity in affected patients.

Recent descriptions of familial nephrogenic diabetes insipidus are generally credited to Forssman [1,2], Waring, Kajdi, and Tappan [3], and Williams and Henry [4]. In 1942, Forssman [1] described hereditary diabetes insipidus in patients from two kindreds involving five and three generations, respectively. The urinary concentrating defect was not amenable to treatment with injections of posterior pituitary lobe extracts, and the pattern of heredity resembled that described by McIlraith (Fig. 86-2). Forssman, like McIlraith [7], concluded that the disorder involved recessive, sex-linked transmission.

In 1945, Forssman [2] published an analysis of the existing literature on hereditary diabetes insipidus together with data acquired on five different kindreds having 32 possible male patients with the disorder; 16 of these patients were studied personally by him. He established that male-to-male transmission did not occur, that descendents of phenotypically normal males were healthy, that polyuria invariably had its onset in infancy, that daily urine volumes in adults exceeded 4 liters, that urinary specific gravities after water deprivation were in the range of 1.003 to 1.008, and that female carriers frequently had unusual thirst, nocturnal water consumption, and impaired urinary concentrating ability following water deprivation. In three affected males from one kindred, water depriva-

MAJOR COMPONENTS OF THE WATER HOMEOSTASIS SYSTEM

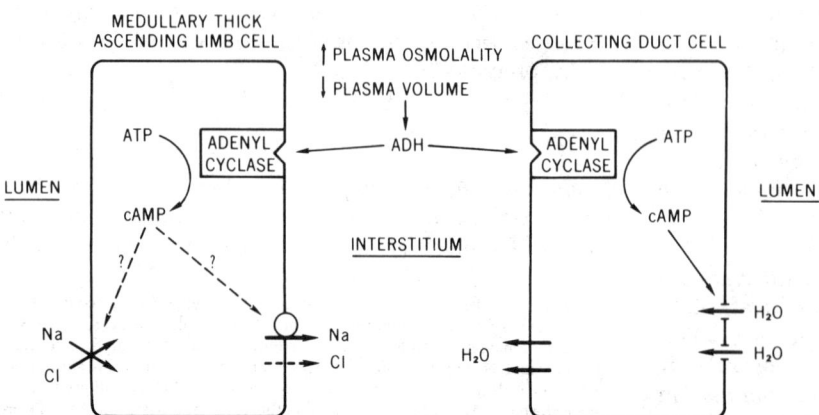

Figure 86-1 The major components of the water homeostasis system.

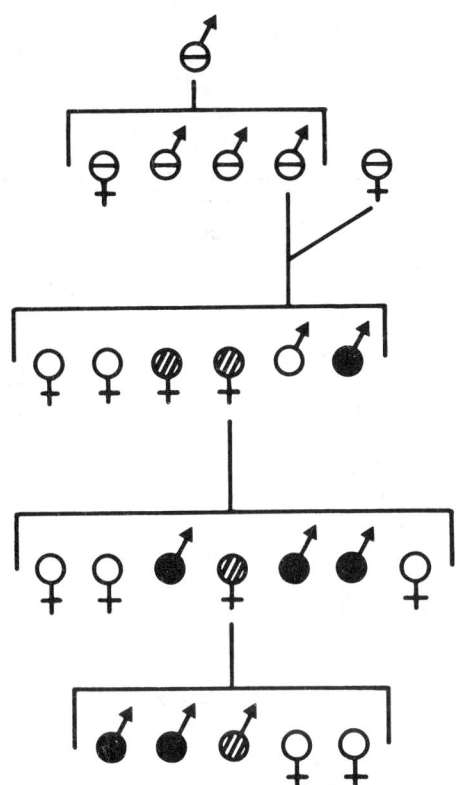

● "affected with extreme thirst"
◑ "slightly affected"
○ "not affected"
⊖ "not affected so far as known"

Figure 86-2 McIlraith's [7] pedigree for hereditary diabetes insipidus involving three generations within a kindred.

tion combined with injections of posterior pituitary lobe extracts failed to reduce urine volume or increase urine specific gravity. In 1947, Williams and Henry [4] applied the term *nephrogenic diabetes insipidus* to the disease, stressing the fact that renal tubular insensitivity to ADH was the primary pathophysiologic disturbance.

Clinical Manifestations

Little can be added to the descriptions provided by Forssman [1, 2], Waring et al. [3], and Williams and Henry [4]. The narrative by Waring et al. [3], published in abstract form, summarizes eloquently and succinctly the main clinical and pathophysiologic features of the disease:

> The syndrome is characterized by onset shortly after birth . . . polydipsia and polyuria which do not respond to pitressin . . . high values for serum sodium and chloride . . . rapid dehydration if fluids are reduced or withheld . . . inability to excrete urine of high specific gravity . . . familial incidence and occurrence in boys only (?).
>
> The presenting complaints were unexplained fever, failure to gain weight and constipation . . . . The bouts of dehydration are usually not associated with acidosis.

The thirst of one of the patients studied was satisfied only when five to six times the normal requirement of fluid was offered. The levels of serum sodium and chloride decreased to normal, and the infant remained afebrile on this high fluid intake . . . . With total restriction of fluids the infant became severely dehydrated within twelve hours; the flow of urine virtually ceased in ten hours; the temperature rose, and the serum sodium and chloride increased greatly . . . . The dehydration could be corrected rapidly by giving water.

Pitressin was given until toxic reactions were seen without any alteration in fluid intake or output.

Renal clearances done under good conditions of hydration showed normal values for mannitol, urea, phosphates and paraaminohippuric acid at high and low levels . . . . Only 70 to 80% of filtered water, as against 99.5 per cent of the filtered sodium and 98.8 per cent of the chloride, was reabsorbed in the renal tubules. Administration of ammonium chloride . . . revealed that the children could excrete acid urine.

In short, the clinical picture in dehydrated patients with nephrogenic diabetes insipidus is one of volume contraction, hypernatremia, and hyperthermia, attended by potentially lethal effects, particularly on the central nervous system. Because of the relatively nonspecific nature of symptoms in early stages of the disease, the disorder may be difficult to identify in the first few months of life. Indeed, a number of authors [2, 4, 9] have called attention to the fact that the disease has been unrecognized during infancy even in kindreds with long family histories of "water babies."

The following considerations illustrate the extreme degree of volume contraction that may occur in affected infants. During the first 6 months of life, body water content is approximately 12 liters per square meter of body surface area [10], and the glomeruler filtration rate ranges between 25 and 40 ml/min per square meter of body surface area [11]; thus, a 5-kg-male infant with body surface area of 0.3 m^2 has a body water content of approximately 4.0 liters and a glomeruler filtration rate of 7.5 to 12 ml/min. If he were affected with severe familial nephrogenic diabetes insipidus where 20 percent of filtered water was excreted, his obligatory urine loss would be 2.0 to 3.5 liters daily, or about 50 to 85 percent of total body water. Small wonder, then, that infants suffering from the disease are markedly susceptible to volume depletion, hyperthermia, and hypernatremia, particularly since they are unable to regulate their own fluid intake.

Mental and Physical Retardation Many authors have commented on the mental and physical retardation that may accompany hereditary nephrogenic diabetes insipidus [2, 4, 8, 9, 12–19], but it has also been well documented [2, 4, 8, 9, 12, 16–20] that children with the disorder may have normal intelligence and physical maturation. Forssman [16] noted a close correlation between repeated bouts of dehydration during infancy and subsequent mental dullness; in patients provided with "a generous supply of fluid" during infancy, growth and maturation were normal. Hillman et al. [19] observed an infant with the disease who, when offered a normal diet, became so fatigued from water ingestion that he could neither sleep nor eat normally; his mental performance and growth rate improved dramatically by reducing dietary salt and protein intake and providing caloric supplementation in the form of fat and carbohydrate. Finally, Reuss et al. [12] carried out psychologic testing in children with nephrogenic diabetes insipidus and documented that patients wih mental retardation uniformly showed signs of organic brain damage. All these observations are in accord with the view [2, 9, 12, 16–19] that physical and mental retardation in familial nephrogenic diabetes insipidus are either the consequence of inadequate caloric ingestion, in the case of growth retardation, or the effects of hypernatremia, in the case of mental impairment.

It is well established that hypernatremia may cause irreversible damage to the central nervous system, particularly in infants. In one series of 50 hypernatremic children the acute mortality was 20 percent, and 37 percent of the survivors had abnormalities on neurologic examination, intelligence testing, or electroencephalography [21]. Likewise, in 100 infants who developed hypernatremic encephalopathy, brain damage developed in 16 patients, 8 of whom subsequently died [22].

Studies in experimental animals confirm that neurologic damage due to brain shrinkage is the major consequence of the hyperosmolar state. Since elevation of body osmolality with solute that permeates cells readily, such as urea in azotemic states, does not produce the neurologic picture of hyperosmolality but hypertonicity with impermeate solutes such as NaCl and glucose does, it is apparent that osmotic shrinkage of brain cells underlies the production of neurologic dysfunction [23].

Renal Function The cardinal abnormality in familial nephrogenic diabetes insipidus is the failure of collecting ducts to increase their water permeability in response to ADH, resulting in the excretion of urine that is hypotonic to plasma. Williams and Henry [4] showed clearly that the concentrating defect is due to end-organ refractorines to ADH, since doses of pitressin sufficient to cause abdominal cramps and cutaneous blanching had no effect on urine volume and concentration. Also, patients who received parenteral injections of pitressin excreted a greater fraction of antidiuretic activity in the urine than normal individuals [24], making it unlikely that abnormally rapid inactivation of the hormone is responsible for the manifestations of the disease.

The concentrating defect in nephrogenic diabetes insipidus often seems to be more severe than in pituitary diabetes insipidus. In Brattleboro strain rats having hereditary hypothalamic diabetes insipidus, urinary hypertonicity in the absence of ADH occurs when the glomerular filtration rate (GFR) is severely reduced [25], but it can also occur with little or no reduction in GFR if renal blood flow is reduced [26]. The suggested mechanism [26] for the formation of hypertonic urine under these conditions involves a striking reduction in the volume of fluid delivered to distal tubules and collecting ducts, so that, in the absence of ADH, the removal of even small amounts of water from collecting ducts results in at least partial equilibration of collecting duct fluid with the renal medullary interstitium, and hence the generation of urine that is hypertonic to plasma. In one patient with familial nephrogenic diabetes insipidus [27], in whom severe reductions in glomerular filtration rate and virtual cessation of urine flow were produced by induced hypotension, the urine became isotonic but not hypertonic to plasma. Other patients with this disease, however, are able to produce urine hypertonic to plasma with reductions in GFR of approximately 50 percent [28].

Four other disturbances in renal structure or function, or in other epithelial transport processes, have been noted in familial nephrogenic diabetes insipidus. Studies in six patients [4, 13, 27, 29] showed renal plasma flow to be reduced while glomeruler filtration rate was normal, resulting in an elevated filtration fraction. It was proposed [29] that the rise in filtra-

tion fraction was the consequence of renal vasoconstriction produced by high concentrations of circulating ADH.

Hyperuricemia has been observed in seven adults with familial nephrogenic diabetes insipidus [27, 29], two of whom developed clinical gout. Urinary clearances of uric acid were reduced while glomerular filtration rates were normal. This suggested that, in adult patients, the disease may be accompanied by a renal tubular defect in uric acid excretion. Since children with familial nephrogenic diabetes insipidus had normal serum uric acid concentrations, Gorden et al. [29] proposed that such a defect is acquired rather than congenital and possibly is related to an elevated filtration fraction or to urinary tract dilatation.

Also, microdissection of autopsy specimens from children with the disease revealed shortening of proximal convoluted tubule segments [30]. It is difficult to reconcile these anatomic findings with the concentrating defect occurring in more terminal nephron segments.

Finally, infants and children with the disorder have increased NaCl concentrations in sweat [31, 32]. The excess salt concentrations in sweat are not reduced by administration of 9-alpha-fluorohydrocortisone [32].

In all other respects, renal function in the disease appears to be normal. In the absence of dehydration or hydronephrosis, plasma electrolytes and plasma acid-base balance are normal, as are the glomerular filtration rate, glucose and amino acid reabsorptive rates, phosphate excretion, and urinary acidifying ability [3, 4, 13, 14, 17, 19, 27, 29, 33, 34].

Radiographic Manifestations

Striking dilatation of the urinary tract may occur in familial nephrogenic diabetes insipidus [28, 35–37]. The dilation progresses in some instances to massive hydroureter, hydronephrosis, and a urinary bladder capacity of 1000 ml. Urinary tract dilatation also occurs in pituitary forms of diabetes insipidus [36]. Moreover, in inbred mice having primary polydipsia and polyuria, hydronephrosis frequently occurs in male but not female animals; possibly because of a relatively long urethra, male animals accommodated less well than female animals to polyuria [38]. According to these views, patients with nephrogenic diabetes insipidus may develop hydronephrosis whenever urinary flow rates exceed the normal emptying capacity of the bladder [37].

Serum Vasopressin Concentrations

Early analyses of the relationship between serum concentrations of ADH, plasma osmolality, and plasma volume were hampered by the lack of specific methods for measuring serum arginine vasopressin levels. Rather, serum ADH concentrations were estimated by bioassay procedures [39] or inferred from the formation of urine hypertonic to plasma following hypertonic NaCl administration or sustained hydropenia [23]. Using a variety of bioassay procedures, a number of workers provided evidence that either the serum or urine of patients with familial nephrogenic diabetes insipidus contained normal to excessive amounts of antidiuretic activity [13, 23, 40, 41].

Robertson and his associates, using a specific radioimmunoassay for arginine vasopressin (AVP) capable of detecting reproducibly plasma AVP concentrations as low as 0.5 pg/ml, have analyzed systematically the relative contributions of blood osmolality and blood volume in regulating plasma AVP concentrations [42–44]. Two of their observations are particularly noteworthy. First, as shown in Fig. 86-3 [42], both in normal subjects and in patients with nephrogenic diabetes insipidus, serum osmolalities greater than 280 mosmol/kg result in near-linear increments in serum AVP concentrations, while in pituitary diabetes insipidus, plasma AVP concentrations change neglibibly or not at all in response to an osmotic challenge. Second, as shown in Fig. 86-4 [42, 44], normal subjects and patients with either primary polydipsia or pituitary diabetes insipidus exhibit a near-linear relationship between urine osmolality and plasma AVP concentrations, while patients with nephrogenic diabetes excrete a consistently hypotonic urine despite fifteenfold variations in plasma AVP levels. These observations [42, 44] provide strong support for the hypothesis [1–4] that familial nephrogenic diabetes insipidus is characterized by end-organ unresponsiveness to ADH.

Hereditary

The hereditary patterns observed by McIlraith ([7]; Fig. 86-2), Forssman [1, 2], and Williams and Henry [4] were interpreted as indicating that familial nephrogenic diabetes insipidus is transmitted as a sex-linked recessive characteristic. Consistent with this view are the observations that male patients with the disorder exhibit complete unresponsiveness to vasopressin [1–4, 9, 13–15, 17–20, 23, 30, 33, 45] and that male-to-male transmission is rare (Fig. 86-2; [1–4]). However, incomplete forms of the disease occur in female sibs, female "carriers" (Fig. 86-2), and female relatives of affected males [1, 2, 7, 13, 23, 33, 45, 46, 47]. And, in families having no evidence of paternal involvement, several females have been reported in

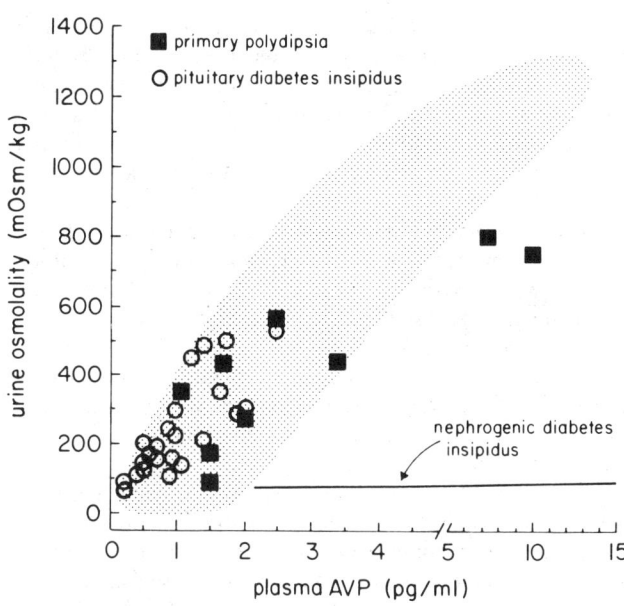

Figure 86-4 The relationship between plasma AVP concentrations and urine osmolality. (*Adapted from Robertson et al.* [42, 44].)

whom the disease was as severe as that observed in males [13, 34, 48]. On the basis of these observations, it appears that familial nephrogenic diabetes insipidus is an X-linked disorder with variable degrees of manifestation, or "penetration," in heterozygous females. If so, mothers and half of the sisters of affected males should either be carriers of the disease or exhibit some form of the disease (Fig. 86-2). In families evaluated with this question in mind, approximately two-thirds of the female relatives of males having the complete disorder failed to concentrate urine normally following dehydration [23, 45]. The interpretation of certain published pedigrees as examples of autosomal inheritance with some degree of sex limitation contains sufficient discrepancies to discount such a pattern of inheritance [23].

In a retrospective analysis of their patients, Bode and Crawford [49] deduced that most North American patients with the disease were descendants of the "Ulster Scot" clan, who reached Nova Scotia in 1761 on the ship *Hopewell*. Among these people, there is a long tradition of "water drinkers" that conforms to the inheritance pattern of a sex-linked recessive trait. Nakano [46] described nephrogenic diabetes insipidus in a Samoan-Caucasian family residing in Hawaii; the family history was traced back to a heterozygous Samoan woman carrier. Familial nephrogenic diabetes insipidus has also been described in an Australian aboriginal kindred having no Caucasian ancestry [47]. Thus, future studies of North American families with the disease may indicate a more general distribution of the disorder than supposed by Bode and Crawford [49].

WATER HOMEOSTASIS

In normal individuals having widely disparate salt and water intakes, plasma osmolality is virtually constant. Although the range of normal values in the population is 285 to 295 mosmol/kg H_2O, the value of plasma osmolality in an individual varies by only 1 to 2 percent. Because plasma osmolality

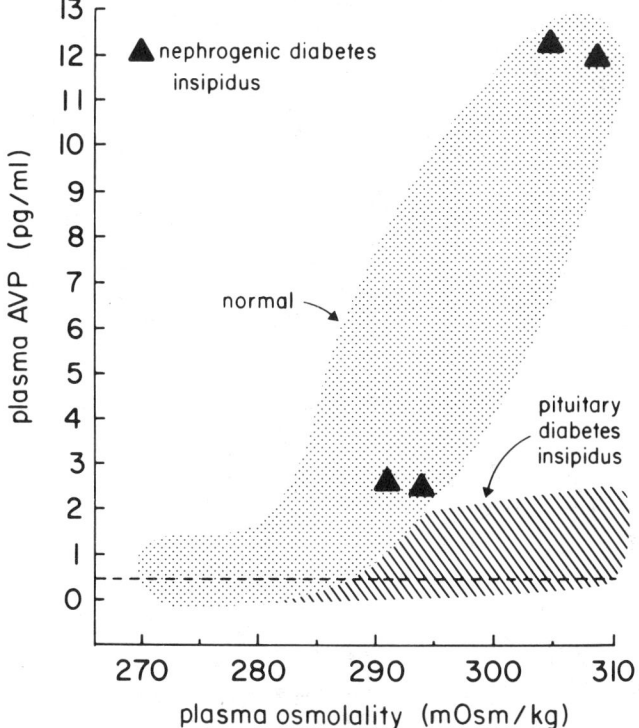

Figure 86-3 The relationship between plasma AVP concentrations and plasma osmolality. (*Adapted from Robertson et al.* [42, 44].)

expresses the ratio of aqueous solutes to total body water, invariance of plasma osmolality in the presence of nonisotonic solute and water ingestion depends on the ability of the kidney to dissociate solute and water excretion: one excretes urine which is either hypotonic to plasma, in the case of relative water excess, or hypertonic to plasma, in the case of relative water deficit.

Since proximal tubular absorption of glomerular ultrafiltrate is an isotonic process, the independent modulation of solute and water excretion is effected by transport phenomena occurring in more distal nephron sites. Stated briefly, the ability to excrete urine as dilute as 50 mosmol/kg H_2O or as concentrated as 1400 mosmol/kg H_2O depends on the following processes. Solute (NaCl) absorption in the water-impermeable ascending limbs of Henle results in dilution of luminal fluid and enrichment of the hypertonic medullary interstitium. In the absence of ADH, the dilute fluid passes unchanged through water-impermeable distal convoluted tubules and collecting ducts, yielding a dilute urine. In the presence of ADH, the water permeability of collecting ducts increases by at least tenfold, thus allowing equilibration of luminal fluid with the hypertonic interstitium and consequently the production of concentrated urine. Glomerular filtration rate and the rate of proximal tubular absorption of glomerular filtrate also influence the final osmolality of urine by varying the magnitude of solute and water delivered to more distal nephron segments.

Antidiuretic Hormone

Chemistry The hormones elaborated by most mammalian neurohypophyses include oxytocin and AVP (Fig. 86-5). Du Vigneaud has summarized the history and details of the epochal work that started with the isolation of oxytocin and arginine vasopressin from beef pituitary glands and lysine vasopressin from hog glands and that led to their eventual chemical synthesis [50].

As shown in Fig. 86-5, both oxytocin and arginine vasopressin are octapeptides having molecular weights of approximately 1100. A sulfhydryl bond between the cysteine residues at positions 1 and 6 forms a single cystine moiety yielding a ring composed of 20 atoms in both molecules. In all mammals with the exception of hogs and other members of the suborder Suina, arginine vasopressin is the antidiuretic hormone; lysine vasopressin, which contains lysine rather than arginine in the 8 position, occurs in Suina species [51]. The antidiuretic hormone among lower vertebrates is arginine vasotocin, which contains the same three C-terminal acyclic amino acids as arginine vasopressin and the tocin ring structure of oxytocin [50, 51].

At least nine neurohypophyseal octapeptides have been isolated from vertebrates [52], and there exist hundreds of synthetic analogues of arginine vasopressin. All these agents share, to varying degrees, uterotonic, vasoconstrictor, and antidiuretic activities. A comparison of oxytocin and arginine vasopressin (Fig. 86-5) indicates that these peptides differ at positions 3 and 8. These structural differences confer rather different biologic activities on the hormones: arginine vasopressin has nearly comparable pressor and antidiuretic activities, both of which are 100 times greater than those of oxytocin, while oxytocin is about 20 times more uterotonic than arginine vasopressin [50]. In the present context we shall consider some of the structural features of neurohypophyseal peptides, with particular emphasis on those which determine antidiuretic activity and specificity.

All analogues of arginine vasopressin and oxytocin synthesized to date have some detectable antidiuretic activity [53, 54]. Antidiuretic activity in the intact animal depends on the

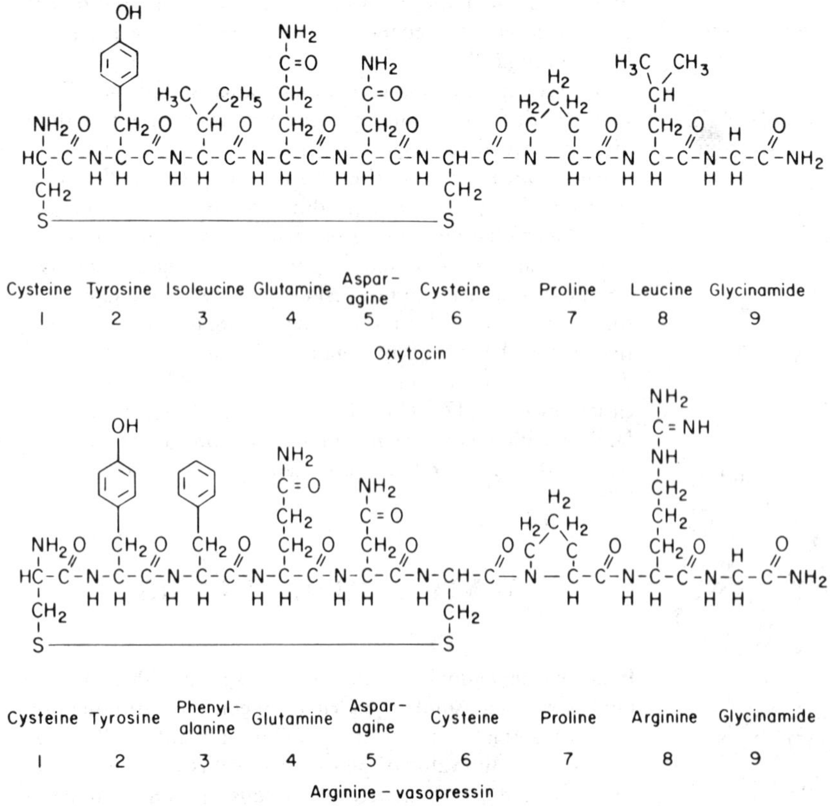

Cysteine	Tyrosine	Isoleucine	Glutamine	Aspar-agine	Cysteine	Proline	Leucine	Glycinamide
1	2	3	4	5	6	7	8	9

Oxytocin

Cysteine	Tyrosine	Phenyl-alanine	Glutamine	Aspar-agine	Cysteine	Proline	Arginine	Glycinamide
1	2	3	4	5	6	7	8	9

Arginine – vasopressin

Figure 86-5 The structures of oxytocin and arginine vasopressin.

ability of a peptide to bind to the renal receptor, to stimulate the adenyl cyclase system, and to resist metabolic degradation [54]. Thus, peptides that activate adenyl cyclase very poorly may still produce a maximal antidiuretic response in the whole animal [54, 55]. Moreover, these compounds exhibit nonlinear coupling of binding affinity and enzyme activation, that is, a very low receptor occupancy rate may give near maximal adenyl cyclase stimulation [57–59]. In a system of isolated bovine renal membrane fractions, vasopressin analogues whose receptor binding affinities varied over five orders of magnitude all produced full activation of adenyl cyclase [56]. Biologic activity is a function of the same phenomenon. For AVP, occupancy of as few as 2.5 percent of receptors by hormone may produce as little as 5 percent of maximal adenyl cyclase activation yet result in full antidiuretic activity [54].

Studies of receptor affinity and adenyl cyclase activation in vitro demonstrate that deamination of position 1 reduces affinity and activation [57], yet this modification enhances strikingly both antidiuretic activity and specificity in vivo [60]. Substitution of the D-arginine enantiomorph for L-arginine in position 8 results in reduced receptor affinity [57] but produces a remarkable specificity for antidiuretic as opposed to vasopressor activity in the whole animal [60]. Furthermore, replacement of one sulfur atom with a methylene group (termed 1-carba substitution) preserves receptor affinity in oxytocin analogues [58] and enhances affinity in vasopressin analogues [57]. Reduction in ring size to 19 members decreases affinity and activity in both molecules [57, 58], while an increase in ring size to 21 members either enhances or little affects these characteristics [57, 58]. Finally, the presence of a basic side chain (positions 7 to 9) contributes to increased receptor affinity [57, 58] but is not necessary for adenyl cyclase activation [59]. Given these apparent discrepancies between observations in vitro and in vivo, it is clear that metabolic stability plays an important role in determining in vivo antidiuretic activity [55, 57, 60–62].

Inactivation of oxytocin depends in part on proteolytic cleavage of the disulfide bond bridging positions 1 and 6 [63], but "dicarba" analogues of arginine vasopressin containing 1,6—CH_2—CH_2— methylene rather than —S—S— disulfide bridges have a substantially longer antidiuretic effect than arginine vasopressin [64]. Similarly, substitution of a single methylene for the cysteine sulfur at positions 1 or 6 enhances both receptor affinity and antidiuretic activity, so long as ring size is not changed [57, 62].

Two other modifications of arginine vasopressin endow marked prolongation of antidiuretic activity and concomitantly increase the specificity of antidiuretic versus vasopressor activity. First, deamination of the 1-hemicystine residue to 1-deaminoarginine vasopressin (dAVP) increases antidiuretic activity fourfold but does not affect pressor activity and results in an antidiuretic/pressor activity ratio of 3.8 for dAVP [60, 61, 64]. Second, substitution of lipophilic amino acids for glutamine in position 4, for example, valine to produce 4-valine AVP (VAVP), or threonine to produce 4-threonine AVP derivatives (dTAVP, dTDAVP), yields further prolongation of antidiureses and specificity for antidiuretic activity [60, 61, 65].

A final substitution has been shown to reduce pressor activity markedly in octapeptides and, in combination with the modifications described above, to yield compounds with remarkably potent antidiuretic capability. Replacement of L-arginine in position 8 with D-arginine (D-arginine vasopressin; DAVP) reduces antidiuretic activity far less than pressor activity, so that the antidiuretic/pressor activity ratio of DAVP is 28 [60, 63]. Walter et al. [66] have interpreted these findings as indicative of a more stringent requirement for complementary charge interaction at pressor than at antidiuretic receptor sites.

These structural modifications of AVP have cumulative effects. Thus, in comparison to AVP: 1-deamino-[8-D-arginine]-vasopressin (dDAVP) has a longer duration of action, three times the antidiuretic effect, and reduced pressor activity [60, 61, 64]; 1-deamino-4-valine-[8-D-arginine]-vasopressin (dVDAVP) has a more prolonged duration of action, four times the antidiuretic potency, and undetectable pressor effects, making it the most specific antidiuretic peptide reported [60, 64, 66]; and 1-deamino-6-carba-[8-D-arginine]1-vasopressin (dCDAVP) has a very prolonged duration of action referable to reduced proteolysis [63, 64], greater antidiuretic potency, and slight pressor activity [62, 64]. All three of these agents, dDAVP, dVDAVP, and dCDAVP, are useful in the treatment of pituitary diabetes insipidus [64, 67] but are not known to affect nephrogenic diabetes insipidus.

Finally, it is clear that molecular characterization of the antidiuretic and pressor activities of AVP and its analogues will require an understanding of the conformations of neurohypophyseal peptides. Urry and Walter [68] have proposed that the conformation of oxytocin includes a two-β-turn structure, one β-turn involving the 20-membered tocin ring (Fig. 86-5) and the second β-turn involving the C-terminal acyclic amino acid sequence; conformational stability is achieved by hydrogen bonding of asparagine (residue 5), both within the first β-turn and with leucine in position 8. Walter et al. [69] have proposed a comparable conformation for the ring component of lysine vasopressin but a more flexible conformation for the acyclic amino acid sequence. Substitution in neurohypophyseal hormones with D-amino acids allows manipulation of the topochemical orientation of CO and NH groups of the ring structure. Studies with these analogues have led to further emphasis on molecular configuration and to a proposal that the Asn^5 and Tyr^2 residues play critical roles in biologic activity through nonionic interactions between the receptor and the CO and NH groups of these amino acids [59, 70].

Although there are analogues of AVP that effectively antagonize the pressor response to vasopressin in vivo [71], all AVP analogues synthesized until recently had some agonist activity for antidiuresis [53]. Now four analogues of AVP have been produced that effectively block the antidiuresis of AVP. The most potent antagonist, $d(CH_2)_5Tyr(ET)VAVP$, when injected into normal rats, caused a water diuresis comparable to that in homozygous Brattleboro rats which lack ADH entirely [53]. The production of an octapeptide antagonistic to AVP does not occur in nephrogenic diabetes insipidus, as these patients have circulating hormone that is immunologically [42, 44] and biologically [41] identical to arginine vasopressin.

Biosynthesis, Storage, and Release   The relationships between the hypothalamus, the posterior pituitary gland, and antidiuretic hormone production derive largely from the work of Scharrer and Scharrer [72], who showed that nerve endings in the posterior pituitary gland have their origin in cell bodies located in the supraoptic and paraventricular nuclei of the hypothalamus, that these nerve cells contain dense granules (neurosecretory granules), and that there is a close correlation between the number of neurosecretory granules and the state of hydration in a number of mammalian species. Because neurosecretory granules accumulate on the hypothalamic rather than pituitary side of axons following transection of the neurohypophyseal tract, the Scharrers [72] proposed that a precursor of ADH is synthesized in supraoptic and paraventricular hypothalamic nuclei and "packaged" in neurosecretory granules that are carried by axoplasmic streaming to nerve endings in the posterior pituitary gland.

At least two lines of evidence provide strong support for this hypothesis. First, in Brattleboro strain rats having hereditary hypothalamic diabetes insipidus, the hypothalamus, neurohypophyseal tract, and posterior pituitary gland contain little or no antidiuretic hormone or neurosecretory granules [73]. Second, guinea pig hypothalamus, but not pituitary gland, is capable of incorporating ^{35}S-cysteine into vasopressin [74, 75]. From an analysis of the kinetics of tracer incorporation into vasopressin and neurosecretory granules, and the effects of the protein synthesis inhibitor puromycin on this process, Sachs et al. have suggested that a bound, inactive hormone precursor protein is synthesized at sites remote from neurosecretory granules; following proteolytic cleavage, ADH and a hormone-specific binding protein (described below) become incorporated into neurosecretory granules [74, 75].

Within neurosecretory granules, ADH is complexed to a specific binding protein, termed neurophysin A or neurophysin II [74–76]. As indicated above, both ADH and neurophysin A may originate from a common, biologically inactive precursor [74, 75]. Oxytocin-secreting neurohypophyseal cells contain neurosecretory granules in which oxytocin is complexed to another specific carrier protein, termed neurophysin B or neurophysin I [75]. Both of these carrier proteins are single polypeptide chains containing 90 to 100 amino acids and having molecular weights of approximately 10,000 [75, 77]. Each of the polypeptide chains exists in equilibrium with its corresponding dimer or higher oligomer [75, 77].

Current evidence, including freeze-fracture and electron microscopy studies, indicates that neurohypophyseal secretion occurs by exocytosis, a quantal process [76]. The exocytotic events involve fusion of membranes from neurosecretory granules with plasma membranes, granule opening at the site of fusion, and release of granule material, including ADH and neurophysin A, into the extracellular space [76]. Since not all the ADH-neurophysin complexes within the posterior pituitary gland are readily available for release, ADH and neurophysin A may be segregated into two pools, a readily released pool and a storage pool [78]. The readily released pool constitutes ADH-neurophysin complexes within neurosecretory granules that are located adjacent to plasma membranes, while the storage pool contains ADH-neurophysin complexes in granules remote from plasma membranes.

The stimuli for exocytosis of neurosecretory granules depend in part on changes in axonal plasma membrane permeability to calcium. It seems probable that stimulation of chemosensitive areas in ADH-producing hypothalamic cells, possibly by cholinergic nerve fibers [79], results in cellular excitation, partial membrane depolarization, and the subsequent generation of sodium-dependent, tetrodotoxin-sensitive [80] action potentials. The latter result in a rapid calcium influx into nerve endings, due to an increase in the permeability of axonal membranes to calcium attendant upon depolarization [76, 81]. The calcium entry, in turn, activates, by an as yet unidentified mechanism, exocytosis of neurosecretory granules and release of ADH and neurophysin A into the circulation.

Distribution and Metabolism   Lysine- or arginine-vasopressin entering the circulation is distributed in a volume approximating that of the extracellular space [41, 82]. Nearly all the hormone in the plasma of dogs and humans exists in an unbound form [41, 82] which, because of its relatively low molecular weight, permeates peripheral and glomerular capillaries readily. Comparison of metabolic clearance rates of biologically active AVP, which is capable of binding to high-affinity renal receptors, with inactive, monoiodinated AVP, which does not bind to receptors, indicates a rapid clearance phase for the active hormone, as opposed to the inactive ^{131}I-AVP [83]. Since this discrepancy is seen only at plasma levels of hormone comparable with those required for maximal urinary concentration, this effect is believed due to specific receptor-mediated clearance [83, 84]. Likewise, rapid AVP clearance is seen in the perfused nonfiltering kidney in the dog [85].

At least four sites of proteolytic cleavage for the hormone have been identified. With reference to Fig. 86-5, arginine vasopressin may undergo cleavage within the liver, by rupture of 1,6—S—S—disulfide bond [62, 63]; within the brain, by cleavage at the 6,7 position and subsequent hydrolysis of 9-glycinamide from the tripeptide [86]; in a variety of tissues, by hydrolysis of the peptide bond between the hemicystine residue in position 1 and tyrosine in position 2 [64, 86]; and within the kidney, by proteolysis of the peptide bond between residues 8 and 9, resulting in glycinamide release [87]. A peptidase of 442,000 M.W. that cleaves glycinamide and results in biologic inactivation has been isolated from renal plasma membranes [88].

Renal excretion of antidiuretic hormone is the second method for elimination of circulating hormone and is estimated to account for about one-fourth of total metabolic clearance [82, 83]. Urine from patients with familial nephrogenic diabetes insipidus contains unusually high amounts of antidiuretic material [24].

In humans, total clearances of ADH, representing both metabolic degradation and renal excretion, are in the range of 2 to 4 ml/min per kilogram of body weight, yielding biologic half-lives in the range of 30 to 40 min [83, 89]. These observations [82, 89, 90] indicate that in humans suppression of endogenous ADH release will result in a detectable change from the antidiuretic to a water diuretic state after approximately 30 min.

The Physiologic Control of ADH Release

In order to maintain plasma osmolality at a constant level, ADH secretion from the posterior pituitary gland must vary directly with small changes in plasma osmolality. ADH may also be released when the plasma osmolality is less than normal. The latter occurs in a least two clinical settings: When extracellular fluid volume is either normal or increased with no disturbance in its distribution and when extracellular fluid, primarily blood volume, is either reduced or abnormally distributed.

Disorders in which antidiuresis and body fluid hypotonicity occur in combination with a normal or an expanded extracellular fluid volume include: the syndrome of inappropriate ADH production [91] that occurs with pulmonary neoplasms, other pulmonary disorders, cranial lesions, and possibly acute intermittent porphyria [92]; the administration of drugs that either stimulate ADH release, such as morphine, barbiturates, and clofibrate [94], or enhance hormone activity, such as chlorpropamide [93] and carbamapezine [95]; and endocrinopathies such as myxedema, in which the factors responsible for an inability to excrete an appropriately dilute urine are uncertain [96].

The combination of plasma hypotonicity and excretion of urine that is either isosmotic or hypertonic to plasma also occurs when blood volume is either reduced absolutely or abnormally distributed. This class of conditions includes: contraction of the extracellular fluid space, particularly when coupled to the administration of electrolyte-free solutions [97]; reductions in left atrial pressure following mitral commissurotomy [98]; prolonged mechanical ventilation [99]; and severe congestive heart failure or hepatic cirrhosis. Thus, nonosmotic factors that relate to changes either in total blood volume or in the distribution of extracellular fluid also elicit ADH release. This section will consider the osmotic and nonosmotic stimuli to ADH release and the quantitative relationships between these two variables.

Osmotic Regulation of ADH Release   Verney's classic studies, summarized in his 1947 Croonian lecture [100], delineated the relationship between changes in plasma osmolality and ADH release. His meticulous observations on urine flow and composition in dogs showed that: (1) following water loading, there was a lag period of approximately 15 min before the onset of water diuresis; (2) short-duration (5 to 20 s) injections of hypertonic NaCl or sucrose, but not urea solutions, provoked a prompt antidiuresis that was abolished by removal of the posterior pituitary gland; and, (3) reductions in urine volume during a maximal water diuresis required as little as a 2 percent increase (produced by NaCl or sucrose but not urea) in the osmolality of blood perfusing the internal carotid arteries.

Verney [100] postulated the presence of osmoreceptors, located in the distribution of the internal carotid arteries, that stimulated ADH release when plasma osmolality was raised by solutes to which osmoreceptors were impermeable; the failure of hypertonic urea injections to provoke antidiuresis was interpreted as indicating that these osmoreceptors were freely permeable to urea. McKinley et al. [101] confirmed Verney's results and showed that carotid infusion of hypertonic urea solution led to a higher CSF sodium concentration than either hypertonic saline or sucrose, yet produced only minor antidiuresis compared with the latter two solutions. They postulated that the osmoreceptors must be located in an area of the brain lacking an effective blood-brain barrier [101]. The cerebral osmoreceptors seem to be located in the hypothalamus [23, 101].

Because normal individuals are not ordinarily in a water diuretic state, Verney argued that the maintenance of a normal plasma osmolality requires the tonic secretion of ADH. It is instructive to consider these observations in terms of the relationship between serum osmolality and plasma arginine vasopressin concentrations determined by radioimmunoassay [42]. As shown in Fig. 86-3, for plasma osmolalities below 280 mosmol/kg, plasma AVP levels are in the range of 0.5 to 1.5 pg/ml;[2] above a plasma osmolality of 280 mosmol/kg, plasma AVP rises in proportion to plasma osmolality according to the relationship: plasma AVP = 0.38 (plasma osmolality = 280). Robertson et al. [56, 58] consider a plasma osmolality of 280

mosmol/kg as the "osmotic threshold" for AVP release, a view that coincides nicely with Verney's deduction [100] that maintenance of a normal plasma osmolality depends on the tonic secretion of ADH.

Nonosmotic Regulation of ADH Release   In 1935, Peters [102] recognized the role of ADH in volume regulation by commenting that "in subjects who have become dehydrated . . . volume of body fluids seems to become more important than . . . osmotic pressure as a determinant of renal activity." Leaf and Mamby [103] provided early evidence for an ADH release mechanism not regulated by extracellular fluid tonicity by showing that dehydrated individuals permitted access to solute-free water developed hyponatremia concomitant with urinary hypertonicity. Subsequently, there has accumulated a large body of evidence indicating that volume-mediated release of ADH may occur as a consequence of stimuli arising from "volume receptors," or baroreceptors. Gauer and Henry [104] termed loci in the venous bed of the systemic circulation, the right side of the heart, and the left atrium the "low" pressure baroreceptors, and loci within the systemic arterial system, "high" pressure baroreceptors.

With regard to the relationship between ADH release and low pressure regions of the vascular bed, positive pressure breathing and the upright position produce antidiuresis, while negative pressure breathing produces a water diuresis [23]. The water diuresis produced by negative pressure breathing can be abolished by administering exogenous ADH [23, 105], thereby providing indirect evidence that the diuresis is mediated by suppression of ADH release. Henry et al. [106], finding that balloon distention of the left atrium produced increases in urine volume, concluded that stimulation of left atrial stretch receptors resulted in suppression of ADH release. The afferent pathway was presumed to be the vagus nerve, which affected ADH production in hypothalamic nuclei by pathways traversing the reticular formation in the brainstem [104].

In studies on the role of the arterial bed in regulating ADH release, hemorrhage in experimental animals [23, 43, 107] resulted in increases in a circulating antidiuretic substance, subsequently identified as vasopressin [43, 107]. Experiments that produced relatively small changes in blood volume accompanied by no change in mean arterial pressure resulted in sixfold increases in plasma vasopressin levels measured with bioassay techniques [97, 108]. In trained unanesthetized dogs, the nonosmotic "threshold" for ADH release, estimated by plasma vasopressin bioassays, was a 10 to 15 percent reduction in blood volume [97]. Since blood volume reductions of this magnitude left mean arterial pressure unchanged while central venous pressure fell, one might argue that the nonosmotic stimuli for ADH release originated in the low pressure system [97] or, stated in another way, that high pressure system baroceptors are less sensitive in stimulating ADH release than those in the low pressure system. In support of this view, Gupta et al. [109] noted that aortic arch pressoreceptors were less sensitive in eliciting ADH release than left atrial pressoreceptors.

In short, volume-mediated mechanisms for ADH release may originate from baroceptors in either the high pressure or the low pressure regions of the cardiovascular system. Under most circumstances, the low pressure system is more sensitive than the high pressure system in modulating volume-regulated ADH release. During volume contraction these nonosmotic stimuli to ADH release may override osmotic stimuli.

Conclusions about nonosmotic stimuli to ADH release have been subject to a number of criticisms. Bioassay techniques for

---

[2] The potency of pure arginine vasopressin is approximately 400 units/mg [97]. Thus, a plasma AVP level of 1 pg/ml would correspond to a concentration of approximately 0.4 μU AVP/ml.

plasma vasopressin concentration are neither specific, especially at low levels of hormone concentrations, nor uniform among investigators [23]. However, specific radioimmunoassays for vasopressin [43, 110] provide a measure of the sensitivity for nonosmotic release of antidiuretic hormone. In the rat, isoosmotic volume contraction produced by intraperitoneal glycerol stimulated vasopressin release at a "threshold" of about 8 percent plasma volume contraction [43]. Acute plasma volume contraction in humans produced by hemofiltration, resulted in detectable rises in plasma vasopressin concentrations at as little as 2.5 percent volume reduction [110].

Agents having systemic hemodynamic effects, which might be expected to affect baroreceptor activity, also modify urinary concentrating ability. Thus, the cholinergic agent acetylcholine [111] and beta-adrenergic agents such as isoproterenol [112] provoke antidiuresis, while alpha-adrenergic agents inhibit vasopressin antidiuresis [112, 113]. It has also been argued that the effects of adrenergic agents on water excretion depend on interactions with renal tubular cells [112] rather than on systemic hemodynamic effects. Thus, Handler et al. [114] have shown that norepinephrine inhibits the water permeability response of toad urinary bladder to vasopressin, and Kurokawa and Massry [115] have shown that norepinephrine may inhibit vasopressin-stimulated cyclic 3',5'-adenosine monophate (cAMP) production by the renal medulla. Taken together, these considerations create uncertainty in assessing the nature of nonosmotic stimuli to ADH release.

Schrier et al. [116] have provided evidence for a hemodynamic role of alpha- and beta-adrenergic agents in mediating vasopressin release as their sole means of affecting renal water excretion. Thus, the beta agonist isoproterenol caused antidiuresis in normal rats but not in the Brattleboro strain of rat that lacks endogenous antidiuretic hormone [117]. Likewise, isoproterenol increased renal medullary cAMP concentrations in normal but not Brattleboro rats [118]. Both results lead to the conclusion that beta-adrenergic stimulation modulates renal water excretion via the release of endogenous vasopressin. Norepinephrine, a primary alpha agonist, reduced urine osmolality and renal medullary cAMP in normal, hydropenic rats [117] but had no effect on antidiuresis in Brattleboro rats receiving an exogenous vasopressin infusion. Measurements in vitro of diffusional water permeability of rat collecting ducts and cAMP content of rat renal papillae failed to show any effect of alpha- or beta-adrenergic agonists on either parameter in the absence of ADH [118], thus excluding a primary tubular effect of these agents. These results demonstrate that alpha-adrenergic stimulation modulates renal water excretion via suppression of endogenous vasopressin release.

Carotid baroreceptor denervation abolished the antidiuretic effect of isoproterenol [119] and the diuretic effect of norepinephrine [120] while cervical vagotomy had no effect. This suggests that the "high" pressure arterial baroreceptors rather than "low" pressure left atrial receptors respond to adrenergic stimuli in the modulation of vasopressin release and renal water excretion.

Nonosmotic mechanisms for ADH release may also depend on the renin-angiotensin system [23]. In unanesthetized dogs, both renin and angiotensin II increased plasma ADH levels estimated by bioassay [121], and comparable results, by use of a double antibody radioimmunoassay for measuring plasma AVP concentrations, were obtained in humans [122]. More recent studies in human subjects demonstrate a reduced sensitivity to volume-mediated vasopressin release, measured by

radioimmunoassay, in nephrectomized patients, who lack circulating renin and angiotensin II, compared with patients having kidneys and an intact renin-angiotensin system [110]. Treatment of nonnephrectomized patients with the angiotensin II converting enzyme inhibitor captopril produced a decrease in volume-mediated vasopressin release to the level seen in nephrectomized patients [110]. Finally, intracerebroventricular infusion of the angiotensin II antagonist saralasin in trained dogs with cannulae chronically implanted in the third ventricle abolished the rise in plasma vasopressin concentrations seen in dogs given isoproterenol, while a rise in plasma renin activity was unimpeded [118]. These latter studies strongly suggest a role for physiologic concentrations of angiotensin II in mediating the vasopressin release of hemodynamic stimuli.

Quantitative Aspects of Osmotic and Nonosmotic Stimuli to ADH Release   The preceding discussion establishes that the regulation of plasma AVP concentrations depends on both osmotic [100, 101] and volume-mediated, nonosmotic stimuli [97, 103, 104, 110, 116]. Dunn et al. [43] have provided a quantitative analysis of the interplay between these two sets of stimuli and plasma AVP levels estimated by radioimmunoassay. Figure 86-6, adapted from their work in the rat [43], shows that, so long as blood volume is maintained within 10 percent of normal, plasma AVP concentrations vary linearly with changes in serum osmolality. When blood volume is isosmotically reduced by more than 10 percent, plasma AVP concentrations rise in a near-exponential fashion to levels approximately twice greater than those produced by raising serum osmolality isovolemically. These observations were confirmed in humans, in whom the "volume threshold" for ADH release is reached when blood volume is reduced by 7 to 10 percent [123, 124]. These quantitative data [43, 123, 124] sup-

Figure 86-6   The relationship between blood volume, plasma osmolality, and plasma AVP concentrations. (Adapted from Dunn et al. [43].)

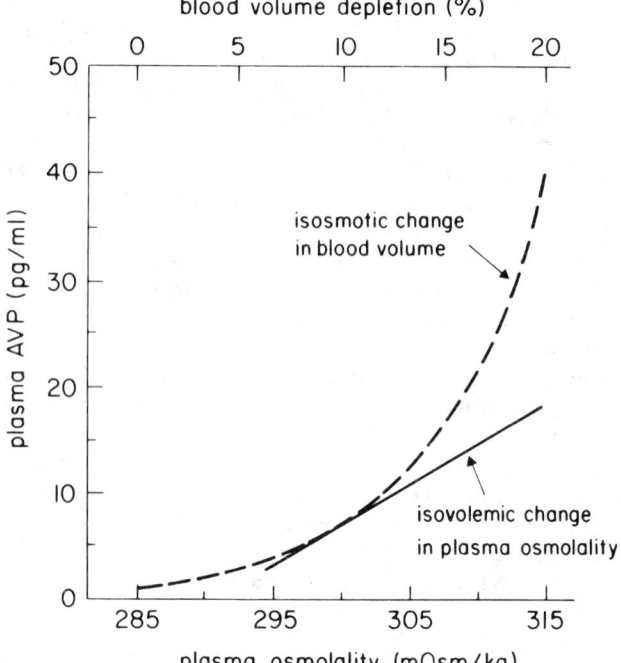

OSMOTIC AND NON-OSMOTIC CONTROL OF PLASMA AVP

port the view [23, 97, 102–104, 116] that, in the setting of volume contraction, nonosmotic stimuli are the predominant forces regulating ADH release.

RENAL CONCENTRATING AND DILUTING MECHANISMS

The Countercurrent Multiplication System

The ability to concentrate the urine coincides, from the evolutionary standpoint, with the appearance of a unique and deceptively simple appearing structure, the loop of Henle. Moreover, the ability among mammals to concentrate the urine correlates fairly well with both the number of loops of Henle which penetrate deep into the inner medullary or papillary area, so-called long loops, and to the ratio of medullary to cortical thickness: the larger the number of long loops and the higher the medullary-to-cortical-thickness ratio, the greater the ability of the mammal to concentrate the urine. Humans appear to have only a modest ability to concentrate the urine, having only one-eighth of their nephrons associated with long loops and a medullary-to-cortical-thickness ratio of 1.6.

It is widely believed that dilution or concentration of urine depends on counterflow mechanisms operating within the renal medulla. Hirokawa [125] provided evidence for this hypothesis in 1908, by noting that the osmolality of the renal medulla exceeded that of the cortex and that medullary hypertonicity increased in proportion to the degree of urinary concentration.

Modern views of renal concentrating and diluting mechanisms have their origin in the work of Kuhn and Ryffel [126], who considered the descending and ascending limbs of Henle as parallel tubes joined by a hairpin turn and that oppositely directed flows in the two tubes permit small differences in osmolality between fluid in the descending and ascending limbs at any level of the renal medulla (the so-called single effect) to be amplified manyfold along the length of the loop of Henle. In 1951, Wirz, Hargitay, and Kuhn [127] showed conclusively that renal medullary fluid within the interstitium, blood vessels, and renal tubules became progressively hypertonic in going from renal cortex to papillary tip, and Hargitay and Kuhn [128] recognized that the loop of Henle might function as a countercurrent multiplier (i.e., the loop itself would provide the driving force for generating both loop and medullary hypertonicity) either by abstracting water in excess of solute from descending limbs or by abstracting solute in excess of water from ascending limbs or both.

Gottschalk and his colleagues provided confirmation for the countercurrent hypothesis. They found that urine in Henle's loop at the papillary tip was as concentrated as that in the collecting duct during antidiuresis [129]. Fluid entering the early distal convolution was hypotonic to plasma in both the absence and presence of ADH [129, 130], and approximately 20 percent of glomerular filtrate was absorbed in Henle's loop [130, 131]. Since proximal tubular fluid absorption is an isotonic process, Gottschalk reasoned that the combination of fluid absorption in Henle's loop and early distal tubular fluid hypotonicity meant that, during transit through the loop, more solute than water was removed from tubular fluid and there-

fore the single effect driving the countercurrent multiplier was solute abstraction from ascending limbs [130, 131].

Thus, the countercurrent multiplication process results from the integrated effect of specialized transport events inherent in different segments of the loop of Henle. The development by Burg and his coworkers [132] of a system for perfusing nephron segments isolated from rabbit kidney has permitted a direct way of assessing the transport properties of virtually all portions of the nephron in vitro. Table 86-1 summarizes the passive transport properties in vitro of those rabbit nephron segments which participate directly in the countercurrent multiplication system and the effects of ADH on certain of these segments.

Kokko and Rector [133] have integrated these data into a model which provides two spatially distinct sites for countercurrent multiplication: an active step in the outer medulla and a passive step in the inner medulla. The salient features of this model, illustrated schematically in Fig. 86-7, may be qualitatively described in the following way. The first multiplication step depends on transport producing NaCl efflux from water-impermeable thick ascending limbs; thus, fluid entering the distal tubule is both hypotonic and salt-poor. During antidiuresis, ADH-enhanced water abstraction from urea-impermeable cortical and outer medullary collecting ducts results in accumulation of urea in fluid entering papillary collecting ducts. Since the latter are urea permeable, passive urea transport down a chemical gradient from tubular fluid to medullary interstitium contributes to medullary hypertonicity,

Figure 86-7 A schematic diagram of Kokko and Rector's [133] model for countercurrent multiplication. The arrows indicate the relative magnitudes of solute and water movement in the various nephron segments. With the exception of active NaCl transport in the thick ascending limb, all water and solute fluxes are passively driven. The thickened walls of the ascending limb of Henle indicate water impermeability. The broken walls indicate the collecting duct ADH-sensitive water permeability. Isotonic fluid entering the thin descending limb is concentrated primarily by water abstraction; at the tip of Henle's loop, NaCl accounts for approximately 90 percent of tubular fluid osmolality. In the thin ascending limb, countercurrent multiplication and dilution of tubular fluid occur because NaCl efflux from lumen to interstitium exceeds urea influx from interstitium to lumen. In the thick ascending limb, active NaCl transport account for countercurrent multiplication and dilution of tubular fluid. In the presence of ADH, urea accumulates in the cortical and outer medullary collecting ducts and enters the interstitium from the inner medullary collecting duct.

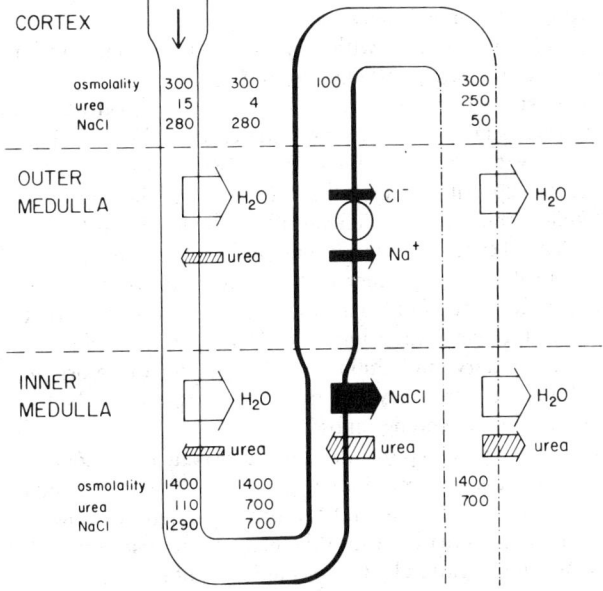

thereby providing a second, but in this case passive, multiplication step. Simultaneously, osmotic equilibration of papillary collecting duct fluid with the medullary interstitium results in the formation of hypertonic urine.

Kokko and Rector [133] have rationalized the progressive concentration and dilution of tubular fluid in descending and ascending thin limbs, respectively, entirely in terms of passive flows. Consider, for example, a medulla whose osmolality ranges from 300 mosmol/kg at the corticomedullary junction to 1400 mosmol/kg at the papillary tip (Fig. 86-7). In keeping with tissue analyses [134], approximately half of the medullary hypertonicity is assigned to NaCl and the remainder to urea. Isotonic fluid containing 280 mosmol/kg NaCl entering the highly water-permeable but urea- and Na$^+$-impermeable descending thin limb is concentrated almost entirely by water abstraction, and so fluid entering the ascending thin limb has a higher NaCl concentration and a lower urea concentration than the medullary interstitium. These passive driving forces between lumen and interstitium, coupled with the fact that the thin ascending limb is more permeable to NaCl than to urea, poise the system for fluid dilution. As fluid moves up the water-impermeable ascending thin limb, passive NaCl efflux from lumen to interstitium exceeds passive urea influx from interstitium to tubular fluid and, concomitantly, urea recycling from papillary collecting ducts through the interstitium to ascending thin limbs. Finally, the process begins again by active NaCl transport from the thick ascending limb.

There is theoretical support for this view. Stephenson [135] considers vasa recta loops to be sufficiently permeable to water and solutes that they can be treated as a single tube, or "central core," which is open at the cortical end, closed at the papillary end, and aligned in parallel with the loop of Henle and the collecting duct. His calculations indicate that, for nephron segments having relative permeabilities for urea, salt, and water similar to those listed in Table 86-1, the combination of passive salt efflux from ascending thin limbs and passive urea efflux from medullary collecting ducts could raise the osmolality of the central core and hence provide a driving force for water abstraction from thin descending limbs and collecting ducts. Stephenson's equations, like the model of Kokko and Rector (Fig. 86-7; [133]), link active salt transport in the outer medulla and cortex and urea impermeability in cortical and outer medullary collecting ducts into a mechanism for urea recycling in the inner medulla.

Not all workers agree with such models for countercurrent multiplication, particularly in regard to four major considerations. First, Kokko and Rector [133] have proposed that 96 percent of osmotic equilibration of descending thin limb fluid is due to water abstraction and only 4 percent to urea entry; thus, NaCl contributes more than 90 percent to the osmolality of fluid reaching the papillary bend of Henle's loop. In contrast, Pennell et al. [136] have found that, in the rat, addition of urea contributes 40 percent to the increase in osmolality in ascending thin limb fluid. These workers therefore argue that, if urea in tubular fluid at the tip of Henle's loop equilibrates with the papillary interstitium, there exists little or no driving force for passive urea recycling from collecting ducts and interstitium to thin ascending limbs.

Second, the pelvic epithelium may participate in the concentrating process by promoting urea and water exchange between the pelvic urine and the papillus, thereby allowing recirculation of urea back into the papillary interstitium. The original demonstration by Gertz et al. [137] of these processes has been extended recently by others [138, 139].

Third, Morel and his coworkers, in an elegant series of studies, have demonstrated ADH-dependent adenylate cyclase activity, not only in the cortical and medullary collecting ducts, but also in both the ascending thin limb and the medullary thick ascending limb (see Ref. 140 for a review of these data), and have suggested that ADH may augment NaCl transport in these segments. This suggestion that ADH might regulate countercurrent multiplication is not new since Wirz [141] and subsequently others [142–144] suggested that ADH might regulate the rate of solute absorption in the ascending limb of Henle, on the basis of finding increased medullary and papillary NaCl concentrations during antidiuresis as compared with water diuresis. This hypothesis has recently gained a great deal of support. A number of workers [145–147] have demonstrated an ADH-mediated increase in salt absorption by the mouse medullary thick ascending limb (mTALH) but not the cortical thick ascending limb [147]. In addition, Hebert et al. [147] have shown that NaCl transport by the mouse medullary thick ascending limb involves the energy-dependent cotransport of NaCl across luminal plasma membranes through cells into the outer medullary interstitium. In other words, chloride entry into medullary thick ascending limb cells appears to be a secondary active transport process, where luminal Cl$^-$ entry into cells is dependent upon the transcellular electrochemical sodium gradient that is maintained by the basolateral membrane (Na$^+$ + K$^+$)-ATPase. Thus it is likely that ADH, at least in some species, can enhance countercurrent multiplication by increasing the rate of NaCl absorption by the medullary thick ascending limb of Henle.

Although ADH increases net NaCl absorption in vitro, mechanisms for modulating this effect must be present since ADH appears to have little effect on external NaCl balance in vivo [148]. Two separate mechanisms may account for the effect of ADH on enhancing countercurrent multiplication while not affecting net NaCl absorption. First, ADH does not alter the passive permeability properties of the medullary thick ascending limb [147]; thus the increase in medullary salt concentration during antidiuresis will necessarily increase dramatically NaCl backleak from the interstitium to tubular fluid, particularly since the medullary thick limb is remarkably leaky to sodium and chloride [147, 149].

In addition, Hebert et al. [150] have recently demonstrated that increasing peritubular osmolality with urea results in a reduction in the ADH- and cAMP-stimulated pump rate. This change in NaCl pump rate appears to be the direct result of the increase in peritubular urea and not to either reductions in cell volume or the transtubular urea gradient. Thus the ADH-mediated increase in the steady-state outer medullary osmolality results in both an increased NaCl backleak and, because of passive urea accumulation in the interstitium, a modulation of the ADH-stimulated NaCl pump rate in the medullary thick ascending limb. These modulation systems could account for the maintenance of medullary hypertonicity and the diluting power of the medullary thick ascending limb without affecting external salt balance.

Fourth and finally, in accord with the ADH-dependent adenylate cyclase activity and the hypothesis of countercurrent multiplication suggested originally by Wirz (see [141] above), Marsh and Azen [151] have found that the Na$^+$ concentration in the thin ascending limb of the hamster is either the same or less than that in the ascending vasa recta, and by assuming that the latter was in equilibrium with interstitial fluid, these workers concluded that active Na$^+$ transport contributes at least in part to inner medullary hypertonicity. In short, the countercur-

Table 86-1 Passive transport coefficients of isolated rabbit nephron segments*

Segment	P_f	$P_{D_{urea}}$	$P_{D_{Na}}$	$P_{D_{Cl}}$	σ_{urea}	σ_{NaCl}
		$cm\ sec^{-1} \times 10^4$				
Descending thin limb	2400	0.15	0.16		0.95	0.96
Ascending thin limb	12	0.70	2.5	12		
Ascending thick limb	11	0.10	0.6	0.1		
Distal convoluted tubule						
−ADH	$\simeq 0$					
+ADH	$\simeq 0$					
Cortical collecting tubule						
−ADH	20	0.03			1.0	1.0
+ADH	186	0.03			1.0	1.0
Outer medullary collecting tubule						
−ADH	15				1.0	1.0
+ADH	190				1.0	1.0
Papillary collecting duct						
−ADH		0.22				
+ADH	65	0.24				

* The passive transport coefficients listed in this table include:

P_f (cm sec $^{-1}$): The permeability coefficient for net water flow, determined from transepithelial water flows produced by osmotic water flows.

P_{D_i} (cm sec $^{-1}$): The permeability coefficient of the ith solute estimated from transepithelial tracer fluxes.

σ_i: The membrane reflection coefficient of the ith solute, defined as the ratio of the observed osmotic pressure difference produced by the solute across the membrane to that predicted from cryoscopically measured osmolalities. For a given membrane, a wholly impermeant solute has a unity reflection coefficient, while a solute crossing the membrane as readily as water has a zero reflection coefficient.

SOURCE: [23].

rent multiplier model of Kokko and Rector [133], which derives largely from the characteristics of isolated rabbit nephron segments in vitro, is not entirely supported by micropuncture results in the rat [136] and hamster [151] in vivo, and the studies in mouse in vitro [145–147].

The Countercurrent Exchange System In the steady state, net solute and water removal by medullary blood flow must be exactly equal to the net amount of solute and water absorbed by medullary nephron segments. At the same time, maintenance of a hypertonic medullary interstitium requires that the rate of solute removal by medullary blood flow be reduced sufficiently to prevent equilibration of medullary interstitial fluid with isotonic plasma. As previously emphasized [23] these requirements are satisfied by countercurrent exchange processes within medullary capillary loops.

The efferent arterioles of juxtamedullary glomeruli branch into peritubular capillary networks. These networks form long loops which descend into the medulla in parallel with descending and ascending limbs of Henle's loop, have hairpin turns at the same medullary level as the associated loop of Henle, and are connected at several levels of the medulla by branches of the capillary plexus [152]. Thus, like the loop of Henle, the vasa recta is a counterflow system in which blood courses in opposite directions in descending and ascending segments. In descending vasa recta, water leaves the blood and solute enters, so that the osmolality at the bend of the vasa recta is the same as that of the tip of the loop of Henle, and presumably also of

the medullary interstitium, at the same point [23, 135]. As blood flows from the tip of the vasa recta back to venules in the inner cortex, it gains water and loses salt to the progressively less hypertonic medullary interstitium. The water lost and solute gained by the descending vasa recta results in water gain and solute loss in the ascending vasa recta, a process requiring no energy input other than the hydrostatic pressure of the blood. The net effect of this countercurrent exchange in the vasca recta is to reduce both the rate of solute loss from the medulla, with respect to a linear blood flow system, and the energy expenditure required to maintain a hypertonic medulla.

Effects of Filtration Rate and Solute Excretion Factors other than antidiuretic hormone and counterflow processes within the renal medulla also affect urinary concentration and dilution. For example, as illustrated in Table 86-1, the water permeability of the collecting duct, even in the absence of ADH, is clearly finite rather than zero. Thus, by varying the rate of fluid delivery to collecting ducts, and hence the time available for water efflux from the latter, the rate of glomerular filtration (GFR) can influence directly the final osmolality of urine. This effect has been documented in hypophysectomized dogs [23] and in Brattleboro rats with hypothalamic diabetes insipidus [25]. In both instances severe reductions in GFR result in the formation of hypertonic urine in the absence of ADH. Presumably, in the presence of very slow urine flow rates in the collecting duct, there is at least partial osmotic equilibration of urine with the medullary interstitium. Conversely, increased glomerular filtration rates produced by sustained expansion of the extracellular fluid volume can result in a hypoosmotic urine even when high levels of vasopressin are maintained by infusion [23].

On the other hand, the recent data of Edwards et al. [26] indicate that severe reductions in GFR are not necessary for urine osmolality to increase in these circumstances. Brattleboro rats can increase urinary osmolality two- to threefold consequent to partial aortic clamping that produces minimal or no decrease in GFR. This increase in urinary osmolality could not be related to alterations in filtration fraction, which would modulate solute delivery to the loop of Henle and collecting ducts, but may have been due to enhancement of inner medullary osmolality resulting from increased urea sequestration.

In clinical terms, the nature and rate of solute excretion have a greater influence on urinary osmolality than glomerular filtration rate. A filtered but nonabsorbed solute like mannitol acts as an osmotic diuretic and reduces fluid absorption within the proximal tubule, so that a progressively greater amount of isosmotic fluid containing nonabsorbed solute enters the loop of Henle. As a consequence, the capacity of the loop of Henle and collecting duct to modify the osmolality of urine is reduced. Thus, in hydropenic individuals receiving ADH, urine osmolality falls during osmotic diuresis [23]. Alternatively, both in patients with nephrogenic diabetes insipidus [34] and in normal subjects undergoing water diuresis [23], urine osmolality rises during progressive osmotic diuresis.

The effect of osmotic diuresis on urine composition may also be viewed by considering solute excretion in terms of the osmolar clearance (C_{osm}, ml/min), which can be regarded as the urinary flow rate required to produce a urine isotonic to plasma. In antidiuresis, a volume of solute-free water, termed *negative free-water clearance*, is removed from urine, and the urinary flow rate $\dot{V}$ is less than C_{osm}. In water diuresis, the urinary flow rate $\dot{V}$ exceeds C_{osm}; the difference between $\dot{V}$ and C_{osm}, termed *positive free-water clearance*, is the amount of solute-free water excreted. During progressive osmotic diuresis, an increasingly greater volume of isotonic fluid containing nonabsorbed solute escapes proximal tubular absorption and is delivered to the loop of Henle. As a consequence, C_{osm} becomes sufficiently large that, even if the magnitude of either positive (during water diuresis) or negative (during antidiuresis) free-water clearance stays unchanged, urine osmolality approaches isotonicity.

These considerations are germane to the apparent isosthenuria of chronic renal disease, which may be due to high rates of solute excretion per nephron [23]. In an azotemic individual, the rate of urea excretion per nephron is strikingly increased, and, in direct analogy to the administration of mannitol to normal subjects, the ability of remaining nephrons to alter the osmolality of urine is reduced, even when these residual nephrons remain ADH-sensitive [23].

Effect of ADH on Solute and Water Permeability

Morphologic observations of the response of the collecting tubule to ADH have confirmed that the final or rate-limiting site of ADH action on water permeability is at the apical epithelial membrane [153–155] and that ADH increases the rate of water permeation through these surfaces [155, 156].

In amphibian species arginine vasotocin plays a comparable role in maintaining water homeostasis. Frogs abstract water

osmotically from pond water (essentially solute-free water) through the skin to blood. Either arginine vasotocin or exogenous arginine vasopressin increases the rate of water permeation through outer, or water-facing, plasma membranes of frog skin [157]. In the toad, final urinary concentration occurs in the bladder. The ADH-sensitive, rate-limiting sites for water transport in this epithelium are the urinary, or mucosal, plasma membranes [158]. In both of these amphibian epithelia, ADH also increases transepithelial Na^+ flux and the permeation rates for certain solutes, notably urea and other small amides [23, 159, 160]. Thus, it was proposed that Na^+, urea, and water transport in these tissues involves permeation through identical ADH-sensitive, rate-limiting sites in urinary plasma membranes [23, 159, 160].

However, in toad urinary bladder, ADH-mediated increments in Na^+, urea, and water transport are completely dissociable [161, 162]. Moreover, ADH-dependent increments in the water permeability of mammalian cortical collecting tubules [156, 163] and outer medullary collecting tubules [164] are not accompanied by increments in urea permeability. These observations indicate that Na^+, urea, and water traverse parallel, independent pathways in urinary plasma membranes [165, 166]. By analyzing the kinetics of urea transport in toad urinary bladder, Hays et al. [161, 165, 167] have concluded that urea permeates urinary plasma membranes via a saturable, ADH-sensitive amide carrier pathway.

ADH Increases the Number of Narrow Aqueous Channels in Apical Plasma Membranes of Collecting Ducts

Analysis of water transport through epithelia requires an understanding of the two methods used for evaluating water transport through membranes. In one instance, net water flux is measured when either a hydrostatic or osmotic pressure gradient exists across the membrane. In accord with the Starling hypothesis, net water flow across the membrane is linearly related to the driving force by P_f (cm sec^{-1}), the permeability coefficient for net water flow. Thus, P_f may be computed from the relation between net water flux and hydrostatic or osmotic pressure.

In the second method, the flux of tracer water, e.g., THO, is measured at zero net volume flow. Both solutions bathing a membrane are at the same hydrostatic pressure and are identical in composition. Tracer water molecules in one solution exchange at random (by diffusion) across the membrane with unlabeled water molecules in the other solution, but there is no net water flux. From Fick's first law of diffusion and the tracer appearance rate in the nonlabeled solution, one may compute P_{D_w} (cm sec^{-1}), the permeability coefficient for water diffusion across the membrane. Since P_{D_w} depends on a diffusion process, it may also be defined as:

$$P_{D_w} = \frac{\beta \, D_m}{\Delta X}$$

where β is the partition coefficient for water between aqueous and membrane phases, D_m (cm^2 sec^{-1}) is the diffusion coefficient of water within the membrane, and ΔX is the membrane thickness in centimeters.

In principle, P_f will equal P_{D_w} when net water transport across a given membrane, due to either osmotic or hydrostatic gradients, occurs exclusively by a solubility-diffusion process. But in the vast majority of natural and synthetic membranes, P_f exceeds the apparent value of P_{D_w} [166]. Three classes of explanations have been proposed to account for this disparity.

First, apical membranes might contain pores sufficiently large to permit laminar or quasi-laminar flow during osmosis [168–169]. In this instance the P_f/P_{D_w} ratio exceeds unity because net volume flow varies with r^4 (r = pore radius), while zero volume flow THO diffusion varies with r^2; by combining Fick's first law with Poiseuille's law, an expression may be derived relating the P_f/P_{D_w} ratio to the pore radius. While this formulation is adequate to describe transport processes through amphotericin B–cholesterol pores ($r \simeq 4$ Å) in lipid bilayer membranes [170], the ADH-dependent P_f/P_{D_w} ratio of approximately 13 (Table 86-1) in the case of cortical collecting tubules would require a pore radius of about 13 Å. Yet, cortical collecting tubules are virtually impermeable to small hydrophilic solutes such as urea ($r \simeq 2.2$ Å; cf. Table 86-1).

A second class of explanations accounting for the disparities between P_f and P_{D_w} assumes that the membrane is homogeneous and that the mode of osmotic water transport across apical plasma membranes is diffusional, but that unstirred layers in series with apical membranes impede THO diffusion at zero volume flow but not net volume flow during osmosis [171–173]. These layers may be viewed picturesquely as unmixed, diffusion-limited regions of water interposed between a membrane surface and a well-mixed solution [171]. According to this view, the relation between P_f and P_{D_w} is:

$$\frac{1}{P_{D_w}} = \frac{1}{P_f} + \frac{\beta \, \Delta X}{D_w^\circ}$$

where $1/P_{D_w}$ is the resistance to THO diffusion at zero volume flow; $1/P_f$ is the apical membrane resistance to water diffusion since during osmosis, net water flow to the membrane interface is not impeded by unstirred layers, and P_f provides an accurate index to the rate of water diffusion across the membrane; and $\beta \, \Delta X/D_w^\circ$ is the postapical membrane resistance, where ΔX is the thickness of the cortical collecting tubule (7 μm), D_w° is the free diffusion coefficient for water, and β is equivalent to a tortuosity factor for postapical membrane diffusion resistances. In use of the data in Table 86-1, a β value of approximately 22 would be required to account for the ADH-dependent P_f/P_{D_w} ratio observed in the cortical collecting tubule. However, estimates of the value of β using highly lipophilic solutes, which traverse lipid membranes with ease, indicated that β was approximately 10 for the cortical collecting tubule [174]. Thus, postapical membrane diffusion resistances, which in principle could be due either to diffusion constraints in the cell or bulk solutions, accounted for a part of but not all the P_f/P_{D_w} disparity.

Finally, following the proposal of Lea [175], if apical plasma membranes contained aqueous channels sufficiently narrow to preclude side-by-side passage of water molecules, water transport would follow single-file kinetics so that $P_f/P_{D_w} = n_w$, where n_w is the number of water molecules in a channel. Combining this relation with Eq. 2 yields:

$$\frac{1}{P_{D_w}} = \frac{n_w}{P_f} + \frac{\beta \, \Delta X}{D_w^\circ}$$

which expresses the effects of postapical membrane diffusion resistances and the single-file effect on the P_f/P_{D_w} ratio. Hebert and Andreoli [174] have recently evaluated this relation in cortical collecting tubules in the presence and absence of ADH. They found that such an explanation was adequate to explain the P_f to P_{D_w} disparity in the cortical collecting tubule, where n_w was 6 (H_2O molecules per channel) and β was approximately ten.

These data [174], and those of Al-Zahid et al. [176], are compatible with the hypothesis that the main route for water transport across apical plasma membranes in the cortical collecting tubule is through narrow aqueous channels which allow for the single-file diffusion of water but effectively exclude urea, and that ADH increases the number of such channels in apical plasma membranes. In fact, Kachadorian and his coworkers [177] have demonstrated a close relationship between the hydro-osmotic effects of ADH in anuran epithelia and the presence of apical intramembranous particle aggregates; they suggest that these aggregates, which are independent of ADH-induced apical membrane fluidity changes, probably represent these water channels [178]. Similar intramembranous particle clusters are observed to appear in mammalian collecting ducts in a dose-related fashion when ADH is added [179].

Intracellular Mediators of ADH Action   It is widely accepted that the effects of ADH on transport processes in hormone-sensitive epithelia are mediated by cAMP in accord with the second-messenger hypothesis [180]. ADH binds to receptors on basolateral surfaces of responsive epithelial cells and produces an adenyl cyclase-mediated acceleration of cAMP synthesis from ATP. Evidence for this chain of events was provided by Orloff and Handler et al. [181, 182], who observed that, in toad bladder, cAMP or theophylline, an inhibitor of cyclic nucleotide phosphodiesterase, brought about changes in NA^+ and water transport identical to those observed with ADH. This finding has been documented by subsequent work in a number of intact tissues, including isolated rabbit cortical collecting tubules [156, 183] and mouse medullary thick ascending limbs [140, 145–147], and the rabbit kidney in vivo [184].

In accord with this view, ADH raises adenyl cyclase activity in tissue slices, cell homogenates, and membrane fractions of mammalian renal medulla [185–187], but not in comparable preparations from mammalian renal cortex [188]. The receptor-ADH interaction is both tissue- and hormone-specific [54, 189] and localized to basolateral rather than urinary membranes [190]. And cellular adenyl cyclase activity is proportional to the degree of hormone binding on receptor sites [54, 56, 191].

Orloff and Handler [192] have pointed out that modulation of ADH effects may occur at one or any combination of four steps: hormone-receptor interactions on basolateral membranes; adenyl cyclase activity; cAMP dephosphorylation catalyzed by cyclic nucleotide phosphodiesterase; and the coupling of cAMP to cellular mechanisms responsible for changes in transport processes in urinary membranes. A schematic illustration of these events is shown in Fig. 86-8. Since the events occurring between hormone binding to receptor sites and activation of adenyl cyclase activity are not known, the relationship between ADH, cAMP, and transport processes in ADH-responsive epithelia may be viewed in the context of two steps: adenyl cyclase activation, beginning with hormone binding and resulting in intracellular cAMP formation; and the link between cAMP and membrane permeability changes. Thus any agent, drug, or hormone that interferes with either of these steps may alter both urinary dilution and concentration. For example, endogenously produced renal prostaglandins modulate ADH activity by affecting the adenyl cyclase activation

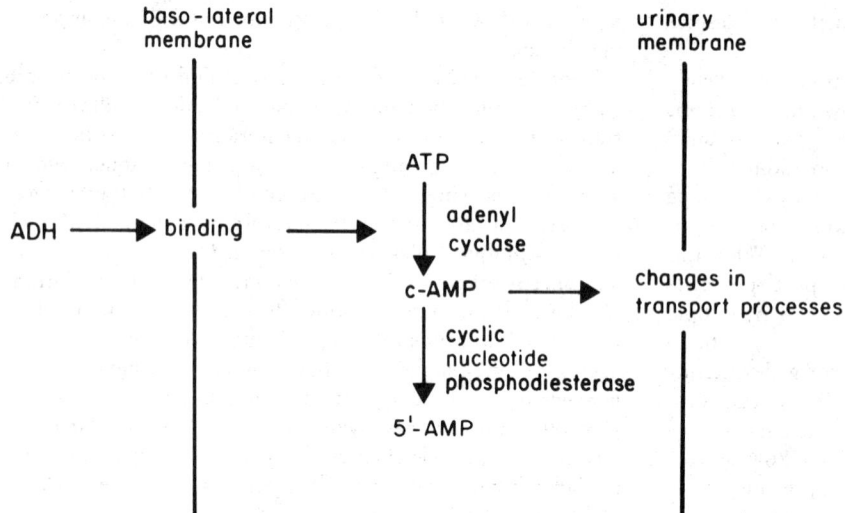

Figure 86-8 The major events regulating ADH activity in hormone-responsive epithelial cells.

step. Prostaglandins inhibit vasopressin-stimulated hydro-osmotic water flow in both toad bladder [193] and cortical collecting tubule [194]. In both epithelia, endogenous prostaglandin synthesis increases in the presence of ADH and diminishes the activity of vasopressin-stimulated adenyl cyclase [195, 196]. Studies in dogs and humans in vivo indicate that suppression of renal prostaglandin synthesis dramatically increases the maximum urinary osmolality achieved after an infusion of vasopressin [197, 198]. Furthermore, several workers have demonstrated increased rates of urinary prostaglandin excretion in patients with nephrogenic diabetes insipidus [199–201].

In regard to the latter step, cAMP alteration of urinary membrane transport processes in ADH-sensitive cells may involve the kinetics of membrane-bound protein phosphorylation-dephosphorylation reactions. Handler and Orloff [202] have proposed that a protein kinase (EC 2.7.1.37) is both activated by cAMP and coupled to specific and separate protein components involved in the water, urea, and Na^+ permeability response to ADH. Colchicine and vinblastine inhibit the antidiuretic response to ADH during water diuresis, with no change in total solute excretion [203]. The inhibition induced by these agents appears to be subsequent to cAMP production and protein phosphorylation reactions [203] and may involve microtubules [204].

PATHOGENESIS

Vasopressin-resistant hyposthenuria or isosthenuria may be due to three types of disturbances:

1. The renal tubules may be ADH-responsive, and negative free-water formation may be normal, but the urine osmolality approaches isotonicity because the volume of isotonic fluid entering the loop of Henle is increased. This mechanism may account for the isosthenuria of chronic renal disease [23].

2. The renal tubule may be ADH-responsive but the renal countercurrent multiplication and exchange systems fail to generate an appropriately hypertonic medullary interstitum; thus, the osmotic driving force for negative free-water formation is either reduced or abolished. Such a disturbance may contribute to the ADH-responsive concentrating defect in a

number of disorders including sickle-cell disease [205]; in normal individuals subjected to prolonged water ingestion [206]; or in patients with pituitary diabetes insipidus, who exhibit a transient inability to concentrate urine maximally following exogenous vasopressin administration [23]; hypokalemia and hypercalcemia, wherein renal papillary Na^+ and total solute concentrations are reduced [23, 207]; and obstructive uropathy associated with hydronephrosis which produces significant reductions in papillary and medullary solute concentrations [208].

3. The volume of isotonic fluid entering the loop of Henle and the countercurrent multiplication and exchange systems are normal, but the renal tubule is unresponsive to ADH.

Following Williams and Henry [4], the term *nephrogenic diabetes insipidus* should be applied to disorders in which renal tubular unresponsiveness to ADH, without disturbances either in solute delivery to the loop of Henle or in countercurrent multiplication or exchange processes, is reponsible for polyuria and hyposthenuria. Thus, with regard to Fig. 86-8, nephrogenic diabetes insipidus may be due to an inability of ADH to raise cellular cAMP concentrations, to an inability of cAMP to increase the water permeability of luminal membranes, or to a combination of these two disorders.

Familial Nephrogenic Diabetes Insipidus

In normal individuals or patients with pituitary diabetes insipidus, exogenous ADH can increase the rate of urinary cAMP excretion [209]. In some patients with familial nephrogenic diabetes insipidus, comparable doses of ADH do not increase rates of urinary cAMP excretion [209, 210]. However, in two groups of children with nephrogenic diabetes insipidus [200, 211] both basal and ADH-stimulated rates of urinary cAMP excretion exceeded those of normal children. These disparate results led to the postulate that familial nephrogenic diabetes insipidus is a heterogeneous disorder produced by either a defect in hormone receptor adenyl cyclase stimulation or a defect beyond the generation of cAMP [211]. Further confusing the issue is the finding by Uttley et al. [212] that total urinary cAMP excretion following vasopressin was the same in patients with familial nephrogenic diabetes insipidus as in normal persons. These authors suggest that measurement of urinary cAMP is futile as an investigative tool in these patients since even in normal persons vasopressin increases urinary cAMP excretion only two- to threefold as opposed to the twenty- to thirtyfold increase seen with parathyroid hormone [213]. Finally, the effect of vasopressin on renal tubule cellular accumulation of cAMP in familial nephrogenic diabetes insipidus is totally unknown. Patients with familial nephrogenic diabetes insipidus can raise plasma cortisol concentrations in response to ADH, a finding interpreted to indicate that vasopressin stimulation of extrarenal, i.e., pituitary, cAMP formation is intact in the disease [214].

Hereditary diabetes insipidus occurs in selected strains of mice, some of which exhibit vasopressin unresponsiveness [215, 216]. In the genotypic strain termed DI +/+ severe, stimulation of medullary adenyl cyclase activity by vasopressin is markedly reduced. The defect seems specific, since the basal level of renal medullary adenyl cyclase activity is normal, as is the stimulation of renal cortical adenyl cyclase activity by parathyroid hormone [217]. Further studies in these mice indicate that vasopressin-stimulated adenyl cyclase activity is modestly reduced in medullary collecting tubule (MCT) segments and severely reduced in medullary ascending limb (MAL) segments when compared with activity in normal mice [218]. Medullary collecting tubule cAMP phosphodiesterase activity was markedly higher in DI +/+ mice than in normal mice, the net result being failure of vasopressin-stimulated cellular cAMP accumulation in cells of either MCT or MAL of the nephrogenic diabetes insipidus mice [218]. These studies may bear on the pathogenesis of familial nephrogenic diabetes insipidus of humans.

Acquired Nephrogenic Diabetes Insipidus

Vasopressin-resistant hyposthenuria associated with otherwise normal or nearly normal renal function may occur as a complication of drug therapy or in association with systemic diseases. Appropriately termed *acquired nephrogenic diabetes insipidus*, this condition is to be distinguished from the rare familial disorder described earlier.

Drug-induced Nephrogenic Diabetes Insipidus A number of reports [219–221] have documented the occurrence of vasopressin-unresponsive hyposthenuria in patients receiving demethylchlortetracycline. Both the concentrating defect and vasopressin-unresponsiveness are reversible and disappear shortly after discontinuance of the antibiotic therapy. The glomerular filtration rate in these patients is generally normal, as is the ability for maximal urinary dilution (positive free-water formation), indicating that solute abstraction from the loop of Henle is probably unimpaired [221].

In toad urinary bladder, contraluminal (serosal) demethylchlortetracycline inhibited the water permeability increase produced by either vasopressin or cAMP [221]. Although other tetracyclines can inhibit ADH or cAMP enhancement of water permeation in toad bladder [222], only demethylchlortetracycline has caused clinical nephrogenic diabetes insipidus in humans. This may relate to specific binding of demethylchlortetracycline to a specific cell protein of approximately 100,000 daltons as shown in toad bladder epithelium [223]. Likewise, in human renal medulla, demethylchlortetracycline noncompetitively inhibited basal adenyl cyclase activity, ADH-stimulated adenyl cyclase activity, and cAMP-dependent protein kinase activity, but did not affect cyclic nucleotide phosphodiesterase activity [224]. These observations in vitro

[221–224] suggest that demethylchlortetracycline-induced nephrogenic diabetes insipidus may be due to inhibition of both cAMP accumulation and the action of cAMP on urinary membranes.

Nephrogenic diabetes insipidus may also be produced by volatile fluorocarbon anesthetics. Methoxyflurane anesthesia is complicated by a full spectrum of renal injury, ranging from vasopressin-resistant polyuria and hyposthenuria to acute tubular necrosis [225]. Both fluoride and oxalic acid, which are metabolic products of methoxyflurane, contribute to the nephrotoxicity of the anesthetic [226]. The polyuric state is related to the markedly increased serum concentration and urinary excretion of inorganic fluoride [227]. Sodium fluoride causes a vasopressin-resistant polyuria in dogs [228], and in rat inorganic fluoride seems to reduce collecting duct water permeability without affecting salt transport in the ascending limb [229].

Finally, serum lithium concentrations of 0.5 to 1.5 meq/liter, which are generally regarded as being in the therapeutic range for affective disorders, produce vasopressin-resistant diabetes insipidus [230–232]. Nephrogenic diabetes insipidus has been observed in 12 to 30 percent of patients receiving lithium therapy [223, 232]; the defect is usually reversible, and urinary concentrating ability returns toward normal when lithium is discontinued [230, 232]. Patients on chronic lithium therapy tend to have higher levels of plasma antidiuretic hormone for a given plasma osmolality [233].

In toad urinary bladder, 11 meq/liter lithium in mucosal (urinary) solutions inhibited the stimulation of water transport produced by vasopressin but not that produced by cAMP [231]. Furthermore, lithium specifically inhibited ADH-activated adenyl cyclase in mammalian renal medulla [234, 235]. This inhibition is seen in both medullary thick ascending limbs and collecting ducts with acute introduction of lithium, but only in medullary collecting ducts in animals chronically treated with lithium [236]. Accordingly, it was proposed that lithium-induced nephrogenic diabetes insipidus was the consequence of an effect proximal to cAMP action [231, 234–236].

Lithium-induced polyuria may also depend on other factors. In the rat, chronic lithium administration produced a polyuria which was unresponsive to either vasopressin or dibutyryl cAMP, while both agents enhanced urinary concentrating ability in rats with hereditary hypothalamic diabetes insipidus [232]. Finally, lithium has been thought to cause primary polydipsia because it stimulates water ingestion and increases polyuria in normal rats [237] and in rats with hereditary hypothalamic diabetes insipidus [238]. Thus the lithium-induced polyuria observed clinically may be the consequence of three effects of the cation: Inhibition of vasopressin-stimulated cAMP formation [231, 234–236]; interference with the action of cAMP on water transport in collecting ducts [232]; and primary polydipsia [237, 238].

Nephrogenic Diabetes Insipidus in Systemic Diseases In rare instances, vasopressin-resistant polyuria may occur in association with amyloidosis [239, 240]. In one such patient, amyloid deposits were localized primarily to the basement membranes of medullary collecting ducts, without involvement of the loops of Henle [239]. In eight patients with Sjögren's syndrome, four had persistent hyposthenuria out of proportion to mild reductions in glomerular filtration rate. In the one patient tested, maximal urinary concentration following vasopressin administration was impaired [241]. The factors responsible for the renal concentrating defect observed in these conditions are not understood.

Diagnosis

The diagnostic characteristics of familial nephrogenic diabetes insipidus include onset during infancy, a positive family history, persistent thirst, polyuria and hyposthenuria that are unresponsive to vasopressin, and serum arginine vasopressin levels that vary appropriately with changes in serum osmolality (Fig. 86–3). Although other abnormalities, e.g., hydronephrosis [35–37] or hyperuricemia [27, 29], may occasionally be present, vasopressin-unresponsive polyuria is the characteristic feature of the disorder. In the absence of dehydration, renal function is normal. Likewise, acquired nephrogenic diabetes insipidus, either drug-induced or accompanying systemic disorders (see above), is characterized by vasopressin-resistant polyuria.

As indicated previously, renal concentrating defects and apparent vasopressin resistance may occur in a number of other settings. For convenience, these may be classified into three major groups: Disorders in which the concentrating defect is largely due to relatively high rates of solute excretion, including primarily chronic renal failure [23]; disorders in which impairment of the renal countercurrent and exchange systems is a major factor contributing to the concentrating defect, including sickle-cell disease [205], prolonged water ingestion [23, 206], hypokalemia [207], hypercalcemia [23, 207], and obstructive uropathy [208]; and disorders having a renal concentrating defect of uncertain cause [23], including juvenile nephronophthisis, medullary cystic disease, cystic disease of the kidney, cystinosis, and pyelonephritis. In most of these conditions, the characteristic findings of the underlying disorder generally preclude error in diagnosis.

Treatment

There is no specific therapy for the disorder. Adequate hydration, easily achieved by oral intake in children and adults but sometimes requiring parenteral supplementation in infants, is essential to prevent the damaging effects of hypernatremia and circulatory collapse, particularly in children. Although polyuria may be minimized by reducing solute intake, this is rarely necessary except in children.

The therapy of the acute episode of dehydration may differ from that in other situations. If sufficient water can be administered orally, hyperosmolality of body fluids is easily overcome. Parenteral therapy with 5 percent dextrose in water may aggravate the hypertonic state of nephrogenic diabetes insipidus if the rate of glucose infusion exceeds the rate of metabolic utilization of glucose so that glycosuria occurs. This osmotic diuresis will increase salt-free water excretion and further the development of hyperosmolality and cellular dehydration. Especially in children, 3 percent dextrose in water or 35 to 50 meq/liter NaCl solution may be required.

Neither arginine vasopressin, Pitressin, nor any of its analogues, lysine vasopressin nor DDAVP, has any effect in the disease. Obviously, drugs that stimulate endogenous ADH release, such as clofibrate [94], are ineffectual, as are agents, such as chlorpropamide, that enhance the tubular activity of ADH [93].

Inhibitors of prostaglandin synthesis with the drugs ibuprofen [242], indomethacin [200, 201, 242], or aspirin [201] reduce urine volume and slightly increase urine osmolality in children with nephrogenic diabetes insipidus. The effect appears to be secondary to a reduction in delivery of solute to the distal tubule and not to an amelioration of prostaglandin antagonism to the tubular action of ADH [200, 201].

Parenteral administration of cAMP [243, 244], or of the potent analogues dibutyryl cAMP [244] and 8-p-chlorophenylthio cAMP [245], fails to decrease urine volume or increase urine osmolality. There is actually an increase in urine volume in children with nephrogenic diabetes insipidus given dibutyryl cAMP that is probably due to its proximal tubular phosphaturic and natriuretic effect, the result being increased solute delivery to the distal tubule [244].

Diuretics such as chlorothiazide are useful therapeutic agents. Crawford and Kennedy [246] first noted that chronic administration of these derivatives to patients with diabetes insipidus resulted in a marked reduction in urine flow and a moderate increase in urine concentration. The observed increase in urine concentration provided by chlorothiazide is in accord with its effect in normal animals and humans during water diuresis [23], when the drug interferes with sodium chloride absorption in distal portions of the nephron, thereby reducing the formation of solute-free water. This effect alone cannot account for the reduction in urine flow. Instead, chlorothiazide-induced reductions in urine volume are also referable to an increased proximal fractional absorption of glomerular filtrate [23]. Enchanced absorption of isosmotic fluid in the proximal nephron may be related to the mild degree of sodium depletion induced by the drug [23].

This increase in isosmotic proximal tubular fluid absorption results in a decrease in the volume of fluid delivered to the distal nephron, the site of defective water absorption, and, therefore, to a reduction in urine volume. Furthermore, once a sodium deficiency is achieved by the diuretic agent, antidiuresis persists without further drug administration as long as the sodium deficiency is maintained by salt restriction [23]. When salt losses are restored, polyuria rapidly returns.

Similar results obtain with regulation of total dietary solute in patients with nephrogenic diabetes insipidus. A diet low in NaCl and protein has caused a greater than twofold reduction in urine volume in one patient [247].

REFERENCES

1. FORSSMAN HH: Om ärftlighetsgången vid diabetes insipidus. *Nord Med* 16:3211, 1942
2. FORSSMAN H: On Hereditary diabetes insipidus. *Acta Med Scand* 121 [Suppl] 159:9, 1945
3. WARING AJ, KAJDI L, TAPPAN V: A congenital defect of water metabolism. *Am J Dis Child* 69:323, 1945
4. WILLIAMS RH, HENRY C: Nephrogenic diabetes insipidus: Transmitted by females and appearing during infancy in males. *Ann Intern Med* 27:84, 1947
5. LA COMBE LU: De la polydipsie. L'Expèrance. *J Méd Chir* 7:305, 1841
6. WEIL A: Über die hereditäre Form des Diabetes insipidus. *Arch F Pathol Anat* 95:70, 1884.
7. MCILRAITH CH: Notes on some cases of diabetes insipidus with marked family and hereditary tendencies. *Lancet* 2:767, 1892
8. DE LANGE C: Über erblichen Diabetes insipidus. *Jahrb F Kinderheilkunde* 145:1, 1935
9. ELLBORG A, FORSSMAN H: Nephrogenic diabetes insipidus in children. *Acta Paediatr* 44:209, 1955
10. FRISS-HANSEN B: Body water compartments in children: Changes during growth and related changes in body composition. *Pediatrics* 28:169, 1961

11. EDELMAN CM JR, BARNETT HL: Pediatric nephrology, in Strauss MB, Welt LG (eds): *Diseases of the Kidney*, 2d ed. Boston, Little, Brown, 1971, p 1349

12. RUESS AL, ROSENTHAL IM: Intelligence in nephrogenic diabetes insipidus. *Am J Dis Child* 105:358, 1963

13. DANCIS J, BIRMINGHAM JR, LESLIE SH: Congenital diabetes insipidus resistant to treatment with pitressin. *Am J Dis Child* 75:316,1949

14. GUARD HL: Pitressin resistant diabetes insipidus nephrogenic function defect. *Med Bull US Army* 10:185, 1953

15. KAO MY, STEINER MM: Diabetes insipidus in infancy resistant to pitressin. *Pediatrics* 12:400, 1953

16. FORSSMAN H: Is hereditary diabetes insipidus of nephrogenic type associated with mental deficiency? *Acta Psychiatr Neurol Scand* 30:577, 1955

17. KIRMAN BH, BLACK JA, WILKINSON RH, EVANS PR: Familial pitressin-resistant diabetes insipidus with mental defect. *Arch Dis Child* 31:59, 1955

18. GAUTIER E, SIMPKISS M: The management of nephrogenic diabetes insipidus in early life. *Acta Paediatr* 46:354, 1957

19. HILLMAN DA, NEYZI O, PORTER P, CUSHMAN A, TALBOT NB: Renal (vasopressin-resistant) diabetes insipidus: Definition of the effects of a homeostatic limitation in capacity to conserve water on the physical, intellectual and emotional development of a child. *Pediatrics* 21:430, 1958

20. WALKER NF, RANCE CP: Inheritance of nephrogenic diabetes insipidus. *Am J Hum Genet* 6:354, 1954

21. MORRIS-JONES PH, HOUSTON IB, EVANS RC: Prognosis of the neurological complications of acute hypernatremia. *Lancet* 2:1385, 1967

22. MACAULEY D, WATSON M: Hypernatraemia in infants as a cause of brain damage. *Arch Dis Child* 42:485, 1967

23. ANDREOLI TE, SCHAFER JA: Nephrogenic diabetes insipidus, in Stanbury JB, Wyngaarden JB, Fredrickson DS (eds): *Metabolic Basis of Inherited Disease*, 4th ed. New York, McGraw-Hill, 1978, p 1634

24. DICKER SE, EGGLETON MG: Hyaluronidase and antidiuretic activity in urine of man. *J Physiol* 154:378, 1960

25. GELLAI M, EDWARDS BR, VALTIN H: Urinary concentrating ability during dehydration in the absence of vasopressin. *Am J Physiol* 237:F100, 1979

26. EDWARDS BR, GALLAI M, VALTIN H: Concentration of urine in the absence of ADH with minimal or no decrease in GFR. *Am J Physiol* 239:F84, 1980.

27. CUTLER RE, KLEEMAN CR, MAXWELL MH, DOWLING JT: Physiologic studies in nephrogenic diabetes insipidus. *J Clin Endocrinal Metab* 22:827, 1962

28. McCONNELL RF, LORENTZ WB, BERGER M, SMITH EH, CARVAJAL HF, TRAVIS LB: The mechanism of urinary concentration in neophrogenic diabetes insipidus. *Pediatr Res* W:33, 1977

29. GORDEN P, ROBERTSON GL, SEEGMILLER JE: Hyperuricemia, a concomitant of congenital vasopressin-resistant diabetes insipidus in the adult. Studies of uric acid metabolism and plasma vasopressin. *N Engl J Med* 284:1057, 1971

30. DARMADY E, OFFER J, PRINCE J, STRANACK F: The proximal convoluted tubule in the renal handling of water. *Lancet* 2:1254, 1964

31. WEBER JW, GAUTIER E: Pitressinresistenter Diabetes insipidus. Therapie mit Silidiuretica. *Helv Paediatr Acta* 16:565, 1961

32. LOBECK CC, BARTA RA, MANGOS JA: Study of sweat in pitressin-resistant diabetes insipidus. *J Pediatr* 62:868, 1963

33. WEST JR, KRAMER JG: Nephrogenic diabetes insipidus. *Pediatrics* 15:424, 1955

34. ORLOFF J, WALSER M: Water and solute excretion in pitressin-resistant diabetes insipidus. *Clin Res Proc* 4:136, 1956

35. TEN BENSEL RW, PETERS ER: Progressive hydronephrosis, hydroureter, and dilatation of the bladder in siblings with congenital nephrogenic diabetes insipidus. *J Pediatr* 77:439, 1970

36. MANSON AD, YALOWITZ PA, RANDALL RV, GREENE LF: Dilatation of the urinary tract associated with pituitary and nephrogenic diabetes insipidus. *J Urol* 103:327, 1970

37. SHAPIRO SR, WOERNER S, ADELMAN RD, PALMER JM: Diabetes insipidus and hydronephrosis. *J Urol* 119:715, 1978

38. SILVERSTEIN E, SOKOLOFF L, MICKELSEN O, JAY GE JR: Primary polydipsia and hydronephrosis in an inbred strain of mice. *Am J Pathol* 38:143, 1961

39. SAWYER WH: Biological assays for neurohypophysial principles in tissues and in blood, in Harris GW, Donovan BT (eds): *The Pituitary Gland*. Berkeley, University of California Press, 1966, p 288

40. DICKER SE, EGGLETON MG: Nephrogenic diabetes insipidus. *Clin Sci* 24:81, 1963

41. HOLLIDAY MA, BURSTIN C, HARRAH J: Evidence that the antidiuretic substance in the plasma of children with nephrogenic diabetes insipidus is antidiuretic hormone. *Pediatrics* 32:384, 1963

42. ROBERTSON GL, MAHR EA, ATHAR S, SINHA T: Development and clinical application of a new method for the radioimmunoassay of arginine vasopressin in human plasma. *J Clin Invest* 52:2340, 1973

43. DUNN FL, BRENNAN TJ, NELSON AE, ROBERTSON GL: The role of blood osmolality and volume in regulating vasopressin secretion in the rat. *J Clin Invest* 52:3212, 1973

44. ROBERTSON GL: Vasopressin in osmotic regulation in man. *Annu Rev Med* 25:315, 1974

45. SCHOEN EJ: Renal diabetes insipidus. *Pediatrics* 26:808, 1960

46. NAKANO KK: Familial nephrogenic diabetes insipidus. *Hawaii Med J* 28:205, 1969

47. SCHULTZ P, LINES DR: Nephrogenic diabetes insipidus in the Australian aboriginal kindred. *Humangenetik* 26:79, 1975

48. CRAWFORD JD, KENNEDY GC: Chlorothiazide in diabetes insipidus. *Nature* 183:891, 1959

49. BODE HH, CRAWFORD JD; Nephrogenic diabetes insipidus in North America—the Hopewell hypothesis. *N Engl J Med* 280:750, 1969

50. DU VIGNEAUD V: Hormones of the mammalian posterior pituitary gland and their naturally occurring analogues. *Johns Hopkins Med J* 124:53, 1969

51. SAWYER WH: Evolution of antidiuretic hormones and their functions. *Am J Med* 42:678, 1967

52. SAWYER WH: Evolution of neurohypophyseal hormones and their receptors. *Fed Proc* 36:1842, 1977

53. SAWYER WH, PANG PKT, SETO J, McENROE M, LAMMEK B, MANNING M: Vasopressin analogs that antagonize antidiuretic responses by rats to the antidiuretic hormone. *Science* 212:49, 1981

54. BUTLEN D, GUILLON G, RAJERISON RM, JARD S, SAWYER WH, MANNING M: Structural requirements for activation of vasopressin-sensitive adenylate cyclase, hormone binding, and antidiuretic actions: Effects of highly potent analogues and competitive inhibitors. *Mol Pharmacol* 14:1006, 1978

55. BARTH T, RAJERISON MR, ROY C, JARD S: Activation of rat kidney adenylate cyclase by vasopressin analogues: Lack of correlation with antidiuretic activity. *Mol Cell Endocrinol* 2:81, 1975

56. HECHTER O, TERADA S, SPITSBERG V, NAKAHARA T, NAKAGAWAGA SH, FLOURET G: Neurohypophyseal hormone-responsive renal adenylate cyclase. III. Relationship between affinity and intrinsic activity in neurohypophyseal hormones and structural analogs. *J Biol Chem* 253:3230, 1978

57. ROY C, BARTH T, JARD S: Vasopressin-sensitive kidney adenylate cyclase. Structural requirements for attachment to the receptor and enzyme activation: Studies with vasopressin analogues. *J Biol Chem* 250:3149, 1975

58. ROY C, BARTH T, JARD S: Vasopressin-sensitive kidney adenylate cyclase. Structural requirements for attachment to the receptor and enzyme activation: Studies with oxytocin analogues. *J Biol Chem* 250:3157, 1975

59. HECHTER O, TERADA S, NAKAHARA T, FLOURET G, BERGMAN RN: Neurohypophyseal hormone-responsive renal adenylate cyclase. II. Relationship between hormonal occupancy of neurohypophyseal hormone receptor sites and adenylate cyclase activation. *J Biol Chem* 253:3219, 1978

60. SAWYER WH, ACOSTA M, BALASPIRI L, JUDD J, MANNING M: Structural changes in the arginine vasopressin molecule that enhance antidiuretic activity and specificity. *Endocrinology* 94:1106, 1974

61. SAWYER WH, ACOSTA M, MANNING M: Structural changes in the arginine vasopressin molecule that prolong its antidiuretic action. *Endocrinology* 95:140, 1974

62. BARTH T, KREJČI I, KUPKOVÁ B, JOŠT K: Pharmacology of cyclic analogues of deamino-oxytocin not containing a disulphide bond (carba analogues). *Eur J Pharmacol* 24:183, 1973

63. KODIA M, GLASS JD, SCHWARTZ IL, WALTER R: Mechanism of inactivation of oxytocin by rat kidney enzymes. *Endocrinology* 88:633, 1971

64. CORT, JH, SCHÜCK O, STŘIBRNÁ J, ŠKOPKOVÁ J, JOŠT K, MULDER JL: Role of the disulfide bridge and the C-terminal tripeptide in the antidiuretic action of vasopressin in man and the rat. *Kidney Int* 8:292, 1975

65. MANNING M, BALASPIRI L, MOEHRING J, HALDAR J, SAWYER WH: Synthesis and some pharmacological properties of deamino [4-threonine, 8-D-arginine] vasopressin and deamino [8-D-arginine] vasopressin, highly potent and specific antidiuretic peptides, and [8-D-arginine] vasopressin and deamino-arginine vasopressin. *J Med Chem* 19:842, 1976

66. WALTER R, SCHWARTZ IL, DARNELL JH, URRY DW: Relation of the conformation of oxytocin to the biology of neurohypophyseal hormones. *Proc Natl Acad Sci USA* 68:1355, 1971

67. EDWARDS RW, KITAU MJ, CHARD T, BESSER GM: Vasopressin analogue DDAVP in diabetes insipidus: Clinical and laboratory studies. *Br Med J* 3:375, 1973

68. URRY DW, WALTER R: Proposed conformation of oxytocin in solution. *Proc Natl Acad Sci USA* 68:956, 1971

69. WALTER R, GLICKSON JD, SCHWARTZ IL, HARVAN RT, MEIENHOFFER J, URY DW: Conformation of lysine vasopressin: A comparison with oxytocin. *Proc Natl Acad Sci USA* 69:1920, 1972

70. HECHTER O, KATO T, NAKAGAWA SH, YANG F, FLOURET G: Contribution of the peptide backbone to the action of oxytocin analogs. *Proc Natl Acad Sci USA* 72:563, 1975

71. KRUSZYNSKI M, LAMMEK B, MANNING M, SETO J, HALDAR J, SAWYER

WH: [1-[(β-mercapto-β, β-cyclopenta methylene propionic acid)], [2-(0-methyl) tyrosine] arginine vasopressin and [1-(β-mercapto-β, β-cyclopenta methylene propionic acid)] arginine vasopressin, highly potent antagonists of the vasopressor response to arginine vasopressin. *J Med Chem* 23:364, 1980

72. SCHARRER E, SCHARRER B:Hormones produced by neurosecretory cells. *Recent Prog Horm Res* 10:183, 1954

73. SAWYER WH, VALTIN H, SOKOL HW: Neurohypophysial principles in rats with familial hypothalamic diabetes insipidus (Brattleboro strain). *Endocrinology* 74:153, 1964

74. SACHS H, FAWCETT CP, TAKABATAKE Y, PORTANOVA R: Biosynthesis and release of vasopressin and neurophysin. *Recent Prog Horm Res* 25:447, 1969

75. PICKERING BT, JONES CW: The neurophysins, in Li CH (ed): *Hormonal Protein and Peptides*, vol V. New York, Academic, 1978, p 103

76. DREIFUSS JJ: A review on neurosecretory granules: Their contents and mechanisms of release. *Ann NY Acad Sci* 248:184, 1975

77. BRESLOW E: On the mechanism of binding of neurohypophyseal hormones and analogs to neurophysins. *Ann NY Acad Sci* 248:423, 1975

78. SACHS H, HALLER EW: Further studies on the capacity of the neurohypophysis to release vasopressin. *Endocrinology* 83:251, 1968

79. ABRAHAMS VC, KOELLE GB, SMART P: Histochemical demonstration of cholinesterases in the hypothalamus of the dog. *J Physiol (London)* 139:137, 1957

80. DREIFUSS JJ, KALNINS I, KELLY JS, RUF KB: Action potentials and release of neurohypophysial hormones in vitro. *J Physiol (London)* 215:805, 1971

81. NORDMANN JJ, DYBALL REJ: Effects of veratridine on Ca fluxes and the release of oxytocin and vasopressin from the isolated rat neurohypophysis. *J Gen Physiol* 72:297, 1978

82. BAUMAN G, DINGMAN JF: Distribution, blood transport, and degradation of antidiuretic hormone in man. *J Clin Invest* 57:1109, 1976

83. WEITZMAN RE, FISHER DA: Arginine vasopressin metabolism in dogs. I. Evidence for a receptor-mediated mechanism *Am J Physiol* 235:E591, 1978

84. WILSON KC, WEITZMAN RE, FISHER DA: Arginine vasopressin metabolism in dogs. II. Modeling and systems analysis. *Am J Physiol* 235:E598, 1978

85. SHADE RE, SHARE L: Renal vasopressin clearance with reduction in renal blood flow in the dog. *Am J Physiol* 232:F341, 1977

86. MARKS N, ABRASH L, WALTER R: Degradation of neurohypophyseal hormones by brain extracts and purified brain enzymes. *Proc Soc Exp Biol Med* 142:455, 1973

87. WALTER R, BOWMAN RH: Mechanism of inactivation of vasopressin and oxytocin by the isolated perfused rat kidney. *Endocrinology* 92:189, 1973

88. NARDACCI NJ, MUKHOPADHYAY S, CAMPBELL BJ: Partial purification and characterization of the antidiuretic hormone-inactivating enzyme from renal plasma membranes. *Biochim Biophys Acta* 377:146, 1975

89. CZACZKES JW, KLEEMAN CR, KOENIG M: Physiologic studies of antidiuretic hormone by its direct measurement in human plasma. *J Clin Invest* 43:1625, 1964

90. NITSCHKE U, BALZAR H: Die Inaktivierung von infundiertem Vasopressin bei Diabetes insipidus-Probanden. *Acta Endocrinol* 62:270, 1969

91. BARTTER FC, SCHWARTZ WB: The syndrome of inappropriate secretion of antidiuretic hormone. *Am J Med* 42:790, 1967

92. NIELSEN B, THORN NA: Transient excess urinary excretion of antidiuretic material in acute intermittent porphyria with hyponatremia and hypomagnesemia. *Am J Med* 38:345, 1965

93. WEISSMAN PN, SHENKMAN L, GREGERMAN RI: Chlorpropamide hyponatremia: Drug-induced inappropriate antidiuretic-hormone activity. *N Engl J Med* 284:65, 1971

94. MOSES AM, HOWANTZ J, VAN GEMERT M, MILLER M: Clofibrate-induced antidiuresis. *J Clin Invest* 53:535, 1973

95. MEINDERS AE, CEJKA V, ROBERTSON GL: The antidiuretic action of carbamazepine in man. *Clin Sci Mol Med* 47:289, 1974

96. DISCALA VA, KINNEY MJ: Effects of myxedema on the renal diluting and concentrating mechanism. *Am J Med* 50:325, 1971

97. SHARE L: Vasopressin, its bioassay and the physiological control of its release. *Am J Med* 42:701, 1967

98. SHU'AYB WA, MORGAN WH, ZIMMERMANN B: Studies of the mechanism of antidiuretic hormone secretion and the post-commissurotomy dilutional syndrome. *Ann Surg* 162:690, 1965

99. SLADEN A, LAVER MB, PONTOPPIDAN H: Pulmonary complications and water retention in prolonged mechanical ventilation. *N Engl J Med* 279:448,1968

100. VERNEY EB: The antidiuretic hormone and the factors which determine its release. *Proc R Soc Lond* (Series B) 135:25, 1947

101. MCKINLEY MJ, DENTON DA, WEISINGER RS: Sensors for antidiuresis and thirstormoreceptors or CSF sodium detectors? *Brain Res* 141:89, 1978

102. PETERS JP: *Body Water. The Exchange of Fluids in Man.* Springfield, Ill. Charles C Thomas, 1935, p. 284

103. LEAF A, MAMBY AR: An antidiuretic mechanism not regulated by extracellular fluid tonicity. *J Clin Invest* 31:60, 1952

104. GAUER OH, HENRY JP: Circulatory basis of fluid volume control. *Physiol Rev* 43:423, 1963

105. MURDAUGH HV, SIEKER HO, MANFREDI F: Effect of altered intrathoracic pressure on renal hemodynamics, electrolyte excretion and water clearance. *J Clin Invest* 38:834, 1959

106. HENRY JP, GAUER OH, REEVES JL: Evidence of the atrial location of receptors influencing urine flow. *Circ Res* 4:85, 1956

107. WEINSTEIN H, BERNE RM, SACHS H: Vasopressin in blood: Effect of hemorrhage. *Endocrinology* 66:712, 1960

108. SHARE L: Acute reduction in extracellular fluid volume and the concentration of antidiuretic hormone in blood. *Endocrinology* 69:925, 1961

109. GUPTA PD, HENRY JP, SINCLAIR R, VON BAUMGARTEN R: Responses of atrial and aortic baroreceptors to nonhypotensive hemorrhage and to transfusion. *Am J Physiol* 211:1429, 1966

110. CAILLENS H, PRUSZCZYNSKI W, MEYRIER A, ANG K-S, ROUSSELET F, ARDAILLOU R: Relationship between change in volemia at constant osmolality and plasma antidiuretic hormone. *Mineral Electrolyte Metab* 4:161, 1980

111. GROSSMAN SP: Direct adrenergic and cholinergic stimulation of hypothalamic mechanisms. *Am J Physiol* 202:872, 1962

112. KLEIN LA, LIBERMAN B, LAKS M, KLEEMAN CR: Interrelated effects of antidiuretic hormone and adrenergic drugs on water metabolism. *Am J Physiol* 221:1657, 1971

113. FISHER DA: Norepinephrine inhibition of vasopressin antidiuresis. *J Clin Invest* 47:540, 1968.

114. HANDLER JS, BENSINGER R, ORLOFF J: Effect of adrenergic agents on toad bladder response to ADH, 3′,5′-AMP, and theophylline. *Am J Physiol* 215:1024, 1968

115. KUROKAWA K, MASSRY SG: Interaction between catecholamines and vasopressin on renal medullary cyclic AMP of rat. *Am J Physiol* 225:825, 1973

116. SCHRIER RW, BERL T, ANDERSON RJ, MCDONALD KM: Non-osmotic regulation of renal water excretion. *Trans Am Clin Climatol Assoc* 87:161, 1976

117. MCDONALD KM, KURUVILA KC, AISENBREY GA, SCHRIER RW: Effect of alpha and beta adrenergic stimulation on renal water excretion and medullary cyclic AMP in intact and diabetes insipidus rats. *Kidney Int* 12:96, 1977

118. RAYSON BMR, RAY C, MORGAN T: A study of the interaction of catecholamines and antidiuretic hormone on water permeability and the cyclic AMP system in isolated papillae of the rat. *Pflügers Arch* 373:99, 1978

119. BERL T, CADNAPAPHORNCHAI P, HARBOTTLE JA, SCHRIER RW: Mechanism of stimulation of vasopressin release during beta adrenergic stimulation with isoproterenol. *J Clin Invest* 53:857, 1974

120. BERL T, CADNAPAHORNCHAI P, HARBOTTLE JA, SCHRIER RW: Mechanism of suppression of vasopressin during alpha-adrenergic stimulation with norepinephrine. *J Clin Invest* 53:219, 1974

121. BRENNAN LA, BONJOUR JP, MALVIN RL: ADH levels during salt depletion in dogs. *Eur J Clin Invest* 2:43, 1971

122. UHLICH E, WEBER P, GRÖSCHEL-STEWART U: Angiotensin-stimulated vasopressin release in man; radioimmunologically determined plasma levels of vasopressin. *Acta Endocrinol [Suppl]* 184:52, 1974

123. GOETZ KL, BOND GC, SMITH WE: Effect of moderate hemorrhage in humans on plasma ADH and renin. *Proc Soc Exp Biol Med* 145:277, 1974

124. ROBERTSON GL, ATHAR S: The interaction of blood osmolality and blood volume in regulating plasma vasopressin in man. *J Clin Endocrinol Metab* 42:613, 1976

125. HIROKAWA W: Ueber den osmotischen Druck des Nierenparenchyms. Hofmeisters *Beitr Physiol Pathol* 11:458, 1908

126. KUHN W, RYFFEL K: Herstellung konzentrierter Lösungen aus verdünnten durch blosse Membranwirkung. Ein Modellversuch zur Funktion der Niere. *Z Physiol Chemie* 276:145, 1942

127. WIRZ VH, HARGITAY B, KUHN W: Lokalisation des Konzentrierungsprozesses in der Niere durch direkte Kryoskopie. *Helv Physiol Acta* 9:196, 1951

128. HARGITAY B, KUHN W: Das Multiplikationsprinzip als Grundlage der Harnkonzentrierung in der Niere. *Z Elektrochem* 55:539, 1951

129. GOTTSCHALK CW, MYLLE M: Micropuncture study of the mammalian urinary concentrating mechanism: Evidence for the countercurrent hypothesis. *Am J Physiol* 4:927, 1959

130. GOTTSCHALK CW: Micropuncture studies of tubular function in the mammalian kidney. *Physiologist* 4:35, 1961

131. GOTTSCHALK CW: Osmotic concentration and dilution of the urine. *Am J Med* 36:670, 1964

132. BURG M, GRANTHAM J, ABRAMOW M, ORLOFF J: Preparation and study of fragments of single rabbit nephrons. *Am J Physiol* 210:1293, 1966

133. KOKKO JP, RECTOR FC JR: Countercurrent multiplication system without active transport in inner medulla. *Kidney Int* 2:214, 1972

134. VALTIN H: Sequestration of urea and nonurea solutes in renal tissues of rats with hereditary hypothalamic diabetes insipidus: Effect of vasopressin and dehydration on the countercurrent mechanism. *J Clin Invest* 45:337, 1966

135. STEPHENSON JL: Concentration of urine in a central core model of the renal counterflow system. *Kidney Int* 2:85, 1972

136. PENNELL JP, LACY FB, JAMISON RL: An in vivo study of the concentrating process in the descending limb of Henle's loop. *Kidney Int* 5:337, 1974

137. GERTZ KH, SCHMIDT-NIELSON B, PAGEL D: Exchange of water, urea and salt between the mammalian renal papilla and the surrounding urine. *Fed Proc* 25:327, 1966

138. SCHULTZ W, SCHNERMANN J: Pelvic urine composition as a determinant of inner medullary solute concentration and urine osmolality. *Pflügers Arch* 334:154, 1972

139. BONVENTRE JV, KARNOVSKY MJ, LECHENE CP: Renal papillary epithelial morphology in antidiuresis and water diuresis. *Am J Physiol: Renal Fluid Electrolyte Physiol* 4:F69, 1978

140. MOREL F: Sites of hormone action in the mammalian nephron. *Am J Physiol: Renal Fluid Electrolyte Physiol* 9:F159, 1981

141. WIRZ H: The location of antidiuretic action in the mammalian kidney, in Heller H (ed): *The Neurohypophysis. Proc. 8th Symposium of the Colston Research Soc*, New York, Academic, 1957, p 157

142. KESSLER RH: Acute effects of brief ureteral stasis on urinary and renal papillary chloride concentration. *Am J Physiol* 199:1215, 1960

143. PERLMUTT JH: Influence of hydration on renal function and medullary sodium during vasopressin infusion. *Am J Physiol* 202:1098, 1962

144. RUIZ-GUIÑAZÚ A, ARRIZURIETA EE, YELINEK L: Electrolyte, water, and urea content in dog kidneys in different states of diuresis. *Am J Physiol* 206:725, 1964

145. HALL DA, VARNEY DM: Effect of vasopressin on electrical potential difference and chloride transport in mouse medullary thick ascending limbs of Henle's loop. *J Clin Invest* 66:792, 1980

146. SASAKI S, IMAI M: Effects of vasopressin on water and NaCl transport across the *in vitro* perfused medullary thick ascending limbs of Henle's loop of mouse, rat and rabbit kidneys. *Pflügers Arch* 383:215, 1980

147. HEBERT SC, CULPEPPER RM, ANDREOLI TE: NaCl transport in mouse medullary thick ascending limbs. I. Functional nephron heterogeneity and ADH-stimulated NaCl cotransport. *Am J Physiol* 10:F412, 1981

148. PETERS G, ROCH-RAMEL F: Renal effects of posterior pituitary peptides and their derivatives, in *Pharmacology of the Endocrine System and Related Drugs: The Neurohypophysis*. New York, Pergamon, 1970, p 229

149. ROCHA AS, KOKKO JP: Sodium chloride and water transport in the medullary thick ascending limb of Henle. Evidence for active chloride transport. *J Clin Invest* 52:612, 1973

150. HEBERT SC, CULPEPPER RM, ANDREOLI TE: NaCl transport in mouse medullary thick ascending limbs. III. Modulation of the ADH effect by peritubular osmolality. *Am J Physiol: Renal Fluid Electrolyte Physiol* 10:F443, 1981

151. MARSH DJ, AZEN SP: Mechanism of NaCl reabsorption by hamster thin ascending limbs of Henle's loop. *Am J Physiol* 228:71, 1975

152. MOFFAT DB, FOURMAN J: The vascular pattern of the rat kidney. *J Anat* 97:543, 1963

153. GANOTE CE, GRANTHAM JJ, MOSES HL, BURG MB, ORLOFF J: Ultrastructural studies of vasopressin effect on isolated perfused renal collecting tubules of the rabbit. *J Cell Biol* 36:355, 1968

154. GRANTHAM JJ, GANOTE CE, BURG MB, ORLOFF J: Paths of transtubular water flow in isolated renal collecting tubules. *J Cell Biol* 41:562, 1968

155. SCHAFER JA, ANDREOLI TE: Cellular constraints to diffusion: The effect of antidiuretic hormone on water flows in isolated mammalian collecting tubules. *J Clin Invest* 51:1264, 1972

156. GRANTHAM JJ, BURG MB: Effect of vasopressin and cyclic AMP on permeability of isolated collecting tubules. *Am J Physiol* 211:255, 1966

157. MACROBBIE EAC, USSING HH: Osmotic behavior of epithelial cells of frog skin. *Acta Physiol Scand* 53:348, 1961

158. MAFFLY RH, HAYS RM, LAMDIN E, LEAF A: The effect of neurohypophyseal hormones on the permeability of the toad bladder to urea. *J Gen Physiol* 39:630, 1960

159. HAYS RM, LEAF A: Studies on the movement of water through the isolated toad bladder and its modification by vasopressin. *J Gen Physiol* 45:904, 1962

160. LEAF A, HAYS RM: Permeability of the isolated toad bladder to solutes and its modification by vasopressin. *J Gen Physiol* 45:921, 1962

161. LEVINE S, FRANKI N, HAYS RM: Effect of phloretin on water and solute movement in the toad bladder. *J Clin Invest* 52:1435, 1973

162. LEVINE SD, LEVINE RD, WORTHINGTON RE, HAYS RM: Selective inhibition of osmotic water flow by methoxyfluorane and halothane. *Clin Res* 23:432, 1975

163. SCHAFER JA, TROUTMAN SL, ANDREOLI TE: Osmosis in cortical collecting tubules: ADH-independent osmotic flow rectification. *J Gen Physiol* 64:228, 1974

164. SCHAFER JA, ANDREOLI TE: The effect of antidiuretic hormone on solute flows in mammalian collecting tubules. *J Clin Invest* 51:1279, 1972

165. HAYS RM, LEVINE SD: Vasopressin. *Kidney Int* 6:307, 1974

166. ANDREOLI TE, SCHAFER JA: Mass transport across cell membranes: The effects of antidiuretic hormone on water and solute flow in epithelia. *Annu Rev Physiol* 39:451, 1976

167. LEVINE S, FRANKI N, HAYS RM: A saturable, vasopressin-sensitive carrier for urea and acetamide in the toad bladder epithelial cell. *J Clin Invest* 52:2083, 1973

168. PAPPENHEIMER JR, RENKIN EM, BONERO LM: Filtration, diffusion, and molecular sieving through peripheral capillary membranes. *Am J Physiol* 167:13, 1951

169. KOEFOED-JOHNSON V, USSING HH: The contributions of diffusion and flow to the passage of D_2O through living membranes. *Acta Physiol Scand* 28:60, 1953

170. HOLZ R, FINKELSTEIN A: The water and nonelectrolyte permeability induced in thin lipid membranes by the polyene antibiotics nystatin and amphotericin B. *J Gen Physiol* 56:125, 1970

171. DAINTY J: Water relations of plant cells. *Adv Bot Res* 1:279, 1963

172. CASS A, FINKELSTEIN A: Water permeability of thin lipid membranes. *J Gen Physiol* 50:1765, 1967

173. ANDREOLI TE, TROUTMAN SL: An analysis of unstirred layers in series with "tight" and "porous" lipid bilayer membranes. *J Gen Physiol* 57:464, 1971

174. HEBERT SC, ANDREOLI TE: Interactions of temperature and ADH on transport processes in cortical collecting tubules. *Am J Physiol: Renal Fluid Electrolyte Physiol* 7:F470, 1980

175. LEA EJA: Permeation through long narrow pores. *J Theor Biol* 5:102, 1963

176. AL-ZAHID G, SCHAFER JA, TROUTMAN SL, ANDREOLI TE: The effect of antidiuretic hormone on water and solute permeation and the activation energies for these processes, in mammalian cortical collecting tubules: Evidence for parallel ADH-sensitive pathways for water and soluble diffusion in luminal plasma membranes. *J Memb Biol* 31:103, 1977

177. KACHADORIAN WA, WADE JB, UITERWYK LC, DISCALA VA: Membrane structural and functional responses to vasopressin in toad bladder. *J Memb Biol* 30:381, 1977

178. KACHADORIAN WA, MULLER J, RUDICH S, DISCALA VA: Relation of ADH effects to altered membrane fluidity in toad urinary bladder. *Am J Physiol* 240:F63, 1981

179. HARMANCI MC, STEIN P, KACHADORIAN WA, VALTIN H, DISCALA VA: Vasopressin and collecting duct intramembraneous particle clusters: A dose-responsive relationship. *Am J Physiol: Renal Fluid Electrolyte Physiol* 8:F560, 1980

180. SUTHERLAND EW: The biological role of adenosine-3'5'-phosphate. *Harvey Lect* 57:17, 1962

181. ORLOFF J, HANDLER JS: The similarity of effects of vasopressin adenosine-3',5'-monophosphate (cyclic AMP) and theophylline on the toad bladder. *J Clin Invest* 41:702, 1962

182. MENDOZA SA, HANDLER JS, ORLOFF J: Effect of inhibitors of sodium transport on response of toad bladder to ADH and cyclic AMP. *Am J Physiol* 219:1440, 1970

183. GRANTHAM JJ, ORLOFF J: Effect of prostaglandin E_1 on the permeability response of the isolated collecting tubule to vasopressin, adenosine 3',5'-monophosphate and theophylline. *J Clin Invest* 47:1154, 1968

184. BARRACLOUGH MA, JONES NF: Effects of adenosine 3',5'-monophosphate on renal function in the rabbit. *Br J Pharmacol* 40:334, 1970

185. CAMPBELL BJ, WOODWARD G, BORBERG V: Calcium-mediated interactions between antidiuretic hormone and renal plasma membranes. *J Biol Chem* 247:6167, 1972

186. DOUSA TP: Effect of renal medullary solutes on vasopressin-sensitive adenyl cyclase. *Am J Physiol* 222:657, 1972

187. DOUSA TP, WALTER R, SCHWARTZ IL, SANDS H, HECHTER O: Role of cyclic AMP in the action of neurohypophyseal hormones on kidney. *Adv Cyclic Nucleotide Res* 1:121, 1972

188. CHASE IR, AURBACH GD: Renal adenyl cyclase: Anatomically separate sites for parathyroid hormone and vasopressin. *Science* 159:545, 1968

189. BOCKAERT J, ROY C, RAJERISON R, JARD S: Specific binding of (^{3}H) lysine-vasopressin to pig kidney plasma membranes. Relationship of receptor occupancy to adenylate cyclase activation. *J Biol Chem* 248:5922, 1973

190. SCHWARTZ IL, SHLATZ LJ, KINNE-SAFFRAN E, KINNE R: Target cell polarity and membrane phosphorylation in relation to the mechanism of action of antidiuretic hormone. *Proc Natl Acad Sci* 71:2595, 1974

191. RAJERISON R, MARCHETTI J, ROY C, BOCKART J, JARD S: The vasopressin-sensitive adenylate cyclase of the rat kidney. *J Biol Chem* 249:6390, 1974

192. ORLOFF J, HANDLER JS: The role of adenosine 3',5'-phosphate in the action of antidiuretic hormone. *Am J Med* 42:757, 1967

193. ORLOFF J, HANDLER JS, BERSTROM S: Effect of prostaglandin (PGE) on the permeability response of the toad bladder to vasopressin, theophylline and adenosine 3'−5'-monophosphate. *Nature* 205:397, 1965

194. GRANTHAM JJ, ORLOFF J: Effect of prostaglandin E₁ on the permeability response of the isolated collecting tubule to vasopressin, adenosine 3'–5'-monophosphate and theophylline. J Clin Invest 47:1154, 1968

195. ORLOFF J, ZUSMAN R: Role of prostaglandin E (PGE) in the modulation of the action of vasopressin on water flow in the urinary bladder of the toad and mammalian kidney. J Memb Biol 40:279, 1978

196. JACKSON BA, EDWARDS RM, DOUSA TP: Vasopressin-prostaglandin interactions in isolated tubules from rat outer medulla. J Lab Clin Med 96:119, 1980

197. ANDERSON RJ, BERL T, McDONALD KM, SCHRIER RW: Evidence for an in vivo antagonism between vasopressin and prostaglandins in the mammalian kidney. J Clin Invest 56:420, 1975

198. TÓTH-FEJES G, MAGYAR A, WALTER J: Renal response to vasopressin after inhibition of prostaglandin synthesis. Am J Physiol 232:F416, 1977

199. FICHMAN M, ZIA P, ZIPSER R: Contribution of urine volume to the elevated urinary prostaglandin E in Bartter's syndrome and central and nephrogenic diabetes insipidus, in Samuelson B, Ramwell P, Paoletti R (eds): Advances in Prostaglandin and Thromboxane Research, New York, Raven, 1980, p 1193

200. USBERTI M, DECHAUX M, GUILLOT M, SELIGMANN R, PAULOVITCH H, LOIRAT C, SACHS C, BROYER M: Renal prostaglandin E₂ in nephrogenic diabetes insipidus: Effects of inhibition of prostaglandin synthesis by indomethacin. J Pediatr 97:476, 1980

201. BLACHAR Y, ZADIK Z, SHEMESH M, KAPLAN BS, LEVIN S: The effect of inhibition of prostaglandin synthesis on free water and osmolar clearances in patients with hereditary nephrogenic diabetes insipidus. Int J Pediatr Nephrol 1:48, 1980

202. HANDLER JS, ORLOFF J: Factors involved in the action of cyclic AMP on the permeability of mammalian kidney and toad urinary bladder. Ann NY Acad Sci 185:345, 1971

203. DOUSA TP, BARNES LD: Effects of colchicine and vinblastine on the cellular action of vasopressin in mammalian kidney. J Clin Invest 54:252, 1974

204. TAYLOR A, MAMELAK M, REAVEN E, MAFFLY R: Vasopressin: Possible role of microtubules and microfilaments in its action. Science 181:347, 1973

205. VAN EPS LWS, PINEDO-VEELS C, DE VRIES GH, DE KONING J: Nature of concentrating defect in sickle-cell nephropathy. Lancet 1:450, 1970

206. DE WARDENER HE, HERXHEIMER A: The effect of a high water intake on the kidney's ability to concentrate the urine in man. J Physiol 139:42, 1957

207. BENNETT CM: Urine concentration and dilution in hypokalemic and hypercalcemic dogs. J Clin Invest 49:1447, 1970

208. EKNOYAN G, SUKI WN, MARTINEZ-MALDONADO M, ANHALT MA: Chronic hydronephrosis: Observations on the mechanism of the defect in urine concentration. Proc Soc Exp Biol Med 134:634, 1970

209. FICHMAN MP, BROOKER G: Deficient renal cyclic adenosine 3'–5' monophosphate production in nephrogenic diabetes insipidus. J Clin Endocrinol Metab 35:35, 1972

210. BELL NH, CLARK CM, AVERY S, SINHA T, TRYGSTAD CW, ALLEN DO: Demonstration of a defect in the formation of adenosine 3',5'-monophosphate in vasopressin-resistant diabetes insipidus. Pediatr Res 8:223, 1974

211. MONN E, OSNES JB, ØYE I: Basal and hormone-induced urinary cyclic AMP in children with renal disorders. Acta Pediatr Scand 65:739, 1976

212. UTTLEY WS, ATKINSON B, ADAMS A, SHIRLING D: Cyclic adenosine monophosphate excretion in urine of patients and carriers of congenital nephrogenic diabetes insipidus. J Inher Metab Dis 1:75, 1978

213. CHASE LR, AURBACH GD: Renal adenyl cyclase; anatomically separate sites for parathyroid hormone and vasopressin. Science 159:545, 1968

214. SOBER AJ, GORDEN P: Pituitary responsiveness to aqueous vasopressin in patients with congenital vasopressin-resistant diabetes insipidus. J Clin Endocrinol Metab 35:924, 1972

215. NAIK DV, VALTIN H: Hereditary vasopressin-resistant urinary concentrating defects in mice. Am J Physiol 217:1183, 1969

216. VIRGO NS, MILLER JR: Hereditary vasopressin-resistant diabetes insipidus in SWV mice. Can J Physiol Pharmacol 52:995, 1974

217. DOUSA TP, VALTIN H: Cellular action of antidiuretic hormone in mice with inherited vasopressin-resistant urinary concentrating defects. J Clin Invest 54:753, 1974

218. JACKSON BA, EDWARDS RM, VALTIN H, DOUSA TP: Cellular action of vasopressin in medullary tubules of mice with hereditary nephrogenic diabetes insipidus. J Clin Invest 66:110, 1980

219. HAYEK A, RAMIREZ J: Demeclocycline-induced diabetes insipidus. JAMA 229:676, 1974

220. WILSON DM, PERRY HO, SAMS WM JR, DOUSA TP: Selective inhibition of human distal tubular function by demeclocycline. Curr Ther Res 15:734, 1973

221. SINGER I, ROTENBERG D: Demeclocycline-induced nephrogenic diabetes insipidus. Ann Intern Med 79:679, 1973

222. FELDMAN HA, SINGER I: Comparative effects of tetracyclines on water flow across toad urinary bladders. J Pharmacol Exp Ther 190:358, 1974

223. SINGER I, FORREST JN: Drug-induced states of nephrogenic diabetes insipidus. Kidney Int 10:82, 1976

224. DOUSA TP, WILSON DM: Effects of demethylchlortetracycline on cellular action of antidiuretic hormone in vitro. Kidney Int 5:279, 1974

225. COUSINS MJ, MAZZE RI: Methoxyflurane nephrotoxicity. JAMA 225:1611, 1973

226. MAZZE RI, COUSINS MJ, KOSEK JC: Dose-related methoxyflurane nephrotoxicity in rats: A biochemical and pathologic correlation. Anesthesiology 36:571, 1972

227. COUSINS MJ, MAZZE RI, KOSEK JC, HITT BA, LOVE FV: The etiology of methoxyflurane nephrotoxicity. J Pharmacol Exp Ther 190:530, 1974

228. FRASCINO JA, O'FLAHERTY J, OLMO C, RIVERA S: Effect of inorganic fluoride on the renal concentrating mechanism. Possible nephrotoxicity in man. J Lab Clin Med 79:192, 1972

229. WALLIN JD, KAPLAN RA: Effect of sodium fluoride on concentrating and diluting ability in the rat. Am J Physiol 232:F335, 1977

230. LEE RV, JAMPOL LM, BROWN WV: Nephrogenic diabetes insipidus and lithium intoxication - complications of lithium carbonate therapy. N Engl J Med 284:93, 1971

231. SINGER I, ROTENBERG D, PUSCHETT JB: Lithium-induced nephrogenic diabetes insipidus: In vivo and in vitro studies. J Clin Invest 51:1081, 1972

232. FORREST JN JR, COHEN AD, TORETTI J, HIMMELHOCH JM, EPSTEIN FH: On the mechanism of lithium-induced diabetes insipidus in man and the rat. J Clin Invest 53:1115, 1974

233. PADFIELD PL, PARK SJ, MORTON JJ, BRAIDWOOD AE: Plasma levels of antidiuretic hormone in patients receiving prolonged lithium therapy. Br J Psychiat 130:144, 1977

234. DOUSA TP: Interaction of lithium with vasopressin-sensitive cyclic AMP system of human renal medulla. Endocrinology 95:1359, 1974

235. GEISLER A, WRAAE O, OLESEN OV: Adenyl cyclase activity in kidneys of rats with lithium-induced polyuria. Acta Pharmacol Toxicol 31:203, 1972

236. JACKSON BA, EDWARDS RM, DOUSA TP: Lithium-induced polyuria: Effect of lithium on adenylate cyclase and adenosine 3',5'-monophosphate phosphodiesterase in medullary ascending limb of Henle's loop and in medullary collecting tubules. Endocrinology 107:1693, 1980

237. GALLA JN, FORREST JN, HECHT B, KASHGARIAN M, HAYSLETT JP: Effect of lithium on water and electrolyte metabolism. Yale J Biol Med 48:305, 1975.

238. HOCHMAN S, GUTMAN Y: Lithium: ADH antagonism and ADH independent action in rats with diabetes insipidus. Eur J Pharmacol 28:100, 1974

239. CARONE FA, EPSTEIN FH: Nephrogenic diabetes insipidus caused by amyloid disease: Evidence in man of the role of the collecting ducts in concentrating urine. Am J Med 29:539, 1960

240. DORHOUT MEES EJ, DEPLANQUE BA, HELDERS J, KOOIKER CJ: Renal amyloidosis presenting as water losing syndrome. Nephron 5:31, 1968

241. KAHN M, MERRITT AD, WOHL MJ, ORLOFF J: Renal concentrating defect in Sjören's syndrome. Ann Intern Med 56:883, 1962

242. FICHMAN M, ZIPSER R, KAYE Z, LEE A, ZIA P: Antidiuresis with suppression of elevated urinary prostaglandin E (PGE) by ibuprofen in nephrogenic diabetes insipidus (NDI) and 1-desamino-8-D-arginine vasopressin (DDAVP) in primary diabetes insipidus (DI). (abstr) VIIth Int Congress of Nephrol: Q-2, Montreal, June 18–23, 1978

243. JONES NF, BARRACLOUGH MA, BARNES N, COTTOM DG: Nephrogenic diabetes insipidus: Effects of 3,5, cyclic-adenosine monophosphate. Arch Dis Child 47:794, 1972

244. PROESMANS W, EGGERMONT E, VANDERSCHUEREN-LODEWEYCKX M, TIDDENS H, EECKELS R: The effect of exogenous 3':5'-adenosine monophosphate on urinary output in children with vasopressin-resistant diabetes insipidus. Pediatr Res 9:509, 1975

245. STERN P, VALTIN H: Lack of clear-cut antidiuretic effect on 8-p-chlorophenylthio cyclic AMP. Mineral Electrolyte Metab 1:330, 1978

246. CRAWFORD JD, KENNEDY GC: Chlorothiazide in diabetes insipidus. Nature 183:891, 1959

247. BLALOCK T, GERRON G. QUITER E, RUDMAN D: Role of diet in the management of vasopressin-responsive and -resistant diabetes insipidus. Am J Clin Nutr 30:1070, 1977

87

CYSTIC FIBROSIS

RICHARD C. TALAMO

BERYL J. ROSENSTEIN

RONALD W. BERNINGER

1. Cystic fibrosis (CF) is the most common lethal or semi-lethal genetic disease in the Caucasian population, with prevalence of about 1:2000 live births in the United States. It is inherited in an autosomal recessive pattern. Heterozygotes are clinically unaffected. No reliable screening test is yet available for the CF gene, for prenatal diagnosis, or for heterozygote detection.

2. Clinically, CF is a generalized disease of exocrine glands. Unusually thick mucous secretions in many organs are associated with (a) chronic obstructive lung disease with predominant airways involvement, recurrent and persistent infections, especially with Pseudomonas and Staphylcoccus, leading to respiratory failure and death, often accompanied by cor pulmonale; (b) exocrine pancreatic insufficiency with steatorrhea and azotorrhea; (c) intestinal obstruction in the neonate (meconium ileus) or later in life; (d) cirrhosis of the liver; (e) infertility, especially in males; and (f) abnormally high sweat sodium and chloride, resulting from failure of salt reabsorption in sweat gland ducts.

3. Diagnosis is made by the clinical features of chronic lung disease, pancreatic insufficiency, and postive family history and is confirmed by abnormal sweat test results, showing elevated sodium or chloride concentrations, or both.

4. Treatment involves a comprehensive team approach which deals with the pulmonary disease, the pancreatic insufficiency, and other gastrointestinal manifestations, as well as the psychosocial problems imposed by the disease.

5. Prognosis has greatly improved, leading to large numbers of adolescent and adult patients.

6. The metabolic defect remains unknown, yet many clues are available. Large numbers of potential "genetic markers" have been studied. Molecules of up to 10,000 daltons are present in the plasma or other extracellular fluids of CF homozygotes and heterozygotes. These molecules inhibit sodium transport or induce mucus production and alter ciliary function. Lectinlike substances appear to be present in some body fluids, and deficiency in an arginine esterase enzymatic activity has been described. Abnormalities are present in polyamine metabolism, and a "CF protein" has been demonstrated by isoelectric focusing.

7. CF cells are characterized in studies in vitro by increased amounts of glycogen, abnormalities in fucose handling, and abnormalities in some ion transport systems, especially the Ca^{2+}-Mg^{2+} ATPase.

8. Abnormalities in autonomic nervous system function have been found in clinical studies.

9. Several of the clinical features of CF are available for study in various animal models, such as the chronically reserpinized rat, but a perfect animal model has not yet been found.

Cystic fibrosis (CF) is the most common lethal or semilethal genetic disease affecting Caucasians. It is transmitted in an autosomal recessive manner. The triad of chronic obstructive pulmonary disease, pancreatic exocrine deficiency, and abnormally high sweat electrolytes is present in most patients. It is the major cause of chronic debilitating pulmonary disease and pancreatic exocrine deficiency during the first three decades of life in the United States and accounts for a significant number of cases of neonatal intestinal obstruction. Heterozygotes have no recognizable clinical symptoms.

Although mentioned in folklore and early medical literature, CF was first reported by Fanconi [1] in 1936. Initially, it was thought to involve primarily the pancreas, but soon researchers realized that many of the clinical and pathologic findings might be explained by a generalized defect in mucous secretion [2]. With the discovery of the sweat gland defect in 1953 [3], it became apparent that there are abnormalities of all the exocrine glands. The basic biochemical defect is unknown. Most of the clinical manifestations can be related to abnormal secretions which result in obstruction of organ passages and abnormal function of the eccrine sweat glands [4]. The name of the disease is derived from the characteristic histologic changes seen in the pancreas (Fig. 87-1).

In this chapter we consider the clinical features and basic research aspects of CF, emphasizing the more recent literature that has appeared since the previous edition of this text. Earlier reviews [4, 5] and texts [6, 7] are also available.

CLINICAL FEATURES

Pulmonary Manifestations

General The respiratory tract is invariably involved, and pulmonary complications usually dominate the clinical picture. Autopsy studies suggest that the lungs are normal at birth [8]. The earliest histologic changes consist of dilatation, hypertrophy, and hyperplasia of the tracheobronchial submucosal glands [9, 10]. It has not been proved that the physical properties of uninfected CF mucus are altered, although it is thought that such secretions give rise to obstruction. The initial pulmonary lesion is obstruction of the small airways [10]. Secondary to obstruction, there is bronchiolitis and mucopurulent plugging of the airways [10, 11]. Bronchial changes are more common than parenchymal changes. The epithelium shows stratification, squamous metaplasia, loss of cilia, and goblet cell hyperplasia [11]. These changes are seen in 50 percent of infants who die before 4 months of age [11]. Squamous metaplasia and loss of cilia contribute to retention of secretions. Bronchiectasis is present in almost all patients past the age of 4 months. It is progressive with age and is especially striking in older patients [10, 11]. Although there is dilatation of air spaces, rarely is there more than minimal true emphysema, with destruction of alveolar walls [10, 11].

Fifty percent of patients present with pulmonary manifestations, usually consisting of chronic cough and wheezing in association with recurrent or chronic infection. Young infants may present with atelectasis, often involving the right upper lobe [12], or a severe bronchiolitic syndrome [13]. Other findings include a barrel-chest deformity, growth retardation, cyanosis, digital clubbing, and pulmonary hypertrophic osteoarthropathy. There is progressive shortness of breath and exercise intolerance. The course is characterized by chronic suppurative bronchitis, with exacerbations and airway obstruction. Pulmonary involvement progresses at a variable rate but eventually leads to respiratory or cardiac failure or both.

Pulmonary Function Airway obstruction, air trapping, and ventilation-perfusion inequalities are the most important functional changes in CF [14, 15]. The lungs may be physiologically normal at birth [16]. The initial functional abnormality is impairment of intrapulmonary gas distribution due to obstruction of the small airways [17–20]. Hypoxemia is due to alveolar hypoventilation, ventilation-perfusion inequalities, impaired diffusion, and right-to-left intrapulmonary shunts [15, 21]. Small airway obstruction is followed by air trapping [15], progressive loss of lung elastic recoil [22], and ventilation-perfusion inequalities [15]. Later, there is large airway obstruction because of dynamic compression of the airways during forced expiration [23] and, finally, increased resistance during quiet breathing resulting from intraluminal obstruction [23]. Other abnormalities include increases in airway resistance, residual volume, and the ratio of residual volume to total lung capacity and decreases in vital capacity and lung compliance [14]. Because of trapped gas, lung volume is more accurately measured by plethysmography than helium dilution [17]. There is wide variation in the long-term course of pulmonary function in CF [24]. Some patients retain near-normal function over a 5- to 7-year period. In general, there is an exponential decline in function of approximately 8 percent per year, with a steeper rate of decline in females than in males.

Radiographic Changes Hyperinflation and bronchial wall thickening are the earliest radiographic findings. Persistent air trapping in infancy is highly suggestive of CF [25]. Subsequent changes include areas of infiltrate, atelectasis, and hilar adenopathy. The upper lobes and middle lobe are often most severely involved. With advanced disease there are bleb formation, extensive bronchiectasis, and pulmonary artery and cardiac enlargement [25] (Fig. 87-2). Branching, fingerlike opacifications, representing mucoid impaction of the bronchi,

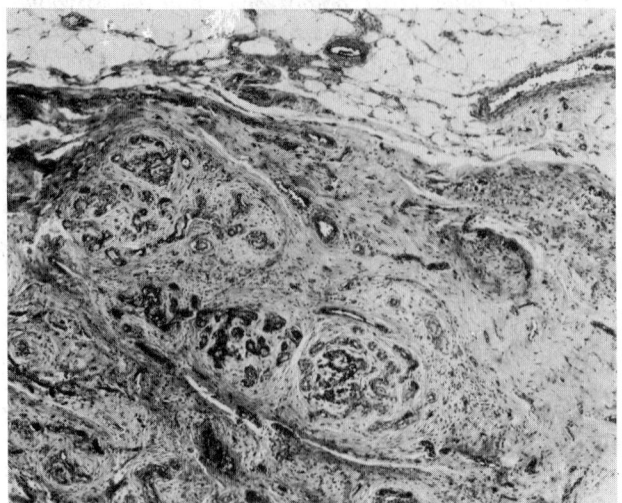

Figure 87-1 Histologic section of pancreas from 12-year-old girl which shows changes typical of CF, including: extensive fibrosis of acini, dilatation of ductules, plugs within acini, and focal acinar calcifications (H & E, ×310).

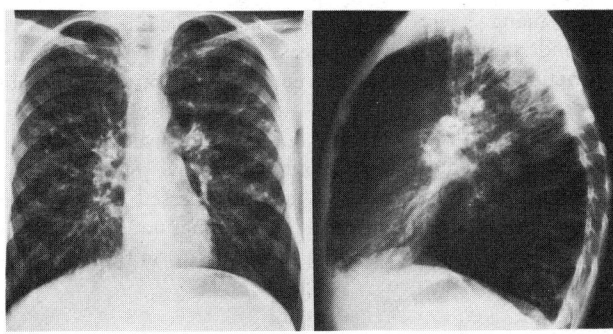

Figure 87-2 Advanced changes of CF seen on this chest radiograph include: hyperinflation, bronchial wall thickening due to bronchiectasis, mucous plugs, and enlarged hila probably due to large pulmonary arteries.

are characteristic of CF [26]. Ventilation-perfusion scans usually demonstrate focal areas of inequality [27] and may be useful in selecting candidates for lung resection. Bronchography is rarely indicated [5].

Infection The major pulmonary problem is chronic infection, particularly with *Staphylococcus aureus* and *Pseudomonas aeruginosa* [28–30]. Infection tends to remain localized to the respiratory tract. Septicemia and extrapulmonary infections are rare [29–32]. Initially, *S. aureus* was the most significant pathogen, but in recent years it has been replaced by *P. aeruginosa* [33]. With advanced disease, over 80 percent of patients consistently harbor *Pseudomonas* strains, the majority of which are heavy slime producers known as mucoid variants and are rarely found in other diseases [29, 30, 33]. Once established, *Pseudomonas* is virtually impossible to eradicate [30]. Precipitins against *P. aeruginosa* are found predominantly in those patients harboring mucoid strains and are associated with a more severe course [29]. The peculiar susceptibility of these patients to infection with mucoid *Pseudomonas* variants is not understood. It may be related to the antibiotic suppression of other bacteria and the antiphagocytic properties of mucoid substance [33, 34]. Systemic defense mechanisms are intact [29] (see below). There is no evidence of a generalized defect in mucociliary clearance [35], although it may be altered secondary to bronchial obstruction. There may be impairment of local immunity in the lung [29]. Pulmonary alveolar macrophages are intrinsically normal, but phagocytosis and killing of *P. aeruginosa* can be inhibited in the presence of CF serum [36]. There is progressive and specific lymphocyte unresponsiveness to *P. aeruginosa* in patients in poor clinical condition [37]. No specific phage types of *S. aureus* have been associated with CF. Thymidine-dependent strains have been reported [38]. The development of staphylococcal precipitins can be prevented by continuous antistaphylococcal chemotherapy [39]. The role of other pathogens in CF is less well-defined. In one study, one-third of respiratory exacerbations were associated with serologic evidence of a respiratory virus infection [40]. *Haemophilus influenzae,* especially type I, is frequently isolated [41], and precipitins against *Haemophilus* have been demonstrated in up to 80 percent of patients [42]. The role of this organism is still unclear. *Candida* colonization of the tracheobronchial tree is common, but pulmonary candidiasis is rare [43].

Allergy The role of allergy in CF is not well-defined. Chronic cough, wheezing, rhinitis, and nasal polyps are com-

mon to both CF and allergy [44]. Depending on the criteria used, the prevalence of atopy in patients with CF ranges from 10 to 70 percent [44–48]. The higher figures are attributable to a high incidence of mold sensitivity [46, 47]. There is controversy as to whether coexisting atopy moderates [44] or worsens [45, 46] the underlying pulmonary disease. Serum precipitins and positive skin test results to *Aspergillus fumigatus* are common [45–47], and through use of selective media, this organism can be cultured from up to 57 percent of patients [46]. The significance of fungi in the pathogenesis of lung injury is not clear, but allergic bronchopulmonary aspergillosis has been described in a few patients [5, 46]. Type III mediated complement-dependent histamine release secondary to *Pseudomonas* infection might be responsible for allergic-inflammatory lung damage [49]. Immune complexes have been detected in sputum, lung, and serum samples from patients with advanced disease [50]. Cutaneous necrotizing venulitis may occur in association with these complexes [51]. Although serum immunoglobulins are normal or elevated in older patients [52], hypogammaglobulinemia-G has been reported in younger patients with less severe pulmonary involvement [53]. This suggests that progression of lung disease may be due, in part, to a hyperimmune response.

Treatment Treatment of the pulmonary manifestations of CF is directed at clearance of excess mucus from the tracheobronchial tree and aggressive antimicrobial therapy. Except in the case of acute respiratory illnesses, guidelines for the use of antibiotics in patients with CF are not well established [5]. In some centers, patients are maintained continuously on one or more agents, usually directed against *S. aureus, H. influenzae,* or both. In other centers, antimicrobial therapy is used only for respiratory exacerbations. Patients who do not respond to outpatient management are usually hospitalized for intensive antibiotic therapy, primarily directed against *Pseudomonas*. This approach is supported by the results of double-blind trials [54, 55]. Patients with CF show enhanced renal excretion of some penicillins and may require large doses to achieve optimal serum levels [56]. They may also require high doses of aminoglycosides to achieve acceptable serum concentrations [57].

Chest physiotherapy is used to enhance the removal of bronchial secretions. Treatments are carried out several times each day, depending on the degree of pulmonary involvement. Physical activity may be a useful adjunct to physiotherapy [58]. Although a variety of aerosolized agents have been used in CF, evidence to support their efficacy is largely anecdotal [59]. In some patients these agents may lead to reflex bronchoconstriction and worsening of pulmonary function. There are no data to document the efficacy of bland aerosols and aerosolized antimicrobials [59]. Earlier reports of improved pulmonary function following the use of nocturnal mist tent therapy [60] have not been confirmed [61], and this form of therapy has largely been abandoned. Aerosolized bronchodilators may be useful. The response of CF patients is highly variable [62], and these agents should be used only after documenting a beneficial response by pulmonary function testing.

There are no data to support the use of oral expectorants. Tracheobronchial lavage has been used in an effort to remove bronchial secretions [63], but, in a controlled trial, it was no more effective than conventional therapy [64]. Therapeutic bronchoscopy has been performed in patients with lobar and segmental atelectasis, but the results are no better than those obtained with intensified medical therapy alone [65]. Intermittent positive pressure breathing may worsen chest overinflation and is usually contraindicated. Surgical treatment of pulmonary complications is rarely undertaken since lung involvement is usually generalized, but lobectomy or segmental resection may be useful in selected cases of persistent atelectasis and localized bronchiectasis [66]. In general, assisted ventilation is not indicated for CF patients with respiratory failure [67]. Its use should be restricted to the occasional patient with good base line status in whom acute respiratory failure develops, or it should be used in association with pulmonary surgery.

Complications

PNEUMOTHORAX In patients with advanced lung disease, pneumothorax, hemoptysis, and cor pulmonale are frequent complications [68]. The overall incidence of pneumothorax is 2 to 10 percent [69–71] and in adults is as high as 16 percent [68]. Occasionally, a tension pneumothorax occurs which may lead to sudden death [71]. Conventional therapy, consisting of closed thoracotomy drainage and the intrapleural installation of sclerosing agents, has been associated with persistent air leaks, prolonged hospitalization, and a high rate of recurrence [69–71]. Because of these complications, open thoracotomy with pleural abrasion and resection of blebs has been recommended as an alternative for initial therapy [69, 70].

HEMOPTYSIS Massive hemoptysis is a serious complication associated with significant mortality [72], a high recurrence rate [73], and poor prognosis [68, 73]. In one series, mean survival from the initial episode was 3.3 years [68]. Bleeding is due to erosion of the bronchial arteries into a bronchus, often in association with an exacerbation of the underlying pulmonary infection [72]. The site of bleeding is best localized by bronchoscopy [74]. In patients with protracted or recurrent episodes of bleeding, segmental resection [74], bronchial artery ligation [74], and endobronchial balloon tamponade [75] have been used successfully. More recently, bleeding has been effectively controlled by percutaneous catheter embolization of the involved bronchial arteries [76].

COR PULMONALE Manifested by hypertrophy of the right ventricle, cor pulmonale is seen in 70 percent of patients dying with CF and occurs in almost one-half of patients surviving past age 15 [77]. Chronic alveolar hypoxia and hypoxemia probably serve as a stimulus to reflex vasoconstriction [78] and medial hypertrophy of the pulmonary arterioles [9]. Severe cor pulmonale has been consistently associated with P_aO_2 values of less than 50 mmHg [79]. Clinically, it may be difficult to recognize cor pulmonale and right-sided failure. Peripheral edema is present in only two-thirds of cases [77] and is often a late manifestation. The electrocardiogram and vectorcardiogram do not consistently correlate with the presence of right ventricular hypertrophy [77, 80]. Aside from the direct measurement of pulmonary artery pressure, echocardiography is the most practical and reliable means of documenting cor pulmonale and following its course [80, 81]. Cardiac function can be further assessed noninvasively by means of radionuclide angiography [82]. Left ventricular hypertrophy and dysfunction may also be present [77, 80, 82], especially in patients with advanced disease. Areas of necrosis and fibrosis are present in the left ventricle of some patients [9, 83], but the clinical significance of these findings is not known.

The management of right-sided failure includes therapy of the underlying pulmonary disease along with diuretics, salt-restriction, digitalis, and oxygen [77]. The results have not been favorable. Mean survival after the onset of cardiac dilatation is 8 months [77] and has not been improved with the use of digitalis. In adults with chronic obstructive pulmonary disease, pulmonary hypertension may be reversed by long-term continuous oxygen therapy [84], but this has not been demonstrated in CF, and the role of oxygen therapy in these patients remains poorly defined.

Upper Respiratory Tract Manifestations

The upper respiratory tract is usually affected, secondary to hyperactive mucus-secreting glands and hypertrophy and edema of the mucous membranes [85]. Radiographic evidence of opacification of the paranasal sinuses is present in almost all patients [86] and may be helpful diagnostically. Clinically significant sinusitis is less common. Nasal obstruction due to nasal polyps has been reported in 6 to 24 percent of patients [68, 85, 87]. Polyps occur at a much younger age in patients with CF as compared with those with underlying atopy [87], and the polyps from these two groups can be differentiated histologically [88]. The incidence of hearing problems is variable, depending on the criteria used [89, 90], but is probably no higher than in the general population [90].

Gastrointestinal Manifestations

Pancreas Morphologic changes in the pancreas vary and, in general, are more severe with increasing age [9]. Diagnostic pancreatic lesions may be absent at all ages, especially in newborns [91]. The earliest pancreatic lesion is focal inspissation of eosinophilic material in acini and ductules, with flattening of the epithelium. This leads to progressive dilatation of the acini and ductules, atrophy of acinar tissue, and eventually fibrosis (Fig. 87-1). Inflammation is not prominent.

The most prominent gastrointestinal manifestations result from the loss of pancreatic enzyme activity and consequent intestinal malabsorption of fats and proteins and, to a lesser extent, carbohydrates. Complete loss of pancreatic enzyme activity is seen in 80 to 85 percent of patients [92]. Loss of function may be progressive [93]. Clinical manifestations include poor or absent weight gain, abdominal distention, lack of subcutaneous fat and muscle tissue, passage of frequent pale, bulky, foul-smelling, and often oily stools, and rectal prolapse [92]. Steatorrhea and azotorrhea are pronounced. Although many infants appear to have a voracious appetite, caloric intake is often deficient [94]. In older patients there may be absence of a pubertal growth spurt and delayed maturation [95]. In general, growth retardation correlates most closely with the degree of pulmonary involvement [95]. There is no correlation between the degree of pancreatic achylia and pulmonary manifestations. Adolescents and young adults with residual pancreatic function may have recurrent episodes of pancreatitis, sometimes as the presenting manifestation [96].

Tests of fat absorption, including 72-h fecal fat excretion, provide an indirect assessment of pancreatic exocrine function. The most direct measure of exocrine function involves analysis of duodenal fluid before and after the intravenous injection of pancreozymin and secretin [97]. In patients with CF, volume and bicarbonate secretion (ductular activity) are grossly reduced, irrespective of the presence of steatorrhea [97]. In those patients with steatorrhea, enzyme secretion (acinar activity) is virtually absent. Ductular activity is more regularly affected than acinar activity [97]. This differs from other forms of exocrine pancreatic insufficiency in which enzyme secretion is more affected than water and bicarbonate secretion. Less invasive means of assessing pancreatic enzyme function include: (1) measurement of stool trypsin and chymotrypsin [98], (2) demonstration of a quantitative decrease in serum pancreatic isoamylase [99] or a relative diminution of serum pancreatic isoamylase bands when compared with salivary isoamylase bands [100], and (3) the urinary excretion of *p*-aminobenzoic acid after the oral administration of synthetic chymotrypsin substrates containing *p*-aminobenzoic acid [101].

TREATMENT   Pancreatic enzyme supplements, consisting of animal pancreas, constitute the primary therapy of the pancreatic enzyme deficiency [92]. The most effective preparations consist of pancrelipase in pH-sensitive enteric-coated microspheres [102]. Following enzyme replacement, there is a reduction in the amount of both fat and nitrogen in the stools [103], although the values do not return to normal. Enzyme dosage is empirical. Complications of enzyme therapy include oral and perianal inflammation and, in parents exposed to powdered pancreatic extracts, the occurrence of immediate hypersensitivity reactions [104]. Hypersensitivity reactions are rare in patients themselves. The high purine content of pancreatic enzymes may lead to hyperuricosuria [105] and hyperuricemia [106] in patients taking large dosages. At autopsy, renal fibrosis and nonspecific renal tubular changes have been seen in some patients [107]. The persistence of steatorrhea, after enzyme replacement, may be due to enzyme inactivation by gastric acidity [108]. Addition of the H_2 receptor antagonist, cimetidine, may result in significant reduction in fecal fat and nitrogen excretion [109].

Effective enzyme therapy has resulted in less need for a low fat diet, although there is usually some attempt at fat reduction. Adequate calories must be provided to compensate for stool losses. Polycose and medium-chain triglyceride supplements can be used to increase caloric intake [94]. Artificial diets and supplements consisting of beef serum hydrolysate, glucose polymer, and medium-chain triglyceride have been associated with improved nutritional status [110] but have not been objectively evaluated. Secondary to pancreatic insufficiency and reduced dietary intake of fats, patients have low serum lipid levels and may be deficient in linoleic acid [111]. The clinical significance of this deficiency is not clear. Results of oral and intravenous supplementation with essential fatty acids have been inconclusive [111–114]. Early reports of decreases in sweat sodium concentrations after fatty acid supplements [111, 112] have not been confirmed [113, 114].

VITAMIN DEFICIENCY   With pancreatic achylia there is malabsorption of the fat-soluble vitamins. Low serum vitamin A levels are due to steatorrhea and a depression of retinol-carrier protein and retinol-binding protein [115]. Xerophthalmia and night blindness occur rarely, usually in association with hepatic involvement [116]. A bulging fontanelle, secondary to vitamin A deficiency, may be the presenting manifestation in infancy [117]. Overt rickets is rare [118], but a significant reduction in vitamin D biologic activity, with associated secondary hyperparathyroidism and reduced bone mineral content, is common [119]. Serum levels of 25-hydroxyvitamin A

are variable but may be reduced [119–121], and significant demineralization is present in up to 44 percent of patients [122]. Severe bleeding associated with hypoprothrombinemia and deficiency of clotting factors II, VII, IX, and X may occur in infants secondary to vitamin K deficiency [123, 124]. The diagnosis of CF should be considered in any infant with hypoprothrombinemia. In all patients with pancreatic achylia, there is a marked reduction in plasma α-tocopherol levels [125]. Red blood cells show increased peroxide-induced hemolysis and a moderate decrease in survival [125], although usually not sufficient to produce hemolytic anemia. Histologic evidence of vitamin E deficiency consists of focal necrosis of striated muscles and ceroid pigment deposition in intestinal smooth muscle [9]. There is severe depression of vitamin B_{12} absorption, which can be corrected by pancreatic enzymes [126]. Clinical manifestations of B_{12} deficiency are rare [127]. The requirements for other water-soluble vitamins are not well-defined. Vitamin deficiencies can be prevented by the daily administration of a water-miscible vitamin preparation [94]. Vitamin K is given prior to surgery and with hemoptysis or intensive antibiotic therapy. The clinical significance of vitamin E deficiency is not clear, but reversal of the hematologic abnormalities can be achieved with daily supplements [125].

HYPOPROTEINEMIA AND EDEMA   The syndrome of edema and hypoproteinemia, due to the defective digestion and absorption of protein secondary to pancreatic enzyme deficiency, may be the presenting manifestation in up to 8 percent of patients with CF [128, 129]. It is seen most often in infants 1 to 6 months of age who have been breast fed or given a soy-based formula. This may be related to an inadequate composition of soy protein [130] or to the presence of a trypsin inhibitor [131]. Other laboratory findings include elevation of liver enzymes and anemia [128, 129]. Falsely negative sweat test results can be seen in the presence of edema [128, 129]. Treatment consists of the use of an elemental formula or the addition of pancreatic enzymes to a cow's milk formula.

CARBOHYDRATE INTOLERANCE   In addition to pancreatic exocrine dysfunction, up to 40 percent of patients show carbohydrate intolerance [132] which progresses to frank diabetes in 1 to 2 percent of cases [133, 134]. The incidence of carbohydrate intolerance increases with age [132], but diabetes has been seen as early as 6 months [134]. Fasting hyperglycemia and glycosuria are present in 8 percent of adults [68]. Diabetes in these patients is characterized by insidious onset, mild clinical course, and absence of ketoacidosis [68, 132]. Retinopathy, nephropathy, neuropathy, and vascular changes are rarely seen [132, 135]. Histologically, the islets may show fragmentation, and they are surrounded and separated by bands of dense collagenous tissue [132]. Both beta and alpha cell functions are impaired. There is insulinopenia, with an absent or sluggish response to glucose [134, 136], along with a diminished capacity for glucagon secretion [137, 138]. Insulin output after tolbutamide or glucagon challenge is variable but subnormal [132, 136]. The mild course of diabetes in these patients may be due to a compensatory enhancement of peripheral tissue sensitivity to insulin, possibly related to an observed increase in the number of insulin receptor sites [139]. There may also be a decrease in the release of glucagonlike substances from the intestine [134]. The diabetes is usually easily managed by modest dietary changes along with low doses of insulin. Oral hypoglycemic agents have not been useful [5].

Meconium Ileus Meconium ileus, in which there is obstruction of the distal ileum by inspissated, tenacious meconium, occurs in 7 percent of newborn infants with CF [140]. With rare exceptions [141], meconium ileus is always associated with CF. The pathogenesis of the obstruction is unclear. It may be related to a deficiency of proteolytic enzymes *or* to secretion of abnormal mucoproteins by the goblet cells of the small intestine [142]. In 25 percent of infants with a history of meconium ileus there are no morphologic lesions of the pancreas [91]. Clinically, infants present with evidence of intestinal obstruction [143, 144] (Fig. 87-3). Associated intestinal complications, including small-bowel atresias, volvulus, and perforation/peritonitis, are present in 45 to 50 percent of the cases [143, 144]. There may be a tendency for meconium ileus to recur in the same family [145]. A delay in the passage of meconium and distal colonic obstruction secondary to the meconium plug syndrome may also be presenting manifestations of CF and are indications for a sweat test [146]. In uncomplicated cases of meconium ileus, the meconium can be removed nonoperatively by the use of Gastrografin enemas [147]. In patients in whom this procedure is unsuccessful, and in those with complications, it may be necessary to resect the involved segment of bowel [143, 144]. In some cases, mucolytics are used intraoperatively to liquefy the inspissated meconium [148] and may eliminate the need for intestinal resection. Patients who survive the newborn period have a prognosis similar to those patients without meconium ileus [143, 144].

Intestinal Complications After the newborn period, there are a variety of intestinal complications [92, 145]. Radiographically, duodenal abnormalities have been noted in 84 percent of patients, consisting of thickened mucosal folds, nodular filling defects, and mucosal smudging [149]. Although there is mucus hyperplasia of Brunner's glands, there is no correlation between the microscopic appearance of the duodenum and the radiographic findings [149]. Clinically, duodenal ulcers have been reported in only a small number of patients [92]. Radiographic abnormalities of the small bowel are uncommon [149], and the histology of the small bowel is normal [150, 151]. Decreased peptide hydrolase activity and decreased tissue accumulation of phenylalanine and cycloleucine [151] suggest that impairment of protein digestion may be partly of mucosal origin. This may be related to a thickened mucinous cover [152]. In 25 percent of patients there is a significant reduction in lactase activity [150, 151], probably as a

secondary phenomenon. Postprandial disacchariduria was found in 21 of 23 patients [153]. Most of the patients with lactase deficiency have been tolerant of milk [150, 151]. Both coeliac disease [154] and regional enteritis [155] have been reported in patients with CF.

As a result of the abnormal behavior of the secretions of the intestinal glands and the deficiency of pancreatic enzymes, the intestinal contents tend to be abnormally thick and puttylike and may lead to a variety of late intestinal complications [92, 145, 156]. There may be recurrent episodes of partial or complete obstruction of the small or large bowel, often preceded or accompanied by colicky abdominal pain and a palpable mass in the right lower quadrant. This symptom complex, referred to as *meconium ileus equivalent,* occurs in as many as 21 percent of older patients [68]. In uncomplicated cases, enemas with hyperosmolar contrast material (e.g., Gastrografin) may be therapeutic as well as diagnostic [156]. Other forms of therapy include increased amounts of pancreatic enzyme, wetting agents, the oral administration of mucolytics such as N-acetylcysteine, and enemas containing pancreatic enzymes or mucolytics [92, 145, 156]. Most episodes can be managed without surgical intervention. Precipitated by the abnormal intestinal contents, there may be episodes of small-bowel volvulus or intussusception. This latter complication occurs in 1 percent of older patients and may be the presenting manifestation. Episodes tend to be recurrent and may be associated with chronic symptoms [157]. Hydrostatic reduction should be attempted, although surgery may be necessary.

The diagnosis of CF can be suggested by the histology of the appendix [158]. Goblet cells are increased in number and distended with mucus, and eosinophilic casts may fill the crypts and extend into the lumen. Mucoid impaction of the appendix may present as a right lower quadrant mass, in the absence of other symptoms [159]. Recurrent episodes of rectal prolapse occur in up to one-quarter of patients, most often between the ages of 1 to 2 years and usually before the diagnosis is established [160]. It is probably related to the presence of frequent bulky stools, malnutrition, and paroxysmal cough. The prolapse is usually partial and easily treated by manual reduction. The diagnosis of CF should be considered in every patient with rectal prolapse. There is increased mucus within the goblet cells of the rectum [161], and histologic abnormalities on rectal biopsy material have been used as a diagnostic aid.

Hepatobiliary System The liver is extensively involved in CF. Focal biliary cirrhosis, characterized by the inspissation of amorphous eosinophilic material in the intrahepatic bile ducts, bile duct proliferation, inflammatory reaction, a variable degree of fibrosis, and focal distribution, is pathognomonic of CF [2, 162] (Fig. 87-4). It is associated with and probably due to an excessive accumulation of biliary mucus. This lesion is present in 25 percent of patients [2, 162] and may appear as early as 3 days of age [163]. It usually produces no clinical manifestations, but secondary to the intrahepatic bile stasis there may be prolonged neonatal jaundice [164]. One-half of such cases occur in association with meconium ileus. The excessive biliary mucus may decrease with increasing age [162]. In 4 to 6 percent of patients the focal biliary cirrhosis progresses to a multilobular biliary cirrhosis which consists of groups of normal-appearing lobules surrounded by dense fibrous septa containing proliferating bile ducts with eosinophilic concretions [162, 165, 166]. This lesion is specific for CF.

Figure 87-3 Newborn with intestinal obstruction. Abdomen film *(left)* shows distended bowel loops with "bubbly" pattern of inspissated meconium in terminal ileum *(arrow).* Barium enema *(right)* shows a microcolon from disuse secondary to intrauterine obstruction.

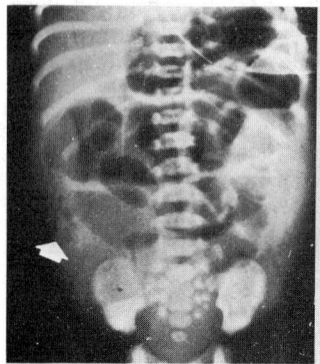
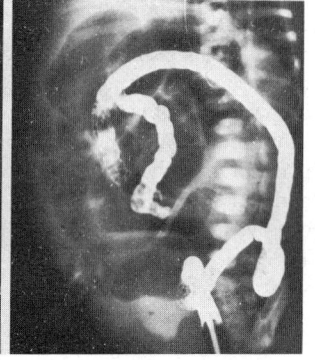

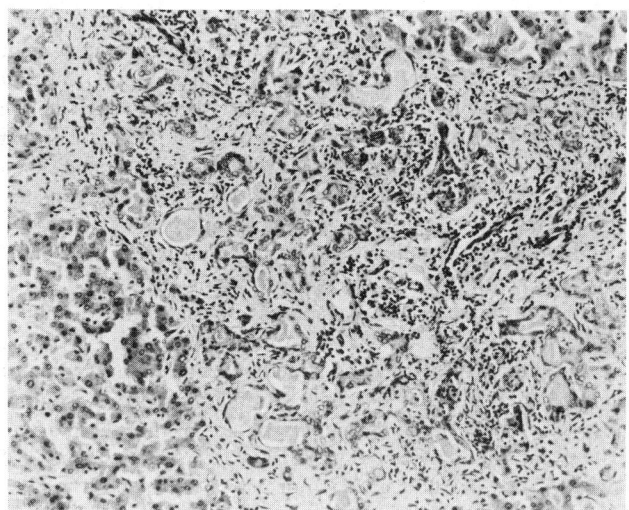

Figure 87-4 Histologic section of liver from 12-year-old girl with CF which shows focal biliary cirrhosis. The periportal area shows fibrosis, chronic inflammation, and bile duct proliferation with intracanalicular bile plugs (H & E, ×620).

The islands of normal hepatic tissue are sufficient to maintain adequate liver function, but the distortion of the liver parenchyma by fibrosis and regenerative nodules may lead to portal hypertension which is manifest clinically in 2 to 3 percent of all patients [166–168] and in 5 percent of adults [68] by hepatosplenomegaly, esophageal varices, and hypersplenism. Liver failure is rare, and liver function tests are generally normal until late in the course [167, 168]. A high total serum alkaline phosphatase value is suggestive of underlying cirrhosis [169]. Liver involvement may be documented at an early stage by scintiscan and computerized tomography [170]. Fatty infiltration of the liver is common in older children [9, 165], and it may present clinically as massive hepatomegaly [167, 168]. In some patients liver complications may be the dominant and, at times, presenting feature [167]. Liver complications are seen only in those patients with pancreatic insufficiency, and there may be a familial pattern to their occurrence [92, 171]. There is no specific therapy for the liver complications. In patients with portal hypertension, portal-systemic shunting and splenectomy may be useful [167, 171]. It is not clear whether surgery should be performed prophylactically or only after an episode of bleeding. The long-term results depend on the degree of underlying pulmonary disease [171]. Post-shunt encephalopathy and hepatic failure are not a problem [167].

Abnormalities of the gallbladder are common but do not correlate with underlying cirrhosis [172, 173]. At autopsy, the gallbladder is abnormal in 30 percent of cases [172]. It is often hypoplastic and filled with thick colorless mucus (white bile). Calculi, nonvisualization, and structural abnormalities are present in up to 45 percent of cholecystograms, but symptoms referable to gallbladder disease are uncommon [173].

Bile Acid Metabolism   Bile acid metabolism is altered in CF [174–177]. In those patients with steatorrhea, there may be a sevenfold increase in fecal bile acid excretion [175], equal to that observed after ileal resection. This is probably due to interference with bile acid absorption at the level of the ileum [175]. There is little correlation between fecal bile acid and fecal fat excretion [176, 177]. Interruption of the enterohepatic circulation is best explained by the binding of bile acids to maldigested protein, fibers, or carbohydrate rather than within the lipid phase alone [177]. Bile acid precipitation secondary to a reduced jejunal pH [178] and a cellular defect of the intestinal mucosa [179] may contribute to decreased absorption. Bile acid losses lead to contraction of the bile acid pool [177], which may lead to further impairment of fat absorption. There is a marked decrease in fecal bile acid output following enzyme therapy, although large amounts continue to be excreted [177]. This may explain the failure of enzyme replacement to totally eliminate steatorrhea. Kinetic studies show that bile acid turnover is accelerated but that with pancreatic enzyme therapy there is a reduction in the turnover rate and enlargement of the bile acid pool (both primary and secondary bile acid fractions) [177]. This suggests that the hepatic mechanisms for the regulation of bile acid synthesis are intact [177].

Genitourinary Tract

The reproductive system is involved in both males and females with CF. Aspermia and infertility are seen in 98 percent of adult males [68, 180]. There is mechanical obstruction of sperm transport secondary to absence or atresia of the vas deferens, along with associated abnormalities of the epididymis and seminal vesicle [181, 182]. Ejaculate volume is decreased and shows increased acidity [181]. There are a decrease in fructose concentration and an increase in citric acid concentration and acid phosphatase activity [181]. Histologically, the testes show active but decreased spermatogenesis. The prostate is normal. It is unclear whether the defect in the Wolffian duct structures is due to anomalous development or to progressive obstruction and obliteration secondary to the presence of abnormal secretions. The frequent autopsy finding of normal genital tract fragments in newborn infants supports the latter hypothesis [183]. These defects appear to be specifically related to CF and may be the most consistent pathologic feature of the disease in early life [182]. An increased incidence of abnormalities associated with testicular descent, i.e., hernia, hydrocele, and undescended testes, reflecting altered development of Wolffian duct–derived structures, has also been reported [184]. All postpubescent males should have their semen analyzed for purposes of counseling.

Although fertility is decreased, many women with CF have borne children [68]. Histologically, there is excessive cytoplasmic and extracellular cervical mucus [185], and there is often plugging of the cervical os by tenacious, dehydrated mucus [185, 186]. This probably acts as a barrier to sperm penetration. The ovaries and endometrium are normal. Among women who become pregnant there is an increased incidence of spontaneous abortion, prematurity, and stillbirths, possibly related to maternal hypoxemia [68, 187]. Endocervical polyps have been described in patients taking oral contraceptives [188]. The development of secondary sex characteristics and menarche may be delayed by several years [189], depending on the underlying nutritional and pulmonary status.

Other Organ Systems

Ocular abnormalities in CF include visual field defects, venous engorgement and tortuosity, hyperemia, and blurring of the nerve head [190]. Acute hemorrhagic retinopathy may occur during exposure to high altitude [191]. Optic atrophy and neuritis with impaired visual acuity have been observed in patients on long-term chloramphenicol therapy [192]. Increased intracranial pressure, manifested by a bulging fontanelle, has been seen in infants with severe respiratory distress [193], in association with vitamin A deficiency [117], and following therapy of malnutrition [194]. Brain abscesses have been reported in young adults [195]. Posterior column degeneration, in most cases limited to the fasciculus gracilis, was present in 19 percent of patients dying after 5 years of age [196]. EEG abnormalities are present in a small percentage of patients, probably as coincidental findings [197]. Intellectual development and school performance are normal, even in those patients who were severely malnourished during infancy [198]. Recurrent transient episodes of seronegative arthritis may occur [199], and seropositive rheumatoid arthritis has also been observed [200].

In the thyroid gland, there is excessive accumulation of lipofuscin pigment in the follicular epithelial cells [201]. In patients treated with iodide, there is a high incidence of goiter, often in association with clinical or laboratory evidence of hypothyroidism [202, 203]. There may be a defect in peripheral deiodination [203]. TSH reserve and response to TSH stimulation are normal [204]. In view of the lack of documentation of the efficacy of iodide as a mucolytic or expectorant, it probably should not be used in patients with CF. Isolated growth hormone deficiency has been documented in two patients, probably as a coincidental finding [205]. In general, growth hormone levels are normal [132].

Salivary Glands

The mucus-secreting salivary glands, i.e., submandibular, sublingual, and submucosal, show morphologic changes similar to those in the pancreas, including dilated ducts with inspissated secretions [9] and eventually atrophy of the acini and fibrosis [206]. The serous-secreting parotid gland shows no morphologic changes. Enlarged submaxillary glands are palpable in over 90 percent of patients [207]. Abnormalities of submaxillary saliva include a decrease of flow rate [208–210], an increase in calcium and protein concentration [208–210], and the appearance of turbidity after physiologic reflex stimulation [210]. The sodium and chloride concentration of the large salivary glands may be normal or slightly elevated [208–211]. A significant elevation in sodium concentrations has been demonstrated in small salivary gland saliva [212]. This is the only exocrine gland, apart from the sweat gland, that consistently exhibits a sodium abnormality in CF. There have been no important clinical problems related to the salivary glands.

Sweat Glands

An abnormality of eccrine sweat gland function resulting in elevated sweat concentrations of sodium, chloride, and potassium is the most constant clinical laboratory finding in CF. Rarely, the diagnosis has been established in patients with normal [213] to intermediate-range sweat electrolyte [214] concentrations. The sweat gland abnormality is unrelated to the severity of the pulmonary and gastrointestinal manifestations [3]. The high concentration of electrolytes in sweat is due to

decreased transductal reabsorption of sodium and chloride [215, 216], probably related to a component of precursor sweat that acts intraluminally to inhibit sodium transport [216]. The inhibitory factor has been demonstrated in the sweat of CF patients using retrograde perfusion of sweat glands in situ [217], and in the sweat [218] and mixed saliva [219] of CF patients using the rat parotid as an experimental model. The sweat gland is otherwise normal physiologically. In children the sweat glands respond appropriately to exogenous aldosterone and to dietary sodium restriction, although the magnitude of the fall in sweat sodium concentrations is smaller than in normal persons [220]. Adults with CF fail to retain significant quantities of sweat sodium during administration of aldosterone [220]. Individual variability in sweat sodium responses limits the diagnostic usefulness of this observation. The sweat rate in CF is not increased [3, 221]. The number of sweat glands per unit area is normal [222]. In both normal persons and patients with CF, the concentrations of sodium and chloride in sweat increase in a linear fashion with increasing sweat rates [221, 223]. The reabsorptive maximum in the CF sweat gland is reached at a distinctly lower secretory rate [221]. Morphologically, the eccrine sweat glands are normal [224].

Clinically, the sweat gland abnormality has important implications. Patients may have a "salty taste" or show salt crystal formation, findings which are highly suggestive of CF. They may also develop dehydration with massive salt depletion [225]. This picture (heat prostration) was first observed during a heat wave and led to the discovery of the sweat gland defect [3]. It has also been observed in cold weather [226], probably as the result of chronic salt loss. In arid climates, chronic metabolic aklalosis and electrolyte depletion, unassociated with the heat prostration syndrome, may be a common presenting manifestation of CF [227]. The apocrine sweat glands may show dilatation and retained secretions [228]. These changes are difficult to evaluate, since they occur more frequently with increasing age and are similar to changes seen in some normal adults.

Diagnosis

Although the diagnosis of CF is usually considered on the basis of characteristic pulmonary and gastrointestinal findings, or a positive family history, documentation of an elevated sweat electrolyte concentration is required for confirmation (Table 87-1). The only acceptable sweat test method is the quantitative pilocarpine iontophoresis sweat test (Gibson-Cooke) [229] in which localized sweating is stimulated by the iontophoresis of pilocarpine into the skin, a sufficient volume of sweat (> 100 mg) is collected, and the electrolyte composition is measured by accepted techniques. The chloride concentration is usually measured, since it best discriminates between normal individuals and those with CF [5]. A chloride concentration greater than 60 meq/liter is consistent with the diagnosis of CF. The sweat chloride concentration can also be measured by applying a chloride ion electrode directly to the sweating skin [230] or by measuring the conductivity of sweat [231]. While these methods may be of some value in screening, they have been associated with an unacceptably high rate of false positive and false negative results [232, 233] and should never be the basis of a definitive diagnosis. The sweat electrolyte abnormal-

Table 87-1 Indications for sweat testing

Pulmonary/upper respiratory	Gastrointestinal	Metabolic/other
Chronic cough	Meconium ileus	Positive family history
Recurrent/chronic pneumonia	Meconium plug syndrome	Failure to thrive
Wheezing/ hyperinflation	Prolonged neonatal jaundice	Salty taste/salt crystals
Tachypnea/ retractions	Steatorrhea	Salt depletion syndrome
Atelectasis (especially right upper lobe)	Rectal prolapse	Metabolic alkalosis
Bronchiectasis	Mucoid-impacted appendix	Hypoprothrombinemia
Hemoptysis	Late intestinal obstruction	Vitamin A deficiency (bulging fontanelle)
Mucoid *Pseudomonas* infection	Recurrent intussusception	Aspermia/absent vas deferens
Nasal polyps	Cirrhosis/portal hypertension	Scrotal calcifications
Pansinusitis	Recurrent pancreatitis	Hypoproteinemia/edema
Digital clubbing		

ity is present from birth and persists throughout life. A volume of sweat sufficient for analysis may be difficult to obtain in the neonatal period, and sweat sodium concentrations have been elevated in some normal infants on the first postnatal day [234].

Elevated concentrations of sweat electrolytes have been reported in other conditions, including: adrenal insufficiency, ectodermal dysplasia, nephrogenic diabetes insipidus, type I glycogen storage disease, hypothyroidism, mucopolysaccharidoses, and fucosidosis [5]. Most of these disorders can be easily differentiated on the basis of characteristic clinical features. Normal sweat electrolyte concentrations have been reported in some patients with CF in the presence of edema and hypoproteinemia [128, 129]. Values became abnormal with resolution of the edema. Most false positive and false negative results are due to technical errors, including inadequate sweat collection and failure to interpret test results correctly [232]. Physiologic variables such as sweating rate, salt intake, and acclimatization may affect the concentration of sweat electrolytes but do not usually interfere with the diagnostic value of the test [235]. Although sweat electrolyte concentrations increase slightly after the age of 15 to 20 years, they remain excellent discriminants for CF in older patients [68]. The sweat test is not useful in diagnosing CF heterozygotes.

Intermediate sweat chloride concentrations in the range of 40 to 60 meq/liter have been reported in patients with chronic pulmonary disease and normal pancreatic function (*atypical cystic fibrosis*) [214]. Borderline sweat electrolyte values are otherwise unusual. In such instances, a change in sweat electrolyte concentration in response to salt restriction or mineralocorticoid administration cannot be used as a reliable differential test [220]. Ancillary findings such as radiographic evidence of pansinusitis, aspermia, or the isolation of a mucoid *Pseudomonas* from the respiratory tract may be helpful [214]. The diagnosis of CF should not be based solely on an elevated sweat electrolyte concentration but should be made only when

associated with pancreatic exocrine deficiency, chronic pulmonary disease, meconium ileus, or a positive family history.

Prevalence and Genetics

Estimates of the prevalence of CF were reviewed in detail in the previous edition of this text. In Caucasian populations the prevalence ranges from 1:1900 to 1:15,000 live births. A reasonable estimate for Caucasians in the United States is 1:2000, with a carrier rate of 1:20. Many other ethnic groups have been studied. The CF gene is rare in both American and African blacks, and its prevalence is 1:90,000 among Hawaiians.

Autosomal recessive inheritance is suggested by most studies of CF genetics, as reviewed previously in detail [236]. Much evidence supports the likelihood of a single mutant allele, although data in favor of genetic heterogeneity are accumulating from biochemical and cell culture studies [237, 238]. Heterozygote advantage has been proposed as an attractive hypothesis for maintenance of CF genes at a high level in the Caucasian population [239]. It will be possible to confirm this phenomenon only when a valid method for heterozygote identification becomes available.

Coincidental occurrence of CF has been reported with several other genetic diseases, including protease inhibitor (Pi) Z α-1-antitrypsin deficiency, Down's syndrome, cri-du-chat syndrome (partial deletion of the short arm of chromosome number 5), agammaglobulinemia, isolated IgA deficiency, thymic alymphoplasia, and the Wiskott-Aldrich syndrome [240].

Screening Screening for CF has been advocated on the observation of improved clinical outcome in response to early intervention [241], as a means of providing information for genetic counseling, and for purposes of enumeration and research. The sweat test has not been useful for screening because of high cost and difficulty in obtaining an adequate quantity of sweat in the newborn period. The most widely used screening tests are those based on the presence of increased amounts of albumin or protein in meconium and which reflect a reduction or absence of pancreatic proteolytic enzymes [242]. Increased concentrations of protein can be detected semiquantitatively with a tetrabromophenolphthalein test strip [243] or by quantitative electroimmunoassay [244]. Unfortunately, these tests will not detect the 15 to 20 percent of patients with normal pancreatic function. Additional problems include occasional false negative values in patients with pancreatic insufficiency [245] and false positive values in the presence of prematurity or melena [242]. The simultaneous measurement of β-D-fucosidase and lactase in meconium may increase the specificity of the test [246]. A recently proposed method for screening is the use of a dried blood spot assay for immunoreactive trypsin [247] (see below).

Prenatal Diagnosis and Heterozygote Detection In the absence of identification of the basic biochemical defect, reliable prenatal diagnosis and heterozygote screening are not available. Bioassays for sodium transport inhibitory factors and mucociliary factors have been difficult to standardize and have no role in heterozygote screening or genetic counseling [235]. Studies showing increased steroid and ouabain resistance [248] or abnormal sodium transport [249] in fibroblasts from CF homozygotes and heterozygotes were not reproducible [249a]. Preliminary results demonstrate that decreased amniotic fluid protease activity may be useful for intrauterine detection [250].

General Therapy

Because of the multisystem involvement, frequency of complications, psychosocial burdens, and potentially poor prognosis, a comprehensive and intensive therapy program is essential. Patients need to be followed at intervals of 2 to 3 months by an available and experienced physician, in conjunction with nursing, nutrition, physical-respiratory therapy, and counseling personnel. Psychosocial support for the patient and other family members is especially important at the time of diagnosis, with exacerbations, and during the terminal phase of the disease. Vocational, educational, financial, and premarital counseling can help the increasing number of adult survivors make a smooth transition to independent living. The goals of therapy include maintenance of adequate nutritional status, prevention or aggressive therapy of pulmonary complications, encouragement of a reasonable level of physical activity, and provision of adequate psychosocial support. With appropriate support, most patients are able to make an age-appropriate adjustment in both home and school [251].

Course and Prognosis

The course of the disease is exceedingly variable from patient to patient. This may possibly be related to genetic heterogeneity. Prognosis is largely determined by the degree of pulmonary involvement. Improved prognosis has been related to early diagnosis [252] and institution of a comprehensive treatment program prior to the onset of irreversible pulmonary changes [189, 241]. Several clinical scoring systems [253, 254] are available for the longitudinal assessment of patients, for prognostic counseling, and for classifying patients for clinical studies. There has been steady improvement in prognosis over the past three decades. In 1950, survival past infancy was unusual. By 1978 the median age at time of death was 13.9 years [255]. Life-table analyses indicate that median survival from birth increased from 14 years in 1969 to 21 years in 1978 [255] (Fig. 87-5). In 1978, 18 percent of all patients under care at specialized CF centers were at least 18 years of age. There is a trend toward poorer early survival but better late survival among black patients [256]. For reasons that are not clear, the survival of male patients at every age appears better than that of female patients [255], although in recent years the gap has narrowed.

BASIC SCIENCE OF CYSTIC FIBROSIS

Immunology, Immunopathology, and Host Defense

There is an unusual relationship of host and infection in CF patients, in that chronic bacterial infection is responsible for

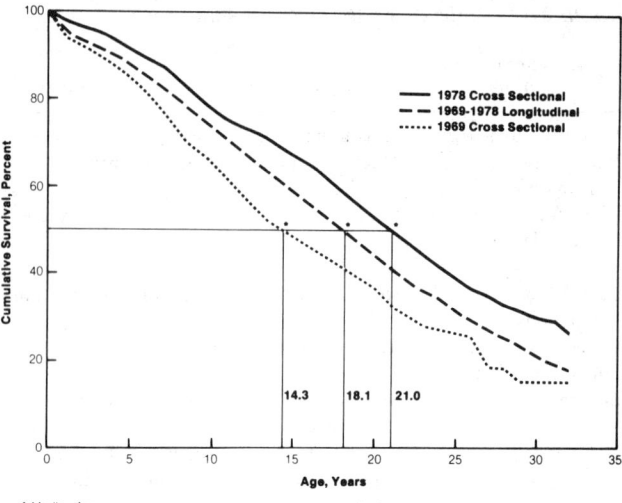

* Median Age

Figure 87-5 Survival curves for United States patients with normal birth. (*From the 1978 report of the Patient Registry* [255] *by permission of the Cystic Fibrosis Foundation.*)

much of the morbidity and mortality in the disease, yet in most cases infection remains localized to the lung [5]. Only occasionally does septicemia occur [31, 32].

B-Cell System   Studies of the B-cell system have demonstrated that cystic fibrosis patients can form all classes of immunoglobulins and that serum levels of IgG, IgA, and IgM generally increase with the duration of the disease [52]. Patients with CF can make antibodies to a variety of common respiratory tract bacterial pathogens [42, 257, 258]. Large numbers of precipitins are found in the circulation of patients with cystic fibrosis who are chronically colonized by *Pseudomonas* [259], and some patients demonstrate evidence for *Pseudomonas*-specific IgE [49]. In a study of immunologic function in 419 patients with CF, the most striking finding was that 22 percent of the 154 patients under 10 years of age had levels of IgG below the limits of a large, age-related control population [53]. Response to tetanus toxoid was adequate in a small subgroup of patients, and the catabolic rate of labeled IgG was normal. In the group of patients under 10 years of age, low levels of serum IgG correlated significantly with better pulmonary function, while high levels of IgG correlated with poor pulmonary function, more chest x-ray abnormalities, and more sputum cultures positive for *P. aeruginosa*. The implication of this study is that, as the host responds to the presence of the continued infection, the immunoglobulin response may become involved in lung tissue damage, perhaps mediated by immune complexes in a type III hypersensitivity reaction [50, 53, 260–262]. The secretory immune system is present in CF, although a larger than normal number of patients have free secretory component in their serum. This suggests that there may be some defect in the synthesis of secretory IgA [263]. A transient deficiency of serum IgA has been found in some CF patients, and in others, secretory component was absent from the saliva [263].

T-Cell System   No specific primary abnormality has been found in the T-cell system in CF. Normal numbers and percentages of T cells have been found in most studies, with some increase in the absolute number of T cells in patients with chronic *Pseudomonas* infection [264, 265]. Abnormalities in specific T-cell function have been identified in patients with far-advanced pulmonary disease [266–268]. Thirteen patients with low clinical scores were found to have a far lower response to *Pseudomonas* in vitro than either normal controls or CF patients with good clinical scores. The serum of patients with advanced disease had a significant inhibitory effect on the T-cell response in vitro to *Pseudomonas* of autologous cells. In contrast, peripheral blood lymphocytes of newly diagnosed CF patients with good clinical scores do respond well in vitro to *Pseudomonas*. In the same group of patients, lymphocyte responses to *Klebsiella*, *Serratia*, and *Proteus* in vitro were found to be depressed.

Complement While some abnormalities in the serum level of specific complement components, especially C3, have been found by some investigators [269], most studies show no abnormalities [270–272]. Consumption of C3 was studied in a hemolytic assay in order to demonstrate that patients with CF have normal C3 activation by *Pseudomonas* or *Staphylococcus* [273]. These experiments demonstrate that in the later components of the complement system, which are very important to host resistance to bacterial infection, there is no gross abnormality in response to activation by at least two species of bacteria that are clinically important in the disease. These results may indicate a combination of classic and alternative complement pathway activation. Other studies have demonstrated specifically that both the classic and alternative complement pathways are intact in CF patients [274, 275]. Several specific complement components, C1q, C3c, C4, and C5, as well as factor B, were found to be normal in CF.

Neutrophils With regard to neutrophil function, numbers of circulating neutrophils are normal or appropriately elevated in association with pulmonary infection in patients with CF. Some evidence for an opsonic defect was found in one study using rabbit alveolar macrophages [276]. Thus, six of nine sera from CF patients did not support the normal phagocytosis of *Pseudomonas*. A possible quantitative or functional defect of a serum immunoglobulin was postulated but never confirmed. While nitroblue tetrazolium (NBT) test results have generally been normal in CF, some authors have found a decreased phagocytic rate in CF neutrophils [277]. In other studies, selective inhibition of phagocytic and bactericidal activities of rabbit alveolar macrophages by serum from patients with CF has been found [278]. This inhibition seemed to be specific for *Pseudomonas*, but CF peripheral blood neutrophils were found by the same investigators to have normal phagocytic and bactericidal activity against *Pseudomonas*. Chemotaxis of neutrophils and monocytes was normal in clinically stable CF patients, as well as in patients having an acute exacerbation of their pulmonary disease [279]. Alveolar macrophages have been studied from the lungs of three CF patients [36]. These cells could phagocytose *Pseudomonas* in the environment of normal serum, but CF serum inhibited phagocytosis of *Pseudomonas* by both normal and CF macrophages. This was specific for *Pseudomonas*, with normal results against *Staphylococcus*.

Protease Inhibitors

The protease inhibitors are potent control proteins whose role is to prevent the constant or inappropriate activation of the several cascade enzyme systems (kallikrein-kinin, complement, coagulation, fibrinolysis) or to inhibit tissue destruction by proteolytic enzymes released in the normal course of the life cycle of cells in certain tissues (e.g., elastase is released normally as neutrophils die in the pulmonary circulation.) Seven major protease inhibitors have been identified in human serum, many of which also appear in a variety of body secretions [280]. A few of these proteins have been studied in great detail in CF, in searches for an uninhibited tissue-damaging enzyme or a cascade enzyme system out of control.

Alpha-2-macroglobulin is a high molecular weight protease inhibitor with strong activity against trypsin and other serine proteases such as kallikrein, collagenase, plasmin, and thrombin. While α-2-macroglobulin levels have been normal in the serum or plasma of CF patients and decrease with age, early studies showed the absence of an α-2-macroglobulin–protease complex in CF plasma [281]. In addition to decreased binding with trypsin, α-2-macroglobulin was shown in some studies to have reduced binding for papain and thrombin [282]. Intermediate values were found in CF obligate heterozygotes. In the same laboratories, purified α-2-macroglobulin was found to be antigenically similar in CF and normal plasma, but the formation of trypsin–α-2-macroglobulin complexes was diminished in CF [283]. No fragmentation of the α-2-macroglobulin from CF patients was observed [284]. Thus, the gradual conversion of normal trypsin–α-2-macroglobulin complexes into fragments appeared to be deficient in CF. Further, CF α-2-macroglobulin was found to have a 40 percent decrease in its sialic acid content and to have defective binding to concanavalin A and wheat-germ agglutinin [285]. Thus, the suggestion of an abnormal carbohydrate portion was made. In contrast, other studies have demonstrated a normal two-dimensional gel electrophoretic pattern of CF α-2-macroglobulin after complete denaturation [286]; an increased molar binding ratio of trypsin to α-2-macroglobulin was found in a different group of CF patients [287]. Along with other children and adults with chronic lung disease, the plasmin–α-2-macroglobulin interaction in CF plasma was normal [288].

Purified α-2-macroglobulin had normal gel electrophoretic patterns and identical subunit molecular weights and trypsin cleavage products [289]. Isoelectric focusing and shifts in isoelectric point after trypsin binding were not abnormal when purified CF α-2-macroglobulin was studied [289], and trypsin-binding capacities of control and CF α-2-macroglobulin were similar [289], as was the esterolytic activity of the trypsin–α-2-macroglobulin complex [289]. In another investigation, purified α-2-macroglobulin showed normal proteolytic subunit cleavage after reaction with trypsin when CF α-2-macroglobulin was studied [290]. In a series of studies, trypsin-binding IgG was identified in serum from CF patients and their mothers, with a high correlation between this finding and the use of oral pancreatic enzyme preparations containing porcine trypsin [291, 292]. A competition between α-2-macroglobulin and antitrypsin antibodies for binding with trypsin was demonstrated in the plasma of both CF patients and rabbits immunized against trypsin [293]. It was suggested that this finding might explain some of the earlier results showing decreased formation of α-2-macroglobulin–trypsin complexes in CF plasma. Alpha-2-macroglobulin from CF plasma has been shown to have increased binding of concanavalin A when compared with that from normal persons or patients with chronic lung disease other than CF [294]. This finding was also characteristic of obligate heterozygotes who had values intermediate between control subjects and CF patients. This increased binding was also true of IgG and IgM as well as the α-2-macroglobulin in CF plasma.

Alpha-1-antitrypsin function, concentration, and genetic typing for protease inhibitor (Pi) types have been studied extensively for abnormalities in patients with CF and their obligate heterozygote parents [240]. No genetic, quantitative, or functional abnormalities have been found, although α-1-antitrypsin levels do increase significantly with age and progression of the chronic pulmonary disease of CF.

Cystic Fibrosis Factors and Other Genetic Markers

A search has taken place over the past 15 years for biologically active substances or biochemical markers which might be useful in identification of the CF basic defect or detection of the CF gene. Although hampered in some cases by unreliable assays and conflicting results, these studies are of some interest and demonstrate some progress.

Sodium Transport Inhibitors   Early studies looked for abnormal materials in CF secretions that could alter sodium transport. Perfusion of the rat parotid gland with either sweat [218] or saliva [219] from CF homozygotes causes a marked inhibition of sodium reabsorption when compared with sweat or saliva from control patients, as measured by a high sodium concentration in pilocarpine-stimulated saliva. Microperfusion of single human sweat glands has shown that inhibition of sodium reabsorption is caused intraluminally by the sweat from CF homozygotes [216, 217] and not in the sweat gland coil [215]. Inhibition of sodium reabsorption in the rat parotid is specifically caused by submandibular, sublingual, and submucosal gland secretions (but not parotid secretions) from CF homozygotes compared with control secretions [295]. Submaxillary and parotid saliva from the chronically reserpinized rat, an animal model for certain clinical aspects of CF, inhibits sodium reabsorption in the rat parotid gland [296]. Although the retrograde perfusion assay of the rat parotid gland is technically difficult and time-consuming, the assay can be standardized and quantitated [295]. The factor or factors present in CF sweat and saliva as well as saliva from the chronically reserpinized rat are both heat-labile and inactivated by freeze-thaw cycles, and they lose 20 to 40 percent of their sodium transport inhibitory activity when stored at 4°C for 24 h [218, 219, 296]. The factor or factors in the saliva of patients with CF appear to be a positively charged (basic) molecule, since addition of heparin to a saline-saliva mixture removes the inhibitor of sodium reabsorption [297]. Other basic materials, like protamine sulfate, polyornithine, polyethyleneimine, arginine-rich histone, and polylysine, also inhibit sodium reabsorption in the rat parotid gland, while heparin removes the activity of these substances.

The rat jejunum has been used in a bioassay to determine the effects of various sera and biologic fluids on sodium-dependent glucose transport. Sera from either CF homozygotes or heterozygotes effected a decrease (inhibition) of short-circuit current in the presence of glucose, relative to control sera [298–300], but there was a large overlap among the groups in all studies. The inhibitory substance or substances in the serum are heat-labile and not related to drug therapy [298]. An assay using everted rat jejunal rings, coupled with measurement of uptake

of labeled methyl-glucose, showed similar results [301]. In plasma the inhibitory substance or substances are nondialyzable. Saliva from CF homozygotes was found to inhibit short-circuit current in the rat colon relative to control saliva [302]. These results correlated with inhibition of sodium reabsorption in the rat parotid gland assay [302]. No inhibition of glucose transport is caused by sera from CF homozygotes or heterozygotes when rat brush-border membrane vesicles are substituted for the rat jejunum. This finding suggests that sodium transport inhibition by a serum factor or factors may be detectable only in certain epithelial tissues such as ducts of salivary and sweat glands and the colon [303].

Factors that influence sodium transport may also be present in cells or tissues in vivo. Fibroblasts from patients with CF accumulate less sodium ion in the presence of ouabain in a tissue culture system than do normal cells [249]. Parotid acinar cells isolated from CF patients contain more sodium ion than parotid acinar cells isolated from controls [304]. The cause of this sodium accumulation has not been determined and may or may not be related to any of the sodium transport inhibition factor(s) present in serum, saliva, or sweat from patients with CF.

Mucociliary Substances   Because of the thickened mucus secretions and a question of abnormal ciliary function in CF, investigators have searched for substances that could alter mucus production or ciliary function. Sera from CF homozygotes and obligate heterozygotes contain one or more substances that inhibit the motility of rabbit tracheal cilia in tissue culture [305]. This work has been replicated in other laboratories, and experimental conditions have been improved to make the assay more reproducible [306, 307]. The ciliary activity of this assay was recently quantitated by use of laser light–scattering spectroscopy techniques [308].

Other mucociliary assays have also been developed. Sera from CF patients and heterozygotes inhibit ciliary activity in gills from the oyster *Crassastrea virginica* [309] or in gills from the freshwater mussel *Unio* [310]. In a similar fashion, plasmas from CF homozygotes and heterozygotes inhibited gill cilia of the freshwater mussel *Dreissensia* [311]. On the other hand, CF sera could not be differentiated from control sera by use of either the rabbit tracheal explant assay or the lateral cilia of the sea mussel *Mytilus edulis* [312]. Tracheal ring explants from hamsters, rabbits, and guinea pigs displayed a decrease in ciliary activity when exposed to CF homozygous sera [313]. Sera from CF homozygotes and controls were reported as ciliotoxic in chicken and rabbit tracheal ring explants [314]. In another bioassay, mouse sperm motility was inhibited by sera from CF homozygotes and heterozygotes [315].

Sera from CF homozygotes and heterozygotes induce mucus production in several bioassays. The free-swimming urn cell complex, obtained from the coelomic cavity of the marine invertebrate *Sipunculus nudus*, secretes a cohesive mucus tail when exposed to sera from CF homozygotes or heterozygotes [316, 317]. Isolated acini from the rat submandibular gland secrete more glycoprotein when allowed to interact with CF homozygous and heterozygous sera [318]. CF homozygous and heterozygous sera stimulated a calcium-dependent potassium efflux from rat submandibular gland slices [319]. Experiments in humans in vivo showed that CF sera inhibited nasal mucociliary clearance only when local inflammation, induced by topical application of anti-IgE, was present [320]. CF sera with high mucociliary tracheal transport rates in vivo caused rapid mucus production and ciliary dyskinesia in the rabbit tracheal explant assay [35].

Attempts have been made to characterize these inhibitors, as well as to determine their presence in biological fluids, cells, and tissues. Different experimental results from various laboratories using the "same" bioassay have resulted from: (1) subtle or gross differences in handling of samples; (2) different tissue culture, maintenance, and selection criteria for bioassay tissue; (3) different bioassay procedures; (4) seasonal, geographical, natural, or supplier variations of experimental organisms; (5) different reagents or equipment; and (6) individual reading and scoring differences.

When the original rabbit trachea ciliary assay was used, the inhibitory material was found to be heat-labile, nondialyzable, and precipitated with euglobulins [305]. Subsequent work with CF sera using the modified rabbit trachea ciliary assay indicated that a substance with a molecular weight of 1000 to 10,000 was associated with IgG, which was necessary to cause ciliary inhibition [321]. Other workers have verified that sera from CF homozygotes and heterozygotes contain a ciliary dyskinesia factor bound to IgG [322]. A 5000-M.W. factor could be dissociated from serum IgG from CF heterozygotes or homozygotes by acidification with EDTA [323]. The factor could also be isolated from CF heterozygote or homozygote sera using protein A-Sepharose to bind IgG subclasses 1, 2, and 4 and the factor, followed by elution at acid pH [324]. This positively charged, 4000- to 6000-M.W. factor is acid-stable, dissociates from IgG at acid pH, is found in biologic fluids from CF homozygotes and heterozygotes, and does not require IgG to produce ciliary dyskinesia [324]. Treatment of normal sera with either epsilon aminocaproic acid (EACA) [325] or EDTA [323] results in production of ciliary dyskinesia activity. EACA generates anaphylatoxin C3a from normal serum [326]. All EDTA-treated sera had the same small molecular weight substance, but it is different from the 5000-M.W. factor present in CF homozygous and heterozygous sera [323].

Initial studies with sera from normal persons and control patients with various diseases indicated that the ciliary dyskinesia activity was specific for sera from CF heterozygotes and homozygotes [305]. The serum substances detected by the rabbit tracheal assay show no correlation with age, sex [307], or a wide variety of clinical features [327]. Recent work has shown that sera from patients with asthma and pulmonary and autoimmune diseases can also cause ciliary dyskinesia in the rabbit tracheal assay [325]. The inhibitory factor in the sera of patients with asthma can be differentiated from the 5000-M.W. factor in CF homozygous and heterozygous sera by two chromatographic procedures and lack of reaction with anti-C3a in the latter case [322, 323].

PHA stimulated lymphocytes, long-term lymphoid cells, and fibroblasts, all from CF homozygotes and heterozygotes, secrete a 1000- to 10,000-M.W. substance which requires added IgG to cause ciliary inhibition in the rabbit trachea [325, 328]. CF homozygous and heterozygous lymphocytes and lymphoid cells also secrete three low molecular weight substances, although IgG is not needed to cause ciliary inhibition in the rabbit trachea [324]. Monocyte-macrophages from CF heterozygotes and homozygotes secrete all three low molecular weight substances, one of which is C3a and another has a molecular weight of 4000 to 6000, is also secreted by CF heterozygous and homozygous T cells, and is also found in CF homozygous and heterozygous sera [324, 329]. B or "null" lymphocytes do not secrete these substances [329]. Amniotic fluids from pregnant CF homozygotes and heterozygotes also cause dyskinesia after addition of IgG [325].

The calcium ionophore A 23187 causes ciliary dyskinesia and mucus secretion similar to CF sera when tested in rabbit tracheal explants [330]. CF homozygous or heterozygous sera, isolated CF IgG, or the calcium ionophore A 23187 quantitatively increase mucus secretion in the rabbit tracheal explants relative to control sera or IgG [331]. CF sera or IgG increase ^{45}Ca uptake in rabbit tracheal explants relative to control sera or IgG. There is no difference between CF homozygous and heterozygous sera and control sera in ATPase or ATP usage by the rabbit tracheal explants [332].

The mechanism of action of these serum mucociliary inhibitors has been investigated in the rabbit tracheal explant assay. Initial reports described ciliary dyskinesia [305, 306]. Subsequent work noted an increase in ciliary beat frequency followed by ciliary dyskinesia and subsequent tissue destruction [307]. Work with laser light-scattering spectroscopy [308] verified the first two parts of the sequence, and other studies [333–335] have documented ultrastructural changes. High-speed cinemicrographic studies showed that CF sera did not cause ciliary dyskinesia [336]. Other workers have observed that serum causes an agglutination of the tracheal cilia [312]. It is not clear at this time whether the ciliary dyskinesia is a secondary effect of cytotoxicity and mucus production.

The mucociliary substance in the serum of CF homozygous and heterozygous patients, detected by the oyster gill assay is nondialyzable, heat-labile, cationic, associated with IgG [309, 337], and precipitable by Rivanol [338]. Control sera, including sera from patients with allergic rhinitis and bronchial asthma, do not cause significant ciliary dyskinesia [309]. Age, sex, or clinical features do not correlate with this factor [309]. Acid citrated-dextrose plasmas from CF homozygotes or heterozygotes also cause dyskinesia [339], but activity is lost in the presence of heparin [340]. The inhibitory serum factor is associated with IgG with a pI of 8.5 [341, 342] but mainly with IgG$_1$ and has a pI of 9.1 to 9.3 [343]. The 6000- to 11,000-M.W. factor can be dissociated from CF homozygous and heterozygous IgG with guanidinium chloride [344]. Added IgG is not required to induce dyskinesia in the oyster assay.

Saliva from CF patients also causes ciliary inhibition, whereas control saliva has no effect [309]. Incubation of saliva from CF patients with heparin overnight removes the ciliary inhibition [340]. Treatment of eight CF patients with systemic heparin resulted in partial or total loss of the ciliary dyskinesia factor in their sera and parotid salivas, with a subsequent return of dyskinesia activity within 24 to 48 h after heparin was stopped [345]. The ciliostatic salivary factor is associated with alpha-amylase in saliva, is dialyzable, and inhibits a mammalian glycogen debranching enzyme [346]. The salivary substance has a molecular weight of less than 12,000 and is quite labile in terms of pH and temperature [347]. Inhibition of the debranching enzyme is similar to that seen with hydroxyalkylamines and polyamine metabolites.

The oyster ciliary dyskinesia factor has also been detected in the media of fibroblasts from CF homozygotes and heterozygotes [348]; it has a molecular weight of 4500 to 10,000 [349] and can bind to IgG$_1$, IgG$_2$, or β_2-microglobulin or glass [350]. This factor increases linearly in the media with increasing fibroblast number [351] and can be inactivated by heat or treatment with pepsin or papain [352]. The association of the dyskinesia factor with IgG$_1$ and IgG$_2$ is not an antigen-antibody reaction since immunoglobulin fragments containing antibody sites fail to bind the factor, but IgG_1 heavy chain does bind it [350]. Native CF IgG cannot bind the ciliary factor as well as either native normal IgG or CF IgG which has been treated with guanidinium chloride [353]. The ciliary factor has also been detected in medium from amniotic cells from a fetus of a CF heterozygote but not in medium from amniotic cells of two normal fetuses [354]. Urine from CF heterozygotes and homozygotes also contains a ciliary dyskinesia factor detected by the oyster gill [355]. Polycations also cause dyskinesia [309].

The mechanism of interaction of ciliary dyskinesia factor with the oyster gill cilia has been investigated. The dyskinesia is not caused by an antigen-antibody reaction; antibody to oyster cilia failed to induce ciliary dyskinesia [356]. Scanning and transmission electron microscopic studies indicated that either sera or active fractions from sera of CF homozygotes or heterozygotes stimulated the production of mucus and caused ultrastructural changes [357]. No differences in ATPase or ATP utilization were detected in homogenized oyster gill or minced oyster gill when sera from normal persons or CF homozygotes and heterozygotes were tested [332]. The oyster ciliary dyskinesia factor may be linked to human chromosome 4, as determined in a study of a series of hybrids between CF homozygous fibroblasts and mouse cells [358].

A ciliary dyskinesia factor, detected in CF plasma by the freshwater mussel *Dreissensia*, was found to be heat-labile, inactivated by freezing or storage in glass, but stable when stored for several months at 2°C [311]. In contrast to the above ciliary dyskinesia factors, the mucus-stimulating substance detected by the urn cell complex assay is released or generated when sera from CF homozygotes and heterozygotes, diluted with seawater, are heated at 85°C for 10 min [316]. The active material binds to protein A-Sepharose and can be separated from inactive IgG by treatment with 8 *M* urea in starting buffer and subsequent elution of the inactive IgG with acetic acid.

Lectinlike Substances   The behavior of CF serum in lymphocyte culture suggested the presence of a lectinlike activity in CF homozygous and heterozygous sera. A hemagglutination assay has been used to demonstrate this activity [359]. The material is associated mainly with IgM and occasionally with IgG in sera from CF homozygotes. The lectinlike material could be dissociated by acidification at pH 5.0. Gel filtration indicated molecular weights of 460 (monomer?) and 780 (dimer?), and activity could be inhibited by fructose and other saccharides as well as by a variety of drugs used to treat CF patients. Control sera had similar materials which were present in much lower titer and not inhibited by fructose. Addition of euglobulin is necessary to detect the lectinlike activity.

A lectin of molecular weight 3500 to 10,000 was found bound to IgM and could be isolated on a fructose-Sepharose column from CF homozygous and heterozygous sera but not from control sera [360]. The interaction of the lectin with the fructose column is calcium- and magnesium-dependent. The molecule is slightly positively charged at pH 8.4.

Arginine Esterases   The cascade enzyme systems involving coagulation, kallikrein-kinin, and fibrinolysis have been studied in CF, in search of excesses or a deficiency of enzyme activity. The arginine esterase activity of CF plasmas treated with chloroform-ellagic acid was shown to be quantitatively less and qualitatively different from similarly treated control

plasmas by ion exchange chromatography and isoelectric focusing [361, 362]. Other investigators, using the same or similar assays, were not able to confirm this observation [363, 364], but a deficiency of arginine esterase activity was substantiated in other laboratories [365, 366]. Further work demonstrated a deficiency of proteolytic activity in the plasma of patients with CF [367], associated with a deficiency of a protease–α-2-macroglobulin complex in CF homozygous and heterozygous plasmas [281, 368]. The deficiency of protease activity in CF sera can be demonstrated by the active site titrant 4-methylumbelliferylguanidinobenzoate (MUGB) in both chloroform-ellagic acid–activated plasma and unactivated plasma obtained from CF homozygotes and heterozygotes [369, 370].

A decrease in MUGB activity in second trimester CF amniotic fluid has been documented [371, 372], while there is no difference in MUGB activity between control and other abnormal second trimester amniotic fluids [372–374]. Gel filtration of control amniotic fluid resulted in two MUGB activities with molecular weights of 200,000 and 100,000 [375]. The latter could be generated by rechromatographing the 200,000-M.W. material. In contrast, CF amniotic fluid showed one MUGB activity peak with 100,000 M.W. [375]. Rechromatography resulted in generation of a MUGB-active 50,000-M.W. peak. Furthermore, isoelectric focusing of control amniotic fluid resulted in five MUGB bands, whereas four MUGB bands were detected in CF amniotic fluid between pI 5.1 and 5.4 [372]. Centrifugation or dialysis did not affect the MUGB activity in either control or CF amniotic fluids. By use of a combination of the MUGB activity, gel filtration, and isoelectric focusing, the outcomes of 13 at-risk pregnancies, 3 of which proved to have CF, were correctly predicted [250].

Arginine esterase deficiency has also been detected in CF saliva [376, 377]. Decrease in MUGB activity has been found in cultures from CF fibroblasts relative to control fibroblasts [378]. The arginine esterase activity and isoelectric focusing patterns were normal in tissue extracts of CF livers compared with control livers [379].

Polyamines   Polyamines, as small, ubiquitous, charged molecules associated with cell division and growth, have been studied extensively for their potential involvement in the pathogenesis of CF. Fibroblasts and lymphocytes from CF homozygotes and heterozygotes incorporate less radiolabeled methylmethionine into RNA than control fibroblasts or lymphocytes [380, 381]. No difference in the activity of the following enzymes in vitro between CF homozygous and control fibroblasts have been noted: (1) diamine oxidase [382]; (2) basal or putrescine-stimulated *S*-adenosyl methionine decarboxylase activity [383]; (3) ornithine decarboxylase activity or putrescine inhibition of ornithine decarboxylase activity [383]; and (4) tRNA and rRNA methylation [384]. There are no differences of inhibition of the proliferation of CF homozygous and control fibroblasts in vitro in the presence of either spermidine or spermine [385]. No difference was observed in uptake of methionine [386] or putrescine [387, 388] between CF homozygous and control fibroblasts.

Spermidine and spermine have been detected in blood [389, 390] as well as in bile and duodenal fluids from both CF homozygotes and control subjects but not in sweat or saliva [389]. Control and CF sweat do contain putrescine [384]. The concentrations and ratio of spermidine to spermine in CF homozygous blood have been shown to be similar to control blood by several investigators [389, 391], while others have found the blood concentration of spermidine to be elevated in CF [392, 393] or the concentration of spermine to be decreased, [390, 393], resulting in a higher ratio of spermidine to spermine in CF homozygotes compared with controls. Blood concentrations of spermidine and spermine in females vary with the menstrual cycle [390, 392]. Spermidine and spermine are found mainly in erythrocytes in CF and control blood and are also detected in lymphocytes and granulocytes, with the spermidine-to-spermine ratio higher in erythrocytes from CF patients as compared with controls [393]. Putrescine and spermine have been quantitated in CF and control urine [392]. Serum levels of putrescine, spermidine, spermine, and plasma diamine oxidase activity are similar in CF children and age-matched controls, although higher in children and CF adult homozygotes and heterozygotes in comparison with adult controls [394].

Other studies have shown that 70 percent of radiolabeled spermidine is conjugated within 4 min in control plasma compared with no detectable conjugation in plasma from CF homozygotes, with subsequent urinary excretion of 11 to 13 percent of the radiolabel in CF homozygotes compared with 60 to 76 percent of the radiolabel for controls within 72 h [395, 396]. CF homozygotes excreted higher levels of putrescine, spermidine, and spermine per milligram creatine in urine than controls [397]. Plasma (with or without added spermidine) or sera, each from CF homozygotes, caused a greater inhibition of transport of radiolabeled methyl-D-glucose in everted rat jejunal rings than control plasma [301]. The inhibitory effect was not lost by dialysis but could be abolished by incubation of the CF homozygote plasma with fresh bovine serum. Addition of spermidine to control plasma, but not buffer alone, induced an inhibition of glucose transport in this system.

Other Proteins and Bioassays   Other techniques which might be used to differentiate CF homozygotes and perhaps heterozygotes from controls have been studied. Isoelectric focusing of sera demonstrated that a band at pI 5.48 was detected in control and CF heterozygote sera but not in CF homozygote sera, whereas a band at pI 8.41 was found in CF homozygous and heterozygous sera but not control sera [398]. The substance at pI 5.48 was later found in one-half or more of all sera tested [368, 399] and subsequently shown to be a fragment of α-2-macroglobulin generated by proteolytic cleavage [368]. Several investigators were not able to detect the CF-specific band at or near pI 8.41 [400–402], but others have confirmed the finding [403–405]. Refinements in the isoelectric focusing technique itself indicated that the CF-specific band has a pI 8.57 ± 0.02 and that all the details concerning collection, storage, processing, etc., of sera must be strictly followed [406, 407]. Additional evidence that the band at pI 8.57 may be CF-specific was obtained by production of an antibody in guinea pigs to the pH 8.3 to 8.6 region of an isoelectric focusing gel of CF homozygote sera [408]. An absorbed, but weak, antibody was used in a rocket immunoelectrophoresis assay to distinguish quantitatively sera from CF homozygotes, heterozygotes, and controls. An antibody was also developed in mice, as well as in a hybridoma, using purified material obtained by subjecting CF homozygous sera to a protein A-Sepharose column followed by isoelectric focusing and using the pH 8.5 to 8.6 region as an antigen [409]. Quantitative differences among the various sera could be shown by rocket immunoelectrophoresis or counterimmunoelectrophoresis using the absorbed antibody. Additional studies with larger numbers of patients and various controls must be done to determine whether the reported antibodies are truly CF-specific.

Another technique consists of the initial isoelectric focusing of sera followed by disc electrophoresis to enhance detection of a CF-specific protein [400], but another group could not reproduce or improve this procedure [402]. CF heterozygotes may be missing one or more of three bands between pI 7.85 and 8.10 usually found in CF homozygous and control sera by isoelectric focusing [410]. Polyacrylamide gel electrophoresis of CF and control sweat at pH 2.3 showed that the CF sweat contains at least one more band than control sweat and at pH 8.9 the CF sweat occasionally had one more band than control sweat [411].

Several other bioassays have been reported in the literature. Diluted CF homozygous or heterozygous sera cause a decreased rate of cytolysis of *Colpidium striatum*, a protozoan ciliate. The active component is associated with IgG [412]. CF homozygous and heterozygous sera also cause an agglutination of *Proteus vulgaris*. The active material is heat-labile and is destroyed by treatment with pronase or antibody to whole human serum, but not by antibody to human IgG or IgA [413]. The studies with *P. vulgaris* have not been replicated in other laboratories [414, 415]. Frog gastric mucosa exhibited large increases in short-circuit current as well as hydrogen ion and chloride ion transport when exposed to CF homozygous plasmas relative to control plasma. The active component has a molecular weight of less than 10,000 and is heat-labile [416]. Saliva from CF homozygotes and heterozygotes interfered with oxygen consumption by nauplii of brine shrimp (*Artemia salina*) [417]. Parotid saliva from CF homozygotes, and to a lesser extent from heterozygotes, caused an initial reduction of zeta potential (a measure of the net charge on negatively charged colloidal particles) of mucus in vitro, followed by an increase in zeta potential relative to control parotid saliva [418, 419]. Purified IgG from CF homozygotes, and to a lesser degree from heterozygotes, caused a long-term increase in zeta potential [420].

A comprehensive table of the various factor assays and properties is available in another review [421] and is updated in Table 87-2.

Serum alpha-fetoprotein levels were increased in CF homozygotes and heterozygotes [422, 423], but other workers in larger studies failed to confirm this finding [424–427]. Carcinoembryonic antigen is elevated in the serum or plasma of CF patients and heterozygotes [428, 429] as well as in CF saliva [430] but is present in normal levels in CF urine [428]. Low serum concentrations of low density and high density lipoproteins have been reported for CF homozygotes but not for heterozygotes [431]. The urinary cyclic nucleotides adenosine 3',5'(cyclic) monophosphate and guanosine 3',5'(cyclic) monophosphate are elevated in adult male CF patients relative to adult male controls, when normalized to either creatinine or body surface area [432, 433]. Serum immunoreactive trypsin is high in neonates with CF [247, 434, 435] and low in older CF patients [434, 436, 437]. Each study compared levels in CF with healthy control subjects and those with a variety of diseases.

Several groups have reported that total serum amylase is normal in CF patients [100, 438, 439]. While the total serum amylase level in CF patients was normal, this was a result of low pancreatic isoamylases and elevated salivary isoamylases [440]. Other investigators have found that the total serum

Table 87-2 Comparison of CF factors detected by bioassays*

Assay	Property			IgG	
	Mol. wt. ×10⁻³	Inactivated by	Net charge	Bound	Needed for assay
A. Sodium transport inhibitors					
1. Rat parotid gland		Heat, freeze-thaw, storage at 4°C			
		Heat, freeze-thaw, storage at 4°C, heparin	+		
2. Rat jejunum		Heat			
3. Rat colon					
B. Mucociliary substances					
1. Rabbit trachea		Heat			
2. Modified rabbit trachea	1–10		+	Yes	Yes
	1–10	Antihuman IgG		No	Yes
	4–6		+	Yes, IgG$_1$, IgG$_2$, and IgG$_4$	No
3. Tracheal rings					
4. *Crassostrea virginica*	6–11	Freeze-thaw, heat, heparin	+	Yes, IgG$_1$	No
	4.5–10	Papain, pepsin, heat, storage at room temperature Heparin	+	Can be if available, IgG$_1$ and IgG$_2$	No
	5–10		+		
	<12	pH, heat, storage at any temperature		No	No
C. Mucus production					
1. Urn cell complex				Yes	
2. Isolated rat submandibular acini					
D. Others					
1. Ca²⁺ dependent K⁺ efflux in rat submandibular slices					
2. Lectin like substances	0.46 and 0.78			Sometimes	
	3.5–10		+	No	
3. Cytolysis of *Colpidium striatum*		Heat, incubation with BSA-anti-BSA		Yes	Yes
4. Agglutination of *Proteus vulgaris*		Heat, pronase, antibody to whole human serum, Freeze-thaw		No	No
5. H⁺ and Cl⁻ transport in frog gastric mucosa	<10	Heat			
6. O₂ consumption by nauplii of *Artemia salina*					
7. Reduction of zeta potential		Heat, glass	+		

* Blank spaces indicate that no information is available.

Table 87-2 Comparison of CF factors detected by bioassays (*Continued*)*

Detected in CF fluids	Comments	References
Sweat		218
Saliva	Inhibition by submandibular, sublingual, and submucosal secretions	219, 295, 297
Serum, plasma		298–301
Saliva	Correlation with Na⁺ transport inhibition in rat parotid	302
Serum	Precipitates with euglobulins	305
Serum, purified IgG	CF serum and CF IgG cause increase of $^{45}Ca^{2+}$ uptake	306, 321, 331
Media from fibroblasts, amniotic fluid cells, long-term lymphocytes, PHA-stimulated leukocytes		325, 326, 328
Serum, media from peripheral blood leukocytes, lymphoid cells, T lymphocytes, monocytes	Dissociated from IgG at pH 3.0 or by EDTA	323, 324, 329
Serum		313
Serum, plasma	Dissociated by guanidinium hydrochloride, precipitated by Rivanol	309, 337, 338, 340, 343, 344, 353
Media of fibroblasts	Also bound by β₂-microglobulin	348–350, 352
Saliva, parotid saliva		309, 340
Urine		355, 421
Saliva	Associated with α-amylase, causes inhibition of mammalian debranching enzyme	346, 347
Serum		316
Serum		318
Serum		319
Serum	Euglobulin required in assay, associated with IgM, dissociated at pH 5.0, inhibited by fructose	359
Serum	Associated with IgM, dissociated by NaCl or binding to fructose-sepharose	360
Serum		412
Serum		413
Plasma		416
Saliva		417
Parotid saliva		418–420

amylase in CF patients with pancreatic insufficiency is decreased because of low pancreatic isoamylases but that the salivary isoamylases are the same as controls [99, 441]. Serum amylase activity is increased in 36 percent of CF patients, the exact level being related to age and sex [442]. CF homozygotes with steatorrhea have the same total serum amylase level as controls, but only salivary isoamylases are present [443]. In contrast, CF patients without steatorrhea have a higher total serum amylase level, made up of higher salivary and pancreatic isoamylases, than either control subjects or CF homozygotes with steatorrhea [443]. Another report found similar results, but also found that the salivary isoamylases were elevated in saliva from CF patients with and without pancreatic insufficiency [444]. Three-fourths of the CF patients have a serum amylase pattern different from control subjects by polyacrylamide electrophoresis [438], whereas CF and heterozygote parotid salivas have fast isoamylases, but there is no difference in protein content or activity relative to those in control subjects [445]. In heterozygotes, while the serum amylase activity is normal [444, 446], the pancreatic isoenzymes are elevated [440, 444, 446], and the salivary isoenzymes are normal [440, 446]. Amylase activity in sweat from CF patients is comparable with that of age-matched controls [439].

Many glycosidases have been reported to be similar in CF and control sera [447, 448]. Alpha-L-fucosidase has been reported to be low in the sera of CF patients relative to that in age-matched control subjects [448], but other investigators did not detect this difference [447, 449]. Alpha-L-fucosidase activity in CF serum has normal isoelectric focusing profiles, kinetics, pH optimum curves, and temperature stabilities [449].

It is possible to use the heat inactivation of plasma alpha-mannosidase and plasma acid phosphatase to differentiate CF patients from heterozygotes and controls [450], but other investigators have failed to reproduce this observation [451, 452]. Serum alpha-glucosidase is elevated in CF homozygotes but not in heterozygotes [447]. The activity of serum glutathione reductase is elevated in CF homozygotes [453]. The serum ribonuclease activity is normal in CF patients and heterozygotes [454], but the acid-stable and thermostable ribonuclease activity in saliva is elevated in CF patients and heterozygotes [455].

Cellular Structure and Function

Much information has been gained from the structural and functional analysis of single CF cell types in tissue culture. Although many attempts have been made to identify a specific genetic metabolic defect, this has not yet been achieved. Many reasonable potential defects have been ruled out, and others still remain possible as a result of such work.

Fibroblasts   Early studies showed that the cytoplasm of CF fibroblasts stained metachromatically [456], similar to the findings in several other inborn metabolic diseases. Many studies since that time have failed to confirm the consistent presence of metachromasia in CF fibroblasts [457]. It has been found in some laboratories that fibroblasts from some CF families are metachromatic, while others are ametachromatic [458]. An accumulation of glycogen has been found in the cytoplasm of CF fibroblasts but not as a finding specific to CF [459]. Some investigators have demonstrated an accumulation of all types of glycosaminoglycans in CF cells [460],

whereas other studies have found normal amounts. Unconfirmed findings in CF fibroblasts in tissue culture include the following: (1) failure of normal amounts of collagen to be produced [461]; (2) an abnormal cell-doubling time [462]; (3) an increase in the fluidity of cell membranes [463]; (4) characteristic changes in peaks on gas-liquid chromatography after pyrolysis of cell membranes [464]; and (5) decreases in colchicine-binding activity and tyrosyl tubulin ligase activity [465].

Many investigators have found that factors may be produced and secreted into the CF fibroblast culture medium which alter ciliary motility and induce the production of mucus in various bioassay systems (see above). Preliminary studies using CF fibroblast-mouse hybrids, have attempted to localize this biologic activity on one of the autosomes [358].

Many hydrolytic enzymes have been studied in CF fibroblasts. Activities which have been found normal include alpha-D-mannosidase [466] and beta-N-acetyl glucosaminidase [467]. While some abnormalities have been found in the carboxypeptidase A and B enzymes, these enzymes are probably normal [468]. On the contrary, it was reported that the heat inactivation of alpha-mannosidase could be used to distinguish CF patients from heterozygotes and normal persons [469]. Induction of alkaline phosphatase activity with Tamm-Horsfall glycoprotein, isoproterenol, and theophylline in fibroblast cultures has been reported to result in differentiation of CF fibroblasts from heterozygote and control fibroblasts [470–472]. It was subsequently found that a medium conditioned by normal fibroblasts inhibits the alkaline phosphatase induction by Tamm-Horsfall glycoprotein in CF fibroblasts [473]. Induction of alkaline phosphatase activity by Tamm-Horsfall glycoprotein, isoproterenol, and theophylline in CF fibroblasts has not been substantiated by other groups [474–476], and no difference of alkaline phosphatase localization, intensity, or activity between CF and control fibroblasts has been found [474]. A double-blind study was carried out twice, once successfully [477] and once unsuccessfully [478]. Alpha-L-fucosidase has been found to be normal by some investigators [479], while others have found an increase in levels as well as unusual predominance of isoenzymes with high isoelectric points [480].

Cell surface glycoproteins appear to be labeled normally and to be taken up and shed normally by CF fibroblasts [481]. These cells are able to synthesize complex carbohydrate side chains, as shown by their ability to glycosylate a viral glycoprotein [482].

Normal methionine transport [386], normal composition and metabolism of linoleic and arachidonic acids [483], and normal thymidine and uridine uptake [484] have also been found.

A finding of considerable potential importance is that the membrane magnesium-calcium ATPase activity is significantly decreased in CF fibroblasts [485].

Other recent findings include the possible presence of an abnormal high molecular weight membrane protein [480] and decreased inhibition of the endocytosis of horseradish peroxidase when cells are stimulated by dimethylsulfoxide or 7-ketocholesterol [480].

In an extensive study of CF fibroblasts by light and electron microscopy, as well as by a variety of cytochemical techniques, a normal number of cytoplasmic bodies containing acidic complex carbohydrate and acid phosphatase were found [457]. Other findings included the absence of intense metachromasia, normal fine structural morphology, and normal staining for neutral, sialic acid–rich and sulfated complex carbohydrate. Thus, there were no findings that might provide a basis for the CF fibroblast metachromasia demonstrated originally.

Lymphocytes and Lymphoblasts CF peripheral blood lymphocytes have been studied extensively in tissue culture. Their plasma membranes have a normal staining pattern on sodium dodecyl sulfate gel electrophoresis [486], a normal phospholipid and total membrane lipid composition [486], and a normal quantity of glucose [486]. The carbohydrate composition of glycopeptides released from the surface of these cells by papain was normal [486], and cellular glycosaminoglycans have been found in normal amounts in these cells.

Abnormalities in the metabolism of cyclic AMP have been demonstrated in cultured lymphocytes. Less cAMP is produced by CF cells than by those from patients with bronchiectasis or normal subjects, in response to stimulation by isoproterenol [487]. Basal activity of adenylate cyclase is normal. The decreased amount of cAMP is not caused by the plasma of CF patients.

Abnormalities in handling of fucose are characteristic of CF lymphocytes in tissue culture. There is a decrease in alpha-L-fucosidase activity caused by an absolute decrease in the amount of enzyme, with normal isoenzymes and a normal subunit molecular weight [488].

CF lymphocytes secrete three different ciliary dyskinesia substances into the tissue culture medium [329]. Only one of these is specific for CF. The T lymphocytes synthesize only this specific substance.

Erythrocytes CF erythrocytes have abnormalities in their fatty acid content, which are probably due to the pancreatic insufficiency characteristic of the disease [489].

Inside-out vesicles of CF erythrocytes show a significantly decreased uptake of calcium [490]. Early studies have previously shown abnormalities in various ATPase enzymes [5].

Monocytes Circulating CF monocytes have increased numbers of insulin receptors and altered insulin affinity [491].

Liver Chronic liver disease is a clinical feature in many patients with CF. Nevertheless, several enzymes have been demonstrated to be normal in CF liver, including neuraminidase, mannosidase, and N-acetyl-glucosaminidase [492]. While the alpha-L-fucosidase has been found to be normal in some studies, others have demonstrated normal properties along with a decrease in certain components of the carbohydrate side chains of the enzyme [493]. Sialyl transferase has been shown to demonstrate deficient or absent basic isoenzyme forms [494].

Parotid Acinar Cells A recent study of parotid acinar cells from nine CF patients and five control subjects demonstrated normal ATP levels and oxygen consumption in the CF cells, with normal morphology on electron microscopy [304]. The CF cells were larger than those obtained from the control subjects and had higher concentrations of amylase, calcium, and sodium than control cells, as well as a lower potassium level. CF cells had increased cAMP and decreased cGMP. This was the first report of specific intracellular levels of components in a secretory tissue from patients with CF.

Exocrine Gland Structure and Function

Sweat Gland The original discovery that sweat from CF patients exhibits significantly elevated sodium and chloride concentrations [3] and, to a lesser extent, increased potassium concentrations has been verified many times. While bicarbonate is elevated in CF sweat [495], calcium and magnesium concentrations do not differ significantly from control sweat concentrations [496]. No difference in osmolality or the concentrations of sodium and chloride is detected in the primary secretions of sweat glands from patients with CF and normal subjects [215]. Experiments with single sweat glands from both CF patients and healthy persons indicate that the sweat from CF patients contains one or more very labile substances which inhibit the reabsorption of sodium intraluminally [216–218].

Salivary Glands Previous studies reported a variety of experimental results for salivary glands [497]. More recent studies employing improved experimental techniques show that stimulated CF parotid gland saliva has significantly higher calcium concentrations than control saliva while flow rate, amylase, and sodium were, in fact, higher but not significantly so [498]. Inorganic phosphate and potassium were similar. Variations in concentrations of sodium, potassium, calcium, and chloride ions, in addition to protein, IgG, IgA, and secretory IgA between stimulated and unstimulated parotid gland saliva, have been documented for both CF homozygotes and normal persons [499]. Two types of turbidity have been described for parotid saliva from subjects [500]. A reversible, rapid-forming cold-dependent turbidity consisting mostly of protein, and a slow-forming, nonreversible turbidity made up of Ca^{2+}, inorganic phosphate, and protein have been described. Microscopic examination revealed that the two types of turbidity each had discrete, electron-dense crystals. The cold type material also had amorphous round particles [501].

A serum factor may be responsible for the parotid gland changes in CF homozygotes. Thus, intraperitoneal injections of CF homozygous sera caused structural alterations and an increased mitotic rate in parotid glands of adult rats but had no effect on the pancreas [533].

Turbidity is present in submaxillary gland saliva from CF homozygotes [4]. The turbidity is caused by a 12,000-M.W. phosphoprotein, which has been purified and characterized and is precipitated with calcium ion at basic pH [502].

CF submandibular saliva has elevated concentrations of calcium, sodium, chloride, protein, and amylase specific activity but normal concentrations of magnesium, inorganic phosphate, potassium, copper, and zinc [209, 503]. Crude-control submandibular secretion contains 21 proteins [504].

More radiolabeled fucose is incorporated into glycoprotein acceptors purified from CF saliva in the presence of either CF or control plasma [505]. While the fucosyl transferase activity was not different, the isoelectric focusing patterns of the glycoprotein acceptors were different [505]. No differences were observed in an ultrastructural and histochemical study of CF and control autonomic nerve fibers in labial salivary glands [506].

Mucous Glands Many studies have been done on CF tissues or glands and crude secretion mixtures [507]. There are no differences in histology or acid and neutral mucins in the tracheobronchial mucous glands from young CF homozygotes and age-matched control subjects, with and without pulmonary infection [8]. Lipids account for 30 to 40 percent of the dry insoluble material from pulmonary lavages of CF homozygotes and patients with asthma [508]. CF tracheobronchial secretions contain a more highly sulfated component [509]. The sulfate groups are probably attached to C-6 of the D-galactose residues [510]. Sputum from children with CF contains acidic mucins which have more sulfate than sialic acid, but large carbohydrate chains, as do patients with other bronchial diseases [511]. The ionic content in sputum of CF homozygotes with bacterial infections is different from that of cancer patients [512].

The composition of CF nasal secretion was similar to control secretion except that calcium was significantly elevated [513]. Tissue culture of nasal polyp epithelium from CF homozygotes and patients with allergic rhinitis resulted in glycoprotein secretions from the CF epithelium, with a higher-labeled sulfate per labeled glucosamine and similar relative amounts of fucose and sialic acid [514].

Rectal biopsy specimens in tissue culture from CF homozygotes, healthy sibs, and control subjects all exhibited normal synthesis, transport, and secretion of epithelial glycoprotein [515], but histologic changes were observed in the CF biopsy specimens [516]. Purified rat intestinal goblet cell mucin showed a decreased solubility in the presence of elevated calcium levels which was reversible by EDTA [517]. Small-intestinal biopsy specimens revealed a correlation between the degree of mucus present and the severity of steatorrhea, as well as the number of cells containing vasoactive intestinal peptide [518]. Glycopeptides from CF meconium had a higher fucose content than control meconium [519].

Autonomic Nervous System Function   Early clinical descriptions of CF suggested that many of its features resembled the effects of autonomic agents, especially pilocarpine, in experimental animals. Many studies of CF in humans are difficult to perform for experimental or ethical reasons.

No true animal model for CF exists, but several experimental animal models mimic one or more clinical features of the disease. Treatment of rats with isoproterenol and pilocarpine induced an increase in bronchial submucosal gland size and the number of goblet cells, as seen in CF [520]. The chronically reserpinized rat exhibits the following "clinical features" which are similar to those seen in humans with CF: (1) submaxillary gland morphology and ultrastructural changes [521] with increased sodium, calcium, protein, and carbohydrate concentrations [522]; (2) sodium reabsorption inhibition in the rat parotid gland assay [296] and inhibition of ciliary activity in the freshwater mussel Unio by saliva [522]; (3) increased pulmonary mucous glycoproteins [523, 524]; and (4) alterations in pancreatic secretions [525]. Chronic administration of isoproterenol to rats causes similar effects in the submaxillary gland [526]. Pancreatic secretions from reserpinized rabbits show alterations suggestive of human CF [527]. The chronically reserpinized mouse has decreased pulmonary clearance of S. aureus, as do CF homozygotes [528].

A mouse model with cribriform degeneration (cri) of the central nervous system [529], which is inherited in an autosomal recessive fashion like CF, has other "clinical features" similar to CF: (1) a defect in sodium transport in the parotid and sweat glands [530]; (2) serum of cri homozygotes has ciliotoxic activity similar to CF homozygote sera in a mouse sperm assay

[315]; and (3) decreased pulmonary clearance of S. aureus [531] with a high number of neutrophils in lung lavage fluid [532].

Possibilities for Identification of the Metabolic Defect

In spite of the extensive and varied research approaches used in the search for the metabolic defect in CF, there is little evidence that an answer is close at hand. Any potential defect must account for the following:

1. The generalized dysfunction of exocrine glands, which is present at or before birth. Evidence of disease during intrauterine life is: (a) obliteration of the vas deferens in CF males at the time of birth, and (b) the clinical variant of meconium ileus in the newborn, in which abnormal gut contents result in intestinal obstruction and occasional perforation with atresia.

2. The sweat defect, in which the sweat duct fails to reabsorb sodium and choride normally.

3. The abnormally thick mucus secretions, which are presumably responsible for the obstruction in many organs and tissues.

4. The presence of factors in various body fluids which disturb salt transport and alter mucus production and ciliary function.

5. Various biochemical abnormalities of cells in culture, such as altered α-L-fucosidase, glycogen accumulation, and abnormal Ca^{2+}-Mg^{2+} ATPase.

6. Susceptibility to infection early in life. In fact, a host defect, as yet undiscovered, may predispose the lung to early infection, which secondarily leads to abnormal mucus production and obstructive pulmonary disease.

7. Abnormalities in autonomic nervous system function.

Future basic research in CF must provide more knowledge of exocrine gland function, host defense mechanisms, and the early pathophysiology of the disease. Greater care must be taken in choosing matched normal and disease control subjects and in correlating findings in CF patients with stages of the disease and its complicated treatment regimens.

REFERENCES

1. FANCONI G, UEHLINGER E, KNAUER C: Das coeliakiesyndrom be: Angeborener zystischer pankreas fibromatose und bronkiektasien. Wien Med Wochenschr 86:753, 1936

2. BODIAN M: Fibrocystic Disease of the Pancreas. A Congenital Disorder of Mucus Production—Mucosis. London, Heineman, 1952

3. DISANT'AGNESE PA, DARLING RC, PERERA GA, SHEA E: Abnormal electrolyte composition of sweat in cystic fibrosis of the pancreas: Clinical significance and relationship to the disease. Pediatrics 12:549, 1953

4. DISANT'AGNESE PA, DAVID PB: Research in cystic fibrosis. N Engl J Med 295:481, 534, 597, 1976

5. WOOD RE, BOAT TF, DOERSHUK CF: State of the art: Cystic fibrosis. Am Rev Resp Dis 113:833, 1976

6. MANGOS JA, TALAMO RC (eds): Cystic Fibrosis: Projections into the Future. New York, Stratton Intercontinental Medical Book Corporation, 1976

7. STURGESS JM (ed): Perspectives in Cystic Fibrosis. Toronto, Canadian Cystic Fibrosis Foundation, 1980

8. OPPENHEIMER EH: Similarity of the tracheobronchial mucous glands and epithelium in infants with and without CF. Hum Pathol 12:36, 1981

9. OPPENHEIMER EH, ESTERLY JR: Pathology of cystic fibrosis: Review of the literature and comparison with 146 autopsied cases, in Rosenberg, Bolande (eds): Perspective in Pediatric Pathology, II. Chicago, Year Book, 1975, p 241

10. ESTERLY JR, OPPENHEIMER EH: Observations in cystic fibrosis of the pancreas. III. Pulmonary lesions. *Johns Hopkins Med J* 122:94, 1968

11. BEDROSSIAN CWM, GREENBERG SD, SINGER DB, HANSEN JJ, ROSENBERG HS: The lung in cystic fibrosis. *Hum Pathol* 7:195, 1976

12. DISANT'AGNESE PA: Bronchial obstruction with lobar atelectasis and emphysema in cystic fibrosis of the pancreas. *Pediatrics* 12:178, 1953

13. LLOYD-STILL JD, KHAW KT, SHWACHMAN H: Severe respiratory distress in infants with cystic fibrosis. *Pediatrics* 53:678, 1974

14. COOK CD, HELLIESEN PJ, KULCZYCKI L, BARRIE H, FRIEDLANDER L, AGATHON S, HARRIS GBC, SHWACHMAN H: Studies of respiratory physiology in children. II. Lung volumes and mechanics of respiration in 64 patients with cystic fibrosis of the pancreas. *Pediatrics* 24:181, 1959

15. FEATHERBY EA, WENG TR, CROZIER DN, DUIC A, REILLY BJ, LEVISON H: Dynamic and static lung volumes, blood gas tensions, and diffusing capacity in patients with cystic fibrosis. *Am Rev Resp Dis* 102:737, 1970

16. GODFREY S, MEARNS M, HOWLETT G: Serial lung function studies in cystic fibrosis in the first 5 years of life. *Arch Dis Child* 53:83, 1978

17. LANDAU LI, PHELAN PH: The spectrum of cystic fibrosis: A study of pulmonary mechanics in 46 patients. *Am Rev Resp Dis* 108:593, 1973

18. DEMUTH GR, HOWATT WF, TALNER NS: Intrapulmonary gas distribution in cystic fibrosis. *Am J Dis Child* 103:129, 1962

19. LAMARRE A, REILLY BJ, BRYAN AC, LEVISON H: Early detection of pulmonary function abnormalities in cystic fibrosis. *Pediatrics* 50:291, 1972

20. FOX WW, BUREAU MA, TAUSSIG LA, MARTIN RR, BEAUDRY PH: Helium flow-volume curves in the detection of early small airway disease. *Pediatrics* 54:293, 1974

21. MOSS AJ, DESILETS DT, HIGASHINO SM, RUTTENBERG HD, MARCANO BA, DOOLEY RR: Intrapulmonary shunts in cystic fibrosis. *Pediatrics* 41:438, 1968

22. MANSELL A, DUBRAWSKY C, LEVISON H, BRYAN AC, CROZIER DN: Lung elastic recoil in cystic fibrosis. *Am Rev Resp Dis* 109:90, 1974

23. MELLINS RB, LEVINE OR, INGRAM RH JR, FISHMAN AP: Obstructive disease of the airways in cystic fibrosis. *Pediatrics* 41:560, 1968

24. COREY M, LEVISON H, CROZIER D: Five- to seven-year course of pulmonary function in cystic fibrosis. *Am Rev Resp Dis* 114:1085, 1976

25. WHITE H, ROWLEY WF: Cystic fibrosis of the pancreas: Clinical and roentegenographic manifestations. *Pediatr Clin North Am* 11:139, 1964

26. WARING WW, BRUNT CH, HILMAN BC: Mucoid impaction of the bronchi in cystic fibrosis. *Pediatrics* 39:166, 1967

27. ALDERSON PD, SECKER-WALKER RH, STROMINGER DB, MCALISTER WH, HILL RL, MARKHAM J: Quantitative assessment of regional ventilation and perfusion in children with cystic fibrosis. *Radiology* 111:151, 1974

28. MAY JR, HERRICK NC, THOMPSON D: Bacterial infection in cystic fibrosis. *Arch Dis Child* 47:908, 1972

29. HOIBY N: *Pseudomonas aeruginosa* infection in cystic fibrosis. *Acta Pathol Microbiol Scand* [C] [Suppl] I:262, 1977

30. REYNOLDS HY: *Pseudomonas aeruginosa* infections: Persisting problems and current research to find new therapies. *Ann Intern Med* 82:819, 1975

31. MCCARTHY MM, ROURK MH, SPOCK A: Bacteremia in patients with cystic fibrosis. *Clin Pediatr* 19:746, 1980

32. ROSENSTEIN BJ, HALL DE: Pneumonia and septicemia due to *Pseudomonas cepacia* in a patient with cystic fibrosis. *Johns Hopkins Med J* 147:188, 1980

33. KULCZYCKI LL, MURPHY TM, BELLANTI JA: *Pseudomonas* colonization in cystic fibrosis. *JAMA* 240:30, 1978

34. BALTIMORE RS, MITCHELL M: Immunologic investigations of mucoid strains of *Pseudomonas aeruginosa*: Comparison of susceptibility to opsonic antibody in mucoid and non-mucoid strains. *J Infect Dis* 141:238, 1980

35. YEATES DB, STURGESS JM, KAHN SR, LEVISON H, ASPIN N: Mucociliary transport in trachea of patients with cystic fibrosis. *Arch Dis Child* 51:28, 1976

36. THOMASSEN MJ, DEMKO CA, WOOD RE, TANDLER B, DEARBORN DG, BOXERBAUM B, KUCHENBROD PJ: Ultrastructure and function of alveolar macrophages from cystic fibrosis patients. *Pediatr Res* 14:715, 1980

37. SORENSEN RU, STERN RC, POLMAR SH: Lymphocyte responsiveness to *Pseudomonas aeruginosa* in cystic fibrosis: Relationship to status of pulmonary disease in sibling pairs. *J Pediatr* 93:201, 1978

38. SPARHAM PD, LOBBAN DI, SPELLER DCE: Isolation of *Staphylococcus aureus* from sputum in cystic fibrosis. *J Clin Pathol* 31:913, 1978

39. LAWSON D, PORTER J: Serum precipitins against respiratory tract pathogens in 522 "normal" children, and 48 cases of cystic fibrosis treated with cloxacillian. *Arch Dis Child* 51:890, 1976

40. WRIGHT PF, KHAW KT, OXMAN MN, SHWACHMAN H: Evaluation of the safety of amantadine-HCL and the role of respiratory virus infections in children with cystic fibrosis. *J Infec Dis* 134:144, 1976

41. HOIBY N, KILIAN M: *Haemophilus* from the lower respiratory tract of patients with cystic fibrosis. *Scand J Resp Dis* 57:103, 1976

42. BURNS MW, MAY JR: Bacterial precipitins in serum of patients with cystic fibrosis. *Lancet* 1:270, 1968

43. JENNER BM, LANDAU LI, PHELAN PD: Pulmonary candidiasis in cystic fibrosis. *Arch Dis Child* 54:555, 1979

44. RACHELEFSKY GS, OSHER A, DOOLEY RR, ANK B, STIEHM ER: Coexistent respiratory allergy and cystic fibrosis. *Am J Dis Child* 128:355, 1974

45. WARNER JO, TAYLOR BW, NORMAN AP, SOOTHILL JF: Association of cystic fibrosis with allergy. *Arch Dis Child* 51:507, 1976

46. NELSON LA, CALLERAME ML, SCHWARTZ RH: Aspergillosis and atopy in cystic fibrosis. *Am Rev Resp Dis* 120:803, 1979

47. SILVERMAN M, HOBBS FDR, GORDON IRS, CARSWELL F: Cystic fibrosis, atopy and airways lability. *Arch Dis Child* 53:873, 1978

48. WARREN CPW, TAI E, BATTEN JC, HUTCHCROFT BJ, PEPYS J: Cystic fibrosis—immunological reactions to *A. fumigatus* and common allergens. *Clin Allergy* 1:1, 1975

49. STAHL SP, HORN S, SCHIOTZ PO, PERMIN H, HOIBY N: *Pseudomonas aeruginosa* allergy in cystic fibrosis. *Allergy* 35:23, 1980

50. MOSS RB, LEWISTON NJ: Immune complexes and humoral response to *Pseudomonas aeruginosa* in cystic fibrosis. *Am Rev Resp Dis* 121:23, 1980

51. SOTER NA, MIHM MC JR, COLTEN HR: Cutaneous nectrotizing venulitis in patients with cystic fibrosis. *J Pediatr* 95:197, 1979

52. SCHWARTZ RH: Serum immunoglobulin levels in cystic fibrosis. *Am J Dis Child* 111:408, 1966

53. MATTHEWS WJ JR, WILLIAMS M, OLIPHINT B, GEHA R, COLTEN HR: Hypogammaglobulinemia in patients with cystic fibrosis. *N Engl J Med* 302:245, 1980

54. WIENTZEN R, PRESTIDGE CB, KRAMER RI, MCCRACKEN GH, NELSON JD: Acute pulmonary exacerbations in cystic fibrosis: A double-blind trial of tobramycin and placebo therapy. *Am J Dis Child* 134:1134, 1980

55. HYATT AC, CHIPPS BE, KUMOR KM, MELLITS ED, LIETMAN PS, ROSENSTEIN BJ: A double-blind controlled trial of anti-*Pseudomonas* chemotherapy in acute respiratory exacerbations in patients with cystic fibrosis. *J Pediatr*, in press

56. YAFFE SJ, GERBRACHT LM, MOSOVICH LL, MATTAR ME, DANISH M, JUSKO WJ: Pharmacokinetics of methicillin in patients with cystic fibrosis. *J Infect Dis* 135:828, 1977

57. RABIN HR, HARLEY FL, BRYAN LE, ELFRING GL: Evaluation of a high dose tobramycin and ticarcillin treatment protocol in cystic fibrosis based on improved susceptibility criteria and antibiotic pharmacokinetics, in Sturgess JM (ed): *Perspectives in Cystic Fibrosis*. Toronto, Canadian Cystic Fibrosis Foundation, 1980, p 320

58. ORENSTEIN DM, FRANKLIN BA, GERMANN KJ, HOROWITZ JG, STERN RC, DOERSHUK CF: Running increases respiratory muscle endurance in cystic fibrosis. *Cystic Fibrosis Club Abstracts* 1980, vol 21, p 39

59. TABACHNIK E, LEVISON H: Clinical application of aerosols in pediatrics. *Am Rev Resp Dis* 122:97, 1980

60. MATTHEWS LW, DOERSHUK CF, SPECTOR S: Mist tent therapy of the obstructive pulmonary lesion of cystic fibrosis. *Pediatrics* 39:176, 1967

61. CHANG N, LEVISON H, CUNNINGHAM K: An evaluation of nightly mist tent therapy for patients with cystic fibrosis. *Am Rev Resp Dis* 107:672, 1973

62. LANDAU LI, PHELAN PD: The variable effect of a bronchodilating agent on pulmonary function in cystic fibrosis. *J Pediatr* 82:863, 1973

63. MILLIS RM, YOUNG RC JR, KULCZYCKI LL: Validation of therapeutic bronchoscopic bronchial washing in cystic fibrosis. *Chest* 71:508, 1977

64. SCHIDLOW DV, SIMON D, PALMER J, EVANS B, WILLIAMS JL, TURTZ MG, HUANG NN: Tracheobronchial lavage in cystic fibrosis, in Sturgess JM (ed): *Perspectives in Cystic Fibrosis*. Toronto, Canadian Cystic Fibrosis Foundation, 1980, p 231

65. STERN RC, BOAT TF, ORENSTEIN DM, WOOD RE, MATTHEWS LW, DOERSHUK CF: Treatment and prognosis of lobar and segmental atelectasis in cystic fibrosis. *Am Rev Resp Dis* 118:821, 1978

66. MEARNS MB, HODSON CJ, JACKSON ADM, HAWORTH EM, SELLORS TH, STURRIDGE M, FRANCE NE, REID L: Pulmonary resection in cystic fibrosis. *Arch Dis Child* 47:499, 1972

67. DAVIS PB, DISANT'AGNESE PA: Assisted ventilation for patients with cystic fibrosis. *JAMA* 239:1851, 1978

68. DISANT'AGNESE PA, DAVIS PB: Cystic fibrosis in adults. *Am J Med* 66:121, 1979

69. RICH RH, WARWICK WJ, LEONARD AS: Open thoracotomy and pleural abrasion in the treatment of spontaneous pneumothorax in cystic fibrosis. *J Pediatr Surg* 13:237, 1978

70. STOWE SM, BOAT TF, MENDELSOHN H, STERN RC, TUCKER AS, DOERSHUK CF, MATTHEWS LW: Open thoracotomy for pneumothorax in cystic fibrosis. *Am Rev Respir Dis* 111:611, 1975

71. LUCK SR, RAFFENSPERGER JG, SULLIVAN HJ, GIBSON LE: Management of pneumothorax in children with chronic pulmonary disease. *J Cardiovasc Surg* 74:834, 1977

72. HOLSCLAW DS, GRAND RJ, SHWACHMAN H: Massive hemoptysis in cystic fibrosis. *J Pediatr* 76:829, 1970

73. STERN RC, WOOD RE, BOAT TF, MATTHEWS LW, TUCKER AS, DOERSHUK CF: Treatment and prognosis of massive hemotysis in patients with cystic fibrosis. *Am Rev Resp Dis* 117:825, 1977

74. SCHUSTER SR, FELLOWS KE: Management of major hemoptysis in patients with cystic fibrosis. J Pediatr Surg 12:889, 1977

75. SWERSKY RB, CHANG JB, WISOFF BG, GORVOY J: Endobronchial balloon tamponade of hemoptysis in patients with cystic fibrosis. Ann Thorac Surg 27:262, 1979

76. FELLOWS KE, KHAW KT, SCHUSTER S, SHWACHMAN H: Bronchial artery embolization in cystic fibrosis: Technique and long-term results. J Pediatr 95:959, 1979

77. STERN RC, BURKAT G, HIRSCHFELT SS, BOAT TF, MATTHEWS LW, LIEBMAN J, DOERSHUK CF: Heart failure in cystic fibrosis. Am J Dis Child 134:267, 1980

78. GOLDRING RM, FISHMAN AP, TURINO GM, COHEN HI, DENNING CR, ANDERSON DH: Pulmonary hypertension and cor pulmonale in cystic fibrosis of the pancreas. J Pediatr 65:501, 1964

79. SIASSI B, MOSS AJ, DOOLEY RR: Clinical recognition of cor pulmonale in cystic fibrosis. J Pediatr 78:794, 1971

80. ROSENTHAL A, TUCKER CR, WILLIAMS RG, KHAW KT, STRIEDER D, SHWACHMAN H: Echocardiographic assessment of cor pulmonale in cystic fibrosis. Pediatr Clin North Am 23:327, 1976

81. ALLEN HD, TAUSSIG LM, GAINES JA, SANN DJ, GOLDBERG SJ: Echocardiographic profiles of the long-term cardiac changes in cystic fibrosis. Chest 75:428, 1979

82. CHIPPS BE, ALDERSON PO, ROLAND JA, YANG S, VANASWEGEN A, MARTINEZ CR, ROSENSTEIN BJ: Non-invasive evaluation of ventricular function in cystic fibrosis. J Pediatr 95:379, 1979

83. NEZELOF C, LESEC G: Multifocal myocardial necrosis and fibrosis in pancreatic diseases of children. Pediatrics 63:361, 1979

84. ABRAHAM AS, COLE RB, BISHOP JM: Reversal of pulmonary hypertension by prolonged oxygen administration to patients with chronic bronchitis. Circ Res 23:147, 1968

85. NEELY JG, HARRISON GM, JERGER JF, GREENBERG SD, PRESBERG H: The otolaryngologic aspects of cystic fibrosis. Trans Acad Ophthalmol Otolaryngol 76:313, 1972

86. LEDESMA-MEDINA J, OSMAN MZ, GIRDANY BR: Abnormal paranasal sinuses in patients with cystic fibrosis of the pancreas: Radiological findings. Pediatr Radiol 9:61, 1980

87. SHWACHMAN H, KULCZYCKI LL, MUELLER HL, FLAKE CG: Nasal polyposis in patients with cystic fibrosis. Pediatrics 30:389, 1962

88. OPPENHEIMER EH, ROSENSTEIN BJ: Differential pathology of nasal polyps in cystic fibrosis and atopy. Lab Invest 40:445, 1979

89. KULCZYCKI LL, BURLER JS, McCORD-DICKMAN D, HERER GR: The hearing of patients with cystic fibrosis. Arch Otolaryngol 20:54, 1970

90. FORMAN-FRANCO B, ABRAMSON AL, GORVOY JD, STEIN T: Cystic fibrosis and hearing loss. Arch Otolaryngol 105:338, 1979

91. OPPENHEIMER EH, ESTERLY JR: Cystic fibrosis of the pancreas: Morphologic findings in infants with and without diagnostic lesions. Arch Pathol 96:149, 1973

92. KOPEL FB: Gastrointestinal manifestations of cystic fibrosis. Gastroenterology 62:483, 1972

93. JOHANSEN PG, ANDERSON CM, HADORN B: Cystic fibrosis of the pancreas: A generalized disturbance of water and electrolyte movement in exocrine tissue. Lancet 1:455, 1968

94. CHASE HP, LONG MA, LAVIN MH: Cystic fibrosis and malnutrition. J Pediatr 95:337, 1979

95. SPROUL A, HUANG N: Growth patterns in children with cystic fibrosis. J Pediatr 65:664, 1964

96. SHWACHMAN H, LEBENTHAL E, KHAW KT: Recurrent acute pancreatitis in patients with cystic fibrosis and normal pancreatic enzymes. Pediatrics 55:86, 1975

97. HADORN B, ZOPPI G, SCHMERLING DH, PRADER A, McINTYRE I, ANDERSON CM: Quantitative assessment of exocrine pancreatic function in infants and children. J Pediatr 73:39, 1968

98. BARBERO GJ, SIBINGA MS, MARINO JM, SEIBEL R: Stool trypsin and chymotrypsin. Am J Dis Child 112:536, 1966

99. WOLF RO, TAUSSIG LM, ROSS ME, WOOD RE: Quantitative evaluation of serum pancreatic isoamylases in cystic fibrosis. J Lab Clin Med 87:164, 1976

100. TAUSSIG LM, WOLF RO, WOODS RE, DECKELBAUM RJ: Use of serum amylase isoenzymes in evaluation of pancreatic function. Pediatrics 54:229, 1974

101. NOUSIA-ARVANITAKIS S, ARVANITAKIS C, DESAI N, GREENBERGER NJ: Diagnosis of exocrine pancreatic insufficiency in cystic fibrosis by the synthetic peptide N-benzoyl-L-tyrosyl-P-aminobenzoic acid. J Pediatr 92:734, 1978

102. KHAW KT, AENIYI-JONES S, GORDON D, PALOMBO J: Comparative effectiveness of Viokase, Cotazym and Pancrease in children with cystic fibrosis. Cystic Fibrosis Club Abstracts, April 26, 1977, p 57

103. HARRIS R, NORMAN AP, PAYNE WW: The effect of pancreatin therapy on fat absorption and nitrogen retention in children with fibrocystic disease of the pancreas. Arch Dis Child 30:424, 1955

104. TWAROG FJ, WEINSTEIN SF, KHAW KT, STRIEDER DJ, COLTEN HR: Hypersensitivity to pancreatic extracts in parents of patients with cystic fibrosis. J Allergy Clin Immunol 59:35, 1977

105. STAPLETON FB, KENNEDY J, NOUSIA-ARVANITAKIS S, LINSHAW MA: Hyperuricosuria due to high dose pancreatic extract therapy in cystic fibrosis. N Engl J Med 295:244, 1976

106. DAVIDSON GP, HASSEL FM, CROZIER D, COREY M, FORSTNER GG: Iatrogenic hyperuricemia in children with cystic fibrosis. J Pediatr 93:976, 1978

107. NOUSIA-ARVANITAKIS S, STAPLETON FB, LINSHAW MA, KENNEDY J: Therapeutic approach to pancreatic-extract-induced hyperuricosuria in cystic fibrosis. J Pediatr 90:302, 1977

108. HEIZER WD, CLEVELAND CR, IBER FL: Gastric inactivation of pancreatic supplements. Bull Johns Hopkins Hosp 116:261, 1965

109. COX KL, ISENBERG JN, OSHER AB, DOOLEY RR: The effect of cimetidine on maldigestion in cystic fibrosis. J Pediatr 94:488, 1979

110. ALLAN JD, MASON A, MOSS AD: Nutritional supplementation in treatment of cystic fibrosis of the pancreas. Am J Dis Child 126:22, 1973

111. ROSENLUND ML, SELEKMAN JA, KIM HK, KRITCHEVSKY D: Dietary essential fatty acids in cystic fibrosis. Pediatrics 59:428, 1977

112. ELLIOTT RB: A therapeutic trial of fatty acid supplementation in cystic fibrosis. Pediatrics 57:474, 1976

113. LLOYD-STILL JD, SIMON SH, WESSEL HU, GIBSON LE: Negative effects of oral fatty acid supplementation on sweat chloride in cystic fibrosis. Pediatrics 64:50, 1979

114. CHASE HP, COTTON EK, ELLIOTT RB: Intravenous linoleic acid supplementation in children with cystic fibrosis. Pediatrics 64:207, 1979

115. SMITH FR, UNDERWOOD BA, DENNING CR: Depressed plasma retinolbinding protein levels in cystic fibrosis. J Lab Clin Med 80:423, 1972

116. PETERSEN RA, PETERSEN VS, ROBB RM: Vitamin A deficiency with xerophthalmia and night blindness in cystic fibrosis. Am J Dis Child 116:662, 1968

117. ABERNATHY RS: Bulging fontanelle as presenting sign in cystic fibrosis. Am J Dis Child 130:1360, 1976

118. SCOTT J, ELIAS E, MOULT PJA, BARNES S, WILLS MR: Rickets in adult cystic fibrosis with myopathy, pancreatic insufficiency and proximal renal tubular dysfunction. Am J Med 63:488, 1977

119. HAHN TJ, SQUIRES AE, HALSTEAD LR, STROMINGER DB: Reduced serum 25-hydroxyvitamin D concentration and disordered mineral metabolism in patients with cystic fibrosis. J Pediatr 94:38, 1979

120. WEISMAN Y, REITER E, STERN RC, ROOT A: Serum concentration of 25-hydroxyvitamin D and 24,25-dihydroxyvitamin D in patients with cystic fibrosis. J Pediatr 95:416, 1979

121. HUBBARD VS, FARRELL PM, DISANT'AGNESE PA: 25-Hydroxycholecalciferol levels in patients with cystic fibrosis. J Pediatr 94:84, 1979

122. MISCHLER EH, CHESNEY J, CHESNEY RW, MAZESS RB: Demineralization in cystic fibrosis. Am J Dis Child 133:632, 1979

123. WALTERS TR, KOCH HF: Hemorrhagic diatheses and cystic fibrosis in infancy. Am J Dis Child 124:641, 1972

124. TORSTENSON OL, HUMPHREY GB, EDSON JR, WARWICK WJ: Cystic fibrosis presenting with severe hemorrhage due to vitamin K malabsorption: A report of three cases. Pediatrics 45:857, 1970

125. FARRELL PM, BIERI JG, FRATANTONI JF, WOOD RE, DISANT'AGNESE PA: The occurrence and effects of human vitamin E deficiency. J Clin Invest 60:233, 1977

126. DEREN JJ, AROBA B, TOSKES PP, HANSELL J, SIBINGA MS: Malabsorption of crystalline vitamin B12 in cystic fibrosis. N Engl J Med 288:949, 1973

127. RUCKER RW, HARRISON GM: Vitamin B12 deficiency in cystic fibrosis. N Engl J Med 289:329, 1973

128. FLEISHER DS, DIGEORGE AM, BARNESS LA, CORNFELD D: Hypoproteinemia and edema in infants with cystic fibrosis of the pancreas. J Pediatr 64:341, 1964

129. GUNN T, BELMONTE MM, COLLE E, DUPONT C: Edema as the presenting symptom of cystic fibrosis: Difficulties in diagnosis. Am J Dis Child 132:317, 1978

130. FLEISHER DS, DiGEORGE AM, AUERBACH BH, HUANG NN, BARNESS LA: Protein metabolism in cystic fibrosis of the pancreas. J Pediatr 64:349, 1964

131. MULNE A, McCLUNG HJ, TOKARSKI P: Antitrypsin activity in soy formulas. Pediatr Res 10:358, 1976

132. HANDWERGER S, ROTH J, GORDEN P, DISANT'AGNESE P, CARPENTER DF, PETER G: Glucose intolerance in cystic fibrosis. N Engl J Med 281:451, 1969

133. ROSAN RC, SHWACHMAN H, KULCZYCKI LL: Diabetes mellitus and cystic fibrosis of the pancreas. Am J Dis Child 104:625, 1962

134. MILNER AD: Blood glucose and serum insulin levels in children with cystic fibrosis. Arch Dis Child 44:351, 1969

135. CHAZAN BI, BALODIMOS MC, HOLSCLAW DS, SHWACHMAN H: Microcirculation in young adults with cystic fibrosis: Retinal and conjunctival vascular changes in relation to diabetes. J Pediatr 77:86, 1970

136. WILMHURST EG, SOELDNER JS, HOLSCLAW DS, KAUFMANN RL, SHWACHMAN H, AOKI TT, GLEASON RE: Endogenous and exogenous insulin responses in patients with cystic fibrosis. Pediatrics 55:75, 1975

137. STAHL M, GIRARD J, RUTISHAUSER M, NARS PW, ZUPPINGER K: Endocrine function of the pancreas in cystic fibrosis: Evidence for an impaired

glucagon and insulin response following arginine infusion. *J Pediatr* 84:821, 1974

138. LIPPE BM, SPERLING MA, DOOLEY RR: Pancreatic alpha and beta cell function in cystic fibrosis. *J Pediatr* 90:751, 1977

139. LIPPE BM, KAPLAN SA, NEUFELD ND, SMITH A, SCOTT M: Insulin receptors in cystic fibrosis: Increased receptor number and altered affinity. *Pediatrics* 65:821, 1980

140. *1975 Report on Survival Studies of Patients with Cystic Fibrosis.* Atlanta, Cystic Fibrosis Foundation, 1977

141. DOLAN TF JR, TOULOUKIAN RJ: Familial meconium ileus not associated with cystic fibrosis. *J Pediatr Surg* 9:821, 1974

142. THOMAIDIS TS, AREY JB: Intestinal lesions in cystic fibrosis of the pancreas. *J Pediatr* 63:444, 1963

143. DONNISON AB, SHWACHMAN H, GROSS RE: A review of 164 children with meconium ileus seen at the Children's Hospital Medical Center, Boston. *Pediatrics* 37:833, 1966

144. HOLSCLAW DS, ECKSTEIN HB, NIXON HH: Meconium ileus: A 20-year review of 109 cases. *Am J Dis Child* 109:101, 1965

145. SHWACHMAN H: Gastrointestinal manifestations of cystic fibrosis. *Pediatr Clin North Am* 22:787, 1975

146. ROSENSTEIN BJ: Cystic fibrosis presenting with the meconium plug syndrome. *Am J Dis Child* 132:167, 1978

147. NOBLETT HR: Treatment of uncomplicated meconium ileus by Gastrografin. *J Pediatr Surg* 4:190, 1969

148. MEEKER IA JR, KINCANNON WN: Acetylcysteine used to liquify inspissated meconium causing intestinal obstruction in the newborn. *Surgery* 56:419, 1964

149. TAUSSIG LM, SALDINO RM, DISANT'AGNESE PA: Radiographic abnormalities of the duodenum and small bowel in cystic fibrosis of the pancreas (mucoviscidosis). *Radiology* 106:369, 1973

150. ANTONOWICZ I, REDDY V, KHAW KT, SHWACHMAN H: Lactase deficiency in patients with cystic fibrosis. *Pediatrics* 42:492, 1968

151. MORIN CL, ROY CC, LASALLE R, BONIN A: Small bowel mucosal dysfunction in patients with cystic fibrosis. *J Pediatr* 88:213, 1976

152. FREYE HB, KURTZ SM, SPOCK A, CAPP MP: Light and electron microscopic examination of the small bowel of children with cystic fibrosis. *J Pediatr* 64:575, 1964

153. GRYBOWSKI JD, THAYER WR JR, GABRIELSON IW, SPIRO HM: Disaccharidouria in gastric-intestinal disease. *Gastroenterology* 45:633, 1963

154. TAYLOR B, SOKOL G: Cystic fibrosis and coeliac disease. *Arch Dis Child* 48:692, 1973

155. O'CONNOR J, LAWSON J: Fibrocystic disease of pancreas and Crohn's Disease. *Br Med J* 4:610, 1972

156. MATSESHE JW, GO VLW, DIMAGNO EP: Meconium ileus equivalent complicating cystic fibrosis in postneonatal children and young adults. *Gastroenterology* 72:732, 1977

157. HOLSCLAW DS, ROCMANS C, SHWACHMAN H: Intussusception in patients with cystic fibrosis. *Pediatrics* 48:51, 1971

158. HOLSCLAW DS, ROCMANS C, SHWACHMAN H: Abdominal complaints and appendiceal changes leading to the diagnosis of cystic fibrosis. *J Pediatr Surg* 9:867, 1974

159. DOLAN TF JR, MEYERS A: Mild cystic fibrosis presenting as an asymptomatic distended appendiceal mass: A case report. *Clin Pediatr* 14:862, 1975

160. KULCZYCKI LL, SHWACHMAN H: Studies in cystic fibrosis of the pancreas: Occurrence of rectal prolapse. *N Engl J Med* 259:409, 1958

161. PARKINS RA: The diagnosis of cystic fibrosis by rectal suction biopsy. *Lancet* 2:851, 1963

162. OPPENHEIMER EH, ESTERLY JR: Hepatic changes in young infants with cystic fibrosis: Possible relation to focal biliary cirrhosis. *J Pediatr* 86:683, 1975

163. COOPER HS, OPPENHEIMER EH: Cystic fibrosis manifested as focal biliary cirrhosis in a newborn infant with congenital heart disease. *Johns Hopkins Med J* 135:268, 1974

164. TALAMO RC, HENDREN WH: Prolonged obstructive jaundice. Report of a case in a neonate with meconium ileus and jejunal atresia. *Am J Dis Child* 115:74, 1968

165. CRAIG JM, HADDAD H, SHWACHMAN H: The pathological changes in the liver in cystic fibrosis of the pancreas. *Am J Dis Child* 93:357, 1957

166. DISANT'AGNESE PA, BLANC WA: A distinctive type of biliary cirrhosis of the liver associated with cystic fibrosis of the pancreas. *Pediatrics* 18:387, 1956

167. STERN RC, STEVENS DP, BOAT TF, DOERSHUK CF, IZANT RJ, MATTHEWS LW: Symptomatic hepatic disease in cystic fibrosis: Incidence, course, and outcome of portal systemic shunting. *Gastroenterology* 70:645, 1976

168. SCHWARZ HP, KRAEMER R, THURNHEER U, ROSSI E: Liver involvement in cystic fibrosis. *Helv Paediatr Acta* 33:351, 1978

169. BOAT TF, DOERSHUK CF, STERN RC, MATTHEWS LW: Serum alkaline phosphatase in cystic fibrosis. *Clin Pediatr* 13:505, 1974

170. CUMMINGHAM DG, CHURCHILL RJ, REYNES CJ: Computed tomography in the evaluation of liver disease in cystic fibrosis patients *J Comput Assist Tomogr* 4:151, 1980

171. SCHUSTER SR, SHWACHMAN H, TOYAMA WM, RUBINO A, KHAW KT: The management of portal hypertension in cystic fibrosis. *J Pediatr Surg* 12:201, 1977

172. ESTERLY JR, OPPENHEIMER EH: Observations in cystic fibrosis of the pancreas. I. The gallbladder. *Bull Johns Hopkins Hosp* 110:247, 1962

173. ISENBERG JN, L'HEUREUX PR, WARWICK WJ, SHARP HL: Clinical observations on the biliary system in cystic fibrosis. *Am J Gastroenterol* 65:134, 1976

174. WEBER AM, ROY CC, CHARTRAND L, LEPAGE G, DUFOUR OL, MORIN CL, LASALLE R: Relationship between bile acid malabsorption and pancreatic insufficiency in cystic fibrosis. *Gut* 17:295, 1976

175. WEBER AM, ROY CC, MORIN CL, LASALLE R: Malabsorption of bile acids in children with cystic fibrosis. *N Engl J Med* 289:1001, 1973

176. GOODCHILD MC, MURPHY GM, HOWELL AM, NUTTER SA, ANDERSON CM: Aspects of bile acid metabolism in cystic fibrosis. *Arch Dis Child* 50:769, 1975

177. WATKINS JB, TERCYAK AM, SZCZEPANIK P, KLEIN PD: Bile salt kinetics in cystic fibrosis: Influence of pancreatic enzyme replacement. *Gastroenterology* 73:1023, 1977

178. ZENTLER-MUNRO PL, NORTHFIELD TC, BATTEN JC: The role of bile acid precipitation in fat maldigestion (abstract), in Sturgess JM (ed): *Perspectives in Cystic Fibrosis.* Toronto, Canadian Cystic Fibrosis Foundation, 1980, p 39a

179. FONDACARO JD, HEUBI JE, KELLOGG FW, INGBERG RL: Bile acid malabsorption in cystic fibrosis (abstract), in Sturgess JM (ed)): *Perspectives in Cystic Fibrosis.* Toronto, Canadian Cystic Fibrosis Foundation, 1980, p 14a

180. TAUSSIG LM, LOBECK CC, DISTANT'AGNESE PA, ACKERMAN DR, KATTWINKEL J: Fertility in males with cystic fibrosis. *N Engl J Med* 287:586, 1972

181. KAPLAN E, SHWACHMAN H, PERLMUTTER AD, RULE A, KHAW KT, HOLSCLAW DS: Reproductive failure in males with cystic fibrosis. *N Engl J Med* 279:65, 1968

182. LANDING BH, WELLS TR, WANG CI: Abnormality of the epididymis and vas deferens in cystic fibrosis. *Arch Pathol* 88:569, 1969

183. OPPENHEIMER EH, ESTERLY JR: Observations on cystic fibrosis of the pancreas. V. Developmental changes in the male genital tract. *J Pediatr* 75:806, 1969

184. HOLSCLAW DS, PERLMUTTER AD, JOCKIN H, SHWACHMAN H: Genital abnormalities in male patients with cystic fibrosis. *J Urol* 106:568, 1971

185. OPPENHEIMER EH, ESTERLY JR: Observations on cystic fibrosis of the pancreas. VI. The uterine cervix. *J Pediatr* 77:991, 1970

186. KOPITO LE, KOSASKY HJ, SHWACHMAN H: Water and electrolytes in cervical mucus from patients with cystic fibrosis. *Fertil Steril* 24:512, 1973

187. GRAND RJ, TALAMO RC, DISANT'AGNESE PA, SCHWARTZ RH: Pregnancy in cystic fibrosis of the pancreas. *JAMA* 195:993, 1966

188. DOOLEY RR, BRAUNSTEIN H, OSHER AB: Polypoid cervicitis in cystic fibrosis patients receiving oral contraceptives. *Am J Obstet Gynecol* 118:971, 1974

189. STERN RC, BOAT TF, DOERSHUCK CF, TUCKER AS, PRIMIANO FP JR, MATTHEWS LW: Course of cystic fibrosis in 95 patients. *J Pediatr* 89:406, 1976

190. BRUCE GM, DENNING CR, SPALTER HF: Ocular findings in cystic fibrosis of the pancreas. *Arch Ophthalmol* 63:391, 1960

191. RIMSZA ME, HERNDRIED LS, KAPLAN AM: Hemorrhagic retinopathy in a patient with cystic fibrosis. *Pediatrics* 62:336, 1978

192. LIETMAN PS, DISANT'AGNESE PA, WONG V: Optic neuritis in cystic fibrosis of the pancreas. *JAMA* 189:924, 1964

193. KATZNELSON D: Increased intracranial pressure in cystic fibrosis. *Acta Paediatr Scand* 67:607, 1978

194. ROACH ES, SINAI SH: Increased intracranial pressure following treatment of cystic fibrosis. *Pediatrics* 66:622, 1980

195. FISCHER EG, SHWACHMAN H, WEPSIC JG: Brain abscess and cystic fibrosis. *J Pediatr* 95:385, 1979

196. GELLER A, GILLES F, SHWACHMAN H: Degeneration of fasciculus gracilis in cystic fibrosis. *Neurology* 27:185, 1977

197. SPOCK A, WILSON WP: Electroencephalograms of patients with cystic fibrosis. *Am J Dis Child* 108:144, 1964

198. ELLIS CE, HILL DE: Growth, intelligence, and school performance in children with cystic fibrosis who have had an episode of malnutrition during infancy. *J Pediatr* 87:565, 1975

199. NEWMAN AJ, ANSELL BM: Episodic arthritis in children with cystic fibrosis. *J Pediatr* 94:594, 1979

200. SAGRANSKY DM, GREENWALD RA, GORVOY JD: Seropositive rheumatoid arthritis in a patient with cystic fibrosis. *Am J Dis Child* 134:319, 1980

201. BOREL DM, REDDY JK: Excessive lipofuscin accumulation in the thyroid gland in mucoviscidosis. *Arch Pathol* 96:269, 1973

202. DOLAN TF, GIBSON LE: Complications of iodide therapy in patients with cystic fibrosis. *J Pediatr* 79:684, 1971

203. AZIZI F, BENTLEY D, VAGENAKIS A, PORTNAY G, BUSH JE, SHWACHMAN H, INGBAR SH, BRAVERMAN LE: Abnormal thyroid function in response to iodides in patients with cystic fibrosis. *Trans Assoc Am Physicians* 87:111, 1974

204. SEGALL-BLANK M, VAGENAKIS AG, TREVES S, SHWACHMAN H, INGBAR SH, BRAVERMAN LE: Evaluation of thyroid function and pituitary TSH reserve in patients with cystic fibrosis. *Cystic Fibrosis Club Abstracts,* 1971, p 21

205. HUBBARD VS, DAVIS PB, DISANT'AGNESE PA, GORDEN P, SCHWARTZ RH: Isolated growth hormone deficiency and cystic fibrosis: A report of two cases. *Am J Dis Childd* 134:317, 1980

206. WARWICK WJ, BERNARD B, MESKIN LH: The involvement of the labial mucous salivary gland in patients with cystic fibrosis. *Pediatrics* 34:621, 1964

207. BARBERO GJ, SIBINGA MS: Enlargement of the submaxillary salivary gland in cystic fibrosis. *Pediatrics* 29:788, 1962

208. MANDEL ID, KUTSCHER A, DENNING CR, THOMPSON RH JR, ZEGARELLI EV: Salivary studies in cystic fibrosis. *Am J Dis Child* 113:431, 1967

209. BLOMFIELD J, WARTON LK, BROWN JM: Flow rate and inorganic components of submandibular saliva in cystic fibrosis. *Arch Dis Child* 48:267, 1973

210. CHERNICK WS, BARBERO GJ, PARKINS FM: Studies on submaxillary saliva in cystic fibrosis. *J Pediatr* 59:890, 1961

211. WIESMANN UN, BOAT TF, DISANT'AGNESE PA: Sodium concentration in unstimulated parotid saliva and on oral mucosa of normal subjects and in patients with cystic fibrosis. *J Pediatr* 76:444, 1970

212. WIESMANN UN, BOAT TF, DISANT'AGNESE PA: Flow-rates and electrolytes in minor salivary gland saliva in normal subjects and patients with cystic fibrosis. *Lancet* 2:510, 1972

213. HUFF DS, HUANG NN, AREY JB: Atypical cystic fibrosis of the pancreas with normal levels of sweat chloride and minimal pancreatic lesions. *J Pediatr* 94:237, 1979

214. STERN RC, BOAT TF, ABRAMOWSKY CR, MATTHEWS LW, WOOD RE, DOERSHUK CF: Intermediate-range sweat chloride concentration and pseudomonas bronchitis. *JAMA* 239:2676, 1978

215. SCHULZ IJ: Micro puncture studies of the sweat formation in cystic fibrosis patients. *J Clin Invest* 48:1470, 1969

216. MANGOS JA: Microperfusion study of the sweat gland abnormality in cystic fibrosis. *Tex Rep Biol Med* 31:651, 1973

217. KAISER D, DRACK E, ROSSI E: Inhibition of net sodium transport in single sweat glands by sweat of patients with cystic fibrosis of the pancreas. *Pediatr Res* 5:167, 1971

218. MANGOS JA, MCSHERRY NR: Sodium transport: Inhibitory factor in sweat of patients with cystic fibrosis. *Science* 158:135, 1967

219. MANGOS JA, MCSHERRY NR, BENKE PJ: A sodium transport inhibitory factor in the saliva of patients with cystic fibrosis of the pancreas. *Pediatr Res* 1:436, 1967

220. GRAND RJ, DISANT'AGNESE PA, TALAMO RC, PALLAVICINI JC: The effects of exogenous aldosterone on sweat electrolytes. II. Patients with cystic fibrosis of the pancreas. *J Pediatr* 70:357, 1967

221. COHEN LF, FARRELL PM, LUNDGREN DW, DISANT'AGNESE PA: Electrolyte values of sweat obtained by local and whole body collection methods in cystic fibrosis patients. *J Pediatr* 89:429, 1976

222. GIBSON LE, DISANT'AGNESE PA: Studies of salt excretion in sweat. *J Pediatr* 62:855, 1963

223. EMRICH HM, STOLL E, FRIOLET B, COLOMBO JP, RICHTERICH R, ROSSI E: Sweat composition in relation to rate of sweating in patients with cystic fibrosis of the pancreas. *Pediatr Res* 2:464, 1968

224. MUNGER BL, BRUSILOW SW, COOKE RE: An electron microscopic study of eccrine sweat glands in patients with cystic fibrosis of the pancreas. *J Pediatr* 59:497, 1961

225. KESSLER WR, ANDERSEN DH: Heat prostration in fibrocystic disease of the pancreas and other conditions. *Pediatrics* 8:648, 1951

226. DISANT'AGNESE PA: Salt depletion in cold weather in infants with cystic fibrosis of the pancreas. *JAMA* 84:2014, 1960

227. BECKERMAN RC, TAUSSIG LM: Hypoelectrolytemia and metabolic alkalosis in infants with cystic fibrosis. *Pediatrics* 63:580, 1979

228. ESTERLY NB, OPPENHEIMER EH, ESTERLY JR: Observations on cystic fibrosis of the pancreas: The apocrine gland. *Am J Dis Child* 123:200, 1972

229. GIBSON LE, COOKE RE: A test for concentration of electrolytes in sweat in cystic fibrosis of the pancreas utilizing pilocarpine by iontophoresis. *Pediatrics* 23:545, 1959.

230. KOPITO L, SHWACHMAN H: Studies in cystic fibrosis: Determination of sweat electrolytes *in situ* with direct reading electrodes. *Pediatrics* 43:794, 1969

231. SHWACHMAN H, DUNHAM R, PHILLIPS WR: Electrical conductivity of sweat. *Pediatrics* 32:85, 1963

232. ROSENSTEIN BJ, LANGBAUM TS, GORDES E, BRUSILOW SW: Cystic fibrosis: Problems encountered with sweat testing. *JAMA* 240:1987, 1978

233. DENNING CR, HUANG NN, CUASAY LR, SHWACHMAN H, TOCCI P, WARWICK WJ, GIBSON LE: Cooperative study comparing three methods of performing sweat tests to diagnose cystic fibrosis. *Pediatrics* 66:752, 1980

234. HARDY JD, DAVIDSON SHH, HIGGINS MU, POLYCARPOU PN: Sweat tests in the newborn period. *Arch Dis Child* 48:316, 1973

235. Report of the Committee for a Study for Evaluation of Testing for Cystic Fibrosis: *J Pediatr* 88:711, 1976

236. THOMPSON MW: Genetics of cystic fibrosis, in Sturgess JM (ed): *Perspectives in Cystic Fibrosis.* Toronto, Canadian Cystic Fibrosis Foundation, 1980, p 281

237. DANES BS, FLENSBORG EW: Cystic fibrosis: Cell culture studies on a Danish population. *Am J Hum Genet* 23:297, 1971

238. CAUDILL M, SCHAFER I, STJERNHOLM R: Sulphate incorporation of leucocytes from patients with cystic fibrosis. *Lancet* 1:32, 1974

239. HIRSCHHORN K: Genetic studies in disease, in Mangos JA, Talamo RC (eds): *Fundamental Problems in Cystic Fibrosis and Related Diseases.* New York, Intercontinental Medical Book Corporation, 1973, p 11

240. TALAMO RC, STIEHM ER, SCHWARTZ RH: Immunologic aspects of cystic fibrosis, in Mangos JA, Talamo RC (eds): *Cystic Fibrosis: Projections into the Future.* New York, Stratton, 1976, p 195

241. SHWACHMAN H, REDMOND A, KHAW KT: Report of 130 patients diagnosed under 3 months of age over a 20 year period. *Pediatrics* 46:335, 1970

242. HOLSCLAW DS JR, KEITH HH, PALMER J: Meconium screening for cystic fibrosis. *Pediatr Ann* 7:16, 1978

243. STEPHAN U, BUSCH EW, KOLLBERG H, HELLSING K: Cystic fibrosis detection by means of a test strip. *Pediatrics* 55:35, 1975

244. RYLEY HC, NEALE LM, BROGAN TD, BRAY PT: Screening for cystic fibrosis in the newborn by meconium analysis. *Arch Dis Child* 54:92, 1979

245. DESAI N, NOUSIA-ARVANITAKIS S: False negative meconium test results in screening for cystic fibrosis. *J Pediatr* 91:447, 1977

246. SHWACHMAN H, ANTONOWICZ I, MAHMOODIAN A: Studies in meconium. *Am J Dis Child* 132:1112, 1978

247. CROSSLEY JR, ELLIOTT RB, SMITH PA: Dried blood spot screening for cystic fibrosis in the newborn. *Lancet* 1:472, 1979

248. ESPSTEIN J, BRESLOW JL: Increased resistance of cystic fibrosis fibroblasts to ouabain toxicity. *Proc Natl Acad Sci USA* 74:1676, 1977

249. BRESLOW JL, MCPHERSON J, EPSTEIN J: Distinguishing homozygous and heterozygous cystic fibrosis fibroblasts from normal cells by differences in sodium transport. *N Engl J Med* 304:1, 1981

249a. BRESLOW JL, MCPHERSON J: Sodium transport in cystic fibrosis fibroblasts not different from normal. *N Engl J Med* 305:98, 1981

250. NADLER HL, WALSH MMJ: Intrauterine detection of cystic fibrosis. *Pediatrics* 66:690, 1980

251. DOROTAR D, DOERSHUK CF, STERN RC, BOAT TF, BOYER W, MATTHEWS L: Psychosocial functioning of children with cystic fibrosis. *Pediatrics* 67:338, 1981

252. ORENSTEIN DM, BOAT TF, STERN RC, TUCKER AS, CHARNOCK EL, MATTHEWS LW, DOERSHUK CF: The effect of early diagnosis and treatment in cystic fibrosis. *Am J Dis Child* 131:973, 1977

253. SHWACHMAN H, KULCZYCKI LL: Long-term study of one hundred five patients with cystic fibrosis. *Am J Dis Child* 96:6, 1958

254. TAUSSIG LM, KATTWINKEL J, FRIEDEWALD WT, DISANT'AGNESE PA: A new prognostic score and clinical evaluation system for cystic fibrosis. *J Pediatr* 82:380, 1973

255. *1978 Report of the Patient Registry.* Rickville, Md, Cystic Fibrosis Foundation, 1978

256. STERN RC, DOERSHUK CF, BOAT TF, TUCKER AS, PRIMIANO FP JR, MATTHEWS LW: Course of cystic fibrosis in black patients. *J Pediatr* 89:412, 1976

257. SCHIOTZ PO, HOIBY N: Precipitating antibodies against *Haemophilus influenzae* and *Staphylococcus aureus* in sputum and serum from patients with cystic fibrosis. *Acta Pathol Microbiol Scand [B]* 87:345, 1979

258. HOIBY N, HERTZ JB: Precipitating antibodies against *Escherichia coli, Bacteroides fragilis ss. thetaiotaomicron* and *Pseudomonas aeruginosa* in serum from normal persons and cystic fibrosis patients, determined by means of crossed immunoelectrophoresis. *Acta Paediatr Scand* 68:495, 1979

259. HOIBY N, AXELSEN NH: Identification and quantification of precipitins against *Pseudomonas aeruginosa* in patients with cystic fibrosis by means of crossed immunoelectrophoresis with intermediate gel. *Acta Pathol Microbiol Scand* 81:298, 1973

260. SCHIOTZ PO, HOIBY N, JUHL P, PERMIN H, NIELSEN H, SVEHAG SE: Immune complexes in cystic fibrosis. *Acta Pathol Microbiol Scand [C]* 85:57, 1977

261. SCHIOTZ PO, NIELSEN H, HOIBY N, GLIKMANN G, SVEHAG SE: Immune complexes in the sputum of patients with cystic fibrosis suffering from chronic *Pseudomonas aeruginosa* lung infection. *Acta Pathol Microbiol Scand [C]* 86:37, 1978

262. BERDISCHEWSKY M, POLLACK M, YOUNG LS, CHIA D, OSHER AB, BARNETT EV: Circulating immune complexes in cystic fibrosis. *Pediatr Res* 14:830, 1980

263. WALLWORK JC, MCFARLANE H: The SIgA system and hypersensitivity in patients with cystic fibrosis. *Clin Allergy* 6:349, 1976

264. WALLWORK JC, BRENCHLEY P, MCCARTHY J: Some aspects of immunity in patients with cystic fibrosis. *Clin Exp Immunol* 18:303, 1974

265. GIBBONS A, ALLAN JD, HOLZEL A, McFARLANE H: Cell-mediated immunity in patients with cystic fibrosis. *Br Med J* 1:120, 1976

266. SORENSEN RU, STERN RC, POLMAR SH: Cellular immunity to bacteria: Impairment of in vitro lymphocyte responses to *Pseudomonas aeruginosa* in cystic fibrosis patients. *Infect Immun* 18:735, 1977

267. SORENSEN RU, STERN RC, CHASE P, POLMAR SH: Defective cellular immunity to gram-negative bacteria in cystic fibrosis patients. *Infect Immun* 23:398, 1979

268. HARPER TB, GAUMER R, WARING W, BRANNON RB, SALVAGGIO JE: Cell mediated immunity and suppressor t-cell function in children with cystic fibrosis. *Lung* 157:219, 1980

269. CONOVER JH, CONOD EJ, HIRSCHHORN K: Complement components in cystic fibrosis. *Lancet* 2:1501, 1973

270. LIEBERMAN J: Complement components in cystic fibrosis. *Lancet* 1:1230, 1974

271. SCANLIN TF, NORMAN ME, ROSENLUND ML: C3 in cystic fibrosis. *Lancet* 1:1382, 1974

272. LYRENE RK, POLHILL RB JR, GUTHRIE LA, TILLER RE: Alternative complement pathway activity in cystic fibrosis. *J Pediatr* 91:681, 1977

273. BUESCHER ES, WINKELSTEIN JA: The ability of bacteria to activate the terminal complement components in serum of patients with cystic fibrosis. *J Pediatr* 93:530, 1978

274. STRAUSS RG: Complement in cystic fibrosis. *Helv Paediatr Acta* 34:429, 1979

275. SCHIOTZ PO, SORENSEN H, HOIBY N: Activated complement in the sputum from patients with cystic fibrosis. *Acta Pathol Microbiol Scand* [C] 87:1, 1979

276. BIGGAR WD, HOLMES B, GOOD RA: Opsonic defect in patients with cystic fibrosis of the pancreas. *Proc Natl Acad Sci* 68:1716, 1971

277. BÖHME B: Phagozytosedefekt der granulozyten bei zystischer fibrose. *Helv Paediatr Acta* 27:607, 1972

278. BOXERBAUM B, KAGUMBA M, MATTHEWS LW: Selective inhibition of phagocytic activity of rabbit alveolar macrophages by cystic fibrosis serum. *Am Rev Resp Dis* 108:777, 1973

279. CHURCH JA, KEENS TG, WANG CI, O'NEAL M, RICHARDS W: Normal neutrophil and monocyte chemotaxis in patients with cystic fibrosis. *J Pediatr* 95:272, 1979

280. MÜLLERTZ S: Natural inhibitors of fibrinolysis, in Davidson JF, Rowan RM, Samama MM, Desnoryers PC (eds): *Progress in Chemical Fibrinolysis and Thrombolysis.* New York, Raven Press, 1978, vol 3, p 213

281. SHAPIRA E, RAO GJS, WESSEL HU, NADLER HL: Absence of an α_2-macroglobulin-protease complex in cystic fibrosis. *Pediatr Res* 10:812, 1976

282. SHAPIRA E, BEN-YOSEPH Y, NADLER HL: Decreased formation of α_2-macroglobulin-protease complexes in plasma of patients with cystic fibrosis. *Biochem Biophys Res Commun* 71:864, 1976

283. SHAPIRA E, MARTIN CL, NADLER HL: Comparison between purified α_2-macroglobulin preparations from normal controls and patients with cystic fibrosis: Kinetic and structural properties of the complex with bovine trypsin. *J Biol Chem* 252:7923, 1977

284. SHAPIRA E, BEN-YOSEPH Y, NADLER HL: Abnormal breakdown of α_2-macroglobulin-trypsin complex in cystic fibrosis. *Clin Chim Acta* 78:359, 1977

285. BEN-YOSEPH Y, DeFRANCO CL, NADLER HL: Decreased sialic acid and altered binding to lectins of purified α_2-macroglobulin from patients with cystic fibrosis. *Clin Chim Acta* 99:31, 1979

286. COMINGS DE, LEFEVER LC, BEN-YOSEPH Y, NADLER HL: Normal two-dimensional gel electrophoresis of α_2-macroglobulin in cystic fibrosis. *Am J Hum Genet* 32:273, 1980

287. SCHIDLOW DV, KUEPPERS F: Trypsin bindings activity of alpha$_2$-macroglobulin in cystic fibrosis and other lung diseases. *Am Rev Resp Dis* 121:31, 1980

288. CHOY H, APPLEGARTH DA, DAVIDSON AGF, WONG LTK: Anti-plasmin (α_2-macroglobulin) activity of plasma from cystic fibrosis patients. *Biochem Biophys Res Commun* 82:1325, 1978

289. PARSONS M, ROMEO G: Cystic fibrosis α_2-macroglobulin protease interaction in vitro. *Clin Chim Acta* 100:215, 1980

290. BURDON MG: Normal subunit cleavage of alpha-2-macroglobulin in cystic fibrosis. *Clin Chim Acta* 100:225, 1980

291. ROMEO G, PARSON M, BOSSEN A, BLESSING-MOORE J, CAVALLI-SFORZA L: Trysin-binding IgG in cystic fibrosis. *Nature* 274:909, 1978

292. ROMEO G, PARSONS M, BOSSEN A, BLESSING-MOORE J, CAVALLI- SFORZA LL: Binding of ^{125}I-labeled proteinases to plasma proteins in cystic fibrosis. *Pediatr Res* 13:1030, 1979

293. ROMEO G, DENARO M, PARSONS M: Competition for trypsin binding between α_2-macroglobulin and antitrypsin antibodies in cystic fibrosis. *J Lab Clin Med* 95:116, 1980

294. SHAPIRA E, MENENDEZ R: Increased binding of concanavalin A to α_2-macroglobulin, IgM and IgG from cystic fibrosis plasma. *Biochem Biophys Res Commun* 93:50, 1980

295. TAYLOR A, MAYO JW, BOAT TF, MATTHEWS LW: Standardized assay for

296. MARTINEZ JR, MARTINEZ AM, GARRETT L, KORMAN P: Chronically reserpinized rat as a model for cystic fibrosis: Na$^+$ transport inhibitory effect in submaxillary saliva. *Pediatr Res* 13:1156, 1979

297. MANGOS JA, McSHERRY NR: Studies on the mechanism of inhibition of sodium transport in cystic fibrosis of the pancreas. *Pediatr Res* 2:378, 1968

298. ARAKI H, FIELD M, SHWACHMAN H: A new assay for cystic fibrosis factor: Effect of sera from patients with cystic fibrosis in the in vitro electrical properties of rat jejunum. *Pediatr Res* 9:932, 1975

299. GILMORE JP, DAVIS M, GIBBS GF: Influence of cystic fibrotic and heterzygous serum on rat jejunum. *Proc Soc Exp Biol Med* 157:70, 1978

300. TUCKER RD, GIBBS GE, CHRISTENSEN MB: Cystic fibrosis serum effect on the short circuit current of rat jejunum. *Pediatr Res* 13:1371, 1979

301. ARVANITAKIS S, MANGOS J, McSHERRY NR, RENNERT O: Effect of polyamines and cystic fibrosis serum on glucose transport. *Tex Rep Biol Med* 34:175, 1976

302. WILL PC, TAYLOR A, LEBOWITZ JL, DEARBORN DG, HOPFER U: Saliva from patients with cystic fibrosis inhibits amiloride-sensitive sodium transport. *Pediatr Res* 14:1245, 1980

303. WILL PC, BOAT TF, HOPFER U: Evidence against a specific effect of serum from patients with cystic fibrosis on sodium-dependent glucose transport in the rat jejunum. *Pediatr Res* 13:1129, 1979

304. MANGOS JA, DONNELLY WH: Isolated parotid acinar cells from patients with cystic fibrosis. Morphology and composition. *J Dent Res* 60:19, 1981

305. SPOCK A, HEICK HMC, CRESS H, LOGAN WS: Abnormal serum factor in patients with cystic fibrosis of the pancreas. *Pediatr Res* 1:173, 1967

306. CONOVER JH, BONFORTE RJ, HATHAWAY P, PACIUS S, CONOD EJ, HIRSCHHORN K, KOPEL FB: Studies on ciliary dyskinesia factor in cystic fibrosis. I. Bioassay and heterozygote detection in serum. *Pediatr Res* 7:220, 1973

307. WILSON GB, MONSHER MT, FUDENBURG HH: Studies on cystic fibrosis using isoelectric focusing. III. Correlation between cystic fibrosis protein and ciliary dyskinesia activity in serum shown by a modified rabbit tracheal bioassay. *Pediatr Res* 11:143, 1977

308. VERDUGO P, HINDS TR, VINCENZI FF: Laser light-scattering spectroscopy: Preliminary results on bioassay of cystic fibrosis factor(s). *Pediatr Res* 13:131, 1979

309. BOWMAN BH, LOCKHART LH, McCOMBS ML: Oyster ciliary inhibition by cystic fibrosis factor. *Science* 165:325, 1969

310. ADSHEAD PC, MARTINEZ JR, KILBURN KH, HESS RA: Ciliary inhibition and axonemal microtubule alterations in freshwater mussels. *Ann NY Acad Sci* 253:192, 1975

311. BESLEY GTN, PATRICK AD, NORMAN APL: Inhibition of the motility of gill cilia of *Dreissenia* by plasma of cystic fibrosis patients and their parents. *J Med Genet* 6:278, 1969

312. SANDERSON MJ, SLEIGH MA: Serum proteins agglutinate cilia and modify ciliary coordination. *Pediatr Res* 15:219, 1981

313. GABRIDGE MG, BRIGHT MJ, AGEE CC, NICKERSON JM, HENDERSON NS: Development of an improved tracheal explant bioassay for the detection of the ciliary dyskinesia factor in cystic fibrosis serum. *Pediatr Res* 13:31, 1979

314. CHERRY JD, RODEN VJ, REJENT AJ, DORNER RW: The inhibition of ciliary activity in tracheal organ cultures by sera from children with cystic fibrosis and control subjects. *J Pediatr* 79:937, 1971

315. PIVETTA OH, LABAL ML, SORDELLI DO: Serum ciliotoxic activity in mutant mice with some hereditary alterations resembling cystic fibrosis. *Pediatr Res* 13:1160, 1979

316. KURLANDSKY LE, BERNINGER RW, TALAMO RC: Mucus-stimulating activity in the sera of patients with cystic fibrosis: Demonstration and preliminary fractionation. *Pediatr Res* 14:1263, 1980

317. BANG BG, BANG FB: Mucus-stimulating substances in human body fluids assayed in an invertebrate mucous cell system. *Johns Hopkins Med J* 145:209, 1979

318. FLEMING N, STURGESS JM: Stimulation of glycoprotein secretion in dispersed rat submandibular gland acini by cystic fibrosis serum. *Experientia* 37:139, 1981

319. BOGART BI, PICARELLI J, GAERLAN PF, DENNING CR: CF serum induced K$^+$ efflux from rat submandibular gland tissue slices: A calcium dependent parameter, in Sturgess JM (ed): *Perspectives in Cystic Fibrosis.* Toronto, Canadian Cystic Fibrosis Foundation, 1980, p 29

320. ROSSMAN C, DOLOVICH J, DOLOVICH M, WILSON W, NEWHOUSE M: Cystic fibrosis-related inhibition of mucociliary clearance in vivo in man. *J Pediatr* 90:579, 1977

321. CONOD EJ, CONOVER JH, GAERLAN P: Separation of serum ciliary dyskinesia substances from cystic fibrosis subjects. *Pediatr Res* 11:45, 1977

322. WILSON GB, FUDENBERG HH: Ciliary dyskinesia factors in cystic fibrosis and asthma. *Nature* 266:463, 1977

323. WILSON GB, FUDENBERG HH: Studies on cystic fibrosis using isoelectric focusing. IV. Distinction between ciliary dyskinesia activity in cystic fibro-

sis and asthmatic sera and association of cystic fibrosis protein with the activity in cystic fibrosis serum. *Pediatr Res* 11:317, 1977

324. WILSON GB, FUDENBURG HH: Separation of ciliary dyskinesia substances found in serum and secreted by cystic fibrosis leukocytes and lymphoid cell lines, using protein A-sepharose CL-4B. *J Lab Clin Med* 92:463, 1978

325. CONOVER JH, CONOD EJ, HIRSCHHORN K: On the nature of the defect in cystic fibrosis. *Tex Rep Biol Med* 34:45, 1976

326. CONOVER JH, CONOD EJ, HIRSCHHORN K: Studies on ciliary dyskinesia factor in cystic fibrosis. IV. Its possible identification as anaphylatoxin (C3a)-IgG complex. *Life Sci* 14:253, 1974

327. NAGY EC, KHAN S, STURGESS JM: Serum factor in cystic fibrosis: Correlation with clinical parameters. *Pediatr Res* 13:729, 1979

328. CONOVER JH, BERATIS NG, CONOD EJ, AINBENDER E, HIRSCHHORN K: Studies on ciliary dyskinesia factor in cystic fibrosis. II. Short-term leukocyte cultures and long-term lymphoid lines. *Pediatr Res* 7:224, 1973

329. WILSON G, BAHM VJ: Synthesis and secretion of cystic fibrosis ciliary dyskinesia substances by purified sub-populations of leukocytes. *J Clin Invest* 66:1010, 1980

330. BOGART BI, CONOD EJ, CONOVER JH: The biologic activities of cystic fibrosis serum. I. The effects of cystic fibrosis sera and calcium ionophore A 23187 on rabbit tracheal explants. *Pediatr Res* 11:131, 1977

331. BOGART BI, CONOD EJ, GAERLAN PF, DENNING CR, CONOVER J: Biological activities of cystic fibrosis serum. III. CF serum induced uptake of $^{45}Ca^{++}$ by rabbit tracheal explants. *Biochem Biophys Res Commun* 88:1398, 1979

332. FARRELL PM, FOX GN, SPICER SS: Determination and characterization of ciliary ATPase in the presence of serum from cystic fibrosis patients. *Pediatr Res* 10:127, 1976

333. CZEGLEDY-NAGY E, STURGESS JM: Cystic fibrosis: Effects of serum factors on mucus secretion. *Lab Invest* 35:588, 1976

334. KENNEDY JR, ALLEN PL: Cystic fibrosis serum effects on rabbit tracheal epithelium: An ultrastructural analysis. *Pediatr Res* 14:1173, 1980

335. BOGART BI, CONOD EJ, GAERLAN PF, CONOVER J: The biologic activities of cystic fibrosis serum. II. Ultrastructural aspects of the effect of cystic fibrosis sera and calcium ionophore A23187 on rabbit tracheal explants. *Pediatr Res* 12:15, 1978

336. CHEUNG ATW, JAHN TL: High speed cinemicrographic studies on rabbit tracheal ciliated epithelia: Cytolytic effect of cystic fibrosis serum on tracheal epithelial cells. *Pediatr Res* 10:144, 1976

337. BOWMAN BH, MCCOMBS ML, LOCKHART LH: Cystic fibrosis: Characterization of the inhibitor to ciliary action in oyster gills. *Science* 167:871, 1970

338. MCCOMBS ML, BOWMAN BH: Rivanol treatment of cystic fibrosis serum: Effect of supernatant upon ciliary action. *Clin Genet* 1:171, 1970

339. HARPER BL, BARNETT DR, BISSETT JD: Immunochemical studies of the plasma and cultured fibroblast media fractions containing the cystic fibrosis ciliary inhibitor. *Tex Rep Biol Med* 34:73, 1976

340. DOGGETT RG, HARRISON GM: Cystic fibrosis: Reversal of ciliary inhibition in serum and saliva by heparin. *Tex Rep Biol Med* 31:685, 1973

341. SCHMOYER IR, BROOKS SP, FISCHER JF: Isolation and characterization of a ciliary dyskinetic factor from cystic fibrosis heterozygous serum. *Life Sci* 11:1037, 1972

342. SCHMOYER IR, FISCHER JF, BROOKS SP: Fractionation of oyster cilia inhibitor from cystic fibrosis heterozygote serum. *Biochem Biophys Res Commun* 46:1923, 1972

343. BARNETT DR, SCHANFIELD MS, MCCOMBS ML, BOWMAN BH: Isoelectric focusing and IgG allotyping of the serum fraction containing the cystic fibrosis ciliary inhibitor. *Tex Rep Biol Med* 31:709, 1973

344. BOWMAN BH, LANKFORD BJ, FULLER GM, CARSON SD, KUROSKY A, BARNETT DR: Cystic fibrosis: The ciliary inhibitor is a small polypeptide associated with immunoglobulin G. *Biochem Biophys Res Commun* 64:1310, 1975

345. DOGGETT RG, HARRISON GM, PATRICK TA: Cystic fibrosis: *In vivo* reversal of the ciliostatic character of serum and parotid secretions by heparin. *Nature [New Biol]* 243:250, 1973

346. GILLARD BK, FEIG SA, HARRISON GM, NELSON TE: Cystic fibrosis: Enzymatic detection of a cilostatic factor. *Pediatr Res* 10:907, 1976

347. IMPERO JE, HARRISON GM, NELSON TE: Cystic fibrosis: Isolation and physical properties of a salivary cystic fibrosis factor. *Pediatr Res* 12:108, 1978

348. BOWMAN BH, BARNETT DR, MATALON R, DANES BS, BEARN AG: Cystic fibrosis: Fractionation of fibroblast media demonstrating ciliary inhibition. *Proc Natl Acad Sci USA* 70:548, 1973

349. BARNETT DR, KUROSKY A, BOWMAN BH, HUTCHISON T, SCHMOYER I, CARSON SD: Cystic fibrosis: Molecular weight estimation of the ciliary inhibitor. *Tex Rep Biol Med* 31:703, 1973

350. DANES BS, LITWIN SD, HÜTTERORTH TH, CLEVE H, BEARN AG: Characterization of cystic fibrosis factor and its interaction with human immunoglobulin. *J Exp Med* 137:1538, 1973

351. BARNETT DR, BARRANCO SC, LOCKHART LH, LANKFORD BJ, MEYNE J, BOWMAN BH: Cystic fibrosis: Growth kinetics and production of the ciliary inhibitor by cultured fibroblasts. *Tex Rep Biol Med* 31:691, 1973

352. BARNETT DR, KUROSKY A, BOWMAN BH, BARRANCO SC: Loss of the ciliary inhibitory effect of the cystic fibrosis factor following proteolytic digestion and heat denaturation. *Tex Rep Biol Med* 31:697, 1973

353. CARSON SD, HARPER BL, BARNETT DR, KUROSKY A, LANKFORD BJ, BOWMAN BH: Electrophoretic studies of the cystic fibrosis ciliary inhibitor and its interaction with immunoglobulin G. *Tex Rep Biol Med* 31:209, 1976

354. BOWMAN BH, LOCKHART LH, HERZBERG VL, BARNETT DR, ARMSTRONG D, KRAMER J: Cystic fibrosis: Synthesis of ciliary inhibitor by amniotic cells. *Clin Genet* 4:461, 1973

355. BOWMAN BH, LANKFORD BJ, MCNEELY MC, CARSON SD, BARNETT DR, BERG K: Cystic fibrosis: Studies with the oyster ciliary assay. *Clin Genet* 12:333, 1977

356. HERZBERG V, CALVERT L, BOWMAN BH: Evidence that the ciliary inhibitor of cystic fibrosis is not an antibody. *J Clin Invest* 52:2732, 1973

357. BAUR, PS, BRINKLEY DR, BOWMAN BH: Effect of cystic fibrosis serum ciliary inhibitor on oyster gill ultrastructure: Analysis by scanning and transmission electron microscopy. *Tex Rep Biol Med* 34:155, 1976

358. MAYO BJ, KLEBE RJ, BARNETT DR, LANKFORD BJ, BOWMAN BH: Somatic cell genetic studies of the cystic fibrosis mucociliary inhibitor. *Clin Genet* 18:379, 1980

359. LIEBERMAN J, KANESHIRO W, COSTEA N: Characteristics of a new screening test for detecting the cystic fibrosis gene: Assay of a serum lectin, in Sturgess JM (ed): *Perspectives in Cystic Fibrosis*. Toronto, Canadian Cystic Fibrosis Foundation, 1980, p 308

360. NORDSTROM OV, BLOMFIELD J, BROWN JM: Isolation and characteristics of a fructose specific lectin from cystic fibrosis homozygote and heterozygote serum, in Sturgess JM (ed): *Perspectives in Cystic Fibrosis*. Toronto, Canadian Cystic Fibrosis Foundation, 1980, p 303

361. RAO GJS, POSNER LA, NADLER HL: Deficiency of kallikrein activity in plasma of patients with cystic fibrosis. *Science* 177:610, 1972

362. RAO GJS, NADLER HL: Arginine esterase in cystic fibrosis of the pancreas. *Pediatr Res* 8:684, 1974

363. LIEBERMAN J: Plasma arginine esterase activity in cystic fibrosis. *Am Rev Resp Dis* 109:399, 1974

364. GOLDSMITH GH, STERN RC, SAITO H, RATNOFF OD: Normal plasma arginine esterase and the Hageman factor (factor XII)-prekallikrein-kininogen system in cystic fibrosis. *J Lab Clin Med* 89:131, 1977

365. COBURN MD, COBURN LA, SOLOMONS CC: Plasma arginine esterase activity in cystic fibrosis. *Am Rev Resp Dis* 110:368, 1974

366. CHAN KYH, APPLEGARTH DA, DAVIDSON AGF: Plasma arginine esterase activity in cystic fibrosis of the pancreas. *Clin Chim Acta* 74:71, 1977

367. RAO GJS, NADLER HL: Deficiency of arginine esterase in cystic fibrosis of the pancreas. Demonstration of the proteolytic nature of the activity. *Pediatr Res* 9:739, 1975

368. WILSON GB, FUDENBERG HH: Studies on cystic fibrosis using isoelectric focusing. II. Demonstration of deficient proteolytic cleavage of α_2-macroglobulin in cystic fibrosis plasma. *Pediatr Res* 10:87, 1976

369. RAO GJS, PLATT WM, NADLER HL: Reaction of 4-methylumbelliferylguanidinobenzoate with proteases in plasma of patients with cystic fibrosis. *Enzyme* 23:314, 1978

370. WALSH-PLATT M, RAO GJS, NADLER HL: Protease deficiency in plasma of patients with cystic fibrosis: Reduced reaction of 4-methylumbelliferylguanidinobenzoate with plasma of patients with cystic fibrosis. *Enzyme* 24:224, 1979

371. WALSH MM, NADLER HL: Methylumbelliferylguanidinobenzoate reactive proteases in amniotic fluid: Possible marker for cystic fibrosis. *Lancet* 1:622, 1979

372. WALSH MMJ, NADLER HL: 4-methylumbelliferylguanidinobenzoate-reactive proteases in human amniotic fluid: Promising marker for the intrauterine detection of cystic fibrosis. *Am J Obstet Gynecol* 137:987, 1980

373. BROCK DJH, HAYWARD C: Methylumbelliferylguanidinobenzoate reactive proteases and prenatal diagnosis of cystic fibrosis. *Lancet* 1:1245, 1979

374. WALSH MMJ, RAO GJS, NADLER HL: Reaction of 4-methylumbelliferylguanidinobenzoate with proteases in human amniotic fluid. *Pediatr Res* 14:353, 1980

375. NADLER HL, WALSH MMJ: Prenatal detection of cystic fibrosis on amniotic fluid. *Lancet* 2:96, 1980

376. RAO GJS, NADLER HL: Deficiency of trypsin-like activity in saliva of patients with cystic fibrosis. *J Pediatr* 80:573, 1972

377. SCHÖNI M, KAISER D, DRACK E, EXMACHER U: Excretion of trypsinlike activity, electrolytes and protein in mixed and parotid saliva of patients with cystic fibrosis of the pancreas. *Eur J Clin Invest* 5:153, 1975

378. PLATT MW, RAO GJS, NADLER HL: Reaction of 4-methylumbelliferylguanidinobenzoate with cultivated skin fibroblasts derived from patients with cystic fibrosis. *Pediatr Res* 12:874, 1978

379. CALLAHAN JW, LEUNG A: Arginine esterase and lysosomal hydrolases in liver from cystic fibrosis subjects. *Pediatr Res* 11:1166, 1977

380. RENNERT OM, FRIAS JL, JULIUS RL, LAPOINTE D: The detection of the heterozygote and homozygote in cystic fibrosis by short term lymphocyte culture studies: A defect in RNA methylation. *Clin Pediatr* 11:351, 1972

381. RENNERT OM, JULIUS RL, LaPOINTE D: RNA methylation: A possible genetic marker in cystic fibrosis. *Pediatrics* 50:485, 1972

382. GAHL WA, PITOT HC: Diamine oxidase activity in fibroblasts from normal and cystic fibrosis patients. *Pediatr Res* 14:118, 1980

383. BUEHLER B, WRIGHT R, SCHOTT S, DARBY B, RENNERT OM: Ornithine decarboxylase and S-adenosyl methionine decarboxylase in skin fibroblasts of normal and cystic fibrosis patients. *Pediatr Res* 11:186, 1977

384. FARRELL PM, LUNDGREN DW: Recent observations concerning RNA methylation and polyamine metabolism in cystic fibrosis, in Mangos JA, Talamo RC (eds): *Cystic Fibrosis: Projections into the Future*. New York, Stratton Intercontinental Medical Book Corporation, 1976, p 223

385. GAHL WA, CHANGUS JE, PITOT HC: The effect of spermidine and spermine on proliferation *in vitro* of fibroblasts from normal and cystic fibrosis patients. *Pediatr Res* 10:531, 1976

386. SULLIVAN JL, KELLY JC, ROESS WB, DEBUSK AG: Membrane function in cystic fibrosis. II. Methionine transport in normal and cystic fibrosis fibroblasts. *Biochem Genet* 15:1125, 1977

387. LUNDGREN DW, HANKINS JM, ULANE MM, WILLISON JW: Putrescine uptake in cystic fibrosis fibroblasts. *J Pediatr* 90:1034, 1977

388. KELLY JC, DEBUSK AG: Membrane function in cystic fibrosis. I. Putrescine transport in normal and cystic fibrosis fibroblasts. *Biochem Genet* 15:695, 1977

389. McEVOY FA, HARTLEY CB: Polyamines in cystic fibrosis. *Pediatr Res* 9:721, 1975

390. LUNDGREN DW, FARRELL PM, DISANT'AGNESE PA: Polyamine alterations in blood of male homozygotes and heterozygotes for cystic fibrosis. *Clin Chim Acta* 62:357, 1975

391. BERRY HK, DENTON MD, GLAZER HS, KELLOGG FW: Normal polyamines in blood of homozygotes for cystic fibrosis, in Campbell RA, Morris DR, Bartos D, Daves GD, Bartos F (eds): *Advances in Polyamine Research*. New York, Raven Press, 1978, vol 2, p 307

392. RENNERT OM, FRIAS J, SHULKA JB: Polyamine metabolism in cystic fibrosis. *Tex Rep Biol Med* 34:187, 1976

393. COHEN LF, LUNDGREN DW, FARRELL PM: Distribution of spermidine and spermine in blood from cystic fibrosis and control subjects. *Blood* 48:469, 1976

394. BAYLIN SB, ROSENSTEIN BJ, MARTON LJ, LOCKWOOD DH: Age-related abnormalities of circulating polyamines and diamine oxidase activity in cystic fibrosis heterozygotes and homozygotes. *Pediatr Res* 14:921, 1980

395. ROSENBLUM MG, DURIE BGM, BECKERMAN RC, TAUSSIG LM, RUSSELL: Cystic fibrosis: Decreased conjugation and excretion of (^{14}C) spermidine. *Science* 200:1496, 1978

396. ROSENBLUM MG, DURIE BGM, SALMON SE, RUSSELL DH: Metabolism of (^{14}C) spermidine and (^{14}C) putrescine in normal volunteers and in cancer patients. *Cancer Res* 38:3161, 1978

397. RUSSELL DH, ROSENBLUM MG, BECKERMAN RC, DURIE BGM, TAUSSIG LM, BARNETT DR: Altered polyamine metabolism in cystic fibrosis. *Pediatr Res* 13:1137, 1979

398. WILSON GB, JAHN TL, FONSECA JR: Demonstration of serum protein differences in cystic fibrosis by isoelectric focusing in thinlayer polyacrylamide gels. *Clin Chim Acta* 49:79, 1973

399. FORSTNER G, KOHELL A, FORSTNER J: Isoelectric focusing of serum in cystic fibrosis: Failure to distinguish homozygote and heterozygote sera. *Clin Chim Acta* 70:459, 1976

400. ALTLAND K, SCHMIDT SR, KAISER G, KNOCHE W: Demonstration of a factor in the serum of homozygotes and heterozygotes for cystic fibrosis by a non-biological technique. *Humangenetik* 28:207, 1975

401. SMITH QT, HAMILTON MJ, SHAPIRO BL: Letter to the editor. *Pediatr Res* 10:999, 1976

402. THOMAS JM, MERRITT AD, HODES ME: Electrophoretic analysis of serum proteins in cystic fibrosis. *Pediatr Res* 11:1148, 1977

403. SCHOLEY J, APPLEGARTH DA, DAVIDSON AGF, WONG LTK: Letter to the editor: Detection of cystic fibrosis protein by electrofocusing. *Pediatr Res* 12:800, 1978

404. TULLY GW, NEVIN GB, YOUNG IR, NEVIN NC: Letter to the editor: Detection of cystic fibrosis protein by isoelectric focusing of serum. *Pediatr Res* 13:1078, 1979

405. NEVIN GB, NEVIN NC, REDMOND AO, YOUNG IR, TULLY GW: Detection of cystic fibrosis homozygotes and heterozygotes by serum isoelectrofocusing. *Hum Genet* 56:387, 1981

406. WILSON GB, ARNAUD P, FUDENBERG, HH: Improved method for detection of cystic fibrosis protein in serum using the LKB multiphor electrofocusing apparatus. *Pediatr Res* 11:986, 1977

407. WILSON GB: Cystic fibrosis protein, a confirmed diagnostic marker for detecting heterozygote carriers: Significance in relation to future screening and to a proposed defect in alpha$_2$-macroglobulin. *Pediatr Res* 13:1079, 1979

408. MANSON JC, BROCK DJH: Development of a quantitative immunoassay for the cystic fibrosis gene. *Lancet* 1:330, 1980

409. WILSON GB: Monospecific antisera, hybridoma antibodies, and immunoassays for cystic fibrosis protein. *Lancet* 2:313, 1980

410. WILSON GB, FUDENBERG HH: Studies on cystic fibrosis using isoelectric focusing. I. An assay for detection of cystic fibrosis homozygotes and heterozygote carriers from serum. *Pediatr Res* 9:635, 1975

411. SCHRÖDER CP, EMRICH HM: Ultramicroelectrophoresis of protein in sweat from patients with cystic fibrosis of the pancreas and controls. *Eur J Pediatr* 128:49, 1978

412. WILSON GB, JAHN TL: Decreased rate of cytolysis of *Colpidium striatium* by cystic fibrosis serum. I. Bioassay and evidence of the possible involvement of a CF factor—IgG complex. *Life Sci* 15:551, 1974

413. COHEN FL, DANIEL WL: Effects of cystic fibrosis sera on *Proteus vulgaris* motility. *J Med Genet* 11:253, 1974

414. BURDON MG, STUART AB: The agglutination of *Proteus vulgaris* by cystic fibrosis serum: A re-examination. *Clin Genet* 17:249, 1980

415. WANG A, TURNER MW, SOOTHILL JF, WARNER JO, NORMAN AP: *Proteus vulgaris* agglutination by cystic fibrosis sera. *Arch Dis Child* 55:130, 1980

416. MORRISSEY SM, TYMVIOS MC: The effect of cystic fibrosis and noncystic fibrosis plasma on electrophysiological responses in isolated frog gastric mucosa. *Monogr Paediatr* 10:102, 1979

417. BARGMAN GJ: Larval brine shrimp (nauplii): A potentially useful model to study cystic fibrosis. *Tex Rep Biol Med* 34:37, 1976

418. LITT M, KHAN MA, KWART H: Parotid secretions in cystic fibrosis: Effect on zeta potential of tracheal mucus. *Biochem Biophys Res Commun* 43:919, 1971

419. LITT M, KHAN MA: Detection of cystic fibrosis heterozygotes using the zeta potential method. *Tex Rep Biol Med* 34:151, 1976

420. KHAN MA, LITT M, KWART H, ROSENLUND ML: Measurement of colloid zeta potential as a test for cystic fibrosis secretion factor. *Tex Rep Biol Med* 31:665, 1973

421. BOWMAN BH: Factors related to cystic fibrosis, in Mangos JA, Talamo RC (eds): *Cystic Fibrosis: Projections into the Future*. New York, Stratton Intercontinental Medical Book Corporation, 1976, p 277

422. CHANDRA RK, MADHAVANKUTTY K, WAY RC: Serum alpha-fetoproetin levels in patients with cystic fibrosis and their parents and siblings. *Br Med J* 1:714, 1975

423. SMITH JA: Serum alpha-fetoprotein in cystic fibrosis. *Br Med J* 2:392, 1975

424. KNÖPFLE G, ROTTHAUWE HW, LEHMANN FG: Serum alpha$_1$-fetoprotein in cystic fibrosis. *Eur J Pediatr* 122:241, 1976

425. BISWAS S, NORMAN AP, BAFFOE G, GRAVES L: Prolactin, growth hormone and alpha-feto-protein in children with cystic fibrosis. *Clin Chim Acta* 69:541, 1976

426. LÜCKING T, MARISS P: Alpha-fetoprotein und cystische fibrose. *Klin Wochenschr* 54:391, 1976

427. BROCK DJH, BARRON L, MANSON J, McCRAE WM: Serum alpha-fetoprotein in cystic fibrosis of the pancreas. *Clin Chim Acta* 82:101, 1978

428. WU JT, HERBST JJ, BRAY PF: Elevated plasma levels of carcinoembryonic antigen in cystic fibrosis. *Pediatr Res* 10:235, 1976

429. WILSON GB, BURDASH NM, ARNAUD P. MONSHER MT, FUDENBERG HH: Carcino-embryonic antigen and cystic fibrosis protein in blood from cystic fibrosis homozygotes and heterozygote carriers. *Scand J Immunol* 5:829, 1976

430. MACSWENN JM, GILLESPIE CT: Salivary carcinoembryonic antigen (CEA) in cystic fibrosis. *Pediatr Res* 14:187, 1980

431. VAUGHAN WJ, LINDGREN FT, WHALEN JB, ABRAHAM S: Serum lipoprotein concentrations in cystic fibrosis. *Science* 199:783, 1978

432. MURAD F, MOSS WM, JOHANSON AJ, SELDEN RF: Urinary excretion of adenosine 3', 5'-monophosphate in normal children and those with cystic fibrosis. *J Clin Endocrinol Metab* 40:552, 1975

433. DAVIS PB: Urinary cyclic nucleotides in adult male cystic fibrosis patients. *Clin Chim Acta* 87:285, 1978

434. KING DN, WALSH MP, HEELEY AF, KUZEMKO JA: Sensitive trypsin assay for dried-blood specimens as a screening procedure for early detection of cystic fibrosis. *Lancet* 2:1217, 1979

435. APPLEGARTH DA, DAVIDSON AGF, KIRBY LT, BRIDGES M, SORENSEN P, WONG LT-K, HARDWICK DF: Dried blood spot screening for cystic fibrosis. *Lancet* 2:1236, 1979

436. DUFFY MJ, McGARRY Y, HYNES N, DUFFY GJ, TOBIN MJ, FITZGERALD MX: Decreased immunoreactive trypsin levels in sera from cystic fibrosis patients. *Clin Chim Acta* 103:233, 1980

437. DANDONA P, HODSON M, BELL J, RAMDIAL L, BELDON I, BATTEN JC: Serum immunoreactive trypsin in cystic fibrosis. *Thorax* 36:60, 1981

438. TOWNES PL, MOORE WD, WHITE MR: Amylase polymorphism: Studies of sera and duodenal aspirates in normal individuals and in cystic fibrosis. *Am J Hum Genet* 28:378, 1976

439. NIKOLAJEK WP, EMICH HM: α-Amylase activity in sweat and serum of patients with cystic fibrosis of the pancreas. *Eur J Pediatr* 122:289, 1976

440. SKUDE G, KOLLBERG H: Serum isoamylases in cystic fibrosis. *Acta Paediatr Scand* 65:145, 1976

441. KENNY D, COOKE A, TEMPANY E, McGEENEY KF: Activity of serum α-amylases in cystic fibrosis. *Clin Chim Acta* 89:429, 1978

442. GILLARD BK, MARKMAN HC, FEIG SA: Differences between cystic fibrosis and normal saliva α-amylase as a function of age and sex. Pediatr Res 12:868, 1978

443. DAVIDSON GP, KOHEIL A, FORSTNER GG: Salivary amylase in cystic fibrosis: A marker of disordered autonomic function. Pediatr Res 12:967, 1978

444. GILLARD BK, SIMBALA JA, FEIG SA: Serum amylase isoenzymes in cystic fibrosis patients. Evidence for a generalized defect in exocrine gland secretory regulation. Pediatr Res 14:1168, 1980

445. DOERING KM, ARGLEBE C, LUBAHN H, CHILLA R: "Fast isoamylases" in the parotid saliva of children with cystic fibrosis and heterozygous carriers. Eur J Pediatr 126:185, 1977

446. SCHIOTZ PO, MAGID E: Serum pancreatic isoamylases in the diagnosis of cystic fibrosis heterozygotes: A non-valuable test. Clin Genet 11:43, 1977

447. CASOLA L, DIMATTEO G, ROMANO M, RUTIGLIANO B, MASTELLA G: Glycosidases in serum of cystic fibrosis patients. Clin Chim Acta 94:83, 1979

448. SCANLIN TF, MATACIC SS, GLICK MC: Abnormal distribution of α-L-fucosidase in cystic fibrosis: Decreased activity in serum. Clin Chim Acta 91:197, 1979

449. ALHADEFF JA, WATKINS P: Cystic fibrosis serum α-L-fucosidase: Confirmation of normal activity levels and normal kinetic and isoelectric focusing properties. Clin Chim Acta 105:131, 1980

450. HÖSLI P, VOGT E: Detection of cystic fibrosis homozygotes and heterozygotes with plasma. Lancet 2:543, 1979

451. HARRIS A, BENSON PF, FENSOM AH: Detection of cystic fibrosis with plasma hydrolases. Lancet 2:1371, 1979

452. PATRICK AD, ELLIS RB: Plasma hydrolases in cystic fibrosis. Lancet 2:1015, 1979

453. SHAPIRO BL, SMITH QT, WARWICK WJ: Serum glutathione reductase and cystic fibrosis. Pediatr Res 9:885, 1975

454. GAHL WA, CHESNEY J, PITOT HC: Serum ribonuclease levels in patients with cystic fibrosis. Biochem Med 19:294, 1978

455. BARDON A, SHUGAR D: Properties of purified salivary ribonuclease, and salivary ribonuclease levels in children with cystic fibrosis and in heterozygous carriers. Clin Chim Acta 101:17, 1980

456. DANES BS, BEARN AG: A genetic cell marker in cystic fibrosis of the pancreas. Lancet 1:1061, 1968

457. SPICER SS, DISANT'AGNESE, VINCENT RA JR, ULANE M: Ultrastructural and cytochemical comparison of cultured normal and cystic fibrosis fibroblasts. Exp Mol Pathol 33:104, 1980

458. DANES BS, HODSON ME, BATTEN J: Cystic fibrosis: Evidence for a genetic compound from a family study in cell culture. Clin Genet 11:83, 1977

459. PALLAVICINI JC, WIESMANN U, UHLENDORF WB, DISANT'AGNESE PA: Glycogen content of tissue culture fibroblasts from patients with cystic fibrosis and other heritable disorders. Pediatrics 77:280, 1976

460. MATALON R, DORFMAN A: Acid mucopolysaccharides in cultured fibroblasts of cystic fibrosis of the pancreas. Biochem Biophys Res Commun 33:954, 1968

461. HOUCK JC, SHARMA VK: Functional failures of "fibrocytic" fibroblasts. Proc Soc Exp Biol Med 135:369, 1970

462. HOUCK JC, CHENG FL: Defects in the cell cycle of fibroblasts obtained from patients with cystic fibrosis. Proc Soc Exp Biol Med 147:167, 1974

463. CHRISTIAN ST, MONTI JA, FINLEY WH: Membrane fluidity in normal and cystic fibrosis fibroblasts. Biochem Biophys Res Comm 79:966, 1977

464. REINER EJ, MORAN TF: High-performance pyrolis-gas chromatography: Potential for differentiating cystic fibrosis cells. J Chromatrogr 221:371, 1980

465. FORREST GL: Colchinine binding activity and tyrosyl tubulin ligase activity in normal and cystic fibrosis fibroblasts. Biochem Biophys Res Commun 98:324, 1981

466. BUTTERWORTH J: Intracellular and extracellular α-D-mannosidase activity of cultured skin fibroblasts: Relationship to cystic fibrosis. Clin Chim Acta 108:347, 1980

467. WILLCOX P: Secretion of β-N-acetylglucosaminidase isoenzymes by cultured cystic fibrosis fibroblasts. Clin Chim Acta 91:81, 1979

468. GUY GJ, BUTTERWORTH J: Carboxypeptidase A activity of cultured skin fibroblasts and relationship to cystic fibrosis. Clin Chim Acta 87:63, 1978

469. HÖSLI P, VOGT E: Cystic fibrosis: Decreased thermostability of α-mannosidase in crude extracellular fluids of patients and carriers. FEBS Lett 104:271, 1979

470. HÖSLI P, ERICKSON RP, VOGT E: Prospects for prenatal diagnosis of cystic fibrosis: Induction of biochemical abnormalities in fibroblasts from patients with cystic fibrosis by a urinary glycoprotein. Biochem Biophys Res Commun 73:209, 1976

471. HÖSLI P, VOGT E: Cystic fibrosis: Leakage of lysosomal enzymes and of alkaline phosphatase into the extracellular space. Biochem Biophys Res Commun 79:741, 1977

472. HÖSLI P, VOGT E: Reliable detection of cystic fibrosis in skin-derived fibroblast cultures. Hum Genet 41:169, 1978

473. CAREY WF, HÖSLI P: Inhibition of Tamm-Horsfall glycoprotein induction of alkaline phosphatase in cystic fibrosis fibroblasts by medium conditioned by normal cells. Aust J Exp Biol Med Sci 57:225, 1979

474. MAYAHARD H, CHANG JP: Electron microscopic study of acid phosphatase activity in cultured human cystic fibrosis fibroblasts. Acta Histochem Cytochem 11:449, 1978

475. WIJCIK L, BUCHWALD M, RIORDAN JR: Induction of alkaline phosphatase in cultured human fibroblasts. Comparison of normal cells and those from patients with cystic fibrosis. Biochim Biophys Acta 585:374, 1979

476. AITKEN DA, HOOGEVEEN A: Alkaline phosphatase activity of normal and cystic fibrosis fibroblasts. J Med Genet 17:187, 1980

477. HÖSLI P, KOLLBERG H, VOGT E: Reliable diagnosis of the major type of cystic fibrosis with fibroblast cultures. Acta Paediatr Scand 67:617, 1978

478. DISANT'AGNESE PA, DAVIS PA: Recent research in cystic fibrosis. Monogr Paediatr 10:66, 1979

479. BUTTERWORTH J, GUY GJ: Primary amniotic fluid cell, skin fibroblast and liver α-+l-fucosidase and its relation to cystic fibrosis. Clin Chim Acta 92:109, 1979

480. SCANLIN TF, GLICK MC: Dynamic and structural aspects of cystic fibrosis fibroblast membranes, in Sturgess JM (ed): Perspectives in Cystic Fibrosis. Toronto, Canadian Cystic Fibrosis Foundation, 1980, p 44

481. OWEN E: Surface labeling of human skin fibroblasts of healthy and cystic fibrosis subjects. J Mol Med 3:203, 1978

482. HUNT LA, SUMMERS DF: Glycosylation of VSV glycoprotein is similar in cystic fibrosis, heterozygous carrier, and normal human fibroblasts. J Supramol Struct 7:213, 1977

483. CHASE HP, DABIERE CS, ELLIOTT RB: Fibroblast fatty acids in cystic fibrosis. Metabolism 29:365, 1980

484. LIMBOSCH S, POLIARD A, GEFFEL RV: Nucleoside uptake in normal and cystic fibrosis fibroblasts in vitro. Clin Chim Acta 102:11, 1980

485. ANSAH T-A, KATZ S: Characterization of a plasma membrane enriched fraction of human skin fibroblasts derived from cystic fibrosis patients and age matched control. Proc West Pharmacol Soc 23:389, 1980

486. MALER T, RIORDAN JR: Isolation and characterization of the plasma membranes of cultured lymphoblasts from patients with cystic fibrosis and normal individuals. Biochim Biophys Acta 598:1, 1980

487. DAVIS PB, LAUNDON SC: Adenylate cyclase in leukocytes from patients with cystic fibrosis. J Lab Clin Med 96:75, 1980

488. MALER T, DUTHIE M, ALON N, RIORDAN JR: α-L-Fucosidase is quantitatively reduced in cultured lymphoblasts from patients with cystic fibrosis. J Biol Chem 256:1420, 1981

489. HUBBARD VS, DUNN GD: Fatty acid composition of erythrocyte phospholipids from patients with cystic fibrosis. Clin Chim Acta 102:115, 1980

490. ANSAH T-A, KATZ S: Evidence for a Ca^{2+}-transport deficiency in patients with cystic fibrosis. Cell Calcium 1:195, 1980

491. LIPPE BM, KAPLAN SA, NEUFELD ND, SMITH A, SCOTT M: Insulin receptors in cystic fibrosis: Increased receptor number and altered affinity. Pediatrics 65:1018, 1980

492. ALHADEFF JA: Lysosomal hydrolases in cystic fibrosis livers. Clin Chim Acta 89:469, 1978

493. ALHADEFF JA, WATKINS P, FREEZE H: Purification and characterization of altered cystic fibrosis liver α-L-fucosidase. Clin Genet 13:417, 1978

494. ALHADEFF JA, CIMINO G: Cystic fibrosis liver sialyltransferase. Clin Genet 13:207, 1978

495. KAISER D, DRACK E: Diminished excretion of bicarbonate from the single sweat gland of patients with cystic fibrosis of the pancreas. Eur J Clin Invest 4:261, 1974

496. PAUNIER L, GIRARDIN E, SIZONENKO PC, WYSS M, MEGEVAND A: Calcium and magnesium concentration in sweat of normal children and patients with cystic fibrosis. Pediatrics 52:446, 1973

497. DEARBORN DG: Water and electrolytes of exocrine secretions, in Mangos JA, Talamo RC (eds): Cystic Fibrosis: Projections into the Future. New York, Stratton Intercontinental Medical Book Corporation, 1976, p 179

498. BLOMFIELD J, RUSH AR, ALLARS HM, BROWN JM: Parotid gland function in children with cystic fibrosis and child control subjects. Pediatr Res 10:574, 1976

499. HEIN J, DAVID A, GRIMM J, GOTTSCHALK B: Protein, IgA, secretory IgA, IgG and electrolytes as parameters of parotid gland function in children with cystic fibrosis. Monogr Paediatr 10:135, 1979

500. ALLARS HM, BLOMFIELD J, RUSH AR, BROWN JM: Colloid and crystal formation in parotid saliva of cystic fibrosis patients and non-cystic fibrosis subjects. I. Physiochemistry. Pediatr Res 10:578, 1976

501. ALLARS HM, COCKAYNE DJH, BLOMFIELD J, RUSH AR, VAN LENNER EW, BROWN JM: Colloid and crystal formation in parotid saliva of cystic fibrosis patients and non-cystic fibrosis subjects. II. Electron microscopy and electrophoresis. Pediatr Res 10:584, 1976

502. BOAT TF, WIESMAN UN, PALLAVICINI JC: Purification and properties of the calcium-precipitable protein in submaxillary saliva of normal and cystic fibrosis subjects. Pediatr Res 8:531, 1974

503. MAYO JW, WALLACE WM, MATTHEWS LW, CARLSON DM: Quantitation of submandibular proteins resolved from normal individuals and children with cystic fibrosis. *Arch Biochem Biophys* 175:507, 1976

504. MAYO JW, CARLSON DM: Protein composition of human submandibular secretions. *Arch Biochem Biophys* 161:134, 1974

505. GUHA AK, KUTTY KM, CHANDRA RK, WAY RC: A study of the salivary glycoprotein in cystic fibrosis patients and controls: Fucose incorporation and protein pattern. *Clin Biochem* 10:153, 1977

506. BOLANDE RP, TOWLER WF: Terminal nervous system in cystic fibrosis. *Arch Pathol* 95:172, 1973

507. ALHADEFF JA: Glycoproteins and cystic fibrosis: A review. *Clin Genet* 14:189, 1978

508. SAHU S, LYNN WS: Lipid composition of airway secretions from patients with asthma and patients with cystic fibrosis. *Am Rev Resp Dis* 115:233, 1977

509. BOAT TF, CHENG PW, IYER RN, CARLSON DM, POLONY I: Human respiratory tract sections: Mucous glycoproteins of nonpurulent tracheobronchial secretions, and sputum of patients with bronchitis and cystic fibrosis. *Arch Biochem Biophys* 177:95, 1976

510. ROUSSEL P, LAMBLIN G, DEGAND P, WALKER-NASIER E, JEANLOZ RW: Heterogeneity of the carbohydrate chains of sulfated bronchial glycoproteins isolated from a patient suffering from cystic fibrosis. *J Biol Chem* 250:2114, 1975

511. LAMBLIN G, LHERMITTE M, LAFITTE JJ, FILLIAT M, DEGAND P, ROUSSEL P: Comparative study of bronchial mucins isolated from the sputum of patients suffering from cystic fibrosis or other chronic bronchial diseases. *Bull Eur Physiopathol Resp* 13:175, 1977

512. KILBOURN JP: Letter to the editor: Bacterial flora and ion content of cystic fibrosis sputum. *Pediatr Res* 14:259, 1980

513. LORIN MI, GAERLAN PF, MANDEL IO, DENNING CR: Composition of nasal secretion in patients with cystic fibrosis. *J Lab Clin Med* 88:114, 1976

514. BOAT TF, KLEINERMAN JI, CARLSON DM, MALONEY WH, MATTHEWS LW: Human respiratory tract secretions. I. Mucous glycoproteins secreted by cultured nasal polyp epithelium from subjects with allergic rhinitis and with cystic fibrosis. *Am Rev Resp Dis* 110:428, 1974

515. NEUTRA MR, GRAND RJ, TRIER JS: Glycoprotein synthesis, transport, and secretion by epithelial cells of human rectal mucosa. Normal and cystic fibrosis. *Lab Invest* 36:535, 1977

516. NEUTRA MR, TRIER JS: Rectal mucosa in cystic fibrosis: Morphological features before and after short term organ culture. *Gastroenterology* 75:701, 1978

517. FORSTNER JF, FORSTNER GG: Effects of calcium on intestinal mucin: Implications for cystic fibrosis. *Pediatr Res* 10:609, 1976

518. JOHNSON C, BUCHANAN K, SHAW C, REDMOND A: Vasoactive intestinal peptide and abnormal mucus accumulation in the small bowel of patients with cystic fibrosis, in Sturgess JM (ed): *Perspectives in Cystic Fibrosis*. Toronto, Canadian Cystic Fibrosis Foundation, 1980, p 97

519. CLAMP JR, GOUGH M: Study of the oligosaccharide units from mucus glycoproteins of meconium from normal infants and from cases of cystic fibrosis with meconium ileus. *Clin Sci* 57:445, 1979

520. STURGESS J, REID L: The effect of isoprenaline and pilocarpine on (a) bronchial mucus-secreting tissue and (b) pancreas, salivary glands, heart, thymus, liver and spleen. *Br J Exp Pathol* 54:388, 1973

521. MARTINEZ JR, ADELSTEIN E, QUISSEL D, BARBERO GJ: The chronically reserpinized rat as a possible model for cystic fibrosis. I. Submaxillary gland morphology and ultrastructure. *Pediatr Res* 9:463, 1975

522. MARTINEZ JR, ADSHEAD PC, QUISSELL DO, BARBERO GJ: The chronically reserpinized rat as a possible model for cystic fibrosis. II. Composition and cilioinhibitory effects of submaxillary saliva. *Pediatr Res* 9:470, 1975

523. MAWHINNEY TP, FEATHER MS, MARTINEZ JR, BARBERO GJ: The chronically reserpinized rat as an animal model for cystic fibrosis. I. Acute effect of isoproterenol and pilocarpine upon pulmonary lavage fluid. *Pediatr Res* 13:760, 1979

524. THOMPSON FE, QUISSELL DO, WILLIAMS CH, MARTINEZ JR: The chronically reserpinized rat as a possible animal model for cystic fibrosis. IV. The protein composition of pulmonary lavage fluid. *Pediatr Res* 10:632, 1976

525. PERLMUTTER J, MARTINEZ JR: The chronically reserpinized rat as a possible model for cystic fibrosis. VII. Alterations in the secretory response to cholecystokinin and to secretin from the pancreas *in vivo*. *Pediatr Res* 12:188, 1978

526. WOOD DL, MARTINEZ JR: The chronically reserpinized rat as a possible model for cystic fibrosis. VI. Synergistic effects of isoproterenol on Ca^{++} and protein in the submaxillary gland. *Pediatr Res* 11:827, 1977

527. SHIFFMAN ML, GILLON MJ, GALEY WR: Water and electrolyte secretion by the pancreas of the reserpinized rabbit: A model for cystic fibrosis, in Sturgess JM (ed) *Perspectives in Cystic Fibrosis*. Toronto, Canadian Cystic Fibrosis Foundation, 1980, p 92

528. SORDELLI DO, CASSINO RJJ, PIVETTA OH: Animal model for cystic fibrosis: Pulmonary clearance of *Staphylococcus aureus* in mice treated with reserpine. *Life Sci* 24:2003, 1979

529. GREEN MC, SIDMAN RL, PIVETTA OH: Cribriform degeneration (cri): A new recessive neurological mutation in the mouse. *Science* 176:800, 1972

530. KAISER D, PIVETTA O, RENNERT OM: Autosomal recessively inherited electrolyte excretory defect in the parotid of the "cribriform degeneration" mouse mutant — possible analogy to cystic fibrosis. *Life Sci* 15:803, 1974

531. PIVETTA OH, SORDELLI DO, LABAL ML: Pulmonary clearance of *Staphylococcus aureus* in mutant mice with some hereditary alterations resembling cystic fibrosis. *Pediatr Res* 11:1133, 1977

532. PIVETTA OH, CASSINO RJJ, SORDELLI DO: Pulmonary cell response to bacterial challenge in mutant mice with some hereditary alterations resembling cystic fibrosis. *Life Sci* 26:1349, 1980

533. SCHNEYER CA, WILBORN WH: Effects of cystic fibrosis serum on the rat parotid gland. *Cell Tissue Res* 169:111, 1976

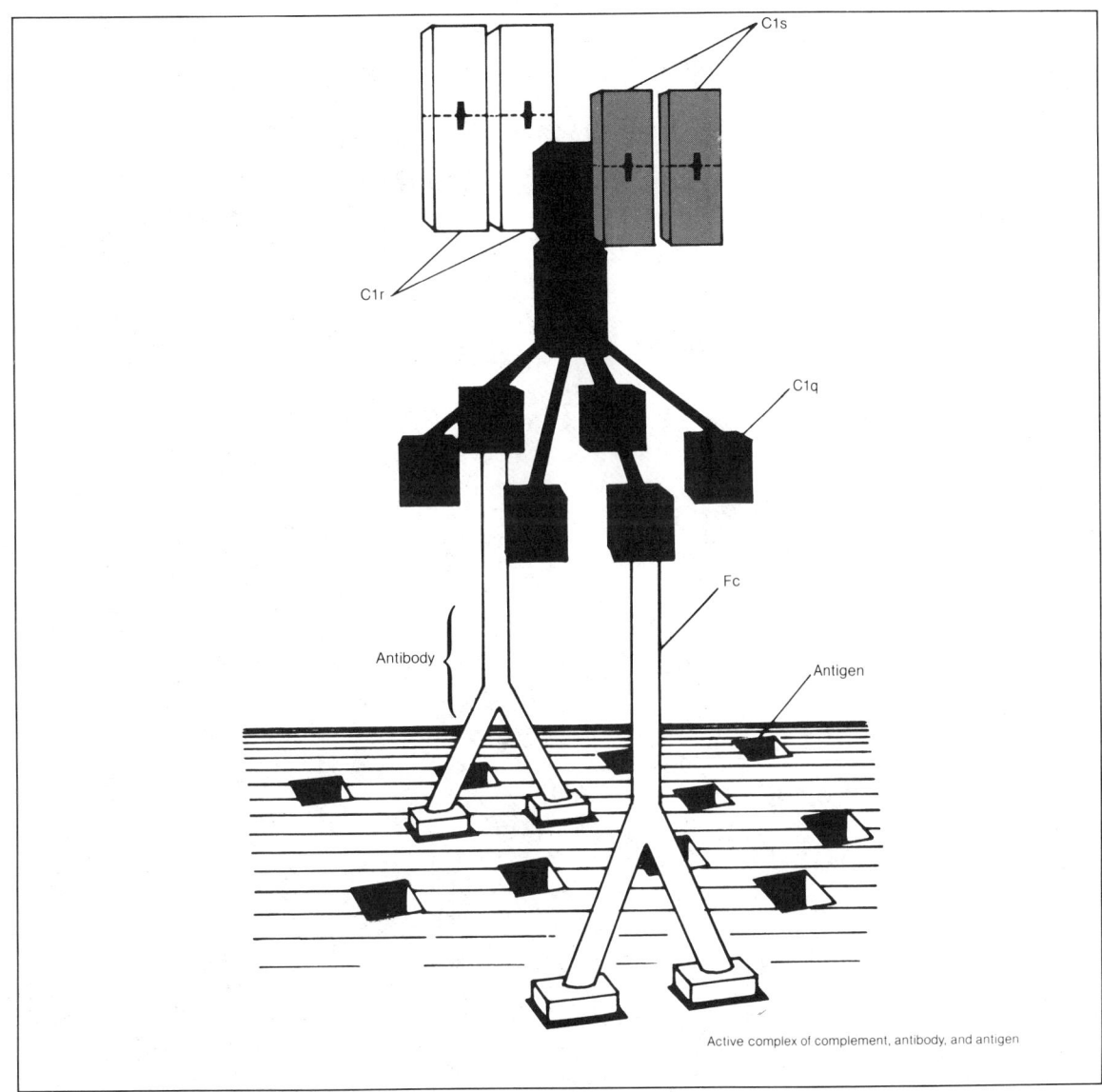

PART 13

Active complex of complement, antibody, and antigen

DISORDERS OF THE IMMUNE AND OTHER DEFENSE MECHANISMS

88

GENETIC DEFECTS IN GAMMA GLOBULIN SYNTHESIS

FRED S. ROSEN

1 *The immunoglobulins of human serum can be subdivided into five major classes: gamma G, gamma A, gamma M, gamma D, and gamma E. Four subclasses of gamma G and two subclasses of Gamma A have been identified. Chemical, genetic, and metabolic differences among the various classes and subclasses have been found. From 12 to 15 closely linked cistrons may control the synthesis of the immunoglobulins.*

2 *An X-linked disease, agammaglobulinemia, is characterized by recurrent pyogenic infections, failure to synthesize antibodies, and absence from the serum of all immunoglobulins. In affected males, plasma cells, which synthesize the immunoglobulins, are found to be absent from lymphoid tissue, bone marrow, spleen, and intestine. A form of the disease in which the onset of agammaglobulinemia is late, occurs in family clusters, but the genetic transmission of the defect is not clarified. Partial defects in immunoglobulin synthesis have been described. Gamma globulin replacement therapy offers adequate prophylaxis against recurrent infection in this group of syndromes.*

3. *A second large group of agammaglobulinemias is accompanied by lymphopenia, failure of normal thymic embryogenesis, an absence of cellular immunity, and is usually fatal. Patients are susceptible to bacterial, fungal, and viral infections. This defect may be transmitted as an X-linked or as an autosomal reces-sive phenomenon. The enzyme adenosine deaminase is absent in a number of patients with the autosomal recessive form of the disease. A number of variants of lymphopenic agammaglobulinemia have been described. Normal immunologic reactivity has been established in affected infants by transplants of histo-compatible bone marrow.*

In 1937 Tiselius first designated the gamma globulins as a distinct group of serum proteins which migrate most slowly toward the anode in an electrophoretic field [1]. In the following year Tiselius and Kabat [2] showed that the antibodies in serum are associated with the gamma globulin fraction. Although it became known during the next two decades that immunization resulted in a heterogeneous antibody response, in that gamma globulins of various molecular weights of "fast" or "slow" mobilities could be elicited, it was not appreciated until the late 1950s that the gamma globulins could be subdivided into various classes. At the present time, five classes of gamma globulins are recognized: IgG, IgA, IgM, IgD, and IgE. These classes of immunoglobulins are related to one another, in that they share a basic structural plan of four polypeptide chains that are symmetrically arranged about the long axis of the molecule. Two of the four polypeptide chains are common to all classes of immunoglobulins. An understanding of the structural relationships among the gamma globulin classes was made possible by the studies of Porter in 1959 [3]. These led to a hypothetical molecular model which has been verified experimentally and by direct visualization with the electron microscope and by x-ray diffraction.

STRUCTURE OF GAMMA GLOBULIN

In 1959 Porter reported that rabbit gamma globulin could be split into three fragments by the enzyme papain, in the presence of cysteine. Two of these are identical and contain the combining sites for antigen, and a third can be crystallized and does not bind antigen [3]. The two identical fragments are designated Fab (for "antigen binding"), and the third, Fc (for "crystallizable"). Fc fragments have a molecular weight of 48,000, and Fab fragments, 52,000. Thus upon papain digestion 1 mol of gamma globulin yields 1 mol of Fc fragments and 2 mol of Fab fragments. The molecular weight of the intact molecule is approximately 150,000.

In 1961 Edelman and Poulik reduced gamma globulin with mercaptoethanol in the presence of urea. By subsequent gel filtration in acid solution, two types of polypeptide chains could be separated [4]. *Heavy chains* (H chains) have a molecular weight of 53,000 to 70,000. The *light chains* (or L chains) have a molecular weight of 22,000. It was determined that Fab fragments are composed of L chains and portions of H chains, and that Fc fragments are composed only of parts of H chains (Fig. 88-1).

In contrast to the plant enzyme papain, animal proteases such as trypsin, chymotrypsin, and pepsin digest the Fc fragment into small peptides while the two Fab fragments remain joined together and retain bivalent antibody activity in a molecule of 100,000 molecular weight. This type of altered molecule is designated F(ab')$_2$ [5].

L chains, with a single minor exception, are covalently linked by a disulfide bond to H chains through the ultimate or penultimate amino acid residue at the carboxy terminus of the L chains, which is a cysteine residue. Variable numbers of disulfide bonds link the H chains together (see Table 88-1); depending on the class or subclass of immunoglobulin, there may be two to five inter-H chain disulfides [6].

The Bence Jones protein found in the urine of patients with multiple myeloma is composed of L chains or dimers of L chains [7]. When rabbits are immunized with individual Bence Jones proteins, two types of antisera to L chains can be obtained. The two types of L chains recognized by such antisera are designated as kappa (κ) and lambda (λ) L chains. All

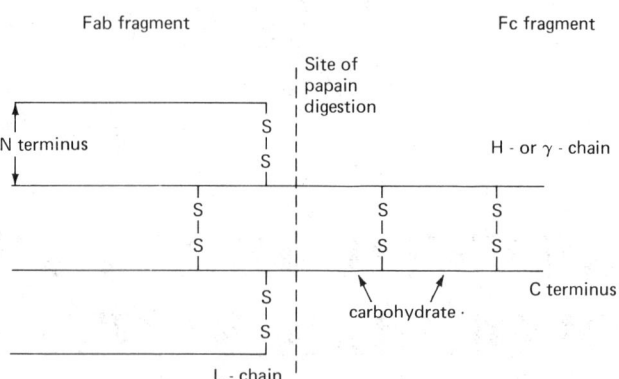

Figure 88-1   A schematic representation of the γ-globulin molecule. (*By R. R. Porter*)

immunoglobulin molecules, regardless of class or subclass, contain L chains of the kappa or lambda type. No individual molecule contains a mixture of the two, so that each immunoglobulin molecule or molecular subunit contains either two κ chains or two λ chains [8].

The amino acid sequences of a number of Bence Jones L chains of both kappa and lambda type have been worked out [9]. From these sequence data, analogies between the C-terminal halves (residues 106 to 212) of the L chains are quite apparent, whereas the N-terminal halves (residues 1 to 105) exhibit considerable variability. The adjacent N-terminal portions of H chains also are highly variable in their amino acid sequences, whereas the remainder of the H chains of various subclasses have constant homologies. The specific activity of the antibody molecule, i.e., its ability to combine with an antigen, resides in the variable portion of the Fab fragment, called the *V region*. No more than 5 percent of the entire molecule is occupied by the combining site. It is not certain how the antigen dictates this structural alteration to render gamma globulin molecules into specific antibodies. The remainder of the immunoglobulin is divisible into domains which are constant in that they exhibit little chemical variation in their amino acid sequence in various immunoglobulin classes. In fact, amino acid sequence analyses would indicate that the *constant (C) domains* have resulted from gene reduplications (Fig. 88-2). At least several biologic functions have been associated with the constant domains of the H chains of IgG (C_{H^2} and C_{H^3}). Complement fixation appears to be a property of the C_{H^2} domain, whereas the effector site for the phagocytic receptors resides in the C_{H^3} domain. Elaborations of the theories of antibody formation can be found in several reviews [10–12].

Before it was learned that there are two types of L chains, different classes of immunoglobulins were recognized by virtue of certain antigenic differences. It was first shown that the

Table 88-1   Physicochemical properties of the immunoglobulins

Immunoglobulin	Sedimentation coefficient, S	Approximate mol wt × 10³	Carbohydrate content	Heavy chains	Total S–S interchain bonds	Molecular formulas
IgG	6.6	150	2.8	γ$_1$	4	γ1$_2$κ$_2$; γ1$_2$λ$_2$
				γ$_2$	6	γ2$_2$κ$_2$; γ2$_2$λ$_2$
				γ$_3$	14	γ3$_2$κ$_2$; γ3$_2$λ$_2$
				γ$_4$	4	γ4$_2$κ$_2$; γ4$_2$λ$_2$
IgA	7, 9, 11, 15	170(n)	10	α$_1$	4	(α1$_2$κ$_2$)$_n$; (α1$_2$λ$_2$)$_n$
				α$_2$	3 or 4	(α2$_2$κ$_2$)$_n$; (α2$_2$λ$_2$)$_n$
IgM	18.6	900	10.2		26	(μ$_2$κ$_2$)$_5$; (μ$_2$λ$_2$)$_5$
IgD	7	160	10		3	δ$_2$λ$_2$; δ$_2$κ$_2$
IgE	7, 9	190	12		4	ε$_2$λ$_2$; ε$_2$κ$_2$

serum of boys with X-linked agammaglobulinemia lacked three classes of globulins, IgG, IgA, and IgM, when the serum was examined with horse antiserum to human serum [13], and that the myeloma globulins and macroglobulins of Waldenström's disease were related to one or another of these three classes of globulins [14] (Table 88-2). Subsequently, a fourth class, IgD, was found in certain myeloma patients whose M component was unrelated to the then-known three [15]. And, lastly, a fifth class, IgE, has been identified with reaginic activity in humans [16]. The differences among classes of the immunoglobulins reside in their H chains. The H chains are also designated by Greek letters for each immunoglobulin, thus: IgG = γ, IgA = α, IgM = μ, IgD = δ, and IgE = ϵ. By analogy with hemoglobin, a molecular formula for each immunoglobulin can be annotated (Table 88-1).

CLASSES AND SUBCLASSES OF IMMUNOGLOBULINS

Pertinent physicochemical data for immunoglobulins are given in Table 88-1. Table 88-2 contains quantitative and metabolic information on each of the immunoglobulin classes [17].

Gamma G Globulin

From 75 to 85 percent of the serum antibodies are contained in the IgG class. Antibodies to the pyogenic bacteria and viruses and antitoxins are principally in the IgG fraction.

Gamma G globulin contains 2.8 percent carbohydrate by weight. This is contained in two symmetrically arranged units attached to an asparagine residue of the H chain at amino acid residue 297 from the N-terminus [18].

The human placenta efficiently transports IgG from the maternal to fetal circulation, whereas the other immunoglobulins are almost completely excluded from the fetus. The mechanism for this active transport involves recognition of the Fc fragment [19].

Four subclasses of IgG globulin have been recognized by means of antigenic differences in individual IgG myeloma proteins. They are designated IgG1, IgG2, IgG3, and IgG4. The frequency distribution of these subclasses in normal serum is

Figure 88-2 Diagrammatic representation of the domains of immunoglobulin G (IgG). V indicates variable domains, and C, constant domains. (*Reprinted with permission from Dr. Blas Frangione.*)

Ig domains

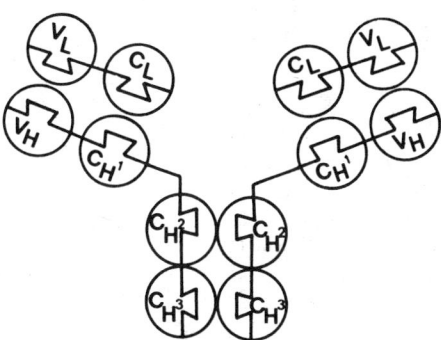

70:18:8:4 [20]. The ability of IgG globulin to fix complement is shared by IgG1, IgG2, and IgG3 but not by IgG4. The property of IgG globulin to fix to the skin receptors, as measured by passive cutaneous anaphylaxis, is contained in the IgG1, IgG3, and IgG4 molecules but not in IgG2. Phagocytic cells have a receptor for IgG1 and IgG3 but not for IgG2 and IgG4. In this case, the effector site has been localized to amino acid residues 407 to 416 of the γ chain of IgG1 [21]. All subclasses cross the placenta. Although the precise chemical localization of most of these functions is not yet known, chemical and genetic differences between the subclasses have been established.

Certain antibodies have been restricted to specific subclasses. For instance, antibodies to the linear polysaccharides are in the IgG2 subclass; anti-Rh, in IgG1 and IgG3; anti-A substance, in IgG1; and anti-factor VIII, principally in IgG4.

Gamma A Globulins

The IgA globulins constitute about 15 percent of the antibodies of human serum. A large spectrum of specificities has been associated with IgA globulins. They have a tendency to polymerize, and about 5 to 10 percent of serum IgA is found as a 9S dimer of the 7S form. Larger aggregates of 11S, 13S, and 15S are also found in serum in smaller amounts. The carbohydrate content of IgA globulin is 10 percent. The sugar is linked to two asparagine residues of the H or α chain. N-acetylgalactosamine is linked to one serine residue of the α chain [22].

Gamma A globulins are encountered in relatively large quantities in saliva, tears, colostrum, succus entericus, and nasal and bronchial secretions. Normal saliva contains 28 mg/dl; colostrum, 151 mg/dl; and tears, 7 mg/dl [23]. Most of the IgA in secretions is 11S globulin, along with lesser amounts of 15S and 7S forms. An additional structural unit is appended to IgA in secretions; it has a molecular weight of approximately 50,000 and has been designated *secretory piece* because of a presumptive function in transporting IgA globulins across mucosal surfaces [24]. This secretory piece is found only in mucosal cells, not in cells which synthesize IgA globulins. Critical evidence for a transport function for this piece is lacking at present. In addition to secretory piece, another polypeptide chain is associated with dimeric or polymeric IgA. It has been designated *J chain* because it appears to join the subunits together. It has a molecular weight of approximately 12,000 [25].

Two subclasses of IgA globulin are known. Not only do the α chains of both subclasses differ, but IgA2 appears to have no inter L-H chain disulfide bonds at all. Hydrogen bonding and other quaternary forces hold L chains of the molecules to the H chains [26].

Gamma A globulins do not fix complement, nor do they cross the placenta. They do neutralize viruses. Local immunization of the nasal mucosa or gastrointestinal tract has been successfully accomplished, with local production of IgA virus-neutralizing globulins. Although infants can synthesize IgA globulins at birth, or in utero if the fetus is stimulated by infection, the serum IgA globulin level rises slowly throughout childhood and does not reach adult levels until the end of the first decade of life.

Gamma M Globulin

Between 5 and 10 percent of serum antibody is encountered in

Table 88-2   Quantitation and metabolism of immunoglobulins in human beings

Immuno-globulin	Serum concentration mg/dl	Percent total body pool in plasma	Half-life, days	Percent plasma pool catabolized/day	Synthetic rate, mg/kg per day
IgG	600–1500	45	23	6.7	33
IgA	200–300	42	5.8	25	24
IgM	75–150	76	5.1	18	6.7
IgD	0–3	75	2.8	37	0.4
IgE	0.05	51	2.5	89	0.016

SOURCE: From Waldmann [17].

a class of immunoglobulins of large molecular size, the macroglobulins. They have a sedimentation coefficient of 19S and a molecular weight of 900,000. In 1957 Deutsch and Morton dissociated IgM globulins with mercaptoethanol into subunits of 6.5S [27]. The subunits, which have a molecular weight of 180,000, are designated IgMs. The intact molecule is composed of five subunits, but each subunit is composed of two L chains and two μ chains and has two combining sites, so that the intact molecule has 10 such combining sites [28]. From electron micrographs it appears that the subunits are arranged in a radial fashion and that the μ chains of the subunits are linked to adjacent subunits by disulfide bonds. The molecule contains 10.2 percent carbohydrate, all attached to the μ chains. The five IgM subunits also appear to be joined by a J chain [29].

A large number of antibody specificities have been associated with IgM. For example, antibodies to the large lipopolysaccharide antigens, such as the Wassermann, Forssman, blood group, and endotoxin antibodies, are principally IgM globulins. The IgM subunits may cross the placenta if they are present as free subunits in maternal serum. Little intact IgM globulin crosses the placental barrier. The fetus, if infected after the twentieth week of gestation, may synthesize considerable amounts of IgM globulins. Ordinarily they become detectable in the first week of extrauterine life and rise rapidly, to achieve adult levels of serum concentration by the age of 6 months.

Approximately one-half of the IgM globulins fix complement. In most detection systems about 1000 times fewer IgM molecules can be measured than other immunoglobulins. This ease of detectability had led to the assumption that IgM antibodies are formed first following an antigenic stimulus, whereas this may in truth be an artifact of the detection system employed.

Gamma D and Gamma E Globulins

The Ishizakas have demonstrated that reaginic antibody in the serum of ragweed sensitive people can be purified and identified with a unique class of immunoglobulins which is designated IgE [30, 31]. These immunoglobulins exhibit all the properties of reaginic antibody in the classic Prausnitz-Küstner test in that they fix to human and monkey skin, are heat-labile, are neutralized by allergens, and mediate histamine release. The discovery of two IgE myelomas has facilitated structural studies of this immunoglobulin class, which is ordinarily present in serum in only trace amounts [32, 33]. A large number of methionine and cysteine residues are present in the ε chain, as well as 11 percent by weight of carbohydrate. Ele-

vated serum levels of IgE globulin have been found in patients with extrinsic asthma, worm infestation, and various allergies [34, 35].

Antibody activity has been associated with IgD globulins. Over 20 patients with IgD myeloma have been reported, but the physiologic significance of this class of globulins is not known.

GENETIC DETERMINANTS OF GAMMA GLOBULINS

As previously intimated, allotypic differences, which are genetically determined, can be found on some immunoglobulin molecules. The known genetic markers are given in Tables 88-3 and 88-4. IgG1 contains the genetic markers G1m(a), G1m(x), G1m(f), and G1m(z) [36]. A γ_1 chain may contain the G1m(a), G1m(x), and G1m(z) markers or the G1m(f) marker. In the latter case, a distinctive peptide is present which replaces the G1m(a) marker peptide, and it is designated G1m(non-a). Thus, G1m(a) and G1m(z) are allelic to G1m(non-a) and G1m(f). The amino acid residue determining the G1m(z) and G1m(f) alleles is located at position 214 of the γ_1 chain, i.e., an arginine for G1m(f) and a lysine for G1m(z). The G1m(a) and G1m(non-a) allelic region is at positions 356 to 358 of the α_1 chain, i.e., Asp-Glu-Leu or Glu-Glu-Met, respectively. IgG2 is known to have one allele, at present designated G2m(n) or G2m(n−). In the IgG3 molecules, two allelic groups are known. One is designated G3m(g), and the other G3m(b). The

Table 88-3   Genetic markers of human immunoglobulins

Immunoglobulin	Marker
IgG1	G1m(a)
	(x)
	(f)
	(z)
IgG2	G2m(n)
IgG3	G3m(b0)
	(b1)
	(b3)
	(b4)
	(b5)
	(g)
IgA2	A2m(1)
	(2)
Kappa chain	Km(1)
	(2)
	(3)

G3m(b) region is complex and can be detected with various antisera. The G3m(b) antigens are designated G3m(b0), G3m(b1), G3m(b3), G3m(b4), and G3m(b5). Although the G3m(b) and G3m(g) determinants are almost never found on the same molecule, the structural determinants are not at the same residues on the γ_3 chain.

IgA1 has no known genetic markers, but two alleles are known for IgA2 and are designated A2m(1) and A2m(2) [37]. IgA2m(1) molecules lack inter-H-L disulfide bridges.

The three alleles of the κ chain occur at the Inv or Km locus. The Km alleles are designated $Km^{1,2}$, Km^1, and Km^3 [38]. $Km^{1,2}$ is associated with a leucine residue at position 191 of the κ chain, whereas Km^3 has a valine at that point. Km^1 is almost always associated with Km^2 in the κ chains of Caucasoids. When Km^1 is present alone, there is a valine-for-alanine substitution at position 153 of the κ chain [39].

The findings of rare Gm complexes has given preliminary evidence for recombination of genes in kindred with offspring whose gamma globulins contain rare gene complexes. It appears that the order of the cistrons may be IgG4-IgG2-IgG3-IgG1 [20].

The extensive homologies in amino acid sequences between the constant portions of the various immunoglobulins have given credence to the hypothesis that this complex system of immunoglobulins has arisen from gene duplications of a single primordial cistron.

In view of the expanding knowledge of the genes which control gamma globulin synthesis, it is somewhat disappointing that only a few patients have been identified in whom there is nonexpression of an allele governing immunoglobulin structure. On the other hand, a spectrum of genetic defects in gamma globulins synthesis results from a failure of development or maturation of cell populations which are involved in the synthesis of immunoglobulins.

It has been known for more than two decades that plasma cells are the site of immunoglobulin synthesis. Plasma cells are normally present in bone marrow, spleen, lymph nodes, tonsils, and inflammatory exudates. A subpopulation of lymphocytes, designated *B lymphocytes*, is the precursor of antibody-forming cells, the "B" indicating their origin from bone marrow or the bursa of Fabricius in avian species. B lymphocytes can be identified, enumerated, and separated from other lymphocytes by virtue of certain distinctive characteristics. In vitro, B lymphocytes can be induced to synthesize and secrete antibodies.

The earliest B lymphocytes are recognized in fetal liver at 12 weeks of human gestation. They subsequently are found in bone marrow, the cortex of lymph nodes and follicles of the spleen as well as in peripheral blood where they compose about 11 percent of the total lymphocyte population. Pre-B cells, the earliest differentiation stage identified, have cytoplasmic μ chains. Subsequently these cells express IgM and then IgM and IgD [40, 41]. Diversification of these IgM, IgD bearing cells leads to surface expression of IgG, IgA, and IgE. At the earliest stages B cells have receptors for C3, Fc, and Epstein-Barr (EB) virus. Infection of B cells with EB virus leads to their transformation into long-term cell lines in vitro. When B cells mature into plasma cells they lose all the aforementioned surface receptors and immunoglobulin [42].

The genetic basis of antibody diversity has been clarified by DNA cloning. The essential elements of the assembly of the genes is shown in Fig. 88-3. The L chains are encoded in three separate genes: a *V gene*, which includes the first two hyper-

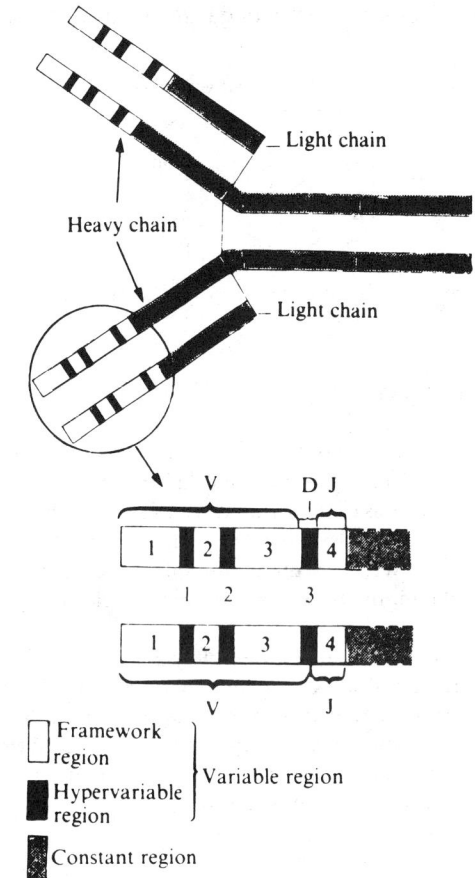

Figure 88-3 Schematic representation of the immunoglobulin genes. (*Reprinted with permission from Miranda Robertson.*)

variable regions and part of the third and the intervening three framework regions; a *J gene*, which encodes the remainder of the third hypervariable region and the fourth framework sequence; and the *C gene*, which encodes the C-terminal half or the constant region. Since there may be 300 to 500 V region genes, and 4 J region genes the capacity for generating diversity in thousands of combinations becomes self-evident. Further complexity is introduced in the H chains by the insertion of a D gene between the V and J regions as is shown in Fig. 88-3. It is now possible to envisage that almost 10^6 various combinants can be formed [43, 44].

X-LINKED AGAMMAGLOBULINEMIA

History

In 1952 Bruton reported the remarkable finding of the absence of gamma globulin from the serum of an 8-year-old boy who had been well up to the age of 4 years, when septic arthritis of the left knee developed. During the next 4 years, the boy had 19 episodes of pneumococcal sepsis, repeated attacks of otitis media, and two bouts of pneumococcal pneumonia. Although these illnesses were successfully treated with antibiotics, immunization with polyvalent pneumococcal vaccines did not protect him or result in the appearance of serum antibodies. Further investigation demonstrated that he was unable to produce

Table 88-4 Characteristics of gamma G globulin subclasses

Immunoglobulin	Caucasoid gene complexes				Complement fixation	Transplacental passage	Fixation to skin	Phagocyte receptors	Frequency distribution
IgG1		x							
	a	a	Non-a	Non-a	+	+	+	+	70
	z	z	f	f					
IgG2	n−	n−	n	n	+	+	0	0	18
IgG3	g	g	b	b	+	+	+	+	8
IgG4					0	+	+	0	4
Frequency of allelic complexes	0.20	0.10	0.52	0.17					

SOURCE: From Natvig et al. [20].

antibodies after typhoid vaccination, and a Schick test remained positive after attempted diphtheria immunization. Free electrophoresis of the serum revealed normal albumin and alpha and beta globulins, but the gamma fraction was undetectable [45]. With adequate intramuscular injections of gamma globulin, the patient has remained well to the present time.

These observations of susceptibility to bacterial infection accompanied by absence of gamma globulin and antibodies from the serum, as well as inability to synthesize antibody following appropriate antigenic stimulation, were confirmed in other patients by other observers within a short time. Over 200 cases of the disease have now been studied.

Clinical Features

Male infants with X-linked agammaglobulinemia usually remain well during the first 9 to 18 months of life, probably because of the passive protection afforded by the maternal gamma globulin. Undue susceptibility to infection becomes evident during the second year of life. Depending on the environment of the child, the presence of older sibs, and other circumstances, the onset of frequent infections may be even further delayed. Almost invariably these children contract infections from the pyogenic organisms, principally staphylococci, pneumococci, streptococci, and *Hemophilus influenzae*. The infections can usually be readily controlled with antimicrobial chemotherapy. Purulent sinusitis, pneumonia, sepsis, meningitis, and furunculosis are the most common types. These infections may recur persistently until proper prophylactic therapy is undertaken. Untreated, many of these children develop chronic progressive bronchiectasis and ultimately die of the pulmonary complications if they survive the innumerable infections.

Agammaglobulinemic children do not have increased susceptibility to the common viral diseases and exanthemas of childhood. They usually sustain measles, mumps, varicella, and rubella in an ordinary fashion [46]. When vaccinated with vaccinia virus, they generally exhibit the usual course of a primary take. They have no unusual infections with enterococci or gram-negative bacilli, nor do they have undue susceptibility to protozoal or mycotic infections. A number of deaths from *Pneumocystis carinii* has been reported in agammaglobulinemic infants and young children. Some agammaglobulinemic children with this parasite have been treated successfully with pentamidine isothionate.

It is particularly noteworthy that in one-third to one-half of these children a condition similar to rheumatoid arthritis of the large joints develops before the diagnosis is established. This complication disappears once replacement therapy with gamma globulin is begun [47].

Other collagen-like diseases have been observed in children with agammaglobulinemia. One of the most distressing and uniformly fatal is a syndrome resembling dermatomyositis [46, 48]. Edema, ligneous induration of the muscles, weakness, and rash over the extensor surfaces of the joints are the salient features. Biopsy and autopsy material show lymphorrhages around the small blood vessels. Similar involvement of the central nervous system has been observed, with progressive and ultimately fatal neurologic disease. Although the distribution of the lymphocytic infiltrates is characteristic of neoplasia, the individual cells of the infiltrate appear to be normal. Neither steroids nor antimetabolites have prevented a fatal outcome. Echo virus has been cultured persistently from the cerebrospinal fluid of several of these patients [49].

Hemolytic anemia, drug eruptions, atopic eczema, poison ivy, allergic rhinitis, and asthma have been observed in agammaglobulinemic patients with high frequency. Wheal and flare reactions cannot be elicited.

Genetics

The study of a large number of kindreds with multiple occurrences of agammaglobulinemia has disclosed an X-linked pattern of inheritance. Besides the occurrence of the disease in brothers, the diagnosis has been established in boys with sisters who subsequently had male children with the disease.

It has not been possible to do extensive linkage studies of the gene. The X-linked blood group Xg(a) is at least three crossover units distant from the agammaglobulinemia gene [50]. The position of the gene in relation to other X-linked traits is not known. The heterozygous female carrier of the gene cannot be detected by currently available methods. The incidence of the defect is not known. No ethnic group has an unusually high incidence of the defect.

Diagnosis

The serum of children with congenital agammaglobulinemia contains less than 100 mg of gamma G globulin per 100 ml. Serum gamma A and gamma M globulins are usually detectable or present in concentrations of less than 1 percent of normal. The small amount of gamma globulin synthesized by these children cannot be differentiated from normal gamma globulin.

The isohemagglutinin levels are low or absent. A positive Schick test in the presence of a history of diphtheria-pertussis-tetanus (DPT) immunization can be used to elicit the defect. Antigenic stimulation with any number of antigens fails to elicit an antibody response. With exquisitely sensitive methods of antibody measurement, very low levels of antibody to certain animal viruses but not to Phi X 174 phage particles can be demonstrated [51]. Apparently, the small amount of gamma globulin present in the serum is not "inert."

Delayed hypersensitivity reactions of both the tuberculin and the skin-contact type are intact, although perhaps quantitatively reduced in some patients. The former can be universally demonstrated with intradermally injected monilia antigen, with killed vaccinia virus after vaccination, or with tuberculin after infection with BCG, and the latter, with 2,4-dinitro-1-chlorobenzene (DNCB) applied to the skin as a patch test after suitable provocation with a vesicant dose of DNCB [52].

Other serum constituents involved in resistance to infection are normal. Serum complement, lysozyme, and properdin system levels, phagocytes, and interferon synthesis are within normal limits.

The diagnosis of X-linked agammaglobulinemia rests on the demonstration of an absence of plasma cells in lymph nodes stimulated with antigen. The basic defect in the disease is, in fact, the absence of plasma cells from the lymph nodes, spleen, intestine, and bone marrow [53]. In addition, there is no normal follicular organization of lymphocytes. The thymus gland is normal.

B lymphocytes are usually, but not always, absent in agammaglobulinemic children [54–57]. Normal numbers of pre-B cells are present in the bone marrow [41]. In rare cases, when B cells are present in the blood, they are unresponsive to mitogenic signals and bear surface IgD and IgM but do not secrete immunoglobulins [58]. Such cells can be transformed by EB virus and maintain their abnormal phenotype in long-term culture. When hybridized with mouse myeloma cells, the hybrid secretes human immunoglobulin H and L chains, thereby demonstrating that the Ig structural genes are intact [59].

Peripheral blood cells respond normally to phytohemagglutinin and to antigenic and allogenic stimuli [60]. Homograft rejection is intact in a few agammaglobulinemic patients who have been studied. Several cases of delayed rejection have been recorded, although normal second-set rejection has been observed. Thus peripheral blood *T lymphocytes,* or thymus-dependent cells, are normal.

Treatment

The injection of gamma globulin has proved to be an effective means of preventing the severe, recurrent, pyogenic infections sustained by these patients. Patients with congenital agammaglobulinemia have received repeated injections at monthly intervals for as long as 16 years without any ill effect or untoward reaction. It was indeed fortuitous that this antigenic material does not produce isosensitization of the immunologically handicapped children.

The dose of gamma globulin that provides effective prophylaxis was found empirically [61]. If the serum level is raised by approximately 200 mg/dl, invasive bacterial infections can be prevented. To achieve the desired level, a newly diagnosed patient is given 1.8 ml, or 300 mg, of gamma globulin per kilogram of body weight, usually in three divided doses of 0.6 ml, or 100 mg/kg. This raises the serum concentration by about 300 mg/dl. Since the half-life of the gamma globulin injected is 30 days or more in these patients, they must receive a monthly injection of 0.6 ml, or 100 mg/kg to maintain the desired level of approximately 200 mg/dl. Smaller doses are ineffective. Preparations suitable for intravenous use will soon be available.

COMMON, VARIED, OR "ACQUIRED" AGAMMAGLOBULINEMIA

Shortly after the initial description of congenital agammaglobulinemia, an acquired form of this disease was described in adults [62, 63]. The acquisition of agammaglobulinemia has been documented in several patients, but close observation has not revealed the cause for this sudden depression of gamma globulin synthesis [64, 65].

This form of agammaglobulinemia has been found equally in males and females. Although there is no clear-cut genetic influence on the occurrence of common varied agammaglobulinemia, multiple cases in a single kindred have been reported [67]. There has been a high incidence of other immunologic abnormalities in relatives of patients with common varied agammaglobulinemia, such as lupus erythematosus, hemolytic anemia, positive rheumatoid factor tests, and thrombocytopenic purpura [68].

Undue susceptibility to pyogenic infection, particularly to recurrent sinusitis and pneumonia, is also a prominent clinical feature of this form of agammaglobulinemia. Patients with chronic progressive bronchiectasis should be prime suspects for the diagnosis.

A prominent and frequent complication of common varied agammaglobulinemia, rarely seen in the congenital disease, is a sprue-like syndrome. Diarrhea, steatorrhea, at times protein-losing enteropathy, and a whole range of malabsorption difficulties afflict more than one-half of all adults with acquired agammaglobulinemia. An intestinal biopsy is rarely rewarding because, more often than not, the characteristic flattening of the villi seen in nontropical sprue is absent, and the biopsy material appears to be perfectly normal. In some instances, nodular lymphoid hyperplasia has been reported [69]. Some of these patients have improved on a gluten-free diet, and others upon elimination of milk from their diet. The most helpful therapy is found only by trial and error. *Giardia lamblia* is very frequently discovered in duodenal biopsies. A short course of metronidazole (Flagyl) therapy usually eliminates the gastrointestinal symptoms [70]. The arthritis so frequently seen in the congenital form of the disease is rarer in the acquired disease.

Another distinguishing feature of the acquired form of the disease is the frequent occurrence of noncaseating granulomas. The lungs, spleen, skin, and liver are most frequently involved. No microorganisms have been found consistently in these lesions. Steroid therapy has been helpful. A number of patients with acquired agammaglobulinemia have splenomegaly, or hepatosplenomegaly, and lymphadenopathy. The complications of hypersplenism have developed in some of these patients. This syndrome has affected multiple members of at least one kindred [71].

Quantitation of immunoglobulins in the serums of patients with common varied agammaglobulinemia usually reveals levels of IgG below 500 mg/dl, higher than those encountered in the serums of children with X-linked disease. Gamma A and gamma M may also be detected in significant quantity in the serums of these patients. The gamma G globulin may show restricted heterogeneity [72].

Lymph nodes lack plasma cells; however, in place of the absent follicles of congenital agammaglobulinemia, abiotrophy of the follicles or striking follicular hyperplasia may be found. Most patients with common varied agammaglobulinemia have B lymphocytes in their blood in normal or increased numbers. In some patients, these B lymphocytes are abnormal in tests in vitro in that they are unresponsive to mitogenic signals from T lymphocytes. Other patients have B lymphocytes which respond normally to the T cell signal by enlargement, division, formation of rough endoplasmic reticulum, and gamma globulin synthesis. The newly synthesized gamma globulin is not secreted [73]. The secretory block is associated with a failure of H chain glycosylation, a penultimate event in normal B lymphocytes prior to gamma globulin secretion [74]. The secretory defect is not corrected by hybridization with mouse myeloma cells [75]. Other patients have been described in whom normal B cells are encountered. The normal functioning of B lymphocytes is suppressed by T cells from such patients [76]. Yet other patients lack T helper cell activity [77] Thus a diverse variety of defects has been uncovered in the B and T lymphocytes of patients with this form of agammaglobulinemia. The biochemical bases for these defects remains to be elucidated.

Patients with primary acquired agammaglobulinemia have an unusually high incidence of "autoimmune" disease, such as pernicious anemia, hemolytic anemia, etc. [78]. Although patients with lymphoma or chronic lymphocytic leukemia may have or may later develop hypogammaglobulinemia, the progression of primary agammaglobulinemia to lymphoreticular malignancy has only rarely been documented. There is a frequent association between thymoma and acquired agammaglobulinemia [80]. Patients with thymoma and agammaglobulinemia may show progressive deterioration of cellular immunity and aregenerative anemia.

THE SELECTIVE IMMUNOGLOBULIN DEFICIENCIES

The advent of immunoelectrophoretic techniques led to a more precise definition of immunoglobulin defects in a number of situations in which the hypogammaglobulinemia involves one or two of the immunoglobulin classes, whereas the others are normal or elevated. Six combinations of the deficits of the three major immunoglobulins are obviously possible, although only two of these have been extensively reported. There have been many attempts to classify these abnormalities, but it is presently more confusing and less helpful to abide by one or

another system of designations than to describe the immuno-electrophoretic findings of the defect under discussion. It has been estimated that about 1 in 200 random hospital admissions has some form of dysgammaglobulinemia or selective immunoglobulin deficiency [80].

Absence of IgA, IgG, Normal or Elevated IgM

One of the common partial immunoglobulin defects is characterized by a deficiency of gamma A and gamma G globulins and increased amounts of gamma M globulin in the serum [81]. Gamma M globulin levels range from 150 to 1000 μg/dl in these patients. In spite of the occasional enormous elevations of the gamma M globulin levels, the gamma M globulin does not form an M component. The gamma M globulin appears to be of normally distributed molecules with antibody activity, particularly those usually associated with the macroglobulins, and to have a normal distribution of kappa and lambda chains. Several, but not all, of these patients have an elevation of the serum gamma D globulins and IgM subunits [82]. Both hereditary and acquired forms of this defect have been observed [83]. In addition to their undue susceptibility to infection, many of these patients acquire thrombocytopenia, neutropenia, renal lesions, and aplastic or hemolytic anemia, presumably manifestations of autoimmune processes. In one patient this was shown to involve the N antigen of the red cell [84]. Administration of exogenous gamma G gobulin has not generally decreased the gamma M globulin levels, although Hitzig has reported that it did ameliorate the severe neutropenia in a boy whom he observed [85], and in another report the IgM level was reduced by exogenous gamma G globulin [86].

The defect can apparently be inherited as an X-linked phenomenon. In one instance four boys of one kindred and two boys of another were reported to have this defect, and identical male twins are known to be affected [87]. A number of the patients have been adult females and older girls, in whom the defect appears to be a primary acquired one [88]. Several patients have died of a diffuse infiltrative process in which plasmacytoid cells proliferated diffusely in the intestine, gallbladder, liver, and other viscera. Enormous unilateral hypertrophy of the tonsil has developed, necessitating removal. B cells are found in normal numbers in the blood. They all have only surface IgM and IgD.

Absence of IgA, Normal IgG, and IgM

The isolated absence of gamma A globulin from the serum occurs in a significant but small proportion of the normal population [89]. Two healthy research workers have found their own serums to lack gamma A globulin [90]. Gamma A deficiency has been associated with steatorrhea and nontropical sprue [91]. These patients lack IgA-producing cells in the lamina propria of the intestinal tract, where IgA-producing cells are found in greatest abundance. Other patients with ataxia telangiectasia lack serum and secretory IgA [92].

Although familial lack of IgA is well documented, the mode of inheritance of the defect is not clearly established [93]. It is not linked to the A2m genotype [94]. Several patients with absent IgA have circulating anti-IgA antibodies. This may result in rapid catabolism of Iga [95] or in plasma transfusion reactions [96, 97]. Gamma A deficiency has been associated with partial deletions of the long arm of chromosome 18, but this is not a regular finding in patients with this chromosomal abnormality. Normal numbers of B cells are present in blood, particularly IgA-bearing B cells.

Selective IgG Subclass Deficiency

A number of patients have been described with recurrent pyogenic infections and selective deficiency of IgG1, IgG2, IgG3, or a combination of these subclasses. Other immunoglobulins are found in normal quantities in the serum [98, 99]. Although the inheritance of these IgG subclass deficiencies is not clear-cut, individuals with deletions of G1m and G3m markers have been encountered [100]. Individuals heterozygous for such deletions have no immunodeficiency disease but may have decreased serum IgG1 or IgG3 levels. In one case, an offspring of parents, one heterozygous for a G1m deletion and the other for a G3m deletion, had symptomatic hypogammaglobulinemia [99]. These immunoglobulin gene deletions are very rare and can account thus far for only a very small portion of patients with immunodeficiency disease. Normal persons who have G3m(b) on their IgG3 have twice the serum concentration of IgG3 as those who have G3m(g) [101].

SEVERE COMBINED IMMUNODEFICIENCY

History

In 1950 Glanzmann and Riniker described two unrelated infants who succumbed to overwhelming infection during the second year of life after a succession of serious infections, including intractable diarrhea, thrush, and a persistent morbilliform rash [102]. Recording persistent and profound lymphopenia in these two infants, they called the disorder *essential lymphocytophthisis*. Several dozen cases of this disease have now been well described [103]. It has been variously designated as "lymphocytosis," "the Swiss type of agammaglobulinemia," "thymic alymphoplasia," "thymic dysplasia," "lymphopenic agammaglobulinemia," etc. At least part of this confusion in terminology results from the fact that different modes of inheritances are fairly clearly established. In the early European descriptions it appeared that the disease was transmitted as an autosomal recessive disorder; there was consanguinity among approximately one-third of parents of affected children [104]. Further studies of affected families in America and Europe strongly suggested an X-linked mode of transmission. This supposition was based on (1) the documentation of affected males in three generations, and (2) the appearance of the disease in sons of a single mother with differing paternities [105, 106]. The fact that the phenocopy can arise from at least two different modes of inheritance probably accounts for the 3:1 ratio of males to females observed in the reported cases.

In 1972 Giblett et al. reported the absence of the enzyme adenosine deaminase in two girls with severe combined immunodeficiency [107]. This enzyme defect is now encountered in approximately one-half the patients with the autosomal recessive form of the disease [108]

Clinical Aspects

For purposes of clinical description it is probably easiest to lump the various genetic types because there is no discernible difference in their clinical course nor, for that matter, in the morbid anatomy of the disease. In any case, infections start early, between 3 and 6 months of age, and a rapid succession of debilitating infections brings about an early demise. Death within the first 2 years of life is the rule. Almost all infants with this disease develop loose, watery, chronic diarrhea. Frequently, stool cultures grow out *Salmonella* or enteropathic *Escherichia coli* strains. Pulmonary infection is also almost universal. Abscess of the lung containing *Pseudomonas aeruginosa* is a common cause of death, as is pneumonitis due to *Pn. carinii*. Extensive moniliasis of the mouth or diaper area persists beyond the neonatal period and is often a first sign of the disease. Thrush is usually present even before any antibiotic therapy. These infants are incapable of limiting and terminating the most benign viral infections. Death has resulted from generalized chickenpox, measles with Hecht's giant-cell pneumonia, and in a few instances from cytomegalovirus and adenovirus infection. Vaccination results in progressive, ultimately fatal, vaccinia infection: BCG inoculation has also resulted in progressive BCG infection. These infants fail to thrive. Lack of weight gain gives the appearance of "runting," which may be aggravated by protein losing enteropathy and severe diarrhea.

Diagnosis

In 1958 the Swiss workers pointed out that agammaglobulinemia is a prominent feature of this disease entity [109, 110]. Serum concentrations of immunoglobulins are very low, and gamma G may exhibit restricted heterogeneity [111]. No antibody synthesis can be detected.

Leukopenia is usually encountered because of the low lymphocyte counts, usually less than 2000 per mm³. The lymphocyte count may be variable and may decline from initial normal neonatal levels (3000 per mm³) to profoundly lymphopenic levels. A single lymphocyte count is, nonetheless, not a reliable index of the disease, since normal counts can be observed occasionally. Electron microscopy reveals that these blood lymphocytes are mostly immature forms resembling lymphoblasts. Indeed they usually bear the thymocyte antigens T9 and T10 [112]. Granulocytes and platelets are normal, but leukocytosis may not occur in the presence of overt infection. Eosinophilia is common, and abnormal granulation of the eosinophils has been reported. The bone marrow is uniformly deficient in plasma cells, lymphocytes, and lymphoblasts. Bone marrow of normal infants contain up to 20 percent of cells in the lymphocytic series. Lymph node biopsy, when feasible, exhibits a complete lack of germinal elements, plasma cells, and lymphocytes. Only the stroma of the node is seen to contain occasional mast cells and eosinophils or, rarely, small collections of lymphoid cells without any apparent organization. Peripheral blood lacks mature B and T cells.

No indicators of delayed sensitivity can be elicited in these infants. They are unresponsive to monilia antigen in the presence of overt, chronic monilia infection. They cannot be sensitized to DNCB. The peripheral blood lymphocytes are completely unresponsive to phytohemagglutinin or allogeneic stimulation. Skin grafts are accepted with no microscopic or macroscopic signs of rejection. At autopsy lymphoid tissue is absent from the spleen, tonsils, appendix, and intestines. The thymus gland is found with difficulty in the neck and has usually failed to descend in the normal manner into the anterior mediastinum. It weighs less than 1 g and is composed of primordial, spindle-shaped cells, occasionally forming swirls or rosettes. No Hassall's corpuscles and few, if any, lymphocytes are found. The dysplasia of the thymus gland is a uniformly characteristic feature of this disease. Adenosine deaminase, an enzyme which converts adenosine to inosine, is universally present in the tissues and serum of all mammalian species; together with adenosine kinase it regulates disposal of adenosine and thus plays a major role in the control of intracellular adenine metabolism. Adenosine deaminase is deficient in the erythrocytes and other tissues of approximately one-half of the infants affected with the autosomal recessive form of severe combined immunodeficiency [98, 99, 113–115]. The enzyme has a common electrophoretic polymorphism [116], which has permitted the detection of a "null" gene in at least two kindred where the obligatory heterozygotes paradoxically were homozygous for erythrocyte adenosine deaminase (ADA) [117, 118]. Although ADA is undetectable in the erythrocytes of affected infants, and is approximately one-half of normal in erythrocytes of heterozygotes, low levels of a mutant enzyme have been observed in fibroblast cultures of skin from affected infants [119]. This finding has made possible prenatal diagnosis by amniocentesis [118].

The gene for ADA has tentatively been assigned to chromosome 20 [120]. The tissue polymorphism of ADA is regulated at the posttranscriptional level, the erythrocyte isoenzyme can be converted to the various tissue forms by incubating erythrocyte ADA with tissues of infants with ADA—severe combined immunodeficiency [121].

The immunodeficiency appears to result from the ADA deficiency. Erythrocytes from ADA-deficient infants incorporate adenosine into AMP, ADP, and ATP, while normal erythrocytes incorporate adenosine principally into IMP. The ADA inhibitor coformycin causes normal erythrocytes to behave like ADA-deficient erythrocytes [122]. Accumulation of adenine nucleotides is toxic to lymphoid precursor cells, as has been shown with other cells in culture [123]. In addition to increased accumulation of ATP in ADA deficiency, there is also increased "trapping" of deoxyadenosine in T cell precursors because these cells have a relatively large amount of deoxyadenosine kinase and a relative deficiency of 5'-nucleotidase [124]. They also accumulate dATP. dATP inhibits ribonucleoside diphosphate reductase, thereby inhibiting DNA synthesis [125, 126]. The toxicity of deoxyadenosine on ADA deficient cells can be revised by deoxycytosine [127]. In addition to the inhibition of ribonucleotide reductase by dATP, increased adenosine concentrations inhibit S-adenosyl homocysteine hydrolase thereby blocking the DNA methylation pathway [128].

Another enzyme in the purine degradation pathway, nucleoside phosphorylase (NP) (which converts inosine to hypoxanthine and guanosine to guanine), has been shown to be deficient in six kindred with a T cell defect [129]. Like ADA deficiency, NP deficiency results in dGTP accumulation and this also inhibits ribonucleotide reductase.

Therapy

Gamma globulin therapy is of no avail in stemming the inex-

orably fatal progress of the defect. Attempts to restore immunologic competence with bone marrow transplants have, in the past, uniformly failed to achieve this end, with development of graft-versus-host disease. This complication has arisen following bone marrow or whole blood transfusion [132]. Transplacentally acquired maternal lymphoid cells may persist for a long time [133].

A characteristic maculopapular rash starting on the face heralds the onset of graft-versus-host disease about 7 days after the administration of histoincompatible immunocompetent cells. The rash spreads rapidly, ultimately involving all skin surfaces, including the palms and soles. Thrombocytopenia, leukopenia, jaundice, and anasarca follow in quick succession, and bone marrow aplasia leads to death from massive hemorrhage by the twelfth to fourteenth day. On the basis of experimental observations it has been reasoned that transplants of bone marrow cells as a source of immunopotential stem cells would restore immunologic competence to these infants. It is apparent from these misadventures that it would be necessary to circumvent the graft-versus-host disease by administering completely histocompatible bone marrow cells. Bone marrow cells from normal sibs who were histocompatible by direct leukocyte typing and by mixed leukocyte culture have been successful [134, 135], both in ADA+ and ADA− cases [115] and in the X-linked recessive form of the disease. Frozen, irradiated red cells have also been transfused to correct ADA deficiency [136].

In the preceding section it has been pointed out that this disease may be inherited by one of several alternative mechanisms and that patients with this disease may exhibit varying degrees of circulating lymphopenia and of lymphoid tissue depletion. The constant pathologic hallmark of the disease resides in the dysplasia of the thymus gland. The immunologic defect appears to result from the maturation failure of immunopotential cells in the bone marrow or from the failure of the thymus anlage to supply some essential factor [137]. In a variant form, so-called reticular dysgenesis [138], the few infants with this disease have died within the first week of life from overwhelming staphylococcal sepsis. In addition to the characteristic thymic dysplasia, lymphopenia, and lymphoid depletion, there are severe neutropenia and depletion of myeloid precursors from the marrow.

At the opposite end of this spectrum are those infants with normal immunoglobulins associated with lymphopenia, lymphoid tissue depletion, and absent cellular immunity [139]. This form of lymphopenia with normal immunoglobulins has often been designated as *Nezelof's syndrome*. Nezelof termed the defect *lymphocytaire normoplasmocytaire et normoglobulinemique*. Indeed, abundant numbers of plasma cells are found in the spleen, intestine, and elsewhere at autopsy, along with the thymic dysplasia and lymphocyte depletion. The clinical course of these infants may be slightly less malignant, but death by the third or fourth year of life has been the rule. A high incidence of Coombs'-positive hemolytic anemia has been encountered in these infants, together with other autoimmune phenomena [140, 141]. Antigenic stimulation with phage particles, bacterial toxins, etc., does not usually result in a normal or even detectable antibody rise. At present it appears that the immune response of these infants is grossly abnormal in spite of normal immunoglobulin levels. All the kindreds reported thus far are consistent with autosomal recessive inheritance. A number of infants have also been reported with only gamma M, or with gamma G and gamma A in their serums [142]. It may be spurious to classify all these variations by the presence of one or another immunoglobulin in the serum, since variations in immunoglobulin pattern have been observed in sibs in an affected kindred.

REFERENCES

1. TISELIUS A: Electrophoresis of serum globulin. II. Electrophoretic analysis of normal and immune serum. *Biochem J* 31:1464, 1937

2. TISELIUS A, KABAT EA: Electrophoresis of immune serum. *Science* 87:416, 1938.

3. PORTER RR: Hydrolysis of rabbit α-globulin and antibodies with crystalline papain. *Biochem J* 73:119, 1959.

4. EDELMAN GM, POULIK MD: Studies on structural units of the α-globulins. *J Exp Med* 113:861, 1961

5. NISONOFF A, WISSLER FC, LIPMAN LM: Properties of a major component of peptic digest of rabbit antibody. *Science* 132:770, 1960

6. FRANCIONE B, MILSTEIN C, PINK JRL: Structural studies of immunoglobulin G. *Nature* 221:145, 1969

7. EDELMAN GM, GALLY JA: Nature of Bence Jones proteins: Chemical similarities to polypeptide chains of myeloma globulins and normal γ globulins. *J Exp Med* 116:207,1962

8. BERNIER GM, CEBRA JJ: Frequency distribution of α-, γ-, κ-, and λ-polypeptide chains in human lymphoid tissues. *J Immunol* 95:246, 1965

9. HILSCHMANN N, CRAIG LC: Amino acid sequence studies with Bence Jones proteins. *Proc Natl Acad Sci USA* 53:1403, 1965.

10. SMITHIES O: Gamma-globulin variability: Genetic hypothesis. *Nature* 199:1231, 1963

11. HAUROWITZ F: Antibody formation and coding problems. *Nature* 205:847, 1965

12. BURNET M: *Self and Non-Self*. London, Cambridge, 1969

13. GITLIN D, HITZIG WH, JANEWAY CA: Multiple serum protein deficiencies in congenital and acquired agammaglobulinemia. *J Clin Invest* 35:1199, 1956

14. HEREMANS JF: Immunochemical studies on protein pathology: Immunoglobulin concept. *Clin Chim Acta* 4:639, 1959

15. ROWE DS, FAHEY JL: New class of human immunoglobulins. I. Unique myeloma protein. *J Exp med* 121:171, 1965

16. ISHIZAKA K, ISHIZAKA T: Physicochemical properties of reaginic antibody. I. Association of reaginic activity with immunoglobulin other than γA or γG globulin. *J Allergy* 37:169, 1966

17. WALDMANN TA: Disorders of immunoglobulin metabolism. *N Engl J Med* 281:1170, 1969

18. EDELMAN GM, CUNNINGHAM BA, GALL WE, COTTLIER PD, RUTISHAUSER U, WAXDAL MJ: The covalent structure of an entire γG immunoglobulin molecule. *Proc Natl Acad Sci USA* 63:78, 1969

19. GITLIN D, KUMATE J, URRUSTI J, MORALES C: Selectivity of human placenta in the transfer of plasma proteins from mother to fetus. *J Clin Invest* 43:1939, 1964

20. NATVIG JB, KUNKEL HG, GEDDE-DAHL T JR: Genetic studies of the heavy chain subgroups of γG globulin, in *Third Nobel Symposium: Gamma Globulins*. Killander J (ed): Stockholm, Almquist & Wiskell, 1967, p 313

21. CICCIMARRA F, ROSEN FS, MERLER E: Localization of the IgG effector site for monocyte receptors. *Proc Natl Acad Sci USA* 72:2081, 1975

22. DAWSON G, CLAMP JR: Investigations on the oligosaccharide units of an A myeloma globulin. *Biochem J* 107:341, 1968

23. CHODIRKER WB, TOMASI TB JR: Gamma globulins: Quantitative relationships in human serum and nonvascular fluids. *Science* 142:1080, 1963

24. CEBRA JJ, SMALL PA JR: Polypeptide chain structure of rabbit immunoglobulins. II. Secretory γA globulin from colostrum. *Biochemistry* 6:503, 1967

25. HALPERN MS, KOSHLAND ME: Novel subunit in secretory IgA. *Nature* 228:1276, 1970

26. GREY HM, ABEL CA, YOUNT WJ, KUNKEL HG: A subclass of human γA-globulins (γA₂) which lacks the disulfide bonds linking heavy and light chains. *J Exp Med* 128:1223, 1968

27. DEUTSCH HF, MORTON JI: Dissociation of human serum macroglobulins. *Science* 125:600, 1957

28. MERLER E, MATSUMOTO S, KARLIN LI: The valency of human γM immunoglobulin antibody. *J Biol Chem* 243:386, 1968

29. MESTECKY J, ZIKAN J, BUTLER WT: Immunoglobulin M and secretory immunoglobulin A: Presence of a common polypeptide chain different from light chain. *Science* 171:1163, 1971

30. ISHIZAKA K, ISHIZAKA T, HORNBROOK MM: Physicochemical properties of reaginic antibody. V. Correlation of reaginic activity with gamma-E-globulin antibody. *J Immunol* 97:840, 1961.

31. ISHIZAKA K, ISHIZAKA T: Identification of gamma E-antibodies as a carrier of reaginic activity. *J Immunol* 97:840, 1966

32. OGAWA M, KOCHWA S, SMITH C, ISHIZAKA K, McINTYRE OR: Clinical aspects of IgE myeloma. *N Engl J Med* 281:1217, 1969

33. JOHANSSON SGO, BENNICH H: Immunological studies of an atypical (myeloma) immunoglobulin. *Immunology* 13:381, 1967

34. JOHANSSON SGO: Raised levels of a new immunoglobulin class in asthma. *Lancet* 2:951, 1967

35. COOMBS RRA, HUNTER A, JONAS WE, BENNICH H, JOHANSSON SGO, PANZANI R: Detection of IgE specific antibody (probably reagin) to castorbean allergen by the red-cell-linked antigen-antiglobulin reaction. *Lancet* 1:1115, 1968

36. NATVIG JB, KUNKEL HG: Genetic markers of human immunoglobulins. *Ser Haematol* 1:66, 1968

37. VYAS GN, FUDENBERG HH: Am(1), the first genetic marker of human immunoglobulin A. *Proc Natl Acad Sci USA* 64:1211, 1969

38. BAGLIONI C, ALESCIO ZONTA L, CIOLI A, CARBONARA A: Chemical basis of the allelic antigenic factor Imᵛ (2) of light chains of human immunoglobulins. *Science* 152:1519, 1966

39. MILSTEIN CP, STEINBERG AG, McLAUGHLIN CL, SOLOMON A: Amino acid sequence change associated with genetic marker Inv (2) of human immunoglobulin. *Nature* 248:160, 1974

40. GATLINGS WE, LAWTON AR, COOPER MD: Immunofluorescent studies of the development of pre-B cells, B lymphocytes and immunoglobulin isotype diversity in human. *Eur J Immunol* 7:804 1977

41. PEARL ER, YOGLER LB, OKOS AJ, CRIST WM, LAWTON AR, COOPER MD: B lymphocyte precursors in human bone marrow: An analysis of normal individuals and patients with antibody deficiency states. *J Immunol* 120:1169, 1978

42. ROSEN A, GERGELY M, JONDAL M, KLEIN G, BUTTON S: Polyclonal Ig production after Epstein-Barr virus infection of human lymphocytes in vitro. *Nature* 267:52, 1977

43. SAKANO H, HÜPPI K, HEINRICH G, TONEGAWA S: Sequences at the somatic recombination sites of immunoglobulin light-chain genes. *Nature* 280:288, 1979

44. GEARHEART PJ, JOHNSON ND, DOUGLAS R, HOOD L: IgG antibodies to phosphorylcholine exhibit more diversity than their IgM counterparts. *Nature* 291:29, 1981

45. BRUTON OC: Agammaglobulinemia. *Pediatrics* 9:722, 1952

46. GITLIN D, JANEWAY CA, APT L, CRAIG JM: Agammaglobulinemia, in Lawrence HS (ed): *Cellular and Humoral Aspects of Hypersensitivity States: Symposium*, New York, Hoeber-Harper, 1959, pp 375–441.

47. JANEWAY CA, GITLIN D, CRAIG JM, GRICE DS: Collagen disease in patients with congenital agammaglobulinemia. *Trans Assoc Am Physicians* 69:93, 1956

48. PAGE AR, HANSEN AE, GOOD RA: Occurrence of leukemia and lymphoma in patients with agammaglobulinemia. *Blood* 21:197, 1963

49. ZIEGLER JB, PENNY R: Total Echo 30 virus infection and amyloidosis in X-linked agammaglobulinemia. *Clin Immunol Immunopathol* 3:347, 1975

50. ROSEN FS, HUTCHINSON GB, ALLEN FH JR: Xg blood groups and congenital hypogammaglobulinemia. *Vox Sang* 10:729, 1965

51. OCHS HD, DAVIS SD, WEDGWOOD RJ: Immunologic responses to bacteriophage ØX174 in immunodeficiency diseases. *J Clin Invest* 50:2559, 1971

52. PORTER HM: Immunologic studies in congenital agammaglobulinemia with emphasis on delayed hypersensitivity. *Pediatrics* 20:958, 1957

53. CRAIG J, GITLIN D, JEWETT T: Response of lymph nodes of normal and congenital agammaglobulinemic children to antigenic stimulation. *Am J Dis Child* 88:626, 1954

54. GREY HM, RABELLINO E, PIROFSKY B: Immunoglobulins on the surface of lymphocytes. IV. Distribution in hypogammaglobulinemia, cellular immune deficiency and chronic lymphatic leukemia. *J Clin Invest* 50:2368, 1971

55. SIEGEL FP, PERNIS B, KUNKEL HG: Lymphocytes in human immunodeficiency states: A study of membrane associated immunoglobulins. *Europ J Immunol* 1:482, 1971

56. GAYL-PICZALSKA KJ, PARK BH, BIGGAR WD, GOOD RA: B and T lymphocytes in primary immunodeficiency disease in man *J Clin Invest* 52:919, 1973

57. GEHA RS, ROSEN FS, MERLER E: Identification and characterization of subpopulations of lymphocytes in human peripheral blood after fractionation on discontinuous gradients of albumin: The cellular defect in X-linked agammaglobulinemia. *J Clin Invest* 52:1726, 1973

58. SCHWABER J, LAZARUS H, ROSEN FS: Restricted classes of immunoglobulin produced by a lymphoid cell line from a patient with agammaglobulinemia. *Proc Natl Acad Sci USA* 75:2421, 1978

59. SCHWABER JF, ROSEN FS: Induction of human immunoglobulin synthesis and secretion in somatic cell hybrids of mouse myeloma and human B lymphocytes from patients with agammaglobulinemia. *J Exp Med* 148:974, 1978

60. COOPERBAND SR, ROSEN FS, KIBRICK S: Studies on the in vitro behavior of agammaglobulinemic lymphocytes. *J Clin Invest* 47:836, 1968

61. JANEWAY CA, ROSEN FS: The gamma globulins. IV. Therapeutic uses of

human gamma globulin. *N Engl J Med* 275:826, 1966

62. PRASAD AS, KOZA DW: Agammaglobulinemia. *Ann Intern Med* 41:629, 1954

63. GRANT GH, WALLACE WD: Agammaglobulinemia. *Lancet* 2:671, 1954

64. CHARACHE P, ROSEN FS, JANEWAY CA, CRAIG JM, ROSENBERG HA: Acquired agammaglobulinemia in siblings. *Lancet* 1:234, 1965

65. ROBBINS JB, EITZMAN DV, ELLIS EF: Immunochemical evidence for development of "acquired" hypogammaglobulinemic state. *N Engl J Med* 274:607, 1966

67. WOLF JK: Primary acquired agammaglobulinemia with family history of collagen disease and hematologic disorders. *N Engl J Med* 266:473, 1962

68. FUDENBERG H, GERMAN J L III, KUNKEL HG: Occurrence of rheumatoid factor and other abnormalities in families of patients with agammaglobulinemia. *Arthritis Rheum* 5:565, 1962

69. HERMANS PE, HUIZENCA KA, HOFFMAN HN II, BROWN AL JR, MARKOWITZ H: Dysgammaglobulinemia associated with nodular lymphoid hyperplasia of small intestine. *Am J Med* 40:78, 1966

70. OCHS HD, AMENT ME, DAVIS SD: Giardiasis with malabsorption in X-linked agammaglobulinemia. *N Engl J Med* 287:341, 1972

71. PRASAD AS, REINER E, WATSON CJ: Syndrome of hypogammaglobulinemia, splenomegaly, and hypersplenism. *Blood* 12:926, 1957

72. HONG R, GOOD RA: Limited heterogeneity of gamma globulin in hypogammaglobulinemia. *Science* 156:1102, 1967

73. GEHA RS, SCHNEEBERGER E, MERLER E, ROSEN FS: Heterogeneity of "acquired" or common variable agammaglobulinemia. *N Engl J Med* 291:1, 1974

74. CICCIMARRA F, ROSEN FS, SCHNEEBERGER E, MERLER E: Failure of heavy chain glycosylation of IgG in some patients with common, variable agammaglobulinemia. *J Clin Invest* 57:1386, 1976

75. SCHWABER JF, ROSEN FS: Somatic cell hybrids of mouse myeloma cells and B lymphocytes from a patient with agammaglobulinemia: Failure to secrete human immunoglobulin. *J Immunol* 122:1849, 1979

76. WALDMANN TA, BRODER S, BLAESE RM, DURM M, BLACKMAN M, STROBER W: Role of suppressor T cells in pathogenesis of common variable hypogammaglobulinemia. *Lancet* 2:609, 1974

77. REINHERZ EL, GEHA R, WOHL ME, MORIMOTO C, ROSEN FS, SCHLOSSMAN SF: Immunodeficiency associated with loss of T4+ T-cell function. *N Engl J Med* 304:811, 1981

78. FUDENBERG HH, SOLOMON A: Acquired agammaglobulinemia with autoimmune hemolytic disease. *Vox Sang* 6:68, 1961

79. MACLEAN LD, ZAK SJ, VARCO RL, GOOD RA: Thymic tumor and acquired agammaglobulinemia: Clinical and experimental study of immune response. *Surgery* 40:1010, 1956

80. HOBBS JR: Immune imbalance in dysagammaglobulinemia type IV. *Lancet* 1:110, 1968

81. ROSEN FS, KEVY S, MERLER E, JANEWAY CA, GITLIN D: Recurrent bacterial infection and dysgammaglobulinemia, deficiency of 7S gamma-globulins in presence of elevated 19s gamma globulin: Report of two cases. *Pediatrics* 28:182, 1961

82. GLEICH GJ, UHR JW, VAUGHAN JH: Antibody formation in dysgammaglobulinemia. *J Clin Invest* 45:1334, 1966

83. ROSEN FS, BOUGAS JA: Acquired dysgammaglobulinemia: Elevation of 19s gamma globulin and deficiency of 7S globulin in woman with chronic progressive bronchiectasis. *N Engl J Med* 269:1336, 1963

84. HINZ CF JR, BOYER JT: Dysgammaglobulinemia in adult manifested as autoimmune hemolytic anemia: Serologic and immunochemical characterization of antibody of unusual specificity. *N Engl J Med* 269:1329, 1963

85. HITZIG WH, SCHLAPPER A: Chronic neutropenia and dysgammaglobulinemia: Possible interrelations, in *International Society of Haematology: Abstracts of the 10th Congress*, D-23. Stockholm, Munksgaard, 1964

86. STIEHM ER, FUDENBERG HH: Clinical and immunologic features of dysgammaglobulinemia type 1: Report of case diagnosed in first year of life. *Am J Med* 40:805, 1966

87. JAMIESON WM, KERR MR: Family with several cases of hypogammaglobulinemia. *Arch Dis Child* 37:330, 1962

88. BARTH WF, ASOFSKY R, LIDDY FJ, TAHAKA Y, ROWE DS, FAHEY JL: Antibody deficiency syndrome: Selective immunoglobulin deficiency with reduced synthesis of gamma and alpha immunoglobulin polypeptide chains. *Am J Med* 39:319, 1965

89. BACHMANN R: Studies on serum γA-globulin level. III. Frequency of A-γA globulinemia. *J Clin Lab Invest* 17:316, 1965

90. ROCKEY JH, HANSON LA, HEREMANS JF, KUNKEL HG: Beta-2A aglobulinemia in two healthy men. *J Lab Clin Med* 63:205, 1964

91. CRABBE PA, HEREMANS JF: Selective IgA deficiency with steatorrhea. *Am J Med* 42:319, 1967

92. YOUNG RR, AUSTEN KF, MOSER HW: Abnormalities of serum gamma-1-A globulin and ataxia telangiectasia. *Medicine* 43:423, 1964

93. STOCKER F, AMMANN P, ROSSI E: Selective γ-A globulin deficiency with dominant autosomal inheritance in a Swiss family. *Arch Dis Child* 43:585, 1968

94. VAN LOGHEM E: Familial occurrence of isolated IgA deficiency associated with antibodies to IgA: Evidence against a structural gene defect. *Eur J Immunol* 4:57, 1974

95. STROBER W, WOCHNER RD, BARLOW MH, MCFARLIN DE, WALDMANN TA: Immunoglobulin metabolism in ataxis telangiectasia. *J Clin Invest* 47:1905, 1968

96. VYAS GN, PERKINS HA, FUDENBERG HH: Anaphylactoid transfusion reactions associated with anti-IgA. *Lancet* 2:312, 1968.

97. SCHMIDT AP, TASWELL HF, GLEICH GJ: Anaphylactic transfusion reactions associated with anti-IgA antibody. *N Engl J Med* 280:188, 1969

98. SCHUR P, BOREL H, GELFAND EW, ALPER CA, ROSEN FS: Selective gamma G globulin in patients with recurrent pyogenic infections. *N Engl J Med* 283:631, 1970

99. YOUNT WJ, HONG R, SELIGMANN M, GOOD RA, KUNKEL HG: Imbalances of gamma globulin subgroups and gene defects in patients with primary hypogammaglobulinemia. *J Clin Invest* 49:1957, 1970

100. NATVIG JB, KUNKEL HG: Human immunoglobulins: Classes, subclasses, genetic variants and idiotypes. *Adv Immunol* 16:1, 1973

101. YOUNT WJ, KUNKEL HG, LITWIN SD: Studies of Vi(γ²c) subgroup of gamma globulin. *J Exp Med* 125:177, 1967

102. GLANZMANN E, RINIKER P: Essentielle Lymphocytophthise: Ein neues Krankheitsbuild aus der Säuglingspathologie. *Ann Paediatr* 175:1, 1950

103. HITZIG WH, BARANDUN S, COTTIER H: Die schweizerische Form der Agammaglobulinamie. *Ergeb Inn Med Kinderheilkd* 27:79, 1968

104. HITZIG WH, WILLI H: Hereditäre lymphoplasmocytäre Dysgenesie. *Schweiz Med Wochenschr* 91:1625, 1961

105. GITLIN D, CRAIG JM: The thymus and other lymphoid tissues in congenital agammaglobulinemia. I. Thymic alymphoplasia and lymphocytic hypoplasia and their relation to infection. *Pediatrics* 32:517, 1963

106. MILLER ME: Thymic dysplasia ("Swiss agammaglobulinemia") I. Graft versus host reaction following bone-marrow transfusion. *J Pediatr* 70:730, 1967

107. GIBLETT ER, ANDERSON J, COHEN F, POLLARA B, MEEUWISSEN HJ: Adenosine deaminase deficiency in two patients with severely impaired cellular immunity. *Lancet* 2:1067, 1972

108. MEEUWISSEN HJ, POLLARA B, PICKERING RJ: Combined immunodeficiency disease associated with adenosine deaminase deficiency. *J Pediatr* 86:169, 1975

109. TOBLER R, COTTIER H: Familiare Lymphopenie mit Agammaglobulinämie und schwerer Moniliasis: die "essentielle Agammaglobulinämie schwerer Moniliasis: die "essentielle Agammaglobulinämie. *Helv Paediatr Acta* 13:313, 1958

110. HITZIG WH, BIRO Z, BOSCH H, HUSER HJ: Agammaglobulinämie und Alymphocytose mit Schwund des lymphatischen Gewebes. *Helv Paediatr Acta* 13:551, 1958

111. GEHA RS, SCHNEEBERGER E, GATIEN J, ROSEN FS, MERLER E: Synthesis of an M component by circulating B lymphocytes in severe combined immunodeficiency. *N Engl J Med* 290:726, 1974

112. REINHERZ EL, COOPER MD, SCHLOSSMAN SF, ROSEN FS: Abnormalities of T cell maturation and regulation in human beings with immunodeficiency disorders. *J Clin Invest*, 68:699, 1981

113. KNUDSEN BB, DISSING J: Adenosine deaminase deficiency in a child with severe combined immunodeficiency. *Clin Genet* 4:144, 1973

114. OCHS HD, YOUNT JE, GIBLETT ER, CHEN SH, SCOTT CR, WEDGWOOD RJ: Adenosine deaminase deficiency and severe combined immunodeficiency syndrome. *Lancet* 1:1393, 1973

115. PARKMAN R, GELFAND EW, ROSEN FS, SANDERSON AR, HIRSCHHORN R: Severe combined immunodeficiency and adenosine deaminase deficiency. *N Engl J Med* 292:714, 1975

116. SPENCER N, HOPKINSON D, HARRIS H: Adenosine deaminase polymorphism in man. *Ann Hum Genet* 32:9, 1968

117. SCOTT CD, CHEN SH, GIBLETT ER: Detection of the carrier state in combined immunodeficiency disease associated with adenosine deaminase deficiency. *J Clin Invest* 53:1194, 1974

118. HIRSCHHORN R, BERATIS N, ROSEN FS, PARKMAN R, STERN R, POLMAR S: Adenosine deaminase deficiency in a child diagnosed prenatally. *Lancet* 1:73, 1975

119. HIRSCHHORN R, BERATIS N, ROSEN FS: Characterization of residual enzyme activity in fibroblasts from patients with adenosine deaminase deficiency and combined immunodeficiency: Evidence for a mutant enzyme. *Proc Natl Acad Sci USA* 73:213, 1976

120. TISHFIELD JA, CREAGAN RP, NICHOLS EA, RUDDLE FH: Assignment of a gene for adenosine deaminase to human chromosome 20. *Hum Hered* 24:1, 1974

121. HIRSCHHORN R: Conversion of human erythrocyte-adenosine deaminase activity to different tissue-specific isozymes. *J Clin Invest* 55:661, 1975

122. AGARWAL RP, CRABTREE GW, PARKS RE, NELSON JA, KEIGHTLEY R, PARKMAN R, ROSEN FS, STEIN RC, POLMAR SH: Purine nucleoside metabolism in the erythrocytes of patients with adenosine deaminase deficiency and severe combined immunodeficiency. *J Clin Invest* 57:1025, 1976

123. GREEN H, CHAN TS: Pyrimidine starvation induced by adenosine in fibro-

blasts and lymphoid cells: Role of adenosine deaminase. *Science* 182:836, 1973

124. CARSON DA, KAYE J, SEEGMILLER JE: Lymphospecific toxicity in adenosine deaminase deficiency and purine nucleoside phosphorylase deficiency: Possible role of nucleoside kinase(s). *Proc Natl Acad Sci USA* 74:5677, 1977

125. MOORE EC, HURLBERT RB: Regulation of mammalian deoxyribonucleotide biosynthesis by nucleotides as activators and inhibitors. *J Biol Chem* 241:4802, 1966

126. ULLMAN B, GUDAS LJ, COHEN A, MARTIN DW JR: Deoxyadenosine metabolism and cytotoxicity in cultured mouse T lymphoma cells: a model for immunodeficiency disease. *Cell* 14:365, 1978

127. COHEN A, GUDAS LJ, AMMANN AJ, STAAL GEJ, MARTIN DW JR: Deoxyguanosine triphosphate as a possible toxic metabolite in the immunodeficiency associated with purine nucleoside phosphorylase deficiency. *J Clin Invest* 61:1405, 1978

128. KREDICH NM, HERSHFIELD MS: S-adenosylhomocysteine toxicity in normal and adenosine kinase-deficient lymphoblasts of human origin. *Proc Natl Acad Sci USA* 76:2450, 1979

129. GIBLETT E, AMMANN AJ, WARA D, SANDMAN R, DIAMOND LK: Nucleoside phosphorylase deficiency in a child with severely defective T cell immunity and normal B cell immunity. *Lancet* 1:1010, 1975

130. STOOP JW, ZEGERS BJM, HENDRICK GFM, SIEGENBECK VAN HEUKELON LH, DE BRES PK, WADMAN SK, BALLICUX RE: Purine nucleoside phosphorylase deficiency associated with selective cellular immunodeficiency. *N Engl J Med* 296:651, 1977

131. GELFAND EW, DOSCH H-M, BIGGAR WD, FOX JH: Partial purine nucleoside phosphorylase deficiency. *J Clin Invest* 61:1071, 1978

132. HATHAWAY WE, GITHENS JH, BLACKBURN WR, FULGINITI V, KEMPE CH: Aplastic anemia, histiocytosis, and erythrodermia in immunologically deficient children—probably human runt disease. *N Engl J Med* 273:953, 1965

133. KADOWAKI J, THOMPSON RI, ZUELZER WW, WOOLLEY PV, BROUGH AJ,

GRUBER D: XX/XY lymphoid chimaerism in congenital immunol deficiency syndrome with thymic alymphopenia. *Lancet* 2:1152, 1965

134. GATTI RA, MEUWISSEN HJ, ALLEN HD, HONG R, GOON RA: Immunologic reconstitution of sex-linked lymphopenic immunologic deficiency. *Lancet* 2:1366, 1968

135. DEKONING J, VAN BEKKUM DW, DICKE KA, DOOREN LJ, VON ROOD JJ, RADI J: Transplantation of bone-marrow cells and fetal thymus in an infant with lymphopenic immunological deficiency. *Lancet* 1:1223, 1969

136. POLMAR SH, STERN RC, SCHWARTZ AL, WETZLER CM, CHASE PA, HIRSCHHORN R: Enzyme replacement therapy for adenosine deaminase deficiency and severe combined immunodeficiency. *N Engl J Med* 295:1337, 1976

137. PYKE KW, DOSCH HN, IPP MM, GELFAND EW: Demonstration of an intrathymic defect in a case of severe combined immunodeficiency disease. *N Engl J Med* 293:424, 1975

138. DEVAAL OM, SEYNHAEVE V: Reticular dysgenesis. *Lancet* 2:1123, 1959

139. NEZELOF C, JAMMET ML, LORTHOLARY P, LABRUNE B, LAMY M: L'hypoplasie héréditaire du thymus: sa place et sa responsabilité dans une observation d'aplasia lymphocytaire, normoplasmocytaire et normoglobulinémique du nourrison. *Arch Fr Pediatr* 21:897, 1964

140. SCHALLER J, CHING Y, WILLIAMS CPS, DAVIS SD, LAGUNOFF D, WEDGWOOD RJ: Hypergammaglobulinemia, antibody deficiency, autoimmune haemolytic anemia, and nephritis in an infant with a familial lymphopenic immune defect. *Lancet* 2:825, 1966

141. GOLDMAN AS, HAGGARD ME, MCFEDDEN J, RITZMAN S, HOUSTON EW, BRATCHER RL, WEISS KG, BOX EM, SZEKRENYES JW: Thymic alymphoplasia, lymphoma and dysglobulinemia. Hyper-γ-A, normo-γ-M, hypo-γ, -G, a-γ-D, and γ-E globulinemia, plasmacytosis, normal delayed hypersensitivity, severe allergic reactions, and Coombs positive anemia. *Pediatrics* 39:348, 1967

142. SACREZ R, WILLARD D, LEVY M, MOYER S, BIGEL P: Lymphocytophthisie d'évolution atypique. *Arch Fr Pediatr* 22:975, 1965

89

INHERITED ABNORMALITIES OF THE COMPLEMENT SYSTEM

DAVID N. GLASS

DOUGLAS T. FEARON

K. FRANK AUSTEN

1. The classic complement system and the alternative complement pathway comprise 18 plasma proteins that serve as effectors of immunologically induced inflammation. These proteins normally exist in plasma in inactive form or in a regulated turnover state. When activated, they participate in a series of proteolytic reactions leading to changes in vascular permeability, the attraction of leukocytes, the enchancement of phagocytosis, and damage to cell membranes.

2. Genetically controlled deficiencies have been described for almost all the components of the complement system and for two of the circulating inhibitors of this system. Deficiency of one component, C3, consistently leads to marked impairment of host defenses, manifested in vivo by recurrent pyogenic and gram-negative infections and impaired leukocyte mobilization, and in vitro by absent serum bactericidal, chemotactic, and opsonic enhancing activity. Deficiency of an inhibitor protein, I, allows uncontrolled activation of the alternative complement pathway with secondary C3 and B deficiencies. I deficiency therefore produces clinical manifestations similar to those of C3 deficiency. Deficiencies of the later complement components, C5, C6, C7, and C8, are associated with recurrent Neisserial infections. Bacteremia is frequent owing to the absence of cytolytic complement action.

3. Deficiency of $\overline{C1}$ inhibitor is associated with the syndrome of hereditary angioedema involving the skin, gastrointestinal tract, or upper respiratory tract. This autosomal dominant disease is infrequent, but not rare. Correct diagnosis may avert needless abdominal surgery or death by asphyxiation because effective pharmacologic intervention is now available in the form of attenuated androgens that stimulate $\overline{C1}$ inhibitor ($\overline{C1}$ INH) production.

4. Many of the deficiency states, especially of C2, are associated with an increased frequency of "autoimmune" diseases such as systemic lupus erythematosus, Henoch-Schönlein purpura, polymyositis, and glomerulonephritis. Since genes coding for three of the complement proteins (C2, C4, and B) have been linked to the major histocompatibility complex on the sixth chromosome, the increased susceptibility to these diseases may reflect genetically linked alterations in immune responses. Alternatively, the process of adaptive immunity may require an intact classic (antibody-dependent) complement-activating sequence in order to clear the products of the immune response. In complement-deficient states there may be prolonged circulation of immune complexes, and this may provoke diseases of autoimmunity.

The complement system consists of 18 proteins present in plasma and other body fluids which comprise two pathways for activation, the classic and the alternative, and a final common effector pathway. The alternative pathway is activated by surfaces of cells and particles that express certain biochemical characteristics. Activation of either pathway leads to assembly of highly specific proteolytic enzymes. These enzymes trigger the common effector pathway. The effector pathway produces a range of biologic effects that include opsonization and cytolysis of the activating target, stimulation of chemotactic, secretory, and synthetic functions in leukocytes, and alteration of vascular permeability. By these processes complement activation induces an inflammatory reaction that benefits the host when it is effectively directed at invading microorganisms. However, when it is excessive or directed against host tissue, as occurs in some connective tissue diseases of humans, complement activation can be detrimental.

Since the preparation of the last edition of this text information about the genetic control of complement systems has greatly increased. Genetic polymorphisms leading to heterogeneity of electrophoretic mobility are now recognized for C2 and for C8 [1, 2], in addition to C4 [3], C3, B, C$\overline{1}$ inhibitor (C$\overline{1}$ INH), and C6. The number of known inherited deficiencies of complement proteins has increased from 11 to 13 and now includes C1q and C9 [4–6]. Analysis of defects in host resistance associated with inherited deficiencies of certain complement proteins has yielded information about the relative importance of specific components in vivo. Certain connective tissue diseases, such as systemic lupus erythematosus, have been found unexpectedly to be associated with the inherited complement deficiencies [7]. Moreover, genes coding for three complement proteins, C2, B, and C4, have been linked to the major histocompatability complex. These new findings may link the immune response to the role that complement plays in controlling the effects of the products of that response [8–10].

BIOCHEMISTRY AND BIOLOGIC ACTIVITY

Components of the complement system and some of their physiochemical properties are listed in Table 89–1. The proteins of the classic and effector pathways are designated by letter C and a number: C1, C4, C2, C3, and C5 to C9. Constituent proteins of the alternative pathway are designated by capital letters: B, D, P, H, and I. C3 is an essential component of the alternative activating mechanism, as well as the effector pathway. It has retained a classic nomenclature because it was first recognized as participating in a classic reaction, namely, complement-dependent hemolysis of antibody-sensitized erythrocytes. Cleavage fragments of components are denoted by lower-case letters, as in C3a, C3b, Ba, Bb. Inactive components are signified by the letter i, as in C2ai and Bbi. An overbar, as in C$\overline{1}$, indicates the enzymatically active form of a component.

Classic Activating Pathway

The classic activating pathway (Fig. 89–1) is initiated when C1 binds to antibody in immune complexes and is converted to its active form, C$\overline{1}$. C1 is a Ca^{2+}–dependent molecular complex containing three subcomponents, C1q, C1r, and C1s [11], which are present in a molar ratio of 1:2:2 [12, 13]. Electron microscopic pictures show C1q to have a hexameric structure resembling a bunch of six tulips [14, 15] with the globular head of each monomer connected by a radial strand to a common stem region. The binding sites for the second constant domain of the Fc region of IgG 1–3 [16] and for the fourth constant domain of IgM [17] reside in the globular regions of C1q [18], giving the subcomponent a potential valency of six for antibody. The collagenlike stem region of the molecule provides the site for the Ca^{2+}–dependent attachment of the $(C1r)_2$–$(C1s)_2$ tetramer [19, 20]. On binding to antigen-antibody complexes containing one IgM or at least two IgG molecules, C1q is thought to effect an allosteric change in C1r. This triggers autocatalytic activation of C1r through either an intra- or intermolecular peptide bond cleavage [21], converting it into a disulfide-linked two-polypeptide chain protein [13, 22]. The serine protease site in the light chain of C$\overline{1}$r hydrolyzes a single peptide bond in precursor C1s to yield C$\overline{1}$s, also composed of two polypeptide chains linked by disulfide(s) with a serine protease site in the light chain [23, 24].

C$\overline{1}$s activates C4 and C2 to assemble C4b,2a, which is the classic pathway C3 convertase or C3-cleaving enzyme. C4 consists of three polypeptide chains, α, β, and γ, held together by noncovalent forces as well as by disulfide bonds [25]. The α chain may have the unusual feature of possessing an internal thioester [26]. Cleavage by C$\overline{1}$s of the 9000 M.W. C4a fragment from the α chain [25] apparently exposes this thioester which then mediates stable attachment of the major C4b fragment by an ester or amide bond [27] to the immune complex-bearing C$\overline{1}$. Although this mode of C4b attachment does not discriminate between autologous and heterologous immune complexes or cell surfaces, binding is restricted to structures in the immediate vicinity of C$\overline{1}$ by the extremely short half-life of the nascent ester binding of C4b. The bound C4b reversibly takes up C2 in the presence of Mg^{2+} [28], and the C$\overline{1}$s subcomponent cleaves the latter [29] into its larger C2a and smaller C2b fragments to form C4b,2a. The catalytic site in C2a is capable of cleaving C3 and C5 to activate the effector complement sequence.

Activation of the classic pathway is regulated by the lability of its C3 convertase and by three control proteins, C$\overline{1}$ inhibitor (C$\overline{1}$ INH), C4 binding protein (C4-bp), and C3b/C4b inactivator (I). C4b,2a undergoes rapid temperature-dependent loss of activity by irreversible dissociation of the C2a fragment which becomes C2ai [30]. C$\overline{1}$ INH forms stable 1:1 complexes with C$\overline{1}$r and C$\overline{1}$s by binding near or at the active site on the light chains of these proteins and abolishes their capacities to cleave their natural substrates [31]. The importance of this protease inhibitor in preventing inappropriate complement activation is illustrated by the marked hypercatabolism of C4 that occurs continuously in individuals with hereditary angioedema who are heterozygous for a deficiency in C$\overline{1}$ INH [32]. The C4-bp binds to C4b to mediate three inhibitory effects [33–35]: prevention of uptake of C2 by C4b, accelerated decay-dissociation of C2a already complexed to C4b, and increased susceptibility of C4b to cleavage-inactivation by I. I is a proteolytic enzyme that hydrolyzes the α polypeptide of C4b at two sites [35], leading to a formation of a small fragment of α chain, termed C4d, which remains attached to the immune complex,

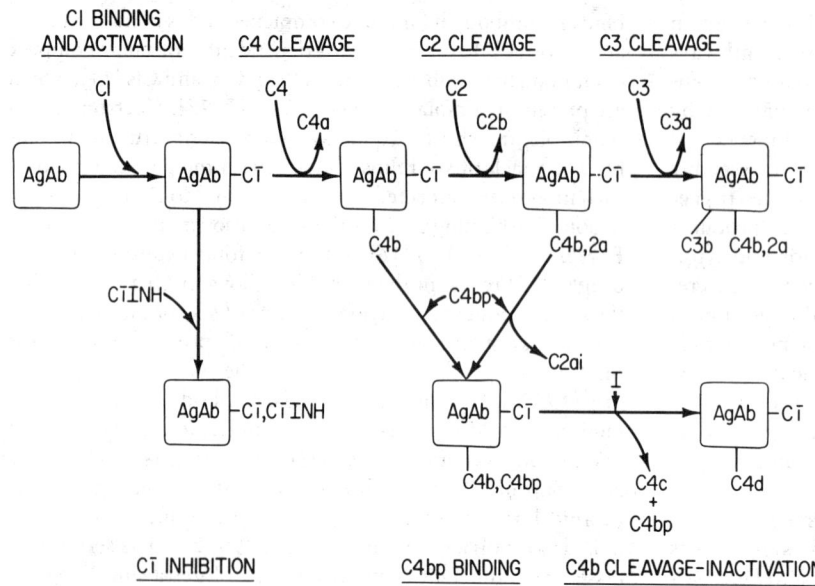

Figure 89-1 The classic pathway of complement activation. An antigen-antibody complex (AgAb) initiates the reaction by binding C1 which then self-activates. The C$\bar{1}$ cleaves C4 and C2 whose major fragments form a bimolecular complex, C4b,2a, the classic pathway C3 convertase. Formation of the C3 convertase is regulated by the control proteins, C$\bar{1}$INH, C4bp, and I.

and a larger C4c fragment, composed of residual α chain and intact β and γ chains, which is released into the fluid phase.

Alternative Activating Pathway

The alternative activating pathway (Fig. 89–2) does not represent simply a redundancy in the complement system, since it can respond directly to certain cell and particle surfaces without their prior sensitization with antibody [36]. Moreover, it has an intrinsic capacity for positive feedback activation of C3 through C9 based on the composition of its "amplification"

C3 convertase, C3b,Bb, which contains C3b, the product of C3 cleavage [37, 38].

Initial cleavage of C3 by the alternative pathway occurs continuously and is independent of the presence of activating substances. It serves only to prime the amplification C3 convertase [39]. The slow interaction in the fluid phase of C3 (which is uncleaved although perhaps chemically altered [40]) with B and D is thought to form the "priming" C3 convertase, C3,Bb. The serine proteolytic site of the Bb subunit [41–43] cleaves small amounts of C3 to release C3a from the α polypeptide and to generate the larger C3b fragment. Coincident with C3b generation and for an extremely short time, an internal thioes-

Table 89-1 Physicochemical characteristics of proteins of the complement system

Name	Molecular Weight	Serum concentration μg/ml	Fragment
Classic activating pathway			
C1q	400,000	70	
C1r	95,000	35	
C1s	85,000	35	
C4	180,000	400	C4a, C4b, C4c, C4d
C2	117,000	25	C2a, C2b
Alternative activating pathway			
C3	185,000	1500	C3a, C3b, C3c, C3d
B	95,000	250	
D	25,000	2	
P	220,000	25	
Effector pathway			
C3			
C5	200,000	85	
C6	128,000	75	C5a, C5b
C7	121,000	55	
C8	153,000	55	
C9	80,000	200	
Control proteins			
C$\bar{1}$ inhibitor	105,000	180	
C4 binding protein	$1.2-1.5 \times 10^6$	250	
I (C3b/C4b inactivator; KAF)	90,000	50	
H (β1H)	150,000	400	

ter within the α polypeptide is capable of forming stable ester linkages to immune complexes and cell surfaces [44–46]. If a suitable acceptor surface is not encountered, the attachment site in C3b decays and the molecule remains in the fluid phase. The C3b bound to bystander surfaces accelerates the activating reaction by rapidly forming a reversible Mg^{2+}-dependent complex with B [47–49]. The latter is cleaved by the serine protease [50–53], D, releasing the Ba fragment and uncovering the C3-cleaving site on the Bb fragment which remains associated with C3b. C3b,Bb amplifies C3 cleavage and catalyzes relatively efficient deposition of newly generated C3b.

The amplification process is regulated by the inherent lability of C3b,Bb, which undergoes rapid spontaneous decay by irreversible dissociation from C3b of the catalytic Bb subunit which becomes inactive Bbi [38, 54]. Amplification is regulated by three proteins, properdin (P), H, and I. P enhances the activity of the amplification C3 convertase by binding to its C3b subunit and retarding decay-dissociation of Bb [54]. H controls formation of C3b,Bb by binding to the C3b subunit and mediating three inhibitory effects: blocking uptake of B [49, 55], accelerating decay-dissociation of bound Bb [56, 57], and making the α polypeptide of C3b susceptible to cleavage by I which generates an inactive form of the protein, iC3b [56, 58]. The alternative activating pathway does not have a protein analogous to C1 INH that inhibits D, and this enzyme normally exists in plasma in its enzymatically active form.

Whether a cell or particle activates the alternative pathway is determined by the relative affinity of bound C3b for B and for H, respectively [49, 59, 60]. C3b that is fixed to the surface of a nonactivator binds H with almost a hundredfold greater affinity ($K_a \simeq 1 \times 10^7\ M^{-1}$) than that with which it binds B ($K_a \simeq 1 \times 10^5\ M^{-1}$) in the presence of 0.5 mM free Mg^{2+}. Fluid phase C3b also appears to complex with H more readily than it does with B. In contrast, C3b on the surface of a cell or particle that activates the alternative pathway binds both proteins with almost equal avidity, its association constant for H decreasing while that for B remains unchanged. With nonactivating surfaces formation of the amplification C3 convertase is impaired because H effectively blocks uptake of B by C3b and promotes irreversible cleavage-inactivation of C3b by I. With activators B can effectively compete with H for binding to C3b, and amplification of C3 cleavage occurs.

A cell surface constituent that regulates the affinity of membrane-associated C3b for H is sialic acid [49, 61–63] which is present in some glycoproteins and glycolipids of cells. Natu-

rally occurring activators of the human alternative pathway such as zymosan, an insoluble derivative of yeast cell walls, and rabbit erythrocytes have absent or diminished amounts of sialic acid on their surfaces, respectively. Enzymatic removal of sialic acid from sheep erythrocytes or chemical cleavage of its polyhyroxylated side chain [61] converts this cell from a nonactivator to an activator of the pathway by decreasing almost a hundredfold the affinity of membrane-bound C3b for H [49]. The capacity of the alternative complement pathway to respond to cells that are relatively deficient in surface sialic acid may be relevant to its apparent role in natural resistance. Most bacteria and all plants lack sialic acid. However, some bacterial species that have capsular sialic acid, such as type III, group B *Streptococcus*, groups B and C *Neisseria meningitidis*, and Kl *Escherichia coli*, are pathogenic for humans.

In a model system, the coupling of heparin glycosaminoglycan to zymosan suppressed the capacity of this microbial material to activate the human alternative pathway by facilitating the regulatory actions of H and I on particle-bound C3b [64]. Because heparin and a closely related mucopolysaccharide, heparan sulfate, can be specifically bound to nucleated cells, and because nucleated cells in culture bear heparin-related polysaccharides, this finding may indicate another mechanism by which mammalian cells modulate activation of the alternative pathway.

Specific antibody augments activation of the human alternative pathway by zymosan [65], rabbit erythrocytes [66], pneumococci [67], streptococci [68], and measles virus-infected HeLa cells [69, 70] independent of any effects on the classic activating pathway. F(ab')₂ fragments are as active as intact IgG, Mg^{2+} but not Ca^{2+} is required, and the reactions can occur in C2-deficient human serum. Several mechanisms may account for the potentiating activity of antibody: Alteration of the target cell surface by covering sialic acid residues, provision of additional binding sites for C3b, either on the antibody molecules themselves or on membrane constituents, and alteration of the spatial distribution of bound C3b to enhance formation of C5 convertase sites [71].

Effector Component Reactions (Fig. 89-3)

The C4b,2a and C3b,Bb enzymes are identical in their substrate specificities. They both cleave C3 at the Arg77-Ser78 bond of the α-polypeptide chain to generate C3a and C3b, and

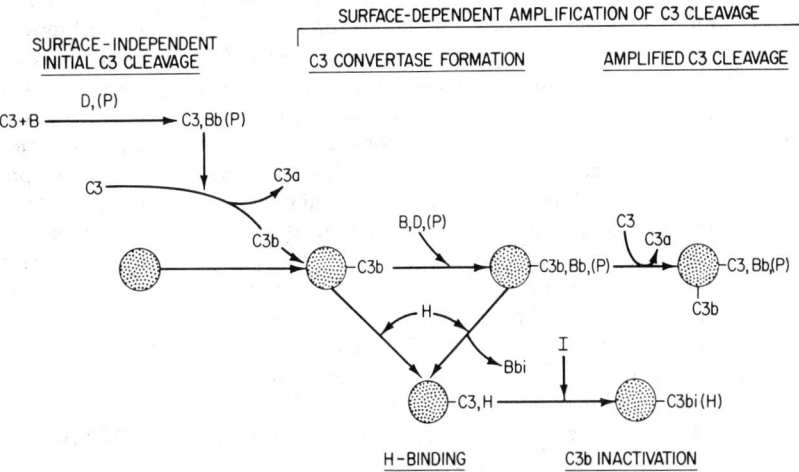

Figure 89-2 The alternative pathway of complement activation. C3b, which is slowly and continuously generated by a "priming" C3 convertase, C3,Bp(P), may attach to bystander cells. If the cell is an activator of the pathway, the amplification C3 convertase, C3b,Bp(P), is formed and catalyzes cleavage and deposition of additional molecules of C3b. In contrast, C3b bound to a nonactivator binds the regulatory protein, H, and is converted to inactive C3bi by I. P is shown in parentheses to indicate that it augments C3 convertase activity but is not required for alternative pathway activation.

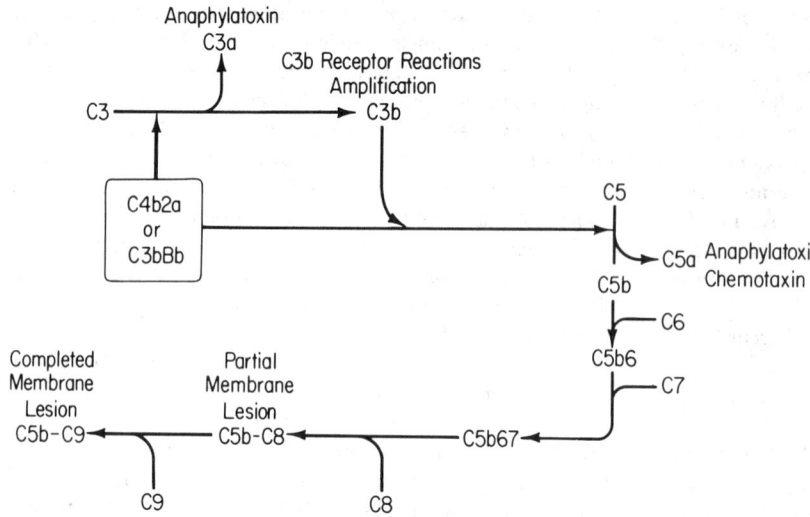

Figure 89-3 The effector sequence of complement which is activated by the C3/C5 convertases of the classic and alternative pathways. Some of the prominent biologic activities associated with cleavage fragments and multimolecular complexes are shown.

C5 at the Arg74-X75 bond of its α-polypeptide chain to generate C5a and C5b fragments. The C3 convertases acquire C5 convertase activity only after C3b has attached to a site on the target that is adjacent to the enzyme [72–75]. This C3b may function by interacting with the substrate C5, rather than with the enzyme because it exhibits an affinity for C5 and C5b,6 [76, 77]. The C5b fragment decays by an unknown mechanism to a cytolytically unreactive form immediately after its release from the generating enzyme into the fluid phase. However, if C5b combines with C6 while it is still associated with the C5 convertase, which is likely as C5 and C6 tend to form a complex in the fluid phase, its cytolytic capacity becomes stabilized [78]. Binding of C7 to C5b,6 creates a trimolecular complex that has exposed hydrophobic sites. Effective insertion into the membrane of the target begins at this stage. Uptake of C8 by membrane-associated C5b-7 apparently leads to further insertion of the complex as unstable transmembrane ion "channels" in synthetic lipid bilayers are formed, and sheep erythrocytes bearing C5b-8 slowly lyse. Binding of as many as five molecules of C9 to a single C5b-8 complex creates a more stable lesion that may lead to rapid lysis of some cells (reviewed in Ref. 79).

C3b Receptors

The biologic activities of the complement proteins are mediated by the capacity of their cleavage fragments to interact either with the target or with specific receptors on cells involved in the inflammatory process. Two components, C4b and C3b, have both activities. They can form covalent attachments to cells and immune complexes and then mediate adherence of those substances to various effector cells which have specific membrane receptors for these complement proteins. C3b receptors also can bind C4b associated with immune complexes, although apparently with lower affinity [80]. The receptors are present in the plasma membranes of human erythrocytes [81], neutrophils [82], eosinophils [83], monocytes and macrophages [84], B lymphocytes [85, 86], mast cells [87, 88], and visceral epithelial cells of the glomerulus [89]. Monocytes and macrophages also have receptors for iC3b [90]. B lymphocytes may express receptors for iC3b and for C3d [86]. The C3b receptor is an integral membrane protein with an apparent molecular weight of 205,000 [91, 92]. It is present predominantly in clusters on neutrophils, monocytes,

and B lymphocytes and exhibits little lateral motion in the plane of the plasma membranes of these cells, suggesting anchorage to subplasmalemmal elements [93].

Neutrophils and resting monocytes and macrophages had been considered to bind but not phagocytize C3b-bearing particles [94, 95]. However, binding of C3b to its receptor was known to enhance synergistically phagocytosis by these cells of particulate targets that carry limited amounts of IgG [82, 94, 95] or lack sialic acid [96]. More recently, the receptor on neutrophils has been shown to mediate rapid absorptive pinocytosis of soluble bivalent anti-C3b receptor antibody independent of Fc receptor interactions [97]. Moreover, mouse macrophages [98, 99] and human monocytes cultured under certain conditions [100] have been found to phagocytize C3b-bearing target cells in the absence of IgG. Internalization of C3b-bearing materials, which is enhanced or mediated by C3b receptors on neutrophils and mononuclear phagocytes, is essential for normal host defense against microbial infection. It may also be important in the clearance of immune complexes.

Several functions of C3b receptors on B lymphocytes have been described or suggested. Depletion of C3 in mice impaired the generation of B memory cells [101]. Incubation of lymphocytes with C3b caused secretion of a lymphokine that was chemotactic for monocytes [102]. Addition of C3c or C3d to culture media inhibited the blastogenic response of human peripheral blood lymphocytes to antigens but not to lectin mitogens [103]. Conversely, addition of anti-C3 antibody to primed mouse spleen cell cultures inhibited the generation of antibody-secreting cells in response to T-dependent antigens [104]. Thus, C3 receptors on B lymphocytes may have some role in the regulation of antibody secretion by these cells, but a clear definition of this role is lacking [105].

C3b receptors on mast cells, like those on neutrophils and monocyte/macrophages, enhance phagocytosis of C3b-bearing bacteria and sheep erythrocytes [87, 88]. The finding that histamine release was not induced by this phagocytic reaction is of interest because C3b-bearing particles induce release of histaminase from granulocytes [106]. Perhaps C3b receptor-dependent events dampen acute hypersensitivity reactions.

Phlogistic Peptides, C3a and C5a

The complete primary structures of the human C3a and C5a

molecules have been delineated, revealing sufficient sequence homology to suggest a common ancestry of the parent proteins, C3 and C5 [107, 108]. Both peptides cause degranulation and release of histamine from mast cells [109, 110], presumably by binding to specific membrane receptors. Subcutaneous injection of these peptides into humans causes a wheal and flare reaction that is blocked by prior administration of H-1 blocking reagents [108]. Serum carboxypeptidase N decreases a hundred- to a thousandfold the histamine-releasing activities of C3a and C5a by cleaving the C-terminal arginine from these peptides. C4a also has spasmogenic activity, but at concentrations several orders of magnitude higher than those required for these activities of C3a and C5a [111].

C5a also induces chemotactic and secretory reactions of polymorphonuclear leukocytes and monocytes. C5a, in nanomolar concentrations, is taken up by specific receptors on neutrophils [112]. When present in a gradient, as would occur when the peptide diffuses away from the site of complement activation, C5a causes directed migration of the cells [113]. Higher concentrations of C5a, particularly in the presence of cytochalasin B, also stimulate noncytotoxic release of lysosomal enzymes [114]. The desArg derivative of C5a retains in vitro chemotactic activity [115] in the presence of a serum cofactor, in contrast to its minimal histamine-releasing and spasmogenic activities [116]. C5a desArg, and perhaps C5a, also induce "stickiness" of granulocyte membranes that may contribute to the adherence of granulocytes to capillary endothelial cells preparatory to migration to the extravascular site of inflammation [117]. Rapid in vivo complement activation also causes leukocytosis. This is believed to be secondary to the elaboration of C3e, a small peptide derived from the α polypeptide of C3, which is capable of releasing granulocytes from the rat femoral bone marrow [118, 119]. Consistent with this thesis is the observation that an individual who genetically lacked C3 did not develop leukocytosis with pyogenic infections [120].

Membrane Attack Complex, C5b-9

There are two means by which the C5b-9 complex can damage membranes. The first is by the formation of a transmembrane channel which appears on electron microscopy as a hollow, thin-walled cylinder of approximately 10 nm internal diameter and 15 nm height. This structure may have a hydrophilic core that allows the passage of salt, water, and small proteins leading to net uptake of water by a cell, with consequent swelling and gross disruption of the membrane. The second means of membrane damage involves the disorganization of the lipid bilayer that occurs when large numbers of amphiphilic C5b-9 complexes are formed in target membranes. Membrane damage by this means may be important for lysis of viruses whose envelope membranes do not function as osmotic barriers (reviewed in Ref. 79).

GENETIC POLYMORPHISMS AND DEFICIENCY STATES

Nomenclature

The nomenclature for genes coding for complement proteins differs in two instances from that used to describe the proteins themselves. The genes determining the structure of B and C4, a single locus for B and two loci for C4, are known as Bf, C4A, and C4B, respectively. Alleles at each complement locus are designated by letter or number (Table 89-3).

Loci for three complement proteins are very closely linked to the genes of the major histocompatability complex (MHC) on the short arm of chromosome six (Fig. 89-4). The MHC contains four principal noncomplement loci defined as HLA-A, B, C, and D. Individual alleles of the loci are numbered by Inter-

Table 89-2 Deficiencies of complement components

Component	Kindreds described	Homozygotes without disease	Associated disease	References
C1q	2	1	Lupuslike syndromes, glomerulonephritis, chronic sepsis, skin disease	[4,5]
C1r	2	2	Lupuslike syndromes, glomerulonephritis, chronic discoid lupus	[258, 259, 262]
C1s	1		Systemic lupus erythematosus	[263]
C2	Many	Yes	Systemic lupus erythematosus, chronic discoid lupus erythematosus, dermatomyositis, vasculitis, Henoch-Schönlein purpura, inflammatory bowel disease, recurrent bacterial infection	[7, 143, 161–172]
C4	2		Systemic lupus erythematosus	[205, 206]
C3	5		Recurrent bacterial infections, nephritis	[120, 245–249]
C5	2	1	Systemic lupus erythematosus, recurrent bacterial infections (Neisseria)	[126, 264]
C6	9	3	Recurrent bacterial infections (Neisseria)	[129, 208, 209, 211–215]
C7	8	4	Raynaud's phenomenon with sclerodactyly, systemic lupus erythematosus, recurrent bacterial infections (Neisseria)	[132, 133, 215, 217 219–221]
C8	5	3	Recurrent bacterial infections (Neisseria), systemic lupus erythematosus, xeroderma pigmentosa	[2, 134, 215, 268, 270]
C9	1	1	None	[6]
C1INH	Many		Hereditary angioedema	[271, 272, 275–280]
I	3	1	Recurrent bacterial infections	[319–321, 323, 324]
P	1	3	Recurrent bacterial infections (Neisseria)	[270a]

* Excluding heterozygous deficiency.

THE HLA REGION: SHORT ARM OF CHROMOSOME SIX

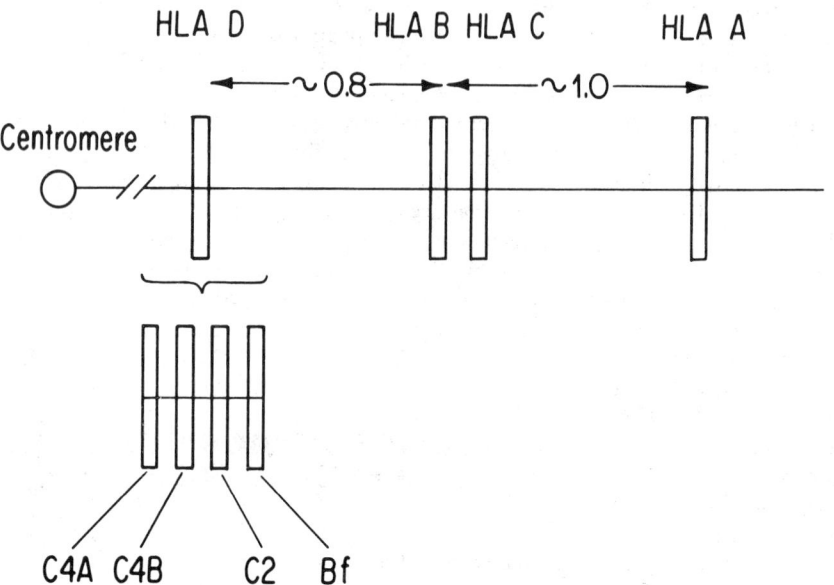

Figure 89-4 The complement loci mapping to the HLA region (short arm of chromosome 6) with approximate distances (recombination units) between the loci.

national Workshop convention in which a provisionally assigned number is noted by a lower case w (workshop). The complete description of an allele includes the region (HLA), the locus (A, B, C, or D), the allele, and provisional status (w) if appropriate, as in HLA-Bw35. The products of the HLA-A, B, and C loci are detected serologically, and those of the HLA-D locus either serologically or by mixed lymphocyte culture (MLC). HLA-D locus products detected serologically are described as HLA-DR.

On the basis of family studies the genes of an individual's

HLA phenotype may usually be assigned to either a maternal or paternal sixth chromosome. The linked genes on each chromosome are then collectively described as a haplotype. In population studies of unrelated individuals some alleles of the different HLA loci occur together more often than would be expected from a random distribution of the alleles in the population at large. The association between particular alleles of different but closely linked HLA loci is described as linkage disequilibrium.

Documented chromosome assignments of the genes deter-

Table 89-3 Major histocompatibility complex–linked complement proteins

Protein	Gene symbol	Common alleles	Gene frequency			Linkage disequilibria	Reference
			Caucasian	Black	Oriental		
C2	C2	C	0.95				1, 140, 141 143–152
		B	0.04			HLA-B15, BfS	
		A	0.01				
		D	<0.01			HLA-A10, HLA-B18, HLA-Dw2 BfS, C4A4,C4B2	
B	Bf	S	0.81	0.44	0.89	C2D, HLA-B7, HLA-B8, HLA-B-27, HLA-DR2	173, 189
		F	0.17	0.51	0.11	HLA-A3, HLA-Bw35	178–188
		F1	0.01	0.05		HLA-B18, HLA-DR3	
		S1	0.01			HLA-B12, HLA-B13, HLA-B14 HLA-Bw21	
C4	C4A	A1					3
		A2	0.08				
		A3	0.70				
		A4	0.05			C4B2, C2D	
		A5	<0.01				
		A6	0.05				
		AQ0	0.10				
C4	C4B	B1	0.76				3
		B2	0.10			C4A4, C2D	
		B3					
		BQ0	0.14				

mining the complement proteins have been made only for the MHC-linked group, C2, B, and C4. Genes for C6 and C7 are known to be closely linked; their chromosome is unknown. The genes for the remaining complement components have been neither assigned chromosomes [121–135] nor linked to genes for other proteins with the exception of C3. The gene or genes for C3 may be linked to those determining familial hypercholesterolemia (see Chap. 33) and for the Lewis blood group substance.

The MHC-linked Complement Proteins

The complement loci linked to HLA, one locus each for C2 and for B and two loci for C4, map close to HLA-D (Fig. 89-4). There is evidence suggesting the Bf locus maps on the HLA-B side of HLA-D [136, 137]. The recombination fraction between the complement loci and HLA-B has been estimated to be approximately 0.8 recombination unit [138]. Crossovers have not been identified between the four MHC-linked complement loci that have products which are polymorphic on electrophoresis. There is some evidence for an MHC-associated mechanism regulating levels of C2 and C4 in that individuals with HLA-Dw2 have been shown to have lower levels of C2 and C4 than those without the antigen [139].

C2 Polymorphism of C2 is demonstrated by isoelectric focusing combined with an assay for C2 functional activity [1, 140]. The majority of individuals are homozygous for the variant designated C2C (or C2-1), frequency 0.95 (Table 89-3). Inheritance has been shown to be on an autosomal codominant basis, as in the family illustrated in Fig. 89-5, which also demonstrates linkage between HLA and C2 genes. The common allele C2C, and the rarer variant C2B, have similar levels of hemolytic C2 activity [141]. The silent or null gene for C2 (designated C2D) is allelic with those coding for the structural variants and has a frequency of less than 0.01 in blood donors [142, 143]. The genes most frequently associated with C2D are HLA-A10 (Aw24), HLA-B18, and HLA-Dw2 [9, 144–148]. In addition to HLA genes, C2D is found to be in linkage disequilibrium with alleles of other MHC-linked loci, specifically with BfS, the electrophoretically slow allele of B, and with the C4 alleles, C4A4 and C4B2 [149, 150]. In at least three pop-

ulation studies, C2B is reported to be in linkage disequilibrium with HLA-B15 [141, 151, 152].

After the initial report in 1960 of an isolated single deficiency of C2, the genetic nature of the deficiency was defined in another family and in the family of the initial proband by hemolytic C2 assay which revealed heterozygous family members [153–155]. Hemolytic C2 assays of C2-deficient persons have ranged from less than 0.1 to 4 percent of the normal mean [156, 157], and there is no detectable C2 protein by immunoassay [158, 159]. Serums from heterozygous-deficient individuals have a low or low-normal CH50 level, and usually a half-normal level of C2 measured both by immunochemical and by functional assay [143, 147]. C2-deficient serum is impaired in antibody-dependent bactericidal assays but not in antibody-independent alternative complement pathway-mediated killing. Monocytes from homozygous C2-deficient individuals produce lower than expected amounts of C2 [160].

The probands of the first three C2D kindreds were healthy [154–157]. However, in a review of 38 homozygous C2-deficient individuals, 14 were reported to have systemic lupus erythematosus (SLE) or discoid lupus [165]. Heterozygous C2 deficiency is also increased in frequency in patients with SLE [143] (Table 89-4). Other chronic inflammatory diseases associated with homozygous C2 deficiency include anaphylactoid purpura, dermatomyositis, vasculitis, glomerulonephritis, inflammatory bowel disease, and rarely recurrent bacterial infections [161–172].

B Agarose gel electrophoresis of whole serum followed by immunochemical or functional hemolytic assay for B demonstrates a genetically determined heterogeneity of this alternative pathway protein [173, 174]. At least 20 electrophoretic variants are described, with two alleles designated BfS and BfF being common in all populations, although there are substantial differences among racial groups (Table 89-3). In North American populations the gene BfS occurs with a frequency of 0.81 in Caucasians, 0.44 in blacks, and 0.89 in Orientals, whereas BfF is found in 0.17 of Caucasians, 0.51 of blacks, and 0.11 of Orientals. Similar differences among racial groups have also been reported in South African populations [175]. Inheritance is on an autosomal codominant basis. A silent or null gene has not been described, but there is a rare allele giving normal levels of B protein which is dysfunctional [177]. Low

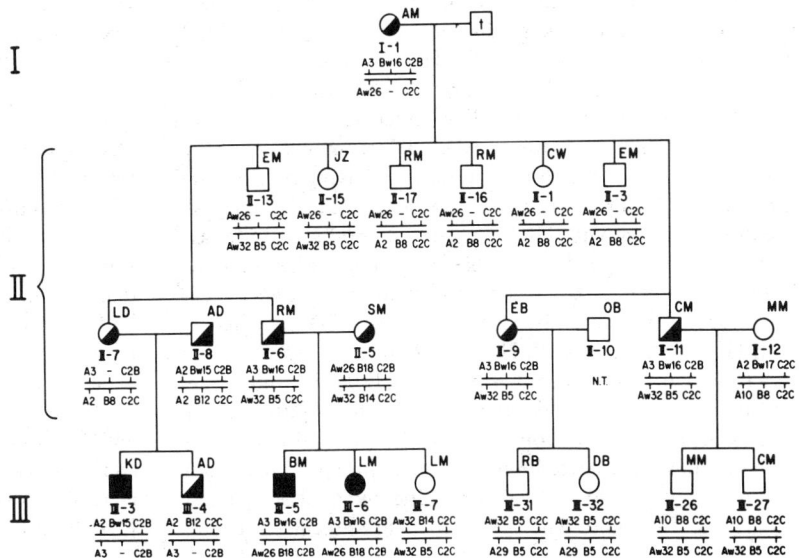

Figure 89-5 The inheritance of C2 and HLA-A and B alleles, in a kindred studied over three generations, showing HLA and C2 haplotypes. C2BC individuals are half shaded, and C2B individuals are completely shaded. (From [141].) (Reprinted by permission of the University of Chicago Press.)

serum levels of B which do not appear to have a primary inherited basis may occur in homozygous and heterozygous C2-deficient individuals [143, 166, 172].

Population studies show linkage disequilibria between Bf alleles and HLA and HLA-linked complement components (Table 89-3). BfS is associated more commonly than expected with HLA-B7, HLA-B8, HLA-B27, HLA-DR2, and C2D, whereas BfF is associated with HLA-A3 and HLA-Bw35. The rare variant BfF1 is associated with HLA-B18 and HLA-DR3, and BfS1 is associated with HLA-B12, HLA-B13, HLA-B14, and HLA-Bw21 [149, 178–188]. The Bf HLA linkage studies have mostly been carried out in populations of North European extraction. An increased frequency of the F1 allele of Bf is present in populations of individuals with diabetes, particularly those with onset of insulin-dependent diabetes before the age of 20 (see Chap. 4) [189, 190] (Table 89-4).

C4 By crossed antigen-antibody electrophoresis C4 was shown to have a complex polymorphism, some of, but not all, the variants being allelic [191, 192]. Electrophoretic techniques did not allow the polymorphism of C4 to be explained in terms of a single locus [191, 195]. Subsequently, the red blood cell group substances, Chido and Rodgers [196], were inferred to be components of C4 because Rodgers-positive, Chido-negative persons were shown to have only the faster-migrating C4 bands, whereas serum of Chido-positive, Rodgers-negative persons typed for the more slowly migrating C4 bands. Serum from a C4-deficient individual was negative for Chido and Rodgers blood group substances. Immobilized anti-human C4 antibody removed C4 activity as well as Chido and Rodgers antigens from serum and purified human C4 neutralized antibodies to Chido and to Rodgers. Evidence had been presented previously demonstrating that both Chido and Rodgers were products of HLA-linked loci but were not allelic [197, 198]. The two-locus inheritance pattern for C4, in which Rodgers is now designated C4A and Chido is termed C4B, is thus linked to HLA [199]. The genes for C4 in the mouse are also linked to the MHC of that species, the H2 region [200–203].

With desialation of plasma before crossed antigen-antibody electrophoresis, seven variants are now described for C4A and four for C4B including silent or null alleles at each locus (Table 89-3). The frequencies of the null alleles C4AQ0 (0.11) and C4BQ0 (0.135) are higher than those of the null genes so far described for other complement components. These closely linked C4 loci show linkage disequilibrium between C4BQ0 with C4A3 and C4A4 with C4B2. The association of C4BQ0 with C4A3 makes the occurrence of the haplotype C4AQ0,C4BQ0 less common than anticipated from the frequency of the null genes themselves [3]. This may account for the rarity of C4D, with only two persons having been recognized [205,206]. Products of the slow or C4B locus are in linkage disequilibrium with HLA-B8, and the products of the fast or C4A locus are in linkage disequilibrium with HLA-B12 [199]. C4A4 and C4B2, in linkage disequilibrium with each other, are also commonly associated with C2D and, hence, with HLA-A10, HLA-B18, HLA-Dw2, and BfS [150].

Serum from a child with C4 deficiency [206] had undetectable immunochemical and functional C4 activity [207]. Other defects in immune function in this child included poor antibody response to a bacteriophage type, failure to switch from IgM to IgG production, and abnormalities in lymphocyte function [207]. This child, who died, experienced recurrent bacte-

rial and viral infections and, like the other C4-deficient patient, had SLE.

C6 and C7 Linkage Group

Combined C6 and C7 deficiency has been observed in a healthy 67-year-old male with antigenic and functional serum levels of C6 and C7 which were 1 to 5 percent and 3 to 9 percent of normal, respectively [208]. Family members partially deficient in C6 were also partially deficient in C7. A second kindred with members exhibiting half-normal levels of C6 and C7, presumably heterozygotes, lacks a homozygous member [209]. In both kindred normal levels of one component were accompanied by normal levels of the other [208, 209]. These two families provide evidence for very close linkage between C6 and C7. The C6 and C7 loci are not within mapping distance of HLA, and the chromosomal assignment is unknown.

C6 Genetically determined variants of C6 are detected either by agarose gel electrophoresis with immunofixation or by isoelectric focusing with functional assay. The common variants are designated A (acidic) or B (basic). Inheritance is autosomal codominant [210] (Table 89-5). C6A and C6B have frequencies of 0.61 and 0.37, respectively, in Caucasians, blacks, and Orientals. A silent or null gene for C6 is allelic with the structural variants [209].

Deficiency of C6 has been described in 11 kindreds, 7 of whom are black. The first case was an 18-year-old black female presenting with an episode of gonococcemia and a past history of good health [211]. Detection of additional probands has followed gonococcal or meningococcal sepsis. This suggests selection because of exposure and an impaired serum bactericidal capacity. Homozygotes are antigenically and functionally deficient in C6, while heterozygotes have half-normal levels. Although bactericidal activity is impaired, C6-deficient serum does sustain the generation of chemotactic and opsonic factors elaborated at the C3 and C5 cleavage stages. The clotting defect manifested by C6-deficient rabbit blood in response to materials that also activate complement was not observed in C6-deficient human blood [212, 213]. In addition to the prominence of Neisserial infections [214, 215], other C6-deficient individuals have recurrent pulmonary infections, chronic brucellosis, and toxoplasmosis. Two of the homozygotes and all heterozygous-deficient individuals are free of recurrent infections [129, 209].

C7 Polymorphism of C7 was not recognized by agarose electrophoresis. However, isoelectric focusing of 1200 serums revealed two rare variants, one present in 4 and the other in 9 of the serums tested [216]. Inheritance is autosomal codominant. The relationship between the null gene for C7 and these rare variants is not known. There are eight kindreds with C7-deficient probands and heterozygous family members with half-normal serum C7 levels; inheritance is autosomal codominant.

Serum from an individual with C7 deficiency, a 13-year-old healthy male with less than 0.002 percent of the normal mean level of this component [217, 218], was opsonic for Staphylococcus albus and sustained zymosan or endotoxin-induced generation of chemotactic activity. Bactericidal activity against E. coli and Klebsiella pneumoniae was absent. A substance

Table 89-4   Diseases associated with altered frequencies of complement component alleles*

Protein	Disease	Allele	Frequency	(Control)	References
C2	Systemic lupus erythematosus	C2D	0.06	(0.01)	143
B	Juvenile onset diabetes mellitus	F1	0.06	(0.03)	189,190
C3	Rheumatoid arthritis	F	0.29	(0.19)	235
	Hepatitis	F†	4/52	(6/21)	236
	Arteriosclerosis	F	0.27	(0.20)	237

* Excluding homozygosity of null alleles.
† Frequency of FF inferred from phenotypes.

that inactivates the hemolytic activity of normal C7, fluid phase and cell-bound, is observed more readily in C7-deficient serum than in normal serum [132, 217]. It most likely represents the C5b,6 complex first described as interacting with C7 in reactive lysis [78]. Indeed, in a 42-year-old white C7-deficient female with Raynaud's phenomenon, sclerodactyly, telangiectasia, and hemolytic levels of C7 ranging between 0.4 and 3 percent of the normal, the C5b,6 has been directly identified [219]. Other clinical problems associated with C7 deficiency include Neisserial infection in three of the eight C7-deficient probands and ankylosing spondylitis and SLE in two further probands [133, 215, 220, 221].

C3 Linkage Group

C3   Figure 89-6 shows 7 of the known variations in mobility of C3 in human plasma; more than 27 allelic variants are described [222–227]. Isolated radiolabeled allotypes maintain their inherent mobilities following reintroduction to serum, and similar differences in mobilities persist following cleavage to C3c. Mobilities are designated with reference to those of the common allotypes, F and S.

Inheritance of the known allotypes is consistent with autosomal codominance. The concentrations of the two gene products in serum from heterozygotes are approximately equal. For Caucasians, the gene frequencies of S and F are 0.75 and 0.25, for blacks 0.90 and 0.10, and for Orientals, 0.98 and 0.02 (Table 89-4). Linkage to histocompatibility antigens is not seen, and data from many kindreds suggest linkage between C3 and the gene(s) for familial hypercholesterolemia [228] and

Lewis blood group substance [229]. In the mouse C3 is linked to H2, the MHC of that species, at a distance of 10 to 11 recombination units [230, 231]. There is some evidence in the mouse that an additional H2-linked locus determines the levels of C3 [232].

No differences in antigenicity are observed among the C3 allotypes when analyzed with antiserums prepared against FS or F1F, and no differences have been found in sedimentation on sucrose density gradients. Variations in the mobility of C3 do not influence its activity as assessed by hemolytic titrations but may alter the capacity to promote immune adherence [233,234]. After orthotopic transplantation of the liver, the change in variants from that of the recipient (FS) to that of the donors (SS) indicates that the liver is the primary site of C3 synthesis in human beings [239].

Abnormal but unconfirmed distributions of C3 variants have been described in disease states. Scandinavian patients with rheumatoid arthritis have a C3F frequency of 0.287, as compared with 0.191 in blood donors. An increase in the C3F allele of comparable degree has been shown in studies of patients with hepatitis, with atherosclerosis, and with cystic fibrosis [235–238] (Table 89-4). A variant of C3F with reduced synthesis [240] has been observed in one individual with arthritis and glomerulonephritis [241]. A silent or null gene, C3D, allelic with the other allotypes, was first observed in family members with half-normal levels of C3 and only a single allotype [242] and was subsequently confirmed by the finding of a homozygote with absent C3 and severe recurrent infections [120, 243].

The first homozygote for C3 deficiency (Fig. 89-7) had less than 0.1 and 0.01 percent of the normal mean C3 level by

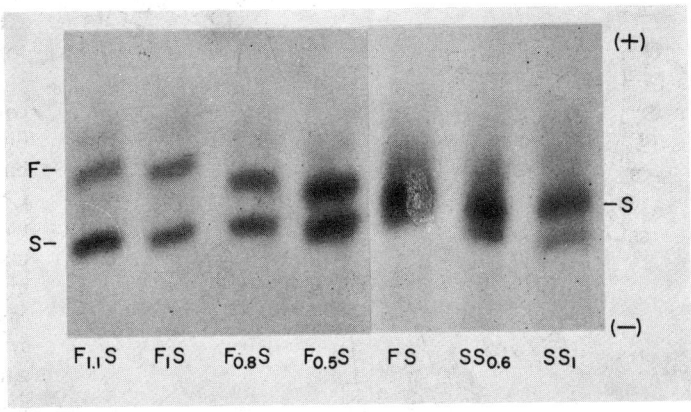

Figure 89-6   Appearance of seven of the allotypes of C3 following prolonged agarose electrophoresis. *(Courtesy of Dr. C. Alper.)*

Table 89-5   Alleles of the non-major histocompatibility complex–linked complement proteins

Protein	Common alleles	Frequency			Reference
		Caucasian	Black*	Oriental	
C6	A	0.61	0.56	0.59	210
	B	0.37	0.38	0.35	
	R	0.015	0.06	0.05	
C3	S	0.75	0.90	0.98	223
	F	0.25	0.10		
C8	A	0.65	0.70	0.66	2
	B	0.35	0.25	0.35	
	A1	0.003	0.05		

* North American.

functional and by immunochemical assay. Total hemolytic complement, and bactericidal, chemotactic, and opsonic activities were absent, as was the response to zymosan activation of the alternative pathway. Immune adherence was one-third normal, presumably owing to the capacity of C4 to mediate this phenomenon. Each of these in vitro abnormalities is correctable by reconstitution of serum with highly purified C3.

Defects in complement-dependent opsonization and cytolysis are attributable to the functional requirements for C3b in opsonization, C5 convertase formation, and amplification convertase formation. The diminished systemic and local accumulation of leukocytes in response to inflammation suggests a role for C3 in mobilization of circulating leukocytes. The monocytes of two C3-deficient patients in culture produced 25 percent of the amount of C3 generated by monocytes from sibs

Figure 89-7   Partial pedigree of a kindred with C3 deficiency. Males are symbolized by squares, females by circles. Half-blackened symbols represent heterozygotes, and the proposita, who is homozygous, is shown as a fully blackened circle and indicated by an arrow. *(Reproduced with permission of Dr. Fred Rosen.)*

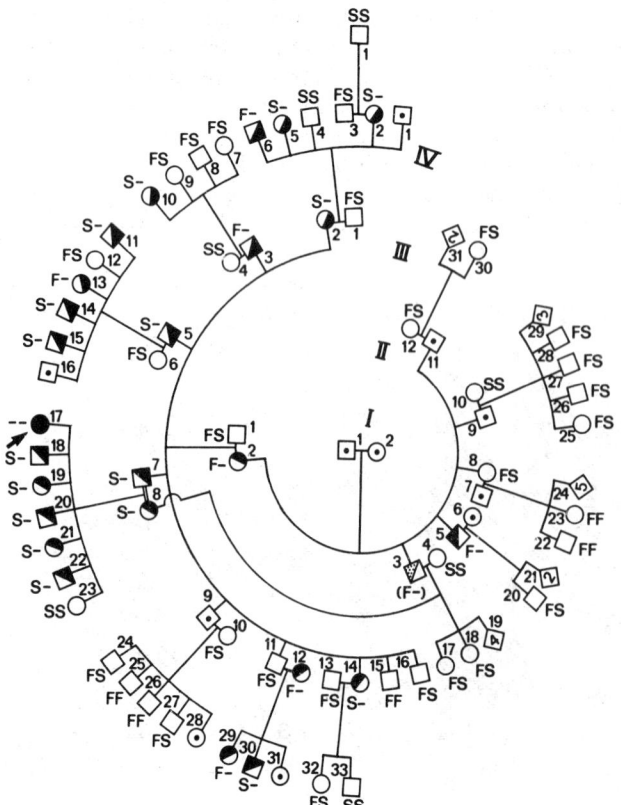

with normal amounts of C3 in serum. This level of monocyte C3 synthesis is in contradistinction to the serum levels of less than 1 percent of normal [244].

Several kindreds with homozygous and heterozygous C3 deficiency have been reported [245–249]. The probands have recurrent infections with both gram-positive and gram-negative bacteria resulting in severe furunculosis, pneumonia, meningitis, and septic arthritis. Three homozygous C3-deficient members of one kindred have nephritis in addition to recurrent infection. A renal biopsy in a sib with heterozygous C3 deficiency showed mesangiocapillary glomerulonephritis [249].

Complement Proteins Not Part of Established Linkage Groups

C1q   Three children have been described with persistently low C1q levels and associated diseases including: SLE at the age of 18 months and subsequent recurrent infections including bacterial meningitis [250]; chronic skin disease, sepsis, and mesangioproliferative glomerulonephritis at age 10 [4]; and SLE with glomerulonephritis at age 4 [5]. Only in the last instance was an acquired deficiency excluded and a genetic basis established [5]. The serum of the proband sustained no antibody-dependent hemolysis but functioned normally in alternative complement pathway–mediated hemolysis. Specific functional C1 activity was less than 1 percent of normal. Since functional activity of C1 was restored by the addition of purified C1q, the other subcomponents of C1, namely C1r and C1s, evidently were normal. The serum of the proband gives an immunoprecipitin line of partial identity with normal C1q; this indicates that the functional defect is associated with some antigenic deletion. One of the proband's sisters who is well has similar findings, and both parents have normal and abnormal C1q present in their serum consistent with a heterozygous state for the altered C1q protein.

Serum levels of C1q are modestly reduced in patients with congenital sex-linked agammaglobulinemia [251] and are diminished to the range of 10 to 25 percent of normal in combined immunodeficiency disease [252, 253]. Levels of C1s, C1r, and of other components are in the normal range or elevated [254]. After reconstitution of immune function by bone marrow transplantation, serum C1q levels returned to normal in four of five patients with combined immunodeficiency disease [255]. C1q deficiency is not a primary defect in biosynthesis since metabolic studies of radiolabeled C1q in hypogammaglobulinemia indicate markedly increased volume of distribution of the isotopically labeled C1q, an elevated fractional catabolic rate, and a normal synthetic rate [257]. It is postulated that C1q forms a loose complex with IgG and is thereby maintained within the intravascular space and protected from extravascular catabolism, and that this accounts for the direct correlation between serum IgG and C1q levels [256].

C1r   The initial description of a C1r-deficient individual with glomerulonephritis did not include family studies [258], but two kindreds with C1r-deficient probands have subsequently been documented [259–261]. In one family the proband has seronegative SLE, a sister has recurrent infections and arthralgias, and three other sibs have died, one at age 12 with SLE and the other two in infancy with gastroenteritis of unknown cause. Homozygous affected individuals have no detectable total hemolytic complement activity or immunochemical C1r, while levels of C1s are approximately 40 percent of normal, and all other complement components, including C1q, are normal or elevated. The activity of the alternative complement pathways, as assessed by endotoxin or cobra venom factor activation, is normal. Family studies have identified heterozygotes with 60 to 90 percent of normal mean C1r levels, with an autosomal codominant mode of inheritance. In a second family with four homozygous C1r-deficient individuals, the proband and a sister have discoid lupus erythematosus and polyarthritis, while the other two sibs are healthy. C1 activity is absent and C1r is immunochemically undetectable. The levels of C1s measured immunochemically were approximately 50 percent or less of the normal mean; it is not known if the low levels of C1s in these two kindreds represent a second genetically determined deficiency or are a consequence of low C1r levels.

C1s   Isolated deficiency of C1s has been reported in a 6-year-old girl with seropositive SLE. No family studies were performed, and the genetic basis of the deficiency was not established. The plasma of the patient contained free C1q and C1r subunits, which were incorporated into macromolecular C1 upon the addition of purified C1s [263].

C5   Isolated C5 deficiency has been recognized in two kindreds, each containing two homozygotes. In the first, the proband, a 20-year-old black female, had seropositive SLE manifested by Raynaud's phenomenon, arthritis, hemolytic anemia, and membranous glomerulonephritis with associated recurrent pyogenic infections. [264]. Addition of purified human C5 restored the whole complement titer (CH50) to normal. Serum bactericidal activity against unsensitized *Salmonella typhi* was absent in the proband and severely impaired in the other homozygote, a half-sister [265]. A second kindred with a C5-deficient proband and a similarly affected twin sister presented because the homozygotes experienced recurrent gonococcal infections [126]. Both kindreds contain some members with hemolytic activities for C5 in the half-normal range, as in autosomal codominant inheritance. Two children with a syndrome composed of infection and eczema, apparently similar to the syndrome designated Leiner's disease, are thought to have a functional abnormality of C5 [266]. This is based upon a relatively selective defect in opsonization of certain particles, such as a baker's yeast or rice starch but not of others, in the presence of hemolytically functional and antigenic C5 [267].

C8   A polymorphism of C8 protein in serum can be demonstrated with the use of isoelectric focusing and a hemolytic assay to locate functional protein [2]. The common alleles in

Caucasians and Orientals, designated C8A and C8B, have similar gene frequencies of 0.65:0.35 and 0.66:0.35 (Table 89-5). Blacks have a distribution of 0.70 for C8A, 0.25 for C8B, and 0.05 for a third allele designated C8A1. C8A1 is present in Caucasians with a frequency of 0.003. Inheritance is autosomal codominant, and the silent or null allele is deduced to be allelic with the electrophoretically determined alleles.

The initial patient recognized to have a selective C8 deficiency was a 23-year-old black woman with prolonged gonococcal septicemia [268]. Whole-complement hemolytic activity (CH50) and C8 levels measured by functional and immunochemical assays were undetectable. Approximately half-normal levels of C8 were present in the proband's parents and in her children. Bactericidal activity, tested with the patient's own strain of *N. gonorrhoeae,* was absent, and both bactericidal activity and CH50 hemolytic activity were rendered normal by the addition of purified C8. C8-deficient serum allows normal opsonization of yeast, staphylococci, and *N. meningitidis* [269] because only activating components and C3 are involved. Two additional C8-deficient probands presented with gonococcal and meningococcal sepsis, and a fourth presented with SLE [215, 270]. In a fifth kindred, from North Africa, three homozygous-deficient members did not have associated disease, while two heterozygous-deficient sibs had xeroderma pigmentosa [134].

C9   Isolated C9 deficiency has been observed in the serum of two Caucasian males, one age 76 years and healthy and the other age 67 years with diabetes mellitus [6]. Their CH50 levels were 33 and 40 percent of normal, respectively. The homozygous-deficient serums lack C9 by immunochemical assay and are less than 0.1 percent of normal in a specific functional assay. In family studies, heterozygous deficiency was defined in members with approximately half-normal levels; inheritance was consistent with autosomal codominance. Killing of bacteria or lysis of antibody-coated sheep cells occurs in the present of C9-deficient serum although at a reduced rate, owing to the fact that the C5-8 terminal complex has some capacity to disrupt a cell membrane [79].

D   Electrophoretic variation in the mobility of alternative pathway protein D has been described with the use of a functional assay. The basis for the elecrtrophoretic heterogeneity has not yet been established [174].

P   Familial deficiency of properdin (P) has been reported in a Swedish family, and an X-linked mode of inheritance has been postulated. One of the P-deficient individuals had Neisserial infection [270a].

C̄1 Inhibitor (C̄1 INH) Deficiency: Hereditary Angioedema (HAE)

Osler distinguished the hereditary form of angiodema in 1888 [271]. His summary of the history of this disease in five generations of one family called attention to most of the important clinical features of hereditary angioedema (HAE), including the prominence of gastrointestinal disturbances and the propensity for sudden death due to upper respiratory obstruction. The autosomal dominant mode of inheritance was further documented in a kindred of 64 individuals, with 28 affected, of whom 15 had died from the acute complications of the disease [272]. The excessive cutaneous response of patients with HAE to the intracutaneous injection of kallikrein [273] suggested the absence of a control protein. This proved to be the inhibitor of the first component of complement, C1̄ INH [274]. C1̄ INH is lacking in the majority of kindreds, but in some it is present antigenically, although in a nonfunctional form [275].

Clinical Aspects Recurrent bouts of acute, circumscribed, and transient edema of the skin are usually the chief complaint of patients with HAE [276–279]. The skin of any part of the body can be involved, but the most common site is either an area of the face or an extremity. Attacks may rarely be heralded by a transient serpiginous erythema or mottling of the skin, but characteristically no changes in the hue or temperature of the involved areas are detectable. The edema usually spreads centripetally from a single site on the body. The simultaneous appearance of multiple, discrete areas of swelling during a single attack is distinctly unusual. The lesions range in size from an area a few centimeters in diameter to involvement of most of an extremity. The localized edema does not itch and cannot be pitted. The swelling may progress for up to 24 or 48 h and then usually subsides over the next 2 or 3 days.

Edema of the wall of the gut, which has been observed by both x-ray and at laparotomy, may lead to severe abdominal pain and profuse vomiting, resembling acute obstruction of the bowel. Watery diarrhea may also occur. The symptoms may be sufficiently severe as to lead to surgical intervention; healed laparotomy scars are a frequent physical finding among patients with HAE. Clinical signs of peritonitis, fever, and marked leukocytosis are not present. Improvement usually occurs within 48 h so that supportive therapy is all that is required. Gastrointestinal attacks may accompany episodes of subcutaneous edema or may occur independently of them. A history of severe, self-limited attacks of abdominal pain accompanied by vomiting or diarrhea or both is so characteristic of HAE that its presence in any patient with angioedema should alert the physician to the possibility of this diagnosis.

Another common feature of HAE is submucosal edema of the upper respiratory tract, which may progress to laryngeal edema with death by asphyxiation. A tracheostomy scar is another common physical finding in this disease. Among affected members of large kindreds, mortality rates due to respiratory obstruction have ranged from as low as 6 percent to as high as 54 percent. Attacks may begin on the face or buccal mucosa and progress to involve the glottis and larynx within a few hours, resulting in increasing hoarseness and laryngeal stridor. The frequency of this life-threatening complication makes it important to distinguish HAE from other more common nonfamilial forms.

Ordinarily there is no periodicity to the attacks of HAE. Some patients have episodes of swelling on an average of once weekly. Others report only a few attacks during their entire lifetimes. Although attacks of angioedema may occur during early childhood, most members of previously undiagnosed kindreds come to the physician's attention at about the onset of puberty. Bouts of edema appear to be most frequent during the reproductive years and occur less often during later life. Exceptions to this are not rare, and the onset of attacks at age 58 in a woman documented to have the biochemical lesion of HAE has been reported [280].

Most patients cite local trauma as a factor which commonly precipitates attacks of angioedema. Dental extractions and tonsillectomies are prone to precipitate severe edema of the oro-

pharynx and glottis, and death has occurred postoperatively. Episodes of pharyngitis are also hazardous. Although many patients assert that exposure to one or another food or allergen is associated with attacks of angioedema, these impressions are difficult to substantiate by skin testing or reexposure to the suspected food. It is not surprising that a lifetime of recurrent swellings, some of which may be potentially asphyxiating, and of unexplained recurrent abdominal pain and gastrointestinal upset should be accompanied by anxiety and frustration. Because there is little objective evidence to suggest that emotional factors have a primary role in the pathogenesis of this disease, we prefer the term *hereditary angioedema* to the older name.

The absence of family history of cutaneous angioedema does not exclude the diagnosis of HAE. Relevant history may include young relatives who have died suddenly of obscure causes or familial complaints related to the gastrointestinal tract. Occasional cases may represent spontaneous mutations. Although HAE is usually considered a rare entity, during the past 10 years we have become aware of 198 affected individuals in 81 kindreds. Other workers in the field have had similar experience.

Pathology The pathologic alterations occurring in HAE have been observed in tissues obtained by skin and peroral jejunal biopsy, laparotomy, and postmortem examination [281]. Skin changes consisting of subcutaneous edema and discontinuity of the postcapillary venules were apparent on electron microscopic examination. There was upper respiratory tract involvement revealing submucosal laryngeal edema; spongiosis of the mucosal epithelial cells with cytoplasmic vacuole formation was also prominent. Diffuse edema and hemorrhage of the lungs occurs, presumably secondary to asphyxiation. Jejunal tissue may show edema of the *lamina propria,* particularly of the superficial portion of the villi, giving a club-shaped appearance; submucosal edema may also be present. The mucocutaneous and visceral tissue findings in HAE can be distinguished from those of fatal systemic anaphylaxis, wherein the involved organs contain an inflammatory infiltrate, frequently with prominence of eosinophils.

Laboratory Diagnosis Deficiency of the function of C1̄ INH can be demonstrated by functional measurements of the inhibitor [282] or can be suspected by measuring the consequence of its absence, i.e., reductions in the serum levels of the substrates of C1, C4 [283], and C2 [284]. Of these, the C4 immunoassay is the simplest screening test available. Less than 1 percent of individuals affected with HAE have C4 protein levels within two standard deviations of the normal mean. Although a normal C4 protein level virtually excludes the diagnosis of HAE, reduced levels are not specifically diagnostic of this disease. Because of its ease of performance, radial immunodiffusion for C1̄ INH protein is utilized to confirm the diagnosis (Fig. 89-8). A serum C1̄ INH protein level of less than 80 μg/ml is present in all individuals with HAE. Approximately 15 percent of kindreds will have a genetic variant form of the disease, in which there are normal serum concentrations of antigenically intact, functionless C1̄ INH protein [257]; thus a functional measurement of C1̄ INH activity is needed to confirm the diagnosis in this group [285].

Treatment Prophylaxis of attacks of angioedema has been achieved by administration of inhibitors of the conver-

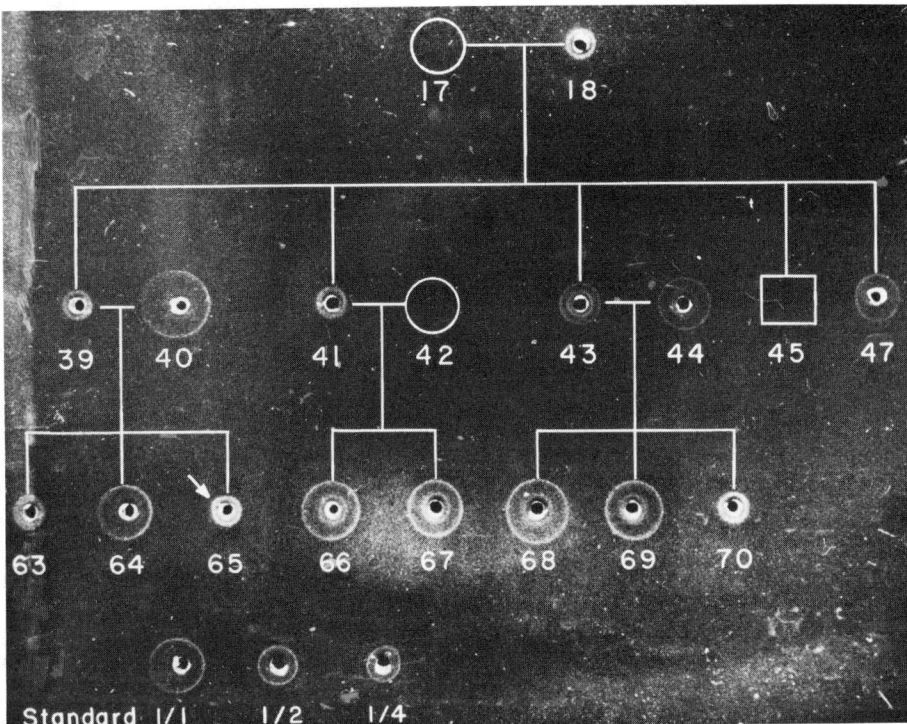

Figure 89-8 Radial immunodiffusion measurements of C̄1INH protein in a kindred with hereditary angioedema. Antibody specific for C̄1INH was incorporated in an agarose gel, and samples of serums placed in holes cut in the gel, arranged in the shape of the pedigree. The size of the precipitin rings which surround the holes is proportional to the concentration of C̄1INH protein in the serums.

sion of plasminogen to plasmin. Although epsilon-aminocaproic acid [286, 287] and tranexamic acid [288] have been used for this purpose, anabolic steroids [289–296] are now preferred. The former drugs do not alter the plasma levels of C̄1 INH or C4. By their effects on the fibrinolytic system they are believed to impair the generation of the presumptive vasoactive peptide mediator. In contrast, anabolic steroids, such as methyltestosterone [289, 290], or 17-α-alkylated derivatives with attenuated androgenic effects, such as oxymethalone [291–293], danazol [294, 295], and stanozolol [295, 296], stimulate synthesis of normal C̄1 INH in these patients. Secondarily, they increase the plasma concentration of C4, reflecting the more effective regulation of C1 by the increased levels of inhibitor. Use of these agents over long periods of time requires consideration of their side effects which include impairment of growth rate in children, masculinization of women, and hepatic dysfunction. Therefore, it is critical to establish the lowest dose that is clinically effective [293, 296], which may represent a compromise between disease suppression and adverse effects. This is particularly important in women of childbearing age or during pregnancy and in children during their growth period.

No specific therapy is available to interrupt ongoing attacks of HAE. A variety of remedies has been tried, but their efficacy is unclear because of the self-limited nature of the attacks. Plasma transfusions have been reported to arrest an attack already in progress [279, 297], although there are theoretical reasons why such therapy might be hazardous [298]. These hazards may be circumvented by use of partially purified C̄1 INH [299], but this is not generally available. Preoperative treatment with epsilon-aminocaproic acid [300] or tranexamic acid [301] has been used to suppress intra- and postoperative attacks of angioedema. Recently, protection has been afforded by administration of high doses of stanozolol for several days prior to operation. This would seem the most rational approach, since it can be monitored by immunochemical measurements of serum levels of C̄1 INH or C4, or both.

Pathogenesis of Edema Attacks of angioedema are associated with an increase in activated serum C̄1, as reflected by increases in the capacity of serum to hydrolyze synthetic amino acid ester substrates [302] or by a further decline in serum levels of the natural substrates of C̄1, namely, C4 and C2 [284]. Even in asymptomatic patients with HAE radiolabeled C4 is catabolized three to five times more rapidly than in normal subjects [303]. This reflects the continuous presence of some activated and uninhibited C1. Although plasma levels of the terminal complement components are maintained within normal limits, moderate hypercatabolism of C3 has been observed, presumably due to the generation of some C4b,2a by the action of C̄1 on C4 and C2 [303]. C̄1s is the activated subunit form of C1. When purified C̄1s is injected into the skin of normal volunteers, an intense wheal develops. Intradermal injection of C̄1s in HAE patients precipitates a full-blown local attack of angioedema, while no response to intradermal C̄1s is observed in subjects with homozygous C2 deficiency. It can be inferred from these studies that C̄1 INH limits the capacity of C̄1 to induce permeability changes, that C2 is an essential ingredient of the reaction [304], and that attacks are associated with further C1 activation.

The mechanism for the episodic activation of C1 in HAE remains unclear. C̄1 inhibitor impairs the capacity of active Hageman factor or its fragments to induce the conversion of prekallikrein to kallikrein and of precursor plasma thromboplastin antecedent (PTA) to its active form [305]. In addition, kallikrein, plasmin, and PTA are directly inhibited by C̄1 INH [306]. The spontaneous attacks may reflect episodic activation of Hageman factor, with subsequent conversion of prekallikrein to kallikrein and of plasminogen to plasmin, enzymes which inactivate and activate C1, respectively [307, 308]. Plasma obtained from patients with HAE during asymptomatic intervals spontaneously generates smooth-muscle contracting activity when incubated in vitro. Generation of this activity is inhibited in the presence of antibody to C4 or to C2 [309]. A heat-stable polypeptide has been isolated from the incubated plasma that is clearly distinguishable from bradykinin on the basis of a paucity of aromatic amino acid residues, susceptibility to inactivation by trypsin, and production of a pressor effect in the rat. In vitro combinations of purified C1s, C4, C2, and plasmin [310] have produced low molecular weight fragments similar in amino acid composition to this polypeptide, but as yet this material has not been fully characterized.

Urinary histamine levels are increased during attacks of angioedema [311], which may reflect the release of C3a anaphylatoxin by C4b,2a. Histamine does not appear to have a central role, since antihistamines do not affect the course of the disease, but a direct effect of anaphylatoxin has not been excluded. The failure of a homozygous C3-deficient patient to develop a cutaneous wheal following the intradermal injection of C1s [243] suggests that C3a or C5a may be involved. These components may act by inducing production of arachidonic acid-derived mediators [312].

Properties of the Abnormal Gene Products   Over 100 kindreds with HAE have been observed without apparent racial selectivity. In all instances, the deficiency in C1 INH appears to be transmitted as an autosomal dominant trait, affected individuals being heterozygotes. Immunofluorescent studies with antibody directed against C1 INH have demonstrated specific fluorescence in 5 to 10 percent of the hepatocytes of normal individuals, but few if any fluorescent cells were observed in liver biopsy specimens from two patients with HAE [313]. The catabolic rate for C1 INH, as measured with purified and radiolabeled C1 INH, was normal. Therefore, the rate of synthesis of C1 INH, calculated from serum levels and catabolic rates, appears to be depressed in HAE [314].

In general the nonfunctional inhibitor proteins are antigenically identical to normal C1 INH [275]. However, the variant protein of a given kindred may exhibit genetically determined abnormalities in electrophoretic mobility, capacity to bind C1s, and ability to inhibit C1s-induced esterolysis [315]. In two kindreds with immunochemically supranormal levels of nonfunctional C1 INH protein, complexes of this protein and serum albumin were observed [275, 316]. Chemical studies of a single variant C1 INH protein purified from plasma indicate a molecular weight which exceeds that of normal C1 INH by about 3 percent, and small differences in amino acid composition, particularly with respect to phenylalanine and acidic amino acids [317]. Patients with abnormal nonfunctional C1 INH, like those with absent protein, respond to androgen treatment with increased levels of normal and functional inhibitor [290, 291, 293–296]. This increase is presumably due to an androgen-induced increase in the synthesis of the protein specified by the normal allele at the C1 INH locus in these heterozygous individuals.

C3b Inactivator (I) Deficiency

Three kindreds with C3b inactivator (I) deficiency have been described. The initial proband was a 26-year-old male with Klinefelter's syndrome and recurrent pyogenic infections including pneumonia, streptococcal and meningococcal septicemia, sinusitis, mastoiditis, and otitis media. His serum was deficient in bactericidal activity for gram negative organisms, opsonization of pneumococci, and generation of chemotactic activity [318, 319]. There was a marked deficiency of B and of C3. Most of the immunoreactive C3 present in the patient's plasma was in the form of C3b rather than C3c and C3d, which are the forms observed in serum of patients with intense cleavage of C3. Metabolic studies with radioiodinated C3 indicated a fractional catabolic rate approximately five times the normal mean value. The synthetic rate was normal. A chronic hemolytic anemia, associated with erythrocytes coated with C3b, was attributed to the inability of the patient's serum to inactivate C3b on the erythrocytes [320]. Specific immunochemical measurement of I established the patient as homozygous for a deficiency in this protein. Certain family members were identified as heterozygous, on the basis of an approximately one-half normal serum concentration [321].

It is now assumed that there is in normal plasma a low grade interaction between C3 and B to form a complex which presents B for cleavage activation by D. The resulting intermediate, C3Bb, then cleaves C3 to C3b. The latter associates with B more avidly to permit D cleavage activation of the amplification C3 convertase, C3b,Bb. Under normal circumstances C3b,Bb in the fluid phase is inactivated by H and I before cleavage of additional C3 can occur. H dissociates Bb from C3b, and C3b is then inactivated by I. The findings in the initial proband, and in two others with meningitis as a clinical presentation [323, 324], indicate that I is a major control protein of the system and that in its absence the sequence progresses spontaneously to secondary cleavage-depletion of C3 and B.

IMMUNOBIOLOGIC IMPLICATIONS

Complement Proteins and Their Mechanism of Evolution

Structural and functional homologies between components of the two activating pathways, classic and alternative, suggest that they may have evolved through a process of gene duplication. Classic and alternative pathway C3 convertases are both bimolecular complexes. The catalytic subunits, C2a and Bb, have identical substrate specificities and similar amino acid compositions [325, 326]. Both are derived from proteins encoded by loci that are closely linked within the HLA complex. These proteases function only when complexed with C4b and C3b, respectively. Both C4b and C3b are bound by covalent esterlike attachments to glycoprotein complexes and cell membranes. Although C3 and C4 are not genetically linked in humans, C3 in the mouse maps close to the MHC, which is the region within which the genes for C4 are coded. Since the activation peptides, C3a and C5a, demonstrate about one-third homology in primary structure [327], the respective parent molecules may also have evolved by gene reduplication. The close linkage between C6 and C7 may be similarly interpreted, the genes for both proteins being duplications from a common precursor; alternatively, one protein may have evolved from the other.

Contribution of the Complement System to Host Defense

Although the initial and subsequent probands with homozygous I deficiency experienced recurrent infections, the allocation of the susceptibility to C3 deficiency was not clear because the B deficiency impaired the function of the alternative complement pathway. The finding of homozygous C3-deficient individuals with similar recurrent bacterial infections, both Neisserial and pyogenic, made clear the central role of C3 in the maintenance of normal host defenses. C3 would not only be critical to a bactericidal reaction, with or without C3b-dependent amplification, but would also be critical to phagocytosis enhancement through the presence of the C3b receptor on neutrophilic and monocytic leukocytes. In addition, the progression of the complement sequence has a role in systemic and local leukocyte mobilization.

Patients deficient in the terminal complement components appear to be susceptible to infections in which there is gram-negative bacteremia, such as those produced by Neisserial organisms. Of 38 homozygous C5-, 6-, 7-, and 8-deficient individuals, 21 experienced such infections, suggesting the importance of the bactericidal reactions in controlling this class of microorganism. Just as the deficiencies in C3 and in terminal components have revealed the clinical importance of certain complement components in aspects of host defense, the absence of such a disease susceptibility in the substantial numbers who have homozygous C2 deficiency serves to emphasize the importance of the alternative activating pathway relative to the classic.

Association of Deficiency States with Rheumatic Diseases

The apparent increased frequency of diseases such as SLE, Henoch-Schönlein purpura, or polymyositis in individuals with complement deficiencies would not have been predicted from the postulated role of complement as a mediator of inflammation in these rheumatic diseases. If anything, a protective effect might have been expected. With the exception of single C5-, C7-, and C8-deficient individuals, all instances of association between rheumatic diseases and complement deficiency have involved proteins of the classic activating pathway. There is even a report of SLE occurring in patients with hypercatabolism of C4 and C2 due to C1 inhibitor deficiency [328].

Since C1 and C4 have been demonstrated to increase the efficiency of antibody in the neutralization of certain viruses, the most direct explanation for the association would involve failure of neutralization of the etiologic agent [329]. An attractive alternative would invoke failure of clearance of antigen-antibody complexes irrespective of the nature of the antigen. In animal models the failure to clear viral antibody has been shown to be important in the pathogenesis of immune complex disease [330]. The latter view would argue that while the alternative pathway is essential for host defense, irrespective of adaptive immunity, the adaptive immunity augmentation afforded by the classic activating pathway is important for the need to clear the products of the immune response.

The location of the genes controlling the C2, B, and C4 polymorphisms in the major histocompatibility complex affords yet another explanation. In the mouse and guinea pig [331] genes controlling immune responsiveness (Ir) to certain synthetic antigens are located in or near the histocompatability complex (see Chap. 3). A similar linkage of Ir genes to histocompatibility complexes has been demonstrated in rhesus monkeys and seems likely in the human. The products of the HLA-D locus are most likely to function as Ir genes, and it is to

this locus that the four complement loci are most closely linked. Association between rheumatic disease and complement deficiencies may result from linkage disequilibrium between a silent or null allele for the complement component and an allele of an Ir gene locus. The association between Ir genes and disease may be primary and that with the complement allele secondary. There is some evidence for this. C2D in homozygous and in heterozygous form occurs in increased frequency in patients with SLE, as does HLA-DR2 [143, 332]. HLA-DR2 is in linkage disequilibrium with C2D, and more patients with SLE have HLA-DR2 than C2D. The greater frequency of HLA-DR2 in SLE and the marginal effect of heterozygous C2 deficiency on complement function suggest that the important association with respect to pathogenesis may be with the HLA-D region allele, rather than with the complement component allele. On the other hand, rheumatic diseases are also associated with component deficiencies that are not coded for in the major histocompatibility region, namely, C1r, C1s, and C1 INH. These associations may represent selection bias resulting from the type of population screened for complement polymorphism. Alternatively, the association may indicate that impaired clearance alone may be sufficient to increase disease susceptibility.

REFERENCES

1. ALPER CA: Inherited structural polymorphism in human C2: Evidence for genetic linkage between C2 and Bf. *J Exp Med.,* 144, 1111, 1976.
2. RAUM D, SPENCE MA, BALAVITCH D, TIDEMAN S, MERRITT AD, TAGGART RT, PETERSEN BHJ, DAY NK, ALPER CA: Genetic control of the eighth component of complement. *J Clin Invest* 64:858, 1979
3. AWDEH ZL, ALPER CA: Inherited structural polymorphism of the fourth component of human complement. *Proc Natl Acad Sci USA* 77, 3576, 1980
4. BERKEL LI, LOOS M, SANAL O, MAUFF G, GUNGEN G, ÖRS U, ERSOY F, YEGIN O: Clinical and immunological studies in a case of selective complete C1q deficiency. *Clin Exp Immunol* 38:52, 1979
5. THOMPSON RA, HAENEY M, REID KBM, DAVIES JG, WHITE RHR, CAMERON AH: A genetic defect of the C1q subcomponent of complement associated with childhood (immune complex) nephritis. *N Engl J Med* 303:22, 1980
6. LINT TF, ZEITZ HJ, GEWURZ H: Inherited deficiency of the ninth component of complement in man. *J Immunol* 125:2252, 1980
7. AGNELLO V, DEBRACCO MME, KUNKEL HG: Hereditary C2 deficiency with some manifestations of systemic lupus erythematosus. *J Immunol* 108:837, 1972
8. ALLEN FH JR: Linkage of HL-A and GBG. *Vox Sang* 27:382, 1974
9. FU SM, KUNKEL HG, BRUSMAN HP, ALLEN FH JR, FOTINO M: Evidence for linkage between HL-A histocompatibility genes and those involved in the synthesis of the second component of complement. *J Exp Med* 140:1108, 1974
10. OCHS HS, ROSENFELD SI, THOMAS ED, GIBLETT ER, ALPER CA, DUPONT D, SCHALLER JG, GILLILAND BC, HANSEN JA, WEDGWOOD RJ: Linkage between the gene (or genes) controlling synthesis of the fourth component of complement and the major histocompatibility complex. *N Engl J Med* 296:470, 1977
11. LEPOW IH, NAFF GB, TODD EW, PENSKY J, HINZ CF: Chromatographic resolution of the first component of human complement into three activities. *J Exp Med* 117:983, 1963
12. NAGASAWA S, TAKAHASHI K, KOYAMA J: Isolation of a complex of the subcomponents of complement, C1r-C1s, from ACD-human plasma. *FEBS Lett* 41:280, 1974
13. GIGLI I, PORTER RR, SIM RB: The unactivated form of the first component of human complement, C1. *Biochem J* 157:541, 1976
14. SHELTON E, YONEMASU K, STROUD RM: Ultrastructure of human complement component, C1. *Proc Natl Acad Sci USA* 69:65, 1972
15. KNOBEL HR, VILLIGER W, ISLIKER H: Chemical analysis and electron microscopy studies of human C1q prepared by different methods. *Eur J Immunol* 5:78, 1975
16. ELLERSON JR, YASMEAN D, PAINTER RH, DORRINGTON KJ: A fragment corresponding to the C_H2 region of IgG with complement-fixing activity. *FEBS Lett* 24:318, 1972
17. HURST MM, VOLANAKIS JE, HESTER RB, STROUD RM, BENNETT JC: The

structural basis for binding of complement by immunoglobulin M. *J Exp Med* 140:1117, 1974

18. KNOBEL HR, HEUSSER C, RODRICK ML, ISLIKER H: Enzymatic digestion of the first component of human complement. *J Immunol* 112:2094, 1974

19. REID KBM: Isolation by partial pepsin digestion of the three collagen-like regions present in subcomponent Clq of the first component of human complement. *Biochem J* 155:5, 1976

20. REID KBM, SIM RB, FAIERS AP: Inhibition of the reconstitution of the haemolytic activity of the first component of human complement by a pepsin derived fragment of the subcomponent Clq. *Biochem J* 161:239, 1977

21. LIN TY, FLETCHER DS: Activation of a complex of Clr and Cls subcomponents of human complement Cl by the third subcomponent Clq. *J Biol Chem* 255:7756, 1980

22. ZICCARDI RJ, COOPER NR: Activation of Clr by proteolytic cleavage. *J Immunol* 116:504, 1976

23. VALET G, COOPER NR: Isolation of the proenzyme forms of Clr and Cls from human serum. *J Immunol* 111:292, 1973

24. SAKAI K, STROUD RM: Purification, molecular properties and activation of Cl proesterase, Cl. *J Immunol* 110:1010, 1973

25. SCHREIBER RD, MÜLLER-EBERHARD HJ: Fourth component of human complement: Description of a three polypeptide chain structure. *J Exp Med* 140:1324, 1974

26. JANATOVA J, TACK BF: Structural requirements for hemolytic function of the fourth component of human complement and autocatalytic cleavage of its α-chain. *Fed Proc* 40:1020, 1981

27. LAW SK, LICHTENBERG NA, HOLCOMBE FH, LEVINE RP: Interaction between the labile binding sites of the fourth (C4) and fifth human complement proteins and erythrocyte cell membranes. *J Immunol* 125:634, 1980

28. MÜLLER-EBERHARD HJ, POLLEY MJ, CALCOTT MA: Formation and functional significance of a molecular complex derived from the second and fourth components of human complement. *J Exp Med* 125:359, 1967

29. NAGASAWA S, STROUD RM: Cleavage of C2 by C1s into the antigenically distinct fragments, C2a and C2b: Demonstration of binding of C2b to C4b. *Proc Natl Acad Sci USA* 74:2998, 1977

30. MAYER MM: Mechanism of haemolysis by complement, in Wolstenholme GEW, Knight J (eds): *Ciba Foundation Symposium on Complement.* London, J.A. Churchill 1965, p 4

31. HARPEL PC, COOPER NR: Studies on human plasma C1 inactivator-enzyme interactions. I. Mechanisms of interaction with C1s, plasmin, and trypsin. *J Clin Invest* 55:593, 1975

32. RUDDY S, CARPENTER CB, CHIN KW, KNOSTMAN JN, SOTER NA, GÖTZE O, MÜLLER-EBERHARD HJ, AUSTEN KF: Human complement metabolism: An analysis of 144 studies. *Medicine* 54:165, 1975

33. FUKITA T, GIGLI I, NUSSENZWEIG V: Human C4-binding protein. II. Role in proteolysis of C4b by C3b inactivator. *J Exp Med* 148:1044, 1978

34. GIGLI I, FUJITA T, NUSSENZWEIG V: Modulation of the classical pathway C3 convertase by the plasma proteins, C4-binding protein and C3b inactivator. *Proc Natl Acad Sci USA* 76:6596, 1979

35. NAGASAWA S, ICHIHARA C, STROUD RM: Cleavage of C4b by C3b inactivator: Production of a nicked form of C4b,C4b′: As an intermediate cleavage product of C4b by C3b inactivator. *J Immunol* 125:578, 1980

36. PILLEMER L, BLUM L, LEPOW IH, ROSS OA, TODD EW, WARDLAW AC: The properdin system and immunity. I. Demonstration and isolation of a new serum protein, properdin, and its role in immune phenomena. *Science* 120:279, 1954

37. MÜLLER-EBERHARD HJ, GÖTZE O: C3 proactivator convertase and its mode of action. *J Exp Med* 135:1003, 1972

38. FEARON DT, AUSTEN KF, RUDDY S: Formation of a hemolytically active cellular intermediate by the interaction between properdin factors B and D and the activated third component of complement. *J Exp Med* 138:1305, 1973

39. FEARON DT, AUSTEN KF: Initiation of C3 cleavage in the alternative complement pathway. *J Immunol* 115:1357, 1975

40. PANGBURN MK, MÜLLER-EBERHARD HJ: Relation of a putative thioester bond in C3 to activation of the alternative pathway and the binding of C3b to biological targets of complement. *J Exp Med* 152:1102, 1980

41. MEDICUS RG, GÖTZE O, MÜLLER-EBERHARD, HJ: The serine protease nature of the C3 and C5 convertases of the classical and alternative complement pathways. *Scand J Immunol* 5:1049, 1976

42. NIEMANN MA, MOLE JE: Complement factor B: A novel class of serine protease. *Fed Proc* 39:1997, 1980

43. CHRISTIE DL, GAGNON J, PORTER RR: Partial sequence of human complement component factor B: Novel type of serine protease. *Proc Natl Acad Sci USA* 77:4923, 1980

44. LAW SK, LEVINE RP: Interaction between the third complement protein and cell surface macromolecules. *Proc Natl Acad Sci USA* 74:2701, 1977

45. LAW SK, LICHTENBERG NA, LEVINE RP: Evidence for an ester linkage

46. TACK BF, HARRISON RA, JANATOVA J, THOMAS M, PRAHL JW: Evidence for the presence of an internal thiol ester in the third component of complement. *Proc Natl Acad Sci USA* in press

47. DAHA, MR, FEARON DT, AUSTEN KF: Isolation of alternative pathway C3 convertase containing uncleaved B and formed in the presence of C3 nephritic factor (C3NeF). *J Immunol* 116:568, 1976

48. VOGT W, DAMES W, SCHMIDT G, DIEMINGER L: Complement activation by the properdin system: Formation of a stoichiometric C3 cleaving complex of properdin factor B with C3b. *Immunochemistry* 14:201, 1977

49. KAZATCHKINE MD, FEARON DT, AUSTEN KF: Human alternative complement pathway: Membrane-associated sialic acid regulates the competition between B and β1H for cell-bound C3b. *J Immunol* 122:75, 1979

50. FEARON DT, AUSTEN KF, RUDDY S: Properdin factor D: Characterization of its active site and isolation of the precursor form. *J Exp Med* 139:355, 1974

51. LESAVRE PH, MÜLLER-EBERHARD HJ: Mechanism of action of factor D of the alternative complement pathway. *J Exp Med* 148:1498, 1978

52. VOLANAKIS JE, BHOWN AS, BENNETT JC, MOLE JE: Partial amino acid sequence of human factor D: Homology with serine proteases. *Proc Natl Acad Sci USA* 77:1116, 1980

53. DAVIS AE III: Active site amino acid sequence of human factor D. *Proc Natl Acad Sci USA* 77:4938, 1980

54. FEARON DT, AUSTEN KF: Properdin: Binding to C3b and stabilization of the C3b-dependent C3 convertase. *J Exp Med* 142:856, 1975

55. CONRAD DH, CARLO JR, RUDDY S: Interaction of β1H globulin with cell-bound C3b: Quantitative analysis of binding and influence of alternative pathway components on binding. *J Exp Med* 147:1792, 1978

56. WHALEY K, RUDDY S: Modulation of the alternative complement pathway by β1H globulin. *J Exp Med* 144:1147, 1976

57. WEILER JM, DAHA MR, AUSTEN KF, FEARON DT: Control of the amplification convertase of complement by the plasma protein, β1H. *Proc Natl Acad Sci USA* 73:3268, 1976

58. PANGBURN MK, SCHREIBER RD, MÜLLER-EBERHARD HJ: Human complement C3b inactivator: Isolation, characterization and demonstration of an absolute requirement for the serum protein β1H for cleavage of C3b and C4b in solution. *J Exp Med* 146:257, 1977

59. FEARON DT, AUSTEN KF: Activation of the alternative complement pathway due to resistance of zymosan-bound amplification convertase to endogenous regulatory mechanisms. *Proc Natl Acad Sci USA* 74:1683, 1977

60. FEARON DT, AUSTEN KF: Activation of the alternative complement pathway with rabbit erythrocytes by circumvention of the regulatory action of endogenous control proteins. *J Exp Med* 146:22, 1977

61. FEARON DT: Regulation by membrane sialic acid of β1H-dependent decay. Dissociation of amplification C3 convertase of the alternative complement pathway. *Proc Natl Acad Sci USA* 75:1971, 1978

62. PANGBURN MK, MÜLLER-EBERHARD HJ: Complement C3 convertase: Cell surface restriction of β1H control and generation of restriction on neuraminidase-treated cells. *Proc Natl Acad Sci USA* 75:2416, 1978

63. NYDEGGER UE, FEARON DT, AUSTEN KF: Autosomal locus regulates inverse relationship between sialic acid content and capacity of mouse erythrocytes to activate human alternative complement pathway. *Proc Natl Acad Sci USA* 75:6078, 1978

64. KAZATCHKINE MD, FEARON DT, SILBERT JE, AUSTEN KF: Surface-associated heparin inhibits zymosan-induced activation of the human alternative complement pathway by augmenting the regulatory action of the control proteins on particle-bound C3b. *J Exp Med* 150:1202, 1979

65. SCHENKEIN HA, RUDDY S: The role of immunoglobulins in alternative complement pathway activation by zymosan. I. Human IgG with specificity for zymosan enhances alternative pathway activation by zymosan. *J Immunol* 126:7, 1981

66. POLHILL RB, NEWMAN JL, PRUITT KM, JOHNSON RB: Kinetic assessment of alternative complement assay in a hemolytic system. II. Influence of antibody in alternative pathway activation. *J Immunol* 121:371, 1978

67. WINKELSTEIN JA, SHIN HS, WOOD WB JR: Heat labile opsonins to pneumococcus. III. Participation of immunoglobulin and of the alternative pathway of C3 activation. *J Immunol* 108:1681, 1972

68. EDWARDS MS, NICHOLSON-WELLER A, BAKER CJ, KASPER DL: The role of specific antibody in alternative complement pathway mediated opsono-phagocytosis of type III, group B streptococcus. *J Exp Med* 151:1275, 1980

69. PERRIN LH, JOSEPH BS, COOPER NR, OLDSTONE MBA: Mechanism of injury of virus-infected cells by antiviral antibody and complement: Participation of IgG, F(ab′)₂ and the alternative pathway. *J Exp Med* 143:1027, 1976

70. SISSONS JGP, COOPER NR, OLDSTONE MBA: Alternative complement pathway mediated lysis of measles virus infected cells. Induction by IgG antibody bound to individual viral glycoproteins and comparative efficacy of F(ab′)₂ and Fab′ fragments. *J Immunol* 123:2144, 1979

71. MOORE FD JR, FEARON DT, AUSTEN KF: IgG on mouse erythrocytes aug-

ments activation of the human alternative complement pathway by enhancing deposition of C3b. *J Immunol* 126:1805, 1981

72. SHIN HS, PICKERING RJ, MAYER MM: The fifth component of the guinea pig complement system. III. Dissociation and transfer of C5b, and the problable site of C5b fixation. *J Immunol* 106:480, 1971

73. COOPER NR, MÜLLER-EBERHARD HJ: The reaction-mechanism of human C5 in immune hemolysis. *J Exp Med* 132:775, 1970

74. DAHA MR, FEARON DT, AUSTEN KF: C3 requirements for formation of alternative pathway C5 convertase. *J Immunol* 117:630, 1976

75. VOGT W, SCHMIDT G: Hydrolytic activation of the fifth component of complement (C5) by C3 convertases depends on its binding to surface-fixed C3b; specific interference with binding by properdin, factor B or propamidine leads to inhibition of C5 cleavage and utilization. *J Immunol* 120:1801, 1978

76. HAMMER CH, ABRAMOVITZ AS, MAYER MM: A new activity of complement component C3: Cell-bound C3b potentiates lysis of erythrocytes by C5b,6 and terminal components. *J Immunol* 117:830, 1976

77. ISENMAN DE, PODACK ER, COOPER NR: The interaction of C5 with C3b in free solution: A sufficient condition for cleavage by a fluid phase C3/C5 convertase. *J Immunol* 124:326, 1980

78. LACHMANN PJ, THOMPSON RA: Reactive lysis: The complement-mediated lysis of unsensitized cells. II. The characterization of activated reactor as C56 and participation of C8 and C9. *J Exp Med* 131:643, 1970

79. MAYER MM, MICHAELS DW, RAMM LE, SHIN ML, WHITLOW MB, WILLOUGHBY JB: Membrane damage by complement. CRC Critical Reviews in Immunology, 2:133, 1981

80. COOPER N: Immune adherence by the fourth component of complement. *Science* 165:396, 1969

81. NELSON DS: Immune adherence. *Adv Immunol* 3:131, 1963

82. GIGLI I, NELSON RA JR: Complement-dependent immune phagocytosis. I. Requirements for C'1, C'4 and C'3. *Exp Cell Res* 51:45, 1968

83. GUPTA S, ROSS GD, GOOD RA, SIEGAL FP: Surface markers of human eosinophils. *Blood* 48:755, 1976

84. HUBER H, POLLEY MJ, LINSCOTT W, FUDENBERG HH, MÜLLER-EBERHARD HJ: Human monocytes: Distinct receptor sites for the third component of complement and for immunoglobulin G. *Science* 162:1281, 1968

85. EDEN A, MILLER GW, NUSSENZWEIG V: Human lymphocytes bear membrane receptors for C3b and C3d. *J Clin Invest* 52:3239, 1973

86. ROSS GD, POLLEY MJ: Specificity of human lymphocyte complement receptors. *J Exp Med* 141:1163, 1975

87. SHER A, HEIN A, MOSER G, CAULFIELD JP: Complement receptors promote phagocytosis of bacteria by rat peritoneal mast cells. *Lab Invest* 41:490, 1979

88. VRANIAN G, CONRAD D, RUDDY S: C3 mediates phagocytosis by rat peritoneal mast cells. *J Immunol* 124:1544, 1980

89. GELFAND MC, FRANK MM, GREEN I: A receptor for the third component of complement in the human renal glomerulus. *J Exp Med* 142:1029, 1975

90. CARLO JR, RUDDY S, STRUELER EJ, CONRAD DH: Complement receptor binding of C3b-coated cells treated with C3b inactivator, β1H and trypsin. *J Immunol* 123:523, 1979

91. FEARON DT: Regulation of the amplification C3 convertase of human complement by an inhibitory protein isolated from human erythrocyte membranes. *Proc Natl Acad Sci USA* 76:5867, 1979

92. FEARON DT: Identification of the membrane glycoprotein that is the C3b receptor of the human erythrocyte, polymorphonuclear leukocyte, B lymphocyte and monocyte. *J Exp Med* 152:20, 1980

93. PETTY HR, SMITH LM, FEARON DT, McCONNELL HM: Lateral distribution and diffusion of the C3b receptor of complement, HLA antigens and lipid probes in peripheral blood leukocytes. *Proc Natl Acad Sci USA* 77:6587, 1980

94. MANTOVANI B, RABINOVITCH M, NUSSENZWEIG V: Phagocytosis of immune complexes by macrophages. Different roles of the macrophage receptor sites for complement (C3) and for immunoglobulin. *J Exp Med* 135:780, 1972

95. MANTOVANI B: Different roles of IgG and complement receptors in phagocytosis by polymorphonuclear leukocytes. *J Immunol* 115:15, 1975

96. CZOP JK, FEARON DT, AUSTEN KF: Membrane sialic acid on target particles modulates their phagocytosis by a trypsin-sensitive mechanism on human monocytes. *Proc Natl Acad Sci USA* 75:3831, 1978

97. FEARON DT, KANEKO I, THOMSON GT: Membrane distribution and adsorptive endocytosis by C3b receptors on human polymorphonuclear leukocytes. *J Exp Med* 153:1615, 1981

98. BIANCO C, GRIFFIN FM JR, SILVERSTEIN SC: Studies of the macrophage complement receptor function upon macrophage activation. *J Exp Med* 141:1278, 1975

99. GRIFFIN JA, GRIFFIN FM JR: Augmentation of macrophage complement receptor function in vitro. I. Characterization of the cellular interactions required for the generation of a T-lymphocyte product that enhances macrophage complement receptor function. *J Exp Med* 150:653, 1979

100. NEWMAN SL, MUSSON RA, HENSON PM: Development of functional complement receptors during in vitro maturation of human monocytes into macrophages. *J Immunol* 125:2236, 1980

101. KLAUS GGB, HUMPHREY JH: The generation of memory cells. I. The role of C3 in the generation of B memory cells. *Immunology* 33:31, 1977

102. SANDBERG AL, WAHL SM, MERGENHAGEN SE: Lymphokine production by C3b stimulated B cells. *J Immunol* 115:139, 1975

103. SCHENKEIN HA, GENCO RJ: Inhibition of lymphocyte blastogenesis by C3c and C3d. *J Immunol* 122:1126, 1979

104. FELDMANN M, PEPYS MB: Role of C3 in in vitro lymphocyte cooperation. *Nature* 249:159, 1974

105. PEPYS MB: Role of complement in the induction of immunological responses. *Transplant Rev* 32:93, 1976

106. HERMAN JJ, ROSNER IK, DAVIS AE, ZEIGER RS, ARNAOUT MA, COLTEN HR: Complement-dependent histaminase release from human granulocytes *J Clin Invest* 63:1195, 1979

107. HUGLI TE: Human anaphylatoxin (C3a) from the third component of complement. *J Biol Chem* 250:8293, 1975

108. HUGLI TE: Complement anaphylatoxins as plasma mediators, spasmogens and chemotaxins, in Bing DH (ed): *The Chemistry and Physiology of the Human Plasma Proteins.* New York, Pergamon, 1979, pp 255–280

109. DIAS DA SILVA W, LEPOW IH: Complement as a mediator of inflammation. II. Biological properties of anaphylatoxin prepared with purified components of human complement. *J Exp Med* 125:921, 1967

110. COCHRANE CG, MÜLLER-EBERHARD HJ: The derivation of two distinct anaphylatoxin activities from the third and fifth components of human complement. *J Exp Med* 127:371, 1968

111. GORSKI JP, HUGLI TE, MÜLLER-EBERHARD HJ: C4a: The third anaphylatoxin of the human complement system. *Proc Natl Acad Sci USA* 76:5299, 1979

112. CHENOWETH DE, HUGLI TE: Demonstration of specific C5a receptor on intact human polymorphonuclear leukocytes. *Proc Natl Acad Sci USA* 75:3943, 1978

113. SHIN HS, SNYDERMAN R, FRIEDMAN E, MELLORS A, MAYER MM: Chemotactic and anaphylatoxic fragment cleaved from the fifth component of guinea pig complement. *Science* 162:361, 1968

114. BECKER EL, SHOWELL JH, HENSON PM, HSU LS: The ability of chemotactic factors to induce lysosomal enzyme release. I. The characteristics of release, the importance of surfaces, and the relationship of enzyme release to chemotactic responsiveness. *J Immunol* 112:2047, 1974

115. FERNANDEZ HN, HENSON PM, OTANI A, HUGLI TE: Chemotactic response to human C3a and C5a anaphylatoxins. I. Evaluation of C3a and C5a leukotaxis in vitro and under simulated in vivo conditions. *J Immunol* 120:109, 1978

116. PEREZ HD, GOLDSTEIN IM, CHERNOFF D, WEBSTER RO, HENSON DM: Chemotactic activity of C5a-DesArg: Evidence for a requirement for an anionic peptide "helper factor" and inhibition by a cationic protein in serum from patients with systemic lupus erythematosus. *Mol Immunol* 17:163, 1980

117. O'FLAHERTY JT, CRADDOCK PR, JACOB AS: Effect of intravascular complement activation on granulocyte adhesiveness and distribution. *Blood* 51:731, 1978

118. ROTHER K: Leukocyte mobilizing factor: A new biological activity derived from the third component of complement. *Eur J Immunol* 2:550, 1972

119. GHEBREHIWET B, MÜLLER-EBERHARD HJ: C3e: An acidic fragment of human C3 with leukocytosis-inducing activity. *J Immunol* 123:616, 1979

120. ALPER CA, COLTEN HR, ROSEN FS, RABSON AR, MACNAB GM, GEAR JSS: Homozygous deficiency of C3 in a patient with repeated infections. *Lancet* 2:1179, 1972

121. DAY NK, RUBINSTEIN P, DEBRACCO M, MONCADA B, HANSEN JA, DUPONT B, THOMSEN M, SVEJGAARD A, JERSILD C: Hereditary C1r deficiency: Lack of linkage to the HL-A region in two families, in Kissmeyer-Nielsen (ed): *Histocompatibility Testing,* Copenhagen, Munksgaard 1975, p 960

122. MITTAL KK, WOLSKI KP, LIM D, GEWURZ A, GEWURZ H, SCHMID FR: Genetic independence between HLA system and deficits in the first and sixth components of complement. *Tissue Antigens* 7:97, 1976

123. GEDDE-DAHL T JR, TEISBERG P, THORSBY E: C3 polymorphism: Genetic linkage relations. *Clin Genet* 6:66, 1974

124. LAMM LU, THORSEN I-L, PETERSEN GB, JORGENSEN J, HENNINGSEN K, BECH B, KISSMEYER-NIELSEN F: Data on the HL-A linkage group. *Ann Hum Genet* 38:383, 1975

125. ROSENFELD SI, WEITKAMP LR, COUNTRYMAN, JK: Non-linkage for a locus of human complement C5 deficiency to the complement C6 structural locus. *Immunogenetics* 7:95, 1978

126. SNYDERMAN R, DURACK DT, McCARTY GA, WARD FE, MEADOWS L: Deficiency of the fifth component of complement in human subjects. Clinical, genetic and immunologic studies in a large kindred. *Am J Med* 67:638, 1979

127. HOBART MJ, LACHMANN PJ: Allotypes of complement components in man. *Transplant Rev* 32:26, 1976

128. OLVING JH, OLAISEN B, GEDDE-DAHL T JR, TEISBERG P: Genetic linkage relations of the sixth component of complement (C6). *Hum Genet* 46:181, 1979

129. DELAGE JM, LEHNER-NETSCH G, LAFLEUR R, SIMARD J, BRUN G, PROCHAZKA E: Simultaneous occurrence of both C6 and C2 deficiency in a French Canadian family. *Immunology* 37:419, 1979

130. KAGAN E, MAIER GMG, NURSE GT, MULLER K, RABSON AR: Further evidence for independent segregation of the HLA system and a structural gene for the sixth component of complement (C6). *Tissue Antigens* 14:15, 1979

131. RITTNER C, OPFERKUCH W, WELLEK B, GROSSE-WILDE H, WERNET P: Lack of linkage between gene(s) controlling the synthesis of the seventh component of complement and the HLA region on chromosome no. 6 in man. *Hum Genet* 34:137, 1976

132. NEMEROW L, GEWURZ H, OSOFSKY A, LINT TF: Inherited deficiency for the seventh component of complement associated with nephritis. *J Clin Invest* 61:1602, 1978

133. DELAGE JM, BERGERON P, SIMARD J, LEHNER-NETSCH G, PROCHAZKA E: Hereditary C7 deficiency. Diagnosis and HLA studies in a French-Canadian family. *J Clin Invest* 60:1061, 1977

134. GIRALDO G, DEGOS L, BETH E, SASPORTES M, MARCELLI KA, GHARBI R, DAY NK: C8 deficiency in a family with xeroderma pigmentosum. Lack of linkage to the HLA region. *Clin Immunol Immunopathol* 8:377, 1977

135. HAENEY MR, THOMPSON RA, FAULKNER J, MACKINTOSH P, BALL AP: Recurrent bacterial meningitis in patients with genetic defects of terminal complement components. *Clin Exp Immunol* 40:16, 1980

136. RAUM D, AWDEH Z, GLASS D, YUNIS E, ALPER C: The location of C2, C4, and Bf relative to HLA-B and HLA-D. *Immunogenetics*, 12:473, 1981

137. HAWKINS BR, DANILOVS JA, O'NEILL GJ: Analysis of recombinant families, in Terasaki P (ed): *Histocompatability Testing 1980*. Los Angeles, University of California, 1980, vol 1, p 148

138. WEITKAMP L, FRANCKE U: Report of the committee on the genetic constitution of chromosome 6. *Cytogenet Cell Genet* 22:92, 1978

139. NERL C, GROSSE-WILDE H, VALET G: Association of low C2 and C4 serum levels with the HLA Dw2 allele in healthy individuals. *J Exp Med* 148:704, 1978

140. MEO T, ATKINSON JP, BERNOCO M, BERNOCO D, CEPPELLINI R: Structural heterogeneity of C2 complement protein and its genetic variants in man: A new polymorphism of the HLA region. *Proc Natl Acad Sci USA* 74:1672, 1977

141. RAUM D, GLASS D, CARPENTER CB, SCHUR PH, ALPER CA: Mapping of the structural gene of the second component of complement with respect to the human major histocompatibility complex. *Am J Hum Genet* 31:35, 1979

142. PARISER KM, RAUM D, BERKMAN EM, ALPER CA, AGNELLO B: Evidence for a silent or null gene in hereditary C2 deficiency. *J Immunol* 121:2580, 1978

143. GLASS D, RAUM D, GIBSON D, STILLMAN JS, SCHUR PH: Inherited deficiency of the second component of complement. Rheumatic disease associations. *J Clin Invest* 58:853, 1976

144. FU SM, STERN R, KUNKEL HG, DUPONT B, HANSEN JA, DAY NK, GOOD RA, JERSILD C, FOTINO M: Mixed lymphocyte culture determinants and C2 deficiency: LD7a associated with C2 deficiency in four families. *J Exp Med* 142:495, 1975

145. DAY NK, L'ESPERANCE P, GOOD RA, MICHAEL AF, HANSEN JA, DUPONT B, JERSILD C: Hereditary C2 deficiency: Genetic studies and association with the HL-A system. *J Exp Med* 141:1464, 1975

146. WOLSKI KP, SCHMID FR, MITTAL KL: Genetic linkage between HL-A system and a deficit of the second component (C2) of complement. *Science* 188:1020, 1975

147. GIBSON DJ, GLASS D, CARPENTER CB, SCHUR PH: Hereditary C2 deficiency: Diagnosis and HLA gene complex associations. *J Immunol* 116:1065, 1975

148. MAHOWALD ML, DALMASSO AP, PETZEL RA, YUNIS EJ: Linkage relationship of C2 deficiency, HLA and glyoxalose 1 loci. *Vox Sang* 37:321, 1979

149. RAUM D, GLASS D, CARPENTER CB, ALPER CA, SCHUR PH: The chromosomal order of genes controlling the major histo-compatibility complex, properdin factor B, and deficiency of the second component of complement. *J Clin Invest* 58:1240, 1976

150. AWDEH Z, RAUM D, GLASS D, AGNELLO V, SCHUR PH, JOHNSTON RB, GELFAND EN, BALLOW M, YUNIS E, ALPER CA: Complement-HLA haplotypes in C2 deficiency. *J Clin Invest* 67:581, 1981

151. MEO T, ATKINSON J, BERNOCO M, BERNOCO D, CEPPELLINI R: Mapping of the HLA locus controlling C2 structural variants and linkage disequilibrium between alleles C2² and Bw15. *Eur J Immunol* 7:916, 1976

152. OLAISEN B, TEISBERG P, GEDDE-DAHL T, JR, THORSBY E: Genetic polymorphism of the second component of human complement (C2). *Hum Genet* 42:301, 1978

153. SILVERSTEIN AM: Essential hypocomplementemia: Report of a case. *Blood* 16:1338, 1960

154. KLEMPERER MR, WOODWORTH HC, ROSEN FS, AUSTEN KF: Hereditary deficiency of the second component of complement (C'2) in man. *J Clin Invest* 45:880, 1966

155. KLEMPERER MR, AUSTEN KF, ROSEN FS: Hereditary deficiency of the second component of complement (C2) in man: Further observations on a second kindred. *J Immunol* 98:72, 1967

156. COOPER NR, TEN BENSEL R, KOHLER PF: Studies of an additional kindred with hereditary deficiency of the second component of human complement (C2) and description of a new method for the quantitation of C2. *J Immunol* 101:1176, 1968

157. RUDDY S, KLEMPERER MR, ROSEN FS, AUSTEN KF, KUMATE J: Hereditary deficiency of the second component of complement (C2) in man: Correlation of C2 haemolytic activity with immunochemical measurements of C2 protein. *Immunology* 18:943, 1970

158. POLLEY MJ: Inherited C'2 deficiency in man: Lack of immunochemically detectable C'2 protein in serums from deficient individuals. *Science* 161:1149, 1968

159. KLEMPERER MR: Hereditary deficiency of the second component of complement in man: An immunochemical study. *J Immunol* 102:168, 1969

160. EINSTEIN LP, ALPER CA, BLOCH KJ, HERRIN JT, ROSEN FS, DAVID JR, COLTEN HR: Biosynthetic defect in monocytes from human beings with genetic deficiency of the second component of complement. *N Engl J Med* 292:1169, 1975

161. DAY NK, GEIGER H, MCLEAN R, MICHAEL A, GOOD RA: C2 deficiency: Development of lupus erythematosus. *J Clin Invest* 52:1601, 1973

162. OSTERLAND CK, ESPINOZA L, PARKER LP, SCHUR PH: Inherited C2 deficiency and systemic lupus erythematosus: Studies on a family. *Ann Intern Med* 82:323, 1975

163. STERN R, FU SM, FOTINO M, AGNELLO V, KUNKEL HG: Hereditary C2 deficiency. Association with skin lesions resembling the discoid lesions of systemic lupus erythematosus. *Arthritis Rheum* 19:517, 1976

164. WILD JH, ZVAIFLER MJ, MÜLLER-EBERHARD HJ, WILSON CB: C3 metabolism in a patient with a deficiency of the second component of complement and discoid lupus erythematosus. *Clin Exp Immunol* 24:238, 1976

165. ANGNELLO V: Complement deficiency states. *Medicine* 57:1, 1978

166. SUSSMAN M, JONES JS, ALMEIDA JD, LACHMANN PJ: Deficiency of second component of complement associated with anaphylactoid purpura and presence of mycoplasma in the serum. *Clin Exp Immunol* 14:531, 1973.

167. GELFAND EW, CLARKSON JO, MINTA JO: Selective deficiency of the second component of complement in a patient with anaphylactoid purpura. *Clin Immunol Immunopathol* 4:269, 1975

168. LEDDY JP, GRIGGS RC, KLEMPERER MR, FRANK MM: Hereditary complement (C2) deficiency with dermatomyositis. *Am J Med* 58:83, 1975

169. FRIEND P, REPINE JF, KIM Y, CLAWSON CC, MICHAEL AF: Deficiency of the second component of complement (C2) with chronic vasculitis. *Ann Intern Med* 83:813, 1975

170. KIM Y, FRIEND PS, DRESNER IG, YUNIS EJ, MICHAEL AF: Inherited deficiency of the second component of complement (C2) with membranoproliferative glomerulonephritis. *Am J Med* 62:765, 1977

171. SLADE JD, LUSKIN AT, GEWURZ H, KRAFT SC, KIRSNER JB, ZEITZ HJ: Inherited deficiency of second component of complement and HLA haplotype A10B18 associated with inflammatory bowel disease. *Ann Intern Med* 88:796, 1978

172. NEWMAN SL, VOGLER LB, FEIGIN RD, JOHNSTON RB JR: Recurrent septicemia associated with congenital deficiency of C2 and partial deficiency of factor B and the alternative complement pathway. *N Engl J Med* 299:290, 1978

173. ALPER CA, BOENISCH T, WATSON L: Genetic polymorphism in human glycine-rich beta-glycoprotein. *J Exp Med* 135:68, 1972

174. MARTIN A, LACHMANN PJ, HALBWACHS L, HOBART MJ: Haemolytic diffusion plate assays for factors B and D of the alternative pathway of complement activation. *Immunochemistry* 13:317, 1976

175. MAUFF G, GAUCHEL FD, HITZEROTH HW: Polymorphism of properdin factor B in South African, Negroid, Indian and Colored populations. *Hum Genet* 33:319, 1976

176. HAUPTMAN G, TANGIO MM, MAYER S: Bf polymorphism: Study of a new variant (Fo. 55). *Hum Genet* 33:275, 1976

177. MAUFF C, HAUPTMANN G, DAHA M, FEDERMANN G: Partial congenital inactivity of properdin factor B. *Eighth International Complement Workshop*. *J Immunol* 124:1531, 1980 (abstract)

178. OLAISEN B, TEISBERG P, GEDDE-DAHL T JR, THORSBY E: The Bf locus in the HLA region of chromosome 6: Linkage and association studies. *Hum Genet* 30:291, 1975

179. BENDER K, MAYEROVA A, FRANK R, HILLER C, WIENKER T: Haplotype analysis of the linkage group HLA-A: HLA-B: Bf and its bearing on the interpretation of the linkage disequilibrium. *Hum Genet* 36:191, 1977

180. ALBERT ED, RITTNER C, SCHOLZ S, KUNTZ B, MICKEY MR: Three-point association of HLA-A, B, Bf haplotypes deduced in 200 parents of 100 families. *Scand J Immunol* 6:459, 1977

181. ARNASON A, LARSEN B, MARSHALL WH, EDWARDS JH, MACKINTOSH P, OLAISEN B, TEISBERG P: Very close linkage between HLA-B and Bf inferred from allelic association. *Nature* 268:527, 1977

182. ARNASON A, THORSTEINSSON J, SIGURBERGSSON K: Ankylosing spondylitis, HLA-B27 and Bf. *Lancet* 1:339, 1978

183. MIGONE N, MALAVASI F, BOSCHIS D, MODENA V: Bf polymorphism and ankylosing spondylitis. *Lancet* 2:163, 1978

184. WELLS LJ, EDWARDS JH, WEBLEY M, JAMES DCO, BREWERTON DA, MACKINTOSH P, MEAKIN M: Ankylosing spondylitis, HLA, and Bf. *Lancet* 1:104, 1979

185. LARSEN B, ARNASON A, BARNARD JM, BUEHLER SK, EDWARDS JH, MARSHALL WH: Bf types of HLA haplotyped individuals in an isolated New Foundland population. *Tissue Antigens* 10:403, 1977

186. DAUSSETT J, LEGRAND L, LEPAGE V, CONTU L, MARAKI-BARGE A, WILDLOECHER J, BENAJAM A, MEO T, DEGOS L: A haplotype study of HLA complex with special reference to the HLA-DR series and to Bf C2 and glyoxalase 1 polymorphisms. *Tissue Antigens* 12:297, 1978

187. BERTRAM J, BAUR MP: HLA-A, B, Bf three point association of 1,072 haplotypes in a German population. *Tissue Antigens* 14:317, 1979

188. STEWART GJ, BASTEN A, KIRK RL: Strong linkage disequilibrium between HLA-DW2 and Bfs in multiple sclerosis and in the normal population. *Tissue Antigens* 14:86, 1979

189. RAUM D, ALPER CA, STEIN R, GABBAY KH: Genetic marker for insulin-dependent diabetes mellitus. *Lancet* 1:1208, 1979

190. RAUM D, DONALDSON VH, ROSEN FS, ALPER CA: Genetics of complement, *Curr Top Hematol* 3:111, 1980

191. ROSENFELD SI, RUDDY S, AUSTEN KF: Structural polymorphism of the fourth component of human complement. *J Clin Invest* 48:2283, 1969

192. BACH S, RUDDY S, AUSTEN KF: Electrophoretic polymorphism of the fourth component of human complement (C4) in paired maternal and foetal plasmas. *Immunology* 21:869, 1971

193. TEISBERG P, OLAISEN B, JONASSEN R, GEDDE-DAHL T JR, THORSBY E: The genetic polymorphism of the fourth component of human complement: Methodological aspects and a presentation of linkage and association data related to its location in the HLA region. *J Exp Med* 146:1380, 1977

194. MAUFF G, BENDER K, FISCHER B: Genetic polymorphism of the fourth component of human complement. *Vox Sang* 34:296, 1978

195. OLAISSEN B, TEISBERG P, NORDHAGEN R, MICHAELSEN T, GEDDE-DAHL T JR: Human C4 locus is duplicated on some chromosomes. *Nature* 279:736, 1979

196. O'NEILL GJ, YANG SY, TEGOLI J, BERGER R, DUPONT B: Chido and Rodgers blood groups are distinct antigenic components of human C4. *Nature* 273:668, 1978

197. MIDDLETON J, CROOKSTON MC, FALK JA, ROBSON EB, COOK PJL, BATCHELOR JR, BODMER J, FERRARA GB, FESTENSTEIN H, HARRIS R, KISSMEYER-NIELSEN F, LAWLER SD, SACHS JA, WOLFE E: Linkage of Chido and HLA. *Tissue Antigens* 4:366, 1974

198. GILES CM, GEDDE-DAHL T JR, ROBSON EB, THORSBY E, OLAISEN B, ARNASON A, KISSMEYER-NIELSEN F, SCHREUDER I: Rgᵃ (Rodgers) and the HLA region: Linkage and associations. *Tissue Antigens* 8:143, 1976

199. O'NEILL GJ, YANG SY, DUPONT B: Two HLA-linked loci controlling the fourth component of human complement. *Proc Natl Acad Sci USA* 75:5165, 1978

200. DEMANT P, CAPKOVA J, HINZOVA E, VORACOVA B: The role of the histocompatibility-2-linked Ss-Slp region in the control of mouse complement. *Proc Natl Acad Sci USA* 70:863, 1973

201. CURMAN B, ÖSTBERG L, SANDBERG L, MALMHEDEN-ERIKSON I, STÅLENHEIM G, RASK L, PETERSON PA: H-2 linked Ss protein is C4 component of complement. *Nature* 258:242, 1975

202. LACHMANN PJ, GRENNAN D, MARTIN A, DEMANT P: Identification of Ss protein as murine C4. *Nature* 258:242, 1975

203. MEO T, KRASTEFF T, SCHREFFLER DC: Immunochemical characterization of murine H-2 controlled Ss (serum substance) protein through identification of its human homologue as the fourth component of complement. *Proc Natl Acad Sci USA* 72:4536, 1975

204. AWDEH ZL, RAUM D, ALPER CA: Genetic polymorphism of human complement C4 and detection of heterozygotes. *Nature* 282:205, 1979

205. HAUPTMANN G, GROSSHANS E, HEID E, MAYER S, BASSET A: Lupus erythemateux aigu avec deficit complet de la fraction C4 du complement. *Nouv Presse Med* 3:881, 1974

206. SCHALLER JG, GILLILAND BG, OCHS HD, LEDDY JP, AGODOA LCY, ROSENFELD SI: Severe systemic lupus erythematosus with nephritis in a boy with deficiency of the fourth component of complement. *Arthritis Rheum* 20:1519, 1977

207. JACKSON CG, OCHS HS, WEDGEWOOD RJ: Immune response of a patient with deficiency of the fourth component of complement and systemic lupus erythematosus. *N Engl J Med* 300:1124, 1979

208. LACHMAN PJ, HOBART MJ, WOO P: Combined genetic deficiency of C6 and C7 in man. *Clin Exp Immunol* 33:193, 1978

209. GLASS D, RAUM D, BALAVITCH D, KAGAN E, RABSON A, SCHUR PH, ALPER CA: Inherited deficiency of the sixth component of complement: A silent or null gene. *J Immunol* 120:538, 1978

210. HOBART MJ, LACHMANN PJ, ALPER CA: Polymorphism of human C6, in Peeters H (ed): *Protides of the Biological Fluids*. New York, Pergamon, 1975, pp 575–580.

211. LEDDY JP, FRANK MM, GAITHER T, BAUM J, KLEMPERER MR: Hereditary deficiency of the sixth component of complement in man. I. Immunochemical, biologic, and family studies. *J Clin Invest* 53:544, 1974

212. HEUSINKVELD RS, LEDDY JP, KLEMPERER MR, BRECKENRIDGE RT: Hereditary deficiency of the sixth component of complement in man. *J Clin Invest* 53:554, 1974

213. ZIMMERMAN TS, MÜLLER-EBERHARD HJ: Blood coagulation initiation by a complement-mediated pathway. *J Exp Med* 134:1601, 1971

214. LIM D, GEWURZ A, LINT TF, GHAZE M, SEPHERI B, GEWURZ H: Absence of the sixth component of complement in a patient with repeated episodes of meningococcal meningitis. *J Pediatr* 89:42, 1976

215. PETERSEN BH, LEE TJ, SNYDERMAN R, BROOKS GF: *Neisseria meningitidis* and *Neisseria gonorrhoeae* bacteremia associated with C6, C7, C8 deficiency. *Ann Intern Med* 90:917, 1979

216. HOBART MJ, JOYSEY V, LACHMANN PJ: Inherited structural variation and linkage relationships of C7. *J Immunogenet* 5:157, 1978

217. WELLEK B, OPFERKUCH W: A case of deficiency of the seventh component of complement in man. Biological properties of a C7-deficient serum and description of a C7-inactivating principle. *Clin Exp Immunol* 19:223, 1975

218. HANNEMA AJ, PONDMAN KW, DÖHMANN U, GADNER H, DOOREN LJ: C7 deficiency in man, in Peeters H (ed): *Protides of the Biological Fluids*. Pergamon, New York, 1975 pp 581–584

219. BOYER JT, GALL EP, NORMAN ME, NILSSON UR, ZIMMERMAN TS: Hereditary deficiency of the seventh component of complement. *J Clin Invest* 56:905, 1975

220. LEE TJ, UTSINGER PD, SNYDERMAN R, YOUNT WJ, SPARLING PF: Familial deficiency of the seventh component of complement associated with recurrent bacteremic infections due to Neisseria. *J Infect Dis* 138:359, 1978

221. ZEITZ HJ, MILLER GW, ALI MA, LINT TF: Deficiency of C7 with systemic lupus erythematosus (SLE) and solubilization of immune complexes in complement (C)-deficient sera. *Clin Res* 26:716A, 1978

222. WIEME RJ, DEMEULENAERE L: Genetically determined electrophoretic variant of the human complement component C′3. *Nature* 214:1042, 1967

223. ALPER CA, PROPP RP: Genetic polymorphism of the third component of human complement. *J Clin Invest* 47:2181, 1968

224. AZEN EA, SMITHIES O: Genetic polymorphism of C′3 (βlc-globulin) in human serum. *Science* 162:905, 1968

225. AZEN EA, SMITHIES O, HILLER O: High voltage starch-gel electrophoresis in the study of post-albumin proteins and C′3 (βlc-globulin) polymorphism. *Biochem Genet* 3:215, 1969

226. ALPER CA, AZEN EA, GESERICK G, GOEDDE HW, RITTNER C, TEISBERG P, WIEME R: Statement on the polymorphism of the third component of complement in man (C3). *Vox Sang* 25:18, 1973

227. RITTNER C, RITTNER B: Description of three hitherto unknown C3 variants: F 0.6, F 0.7 and S 2.4 (old nomenclature). *Vox Sang* 25:17, 1973 (abstract)

228. BERG K, HEIBERG A: Linkage between familial hypercholesterolemia with xanthomatosis and the C3 polymorphism confirmed. *Cytogenet Cell Genet* 22:621, 1978

229. WEITKAMP LR, JOHNSTON E, GUTTORMSEN SA: Probable genetic linkage between loci for Lewis blood-group and complement-C3. *Cytogenet Cell Genet* 23:183, 1979

230. DA SILVA FP, HOECKER GF, DAY NK, VIENNE K, RUBINSTEIN P: Murine complement component 3: Genetic variation and linkage to H-2. *Proc Natl Acad Sci USA* 75:963, 1978

231. NATSUUME-SAKAI S, HAYAKAWA J, TAKAHASHI M: Genetic polymorphism of murine C3 controlled by a single co-dominant locus in chromosome 17. *J Immunol* 121:491, 1978

232. FERREIRA A, NUSSENZWEIG V: Genetic control of complement (C3) levels of the third component of complement and the H-2 complex. *J Exp Med* 141:513, 1975

233. COLTEN HR, ALPER CA: Hemolytic efficiencies of genetic variants of human C3. *J Immunol* 108:1184, 1972

234. ARVILOMMI H: Capacity of complement C3 phenotypes to bind on to mononuclear cells in man. *Nature* 251:740, 1974

235. BRONNESTAM R: Studies of the C3 polymorphism. Relationship between C3 phenotypes and rheumatoid arthritis. *Hum Hered* 23:206, 1973

236. FARHUD DD, ANANTHAKRISHNAN R, WALTER H: Association between C′3 phenotypes and various diseases. *Hummangenetik* 17:57, 1972

237. SORENSEN H, DISSING J: Association between C3 F gene and atherosclerotic vascular diseases. *Hum Hered* 25:279, 1975

238. DISSING J, LUND J, SORENSEN H: C3 polymorphism in a group of old arteriosclerotic patients. *Hum Hered* 22:466, 1972

239. ALPER CA, JOHNSON AM, BIRTCH AG, MOORE FD: Human C3: Evidence for the liver as the primary site of synthesis. *Science* 163:286, 1969

240. ALPER CA, ROSEN FS: Studies of a hypomorphic variant of human C3. *J Clin Invest* 50:324, 1971

241. McLean RH, Weinstein A, Damjanov I, Rothfield N: Hypomorphic variant C3, arthritis and chronic glomerulonephritis. *J Pediatr* 93:937, 1978

242. Alper CA, Propp RP, Klemperer MR, Rosen FS: Inherited deficiency of the third component of human complement (C'3). *J Clin Invest* 48:553, 1969

243. Alper CA, Colten HR, Gear JSS, Rabson AR, Rosen, FS: Homozygous C3 deficiency: The role of C3 in antibody production, C1s induced vasopermeability and cobra venom-induced passive hemolysis. *J Clin Invest* 57:222, 1976

244. Einstein LP, Hansen PJ, Ballow M, Davis AE III, Davis JS IV, Alper CA, Rosen FS, Colten HR: Biosynthesis of the third component of complement (C3) in vitro by monocytes from both normal and homozygous C3-deficient humans. *J Clin Invest* 60:963, 1977

245. Ballow M, Shira JE, Harden L, Yang SY, Day NK: Complete absence of the third component of complement in man. *J Clin Invest* 56:703, 1975

246. Grace HJ, Brereton-Stiles GG, Vos GH, Schonland M: A family with partial and total deficiency of complement C3. *S Afr Med J* 50:139, 1976

247. Davis AE III, Davis JS IV, Rabson AR, Osofsky SG, Colten HR, Rosen FS, Alper CA: Homozygous C3 deficiency: Detection of C3 by radioimmunoassay. *Clin Immunol Immunopathol* 8:543, 1977

248. Osofsky SG, Thompson BH, Lint TF, Gewurz H: Hereditary deficiency of the third component of complement in a child with fever, skin rash and arthralgias: Response to transfusion of whole blood. *J Pediatr* 90:180, 1977

249. Pussell BA, Bourke E, Nayef M, Morris S, Peters DK: Complement deficiency and nephritis. *Lancet* 1:675, 1980

250. Wara DW, Reiter E, Doyle NE, Gewurz H, Ammann AJ: Persistant Clq deficiency in a patient with systemic lupus erythematosus-like syndrome. *J Pediatr* 86:743, 1975

251. Müller-Eberhard HJ, Kunkel HG: Isolation of a thermolabile serum protein which precipitates gamma globulin aggregates and participates in immune hemolysis. *Proc Soc Exp Biol Med* 106:291, 1961

252. O'Connell EJ, Enriquez P, Linman JW, Gleich GJ, McDuffie FC: Absence of first component of complement in man: Association with thymica lymphoplasia and defective inflammatory response. *J Lab Clin Med* 70:715, 1967

253. Gewurz H, Pickering RJ, Christian CL, Snyderman R, Mergenhagen SE, Good RA: Decreased C'1q protein concentration and agglutinating activity in agammaglobulinaemia syndromes: An inborn error reflected in the complement system. *Clin Exp Immunol* 3:437, 1968

254. Stroud RM, Nagaki K, Pickering RJ, Gewurz H, Good RA, Cooper MD: Subunits of the first complement component in immunologic deficiency syndromes: Independence of C1s and C1. *Clin Exp Immunol* 7:133, 1970

255. Ballow M, Day NK, Biggar WD, Park BH, Yount WJ, Good RA: Reconstitution of Clq after bone marrow transplantation in patients with severe combined immunodeficiency. *Clin Immunol Immunopathol* 2:28, 1973

256. Kohler PF, Müller-Eberhard HJ: Complement-immunoglobulin relation: Deficiency of C'1q associated with impaired immunoglobulin G synthesis. *Science* 163:474, 1969

257. Kohler PF, Müller-Eberhard HJ: Metabolism of Clq: Studies in hypogammaglobulinemia, myeloma, and systemic lupus erythematosus. *J Clin Invest* 51:868, 1972

258. Pickering RJ, Naff GB, Stroud RM, Good RA, Gewurz H: Deficiency of C1r in human serum. Effects on the structure and function of macromolecular C1. *J Exp Med* 131:803, 1970

259. Day NK, Geiger H, Stroud R, deBracco M, Moncada B, Windhorst D, Good RA: Clr deficiency: An inborn error associated with cutaneous and renal disease. *J Clin Invest* 51:1102, 1972

260. Moncada B, Day NK, Good RA, Windhorst DB: Lupus erythematosus-like syndrome with a familial defect of complement. *N Engl J Med* 286:689, 1972

261. deBracco MME, Windhorst D, Stroud RM, Moncada B: The autosomal recessive mode of inheritance of Clr deficiency in a large Puerto Rican family. *Clin Exp Immunol* 16:183, 1974

262. Lee SL, Wallace SL, Barone R, Blum L, Chase PH: Familial deficiency of two units of the first component of complement (C1r and C1s) associated with a lupus-erythematosus-like disease. *Arthritis Rheum* 21:958, 1978

263. Pondman KW, Hannema A, Cormane R, Stoop JW: Ongewone complementdeficientie bij een patient met lupus erythematosus dis seminatus. *Ned Tijdschr Geneeskd* 113:1462, 1969

264. Rosenfeld SI, Kelly ME, Leddy JP: Hereditary deficiency of the fifth component of complement in man. I. Clinical, immunochemical, and family studies. *J Clin Invest* 57:1626, 1976

265. Rosenfeld SI, Baum J, Steigbigel RT, Leddy JP: Hereditary deficiency of the fifth component of complement in man. II. Biological properties of C5-deficient human serum. *J Clin Invest* 57:1635, 1976

266. Miller ME, Seals J, Kaye R, Levitsky LC: A familial, plasma associated defect of phagocytosis: A new cause of recurrent bacterial infections. *Lancet* 2:60, 1968

267. Miller ME, Nilsson UR: A familial deficiency of the phacogytosis-enhancing activity of serum related to a dysfunction of the fifth component of complement (C5). *N Engl J Med* 282:354, 1970

268. Petersen BH, Graham JA, Brooks GF: Human deficiency of the eighth component of complement. The requirement of C8 for serum *Neisseria gonorrhoeae* bactericidal activity. *J Clin Invest* 57:283, 1976

269. Nicholson A, Lepow IH: Host defense against *Neisseria meningitidis* requires a complement-dependent bactericidal activity. *Science* 205:298, 1979

270. Jasin HE: Absence of the eighth component of complement in association with systemic lupus erythematosus-like disease. *J Clin Invest* 60:709, 1977

270a. Braconier JH, Sjöholm AG, Söderström C: Deficiency of properdin in a family with fulminant meningococcal infections. Abstracts of the IX International Complement Workshop. *Mol Immunol*, in press

271. Osler W: Hereditary angioneurotic edema. *Am J Med Sci* 95:362, 1888

272. Crowder JR, Crowder TR: Five generations of angioneurotic edema. *Arch Intern Med* 20:840, 1917

273. Landerman NS, Webster ME, Becker EL, Ratcliffe HE: Hereditary angioneurotic edema. II. Deficiency of inhibitor for serum globulin permeability factor and/or plasma kallikrein. *J Allergy* 33:330,1962

274. Donaldson VH, Evans RR: A biochemical abnormality in hereditary angioneurotic edema: Absence of serum inhibitor of C'1-esterase. *Am J Med* 35:37, 1963

275. Rosen FS, Charache P, Pensky J, Donaldson V: Hereditary angioneurotic edema: Two genetic variants. *Science* 148:957, 1965

276. Spaulding WB: Hereditary angioneurotic edema in two families. *Can Med Assoc J* 73:181, 1955

277. Landerman NS: Hereditary angioneurotic edema. I. Case reports and review of the literature. *J Allergy* 33:316, 1972

278. Donaldson VH, Rosen FS: Hereditary angioneurotic edema: A clinical survey. *Pediatrics* 37:1017, 1966

279. Beck P, Wills D, Davies GT, Lachmann PJ, Sussman M: A family study of hereditary angioneurotic oedema. *Q J Med* 42:317, 1973

280. Thorvaldsson SE, Sedlack RE, Gleich GJ, Ruddy S: Angioneurotic edema and deficiency of C1 esterase inhibitor in a 61-year old woman. *Ann Intern Med* 71:353, 1969

281. Sheffer AL, Craig JM, Willms-Kretchmer K, Austen KF, Rosen FS: Histopathological and ultrastructural observations on tissues from patients with hereditary angioneurotic edema. *J Allergy* 47:292, 1971

282. Levy LR, Lepow IH: Assay and properties of a serum inhibitor of C1-esterase. *Proc Soc Exp Med* 101:608, 1959

283. Ruddy S, Gigli I, Sheffer AL, Austen KF: The laboratory diagnosis of hereditary angioedema, in Rose B, Richter M, Sehon A, Frankland AW (eds): *Allergology, Proceedings of the 6th International Congress of Allergology.* Amsterdam, Excerpta Medica, 1968, pp 351–359

284. Austen KF, Sheffer AL: Detection of hereditary angioneurotic edema by demonstration of a reduction in the second component of human complement. *N Engl J Med* 272:649, 1965

285. Gigli I, Ruddy S, Austen KF: The stoichiometric measurement of the serum inhibitor of the first component of complement by the inhibition of immune hemolysis. *J Immunol* 100:1154, 1968

286. Lundh B, Laurell A-B, Wetterqvist H, White T, Granerus G: A case of hereditary angioneurotic oedema, successfully treated with ε-aminocaproic acid. *Clin Exp Immunol* 3:733, 1968

287. Frank MM, Sargeant JS, Kane MA, Alling DW: Epsilon aminocaproic acid therapy of hereditary angioneurotic edema: A double blind study. *N Engl J Med* 286:808, 1972

288. Sheffer AL, Austen KF, Rosen F: Tranexamic acid therapy in hereditary angioneurotic edema. *N Engl J Med* 287:452, 1972

289. Spaulding WB: Methyl testosterone therapy for hereditary episodic edema (hereditary angioneurotic edema). *Ann Intern Med* 53:739, 1960

290. Sheffer AL, Fearon DT, Austen KF: Methyltestosterone therapy in hereditary angioedema. *Ann Intern Med* 86:306, 1977

291. Rosse WE, Logue GL, Silberman HR, Frank MM: The effect of synthetic androgens in hereditary angioneurotic edema: Alteration of C1 inhibitor and C4 levels. *Trans Assoc Am Physicians* 89:122, 1976

292. Davis PS, Davis FB, Charache P: Long-term therapy of hereditary angioedema (HAE). *Johns Hopkins Med J* 135:391, 1974

293. Sheffer AL, Fearon DT, Austen KF: Clinical and biochemical effects of impeded androgen (oxymethalone) therapy of hereditary angioedema. *J Allergy Clin Immunol* 64:275, 1979

294. Gelfand JA, Sherins RJ, Alling DW, Frank MM: Treatment of hereditary angioedema with danazol: Reversal of clinical and biochemical abnormalities. *N Engl J Med* 295:1444, 1976

295. Agostini A, Cicardi M, Martignoni GC, Bergamaschini L, Marasini B: Danazol and stanozolol in long-term prophylactic treatment of hereditary angioedema. *J Allergy Clin Immunol* 65:75, 1980

296. SHEFFER AL, FEARON DT, AUSTEN KF: Clinical and biochemical effects of stanozolol therapy for hereditary angioedema. *J Allergy Clin Immunol* 68:181, 1981

297. PICKERING RJ, KELLY JR, GOOD RA, GEWURZ H: Replacement therapy in hereditary angioedema: Successful treatment of two patients with fresh frozen plasma. *Lancet* 1:326, 1969

298. ROSEN FS, AUSTEN KF: The "neurotic edema" (hereditary angioedema). *N Engl J Med* 280:1356, 1969

299. GADEK JE, HOSEA SW, GELFAND JA, SANTAELLA M, WICKERHAUSER M, TRIANTAPHYLLOPOULOS DC, FRANK MM: Replacement therapy in hereditary angioedema. *N Engl J Med* 302:542, 1980

300. PENCE HL, EVANS R, GUERNSEY L II, GERHARD RC: Prophylactic use of epsilon-aminocaproic acid for oral surgery in a patient with hereditary angioneurotic edema. *J Allergy Clin Immunol* 53:298, 1974

301. SHEFFER AL, FEARON DT, AUSTEN KF, ROSEN FS: Tranexamic acid: Preoperative prophylactic therapy for patients with hereditary angioneurotic edema. *J Allergy Clin Immunol* 60:38, 1977

302. DONALDSON VH, ROSEN FS: Action of complement in hereditary angioneurotic edema: The role of C'1 esterase. *J Clin Invest* 43:2204, 1964

303. CARPENTER CB, RUDDY S, SHEHADEH I, MÜLLER-EBERHARD HJ, MERRILL JP, AUSTEN KF: Complement metabolism in man: Hypercatabolism of the fourth (C4) and third (C3) components in patients with renal allograft rejection and hereditary angioedema (HAE). *J Clin Invest* 48:1495, 1969

304. KLEMPERER MR, DONALDSON VH, ROSEN FS: Effect of C'1 esterase on vascular permeability in man: Studies in normal and complement-deficient individuals and in patients with hereditary angioneurotic edema. *J Clin Invest* 47:604, 1968

305. SCHREIBER AD, KAPLAN AP, AUSTEN KF: Inhibition by C1INH of Hageman factor fragment activation of coagulation, fibrinolysis, and kinin-generation. *J Clin Invest* 52:1402, 1973

306. RATNOFF OD, PENSKY J, OGSTON D, NAFF GB: The inhibition of plasma kallikrein, plasma permeability factor, and the C'1r subcomponent of the first component of complement by serum C'1 esterase inhibitor. *J Exp Med* 129:315, 1969

307. RATNOFF OD, NAFF GB: The conversion of C'1s to C'1 esterase by plasmin and trypsin. *J Exp Med* 125:337, 1967

308. COOPER WR, MILES LA, GRIFFIN JH: Effects of plasma kallikrein and plasmin on the first complement component. *J Immunol* 124:1517, 1980

309. DONALDSON VH, RATNOFF OD, DIAS DA SILVA W, ROSEN FS: Permeability-increasing activity in hereditary angioneurotic edema plasma. II. Mechanism of formation and partial characterization. *J Clin Invest* 48:642, 1969

310. DONALDSON VH, ROSEN FS, BING DH: Role of the second component of complement and plasmin in kinin release in hereditary angioneurotic edema. *Trans Assoc Am Phys* 90:174, 1977

311. GRANERUS G, HALLBERG L, LAURELL AB, WETTERQVIST H: Studies on the histamine metabolism and the complement system in hereditary angioneurotic edema. *Acta Med Scand* 182:11, 1967

312. WILLIAMS TJ, JOSE PJ: Mediation of increased vascular permeability after complement activation. *J Exp Med* 153:136, 1981

313. JOHNSON AM, ALPER CA, ROSEN FS, CRAIG JM: C1 inhibitor: Evidence for decreased hepatic synthesis in hereditary angioneurotic edema. *Science* 173:553, 1971

314. BRACKERTZ D, ISLER E, KUEPPERS F: Half-life of C1INH in hereditary angioneurotic oedema (HAE). *Clin Allergy* 5:89, 1975

315. ROSEN FS, ALPER CA, PENSKY J, KLEMPERER MR, DONALDSON VH: Genetically determined heterogeneity of the C1 esterase inhibitor in patients with hereditary angioneurotic edema. *J Clin Invest* 50:2143, 1971

316. LAURELL A-B, LINDEGREN J, MALMROS I, MARTENSSON H: Enzymatic and immunochemical estimation of C1 esterase inhibitor in sera from patients with hereditary angioneurotic edema. *Scand J Clin Lab Invest* 24:221, 1969

317. HARPEL PC, HUGLI TE, COOPER NR: Studies of human plasma C1 inactivator enzyme interactions. II. Structure features of an abnormal C1 inactivator from a kindred with hereditary angioneurotic edema. *J Clin Invest* 55:605, 1975

318. ALPER CA, ABRAMSON N, JOHNSTON RB JR, JANDL JH, ROSEN FS: Studies in vivo and in vitro on an abnormality in the metabolism of C3 in a patient with increased susceptibility to infection. *J Clin Invest* 49:1975, 1970

319. ALPER CA, ABRAMSON N, JOHNSTON RB JR, JANDL JH, ROSEN FS: Increased susceptibility to infection associated with abnormalities of complement-mediated functions and of the third component of complement (C3). *N Engl J Med* 282:349, 1970

320. ABRAMSON N, ALPER CA, LACHMANN PJ, ROSEN FS, JANDL JH: Deficiency of C3 inactivator in man. *J Immunol* 107:19, 1971

321. ALPER CA, ROSEN FS, LACHMANN PJ: Inactivator of the third component of complement as an inhibitor in the properdin pathway. *Proc Natl Acad Sci USA* 69:2910, 1972

322. ZIEGLER JB, ALPER CA, ROSEN FS, LACHMANN PJ, SHERINGTON L: Restoration by purified C3b inactivator of complement-mediated function in vivo in a patient with C3b inactivator deficiency. *J Clin Invest* 55:668, 1975

323. THOMPSON RA, LACHMANN PJ: A second case of human C3b inhibitor (KAF) deficiency. *Clin Exp Immunol* 27:23, 1977

324. ENG RHK, SELIGMAN SJ, ARNAOUT MA, ALPER CA: Variable expression of homozygous C3b inactivator deficiency. *Clin Res* 26:394 (abstract) 1978

325. KERR MA, PORTER RR: The purification and properties of the second component of human complement. *Biochem J* 171:99, 1979

326. NGAN B, MINTA JO: Analysis of the peptide maps of human C2 and factor B: Evidence for structural homology and common ancestry. *J Immunol* 120:1788, 1978

327. FERNANDEZ HN, HUGLI TE: Chemical evidence for common genetic ancestry of complement components C3 and C5. *J Biol Chem* 252:1826, 1977

328. KOHLER PF, PERCY J, CAMPION WM, SMYTH CJ: Hereditary angioedema and "familial" lupus erythematosus in identical twin boys. *Am J Med* 56:406, 1974

329. DANIELS CA, BORSOS T, RAPP HJ, SNYDERMAN R, NOTKINS AL: Neutralization of sensitized virus by purified components of complement. *Proc Natl Acad Sci USA* 65:528, 1970

330. DIXON F, CROKER B, DEL VILLANO B, JENSEN F, LERNER R: Oncornavirus infection and "auto" immune complex disease of mice, in Brent L, Holborow J (eds): *Progress in Immunology II*. Amsterdam, North-Holland, 1974, vol V, pp 49–55

331. BENACERRAF B, MCDEVITT HO: Histocompatibility-linked immune response genes. *Science* 175:273, 1972

332. REINERTSEN JL, KLIPPEL JH, JOHNSON AH, STEINBERG AD, DECKER JL, MANN DL: B-lymphocyte alloantigens associated with systemic lupus erythematosus. *N Engl J Med* 299:515, 1978

90

CHRONIC GRANULOMATOUS DISEASE AND OTHER DISORDERS OF OXIDATIVE KILLING BY PHAGOCYTES

BERNARD M. BABIOR

CAROL A. CROWLEY

1. Phagocytes employ powerful microbicidal oxidants for the destruction of ingested microorganisms. These oxidants are produced during a metabolic event known as the respiratory burst. The burst is initiated by the activation of a plasma membrane-bound flavoprotein oxidase, dormant in resting cells, which catalyzes the production of superoxide (O_2^-) according to the reaction: $NADPH + 2\ O_2 \rightarrow NADP + 2\ O_2^-$. Part of the O_2^- produced in this reaction dismutes to form H_2O_2. Subsequent reactions involving O_2^- and H_2O_2 lead to the formation of highly reactive oxidizing radicals such as $OH^{\cdot}$ which are used by phagocytes as microbicidal agents. H_2O_2 also serves to oxidize Cl^- to OCl^- in a reaction catalyzed by myeloperoxidase. The OCl^- produced in this reaction is also employed by phagocytes as a microbicidal agent and probably constitutes the most potent such agent manufactured by these cells.

2. Phagocytes possess several means of defending themselves against endogenously produced oxidants. The most important of these is a glutathione-dependent system whose enzymatic components are glutathione peroxidase and glutathione reductase. The net effect of this system is to reduce H_2O_2 to water at the expense of NADPH, which is oxidized to NADP. This NADP is reconverted to NADPH by the hexose monophosphate shunt, as is the NADP generated in the O_2^--forming reaction described above. Other antioxidant constitu-

ents of phagocytes include superoxide dismutase, catalase, and certain low molecular weight oxidant scavengers.

3. Several inherited abnormalities affect the oxygen-dependent microbicidal systems of phagocytes. Clinically, the most important of these abnormalities is chronic granulomatous disease. This is a group of conditions in which phagocytes cannot manufacture O_2^-, either because the O_2^--forming oxidase cannot be activated or (much less commonly) because the oxidase itself is defective. The most common form of the disease is transmitted in an X-linked recessive manner, but autosomal recessive varieties are also seen. Affected patients suffer frequent, severe, and protracted bacterial and fungal infections involving the deep subcutaneous tissues, lymph nodes, lungs, liver, and other organ systems. Management involves antibiotic prophylaxis and vigorous treatment of infections; bone marrow transplantation has been used with some success. A clinical picture similar to that of chronic granulomatous disease has been reported to accompany the characteristic hemolytic anemia in patients with very severe glucose-6-phosphate dehydrogenase deficiency.

4. Other inherited abnormalities of the oxygen-dependent microbicidal systems include myeloperoxidase deficiency, a common condition characterized by a mild

impairment in bacterial killing by phagocytes; glutathione reductase deficiency, associated with hemolytic anemia and an abbreviated respiratory burst but no significant microbicidal abnormality; and glutathione synthetase deficiency, which in its severe form leads to oxoprolinuria and a metabolic acidosis but only a mild microbicidal defect. Bacterial infections attributable to impaired phagocytic function are distinctly unusual in these conditions.

HISTORY

The initial observations relating oxygen to microbial killing by phagocytes were published in 1933 [1], some 50 years after Metchnikoff had discovered the role of these cells in host defense [2]. In that year, Baldridge and Gerard, studying the metabolism of canine neutrophils, reported that oxygen uptake by these cells rose by a factor of 2 to 4 when they were engaged in the phagocytosis of *Sarcina lutea*. This rise in oxygen uptake was attributed to the additional substrate oxidation required to provide energy for phagocytosis. Little further attention was paid to this report until 1959, when the real meaning of Baldridge and Gerard's experiments was elucidated by Karnovsky's crucial finding that the increase in oxygen uptake associated with phagocytosis was not blocked by cyanide [3]. This meant that the alteration in oxygen uptake was not connected with energy production, because oxygen consumption related to ATP formation would have been abolished by CN^- under the conditions used in Karnovsky's experiments. Oxygen was therefore being used by the phagocyte for some other purpose.

This purpose was discovered by Quastel [4]. He confirmed Karnovsky's findings and reported, in addition, that phagocytosing neutrophils liberated H_2O_2 into the surrounding medium. He postulated that this H_2O_2 was generated from the oxygen taken up by phagocytes in response to particle stimulation and that it functioned as an antimicrobial agent. Karnovsky and his associates had previously discovered that phagocytes engaged in particle uptake augmented their rate of glucose oxidation via the hexose monophosphate shunt [5]. It was logical to conclude that the reducing equivalents used in H_2O_2 production were provided by the hexose monophosphate shunt. Thus the outline of the metabolic event now known as the *respiratory burst* was formulated:

Reduced pyridine nucleotide + O_2 $\longrightarrow$
$\qquad$ oxidized pyridine nucleotide + H_2O_2

The importance of the respiratory burst in the destruction of microorganisms was firmly established by the study of the inherited condition known as *chronic granulomatous disease* (CGD). This disease, first described in 1957 by Good and his associates and by Landing and Shirkey [6, 7] is characterized by an unusual susceptibility to infections by certain species of bacteria and fungi. The underlying basis for this defect in host defense was discovered independently by Good and coworkers [8] and by Baehner and Nathan [9], who showed that CGD phagocytes fail to undergo the respiratory burst during particle ingestion. By these findings, the respiratory burst was securely tied to antimicrobial defenses in vivo, verifying Quastel's original hypothesis.

The studies performed up to that time had thus clearly shown that upon exposure to particles, phagocytes converted oxygen to H_2O_2, which was used for the destruction of microorganisms. H_2O_2 itself, however, is only weakly microbicidal, in part at least because microorganisms are well-defended against this oxidant by catalase and other H_2O_2-destroying metabolic systems. It was soon shown that, rather than being employed directly against microorganisms, H_2O_2 served as a precursor for the formation of much more potent microbicidal agents.

The first demonstration that this was the case was the discovery by Klebanoff of the role of myeloperoxidase in oxygen-dependent microbial killing by phagocytes. This enzyme had been recognized as a constituent of phagocytes since 1941, when it was discovered by Agner [10], but it was only when Klebanoff showed that halide ion was necessary for the expression of microbicidal activity that its function was established [11, 12]. Present evidence indicates that the function of myeloperoxidase is to catalyze the oxidation of Cl^- by H_2O_2 to generate HOCl, a very potent antimicrobial agent.

Two years after Klebanoff's discovery, the first patient with inherited myeloperoxidase deficiency was reported [13]. Studies in this patient provided the first clue to the existence of another oxygen-dependent microbicidal system, one that did not require myeloperoxidase. The evidence leading to this conclusion was that this patient had very little trouble with infection, in contrast to patients with chronic granulomatous disease, in whom the inability to express a respiratory burst led to recurrent, severe, and prolonged bacterial infections. There appeared to be an oxygen-dependent microbicidal mechanism that was preventing bacterial infections in patients with myeloperoxidase deficiency but was inoperative in patients with chronic granulomatous disease.

The nature of the second oxygen-dependent microbicidal system was revealed by the discovery that phagocytes manufacture O_2^- during the respiratory burst [14]. O_2^- is the primary compound formed in the respiratory burst, giving rise in secondary reactions to H_2O_2 and all the other oxidants generated during this event. Among these other oxidants are reactive oxidizing radicals currently thought to be produced by the reaction of O_2^- with peroxides formed as a consequence of these secondary reactions. These reactive oxidants appear to be the microbicidal agents active in the second microbicidal system.

It is evident from the foregoing that oxygen-dependent killing by phagocytes is a complex process involving special chemical and metabolic pathways, some of which are unique to phagocytic cells. These pathways and the inherited diseases that affect them are the subjects of this chapter.

NORMAL MECHANISMS OF OXYGEN-DEPENDENT KILLING BY PHAGOCYTES

In functional terms, the mechanism of oxygen-dependent killing by phagocytes can be divided into three components: (1) Reduction of oxygen to O_2^- and H_2O_2, a metabolic event generally known as the respiratory burst; (2) conversion of respiratory burst products to potent microbicidal oxidants; and (3) destruction of those respiratory burst products which leak into the cytoplasm of the phagocyte by the antioxidant systems of the cell. Inherited deficiencies involving each of these components have been described. Before discussing these, a review of normal oxygen-dependent killing will be presented.

The Respiratory Burst

The respiratory burst is the critical element of the oxygen-dependent killing mechanism, for it is during this event that the oxygen-containing precursors of the microbicidal oxidants are generated, and without these precursors no oxygen-dependent killing can take place. The respiratory burst consists of a series of changes in oxygen metabolism that occur when a phagocyte is exposed to an appropriate stimulus. During this event, which lasts from a few minutes to an hour or so depending on the stimulus and cell type [3, 15–21], oxygen uptake increases dramatically (accounting for the term *respiratory burst*) [1, 6, 22–26]. Oxidation of glucose via hexose monophosphate shunt also rises sharply [3–5, 27–31], and O_2^- [15, 18–21, 32–42] and H_2O_2 [4, 17a, 33, 37, 39, 43–47] are generated in large quantities. The burst has been demonstrated in neutrophils, eosinophils, and mononuclear phagocytes, although its activity in the last depends on the stage of development of the cell, being very active in monocytes and in "activated" macrophages but weak in resident peritoneal macrophages [18, 34, 48, 49]. A very brief respiratory burst has also been reported to occur in basophils [21].

The biochemical basis for the respiratory burst is the activation of an enzyme, dormant in unstimulated cells, which catalyzes the reduction of oxygen to O_2^- at the expense of a reduced pyridine nucleotide [50–55]. For reasons to be discussed below, it appears that the physiologic electron donor is NADPH. The O_2^--forming reaction may therefore be written

$$NADPH + 2 O_2 \longrightarrow NADP^+ + 2 O_2^- + H^+$$

and the enzyme that catalyzes the reaction is the *NADPH oxidase*.

The H_2O_2 generated during the respiratory burst appears to arise exclusively by the dismutation of O_2^- [37, 39]. This dismutation is a rapid spontaneous reaction ($k = 4 \times 10^5\ M^{-1}$ s^{-1} at pH 7.0) [56] which can be further accelerated by superoxide dismutase ($k = 2.4 \times 10^9\ M^{-1}\ s^{-1}$ for the reaction between O_2^- and superoxide dismutase at 25°C) [57], an enzyme which will be discussed in more detail below.

$$2 O_2^- + 2 H^+ \longrightarrow H_2O_2 + O_2$$

In human neutrophils stimulated by opsonized staphylococci [37] or IgG-coated latex [46] about 50 to 70 percent of the O_2^- is converted to H_2O_2; the rest of the O_2^- has not been explicitly accounted for, but it presumably reacts with other components in the phagocyte or the extracellular medium. The stoichiometric relationship between O_2^- and H_2O_2 has not been examined with other classes of phagocytes.

Hexosemonophosphate shunt activation results from an increase in the rate of oxidation of NADPH during the respiratory burst. This increase in NADPH oxidation has been documented by measurements of pyridine nucleotide levels in resting and activated neutrophils (Table 90-1) [58, 58a]. It is accounted for by two processes: (1) the consumption of NADPH in the O_2^--generating reaction and (2) the operation of a glutathione-dependent H_2O_2-consuming system which composes one of the antioxidant defenses of the phagocyte [45, 60–66]. These processes deplete NADPH, which must be restored if the respiratory burst is to continue in operation. Restoration is accomplished by the first two reactions of the hexosemonophosphate shunt. These are reactions in which $NADP^+$ is converted to NADPH [59, 67]. They are catalyzed successively by glucose-6-phosphate dehydrogenase (see Chap. 74):

Glucose-6-phosphate + NADP $\longrightarrow$

6-phosphogluconate + NADPH

and 6-phosphogluconate dehydrogenase:

6-Phosphogluconate + NADP $\longrightarrow$

ribulose-5-phosphate + NADPH + CO_2

Subsequent reactions involve a complex series of sugar phosphate interconversions which result eventually in the catabolism of the 5-carbon sugar via the glycolytic pathway [68–70].

In some species the operation of the hexosemonophosphate shunt is reinforced by the action of the enzyme NAD kinase, which catalyzes the phosphorylation of NAD to NADP [58a, 58b]. This kinase compensates for the increase in NADPH oxidation imposed by the respiratory burst by increasing the total quantity of phosphorylated pyridine nucleotides (NADP + NADPH) in the activated neutrophil. As a consequence, the concentration of NADPH remains almost the same as it was in the resting cell, though the concentration of NADP rises sharply [58a]. The activity of this enzyme is likely to be an important factor in maintaining a vigorous respiratory burst, since burst activity has been shown to be closely tied to the intracellular concentration of NADPH [59].

It was stated above that the physiologic electron donor for the O_2^--forming reaction is NADPH. This has been a controversial topic for many years, some experts arguing in favor of NADPH [50–55, 70a, 71–78] and others arguing for NADH [44, 79–85]. We believe that NADPH is the electron donor in vivo for three reasons. First, the fall in the NADPH/NADP ratio substantially exceeds the fall in the NADH/NAD ratio during the respiratory burst [58, 58a]. Second, phagocytes with impaired NADPH production due to severe glucose-6-phosphate dehydrogenase deficiency cannot express the respiratory burst [86–88]. This means that if NADH were the physiologic electron donor, it would, in turn, have to obtain reducing equivalents from NADPH in a reaction rapid enough to sustain the respiratory burst. This is unlikely because, even though enzymes capable of catalyzing this sort of reaction are present in human neutrophils [87, 87a], the pyridine nucleotide ratios indicate that, in the neutrophil, the NAD $\rightleftharpoons$ NADH and NADP $\rightleftharpoons$ NADPH couples do not equilibrate with each other. Third, the enzyme likely to be responsible for O_2^- production by phagocytes shows a marked preference for NADPH [51, 53, 55, 71–78]. A full discussion of the entire issue may be found in Ref. 89 to 92.

Activation One of the most puzzling aspects of the respiratory burst is the mechanism by which it is activated. Although many of the properties of the activation sequence are known, full understanding of this process at a biochemical level has not yet been achieved. Any biochemical explanation of the activation process will have to incorporate the following facts:

1. Activation is a multiple-step process. This is indicated by the reproducible lag of 30 to 60 s between exposure of phagocyte to a stimulus and the onset of the respiratory burst [40, 47,

Table 90-1 Pyridine nucleotide concentrations in neutrophils

| | Concentration, mM | | | | |
| | Resting | | | Phagocytosing | |
Pyridine nucleotide	Human[*]	Guinea pig	Horse	Guinea pig	Horse
NAD	0.23	0.56	0.42	0.58	0.30
NADH	0.067	0.079	0.26	0.076	0.27
NADP	0.053	0.041	0.050	0.084	0.23
NADPH	0.067	0.35	0.070	0.27	0.047

[*] Concentrations of pyridine nucleotides in human cells were calculated from the data of Baehner and Karnovsky [81], assuming a cell volume of 0.36 pl. Concentrations of pyridine nucleotides in guinea pig cells were taken from Selvaraj and Sbarra [58], and in horse cells from Heyneman and Bauwens-Monbaliu [58a].

54, 93–95]. Moreover, the existence of patients in whom the respiratory burst can be activated by some stimuli but not by others [96, 97] suggests at least two points of entry into the activation sequence.

2. Activation can be accomplished by a remarkably large number of stimuli. Some are particulate—for example, latex beads [14, 32, 33, 47, 73, 76], opsonized zymosan [19, 25, 36, 40, 98], and opsonized bacteria [15, 37, 47]—but many are soluble [3, 26, 28, 35, 40, 42, 93, 95, 98–119]. Furthermore, the soluble stimuli differ widely in structure. They include substances as simple as F^- [3, 99, 100] and as complex as N-formylmethionylleucylphenylalanine (f–Met–Leu–Phe) [42, 95, 103–106] and cytochalasin E [115, 116]. A partial list of the soluble agents known to activate the respiratory burst is given in Table 90-2.

3. Activation appears to be an energy-requiring process. Cells exposed to stimuli under conditions that block both glycolysis and mitochondrial oxidation are unable to express a respiratory burst [94, 120].

4. F^- is able to activate the respiratory burst in a reversible fashion [99]. O_2^- production by neutrophils stimulated with F^- stops when F^- is removed and resumes when F^- is added again. This reversibility would seem to rule out an activation mechanism involving limited proteolysis. Nevertheless, it has been found that activation is prevented by inhibitors of proteolysis such as DFP and soybean trypsin inhibitor [116, 121], suggesting that limited proteolysis may indeed play a role in the activation mechanism. It is not known how these seemingly conflicting findings can be reconciled.

5. Extracellular calcium is required for respiratory burst activation by many stimuli [93, 99, 105, 117]. Phorbol myristate acetate, however, can activate in the absence of extracellular calcium [94].

6. Activation can occur without phagocytosis or degranulation. All that is necessary is contact of the stimulus with the surface of the phagocyte [35, 99].

7. A transient change in the membrane potential takes place within 5 s after exposure of the cell to a stimulus, well before the onset of the respiratory burst (Fig. 90-1) [93, 122, 123]. Whether this potential change is related to the burst is unclear. Such a relationship has been suggested by the finding that neutrophils from several patients whose phagocytes are congenitally incapable of expressing a burst also fail to show a potential change when exposed to certain stimuli (e.g., phorbol myristate acetate—see below) [122, 123]. On the other hand, the response of the transmembrane potential to a burst-activating calcium ionophore is normal in the congenitally defective

phagocytes, even though the ionophore is completely unable to elicit a burst from these cells [123].

Taken together, these findings imply a complex mechanism of activation which is tightly regulated in order to ensure that the burst is expressed only at appropriate times and places. The molecular details of this mechanism remain to be elucidated.

Termination The respiratory burst is a transient event, lasting on the average only 10 to 20 min [3, 15–21] (Fig. 90-2). The termination of the burst seems to be due to the destruction of the O_2^--forming oxidase by the microbicidal mechanisms of the cell [16]. Both oxygen-dependent and oxygen-independent mechanisms participate in the destruction of the oxidase, the oxygen-dependent mechanisms being more effective in this regard.

The O_2^--forming Enzyme The identity of the enzyme responsible for the first reaction in the respiratory burst has been the subject of many investigations and some controversy since the discoveries made by Karnovsky [3] and Quastel [4]. The present evidence strongly favors a particulate NADPH oxidase as the respiratory burst enzyme. This oxidase was first reported by Iyer and Quastel in 1963 [71], and its existence has been confirmed by many other groups [19, 50–55, 72–78, 124, 125]. It has been found in homogenates of human [50–53, 55, 76–78] and guinea pig [53, 54, 71–75] neutrophils as well as human eosinophils [19]. Little or no activity is found in preparations from unstimulated cells, but homogenates from phagocytes stimulated with opsonized zymosan [50, 51, 126] or phorbol myristate acetate [55, 127] are able to catalyze the production of large quantities of O_2^-. Either pyridine nucleotide can be used as electron donor for this O_2^--forming reaction, but enzymes from both human and guinea pig cells seem to prefer NADPH, since the K_m for this nucleotide has been reported to be ten- to thirtyfold lower than the K_m for NADH [51, 54, 55, 125, 126] (Table 90-3).

Several lines of evidence, including subcellular fractionation

Table 90-2 Soluble agents that provoke the respiratory burst

Phorbol myristate acetate	Antineutrophil antibodies
Fluoride	Anionic detergents
C5a	Phospholipase C
Cytochalasin E	Fatty acids
A23187 (a calcium ionophore)	Wheat germ agglutinin
FMetLeuPhe and other N-formylated chemotactic peptides	Leukocytic pyrogen

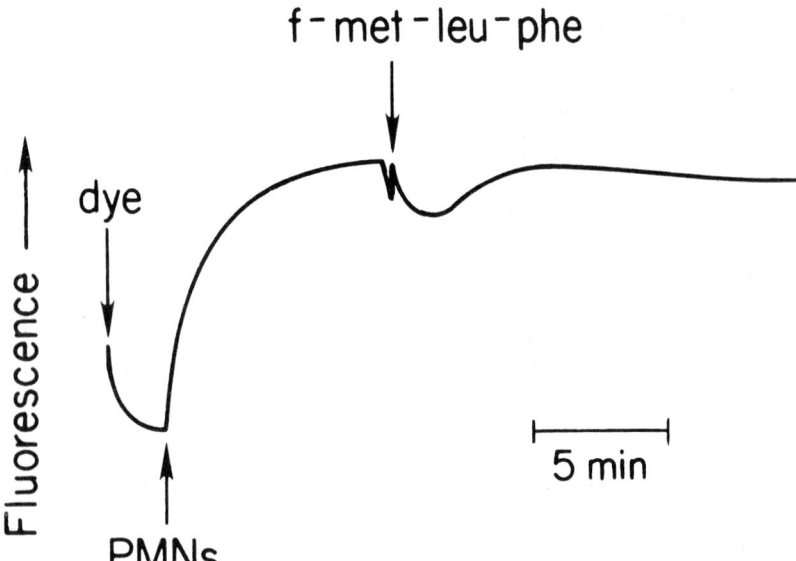

Figure 90-1 Membrane potential changes which precede the respiratory burst, as measured by changes in the fluorescence of a potential-sensitive cyanine dye. A downward deflection represents depolarization.

experiments, indicate that the NADPH oxidase is situated in the plasma membrane of the phagocyte [53, 54, 82, 85, 127, 128]. This is an ideal location for the oxidase, since during phagocytosis, plasma membrane invaginates to become the wall of the phagosome, placing the enzyme in a position to deliver oxidants into the phagocytic vesicle with maximum efficiency. The oxidase does not appear to cross the membrane, but seems to be situated in its inner half with the portion containing the pyridine nucleotide binding site extending into the cytoplasm [17a, 128a].

The enzyme has been solubilized by the use of detergents [124–126]. Using the soluble enzyme, investigators have been able to determine other properties, such as a requirement for FAD [129, 130, 130a] (K_m = 0.06 μM) and a reduced -SH group [126, 130] as well as for phospholipid [126]. The phospholipid requirement can be fulfilled by phosphatidylethanolamine, but not by phosphatidylserine or lecithin. With respect to its electron acceptor, the enzyme appears to be absolutely specific for oxygen, failing to transfer electrons from NADPH to several artificial electron acceptors which have been shown to function with other flavoenzymes [130].

The possibility has been raised that the O_2^--forming oxidase actually consists of an electron transport chain in which the flavoenzyme is only one component. A neutrophil quinone has been proposed as another member of this hypothetical electron transport chain [130b–130d]. Because this quinone is found primarily in the granules of resting neutrophils while the O_2^--forming apparatus of activated neutrophils is located in the plasma membrane, it has been proposed that the quinone is transferred to the plasma membrane during the degranulation that accompanies activation, an event that would result in the assembly of the entire electron transport chain in the membrane of the activated cell. Such a transfer could not occur during the activation of the respiratory burst by F^-, because this agent provokes the respiratory burst without causing degranulation [99]; this does not however exclude a role for the quinone in O_2^- production, because a small fraction of the quinone is native to the plasma membrane where it could serve as an electron carrier without the need for translocation. Offering support for a role for a quinone in the respiratory burst are studies showing that exogenous quinones and quinonelike compounds can alter rates of oxygen consumption and O_2^-

production in stimulated neutrophils, as well as work showing the presence in human neutrophils of a pyridine nucleotide dehydrogenase that can employ quinones as electron acceptors [130e]. Further study is necessary, however, before the participation of quinones in the O_2^--forming reaction can be regarded as conclusively proven.

Evidence supporting the participation of the particulate NADPH oxidase in the respiratory burst includes the fact that the enzyme is activated concomitantly with activation of the respiratory burst in intact phagocytes [25, 50, 51, 54, 55] and the demonstration that oxygen uptake by intact neutrophils during the respiratory burst can be accounted for quantitatively by the activity of the oxidase [125]. The strongest evidence concerning this point has to do with the very low levels of oxidase activity in the neutrophils of patients with chronic granulomatous disease [50–53, 55, 125, 129].[1] This will be discussed in the subsequent section on the biochemical defect in that condition. Also to be discussed in that section is evidence suggesting the involvement of a b-type cytochrome in O_2^- production.

Oxygen-dependent Microbicidal Systems

Of the two respiratory burst products, H_2O_2 is only weakly microbicidal [131, 132], and O_2^- appears to have no microbicidal activity whatsoever [32, 133–137]. The major function of these compounds is to serve as precursors of the very powerful oxidants actually employed by phagocytes for killing. These lethal oxidants are formed from the respiratory burst products by two distinct pathways. One of the pathways requires myeloperoxidase, and the other does not.

The Myeloperoxidase-dependent Killing System Myeloperoxidase is a heme-containing enzyme which is present in very large quantities [138] in the azurophil granules of neutrophils [139–142] (Fig. 90-3). The enzyme is also

---

[1] Other pyridine nucleotide oxidases have been postulated to be responsible for the respiratory burst in phagocytes. Levels of these oxidases are normal [8, 76, 78] or only partly decreased [81, 83] in CGD. The only oxidase whose activity in CGD cells is reduced in proportion to the reduction in respiratory burst activity is the NADPH oxidase described in this section. For a full discussion of this topic, see Ref. 89 to 92.

Table 90-3 Michaelis constants for the oxidation of reduced pyridine nucleotides by the NADPH oxidase of neutrophils

| Species | K_m, mM | |
	NADPH	NADH
Human	0.033	0.93
Guinea pig	0.046	0.58

present in the juvenile forms of mononuclear phagocytes (monocytes and early activated macrophages) [143–146] but disappears from mononuclear phagocytes which have reached their fully mature activated state [143–145]. Eosinophils lack this enzyme, containing instead a unique peroxidase which is structurally and functionally distinct from myeloperoxidase [147].

Human myeloperoxidase has been purified by several groups [148–150], but there is little agreement as to its structure. Its molecular weight has been variously reported as 118,000, 144,000 and 153,000. It is composed of several subunits, but there is disagreement about their number and molecular weights. All agree, however, that the enzyme contains two iron porphyrin groups [151]. These appear to be attached to the protein by covalent links [151, 152]. The optical absorption bands of myeloperoxidase are at longer wavelengths than those of most peroxidases [148b, 153–155], giving it its characteristic green color. This peculiar spectrum may reflect the fact that the prosthetic group is an unusual type of heme substituted with a peripheral aldehyde residue [152]. The reactions catalyzed by myeloperoxidase are generally typical of those catalyzed by other peroxidases. Oxidations by hydrogen peroxide are the most characteristic of these. Substrates for these oxidations include phenols and aromatic amines, their colored oxidation products serving as the basis for assays of myeloperoxidase (e.g., the oxidation of guaiacol to tetraguaiacol [156]); halide ions, which are converted to hypohalous

acids or their chemical equivalents [157, 158]; and amino acids and peptides (see below).

$$X^- + H_2O_2 + H^+ \longrightarrow XOH + H_2O,$$

$$X^- = Cl^-, Br^-, I^-$$

The enzyme also catalyzes the so-called peroxidase-oxidase reactions, a group of oxidations that proceed in the absence of added H_2O_2 [159]. These oxidations take place by highly complex free-radical chains which are initiated by the small amounts of H_2O_2 that arise spontaneously in the reaction mixtures but, once started, employ oxygen, not H_2O_2, as the oxidizing agent. The ability of myeloperoxidase to catalyze NADH oxidation by the peroxidase-oxidase mechanism [160–162] led for a time to the belief that myeloperoxidase was the respiratory burst oxidase, but this is no longer considered to be the case [163, 164].

The substrate that is most relevant in biologic terms is the chloride ion. This ion is readily oxidized to OCl^- by H_2O_2, the equilibrium constant for the reaction

$$H_2O_2 + Cl^- \longrightarrow H_2O + OCl^-$$

being about 10^3 at pH 7 as calculated from oxidation-reduction potentials [165]. Myeloperoxidase catalyzes this oxidation, as well as the oxidations of Br^- and I^- [166] and the pseudohalide SCN^- [167].

The kinetics of halide oxidation are complex, because the affinity of the enzyme for each substrate (halide and H_2O_2) is affected by the concentration of the other [168] as well as by pH [169]. Furthermore, Cl^- at least is an inhibitor of the enzyme at high concentrations ($>0.1\ M$). A precise K_m for

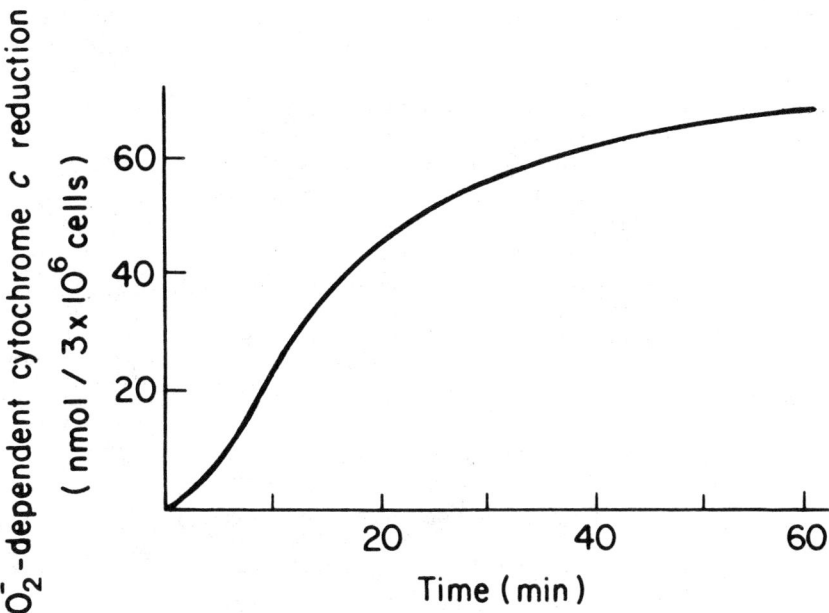

Figure 90-2 The course of the respiratory burst. O_2^- production by *Escherichia coli*-stimulated human neutrophils as a function of time.

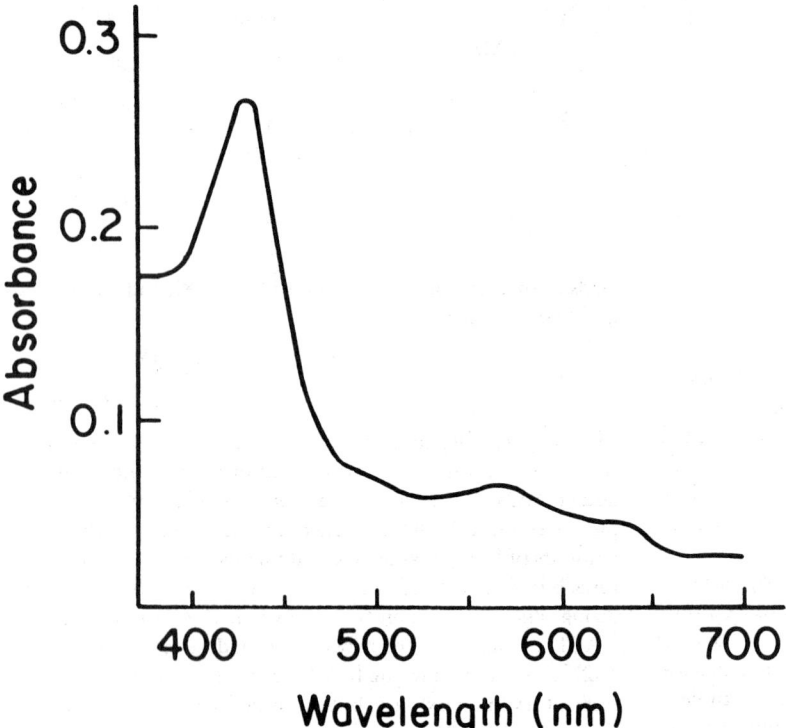

Figure 90-3 Spectrum of myeloperoxidase from human neutrophils. The spectrum of 2.8 μM myeloperoxidase at pH 7.4 is shown.

Cl^- that can be used to interpret the behavior of myeloperoxidase in vivo is therefore difficult to specify. Under conditions that seem reasonable approximations of those in the phagocyte (pH 5.0 to 5.5 and H_2O_2 at ca. 1 mM), myeloperoxidase-dependent oxidations are rapid at Cl^- concentrations in the vicinity of 0.1 M.

Other properties of myeloperoxidase that are pertinent to its function are its cationic nature, which causes it to adhere to negatively charged surfaces such as those of bacteria [10, 148], and its low pH optimum (Fig. 90-4) [169], which augments its activity under the acidic conditions prevailing in the phagosome. The enzyme is inhibited strongly by heme enzyme reagents such as CN^- and N_3^- [12, 131, 166, 170] as well as by certain sulfur-containing compounds such as the antithyroid agent methimazole [16, 170].

Most significant is the fact that myeloperoxidase together with H_2O_2 and a halide ion constitutes an unusually powerful microbicidal system [11, 12, 131, 167, 170–172], amplifying the antimicrobial potency of H_2O_2 by a factor of 50 [131]. The effectiveness of the various halide ions in the peroxide-halide-myeloperoxidase microbicidal system, as measured by the concentration required to kill half the bacteria under defined conditions, declines in the order $I^- > Br^- > Cl^-$ (Fig. 90-5) [166]. Cl^- is present in human neutrophils in concentrations sufficient for use by myeloperoxidase [173], in contradistinction to Br^- and I^-, which, though theoretically better substrates, are for practical purposes unavailable to the enzyme since their concentrations in the cytoplasm are exceedingly low. It is therefore highly likely that the physiologic substrate for myeloperoxidase is Cl^-.

It is probable that the microbicidal activity of the peroxide-halide-myeloperoxidase system is mediated by OCl^-.[2] The components necessary for its production—namely, myeloperoxidase, H_2O_2, and Cl^-—are all found in high concentrations in phagocytic vesicles. The antiseptic properties of OCl^- have been recognized for a long time and are exploited in such processes as the purification of water for drinking and swimming.

Finally, direct evidence for the use of OCl^- as an antimicrobial agent by phagocytes has been provided by two observations: (1) The demonstration that neutrophils convert Cl^- to chlorine gas [157], probably by the well-known reaction between Cl^- and OCl^- that takes place under acidic conditions

$$Cl^- + OCl^- + 2\,H^+ \longrightarrow Cl_2 + H_2O$$

and (2) the finding that neutrophils mediate the incorporation of chloride into macromolecules during the ingestion of bacteria [168, 169, 181],[3] a reaction in which OCl^- can serve as the halogenating agent.

The chemical basis for the microbicidal action of OCl^- is not known. The compound can oxidize a variety of biologically significant substances, and one or more of these oxidations might prove to be pertinent to its in vivo activity. Amines of all kinds are oxidized to chloramines. Ammonia is converted to monochloroamine, a potent oxidant whose microbicidal activity exceeds that of OCl^-, possibly because its lipid solubility gives it readier access to the interior of the microorganism [186a]:

$$HN_4^+ + OCl^- \longrightarrow NH_2Cl + H_2O$$

[2] Singlet oxygen, an electronically excited form of molecular oxygen that reacts rapidly with certain biologically significant chemical groups such as the imidazole ring and the double bond of unsaturated fatty acids [174], has been proposed as a microbicidal agent on the basis of studies of phagocyte chemiluminescence and experiments with singlet oxygen quenchers and trapping reagents [175–178]. The evidence supporting a role for singlet oxygen is ambiguous, however, because the methods used to date for the detection of singlet oxygen lack specificity [179, 180]. In particular, it has been pointed out that the data used to support the production of singlet oxygen by phagocytes can be used equally well as evidence for OCl^- production. In view of this, we believe that judgment should be reserved regarding the participation of singlet oxygen in oxygen-dependent microbial killing by phagocytes.

[3] Most of the work on halogenation of macromolecules by the myeloperoxidase system has been performed with I^- as halide, and the incorporation of radioactive I^- into trichloroacetic acid-precipitable material has been used as a test of the function of the peroxide-halide-myeloperoxidase system in phagocytes [11–13, 158, 166, 170, 182–185]. In whole neutrophils the incorporation of I^- into macromolecules has been shown to take place primarily in the phagocytic vesicles and their contents [186].

Amino acids are oxidized to aldehydes with the liberation of CO_2 and NH_3 by a reaction which goes through a monochloroamine intermediate [187–189]:

$$NH_2 \qquad\qquad HNCl \qquad\qquad CO_2$$
$$| \qquad\qquad\qquad | \qquad\qquad\qquad$$
$$RCH—COOH + OCl^- \dashrightarrow RCH—COOH \longrightarrow RCHO + NH_4Cl$$

A similar reaction with taurine proceeds only as far as the chloramine, which in this case is rather stable and unreactive [190]. The high concentrations of taurine in neutrophils [191] suggest that it may play an antioxidant role in this cell as a scavenger of OCl^-. A dichloroamine can also be formed whose further reactions generate nitriles (HCN, in the case of glycine), CO_2, and HCl [189, 192].

$$NH_2 \qquad\qquad NCl_2 \qquad\qquad CO_2$$
$$| \qquad\qquad\qquad | \qquad\qquad\qquad$$
$$RCH—COOH + 2OCl^- \longrightarrow RCH—COOH \longrightarrow RC{\equiv}N + 2HCl$$

Peptide N-terminal dichloroamines cleave at the N-terminal peptide bond [193],

$$NH_2 \qquad\qquad NCl_2 \qquad\qquad CO_2$$
$$| \qquad\qquad\qquad | \qquad\qquad\qquad$$
$$RCH—C—NHR' \longrightarrow RCH—C—NHR' \longrightarrow RC{\equiv}N + NH_2R'$$
$$\| \qquad\qquad\qquad \| \qquad\qquad\qquad$$
$$O \qquad\qquad\qquad O$$

a process whose implications in vivo are clear. Tyrosine is halogenated [194]. Methionine is oxidized to methionine sulfoxide [194a],

$$CH_3—S—CH_2CH_2CHNH_2COOH + OCl^- \longrightarrow$$

$$O$$
$$\|$$
$$CH_3—S—CH_2CH_2CHNH_2COOH$$

a reaction that has been postulated to regulate chemotaxis by the oxidative inactivation of methionine-containing chemotactic peptides such as N-FMetLeuPhe [195, 196]. Mercaptans are also oxidized by OCl^-, initially to sulfenic acids [197] and perhaps subsequently to higher sulfur acids [198]

Figure 90-4 Activity of myeloperoxidase as a function of pH. The optimum varies with the concentration of Cl^-.

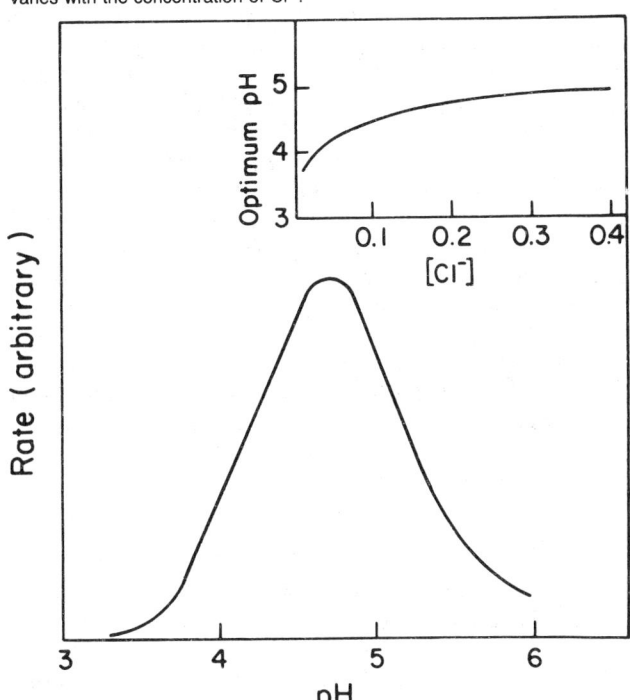

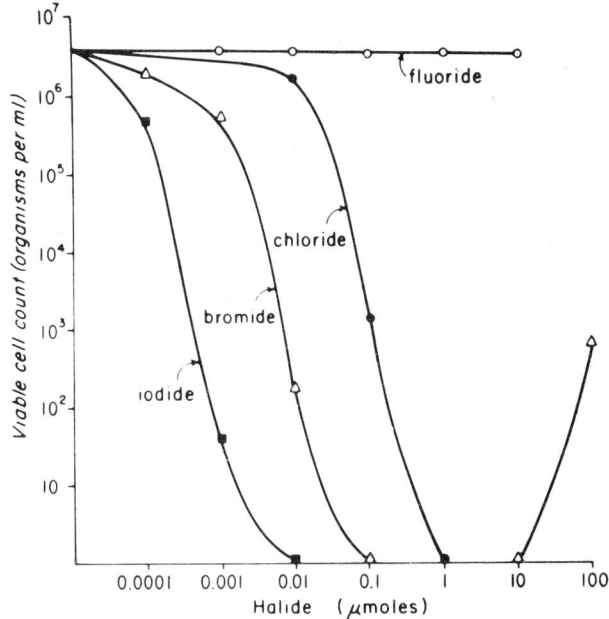

Figure 90-5 Potency of the halides in the microbicidal peroxide-halide-myeloperoxidase system. *(Reproduced with permission from the Journal of Bacteriology.)*

$$R—SH + OCl^- \longrightarrow R—S—OH \longrightarrow \longrightarrow R—SO_3^=$$

On a macromolecular scale, the peroxide-halide-myeloperoxidase system has been shown to decarboxylate proteins ingested by neutrophils [199], and to potentiate tissue damage during inflammation by inactivating α1-antiproteinase, the major circulating inhibitor of the neutral protease released by neutrophils at inflammatory sites [200–200b]. OCl^- destroys a number of types of enzymes: $-SH$ requiring enzymes, heme enzymes, and enzymes with iron-sulfur centers; its effect on the iron-sulfur enzymes is particularly rapid [200c]. As to its mechanism of killing, both increased cell wall permeability [200d] and a fall in the intracellular concentration of reduced sulfhydryl compounds [198] has been found to correlate with bacterial death during exposure to the peroxide-halide-myeloperoxidase system. A deeper understanding of the killing process awaits the further characterization of the alterations in the macromolecular constituents of organisms exposed to this OCl^--generating system.

Oxidizing Radicals   In the context of the oxygen-dependent killing mechanisms of phagocytes, the term *oxidizing radicals* refers to a group of compounds produced during the respiratory burst which are characterized by unusually high reactivity and the presence of an unpaired electron. These compounds appear to be essential components in a myeloperoxidase-independent but oxygen-requiring microbicidal system. They have been detected by their ability to release hydrocarbons from compounds containing carbon-sulfur bonds [201–207, 207a],

$$CH_3SCH_2CH_2CHO + OH^\cdot \longrightarrow$$
$$\tfrac{1}{2}CH_3\,SSCH_3 + HCOOH + CH_2{=}CH_2 \uparrow$$

$$CH_3SCH_3 + OH^\cdot \longrightarrow CH_3^\cdot + CH_3S—OH$$
$$\| \qquad\qquad RH \qquad\qquad \|$$
$$O \qquad\qquad R^\cdot \qquad\qquad O$$
$$CH_4 \uparrow$$

an oxidation that can be accomplished by a variety of radicals including hydroxyl (OH$^{\cdot}$), alkoxyl (OR$^{\cdot}$), acyl (R—COO$^{\cdot}$), and alkyl (R$^{\cdot}$) [208], but not by the rather unreactive O$_2^-$ radical [201]. Of these, only OH$^{\cdot}$ has been identified specifically, by a spin-trapping technique [209, 210], but the production of at least some of the others seems highly probable given the nature of the system in which the radicals are generated.

The reactions which generate oxidizing radicals are not clearly defined. A likely mechanism at least for OH$^{\cdot}$ production would be the reaction between O$_2^-$ and H$_2$O$_2$, the Haber-Weiss reaction [211–213]. This is catalyzed by transition metal ions such as Fe and yields OH$^{\cdot}$ at a respectable rate:

$$H_2O_2 + Fe^{2+} \longrightarrow OH^{\cdot} + Fe^{3+} + OH^-$$

$$O_2^- + Fe^{3+} \longrightarrow O_2 + Fe^{2+}$$

Evidence suggests that some phagocytes may also use other mechanisms for oxidizing radical production. Both radical-mediated release of ethylene from thioethers and OH$^{\cdot}$ production as measured by spin trapping are blocked by superoxide dismutase, implicating O$_2^-$ in oxidant formation, but catalase has only a variable effect on these reactions [202–207, 209, 210]. This indicates that OH$^{\cdot}$ can be produced in phagocytes by an H$_2$O$_2$-independent route and suggests in addition that ethylene release may in part be due to oxidants other than OH$^{\cdot}$. A further complication regarding the route of production of oxidizing radicals is the finding that ethylene release in response to activation of the burst is sharply reduced, although not abolished, in myeloperoxidase-deficient cells [214, but see 210]. This result implicates myeloperoxidase in the generation of at least some fraction of the radicals responsible for ethylene production. Paradoxically, ethylene production is stimulated by N$_3^-$, a potent inhibitor of myeloperoxidase [205, 214]. This could reflect the formation of the highly reactive NO$^{\cdot}$ radical, known to be made by the heme enzyme-catalyzed oxidation of N$_3^-$ by H$_2$O$_2$ [215].

Regardless of the mechanisms by which these oxidizing radicals are produced, their ability to kill microorganisms has been clearly shown both in model systems [133–135, 137, 216] and in experiments with phagocytes [32, 217]. The best of the models is the xanthine oxidase-acetaldehyde system, which has been shown both to produce OH$^{\cdot}$ and to use this oxidant for the destruction of bacteria [137]. A role for oxidizing radicals in microbial killing in vivo is strongly indicated by the finding that, under appropriate circumstances, bacterial killing by neutrophils is strongly inhibited by the enzyme-catalyzed destruction of either H$_2$O$_2$ or O$_2^-$, the substrates for OH$^{\cdot}$ production by the Haber-Weiss reaction, or by the addition of OH$^{\cdot}$ scavengers [32, 217]. Studies of the effects of activated phagocytes on endothelial cells, erythrocytes [218, 219], and synovial fluid [220] suggest that oxidizing radicals are also responsible for some of the tissue damage that occurs during inflammation.

Even fewer details are known about the biochemical mechanisms of damage by oxidizing radicals than are known about the peroxide-halide-myeloperoxidase system discussed above. Because of the exceedingly great reactivity of many of these radicals [221], the damage is likely to affect many cellular constituents. For example, membrane damage may occur owing to the peroxidation of constituent phospholipids [222–224]. Lipid peroxidation is a likely consequence of oxidizing radical production and in fact has been demonstrated in phagocytizing systems [225, 226]. Damage to nucleic acids is another possibility. O$_2^-$-forming systems have been shown to induce single-strand breaks in double-stranded DNA, almost certainly due to the OH$^{\cdot}$ generated as a by-product in such systems [227–231]. DNA damage by this mechanism could conceivably take place in microorganisms ingested by phagocytes, although this has not yet been demonstrated experimentally. Potentially harmful oxidations of nucleotides and amino acids have been shown to be mediated by OH$^{\cdot}$, and sulfhydryl compounds are likely to be targets of oxidizing radicals as well [221]. Which if any of the above are actually involved in microbial killing remains to be determined.

Antioxidant Systems of Phagocytes

In addition to destroying ingested organisms, the oxidants produced during the respiratory burst may damage host cells and tissues, including the phagocytes themselves. Therefore, phagocytes are supplied with a series of effective systems to trap or destroy the oxidants before they do harm.

Superoxide Dismutases Superoxide dismutases are enzymes that catalyze the conversion of O$_2^-$ to oxygen and H$_2$O$_2$ [232].

$$2\, O_2^- + 2\, H^+ \longrightarrow O_2 + H_2O_2$$

This reaction also occurs spontaneously, and its rate constant is rather high at physiologic pH values ($k = 4 \times 10^5\ M^{-1}\ s^{-1}$) [56]. The spontaneous reaction is bimolecular, implying that even at low rates of production tissue O$_2^-$ concentrations could rise to unacceptable levels before the rate of spontaneous dismutation would equal the rate of O$_2^-$ generation (Fig. 90-6). The superoxide dismutases operate on one O$_2^-$ molecule at a time, thus maintaining tissue O$_2^-$ concentrations at negligible levels. This is the most likely explanation for the presence of superoxide dismutases in tissues, even though spontaneous dismutation is facile.

Human tissues contain two types of superoxide dismutase: a dimeric protein of molecular weight 33,000 containing one copper and one zinc per subunit [233] and an 85,000-dalton tetramer containing one manganese per subunit [234]. Both types are found in neutrophils, although the total concentration of dismutase in this cell is low [19, 235], amounting to only 15 percent of that in red blood cells [236–238] and less than 5 percent of that in liver [234] when expressed as units per gram wet weight of tissue. These concentrations are nevertheless sufficient, since resting neutrophils consume very little oxygen and produce almost no O$_2^-$, while activated neutrophils are suicide cells for which long-term protection from oxidant damage would be superfluous. Eosinophils similarly contain comparatively low concentrations of dismutase [19].

Catalase Catalase, a large (263,000 M.W.) tetrameric heme enzyme containing one prosthetic group per subunit [239], has been found in several human tissues—polymorphonuclear leukocytes, erythrocytes, and liver [239, 240]—and is probably present in all. It catalyzes the conversion of H$_2$O$_2$ to oxygen and water:

$$2\, H_2O_2 \longrightarrow O_2 + H_2O$$

At high concentrations, H$_2$O$_2$ is rapidly destroyed by catalase. Because the reaction rate is strictly proportional to H$_2$O$_2$ concentration, catalase-mediated destruction of H$_2$O$_2$ is inefficient at the low peroxide levels likely to be present in tissues

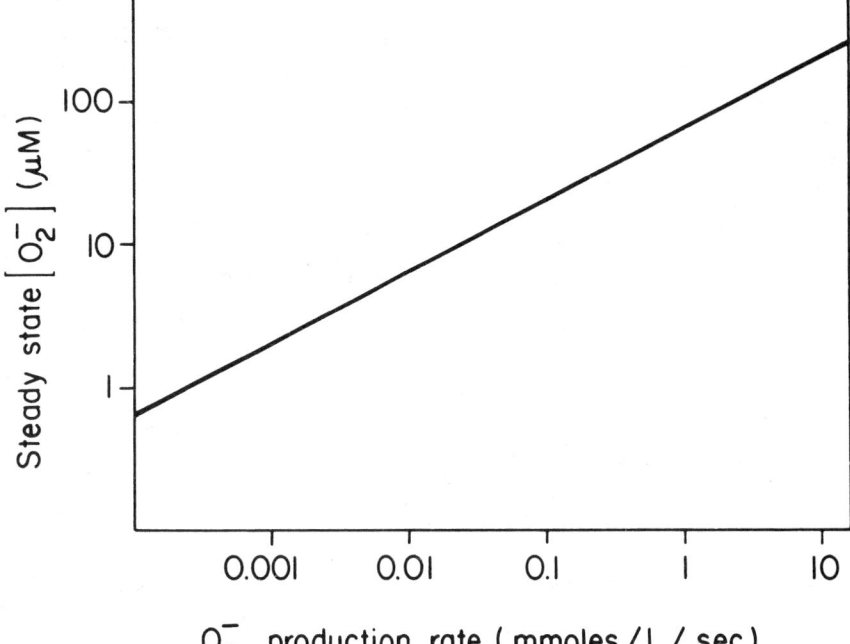

Figure 90-6 Steady state concentration of O_2^- at physiologic pH as a function of the rate of O_2^- production, assuming that all O_2^- consumption occurs by spontaneous dismutation. The rate constant for 10^7 fully stimulated packed neutrophils, which occupy a volume of about 4 μl, is approximately 4 mmoles/(liter · s), assuming negligible diffusion of O_2^- out of the mass of cells.

[241]. It is probable that catalase serves a backup role in antioxidant defenses, functioning mainly when the load of H_2O_2 imposed on a cell is too great to be handled by the glutathione-dependent system which represents the primary H_2O_2-neutralizing pathway of the cell [242].

Glutathione-dependent Destruction of H_2O_2 Most of the H_2O_2 to which phagocytes are exposed, including that which leaks into the cytoplasm during the respiratory burst, is destroyed by a glutathione-requiring coupled enzyme system whose ultimate effect is to reduce H_2O_2 to water at the expense of NADPH [60–62]. The reactions are as follows:

$$2\ GSH + H_2O_2 \longrightarrow GSSG + 2\ H_2O$$

catalyzed by glutathione peroxidase, and

$$GSSG + NADPH + H^+ \longrightarrow 2\ GSH + NADP^+$$

catalyzed by glutathione reductase. In this pathway, glutathione cycles between its oxidized and reduced states, serving as a catalyst for H_2O_2 reduction. The NADP is re-reduced by the hexose monophosphate shunt, just as is the NADP generated in the O_2^--forming reaction. A substantial fraction of the hexose monophosphate shunt activity expressed during the respiratory burst is attributable to this glutathione-dependent H_2O_2-consuming pathway [45].

The two enzymes of the pathway have been well studied in animals and to a lesser extent in humans. Glutathione reductase is a flavoenzyme, employing FAD as the physiologic cofactor [243, 244]. It is an efficient catalyst [245], showing Michaelis constants for NADPH and GSSG of 16 and 96 μM, respectively, and a turnover number of 400 s⁻¹. Structural studies have shown the enzyme to be a dimeric protein of 115,000 M.W. [243].

Glutathione peroxidase, a tetramer of 84,000 M.W. [246, 247], is remarkable in that it is one of the few enzymes that contain selenium. The selenium has been shown to be present in selenocysteine, one residue of which is present in each subunit [247, 248]. The enzyme catalyzes the reduction not only

of H_2O_2, but also of alkyl hydroperoxides, including the hydroperoxides formed during the autoxidation of polyunsaturated fatty acids [249–251]:

$$ROOH + 2\ GSH \longrightarrow ROH + H_2O + GSSG$$

A second glutathione peroxidase, free of selenium, has been found in rat liver [250, 251]. This second enzyme does not appear to occur in phagocytes [252].

During the respiratory burst there appears to be only a modest alteration in the levels of reduced and oxidized glutathione in neutrophils (Fig. 90-7) [64, 65, but see 252a]. Thus, despite what is probably a vigorous oxidation of GSH to GSSG by H_2O_2, a reaction which is rapid even in the absence of a catalyst [44] and is accelerated further by glutathione peroxidase, the antioxidant capacity of the glutathione system remains high. The behavior of the glutathione pool under these conditions provides further evidence as to the efficiency of glutathione reductase.

Low Molecular Weight Antioxidants Neutrophils contain three compounds to which an enzyme-independent antioxidant role might be attributed: taurine, ascorbic acid, and α-tocopherol (vitamin E). Taurine reacts with OCl⁻ to form a stable nonreactive N-chloroamine (see above) [190] and on these grounds may be considered an antioxidant because of its ability to scavenge the highly reactive OCl⁻ moiety. Ascorbic acid is a nonspecific radical scavenger, reacting with potent oxidants such as OH˙ to generate the innocuous ascorbate semiquinone radical, which in turn can donate its odd electron to a second oxidizing radical to yield dehydroascorbate:

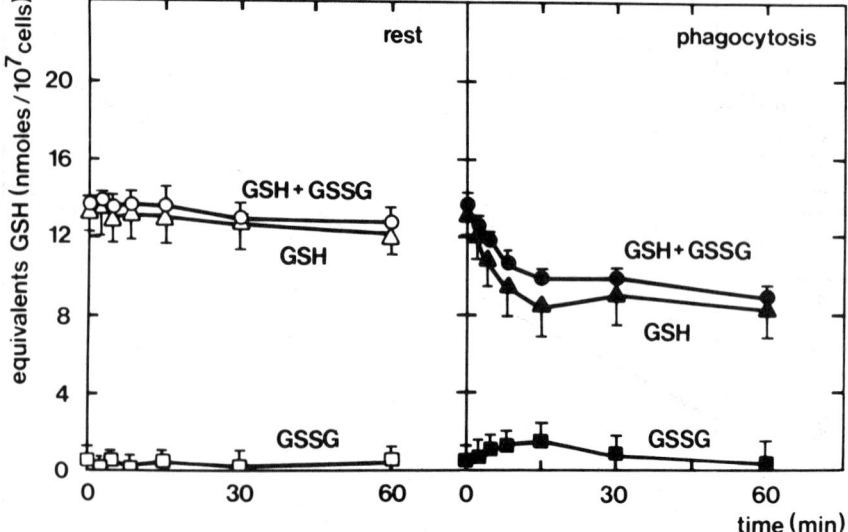

Figure 90-7 Changes in glutathione concentration during the respiratory burst in human neutrophils. *(Reproduced with permission from Blood; Journal of Hematology.)*

Neutrophils contain an enzyme that can convert dehydroascorbate back to ascorbate; this implies the existence of a radical scavenging system based on the cyclic oxidation and re-reduction of ascorbic acid [63, 252b], but direct evidence that ascorbate serves in this capacity is not yet available. α-Tocopherol is also an efficient scavenger of oxidizing radicals:

There is abundant evidence that α-tocopherol functions as an antioxidant in phagocytes [253–255].

A scheme summarizing the metabolic pathways involved in the respiratory burst of normal phagocytes appears as Fig. 90-8.

INHERITED ABNORMALITIES OF OXYGEN-DEPENDENT KILLING BY PHAGOCYTES

Chronic Granulomatous Disease

Chronic granulomatous disease (CGD) is a congenital immunodeficiency syndrome characterized by failure of the respiratory burst in phagocytic cells. This metabolic abnormality results in impaired phagocyte microbicidal capacity. The genetics, clinical manifestations, and laboratory features of CGD have been well described during the past two decades. The molecular defect in CGD, however, is incompletely understood.

Genetics Two inheritance patterns are noted in families of patients with CGD. The majority of cases are X-linked, but some appear to be autosomal recessive.

The existence of an X-linked form of CGD is indicated by several lines of evidence. First, the disease shows a definite male predominance: of 168 cases reported through 1977, more than 80 percent were male [256]. Second, the condition has been described in maternal cousins and half-brothers with different fathers [257]. The strongest evidence for X-linked inheritance is the identification of a carrier state in mothers and sisters of many affected males [257, 258]. Bactericidal and metabolic testing of the neutrophils of such relatives has revealed a spectrum of functional capabilities ranging from near normal to profoundly deficient [258], consistent with the Lyon hypothesis of random inactivation of one X chromosome in female cells [259]. Slide tests which permit the identification of the specific metabolic defect in individual neutrophils have confirmed the presence in CGD carriers of two distinct populations of neutrophils: one with normal metabolic (and presumably functional) capabilities and another with the metabolic abnormalities characteristic of patients with CGD [260].

The majority of carrier females are healthy and do not suffer from recurrent or unusually severe infections despite the fact that a subpopulation of their neutrophils is defective. However, one CGD carrier with a high percentage of abnormal phagocytes and chronic Salmonellosis [261], and several carriers have been reported to develop an illness resembling lupus erythematosus [262].

The first females with full-blown CGD were reported in 1968 [263, 264]. Since then it has become clear that not all cases of CGD are X-linked. Some affected females have been accounted for on the basis of an X-linked mode of transmission with chance inactivation of most of or all the normal X chromosomes in the neutrophils of the heterozygote [264a]. But the occurrence of the disease in female sibs [260, 265] and of consanguinity in the family of an affected female [263], as well as failure to detect the carrier state in the mothers of some CGD patients of both sexes [260, 263–267], suggests transmission by an autosomal recessive gene in some families. In most cases presumed to be autosomal recessive, both parents have had normal neutrophil function [263–269]. One group of investigators, however, reported an intermediate degree of neutrophil dysfunction in both parents of some affected children [270, 271]. Occasional cases of CGD have been reported in which family studies do not conform to either X-linked or autosomal recessive inheritance [272]. Spontaneous gene mutation cannot be excluded in isolated cases of CGD in which no carrier parent can be identified.

In summary, the majority of cases of CGD appear to be transmitted in an X-linked fashion, while the rest display an autosomal recessive pattern of inheritance. Other forms of inheritance and spontaneous gene mutation are rare, if they occur at all.

Clinical Course The major clinical manifestation of CGD is susceptibility to infection. Infectious episodes are frequent, severe, and often prolonged. In this regard CGD patients resemble children with other immunodeficiency syndromes. In addition, CGD patients often develop inflammatory masses of characteristic pathology (Fig. 90-9) which may grow large enough to compress or obstruct vital organs, a unique feature of this illness which may be related to the prolonged survival of infecting microorganisms within phagocytes. Patients with CGD often display the nonspecific effects of chronic inflammatory illness, including failure to thrive, reticuloendothelial hyperplasia, hypergammaglobulinemia, and anemia. Although the disorder is incurable, better supportive medical care has improved the outlook for patients with CGD, a disease thought at one time to have a uniformly fatal outcome during childhood.

AGE AT ONSET Most patients with CGD will begin to experience recurrent severe infections during the first year of life. Of the patients reviewed through 1977 [256], 78 percent had developed their first symptoms by 1 year of age. Indeed, cases have presented with infection as early as the first week of life [256].

On the other hand, there have been several reports of patients with CGD who have had no significant infections until after the age of 6 and who were not diagnosed until adolescence or adulthood [273–276]. It is now recognized that CGD is not invariably a severe disorder presenting during infancy and resulting in death during childhood. In some patients the disorder is relatively mild, causing few problems even before prophylactic antibiotics and aggressive management of infections favorably alter the course. The reason for the wide variation in clinical severity is not known. Other genetic factors which potentiate nonoxidative killing mechanisms of phagocytes or other aspects of host defense may play a role. For example, a family has been reported in which four adult male

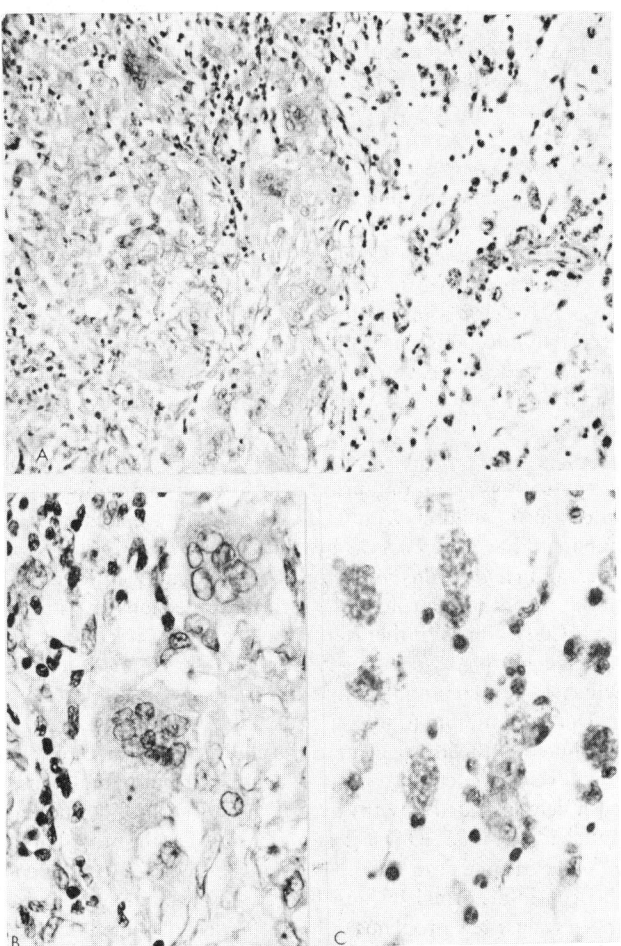

Figure 90-9 Pathology of chronic granulomatous disease. Pathologic specimen from the enlarged thymus of a 4-year-old male with CGD. *A.* Low-power view of an area of granulomatous inflammation demonstrating both giant cells and histiocytes containing pigmented material. *B.* Higher-power view of a cluster of multinucleate giant cells. *C.* High-power view of the characteristic histiocytes containing pigmented lipid material; the exact nature and origin of this material are unknown.

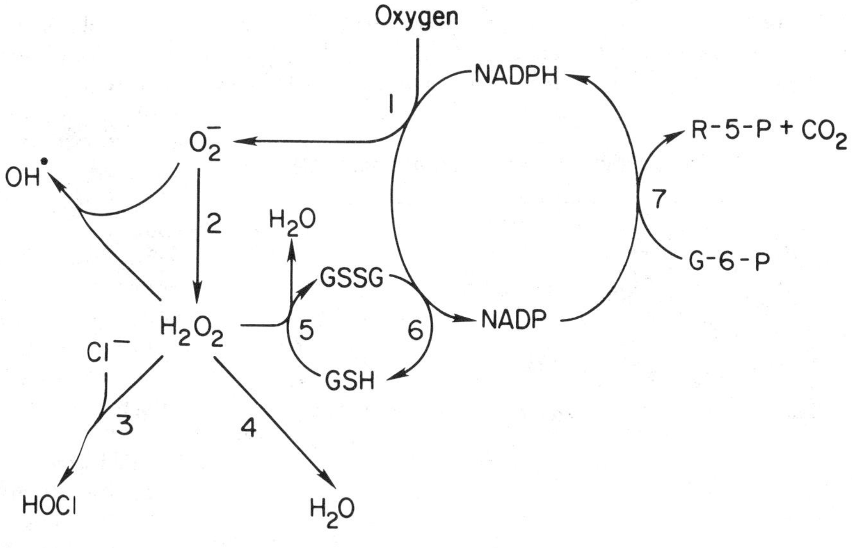

Figure 90-8 The respiratory burst: Pathways of oxygen metabolism. Enzymes are indicated by numerals as follows: 1, NADPH oxidase; 2, superoxide dismutase; 3, myeloperoxidase; 4, catalase; 5, glutathione peroxidase; 6, glutathione reductase; 7, glucose-6-phosphate dehydrogenase and 6-phosphogluconate dehydrogenase.

sibs with confirmed X-linked CGD had relatively mild clinical courses [277]. Although the neutrophils from these patients showed the characteristic severe metabolic abnormalities of CGD (see below), their bacterial killing was somewhat more efficient than that of cells from most CGD patients. This difference was not explained, but it does suggest that an inherited factor may have modified the course of the disease in these brothers.

Thus, most cases of CGD are recognized during infancy or early childhood. Most of the reported cases in which the diagnosis was delayed until adolescence or later had a history of recurrent infections since childhood. The natural history of the disorder is variable, ranging from rapidly fatal to compatible with life into middle age even without aggressive medical intervention.

PATHOGENS   The organisms which most commonly cause infections in children with CGD are listed in Table 90-4. It is apparent that *Streptococcus pyogenes*, *Streptococcus pneumoniae*, and *Hemophilus influenza*, the usual pathogens of childhood, do not play a role in the recurrent infections of patients with CGD. On the other hand, these patients are frequently infected by *Staphylococcus aureus* and the enteric bacteria, which do not commonly cause disease in normal children.

The susceptibility to infections in patients with CGD can be attributed to the impairment in the ability of their neutrophils to kill certain microorganisms. This impairment in ability has been demonstrated in vitro by using *S. aureus* [278] and enteric bacteria [185, 278] as test organisms. On the other hand, CGD neutrophils can kill other pathogenic species (e.g., streptococci) in a normal fashion [279]. This explains why these species cause few problems in CGD. It was postulated that the selective nature of the killing defect could be attributed to the ability of susceptible bacteria to generate sufficient hydrogen peroxide within the phagocytic vacuole to compensate for the deficient H_2O_2 production of the CGD neutrophils [185]. Support for this hypothesis was provided by the demonstration that catalase-producing bacteria, which excrete no detectable H_2O_2, were not killed by CGD neutrophils, whereas catalase-negative organisms, which excrete H_2O_2 into their environment, were killed in a normal manner [280]. Indeed, it has been possible to correct the killing defect of CGD neutrophils in vitro by experimentally introducing a H_2O_2-generating system (glucose oxidase–coated latex particles) into the defective cells [281].

In addition to catalase-positive bacteria, certain fungi are frequent pathogens in CGD patients [281a] (see Table 90-4). *Candida albicans* infections are common; a defect in the killing

Table 90-4   Most common infecting organisms in CGD

Bacteria
  Staphylococcus aureus
  Escherichia coli
  Salmonellae
  Pseudomonas
  Mycobacteria
  Nocardia species
  Klebsiella - Enterobacter - Serratia

Fungi
  Candida albicans
  Aspergillus sp.

of this fungus by CGD neutrophils has been demonstrated [282]. *Aspergillus* infections are also frequent in CGD [283–285], and their incidence may be rising because of the more widespread use of effective prophylactic medications to prevent bacterial and candidal infections [285].

Species of mycobacteria and *Nocardia* have been reported to cause serious infections in CGD patients [274, 286–289]. *Pneumocystis carinii* pneumonia has been described in one patient [290].

Thus, patients with CGD are frequently infected by microorganisms which are unusual pathogens in children. The predominant offenders are *S. aureus*, enteric bacteria, *Candida*, and *Aspergillus* species.

ORGAN SYSTEMS   Patients with CGD can develop infections in almost any location, but some sites are more frequently involved than others. The skin, which is always challenged by contact with microorganisms, is often affected early in the course of the disease [291]. Pyogenic dermatitis, furunculosis, and subcutaneous abscesses are common manifestations. In addition, many patients develop an infectious eczematoid dermatitis, especially on the face.

Like the skin, the mucous membranes of the mouth and intestinal tract are teeming with microorganisms which may invade through the mucosa and cause disease in children with neutrophil dysfunction. Recurrent stomatitis is a characteristic feature of CGD, and esophagitis, frequently due to *Candida* species, is occasionally seen. The latter may result in stricture formation, giving rise to dysphagia and regurgitation (see Fig. 90-10). Chronic enteritis and colitis have been demonstrated in many patients by radiologic studies or biopsy [292, 293] and often cause symptoms such as abdominal discomfort and recurrent diarrhea, with or without frank malabsorption. Intestinal obstruction from large inflammatory masses [294] has been reported, as has abscess formation, especially around the rectum. Although the stomach is normally sterile, children with CGD have a predilection for developing granulomatous inflammation of the wall of the gastric antrum resulting in annular narrowing of the lumen [295]. This frequently leads to persistent vomiting and failure to thrive. Figure 90-11 demonstrates the characteristic radiologic abnormality of this peculiar condition, which may develop at a very young age and be the presenting feature of CGD.

The reticuloendothelial system is also a common site of infection. Lymphadenopathy is very common among children with CGD, as are splenomegaly and hepatomegaly. Suppurative lymphadenitis which drains spontaneously or requires surgical intervention is often seen early in the course of the disease. The offending microorganisms are usually *S. aureus* or enteric bacteria. Hepatic and perihepatic abscesses were reported in over one-third of the 168 cases reviewed by Johnston [256]. The frequent reticuloendothelial involvement in CGD and its characteristic histologic appearance may be due to the escape of viable microorganisms from defective neutrophils followed by their ingestion by macrophages in the lymph nodes, spleen, and liver. Because these macrophages share the oxidative killing defect of the circulating neutrophils, they, too, are unable to destroy the bacteria efficiently [296]. Viable microorganisms persisting within the macrophages induce hyperplasia, chronic inflammation, and granuloma formation. These bacteria may proliferate to such an extent that necrosis and abscess formation result.

Osteomyelitis is another common problem in children with

involved, but metacarpals and metatarsals are unusually common sites. Multiple bones are frequently involved simultaneously or sequentially. Causative organisms include all those to which children with CGD are susceptible, but *Serratia marcescens* is particularly common as a cause of osteomyelitis.

Pneumonia and pulmonary abscesses are also seen frequently in patients with CGD. Pneumonia may be bronchial, lobar, or interstitial and is often associated with enlarged hilar lymph nodes. Unusual pulmonary manifestations in CGD include caseating granulomata and areas of consolidation which appear encapsulated on x-ray [298, 299]. Enteric bacteria, *S. aureus*, and *Aspergillus* species often cause serious pulmonary infections in patients with CGD, but pneumococcal pneumonia is not a particular problem. Pleural effusions may occur as complications of pulmonary infections or subdiaphragmatic abscesses.

Genitourinary complications of CGD include granulomatous cystitis [300–302], pyelonephritis, renal abscesses [303], and obstructive uropathy due to granulomatous masses in the bladder wall or in the perirectal area (Fig. 90-12). Immune complex glomerulonephritis, attributed to prolonged antigenic stimulation from a chronic *S. aureus* infection, has been reported in a patient with CGD [304]. Renal amyloidosis has also been reported [305].

Less common problems in CGD include eye lesions [306], thyroiditis [285], and peritonitis. Meningitis and septicemia, often due to *Salmonella* [256, 307], can be life-threatening.

The frequency of infections in CGD varies from one patient to another, but recurrent, unusually severe, and prolonged infections are the rule. After the institution of prophylactic antibiotics, which is now common practice in CGD, acute febrile illnesses are less frequent, but large inflammatory masses which may cause discomfort or obstructive symptoms become a serious problem (Fig. 90-13). Biopsy and culture of such masses may or may not reveal the pathogenic organism [308].

Laboratory Features

GENERAL   Children with CGD are usually evaluated during infancy or early childhood because of recurrent, severe infections with unusual pathogens. The blood counts reveal a mild anemia in about 75 percent of cases [309]. The red blood cell morphology may be either normochromic, normocytic or hypochromic, microcytic. Other features are consistent with anemia due to chronic inflammatory disease. There are normal to increased numbers of morphologically normal neutrophils and monocytes. During acute infections there is an appropriate leukocytosis and left shift.

Studies of B-lymphocyte and plasma cell function are normal. Serum concentrations of immunoglobulins are usually elevated with normal proportions of the subclasses. Primary and anamnestic antibody response to antigenic stimulation is normal [310]. Tests of T-lymphocyte function [310], such as skin tests, as well as complement levels and the ability of CGD serum to opsonize particles, are also normal.

TESTS OF PHAGOCYTE FUNCTION   In most cases studied, CGD neutrophils have been shown to be capable of normal chemotactic response both in vivo (Rebuck skin window) [310] and in vitro (two-compartment chamber assays) [311, 312]. Several cases of CGD have been reported in which a

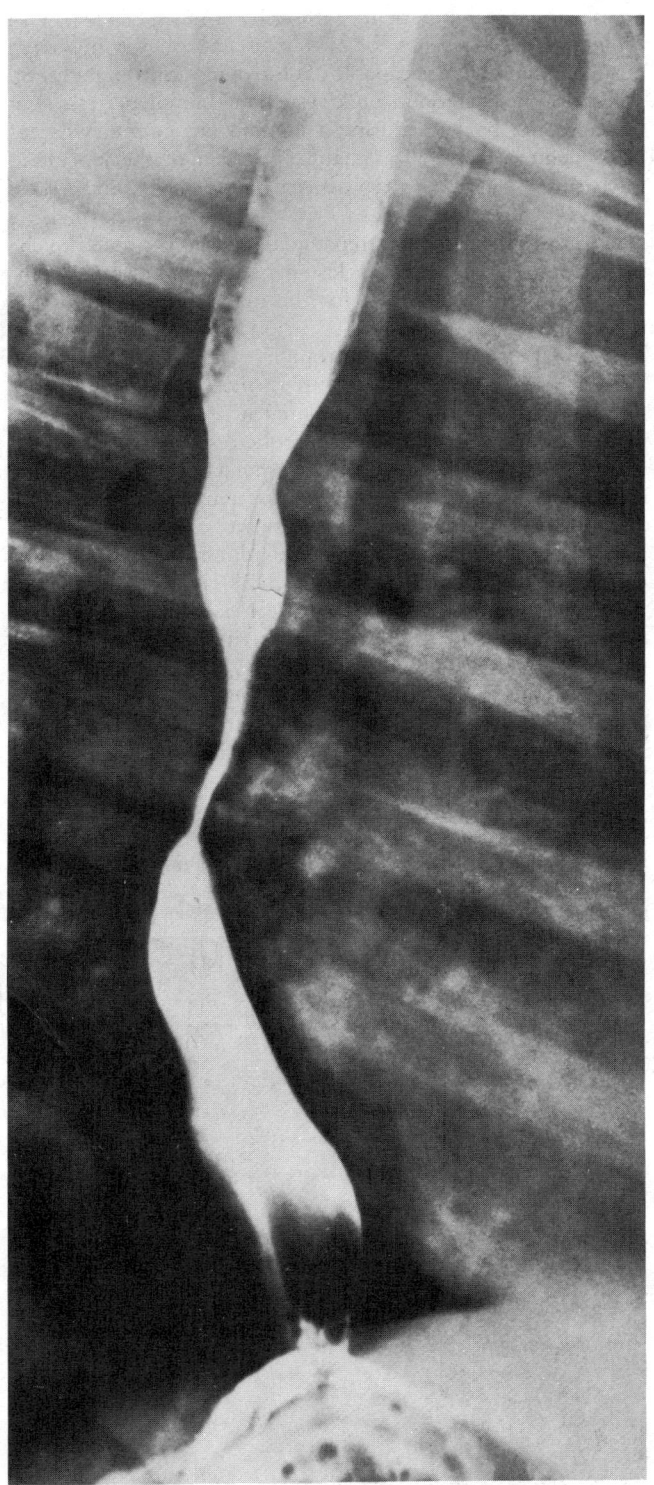

Figure 90-10 Esophageal stricture in a patient with CGD. Roentgenogram from the upper GI series of a boy with X-linked CGD showing fixed narrowing of the midesophagus. This stenotic area coexisted with evidence of active *Candida* esophagitis. Management consisted of surgical dilatation and amphotericin B. Esophageal narrowing can also be due to extrinsic compression by inflammatory masses (see Fig. 90-13).

CGD. As early as 1969 the clinical and radiologic characteristics of bone findings in CGD were well described [297]. Clinical signs of inflammation (i.e., swelling and erythema of the overlying skin) may not be prominent. Any bone may be

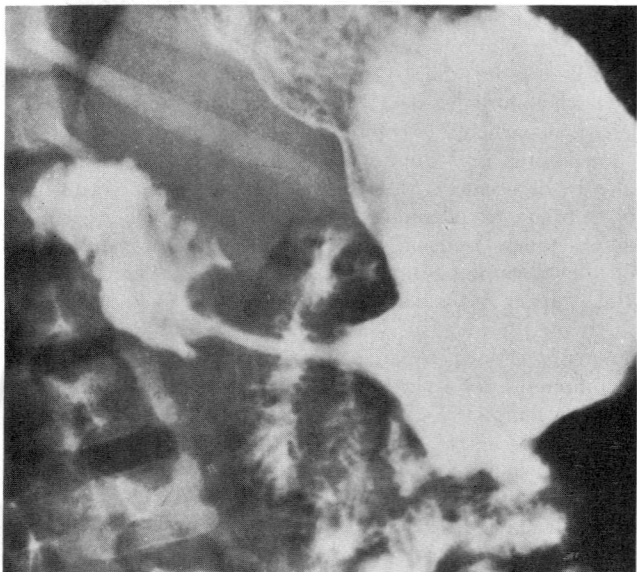

Figure 90-11 Gastric antral lesion in a patient with CGD. Characteristic roentgenographic appearance of the gastric antral lesion in a 4-year-old boy with X-linked CGD who presented with persistent vomiting. There is a concentric prepyloric narrowing which was associated with delayed gastric emptying. Biopsy of the lesion revealed granulomatous inflammation. Cultures for bacteria and fungi were negative. The patient was managed conservatively with small, frequent feedings. The lesion spontaneously improved over 1 year.

defect in neutrophil chemotaxis was detected in addition to the more characteristic metabolic abnormalities of the disease [311, 313, 314]. In some, the chemotactic abnormality was due to a circulating inhibitor [311, 313]. In general, however, chemotaxis is normal in patients with CGD.

Phagocytosis by CGD neutrophils is normal. This has been demonstrated with bacteria [278], latex spherules [281], and opsonized lipopolysaccharide-coated oil droplets [315, 316]. Furthermore, indirect evidence of normal phagocytosis by CGD neutrophils is provided by the fact that the increased lecithin synthesis which is associated with phagocytosis proceeds normally in CGD neutrophils [317].

Several early investigators proposed that the fundamental abnormality of CGD was failure of degranulation [8]. They noted that, although granule contents were normal, there was morphologic evidence of an inability to empty the granule enzymes and other microbicidal substances into a phagocytic vacuole [8, 278, 279, 318]. They postulated that the ability of bacteria to survive and proliferate in CGD neutrophils was secondary to faulty fusion of granules and inadequate release of lysosomal enzymes into the phagocytic vacuoles. Subsequently, however, other investigators found that degranulation was normal in CGD [163, 266, 316, 317, 319, 320]. Kinetic studies using biochemical methodology showed that, although degranulation in CGD neutrophils was initially relatively slow, it had reached normal levels by 15 min [321]. It is now agreed that abnormal degranulation is not the primary defect in neutrophils from patients with CGD.

Thus, in most cases of CGD, tests of the earlier steps of phagocyte function, including chemotaxis, particle ingestion, and degranulation, are normal. Consistently abnormal, however, are studies of intracellular bacterial killing and of the metabolic response to phagocytosis.

Intracellular killing of certain species of microorganisms is grossly abnormal in patients with CGD [185, 278, 318]. With *S. aureus, A. aerogenes,* or *S. marcescens,* neutrophils from normal individuals are capable of destroying approximately 80 percent of the bacteria in a test system containing plasma, neutrophils, and bacteria during a 60 min incubation, whereas CGD neutrophils kill less than 20 percent of the inoculum. Intracellular killing of streptococcal species [279] and *Lactobacillus acidophilus* [185] by CGD neutrophils is normal. As mentioned above, this discrepancy has been attributed to the production by the latter (catalase-negative) organisms of sufficient H_2O_2 to compensate for the metabolic defects of the CGD phagocytes [280].

The inability of CGD neutrophils to kill catalase-positive bacteria can be ascribed to failure of these cells to undergo a normal respiratory burst, an essential step in the generation of microbicidal agents [8]. The metabolic responses to phagocytosis which are known to play a role in bacterial killing include increased oxygen consumption, production of H_2O_2 and O_2^-, and augmented activity of the hexose monophosphate (HMP) shunt. All these responses are greatly diminished in phagocytosing CGD neutrophils [8, 50, 322, 323]. A primary defect in the HMP shunt in CGD cells has been excluded by the demonstration of normal HMP shunt activity induced by methylene blue (methylene blue oxidizes NADPH, and the resultant increased concentration of $NADP^+$ stimulates the shunt) [8]. Thus the failure of HMP shunt activation in CGD neutrophils is secondary to failure to utilize NADPH during the respiratory burst.

Figure 90-12 Obstructive uropathy in a patient with CGD. Intravenous pyelogram of a boy with X-linked CGD demonstrating hydronephrosis and hydroureter on the left side. The obstruction was due to compression by a large inflammatory mass in the pelvis between the rectum and the bladder.

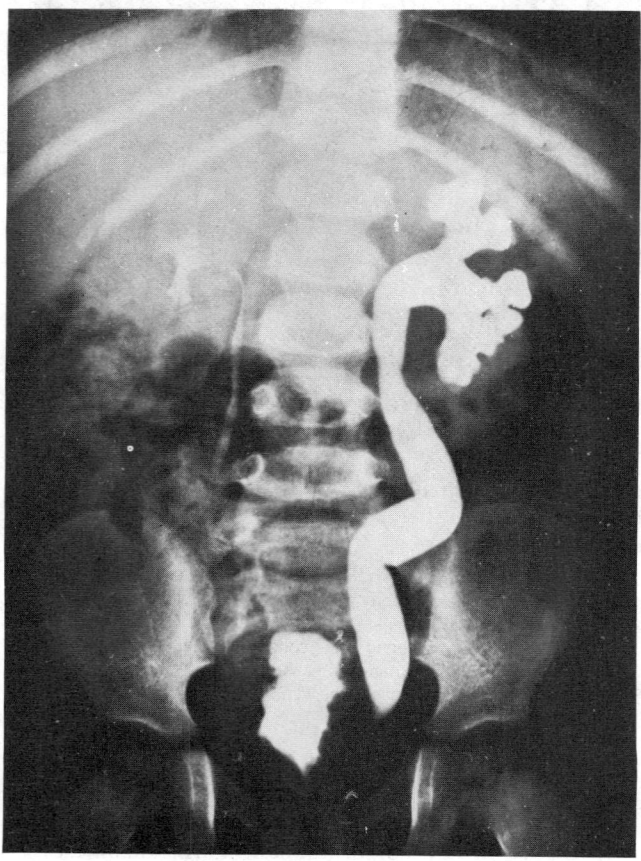

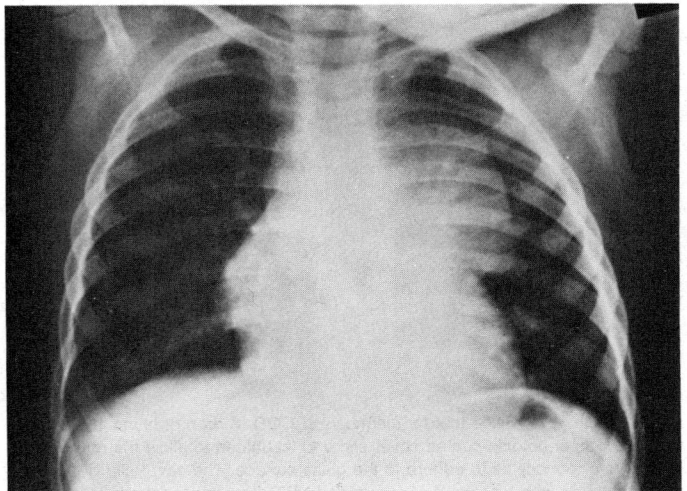

Figure 90-13 Mediastinal mass in a patient with CGD. Chest roentgenogram of a 4-year-old male with CGD who presented with dysphagia and regurgitation. The mass originated in the left anterior mediastinum and extended posteriorly to compress the esophagus. The large mass was excised completely and the symptoms were immediately relieved. Pathology revealed cyst formation and granulomatous inflammation with pigmented histiocytes. Cultures were negative for bacteria and fungi. *(Reproduced with permission of the editors from American Journal of Diseases of Childhood.)*

Other laboratory features of CGD are also secondary to the failure of the respiratory burst reactions. Inability of CGD neutrophils to fix iodide to phagocytosed catalase-positive bacteria is due to failure to generate the H_2O_2 necessary for the myeloperoxidase-H_2O_2-halide antimicrobial system, which normally results in incorporation of the halide into bacterial protein [185]. CGD neutrophils can fix iodide to living, but not heat-killed, catalase-negative bacteria. Presumably the living catalase-negative organisms produce enough H_2O_2 to participate in the myeloperoxidase-dependent reactions, which can then proceed normally in CGD cells.

Similarly, the failure of CGD neutrophils to exhibit chemiluminescence is secondary to the abnormal respiratory burst [324, 325]. Chemiluminescence is light emission by electronically excited molecules which are generated during a chemical reaction. Chemiluminescence by human neutrophils occurs with phagocytosis and is due to electronically excited substances formed during oxidations mediated by respiratory burst products [52, 326]. None of these reactions can be carried out by CGD neutrophils. Consequently, chemiluminescence during phagocytosis is virtually absent.

An indirect but accurate and simple means of assessing the integrity of the respiratory burst is the measurement of nitroblue tetrazolium (NBT) dye reduction by stimulated neutrophils [263]. Normal neutrophils, activated by a suitable stimulus in the presence of NBT, will reduce the yellow dye to insoluble purple formazan by means of the O_2^- produced during the respiratory burst. Neutrophils from patients with CGD fail to reduce the dye. This observation has formed the basis of screening tests for CGD [260, 263]. An example is the endotoxin-stimulated NBT slide test [260] in which individual granulocytes are evaluated microscopically for their ability to reduce NBT (Fig. 90-14).

Chronic granulomatous disease has been diagnosed prenatally by a modification of the NBT slide test performed on fetal blood samples obtained by placental-vessel puncture [327].

OTHER LABORATORY FEATURES It was noted in 1971 that the erythrocytes of some patients with X-linked CGD possess the rare McLeod phenotype (weak Kell antigens) [328]. An X-linked antigen related to the Kell blood group system, designated Kx, and thought to be the precursor of the antigens in the Kell complex, is missing from the red blood cell membrane of these patients. Kx, also present in neutrophils and mono-

cytes from normal individuals, is absent from the leukocytes of the same CGD patients [329, 330]. The association between the McLeod phenotype and CGD is thought to be due to linkage between the gene responsible for the biosynthesis of the substance utilized in the production of the Kell complex and the gene whose dysfunction causes X-linked CGD.

The Metabolic Defect in CGD Phagocytes from patients with CGD cannot express a respiratory burst because of an abnormality in the complex apparatus that is responsible for the critical O_2^--forming reaction of the burst. Numerous studies have shown that homogenates of CGD phagocytes incubated with the usual concentrations of reduced pyridine nucleotides (ca. 0.1 mM) display gross deficiencies in O_2^- formation, their O_2^- production rates ranging from zero to at most a few percent of the O_2^- production rates of normal preparations [50–53, 55, 76-78, 331]. The defect is thus expressed as a deficiency in the O_2^--forming NADPH oxidase of the phagocyte plasma membrane. The active oxidase itself, however, is generated from a dormant precursor by an activation process that appears to require at least two sequential steps [96, 97], each presumably catalyzed by a different enzyme. Thus, the deficiency in oxidase activity seen in CGD could theoretically result from a lesion in any one of these elements. Present evidence suggests that most cases of CGD are due to defects in the activating apparatus, although at least one patient seems to have an abnormal oxidase [331a].

The most common form of CGD is the X-linked variety. Studies to date have suggested that a defect in activation is the explanation for the respiratory burst abnormality in this condition. When normal phagocytes are exposed to an activating stimulus, alterations in transmembrane potentials seem to take place whose nature depends on the stimulus employed: phorbol myristate acetate causes a depolarization followed by a return toward base line potentials,[4] while the chemotactic peptide FMetLeuPhe and the calcium ionophore A23187 cause depolarization exclusively [122, 123] (Fig. 90-15). With FMetLeuPhe and A23187, these potential changes precede the onset of the respiratory burst, but they sometimes follow the onset of the burst when phorbol is used as the stimulus. Cells from patients with X-linked CGD do not depolarize in response to

---

[4] At least part of the apparent return to baseline potentials has recently been shown to be an artifact [331b].

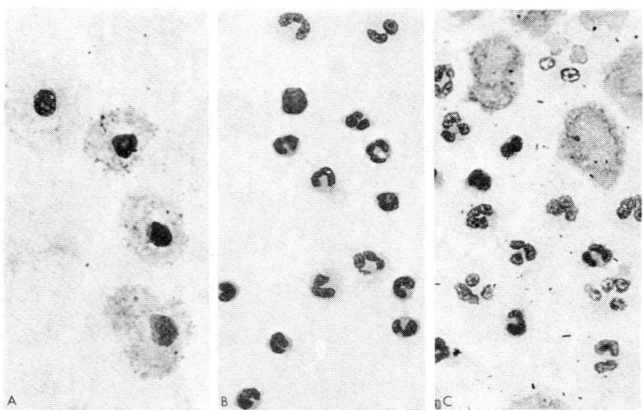

Figure 90-14 NBT slide test for diagnosis of CGD. A drop of blood is placed on an endotoxin-coated cover slip and incubated to allow the granulocytes and monocytes to adhere to the glass surface. The cover slip is then incubated with a solution of serum and NBT dye, then washed, fixed, counterstained, and mounted. *A.* Normal control; all the granulocytes are NBT-positive and appear as large, degenerated cells with pale-blue cytoplasm. *B.* CGD patient; none of the granulocytes are NBT-positive. The neutrophils retain their typical morphologic appearance and contain no blue (reduced) dye. *C.* Carrier of CGD. Two populations of cells coexist. Some granulocytes are NBT-positive and others are negative.

FMetLeuPhe or phorbol myristate acetate [122, 123], though the response to A23187 is normal [123]. The delay in depolarization with phorbol and the normality of the depolarization response in A23187-treated CGD cells are findings that dissociate the membrane potential change from the activation of the oxidase. Thus both phenomena are consequences of a third event, hitherto undetected, but the fact that membrane potential changes and O_2^- production are both altered under some circumstances suggests that CGD in these patients is due to a defect in the activation process rather than in the oxidase itself.

An interesting finding that may be related to the activation defect in X-linked chronic granulomatous disease is the absence of a low potential [332] b-type cytochrome from the plasma membrane of phagocytes from some [333, 333a, 334] but not all [334, 335] patients with this condition. This cytochrome, a major component of the plasma membrane according to one group of workers [332, 335a] but located mainly in the granules according to another [130c], is detected by the appearance of peaks at 429, 530, and 559 nm in the difference spectrum of dithionite-reduced vs. unreduced neutrophil membranes [336, 337]. With preparations from some CGD cells this difference spectrum is not seen, indicating that the cytochrome is probably missing from these cells. It is unlikely that this cytochrome is directly responsible for O_2^- production, because it is not reduced by either NADH or NADPH [130a, 332]. Further evidence against the direct participation of the cytochrome in respiratory burst O_2^- production is the fact that it forms a tight complex with carbon monoxide [332, 336, 337], an agent that has no effect on the respiratory burst [338]. Nevertheless, the possibility that the cytochrome plays some role in the respiratory burst is intriguing in view of its connection with chronic granulomatous disease. The nature of this role remains to be determined.

Another category of patients with CGD are those whose cells produce O_2^- in response to some but not other stimuli [96, 97]. In these patients the case for a defect in activation is solid. The ability of cells from these patients to express a re-

spiratory burst, albeit under restricted circumstances, shows that the oxidase is present and functioning normally. The fact that some stimuli can trigger the burst while others cannot places the metabolic lesion in the activation apparatus—specifically, in the portion of the activating apparatus that responds exclusively to those stimuli which fail to activate the defective cells.

Finally, a patient has been described in whom the oxidase itself appears to be defective. Neutrophils from this patient, a 5-year-old male, are able to respond to stimuli but generate O_2^- at less than 5 percent the normal rate. Studies with the cell-free O_2^--forming system from this patient have shown that the K_m of the oxidase for NADPH is about 10 times the normal value. The disease in this patient can thus be attributed to a low affinity oxidase which cannot generate adequate quantities of oxidants from physiologic concentrations of NADPH [331a]. This patient not only provides the first example of CGD in which the lesion resides in the oxidase itself, but also indicates that phagocytes probably contain only one O_2^--forming respiratory burst oxidase.

These forms of CGD are classified in Table 90-5, and a scheme rationalizing their biochemical features is presented in Fig. 90-16. This scheme is hypothetical, the sole purpose being to provide a logical interpretation of the largely indirect biochemical observations available at present. Further investigation will establish the extent to which it corresponds to reality.

Treatment   The management of CGD is supportive and directed at the prevention and treatment of infections. Presently there is no method available for correcting the neutrophil abnormality in vivo. Prophylactic oral antibiotics are usually prescribed for CGD patients. In our experience, the combination of a penicillinase-resistant penicillin plus trimethoprim-sulfamethoxazole and the anticandidal agent nystatin has been associated with decrease in the incidence of acute bacterial and candidal infections. No prospective controlled studies have been carried out.

Acute bacterial infections must be treated with an appropriate antibiotic. Every attempt must be made to identify the offending microorganism(s) and determine its (their) sensitivity. Aspiration or biopsy of infected sites is recommended. Antibiotics must be given parenterally in high doses for prolonged periods of time (6 to 8 weeks) in order to prevent relapses as viable microorganisms are released from degenerating phagocytes. Granulocyte transfusions have been administered to some patients with bacterial [339, 340], fungal [284], and other [290] infections. Their efficacy in CGD has not been established, but it seems reasonable to administer them to seriously ill, acutely infected patients.

Patients with large inflammatory masses which cause pain or obstructive symptoms generally benefit from surgical

Table 90-5   A classification of chronic granulomatous disease

Type	Defect	Transmission
1	Failure of activation by all stimuli	X-linked, ? autosomal recessive
2	Failure of activation by some stimuli	Autosomal recessive
3	Abnormal NADPH oxidase	X-linked

removal of the mass. Often no infecting microorganism can be found by pathologic examination or culture [308].

Bone marrow transplantation has been employed with limited success in selected cases [341].

Leukocyte Glucose-6-Phosphate Dehydrogenase Deficiency

Patients with severe leukocyte G-6-PD deficiency have increased susceptibility to infections and abnormal phagocytic function resembling that of patients with CGD [87, 88]. Clinically significant *leukocyte* G-6-PD deficiency, however, is very rare compared with clinically significant *erythrocyte* G-6-PD deficiency, which is a relatively common cause of hemolytic anemia (see Chap. 74). This discrepancy arises from the properties of the various mutant enzymes.

G-6-PD in leukocytes and G-6-PD in erythrocytes are under the control of the same gene [342]. Therefore, the leukocytes of an individual with one of the many erythrocyte G-6-PD vari-

ants will contain the same variant enzyme. The degree to which leukocyte function is impaired in G-6-PD deficiency depends on the properties of the variant.

In some instances, the properties of the variant enzyme are such that leukocyte function is unaffected. This is the case, for example, in the common A− type of G-6-PD deficiency seen in black patients. The enzyme in these individuals is normal in function and is synthesized in normal amounts but is moderately unstable. With this variant, erythrocyte G-6-PD activity is reduced because of the decay of the enzyme during the aging of the long-lived red blood cell. The neutrophil has a life-span which is too short to allow clinically significant decay of this mildly unstable variant.

There are other G-6-PD variants which, because of severe functional defects, low rates of synthesis, or marked instability, show extremely low levels within neutrophils as well as erythrocytes. In these cases, neutrophil function may be impaired owing to the deficiency of G-6-PD. The deficiency must be very marked for this to occur, because neutrophils contain a great excess of G-6-PD activity over that which is required to produce enough NADPH to sustain the respiratory burst. Even individuals with only 20 percent of expected leukocyte G-6-PD activity show no susceptibility to infections [343] and have normal metabolic and bactericidal capability [343, 344]. One individual with leukocyte G-6-PD activity of 5 percent did have abnormal leukocyte function in vitro but did not have a history of recurrent or unusually severe infections [86].

For the foregoing reasons, clinically significant leukocyte G-6-PD deficiency is extremely rare. Only four such patients, including three brothers, have been reported. All had undetectable levels of leukocyte G-6-PD activity [87, 88]. Three had recurrent infections which began during adolescence or adulthood. The fourth did not have frequent infections, but had not yet reached adolescence. Only one of the patients had serious, life-threatening infections. The pathogenic organisms, when identified, were similar to those which affect patients with CGD. All these patients had extremely low levels of *erythrocyte* G-6-PD activity, with consequent congenital nonspherocytic hemolytic anemia. Thus, severe leukocyte G-6-PD deficiency, like CGD, is characterized clinically by susceptibility to infections by catalase-positive microorganisms, although infections are less frequent and less severe than in patients with CGD. Leukocyte G-6-PD deficiency is X-linked and is always associated with severe erythrocyte G-6-PD deficiency.

Neutrophil function tests in such patients are similar to those in CGD [87, 88]. G-6-PD deficiency neutrophils exhibit normal particle ingestion and degranulation. Bactericidal assays reveal defective killing of catalase-positive bacteria but normal killing of catalase-negative species. Reduction of NBT dye is decreased. The metabolic accompaniments of phagocytosis, such as oxygen consumption, hydrogen peroxide production, and HMP shunt stimulation, do not occur. In contrast to the situation in CGD, there is no HMP shunt augmentation by methylene blue, indicating a defect in the shunt itself [87].

The presence of severe leukocyte G-6-PD deficiency may be suspected on demonstrating low erythrocyte G-6-PD activity in a patient with recurrent infections and failure of the respiratory burst. The diagnosis is confirmed by assay of the enzyme in the patient's leukocytes. Management is directed at prevention and early aggressive treatment of infections. It should be noted that sulfonamides and certain other anti-

Figure 90-15 Membrane potential changes occurring on exposure of normal and CGD neutrophils to various respiratory burst stimuli.

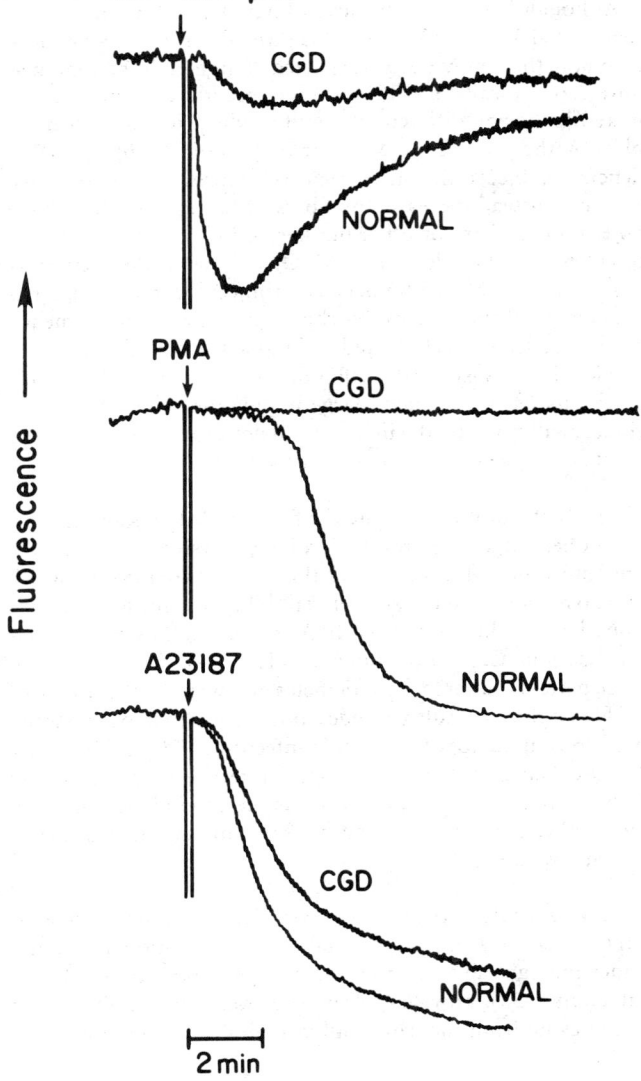

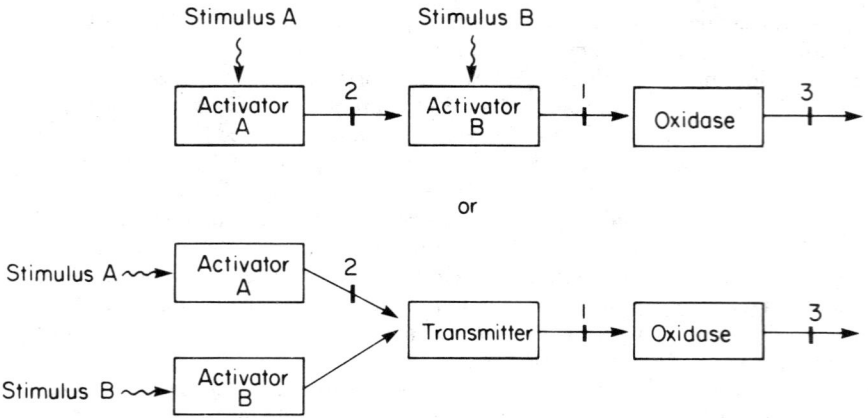

Figure 90-16 Possible sites of enzymatic lesions in various types of chronic granulomatous disease.

microbial drugs may exacerbate the hemolytic process in G-6-PD–deficient patients.

Metabolic Basis of the Functional Abnormalities in G-6-PD Deficiency   The CGD-like phenotype in severe glucose-6-phosphate dehydrogenase deficiency almost certainly results from the inability of the deficient cells to maintain normal intracellular NADPH levels during the respiratory burst. NADPH in phagocytes is provided mainly by the HMP shunt, a metabolic pathway whose activity depends on the level of activity of its first enzyme, glucose-6-phosphate dehydrogenase. In normal human phagocytes undergoing a respiratory burst, this enzyme is capable of supplying NADPH at a rate sufficient both to maintain O_2^- production and to support the antioxidant systems of the cell. With reduced levels of G-6-PD, the regeneration of NADPH will not keep up with its consumption during a full respiratory burst, and intracellular NADPH will drop rapidly.[5] As the NADPH concentration falls, the respiratory burst will slow until a concentration is reached at which the consumption of NADPH is equal to its production. This sequence of events explains why neutrophils containing G-6-PD at 5 percent of normal levels showed both a major reduction in NADPH concentration and a sharply decreased respiratory burst [86]. It is, therefore, not unexpected that sufficiently low levels of leukocyte G-6-PD will lead to a clinical syndrome resembling CGD.

Myeloperoxidase Deficiency

Myeloperoxidase (MPO) deficiency is an inherited condition characterized by the total absence of this heme-containing enzyme from the azurophil granules of neutrophils and mononuclear phagocytes. This results in an impairment of the in vitro microbicidal capacity of the phagocytes. Despite the laboratory abnormality, individuals with MPO deficiency are usually healthy and do not suffer from recurrent or severe infections unless there are additional predisposing factors.

Incidence and Genetics   MPO deficiency is inherited as an autosomal recessive trait. This has been demonstrated in several family studies [13, 345], the most comprehensive of which involved 28 relatives of an MPO-deficient Portuguese

woman [345]. In this family the proband had no detectable MPO in her neutrophils or monocytes. Her parents, children, and several other close relatives had values which were intermediate between those of the patient and a control population. The authors concluded on the basis of this large family study that MPO deficiency is an autosomal recessive condition, a conclusion which had been suggested by previous studies of nine relatives of another proband [13] and is consistent with subsequent investigations [346–346b].

Although fewer than 20 cases of MPO deficiency have been reported [13, 165, 328, 345–351], the disorder may be more common than previously suspected. Large-scale screening is now economically feasible using a recently developed automated leukocyte differential counter which identifies neutrophils by the presence of MPO activity [346–346b]. In MPO-deficient subjects, this instrument recognizes few neutrophils, showing instead increased numbers of large cells which have no enzyme activity or other marker and which appear to represent neutrophils devoid of MPO. Following the identification of a possible MPO-deficient subject by the automated counter, confirmation by biochemical assay or other means can be carried out. This rapid technique has already identified previously unsuspected MPO-deficient individuals [346–346b]. Its use in screening large populations of healthy individuals will generate the information necessary to calculate the exact incidence of MPO deficiency.

Clinical Course   Despite the fact that MPO is an essential component of an important microbicidal system in the neutrophil, most individuals who lack this enzyme are in good health and do not show an unusual susceptibility to infections. Exceptions have included a few MPO-deficient adults who developed serious C. albicans infections [13, 345, 346b]. Some of these patients suffered from diabetes and were on therapy with oral hypoglycemic sulfonamides, both of which may constitute predisposing factors to Candida infections [345, 352]. Other MPO-deficient patients developed infections of underlying skin disorders. Striking, however, is the general well-being of most MPO-deficient individuals. This is in marked contrast to patients with CGD.

Laboratory Features   Neutrophils from individuals with MPO deficiency appear normal with conventional staining under the light and electron microscopes. Special histochemical stains [353], however, clearly demonstrate the absence of this enzyme from the azurophil granules. Investigation of the

---

[5] The normal neutrophil contains only enough NADPH to support a full respiratory burst for 10 s, in the absence of a regenerating system.

neutrophil function of MPO-deficient subjects has revealed normal chemotaxis [13, 349], normal phagocytosis of bacteria and fungi [13, 349], a normal complement of other granule enzymes, and normal degranulation [13].

Bacterial killing is delayed compared with normal cells but is ultimately complete [13, 170, 171, 346a]. This is shown in Fig. 90-17 which compares killing of *S. aureus* by MPO-deficient neutrophils with that of normal and CGD cells. During the first hour of incubation MPO-deficient neutrophils killed only 15 percent of the bacteria killed by normal control neutrophils over the same interval. After 3 h there were no significant differences between the two assays with respect to the number of viable bacteria. This was in contrast to the results obtained with CGD cells, in which bacteria survived within the phagocytes for long periods of time.

Fungicidal activity of MPO-deficient neutrophils is more seriously impaired than bactericidal activity [13]. During the first hour of incubation with *Candida* species, MPO-deficient neutrophils killed virtually none of the fungi, whereas normal neutrophils killed about a third of the original number. In neither case was there significant fungicidal activity after 1 h of incubation. Despite the failure to kill the *Candida*, MPO-deficient neutrophils are capable of inhibiting their intracellular germination. CGD neutrophils lack this candidastatic effect [354].

The ability of MPO-deficient neutrophils to fix radioactive I⁻ to ingested microorganisms in vitro is virtually absent [12, 170, 182, 184, 349]. This is similar to the situation in CGD. In the latter condition, iodination is defective because the neutrophils fail to generate the necessary hydrogen peroxide, whereas in MPO deficiency the iodination defect results from the lack of the enzyme required to catalyze the halogenation reaction. Thus, the important $MPO-H_2O_2$-halide microbicidal system is totally nonfunctional in both MPO-deficient and CGD neutrophils. Yet the bactericidal and candidastatic defects in CGD are much more severe than in MPO deficiency, an in vitro obser-

vation which is entirely borne out clinically. It has been postulated that MPO-independent oxygen-requiring microbicidal systems, which kill slowly but completely, are responsible for the mildness of the microbicidal defect in MPO deficiency (see below) [170].

The respiratory burst is exaggerated in MPO-deficient cells [170, 326, 355]. The rates of oxidant formation are initially comparable in normal and MPO-deficient cells, but in the latter, oxidant production continues for a longer period of time than in normal cells. This results in substantial increases in total oxygen consumption, superoxide and hydrogen peroxide production, and HMP shunt activity in MPO deficiency (Fig. 90-18) [170, 326].

In contrast, chemiluminescence in MPO-deficient cells is initially decreased, indicating a role for MPO in light-emitting oxidation reactions [326]. By 90 min, however, light emission by MPO-deficient cells is greater than normal, presumably because of the protracted respiratory burst in these cells. Both MPO-dependent and MPO-independent reactions seem to play a role in chemiluminescence by phagocytosing neutrophils. In CGD, neither of these types of light-emitting reactions can occur, since both are contingent on a normal respiratory burst.

The Metabolic Defect in Myeloperoxidase Deficiency

In physiologic terms the most significant abnormality in myeloperoxidase-deficient cells is their inability to generate the potent antimicrobial oxidant OCl⁻. Failure to manufacture this agent leads to the characteristic microbicidal defect in these cells [170]. This defect has been reproduced in a model system which uses xanthine oxidase and acetaldehyde to generate O_2^- radicals [137]. When *S. aureus* are added to this model system, they are killed slowly but thoroughly, survival falling to 1 percent after an hour of incubation. Bacterial killing is greatly accelerated by the addition of myeloperoxidase (Fig. 90-19). A striking similarity is seen between rates of killing by normal and myeloperoxidase-deficient neutrophils on one hand and the complete and myeloperoxidase-deficient model system on the other. This similarity, and the contrast between the susceptibility of *S. aureus* to myeloperoxidase-deficient cells and their resistance to CGD cells, provide strong evidence for the importance of oxidizing radicals as a backup system for bacterial killing, serving as the primary oxygen-dependent microbicidal system when the more potent myeloperoxidase-dependent system is lacking.

One organism against which oxidizing radicals seem not to be very effective is *C. albicans*. As mentioned above, myeloperoxidase-deficient cells kill this organism poorly even in long incubations [13, 356], a result to be contrasted with that seen with *S. aureus*. OCl⁻ thus seems to be the critical microbicidal oxidant for the destruction of this fungus, with secondary killing mainly by relatively ineffective cationic proteins which do not require oxygen for their activity [356]. This may explain the susceptibility of certain myeloperoxidase-deficient patients to infections by *C. albicans*.

In MPO deficiency, the microbicidal oxidizing radicals may be present in greater than usual amounts because of the increase in respiratory burst activity seen in this condition [170, 326, 355]. This increase in the burst is probably secondary to the improved survival of the O_2^--forming oxidase that results from the absence of myeloperoxidase from these cells [16]. Measurements of oxidase survival have not been made

Figure 90-17 The defect in microbial killing in myeloperoxidase-deficient neutrophils.

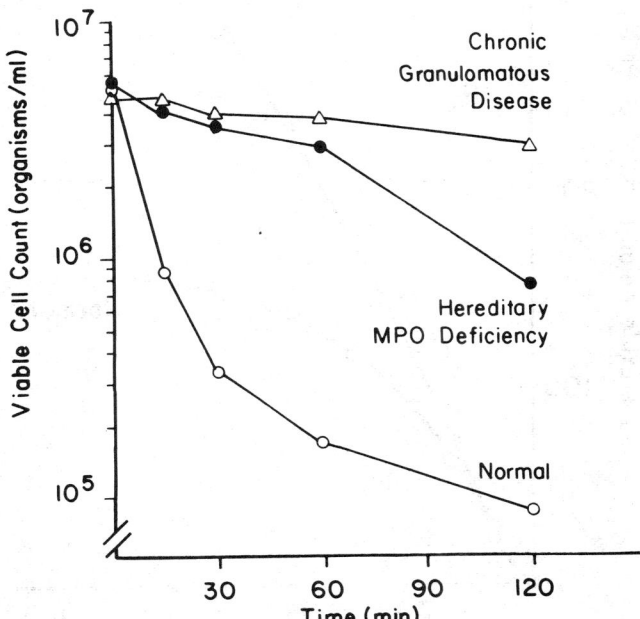

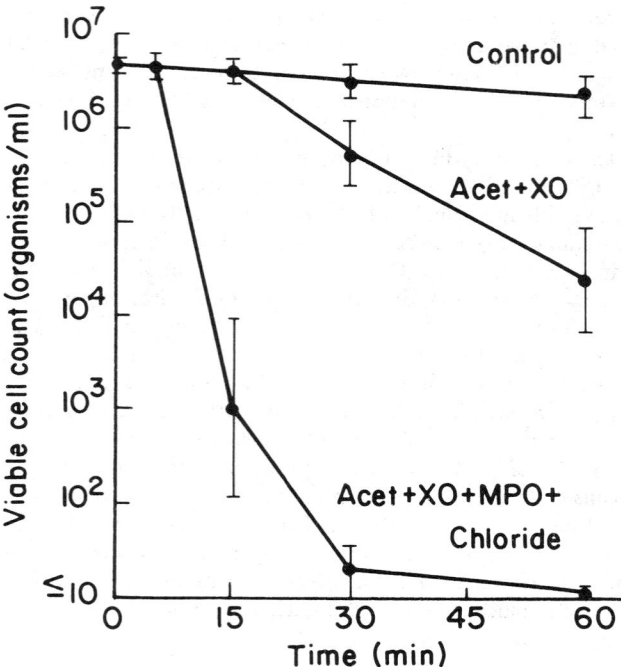

Figure 90-18 Microbicidal activity of xanthine oxidase plus acetaldehyde in the absence and presence of myeloperoxidase.

with myeloperoxidase-deficient neutrophils themselves, but inhibitors of myeloperoxidase are known to provide the O_2^--forming enzyme with substantial protection against oxygen-mediated inactivation. The fact that the respiratory burst is augmented in MPO-deficient cells may thus offset, at least in part, the microbicidal defect resulting from the absence of this potent antimicrobial enzyme from the phagocyte.

Other manifestations of myeloperoxidase activity are also absent from myeloperoxidase-deficient cells. The incorporation of radioactive I^- into proteins does not take place [12, 170, 182, 184] (see above) because the cells cannot oxidize I^-. Reactions which probably involve OCl^- as the oxidant also fail to occur. These include the oxidation of phenols and aromatic amines such as guaiacol, benzidine, and dianisidine, whose colored reaction products have been used to quantify myeloperoxidase activity, and the coupling of estrogens to macromolecules [357], a reaction that might involve an initial oxidation of the phenolic A ring followed by nonenzymatic addition of the reactive product to suitable amino acid residues. The release of ethylene from 2-keto-4-methylthiobutyric acid, an index of oxidizing radical production, is also decreased by a factor of 10 [214]; the biochemical basis for this finding has been discussed (see page 1958).

Despite many functional studies on myeloperoxidase-deficient cells, little is known about the defect in enzymologic terms. In one patient with hereditary myeloperoxidase deficiency, the enzyme was missing by both functional and immunologic assays, and the characteristic spectrum of its heme moiety was not seen [147]. The protein was therefore completely absent from the cells, indicating either a failure of synthesis or the production of a highly unstable variant that was inactivated and destroyed rapidly enough to leave no traces of its presence. Studies on the nature of the enzymologic defect in more recently reported patients remain to be published.

Treatment   There is no specific treatment for MPO defi-

ciency, although the tendency of some of these individuals to develop *Candida* infections should be recognized.

Glutathione Reductase Deficiency

The glutathione system has a role in protecting phagocytes against oxidative damage by the highly reactive compounds which are generated during the respiratory burst. In the process of detoxifying these compounds, glutathione (GSH) is oxidized to its dimer, GSSG. Glutathione reductase catalyzes the reconversion of GSSG to GSH, thereby maintaining the levels of reduced glutathione in the phagocyte.

Many patients have been reported with partial deficiencies of glutathione reductase, but in most of these the low enzyme activity seems to have resulted from dietary riboflavin deficiency with consequent depletion of the flavin cofactor of the enzyme [244]. One family has been reported, however, in which decreased glutathione reductase activity was due to a true enzyme deficiency [358, 359]. In this family the levels of glutathione reductase in the neutrophils and monocytes of the three children were reduced to 10 to 15 percent of normal. The parents, who were first cousins, each had half of the normal activity of this enzyme. The erythrocytes of the family members showed similar but more severe decreases in glutathione reductase. Glutathione reductase activity did not improve following the administration of riboflavin in vivo or the addition of FAD to the reaction mixture in vitro, thus excluding riboflavin deficiency as a cause of the abnormality. These findings

Figure 90-19 O_2^- production by myeloperoxidase-deficient neutrophils.

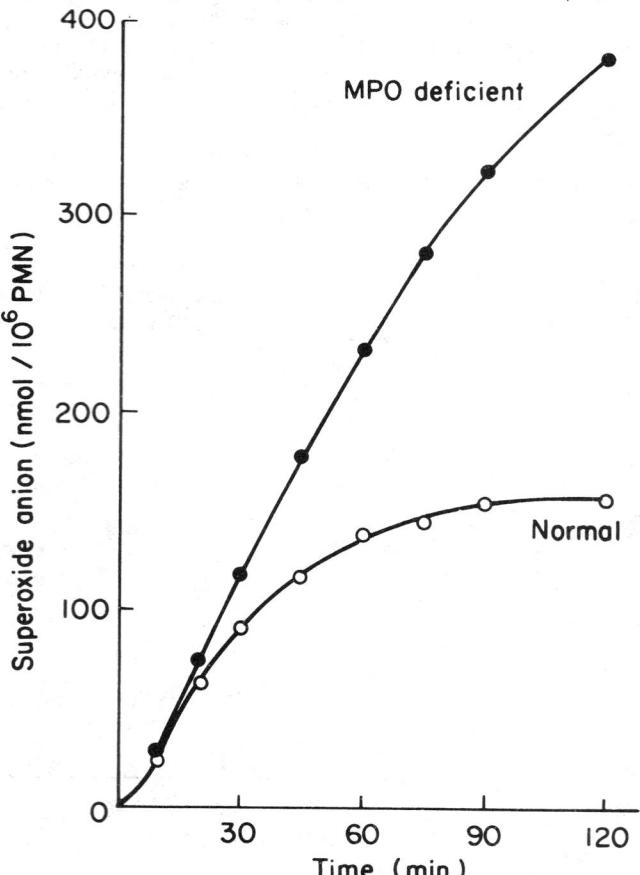

suggest that the glutathione reductase in erythrocytes and leukocytes is encoded by the same gene and that the enzyme deficiency is inherited as an autosomal recessive trait.

As to clinical manifestations, none of the family members had unusually frequent or severe bacterial infections. The two older sibs had juvenile cataracts and deafness. Although none had chronic hemolytic anemia, one sib developed a hemolytic crisis following the ingestion of fava beans.

The neutrophils of the glutathione reductase–deficient subjects were normal in appearance and showed normal chemotaxis, phagocytosis, and degranulation. Microbicidal capacity was normal at low ratios of bacteria to neutrophils but was moderately impaired at bacteria/neutrophil ratios of 18:1 and greater [359].

The major functional abnormality involved the respiratory burst [359]. Oxygen consumption and H_2O_2 production during phagocytosis by glutathione reductase–deficient neutrophils were normal for the first 5 min but thereafter fell rapidly to zero, in contrast to normal phagocytosing cells in which these proceed at a rapid rate for more than 15 min. Similarly, iodination of zymosan particles, which depends on the availability of H_2O_2, was initially normal and then decreased rapidly. HMP shunt activity did not achieve a rate comparable with that of normal cells during the early postphagocytic period. In addition, it diminished more quickly than normal. The HMP shunt was adequately stimulated by methylene blue, ruling out a primary defect in the shunt itself as the cause of its decreased activity in glutathione reductase–deficient cells. Paradoxically, O_2^- production over 30 min was normal. The explanation for this paradox lies in the method of assay, as will be seen below, and provides the key to the pathophysiology of the respiratory burst abnormality seen in this condition.

Metabolic Basis of Functional Abnormality on Glutathione Reductase Deficiency

The functional abnormality in the neutrophils from patients with glutathione reductase deficiency seems to reflect the inability of these cells to deal normally with H_2O_2 [359]. When the respiratory burst in these cells was measured by a technique that prevented the accumulation of H_2O_2 (the cytochrome c assay for O_2^- production, a method in which the O_2^- is prevented from undergoing dismutation and instead is converted exclusively to oxygen), it was of normal duration. Other methods of measuring the respiratory burst permitted H_2O_2 to accumulate. When the burst was measured by these methods, it lasted only 3 to 5 min. Furthermore, incubation of these cells with H_2O_2 prior to activation led to a substantial attenuation of the respiratory burst, an effect not seen with normal neutrophils. It seems likely that the abbreviated burst was due to the accumulation of endogenously manufactured H_2O_2 in the defective cell, leading to inactivation of the O_2^--forming oxidase, which has been shown experimentally to be highly susceptible to oxidative destruction [16].

Accumulation of H_2O_2 in the defective cell is probably due to a deficiency in GSH that develops during the course of the respiratory burst [66]. The primary H_2O_2-detoxifying enzyme in the cytoplasm of the phagocyte is glutatione peroxidase, the activity of which results in conversion of GSH to GSSG. In the normal cell GSSG formed in this reaction is rapidly converted back to GSH by the action of glutathione reductase, and so levels of GSH and GSSG remain relatively constant even during the respiratory burst. In deficient cells, GSH levels fell rapidly during the respiratory burst (Fig. 90-20) because the activ-

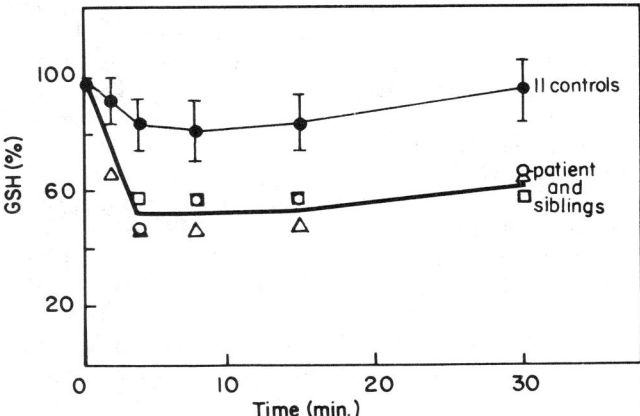

Figure 90-20 Glutathione levels during the respiratory burst in glutathione reductase–deficient neutrophils.

ity of glutathione reductase was not great enough to maintain a normal concentration of GSH in the face of the oxidative challenge posed by the burst. It is probable that when the GSH level fell sufficiently, the glutathione peroxidase reaction could no longer keep up with H_2O_2 load entering the cytoplasm. H_2O_2 then accumulated, and the respiratory burst oxidase was inactivated.

Glutathione Synthetase Deficiency

Abnormalities in the glutathione system may result from decreased synthesis of glutathione, a tripeptide synthesized in two energy-dependent steps as shown below:

$$\text{Glutamic acid + cysteine + ATP} \longrightarrow \gamma\text{-glutamyl-cysteine + ADP}$$

$$\gamma\text{-Glutamyl-cysteine + ATP} \longrightarrow \text{glutathione + ADP}$$

The first step is catalyzed by γ-glutamyl-cysteine synthetase and the second by glutathione synthetase. Deficiency of the latter enzyme leads to a disorder in which phagocyte function may be impaired [254, 360–362].

Congenital glutathione synthetase deficiency is inherited as an autosomal recessive disorder. It gives rise to two distinct clinical syndromes whose differences have been attributed to genetic heterogeneity among the glutathione synthetase mutations [360]. One type causes isolated congenital hemolytic anemia due to low levels of glutathione in erythrocytes. In this variant, leukocyte glutathione is only slightly reduced. This type of glutathione synthetase deficiency is due to an unstable mutant enzyme that reaches functionally inadequate levels only in the erythrocytes. This situation is analogous to that of the unstable G-6-PD variants (see above).

Patients with the second type of glutathione synthetase deficiency, which can be caused by at least two different mutant enzymes [361], have a clinically more severe disorder and show significant abnormalities of leukocyte glutathione metabolism. Their major clinical manifestation is a severe metabolic acidosis due to extremely high levels of 5-oxoproline in the plasma. Large amounts of this metabolite are also excreted in the urine [361]. The increased production of 5-oxoproline results from overactivity of γ-glutamyl-cysteine synthetase, the first enzyme in the glutathione synthetic pathway. Its increased activity is caused by diminished intracellular levels of glutathione, the feedback inhibitor of the enzyme. The consequence is an accumulation of γ-glutamyl-cysteine, the substrate for glutathione synthetase. This compound cannot be converted to glutathione because of the deficiency of glutathione synthetase, and so it is metabolized via an alternative pathway to 5-oxoproline, whose accumulation causes severe acidosis (see Chap. 17).

Another manifestation in these patients is a congenital hemolytic anemia. This anemia is similar to that seen in the other type of glutathione synthetase deficiency.

Abnormalities of leukocyte glutathione metabolism have been demonstrated in several patients with the oxoprolinuric type of glutathione synthetase deficiency [254, 360–362]. Glutathione synthetase activity and the levels of reduced glutathione are very low in the leukocytes of individuals with this disorder. Neutrophil function studies were performed in one such patient, who had frequent episodes of otitis media accompanied on several occasions by severe neutropenia [254]. These studies revealed normal chemotaxis, phagocytosis, NBT dye reduction, and HMP shunt stimulation. Following phagocytosis, excessive hydrogen peroxide was released into the extracellular medium, suggesting impaired ability to detoxify this oxidant compound. Fixation of radioactive iodide to protein was reduced to 25 percent of normal. Bacterial killing capacity was also decreased.

Because vitamin E has a role in detoxifying oxidant compounds and preventing damage to neutrophils during phagocytosis, a therapeutic trial of vitamin E (400 IU of alphatocopherol daily by mouth) was given to this patient [254]. The functional abnormalities of the granulocytes were corrected, and the episodes of infection and neutropenia ceased. Accordingly, vitamin E should be considered as treatment in symptomatic patients with severe glutathione synthetase deficiency. The metabolic acidosis has been successfully managed with oral sodium bicarbonate [361].

Metabolic Basis of Functional Abnormalities in Oxoprolinuric Glutathione Synthetase Deficiency. Contrary to the situation in glutathione reductase deficiency, the respiratory burst in glutathione synthetase deficiency is intact [256, 364]. This may be related to the fact that glutathione, although present at greatly diminished levels, can be maintained in the reduced form by the action of glutathione reductase, thereby affording adequate protection against oxidant stress. The functional abnormalities in this condition appear rather to result from defects in the behavior of microtubules. Microtubules are cytoskeletal elements whose purpose seems to be to impose spatial organization on cell motility and the locations and movements of subcellular organelles [363–369]. Their arrangement within the cell is fluid, and they assemble and reassemble to form networks of varying configurations depending on the activity in which the cell is engaged. This process of assembly and disassembly is connected in some way with glutathione metabolism [63, 65]. In glutathione synthetase–deficient neutrophils, microtubule assembly is disrupted [254, 362, 370], presumably because the glutathione which is required for orderly microtubule behavior is not present in sufficient amounts. It is thought that the abnormalities in motility, granule function, and bacterial killing that are observed in this condition are attributable to the disruption in microtubule function that occurs as a result of the abnormality in glutathione production.

Other Disorders of Neutrophil Function

Reports that have been questioned on technical grounds [371]

have stated that glutathione peroxidase deficiency causes a clinical picture resembling chronic granulomatous disease [318, 372, 373]. The questions raised about these reports, together with animal experiments showing that total glutathione peroxidase deficiency induced by selenium deprivation is compatible with a normal respiratory burst [252, 374], suggest that judgment should be reserved as to whether this condition causes neutrophil dysfunction.

A study was carried out on neutrophil function in a patient with congenital acatalasia [242]. The only abnormality found in these cells was an unusual susceptibility to damage by exogenous H_2O_2. The respiratory burst was entirely normal, as were other neutrophil functions including chemotaxis, phagocytosis, degranulation, and bacterial killing. These findings confirm that the glutathione reductase–glutathione peroxidase system is primarily responsible for the destruction of endogenously generated H_2O_2.

Supported in part by USPHS Grant NO. AI 11827.

REFERENCES

1. BALDRIDGE CW, GERARD RW: The extra respiration of phagocytosis. *Am J Physiol* 103:235, 1933
2. METCHNIKOFF E: Untersuchungen über die intracellulare verdauung bei wirbellosen thieren. *Arb Zoologischen Inst Univ Wien*, 5:141, 1883
3. SBARRA AJ, KARNOVSKY ML: The biochemical basis of phagocytosis. I. Metabolic changes during the ingestion of particles by polymorphonuclear leukocytes. *J Biol Chem* 234:1355, 1959
4. IYER GYN, ISLAM MF, QUASTEL JH: Biochemical aspects of phagocytosis. *Nature* 192:535, 1961
5. STÄHELIN H, KARNOVSKY ML, FARNHAM AE, SUTER E: Studies on the interaction between phagocytes and tubercle bacilli. III. Some metabolic effects in guinea pigs associated with infection with tubercle bacilli. *J Exp Med* 105:265, 1957
6. BERENDES H, BRIDGES RA, GOOD RA: A fatal granulomatosis of childhood: The clinical study of a new syndrome. *Minn Med* 40:309, 1957
7. LANDING BH, SHIRKEY HS: Syndrome of recurrent infection and infiltration of viscera by pigmented lipid histiocytes. *Pediatrics* 20:431, 1957
8. HOLMES B, PAGE AR, GOOD RA: Studies of the metabolic activity of leukocytes from patients with a genetic abnormality of phagocyte function. *J Clin Invest* 46:1422, 1967
9. BAEHNER RL, NATHAN DG: Leukocyte oxidase: Defective activity in chronic granulomatous disease. *Science* 155:835, 1967
10. AGNER K: Verdoperoxidase. A ferment isolated from leucocytes. *Acta Physiol Scand* 2(Suppl. 8) 1, 1941
11. KLEBANOFF SJ: A peroxidase-mediated antimicrobial system in leukocytes. *J Clin Invest* 46:1078, 1967
12. KLEBANOFF SJ: Iodination of bacteria: A bactericidal mechanism. *J Exp Med* 126:1063, 1967
13. LEHRER RI, CLINE MJ: Leukocyte myeloperoxidase deficiency and disseminated candidiasis: The role of myeloperoxidase in resistance to Candida infection. *J Clin Invest* 48:1478, 1969
14. BABIOR BM, KIPNES RS, CURNUTTE JT: Biological defense mechanisms: The production by leukocytes of superoxide, a potential bactericidal agent. *J Clin Invest* 52:741, 1973
15. CURNUTTE JT, BABIOR BM: Biological defense mechanisms. The effect of bacteria and serum on superoxide production by granulocytes. *J Clin Invest* 53:1662, 1974
16. JANDL RC, ANDRÉ-SCHWARTZ J, BORGES-DUBOIS L, KIPNES RS, McMURRICH BJ, BABIOR BM: Termination of the respiratory burst in human neutrophils. *J Clin Invest* 61:1176, 1978
17. SEGAL AW, COADE SB: Kinetics of oxygen consumption by phagocytosing human neutrophils. *Biochem Biophys Res Commun* 84:611, 1978
17a. BADWEY JA, CURNUTTE JT, ROBINSON JM, LAZDINS JR, BRIGGS RT, KARNOVSKY MJ, KARNOVSKY ML: Comparative aspects of oxidative metabolism of neutrophils from human blood and guinea pig peritonea: Magnitude of the respiratory burst, dependence upon stimulating agents, and localization of the oxidases. *J Cell Physiol* 105:541, 1980
18. JOHNSTON RB JR: Oxygen metabolism and the microbicidal activity of macrophages. *Fed Proc* 37:2759, 1978
19. TAUBER AI, GOETZL EJ, BABIOR BM: Unique characteristics of superoxide production by human eosinophils in eosinophilic states. *Inflammation* 3:261, 1979

20. DeChatelet LR, Shirley PS, McPhail LC, Huntley CC, Muss HB, Bass DA: Oxidative metabolism of the human eosinophil. *Blood* 50:525, 1977

21. Henderson WR, Kaliner M: Immunologic and nonimmunologic generation of superoxide from mast cells and basophils. *J Clin Invest* 61:187, 1978

22. Oren R, Farnham AE, Saito K, Milofsky E, Karnovsky ML: Metabolic patterns in three types of phagocytic cells. *J Cell Biol* 17:487, 1963

23. Baehner RL, Johnston RB Jr: Metabolic and bactericidal activities of human eosinophils. *Br J Haematol* 20:277, 1971

24. Weening RS, Roos D, Loos JA: Oxygen consumption of phagocytizing cells in human leukocyte and granulocyte preparations: A comparative study. *J Lab Clin Med* 83:570, 1974

25. Gabig TG, Bearman SI, Babior BM: Effects of oxygen tension and pH on the respiratory burst of human neutrophils. *Blood* 53:1133, 1979

26. Cohen MS, Metcalf JA, Root RK: Regulation of oxygen metabolism in human granulocytes: Relationship between stimulus binding and oxidative response using plant lectins as probes. *Blood* 55:1003, 1980

27. Zatti M, Rossi F: Relationship between glycolysis and respiration in surfactant-treated leukocytes. *Biochim Biophys Acta* 148:553, 1967

28. Repine JE, White JG, Clawson CC, Holmes BH: The influence of phorbol myristate acetate on oxygen consumption by polymorphonuclear leukocytes. *J Lab Clin Med* 83:911, 1974

29. Stjernholm R, Manek RC: Carbohydrate metabolism in leukocytes. XIV. Regulation of pentose cycle activity and glycogen metabolism during phagocytosis. *J Reticuloendothel Soc* 8:550, 1970

30. Davidson WD, Tanaka KR: Instantaneous and continuous measurement of phagocytosis stimulated glucose oxidation in human granulocytes by an ionization chamber method. *Br J Haematol* 25:783, 1973

31. Stossel TP, Mason RJ, Hartwig J, Vaughan M: Quantitative studies of phagocytosis by polymorphonuclear leukocytes: Use of emulsions to measure the initial rate of phagocytosis. *J Clin Invest* 51:615, 1972

32. Johnston RB, Keele BB, Misra HP, Lehmeyer JE, Webb LS, Baehner RL, Rajagopalan KV: The role of superoxide anion generation in phagocytic bactericidal activity. Studies with normal and chronic granulomatous disease leukocytes. *J Clin Invest* 55:1357, 1975

33. Weening RS, Wever R, Roos D: Quantitative aspects of the production of superoxide radicals by phagocytizing human granulocytes. *J Lab Clin Med* 85:245, 1975

34. Drath DB, Karnovsky ML: Superoxide production by phagocytic leukocytes. *J Exp Med* 141:257, 1975

35. Goldstein IM, Roos D, Kaplan HB, Weissmann G: Complement and immunoglobulins stimulate superoxide production by human leukocytes independently of phagocytosis. *J Clin Invest* 46:1155, 1975

36. Sagone AL Jr, King GW, Metz EN: A comparison of the metabolic response to phagocytosis in human granulocytes and monocytes. *J Clin Invest* 57:1352, 1976

37. Root RK, Metcalf JA: H_2O_2 release from human granulocytes during phagocytosis: Relationship to superoxide anion formation and cellular catabolism of H_2O_2: Studies with normal and cytochalasin B treated cells. *J Clin Invest* 60:1266, 1977

38. Klebanoff SJ, Durack DT, Rosen H, Clark RA: Functional studies on human peritoneal eosinophils. *Immun* 17:167, 1977

39. Nathan CF, Root RK: Hydrogen peroxide release from mouse peritoneal macrophages. Dependence on sequential activation and triggering. *J Exp Med* 146:1648, 1977

40. Cohen HJ, Chovaniec ME: Superoxide generation by digitonin-stimulated guinea pig granulocytes. A basis for a continuous assay for monitoring superoxide production and for the study of the activation of the generating system. *J Clin Invest* 61:1081, 1978

41. Diaz P, Jones DG, Kay AB: Histamine-coated particles generate superoxide (O_2^-) and chemiluminescence in alveolar macrophages. *Nature* 278:454, 1979

42. Holian A, Daniele RP: Stimulation of oxygen consumption and superoxide anion production in pulmonary macrophages by N-formylmethionyl peptides. *FEBS Lett* 108:47, 1979

43. Paul BB, Sbarra AJ: The role of the phagocyte in host parasite interactions. XIII. The direct quantitative estimation of H_2O_2 in phagocytizing cells. *Biochim Biophys Acta* 156:168, 1968

44. Baehner RL, Gilman N, Karnovsky ML: Respiration and glucose oxidation in human and guinea pig leukocytes: Comparative studies. *J Clin Invest* 49:692, 1970

45. Baehner RL, Murrmann SK, Davis J, Johnston RB Jr: The role of superoxide anion and hydrogen peroxide in phagocytosis-associated oxidative metabolic reactions. *J Clin Invest* 56:571, 1975

46. Homan-Müller JWT, Weening RS, Roos D: Production of hydrogen peroxide by phagocytizing human granulocytes. *J Lab Clin Med* 85:198, 1975

47. Root RK, Metcalf J, Oshino N, Chance B: H_2O_2 release from human granulocytes during phagocytosis. I. Documentation, quantitation, and some regulating factors. *J Clin Invest* 55:945, 1975

48. Johnston RB Jr, Godzik CA, Cohn ZA: Increased superoxide anion production by immunologically activated and chemically elicited macrophages. *J Exp Med* 148:115, 1978

49. Pabst MJ, Johnston RB Jr: Increased production of superoxide anion by macrophages exposed in vitro to muramyl dipeptide or lipopolysaccharide. *J Exp Med* 151:101, 1980

50. Curnutte JT, Kipnes RS, Babior BM: Defect in pyridine nucleotide dependent superoxide production by a particulate fraction from the granulocytes of patients with chronic granulomatous disease. *N Engl J Med* 293:628, 1975

51. Babior BM, Curnutte JT, McMurrich BJ: The particulate superoxide-forming system from human neutrophils. Properties of the system and further evidence supporting its participation in the respiratory burst. *J Clin Invest* 58:989, 1976

52. McPhail LC, DeChatelet LR, Johnston RB Jr: Generation of chemiluminescence by a particulate fraction isolated from human neutrophils. *J Clin Invest* 63:648, 1979

53. Cohen HJ, Newburger PE, Chovaniec ME: NAD(P)H-dependent superoxide production by phagocytic vesicles from guinea pig and human granulocytes. *J Biol Chem* 255:6584, 1980

54. Cohen HJ, Chovaniec ME, Davies WA: Activation of the guinea pig granulocyte NAD(P)H-dependent superoxide generating enzyme: Localization in a plasma membrane enriched particle and kinetics of activation. *Blood* 55:355, 1980

55. Suzuki Y, Lehrer RI: NAD(P)H oxidase activity in human neutrophils stimulated by phorbol myristate acetate. *J Clin Invest* 66:1409, 1980

56. Bielski BH, Allen AO: Mechanism of the disproportionation of superoxide radicals. *J Phys Chem* 81:1048, 1977

57. Fielden EM, Roberts PB, Bray RC, Lowe DT, Mautner GN, Rotilio G, Calabrese L: The mechanism of action of superoxide dismutase from pulse radiolysis and electron paramagnetic resonance. *Biochem J* 139:49, 1974

58. Selvaraj RJ, Sbarra AJ: The role of the phagocyte in host-parasite interactions. VII. Di- and triphosphopyridine nucleotide kinetics during phagocytosis. *Biochim Biophys Acta* 141:243, 1967

58a. Heyreman RA, Bauwens-Monbaliu D: Kinetics of nicotinamide adenine dinucleotides in oleate-stimulated polymorphonuclear leukocytes. *FEBS Lett* 127:87, 1981

58b. DeChatelet LR, McCall CE, Cooper MR, Shirley PS: NAD kinase in human polymorphonuclear leukocytes. *J Reticuloendothel Soc* 12:387, 1972

59. Beck WS: Occurrence and control of the phosphogluconate oxidation pathway in normal and leukemic leukocytes. *J Biol Chem* 232:271, 1958

60. Reed PW: Glutathione and the hexose monophosphate shunt in phagocytizing and hydrogen peroxide-treated rat leukocytes. *J Biol Chem* 244:2459, 1969

61. Strauss RR, Paul BB, Jacobs AA, Sbarra AJ: The role of the phagocyte in host-parasite interactions. XIX. Leukocytic glutathione reductase and its involvement in phagocytosis. *Arch Biochem Biophys* 135:265, 1969

62. Vogt MT, Thomas C, Vassallo CL, Basford RE, Gee JBL: Glutathione-dependent peroxidative metabolism in the alveolar macrophage. *J Clin Invest* 50:401, 1971

63. Oliver JM, Albertini DF, Berlin RD: Effects of glutathione-oxidizing agents on microtubule assembly and microtubule-dependent surface properties of human neutrophils. *J Cell Biol* 71:921, 1976

64. Stankova L, Rigas AD, Keown P, Bigley R: Leukocyte ascorbate and glutathione: Potential capacity for inactivating oxidants and free radicals. *J Reticuloendothel Soc* 21:97, 1977

65. Burchill BR, Oliver JM, Pearson CB, Leinbach ED, Berlin RD: Microtubule dynamics and glutathione metabolism in phagocytizing human polymorphonuclear leukocytes. *J Cell Biol* 76:439, 1978

66. Voetman AA, Loos JA, Roos D: Changes in the levels of glutathione in phagocytizing human neutrophils. *Blood* 55:741, 1980

67. Beck WS: The control of leukocyte glycolysis. *J Biol Chem* 232:251, 1958

68. Noble EP, Stjernholm RL, Weisberger AS: Carbohydrate metabolism in leukocytes. I. The pathway of two- and three-carbon compounds in the rabbit polymorphonuclear leukocyte. *J Biol Chem* 235:1261, 1960

69. Stjernholm R, Noble EP: Carbohydrate metabolism in leukocytes. II. The pathway of ribose and xylose metabolism in the rabbit polymorphonuclear leukocyte. *J Biol Chem* 236:614, 1961

70. Wood HG, Katz J, Landau BR: Estimation of pathways of carbohydrate metabolism. *Biochem Z* 238:809, 1963

70a. Nakamura M, Baxter CR, Masters BSS: Simultaneous demonstration of phagocytosis-connected oxygen consumption and corresponding NAD (P)H oxidase activity: Direct evidence for NADPH as the predominant electron donor to oxygen in phagocytizing human neutrophils. *Biochem Biophys Res Comm* 98:743, 1981

71. Iyer GYN, Quastel JH: NADPH and NADH oxidation by guinea pig polymorphonuclear leucocytes. *Can J Biochem Physiol* 41:427, 1963

72. Rossi F, Zatti M: Biochemical aspects of phagocytosis in polymorphonuclear leucocytes. NADH and NADPH oxidation by the granules of resting and phagocytizing cells. *Experientia* 20:21, 1964

73. Patriarca P, Cramer R, Moncalvo S, Rossi F, Romeo D: Enzymatic basis of metabolic stimulation in leucocytes during phagocytosis: The role of activated NADPH oxidase. *Arch Biochem Biophys* 145:255, 1971

74. Paul BB, Strauss RR, Jacobs AA, Sbarra AJ: Direct involvement of NADPH oxidase with the stimulated respiratory and hexosemonophosphate shunt activities in phagocytizing leukocytes. *Exp Cell Res* 73:456, 1972

75. Patriarca P, Dri P, Kakinuma K, Tedesco F, Rossi F: Studies on the mechanism of metabolic stimulation in polymorphonuclear leukocytes during phagocytosis. I. Evidence for superoxide anion involvement in the oxidation of NADPH. *Biochim Biophys Acta* 385:380, 1975

75a. Bellavite P, Berton G, Dri P: Studies on the NADPH oxidation by subcellular particles from phagocytising polymorphonuclear leucocytes. Evidence for the involvement of three mechanisms. *Biochim Biophys Acta* 591:434, 1980

76. Hohn DC, Lehrer RI: NADPH oxidase deficiency in X-linked chronic granulomatous disease. *J Clin Invest* 55:707, 1975

77. McPhail LC, DeChatelet LR, Shirley PS: Further characterization of NADPH oxidase activity of human polymorphonuclear leukocytes. *J Clin Invest* 58:774, 1976

78. Iverson D, DeChatelet LR, Spitznagel JK, Wang P: Comparison of NADH and NADPH oxidase activities in granules isolated from human polymorphonuclear leukocytes with a fluorimetric assay. *J Clin Invest* 59:282, 1977

78a. Hoffman M, Autor AP: Production of superoxide anion by an NADPH-oxidase from rat pulmonary macrophages. *FEBS Lett* 121:352, 1980

79. Evans WH, Karnovsky ML: A possible mechanism for the stimulation of some metabolic functions during phagocytosis. *J Biol Chem* 236:30, 1961

80. Cagan RH, Karnovsky ML: Enzymatic basis of the respiratory stimulation during phagocytosis. *Nature* 204:255, 1965

81. Baehner RL, Karnovsky ML: Deficiency of reduced nicotinamide-adenine dinucleotide oxidase in chronic granulomatous disease. *Science* 162:1277, 1968

82. Briggs RT, Drath DB, Karnovsky ML, Karnovsky MJ: Localization of NADH oxidase on the surface of human polymorphonuclear leukocytes by a new cytochemical method. *J Cell Biol* 67:566, 1975

83. Segal AW, Peters TJ: Characterization of the enzyme defect in chronic granulomatous disease. *Lancet* 1:1363, 1976

84. Briggs RT, Karnovsky ML, Karnovsky MJ: Hydrogen peroxide production in chronic granulomatous disease: A cytochemical study of reduced pyridine nucleotide oxidases. *J Clin Invest* 59:1088, 1977

85. Badwey JA, Karnovsky ML: Production of superoxide and hydrogen peroxide by an NADH-oxidase in guinea pig polymorphonuclear leukocytes. *J Biol Chem* 254:11530, 1979

86. Baehner RL, Johnston RB Jr, Nathan DG: Comparative study of the metabolic and bactericidal characteristics of severely glucose-6-phosphate dehydrogenase deficient polymorphonuclear leukocytes and leukocytes from children with chronic granulomatous disease. *J Reticuloendothel Soc* 12:150, 1972

87. Cooper MR, DeChatelet LR, McCall CE, LaVia MF, Spurr CL, Baehner RL: Complete deficiency of leukocyte glucose-6-phosphate dehydrogenase with defective bactericidal activity. *J Clin Invest* 51:769, 1972

87a. Shirley PS, Campbell TL, Cheadle E, DeChatelet LR: Transhydrogenase activity in human leukocytes. *J Reticuloendothel Soc* 25:575, 1979

88. Gray GR, Stomatoyannopoulos G, Naiman SC, Kilman NR, Klebanoff SJ, Austin T, Yoshida A, Robinson GCF: Neutrophil dysfunction, chronic granulomatous disease, and nonspherocytic hemolytic anemia caused by complete deficiency of glucose-6-phosphate dehydrogenase. *Lancet* 2:530, 1973

89. Karnovsky ML: Chronic granulomatous disease—pieces of a cellular and molecular puzzle. *Fed Proc* 32:1527, 1973

90. Cheson BD, Curnutte JT, Babior BM: The oxidative killing mechanisms of the neutrophil. *Prog Clin Immunol* 3:1, 1977

91. Babior BM: Oxygen-dependent microbial killing by phagocytes. *N Engl J Med* 298:659, 1978

92. Badwey JA, Karnovsky ML: Active oxygen species and the functions of phagocytic leukocytes. *Annu Rev Biochem* 49:695, 1980

93. Korchak HM, Weissmann G: Changes in membrane potential of human granulocytes antecede the metabolic responses to surface stimulation. *Proc Natl Acad Sci* 75:3818, 1978

94. Newburger PE, Chovaniec ME, Cohen HJ: Activity and activation of the granulocyte superoxide-generating system. *Blood* 55:85, 1980

95. Smolen JE, Korchak HM, Weissmann G: Initial kinetics of lysosomal enzyme secretion and superoxide anion generation by human polymorphonuclear leukocytes. *Inflammation* 4:145, 1980

96. Weening RS, Roos D, Weemaes CMR, Homan-Müller JWT, van Schaik MLJ: Defective initiation of the metabolic stimulation in phagocytizing granulocytes: A new congenital defect. *J Lab Clin Med* 88:757, 1976

97. Harvath L, Anderson BR: Defective initiation of oxidative metabolism in polymorphonuclear leukocytes. *N Engl J Med* 300:1130, 1979

98. DeChatelet LR, Shirley PS, Johnston RB Jr: Effect of phorbol myristate acetate on the oxidative metabolism of human polymorphonuclear leukocytes. *Blood* 47:545, 1976

99. Curnutte JT, Babior BM, Karnovsky ML: Fluoride-mediated activation of the respiratory burst in human neutrophils. A reversible process. *J Clin Invest* 63:637, 1979

100. Harvath L, Amirault HJ, Andersen BR: Chemiluminescence of human and canine polymorphonuclear leukocytes in the absence of phagocytosis. *J Clin Invest* 61:1145, 1978

101. Hoidal JR, Repine JE, Beall GD, Rasp FL Jr, White JG: The effect of phorbol myristate acetate on the metabolism and ultrastructure of human alveolar macrophages. *Am J Pathol* 91:469, 1976

102. Goetzl EJ, Austen KF: Stimulation of human neutrophil leukocyte aerobic glucose metabolism by purified chemotactic factors. *J Clin Invest* 53:591, 1974

103. Simchowitz L, Atkinson JP, Spilberg I: Stimulus-specific deactivation of chemotactic factor-induced cyclic AMP response and superoxide generation by human neutrophils. *J Clin Invest* 66:736, 1980

104. Boxer LA, Yoder M, Bonsib S, Schmidt M, Ho P, Jersild R, Baehner RL: Effects of a chemotactic factor, N-formylmethionyl peptide, on adherence, superoxide anion generation, phagocytosis, and microtubule assembly of human polymorphonuclear leukocytes. *J Lab Clin Med* 93:506, 1979

105. Simchowitz L, Spilberg I: Generation of superoxide radicals by human peripheral neutrophils activated by chemotactic factor. Evidence for the role of calcium. *J Lab Clin Med* 93:583, 1979

106. Hatch GE, Gardner DE, Menzel DB: Chemiluminescence of phagocytic cells caused by N-formylmethionyl peptides. *J Exp Med* 147:182, 1978

107. Graham RC Jr, Karnovsky MJ, Shafer AW, Glass EA, Karnovsky ML: Metabolic and morphological observations on the effect of surface-active agents on leukocytes. *J Cell Biol* 32:629, 1967

108. Rossi F, Zatti M: Mechanism of the respiratory stimulation in saponine-treated leukocytes. The KCN-insensitive oxidation of NADPH. *Biochim Biophys Acta* 153:296, 1968

109. Evans WH, Mueller PS: Effects of palmitate on the metabolism of leucocytes from guinea pig exudate. *J Lipid Res* 4:39, 1963

110. Kakinuma K: Effects of fatty acids on the oxidative metabolism of leukocytes. *Biochim Biophys Acta* 348:76, 1974

111. Kakinuma K, Minakami S: Effects of fatty acids on superoxide radical generation in leukocytes. *Biochim Biophys Acta* 538:50, 1978

112. Patriarca P, Cramer R, Marussi M, Moncalvo S, Rossi F: Phospholipid splitting and metabolic stimulation in polymorphonuclear leukocytes. *J Reticuloendothel Soc* 10:251, 1971

113. Rossi F, Zatti M, Patriarca P, Cramer R: Effect of specific antibodies on the metabolism of guinea pig polymorphonuclear leukocytes. *J Reticuloendothel Soc* 9:67, 1971

113a. Hafeman DG, Lewis JT, McConnell HM: Triggering of the macrophage and neutrophil respiratory burst by antibody bound to a spin-label phospholipid hapten in model lipid bilayer membranes. *Biochem* 19:5387, 1980

114. Yasaka T, Kambara T: Different effect of concanavalin A and its succinylated derivative on superoxide release in peritoneal macrophages. *Biochim Biophys Acta* 585:229, 1979

115. Nakagawara A, Minakami S: Role of cytoskeletal elements in cytochalasin E-induced superoxide production by human polymorphonuclear leukocytes. *Biochim Biophys Acta* 584:143, 1979

116. Kitagawa S, Takaku F, Sakamoto S: Evidence that proteases are involved in superoxide production by human polymorphonuclear leukocytes and monocytes. *J Clin Invest* 65:74, 1980

117. Romeo D, Zabucchi G, Miani N, Rossi F: Ion movement across leukocyte plasma membrane and excitation of their metabolism. *Nature* 253:542, 1975

118. Matsumoto T, Takeshige K, Minakami S: Inhibition of phagocytotic metabolic changes of leukocytes by an intracellular calcium-antagonist 8-(N, N-diethylamino)-octyl-3,4,5-trimethoxybenzoate. *Biochem Biophys Res Comm* 88:974, 1979

118a. Takeshige K, Minakami S: Involvement of calmodulin in phagocytotic respiratory burst of leukocytes. *Biochem Biophys Res Comm*: 99:484, 1981

119. Klempner MS, Dinarello CA, Henderson WR, Gallin JI: Stimulation of neutrophil oxygen-dependent metabolism by human leukocytic pyrogen. *J Clin Invest* 64:996, 1979

120. Cohen HJ, Chovaniec ME: Superoxide production by digitonin-stimulated guinea pig granulocytes. The effects of N-ethylmaleimide, divalent cations, and glycolytic and mitochondrial inhibitors on the activation of the superoxide generating system. *J Clin Invest* 61:1088, 1978

121. GOLDSTEIN BD, WITZ G, AMORUSO M, TROLL W: Protease inhibitors antagonize the activation of polymorphonuclear leukocyte oxygen consumption. *Biochem Biophys Res Comm* 88:854, 1979

122. WHITIN JC, CHAPMAN CE, SIMONS ER, CHOVANIEC ME, COHEN HJ: Correlation between membrane potential changes and superoxide production in human granulocytes stimulated by phorbol myristate acetate. *J Biol Chem* 255:1874, 1980

123. SELIGMANN BE, GALLIN JI: Use of lipophilic probes of membrane potential to assess human neutrophil activation. Abnormality in chronic granulomatous disease. *J Clin Invest* 66:493, 1980

124. GABIG TG, KIPNES RS, BABIOR BM: Solubilization of the O_2^--forming activity responsible for the respiratory burst in human neutrophils. *J Biol Chem* 253:6663, 1978

125. GABIG TG, BABIOR BM: The O_2^--forming oxidase responsible for the respiratory burst in human neutrophils. Properties of the solubilized enzyme. *J Biol Chem* 254:9070, 1979

126. TAUBER AI, GOETZL EJ: Structural and catalytic properties of the solubilized superoxide-generating activity of human polymorphonuclear leukocytes. Solubilization, stabilization in solution, and partial characterization. *Biochemistry* 25:5576, 1979

127. DEWALD B, BAGGIOLINI M, CURNUTTE JT, BABIOR BM: Subcellular localization of the superoxide-forming enzyme in human neutrophils. *J Clin Invest* 63:21, 1979

128. GOLDSTEIN IM, CERQUEIRA M, LIND S, KAPLAN HB: Evidence that the superoxide-generating system of human leukocytes is associated with the cell surface. *J Clin Invest* 59:249, 1977

128a. BABIOR GL, ROSIN RE, McMURRICH BJ, PETERS WA, BABIOR BM: Arrangement of the respiratory burst oxidase in the plasma membrane of the neutrophil. *J Clin Invest* 67:1724, 1981

129. BABIOR BM, KIPNES RS: Superoxide-forming enzyme from human neutrophils: Evidence for a flavin requirement. *Blood* 50:517, 1977

130. BABIOR BM, PETERS WA: The O_2^--producing enzyme of human neutrophils: Further properties. *J Biol Chem* 256:2321, 1981

130a. LIGHT DR, WALSH C, O'CALLAGHAN A, GOETZL EJ, TAUBER AI: Characteristics of the cofactor requirements for the superoxide-generating NADPH oxidase of human polymorphonuclear leukocytes. *Biochem* 20:1468, 1981

130b. MILLARD JA, GERARD KW, SCHNEIDER DL: The isolation from rat peritoneal leukocytes of plasma membranes enriched in alkaline phosphatase and a b-type cytochrome. *Biochem Biophys Res Comm* 90:321, 1979

130c. SLOAN EP, CRAWFORD DR, SCHNEIDER DL: Isolation of plasma membrane from human neutrophils and determination of cytochrome b and quinone content. *J Exp Med* 153:1316, 1981

130d. CRAWFORD DR, SCHNEIDER DL: Evidence that a quinone may be required for the production of superoxide and hydrogen peroxide in neutrophils. *Biochem Biophys Res Comm* 99:1277, 1981

130e. KARNOVSKY ML, BADWEY JA, TAUBER AI: How, where and why phagocytic leukocytes produce superoxide and peroxide, in Bloch K, Bolis L, Tosteson DC (eds): *Membranes, Molecules, Toxins and Cells*, PSG, Inc., Boston, p 163

131. McRIPLEY RJ, SBARRA AJ: Role of the phagocyte in host-parasite interactions. XII. Hydrogen peroxide-myeloperoxidase bactericidal system in the phagocyte. *J Bacteriol* 94:1425, 1967

132. DRATH DB, KARNOVSKY ML: Bactericidal activity of metal-mediated peroxide-ascorbate systems. *Infect Immun* 10:1077, 1974

133. GREGORY EM, YOST FJ JR, FRIDOVICH I: Superoxide dismutase of *Escherichia coli*: Intracellular localization and functions. *J Bacteriol* 115:987, 1973

134. GREGORY EM, FRIDOVICH I: Oxygen metabolism in *Lactobacillus plantarum*. *J Bacteriol* 117:166, 1974

135. BABIOR BM, CURNUTTE JT, KIPNES RS: Biological defense mechanisms: Evidence for the participation of superoxide in bacterial killing by xanthine oxidase. *J Lab Clin Med* 85:235, 1975

136. MANDELL GL: Catalase, superoxide dismutase, and virulence of *Staphylococcus aureus*. In vitro and in vivo studies with emphasis on staphylococcal-leukocyte interaction. *J Clin Invest* 55:561, 1975

137. ROSEN H, KLEBANOFF SJ: Bactericidal activity of a superoxide anion-generating system. A model for the polymorphonuclear leukocyte. *J Exp Med* 149:27, 1979

138. SCHULTZ J, KAMINKER K: Myeloperoxidase of the leucocyte of normal human blood. I. Content and localization. *Arch Biochem Biophys* 96:465, 1962

139. SCHULTZ J, CORLIN R, ODDI F, KAMINKER K, JONES W: Myeloperoxidase of the leucocyte of normal human blood. *Arch Biochem Biophys* 111:73, 1965

140. BAINTON DF, FARQUHAR MG: Differences in enzyme content of azurophil and specific granules of polymorphonuclear leukocytes. II. Cytochemistry and electron microscopy of bone marrow cells. *J Cell Biol* 39:299, 1968

141. MICHELL RH, KARNOVSKY MJ, KARNOVSKY ML: The distributions of some granule-associated enzymes in guinea pig polymorphonuclear leukocytes. *Biochem J* 116:207, 1970

142. BRETZ U, BAGGIOLINI M: Biochemical and morphological characterization of azurophil and specific granules of human neutrophilic polymorphonuclear leukocytes. *J Cell Biol* 63:251, 1974

143. van FURTH R, HIRSCH JG, FEDORKO ME: Morphology and peroxidase cytochemistry of mouse promonocytes, monocytes, and macrophages. *J Exp Med* 132:794, 1970

144. van der MEER JWM, REELEN RHJ, FLUITSMA DM, van FURTH R: Ultrastructure of mononuclear phagocytes developing in liquid bone marrow cultures. *J Exp Med* 149:17, 1979

145. BAINTON DF, GOLDE DW: Differentiation of macrophages from normal human bone marrow in liquid culture. Electron microscopy and cytochemistry. *J Clin Invest* 101:1555, 1978

146. BOS A, WEVER R, ROOS D: Characterization and quantification of the peroxidase in human monocytes. *Biochim Biophys Acta* 525:37, 1978

147. SALMON SE, CLINE MJ, SCHULTZ J, LEHRER RI: Myeloperoxidase deficiency. Immunologic study of a genetic leukocyte defect. *N Engl J Med* 282:250, 1970

148. SCHULTZ J, SHMUKLER WH: Myeloperoxidase of the leucocyte of normal human blood. II. Isolation, spectrophotometry and amino acid analysis. *Biochemistry* 3:1234, 1964

148a. OLSSON I, OLOFSSON T, ODEBERG H: Myeloperoxidase-mediated iodination in granulocytes. *Scand J Haematol* 9:483, 1972

148b. BAKKENIST ARJ, WEVER R, VULSMA T, PLAT H, VAN GELDER BF: Isolation procedure and some properties of myeloperoxidase from human leucocytes. *Biochim Biophys Acta* 524:45, 1978

149. ANDREWS PC, KRINSKY NI: The reductive cleavage of myeloperoxidase in half, producing enzymically active hemi-myeloperoxidase. *J Biol Chem* 256:4211, 1981

150. MATHESON NR, WONG PS, TRAVIS J: Isolation and properties of human neutrophil myeloperoxidase. *Biochem* 20:325, 1981

151. HARRISON JE, SCHULTZ J: Myeloperoxidase: Confirmation and nature of heme-binding inequivalence. Resolution of a carbonyl-substituted heme. *Biochim Biophys Acta* 536:341, 1978

152. WU NC, SCHULTZ J: The prosthetic group of myeloperoxidase. *FEBS Lett* 60:141, 1975

153. ODAJIMA T, YAMAZAKI I: Myeloperoxidase of the leukocyte of normal blood. IV. Some physiochemical properties. *Biochim Biophys Acta* 284:360, 1972

154. CHIANG R, MAKINO R, SPOMER WE, HAGER LP: Chloroperoxidase: P-456 type absorption in the absence of sulfhydryl groups. *Biochem* 14:4166, 1975

155. ARAISO T, MIYOSHI K, YAMAZAKI I: Mechanisms of electron transfer from sulfite to horseradish peroxidase–hydroperoxide compounds. *Biochemistry* 15:3059, 1976

156. MAEHLY AC: The assay of catalase and peroxidases. Part I. General assay methods. *Methods Biochem Anal* 1:358, 1953

157. HARRISON JE, SCHULTZ J: Studies on the chlorinating activity of myeloperoxidase. *J Biol Chem* 251:1371, 1976

158. MORRISON M, SCHONBAUM GR: Peroxidase-catalyzed halogenation. *Annu Rev Biochem* 45:861, 1976

159. YAMAZAKI I, YOKOTA K: Oxidation states of peroxidase. *Mol Cell Biochem* 2:39, 1973

160. ROBERTS J, QUASTEL JH: Oxidation of reduced triphosphopyridine nucleotide by guinea pig polymorphonuclear leucocytes. *Nature* 202:85, 1964

161. ODAJIMA T: Myeloperoxidase of the leukocyte of normal blood. II. The oxidation-reduction reaction mechanism of the myeloperoxidase system. *Biochim Biophys Acta* 235:52, 1971

162. TAKANAKA K, O'BRIEN PJ: Mechanisms of H_2O_2 formation by leukocytes. Properties of the NAD(P)H oxidase activity of intact leukocytes. *Arch Biochem Biophys* 169:436, 1975

163. BAEHNER RL, KARNOVSKY MJ, KARNOVSKY ML: Degranulation of leukocytes in chronic granulomatous disease. *J Clin Invest* 48:187, 1969

164. PATRIARCA P, CRAMER R, TEDESCO F, KAKINUMA K: Studies on the mechanism of metabolic stimulation in polymorphonuclear leucocytes during phagocytosis. II. Presence of the $NADPH_2$ oxidizing activity in a myeloperoxidase-deficient subject. *Biochim Biophys Acta* 385:387, 1975

165. WEAST RC (ed): *Handbook of Chemistry and Physics*, 50th ed. Cleveland, Chemical Rubber Co., D-109, 1969

166. KLEBANOFF SJ: Myeloperoxidase-halide-hydrogen peroxide antibacterial system. *J Bacteriol* 95:2131, 1968

167. KLEBANOFF SJ, CLEM WH, LUEBKE RG: The peroxide-thiocyanate-hydrogen peroxide antimicrobial system. *Biochim Biophys Acta* 117:63, 1966

168. ZGLICZYNSKI JM, SELVARAJ RJ, PAUL BB, STELMASZYNSKA T, POSKITT PKF, SBARRA AJ: Chlorination by the myeloperoxidase-H_2O_2-Cl^- antimicrobial system at acid and neutral pH. *Proc Soc Exp Biol Med* 154:418, 1977

169. STELMASZYNSKA T, ZGLICZYNSKI JM: Myeloperoxidase of human neutrophilic granulocytes as chlorinating enzyme. *Eur J Biochem* 45:305, 1974

170. KLEBANOFF SJ, HAMON CB: Role of myeloperoxidase-mediated antimicrobial systems in intact leukocytes. *J Reticuloendothel Soc* 12:170, 1972

171. KLEBANOFF SJ: Myeloperoxidase: contribution to the microbicidal activity of intact leukocytes. *Science* 169:1095, 1970

172. REST RF, SPITZNAGEL JK: Myeloperoxidase-Cl⁻-H₂O₂ bactericidal system: Effect of bacterial membrane structure and growth conditions. *Infect Immun* 19:1110, 1978

173. BARON DN, AHMED SA: Intracellular concentrations of water and of the principal electrolytes determined by the analysis of isolated human leucocytes. *Clin Sci* 37:205, 1969

174. KRINSKY NI: Biological roles of singlet oxygen, in Wasserman HH, Murray RW (eds): *Singlet Oxygen*. New York, Academic, 1979, p 597

175. ALLEN RC, STJERNHOLM RL, STEELE RH: Evidence for the generation of an electronic excitation state(s) in human polymorphonuclear leukocytes and its participation in bactericidal activity. *Biochem Biophys Res Comm* 47:679, 1972

176. KRINSKY NI: Singlet excited oxygen as a mediator of the antibacterial action of leukocytes. *Science* 186:363, 1974

177. ROSEN H, KLEBANOFF SJ: Formation of singlet oxygen by the myeloperoxidase-mediated antimicrobial system. *J Biol Chem* 252:4803, 1977

178. PIATT J, O'BRIEN PJ: Singlet oxygen formation by a peroxidase, H₂O₂ and halide system. *Eur J Biochem* 93:323, 1979

179. CHESON BD, CHRISTENSEN RL, SPERLING R, KOHLER BE, BABIOR BM: The origin of the chemiluminescence of phagocytosing granulocytes. *J Clin Invest* 58:789, 1976

180. HELD AM, HURST JK: Ambiguity associated with use of singlet oxygen trapping agents in myeloperoxidase-catalyzed oxidations. *Biochem Biophy Res Comm* 81:878, 1978

181. ZGLICZYNSKI JM, STELMASZYNSKA T: Chlorinating ability of human phagocytosing leucocytes. *Eur J Biochem* 56:157, 1975

182. PINCUS SH, KLEBANOFF SJ: Quantitative leukocyte iodination. *N Engl J Med* 284:744, 1971

183. SIMMONS SR, KARNOVSKY ML: Iodinating ability of various leukocytes and their bactericidal activity. *J Exp Med* 138:44, 1973

184. KLEBANOFF SJ, CLARK RA: Iodination by human polymorphonuclear leukocytes: A re-evaluation. *J Lab Clin Med* 89:675, 1977

185. KLEBANOFF SJ, WHITE LR: Iodination defect in the leukocytes of a patient with chronic granulomatous disease of childhood. *N Engl J Med* 280:460, 1969

186. ROOT RK, STOSSEL TP: Myeloperoxidase-mediated iodination by granulocytes. Intracellular site of operation and some regulating factors. *J Clin Invest* 53:1207, 1974

186a. THOMAS EL: Myeloperoxidase-hydrogen peroxide-chloride antimicrobial system: Effect of exogenous amines on antibacterial action against *E. coli*. *Infect Immun* 25:110, 1979

187. ZGLICZYNSKI JM, STELMASZYNSKA T, OSTROWSKI W, NASKALSKI J, SZYNAJD J: Myeloperoxidase of human leukemic leukocytes: Oxidation of amino acids in the presence of hydrogen peroxide. *Eur J Biochem* 4:540, 1968

188. STRAUSS RR, PAUL BB, JACOBS AA, SBARRA AJ: Role of the phagocyte in host-parasite interactions. XXII. H₂O₂-dependent decarboxylation and deamination by myeloperoxidase and its relationship to antimicrobial activity. *J Reticuloendothel Soc* 7:754, 1970

189. PEREIRA WE, HOYANO Y, SUMMONS RE, BACON VA, DUFFIELD AM: Chlorination studies. II. The reaction of aqueous hypochlorous acid with α-amino acids and dipeptides. *Biochim Biophys Acta* 313:170, 1973

190. NASKALSKI JW: Myeloperoxidase inactivation in the course of catalysis of chlorination of taurine. *Biochim Biophy Acta* 485:291, 1977

191. HOUPERT Y, TARALLO P, SIEST G: Quantitative determination of granulocytic amino acids in healthy men and women. *Clin Chim Acta* 69:383, 1976

192. ZGLICZYNSKI JM, STELMASZYNSKA T: Hydrogen cyanide and cyanogen chloride formation by the myeloperoxidase-H₂O₂-Cl⁻ system. *Biochim Biophys Acta* 567:309, 1979

193. STOLC V: Characterization of iodoproteins secreted by phagocytosing human polymorphonuclear leukocytes. *J Biol Chem* 254:1273, 1979

194. STOLC V: Release of monoiodotyrosine and iodoprotein from human leukocytes. *J Clin Endocrinol Metab* 37:397, 1973

195. TSAN MF, CHEN JW: Oxidation of methionine by human polymorphonuclear leukocytes. *J Clin Invest* 65:1041, 1980

195a. CLARK RA, KLEBANOFF SJ: Chemotactic factor inactivation by the myeloperoxidase-hydrogen peroxide-halide system. *J Clin Invest* 64:913, 1979

196. CLARK RA, SZOT S, VERIKATASUBRAMANIAN K, SCHIFFMANN E: Chemotactic factor inactivation by myeloperoxidase-mediated oxidation of methionine. *J Immunol* 124:2020, 1980

197. THOMAS EL, AUNE TM: Peroxidase-catalyzed oxidation of protein sulfhydryls mediated by iodine. *Biochemistry* 16:3581, 1977

198. THOMAS EL: Myeloperoxidase, hydrogen peroxide, chloride antimicrobial system: Nitrogen-chlorine derivatives of bacterial components in bactericidal action against *Escherichia coli*. *Infect Immun* 23:522, 1979

199. ADENIYI-JONES SK, KARNOVSKY ML: Oxidation decarboxylation of free and peptide-linked amino acids in phagocytizing guinea pig granulocytes. *J Clin Invest* 68:365, 1981

200. MATHESON NR, WONG PS, TRAVIS J: Enzymatic inactivation of human alpha-1-proteinase inhibitor by neutrophil myeloperoxidase. *Biochem Biophys Res Comm* 88:402, 1979

200a. JOHNSON D, TRAVIS J: The oxidative inactivation of human α-1-proteinase inhibitor. Further evidence for methionine at the reactive center. *J Biol Chem* 254:4022, 1979

200b. CARP H, JANOFF A: In vitro suppression of serum elastase-inhibitory capacity by reactive oxygen species generated by phagocytosing polymorphonuclear leukocytes. *J Clin Invest* 63:793, 1979

200c. ALBRICH JM, McCARTHY CA, HURST JK: Biological reactivity of hypochlorous acid: Implications for microbicidal mechanisms of leukocyte myeloperoxidase. *Proc Natl Acad Sci* 78:210, 1981

200d. SIPS HJ, HAMERS MN: Mechanism of the bactericidal action of myeloperoxidase: Increased permeability of the *Escherichia coli* cell envelope. *J Immunol* 31:11, 1981

201. BEAUCHAMP C, FRIDOVICH I: A mechanism for the production of ethylene from methional: The generation of hydroxyl radical by xanthine oxidase. *J Biol Chem* 245:4641, 1970

202. TAUBER AI, BABIOR BM: Evidence for hydroxyl radical production by human neutrophils. *J Clin Invest* 60:374, 1977

203. WEISS SJ, KING GW, LoBUGLIO AF: Evidence for hydroxyl radical generation by human monocytes. *J Clin Invest* 60:370, 1977

204. WEISS SJ, RUSTAGI PK, LoBUGLIO AF: Human granulocyte generation of hydroxyl radical. *J Exp Med* 147:316, 1978

205. TAUBER AI, GABIG TG, BABIOR BM: Evidence for production of oxidizing radicals by the particulate O₂⁻-forming system from human neutrophils. *Blood* 53:666, 1979

206. REPINE JE, EATON JW, ANDERS MW, HOIDAL JR, Fox RB: Generation of hydroxyl radical by enzymes, chemicals, and human phagocytes in vitro. Detection with the anti-inflammatory agent, dimethyl sulfoxide. *J Clin Invest* 64:1652, 1979

207. DRATH DB, KARNOVSKY ML, HUBER GL: Hydroxyl radical formation in phagocytic cells of the rat. *J Appl Physiol* 46:136, 1979

207a. TAKANAKA V, O'BRIEN PJ: Generation of activated oxygen species by polymorphonuclear leukocytes. *FEBS Lett* 110:283, 1980

208. PRYOR WA, TANG RH: Ethylene formation from methional. *Biochem Biophys Res Comm* 81:498, 1978

209. GREEN MR, HILL HAO, OKOLOW-ZUBKOWSKA MJ, SEGAL AW: The production of hydroxyl and superoxide radicals by stimulated human neutrophils—measurements by EPR spectroscopy. *FEBS Lett* 100:23, 1979

210. ROSEN H, KLEBANOFF SJ: Hydroxyl radical generation by polymorphonuclear leukocytes measured by electron spin resonance spectroscopy. *J Clin Invest* 64:1725, 1979

211. HABER F, WEISS J: The catalytic decomposition of hydrogen peroxide by iron salts. *Proc R Soc Edinburgh Sect A (Math Phys Sci)* 147:332, 1934

212. HALLIWELL B: Superoxide-dependent formation of hydroxyl radicals in the presence of iron salts. *FEBS Lett* 96:238, 1978

213. McCORD JM, DAY ED Jr: Superoxide-dependent production of hydroxyl radical catalyzed by iron-EDTA complex. *FEBS Lett* 86:139, 1978

214. KLEBANOFF SJ, ROSEN H: Ethylene formation by polymorphonuclear leukocytes. *J Exp Med* 148:490, 1978

215. CRAVEN PA, DeRUBERTIS FR: Restoration of the responsiveness of purified guanylate cyclase to nitrosoguanidine, nitric oxide, and related activators by heme and hemoproteins. *J Biol Chem* 253:8433, 1978

216. VAN HEMMEN JJ, MEULING WJA: Inactivation of *Escherichia coli* by superoxide radicals and their dismutation products. *Arch Biochem Biophys* 182:743, 1977

217. MURRAY HW, COHN ZA: Macrophage oxygen-dependent antimicrobial activity. I. Susceptibility of *Toxoplasma gondii* to oxygen intermediates. *J Exp Med* 150:938, 1979

218. WEISS SJ, LoBUGLIO AF, KESSLER HB: Oxidative mechanisms of monocyte-mediated cytotoxicity. *Proc Natl Acad Sci* 77:584, 1980

219. KATZ P, SIMONE CB, HENKART PA, FAUCI AS: Mechanisms of antibody-dependent cellular cytotoxicity. The use of effector cells from chronic granulomatous disease patients as investigative probes. *J Clin Invest* 65:55, 1980

220. McCORD JM: Free radicals and inflammation: Protection of synovial fluid by superoxide dismutase. *Science* 185:529, 1974

221. DORFMAN LM, ADAMS GE: Reactivity of the hydroxyl radical in aqueous solutions. NSRDS-NBS 46 Washington, D.C., Government Printing Office, 1972

222. SAPRIN AN, PIETTE LH: Spin trapping and its application in the study of lipid peroxidation and free radical production with liver microsomes. *Arch Biochem Biophys* 180:480, 1977

223. LAI CS, PIETTE LH: Spin-trapping studies of hydroxyl radical production involved in lipid peroxidation. *Arch Biochem Biophys* 190:27, 1978

224. SVINGEN BA, BUEGE JA, O'NEAL FO, AUST SD: The mechanism of NADPH-dependent lipid peroxidation. The propagation of lipid peroxidation. *J Biol Chem* 254:5892, 1979

225. STOSSEL TP, MASON RJ, SMITH AL: Lipid peroxidation by human blood phagocytes. *J Clin Invest* 54:638, 1974

226. SHOHET SB, PITT J, BAEHNER RL, POPLACK DG: Lipid peroxidation in the killing of phagocytized pneumococci. *Infect Immun* 10:1321, 1974

227. WHITE HL, WHITE JR: Interaction of streptonigrin with DNA in vitro. *Biochim Biophys Acta* 132:648, 1966

228. MIZUNO NS, GILBOE DP: Binding of streptonigrin to DNA. *Biochim Biophys Acta* 224:319, 1970

229. CONE R, HASAN SK, LOWN JW, MORGAN AR: The mechanism of the degradation of DNA by streptonigrin. *Can J Biochem* 54:219, 1976

230. LOWN JW, BEGLEITER A, JOHNSON D, MORGAN AR: Studies related to antitumor antibiotics. Part V. Reactions of mitomycin C with DNA examined by ethidium fluorescence assay. *Can J Biochem* 54:110, 1976

231. LOWN JW, SIM SK, MAJUMDAR KC, CHANG RY: Strand scission of DNA by bound adriamycin and daunorubicin in the presence of reducing agents. *Biochem Biophys Res Comm* 76:705, 1977

232. FRIDOVICH I: Superoxide dismutase. *Adv Enzymol* 41:35, 1974

233. BANNISTER WH, ANASTASI A, BANNISTER JV: Human erythrocyte superoxide dismutase (erythrocuprein), in Michelson AM, McCord JM, Fridovich I (eds): *Superoxide and Superoxide Dismutases*. London, Academic, 1977, p 107

234. MCCORD JM, BOYLE JA, DAY ED JR, RIZZOLO LJ, SALIN ML: A manganese-containing superoxide dismutase from human liver, in Michelson AM, McCord JM, Fridovich I (eds): *Superoxide and Superoxide Dismutases*. London, Academic, 1977, p 129

235. SALIN ML, MCCORD JM: Superoxide dismutase in polymorphonuclear leukocytes. *J Clin Invest* 54:1005, 1974

236. WINTERBOURN CC, HAWKINS RE, BRIAN M, CARRELL RW: The estimation of red cell superoxide dismutase activity. *J Lab Clin Med* 85:337, 1975

237. CONCETTI A, MASSEI P, ROTILIO G, BRUNORI M, RACHMILEWITZ EA: Superoxide dismutase in red blood cells: Method of assay and enzyme content in normal subjects and in patients with β-thalassemia (major and intermedia). *J Lab Clin Med* 87:1057, 1976

238. MICHELSON AM, PUGET K, DUROSAY P: Clinical aspects of the dosage of erythrocuprein, in Michelson AM, McCord JM, Fridovich I (eds): *Superoxide and Superoxide Dismutases*. London, Academic, 1977, p 468

239. AEBI H, WYSS SR, SCHERZ B, SKVARIL F: Heterogeneity of erythrocyte catalase. II. Isolation and characterization of normal and variant erythrocyte catalases and their subunits. *Eur J Biochem* 48:137, 1974

240. OLOFSSON T, OLSSON I: Purification of human granulocyte catalase in chronic myeloid leukemia. *Biochim Biophys Acta* 482:301, 1977

241. NICHOLLS P, SCHONBAUM GR: *Catalases*, in Boyer PD, Lardy H, Myrbäck K (eds): *The Enzymes*, 2d ed. Academic, New York, 1963, p 198

242. ROOS D, WEENING RS, WYSS SR, AEBI HE: Protection of human neutrophils by endogenous catalase. Studies with cells from catalase-deficient individuals. *J Clin Invest* 65:1515, 1980

243. STAAL GEJ, VISSER J, VEEGER C: Purification and properties of glutathione reductase of human erythrocytes. *Biochim Biophys Acta* 185:39, 1969

244. BEUTLER E: Effect of flavin compounds on glutathione reductase activity: In vivo and in vitro studies. *J Clin Invest* 48:1969, 1957

245. SCOTT EM, DUNCAN IW, EKSTRAND V: Purification and properties of glutathione reductase of human erythrocytes. *J Biol Chem* 238:3928, 1963

246. FLOHÉ L, EISELE B, WENDEL A: Glutathion-peroxidase. I. Reindarstellung und molekulargewichtsbestimmungen. *Z Physiol Chem* 352:151, 1971

247. FLOHÉ L, GUNZLER WA, SCHOCK HH: Glutathione peroxidase: A selenoenzyme. *FEBS Lett* 32:132, 1973

248. FORSTROM JW, ZAKOWSKI JJ, TAPPEL AL: Identification of the catalytic site of rat liver glutathione peroxidase as selenocysteine. *Biochemistry* 17:2639, 1978

249. SPLITTGERBER AG, TAPPEL AL: Steady state and pre-steady state kinetic properties of rat liver selenium-glutathione peroxidase. *J Biol Chem* 254:9807, 1979

250. BURK RF, NISHIKI K, LAWRENCE RA, CHANCE B: Peroxide removal by selenium-dependent and selenium-independent glutathione peroxidases in hemoglobin-free perfused rat liver. *J Biol Chem* 253:43, 1978

251. SHREVE MR, MORRISSEY PG, O'BRIEN PJ: Lipid and steroid hydroperoxides as substrates for the non-selenium-dependent glutathione peroxidase. *Biochem J* 177:761, 1979

252. BASS DA, DECHATELET LR, BURK RF, SHIRLEY P, SZJEDA P: Polymorphonuclear leukocyte bactericidal activity and oxidative metabolism during glutathione peroxidase deficiency. *Infect Immun* 18:78, 1977

252a. MENDELSON DS, METZ EN, SAGONE AL: Effect of phagocytosis on the reduced soluble sulfhydryl content of human granulocytes. *Blood* 50:1023, 1977

252b. BIGLEY RH, STANKOVA L: Uptake and reduction of oxidized and reduced ascorbate by human leukocytes. *J Exp Med* 139:1084, 1974

253. BAEHNER RL, BOXER LA, ALLEN JM, DAVIS J: Autoxidation as a basis for altered function by polymorphonuclear leukocytes. *Blood* 50:327, 1977

254. BOXER LA, OLIVER JM, SPIELBERG SP, ALLEN JM, SCHULMAN JD: Protection of granulocytes by vitamin E in glutathione synthetase deficiency. *N Engl J Med* 301:901, 1979

255. BOXER LA, HARRIS RE, BAEHNER RL: Regulation of membrane peroxidation in health and disease. *Pediatrics (Suppl)* 64:713, 1979

256. JOHNSTON RB JR, NEWMAN SL: Chronic granulomatous disease. *Pediatr Clin North Am* 24:365, 1977

257. WINDHORST DB, PAGE AR, HOLMES B, QUIE PG, GOOD RA: The pattern of genetic transmission of the leukocyte defect in fatal granulomatous disease of childhood. *J Clin Invest* 47:1026, 1968

258. REPINE JE, CLAWSON CC, WHITE JG, HOLMES B: Spectrum of function of neutrophils from carriers of sex-linked chronic granulomatous disease. *J Pediatr* 87:901, 1975

259. LYON MF: Sex chromatin and gene action in the mammalian X-chromosome. *Am J Hum Genet* 14:135, 1962

260. OCHS HD, IGO RP: The NBT slide test: A simple screening method for detecting chronic granulomatous disease and female carriers. *J Pediatr* 83:77, 1973

261. MOELLERING RC, WEINBERG AN: Persistent Salmonella infection in a female carrier for chronic granulomatous disease. *Ann Intern Med* 73:595, 1970

262. SCHALLER J: Illness resembling lupus erythematosus in mothers of boys with chronic granulomatous disease. *Ann Intern Med* 76:747, 1972

263. BAEHNER RL, NATHAN DG: Quantitative nitroblue tetrazolium test in chronic granulomatous disease. *N Engl J Med* 278:971, 1968

264. QUIE PG, KAPLAN EL, PAGE AR, GRUSKAY FL, MALAWISTA SE: Defective polymorphonuclear leukocyte function and chronic granulomatous disease in two female children. *N Engl J Med* 278:976, 1968

264a. MILLS EL, RHOLL KS, QUIE PG: X-linked inheritance in females with chronic granulomatous disease. *J Clin Invest* 66:332, 1980

265. AZIMI PH, BODENBENDER JG, HINTZ RL, KONTRAS SB: Chronic granulomatous disease in three female siblings. *JAMA* 206:2865, 1968

266. DOUGLAS SD, DAVIS WC, FUDENBERG HH: Granulocytopathies: Pleomorphism of neutrophil dysfunction. *Am J Med* 46:901, 1969

267. KOCH C, SOGAARD H, CHRISTENSEN MF: Inheritance of chronic granulomatous disease in females. *Acta Paediatr Scand* 62:659, 1973

268. KONTRAS SB, BASS JC: Chronic granulomatous disease. *Lancet* 1: 646, 1979

269. ELGEFORS B, OLLING S, PETERSON H: Chronic granulomatous disease in three siblings. *Scand J Infect Dis* 10:79, 1978

270. THOMPSON EN, CHANDRA RK, COPE WA, SOOTHILL JF: Leucocyte abnormality in both parents of a patient with chronic granulomatous disease. *Lancet* 2:799, 1969

271. CHANDRA RK, COPE WA, SOOTHILL JF: Chronic granulomatous disease: Evidence of an autosomal mode of inheritance. *Lancet* 1:71, 1969

272. BJÖRKSTEN B, LUNDMARK KM: Abnormal nitroblue tetrazolium test in relatives of a female with chronic granulomatous disease. *Scand J Infect Dis* 4:167, 1972

273. BALFOUR HH JR, SHEHAN JJ, SPEICHER CE, KAUDER E: Chronic granulomatous disease of childhood in a 23-year-old man. *JAMA* 217:960, 1971

274. CHUSID MJ, PARRILLO JE, FAUCI AS: Chronic granulomatous disease: Diagnosis in a 27-year old man with *Mycobacterium fortuitum*. *JAMA* 233:1295, 1975

275. BIGGAR WD, BURON S, HOLMES B: Chronic granulomatous disease in an adult male: A proposed X-linked defect. *J Pediatr* 88:63, 1976

276. PERRY HB, BOULANGER M, PENNOYER D: Chronic granulomatous disease in an adult with recurrent abscesses. *Arch Surg* 115:200, 1980

277. DILWORTH JA, MANDELL GL: Adults with chronic granulomatous disease of childhood. *Am J Med* 63:233, 1977

278. HOLMES B, QUIE PG, WINDHORST DB, GOOD RA: Fatal granulomatous disease of childhood: An inborn abnormality of phagocytic function. *Lancet* 1:1225, 1966

279. KAPLAN EL, LAXDAL T, QUIE PG: Studies of polymorphonuclear leukocytes from patients with chronic granulomatous disease of childhood: Bactericidal capacity for streptococci. *Pediatrics* 41:591, 1968

280. MANDELL GL, HOOK EW: Leukocyte bactericidal activity in chronic granulomatous disease: Correlation of bacterial hydrogen peroxide production and susceptibility to intracellular killing. *J Bact* 100:531, 1969

281. JOHNSTON RB JR, BAEHNER RL: Improvement of leukocyte bactericidal activity in chronic granulomatous disease. *Blood* 35:350, 1970

281a. COHEN MS, ISTURIZ PE, MALECH HL, ROOT RK, WILFERT CM, GUTMAN L, BUCKLEY RH: Fungal infection in chronic granulomatous disease. The importance of the phagocyte in defense against fungi. *Am J Med* 71:59, 1981

282. OH MK, RODEY GE, GOOD RA, CHILGREN RA, QUIE PG: Defective candidacidal capacity of polymorphonuclear leukocytes in chronic granulomatous disease of childhood. *J Pediatr* 72:300, 1969

283. HALAZUN JF, ANAST CS, LUKENS JN: Thyrotoxicosis associated with *Aspergillus* thyroiditis in chronic granulomatous disease. *J Pediatr* 80:106, 1972

284. RAUBITSCHEK AA, LEVIN AS, STITES DP, SHAW EB, FUDENBERG HH: Normal granulocyte infusion therapy for aspergillosis in chronic granulomatous disease. *Pediatrics*, 51:230, 1973

285. BUJAK JS, KWON-CHUNG KJ, CHUSID MF: Osteomyelitis and pneumonia

in a boy with chronic granulomatous disease of childhood caused by a mutant strain of *Aspergillus nidulans*. *Am J Clin Path* 61:361, 1974

286. BUJAK JS, OTTESEN EA, DINARELLO CA, BRENNER VJ: Nocardiosis in a child with chronic granulomatous disease. *J Pediatr* 83:98, 1973

287. IDRISS ZH, CUNNINGHAM RJ, WILFERT CM: Nocardiosis in children: Report of three cases and review of the literature. *Pediatrics* 55:479, 1975

288. ESTERLY JR, STURNER WO, ESTERLY NB, WINDHORST DB: Disseminated BCG in twin boys with presumed chronic granulomatous disease of childhood. *Pediatrics* 48:141, 1971

289. VERRONEN P: Presumed disseminated BCG in a boy with chronic granulomatous disease of childhood. *Acta Paediatr Scand* 63:627, 1974

290. PEDERSEN KF, JOHANSEN KS, ROSENKVIST J, TYGSTRUP I, VALERIUS N: Refractory *Pneumocystis carinii* infection in chronic granulomatous disease: Successful treatment with granulocytes. *Pediatrics* 64:935, 1979

291. WINDHORST DB, GOOD RA: Dermatologic manifestations of fatal granulomatous disease of childhood. *Arch Dermatol* 103:351, 1971

292. AMENT ME, OCHS HD: Gastrointestinal manifestations of chronic granulomatous disease. *N Engl J Med* 288:382, 1973

293. STY JR, CHUSID MJ, BABBITT, DP, WERLIN SL: Involvement of the colon in chronic granulomatous disease of childhood. *Radiology* 132:618, 1979

294. HARRIS BH, BOLES TE: Intestinal lesions in chronic granulomatous disease of childhood. *J Pediatr Surg* 8:955, 1973

295. GRISCOM NT, KIRKPATRICK JA, GIRDANY BR, BERDON WE, GRAND RJ, MACKIE GG: Gastric antral narrowing in chronic granulomatous disease of childhood. *Pediatrics* 54:456, 1974

296. HOIDAL JR, FOX RB, REPINE JE: Defective oxidative metabolic responses in vitro of alveolar macrophages in chronic granulomatous disease. *Am Rev Resp Dis* 20:613, 1979

297. WOLFSON JJ, KANE WJ, LAXDAL SD, GOOD RA, QUIE PG: Bone findings in chronic granulomatous disease of childhood. *J Bone Joint Surg* 51:1573, 1969

298. WOLFSON JJ, QUIE PG, LAXDAL SD, GOOD RA: Roentgenologic manifestations in children with a genetic defect of polymorphonuclear leukocyte function. *Radiology* 1:37, 1968

299. GOLD RH, DOUGLAS SD, PREGER L, STEINBACH HL, FUDENBERG HH: Roentgenographic features of the neutrophil dysfunction syndromes. *Radiology* 92:1045, 1969

300. KONTRAS SB, BODENBENDER JG, McCLAVE C, SMITH JP: Interstitial cystitis in chronic granulomatous disease. *J Urol* 105:575, 1971

301. CYR WL, JOHNSON H, BALFOUR J: Granulomatous cystitis as a manifestation of chronic granulomatous disease of childhood. *J Urol* 110:357, 1973

302. YOUNG AK, MIDDLETON RG: Urologic manifestations of chronic granulomatous disease of infancy. *J Urol* 123:119, 1980

303. FORBES GS, HARTMAN GW, BURKE EC, SEGURA JW: Genitourinary involvement in chronic granulomatous disease of childhood. *Am J Roentgenol* 127:683, 1976

304. VAN RHENEN DJ, KOOLEN MI, FLETKAMP-VROOM TM, WEENING RS: Immune complex glomerulonephritis in chronic granulomatous disease. *Acta Med Scand* 206:233, 1979

305. DESEIGNEUX R, KANFER A, TERRIOUX P, SRAER JD, WHITWORTH JA: Renal amyloidosis in chronic granulomatous disease. *Br med J* 4:230, 1974

306. MARTYN LJ, LISCHNER HW, PILEGGI AJ, HARLEY RD: Chorioretinal lesions in familial chronic granulomatous disease of childhood. *Am J Ophthalmol* 73:403, 1972

307. LAZARUS GM, NEU HC: Agents responsible for infection in chronic granulomatous disease of childhood. *J Pediatr* 86:415, 1975

308. EMMENS R, WHITTEN DM, DARLING D, LEAPE L: Thymic cyst causing dysphagia: Report of a case in a 4-year-old boy with chronic granulomatous disease. *Am J Dis Child* 133:219, 1979

309. JOHNSTON RB JR, BAEHNER RL: Chronic granulomatous disease: Correlation between pathogenesis and clinical findings. *Pediatrics*, 48:730, 1971

310. BRIDGES RA, BERENDES H, GOOD RA: A fatal granulomatous disease of childhood. *Am J Dis Child* 97:387, 1959

311. WARD PA, SCHLEGEL RJ: Impaired leucotactic responsiveness in a child with recurrent infections. *Lancet* 2:344, 1969

312. SNYDERMAN R, PIKE MC, ALTMAN LC: Abnormalities of leukocyte chemotaxis in human disease. *Ann NY Acad Sci* 256, 386, 1975.

313. CLARK RA, KLEBANOFF SJ: Chronic granulomatous disease: Studies of a family with impaired neutrophil chemotactic, metabolic and bactericidal function. *Am J Med* 65:941, 1978

314. EDELSON PJ, STITES DP, GOLD S, FUDENBERG HH: Disorders of neutrophil function: Defects in the early stages of the phagocytic process. *Clin Exp Immunol* 13:21, 1973

315. STOSSEL TP: Evaluation of opsonic and leukocyte function with a spectrophotometric test in patients with infection and with phagocytic disorders. *Blood* 42:121, 1973

316. STOSSEL TP, ROOT RK, VAUGHAN M: Phagocytosis in chronic granuloma-

tous disease and the Chediak-Higashi syndrome. *N Engl J Med* 286, 120, 1972

317. ELSBACH P, ZUCKER FD, SANSARICO C: Increased lecithin synthesis during phagocytosis by normal leukocytes and by leukocytes of a patient with chronic granulomatous disease. *N Engl J Med* 280:1319, 1980

318. QUIE PG, WHITE JG, HOLMES B, GOOD RA: In vitro bactericidal capacity of human polymorphonuclear leukocytes: Diminished activity in chronic granulomatous disease of childhood. *J Clin Invest* 46:668, 1967

319. KAUDER E, KAHLE LL, MORENO H, PARTIN JC: Leukocyte degranulation and vacuole formation in patients with chronic granulomatous disease of childhood. *J Clin Invest* 47:1753, 1968

320. MANDELL GL, HOOK EW: Leukocyte function in chronic granulomatous disease of childhood: Studies on a 17-year-old boy. *Am J Med* 47:473, 1969

321. GOLD SB, HANES DM, STITES DP, FUDENBERG HH: Abnormal kinetics of degranulation in chronic granulomatous disease. *N Engl J Med* 291:332, 1974

322. HOLMES B, PAGE AR, WINDHORST DB, QUIE PG, WHITE JG, GOOD RA: The metabolic pattern and phagocytic function of leukocytes from children with chronic granulomatous disease. *Ann NY Acad Sci* 155:888, 1968

323. CURNUTTE JT, WHITTEN DM, BABIOR BM: Defective superoxide production by granulocytes from patients with chronic granulomatous disease. *N Engl J Med* 290:593, 1974

324. STJERNHOLM RL, ALLEN RC, STEELE RH, WARING WW, HARRIS JA: Impaired chemilumenescence during phagocytosis of opsonized bacteria. *Infect Immun* 7:313, 1973

325. ALLEN RC, STJERNHOLM RL, REED MA, HARPER TB, GUPTA S, STEELE RA, WARING WW: Correlation of metabolic and chemiluminescent responses of granulocytes from three female siblings with chronic granulomatous disease. *J Infect Dis* 136:510, 1977

326. ROSEN H, KLEBANOFF SJ: Chemiluminescence and superoxide production by myeloperoxidase-deficient leukocytes. *J Clin Invest* 58:50, 1976

327. NEWBURGER PE, COHEN HJ, ROTHCHILD S, HOBBINS JC, MALAWISTA SE, MAHONEY MJ: Prenatal diagnosis of chronic granulomatous disease. *N Engl J Med* 300:178, 1979

328. GIBLETT ER, KLEBANOFF SJ, PINCUS SH, SWANSON J, PARK BH, McCULLOUGH J: Kell phenotypes in chronic granulomatous disease: A potential transfusion hazard. *Lancet* 1:1235, 1971

329. MARSH WL, URETSKY SC, DOUGLAS SD: Antigens of the Kell blood group system on neutrophils and monocytes: Their relation to chronic granulomatous disease. *J Pediatr* 87:1117, 1975

330. MARSH WL, ØYEN R, NICHOLS ME: Kx antigen, the McLeod phenotype, and chronic granulomatous disease: Further studies. *Vox Sang* 31:356, 1976

331. McPHAIL LC, DeCHATELET LR, SHIRLEY PS, WILFERT C, JOHNSTON RB, JR, McCALL CE: Deficiency of NADPH oxidase activity in chronic granulomatous disease. *J Pediatr* 90:213, 1977

331a. LEW PD, SOUTHWICK FS, STOSSEL TP, WHITIN JC, SIMONS E, COHEN HJ: A variant of chronic granulomatous disease: Deficient oxidative metabolism due to a low-affinity NADPH oxidase. *N Engl J Med* 305:1329, 1981

331b. WHITIN JC, CLARK RA, SIMONS ER, COHEN HJ: Effects of the myeloperoxidase system on fluorescent probes of granulocyte membrane potential. *J Biol Chem* 256:8904, 1981

332. CROSS AR, JONES OTG, HARPER AM, SEGAL AW: Oxidation-reduction properties of the cytochrome *b* found in the plasma membrane fraction of human neutrophils: A possible oxidase in the respiratory burst. *Biochem J* 194:599, 1981

333. SEGAL AW, WEBSTER D, JONES OTG, ALLISON AC: Absence of a newly described cytochrome b from neutrophils of patients with chronic granulomatous disease. *Lancet* 2:446, 1978

333a. SEGAL AW, JONES OTG: Absence of cytochrome b reduction in stimulated neutrophils from both female and male patients with chronic granulomatous disease. *FEBS Lett* 110:111, 1980

334. BORREGAARD N, JOHANSEN KS, ESMANN V: Quantitation of superoxide production in human polymorphonuclear leukocytes from normals and 3 types of chronic granulomatous disease. *Biochem Biophys Res Comm* 90:214, 1979

335. BORREGAARD N, JOHANSEN KS, TAUDORFF E, WANDALL JH: Cytochrome b is present in neutrophils from patients with chronic granulomatous disease. *Lancet* 2:949, 1979

335a. SEGAL AW, JONES OTG: Rapid incorporation of the human neutrophil plasma membrane cytochrome b into phagocytic vesicles. *Biochem Biophys Res Comm* 92:710, 1980

336. SHINAGAWA Y, TANAKA C, TERAOKA A, SHINAGAWA Y: A new cytochrome in neutrophilic granules of rabbit leucocyte. *J Biochem* 59:622, 1966

337. SEGAL AW, JONES OTG: The subcellular distribution and some properties of the cytochrome b component of the microbicidal oxidase system of human neutrophils. *Biochem J* 182:181, 1979

338. NAKAMURA M, NAKAMURA MA, OKAMURA J, KOBAYASHI Y: A rapid and quantitative assay of phagocytosis-connected oxygen consumption by leukocytes in whole blood. *J. Lab. Clin. Med.*, 91, 568, 1978.

339. Chusid MJ, Tomasulo PA; Survival of transfused normal granulocytes in a patient with chronic granulomatous disease. *Pediatrics* 61:556, 1978

340. Chusid MJ, Shea M, Sarff L: Determination of posttransfusion granulocyte kinetics by chemiluminescence in chronic granulomatous disease. *J Lab Clin Med* 95:155, 1980

341. Westminster Hospitals Bone Marrow Transplant Team: Bone marrow transplant from an unrelated donor for chronic granulomatous disease. *Lancet* 1:210, 1977

342. Yoshida A, Stamatoyannopoulos G, Motulsky AG: Biochemical genetics of glucose-6-phosphate dehydrogenase variation. *Ann NY Acad Sci* 155:868, 1968

343. Ramot B, Fisher S, Szemberg A, Adam A, Sheba C, Gafni D: A study of subjects with erythrocyte glucose-6-phosphate dehydrogenase deficiency. II. Investigation of leukocyte enzymes. *J Clin Invest* 38:2234, 1959

344. Rodey GE, Jacob HS, Holmes B, McArthur JR, Good RA: Leukocyte glucose-6-phosphate dehydrogenase levels and bactericidal activity. *Lancet* 1:355, 1970

345. Cech P, Papathanassiou A, Boreux G, Roth P, Miescher P: Hereditary myeloperoxidase deficiency. *Blood* 53:403, 1979

346. Kitahara M, Simonian Y, Eyre HJ: Neutrophil myeloperoxidase: A simple reproducible technique to determine activity. *J Lab Clin Med* 93:232, 1979

346a. Vitahara M, Egre HJ, Simonian Y, Atkin CL, Hasstedt SJ: Hereditary myeloperoxidase deficiency. *Blood* 57:888, 1981

346b. Parry MF, Root RK, Metcalf JA, Delaney KK, Kaplow LS, Richar WJ: Myeloperoxidase deficiency. Prevalence and clinical significance. *Ann Int Med* 95:293, 1981

347. Grignaschi VJ, Sperperato A, Etcheberry M, Macario A: Un nueva cuarda citoquimico: negatividad espontanea de las reacciones, de peroxidasas, oxidasas y lipido en la progenie neutrophilay en los monocitos, de dos hermanos. *Rev Assoc Med Argent* 77:218, 1963

348. Undritz E: Die Alius-Grignaschi-Anomalie: Der erblichkonstitutionelle peroxydase defekt der neutrophilen und monozyten. *Blut* 14:129, 1968

349. Stendahl O, Lindgren S: Function of granulocytes with a deficient myeloperoxidase-mediated iodination in a patient with a generalized pustular psoriasis. *Scand J Haematol* 16:144, 1976

350. Huhn D, Belohradsky BH, Haas R: Familiärer myeloperoxidasedefekt und akute myeloische leukämie. *Acta Haematol* 59:129, 1978

351. Robertson CF, Thong YH, Hodge GL, Cheney K: Primary myeloperoxidase deficiency associated with impaired neutrophil margination and chemotaxis. *Acta Paediatr Scand* 68:915, 1979

352. Lehrer RI: Inhibition by sulfonamides of the candidacidal activity of human neutrophils. *J Clin Invest* 50:2498, 1971

353. Kaplow LS: Simplified myeloperoxidase stain using benzidine dihydrochloride. *Blood* 26:215, 1965

354. Lehrer RI: Measurement of candidacidal activity of specific leukocyte types in mixed cell populations. *Infect Immun* 2:42, 1970

355. Klebanoff SJ, Pincus SH: Hydrogen peroxide utilization in myeloperoxidase-deficient leukocytes: A possible microbicidal control mechanism. *J Clin Invest* 50:2226, 1971

356. Lehrer RI: Functional aspects of a second mechanism of candidacidal activity by human neutrophils. *J Clin Invest* 51:2566, 1972

357. Klebanoff SJ: Estrogen binding by leukocytes during phagocytosis. *J Exp Med* 145:983, 1977

358. Loos H, Roos D, Weening R, Houwerzijl J: Familial deficiency of glutathione reductase in human blood cells. *Blood* 48:53, 1976

359. Roos D, Weening RS, Voetman AA, van Schaik MLJ, Bot AAM, Meerhof LJ, Loos JA: Protection of phagocytic leukocytes by endogenous glutathione: Studies in a family with glutathione reductase deficiency. *Blood* 53:851, 1979

360. Spielberg SP, Corash LM, Butler JD, Tietze F, Rogers L, Schulman JD: Biochemical heterogeneity in glutathione synthetase deficiency. *J Clin Invest* 61:1417, 1978

361. Spielberg SP, Kramer LI, Goodman SI, Butler J, Tietze F, Quinn P, Schulman JD: 5-Oxoprolinuria: Biochemical observations and case report. *J Pediatr* 91:237, 1977

362. Spielberg SP, Boxer LA, Oliver JM, Allen JM, Schulman JD: Oxidative damage to neutrophils in glutathione synthetase deficiency. *Br J Haematol* 42:215, 1979

363. Ryan GB, Borysenko JZ, Karnovsky MJ: Factors affecting the redistribution of surface-bound concanavalin A on human polymorphonuclear leukocytes. *J Cell Biol* 62:351, 1974

364. Malech HL, Root RK, Gallin JI: Structural analysis of human neutrophil migration. *J Cell Biol* 75:666, 1977

365. Allan RB, Wilkinson PC: A visual analysis of chemotactic and chemokinetic locomotion of human neutrophil leucocytes. Use of a new chemotaxis assay with *Candida albicans* as gradient source. *Exp Cell Res* 111:191, 1978

366. Hoffstein S, Goldstein IM, Weissmann G: Role of microtubule assembly in lysosomal enzyme secretion from human polymorphonuclear leucocytes: a reevaluation. *J Cell Biol* 73:242, 1977

367. Henson PM, Zanolari B, Schwartzman NA, Hong SR: Intracellular control of human neutrophil secretion. I. C5a-induced stimulus-specific desensitization and the effects of cytochalasin B. *J Immunol* 121:851, 1978

368. Malawista SE, Oliver JM, Rudolph SA: Microtubules and cyclic AMP in human leukocytes: On the order of things. *J Cell Biol* 77:881, 1978

369. Berlin RD, Oliver JM: Analogous ultrastructure and surface properties during capping and phagocytosis in leukocytes. *J Cell Biol* 77:789, 1978

370. Oliver JM, Spielberg, SP, Pearson CB, Schulman JD: Microtubule assembly and function in normal and glutathione synthetase-deficient polymorphonuclear leukocytes. *J Immunol* 120:1181, 1978

371. Babior BM: Oxygen-dependent microbial killing by phagocytes. *N Engl J Med* 298:721, 1978

372. Holmes B, Park BH, Malawista SE, Quie PG, Nelson DL, Good RA: Chronic granulomatous disease in females: A deficiency of leukocyte glutathione peroxidase. *N Engl J Med* 283:217, 1970

373. Matsuda I, Oka Y, Taniguchi N, Furuyama M, Kodama S, Arashima S, Mitsuyama T: Leukocyte glutathione peroxidase deficiency in a male patient with chronic granulomatous disease, *J Pediatr* 88:581, 1976

374. McCallister J, Harris RE, Baehner RL, Boxer LA: Alteration of microtubule function in glutathione peroxidase-deficient polymorphonuclear leukocytes. *J Reticuloendothel Soc* 27:59, 1980

91

THE IMMOTILE-CILIA SYNDROME INCLUDING KARTAGENER'S SYNDROME

BJÖRN A. AFZELIUS

BJÖRN MOSSBERG

1. The immotile-cilia syndrome is a genetically determined disorder characterized by immotility or poor motility of the cilia in the airways and elsewhere. Spermatozoa also are either immotile or poorly motile.

2. Kartagener's syndrome is a subgroup of the immotile-cilia syndrome and is further characterized by situs inversus viscerum. Situs inversus, bronchiectasis, and chronic sinusitis form the classic Kartagener's triad.

3. The reason for the ciliary immotility can usually be seen with an electron microscopic investigation of a ciliated mucosal biopsy or of an ejaculate. Certain specific defects in the ciliary axoneme can be found and are pathognomic of the syndrome. These defects include missing dynein arms, abnormally short dynein arms, short spokes with no central sheath, missing central microtubules, and displacement of one of the nine peripheral microtubular doublets. Certain other ciliary abnormalities, such as compound cilia, may also be present but are not specific. Cilia may also be oriented randomly. Cilia from epithelia and sperm tails will exhibit the same defects in the same patient. The functional capacity of the cilia can be evaluated by light microscopic examination of living cilia or spermatozoa, or by measurements of mucociliary transport.

4. The clinical consequences of the immotile-cilia syndrome include chronic cough and expectoration of mucoid, mucopurulent, or purulent sputum, bronchiectasis, chronic rhinitis and nasal polyposis, chronic or recurrent maxillary sinusitis, and often an agenesis of the frontal sinuses. Otosalpingitis and otitis are common. Obstructive lung disease may develop early in life and is expressed as chronic air flow limitation. The clinical manifestations date from early childhood. Neonatal asphyxia may occur.

5. Males are usually sterile. Females may have normal fertility.

6. Treatment is symptomatic and directed against complications in the upper and lower respiratory tract. Physiotherapy with postural drainage should probably be started early in life. With modern care and abstinence from smoking the prognosis in the immotile-cilia syndrome is good.

7. The immotile-cilia syndrome clearly is a heterogeneous disease. Many genes participate in the construction of a cilium, and an error in a number of them will prevent the cilia from working properly. The inheritance in most cases is autosomal recessive. Half the affected sibs have situs inversus in families in which the immotile-cilia syndrome occurs. Presumably chance alone decides between situs inversus and situs solitus in homozygotes of the immotile-cilia syndrome.

In a paper in 1933 Manes Kartagener published the case histories of four persons who all had situs inversus totalis, bronchiectasis, and chronic sinusitis [1]. This combination of symptoms has later come to be known under the name *Kartagener's syndrome* or *Kartagener's triad*. In the Soviet Union it is usually called *Siewert's* or *Zivert's syndrome*. Siewert wrote a description of a person with situs inversus combined with bronchiectasis, initially (1902) in Russian and somewhat later in German [2].

Kartagener's paper, entitled "Zur Pathogenese der Bronchiektasien," is an attempt to explain the genesis of bronchiectases. Kartagener wrote, "In transposition of the viscera there is often a weakness of the bronchi, possibly due to a deficiency of elastic tissue, which renders those with it liable to develop bronchiectasis."

The frequent association between bronchiectasis and situs inversus has been confirmed by numerous investigators, but the explanation given by Kartagener has been superseded by another theory of pathogenesis: Kartagener's syndrome is caused by a structural abnormality of the cilia on embryonic cells and on ciliated epithelia. Because of this abnormality the cilia are immotile or poorly motile [3], and, hence, they are nonfunctional. Ciliary immotility is associated with situs inversus in only about half the cases; thus there are about as many cases with bronchiectasis and chronic sinusitis (due to ciliary defects) but without situs inversus as there are with Kartagener's syndrome.

For this reason, and because situs inversus per se usually has no serious implications, this chapter will treat the *immotile-cilia syndrome* in its entirety and will include Kartagener's syndrome as a subgroup of the immotile-cilia syndrome.

PREVALENCE

Most authors estimate the prevalence of Kartagener's syndrome at 1:30,000 to 1:60,000 [4, 5]. Different values will be obtained depending on how strictly the investigator adheres to the original definition. For example, a generalized bronchitis rather than bronchiectasis may be regarded as part of Kartagener's triad. Bronchiectasis is not congenital but develops during life.

The prevalence of the immotile-cilia syndrome can be estimated from the following data. Situs inversus has a prevalence in Europe and the United States of 1:8000 to 1:11,000 [4, 6]. Roughly a fourth to a fifth of all persons with situs inversus also have bronchiectasis [6]. A somewhat higher fraction has generalized bronchitis but not (yet) bronchiectasis. Over 90 percent of all cases of bronchiectasis have chronic sinusitis [6]. This gives a figure of the prevalence of Kartagener's syndrome in the order of 1:40,000. If it is true, as assumed [3], that 50 percent of patients with the immotile-cilia syndrome have situs inversus, then the prevalence of this syndrome will be twice that of Kartagener's syndrome, or about 1:20,000.

A somewhat higher value for the prevalence may be found among newborns, since infants with Kartagener's syndrome probably have an increased mortality.

The prevalence of situs inversus or of Kartagener's syndrome may vary in different countries, such as Japan, where consanguine marriages are common. Situs inversus is found with a prevalence of 1:5000 in Israel [7] and 1:4100 in Japan

[8]. Yet, Kartagener's syndrome seems rarer in Israel than in Europe and the United States.

Geographic and Racial Distribution

Kartagener's syndrome has been described in all major races and from most countries with medical journals. Detailed pedigrees have been published from Germany [9–11], Great Britain [12], France [13], the United States [14–16], Israel [17], Japan [8], and other countries. In all these publications it was remarked that one or several sibs of the propositus had the same bronchial and sinusoidal symptoms as the propositus but had no situs inversus. Sometimes these sibs have been claimed to have an "incomplete Kartagener's syndrome." The equal number of affected sibs with and without situs inversus speaks in favor of the opinion [3] that the immotile-cilia syndrome is inherited as a recessive disorder and that chance alone determines whether the viscera take up the normal or the reversed position during embryogenesis.

The Polynesian population of New Zealand may be a special case. According to Wakefield and Waite [18] 12 Polynesians were diagnosed as having the immotile-cilia syndrome, and none of them had situs inversus. Bronchiectasis is relatively common among the Polynesians in New Zealand, Samoa, and elsewhere, and they may have a particular form of the immotile-cilia syndrome that does not involve a risk of situs inversus [18].

CILIA IN THE HUMAN BODY

The symptoms of the immotile-cilia syndrome and of its subgroup, Kartagener's syndrome, cannot be understood without a knowledge of the distribution in the body of cilia of the normal ciliary anatomy.

Cilia and sperm tails are outgrowths from centrioles (basal bodies) with an architecture as shown in Fig. 91-1. The central axis is called the *axoneme* and consists of nine microtubular doublets in a ring around two single microtubules. These 11 units are joined by three types of bonds: (1) Two rows of arms along each doublet. The outer arms have a complex structure, while the inner arms are somewhat shorter and simpler. The arms are composed of the major ATPases that are responsible for the ciliary work; they are proteins, called *dynein*. (2) Nexin links which also connect the doublets and which are presumed to act like resistant elastic bonds that keep the axoneme together. (3) Spokes which extend from the outer doublets to a *central sheath* that surrounds the two central microtubules.

The two main protein components of the cilium are tubulin and dynein, which make up the microtubules and the dynein arms, respectively. There is a functional analogy between the tubulin-dynein system in cilia and the actin-myosin system in muscles (or in most other contractile systems in nonmuscular cells). Thus, the dynein arms are structures which are instrumental in the sliding of microtubules during ciliary work, as are myosin filaments during muscle contraction. Like myosin, the dynein molecule has a high molecular weight and is an ATPase. The dynein arms can thus be considered to provide the motor force for beating of cilia.

The nexin links presumably are responsible for the mainte-

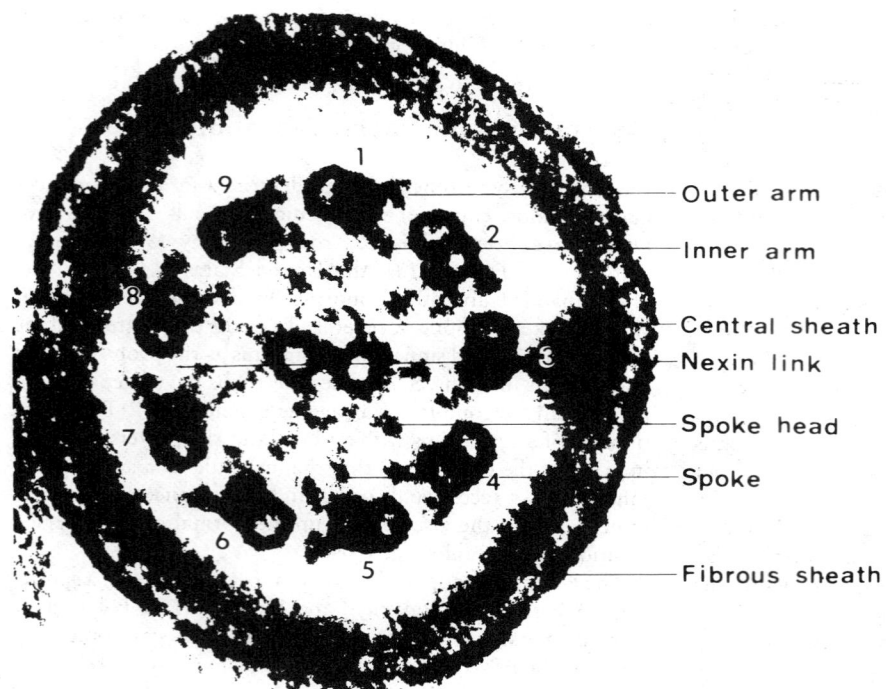

Outer arm

Inner arm

Central sheath

Nexin link

Spoke head

Spoke

Fibrous sheath

Figure 91-1 Electron micrograph of a transversely sectioned human sperm tail from a healthy man. The central part of the sperm tail has the same structure as that of a cilium. There are nine outer microtubular doublets in a ring around two central microtubules. The terms used for some of the components are given. (*Reproduced by permission of Journal of Ultrastructure Research [25]*).

nance of axoneme structure during sliding. They seem to limit the sliding by being stretchable only to a certain degree. It has also been suggested that the nexin links pull the doublets together in the initial phase of bend induction, allowing the dynein arms to interact with adjacent doublets.

The spokes may interact with the central sheath at the start of bending as a part of the mechanism for converting sliding into bending. It also appears probable that the spokes give the cilium a certain rigidity, preventing it from making sharp nicks, while allowing it to bend. Further details of the ciliary machinery and its mode of action can be found in Refs. 4 and 19 to 21.

Ciliated epithelia are found in the following places in the human body: the upper airways (i.e., the nasal passages, the paranasal sinuses, the eustachian tubes, the middle ear mucosa, and the pharynx down to the orifice of the esophagus); the lower airways (i.e., the trachea, the primary and secondary bronchi, and the bronchioles down to the respiratory bronchioles); the ependymal lining of the brain and central canal of the spinal cord; the endometrial lining of the deeper parts of the cervix; the oviduct; and the ductuli efferentes on the border between the testis and epididymis.

Some epithelia have a single cilium per cell, sometimes called a primary cilium, a solitary cilium, or a monocilium. This is true of the inner corneal endothelium, the trabecular meshwork, and the choroid of the eye [22] as well as of several of the embryonic epithelia [4]. Whether the primary cilia are capable of motility is unknown.

Certain sensory cells carry a sensory hair that is a modified cilium. The tail of the human spermatozoon has an axoneme that has the typical structure of a cilium.

Our knowledge about the normal functions of the cilia is incomplete. The epithelium of the upper and lower airways and of the middle ear is a mixture of ciliated and nonciliated cells. Some of the nonciliated cells secrete a serous fluid which forms a 5-μm-thick layer in which the cilia beat. The goblet cells and the mucous glands secrete a mucus which forms a

blanket overlying the ciliary tips that also is about 5 μm wide and that is either patchy or continuous [19]. The ciliary beating moves the mucous blanket toward the esophagus and the mucus is swallowed. The speed of the movement of the mucous blanket is in the order of 2 mm/min in the lung and 10 mm/min in the trachea; its volume is about 0.5 ml per kilogram of body weight per day [21]. The mucous blanket traps inhaled particles and endogenous debris which are then eliminated by the mucociliary clearance mechanism.

The role of cilia in the oviducts, the ductuli efferentes, and the ependyma of the central nervous system is largely speculative. Similarly, nothing is known about the role of single cilia on monociliated epithelia.

Ultrastructure of Cilia and Sperm Tails in the Immotile-Cilia Syndrome

The essential feature of the immotile-cilia syndrome, including Kartagener's syndrome, is the abnormal structure and function of cilia. Most, if not all, clinical data of this syndrome can be explained by this single feature.

Cilia or sperm tails from more than 150 persons with the immotile-cilia syndrome have been examined, and the data from different laboratories are in essential agreement [23–29]. Different types of ciliary abnormalities are recorded, and it is evident that the immotile-cilia syndrome is a heterogeneous disease. The following subgroups can be defined:

1. Both rows of dynein arms are missing [3, 4, 25, 29, 31, 39, 45] (Fig. 91-2).

2. The inner dynein arms are missing, and the outer dynein arms are short [24, 28].

3. The inner arms, the nexin links, and the spokes are missing, the circle of microtubular doublets is disrupted, and the outer arms are prominent [25, 28].

4. The outer dynein arms are missing [25] (Fig. 91-3).

5. The spokes or the spoke heads and central sheath are missing [4, 25, 26] (Fig. 91-4).

6. The central microtubules are very short or absent, and one of the nine microtubular doublets is transposed to a central position [27].

7. Cilia have normal ultrastructure with respect to microtubules, dynein arms, spokes, and central sheath [30], but in the light microscope they can be seen to be immotile.

8. Cilia may perhaps even be completely lacking [24].

Other subgroups may well exist. In most cases the cilia are oriented randomly. This alone would seem to exclude coordinated activity [4] (Figs. 91-5 and 91-6). It is of interest that about half the cases within each of the six first subgroups have situs inversus.

In at least 30 cases cilia from two or more different types of epithelia or sperm tails and cilia from the same person with the immotile-cilia syndrome have been examined [24, 31], and it has appeared that all cilia and sperm tails display the same type of defect. The defect often is more easily studied in an ejaculate than in cilia from the nasal or endometrial mucosa.

Ciliary abnormalities other than those listed above have been described in patients with infections, allergies, or conditions other than the immotile-cilia syndrome. These include the clumping of several axonemes within a common limiting membrane (into what have been called compound cilia or multicilia), or the presence of supernumerary or missing microtubules in the axoneme [32, 33]. These types of ciliary abnormalities therefore are not diagnostic of the immotile-cilia syndrome but may be due to nonspecific damage to the cilia.

Motility of Cilia and Sperm Tails

The immotile-cilia syndrome is due to the cilia being immotile or poorly motile. This feature can be examined by different means:

A freshly collected ejaculate can be examined and sperm

Figure 91-2 The sperm tail of a man with the immotile-cilia syndrome. In this man the sperm tails and the cilia are characterized by a total or nearly total lack of both the outer and inner dynein arms.

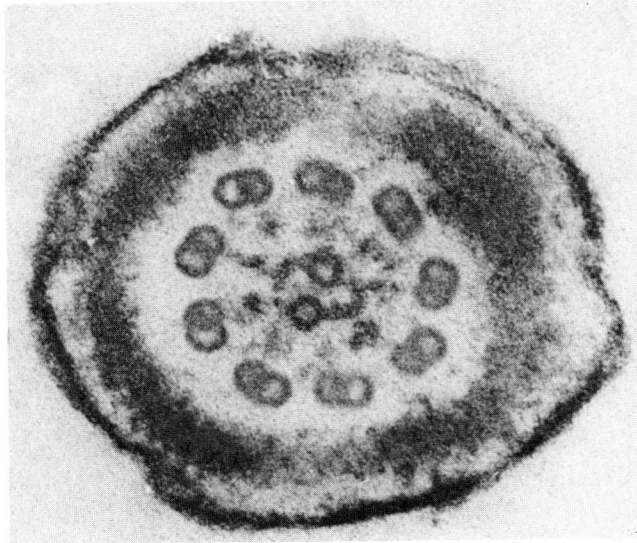

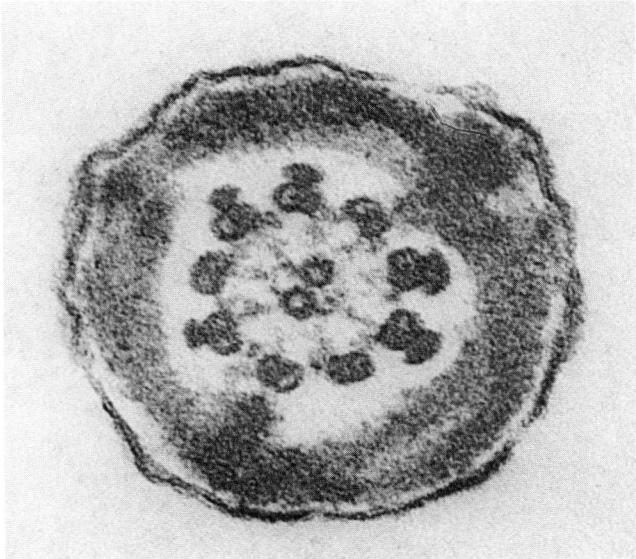

Figure 91-3 The sperm tail of a man with the immotile-cilia syndrome and characterized by the presence of inner dynein arms but no, or very few, outer dynein arms. The spermatozoa had some degree of motility.

motility evaluated. Sperm immotility (or poor motility) is closely correlated with ciliary dysfunction when the spermatozoa have a normal light microscopic appearance [31]. Other conditions in which spermatozoa are immotile have to be excluded: exposure of the ejaculate to cold, immobilization by antibodies, necrospermia (i.e., dead spermatozoa), and certain disorders in which the spermatozoa are grossly abnormal [31].

Biopsies or brushings from the ciliated epithelium of the nasal cavity, the bronchus, the middle ear, nasal polyps, or the endometrium can be examined with the phase contrast or the interference contrast microscope [23, 34, 35]. Cilia from healthy persons will beat as long as the culture medium is aerated; those from the immotile-cilia syndrome will either be completely immotile [23, 24, 34] or else show erratic movements [35–37].

Biopsies that have been fixed and prepared for scanning electron microscopy may also have diagnostic value. Whereas the ciliary tips from healthy epithelia all point in the same general direction, those from patients with the immotile-cilia syndrome lack an ordered orientation [34].

Mucociliary transport can be measured. The earliest demonstration of nonfunctioning cilia in the tracheobronchial tract came from such measurements performed on two patients with Kartagener's syndrome [38]. They inhaled a radioactively tagged test aerosol, and the radioactivity in the lungs was measured during 2 h. Mucociliary transport is extremely slow and probably absent in patients with the immotile-cilia syndrome [27, 39]. Coughing can partly compensate for the defective transport [39].

An alternative method for demonstrating mucociliary transport includes direct observation of visible or radioopaque particles deposited in the nose or trachea, or the application of saccharin particles to the nose followed by measurement of the time until the saccharin is tasted.

Certain investigators have stressed that the term *immotile-cilia syndrome* is unsuitable, because the cilia from some patients have some degree of ciliary motility [35–37]. The term

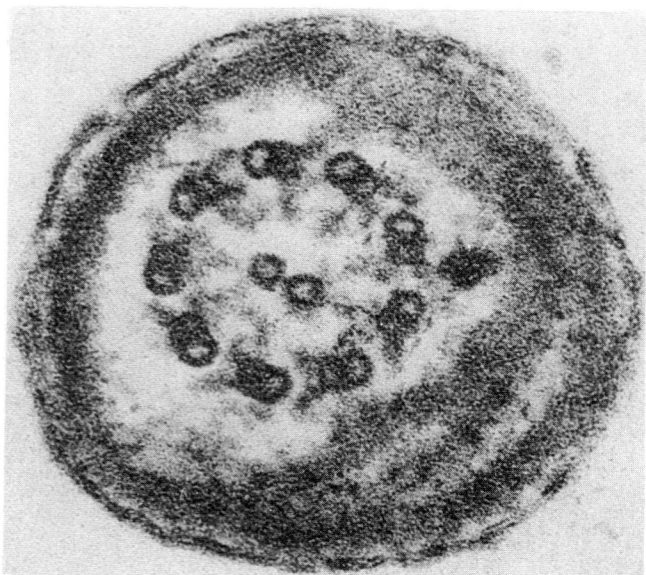

Figure 91-4   The sperm tail of a man with the immotile-cilia syndrome and characterized by abnormally short spokes and defective central sheath.

dyskinetic ciliary syndrome has been proposed. Others have suggested *abnormal-cilia syndrome*. The existence of a clinical entity characterized by a ciliary insufficiency has not been challenged. In some cases the cilia show a pendulous movement rather than the usual rather complex normal ciliary strokes. In these patients the cilia are functionally incompetent, and, accordingly, it seems reasonable to include these functionally defective cilia, which are incapable of mucus transport, in the entity *immotile-cilia syndrome*. The syndrome could logically be given the code number 748.70 in the International Classification of Diseases.

Situs Inversus and Embryonic Cilia

The following explanation has been suggested for the association between ciliary immotility and situs inversus [3]. Embryonic epithelia often carry a single cilium per cell. In the normal course of events these cilia are assumed to beat and, by their beatings, cause the heart to be moved to the left side and the liver to the right side of the body. With no ciliary work, chance alone will decide whether the visceral asymmetry will be the normal one or the reversed one. The validity or invalidity of this assumption can be tested only when suitable animal models are examined, such as the mouse strain described by Layton [40].

GENETIC CONSIDERATIONS

An examination of published pedigrees [8–17] shows that the immotile-cilia syndrome is inherited as a recessive autosomal trait. Half of the affected persons have situs inversus. As a consequence, one-eighth of the offspring of a mating between two heterozygotes will have situs inversus. It is believed that chance alone decides between situs inversus and situs solitus

(normal asymmetry) in homozygotes of the immotile-cilia syndrome.

One of the pedigrees published by Katsuhara is more compatible with a dominant mode of inheritance than with the recessive one [8]. It shows a woman, her daughter, and a granddaughter, but none of their sibs, with immotile-cilia syndrome. Presumably there are both recessive and dominant modes of inheritance of this disease, although the dominant form(s) are rare.

The primary gene products may be those proteins that are seen to be missing in the cilia: dyneins, nexin, spoke proteins, etc. Alternatively, they may be proteins that are responsible for the binding of the dyneins (nexin, etc.) to the microtubules, for their incorporation into the axonemal framework, or for their transport from the site of synthesis to the site of action.

Figure 91-5   Cilia from the bronchial mucosa from a person who has normal cilia. It is to be noted that the cilia have an ordered orientation best seen in the orientation of the two central microtubules.

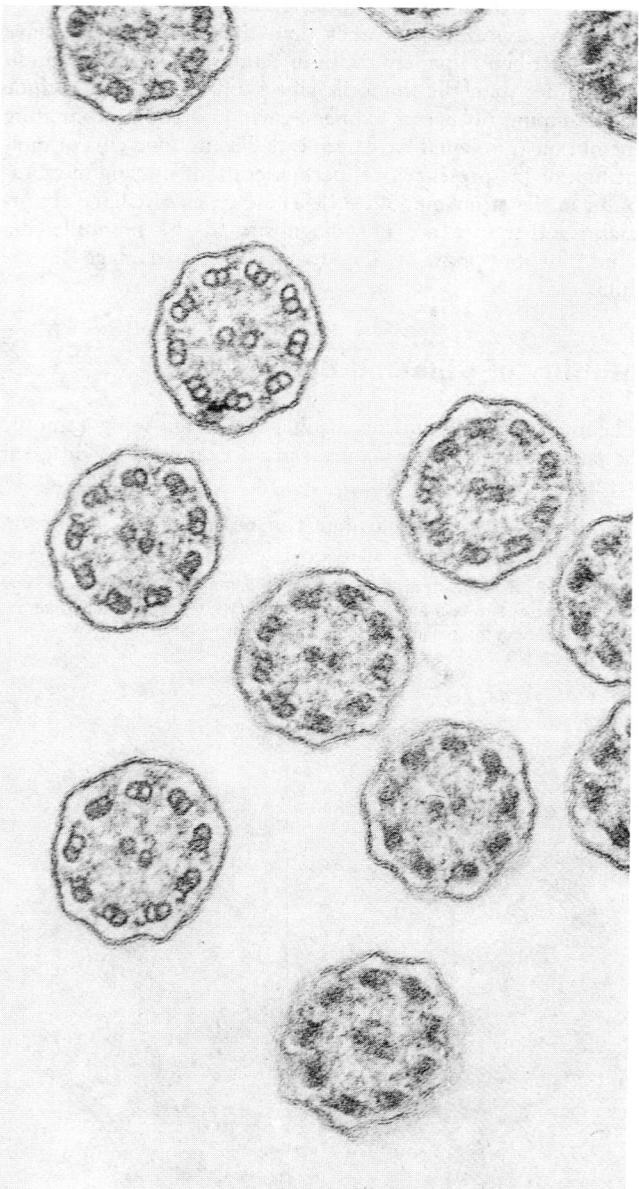

Well over 100 different polypeptides have been identified within the ciliary axoneme of lower organisms [41]. It is likely that genes responsible for different subgroups of the immotile-cilia syndrome are located on many chromosomes in humans. Attempts to localize the (assumed single) gene for Kartagener's syndrome have been completely unsuccessful. Conclusive results will probably be obtained only when definitive studies are restricted to one family, and these results may not necessarily be extended to other families.

Chromosomal studies on several patients have almost always disclosed a normal karyotype [5]. Richer et al. [42] reported a man with the immotile-cilia syndrome and trisomy 12 mosaicism.

Males and females are equally affected. Males with the syndrome have immotile spermatozoa and are sterile. Male sterility can also be observed in most, but not all, published pedigrees. No proofs of paternity are given in the papers by Finkler [7], Logan et al. [16], and Heuckenkamp et al. [43], and male fertility in these families is thus not fully documented. It is conceivable that some subgroups of the immotile-cilia are characterized by cilia which have poor motility owing to defective proteins needed for ciliary coordination or orientation. In these cases the spermatozoa might be normally motile, and males might be fertile.

In a Norwegian population 5 percent of all children with Kartagener's syndrome had parents that were first cousins, and 16 percent had parents that were second cousins [44]. Among the population in general 0.5 percent of parents are first cousins.

CLINICAL FEATURES

Diagnosis

For clinical purposes the diagnosis of the immotile-cilia syndrome can be regarded as established in (1) patients with complete Kartagener's syndrome; (2) men without situs inversus but a typical clinical history (chronic bronchitis and rhinitis since early childhood) and with living but immotile spermatozoa; (3) patients without situs inversus but with typical clinical signs and sibs with the complete Kartagener's syndrome; (4) those without situs inversus but with the clinical signs, if a nasal or bronchial biopsy shows the characteristic defects of the cilia.

Patients with situs inversus accompanied by other types of respiratory tract disease, such as asthma and atopic rhinitis, which are not caused by immotile cilia, should not be confused with patients with the immotile-cilia syndrome.

Respiratory Tract

In the immotile-cilia syndrome respiratory tract disease usually can be traced back to early childhood. In some there is a history of neonatal asphyxia [39]. Chronic cough and expectoration of mucoid, mucopurulent, and at times purulent sputum are prominent. Chronic rhinitis is often complicated by nasal polyposis. Chronic or recurrent maxillary sinusitis is almost always present, and the frontal sinuses often fail to develop.

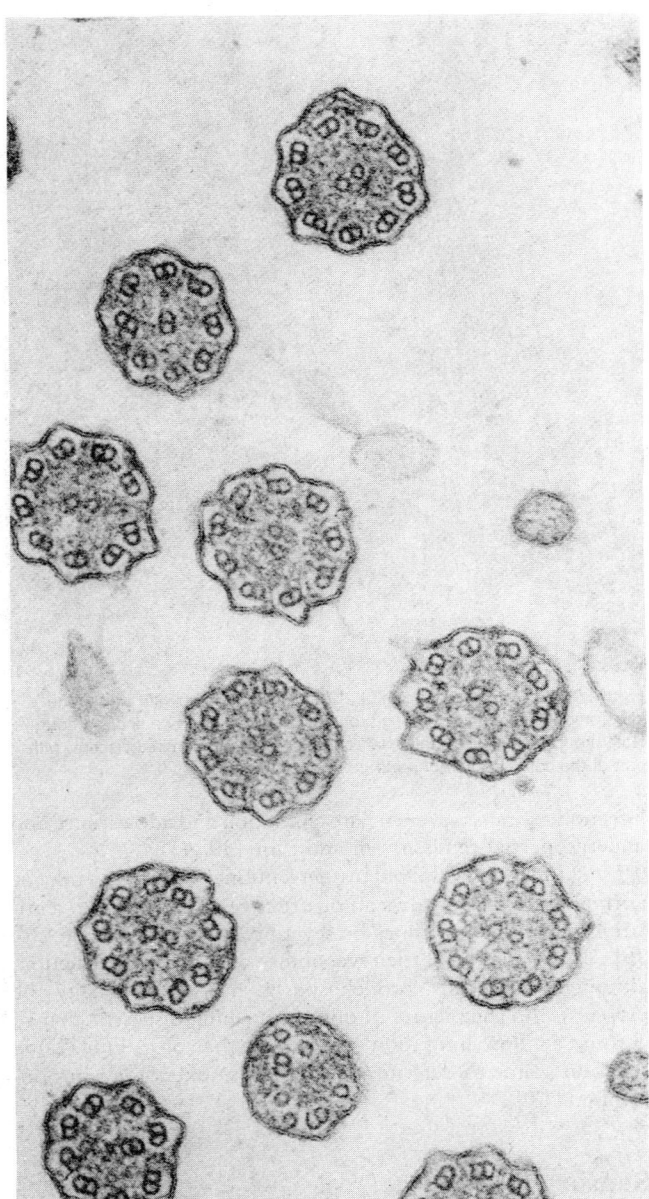

Figure 91-6 Cilia from the bronchial mucosa from a man with the immotile-cilia syndrome. The dynein arms are largely missing, and there is no fixed orientation of the cilia.

Chronic or recurrent otosalpingitis or otitis media is frequent. At times when there is no apparent infection, the sedimentation rate may be normal and sputum cultures may fail to reveal specific pathogens. Serum immunoglobulins are usually normal [30, 39, 45, 47].

Bronchiectases are probably not present at birth but may be acquired during childhood or adolescence (Figs. 91-7 and 91-8). These usually develop in dependent parts of the lungs, may be cylindrical or saccular, and on histologic examination show nonspecific inflammation. The changes are not different from bronchiectases from other causes [46]. When bronchiectasis develops, there may be marked worsening of symptoms, with increased expectoration, infectious episodes with fever, hemoptysis, and development of clubbed fingers. In some patients the symptoms of upper and lower respiratory tract

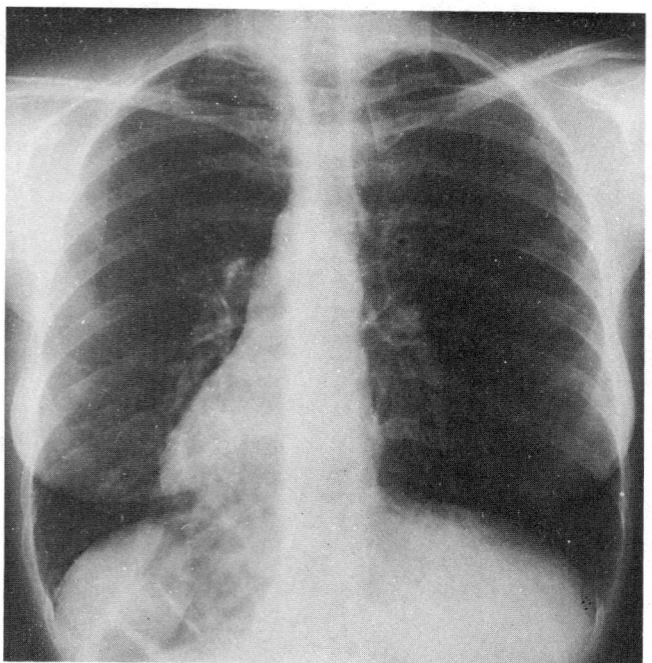

Figure 91-7 Chest radiograph of a 32-year-old woman with Kartagener's syndrome. Changes suggesting bronchiectasis are seen behind the heart. Note the transposition of the heart and also of the abdominal viscera, with part of the colon to the right and the liver to the left.

infection are most severe in late childhood and adolescence and undergo partial remission in adult life [39, 45].

Lung function evaluated by conventional spirometry may be normal but usually shows an obstructive impairment of ventilation which may at times be severe by the third decade [36, 39]. Usually there is little reversibility of airways obstruction, although significant bronchospasm may occasionally be present [39]. The picture of obstructive lung disease is that of chronic air flow limitation rather than that of asthma. Lung function seems to deteriorate faster in smokers than in non-smokers. [39].

Sensory Organs

A moderate decrease in hearing is common and may be regarded as a consequence of chronic otitis [48–50]. Congenital deafness has also been recorded [1, 5, 51] and may be coincidental. The eustachian tubes may be obstructed and the mastoid air cells may be poorly aerated. A decrease in hearing ability may be caused by fluid in the middle ear. The sense of balance seems not to be affected in the majority of cases [5].

Examination of the eyes of 10 patients with the syndrome showed corneal abnormalities in 9 [52] but no other consistent abnormalities. These abnormalities may be secondary to a developmental disturbance. It may be remembered that the corneal endothelium is a monociliated epithelium.

Some patients have been described who suffer from both Kartagener's syndrome and either retinitis pigmentosa [54] or a pigmented degeneration of the retina [53]. This is interesting because Fox et al. [55] have claimed that abnormalities in the ultrastructure of human nasal cilia are found in persons suffering from retinitis pigmentosa.

Most subjects with inborn ciliary immotility are anosmic or have a poor sense of smell.

Central Nervous System

In the literature on the syndrome one often notes that some of the patients suffer from dull headaches, endogenous depression [4], or schizophrenia [56]. In the Swedish case reports two-thirds of the patients complained of chronic headaches, and many had sought medical advice for this complaint. The headaches persist even during periods free of sinusitis or other infections.

It may be that patients with the immotile-cilia syndrome run a higher-than-normal risk of hydrocephalus. This possibility is suggested by two observations. Ciliary defects are found in *hpy/hpy* mice, as well as hydrocephalus and polydactyly [57]. Also, occasional patients with Kartagener's syndrome have died from hydrocephalus [54, 58]. It may be assumed that ependymal cilia normally keep the aqueduct patent and that the risk of stenosis is increased with ciliary immotility.

The brains of seven persons with the immotile-cilia syndrome have been examined by means of computer tomography. In two or three of these a slight enlargement of the ventricular system and also the sulci was found [4]. The brain does not seem to mirror the situs inversus in persons having Kartagener's syndrome; only 3 of 36 patients (8 percent) were left-handed [4].

Reproductive Organs

Women with the immotile-cilia syndrome seem to be normally fertile [59, 60], which is remarkable in light of the fact that the oviducts have a ciliated mucosa and that the ciliary beats generally are believed to transport the egg. There are no records of ectopic pregnancies, an increased prevalence of abortions, or salpingitis or any other peculiarity, except for some cases of genital hypoplasia [4, 5].

Whether all men are sterile is still an open question. Since most men produce an ejaculate that contains spermatozoa, the ducts from the testes to the vasa efferentes are known to be open. Some patients have hydrocele [61] or are azoospermic [35] or oligospermic [36, 38]. In one patient the amount of the protein carboxyl-methylase has been measured in spermatozoa and found to be decreased [62]. This enzyme plays a role in chemotactic responses in bacteria and may also be involved in animal cell motility.

Cardiovascular System

Persons with Kartagener's syndrome have dextrocardia. Whereas heart malformations are common in dextrocardia, a normal (albeit mirrored) heart is the rule in Kartagener's syndrome. A few malformations of the heart have been recorded, as well as some instances of incomplete situs inversus [5].

Leukocytes

The capacity of the leukocytes to orient and to migrate in a chemotactic gradient has been examined in an attempt to find out whether defects in cell motility are restricted to spermatozoa and ciliated cells have a more general occurrence. It has then been found that the chemotactic migration indeed is significantly reduced in some, but not all, persons investigated,

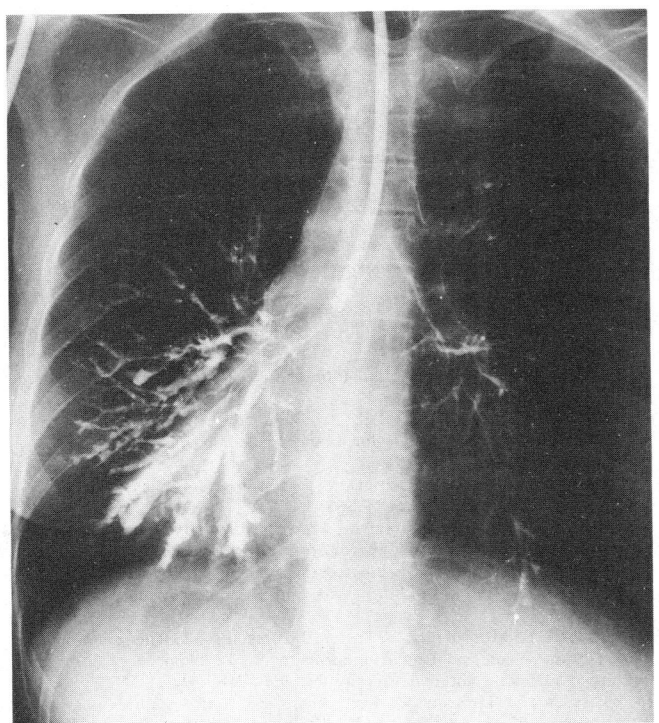

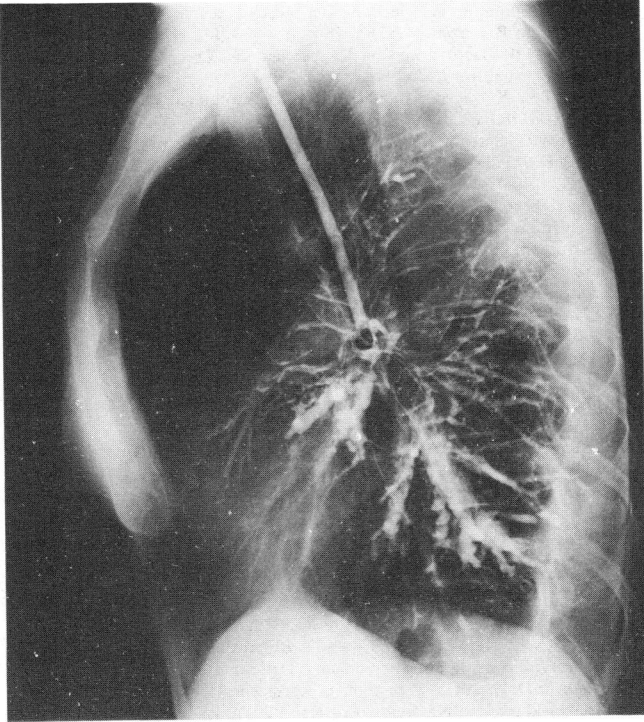

Figure 91-8 A and B. Bronchography of the right lung from the same patient as in Fig. 91-7. Large bronchiectasis is seen in the lower lobe and in the right-sided lingula segment of the upper lobe.

and also, that the capacity to orient is hampered [63]. Whether this decreased motility is a primary phenomenon and one which will explain why persons with the immotile-cilia syndrome have frequent infections, or whether it is a consequence of the chronic infections is at present unknown. Most persons with the immotile-cilia syndrome do not appear to have more infections than normal at sites outside the airways.

Developmental Anomalies

An extensive list of malformations and diseases that have been observed in patients suffering from Kartagener's syndrome is found in Ref. 5. It is likely that the simultaneous occurrence of a certain disease and the syndrome in many cases is purely coincidental. In other instances a disease or an anomaly may be a direct or indirect consequence of the ciliary malfunction. If so, one might expect to find the anomaly in several patients. Some of the congenital cardiac malformations may belong to this category. So may polydactyly, which has been noted in some patients [64, 65] and which is also characteristic of *hpy/hpy* mice, a strain in which cilia are abnormal [57].

TREATMENT AND PROGNOSIS

Treatment is symptomatic and is directed against complications in the upper and lower respiratory tracts. There is no method available to restore ciliary and spermatozoal motility *in situ*.

Antibiotics or chemotherapeutic agents are usually given when there are signs of infections. Since no particular bacteria have been found to be associated with the syndrome, general guidelines are followed when choosing antibiotic therapy.

The value of mucolytics is uncertain, but they may be tried in selected cases. Bronchodilators (beta₂-adrenergics, methylxanthines, or both) may be valuable when there is airway obstruction with a component of bronchospasm. In these patients, beta-adrenergic drugs do not promote mucociliary clearance as they do in healthy persons [38].

Physiotherapy with postural drainage is often important and should probably be started as early in life as possible to prevent complications, such as bronchiectasis.

Surgical intervention against maxillary sinusitis, middle ear disease, or nasal polyposis is often necessary and valuable. Thoracic surgical intervention against bronchiectasis is sometimes indicated. In one series of 14 subjects, bronchiectasis was demonstrated in 9, and 6 of them had undergone resectional surgery [39]. In half of these operation had resulted in a definite clinical improvement. Selection for surgery should be made on the basis of a careful individual evaluation following general guidelines. The symptoms of chronic bronchitis are not cured by resectional surgery. Abandonment of smoking is a most important preventive measure, as smoking probably greatly accelerates deterioration of lung function [39].

Without access to antibiotics the average life span is probably somewhat reduced owing to severe respiratory tract infections, particularly in childhood and adolescence. The frequent and early development of chronic obstructive pulmonary disease and the possible development of respiratory insufficiency also tend to reduce the average life span. Whether there is an increased risk of lung cancer in the syndrome is not known.

Most persons with the syndrome seem to live an active life [39, 45]. General physical and mental development is not retarded by the chronic disease. Situs inversus usually is not combined with congenital malformations. Kartagener's syndrome has been described in old age [66]. With modern medical care and abstinence from smoking the prognosis may therefore be encouraging or even excellent.

REFERENCES

1. KARTAGENER M: Zur Pathogenese der Bronchiektasien: Bronchiektasien bei Situs viscerum inversus. *Beitr Klin Tuberk* 83:489, 1933

2. SIEWERT AK: Ueber einen Fall von Bronchiectasie bei einem Patienten mit Situs inversus viscerum. *Berl Klin Wochenschr* 41:139, 1904

3. AFZELIUS BA: A human syndrome caused by immotile cilia *Science (Washington)* 193:317, 1976

4. AFZELIUS BA: The immotile-cilia syndrome and other ciliary diseases. *Intern Rev Exp Pathol* 19:1, 1979

5. ROTT H-D: Kartagener's syndrome and the syndrome of immotile cilia. *Hum Genet* 46:249, 1979

6. ADAMS R, CHURCHILL ED: Situs inversus, sinusitis and bronchiectasis. *J Thorac Surg* 7:206, 1937

7. FINKLER E: Kartageners Syndrom. Ein kasuistischer Beitrag. *Schweiz Med Wochenschr* 86:631, 1956

8. KATSUHARA K, KAWAMOTO S, WAKABAYASHI T, BELSKY JL: Situs inversus totalis and Kartagener's syndrome in a Japanese population. *Chest* 61:56, 1972

9. KARTAGENER M, HORLACHER A: Zur Pathogenese der Bronchiektasien, Situs viscerum inversus und polyposis nasi in einem Falle familiarer Bronchiektasien. *Beitr Klin Tuberk* 87:331, 1935

10. WEINAUG P: Ein Fall von Kartagener-Syndrom bei Geschwistern. *Z Erkr Atmungsorgane* 134:454, 1971

11. ROTT H-D, WARNATZ H, PASCH-HILGERS R, WEIKL A: Kartagener's syndrome in sibs. Clinical and immunological investigations. *Hum Genet* 43:1, 1978

12. KNOX G, MURRAY S, STRANG L: A family with Kartagener's syndrome: linkage data. *Ann Hum Genet (London)* 24:137, 1960

13. MONNET P: Situs inversus and bronchopulmonary disease in the neonatal period. *Arch Fr Pediatr* 35:607, 1978

14. PERONE PM: Situs viscerum inversus, bronchiettasie e sinusiti: Tre casi di sindrome di Kartagener. *Arch Ital Otol* 67:653, 1956

15. OVERHOLT EL, BANMAN DF: Variants of Kartagener's syndrome in the same family. *Ann Intern Med* 48:574, 1958

16. LOGAN WD, ABBOTT OA, HATCHER CR: Kartagener's triad. *Dis Chest* 48:613, 1965

17. GUGGENHEIM F: Kartagener's syndrome in an Arab family. *Isr J Med Sci* 7:1079, 1971

18. WAKEFIELD SJ, WAITE D: Abnormal cilia in Polynesians with bronchiectasis. *Am Rev Resp Dis* 121:1003, 1980

19. SLEIGH M: The nature and action of respiratory tract cilia, in Brain JD, Procter DF, Reid LM (eds): *Respiratory Defence Mechanisms*, Monograph 3 of *Lung Biology in Health and Disease*. New York, Dekker, 1977, p 247

20. SATIR P: Basis of flagellar motility in spermatozoa. Current status, in Fawcett DW, Bedford JM (eds): *The Spermatozoon*, Baltimore, Urban and Schwarzenberg, 1979, p 81

21. STURGESS J: Mucous secretion in the respiratory tract. *Pediatr Clin North Am* 26:481, 1979

22. SVEDBERGH B, BILL A: Scanning electron microscopic studies of the corneal epithelium in man and monkeys. *Acta Ophthalmol* 50:321, 1972

23. GRIMFIELD JA, TOURNIER G, JOUANNET P, BISSON JP, SALOMON JL, BACULARD A, GERBEAUX J: Immotile cilia syndrome in infants and children. *Thorax* 34:709, 1979

24. JAHRSDOERFER R, FELDMAN PS, RUBEL EW, GUERRANT JL, EGGLESTON PA, SELDEN RF: Otitis media and the immotile cilia syndrome. *Laryngoscope* 89:769, 1979

25. AFZELIUS BA, ELIASSON R: Flagellar mutants in man: On the heterogeneity of the immotile-cilia syndrome. *J Ultrastruct Res* 69:43, 1979

26. STURGESS JM, CHAO J, WONG J, ASPIN N, TURNER JAP: Cilia with defective radial spokes. A cause of human respiratory disease. *N Engl J Med* 300:53, 1979

27. STURGESS JM, CHAO J, TURNER JAP: Transposition of ciliary microtubules. Another cause of impaired ciliary motility. *N Engl J Med* 303:318, 1980

28. SCHNEEBERGER EE, McCORMACK J, ISSENBERG H, SCHUSTER SR, GERALD PS: Heterogeneity of ciliary morphology in the immotile-cilia syndrome in man. *J Ultrastruct Res* 73:34, 1980

29. PEDERSEN H, REBBE H: Absence of arms in the axoneme of immobile human spermatozoa. *Biol Reprod* 12:541, 1975

30. HERZON FS, MURPHY S: Normal ciliary ultrastructure in children with Kartagener's syndrome. *Ann Otol Rhinol Laryngol* 89:81, 1980

31. CAMNER P, AFZELIUS BA, ELIASSON R, MOSSBERG B: Relation between abnormalities of human sperm flagella and respiratory tract disease. *Int J Androl* 2:211, 1979

32. KONRADOVA V, HLOUSKOVA Z, TOMANEK A: Atypical kinocilia in human epithelium from large bronchus. *Folia Morphol (Prague)* 23:293, 1975

33. TAKASAKA T, SATO M, ONODERA A: Atypical cilia in the human nasal mucosa. *Ann Otol Rhinol Laryngol* 89:37, 1980

34. VEERMAN AJP, VANDELDEN L, FEENSTRA L, LEENE W: The immotile cilia syndrome—phase contrast light microscopy, scanning and transmission electron microscopy. *Pediatrics* 65:698, 1980

35. RUTLAND J, COLE PJ: Non-invasive sampling of nasal cilia for measurement of beat frequency and study of ultrastructure. *Lancet* 2:564, 1980

36. ROSSMAN CM, FORREST JB, LEE RMKW, NEWHOUSE MT: The dyskinetic cilia syndrome—ciliary motility in immotile cilia syndrome. *Chest* 78:580, 1980

37. PEDERSEN M, MYGIND N: Ciliary motility in the immotile cilia syndrome. *Br J Dis Chest* 74:239, 1980

38. CAMNER P, MOSSBERG B, AFZELIUS BA: Evidence for congenitally nonfunctioning cilia in the tracheobronchial tract in two subjects. *Am Rev Resp Dis* 112:807, 1975

39. MOSSBERG B, AFZELIUS BA, ELIASSON R, CAMNER P: On the pathogenesis of obstructive lung disease: A study in the immotile-cilia syndrome. *Scand J Resp Dis* 59:55, 1978

40. LAYTON WM: Random determination of a developmental process. *J Hered* 67:336, 1976

41. HUANG B, PIPERNO G, LUCK DJL: Paralyzed flagella mutants of Chlamydomonas reinhardtii. Defective for axonemal doublet microtubular arms. *J Biol Chem* 254:3091, 1979

42. RICHER C-L, BLEAU G, CHAPDELAINE A: Trisomy 12 mosaicism in an infertile man. *Can J Genet Cytol* 19:565, 1977

43. HEUCKENKAMP PU, MARSHALL M, MEIER J, PARRISIUS, ZÖLLNER N: Das Kartagener-syndrom. *Dtsch Med Wochenschr* 97:1458, 1972

44. TORGERSEN J: Genic factors in visceral asymmetry and in the development and pathologic changes of lungs, heart and abdominal organs. *Arch Pathol* 47:566, 1949

45. ELIASSON R, MOSSBERG B, CAMNER P, AFZELIUS BA: The immotile-cilia syndrome. A congenital ciliary abnormality as an etiologic factor in chronic airway infections and male sterility. *N Engl J Med* 297:1, 1977

46. MOSSBERG B, HANNGREN Å: Kartagener's syndrome—a ciliary immotility syndrome. *Mt Sinai J Med* 44:837, 1977

47. ROOKLIN AR, McGEADY SJ, MIKAELIAN DO, SORIANO RZ, MAUSMANN HC: The immotile cilia syndrome—a cause of recurrent pulmonary disease in children. *Pediatrics* 66:526, 1980

48. HOLMES LB, BLENNERHASSETT JB, AUSTEN KF: A reappraisal of Kartagener's syndrome. *Am J Med Sci* 255:13, 1968

49. SETHI BR: Kartagener's syndrome and its otological manifestations. *J Laryngol Otol* 89:183, 1975

50. HOWELL JT, SCHOCHTET SS, GOLDMAN AS: Ultrastructural defects of respiratory tract cilia associated with chronic infections. *Arch Pathol Lab Med* 104:52, 1980

51. LAKE K, SHARMA OP: Kartagener's syndrome and deaf-mutism: An unusual association. *Chest* 64:661, 1973

52. SVEDBERGH B, JOHNSSON V, AFZELIUS BA: Immotile-cilia syndrome and the cilia of the eye. *Albrecht von Graefes Arch Klin Exp Ophthalmol* 1981, in press

53. SEGAL P, KIKIELA M, MRZYGLOD B, ZEROMSKA-ZBIERSKA I: Kartagener's syndrome with familial eye changes. *Am J Ophthalmol* 55:1043, 1963

54. CHILD AH: Personal communication

55. FOX B, BULL TB, ARDEN GB: Variations in the ultrastructure of human nasal cilia including abnormalities found in retinitis pigmentosa. *J Clin Pathol* 33:327, 1980

56. GLICK ID, GRAUBERT DN: Kartagener's syndrome and schizophrenia: A report of a case with chromosomal studies. *Am J Psych* 121:603, 1964

57. BRYAN JHD, CHANDLER DB: Tracheal ciliary defects in mice homozygous for a recessive pleiotropic mutation, hydrocephalus-polydactyly. *J Cell Biol* 79:281a, 1978

58. BERGSTROM WH, COOK CD, SCANELL JG, BERENBERG W: Situs inversus, bronchiectasis and sinusitis. *Pediatrics* 6:573, 1950

59. AFZELIUS BA, CAMNER P, MOSSBERG B: On the function of cilia in the female reproductive tract. *Fertil Steril* 29:72, 1978

60. BLEAU G, RICHER C-L, BOUSQUET D: Absence of dynein arms in cilia of endocervical cells in a fertile woman. *Fertil Steril* 30:362, 1978

61. PELLNITZ D, HEYLAND S: Beitrag zur Kartagenerschen Trias (Situs inversus, Bronchiektasis und Nasenpolypen) HNO 3:41, 1952

62. GAGNON C, SHERINS RJ, MANN T, BARDIN W, AMELAR RD, DUBIN L: Deficiency of protein carboxyl-methylase in spermatozoa of necrospermic patients, in Steinberger A, Steinberger E (eds): *Testicular Development, Structure, and Functions.* New York, Raven, 1980, p 491

63. AFZELIUS BA, EWETZ L, PALMBLAD J, UDEN A-M, VENIZELOS N: Structure and function of neutrophil leukocytes from patients with the immotile-cilia syndrome. *Acta Med Scand* 208:145, 1980

64. CONWAY DJ: A congenital factor in bronchiectasis. *Arch Dis Child* 26:253, 1951

65. SIELICKA-ZUBER L, FICER J: Zespól Kartagener. *Przegl Dermatol (Warsaw)* 61:171, 1974

66. AMJAD H, RICHBURG FD, ADLER E: Kartagener's syndrome. Case report in an elderly man. *JAMA* 227:1420, 1974

LIST OF ABBREVIATIONS

ACAT: Acyl CoA:cholesterol acyl-transferase
ADA: Adenine deaminase
ADH: Antidiuretic hormone
AdoCbl: Adenosylcobalamin
AGA: N-Acetylglutamate
AGS: N-Acetylglutamate synthetase
AIC: 5-Aminoimidazole-4-carboxamide
AIP: Acute intermittent porphyria
ALA: δ-Aminolevulinic acid
Ald: Aldolase
AMP: Adenosine monophosphate
Apo A-I: Apolipoprotein A-I
Apo A-II: Apolipoprotein A-II
Apo A-III: Apolipoprotein A-III
Apo B: Apolipoprotein B
Apo C-I: Apolipoprotein C-I
Apo C-II: Apolipoprotein C-II
Apo C-III: Apolipoprotein C-III
Apo D: Apolipoprotein D
Apo E: Apolipoprotein E
APRT: Adenine phosphoryribosyltransferase
AROA: Autosomal recessive ocular albinism
ASA: Argininosuccinate
ASAL: Argininosuccinate lyase
ASAS: Argininosuccinate synthetase
AT: L-(αS, $5S$)-α-Amino-3-chloro-4,5-dihydro-5-isoxazoleacetic acid
AVP: Arginine vasopressin

BCAA: Branched-chain amino acids
BCKA: Branched-chain keto acids
BCKDH: Branched-chain keto acid dehydrogenase
BSP: Bromsulfothalein

C_1 INH: C_1 inhibitor
C4-BP: C4 binding protein
CAH: Congenital adrenal hyperplasia
CAP: Carbamyl phosphate
CE: Cholesteryl ester
CEP: Congenital erythropoietic porphyria

CESD: Cholesteryl ester storage disease
CF: Cystic fibrosis
CGD: Chronic granulomatous disease
CHS: Chediak-Higashi Syndrome
CML: Cell-mediated lympholysis
CN Cbl: Cyanocobalamin
CP: Carbamoyl phosphate
CPK: Creatinine phosphokinase
C/PL: Cholesterol to phospholipid ratio
CPPD: Calcium pyrophosphate dihydrate
CPS: Carbamoyl phosphate synthetase
CPS I: Carbamyl phosphate synthetase I
CPS II: Carbamyl phosphate synthetase II
CRM: Cross-reacting material
cRTA: Complete renal tubular acidosis
CS: Cholesterol sulfate
CSF: Cerebrospinal fluid
CTX: Cerebrotendinous xanthomatosis
Cyclic AMP: Cyclic adenosine-3′-5′-monophosphate

dAVP: Deaminoarginine vasopressin
DBH: Dopamine β-hydroxylase
dCDAVP: 1-Deamino-6-carba-[8-D-arginine] 1-vasopressin
2,8-DHA: 2,8-Dihydroxyadenine
DHEA: Dihydroepiandosterone
DHEAS: Dehydroepiandosterone sulfate
DHF: Dihydrofolic acid
DLT: Dihydrolipoyltransacetylase
DMD: Duchenne's muscular dystrophy
DNA: Deoxyribonucleic acid
DNPH: Dinitrophenylhydrazine
DOC: Deoxycorticosterone
Dol-P: Dolichol phosphate
DOVA: γ δ-Dioxovalerate
2,3 DPG: 2,3-Diphosphoglycerate
DR: Dihydrotestosterone-receptor
DTT: Dithiothreitol

E_1: Branched chain keto acid decarboxylase
E_2: Dihydrolipoyl transacetylase
E_3: Dihydrolipoyl dehydrogenase
EA-TDA: 2-Ethylamino-1,3,4-thiadiazole
EDTA: Ethylenediaminetetraacetate
ELB: Early labeled peak (of bilirubin)
elF: Elongation factor
EMA: Ethylmalonic-adipic aciduria
EMG: Electron myography
EPP: Erythropoietic protoporphyria
ER: Endoplasmic reticulum
ESR: Electron spin resonance

FABP: Folate-binding protein
FFA: Fumarylacetoacetate hydrolyase
FGAM: Phosphoribosylformyglycinamidine
FIGLU: Formiminoglutamic acid
N-FMetLeuPhe: N-Formylmethionyl-leucyl-phenylalanine
FS: Fanconi syndrome
FSH: Facioscapulohumeral muscular dystrophy

G-6-PD: Glucose-6-phosphate dehydrogenase
GA II: Glutaric aciduria Type II
GABA: γ-Aminobutyric acid
Gal-Gal-Cer: Galabiosylceramide
Gal-Gal-Glc-Cer: Globotriaosylceramide
GalNAC: (N-Acetylgalactosamine)
GC: Gas chromatography
GERL: Golgi endoplasmic reticulum-like
G/F protein: Nucleotide binding protein
GFR: Glomerular filtration rate
Glc-Cer: Glucosylceramide
GlcNAC: N-Acetylglucosamine
GMP: Guanosine monophosphate
GPI: Glucosephosphate isomerase
GSH: Glutathione
GSH-P_x: Glutathione peroxidase
GSSG: Oxidized glutathione

GSSG-R:	Glutathione reductase	MCH:	Mean corpuscular hemoglobin	PKU:	Phenylketonuria
GTP:	Guanosine triphosphate			PLT:	Primed lymphocyte typing
		MCHC:	Mean corpuscular hemoglobin concentration	PNP:	Purine nucleoside phosphorylase
8-HA:	8-Hydroxyadenine	MCPA CoA:	Methylene-cyclopropylacetyl CoA	PP:	Pentose phosphate
HAE:	Hereditary angioedema			PP-ribose-P:	Phosphoribosylpyrophosphate
hCG:	Human chorionic gonadotropin	MCV:	Mean corpuscular volume	PRA:	Plasma renin activity
		MeCbl:	Methylcobalamin	PTH:	Parathyroid hormone
HCP:	Hereditary coproporphyria	MeH₄folate:	N⁵Methyltetrahydrofolate	PZA:	Pyrazinoic acid
HDL:	High-density lipoprotein	MHC:	Histocompatability complex		
HEP:	Hepatoerythrocytic porphyria	MLC:	Mixed lymphocyte culture		
		MLD:	Metachromatic leukodystrophy	R-5-P:	Ribose-5-phosphate
Hex B:	Hexosaminidase B			RBW:	Renal bicarbonate wasting
Hex A:	Hexosaminidase A	MLR:	Mixed lymphocyte response	RER:	Rough endoplasmic reticulum
HFI:	Hereditary fructose intolerance	MODY:	Maturity onset diabetes of the young		
HK:	Hexokinase	MPO:	Myeloperoxidase	RNA:	Ribonucleic acid
HLA:	Human leukocyte antigens	MS:	Mass spectrometry	mRNA:	Messenger RNA
HMG CoA:	3-Hydroxy-3 methylglutaryl CoA	β-MSH:	β-Melanocyte-stimulating hormone	tRNA:	Transfer RNA
				RTA:	Renal tubular acidosis
HMG-CoA reductase:	3-Hydroxy-3 methylglutaryl coenzyme A reductase	MSUD:	Maple syrup urine disease		
		4MU-β-D galactoside:	4-Methylumbelliferyl-β-galactoside		
HPP:	Hereditary pyropoikilocytosis	MyD:	Myotonic dystrophy	SA:	Sialic acid
				SAM:	S-adenosylmethionine
HPRT:	Hypoxanthine-guanine phosphoribosyltransferase			SCE:	Sister chromatic exchange
				SCID:	Severe combined immunodeficiency disease
HPS:	Hermansky-Pudlak Syndrome	NAG:	N-Acetylglutamate	SDS-PAGE:	Sodium dodecyl sulfate polyacrylamide gel electrophoresis
		NBT:	Nitroblue tetrazolium		
HS:	Hereditary spherocytosis	NP:	Nucleotide phosphorylase		
HSD:	Hydroxysteroid dehydrogenase	N Protein:	Nucleotide-binding protein	SER:	Smooth endoplasmic reticulum
				SGOT:	Serum glutamic oxaloacetic transaminase
ICW:	Intracellular water			SHBG:	Sex-hormone-binding globulin
IDL:	Intermediate density lipoproteins	OA:	Ocular albinism		
		OAT:	Ornithine aminotransferase	SK:	Streptokinase
IF:	Intrinsic factor	OCA:	Oculocutaneous albinism	SLE:	Systemic lupus erythematosus
IgA:	Gamma A globulin	OCT:	Ornithine carbamoyl transferase		
IgG:	Gamma G globulin				
IgM:	Gamma M globulin	ODC:	Orotidine-5'-phosphate decarboxylase		
IMP:	Inosinic acid				
iRTA:	Incomplete renal tubular acidosis	OEC:	Oxygen equilibrium curve	T₃:	Triiodothyronine
		OF:	Osmotic fragility	rT₃:	3-3'-5'-Triiodothyronine
		18-OHB:	18-Hydroxycorticosterone	T₄:	Thyroxine
		OH-Cbl:	Hydroxycobalamin	TAT:	Tyrosine aminotransferase
KGDH:	2-Ketoglutarate dehydrogenase	3-OMG:	3-O-methyl-D-glucose	TBG:	Thyroxine-binding globulin
		OMP:	Orotidine-5'-phosphate	TBPA:	Thyroxine-binding prealbumin
KIC:	2-Ketoisocaproic acid	OPRT:	Orotate phosphoribosyltransferase		
KIV:	2-Ketoisovaleric acid			TC I:	Transcobalamin I
KMV:	2-Keto-3-methylvaleric acid			TC II:	Transcobalamin II
				TCDD:	2,3,7,8-Tetrachlorodibenzo-p-dioxin
LAD:	Dihydrolipoyl dehydrogenase	P5C:	Pyrroline-5-carboxylic acid	TeBG:	Testosterone-binding globulin
		PAH:	Para-aminohippuric acid		
LASS:	Labile aggregation-stimulating substance	PAPS:	Phosphoadenosylphosphosulfate	THF:	Tetrahydrofolic acid
		PBG:	Porphobilinogen	dTMP:	Thymidylate
LCAT:	Lecithin:cholesterol acyltransferase	PC:	Phosphorylcholine	TPI:	Triose phosphate isomerase
		PCT:	Porphyria cutanea tarda	TPP:	Thiamine pyrophosphate
LDH:	Lactate dehydrogenase	PDH:	Pyruvate dehydrogenase	TR:	Testosterone receptor
LDL:	Low density lipoproteins	PDHC:	Pyruvate dehydrogenase complex	TRH:	Thyrotropin-releasing hormone
LG:	Limb girdle				
LH:	Luteinizing hormone	PEA:	Phosphorylethanolamine	TRP:	Tubular reabsorption of phosphate
LPL:	Lipoprotein lipase	PFK:	Phosphofructokinase		
		PGK:	Phosphoglycerate kinase	TSD:	Tay-Sachs disease
		PHA:	Phyto-hemagglutinin	TSH:	Thyrotropin
MA:	Maleic acid	PHLA:	Post-heparin plasma lipolytic activity	TXA₂:	Thromboxane A₂
MAA:	Maleylacetoacetate hydrolyase			Ty-neg:	Tyrosinase-negative (oculocutaneous albinism)
		PHPAA:	p-Hydroxyphenylacetic acid		

UDP:	Uridine diphosphate	VDDR:	Vitamin D – dependent rickets	vWF:	von Willebrand factor
dUMP:	Uridylate	VIP:	Vasointestinal peptide		
		VLDL:	Very low density lipoprotein	XMP:	Xanthylic acid
		VP:	Variegate porphyria	XOAN:	X-linked ocular albinism (Nettleship)
VAVP:	4-Valine arginine vasopressin	WD:	Wolman's disease	XP:	Xeroderma pigmentosum

INDEX